MW01056075

BRANT AND HELMS' FUNDAMENTALS OF DIAGNOSTIC RADIOLOGY

FIFTH EDITION

SECTION EDITORS

SECTION I
BASIC PRINCIPLES

William E. Brant, MD, FACR
Professor Emeritus
Department of Radiology and Medical Imaging
University of Virginia School of Medicine
Charlottesville, Virginia

SECTION II
NEURORADIOLOGY

Erik H. L. Gaensler, MD
Clinical Professor
Department of Radiology and Biomedical Imaging
University of California, San Francisco
Neuroradiologist
Bay Imaging Consultants

Jerome A. Barakos, MD
Director of Neuroimaging
Department of Radiology
California Pacific Medical Center
San Francisco, California

SECTION III
CHEST

Jeffrey S. Klein, MD, FACR
A. Bradley Soule and John P. Tampas Green and Gold Professor of Radiology
Department of Radiology
Larner College of Medicine at the University of Vermont
Burlington, Vermont

SECTION IV
BREAST RADIOLOGY

Brandi T. Nicholson, MD, FSBI
Associate Professor
Department of Radiology and Medical Imaging
University of Virginia School of Medicine
Charlottesville, Virginia

SECTION V
CARDIAC RADIOLOGY

Seth Kligerman, MD
Associate Professor
Division Chief of Cardiothoracic Radiology
Department of Radiology
University of California, San Diego
San Diego, California

SECTION VI
VASCULAR AND INTERVENTIONAL RADIOLOGY

Juan C. Camacho, MD
Assistant Attending Radiologist Interventional Radiology
Memorial Sloan Kettering Cancer Center
Assistant Professor
Department of Radiology
Weill Cornell Medical College
New York, New York

Akhilesh K. Sista, MD, FSIR
Associate Professor and Section Chief
Vascular Interventional Radiology
Department of Radiology
New York University School of Medicine
New York, New York

SECTION VII
GASTROINTESTINAL TRACT

William E. Brant, MD, FACR
Professor Emeritus
Department of Radiology and Medical Imaging
University of Virginia School of Medicine
Charlottesville, Virginia

SECTION VIII
GENITOURINARY TRACT

William E. Brant, MD, FACR
Professor Emeritus
Department of Radiology and Medical Imaging
University of Virginia School of Medicine
Charlottesville, Virginia

SECTION IX
ULTRASONOGRAPHY

William E. Brant, MD, FACR
Professor Emeritus
Department of Radiology and Medical Imaging
University of Virginia School of Medicine
Charlottesville, Virginia

SECTION X
MUSCULOSKELETAL RADIOLOGY

Clyde A. Helms, MD
Consultant
Department of Radiology
Duke University Medical Center
Durham, North Carolina
Consultant
Department of Radiology
University of New Mexico
Albuquerque, New Mexico

Emily N. Vinson, MD
Assistant Professor of Radiology
Chief, Division of Musculoskeletal Imaging
Duke University School of Medicine
Durham, North Carolina

SECTION XI
PEDIATRIC RADIOLOGY

Alan S. Brody, MD
Professor of Radiology and Pediatrics
Department of Radiology
Cincinnati Children's Hospital Medical Center
Cincinnati, Ohio

Andrew T. Trout, MD
Radiologist
Department of Radiology
Cincinnati Children's Hospital Medical Center
Cincinnati, Ohio

SECTION XII
NUCLEAR RADIOLOGY

Brett J. Mollard, MD
Body Section Co-Chief
Abdominal Imaging and Nuclear Medicine
TRA Medical Imaging
Tacoma, Washington

BRANT AND HELMS' FUNDAMENTALS OF DIAGNOSTIC RADIOLOGY

FIFTH EDITION

EDITORS

JEFFREY S. KLEIN, MD, FACR

A. Bradley Soule and John P. Tampas Green and Gold
Professor of Radiology
Department of Radiology
Larner College of Medicine at the University of Vermont
Burlington, Vermont

WILLIAM E. BRANT, MD, FACR

Professor Emeritus
Department of Radiology and Medical Imaging
University of Virginia School of Medicine
Charlottesville, Virginia

CLYDE A. HELMS, MD

Consultant
Department of Radiology
Duke University Medical Center
Durham, North Carolina
Consultant
Department of Radiology
University of New Mexico
Albuquerque, New Mexico

EMILY N. VINSON, MD

Assistant Professor of Radiology
Chief, Division of Musculoskeletal Imaging
Duke University School of Medicine
Durham, North Carolina

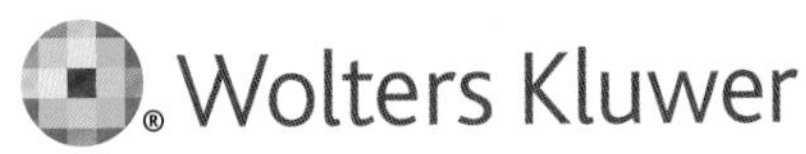

Philadelphia • Baltimore • New York • London
Buenos Aires • Hong Kong • Sydney • Tokyo

Acquisitions Editor: Sharon Zinner
Editorial Assistant: Dave Murphy
Marketing Manager: Julie Sikora
Production Project Manager: Joan Sinclar
Design Coordinator: Stephen Druding
Manufacturing Coordinator: Beth Welsh
Prepress Vendor: Aptara, Inc.

5th edition

9 8 7 6 5 4 3 2 1

Printed in China

978-1-4963-6738-9
1-4963-6738-3
Library of Congress Cataloging-in-Publication Data
available upon request

shop.lww.com

CCS0918

To my wife, Dr. Judy Tam, for her love, support, and encouragement, and our children, Joshua, Benjamin and Jessica, for reminding me what is most important in life.

—Jeffrey S. Klein, MD, FACR

I dedicate this 5th edition of our textbook to my wife, Barbara, whose love, immense patience and support makes my work on it possible, to our 10 grandchildren: Sophia, Grayson, and Noah; Danielle; Finn and Josie; Evan and Katie; Dylan and Amelia, and to the memory of my daughter, Rachel.

—WEB

To Jennifer Pohl who is the finest person I have ever known and has made me a better person in every way.

—Clyde A. Helms, MD

To my husband, Stephen, and our children, Allison and Matthew, who have given me all the best things in life. I wish the same for them, always.

—ENV

CONTRIBUTORS

Eric T. Aaltonen, MD, MPH
Assistant Professor
Vascular Interventional Radiology
Department of Radiology
New York University School of Medicine
New York, New York

Sarah H. Allgeier, MD, PhD
Fellow
Vascular Interventional Radiology
Department of Radiology
Medical University of South Carolina
Charleston, South Carolina

Jason J. Bailey, MD
Nuclear Medicine and Abdominal Radiologist
CMI Radiology Group
Fresno, California

Jerome A. Barakos, MD
Director of Neuroimaging
California Pacific Medical Center Sutter Health
Sutter Pacific Epilepsy Program

Spencer Behr, MD
Associate Professor of Clinical Radiology
Department of Radiology and Biomedical Imaging
University of California, San Francisco
San Francisco, California

Stephen Bracewell, MD
Resident Physician
Department of Radiology
Medical University of South Carolina
Charleston, South Carolina

William E. Brant, MD, FACR
Professor Emeritus
Department of Radiology and Medical Imaging
University of Virginia School of Medicine
Charlottesville, Virginia

Alan S. Brody, MD
Professor of Radiology and Pediatrics
Department of Radiology
Cincinnati Children's Hospital
University of Cincinnati College of Medicine
Cincinnati, Ohio

Richard K. J. Brown, MD, FACR
Professor, Department of Radiology
Director of Clinical Nuclear Medicine and Molecular Imaging
University of Michigan Health System
Ann Arbor, Michigan

Juan C. Camacho, MD
Assistant Attending Radiologist
Interventional Radiology
Memorial Sloan Kettering Cancer Center
Assistant Professor
Department of Radiology
Weill Cornell Medical College
New York, New York

Nancy A. Chauvin, MD
Associate Professor
Department of Radiology
Penn State College of Medicine
Hershey, PA

Nathaniel A. Chuang, MD
Associate Clinical Professor
Department of Radiology
University of California, San Diego
Neuroradiologist
San Diego Imaging Medical Group
San Diego, California

Marc G. Cote, DO, FACOI, FACP
Assistant Dean for Clinical Education
Associate Professor of Internal Medicine
Pacific Northwest University of Health Sciences
College of Osteopathic Medicine
Yakima, Washington

Bradley Fehrenbach, MD
Nuclear Radiologist
Diversified Radiology
Denver, Colorado

Robert R. Flavell, MD, PhD
Assistant Professor in Residence
Department of Radiology and Biomedical Imaging
Section of Nuclear Medicine
University of California, San Francisco
San Francisco, California

Robert J. Fleck, Jr., MD
Associate Professor
Department of Radiology
Cincinnati Children's Hospital Medical Center
University of Cincinnati
Cincinnati, Ohio

Carl Gunnar Forsberg, MD
Resident Physician
Department of Radiology
Medical University of South Carolina
Charleston, South Carolina

Erik H. L. Gaensler, MD
Clinical Professor
Department of Radiology and Biomedical Imaging
University of California, San Francisco
Neuroradiologist
Bay Imaging Consultants

Arpit Gandhi, MD
Radiology resident
Christiana Care Health System
Newark, Delaware

Alisa D. Gean, MD
Professor Emeritus
Department of Radiology and Biomedical Imaging
University of California, San Francisco
San Francisco, California

Curtis E. Green, MD
Professor of Radiology and Cardiology
Department of Radiology
Larner College of Medicine at the University of Vermont
Burlington, Vermont

Marcelo Guimaraes, MD, FSIR
Professor and Director
Vascular Interventional Radiology
Department of Radiology
Medical University of South Carolina
Charleston, South Carolina

Aishwarya Gulati, MD
Resident Physician
Department of Internal Medicine
Carle Foundation Hospital
Urbana, Illinois

Kate Hanneman, MD, MPH, FRCPC
Assistant Professor
Department of Medical Imaging, Toronto General Hospital
University of Toronto
Toronto, Canada

Peter A. Harri, MD
Assistant Professor
Abdominal Imaging
Department of Radiology and Imaging Sciences
Emory University School of Medicine
Atlanta, Georgia

Heather Hartung, RN-BSN
RN Patient Navigator
Vascular Interventional Radiology
Medical University of South Carolina
Charleston, South Carolina

Clyde A. Helms, MD
Consultant
Department of Radiology
Duke University Medical Center
Durham, North Carolina
Consultant
Department of Radiology
University of New Mexico
Albuquerque, New Mexico

Cash Jeremy Horn, MD
Assistant Professor
Vascular Interventional Radiology
Department of Radiology
New York University School of Medicine
New York, New York

Michael J. Horowitz, MD, PhD
Cardiothoracic Imaging Fellow
Department of Radiology
UC San Diego Medical Center
San Diego, California

Albert Hsiao, MD, PhD
Assistant Professor
Department of Radiology
UC San Diego
La Jolla, California

Kathleen Jacobs, MD
Assistant Professor
Department of Radiology
University of California, San Diego
San Diego, California

Blaise V. Jones, MD
Chief, Neuroradiology
Cincinnati Children's Hospital Medical Center
Professor
University of Cincinnati School of Medicine
Cincinnati, Ohio

Vivek Kalia, MD, MPH, MS
Assistant Professor of Radiology
Department of Radiology
Division of Musculoskeletal Radiology
University of Michigan Health System
Ann Arbor, Michigan

Asef Khwaja, MD
Assistant Professor of Radiology
Department of Radiology
The Children's Hospital of Philadelphia. Perelman School of Medicine at the University of Pennsylvania
Philadelphia, Pennsylvania

Jeffrey S. Klein, MD, FACR
A. Bradley Soule and John P. Tampas Green and Gold
Professor of Radiology
Department of Radiology
Larner College of Medicine at the University of Vermont
Burlington, Vermont

Seth Kligerman, MD
Associate Professor
Division Chief of Cardiothoracic Radiology
Department of Radiology
University of California, San Diego
San Diego, California

Nima Kokabi, MD
Assistant Professor
Interventional Radiology and Image-guided Medicine
Department of Radiology and Imaging Sciences
Emory University School of Medicine
Atlanta, Georgia

Kelly K. Koeller, MD, FACR
Associate Professor
Department of Radiology
Mayo Clinic
Rochester, MN and
Chief, Neuroradiology
American Institute for Radiologic Pathology
Silver Spring, Maryland

Tuong H. Le, MD, PhD
Brain and Spine Imaging Consultants (BASIC)
Dallas, Texas

Jay S. Leb, MD
Assistant Professor
Department of Radiology
Columbia University Medical Center
New York, New York

Clayton Li, MD
Resident Physician
Department of Radiology
New York University School of Medicine
New York, New York

Jeffrey P. Lin, MD, PhD
Nuclear Radiologist
TRA Medical Imaging
Tacoma, Washington

Camilla E. Lindan, MD
Assistant Clinical Professor
Department of Radiology
University of California San Francisco
Department of Diagnostic Imaging
Kaiser Hospital, San Francisco, California

Louis G. Martin, MD, FACR, FSIR
Emeritus Professor
Interventional Radiology and Image-guided Medicine
Department of Radiology and Imaging Sciences
Emory University School of Medicine
Atlanta, Georgia

Meredith McDermott, MD
Assistant Professor
Vascular Interventional Radiology
Department of Radiology
New York University School of Medicine
New York, New York

Pardeep K. Mittal, MD, FACR
Professor
Body Imaging
Department of Radiology and Imaging
Medical College of Georgia
Augusta, Georgia

Brett J. Mollard, MD
Body Section Co-Chief
Abdominal Imaging and Nuclear Medicine
TRA Medical Imaging
Tacoma, Washington

Govind Mukundan, MD
Neuroradiology Section
Sutter Imaging
Sacramento, California

Christopher A. Mutch, MD, PhD
Radiologist
Bay Imaging Consultants
Walnut Creek, California

Usha D. Nagaraj, MD
Assistant Professor of Clinical Radiology and Pediatrics
Cincinnati Children's Hospital Medical Center/ University of Cincinnati College of Medicine
Cincinnati, Ohio

Jonathan V. Nguyen, MD
Assistant Professor
Department of Radiology
University of Virginia Health System
Charlottesville, Virgina

Brandi T. Nicholson, MD, FSBI
Associate Professor
Department of Radiology and Medical Imaging
University of Virginia School of Medicine
Charlottesville, Virginia

Walter L. Olsen, MD, FACR
San Diego Imaging Medical Group
San Diego, California

Amish Patel, MD
Assistant Professor
Vascular Interventional Radiology
Department of Radiology
New York University School of Medicine
New York, New York

Jonathan David Perry, MD
Chief Resident
Department of Radiology
Medical University of South Carolina
Charleston, South Carolina

Jennifer Pohl, PhD, MD
Associate Professor
Department of Radiology
University of New Mexico
Albuquerque, New Mexico

Derk D. Purcell, MD
Assistant Clinical Professor
Department of Radiology and Biomedical Imaging
University of California, San Francisco
California Pacific Medical Center
San Francisco, California

Carrie M. Rochman, MD
Assistant Professor
Department of Radiology and Medical Imaging
University of Virginia Health System
Charlottesville, Virginia

Howard A. Rowley, MD
Joseph Sackett Professor of Radiology
Professor of Radiology, Neurology, and Neurosurgery
University of Wisconsin
Madison, Wisconsin

Claudio Schonholz
Professor
Vascular Interventional Radiology
Department of Radiology
Medical University of South Carolina
Charleston, South Carolina

David J. Seidenwurm, MD
Network Medical Director
Quality Committee Chair
Sutter Medical Foundation
Sacramento, California

Robert Y. Shih, MD
Assistant Professor
Department of Radiology
Uniformed Services University
Bethesda, Maryland

Akhilesh K. Sista, MD, FSIR
Associate Professor and Section Chief Vascular Interventional Radiology
Department of Radiology
New York University School of Medicine
New York, New York

Ethan A. Smith, MD
Associate Professor
Department of Radiology
Cincinnati Children's Hospital Medical Center
University of Cincinnati College of Medicine
Cincinnati, Ohio

Divya Sridhar, MD
Assistant Professor
Vascular Interventional Radiology
Department of Radiology
New York University School of Medicine
New York, New York

Judy K. Tam, MD
Associate Professor of Radiology
Department of Radiology
Larner College of Medicine at the University of Vermont
Burlington, Vermont

Anobel Tamrazi, MD, PhD
Interventional Radiology
Palo Alto Medical Foundation
Redwood City, California

Bedros Taslakian, MD
Assistant Professor
Vascular and Interventional Radiology
Department of Radiology
New York University School of Medicine
New York, New York

Andrew T. Trout, MD
Associate Professor of Radiology
Cincinnati Children's Hospital Medical Center
Cincinnati, Ohio

Emily N. Vinson, MD
Assistant Professor of Radiology
Chief, Division of Musculoskeletal Imaging
Duke University School of Medicine
Durham, North Carolina

Vibhor Wadhwa, MD
Radiology Resident
Department of Radiology
University of Arkansas for Medical Sciences
Little Rock, Arkansas

Alyssa T. Watanabe, MD
Clinical Associate Professor
Neuroradiology Division
USC Keck School of Medicine
Los Angels, California

Elizabeth Weihe, MD
Associate Professor
Department of Radiology
University of California-San Diego
San Diego, California

Ricardo Tadayoshi Barbosa Yamada, MD
Assistant Professor
Vascular Interventional Radiology
Department of Radiology
Medical University of South Carolina
Charleston, South Carolina

PREFACE

Much has changed in radiology since *Fundamentals of Diagnostic Radiology* by Brant and Helms was first conceived in the late 1980s as an aide to radiology residents studying for their radiology oral board examinations. In the past 30 years, the amount of information dispensed during radiology residency has increased dramatically, and there has been an explosion in technology including advances in multidetector and coned-beam computed tomography, magnetic resonance imaging, nuclear medicine, and ultrasound. The past 10 to 15 years have seen the development of new imaging modalities including digital tomosynthesis, dual-energy subtraction radiography, functional/metabolic imaging, and the birth of interventional oncology with new image-guided treatment techniques including thermal tumor ablation and targeted transcatheter treatment of neoplasms. In the United States an examination taken by residents in their 36th month of training has in part replaced the old oral examinations for those seeking diagnostic radiology certification by the American Board of Radiology. Despite a multitude of online sources of information for radiology residents, there remains a need for basic, high-quality introductory material that spans all diagnostic radiology subspecialties.

This fifth edition of *Brant and Helms' Fundamentals of Diagnostic Radiology* contains significantly expanded and revised sections dedicated to breast radiology, cardiac imaging, vascular/interventional radiology, pediatric radiology, and nuclear medicine that reflect the growing fund of knowledge in these subspecialties and their increased importance in radiology resident curricula. We are fortunate to have six new section editors who have contributed their expertise to this new edition and have invited contributions from many recently trained radiologists in creating an updated version of core material. Dr. Brandi T. Nicholson, a breast radiologist and Associate Residency Program Director for the diagnostic residency program at the University of Virginia Health System has created a section that covers screening, diagnostic, and interventional breast radiology. Dr. Seth Kligerman, Section Chief of Cardiothoracic Imaging at the University of California, San Diego, shares his knowledge and experience in cardiovascular imaging in a significantly expanded Cardiac section. The Vascular and Interventional Radiology section, edited by Drs. Akhilesh Sista of NYU Langone Medical Center and Juan Camacho of the Memorial Sloan Kettering Cancer Center in New York provides a thorough introduction to the spectrum of image-guided vascular and nonvascular interventions including the interventional treatment of hepatic malignancies. Drs. Alan Brody and Andrew Trout of the Cincinnati Children's Hospital Medical Center have significantly revised the section on Pediatric Radiology. The Nuclear Medicine section, edited by Dr. Brett J. Mollard of Diagnostic Imaging Northwest, is completely revised with a more condensed review of common nuclear medicine topics.

Those familiar with previous editions will recognize editors and authors Drs. William Brant and Clyde Helms, who developed the concept of *Fundamentals of Diagnostic Radiology* 30 years ago. For this fifth edition, Bill has updated his introductory chapter on diagnostic imaging methods and contributed updated material on gastrointestinal and genitourinary radiology and ultrasound. Clyde has updated his section on Musculoskeletal Imaging along with Dr. Emily Vinson, Division Chief of Musculoskeletal Imaging at Duke University Medical Center, who now joins as an editor of Fundamentals. Drs. Erik Gaensler and Jerome Barakos have returned to edit the revised Neuroradiology section. Dr. Jeffrey Klein, along with colleagues from the Larner College of Medicine at the University of Vermont, provides an updated section on Chest Radiology and is now a senior editor of *Brant and Helms' Fundamentals of Diagnostic Radiology*.

The editors of Fundamentals would like to acknowledge the efforts of the staff of Wolters Kluwer who have supported this new edition and helped guide it to successful completion. Sharon Zinner, Senior Acquisitions Editor at Wolters Kluwer Health, has lent her steady hand and vast experience with radiology textbooks to this major revision. David Murphy, Senior Managing Editor at Wolters Kluwer Health, has kept everyone on task over the past 2 years. Indu Jawwad, Senior Project Manager and Joan Sinclair, Production Manager, have worked closely with the editors and authors during the proofing and final editing stages of the book.

—Jeffrey S. Klein, MD, FACR
—William E. Brant, MD, FACR
—Clyde A. Helms, MD
—Emily N. Vinson, MD

CONTENTS

SECTION VI
VASCULAR AND INTERVENTIONAL RADIOLOGY

SECTION EDITORS: Juan C. Camacho and Akhilesh K. Sista

SECTION VII
GASTROINTESTINAL TRACT

SECTION EDITOR: William E. Brant

SECTION VIII
GENITOURINARY TRACT

SECTION EDITOR: William E. Brant

SECTION IX
ULTRASONOGRAPHY

SECTION EDITOR: William E. Brant

SECTION X
MUSCULOSKELETAL RADIOLOGY

SECTION EDITORS: Clyde A. Helms and Emily N. Vinson

SECTION XI
PEDIATRIC RADIOLOGY

SECTION EDITORS: Andrew T. Trout and Alan S. Brody

SECTION XII
NUCLEAR RADIOLOGY

SECTION EDITOR: Brett J. Mollard

LIST OF UNIVERSAL ABBREVIATIONS

Abbreviations for use throughout Klein/Brant/Helms/Vinson, *Fundamentals of Diagnostic Radiology*, 5th Edition.

AIDS	Acquired immunodeficiency Syndrome
CNS	Central nervous system
CT	Computed tomography
CSF	Cerebrospinal fluid
CXR	Conventional chest radiograph
DWI	Diffusion weighted imaging (MR)
FDG	18-F-fluorodeoxyglucose
GRE	Gradient-echo MR imaging
GI	Gastrointestinal
HIV	Human immunodeficiency virus
HRCT	High resolution chest CT
HU	Hounsfield unit – a reference scale for CT
IV	Intravenous
LA	Left atrium
LV	Left ventricle
MDCT	Multi-detector computed tomography
MR	Magnetic resonance imaging
PA	Pulmonary artery
PET	Positron emission tomography
PET-CT	Positron emission tomography – computed tomography
SPECT	Single-photon emission computed tomography
RA	Right atrium
RV	Right ventricle
T1WI	T1-weighted image (MR)
T2WI	T2-weighted image (MR)
US	Ultrasound

SECTION I

BASIC PRINCIPLES

SECTION EDITOR: William E. Brant

CHAPTER 1 ■ DIAGNOSTIC IMAGING METHODS

WILLIAM E. BRANT

Diagnostic radiology is a dynamic specialty that continues to undergo rapid change with ongoing advancements in utilization and technology. Not only has the number of imaging methods increased, but each one continues to undergo improvement and refinement of its use in medical diagnosis. This chapter reviews the basics of the major diagnostic imaging methods and provides the basic principles of image interpretation for each method. Contrast agents commonly used in diagnostic radiology are discussed. The basics of nuclear radiology are discussed in later chapters.

CONVENTIONAL RADIOGRAPHY

Conventional radiographic examination of the human body dates back to the genesis of diagnostic radiology in 1895 when Wilhelm Roentgen produced the first x-ray film image of his wife's hand. Conventional radiography remains fundamental to the practice of diagnostic imaging.

Image Generation. X-rays are a form of radiant energy similar in many ways to visible light. X-rays differ from visible light in that they have a very short wavelength and are able to penetrate many substances that are opaque to light. The x-ray beam is produced by bombarding a tungsten target with an electron beam within an x-ray tube.

Film Radiography. Conventional film radiography utilizes a screen-film system within a film cassette as the x-ray detector. As x-rays pass through the human body they are attenuated by interaction with body tissues (absorption and scatter) and produce an image pattern on film that is recognizable as human anatomy. X-rays transmitted through the patient bombard a fluorescent particle–coated screen within the film cassette causing a photochemical interaction that emits light rays, which expose photographic film within the cassette (Fig. 1.1). The film is removed from the cassette and developed by an automated chemical film processor. The final product is an x-ray image of the patient's anatomy on a film (Fig. 1.2).

Computed radiography (CR) is a filmless system that eliminates chemical processing and provides digital radiographic images. CR substitutes a phosphor imaging plate for the film-screen cassette. CR cassette sizes match those available for traditional film-screen cassettes. The same gantry, x-ray tube, and exposure control systems, and cassette holders used in conventional radiography are utilized for CR. The phosphor-coated imaging plate interacts with x-rays transmitted through the patient to capture a latent image. The phosphor plate is placed within a reading device that scans the plate with a helium-neon laser, emitting light, which is captured by a photomultiplier tube and processed into a digital image. The CR receptor is erased with white light and is used repeatedly. The digital image is transferred to a computerized picture archiving and communication system (PACS). The PACS stores and transmits digital images via computer networks to give physicians and healthcare providers in many locations simultaneous instant access to the diagnostic images.

Digital radiography (DR) provides a filmless and cassetteless system for capturing x-ray images in digital format. DR substitutes a fixed electronic detector or charge-coupled device (CCD) for the film-screen cassette or phosphor imaging plate. Direct read-out detectors produce an immediate digital radiographic image. Most DR detectors are installed in a fixed gantry limiting the ability of the system to obtain images portably at the patient's bedside. CR is generally used for that purpose in a digital imaging department. Direct digital image capture is particularly useful for angiography providing rapid digital image subtraction and for fluoroscopy and image-guided interventional procedures capturing video images with low, continuous radiation.

Fluoroscopy enables real-time radiographic visualization of moving anatomic structures. A continuous x-ray beam passes through the patient and falls onto a digital radiographic system. The digital images are displayed in real time on a television monitor, and are recorded digitally as a movie clip or as a series of images. Fluoroscopy is extremely useful to evaluate motion such as swallowing, intestinal peristalsis, movement of the diaphragm with respiration, and cardiac action. Fluoroscopy is also used to perform and monitor continuously radiographic procedures such as barium studies, catheter placements, and other interventional procedures. Video and static fluoroscopic images are routinely stored in digital format on a PACS for retrospective interpretation and documentation.

Conventional angiography involves the opacification of blood vessels by intravascular injection of iodinated contrast agents. ***Conventional arteriography*** uses small flexible

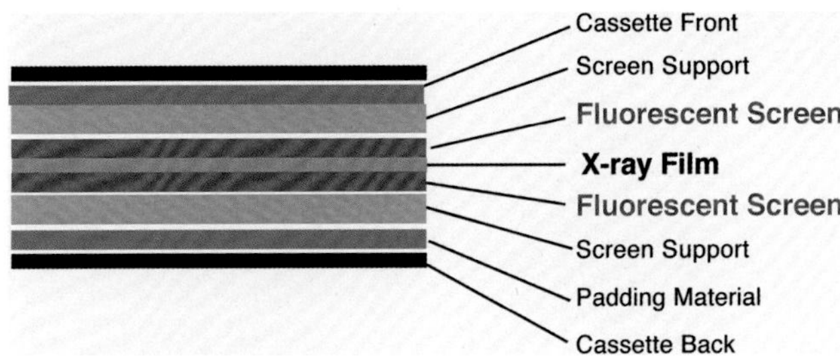

FIGURE 1.1. **X-Ray Film Cassette.** Diagram demonstrates a sheet of x-ray film between two fluorescent screens within a light-proof cassette.

catheters that are placed in the arterial system usually via puncture of the femoral artery in the groin. With the use of fluoroscopy for guidance, catheters of various sizes and shapes can be manipulated selectively into virtually every major artery. Contrast injection is performed by hand or by mechanical injector and is accompanied by digital computer acquisition (DR) of the fluoroscopic image. The result is a timed series of images depicting contrast flow through the artery injected and the tissues perfused. ***Conventional venography*** is performed by contrast injection of veins via distal puncture or selective catheterization.

Naming Radiographic Views. Most radiographic views are named on the basis of the direction that the x-ray beam passes through the patient. A posteroanterior (PA) chest radiograph is one in which the x-ray beam passes through the back of the patient and exits through the front of the patient to expose an x-ray detector positioned against the patient's chest. An anteroposterior (AP) chest radiograph is exposed by an x-ray beam passing through the patient from front to back. A craniocaudad (CC) mammogram is produced by passing a beam through the breast in a vertical, cranial to caudad, direction with the patient standing or sitting. Views are additionally named by identifying the position of the patient. Erect, supine, or prone views may be specified. A right lateral decubitus view of the chest is exposed with a horizontal x-ray beam passing through the chest of a patient lying on his or her right side. Radiographs taken during fluoroscopy are named on the basis of the patient's position relative to the fluoroscopic table because the x-ray tube is positioned beneath the table. A right posterior oblique (RPO) view is taken with the patient lying with the right side of his or her back against the table and the left side elevated away from the table. The x-ray beam generated by the x-ray tube located beneath the table passes through the patient to the x-ray detector located above the patient.

Principles of Interpretation. Conventional radiographs demonstrate five basic radiographic densities: air, fat, soft tissue, bone, and metal (or x-ray contrast agents). Air attenuates very little of the x-ray beam, allowing nearly the full force of the beam to pass through the patient and blacken the radiographic image. Bone, metal, and radiographic contrast agents attenuate a large proportion of the x-ray beam, allowing very little radiation through to blacken the image. Thus, bone, metallic objects, and structures opacified by x-ray contrast agents appear white on radiographs. Fat and soft tissues attenuate intermediate amounts of the x-ray beam, resulting in proportional degrees of image blackening (shades of gray). Soft tissue attenuates more radiation than fatty tissues. Thick structures attenuate more radiation than thin structures of the same composition. Anatomic structures are seen on radiographs when they are outlined in whole or in part by tissues of different x-ray attenuation. Air in the lung outlines pulmonary vascular structures, producing a detailed pattern of the lung parenchyma (Fig. 1.3). Fat within the abdomen outlines the margins of the liver, spleen, and kidneys, allowing their visualization (Fig. 1.2B). The high density of bones enables visualization of bone details through overlying soft tissues (Figs. 1.2B and 1.3). Metallic objects such as surgical clips are usually clearly seen because they highly attenuate the x-ray beam. Radiographic contrast agents are suspensions of iodine or barium compounds that highly attenuate the x-ray beam and are used to outline anatomic structures. Disease states may obscure normally visualized anatomic structures by silhouetting their outline. Pneumonia in the right middle lobe of the lung replaces air in the alveoli with fluid and pus silhouetting the right heart border (Fig. 1.4).

CROSS-SECTIONAL IMAGING TECHNIQUES

CT, MR, and US are techniques that produce cross-sectional images of the body. All three interrogate a three-dimensional volume or slice of patient tissue to produce a two-dimensional image. The resulting image is made up of a matrix of picture elements (*pixels*), each of which represents a volume element (*voxel*) of patient tissue. The tissue composition of the voxel is averaged (*volume averaged*) for display as a pixel. CT and MR assign a numerical value to each picture element in the matrix. The matrix of picture elements that make up each image is usually between 256 × 256 (65,536 pixels) to 1,024 × 1,024

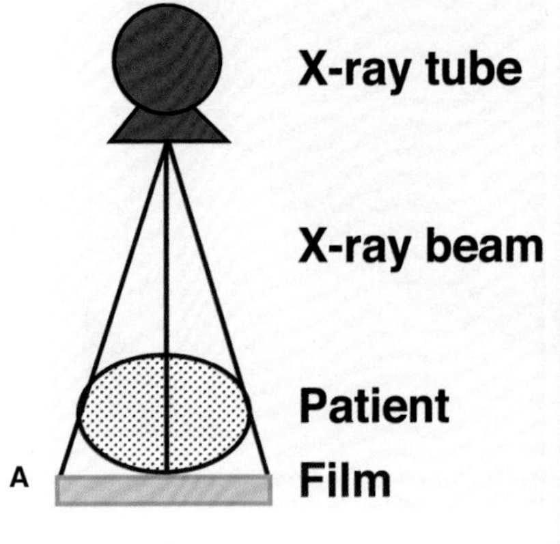

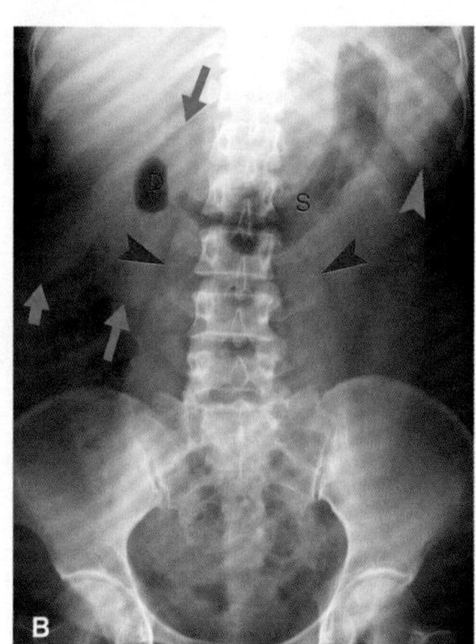

FIGURE 1.2. **Conventional Radiography. A:** Diagram of an x-ray tube producing x-rays that pass through the patient and expose the radiographic film. For digital radiography a phosphor imaging plate or fixed electronic detector takes the place of the film cassette. **B:** Supine AP (anteroposterior) radiograph of the abdomen reveals the patient's anatomy because anatomic structures differ in their capacity to attenuate x-rays that pass through the patient. The stomach (*S*) and duodenum (*D*) are visualized because air in the lumen is of lesser radiographic density than the soft tissues that surround the GI tract. The right kidney (between *thin blue arrows*), edge of the liver (*fat blue arrow*), edge of the spleen (*blue arrowhead*), and both psoas muscles (*red arrowheads*) are visualized because lower attenuation fat outlines the soft tissue density of these structures. The bones of the ribs, spine, pelvis, and hips are clearly seen through the soft tissues because of their high radiographic density.

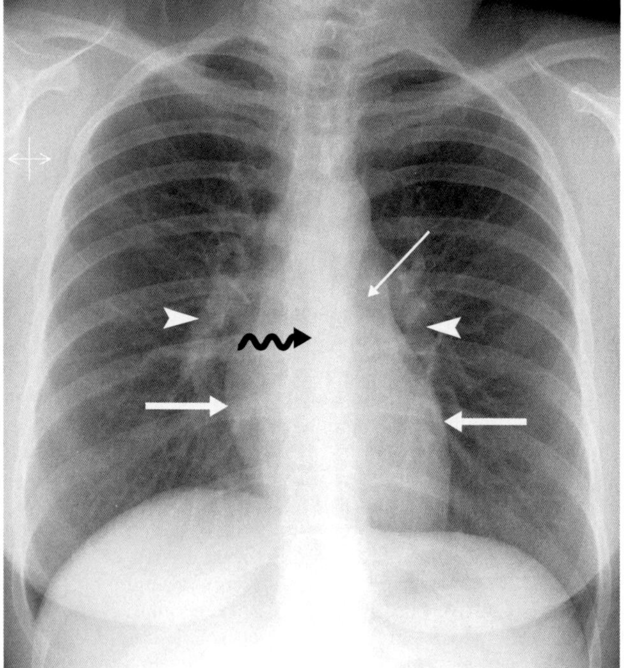

FIGURE 1.3. **Erect PA Chest Radiograph.** The pulmonary arteries (*arrowheads*) are seen in the lung because the vessels are outlined by air in alveoli. Both cardiac border (*fat arrows*) are crisply defined by adjacent air-filled lung. The left main bronchus (*skinny arrow*) is seen because its air-filled lumen is surrounded by soft tissue of the mediastinum. The azygoesophageal recess (*squiggly arrow*) is well defined by air-filled lung of the right lower lobe.

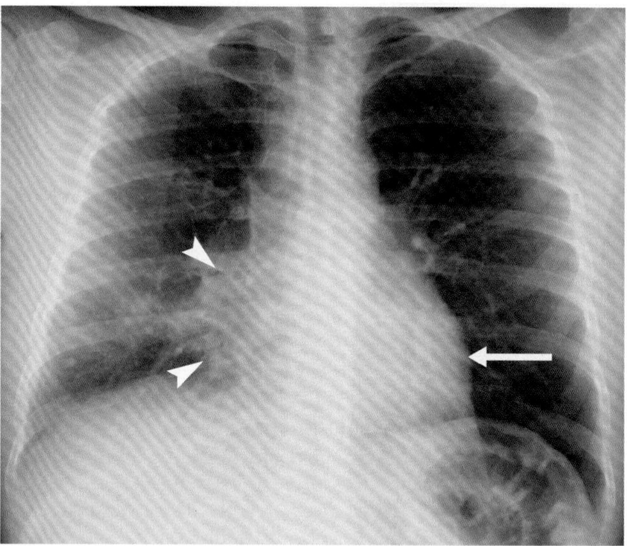

FIGURE 1.4. **Right Middle Lobe Pneumonia.** PA erect chest radiograph demonstrates pneumonia (*arrowheads*) in the right middle lobe replacing the lucency of air in the lung with soft tissue density and silhouetting the right heart border. Note the normal sharp definition of the left heart border (*arrow*) defined by the normal air-containing lingula.

(1,048,576 pixels) determined by the specified acquisition parameters (Fig. 1.5).

To produce an anatomic image, shades of gray are assigned to ranges of pixel values. For example, 16 shades of gray may be divided over a *window width* of 320 pixel values (Fig. 1.6). Groups of 20 pixel values are each assigned one of the 16 gray shades. The middle gray shade is assigned to the pixel values centered on a selected *window level*. Pixels with values greater than the upper limit of the window width are displayed white, and pixels with values less than the lower limit of the window width are displayed black. To analyze optimally all of the anatomic information of any particular slice, the image is viewed at different window-width and window-level settings optimized for bone, air-filled lung, soft tissue, and so forth (Fig. 1.7).

The digital images obtained by CT, MR, and US examination are ideal for storage and access on PACS. Current PACS allow a broad range of image manipulation while viewing and interpreting images. Among the features that can be used are scrolling, interactive alterations in window width and window level, magnification, fusing of images from different modalities, reformatting serial images in different anatomic planes, creating three-dimensional reconstructions, and marking key images that summarize major findings.

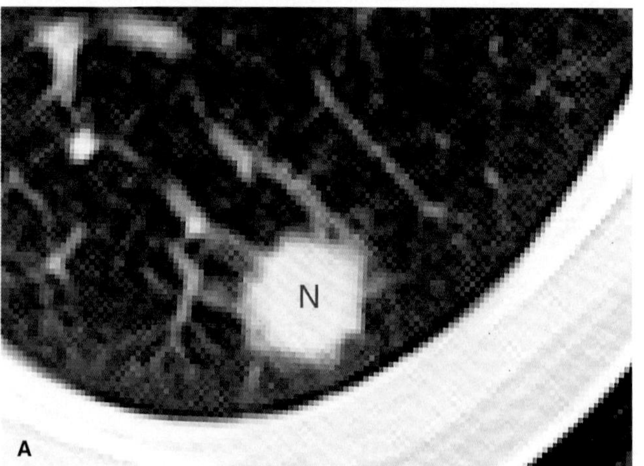

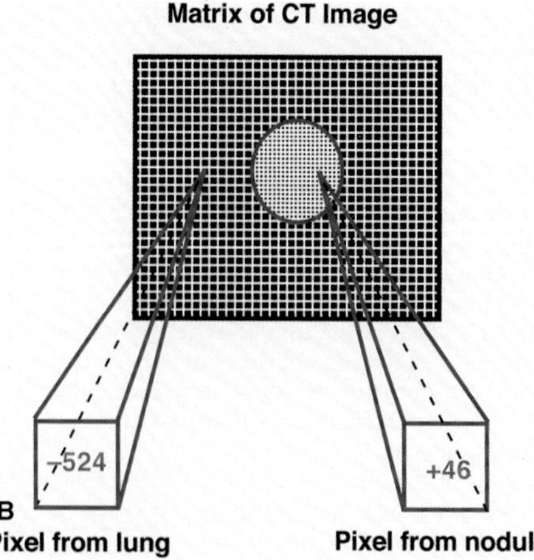

FIGURE 1.5. **Image Matrix. A:** Magnified CT image of a pulmonary nodule (*N*). The pixels that make up the image are evident as tiny squares within the image. The window width is set at 2,000 H with a window level of –600 H to accentuate visualization of the white soft tissue nodule on a background of gray, air-filled lung. **B:** Diagram of the matrix that constitutes the CT image. A pixel from air-filled lung with a calculated CT number of –524 H is gray, whereas a pixel from the soft tissue nodule with a calculated CT number of +46 H is white.

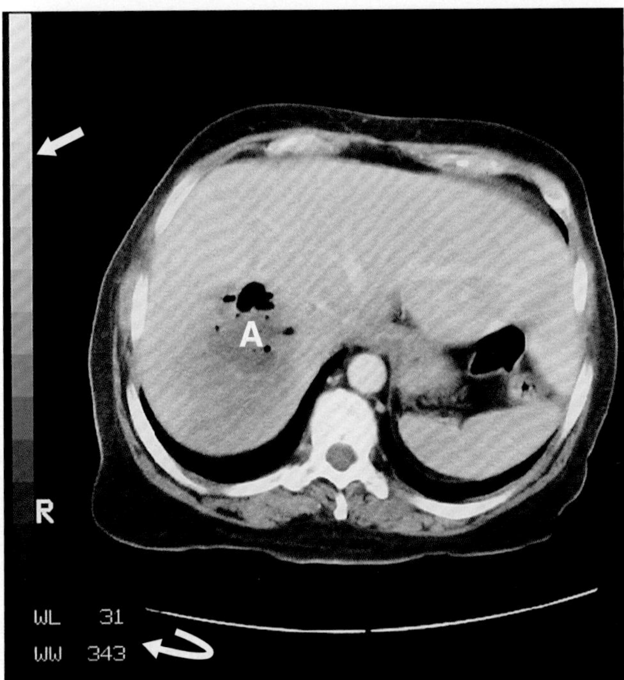

FIGURE 1.6. **Gray Scale.** A CT image of the abdomen includes a gray scale (*straight arrow*) along its left edge. Each individual pixel in the CT image is assigned a shade of gray depending on its calculated CT number (H unit) and the window width and window level (WW, WL, *curved arrow*) selected by the CT operator. Pure white and pure black are at the top and bottom of the gray scale. *R* indicates the patient's right side. Cross-sectional images in the transverse plane are routinely viewed from "below," as if standing at the patient's feet. This orientation allows easy correlation with conventional radiographs, which are routinely viewed as if facing the patient with the patient's right side to the viewer's left. This patient has an abscess (*A*) in the liver.

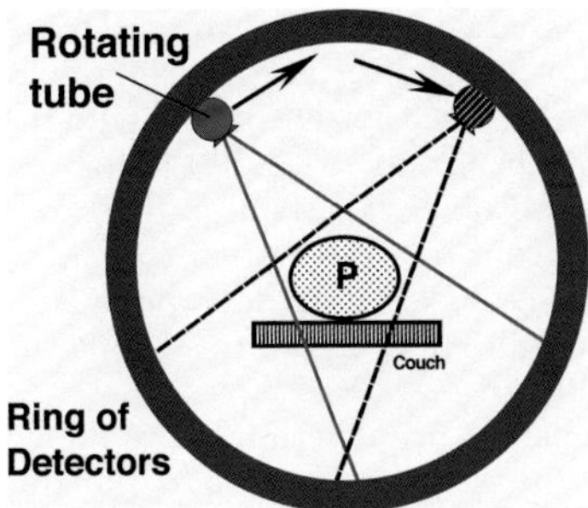

FIGURE 1.8. **Computed Tomography.** Diagram of a CT scanner. The patient (P) is placed on an examination couch within the core of the CT unit. An x-ray tube rotates around the patient, producing pulses of radiation that pass through the patient. Transmitted x-rays are detected by a bank of radiation detectors opposite the x-ray tube. X-ray transmission data are sent to a computer, which uses an assigned algorithm to calculate the matrix of CT numbers used to produce the anatomic cross-sectional image. With helical CT scan technique, the patient couch moves the patient continuously through the rotating x-ray beam. With multidetector CT, multiple image slices are obtained simultaneously as the patient is moved through the scanner.

Computed Tomography

CT uses a computer to reconstruct mathematically a cross-sectional image of the body from measurements of x-ray transmission through thin slices of patient tissue. A narrow, well-collimated beam of x-rays is generated on one side of the patient (Fig. 1.8). The x-ray beam is attenuated by absorption and scatter as it passes through the patient. Sensitive detectors on the opposite side of the patient measure x-ray transmission through the slice. These measurements are systematically repeated many times from different directions while the x-ray tube is pulsed as it rotates around the patient. CT numbers are assigned to each pixel in the image by a computer algorithm that uses as data these measurements of transmitted x-rays. CT pixel numbers are proportional to the difference in average x-ray attenuation of the tissue within

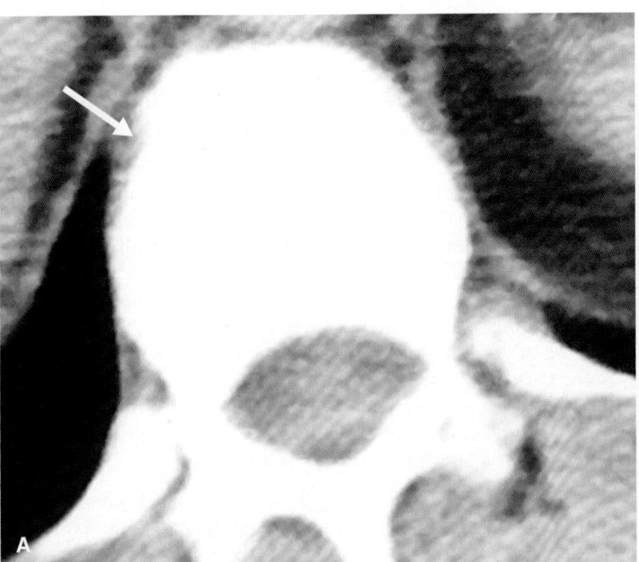

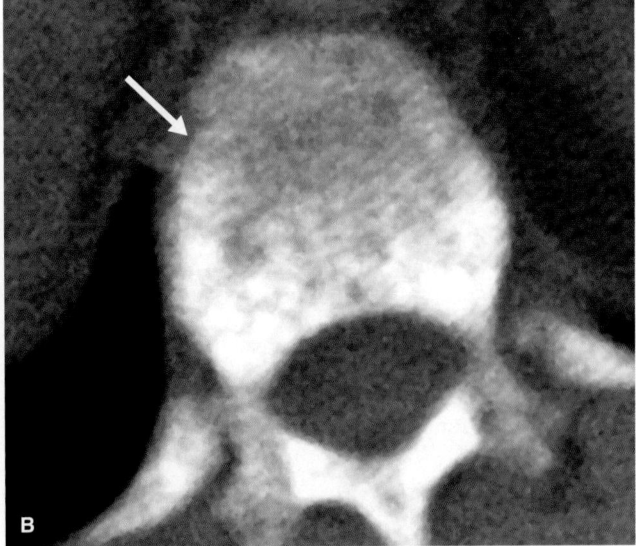

FIGURE 1.7. **CT Windows. A:** A CT image of a lower thoracic vertebral body photographed with "soft tissue windows" (window width = 482 H, window level = –14 H) portrays a thoracic vertebra (*arrow*) entirely white with no bone detail. **B:** The same CT image rephotographed with "bone windows" (window width = 2,000 H, window level = 400 H) demonstrates destructive changes in the vertebral body (*arrow*) owing to metastatic lung carcinoma.

the voxel compared with that of water. A Hounsfield unit (H) scale, named for Sir Godfrey Hounsfield, the inventor of CT, is used. Water is assigned a value of 0 H, with the scale extending from −1,000 H for air to +3,000 H for very dense bone. H units are not absolute values but, rather, are relative values that may vary from one CT system to another. In general, cortical bone is +700 H, cancellous bone is +3,000 H, soft tissue is +40 to +80 H, fat is −90 to −120 H, lung is −500 H, and air is −1,000 H.

Voxel dimensions are determined by the computer algorithm chosen for reconstruction and the thickness of the scanned slice. Most CT units allow slice-thickness specifications between 0.5 and 10 mm. Data for an individual slice are routinely acquired in 1 second or less. Advantages of CT compared with MR include rapid scan acquisition, superior bone detail, and demonstration of calcifications. CT scanning is generally limited to the axial plane; however, images may be reformatted in sagittal, coronal, or oblique planes, or as three-dimensional images. Multidetector CT allows the acquisition of cube-shaped isotropic voxels of equal length on all three sides. Isotropic voxels allow direct image reconstruction in any plane without loss of resolution.

Conventional CT (single-slice CT) obtains image data one slice at a time. The patient holds his or her breath, a slice is taken, the patient breathes, the table moves, and the sequence is repeated. This technique requires at least two to three times the total scanning time of helical CT for any given patient scan volume, making optimization of scanning during maximum contrast more difficult. Minor changes in lung volume with each breath-hold may make substantial changes in the chest and abdomen anatomy scanned, resulting in "skip" areas. Conventional scanners have largely been replaced by multidetector helical CT scanners.

Helical CT, also called spiral CT, is performed by moving the patient table at a constant speed through the CT gantry while scanning continuously with an x-ray tube rotating around the patient. A continuous volume of image data is acquired during a single breath-hold. This technique dramatically improves the speed of image acquisition, enables scanning during optimal contrast opacification, and eliminates artifacts and errors caused by misregistration and variations in patient breathing. The entire liver may be scanned in a single breath-hold; the entire abdomen and pelvis, in one or two breath-holds, all with optimal timing for organ opacification following intravenous contrast administration. Volume acquisition enables retrospective reconstruction of multiple overlapping slices, improving visualization of small lesions and allowing high-detail three-dimensional CT angiography (Fig. 1.9). Scans can be obtained during multiple phases of organ enhancement; arterial, venous, parenchymal, delayed.

Multidetector helical CT (MDCT) was a major technical advance in CT imaging, utilizing the principles of the helical scanner but incorporating multiple rows of detector rings. This allows acquisition of multiple slices per tube rotation increasing the area of the patient that can be covered in a given time by the x-ray beam. Available systems have moved quickly from 2-slice to 256 to 320-slice, which can cover over 400 mm of patient length for each 1-second or less rotation of the tube. The key advantage of MDCT is speed. MDCT is many times faster than single-slice helical CT. For body scanning 1-mm slices can be obtained creating isotropic voxels (1 × 1 × 1 mm) allowing image reconstruction in any anatomic plane without loss of resolution. Broad area coverage allows for high detail CT angiography and "virtual" CT colonoscopy and bronchoscopy. Nothing is free, however, and a significant disadvantage of MDCT is radiation dose, which can be three to five times higher with MDCT than with single-slice CT. Thin slices and multiple acquisitions add great diagnostic capability but at the cost of increased radiation dose to the patient.

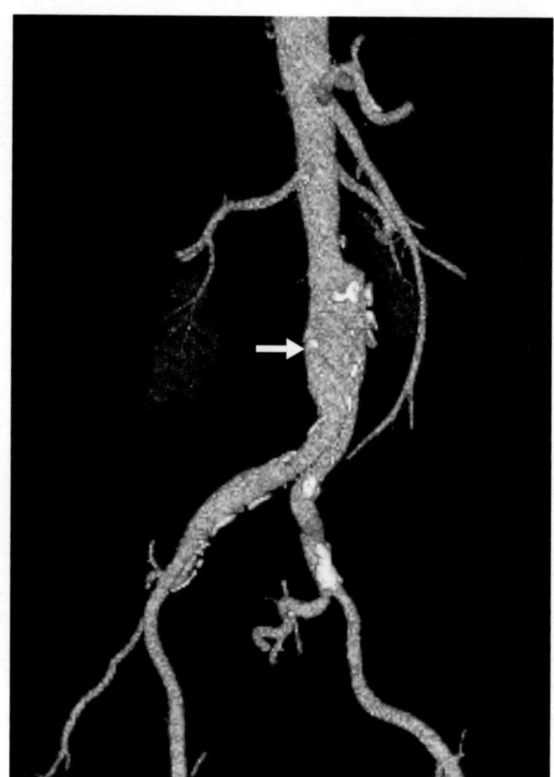

FIGURE 1.9. **CT Angiogram.** A three-dimensional, shaded surface display, angiogram image of the aorta and its branches was created from a series of axial plane MDCT images obtained during rapid bolus IV contrast agent administration. Intravenous contrast injection greatly increases the CT numbers of the arteries allowing removal of structures with lower CT density from the image by "thresholding." Only pixels with CT numbers higher than a specified threshold value are displayed. Computer algorithms create a "virtual" three-dimensional image from data provided by many overlapping axial slices. The three-dimensional image can be rotated and viewed from any desired angle on a computer monitor. "Shading," simulating light cast from a remote light source, enhances the three-dimensional visual effect. This patient has advanced atherosclerosis (atherosclerotic plaques are shown in white) and a small aneurysm (*arrow*) of the infrarenal abdominal aorta. The enhanced kidneys are partially shaded red.

CT fluoroscopy is another advancement in CT technology that allows for real-time CT imaging. This technique dramatically improves the ability to perform percutaneous image-guided interventions quickly and at a generally moderate radiation dose. The operator can step on a floor pedal while moving the CT table or observing patient motion. Rapid image reconstruction provides real-time images of anatomy, lesions, and needle or catheter placement. CT fluoroscopy is now routinely used to guide biopsy, drainage, and interventional procedures anywhere in the body. It is particularly useful in guidance of needle placements where there is physiologic motion such as in the chest and abdomen.

Dual-energy CT (dual-source CT) utilizes two x-ray sources and two x-ray detectors to simultaneously interrogate tissues to determine how tissue behaves at different radiation energies. This technique adds information about tissue composition. Differences in fat, soft tissue, and contrast agents at different energy levels expand lesion conspicuity and characterization. Image data can be captured in half the time required for conventional MDCT. This vastly improves the ability to image the heart without the use of potentially dangerous beta-blockers to slow the heart rate. The chemical composition of urinary calculi can be determined allowing selection of medical versus surgical treatment.

Contrast Administration in CT. Intravenous iodine-based contrast agents are administered intravenously during CT to enhance density differences between lesions and surrounding parenchyma, to demonstrate vascular anatomy and vessel patency, and to characterize lesions by their patterns of contrast enhancement. Optimal use of intravenous contrast depends upon the anatomy, physiology, and pathology of the organ of interest. In the brain the normal blood–brain barrier of tight neural capillary endothelial junctions prevents access of contrast into the neural extravascular space. Defects in the blood–brain barrier associated with tumors, stroke, infection, and other lesions enable contrast accumulation within abnormal tissue, improving its visibility. In nonneural tissues, the capillary endothelium has loose junctions, enabling free access of contrast into the extravascular space. Contrast administration and timing of CT scanning must be carefully planned to optimize differences in enhancement patterns between lesions and normal tissues. For example, most liver tumors are predominantly supplied by the hepatic artery, whereas the liver parenchyma is predominantly supplied by the portal vein (~70%), with a lesser contribution from the hepatic artery (~30%). Contrast given by bolus injection in a peripheral arm vein will arrive earliest in the hepatic artery and enhance (i.e., increase the CT density of) many tumors to a greater extent than the liver parenchyma. Maximal enhancement of the liver parenchyma is delayed 1 to 2 minutes until the contrast has circulated through the intestinal tract and spleen and is returned to the liver via the portal vein. Differentiation of tumor and parenchyma by contrast enhancement can thus be maximized by giving an IV bolus of contrast and by performing rapid CT scanning of the liver early during maximum arterial enhancement and delayed scanning during maximum portal venous enhancement. MDCT is ideal for this early and rapid scanning of the liver. Oral or rectal contrast is generally required to opacify the bowel for CT scans of the abdomen and pelvis. Bowel without intraluminal contrast may be difficult to differentiate from tumors, lymph nodes, and hematoma.

CT Artifacts. Artifacts refer to components of the image that do not faithfully reproduce actual anatomic structures because of distortion, addition, or deletion of information. Artifacts degrade the image and may cause errors in diagnosis.

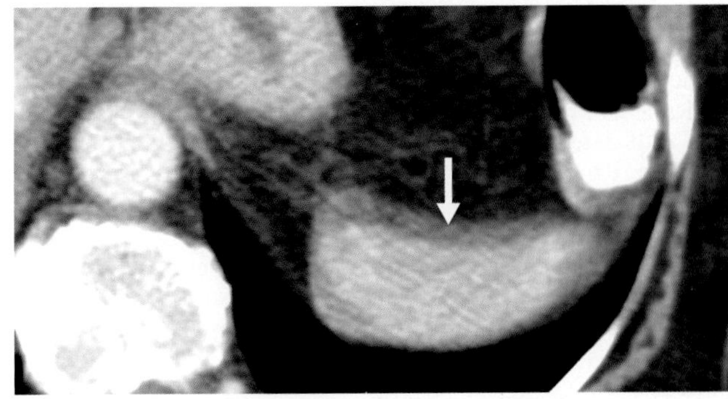

FIGURE 1.11. **Motion Artifact.** Breathing motion during image acquisition duplicates the margin (*arrow*) of the spleen simulating a subcapsular hematoma in this patient imaged because of abdominal trauma.

Volume averaging is present in every CT image and must always be considered in image interpretation. The displayed two-dimensional image is created from data obtained and *averaged* from a three-dimensional volume of patient tissue. Slices above and below the image being interpreted must be examined for sources of volume averaging that may be misinterpreted as pathology.

Beam hardening artifact results from greater attenuation of low-energy x-ray photons than high-energy x-ray photons as they pass through tissue. The mean energy of the x-ray beam is increased (the beam is "hardened"), resulting in less attenuation at the end of the beam than at its beginning. Beam-hardening errors are seen as areas or streaks of low density (Fig. 1.10) extending from structures of high x-ray attenuation such as the petrous bones, shoulders, and hips, or concentrations of contrast agents.

Motion artifact results when structures move to different positions during image acquisition. Motion occurs as a result of voluntary or involuntary patient movement, breathing, heartbeat, vessel pulsation, or peristalsis. Motion is demonstrated in the image as prominent streaks from high- to low-density interfaces or as blurred or duplicated images (Fig. 1.11).

Streak artifacts emanate from high-density sharp-edged objects such as vascular clips and dental fillings (Fig. 1.12).

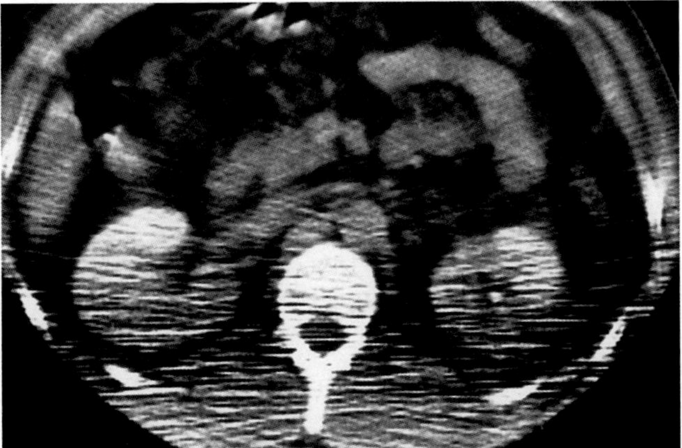

FIGURE 1.10. **Beam Hardening Artifact.** A CT image of the abdomen is severely degraded by beam hardening artifact that produces dark streaks across the lower half of the image. The artifact was caused by marked attenuation of the x-ray beam by the patient's arms, which were kept at his sides owing to injury.

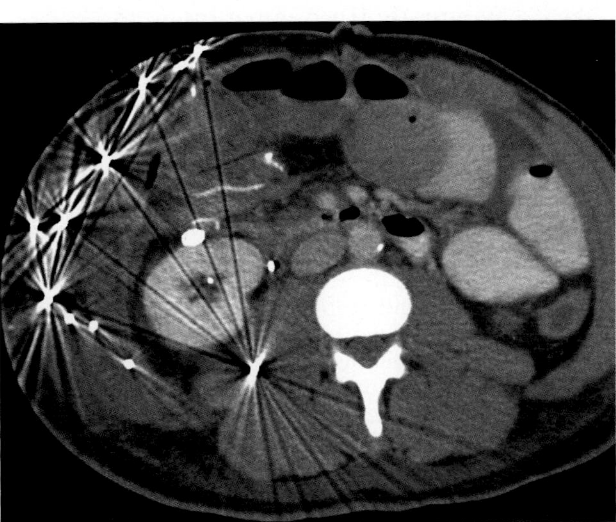

FIGURE 1.12. **Streak Artifact.** Shotgun pellets produce severe streak artifact on this CT image.

Reconstruction algorithms cannot handle the extreme differences in x-ray attenuation between very dense objects and adjacent tissue.

Ring artifacts occur when the CT scanner is out of calibration and detectors give erroneous readings at each angle of rotation. Ring artifacts are seen as high- or low-density circular rings in the image.

Quantum mottle artifacts produce noise in the image seen as salt and pepper pattern of random dark and light specks throughout the image. The image noise results from insufficient x-ray transmission data caused by inappropriate radiation settings for the location of scanning and the size of the patient.

Principles of CT Interpretation. Like all imaging analysis, CT interpretation is based on an organized and comprehensive approach. CT images are viewed in sequential anatomic order, examining each slice with reference to slices above and below. This image analysis is made dramatically easier by viewing CT images on a PACS workstation. The interpreting physician can scroll up and down the stacked image display. The radiologist must seek to develop a three-dimensional concept of the anatomy and pathology displayed. This analysis is fostered by the availability of images obtained or reconstructed in coronal and sagittal, as well as axial planes. The study must be interpreted with reference to the scan parameters, slice thickness and spacing, administration of contrast, timing of scanning relative to contrast enhancement, and presence of artifacts. Axial images are oriented so that the observer is looking at the patient from below. The patient's right side is oriented on the left side of the image. Optimal bone detail is viewed at "bone windows," generally a window width of 2,000 H and a window level of 400 to 600 H. Lungs are viewed at "lung windows" with a window width of 1,000 to 2,000 H and window levels of –500 to –600 H. Soft tissues are examined at window width 400 to 500 H and window level 20 to 40 H. Narrow windows (width = 100 to 150 H, level = 70 to 80 H) increase image contrast and aid in the detection of subtle liver and spleen lesions. PACS workstation viewing of digital images allows the interpreter to actively manipulate the image, magnify, change image brightness and contrast, measure attenuation, and to create oblique and three-dimensional image reconstructions to optimize interpretation.

Magnetic Resonance Imaging

MR is a technique that produces tomographic images by means of magnetic fields and radiowaves. Although CT evaluates only a single tissue parameter, x-ray attenuation, MR analyzes multiple tissue characteristics including hydrogen (proton) density, T1 and T2 relaxation times of tissue, and blood flow within tissue. The soft tissue contrast provided by MR is substantially better than for any other imaging modality. Differences in the density of protons available to contribute to the MR signal discriminate one tissue from another. Most tissues can be differentiated by significant differences in their characteristic T1 and T2 relaxation times. T1 and T2 are features of the three-dimensional molecular environment that surrounds each proton in the tissue imaged. T1 is a measure of a proton's ability to exchange energy with its surrounding chemical matrix. It is a measure of how quickly a tissue can become magnetized. T2 conveys how quickly a given tissue loses its magnetization. Blood flow has a complex effect on the MR signal that may decrease or increase signal intensity within blood vessels.

The complex physics of MR is beyond the scope of this book but is reviewed in detail in the text *Essentials of Body MRI*. In simplest terms, MR is based on the ability of a small number of protons within the body to absorb and emit radiowave energy when the body is placed within a strong magnetic field. Different tissues absorb and release radiowave energy at different, detectable, and characteristic rates. MR scans are obtained by placing the patient in a static magnetic field 0.02 to 3 Tesla (T) in strength, depending on the particular MR unit used. Scanners using a magnetic field of 1.5 T are most common. MR scanners at 4 T, 7 T, 8 T, and 9.4 T are being developed. Low-field strength systems (<0.1 T), midfield systems (0.1 to 1.0 T), and high-field systems (1.5 T and 3.0 T) each have their own advantages and disadvantages. The choice of unit for imaging is based on preference and local availability. A small number of tissue protons in the patient align with the main magnetic field and are subsequently displaced from their alignment by application of radiofrequency (RF) gradients. When the RF gradient is terminated, the displaced protons realign with the main magnetic field, releasing a small pulse of energy that is detected, localized, and then processed by a computer algorithms similar to those used in CT to produce cross-sectional tomographic anatomic images. Slice location is determined by application of a slice selection gradient of gradually increasing intensity along the z-axis, defined as being parallel to the direction of the scanner's static magnetic field. The small energy pulses released by tissue protons are further localized by "frequency-encoding" in one direction (x-axis) and "phase-encoding" in the other direction (y-axis). Images can be obtained in any anatomic plane by adjusting the orientation of the x-axis, y-axis, and z-axis magnetic field gradients. Because the MR signal is very weak, prolonged imaging time is often required for optimal images. Standard spin-echo sequences produce a batch of images in 10 to 20 minutes. Rather than obtaining data for each image one slice at a time, many spin-echo MR sequences obtain data for all slices in the imaged tissue volume throughout the entire imaging time. Thus, motion caused by breathing and cardiac and vascular pulsation may degrade the image substantially. MR has advanced to rapid imaging breath-hold techniques using gradient recalled echo (GRE), echo train, and echo-planar sequences. Continued rapid-paced technologic improvements are making MR acquisition times comparable with those for CT.

Present MR technology relies on a variety of MR sequence techniques, with many variations used by different MR manufacturers (Fig. 1.13). Acronyms rule.

Spin-echo (SE) pulse sequences produce standard T1-weighted images (WI), T2WI, and proton density–weighted images. T1WI emphasize differences in the T1 relaxation times between tissues, while minimizing differences in T2 times. On the resultant image tissues with short T1 values are relatively bright (high signal intensity), while those with long T1 times are relatively dark (low signal intensity). T1WI usually provide the best anatomic detail and are good for identifying fat, subacute hemorrhage, and proteinaceous fluids. T2WI emphasize differences in the T2 relaxation times of tissues while minimizing differences in T1 times. Tissues with long T2 times are relatively bright, while those with short T2 times are relatively dark. T2WI usually provide the most sensitive detection of edema and pathologic lesions. Proton density–weighted images accentuate proton density differences in tissues and are most useful in brain imaging.

Two major components of MR instrument settings selected by the operator for SE sequences are TR and TE. The time between administered RF pulses, or the time provided for protons to align with the main magnetic field, is TR (time of repetition). The time provided for absorbed radiowave energy to be released and detected is TE (time of echo). Spin-echo T1WI are obtained by selecting short TR (~500 ms) and short TE

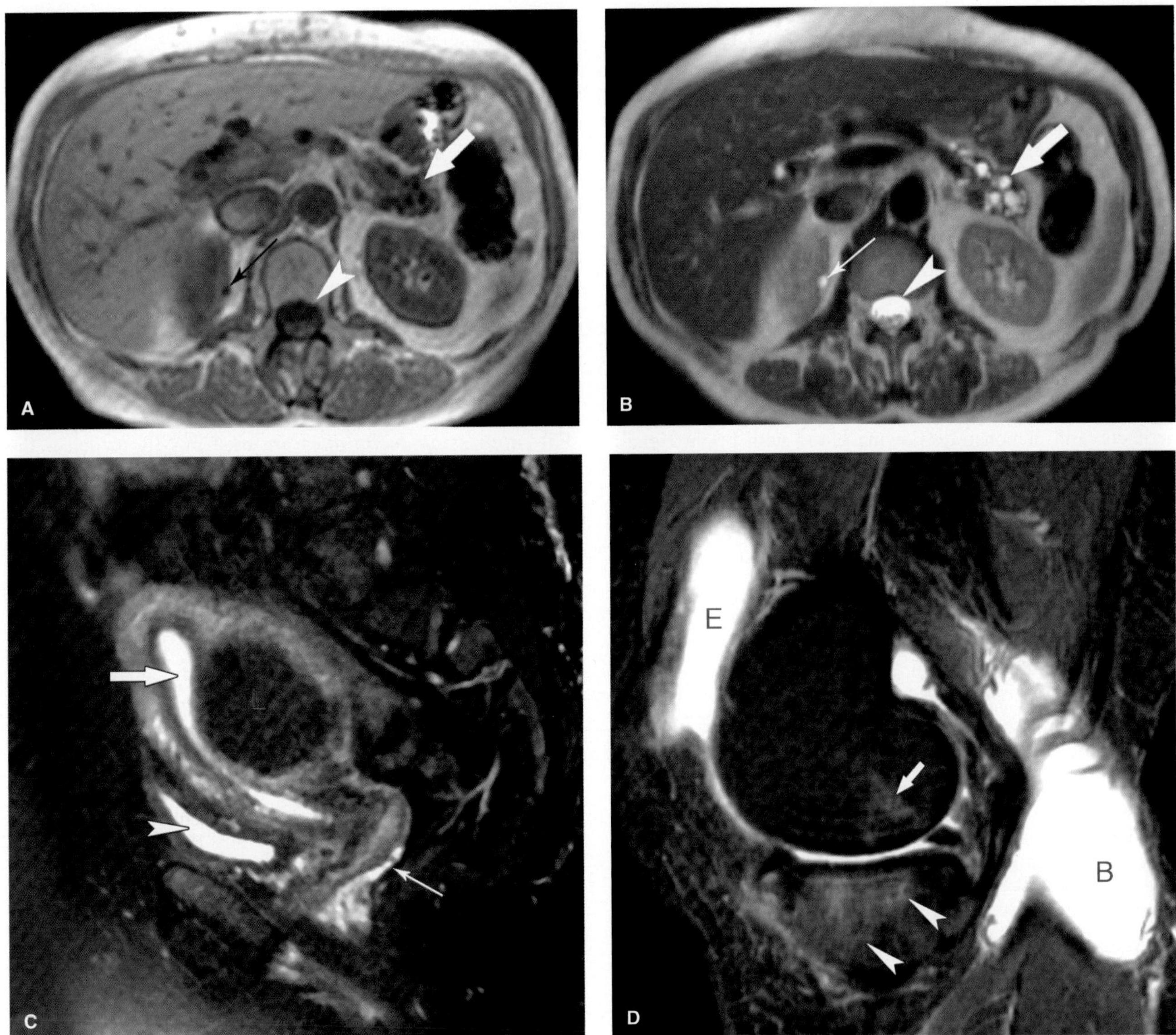

FIGURE 1.13. **MR Sequences.** Gradient recall in-phase T1WI, **A**, and HASTE T2WI, **B**, taken at the same slice location demonstrates dark signal in free water on T1WI and bright signal of free water on T2WI. Note the improved conspicuity of the cystic lesion (*thick arrows*) of the pancreas on the T2WI compared to the T1WI. The cerebrospinal fluid (*arrowheads*) in the spinal canal also shows marked increase in signal on T2WI. A tiny cyst (*skinny arrows*) in the right kidney is confirmed as benign by showing the signal intensities of simple free water (dark on T1WI, bright on T2WI). **C:** Sagittal turbo spin-echo (TSE) T2WI with fat saturation shows a low signal leiomyoma (*L*) and bright signal from fluid in the endometrial canal (*thick arrow*) and from urine in the bladder (*arrowhead*). A small amount of fluid is evident in the cul-de-sac (*skinny arrow*), a normal finding in a woman of child-bearing age. Note the lack of signal from fat as compared to **B**, the T2WI without fat saturation. **D:** Sagittal plane STIR image of the knee accentuates bright signal from free water in the knee effusion (*E*), Baker cyst (*B*), and bone bruise edema in the femoral condyle (*arrow*) and tibial plateau (*arrowheads*).

(~20 ms) settings. Spin-echo T2WI use a long TR (≥2,000 ms) and long TE (≥70 ms). Proton density–weighted images use a long TR (2,000 to 3,000 ms) and a short TE (25 to 30 ms) to minimize T1 and T2 effect and accentuate hydrogen-density differences in tissues.

Multiple spin-echo sequences, also known as echo-train, rapid-acquisition relaxation-enhanced (RARE), fast spin-echo (FSE), or turbo spin-echo (TSE) sequences, significantly reduce image acquisition time. Signal intensity is less than with SE sequences and image blurring occurs. Fat is bright on T2WI impairing detection of pathology, such as edema in fat adjacent to an inflammatory process. Addition of fat-suppression techniques counters this effect. Fast low-angle acquisition with relaxation enhancement (FLARE) and half-Fourier acquisition single-shot turbo spin echo (HASTE) are variations of this technique.

Inversion recovery (IR) pulse sequences are used mainly to emphasize differences in T1 relaxation times of tissues. A delay time, TI (time of inversion) is added to the TE and TR instrument settings selected by the operator. Standard IR sequences, using a long TI, produce T1WI. Tissues with short T1 times yield a brighter signal. *Short TI inversion recovery* (STIR) sequences are the most commonly used. This sequence achieves additive T1-weighted, T2-weighted, and proton density weighted contrast to increase lesion conspicuity. With STIR sequences, all tissues with short T1 relaxation times, including fat, are suppressed, whereas tissue with high water content, including many pathologic lesions, are accentuated, yielding a bright signal on a dark background of nulled short-T1 tissue. STIR images more closely resemble strongly T2WI.

Gradient recalled echo (GRE) pulse sequences are used to perform fast MR and MR angiography. Rapid image sequences are particularly useful in body MR to minimize motion artifact of breathing, heartbeat, vessel pulsation, and bowel peristalsis. T1-weighted GRE sequences have completely replaced SE T1-weighted sequences in body MR imaging. Partial "flip angles" of less than 90 degrees are used to decrease the time to signal recovery. Signal intensity arising from T2 relaxation characteristics of tissue is strongly affected by imperfections in the magnetic field on GRE images. Magnetization decay time with GRE imaging is termed T2* ("T2 star") and is much shorter than the "true" T2 decay times seen with SE imaging. T2*-weighted imaging are used to depict hemorrhage, calcification, and iron deposition in tissues. GRE images are characteristically low in image contrast, have more prominent artifacts, and demonstrate flowing blood with bright signal. T1-, T2-, T2*-, and proton density–image weighting is determined by the combination of flip angle, TR, and TE settings. Fast GRE techniques include fast low-angle shot (FLASH), gradient-recalled acquisition in steady state (GRASS), and true fast imaging with steady-state precession (FISP), snapshot FLASH, rapid acquisition with gradient echo (RAGE) and magnetization prepared RAGE (MPRAGE).

Echo-planar imaging is a very fast MR technique that can produce single-slice images in 20 to 100 ms. All spatial encoding information is obtained after a single RF excitation, compared with the multiple RF excitations separated by TR intervals required for conventional MR. Motion artifact is virtually eliminated, and moving structures can be "freeze-frame" imaged. Special hardware is required for echo-planar imaging, but standard SE, GRE, and IR pulse sequences can be obtained. Echo-planar imaging overcomes many of the time and motion limitations of conventional MR and enables expansion of MR to new areas such as blood perfusion and cortical activation of the brain.

Diffusion-weighted imaging (DWI) sequences are designed to detect alteration in the random (brownian) motion of water molecules within tissues. DWI measures diffusion, the mean path length traveled by water molecules within a specific time interval. DWI techniques were initially applied to neuroradiology particularly in detection of acute cerebral ischemia but have become increasing useful in body imaging for tumor detection, tumor characterization, and evaluation of tumor response to treatment.

Diffusion-tensor imaging (DTI) and fiber tractography demonstrate the orientation and integrity of white matter fibers particularly useful in diagnosis of diseases of the corpus callosum and in cortical dysplasia. DTI also has application in imaging muscle fibers in the heart and musculoskeletal system.

MR spectroscopy provides demonstration of relative tissue metabolite concentrations based on chemical shift phenomena. Choline, creatine, citrate, lactate, and other metabolites change in different pathologic conditions. For example, in the breast peaks of choline suggest malignancy. MR spectroscopy has expanding utility in diagnosis of conditions in the brain, breast, abdominal organs, and musculoskeletal system.

Fat-suppression techniques are used in MR to detect the presence of fat or to suppress signal from fat to enhance detection of pathology (tumor invasion into fat or edema in fat).

Fat-saturation technique takes advantage of the difference in resonance frequencies of water and fat. Signal from fat is suppressed while the image is produced from the remaining signal of water. Fat-saturation technique modifies only the signal of fat without modifying signal characteristics of other tissues. It can be used effectively with contrast-enhanced images. This technique is highly sensitive to magnetic field inhomogeneity and misregistration artifacts, and does not work well with low-field magnets. The technique is optimal for suppressing signal from macroscopic fat within adipose tissue (Fig. 1.13C).

Short TI Inversion Recovery (STIR) provides global homogeneous fat suppression but suppresses all tissues with very short T1, including tissue enhanced by administration of intravenous gadolinium, mucoid tissue, hemorrhage, and proteinaceous fluid (Fig. 1.13D). It can be used with low-field magnets and is insensitive to inhomogeneities in the magnetic field.

Chemical shift imaging (opposed phase MR) is fast, reliable, and optimal for detection of small amounts of fat such as intracellular fat in adrenal adenomas and fatty-infiltrated hepatocytes in the liver (Fig. 1.14). Resonance frequency of water is different (faster than) that of fat. In-phase (IP) images add signal from fat and water. Opposed phase (out-of-phase

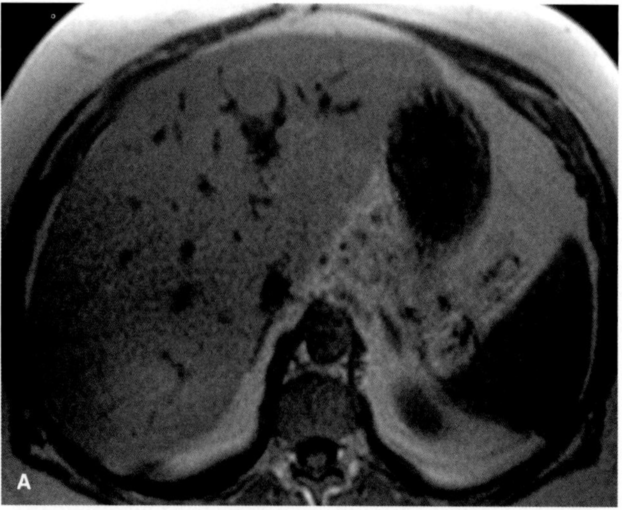

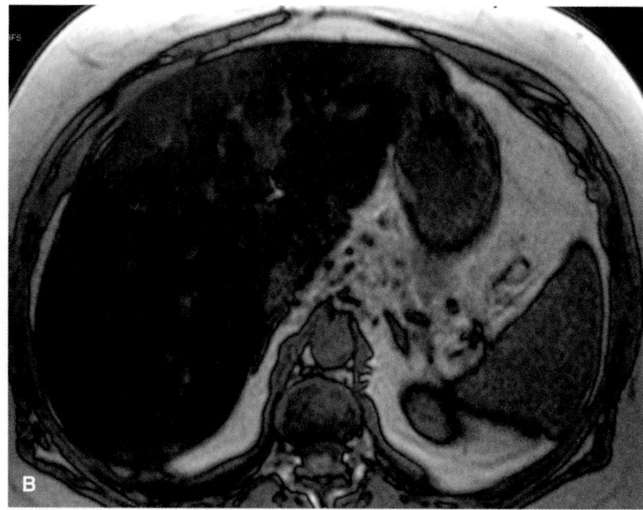

FIGURE 1.14. **Opposed Phase Fat-Suppression Technique.** Compare the in-phase image of the liver, **A**, with the opposed phase image of the liver, **B**. The dramatic darkening of the liver on the opposed phase image is indicative of diffuse fatty infiltration. The signal from fat within hepatocytes is subtracted from the total signal including fat and water on the in-phase image.

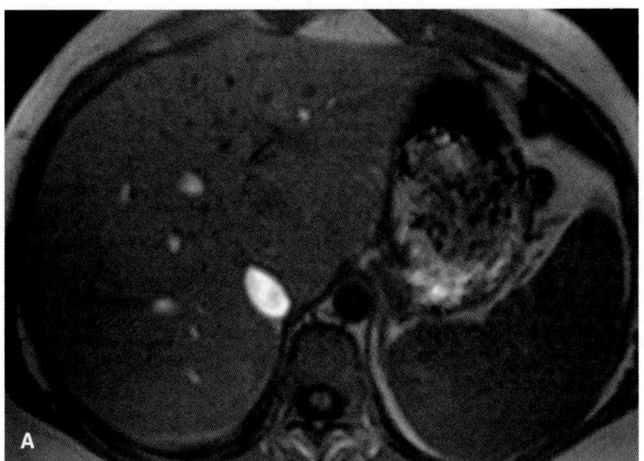

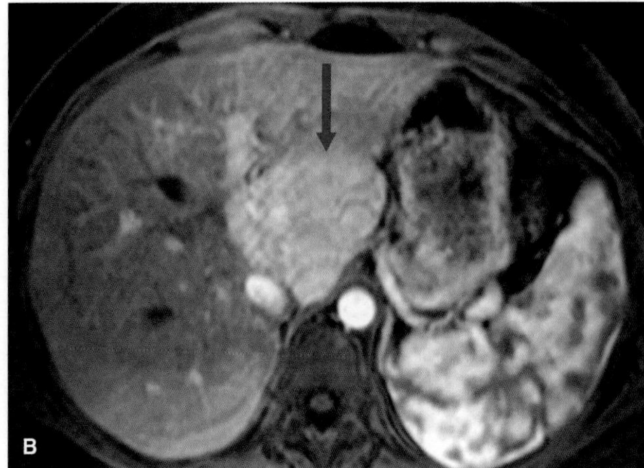

FIGURE 1.15. **Contrast Administration in MR.** Intravenous administration of gadolinium chelate dramatically increases the conspicuity of the liver mass (*arrow*) on an early postcontrast image, **B**, compared to a noncontrast image, **A**. The mottled enhancement of the spleen is caused by the relatively slow diffusion of contrast through the splenic sinusoids.

[OP]) images subtract water signal from fat signal. The presence of fat within cells is demonstrated by a distinct drop in signal intensity on the OP image compared to the IP image. Chemical shift imaging is characterized by two distinctive edge artifacts. The technique results in spatial misregistration of fat signal resulting in alternating bands of bright and dark signal at water/fat interfaces in the frequency-encoded direction. The second artifact is a thin black line at interface between fat and water laden tissue (e.g., the interface between the kidney and perinephric fat) has been termed the "india ink artifact." This artifact is useful in identification of the OP image and may additionally be used to identify fatty tumors such as angiomyolipomas. The india ink artifact occurs along the entire border between fat and water (fat/organ, fat/muscle), not only in the frequency-encoded direction. The artifact results from the presence of fat and water molecules in the same voxel resulting in loss of signal by phase cancellation in all directions. Adipose tissue contains abundant fat and little water so the signal is minimally reduced on OP images. However, tissue with low fat content but high water content (adrenal adenomas, fat-infiltrated hepatocytes) shows a prominent loss of signal on OP images compared to IP images. The obvious limitation is that opposed phase MR does not suppress signal from adipose tissue (Fig. 1.14B).

Advantages of MR include its outstanding soft tissue contrast resolution, ability to provide images in any anatomic plane, and absence of ionizing radiation. MR is limited in its ability to demonstrate dense bone detail or calcifications, has long imaging times for many pulse sequences, limited spatial resolution compared with CT, limited availability in some geographic areas, and is expensive. Because of the physically confining space for the patient within the magnet, a number of patients experience symptoms of claustrophobia and require sedation or are simply unable to tolerate MR scanning. "Open" magnet design aids in the MR imaging of very large and claustrophobic patients but these units are generally of lower-field strength and lack the resolution of the high-field strength "tube" magnets.

Contrast Administration in MR. Gadolinium chelates are used, similar to the use of iodinated contrast agents in CT, to identify blood vessels and confirm their patency, to identify regions of disruption of the blood–brain barrier, to enhance organs to accentuate pathology (Fig. 1.15), and to document patterns of lesion enhancement. Gadolinium is a rare-earth heavy metal ion with paramagnetic effect that shortens the T1 and T2 relaxation times of hydrogen nuclei within its local magnetic field. Gadolinium is important in providing high-quality MR angiographic studies by enhancing the signal differences between blood vessels and surrounding tissues. At recommended doses, gadolinium shortens T1 to a much greater extent than it shortens T2. Increases in signal intensity resulting from T1 shortening resulting from concentrations of gadolinium are best seen on T1WI. However, when very high tissue concentration is reached, such as in the renal collecting system, T2 shortening causes a significant loss of signal intensity that is best seen on T2WI. Like iodinated contrast agents used in CT and radiography, gadolinium-based agents have potential adverse effects that must be considered before administration to patients.

Safety Considerations. The MR environment creates potential risks not only to the patient being imaged but also accompanying family members and healthcare personnel. MR is contraindicated in patients who have electrically, magnetically, or mechanically activated implants including cardiac pacemakers, insulin pumps, cochlear implants, neurostimulators, bone-growth stimulators, and implantable drug infusion pumps. Patients with intracardiac pacing wires or Swan–Ganz catheters are at risk for RF current-induced cardiac fibrillation and burns. Ferromagnetic implants such as cerebral aneurysm clips, vascular clips, and skin staples are at risk for rotation and dislodgment, burns, and induced electrical currents. Bullets, shrapnel, and metallic fragments may move and cause additional injury or become projectiles in the magnetic field. Metal workers and patients with a history of penetrating eye injuries should be screened with radiographs of the orbits to detect intraocular metallic foreign bodies that may dislodge, tear the retina, and cause blindness. Certain transdermal-medicated patches contain traces of aluminum and other metals in the adhesive backing. If worn during MR imaging skin burns may occur at the patch site. A variety of implantable devices have been confirmed to be safe for MR, including nonferromagnetic vascular clips and staples, orthopedic devices composed of nonferromagnetic materials, and a variety of noncardiac implantable pacemakers and stimulators. Each device must be checked for its MR compatibility. Prosthetic heart valves with metal components and stainless steel Greenfield filters are considered safe because the in vivo forces affecting them are stronger than the deflecting forces of the electromagnetic field. No convincing body of evidence indicates that short-term exposure to the electromagnetic fields of MR harms the developing

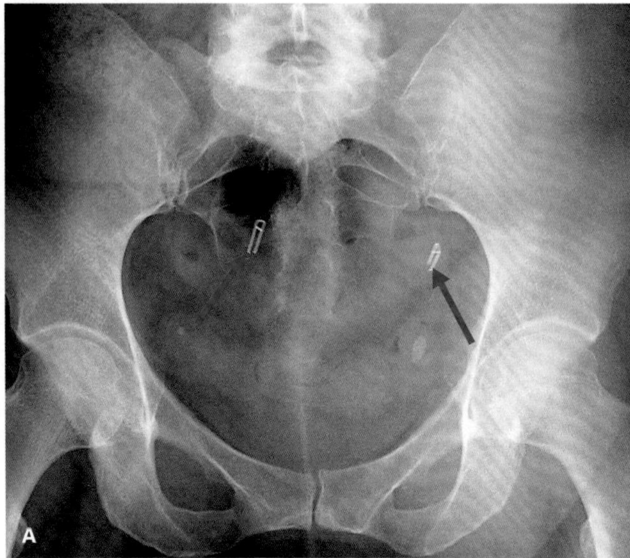

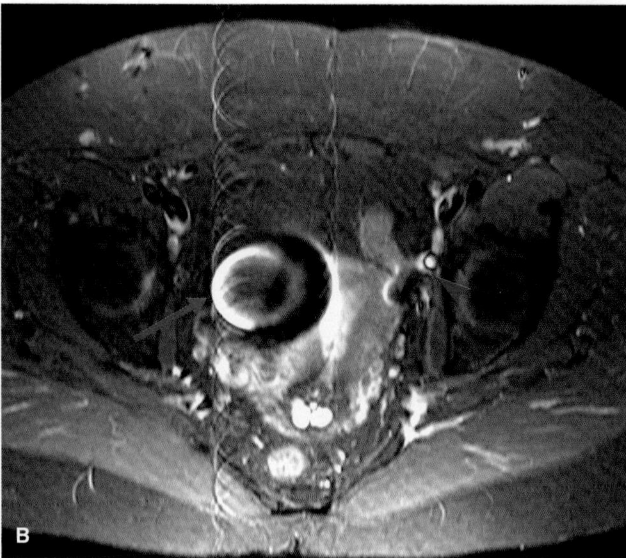

FIGURE 1.16. **Magnetic Susceptibility Artifact.** Radiograph of the pelvis, **A**, and axial plane T2-weighted MR image, **B**, in the same patient show the artifact (*red arrow, red arrowhead*) produced by metallic clips (*blue arrows*) used for tubal ligation. The dramatic increase in artifact on the right side (*red arrow*) as compared to the left side (*red arrowhead*) is caused by proximity of the right-sided clip to a blood vessel creating pulsatile motion of the clip.

fetus, although it is not possible to prove that MR is absolutely safe in pregnancy. Pregnant patients can be scanned, provided the study is medically indicated. In the event of a cardiac arrest the patient must be removed from the MR magnet room to run cardiopulmonary resuscitation.

MR Artifacts. Artifacts are intrinsic to MR technique and must be recognized to avoid mistaking them for disease.

Magnetic susceptibility artifact is caused by focal distortions in the main magnetic field resulting from the presence of ferromagnetic objects such as orthopedic devices, surgical clips and wires, dentures, metallic foreign bodies in the patient, and ingested material, such as various forms of iron tablets. The artifact is seen as areas of signal void at the location of the metal implant (Fig. 1.16), often with a rim of increased intensity and a distortion of the image in the vicinity.

FIGURE 1.17. **Motion Artifact.** Pulsations of the aorta (*arrow*) produce numerous ghosts of the aorta in the phase-encoded direction. Swapping the phase-encoded direction with the frequency-encoded direction will enable evaluation of the left lobe of the liver.

Motion artifact is common in MR when image acquisition time is long. Random motion produces blurring of the image. Periodic motion, such as that caused by pulsating blood vessels, causes ghosts of the moving structures (Fig. 1.17). Motion artifacts are most visible along the phase-encoded direction. Swapping phase- and frequency-encoded directions may make the artifacts less bothersome.

Chemical shift misregistration occurs at interfaces between fat and water. Protons bound in lipid molecules experience a slightly lower magnetic influence than protons in water when exposed to an externally applied gradient magnetic field, resulting in misregistration of signal location. The artifact is seen as a line of high-signal intensity on one side of the fat–water interface and a line of signal void at the opposite side of the fat–water interface (Fig. 1.18). Evaluation of the bladder wall and renal margins is difficult in the presence of this artifact.

Truncation error occurs adjacent to sharp boundaries between tissues of markedly different contrast. The artifact is attributable to inherent errors in the Fourier transform technique of image reconstruction. The artifact appears as

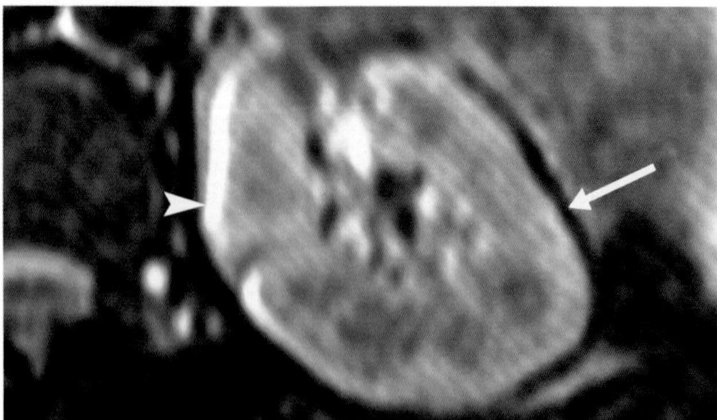

FIGURE 1.18. **Chemical Shift Artifact.** Chemical shift misregistration between fat and kidney tissue produces a high-density band (*arrowhead*) on the medial aspect of the left kidney and a low-density band (*arrow*) on its lateral aspect.

TABLE 1.1

RULES OF MR SOFT TISSUE CONTRAST

T1-Weighted Images		
Short T1 tissue	⇒	High signal
Long T1 tissue	⇒	Low signal
T2-Weighted Images		
Short T2 tissue	⇒	Low signal
Long T2 tissue	⇒	High signal

regularly spaced alternating parallel bands of bright and dark signal. It may simulate a syrinx of the spinal cord or a meniscal tear in the knee.

Aliasing, or image wraparound, artifact occurs when anatomy outside the designated field of view but within the image plane is mismapped onto the opposite side of the image, for instance, on a midline sagittal brain MR, the patient's nose may be artifactually displayed over the area of the posterior fossa. Aliasing may be eliminated by increasing the field of view (at the expense of loss of image resolution) or by increasing the number of phase-encoding steps outside the field of view (oversampling).

Principles of MR Interpretation. Outstanding soft tissue contrast is obtained in MR by designing imaging sequences that accentuate differences in T1 and T2 tissue relaxation times. Sequences that accentuate differences in proton density are fruitful in brain imaging but are generally less useful for extracranial soft tissue imaging, in which proton density differences are small. Interpreting MR depends on a clear understanding of the biophysical basis of MR tissue contrast. Water is the major source of the MR signal in tissues other than fat. Mineral-rich structures such as bone and calculi, and collagenous tissues such as ligaments, tendons, fibrocartilage, and tissue fibrosis, are low in water content and lack mobile protons to produce an MR signal. These tissues are low in signal intensity on all MR sequences. Water in tissue exists in at least two physical states: *free water* with unrestricted motion and *bound water* with restricted motion owing to hydrogen bonding with proteins. Free water is found mainly in extracellular fluid, whereas bound water is found mainly in intracellular fluid. Intracellular water is both bound and free and is in a condition of rapid exchange between the two states.

Free water has long T1 and T2 relaxation times, resulting in low signal intensity on T1WI and high signal intensity on T2WI (Table 1.1). Organs with abundant extracellular fluid, and therefore large amounts of free water, include kidney (urine); ovaries and thyroid (fluid-filled follicles); spleen and penis (stagnant blood); and prostate, testes, and seminal vesicles (fluid in tubules) (Table 1.2). Edema is an increase in extracellular fluid and tends to have the effect of prolonging T1 and T2 relaxation times in affected tissues. Most neoplastic tissues have an increase in extracellular fluid as well as an increase in the proportion of intracellular free water, resulting in their visualization with bright signal intensity on T2WI. In organs, such as the kidney, that are also rich in extracellular or free water, neoplasms may appear isointense or hypointense compared with the bright normal parenchyma on T2WI. Neoplasms that are hypocellular or fibrotic have low signal intensity on T2WI because fibrous tissue dominates their signal characteristics. Simple cysts, cerebrospinal fluid, urine in the bladder, and bile in the gallbladder all reflect the signal characteristics of free water.

Proteinaceous Fluids. The addition of protein to free water has the effect of shortening the T1 relaxation time, thus

TABLE 1.2

MR SIGNAL STRENGTH OF TISSUES AND BODY FLUIDS

■ TISSUE/BODY FLUID	■ EXAMPLES	■ T1WI SIGNAL	■ T2WI SIGNAL
Gas	Air in the lung Gas in the bowel	Absent	Absent
Mineral rich tissue	Cortical bone Calculi	Absent	Absent
Collagenous tissue	Ligaments, tendons Fibrocartilage, scar tissue	Low	Low
Fat	Adipose tissue Fatty bone marrow	High	Intermediate to high
High bound water tissue	Liver, pancreas, adrenal Muscle, hyaline cartilage	Low	Low to intermediate
High free water tissue	Kidney, testes, prostate Seminal vesicles, ovary Thyroid, spleen, penis Bladder, gallbladder, edema	Low	High
Fluid	Urine, bile Simple cysts	Black	White
Proteinaceous fluid	Complicated cyst, abscess Synovial fluid, nucleus pulposus	Intermediate	High
Brain tissue/fluid	Gray matter White matter Ventricles/cerebrospinal fluid	Low High Black	High Low White

Modified from Mitchell DG, Burk DL Jr, Vinitski S, Rifkin MD. The biophysical basis of tissue contrast in extracranial MR imaging. *AJR Am J Roentgenol* 1987;149:831–837 and Atlas SW, ed. *Magnetic Resonance Imaging of the Brain and Spine*. 4th ed. Philadelphia, PA: Lippincott Williams & Wilkins; 2009.

brightening the signal on T1WI. T2 relaxation is also shortened, but the T1 shortening effect is dominant even on T2WI. Therefore, proteinaceous fluid collections remain high in signal intensity on T2WI. Proteinaceous fluids include synovial fluid, complicated cysts, abscesses, many pathologic fluid collections, and necrotic areas within tumors.

Soft tissues with a predominance of intracellular bound water have shorter T1 and T2 times than do tissues with large amounts of extracellular water. These tissues, including the liver, pancreas, adrenal glands, and muscle, have intermediate signal intensities on both T1WI and T2WI. Intracellular protein synthesis shortens T1 even more; therefore, muscle, being less active in protein synthesis, is lower in signal intensity on T1WI than are organs with more active protein synthesis. Benign lesions with a predominance of normal cells, such as focal nodular hyperplasia in the liver, tend to remain isointense with their surrounding normal parenchyma on all imaging sequences. Hyaline cartilage has a predominance of extracellular water, but the water is extensively bound to a mucopolysaccharide matrix. Its signal characteristics resemble cellular soft tissues, and it is intermediate in strength on most imaging sequences. Organs with high free water content such as the kidney, testis, prostate, and seminal vesicles reflect free water signal and are low signal on T1WI and high signal on T2WI.

Fat. Protons in fat are bound to hydrophobic intermediate-sized molecules and exchange energy efficiently within their chemical environment. T1 relaxation time is short, resulting in high signal on T1WI. T2 of fat is shorter than T2 of water, resulting in lower signal intensity for fat, relative to water, on strongly T2WI. On images with lesser degrees of T2 weighting, T1 effect predominates and fat appears isointense or slightly hyperintense compared with water. Specialized fat-saturation imaging sequences are used to reduce the signal intensity of fat and enhance the visibility of edema and pathologic processes within fat. STIR sequences suppress signals from all tissues with short T1 times, including fat and gadolinium contrast agents.

Flowing Blood. The MR signal of slow-moving blood, such as in the spleen, venous plexuses, and cavernous hemangiomas, is dominated by the large amount of extracellular free water present, resulting in low signal on T1WI and high signal on T2WI. Higher-velocity blood flow, however, alters the MR signal in complex ways depending on multiple factors. Protons may move out of the imaging plane between RF absorption and RF release, resulting in high-velocity signal loss. Alternatively, blood may be replaced by fully magnetized blood from outside of the image volume, resulting in flow-related enhancement. Flow-related enhancement predominates in GRE imaging, resulting in bright signal intensity ("white blood") for flowing blood, whereas high-velocity signal loss predominates in spin-echo imaging, resulting in signal void ("black blood") in areas of flowing blood.

Hemorrhage. MR of hemorrhage depends on the age of the hemorrhage, the physical and oxidative state of hemoglobin, the location of the hemorrhage, and whether the source of hemorrhage was arterial or venous (Table 1.3). Hemorrhage in the first few hours (hyperacute) is high in free water content and thus has low signal on T1WI and high signal on T2WI. Immediately following intraparenchymal arterial hemorrhage, red blood cells are saturated with oxygen and contain oxyhemoglobin, which is not paramagnetic and has little effect on the MR signal from surrounding water protons. Hemorrhage from a venous source contains deoxyhemoglobin, which is paramagnetic and does affect signal from surrounding water protons. Intracellular deoxyhemoglobin selectively shortens T2, reducing signal intensity on T2WI. Thus, acute hemorrhage from a venous source is not as bright on T2WI as is acute hemorrhage from an arterial source. Within a few hours, red blood cells, from either arterial or venous sources, desaturate and contain predominantly deoxyhemoglobin. The most hypoxic and desaturated portions of the hematoma have the lowest signal. The dark hematoma at this stage is often surrounded by high intensity owing to encircling serum and edema. By approximately 1 week, intracellular deoxyhemoglobin is converted to intracellular methemoglobin beginning at the periphery of the clot. Intracellular methemoglobin is paramagnetic but has restricted motion and is heterogeneous in distribution, shortening T1 and selectively shortening T2, resulting in high signal on T1WI and low signal on T2WI. Lysis of red blood cells at 1 week to 1 month increases access of methemoglobin to water molecules, enhancing the T1 shortening effect. T1 shortening predominates over T2 shortening even on T2WI, resulting in high signal on both T1WI and T2WI. The more dilute the concentration of extracellular methemoglobin (the more water that is present), the higher the signal intensity on T2WI. Areas of low signal intensity on T2WI correspond to retracted clot with intact red cell membranes.

TABLE 1.3

MR OF HEMORRHAGE

■ AGE	■ DOMINANT COMPONENT	■ T1WI SIGNAL	■ T2WI SIGNAL
Hyperacute (<12 hours)			
Arterial	Free water + Oxyhemoglobin	Low	High
Venous	Free water + Deoxyhemoglobin	Low	Less bright than arterial hemorrhage
Acute (hours to days)	Deoxyhemoglobin	Low	Low
Early subacute (few days)	Intracellular deoxyhemoglobin	High	Low
Late subacute (4–7 days to 1 month)	Intracellular methemoglobin	High	High
Chronic (weeks to years)	Hemosiderin and ferritin	Low	Black
Scar	Hemosiderin	Black	Black

Modified from Mitchell DG, Burk DL Jr, Vinitski S, Rifkin MD. The biophysical basis of tissue contrast in extracranial MR imaging. *AJR* 1987;149:831–837 and Brant WE, de Lange EE, eds. *Essentials of Body MRI.* New York: Oxford University Press; 2012.

At approximately the same time as lysis of red blood cells is occurring centrally within the clot, releasing free methemoglobin, hemosiderin is being ingested by macrophages at the periphery of the clot. Hemosiderin is highly paramagnetic, but water insolubility precludes close interaction with water, thus restricting T1 shortening. Limited motion of hemosiderin in its intracellular location causes local inhomogeneous magnetic susceptibility and T2 shortening. The result is low signal on both T1WI and T2WI. Edema surrounding the hypointense band of hemosiderin produces a concentric outer rim of hyperintensity on T2WI as long as edema is present. Hemosiderin-laden macrophages quickly enter the bloodstream, removing hemosiderin from hematoma in nonneural tissues and in areas of the brain where the blood–brain barrier is destroyed, such as in areas of hemorrhage into tumor. Where the blood–brain barrier is quickly repaired, the hemosiderin may remain in brain tissue for long periods and be seen as persisting low intensity. Differentiation of hematoma from other tissues generally requires at least two pulse sequences. Different areas of the hematoma may show signal intensity effects dominated by components in differing stages of evolution.

Ultrasonography

US imaging is performed by using the pulse-echo technique (Fig. 1.19). The US transducer converts electrical energy to a brief pulse of high-frequency sound energy that is transmitted into patient tissues. The US transducer then becomes a receiver, detecting echoes of sound energy reflected from tissue. The depth of any particular echo is determined by accurating measuring the round-trip time of flight for the transmitted pulse and the returning echo and by calculating the depth of the reflecting tissue interface by assuming an average speed of sound in tissue of 1,540 m/s. The US instrument assumes that all returning echoes originate from along the line of sight of the transmitted pulse. The composite image is produced by interrogating tissue in the field of view with multiple closely spaced US pulses. The shape and appearance of the resulting image depend on the design of the particular transducer used (Fig. 1.20). Modern US units operate sufficiently quickly to produce nearly real-time images of moving patient tissue, enabling assessment of respiratory and cardiac movement, vascular pulsations, peristalsis, and the moving fetus. Most medical imaging is performed using US transducers that produce sound pulses in the frequency range of 1 to 17 MHz. Higher frequencies (10 to 17 MHz) yield the greatest spatial resolution but are restricted by limited penetration. Lower frequencies (1 to 3.5 MHz) enable better penetration of tissues

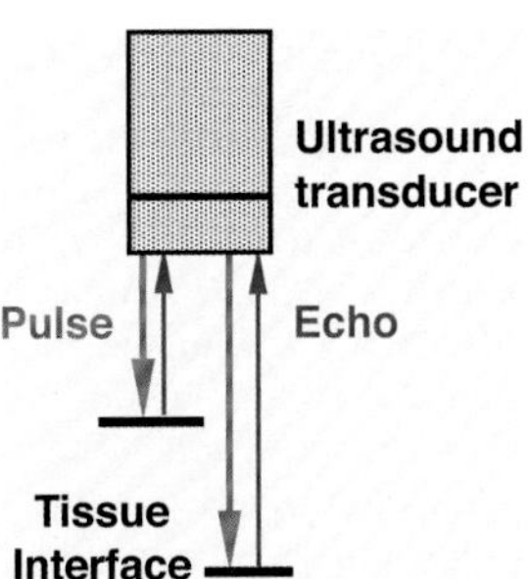

FIGURE 1.19. **US Pulse-Echo Technique.** The US transducer transmits a brief pulse of US energy into tissue. The transmitted US pulse encounters tissue interfaces that reflect a portion of the US beam back to the transducer. The depth of the tissue interface is determined by the round-trip time of flight for the transmitted pulse and the returning echo, assuming an average speed of 1,540 m/s for sound transmission in human tissue.

but at the cost of poorer resolution. Broad band transducers offer a range of sound frequencies to optimize penetration and image resolution. High-frequency transducers are routinely used for endoluminal applications; examination of superficial structures such as thyroid, breast, and testes; and examination of infants, children, and small adults. Lower-frequency transducers are used for most abdominal, pelvic, and obstetric applications.

US examinations are performed by applying the US transducer directly onto the patient's skin using a water-soluble gel as a coupling agent to ensure good contact and transmission of the US beam. Images are produced in any anatomic plane by adjusting the orientation and angulation of the transducer and the position of the patient. The standard orthogonal planes—axial, sagittal, and coronal—provide the easiest recognition of anatomy but may not be optimal for demonstration of all anatomic structures. The quality of all US examinations depends heavily on the skill and diligence of the sonographer. US examinations generally provide the most diagnostic information when they are directed at solving a particular clinical problem.

Visualization of anatomic structures by US is limited by bone and by gas-containing structures such as bowel and lung. Sound energy is nearly completely absorbed at interfaces between soft tissue and bone, causing an acoustic shadow with limited visualization of structures deep to the bone surface. Soft tissue–gas interfaces cause nearly complete reflection of the sound beam, eliminating visualization of deeper structures. Optimal visualization of many organs is performed through "acoustic windows" that allow adequate sound transmission. The liver is imaged through the windows of the intercostal spaces. The pancreas is visualized through the window of the left lobe of the liver. Pelvic organs are examined through the urine-filled bladder, which displaces the gas-filled bowel out of the pelvis. US visualization of structures in the chest depends on finding windows between bone and air-filled lung. US examination may also be limited by surgical wounds, dressings, and skin lesions, which preclude firm transducer contact with the skin. Endoluminal techniques obviate many of the problems of surface scanning. Endovaginal transducers allow close and highly detailed visualization of the uterus and ovaries without intervening tissues. Endorectal transducers enable intimate examination of the prostate gland and rectum. Endoscopic US provides detailed images of the mediastinum, heart, and pancreas viewed through the esophagus or upper gastrointestinal tract.

Doppler US is an important adjunct to real-time gray-scale anatomic imaging. The Doppler effect is a shift in the frequency of returning echoes, compared with the transmitted pulse, caused by reflection of the sound wave from a moving object. In medical imaging, the moving objects of interest are red blood cells in flowing blood. If blood flow is relatively away from the face of the transducer, the echo frequency is shifted lower. If blood flow is relatively toward the face of the transducer, the echo frequency is shifted higher. The amount of frequency shift is proportional to the relative velocity of the moving red blood cells.

Doppler US can detect not only the presence of blood flow but can also determine its direction and velocity. The Doppler frequency shift is in the audible range, producing a sound of blood flow that has additional diagnostic value. *Pulsed Doppler* uses a Doppler sample volume that is time-gated to interrogate only a select volume of patient tissue for the Doppler shift. *Duplex Doppler* combines real-time gray-scale imaging with pulsed Doppler to enable accurate placement of the Doppler sample volume in visualized blood vessels or specific areas of interest. *Color Doppler* combines gray scale and color-coded Doppler information in a single image (Fig. 1.21). Stationary

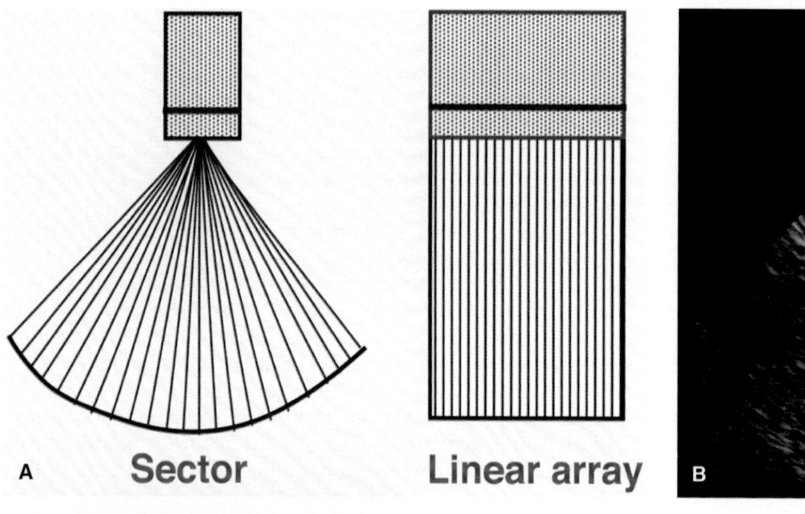

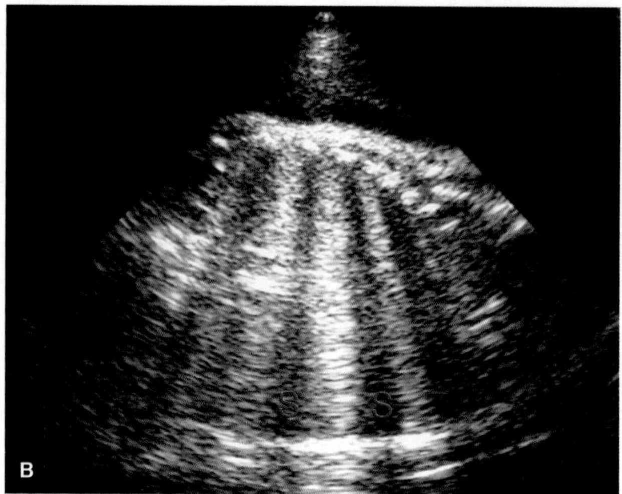

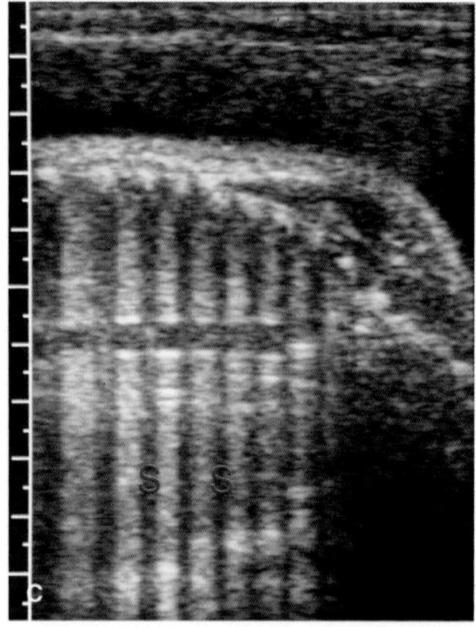

FIGURE 1.20. Sector Versus Linear Array US Transducers. A: Diagram of the diverging US beams transmitted by a sector transducer (**left**) and the parallel US beams transmitted by linear array transducer (**right**). Sector transducers have the advantage of wider field of view in the far field, whereas linear array transducers have a wider field of view in the near field. **B:** Sector transducer image of a fetus shows prominent shadowing (*S*) from the fetal ribs. Note how the width of the shadows expands with increasing depth because of the diverging US beams. **C:** Linear array transducer image of the same fetus shows parallel nonwidening shadows (*S*) from the fetal ribs. Note the improved visualization of the near field.

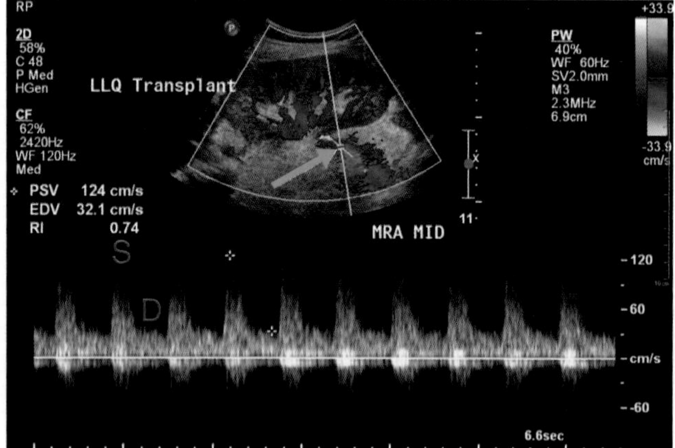

FIGURE 1.21. Color and Spectral Doppler of a Transplant Kidney. The color image at the top shows normal perfusion of the transplant kidney with the arteries displayed in red (toward the transducer) and the veins displayed in blue (away from the transducer). Spectral Doppler at the bottom shows normal pulsatility of the main artery to the transplant kidney with flow into the kidney throughout the cardiac cycle. High-velocity flow is evident in systole (*S*) with lower-velocity flow throughout diastole (*D*). The *green arrow* shows placement of the sample volume from which the spectral Doppler signal was obtained.

tissue with echoes having no Doppler shift are displayed in shades of gray, whereas blood flow and moving tissue producing echoes having a detectable Doppler shift are displayed in color. Blood flow relatively toward the transducer face is routinely displayed in shades of red, whereas blood flow relatively away from the transducer face is displayed in shades of blue. Lighter-color shades imply higher-flow velocities. Doppler US is discussed in further detail in Chapter 54.

Tissue Harmonic Imaging. Harmonic sound waves occur at sound frequencies that are integer multiples of the frequency of the primary sound wave. Harmonic US instrumentation filters out the frequency of the primary sound wave and generates diagnostic images from the second harmonic of the primary wave. The advantages of tissue harmonic imaging (THI) are reduction in artifacts caused by side lobes, grating lobes, and reverberation as well as improved signal to noise ratio. *Differential THI* utilizes two pulses transmitted into tissue simultaneously. The primary frequencies of both pulses are cancelled out and the second harmonic frequency of both pulses, as well as the frequency difference between the two pulses, are used to create the US image. Both forms of THI improve image detail, reduce noise, improve margin sharpness, and improve US penetration. THI is used for improved detection and characterization of breast lesions, lymph nodes, thyroid nodules, focal abnormalities of the liver and pancreas, and differentiation of cysts and solid lesions in the kidneys. THI is also utilized for US contrast agent applications using microbubbles.

Elastography. US elastography is a US imaging technique based on detecting differences in tissue stiffness. Various neoplastic, pathologic, and physiologic processes change the elasticity of normal tissues. Elasticity describes the propensity of tissue to resist deformation from an applied force and to return to its original shape when the force is removed. Many solid tumors are stiffer than surrounding healthy tissue. Fibrotic changes in the liver are stiffer than normal liver parenchyma. Diseased tendons are softer than normal tendons. Two types of US elastographic evaluation are in common use: strain elastography and shear wave elastography. *Strain elastography* measures physical tissue displacement by manually pressing the US transducer on the lesion or tissue, or by observing compression of tissue by physiologic motion such as heart beat or respiration. Tissue displacement is measured by Doppler tracking, radiofrequency echo tracking, or both, depending on the instrument manufacturer. *Shear wave elastography* measures the speed of shear waves produced by tissue displacement. Shear waves are waves of acoustic energy that propagate perpendicular to a compression force in elastic tissue. Tissue compression is achieved by producing a short-duration, high-intensity acoustic pulse, termed acoustic radiation force impulse (ARFI). Elastography is used to measure the degree of fibrosis in chronic liver disease, to assist in differentiation of benign from malignant lesions in the breast, liver, thyroid, kidney, prostate and other tissues, and to characterize various pathologic conditions and traumatic injuries to the musculoskeletal system.

US Artifacts. Artifacts are extremely common in US imaging and must be recognized to avoid diagnostic errors. Some artifacts, such as acoustic shadowing and enhancement, are diagnostically useful.

Acoustic shadowing is produced by nearly complete absorption, or by complete reflection, of the US beam, obscuring deeper tissue structures. Acoustic shadows are produced by gallstones (Fig. 1.22), urinary tract stones, bone, metallic objects, and gas bubbles. The presence of acoustic shadowing aids in the identification of all types of calculi.

Acoustic enhancement refers to the increased intensity of echoes deep to structures that transmit sound exceptionally well such as cysts (Fig. 1.23), fluid-filled bladder and gallbladder, and some homogeneous solid masses such as lymphoma-replaced lymph nodes. The presence of acoustic enhancement aids in the identification of cysts and fluid-filled structures.

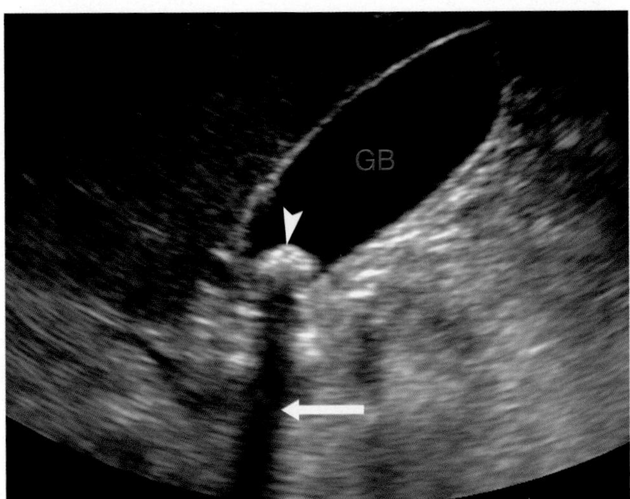

FIGURE 1.22. Acoustic Shadowing. A gallstone (*arrowhead*) at the neck of the gallbladder (GB) produces a dark acoustic shadow (*arrow*) by absorption of the US beam. Demonstration of acoustic shadowing is important in the US diagnosis of biliary and renal calculi.

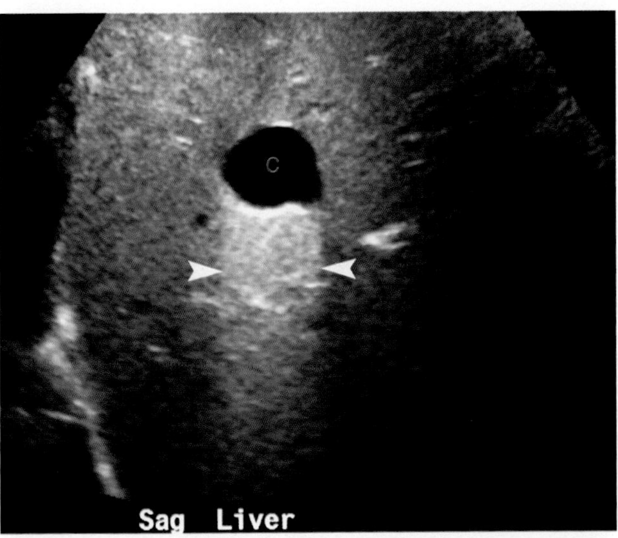

FIGURE 1.23. Acoustic Enhancement. US image of a cyst (*c*) in the liver demonstrates acoustic enhancement (*arrowheads*) as a band of bright echoes deep to the cyst.

Reverberation artifact is caused by repeated reflections between strong acoustic reflectors. Returning echoes are re-reflected into tissues, producing multiple echoes of the same structures that are portrayed on the image progressively deeper in tissue because of prolonged time of flight of echoes eventually returning to the transducer. Reverberation artifact is seen as repeating bands of echoes of progressively decreasing intensity at regularly spaced intervals.

Mirror image artifact is commonly evident when examining the upper abdomen and diaphragm. Multipath reflection from the strong sound reflection produced by the air-filled lung surface above the curving diaphragm results in depiction of liver or spleen tissue pattern both below and above the diaphragm (Fig. 1.24).

Ring down, or comet tail, artifact is seen as a pattern of tapering bright echoes trailing from small bright reflectors such as air bubbles and cholesterol crystals. The artifact may result from vibrations of the reflector or multiple short-path reverberations. Comet tail artifacts are used to identify precipitated cholesterol crystals associated with adenomyomatosis of the gallbladder and to identify precipitated thyroid colloid in benign colloid cysts.

Twinkle is an artifact of intrinsic machine noise seen with color Doppler (Fig. 1.25). Twinkling artifact appears as a random pattern of various colors displayed on highly reflective objects such as calculi. Twinkle artifact is more sensitive for detection of stones than is acoustic shadowing. Twinkle artifact is highly dependent on machine settings and is most pronounced when the reflecting surface is rough.

Principles of US Interpretation. Interpretation of US examination is best performed by the radiologist who has studied the images produced by the sonographer and who, with transducer in hand, has personally examined the patient. US in the hands of a skilled physician is a dynamic extension of physical examination. The examining physician has the opportunity to query the patient regarding current and past symptoms, previous surgery, and pertinent medical history. Suspected masses can be palpated as well as examined by US. Artifacts are more

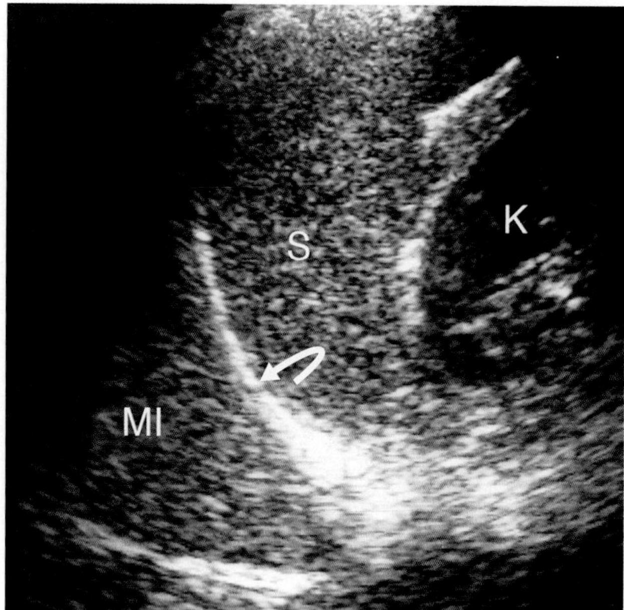

FIGURE 1.24. **Mirror-Image Artifact.** Longitudinal image of the left upper quadrant of the abdomen demonstrates the spleen (*S*), diaphragm (*arrow*), and artifactual mirror image (*MI*) of the spleen above the diaphragm. K, left kidney.

easily differentiated from true components of the image by real-time examination. Active examination enables rapid assessment of three-dimensional anatomic relationships. The real-time US examination yields thousands of images within a few minutes. The static images and short video clips recorded in PACS serve only to document the dynamic real-time examination. All questions in interpretation should be answered by active sonographic examination.

Fluid-containing structures such as cysts, dilated calyces and ureters, and the distended bladder and gallbladder characteristically demonstrate well-defined walls, absence of internal echoes, and distal acoustic enhancement. Solid tissue demonstrates a speckled pattern of tissue texture with definable blood vessels, best demonstrated by color Doppler. Fat is usually highly echogenic, whereas solid organs such as liver, pancreas,

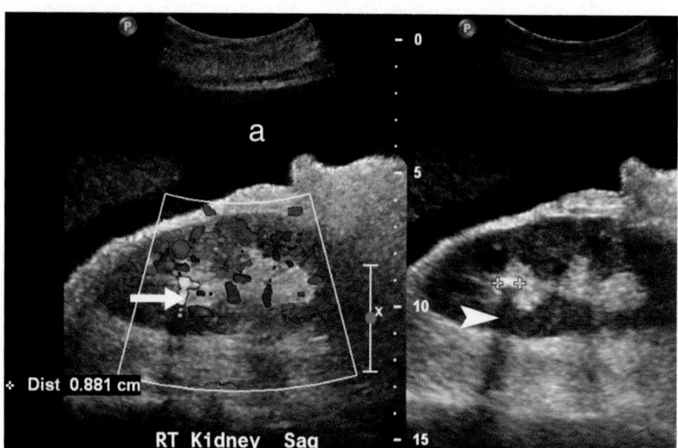

FIGURE 1.25. **Twinkle Artifact.** The gray scale image of the right kidney on the right shows a kidney stone (between *cursors*, +) casting an acoustic shadow (*arrowhead*). On the left the same image utilizing color Doppler shows blood flow in the kidney in red and blue colors and the amorphous color signal of the twinkle artifact (*arrow*) emanating from the stone. This patient also has ascites (*a*).

and kidney demonstrate lower degrees of echogenicity. Lesions within or arising from organs demonstrate mass effect with alteration of organ contour and displacement of blood vessels and with alteration in tissue echogenicity and texture. Lesions of lower echogenicity (lower-intensity echoes) than surrounding parenchyma are termed *hypoechoic*, and lesions of greater echogenicity (higher-intensity echoes) than surrounding parenchyma are called *hyperechoic*. The term *anechoic* refers to the complete absence of echoes, such as within simple cysts. Cystic structures containing fluid having echoes such as blood, pus, or mucin may cause confusion in the sonographic differentiation of cystic and solid lesions. Echo-containing cystic structures demonstrate the absence of internal blood vessels, fluid–fluid layering, shifting contents with transducer compression or change in patient position, and well-defined walls. Acoustic enhancement might or might not be present.

US Biosafety Considerations. While US is generally considered to be safe at the low-energy output routinely used in diagnostic imaging, adverse effects can be demonstrated at higher-energy levels including those used for Doppler evaluation. Potential adverse effects include deposition of heat, tissue cavitation, and chemical reactions induced by oxygen radicals. Special consideration must be given to the fetus especially during the vulnerable first trimester. Doppler US should never be used to document fetal heart motion and care should be taken to keep the first trimester fetus out of the direct Doppler beam during diagnostic examinations. The lowest possible acoustic power setting should always be used. US should be utilized for medical diagnosis only, and not for entertainment. High-intensity focused US is used to destroy tissue in the treatment of both malignant and benign diseases.

RADIOGRAPHIC CONTRAST AGENTS

Iodinated Contrast Agents

Water-soluble contrast agents (Table 1.4), consisting of molecules containing atoms of iodine, are used extensively for intravascular applications in CT, urography, angiography, arthrography, cystography, fistulography, and opacification of the lumen of the gastrointestinal tract. With the ever-expanding use of CT, the number of patients exposed to iodinated contrast agents continues to increase. Fortunately, the risk of adverse reaction is low, but real risk is inherent in their use. Any contrast agent administration, regardless of dose or route of administration, carries a finite risk of mild to life-threatening reaction. Provision for prompt treatment of any adverse reaction to contrast agents is essential. Older, cheaper, high-osmolar ionic agents have been near completely replaced in most applications by newer but more expensive, low-osmolar agents because of safety considerations.

Ionic contrast agents (high-osmolality contrast agents) had been considered safe and effective for more than 70 years. Ionic media are acid salts that dissociate in water into an iodine-containing negatively charged anion (diatrizoate, iothalamate) and a positively charged cation (sodium or meglumine). To achieve a sufficient concentration of iodine for radiographic visualization, ionic agents are markedly hypertonic (approximately six times the osmolality of plasma). High osmolality and viscosity cause significant hemodynamic, cardiac, and subjective effects including vasodilatation, heat, pain, osmotic diuresis, and decreased myocardial contractility.

Nonionic contrast agents (low-osmolality contrast agents) have an osmolality reduced to one to two times that of blood, resulting in a significant decrease in the already low incidence

TABLE 1.4

STAGES OF CHRONIC KIDNEY DISEASE

■ STAGE	■ DESCRIPTION	■ GLOMERULAR FILTRATION RATE (GFR) (mL/min/1.73 m^2)
Stage 1	Kidney damage with normal or increased GFR	>90
Stage 2	Mild reduction in GFR	60–89
Stage 3A Stage 3B	Moderate reduction in GFR	45–59 30–44
Stage 4	Severe reduction in GFR	15–29
Stage 5	Kidney failure	<15

Chronic kidney disease is defined as kidney damage or a decreased glomerular filtration rate of less than 60 mL/min/1.73 m^2 for 3 or more months.
Kidney Disease: Improving Global Outcomes (KDIGO). Levin A, Stevens PE. Summary of KDIGO 2012 CKD Guideline: behind the scenes, need for guidance, and a framework for moving forward. *Kidney Int* 2014;85:49–61.

of adverse reactions. Reduction in osmolality is achieved by making compounds that are nonionic monomers. Reduced osmolality results in less hemodynamic alteration on contrast injection. Nonionic contrast agents continue to be significantly more expensive than ionic contrast agents.

All iodinated contrast agents have a chemical structure based on a benzene ring containing three iodine atoms. Following IV injection, contrast media are distributed quickly into the extracellular space. Excretion is by renal glomerular filtration. Vicarious excretion through the liver, biliary system, and intestinal tract occurs when renal function is impaired.

Adverse side effects are uncommon reported in 0.2% to 0.7% of patients receiving nonionic lower-osmolality agents. The mortality incidence estimated for intravascular use of low-osmolality iodinated contrast agents is 1 fatality per 170,000 contrast media administrations. The precise pathophysiology of adverse reactions to contrast agents is unknown. However, an increasing body of evidence suggests that a true allergic reaction mediated by IgE is a likely precipitating event. Triggering of mast cells to release histamine is related to severe reactions. Accurate prediction of contrast reactions is not possible but patients with a history of previous contrast reaction are clearly at higher risk, up to five times increased risk. A history of asthma or significant allergic reactions to other allergens also increases the risk. Cardiovascular effects are more common and more severe in patients with cardiac disease. Patient-reported "allergy" to shellfish is no longer considered a risk factor.

Mild adverse effects are most common. Nausea, vomiting, urticaria, pruritus, mild cutaneous edema, feeling of warmth with injection, and pain at the injection site occur with greater frequency following injection of ionic agents and is related to their higher osmolality. Similar reactions to low-osmolality agents are rare. Most mild reactions do not require treatment. Patients should be observed for 20 to 30 minutes to ensure that the reaction does not become more severe.

Moderate reactions are not life threatening but commonly require treatment for symptoms. Patients with severe hives, vasovagal reactions, bronchospasm, prolonged nausea or vomiting, and mild laryngeal edema should be monitored until symptoms resolve. Diphenhydramine is effective for relief of symptomatic hives. Beta-agonist inhalers help with bronchospasm, and epinephrine is indicated for laryngeal spasm. Leg elevation is indicated for vasovagal reactions and hypotension.

Severe, potentially life-threatening, side effects nearly always occur within the first 20 minutes following intravascular injection. These are rare but must be recognized and treated immediately. The risk of death precipitated by intravenous injection of iodinated contrast is conservatively estimated at 1 in 170,000. Severe bronchospasm or severe laryngeal edema may progress to loss of consciousness, seizures, and cardiac arrest. Complete cardiovascular collapse requires life-support equipment and immediate cardiopulmonary resuscitation. Cardiotoxic effects include hypotension, dysrhythmias, and precipitation of acute congestive heart failure.

Local Adverse Effects. Venous thrombosis may occur as a result of endothelial damage precipitated by intravenous infusion of contrast. Extravasation of contrast at the injection site is associated with pain, edema, skin slough, or deeper tissue necrosis. If extravasation occurs the affected limb should be elevated. Warm compresses may help absorption of contrast agent, while cold compresses seem more effective at reducing pain at the injection site.

Postcontrast Acute Kidney Injury. Deterioration in renal function that occurs within 48 hours of intravascular contrast administration has been termed postcontrast acute kidney injury (PC-AKI). The term encompasses all causes of acute kidney injury (AKI) whether or not it is caused by contrast administration. ***Contrast-induced nephropathy*** (CIN) is the specific term applied to those rare cases of PC-AKI believed caused by a toxic effect of contrast agent. AKI is defined by the Acute Kidney Injury Network as having one of the following criteria occurring within 48 hours of nephrotoxic event:

- Rise in absolute serum creatinine ≥0.3 mg/dL.
- Percentage increase in serum creatinine ≥50%.
- Reduction in urine output to ≤0.5 mL/kg/hr for at least 6 hours.

While the exact cause of CIN is uncertain pathogenic factors may include vasoconstriction of renal vessels, direct toxicity to the renal tubules, osmotic injury, and chemotoxicity. Intra-arterial administration of contrast agent, especially cardiac angiography, carries a higher risk of CIN than does intravenous contrast administration. The typical clinical course of PC-AKI is transient asymptomatic elevation of serum creatinine within 24 hours of intravascular contrast injection. Serum creatinine levels peak within 4 days, and most return to baseline within 7 to 10 days. However, in some patients permanent renal dysfunction occurs.

Prominent risk factors for PC-AKI include pre-existing chronic severe renal insufficiency and diabetes mellitus. Other less prominent risk factors include dehydration, advanced age, hypertension, multiple myeloma, and patients who receive multiple contrast agent administrations over a short period of time (24 hours). Patients with pre-existing cardiovascular disease are at increased risk of cardiovascular adverse effects.

Serum creatinine concentration measurement alone is an insensitive indicator of kidney function. Serum creatinine levels are affected by the patient's age, gender, muscle mass, and nutritional status. The commonly used cutoff value of ≥1.5 mg/dL fails to identify 40% of patients at risk for CIN. Glomerular filtration rate (GFR) is generally accepted as the best indicator of renal function. Several well-validated formulas have been developed to provide an estimated glomerular filtration rate (eGFR) calculated from measured serum creatinine concentration. The eGFR has been widely accepted as an excellent rapidly obtained estimate of renal function. Serum creatinine concentration can now be determined within

TABLE 1.5

SELECTED LIST OF IODINATED CONTRAST AGENTS

NAME (CONCENTRATION IN mg CONTRAST/mL)	PRODUCT	IODINE (mg/mL)	VISCOSITY AT 25°C (cp OR mPa.s)[a]	OSMOLALITY (mOsm/kg H_2O)
Nonionic				
Iohexol (300)	Omnipaque™ 300 (GE Healthcare)	300	11.8	672
Iopamidol (612)	Isovue 300™ (Bracco)	300	8.8	616
Iopromide	Ultravist 300™ (Bayer Healthcare)	300	9.2	607
Ioxilan (623)	Oxilan 300™ (Guerbet)	300	9.4	610
Ioversol (640)	Optiray 300™ (Mallinckrodt)	300	8.2	651
Iodixanol (652)	Visipaque 320™ (GE Healthcare)	320	26.6	290
Ionic				
Iothalamate (600)	Conray™ (Covidien)	282	4	1,400
Ioxaglate meglumine/sodium (589)	Hexabrix™ (Guerbet)	320	15.7	~600
Diatrizoate meglumine/sodium (760)	MD-76™ (Mallinckrodt)	370	16.4	1,551

[a]cp, centipoise; mPa.s, millipascal-second.
Modified from Appendix A—Contrast Media Specifications, ACR Manual on Contrast Media—Version 10.2, 2016.

minutes by point-of-care testing. The most commonly used calculation for eGFR is the Modification of Diet in Renal Disease (MDRD) formula(32). The eGFR value is then applied to estimate the stage and severity of kidney disease (Table 1.5). A stable baseline eGFR >45 mL/min/1.73 m^2 is not a risk factor for CIN. For patients with a stable baseline eGFR of 30 to 44 mL/min/1.73 m^2 risk of CIN is very low. Patients with stage IV and stage V chronic kidney disease and eGFR below 30 mL/min/1.73 m^2 have distinct, though still low, risk of CIN.

The American College of Radiology suggests that the following risk factors are indications for renal function assessment before intravascular use of iodinated contrast media:

- Age >60 years.
- History of kidney disease including: dialysis, kidney transplant, single kidney, renal cancer, and renal surgery.
- History of hypertension requiring medical therapy.
- History of diabetes mellitus.
- Use of metformin or metformin-containing drug combinations.

Accepted screening for renal function assessment includes determination of serum creatinine and calculation of eGFR. Patients without the listed risk factors do not require renal function screening. Patients with end-stage chronic kidney disease who are anuric can receive contrast agents without risk of further renal damage because their kidneys no longer function. Those with oliguric end-stage renal disease may become anuric on exposure to intravascular contrast. Patients on dialysis could theoretically become volume overloaded by the osmotic load of contrast agents, and those dialysis patients with severe underlying cardiac dysfunction could become further impaired. Because low-osmolality contrast agents are readily cleared by dialysis, dialysis may be scheduled soon after contrast administration to limit adverse effects.

Adequate hydration is essential in the prevention of contrast-induced nephropathy. Patients should be encouraged to drink several liters of fluid over the 12 to 24 hours before and after intravascular contrast administration.

Metformin (Glucophage®, Fortamet®, Glumetza®, Riomet®) is an oral antihyperglycemic agent used to treat type II diabetes mellitus. It may precipitate potentially fatal lactic acidosis in the presence of renal impairment. Patient mortality if this occurs is reported as 50%. Metformin itself is not a risk factor for PC-AKI, but contrast media administration in the presence of metformin may precipitate AKI and risk of lactic acidosis. The U.S. Food and Drug Administration recommends temporarily withholding metformin in patients receiving iodinated contrast agents for radiographic studies. Metformin should be discontinued for 48 hours after contrast administration and reinstated only after renal function has been reevaluated and found to be normal. Withholding metformin is not necessary following gadolinium administration in the smaller doses used for MR.

Premedication regimens have been proven to decrease, but not eliminate, the frequency of acute allergic-like contrast reactions. See the American College of Radiology Manual on Contrast Media for the latest recommendations on premedication strategies.

Recommendations for safe use of iodinated contrast agents

- Ensure that intravascular contrast agents are truly necessary for each radiographic examination where contrast administration is a consideration.
- Use the minimum effective dose of contrast agent for every examination.
- Use premedication regimens for patients who are considered high risk for adverse reactions including: (a) previous history of adverse reaction to contrast agents administered intravascularly (sensation of heat, flushing, or a single episode of nausea or vomiting does not increase the risk); (b) a clear history of asthma or allergies (atopic individuals). (A history of specific allergies to shellfish or iodine is not reliable as a predictor of contrast reaction.)
- Measure serum creatinine and calculate eGFR in, at a minimum, patients who fall into the following categories: known kidney disease; family history of renal failure; diabetes treated with insulin or other drugs; paraproteinemia syndromes (multiple myeloma); patients on nephrotoxic drugs;

known cardiac dysfunction including severe congestive heart failure, severe arrhythmias, unstable angina, recent myocardial infarction, or pulmonary hypertension; sickle cell disease; all hospitalized patients. Stratify patient risk by reference to the stage of kidney disease (Table 1.5).

- Encourage oral hydration in every patient receiving contrast agents and consider intravenous hydration with normal saline before and after intravenous contrast administration in patients at increased risk for PC-AKI.
- N-acetylcysteine administration may be somewhat effective in preventing contrast-induced nephropathy. See the American College of Radiology Manual on Contrast Media for the latest recommendations on N-acetylcysteine administration.
- Patients on chronic dialysis are at risk for adverse effect of the osmotic load of contrast and its direct toxicity on the heart. Since contrast agents are readily cleared from the blood by dialysis, dialysis on the same day as contrast administration is prudent.
- Determine if patients are taking metformin before administering iodinated contrast agents. Follow recommendations in the American College of Radiology Manual on Contrast Media.
- Administration of iodinated contrast agents to children requires special considerations of contrast osmolality and viscosity, treatment of adverse reactions, and prevention of PC-AKI. Breastfeeding mothers can safely receive contrast agents.
- Use of contrast agents in pregnant women should be avoided if possible. Contrast agents cross the placenta and enter the fetal circulation. The safety of contrast agents for the patient and the fetus is not established. If contrast agents must be administered, the American College of Radiology recommends obtaining written informed consent from the mother.
- Recommendations for treatment of adverse reactions to contrast agents is covered in American College of Radiology Manual on Contrast Media.

Magnetic Resonance Imaging Intravascular Contrast Agents

Gadolinium chelates are the most commonly used MR contrast agents (Table 1.6). They enhance tissue on MR by paramagnetic effect produced by the presence of gadolinium within the molecule. Available gadolinium contrast agents approved for use in the United States or Europe include ionic and nonionic, macrocyclic and linear chelates listed in Table 1.5. While the agents differ in osmolality and viscosity, their distribution and elimination are very similar to the water soluble iodine-based contrast agents used in CT. Gadolinium chelates are injected intravenously, diffuse rapidly into the extracellular fluid and blood pool spaces, and are excreted by glomerular filtration. Approximately 80% of the injected dose is excreted within 3 hours. MR imaging is usually performed immediately after injection.

Immediate adverse reactions to gadolinium agents administered at the 0.1 to 0.2 mmol/kg doses used for MR are quite uncommon (0.07% to 2.4%). Mild reactions of nausea, vomiting, headache, warmth or coldness at the injection site, paresthesias, dizziness, or itching are most common. More severe reactions include bronchospasm, wheezing, hypotension, tachycardia, and dyspnea. Life-threatening reactions are rare (<0.01%). Only 55 severe reactions were reported in a survey of 20 million doses administered. Gadolinium has no nephrotoxicity at doses used for MR. Treatment for adverse reactions to gadolinium agents is essential the same as that for iodinated agents. See the American College of Radiology Manual on Contrast Media for current recommendations.

Risk Factors. Patients with a history of acute adverse reactions have about eight times increased risk of a subsequent reaction. Patients with a history of asthma or severe allergies have a mild increased risk. Patients with a history of adverse reactions to iodinated contrast agents are not at increased risk for adverse reactions to gadolinium agents. Since many different chemical forms of gadolinium agents are available it is prudent to switch to a different agent for patients with a history of prior reactions.

Serum Calcium. Two gadolinium chelates, gadodiamide and gadoversetamide, have been identified as causing interference with colorimetric methods of determining serum calcium levels leading to an erroneous diagnosis of hypocalcemia. Gadopentetate and gadobenate chelates have been shown to generate no interference with colorimetric measurements of serum calcium.

TABLE 1.6

GADOLINIUM-BASED INTRAVASCULAR CONTRAST AGENTS

NAME	PRODUCT	OSMOLALITY mOsm/kgH_2O	RELAXIVITY[a] 1.5 T T1/T2
Nonionic			
Gadoteridol	Prohance™ (Bracco)	630	4.1/5.0
Gadodiamide[b]	Omniscan™ (GE Healthcare)	789	4.3/5.2
Gadoverstamide[b]	Optimark™ (Mallinckrodt)	1,110	4.7/5.2
Gadobutrol	Gadovist/Gadavost™ (Bayer Healthcare)	1,603	5.2/6.1
Ionic			
Gadopentetate[b]	Magnevist™ (Bayer Healthcare)	1,960	4.1/4.6
Gadobenate	Multihance™ (Bracco)	1,970	6.3/8.7
Gadoxetate	EOVIST/Primovist™ (Bayer HealthCare)	688	6.9/8.7
Gadoterate	Dotarem™ (Guerbet)	1,350	3.6/4.3
Gadofosveset	Ablavar/Vasovist™ (Lantheus)	825	19/34

[a]Relaxivity of MR contrast agents refers to the degree to which the agent can enhance longitudinal (T1) or transverse (T2) water relaxation rate constant normalized to the concentration of the contrast agent.
[b]These three agents (*in italic*) are associated with the highest risk of developing NSF. They account for 97% of all reported cases.
Modified from Appendix A—Contrast Media Specifications, ACR Manual on Contrast Media—Version 10.2, 2016.

Nephrogenic Systemic Fibrosis. For many years gadolinium-based MR contrast agents were considered to be among the safest drugs in medical practice. Gadolinium contrast–enhanced MR was frequently recommended as a substitute for iodinated contrast-enhanced CT in patients with impaired renal function and concern for contrast-induced nephropathy. In 1997, a new, rare, sclerosing skin disease was recognized in patients with chronic renal failure. Identification of additional cases led to the recognition that the disease was not confined to the skin but could affect multiple organs including the liver, lungs, muscles, and heart. The name nephrogenic systemic fibrosis (NSF) was applied to the condition. In 2006, publications appeared linking NSF to the use of gadolinium in patients with impaired renal function. Cases were being recognized worldwide. Signs of NSF were recognized within hours to within 30 days of exposure to gadolinium agents. Clinically, NSF varies in its manifestations from patient to patient and over time. Skin changes start as an erythematous rash with nonpitting swelling and intense itching of affected areas. Pain, dysesthesias, and hyperesthesias develop. Intense neuropathy leads to difficulty walking and painful disability. The dermis becomes thickened, hardened, and inflexible leading to contractures that impair joint mobility. Affected skin becomes hyperpigmented. Severe cases lead to complete disability with patients being unable to walk, bathe, or care for themselves. Radiographic findings in patients with NSF include skin thickening, infiltration of subcutaneous tissues, joint contractures, and on bone scintigraphy diffuse soft tissue uptake of radionuclide. To date, no curative treatment exists for this disease. The great majority of cases (>95%) have occurred in patients with stage 5 chronic kidney disease (eGFR <15 cc/min/1.73 m^2) and no cases have occurred in patients with normal renal function (eGFR >60 cc/min/1.73 m^2). It is currently estimated that patients with chronic kidney disease, stage 4 and 5 (eGFR <30 mL/min/1.73 m^2), have a 1% to 7% chance of developing NSF after intravascular administration of gadolinium-based contrast agents. Patients at specific risk of NSF include those on dialysis of any form and those with AKI.

Any age group may be affected. Published cases have been associated with administration of gadodiamide (~70%), gadopentetate dimeglumine (~25%), and gadoversetamide (~5%). The incidence of disease is distinctly highest with gadodiamide approaching 15% of patients with end-stage renal disease or on dialysis who received high doses (40 mL) of the agent. Gadolinium is never found in normal biologic tissue in patients who have never received gadolinium contrast agents but is present in its free and highly toxic ionic form in affected tissues of patients with NSF.

Gadolinium in free ionic form is a potent toxin. Gadolinium contrast agents bind (or chelate) the ion to a ligand molecule to make the agents relatively safe for human use. In patients with normal renal function the chelate is quickly excreted in the urine. However, in patients with impaired renal function the chelate remains in the body for a much longer time. The three agents found to have the highest association with NSF are also those with the least stable binding of gadolinium to the ligand molecule. Ionic gadolinium distributes to the skin and other tissues when freed from the ligand. These agents also have the greatest stimulatory effect on human fibroblast proliferation. Use of high doses of gadolinium for MR angiographic and body imaging applications increases the risk of NSF.

Recent studies indicate that gadolinium may be retained indefinitely within brain, skin, and bones of patients without renal impairment who receive multiple doses of gadolinium agents. Adults and children with multiple sclerosis who undergo multiple gadolinium-enhanced MR examinations are especially at risk. In the brain gadolinium concentrates most within the basal ganglia. Retained gadolinium in tissues appears to be dependent on dose and independent of renal impairment. To date, no adverse effects of this gadolinium deposition has been reported but the long-term effects are unknown.

Guidelines for avoiding NSF and safe use of MR contrast agents have been issued by the American College of Radiology. All patients should be screened for potential renal impairment prior to receiving gadolinium-based contrast agents. Risk factors for renal impairment are the same as those listed in the section on iodinated contrast agents. At-risk patients should undergo blood testing for serum creatinine and eGFR calculation. Patients with eGFR <30 mL/min/1.73 m^2, on any form of dialysis, or with AKI are at increased risk for NSF and gadolinium contrast administration should be avoided in most cases. Patients with chronic kidney disease stage 1 or 2 (eGFR >60 mL/min/1.73 m^2), are not considered at risk for NSF and gadolinium agents may be safely administered. Only a few NSF cases have been reported in children, and none under 6 years of age. However, the ACR recommends that the same guidelines be followed in children as in adults.

The minimum dose of gadolinium contrast agent that generates a diagnostic MR examination should be utilized in all patients. The reason for the examination and the use of gadolinium contrast agent should be documented in all cases. Especially in patients determined to be at risk for NSF the contrast agent chosen should not be one of the three linear agents reported to be at highest risk for NSF (Table 1.6). In pregnant patients, gadolinium agents should be used only with great cautions. Like iodinated contrast agents gadolinium agents readily cross the placenta and enter fetal circulation appearing in the fetal bladder within 11 minutes following maternal intravenous administration. Excretion by the fetus into the amniotic fluid may recirculate the gadolinium agent as the fetus swallows amniotic fluid. While there have been no reportable adverse effects to the fetus nor any cases of NSF in pregnant patients, the effect on the fetus remains unknown. The benefit of gadolinium contrast administration in pregnant patients must be weighed against the unknown effect on the fetus. If a gadolinium agent is administered, it should be at the lowest dose to achieve a diagnostic examination.

Gastrointestinal Contrast Agents

Barium sulfate is the standard opaque contrast agent for routine fluoroscopic contrast studies of the upper and lower GI tract. Current formulations provide excellent coating of the GI mucosa. "Thin," more fluid, suspensions are used for single-contrast studies, whereas "thick," more viscous, suspensions coat the mucosa for double-contrast examinations. Barium preparations are remarkably well tolerated. Aspiration of barium rarely causes a clinical problem. Small amounts are cleared from the lungs within hours; however, huge amounts may result in pneumonia. Suspected allergic reactions including hives, respiratory arrest, and anaphylaxis have been rarely reported. Allergic reactions to latex used in enema balloons and rectal examination gloves are more common than reactions to the barium products themselves. The major risk from the use of barium sulfate is barium peritonitis resulting from the spill of barium into the peritoneal cavity as a result of perforations of the GI tract. Barium deposits act as foreign bodies, inducing fibrin deposition and massive ascites. Bacterial contamination from intestinal contents can lead to sepsis, shock, and death in up to 50% of patients. Esophageal leak may cause mediastinitis.

Gas Agents. Air and carbon dioxide gas are effective and inexpensive contrast agents for both CT and fluoroscopic studies. A number of effervescent powders, granules, and tablets that release carbon dioxide on contact with water are routinely used. These preparations are excellent for distending the stomach for CT or barium studies. Air injected directly into the GI tract via a nasogastric or enema tube may be used to distend the stomach or colon.

Water-soluble iodinated contrast media opacify the bowel lumen by passive filling, rather than mucosal coating, and are considered by most radiologists to be inferior to barium agents for routine fluoroscopic GI studies. Because of the high mortality associated with barium peritonitis, however, water-soluble agents are indicated when GI tract perforation is suspected. Water-soluble agents are quickly reabsorbed through the peritoneal surface if perforation is present. Dilute solutions (2% to 5%) of ionic agents are routinely used in CT to opacify the GI tract. Ionic contrast agents stimulate intestinal peristalsis, which promotes faster opacification of the distal bowel on CT and may be useful in the postoperative patient with ileus. The major risk of oral water-soluble agents is aspiration, which may cause chemical pneumonitis. Low-osmolar agents may be safer and are preferred when aspiration is deemed a risk. Large volumes of hypertonic water-soluble agents in the GI tract draw water into the gut and may result in hypovolemia, shock, and even death, especially in infants and debilitated adults.

Ultrasound Intravascular Contrast Agents

US contrast agents are available to improve US characterization of tissue and lesion vascularity, similar to the use of intravascular contrast agents in CT and MR. US contrast agents consist of microbubbles of air or perfluorocarbon gas encased within a thin shell made of protein, lipid, or polymers. Their size, slightly smaller than red blood cells, keeps the microbubbles within the vascular system and allows them to flow through the pulmonary circulation to the systemic circulation following peripheral intravenous injection. The contrast thus acts as a blood pool agent. The gas diffuses through its shell resulting in disappearance of the microbubbles with a half-life in blood of a few minutes. No adverse bioeffects of the agents have been reported. A variety of US imaging techniques, some requiring additional software or hardware, are utilized for contrast agent imaging. These include power and spectral Doppler, harmonic imaging, and pulse-inversion imaging. The microbubbles interact with the imaging technique, oscillate at a resonant frequency, and can be made to abruptly disrupt to improve the signal from the contrast agent. Imaging is performed in arterial and venous phases. Contrast washout or sustained enhancement of lesions can be assessed. In 2016, the U.S. Food and Drug Administration approved the first ultrasound contrast agent for use in the liver and in 2017 in the urinary tract for evaluation of vesicoureteral reflux in pediatric patients.

RADIATION RISK AND ENSURING PATIENT SAFETY

While the benefits of using ionizing radiation for medical diagnosis are enormous and continue to expand, attention must be paid to the risks associated with the use of ionizing radiation. As CT has improved dramatically in capability to provide accurate medical diagnosis, its use has skyrocketed. It is estimated that as many as 72 million CT scans are now performed annually in the United States with worldwide use approaching 300 million CT scans annually. In the United States, an estimated 7 million CT scans are performed on pediatric patients. This use exposes a significant portion of the world population to increased radiation over naturally occurring radiation exposures. Currently, medical imaging is estimated to account for up to 48% of the total radiation exposure to the population, up from 15% estimated in 1987. CT alone accounts for 24% of the total radiation exposure to the population. Of particular concern is the use of ionizing radiation, especially CT scanning, in children, pregnant women, and repeatedly in chronically ill patients, especially those of a young age. The potential risks of exposure to ionizing radiation include induction of malignancy, genetic mutations, and congenital malformations. Known clinically apparent adverse effects include transient and permanent skin reactions, which are seen at radiation doses achieved during fluoroscopically guided interventional procedures.

Data on the risk of the low doses of ionizing radiation used for diagnostic radiology is imperfect and controversial. Risk estimates for low dose radiation is derived primarily from data on survivors of high radiation exposure from the atomic explosions in Hiroshima and Nagasaki in 1945. Additional data come from high-level exposures from nuclear accidents such as Chernobyl in 1986. There continues to be no direct evidence that low-level radiation causes cancer or birth defects. All concern is based upon estimates of risk. The most conservative estimate of risk uses a linear model without threshold based on high-level exposure data that indicate a small but finite risk of developing cancer, especially in children as a result of CT scanning and other medical imaging using ionizing radiation. These risk estimates assume the absence of a threshold dose below which no harm may occur. Many experts believe a threshold dose rather than linear, no threshold, extrapolation is the correct model. Nonetheless, using the linear extrapolation method, estimated life-time risk for a 1-year old undergoing an abdominal CT scan is 0.18% and for a head CT 0.07%. However, this added risk is minute compared to the estimated 23% individual risk of developing cancer in one's lifetime. This very conservative and highly significant overestimate of risk must be balanced against the benefit of achieving a proper diagnosis by use of CT. In many instances the immediate benefit dramatically outweighs the minute risk. There is no marker currently available that allows differentiation of a cancer caused by radiation exposure from one that occurs naturally. Additional cancers possibly related to radiation exposure have a latency period of 30 to 40 years. Patients over age 50 and those already with cancer and who receive repeated CT scans are not likely to experience additional radiation-induced cancers.

Radiation Dose. In a study of nearly 1 million adults CT and nuclear medicine procedures accounted for 75% of cumulative effective radiation dose. CT accounts for 10% of all x-ray based procedures but contributes two-thirds of the total medically related radiation exposures to patients. A CT of the abdomen may have 200 to 250 times the radiation dose of a chest radiograph. A CT pulmonary angiogram delivers 2.0 rads (20 mGy) per breast compared to 0.30 rads (3 mGy) per breast for a mammogram. Estimated average doses for a variety of common diagnostic imaging procedures utilizing ionizing radiation are listed in Table 1.7.

Pregnancy and Radiation. In pregnancy the radiation risk to the fetus is magnified by the small size of the developing human with rapid growth and extremely active cell division. Potential harmful effects of ionizing radiation to the fetus include: prenatal death (especially in very early pregnancy), intrauterine growth retardation, mental retardation, organ malformation, and development of cancer during childhood. The risk of each effect depends upon the gestational age at the time of exposure and the total fetal dose delivered throughout gestation. Radiation risk is highest in the first trimester, diminishes in the second trimester, and is lowest in the third trimester. If the uterus is outside the field of view of the x-ray beam, the fetus receives only scatter radiation and the radiation dose is minimal. If the fetus is exposed to the direct x-ray

TABLE 1.7

RADIATION DOSE ESTIMATES TO THE PATIENT FROM DIAGNOSTIC EXAMINATIONS

■ DIAGNOSTIC EXAMINATION	■ ESTIMATED EFFECTIVE DOSE (16 SLICE SCANNER FOR CT) mGy
Head CT	2
Chest CT routine	8–10
CT pulmonary angiogram	15
Abdomen CT	10
Pelvis CT	10
Ventilation/Perfusion radionuclide scan	1
Chest radiograph (PA view) with grid	0.20
Chest radiograph (lateral view) with grid	0.75
Abdomen (AP)	5
Cervical spine radiograph (AP)	1.20
Thoracic spine radiograph (AP)	3.50
Thoracic spine radiograph (lateral)	10.00
Lumbar spine radiograph (AP)	5.00
Lumbar spine radiograph (lateral)	15.00
Pelvis radiograph	5.00
Hip radiograph	5.00
Background Radiation	
Exposure at sea level	3 mGy/yr
Exposure at 5,000 ft altitude (Denver)	10 mGy/yr
Seven-hour airplane flight	0.05 mGy

PA, posteroanterior view; AP, anteroposterior view; 10 mGy, 1 rad. Data from Fazel R, Krumholz HM, Wang Y, et al. Exposure to low-dose ionizing radiation from medical imaging procedures. *NEJM* 2009;361:849–857; Parry RA, Glaze SA, Archer BR. Typical patient radiation doses in diagnostic radiology. *Radiographics* 1999; 19:1289–1302.

TABLE 1.8

RADIATION DOSE ESTIMATES TO THE FETUS FROM DIAGNOSTIC EXAMINATIONS

■ DIAGNOSTIC EXAMINATION	■ ESTIMATED FETAL DOSE (16 SLICE SCANNER FOR CT) mGy
Head CT	0–0.1
Chest CT routine	0.2
CT pulmonary angiogram	0.2–0.6
Abdomen CT	4
Abdomen & pelvis CT	12–25
Stone protocol CT (low dose)	10–12
CT arteriogram—aorta	34
Extremity radiograph	<0.001
Chest radiographs (PA, lateral)	0.002
Cervical spine radiographs (AP, lateral)	<0.001
Thoracic spine radiographs (AP, lateral)	0.003
Lumbar spine radiographs (AP, lateral)	1–3.4
Pelvis radiograph	1.7
Hip radiograph	1.3
Barium enema	7–39

PA, posteroanterior view; AP, anteroposterior view; 10 mGy, 1 rad. Data from McCollough CH, Schueler BA, Atwell TD, et al. Radiation exposure and pregnancy: when should we be concerned. *Radiographics* 2007;27:909–918; Patel SJ, Reede DL, Katz DS, Subramaniam R, Amorosa JK. Imaging the pregnant patient for non-obstetric conditions: algorithms and radiation dose considerations. *Radiographics* 2007;27:1705–1722; and Wieseler KM, Bhargava P, Kanal KM, et al. Imaging in pregnant patients: examination appropriateness. *Radiographics* 2010;30:1215–1233.

beam within the field of view, dose depends on thickness of the patient, depth of the conceptus from the skin, x-ray technique, and direction of the beam (Table 1.8). In the first 2 weeks of pregnancy radiation exposure has an all or none effect. Radiation may terminate the pregnancy or the embryo may recover completely. At 3 to 8 weeks after conception organogenesis is at its maximum and radiation exposure may cause organ malformation. The central nervous system is most sensitive from 8 to 15 weeks of gestation. Significant exposure at this time may cause mental retardation microcephaly. In the third trimester the fetus is much less radiosensitive and functional impairments and organ malformations are unlikely. The National Council on Radiation Protection and Measurement has set 50 mGy (5 rads) as the cumulative maximum "acceptable" fetal dose during the entire pregnancy. Below this threshold it is very unlikely that any adverse effect on the fetus will be detectable. No diagnostic study exceeds this dose (Table 1.8). However, repeated exposure to ionizing radiation during gestation can certainly exceed this dose and harm the fetus. The risk becomes significant above 100 mGy. The International Commission on Radiological Protection states that "fetal doses below 100 mGy should not be considered a reason for terminating a pregnancy. At fetal doses above this level, there can be fetal damage, the magnitude and type of which is a function of dose and stage of pregnancy."

Children and Radiation. Many (up to 11%) diagnostic examinations utilizing ionizing radiation are performed on infants and children who are more susceptible to the adverse effects of radiation. These considerations mandate a responsibility for the radiologist and the ordering physician to limit CT to definitive indications, provide dose efficient CT imaging protocols, offer alternative imaging techniques especially for young children who are at the greatest risk from radiation, work with manufacturers to limit radiation dose, and educate patients and healthcare providers on the potential risk of low-dose radiation.

Skin Reactions. At radiation doses higher than 5 Gy, a dose that is achieved during complex and prolonged fluoroscopically guided interventional procedures, clinically noticeable changes in the skin and hair may occur. Skin reactions include erythema, epilation, desquamation, dermal atrophy, and telangiectasia. Changes may be transient or permanent depending upon the dose. Specialized wound care may be needed if skin dose exceeds 10 Gy.

Radiation Protection Actions

- All diagnostic imaging utilizing ionizing radiation must use the principle "As Low As Reasonably Achievable" (ALARA) with respect to dose and technique. Optimal dose is the goal. Too low a radiation dose resulting in a nondiagnostic examination will not provide the diagnosis and may impair the patient's proper treatment. Too high a radiation dose provides unnecessary exposure. Pediatric-specific protocols and protocols based on the size of the patient should be utilized.
- The referring physician and radiologist must weigh the risk of exposure to ionizing radiation needed to perform the examination against the expected benefit to be derived from the diagnostic information.
- Unnecessary imaging utilizing ionizing radiation, especially CT scans, must be eliminated.
- The American College of Radiology, through panels of experts, has developed Appropriateness Criteria to serve as guidelines for employing the most appropriate imaging test for a wide range of specific clinical conditions. These serve to promote the most efficacious use of radiology.
- The Image Gently program is an initiative of the Alliance for Radiation Safety in Pediatric Imaging offering guidelines that intend to lower radiation exposures of children undergoing diagnostic imaging.
- Each examination must be tailored specifically to the needs of the patient.
- Use alternative imaging methods, such as MR or US, whenever appropriate.
- In pregnancy, avoid radiation exposure to the embryo in the first trimester of pregnancy. Women of child bearing age must be queried as to the possibility of pregnancy prior to radiation exposure, especially if the uterus is to be directly exposed. Uncertain answers should be followed with a pregnancy test.
- Limit the radiation field of view to the area of concern—avoid direct exposure of the unshielded uterus.
- Radiography involves a less collimated x-ray beam resulting in more scattered radiation in the room. The pelvis should be shielded with lead when performing radiography of other body parts.
- In pregnancy, radiographic, fluoroscopic, and CT examination of areas of the body that do not expose the uterus to the direct x-ray beam deliver minimal radiation dose to the fetus (Table 1.8).
- CT involves a tightly collimated beam with very little scatter radiation in the room. Radiation exposure from other than the direct x-ray beam comes from scatter within the patient. Shielding the pelvis has little protective effect and is unnecessary.
- US and MR should be the initial imaging considerations for evaluation of pregnant patients with acute conditions. CT may prove to be the appropriate diagnostic test. A single CT scan can be performed with the knowledge that no evidence exists that a single limited CT examination causes harm to the fetus.
- No harmful effect to the fetus has been demonstrated to date from clinical MR examinations at 1.5 T and below.
- In pregnancy both the mother and the fetus are your patients. While appropriate caution regarding use of ionizing radiation for diagnostic imaging should be utilized, potential benefit to both mother and infant must be considered. The fetus may not survive if the mother does not survive.
- Avoid the use of contrast agents in pregnancy for either CT or MR whenever possible. Neither iodinated contrast agents nor gadolinium agents are approved for use in pregnancy. Contrast agents should be used only if critical to the health of the mother.

RADIOLOGY REPORTING

An essential skill of the radiologist is preparation of the radiology report describing imaging findings and their importance and coming to a conclusion as decisive as possible. The radiology report must be accurate, comprehensive, concise, and clearly understandable. It is a medical-legal document that is a vital element of the patient's medical record. It is essential for accurate billing and reimbursement. We must never forget that the images we interpret are those of a living, breathing, important human being. Effective timely communication is essential.

The following are essential components of a radiology report:

- Demographics: patient name; medical record number; ordering physician or healthcare provider; name, date, and time of the examination; components of the examination, location of the facility where the examination was performed; name and contact information of the interpreting radiologist.
- Clinical information: indications which justify the examination and are essential to determining the relevance of findings.
- Findings: pathologic and important normal findings using pertinent medical terminology. Comparison should be made to pertinent studies previously obtained. The clinical question asked should be answered as explicitly as possible.
- Limitations: State factors that compromise the examination or procedure. State any significant complications or patient adverse reactions.
- Impression/conclusion/diagnosis: A specific diagnosis should be rendered whenever possible. Give a differential diagnosis whenever appropriate. Recommend or suggest additional or follow-up studies when clinically appropriate.
- Critical findings must be communicated to requesting healthcare provider as soon as possible. Documentation of the communication should be included in the final report.
- Consider providing the patient with the final report. This has become the standard in many breast imaging, and other, radiology practices.

Suggested Readings

ACR Expert Panel on MR Safety; Kanal E, Barkovich AJ, Bell C, et al. ACR guidance document on MR safe practices: 2013. *J Magn Reson Imaging* 2013;37:501–530.

American College of Radiology. *ACR Practice Parameter for Communication of Diagnostic Imaging Findings*. Resolution 11, Revised 2014. Reston, VA: American College of Radiology; 2014:1–9.

American College of Radiology Committee on Drugs and Contrast Media. *Manual on Contrast Media. Version 10.2*. Reston, VA: American College of Radiology; 2016.

American College of Radiology; Hendrick RE. MRI terminology glossary. https://www.acr.org/~/media/ACR/Documents/PDF/QualitySafety/Resources/GlossaryOfMRTerms.pdf

Amis ES Jr, Butler PF, Applegate K, et al. American College of Radiology white paper on radiation dose in medicine. *J Am Coll Radiol* 2007;4:272–284.

Anvari A, Forsberg F, Samir AE. A primer on the physical principles of tissue harmonic imaging. *Radiographics* 2015;35:1955–1964.

Bioeffects Committee of the American Institute of Ultrasound in Medicine. American Institute of Ultrasound in Medicine consensus report on potential bioeffects of diagnostic ultrasound. *J Ultrasound Med* 2008;27:503–515.

Boone JM. Multidetector CT: opportunities, challenges, and concerns associated with scanners with 64 or more detector rows. *Radiology* 2006;241:334–337.

Brant WE. *The Core Curriculum: Ultrasound*. Philadelphia, PA: Lippincott Williams & Wilkins; 2001.

Brant WE, de Lange EE, eds. *Essentials of Body MRI*. New York: Oxford University Press; 2012.

Bushberg JT, Seibert JA, Leidholdt EMJ, Boone JM. *The Essential Physics of Medical Imaging*. 3rd ed. Philadelphia, PA: Lippincott Williams & Wilkins—Wolters Kluwer; 2012.

Carroll QB. *Radiography in the Digital Age: Physics-Exposure-Radiation Biology*. Springfield, IL: Charles C. Thomas Publisher; 2011.

Cibull SL, Harris GR, Nell DM. Trends in diagnostic ultrasound acoustic output from data reported to the US Food and Drug Administration for device indications that include fetal applications. *J Ultrasound Med* 2013;32: 1921–1932.

Cody DD, Mahesh M. Technological advances in multi-detector CT with a focus on cardiac imaging. *Radiographics* 2007;27:1829–1827.

Coursey CA, Nelson RC, Boll DT, et al. Dual-energy multidetector CT: how does it work, what can it tell us, and when can we use it in abdominopelvic imaging? *Radiographics* 2010;30:1037–1055.

Dance DR, Christofides S, Maidment ADA, et al. *Diagnostic Radiology Physics: A Handbook for Teachers and Students*. Vienna: International Atomic Energy Agency; 2014.

Denham SL, Alexander LF, Robbin ML. Contrast-enhanced ultrasound: practical review for the assessment of hepatic and renal lesions. *Ultrasound Q* 2016;32:116–125.

Hendee WR, O'Connor MK. Radiation risks of medical imaging: separating fact from fantasy. *Radiology* 2012;264:312–321.

Huang SY, Seethamraju RT, Patel P, et al. Body MR imaging, artifacts, k-space, and solutions. *Radiographics* 2015;35:1439–1460.

Johnson TRC. Dual-energy CT: general principles. *AJR* 2012;198:S3–S8.

Körner M, Weber CH, Wirth S, et al. Advances in digital radiography: physical principles and system overview. *Radiographics* 2007;27:675–686.

Morelli JN, Runge VM, Attenberger U, et al. An image-based approach to understanding the physics of MR artifacts. *Radiographics* 2011;31:849–866.

Paulsen EK, Sheafor DH, Enterline DS, et al. CT fluoroscopy-guided interventional procedures: techniques and radiation dose to radiologists. *Radiology* 2001;220:161–167.

Pooley RA, McKinney JM, Miller DA. The AAPM/RSNA physics tutorial for residents: digital fluoroscopy. *Radiographics* 2001;21:521–534.

Prabhu SJ, Kanal K, Bhargava P, Vaidya S, Dighe MK. Ultrasound artifacts: classification, applied physics with illustrations, and imaging appearances. *Ultrasound Q* 2014;30:145–157.

Raman SP, Mahesh M, Blasko RV, Fishman EK. CT scan parameters and radiation dose: practical advice for radiologists. *J Am Coll Radiol* 2013;10:840–846.

Sigrist RMS, Liau J, Kaffas AE, Chammas MC, Willmann JK. Ultrasound elastography: review of techniques and clinical applications. *Theranostics* 2017;7:1303–1329.

Tirada N, Dreizin D, Khati NJ, Akin EA, Zeman RK. Imaging pregnant and lactating patients. *Radiographics* 2015;35:1751–1765.

Williams MB, Krupinski EA, Strauss KJ, et al. Digital radiography image quality: image acquisition. *J Am Coll Radiol* 2007;4:371–388.

SECTION II

NEUROradiology

SECTION EDITORS: Erik H. L. Gaensler and Jerome A. Barakos

CHAPTER 2 ■ INTRODUCTION TO BRAIN IMAGING

GOVIND MUKUNDAN AND DAVID J. SEIDENWURM

This chapter provides an atlas of neuroanatomy and a discussion of the principles of brain imaging and interpretation. Brain anatomy is shown on 3T MR T2-weighted images in axial plane (Figs. 2.1 to 2.8), on 3T MR T1-weighted images in coronal plane (Figs. 2.9 to 2.16), and on 3T MR T1-weighted images in the sagittal plane (Figs. 2.17 and 2.18). Examples of ultrafast MR FIESTA (fast imaging employing steady-state acquisition) images are shown in Figures 2.19 and 2.20, as well as susceptibility-weighted images (SWIs) in Figure 2.21. Examples of functional MR imaging (fMRI) are shown in Figure 2.22, MR 3T diffusion tensor image in Figure 2.23, and diffusion white matter tractography in Figure 2.24. Stroke imaging intervention case showing continuum of neuroimaging is shown in Figure 2.25A to F.

LOOKING AT THE BRAIN

A few simple principles can be employed to ensure that no neurosurgical emergency is missed, even on a first cursory look at an emergency CT scan at midnight.

Midline. The middle of the patient's brain should be in the middle of the patient's head and the two sides of the brain should look alike (Figs. 2.1 to 2.5). While there are important functional asymmetries between the right and left hemispheres, the anatomic differences are subtle and play no role in clinical neuroradiology. Any shift of midline structures is presumed to represent a mass lesion on the side from which the midline is displaced. For practical purposes, there are no "sucking" brain wounds that draw the midline toward themselves. If the interventricular septum and third ventricle are located in the midline, no subfalcine herniation is present (Fig. 2.5).

Symmetry of the brain is the key to radiologic evaluation. Only experience teaches how much asymmetry is within the range of normal variation. In general, the sulcal pattern should be symmetric. The sulci on one side are the same size as the corresponding sulci on the other. The anterior interhemispheric fissure should be visualized. Loss of sulci may result from compression owing to mass or opacification of CSF following subarachnoid hemorrhage or, less commonly, meningitis or spreading of a CSF-borne tumor. The sulci extend to the inner table of the skull. In older patients, some atrophy is normal. Significant medial displacement of the sulci may represent compression resulting from an extracerebral fluid collection, such as a subdural or epidural hematoma. Because these may be bilateral and similar in density to the brain, care needs to be taken in evaluating the periphery of the brain.

Basal Cisterns. More subtle, but more important, signs of intracranial mass include distortion of the CSF spaces of the posterior fossa and base of the brain. The key structures here are the quadrigeminal plate cistern and the suprasellar cistern (Figs. 2.6, 2.10, and 2.16). Because these CSF spaces are traversed by important neural structures, careful attention to these regions is essential. The quadrigeminal plate cistern in the axial plane has the appearance of a symmetric smile. Any asymmetry must be suspect, and abnormality of this cistern may represent rotation of the brainstem resulting from transtentorial herniation, effacement of the cistern on account of cerebellar or brainstem mass, or opacification of the cistern as in subarachnoid hemorrhage.

The suprasellar cistern looks like a pentagon, the Jewish star, or the Hindu Shatkona, depending upon the angulation of the scan through it (Fig. 2.6). The five corners of the pentagon are the interhemispheric fissure anteriorly, the sylvian cisterns anterolaterally, and the ambient cisterns posterolaterally. The sixth point of the superimposed Jewish star or Shatkona is in the interpeduncular fossa posteriorly. The cistern has the density of CSF and the structure is symmetric. The anatomic continuations of the cistern are the same density as CSF. Significant asymmetry may be a result of uncal herniation. Central mass may be the result of a sellar or suprasellar tumor. Opacification of the cistern may be the result of subarachnoid hemorrhage or meningitis.

Ventricles. The final structure that must be evaluated in a quick review of a brain scan is the ventricular system. It is best to start with the fourth ventricle in the posterior fossa, because it is the hardest to see on CT. Asymmetry or shift of the fourth ventricle may be the only sign of significant intracranial masses. Because of the shape of the fourth ventricle, some asymmetry in appearance may reflect the patient's position in the scanner.

The overall size of the ventricular system is assessed next. Enlargement of the lateral ventricles and third ventricle in the setting of headache, or with signs of intracranial mass, may represent hydrocephalus, a potentially fatal yet easily treatable condition. Hydrocephalus is distinguished from enlargement of the ventricular system as the result of atrophy by a discrepancy in the degree of ventricular and sulcal enlargement, and by a characteristic pattern of frontal horn and temporal horn enlargement and a round appearance of the anterior portion of the third ventricle.

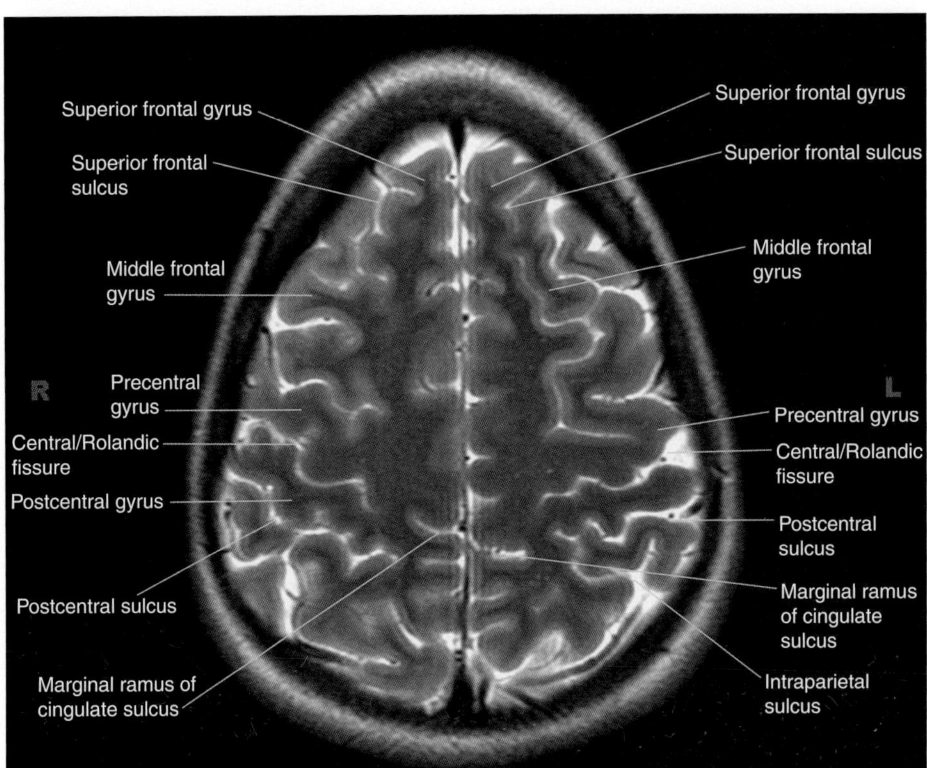

FIGURE 2.1. Brain MR. Cerebral hemispheres. Axial plane T2-weighted image at 3T.

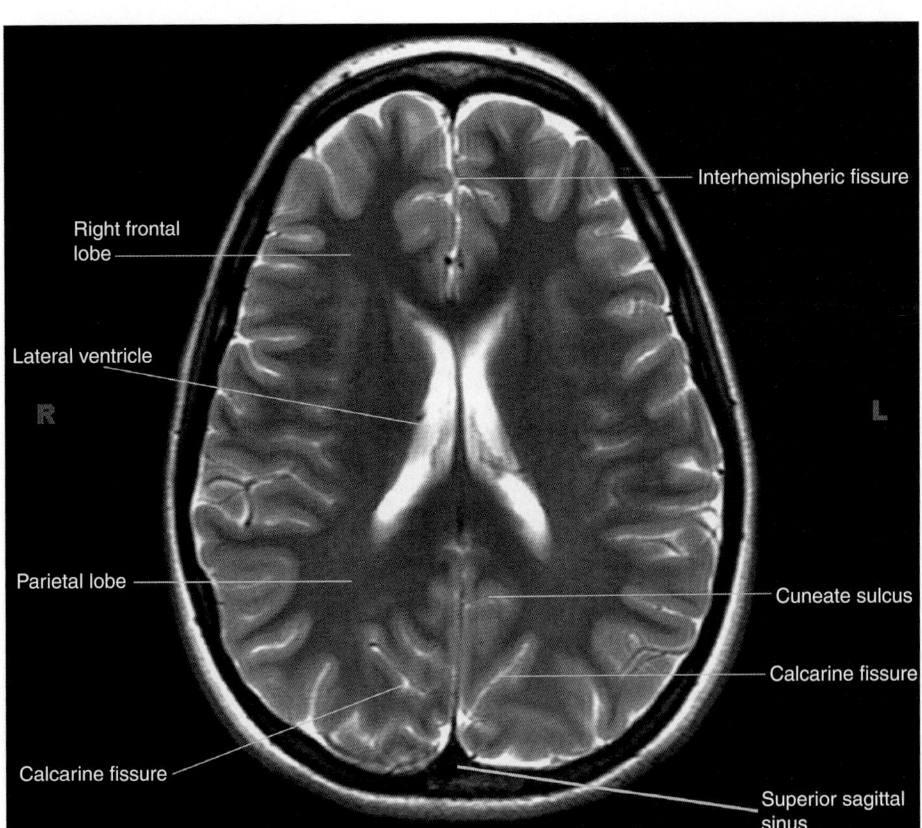

FIGURE 2.2. Brain MR. Body of the lateral ventricles. Axial plane T2-weighted image at 3T.

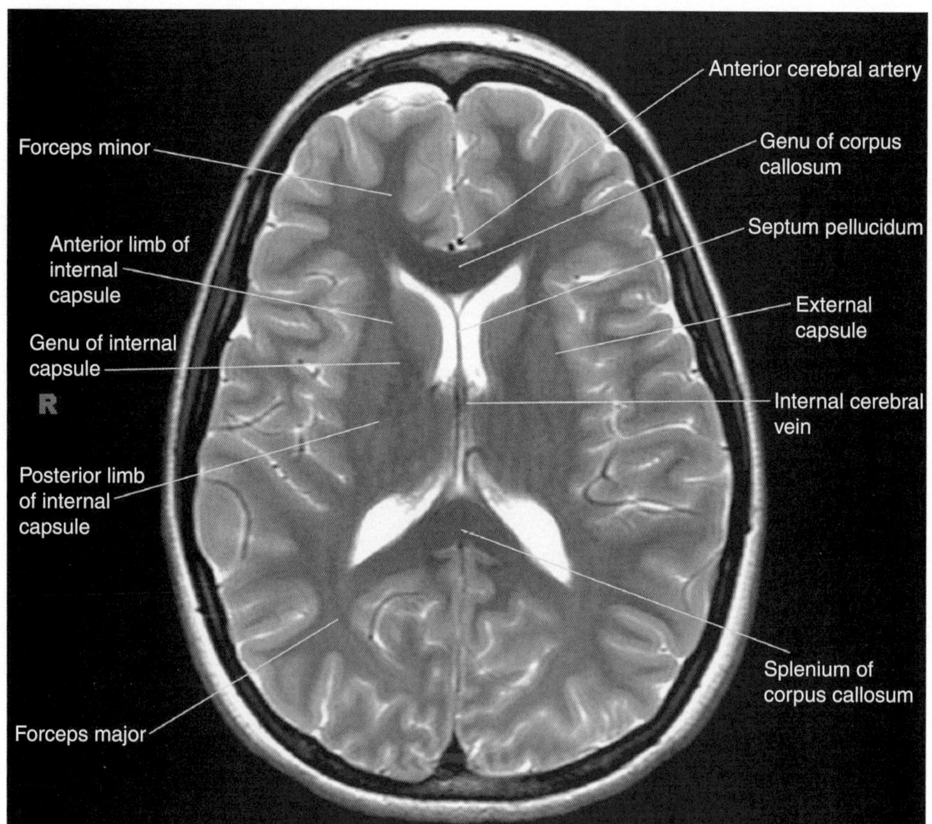

FIGURE 2.3. **Brain MR.** Internal cerebral veins. Axial plane T2-weighted image at 3T.

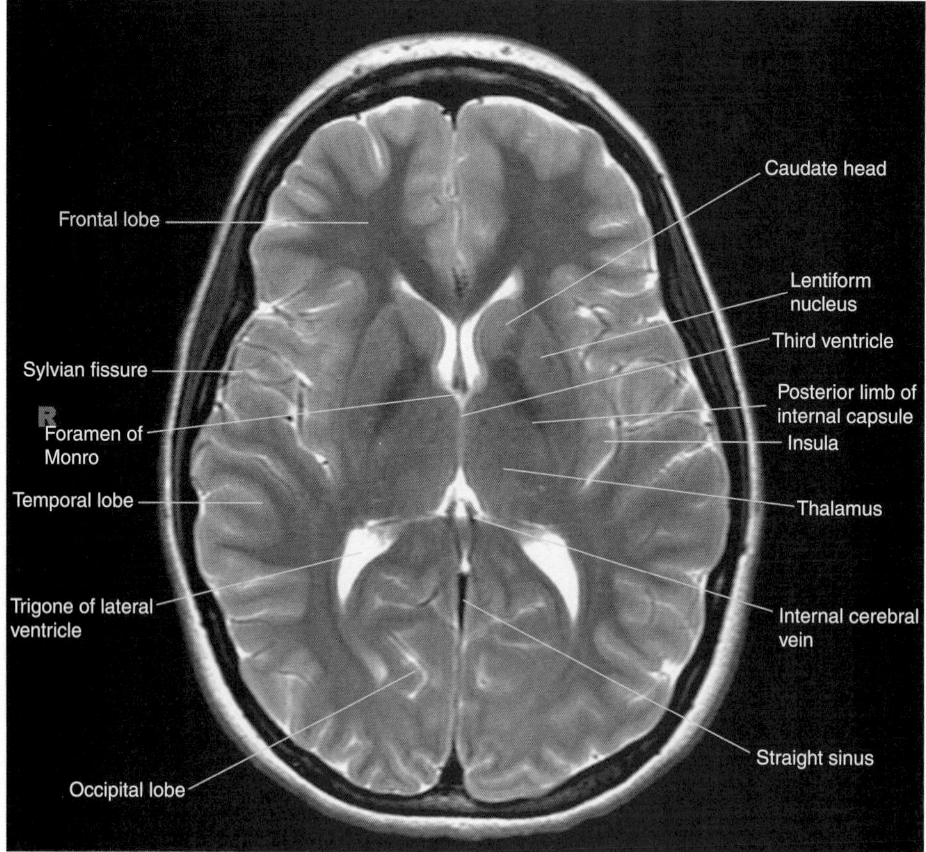

FIGURE 2.4. **Brain MR.** Foramina of Monro. Axial plane T2-weighted image at 3T.

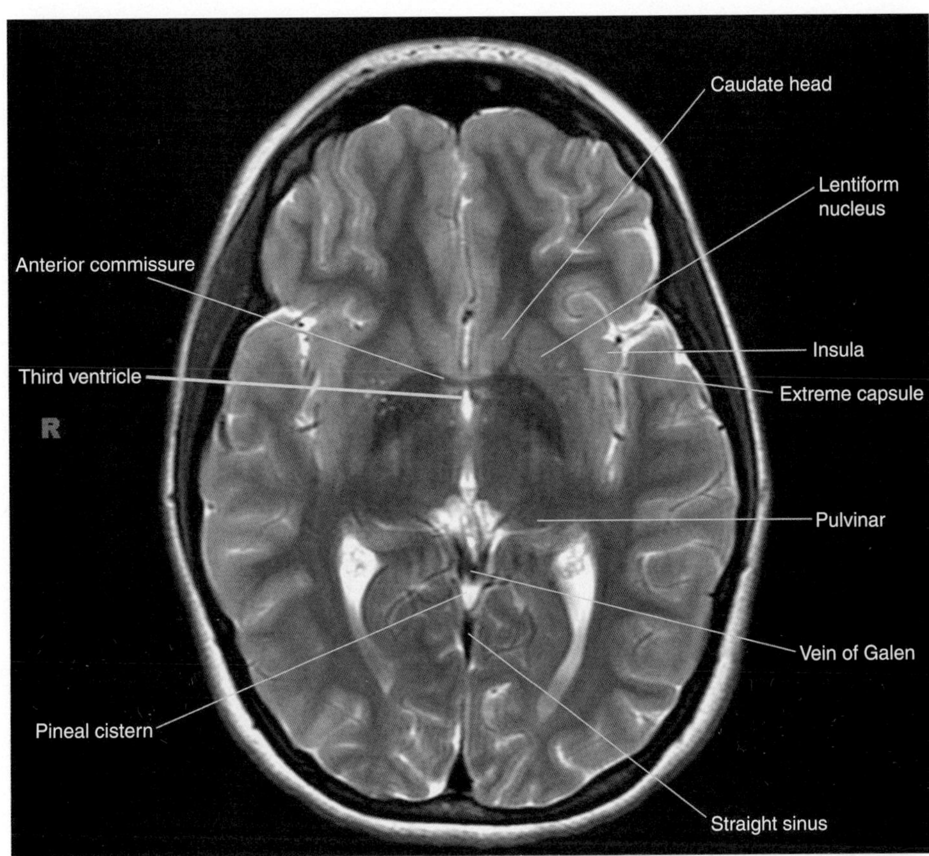

FIGURE 2.5. **Brain MR.** Third ventricle. Axial plane T2-weighted image at 3T.

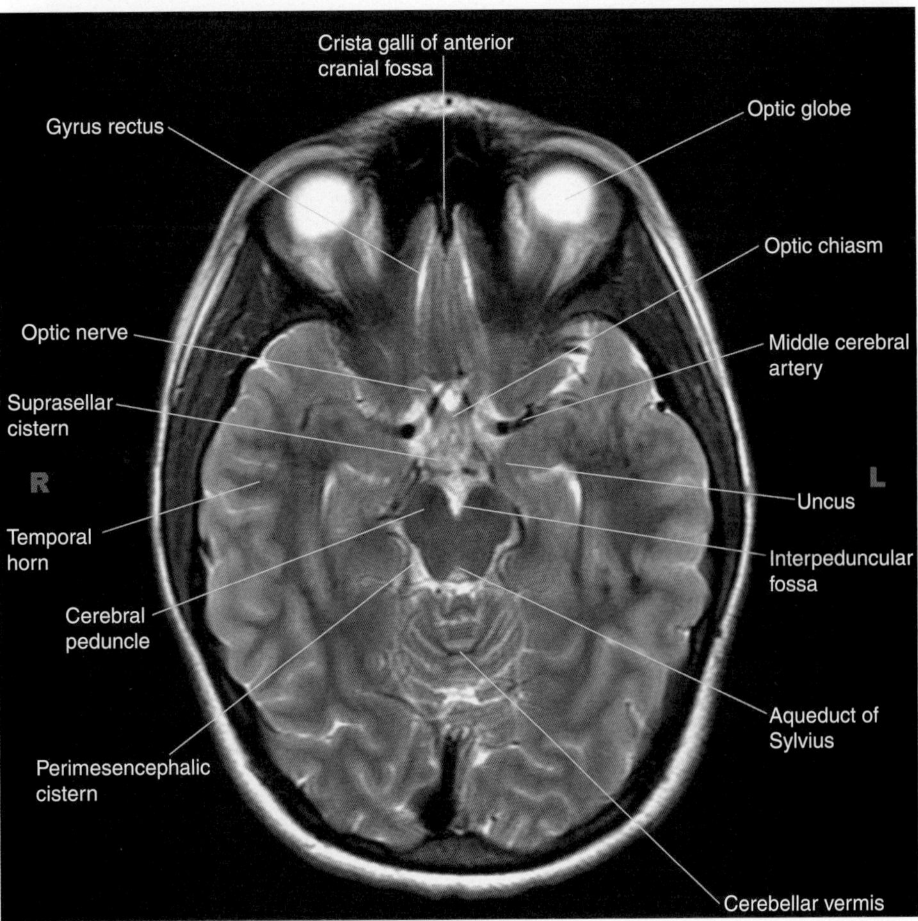

FIGURE 2.6. **Brain MR.** Suprasellar cistern. Axial plane T2-weighted image at 3T.

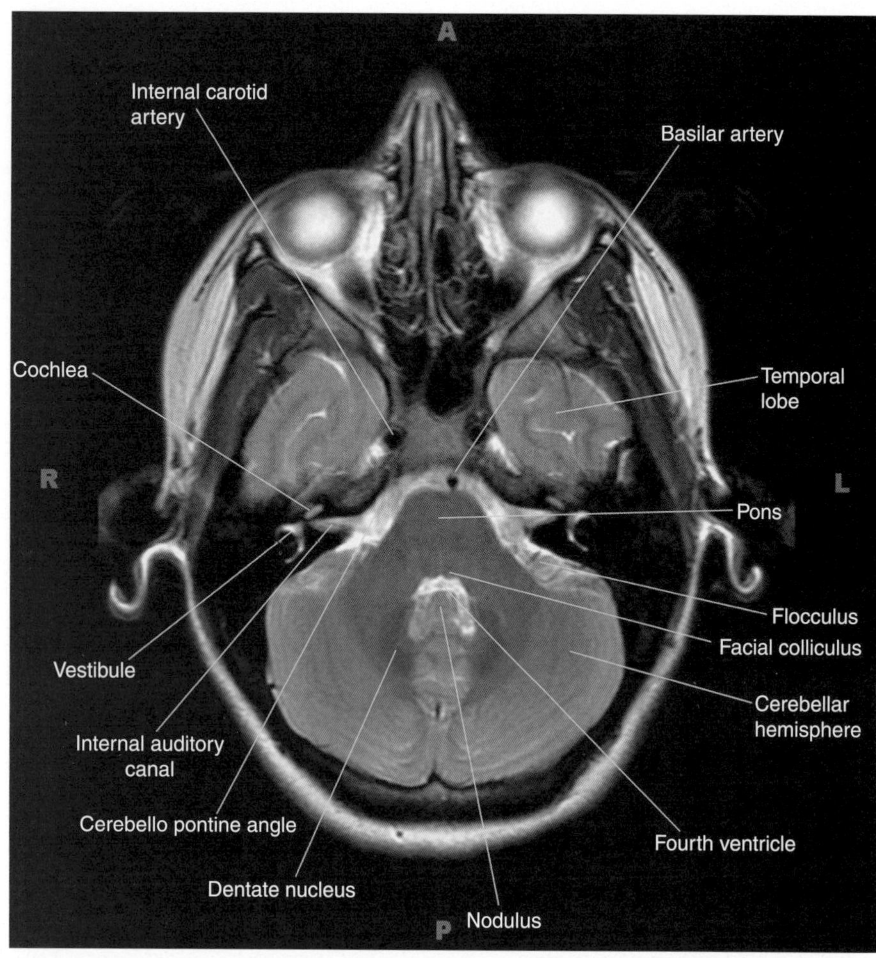

FIGURE 2.7. Brain MR. Fourth ventricle. Axial plane T2-weighted image at 3T.

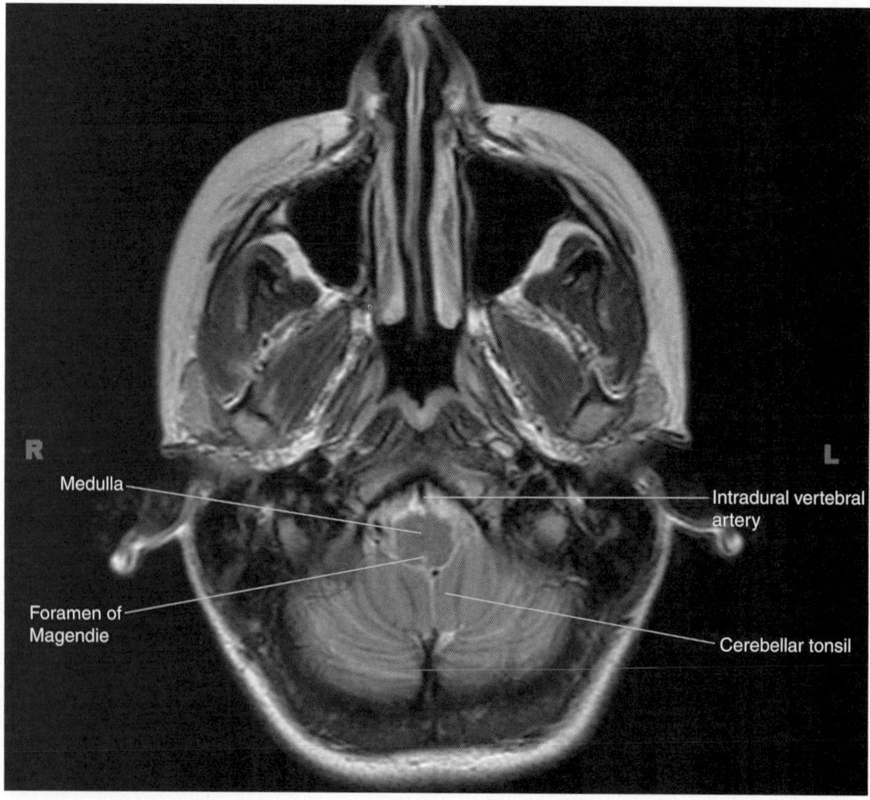

FIGURE 2.8. Brain MR. Medulla. Axial plane T2-weighted image at 3T.

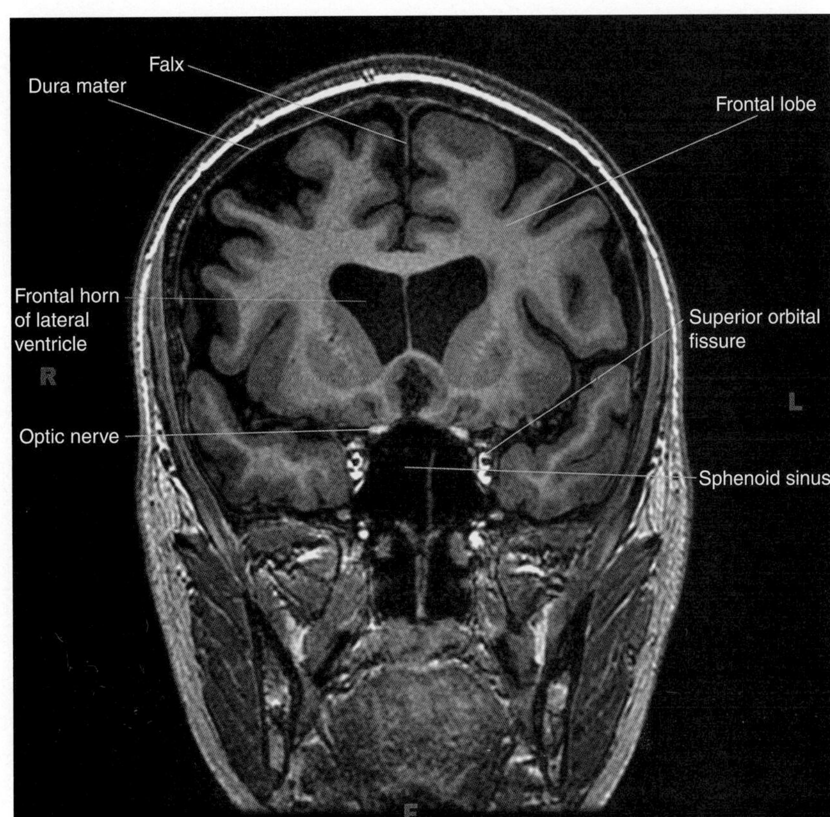

FIGURE 2.9. **Brain MR.** Frontal lobes. Coronal plane T1-weighted image at 3T.

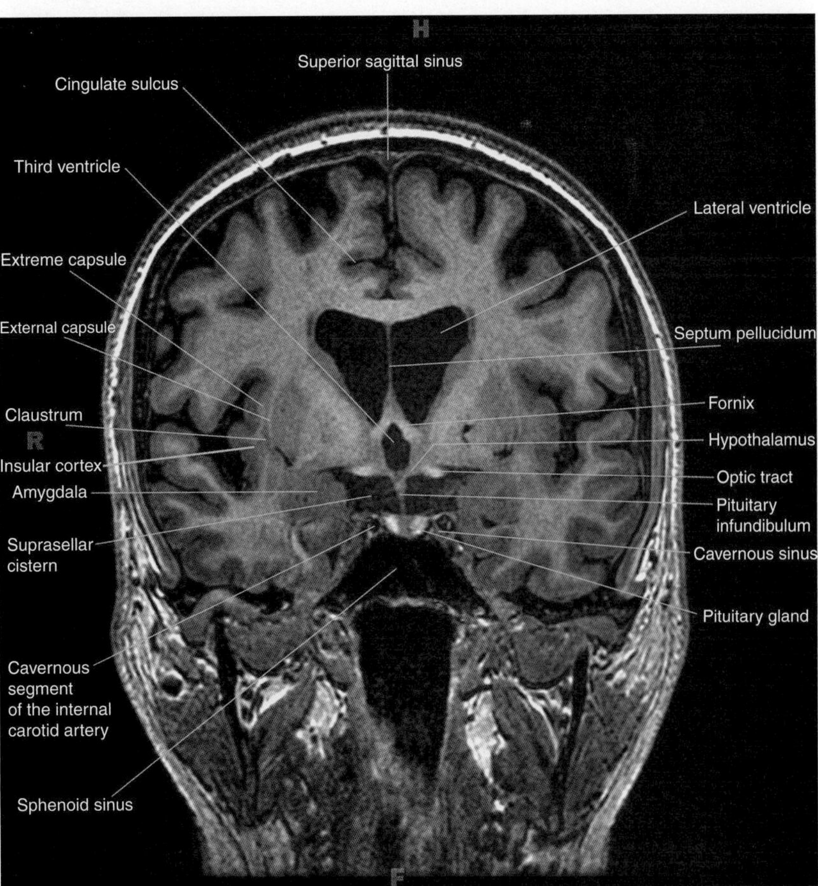

FIGURE 2.10. **Brain MR.** Pituitary infundibulum. Coronal plane T1-weighted image at 3T.

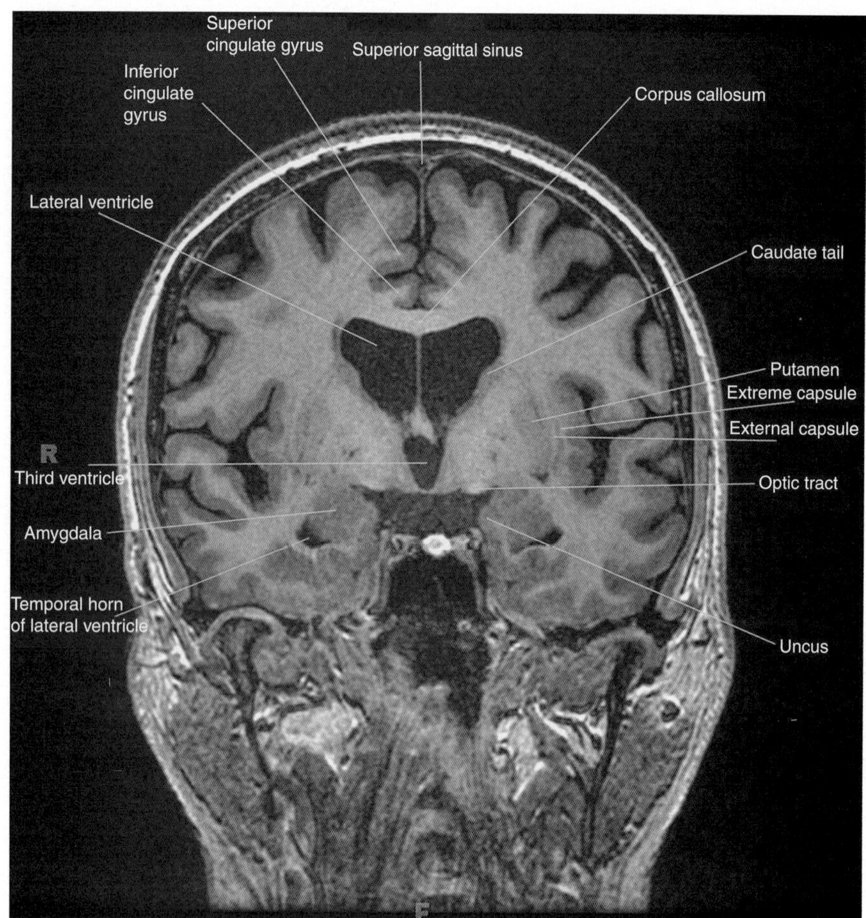

FIGURE 2.11. Brain MR. Optic tracts. Coronal plane T1-weighted image at 3T.

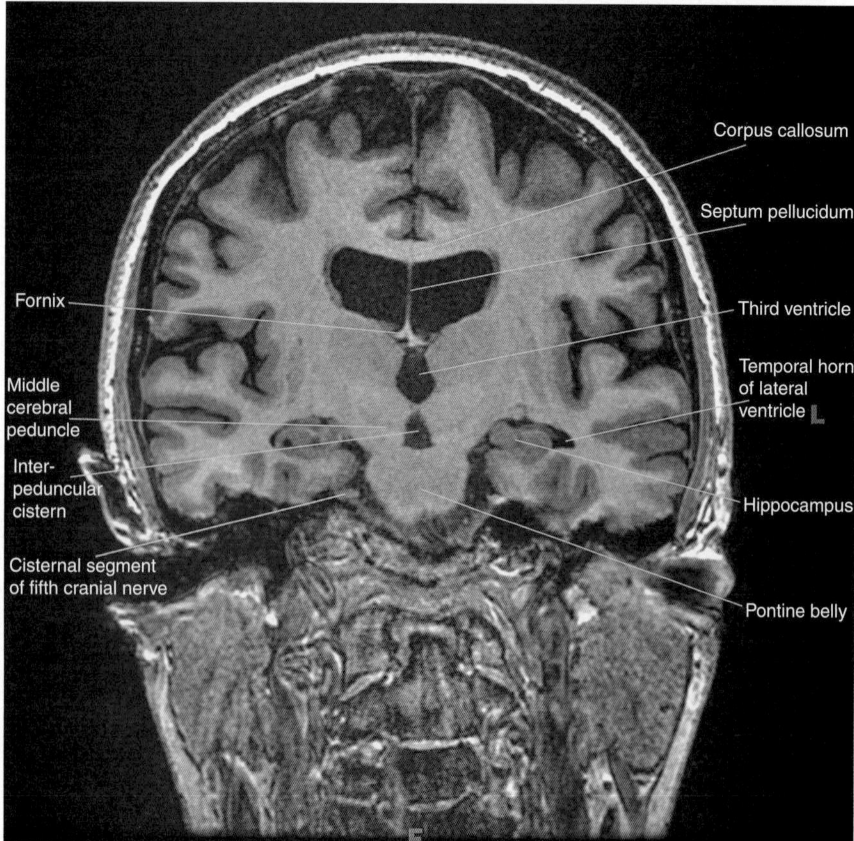

FIGURE 2.12. Brain MR. Third ventricle. Coronal plane T1-weighted image at 3T.

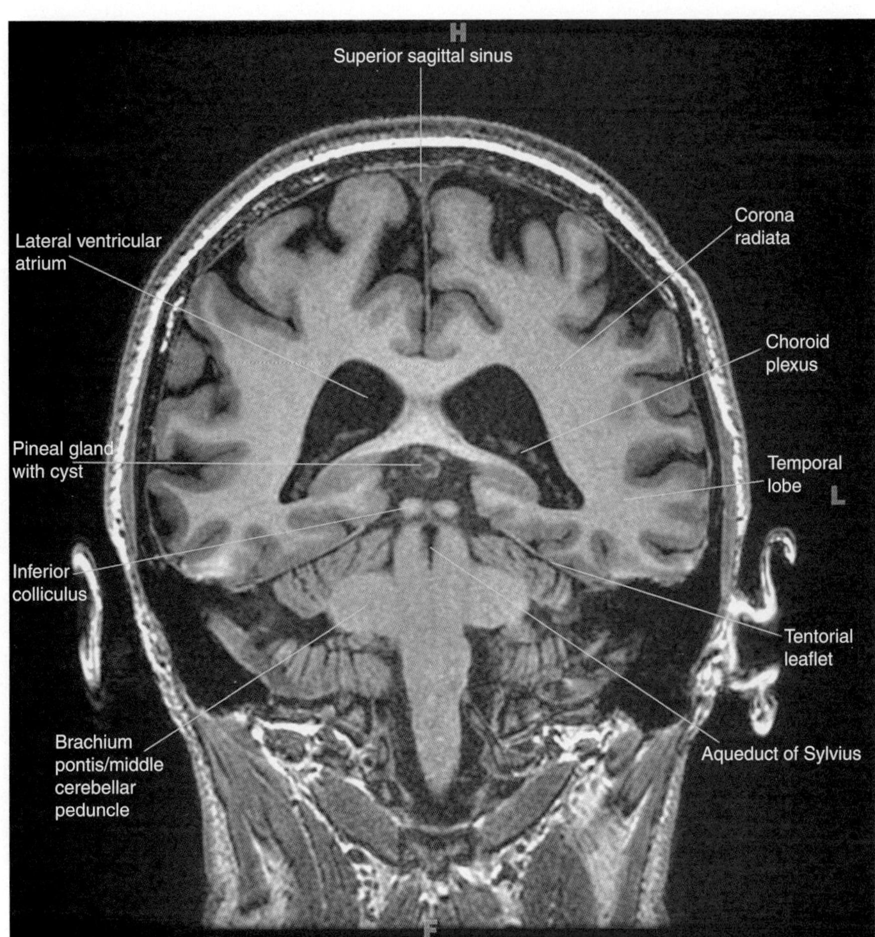

FIGURE 2.13. **Brain MR.** Middle cerebellar peduncle. Coronal plane T1-weighted image at 3T.

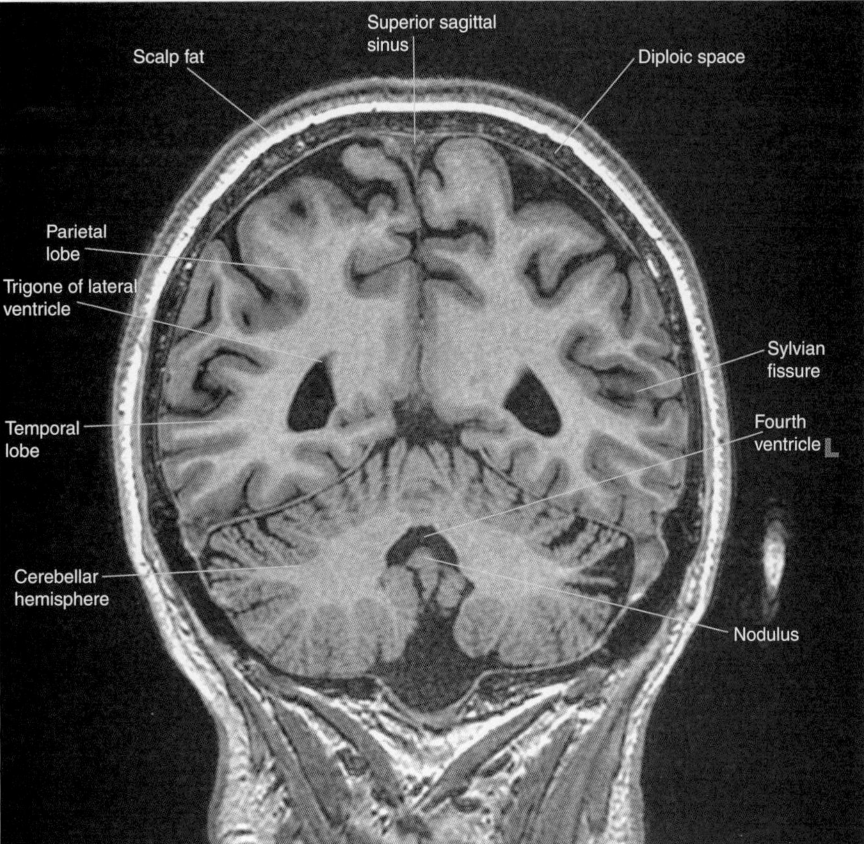

FIGURE 2.14. **Brain MR.** Fourth ventricle. Coronal plane T1-weighted image at 3T.

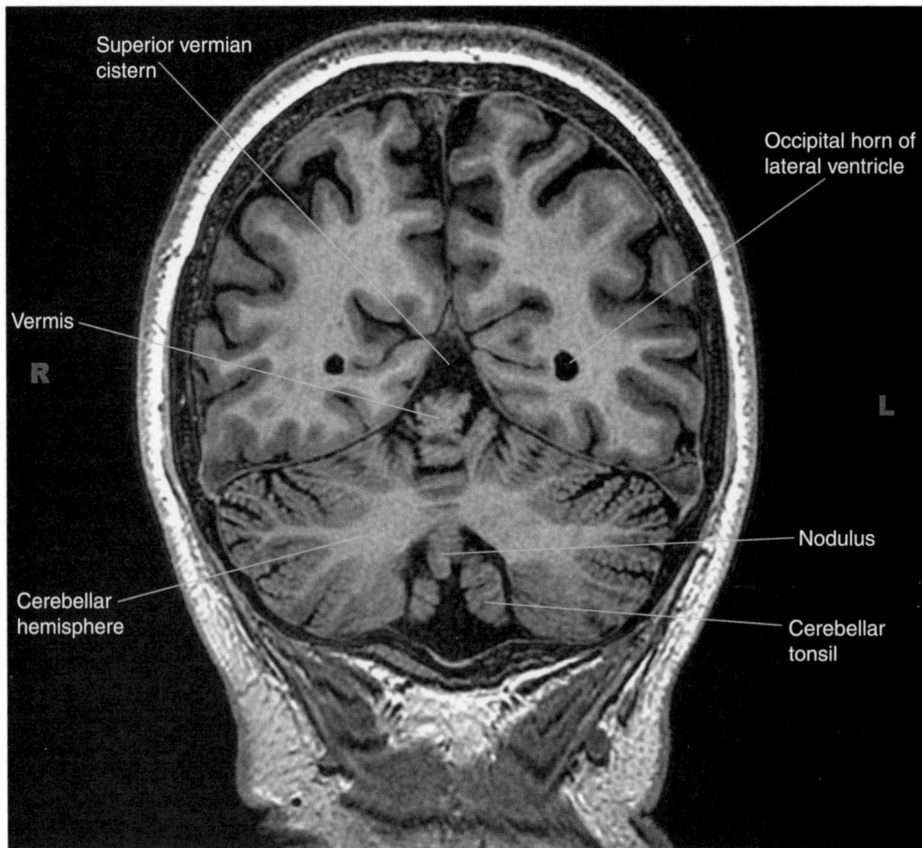

FIGURE 2.15. **Brain MR.** Occipital horns of the lateral ventricles. Coronal plane T1-weighted image at 3T.

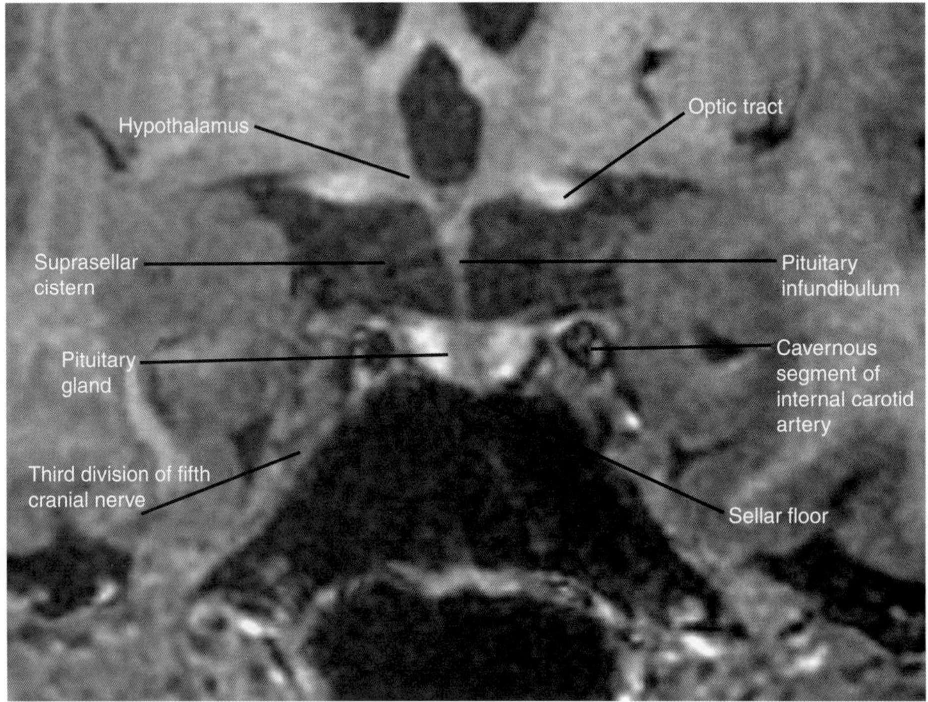

FIGURE 2.16. **Brain MR.** Pituitary gland. Coronal plane magnified T1-weighted image at 3T.

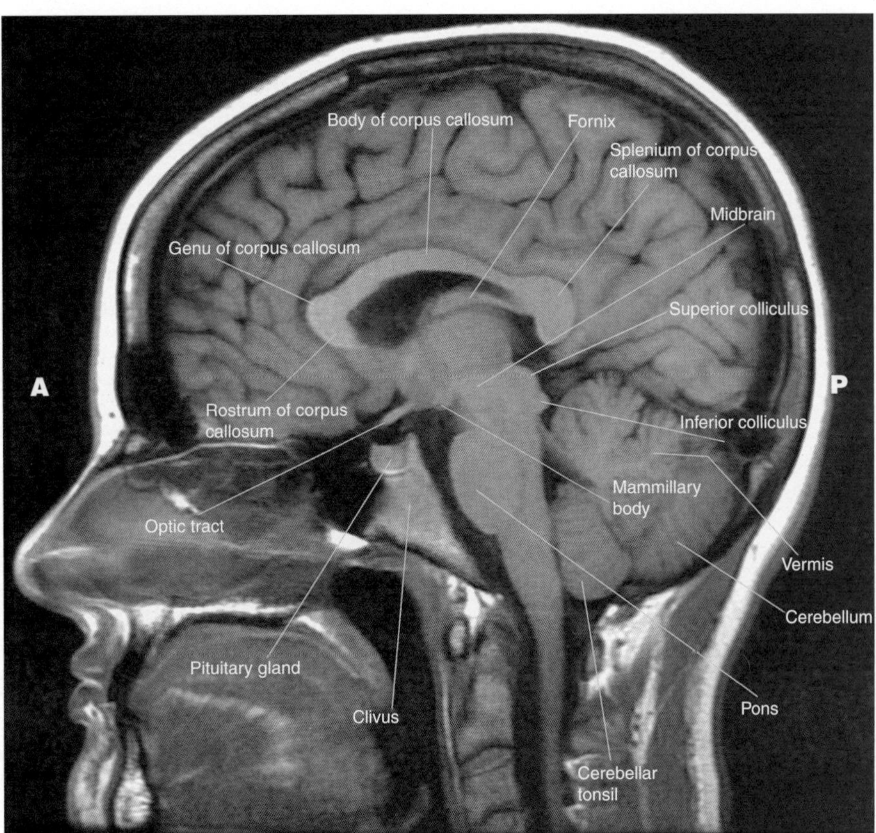

FIGURE 2.17. Brain MR. Sagittal midline. T1-weighted image at 3T.

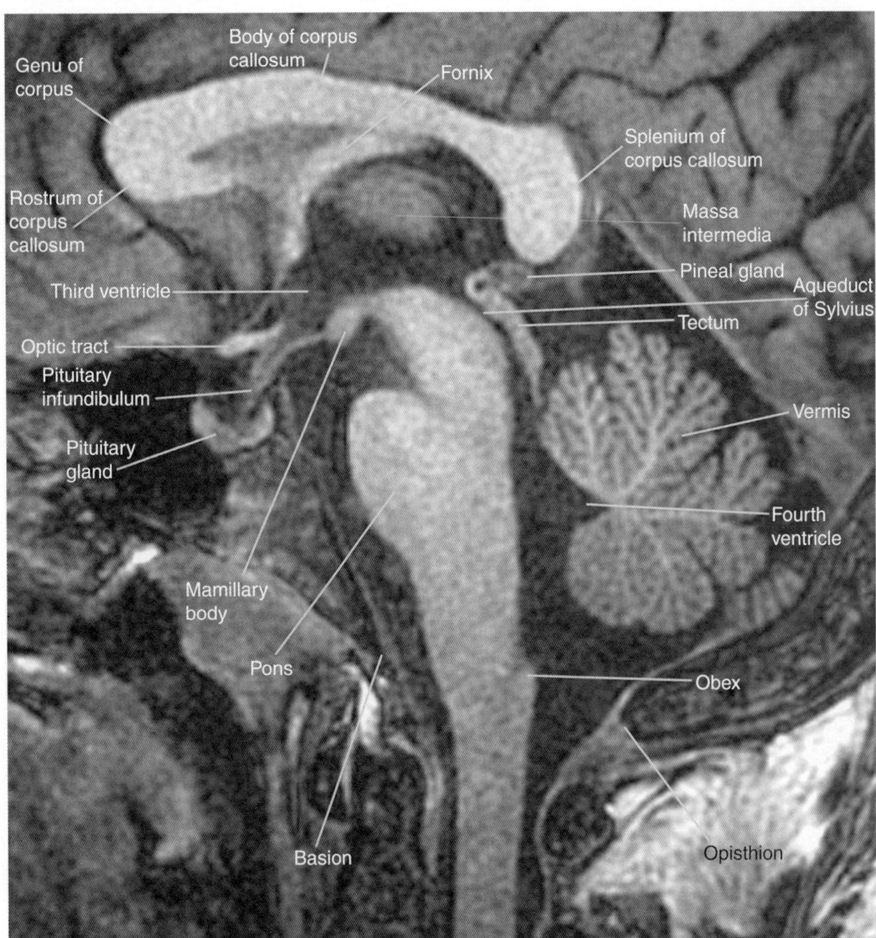

FIGURE 2.18. Brain MR. Pituitary infundibulum. Sagittal plane T1-weighted image at 3T.

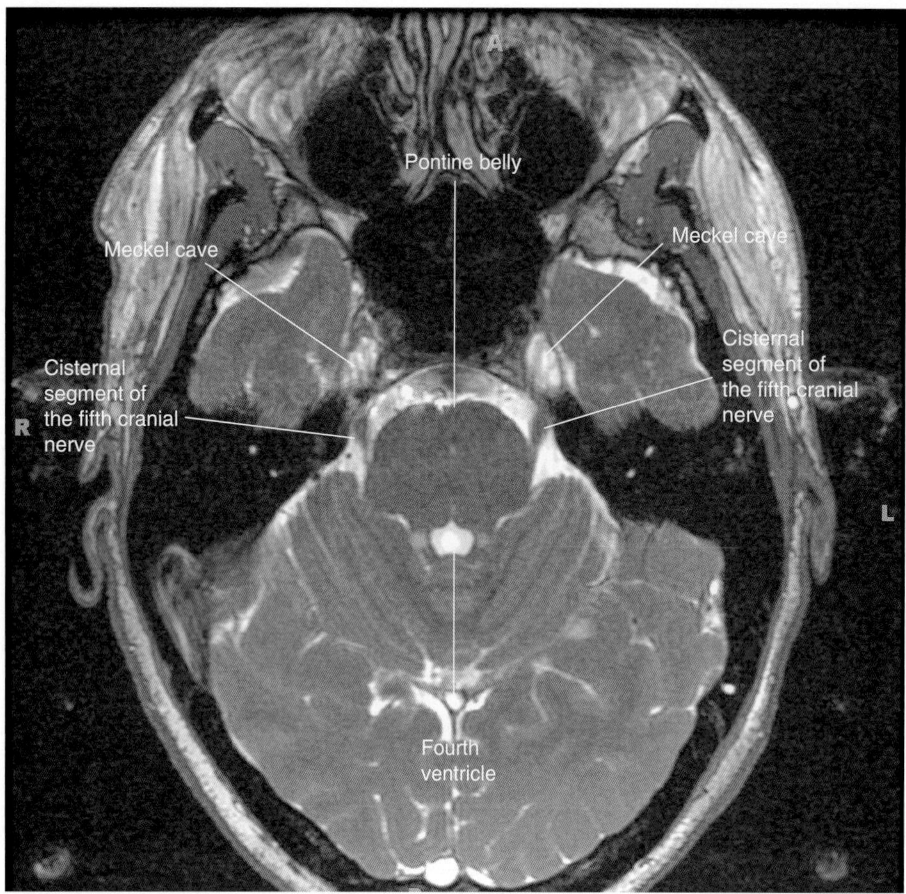

FIGURE 2.19. **Brain MR.** Fifth cranial nerves. Axial plane FIESTA image at 3T.

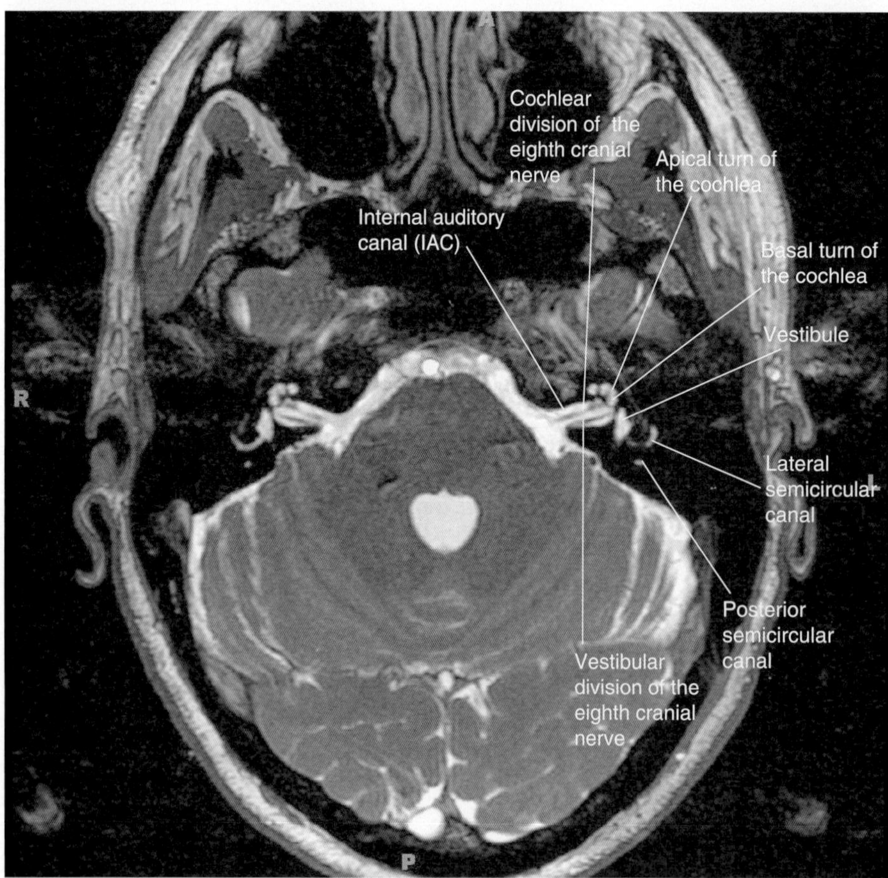

FIGURE 2.20. **Brain MR.** Internal auditory canals. Axial plane FIESTA image at 3T.

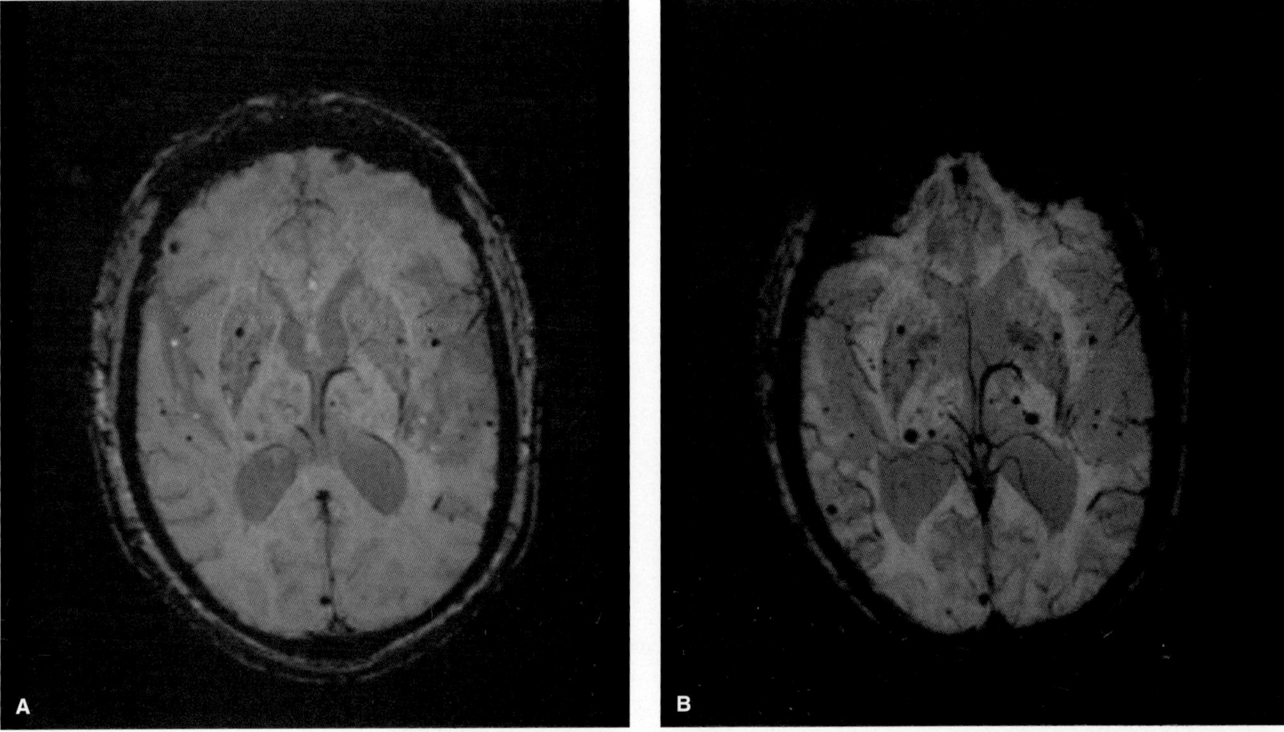

FIGURE 2.21. **Brain MR.** Level of the basal ganglia showing microhemorrhages. **A:** Axial plane susceptibility-weighted image (SWI) at 3TWE. **B:** Axial plane SWI at maximum intensity.

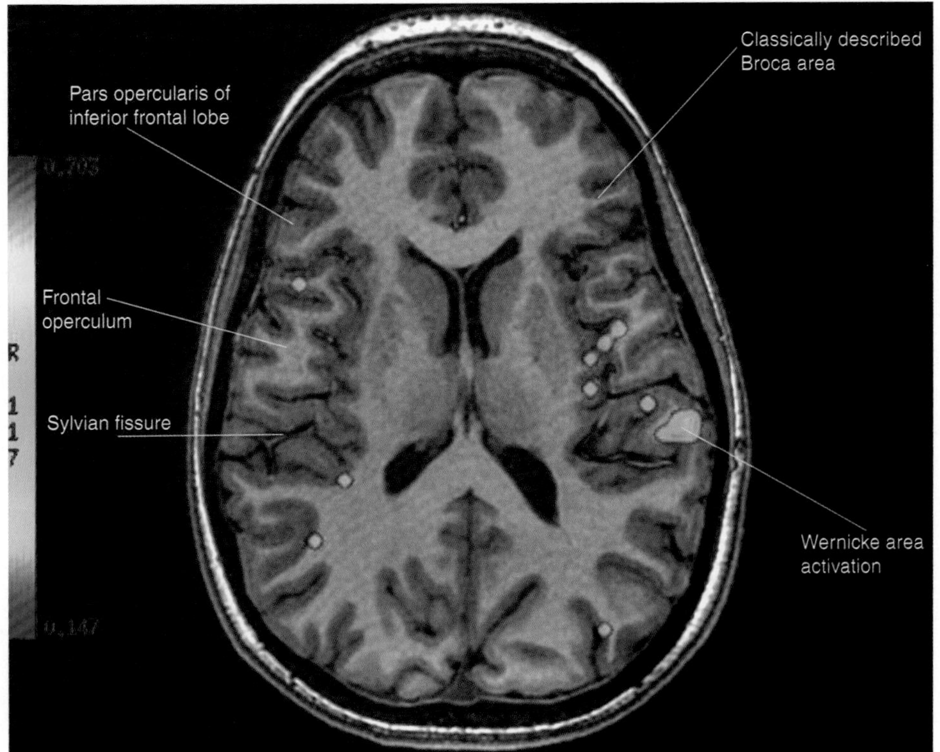

FIGURE 2.22. **Functional Brain MR.** Left hemispheric Wernicke area activation with semantic decision task paradigm. Blood oxygen level–dependent (BOLD) sequence derived data overlaid on FSPGR anatomic sequence acquired at 3T.

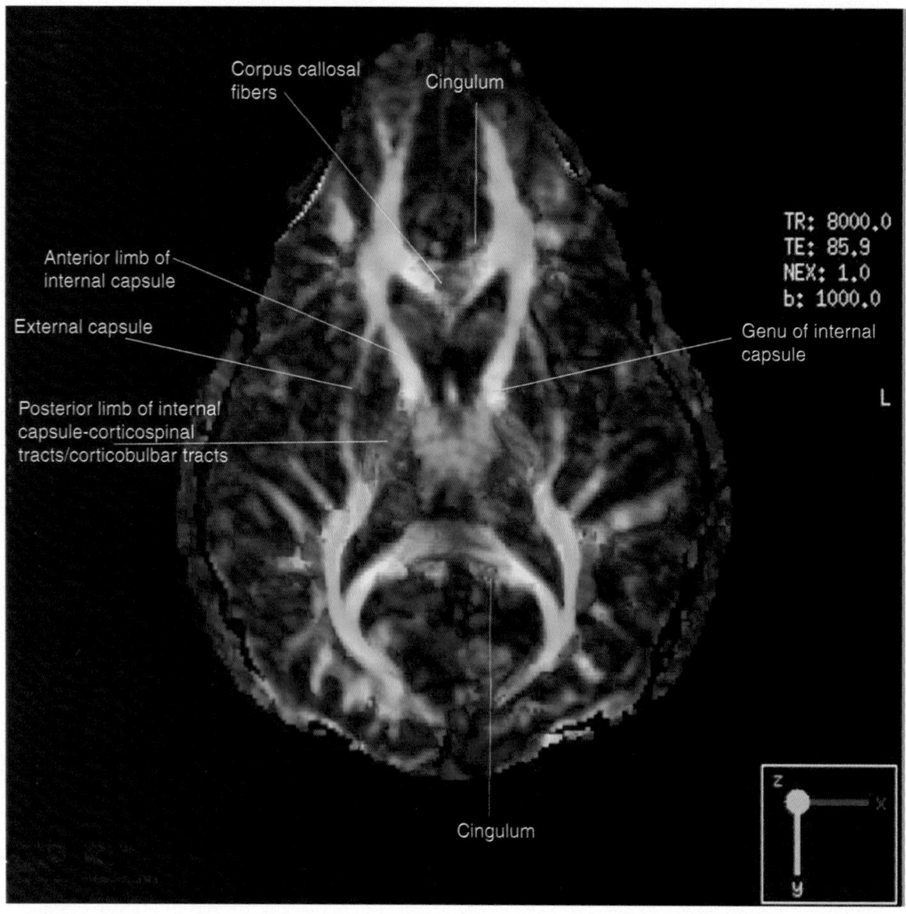

FIGURE 2.23. Diffusion Tensor Imaging. White matter tracts at the level of the internal capsule. Color-encoded fractional anisotropy maps derived from diffusion tensor data at 3T.

Emergency CT Checklist. When confronted with a CT scan under emergency conditions, radiologists must ask themselves these five questions.

1. Is the middle of the brain in the middle of the head?
2. Do the two sides of the brain look alike?
3. Can you see the smile and the pentagon or Jewish star/Shatkona?
4. Is the fourth ventricle in the midline and more or less symmetrical?
5. Are the lateral ventricles huge, with effaced sulci?

If a radiologist can give the right answers to these five questions, there is no neurosurgical emergency. This approach leaves many important diagnoses unmade, but the diseases are either untreatable or treatment can safely be delayed several hours. It is important to note that thrombolysis candidates require close scrutiny of the basal ganglia and cortex for signs of early ischemia as well as global, acute hemorrhage. When stroke triage is performed, specialized imaging techniques such as perfusion CT and CT angiography (CTA) often follow the initial screening CT in a stroke imaging bundle. In an increasing number of centers, MR stroke triage is performed, provided that the clinical suspicion of intracranial hemorrhage is very low and no contraindication to MR is known.

Midline Structures. The anatomy of the midline of the brain is extremely complex, and because the structures are not duplicated, principles of symmetry cannot be applied. The midline anatomy must be learned in detail. There are three prime areas to study.

Suprasellar Region. The first is the suprasellar and sellar regions. On virtually every MR examination it is possible to localize the sella turcica, the pituitary gland, pituitary infundibulum, optic chiasm, anterior third ventricle, mammillary bodies, and anterior interhemispheric fissure. Important vascular structures are also seen in this region. The tip of the basilar artery and the posterior cerebral arteries are seen posteriorly, and the anterior cerebral arteries are visualized anterior and superior to the sella (Fig. 2.10). The anterior cerebral arteries travel in the interhemispheric fissure. Slightly off the midline, the "S-" shaped carotid siphons and the posterior communicating arteries are visualized. Parallel to the course of the posterior communicating artery (Pcomm), we frequently see the third cranial nerve. In the parasagittal location, near the optic chiasm, we see the optic nerve anteriorly and the optic tract posteriorly.

Pineal Region. The next important region to study in the midline is the pineal region. It is crucial to identify the midbrain, the midbrain tegmentum (frequently with a small lucency representing the decussation of the superior cerebellar peduncle), the aqueduct of Sylvius, the midbrain tectum with superior and inferior colliculi, the pineal gland, and the superior cerebellar vermian lobules. If the precentral cerebellar vein can be seen in the superior vermian cistern, a mass here is unlikely.

Craniocervical Junction. Historically, the craniocervical junction was a relative blind spot to the neuroradiologist,

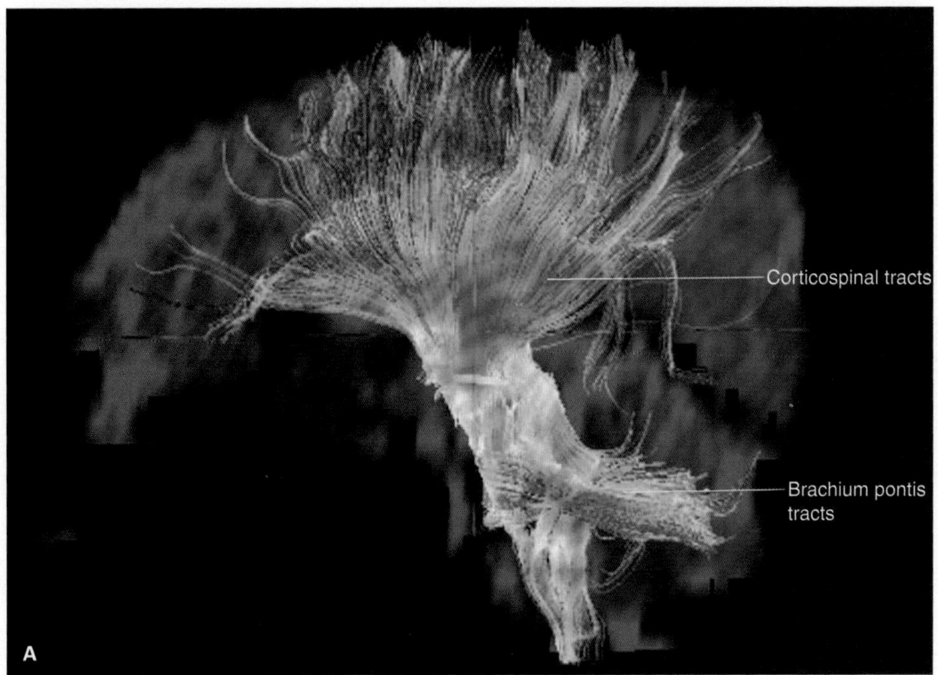

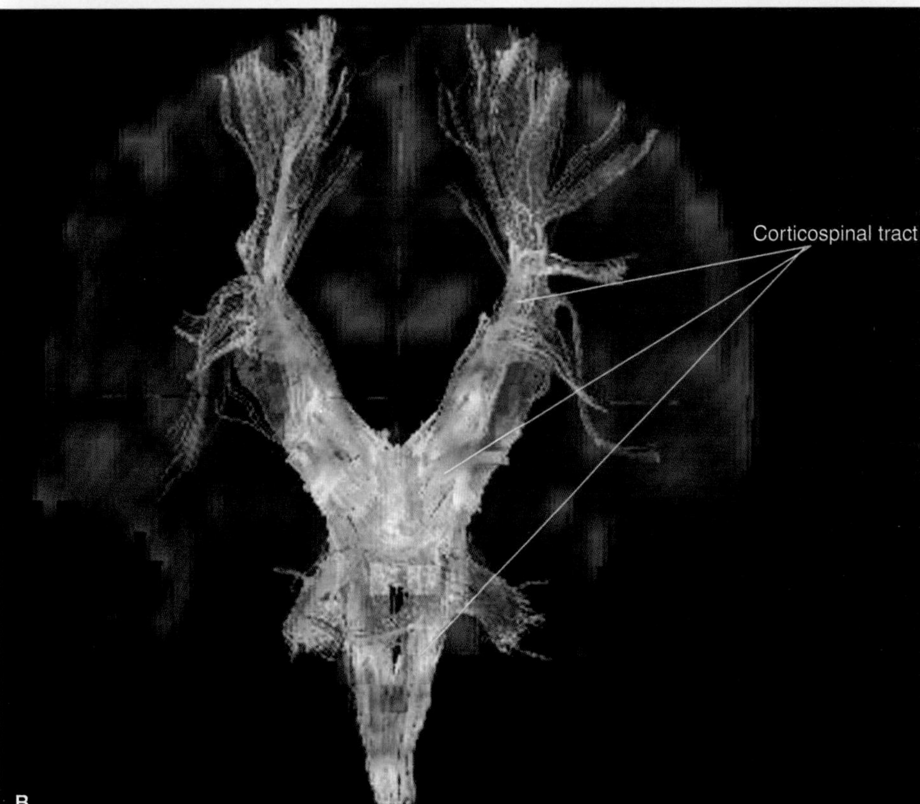

FIGURE 2.24. Corticospinal Tracts. **A:** White matter tractography. Sagittal projection. **B:** Coronal projection.

but this is no longer true, so it is particularly important to study this region. The anterior arch of C1, the odontoid process, and the cervical occipital ligaments are seen anteriorly. The sharp inferior edge of the clivus marks the anterior lip of the foramen magnum. The posterior lip is marked by the cortical margin of the occipital bone. The cerebellar tonsils should project no more than 5 mm below a line drawn between the anterior and posterior lips of the foramen magnum. The obex, the most posterior projection of the dorsal medulla, should lie above this imaginary line. The only structures visible at this level within the calvarium and spinal canal are the cervical medullary junction and a tiny bit of cerebellar tonsillar tissue. Any other soft tissue in this location is pathologic.

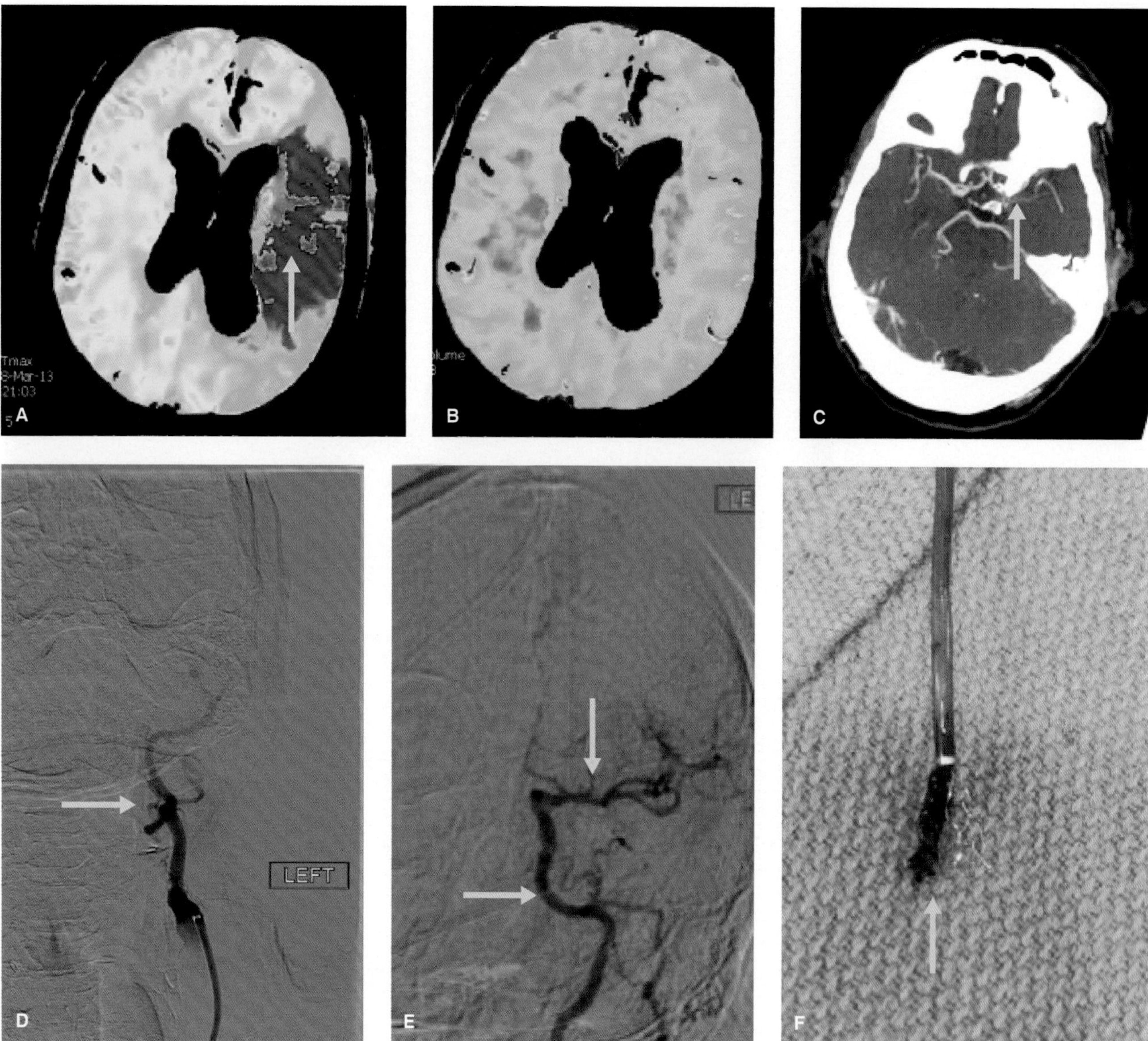

FIGURE 2.25. Gamut of Stroke Imaging Intervention. A 92-year-old male 1 hour after sudden onset of aphasia and right hemiplegia. Complete recovery after mechanical thrombectomy. **A:** CT perfusion, Tmax image showing large penumbra corresponding to a large part of the left MCA territory (*blue arrow*). **B:** CT perfusion, CBV (blood volume) image showing no significant flow stasis (infarct correlate) showing mismatch. **C:** CT angiogram, axial image at the level of the MCA trunks shows large thrombus in the left M1 MCA extending to the proximal M2 branches (*blue arrow*). This extended to the ICA origin. **D:** Left carotid artery angiogram showing left ICA occlusion from origin (*blue arrow*). **E:** Left carotid artery angiogram following successful mechanical thrombectomy shows complete left anterior circulation recanalization (*blue arrows*). **F:** Large thrombus retrieved from the left MCA. Note that distal thrombus shape matches that of the distal M1 and proximal M2 branches (*blue arrow*). (Courtesy Lotfi Hacein-Bey, MD.)

CURRENT NEUROIMAGING OPTIONS

With the bewildering and ever-increasing array of examinations available for imaging the brain, it seems a hopeless task to decide which of them is best for a given clinical situation. To make matters easier, we can eliminate two from the start. Plain radiography is useless in patient management and is only of value in the documentation of fracture for medical/legal reasons. Nuclear medicine brain scans are useful in certain specialized settings, such as medically refractory epilepsy, movement disorders and dementia, in which PET scans play important roles (see Chapter 64). We still must decide between CT, MR, US, and angiography in the evaluation of the acute neurologic patient.

The radiologist also needs to decide whether to give intravenous contrast material and which special CT and MR techniques to employ. Angiography is used in the acute setting based upon the appropriate combination of CT, MR, and clinical findings. US may be used as the first test in infants, or for evaluation of the carotids, or with transcranial techniques for evaluation of the intracranial vessels after initial imaging triage. Therefore, the only contenders for the "first test" for the brain are MR and CT. A standard MR examination generally consists of a T1-weighted sequence, a

T2-weighted sequence, diffusion-weighted imaging (DWI), and fluid-attenuated inversion recovery (FLAIR) and may be supplemented by T1-weighted images with gadolinium-based contrast agents. SWIs may be obtained as indicated as well for blood products. A standard CT examination consists of axial images reviewed at brain and bone windows and may be supplemented by repeat images with intravenous iodinated contrast. In centers employing advanced stroke therapies, CT perfusion and CTA supplement diagnostic triage.

As a general rule in brain imaging, CT is performed for acute neurologic illness and MR for the more chronic and subacute cases. That is, if the onset of neurologic symptoms referable to the brain was within 24 to 48 hours, start with a CT. If the problem is older than 2 days, start with an MR. If the CT or MR suggests a primary vascular lesion, such as an arteriovenous malformation (AVM) or aneurysm, do an MR or CT angiogram and/or catheter angiogram. MR angiography (MRA) is best for screening for AVMs and CTA for problem solving and aneurysm treatment planning. Catheter angiography is generally reserved for endovascular treatment since virtually all diagnoses are made noninvasively. If the CT or MR suggests tumor or abscess, give contrast. If the CT or MR fails to demonstrate an acute infarct and the symptoms suggest a transient ischemic attack or stroke, do a carotid Doppler US, or MRA, or CTA. Always use NASCET method to document stenosis. Don't use intravenous iodinated contrast for CT in the acute setting unless brain abscess or tumor is a strong consideration or if needed for your stroke triage protocol. Give gadolinium for MR whenever there is a clinical finding that suggests a specific neurologic localization, a seizure, or a strong history of cancer or infectious disease. Exceptions to these general guidelines are few. Follow the rules and you'll be doing the right thing in the majority of cases. Sometimes an MR will be required to clarify a questionable finding on CT. Also, remember that some patients are simply too sick to study easily with MR. These include multisystem trauma patients or those who require assisted ventilation. Patients who cannot hold still, such as children or highly agitated adults, must be sedated for MR. Sedation carries its own set of risks, which must be weighed carefully, and properly trained personnel and appropriate monitoring are essential. Radiation risks of CT and NSF risks of gadolinium should not alter imaging approaches for acute neurologic syndromes as the benefits usually vastly outweigh these risks.

MR spectroscopy, MR and CT angiography and perfusion techniques, and MR diffusion techniques are now routine in neuroradiology practice.

Proton MR spectroscopy shows the distribution of brain metabolites based upon the chemical shift of the protons within them, which is a property determined by the chemical environment of the protons in question. This is the form of magnetic resonance analysis you learned in organic chemistry! Please refer to Chapters 5 and 7 to see spectroscopy in action, analyzing tumor and white matter cases, respectively. In practice, three normal metabolites are the most interesting: choline, which is a marker for cell membranes and hence a marker for cellular turnover; N-acetyl aspartate (NAA), which is a compound found only in neurons and therefore a marker of neuronal density; and creatine, which is evenly distributed in many types of cells and serves as a reference standard.

Choline may be considered a tumor marker. If an intracranial mass is indeterminate with respect to etiology, elevation of the choline-to-creatine ratio may help to distinguish radiation necrosis from recurrent tumor or infection. Another use of the choline peak is tumor grading. Since the prognosis of a primary brain tumor is determined by the highest histologic grade of tissue within it, and histologic grade correlates with choline-to-creatine ratio, biopsy of the site with the highest choline-to-creatine ratio is likely to reflect the histologic grade of the tumor. Biopsy targeted by MR spectroscopy will better reflect the true nature of the lesion. This rule is not perfect; for example, if the choline peak is sky high, think of a meningioma. Demyelinating processes such as multiple sclerosis can also present with elevated choline peaks.

A decrease in the NAA-to-creatine ratio is seen in a variety of conditions that are associated with neuronal death. Focally decreased NAA is seen in mesial temporal sclerosis and infarcts. Global depletion of NAA can be seen in multiple sclerosis and dementing diseases such as Alzheimer disease (AD), which also demonstrates elevated myoinositol. Any space-occupying mass that replaces brain will also have a small NAA peak. Abscesses and metastatic lesions will have lower NAA-to-creatine ratios than primary brain tumors, which tend to infiltrate rather than replace brain. Markedly elevated NAA levels are seen in Canavan disease as a result of a specific defect in the enzyme that metabolizes it. The NAA accumulates, producing a distinct spectroscopic pattern.

Elevated levels of abnormal metabolites are sometimes present in the brain. A nonspecific necrosis peak is seen in malignant tumors, infections, and some active demyelinating lesions. Amino acid peaks can be seen in intracranial infections. A characteristic doublet peak of lactic acid can help make the diagnosis of ischemia. This has been useful in infants with suspected hypoxemic ischemic encephalopathy. This may also aid in diagnosis of mitochondrial encephalopathies.

Noninvasive angiographic techniques are now routinely used. CTA depends upon the rapid bolus injection of iodinated contrast, rapid imaging with a multidetector spiral CT, and rapid data processing to produce clinically useful images of the cerebral vessels. Two major classes of images are produced with these studies: relatively thick cross-sectional images using maximum intensity projection (MIP) and shaded three-dimensional surface renderings. Because reconstruction techniques are time consuming, bone is hard to distinguish from vessels, and venous contamination can be problematic, it is best to go where the climate suits your clothes when interpreting CTA. Look at the MIP images most likely to answer your clinical question and remember that CTA is a problem-solving technique rather than a screening method. In subarachnoid hemorrhage, use the sagittal MIP for the carotid ophthalmic aneurysm, the Pcomm and the posterior inferior cerebellar artery (PICA) origin, the coronal MIP for the anterior communicating artery (Acomm), carotid "T" and basilar tip, and the axial MIP for the Acomm and Pcomm. Remember that the middle cerebral artery (MCA) is a relative blind spot so it must be inspected carefully on all images. Once an aneurysm is found, the shaded surface renderings are invaluable in treatment planning, especially in determining the configuration of the neck and sizing the aneurysm for coil selection. In suspected infarct, use the symptoms as a guide and carefully follow the appropriate vessels to an abrupt halt or significant narrowing. A vessel segment ought to reside completely within the MIP volume to be analyzed accurately. Be careful not to misinterpret a vessel leaving the slice as an obstruction or one curving partly outside the slice as a stenosis. Confirm the degree of stenosis by viewing the vessel in cross section.

MRA is harder to obtain but easier to read. There is inherently greater contrast between the vessel and the surrounding tissues. Noncontrast MRA techniques depend upon the phenomenon of *flow-related enhancement,* in which moving spins behave differently than stationary spins. Images are created by choosing parameters that increase the signal of the flowing blood. First-pass gadolinium-enhanced MRA provides superior quality images that enhance diagnostic confidence but not necessarily accuracy. Both source images and MIP reconstructions of user-defined volumes are reviewed. Separate images of the anterior and posterior cerebral circulations are performed and the right and left carotid systems are viewed separately. Because the vessels are viewed in isolation, the conspicuity of aneurysms and other vascular lesions is excellent, though artifacts resulting from patient motion, in-plane vascular flow, and susceptibility artifacts can be problematic. MRA is most useful when patients are not acutely ill. Intracranial vascular stenoses and aneurysms are reliable depicted. Both MRA and CTA are very useful extracranially as well. However, it should be noted that CTA has a higher resolution when compared to MRA and thus is often used to problem solve questionable MRA findings.

Diffusion-weighted imaging (DWI) has greatly enhanced the ability of MRI to diagnose cerebral infarct early and accurately. This technique exploits the phenomenon of diffusion, which is related to Brownian motion at the molecular level. DWI takes advantage of the fact that intracellular water molecules are much more limited in their movement than extracellular ones, because they quickly bump into the cell membrane that contains them. The more restricted the movement of water, the brighter it will be on DWI sequences. In stroke, ischemic areas tend to swell following osmosis of free water into the dying cells, and these areas become bright on DWI as a result of the increased ratio of intracellular to extracellular water. This change on DWI precedes changes on T2 and FLAIR, making DWI a key sequence in the early detection of stroke. CSF contains the least-restricted water in the brain and will be dark on DWI. Low signal on DWI therefore distinguishes arachnoid cysts from intracranial epidermoid cysts.

Tumor, trauma, and infection can have an ambiguous appearance on DWI, as both intracellular and extracellular water may increase. Fortunately, the T2 effects of extracellular edema can be accounted for and "subtracted" out using apparent diffusion coefficient (ADC) maps. Please refer to the examples in Chapter 4, as a picture is worth a thousand words in understanding this complicated and powerful tool that has become routine part of daily practice. Restricted diffusion has been well described in the literature in multiple sclerosis/other demyelinating processes, brain abscess and highly cellular high-grade primary brain tumors, metastatic disease and lymphoma. Restricted diffusion in higher-grade tumors can be particularly useful in solidifying the diagnosis and giving the referring clinician a better idea of the grade of the tumor being evaluated.

The diffusion phenomenon has also been exploited in MRI to map white matter tracts for surgical treatment planning and other purposes. This tool, *diffusion tensor imaging* (DTI) (Fig. 2.23) exploits the fact that within elongated cell processes such as axons, water can diffuse more freely "down the tube" than "sideways," allowing for reconstruction of white matter tracts or "tractography" (Figs. 2.23 and 2.24A–B).

MR and CT perfusion techniques are extremely useful for the depiction of regions of relatively diminished flow in ischemic cerebral tissue and perfusion. Most MR perfusion scans rely on a first-pass bolus gadolinium injection, during which the brain is imaged sequentially. Because the gadolinium is paramagnetic, the signal on highly T2*-weighted images is decreased in a manner proportional to perfusion. The abnormally perfused brain does not demonstrate this flow-related phenomenon as much or as soon. In the acute stroke patient, a delay of the time to peak that is greater than 6 seconds strongly suggests ischemia. Other perfusion parameters are also employed. CT perfusion relies on the principle that perfused areas of the brain will attenuate the x-ray beam more than the ischemic brain during an iodinated contrast injection. This is because more of the contrast agent will reach the normal brain sooner than it will reach the abnormal brain. Sequential scans are performed, and the time to peak enhancement and other parameters can be calculated. Delayed arrival of contrast and transit of contrast documents ischemia, and other parameters may predict infarct.

MR perfusion techniques also play an important role in the management of primary brain tumors by predicting the most malignant portion of the tumor, which determines the biologic nature of the lesion and the patient's prognosis. Increased relative cerebral blood volume within a tumor appears to correlate with tumor angiogenesis and hence tumor grade. Areas of increasing abnormality on perfusion-weighted MR examinations correlate well with areas of increasing malignancy. Biopsy and treatment guided by these images promise to improve prognosis and outcome in patients with astrocytoma and other brain tumors. Caveats include newer angiogenesis modifying chemotherapeutic agents that can alter the CBV of treated high-grade tumors as well as vascular tumors such as oligodendrogliomas that can appear to mimic higher-grade tumors.

Hemorrhage-Sensitive Sequences: T2*- Versus Susceptibility-Weighted Imaging. While noncontrast CT is still considered superior for detection of acute subarachnoid hemorrhage, there are MR options for parenchymal hemorrhage, found in diverse pathologies from trauma, hypertensive/ischemic hemorrhage, amyloid angiopathy, vasculitis through melanoma, and hemorrhagic metastases. The most common is the T2* or gradient recalled echo sequence without the 180 degree refocusing pulse, thus allowing the signal to decay in the presence of paramagnetic blood products like hemosiderin. This option is available on almost all MR scanners. The other option is SWI, which is a more complex sequence long TE 3D gradient echo sequence with flow compensation using both magnitude and filtered phase data. This is more sensitive than T2* imaging for blood, and phase data can differentiate between blood products and calcification. The sensitivity of the sequence together with exquisite venous visualization makes the use of maximal intensity projections (MIPs) very useful in separating normal veins from pathology (Fig. 2.21).

Functional MR imaging (fMRI) refers to studies of the brain using blood oxygen level–dependent imaging (BOLD) (Figs. 2.22). These images rely upon the interesting fact that neuronal activation, for example, over the hand motor colliculus, increases local blood flow and oxyhemoglobin content in excess of tissue oxygen requirements (1). Thus the local increase in oxy to deoxyhemoglobin ratio produces changes in magnetic susceptibility that are measurable on fMRI sequences and correlate well with neuronal activity. By comparing images captured during sensory stimulation, motor activity, or higher cortical tasks with those obtained while the patient is in a resting or control condition, one can create images highlighting the area or areas of the brain that are responsible for the brain function in question. Reliable localization of motor and language functions assists in planning surgery for epilepsy and brain tumors. fMRI has become an essential technique for basic neurobehavioral and neurophysiologic research. The potential for this powerful technique has only begun to be explored.

IMAGING STRATEGY FOR COMMON CLINICAL SYNDROMES

While an almost infinite variety of clinical symptoms may be related to the CNS, most patients can be divided into a limited number of categories (Table 2.1).

TABLE 2.1

PREFERRED INITIAL IMAGING STUDY BY CLINICAL PRESENTATIONS

CLINICAL PRESENTATION	CT WITHOUT CONTRAST	CT WITH CONTRAST	MR WITHOUT CONTRAST	MR WITH CONTRAST
Trauma	XX			
Stroke	XX			
Seizure	X	X	X	XX
Infection	X	X	X	XX
Cancer	X	X	X	XX
Acute headache	XX			
Chronic headache			XX	
Dementia			XX	
Coma	XX			

XX, best study; X, acceptable study (depends on circumstances).

Acute trauma patients have perhaps the most dramatic presentation. A noncontrast-enhanced CT scan is preferred, because CT can be obtained quickly and on virtually any patient. Furthermore, CT scanners are almost universally available in hospital emergency rooms. The most important abnormalities to be detected are extracerebral hematomas. These lesions produce devastating neurologic symptoms that can be completely reversed if treated early. Intracerebral contusions are of secondary interest because they are more difficult to treat surgically, and the results of treatment are less encouraging.

Posttraumatic Encephalopathy/Chronic Traumatic Encephalopathy. This diagnosis has no clearly defined imaging criteria in the literature besides parenchymal hemorrhages best seen on gradient echo MR sequence or SWI denoting hemorrhagic contusions/diffuse axonal injury. It is crucial to evaluate the clinical and imaging features of traumatic brain injury, especially in mild cases, and distinguish among various mechanisms of injury both in civilian and military contexts. The difficulty in developing nonhemorrhagic imaging criteria largely stems from multiple confounding clinical comorbidities and defining common pre-existing white matter disease burden. Numerous techniques are valuable at the group level for research purposes, but none has been satisfactorily validated at the level of the individual patient.

Stroke. Noncontrast CT scan is the preferred initial imaging study. The majority of strokes are bland infarcts, and in the acute phase, the CT scan is normal or nearly normal. In these patients we search for evidence of hemorrhage. A cerebral hematoma presenting as a stroke suggests hypertensive encephalopathy or amyloid angiopathy, depending upon the distribution of the lesion and the age of the patient. Subarachnoid hemorrhage requires further workup by MR and/or angiography to search for an aneurysm or AVM. If no hemorrhage is seen, a bland infarct is presumed to be present but, as yet, occult to CT scanning. The absence of hemorrhage visible on CT allows the clinician to perform anticoagulation or thrombolytic therapy to prevent progression or even reverse the neurologic deficit.

Prethrombolytic and Prethrombectomy Evaluation. Recent developments in stroke therapy require further attention to the examination of patients considered for acute thrombolysis, because hemorrhagic complications are more common when early signs of large infarcts are present on the initial CT or, by inference, MR. Loss of gray/white distinction, low attenuation in the basal ganglia, and poor definition of the insula on CT may contraindicate thrombolytic therapy.

A simple set of questions to ask when evaluating a noncontrast CT in the acute stroke syndrome setting:

1. Are there signs of an acute infarct? How big?
2. Is there acute blood?
3. Is there a hyperdense artery, for example, MCA, suggesting a large vessel clot?

In some centers, stroke triage is performed to evaluate the potential for salvaging an ischemic brain. The point is to distinguish brain that is irreversibly damaged from that which is merely temporarily starved for blood flow, and to visualize the offending vascular lesion directly. Local factors determine whether CT or MR is preferred. MR is clearly superior in depicting irreversible infarct sooner and provides an enormous amount of useful physiologic data relatively rapidly, and gadolinium contrast is safer than iodinated contrast and without the cumulative radiation dose associated with CT. CT, however, is more readily available within the stroke treatment time window, is almost never contraindicated, detects virtually all acute hemorrhage, and provides almost all of the information potentially available with MRI rapidly and safely.

CT techniques rely on the usually valid inference that visible parenchymal changes are irreversible, and that, conversely, some areas of diminished blood flow might be saved if the plain CT appears normal. A CT perfusion study demonstrating asymmetry corresponding to clinical symptoms may thus define an "ischemic penumbra" if one mentally subtracts the abnormal plain CT volume from the abnormally perfused volume of brain. One can compare multiple perfusion parameter maps to refine this assessment. Relative cerebral blood volume appears to correlate with infarct, allowing a mismatch between perfusion time and volume to suggest the ischemic penumbra.

A quick CTA can show the vascular occlusion directly, essential for selection of patients for mechanical thrombectomy. This is of particular importance for treatment if involving a large vessel, given the recent evidence of benefit of large vessel thrombectomies in the DAWN and DEFUSE trials (see image vignette in Fig. 2.25A to F and references at the end of this chapter).

MR techniques can be used similarly. Highly T2*-weighted sequences are used to exclude hemorrhage, DWI defines infarcted tissue, and perfusion scans show areas of diminished blood flow. By subtracting the volume of abnormal diffusion from the volume of abnormal perfusion, the area of "diffusion–perfusion mismatch" representing the penumbra of potentially salvageable brain is defined. MRA defines the vascular lesion directly.

Use these techniques cautiously, validate them in your institution with the stroke team, and remember to keep your protocol as simple as possible. Keep in mind that the exclusion of hemorrhage in this population is critical, careful MRI protocol design and interpretation are essential if MRI is the primary stroke imaging modality.

Seizure patients present interesting problems for the radiologist. If it is the patient's first seizure, an intracranial tumor, infection, or other acute process must be excluded. For this reason, contrast-enhanced MR or contrast-enhanced CT is the preferred approach. If the patient is in the immediate postictal state, or if a residual neurologic deficit is present at the time of imaging, a noncontrast CT scan should be obtained as the first study.

If the seizure disorder is chronic, and particularly if it is refractory to medical therapy, then a detailed MR examination, including high-resolution coronal images of the medial temporal lobes and other clinically suspected abnormal brain structures, is performed. It is preferable to perform this study with the knowledge of clinical seizure semiology and results of EEG testing for the most accurate interpretation.

Infection and Cancer. For patients in whom infectious disease or cancer is a consideration, contrast-enhanced MR is the preferred study. Parenchymal tumor or metastatic disease will be demonstrated with this study, and contrast-enhanced MR has the advantage of depicting meningeal diseases much better than any other imaging modality. In some centers and under certain clinical conditions, contrast-enhanced CT is performed rather than MR. It is difficult to quantify the clinical impact of this choice of imaging strategy. It can be justified on grounds of economic cost and considerable clinical experience. Occasionally, a noncontrast CT will demonstrate punctate calcifications that are overlooked on contrast-enhanced CT or MRI.

Headache is a frequent indication for imaging of the brain. Patients with severe, acute headaches should be imaged with noncontrast head CT. Severe acute headaches may be the result of subarachnoid hemorrhage, acute hydrocephalus, or an enlarging intracranial mass. The chronic headache patient is generally evaluated by MR scanning. If the headache is not accompanied by local neurologic symptoms, a noncontrast MR scan is usually sufficient. However, if the headache is associated with focal neurologic complaints, then gadolinium-enhanced MR scanning is indicated. When chronic headache is the sole presenting complaint, the yield of imaging is low and guidelines suggest that imaging may be superfluous.

Coma. It is crucial to distinguish between a patient with an acute confusional state or coma and a patient who is chronically demented. The comatose or acutely confused patient should be imaged to detect an intracranial hemorrhage. These patients are studied urgently with noncontrast CT. However, the majority of patients who present in this manner will not have an acute structural lesion of the brain. Many will be comatose owing to metabolic abnormalities of the brain. An acute infarct may be present, but this may be invisible on CT, particularly in the brainstem.

Dementia. The chronic dementia patient is generally studied by noncontrast MR as a screening examination for large frontal masses, hydrocephalus, and other treatable abnormalities that may cause a clinical picture that is indistinguishable from AD. MR may also demonstrate small-vessel ischemic changes in the cerebral white matter and small infarcts, which also may clinically mimic AD. If these findings are not present, and the clinical picture is correct, the clinician may offer a diagnosis of AD. PET studies may play a role in assessing prognosis and guiding therapy, especially in the clinical setting of mild cognitive impairment.

ANALYSIS OF THE ABNORMALITY

When an abnormality is detected, the goal of the radiologist is to categorize the finding and, if possible, make a specific diagnosis. Given the large number and relatively infrequent specific findings of neurologic diseases, it is essential to adopt a systematic analytic method to narrow the range of differential diagnostic possibilities. Armed with an amalgam of basic clinical, anatomic, and pathologic knowledge, we can create such a system.

The central question in lesion analysis is the presence of mass or atrophy. Once the brain has completed its development, any injury resulting in tissue loss is permanent. While functional recovery can occur, tissue loss is virtually never restored. Whenever focal or diffuse tissue loss is identified, a strong inference is drawn that the lesion is permanent and untreatable. On the other hand, if the brain is expanded, with normal structures displaced away from the lesion, the lesion is probably active and potentially treatable. Therefore, the urgency for specific diagnosis is greater.

Mass. The concept of mass effect is an essential starting point. A mass is recognized by displacement of normal structures away from the abnormality. The term *mass* is used in a sense that differs somewhat from our understanding of mass in physics, where the central feature of mass is its gravitational affect. The term *mass* in neuroradiology is employed in the sense of an object occupying space. Since two solid objects cannot coexist in the same space, the mass displaces normal cerebral structures away from it. The normal midline structures may be shifted contralateral to the mass. The sulci adjacent to the mass may be effaced, since the CSF in the sulci is displaced by the mass. Similarly, ipsilateral ventricular structures may be compressed by a mass, rendering the ipsilateral ventricle smaller than the contralateral ventricle. These specific points might be summarized by the question: is there too much tissue within the skull?

Atrophy or Volume Loss. Conversely, an atrophic lesion is recognized by widening of the ipsilateral sulci or enlargement of the ventricle adjacent to the lesion. We may ask the question: is there too little brain? It is important to note that we have not listed shift of the midline toward the side of the lesion as a sign of atrophy. Shift ipsilateral to an atrophic lesion is very unusual and is only seen commonly in congenital hemiatrophy. Even if a complete hemispherectomy is performed, shift of the midline toward the side of the hemispherectomy defect is almost always a sign of mass in the remaining cerebral hemisphere or an extra-axial mass compressing it.

When a pattern of diffuse cerebral atrophy is encountered, the first question we must ask is: what is the patient's age? If the patient is over 65 and has normal cognitive function, a diagnosis of age-appropriate cerebral atrophy can be made. Experience teaches us the range of normal to be expected for each age group. If the patient is demented, a diagnosis of AD may be made on clinical grounds. It has been recently suggested that specific neuroradiologic features of AD exist, such as focal atrophy of the hippocampal regions of the medial temporal lobe, but this has yet to be confirmed prospectively with sufficient reliability. PET scanning may sometimes be useful in this setting. If the patient is below 65 years of age, a large number of relatively rare conditions (discussed in Chapter 7) must be considered.

Reversible Atrophy. It is most important for the radiologist to consider the three common causes of reversible cerebral atrophy. They are related to dehydration and starvation. Patients with Addison disease, high-dose steroid therapy or other causes of dehydration or abnormal fluid balance may occasionally present with a CT picture of atrophy. With treatment, a more normal appearance of the brain can be restored. Nutritional causes of reversible cerebral atrophy exist in anorexia nervosa and bulimia. The relative contribution of dehydration and starvation in these conditions is difficult to determine. Alcoholism may also occasionally result in reversible "cerebral atrophy." Although the neurotoxic effects of alcohol are not reversible, it has been hypothesized that the accompanying nutritional deficiencies may be corrected, restoring a more normal appearance to the brain on imaging studies.

Mass Lesion: Intra-Axial or Extra-Axial. Should a mass be identified, the first question we must ask is: Is the mass *intra-axial,* within the brain and expanding it, or *extra-axial,* outside the brain and compressing it? This distinction is usually obvious, but in some cases it is very difficult. Intra-axial masses are more dangerous to the patient and less easily treated than extra-axial masses. Therefore, we prefer to orient our approach to detect extra-axial masses reliably. Intra-axial masses are, most commonly, metastases, intracranial hemorrhages, primary intracranial tumors such as glioblastoma, and brain abscesses. Extra-axial masses are, most commonly, subdural or epidural hematomas, meningiomas, metastases, neuromas, and dermoid or epidermoid cysts.

To distinguish an intra-axial from an extra-axial mass, concentrate on the margins of the mass. Just as the beach is more interesting than the open sea, the interface between the mass and the surrounding brain is more interesting than the center of the mass. Extra-axial masses generally possess a broad dural surface. In contrast, intra-axial masses are surrounded completely by brain. In the posterior fossa, the most reliable sign of an extra-axial mass is widening of the ipsilateral subarachnoid space. The cerebellum and brainstem are displaced away from the bony margins of the calvarium by the mass. In contrast, intra-axial masses demonstrate a narrow ipsilateral subarachnoid space. In the supratentorial compartment, we evaluate a mass somewhat differently. With an intra-axial mass, the gyri are expanded and the CSF spaces are compressed. The CSF spaces adjacent to an extra-axial mass, on the other hand, become larger as we approach the mass.

With the multiplanar capability of MR we are frequently able to visualize direct displacement of the brain away from the dura by an extra-axial mass. When gadolinium is administered, extra-axial masses frequently show dural enhancement, whereas this is less common with intra-axial masses. Extra-axial masses tend to enhance homogeneously, for example, meningioma or neuroma, or not at all, for example, extracerebral hematomas and cysts. Intra-axial lesions tend to enhance in a ring-like or irregular fashion. In general, intra-axial masses have more surrounding edema than extra-axial masses of the same size.

Solitary or Multiple. Once a mass is identified and its location within or outside the brain is established, the next question we ask is: is this a solitary lesion, or are there multiple lesions? The implication is that a single lesion is more likely to be the result of isolated primary cerebral disease and that multiple lesions are more likely to be manifestations of widespread or systemic diseases. A single ring-enhancing lesion within the brain may suggest a glioblastoma. Multiple ring-enhancing lesions within the brain more likely represent metastases or abscesses. If a single infarct is identified, it is likely to be caused by a lesion within the carotid circulation ipsilateral to the lesion. If multiple infarcts are seen, they may represent border-zone infarcts resulting from global hypoperfusion or they may be a result of a cardiac source of emboli.

Gray Matter or White Matter. If a lesion within the brain is primarily manifest by lucency on CT or increased signal on the T2-weighted MR, the most important question is whether the lesion involves gray matter, white matter, or both. Diseases primarily involving white matter without mass effect are attributable to a wide array of causes (see Chapter 7). Lesions involving gray matter are usually a result of infarct, trauma, or encephalitis. If the lesion has mass effect, these conditions are likely acute. If the lesion is atrophic, it is likely chronic.

If the white matter is exclusively involved and the lesion is expansile, a pattern of edema is most likely present. Usually this will represent vasogenic edema caused by an intracerebral mass. The frond-like pattern of white matter extension and mass effect is typical. This form of edema results from disturbances in tight capillary junctions that occur in association with cerebral tumors, abscesses, or hematomas. This type of edema tends to progress relatively slowly and persist over time. If there is relatively more edema compared to the size of the lesion, a tumor or abscess is considered to be more likely than a hematoma.

If there is white matter expansion and increased T2 signal on MR or lucency on CT with gray matter involvement, cytotoxic edema is present. Cytotoxic edema results from increased tissue water content following the neuropathologic response to cell death. In these cases, infarct, trauma, or encephalitis should be considered. This is called the *gray matter pattern.*

Lesion Distribution. When a gray matter pattern is identified, the distribution of the gray matter abnormality allows us to distinguish among infarct, trauma, and encephalitis. Infarcts are distributed according to vascular patterns described in Chapter 4. For example, if a wedge-shaped lesion involves the opercula of the sylvian fissure and the underlying white matter and basal ganglia, a diagnosis of MCA territory infarct is made. Similarly, if the medial aspect of the cerebral hemisphere anteriorly and over the convexity is involved, an anterior cerebral infarct is diagnosed. If the area of involvement falls between two major vascular territories, a border-zone or "watershed" infarct is likely. With multiple border-zone infarcts, global hypoperfusion because of cardiac arrest must be suspected. If the deep gray matter structures bilaterally are involved, pure anoxia owing to carbon monoxide poisoning or respiratory arrest should be considered. These pure patterns are somewhat idealized, because hypoxemia and ischemia are frequently associated.

Traumatic lesions are also distributed in a characteristic fashion (see Chapter 3). Because of the transmission of forces through the brain and the relationship of the brain to the surrounding skull, traumatic lesions tend to occur at the orbital frontal and frontal polar regions, the temporal poles, and the occipital poles in acceleration/deceleration injuries. A direct blow produces injury beneath the site of blow and opposite the site. The lesion opposite the blow is called the *contrecoup injury*. Penetrating brain wounds are distributed according to the path of the missile or the location of the trauma.

Herpes simplex encephalitis is also distributed in a characteristic fashion. This disease spreads from the oral and nasal mucosa to the trigeminal and olfactory ganglion cells and then transdurally to the brain. The most common locations for involvement are the medial temporal lobes adjacent to the trigeminal ganglia and the orbital frontal regions adjacent to the olfactory bulbs. Other forms of encephalitis are less common and are diagnosed by typical clinical presentation, characteristic CSF findings, cultures, and mixed gray and white matter pattern of involvement at other sites.

Contrast Enhancement. The next question we ask about a cerebral abnormality is whether or not it is associated with abnormal contrast enhancement. Enhancement of the brain parenchyma means that the blood–brain barrier has broken down and that the process is biologically active. In the astrocytoma tumor line, an increase in enhancement correlates with higher tumor grade. However, enhancement does not imply malignancy. Infarcts, hemorrhages, abscesses, and encephalitis all can demonstrate contrast enhancement. However, in these nonneoplastic processes, enhancement appears only in the acute phase and resolves with time.

Signal Intensity or Attenuation Pattern. You will note that we have saved patterns of signal intensity for last. These patterns are specific to the imaging modality or MR pulse sequence employed and are therefore the least generally applicable and to a great extent, the least reliable radiologic findings. Knowledge of the physical basis for imaging with CT and MR is necessary to understand the pattern of signal intensities within the brain. However, as a starting point, one need only know that if an abnormality is white on CT or white on T1 MR or black on T2 MR, hemorrhage must be considered. Also, if the brain is as bright as a light bulb on diffusion-weighted MR images, infarct is suggested. This topic is discussed extensively elsewhere.

Suggested Readings

Albers GW, Marks MP, Kemp S, et al. Thrombectomy for stroke at 6 to 16 hours with selection by perfusion imaging. *N Engl J Med* 2018;378(8):708–718.

Atlas S, ed. *Magnetic Resonance Imaging of the Brain and Spine*. Philadelphia, PA: Lippincott Williams & Wilkins, 2002.

Brodal P. *The Central Nervous System: Structure and Function*. 1st ed. New York: Oxford University Press; 1992.

Burger PC. *Surgical Pathology of the Nervous System and Its Coverings*. New York: Churchill-Livingstone; 2002.

Davis RL, Robertson DM. *Textbook of Neuropathology*. 3rd ed. Baltimore, MD: Williams & Wilkins; 1997.

DeGroot J. *Correlative Neuroanatomy*. 21st ed. Norwalk, CT: Appleton & Lange; 1991.

Escourolle R, Poirier J, Gray F. *Manual of Basic Neuropathology*. 4th ed. London: Butterworth-Heinemann; 2003.

Fox PT, Raichle ME. Focal physiological uncoupling of cerebral blood flow and oxidative metabolism during somatosensory stimulation in human subjects. *Proc Natl Acad Sci USA* 1986;83(4):1140–1144.

Grossman RI, Yousem DM. *Neuroradiology: The Requisites*. St. Louis, MO: Mosby; 2003.

Nogueira RG, Jadhav AP, Haussen DC, et al. Thrombectomy 6 to 24 hours after stroke with a mismatch between deficit and infarct. *N Engl J Med* 2018;378(1):11–21.

Osborn A. *Diagnostic Imaging: Brain*. Salt Lake City, UT: AMIRSYS; 2004.

Plum F, Posner JB. *The Diagnosis of Stupor and Coma*. 3rd ed. Philadelphia, PA: FA Davis; 1980.

Shams S, Martola J, Cavallin L, et al. SWI or T2*: Which MRI sequence to use in the detection of cerebral microbleeds? The Karolinska Imaging Dementia Study. *AJNR Am J Neuroradiol* 2015;36(6):1089–1095.

Sox HC, Blatt MA, Higgins MC, Marton KI. *Medical Decision Making*. Boston, MA: Butterworths; 1988.

Von Kummer R, Bozzao L, Manalfe C. *Early CT Diagnosis of Hemispheric Brain Infarction*. Berlin: Springer; 1995.

CHAPTER 3 ■ CRANIOFACIAL TRAUMA

ALISA D. GEAN, TUONG H. LE, AND CHRISTOPHER A. MUTCH

HEAD TRAUMA

Imaging Strategy

CT and MRI constitute the bulk of traumatic craniofacial imaging studies. These modalities each play different roles and have relative advantages and disadvantages. **Noncontrast multidetector CT** (MDCT) is typically the initial imaging modality of choice[1–3] as it is widely available, fast, and very sensitive for detecting abnormalities that would require emergent neurosurgical attention, namely acute intracranial hemorrhage, herniation, and hydrocephalus. MDCT also excels in the detection of skull fractures and radiopaque foreign bodies (e.g., bullet fragments). Intravenous contrast medium is not used in the initial evaluation because it may mimic or mask underlying hemorrhage. CT images must be reviewed using multiple windows. A narrow window width is used to evaluate the brain, a slightly wider window width is used to exaggerate contrast between extra-axial collections and the adjacent skull, and a very wide window is used to evaluate the skull itself.

MRI has traditionally been less desirable than CT in the acute setting because of the longer examination times, difficulty in managing life-support and other monitoring equipment, and inferior demonstration of bone detail. MR also requires additional safety screening for metallic foreign bodies (especially the setting of penetrating trauma) and incompatible medical devices. MRI, however, has been shown to be comparable or superior to CT in the detection of acute epidural and subdural hematomas and nonhemorrhagic brain injury.[4,5] MR is also more sensitive to brainstem injury and to subacute and chronic hemorrhage, especially with fluid-attenuated inversion recovery (FLAIR), gradient-recalled echo (GRE) T2*-weighted, and susceptibility-weighted imaging (SWI).[6–8] SWI is particularly sensitive to blood products and can often identify small areas of hemorrhage undetectable on GRE sequences or even CT.[9] Diffusion-weighted and diffusion tensor imaging have improved detection of both acute and chronic neuronal injury.[10–13] In the majority of cases, MR is the modality of choice for patients with subacute and chronic head injury and is recommended for patients with acute head trauma when neurologic findings are unexplained by CT. MR is also more accurate in predicting long-term prognosis. With the continued development in faster imaging sequences and greater scanner availability, the role of MR in the evaluation of acute head trauma will continue to increase.

Cases in which there are known or suspected vascular injuries may require specialized vascular imaging. Noninvasive techniques include **CT and MR angiography** and some cases may require catheter cerebral angiography for diagnosis and treatment.

In the past, **skull radiographs** were often obtained in the initial evaluation of trauma, particularly in children; though, this has fallen out of favor as there can be significant intracranial injury without a detectable abnormality on skull films. Patients who are judged to be at low risk for intracranial injury on the basis of a careful history and physical examination should be observed, and patients at high risk should be imaged by CT. The decision to obtain imaging in the setting of trauma is typically made using clinical guidelines such as the Canadian CT Head Rules, New Orleans Criteria or National Emergency X-Ray Utilization Study II (NEXUS II).[14–16]

Scalp Injury

When interpreting CT scans for head trauma, it is helpful to begin by examining the extracranial structures for evidence of scalp injury or radiopaque foreign bodies. Scalp soft tissue swelling is often the only reliable evidence of the site of impact. The subgaleal hematoma is the most common manifestation of scalp injury and can be recognized on CT or MR

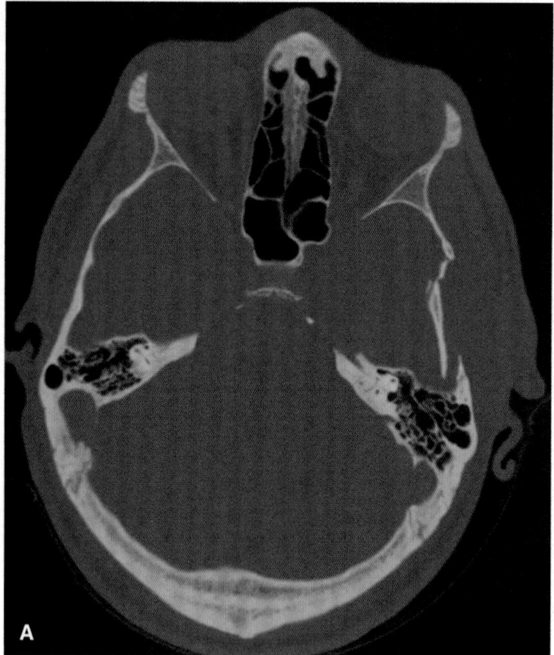

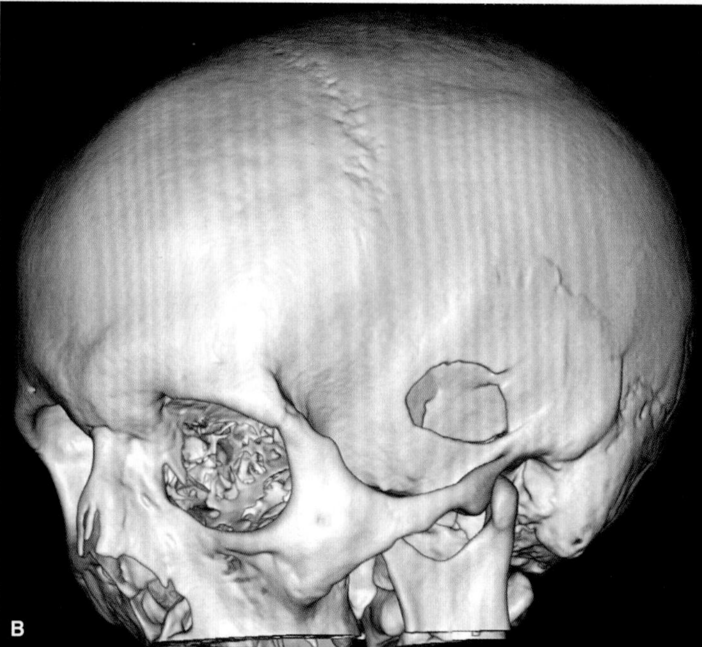

FIGURE 3.1. **Depressed Skull Fracture.** Axial bone window CT image (**A**) and 3D reconstruction (**B**) of the same CT demonstrate a comminuted depressed fracture of the left temporal bone.

as focal soft tissue swelling of the scalp located beneath the subcutaneous fibrofatty tissue and above the temporalis muscle and calvarium.

Skull Fractures

Nondisplaced linear fractures of the calvarium are the most common type of skull fracture. They may be difficult to detect on CT scans, especially when the fracture plane is parallel to the plane of section. Fortunately, isolated linear skull fractures do not require treatment. Surgical management is usually indicated for depressed and compound skull fractures, both of which are seen better on CT scans than on plain films (Fig. 3.1). Depressed fractures are frequently associated with an underlying contusion. Intracranial air ("pneumocephalus") may be seen with compound skull fractures or fractures involving the paranasal sinuses. Thin-section CT using a bone algorithm and multiplanar reformats is the best method to evaluate fractures in critical areas, such as the skull base, orbit, or facial bones. Thin sections can also be helpful to evaluate the degree of comminution and depression of bone fragments.

Temporal Bone Fractures

Thin-section, high-resolution CT scanning has led to a dramatic improvement in the ability to detect and characterize temporal bone fractures. Patients with fractures of the temporal bone may present with deafness, facial nerve palsies, vertigo, dizziness, or nystagmus. Clinical symptoms are often masked in the presence of other serious injuries. Physical signs of temporal bone fracture include hemotympanum, CSF otorrhea, and ecchymosis over the mastoid process ("Battle sign"). Temporal bone fractures may be first suspected on standard head CT scans performed to exclude intracranial injury. Findings such as opacification of the mastoid air cells, fluid in the middle ear cavity, pneumocephalus, or occasionally, pneumolabyrinth (Fig. 3.2) should raise the suspicion of a temporal bone fracture. Optimal evaluation of a suspected temporal bone fracture requires thin-section MDCT (typically submillimeter) with axial and coronal reformats using a bone algorithm.

Fractures of the temporal bone can be classified either according to their orientation relative to the long axis of the petrous bone[17] or according to their involvement of the otic capsule.[18,19] On the basis of the older Ulrich classification, if the fracture parallels the long axis of the petrous pyramid, it is termed a "longitudinal" fracture; fractures perpendicular to the long axis of the petrous bone are termed "transverse" fractures. "Mixed" fracture types also occur.

The longitudinal temporal bone fracture (Fig. 3.3) represents 70% to 90% of temporal bone fractures.[20] It results from a blow to the side of the head. Complications include conductive hearing loss, dislocation or fracture of the ossicles (Figs. 3.3 and 3.4), and CSF otorhinorrhea. Facial nerve palsy

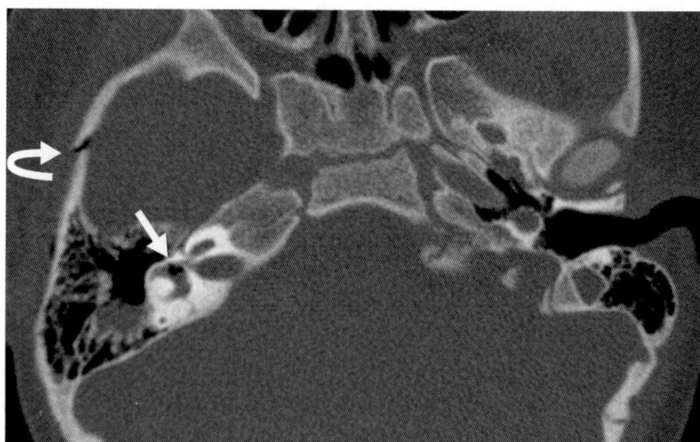

FIGURE 3.2. **Pneumolabyrinth.** Axial bone window CT image at the level of the right otic capsule shows abnormal gas within the right vestibular apparatus compatible with pneumolabyrinth (*straight arrow*). There is also a minimally displaced fracture of the right squamous temporal bone (*curved arrow*).

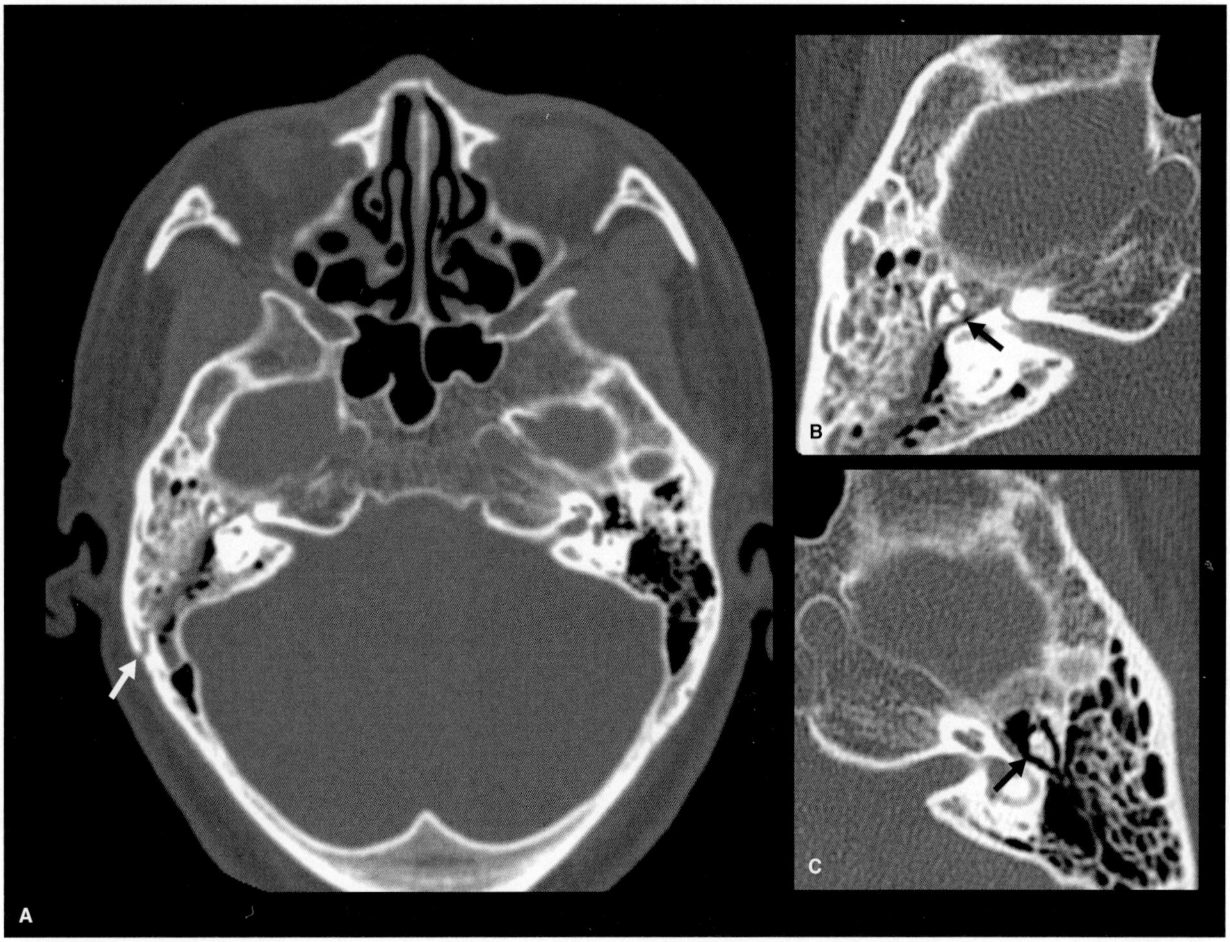

FIGURE 3.3. **Longitudinal Temporal Bone Fracture.** Longitudinal right temporal bone fracture is detected on noncontrast CT (**A**, *white arrow*). There is associated hemorrhage in the right mastoid air cells and middle ear cavity. High-resolution reformats of the temporal bones were then obtained, which demonstrate mild right malleo-incal dislocation (**B**, *black arrow*) when compared to the normal malleo-incal relationship on the left (**C**, *black arrow*). This fracture spares the otic capsule.

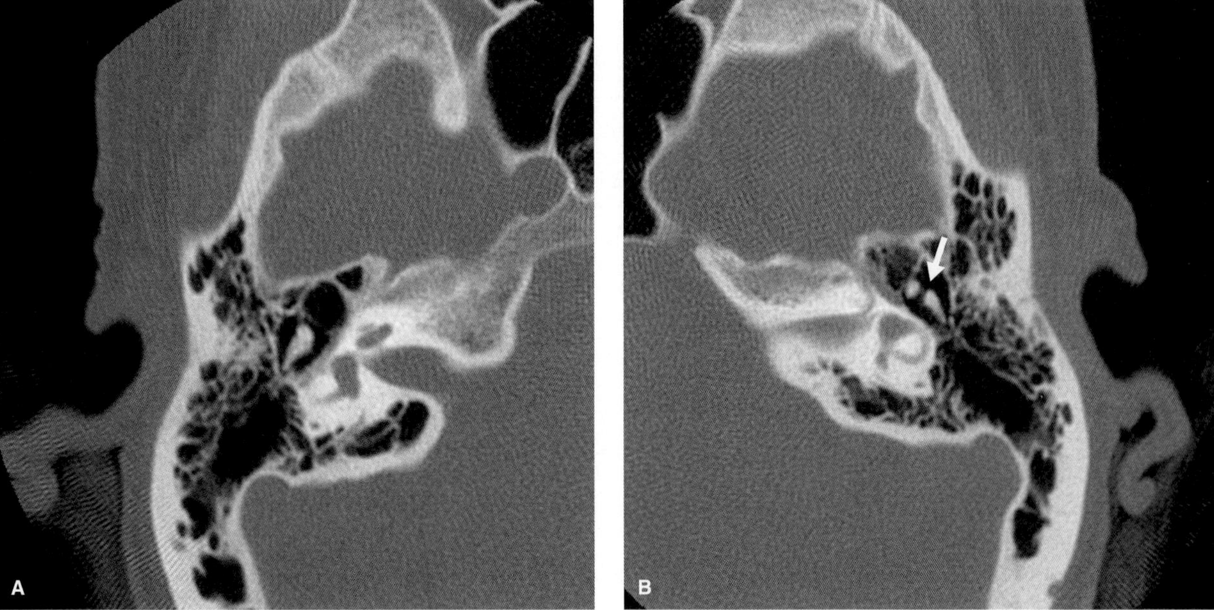

FIGURE 3.4. **Ossicular Dislocation.** Axial high-resolution CT images through the bilateral temporal bones reveal more pronounced left malleo-incal dislocation (*arrow*, **B**). Normal right ossicular alignment is shown on the right for comparison (**A**).

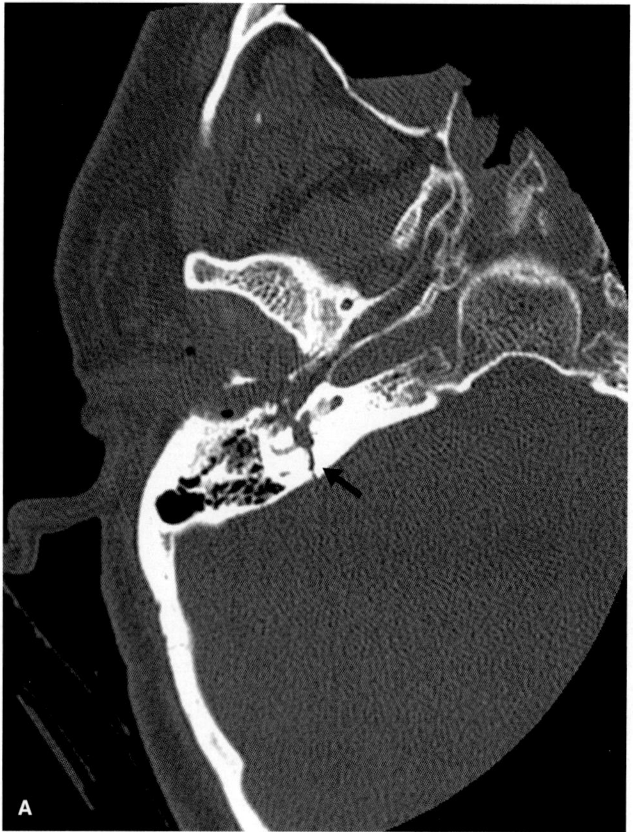

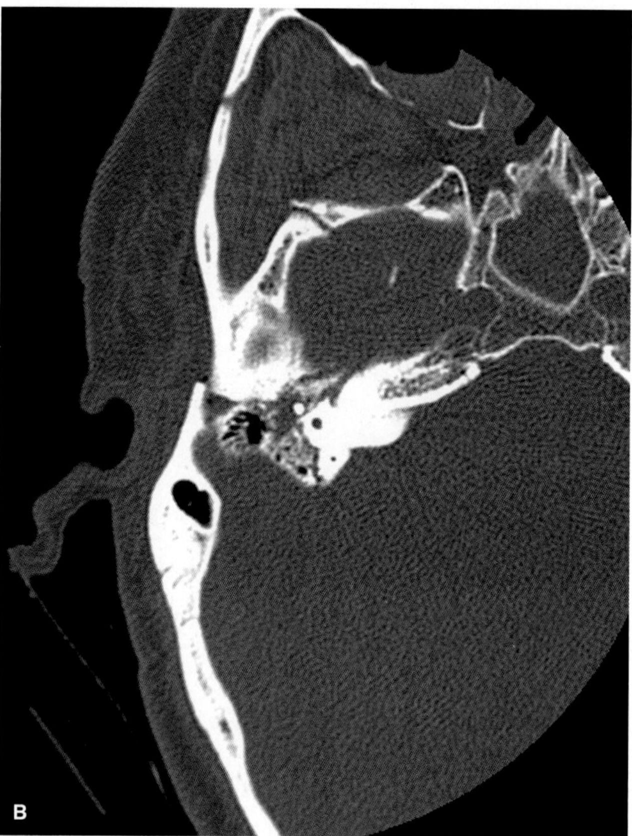

FIGURE 3.5. **Otic Capsule Violating Temporal Bone Fracture.** Axial CT images through the right temporal bone demonstrate a comminuted transverse fracture violating the otic capsules. (**A**) A fracture line (*black arrow*) is noted extending from the vestibule posteriorly into the posterior fossa intracranial cavity. (**B**) A slightly more superior image on the right reveals extension into the middle cranial fossa as well. There is also fluid in the middle ear cavity and mastoid air cells. The head of the malleolus is visualized but is not associated with the incus.

may occur, but it is often delayed and incomplete. Sensorineural hearing loss is uncommon.

The transverse temporal bone fracture usually results from a blow to the occiput or frontal region. Complications are usually more severe and include sensorineural hearing loss, severe vertigo, nystagmus, and perilymphatic fistula. Facial palsy is seen in 30% to 50% of these cases and is often complete.[20] Transverse fractures may also involve the carotid canal or jugular foramen, causing injury to the carotid artery or jugular vein.

Mixed and oblique fracture types also occur, and the simple classification of fractures as longitudinal or transverse may not be sufficient.[21] *Otic capsule–sparing* fractures run anterolateral to the otic capsule and are usually caused by direct blows to the temporoparietal region. With *otic capsule–violating* fractures, the cochlea and the semicircular canals are damaged (Fig. 3.5). These fractures are the results of direct impacts to the occipital region. Compared with otic-sparing fractures, patients with otic capsule–violating fractures are 2 to 5 times more likely to develop facial nerve injury, 4 to 8 times more likely to develop CSF leak, and 7 to 25 times more likely to experience hearing loss, as well as more likely to sustain intracranial injuries such as epidural hematoma and subarachnoid hemorrhage.[18,19]

Head Injury Classification

Classification of Head Injury. Traumatic head injury can be divided into primary and secondary forms. Primary lesions are those that occur as a direct result of a blow to the head. Secondary lesions occur as a consequence of primary lesions, usually as a result of mass effect or vascular compromise. Secondary lesions are often preventable, whereas primary injuries, by definition, have already occurred by the time the patient arrives in the emergency department.

Primary lesions include epidural, subdural, subarachnoid, and intraventricular hemorrhage, as well as diffuse axonal injury (DAI), cortical contusions, intracerebral hematomas, and subcortical gray matter injury. Direct injury to the cerebral vasculature is another type of primary lesion.

Secondary lesions include cerebral swelling, brain herniation, hydrocephalus, ischemia or infarction, CSF leak, leptomeningeal cyst, and encephalomalacia.

Brainstem injury, which is also divided into primary and secondary forms, is discussed later in this chapter.

Primary Head Injury: Extra-Axial

Epidural hematomas are usually arterial in origin and often result from a skull fracture that disrupts the middle meningeal artery. The developing hematoma strips the dura from the inner table of the skull, forming an ovoid mass that displaces the adjacent brain (Figs. 3.6 and 3.7). They may occur from stretching or tearing of meningeal arteries without an associated fracture, especially in children. Overall, skull fractures are seen in 85% to 95% of cases. In approximately a third of patients with an epidural hematoma, neurologic deterioration occurs after a lucid interval.[22]

Most epidural hematomas are temporal or temporoparietal in location, though frontal and occipital hematomas can

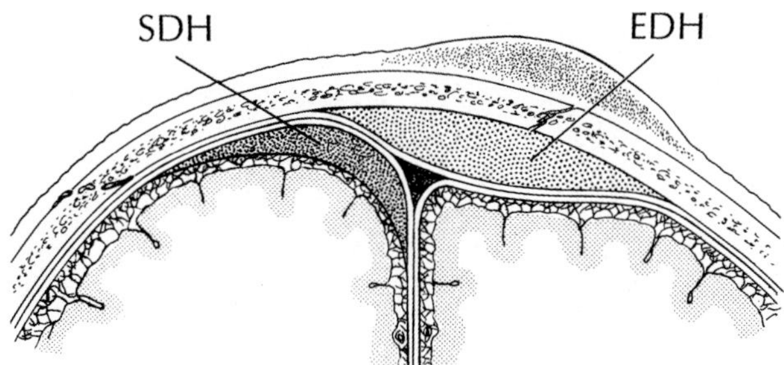

FIGURE 3.6. **Epidural Versus Subdural Hematoma.** Axial diagram of the brain surface in the frontal region demonstrates the characteristic locations of the epidural hematoma (EDH) compared with the subdural hematoma (SDH). Note how the EDH is located above the outer dural layer and the SDH is located beneath the inner dural layer. Only the EDH can cross the falx cerebri. (Reprinted with permission from Gean AD. *Imaging of Head Trauma*. Philadelphia, PA: Lippincott Williams & Wilkins; 1994:76.)

also occur. Venous epidural hematomas are less common than arterial epidural hematomas and tend to occur at the vertex, posterior fossa, or anterior aspect of the middle cranial fossa. Venous epidural hematomas usually occur as a result of disrupted dural venous sinuses (Fig. 3.8).

On CT, acute epidural hematomas appear as well-defined, high attenuation lenticular or biconvex extra-axial collections (Fig. 3.6). Associated mass effect with sulcal effacement and midline shift is frequently seen. Bone windows usually demonstrate an overlying linear skull fracture (Fig. 3.7). Because epidural hematomas exist in the potential space between the dura and inner table of the skull, they usually will not cross cranial sutures, where the periosteal layer of the dura is firmly attached (Fig. 3.6). Near the vertex, the periosteum forms the outer wall of the sagittal sinus and is less tightly adherent to the sagittal suture. Therefore, vertex epidurals, which are usually of venous origin from disruption of the sagittal sinus, can cross midline. Epidural hematomas are external to and thus not bounded by dural reflections including the tentorium (Fig. 3.8). Occasionally, an acute epidural hematoma will appear heterogeneous, containing irregular areas of lower attenuation. This finding may indicate active extravasation of fresh unclotted blood into the collection and warrants immediate surgical attention.

Subdural hematomas are typically venous in origin, resulting from stretching or tearing of cortical veins that traverse the subdural space en route to the dural sinuses (Fig. 3.6). They may also result from disruption of penetrating branches of superficial cerebral arteries. Because the inner dural layer and arachnoid are not as firmly attached as the structures that make up the epidural space, the subdural hematoma typically extends over a much larger area than the epidural hematoma. Patients with a subdural hematoma commonly present after acute deceleration injury from a motor vehicle accident or fall. The same mechanism can cause cortical contusions and DAI, which are frequently seen in association with acute subdural hematomas.

On axial CT, acute subdural hematomas appear as crescent-shaped extra-axial collections of high attenuation (Fig. 3.9). Most subdural hematomas are supratentorial, located along the convexity. They are also frequently seen along the falx and tentorium. Because dural reflections form the falx cerebri and tentorium, subdural collections will not cross these structures (see Fig. 3.6). Unlike epidural hematomas, subdural hematomas can cross sutural margins and, in fact, are frequently seen layering along the entire hemispheric convexity from the anterior falx to the posterior falx. Diffuse swelling of the underlying hemisphere is common with subdural hematomas. Because of this, there may be more mass effect than would be expected by the size of the collection and there may be little or no reduction in midline shift after evacuation of a hemispheric subdural hematoma.

The CT appearance of subdural hematomas changes with time. The density of an acute subdural hematoma initially increases because of clot retraction. By the time most acute subdural hematomas are imaged, the collection is hyperdense, measuring 50 to 60 HU, relative to normal brain, which measures 18 to 30 HU. The density will then progressively decrease as protein degradation occurs within the hematoma. Occasionally, acute subdural blood may be

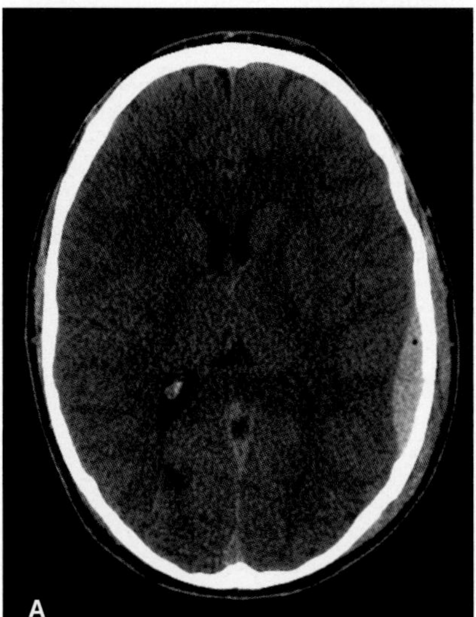

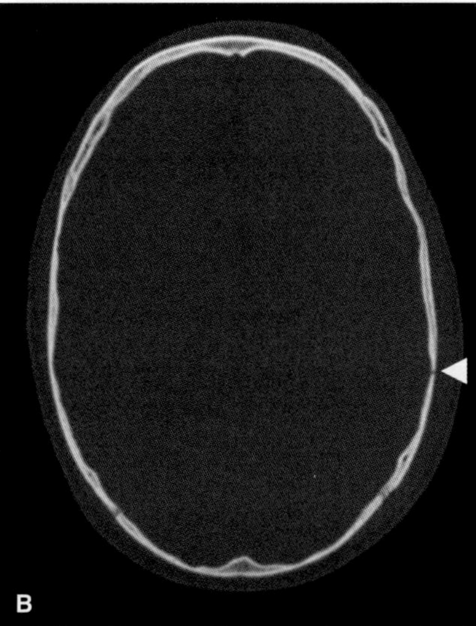

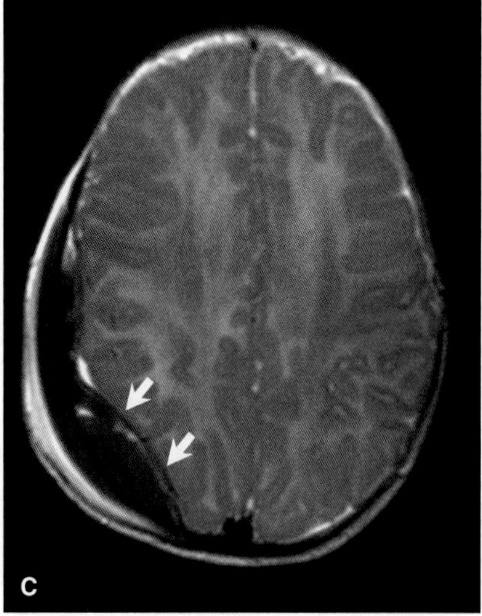

FIGURE 3.7. **Epidural Hematoma.** Noncontrast CT (**A, B**) performed on a young man who was "found down" with altered mental status. Note the classic biconvex hyperdense epidural hematoma with an overlying nondisplaced calvarial fracture (*arrowhead*). There is a small focus of pneumocephalus within the hemorrhage. Axial T2WI (**C**) from a "rapid" MR protocol in a 3-month-old infant who was dropped onto concrete reveals a right parietal biconvex low signal epidural collection. Note the position of the dura (the thin black line deep to the collection denoted by *white arrows*) deep to the hematoma verifying that the collection is located in the epidural space.

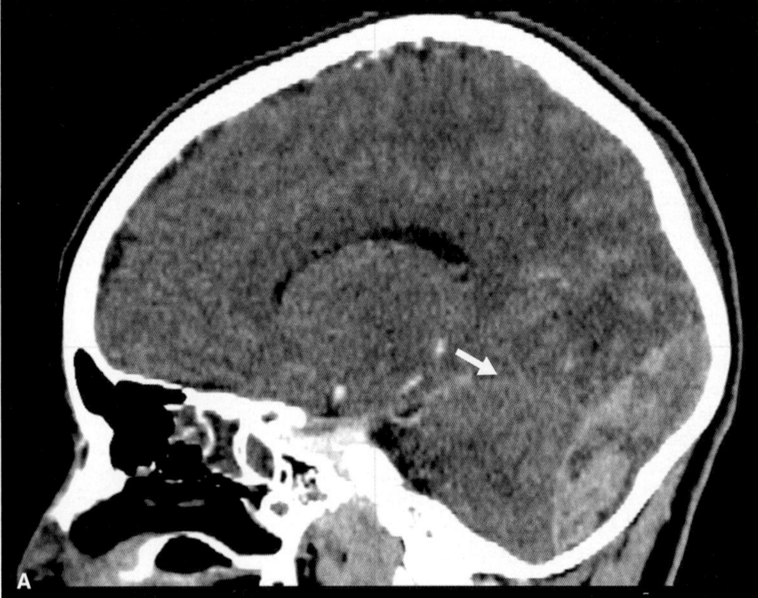

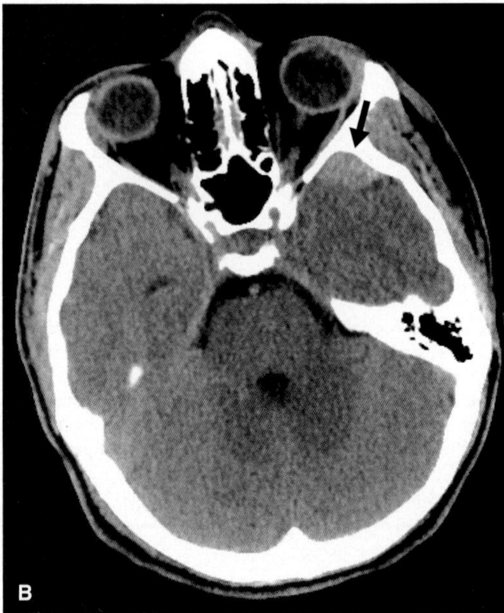

FIGURE 3.8. **Epidural Hematomas.** Sagittal reformatted image from a noncontrast CT of a 13 year old with a posterior fossa heterogeneous density epidural hematoma (**A**). These images demonstrate how the hematoma crosses the plane of the tentorium cerebelli (*arrow*) into the posterior fossa, characteristic of epidural hematomas (unlike subdural hematomas) as they are not constrained by dural boundaries. Noncontrast CT from a different patient (**B**) following assault reveals a high-density right sphenoparietal venous epidural hematoma (*black arrow*) along the anterior margin of the middle cranial fossa. In contrast to arterial epidural hematomas, venous epidural hematomas bleed under lower pressure and are therefore less likely to increase in size.

isodense (Fig. 3.10A) or hypodense in patients with severe anemia or active extravasation ("hyperacute" subdural hematoma). Rebleeding during evolution of a subdural hematoma causes a heterogeneous appearance from the mixture of fresh blood and partially liquefied hematoma. A sediment level or "hematocrit effect" may be seen either from rebleeding or in patients with clotting disorders (Fig. 3.11). Chronic subdural hematomas have low attenuation values similar to CSF. On noncontrast CT scans, it can be difficult to distinguish them from prominent subarachnoid space secondary to cerebral atrophy. Contrast enhancement can help by demonstrating an enhancing capsule or displaced cortical veins (Fig. 3.10B).

During the transition from acute to chronic subdural hematomas, an isodense phase occurs, usually between several days and 3 weeks after the acute event. Although the subdural hematoma itself is less conspicuous during this isodense phase, there are indirect signs on a noncontrast CT scan that should lead to the correct diagnosis. These include effacement of sulci, effacement or distortion of the white matter ("*white matter buckling*"), abnormal separation of the gray–white matter junction from

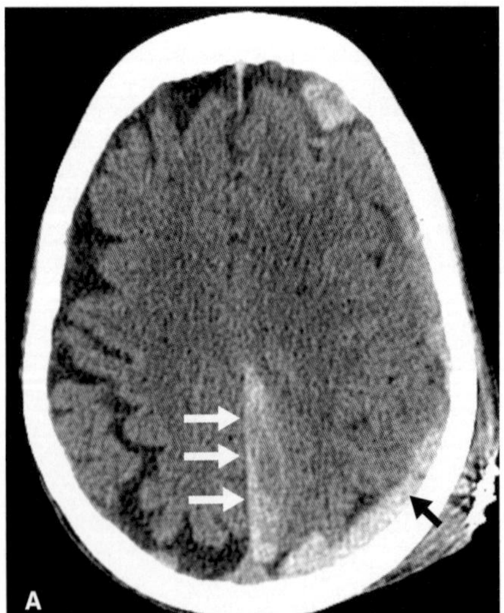

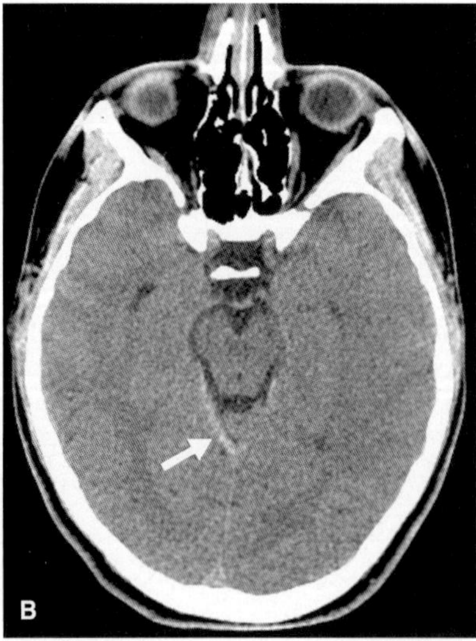

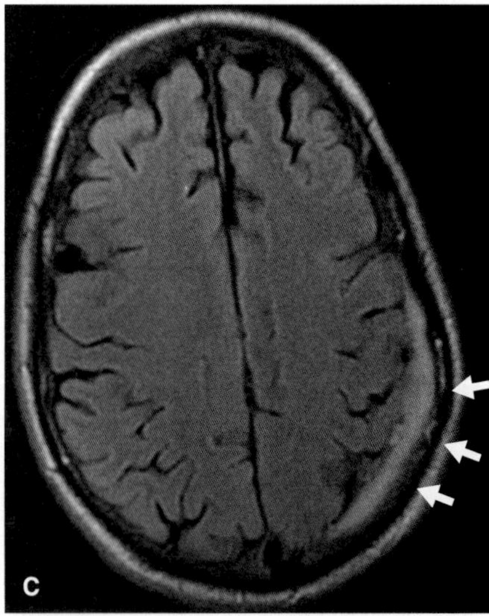

FIGURE 3.9. **Acute Subdural Hematoma.** Noncontrast CT (**A**) obtained after a fall in an elderly woman with a left parietal scalp laceration shows acute hemorrhage along the left convexity (*black arrow*) and left falx cerebri (*white arrows*). Note that subdural hematoma does not cross the dural sinus to extend to the other side of the falx. Noncontrast CT (**B**) from a younger patient following a motor vehicle accident reveals a subtle subdural hematoma along the right tentorium cerebelli (*white arrow*), a common location. Axial T2/FLAIR MR image (**C**) from a different man after head injury illustrates the excellent contrast difference on MR between the FLAIR hyperintense subdural hematoma (*white arrows*) and the adjacent hypointense calvarium.

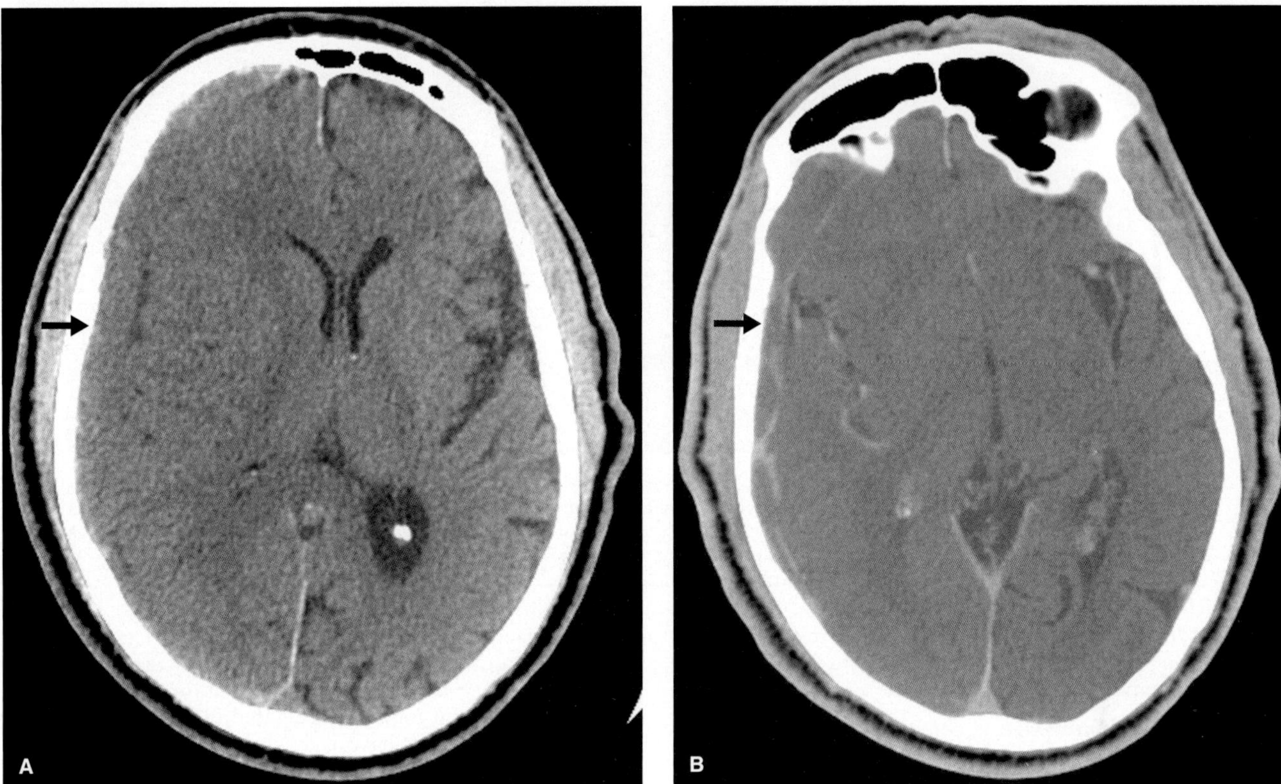

FIGURE 3.10. **Subacute Subdural Hematoma.** Noncontrast CT (**A**) performed on an 82-year-old man following a fall reveals a right convexity subdural hematoma (*arrow*), isodense to the adjacent cortex compatible with subacute age. Postcontrast imaging is generally not required for evaluation of a subdural hematoma; however, it was obtained in this case. The postcontrast CT (**B**) demonstrates peripheral enhancement of the collection (*arrow*) without evidence of active extravasation, again compatible with subacute injury.

the inner table of the skull ("*thick gray matter mantle*"), distortion of the ventricles, and midline shift (Fig. 3.10).

The MR appearance of subdural hematomas depends on the biochemical state of hemoglobin, which varies with the age of the hematoma. Acute subdural hematomas are isointense to brain on T1WI and hypointense on T2WI. MR is particularly helpful during the subacute phase, when the subdural hematoma may be isodense or hypodense on CT scans. T1WI will demonstrate high signal intensity caused by the presence of methemoglobin in the subdural collection. This high signal clearly distinguishes subdural hematomas from most nonhemorrhagic fluid collections. The T2 signal increases and the T1 signal gradually decreases as the hemorrhage ages in chronic subdural hematomas (Fig. 3.11). MR also reveals that subacute subdural hematomas frequently have a lentiform or biconvex appearance when seen in the coronal plane, rather than the crescent-shaped appearance that is characteristic on axial CT scans. The multiplanar capability of MR scanning is

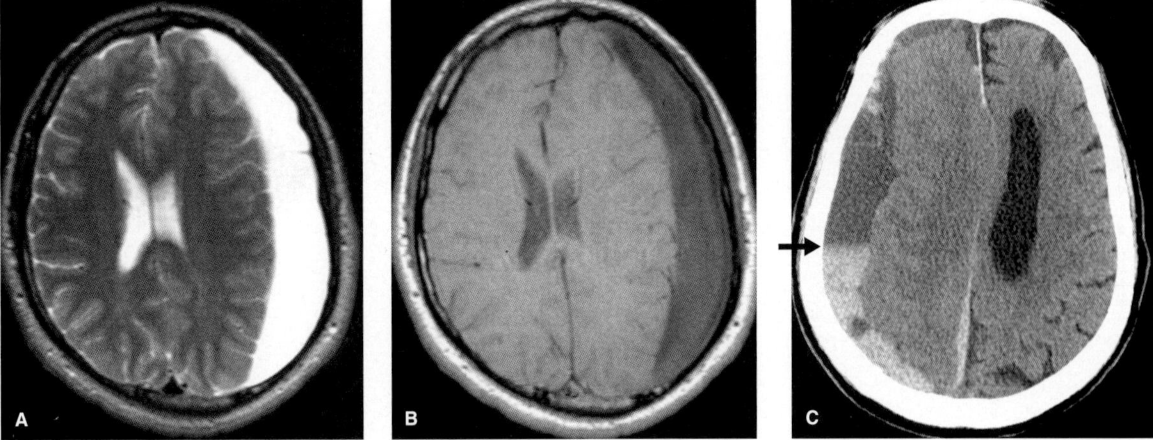

FIGURE 3.11. **Chronic Subdural Hematoma.** Axial MR T2WI (**A**) and T1WI (**B**) from a 22-year-old patient with headaches and a remote history of head trauma reveal a chronic left convexity hematoma. Axial noncontrast CT (**C**) from a different patient, a 73-year-old man with left-sided weakness, shows the appearance of a mixed-density, "acute-on-chronic" subdural hematoma along the right convexity and falx cerebri with subfalcine herniation. Note the dependent layering of the acute, denser blood products within the chronic, hypodense collection; this is often referred to as the "hematocrit sign" (*arrow*).

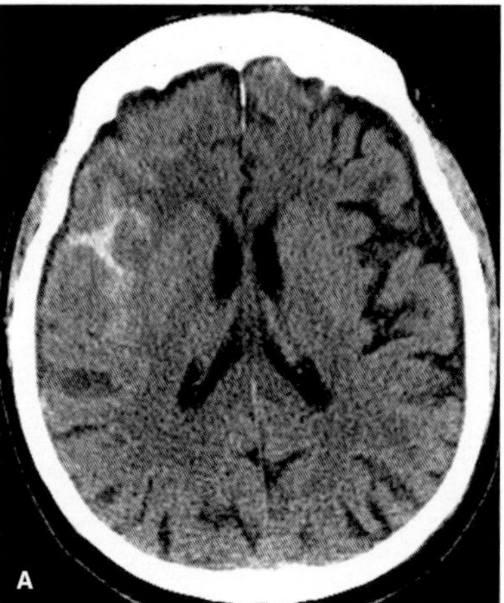

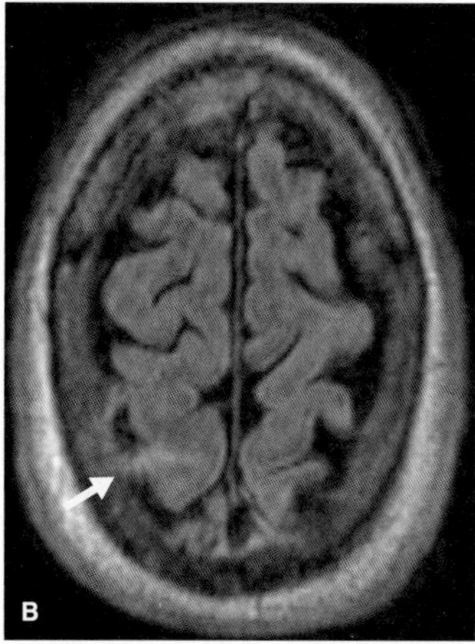

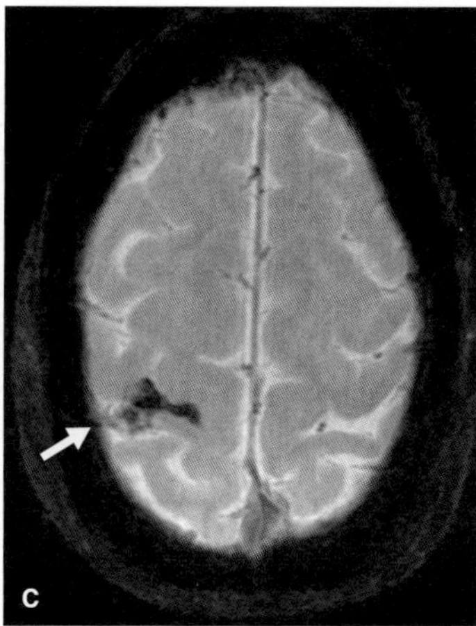

FIGURE 3.12. Subarachnoid Hemorrhage. Noncontrast CT axial image (**A**) shows high attenuation material within the sulci and right sylvian fissure consistent with subarachnoid hemorrhage. MRI performed 3 days following a fall in a different patient demonstrates MR sensitivity for small amounts of subarachnoid hemorrhage (*white arrows*) which does not suppress like normal CSF on FLAIR imaging (**B**) and appears markedly hypointense on SWI (**C**).

helpful in identifying small convexity and vertex hematomas that might not be detected on axial CT scans because of the similar attenuation of the adjacent bone.

Subarachnoid hemorrhage is common in head injury but is rarely large enough to cause a significant mass effect. It results from the disruption of small subarachnoid vessels or direct extension into the subarachnoid space by a contusion or hematoma. On CT, subarachnoid hemorrhage appears as linear areas of high attenuation within the cisterns and sulci (Fig. 3.12). Subarachnoid collections along the convexity or tentorium can be differentiated from subdural hematomas by their extension into adjacent sulci. Occasionally, the only finding is apparent effacement of sulci when the sulci are filled with small amounts of blood. In patients who are found unconscious after an unwitnessed event, detection of subarachnoid hemorrhage may indicate a ruptured aneurysm, rather than trauma, as the primary cause. In such cases, contrast-enhanced CT angiography and/or conventional catheter angiography needs to be considered.

Hyperacute subarachnoid hemorrhage is traditionally more difficult to detect on conventional MR than it is on CT scans because it can be isointense to brain parenchyma on T1-weighted (T1W) and T2-weighted (T2W) images. However, FLAIR and SWI have been shown to be more sensitive than CT in detecting acute subarachnoid blood (Figs. 3.12 and 3.13).[23] Subacute subarachnoid hemorrhage may be better appreciated on MR because of its high signal intensity at a time when the blood is isointense to CSF on CT.[24] Chronic hemorrhage on MR scans may show hemosiderin staining in the subarachnoid space, which appears as areas of markedly decreased signal intensity on T1- and T2W sequences ("superficial hemosiderosis"). Subarachnoid hemorrhage may lead to subsequent hydrocephalus by impaired CSF resorption at the level of arachnoid villi.

Intraventricular hemorrhage is commonly seen in patients with head injuries and can occur by several mechanisms. First, it can result from rotationally induced tearing of subependymal veins on the surface of the ventricles.[25] Another mechanism is

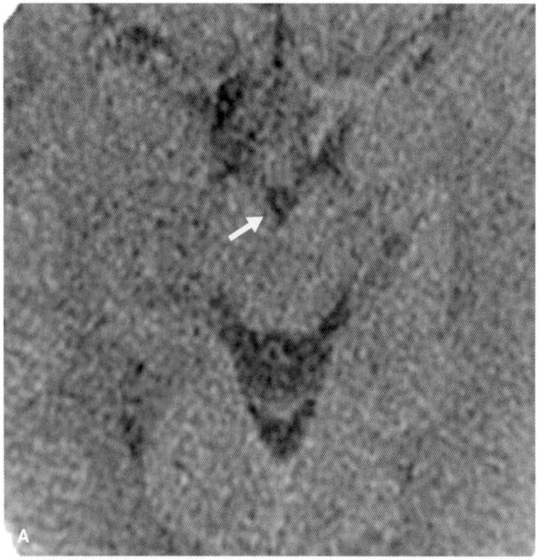

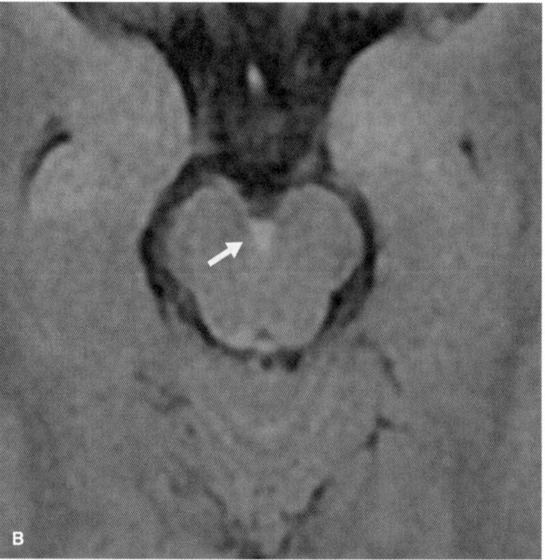

FIGURE 3.13. Noncontrast CT (**A**) and FLAIR MR (**B**) images obtained the same day in a 33-year-old woman following a motor vehicle crash. The trace interpeduncular subarachnoid hemorrhage (*arrow*) is not apparent on CT but is visible on MR, highlighting the greater sensitivity of MR to blood products.

by direct extension of a parenchymal hematoma into the ventricular system.[22] Third, intraventricular blood can result from retrograde flow of subarachnoid hemorrhage into the ventricular system through the fourth ventricular outflow foramina. Patients with intraventricular hemorrhage are at risk for subsequent hydrocephalus by obstruction either at the level of the aqueduct or arachnoid villi.

On CT, intraventricular hemorrhage appears as hyperdense material, layering dependently within the ventricular system (see Fig. 3.18). Tiny collections of increased density layering in the occipital horns may be the only clue to intraventricular hemorrhage.

Primary Head Injury: Intra-Axial

Diffuse axonal injury (DAI) is one of the most common types of primary neuronal injuries in patients with severe head trauma. As the name implies, DAI is characterized by widespread disruption of axons that occurs at the time of an acceleration or deceleration injury. The affected areas of the brain may be distant from the site of direct impact; in fact, direct impact is not necessary to cause this type of injury.

The incidence of DAI was likely underestimated until recently because of the difficulty in visualizing these lesions on existing imaging studies as well as on histologic specimens. DAI is much better seen by MR than CT.[5] This factor accounts to a large degree for the increased success of MR at explaining neurologic deficits after trauma and in predicting long-term outcome. Though MR has improved the detection of DAI in patients suffering head trauma, the incidence of this form of injury is probably still underestimated. Newer imaging methods, such as diffusion-weighted and diffusion tensor imaging with three-dimensional tractography, have shown potential in improving the detection of white matter injury in both acute and chronic DAI.[10–13]

Patients with DAI are most commonly injured in high-speed motor vehicle crashes. These lesions have not been seen as a consequence of simple falls, such as when a patient falls from the standing position. Loss of consciousness typically starts immediately after the injury and is more severe than in patients with cortical contusions or hematomas.

CT findings in DAI can be subtle or absent. Most common is the finding of small, petechial hemorrhages at the gray–white junction of the cerebral hemispheres or corpus callosum (Fig. 3.14A). Ill-defined areas of decreased attenuation on CT may occasionally be seen with nonhemorrhagic lesions.

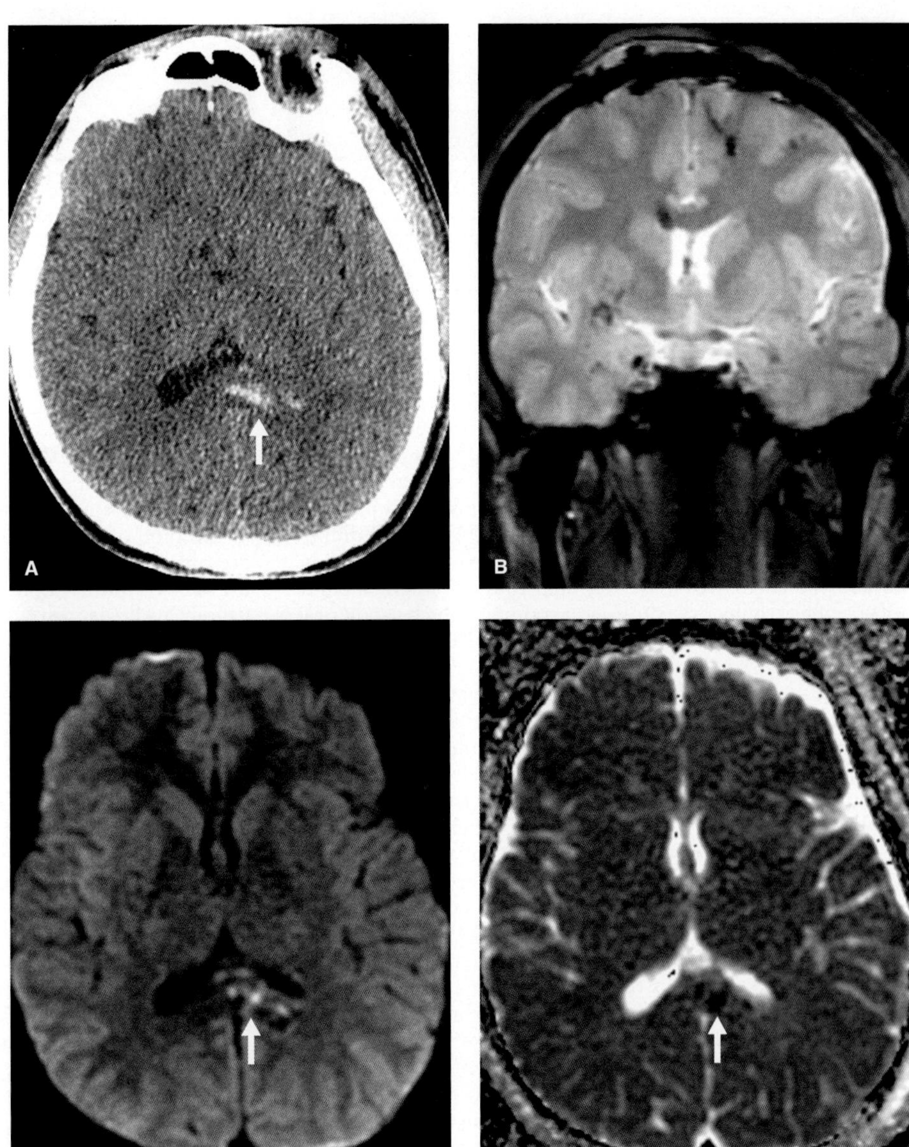

FIGURE 3.14. Acute Diffuse Axonal Injury. CT and MR images from a patient who presented with altered mental status following an assault. Noncontrast CT (**A**) shows multiple areas of hemorrhagic axonal shearing injury involving the splenium of the corpus callosum (*arrow*). This area (*arrows*) shows increased susceptibility on MPGR (**B**) and reduced diffusion (**C**), low ADC value (**D**) on MRI performed the same day. The coronal MPGR image (**B**) also reveals numerous additional white matter shear injuries (low signal) compatible with diffuse axonal injury.

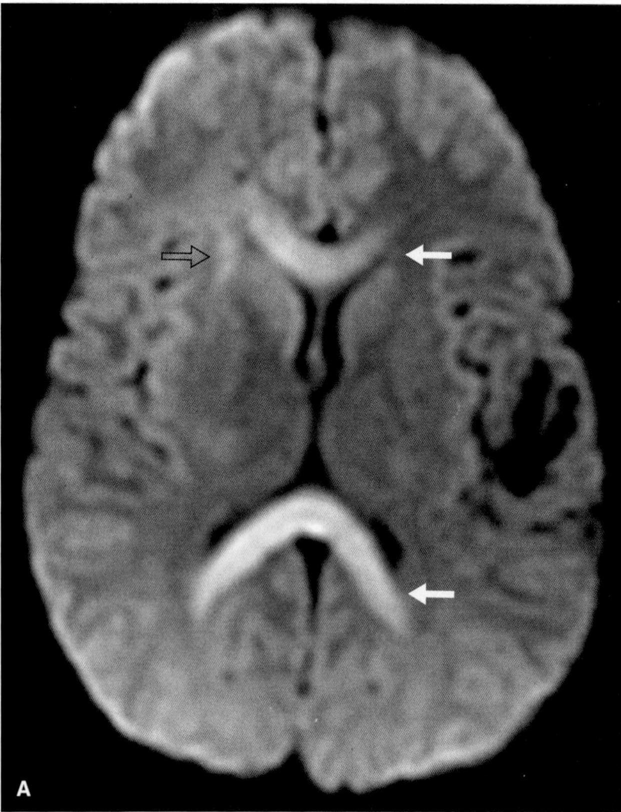

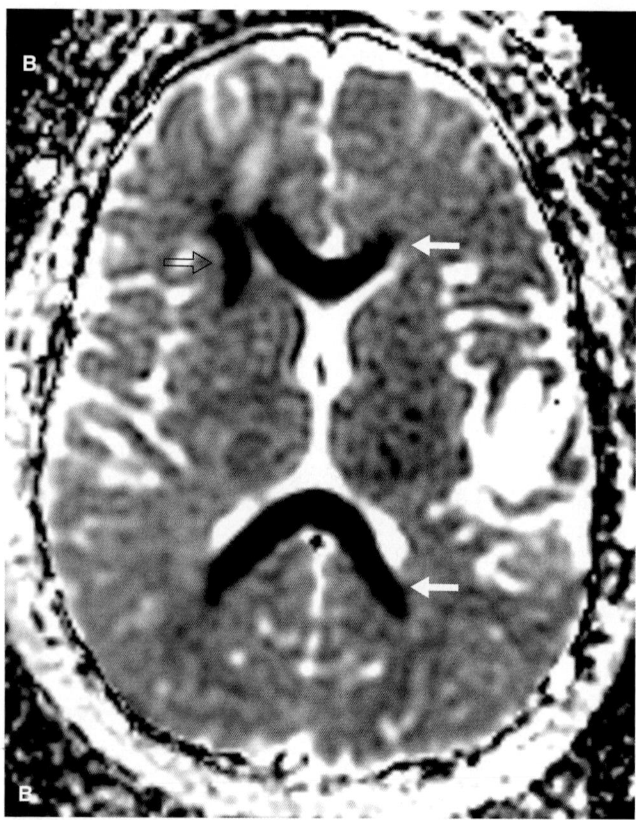

FIGURE 3.15. **Severe Diffuse Axonal Injury.** MR DWI (**A**) and ADC map (**B**) from 23 year old with head trauma after a motorcycle accident show marked reduced diffusion in the genu and splenium (*filled arrows*) of the corpus callosum, also consistent with a combination of Wallerian degeneration and traumatic axonal injury. The entire right frontal lobe white matter shows abnormal signal with a more focal insult to the anterior subinsular region (*open arrows*).

On MR, nonhemorrhagic DAI lesions appear as small foci of T2 prolongation (increased signal) on FLAIR images or low ADC on diffusion-weighted images within the white matter (Figs. 3.14 and 3.15). Hemorrhagic DAI appears as low signal on gradient echo (GRE) or SWI. The lesions tend to be multiple, with as many as 15 to 20 lesions seen in patients with severe head injury. The conspicuity of DAI on MR diminishes over weeks to months as the damaged axons degenerate and the edema resolves. Residual findings might include nonspecific atrophy or hemosiderin staining, which can persist for years and is especially obvious on SWI or GRE images (Fig. 3.16).

DAI is seen in characteristic locations that correlate with the severity of the trauma. Patients with the mildest forms of injury have lesions confined to the frontal and temporal white matter, near the gray–white junction. The lesions typically involve the parasagittal regions of the frontal lobes and periventricular regions of the temporal lobes. Patients with more severe trauma have DAI involving lobar white matter as well as the corpus callosum, especially the posterior body and splenium (Figs. 3.14 and 3.15). The corpus callosum accounts for approximately 20% of all DAI lesions.[22] Initially thought to be caused by direct impact from the falx, experimental work shows that injury to the corpus callosum is most commonly caused by rotational shear forces, like all forms of DAI.[26] The corpus callosum may be particularly susceptible to DAI because the falx prevents displacement of the cerebral hemispheres. DAI of the corpus callosum is almost always seen in association with lesions in the lobar white matter. DAI in the most severe cases involves the dorsolateral aspect of the midbrain and upper pons, in addition to the lobar white matter and corpus callosum (see Brainstem Injury).

Cortical contusions are areas of focal brain injury primarily involving superficial gray matter. Patients with cortical contusions are much less likely to have loss of consciousness at the time of injury than are patients with DAI. Contusions are also associated with a better prognosis than DAI. They are very common in patients with severe head trauma and are usually well seen on CT scans. Contusions characteristically occur near bony protuberances of the skull and skull base. They tend to be multiple and bilateral and are more commonly hemorrhagic than DAI. Common sites are the temporal lobes above the petrous bone or posterior to the greater sphenoid wing, and the frontal lobes above the cribriform plate, planum sphenoidale, and lesser sphenoid wing (Fig. 3.17A–C,F). Less than 10% of lesions involve the cerebellum (Fig. 3.17D–F).[11] Contusions can also occur at the margins of depressed skull fractures.

The CT appearance of cortical contusions characteristically varies with the age of the lesion. Many nonhemorrhagic lesions are initially poorly seen but become more obvious during the first week because of associated edema. Hemorrhagic lesions are seen as foci of high attenuation within superficial gray matter (Fig. 3.17A,D). These may be surrounded by larger areas of low attenuation secondary to surrounding edema. During the first week, the characteristic CT pattern of mixed areas of hypodensity and hyperdensity ("salt-and-pepper" pattern) becomes more apparent. Occasionally, surgical decompression of the contused brain is required to alleviate severe mass effect. Areas of prior contusion can often be recognized as foci

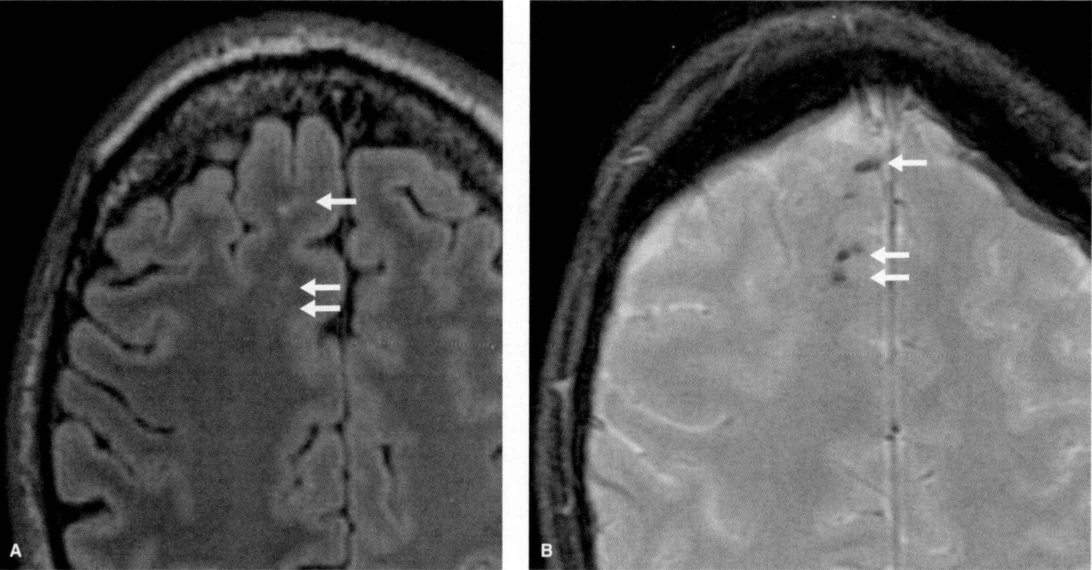

FIGURE 3.16. MR Appearance of Chronic Traumatic Axonal Injury. MR images from a 31-year-old man who suffered mild TBI 2 months prior to imaging reveal subtle hyperintense subcortical white matter lesions (*arrows*) on T2/FLAIR images (**A**) in the medial right frontal lobe. These lesions (*arrows*) are more pronounced on SWI where they appear as low signal (**B**).

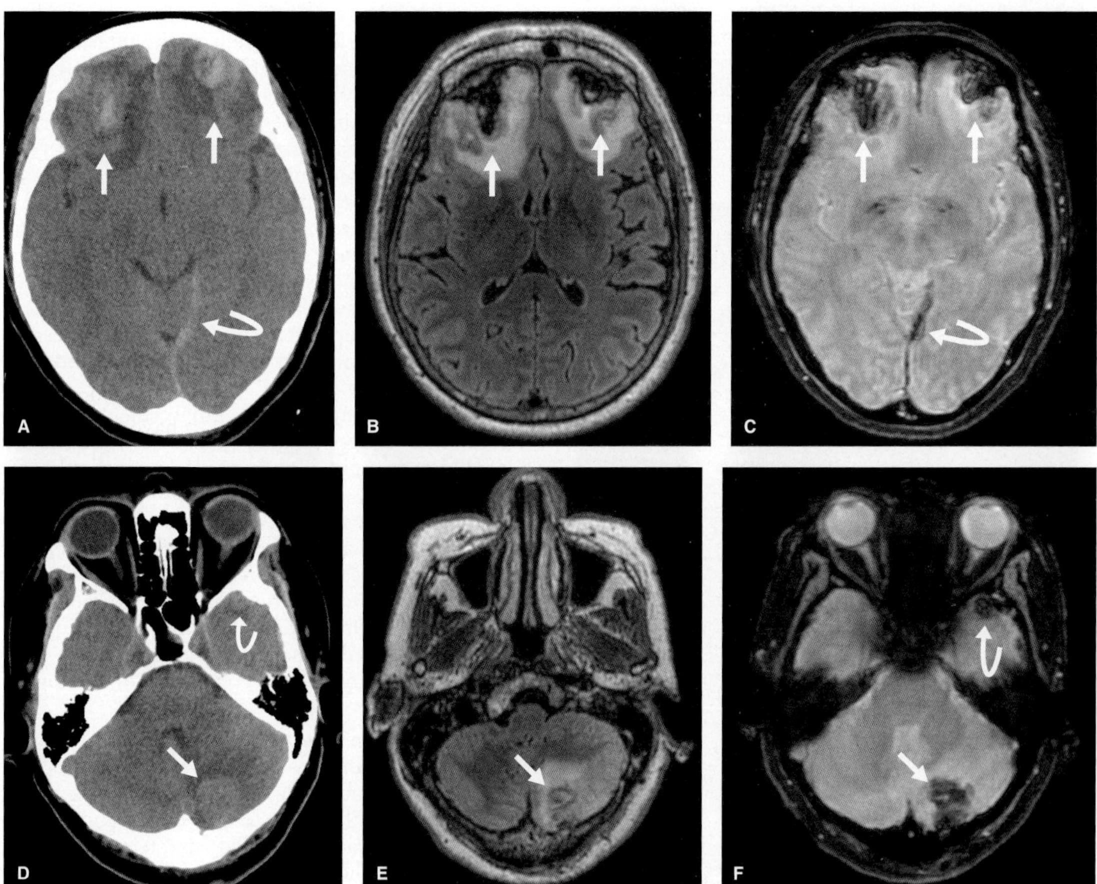

FIGURE 3.17. Hemorrhagic Cortical Contusion. CT and MR imaging in a middle-aged female following a fall in which the back of her head hit a pavement. Noncontrast CT (**A, D**), FLAIR (**B, E**), and susceptibility-weighted MR (**C, F**) images show left cerebellar (**D–F**, *arrows*) and large bifrontal (**A–C**, *straight arrows*) hemorrhagic contusions compatible with coup and contrecoup injuries, respectively. There is also a contrecoup contusion in the left anterior temporal lobe (**D, F**, *curved arrow*). These lesions have a classic appearance on CT and MR with low signal on SWI (**C, F**) and increased density on CT (**A, D**). There is significant surrounding vasogenic edema, which is hyperintense on FLAIR images (**B, E**) and hypodense on CT (**A, D**). Also note the increased prominence of the left tentorial subdural hematoma (*curved arrow*) on MR SWI (**C**) compared to CT (**A**).

of encephalomalacia within the same characteristic locations just described.

On MR imaging, contusions appear as poorly marginated areas of increased signal on FLAIR and T2W sequences (Fig. 3.17E,F). They are recognized because of their characteristic distribution in the frontal and temporal lobes and often have a "gyral" morphology. Hemorrhage causes heterogeneous signal intensity that varies depending on the age of the lesion. Hemosiderin staining from hemorrhage of any cause leads to markedly decreased signal intensity particularly on GRE or SWI (Fig. 3.17C,F). This signal loss can persist indefinitely as a marker of prior hemorrhage.

Intracerebral Hematoma. Occasionally, intraparenchymal hemorrhage is seen that is not necessarily associated with cortical contusion but rather represents shear-induced hemorrhage from the rupture of small intraparenchymal blood vessels. This lesion is known simply as an intracerebral hematoma. Intracerebral hematomas tend to have less surrounding edema than cortical contusions because they represent bleeding into areas of relatively normal brain. Most intracerebral hematomas are located in the frontotemporal white matter, although they can also occur in the basal ganglia (Fig. 3.18). They are often associated with skull fractures and other primary neuronal lesions, including contusions and DAI. In the absence of other significant lesions, patients with intracerebral hematomas can remain lucid after their injury. When symptoms develop, they commonly result from the mass effect associated with an expanding hematoma. In cases where CT angiography is also performed, active extravasation of contrast into the hematoma (often termed the "spot sign") predicts future expansion of the hematoma and worsens clinical outcome. Intracerebral hematomas can also present late secondary to delayed hemorrhage, which is another cause of clinical deterioration during the first several days after head trauma.

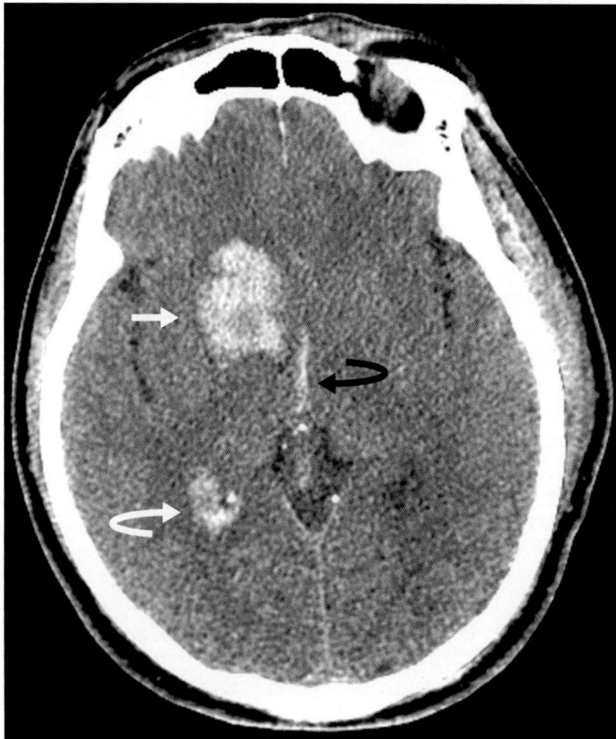

FIGURE 3.18. Intracerebral Hematoma. Axial CT scan demonstrates a high attenuation mass (*straight arrow*) within the right basal ganglia compatible with an acute intracerebral hematoma. There is intraventricular extension of hemorrhage into the right lateral ventricle (*white curved arrow*) and third ventricle (*black curved arrow*).

Subcortical gray matter injury is an uncommon manifestation of primary intra-axial injury and is seen as multiple, petechial hemorrhages primarily affecting the basal ganglia and thalamus. These represent microscopic perivascular collections of blood that may result from disruption of multiple small perforating vessels. These lesions are typically seen following severe head trauma.

Vascular injuries as causes of intra- and extra-axial hematomas were discussed previously. Other types of traumatic vascular injuries include arterial dissection (Fig. 3.19) or occlusion, pseudoaneurysm formation (Fig. 3.20), and the acquired arteriovenous fistula (Fig. 3.21). Arterial injury commonly accompanies fractures of the base of the skull. The internal carotid is the most often injured artery, especially at sites of fixation. These include its entrance to the carotid canal at the base of the petrous bone and at its exit from the cavernous sinus below the anterior clinoid process (Fig. 3.20).

MR findings of vascular injury include the presence of an intramural hematoma (best seen on T1W with fat suppression, Fig. 3.19A) or intimal flap with dissection, or the absence of normal vascular flow void with occlusion. An associated parenchymal infarction might also be seen. MR angiography is also useful in evaluating patients with suspected traumatic vascular injury (Fig. 3.19B,C). Conventional angiograms are often needed to confirm and delineate dissections and may also show spasm or pseudoaneurysm formation in injuries to the vessel wall.

The carotid cavernous fistula (CCF) is a communication between the cavernous portion of the internal carotid artery and the surrounding venous plexus. The lesion typically follows a full-thickness arterial injury, resulting in venous engorgement of the cavernous sinus and its draining tributaries (e.g., the ipsilateral superior ophthalmic vein and inferior petrosal sinus). Findings may be bilateral because venous channels connect the cavernous sinuses. The CCF most often results from severe head injury. Skull base fractures, especially those involving the sphenoid bone, indicate patients at increased risk for associated cavernous carotid injury. The CCF may also result from ruptured cavernous carotid aneurysms. On CTA or MR, the CCF may manifest as enlarged superior ophthalmic vein, cavernous sinus, and petrosal sinus flow voids. There may be evidence of proptosis, swelling of the preseptal soft tissues, and enlargement of the extraocular musculature. Diagnosis usually requires selective carotid angiography with rapid filming to demonstrate the site of communication (Fig. 3.21). On occasion, patients present with findings weeks or months after the initial trauma.

Dural fistulas are also associated with trauma. For example, they may be caused by laceration of the middle meningeal artery with resultant meningeal artery to meningeal vein fistula formation. Drainage via meningeal veins prevents formation of an epidural hematoma. Patients may be asymptomatic or present with nonspecific complaints, including tinnitus.

Mechanisms of Primary Head Injuries. Early research suggested that head injuries could be explained by areas of parenchymal compression and rarefaction caused by direct impact. Many authors still use the terms "coup" and "contrecoup" to describe intracranial lesions that characteristically occur on the side of and on the opposite the side of a blow to the head, respectively. However, Gentry et al. have questioned the use of these terms, which they feel incorrectly imply that neuronal injury is caused by compression and rarefaction strains subsequent to direct impact.[22]

Gennarelli et al. have shown in a primate model that all major types of intra-axial lesions, as well as subdural hematomas, can be produced purely by rotational acceleration of the head without direct impact.[26] Only skull fractures and epidural

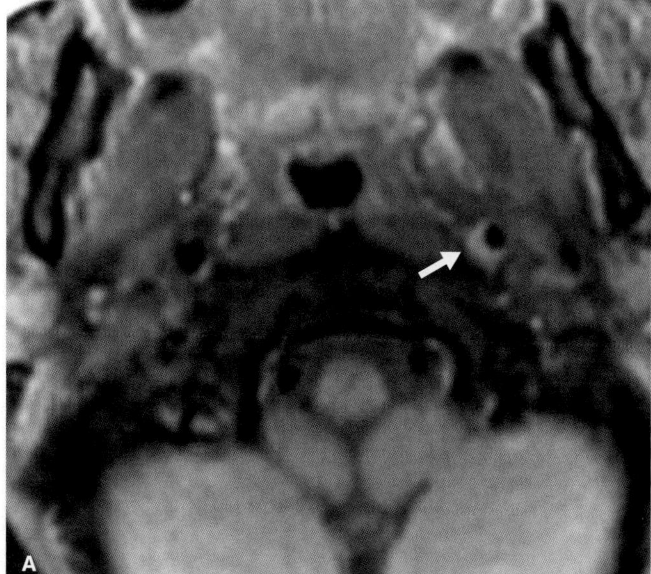

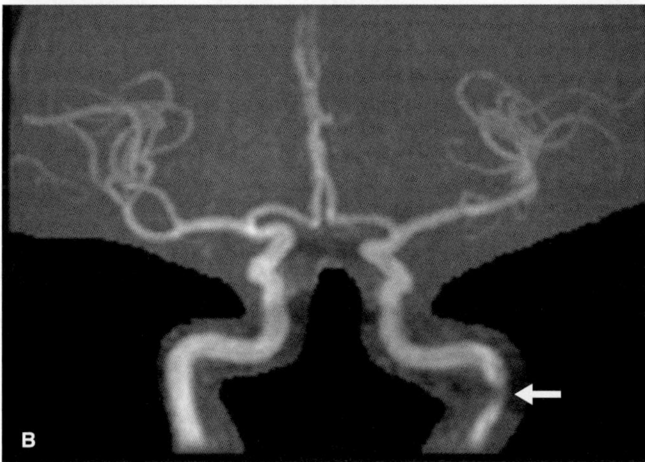

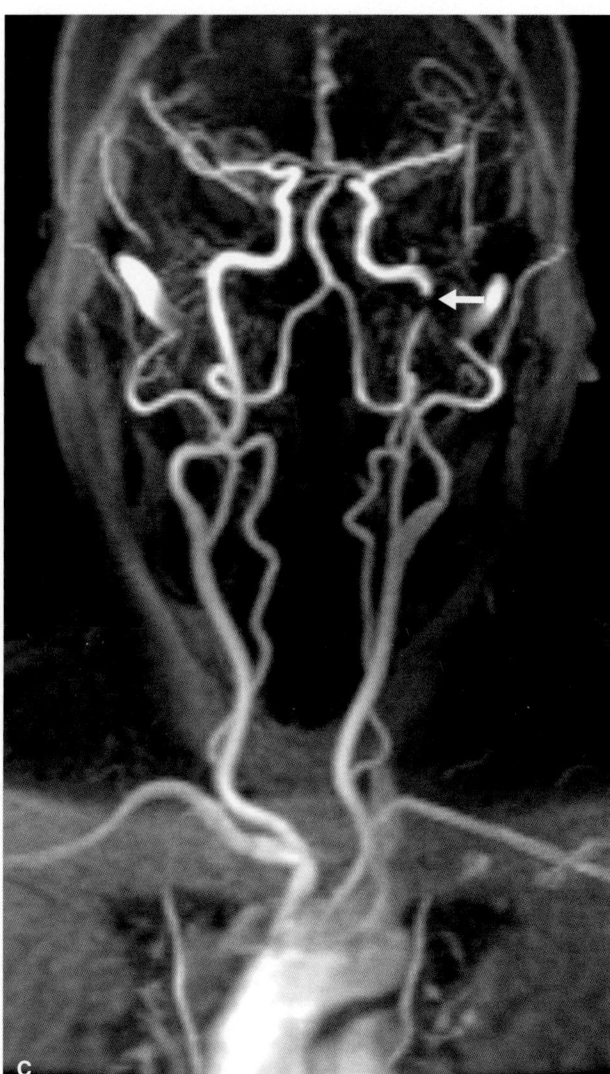

FIGURE 3.19. Carotid Artery Dissection. T1-weighted fat-suppression MR image (**A**) demonstrates crescentic T1 hyperintensity of an intramural hematoma (*arrow*) following acute dissection of the left internal carotid artery. Time-of-flight noncontrast MRA (**B**) of the same patient reveals focal narrowing (*arrow*) of the left internal carotid at the skull base, a common location for traumatic dissection. Contrast-enhanced MRA of the head and neck (**C**) also shows corresponding stenosis at the site of the skull base left internal carotid dissection (*arrow*).

hematomas require a physical blow to the head. Rotational acceleration causes damage by shear forces, rather than by compression–rarefaction strain. Compression–rarefaction strain is not felt to play a significant role in most head injuries.

The character of the accelerational force influences the type of injury produced. Cortical contusions and intracranial hematomas are more severe when the period of acceleration or deceleration is very short, whereas DAI and gliding contusions are associated with a longer acceleration or deceleration injury. Thus, DAI is more common in motor vehicle accidents while contusions and hematomas are more frequent in falls.

Secondary Head Injury

Diffuse cerebral swelling is a common manifestation of head trauma. It may occur either because of an increase in cerebral blood volume or an increase in tissue fluid content. Hyperemia refers to an increase in blood volume, whereas cerebral edema refers to an increase in tissue fluid. Both lead to generalized mass effect with effacement of sulci, suprasellar and quadrigeminal plate cisterns, and compression of the ventricular system. Effacement of the brainstem cisterns indicates severe mass effect and may herald impending transtentorial herniation.

Cerebral swelling from hyperemia is most commonly seen in children and adolescents. The pathogenesis is poorly understood but appears to be the result of loss of normal cerebral autoregulation. Hyperemia is recognized on CT as ill-defined mass effect, effacement of sulci, and normal attenuation of brain. Acute subdural hematomas are often associated with unilateral swelling of the ipsilateral hemisphere.

Diffuse cerebral edema occurs secondary to tissue hypoxia. Because of the increase in tissue fluid, edema causes decreased attenuation on CT images with loss of gray–white differentiation. The cerebellum and brainstem are usually spared and may appear hyperdense relative to the cerebral hemispheres (Fig. 3.22). Often, the falx and cerebral vessels appear dense, mimicking acute subarachnoid hemorrhage. Focal areas of edema are frequently seen in association with cortical contusions and may contribute significantly to mass effect.

Brain Herniation. Several forms of herniation are seen secondary to mass effect produced by primary intracranial injury. These are not specific for head trauma and can be seen secondary to

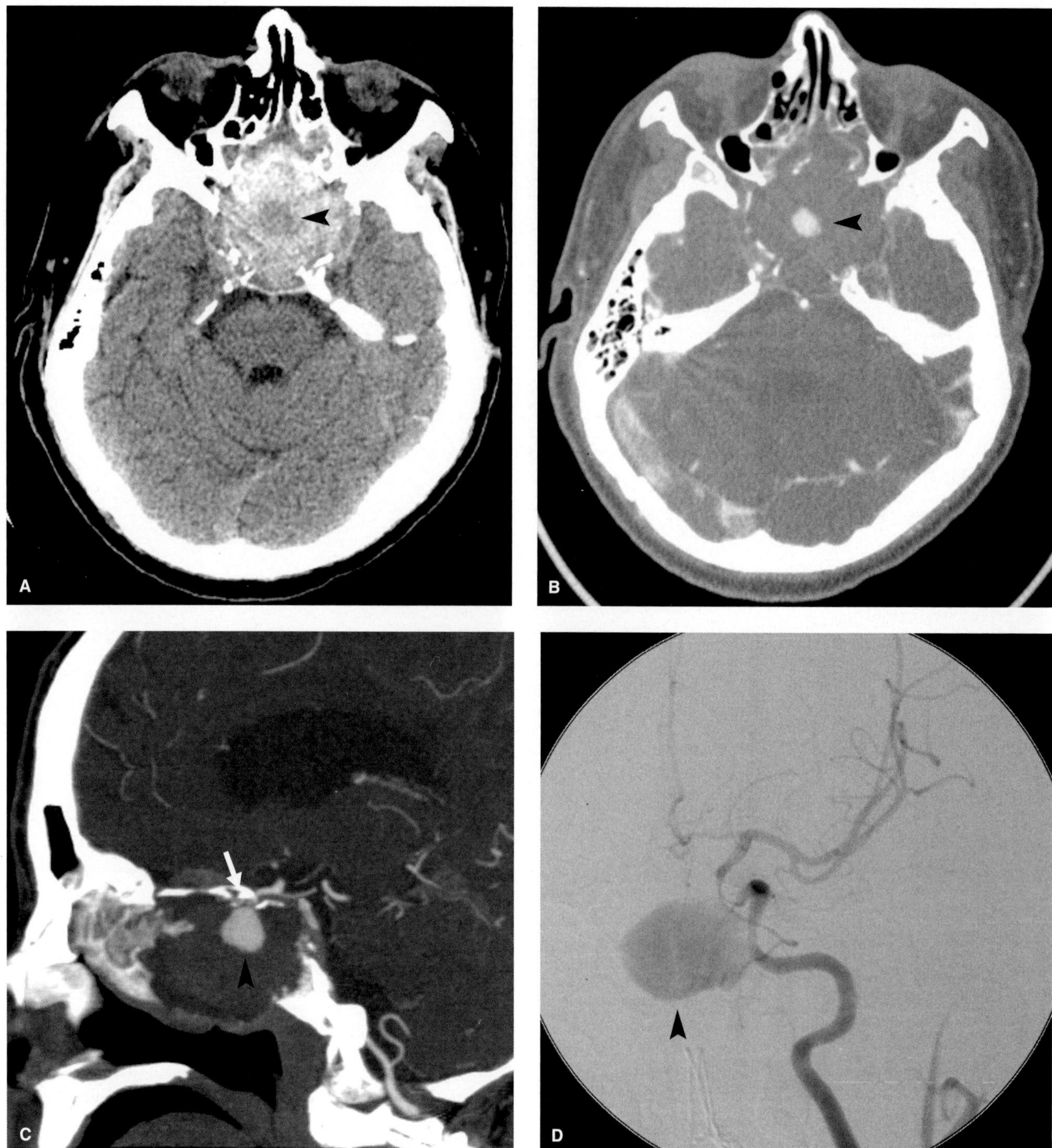

FIGURE 3.20. Posttraumatic Pseudoaneurysm. This 43-year-old man presented with headache and visual symptoms 3 months after suffering facial fractures in a motor vehicle accident. Noncontrast CT reveals a large hyperdense mass within the anterior skull base (**A**) eroding the sphenoid bone, sella, and the orbits. Axial (**B**) and sagittal (**C**) reformatted CT angiography images performed the same day show the central area of the mass enhancing (*arrowhead*) to the same extent as the adjacent intracranial arteries (**C**). In addition, there is an apparent narrow-necked connection (*arrow*) between the enhancing portion and the left cavernous internal carotid artery (**C**), consistent with a pseudoaneurysm. Note that the central low density (**A**, *arrowhead*) within the higher-density thrombosed portion of the pseudoaneurysm correlates with the central nonthrombosed enhancing area (**B**, *arrowhead*) on the postcontrast images. Catheter angiography (**D**), imaged following injection of the left internal carotid artery, again demonstrates the pseudoaneurysm (*arrowhead*) which was subsequently treated with endovascular coil embolization.

mass effect produced by other causes as well, including intracranial hemorrhage, infarction, or neoplasm (Fig. 3.23).

Subfalcine herniation, in which the cingulate gyrus is displaced across the midline under the falx cerebri, is the most common form of brain herniation (Fig. 3.11). Compression of the adjacent lateral ventricle may be seen on CT scans, as well as enlargement of the contralateral ventricle from obstruction at the level of the foramen of Monro. Both anterior cerebral arteries (ACAs) may be displaced to the contralateral side.

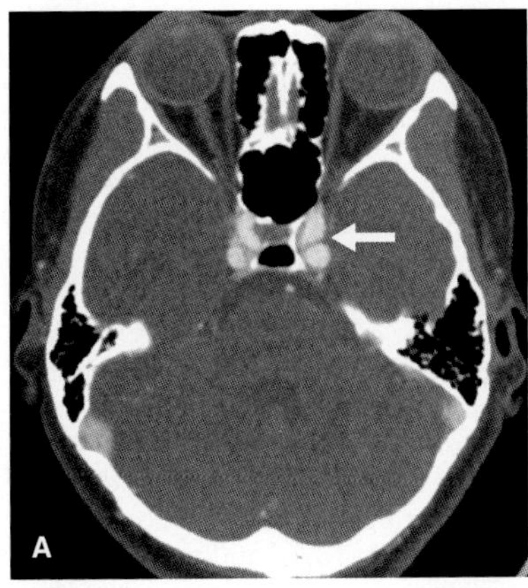

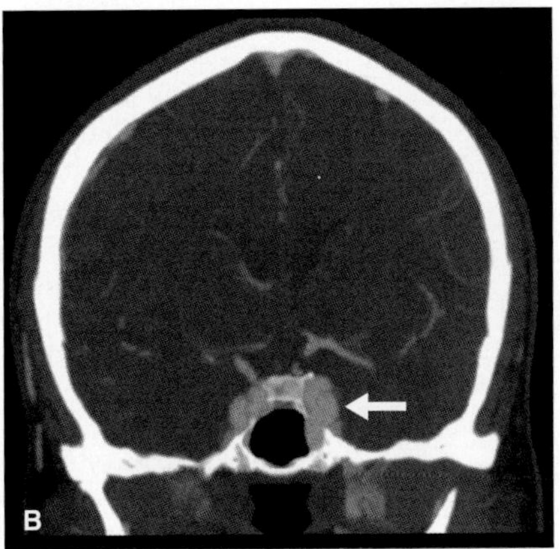

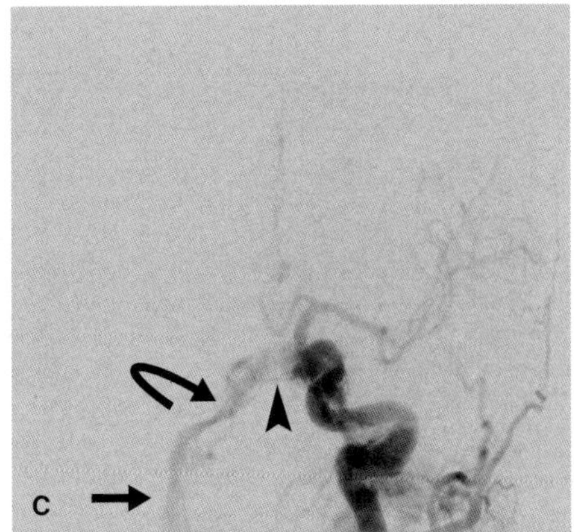

FIGURE 3.21. **Carotid Cavernous Fistula.** Axial (**A**) and coronal (**B**) images from a CTA of the head reveal fullness in the left greater than right cavernous sinus (*arrows*). Subsequent left common carotid angiogram (**C**) in the same patient shows abnormal early opacification of the cavernous sinus (*arrowhead*), inferior petrosal sinus (*curved arrow*), and jugular vein (*arrow*) during the early-arterial phase.

These patients are at risk of ACA infarction in the distribution of the callosomarginal branch of the ACA, where it becomes trapped against the falx.

Uncal herniation, in which the medial aspect of the temporal lobe is displaced medially over the free margin of the tentorium, is also common (Fig. 3.24). Uncal herniation causes focal effacement of the ambient cistern and the lateral aspect of the suprasellar cistern. Rarely, displacement of the brainstem causes compression of the contralateral cerebral peduncle against the tentorial margin, resulting in peduncular hemorrhage or infarction. The focal impression on the cerebral peduncle is known as "Kernohan notch." Mass effect on the third cranial nerve and compression of the contralateral cerebral peduncle cause a recognizable clinical syndrome characterized by a blown pupil with ipsilateral hemiparesis.

Transtentorial Herniation. The brain can herniate either downward or upward across the tentorium. Descending transtentorial herniation is recognized by effacement of the suprasellar and perimesencephalic cisterns. Pineal calcification, usually seen at about the same level as calcified choroid plexus in the trigones of the lateral ventricles, is displaced inferiorly. Large posterior fossa hematomas can cause ascending transtentorial herniation, in which the vermis and portions of the cerebellar hemispheres can herniate through the

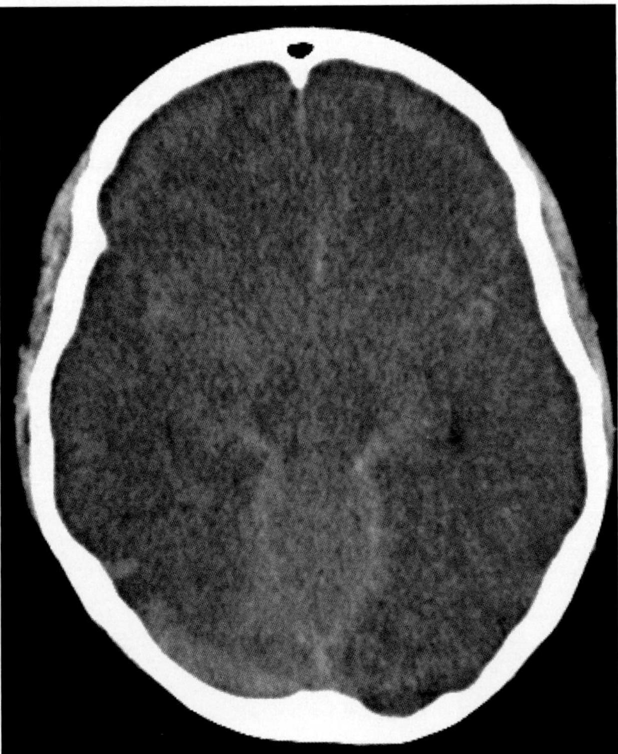
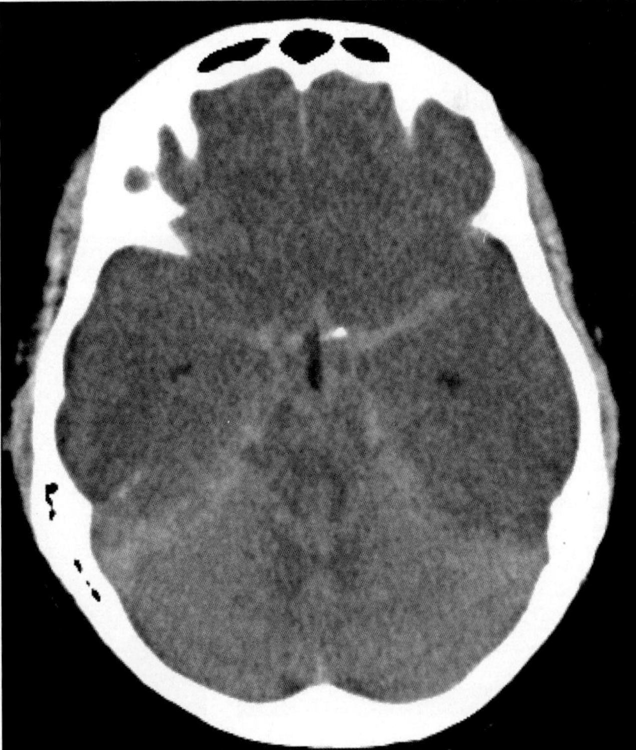

FIGURE 3.22. **Diffuse Cerebral Edema.** Noncontrast CT scan of a patient following strangulation shows diffuse decrease in attenuation of the cerebral hemispheres with loss of gray–white differentiation indicating diffuse cerebral edema. Sparing of the brainstem and cerebellum causes these structures to appear dense relative to the rest of the brain. The relative increased density of the subarachnoid spaces has led to this appearance being described as "pseudosubarachnoid hemorrhage."

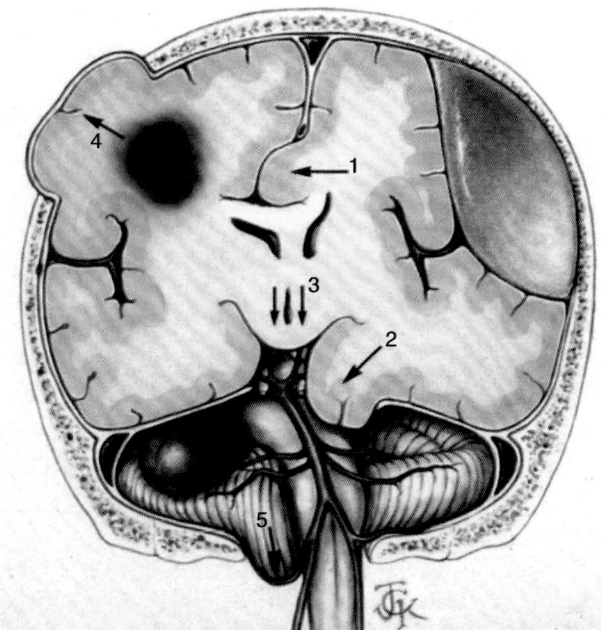

FIGURE 3.23. Diagram of the Major Types of Brain Herniations. (1) Subfalcine herniation. (2) Uncal herniation. (3) Descending transtentorial herniation. (4) External herniation. (5) Tonsillar herniation. (Reprinted with permission from Gean AD. *Imaging of Head Trauma*. Philadelphia, PA: Lippincott Williams & Wilkins; 1994:264.)

tentorial incisura. This is much less common than descending transtentorial herniation. Posterior fossa hematomas can also cause herniation of the cerebellar tonsils downward through the foramen magnum. Finally, external herniation can occur in which swelling or mass effect causes the brain to herniate through a calvarial defect. This can be posttraumatic or occur at the time of craniotomy and prevent closure of the skull flap.

Hydrocephalus can occur after subarachnoid or intraventricular hemorrhage as a result of either impaired CSF reabsorption at the level of the arachnoid granulations or obstruction at the level of the aqueduct or fourth ventricular outflow foramina. Mass effect from cerebral swelling or an adjacent hematoma can also cause hydrocephalus by compression of the aqueduct or outflow foramina of the fourth ventricle. Asymmetrical lateral ventricular dilatation can be produced by compression of the foramen of Monro.

Ischemia or Infarction. Posttraumatic ischemia or infarction can result from raised intracranial pressure, embolization from a vascular dissection, or direct mass effect on cerebral vasculature from brain herniation or an overlying extra-axial collection. In addition, patients may suffer diffuse ischemic damage from acute reduction in cerebral blood flow or from hypoxemia secondary to respiratory arrest or status epilepticus. Patterns of infarction from focal mass effect include ACA infarction from subfalcine herniation, posterior cerebral artery infarction from uncal herniation (Fig. 3.24), and posterior inferior communicating artery infarction from tonsillar herniation. Ischemia or infarction secondary to globally reduced cerebral perfusion tends to occur in characteristic "watershed zones" and is not specific for trauma (see Chapter 4).

CSF leak requires a dural tear and can occur after calvarial or skull base fractures. CSF rhinorrhea occurs subsequent to fractures in which communication develops between the subarachnoid space and the paranasal sinuses or middle ear cavity. CSF otorrhea occurs when communication between the subarachnoid space and middle ear occurs in association with disruption of the tympanic membrane. CSF leaks can be difficult to localize and can lead to recurrent meningeal infection. Radionuclide cisternography is highly sensitive for the presence of CSF extravasation; however, CT scanning with intrathecal contrast is required for detailed anatomic localization of the defect (Fig. 3.25).

Leptomeningeal cyst or "growing fracture" is caused by a traumatic tear in the dura, which allows an outpouching of arachnoid to occur at the site of a suture or skull fracture. This leads to progressive, slow widening of the skull defect or suture, presumably as a result of CSF pulsations. The leptomeningeal cyst appears as a lytic skull defect on CT or plain skull films (Fig. 3.26), which can enlarge over time. On MRI, it follows CSF signal on all pulse sequences.

Encephalomalacia. Focal encephalomalacia consists of tissue loss with surrounding gliosis and is a frequent manifestation

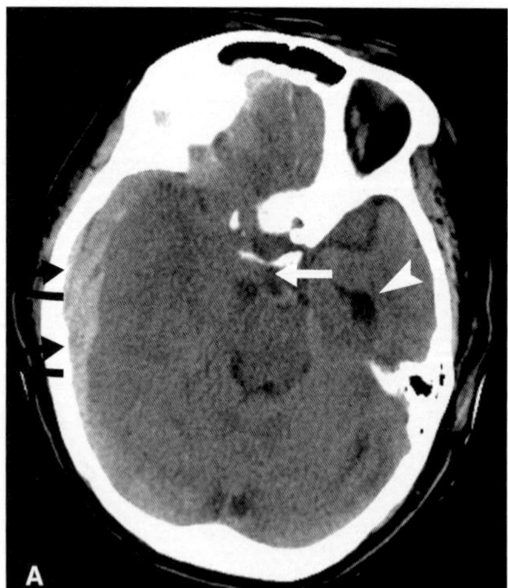

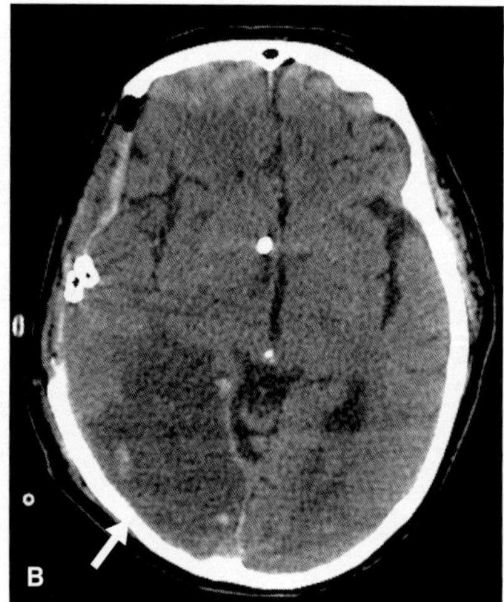

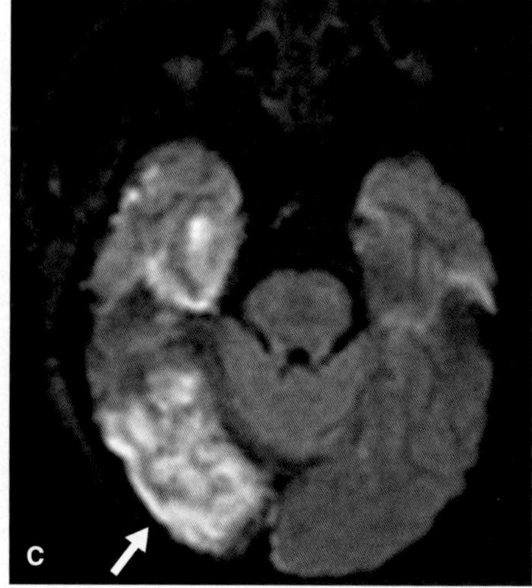

FIGURE 3.24. Uncal Herniation. Serial imaging of a 74-year-old woman following traumatic brain injury. The preoperative noncontrast CT image (**A**) demonstrates mass effect from a right holohemispheric subdural hematoma (*curved arrows*) resulting in pronounced right uncal herniation (*arrow*) and trapping of the temporal horn of the left lateral ventricle (*arrowhead*). Postoperative noncontrast CT obtained later the same day (**B**) reveals a decompressive craniectomy, ventricular drain placement, and a new large hypodensity involving the territory of the right posterior cerebral artery territory (*arrow*), compatible with infarct. Diffusion-weighted MRI (**C**) obtained 4 days after initial injury confirms the right PCA territory infarct (*arrow*), secondary to compression of the proximal PCA by the previously herniated right uncus.

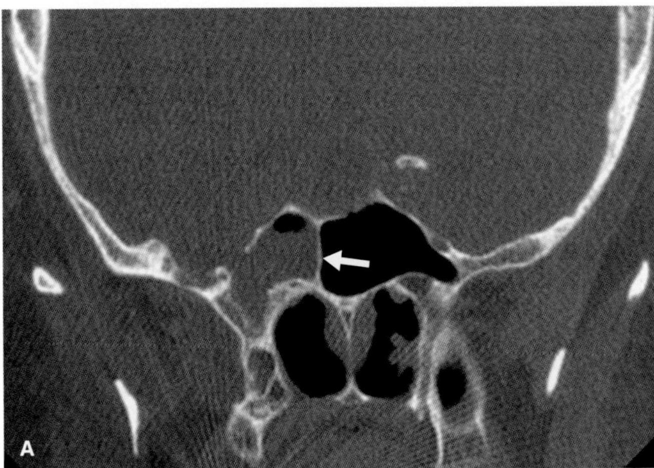

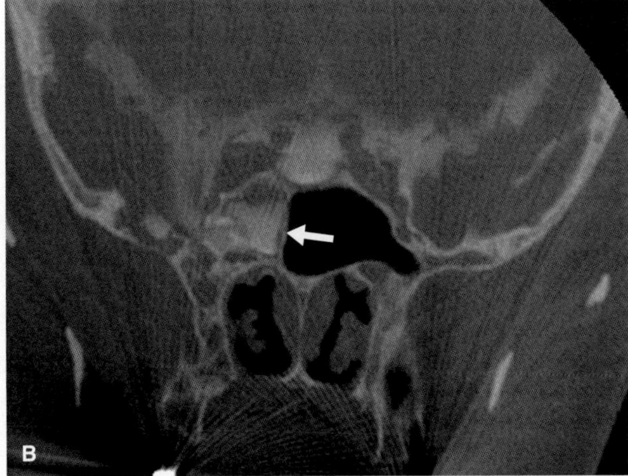

FIGURE 3.25. CSF Leak. A 55-year-old female with a history of remote trauma and meningitis. Coronal reformatted image from initial noncontrast CT (**A**) reveals near-complete opacification right sphenoid sinus (*arrow*) with a large bony defect between the lateral wall of the right sphenoid sinus and the middle cranial fossa. CT cisternography following intrathecal injection of contrast agent (**B**) confirms abnormal leakage of CSF contrast from the middle cranial fossa into the sphenoid sinus (*arrow*).

of remote head injury. It may be asymptomatic or serve as a potential seizure focus. CT demonstrates fairly well-defined areas of low attenuation with volume loss. There may be dilation of adjacent portions of the ventricular system. Encephalomalacia will follow CSF signal on MR sequences, except for gliosis, which appears as increased signal intensity on both FLAIR and T2WI. The appearance of encephalomalacia is not specific for posttraumatic injury, but the locations are characteristic: anteroinferior frontal and temporal lobes. Focal volume loss along the white matter tracts associated with cell death is known as Wallerian degeneration and may be seen on CT and especially MR studies.

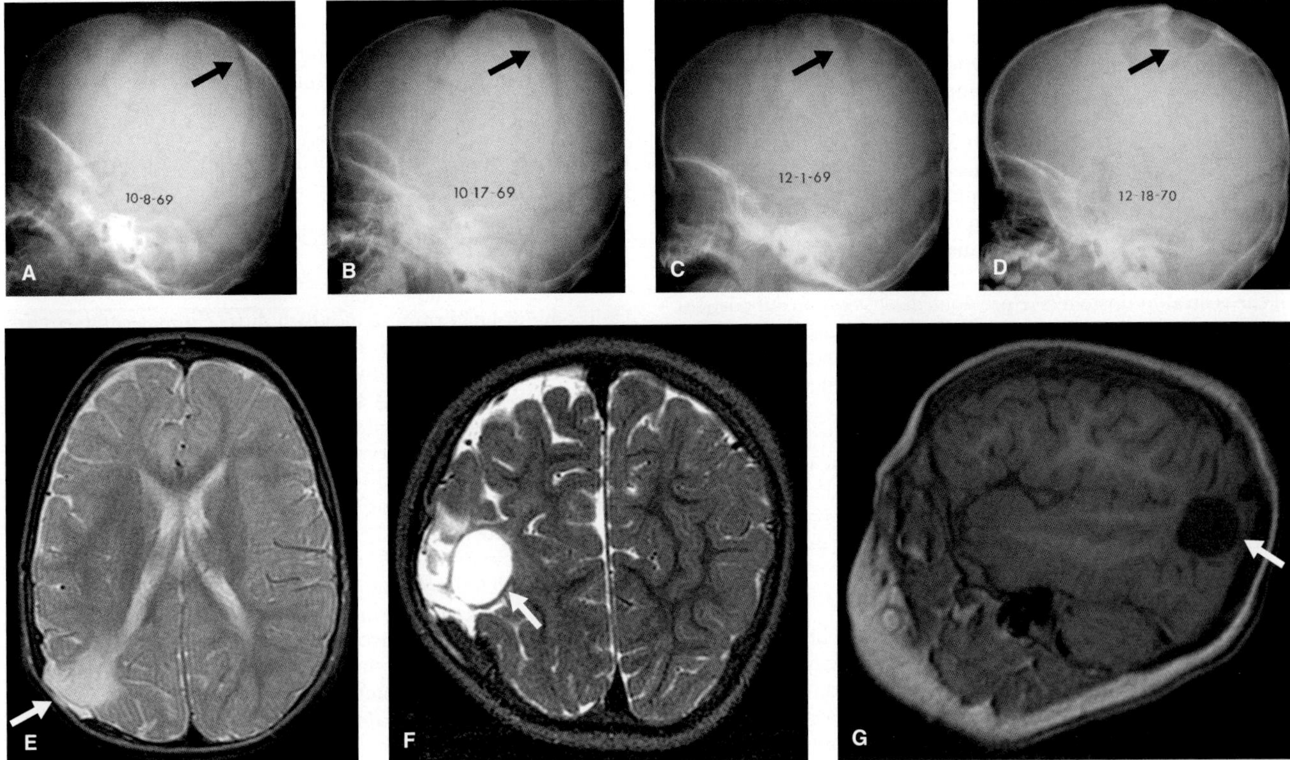

FIGURE 3.26. Leptomeningeal Cyst. Lateral skull radiograph (**A**) from a 6-month-old infant who presented with unconsciousness shows a slightly diastatic fracture (*black arrow*) of the parietal bone. Follow-up radiographs at 2 weeks (**B**) and 6 weeks (**C**) show progressive widening of the fracture (*black arrows*). The chronic leptomeningeal cyst (**D**, *black arrow*), which has resulted, appears as a lobulated lytic lesion with scalloped margins. MRI (**E–G**) from a different 13 month old who had fallen from her mother's arms 9 months earlier. Axial (**E**) and coronal (**F**) T2WI and sagittal T1WI (**G**) reveal a cystic lesion (*white arrows*) with surrounding encephalomalacia in the right temporoparietal cortex, which extends into a defect in the overlying parietal bone compatible with a chronic leptomeningeal cyst. Note that the cyst follows CSF signal on both T1WI and T2WI.

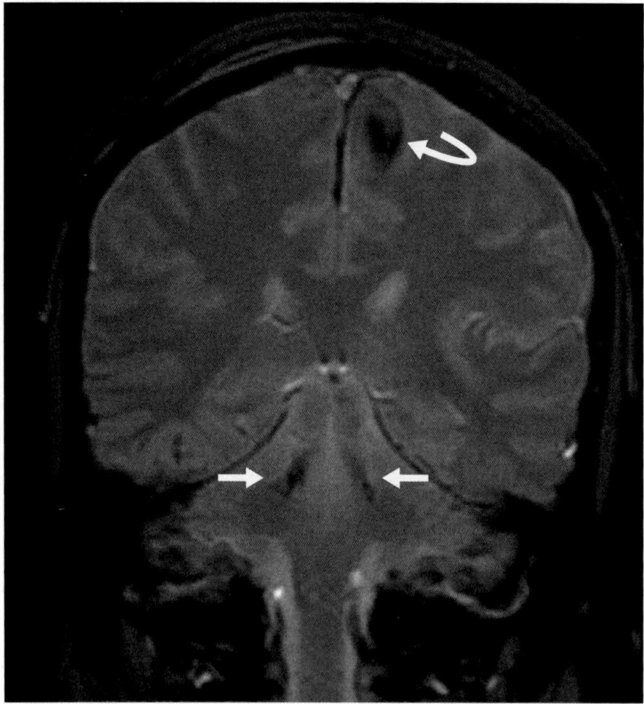

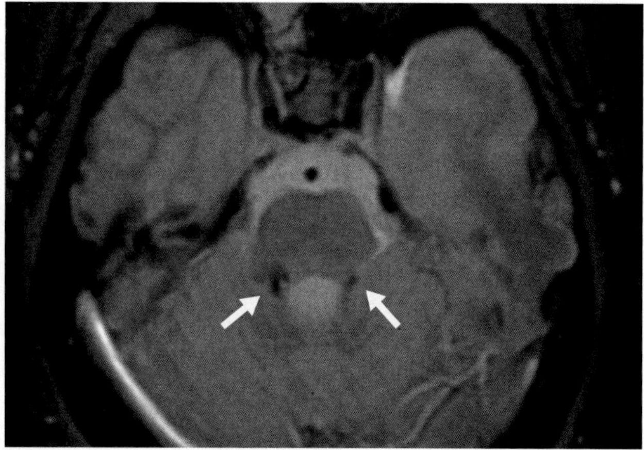

FIGURE 3.27. **Primary Brainstem Injury.** Coronal and axial GRE MR images from a 23 year old, following a severe motorcycle crash resulting in severe diffuse axonal injury. Note the *arrows* of increased susceptibility (low signal at *arrows*) involving the bilateral superior cerebellar peduncles, a common site for brainstem traumatic axonal injury. The coronal image also reveals supratentorial injuries including a small parafalcine subdural hematoma and subcortical axonal injury (*curved arrow*).

Brainstem Injury

Primary. The most common form of primary brainstem injury is DAI, which affects the dorsolateral aspect of the midbrain and upper pons (Fig. 3.27). The superior cerebellar peduncles and the medial lemnisci are particularly vulnerable. Both the location and lack of sufficient amounts of hemorrhage make this lesion difficult to diagnose on CT scans. Brainstem DAI is nearly always seen in association with lesions of the frontal or temporal white matter and corpus callosum. This distinguishes brainstem DAI from a rare form of primary injury caused by direct impact of the free margin of the tentorium on the brainstem. Primary brainstem injury may also occur in the form of multiple petechial hemorrhages in the periaqueductal regions of the rostral brainstem (see previous discussion on subcortical gray matter injury). These petechial hemorrhages are not associated with DAI, although they occur in a similar distribution. This form of injury represents disruption of penetrating brainstem blood vessels by shear strain and carries a grim prognosis.

An extremely rare form of indirect primary brainstem injury is the pontomedullary separation or rent. As the name implies, this represents a tear in the ventral surface of the brainstem at the junction of the pons and medulla. There is a spectrum of severity ranging from a small tear to complete avulsion of the brainstem. Pontomedullary separation can occur without associated diffuse cerebral injury. This lesion is usually fatal.

Secondary brainstem injury includes infarction, hemorrhage, or compression of the brainstem as a result of adjacent or systemic pathology. Brainstem infarction from hypotension-induced cerebral hypoperfusion is usually seen in conjunction with supratentorial ischemic injury. The brainstem may be relatively spared in hypoxic injury. Mechanical compression of the brainstem usually occurs in the setting of uncal herniation. There may be visible displacement or a change in the overall shape of the brainstem as a result of the mass effect. Neurologic injury caused by brainstem compression may be reversible in the absence of intrinsic brainstem lesions.

Brainstem lesions that occur as a result of downward herniation, or hypoxia or ischemia, usually involve the ventral or ventrolateral aspect of the brainstem, in contrast to primary brainstem lesions, which are most common in the dorsolateral aspect of the brainstem. A characteristic secondary brainstem lesion is the Duret hemorrhage. This is a midline hematoma in the tegmentum of the rostral pons and midbrain seen in association with descending transtentorial herniation. It is believed to result from stretching or tearing of penetrating arteries as the brainstem is caudally displaced (Fig. 3.28). The brainstem infarct is another type of secondary brainstem injury that typically occurs in the central tegmentum of the pons and midbrain.

Penetrating Trauma

Unlike blunt head trauma in which diffuse injury often occurs secondary to acceleration-induced shear strain, in penetrating injury the damage is defined by the trajectory of the object. Penetrating sharp objects such as knives or glass cause tissue laceration along their course with resultant bleeding or infarction from vascular injury. Plain films or CT can be used to confirm and localize radiopaque intracranial foreign bodies. Leaded glass and metal are hyperdense on CT scans, whereas wood is hypodense.

Gunshot wounds are among the most common causes of penetrating head trauma. They can cause the type of injuries seen in nonpenetrating trauma as well, because significant blunt force occurs from the bullet's impact on the skull. Metallic foreign bodies such as bullet fragments often cause significant streak artifact, which can obscure underlying injury. Tilting the CT gantry to change the plane of section helps minimize this artifact. The entry and exit sites can often be distinguished by the direction of beveling of the calvarial defect or from the pattern of calvarial fracture. The bullet path can often be recognized on CT as a linear hemorrhagic strip (Fig. 3.29). Gunshot wounds in which the bullet crosses the midline or in which small fragments are seen displaced from the main bullet are associated with a poorer prognosis.

Additional complications of penetrating injury are caused by associated skull fractures and dural lacerations

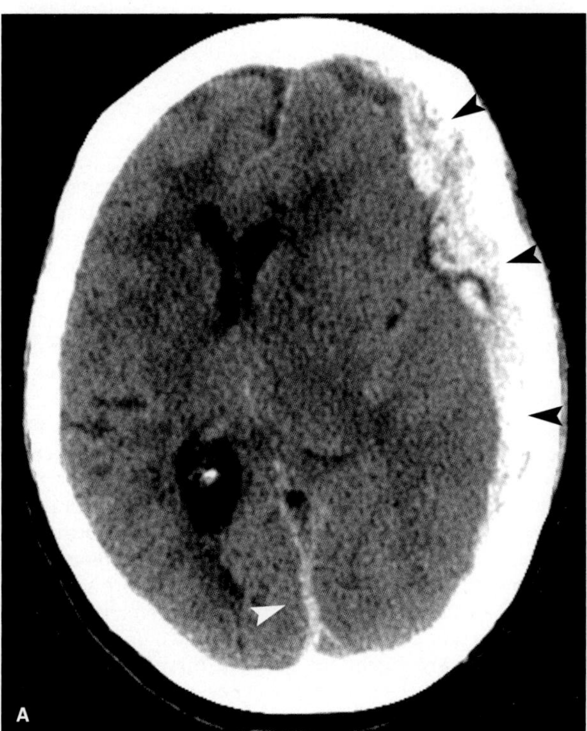

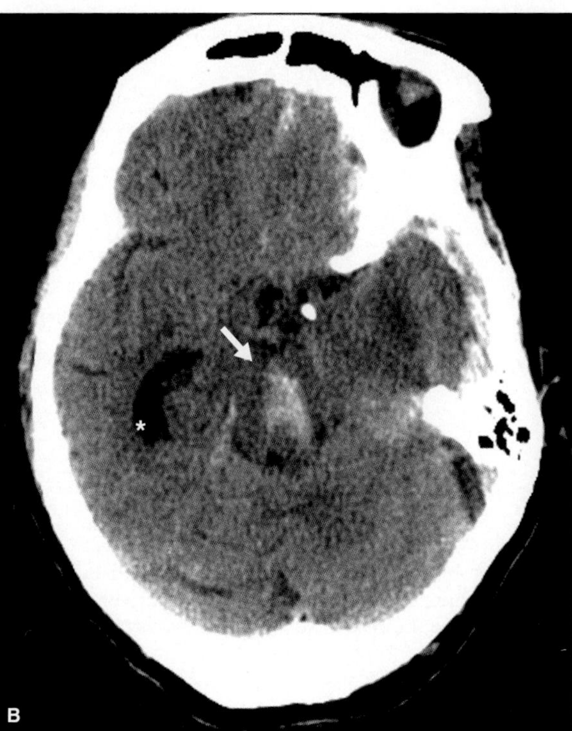

FIGURE 3.28. **Duret Hemorrhage.** Axial noncontrast CT images from an 80-year-old female reveal left convexity holohemispheric (**A**, *black arrowheads*) and parafalcine subdural (**A**, *white arrowheads*) hematomas. Secondary complications related to mass effect include subfalcine herniation (**A**), left uncal and downward transtentorial herniation (**B**), trapping of the temporal horn (*asterisk*) of the right lateral ventricle secondary, and acute hemorrhage in the midbrain (not shown) and pons (**B**), known as Duret hemorrhage (*arrow*). Duret hemorrhage is a type of secondary brainstem injury that occurs in association with downward transtentorial herniation and can be distinguished from most primary brainstem injuries by its midline location (compare with Fig. 3.27).

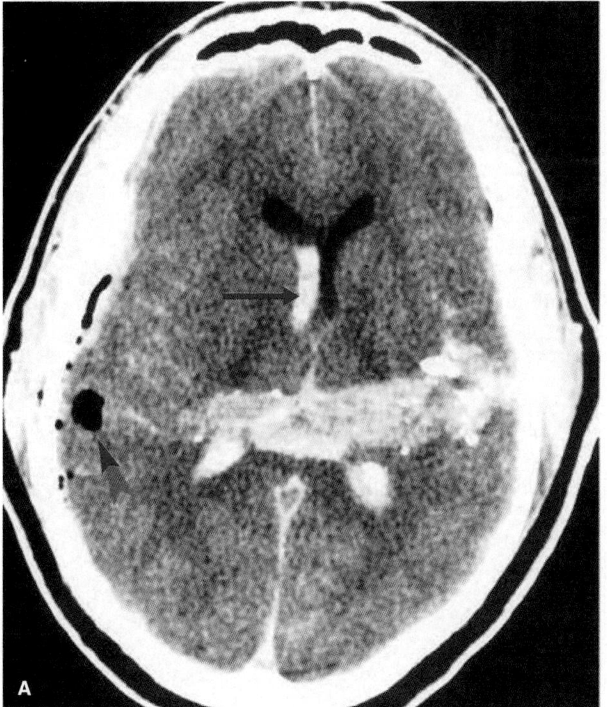

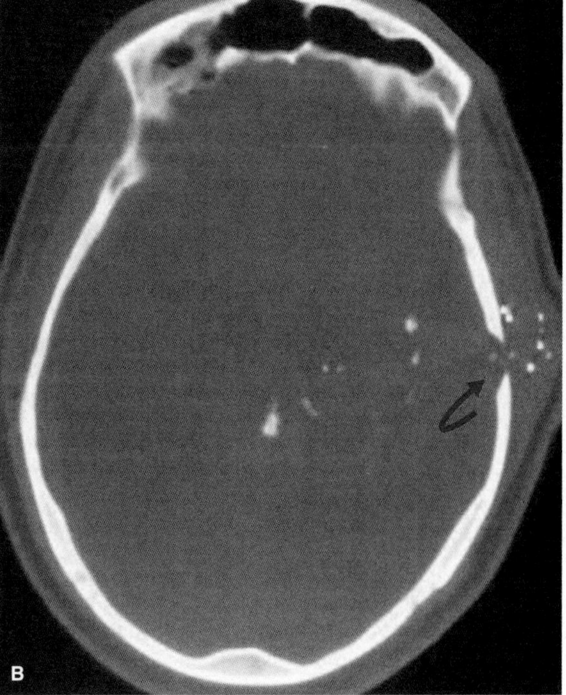

FIGURE 3.29. **Gunshot Wound. A:** Noncontrast CT scan shows hemorrhage delineating the bullet's path in this despondent southpaw. There is associated intraventricular (*arrow*) and subarachnoid hemorrhage as well as pneumocephalus (*arrowhead*) and a right subdural hematoma. **B:** Bone window shows the typical beveled entry site (*curved arrow*) and scattered bullet fragments along the trajectory. (Reprinted with permission from Gean AD. *Imaging of Head Trauma*. Philadelphia, PA: Lippincott Williams & Wilkins; 1994:193.)

TABLE 3.1

THE GLASGOW COMA SCALE[a]

■ EYE OPENING	■ BEST MOTOR	■ BEST VERBAL
4—spontaneous	6—obeys	5—oriented
3—to voice	5—localizes	4—confused
2—to pain	4—withdraws	3—inappropriate words
1—none	3—abnormal flexion	2—incomprehensible words
	2—extensor posturing	1—nothing
	1—flaccid	

[a]The total score is the sum of the scores in each category.

with resultant pneumocephalus, CSF leaks, and infection. Fragments of bone, skin, or hair that may be driven intracranially also increase the risk of subsequent abscess formation.

Predicting Outcome After Acute Head Trauma

The Glasgow coma scale (GCS), which stratifies patients with acute head trauma on the basis of clinical findings including level of consciousness, brainstem reflexes, and response to pain, helps standardize assessment of the severity of injury (Table 3.1). Mild head injury refers to a GCS of 13 to 15, moderate head injury refers to a GCS of 9 to 12, and severe head injury is defined as a GCS of 8 or below. Although there is a direct correlation between the initial GCS score and subsequent morbidity and mortality, the GCS is limited in its ability to predict long-term outcome. Likewise, CT findings, although valuable in identifying injuries requiring acute intervention, do not correlate well with prognosis. There is growing evidence, however, that MR will be helpful in determining a patient's prognosis after severe head injury.[11,27,28] This reflects the advantage of MR over CT in detecting brainstem injury and DAI. MR studies have shown good correlation between initial GCS and the number and distribution of DAI lesions. Numerous DAI lesions and the presence of DAI in the corpus callosum or brainstem are associated with more severe clinical findings and low initial scores on the GCS. Perhaps more important is the finding that the number of DAI lesions and the presence of brainstem injury or corpus callosum DAI are associated with poor long-term outcome.[29] The number of cortical contusions is not related to outcome, except in cases with significant mass effect. There is also a poor correlation between the presence of an isolated epidural or subdural hematoma and long-term outcome, unless transtentorial herniation is also present.

Child Abuse

Nonaccidental trauma accounts for at least 80% of deaths from head trauma in children younger than 2 years of age.[30] It is important to consider the possibility of child abuse and to recognize the characteristic features in these suspected cases.

Skull fractures represent the second most common skeletal injury in child abuse after long bone fracture. They are only found in approximately 50% of children with intracranial injuries from abuse.[31,32] In patients with suspected intracranial injury, CT should be the initial imaging study. Skull films are rarely indicated, except perhaps for documentation of cranial injury in neurologically intact children with suspected child abuse.

Subdural hematomas are the most commonly recognized intracranial complication from child abuse. The association of subdural hematomas and retinal hemorrhages in children with metaphyseal long bone fractures was described as "whiplash shaken injury" by Caffey in 1946.[33] The mechanism was thought to be one of violent shaking, with generation of rotational and shear forces intracranially because of the weak neck musculature. The mechanism might include impact against a soft object such as a mattress, which has been shown experimentally to increase the forces produced into the range that could cause coma, subdural hematomas, and primary brain injury, leading to the term "shaken impact injury."[34]

Subdural hematomas in child abuse often are found in the posterior interhemispheric fissure. These are seen on CT as hyperdense collections with a flat medial border along the falx and an irregular convex lateral border. Subdural hematomas may also be found along the convexity, over the tentorial surface, at the skull base, or in the posterior fossa. Occasionally, low-density extra-axial fluid collections are seen in infants without any clear precipitating trauma or infection. These most often represent dilated CSF spaces, known as "benign enlargement of the subarachnoid space of infancy," but can mimic chronic subdural hematomas. They occur in neurologically intact infants 3 to 6 months old who present with enlarging head circumference. In this setting, they require no treatment and usually regress by age 2 years. An old term for this condition, "external hydrocephalus," has been abandoned by many because it fails to convey the benign nature of the condition. Epidural hematomas are not frequently seen in child abuse.

The most common intra-axial manifestation of head injury related to child abuse is diffuse brain swelling. The initial swelling is believed to be caused by vasodilation associated with loss of autoregulation. At this stage, the injury may be reversible despite dramatic findings on CT. CT scans show global effacement of the subarachnoid space and compressed ventricles. As the brain becomes edematous, the normal attenuation of gray and white matter may appear indistinguishable or even reversed. The cerebral hemispheres will demonstrate diffusely decreased attenuation. The brainstem, cerebellum, and possibly deep gray matter structures may be spared (Fig. 3.22). Cerebral edema in the setting of shaking injury can also occur secondary to respiratory depression, apnea, and hypoxia. The other manifestations of intra-axial injury previously described in this chapter may also be seen in child abuse, including DAI and brainstem injury. Cortical contusions occur but are considered less common, possibly because the inner surface of the skull is relatively smooth in children. In infants, head trauma may lead to tears at the gray–white junction, especially in the frontal and temporal lobes.

Multiple injuries of various ages also strongly suggest child abuse. Chronic sequelae of head injury in children include chronic subdural collections (which may occasionally calcify), global cerebral atrophy, and encephalomalacia. Although CT is the modality of choice for the evaluation of acute head injury in children, MR can help identify subdural collections of various ages or hemosiderin deposits from prior hemorrhages. The ability of MR to identify these remote intracranial hemorrhages makes it an important tool in the evaluation of suspected child abuse. In some centers, it has been proposed as a necessary complement to the skeletal series. MR is also recommended when patients are clinically stable after head injury, to help determine the full extent of injury and prognosis. "Rapid" MRI examinations with limited sequences and imaging time reduced to 3 to 4 minutes may help with this in the future, but further studies are required to ensure diagnostic accuracy is on par with CT and standard MR imaging.[35]

FACIAL TRAUMA

Imaging Strategy

CT. MDCT has also supplanted plain film radiography as the modality of choice for the evaluation of facial fractures as it provides excellent bony detail. Volumetric acquisitions allow for submillimeter-slice thickness and multiplanar reformation from a single acquisition. Coronal reformats are particularly useful for evaluation of the orbits, palate, and cranial floor. The volumetric CT data can also be used to create three-dimensional reconstructions which can be useful in the evaluation of complex fractures or preoperative planning. Soft tissue windows are used for the evaluation of complications such as orbital hematoma, extraocular muscle entrapment, or optic nerve impingement. Contrast is unnecessary except in the rare circumstance in which vascular injury is being considered.

Plain Films. While employed less commonly than in the past, facial fractures can often be diagnosed by plain films and are still sometimes obtained in less complicated cases. Four views are usually adequate in the plain film evaluation of acute facial trauma. These are the Caldwell view, a shallow Waters view, a cross-table lateral view, and a submental vertex view. The lateral and submental vertex views are both obtained with a horizontal beam, thus enabling the detection of air–fluid levels.

MR. The facial bones are difficult to visualize on MR scanning because they and the adjacent aerated sinuses are relatively void of signal. MR may be useful for injuries to orbital contents including the optic nerve, globe, and extraocular muscles. It is also useful for assessing potential vascular complications such as arterial dissections, pseudoaneurysms, and arteriovenous fistulas, and it is the best way to evaluate trauma to the temporomandibular joint.

Angiography may be indicated when clinical or radiographic evidence suggests a vascular injury. Vascular injuries are more frequent with penetrating trauma, such as that occurring from gunshot or stab wounds. Fractures that extend through the carotid canal also predispose to vascular injury and may require angiographic evaluation.

Soft Tissue Findings

Indirect signs of facial injury on CT and plain films can help provide objective evidence of trauma, localize the site of impact, and direct attention to areas of potential bony injury.

Paranasal sinus opacification suggests the presence of an associated fracture, particularly when air–fluid levels are seen. Fluid levels are most commonly seen in the maxillary sinus but may also be seen in the frontal or sphenoid sinuses. The ethmoids may become opacified with acute hemorrhage but are less likely to demonstrate fluid levels on plain films, probably because they contain internal septations.

Air in the soft tissues is also suggestive of associated fractures, depending on location. Orbital emphysema is most commonly caused by fracture of the thin medial orbital wall. Orbital floor blow-out fractures can also cause orbital emphysema (Fig. 3.30).

Occasionally, facial images reveal important findings unrelated to fracture of the facial bones. For example, the films should be scrutinized for the presence of foreign bodies that may not be clinically apparent. The craniocervical junction and upper cervical spine should be examined when included in the study. Nasopharyngeal and prevertebral soft tissue swelling can indicate hemorrhage from cervical or skull base fractures. Pneumocephalus or depressed skull fractures are also occasionally seen.

Nasal Fractures

Nasal bone fractures are the most common fractures of the facial skeleton. They can occur as an isolated injury or in association with other facial fractures. Nasal trauma frequently

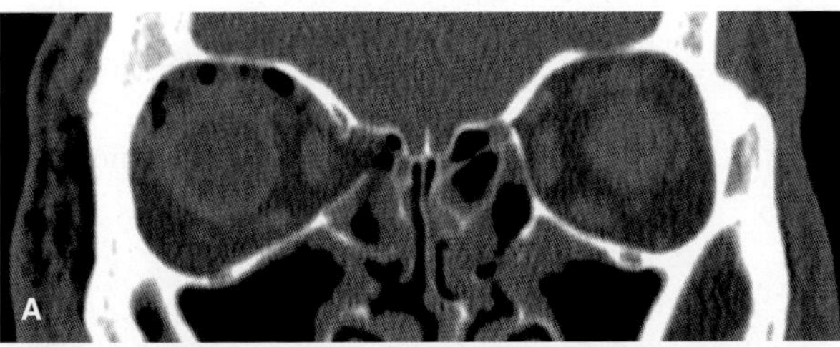

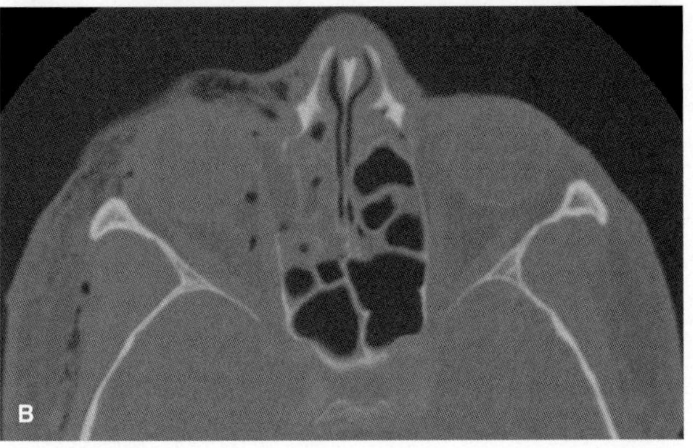

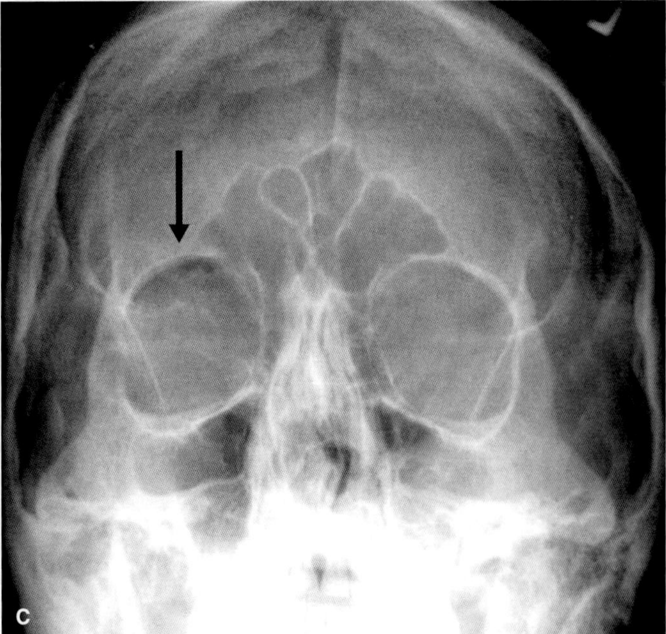

FIGURE 3.30. Medial Orbital Wall Fracture. Coronal (**A**) and axial (**B**) CT images through the orbits reveal discontinuity of the right lamina papyracea that forms the medial orbital wall. There is herniation of orbital fat through the defect into the right ethmoid air cells (**A**) and gas from the sinus is visualized within the orbit (orbital emphysema). AP skull radiograph (**C**) in a different patient reveals right orbital emphysema (*arrow*). Subtle fractures are more difficult to appreciate on plain films, but the presence of orbital emphysema should prompt further evaluation with CT.

results in a depressed fracture of one of the paired nasal bones, without associated ethmoidal injury. An anterior blow can fracture both nasal bones as well as the nasal septum. Associated fractures of the frontal process of the maxilla can be seen. Cartilaginous nasal injury cannot be diagnosed radiographically.

Nasal fractures are usually clinically evident and do not require radiologic diagnosis. Films of the nasal bone may document injury but are generally not useful for patient management and are often unnecessary. Fractures of the nasal bone may be transverse or longitudinal. Longitudinal fractures can be confused with the nasomaxillary suture and nasociliary grooves, which have the same orientation. Transverse fractures of the nasal bone are more common and are easily detected because they are oriented perpendicular to the normal suture line.

When films are obtained, remember to look for fractures of the anterior nasal spine of the maxilla, which may be associated with nasal fractures. One potentially serious injury that can be suggested on plain films or CT is a septal hematoma. Trauma to the septal cartilage may lead to hematoma formation between the perichondrium and cartilage, which can cause cartilage necrosis by disrupting the vascular supply. An organized hematoma can also cause breathing difficulty and may predispose to septal abscess formation.

Maxillary and Paranasal Sinus Fractures

Fracture of the maxillary alveolus is the most common isolated maxillary fracture. It frequently results from a blow to the chin that drives the teeth of the mandible into the maxillary dental arch. These fractures are usually demonstrated by dental films or panorex (panoramic radiographs) but can be seen on CT if the scan is extended inferior to the level of the palate. Associated fractures of the mandible are common with this form of injury, as predicted by the mechanism.

Fractures of the palatine process of the maxilla and horizontal plate of the palatine bone commonly occur in the sagittal plane near the midline. Palate fractures may also be seen in association with complex fractures of the midface (Fig. 3.31).

The most common isolated sinus fracture involves the anterolateral wall of the maxillary antrum. The fracture may be seen directly or may be suspected by the finding of a maxillary sinus fluid level in the setting of acute trauma.

Isolated frontal sinus fractures can also occur and may be more serious if they extend intracranially. Frontal sinus fractures may be linear or comminuted and depressed. Open (compound) frontal sinus fractures involve the posterior sinus wall. These can lead to CSF rhinorrhea and recurrent meningitis or intracerebral abscess formation. Pneumocephalus may be seen in association with these fractures. Fractures of the medial wall and superior rim of the orbit frequently involve the frontal sinus.

Fractures of the sphenoid sinus are often seen in association with fractures of the orbital roof, nasoethmoid complex, midface, or temporal bone. Nondisplaced sphenoid sinus fractures may be subtle on CT. Angiography should be considered if there is a suspicion of associated vascular injury involving the cavernous portion of the internal carotid artery.

Orbital Trauma

Fractures. The orbit is involved in a number of facial fractures including the tripod, Le Fort, and nasoethmoidal complex

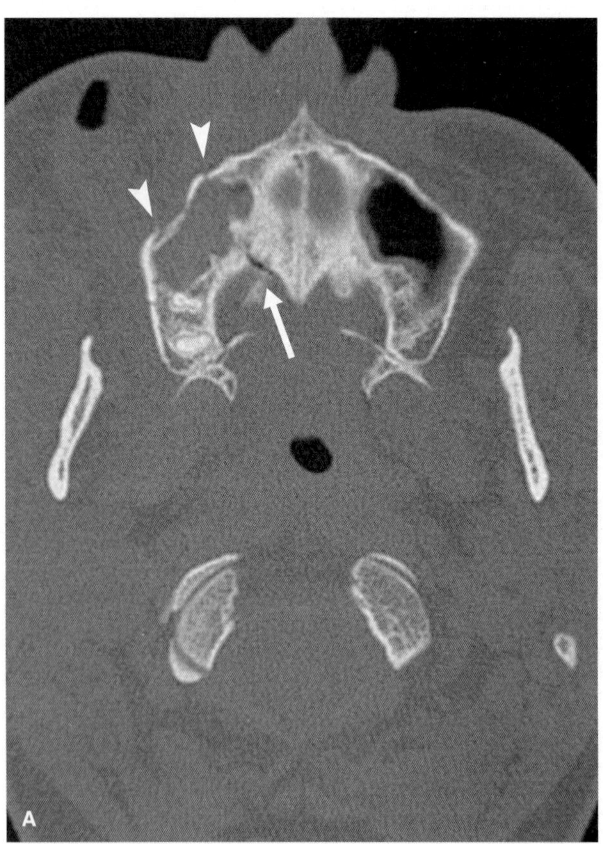

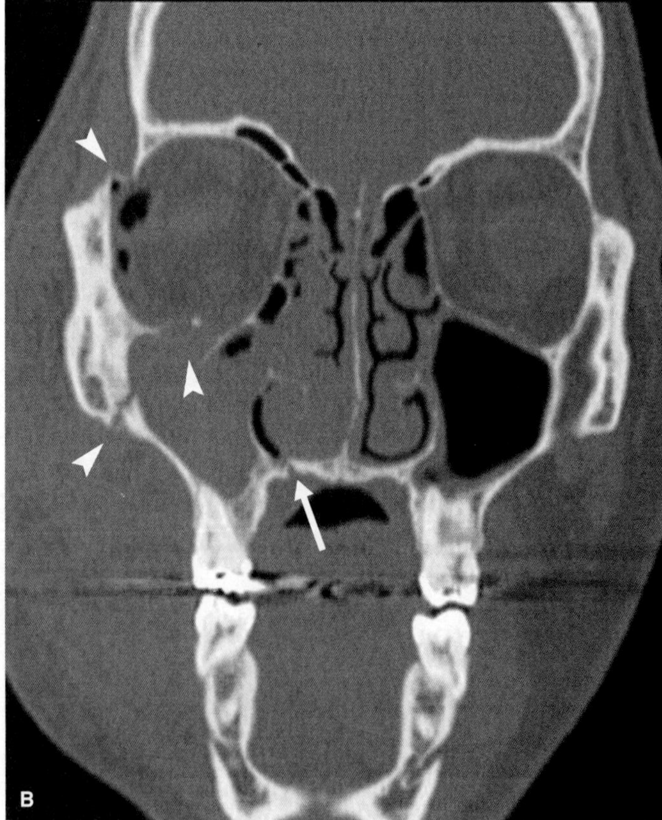

FIGURE 3.31. Palate Fracture. Axial (**A**) and coronal (**B**) CT images reveal a minimally displaced fracture of the right aspect of the hard palate (*arrows*). There are also multiple additional right facial fractures including a right zygomaticomaxillary complex fracture (*arrowheads*). Right-sided orbital emphysema and hemorrhage in the right maxillary sinus are also present.

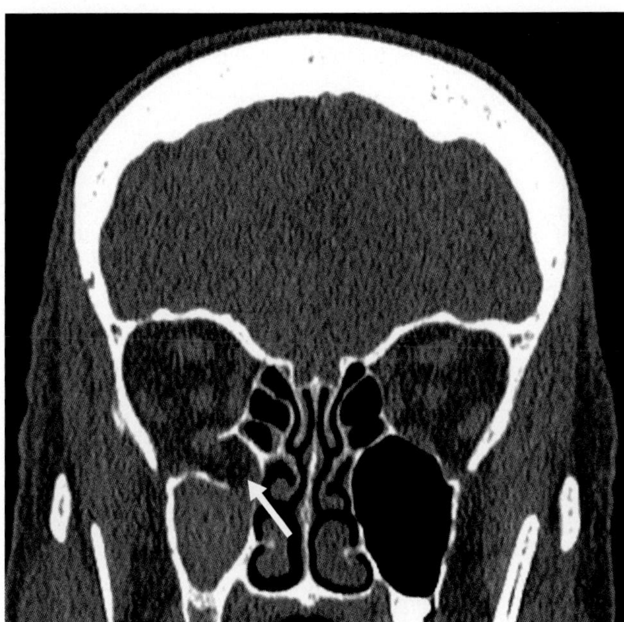

FIGURE 3.32. **Orbital Floor Fracture.** Coronal reformat CT reveals fracture of the right inferior orbital wall with herniation of orbital fat into the defect (*arrow*). The right inferior rectus muscle is also partially herniated and appears mildly enlarged compared to the contralateral left inferior rectus. This appearance is concerning for extraocular muscle entrapment.

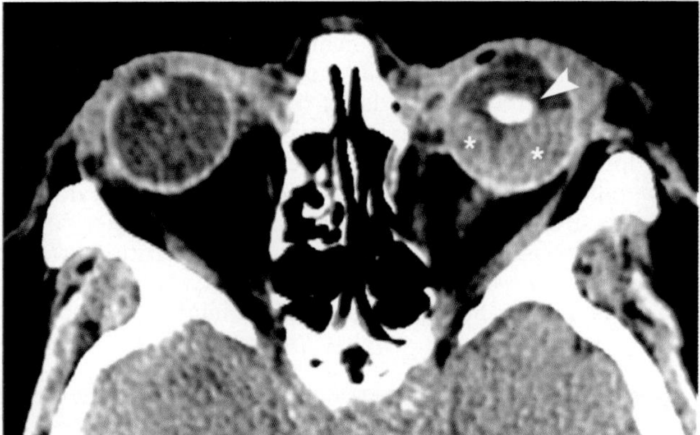

FIGURE 3.33. **Globe Trauma.** Axial CT image through the orbits after trauma to the left globe reveals posterior dislocation of the lens (*arrowhead*) with retinal detachment and a hyperdense subretinal hematoma (*asterisk*).

fractures. Isolated orbital wall fractures usually involve either the medial wall or orbital floor. Medial wall fractures are detected on plain films by the presence of orbital emphysema and opacification of the adjacent ethmoid air cells. Medial wall fractures can be directly visualized well with axial or coronal CT scans. Bone displacement is usually minimal, and muscle entrapment is unusual.

Orbital floor fractures are usually linear when seen in association with other facial fractures. These are rarely associated with entrapment. Comminuted orbital floor fractures, or blow-out fractures, may be seen as an isolated injury and result from a direct blow to the eye. Intraorbital pressure is acutely increased and relieved by fracture through the orbital floor (Fig. 3.32). The orbital rim remains intact in pure blow-out fractures. Blow-out fractures are often associated with herniation of orbital contents through the fracture. When the inferior rectus muscle is compromised, patients will experience persistent vertical diplopia. Mild or transient diplopia can occur simply because of periorbital edema or hemorrhage. Rarely, fragments from an orbital floor fracture buckle upward into the orbit, an injury referred to as a "blow-in" fracture.

Plain film findings suggestive of orbital floor blow-out fractures include orbital emphysema, a fluid level in the ipsilateral maxillary sinus, indistinct orbital floor on Waters view, and soft tissue representing prolapsed orbital contents in the superior aspect of the maxillary sinus. A bony spicule may be seen in the antrum, representing the inferiorly displaced fracture fragment. Blow-out fractures are best seen on coronal CT images (Fig. 3.32).

Soft Tissue Injury. Blunt traumatic injury to the globe can manifest as traumatic globe rupture, lens dislocation, or hemorrhage (Fig. 3.33). Subretinal hemorrhage appears as biconvex high-density collections along the posterior aspect of the globe, bounded by the optic nerve (Fig. 3.33).

Penetrating foreign bodies such as bullets, metal fragments, glass, or other sharp objects account for a significant amount of traumatic injury to the orbit. Thin-section MDCT is the method of choice for confirming the presence of foreign bodies and for this localization. CT can usually clearly define the relationship of bone fragments or foreign bodies to critical structures such as the optic nerve, globe, or extraocular muscles (Fig. 3.34). MR carries a potential risk of further injury by causing motion of intraocular ferromagnetic metal.

Traumatic optic neuropathy is seen in a significant number of patients with severe head trauma and occasionally occurs in patients with relatively minor deceleration injury. Damage may be maximal initially, with unilateral blindness or decreased acuity, or may worsen in the first few days after the

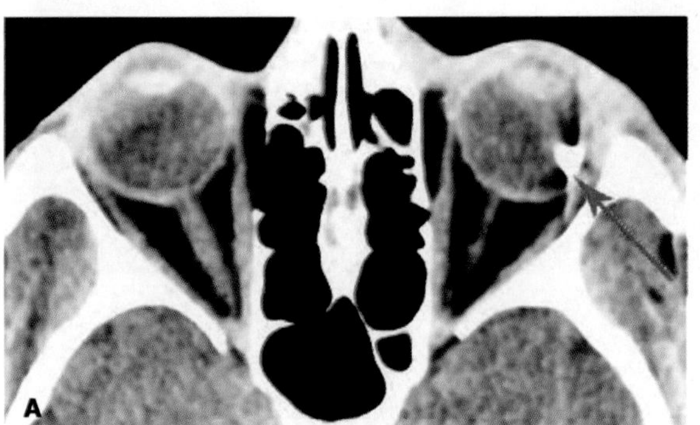

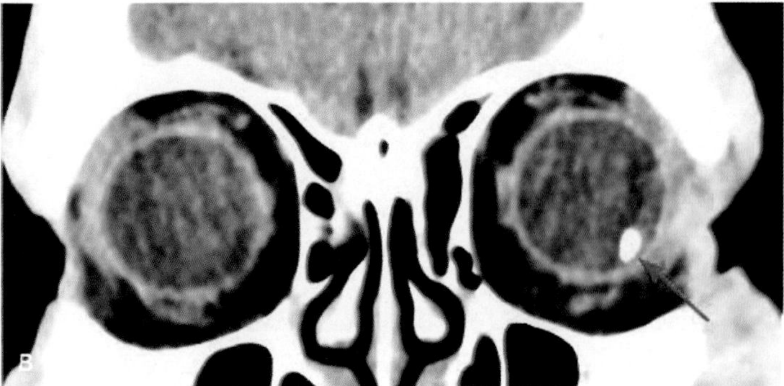

FIGURE 3.34. **Intraocular Metallic Foreign Body.** Axial (**A**) and coronal (**B**) CT scans confirm the presence of a metallic foreign body (*arrows*) in the left globe.

injury. When delayed worsening occurs, secondary optic nerve compression from edema or hemorrhage in the optic nerve sheath should be considered. Imaging studies, particularly CT scans, are indicated to detect fractures through the optic canal or orbital apex. Rarely, displaced fractures are responsible for direct injury to the optic nerve sheath. More commonly, these fractures are nondisplaced but serve as evidence of severe stress transmitted to the orbital apex. Primary optic nerve injury may occur as a result of deceleration strain, causing damage to the delicate meningeal vessels or direct neural disruption. Secondary optic nerve injury may occur as a result of swelling of the optic nerve within the rigid bony canal, with subsequent mechanical compression and vascular compromise.

Fractures of the Zygoma

The zygoma, or "cheekbone," is one of the most common sites of injury in fractures that involve multiple facial bones. Zygomatic arch fractures may occur as an isolated finding, or as part of a zygomaticomaxillary complex ("tripod,"

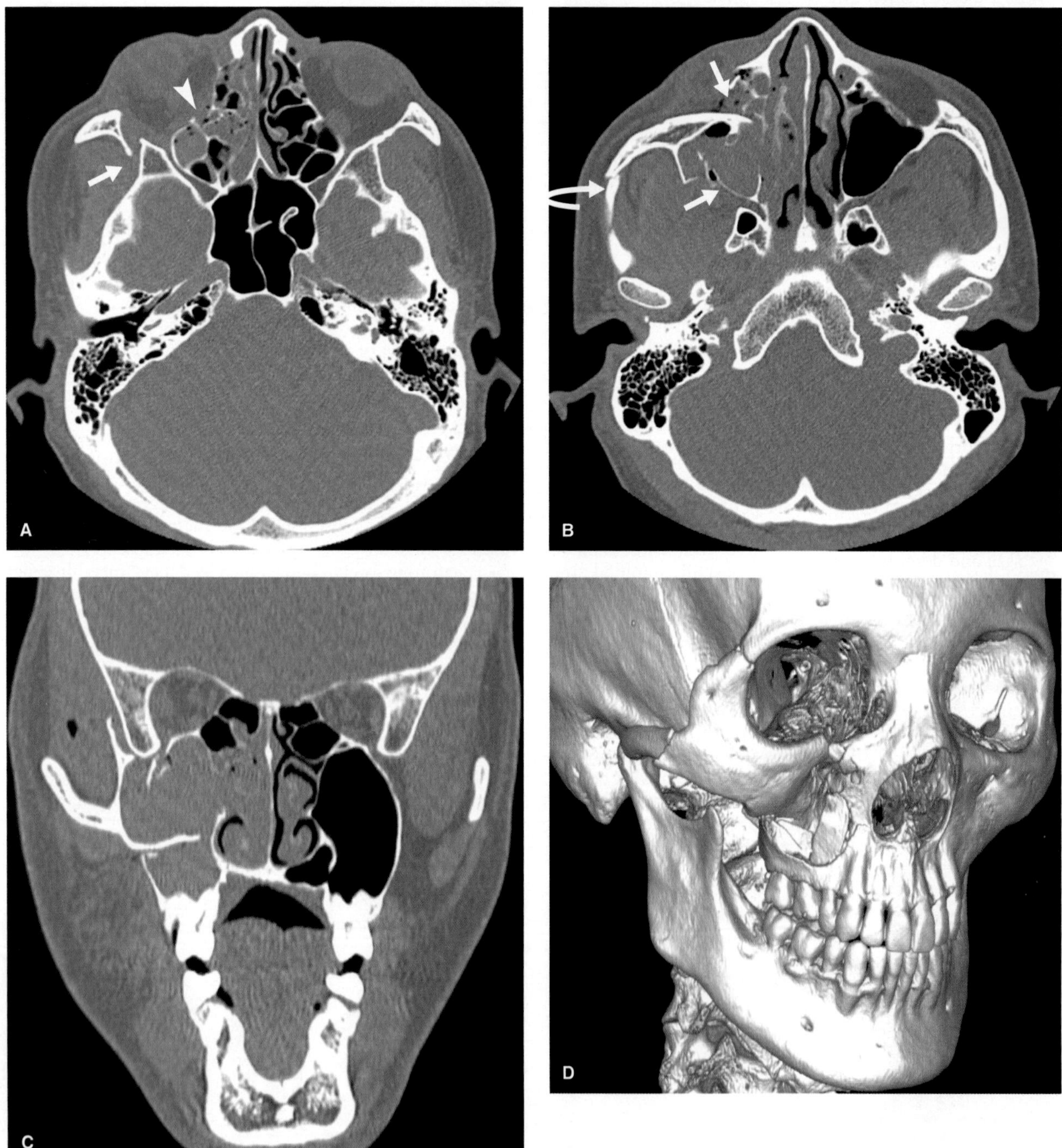

FIGURE 3.35. Zygomaticomaxillary Complex Fracture. Axial (**A**, **B**) and coronal CT reformats reveal right-sided fractures through the lateral orbital wall/zygoma (**A**, *arrow*), orbital floor (**A**, *arrowhead*), zygomatic arch (**B**, *curved arrow*), and anterior and posterior walls of the right maxillary sinus (**B**, *arrows*). Coronal reformat (**C**) and 3D reconstructions (**D**) provide excellent perspective of the displaced fracture and resultant deformity of the right inferolateral orbit.

"quadripod," or "trimalar") fracture. Comminution and depression are frequently seen with zygomatic arch fractures. On plain films, the zygomatic arch is best evaluated on the submental vertex view. Deformity of the arch is a frequent finding in populations with a high incidence of facial trauma, and clinical examination may be required to differentiate acute from chronic injury.

Zygomaticomaxillary complex fractures usually result from a blow to the face. The zygoma articulates with the frontal, maxillary, sphenoid, and temporal bones. Fractures are somewhat variable, but typically involve the zygomatic arch, zygomaticofrontal suture, infraorbital rim, orbital floor, lateral wall of the maxillary sinus, and lateral wall of the orbit. Injury to the infraorbital nerve is common, secondary to fracture of the infraorbital rim at the infraorbital foramen. Diastasis of the zygomaticofrontal suture may injure the lateral canthal ligament or suspensory ligaments of the globe. Many of the fractures associated with this injury can be seen on plain films but are better demonstrated by CT scan (Fig. 3.35). Associated findings on plain films include opacification of the ipsilateral maxillary antrum and posterior displacement of the body of the zygoma on the submental vertex view with overlying soft tissue swelling.

Fractures of the Midface (Le Fort Fractures)

Complex fractures of the facial bones are frequently classified according to the method of Le Fort, who developed his theory by inflicting facial trauma on cadavers and analyzing the results. He described three general patterns of fractures that differ in location of the fracture plane across the face (Fig. 3.36).[36] The three Le Fort fractures initially described are bilateral processes. All involve the pterygoid plates, which help anchor the facial bones to the skull. Although there is great variability in complex facial fractures, and the classic Le Fort injuries are rarely seen in their pure form, they remain a convenient way to categorize and describe basic patterns of injury. Frequently, similar patterns of injury are seen on one side only and are known as "hemi–Le Fort" injuries. Combinations also occur, such as a Le Fort I pattern on one side and a Le Fort II pattern on the other.

Le Fort I, or "floating palate," fracture is a horizontal fracture through the maxillary sinuses. It extends through the nasal septum and walls of the maxillary sinuses into the inferior aspect of the pterygoid plates. The fracture plane is parallel to the plane of axial CT images but is recognized by the fracture of all walls of both maxillary sinuses (Fig. 3.37). It is well seen in the coronal plane. There may be an associated midpalatal or maxillary split fracture. The Le Fort I fracture is more often seen in the pure form than is either the Le Fort II or Le Fort III fractures. It occasionally may be accompanied by a unilateral zygomaticomaxillary complex fracture.

Le Fort II, or "pyramidal," fracture describes a fracture through the medial orbital and lateral maxillary walls. It begins at the bridge of the nose and extends in a pyramidal fashion through the nasal septum, frontal process of the maxilla, medial wall of the orbit, inferior orbital rim, superior, lateral, and posterior walls of the maxillary antrum, and midportion of the pterygoid plates. The zygomatic arch and lateral orbital walls are left intact. The Le Fort II is usually associated with posterior displacement of the facial bones, resulting in a "dish-face" deformity and malocclusion. The infraorbital nerve is frequently injured. Le Fort II fractures are rarely seen in the pure form.

Le Fort III fracture, or "craniofacial disjunction," is a horizontally oriented fracture through the orbits. It begins near the nasofrontal suture and extends posteriorly to involve the nasal septum, medial and lateral orbital walls, zygomatic arch, and base (superior aspect) of the pterygoid plates. Patients with a Le Fort III fracture also have dish-face deformity and malocclusion. Injury to the infraorbital nerve is less commonly seen with Le Fort III than with Le Fort II fractures. A recognizable feature on plain films is the elongated appearance of the orbits on Waters and Caldwell views.

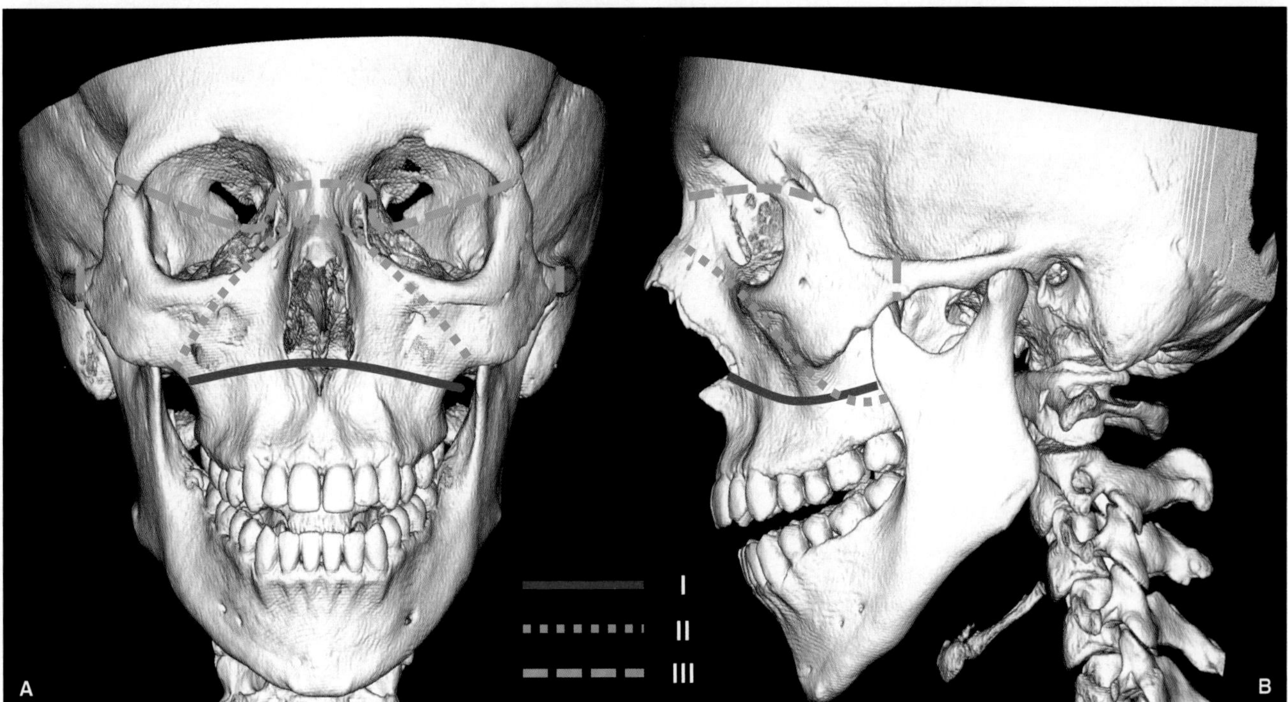

FIGURE 3.36. **Diagram of Le Fort Fractures.** Frontal (**A**) and lateral (**B**) projections of a 3D reconstruction of a facial CT demonstrate the patterns of facial fractures as originally described by Le Fort.

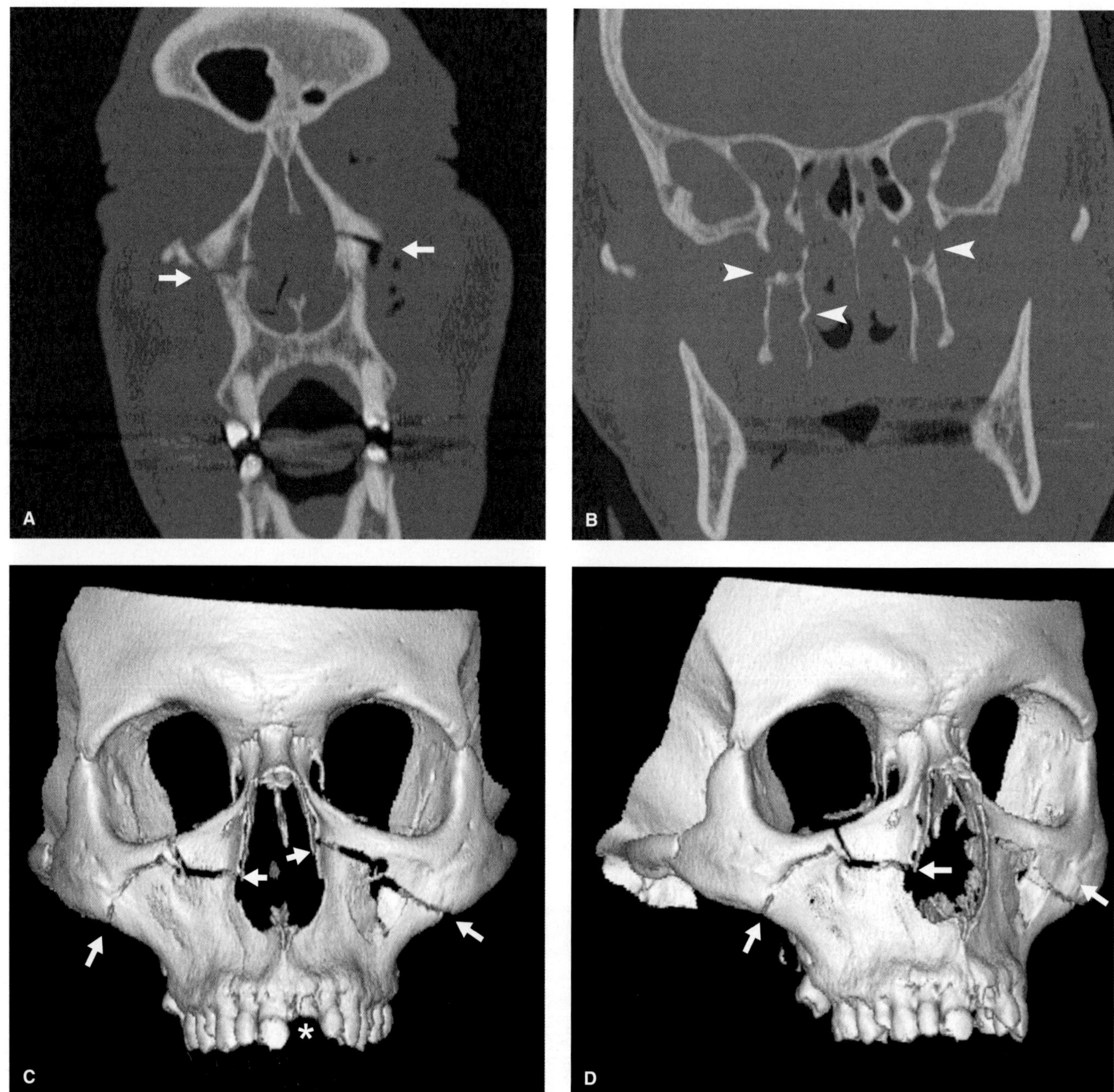

FIGURE 3.37. Le Fort I Fracture. Coronal CT reformats through the anterior (**A**) and posterior (**B**) aspects of the maxillary sinuses reveal fractures extending through all walls of the maxillary sinuses extending through the pterygoid plates (**B**, *arrowheads*). This injury is often best appreciated on coronal images as the fracture lines can often run parallel to axial images. These fractures (*arrows*) disrupt all three vertical buttresses of the maxilla (nasomaxillary, zygomaticomaxillary, and pterygomaxillary) and can lead to the "floating maxilla" appearance, which is well demonstrated on AP (**C**) and oblique (**D**) 3D reconstructions. Note that the left maxillary central incisor has also been avulsed (*asterisk*).

When interpreting CT scans obtained for facial trauma, it is probably best to describe the specific bones that are fractured on either side of the face. When appropriate, the Le Fort injury that best describes the distribution of fractures may also be used to categorize complex fractures.

Nasoethmoidal Fractures

Nasoethmoidal complex injuries describe the constellation of findings seen as a result of a blow to the midface between the eyes. This term encompasses a wide variety of different fracture complexes that are best described by listing the specific fractures seen on CT scans. These injuries may include fractures of the lamina papyracea, inferior, medial, and supraorbital rims, frontal or ethmoid sinuses, orbital roofs, nasal bone and frontal process of the maxilla, and sphenoid bone (Fig. 3.38). These fractures have also been called orbitoethmoid or nasoethmoid–orbital fractures because of the importance of the often-associated orbital injuries. There may be associated fractures of the skull base and clivus. Other findings include orbital and intracranial air, opacification of the ethmoid and frontal sinuses, and depression of the midface. Nasoethmoidal fractures can be suspected on plain films when the lateral view shows posterior displacement of the nasion. Thin-section CT helps evaluate the extent of the injury and

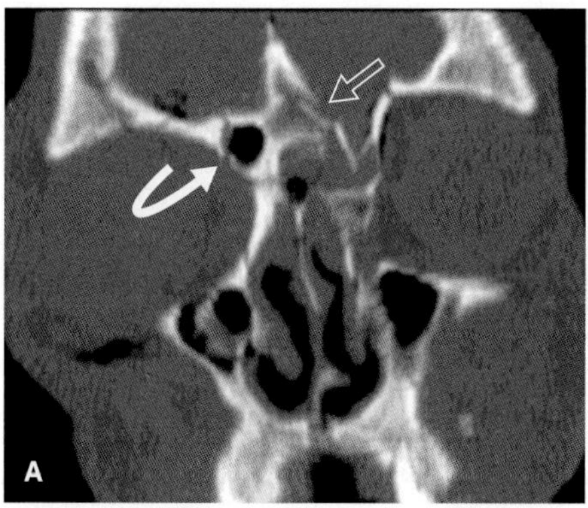

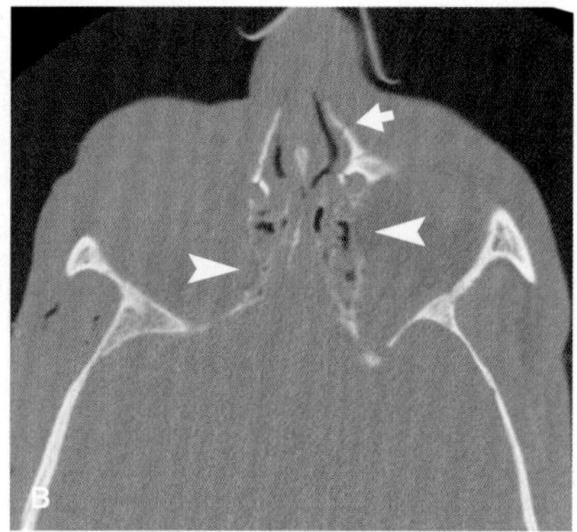

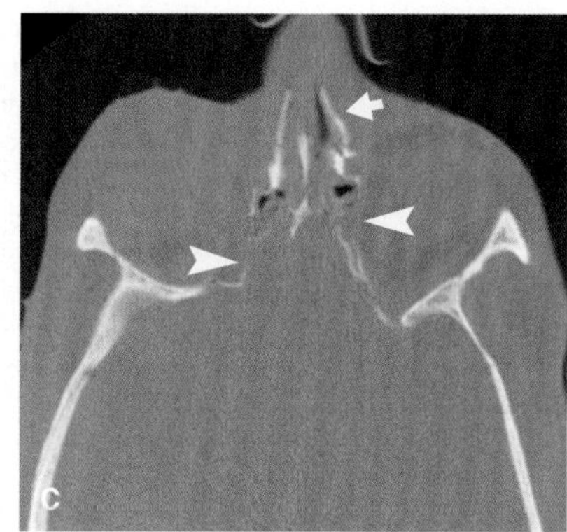

FIGURE 3.38. **Naso-Orbitoethmoid Complex Fracture.** Coronal (**A**) and axial (**B, C**) CT images demonstrate a depressed fracture involving the root of the nose (*open arrow*), nasal bones (*arrows*), nasal lacrimal duct (*curved arrow*), and anterior ethmoids. Bilateral fractures of the medial orbital walls are also present (*arrowheads*) with orbital emphysema. Fracture also extends through the roofs of the orbits with a small amount of pneumocephalus (**A**).

helps localize bony fragments that might encroach on the optic nerve or canal.

Complications of nasoethmoidal complex fractures depend on the location and extent of injury. Patients with fractures involving the floor of the anterior cranial fossa are prone to develop CSF leaks because of the high frequency of associated dural lacerations. The olfactory nerves are frequently injured when fractures extend to the cribriform plate. As mentioned earlier, orbital injuries are often seen as a component of naso-ethmoid fractures. The globes or optic nerves may be damaged by displaced medial orbital wall fracture fragments.

Mandibular Fractures

Mandibular fractures are extremely common in patients with maxillofacial injury. CT is again the most sensitive study and typically the initial imaging study obtained, though, plain films can still be used in the initial evaluation of patients with suspected mandibular injury. The mandibular series includes PA, lateral, Towne, and bilateral oblique projections. Panoramic radiographs (panorex films) can also be used to evaluate mandibular injury.

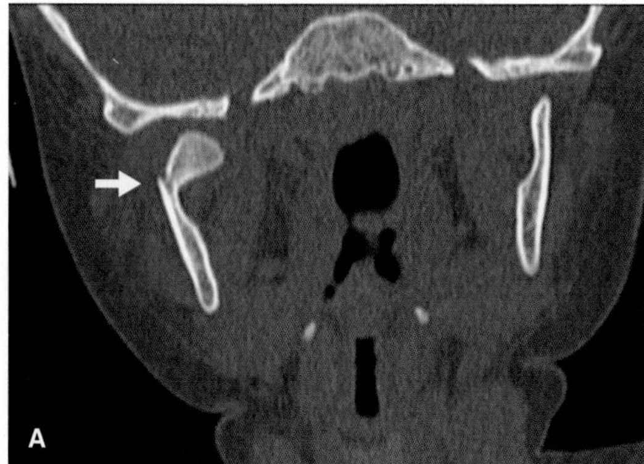

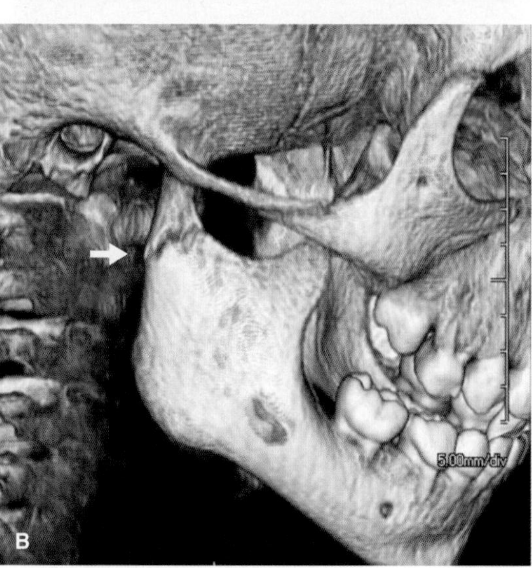

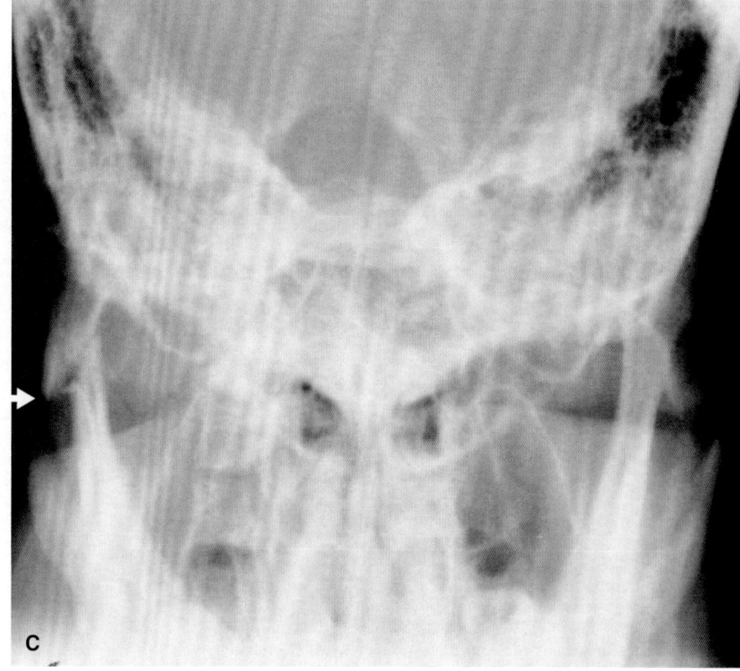

FIGURE 3.39. **Mandibular Condylar Fracture.** Coronal reformat CT (**A**) and 3D reconstruction (**B**) from a 2.5 year old after trauma to the right face reveal a displaced right mandibular condyle fracture (*arrows*). Radiograph in Towne projection (**C**) from a different adult patient with a similar injury shows a displaced right subcondylar fracture (*arrow*).

Mandibular fractures can be considered either simple or compound. Simple fractures are most common in the ramus and condyle and do not communicate externally or with the mouth. Compound fractures are those that communicate internally through a tooth socket or externally through a laceration. Fractures of the body of the mandible are almost always compound fractures. Pathologic mandibular fractures can occur at sites of infection or neoplasm. Mandibular fractures are frequently multiple or bilateral, and such fractures often involve the condyle (Fig. 3.39). Subcondylar fractures may be recognized on plain films by the "cortical ring" sign, a well-corticated density seen above the condylar neck on lateral views because of the horizontal axis of the fragment. A common pattern of injury is a unilateral condylar fracture with a contralateral fracture of the mandibular angle. The mandibular angle is also the most common site of isolated injury. Fractures of the ramus and coronoid processes are rare. Fractures through the symphysis or parasymphyseal region are common but difficult to diagnose on plain films because of the obliquity of the fracture plane. Fractures involving the dentoalveolar complex are also often missed on mandibular series and require intraoral dental films or CT for evaluation. Bilateral fractures through the mandibular body or comminuted fractures can lead to airway obstruction from posterior displacement of the tongue and free mandibular fragment.

References

1. Wintermark M, Sanelli PC, Anzai Y, Tsiouris AJ, Whitlow CT. Imaging evidence and recommendations for traumatic brain injury: advanced neuro- and neurovascular imaging techniques. *AJNR Am J Neuroradiol* 2015;36(2):E1–E11.
2. Ryan ME, Palasis S, Saigal G, et al. ACR Appropriateness Criteria head trauma—child. *J Am Coll Radiol* 2014;11(10):939–947.
3. Shetty VS, Reis MN, Aulino JM, et al. ACR Appropriateness Criteria head trauma. *J Am Coll Radiol* 2016;13(6):668–679.
4. Gentry LR, Godersky JC, Thompson B, Dunn VD. Prospective comparative study of intermediate-field MR and CT in the evaluation of closed head trauma. *AJR Am J Roentgenol* 1988;150:673–682.
5. Orrison WW, Gentry LR, Stimac GK, Tarrel RM, Espinosa MC, Cobb LC. Blinded comparison of cranial CT and MR in closed head injury evaluation. *AJNR Am J Neuroradiol* 1994;15:351–356.
6. Noguchi K, Ogawa T, Seto H, et al. Subacute and chronic subarachnoid hemorrhage: diagnosis with fluid-attenuated inversion-recovery MR imaging. *Radiology* 1997;203:257–262.
7. Woodcock RJ, Short J, Do HM, Jensen ME, Kallmes DF. Imaging of acute subarachnoid hemorrhage with a fluid-attenuated inversion recovery sequence in an animal model: comparison with non-contrast-enhanced CT. *AJNR Am J Neuroradiol* 2001;22:1698–1703.
8. Haacke EM, Xu Y, Cheng YC, Reichenbach JR. Susceptibility weighted imaging (SWI). *Magn Reson Med* 2004;52:612–618.
9. Tong KA, Ashwal S, Holshouser BA, et al. Hemorrhagic shearing lesions in children and adolescents with posttraumatic diffuse axonal injury: improved detection and initial results. *Radiology* 2003;227:332–339.
10. Alsop DC, Murai H, Detre JA, McIntosh TK, Smith DH. Detection of acute pathologic changes following experimental traumatic brain injury using diffusion-weighted magnetic resonance imaging. *J Neurotrauma* 1996;13: 515–521.
11. Huisman TA, Schwamm LH, Schaefer PW, et al. Diffusion tensor imaging as potential biomarker of white matter injury in diffuse axonal injury. *AJNR Am J Neuroradiol* 2004;25:370–376.
12. Arfanakis K, Haughton VM, Carew JD, Rogers BP, Dempsey RJ, Meyerand ME. Diffusion tensor MR imaging in diffuse axonal injury. *AJNR Am J Neuroradiol* 2002;23:794–802.
13. Liu AY, Maldjian JA, Bagley LJ, Sinson GP, Grossman RI. Traumatic brain injury: diffusion-weighted MR imaging findings. *AJNR Am J Neuroradiol* 1999;20:1636–1641.
14. Stiell IG, Wells GA, Vandemheen K, et al. The Canadian CT Head Rule for patients with minor head injury. *Lancet* 2001;357:1391–1396.
15. Mower WR, Hoffman JR, Herbert M, et al. Developing a decision instrument to guide computed tomographic imaging of blunt head injury patients. *J Trauma* 2005;59:954–959.
16. Haydel MJ, Preston CA, Mills TJ, Luber S, Blaudeau E, DeBlieux PM. Indications for computed tomography in patients with minor head injury. *N Engl J Med* 2000;343:100–105.
17. Ulrich K. Verletzungen des Gehorlorgans bei Schadelbasisfrakturen: eine histologische und klinische Studie. *Acta Otolaryngol Suppl* 1926;6:1–150.
18. Dahiya R, Keller JD, Litofsky NS, Bankey PE, Bonassar LJ, Megerian CA. Temporal bone fractures: otic capsule sparing versus otic capsule violating clinical and radiographic considerations. *J Trauma* 1999;47:1079–1083.
19. Little SC, Kesser BW. Radiographic classification of temporal bone fractures: clinical predictability using a new system. *Arch Otolaryngol Head Neck Surg* 2006;132:1300–1304.
20. Gentry LR. Temporal bone trauma: current perspective for diagnostic evaluation. *Neuroimaging Clin N Am* 1991;1:319–340.
21. Ghorayeb BY, Yeakley JW. Temporal bone fractures: longitudinal or oblique? The case for oblique temporal bone fractures. *Laryngoscope* 1992;102:129–134.
22. Gentry LR. Imaging of closed head injury. *Radiology* 1994;191:1–17.
23. Verma RK, Kottke R, Andereggen L, et al. Detecting subarachnoid hemorrhage: comparison of combined FLAIR/SWI versus CT. *Eur J Radiol* 2013;82:1539–1545.
24. Stuckey SL, Goh TD, Heffernan T, Rowan D. Hyperintensity in the subarachnoid space on FLAIR MRI. *AJR Am J Roentgenol* 2007;189:913–921.
25. Gentry LR, Thompson B, Godersky JC. Trauma to the corpus callosum: MR features. *AJNR Am J Neuroradiol* 1988;9:1129–1138.
26. Gennarelli TA, Thibault LE, Adams JH, Graham DI, Thompson CJ, Marcincin RP. Diffuse axonal injury and traumatic coma in the primate. *Ann Neurol* 1982;12:564–574.
27. Shanmuganathan K, Gullapalli RP, Mirvis SE, Roys S, Murthy P. Whole-brain apparent diffusion coefficient in traumatic brain injury: correlation with Glasgow Coma Scale score. *AJNR Am J Neuroradiol* 2004;25:539–544.
28. Yuh EL, Cooper SR, Mukherjee P, et al. Diffusion tensor imaging for outcome prediction in mild traumatic brain injury: a TRACK-TBI study. *J Neurotrauma* 2014;31:1457–1477.
29. Moen KG, Brezova V, Skandsen T, Håberg AK, Folvik M, Vik A. Traumatic axonal injury: the prognostic value of lesion load in corpus callosum, brain stem, and thalamus in different magnetic resonance imaging sequences. *J Neurotrauma* 2014;31:1486–1496.
30. Bruce DA, Zimmerman RA. Shaken impact syndrome. *Pediatr Ann* 1989; 18:482–484, 486–489, 492–494.
31. Merten DF, Osborne DR, Radkowski MA, Leonidas JC. Craniocerebral trauma in the child abuse syndrome: radiological observations. *Pediatr Radiol* 1984;14:272–277.
32. Zimmerman RA, Bilaniuk LT. Pediatric head trauma. *Neuroimaging Clin N Am* 1994;4:349–366.
33. Caffey J. Multiple fractures in the long bones of infants suffering from chronic subdural hematoma. *Am J Roentgenol Radium Ther* 1946;56:163–173.
34. Duhaime AC, Gennarelli TA, Thibault LE, Bruce DA, Margulies SS, Wiser R. The shaken baby syndrome. A clinical, pathological, and biomechanical study. *J Neurosurg* 1987;66:409–415.
35. Cohen AR, Caruso P, Duhaime AC, Klig JE. Feasibility of "rapid" magnetic resonance imaging in pediatric acute head injury. *Am J Emerg Med* 2015; 33:887–890.
36. Le Fort R. Etude experimentale sur les fractures de la machoire superieure, parts I, II, III. *Revue Chirurgio* 1901;23:208–227.

Suggested Readings

Intracranial Injury

Gean AD. *Brain Injury: Applications From War and Terrorism*. Philadelphia, PA: Wolters Kluwer Health; 2014: p. 338.

Wintermark M, Sanelli PC, Anzai Y, Tsiouris AJ, Whitlow CT. Imaging evidence and recommendations for traumatic brain injury: advanced neuro- and neurovascular imaging techniques. *AJNR Am J Neuroradiol* 2015;36(2):E1–E11.

Wintermark M, Sanelli PC, Anzai Y, Tsiouris AJ, Whitlow CT. Imaging evidence and recommendations for traumatic brain injury: conventional neuroimaging techniques. *J Am Coll Radiol* 2015;12:e1–e14.

Cranial and Skull Base Injury

Kennedy TA, Avey GD, Gentry LR. Imaging of temporal bone trauma. *Neuroimaging Clin N Am* 2014;24(3):467–486, viii.

Head Trauma in Child Abuse

Choudhary AK, Servaes S, Slovis TL, et al. Consensus statement on abusive head trauma in infants and young children. *Pediatric Radiology [electronic article]* 2018. Available from https://doi.org/10.1007/s00247-018-4149-1.

Facial Trauma

Uzelac A, Gean AD. Orbital and facial fractures. *Neuroimaging Clin N Am* 2014;24(3):407–424, vii.

CHAPTER 4 ■ CEREBROVASCULAR DISEASE

HOWARD A. ROWLEY

Stroke is a clinical term applied to any abrupt nontraumatic brain insult—literally "a blow from an unseen hand." Strokes are caused by either brain infarction (75%) or hemorrhage (25%), and must be distinguished from other conditions causing abrupt neurologic deficits. *Infarction* is a permanent injury which occurs when tissue perfusion is decreased long enough to cause necrosis, typically due to occlusion of the feeding artery. *Transient ischemic attacks* (TIAs) are classically defined as transient neurologic symptoms or signs lasting less than 24 hours, which may serve as a "warning sign" of an infarction occurring in the next few weeks or months. TIAs are often due to temporary occlusion of a feeding artery. Even though signs and symptoms may be transient, a TIA patient is considered to have had a stroke if imaging confirms an acute lesion. *Hemorrhage* is seen when blood ruptures through the arterial wall, spilling into the surrounding parenchyma, subarachnoid space, or ventricles.

Stroke is the third leading cause of death in the United States and major source of long-term disability among survivors. The approach to treatment of ischemic stroke has been largely preventative or supportive in the past, but approval of intravenous (IV) thrombolysis for acute stroke and proven outcome benefits of endovascular devices have made rapid imaging and intervention a critical part of stroke management. The patient with hemorrhage may harbor an aneurysm, vascular malformation, or other condition, each having important differences in treatment options. The radiologist plays a critical role in the triage and evaluation of all stroke patients. Selection of the proper imaging protocol, recognition of early ischemic changes, differentiation of stroke from other brain disorders, and recognition of important stroke subtypes can have a significant impact on therapy and outcome.

This chapter reviews the pathophysiology of stroke, the time course of findings on computed tomography and magnetic resonance imaging, patterns of arterial and venous occlusions, and overall radiologic approach to evaluation of the stroke patient.

ISCHEMIC STROKE

Etiology. Despite our best clinical efforts, no clear source is ever identified in up to a quarter of patients with brain infarction. Among those with an established mechanism, about two-thirds of infarcts are caused by thrombi and one-third by emboli. Thrombi are formed at sites of abnormal vascular endothelium, typically over an area of atherosclerotic plaque or ulcer. Small vessel thrombi frequently occur in "end-arteries" of the brain, accounting for about one-fifth of infarcts ("lacunes"). Emboli may arise from the heart, aortic arch, carotid arteries, or vertebral arteries, causing infarction by distal migration and occlusion. There is obviously overlap between the thrombotic and embolic groups, since the majority of emboli begin as thrombi somewhere more proximal in the cardiovascular tree (hence the practical term, "thromboembolic disease"). Vasculitis, vasospasm, coagulopathies, global hypoperfusion, and venous thrombosis each account for 5% or fewer of acute strokes, but are important to recognize due to differing treatment and prognosis. A given patient's age, medical history, and type of stroke seen will help establish the major etiologic considerations (Table 4.1).

Pathophysiologic Basis for Imaging Changes

Brain Metabolism and Selective Vulnerability. Neurons lead a precarious life. The brain consumes 20% of the total cardiac output to maintain its minute-to-minute delivery of glucose and oxygen. Since there are no significant long-term energy stores (e.g., glycogen, fat), disruption of blood flow for even a few minutes will lead to neuronal death. The extent of injury depends on both the duration and degree of ischemia. Minor reduction in perfusion is initially compensated for by increased extraction of substrate, but injury becomes inevitable below a critical flow threshold (10 to 20 mL/100 g tissue/min vs. normal 55 mL/100 g tissue/min).

TABLE 4.1

DIFFERENTIAL DIAGNOSIS OF ISCHEMIC STROKE BY AGE

■ PEDIATRIC	■ YOUNG ADULT	■ ELDERLY
Congenital heart disease	Cardiac emboli	Atherosclerosis
Blood dyscrasias	Atherosclerosis	Cardiac emboli
Meningitis	Drug abuse	Coagulopathy
Arterial dissection	Arterial dissection	Amyloid
Trauma	Coagulopathy	Vasculitis
ECMO	Vasculitis	Venous thrombosis
Venous thrombosis	Venous thrombosis	

ECMO, extracorporeal membrane oxygenation.

Certain cell types and neuroanatomic regions show selective vulnerability to ischemic injury. Gray matter normally receives three to four times more blood flow than white matter, and is therefore more likely to suffer under conditions of oligemia. Some subsets of neurons (e.g., cerebellar Purkinje cells, hippocampal CA-1 neurons) are injured more readily than others, possibly due to greater concentrations of receptors for excitatory amino acids. The slower metabolizing capillary endothelial cells and white matter oligodendrocytes are more resistant to ischemia than gray matter, but will also die when deprived of nutrients. Cells served by penetrating end-arteries or those residing in the watershed zone between major territories have no alternate route for perfusion, and are therefore more prone to infarction. Damage will likely be more severe in a patient with an incomplete circle of Willis than in one with a complete arterial collateral pathway.

Imaging Findings in Acute Ischemia. Ischemia causes a cascade of cellular level events leading to the gross pathologic changes detected in clinical imaging. Failure of membrane pumps permits efflux of K^+ and simultaneous influx of Ca^{2+}, Na^+, and water. This leads to cellular ("cytotoxic") edema, observed clinically as increased water content in the affected region. *Changes in brain water are key to understanding signs of infarction by CT and MR.* Even a small increase in water content causes characteristic decreased attenuation on CT, low signal on T1-weighted MR, and high signal on T2- and diffusion-weighted MR. Cytotoxic edema peaks 3 to 7 days post infarction and is maximum in the gray matter. A smaller component of vasogenic edema also develops as the more resistant capillary endothelial cells lose integrity. (In contrast, tumor-associated edema is primarily vasogenic and preferentially affects the white matter—see Chapter 5.)

Careful inspection of CT and MR images done within minutes to a few hours after vessel occlusion can give clues to ischemic injury, even before gross tissue edema or mass effect are seen. These "hyperacute" signs primarily relate to morphologic changes in the vessels or physiology of perfusion rather than density or signal changes in the parenchyma. On CT, the actual thrombus may occasionally be seen in larger intracranial branches, resulting in the "hyperdense artery sign" (Fig. 4.1). On MR, the normal black signal of flowing blood within the

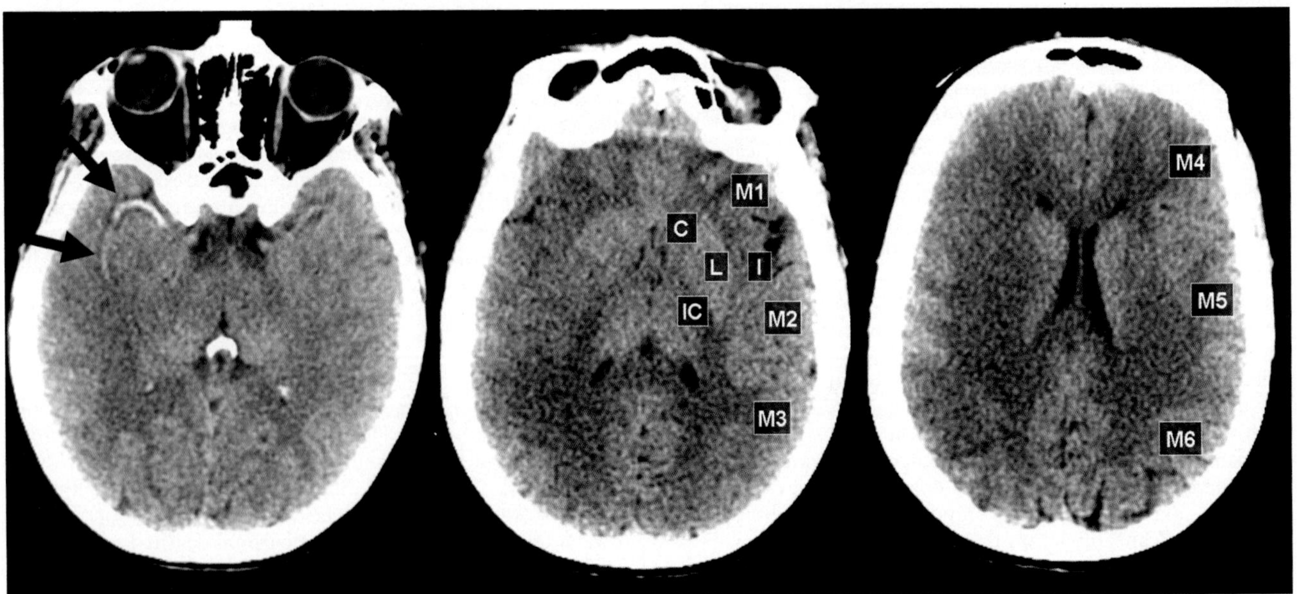

FIGURE 4.1. Hyperdense Artery Sign and Early Edema on CT. Three hours post occlusion, high density indicative of thrombus is seen in the proximal right middle cerebral artery (*arrows*). Extensive right hemisphere edema is already present. The 10 regions scored by ASPECTS are shown in the normal left hemisphere. The ASPECT score is only 3, with points off for low attenuation in the right insula, posterior lentiform nucleus, M1, M2, M3, M4, and M5 cortical regions. Edema involves more than 1/3 MCA territory and ASPECTS is much lower than 7, both predicting a poor candidate for acute thrombolysis. For a tutorial on ASPECT scoring, see: www.aspectsinstroke.com.

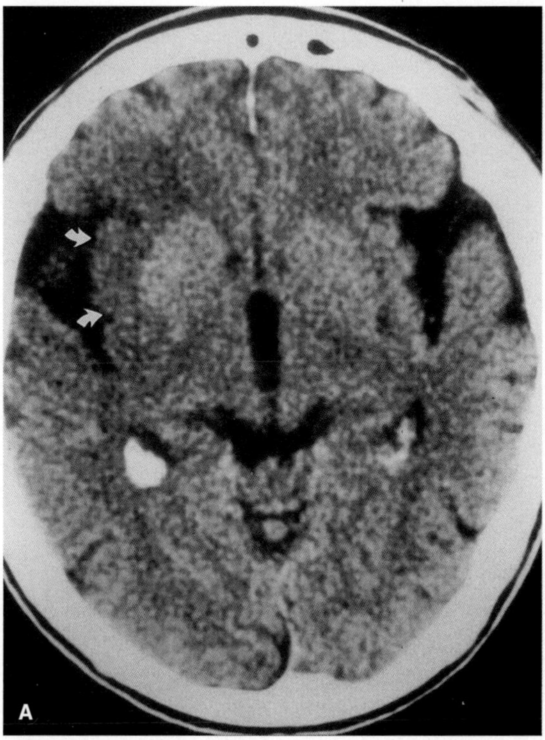

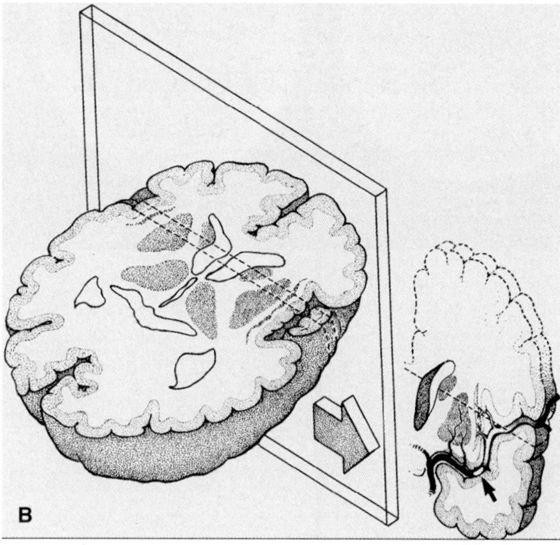

FIGURE 4.2. **Insular Ribbon Sign. A:** A noncontrast CT done 4 hours after right MCA occlusion shows decreased attenuation and loss of gray-white borders in the right insular region (*arrows*). **B:** Diagram of the insula in transverse and coronal planes. The insular cortex, claustrum, and extreme capsule are infarcted due to occlusion of the MCA (*arrow*) beyond the lateral lenticulostriate vessels. (From Truwit CL, Barkovich AJ, Gean-Marton A, Hibri N, Norman D. Loss of the insular ribbon: another early CT sign of acute middle cerebral artery infarction. *Radiology* 1990;176:801–806.)

lumen ("flow void") is immediately lost and may be replaced by abnormal signal representing clot or slow flow.

Acute MCA Ischemia on CT: Insular Ribbon and Lentiform Nucleus Edema. CT scans done within 6 hours of middle cerebral artery (MCA) occlusion will commonly exhibit the "insular ribbon sign," a subtle but important blurring of the gray-white layers of the insula due to early edema (Fig. 4.2). Early edema may also be most conspicuous in the putamen in proximal MCA occlusions (lentiform nucleus edema sign). MR examinations in the first few hours may show a similar loss of gray-white borders and slight crowding of sulci in areas destined to undergo infarction. However, the most sensitive imaging sequence for detection of brain ischemia is diffusion-weighted MR imaging, which may turn positive minutes after infarction begins, well before the CT shows even subtle signs. Hyperintense signal on diffusion-weighted images (DWIs) ("light-bulb sign") precedes T2 hyperintensity, which typically develops at 6 to 12 hours post ictus (Fig. 4.5).

Imaging Triage for Emergency Stroke Intervention

Careful but rapid interpretation of CT scans is particularly important in patients who are candidates for IV thrombolytic drug treatment (e.g., tissue plasminogen activator [t-PA]), intra-arterial (IA) endovascular intervention, or combined treatment. IV t-PA is front line therapy for patients within 4.5 hours of symptom onset, and patients with favorable imaging may also be selected for endovascular thrombectomy up to at least 24 hours, sometimes using a bridging approach of IV followed by IA therapy. The screening CT is examined to exclude patients with brain hemorrhage, masses, or other structural abnormalities that contraindicate thrombolysis. Patients with extensive edema on their initial CT scan likely have an extensive "core" area of infarction already, simultaneously reducing their likelihood of benefit and increasing their risk for reperfusion hemorrhage. Previous guidelines suggested patients with edema affecting more than one-third of the MCA territory should be excluded from reperfusion therapies, but no strict cut-off value of baseline edema is universally agreed upon. Many centers have adopted a simple 10-point scoring system (ASPECTS) to provide a quantitative method of assessment and fast communication within the stroke team (Fig. 4.1). Patients with unfavorable low ASPECTS (~ <7) are excluded from some treatment algorithms, while those with "good" ASPECTS (~7–10) indicative of limited edema (e.g., isolated insular ribbon sign or limited lentiform nucleus edema alone) are considered appropriate for thrombolysis. Current work suggests that perfusion-sensitive CT and MR techniques may also be useful in identifying ischemic but still salvageable tissue (ischemic penumbra) to successfully guide selection of patients for stent retriever therapy beyond 4.5 hours (Figs. 4.3 to 4.6).

Diffusion-Weighted MR in Acute Ischemia. DWI uses a novel form of MR tissue contrast to detect ischemic changes within minutes of stroke onset. DWIs are acquired by applying a strong gradient pair that sensitizes the images to microscopic (Brownian) water motion. Brain water diffusion rates fall rapidly during acute ischemia, recovering to normal over days or weeks in infarcted tissues. Since random water motion is slowed down in areas of acute ischemia, the early infarct stands out as bright signal on DWI, compared to dark signal (dephasing) in the normal areas. Acute stroke patients may show clear DWI changes hours before any abnormality can be seen on spin-echo T2-weighted MR (Fig. 4.5). This can also be a useful way to distinguish new ischemic areas (high signal

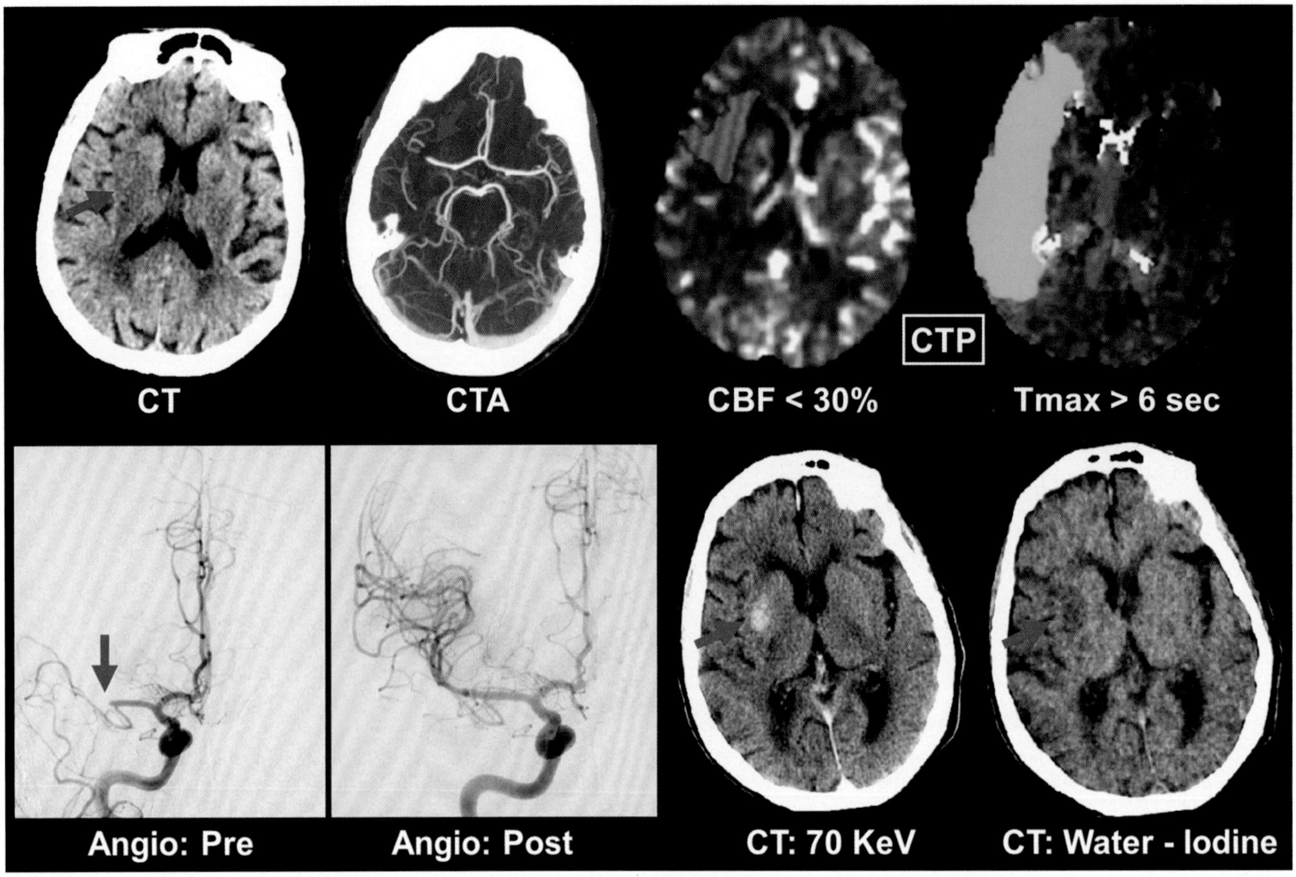

FIGURE 4.3. **Multimodal CT-Based Stroke Triage and Endovascular Intervention.** This 78-year-old woman developed abrupt left hemiplegia 2 days after hemicolectomy for colon cancer. She had atrial fibrillation and prior embolic strokes, but her usual oral anticoagulants were withheld for surgery. CT shows low attenuation in the right lentiform nucleus and posterior limb of internal capsule (*arrow*), with ASPECTS = 8. CTA confirms right M1 occlusion (*arrow*) with poor distal collateral flow. CT perfusion (CTP) processed with RAPID software (iSchemaView) shows a favorable "target mismatch" pattern: small low CBF volume = 6 mL (*shaded pink*), with significantly prolonged Tmax transit times = 92 mL (*shaded green*), for a calculated mismatch volume (putative penumbra) = 86 mL. Given the favorable ASPECTS, a small "core" infarct, large putative penumbra, and accessible proximal clot, she underwent emergent thrombectomy. At angiography the M1 occlusion was confirmed (AP view, right carotid injection; *arrow*) and then promptly recanalized using a stent retriever. Postprocedure dual-energy CT using low KeV shows stippled density in the lentiform nucleus indicative of benign angiographic iodine contrast retention ("stain") in the ischemic core (*arrow*), with small bland infarct (no hemorrhage) confirmed on the water density images with iodine density subtracted.

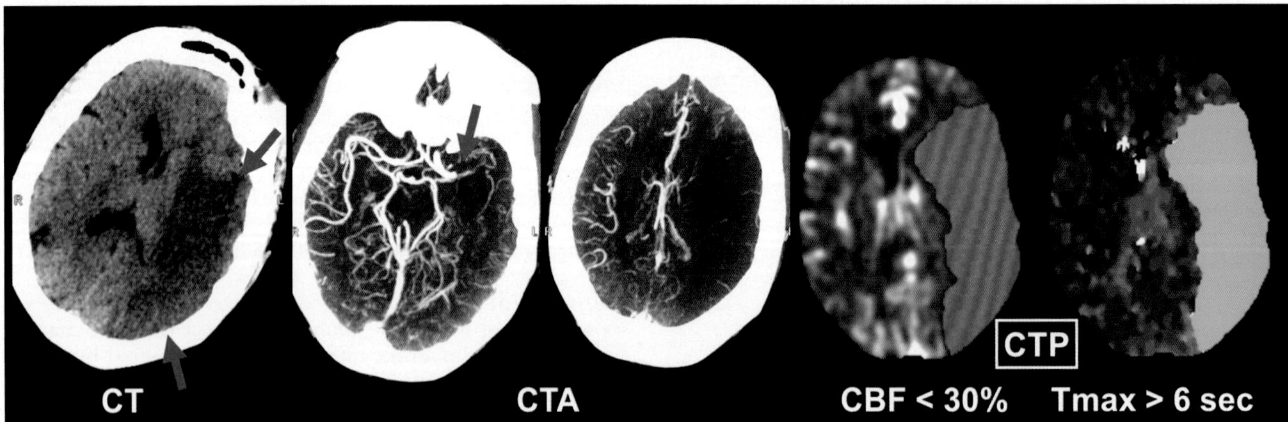

FIGURE 4.4. **CT Stroke Triage; Futile/"Malignant" Pattern, Unsuitable for Intervention.** This 62-year-old woman was transferred with stroke of unknown onset time. CT shows a very large area of well-developed left MCA infarction (*arrows*; ASPECTS = 1), a small old right parietal infarct, and old right basal ganglia lacunes. CTA shows a proximal left M1 segment MCA occlusion (*arrow*) with poor distal collateral filling. CT perfusion maps (RAPID software) depict an essentially matched/completed large infarct, with low CBF core = 135 mL (*shaded pink*) and prolonged Tmax transit times = 153 mL (*shaded green*). Although the clot is proximal and technically accessible, this is a poor candidate for intervention due to combined negative features of large core infarction (low ASPECTS and large volume of low CBF), matching severe Tmax region (indicative of no significant penumbra to salvage), and poor collaterals on CTA.

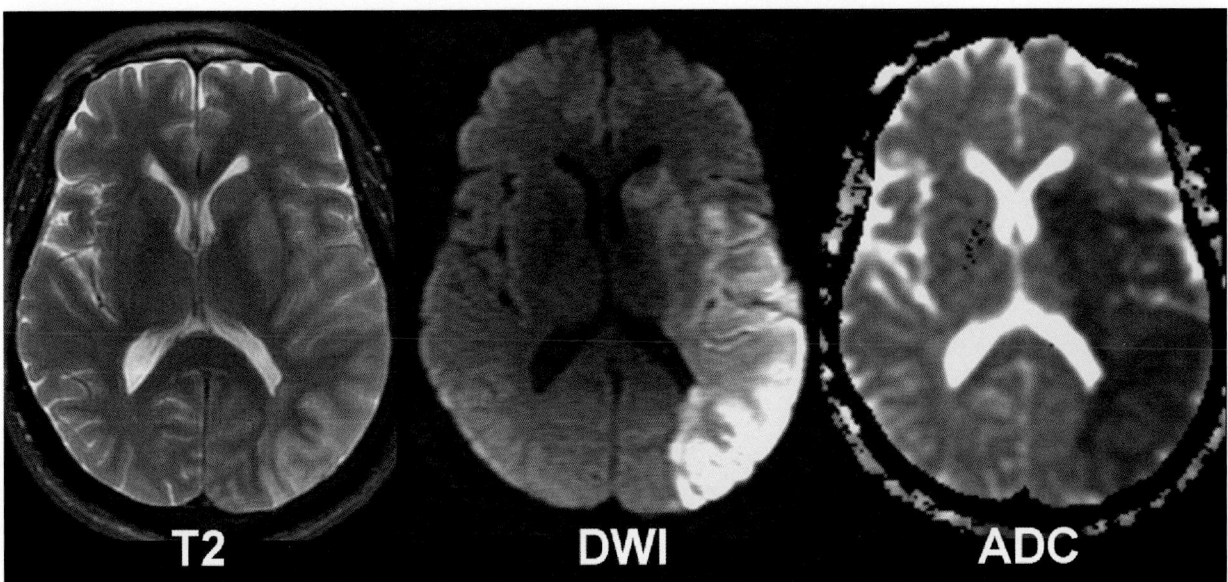

FIGURE 4.5. **Edema in Stroke of Unknown Onset Time.** This patient was found unresponsive with unknown time of symptom onset. Edema is detected as high signal intensity and mild sulcal effacement in the left MCA territory on T2-weighted transverse images, and there is a loss of flow voids in the left sylvian MCA branches. Hyperintensity on DWI and hypointensity on ADC maps are characteristic of cytotoxic edema in acute ischemia. These images suggest the stroke is approximately 4 to 8 hours old. Recent wake-up stroke trials show that if T2/FLAIR is negative, with only a small diffusion positive lesion, this indicates an early infarct, and the patient may be a candidate for IV TPA (based on the "tissue clock"—not the "ticking clock").

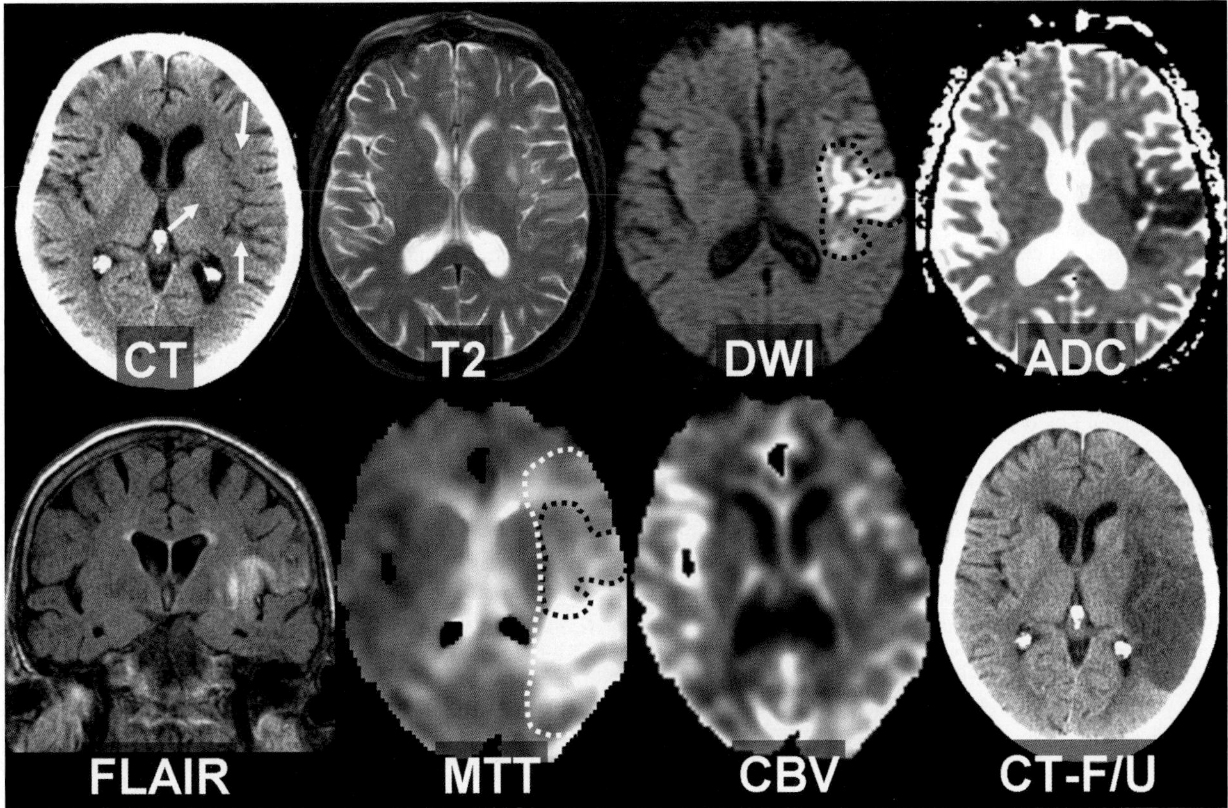

FIGURE 4.6. **Diffusion–Perfusion Mismatch in Acute Ischemia.** This 86-year-old woman with a history of atrial fibrillation developed sudden right hemiplegia and aphasia. **A:** The noncontrast CT shows subtle low attenuation in the left putamen, insula, and sylvian cortex (*arrows*). On T2WI, the cortical gray matter shows mild edema, confirmed to represent cytotoxic edema on DWI and ADC. FLAIR shows cortical edema and stasis in the left MCA. Perfusion-weighted images (MTT, mean transit time; and CBV, cerebral blood volume) show a larger area at risk extending into the parietal lobe (MTT defect in *white dashes*; DWI lesion superimposed in *black dashes*). The hypoperfused tissue not yet infarcted is considered tissue at risk, or the ischemic penumbra. Diffusion lesions tend to "grow into"; severe surrounding perfusion lesions if untreated. Follow-up CT shows extension of infarction into the penumbral tissue identified by MTT.

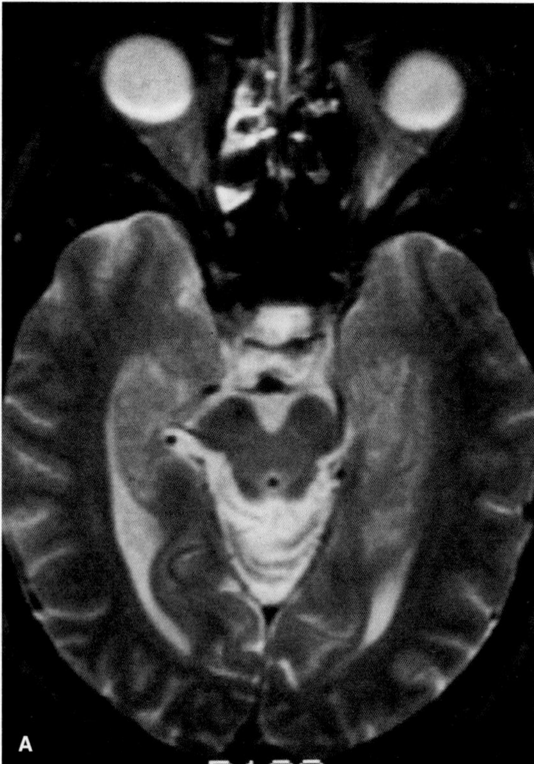

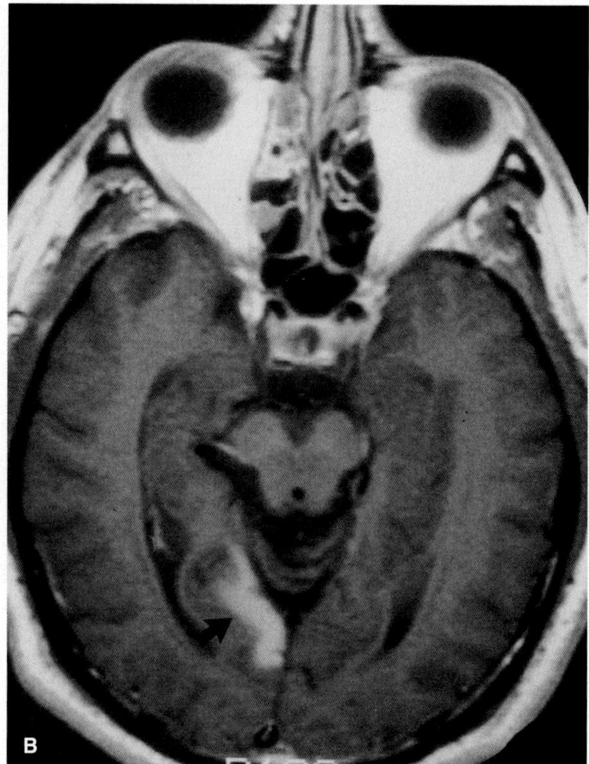

FIGURE 4.7. **Fogging Effect and Gyral Enhancement in Subacute Infarction.** As edema and mass effect subside, but before development of atrophy, infarcts may be inconspicuous on unenhanced CT or MR images. **A:** T2WI is essentially normal in the occipital regions 13 days after right posterior cerebral artery infarction. **B:** T1WI after gadolinium shows enhancement of the infarcted deep right occipital cortex (*arrow*).

on DWI) from older lesions (normal or low signal on DWI). By using a series of different diffusion gradient strengths, the process may also be quantified in an apparent diffusion coefficient (ADC). The ADC reflects "pure" diffusion behavior, free of any underlying T2 contributions ("shine through" or "dark through"). DWI acquisition is facilitated using echo-planar MR systems with their inherently faster, stronger gradients and rapid digitization equipment.

FLuid Attenuated Inversion Recovery (FLAIR) in Ischemia. FLAIR allows T2 weighting of the parenchyma while simultaneously suppressing free water signal from the cerebrospinal fluid (CSF). These techniques increase conspicuity of T2 changes in ischemia. FLAIR is not inherently better than T2 MR for early detection of ischemia, but may be particularly helpful in detecting small lesions in the cortex and is critical for exclusion of acute subarachnoid hemorrhage (SAH) using MRI.

Subacute and Chronic Ischemia. In the subacute phase, edema leads to mass effect, ranging from slight sulcal effacement to marked midline shift with brain herniation, depending on the size and location of infarct. These changes peak at 3 to 7 days, with progressive brain softening (encephalomalacia) ensuing thereafter. One potential imaging pitfall, the "fogging effect," may be encountered on CTs done during the 2nd week after infarction as edema and mass effect are subsiding. At this stage, decrease in edema and accumulation of proteins from cell lysis balance one another such that brain morphology and density in the injured region can be nearly normal by CT. Fogging effects are much less of a problem on MR due to its greater tissue sensitivity, particularly when contrast is used (Fig. 4.7). Edema or mass effect that persists beyond 1 month effectively rules out simple ischemia, and should raise the possibility of recurrent infarction or an underlying tumor.

In the weeks and months following infarction, macrophages remove dead tissue, leaving a small amount of gliotic scar and encephalomalacia behind. CSF takes up the space previously occupied by brain. The affected corticospinal tract atrophies (Wallerian degeneration) leading to a shrunken appearance of the ipsilateral cerebral peduncle. If hemorrhage accompanied the infarct, hemosiderin may be seen grossly or detected as signal hypointensity by T2-weighted images (T2WI). Widening of adjacent sulci and "ex-vacuo" dilatation of the ventricle occurs adjacent to the infarcted area (Fig. 4.8).

Hemorrhagic Transformation of Infarction

Reperfusion into infarcted capillary beds may secondarily lead to gross or microscopic hemorrhage, seen in up to half of infarcts. In most cases this takes the form of microscopic leakage (diapedesis) of red blood cells, but on rare occasions a frank hematoma will form. Physical disruption of the capillary endothelial cells, loss of vascular autoregulation, and anticoagulation or thrombolytic use may all contribute to the development of these hemorrhages. Patients may develop headaches at the time of bleeding, but commonly have no new symptoms, presumably because the hemorrhage occurs within brain areas that are already dead or dysfunctional. Hemorrhagic infarction is confined to the territory of the infarcted vessel, whereas primary hemorrhage does not necessarily respect vascular boundaries. Intraventricular extension is uncommonly seen with hemorrhagic transformation and should raise the possibility of another process (such as hypertensive bleed or a ruptured arteriovenous malformation [AVM]).

The peak time for hemorrhagic transformation is at about 1 to 2 weeks post infarction. It is usually manifest as

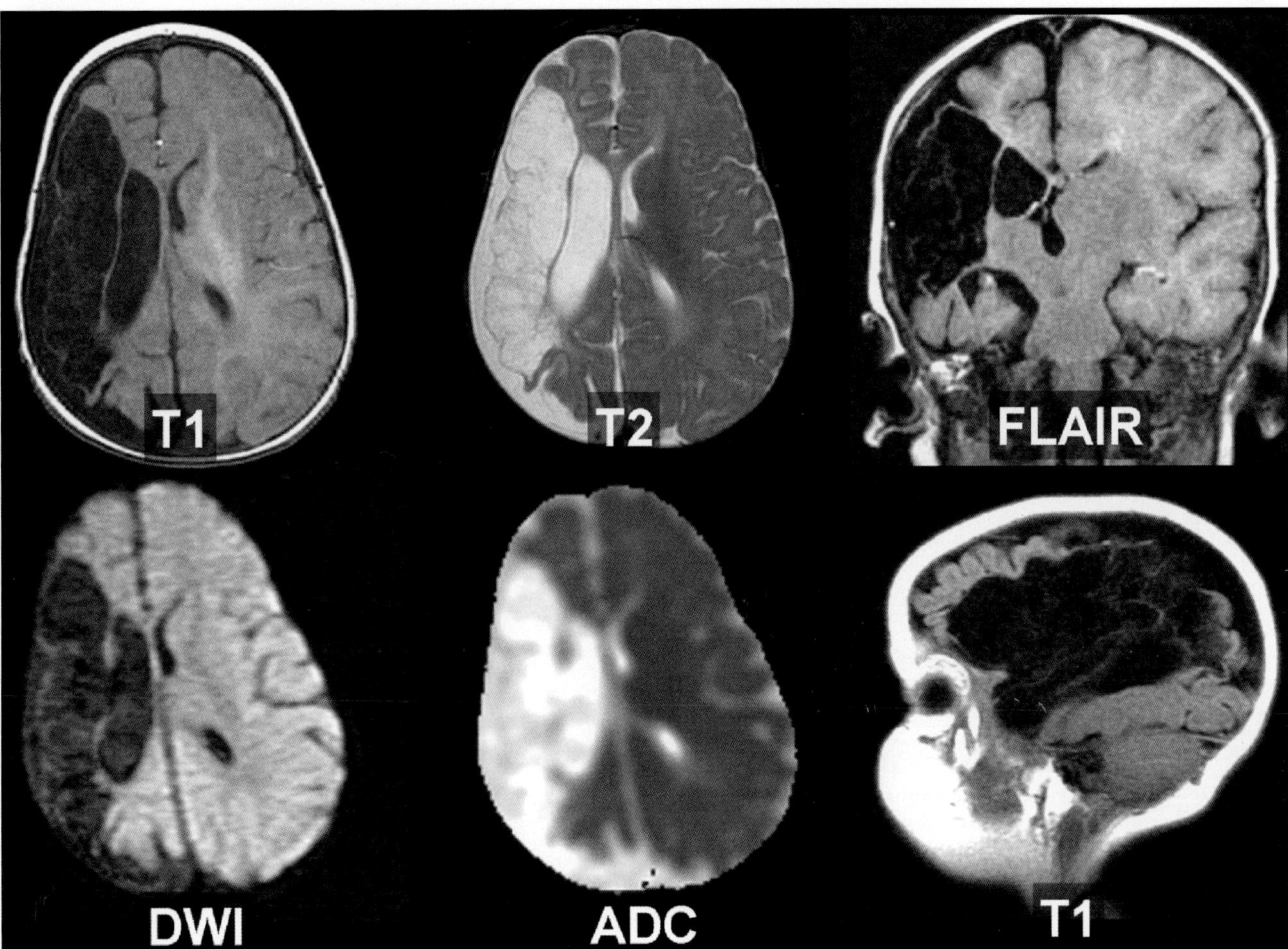

FIGURE 4.8. Chronic Infarction. Cystic encephalomalacia is present in the right MCA territory on MR in a 7 month old with neonatal infarction. Note cystic changes approach CSF on all sequences, including DWI and ADC, with minimal gliosis. There is volume loss with widening of the ipsilateral ventricle (ex-vacuo dilatation).

a serpiginous line of petechial blood following the gyral contours of the infarcted cortex. These dots of hemorrhage are often patchy and discontinuous. On CT a faint line of high attenuation is observed, and on MR bright signal is seen along the affected gyrus on the unenhanced T1WI because of methemoglobin (Fig. 4.9). (Alternate explanations for this bright signal have been offered, including laminar necrosis or calcification related to infarction; the practical point is to recognize this appearance as a feature of ischemia.) The petechial gyral pattern is not seen in primary brain hemorrhage and can be helpful in confirming the underlying ischemic etiology of a suspicious lesion. This is considered a normal part of the evolution of an infarct. Management in the presence of petechial hemorrhage is controversial, but many neurologists continue anticoagulation if there is a well-documented embolic source.

More extensive hemorrhagic transformation of the infarcted tissue may lead to the formation of a gross parenchymal hematoma. Here, the blood does not conform to a gyrus and may form a clot indistinguishable from a primary hematoma. Large cortical infarcts are at somewhat higher risk for this type of change, compared with limited cortical or subcortical lesions. Catastrophic hemorrhagic transformation can also follow thrombolysis, particularly when treatment is delayed or the baseline CT shows extensive edema. In contrast to the petechial gyral transformation described above, gross parenchymal hematomas tend to occur earlier and are more commonly associated with clinical deterioration. Confluent hematomas seen on infarct follow-up studies should be reported promptly since anticoagulation therapy is contraindicated, even when the finding is incidental.

Use of Contrast in Ischemic Stroke

CT Triage. A noncontrast CT remains the initial radiologic examination of choice for emergency triage of suspected acute stroke. It serves to rule out hemorrhage, may define patterns and extent of ischemic injury, shows areas of abnormal vascular calcification (e.g., giant aneurysms), and excludes mass lesions. This is important first-line information needed by the clinician faced with determining the need for lumbar puncture, vascular surgery, anticoagulation, thrombolysis, cardiac evaluation, or other therapies—especially IV t-PA. Advanced triage protocols now prospectively incorporate CTA and often perfusion examinations to help refine selection of patients for IV t-PA, endovascular therapy, or combinations. Advanced imaging should be incorporated during the initial imaging session to enable an accurate diagnosis, avoid delay, and individualize therapeutic choices. Given the urgency of stroke and the low toxicity of modern iodinated contrast agents, contrast-enhanced examinations need not wait for renal function screening—stroke victims are treated like a trauma patient. All acute stroke CTs should be reviewed as highest priority, real time on the scanning console or PACS system to immediately

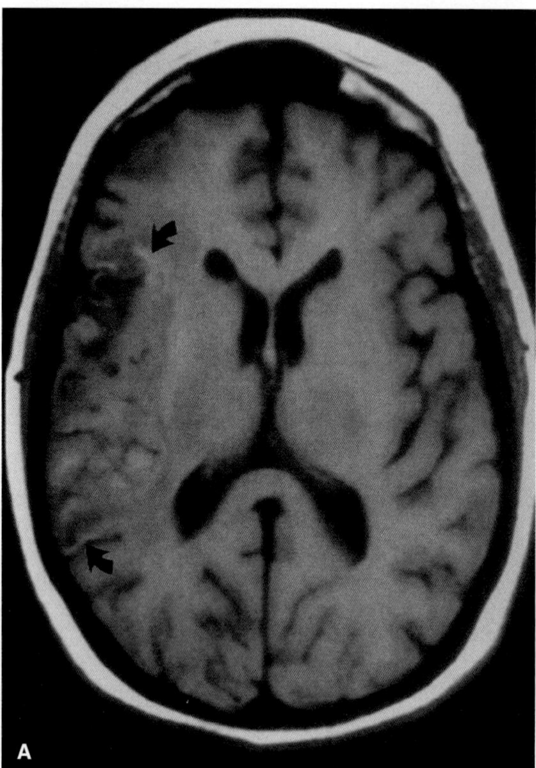

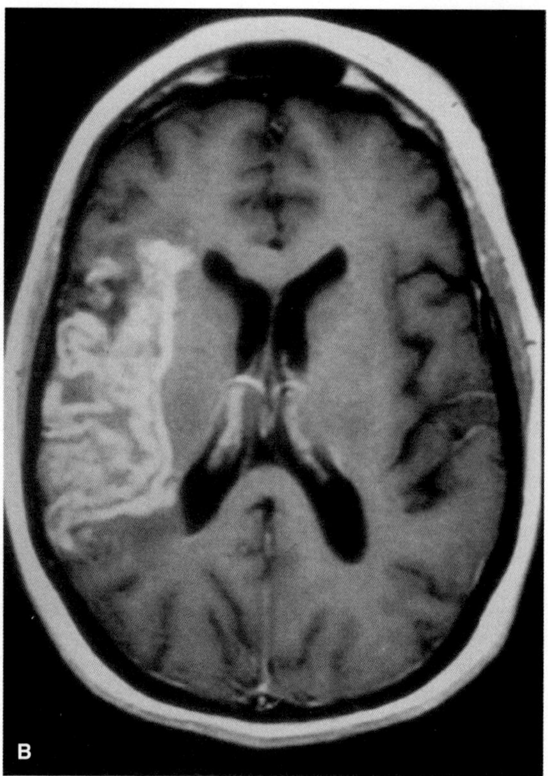

FIGURE 4.9. **Petechial Hemorrhage and Gyral Enhancement in Subacute Infarction. A:** Precontrast T1WI shows mild effacement of sulci in the right MCA territory. A few subtle areas of bright signal intensity scattered along the cortex indicate areas of petechial hemorrhage or laminar necrosis (*arrows*). **B:** Postcontrast T1WI demonstrates marked gyral enhancement, a hallmark of subacute infarction.

exclude hemorrhage or large infarcts so that IV t-PA decisions can be made. If endovascular therapy is available, CTA and CT perfusion are best done immediately after the noncontrast CT—without taking the patient off the scanner—to help determine suitability. A postcontrast head CT is normally acquired last in the stroke protocol, since a nonstroke lesion such as a tumor, abscess, or an isodense subdural hematoma might be shown to better advantage with contrast. Although MRI with diffusion sequences is arguably better than CT for acute stroke triage, the speed and 24/7 practicality of CT win out as the modality of choice in most centers.

An intact blood–brain barrier normally excludes contrast from the brain. Leakage of macromolecular contrast agents through damaged vessels leads to local accumulation of iodine, seen as high attenuation (enhancement) of infarcted parenchyma. Blood–brain barrier breakdown underlies both hemorrhagic transformation and contrast enhancement of infarctions. Not surprisingly, then, these processes are seen at roughly the same time and often in combination. As with petechial gyral hemorrhage, a gyral pattern of enhancement (by CT or MR) is highly specific evidence of an underlying infarction. CT-detected enhancement of infarcted brain parenchyma typically begins at about 1 week, peaks at 7 to 14 days, often assumes a gyral pattern, and is less commonly observed in subcortical regions. Enhancement is seen in about half of patients during the 1st week and in about two-thirds between weeks 1 and 4. As gliosis ensues and the blood–brain barrier is repaired, enhancement fades and then resolves by 3 months.

MR Contrast. Most of the comments regarding the strategy, pathophysiology, and enhancement patterns for CT also generally hold true for contrast in MR. IV gadolinium contrast agents are very well tolerated by stroke patients and may give valuable information not readily available from the noncontrast MR. Stasis of gadolinium within vessels or leakage of contrast through an abnormal blood–brain barrier will shorten T1 relaxation of adjacent protons, leading to hyperintensity (enhancement) on T1WI. As with CT, a noncontrast MR sequence is mandatory before contrast is given since enhancement and subacute blood both appear hyperintense on T1WI. (This will be discussed in the "Hemorrhage" section.) An IV bolus of contrast may also be captured dynamically using rapid imaging techniques to produce a family of perfusion-weighted images to help identify ischemic regions.

Intravascular enhancement on MR is commonly seen in the infarcted territory during the 1st week. This may be due to slow flow or vasodilatation leading to stasis of gadolinium, likely in both arteries and veins. The intravascular enhancement pattern may be detected within minutes of vessel occlusion, is seen in a majority of cortical infarcts at 1 to 3 days, and resolves by 10 days. The proximal trunks of more distally occluded arteries and leptomeningeal cortical channels are most prominently involved (Fig. 4.10). The area of vascular enhancement may extend beyond the T2 hyperintensity, possibly indicating recruitment of collateral supply at the ischemic border. Meningeal enhancement which attends meningitis, and dural enhancement seen postoperatively can superficially resemble intravascular enhancement, but the distinction should be obvious on clinical grounds. MR intravascular enhancement helps identify early strokes, indicates ongoing slow flow, and has no obvious CT counterpart.

MR parenchymal enhancement occurs in a similar pattern to that seen on CT (and with the same time course seen by nuclear medicine infarct scans of the past). It may occur as early as day 1, but more typically begins after the 1st week, a time when intravascular enhancement is waning. Reperfusion

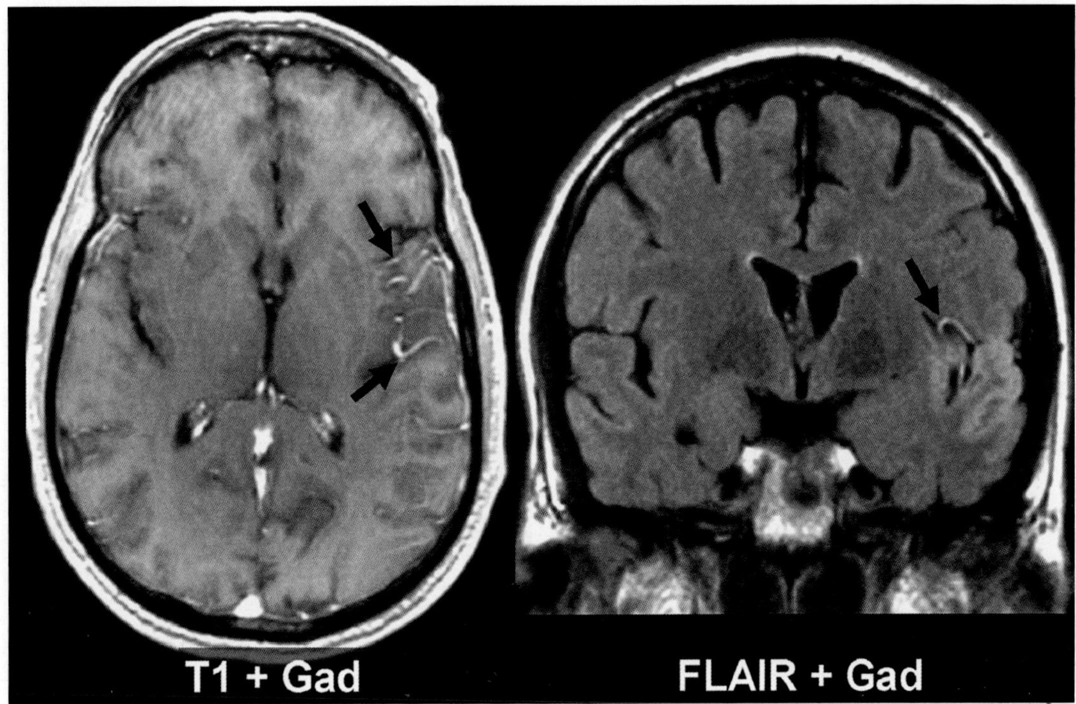

FIGURE 4.10. **Intravascular Stasis and Enhancement in Acute Infarction.** Postcontrast T1 and FLAIR images in acute left MCA infarction. Mild sulcal effacement and prominent enhancement of sylvian branches of the MCA (*arrows*) are evident on T1. As seen here, FLAIR can show similar vascular signs of stasis, either before or after contrast. Intravascular enhancement is typically seen only during the first 10 days after stroke.

after thrombolysis can lead to early enhancement. Virtually all cortical infarcts enhance by MR at 2 weeks. Elster has summarized this in his Rule of 3s: MR parenchymal enhancement peaks at 3 days to 3 weeks and resolves by 3 months.

The imaging time course for CT and MR examinations in brain infarction are summarized in Table 4.2.

Pattern Recognition in Ischemic Stroke

Familiarity with the major vascular territories can help distinguish between infarction and other pathologic processes. The clinical time course and localization should be consistent with the imaging findings, and all should correspond to a known vascular distribution. Stroke localization is not necessarily synonymous with "focal." An ischemic event may cause a pattern of damage which is diffuse (hypoxic-ischemic injury), multifocal (vasculitis, emboli), or focal (single embolism or thrombus). The vessels causing stroke may be large or small, and may be on either the arterial or venous side. There is no such thing as a "funny" stroke; if it does not fit a vascular territory then the differential diagnosis changes (Fig. 4.11).

The relation of vascular anatomy to functional neuroanatomy is at the heart of clinicoradiologic correlation in stroke.

TABLE 4.2

IMAGING TIME COURSE AFTER BRAIN INFARCTION

■ TIME	■ CT	■ MR
Minutes	No changes	Absent flow void Arterial enhancement (days 1–10) DWI: high signal
2–6 hours	Hyperdense artery sign Insular ribbon sign	Brain swelling (T1) Subtle T2 hyperintensity
6–12 hours	Sulcal effacement +/– Decreased attenuation	T2 hyperintensity
12–24 hours	Decreased attenuation	T1 hypointensity
3–7 days	Maximum swelling	Maximum swelling
3–21 days	Gyral enhancement (peak: 7–14 days)	Gyral enhancement (peak: 3–21 days) Petechial methemoglobin
30–90 days	Encephalomalacia Loss of enhancement Resolution of petechial blood	Encephalomalacia Loss of enhancement Resolution of petechial blood

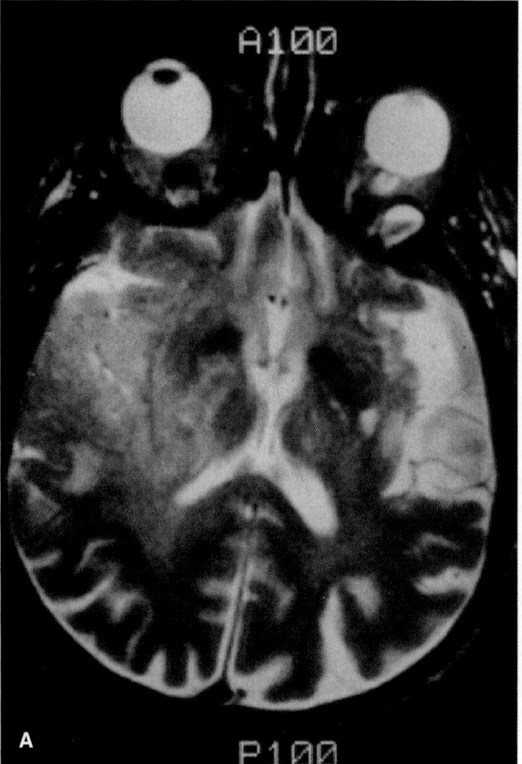

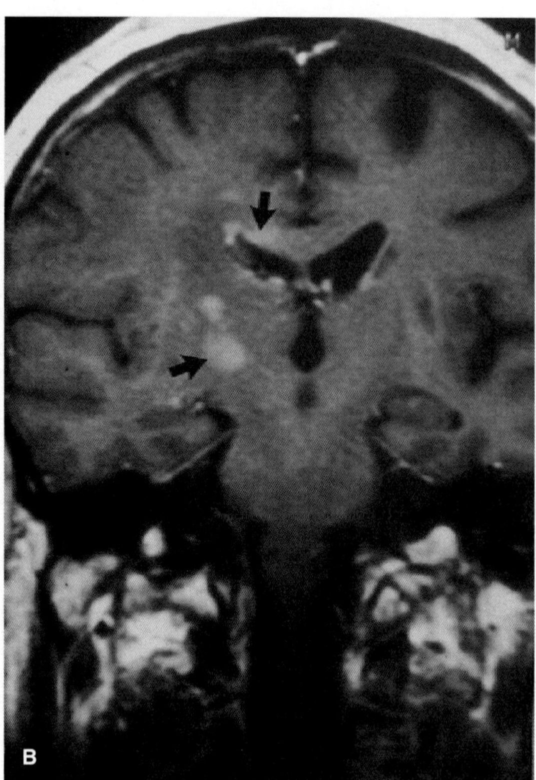

FIGURE 4.11. **Glioblastoma Mimicking a Stroke. A:** T2-weighted axial section shows edema primarily in the right MCA territory, but with additional involvement of the medial temporal lobe, thalamus, and periatrial regions. **B:** Postcontrast coronal T1WI shows patchy, nodular areas of enhancement in the basal ganglia and periventricular regions (*arrows*). Even with a strong clinical history for stroke-like onset, the nonvascular distribution and atypical enhancement pattern effectively exclude underlying infarction. When in doubt, follow-up imaging studies will usually clarify the diagnosis.

Classically strokes and TIAs are divided into anterior (carotid territory) or posterior (vertebrobasilar territory) events. Patients with anterior circulation ischemia have been shown to benefit from carotid endarterectomy when the carotid is narrowed by at least 70% compared to its normal diameter. Surgery has not been proven beneficial for patients with lesser degrees of carotid stenosis or those with posterior territory TIAs, who therefore usually receive medical therapy (e.g., anticoagulation). Ischemia in the carotid territory may cause visual changes, aphasia, or sensorimotor deficits due to retinal, cortical, or subcortical damage. Vertebrobasilar strokes are more likely to cause syncope, ataxia, cranial nerve findings, homonymous visual field deficits, and facial symptoms opposite those of the body. A given deficit can be predicted from the known functional topography of the cortex and its connections through the internal capsule (Fig. 4.12).

The patterns of injury observed after occlusion of large arteries in the anterior and posterior circulations, small arteries in any region, and of the dural venous channels are reviewed in turn.

Anterior (Carotid) Circulation

Internal Carotid Artery (ICA). Thromboembolic disease in the ICA may cause TIAs or infarction in its MCA or anterior cerebral artery (ACA) branches or in the watershed zone between them. Embolic occlusion of the ophthalmic branch of the ICA may cause transient monocular blindness (*amaurosis fugax*). Observation of any of these patterns should prompt imaging of the carotid arteries. The extent and distribution of ischemia observed depends on the time course of occlusion, degree of oligemia, and available collateral supply. Complete carotid occlusions are occasionally found in asymptomatic patients with a well-developed collateral supply.

Atherosclerotic disease near the carotid bifurcation is responsible for the majority of ischemic events in the ICA territory. Arterial dissection, trauma, fibromuscular dysplasia, tumor encasement, prior neck radiotherapy, and connective tissue diseases may also cause significant carotid narrowing (Fig. 4.13). Hemodynamic effects begin to be seen when there is >80% reduction in area or >60% decrease in diameter. Lesions causing less severe narrowing may nonetheless become symptomatic when they serve as a nidus for thrombus formation or are unmasked by hypotension. Studies have shown a clear benefit of endarterectomy in symptomatic patients with >70% stenosis but not for those with <30% narrowing. In many centers, carotid stents are now used in place of surgery, especially for high-risk patients.

Noninvasive screening of the carotid arteries may be achieved with either US, MR angiography (MRA), or CT angiography (CTA). The choice of modality depends on the abilities of the available personnel and equipment. Sensitivity and specificity are as high as 85% to 90% for each of these techniques. These methods noninvasively identify patients with hemodynamically significant disease who might then be referred for conventional angiography or directly to intervention. US is the most commonly employed screening examination in most centers. It has the advantage of portability, generally lower costs, and can be performed in patients with contraindications to MR/MRA. US is more operator dependent than MRA and is unable to reliably assess portions of the distal ICA near the skull base. CTA provides excellent visualization from the arch to intracranial circulation, but at the small risk of contrast

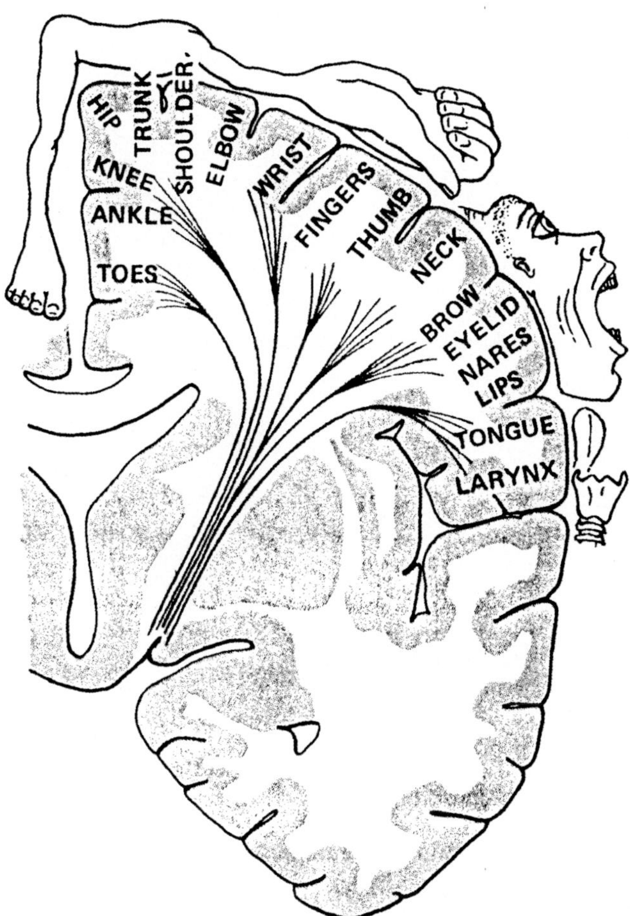

FIGURE 4.12. **Homunculus.** A coronal section through the precentral (motor) cortex depicts the topographic representation of the opposite side of the body. The face and hand areas are served by the MCA territory, the leg by the ACA. (From Gilman S, Winans SS. *Essentials of Clinical Neuroanatomy & Neurophysiology*. Philadelphia, PA: F.A. Davis Company; 1982.)

toxicity and radiation exposure. MRA can evaluate the entire course of the carotid and may be quickly performed in conjunction with the patient's brain MR study. It is a particularly good method for screening pediatric or elderly patients in whom conventional angiography may be technically more difficult.

Selective common carotid angiography remains the gold standard for preprocedure carotid artery evaluation, but is being replaced by noninvasive studies in many centers. The study should cover the entire ICA, including cervical and cranial portions. Evaluation of the surgically inaccessible cranial segments (petrous, cavernous, and supraclinoid) is necessary to exclude high-grade intracranial stenoses or "tandem" lesions which might contraindicate endarterectomy.

Anterior Cerebral Artery. The terminal bifurcation of the ICA is into the anterior and middle cerebral arteries (Fig. 4.14). The ACA is divided into three subgroups: *medial lenticulostriates* serve the rostral portions of the basal ganglia; *pericallosal* branches supply the corpus callosum; and *hemispheric* branches serve the medial aspects of the frontal and parietal lobes (Fig. 4.15). About 5% of infarcts involve the ACA.

The medial lenticulostriates penetrate the anterior perforating substance to give variable supply the anterior-inferior aspect of the internal capsule, putamen, globus pallidus, caudate head, and portions of the hypothalamus and optic chiasm. The largest of these vessels supplies the caudate head/anterior internal capsule region and is recognized as our friend, the recurrent artery of Heubner. Infarction in the medial lenticulostriate territory may cause problems with speech production (motor aphasia), facial weakness, and disturbances in mood and judgment.

Above the takeoff of the lenticulostriates, the ACAs are interconnected by the anterior communicating artery. Each ACA ascends further, giving off branches to the frontal pole (orbitofrontal and frontopolar arteries). The ACAs terminate as a bifurcation into the (lower) pericallosal and (upper) callosomarginal branches. These arteries run parallel to the corpus callosum from front to back, giving supply to the medial cortex of the frontal and parietal lobes. As its name would imply the pericallosal artery courses around and feeds the corpus callosum. ACA branching patterns are quite variable from one patient to the next, with about 10% having only one pericallosal branch which supplies both hemispheres, an "azygos" ACA (Fig. 4.16).

Unilateral damage in the ACA hemispheric branches will cause preferential leg weakness on the opposite side of the body (Table 4.3). Bilateral ACA infarctions lead to incontinence and an awake but apathetic state known as akinetic mutism. Infarction of the corpus callosum can cause a variety of interhemispheric disconnection syndromes.

Middle Cerebral Artery. The MCA supplies more brain tissue than any other intracranial vessel and is host to almost two-thirds of infarcts. Its offspring are the *lateral lenticulostriates* which supply most of the basal ganglia region and the *hemispheric branches* which serve the lateral cerebral surface (Figs. 4.4 and 4.17).

The lateral lenticulostriates arise from the proximal MCA as numerous small perforating end-arteries distributed to the putamen, lateral globus pallidus, superior half of the internal capsule and adjacent corona radiata, and majority of the caudate. Isolated vascular lesions of the globus pallidus or putamen are commonly asymptomatic or may affect contralateral muscle tone and motor control. Lesions of the internal capsule or corona radiata may cause pure or mixed sensory and motor deficits on the opposite side of the body. Interruption of visual connections to the lateral geniculate nucleus results in a subtle type of contralateral homonymous hemianopsia. Rarely, the arcuate fasciculus pathway from Wernicke to Broca speech areas may be selectively infarcted, leading to a conduction aphasia (inability to repeat or read aloud, despite preserved comprehension and fluency).

The MCA loops laterally through the insula where it bifurcates or trifurcates into its major cortical branches (Fig. 4.14). The insula itself is supplied by hemispheric branches, not by the lateral lenticulostriates. When the proximal MCA is occluded, this insular region is farthest from any potential collateral supply, probably explaining the early appearance of edema which gives rise to the "insular ribbon sign" (Fig. 4.2). The anterior hemispheric branches of the MCA supply the anterolateral tip of the temporal lobe (anterior temporal artery), the frontal lobe (operculofrontal arteries), and the motor and sensory strips (central sulcus arteries). Posterior hemispheric branches of the MCA supply the parietal lobe behind the sensory strip (posterior parietal artery), the posterolateral parietal and lateral occipital lobes (angular artery), and the majority of the temporal lobe (posterior temporal artery).

Occlusion of the rostral MCA branches of the dominant hemisphere will cause a motor (Broca) aphasia in which comprehension remains intact. Posterior branches in the dominant hemisphere supply Wernicke area, causing a receptive aphasia when occluded. Posterior temporal branch occlusion may interrupt visual radiations, causing contralateral homonymous field defects. Involvement of either hemisphere's precentral

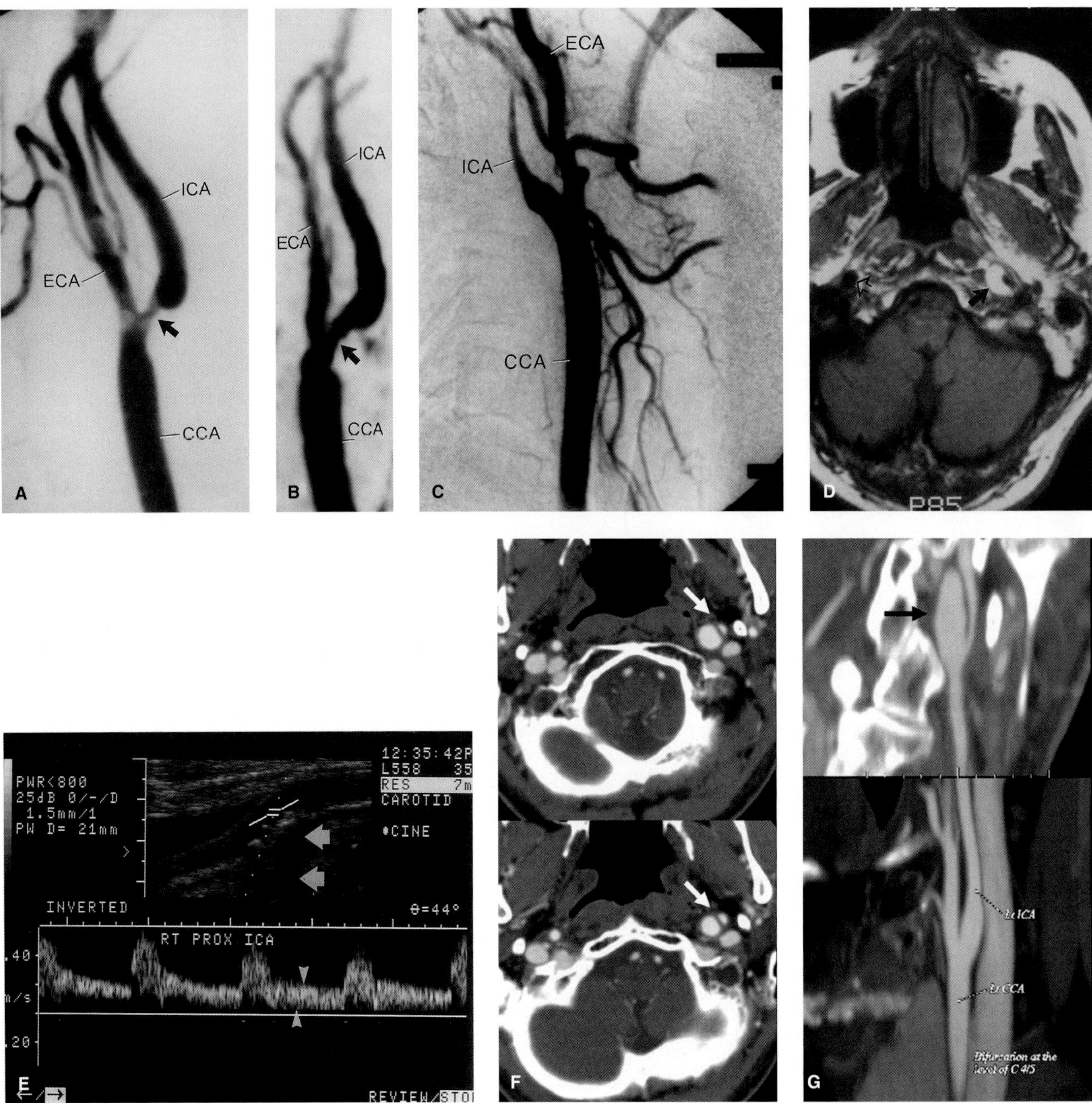

FIGURE 4.13. **Carotid Disease. A:** Atherosclerosis. Lateral view of the carotid bifurcation by conventional digital subtraction angiography. The diameter of the proximal ICA (*arrow*) is reduced approximately 60% compared with its normal caliber above. *CCA*, common carotid artery; *ICA*, internal carotid artery; *ECA*, external carotid artery and its branches. **B:** Atherosclerosis. Lateral maximum intensity projection from a 2D time-of-flight MR angiogram in the same patient shows a very similar pattern of proximal narrowing (*arrow*). **C:** Carotid dissection with a tapering occlusion in the ICA just above the bifurcation. **D:** Carotid dissection in another patient shows the "mural crescent sign" indicative of intramural thrombus in the petrous portion of the left ICA (*arrow*). Note the normal caliber flow void and scant amounts of fat surrounding the normal right ICA (*open arrow*) on T1WI. **E:** Carotid US shows calcified plaque with acoustic shadowing (*arrows*), vessel narrowing, and spectral broadening (between *arrowheads*) in a case of atherosclerosis. **F** and **G:** CTA of carotid dissection with pseudoaneurysm. Source images (**F**) show a flap (*white arrows*) between the narrowed native lumen and the medially situated pseudoaneurysm. Thick slab 2D reconstructions (**G**) show a normal carotid bifurcation and distal cervical "wind-sock" pseudoaneurysm (*black arrow*).

gyrus (motor strip) will produce contralateral weakness which affects face and arm more than leg (Fig. 4.12). Contralateral cortical sensory loss occurs when the primary or association sensory cortex behind the central sulcus is affected. In the nondominant right hemisphere, posterior MCA infarcts commonly cause confusional states, bizarre impairment in visuospatial abilities, and sometimes neglect (or nonrecognition) of the left body. Complete occlusion of the MCA beyond the lenticulostriates causes a combination of these deficits: contralateral face and arm hemiparesis, field defect, and either neglect or global aphasia, depending on which hemisphere is affected. Leg weakness may also be seen when the MCA stem is occluded, because of internal capsule involvement. These relationships are summarized in Table 4.3.

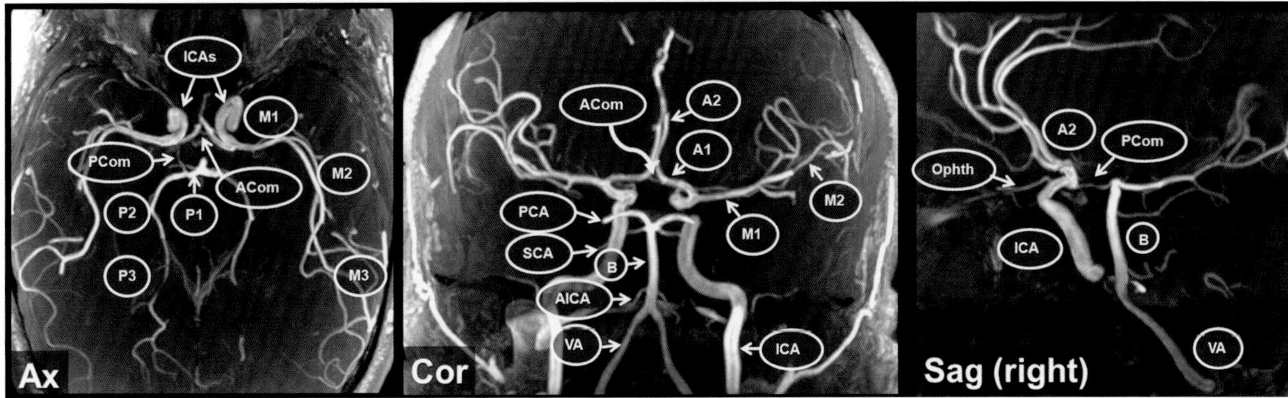

FIGURE 4.14. **MR Angiography of the Normal Circle of Willis and Its Branches.** 3D time-of-flight (TOF) MRA images processed into thick maximum intensity projections (MIPs) in three planes show major branches of the anterior (carotid) and posterior (vertebrobasilar) circulation. Ax, Axial/submentovertex projection outlines the relationship of the major vessels to the circle of Willis. We are looking "down the barrel" of the internal carotid arteries (ICA) and basilar artery. Small right posterior communicating artery (PCom) and small anterior communicating artery (ACom) are present, giving potential collateral routes around the circle. The anterior cerebrals project between the ICAs. Cor, coronal/anterior projection depicts the normal internal carotid arteries (ICA) with bifurcation into the ACA and MCA intracranial branches, numbered sequentially for distal branching order (e.g., M1, M2, M3, etc., proceeding proximal to distal). The paired vertebral arteries (VA) form the single basilar (B) which terminates in paired posterior cerebral arteries (PCA), giving off the cerebellar arteries (SCA, superior cerebellar; AICA, anterior inferior cerebellar artery; and PICA, posterior inferior cerebellar artery—not shown here) along the way. Sagittal (sag)/lateral projection shows a single right PCom extending posteriorly and the ophthalmic artery (Ophth) coursing anteriorly.

Posterior (Vertebrobasilar) Circulation

Vertebral Arteries. The vertebral arteries usually originate from the subclavian arteries, ascend straight upward in the transverse foramina of C6–C3, turn sharply through the C2–C1-foramen magnum levels and unite anterior to the low medulla to form the basilar artery (Fig. 4.18). Atherosclerotic narrowing commonly affects the vertebral arteries at their origins and may affect the basilar artery over variable lengths. Narrowing of the cervical portion of the vertebrals may be due to compressive uncovertebral osteophytes. Rapid head turning (e.g., motor vehicle accidents) may stretch the vertebrals at the C1–C2 level, leading to arterial dissection. Any of these conditions may cause vertebrobasilar ischemia via thrombotic or embolic mechanisms. Anticoagulation and antiplatelet agents remain the mainstay of treatment for vertebrobasilar ischemia.

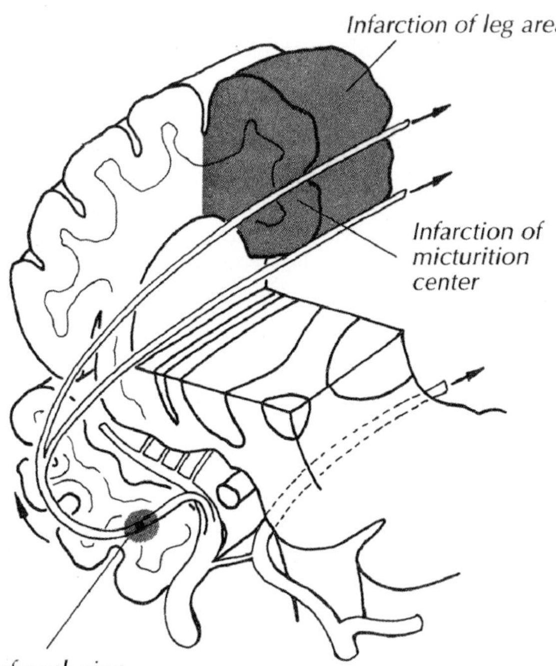

FIGURE 4.15. **Anterior Cerebral Artery Occlusion.** An ACA occlusion causes infarction of the paramedian frontal cortex responsible for motor and sensory function of the opposite leg (*stippled area*). If bilateral, incontinence and akinetic mutism may also be seen. Arrows indicate direction of blood flow. (From Patten J. *Neurological Differential Diagnosis*. New York: Springer Verlag; 1996.)

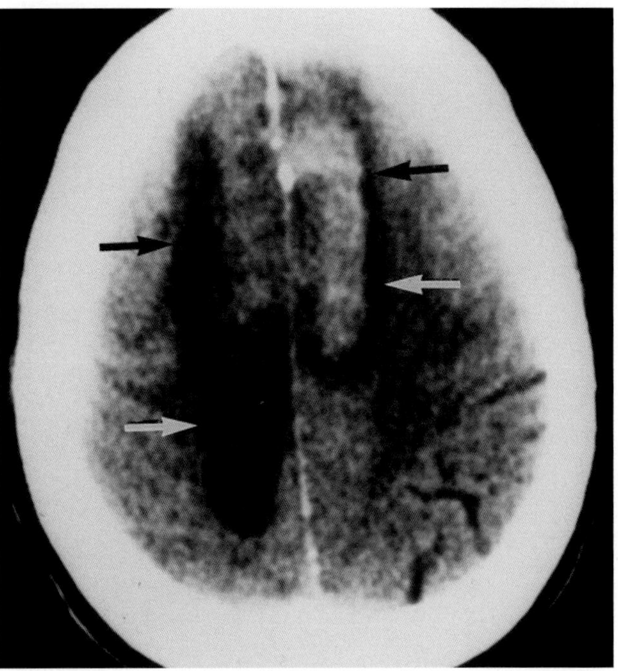

FIGURE 4.16. **Hemorrhagic Infarction.** Hemorrhagic infarction in a bilateral ACA distribution (*arrows*) shown by noncontrast CT. This was an embolic stroke, presumably occluding an azygos ACA.

TABLE 4.3

FUNCTIONAL VASCULAR ANATOMY[a]

VESSEL	BRANCH	SIDE	DEFICIT/SYNDROME
ACA	Hemispheric	Either	Leg weakness
		Both	Incontinence, akinetic mutism
	Medial lenticulostriates	Either	Facial weakness
		Left	Dysarthria; ± motor aphasia
MCA	Hemispheric	Either	Face and arm > leg weakness
		Left	Motor aphasia (anterior lesion)
			Receptive aphasia(posterior lesion)
			Global aphasia (total MCA)
		Right	Neglect syndromes
			Visuospatial dysfunction
	Lateral lenticulostriates	Either	Variable lacunar syndromes
PCA	Hemispheric	Either	Hemianopsia
		Both	Cortical blindness
			Memory deficits
	Thalamoperforators	Either	Somnolence
			Sensory disturbances
Cerebellar	PICA, AICA, or SCA	Either	Ataxia, vertigo, vomiting
			Coma if mass effect
			± Brainstem deficits
Watershed	ACA/MCA/PCA	Either	Man in a barrel syndrome
		Bilateral	Severe memory problems

[a]Assumes left hemisphere language dominance.
PICA, posterior inferior cerebellar artery; AICA, anterior inferior cerebellar artery; SCA, superior cerebellar artery; ACA, anterior cerebral artery; MCA, middle cerebral artery; PCA, posterior cerebral artery.

Angioplasty or stenting are sometimes feasible for correction of atherosclerotic lesions, but are usually reserved for medically refractory cases.

Basilar Artery. The basilar is formed by the union of the two vertebral arteries. As it ascends between the clivus and brainstem,

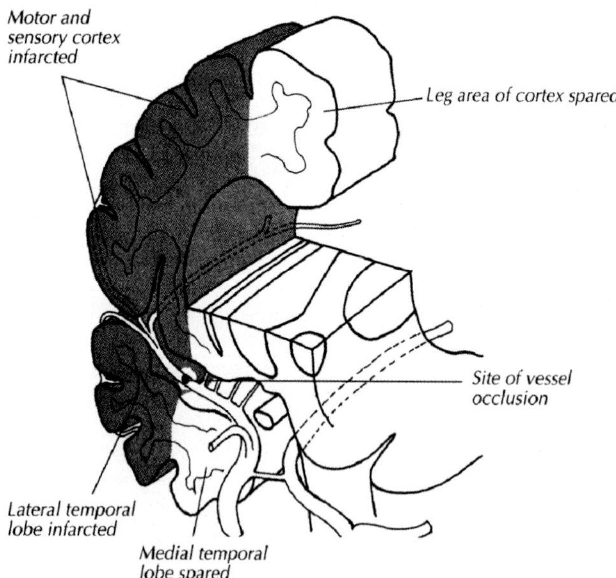

FIGURE 4.17. **Middle Cerebral Artery Occlusion.** An MCA occlusion distal to the lateral lenticulostriates causes infarction of the motor and sensory cortex of the arm and face (*stippled area*). More proximal occlusion will also affect the internal capsule, potentially adding leg deficits. (From Patten J. *Neurological Differential Diagnosis*. New York: Springer Verlag; 1996.)

it sends large branches to the cerebellum and smaller perforating vessels to the brainstem. The basilar ends at its bifurcation into the posterior cerebral arteries just above the tentorium cerebelli. Occlusion of the basilar artery itself is usually rapidly fatal, due to infarction of respiratory and cardiac centers in the medulla. Occlusion of the perforating end-arteries from the basilar artery causes focal brainstem infarction, usually manifest as cranial nerve dysfunction, ataxia, somnolence, and crossed motor or sensory deficits. These lesions characteristically respect the midline of the brainstem and often extend to the ventral surface (Fig. 4.19). Metabolic disturbances (e.g., central pontine myelinolysis) and hypertensive hemorrhages (most commonly in the pons) tend to be more centrally or diffusely located. Large or multiple lesions in the pons can cause a nightmarish syndrome of quadriparesis with intact cognition, the "locked in" state.

Posterior Cerebral Artery (PCA). The basilar artery ends at its bifurcation into the PCAs at the midbrain level, just above the tentorial hiatus. The major branches of the PCA include midbrain and thalamic *perforating vessels*, *posterior choroidal arteries*, and *cortical branches* to the medial temporal and occipital lobes (Fig. 4.20). Ten to 15% of infarcts occur in the PCA territory.

The proximal segments of the PCAs sweep posterolaterally around the midbrain, giving off small perforating branches to the mesencephalon and thalamus along the way. Midbrain infarction causes loss of the pupillary light responses, impaired upgaze, and somnolence due to damage of the quadrigeminal plate, third cranial nerve nuclei, and reticular activating formation, respectively. Proximal PCA perforators also supply the majority of the thalamus and sometimes portions of the posterior limb of the internal capsule. Thalamic infarction may cause a variety of disturbances, but contralateral sensory loss is the most common problem.

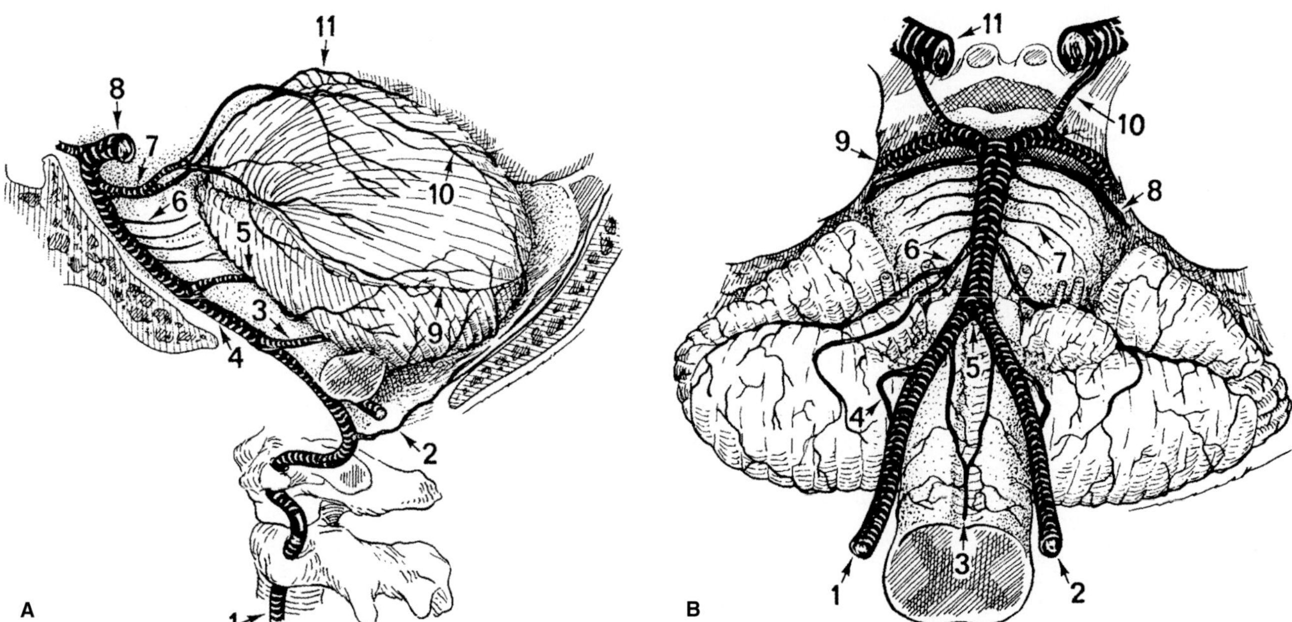

FIGURE 4.18. **Vertebrobasilar Arteries. A:** Lateral view. 1, left vertebral; 2, posterior meningeal; 3, posterior inferior cerebellar (PICA); 4, basilar; 5, anterior inferior cerebellar artery (AICA); 6, pontine perforators; 7, superior cerebellar artery (SCA); 8, posterior cerebral artery (PCA); 9, branches of the SCA and AICA in the horizontal fissure of the cerebellum; 10, SCA hemispheric branches; 11, superior vermian branches. **B:** Anterior view. 1, right vertebral; 2, left vertebral; 3, anterior spinal; 4, PICA; 5, basilar; 6, AICA; 7, pontine; 8, SCA; 9, PCA; 10, posterior communicating; 11, ICA. (From Osborn AG. *Introduction to Cerebral Angiography*. Philadelphia, PA: Harper & Row; 1980.)

The posterior choroidal arteries arise from the proximal PCA to supply the choroid plexus of the third and lateral ventricles, pineal gland, and regions contiguous with the third ventricle. Isolated posterior choroid infarctions are rare due to rich collateral supply through the choroid plexus. PCA cortical branches supply the inferomedial temporal lobe (inferior temporal arteries), superior occipital gyrus (parieto-occipital artery), and visual cortex of the occipital lobes (calcarine artery) (Fig. 4.21). Hemispheric PCA occlusions are usually from an embolic source. Inferomedial temporal infarction may cause memory deficits, which are severe when bilateral. Loss of the primary visual cortex causes complete loss of vision in the opposite visual field (homonymous hemianopsia).

In about 20% of patients, one or both of the proximal ("P1") PCA segments may be hypoplastic or absent. In these cases flow is derived from the ICA system via a prominent posterior communicating artery. This is commonly referred to as "fetal origin" of the PCA, since embryologically the PCA develops with the ICA. Since this is a fairly common variation, both vertebral and carotid disease should be considered when evaluating PCA infarctions.

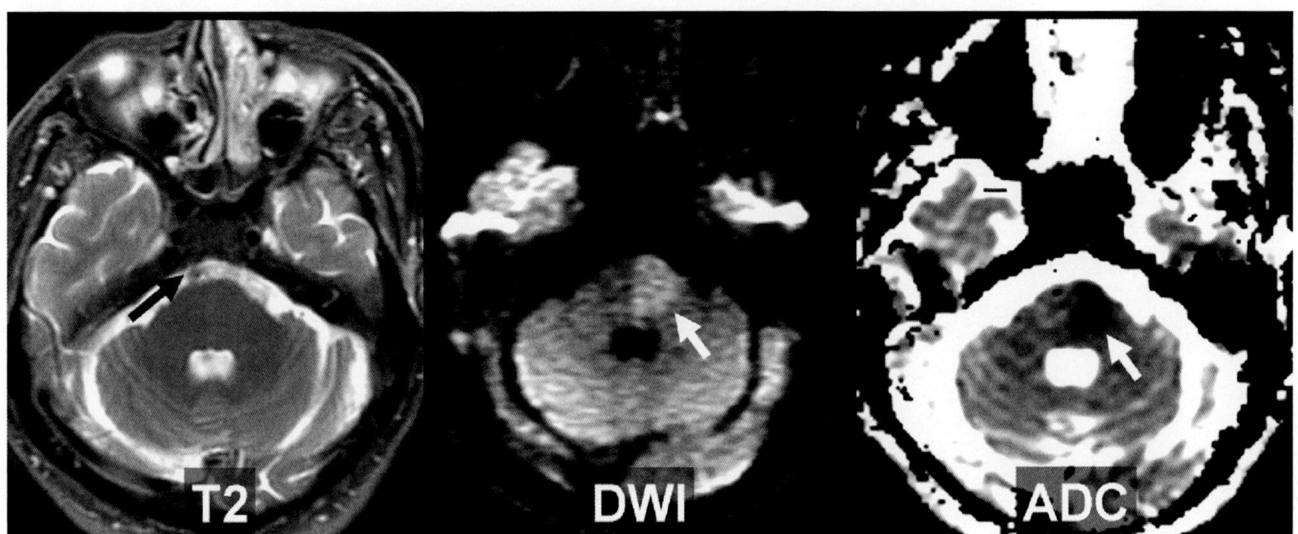

FIGURE 4.19. **Acute Brainstem Infarction.** Although T2 appears normal in the pons, DWI and ADC show a left paramedian pontine infarct (*white arrows*) which respects the midline. Note vessel wall thickening and narrowing of the flow void in the basilar artery on T2 (*black arrow*) due to focal atherosclerosis.

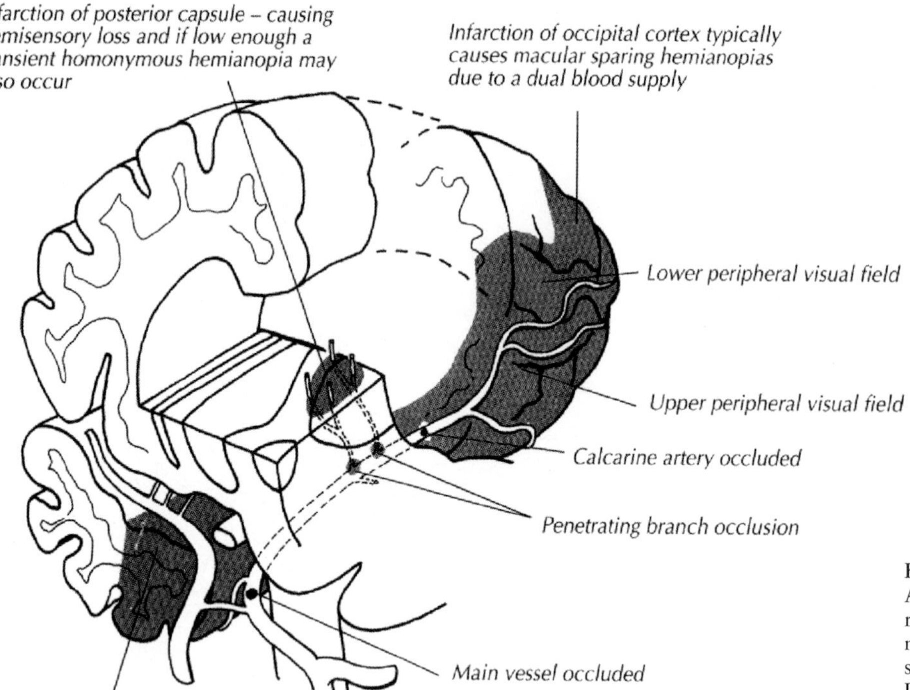

Infarction of posterior capsule – causing hemisensory loss and if low enough a transient homonymous hemianopia may also occur
Infarction of occipital cortex typically causes macular sparing hemianopias due to a dual blood supply
Lower peripheral visual field
Upper peripheral visual field
Calcarine artery occluded
Penetrating branch occlusion
Main vessel occluded
Area of temporal lobe also infarcted by main vessel occlusion but unless bilateral minimal memory deficit occurs

FIGURE 4.20. **Posterior Cerebral Artery Occlusion.** A PCA occlusion results in syndromes of memory impairment, opposite visual field loss, and sometimes hemisensory deficits. (From Patten J. *Neurological Differential Diagnosis*. New York: Springer Verlag; 1996.)

Cerebellar Arteries. Headache, vertigo, nausea, vomiting, and ipsilateral ataxia are the hallmarks of cerebellar stroke; 85% are ischemic and 15% are primary hemorrhages. Clinically it is difficult to distinguish which cerebellar subterritory is involved and whether it derives from infarction or hemorrhage. *Because of clinical urgency, acute evaluation of suspected cerebellar strokes should be performed by CT.* Cerebellar hemorrhages and any infarctions with significant mass effect are neurosurgical emergencies requiring posterior fossa decompression. Multiplanar MR is preferred for evaluation

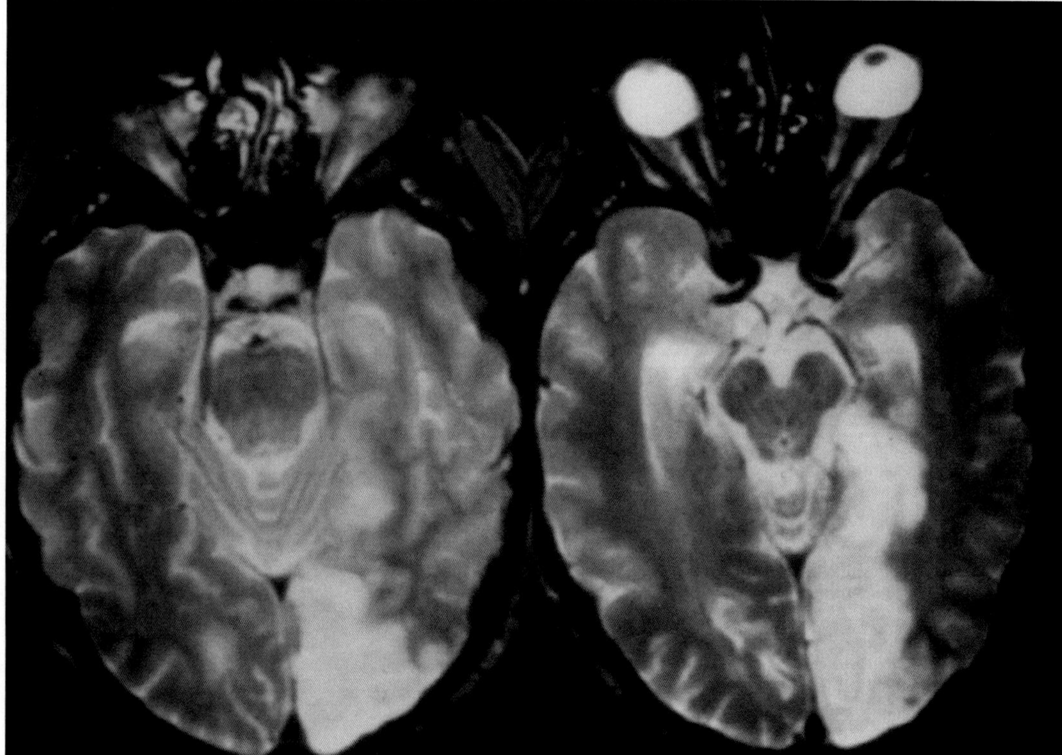

FIGURE 4.21. **Posterior Cerebral Artery Infarction.** Adjacent T2WI shows involvement of the left occipital lobe and medial temporal lobe. The patient presented with a dense right homonymous visual field defect.

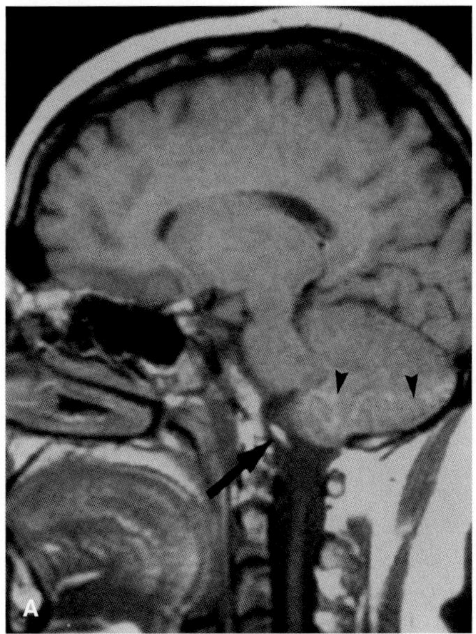

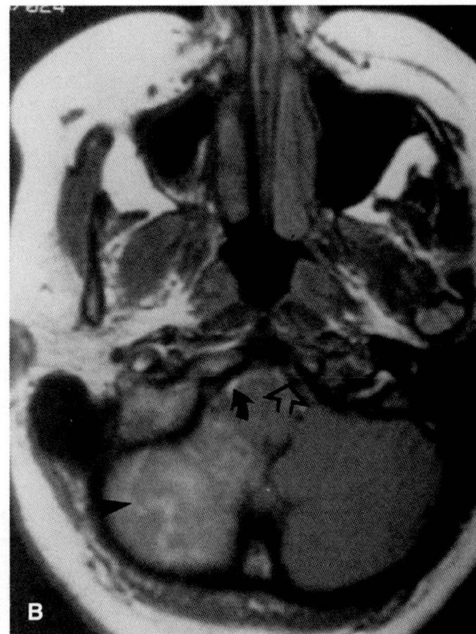

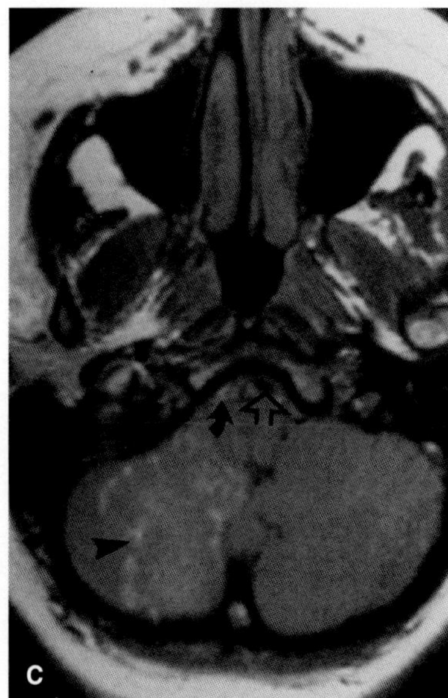

FIGURE 4.22. **Vertebral Dissection With PICA Infarction.** This patient developed neck pain and ataxia following a skiing accident. Sagittal (**A**) and transverse (**B**) T1WI without contrast show high signal in the occluded right vertebral artery (*closed arrows*) with preserved flow void in the left vertebral artery (*open arrows*). Hemorrhagic infarction is seen in the right PICA territory (*arrowheads*).

beyond the acute phase, since beam-hardening artifacts degrade posterior fossa images on CT.

Even though deficits related to the cerebellar territories are hard to distinguish clinically, it is important to recognize characteristic distributions in order to elucidate stroke mechanisms. Luckily, only a *SAP* would forget the correct order of cerebellar branches going from top to bottom: the *s*uperior, *a*nterior inferior, and *p*osterior inferior cerebellar arteries (AICAs) (Fig. 4.18).

Superior Cerebellar Arteries (SCAs). The upper parts of the cerebellum are supplied by the SCA. These arise from the distal basilar as the last large branches beneath the tentorium cerebelli. The SCA territory includes the superior vermis, middle and superior cerebellar peduncles, and superolateral aspects of the cerebellar hemispheres (i.e., the "roof" of the cerebellum). Most SCA infarcts are embolic.

Anterior Inferior Cerebellar Arteries. These arteries arise from the proximal basilar to supply the anteromedial cerebellum and sometimes part of the middle cerebellar peduncle. AICA is usually the smallest of the three major cerebellar hemisphere branches. Occlusion commonly causes ipsilateral limb ataxia, nausea, vomiting, dizziness, and headache.

Posterior Inferior Cerebellar Arteries. The bottom of the cerebellum is supplied by the PICA. The PICA is the first major intracranial branch of the vertebrobasilar system, usually arising from the distal vertebral artery 1 to 2 cm below the basilar origin. Its territory is variable but often includes the dorsolateral medulla, inferior vermis, and posterolateral cerebellar hemisphere. PICA maintains a reciprocal relation with AICA above it. If the PICA is large then the ipsilateral AICA is usually small, and vice versa. This arrangement is sometimes referred to as the AICA–PICA loop. PICA is usually the largest cerebellar hemispheric branch and the most commonly infarcted. Occlusions may occur from extension of a vertebral dissection which began at the C1–C2 level (Fig. 4.22). If only the cerebellar hemisphere is affected, ipsilateral limb ataxia, nausea, vomiting, dizziness, and headache are seen, just as for AICA infarcts. Involvement of the medulla in PICA infarction adds elements of Wallenberg syndrome, including ataxia, facial numbness, Horner syndrome, dysphagia, and dysarthria.

Watershed (Borderzone) Infarction

An episode of transient global hypoperfusion may result in bilateral infarctions in the watershed regions between arterial territories (also referred to as the borderzones). Typical triggering events include cardiac arrest, massive bleeding, anaphylaxis, and surgery under general anesthesia. The borderzones are regions perfused by terminal branches of two adjacent arterial territories (Fig. 4.23). When flow in one or both of the parent vessels falls below a critical level, the brain living in the watershed zone is the first to go. Unilateral watershed damage may be seen when carotid occlusion or stenosis is unmasked by global hypotension. Images show a string of small deep white matter lesions ("rosary bead sign") or damage extending out from the "corners" of the lateral ventricles on higher sections (Fig. 4.24). Characteristic clinical findings include weakness isolated to the upper arms ("man in a barrel syndrome"), cortical blindness, and memory loss.

Small Vessel Ischemia

Lacunes are small subcortical infarcts that may occur in any territory. They account for about 15% to 20% of all strokes. Lacunes are the 2 to 5 mm^3 cavities (literally, "little lakes") left in the brain as the result of occlusion of a penetrating artery causing infarction and ensuing encephalomalacia. Patients usually have a history of longstanding hypertension, leading to lipohyalinosis of the vessels and eventual thrombosis. TIAs precede the stroke in 60% of cases, and a stuttering course is common in the first 2 days. Pure motor or sensory syndromes may occur with these small lesions. Characteristic locations include the lenticular nucleus (37%), pons (16%), thalamus (14%), caudate (10%), and internal capsule/corona radiata (10%) (Fig. 4.25).

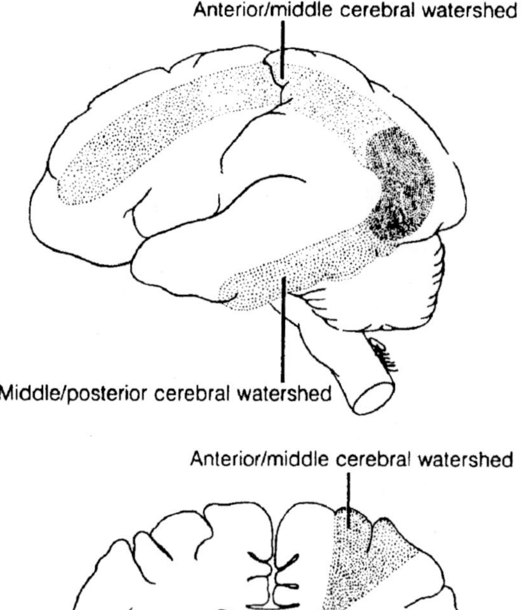

FIGURE 4.23. **Watershed Ischemia.** Stippled brain areas are served by terminal branches of adjacent parent arteries. The watershed zones are at highest risk of infarction when flow is reduced in one or both carotids. (From Simon RP, Aminoff MJ, Greenberg DA, eds. *Clinical Neurology*. Norwalk, CT: Appleton & Lange; 1989.)

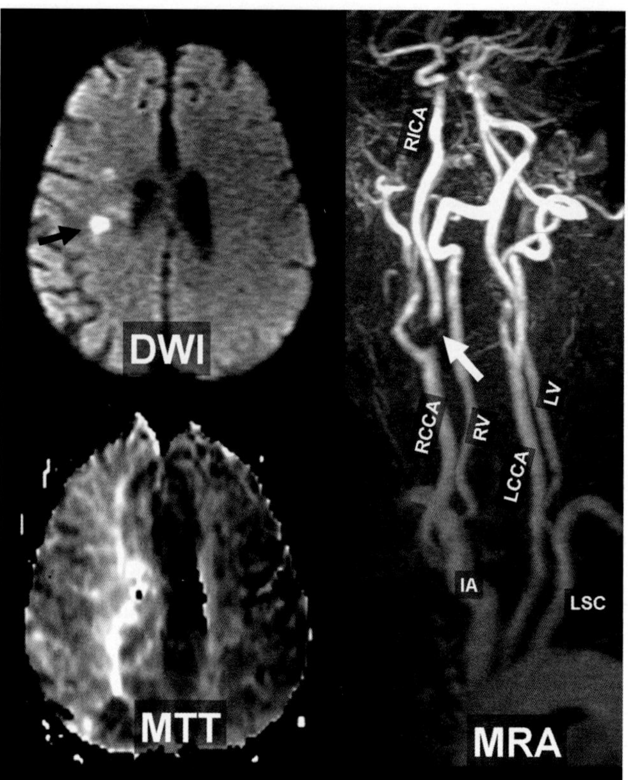

FIGURE 4.24. **Watershed Infarctions.** This patient presented with left body "shaking-limb" TIAs. DWI shows a cluster of lesions in the right corona radiata (*black arrow*). MTT maps indicate long transit times for the entire hemisphere, particularly the deep watershed zones (whiter colors = longer times). Gadolinium-enhanced MRA shows fairly normal great vessel origins, but a critical stenosis of the proximal right ICA with a flow gap (*white arrow*). Mechanisms leading watershed ischemia are debated, but may include distal emboli, local thrombosis due to slow flow, and hemodynamic causes.

Internal capsule lacunes are an especially important subset of lacunes because they are quite common and cause characteristic syndromes. Axonal projections to and from the cortex must funnel through the internal capsule and brainstem where even tiny lacunes may cause major deficits. The internal capsule receives supply from multiple small perforating arteries at the base of the brain, all of which are common sites for lacunar infarction and hypertensive hemorrhages. Its contributors include the ACA and MCA lenticulostriates, the ICA anterior choroidal branch, and PCA thalamogeniculates. Isolated lesions of the anterior limb interrupt connections of the anterior frontal lobe, but are usually clinically silent. Beginning at the genu and working back, the capsule carries corticobulbar, *h*ead, *a*rm, and then *l*eg fibers in a somatotopically organized fashion (Fig. 4.26). (Our little homunculus man, *HAL*, stands in the posterior limb with his head at the genu, reclining with his head directed medially as he enters the cerebral peduncle.) Lesions in the posterior limb are clinically most important since they may cause severe sensory, motor, or mixed deficits. Lesions at the genu may disrupt speech production or swallowing, but generally become apparent only when bilateral.

Lacunes Versus Perivascular Spaces. "Etat lacunaire" refers to a state of multiple lacunar infarctions. The term is still used in the literature and should be distinguished from the term "etat crible" which refers to enlarged perivascular spaces (Virchow–Robin spaces) that may develop around perforating vessels (Fig. 4.27). These normal spaces may simulate lacunes but have no associated neurologic deficit or other clinical relevance. By definition, Virchow–Robin spaces should follow CSF intensity on all MR sequences, have no associated mass effect, and occur along the path of a penetrating vessel. Common locations include the medial temporal lobes and inferior one-third of the putamen and thalamus. Occasionally they may be seen along the course of small medullary veins near the vertex, particularly on T2 images at 3 T. Most perivascular spaces seen on MR are between 1 and 3 mm in diameter, but some may be 5 mm or larger. Enlarged perivascular spaces are observed as a normal variant in all age groups (Fig. 4.28). Both increasing size and frequency are noted with increasing age.

Small Vessel Ischemic Changes. Small foci of T2 hyperintensity are commonly seen scattered throughout the brains of older patients, with or without clinical symptoms. These "UBOs" (unidentified bright objects) can cause considerable consternation. They are commonly associated with patchy or diffuse T2 hyperintensity in the centrum semiovale (Fig. 4.28). Pages could be filled with different authors' terms for related processes: white matter hyperintensities, small vessel ischemic disease, senescent change, Binswanger disease, multi-infarct dementia, and leukoariosis, to name a few. There is no consensus on when these imaging changes should be considered abnormal, and when they simply represent a normal part of the aging process. At one end of the spectrum are patients who have collected enough tiny infarcts over the years to impair brain function. Individually or in small numbers these were

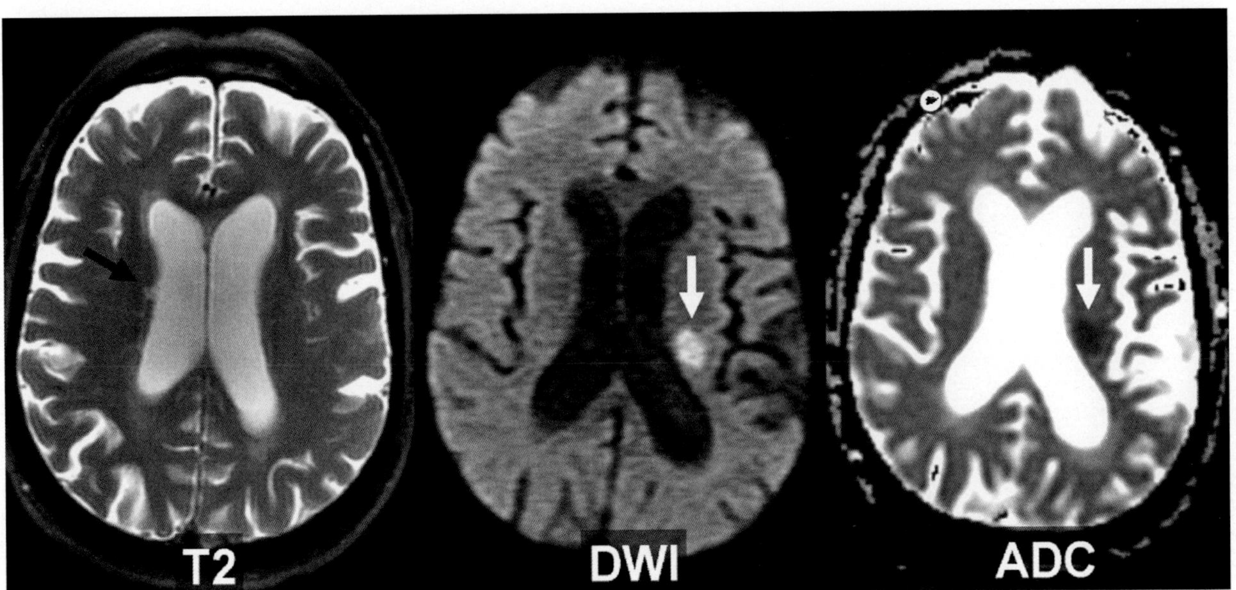

FIGURE 4.25. **Old Versus New Lacunes Distinguished by T2 and DWI.** This patient presented with a pure motor stroke. T2 shows a small old lacune in the right periventricular white matter (*black arrow*) and age-related periatrial white matter changes. The cytotoxic edema of the acute infarct is seen only on DWI and ADC maps (*white arrows*). DWI in an acute infarct may remain hyperintense for about a month, and then evolves toward more water-like signal thereafter.

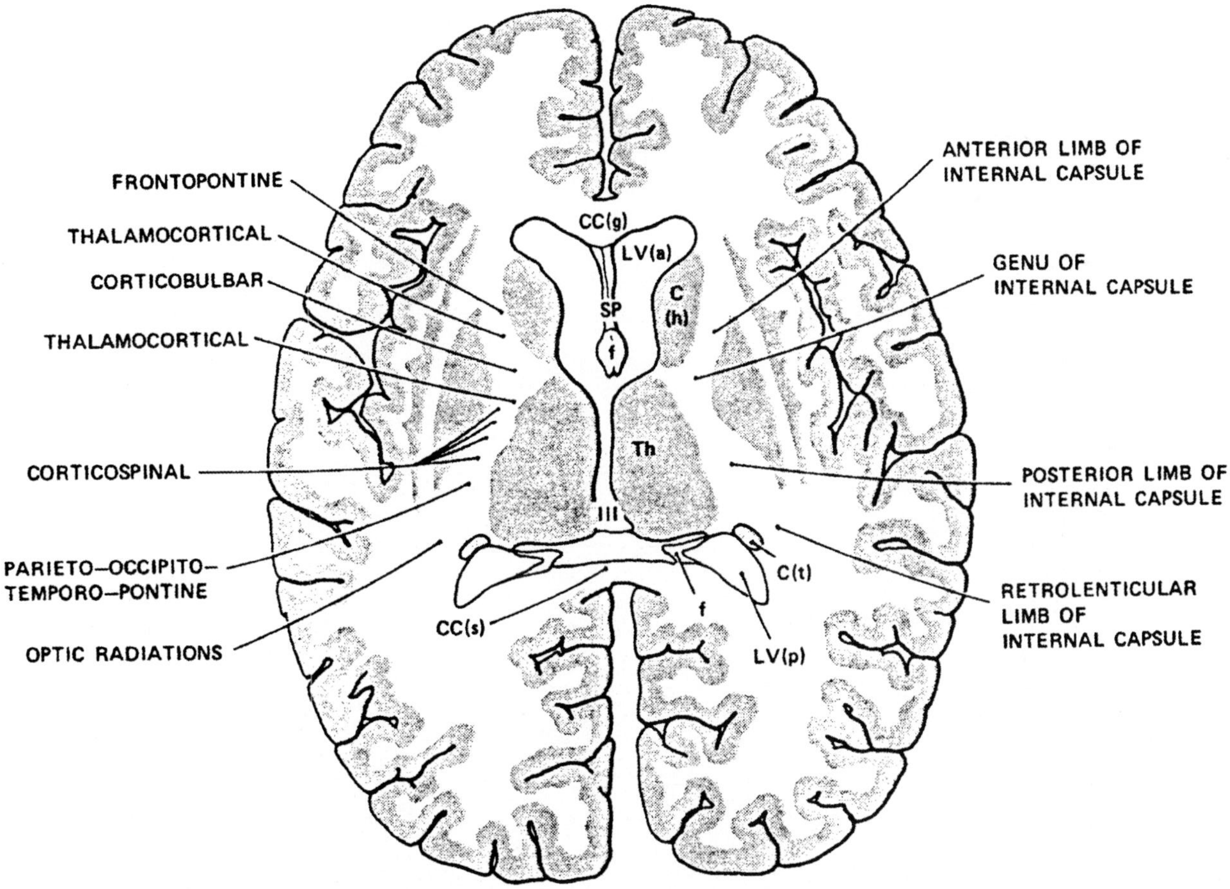

FIGURE 4.26. **Somatotopy of the Internal Capsule.** Transverse diagram showing the main parts of the internal capsule (labeled on the right) and major fiber tracts passing through it (labeled on the left). CC(g), genu of the corpus callosum; CC(s), splenium of the corpus callosum; C(h), caudate head; C(t), caudate tail; f, fornix; LV(a), anterior horn of the lateral ventricle; LV(p), posterior horn of the lateral ventricle; SP, septum pellucidum; Th, thalamus; III, third ventricle. (From Gilman S, Winans SS. *Manter and Gatz's Essentials of Clinical Neuroanatomy & Neurophysiology*. Philadelphia, PA: F.A. Davis Company, 1982.)

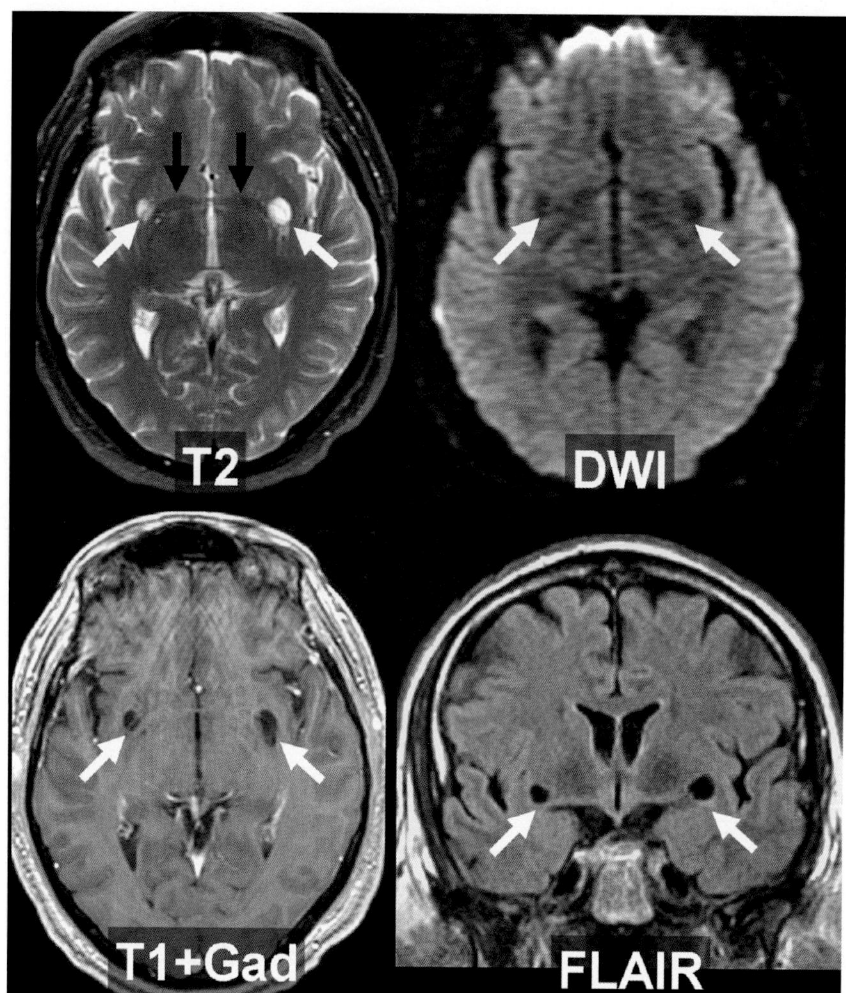

FIGURE 4.27. Virchow–Robin Spaces. All sequences show enlarged but normal perivascular spaces (*white arrows*) which exactly follow CSF intensity. There is no mass effect, and the patient had no symptoms referable to this region. These spaces are commonly seen at the ends of the anterior commissure ("black mustache," *black arrows*) in the anterior inferior basal ganglia. They should not be mistaken for lacunes, which typically show DWI hyperintensity acutely and signs of gliosis on FLAIR chronically.

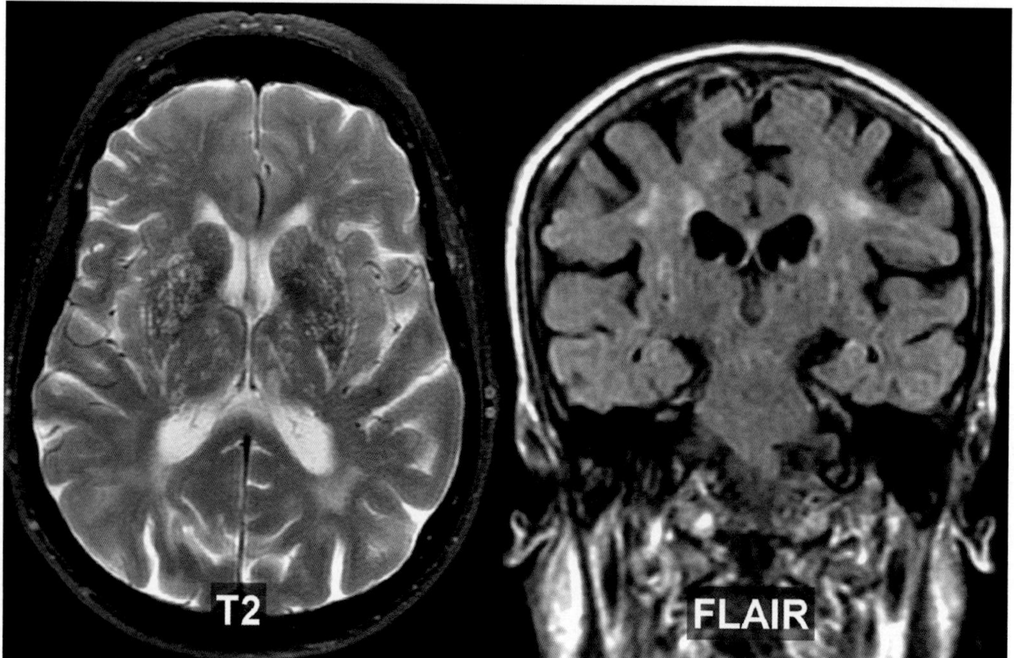

FIGURE 4.28. Small Vessel Ischemic Changes and Perivascular Spaces in Aging. Transverse T2WI at the level of the basal ganglia shows numerous areas of hyperintensity. The radial, linear areas likely represent prominent CSF spaces around small medullary veins ("etat crible"). Coronal FLAIR shows hyperintensity indicative of gliosis limited to just the old ischemic lesions, not seen around the prominent perivascular spaces.

presumably asymptomatic, but in aggregate contribute to a vascular dementia picture. At the other end of the spectrum are perfectly healthy patients who have presumably developed a speck of gliosis or occlusion of an inconsequential tiny vessel as a normal part of aging. The clinical findings must determine which of these patients with small vessel ischemic changes needs further workup.

Vasculitis and Reversible Cerebral Vasoconstriction Syndrome. Patchy inflammatory changes in arterial walls may lead to either large or small vessel stroke. Vasculitis may be triggered by autoimmune disorders, polyarteritis nodosa, and idiopathic processes (e.g., giant cell arteritis). Drug exposure (heroin, amphetamines, serotonin reuptake inhibitors), migraine, and postictal states have been linked to reversible cerebral vasoconstriction syndrome (RCVS), which can mimic vasculitis. RCVS causes irregular beading of vessels, but usually without the inflammatory infiltration of the vessel wall characteristic of vasculitis. Vasculitic infarcts are often scattered across multiple vascular territories and therefore may produce atypical patterns of damage. Varying stages of inflammation, necrosis, fibrosis, and aneurysms may be seen simultaneously.

Cases of suspected vasculitis are evaluated by conventional angiography which provides the highest possible resolution. Views of the intracranial circulation and the external carotid artery are reviewed in search of irregular focal narrowing. High-resolution gadolinium-enhanced black blood MR images with fat saturation can also sometimes show focal arterial wall thickening. Positive sites may then be selected for biopsy confirmation. Sometimes the vessels affected are so small the angiogram is normal. In these cases, skin, nerve, muscle, or random temporal artery biopsy may be required to make the diagnosis. Diagnostic confirmation is important, since many of the vasculitides respond to steroids or cytotoxic drugs, or in the case of RCVS, potential treatment with vasodilators and removal of the underlying trigger.

Venous Infarction

Venous occlusion is an uncommon but important cause of stroke. Characteristically, venous infarcts occur in younger patients who present with headache, sudden focal deficits, and often seizures. Predisposing factors include hypercoagulable states, pregnancy, infection (spread from contiguous scalp, face, middle ear, or sinus), dehydration, meningitis, and direct invasion by tumor. Even though arterial supply is intact, blockage of outflow leads to stasis, deoxygenation of blood, and neuronal death. Continued perfusion into damaged, occluded vessels frequently leads to hemorrhage. Any dural sinus or cortical vein may be affected, but the commonest are superior sagittal, transverse (lateral), straight sinus, and cavernous sinus occlusions, either alone or in combination.

A pattern of hemorrhagic infarction in the deep cortical or subcortical regions is usually present. These lesions tend to be rounded and may spare some overlying cortex, as opposed to the classic wedge-shaped arterial occlusions which grow larger toward the surface. Venous infarctions may also be suspected when there is an apparent infarct not conforming to a known arterial territory (Fig. 4.29).

The venous clot responsible may be seen indirectly as a filling defect in the superior sagittal sinus on contrast-enhanced CT, the "empty delta" sign (Fig. 4.30). The empty delta sign is usually present 1 to 4 weeks after sinus occlusion, but may not be seen in the acute and chronic phases of the disease. Small venous occlusions are not reliably detected by CT. An appearance which mimics the empty delta sign has also been described in up to 10% of normal patients when CT scanning is delayed for more than 30 minutes after contrast infusion. This is probably due to differential blood pool clearance and dural absorption of contrast, effectively highlighting the dural margins of a normal venous sinus.

A combination of spin-echo MR and MR venography probably provide the best imaging evaluation for dural sinus occlusion. On MR, venous sinus thrombosis is suspected when venous flow voids are lost and confirmed when actual clot is observed (Fig. 4.30). Normal but slowly flowing blood can sometimes cause high signal within veins, a potential MR pitfall in the diagnosis of venous occlusion. MR venography can be very helpful in equivocal cases. Whole brain CTA protocols modified to add a slightly longer scan delay after injection also offer an excellent noninvasive evaluation of venous disease. Conventional angiography is now mostly reserved for difficult diagnostic cases or when endovascular intervention is considered.

HEMORRHAGE

Hemorrhage occurs when an artery or vein ruptures, allowing blood to burst forth into the brain parenchyma or subarachnoid

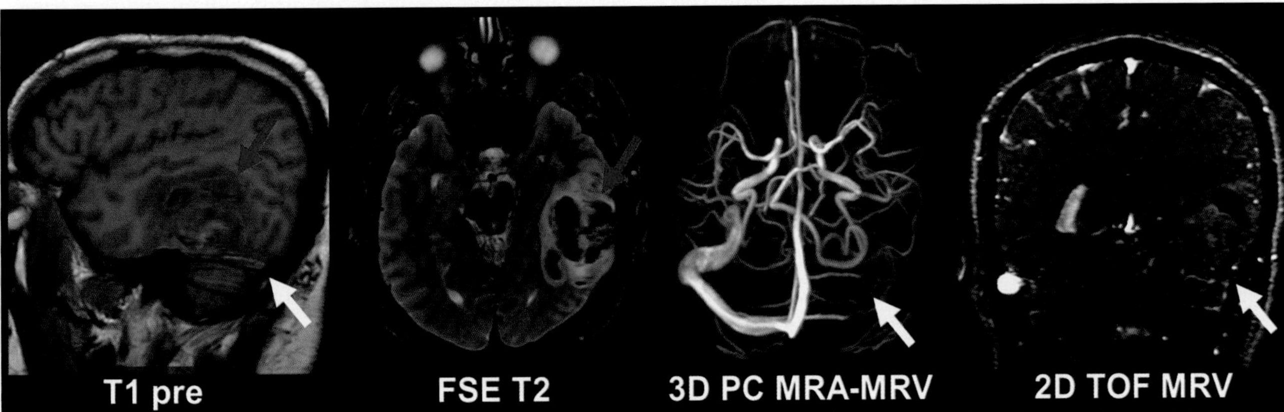

FIGURE 4.29. Transverse Sinus Occlusion With Venous Infarction. Venous infarction from combined left transverse sinus and vein of Labbe occlusions. This previously healthy man presented with abrupt Wernicke (receptive) aphasia. T1- and T2-weighted images show mixed edema and early hemorrhage (consistent with intracellular deoxyhemoglobin—iso on T1, dark on T2) in the posterior inferior left temporal lobe (*red arrows*). This location and appearance is classic for venous infarction in the territory of the vein of Labbe, which occurs when its drainage pathway into the transverse sinus (*white arrows*) becomes thrombosed, as confirmed here on MR venography (3D phase contrast and 2D time of flight).

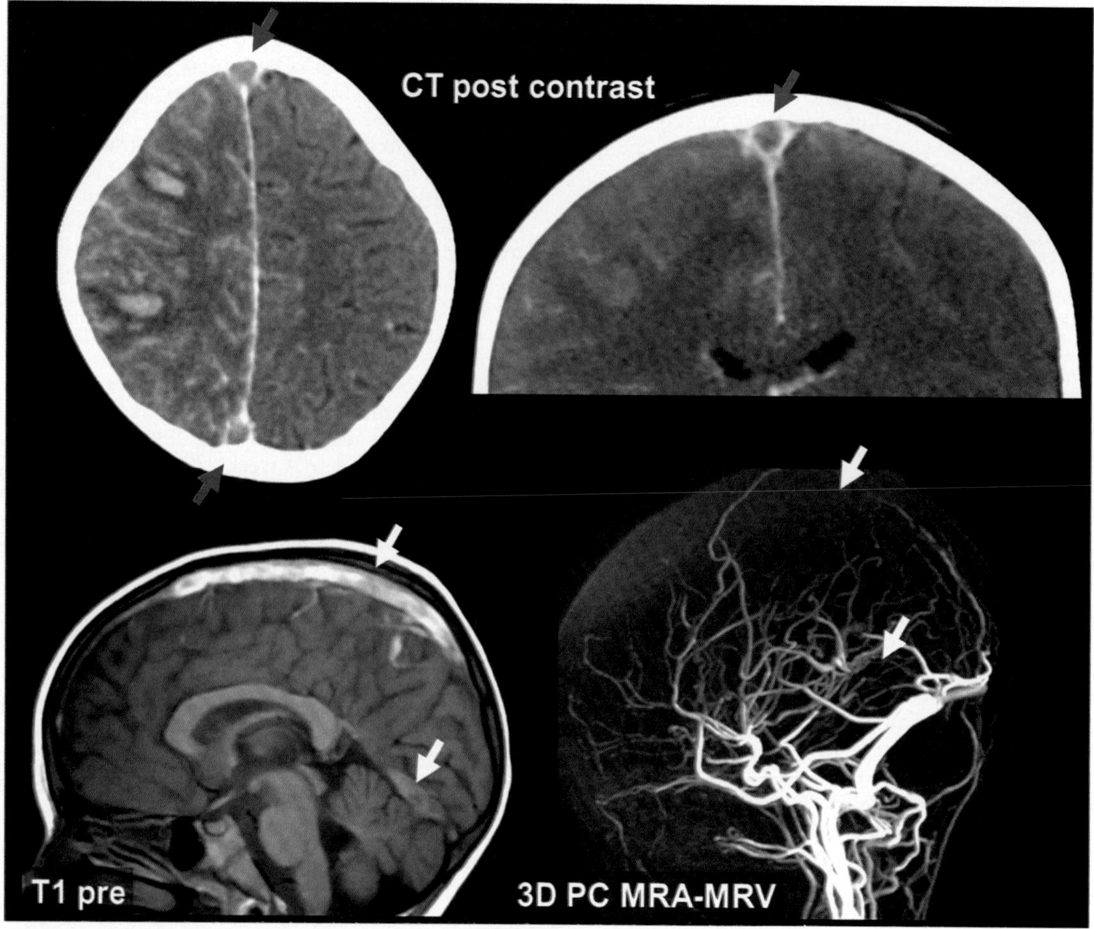

FIGURE 4.30. Venous Sinus Thrombosis Complicated by Hemorrhagic Venous Infarction. This 4-year-old girl recently treated with L-asparaginase for leukemia presented with headache, seizures, and left hemiparesis. CT images (above) show areas of right frontal lobe hemorrhage, edema, and leptomeningeal congestion. Filling defects (clot) outlined by enhancing dura of the superior sagittal sinus are the classic "empty delta sign" of dural sinus thrombosis (*arrows*) in both axial and coronal reconstructions. Follow-up MRI (below) shows T1-bright methemoglobin clot in the superior sagittal sinus (*white arrows*) and isointense signal in the straight sinus; MR venography confirms lack of flow in these sinuses.

spaces. Although mixed patterns occur, hemorrhages are most conveniently divided into subarachnoid and parenchymal categories. Imaging studies are critical in determining the source of bleeding and in showing any associated complications. The location and pattern of hemorrhage help predict what the underlying lesion is and direct further workup.

Imaging of Hemorrhage

Hemorrhages are detected due to increased attenuation on CT and complex signal patterns related to iron oxidation on MR. In both cases, the formation of "clot," which has far less serum and therefore water than whole blood, also plays a role in the imaging findings. *A noncontrast CT remains the test of choice for emergency evaluation of suspected hemorrhage.* Although acute blood can sometimes be challenging to detect on routine MR, sensitivity is excellent when FLAIR is used for SAH and gradient echo T2* sequences are used for parenchymal bleeding. MR is better than CT for detection and characterization of subacute or chronic hemorrhage (Fig. 4.31).

The MR signal generated by blood depends on a complex interplay of hematocrit, oxygen content, type of hemoglobin and chemical state of its iron-containing moieties, tissue pH, protein content of any clot formed, and the integrity of red blood cell membranes. Dominant among these mechanisms is the oxidation state and location of iron species related to hemoglobin. Oxygenated hemoglobin is sequentially converted to deoxyhemoglobin, methemoglobin, and then hemosiderin over time. The magnetic properties of the resultant degradation products change the MR relaxation rates of adjacent protons, allowing the hemorrhage to be detected. A small halo of surrounding edema is common in the subacute phase of parenchymal bleeds, sometimes making interpretation of signal changes quite complex. High-field scanners and gradient echo sequences tend to improve conspicuity of subacute and chronic blood products. The general pattern of MR signal changes seen over time on a 1.5 T magnet is summarized in Table 4.4 and Figure 4.32. Individual cases may of course vary somewhat from these simplified guidelines due to the multiple factors involved.

A brief stroll down physical chemistry lane will help us understand the complicated signal changes seen during the evolution of a hemorrhage. In order to change the signal characteristics of a tissue, hemorrhage must affect T1 or T2 relaxation. The sequential oxidation products of hemoglobin accomplish this due to changes in both magnetic properties and in molecular conformation. Iron within hemorrhage breakdown products changes the effective local magnetic field, a process known as magnetic susceptibility. This change in field is translated

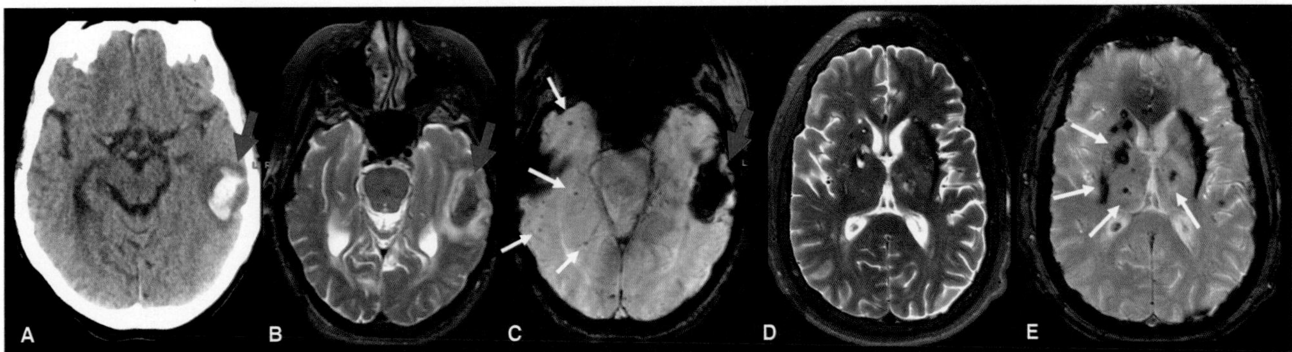

FIGURE 4.31. Amyloid Versus Hypertensive Microbleeds. Amyloid (**A–C**): Noncontrast CT (**A**) and FSE T2 (**B**) show an acute left temporal lobe hematoma (*red arrows*) which blooms darker on T2* (**C**). Key to the diagnosis of amyloid is the identification of numerous additional punctate old hemorrhages (aka "microbleeds") on T2*, distributed peripherally, in the cortex and near the gray-white junction (*white arrows*). Hypertensive hemorrhage (T2, **D**, and T2*, **E**) more typically involves the deep gray structures (*white arrows*), especially the thalami and basal ganglia, often keeping company with lacunes. Although CT can detect large acute hemorrhages from any cause, MRI gradient echo T2* or susceptibility-weighted sequences are required to detect older microbleeds and thereby facilitate differential diagnosis.

into an alteration in signal intensity because of acceleration or slowing of T1 and T2 relaxation rates. Changes in T1 relaxation occur only within a very short range (measured in angstroms) while T2 effects can be seen millimeters away.

Under normal conditions, circulating red blood cells contain a mixture of both oxy- and deoxyhemoglobin forms. During transit through the capillary bed, tissues extract oxygen according to metabolic needs, converting oxyhemoglobin to deoxyhemoglobin in the process.

Neither of these forms have much detectable effect on T1 signal intensity in clinical images, but they may be distinguished due to their opposite effects on T2WI. *Oxyhemoglobin* is a diamagnetic compound containing ferrous (Fe^{+2}) ions, *detected as high signal intensity* on T2WI (particularly first echo). Deoxyhemoglobin also contains Fe^{+2} ions but is a paramagnetic substance. The magnetic susceptibility of deoxyhemoglobin causes accelerated dephasing of spins on T2- or T2*-weighted images (e.g., gradient-recalled echo sequences) which results in signal loss. *Deoxyhemoglobin* is therefore *hypointense* on heavily T2WI. These patterns of altered T2 signals are occasionally encountered on clinical images of acute hemorrhage. These same magnetic susceptibility effects related to the balance of blood oxygenation form the basis for clinical functional MR mapping methods (brain regions activated by a task recruit more blood flow and oxyhemoglobin, detected as a focal *increase* in T2* MR signal).

When hemorrhage occurs, oxyhemoglobin is converted to deoxyhemoglobin at a rate dependent on local pH and oxygen tension. This takes place over hours for parenchymal hematomas but can be considerably delayed when oxygen-containing CSF surrounds subarachnoid blood. This may explain why acute subarachnoid blood is relatively difficult to detect by routine MR, but is readily detectable with FLAIR imaging (signal in bloody CSF is not suppressed). In parenchymal or extraaxial hematomas, further oxidation of deoxyhemoglobin leads to formation of methemoglobin, a ferric (Fe^{+3}) paramagnetic substance. This occurs over several days or longer, parallel in time course to lysis of red blood cells.

Methemoglobin causes a marked acceleration of T1 relaxation, leading to bright signal on T1WI (Fig. 4.30). Methemoglobin contained within intact red cells is able to set up local field gradients between the cell and the protons outside; this magnetic susceptibility leads to signal loss on T2WI. After cell lysis methemoglobin is dispersed throughout the tissue water, the gradient is lost, and T2 relaxation similar to CSF is seen. Bright T1 signal is a helpful indicator of subacute blood products; the appearance on T2 tells you whether this is still early intracellular (dark T2) or later extracellular (bright T2) stage. T2WI of subacute hematomas therefore show a "hematocrit effect": a dependent layer of intact cells exhibiting dark signal and a plasma supernatant showing bright signal.

Further oxidation of hemoglobin and breakdown of the globin molecule leads to accumulation of hemosiderin in the lysosomes of macrophages. Hemosiderin causes the gross rust-colored stain at the edges of an old hematoma seen at surgery or autopsy, even years after the index event. This is a paramagnetic ferric (Fe^{+3}) containing substance that is insoluble in water. As a result, hemosiderin shows no appreciable T1 effects but very prominent T2 shortening (dark signal) due to magnetic susceptibility (T2*) effects. An area of remote

TABLE 4.4

EVOLUTION OF HEMORRHAGE BY MR

■ TIME	■ RBC[a]	■ HEMOGLOBIN STATE	■ T1 SIGNAL	■ T2 SIGNAL
<1 day	Intact	Oxyhemoglobin	Iso/dark	Bright
0–2 days	Intact	Deoxyhemoglobin	Iso/dark	Dark
2–14 days	Intact	Methemoglobin (intracellular)	Bright	Dark
10–21 days	Lysed	Methemoglobin (extracellular)	Bright	Bright
≥21 days	Lysed	Hemosiderin/Ferritin	Iso/dark	Dark

[a]Red blood cells.

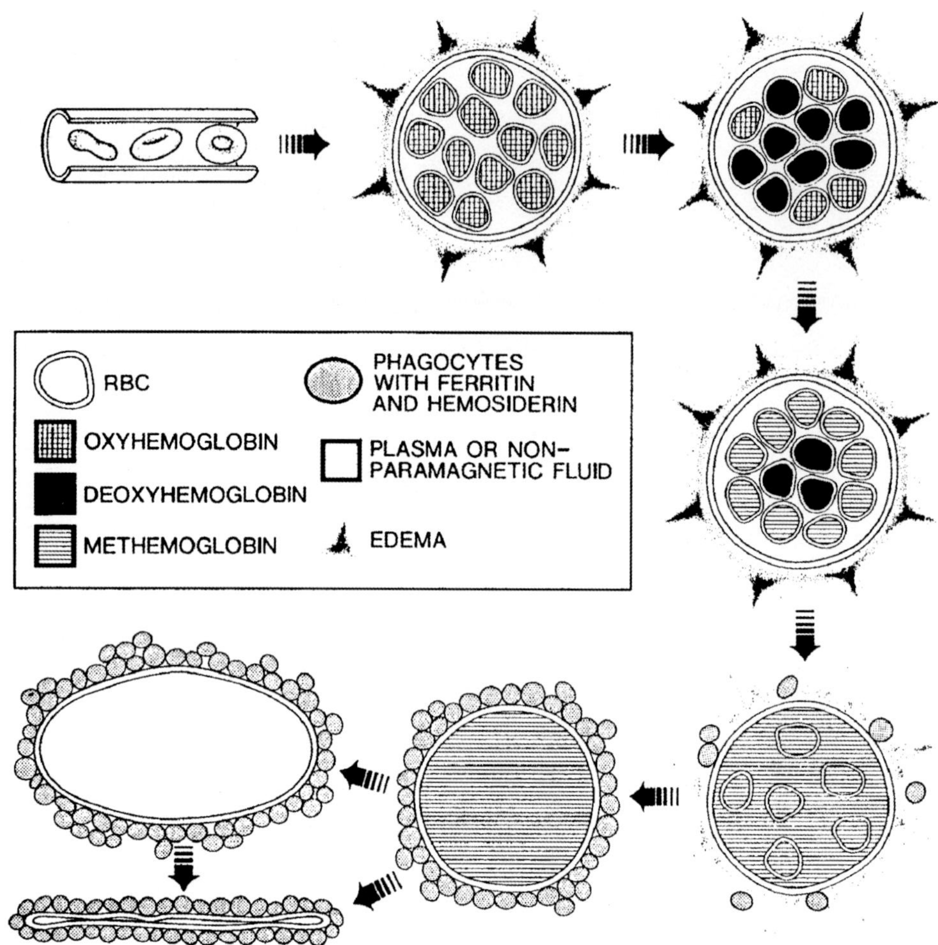

FIGURE 4.32. **Biochemical Evolution of Hemorrhage.** Within minutes of hemorrhage, a hematoma consists of intact red blood cells containing oxyhemoglobin. Over several hours, the clot begins to retract and the hemoglobin is oxidized from oxy- to deoxy- to methemoglobin. Methemoglobin tends to form in a ring which converges from the periphery to the center over time. Red cells lyse, releasing methemoglobin into the surrounding fluid. Macrophages break down the iron products into hemosiderin and ferritin, leaving a stain at the periphery of older hematomas. (From Atlas SW. *Magnetic Resonance Imaging of the Brain and Spine*. New York: Raven Press; 1991.)

hemorrhage will commonly be seen as atrophy alone on CT or T1-weighted MR, but a dark rim along the cleft on T2WI implicates a prior bleed. Occasionally, large or recurrent SAHs will lead to diffuse hemosiderin deposition on the brain surface, a condition known as superficial hemosiderosis (or superficial siderosis).

Subarachnoid Hemorrhage

The subarachnoid space is the CSF-lined compartment which surrounds the blood vessels and communicates with the ventricular system. SAH is most commonly due to aneurysm rupture. AVMs of the brain or spinal cord and vascular malformations involving the dura may also cause SAH, but usually in combination with parenchymal or subdural bleeding, respectively. Previously normal vessels may rupture into the subarachnoid space when damaged by drugs, trauma, or dissection. SAH may also occasionally be seen in patients with marked thrombocytopenia or other severe coagulopathies.

Patients with aneurysms may develop symptoms attributable to either bleeding or local mass effect. Sudden, severe headache is the most common symptom of aneurysm rupture, sometimes described by patients as the worst headache of their life. Unruptured aneurysms or those with limited surrounding hemorrhage may also develop significant mass effect with or without headache. Classic presentations in this regard are the unilateral third nerve palsy due to a posterior communicating artery aneurysm, cavernous sinus syndrome due to an ICA/parasellar aneurysm, and optic chiasmal syndrome (bitemporal field defect) due to an anterior communicating artery aneurysm.

A patient who presents with SAH is very likely to harbor a ruptured congenital (berry) aneurysm (Fig. 4.33). One to 2% of us have aneurysms, thought to occur due to a congenital absence of the arterial media. Probably many of these aneurysms remain asymptomatic, but those greater than 3 to 5 mm are at increased risk for rupture. Berry aneurysms often occur near branch points of the circle of Willis. About 85% sprout from the anterior part of the circle of Willis, while 15% arise in the vertebrobasilar territory. Common locations include branch points near the anterior communicating (33%), middle cerebral (30%), posterior communicating (25%), and basilar (10%) arteries. Less commonly the ophthalmic artery, cavernous ICA, or PICA are to blame. When distal branch aneurysms are seen, an episode of prior trauma or systemic infection should be considered (e.g., bacterial endocarditis with "mycotic" aneurysm). Other conditions associated with aneurysms include atherosclerosis, fibromuscular disease, and polycystic kidney disease. Management depends on the clinical situation, location, and size of the aneurysm. Treatment options include surgical clipping, interventional endovascular coil embolization, and combinations of the two (Fig. 4.34).

Even large acute SAHs easily seen by CT may be entirely missed on routine spin-echo MR. CT is over 90% sensitive for the detection of acute SAH, probably due to the increased density of clotted blood. Use of FLAIR sequences on MR can improve conspicuity of acute blood, but CT is still considered the imaging method of choice when clinical findings suggest the possibility of SAH (Fig. 4.34). SAHs may be quite difficult to detect even by CT when the patient's hematocrit is low, the amount of hemorrhage small, or there is a delay in scanning.

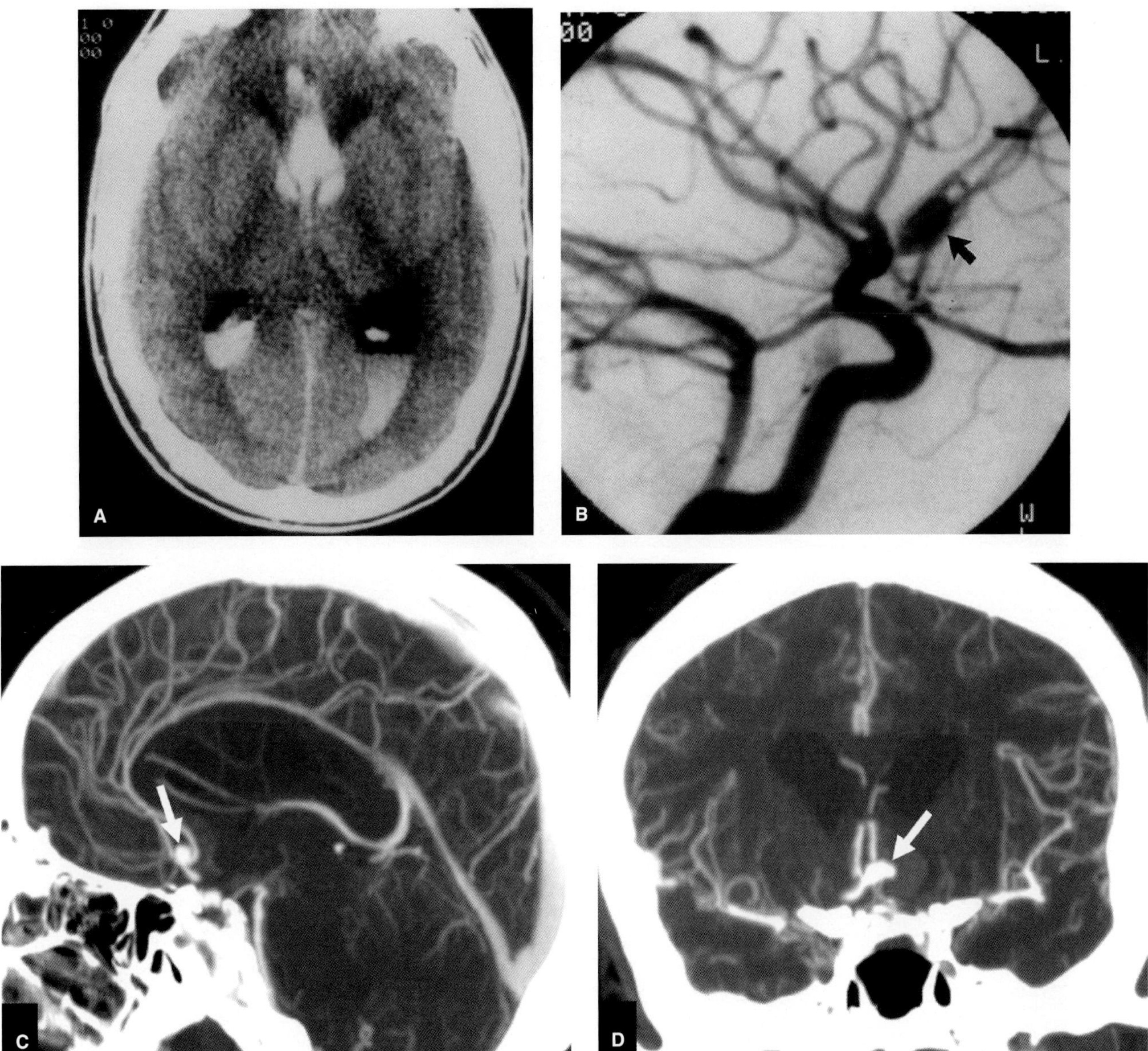

FIGURE 4.33. **Ruptured Anterior Communicating Artery Aneurysm.** This 21-year-old man collapsed immediately after snorting a line of cocaine. **A:** Non-contrast CT shows blood in the interhemispheric fissure and in the dependent portions of the lateral ventricles. Blood in the ventricles, cisterns, or layered in the sulci is subarachnoid by definition. **B:** Lateral view from a digital subtraction angiogram demonstrates a large anterior communicating artery aneurysm (*arrow*). Over half of drug abusers with intracranial hemorrhage will be found to have an underlying aneurysm or AVM. CTA in a similar case showing a ruptured aneurysm (*white arrows*) in sagittal (**C**) and coronal (**D**) thick 2D reconstructions.

In these cases detection of red blood cells or xanthochromia by lumbar puncture may be the only way to confirm a suspected SAH. The most sensitive places to look for SAH on CT are the dependent portions of the subarachnoid space where gravity causes the blood to settle—the interpeduncular fossa, posterior sylvian fissure, and the far posterior aspects of the occipital horns (Fig. 4.35). Prompt scanning is important, since dissolution of subarachnoid blood reduces CT sensitivity to 66% by day 3.

About 15% to 20% of patients with subarachnoid bleeding will have multiple aneurysms. Due to this multiplicity, a CTA or "four-vessel" angiogram is needed on the initial evaluation. When multiple aneurysms are present, the one that is largest or more irregular, has focal mass effect, intra-aneurysmal clot, or shows a change on serial examinations is likely to be the culprit. CTA has become an important front line screening tool for emergent evaluation of SAH, and in most centers, has largely replaced diagnostic angiography. MRA is not yet of proven reliability for the primary workup of a patient presenting with SAH. The combination of MR and MRA probably detects the vast majority of aneurysms greater than 3 mm, making it a reasonable elective screening tool for some at-risk patients (strong family histories, polycystic kidney disease, etc.).

The location of blood in the subarachnoid spaces is imperfectly correlated with the location of a ruptured aneurysm, as subarachnoid blood can layer dependently. Sometimes a parenchymal clot will surround the site of hemorrhage, or thrombus may be seen in the aneurysm itself. When the routine screening CT shows SAH, CTA can be immediately performed to evaluate for aneurysms while the patient is still on the scanner. Within a few days a focus of methemoglobin may

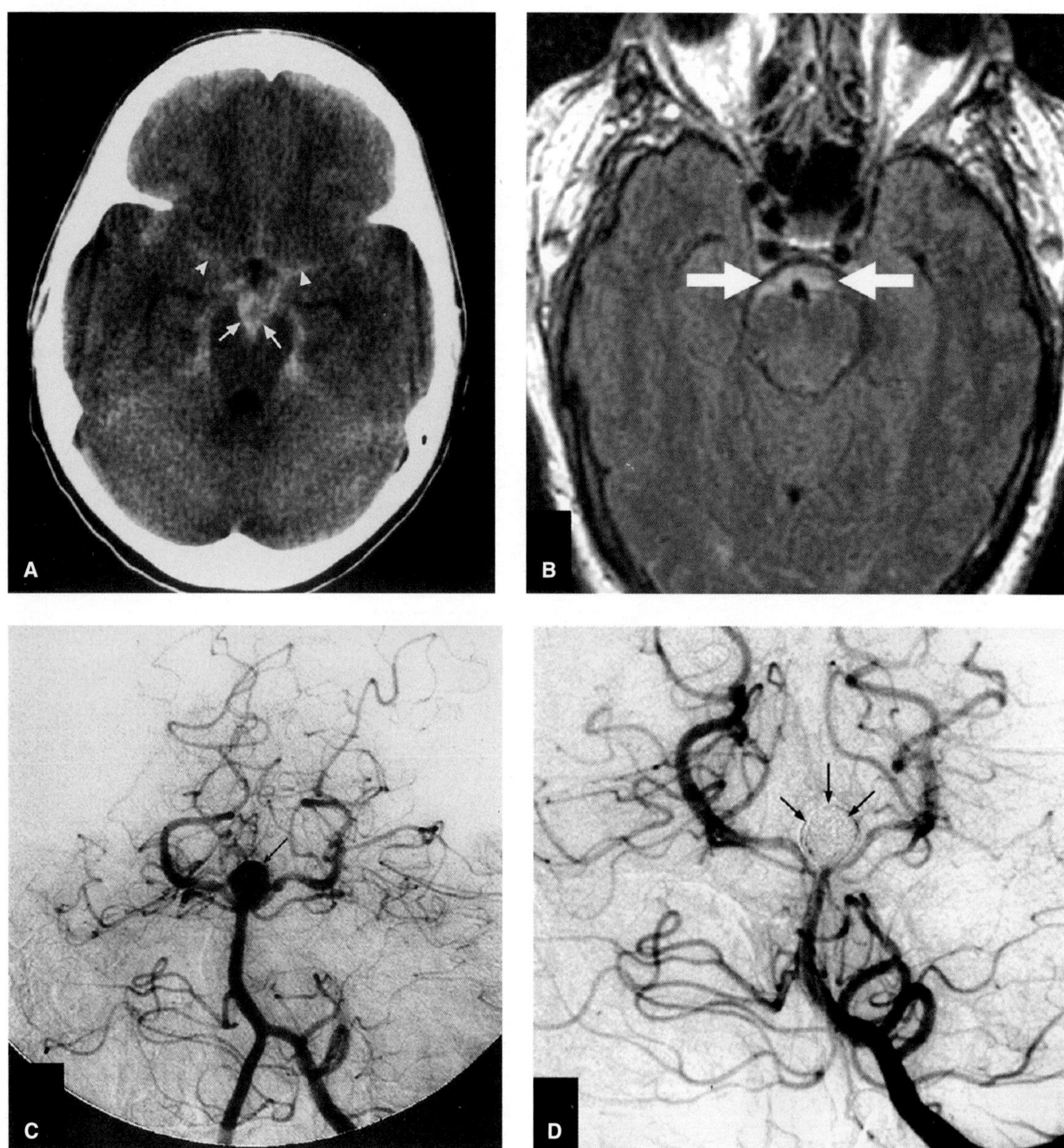

FIGURE 4.34. **Endovascular Coil Treatment of a Basilar Tip Aneurysm.** This 36-year-old patient presented with a severe headache. **A:** A noncontrast CT shows prominent subarachnoid hemorrhage in the interpeduncular fossa (*arrows*) and throughout the basilar cisterns (*arrowheads*). **B:** SAH is commonly missed on routine MR sequences, but is easily visible on T2 FLAIR (*large white arrows*). **C:** Angiogram, frontal view of a left vertebral injection shows a basilar tip aneurysm (*arrow*). **D:** Angiogram following endovascular placement of electrolytically detachable platinum coils shows obliteration of the aneurysm (*arrows*) with preservation of adjacent arterial branches.

sometimes pinpoint the bleeding site on MR. Unless there has been a massive SAH or rebleeding, subarachnoid blood is generally inconspicuous on CT at 1 week.

Evaluation and management of aneurysmal SAH has changed considerably over the past 15 years due to wider application of CTA and endovascular coil embolization. While surgically easily accessible aneurysms are still well treated by traditional open clipping, endovascular coiling has been shown to have overall lower morbidity and mortality. Early clipping or coiling allows more aggressive treatment for vasospasm, a much feared complication seen beginning a few days after SAH. These considerations have lead many centers to screen all acute SAHs using diagnostic CTA, followed by angiography for complex cases or those expected to proceed to coil intervention. Two- and three-dimensional CTA reconstructions of aneurysms can help select and plan either open surgical or endovascular procedures.

Follow-up studies are an integral part of SAH evaluation. The initial or subsequent CT may show communicating hydrocephalus requiring a ventriculostomy or shunt. Episodes of possible rebleeding are evaluated with noncontrast CT. Infarcts may also be seen in patients with elevated intracranial pressure or vasospasm, and are the main pathologic finding in patients whose condition continues to deteriorate after the initial SAH. Posttreatment angiography is used to assess adequacy of clip placement and to rule out vasospasm. Angiography or MRA can be used to follow coiled aneurysms.

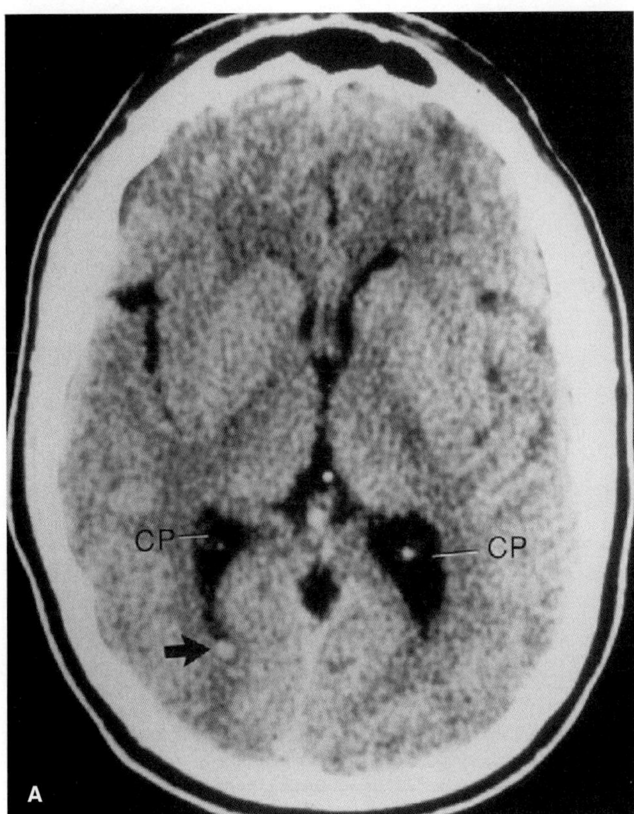

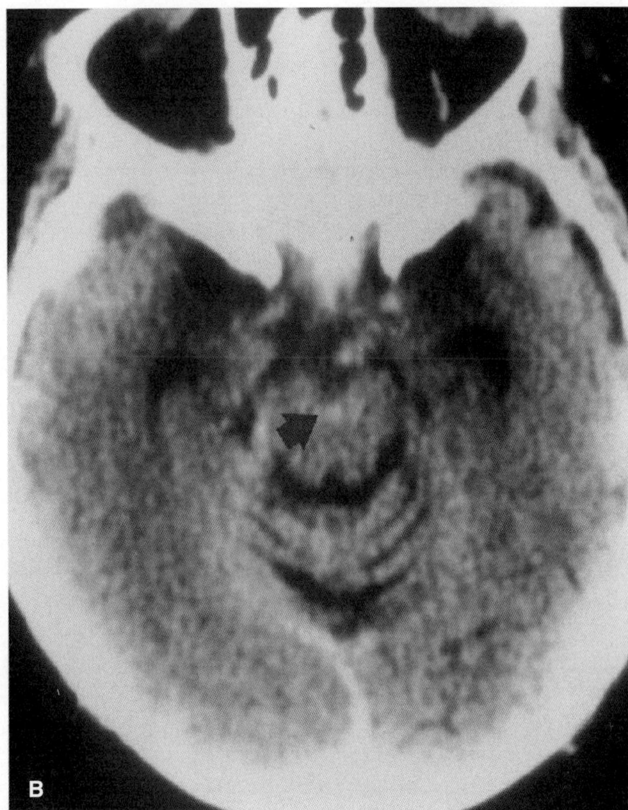

FIGURE 4.35. Subtle Subarachnoid Hemorrhage by CT. The most sensitive areas for detecting SAH are the dependent parts of the occipital horns (**A**, *arrow*) and the interpeduncular fossa (**B**, *arrow*). The choroid plexus at the atrium of the lateral ventricle (**A**, CP) normally appears dense due to calcification or enhancement. The nondependent location of the choroid differentiates it from hemorrhage.

Parenchymal Hemorrhage

Primary intraparenchymal hemorrhage occurs as a result of bleeding directly into the brain substance. Traumatic hemorrhages are not included in this section; they are discussed in Chapter 3. Parenchymal bleeds generally have a higher initial mortality than infarcts, but on recovery show fewer deficits than a similar-sized infarct. This is because hemorrhage tends to tear through and displace brain tissue, but can be resorbed. A similar-sized infarct is made up of dead rather than just displaced neurons. The main differential considerations are hypertensive hemorrhage, vascular malformations, drug effects, amyloid angiopathy, and bloody tumors.

Hypertensive hemorrhages are seen in the putamen (35% to 50%), the subcortical white matter (30%), the cerebellum (15%), thalamus (10% to 15%), and pons (5% to 10%) (Fig. 4.36). As with lacunes, lipohyalinosis of vessels is thought to be the primary predisposing pathologic feature, although miliary aneurysms in the vessel wall may also play a role. Small hypertensive hemorrhages may resolve with few deficits. Bleeds in the posterior fossa, those with a large amount of mass effect, or hemorrhages extending into the ventricular system have a relatively poor prognosis. The pattern of microbleeds sometimes seen in a patient with hemorrhage can help distinguish hypertension from amyloid-related bleeding (Fig. 4.31). Focal contrast extravasation within an acute hematoma on CTA or routine contrast-enhanced images ("spot sign") predicts a high risk of clot expansion over the first several hours after admission, compared to those without a spot sign (Figs. 4.36 and 4.37).

Vascular malformations are far less frequently encountered than hypertension, but are a cause of hemorrhage which must be ruled out, especially in young patients. Vascular malformations develop due to a congenitally abnormal vascular connection which may enlarge over time. The relative frequency of vascular malformations as a cause of intracranial hemorrhage is about 5%. There are four main subtypes: AVMs, cavernous malformations, telangiectasias, and venous malformations.

Arteriovenous malformations are high flow lesions and the most common type of brain vascular malformation. AVMs are an abnormal tangle of arteries directly connected to veins without an intervening capillary network. About 80% to 90% are supratentorial, but any area may be affected. Most patients present with hemorrhage or seizures. AVMs have a 2% to 3% annual risk of bleeding, but the risk may double or triple in the first year after an initial bleed. Treatment depends on the age of the patient, symptoms, and philosophy of the attending physicians. Embolization, surgery, and radiotherapy all may play a role.

Unruptured AVMs typically appear as a jumble of enlarged vessels without mass effect (Fig. 4.38). Noncontrast CT will show a mixed attenuation lesion, sometimes with evidence of calcification. MR demonstrates flow voids or complex flow patterns, sometimes leading to artifacts in the phase-encoding direction. T2- or T2*-weighted images may show dark signal intensity related to the AVM, a sign of prior hemorrhage with hemosiderin deposition. IV contrast usually results in marked enhancement and therefore increased conspicuity of the AVM on both CT and MR studies. Feeding arteries and draining veins may show impressive enlargement well beyond the

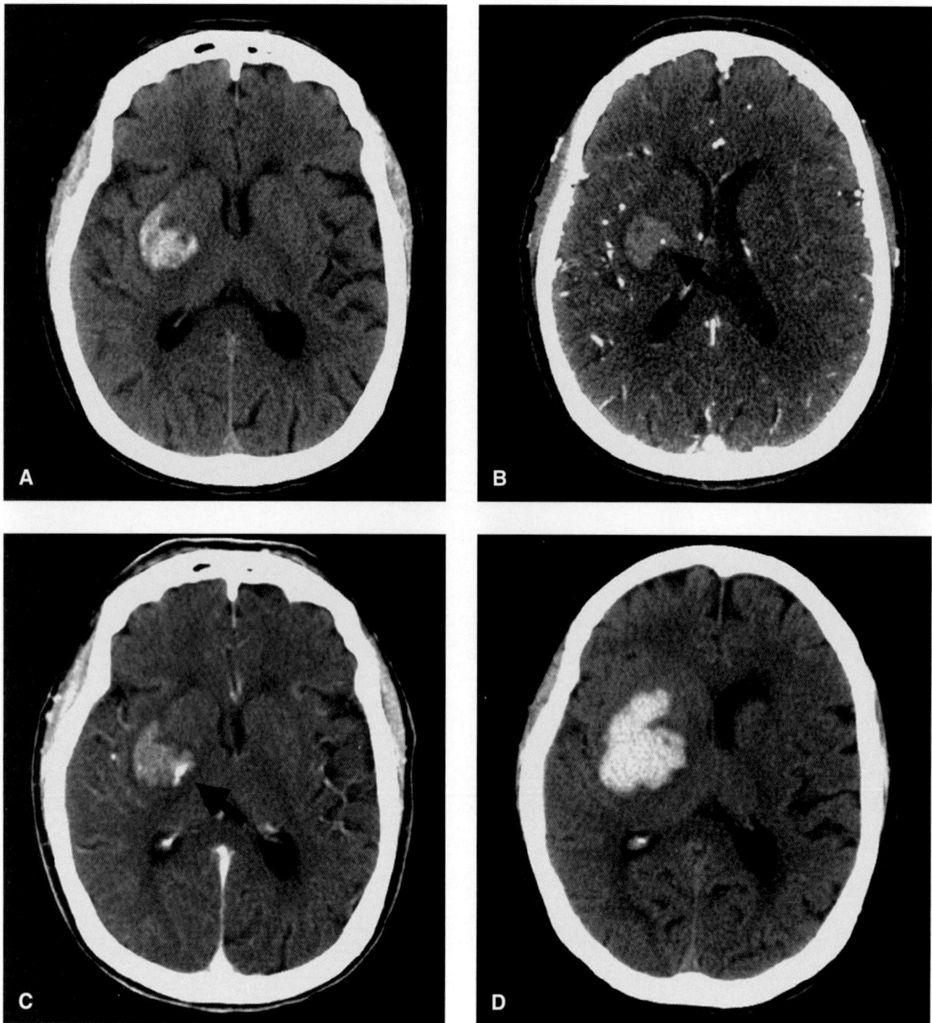

FIGURE 4.36. **Hypertensive Hemorrhage, "Spot Sign" Predicts Clot Expansion.** This patient with a history of hypertension presented with abrupt left hemiparesis. Noncontrast CT (**A**) shows a focal parenchymal hematoma centered in the right putamen. CTA source images (**B**) show a tiny focus contrast extravasation (*arrow*) contained within the hematoma which is even more conspicuous on routine postcontrast images (**C**) obtained 4 minutes after the CTA. Focal spot signs on either CTA or contrast CT suggest active bleeding and therefore high risk of hematoma expansion over the next several hours. (**D**) Follow-up noncontrast CT at 24 hours confirms marked enlargement of the hematoma as well as worsening mass effect.

center (nidus) of the AVM. About 10% of AVMs will develop an associated aneurysm, generally on a feeding artery. Angiography remains the definitive method for evaluation of the AVMs anatomy and dynamic flow patterns.

Telangiectasias are dilated capillary-sized vessels usually diagnosed at autopsy. These are generally small, solitary lesions found incidentally by contrast-enhanced MR, most often in the pons. No treatment is necessary.

Venous malformations (aka developmental venous anomalies, venous angiomas) are congenitally variant veins which drain normal brain. They are seen in about 5% of patients studied by contrast MR but may easily be missed on CT or noncontrast

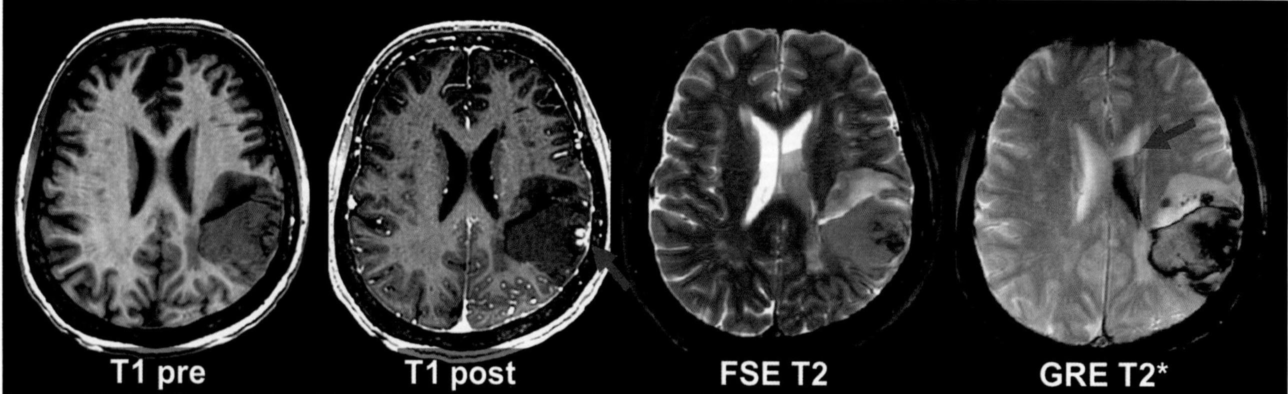

FIGURE 4.37. **Acute Left Parietal Parenchymal Hematoma on MRI.** Signal intensity is isointense on T1 and T2, with heterogeneous dark signal on T2*, indicative of a mixture of oxy- and deoxyhemoglobin (deoxy = dark components, "blooming" due to susceptibility). Focal puddles of contrast enhancement along the lateral margin on T1 postcontrast images (*arrow*) are an MRI "spot sign" indicative of active bleeding with risk of further clot expansion. Additional poor prognostic signs include intraventricular extension (*arrow*, T2*), and clot volume >30 mL (5 × 5 × 4 cm in diameter, for an estimated volume of 50 mL using [A × B × C]/2 rule in this case).

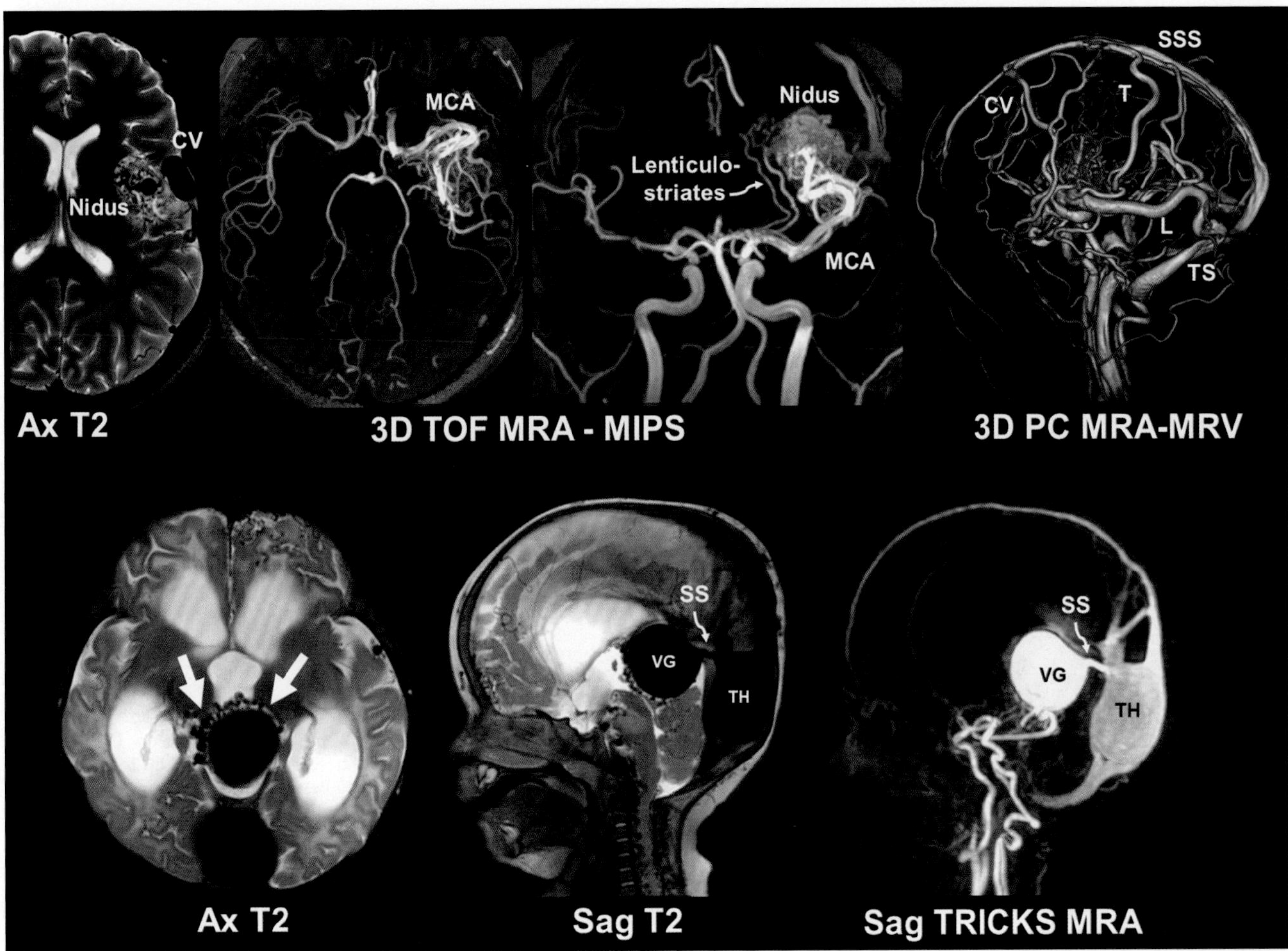

FIGURE 4.38. **High-Flow Vascular Malformations. Top:** Arteriovenous malformation (AVM) with nidus in the left insular region, fed by enlarged MCA branches and drained by engorged cortical veins (CV) including the veins of Trolard (T) and Labbe (L), with prominent superior sagittal sinus (SSS). **Bottom:** Infant girl with enlarging head circumference found to have a vein of Galen malformation, complicated by obstructive hydrocephalus. There is rapid shunting from feeding vessels (*arrows*) into a rounded, enlarged vein of Galen (VG) pouch and outward through a narrow straight sinus (SS) into a massively enlarged torcular herophili (TH).

MR. The classic appearance is of an enlarged enhancing stellate venous complex extending to the ventricular or cortical surface. The contrast-enhanced MR appearance is usually diagnostic, and most will show a dark signal on T2* due to deoxygenated venous blood, such that angiography is rarely if ever needed for confirmation. Although these may rarely bleed, treatment is somewhat controversial since they are very commonly seen in asymptomatic patients and are often the only venous drainage for a brain region.

Cavernous malformations are thin-walled sinusoidal vessels (neither arteries nor veins) which may present with seizures or small parenchymal hemorrhages. These lesions may be asymptomatic and can occur on a familial basis. CT scans and angiography are usually normal. MR will show a reticulated, often enhancing lesion with dark rim (hemosiderin) on T2 (Fig. 4.39). Venous malformations may provide drainage for cavernous malformations, but no arterialized feeding vessels should be seen. Unless recently ruptured, a cavernous malformation should show no mass effect or edema. If all these criteria are met, conventional angiography may be unnecessary.

Hemorrhage due to Coagulopathies. Intracranial hemorrhage may also occur because of blood dyscrasias. Chronic oral anticoagulation increases by eightfold the risk of intracranial hemorrhage. The association is particularly true when the coagulation parameters are extended beyond the recommended therapeutic range and when bleeding occurs in the setting of direct thrombin inhibitors.

Drug-Associated Hemorrhage. Sympathomimetic drugs seem to provide an effective (if unintended) stress test for the presence of brain vascular anomalies (Fig. 4.33). Drugs such as amphetamines and cocaine have been commonly associated with intracranial hemorrhage. Symptoms develop within minutes to hours following the use of the drug. The genesis may be related to transient hypertension or RCVS. Up to 50% of drug abusers who suffer an intracranial hemorrhage have a demonstrable underlying structural cause such as an aneurysm or AVM.

Amyloid angiopathy or "congophilic" angiopathy is an increasingly recognized cause of intracranial hemorrhage, frequently lobar in nature. It is characterized by amyloid deposits in the media and adventitia of medium size and small cortical leptomeningeal arteries. It is not associated with systemic vascular amyloidosis. This angiopathy characteristically affects elderly individuals. Autopsy incidence rises steeply, ranging from 8% in the seventh decade to 22% to 35% in the eighth decade, 40% in the ninth decade, and 58% in persons older than 90. It is rarely seen in patients younger than 55. Cerebral amyloid angiopathy is associated with dementia in about 30% of cases. Systemic hypertension is common in this age group but is not directly

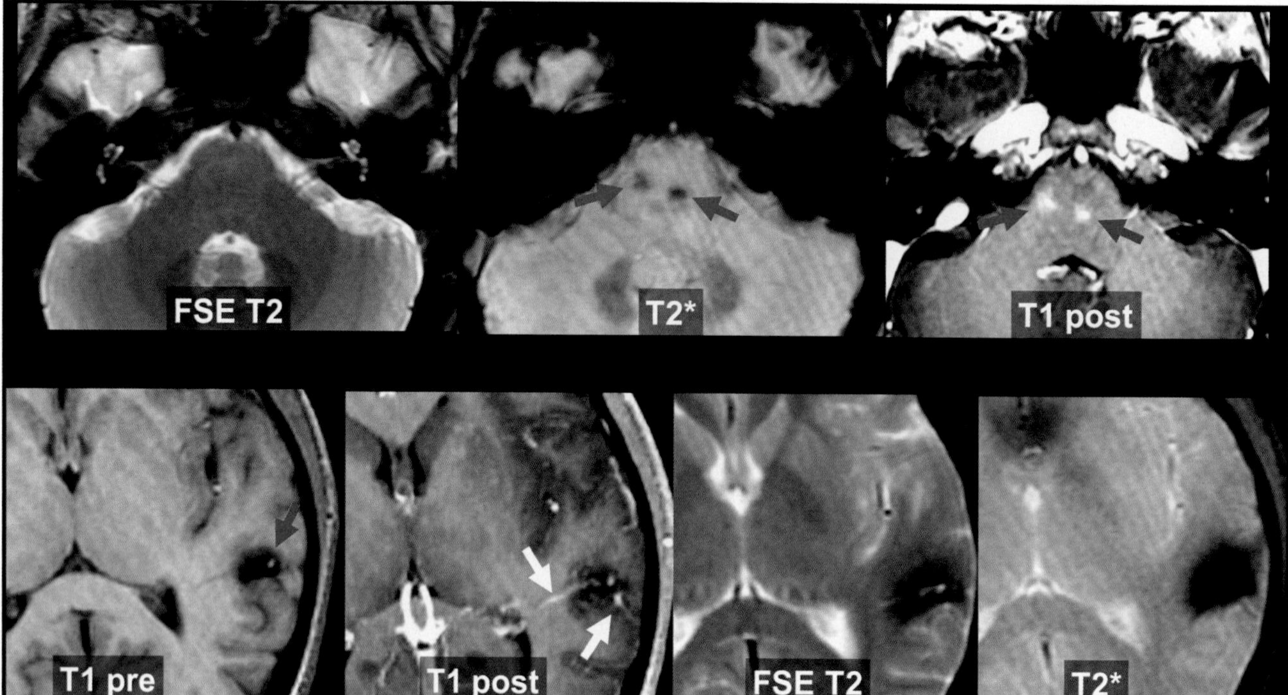

FIGURE 4.39. Low-Flow Vascular Malformations. Top: Incidental pontine capillary telangiectasias. No changes are visible on T2, but focal signal dropout on T2* (SWAN sequence) is indicative of deoxyhemoglobin in slow flowing small veins. These are visible as lacy, focal enhancement on T1-weighted images after gadolinium (*arrows*). These are a "don't touch" lesion that should not be confused with pathology such as metastatic disease or active demyelination. **Bottom:** Developmental venous anomaly (DVA) with associated cavernous malformation (aka, cavernoma). Characteristic "popcorn" lesion on T1 and T2 shows tissue loss and bright foci centrally, with dark periphery (*red arrows*). A small DVA is seen, with small radicles adjacent to the cavernoma and a collector vein passing toward the periatrial ependymal veins (*white arrows*). T2* shows magnification of dark signal ("blooming") due to old iron-containing blood products including hemosiderin. DVAs are usually asymptomatic, but on rare occasions give birth to a cavernous malformation which can rebleed or cause focal symptoms.

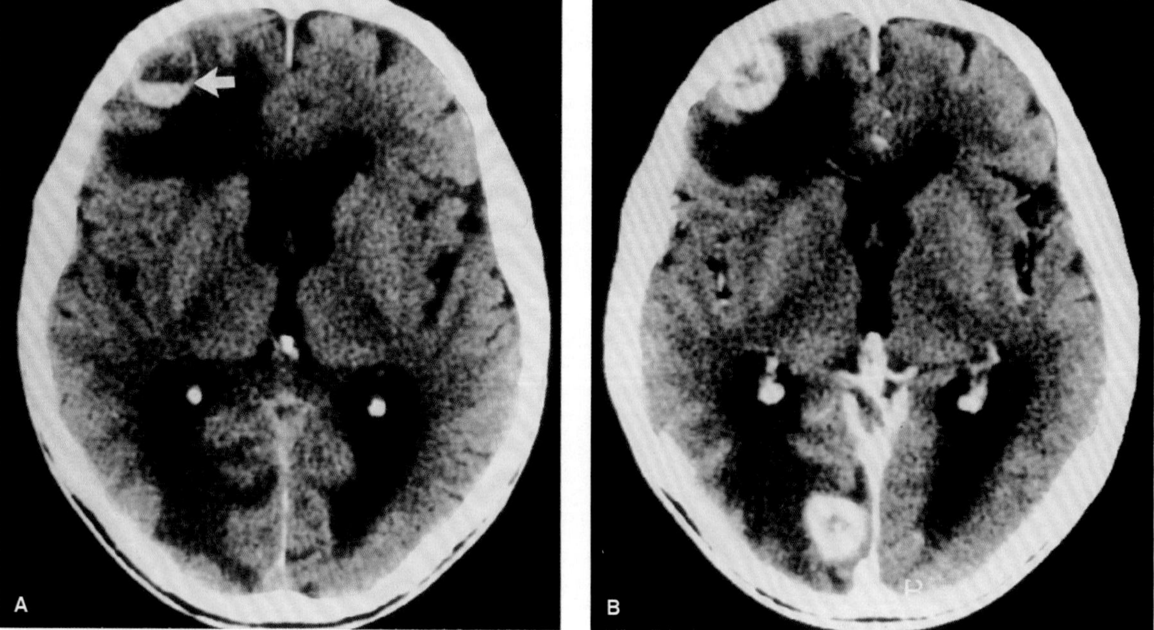

FIGURE 4.40. Hemorrhagic Metastases. This patient with oat cell carcinoma of the lung presented with new onset seizures. The precontrast CT (**A**) shows a rounded bloody mass in the right frontal lobe with a "hematocrit" layer (*arrow*). Marked white matter edema surrounds this lesion and is also seen in the right occipital lobe. Postcontrast scan (**B**) shows irregular ring enhancement of the bloody lesion and a second discrete focus is identified in the occipital lobe. The degree of surrounding edema, focal and irregular enhancement, and nonvascular distribution implicate metastases and not stroke.

TABLE 4.5

FEATURES OF BENIGN VERSUS MALIGNANT INTRACRANIAL HEMORRHAGE

■ SIGN	■ BENIGN	■ MALIGNANT
Evolution of blood products	Peripheral to central	Irregular, complex
Hemosiderin rim	Complete	Delayed, incomplete
Surrounding edema	Minimal/mild	Moderate/severe
Acute enhancement patterns	Minimal (unless AVM)	Moderate/severe

related to cerebral amyloid angiopathy. Widespread, multifocal involvement can be seen in some cases, particularly when T2*-weighted MR sequences are used to make old hemorrhages more conspicuous (Fig. 4.31). Amyloid angiopathy should come to mind when an elderly or demented patient presents with new or recurrent superficial hemorrhages. Pre-existing amyloid "microbleeds" may also be an underlying source for some cases of postthrombolytic hemorrhage.

Primary Hemorrhage Versus Hemorrhagic Neoplasm

Intracranial tumors are an uncommon but well-recognized cause of intracranial hemorrhage. They account for 1% to 2% of bleeds in autopsy series and as high as 6% to 10% in clinical radiologic series. Tumor necrosis, vascular invasion, and neovascularity may contribute to the pathogenesis of hemorrhagic neoplasms. Glioblastomas are the most common primary brain tumors to hemorrhage, while in the metastatic category bronchogenic carcinoma, thyroid, melanoma, choriocarcinoma, and renal cell carcinoma often bleed (Fig. 4.40).

It may be possible to distinguish between a hemorrhagic neoplasm and a primary (benign) intracranial hemorrhage based on the MR findings. Intratumoral bleeds tend to be more complex and heterogeneous than benign hematomas. The expected evolution of blood products is commonly delayed with tumors, possibly due to profound intratumoral hypoxia. If a patient is scanned in the acute phase, lack of enhancement beyond the hematoma strongly supports a primary intracranial hemorrhage. If there is an enhancing component, then lesions such as tumor or AVM must be considered. In the subacute phase, however, a resolving hematoma may develop a thin area of ring enhancement of its own. Both acute hemorrhage and hemorrhagic neoplasms may cause an edematous reaction, although in the tumors edema is more predominant. In a benign intracranial hypertensive bleed, the edema should begin to substantially resolve within a week, while in the presence of a neoplasm it should persist. With a resolving benign hematoma, a fully circumferential hemosiderin ring begins to develop at about 2 to 3 weeks' time on MR. In the hematoma associated with tumor, this hemosiderin ring may be absent or incomplete. These useful differential features are summarized in Table 4.5. Sometimes when the findings are ambiguous, a follow-up examination in 3 to 6 weeks will clarify the diagnosis, avoiding a biopsy.

Suggested Readings

Akbik F, Hirsch JA, Cougo-Pinto PT, Chandra RV, Simonsen CZ, Leslie-Mazwi T. The evolution of mechanical thrombectomy for acute stroke. *Curr Treat Options Cardiovasc Med* 2016;18(5):32. Available from https://doi.org/10.1007/s11936-016-0457-7.

Albers GW, Marks MP, Kemp S, et al. Thrombectomy for stroke at 6 to 16 hours with selection by perfusion imaging. *N Engl J Med* 2018;378(8): 708–718. Available from https://doi.org/10.1056/NEJMoa1713973.

Bracard S, Ducrocq X, Mas JL, et al. Mechanical thrombectomy after intravenous alteplase versus alteplase alone after stroke (THRACE): a randomised controlled trial. *Lancet Neurol* 2016;15(11):1138–1147. Available from https://doi.org/10.1016/S1474-4422(16)30177-6.

Brunnquell CL, Avey GD, Szczykutowicz TP. Objective evaluation of CT time efficiency in acute stroke response. *J Am Coll Radiol* 2018;15(6):876–880. Available from https://doi.org/10.1016/j.jacr.2018.01.011.

Campbell BCV, Donnan GA, Lees KR, et al. Endovascular stent thrombectomy: the new standard of care for large vessel ischaemic stroke. *Lancet Neurol* 2015;14(8):846–854. Available from https://doi.org/10.1016/S1474-4422(15)00140-4.

Cheng-Ching E, Frontera JA, Man S, et al. Degree of collaterals and not time is the determining factor of core infarct volume within 6 hours of stroke onset. *AJNR Am J Neuroradiol* 2015;36(7):1272–1276. Available from https://doi.org/10.3174/ajnr.A4274.

Deipolyi AR, Hamberg LM, Gonzaléz RG, Hirsch JA, Hunter GJ, et al. Diagnostic yield of emergency department arch-to-vertex CT angiography in patients with suspected acute stroke. *AJNR Am J Neuroradiol* 2015;36(2):265–268. Available from https://doi.org/10.3174/ajnr.A4112.

Goyal M, Yu AY, Menon BK, et al. Endovascular therapy in acute ischemic stroke: challenges and transition from trials to bedside. *Stroke* 2016;47(2):548–553. Available from https://doi.org/10.1161/STROKEAHA.115.011426.

Hemphill JC 3rd, Bonovich DC, Besmertis L, Manley GT, Johnston SC, et al. The ICH Score: a simple, reliable grading scale for intracerebral hemorrhage. *Stroke* 2001;32;891–897.

Josephson SA, Dillon WP, Smith WS. Incidence of contrast nephropathy from cerebral CT angiography and CT perfusion imaging. *Neurology* 2005;64(10):1805–1806. Available from https://doi.org/10.1212/01.WNL.0000161845.69114.62.

Jovin TG, Saver JL, Ribo M, et al. Diffusion-weighted imaging or computerized tomography perfusion assessment with clinical mismatch in the triage of wake up and late presenting strokes undergoing neurointervention with Trevo (DAWN) trial methods. *Int J Stroke* 2017;12(6):641–652. Available from https://doi.org/10.1177/1747493017710341.

Lansberg MG, Christensen S, Kemp S, et al. Computed tomographic perfusion to predict response to recanalization in ischemic stroke. *Ann Neurol* 2017;81(6):849–856. Available from https://doi.org/10.1002/ana.24953.

Leach JL, Fortuna RB, Jones BV, Gaskill-Shipley MF. Imaging of cerebral venous thrombosis: current techniques, spectrum of findings, and diagnostic pitfalls. *Radiographics* 2006;S19–S41; discussion S42–S43. Available from https://doi.org/10.1148/rg.26si055174.

Lev MH, Farkas J, Rodriguez VR, et al. CT angiography in the rapid triage of patients with hyperacute stroke to intraarterial thrombolysis: accuracy in the detection of large vessel thrombus. *J Comput Assist Tomogr* 2001;25(4):520–528. Available from https://doi.org/10.1097/00004728-200107000-00003.

McTaggart RA, Ansari SA, Goyal M, et al. Initial hospital management of patients with emergent large vessel occlusion (ELVO): report of the standards and guidelines committee of the Society of NeuroInterventional Surgery. *J Neurointerv Surg* 2017;9(3):316–323. Available from https://doi.org/10.1136/neurintsurg-2015-011984.

Menon BK, Almekhlafi MA, Pereira VM, et al. Optimal workflow and process-based performance measures for endovascular therapy in acute ischemic stroke: analysis of the solitaire FR thrombectomy for acute revascularization study. *Stroke* 2014;45(7):2024–2029. Available from https://doi.org/10.1161/STROKEAHA.114.005050.

Morotti A, Dowlatshahi D, Boulouis G, et al; ATACH-II, NETT, and PREDICT Investigators. Predicting intracerebral hemorrhage expansion with noncontrast computed tomography: The BAT Score. *Stroke* 2018;49(5):1163–1169. Available from https://doi.org/10.1161/STROKEAHA.117.020138

Muir KW, Ford GA, Messow CM, et al. Endovascular therapy for acute ischaemic stroke: The Pragmatic Ischaemic Stroke Thrombectomy Evaluation (PISTE) randomised, controlled trial. *J Neurol Neurosurg Psychiatry* 2017;88(1):38–44. Available from https://doi.org/10.1136/jnnp-2016-314117.

Nogueira RG, Jadhav AP, Haussen DC, et al. Thrombectomy 6 to 24 hours after stroke with a mismatch between deficit and infarct. *N Engl J Med* 2018;378(1):11–21. Available from https://doi.org/10.1056/NEJMoa1706442.

Pexman JH, Barber PA, Hill MD, et al. Use of the Alberta Stroke Program Early CT Score (ASPECTS) for assessing CT scans in patients with acute stroke. *AJNR Am J Neuroradiol* 2001;22(8):1534–1542. Available from https://doi.org/10.1111/j.1747-4949.2009.00337.x.

Powers WJ, Rabinstein AA, Ackerson T, et al. 2018 guidelines for the early management of patients with acute ischemic stroke: a guideline for healthcare professionals from the American Heart Association/American Stroke Association. *Stroke* 2018;49(3):e46–e110. Available from https://doi.org/10.1161/STR.0000000000000158.

Riedel CH, Zimmermann P, Jensen-Kondering U, Stingele R, Deuschl G, Jansen O. The importance of size: successful recanalization by intravenous thrombolysis in acute anterior stroke depends on thrombus length. *Stroke* 2011;42(6):1775–1777. Available from https://doi.org/10.1161/STROKEAHA.110.609693.

Rowley HA. The four Ps of acute stroke imaging: parenchyma, pipes, perfusion, and penumbra. *AJNR Am J Neuroradiol* 2001;22(4):599–600.

Tsai JP, Mlynash M, Christensen S, et al. Time from imaging to endovascular reperfusion predicts outcome in acute stroke. *Stroke* 2018;49(4):952–957. Available from https://doi.org/10.1161/STROKEAHA.117.018858.

Turk AS, Turner R, Spiotta A, et al. Comparison of endovascular treatment approaches for acute ischemic stroke: cost effectiveness, technical success, and clinical outcomes. *J Neurointerv Surg* 2015;7(9):666–670. Available from https://doi.org/10.1136/neurintsurg-2014-011282.

Venema E, Boodt N, Berkhemer OA, et al. Workflow and factors associated with delay in the delivery of intra-arterial treatment for acute ischemic stroke in the MR CLEAN trial. *J Neurointerv Surg* 2018;10(5):424–428. Available from https://doi.org/10.1136/neurintsurg-2017-013198.

CHAPTER 5 ■ CENTRAL NERVOUS SYSTEM NEOPLASMS AND TUMOR-LIKE MASSES

ROBERT Y. SHIH AND KELLY K. KOELLER

Although neoplasms of the central nervous system (CNS) are uncommon, these lesions garner exceptional interest because of the dramatic and sometimes catastrophic alteration they induce in the lives of affected patients. A useful resource for understanding the scope of the problem is the Central Brain Tumor Registry of the United States (CBTRUS), which provides statistical reports on primary CNS tumors across a large population (over 300 million). Based on epidemiologic data from 2009 to 2013, the annual incidence rate is 22 cases per 100,000 people. Approximately one-third of cases are malignant (32%), half of which are glioblastomas (15%). The other two-thirds are nonmalignant (68%), half of which are meningiomas (36%). These numbers do not include secondary CNS tumors (i.e., intracranial metastases from extracranial primary), which become more frequent with increasing age.

TUMOR CLASSIFICATION

In 1926, neurosurgeons Bailey and Cushing published a landmark book: "A Classification of the Tumors of the Glioma Group on a Histogenetic Basis With a Correlated Study of Prognosis." It served as the foundation for modern neuro-oncology and our current World Health Organization (WHO) classification, which continues to categorize CNS tumors based on histogenesis (cell of origin) and prognosis (tumor grade). The CNS WHO classification has undergone four revisions since the first edition of the "Blue Book" in 1979. While the most recent update in 2016 is now the official lexicon, introducing genetically defined entities for the first time, the fourth edition from 2007 remains a useful introduction to the world of CNS tumors.

The 2007 CNS WHO classified CNS tumors into seven broad categories (the 2016 CNS WHO utilizes 17 categories): tumors of neuroepithelial tissue; tumors of cranial and paraspinal nerves; tumors of the meninges; lymphomas and hematopoietic neoplasms; germ cell tumors (GCTs); tumors of the sellar region; and metastatic tumors. The presumed cell of origin directly impacts on tumor nomenclature. For example, if the cellular composition primarily resembles astrocytes, then the tumor is called an astrocytoma (Table 5.1). In addition to a name, each recognized tumor entity is also assigned a WHO grade, from I (least malignant) to IV (most malignant). Grades I and II are considered low-grade; grades III and IV are considered high-grade.

CLINICAL PRESENTATION

Patients with CNS neoplasms may present with headaches, seizures, or focal neurologic deficits. Tumors of the sellar region may also present with endocrinologic deficits. Alternatively, patients may be asymptomatic and present with abnormal findings on a screening study.

Headaches. While the brain parenchyma itself lacks pain receptors, there are nociceptors in the meninges and vessels, which are sensitive to stretch and therefore to any changes in intracranial pressure (ICP). Because space-occupying neoplasms are more likely to cause intracranial hypertension than hypotension, these headaches are usually worse in the supine than the upright position, for example, the onset of severe headaches during or after sleeping at night.

Seizures. Lesions that affect or abut the cerebral cortex, including but not limited to neoplasms, can result in paroxysmal neuronal discharges and therefore seizure activity.

Focal Neurologic Deficits. The nature of the focal neurologic deficits will depend on the location of the neoplasm. For example, a large anterior falcine meningioma next to the frontal lobes may present with cognitive behavioral symptoms, while a diffuse infiltrative brainstem glioma may present with multiple lower cranial nerve palsies.

NEUROIMAGING PROTOCOL

The two primary modalities for neuroimaging evaluation of intracranial neoplasms are computed tomography (CT) and

TABLE 5.1

PATHOLOGIC CLASSIFICATION BY HISTOLOGIC APPEARANCE

■ CATEGORY	■ CELL OF ORIGIN	■ EXAMPLES
Neuroepithelial tumors	Astrocytic Oligodendroglial Ependymal Choroid plexus Neuronal Pineal Embryonal	Diffuse astrocytoma Oligodendroglioma Ependymoma Choroid plexus papilloma Gangliocytoma Pineocytoma Medulloblastoma
Peripheral nerve tumors	Nerve sheath	Schwannoma
Meningeal tumors	Meningothelial Mesenchymal Melanocytic	Meningioma Hemangiopericytoma Melanocytoma
Hematopoietic tumors	Lymphocytic Histiocytic	Primary CNS lymphoma Langerhans cell histiocytosis
Germ cell tumors	Germ cells	Germinoma
Sellar region tumors	Rathke pouch	Craniopharyngioma
Metastatic tumors	Systemic primary	Secondary CNS lymphoma

magnetic resonance imaging (MRI). Position emission tomography (PET) may also be useful in select circumstances.

CT. Head CT is the study of choice for the evaluation of a patient with acute symptoms. It is fast, widely available, and highly effective at detecting potential neurosurgical emergencies, for example, acute hemorrhage, herniation, or hydrocephalus. If a screening head CT uncovers a possible mass, it is usually further evaluated with brain MRI, unless there are safety contraindications (e.g., shrapnel in sensitive locations, some implanted electronic devices). In patients who cannot undergo MRI, or who cannot receive gadolinium-based contrast agents for MRI, a contrast-enhanced head CT may be performed using iodine-based contrast agents.

MRI. Contrast-enhanced brain MRI is the study of choice for the evaluation of a patient with an intracranial neoplasm. It offers superior contrast resolution on both precontrast and postcontrast imaging, when compared with CT. A basic evaluation will include diffusion-weighted imaging (DWI), T2-weighted imaging (often using fluid-attenuated inversion recovery [FLAIR] to null CSF signal), T2*-weighted imaging (gradient echo [GRE] or susceptibility-weighted imaging [SWI]), and pre/postcontrast T1-weighted imaging. More advanced options for tumor analysis include perfusion-weighted imaging (PWI) and proton MR spectroscopy (MRS).

Diffusion. MR diffusion measures diffusion of water molecules and is a standard sequence in most brain protocols. DWI usually involves rapid echo planar imaging (EPI) of the brain with and without a diffusion-sensitizing gradient, often referred to as the b1000 and b0 images. The degree of T2* signal loss from b0 to b1000 correlates with diffusivity, therefore high signal on the b1000 images indicates restricted diffusion. This may be seen in the setting of acute stroke (cytotoxic edema), hypercellular tumors (e.g., lymphoma), and highly viscous fluids. Diffusion tensor imaging (DTI) is a related technique that employs multidirectional diffusion-sensitizing gradients; it is sometimes performed for preoperative white matter tractography.

Perfusion. MR perfusion measures cerebral blood volume (CBV) as a noninvasive marker of tumor vascularity, which usually increases with tumor grade. Dynamic susceptibility contrast (DSC) and dynamic contrast enhanced (DCE) techniques measure T2* and T1 signal changes, respectively, during a bolus injection of intravenous contrast. Arterial spin labeling (ASL) is a noncontrast technique that magnetically labels arterial blood water flowing into the region of interest (brain). DSC is most common and is postprocessed to generate T2* signal curves and relative CBV values, which may assist with differentiating solitary brain metastasis from high-grade glioma, and with differentiating radiation necrosis from recurrent neoplasm.

Spectroscopy. MRS measures chemical shift of nonwater molecules in a region of interest (single or multi voxel) as a noninvasive marker of tumor metabolism. The chemical or frequency shift is measured in parts per million (ppm), calibrated relative to tetramethylsilane (TMS). In normal brain, the main metabolite peaks are choline at 3.2 ppm, creatine at 3.0 ppm, and N-acetylaspartate at 2.0 ppm, which form an upward slope from left to right (i.e., Hunter's angle). Choline/creatine ratio >2 is suggestive of high-grade tumor (Table 5.2).

PET. Although PET using fluorodeoxyglucose (FDG) is commonly utilized for cancer staging outside the CNS, it is less sensitive inside the CNS due to a high natural background uptake of glucose by normal brain tissue, especially gray matter. It may be useful in select circumstances, for example, distinguishing residual/recurrent tumor from radiation-induced changes in the white matter. Alternative radiotracers (e.g., C-11 methionine) may also be useful in select circumstances and can offer better contrast resolution for detection of high-grade tumor, but are mostly limited to medical centers with appropriate expertise and equipment (e.g., on-site cyclotron).

NEUROIMAGING ANALYSIS

After the neuroimaging study has been performed, the detection of an intracranial abnormality should immediately provoke the following three questions:

Mass? The number one question to ask: "Is it a mass?" It is important to remember that a focal abnormality of density/attenuation on CT or signal intensity on MRI indicates a

TABLE 5.2

METABOLITE PEAKS ON MR SPECTROSCOPY

METABOLITE (PPM)	TUMOR MARKER	HIGHER GRADE[a]
Myoinositol (3.5)	Astrocytes	Decrease
Choline (3.2)	Cellularity	Increase
Creatine (3.0)	Energy	Decrease
N-acetylaspartate (2.0)	Neurons	Decrease
Lactate (1.3)	Hypoxia	Increase
Lipids (0.9–1.4)	Necrosis	Increase

[a]This column lists whether a metabolite tends to increase or decrease with higher tumor grade.

"lesion," but does not necessarily equate to a "mass," which by definition must have "mass effect." In other words, it should be expansile, demonstrate volume gain, and displace normal brain structures. There should not be atrophy or volume loss, which would suggest chronic gliosis, rather than a "mass." There are two caveats: (1) it can sometimes be difficult to ascertain volume gain versus volume loss with smaller lesions; and (2) many nonneoplastic diseases may also produce "mass effect" and therefore qualify as a "mass" (Fig. 5.1).

Location? Once the presence of a mass has been determined, the next important question to ask: "Is the mass intra-axial or extra-axial?" Determining the location of a mass, where it is centered, will help to narrow down the likely sites of origin and the differential diagnosis. For the purposes of this chapter, "intra-axial" means inside the pia mater, including both the parenchymal and the ventricular compartments, paralleling the use of "intra-medullary" in the spinal cord (please note that "intra-axial" is sometimes used to refer to the parenchymal compartment alone). Because the brain derives from neuroectoderm, primary intra-axial tumors, both parenchymal and ventricular, are mostly composed of neuroepithelial tissue, with few exceptions.

In contrast, primary extra-axial tumors, located and arising outside the pia mater, are mostly composed of nonneuroepithelial tissue, for example, meningothelial/mesenchymal cells.

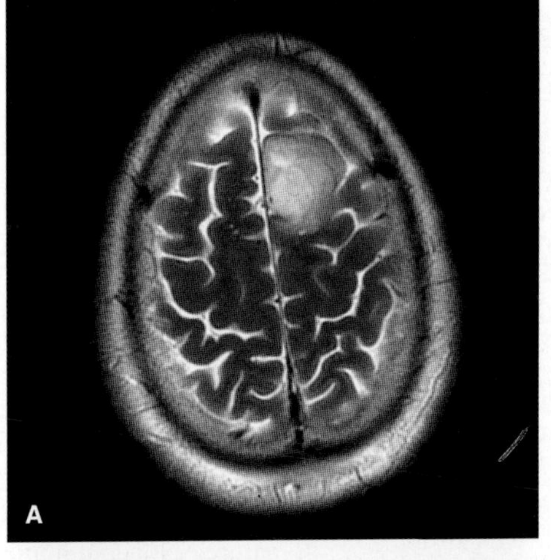

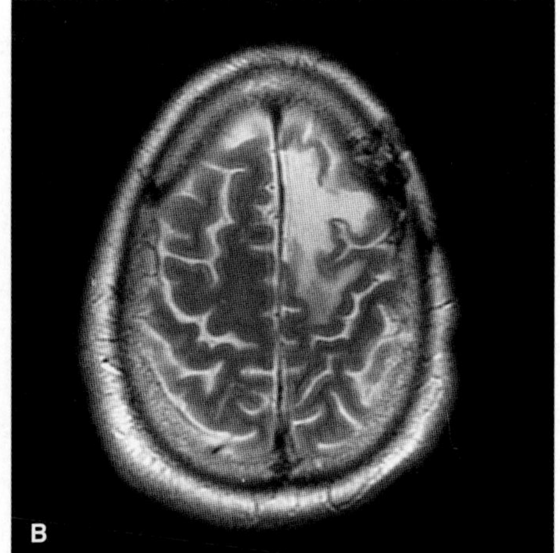

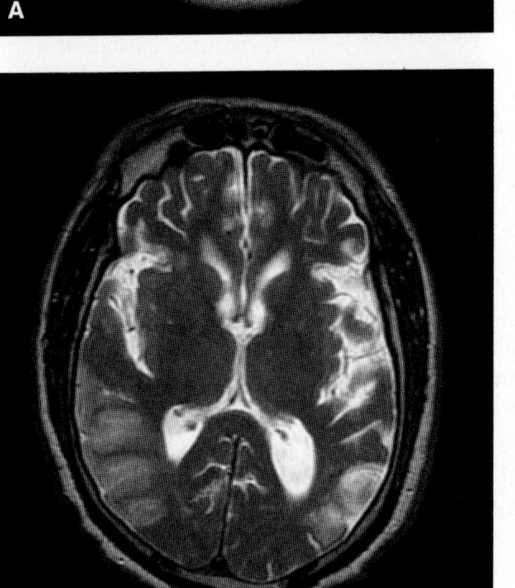

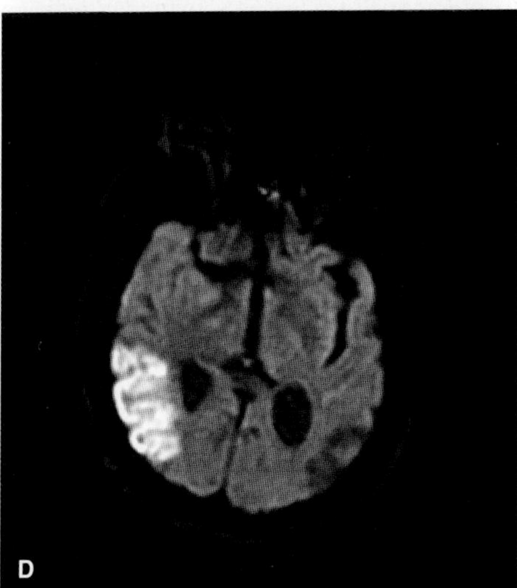

FIGURE 5.1. Is It A Mass? Tumor/Edema Versus Chronic Gliosis. **A:** Axial T2 reveals an expansile lesion in the left frontal lobe with "mass effect." This mass was resected and confirmed as tumor (low-grade oligodendroglioma). **B:** Follow-up axial T2 shows an atrophic lesion at the resection site with volume loss. This represents chronic gliosis. **C:** Axial T2 in a different patient shows an expansile lesion in the right temporal lobe also with "mass effect." This was edema or swelling, in this case from acute stroke. An old stroke (chronic gliosis) can be seen in the left temporal lobe. **D:** Axial DWI confirms restricted diffusion on the right. While this case was fairly straightforward, edema can be mistaken for tumor and vice versa. Chronic gliosis demonstrates volume loss not gain and should not be mistaken for edema or tumor.

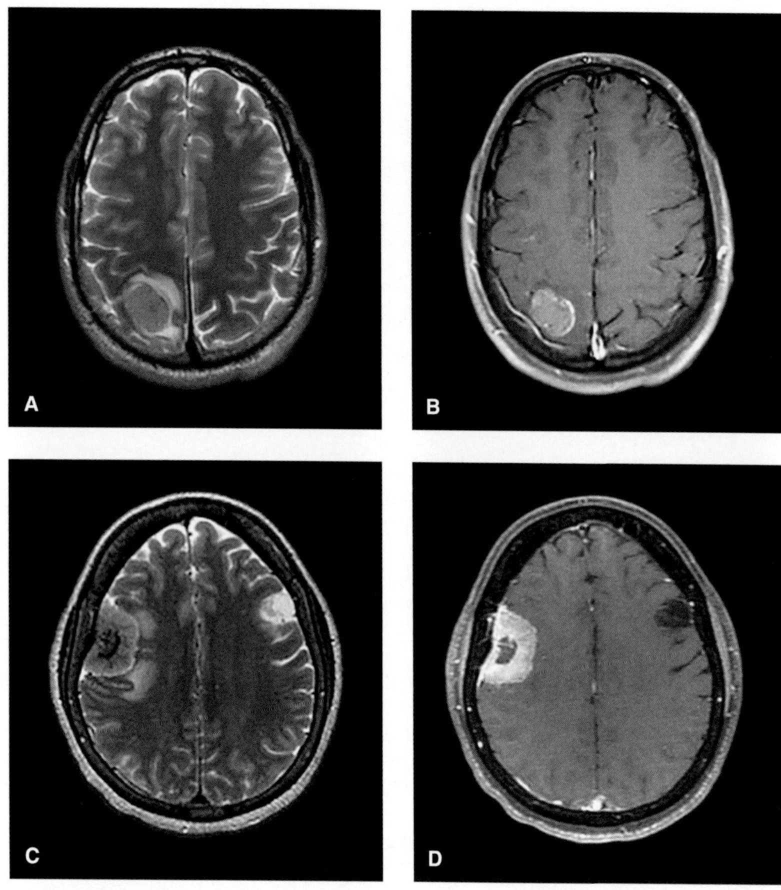

FIGURE 5.2. **Location? Intra-Axial Versus Extra-Axial Compartments. A, B:** Axial T2 and postgadolinium T1 illustrate an enhancing metastasis in the right parietal lobe with a small amount of adjacent edema. This intra-axial mass is surrounded by brain parenchyma and therefore expands the white matter fronds. **C, D:** Axial T2 and postgadolinium T1 uncover an enhancing meningioma at the right frontal convexity with a small amount of adjacent edema (see also chronic gliosis in left frontal lobe). This extra-axial mass is separate from brain parenchyma and therefore buckles or compresses the white matter fronds. Differentiating between intra-axial and extra-axial is critical when analyzing intracranial masses (but not always easy).

On imaging, extra-axial masses are characterized by "white matter buckling" or inward compression of the cortical gray matter and underlying white matter fronds (there may also be a visible intervening CSF cleft). On the other hand, intra-axial masses tend to expand the white matter and thicken its fronds, with a "claw sign" of normal brain parenchyma wrapped around the margins of the mass. The distinction between intra-axial and extra-axial is a critical step in formulating a differential diagnosis for an intracranial tumor (Fig. 5.2), however it can sometimes be difficult or even misleading with lesions centered near the surface of the brain (pia mater).

Imaging Patterns? After a mass has been identified, and its location or compartment has been determined, we can look to other imaging features that may help guide treatment or narrow the differential diagnosis (Table 5.3).

Hemorrhage. Intratumoral hemorrhage is more common in highly vascular neoplasms, such as glioblastoma or oligodendroglioma, as well as certain metastases (Table 5.4). It can be clinically silent or can present acutely due to the sudden increase in mass effect. High attenuation on CT, high signal intensity on T1, and low signal intensity on T2/T2* are imaging markers of possible hemorrhage, although there is some variability depending on the exact phase of blood products. In the setting of a newly diagnosed parenchymal hematoma, a heterogeneous appearance on CT or MRI is worrisome for underlying neoplasm or vascular malformation.

Herniation. Herniation is the protrusion of an anatomic structure from its normal position. With regard to the cerebrum, a mass can cause subfalcine or uncal herniation. Subfalcine herniation is more common and involves partial displacement of a cerebral hemisphere (e.g., cingulate gyrus) across the midline into the contralateral cranial compartment (i.e., "midline shift"). When severe, this can compress or compromise the anterior cerebral arteries. Uncal herniation is less common and involves partial displacement of the medial temporal lobe (e.g., uncus) into the basal cisterns and tentorial hiatus (i.e., transtentorial herniation). When severe, this can compress the ipsilateral posterior cerebral artery, the contralateral midbrain, or the ipsilateral oculomotor nerve ("blown pupil"). With regard to the cerebellum, a mass can cause superior vermian or inferior tonsillar herniation, with potentially devastating mass effect on the brainstem.

Hydrocephalus. Hydrocephalus will also contribute to elevated ICP and may be noncommunicating or communicating in nature. Noncommunicating hydrocephalus is seen with tumor locations that can obstruct CSF flow within the ventricular system, for example, near the foramen of Monro or the aqueduct of Sylvius. Communicating hydrocephalus is seen with diseases that interfere with CSF reabsorption at the arachnoid granulations (e.g., leptomeningeal metastases) and less commonly with choroid plexus tumors that can cause CSF overproduction. Generally speaking, the clinical course informs the degree of urgency for neurosurgical intervention, for example, headaches or deficits rapidly progressive over hours to days require more urgent attention than similar symptoms stable or slowly progressive over months to years.

Low Attenuation on CT. Low attenuation on CT is fairly nonspecific, like high signal intensity on T2, because many tumors have increased water content, compared with normal brain tissue. The differential diagnosis for a low attenuation expansile lesion encompasses both tumor and edema, including edema unrelated to neoplastic disease (e.g., cytotoxic edema from stroke, inflammatory edema from encephalitis). When the clinical history and neuroimaging features are not

TABLE 5.3

RADIOLOGIC CLASSIFICATION BY NEUROIMAGING APPEARANCE

CATEGORY	IMAGING PATTERN	EXAMPLES
Intra-axial tumors (often neuroepithelial)	Nonenhancing mass	Diffuse astrocytoma Oligodendroglioma
	Enhancing mass in adult	Glioblastoma[a] Metastasis
	Enhancing mass in child	Pilocytic astrocytoma Embryonal tumors
	Hyperattenuating mass	Primary CNS lymphoma Embryonal tumors
	Cortical mass	DNET Ganglioglioma
	Ventricular mass	Ependymal tumors Central neurocytoma
	Choroid plexus mass	Choroid plexus tumors Meningioma[a]
	Pineal region mass	Pineal parenchymal tumors Germ cell tumors
Extra-axial tumors (non-neuroepithelial)	Cranial nerve mass (III–XII)	Schwannoma Leptomeningeal disease
	Dural-based mass	Meningioma[a] Mesenchymal tumors
	Sellar region mass	Pituitary adenoma[a] Craniopharyngioma

[a]Glioblastomas, meningiomas, and adenomas together account for 67% of primary CNS tumors.

sufficient to differentiate a possible tumor from ischemic or inflammatory edema, consider a short interval follow-up study to see whether the lesion evolves or resolves over time.

High Attenuation on CT. High attenuation on CT, like low signal intensity on T2, may be caused by blood products, calcifications, proteinaceous fluid, or highly cellular neoplasms. Small round blue cell tumors, including lymphomas and embryonal tumors, are often isodense to hyperdense, relative to normal gray matter. These hypercellular neoplasms are characterized by high nucleus-to-cytoplasm ratios and lower free water content, which also results in lower signal intensity on T2-weighted and apparent diffusion coefficient (ADC) images. Calcifications are best detected by CT and are more frequently encountered in certain tumors (Table 5.5).

High Signal Intensity on T1. Hyperintense signal on the pregadolinium T1-weighted images is relatively uncommon and usually indicates the presence of fat (lipids), blood (methemoglobin), or protein (e.g., melanin). Either low density on CT (negative Hounsfield units) or loss of signal on fat-saturated images can be used to confirm whether the T1 shortening is due to fat or lipids, for example, when making a diagnosis of intracranial dermoid, lipoma, or teratoma.

Low Signal Intensity on T2. As previously mentioned under "high attenuation," T2 hypointensity can be seen with intratumoral calcification or hemorrhage, while lesser degrees of hypointensity (i.e., similar to gray matter) can be seen with highly cellular neoplasms. The latter is worrisome for high-grade malignancies, when the mass is intra-axial, but is most commonly encountered with low-grade meningiomas, when the mass is extra-axial and dural-based.

Enhancement. One of the themes of this section is that different neuroimaging techniques can provide different kinds of information about a tumor, analogous to the wide array of different stains available to the histopathologist. Parenchymal enhancement, whether using iodine- or gadolinium-based contrast agents, tells us about the integrity of the protective blood–brain barrier, which is composed of special endothelium with tight junctions. When the blood–brain barrier is absent or broken, contrast macromolecules are able to leak from the intravascular into the interstitial compartment, resulting in

TABLE 5.4

MNEMONIC FOR HEMORRHAGIC METASTASES[a] ("MR CT BB")

Melanoma
Renal cell carcinoma
Choriocarcinoma
Thyroid carcinoma
Breast carcinoma
Bronchogenic carcinoma (lung)

[a]Glioblastoma, oligodendroglioma, and AT/RT for hemorrhagic primaries.

TABLE 5.5

MNEMONIC FOR CALCIFIED INTRACRANIAL MASSES ("CA COME")

Craniopharyngioma
Astrocytoma, aneurysm
Choroid plexus tumor
Oligodendroglioma[a]
Meningioma
Ependymoma

[a]Highest frequency (>50%).

TABLE 5.6

FIVE POSSIBILITIES IN GLIOBLASTOMA FOLLOW-UP

	ENHANCING LESION[a]	TUMOR BURDEN
Interval stability	Stable	Stable
Tumor response	Decreased	Decreased
Tumor progression	Increased	Increased
Pseudoprogression[b]	Increased	Stable or decreased
Pseudoresponse[c]	Decreased	Stable or increased

[a]If using RANO (Response Assessment in Neuro-Oncology) criteria, response is defined as 50% or more decrease in measurable enhancing lesions (products of long- and short-axis measurements on axial images); progression is defined as 25% or more increase; everything between is stable.
[b]Pseudoprogression occurs in the setting of recent radiation therapy. Possible clues include lack of progression by T2/FLAIR images or clinical status.
[c]Pseudoresponse occurs in the setting of recent antiangiogenic therapy. Possible clues include progression by T2/FLAIR images or clinical status.

parenchymal enhancement. This is a normal finding in specialized tissues without a blood–brain barrier, for example, choroid plexus, pituitary gland, and pineal gland. This is also a normal finding during the healing phase for infarcts and hematomas. When visualized in the neoplastic setting, it is an imaging marker of fenestrated capillaries, which is a benign finding in some low-grade tumors (circumscribed gliomas), but can also be a marker of high-grade microvascular proliferation in other tumors (diffuse gliomas). Nonneuroepithelial tumors (e.g., metastases) lack a blood–brain barrier and generally enhance.

POSTOPERATIVE IMAGING

In the evaluation of a postoperative brain tumor patient, timing is of the essence. It is recognized that vascularized granulation tissue develops within 48 to 72 hours following surgery and enhances after administration of contrast. Therefore, as long as it is safe for the patient, it is ideal to obtain a postoperative contrast-enhanced study, usually MRI, within a 48- to 72-hour window, to minimize the formation of reactive granulation tissue, which can be confused for residual enhancing tumor. This study is used to check for large hematoma or residual tumor, which may necessitate a return to the operating room, and for restricted diffusion along the margin of the resection cavity, which may enhance on follow-up studies in the subacute phase, like other infarcts.

FOLLOW-UP IMAGING

Most low-grade neoplasms are treated by maximal safe resection alone, somewhat dependent on the location of the tumor. Follow-up studies are used to check for any residual or recurrent tumor, for example, any new or enlarging lesions on T2 and postgadolinium images. Most high-grade neoplasms are treated by multimodality therapy, consisting of maximal safe resection, plus radiation and/or chemotherapy. For example, the current standard therapy for glioblastoma is the Stupp protocol: maximal safe resection, followed by fractionated radiation and temozolomide chemotherapy for 6 weeks, followed by adjuvant temozolomide for 6 cycles/months.

Radiation therapy can damage the small vessels and white matter of the brain, which complicates the assessment for residual or recurrent tumor. For example, "pseudoprogression" is the term for a transient radiation-induced enhancing lesion that appears during treatment of glioblastoma, less than 6 months after radiation, difficult to distinguish from true progression (Table 5.6). Radiation necrosis is the term for a more severe permanent tissue injury that happens later, months to years postradiation. A question of treatment effect versus recurrent tumor is usually managed by close follow-up or biopsy; imaging alone cannot provide a definitive answer.

SPECIFIC NEOPLASMS

It is difficult, if not impossible, to guarantee a specific *histologic* diagnosis based entirely on the imaging appearance. However, by taking into account factors such as tumor location (intra-axial, extra-axial, pineal/sellar region) and clinical setting (age, gender, serum/CSF labs), a differential diagnosis can often be limited to just a few likely possibilities, or sometimes a single most likely possibility, especially with relatively common neoplasms like glioblastoma or meningioma. Our primary responsibility in image interpretation is to help guide clinical care in the right direction; "nailing" the diagnosis is of secondary importance, especially when dealing with relatively rare tumors or variants. A tissue diagnosis always remains the gold standard.

Intra-Axial Tumors: Glial

According to the CBTRUS data from 2009 to 2013, approximately 40% of primary CNS tumors are intra-axial, which are predominantly tumors of neuroepithelial tissue, with few exceptions, for example, primary CNS lymphoma (PCNSL) (2%). Because glial cells are more mitotically active than neurons, "gliomas" account for the majority of primary intra-axial tumors and approximately 25% of all primary CNS tumors. There is no standard definition for the term "glioma." For the purposes of this chapter, it will be used broadly to encompass all tumors derived from glial cells: astrocytes, oligodendrocytes, ependymal cells, and choroid plexus epithelium.

Astrocytomas. Astrocytic tumors account for the majority (approximately 75%) of all gliomas. Both astrocytomas and gliomas can be divided into two major groups based on growth pattern: circumscribed versus diffuse (Table 5.7). The circumscribed gliomas demonstrate more well-defined margins on microscopic examination and tend to be more amenable to a surgical cure. They also tend toward lower grade

TABLE 5.7

TWO GROUPS OF GLIOMAS BY GROWTH PATTERN

	■ CIRCUMSCRIBED	■ DIFFUSE/INFILTRATIVE
Cell of origin	Astrocytes Ependymal cells Choroid plexus epithelium	Astrocytes Oligodendrocytes
Age predilection	Pediatric (except subependymoma)	Adult
WHO grade range	I–III	II–IV
Enhancement	Usually enhancing (any grade)	Marker of higher grade tumor
Example	Pilocytic astrocytoma = most common pediatric CNS tumor	Glioblastoma most common primary intra-axial CNS tumor

and younger age at clinical presentation (e.g., pediatric). The diffuse or infiltrative gliomas demonstrate more ill-defined margins on microscopic examination, regardless of the macroscopic appearance on cross-sectional imaging.

Pilocytic Astrocytoma. The most common pediatric CNS tumor and the prototypical example of a circumscribed glioma is the pilocytic astrocytoma (WHO Grade I). The most common location is the cerebellum (60%), followed by the optic pathways/hypothalamus (30%), and then brainstem. The most common age group is children (<20 years old), therefore it is also known as "juvenile" pilocytic astrocytoma, although it can rarely present in adulthood, when it may be an unexpected and more aggressive diagnosis. It is associated with neurofibromatosis type 1 (NF1) and found in 15% ("optic gliomas"). This Grade I tumor has low proliferative activity and excellent prognosis, especially when located in surgically accessible locations (e.g., cerebellum).

Other Circumscribed Astrocytomas. Pilomyxoid astrocytoma (WHO Grade II) is a less common and more aggressive variant of pilocytic astrocytoma that most commonly occurs in the suprasellar region. Subependymal giant cell astrocytoma (WHO Grade I) is a slow-growing tumor located at the foramen of Monro and is associated with tuberous sclerosis. Pleomorphic xanthoastrocytoma (PXA) (WHO Grade II) is a peripherally located cerebral tumor that often involves the cortex/meninges. There is a more aggressive variant called anaplastic PXA (WHO Grade III).

Imaging Patterns. All of the circumscribed astrocytomas possess fenestrated capillaries and are expected to enhance (i.e., nonintact blood–brain barrier). Because the leaky vessels can secrete fluid into surrounding tissues, the most common imaging pattern is a circumscribed enhancing mass, which may be accompanied by internal or adjacent fluid-filled cysts. For this reason, the appearance of a nonenhancing cyst with enhancing mural nodule in the cerebellum is the classic presentation of a pilocytic astrocytoma in a child (Fig. 5.3). This also happens to be a common imaging pattern for hemangioblastoma, however that presents in adulthood.

Diffuse Astrocytoma and Anaplastic Astrocytoma. Diffuse gliomas are infiltrative in nature and fall on a spectrum from low-grade to high-grade. The diffuse astrocytoma (WHO Grade II) is a low-grade astrocytic tumor with low-level proliferative activity. The development of increased cellularity, mitotic activity, or nuclear atypia on histopathology would identify evolution to the anaplastic astrocytoma (WHO Grade III). The 2016 CNS WHO genetically subdivides diffuse gliomas into isocitrate dehydrogenase (IDH) mutant versus wildtype; a majority of diffuse and anaplastic astrocytomas are IDH-mutant, which have better prognosis. Noninvasive detection of IDH-mutant gliomas by spectroscopy (2-hydroxyglutarate) is an example of ongoing research efforts in molecular imaging and precision medicine for neuro-oncology.

Imaging Patterns. The low-grade diffuse astrocytoma and the high-grade anaplastic astrocytoma are discussed together because they share a common imaging pattern. They both tend to present as expansile parenchymal lesions, hypodense on CT and hyperintense on T2, without significant enhancement (intact blood–brain barrier). This pattern can also be seen with oligodendroglioma, which is a less common neoplasm than astrocytoma. It may not be possible to distinguish diffuse from anaplastic astrocytoma before biopsy (Fig. 5.4). Possible clues to the latter include older age (>40 years old) and imaging markers of increased cellularity (decreased diffusion), mitotic activity (increased choline), or tumor vascularity (increased perfusion).

Glioblastoma. Also known by the older term glioblastoma multiforme (GBM), glioblastoma is a Grade IV or malignant astrocytoma and is overall the most common primary intra-axial tumor of the CNS. It accounts for over half of gliomas (55%), compared with the lower grades: anaplastic astrocytoma (6%), diffuse astrocytoma (8%), and pilocytic astrocytoma (5%). It is most common in older adults (>40 years old), although it can present at any age, even infancy. It is a diffuse or infiltrative astrocytic tumor with high-grade features like anaplastic astrocytoma, plus additional development of necrosis and/or microvascular proliferation on histopathology. The necrosis and neovascularity are secondary effects of rapid tumor growth with hypoxia.

The vast majority are IDH-wildtype (>90%), also known as primary glioblastomas, because they tend to present *de novo* in older adults (median age 62 years) by skipping or rapidly progressing through diffuse-anaplastic grades. The rest (<10%) are IDH-mutant or secondary glioblastomas, which tend to develop from lower grade tumors in younger adults (median age 44 years) with a less aggressive clinical course. Another favorable molecular marker is methylation (inactivation) of the gene promoter for the O6-methylguanine-DNA methyltransferase (MGMT) repair enzyme that counteracts the effects of temozolomide chemotherapy. While there are long-term survivors, median survival with treatment is 15 months (31 months for IDH-mutant).

Imaging Patterns. Glioblastoma typically presents as a heterogeneously enhancing parenchymal mass with surrounding vasogenic edema (Fig. 5.5). The heterogeneous enhancement reflects the necrosis and microvascular proliferation seen on histology. The latter lacks a normal blood–brain barrier and

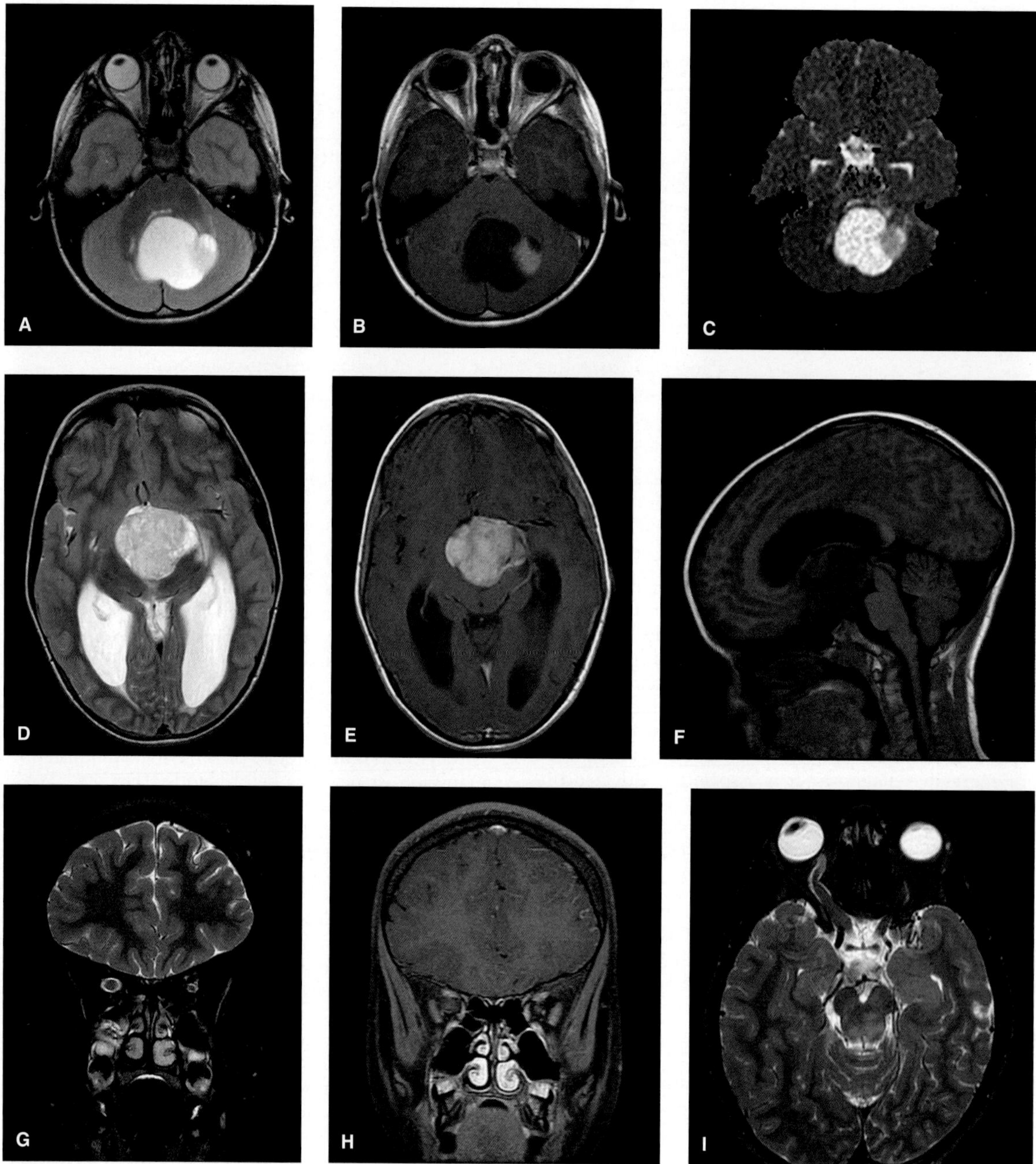

FIGURE 5.3. **Three Examples of Pilocytic Astrocytoma in Different Children. A–C:** Axial T2, axial postgadolinium T1, and axial ADC in a child with headache and intractable vomiting reveal a classic "cyst with nodule" appearance of cerebellar pilocytic astrocytoma. The tumor nodule demonstrates enhancement and increased diffusion. Hemangioblastoma can have a similar appearance, however that presents in adulthood. **D–F:** Axial T2, axial postgadolinium T1, and sagittal T1 in a child with headache and papilledema uncover a mostly solid enhancing mass centered around the suprasellar cistern. A pilocytic astrocytoma in this location is also known as a "hypothalamic-chiasmatic glioma"; differential diagnosis includes pilomyxoid astrocytoma. **G–I:** Coronal T2, coronal postgadolinium T1, and axial T2 in a child with neurofibromatosis type 1 show an enlarged right optic nerve from a nonenhancing pilocytic astrocytoma ("optic glioma"). Children with NF1 can also have focal areas of signal intensity (FASI) in the deep white matter, for example, note the patchy T2 signal abnormality in the midbrain on the axial T2 image.

accounts for the postcontrast enhancing lesion. In addition to central necrosis, there may also be calcification or hemorrhage. Glioblastoma can present as a single enhancing mass, multifocal enhancing masses, or as a combination of both enhancing and nonenhancing tumor. While the first two patterns can also be seen with metastases, the third pattern is highly suspicious for glioblastoma; a biopsy should target the enhancing tumor.

Ring Enhancement. On contrast-enhanced CT and MRI, virtually all glioblastomas will show at least some enhancement, usually in a heterogeneous or ring-like pattern. Many other lesions can present as a ring enhancing mass, to include metastasis and abscess (Table 5.8). The enhancing rim of necrotic tumor, whether glioblastoma or metastasis, tends to be more thick and irregular, while the enhancing capsule of an abscess tends to be more thin and smooth. Also, on DWI, it

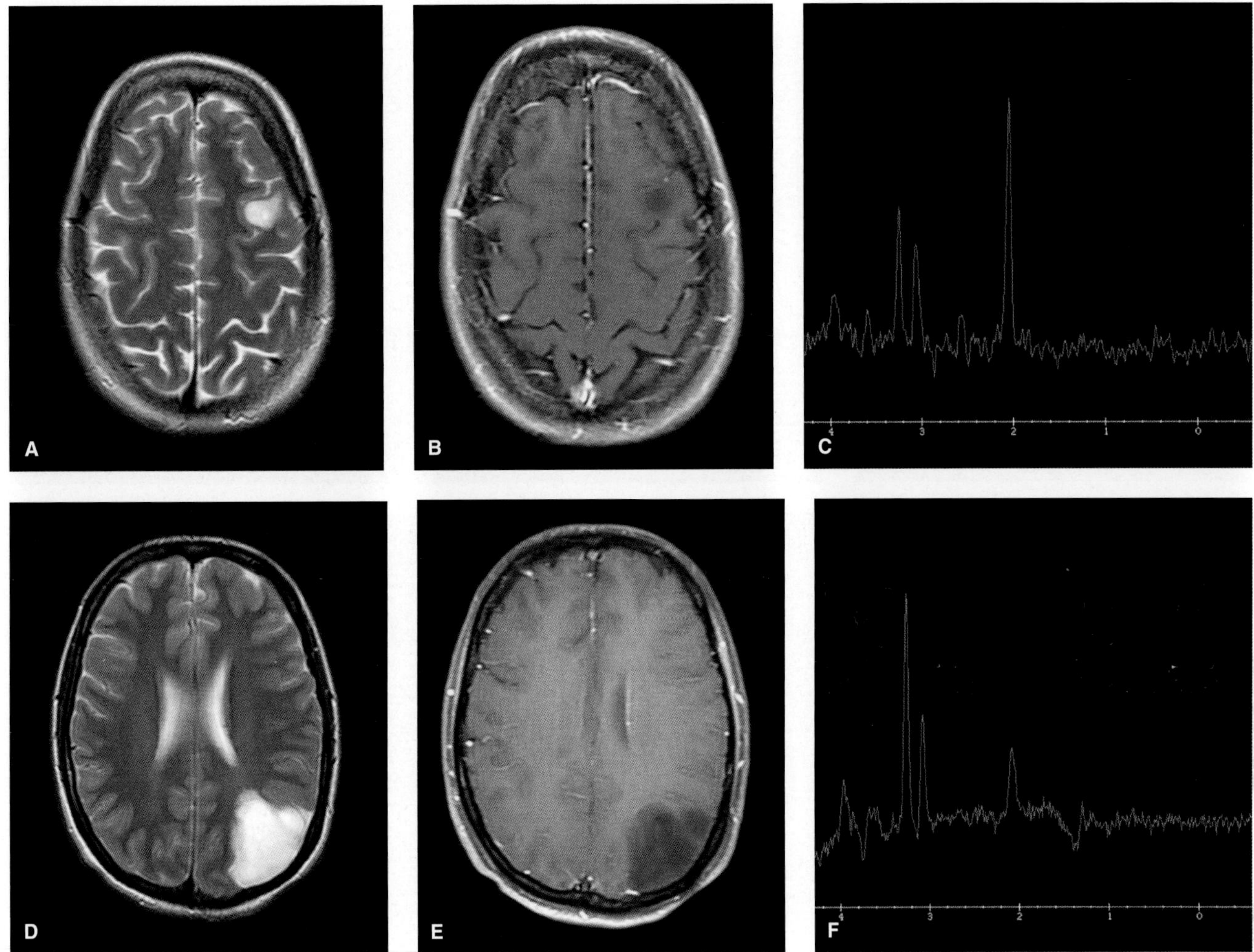

FIGURE 5.4. **Diffuse and Anaplastic Astrocytoma in Two Different Adults. A, B:** Axial T2 and postgadolinium T1 demonstrate a nonenhancing T2 hyperintense mass in the left frontal lobe. **C:** Single voxel spectroscopy reveals minimal elevation of the choline peak (3.2 ppm) relative to the adjacent creatine peak (3.0 ppm). A biopsy confirmed a diffuse astrocytoma (WHO Grade II). **D, E:** Axial T2 and postgadolinium T1 from a different patient also demonstrate a nonenhancing T2 hyperintense mass, this time in the left parietal lobe. **F:** Spectroscopy reveals prominent elevation of the choline peak, which serves as a marker of higher cellularity or mitotic activity. A biopsy confirmed an anaplastic astrocytoma (WHO Grade III) in this case.

is more characteristic to see restricted diffusion in the hypercellular wall of a necrotic tumor versus the purulent contents of a pyogenic abscess (Fig. 5.5). A mass with an incomplete ring of enhancement ("horseshoe" or "open ring" sign) should prompt consideration of a tumefactive demyelinating lesion, rather than neoplasm or abscess.

TABLE 5.8

MNEMONIC FOR RING ENHANCING LESIONS ("MAGIC DR")

<u>M</u>etastasis
<u>A</u>bscess[a]
<u>G</u>lioma (especially glioblastoma)
<u>I</u>nfarct (subacute or healing phase)
<u>C</u>ontusion/hematoma (subacute)
<u>D</u>emyelinating disease
<u>R</u>adiation necrosis

[a]Consider atypical infections, as well as CNS lymphoma, in immunocompromised patients.

Butterfly Glioma. When a diffuse or infiltrative glioma, most commonly a glioblastoma, crosses the corpus callosum to involve both cerebral hemispheres, it can resemble the shape of butterfly wings on axial and coronal imaging (Fig. 5.6). This is colloquially referred to as a "butterfly glioma" (not a defined entity in CNS WHO classification). It is important to recognize that an expansile lesion within the corpus callosum cannot be attributed to vasogenic edema, because the callosal fibers are too tightly packed for interstitial fluid to be transmitted across them. It must represent either an infiltrative neoplasm (e.g., "butterfly glioma" or lymphoma) or direct damage to the white matter of the corpus callosum (e.g., demyelinating lesion or cytotoxic edema).

Brainstem Glioma. In adults, "brainstem glioma" can refer to either a diffuse infiltrative glioma, similar to supratentorial diffuse gliomas but in a less common location, or a focal tectal glioma, which is a low-grade tumor in the midbrain that causes obstructive hydrocephalus (Fig. 5.7). In young children, "brainstem glioma" or "diffuse intrinsic pontine glioma" refers to a diffuse infiltrative glioma with highly aggressive behavior, despite absent or minimal enhancement. In pediatric patients who undergo stereotactic needle biopsy, the most likely diagnosis is "diffuse midline glioma, H3 K27M-mutant," which is

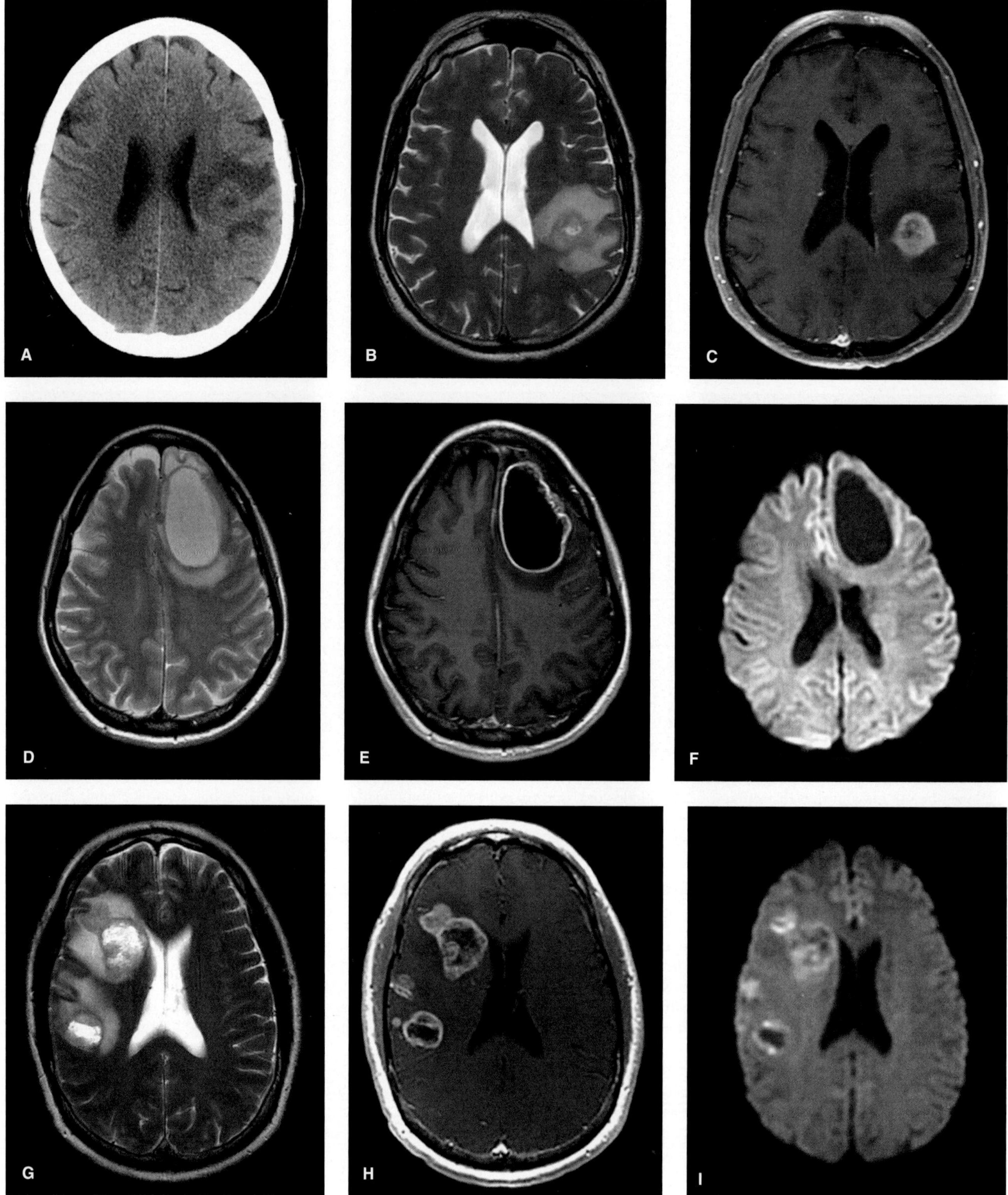

FIGURE 5.5. **Three Examples of Glioblastoma in Different Adult Patients. A:** Head CT shows a ring-like mass with surrounding vasogenic edema in the left frontal lobe. **B, C:** Axial T2 and postgadolinium T1 confirm a heterogeneously enhancing mass (i.e., blood–brain barrier is not intact). The ill-defined margins would favor a glioblastoma over a metastasis. **D, E:** Axial T2 and postgadolinium T1 in a second patient reveal a ring enhancing mass with a greater degree of central or internal necrosis. **F:** On axial DWI, the central nonenhancing fluid does not show restricted diffusion, in contrast to a pyogenic abscess. **G, H:** Axial T2 and postgadolinium T1 in a third patient illustrate multifocal glioblastoma in the right frontal lobe. **I:** On axial DWI, there can be restriction of water molecule diffusion in the solid or enhancing component due to tumor cellularity, in contrast to more free diffusion in the fluid or necrotic portion.

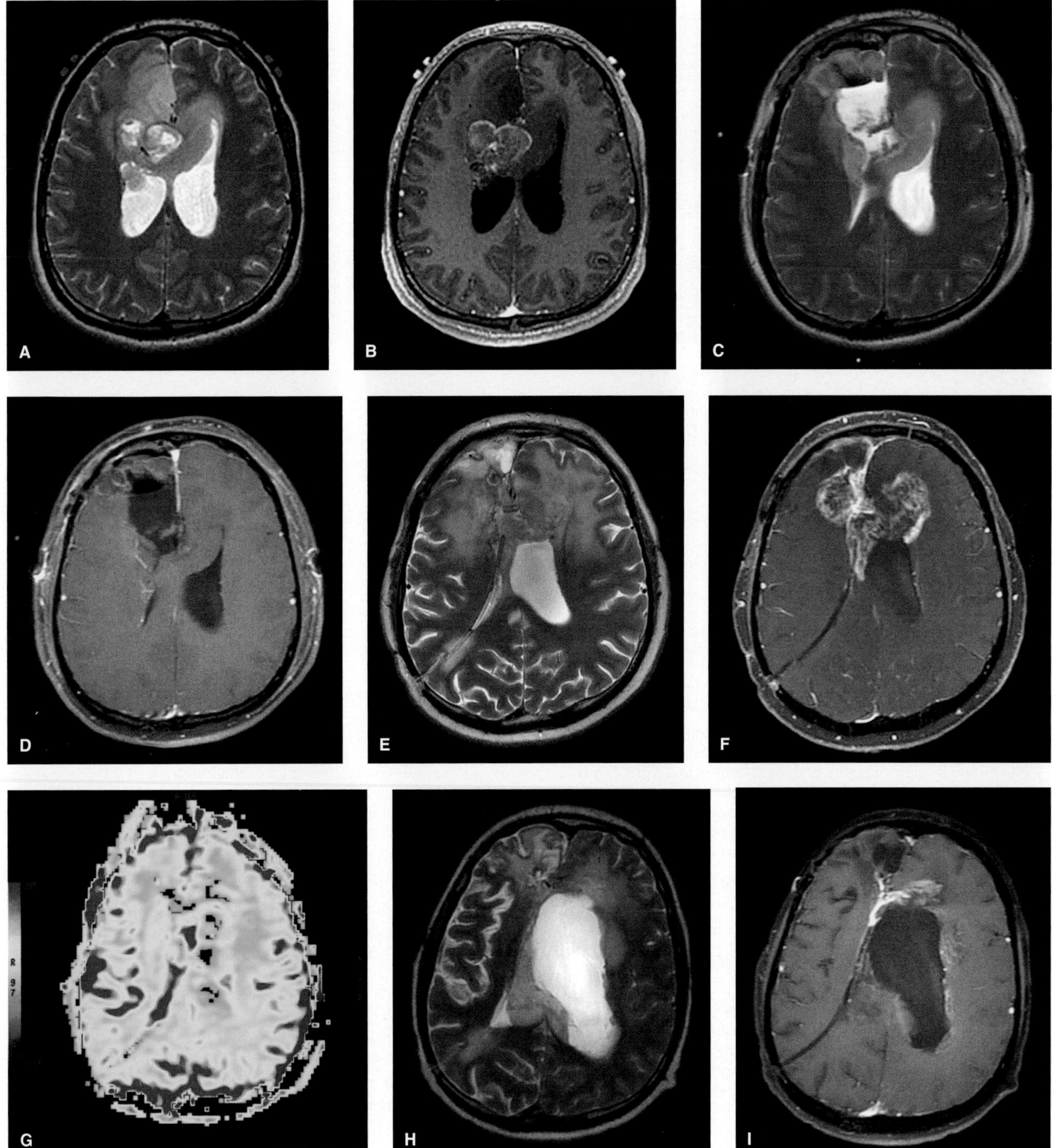

FIGURE 5.6. **"Butterfly Glioma" With Pseudoprogression Then True Progression. A, B:** Axial T2 and postgadolinium T1 reveal a heterogeneously enhancing mass that crosses the genu of the corpus callosum in a young adult patient (preoperative MRI with scalp fiducials). **C, D:** Axial T2 and postgadolinium T1 from the postoperative MRI confirm successful resection of the enhancing component, with residual nonenhancing T2 hyperintense tumor. Tissue diagnosis was glioblastoma, IDH-mutant (most are IDH-wildtype). **E, F:** Axial T2 and postgadolinium T1 from a follow-up MRI after radiation therapy show a new enhancing lesion centered at the genu with a "soap bubble" or "Swiss cheese" pattern. **G:** On perfusion MRI (rCBV map), there was no hypervascularity to suggest recurrent glioblastoma, and this lesion was treated conservatively as probable pseudoprogression. **H, I:** On a study from 1 year later, axial T2 and postgadolinium T1 show that the enhancing lesion at the genu has mostly resolved. Unfortunately, there were new faintly enhancing masses at the medial and lateral walls of the left lateral ventricle.

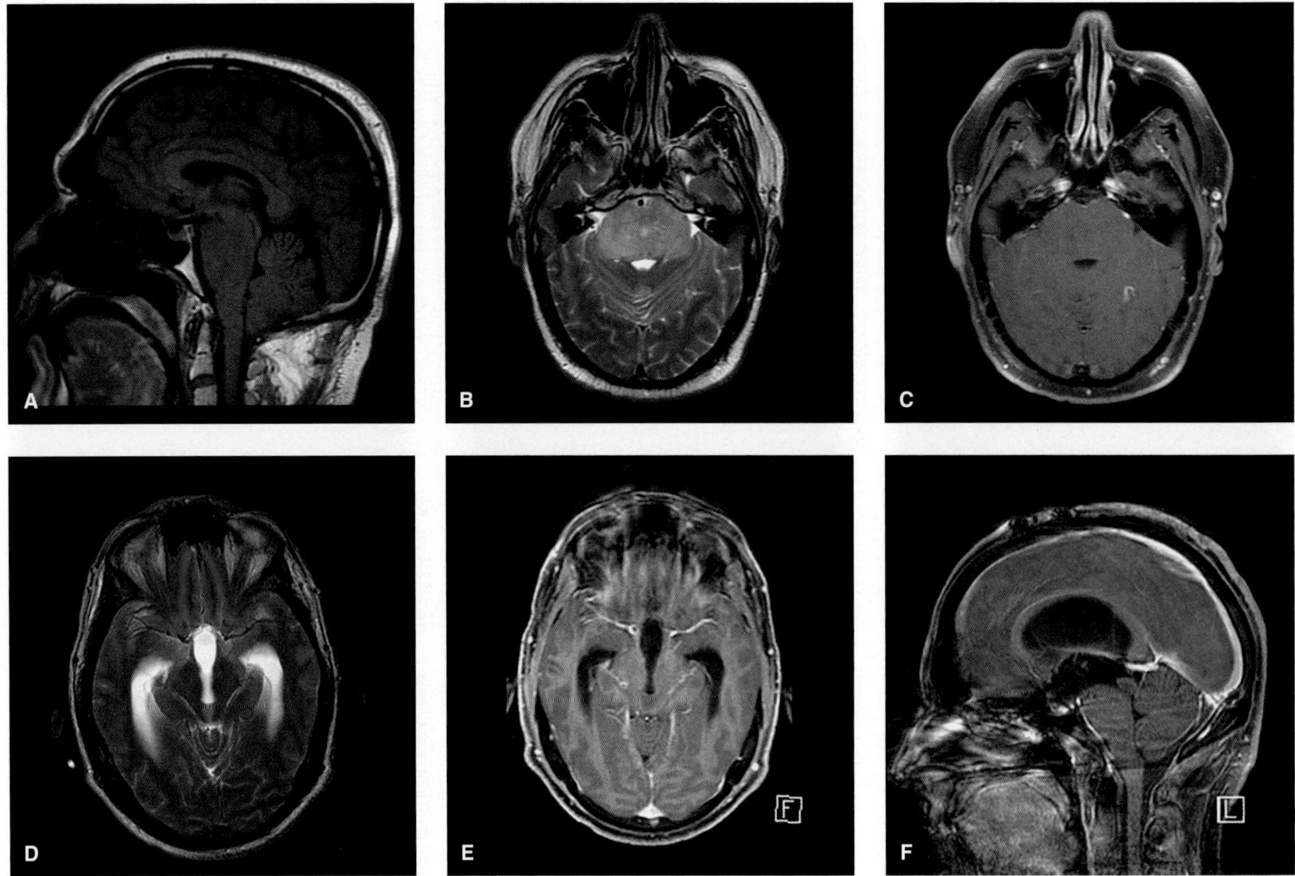

FIGURE 5.7. **Two Examples of Brainstem Gliomas in Different Adult Patients. A–C:** Sagittal T1, axial T2, and axial postgadolinium T1 show a large expansile nonenhancing T2 hyperintense lesion occupying most of the pons. A stereotactic needle biopsy confirmed a diffuse astrocytoma (WHO Grade II). This imaging pattern is known as a diffuse intrinsic pontine glioma (DIPG) and can be associated with much more aggressive behavior in children, despite a similar nonenhancing appearance. **D–F:** Axial T2, axial postgadolinium T1, and sagittal postgadolinium T1 from a different patient reveal a small expansile nonenhancing T2 hyperintense lesion in the dorsal midbrain. This imaging pattern is known as a focal tectal glioma, which is generally low-grade and not biopsied. Treatment is directed at relieving obstructive hydrocephalus.

a new genetically defined entity in the 2016 CNS WHO and is the only other Grade IV glioma aside from glioblastoma.

Gliomatosis Cerebri. This term describes the widespread infiltrative growth of a diffuse glioma, more commonly astrocytoma than oligodendroglioma, to involve at least three lobes of the brain. It is uncommon and was a recognized entity in the 2007 CNS WHO, but has been removed from the 2016 CNS WHO, which favors applying the specific histologic diagnosis (e.g., glioblastoma). Nevertheless, this term may still be encountered in clinical practice.

Oligodendrogliomas. Diffuse gliomas encompass both astrocytomas and oligodendrogliomas. The latter are much less common and account for only 6% of all gliomas. They demonstrate a diffuse growth pattern, just like their astrocytic counterparts, with neoplastic cells infiltrating beyond the macroscopic margins of the tumor. On microscopy, these cells have a "fried egg" appearance due to round nuclei surrounded by clear cytoplasm (fixation artifact). Additional histologic features include microcalcifications and a dense network of branching capillaries ("chicken wire"). The development of increased cellularity, mitotic activity, or nuclear atypia upgrades oligodendroglioma (WHO Grade II) to anaplastic oligodendroglioma (WHO Grade III). The latter may also demonstrate necrosis and/or microvascular proliferation.

Molecular Parameters. Under the 2016 CNS WHO, oligodendrogliomas are now classified using both phenotype and genotype criteria (integrated diagnosis). In addition to the histologic features detailed above, they are also characterized by the following: IDH mutated and 1p/19q codeleted (i.e., loss of chromosomal arms 1p and 19q). These genetic alterations carry a favorable prognosis (Table 5.9), and overall oligodendrogliomas will do better than astrocytomas of equivalent grade. Under the 2007 CNS WHO, oligoastrocytoma and anaplastic oligoastrocytoma were recognized entities ("mixed gliomas"); these relatively imprecise terms are discouraged in the molecular era (astrocytomas are 1p/19q intact, oligodendrogliomas are 1p/19q codeleted).

Imaging Patterns. The imaging appearance of oligodendroglioma overlaps with that of the more common astrocytoma (diffuse). Both will present as expansile infiltrative parenchymal lesions, typically hypodense on CT and hyperintense on T2. Oligodendrogliomas are most commonly located in the frontal lobes and often extend peripherally to involve the cortex. Compared with astrocytomas, oligodendrogliomas are more likely to exhibit calcifications on CT and poorly defined margins with heterogeneous signal intensity on MRI (Fig. 5.8). They are also more vascular tumors; roughly 50% show variable enhancement. It may not be possible to distinguish oligodendroglioma from anaplastic oligodendroglioma. Possible clues to the latter include older age (>40 years old) and imaging markers of increased cellularity (decreased diffusion), mitotic activity (increased choline), or tumor vascularity (increased perfusion).

TABLE 5.9

CLASSIFICATION OF DIFFUSE GLIOMAS BY PHENOTYPE/GENOTYPE

	■ MORE FAVORABLE PROGNOSIS	■ LESS FAVORABLE PROGNOSIS
Phenotype:		
Cell of origin	Oligodendrocyte[a]	Astrocyte
Histologic grade	Low-grade (II)	High-grade (III–IV)
Histologic features	Cytologic atypia alone	Anaplasia Mitotic activity Microvascular proliferation Necrosis
Genotype:		
IDH1 and/or IDH2 gene	Mutant	Wildtype
MGMT gene promoter	Methylated	Unmethylated
1p/19q chromosomes[a]	Codeleted	Intact

[a]Oligodendroglial tumors are molecularly characterized by IDH mutation and 1p/19q codeletion and have a tendency to be more vascular and less aggressive than their astrocytic counterparts.

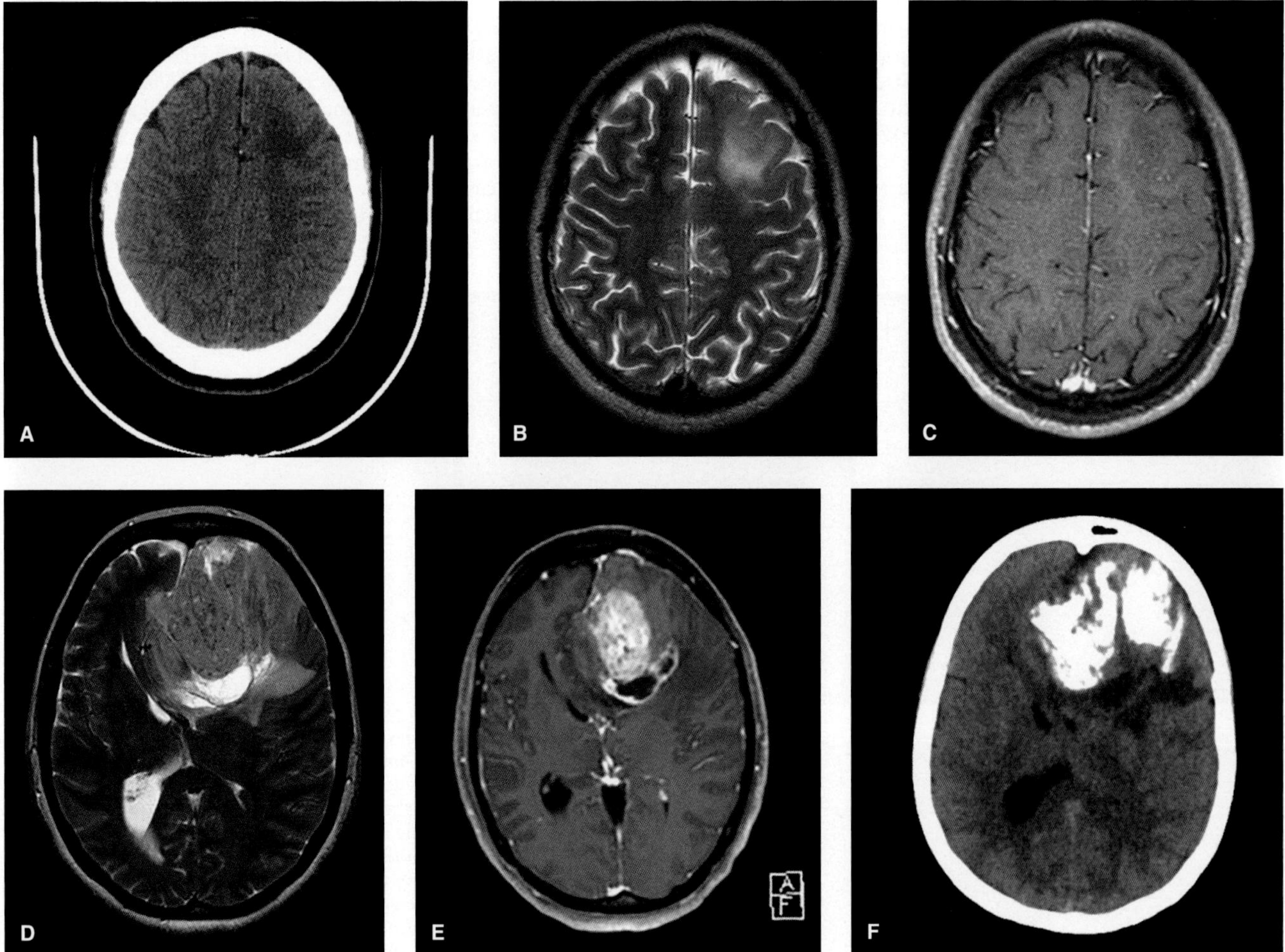

FIGURE 5.8. **Oligodendroglioma and Anaplastic Oligodendroglioma in Adults. A:** Head CT reveals a subtle hypoattenuating lesion in the left frontal lobe. Differential diagnosis includes edema or tumor. **B, C:** Axial T2 and postgadolinium T1 from the subsequent MRI show a nonenhancing T2 hyperintense mass that infiltrates the left frontal cortex and subcortical white matter with ill-defined margins. These descriptors are typical of oligodendroglioma (WHO Grade II), confirmed by excisional biopsy. **D, E:** Axial T2 and postgadolinium T1 from a different adult patient show a much larger and more heterogeneous mass originating in the left frontal lobe with abnormal enhancement. This turned out to be an anaplastic oligodendroglioma (WHO Grade III). **F:** Head CT also shows characteristic calcifications, which were much better depicted on the CT than on the MRI's T2*-weighted gradient echo sequences (not shown).

Ependymomas. Ependymal tumors are also uncommon and account for approximately 7% of all gliomas. Similar to other circumscribed gliomas, they tend to present in the pediatric population (<20 years old). The exception is the subependymoma, which will be discussed separately. The ependymoma (WHO Grade II) and the anaplastic ependymoma (WHO Grade III) arise from the ependymal cells lining the ventricular system and the central canal of the spinal cord, therefore they often present as a fourth ventricular mass in children, less commonly as an intramedullary mass in adults. Curiously, there is a predilection for ependymomas to originate within the brain parenchyma, rather than the lateral-third ventricles, when they present supratentorially. Many of these supratentorial ependymomas share a genetic alteration and are classified as "ependymoma, RELA fusion-positive" under the 2016 CNS WHO. On histopathology, ependymomas will show perivascular pseudorosettes more often than true ependymal rosettes.

Imaging Patterns. The most common pattern for intracranial ependymoma is a heterogeneous enhancing mass within the fourth ventricle in a child (Fig. 5.9). They are soft plastic tumors that frequently extrude out the foramina of Luschka laterally or Magendie inferiorly. They are also capable of paraventricular or transependymal invasion into the brain parenchyma, causing vasogenic edema. Less common sites of origin include the cerebellopontine angles (CPA), the cerebral hemispheres, and the lateral-third ventricles. Regardless of the location, ependymomas are often heterogeneous on CT and MRI, characterized by intratumoral calcification, cystic change, and/or hemorrhage. While choroid plexus tumors can also present as intraventricular enhancing masses in children, they favor the lateral ventricles over the fourth ventricle.

Subependymoma. Immediately underneath the ependymal lining of the ventricular system lies a thin subependymal glial plate. A tumor that arises from this region is termed a subependymoma (WHO Grade I). The most common locations are the inferior fourth ventricle, followed by lateral-third ventricles, followed by spinal cord. These tumors usually present in older adults (age >40 years old), who may be completely asymptomatic or may have obstructive hydrocephalus. Like ependymomas, these tumors trend toward heterogeneity on CT and MRI. Unlike ependymomas, as well as most other ventricular neoplasms, subependymomas are relatively hypovascular and will show less enhancement on postcontrast imaging (Fig. 5.9).

Choroid Plexus Tumors. Since the choroid plexus is formed embryologically by invagination of leptomeninges into the lateral ventricles through the choroidal fissure, choroid plexus epithelium and stroma are derived from ependymal cells and arachnoid mater, respectively. Neoplasms of the choroid plexus epithelium are rare and account for <1% of all gliomas. They usually present in children (age <20 years old) and fall on a spectrum: choroid plexus papilloma (WHO Grade I), atypical choroid plexus papilloma (WHO Grade II), and choroid plexus carcinoma (WHO Grade III). Any grade can be associated with communicating hydrocephalus (from CSF overproduction and/or impaired resorption) as well as CSF dissemination of tumor.

Imaging Patterns. Choroid plexus tumors are intensely enhancing masses with lobulated margins that are usually centered at the atrium or trigone of the lateral ventricle, arising from the choroid plexus glomus (Fig. 5.10), and less commonly in the fourth ventricle. There can be overlap in the imaging appearance of papilloma and carcinoma. The latter accounts for 20% of cases and is often heterogeneous and aggressive with parenchymal invasion.

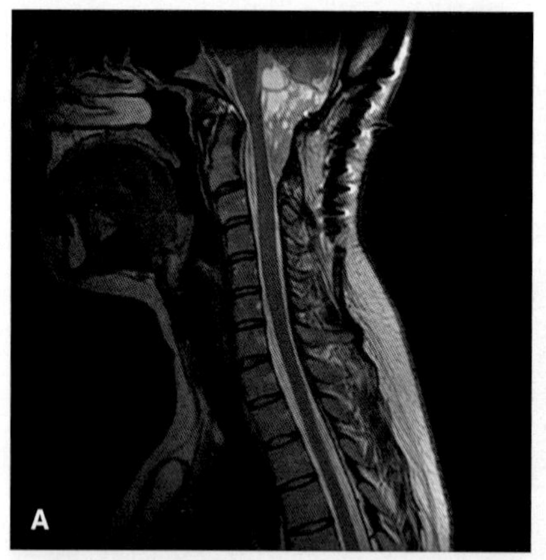

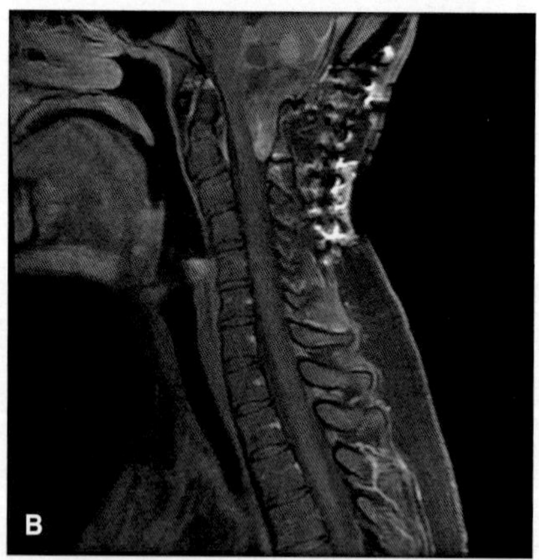

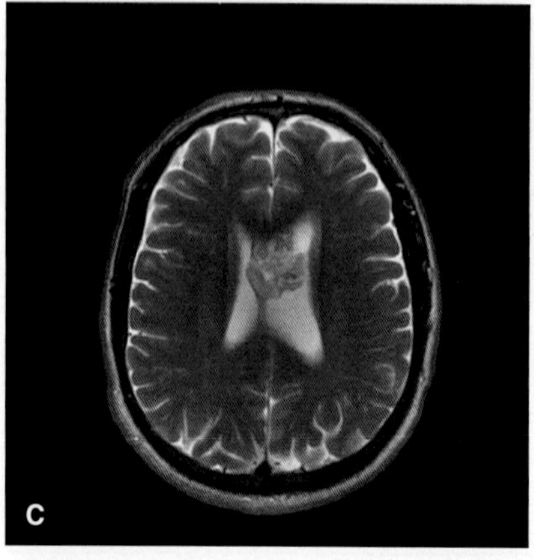

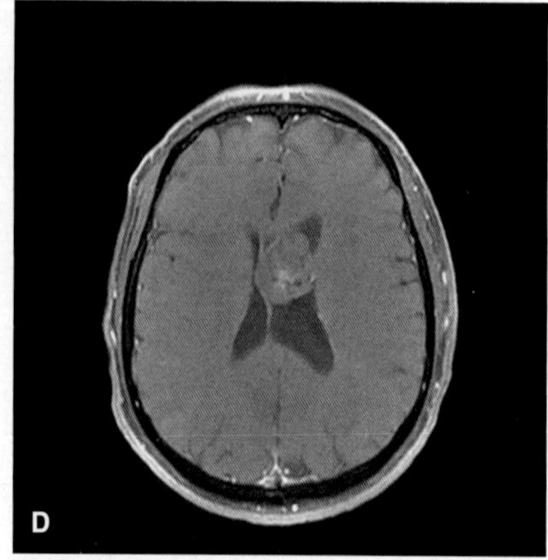

FIGURE 5.9. **Two Examples of Ependymal Tumors in Different Adult Patients. A, B:** Sagittal T2 and postgadolinium T1 from a cervical spine MRI reveal a heterogeneous mass at the inferior aspect of the fourth ventricle, with both solid enhancing and cystic nonenhancing components. This was a young adult with remote history of posterior fossa tumor resection as a child (note postoperative changes in suboccipital soft tissues) and now a recurrent ependymoma (WHO Grade II). **C, D:** Axial T2 and postgadolinium T1 from a different older adult patient (age >40 years old) show a mass arising from the medial wall of the left lateral ventricle (septum pellucidum). This was a subependymoma (WHO Grade I), which often shows little enhancement.

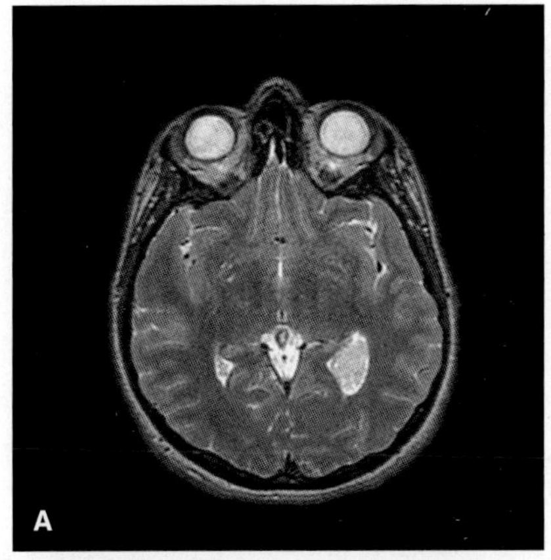

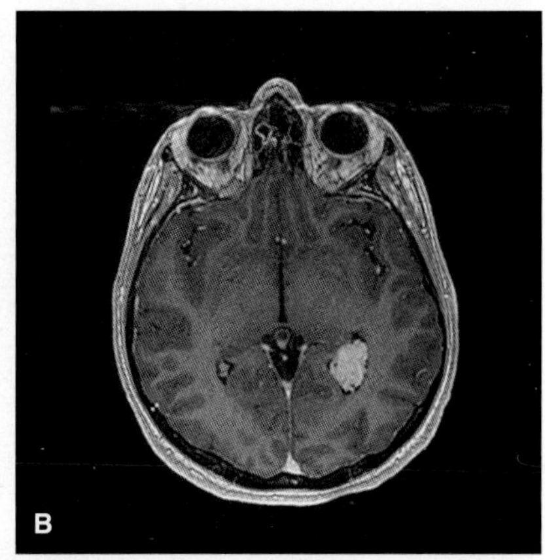

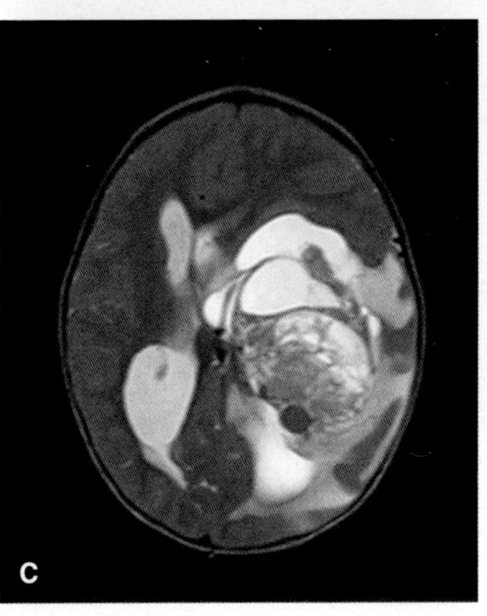

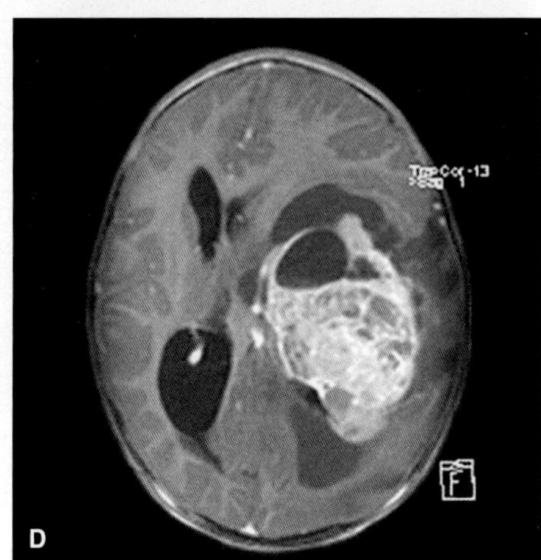

FIGURE 5.10. **Two Examples of Choroid Plexus Tumors in Different Patients. A, B:** Axial T2 and postgadolinium T1 from a young adult reveal a small avidly enhancing mass with lobulated margins in the atrium or trigone of the left lateral ventricle. Because this enlarged over time, it was resected and confirmed to be a choroid plexus papilloma (WHO Grade I). Note how it is centered on the choroid plexus itself, rather than arising from the ventricular wall. **C, D:** Axial T2 and postgadolinium T1 from a young child (different patient) show a much larger and more heterogeneous mass, also centered around the expected location of the left choroid plexus glomus. This was confirmed to be a choroid plexus carcinoma (WHO Grade III).

Intra-Axial Tumors: Nonglial

The vast majority of primary intra-axial tumors are derived from neuroepithelial cells; roughly two-thirds are derived from glial cells, specifically. Nonglial tumors of neuroepithelial origin include neuronal tumors, embryonal tumors, and pineal tumors.

Neuronal and Mixed Neuronal-Glial Tumors. These tumors are characterized by varying degrees of neuronal differentiation (e.g., neurocytes and ganglion cells), often with a glial component too. They generally present in children or young adults (age <40 years old). They are uncommon and account for approximately 1% of all primary CNS tumors.

Dysembryoplastic Neuroepithelial Tumor (DNET). DNET is a benign mixed neuronal-glial (aka glioneuronal) tumor with an excellent prognosis (WHO Grade I), associated with medically refractory partial complex seizures in children or young adults. DNET is identified histologically by the presence of cortical dysplasia and columns of bundled axons lined with oligodendroglial-like cells ("specific glioneuronal unit"). There are cortical neurons "floating" in a mucinous background; the latter correlates with hyperintensity on T2. The typical imaging pattern is a nonenhancing multicystic ("bubbly") mass at the cerebral cortex in a young patient, usually the temporal lobe (Fig. 5.11).

Gangliocytoma and Ganglioglioma. As the name would imply, gangliocytoma is a pure neuronal tumor composed of neoplastic ganglion cells; ganglioglioma is a mixed glioneuronal tumor with neoplastic glial cells as well. Both are low-grade tumors (WHO Grade I) with a good prognosis, although there is a rare variant, the anaplastic ganglioglioma (WHO Grade III), with high-grade features in the glial component. The typical imaging pattern is a partially enhancing mass at the cerebral cortex in a young patient (Fig. 5.11); this is the most common neoplastic etiology for temporal lobe epilepsy. Gangliocytoma and ganglioglioma may arise from gray matter anywhere within the CNS, including the hypothalamus, cerebellum, and spinal cord.

Dysplastic Cerebellar Gangliocytoma (Lhermitte–Duclos Disease). This benign slowly growing neoplasm versus hamartoma of the cerebellum (WHO Grade I) usually presents in young adults with symptoms related to local mass effect. The classic imaging pattern is a nonenhancing mass that expands the cerebellar folia and causes a "striated cerebellum" appearance on MRI. It is frequently associated with Cowden syndrome, an autosomal dominant phakomatosis with multiple hamartomas and mutations in the PTEN (phosphatase and tensin homolog) tumor suppressor gene.

Desmoplastic Infantile Astrocytoma and Ganglioglioma (DIA and DIG). DIA and DIG fall on a histologic spectrum and are both categorized under neuronal tumors, though DIA will not have neoplastic neurons. Like ganglioglioma, they can present as a heterogeneous mixed cystic-solid mass ("cyst and nodule" appearance) involving the cerebral cortex (Fig. 5.11). It may cause a desmoplastic reaction with thickening and enhancement of the overlying meninges, analogous to PXA. Unlike ganglioglioma and PXA, DIG tends to present in infancy (<2 years old), with rapidly progressive macrocephaly. It may appear aggressive, due to its large size and heterogeneity, but it carries a good prognosis (WHO Grade I).

Papillary Glioneuronal Tumor (PGNT) and Rosette-Forming Glioneuronal Tumor (RGNT). These entities were officially introduced and recognized in the 2007 CNS WHO. They are

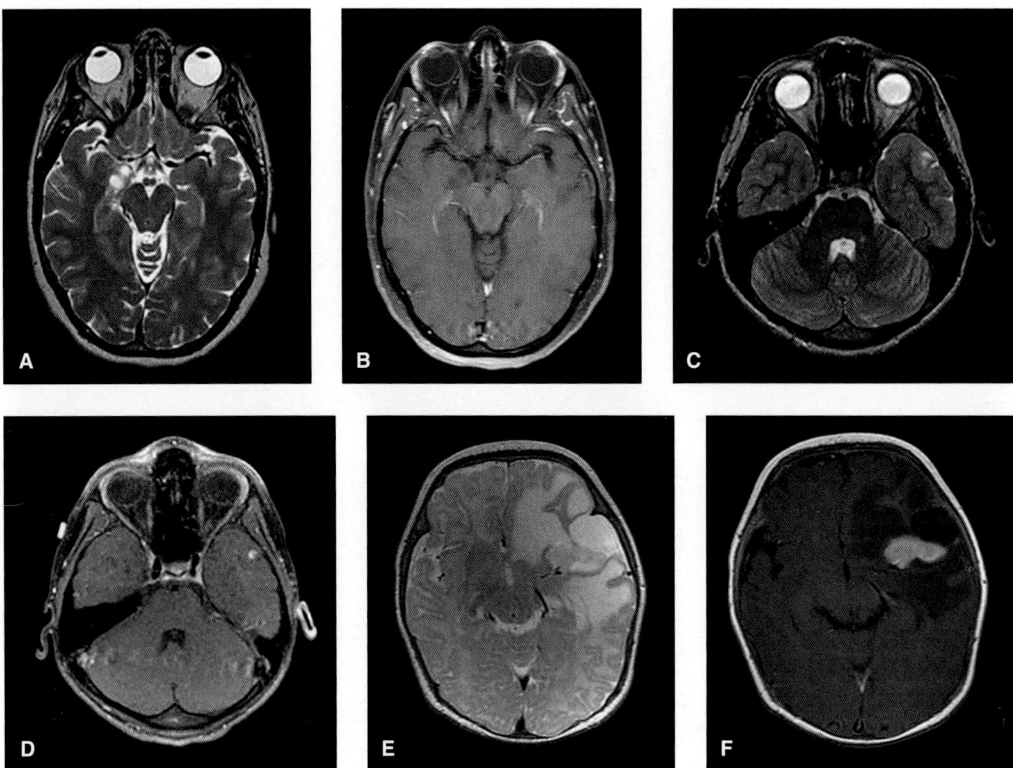

FIGURE 5.11. **Three Examples of Neuronal Tumors in Different Patients. A, B:** Axial T2 and postgadolinium T1 from a young adult with epilepsy uncover a nonenhancing multicystic ("bubbly") mass at the right medial temporal lobe cortex. Biopsy confirmed a DNET (WHO Grade I). **C, D:** Axial T2 and postgadolinium T1 from a different young adult patient with seizures reveal a partially cystic partially enhancing mass at the left lateral temporal lobe cortex. This turned out to be a different neuronal tumor, a ganglioglioma (WHO Grade I). **E, F:** Axial T2 and postgadolinium T1 from an infant with epilepsy and apneic spells demonstrate a much larger partially cystic partially enhancing mass involving the left frontal and temporal lobes. This was a desmoplastic infantile ganglioglioma, which is also a WHO Grade I neuronal tumor.

rare Grade I tumors with mixed glial and neuronal elements. In PGNT, the glial cells form a pseudopapillary arrangement with interpapillary neuronal cells. It presents as a cerebral mixed cystic-solid mass, with predilection for the temporal lobe, similar to ganglioglioma. In RGNT, the glial component resembles a pilocytic astrocytoma, while the neuronal component forms neurocytic rosettes and perivascular pseudorosettes. It also presents as a mixed cystic-solid mass, but is most commonly located in the midline, around the fourth ventricle, or the cerebral aqueduct.

Central Neurocytoma. In contrast with other neuronal tumors, which are parenchymal and often cortical in location, central neurocytoma (WHO Grade II) is a ventricular tumor, with an unclear cell of origin. Histologically, the neurocytes can resemble oligodendrocytes, hence these tumors were initially mistaken for intraventricular oligodendrogliomas. They usually present in young adults (20 to 40 years old) as an intensely enhancing mass arising from the septum pellucidum or lateral ventricular wall, near the foramen of Monro. On T2-weighted images, they have a heterogeneous appearance ("bubbly"). A histologically similar tumor that occurs in the brain parenchyma is called an extraventricular neurocytoma (WHO Grade II).

Embryonal Tumors. These are highly malignant tumors of neuroepithelial origin (WHO Grade IV), which are too poorly differentiated to be categorized as glial or neuronal tumors. There can be significant overlap in the histologic and radiologic appearance of these tumors, which tend to present as hypercellular hyperattenuating masses in children (age <20 years old). They account for approximately 1% of all primary CNS tumors (11% in first two decades).

Medulloblastoma. Infratentorial tumors are more common than supratentorial tumors in children after infancy and before adolescence. As the most common CNS embryonal tumor (constitutes two-thirds of cases), as well as the second most common pediatric CNS tumor (after pilocytic astrocytoma), medulloblastoma is a critical member of the pediatric posterior fossa differential diagnosis (Table 5.10). Most cases manifest in young children, under 10 years of age, and arise in the midline from the cerebellar vermis. When these tumors arise in older children and adults, they have a tendency to be located laterally within the cerebellar hemisphere.

Histologically and Genetically Defined Subtypes. Medulloblastoma has four histologic subtypes (classic, desmoplastic/nodular, medulloblastoma with extensive nodularity [MBEN], and large cell/anaplastic) as well as four genetic subtypes (WNT-activated, SHH-activated, group 3, and group 4), with prognostic implications (Table 5.11). Large cell/anaplastic is the most likely to show CSF dissemination, which is seen in a third of all medulloblastomas.

Imaging Patterns. The most classic appearance of medulloblastoma is a hyperdense mass at the cerebellar vermis in a young child (Fig. 5.12). The hyperattenuation reflects hypercellularity ("small round blue cell tumor"), which also results in lower signal on T2 and ADC images. A hypercellular

TABLE 5.10

MNEMONIC FOR PEDIATRIC POSTERIOR FOSSA TUMORS ("GAME")

	■ TYPICAL LOCATION	■ TYPICAL APPEARANCE
Brainstem Glioma (typically WHO Grade IV)	Pons (diffuse intrinsic pontine glioma, H3.3K27M mutation)	Infiltrative nonenhancing T2 hyperintense expansile mass
Pilocytic Astrocytoma[a] (WHO Grade I)	Cerebellar hemisphere, less common tectum or medulla	Nonenhancing cyst with enhancing mural nodule
Medulloblastoma[a] (WHO Grade IV)	Cerebellar vermis (midline), lateral location in 1/4 cases	High attenuation on CT Low signal on T2/ADC
Ependymoma (typically WHO Grade II)	Fourth ventricle, may ooze out foramen of Luschka/Magendie	Heterogeneous enhancement with cysts and calcifications

[a]Pilocytic astrocytoma (prototypical example of a circumscribed glioma) and medulloblastoma (prototypical example of an embryonal tumor) are the two most common pediatric CNS tumors.

hyperattenuating posterior fossa mass in a child or a young adult should always prompt consideration of medulloblastoma, even if the tumor is off midline.

Other Embryonal Tumors. One-third of CNS embryonal tumors will be diagnosed as atypical teratoid/rhabdoid tumor (AT/RT) and other rarer nonmedulloblastoma entities. AT/RT can present as a heterogeneous hyperattenuating mass anywhere in the CNS, usually in infants or very young children (age <4 years old). It is genetically defined by alterations of INI1, which can be tested by immunohistochemistry. When cases do not meet criteria for medulloblastoma, AT/RT, or other defined entities, "CNS embryonal tumor, not otherwise specified (NOS)" has replaced "CNS primitive neuroectodermal tumor (PNET)" as a new moniker.

Intra-Axial Tumors: Nonneuroepithelial

Since the brain is derived from neuroectoderm, it is relatively uncommon to encounter a primary intra-axial neoplasm of nonneuroepithelial origin. Secondary or metastatic disease will account for the vast majority of nonneuroepithelial intra-axial tumors.

Hemangioblastoma. While medulloblastoma is the most common primary intra-axial posterior fossa mass of childhood, hemangioblastoma is the most common primary intra-axial posterior fossa mass of adulthood, usually presenting in middle age (40 to 60 years old). Despite the suffix "blastoma," this is a benign neoplasm (WHO Grade I), characterized by vacuolated stromal cells with angiogenic potential. It has been categorized as a meningeal and mesenchymal tumor under the 2007 and 2016 CNS WHO classifications. Although most cases are sporadic, approximately 25% of cases are familial and associated with von Hippel–Lindau (VHL) syndrome. These tend to present with multiple tumors at a younger age (20 to 40 years old).

Imaging Pattern. Hemangioblastomas are circumscribed enhancing tumors that can secrete fluid and produce internal or adjacent cysts. Therefore, it can have the same classic "cyst with nodule" appearance in the cerebellum as the pilocytic astrocytoma (Fig. 5.13). Clinical presentation in adulthood and increased vascularity (e.g., flow voids, elevated CBV) favor a hemangioblastoma. The primary differential diagnosis would be hypervascular metastasis, for example, renal cell carcinoma. Fewer than 10% of hemangioblastomas arise outside the posterior fossa, often in the setting of VHL, and also present as pial-based enhancing nodules, with or without cysts.

Primary CNS Lymphoma (PCNSL). Diffuse large B-cell lymphoma is the most common non-Hodgkin lymphoma of adults and can arise in virtually any compartment of the body, including the brain parenchyma. PCNSL typically presents in older adults (age >40 years old) with altered mental status or focal neurologic deficits. Suspicion for PCNSL should prompt lumbar puncture for CSF cytology, followed by stereotactic

TABLE 5.11

MOLECULAR VERSUS HISTOLOGIC SUBTYPES OF MEDULLOBLASTOMA

■ GENOTYPE	■ PHENOTYPE	■ COMMENTS
WNT-activated	Usually classic histology Lateral location (peduncle)	Best prognosis Least common
SHH-activated TP53-mutant	Classic or large cell/anaplastic Midline location (vermis)	Poor prognosis
SHH-activated TP53-wildtype	Desmoplastic/nodular, MBEN Lateral location (hemisphere)	Good prognosis
"Group 3"	Classic or large cell/anaplastic Midline location (vermis)	Worst prognosis
"Group 4"	Classic or large cell/anaplastic Midline location (vermis)	Intermediate prognosis Most common

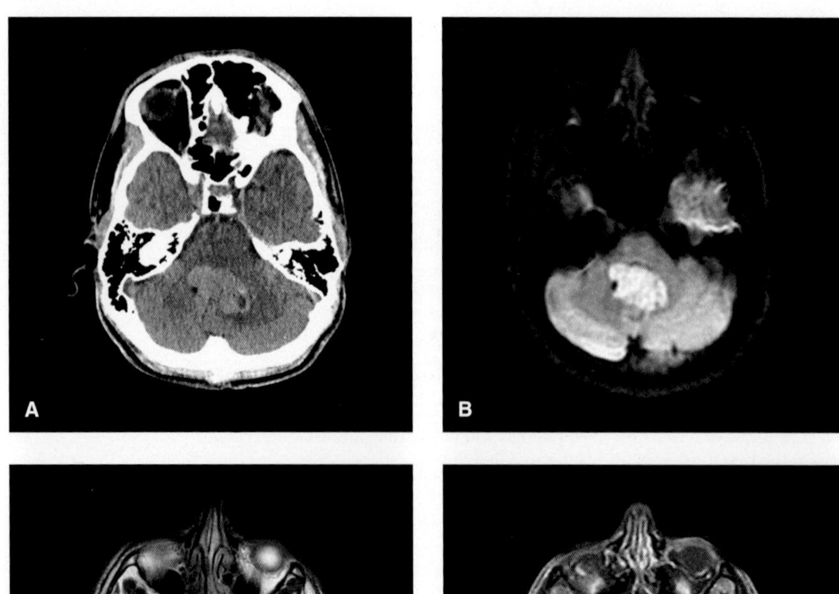

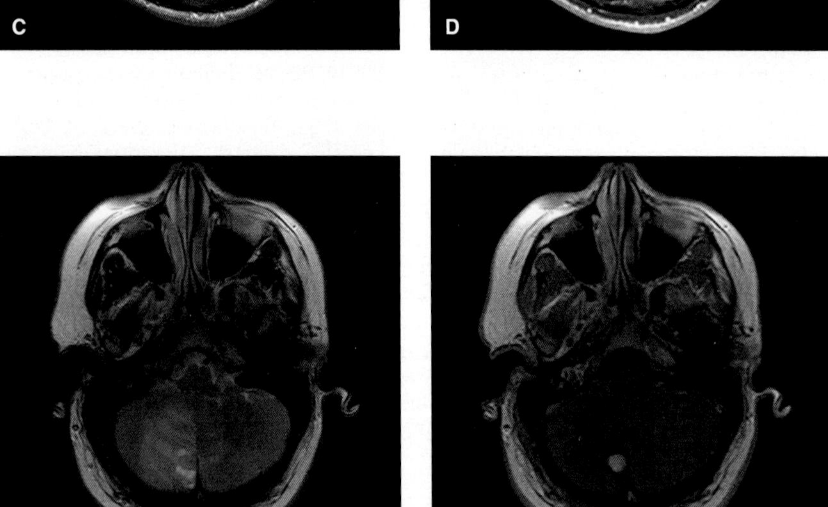

FIGURE 5.12. **Embryonal Tumor (Medulloblastoma) in a Young Patient. A:** Head CT from a young adult with headache reveals a hyperdense or hyperattenuating mass in the midline posterior fossa. **B:** Axial DWI shows restricted diffusion, which is also suspicious for a hypercellular tumor. **C, D:** Axial T2 and postgadolinium T1 confirm an enhancing mass, similar in T2 signal intensity to normal gray matter. Any intra-axial mass with hypercellular features in a young patient should prompt consideration of an embryonal tumor. Medulloblastoma is the most common and originates in the posterior fossa. Tissue diagnosis in this case was medulloblastoma (Grade: IV; histology: classic; genetics: WNT-activated; prognosis: relatively good).

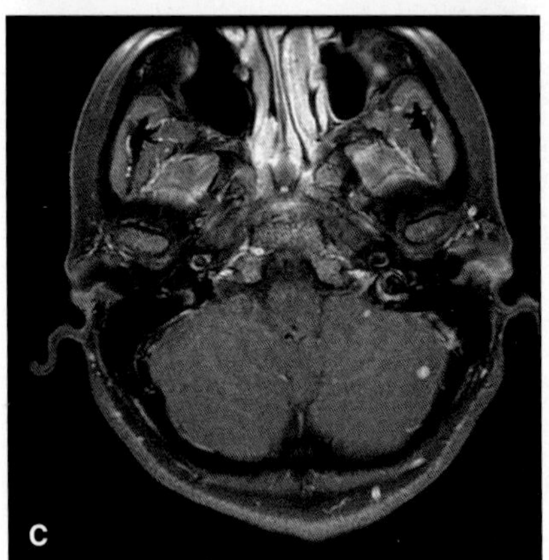

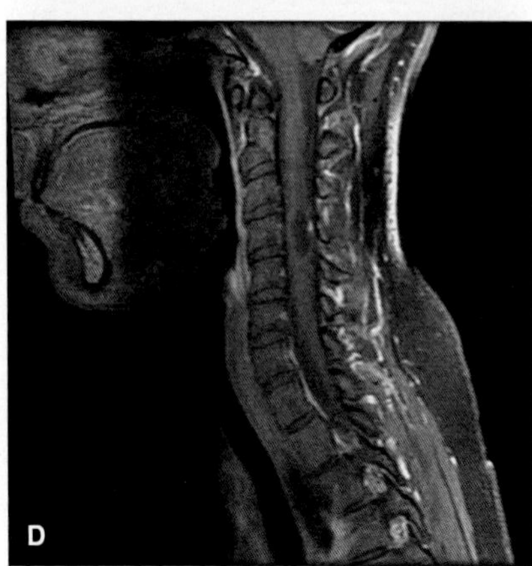

FIGURE 5.13 **Examples of a Mesenchymal Tumor (Hemangioblastoma). A, B:** Axial T2 and postgadolinium T1 reveal a partially cystic partially solid/enhancing mass at the pial surface of the right cerebellar hemisphere, with surrounding vasogenic edema. This was resected and confirmed to be a sporadic hemangioblastoma in an older adult patient. **C, D:** From a younger adult patient with von Hippel–Lindau syndrome, axial postgadolinium T1 of the brain and sagittal postgadolinium T1 of the cervical spine demonstrate three small enhancing nodules at the pial surface of the left cerebellar hemisphere and the cervical spinal cord with an adjacent nonenhancing cyst. These are familial hemangioblastomas in association with VHL.

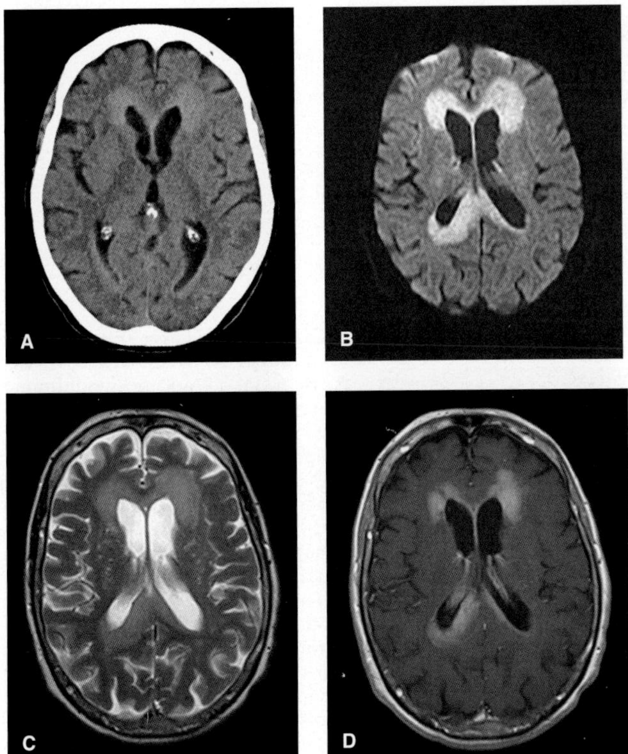

FIGURE 5.14. Primary Central Nervous System Lymphoma (PCNSL). A: Head CT from an elderly patient with progressive dementia reveals abnormal hyperdensity or hyperattenuation in the brain parenchyma adjacent to the lateral ventricles. **B:** Axial DWI shows corresponding restricted diffusion, which is also suspicious for a hypercellular tumor. **C, D:** Axial T2 and postgadolinium T1 confirm a homogeneously enhancing mass, next to CSF spaces (aka "rimphoma"), similar in T2 signal intensity to normal gray matter. This is the classic appearance of primary CNS lymphoma (diffuse large B-cell lymphoma). Immunodeficiency-associated CNS lymphomas can have a different appearance (heterogeneous or weak enhancement).

needle biopsy if negative. Maximal safe resection is not performed for PCNSL, which is primarily treated with chemotherapy. Glucocorticoids can shrink the tumor transiently and sometimes dramatically ("ghost tumor"); withholding steroid therapy before a biopsy may help to maximize sensitivity.

Imaging Patterns. Like embryonal tumors, lymphomas are characterized by high cellular density, high nucleus-to-cytoplasm ratio, and lower free water content. In an immunocompetent patient, the classic imaging pattern of PCNSL is a homogeneously enhancing mass that abuts the CSF spaces and wraps around the ventricles or sulci ("rimphoma"), with homogeneous hyperdensity on CT and corresponding hypointensity on T2/ADC (Fig. 5.14). Other than diffuse gliomas, it is the other neoplasm that can infiltrate the corpus callosum. Many of these classic descriptors do not apply to immunocompromised patients, since AIDS-related or EBV-positive PCNSL tends to present with multifocal heterogeneous lesions and variable or ring-like enhancement. Differential diagnosis includes infection or abscesses in the immunocompromised setting, for example, toxoplasmosis was a primary concern during the HIV/AIDS epidemic.

Metastatic Tumors. Approximately 25% of patients with systemic cancer will develop brain metastases, and approximately 50% of brain metastases are secondary to lung cancer. In the intracranial or intradural compartment, parenchymal metastases are more common (usually supratentorial) than intraventricular, leptomeningeal, or pachymeningeal metastases. While metastases are often multifocal due to hematogenous dissemination, they can also present as solitary masses. Corticosteroids or anticonvulsants may be used to reduce edema or seizures; radiation and surgery are possible treatment modalities for brain metastases.

Imaging Patterns. The classic appearance of metastatic tumor on CT or MRI is one or multiple enhancing masses, with circumscribed margins, located peripherally near the gray–white matter junction, and surrounded by marked vasogenic edema (Fig. 5.15). The enhancement reflects lack of a blood–brain barrier (nonneural tissue); the well-defined margins mirror the histologic appearance; the peripheral location is related to hematogenous dissemination; and the vasogenic edema can be seen with any enhancing lesion (both findings correlate with leaky vessels). If the patient cannot receive gadolinium, noncontrast MRI or contrast-enhanced CT may be performed, although with decreased sensitivity for small or subcentimeter metastases.

Leptomeningeal Disease. Leptomeningeal metastases have many synonyms: CSF/subarachnoid dissemination of tumor, leptomeningeal carcinomatosis, carcinomatous meningitis, neoplastic meningitis, or "drop" metastases when originating from a primary CNS tumor. On imaging, it may appear as thin or nodular enhancement in the subarachnoid spaces, often accompanied by loss of normal CSF nulling on T2 FLAIR images, sometimes complicated by communicating hydrocephalus as well (Fig. 5.15). Delayed postgadolinium images and postgadolinium T2 FLAIR images are ways to increase sensitivity for leptomeningeal disease.

Extra-Axial Tumors

While nonmetastatic tumors arising inside the pia mater are overwhelmingly of neuroepithelial origin, nonmetastatic tumors arising outside the pia mater (extra-axial) tend to be mesenchymal in nature, which reflect the different kinds of tissue they originate from.

Schwannoma. Whereas oligodendrocytes are responsible for myelination in the CNS, Schwann cells form the myelin sheaths in peripheral nerves, including cranial nerves III–XII. Intracranial schwannomas are benign extra-axial neoplasms (WHO Grade I), which arise from the vestibular nerve (CN8) in the vast majority of cases. Less commonly, they may arise from the other cranial nerves (CN5), and rarely, they may arise within the brain parenchyma, possibly originating from peripheral nerves that innervate vessel walls (*nervi vasorum*). Symptoms are dependent on tumor location. Because vestibular schwannomas are the most common posterior fossa tumor in adults, they are the reason for screening MRI in asymmetric sensorineural hearing loss.

Imaging Patterns. Schwannomas are focal encapsulated tumors with spindle-shaped neoplastic Schwann cells on histopathology, which may be organized in a more cellular Antoni A pattern with nuclear palisading ("Verocay bodies"), versus a less cellular Antoni B pattern with cystic degeneration ("ancient change"). This spectrum is reflected on imaging as schwannomas can be heterogeneous in signal intensity, especially when large, although they are generally described as enhancing T2 hyperintense masses along a peripheral nerve. Vestibular schwannomas will often arise within and gradually expand the bony internal auditory canal, while growing medially into the CPA cistern, yielding an "ice cream cone" appearance (Fig. 5.16). Other mass lesions of the CPA are much less common (Table 5.12).

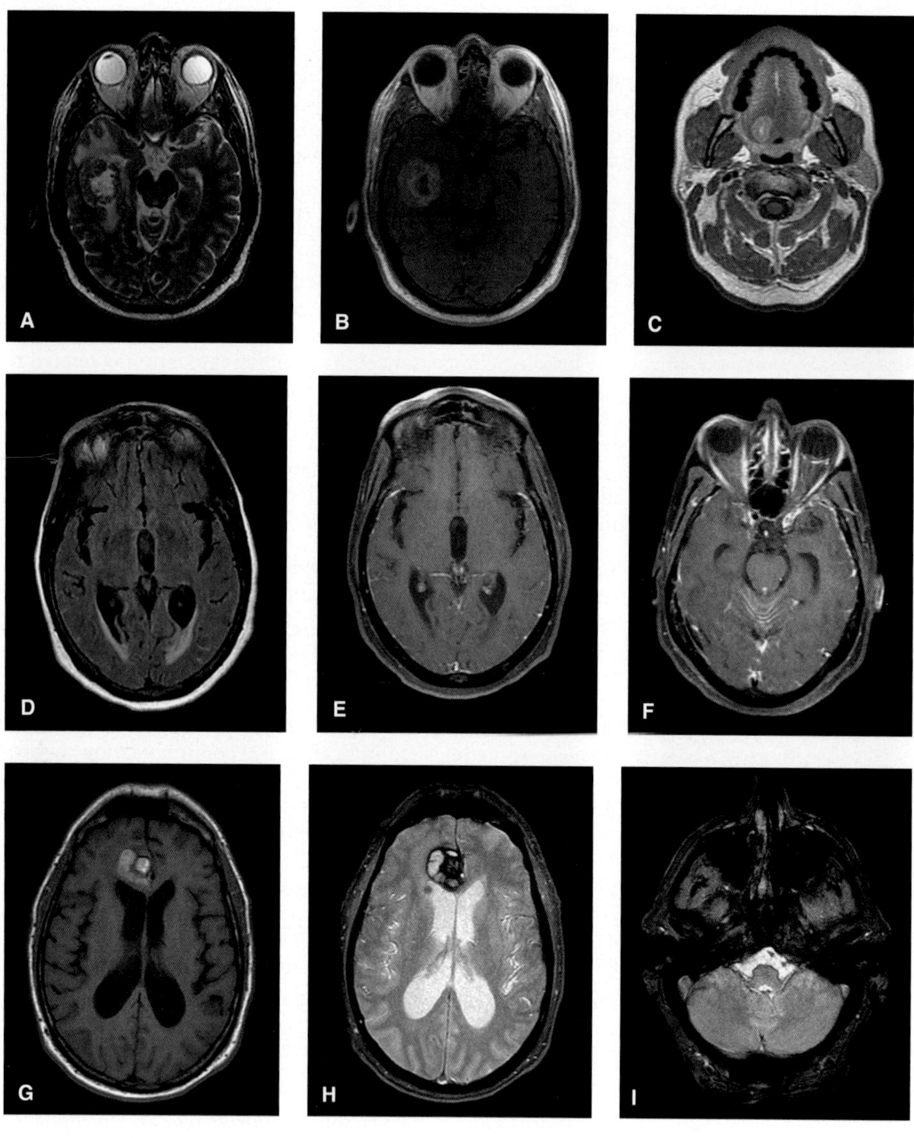

FIGURE 5.15 Three Examples of Secondary or Metastatic Disease. A, B: Axial T2 and postgadolinium T1 reveal a heterogeneously enhancing mass with vasogenic edema in the right temporal lobe. This was a brain metastasis in a patient with known history of leiomyosarcoma. C: Axial postgadolinium T1 at a lower level shows an additional tongue lesion. Metastatic lesions usually have well-defined margins. D, E: Axial FLAIR and postgadolinium T1 from a different patient with known history of breast cancer reveal ventricular enlargement with transependymal edema at the occipital horns. There is also subtle FLAIR signal abnormality and enhancement in the cerebral sulci. F: Axial postgadolinium T1 at a lower level shows abnormal enhancement lining the cerebellar folia. This was a case of leptomeningeal carcinomatosis with communicating hydrocephalus. G, H: Axial T1 and axial GRE from a third patient with known history of melanoma reveal a hemorrhagic mass (T1 hyperintense T2* hypointense) in the right frontal lobe. There was minimal enhancement on postgadolinium images (not shown). I: Axial GRE at a lower level shows superficial siderosis along the surface of the medulla.

Neurofibromatosis Type 2 and Schwannomatosis. Neurofibromatosis type 2 is a misnomer and is characterized by multiple schwannomas (and meningiomas), not neurofibromas. It is autosomal dominant and associated with mutations in the NF2 tumor suppressor gene. Bilateral vestibular schwannomas are diagnostic of NF2. As the name would suggest, schwannomatosis also shows multiple schwannomas, although without the predilection for CN8. It is autosomal dominant and associated with mutations in the SMARCB1 tumor suppressor gene.

Other Peripheral Nerve Sheath Tumors. The 2016 CNS WHO also lists neurofibroma (WHO Grade I), perineurioma (WHO Grade I), and malignant peripheral nerve sheath tumor (WHO Grade II to IV), all of which are rarely encountered in the cranial vault.

Meningioma. Meningiomas are the most common extra-axial tumors and also the most common primary CNS tumors (36%). They are more frequent in females than males (2:1 ratio) and usually present in older adults (age >40 years old). They arise from arachnoid cap cells in the arachnoid mater, which abuts the dura mater on the inside of the skull. Half of the cases present as dural-based masses along the cerebral convexity or the falx cerebri (parasagittal). Other locations include the sphenoid wing, the cavernous sinus, the optic nerve sheath, the olfactory groove, the suprasellar region, the petrous ridge, the tentorium cerebelli, the posterior fossa, the CPA, the foramen magnum, the spinal canal, and the lateral ventricle.

WHO Classification. Benign (Grade I), atypical (Grade II), and anaplastic or malignant (Grade III) account for >90%, ~6%, and ~1% of meningiomas, respectively. Tumor grading is based on the degree of mitotic activity or anaplastic features. A histologic Grade I tumor that breaches the pial barrier (i.e., brain invasion) is considered a Grade II tumor. In addition to these three entities, the WHO classification also lists 13 histologic variants. The most common is transitional, which has features of both meningothelial and fibroblastic meningiomas. Chordoid and clear cell are Grade II meningiomas; papillary and rhabdoid are Grade III meningiomas.

Imaging Patterns. A classic but nonspecific appearance of a meningioma is an enhancing dural-based mass, which may be accompanied by adjacent dural thickening ("dural tail") and osseous changes (e.g., hyperostosis). They tend to be isodense on CT and isointense on T2/ADC to gray matter (Fig. 5.17), which can make them hard to visualize on noncontrast studies when small. They avidly enhance on postcontrast images. If angiography is performed as part of the workup (e.g., preoperative embolization), there is a radial arrangement of the vessels with an early dense tumor blush that persists well into the

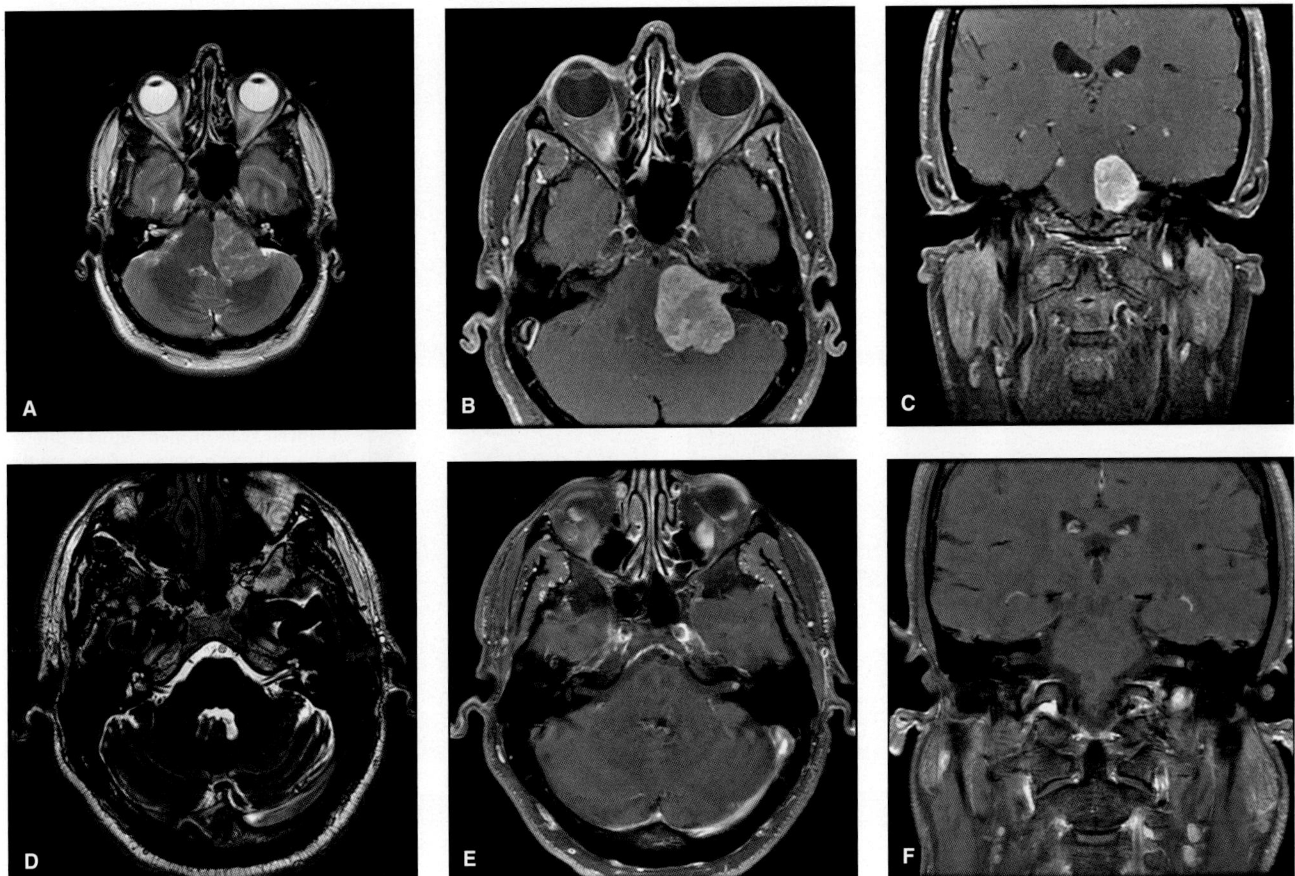

FIGURE 5.16. **Two Examples of Nerve Sheath Tumor (Schwannoma). A:** Axial T2 of the brain from a patient with asymmetric sensorineural hearing loss shows a large extra-axial mass in the left cerebellopontine angle. **B, C:** Axial and coronal postgadolinium T1 of the internal auditory canals (smaller field-of-view) confirm that this mass enhances and involves the left internal auditory canal (IAC). This vestibular schwannoma underwent excisional biopsy. There is a tiny enhancing lesion at the right lateral margin of the midbrain on the coronal image, which could represent another schwannoma. **D:** Screening FIESTA from a different patient with asymmetric hearing loss reveals a subtle round lesion at the fundus of the left IAC. This patient was called back for additional imaging. **E, F:** Axial and coronal postgadolinium T1 clearly show enhancement in this tiny presumed schwannoma (being managed conservatively).

venous phase. This angiographic finding has been called the "mother-in-law sign" because it shows up early and stays late.

Meningiomas can have a rounded globose shape or a flattened *en plaque* morphology. When located at or next to a dural venous sinus, it is important to assess for invasion or involvement, which may restrict the ability to obtain a gross total resection safely. It is not uncommon for a meningioma to evoke vasogenic edema in the adjacent brain parenchyma, especially when it is supplied by internal rather than external carotid artery branches; this alone is not a sign of brain invasion or higher-grade tumor. It can be difficult to distinguish the very common meningioma from the less common higher grades and from other nonmeningothelial causes of dural-based masses (Table 5.13). Biopsy versus observation are the main options.

Ventricular Meningioma. Since the choroid plexus is formed embryologically by invagination of leptomeninges into the lateral ventricles through the choroidal fissure, choroid plexus epithelium and stroma are derived from ependymal cells and

TABLE 5.12

MNEMONIC FOR CEREBELLOPONTINE ANGLE MASSES ("AMEN")

	T1	T2	ADC	ENHANCEMENT
Arachnoid cyst	Hypointense	Hyperintense	Hyperintense	No
Meningioma	Isointense	Isointense	Isointense	Yes
Epidermoid cyst	Hypointense	Hyperintense	Isointense	No
"Neuroma" (i.e., schwannoma)[a]	Hypointense	Hyperintense	Hyperintense	Yes

[a]Vestibular schwannoma used to be called "acoustic neuroma" (another mnemonic = "SAME").

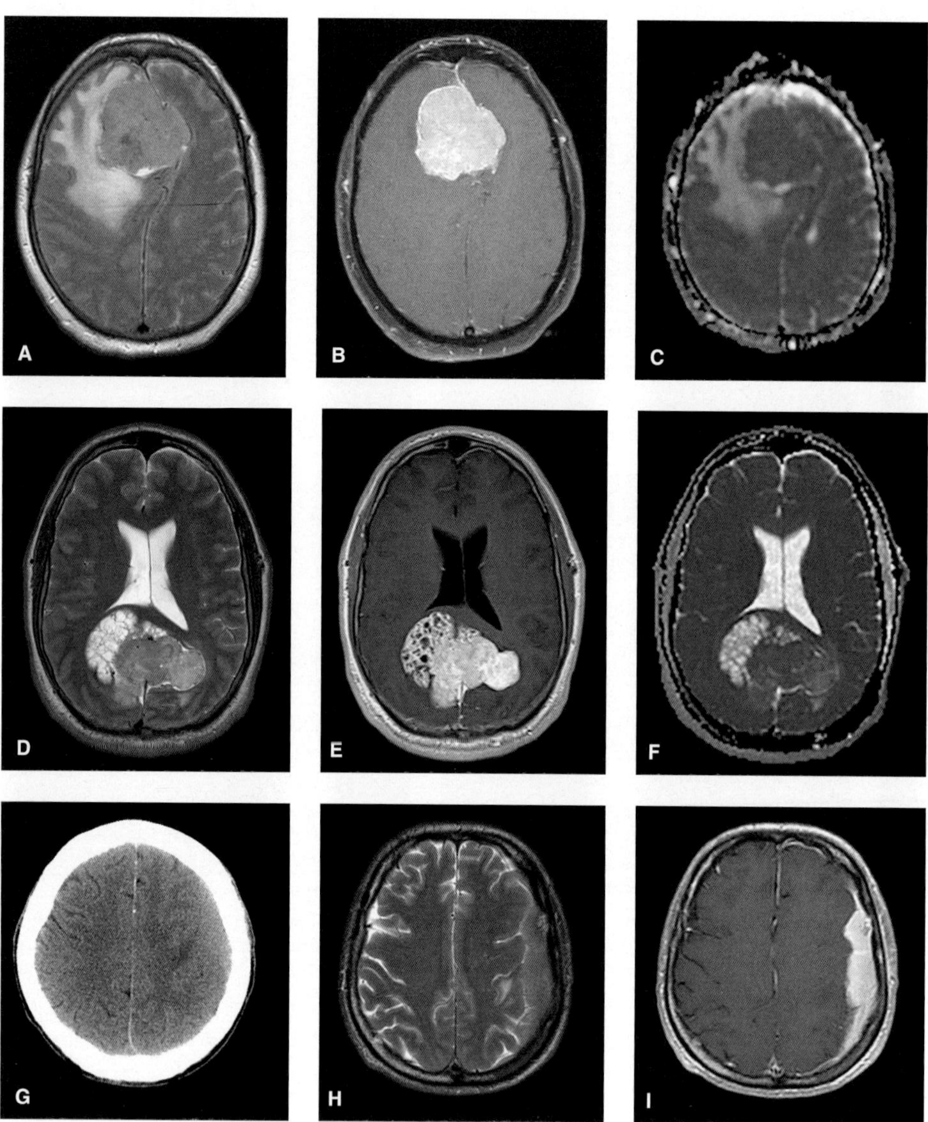

FIGURE 5.17. **Three Different Categories of Dural-Based Tumors. A, B:** Axial T2 and postgadolinium T1 from an older adult female with cognitive symptoms show an enhancing T2 isointense mass arising from the anterior falx, with vasogenic edema in the right frontal lobe. You can see a "CSF cleft sign" at the margins of this extra-axial mass, which turned out to be a meningioma (WHO Grade I). **C:** Relatively low diffusivity or signal intensity on axial ADC is often seen in meningioma due to high cellular density, despite usually being a low-grade tumor. **D–F:** Axial T2, postgadolinium T1, and ADC from a young adult male reveal a lobulated heterogeneously enhancing mass arising from the posterior falx, whose solid enhancing portions are hypervascular and hypercellular (isointense to gray matter on T2/ADC). This turned out to be a hemangiopericytoma (WHO Grade II). **G:** Head CT from an older adult male with sudden onset weakness of the right upper extremity was initially interpreted as an isodense subdural hematoma along the left frontoparietal convexity. **H, I:** Subsequent axial T2 and postgadolinium T1 revealed this to be an enhancing vascularized T2 isointense mass not a hematoma. This turned out to be an extranodal marginal zone lymphoma. Differential diagnosis categories for dural-based neoplasms include meningothelial (meningioma), mesenchymal, and metastatic/hematopoietic.

arachnoid mater, respectively. Arachnoid cap cells are therefore found in normal choroid plexus stroma and may give rise to a very common tumor (meningioma) in a very uncommon location (~1%). An avidly enhancing mass located in the atrium/trigone of a lateral ventricle should prompt consideration of choroid plexus papilloma in a child and intraventricular meningioma in an older adult (Table 5.14).

Hemangiopericytoma. Previously known as "angioblastic meningioma," hemangiopericytoma was officially recognized as a distinct clinicopathologic entity under the 2007 CNS WHO.

TABLE 5.13

SIMPLIFIED APPROACH TO DURAL-BASED MASSES

■ CATEGORIES	■ EXAMPLES
Meningothelial	Meningioma
Mesenchymal	Hemangiopericytoma
Metastatic	Breast, prostate, lung
Hematopoietic	Leukemia, lymphoma
Inflammatory	Sarcoidosis, tuberculosis

This rare tumor has a peak incidence at 30 to 50 years and arises from modified pericapillary smooth muscle cells (pericytes of Zimmerman). Like meningiomas, hemangiopericytoma presents as a dural-based mass; unlike meningiomas, it is an aggressive mesenchymal tumor (sarcoma) with a propensity for local recurrence and distant metastasis. It is also highly cellular and vascular, with irregular branching capillaries on histologic examination ("staghorn vessels").

The 2007 CNS WHO classification included the Grade II hemangiopericytoma and the Grade III anaplastic hemangiopericytoma; the latter was differentiated by increased mitotic activity. These are now recognized as belonging on the same spectrum as the less cellular and more collagenous solitary fibrous tumor, a benign Grade I tumor of the extracranial soft tissues. These three entities share a molecular feature (STAT6 gene fusion) and are listed together as "solitary fibrous tumor/hemangiopericytoma" (Grade I, II, or III) under the 2016 CNS WHO classification.

Imaging Patterns. The overall imaging presentation is often very similar to that of a meningioma (Fig. 5.17), with a few exceptions. In 33% of cases, hemangiopericytomas show a narrow base of attachment to the dura, instead of the broad base seen in the vast majority of meningiomas. It is also typically multilobulated, rather than hemispheric in shape, as seen in most meningiomas. Bone destruction and flow voids are

TABLE 5.14

SIMPLIFIED APPROACH TO VENTRICULAR TUMORS

	SITE OF ORIGIN	AGE PREDILECTION (YEARS)	ENHANCEMENT
Ependymoma	Ependymal lining	<20	Strong
Central neurocytoma	Septum pellucidum	20–40	Strong
Subependymoma	Subependymal plate	>40	Weak
Choroid plexus tumor	Choroid plexus epithelium	<20	Strong
Meningioma	Choroid plexus stroma	>40	Strong
Metastasis	Choroid plexus stroma	>40	Strong

more common in hemangiopericytomas; hyperostosis and calcifications are more common in meningiomas. Spectroscopy can show elevated myoinositol in hemangiopericytomas, versus the alanine peak characteristic of meningiomas.

Meningeal Melanocytoma and Melanoma. There are normal melanocytes in the leptomeninges, as well as the uvea of the eye, which may give rise to primary low-grade melanocytoma or high-grade melanoma. Secondary metastases from cutaneous malignant melanoma are more common. These diseases have a nonspecific imaging pattern, with an intradural enhancing mass, or masses in the setting of meningeal melanocytosis and melanomatosis. Intrinsic T1 hyperintensity may be suggestive and is attributed to melanin or hemorrhage, but is not always present.

Pineal Region Masses

The pineal gland is a small usually subcentimeter "pinecone"–shaped structure, which has been historically described as the "third eye" or the "principal seat of the soul." Its true function is as an endocrine organ that secretes melatonin into the bloodstream, therefore it lacks a blood–brain barrier and normally enhances on postcontrast images. It also normally begins to calcify during adolescence. It is located in the midline at the posterior margin of the third ventricle, just below the splenium of the corpus callosum and just above the tectum of the midbrain. It is common to see internal cysts, which may compress the midbrain/aqueduct when very large. Tumors of the pineal region are rare and account for less than 1% of all primary CNS tumors.

Pineal Parenchymal Tumors. When presented with solid enhancing masses in the pineal region, it is natural to think first of tumors arising from the neuroepithelial cells that compose the pineal gland (pineocytes). These pineal parenchymal tumors range from Grade I to IV.

Pineocytoma. Pineocytomas are WHO Grade I and are circumscribed slow growing tumors that tend to present in adults with symptoms related to local mass effect. They can be cystic or solid in morphology. As typical for low-grade tumors, surgery is the primary treatment.

Pineal Parenchymal Tumor of Intermediate Differentiation (PPTID). PPTIDs are WHO Grade II or III and are more atypical aggressive lobulated enhancing masses that also tend to present in adults. This rare entity was first recognized in the 2000 CNS WHO (third edition).

Pineoblastoma. Pineoblastomas are WHO Grade IV and are highly malignant undifferentiated embryonal tumors of the pineal gland that tend to present in children. They are enhancing and hypercellular in appearance, for example, hyperdense on CT and hypointense on T2/ADC (Fig. 5.18). As for other embryonal tumors, prognosis is poor with propensity for CSF dissemination, and treatment is a multimodal combination of surgery, radiation, and chemotherapy.

Germ Cell Tumors. While germ cells are generally associated with the gonads, intracranial rests may give rise to GCTs of the CNS, which actually constitute the most common type of neoplasm in the pineal region (60%). Similar to their gonadal counterparts, GCTs can be divided into two subcategories: germinoma, also known as dysgerminoma or seminoma, and the nongerminomatous or nonseminomatous GCTs. They tend to occur in children and in the midline, for example, pineal in ~2/3 and suprasellar in ~1/3 of cases. Similar to the hematopoietic and metastatic categories, GCTs do not have a CNS WHO Grade.

Germinoma. Germinomas are the most common intracranial GCTs and have a strong preference for males over females, particularly in the pineal region (10:1 ratio). They are hypercellular with sheets of polygonal germ cells and may be complicated by CSF dissemination. For these reasons, they can be difficult to distinguish from pineoblastomas. It has been noted that germ cell tumors tend to wrap around or "engulf" normal pineal calcifications, while pineal parenchymal tumors tend to displace or "explode" them. Radiation not surgery is the primary treatment modality for biopsy-confirmed germinomas, which have a favorable prognosis (Fig. 5.18).

Other Germ Cell Tumors. Nongerminomatous GCTs (NGGCTs) include embryonal carcinoma, yolk sac tumor (also known as endodermal sinus tumor), choriocarcinoma, teratoma, and mixed germ cell tumors. Like germinoma, these tend to present in children and in pineal or suprasellar locations. Unlike germinoma, these are less common, more aggressive, and more heterogeneous in appearance. A heterogeneous enhancing mass with internal fat density or signal should prompt consideration of a teratoma, given its ability to recapitulate tissues from multiple germ layers. A heterogeneous midline mass in a newborn should prompt consideration of a congenital teratoma, given that these tumors are thought to arise *in utero* (may present at any age).

Tumors Arising From Adjacent Structures. Aside from pineal parenchymal and germ cell tumors, other masses that can project into the pineal region include tentorial meningiomas and exophytic gliomas arising from the splenium superiorly or the tectum inferiorly. There is also the papillary tumor of the pineal region (PTPR), which is a WHO Grade II or III neuroepithelial tumor arising from the subcommissural organ, a small ependymal gland located at the posterior margin of the third ventricle, just below the posterior commissure. It presents as an enhancing mass in adults and can be hard to differentiate from other pineal region tumors (Table 5.15).

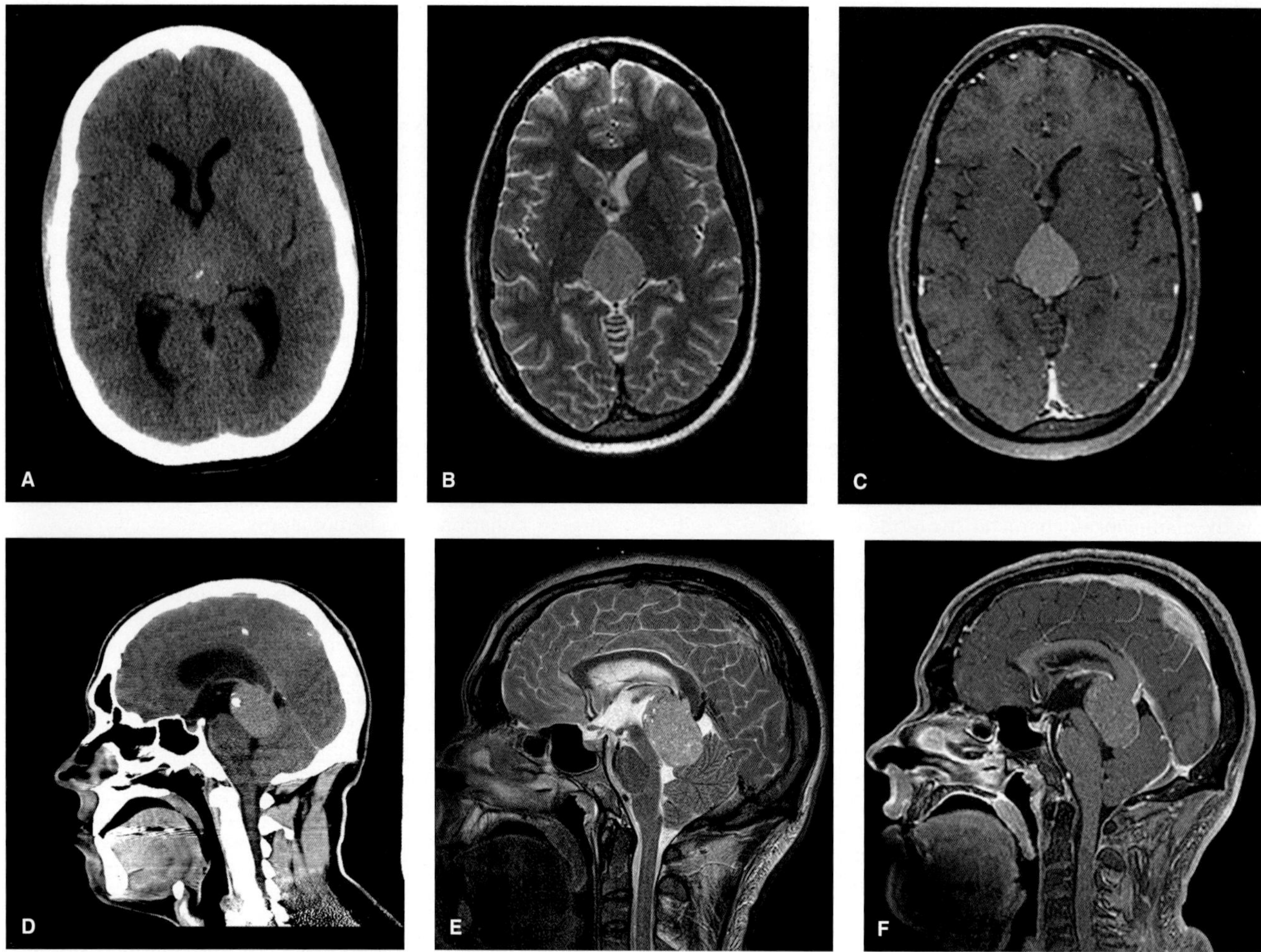

FIGURE 5.18. **Two Different Categories of Pineal Region Tumors. A:** Head CT from a young adult female illustrates an iso- to hyperattenuating mass in the pineal region, located at the posterior margin of the third ventricle. **B, C:** Axial T2 and postgadolinium T1 from preoperative MRI (note the left frontal scalp fiducial) confirm a solid enhancing mass, which was diagnosed as a pineoblastoma (WHO Grade IV). She had presented with obstructive hydrocephalus (note the tip of the ventricular drain in the right frontal horn). **D–F:** Sagittal CT, T2, and postgadolinium T1 in a young adult male who had also presented with hydrocephalus show another hyperattenuating enhancing mass in the pineal region. Unlike the first case, this mass seems to engulf the normal pineal gland calcification and was diagnosed as germinoma, which responded well to radiation therapy. Differential diagnosis categories for pineal region masses include pineal parenchymal (WHO grades I to IV) and germ cell tumors.

TABLE 5.15

SIMPLIFIED APPROACH TO PINEAL REGION MASSES

■ CELL OF ORIGIN	■ NEOPLASMS
Pineal parenchymal tumors	Pineocytoma (Grade I) Pineal parenchymal tumor of intermediate differentiation (Grade II or III) Pineoblastoma (Grade IV)
Germ cell tumors (GCT)	Germinoma Embryonal carcinoma Yolk sac tumor (endodermal sinus) Choriocarcinoma Teratoma (mature or immature) Mixed GCT
Adjacent structures	Papillary tumor of the pineal region Meningioma (e.g., tentorial) Glioma (e.g., tectal)
Nonneoplastic	Vein of Galen malformation

Sellar Region Masses

The sella turcica ("Turkish saddle") is a midline depression at the top of the sphenoid body that holds the pituitary gland. It is separated from the suprasellar cistern superiorly by the diaphragm sellae, which attaches to the tuberculum sellae anteriorly and the dorsum sellae posteriorly. With aging, this dural reflection can weaken and permit the subarachnoid space to herniate inferiorly from the suprasellar cistern into the sella turcica ("empty sella" appearance).

The pituitary stalk (infundibulum) and the posterior pituitary (neurohypophysis) are derived from neuroectoderm and are extensions of the diencephalon. The anterior pituitary (adenohypophysis) is derived from surface ectoderm, specifically from the primitive stomodeum, which also gives rise to the mouth. During development, this tissue forms an epithelial diverticulum, also known as a craniopharyngeal duct or Rathke pouch, which extends from the pharynx into the cranial vault to meet the neurohypophysis and form the adenohypophysis anteriorly.

Pituitary Adenomas. Pituitary adenomas arise from the adenohypophysis and are not listed in the CNS WHO classifications (considered endocrine). According to CBTRUS data from 2009 to 2013, they are one of the three most common primary CNS neoplasms: meningiomas (36%), adenomas (16%), and glioblastoma (15%). They usually present in adulthood, often in young adults (20 to 40 years old). They can be separated by size into microadenomas (<1 cm) and macroadenomas (>1 cm). While macroadenomas can often be detected on standard brain CT or MRI, microadenomas will require dedicated evaluation with a higher resolution sella/pituitary MRI.

Microadenomas are too small to cause local mass effect and therefore present with symptoms of oversecretion or as incidental findings on neuroimaging (or autopsy). Hormonal symptoms will depend on the endocrine cell of origin: lactotrophs make prolactin, somatotrophs make growth hormone (GH), corticotrophs make adrenocorticotropic hormone (ACTH), thyrotrophs make thyroid-stimulating hormone (TSH), gonadotrophs make luteinizing hormone (LH) and follicle-stimulating hormone (FSH), and "null cells" are nonfunctional. Prolactinomas are most common and may produce amenorrhea/galactorrhea in women or decreased libido in men. GH-secreting adenomas are second most common and may produce acromegaly or gigantism. Prolactinomas can be medically treated with dopamine agonists like cabergoline (Fig. 5.19).

Macroadenomas may cause symptoms from local mass effect. Usually, the primary concern is visual loss from compression of the optic nerves, chiasm, or tracts superiorly. Compression of the pituitary gland or stalk may produce hypopituitarism or hyperprolactinemia ("stalk effect"), respectively. Lateral invasion of the cavernous sinuses may produce severe hyperprolactinemia or diplopia from mass effect on cranial nerves. For symptomatic macroadenomas, particularly in the setting of progressive visual loss, surgical debulking or resection can be performed to relieve mass effect, usually by endonasal transsphenoidal approach (Fig. 5.19). The vast majority of adenomas are benign; atypical adenomas and carcinomas are extremely rare.

Imaging Patterns. The pituitary gland is most often evaluated by MRI with thin slice T1- and T2-weighted images in the sagittal and coronal planes. Gadolinium contrast is usually administered to help identify any solid enhancing tumor and to increase sensitivity for microadenomas. Since the endocrine pituitary gland has a hypophyseal portal system, which lacks a blood–brain barrier, it normally demonstrates fairly intense homogeneous enhancement. Therefore, adenomas usually appear as relatively hypoenhancing lesions, when compared with normal pituitary and cavernous sinuses. DCE MRI of the pituitary gland is sometimes performed to help detect microadenomas, which will take up contrast slower than normal tissue.

Because lactotrophs and somatotrophs are located laterally in the pituitary gland, most adenomas will arise laterally as well. Microadenomas may demonstrate mild upward bowing of the superior pituitary margin on one side and may cause mild deviation of the pituitary stalk to the other side. Macroadenomas are much less subtle. They can expand the bony sella turcica, extend superiorly into the suprasellar cistern, and invade laterally into the cavernous sinus. The latter is identified by lateral extension of tumor past the midpoint of the cavernous internal carotid artery flow void on coronal images (Fig. 5.19). Due to high cellularity, these tumors can be hyperdense on CT and hypointense on T2, similar to gray matter. There can also be heterogeneous signal related to tumoral cysts, infarcts, or hemorrhages. When a pituitary macroadenoma suddenly enlarges due to hemorrhage, this acute syndrome is called "pituitary apoplexy."

Craniopharyngioma. Craniopharyngioma is a WHO Grade I tumor that arises from squamous epithelial remnants of the craniopharyngeal duct, also known as Rathke pouch. Therefore, it can occur anywhere between the nasopharynx and the third ventricle, but it is most commonly centered in the suprasellar region (Table 5.16). Adamantinomatous craniopharyngiomas are the most common nonneuroepithelial CNS tumor of childhood. They are characterized by heterogeneity as described by the 90% rule: 90% show cystic change, 90% show calcifications, and 90% show solid or nodular enhancement (Fig. 5.19). They can also present in adulthood.

Papillary craniopharyngiomas are the other type and are less commonly encountered. They tend to present in older adults as a solid enhancing mass. Rathke cleft cysts are nonneoplastic cysts that result from a persistent cleft in Rathke pouch that fails to involute. Like adamantinomatous craniopharyngiomas, they are cystic, often filled with proteinaceous fluid, and are located in the sellar or suprasellar region. Unlike craniopharyngiomas, Rathke cleft cysts will not have solid or nodular enhancement (Fig. 5.19) and are often small and asymptomatic.

Other Sellar Region Masses. Spindle cell oncocytoma is a rare nonendocrine tumor (WHO Grade I) of the adenohypophysis that closely resembles a nonfunctioning macroadenoma. Pituicytoma and granular cell tumor are rare glial tumors (WHO Grade I) that arise from the neurohypophysis or infundibulum. Other neoplastic causes of a thick enhancing infundibulum include germinoma or Langerhans cell histiocytosis in a child and lymphoma or metastases in an adult. Inflammatory causes include meningitis, neurosarcoidosis, and lymphocytic hypophysitis.

TABLE 5.16

MNEMONIC FOR SUPRASELLAR MASSES ("SATCHMO")

Sarcoidosis
Adenoma, Aneurysm
Teratoma/germinoma, Tuberculosis
Craniopharyngioma, Rathke Cleft Cyst
Hypothalamic glioma, Hamartoma, Histiocytosis
Meningioma, Metastasis
Optic pathway glioma

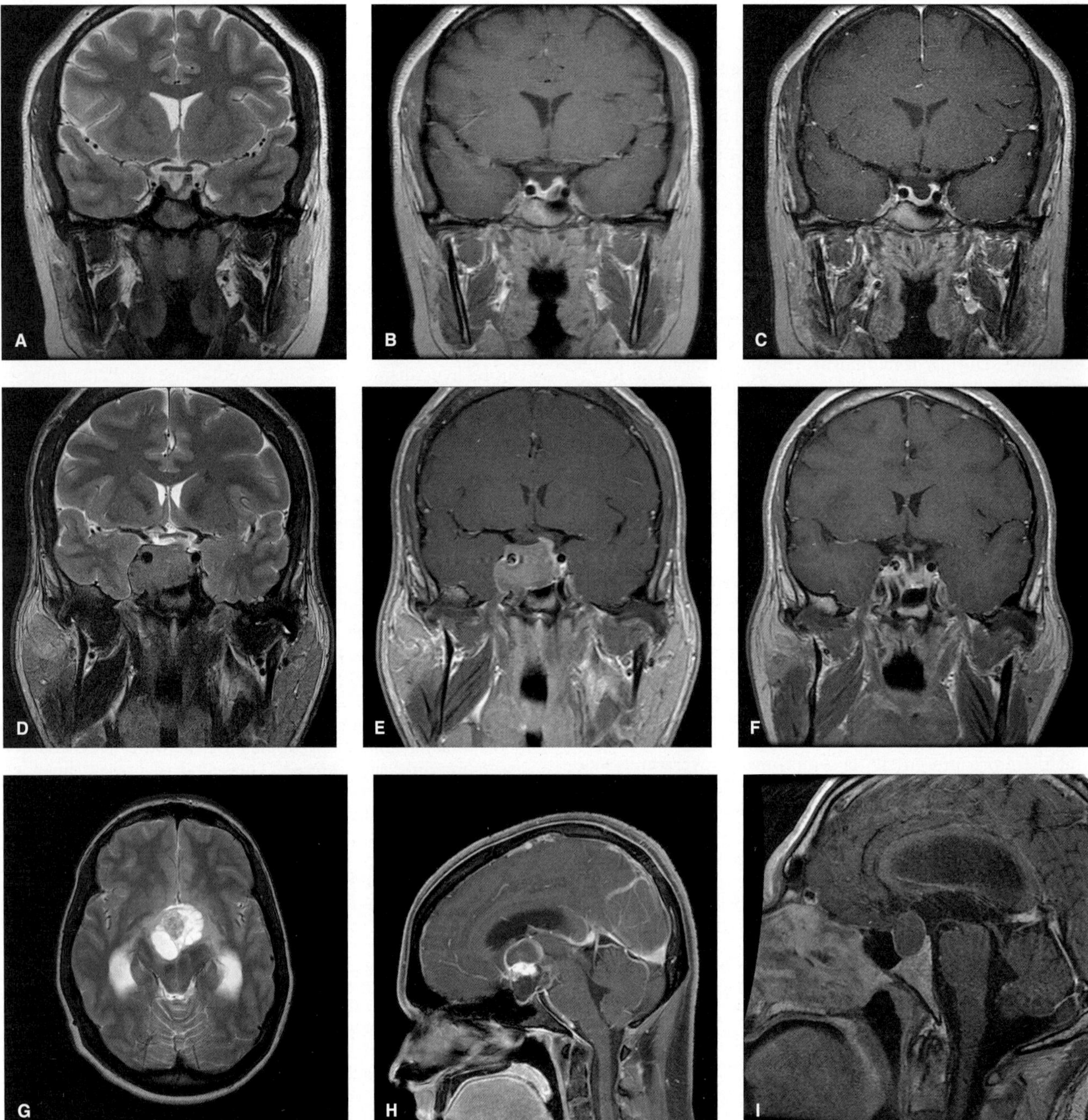

FIGURE 5.19. Three Examples of Sellar Region Tumors (Plus One Cyst). A, B: Coronal T2 and postgadolinium T1 from a young adult female with galactorrhea uncover a subcentimeter T2 hyperintense lesion in the left lateral pituitary, which enhances less avidly than the normal gland. This is a prolactin-secreting microadenoma (microprolactinoma). **C:** Follow-up postgadolinium T1 confirms interval regression of the microadenoma after medical therapy with cabergoline. **D, E:** Coronal T2 and postgadolinium T1 from a young adult male with acromegaly demonstrate a large enhancing T2 hypointense mass that is centered in the right sella turcica and involves the right cavernous sinus. This growth hormone-secreting macroadenoma displaces the more avidly enhancing residual pituitary gland/stalk to the left. **F:** Follow-up postgadolinium T1 after surgical therapy (transsphenoidal resection) depicts a very small amount of residual tumor on the right. **G, H:** Axial T2 and sagittal postgadolinium T1 from a different young adult patient show a mixed cystic-solid enhancing mass that is centered in the suprasellar cistern and causing obstructive hydrocephalus. This is a classic imaging pattern for craniopharyngioma, specifically the adamantinomatous type. **I:** Sagittal postgadolinium T1 from a different patient shows another lesion that can arise from the embryonic craniopharyngeal duct. Unlike the craniopharyngioma, a Rathke cleft cyst is developmental not neoplastic and has no solid enhancement.

Masses of Developmental Origin

All entities in this final section are congenital or developmental, not neoplastic, but are included because they can cause mass effect and may be mistaken for a tumor by the untrained eye/brain. None of the following should demonstrate any solid or nodular enhancement.

Arachnoid Cysts. These thin-walled meningothelial cysts are located in the subarachnoid space and are thought to result from a congenital duplication or splitting of the embryonic arachnoid

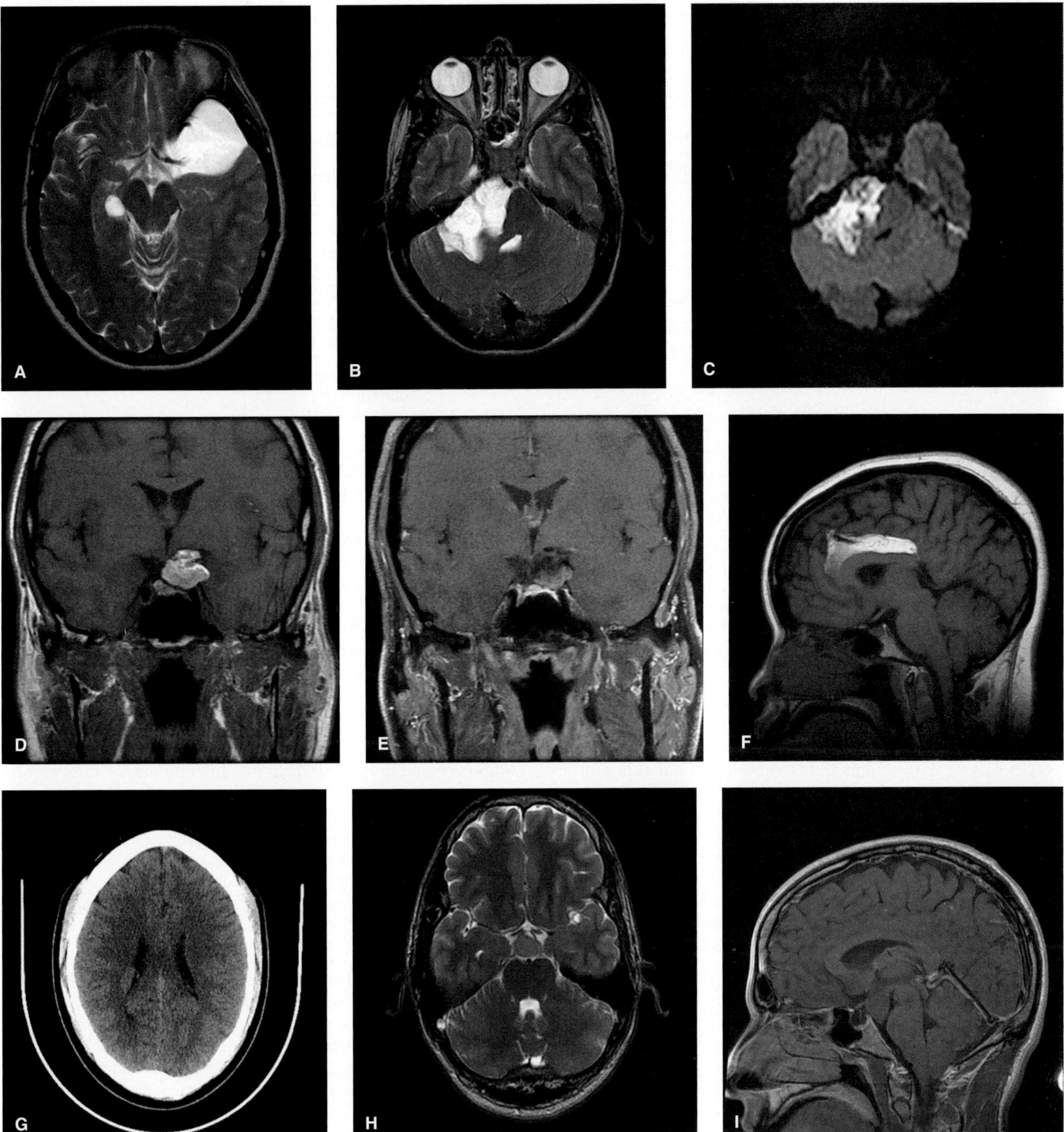

FIGURE 5.20. Six Different "Masses" of Developmental Origin (Not Tumor). A: Axial T2 from the first patient reveals two congenital arachnoid cysts. The larger is at the left middle cranial fossa; the smaller is at the right choroidal fissure; both followed CSF signal on all sequences. **B, C:** Axial T2 and DWI from the second patient demonstrate a large epidermoid cyst in the right cerebellopontine angle (note the traversing cranial nerve V). While epidermoids may resemble a weird arachnoid cyst on some imaging, the characteristic restricted diffusion (relative to normal CSF) is very helpful in making the diagnosis. **D, E:** Coronal T1 and postgadolinium T1 with fat saturation from the third patient show a heterogeneous mass in the left suprasellar cistern with internal fat or lipid signal. This is a dermoid cyst with sebaceous contents. Note the absence of solid or nodular enhancement (not a tumor). **F:** Sagittal T1 from the fourth patient illustrates a pericallosal or interhemispheric lipoma, with a more homogeneous appearance than the previous dermoid cyst. The corpus callosum is mildly hypoplastic (absent splenium). Intracranial lipomas can also occur in the basal cisterns and arise from maldevelopment of the primitive meninges. **G:** Head CT from the fifth patient depicts periventricular or subependymal gray matter heterotopia on the right side. It also followed gray matter signal on subsequent brain MRI (not shown). **H, I:** Axial T2 and sagittal postgadolinium T1 from the sixth patient reveal an exophytic mass at the tuber cinereum of the hypothalamus, which follows gray matter in signal and does not enhance. This is an example of a hypothalamic hamartoma, which is not a neoplasm/tumor.

TABLE 5.17

EPIDERMOID VERSUS DERMOID "TUMORS"

	■ EPIDERMOID	■ DERMOID
Frequency	More common	Less common
Etiology	Ectodermal inclusion cyst	Ectodermal inclusion cyst
Radiology	May resemble CSF in density and signal, except for marked hyperintensity on DWI	Look for internal fat density and signal due to sebum, no solid enhancement
Surgery	"Pearly tumor" due to keratin	Accidental rupture or spillage of the cyst contents can cause chemical meningitis
Pathology	Similar to epidermis (keratinized stratified squamous epithelium)	Epidermoid + dermal adnexa (e.g., sebaceous glands, sweat glands, hair follicles)

during development. Rarely, secondary or acquired arachnoid cysts can also develop as chronic sequelae of prior inflammation (e.g., meningitis, hemorrhage). Arachnoid cysts will follow CSF density or signal on CT and MRI, including DWI (i.e., free diffusion of water molecules). Approximately 50% are seen in the middle cranial fossa, where they may be quite large (Fig. 5.20). Other sites include the cerebral convexities, the basal cisterns, and the posterior fossa. Note that an enlarged retrocerebellar CSF space is often called a mega cisterna magna, unless there is mass effect on the cerebellum and fourth ventricle.

Epidermoid and Dermoid Cysts. During closure of the embryonic neural tube, which is formed from neuroectoderm, the abnormal inclusion of surface or external ectoderm can produce cysts with linings that resemble normal skin epithelium. Epidermoids account for roughly 1% of all intracranial masses and usually present in adulthood (peak age ~40 years); dermoids are much less common and present earlier in life (peak age ~20 years). Both are benign, characterized by slow growth, and lined by squamous epithelium that produces large amounts of keratin. The key histologic distinction between epidermoid and dermoid is that the latter contains skin adnexa or appendages, such as hair follicles and sweat/sebaceous glands (Table 5.17).

Imaging Patterns. There is a tendency for epidermoids to be more lateral (e.g., CPA) and for dermoids to be more midline (e.g., suprasellar cistern), although there is overlap in their presenting locations. The more significant difference is their contents. The imaging pattern of an epidermoid is a lobulated cyst that closely, but not perfectly, resembles CSF density on CT and CSF signal on T1- and T2-weighted images. DWI is the best way to identify and differentiate an epidermoid from a weird arachnoid cyst. Epidermoids are hyperintense on DWI, unlike CSF, and ADC maps will show restricted diffusion relative to CSF (Fig. 5.20). Rarely, epidermoids can be highly proteinaceous and demonstrate an atypical appearance on CT (hyperdense) or MRI (T1 hyperintense); this atypical presentation is called a "white epidermoid."

While dermoids contain keratinous and squamous debris like epidermoids, they also have greasy contents, courtesy of the pilosebaceous units (hair follicle + sebaceous gland). This oily sebum is not true adipose tissue, but follows fat density or signal on CT and MRI (Fig. 5.20), including fat saturation. These are nonneoplastic inclusion cysts and should not demonstrate any solid or nodular enhancement. Dermoids may rupture into the subarachnoid space, producing an aseptic or chemical meningitis, with multiple fatty-type droplets (sebum) on imaging.

Colloid Cyst. Colloid cysts are endodermal inclusion cysts, whose lining resembles bronchial or respiratory epithelium, hence they are filled with mucin and are highly proteinaceous. They are found at the anterosuperior roof of the third ventricle near the foramen of Monro, where they can cause acute hydrocephalus and sudden death. They can also present chronically with paroxysmal headaches and/or neurologic deficits, exacerbated by tilting the head forward (Brun phenomenon), due to ball-valve action of the cyst. The classic imaging pattern is a round hyperdense lesion at the anterior third ventricle near the foramen of Monro on noncontrast CT, with variable signal intensity on T1/T2, depending on level of protein content.

Lipoma. Intracranial lipomas are nonneoplastic masses of true adipose tissue that result from maldifferentiation of the embryonic *meninx primitiva* into fat rather than normal subarachnoid space. They are most common in the interhemispheric fissure (possibly associated with callosal dysgenesis), suprasellar cistern, and quadrigeminal cistern. They are usually asymptomatic with normal traversing blood vessels and cranial nerves; these are not surgical lesions. Lipomas will be entirely composed of fat density or signal, unlike dermoids and teratomas (Fig. 5.20).

Hamartoma of the Tuber Cinereum. Gray matter heterotopia (Greek for "other place") is ectopic nodules of misplaced neurons due to arrested migration during development (Fig. 5.20). These clumps can be mistaken for tumor and are most often found in a periventricular or subependymal location. The abnormal heterotopic gray matter may be asymptomatic or epileptogenic; it should closely follow normal gray matter density or signal on CT and MRI, with possibility of slight T2 hyperintensity related to gliosis. When it occurs in the hypothalamus, usually the tuber cinereum between the optic chiasm and mammillary bodies, it is often called a hamartoma (from Greek for "tragic error"). This unusual location may present with unusual symptoms, for example, gelastic seizures (laughing fits) or precocious puberty. It may be sessile or pedunculated in morphology. It can be differentiated from a chiasmatic-hypothalamic glioma by imaging pattern; on MRI the latter will not follow gray matter signal and will usually enhance (pilocytic astrocytoma).

Suggested Readings

Barajas RF Jr, Cha S. Metastasis in adult brain tumors. *Neuroimaging Clin N Am* 2016;26(4):601–620.

Brandão LA, Poussaint TY. Pediatric brain tumors. *Neuroimaging Clin N Am* 2013;23(3):499–525.

Castillo M. History and evolution of brain tumor imaging: insights through radiology. *Radiology* 2014;273(2 Suppl):S111–S125.
Cha S. Update on brain tumor imaging: from anatomy to physiology. *AJNR Am J Neuroradiol* 2006;27(3):475–487.
Clarke JL, Chang S. Pseudoprogression and pseudoresponse: challenges in brain tumor imaging. *Curr Neurol Neurosci Rep* 2009;9(3):241–246.
Dalesandro MF, Andre JB. Posttreatment evaluation of brain gliomas. *Neuroimaging Clin N Am* 2016;26(4):581–599.
Drake-Pérez M, Smirniotopoulos JG. Extraparenchymal lesions in adults. *Neuroimaging Clin N Am* 2016;26(4):621–646.
Ferguson S, Lesniak MS. Percival Bailey and the classification of brain tumors. *Neurosurg Focus* 2005;18(4):e7.
Given CA 2nd, Stevens BS, Lee C. The MRI appearance of tumefactive demyelinating lesions. *AJR Am J Roentgenol* 2004;182(1):195–199.
Johnson DR, Diehn FE, Giannini C, et al. Genetically defined oligodendroglioma is characterized by indistinct tumor borders at MRI. *AJNR Am J Neuroradiol* 2017;38(4):678–684.
Johnson DR, Guerin JB, Giannini C, Morris JM, Eckel LJ, Kaufmann TJ. 2016 updates to the WHO brain tumor classification system: What the radiologist needs to know. *Radiographics* 2017;37(7):2164–2180.
Koeller KK, Henry JM. From the archives of the AFIP: superficial gliomas: radiologic-pathologic correlation. Armed Forces Institute of Pathology. *Radiographics* 2001;21(6):1533–1556.
Koeller KK, Rushing EJ. From the archives of the AFIP: pilocytic astrocytoma: radiologic-pathologic correlation. *Radiographics* 2004;24(6):1693–1708.
Koeller KK, Rushing EJ. From the archives of the AFIP: oligodendroglioma and its variants: radiologic-pathologic correlation. *Radiographics* 2005;25(6): 1669–1688.
Koeller KK, Shih RY. Extranodal lymphoma of the central nervous system and spine. *Radiol Clin North Am* 2016;54(4):649–671.
Kunschner LJ. Harvey Cushing and medulloblastoma. *Arch Neurol* 2002; 59(4):642–645.
Louis DN, Ohgaki H, Wiestler OD, et al. The 2007 WHO classification of tumours of the central nervous system. *Acta Neuropathol* 2007;114(2): 97–109.
Louis DN, Perry A, Reifenberger G, et al. The 2016 World Health Organization classification of tumors of the central nervous system: a summary. *Acta Neuropathol* 2016;131(6):803–820.
Mabray MC, Cha S. Advanced MR imaging techniques in daily practice. *Neuroimaging Clin N Am* 2016;26(4):647–666.
Mohammadzadeh A, Mohammadzadeh V, Kooraki S, et al. Pretreatment evaluation of glioma. *Neuroimaging Clin N Am* 2016;26(4):567–580.
Ostrom QT, Gittleman H, Xu J, et al. CBTRUS Statistical Report: Primary Brain and Other Central Nervous System Tumors Diagnosed in the United States in 2009–2013. *Neuro Oncol* 2016;18(suppl 5):v1–v75.
Rees JH, Smirniotopoulos JG, Jones RV, Wong K. Glioblastoma multiforme: radiologic-pathologic correlation. *Radiographics* 1996;16(6):1413–1438.
Shih RY, Koeller KK. Embryonal tumors of the central nervous system: from the radiologic pathology archives. *Radiographics* 2018;38(2):525–541.
Shih RY, Smirniotopoulos JG. Posterior fossa tumors in adult patients. *Neuroimaging Clin N Am* 2016;26(4):493–510.
Smith AB, Horkanyne-Szakaly I, Schroeder JW, Rushing EJ. From the radiologic pathology archives: mass lesions of the dura: beyond meningioma-radiologic-pathologic correlation. *Radiographics* 2014;34(2):295–312.
Smith AB, Rushing EJ, Smirniotopoulos JG. From the archives of the AFIP: lesions of the pineal region: radiologic-pathologic correlation. *Radiographics* 2010;30(7):2001–2020.
Smith AB, Smirniotopoulos JG, Horkanyne-Szakaly I. From the radiologic pathology archives: intraventricular neoplasms: radiologic-pathologic correlation. *Radiographics* 2013;33(1):21–43.

CHAPTER 6 ■ CENTRAL NERVOUS SYSTEM INFECTIONS

NATHANIEL A. CHUANG AND WALTER L. OLSEN

Neuroimaging is an important tool used in the evaluation and treatment of infections of the central nervous system (CNS). These infections frequently have dire neurologic consequences and their early diagnosis and management, with the aid of CT and MRI in particular, are crucial. Prior to the widespread availability of CT, pyogenic abscesses of the brain carried a 30% to 70% mortality rate. The mortality rate has since dropped to less than 5%, largely because of the ability of neuroimaging to accurately diagnose and localize abscesses and monitor the efficacy of appropriate interventions. MRI is usually the imaging modality of choice for CNS infections because of its improved sensitivity and specificity compared to CT. However, CT can be preferred for unstable and/or uncooperative patients because it allows much shorter imaging times and easier patient monitoring.

CONGENITAL INFECTIONS

Congenital infections of the fetal and neonatal brain are commonly referred to as the group of TORCH infections, which include: Toxoplasmosis, Other infections (such as syphilis, varicella zoster, lymphocytic choriomeningitis), Rubella, Cytomegalovirus, and Herpes simplex (and HIV). Zika virus is also now recognized as another important prenatal CNS infection. These pathogens can be transmitted transplacentally in utero or during the birth process. They often result in significant brain injury, and congenital brain malformations are more frequently seen with earlier onset of infections in utero due to disruption of the normal CNS development during fetal gestation.

Cytomegalovirus (CMV) is a member of the herpes family of viruses and the most common congenital CNS infection. In utero transmission occurs hematogenously during viral reactivation in seropositive pregnant women (CMV-seropositivity in different populations worldwide ranges between 40% and 100%) or primary infection during pregnancy. Maternal CMV infection results in transplacental transmission to the fetus in 30% to 50% of cases and symptomatic disease in 5%. Postnatal infection can occur via viral shedding in breast milk. Symptomatic neonates may have hepatosplenomegaly, jaundice, cerebral involvement (psychomotor retardation), chorioretinitis, and deafness. The virus preferentially multiplies along the ependyma and germinal matrix resulting in a periventricular pattern of injury and development of dystrophic calcifications. Obstetrical and neonatal cranial US can demonstrate hypoechoic periventricular ring-like zones and the subsequent characteristic hyperechoic periventricular calcifications. CT without contrast best depicts these periventricular calcifications (Fig. 6.1). There are usually no calcifications of the basal ganglia or cortex, as is seen in congenital toxoplasmosis. Loss of periventricular white matter results in cysts, ventriculomegaly, and microcephaly. Infections during the first trimester can result in neuronal migrational anomalies such as heterotopia and lissencephaly and disorders of cortical organization, including schizencephaly, polymicrogyria, and cortical dysplasia, all of which are better shown by MRI. Delayed myelination and cerebellar hypoplasia are also common findings. CNS malformations are less common in patients infected later during gestation but delayed myelination and periventricular white matter lesions are still seen.

Toxoplasmosis follows CMV in frequency among congenital CNS infections and is caused by the parasitic protozoan *Toxoplasma gondii,* which occurs worldwide. Congenital infection results from hematogenous spread after a pregnant woman eats undercooked meat or is exposed to cat feces, both of which can harbor viable oocysts. A necrotizing encephalitis of the fetal brain ensues which can cause severe destruction, especially during the first two trimesters of gestation, but typically no developmental malformations. The infant is usually born with microcephaly, chorioretinitis, and mental retardation. Imaging studies reveal atrophy, dilated ventricles, and dystrophic calcifications (Fig. 6.2). The calcifications are scattered in the white matter, basal ganglia, and cortex. This is in distinction to the primarily periventricular calcifications observed in congenital CMV infection.

Lymphocytic choriomeningitis virus (LCMV) is a rodent-borne arenavirus which can closely mimic toxoplasmosis and CMV on neonatal neuroimaging. Onset of infection in the first trimester often leads to spontaneous abortion. Otherwise, typical clinical presentation at birth includes chorioretinitis

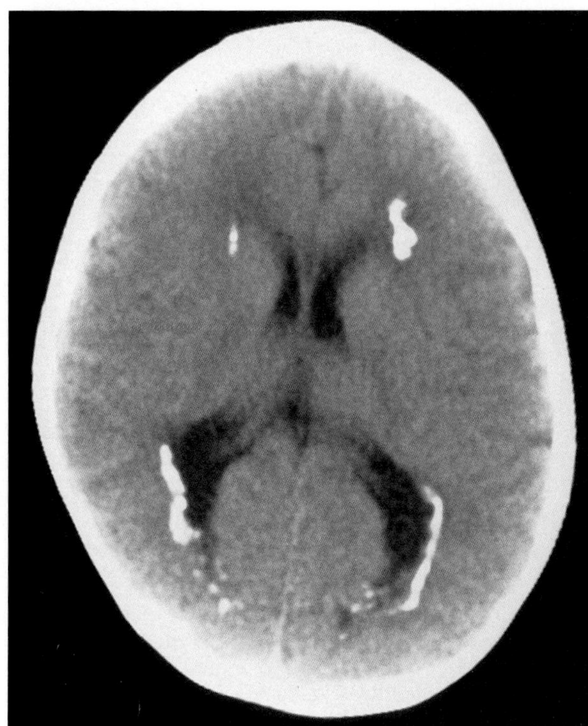

FIGURE 6.1. **Congenital Cytomegalovirus (CMV) Infection.** Nonenhanced CT (NECT) image shows multiple periventricular hyperdense calcifications. The calcifications in congenital CMV infection tend to be periventricular only, as in this case. With congenital toxoplasmosis, calcifications may be found throughout the brain.

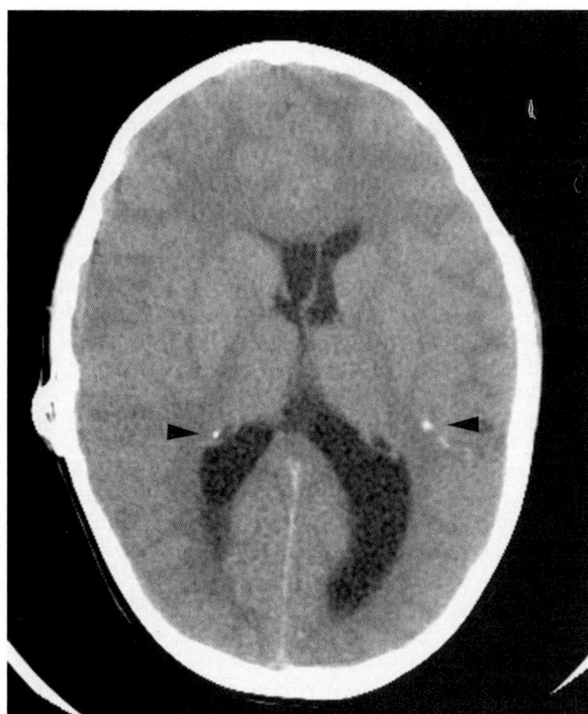

FIGURE 6.2. **Congenital Toxoplasmosis.** NECT image shows hyperdense calcifications at the gray–white matter junction of the left cerebral hemisphere and along the right periventricular region (*arrowheads*). The patient also has ventriculomegaly due to chronic hydrocephalus with a ventriculoperitoneal shunt (not shown).

and either hydrocephalus or microcephaly but with results of accompanying microbiologic and serologic studies being negative for more common congenital pathogens. When present on CT or MRI, cerebral calcifications can be periventricular in location and/or distributed between the white matter, deep gray nuclei, and cortex. White matter volume loss with hypodensity on CT or T2 hyperintensity on MRI may coexist with ventriculomegaly.

Herpes simplex (HSV) encephalitis in neonates most often results from infection during descent through the birth canal when the mother has a genital infection with herpes virus, type 2. Occasionally, there is transplacental transmission before delivery, but this usually results in spontaneous abortion. CNS infection causes a diffuse encephalitis with infarction which is either fatal or has severe neurologic consequences. The infant typically presents with a fever, rash, lethargy, and seizures in the first several weeks of life. CSF analysis reveals pleocytosis, increased protein, and decreased glucose. If the patient survives, varying degrees of microcephaly, mental retardation, microphthalmia, enlarged ventricles, intracranial calcifications, and multicystic encephalomalacia may occur. Early in the course of the encephalitis, cranial US will show areas of increased parenchymal echogenicity. CT may demonstrate diffuse brain swelling or bilateral patchy areas of hypodensity in the cerebral white matter and cortex, with relative sparing of the basal ganglia, thalami, and posterior fossa structures (Fig. 6.3A). These hypodense lesions correspond to areas of T2 hyperintensity on MRI and progress to areas of necrosis and cystic encephalomalacia. Associated hemorrhage, calcifications, and meningeal and patchy parenchymal enhancement can be seen with both CT and MRI (Fig. 6.3B).

Congenital HIV. Infection with human immunodeficiency virus (HIV) can occur transplacentally during childbirth and postnatally via breast feeding. Affected infants are more susceptible to respiratory infections and diarrhea and can present with encephalopathy, developmental delay, and failure to thrive. The opportunistic infections and neoplasms seen in adults with acquired immunodeficiency syndrome (AIDS) are not usually observed in young children. HIV encephalitis primarily affects white matter and basal ganglia resulting in diffuse cerebral volume loss. Symmetric calcifications in the basal ganglia, especially the globi pallidi, are best seen with CT, while MRI allows better demonstration of T2-hyperintense white matter abnormalities. Subtle enhancement of the basal ganglia can occasionally be detected. In some cases, MR angiography (MRA) may reveal an associated vasculopathy with fusiform dilation and ectasia of the intracranial arteries.

Rubella was once a devastating fetal viral infection but is now very uncommon because of widespread immunization of females before child-bearing age. Transplacental transmission takes place during maternal infection with the worst consequences arising from first trimester infections causing diffuse meningoencephalitis, brain infarction, and necrosis. Infants who survive severe infections present with microcephaly, ocular abnormalities, and deafness. CT reveals dystrophic calcifications in the deep gray nuclei and cortex (Fig. 6.4), whereas MRI better demonstrates infarcts, white matter volume loss, and occasionally, delayed myelination.

Zika virus (ZIKV) is a flavivirus which originated in Africa and Southeast Asia and is transmitted by several species of mosquitoes, especially *Aedes aegypti*. Outbreaks in recent years in the Pacific islands and the Americas, particularly in northeastern Brazil, have been associated with markedly elevated incidence of congenital microcephaly and CNS malformations. However, ZIKV infections have been confirmed in infants with CNS malformations both with and without microcephaly. The virus has been isolated from fetal brain

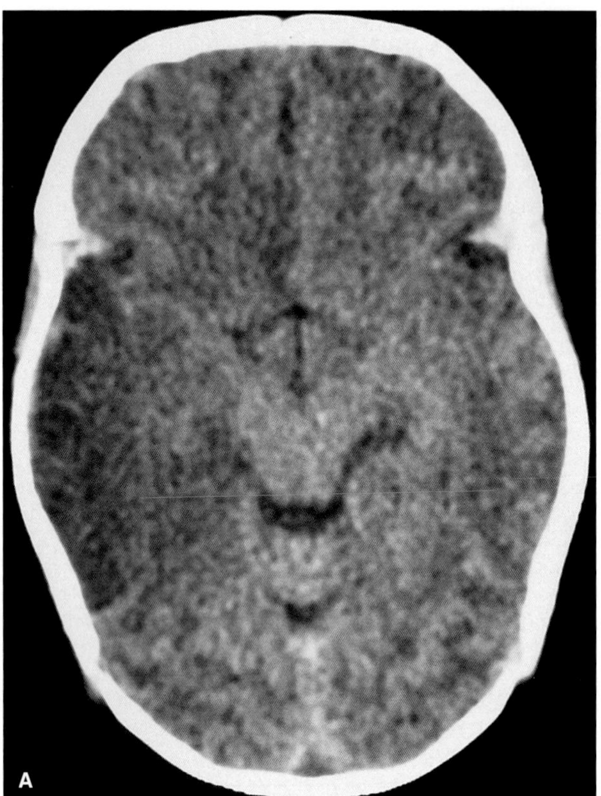

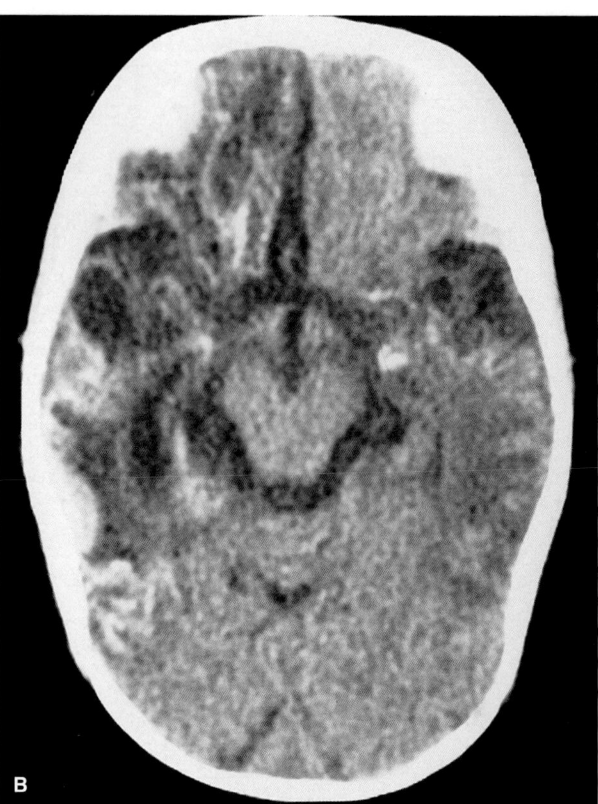

FIGURE 6.3. Neonatal Herpes Encephalitis. A: NECT of a 2-week-old child with acute herpes simplex, type 2, encephalitis shows hypodense swelling in the right temporal lobe and, to a lesser extent, in the frontal and left temporal lobes. **B:** Three weeks later, NECT scan on this same infant reveals multiple areas of cystic encephalomalacia and widespread gray matter calcification, which are typical of late-stage neonatal herpes infection.

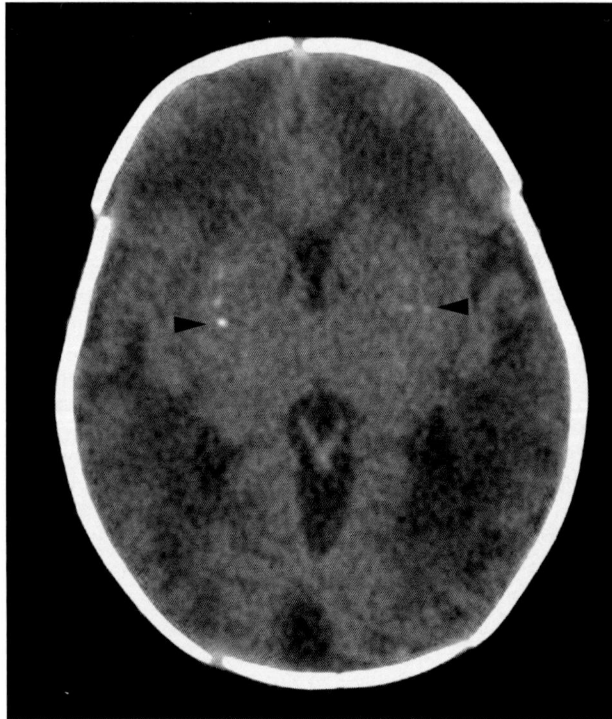

FIGURE 6.4. Congenital Rubella. NECT image in this neonate demonstrates multiple punctate hyperdense calcifications in the bilateral basal ganglia (*arrowheads*) and hypodense white matter.

tissue but unlike CMV does not appear to have a predilection for the germinal matrix. ZIKV impairs cell proliferation and promotes apoptosis and cell death. CT best demonstrates both punctate or linear calcifications which localize predominantly to the gray–white junction in the frontal and parietal lobes and, to a lesser extent, along the deep gray nuclei and periventricular zone. Other typical neuroimaging features are best seen on MRI and can overlap with congenital CMV infection and include brain volume loss, ventriculomegaly, abnormal myelination, callosal dysgenesis, heterotopia, lissencephaly, and polymicrogyria (Fig. 6.5). Cerebellar and brainstem hypoplasia and calcifications are rarer. In patients with severe microcephaly, calvarial deformities such as overriding bones and pointed occiput are frequently present. Serial fetal US after 18 to 20 weeks of gestational age and screening for fetal microcephaly and CNS malformations and calcifications can be considered in pregnant women with suspected Zika virus infection. Fetal MRI can be well utilized to demonstrate complex CNS malformations initially detected by US.

EXTRA-AXIAL INFECTIONS

Subdural and Epidural Infections

Extra-axial pyogenic infections can involve the epidural or subdural spaces. Both epidural and subdural abscesses or empyemas may result from paranasal sinusitis, otomastoiditis, orbital infections, penetrating injuries, surgery, or superinfection of pre-existing extra-axial collections. CT and MR scans show an extra-axial collection with increased density

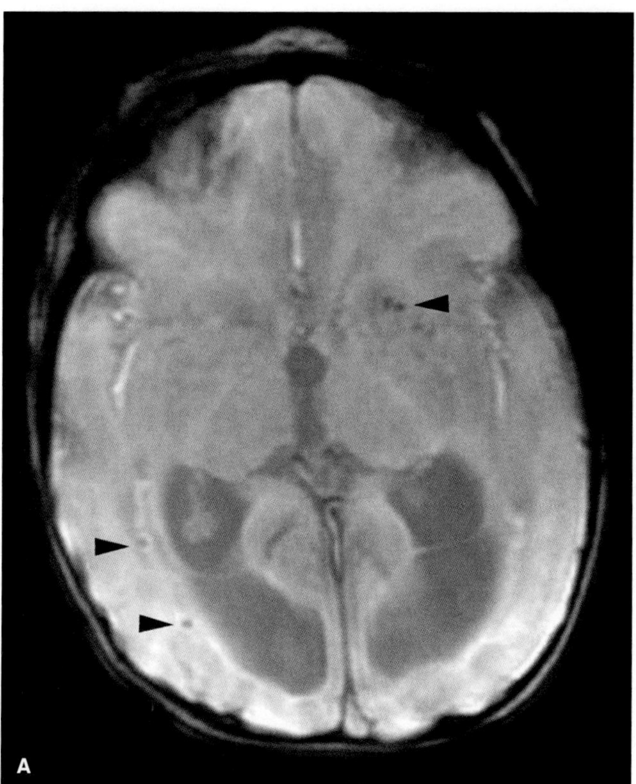

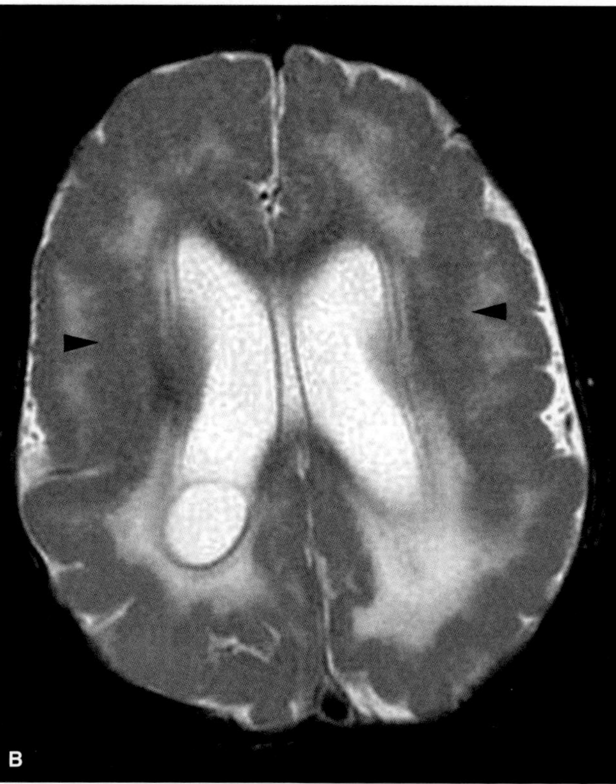

FIGURE 6.5. **Congenital Zika Infection. A:** Transaxial susceptibility weighted image (SWI) in this 8-month-old infant with microcephaly and spasticity demonstrates multiple small, punctate hypointense calcifications along the left basal ganglia and right periventricular region (*black arrowheads*). **B:** T2WI shows diffusely simplified gyral pattern with thick and irregular cortex, consistent with extensive pachygyria and polymicrogyria. Bilateral anterior periventricular and subcortical heterotopia are present (*black arrowheads*). Note the abnormal T2-hyperintense white matter and right posterior subependymal cyst.

(Fig. 6.6) or increased T1 and T2 signal intensity compared to CSF. The margins of the collection usually enhance smoothly with contrast. MRI is more sensitive than CT for both epidural and subdural empyemas because the multiplanar capability of MRI alleviates the problem of partial volume averaging with the calvarium on CT. Cranial US in infants can demonstrate heterogeneous echogenic extra-axial collections and hyperechoic material in the subarachnoid space if the child also has meningitis. Epidural empyemas are generally confined by dural attachments which prevent rapid expansion of epidural abscesses and account for their lentiform shape and convex inner margins. However, subdural empyemas can spread more easily through the subdural space and be more acutely life threatening (Fig. 6.7A,B), thus requiring rapid neurosurgical intervention. Subjacent cerebritis may develop with both entities. Cortical venous thrombosis resulting in venous infarcts is a common result of these infections, and MRI and MR venography (MRV) allow easier detection of venous thrombosis and venous infarcts. Evaluation for adjacent sinusitis or skull abnormalities is also required. Frontal sinusitis in children can be complicated by osteomyelitis, with subperiosteal, epidural, or subdural abscesses. This is referred to as Pott puffy tumor. Subdural empyemas can be hyperintense on diffusion-weighted imaging (DWI), allowing them to be distinguished from subdural effusions (Fig. 6.7C) which can also enhance mildly. Subdural hygromas are identical to CSF in density and signal intensity and do not enhance.

Mild, smooth dural or meningeal enhancement may be seen after craniotomies and in patients with ventriculostomy catheters, especially with MRI (Fig. 6.8). This enhancement can persist for years and should be considered benign in this clinical setting. It most likely reflects a chemical meningitis

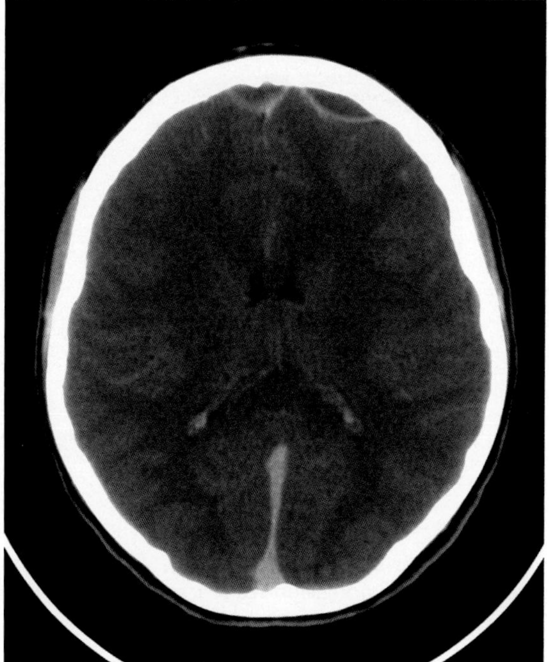

FIGURE 6.6. **Epidural Abscess.** Contrast-enhanced CT (CECT) image in a 13-year-old child presenting with frontal sinusitis and headaches. There are two adjacent anterior frontal lentiform-shaped epidural collections of intermediate-density pus. One of the collections extends across the midline, anterior to the falx. The inner margins of both collections enhance smoothly.

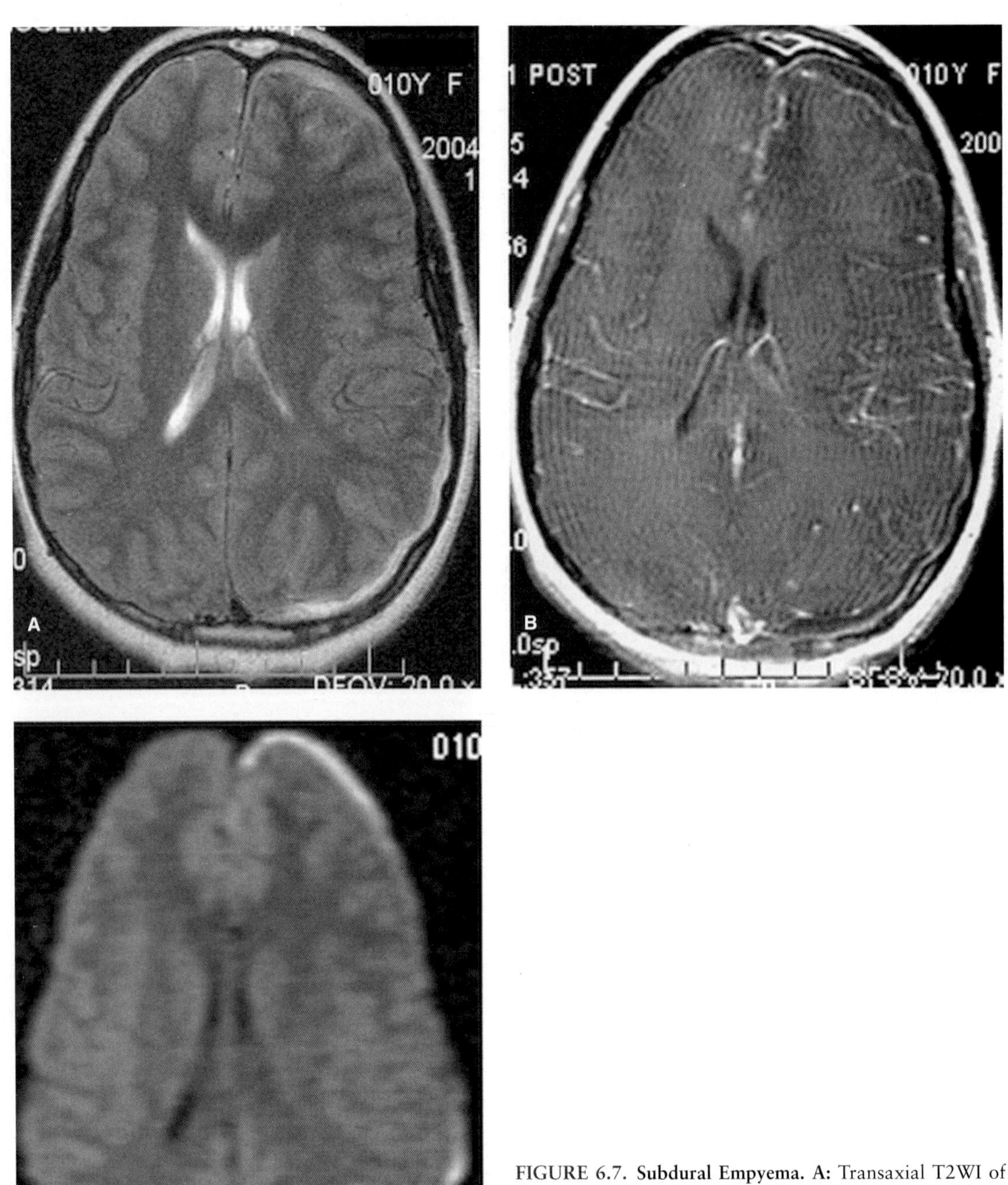

FIGURE 6.7. **Subdural Empyema. A:** Transaxial T2WI of this 8-year-old child shows a thin, hyperintense subdural fluid collection along the left cerebral hemisphere with mass effect. **B:** Contrast-enhanced T1WI shows hypointense left subdural fluid with dural enhancement. **C:** Diffusion-weighted imaging (DWI) shows increased signal intensity of the fluid, indicating an empyema, and not a sterile subdural effusion, which would be hypointense on this sequence.

resulting from perioperative hemorrhage and/or dural scarring. Intracranial hypotension from a spontaneous or iatrogenic CSF leak (including recent lumbar puncture) can also result in smooth symmetric dural enhancement, both intracranially and along the spinal canal.

Meningitis

Meningitis can be caused by bacteria, mycobacteria, fungi, parasites, and viruses. Bacterial meningitis is caused by *Haemophilus influenzae* (in children), *Neisseria meningitidis* (in teens and young adults), and *Streptococcus pneumoniae* (in older adults) in over 80% of cases. Group B streptococcus and *Escherichia coli* meningitis occurs in neonates, while Citrobacter meningitis is seen commonly in premature newborns. The bacteria most commonly enter the meninges during systemic bacteremia but can spread directly from infected sinuses or after surgery or trauma. Patients present with a relatively acute onset of fever, neck stiffness, irritability, and headache, followed by a decline in mental status. CSF studies are usually diagnostic and CT scans performed in the emergency setting

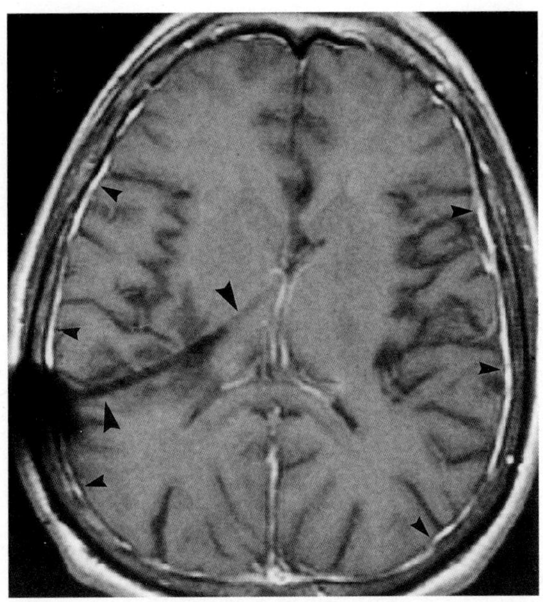

FIGURE 6.8. **Benign Postoperative Meningeal Enhancement.** Several years after brain surgery, contrast-enhanced T1WI reveals smooth but definitely abnormal enhancement of the dura (*small arrowheads*). There were no signs of infection or tumor recurrence. A ventricular shunt tube is seen on the right side (*large arrowheads*).

are frequently normal (Fig 6.9A). The inflammatory exudate caused by the meningitis may produce high density on CT and hyperintensity on FLAIR MR sequences within the subarachnoid spaces and ventricles. Other differential diagnostic considerations include ruptured aneurysm with subarachnoid hemorrhage, leptomeningeal metastases, neurosarcoidosis, and lymphoma. Diffuse cerebral edema is sometimes seen (Fig. 6.9B). If contrast is given, meningeal enhancement can range from being absent or subtle to very thick and extensive.

Neuroimaging is perhaps used more importantly later in the course of meningitis when there are suspected complications such as hydrocephalus, cerebritis or abscess (to be discussed later), arterial or venous infarction, subdural effusion or empyema, and herniation. Communicating hydrocephalus is more typical than the noncommunicating type and reflects impaired CSF resorption by arachnoid granulations. Assessment of arterial and venous infarction with MRI can be done with a combination of diffusion-weighted imaging, MRA, and MRV. Contrast-enhanced CT angiography (CTA) and CT venography (CTV) are also helpful but are associated with increased radiation exposure. Subdural effusions may be seen in infants, especially with *H. influenzae* meningitis. Subdural effusions appear as thin collections along the surface of the brain that are isodense on CT and isointense with CSF on MRI (Fig. 6.10) and may show mild enhancement with contrast agents. These sterile effusions can also be identified with cranial sonography in infants. Echogenic sulci, ventriculomegaly, and abnormal parenchymal echogenicity are visualized by US in infants with bacterial meningitis (Fig. 6.9C).

Tuberculous meningitis is the most common form of CNS tuberculosis. It is usually caused by *Mycobacterium tuberculosis*, but atypical mycobacteria such as *Mycobacterium avium-intracellulare* can rarely be causative. Tuberculous (TB) meningitis occurs in all age groups but particularly in children and the elderly. AIDS patients, prisoners, and immigrants from regions with endemic TB are also affected disproportionately. Approximately 5% to 10% of patients with tuberculosis develop CNS disease. The disease spreads to the meninges hematogenously from the lungs, but the chest radiograph is normal in 40% to 75% of patients. The tuberculin skin test can be deceivingly negative. Clinically, there is usually a subacute or insidious onset of headache, malaise, weakness, apathy, or focal neurologic findings. CSF should demonstrate pleocytosis, elevated protein, and markedly reduced glucose levels. Mycobacterial cultures of CSF may be negative or take weeks to confirm an infection, and polymerase chain reaction (PCR) studies may be more sensitive. Imaging studies will show thickened and enhancing meninges, especially along the basal cisterns (Fig. 6.11), corresponding to a thick gelatinous inflammatory exudate. In contrast, meningeal enhancement in bacterial meningitis is usually more peripherally distributed and less thick when compared to tuberculous and other granulomatous meningitides. The differential diagnosis of tuberculous meningitis includes fungal meningitis, racemose cysticercosis, neurosarcoidosis, and carcinomatous meningitis.

TB meningitis can present with concomitant infection of the brain parenchyma in a miliary pattern or with larger tuberculomas or abscesses, which will be discussed in more detail later. Frequent complications include hydrocephalus or infarcts. The inflammatory exudate in the basal cisterns may extend along perivascular spaces causing an arteritis with irregular narrowing or occlusion of vessels, and infarcts occur most commonly along the distribution of the lenticulostriate and thalamoperforating arteries and in the deep gray nuclei. MRA can be helpful.

Fungal meningitis usually causes thick meningeal enhancement in the basal cisterns, in a similar fashion to tuberculosis (Fig. 6.12). However, in cases of cryptococcal meningitis, the degree of enhancement varies with the immunocompetence of the patient. Hydrocephalus is common but infarcts and extension of fungal infection into the brain substance occur less often than with tuberculous or pyogenic meningitis (except in cases of aspergillosis and mucormycosis). Fungal infections of the brain parenchyma will be discussed in more detail subsequently.

Meningobasal or racemose cysticercosis occurs when the larvae of the pork tapeworm *Taenia solium* infest the subarachnoid space, especially the basal cisterns (parenchymal neurocysticercosis will be discussed later). The larval cysts may grow in grape-like clusters (Latin translation of "clusters" is "racemose") or conform to the shape of the involved cisterns. These cystic lesions are isodense on CT and isointense on MRI, to CSF (Fig. 6.13). No mural nodules (i.e., parasitic scolex) or calcifications are seen, but mural enhancement of the cysts or diffuse meningeal enhancement can be observed. Hydrocephalus is often present.

Intraventricular cysticercosis can be difficult to detect by CT and MRI since the cysts are usually isodense and isointense to CSF. Subtle signal changes (especially on proton-density weighted and fluid-attenuated inversion recovery [FLAIR] sequences) and lack of CSF pulsations within the cyst make them more visible on MRI than CT (Fig. 6.14). Enhancement may or may not be present depending on the stage of disease, similar to the parenchymal form. A mural scolex can often be seen within these cysts. Cysts may obstruct the foramen of Monro, the sylvian aqueduct, or the third and fourth ventricles, resulting in hydrocephalus. Death may result from acute hydrocephalus and ventriculitis follows cyst rupture.

Viral meningitis is caused most commonly by the enteroviruses but can be caused by mumps, Epstein–Barr virus (EBV), togaviruses, lymphocytic choriomeningitis virus, and HIV. Patients usually present with a flu-like illness, fever, headaches, and nuchal rigidity. Most patients do not require treatment and neurologic deficits are uncommon unless infection

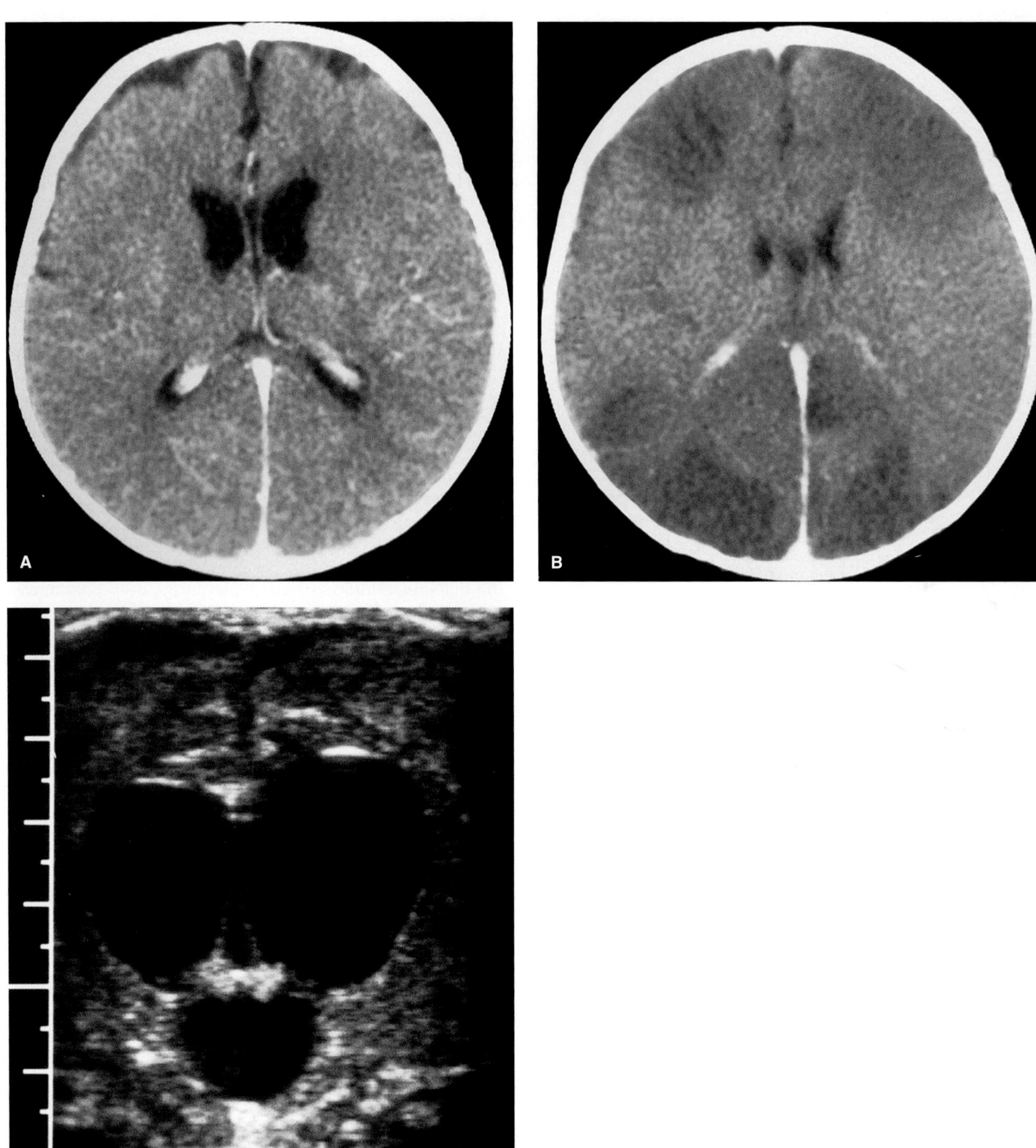

FIGURE 6.9. **Bacterial Meningitis.** **A:** Initial CECT scan on this 3-month-old boy is normal. **B:** CECT scan obtained 1 day later shows marked brain swelling with focal areas of low density representing edema or ischemia in the frontal and occipital lobes. **C:** One month later, an intracranial US shows ventriculomegaly from marked cortical atrophy resulting from widespread cortical destruction.

progresses to encephalitis. Neuroimaging studies are typically normal but mild meningeal enhancement can occur.

Sarcoidosis is a noninfectious granulomatous disease of unclear etiology which involves the CNS in up to 14% of patients at autopsy. Only a minority of cases present with neurologic signs or symptoms such as headaches, cranial neuropathies, pituitary dysfunction, seizures, or other focal neurologic deficits. Aside from biopsy, confirming increased serum and CSF levels of angiotensin-converting enzyme (ACE) and pulmonary involvement are helpful for diagnosis. Neurosarcoidosis primarily affects the leptomeninges, and abnormal

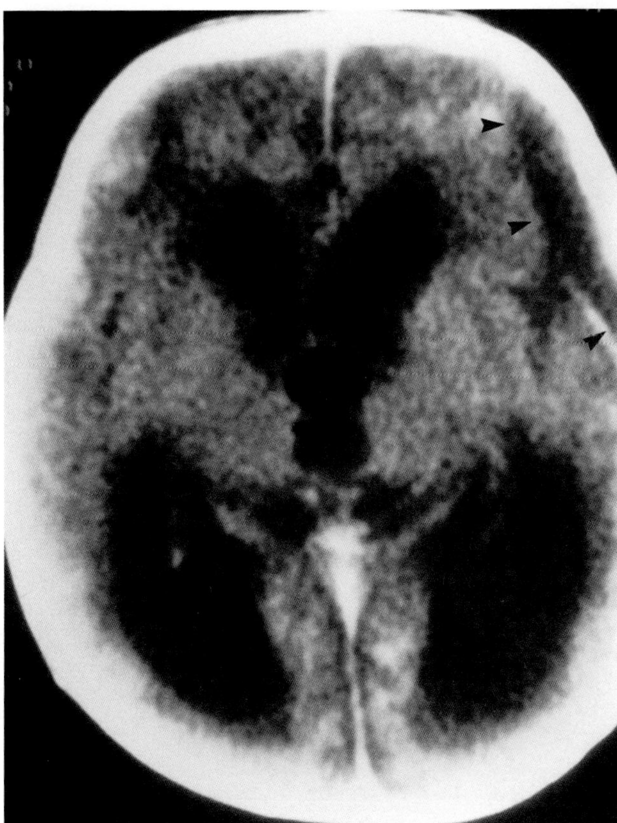

FIGURE 6.10. **Subdural Effusion.** CECT image of this 6 years old with *Haemophilus influenzae* meningitis reveals a subdural collection nearly isodense with CSF (*arrowheads*). Subdural effusions are common with *H. influenzae* meningitis. There is also enlargement of the lateral and third ventricles due to communicating hydrocephalus, which is a common complication of meningitis.

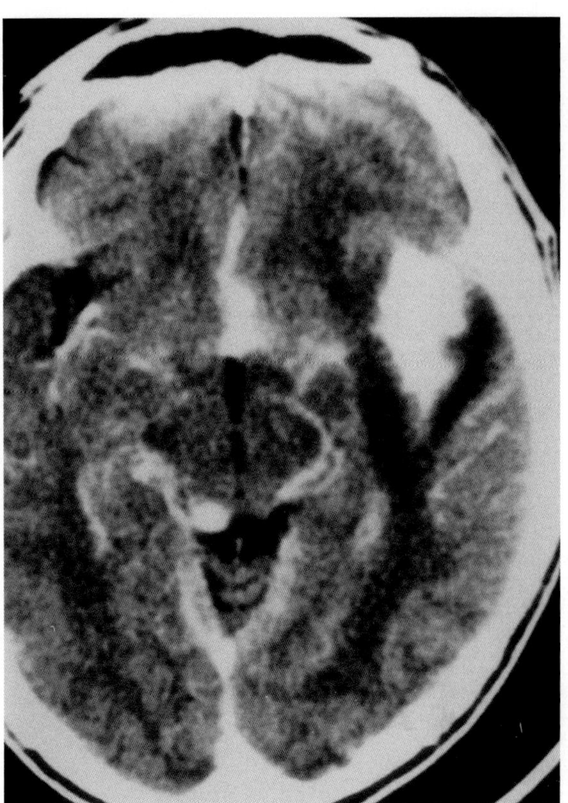

FIGURE 6.11. **Tuberculous Meningitis.** CECT image shows markedly abnormal contrast enhancement in the left sylvian fissure, interhemispheric fissure, ambient cistern, and along the tentorium. This thick, irregular enhancement in the basal cisterns is typical of a pachymeningitis such as tuberculous or fungal meningitis. CT scans in patients with bacterial meningitis are usually normal or may reveal subtle hyperdensity or enhancement in the peripheral sulci.

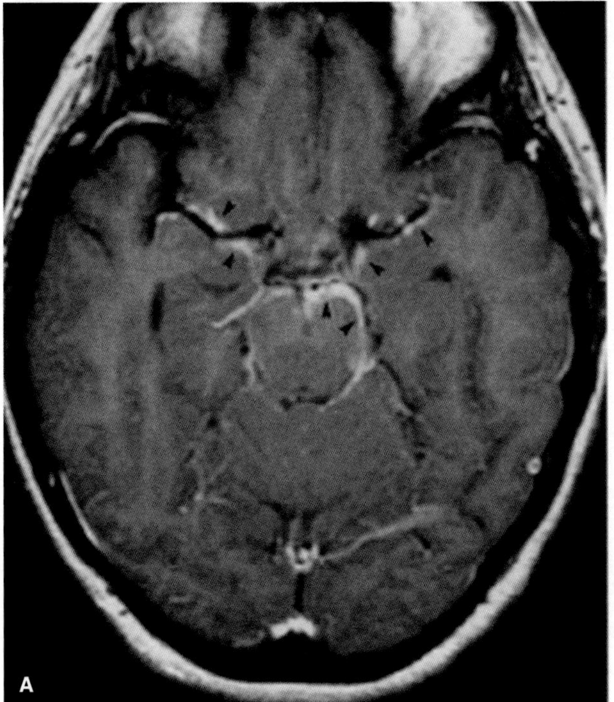

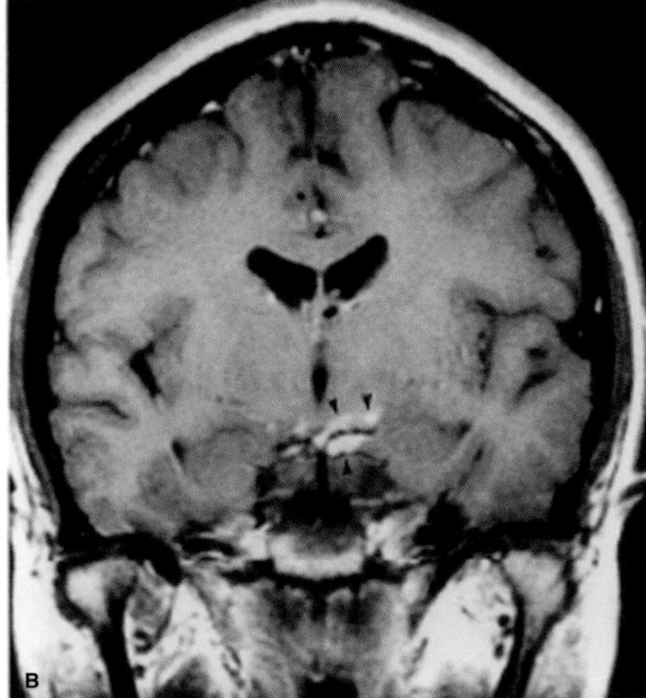

FIGURE 6.12. **Coccidioidomycosis Meningitis.** Contrast-enhanced transaxial (**A**) and coronal (**B**) T1WI reveal abnormal enhancement of the meninges in the basal cisterns (*arrowheads*).

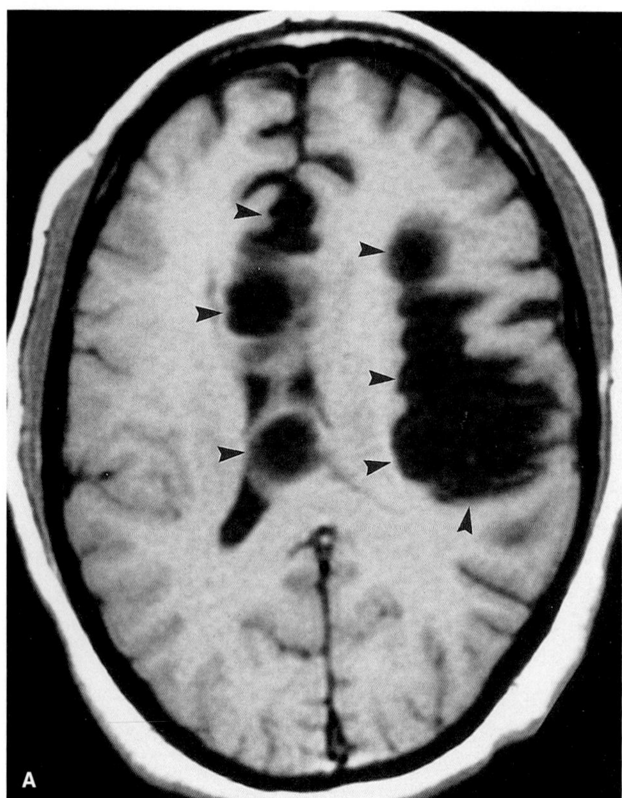

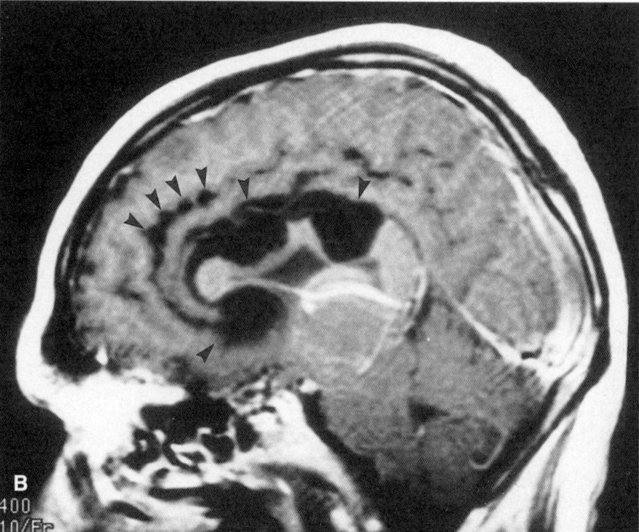

FIGURE 6.13. **Subarachnoid (Racemose) Cysticercosis.** Nonenhanced transaxial T1WI (**A**) and contrast-enhanced sagittal T1WI (**B**) scans show multiple nonenhancing cysts in the left sylvian fissure, callosal sulcus, and cingulate sulcus (*arrowheads*). The corpus callosum is markedly distorted by the cysts. These cysts lack a scolex but grow by proliferation of the cyst wall.

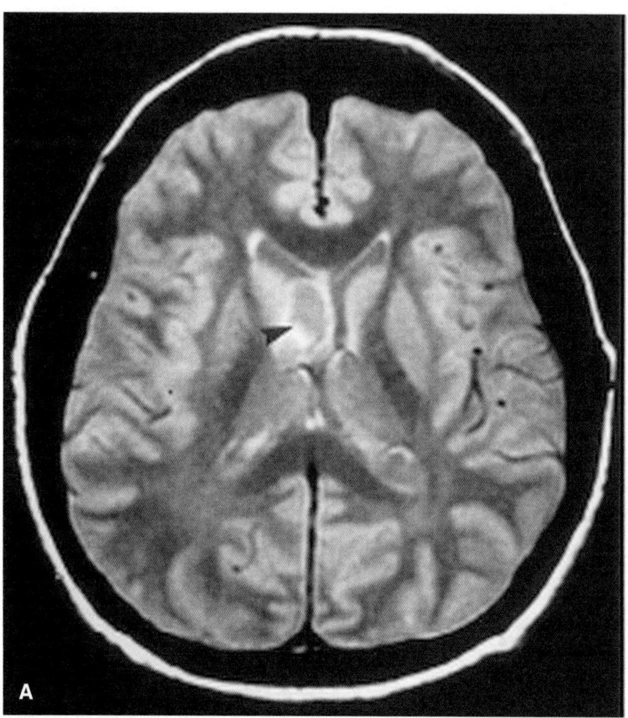

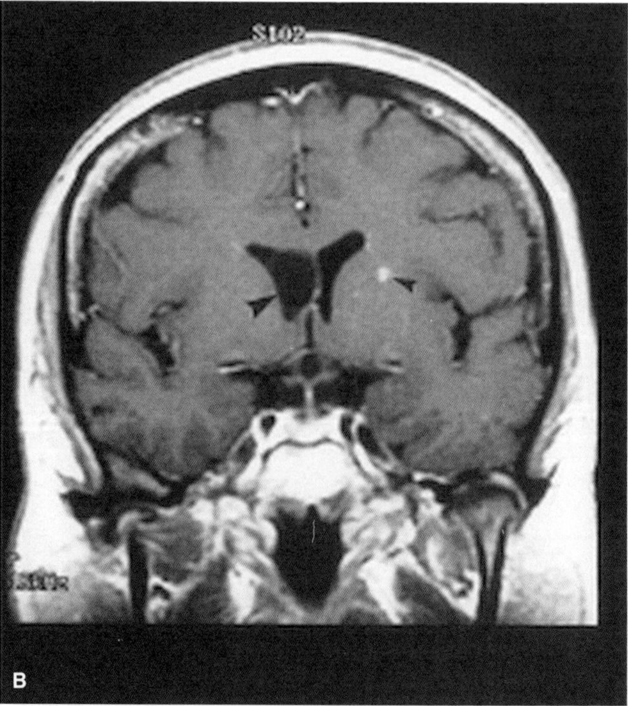

FIGURE 6.14. **Intraventricular Cysticercosis.** Transaxial proton-density weighted image (**A**) and contrast-enhanced coronal T1WI (**B**) show a cystic mass in the frontal horn of the right lateral ventricle (*large arrowheads*). The lesion is slightly hyperintense compared with CSF in the ventricle. The scolex is of high signal intensity in the posterior aspect of the cyst in (**A**). There is also a small parenchymal lesion in the left basal ganglia (*small arrowhead*).

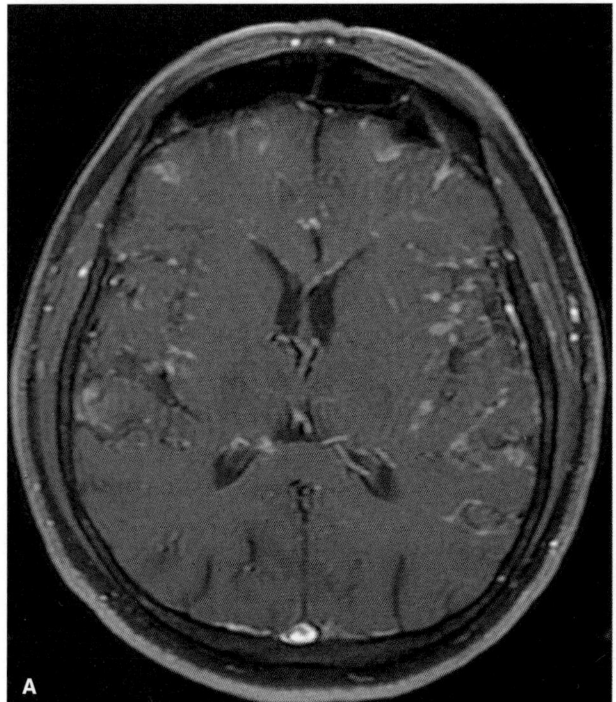

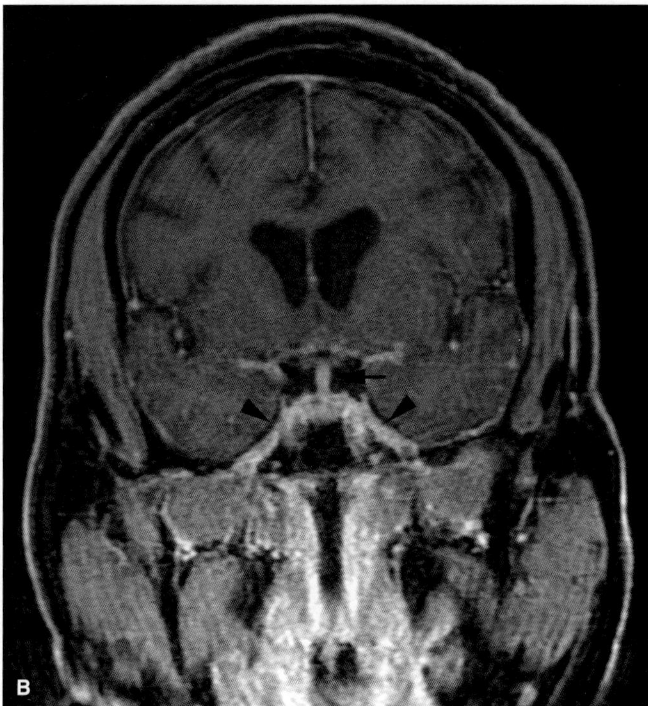

FIGURE 6.15. Neurosarcoidosis. Contrast-enhanced transaxial (**A**) and coronal (B) T1WI show extensive nodular leptomeningeal, mild ependymal, and scattered peripheral cortical enhancement. There is also prominent enhancement and thickening of the hypothalamic infundibulum (*arrow*), pituitary gland, and V2 and V3 divisions of the bilateral trigeminal nerves (*arrowheads*) on (**B**).

leptomeningeal and dural enhancement can be seen with both CT and MRI (Fig. 6.15A). Thickening and enhancement of the cranial nerves and the hypothalamic–pituitary axis are not uncommon (Fig. 6.15B). Focal enhancing intra-axial masses or nonenhancing small white matter lesions may also be present. Calcifications are not typical. Differential diagnosis includes granulomatous CNS infections, metastatic disease, Wegener granulomatosis, and Langerhans cell histiocytosis.

PARENCHYMAL INFECTIONS

Pyogenic Cerebritis and Abscess

Bacterial infections of the brain may develop by direct extension following trauma, surgery, paranasal sinusitis, otomastoiditis, or dental infections. Hematogenously spread infections occur even more frequently, especially in patients with lung infections, endocarditis, or congenital heart disease. Anaerobic bacteria are the most common organisms overall. Infection with *Staphylococcus aureus* is common after surgery or trauma. Gram-negative rod, pneumococcal, streptococcal, listerial, nocardial, and actinomycotic infections also occur with some frequency. With infections resulting from hematogenous spread, the frontal and parietal lobes (middle cerebral artery distribution) are most commonly involved, with the abscess centered at the gray–white junction. The frontal lobes are most commonly affected with spread of sinus infections. The temporal lobes or cerebellum are involved in patients with spread from otomastoiditis.

Clinical symptoms in patients with pyogenic brain infections may be mild or severe. Headache is common. There may be varying degrees of lethargy, obtundation, nausea, vomiting, and fever. Fever is absent more than 50% of the time. Meningeal signs are present in only 30% of patients. Focal neurologic deficits, papilledema, nuchal rigidity, and seizures can develop rapidly, over the course of a few days. This is in distinction to tumors where these symptoms usually develop more slowly. There is often, but not invariably, an elevated white blood cell count. CSF studies are often nonspecific and may not be obtained because of the risk of herniation following lumbar puncture in the setting of a brain mass.

A solitary abscess is usually treated surgically. Often, stereotactic needle aspiration followed by antibiotic therapy is performed, especially if the abscess is in an eloquent area of the brain. If there is significant mass effect or if the lesion is in a relatively "safe" area, a formal drainage or resection is performed. With early cerebritis, small or multiple abscesses, or if the patient is a poor surgical candidate, antibiotic therapy alone is used. Imaging studies should be performed frequently (perhaps weekly) to monitor the efficacy of treatment and to assess for complications such as herniation, infarction, and hydrocephalus.

The imaging appearance of cerebritis and brain abscesses evolves and corresponds with four pathologically described stages:

Early Cerebritis. Within the first few days of infection, the infected portion of the brain is swollen and edematous. Areas of early necrosis are filled with inflammatory polymorphonuclear leukocytes, lymphocytes, and plasma cells. Organisms are present in both the center and the periphery of the lesion which has ill-defined margins. CT scans may be normal or show an area of low density (Fig. 6.16A). On MRI, the lesion is hypointense or isointense on T1WI and hyperintense on T2WI and FLAIR images (Fig. 6.16B,C). There may be mild mass effect and patchy areas of enhancement within the lesion on both CT and MRI. A ring of enhancement is not present at this stage, thus distinguishing it from the later three stages. Unfortunately, these imaging features are nonspecific and can be seen with neoplasms or infarcts. The clinical features are, therefore, most important in making the correct diagnosis. If the diagnosis can be made at this stage, nonsurgical treatment with antibiotics is often effective.

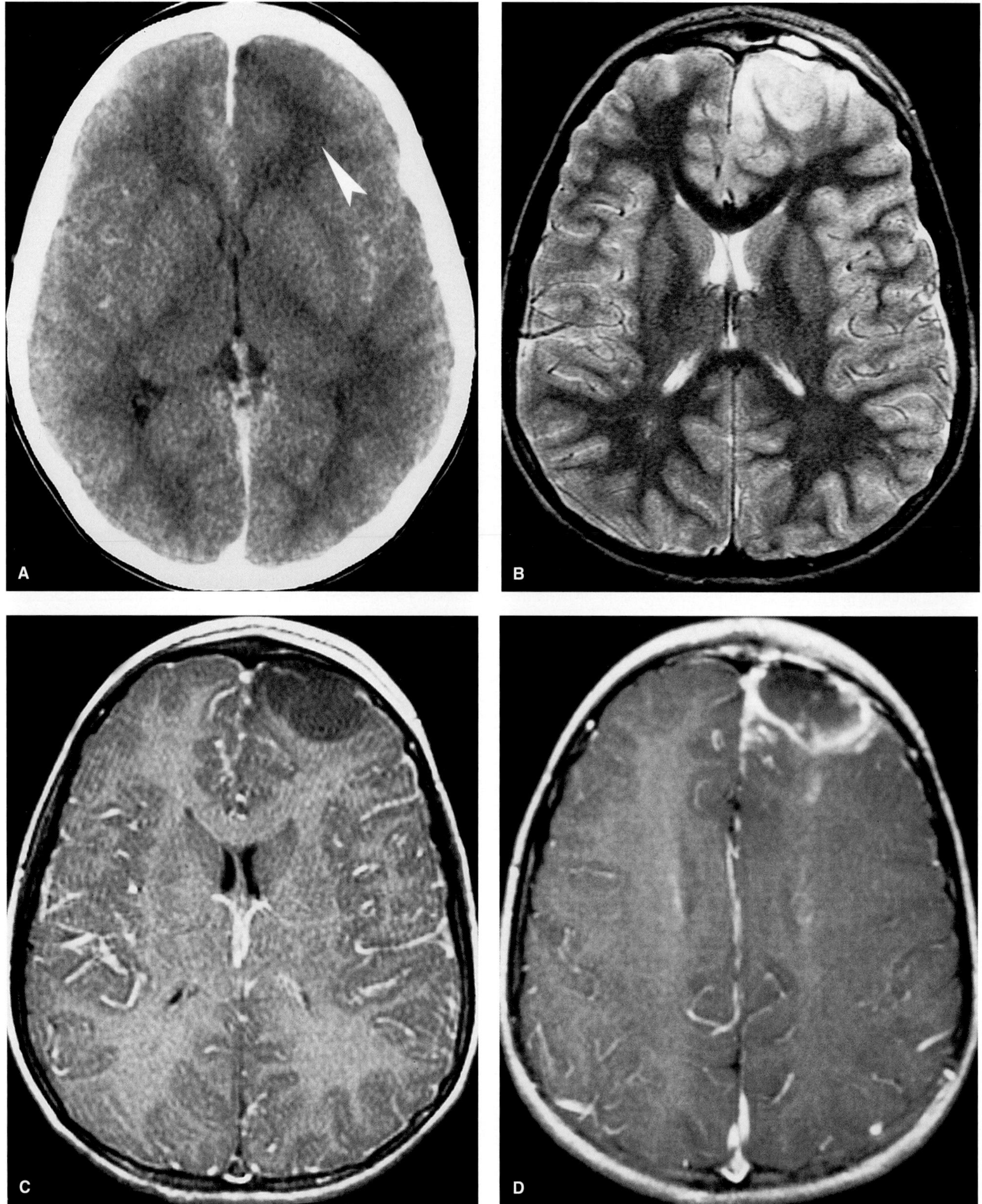

FIGURE 6.16. **Early Cerebritis. A:** CECT scan shows a subtle area of decreased density in the left frontal lobe (*arrowhead*). **B:** Transaxial T2WI obtained the next day shows high signal intensity in the left frontal lobe and left frontal sinusitis. **C:** Contrast-enhanced T1WI shows hypointensity without enhancement, consistent with early cerebritis. **D:** Two weeks later, contrast-enhanced T1WI shows a ring-enhancing abscess with an early capsule.

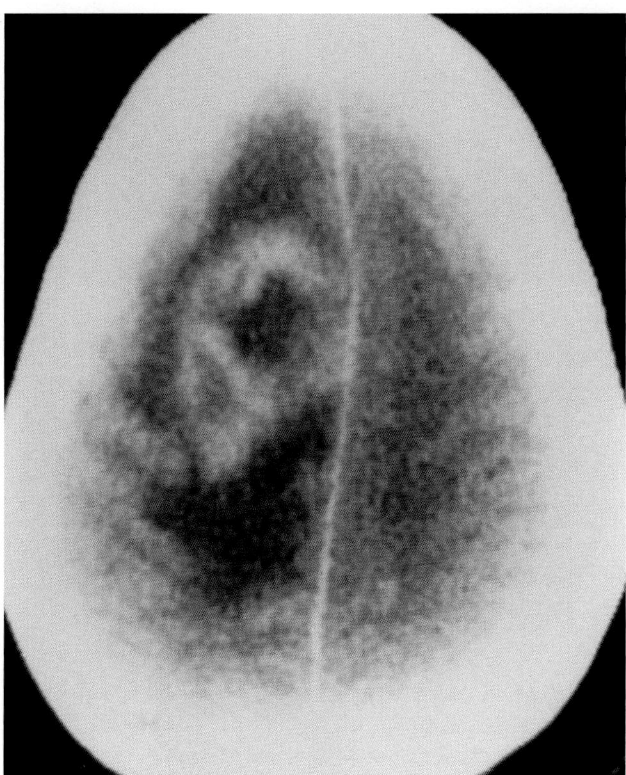

FIGURE 6.17. **Late Cerebritis.** CECT scan demonstrates irregular enhancement peripherally and low density centrally. There is surrounding hypodense vasogenic edema. This is typical of the late cerebritis stage of pyogenic infection.

Late cerebritis occurs within 1 or 2 weeks of infection. Central necrosis progresses and begins to coalesce, with fewer organisms detected pathologically. There is vascular proliferation at the periphery of the lesion, with more inflammatory cells and early granulation tissue, which represent the brain's effort to contain the infection. Not surprisingly, this corresponds to irregular contrast enhancement at the edges of the lesion on imaging studies (Fig. 6.17). Centrally, there is increased hypodensity on CT, hypointensity on T1WI, and hyperintensity on T2WI and FLAIR sequences on MRI. DWI may show some increased signal intensity within the center of the lesion. Scans acquired after a delay following administration of contrast material may show some late central enhancement. There is worsening vasogenic edema present outside the enhancing rim and overall increased mass effect. No discrete T2-hypointense capsule is evident on MRI, as may be observed in some mature abscesses. This stage can also be treated effectively with antibiotic therapy, but distinguishing late cerebritis from an early abscess or tumor can be difficult and surgery is often performed.

Early Capsule. Within 2 weeks, the infection is walled off as a capsule of collagen and reticulin forms along the inflammatory vascular margin of the infection. Macrophages, phagocytes, and neutrophils are also present in the capsule. The necrotic center contains very few organisms. Contrast-enhanced CT and MR scans show a well-defined, usually smooth and thin, rim of enhancement (Fig. 6.16D). The rim tends to be T2 hypointense. Central necrosis again results in hypodensity on CT and T1 hypointensity and T2 hyperintensity on MRI. Prominent surrounding vasogenic edema usually persists. There is reduced diffusion with hyperintensity centrally on DWI.

Late Capsule. In the late capsule stage, the rim of enhancement becomes even better defined and thicker, reflecting more complete collagen in the abscess wall (Fig. 6.18). Multiloculation is common. Prominent increased signal intensity present centrally on DWI is an extremely helpful imaging feature (Fig. 6.19C). The capsule often exhibits characteristic features on MRI that are helpful diagnostically at this stage. On T1WI, the capsule is usually isointense or hyperintense to white matter, and on T2WI, it is usually hypointense to white matter (Fig. 6.19A,B). These signal characteristics suggest paramagnetic T1 and T2 shortening, similar to that seen during the evolution of hematomas (see Chapter 4). However, hemorrhage is not always found pathologically, and these paramagnetic effects may also reflect the presence of free radicals produced by macrophages. Regardless, the MR appearance of the capsule is fairly specific for an abscess. The inner aspect of the enhancing capsule is often (about 50% of the time) thinner than the peripheral aspect (Figs. 6.18C and 6.19D). This reflects relatively decreased blood supply and fibroblast migration centrally compared with cortically. This thin medial rim predisposes to intraventricular rupture of the abscess and resulting ependymitis/ventriculitis (Fig. 6.18C). CT or MR scans reveal enhancement of the ependymal lining of the ventricles and altered density and signal intensity of the intraventricular CSF.

The differential diagnosis of bacterial cerebral abscess includes neoplasm, resolving hematoma, subacute infarct, or demyelination. The clinical features combined with the appearance of prominent central hyperintensity on DWI, smooth complete enhancing rim, significant surrounding vasogenic edema, and T2 hypointensity of the capsule should strongly suggest a brain abscess. Neoplasms typically show irregular enhancement and rarely increased signal intensity on DWI. Resolving hematomas demonstrate the obvious presence of blood products. Subacute infarcts typically present with an appropriate clinical history and gyriform enhancement along a vascular territory. Demyelinating lesions often have an incomplete ring of enhancement and accompanying characteristic white matter lesions. MR spectroscopy (MRS) can assist in confirming a cerebral abscess if a combination of elevated lactate and amino acids is found in the center of the lesion.

Septic Embolus. Infections that begin with a septic embolus may not have the typical appearance of an abscess. The embolus frequently causes an infarct that dominates the imaging findings. Depending on the size of the embolus, there may be a small, rounded area of enhancement or a larger, wedge-shaped cortical infarct. As with other embolic infarcts, hemorrhage may occur. Because the nonviable, infarcted tissue has a poor blood supply, a typical capsule may not form. A thicker, more irregular ring of enhancement that persists within an area of infarction should suggest the diagnosis. Septic emboli may lead to mycotic aneurysm formation, which can result in intraparenchymal or subarachnoid hemorrhage.

Mycobacterial Infections

The most common form of CNS mycobacterial infection is tuberculous meningitis, which has been discussed previously. Focal mycobacterial infection of the brain occurs in two forms: tuberculoma and abscess. A tuberculoma is a granuloma with central caseous necrosis. In contrast, a tuberculous abscess has characteristics similar to those of a pyogenic abscess but usually develops in patients with impaired T-cell immunity.

Tuberculoma. In the early 20th century, one-third of all brain mass lesions in England were tuberculomas. Improved prevention and treatment have made these lesions unusual in industrialized countries. Unfortunately, in developing areas of the world with endemic TB, tuberculomas still account for 15% to 30% of brain masses. In developed countries, tuberculomas usually result from reactivation of quiescent disease, although

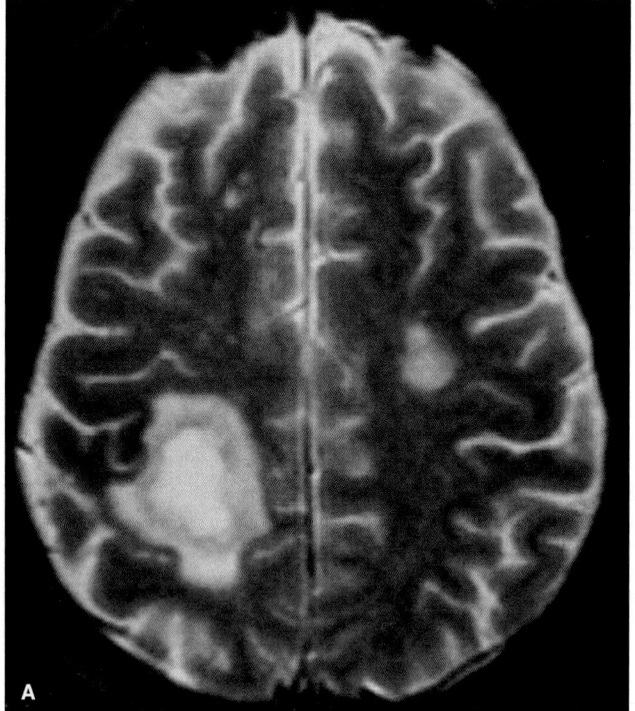

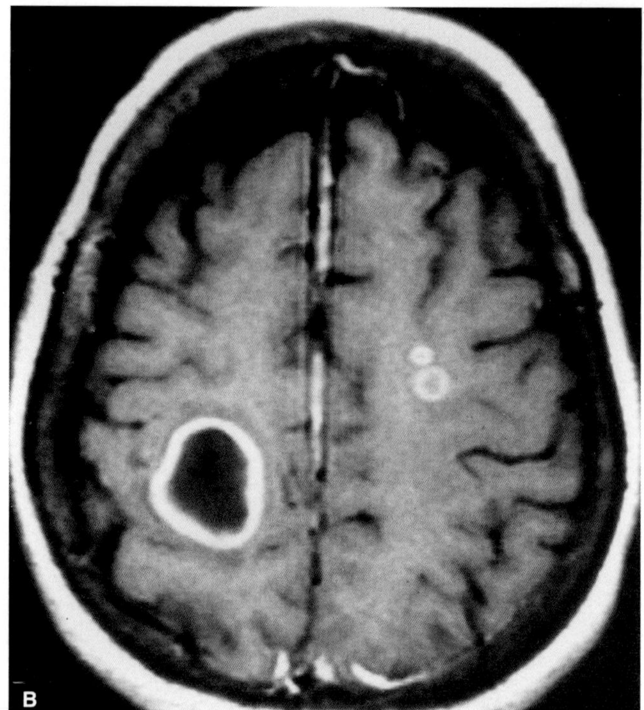

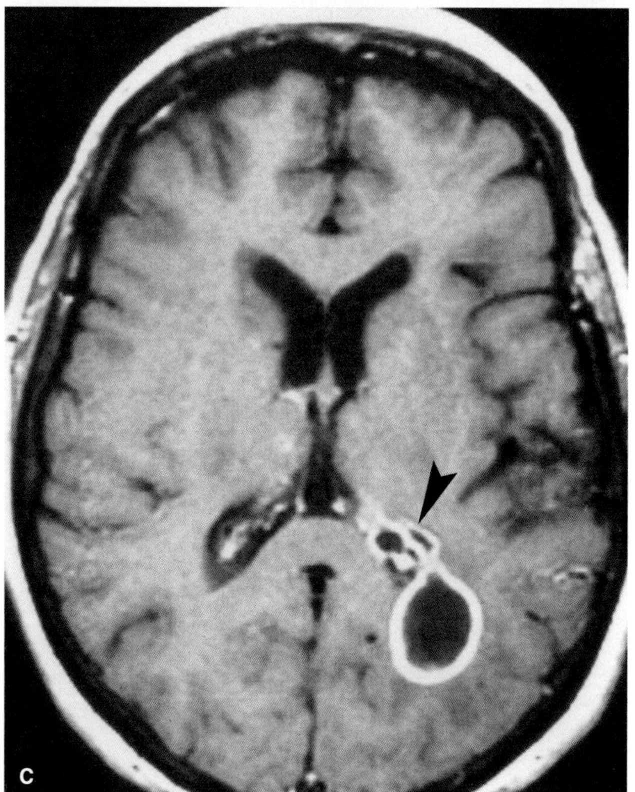

FIGURE 6.18. **Multiple Pyogenic Abscesses. A:** Transaxial T2WI reveals a right parietal lesion with hyperintensity centrally and hypointensity peripherally within the capsule. There is surrounding hyperintense vasogenic edema. Two smaller hyperintense lesions are present on the left. **B:** Contrast-enhanced T1WI shows thin, smooth enhancement of all three lesions. **C:** More inferiorly, the contrast-enhanced T1WI reveals a fourth abscess that has extended into the atrium of the left lateral ventricle (*arrowhead*). The enhancement pattern and intraventricular extension favor the diagnosis of abscess over tumor. These lesions proved to be abscesses that cultured anaerobic streptococci. (Case courtesy of Dr. Vincent Burke, Atherton, California.)

only 50% of patients have a known history of previous tuberculosis. As mentioned before, infection spreads to the brain hematogenously from the lungs. Most tuberculomas are not associated with TB meningitis. Clinical features include headache, seizures, papilledema, and focal neurologic deficits. Fever is seen only rarely. The CSF is almost always abnormal showing pleocytosis with increased protein and decreased glucose, but confirmation of TB by mycobacterial cultures can be difficult. An abnormal chest radiograph is present in up to 50% of patients. These lesions can be treated medically if there are characteristic clinical and imaging features. Surgery is often performed when the diagnosis is in doubt or for medical treatment failures and large lesions.

Most tuberculomas in adults are supratentorial involving the frontal or parietal lobes. Sixty percent of tuberculomas in children are in the posterior fossa, usually the cerebellum.

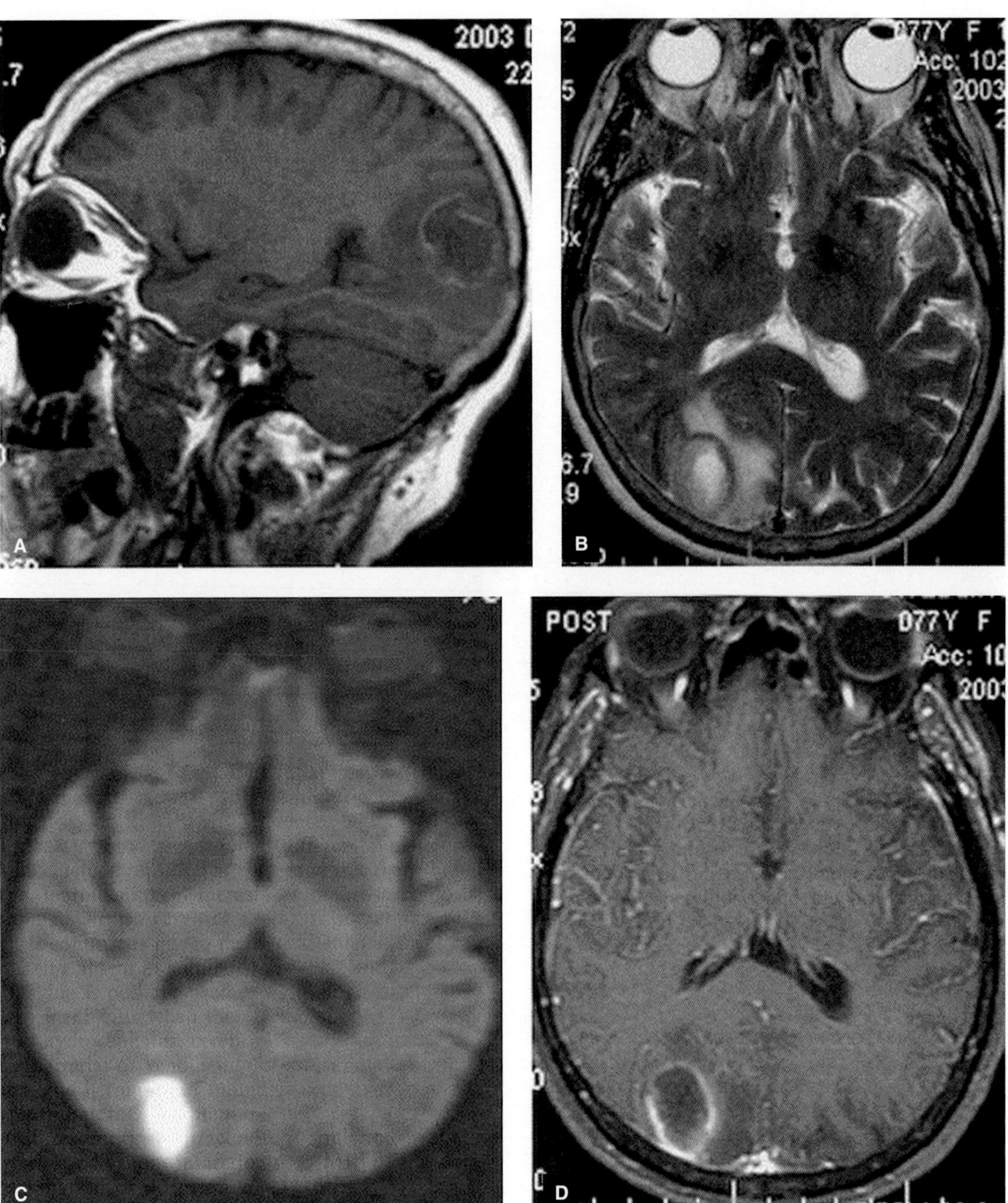

FIGURE 6.19. **Pyogenic Cerebral Abscess.** This case illustrates most of the classic features of a cerebral abscess. **A:** Sagittal T1WI shows high signal in the rim of the abscess as a result of paramagnetic T1 shortening. **B:** Transaxial T2WI shows hypointensity of the rim from T2 shortening with hyperintensity centrally and significant surrounding edema. **C:** DWI shows hyperintensity centrally, a characteristic feature of abscesses that is usually not seen with necrotic tumors. **D:** Contrast-enhanced T1WI shows enhancement of the rim that is thinnest medially, as is often the case with abscesses.

Multiple and miliary lesions are common. CT shows one or more isodense or slightly hyperdense nodules or small mass lesions. Multiple lesions are present about 50% of the time. The center of the tuberculoma is usually denser than the fluidlike center of a bacterial abscess because of caseous necrosis. A "target" appearance, with a central calcification surrounded by rim enhancement, is an uncommon but helpful finding strongly suggesting the diagnosis. Calcification is present in fewer than 5% of cases at the initial diagnosis but is commonly seen with treatment as the lesions resolve. With MRI, tuberculomas may be high or low in signal intensity on T2WI, depending upon the size of the lesion and the water content of the caseous necrosis (Fig. 6.20A). The wall of the tuberculoma is often hypointense on T2WI. There is significant enhancement after gadolinium administration with a solid nodular or thick, ring-shaped appearance (Fig. 6.20B). There may or may not be increased signal intensity centrally on DWI, unlike bacterial infections which usually show reduced diffusion. Surrounding edema is often relatively mild. The differential diagnosis includes neoplasm, bacterial abscess, fungal and parasitic infections, and neurosarcoidosis. However, simultaneous parenchymal abscesses with basilar meningitis should cause a high suspicion for CNS tuberculosis.

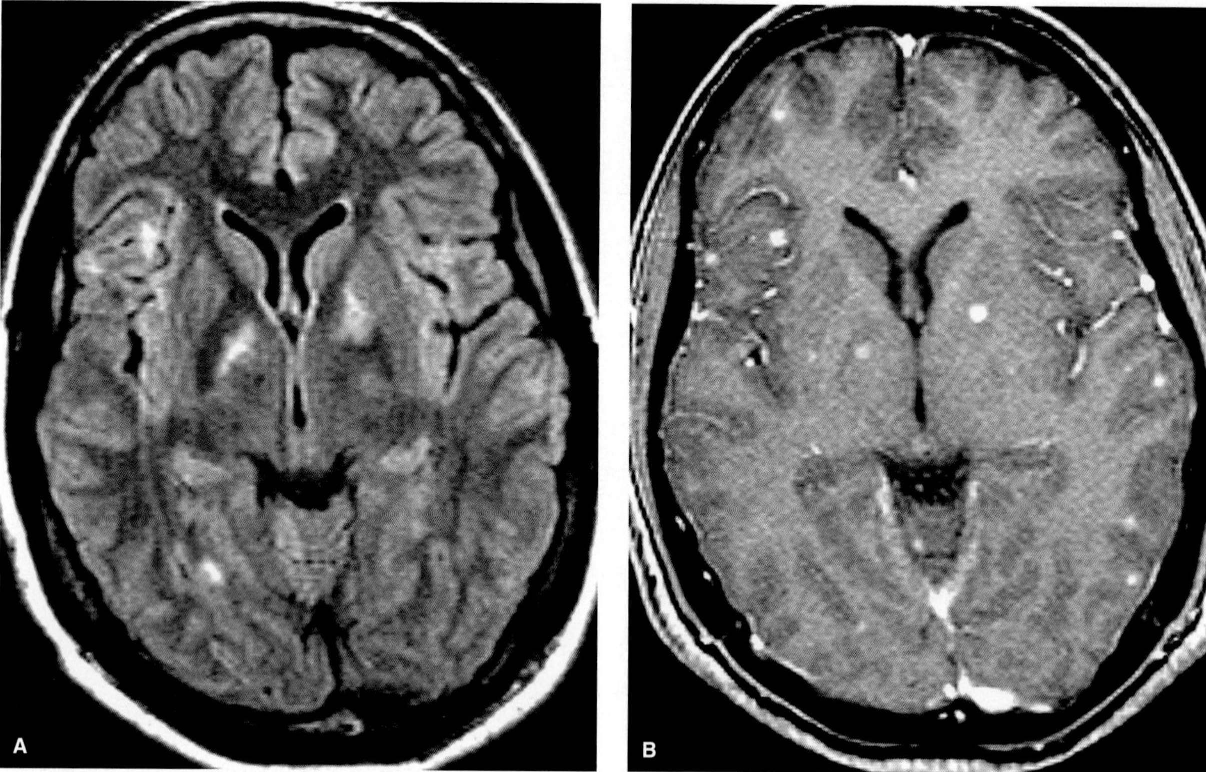

FIGURE 6.20. **Multiple Tuberculomas. A:** Transaxial FLAIR image shows multiple small areas of T2 hyperintensity and mild edema bilaterally. **B:** Contrast-enhanced transaxial T1WI shows multiple small enhancing nodules.

Tuberculous abscess is a rare complication seen primarily in immunocompromised patients. Impaired T-cell function prevents the normal host response required for tuberculoma formation with caseous necrosis. Symptoms develop and lesions grow more rapidly than seen with tuberculomas. The imaging features are similar to that seen with bacterial abscesses. The lesions are often large and multiloculated, in distinction to tuberculomas. Prominent edema and mass effect also distinguish a tuberculous abscess from tuberculoma. Atypical mycobacterial infections are also more common in immunocompromised patients.

Fungal Infections

Fungal infections of the CNS can be grouped into endemic and/or opportunistic categories. Endemic fungal infections are usually geographically restricted. They can occur in both immunocompetent and immunosuppressed patients. Opportunistic fungal infections occur worldwide but usually in immunocompromised patients such as infants, the elderly, or chronically ill. Endemic fungal infections are present predominantly with granulomatous meningitis, as has been discussed, and parenchymal disease is unusual. On the other hand, parenchymal involvement is seen with much higher frequency with opportunistic fungal infections.

Endemic Fungal Infections. The most common endemic fungal infections in the United States are coccidioidomycosis, North American blastomycosis, and histoplasmosis. These infections usually manifest as granulomatous meningitis, as has been discussed, and focal parenchymal lesions are unusual. CNS involvement is a manifestation of disseminated infection, with hematogenous spread, usually from pulmonary disease.

Coccidioidomycosis is caused by the soil fungus *Coccidioides immitis* which occurs in the southwestern United States and Northern Mexico. The spores are inhaled, with outbreaks occurring after groundbreaking for construction projects. Most infected patients are asymptomatic or have mild respiratory symptoms. Less than 1% of patients develop disseminated infection and meningitis. Focal parenchymal granulomas are rare.

Blastomycosis is caused by *Blastomyces dermatitidis* which survives in damp soil along the Ohio and Mississippi River valleys. CNS involvement occurs in 6% to 33% of disseminated infection. Meningitis is the most frequent presentation, but parenchymal abscesses and granulomas occur more frequently than with coccidioidomycosis. Epidural granulomas and abscesses also occur in the head and spine, usually from direct extension from adjacent sites of osteomyelitis. Up to 40% of focal brain lesions are multiple.

Histoplasmosis is usually seen in patients who are asymptomatic or present with a benign pulmonary infection. The causative pathogen is another soil fungus *Histoplasma capsulatum,* which is also found in the Ohio and Mississippi River valleys. Disseminated infection is unusual and only a small percent of disseminated cases involve the CNS, where meningitis is most common. Multiple or solitary granulomas may occur. Abscesses rarely develop.

As seen with CT or MRI, most fungal granulomas are small and show solid or thick rim enhancement (Fig. 6.21) similar to tuberculomas. Fungal abscesses (as sometimes seen with blastomycosis) have an appearance similar to that of the bacterial abscesses. Accompanying meningitis with meningeal enhancement is a common feature. Hydrocephalus is also common, especially with coccidioidomycosis. The differential diagnosis includes TB, multiple bacterial abscesses, septic emboli, parasitic infection, and metastatic disease.

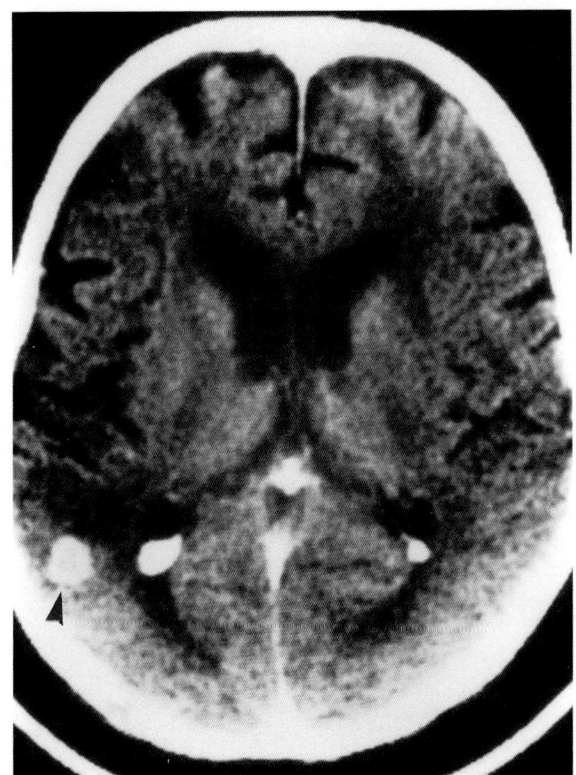

FIGURE 6.21. **Histoplasmosis Granuloma.** This patient had disseminated histoplasmosis with several lesions in the brain and spine. CECT shows a solidly enhancing lesion near the atrium of the right lateral ventricle (*arrowhead*). Most fungal granulomas are small and show either solid or thick rim enhancement. (Case courtesy of Dr. J. R. Jinkins, San Antonio, Texas.)

Opportunistic Fungal Infections. The most common opportunistic fungal CNS infections are cryptococcosis, aspergillosis, mucormycosis, and candidiasis. These usually present as meningitis, but focal parenchymal lesions are unfortunately not uncommon in immunologically vulnerable patients with diabetes, leukemia, lymphoma, AIDS, or organ transplants.

Aspergillosis involves the CNS in 60% to 70% of patients with disseminated disease. The infection may arise from hematogenous spread or by direct and aggressive extension from an infected paranasal sinus, leading to meningitis or meningoencephalitis. The mortality rate with invasive intracerebral aspergillosis is greater than 85%. Parenchymal disease usually takes the form of an abscess which are often multiple and show irregular ring enhancement (Fig. 6.22). The amount of enhancement depends upon the immunocompromised host's ability to fight the infection. The abscesses are frequently T2 hypointense centrally on MRI due to hemorrhage or the presence of heavy metals concentrated by the fungus (Fig. 6.23). Subcortical or cortical infarcts from blood vessel invasion may occur.

Mucormycosis. Mucor invades the brain usually by direct extension from the sinuses, nose, or oral cavity but hematogenous spread also occurs. Almost all patients are diabetic or otherwise immunocompromised. The mortality rate in treated diabetic patients is 65% to 75% and is worse in immunocompromised patients. Like aspergillosis, mucormycosis tends to invade blood vessels. CT and MR studies in patients with CNS mucormycosis will reveal single or multiple mass lesions with the degree of peripheral enhancement and vasogenic edema varying with the patient's immunocompromised state (Fig. 6.24). Smaller lesions will show a solid-enhancement pattern. The lesions are often in the base of the brain, adjacent to diseased sinuses. Infarcts, intra-axial or extra-axial hemorrhage, and meningeal enhancement can be seen with CT and MRI. A lesion with peripheral enhancement, cortical sparing, and a nonvascular distribution is more likely to be a mucormycotic abscess than an infarct, but often it is difficult to distinguish both.

Candidiasis usually causes meningitis but granulomas and small abscesses may occur. Spread to the CNS is usually hematogenous from the lungs or the gastrointestinal tract. In cases of CNS candidiasis, meningeal enhancement or multiple small enhancing granulomas or microabscesses are usually seen. Infarcts, hydrocephalus, and large abscesses may also be identified.

Cryptococcosis is the most frequently reported CNS fungal infection. It preferentially involves immunosuppressed patients, and especially those with AIDS, but cases are also seen in immunocompetent individuals. *Cryptococcus neoformans* is responsible for most cases in immunocompromised patients, whereas *Cryptococcus gattii* is reported mostly in patients with normal immune function. *C. neoformans* is found in high levels in bird excreta and *C. gattii* is associated with tropical and subtropical trees. CNS cryptococcosis in AIDS will also be described later in this chapter. Infection of the CNS occurs via hematogenous spread from the lungs. Serum and CSF studies are valuable in making the diagnosis, since about 90% of the patients have cryptococcal antigen (CrAg) in the CSF and/or antibody in the serum. The usual manifestation is meningitis but granulomas ("cryptococcomas") can occur in about 10% of cases and are usually multiple. CT scans in patients with cryptococcosis are frequently normal or demonstrate only mild meningeal enhancement and/or hydrocephalus. Cryptococcomas are shown as small, usually multiple, solid-enhancing, peripherally located parenchymal nodules with vasogenic edema. Ring-like enhancement and calcifications are occasionally seen. With the improved sensitivity of MRI, parenchymal lesions and meningeal disease are seen more frequently than with CT. Leptomeningeal nodules are often only seen on contrast-enhanced T1WI as multiple tiny enhancing lesions near the basal cisterns and within the sulci. Diffuse meningeal enhancement is unusual. Cryptococcal gelatinous pseudocysts are seen in immunocompromised, especially AIDS patients, and are described in further detail later. Briefly, these are dilated perivascular spaces filled with the organism and mucinous material. They appear as rounded, smoothly marginated lesions in the basal ganglia that are nearly isodense and isointense to CSF (see Fig. 6.41). There is minimal, if any, peripheral edema or enhancement.

Parasitic Infections

Parasitic infections are common throughout much of the developing world but are relatively uncommon in the industrialized nations. The most common infections likely to be encountered in the United States are cysticercosis, echinococcosis, toxoplasmosis, and rarely, amebiasis. CNS involvement in malaria, trypanosomiasis, paragonimiasis, sparganosis, schistosomiasis, and trichinosis is rarely encountered in the United States and will not be discussed. However, it is interesting to note that malaria and amebiasis are the two most common causes of mortality from parasitic infections worldwide.

Cysticercosis is caused by the larvae of the pork tapeworm *Taenia solium*. Transmission occurs via the fecal–oral route. When larvae are ingested, intestinal disease results, and eggs are released into the bowel stream. Humans become the intermediate host if the eggs are ingested by humans instead of pigs. In this situation, the eggs form oncospheres (primary larvae), which hatch in the intestine and are hematogenously distributed throughout the body where they form cysticerci

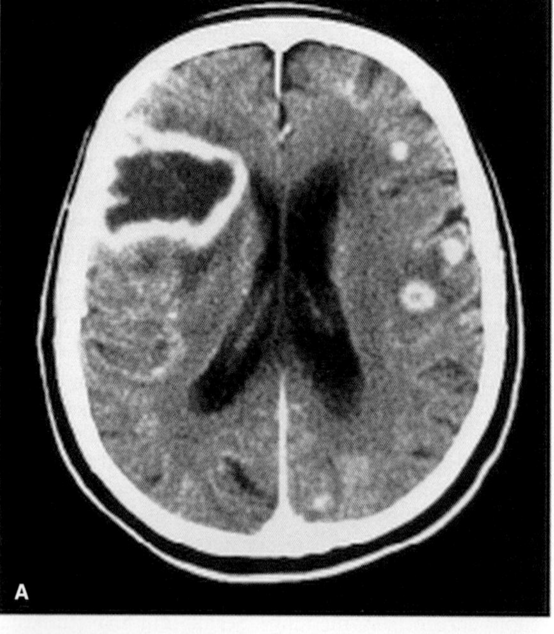

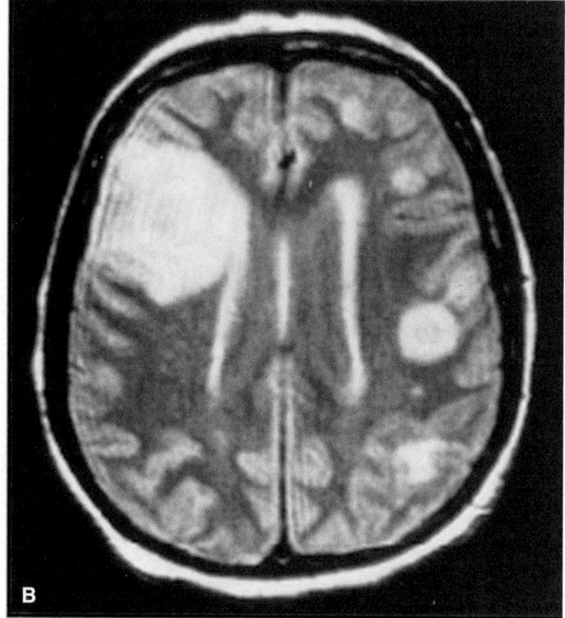

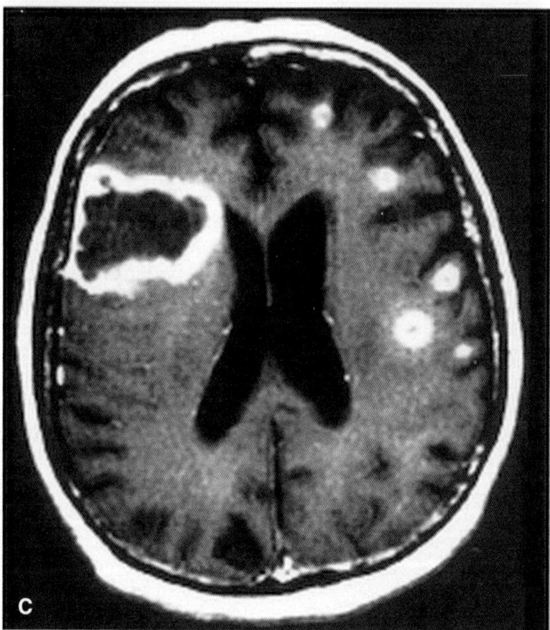

FIGURE 6.22. **Disseminated Aspergillosis.** CECT (**A**), transaxial proton-density weighted sequence (**B**), and contrast-enhanced T1WI (**C**) show a large necrotic mass in the right frontal lobe and several smaller lesions in the left hemisphere. The right frontal lobe lesion was surgically drained and aspergillosis was found. The patient was a poorly controlled diabetic.

(secondary larvae). The cysticerci cannot develop further in humans and they eventually die. Cysticerci that reach the CNS may infest the parenchyma, meninges, ventricles, or spine. This disease is fairly frequently encountered in the southwestern United States, and especially in Latin American immigrants. Patients present with headaches and seizures occur in more than 90% of patients. Neurocysticercosis is the most common cause of seizures in Latin America. Encephalitic symptoms are also common. Serum and CSF serologies are important diagnostic tests. Treatment is with anticysticercal drugs such as praziquantel and albendazole.

Parenchymal cysticercosis is more common than the meningobasal and intraventricular forms of extra-axial infection, already discussed above. Progression of parenchymal neurocysticercosis through various described stages may take place over the course of months and years, and CT and MRI are useful in diagnosis, staging, and monitoring treatment of this infection. At the earliest onset of infestation, neuroimaging shows minimal, if any, edema and/or nodular enhancement. In the *vesicular stage,* viable parasitic cysts appear as small (usually 1 cm or less), solitary or multiple rounded lesions that are hypodense on CT and isointense to CSF on MRI (Fig. 6.25). The lesions are usually peripherally distributed near the gray–white junction or in the gray matter. A small marginal nodule representing the scolex is sometimes seen (Figs. 6.25B and 6.26). There is usually no enhancement or edema. The *colloid stage* ensues when the cyst dies and its fluid leaks into the surrounding brain inciting inflammation. This produces clinical symptoms of acute encephalitis, which may be severe depending on the number of lesions. Imaging studies now reveal ring-enhancing lesions with surrounding vasogenic edema (Fig. 6.26). The colloidal cyst fluid becomes increasingly dense on CT and hyperintense on MRI when compared with CSF. The dead cyst further degenerates in the *nodular granular stage,* becomes smaller and causes less edema, but shows increasing nodular or irregular peripheral enhancement.

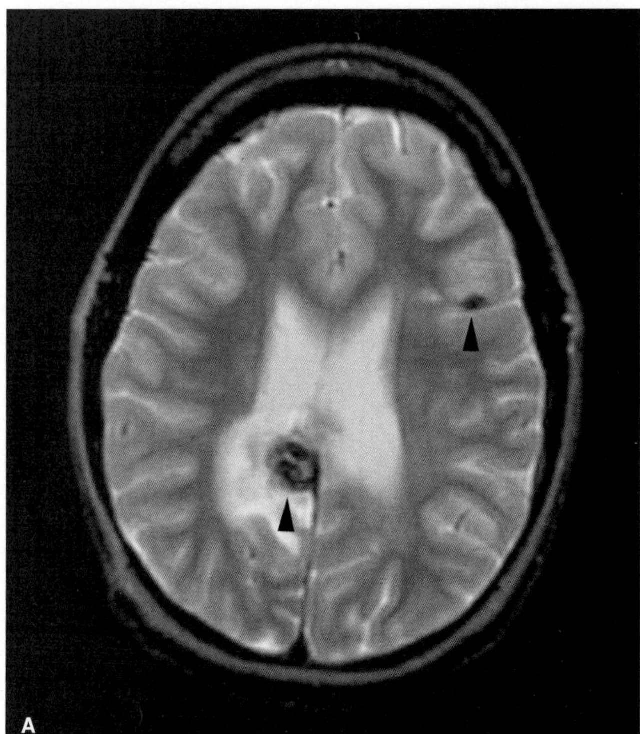

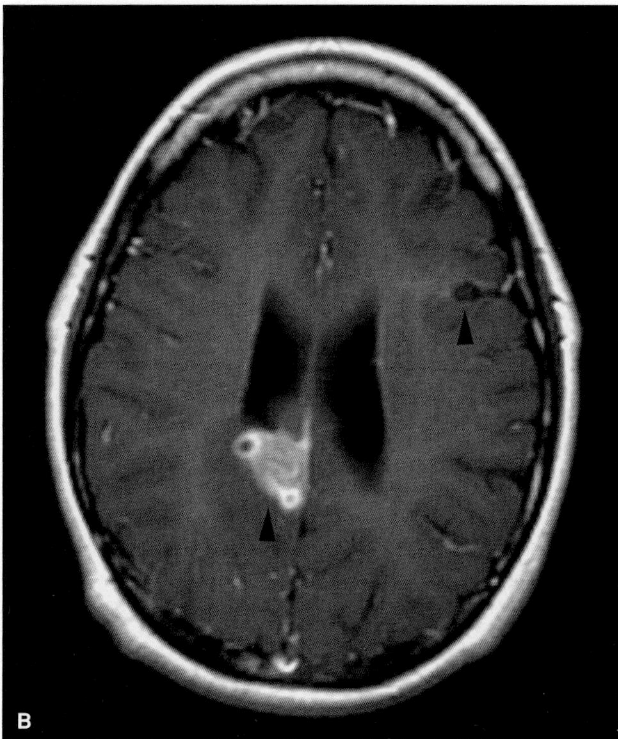

FIGURE 6.23. Disseminated Aspergillosis. A: Transaxial T2WI of this 12-year-old child with leukemia shows two T2-hypointense lesions in the right posterior body of the corpus callosum and at the gray–white matter junction of the left frontal lobe (*arrowheads*). The appearance of the larger right-sided lesion is due to T2 shortening caused by the presence of paramagnetic hemorrhage and/or heavy metals frequently associated with fungal infections. The smaller left frontal lesion was previously treated and is calcified on CT (not shown). **B:** Contrast-enhanced T1WI demonstrates intense enhancement of the larger, active right-sided lesion.

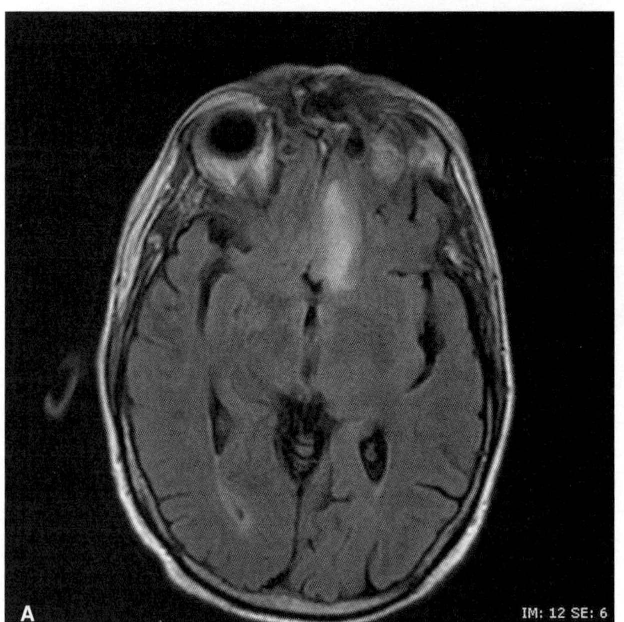

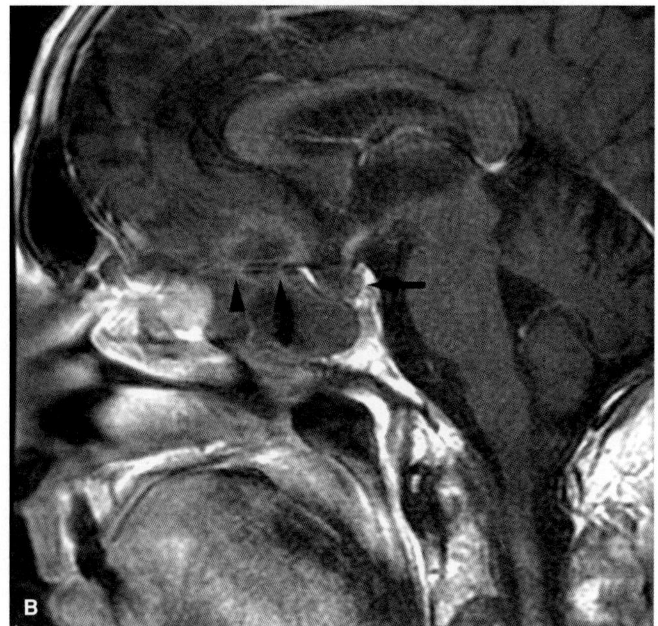

FIGURE 6.24. Mucormycosis. A: Transaxial FLAIR image in this 64-year-old patient with diabetes and leukemia demonstrates T2-hyperintense edema and swelling of the gyrus rectus along the inferomedial left frontal lobe (*arrowhead*), reflecting cerebritis. **B:** Contrast-enhanced sagittal T1WI shows dehiscence of the roof of the ethmoid and sphenoid sinuses with extension of fungal sinus infection intracranially (*arrowheads*). There is mild irregular enhancement of the adjacent gyrus rectus consistent with late cerebritis. Note the lack of normal enhancement of the pituitary gland due to infarction (*arrow*). The patient also exhibited signs of pituitary dysfunction and died within days of presentation despite surgical and antifungal therapy.

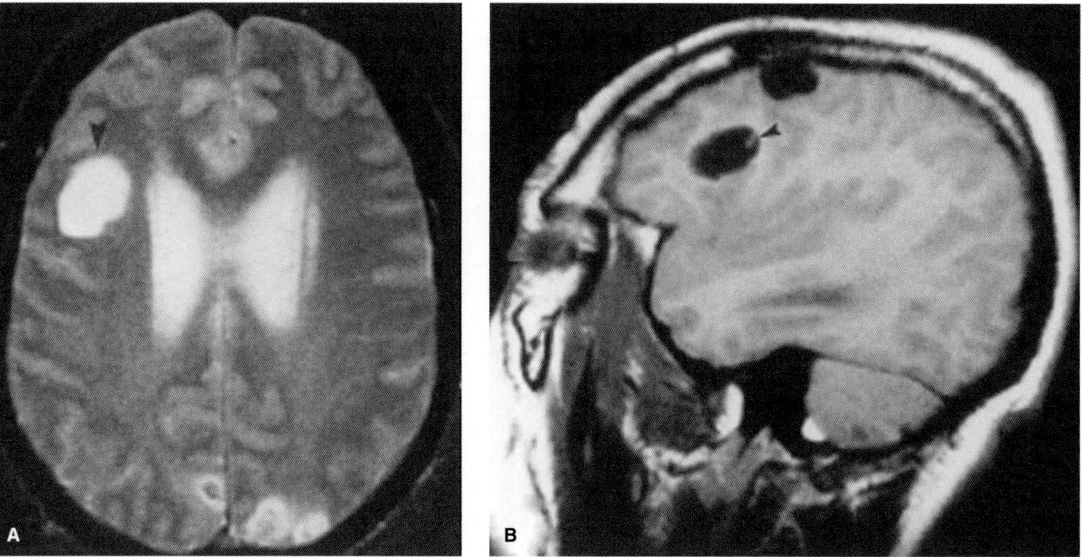

FIGURE 6.25. **Cysticercosis. A:** Transaxial T2WI shows a right frontal lesion isointense with CSF (*arrowhead*). There is no surrounding edema, indicating that this is early in the course of disease. Three smaller lesions are present posteriorly. **B:** Parasagittal T1WI in the same patient shows two cysticercal cysts that are isointense with CSF. A scolex is visible in one of the cysts (*arrowhead*).

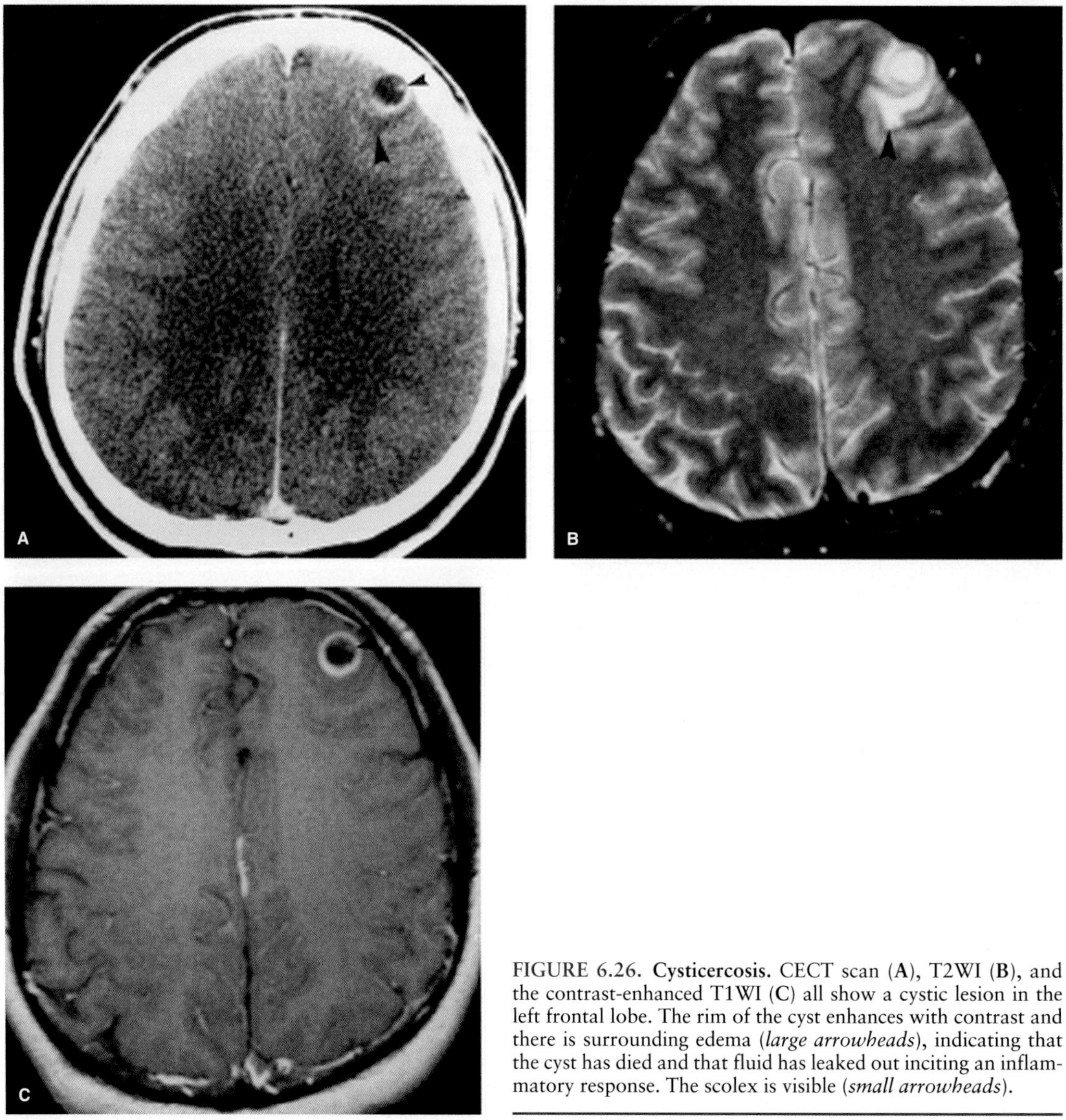

A B C

FIGURE 6.26. **Cysticercosis.** CECT scan (**A**), T2WI (**B**), and the contrast-enhanced T1WI (**C**) all show a cystic lesion in the left frontal lobe. The rim of the cyst enhances with contrast and there is surrounding edema (*large arrowheads*), indicating that the cyst has died and that fluid has leaked out inciting an inflammatory response. The scolex is visible (*small arrowheads*).

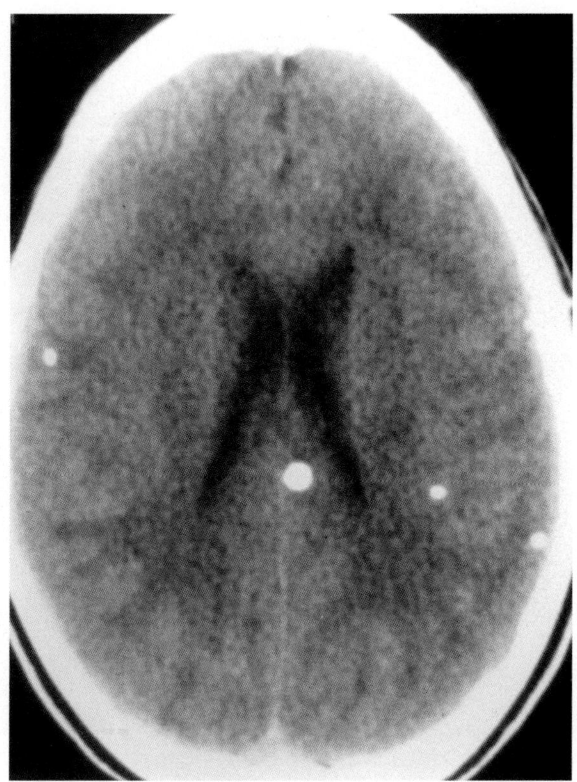

FIGURE 6.27. **Late-Stage Cysticercosis.** NECT scan shows multiple calcifications in the gray matter and gray–white junction, which are typical of old cysticercosis.

In the last *nodular calcified stage,* a dense residual calcification is left with no remaining edema or enhancement. CT without contrast excels at detecting these small, peripherally distributed calcifications (Fig. 6.27). With MRI, the calcifications are best seen on T2*-weighted gradient-recalled echo (GRE) sequences. Once the cyst has degenerated, further drug therapy is not warranted. Differential diagnosis includes metastatic disease, granulomatous infections, or abscesses.

Meningobasal (racemose) and intraventricular cysticercosis have been discussed previously in this chapter (Figs. 6.13 and 6.14). Spinal cysticercosis is usually intradural but can be either intramedullary or extramedullary. Intramedullary lesions are best seen with MRI as solid or ring-enhancing cord lesions, similar to that seen in the brain parenchyma. Extramedullary cysts are analogous to the racemose form and, like most spinal pathology, are best evaluated with MRI.

Echinococcosis, also known as hydatid disease, occurs in South America, Africa, Central Europe, the Middle East, and rarely in the southwestern United States. The etiologic agent is the dog tapeworm *Echinococcus granulosus* and humans are intermediate hosts, as seen in cysticercosis. Hydatid cysts are most frequently present in the lung and liver but the brain is involved in 1% to 4% of cases. Patients usually present with neurologic symptoms related to increased intracranial pressure. The cysts are usually solitary, unilocular or multilocular, large, round, and smoothly marginated. They are most often supratentorial and may rarely have mural calcifications. With CT, the fluid within the cyst is usually isodense with CSF. There is usually no surrounding edema or abnormal contrast enhancement, unless the cyst has ruptured, leading to an inflammatory reaction and more acute presentation. With MRI, the lesions are usually nearly isointense with CSF but can have a T2-hypointense rim.

Toxoplasmosis is caused by the protozoa *T. gondii,* which occurs worldwide. The congenital form has been described above (Fig. 6.2). The acquired form is seen primarily in immunocompromised patients and is very common in AIDS patients and will be outlined later (see Fig. 6.39).

Amebic meningoencephalitis is sometimes seen in the southern United States. *Entamoeba histolytica,* Acanthamoeba, and *Naegleria fowleri* are the most often implicated pathogens. Hematogenous spread to the CNS in patients with amebic infections of the gastrointestinal tract is most common but can also occur following inhalation of particles or exposure through skin wounds. *N. fowleri* enters the nasal cavity of patients swimming in infested freshwater ponds and extend through the olfactory apparatus and cribriform plate into the brain. Severe meningoencephalitis results and is usually fatal. Imaging studies often underestimate the severity of the disease. Early in the infection, there may be meningeal and/or gray matter enhancement. Associated vasculitis and cerebral infarction can occasionally be observed. Later, there is diffuse cerebral edema and hemorrhage may occur. There are a few reports of amebic brain abscesses appearing as single or multiple lesions with solid or ring-like enhancement with surrounding edema (Fig. 6.28). Amebic abscesses are more common in debilitated or immunosuppressed patients.

Spirochete Infections

Neurosyphilis is caused by the sexually transmitted spirochete *Treponema pallidum.* It develops in about 5% of patients who are not treated for the primary infection. Involvement of the CNS usually occurs in the secondary or tertiary stages. This disease is now rare because of the efficacy of antibiotics, namely penicillin. However, neurosyphilis is more likely to develop in HIV-infected patients, and the neurologic symptoms occur after a shorter latency period than in other patients. Patients with neurosyphilis are usually asymptomatic. Symptomatic patients may have headaches, meningitis, cranial neuropathies, ischemic stroke, altered mental status, progressive dementia, or tabes dorsalis (loss of spinal pain sensation and proprioception). Diagnosis can be confirmed via serologic markers or microbiologic culture. Neuroimaging can be normal or demonstrate cerebral volume loss and nonspecific T2-hyperintense white matter lesions on MRI. Meningeal enhancement is unusual but cranial nerve enhancement in patients with syphilitic cranial neuritis has been described. Rarely, gummas (syphylitic granulomas) do develop. These usually appear as small enhancing nodules at the surface of the brain with adjacent meningeal enhancement.

Meningovascular syphilis presents as an acute stroke syndrome or a subacute illness with a variety of symptoms. Pathologically, there is thickening of the meninges and a medium-to-large vessel arteritis. Imaging studies reveal small infarcts of the basal ganglia, white matter, cerebral cortex, or cerebellum (Fig. 6.29A). The infarcts may exhibit patchy or gyriform enhancement and are best seen with MRI. MRA and conventional angiography in patients with meningovascular neurosyphilis reveal multiple segmental constrictions and/or occlusions of large and medium arteries, including the distal internal carotid, anterior cerebral, middle cerebral, posterior cerebral, and distal basilar arteries (Fig. 6.29B).

Lyme disease (or Lyme borreliosis) is a multisystem spirochete infection which is most commonly caused by *Borrelia burgdorferi* in North America. It is spread to humans worldwide via ticks from deer, mice, raccoons, and birds. The disease occurs most frequently on the East Coast but may occur anywhere in the United States. The disease begins as a flu-like illness with a rash and an expanding skin lesion at the tick

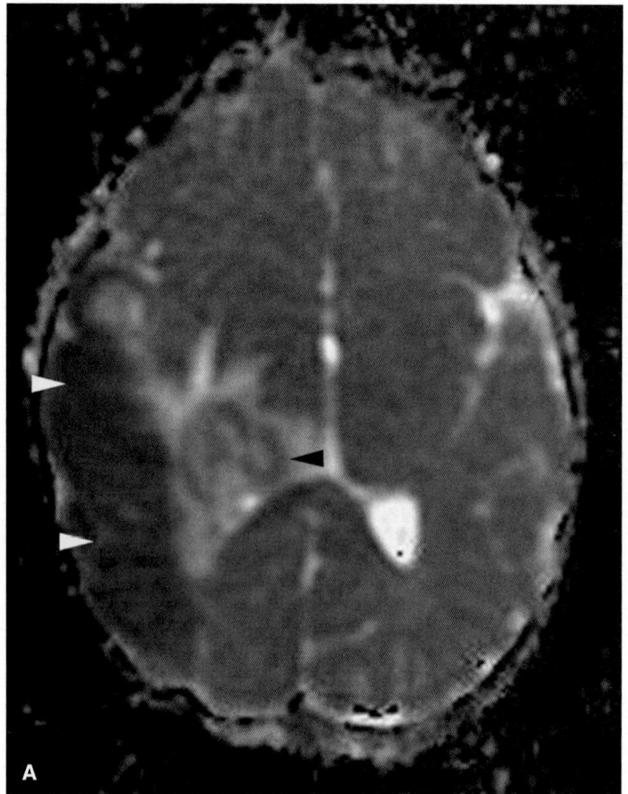

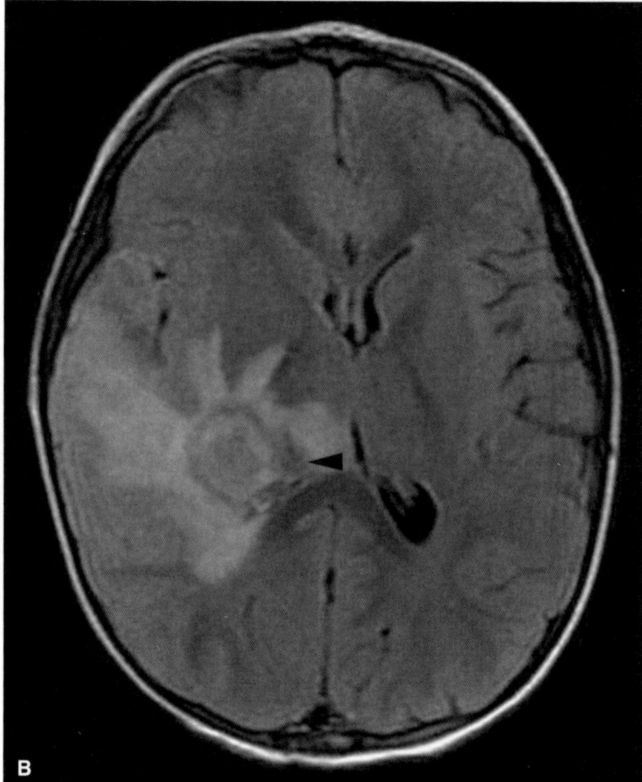

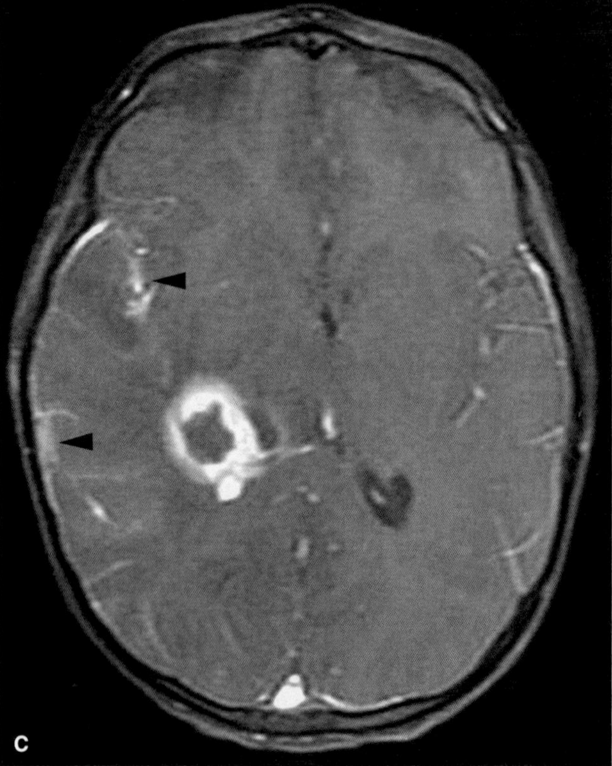

FIGURE 6.28. **Granulomatous Amebic Encephalitis. A:** Transaxial apparent diffusion coefficient map in this 2-year-old child with fatal Balamuthia mandrillaris infection demonstrates irregular necrotic abscess with mixed but not significantly reduced diffusion (*black arrowhead*) along the right periatrial region. Concurrent right middle cerebral artery acute infarct with hypointense reduced diffusion is present (*white arrowheads*). **B:** FLAIR image shows the same amebic abscess (*black arrowhead*) with hypointense, irregular peripheral ring and significant surrounding T2-hyperintense edema. **C:** Contrast-enhanced T1WI reveals thick irregular enhancement around the periphery of abscess. Additional enhancing, thick inflammatory leptomeningeal exudate present along the right sylvian fissure and temporoparietal region (*black arrowheads*) likely contributes to vasculitis and above-described infarct.

bite site. In a minority of patients, cardiac, arthritic, or neurologic symptoms develop. Neurologic abnormalities are found in 10% to 15% of patients. A variety of symptoms including peripheral and cranial neuropathies, radiculopathies, myelopathies, encephalitis, meningitis, pain syndromes, and cognitive and movement disorders have been reported. Treatment with antibiotics and corticosteroids may have variable results. MRI is the modality of choice for imaging these patients. In patients with cranial neuritis, MR scans may show thick, enhancing cranial nerves. Cranial nerves III to VIII can be involved, with the facial nerve most commonly affected. In patients with parenchymal CNS Lyme disease, MR studies show multiple

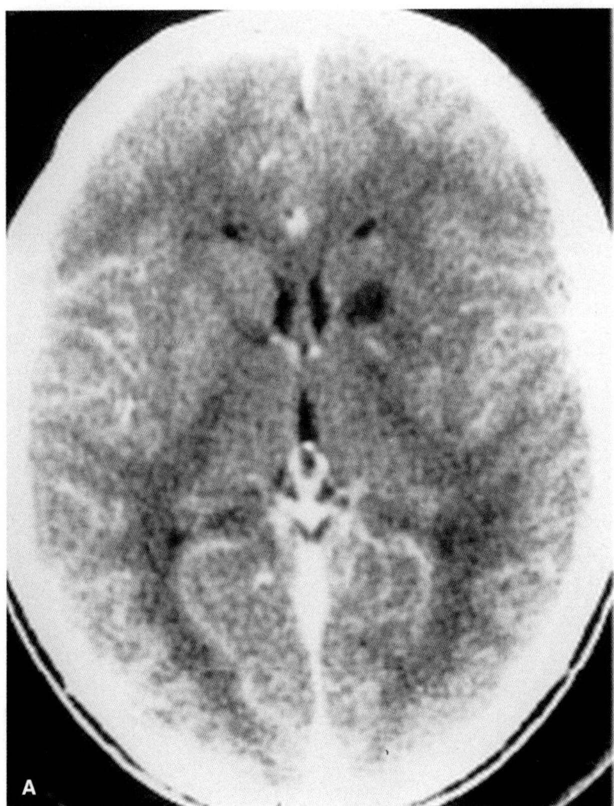

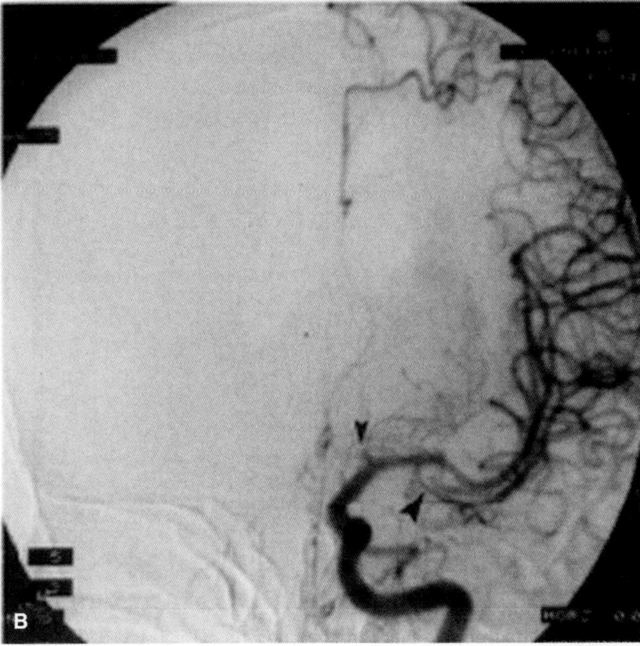

FIGURE 6.29. **Meningovascular Syphilis. A:** CECT scan reveals a small infarct in the left striatal nucleus in this 21-year-old man with meningovascular syphilis. **B:** Frontal projection of a conventional arteriogram of the left internal carotid arteriogram on another patient with meningovascular syphilis shows occlusion of the left anterior cerebral artery (*small arrowhead*) and narrowing of the branches of the left middle cerebral artery (*large arrowhead*). Both patients improved with penicillin therapy.

small white matter lesions, similar to that seen with multiple sclerosis. The lesions can be found in the supratentorial and infratentorial white matter tracts. They often enhance with contrast in a nodular or ring-like pattern, depending on their size. There may be meningeal enhancement. The differential diagnosis includes multiple sclerosis and other demyelinating processes, neurosarcoidosis, or vasculitis.

Viral Infections

Herpes simplex encephalitis occurs in immunocompetent patients of all ages and is the most common cause of sporadic encephalitis. As mentioned above, neonatal herpes encephalitis is caused by the transmission of genital HSV2 from the mother to the infant during vaginal delivery. However, herpes simplex virus type 1 (HSV1) is responsible for the vast majority of cases of encephalitis in other age groups. Herpes infection may cause encephalitis or cranial neuritis. The infection usually is secondary to reactivation of latent HSV1, especially within the trigeminal ganglion. Patients with herpes encephalitis present with fever, headaches, lethargy, mental status changes, aphasia, or other focal neurologic deficits. Seizures and coma may occur. An inconstant but characteristic electroencephalographic (EEG) finding is a localized spiked and slow wave pattern in the temporal lobes. Neuroimaging is a crucial diagnostic tool since CSF studies are often initially nonspecific. Early empiric antiviral therapy with acyclovir even before CSF PCR studies become confirmatory can significantly reduce mortality, but many survivors have permanent neurologic deficits. Mortality in untreated patients can exceed 70%. CT scans may be normal or show poorly defined hypodense regions in one or both temporal lobes (Figs. 6.30 and 6.31A). Since CT findings may not be apparent during the first few days of symptoms, early evaluation with MRI should be strongly encouraged. MRI should show a symmetric or asymmetric gyral pattern of hyperintensity on T2WI and FLAIR images in the temporal lobes with a predilection for the hippocampus and insular cortex but sparing of the subjacent putamen. This is best appreciated on FLAIR sequences (Figs. 6.31B,C and 6.32A). The frontal lobes and cingulate gyrus in particular may also be involved. Swelling with mass effect can be seen. Reduced diffusion on DWI is often present (Fig. 6.32B). Early on, meningeal enhancement may be seen. Parenchymal enhancement or subtle evidence of hemorrhage may present later (Fig. 6.32C). The differential diagnosis includes middle cerebral artery infarction (which follows a vascular distribution), other viral encephalitides, postictal changes, and infiltrating glioma.

Varicella zoster virus (VZV) rarely does cause encephalitis that can be similar to that caused by herpes simplex. Neurologic symptoms typically follow an illness with skin rash, and VZV encephalitis has a more multifocal distribution and less predilection for temporal lobe involvement than seen with HSV1. VZV is also the cause of herpes zoster ophthalmicus which can be complicated by ipsilateral cerebral angiitis causing cerebral infarction and contralateral hemiparesis. Neuroimaging studies show typical infarcts, and angiography shows segmental areas of narrowing and/or beading of large- and medium-sized arteries. Mycotic aneurysms may develop. The brainstem can also be involved. VZV may infect any of

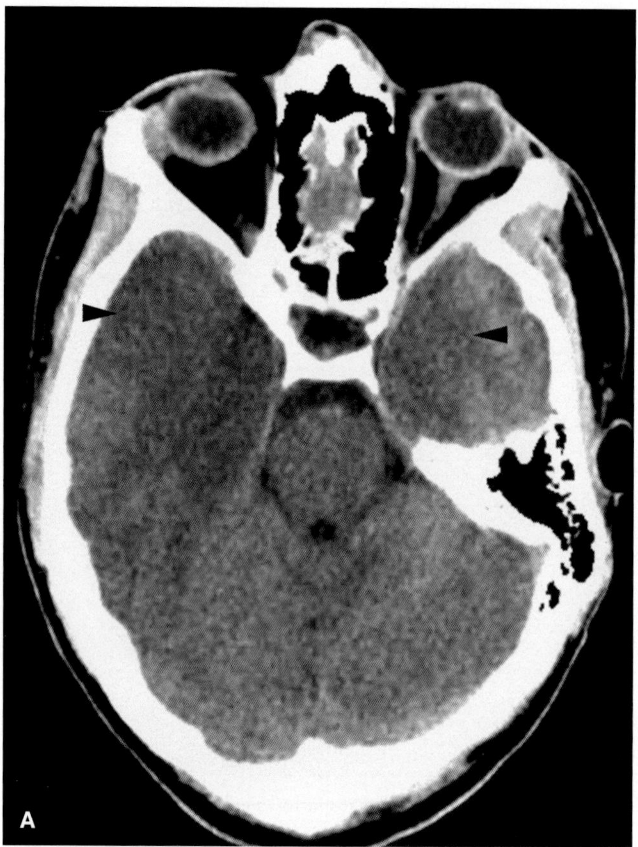

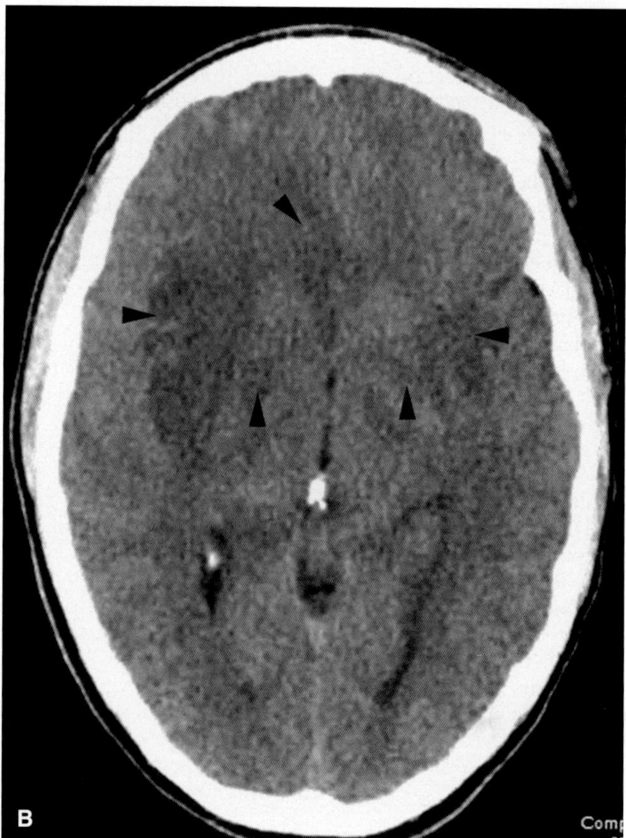

FIGURE 6.30. **Adult Herpes Simplex, Type 1, (HSV1) Encephalitis.** NECT images (**A, B**) demonstrate hypodensity and edema of both temporal and frontal lobes, perisylvian regions, and basal ganglia, right more than left (*black arrowheads*). The appearance is similar to cerebral infarcts, but the clinical presentation is usually distinct.

the cranial nerves, but CNs VII and VIII are most commonly involved and result in herpes zoster oticus (Ramsay Hunt syndrome). Clinically, there is ear pain and facial paralysis accompanied by a vesicular eruption about the ear. CT scans are usually normal but MRI of the internal auditory canals should reveal abnormal enhancement of one or both of these cranial nerves.

Cytomegalovirus encephalitis is unusual, except when encountered in congenital form (Fig. 6.1) or in immunosuppressed adult patients, especially those with AIDS. Both these presentations are described in other sections of this chapter.

Subacute sclerosing panencephalitis (SSPE) is a very rare condition caused by chronic infection by a variant of the measles virus. It typically presents in children and young adults with prior measles infection before the age of 2 years and after an intervening asymptomatic period of up to years. The disease causes progressive dementia, seizures, myoclonus and paralysis, and virtually always leads to death. There is no cure but if diagnosed early enough, lifelong treatment with antivirals and interferon may slow neurologic decline. CSF studies and EEG provide helpful diagnostic information. There is poor correlation between conventional MRI features and the four defined clinical stages of disease. Initial findings can often be normal but can reveal early asymmetric patchy or diffuse swelling with hypodensity and T2 hyperintensity of the cerebral white matter. Enhancement is usually absent. On DWI, inconsistent patterns of reduced diffusion involving cortex, white matter, corpus callosum, internal capsules, thalami, and brainstem have been documented in a small number of cases of early or rapidly progressive SSPE (Fig. 6.33). Other reports have correlated increased diffusion in cerebral white matter with the severity of later clinical stages. In the very late stages, profound cortical atrophy develops. Differential considerations include demyelination, progressive multifocal leukoencephalopathy (PML), and HIV encephalitis.

Encephalitis can be caused by a variety of viruses not already discussed, including EBV, enteroviruses, arboviruses, and mumps. In the United States, St. Louis, California, Western equine, and Eastern equine encephalitides are caused by arboviruses (insect borne) which preferentially affect the deep gray nuclei and brainstem. West Nile virus is a mosquito-borne arbovirus increasingly seen across the United States, which incites a meningoencephalitis of widely variable clinical severity. Japanese encephalitis is caused by a similar virus endemic in Asia. On neuroimaging, both West Nile and Japanese encephalitides can demonstrate symmetric swelling, hypodensity, and T2 hyperintensity of the thalami, basal ganglia, and brainstem (Fig. 6.34). Associated enhancement and reduced diffusion may also be observed. A similar pattern of injury with additional superimposed hemorrhage is seen in acute necrotizing encephalitis in children and has been associated with influenza A and B viruses. Rasmussen encephalitis is a devastating disease of childhood and of unknown etiology. Viral and/or autoimmune encephalitis are implicated. The clinical course is characterized by intractable seizures, progressive neurologic deficits, and frequently, coma. The disease usually affects one cerebral hemisphere. MR studies show focal

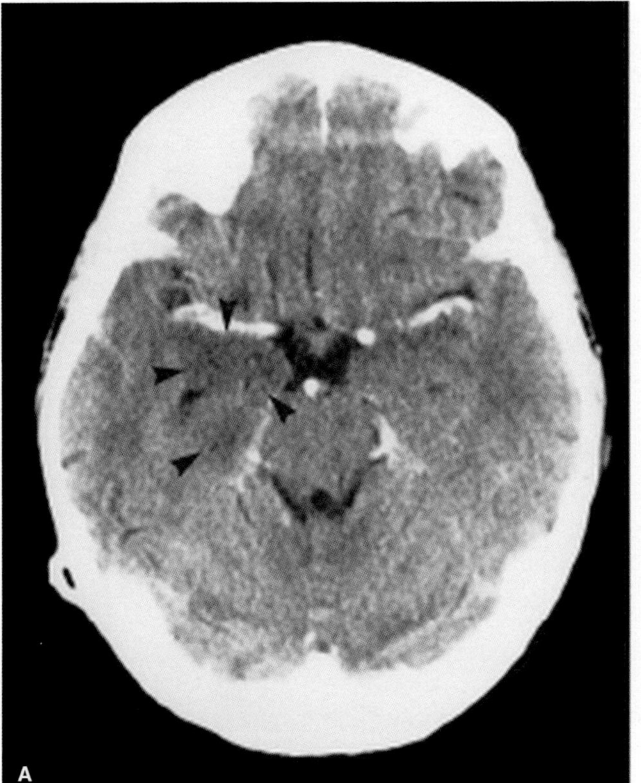

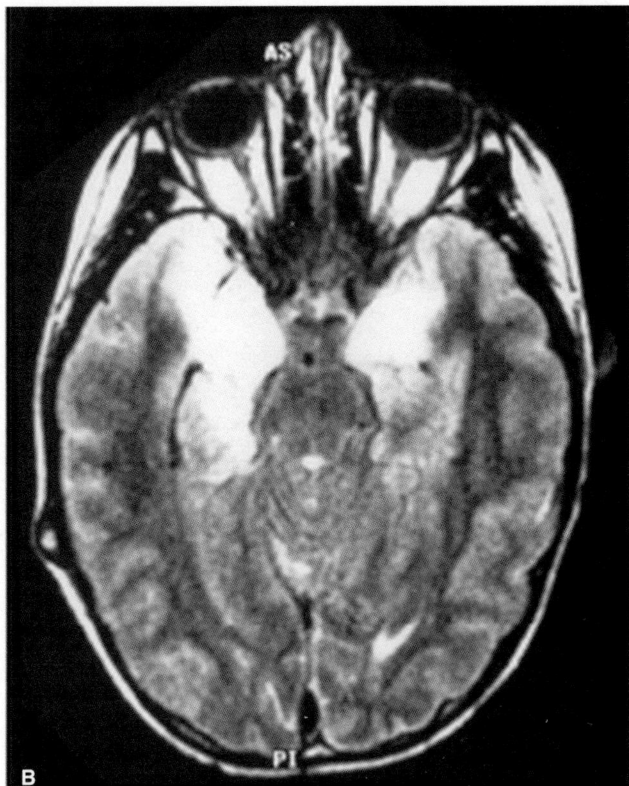

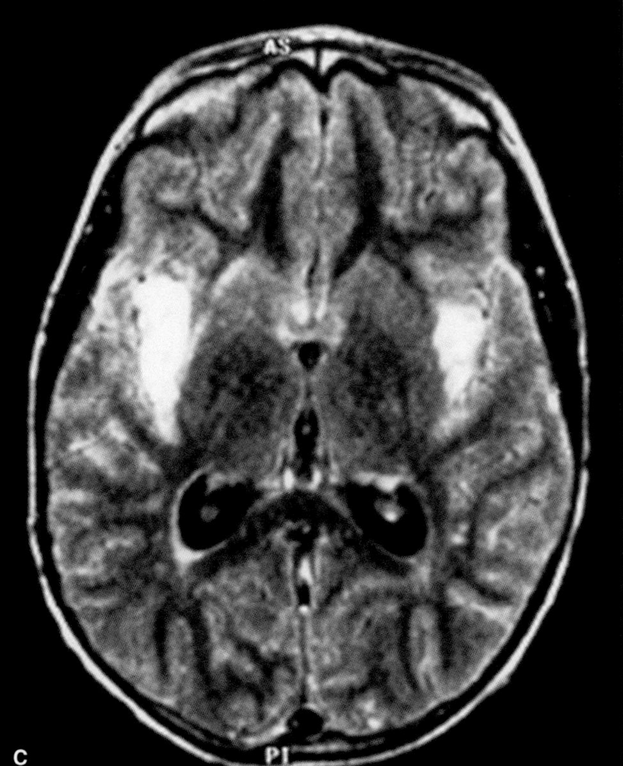

FIGURE 6.31. **HSV1 Encephalitis.** CECT scan (**A**) on this 8-year-old boy with decreased level of consciousness reveals subtle low density in the right temporal lobe (*arrowheads*). Transaxial FLAIR images (**B, C**) obtained on the same day show prominent areas of T2 hyperintensity in both temporal lobes with sparing of the putamina. This case illustrates why MRI is the imaging modality of choice when herpes encephalitis is suspected.

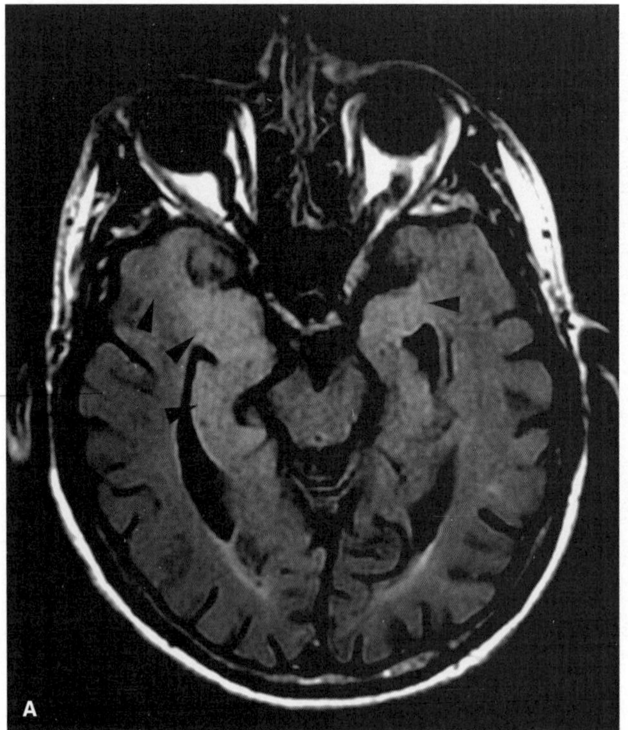

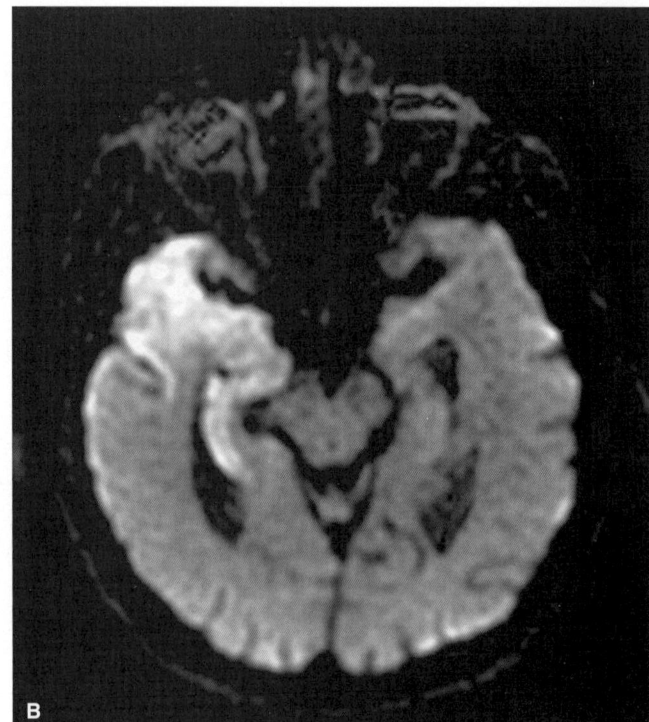

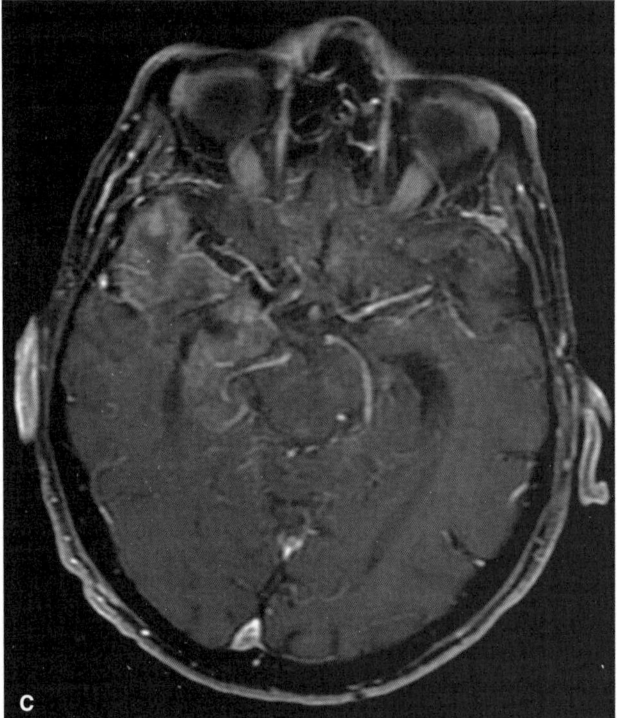

FIGURE 6.32. HSV1 Encephalitis. A: Transaxial FLAIR image of an 83-year-old patient who presented with altered mental status shows T2-hyperintense swelling of the anterior and medial right temporal lobe (including the hippocampus) and the left amygdala (*arrowheads*). **B:** DWI demonstrates corresponding reduced diffusion and hyperintensity of the right temporal lobe. **C:** Contrast-enhanced T1WI obtained 2 weeks later demonstrates development of gyral parenchymal enhancement of the right temporal lobe.

cortical swelling and T2 hyperintensity with minimal, if any, enhancement in the involved hemisphere early on, but these progress to dramatic asymmetric atrophy later. The affected hemisphere has been shown to be hypometabolic by SPECT and PET nuclear scans.

Nonviral pathogens, such as the bacteria *Rickettsia rickettsii* (Rocky Mountain spotted fever), *Listeria monocytogenes,* and *Mycoplasma pneumoniae* are rare causes of encephalitis. Listeria and Mycoplasma have a notable predilection for the brainstem and cerebellum, causing rhombencephalitis.

Cerebellitis is an uncommon infectious or inflammatory process primarily affecting the cerebelllar hemispheres in a symmetric or asymmetric pattern. Numerous associated viral infectious agents have been found including HSV1, VZV, EBV, CMV, human herpesvirus 6 (HHV-6), enteroviruses, measles, mumps, rubella, and influenza A. Bacterial pathogens, such as

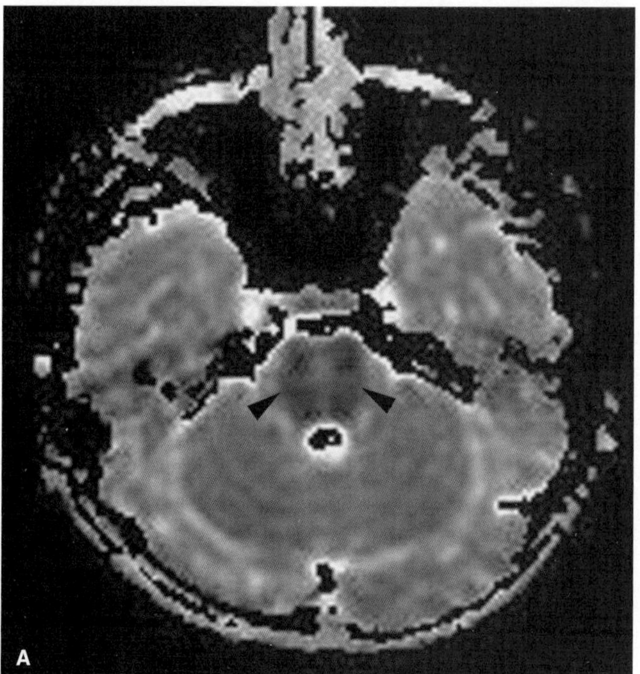

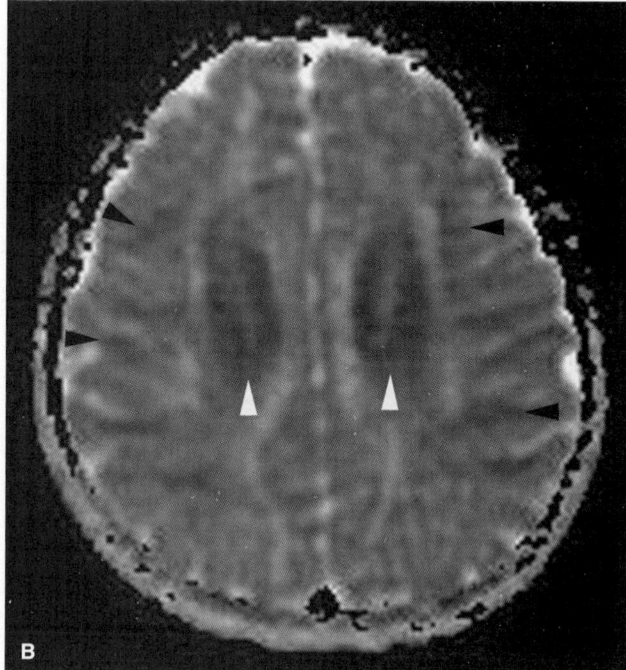

FIGURE 6.33. **Subacute Sclerosing Panencephalitis.** Transaxial apparent diffusion coefficient maps (**A, B**) show extensive symmetric hypointense areas of reduced diffusion in the bilateral pons, frontal and parietal gray–white matter junction and subcortical white matter (*black arrowheads*), and centrum semiovale (*white arrowheads*) at the initial presentation of this child with myoclonus and progressive dementia who was diagnosed with SSPE via serologic markers. On other MR images not shown, there were additional regions of reduced diffusion along the corona radiata, corpus callosum, internal capsules, and midbrain, but the remaining MRI sequences were normal.

Mycoplasma and Listeria, and Lyme disease have also been confirmed in patients with acute cerebellitis. Unfortunately, an etiologic agent is often not established in a large subset of these patients. Children are more commonly afflicted by cerebellitis and present with headaches, vomiting, ataxia, and other cerebellar signs. Hypodensity on CT and T2 hyperintensity on MRI correspond to bilateral or unilateral cerebellar edema and swelling, with occasional brainstem involvement (Fig. 6.35A,C). DWI usually demonstrates mildly increased diffusion (Fig. 6.35B) in contrast to reduced diffusion present in acute cerebellar infarction. Mild leptomeningeal and parenchymal enhancement is typically present (Fig. 6.35D). Mass effect and compression of the fourth ventricle and brainstem can lead to noncommunicating hydrocephalus. Differential diagnosis should include cerebellar infarcts, severe hypoxic–ischemic injury, acute disseminated encephalomyelitis, postvaccination inflammation, Lhermitte–Duclos disease (dysplastic cerebellar gangliocytoma), other neoplasms, or extremely rare toxic or metabolic injuries (e.g., carbon monoxide and mitochondrial disease).

Acute disseminated encephalomyelitis (ADEM) is an acute demyelinating disease that occurs most commonly after a recent viral illness or vaccination but sometimes spontaneously. Autoimmune demyelination is the currently accepted mechanism, and infectious pathogens have not been isolated. Acute symptoms include fever, headache, and meningismus. Seizures, focal neurologic deficits, and coma may develop. The mortality rate ranges between 10% and 20% but if treatment with steroids begins early, most patients make a full recovery. MRI is much more sensitive than CT in detecting the associated white matter lesions which are hypodense and T2 hyperintense and usually multiple (Fig. 6.36). The brainstem, cerebellum, deep gray nuclei, and gray–white matter interface can be involved. The pattern of enhancement is extremely variable. In the absence of gray matter involvement, the imaging appearance can be similar to multiple sclerosis, but patients are mostly children who suffer a monophasic clinical course. The lesions regress with successful treatment, correlating with clinical improvement. Acute hemorrhagic leukoencephalitis is a rare, severe variant of ADEM that is often fatal. The major imaging feature is a rapid progression of white matter lesions over the course of several days. Pathologically, there is perivascular hemorrhagic necrosis, primarily in the centrum semiovale.

Creutzfeldt–Jakob Disease

Creutzfeldt–Jakob disease (CJD) is a transmissible spongiform encephalopathy caused by an infectious proteinaceous particle or "prion." It is a rare, uniformly fatal, and rapidly progressive neurodegenerative disorder. Prions are protease-resistant particles resulting from altered conformation of a normal host cellular protein encoded by the PrP gene. Prions accumulate in the neural tissue and result in cell death. Patients initially present with variable neurologic signs but ultimately develop a rapidly progressive dementia with myoclonic jerks and akinetic mutism. Mortality within the first year has been reported to be >80%. Characteristic periodic sharp waves may be seen on EEG. The sporadic type (sCJD) is seen in the elderly worldwide. Iatrogenic CJD has been reported with prion transmission via neurosurgical tools, corneal transplants, and the use of cadaveric dura mater or pituitary extracts. Imaging with CT is not helpful and is usually normal or shows generalized cerebral volume loss. DWI and FLAIR sequences are most if these patients undergo MRI. Both sequences can demonstrate hyperintensity in the striatum

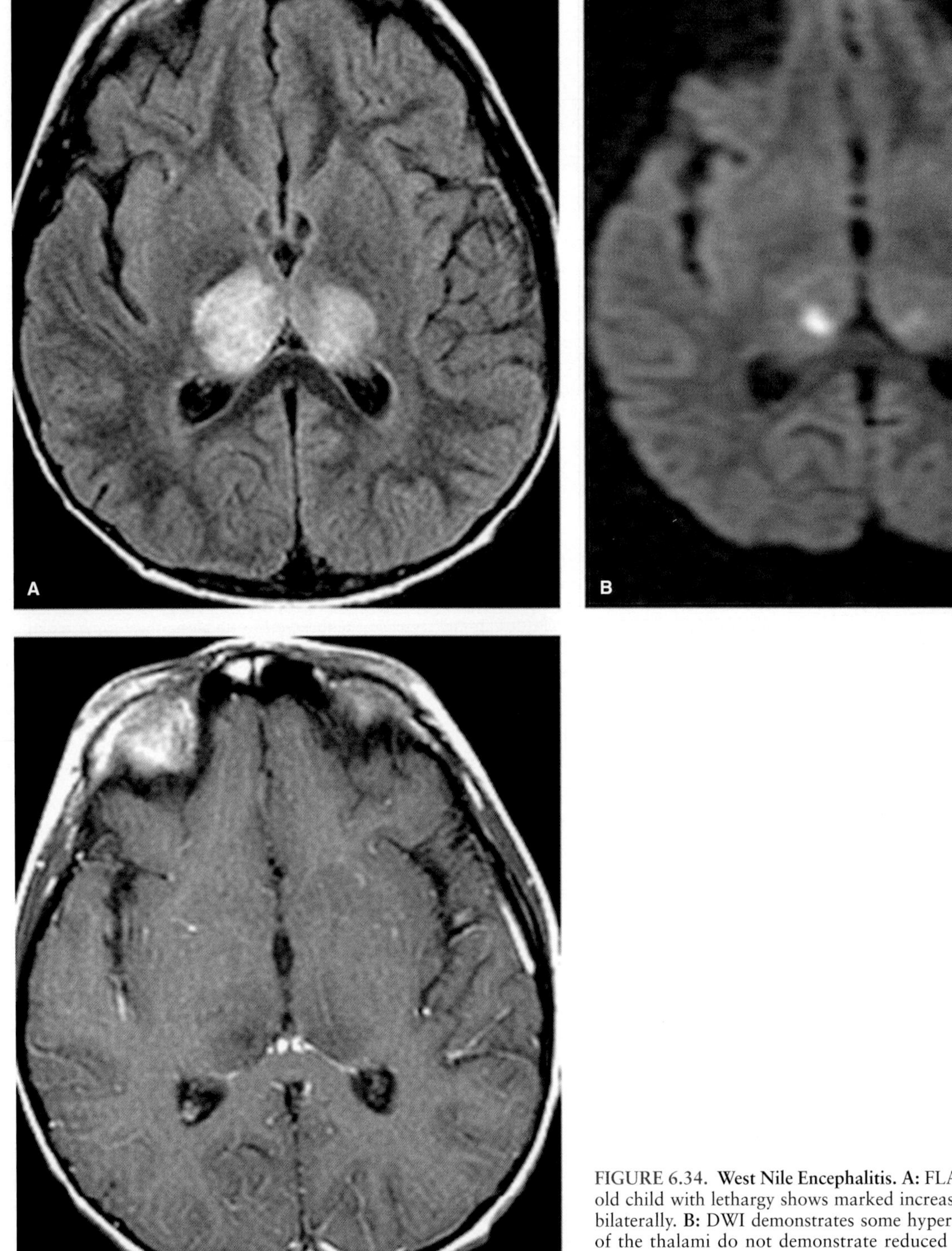

FIGURE 6.34. **West Nile Encephalitis. A:** FLAIR image in this 7-year-old child with lethargy shows marked increased signal in the thalami bilaterally. **B:** DWI demonstrates some hyperintense signal, but most of the thalami do not demonstrate reduced diffusion. **C:** Contrast-enhanced T1WI shows no abnormal contrast. CSF studies were positive for the virus that causes West Nile fever.

(caudate and putaminal nuclei) symmetrically and/or subtle ribbon-like hyperintensity in scattered areas of the cerebral cortex in early cases (Fig. 6.37). These features and cerebral atrophy become more apparent as the patient declines. Lack of enhancement is the rule.

New variant Creutzfeldt–Jakob disease (nvCJD) is linked to bovine spongiform encephalopathy whereby prions are transmitted to humans who eat the meat of infected cows. Patients with nvCJD are generally younger than those with sCJD and most cases have been seen in the United Kingdom. Although the other clinical features are similar to sCJD, MRI shows different findings of symmetric T2 hyperintensity in the posterior and dorsomedial aspects of the thalamic nuclei (i.e., the pulvinar and "hockey-stick" signs). Differential diagnosis

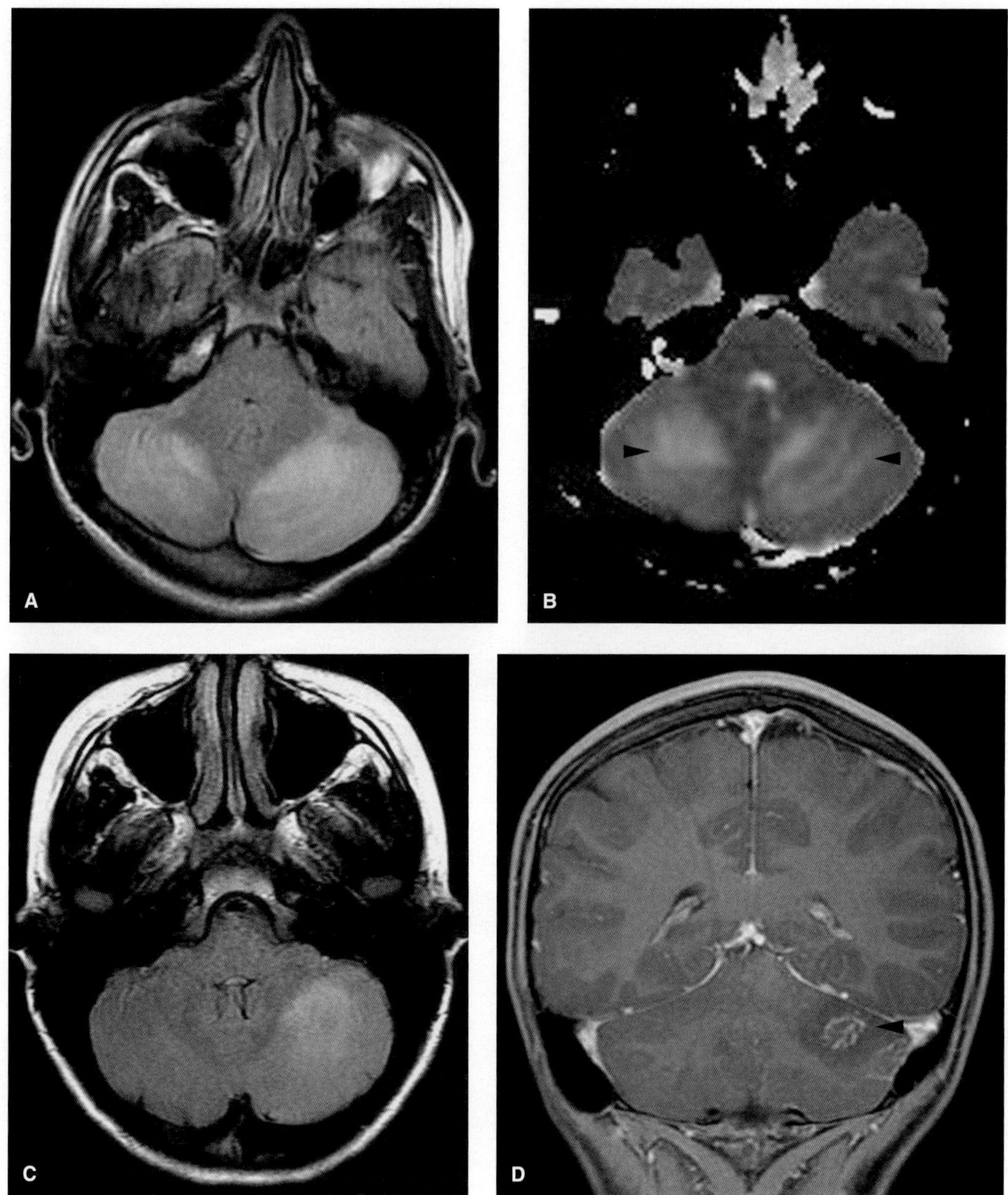

FIGURE 6.35. **Cerebellitis. A:** Transaxial FLAIR image in a child who presented with headaches and vomiting following a viral illness. Significant T2-hyperintense edema and swelling of the bilateral cerebellar hemispheres are depicted. **B:** Apparent diffusion coefficient map shows corresponding hyperintense increased diffusion (*black arrowheads*). No causative infectious pathogen was identified. **C:** Transaxial FLAIR image in a different child with Mycoplasma infection. Asymmetric unilateral T2-hyperintense edema of the left cerebellum. **D:** Contrast-enhanced coronal T1WI shows associated leptomeningeal and parenchymal enhancement (*black arrowhead*).

for CJD includes hypoxic–ischemic encephalopathy, metabolic or toxic injury, or encephalitis.

ACQUIRED IMMUNODEFICIENCY SYNDROME–RELATED INFECTIONS

The CNS is a common site of involvement in patients with AIDS. The incidence of CNS involvement has declined since the introduction of highly active antiretroviral therapy (HAART), yet up to two-thirds of AIDS patients still develop some form of CNS disease. A variety of infections and neoplasms may be diagnosed in these patients. The most common infections include: HIV encephalopathy; toxoplasmosis, cryptococcosis, and other fungal infections; CMV and herpes encephalitis; mycobacterial infection; PML; and meningovascular syphilis. Primary CNS lymphoma is by far the most common tumor, but metastatic lymphoma, gliomas, and rarely, Kaposi sarcoma may also occur.

HIV Encephalopathy. HIV is the etiologic agent in AIDS and primarily infects CD4 lymphocytes but has also been shown to be neurotropic. The virus is found in the brains of up to

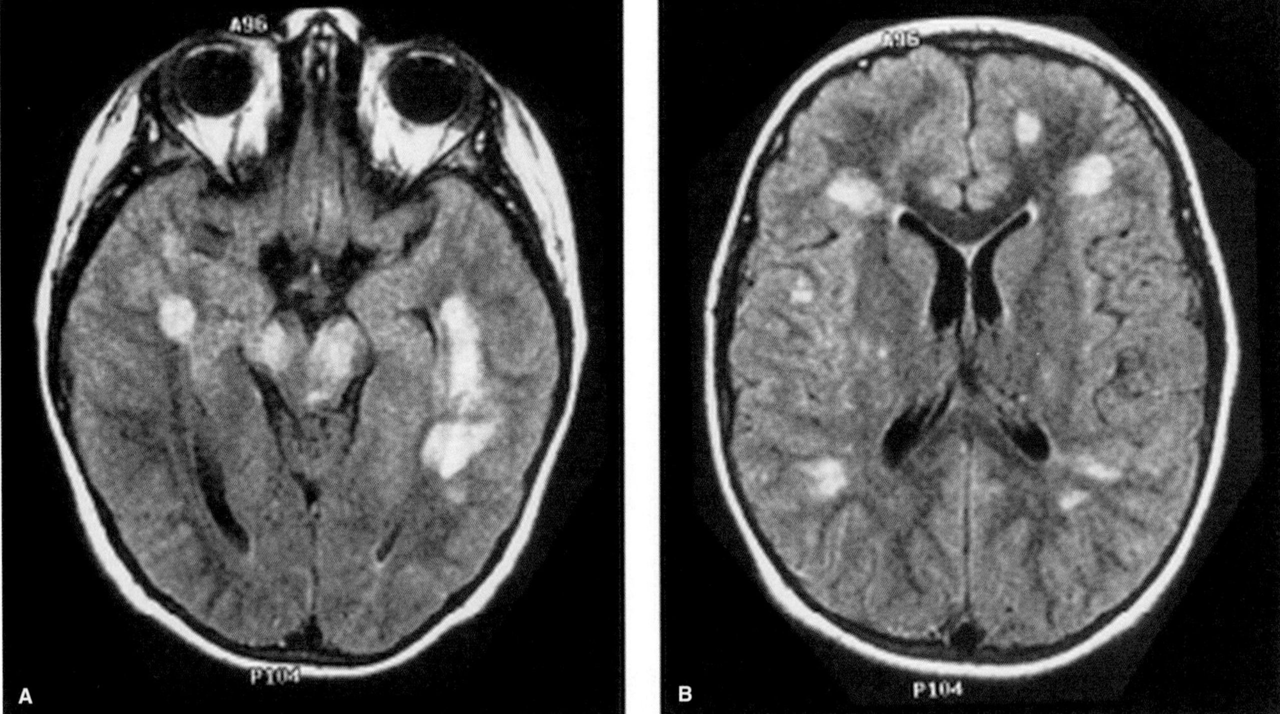

FIGURE 6.36. **Acute Disseminated Encephalomyelitis (ADEM).** Transaxial FLAIR scans (**A, B**) show multiple areas of high signal intensity in the cerebral white matter and midbrain. FLAIR sequences are extremely sensitive for detecting white matter lesions. This 8-year-old child recovered fully after steroid therapy.

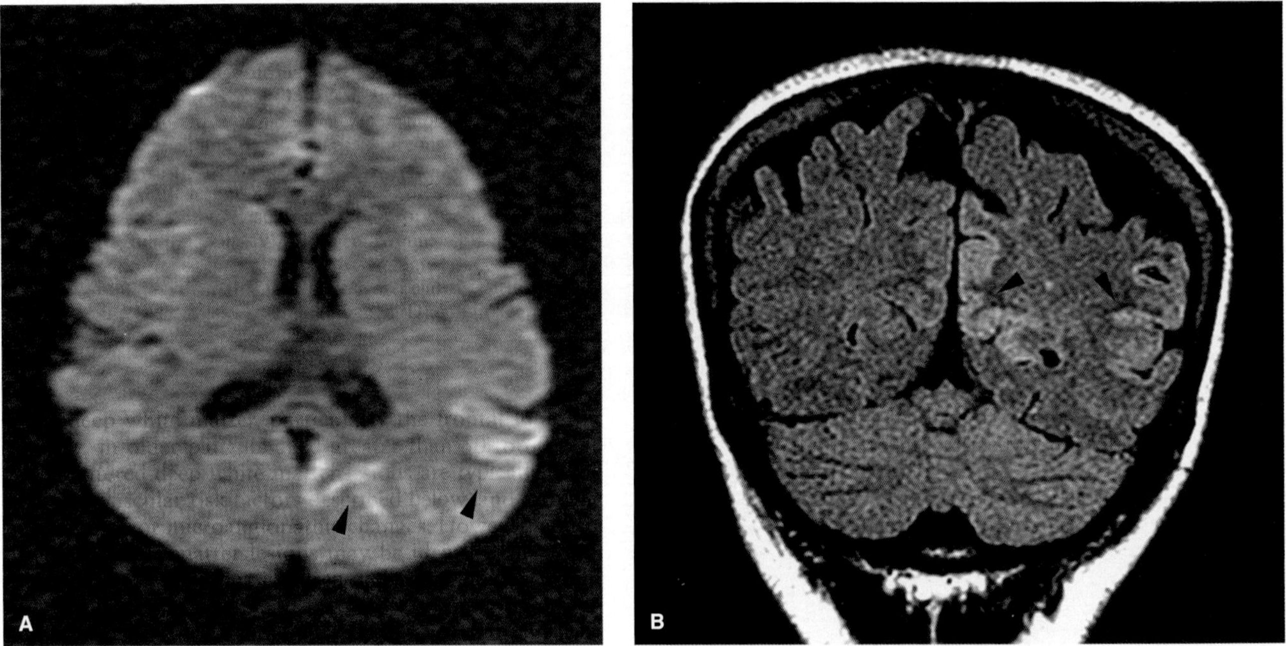

FIGURE 6.37. **Sporadic Creutzfeldt–Jakob Disease. A:** Transaxial DWI in this 41-year-old patient with progressive memory loss demonstrates ribbon-like cortical hyperintensity and reduced diffusion along the left occipital and parietal lobes (*arrowheads*). **B:** Coronal FLAIR image shows corresponding cortical T2 hyperintensity.

90% of AIDS patients at autopsy. Clinical symptoms of brain involvement by HIV occur in a minority of these patients. Primary HIV infection of the brain results in vacuolation of the white matter, with areas of demyelination and multinucleated giant cells. The centrum semiovale is most severely involved, but all white matter tracts, including the brainstem and cerebellum, may be affected. The cortical gray matter is usually spared. Clinically, patients with HIV encephalitis may develop a subcortical dementia with cognitive, behavioral, and motor deterioration. This is known as AIDS dementia complex (ADC) in adults, which is seen in 5% to 30% of various groups of AIDS patients depending on the availability of HAART. On the other hand, HIV-associated progressive encephalopathy (HPE) is used to describe infants and children with HIV encephalitis who exhibit loss of developmental milestones, apathy, failure of brain growth and myelination, and spastic paraparesis. Children with HPE exhibit less frequent CNS opportunistic infections and neoplasms compared to adults with ADC.

Diffuse atrophy is the most common manifestation of HIV infection of the brain on neuroimaging studies (Fig. 6.38). This is largely central atrophy, reflecting the predominant white matter involvement. White matter lesions are also commonly seen in patients with ADC. MRI is significantly more sensitive than CT for detecting these abnormalities. A diffuse, symmetric, ill-defined, often hazy pattern of T2 hyperintensity in the deep and periventricular white matter or multiple small T2-hyperintense white matter lesions are the most common findings. The punctate lesions do not correlate well with symptoms. No mass effect or abnormal contrast enhancement should be seen. The most advanced cases of HIV encephalopathy show extensive bilateral areas of abnormal T2 signal intensity throughout the periventricular white matter, brainstem, and cerebellum (Fig. 6.39). Congenital HIV infection has been described previously. In young children with HIV encephalitis, generalized atrophy and symmetric calcifications in the basal ganglia are the most common observations. White matter hypodensity and T2 hyperintensity are also sometimes seen. These imaging abnormalities often regress if the patient responds clinically to treatment with HAART. Differential diagnosis includes CMV, HSV encephalitis, or PML.

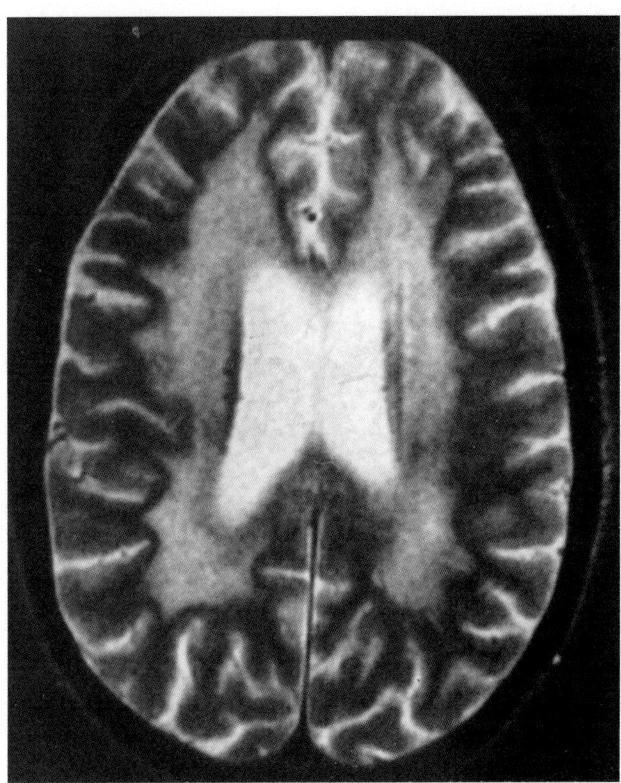

FIGURE 6.39. HIV Encephalopathy. This young patient clinically had AIDS dementia complex. T2WI shows cerebral atrophy with widespread abnormal high signal in the periventricular white matter.

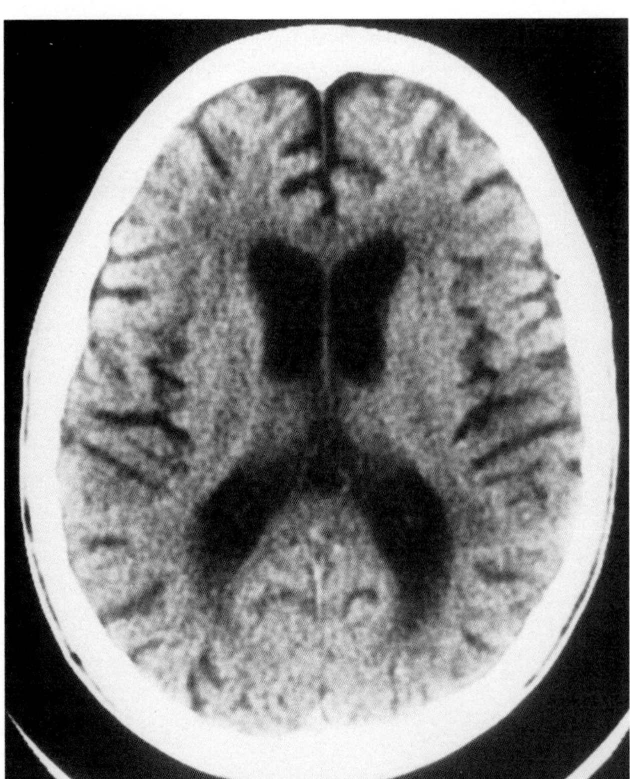

FIGURE 6.38. AIDS-Related Atrophy. NECT scan reveals enlarged ventricles and sulci in this 24-year-old patient with AIDS. This is the most common abnormality found on brain imaging of patients with AIDS. It often correlates with AIDS dementia complex.

Toxoplasmosis is the most common opportunistic CNS infection and brain mass in AIDS patients, occurring in about 13% to 33% of these patients with CNS complications. It occurs in patients with CD4 lymphocyte counts <200 cells/mm^3. *T. gondii,* a protozoan, which is ubiquitous throughout the world and causes subclinical or mild infection in a large percentage of the population. In AIDS, CNS toxoplasmosis results from reactivation of the previously acquired infection. A necrotizing encephalitis usually results with the formation of thin-walled abscesses. Patients present with headache, fever, lethargy, diminished level of consciousness, and focal neurologic deficits, which initially can be confused clinically with the subacute encephalitis of primary HIV infection. Early neuroimaging is therefore important in patient management.

The typical imaging appearance of CNS toxoplasmosis is that of multiple enhancing parenchymal lesions with surrounding vasogenic edema (Figs. 6.40 and 6.41). The lesions are usually relatively small, ranging between 1 and 4 cm in diameter, and exhibit surrounding vasogenic edema often with mass effect. The lesions are hypodense on CT and T1 hypointense on MRI but may have a variable but typically hyperintense signal on T2WI and DWI. Larger lesions usually exhibit ring-like enhancement, while smaller lesions usually enhance solidly. The basal ganglia are a favored site, but white

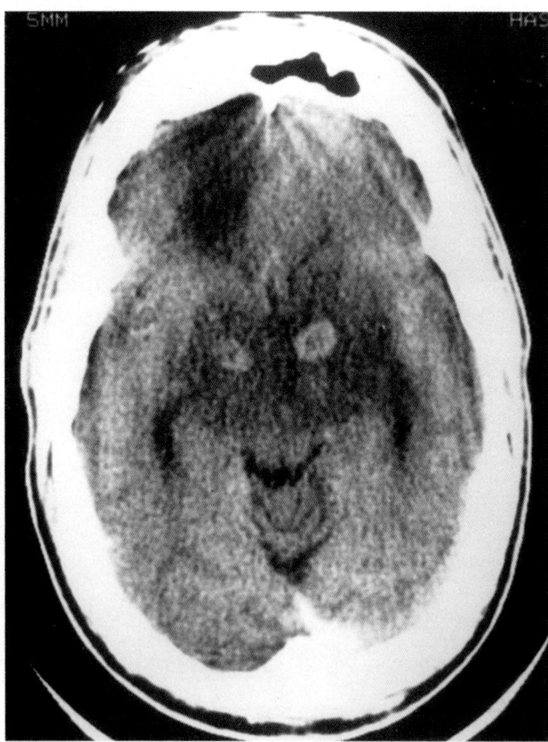

FIGURE 6.40. **Toxoplasmosis.** CECT scan reveals bilateral ring-enhancing lesions in the basal ganglia of this patient with AIDS. There is marked surrounding hypodense edema. The basal ganglia are commonly affected by toxoplasmosis.

matter and cortical lesions are also common. The main differential consideration is primary CNS lymphoma, which will be discussed later. A clinical and imaging response to appropriate antibiotics should distinguish between toxoplasmosis and lymphoma in most cases (Fig. 6.41). Biopsy is considered for atypical cases or when there is no response to antibiotics. Residual calcifications may develop after successful treatment. Other infections or neoplasms which can mimic toxoplasmosis are unusual. Fungal, mycobacterial, and amebic abscesses do occur but bacterial abscesses are rare in AIDS patients.

Fungal Meningitis. Although fungal abscesses and granulomas are unusual, fungal meningitis is a common complication of AIDS occurring in 5% to 15% of patients. CNS cryptococcosis has been discussed previously and is the most common fungal CNS infection in HIV-positive patients. The diagnosis is made when the cryptococcal antigen (CrAg) is detected in serum or CSF. Meningitis is the most frequent presentation but usually mild because of the impaired inflammatory response of the immunocompromised host. As a result, minimal if any meningeal or ependymal enhancement can be seen on neuroimaging studies but hydrocephalus is not uncommon. Cryptococcal gelatinous pseudocysts are particular lesions usually found only in immunocompromised patients, especially AIDS patients (see Fig. 6.42). These are cystic lesions, usually in the basal ganglia where the organism and mucinous deposits have extended beyond the perivascular spaces into the surrounding brain substance. On CT, gelatinous pseudocysts are smooth, round, low-density masses with no contrast enhancement and can mimic old lacunar infarcts. They are better seen with MRI where the lesions are almost isointense or hypointense on T1WI and hyperintense on T2WI with CSF. Mild peripheral edema and enhancement may be present on MRI but almost

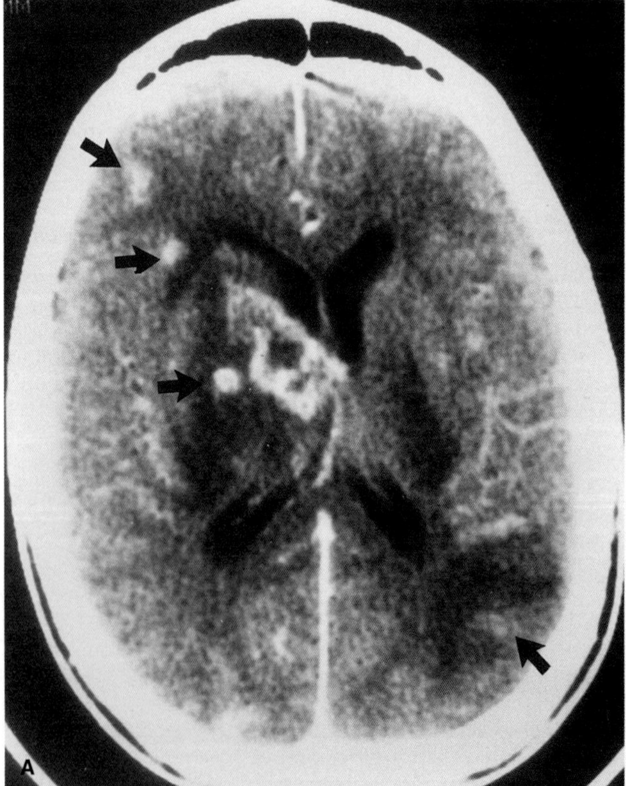

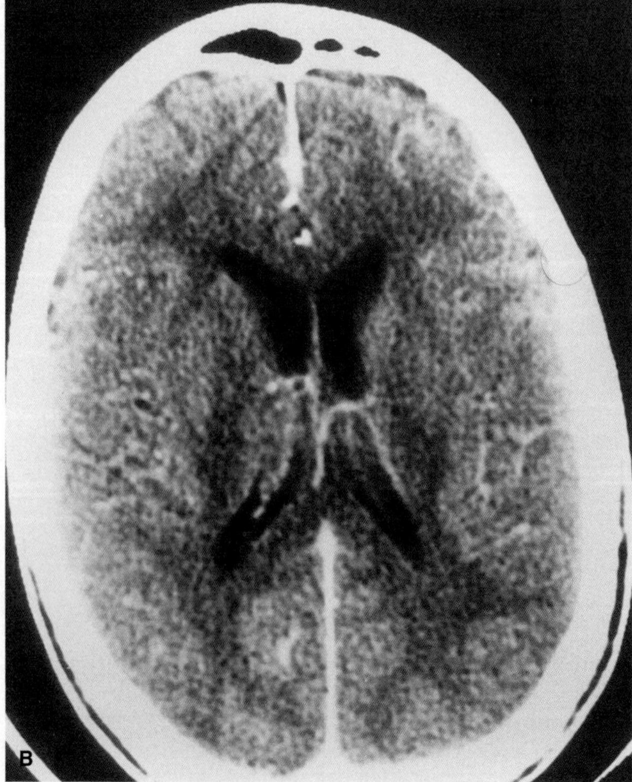

FIGURE 6.41. **Toxoplasmosis. A:** CECT scan shows a large enhancing mass in the right basal ganglia and several other small enhancing lesions (*arrows*). The small size and multiplicity of the lesions favor toxoplasmosis over lymphoma. **B:** Following 2 weeks of antibiotic therapy, CECT scan reveals complete resolution of the lesions, typical for toxoplasmosis.

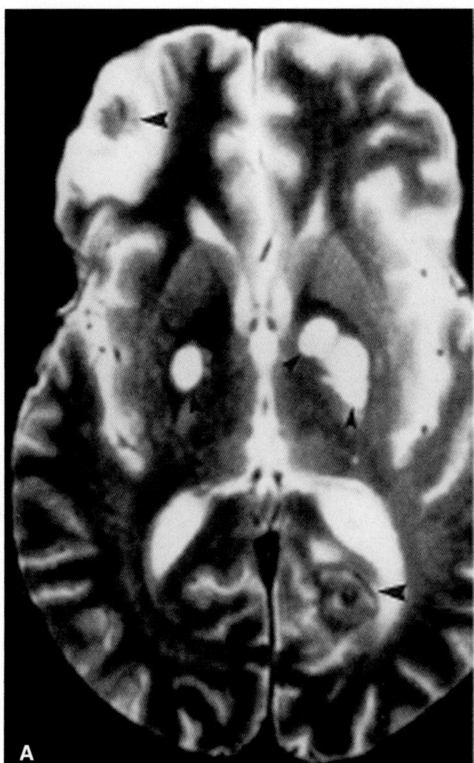

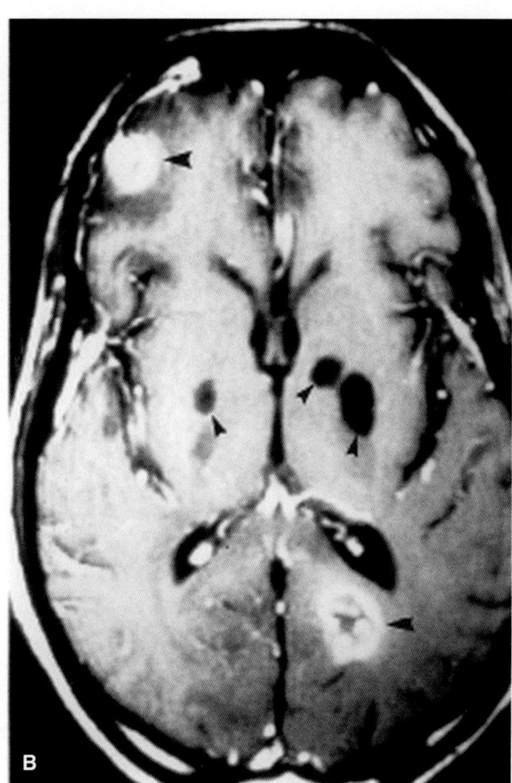

FIGURE 6.42. **Cryptococcosis and Toxoplasmosis. A:** Transaxial T2WI reveals multiple rounded lesions that are isointense to CSF in the basal ganglia (*small arrowheads*). There is no surrounding edema. Darker lesions with surrounding edema are present in the right frontal and left occipital lobes (*large arrowheads*). **B:** Contrast-enhanced T1WI again reveals the basal ganglia lesions to be isointense with CSF (*small arrowheads*). There is no contrast enhancement. The appearance of these lesions is typical of gelatinous pseudocysts of cryptococcosis. These lesions represent dilated perivascular spaces filled with cryptococcus organisms and mucin. The right frontal and left occipital lesions do enhance with contrast (*large arrowheads*) as is typical of toxoplasmosis.

never to the degree seen with toxoplasmosis. Enhancing cryptococcomas are rather unusual in AIDS patients.

Progressive multifocal leukoencephalopathy (PML) is an infection of immunosuppressed patients caused by reactivation of the latent JC polyomavirus ("JC" being the initials of the patient in whom the virus was first described). The incidence of PML in AIDS patients is up to 8% but has decreased in the setting of HAART. It can also occur in other immunosuppressed patients such as transplant recipients and those with leukemia, lymphoma, or congenital immunodeficiencies. It does not occur in patients with normal immunity. It has also been described in multiple sclerosis patients being treated with the monoclonal antibody natalizumab which inhibits lymphocyte migration across the blood–brain barrier. The infection causes multifocal demyelination and necrosis, primarily involving the white matter. Clinical signs include changes in mental status, blindness, aphasia, hemiparesis, ataxia, and other focal neurologic deficits. There is a >90% mortality within 1 year of diagnosis. HAART significantly prolongs survival but can be associated with worsening brain damage by precipitating immune reconstitution inflammatory syndrome (IRIS). AIDS patients with PML usually have CD4 counts <200 cells/mm^3. Routine CSF studies are often normal. A positive CSF PCR result and compatible clinical and appropriate neuroimaging features are used for diagnosis. CT shows one or more hypodense lesions, usually asymmetrically distributed, within the subcortical and deep white matter. On MRI, these exhibit decreased signal intensity on T1WI and increased signal on T2WI, FLAIR, and DWI sequences (Fig. 6.43). The lesions may be solitary or multifocal. Mass effect and contrast enhancement are almost always absent, which are very important distinguishing features. Rarely, both gray and white matter or the basal ganglia are involved, simulating an infarct. The main differential diagnosis in the setting of AIDS is HIV encephalitis which is usually more diffuse, symmetric, and less T2 hyperintense on MRI and does not extend to the gray–white matter junction.

Viral Infection. CMV infection is a common CNS infection in AIDS patients pathologically but does not usually result in frank tissue necrosis and is usually subclinical. There are many cases of pathologically proven CMV brain infection with normal CT and MR scans. CMV meningoencephalitis is occasionally imaged as areas of hyperintensity on T2WI in the immediate periventricular white matter. Subependymal contrast enhancement, if present, is a valuable diagnostic sign. CMV will very rarely present as a ring-enhancing mass. Herpes simplex and varicella viral infections are also only occasionally imaged. Their more benign clinical course and imaging appearance in AIDS may be due to a diminished immune response causing less brain damage.

Intracranial mycobacterial infections occur in a relatively small percentage of AIDS patients. Most of these patients are intravenous drug abusers with pulmonary tuberculosis. Chest radiographs are positive in about 65% of cases. There is a very high mortality rate (nearly 80%) in these patients. CNS infection with *M. avium-intracellulare* is much rarer. Most patients present with meningitis. Imaging studies in these patients reveal communicating hydrocephalus and/or meningeal enhancement.

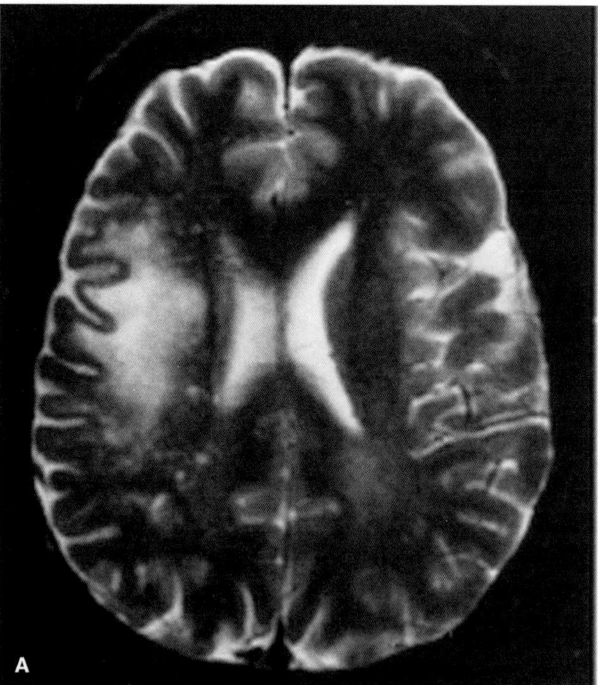

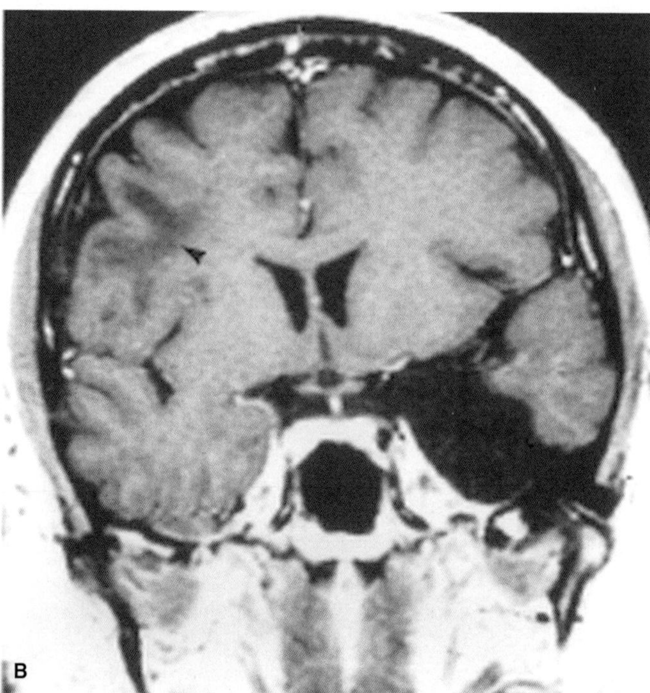

FIGURE 6.43. Progressive Multifocal Leukoencephalopathy (PML). A: Transaxial T2WI demonstrates an area of abnormal hyperintensity in the right corona radiata. There is no significant mass effect. **B:** Contrast-enhanced T1WI shows the lesion to be of low signal intensity (*arrowhead*) and without enhancement. These are typical features of PML, which was proven by biopsy in this patient with AIDS. Incidentally, a left temporal arachnoid cyst can be noted.

Tuberculomas occur in about 25% of patients with HIV-related CNS tuberculosis. AIDS patients have a higher vulnerability for developing tuberculous abscesses than other patients, but these are still seen less frequently than tuberculomas. Tuberculomas are usually smaller and have less edema than tuberculous abscesses.

Primary CNS lymphoma is by far the most common intracranial neoplasm in patients with AIDS. Up to 5% of AIDS patients will develop this tumor but the incidence has subsided with the availability of HAART. It is the main differential diagnostic consideration along with CNS toxoplasmosis when a mass lesion is found in an AIDS patient. Toxoplasmosis is more common than lymphoma and responds to antibiotic therapy. As with toxoplasmosis, these patients present with symptoms of a space-occupying intracranial lesion. Solitary or multiple enhancing mass lesions are found with neuroimaging studies (Fig. 6.44). The lesions are usually centrally located within the deep white matter or basal ganglia, but cortical lesions occur occasionally. There may be subependymal spread or extension across the corpus callosum, which do not usually occur with toxoplasmosis. With CT, the lesions are often isodense or hyperdense compared with white matter. With MRI, there is variable signal intensity which can be isointense or hypointense on T1WI and hypointense or hyperintense on T2WI and FLAIR sequences. The lesions almost always enhance with contrast in either a ring or solid pattern. The imaging appearance is often indistinguishable from that of toxoplasmosis but the size and number of lesions can be helpful. Toxoplasmosis is more frequently multiple, and the lesions are usually smaller than with lymphoma. Lymphoma is favored if lesions demonstrate T2 hypointensity coupled with diffuse, homogeneous contrast enhancement on MRI. Central T2 hyperintensity, a T2-hypointense rim, and ring-like contrast enhancement favor toxoplasmosis. Lymphoma more commonly demonstrates associated reduced diffusion

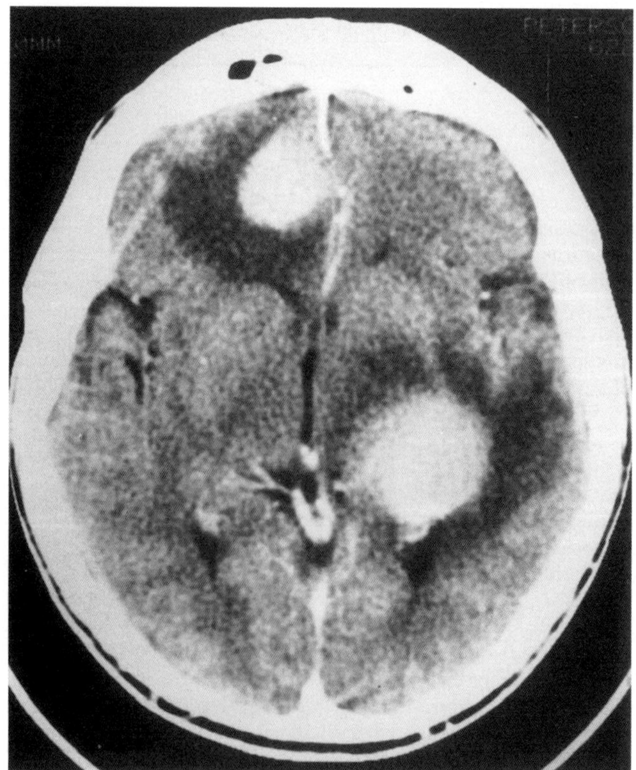

FIGURE 6.44. Primary CNS Lymphoma. CECT scan of a patient with AIDS shows two solidly enhancing masses with surrounding vasogenic edema. The relatively large size and solid enhancement pattern are more compatible with lymphoma than toxoplasmosis, as was proven in this case.

and hyperintensity on DWI, presumably due to hypercellularity. MRS shows increased choline and decreased N-acetyl aspartate (NAA) with lymphoma, while toxoplasmosis shows decreased choline and NAA with increased lipid and lactate.

Suggested Readings

Barkovich AJ, Lindan CE. Congenital cytomegalovirus infection of the brain: imaging analysis and embryologic considerations. *AJNR Am J Neuroradiol* 1994;15(4):703–715.

Becker LE. Infections of the developing brain. *AJNR Am J Neuroradiol* 1992;13(2):537–549.

Boesch C, Issakainen J, Kewitz G, Kikinis R, Martin E, Boltshauser E. Magnetic resonance imaging of the brain in congenital cytomegalovirus infection. *Pediatr Radiol* 1989;19(2):91–93.

Brightbill TC, Ihmeidan IH, Post MJ, Berger JR, Katz DA. Neurosyphilis in HIV-positive and HIV-negative patients: neuroimaging findings. *AJNR Am J Neuroradiol* 1995;16(4):703–711.

Collie DA, Summers DM, Ironside JW, et al. Diagnosing variant Creutzfeldt-Jakob disease with the pulvinar sign: MR imaging findings in 86 neuropathologically confirmed cases. *AJNR Am J Neuroradiol* 2003;24(8):1560–1569.

Dumas JL, Visy JM, Belin C, Gaston A, Goldlust D, Dumas M. Parenchymal neurocysticercosis: follow-up and staging by MRI. *Neuroradiology* 1997;39(1):12–18.

Garrels K, Kucharczyk W, Wortzman G, Shandling M. Progressive multifocal leukoencephalopathy: clinical and MR response to treatment. *AJNR Am J Neuroradiol.* 1996;17(3):597–600.

Kanamalla US, Ibarra RA, Jinkins JR. Imaging of cranial meningitis and ventriculitis. *Neuroimaging Clin N Am* 2000;10(2):309–331.

Kauffman WM, Sivit CJ, Fitz CR, Rakusan TA, Herzog K, Chandra RS. CT and MR evaluation of intracranial involvement in pediatric HIV infection: a clinical-imaging correlation. *AJNR Am J Neuroradiol* 1992;13(3):949–957.

Küker W, Mader I, Nägele T, et al. Progressive multifocal leukoencephalopathy: value of diffusion-weighted and contrast-enhanced magnetic resonance imaging for diagnosis and treatment control. *Eur J Neurol* 2006;13(8):819–826.

Küker W, Nägele T, Schmidt F, Heckl S, Herrlinger U. Diffusion-weighted MRI in herpes simplex encephalitis: a report of three cases. *Neuroradiology* 2004;46(2):122–125.

Lai PH, Ho JT, Chen WL, et al. Brain abscess and necrotic brain tumor: discrimination with proton MR spectroscopy and diffusion-weighted imaging. *AJNR Am J Neuroradiol* 2002;23(8):1369–1377.

Lim CC, Sitoh YY, Hui F, et al. Nipah viral encephalitis or Japanese encephalitis? MR findings in a new zoonotic disease. *AJNR Am J Neuroradiol* 2000;21(3):455–461.

Mader I, Stock KW, Ettlin T, Probst A. Acute disseminated encephalomyelitis: MR and CT features. *AJNR Am J Neuroradiol* 1996;17(1):104–109.

Mishra AM, Gupta RK, Jaggi RS, et al. Role of diffusion-weighted imaging and in vivo proton magnetic resonance spectroscopy in the differential diagnosis of ring-enhancing intracranial cystic mass lesions. *J Comput Assist Tomogr* 2004;28(4):540–547.

Post MJ, Hensley GT, Moskowitz LB, Fischl M. Cytomegalic inclusion virus encephalitis in patients with AIDS: CT, clinical, and pathologic correlation. *AJR Am J Roentgenol* 1986;146(6):1229–1234.

Rafto SE, Milton WJ, Galetta SL, Grossman RI. Biopsy-confirmed CNS Lyme disease: MR appearance at 1.5 T. *AJNR Am J Neuroradiol* 1990;11(3):482–484.

Rosas H, Wippold FJ 2nd. West Nile virus: case report with MR imaging findings. *AJNR Am J Neuroradiol* 2003;24(7):1376–1378.

Sibtain NA, Chinn RJS. Imaging of the central nervous system in HIV infection. *Imaging* 2002;14:48–59.

Soares de Oliveira-Szejnfeld P, Levine D, Melo AS, et al. Congenital brain abnormalities and Zika virus: what the radiologist can expect to see prenatally and postnatally. *Radiology* 2016;281(1):203–218.

Stadnik TW, Demaerel P, Luypaert RR, et al. Imaging tutorial: differential diagnosis of bright lesions on diffusion-weighted MR images. *Radiographics* 2003;23(1):e7.

Thurnher MM, Schindler EG, Thurnher SA, Pernerstorfer-Schon H, Kleibl-Popov C, Rieger A. Highly active antiretroviral therapy for patients with AIDS dementia complex: effect on MR imaging findings and clinical course. *AJNR Am J Neuroradiol* 2000;21(4):670–678.

Tien RD, Chu PK, Hesselink JR, Duberg A, Wiley C. Intracranial cryptococcosis in immunocompromised patients: CT and MR findings in 29 cases. *AJNR Am J Neuroradiol* 1991;12(2):283–289.

Tien RD, Felsberg GJ, Osumi AK. Herpesvirus infections of the CNS: MR findings. *AJR Am J Roentgenol* 1993;161(1):167–176.

Ukisu R, Kushihashi T, Kitanosono T, et al. Serial diffusion-weighted MRI of Creutzfeldt-Jakob disease. *AJR Am J Roentgenol* 2005;184(2):560–566.

Wada R, Kucharczyk W. Prion infections of the brain. *Neuroimaging Clin N Am* 2008;18(1):183–191.

Wasay M, Kheleani BA, Moolani MK, et al. Brain CT and MRI findings in 100 consecutive patients with intracranial tuberculoma. *J Neuroimaging* 2003;13(3):240–247.

Whiteman M, Espinoza L, Post MJ, Bell MD, Falcone S. Central nervous system tuberculosis in HIV-infected patients: clinical and radiographic findings. *AJNR Am J Neuroradiol* 1995;16(6):1319–1327.

Wong AM, Zimmerman RA, Simon EM, Pollock AN, Bilaniuk LT. Diffusion-weighted MR imaging of subdural empyemas in children. *AJNR Am J Neuroradiol* 2004;25(6):1016–1021.

CHAPTER 7 ■ WHITE MATTER AND NEURODEGENERATIVE DISEASES

JEROME A. BARAKOS AND DEREK D. PURCELL

In contrast to gray matter, which contains neuronal cell bodies, white matter is composed of the long processes of these neurons. The axonal processes are wrapped by myelin sheaths, and it is the lipid composition of these sheaths for which white matter is named. In this chapter, a host of diseases characterized by the involvement of white matter are described. This is followed by a discussion of hydrocephalus and neurodegenerative disorders.

The marked sensitivity of T2-weighted images (T2WI) in the detection of pathologic water (edema) and scarring (gliosis), allows white matter lesions to be readily detected, providing high sensitivity to lesion detection. However, the difficulty confronting the radiologist is that a wide gamut of diseases may involve the white matter, and thus white matter lesions are often nonspecific in nature, that is, low specificity. The specificity of lesion characterization arises when combining an understanding of various white matter diseases and their corresponding clinical features with lesion morphology and anatomic distribution. This combination of clinical information and imaging data is the cornerstone of what enables the radiologist to generate an accurate and meaningful differential diagnostic list.

Cerebral white matter diseases are classified into two broad categories: demyelinating and dysmyelinating. *Demyelination* is an acquired disorder that affects normal myelin. The vast majority of white matter diseases, especially in the adult, fall into this category and are the principal focus of this chapter. In contrast, *dysmyelination* is an inherited disorder affecting the formation or maintenance of myelin, and thus is typically encountered in the pediatric population. Dysmyelination is rare and is discussed later in this chapter.

DEMYELINATING DISEASES

Demyelinating disease can be divided into four main categories on the basis of etiology: (1) primary/immune-mediated, (2) ischemic, (3) infectious, and (4) toxic and metabolic (Table 7.1).

Primary Demyelination

Multiple sclerosis (MS) is the classic example of a primary or immune-mediated demyelinating disease and is the most common nontraumatic cause of neurologic disability in young adults. MS is an autoimmune disorder affecting the central nervous system and is a disease characterized by immune dysfunction with the production of abnormal immunoglobulins and T cells, which are activated against myelin and mediate the damage associated with the disease. It is a chronic, relapsing, often disabling disease affecting more than a quarter of a million people in the United States alone. The age of onset is between 20 and 40 years, with only 10% of cases presenting in individuals older than 50 years. There is a female predominance of almost two to one. Although several environmental factors have been associated with MS, such as higher geographic latitudes and upper socioeconomic status, the etiology of MS remains unclear.

Establishing a diagnosis of MS is challenging, because no specific examination, laboratory test, or physical finding, taken in isolation, is unequivocally diagnostic or pathognomonic of this disorder. At the same time, diagnosing a patient with MS is portentous, as there are significant implications on many aspects of their life, including eligibility for health insurance. However, establishing the diagnosis is important because promising therapies are available, including β-interferon and antineoplastic drugs. These agents suppress the activity of the T cells, B cells, and macrophages that are thought to lead the attack on the myelin sheath.

The classic clinical definition of MS is multiple CNS lesions separated in both time and space. Patients may present with virtually any neurologic deficit, but they most commonly present with limb weakness, paresthesia, vertigo, and visual or urinary disturbances. Important characteristics of MS symptoms are their multiplicity and tendency to vary over time. The clinical course of MS is characterized by unpredictable relapses and remissions of symptoms. The diagnosis can be supported with clinical studies, which include visual, somatosensory, or motor-evoked potentials and analysis of CSF for oligoclonal banding, immunoglobulin G index, and presence of myelin basic protein. Histopathologically, active MS lesions represent areas of selective destruction of myelin sheaths and perivenular inflammation, with relative sparing of the underlying axons. These lesions may occur throughout the white matter of the CNS, including the spinal cord. The inflammatory demyelination interrupts nerve conduction and nerve function, producing the symptoms of MS. Note that

TABLE 7.1

CLASSIFICATION OF WHITE MATTER DISEASES

Primary demyelination Multiple sclerosis
Ischemic demyelination Deep white matter ischemia (leukoaraiosis) Lacunar infarcts Vasculitis (including sarcoidosis and lupus) Dissection Thromboembolic infarcts Migrainous ischemia Moyamoya disease Posthypoxic leukoencephalopathy
Infection-related demyelination Progressive multifocal leukoencephalopathy HIV encephalopathy Acute disseminated encephalomyelitis Subacute sclerosing panencephalitis Lyme disease Neurosyphilis
Toxic and metabolic demyelination Central pontine myelinolysis and extrapontine myelinolysis Marchiafava–Bignami disease Wernicke–Korsakoff syndrome Radiation leukoencephalopathy Necrotizing leukoencephalopathy
Dysmyelination (inherited white matter disease) Metachromatic leukodystrophy Adrenal leukodystrophy Leigh disease Alexander disease

histopathologically, the inflammation is a key differentiating feature between MS and other white matter conditions, such as osmotic myelinolysis (central pontine and extrapontine myelinolysis) and posterior reversible encephalopathy syndrome (PRES), which lack inflammatory changes. MRI is the most sensitive indicator in the detection of MS plaques, but imaging findings alone should never be considered diagnostic. In clinically confirmed cases of MS, MRI typically demonstrates lesions in more than 90% of cases. This compares with far less than 50% for CT and 70% to 85% for laboratory tests such as brainstem-evoked potentials and CSF oligoclonal bands. Nevertheless, the ultimate diagnosis rests with the careful combination of clinical symptoms, history, and clinical testing, including MRI.

A variety of T2WI techniques have been described for optimizing the detection of white matter lesions, with T2-fluid–attenuated inversion recovery (FLAIR) sequences leading the way. As the name suggests, FLAIR imaging has the advantage of providing heavy T2 weighting while suppressing signal from CSF. As such, FLAIR images provide improved lesion conspicuity of periventricular lesions, which may otherwise be obscured by the bright signal of CSF on fast spin-echo (FSE) T2WIs. Comparative studies have demonstrated that FLAIR imaging provides the best visualization of supratentorial white matter lesions. However, the FLAIR sequence may have mild limitations when imaging the posterior fossa and spine, partly because of pulsation artifacts. In these anatomic regions, both proton density and short tau inversion recovery (STIR) imaging are valuable.

MS plaques are typically round or ovoid, with a periventricular, juxtacortical, infratentorial, and spinal cord location (Fig. 7.1). Lesions are bright on T2WIs, reflecting either acute lesions with active inflammation/demyelination or chronic lesions with gliotic scarring. Contrast-enhancing lesions and lesions with restricted diffusion on diffusion-weighted imaging (DWI) are indicative of acute lesions with active demyelination and disruption of the blood–brain barrier. In older lesions, without residual inflammatory reaction, abnormal high signal on T2WIs persists, reflecting residual scarring (gliosis). Within the CNS, cells can mount only a limited response to neuronal injury. This scarring typically manifests as a focal proliferation of astroglia at the site of injury, termed "gliosis." In severe cases of MS, actual loss of neuronal tissue may occur and the white matter lesions may have dark signal on T1WIs, often referred to as the "dark lesions" of MS. These lesions are prognostically significant because they reflect actual loss of underlying neuronal tissue rather than simple demyelination and are in keeping with a more advanced stage of this disease. In addition, in chronic cases of MS, there is diffuse loss of deep cerebral white matter, with associated thinning of the corpus callosum and ex vacuo ventriculomegaly.

Although many white matter lesions are nonspecific in nature, the pattern suggestive of MS includes lesions that are periependymal (abutting the ependymal, i.e., ventricular surface), juxtacortical (at the gray–white cortical junction), or lesions involving the posterior fossa structures. The pons is excluded because most pontine lesions are either ischemic in nature or the result of osmotic demyelination, discussed later in this chapter. The periventricular lesions suggestive of MS are often ovoid and aligned perpendicular to the long axis of the ventricles. This pattern is the result of the alignment of the lesions along the perivenular spaces. Additional characteristic features include lesions along the callosal–septal interface, as well as lesions that are confluent in nature and greater than 6 mm in diameter with a periventricular or juxtacortical location.

In addition to the periventricular white matter, the cerebellar and cerebral peduncles, as well as the corpus callosum, medulla, and spinal cord can be involved in MS. Ischemic changes are rare in these locations; as a result, if lesions are located in these areas and are also accompanied by periventricular lesions, this increases the specificity for the diagnosis of a primary demyelinating condition. The pons is excluded from this list of posterior fossa structures due to its proclivity for small-vessel ischemic injury. In contrast, because ischemic changes rarely involve the medulla and cerebellar/cerebral peduncles, the presence of lesions in these areas is a useful differential diagnostic factor in suggesting MS. This is particularly important in patients older than 50 years, because it is difficult to decide whether multifocal white matter lesions are the result of ischemia or a demyelinating process. In addition, MS brainstem lesions are typically peripheral in location, in contrast to ischemic changes which tend to be centrally located.

Although the periependymal, juxtacortical, and posterior fossa location of white matter lesions described above are certainly suggestive of MS, these findings are not pathognomonic of MS as numerous other pathologic conditions outlined below, such as lupus, antiphospholipid syndrome, and other vasculitic/angiopathic conditions may have a similar imaging appearance.

In contrast to the periependymal and posterior fossa white matter lesions discussed above, which are indicative of some form of pathologic demyelinating conditions, many normal patients will have incidental white matter foci typically scattered in the deep white matter. Specifically, with the quality of modern-day MRI and the exquisite sensitivity of sequences such as thin section 3D volume T2-FLAIR, a significant number of MRIs in normal patients will reveal small scattered white matter lesions. In contrast to the morphology of the pathologic lesions discussed above, these incidental lesions are not periependymal or within the posterior fossa, but generally

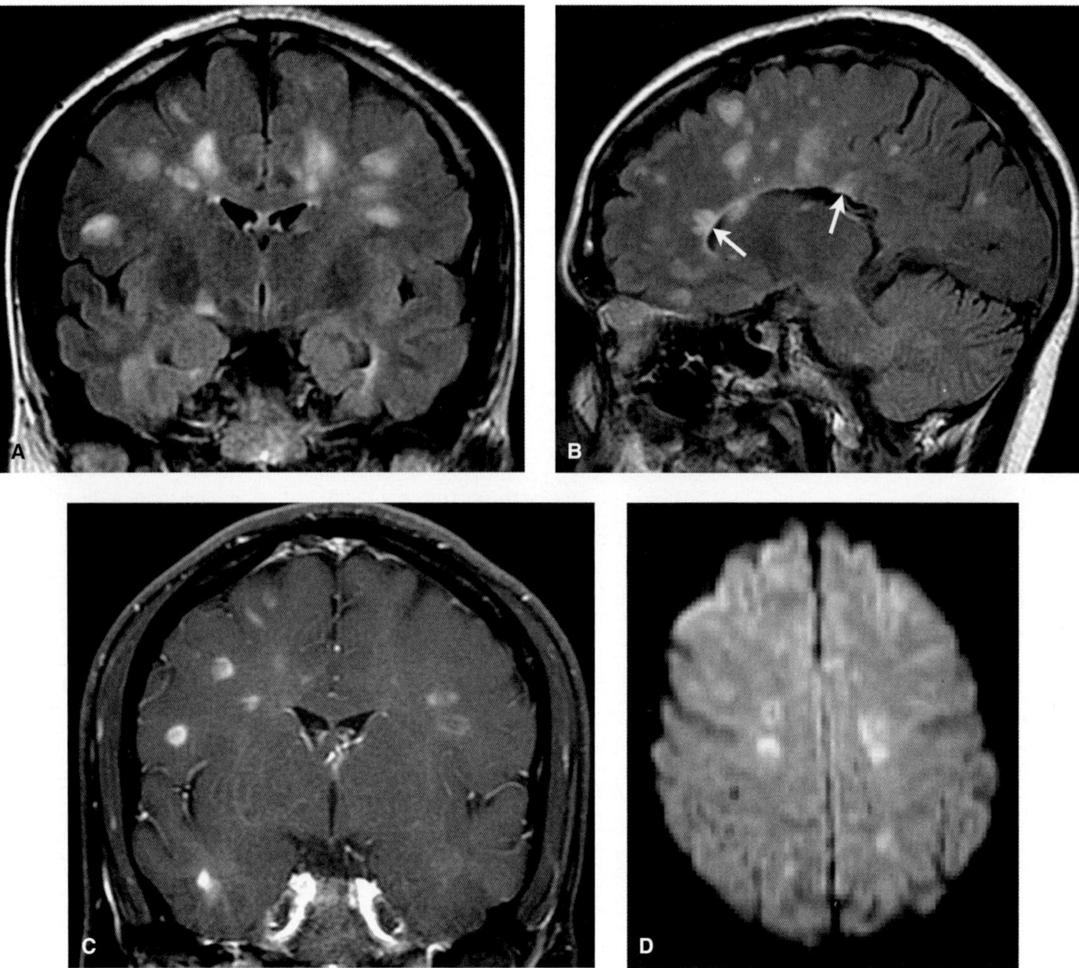

FIGURE 7.1. **Multiple Sclerosis.** Coronal and sagittal fluid-attenuated inversion recovery images (**A, B**), coronal postcontrast fat saturation T1WI (**C**), and axial diffusion-weighted image (**D**). A 26-year-old woman with multiple sclerosis (MS) and a recent flare-up in clinical symptoms demonstrates numerous patchy white matter lesions scattered throughout the subcortical and deep cerebral white matter. Note how many of these lesions have a characteristic flame-shaped configuration with a periependymal or juxtacortical location (*arrows*). Although the periventricular lesions are very suggestive of MS, these lesions are not in and of themselves diagnostic of MS and must be correlated with clinical examination and other clinical studies (visual, somatosensory, or motor-evoked potentials, and analysis of CSF for oligoclonal banding and immunoglobulin G index) before confirming a diagnosis of MS. These lesions may be indistinguishable from other demyelinating conditions, such as acute disseminated encephalomyelitis, and autoimmune/connective tissue disorders such as systemic lupus erythematosus. Note the associated contrast enhancement and restrictive diffusion evident on postcontrast image (**C**) and the diffusion-weighted image (**D**), are in keeping with active foci of demyelination.

in the deep white matter, particularly the frontal lobes. For example, in older patients aged greater than 50 to 60 years, these scattered deep white matter lesions are typically associated with vascular risk factors described below, and are called leukoaraiosis or microangiopathic changes. However, nonspecific deep white matter lesions may be identified in normal young patients, including children and young adults, without any vascular risk factors. In fact, in this young age group, studies have revealed white matter lesions in up to 50%. It is important to note that these incidental lesions are often punctate measuring on the order of 1 to 2 mm, and quite different from the periependymal lesions of MS. In contrast to MS lesions, these incidental hyperintense foci are typically located within the subcortical and deep white matter, often clustered in the frontal lobes and associated with perivascular spaces (Fig. 7.2). These punctate foci may simply represent normal gliosis associated with the perivascular space. It should also be pointed out that these punctate foci of hyperintensity are not associated with traumatic etiology. Chapter 3 highlights the characteristic imaging features of traumatic pathology such as diffuse axonal injury characterized by microbleeds as the hallmark of traumatic pathology.

MS lesions may also present as a large, conglomerate, deep white matter mass that can be mistaken for a neoplasm (Fig. 7.3). These lesions are referred to as tumefactive MS or tumefactive demyelinating lesions (TDL) and differentiation from malignancy may be challenging, with lesions not uncommonly making it to biopsy before the correct diagnosis is established. A useful imaging finding that often differentiates these conglomerate MS plaques from neoplasms is that they often demonstrate a peripheral crescentic rim of contrast enhancement, which represents the advancing leading edge of active demyelination. Additional clues to the diagnosis include paucity of perilesional edema as well as relative lack of mass effect for lesion size. Detecting these unique features and searching carefully for other more characteristic periventricular or posterior fossa lesions are essential clues in distinguishing TDL from neoplasm.

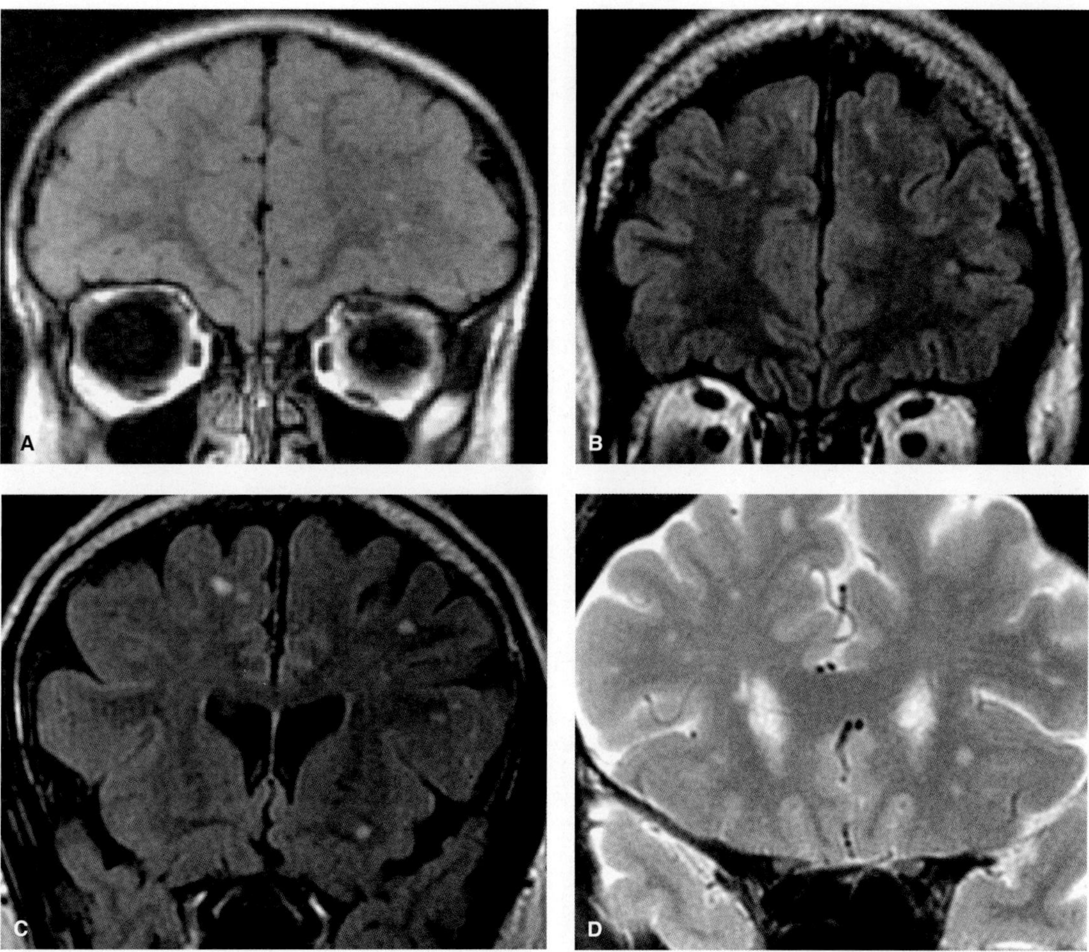

FIGURE 7.2. **Collage: Punctate White Matter Foci Without Underlying Disease.** Series of patients A, B, C, and D (ages 3,12,17 and 21 years) presenting with various benign symptoms in which imaging of the brain was obtained incidentally during MRI of facial and sinus conditions. These tiny punctate foci have been reported in up to 50% of young patients and potentially reflect small foci of nonspecific signal associated with perivascular spaces.

The spinal cord may also be involved with MS, and whenever a focal abnormality of the spinal cord is detected, a demyelinating MS plaque must be in the differential diagnosis. Demyelinating plaques may have mild mass effect as well as contrast enhancement, thus mimicking a neoplasm. Spinal cord MS plaques are typically well defined, less than one to two vertebral segments in the craniocaudal dimension, and less than 50% of the cross-sectional area of the spinal cord often affecting the peripheral white matter. The majority of spinal cord MS lesions (70% to 80%) will have associated plaques in the brain. In the setting of a cord lesion, performing an MRI of the head may confirm the diagnosis, thus avoiding a spinal cord biopsy (see Chapter 9, Fig. 9.36).

Ischemic Demyelination

Age-Related Demyelination. Small-vessel ischemic changes within the deep cerebral white matter are seen with such frequency in middle age (>50 to 60 years) that they are considered a normal part of aging. This represents an arteriosclerotic vasculopathy of the penetrating cerebral arteries. The deep white matter is more susceptible to ischemic injury than gray matter, because it is supplied by long, small-caliber penetrating end arteries, without significant collateral supply. In contrast, cortical gray matter, as well as parts of the brainstem such as the midbrain and medulla, has robust collateral blood supply, thus minimizing the risk of ischemia. The deep penetrating vessels supplying the white matter become narrowed by arteriosclerosis and lipohyalin deposits. The result is the formation of small ischemic lesions, primarily involving the deep cerebral and periventricular white matter as well as the basal ganglia (Fig. 7.4). The cortex, subcortical "U" fibers, central corpus callosum, medulla, midbrain, and cerebellar peduncles are usually spared because of their dual blood supply, which decreases their vulnerability to hypoperfusion. As previously described, if lesions are identified in these locations, a cause other than ischemia should be entertained.

Histologically, areas of infarction demonstrate axonal atrophy with diminished myelin. Early neuropathologists noted the areas of paleness associated with these changes and coined the term "myelin pallor." These white matter changes have received many names over the years, including leukoaraiosis, microangiopathic leukoencephalopathy, and subcortical arteriosclerotic encephalopathy. None of these terms are very satisfying, as they do not accurately reflect all the changes observed histologically and overstate the clinical significance of these lesions. A more appropriate term may simply be "age-related white matter changes." These small ischemic white matter lesions are often asymptomatic, and clinical correlation is always required before a diagnosis of subcortical arteriosclerotic encephalopathy or multi-infarct dementia (Binswanger disease) is made. The white matter infarcts just described differ from lacunar infarcts. Lacunae

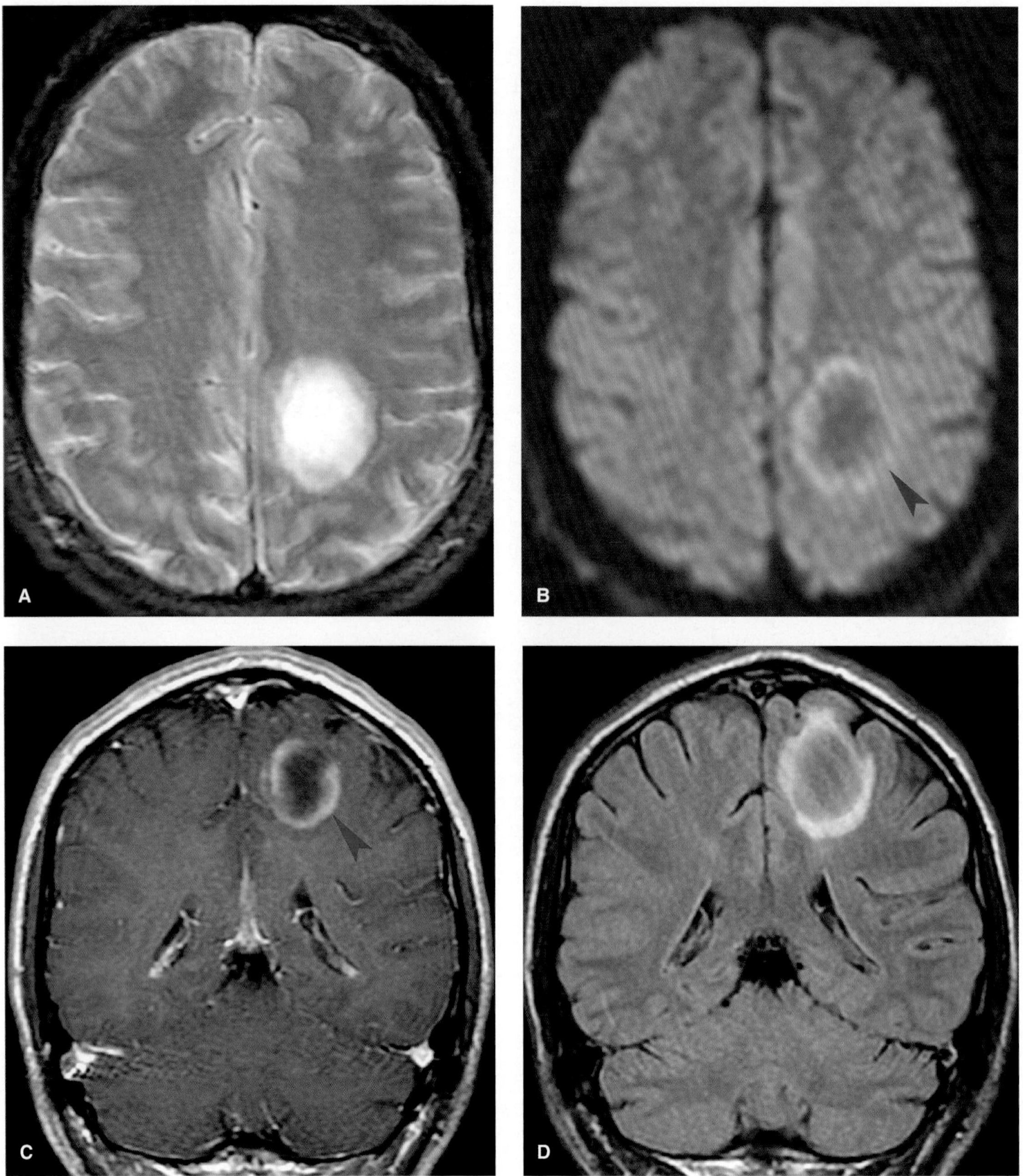

FIGURE 7.3. **Tumefactive Demyelinating Lesion (TDL).** Axial T2WI (**A**), DWI (**B**), coronal postcontrast T1WI (**C**), and fluid-attenuated inversion recovery image (**D**). Images from a 30-year-old woman presenting with transient bouts of right hemiparesis, as well as depression and fatigue. Images reveal a large left parietal mass with a peripheral rim of restricted diffusion and enhancement (*arrowheads*). This lesion could be mistaken for a neoplasm or atypical progressive multifocal leukoencephalopathy and undergo biopsy. The diagnosis of tumefactive MS was confirmed with paraclinical testing, including evoked potentials and CSF oligoclonal bands.

refer to small infarcts (5 to 10 mm) occurring within the basal ganglia, typically the upper two-thirds of the putamen. Both lacunar and deep white matter infarcts have similar etiologies and are the result of disease involving the deep penetrating arteries.

Differentiating white matter lesions related to ischemic changes from MS lesions can be difficult, especially in the older patient. This is important because 10% of patients who present with MS are older than 50 years of age. Laboratory testing such as CSF analysis for oligoclonal bands and history are helpful. In addition, deep white matter infarcts tend to spare the subcortical arcuate fibers and the corpus callosum, both of which can be involved with MS. Involvement of the callosal–septal interface is quite specific for MS.

Nonspecific punctuate white matter lesions (small bright lesions on T2WIs) are more prominent in any patient with a vasculopathy, such as related to atherosclerosis and vascular risk factors (e.g., age, hypertension, diabetes, hyperlipidemia, coronary artery disease, smoking); hypercoagulable conditions; vasculitis (lupus, sarcoid, polyarteritis nodosa, Behçet syndrome); or drug-related vasculopathy. In younger individuals with punctuate white matter lesions, if a definable pathology exists, hypercoagulable states, as well as embolic and vasculitic

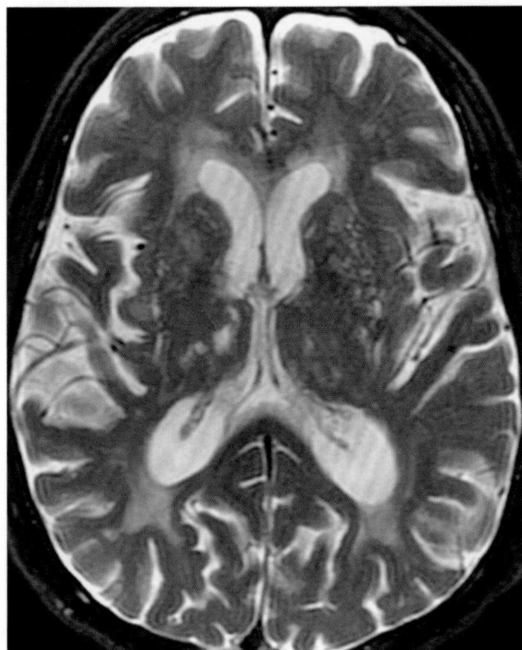

FIGURE 7.4. **Ischemic Demyelination.** This 72-year-old woman presented with forgetfulness. Axial fast spin–echo T2WI reveals diffuse patchy lesions throughout the subcortical and deep white matter. These lesions are in keeping with ischemic demyelination of the deep white matter, with several old lacunar infarcts (*arrow*) of the basal ganglia. Note the ex vacuo ventriculomegaly resulting from loss of deep cerebral white matter.

etiologies, figure prominently (Figs. 7.5 to 7.8). Hypercoagulable conditions include a diverse set of diseases with the common theme of increased risk of microvascular thrombotic disease. Serum testing can be used to evaluate for the presence of these disease conditions, which include homocystinemia, antiphospholipid syndrome, Factor V Leiden, prothrombin gene mutation, and deficiencies of natural proteins that prevent clotting (the anticoagulant proteins such as antithrombin, protein C, and protein S deficiencies). A classic case presentation is that of a young adult female with prior miscarriages presenting with headaches/migraines and ischemic white matter changes. These findings are suggestive of antiphospholipid syndrome (aka phospholipid antibody syndrome), where circulating antiphospholipid antibodies (cardiolipin or lupus anticoagulant antibodies) lead to a hypercoagulable state with resultant white matter and ischemic changes.

In children and the young adult population presenting with small punctate white matter lesions, remember these may simply represent incidental nonspecific foci typically encountered in normal patients. Specifically, as described earlier, in many normal children and young adults, tiny deep white matter hyperintensities are common, having no known etiology despite evaluation for all the conditions outlined above. In this setting, these lesions may simply reflect a small focus of gliosis associated with normal perivascular space or simply the gliotic residue of a remote unspecified insult, such as an immune-mediated postviral condition. However, if pathology is suspected clinically, one should consider conditions such as hypercoagulable states and migrainous ischemia, as well as cardiogenic embolic etiologies. An echocardiogram plays an important role in the evaluation of a potential patent foramen ovale or cardiac valvular vegetation.

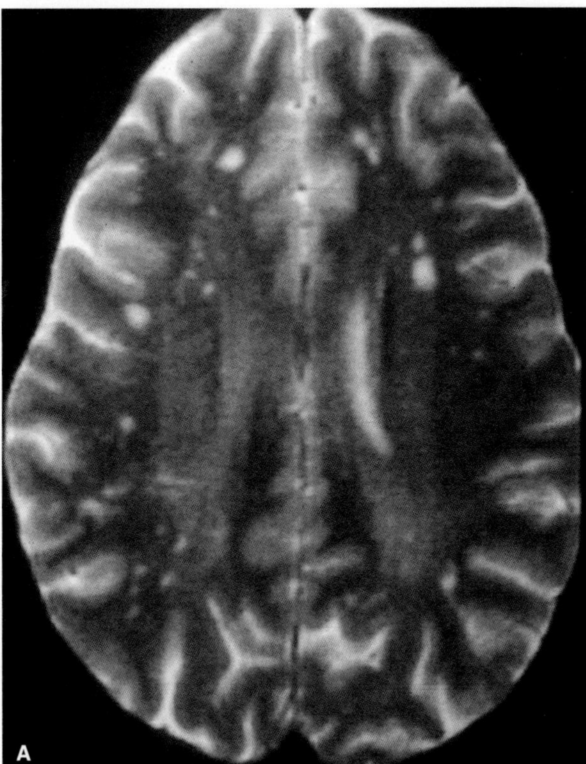

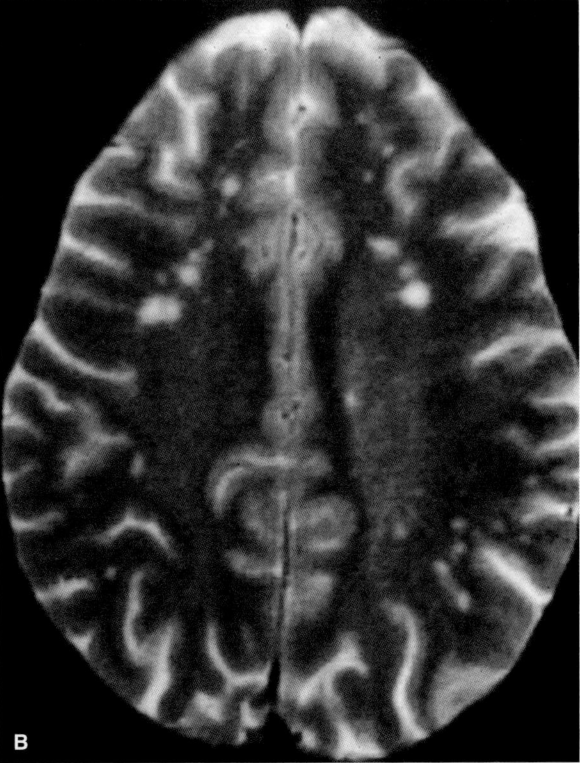

FIGURE 7.5. **Antiphospholipid Antibody Syndrome.** This 32-year-old woman presented with headaches and a history of several miscarriages (**A, B**). T2WIs demonstrate scattered focal subcortical and deep white matter lesions. Although these lesions are nonspecific, serum testing revealed elevated circulating pathogenic immunoglobulins/antibodies specifically targeting DNA and other nuclear constituents collectively termed antibodies to nuclear antigens, for example, lupus anticoagulants and anticardiolipin antibodies. This represents an immune complex disease referred to as antiphospholipid antibody syndrome.

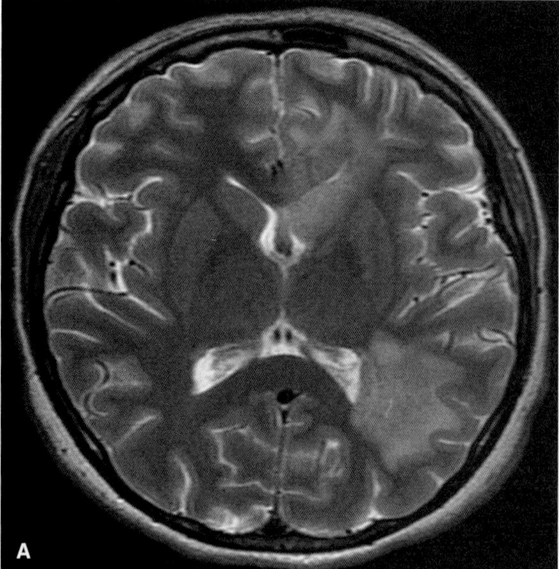

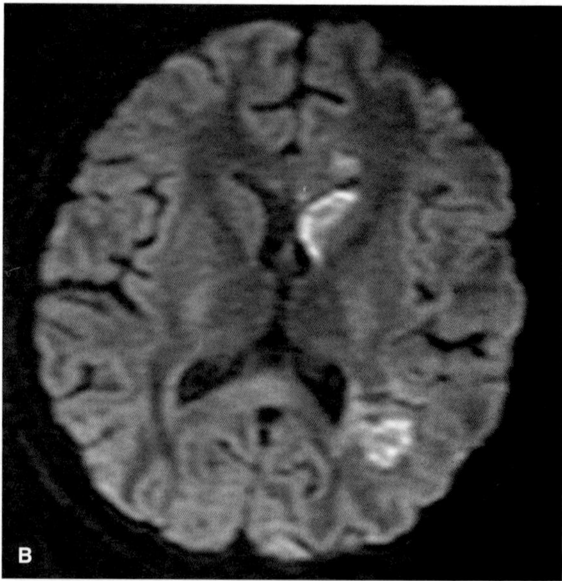

FIGURE 7.6. **Lupus Cerebritis.** Part 1: A 24-year-old woman presented with acute onset of a neuropsychiatric condition. **A:** Axial T2WI and (**B**) DWI showing areas of acute ischemia. Ischemic findings are often nonspecific and a wide range of etiologies must be considered include a diverse range of vasculitic conditions. Vasculitic conditions are classified as primary (confined to the CNS, e.g., primary angiitis of the CNS) or secondary (associated with systemic inflammatory or infectious process). The secondary vasculitides can be divided by the size of involved vessels (large blood vessels: giant cell arteritis; medium blood vessel: polyarteritis nodosa; and variable vessel size: Behçet disease). The secondary vasculitides can also be classified by their associated systemic disease (e.g., SLE, RA, Sjögren's, APLA syndrome, and scleroderma) as well as with known etiologies such as drug-, radiation-, or infection-induced vasculitis.

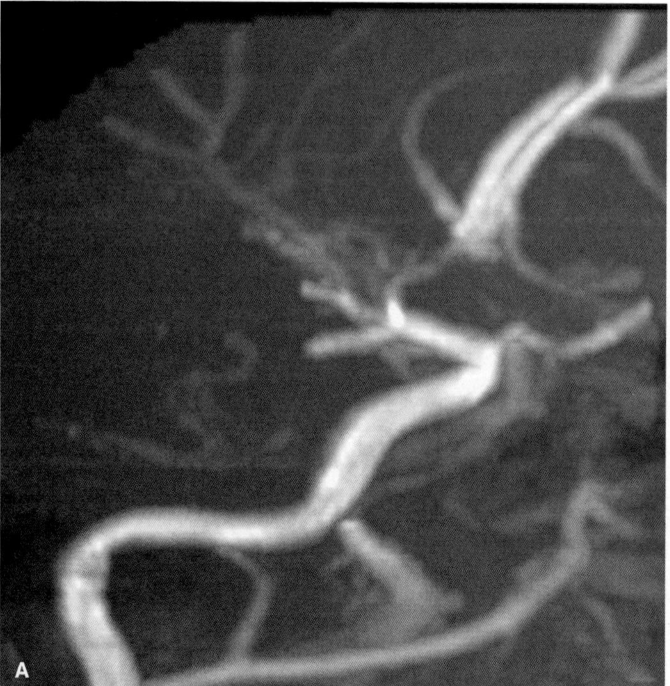

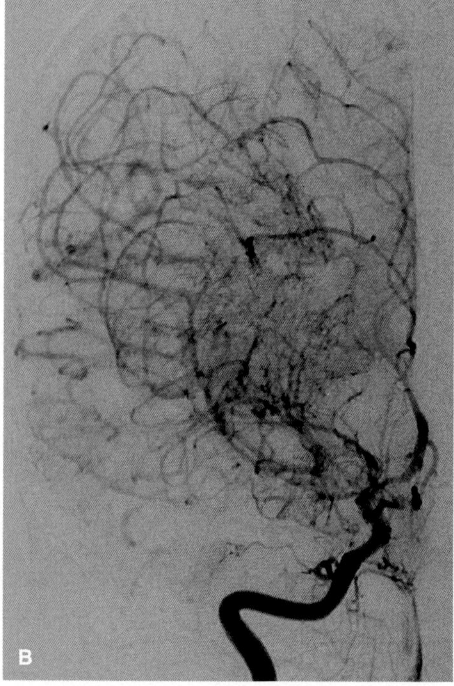

FIGURE 7.7. **Moyamoya Disease.** A 17-year-old presents with episodes of focal motor weakness. T2WI (not shown) showed multiple scattered subcortical white matter hyperintensities. **A.** T1WI shows a left thalamic infarct and a dramatic proliferation of tiny collateral vessels throughout the deep gray matter. **B.** Conventional angiography reveals marked stenosis of the supraclinoid internal carotid artery, with dramatic proliferation of tiny collateral vessels presenting as a "puff of smoke" (the literal Japanese translation of *moyamoya*). The term "moyamoya disease" refers to idiopathic forms of this condition whereas "moyamoya syndrome" is when the underlying etiology is known (e.g., fribromuscular dysplasia, Marfan syndrome, NF1, SLE, Down syndrome, etc.). The cause of the vascular disorder in this child was unknown but can be treated with various external to internal vascular bypass surgeries such as encephaloduroarteriosynangiosis. MRI angiography plays a useful role in assessing the patency of these shunts once surgically completed.

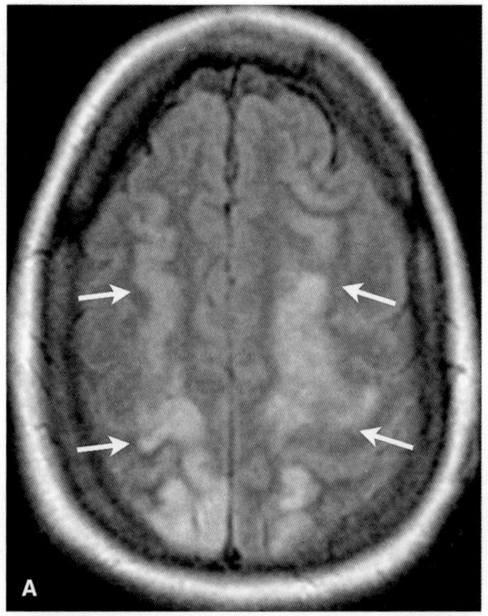

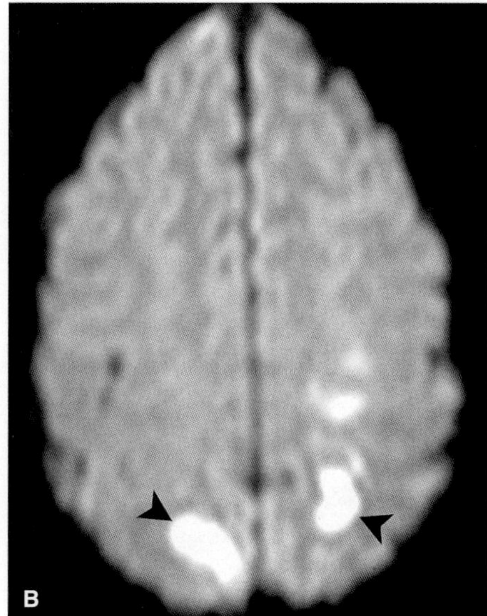

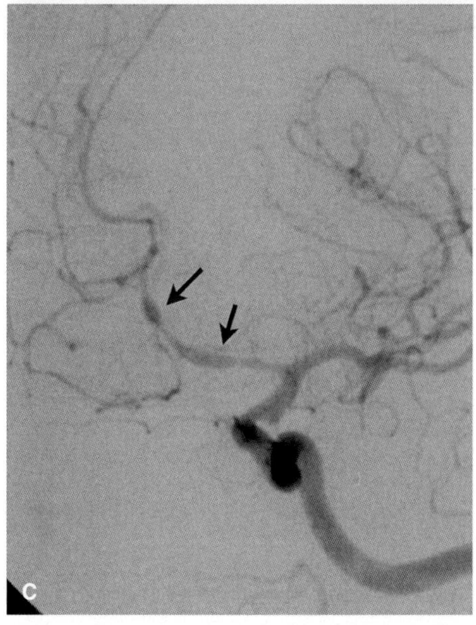

FIGURE 7.8. **Drug-Induced Vasculopathy.** Axial fluid-attenuated inversion recovery image (**A**), diffusion-weighted image (**B**), and angiography (**C**) in a 43-year-old woman who presented with headache, confusion, and weakness. Significant signal abnormalities are noted involving the cortex and subcortical white matter of the high frontoparietal convexities (*arrows* in A) with associated restricted diffusion (*arrowheads* in B). Catheter angiography reveals considerable vascular beading (*arrows* in C). Drug-induced vasculopathy is most commonly seen with methamphetamine and sympathomimetic drugs. Both angiography and brain biopsy each have about 30% false-positive rates.

Ependymitis granularis is a normal anatomic finding that may mimic pathology. Ependymitis granularis consists of an area of high signal on a T2WI along the tips of the frontal horns (Fig. 7.9). These foci of signal range in width from several millimeters to a centimeter. Histologic studies of this subependymal area reveal a loose network of axons with low myelin count. This porous ependyma allows transependymal flow of CSF, resulting in a focal area of T2 prolongation. Unfortunately, this entity has been given a name that sounds more like a disease entity rather than a simple histologic observation. Similarly, with the use of FLAIR imaging, a region of periventricular T2 hyperintensity may be noted about the ventricular trigones as a normal finding. With age as well as significant vascular risk factors, prominent periventricular T2 hyperintensity may be noted along the entire length of the lateral ventricles, and this may be referred to as *senescent periventricular hyperintensity* or *periventricular halo*. This finding may become more prominent with greater degrees of underlying vascular pathology or in the setting of a demyelinating condition such as MS.

Prominent perivascular spaces may also mimic deep white matter or lacunar infarcts. As blood vessels penetrate into the brain parenchyma, they are enveloped by the CSF and a thin sheath of pia. These CSF-filled perivascular clefts are called Virchow–Robin spaces and present as punctate foci of high signal on T2WIs (Fig. 7.10). They are typically located in the centrum semiovale (high cerebral hemispheric white matter) and the lower basal ganglia at the level of the anterior commissure, where the lenticulostriate arteries enter the brain parenchyma. These perivascular spaces are typically 1 to 2 mm in diameter but can be considerably larger. They can be seen as a normal variant at any age but become more prominent with increasing age as atrophy occurs.

An important means for differentiating a periventricular space from a parenchymal lesion is the use of the proton density–weighted (first-echo T2W) or FLAIR images. On the proton density-weighted sequence, CSF has similar signal intensity as white matter. A perivascular space is composed of CSF and will parallel CSF signal intensity on all sequences (i.e., isointense to brain parenchyma on proton-density sequences). In contrast, ischemic lesions, unless cavitated with cystic change, will be bright on the proton-density sequence as a result of the presence of associated gliosis. Both a deep infarct and a perivascular space will be bright on the second-echo T2WI, but only the infarct will remain bright on the first-echo

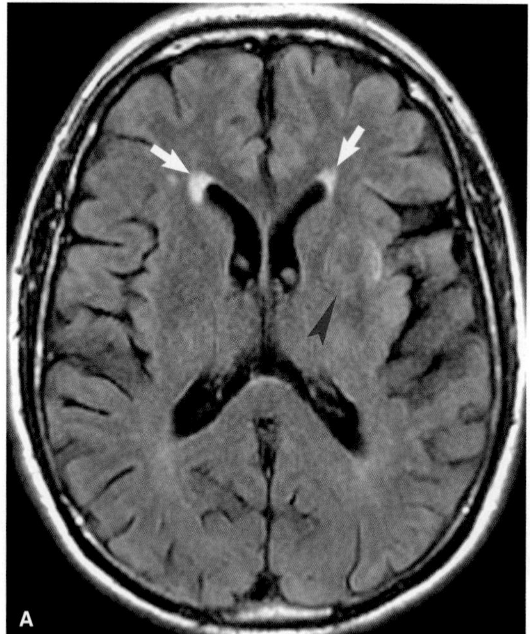
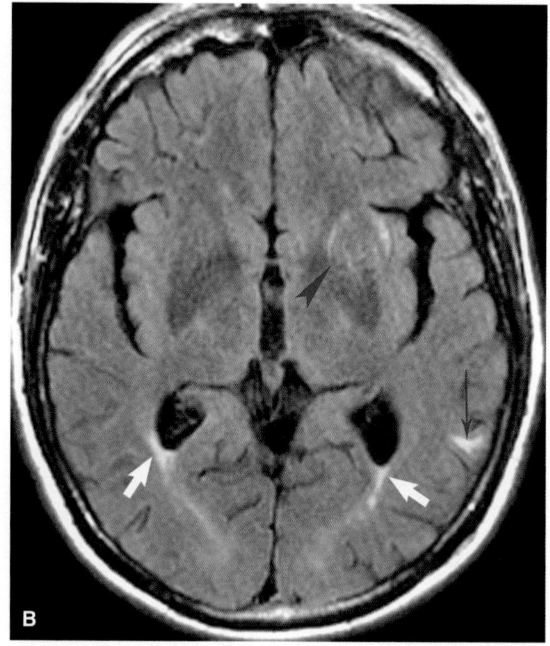

FIGURE 7.9. **Ependymitis Granularis (Normal Finding). A, B:** Axial fluid-attenuated inversion recovery images in a 42-year-old man presenting with headaches. The periventricular hyperintensity noted about the tips of the frontal and occipital ventricular horns is a normal finding (*white arrows*). These areas of periependymal hyperintensity may be exacerbated by any process that results in underlying white matter disease. Note the circular artifact located within the left basal ganglia; it is related to the magnetic susceptibility artifact from the patient's orthodontic braces (*red arrowheads*). One should be aware of artifacts that may mimic pathologic lesions, especially flow and magnetic susceptibility artifacts that can give rise to lesions that are not necessarily contiguous to the cause of the artifact. Incidental note is made of a small focus of subcortical hyperintensity along the left temporoparietal lobe related to a site of posttraumatic gliosis (*red arrow* in **B**).

image. Similarly, on a FLAIR image, because fluid signal is attenuated, only true parenchymal lesions with gliosis will yield abnormal signal. On occasion, however, a small amount of persistent T2 hyperintensity can be associated with perivascular spaces on the proton-density or FLAIR sequences, and this may account for many of the incidental punctate foci of hyperintensities noted in the young. An additional differentiating feature between giant perivascular spaces and lacunae is location. Lacunar infarcts tend to occur in the upper two-thirds of the corpus striatum because they reflect end-arteriole infarcts in the distal vascular distribution. In contrast, periventricular spaces are typically smaller, bilateral, and often symmetric within the inferior third of the striatum, where the vessels enter the anterior perforated substance.

It should also be noted that on occasion a cystic lacunae may present as hyperintense on FLAIR due to the presence of subtle proteinaceous content. In these circumstances, the true cystic nature of this lesion will only become evident on a high-resolution 3D T1-weighted sequence.

CADASIL Disease. Cerebral autosomal dominant arteriopathy with subcortical infarcts and leukoencephalopathy (CADASIL) is an inheritable condition relating to a Notch 3 mutation on chromosome 19. As the name indicates, this condition presents with ischemic changes, often in middle age. The presence of subcortical anterior temporal and medial frontal lesions is relatively specific for this condition (Fig. 7.11). The difference in the anatomic distribution of the white matter involvement in contrast to routine small-vessel ischemic changes, is felt to be CADASIL's effect on slightly larger caliber leptomeningeal vessels.

CNS Vasculitis. CNS vasculitis represents a heterogeneous group of disorders which are associated with inflammation of blood vessels leading to a variety of ischemic manifestations ranging from ischemic brain lesions, cerebral perfusion deficits, intracerebral or subarachnoid hemorrhage to vessel stenosis. The imaging findings of a vasculitis are often nonspecific, and thus it is important to consider a vasculitis whenever encountering ischemic lesions. Many vasculitic conditions are associated with systemic symptoms, and when the CNS findings are part of a systemic disorder the diagnosis is made easier, for example, systemic connective tissue disorders, infection, malignancy, drug use, or radiation therapy. In addition, relevant laboratory tests such as erythrocyte sedimentation rate (ESR), C-reactive protein level, rheumatoid factor, and complement level may be of value in supporting a diagnosis of vasculitis.

Primary Angiitis of the Central Nervous System (PACNS). PACNS is an idiopathic vasculitis limited to the brain and spinal cord typically observed in the fifth and sixth decades of life. This condition is associated with an elevation in inflammatory markers such as ESR. MRI findings are nonspecific but angiography may show segmental irregularity and narrowing of both small- and medium-sized parenchymal and leptomeningeal blood vessels.

Systemic Lupus Erythematosus (SLE). SLE is an autoimmune disorder which presents with white matter lesions (75% of patients) as well as a spectrum of neurologic and neuropsychiatric manifestations such psychosis, stroke, headaches, and neurocognitive deficits. Females are afflicted at a 10:1 ratio compared to males, with a peak age of onset in the second through fourth decades of life. About half of these patients may have associated generalized cerebral atrophy.

Moyamoya Disease. Japanese for "puff of smoke" is a progressive occlusive condition of the supraclinoid or terminal aspects of the internal cerebral arteries. The term "moyamoya disease" is used in idiopathic or familial conditions, whereas

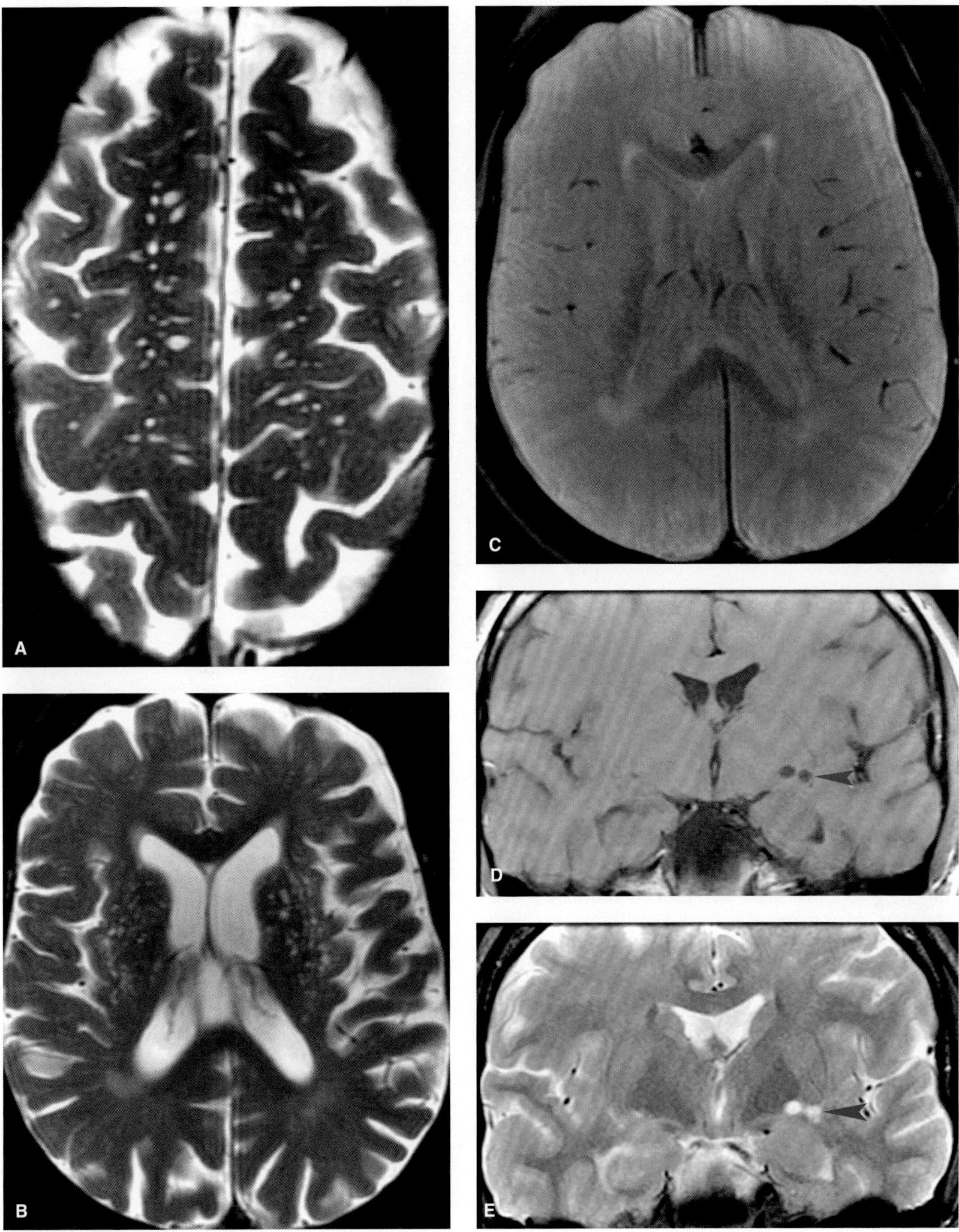

FIGURE 7.10. **Virchow–Robin Spaces.** Small punctuate foci of water signal are noted within the centrum semiovale (**A**) and basal ganglia (**B**), consistent with perivascular spaces. These spaces penetrate the brain parenchyma and reflect perivascular extensions of the pia mater that accompany the arteries entering and the veins emerging from the cerebral cortex. These perivascular spaces are almost imperceptible on the proton density–weighted image (**C**), which helps confirm their identity as water, rather than white matter ischemic gliotic lesions. Although perivascular spaces are typically 1 to 2 mm in diameter, they can be considerably larger. Large perivascular spaces (about 0.5 to 1 cm) are occasionally noted within the caudal aspect of the basal ganglia and referred to as giant perivascular spaces. Coronal T1WI (**D**) and fast spin–echo T2WI (**E**) in a 38-year-old man demonstrate well-rounded, left-sided cysts along the course of the lenticulostriate arteries (*arrowheads*) as they enter the basal ganglia through the anterior perforated substance. An old cavitated lacunar infarction may have a similar appearance but would be distinctly unusual in the inferior portion of the striatum. Note that lacunar infarcts are the result of vessel occlusion and thus occur along the distal extent of the lenticulostriate arteries; therefore, they tend to be located more superiorly within the basal ganglia. In addition, lacunar infarcts may have associated gliotic T2 hyperintensity on proton density and fluid-attenuated inversion recovery images, a finding not seen with giant perivascular spaces.

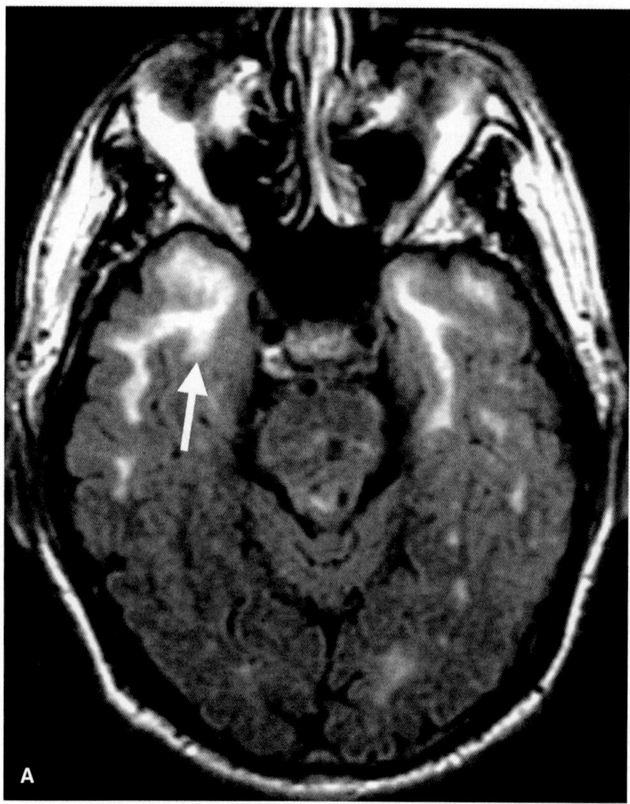

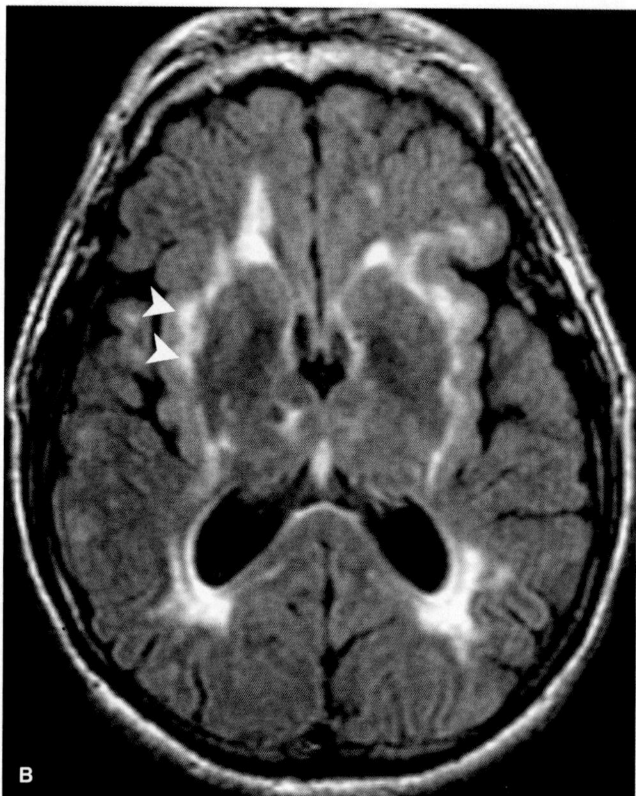

FIGURE 7.11. **CADASIL Disease.** Cerebral autosomal dominant arteriopathy with subcortical infarcts and leukoencephalopathy (CADASIL). **A, B:** Axial fluid-attenuated inversion recovery images. A 52-year-old presenting with early cognitive dysfunction. The involvement of anterior temporal (*arrow*), medial frontal, and external capsule white matter (*arrowheads*) is relatively specific for this condition. In contrast to typical small-vessel ischemic disease, with CADASIL, the involvement of larger leptomeningeal vessels results in a predilection for involvement of the arcuate fibers in these affected regions.

"moyamoya syndrome" is used when there is a known cause such as radiation vasculitis, sickle cell anemia, and Down or Marfan syndrome. Moyamoya disease is a condition of children and young adults with a bimodal age distribution (first peak 4 years of age and second peak 30 to 40 years of age). Characteristic imaging findings include marked narrowing and occlusion of the terminal internal cerebral arteries (usually bilateral, but may be asymmetric and occasionally unilateral), with formation of a diffuse extensive network of tiny collateral vessels throughout the deep gray matter structures. On angiography, the enhancement of these collateral vessels results in a dense blush of contrast, giving rise to the term "puff of smoke."

Infection-Related Demyelination

Various infectious agents may result in white matter disease, either directly or indirectly, and most commonly are viral. Some of the more common agents are described here. For further discussion of virus-induced white matter pathology, see Chapter 6.

Herpes encephalitis is the most common fatal encephalitis. Although this condition is also discussed in Chapter 6, its importance warrants repetition. The form of herpes encephalitis which occurs in children and adults and is caused by herpes simplex virus (HSV) type 1 (oral herpes); this is in contrast to neonatal herpes encephalitis, which is caused by HSV type 2 (genital herpes). Presenting symptomatology is typically nonspecific, and may consist of headache, mild confusion and disorientation, changes in behavior, and difficulty with memory. In more advanced cases there may be fever, mental deterioration, and seizures. As a result of this variable clinical presentation, diagnosis may be difficult. This emphasizes the crucial role of the radiologist in entertaining this diagnosis when appropriate imaging findings are noted. Antiviral treatment is simple and effective, but failure to treat results in 100% mortality. Although the diagnosis may be confirmed by a polymerase chain reaction, detection of herpes DNA in the CSF takes several days and therapy must be instituted on the basis of clinical presentation and imaging results, prior to the return of this test result.

HSV type 1 has a particular predilection for the limbic system, with localization of infection to temporal lobes, insular cortex, subfrontal area, and cingulate gyri (Fig. 7.12). The limbic system is responsible for integration of emotion, memory, and complex behavior, and involvement of these structures accounts for some of the behavioral symptoms at presentation. Imaging reveals primarily T2 hyperintensity of the involved cortex and subcortical structures presenting as encephalitis with variable contrast enhancement. Initially, herpes encephalitis is usually unilateral; however, sequential bilateral involvement is highly suggestive of the disease. Histopathologically, herpes infection is a fulminant necrotizing meningoencephalitis associated with edema, necrosis, hemorrhage, and eventually encephalomalacia. As a result, hemorrhage within the area of involved parenchyma is strongly supportive of this diagnosis.

Acute disseminated encephalomyelitis (ADEM), a postinfectious and postvaccinal encephalomyelitis, typically occurs after a viral illness or vaccination, with measles, rubella, varicella, and mumps being the most common agents. This

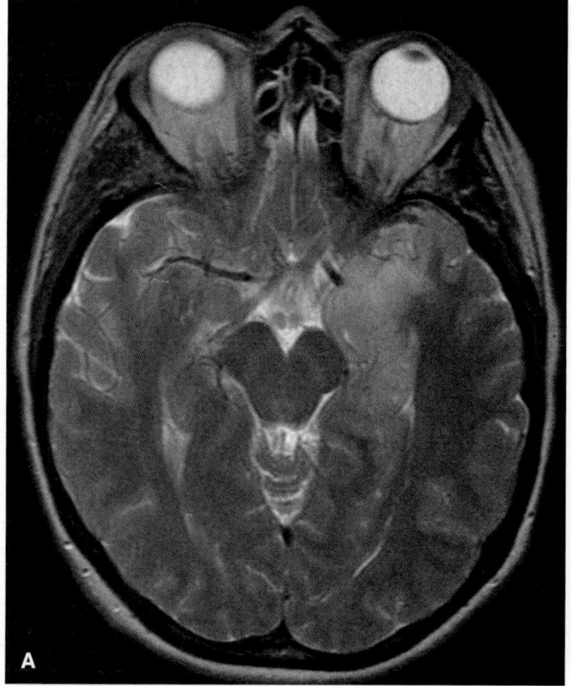

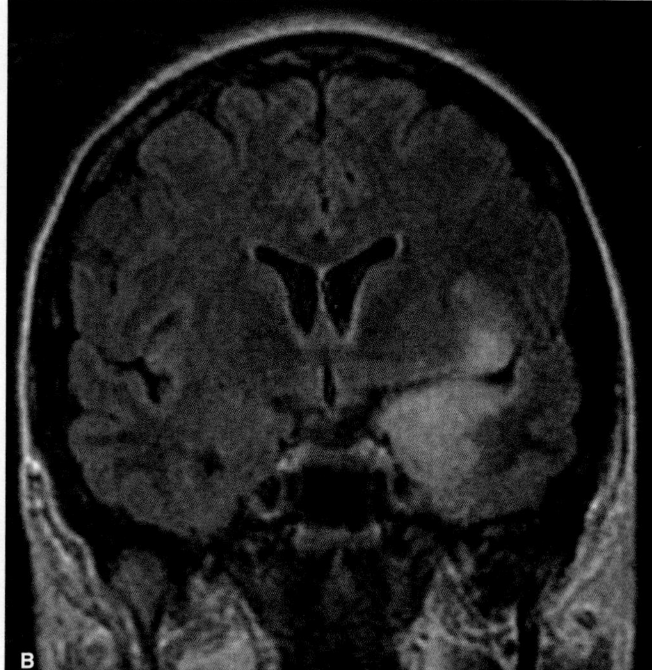

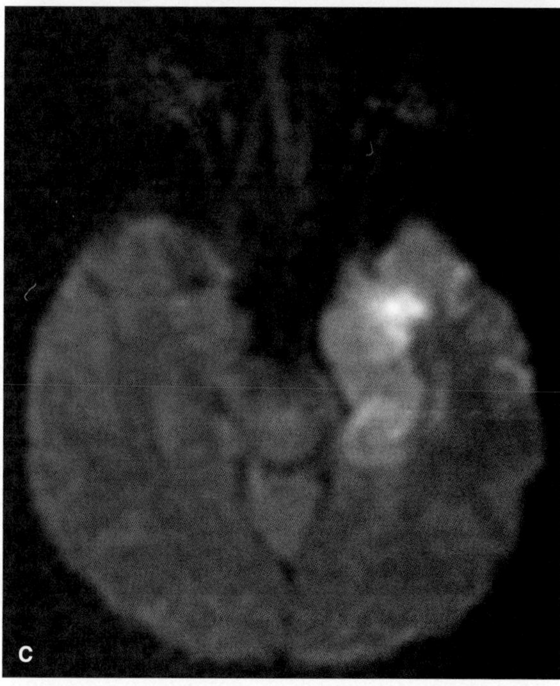

FIGURE 7.12. **Herpes Encephalitis.** A: T2WI. B: T2-FLAIR. C: DWI. Young male presented with confusion, word-finding difficulty, and odd behavior. MRI demonstrates significant abnormality of the left temporal lobe including restricted diffusion. In early stages, the abnormality is typically confined to the insular cortex or medial temporal lobes bilaterally, which is characteristic for herpes encephalitis. The radiologist must have a low threshold for considering this diagnosis when there is abnormality of the temporal lobes, insular cortex, or cingulate gyrus, as failure of treatment results in 100% mortality. Herpes encephalitis represents one of the few conditions in which the radiologist stands to make a life-saving diagnosis which may be easily overlooked by the treating clinicians.

condition is considered an immune-mediated inflammatory demyelinating disease, but sometimes it has no recognized antecedent infection or inciting malady.

It is theorized that the body's antiviral immune reaction cross-reacts with myelin sheaths, resulting in an acute, aggressive form of demyelination. This unintended antiviral response against myelin is a result of shared molecular homology between viral proteins and normal human CNS proteins. Recall that oligodendrocytes are responsible for the formation and maintenance of the myelin sheaths, and their damage results in demyelination.

Demyelinating lesions associated with ADEM typically begin approximately 2 weeks after a viral infection with the abrupt clinical onset of neurologic symptoms, which include decreased levels of consciousness varying from lethargy to coma; convulsions; multifocal neurologic symptoms such as hemiparesis, paraparesis, and tetraparesis; cranial nerve palsies; movement disorders; and seizures. In the majority of cases, there is spontaneous resolution of symptoms, but permanent sequelae can be seen in up to 25% of patients, with some even progressing to death. Although ADEM occurs most commonly in children, persons of any age can be affected. Lesions primarily involve white matter, but gray matter may also be affected. MRI demonstrates multifocal or confluent white matter lesions similar to those of MS (Fig. 7.13). A differential feature is that ADEM is a monophasic illness, unlike MS, which has a remitting and relapsing course. This is a feature often useful in differentiating ADEM from MS. Specifically, if the majority of the identified white matter lesions enhance, this suggests a monophasic demyelinating process (i.e., ADEM).

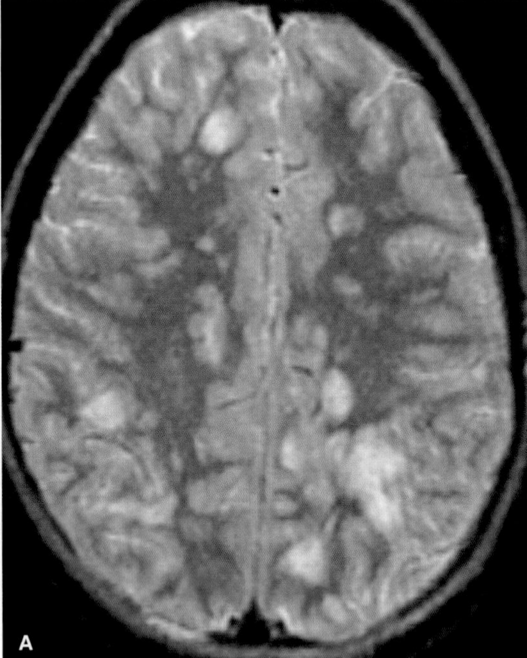

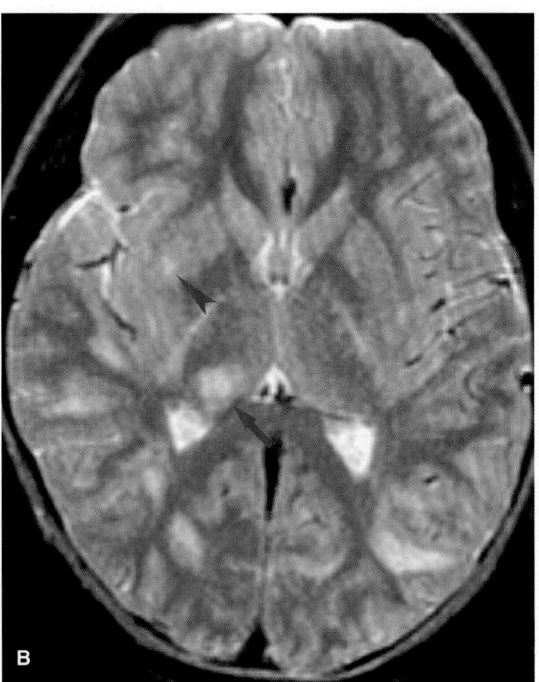

FIGURE 7.13. **Acute Disseminated Encephalomyelitis. A, B:** Axial T2WIs. A 14-year-old boy presented with deteriorating mental status a week following viral gastroenteritis. Imaging reveals multiple patchy subcortical and deep white matter lesions, as well as involvement of deep gray matter structures, including the right putamen (*arrowhead*) and thalamus (*arrow*). Following the administration of contrast, most lesions enhanced (not shown) consistent with an acute demyelinating process. The enhancement of most lesions is suggestive of a monophasic demyelinating process. The patient improved after treatment with high-dose intravenous corticosteroids and intravenous immunoglobulin.

Subacute sclerosing panencephalitis represents a reactivated, slowly progressive infection caused by the measles virus. Children between the ages of 5 and 12 years who have had measles, usually before the age of 3 years, are typically affected. MRI demonstrates patchy areas of periventricular demyelination as well as lesions of the basal ganglia. The disease course is variable and may be rapidly progressive or protracted.

Progressive multifocal leukoencephalopathy (PML) is seen in a wide range of immune-compromised individuals, ranging from those treated with immunosuppressants and cytotoxic agents (e.g., transplant patients, inflammatory arthritis) to patients with AIDS. PML represents a reactivation of a latent JC polyomavirus. This opportunistic infection is usually seen in severely immunocompromised patients with very low T-cell counts, particularly individuals with AIDS, lymphoma, organ transplantation, and disseminated malignancies. The JC virus infects oligodendrocytes, which are the axonal support cells that generate the myelin sheath. As a result, damage to the oligodendrocytes results in widespread demyelination. PML typically involves the deep cerebral white matter, with subcortical U-fiber involvement, but spares the cortex and deep gray matter (Fig. 7.14). Lesions are characterized by a lack of mass effect, contrast enhancement, and hemorrhage and are typically located in the parietooccipital region. These lesions progress rapidly and coalesce into larger confluent asymmetric areas. Although most lesions involve the supratentorial white matter, involvement of gray matter and infratentorial structures (cerebellum and brain-stem) is possible. PML is typically relentlessly progressive, with death typically ensuing within several months from the time of initial diagnosis, although more chronic and indolent cases have been reported.

HIV Encephalopathy. HIV involvement of the brain presents as subacute encephalitis, referred to as *AIDS dementia complex* or *diffuse HIV encephalopathy.* This is characterized clinically by a progressive dementia without focal neurologic signs. HIV encephalopathy does not appear to be the result of a direct infection of the neurons or macroglia (i.e., CNS support cells, astrocytes, oligodendrocytes). Instead, the active HIV infection develops in the microglia (brain macrophages). The cytokines and excitatory compounds that are produced as a result of this infection have a toxic effect on adjacent neurons.

HIV encephalopathy most often results in mild cerebral atrophy without a focal abnormality. Occasionally, HIV encephalopathy causes focal or diffuse white matter hyperintensities on T2WIs. Typically, HIV white matter involvement presents as subtle, diffuse T2 hyperintensity that often is bilateral and relatively symmetric. This supratentorial white matter signal abnormality is ill-defined and often involves a large area, in contrast to the dense lesions that are characteristic of PML. HIV encephalopathy can also present with more focal punctate lesions. HIV lesions do not demonstrate contrast enhancement.

Demyelination may also occur as an indirect result of a viral infection. Specifically, demyelination may follow a viral illness, the result of a virus-induced autoimmune response to white matter. This process may account for many of the incidental punctate foci of T2 hyperintensity noted in the young.

Toxic and Metabolic Demyelination

Central pontine myelinolysis (CPM) is a disorder that results in characteristic demyelination of the central pons. This is most commonly seen in patients with electrolyte abnormalities, particularly involving hyponatremia, that are rapidly corrected, giving rise to the term "osmotic demyelination syndrome." This condition occurs most commonly in children

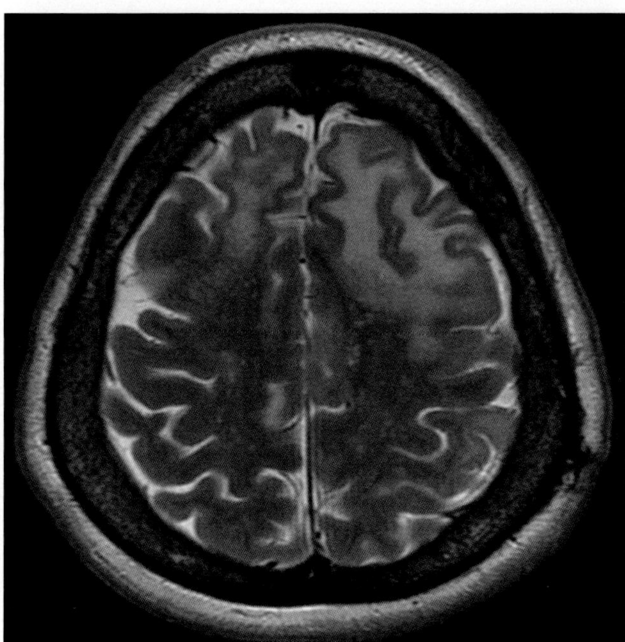

FIGURE 7.14. **Progressive Multifocal Leukoencephalopathy. A:** T2WI. A 32-year-old HIV-positive man presents with cognitive deterioration and mild weakness. Imaging reveals a subcortical focus of abnormality within the high frontal lobes, left greater than right. Characteristic features of this demyelinating process include minimal to no mass effect, even when very large, and essentially no contrast enhancement or hemorrhage. Also note the extension to the subcortical U fibers, that is, to the edge of the subcortical mantle, a characteristic feature of this type of demyelination. A very low T-cell count reflecting an immunocompromised status is also key to the diagnosis. In an immunocompetent patient, differential diagnostic considerations for this type of lesion would include posterior reversible encephalopathy syndrome, which can have a similar imaging appearance, but without such defined subcortical U-fiber extension.

and alcoholics with malnutrition. Occasionally, cases have been associated with diabetes, leukemia, transplant recipients, chronically debilitated patients, and others with conditions resulting in chronic malnutrition. The clinical course is classically described as biphasic, beginning with a generalized encephalopathy caused by the hyponatremia, which usually transiently improves following initial correction of sodium. This is followed by a second neurologic syndrome, which occurs 2 to 3 days following correction or overcorrection of hyponatremia caused by myelinolysis. This latter phase is classically characterized by a rapidly evolving corticospinal syndrome with quadriplegia, acute changes in mental status, and a "locked-in" state in which the patient is mute, unable to move, and occasionally comatose. Patients tend to be extremely ill and often have a very poor prognosis.

The pathophysiology of CPM relates to a disturbance in the physiologic balance of osmolality within the brain tissue. Oligodendroglial cells are most susceptible to CPM-related osmotic stresses, with the distribution of CPM changes paralleling the distribution of oligodendroglial cells within the central pons, thalamus, globus pallidus, putamen, lateral geniculate body, and other extrapontine sites. The mechanism of myelinolysis remains to be completely elucidated, but it appears to be distinct from a demyelinating process like that of MS, in which an inflammatory response predominates. CPM is characterized by intramyelinic splitting, vacuolization, and rupture of myelin sheaths, presumably because of osmotic effects. However, there is preservation of neurons and axons. Note that there is no inflammatory reaction associated with osmotic demyelination, differentiating this process from MS, which is characterized by marked perivascular inflammation. MRI characteristically demonstrates abnormal high signal on T2WI, corresponding to the regions of central pontine demyelination (Fig. 7.15). In addition, extrapontine sites of involvement have been described in this condition, including the white matter of the cerebellum, thalamus, globus pallidus, putamen, and lateral geniculate body, giving rise to the term *extrapontine myelinolysis*.

Posterior reversible encephalopathy syndrome (PRES) is a condition characterized by signal changes within the brain parenchyma, primarily involving the posterior vascular distribution. It has also been referred to as *reversible posterior leukoencephalopathy syndrome (RPLE)*. Patients may present with a wide variety of symptoms including headache, seizures, visual changes, and altered mental status, with MRI revealing relatively symmetric areas of bilateral subcortical and cortical vasogenic edema within the parietooccipital lobes (Fig. 7.16). The leading theory regarding the etiology of this condition is a temporary failure of the autoregulatory capabilities of the cerebral vessels, leading to hyperperfusion, breakdown of the blood–brain barrier, and consequent vasogenic edema, but no acute ischemic changes. Autoregulation maintains a constant blood flow to the brain, despite systemic blood pressure alterations, but this can be overcome at a "breakthrough" point, at which time the increased systemic blood pressure is transmitted to the brain, resulting in brain hyperperfusion. This increased perfusion pressure is sufficient to overcome the blood–brain barrier, allowing extravasation of fluid, macromolecules, and even red blood cells into the brain parenchyma. The preferential involvement of the parietal and occipital lobes is thought to be related to the relatively poor sympathetic innervation of the posterior circulation.

A very diverse set of conditions leads to the characteristic clinical and radiologic presentation of PRES. Conditions include treatment with cyclosporin A or tacrolimus (FK506), acute renal failure/uremia, hemolytic uremic syndrome, eclampsia, thrombotic thrombocytopenia purpura, and treatment with a wide variety of chemotherapeutic agents, including interferon. More recently, similar findings have been noted in the treatment of Alzheimer disease, with the use of various investigational therapeutic agents that target the removal of CNS amyloid. When the imaging findings of PRES are noted in the setting of treatment with an amyloid removing agent, the condition is termed amyloid-related imaging abnormalities (ARIAs).

This diverse set of offending agents suggests a final common etiologic pathway involving either endothelial injury, elevated blood pressure, or a combination of these factors. Associated clinical conditions presumably contribute to this physiologic effect by cytotoxic effects on the vascular endothelium (endotoxins), causing increasing capillary permeability that allows this process to occur at near-normal blood pressures, or by inducing or exacerbating hypertension. Hypertension is often associated with PRES but may be relatively mild and is not universally present, especially in the setting of immunosuppression. Note that this condition is not always reversible and may occasionally result in hemorrhagic infarctions.

Marchiafava–Bignami disease is a rare form of demyelination seen most frequently in alcoholics. This condition was first described in Italian red-wine drinkers, but it has since been reported with other types of alcohol use as well as in nonalcoholics. The disease is characterized by demyelination involving the central fibers (medial zone) of the corpus callosum, although other white matter tracts may be involved, including the anterior and posterior commissures, the centrum semiovale, and the middle cerebral peduncles. This is felt to reflect a form of osmotic demyelination, as discussed earlier in

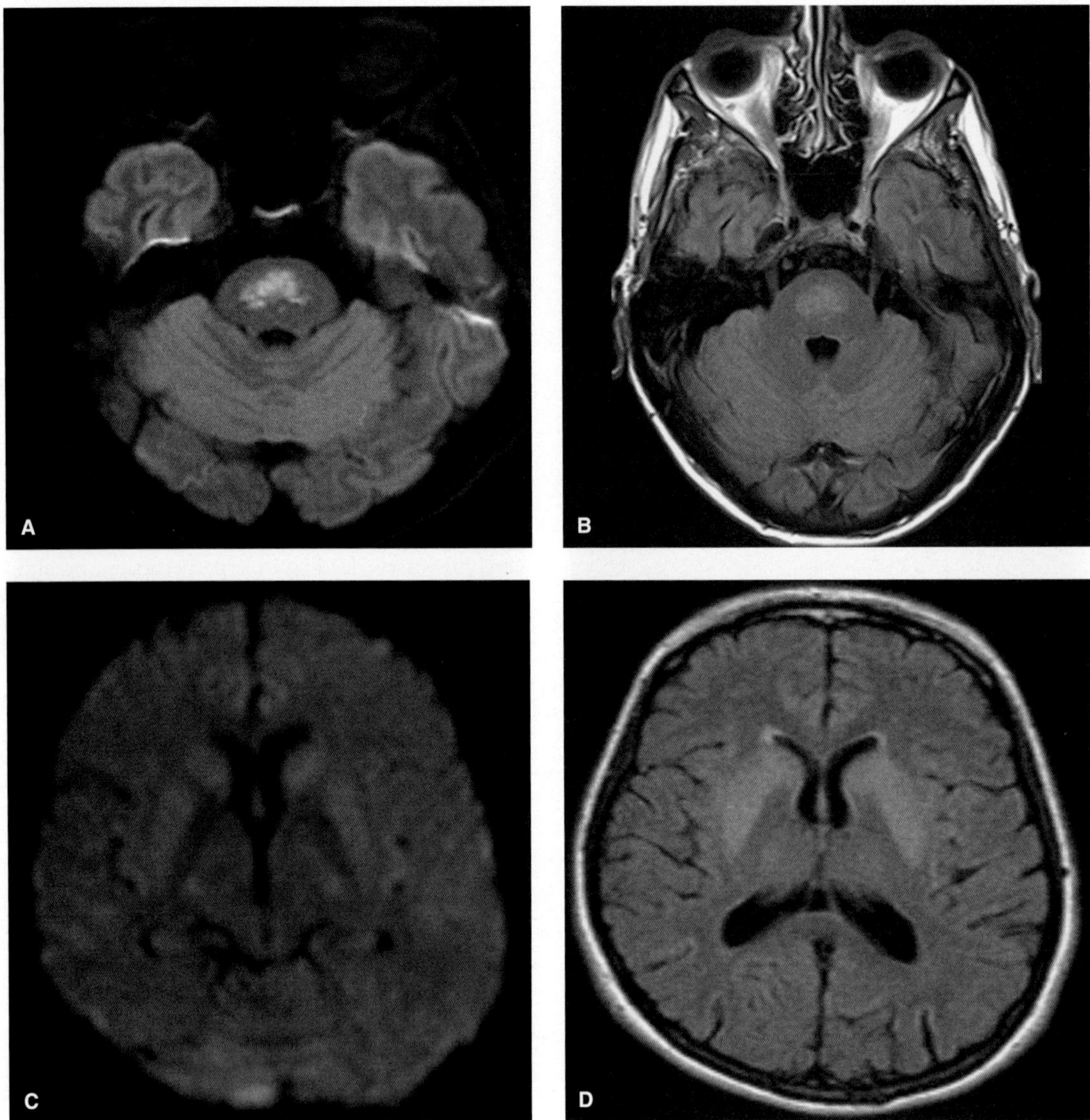

FIGURE 7.15. **Osmotic Demyelination Syndrome: Central Pontine and Extrapontine Myelinolysis (CPM and EPM). A:** Diffusion-weighted image, (**B**) T2-FLAIR. An alcoholic patient was admitted with serum sodium of 110 mEq/mL. After rapid normalization of serum sodium, the patient became comatose. Imaging demonstrates diffuse hyperintensity within the basis pontis with associated restricted diffusion. These findings are in keeping with the acute osmotic changes relating to an osmotic injury. Imaging changes are typically identified first on DWI, several days before appearance on T2WI. Thus, when CPM is a clinical concern, always carefully scrutinize the DWI study. The T2WI changes, in isolation, are most commonly a reflection of long-standing small-vessel ischemic changes. Clinical history is of value in helping to differentiate central pontine myelinolysis from infarction (ischemic demyelination). **C:** Diffusion-weighted image. **D:** T2-FLAIR. Osmotic demyelination may also occur outside of the pons and is described as extrapontine myelinolysis, typically involving the deep gray mater structures (basal ganglia, thalami) and deep white matter tracts (internal, external, and extreme capsule as well as the splenium of the corpus callosum).

extrapontine myelinolysis. Onset is usually insidious, with the most common symptom being nonspecific dementia.

Wernicke encephalopathy and Korsakoff syndrome are metabolic disorders caused by thiamine (B_1 vitamin) deficiency secondary to poor oral intake in severe chronic alcoholics (most common association), hematologic malignancies, or recurrent vomiting in pregnant patients. In fact, this condition may occur in many different non–alcohol-related pathologic conditions that share the common denominator of malnutrition. In general, there is a good clinical response to thiamine administration. As such, thinking of this condition when encountering the characteristic lesions of the deep gray matter and periaqueductal gray may allow early diagnosis of the condition.

Classically, Wernicke encephalopathy is characterized by the clinical triad of acute onset of ocular movement abnormalities, ataxia, and confusion. Korsakoff, a Russian psychiatrist, described the disturbance of memory in long-term alcoholics. Therefore, if persistent learning and memory deficits are present in patients with Wernicke encephalopathy, the symptom complex is termed "Wernicke–Korsakoff syndrome."

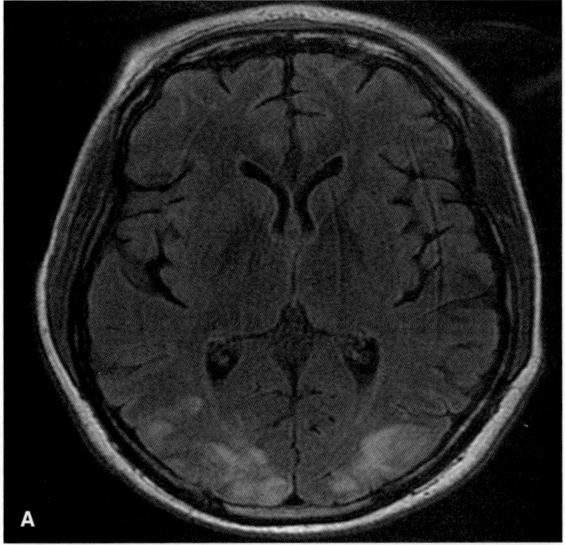

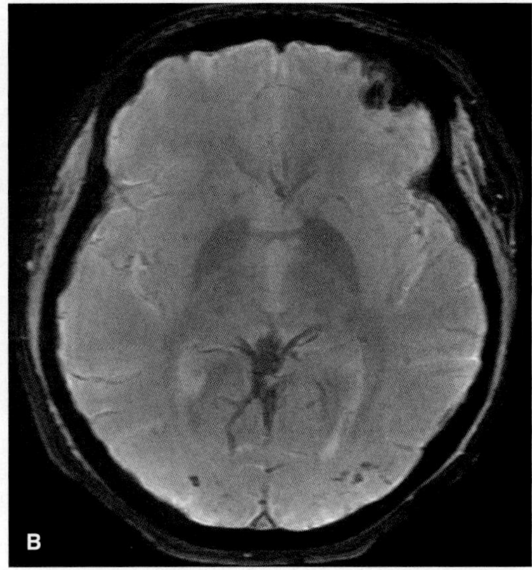

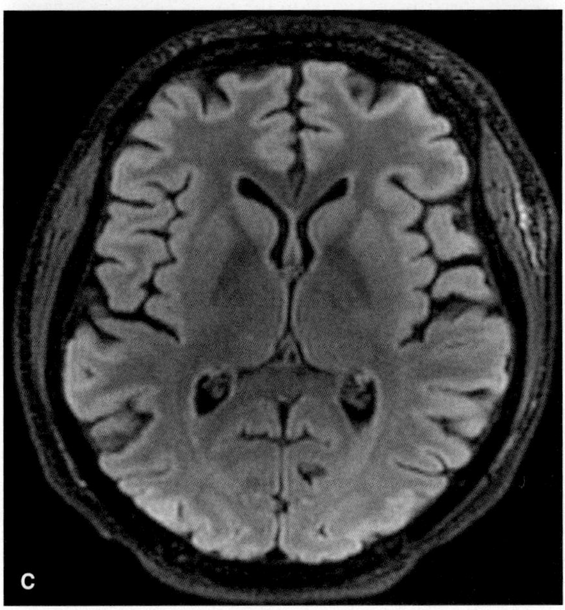

FIGURE 7.16. **Posterior Reversible Encephalopathy Syndrome (PRES).** **A:** T2-FLAIR. A 43-year-old transplant patient who was being treated with cyclosporine presented with visual disturbances and hypertension. T2WIs reveal patchy areas of primarily subcortical signal abnormality, with some cortical involvement, within the parietooccipital lobes, corresponding to the posterior vascular distribution. Imaging findings are consistent with vasogenic edema, as there was no associated restricted diffusion or contrast enhancement (images not shown). These findings are in keeping with transient dysfunction of vascular permeability, the result of a combination of endothelial toxicity and elevated blood pressure. **B:** SWAN. Typically PRES is not associated with cytotoxic edema or parenchymal hemorrhage. However, in more severe cases, this condition may go on to result in varying degrees of hemorrhage (microp-etechial to frank parenchymal hemorrhage) and ischemia. **C:** T2-FLAIR. The treatment for PRES, is typically to remove the offending agent. In this case, both clinical symptoms and imaging findings resolved after the cyclosporine doses were reduced, confirming this as a transient period of leaky capillaries. Note although this condition is often parietal–occipital in location, it may be found anywhere throughout the cerebrum and cerebellum.

In the acute stage of this disease, MRI may reveal T2 hyperintensity or contrast enhancement of the mammillary bodies, basal ganglia, thalamus, and brainstem, with periaqueductal involvement. In contrast, the chronic stage may show atrophy of the mammillary bodies, midbrain tegmentum, as well as dilatation of the third ventricle. Except for the mammillary body involvement, these findings are very similar to the Leigh disease, which supports the notion that enzymatic deregulation in Leigh disease is tied in some fashion to thiamine metabolism.

Radiation Leukoencephalitis. Radiation may result in damage to the white matter secondary to a radiation-induced vasculopathy. Radiation leukoencephalitis usually follows a cumulative dose in excess of 40 Gy delivered to the brain and occurs 6 to 9 months after treatment. Findings consist of areas of abnormal high signal on T2WIs, typically involving confluent areas of white matter extending to involve the subcortical U fibers in the distribution of the irradiated brain (Fig. 7.17). Note that this represents an indirect effect of radiation on the brain and results from an arteritis (endothelial hypertrophy, medial hyalinization, and fibrosis) involving small arteries and arterioles.

Radiation Necrosis and Radiation Arteritis. In contrast to the rather benign nature of radiation leukoencephalitis, radiation necrosis and radiation arteritis are major hazards related to CNS radiation. Both of these radiation effects are strongly dose-related and are less commonly seen today because of greater fractionation of CNS radiation doses. Radiation necrosis may occur several weeks to years after radiation, but it most commonly occurs between 6 and 24 months after radiation. Radiation necrosis is rarely noted at less than 6 months after treatment unless gamma knife is employed. Note that gamma knife is an ablative procedure designed to destroy the targeted tissue and thus may more easily incite frank radiation necrosis. This is in contrast to radiation therapy, which is not ablative in nature. Radiation necrosis can be progressive and fatal. Radiation necrosis typically presents as an enhancing lesion with mass effect and ring enhancement or as multiple

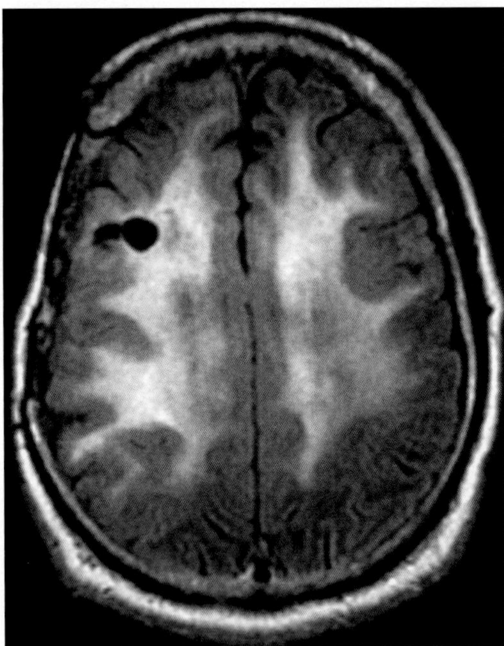

FIGURE 7.17. **Radiation Leukoencephalopathy.** A 62-year-old woman underwent MRI 1 year after whole brain radiation for metastatic CNS breast carcinoma. Axial fluid-attenuated inversion recovery image reveals confluent high signal throughout the periventricular white matter, with residua relating to resection of right frontal metastasis. This finding may be associated with loss of deep cerebral white matter with concomitant ex vacuo ventriculomegaly. Although this condition may result in some degree of neurocognitive deficits, this patient was entirely asymptomatic and was simply returning for a routine follow-up examination.

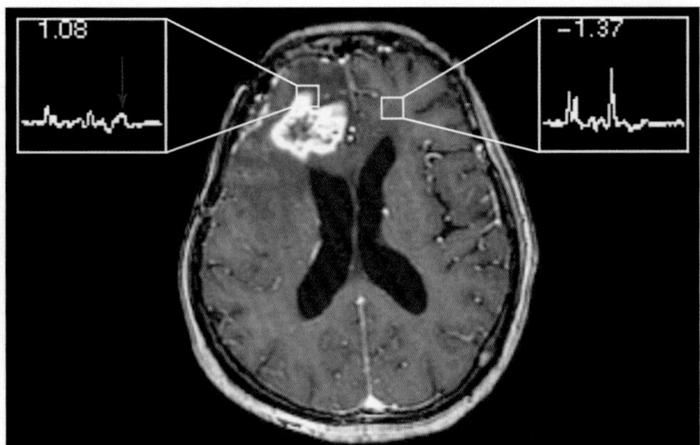

FIGURE 7.18. **Radiation Necrosis.** Axial postgadolinium T1WI with multivoxel MR spectroscopy. A 45-year-old man presented 8 months following resection and irradiation of a right frontal glioma, with development of an enhancing mass lesion within the operative bed. Despite this ominous appearance, this lesion revealed no radioisotope uptake on ^{18}F-2-fluoro-2-d-deoxyglucose PET (not shown). Representative MR spectroscopy voxel in the region of lesion enhancement reveals a small lactate and lipid peak (*arrow*) (0.9 to 1.3 ppm) with reduction in all other major metabolites (choline, creatine, and *N*-acetylaspartate). This can be contrasted with the normal-appearing spectrum from the left frontal lobe. Both PET and MR spectroscopy confirm the diagnosis of radiation necrosis. Serial MR scanning performed at 3-month intervals revealed a slowly regressing lesion that resolved by the 24-month follow-up study.

foci of enhancement, mimicking recurrent neoplasm. Radiation may also induce telangiectasia within the radiation field, which may appear similar to cryptic vascular malformations.

Radiation necrosis is found most commonly in or near the irradiated tumor bed, but it sometimes is more remote from the tumor bed. It is theorized that the partially injured brain parenchyma within and adjacent to the tumor bed is more susceptible to radiation injury, thus accounting for the distribution of radiation necrosis. After resection of a brain neoplasm and subsequent radiation therapy, it can be very difficult to differentiate tumor recurrence from radiation-associated necrosis, because both conditions may continue to grow and demonstrate imaging features characteristic of neoplasm, that is, lesion growth, irregular ring enhancement, edema, and mass effect (Fig. 7.18). If during serial scanning a lesion within the treated tumor bed stabilizes and regresses, this is obviously radiation necrosis, but if the lesion progresses, differentiation between tumor and radiation necrosis is difficult. PET and MR spectroscopy (MRS) are valuable in distinguishing between tumor recurrence and radiation necrosis. With PET scanning, a short-lived radioactive isotope (e.g., ^{18}F fluorodeoxyglucose) that decays by emitting a positron, is combined with glucose, a metabolically active molecule. This tracer mimics glucose and is taken up and retained by tissues with higher than normal metabolic activity, such as tumor recurrence. This is in contrast to radiation necrosis, which is not metabolically active.

Proton (hydrogen) MRS imaging characterizes the metabolite profiles of tumoral and nontumoral brain lesions. This biochemical information helps distinguish areas of tumor recurrence from areas of radiation necrosis. Major brain metabolites include choline (Cho), creatine (Cr), and *N*-acetylaspartate (NAA) (located at 3.2, 3.0, and 2.0 ppm, respectively). Choline reflects cellular density and proliferation, and is often elevated with tumor. Creatine is a normal cellular metabolite and is often stable in a variety of disease conditions. Thus creatine is often used as a denominator in calculating choline and NAA ratios (Cho/Cr and NAA/Cr), which corrects for individual variation and allows for comparison between individual subjects. NAA is a neuronal marker and reflects neuronal density. Loss of the NAA signal is consistent with neuronal loss or damage, which can be seen in a wide variety of disease conditions, including radiation necrosis and even MS.

Large vessels included within the radiation port may undergo radiation-induced endothelial hypertrophy, medial hyalinization, and fibrosis. The net result is a progressive vascular narrowing that may be obliterative in nature. This often involves the cavernous and supraclinoid portions of the carotid arteries in children who have undergone irradiation of the parasellar region for treatment of tumors, for example, craniopharyngiomas or optic and hypothalamic gliomas. The near-complete obliteration of the supraclinoid carotid arteries results in cerebral and striatal ischemic changes. Occasionally, there may be a compensatory proliferation of lenticulostriate collaterals. When performing angiography, these collateral vessels present with a blush, which in Japan has been referred to as *Moyamoya,* meaning "puff of smoke." Moyamoya disease classically refers to a supraclinoid obliterative arteriopathy that occurs primarily in children and is idiopathic in nature (Fig. 7.7).

When methotrexate chemotherapy (intrathecal or systemic) is administered in combination with CNS radiation, these agents may have a synergistic effect in causing marked white matter abnormalities. It is theorized that low-dose radiation alters the blood–brain barrier, allowing increased penetration of methotrexate to neurotoxic levels. This has been noted most frequently in children being treated for leukemia, and two specific conditions have been described. The first has been called *mineralizing microangiopathy,* which is seen in up to one-third of these children. This results in diffuse destructive changes to the brain characterized by symmetric corticomedullary junction and basal ganglia calcifications. There is also diffuse signal abnormality throughout the white matter. A more serious but less common complication of combined radiation and methotrexate therapy is called *necrotizing leukoencephalopathy.* This process results in widespread damage to the white matter, consisting of demyelination, necrosis, and gliosis. MRI reveals large, diffuse, confluent areas of white matter signal abnormality with cortical sparing. Clinically, these children may have symptoms ranging from slight reductions in cognitive function to progressive dementia, seizures, hemiplegia, and coma.

DYSMYELINATING DISEASES

The disease processes that have been described up until this point are demyelinating, as they represent the destruction of normal myelin. In contrast, the *dysmyelinating* conditions, also referred to as leukodystrophies, are disorders in which myelin is abnormally formed or cannot be maintained in its normal state because of an inherited enzymatic or metabolic disorder. Although most of these conditions are not treatable, establishing a diagnosis is valuable in providing a prognosis and enables parental genetic counseling. These conditions are characterized by the progressive destruction of myelin owing to the accumulation of various catabolites, depending on the specific enzyme deficiency. Children often present clinically with progressive mental and motor deterioration. Radiographically, these diseases present with diffuse white matter lesions that are very similar to one another; however, some distinguishing features do exist (Table 7.2). The radiologist may play an important role in the diagnosis of these conditions, because astute interpretation of abnormal imaging findings may allow them to be the first physician to suggest the possibility of a metabolic disease. Factors that are helpful in differentiation between the leukodystrophies include the age of onset and the pattern of white matter involvement. Ultimately, serum biochemical and enzymatic analyses allow a specific diagnosis to be made. Dysmyelinating diseases are rather uncommon, and we will focus on a few of the classic conditions.

Metachromatic leukodystrophy is the most common of the leukodystrophies. It is transmitted by an autosomal recessive pattern and is the result of a deficiency of the enzyme arylsulfatase A. The most common type is an infantile form that becomes apparent at approximately 2 years of age with gait disorder and mental deterioration. There is steady disease progression, with death occurring within 5 years of the time of onset. MRI demonstrates progressive symmetric areas of nonspecific white matter involvement with sparing of the subcortical U fibers. Imaging findings are typically nonspecific.

Adrenal leukodystrophy is a sex-linked recessive condition (peroxisomal enzyme deficiency) occurring only in boys. Typical age of onset is between 5 and 10 years of age. As the name implies, these patients often have symptoms related to the adrenal gland, such as adrenal insufficiency or abnormal skin pigmentation. Adrenal leukodystrophy has a striking predilection for the visual and auditory pathways, presenting with symmetric involvement of the periatrial white matter with extension into the splenium of the corpus callosum (Fig. 7.19). The predilection for periatrial involvement results in early extension to the medial and lateral geniculate nuclei, which represent relays for the auditory and visual pathways, respectively. This accounts for the early presentation of visual and auditory symptomatology in these children.

Leigh disease, also called subacute necrotizing encephalomyelopathy, is a mitochondrial enzyme defect that commonly manifests in infancy or childhood (usually younger than 5 years). Leigh disease has histopathologic findings similar to those of Wernicke encephalopathy (metabolic disorder caused by thiamine [B_1 vitamin] deficiency secondary to poor oral intake in chronic alcoholics); hence the suspicion that it is related to an inborn defect in thiamine metabolism. Clinical findings are extremely variable and often nonspecific. Symmetric focal necrotic lesions are found in the basal ganglia and thalamus as well as in the subcortical white matter (Fig. 7.20). Lesions may also extend into the midbrain, medulla, and posterior columns of the spinal cord. A characteristic finding is involvement of the periaqueductal gray matter. In contrast to Wernicke encephalopathy, there is sparing of the mammillary bodies. In the same family of mitochondrial disorders are two additional encephalopathies, which have the acronyms MELAS (mitochondrial myelopathy, encephalopathy, lactic acidosis, and stroke-like episodes) and MERRF (myoclonic epilepsy and ragged red fibers). These inherited mitochondrial abnormalities are caused by point mutations of mitochondrial DNA or mitochondrial RNA and represent progressive neurodegenerative disorders characterized clinically by strokes, stroke-like events, nausea, vomiting, encephalopathy, seizures, short stature, headaches, muscle weakness, exercise intolerance, neurosensory hearing loss, and myopathy.

TABLE 7.2

DYSMYELINATING DISEASES

■ DISEASE	■ HEAD SIZE	■ AGE OF ONSET (Yr)	■ WHITE MATTER INVOLVEMENT	■ GRAY MATTER INVOLVEMENT
Metachromatic leukodystrophy	Normal	Infantile form: 1–2 Juvenile form: 5–7	Diffusely affected	None
Adrenoleukodystrophy	Normal	5–10	Symmetric occipital and splenium of corpus callosum	None
Leigh disease	Normal	<5	Focal areas of subcortical white matter	Basal ganglia and periaqueductal gray
Alexander disease	Normal to large	≤1	Frontal	None
Canavan disease	Normal to large	≤1	Diffusely affected	Vacuolization of cortical gray matter

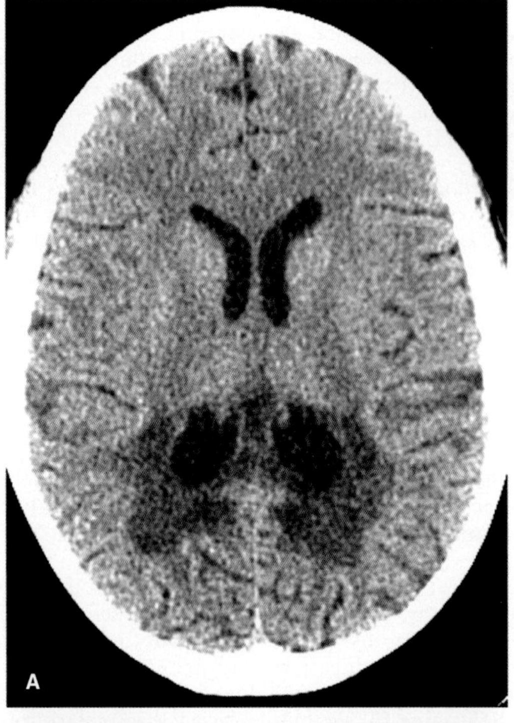

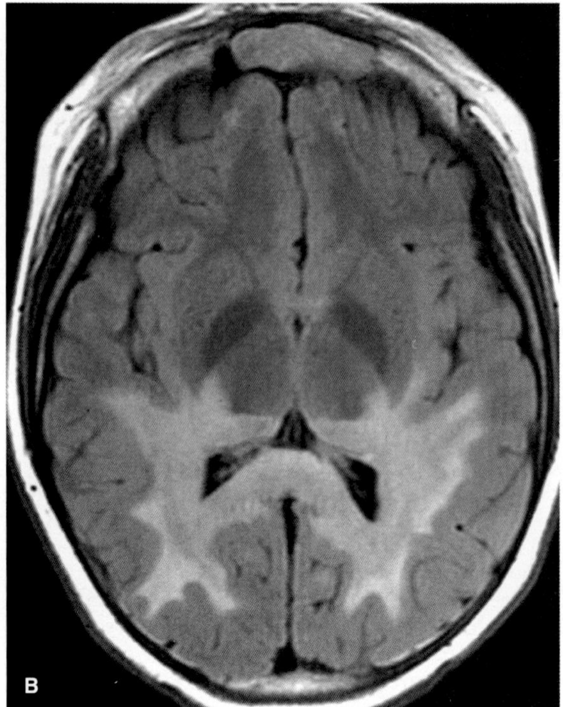

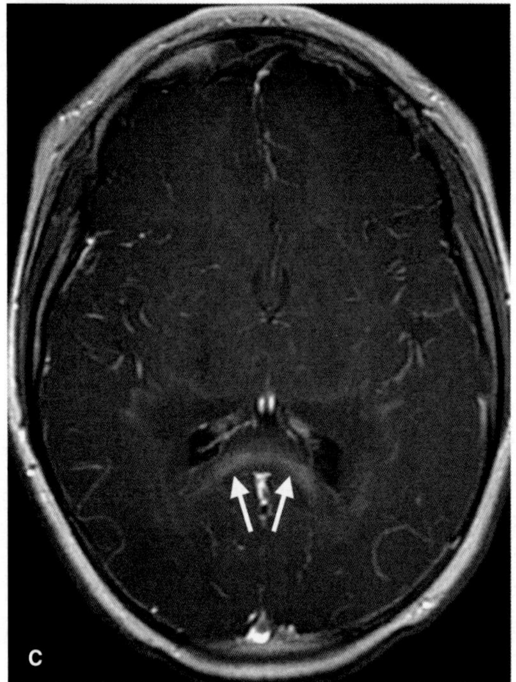

FIGURE 7.19. **Adrenal Leukodystrophy. A:** Axial CT. **B:** Fluid-attenuated inversion recovery image. **C:** Postcontrast T1WI. Two different patients (CT and MRI, respectively) presented with gradual gait disturbance, hearing and visual symptoms, and adrenal insufficiency. Imaging reveals abnormality within the periatrial and occipital white matter extending into the splenium of the corpus callosum. Involvement extends into the region of the medial and lateral geniculate bodies, accounting for the patient's hearing and visual symptoms, respectively. Note the associated contrast enhancement of the splenium (*arrows*) in keeping with an acute phase of metabolic related demyelination.

Alexander and Canavan diseases are the rarest of the leukodystrophies and may appear as early as the first few weeks of life. Patients often have an enlarged brain and have macrocephaly on examination. Typically, these patients present with seizures, spasticity, and delayed developmental milestones. In Alexander disease, white matter lesions often begin in the frontal white matter and progress posteriorly (Fig. 7.21). Canavan disease is caused by a deficiency of the enzyme aspartoacylase, which leads to the buildup of NAA in the brain and subsequent myelin destruction. This results in a pathognomonic MRI spectra consisting of a giant NAA peak.

CEREBROSPINAL FLUID DYNAMICS

In patients with acute hydrocephalus, transependymal flow of CSF may mimic periventricular white matter disease. CSF is produced predominantly by the choroid plexus of the lateral, third, and fourth ventricles. CSF flows from the lateral ventricles into the third ventricle through the foramina of Monro and then by way of the cerebral aqueduct into the fourth ventricle. The CSF leaves the ventricular system via the lateral

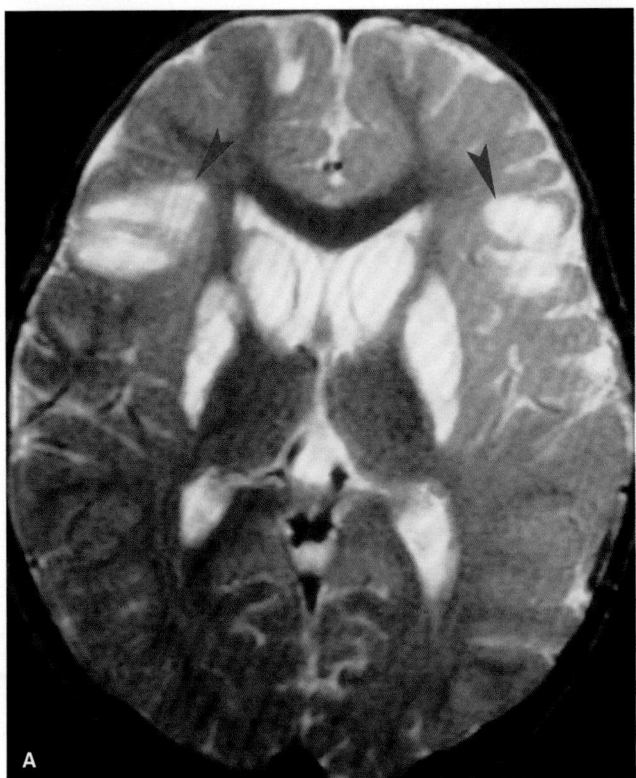

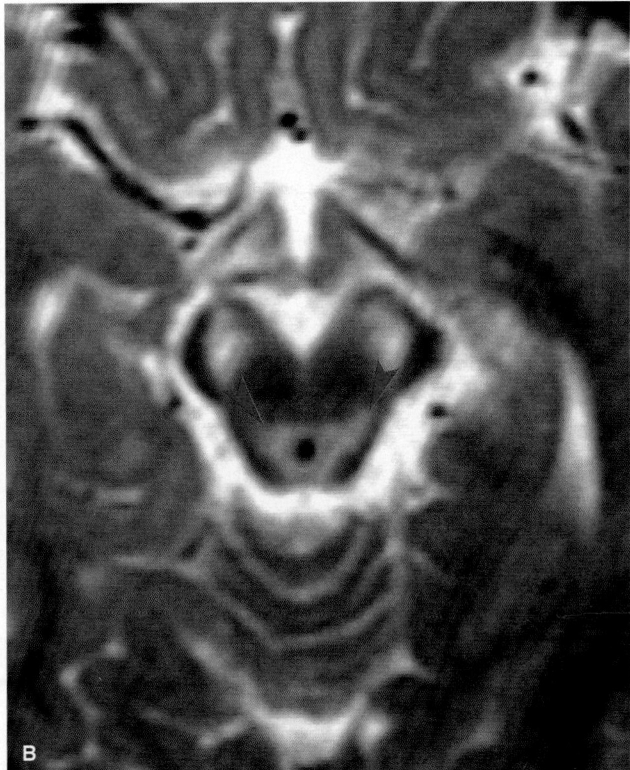

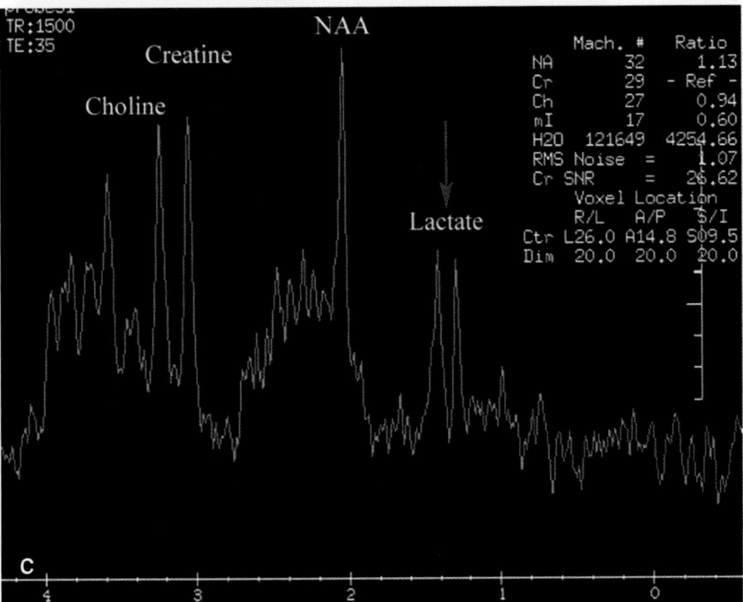

FIGURE 7.20. Leigh Disease. Leigh disease (mitochondrial enzyme defect) in a 3-year-old patient presenting with progressive hypotonia and seizures. **A:** T2WI demonstrates a wide spectrum of gray and white matter lesions reported in Leigh disease, including basal ganglia (globus pallidus, putamen, caudate); brainstem (midbrain and periaqueductal gray); and subcortical white matter involvement (*arrowheads*). **B:** Involvement of the periaqueductal gray matter (*arrowheads*) is quite characteristic for either Leigh disease or Wernicke syndrome. Both conditions are associated with thiamine deficiency; the former is related to mitochondrial enzymatic deficiencies involved with the metabolism of thiamine, and in the latter, it is nutritional. A differentiating feature is involvement of the mammillary bodies in Wernicke syndrome, which is absent in Leigh disease. **C:** MR spectroscopy reveals an elevated lactate peak at 1.3 ppm, which supports the diagnosis of Leigh disease. Mitochondrial enzyme deficiencies associated with Leigh disease include pyruvate dehydrogenase complex, pyruvate carboxylase, and electron transport chain, which result in elevated blood, CSF and CNS lactate, and pyruvate levels.

and medial fourth ventricular foramina (the foramina of Luschka and Magendie, respectively). CSF then travels through the basilar cisterns and over the surfaces of the cerebral hemispheres. The principal site of absorption is into the venous circulation through the arachnoid villi, which project into the dural sinuses, primarily the superior sagittal sinus. Although the principal routes of CSF production and absorption are as outlined, a significant amount of CSF may be both produced and reabsorbed via the ependymal lining of the ventricles. This transependymal flow of CSF can become an important means of CSF reabsorption during ventricular obstruction.

Hydrocephalus is caused by an obstruction of the CSF circulatory pathway and is classified into two principal types: noncommunicating and communicating. *Noncommunicating hydrocephalus* refers to an obstruction occurring within the ventricular system that prevents CSF from exiting the ventricles (Fig. 7.22). In contrast, with *communicating hydrocephalus,* the level of obstruction is beyond the ventricular system, located instead within the subarachnoid space. CSF is able to exit the ventricular system but fails to undergo normal resorption by the arachnoid villi. In theory, with communicating hydrocephalus, most of the ventricular system is

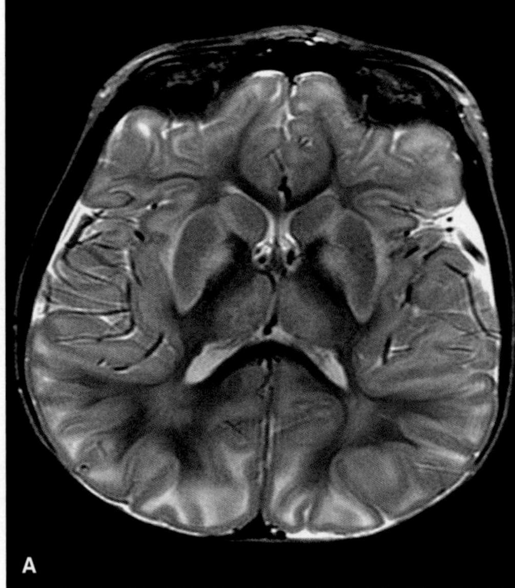

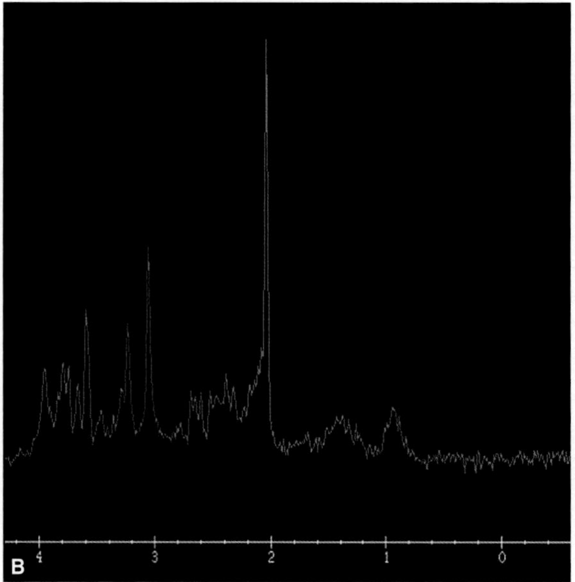

FIGURE 7.21. Canavan Disease. A 22-month-old child presented with progressive spastic quadriparesis and macrocephaly. **A:** Axial T2WI reveals diffuse high signal extending throughout the cerebral white matter involving the subcortical U fibers. This is a nonspecific finding that could reflect an advanced stage of many of the leukodystrophies. **B:** However, the MR spectroscopy reveals a markedly elevated *N*-acetylaspartate (NAA), diagnostic of a deficiency of the enzyme aspartoacylase (Canavan disease), which leads to the buildup of NAA in the brain and subsequent myelin destruction. The mnemonic CaNAAvan may assist in remembering this diagnostic finding.

enlarged, whereas with noncommunicating hydrocephalus, dilation occurs up to the point of obstruction. The fourth ventricle often does not dilate because of the relatively confined nature of the posterior fossa and thus cannot be used as a reliable means by which to differentiate communicating from noncommunicating hydrocephalus. Communicating hydrocephalus will commonly demonstrate supratentorial ventriculomegaly, with a fourth ventricle that appears normal. Although dilation of the fourth ventricle is suggestive of communicating hydrocephalus, it is not a reliable sign, because obstruction at the outlet foramina of the fourth ventricle (Luschka and Magendie) may result in a similar appearance.

In assessing for the presence of hydrocephalus, specific attention should be directed to the third ventricle and the temporal ventricular horns. Convex bowing of the lateral walls and inferior recesses of the third ventricle is characteristic for hydrocephalus. As with fourth ventricular

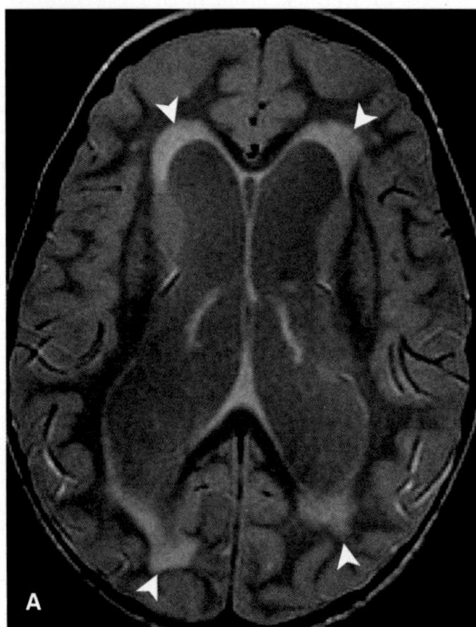

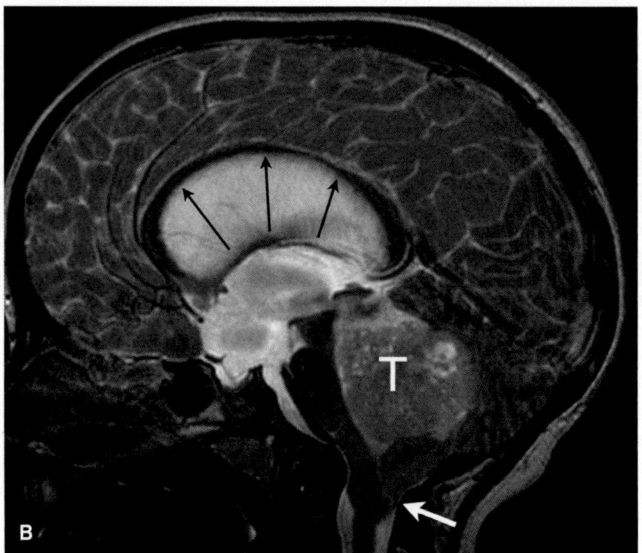

FIGURE 7.22. Hydrocephalus. A: Axial fluid-attenuated inversion recovery image. **B:** Sagittal T2WI. A 6-year-old presenting with chronic headaches. Axial image reveals dilated ventricles with periventricular hyperintensity consistent with transependymal flow of CSF (*arrowheads*). On sagittal imaging, the pressure changes indicative of hydrocephalus include the upward convex bowing of the corpus callosum (*arrow*), downward convex ballooning of the inferior third ventricular recesses which obliterate the suprasellar cistern, and tonsillar ectopia (*white arrow*). The obstructing ependymoma (*T*) is evident as a large mass, which fills the fourth ventricle.

enlargement, however, this finding is seldom present. A far more sensitive indicator of hydrocephalus is enlargement of the temporal horns. The temporal horns sometimes will demonstrate enlargement, even before lateral ventricular involvement is evident. Bowing and stretching of the corpus callosum, easily detected on the sagittal images, is an additional finding that is suggestive of hydrocephalus.

Ex Vacuo Ventriculomegaly. A distinction must be made between hydrocephalus and ex vacuo ventriculomegaly. The latter represents an enlarged ventricular system that is simply the result of parenchymal atrophy. With atrophy, the loss of brain matter results in prominence of all CSF spaces, both the cerebral sulci as well as the ventricles. In contrast with the hydrocephalus, the ventricles are enlarged out of proportion to the sulci. The third ventricle and temporal ventricular horns are particularly helpful in making this distinction. Both of these ventricular spaces are surrounded by tissue that is not typically subject to significant atrophy. The third ventricle is surrounded by the thalamus (gray matter), and there is a relative paucity of white matter within the temporal lobes. This is in contrast to the large amount of white matter surrounding the lateral ventricles, which may undergo atrophy. Enlargement of the third ventricle, with bowing of its lateral and inferior recesses as well as temporal horn enlargement, suggests hydrocephalus.

Subarachnoid hemorrhage and meningitis are the most frequent causes of acute hydrocephalus and may result in either communicating or noncommunicating hydrocephalus, with obstruction at any level of the ventricular system, the basilar cisterns, or the arachnoid villi. The obstruction is caused by adhesions and inflammation, and no obstructing mass is typically detected. Noncommunicating hydrocephalus can be the result of either an acquired or a congenital obstructive process. Benign congenital webs may form across the cerebral aqueduct, resulting in aqueductal stenosis. In addition, the Chiari and Dandy–Walker malformations are believed to represent adhesions occurring during CNS development, at the outlet foramina of the fourth ventricle and posterior fossa. A variety of neoplasms may result in obstructive hydrocephalus, often in very characteristic locations. Colloid cysts typically block the anterior third ventricle, pineal tumors, and tectal gliomas obstruct the aqueduct, and ependymomas and medulloblastomas interrupt CSF flow at the level of the fourth ventricle. Whenever hydrocephalus is detected, it is important to inspect the ventricles for an obstructing mass. A location that should be specifically evaluated is the cerebral aqueduct. On routine axial and sagittal images, a normal pulsatile flow void should be detected; otherwise, the diagnosis of aqueductal stenosis should be considered.

The duration of hydrocephalus affects the imaging findings. In acute hydrocephalus, there is insufficient time for compensatory mechanisms, and a striking amount of transependymal CSF flow will be noted. This results in a dramatic accumulation of high signal in the periventricular white matter on T2WIs. In chronic forms of hydrocephalus, compensatory mechanisms of CNS production and resorption have occurred and the degree of transependymal flow is minimal.

Normal pressure hydrocephalus (NPH) is a chronic, low-level form of hydrocephalus. The classic clinical triad is dementia, gait disturbance, and urinary incontinence. In this condition, the CSF pressure is within normal limits, but a slight gradient exists between the ventricular system and the subarachnoid space because of an incomplete subarachnoid CSF block. This most commonly results from a previous subarachnoid hemorrhage or meningeal infection. The result is diffuse ventriculomegaly that is out of proportion to the degree of sulcal prominence. Differentiating mild hydrocephalus from atrophic ventriculomegaly can be very difficult. Studies suggest that MRI CSF velocity and stroke volume calculations can be used to predict which patients may have favorable response to ventriculoperitoneal shunting. In addition to cross-sectional studies, radioisotope studies may be of value. The classic findings on radioisotope cisternogram are early entry of the radiopharmaceutical into the lateral ventricles, with persistence at 24 and 48 hours, and considerable delay in the ascend to the parasagittal region. Differentiating NPH from atrophic ventriculomegaly can be very difficult, and unfortunately, no imaging study is definitive in making this diagnosis. NPH is not a radiographic diagnosis, and close correlation of clinical and imaging findings is required to establish the diagnosis. The definitive diagnosis of NPH is made on demonstrating clinical improvement following ventricular shunting.

NEURODEGENERATIVE DISORDERS

Neurodegenerative disorders frequently have no known cause and result in progressive neurologic deterioration that is faster than expected given the patient's age.

Alzheimer disease (AD) is the most common neurodegenerative disease and the most common cause of dementia. It is estimated that in the United States alone there are about 4 million people with this disorder. The number of those affected by AD is rapidly increasing as the world's population ages. It is estimated that by the year 2050, the number of people with AD will increase threefold, to about 60 million worldwide, with about 14 million in the United States alone. Although the cause of AD is not clear, histopathologically the disease is characterized by two abnormal structures in the brain: *neuritic plaques* and *neurofibrillary tangles*. Neuritic plaques are composed of tortuous neuritic processes surrounding a central amyloid core, which consists primarily of a small peptide known as β-amyloid, derived from a larger amyloid precursor protein. Neurofibrillary tangles contain an abnormal tau protein that is associated with microtubules. Both plaques and tangles seem to interfere with normal neuronal functioning.

Neuroimaging studies of patients with AD demonstrate diffuse atrophy, with a predilection for the hippocampal formation, temporal lobes, and parietotemporal cortices. As a result, enlargement of the temporal horns, suprasellar cisterns, and Sylvian fissures may be useful in discriminating AD from normal age-related atrophy (Fig. 7.23). A variety of functional imaging modalities (PET as well as perfusion MRI with arterial spin labeling and regional cerebral blood flow calculations) are being used to diagnose and differentiate AD from senescent dementia. Also PET plays an important role in therapeutic drug trials for AD, where numerous ^{18}F-labeled PET ligands (specific for AD-related proteins, such as amyloid) allow not only for the early detection of this disease but also help to identify efficacious treatments by evaluating the early response to drugs, far before any changes in clinical symptoms would be evident.

Parkinson disease is the most common basal ganglia disorder and one of the leading causes of neurologic disability in individuals older than age 60. This disease is characterized clinically by tremor, muscular rigidity, and loss of postural reflexes. About 25% of Parkinson patients also develop dementia. Parkinsonism results from a deficiency of the neurotransmitter dopamine caused by dysfunction of the dopaminergic neuronal system, specifically the pars compacta of the substantia nigra. The loss of these nerve cells results in a decreased concentration

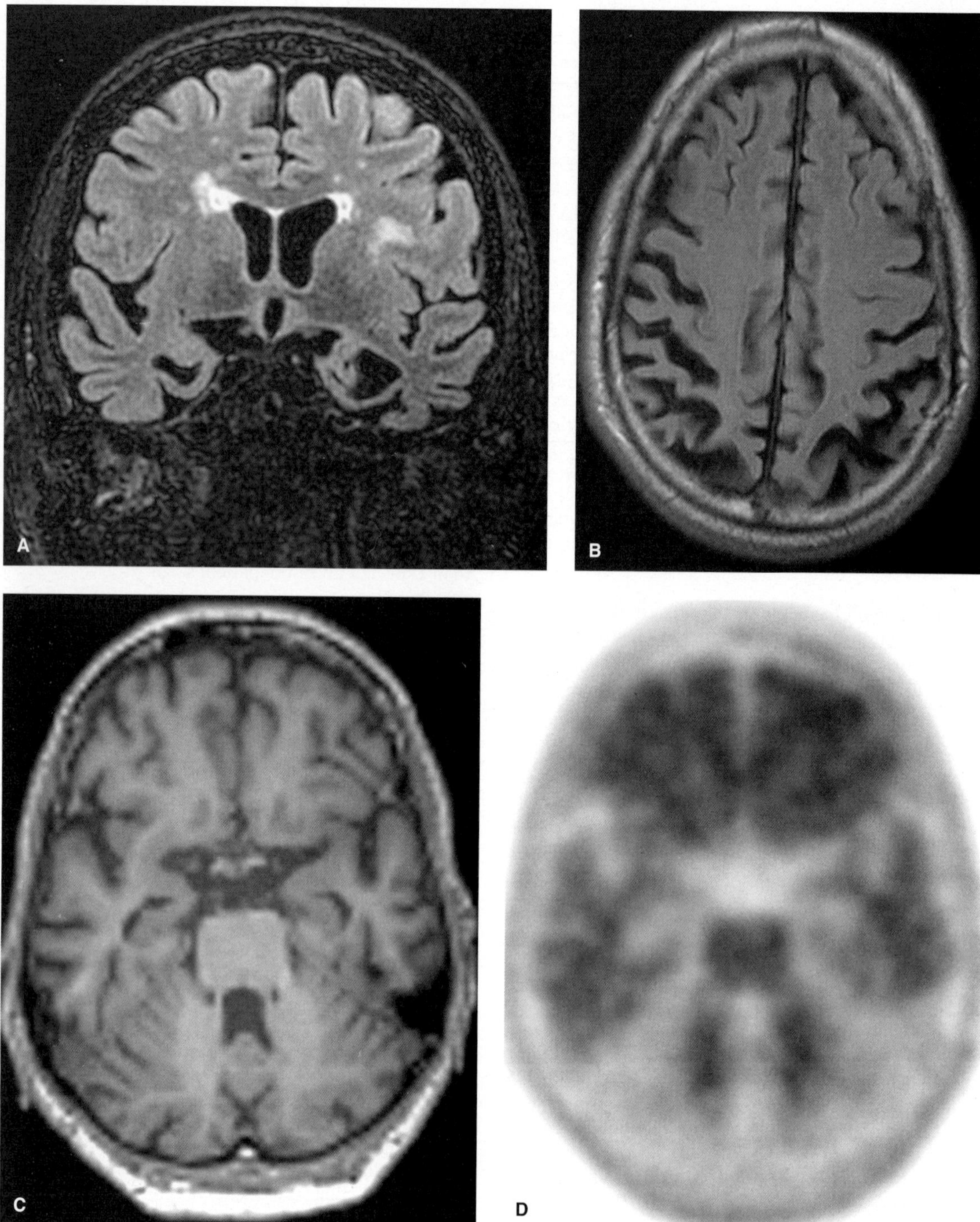

FIGURE 7.23. Alzheimer Disease. A: T2-FLAIR. A 70-year-old man with early dementia reveals prominent temporal lobe and hippocampal atrophy. **B:** T2WI. Alzheimer disease is also characterized by posterior cortical atrophy namely parietal lobe (including the posterior cingulate sulcus, parietooccipital sulcus, and precuneus). Alzheimer disease is a neurodegenerative disorder and the most common pathologic cause of dementia responsible for 60% to 80% of all dementia. Risk factors include advanced age and apolipoprotein E (APOE) ε4 allele carrier status. Disproportionate parietotemporal cortical atrophy relative to the extent of white matter disease, supports the diagnosis of Alzheimer disease rather than a pure ischemic or multi-infarct dementia. Note, however, that Alzheimer disease is associated with a higher incidence of white matter ischemic changes and periventricular halo than corresponding controls. As such the presence of white matter change with parietotemporal atrophy should not detract from suggesting the diagnosis. **C:** T1WI. **D:** Amyloid PET scan. Mild cognitive impairment (MCI). A 50-year-old woman presents with mild memory deficits. MRI imaging is normal without any temporal lobe or parietal lobe atrophy. However, a PET scan using an amyloid tracer, shows abnormal uptake in the cortex (smooth cortical appearance) in keeping with abnormal amyloid accumulation in the brain. This finding is associated with a high likelihood of the development of AD. The early stages of Alzheimer disease are characterized by the accumulation of cerebral amyloid-β (Aβ) within the brain forming neuritic plaques, neurofibrillary tangles. This process occurs two to three decades before these plaques and tangles result in eventual progressive loss of neurons leading to the development of clinical symptoms. As such the use of amyloid PET scanning can help establish the diagnosis at an early stage. This will become important once disease-modifying agents are available in the treatment of AD.

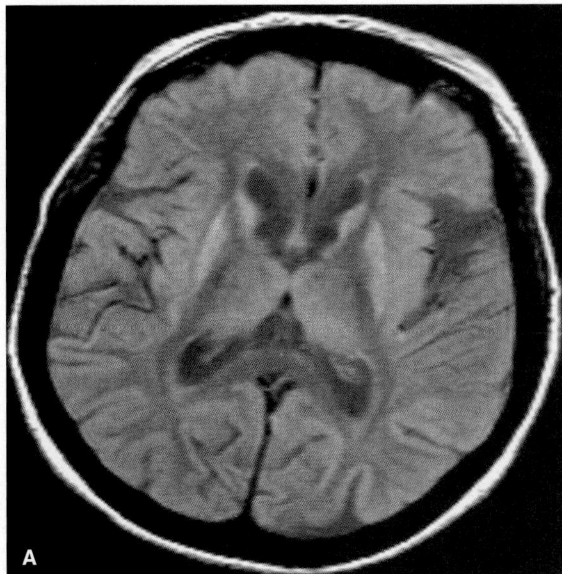

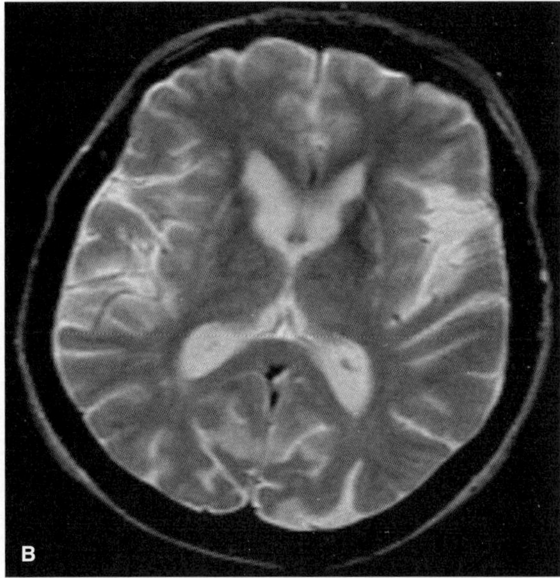

FIGURE 7.24. **Huntington Disease.** Axial (**A**) T2-FLAIR and (**B**) T2W images. A 48-year-old woman who presented with movement and behavioral disorders, had a familial history of similar presentation in her father. Note the hyperintensity and atrophic changes of both the caudate head as well as the putamen. The striking caudate head atrophy results in characteristic enlargement of the frontal horns, which reveal a heart-shaped configuration on coronal imaging. This neurodegenerative condition is autosomal dominant with full penetrance. Involvement of these gray matter structures results in choreoathetosis, with typical onset in the fifth decade of life.

of endogenous striatal dopamine, and after approximately 80% of these cells die, the patient begins to develop symptoms. MRI is relatively insensitive in the detection of this loss of tissue, but it can be used to image patients with movement disorders to exclude other underlying pathologies, such as stroke or tumor. MRI may occasionally reveal thinning of the pars compacta. The substantia nigra is made of the pars compacta (high signal intensity band on T2WIs) posteriorly, which is sandwiched between the pars reticulata anteriorly and the red nuclei posteriorly. With thinning of the pars compacta, the high signal intensity band between the pars reticularis and the red nuclei is lost. However, this finding is only occasionally noted in very severe forms of the disease. In contrast, PET is a more sensitive tool in the study of diseases of the dopaminergic system. Specifically, ^{18}F-labeled PET ligands have been developed for imaging the postsynaptic dopamine D1 and D2 receptor system. The involvement of this receptor system in numerous brain disorders such as schizophrenia, Parkinson disease, and other movement disorders has prompted an intense research in this field. With ^{18}F-labeled levodopa (DOPA), Parkinson patients show a characteristic deficit in putaminal DOPA uptake. The symptoms of Parkinson disease can sometimes be alleviated by treatment with levodopa, which increases the amount of dopamine that is endogenously synthesized, facilitating the activity of the remaining dopaminergic neurons. A variety of parkinsonian syndromes exist, including Parkinson disease, progressive supranuclear palsy, and striatonigral degeneration. Idiopathic Parkinson disease is referred to as *paralysis agitans* and affects 2% to 3% of the population at some time during their life.

The following are degenerative diseases of the extrapyramidal nuclei.

Huntington disease is a progressive hereditary disorder that appears in the fourth and fifth decades of life. This disease is characterized by a movement disorder (typically choreoathetosis), dementia, and emotional disturbance. Huntington disease is inherited in an autosomal dominant pattern with complete penetrance. Although neuroimaging studies demonstrate diffuse cortical atrophy, the caudate nucleus and putamen are most severely affected. Atrophy of the caudate nucleus results in characteristic enlargement of the frontal horns, which take on a heart-shaped configuration (Fig. 7.24).

Wilson disease, also known as hepatolenticular degeneration, is an inborn error of copper metabolism that is associated with hepatic cirrhosis and degenerative changes of the basal ganglia. A deficiency of ceruloplasmin (serum transport protein of copper) results in deposition of toxic levels of copper in various organs. Patients present with varied neurologic and psychiatric findings, including dystonia, tremor, and rigidity. The Kayser–Fleischer ring, an intracorneal deposit of copper, is virtually diagnostic of the disease when present (75% of cases). MRI findings include diffuse atrophy with signal abnormalities involving the deep gray matter nuclei and deep white matter.

In addition to these neurodegenerative diseases, abnormalities of the basal ganglia can have a wide range of causes. Toxins such as carbon monoxide or methanol poisoning may result in signal abnormalities of the basal ganglia, characteristically the globus pallidus and putamen, respectively (Fig. 7.25). Also, infectious conditions such as West Nile virus (WNV) and Creutzfeldt–Jakob disease (CJD) may present with areas of signal abnormality within the basal ganglia. Both of these conditions have become cause of great concern recently, given their increased incidence and unusual modes of transmission (WNV via mosquitoes and CJD via consumption of infected beef products). T1 shortening (high signal on T1WIs) has been described within the basal ganglia and brainstem, associated with hepatic dysfunction, such as hepatic encephalopathy as well as hyperalimentation. The cause of these findings has not been fully determined. Occasionally, faint calcification of the basal ganglia may also appear as high signal on T1WIs. This is the result of the hydration layer effect, where water molecules that are adjacent to the calcification have reduced relaxation times. This same effect causes T1 shortening with proteinaceous fluids. As a result, any condition that results in subtle calcifications within the basal ganglia may demonstrate T1 shortening within the basal ganglia.

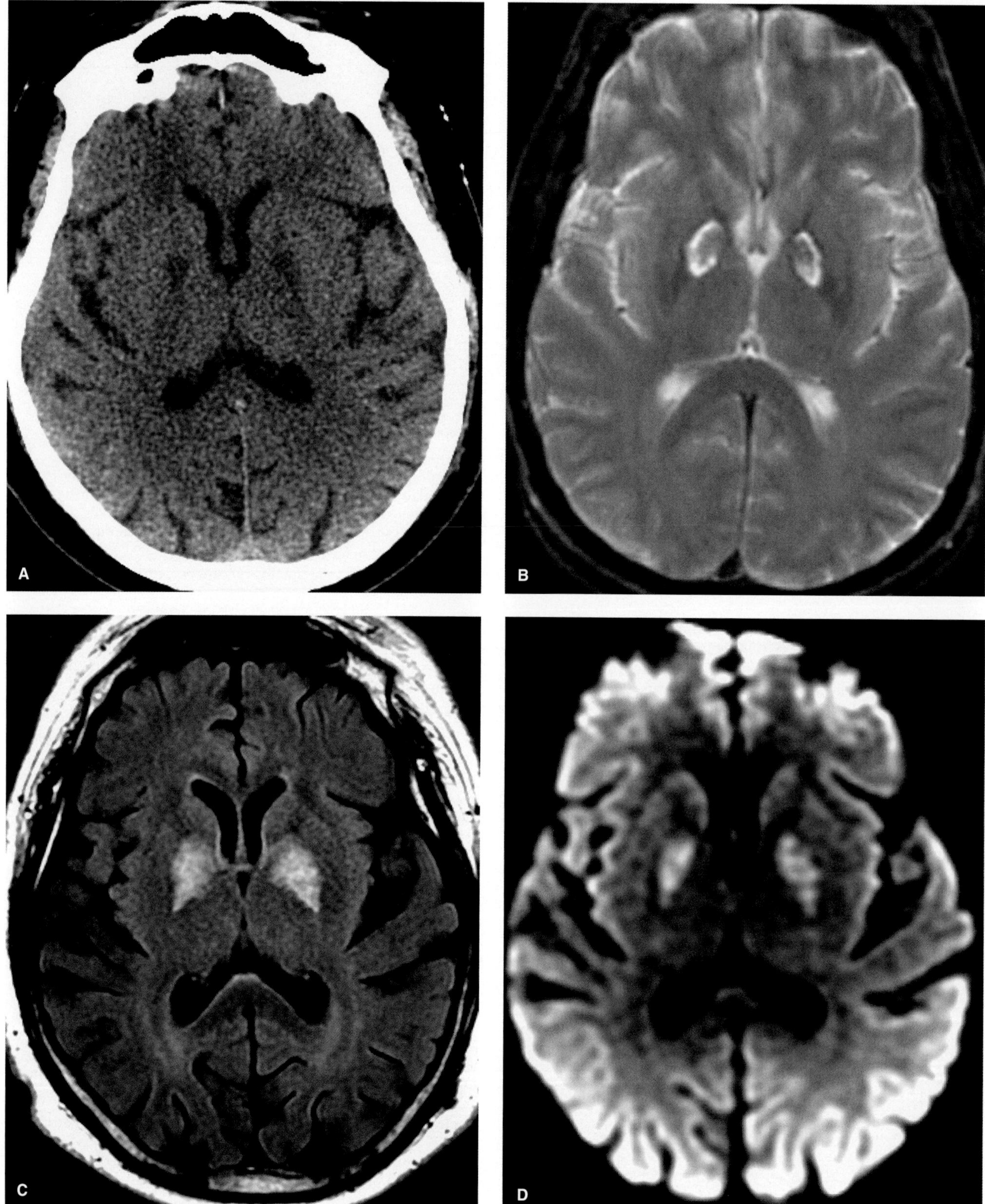

FIGURE 7.25. Carbon Monoxide Toxicity. A: Axial CT. **B:** T2WI. **C:** Fluid-attenuated inversion recovery image. **D:** Diffusion-weighted image. A 55-year-old man presented with confusion following carbon monoxide exposure relating to use of a faulty kerosene heater within a poorly ventilated dwelling. Bilateral hyperintense lesions of the globus pallidus are noted. Bilateral lesions of the basal ganglia can be seen in a variety of insults, including methanol toxicity (putaminal); metabolic conditions such as Wilson disease (hepatolenticular degeneration, a disorder of copper metabolism); Hallervorden–Spatz disease (iron deposition within the globus pallidus); and mitochondrial disorders (Leigh disease and Kearns–Sayre syndrome).

Suggested Readings

Abdel Razek AA, Alvarez H, Bagg S, Refaat S, Castillo M. Imaging spectrum of CNS vasculitis. *Radiographics* 2014;34(4):873–894.

Kartal MG, Algin O. Evaluation of hydrocephalus and other cerebrospinal fluid disorders with MRI: An update. *Insights Imaging* 2014;5(4):531–541.

Martin-Macintosh EL, Broski SM, Johnson GB, Hunt CH, Cullen EL, Peller PJ. Multimodality imaging of neurodegenerative processes: Part 1, The basics and common dementias. *AJR Am J Roentgenol* 2016;207:871–882.

Martin-Macintosh EL, Broski SM, Johnson GB, Hunt CH, Cullen EL, Peller PJ. Multimodality imaging of neurodegenerative processes: Part 2, Atypical dementias. *AJR Am J Roentgenol* 2016;207:883–895.

Sarbu N, Shih RY, Jones RV, Horkayne-Szakaly I, Oleaga L, Smirniotopoulos JG. White matter diseases with radiologic-pathologic correlation. *Radiographics* 2016;36:1426–1447.

Thompson AJ, Banwell BL, Barkhof F, et al. Diagnosis of multiple sclerosis: 2017 revisions of the McDonald criteria. *Lancet Neurol* 2018;17(2):162–173.

CHAPTER 8 ■ HEAD AND NECK IMAGING

JEROME A. BARAKOS AND DERK D. PURCELL

"Head and neck" is a term used collectively to describe the extracranial structures, including the sinonasal cavity, skull base, pharynx, oral cavity, larynx, neck, orbit, and temporal bone. The head and neck region encompasses a tremendous spectrum of tissues in a compact space, with almost every organ system represented, including the digestive, respiratory, nervous, osseous, and vascular systems. Because of this anatomic complexity, the head and neck region is an area approached with considerable trepidation. However, accurate assessment of this area can be accomplished by combining an understanding of the normal anatomy, with familiarity of the scope of pathologic entities that may occur in this region. We will begin our discussion by considering lesions of the paranasal sinuses and nasal cavity. This will be followed by a review of the skull base, the deep spaces of the neck, the lymph nodes, the orbits, and finally congenital head and neck lesions.

Imaging Methods. Both multislice helical/spiral CT and MR can provide exquisite imaging of the normal and pathologic anatomy of the head and neck. Although each modality has advantages and disadvantages, the decision on whether to use CT versus MR for each individual case is often based on considering which technique the patient is more likely to tolerate. For example, if a patient has difficulty handling their oral secretions because of prior head and neck surgery, particularly following tracheotomy or partial glossectomy, they may have significant hardship lying still for the time required for MR scanning. In such cases, the rapid imaging time of CT is more likely to yield a study unmarred by motion artifact. Because calcification is better depicted with CT, this is the modality of choice when looking for obstructing salivary ductal calculi (sialoliths) or for the detection of fractures. A principal drawback with CT is the increasing concern of radiation exposure, especially in the pediatric and young adult population. However, in an older adult, especially with a known malignancy, the potential advantages of CT, including rapid scanning and reduced motion artifact should serve to outweigh any radiation exposure concerns. In contrast, MR provides outstanding sensitivity for the discrimination of soft tissues and often better demonstrates the full extent of pathology. At the same time, the superior tissue contrast discrimination of MR allows for enhanced diagnostic specificity. The direct multiplanar capability of MR may also provide for improved evaluation of pathologic entities. For example, because of the horizontal orientation of the palate, floor of the mouth, and skull base, sagittal and coronal imaging are invaluable in optimally assessing these areas.

PET. The advent of PET imaging has had a profound effect on the evaluation and staging of head and neck malignancies. In combination with either MR or CT imaging, PET has greatly increased the sensitivity and specificity in the evaluation of primary as well as recurrent malignancies. PET is a functional imaging modality based upon the distribution of a glucose analog radioisotope (18-F-fluorodeoxyglucose). Pathologic conditions that have an affinity for glucose will take up this isotope at a greater rate than normal surrounding tissues and thus be identifiable as areas of abnormality (Fig. 8.1).

Lesions found on PET scan are characterized by a standardized uptake value (SUV). The SUV refers to the relative radioactivity of a particular lesion when standardized to the injection dose and adjusted for body weight. As a result, the SUV is an absolute value that can be compared from patient to patient and examination to examination. In general, an SUV of greater than 3 is considered pathologic, but there are many caveats. A wide variety of nonmalignant conditions may give rise to an elevated SUV, most notably infection and postoperative changes. In addition, some neoplasms have poor glucose affinity, resulting in a low SUV. PET alone may be highly sensitive, but it is not very specific. The true benefit of PET is realized when its physiologic/functional information is combined with the high spatial resolution morphologic information of CT and/or MR. In summary, combining PET findings with CT and MR, results in a marked increase in sensitivity and specificity, making this combination a powerful diagnostic tool.

PARANASAL SINUSES AND NASAL CAVITY

Sinusitis. Inflammatory disease is the most common pathology involving the paranasal sinuses and nasal cavity. Mild mucosal thickening, primarily within the maxillary and ethmoid sinuses, is common, even in asymptomatic individuals.

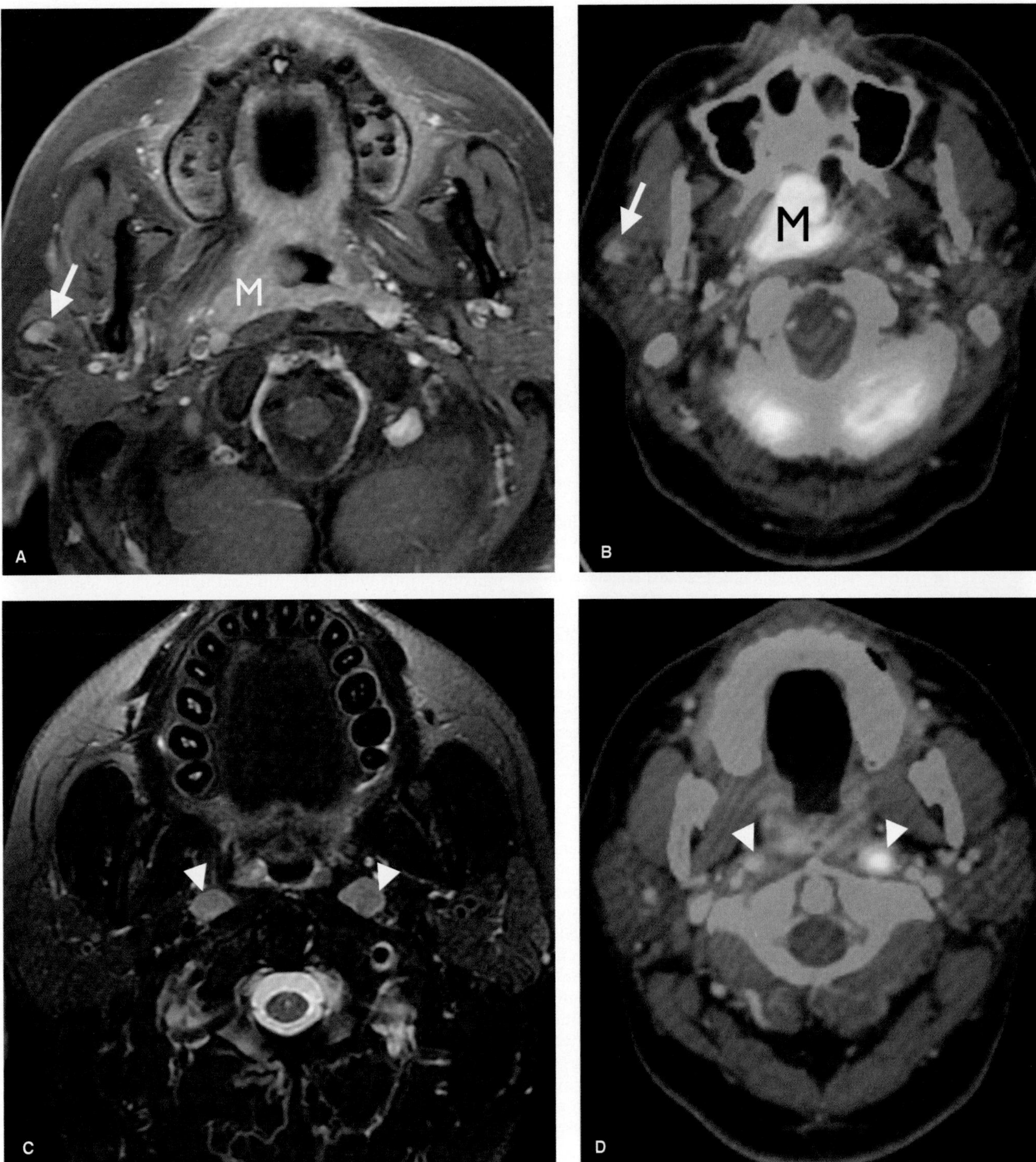

FIGURE 8.1. **MRI and PET-CT. A:** Axial postgadolinium-enhanced fat-suppressed (post-gad fat-sat) T1WI of a 47-year-old man who presented with a right nasopharyngeal mass (M). **B:** Corresponding PET-CT reveals associated abnormal isotope uptake within the mass. However, abnormal isotope uptake is also noted in a subcentimeter right parotid lymph node (*arrow* in Figure A and B). This node could easily be overlooked prospectively during interpretation of the MR. As expected, histology of the nasopharyngeal mass reflected a squamous cell carcinoma, the most common malignancy arising from the head and neck mucosal surfaces. The right parotid lymph node also proved to reflect metastatic disease. C and **D:** Enlarged bilateral retropharyngeal nodes are evident on MR (*arrowheads*), with corresponding abnormal isotope uptake on PET-CT. This case demonstrates the value of staging head and neck malignancies with PET-CT, as well as the increased specificity of combining functional/physiologic imaging (PET) with morphologic imaging (CT/MR).

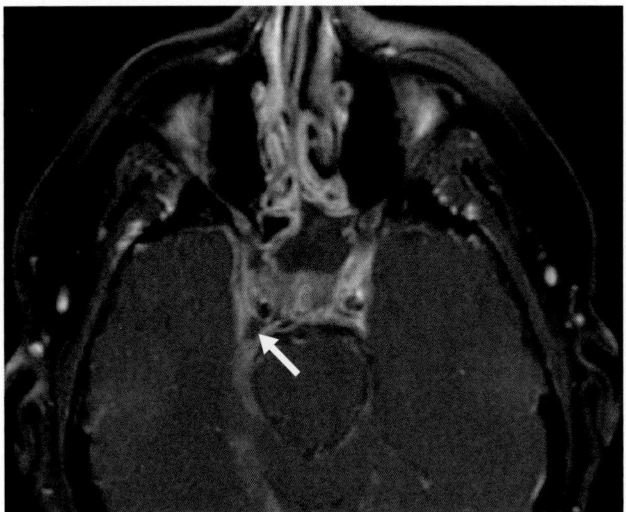

FIGURE 8.2. **Acute Sphenoid Sinusitis With Cavernous Sinus Thrombosis.** A 35-year-old diabetic male presented with a rapidly progressive sinusitis with symptoms of headache and ophthalmoplegia. Axial fat-sat T1WI post contrast. The sphenoid sinus is opacified. Sphenoid sinusitis is of great clinical concern as it may easily extend in a retrograde fashion intracranially owing to the presence of valveless veins. The patient's clinical condition deteriorated rapidly as the infection extended into the cavernous sinus, with resultant cavernous sinus thrombosis. The cavernous sinus thrombosis is characterized by the enlargement of the cavernous sinuses, with bowing/convex outer margins, while frank thrombus (dark signal, with lack of luminal contrast enhancement) is visualized within the posterior right cavernous sinus (*arrow*). Differential diagnostic conditions for enlargement of the cavernous sinuses would include carotid-cavernous fistula and Tolosa–Hunt syndrome (an idiopathic nongranulomatous inflammatory condition of the cavernous sinus).

In contrast, acute sinusitis is characterized by the presence of air–fluid levels or foamy-appearing sinus secretions and is typically caused by a viral upper respiratory tract infection (Fig. 8.2). In chronic sinusitis, changes include mucoperiosteal thickening as well as osseous thickening of the sinus walls. Soft tissue findings suggestive of sinusitis are best detected on T2WIs, as they are often high in signal. An exception is chronic sinus secretions that have become so desiccated that they yield no signal on either T1 or T2WIs and may mimic an aerated sinus. These sinus concretions and the bony wall thickening associated with chronic sinusitis are most easily appreciated on CT. Similar findings of hypointense T1 and T2WI sinus opacification have also been described in chronic noninvasive aspergillus sinusitis and chronic allergic hypersensitivity aspergillus sinusitis.

Endoscopic sinonasal surgery, used for the evaluation and treatment of inflammatory sinonasal disease, is being performed with increasing frequency. Direct coronal sinus CT provides exquisite definition of sinonasal anatomy and provides pre-endoscopic sinus assessment (Fig. 8.3). Knowledge of the anatomy of the lateral wall of the nasal cavity and routes of mucociliary drainage of the paranasal sinuses is critical to understanding patterns of inflammatory sinonasal disease. A major area of mucociliary drainage is the middle meatus, known as the *ostiomeatal unit.* It is important to note that disease limited to the infundibulum of the maxillary ostium will result in isolated obstruction of the maxillary sinus. In contrast, a lesion located in the hiatus semilunaris (middle meatus) results in combined obstruction of the ipsilateral maxillary sinus, anterior and middle ethmoid air cells, and the frontal sinus. This combined pattern of sinonasal disease has been described as the "ostiomeatal pattern" of obstruction. This pattern is significant because it indicates that one's attention should be directed to identifying the offending lesion within the hiatus semilunaris, rather than simply describing the presence of diffuse sinus disease.

Several common complications are associated with sinusitis, including inflammatory polyps, mucous retention cysts, mucoceles, and most importantly cavernous sinus thrombosis.

Inflammatory Polyps. Chronic inflammation leads to mucosal hyperplasia, which results in mucosal redundancy and polyp formation. Most often these polyps blend imperceptibly with the mucoperiosteal thickening and cannot be clearly differentiated. When an antral polyp expands to the point where it prolapses through the sinus ostium, it is referred to as an *antrochoanal* polyp. Although these polyps may not be associated with chronic sinusitis, they are similar to inflammatory polyps in that they represent areas of reactive mucosal thickening. Their characteristic appearance is that of a soft tissue mass extending from the maxillary sinus to fill the ipsilateral nasal cavity and nasopharynx. Often, the ostium of the maxillary sinus will be enlarged secondary to the mass effect of the polyp. The importance in recognizing such a lesion is that if it is surgically snared as if it were a nasal polyp, without regard for its antral stalk, it will recur.

Mucous retention cysts simply represent obstructed mucous glands within the mucosal lining. These lesions have a characteristic rounded appearance, measuring one to several centimeters in diameter, with the maxillary sinus being most commonly involved. These lesions are commonly recognized in asymptomatic individuals.

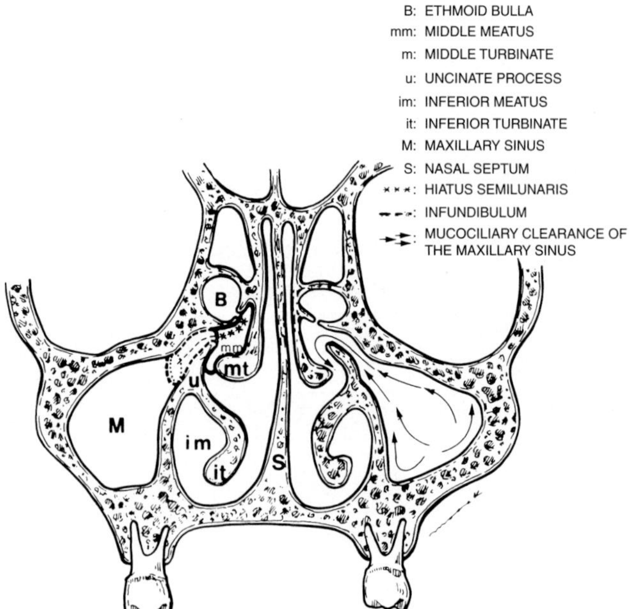

FIGURE 8.3. **Ostiomeatal Unit (OMU).** Line drawing in coronal plane demonstrates the anatomy of the OMU. Lines with *arrows* show the normal route of mucociliary clearance. Infundibular (*dashed line*) and OMU (*solid line*) patterns of obstruction are shown. Coronal CT far surpasses plain sinus films in evaluating problems of the OMU for potential relief through endoscopic surgery. B, ethmoid bulla; M, maxillary sinus; u, uncinate process; mt, middle turbinate; mm, middle meatus; im, inferior meatus; it, inferior turbinate; S, nasal septum. (Reprinted with permission from Babbel RW, Harnsberger HR, Sonkens J, Hunt S. Recurring patterns of inflammatory sinonasal disease demonstrated on screening sinus CT. *AJNR Am J Neuroradiol* 1992;13(3):903–912.)

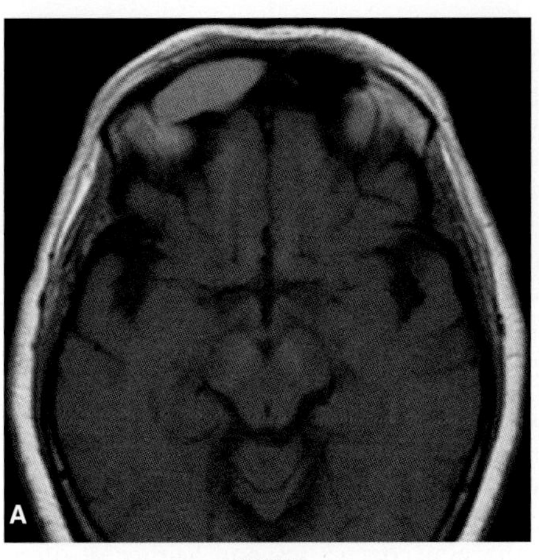

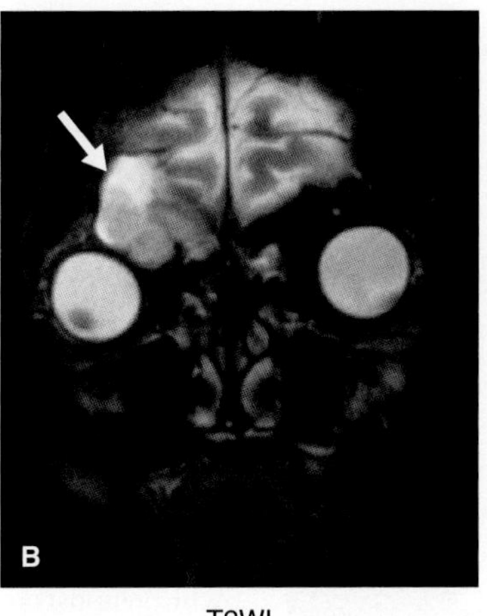

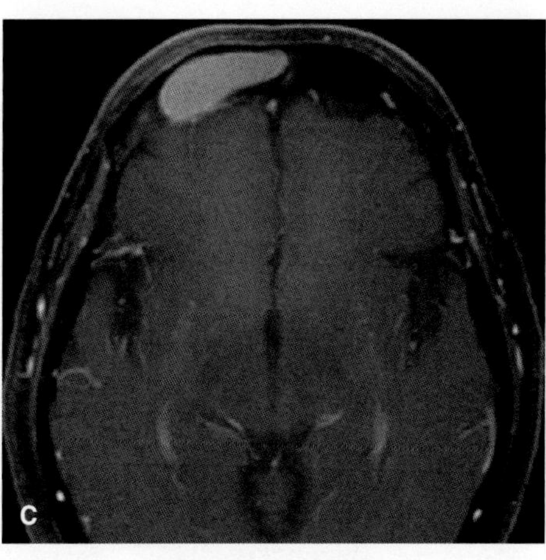

FIGURE 8.4. **Sinus Mucocele. A:** Axial T1WI. **B:** Coronal T2WI. **C:** Axial T1WI postcontrast. Patient presented with frontal headache pain, resulting from mass effect from a frontal sinus mucocele. A mucocele results from chronic obstruction of a paranasal sinus that becomes blocked and converted into a fluid-filled cyst. Over time, this lesion may expand, eroding bone and resulting in proptosis.

Mucocele is similar to a retention cyst, but instead of disease being confined to the single mucous gland, the lesion expands to the point where the entire sinus becomes obstructed. This typically occurs because of a mass obstructing the draining sinus ostium. The characteristic feature of a mucocele is frank expansion of the sinus with associated sinus wall bony thinning and remodeling. The frontal sinus is the sinus most commonly affected, but any sinus may be involved (Fig. 8.4). If the mucocele becomes infected, it demonstrates peripheral enhancement and is referred to as a *mucopyocele.*

Inverting Papilloma. A variety of papillomas occur within the nasal cavity, but most attention has focused on the inverting papilloma. These papillomas are named based on their histologic appearance. In this condition, the neoplastic nasal epithelium inverts and grows into the underlying mucosa. These papillomas are not believed to be associated with allergy or chronic infection because they are almost invariably unilateral in location. Inverting papillomas occur exclusively on the lateral nasal wall, centered on the hiatus semilunaris. Because of their increased association with squamous cell carcinoma, it is recommended that these lesions be surgically resected with wide mucosal margins.

Juvenile nasopharyngeal angiofibromas are typically seen in male adolescents presenting with epistaxis. The tumor arises from fibrovascular stroma of the nasal wall adjacent to the sphenopalatine foramen. This is a benign tumor that can be very locally aggressive. In an adolescent male presenting with a nasal mass and epistaxis, it is important to have a high clinical suspicion for this lesion, because life-threatening hemorrhage may result if a biopsy or limited resection is attempted. The tumor characteristically fills the nasopharynx and bows the posterior wall of the maxillary sinus forward. In fact, the retromaxillary pterygopalatine fossa location is a hallmark feature that should elicit this diagnosis for consideration. Juvenile nasopharyngeal angiofibromas enhance markedly with contrast administration, differentiating them from the rarer lymphangioma. Preoperatively, interventional radiology may play a role in embolization of these lesions, making them less vascular and facilitating surgical resection.

Malignancies. The tissues within the paranasal sinuses and nasal cavity that give rise to malignancies include squamous epithelium, lymphoid tissue, and minor salivary glands. The corresponding malignancies are therefore squamous cell carcinoma, lymphoma, and minor salivary tumors. Because the entire upper aerodigestive tract is lined with squamous epithelium, it follows that *squamous cell carcinoma* is the most common malignancy (80% to 90%) of not only the paranasal sinuses and nasal cavity, but of the entire head and neck. Squamous cell carcinoma of the sinuses is often clinically silent until it is quite advanced. Early symptoms are usually related to obstructive sinusitis. Imaging findings consist of an opacified sinus with associated bony wall destruction. These findings are nonspecific and do not allow differentiation from non-Hodgkin lymphoma or a minor salivary gland malignancy. The presence of constitutional symptoms with prominent head and neck or systemic adenopathy suggests lymphoma, particularly in a child or young adult.

Minor salivary glands are dispersed throughout the upper aerodigestive tract but are most highly concentrated in the palate. Any of these minor salivary glands found throughout the head and neck, may give rise to salivary neoplasms. In contrast to parotid gland salivary neoplasms, the majority of which are benign, most minor salivary neoplasms are malignant. The most common salivary malignancies include adenoid cystic carcinoma, adenocarcinoma, and mucoepidermoid carcinoma.

An *esthesioneuroblastoma* is an additional malignancy that should be mentioned when describing lesions of the nasal cavity. The esthesioneuroblastoma is a tumor that arises from the neurosensory receptor cells of the olfactory nerve and mucosa. Thus, this lesion may originate anywhere from the cribriform plate to the turbinates. This tumor is often quite destructive by the time of diagnosis and is found high within the nasal vault (Fig. 8.5). Involvement of the cribriform plate with extension into the anterior cranial fossa is not uncommon with esthesioneuroblastoma and should suggest this diagnosis.

In assessing the size and extent of sinonasal cavity pathology, it is often difficult to differentiate the offending lesion from associated obstructed sinus secretions. In such instances, fat-suppressed T2WI sequences are of value, because in general, sinus secretions will be brighter than the malignancy, which is often isointense with respect to muscle.

SKULL BASE

The skull base extends from the nose anteriorly to the occipital protuberance posteriorly and is composed of five bones: the ethmoid, sphenoid, occipital, temporal, and frontal bones.

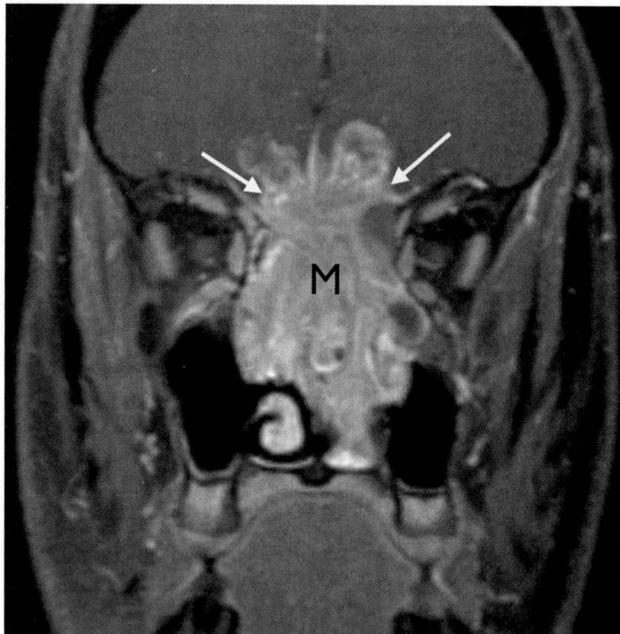

FIGURE 8.5. Esthesioneuroblastoma. Coronal fat-suppressed postgadolinium T1WI. A large destructive mass (M) in the nasal cavity extends through the cribriform plate into the anterior cranial fossa (*arrows*). This degree of frank bony destruction is unusual for squamous cell carcinoma and lymphoma, but characteristic of esthesioneuroblastoma.

The skull base contains many foramina through which both vessels and nerves pass. Because the skull base has an undulating surface with a horizontal orientation, coronal or sagittal images are valuable in its evaluation.

Tumors of the Skull Base

Tumors may arise that are intrinsic to the skull base. In addition, an extrinsic lesion may extend to involve the skull base from either above or below. Any lesion from the paranasal sinuses and nasal cavity already described, may extend to involve the skull base. Other lesions that may extend to involve the skull base include paragangliomas, neural sheath tumors (schwannoma and neurofibroma), and meningiomas. Although various primary malignant neoplasms of the skull base are described later, most malignant lesions of the skull base are metastatic in origin.

Primary malignant neoplasms are relatively uncommon, comprising only about 2% to 3% of skull base tumors. The three most common primary malignant tumors are chordoma, chondrosarcoma, and osteogenic sarcoma. Differentiating these lesions, especially chordomas from chondrosarcomas using both radiologic and histologic criteria can be difficult. Thus the anatomic location of these lesions proves useful in suggesting one lesion over another. *Chordoma* is a bone neoplasm that arises from remnants of the primitive notochord. Classically, this lesion will present as a destructive midline mass centered in the clivus. These tumors may be found anywhere along the craniospinal axis; typically 35% of lesions involve the clivus, 50% the sacrum, and 15% the vertebral bodies. Radiographically, this lesion is characterized as a midline destructive bony lesion with predilection for the sphenooccipital synchondrosis. On a sagittal image, the sphenooccipital synchondrosis is occasionally seen as a horizontal line in the midclivus, midway between sella and basion (tip of clivus). *Chondrosarcomas* are malignant tumors that develop from cartilage. Because the skull base is preformed in cartilage, there is a predilection for chondrosarcoma to involve the skull base. A preferred site of origin is parasellar in location, at the petroclival junction. *Osteogenic sarcoma* is typically the result of prior radiation therapy or malignant transformation of Paget disease.

Although a central destructive clival lesion is characteristic for chordoma and a paraclival destructive bony lesion is suggestive of chondrosarcoma, our differential diagnostic list includes several other bony lesions. The skull base, like any bone, may be affected by metastases, myeloma, plasmacytoma, fibrous dysplasia, and Paget disease. As with any bony lesion, CT helps to differentiate among these diagnostic possibilities. For example, fibrous dysplasia will reveal a smooth, ground-glass appearance on CT, while Paget disease will demonstrate trabecular coarsening, and neither of these conditions will reveal bony destruction.

Lesions of the jugular foramen are most commonly paragangliomas and are discussed under the heading "Carotid Space." Paragangliomas arise from glomus cells derived from the embryonic neural crest, functioning as part of the sympathetic nervous system. As such, they may occur anywhere along the sympathetic fibers of the head and neck, but those involving the skull base, specifically the jugular foramen are referred to as a glomus jugulare. These patients commonly present with pulsatile tinnitus and a conductive hearing loss. CT and MR may play complementary roles in evaluating these lesions. CT often demonstrates "moth-eaten" destruction of the bone surrounding the jugular fossa, with MR revealing the typical heterogeneous "salt-and-pepper" signal related to numerous flow voids. Malignant tumors are often indistinguishable from paragangliomas on CT, but most fail to demonstrate flow voids on MR. Other lesions of the jugular fossa include schwannomas (arising from cranial nerves IX–XI) and meningiomas. These lesions cause a smooth expansion of the jugular foramen with marked enhancement. In addition, schwannomas may demonstrate cystic components.

Temporal Bone

Although a thorough discussion of the temporal bone is beyond the scope of this chapter, we will focus on some highlights. The most common diseases involving the temporal bone are inflammatory in nature and include cholesteatomas. Eustachian tube dysfunction with resultant decreased intratympanic pressure is believed to be the principal defect responsible for inflammatory disease of the middle ear and mastoid.

Cholesteatoma is an epidermoid cyst composed of desquamating stratified squamous epithelium. These cysts enlarge because of the progressive accumulation of epithelial debris within their lumen. They may be either congenital (2%) or acquired (98%). Congenital cholesteatomas originate from epithelial rests within or adjacent to the temporal bone. Acquired cholesteatomas originate from the stratified squamous epithelium of the tympanic membrane. These begin as localized tympanic membrane retraction pockets. The diagnosis of a cholesteatoma is based on the detection of a soft tissue mass within the middle ear cavity, typically with associated bony erosion. The superior portion of the tympanic membrane (pars flaccida) retracts easily and is the most common site for formation of an acquired cholesteatoma. Cholesteatomas arising in this area originate within the Prussak space (superior recess of the tympanic membrane), which is located medial to the pars flaccida between the scutum and the neck of the malleus. Thus, a finding of soft tissue in this region with subtle erosion of the scutum and medial displacement of the ossicles is characteristic of a cholesteatoma. Note that when fluid or inflammatory pathology is present, such as with otitis media, these changes cannot be differentiated from cholesteatoma because they have similar densities.

Although most cholesteatomas can be easily diagnosed otoscopically, the clinician cannot judge the size and full extent of the lesion. As a result, CT plays an important role in determining the size of the lesion, as well as the status of the ossicles, the labyrinth, the tegmen, and the facial nerve. MR has a limited role in the evaluation of erosive lesions of the temporal bone, because poor visualization of osseous landmarks limits localization of the process and it gives little information concerning the status of the ossicles and other bony structures. However cholesteatomas often reveal restricted diffusion (high signal) on diffusion-weighted echo-planar imaging (DW-EPI). Thus MR with diffusion imaging may provide complementary value in the initial diagnosis, or utility in the evaluation of residual or recurrent cholesteatoma.

Cholesterol granuloma, also known as *giant cholesterol cyst,* is a type of granulation tissue that may involve the petrous apex. These lesions represent petrous apex air cells that have become partially obstructed and are filled with cholesterol debris and hemorrhagic fluid. Because of their hemorrhagic components, these lesions are characterized by high signal on both T1WIs and T2WIs. When faced with an opacified petrous apex, differential diagnostic considerations include retained fluid secretions (parallels signal intensity of fluid, dark T1, bright T2, and no enhancement); petrous apicitis (parallels signal intensity of abscess, dark T1, bright T2, and ring enhancement); and non-aerated petrous apex (parallels signal intensity of fatty bone marrow, bright T1, dark T2, and no enhancement).

SUPRAHYOID HEAD AND NECK

When a patient presents with a head and neck mass, the age of presentation is an important consideration when establishing a differential diagnostic list. In the pediatric age group, the majority of lesions (>90%) will be benign and consist of a variety of congenital or inflammatory entities (see "Congenital Lesions"). If a malignancy is encountered, it will most likely be a lymphoma (e.g., Burkitt lymphoma if rapid growth is noted) or rhabdomyosarcoma. In sharp contrast, when an adult presents with a head and neck mass (excluding thyroid lesions), the vast majority of lesions (>90%) will be malignant (Fig. 8.6). In the younger adult (20 to 40 years), the most common malignancy will be lymphoma, and in adults older than 40 years, the most common neck mass will be nodal metastases.

The suprahyoid head and neck is traditionally divided into compartments that include the nasopharynx, oropharynx, and oral cavity. An understanding of the division between these spaces is essential to accurately determine and describe the full extent of mucosal lesions.

The term *nasopharynx* is frequently misused as a nonspecific term to describe any area in the upper aerodigestive tract. In fact, the nasopharynx refers to a very specific portion of the pharynx. The nasopharynx lies above the oropharynx and is divided from the oropharynx by a horizontal line drawn along the hard and soft palates. Posteriorly the nasopharynx is bounded by the pharyngeal constrictor muscles, and anteriorly it is bounded by the nasal cavity at the nasal choana (paired funnel-shaped openings between the nasal cavity and the nasopharynx). Below the hard palate lie the *oral cavity* and *oropharynx*. These two areas are divided by a ring of structures that includes the circumvallate papillae (located along the posterior aspect of the tongue), the tonsillar pillars, and the soft palate.

These traditional compartments (nasopharynx, oropharynx, and oral cavity) are important for describing the spread of superficial, mucosa-based lesions. In contrast to this division, multiple facial planes divide the deep head and neck into spaces that form true compartments. It is important to realize that these deep spaces are unrelated to the traditional division of the head and neck and traverse the neck without regard to the traditional divisions. Therefore, when describing deep head and neck lesions, the traditional pharyngeal subdivisions are of limited value. Most radiologists have adapted a spatial

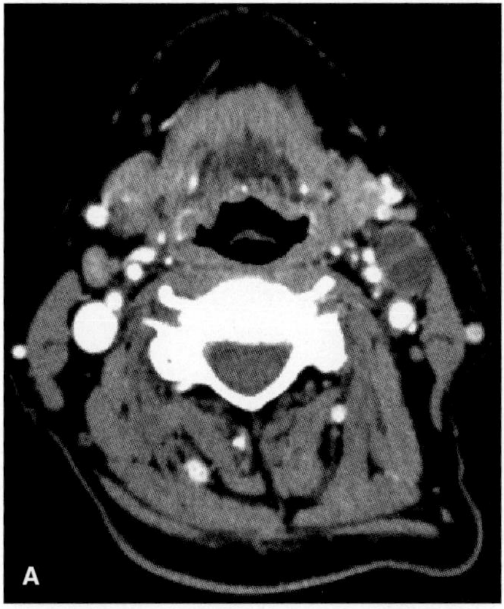

CE-CT

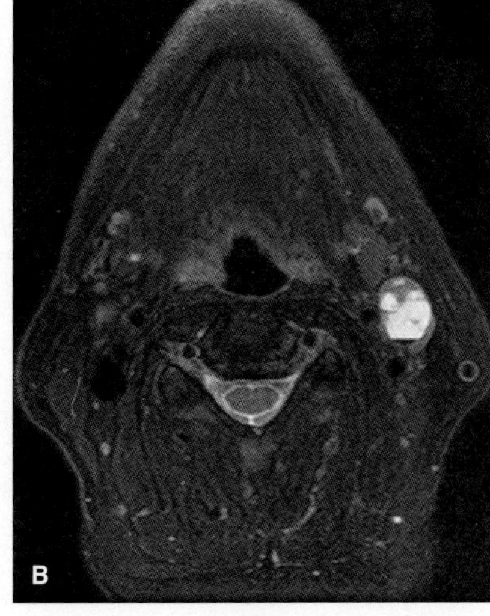

T2WI

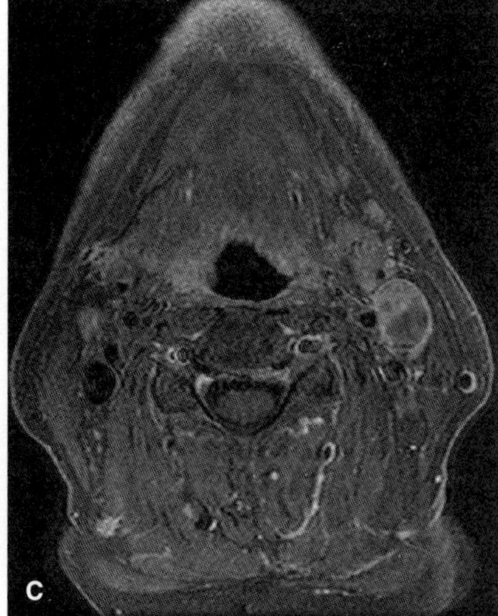

T1WI postcontrast

FIGURE 8.6. **Squamous Cell Carcinoma: Cystic Nodal Metastasis. A:** Contrast-enhanced CT. **B:** Axial T2WI. **C:** Axial post-gad fat-sat T1WI. This 45-year-old patient was referred for a "branchial cleft cyst." Patient had a 4-month history of a left-sided neck mass that would swell during upper respiratory tract infections. Images reveal a multiseptated cystic lesion in the left jugular nodal chain. On biopsy, this proved to be a squamous cell, cystic nodal metastasis. Although this lesion may appear similar to a branchial cleft cyst, the presence of multiple additional nodes is unusual. A branchial cleft cyst may exhibit a thickened wall with septations, depending on current or previous infections.

approach to the head and neck, described as follows and popularized by Dr. Ric Harnsberger.

The deep anatomy of the head and neck is subdivided by layers of the deep cervical fascia into the following spaces: (1) superficial mucosal; (2) parapharyngeal; (3) carotid; (4) parotid; (5) masticator; (6) retropharyngeal; and (7) prevertebral. When evaluating a patient with pathology in the deep head and neck, it is important to determine within which space the pathology lies. Because only a limited number of structures are located within each compartment, these are the structures from which pathology will arise. Therefore, only specific pathology will be found within these separate fascial spaces, markedly limiting the differential diagnosis. For example, the principal structures within the parotid space are the parotid gland and parotid lymph nodes. Consequently, if a parotid space mass is identified, the diagnosis is primarily limited to either a parotid tumor or nodal disease. Each of these seven spaces will be reviewed in detail (Table 8.1). Note that although this spatial division is popular with radiologists, surgeons and otolaryngologists occasionally use different terms, for example, "retrostyloid space" instead of "carotid space."

Superficial Mucosal Space

The superficial mucosal space includes all structures on the airway side of the pharyngobasilar fascia. The principal constituent of this space is the mucosa of the upper aerodigestive tract, which consists of squamous epithelium, submucosal lymphatics, and hundreds of minor salivary glands. The pharyngobasilar fascia represents the superior aponeurosis of the superior pharyngeal constrictor muscle, which inserts into the skull base. This tough fascia separates the mucosal space from the surrounding parapharyngeal space. Lesions originating within the superficial mucosal space may invade deep to the mucosal surface, resulting first in lateral displacement and

TABLE 8.1

DEEP COMPARTMENTS OF THE HEAD AND NECK

■ COMPARTMENT	■ CONTENTS	■ PATHOLOGY
Mucosal	Squamous mucosa Lymphoid tissue (adenoids, lingual tonsils) Minor salivary glands	Nasopharyngeal carcinoma Squamous cell carcinoma Lymphoma Minor salivary gland tumors Juvenile angiofibroma Rhabdomyosarcoma
Parapharyngeal	Fat Trigeminal nerve (V3) Internal maxillary artery Ascending pharyngeal artery	Minor salivary gland tumor Lipoma Cellulitis/abscess Schwannoma
Parotid	Parotid gland Intraparotid lymph nodes Facial nerve (VII) External carotid artery Retromandibular vein	Salivary gland tumors Metastatic adenopathy Lymphoma Parotid cysts
Carotid	Cranial nerves IX–XII Sympathetic nerves Jugular chain nodes Carotid artery Jugular vein	Schwannoma Neurofibroma Paraganglioma Metastatic adenopathy Lymphoma Cellulitis/abscess Meningioma
Masticator	Muscles of mastication Ramus and body of mandible Inferior alveolar nerve	Odontogenic abscess Osteomyelitis Direct spread of squamous cell carcinoma Lymphoma Minor salivary tumor Sarcoma of muscle or bone
Retropharyngeal	Lymph nodes (lateral and medial retropharyngeal) Fat	Metastatic adenopathy Lymphoma
Prevertebral	Cervical vertebrae Prevertebral muscles Paraspinal muscles Phrenic nerve	Abscess/cellulitis Osseous metastases Chordoma Osteomyelitis Cellulitis Abscess

For further discussion, please see Harnsberger HR, Glastonbury CM, Michel MA, Koch BL. *Diagnostic Imaging: Head and Neck*. Salt Lake City, UT: Amirsys Diagnostic Imaging (Lippincott); 2010.

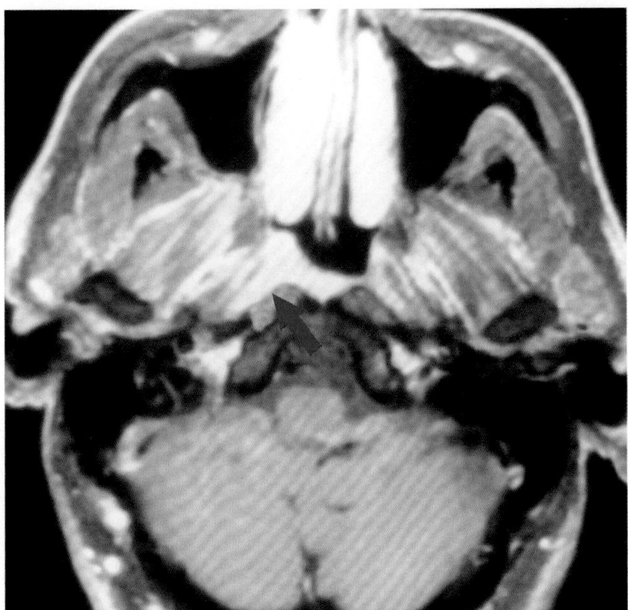

FIGURE 8.7. **Squamous Cell Carcinoma.** Axial post-gad fat-sat T1WI through the level of the nasopharynx. Contrast-enhancing soft tissue fills the right fossa of Rosenmüller (*arrow*). Although this lesion appears confined to the mucosal space without invasion into the underlying parapharyngeal tissues, submandibular nodal metastases were present. This example underscores the point that asymmetries of the mucosal space may represent a malignancy, and careful correlation with physical examination should be suggested by the radiologist.

then obliteration of the parapharyngeal space. However, many early lesions that begin within the mucosal space present as only mild mucosal irregularities or asymmetries (Fig. 8.7). This space is easily evaluated by the clinician and thus the radiologist should have a low threshold for suggesting the presence of abnormalities within this space. In children, there is frequently prominent adenoidal tissue that fills the nasopharynx. Even in adults, following a recent upper respiratory infection, prominent symmetrical mucosal tissue may be noted; this is of little concern as long as there is no invasion of deep facial places and no associated adenopathy (Fig. 8.8).

Benign Lesions. The most common benign lesions arising in the mucosal space are Tornwaldt cysts and lesions related to minor salivary gland tissue. *Tornwaldt cysts* are sharply marginated and are found in the midline with high-signal intensity on T2WIs (Fig. 8.9). They are believed to be remnants of notochordal tissue aberrantly located in the nasopharynx and have an incidence of approximately 1% to 2% in normal patients. Lesions arising from minor salivary glands include retention cysts and benign neoplasms. *Retention cysts* represent obstructed glands similar to those found within the paranasal sinuses. The most common benign neoplasm is the benign mixed cell tumor (pleomorphic adenoma). Both of these lesions present as well circumscribed, rounded lesions that have high-signal intensity on T2WIs.

Malignant Lesions. The most common malignant neoplasms of the mucosal space are squamous cell carcinoma, non-Hodgkin lymphoma, and minor salivary gland malignancies; of these, squamous cell carcinoma is by far the most common. Unfortunately, these malignancies all appear similar on CT and MR. Initially there is mass effect, often associated with lateral compression or obliteration of the parapharyngeal space, followed by invasion of the skull base. An early triad of radiographic findings consists of (1) superficial nasopharyngeal mucosal asymmetry; (2) ipsilateral retropharyngeal adenopathy; and (3) mastoid opacification. Mastoid opacification is an important early warning sign (Fig. 8.10). Mastoid opacification is easily detected on T2WIs and suggests potential dysfunction of the eustachian tube, frequently the result of tumor infiltration of the tensor veli palatini muscles. This finding directs the radiologist to carefully evaluate the mucosa of the nasopharynx. Note that both the nasopharynx

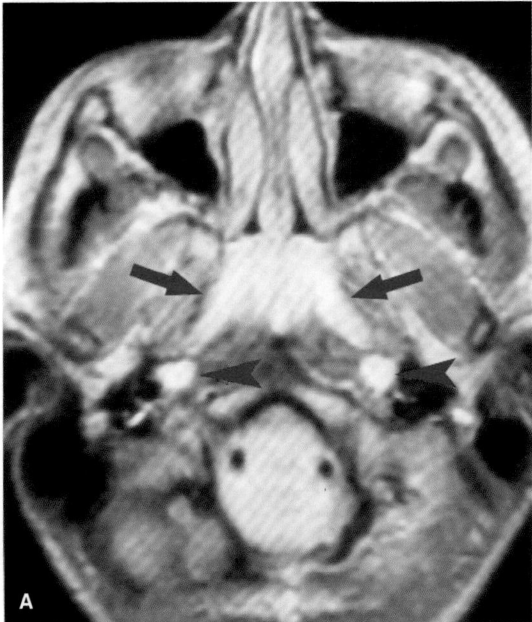

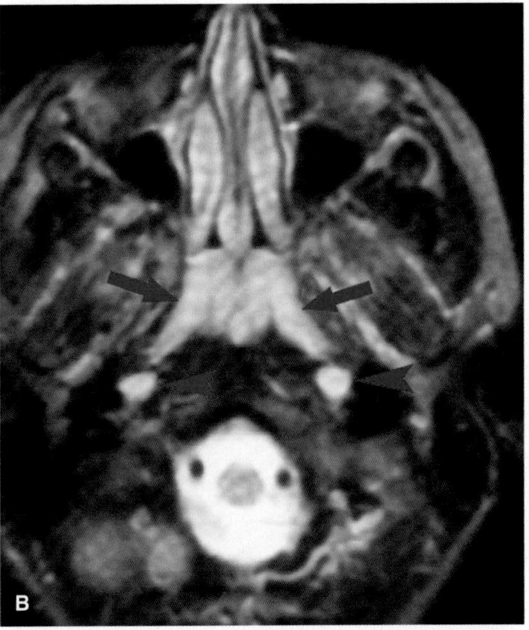

FIGURE 8.8. **Adenoidal Hypertrophy.** Axial proton density and T2WIs in a 5-year-old child. Prominent adenoidal tissue (*arrows*) fills the nasopharynx, expanding the fossa of Rosenmüller bilaterally. In addition, lateral retropharyngeal nodes (*arrowheads*) are clearly visualized. These findings are typical for a normal child, and even common in a young adult especially in association with a recent upper respiratory infection. As always, correlation with clinical history is paramount in helping to formulate the proper differential diagnosis.

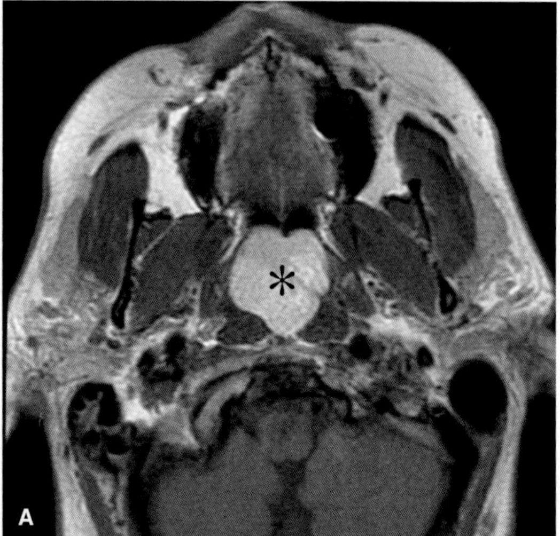

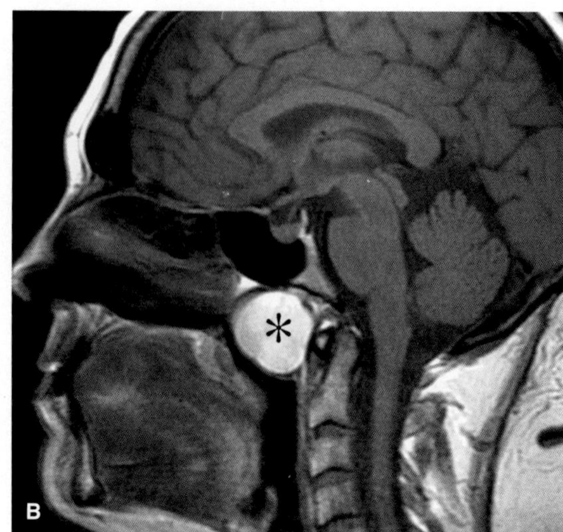

FIGURE 8.9. Tornwaldt Cyst. Axial (**A**) and sagittal (**B**) T1WIs. A well-circumscribed mass (*asterisk*) with intrinsic T1 shortening (high signal intensity on T1WI) appears in the superficial mucosa space. This midline and superficial location is characteristic of a Tornwaldt cyst, a remnant of the primitive notochord. This lesion is found in 1% to 2% of the normal population, typically measuring less than a centimeter in diameter.

and the mastoid air cells are included on every head CT and MR scan, and these areas should not be overlooked on routine head imaging.

The use of fat suppression with both T2WI and contrast-enhanced imaging is useful in improving detection and defining the extent of pathology. This is because the suppression of the intrinsic high signal from fat, provides for improved conspicuity of lesion with inherent T2 hyperintensity or contrast enhancement. Nevertheless, do not underestimate the value of a routine precontrast T1WI, as the normal bright fat planes serve as an invaluable tool allowing detection of infiltrating pathology as the normally bright fat is replaced. In addition, these sequences allow the detection of subtle perineural spread of neoplasms, particularly along cranial nerves extending into the skull base. This is particularly important with adenoid cystic carcinoma, which has a marked propensity for perineural spread and is the most common minor salivary gland malignancy.

Squamous cell carcinoma is the most common malignancy of the upper aerodigestive tract. However, a particular variant of squamous cell carcinoma occurs within the nasopharynx and is termed "nasopharyngeal carcinoma." Nasopharyngeal carcinoma has several unique histologic features that distinguish it from squamous cell carcinoma. Although squamous cell carcinoma is common in the Caucasian population, nasopharyngeal carcinoma is not, with an incidence of about 1 in 100,000 people per year. This is in contrast to rates that are 20 times higher in Asia, particularly in southern regions of China. Although smoking and alcohol abuse are often

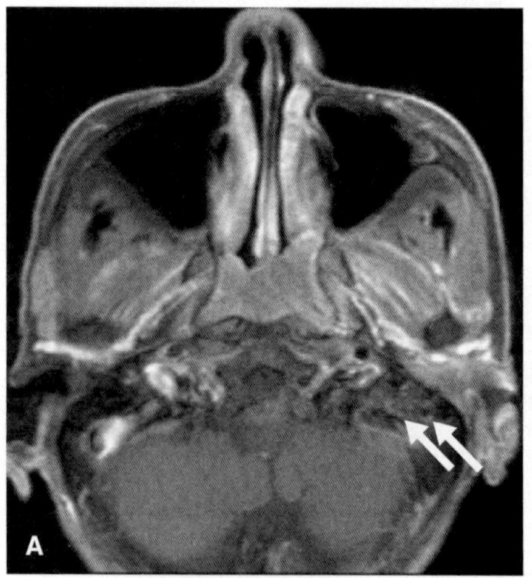

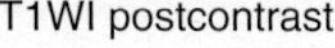

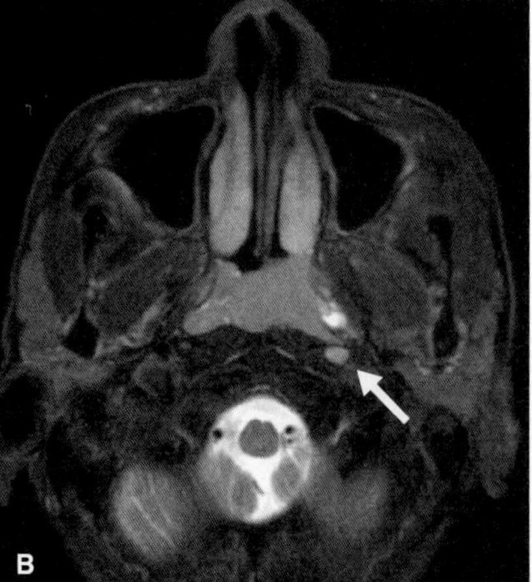

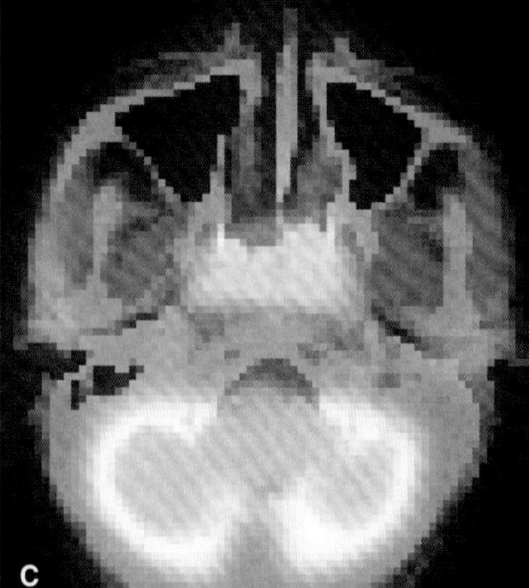

FIGURE 8.10. Nasopharyngeal Malignancy. A: T1W1 post contrast. **B:** Axial T2WI. **C:** FDG PET/CT. Imaging reveals a large mucosal-based mass with avid isotope uptake centered within the left lateral nasopharynx. The triad of nasopharyngeal malignancy consists of (1) mucosal mass of the lateral nasopharynx (fossa of Rosenmüller), (2) lateral retropharyngeal nodes (**B**, *arrow*), and (3) mastoid opacification/effusion (**A**, *arrows*). Mastoid opacification is the result of dysfunction of the eustachian tube, and should always prompt search for the offending nasopharyngeal mass. It should be noted that the nasopharynx and mastoids are included on every CT and MRI of the head, and a brief assessment of the nasopharynx and mastoids can assist the radiologist in identifying an early or unsuspected malignancy.

associated with squamous cell carcinoma, they have no causal association with nasopharyngeal carcinoma. However, both environmental and genetic factors do appear to play a role in the genesis of nasopharyngeal carcinoma. Specifically, immunoglobulin A antibodies to the Epstein–Barr virus have been associated with nasopharyngeal carcinoma.

Lymphoma involving the mucosa cannot be differentiated by imaging from squamous cell or minor salivary gland carcinoma. However, non-Hodgkin lymphoma frequently has systemic manifestations, with extranodal and extralymphatic sites of involvement that are atypical for these other malignancies. Thus, the presence of a mucosal mass in association with bulky supraclavicular and mediastinal adenopathy as well as splenomegaly would be suggestive of lymphoma.

Parapharyngeal Space

The parapharyngeal space is a triangular, fat-filled compartment that extends from the skull base to the submandibular gland region. It is located at the center of the surrounding spaces and is compressed or infiltrated in a characteristic fashion by masses originating from the various spaces. The primary importance of the parapharyngeal space is that it serves as an important landmark of mass effect in the deep face. When a lesion occurs in any of the four surrounding spaces, there will be characteristic impressions on the parapharyngeal fat space, which will suggest the space of tumor origin.

The parapharyngeal space is surrounded by the carotid space posteriorly, the parotid space laterally, the masticator space anteriorly, and the superficial mucosal space medially. Therefore, the parapharyngeal space will be compressed on its medial surface by masses originating from the mucosal surface, displaced anteriorly by carotid sheath masses, displaced medially by parotid masses, and displaced posteriorly and medially by masses within the masticator space. Thus, by assessing the location and displacement pattern of the parapharyngeal space, one can assign a space of origin to a deep facial mass (Fig. 8.11).

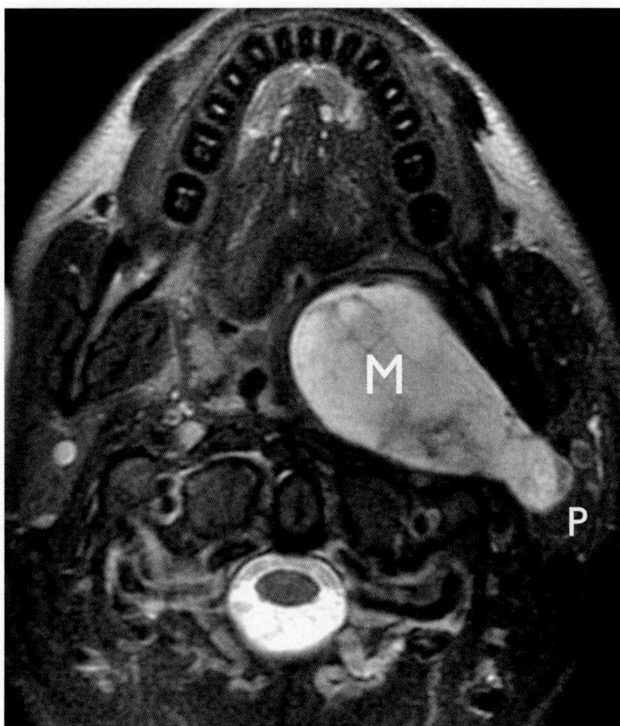

FIGURE 8.11. **Parotid Benign Mixed-Cell Adenoma (Pleomorphic Adenoma).** Axial fat-sat T2WI through the level of the oropharynx. A mass (M) appears to lie in the deep left parapharyngeal space. However this lesion contacts the deep lobe of the parotid gland (P), and is diving deep, displacing the parapharyngeal space medially and the masticator space anteriorly. The stylomandibular notch, identified from the carotid space to the mandible is widened, characteristic of a deep lobe parotid lesion. This is a classic appearance of a deep lobe parotid gland lesion, even though it appears sharply demarcated from the normal parotid tissue (P). Conversely, a lesion originating from the carotid space would result in narrowing of the stylomandibular notch. Note that the failure of fat suppression in the anterior chin (high signal subcutaneous fat anteriorly, while uniform fat suppression is noted in the mid and posterior portion of the image) is a common finding due to the anatomic asymmetry of the cranial–cervical junction.

Carotid Space

Masses of the carotid space deviate the parapharyngeal space anteriorly and will separate or anteriorly displace the carotid and jugular vein. They sometimes displace the styloid process anteriorly, which narrows the stylomandibular notch (the space between the styloid process and the mandible). This is a characteristic feature that distinguishes these lesions from deep parotid space lesions, which widen the stylomandibular notch.

Pseudomasses. When evaluating carotid space tumors, there are several pseudomasses of the carotid space that must be taken into account. These pseudomasses are vascular variants that may be mistaken for masses both clinically and radiographically. Asymmetry of the internal jugular veins is the most common variation in the vascular anatomy of the neck. Marked asymmetry between the size of the left and right jugular veins is common, with the right vein typically being the larger of the two. In addition, the jugular veins may demonstrate considerable variability in the degree of signal within their lumina, ranging from bright to signal void. The intraluminal bright regions should not be mistaken for thrombosis. It is important to follow the signal on serial images to visualize the tubular nature, thus confirming that the signal represents vasculature; otherwise it may easily be mistaken for adenopathy. Tortuosity of the carotid artery may present as a submucosal pulsatile mass in the pharynx. This variation, which is frequently seen in the elderly, is easily detected on CT or MR and obviates the need for further diagnostic workup unless a posttraumatic aneurysm is suspected.

Tumors. Most carotid space masses are benign neoplasms that arise from nerves located within the carotid sheath. The most common lesions are *paragangliomas* (also called *chemodectomas*) and nerve sheath tumors such as *schwannomas* and *neurofibromas*. Paragangliomas are vascular tumors that arise from neural crest cell derivatives. These lesions are named according to the nerves from which they arise and their location of origin. When arising from the carotid body, at the carotid bifurcation, paragangliomas are called *carotid body tumors* (Fig. 8.12). Paragangliomas may also arise from the ganglion of the vagus nerve (glomus vagale tumors), along the jugular ganglion of the vagus nerve (glomus jugulare tumors), and around the Arnold and Jacobson nerves in the middle ear (glomus tympanicum tumors). Despite the use of different names, the imaging features and histology remain the same.

Clinically, patients with paragangliomas present with a painless, slowly progressive neck mass that may be pulsatile with an associated bruit. Because these lesions are located within the carotid sheath, there are often associated slowly progressive cranial neuropathies (cranial nerves IX–XII) (Fig. 8.13). Paragangliomas are often multiple (5% to 10%)

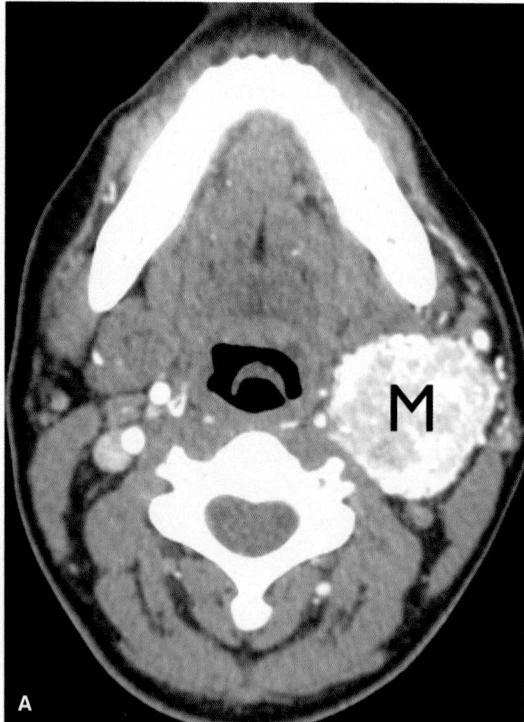

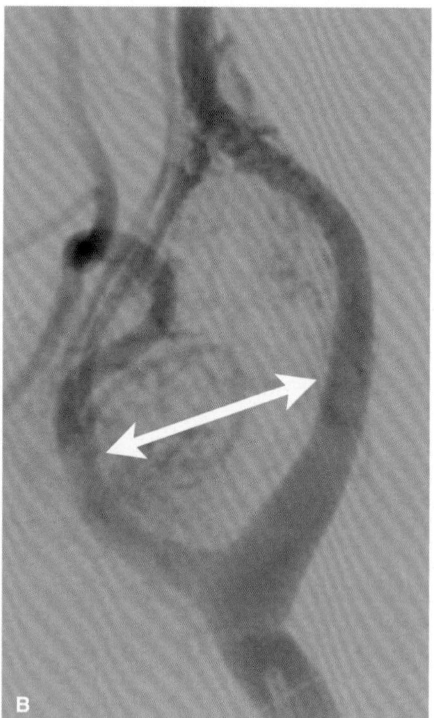

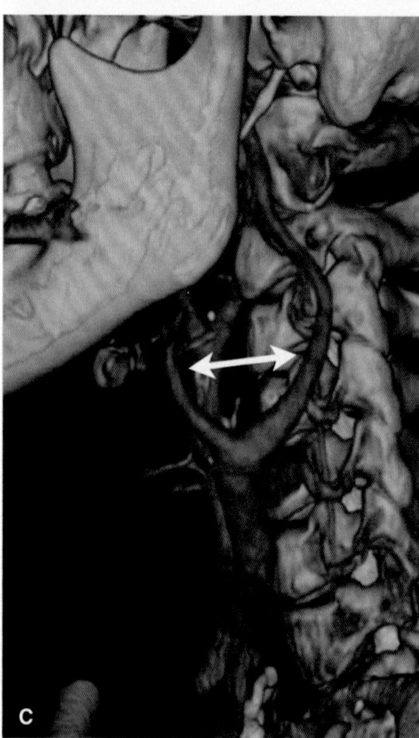

FIGURE 8.12. Carotid Body Tumor. A: Axial arterial phase contrast-enhanced CT. **B:** conventional x-ray angiography. **C:** CT angiography. A vascular mass (M) is identified located between the carotid bifurcation, with splaying of the internal and external carotid arteries (*double-headed arrow*), characteristic of a carotid body tumor. The vascularity and location supports the diagnosis of a paraganglioma, specifically a carotid body tumor. The lesion vascularity typically provides numerous flow voids on MR, yielding a "salt and pepper" appearance. Angiography is helpful in providing preoperative embolization, facilitating surgical resection.

and, in familial cases, are multiple 25% to 33% of the time. Therefore, if a lesion is detected, it is essential to look for others.

Angiographically, paragangliomas are very vascular, with a strong blush in the capillary phase. Treatment often consists of surgical resection. Interventional radiology plays an important role in permitting preoperative embolization, thus reducing blood loss during surgery. On CT and MR scanning, paragangliomas and neuromas are both densely enhancing and are typically indistinguishable. In contrast, on MR, paragangliomas are characterized by multiple flow voids and prominent enhancement, but neuromas usually do not demonstrate flow voids and can be cystic (Fig. 8.14). These features reflect the typically more vascular nature of paragangliomas. Note that these findings are not pathognomonic for paragangliomas, because very vascular schwannomas may also, on occasion, have associated flow voids.

Schwannomas are encapsulated tumors that arise from nerve sheath coverings and do not infiltrate the substance of the nerve. Within the carotid space, schwannomas often arise from the vagus nerve and present as benign neck masses. Schwannomas may occasionally show cystic change and

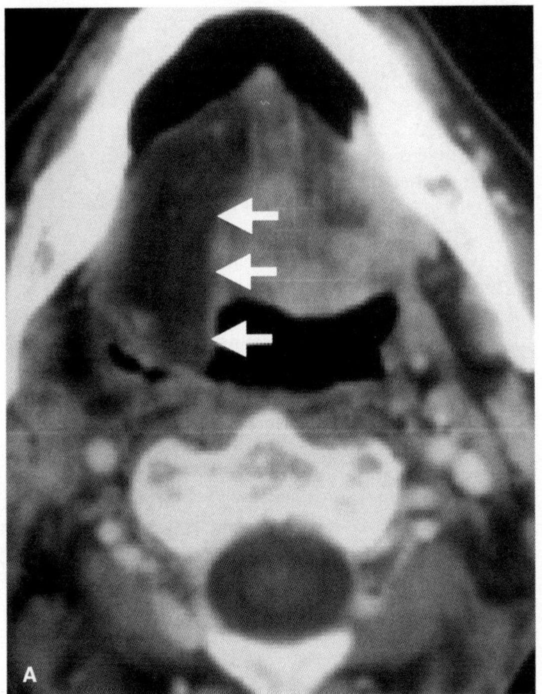

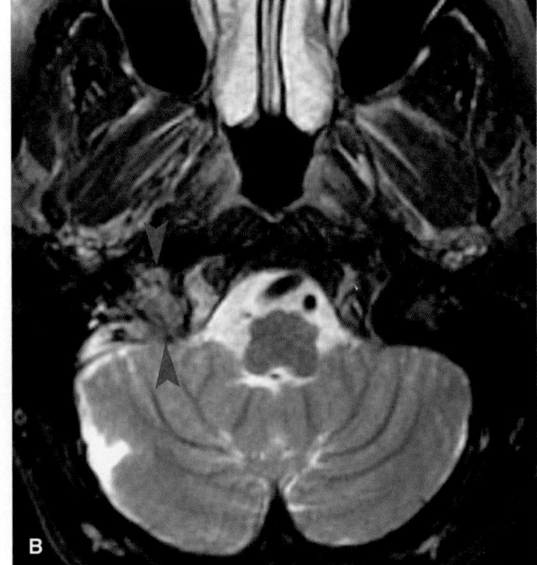

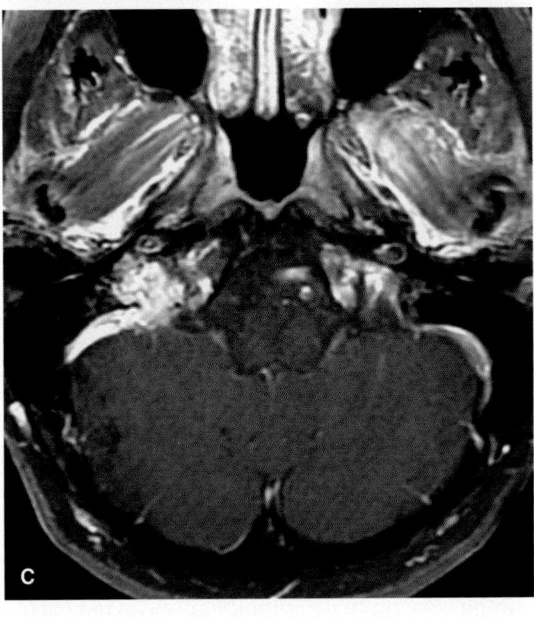

FIGURE 8.13. **Glomus Jugulare Tumor. A:** Axial contrast-enhanced CT. Fatty atrophy of the right tongue (hypoglossal nerve palsy) and patulousness of the right oropharynx (vagus nerve palsy) (*white arrows*) are evident. Dysfunction of multiple lower cranial nerves suggests involvement of the skull base, where cranial nerves IX–XII arise in close proximity. **B:** Axial fat-sat T2WI, and (**C**) post-gad fat-sat T1WI. A contrast-enhancing mass is identified filling the right jugular foramen (*arrowheads*) indicative of a glomus jugulare tumor. **C:** Corresponding slow flow or thrombus is noted in the contiguous sigmoid sinus (*arrow*).

necrosis. In contrast to schwannomas, neurofibromas are not encapsulated and usually occur as multiple lesions that permeate the substance of the nerve fibers.

Lymph nodes are a common source of pathology within the carotid space. In fact, the principal malignancy of the carotid space is squamous cell nodal metastasis. The deep cervical jugular nodal chain is located within the carotid space and serves as the final common efferent pathway of lymphatic drainage from the head and neck. As such, any pathology of the head and neck (metastases, lymphoma, infection, benign hyperplasia) will typically involve the jugular nodal chain and be found within the carotid space.

Parotid Space

Masses arising from the deep lobe of the parotid gland will deviate the parapharyngeal space medially. Unlike carotid space masses, deep parotid masses push the styloid process and carotid vessels posteriorly. This results in characteristic widening of the stylomastoid foramen. The structures within the parotid space that may give rise to pathology include the parotid gland and lymph nodes. The parotid gland is the only salivary gland with lymph nodes contained within its capsule. This reflects the embryogenesis of the parotid gland, the late encapsulation of which results in the presence of lymph nodes within the gland parenchyma (Fig. 8.15). Consequently, pathology of the parotid space includes salivary gland tumors and nodal disease. Normally these intraparotid nodes are subcentimeter and may be difficult to visualize.

Parotid Tumors. Most parotid tumors are benign (80%), and most of these are benign mixed-cell tumors (pleomorphic adenomas). The second most common benign salivary gland tumor is the Warthin tumor. Malignant tumors, which account for 20% of all parotid lesions, include adenocystic carcinoma,

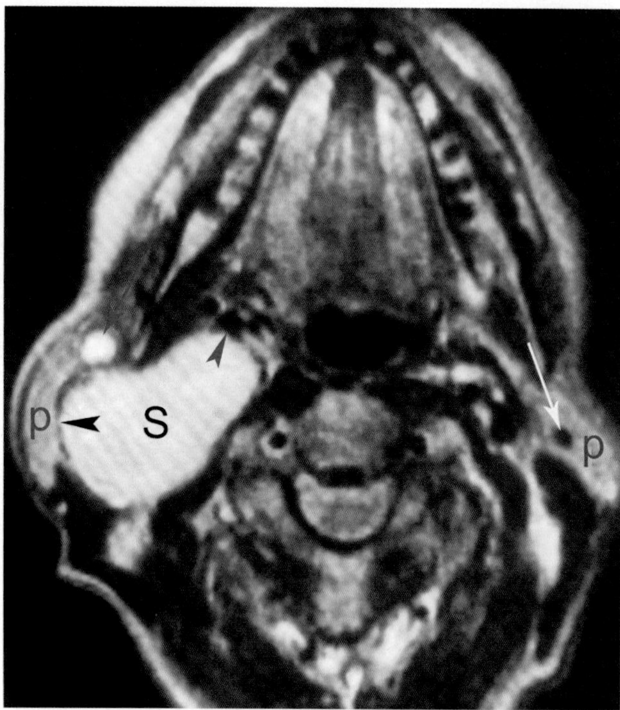

FIGURE 8.14. **Schwannoma.** Axial T2WI through the floor of the mouth. The patient presented with a painless neck mass. A homogeneous mass (*S*) displaces the carotid space anteriorly (*red arrowhead*) and the parotid space (*p*) laterally (*black arrowhead*). Anterior displacement of the carotid artery is characteristic of a carotid space mass. The lack of associated flow voids suggests that this lesion is a nerve sheath tumor, that is, schwannoma of the vagus nerve, as opposed to a paraganglioma. High signal within the right retromandibular vein (*red arrow*) is a result of partial compression. Normal flow void is seen in the opposite retromandibular vein (*white arrow*).

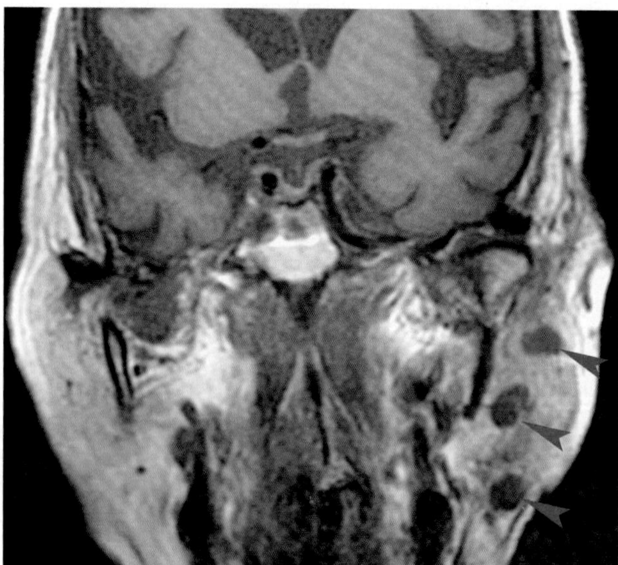

FIGURE 8.15. **Metastatic Lymph Nodes Within the Parotid Gland Capsule.** This 78-year-old man presented with left parotid swelling. Coronal T1WI reveals several enlarged nodes within the left parotid gland (*arrowheads*). The parotid gland serves as the drainage pathway for the posterior auricular scalp and is characterized by its fatty signal intensity. The finding of abnormally enlarged and necrotic intraparotid nodes initiated a search for ipsilateral pathology, which revealed a retroauricular scalp angiosarcoma.

adenocarcinoma, squamous cell carcinoma, and mucoepidermoid carcinoma. MR and CT imaging cannot with certainty differentiate benign from malignant disease. Both may present as well-circumscribed lesions. Tumor homogeneity, indistinct margins, and signal intensity are poor predictors of histology. Nevertheless, benign pleomorphic adenomas are typically well circumscribed and very bright on T2WIs and demonstrate heterogeneous enhancement (Fig. 8.16). Both CT and MR are useful in portraying the relationship of a tumor to surrounding normal anatomy and can demonstrate the location and extent of a parotid mass before biopsy. A feature predictive of malignancy is infiltration into deep neck structures, such as the masticator or parapharyngeal space. Clinical involvement of the facial nerve is another ominous finding suggestive of malignancy.

The presence of multiple lesions within the parotid space may be seen with several conditions, including either inflammatory or malignant adenopathy. Another possibility is the Warthin tumor (benign salivary gland tumor), which is multiple 10% of the time and more common in men. Parotid cysts have been seen in collagen vascular disease (Sjögren syndrome) and also described in patients with AIDS (Fig. 8.17). These parotid cysts, also known as lymphoepithelial cysts, are believed to be the result of partial obstruction of the terminal ducts by surrounding lymphocytic infiltration.

Masticator Space

The masticator space is formed by a superficial layer of the deep cervical fascia that surrounds the muscles of mastication and the mandible. It extends from the angle of the mandible superiorly to the skull base and over the temporalis muscle. The muscles of mastication include the temporalis, the medial and lateral pterygoid, and the masseter. In addition, branches of the trigeminal nerve and the internal maxillary artery are located within this space. Masses in the masticator space displace the parapharyngeal space medially and posteriorly.

Most masses of the masticator space are infectious in origin. They usually result from either dental caries or dental extraction. A mass will often surround the mandible and may extend superiorly along the temporalis muscle. In addition, pseudotumors of the masticator space are common and include accessory parotid glands as well as marked muscle hypertrophy resulting from bruxism. Occasionally, an accessory parotid gland may occur along the anterior surface of the masseter muscle and can be mistaken for a mass. Asymmetry of the muscles of mastication may result from unilateral atrophy, owing to compromise of the mandibular division of the fifth cranial nerve (V3). This is most commonly seen in patients with head and neck neoplasms with perineural extension along the trigeminal nerve.

Primary malignancies of the masticator space are very uncommon. Malignancies of this space most often result from the extension of oropharyngeal or tongue base squamous cell carcinoma to involve the muscles of mastication. In addition, tumor or infection from oropharyngeal or nasopharyngeal lesions may spread along the third division of the fifth cranial nerve, allowing the tumor to ascend through the foramen ovale into the cavernous sinus (Fig. 8.18). From this location, a tumor may extend posteriorly along the cisternal portion of the trigeminal nerve to the brainstem. Primary malignancies of the masticator space include sarcomas arising from muscle, chondroid, or nerve elements. In addition, sarcomas of the bone such as osteosarcoma (Fig. 8.19) and Ewing sarcoma may be seen. Non-Hodgkin lymphoma will occasionally involve the mandible or extraosseous soft tissues of the masticator space.

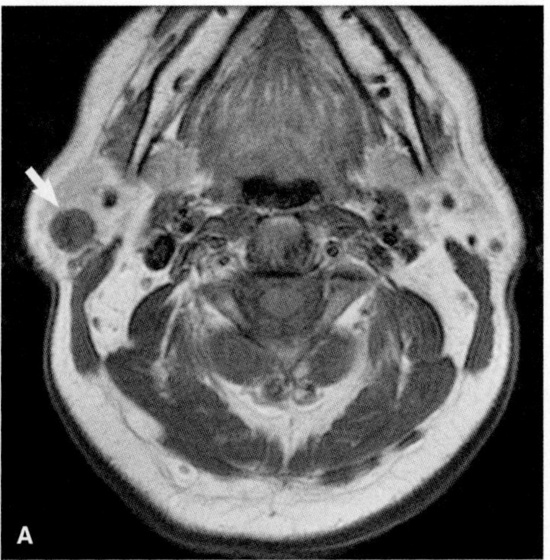

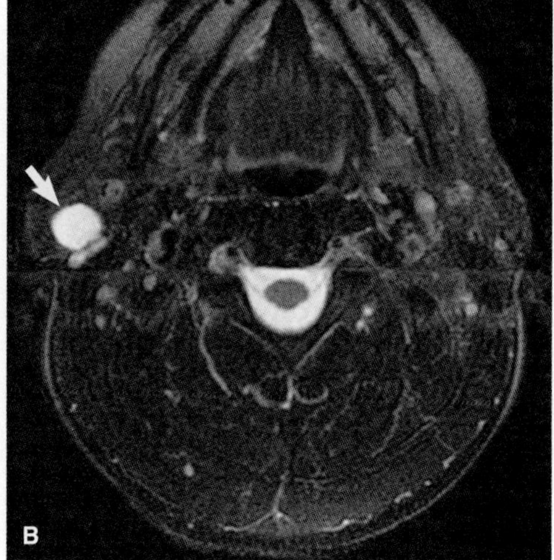

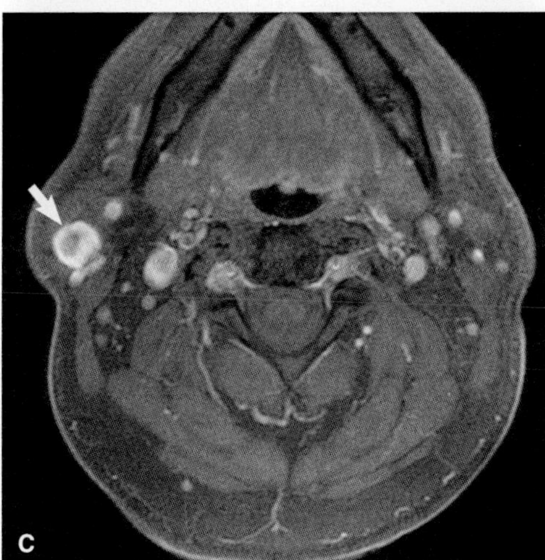

FIGURE 8.16. Benign Pleomorphic Adenoma. **A:** Axial T1WI. **B:** Axial fat-sat T2WI. **C:** Post-gad fat-sat T1WI. The patient presents with a well-circumscribed parotid mass (*arrow*), which is bright on T2WI and demonstrates heterogeneous contrast enhancement. These imaging features are consistent with a benign pleomorphic adenoma, which is the most common parotid lesion, accounting for 80% of all benign parotid tumors.

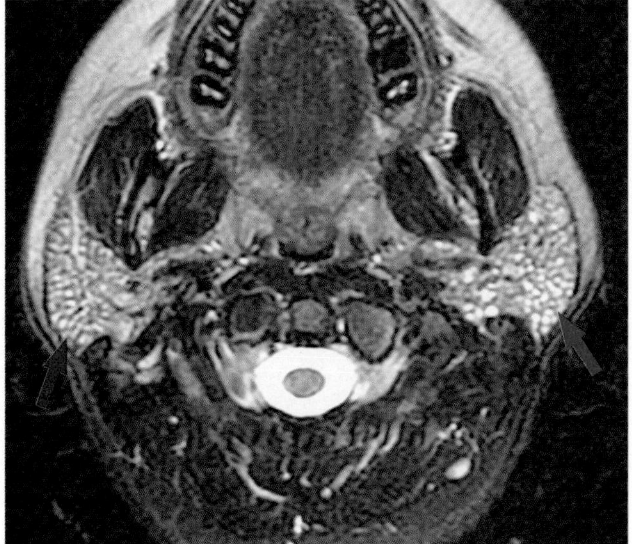

FIGURE 8.17. Benign Lymphoepithelial Cysts in Sjögren Syndrome. Axial T2WI. A 27-year-old woman presented with parotid swelling and complaints of dry eyes and mouth and was diagnosed with Sjögren syndrome, a chronic autoimmune disorder. MR reveals innumerable tiny parotid cysts (*arrows*), reflecting the lymphocytic infiltration of the exocrine glands, which causes lymphatic obstruction and cyst formation. Parotid cysts (benign lymphoepithelial cysts) can be seen in a variety of conditions with lymphocytic infiltration, including AIDS.

Retropharyngeal Space

The retropharyngeal space is a potential space that lies posterior to the superficial mucosal space and pharyngeal constrictor muscles and anterior to the prevertebral space. A mass within this space results in characteristic posterior displacement of the prevertebral muscles. The fascial planes in this area are complex but can be considered as forming a single compartment for simplicity. This space is significant because it serves as a potential conduit for the spread of tumor or infection from the pharynx to the mediastinum (Fig. 8.20). In contrast to the carotid and parotid spaces, in which inflammatory disease and metastases account for a minority of lesions, most lesions of the retropharyngeal space are a result of infection or nodal malignancy. This space is most often involved with nodal malignancy because of lymphoma or metastatic head and neck squamous cell carcinoma. These tumors frequently affect the retropharyngeal nodes, which are divided into a medial and lateral group. The lateral retropharyngeal nodes, also known as nodes of Rouviere, are normal when seen in younger patients but must be viewed with suspicion in individuals older than 30 years. In addition, head and neck infections may sometimes extend into the retropharyngeal space via lymphatics. Because the retropharyngeal space may serve as a conduit, spreading infection into the mediastinum, this space has also been referred to as the "danger space." Neck infections are most often the result of tonsillitis, dental disease, trauma, endocarditis, and systemic infections such as tuberculosis.

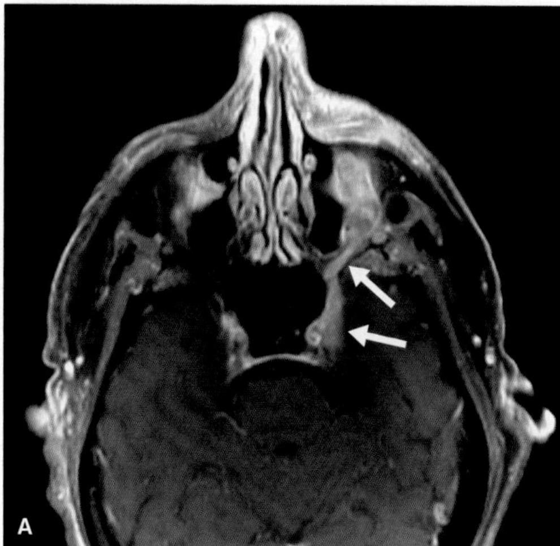

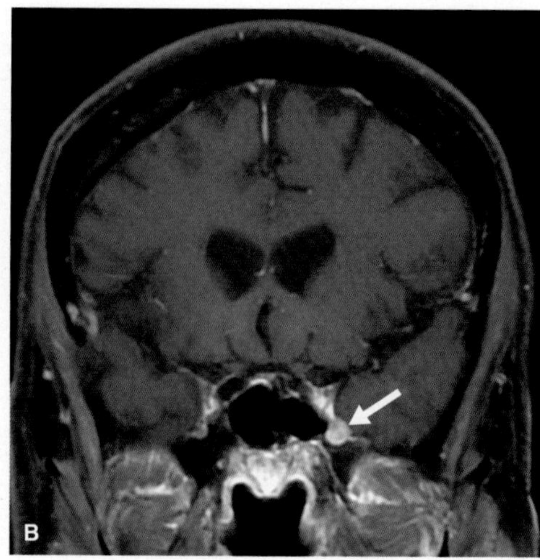

FIGURE 8.18. **Perineural Spread of Disease: Mucormycosis Infection.** A 21-year-old patient presented in diabetic ketoacidosis, with left facial numbness. Perineural spread of disease is noted extending along the anterior cheek all the way to the cavernous sinus. Perineural spread of a neoplasm, such as adenoid cystic carcinoma or squamous carcinoma, would have an identical imaging appearance. **A:** Axial post-gad fat-sat T1WI. **B:** Coronal post-gad fat-sat T1WI through the level of the cavernous sinus. Soft tissue infiltration involves the left malleolar soft tissues, and extends along the maxillary division of the trigeminal nerve (V2) (*arrows*) into the cavernous sinus. On coronal imaging an enlarged V2 nerve is identified extending through the foramen rotundum (*arrow*).

With the advent of antibiotics, infections occur much less commonly but are often seen in immunosuppressed patients. On routine T1WIs and T2WIs it can be difficult to differentiate an abscess from cellulitis, as both can be isointense to muscle on T1 and hyperintense on T2. Gadolinium is of value

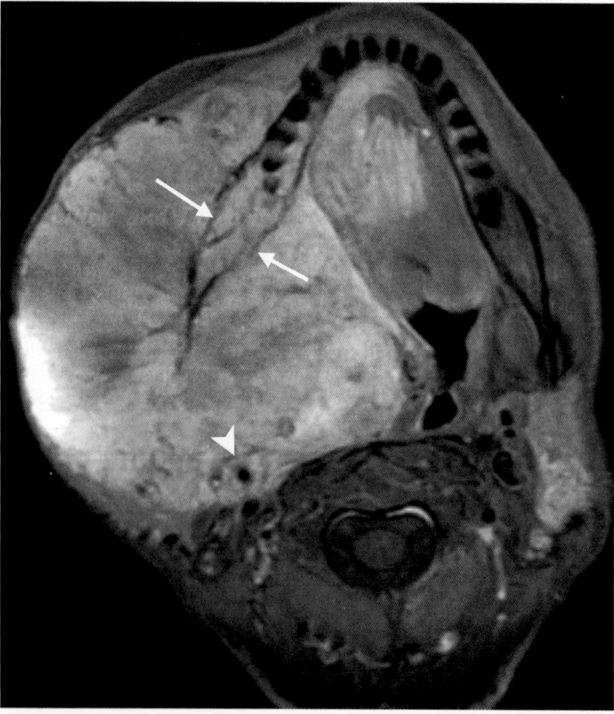

FIGURE 8.19. **Osteosarcoma of the Masticator Space.** Axial post-gad fat-sat T1WI. A 23-year-old man presented with a diffusely infiltrating mass of the right masticator space. This lesion appears to be centered upon the right body of mandible (*arrows*), with extension into all surrounding soft tissue structures. Posterior displacement and encasement of the right carotid artery noted (*arrowhead*).

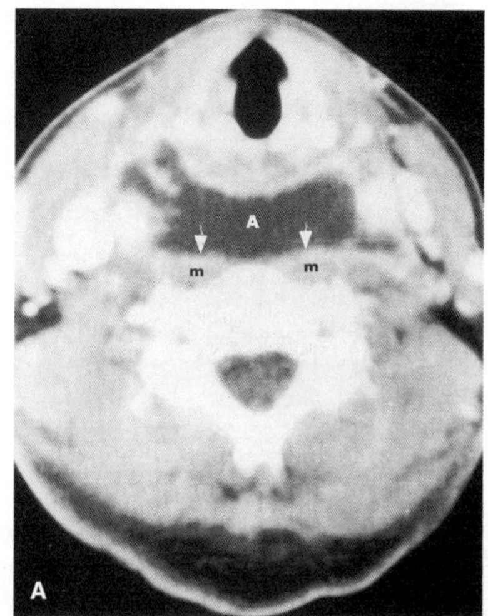

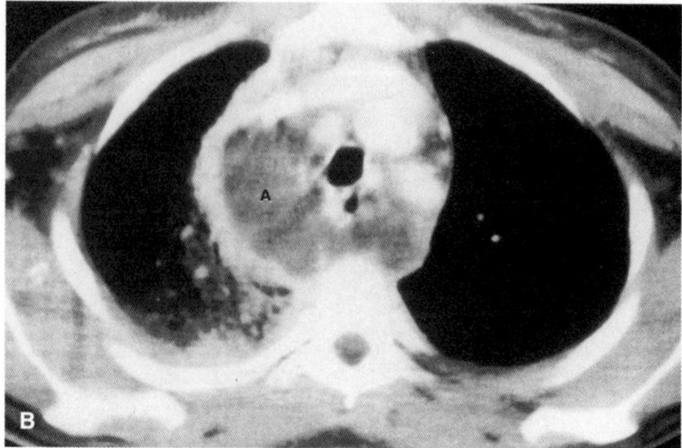

FIGURE 8.20. **Retropharyngeal Abscess.** Axial contrast-enhanced CT through the level of the larynx (**A**) and the upper mediastinum (**B**). A large fluid collection (*A*) extends from the retropharyngeal space into the upper mediastinum. The posterior displacement of the prevertebral muscles (*m*) (*arrows*) identifies this collection as being retropharyngeal as opposed to prevertebral.

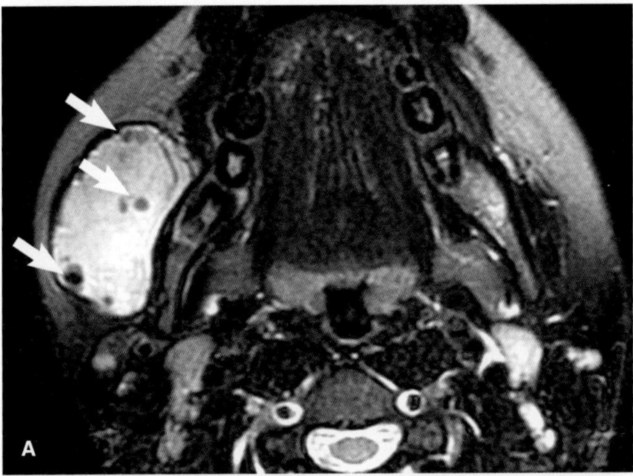

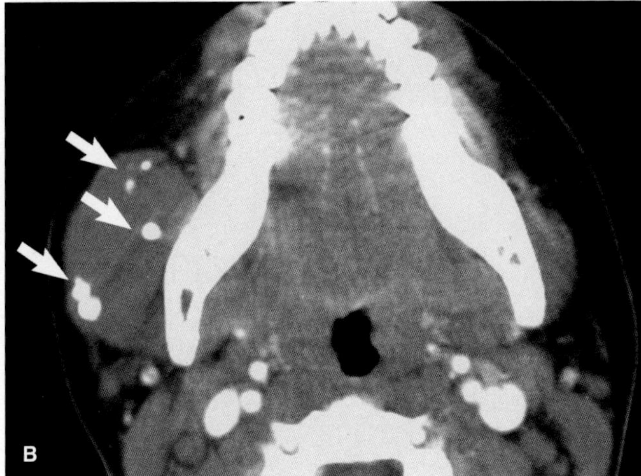

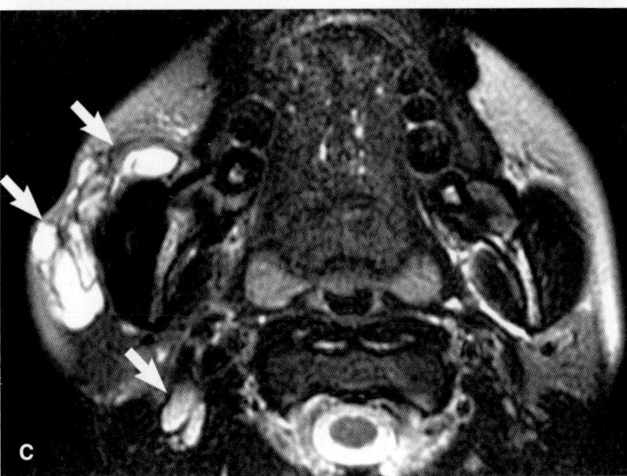

FIGURE 8.21. **Hemangioma. A:** Patient presented with a facial mass, which demonstrates high signal on T2WI with punctuate foci of signal void (*arrows*). **B:** On CT, these foci of low T2 signal prove to be phleboliths (*arrows*), which is essentially pathognomonic of the diagnosis of hemangioma. **C:** In another patient with a similar clinical presentation, a T2WI reveals a multilobulated and multiseptated high signal intensity lesion. The striking well-circumscribed areas of T2 hyperintensity with trans-spatial involvement are typical for a hemangioma (*arrows*). Lymphangiomas may be indistinguishable from this lesion, but often have fluid–fluid levels related to hemorrhage.

in making this differentiation, as an abscess will demonstrate a rim of contrast enhancement surrounding a liquefied center.

Prevertebral Space

The prevertebral space is formed by the prevertebral fascia, which surrounds the prevertebral muscles. Masses of the prevertebral space displace the prevertebral muscles anteriorly. This allows prevertebral lesions to be easily differentiated from retropharyngeal processes, which will displace these muscles posteriorly. The structures that give rise to most pathologies in this space are the cervical vertebral bodies. Any process that involves the vertebral bodies, such as tumor (metastasis, chordoma, etc.) or osteomyelitis, may extend anteriorly to involve this space.

Trans-Spatial Diseases

Occasionally, masses may not be localized to one of the spaces described above. Such masses are often secondary to lesions involving anatomic structures that normally traverse spaces of the head and neck, for example, lymphatics, nerves, and vessels. Examples include the following three categories: (1) lymphatic masses (lymphangioma); (2) neural masses (neurofibroma, schwannoma, perineural spread of tumor); and (3) vascular masses (hemangioma). Differentiation between these subtypes can occasionally be made by virtue of signal intensity characteristics. For instance, neurofibromas may have a characteristic low-intensity center on T1 and often involve more than one peripheral nerve. This is distinctly different from both lymphatic and vascular masses. Lymphangiomas and hemangiomas are congenital abnormalities that look quite similar on MR. Both entities have increased signal intensity on T2WIs and are infiltrative. Hemangiomas may have phleboliths, which may be easily detected on CT (Fig. 8.21). Lymphangiomas tend to have heterogeneous signal intensity with evidence of blood degradation products. Both entities should be considered in a patient with a history of chronic facial swelling and who shows CT or MR evidence of an infiltrative process that traverses several spaces.

Perineural Disease. Perineural spread of disease allows tumor or infection to gain access into noncontiguous spaces of the head and neck. The complex system of cranial nerves coursing through the skull base serves as a conduit for the spread of tumor and infection. Fungal infections (Fig. 8.18), squamous cell carcinoma, and adenoid cystic carcinoma have a particular proclivity for perineural spread of disease, which serves as a hallmark of these diseases. If a patient with a known head and neck primary neoplasm or immunocompromised status (susceptible to fungal infections) presents with facial numbness or dysesthesias, this is highly suggestive of perineural spread of disease, and careful attention must be paid to imaging of the cranial nerves of the skull base.

LYMPH NODES

Once a primary neoplasm of the head and neck is detected, the assessment of lymph nodes is a vital part of tumor staging.

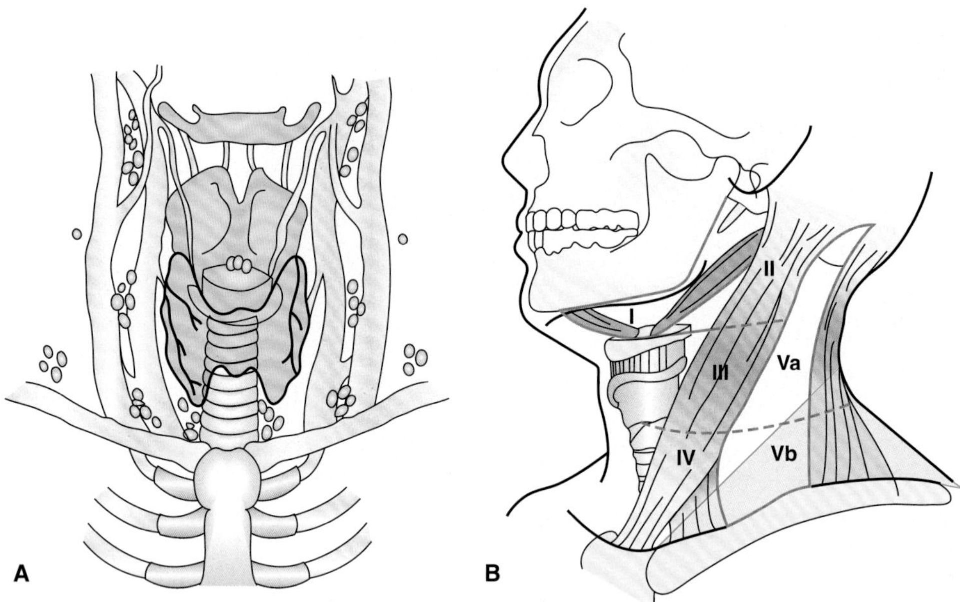

FIGURE 8.22. **The Thyroid Gland and Lymphatic Node Basins. A:** Schematic representation of the lymphatic node basins of the neck. The lateral neck lymph node compartments (levels II to V) and the central neck compartment (level IV). **B:** Schematic illustration of the anatomic borders of the central neck compartment (level VI). The superior margin is at the level of the hyoid bone, the inferior margin is at the level of the brachiocephalic vessels, and the lateral margins are at the medial aspect of the common carotid arteries (**A**). The central neck (level VI) contains the precricoid (Delphian), pretracheal, paratracheal, and perithyroidal nodes, including those along the recurrent laryngeal nerves, and the external branch of the superior laryngeal nerve. The parathyroid glands are also normally located in the central neck (**B**). (From DeVita VT, Lawrence T, Rosenberg S, eds. *DeVita, Lawrence, and Rosenberg's Cancer: Principles and Practice of Oncology.* Philadelphia, PA: Wolters Kluwer Health; 2015, with permission.)

The presence of a single ipsilateral malignant node reduces the patient's expected survival by 50%, with extracapsular nodal extension reducing survival by an additional 25%. Thus, the detection of nodal disease is critical for both prognosis and therapy. CT, MR, and PET all play a vital role in the staging of head and neck neoplasms, because clinically, it is difficult to determine the full size of the primary neoplasm and its associated nodal extension. At least 15% of malignant nodes are clinically occult because of their deep location (e.g., retropharyngeal nodes) and thus are not palpable by the clinician. The overall error rate in assessing the presence of adenopathy by palpation is between 25% and 33%. Thus, PET combined with either CT or MR is vital in obtaining the most accurate pretreatment planning information.

There are at least 10 major lymph node groups in the head and neck. Knowledge of the location of these cervical lymph node chains and the usual modes of spread of head and neck disease is essential for successful analysis of CT and MR scans. The lymph nodes of the neck have been divided into seven levels, I through VII (Fig. 8.22). This classification is used generally for the staging of squamous cell carcinoma. Of note, this system does not include some important nodal groups such as the retropharyngeal, parotid, and supraclavicular space as well as occipital nodes. We will focus on the principal lymph node group of the neck: the internal jugular chain. The internal jugular nodal chain serves as the final common afferent pathway for lymphatic drainage of the entire head and neck. This nodal chain follows the oblique course of the jugular vein beneath and adjacent to the anterior border of the sternocleidomastoid muscle. The jugulodigastric node is the highest node of the internal jugular chain. It is located where the posterior belly of the digastric muscle crosses this chain, near the level of the hyoid bone. The jugulodigastric lymph node is immediately posterior to the submandibular gland and provides lymphatic drainage from the tonsil, oral cavity, pharynx, and submandibular nodes.

Most lymph nodes of the head and neck should be equal to or less than 1 cm in short-axis except the jugulodigastric and submandibular nodes which may normally measure up to 1.5 cm in diameter. When an enlarged node is encountered on CT or MR, differentiation between a benign reactive node and a malignant one can be difficult. Several features that suggest malignancy are (1) peripheral nodal enhancement with central necrosis, (2) extracapsular spread with infiltration of adjacent tissues, and (3) a matted conglomerate mass of nodes. Nodal size itself is a less reliable indicator of malignancy, but it is used because the other more reliable differentiating features are frequently not present. If size criteria alone are used, approximately 70% of enlarged nodes are secondary to metastatic disease and 30% are caused by benign reactive hyperplasia. Note that the features described as characteristic for malignancy are the same as those for infection, and the two cannot be differentiated by imaging. Fortunately, this distinction is often easily made clinically.

PET scanning plays a vital role in the staging of any head and neck malignancy. Because metastatic nodes, regardless of size, are typically very glucose avid, PET provides exquisite sensitivity and specificity in the detection of cervical metastatic nodal disease. A lymph node that appears normal by size criteria on MR or CT may in fact be malignant if hot on PET scan. The converse is also true; an enlarged lymph node on MR or CT may in fact be benign reactive in nature, if cold on PET.

Lymph nodes can be accurately detected with either multislice helical CT or MR, and the decision regarding which technique to use should be based upon the imaging the patient is most likely to tolerate. Head and neck oncology patients often have respiratory and swallowing issues that prevent them from keeping sufficiently still for satisfactory MR scans. In

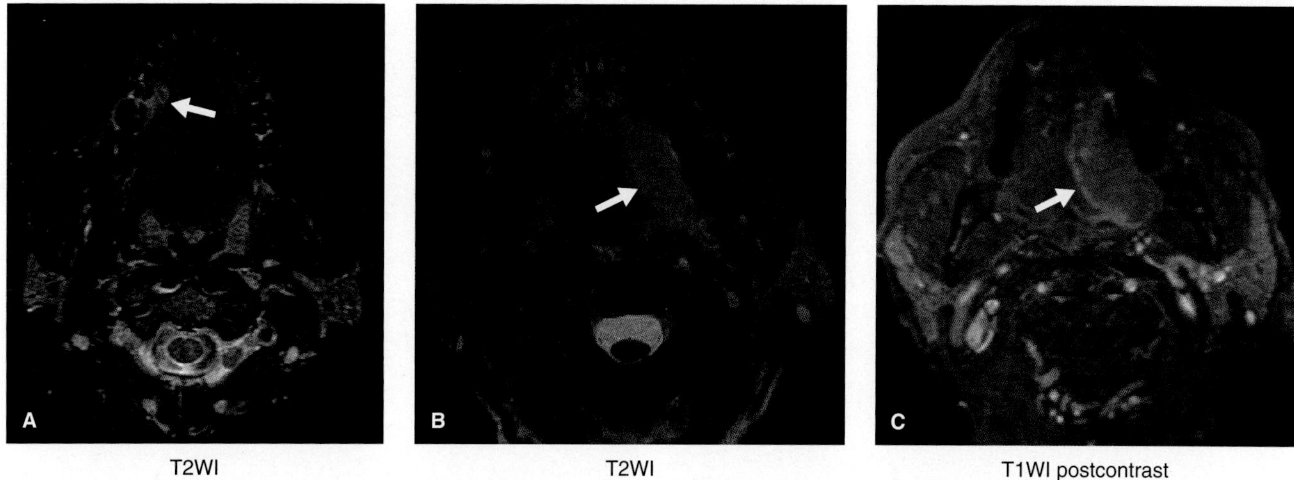

FIGURE 8.23. **Squamous Cell Carcinoma of the Tongue, Two Examples.** Case 1 Axial T2WI (**A**): A small right anterior lateral tongue lesion is noted (*arrow*). Early stage tongue cancers typically have an excellent outcome with the presence of occult metastases as the main predictor of survival outcome. Case 2 Axial T2WI (**B**) and axial post-gad fat-sat T1WI (**C**) through the level of the oropharynx. A large left tongue base squamous cell carcinoma mass extends deep into the intrinsic tongue musculature (*arrow* in figure **B** and **C**). Associated metastatic adenopathy is common in this setting and inspection for abnormal lymph nodes should be carefully performed.

contrast, multislice CT provides for rapid thin-section imaging of the neck with minimal motion artifact. With MR imaging, lymph nodes are well visualized on fat-suppressed FSE T2WIs, as well as precontrast T1WIs and postcontrast fat-suppressed T1WIs. Normal lymph nodes demonstrate homogeneous signal intensity, whether on precontrast or postcontrast T1WIs or T2WIs. Any heterogeneity in signal, especially in the presence of cystic change or necrosis, is consistent with metastatic disease (Figs. 8.6 and 8.23). Note that a fatty central hilus is a normal finding. Shape is also a differentiating feature, as a rounded shape suggests neoplastic nodal infiltration with associated nodal expansion. In contrast, if a node is enlarged but maintains its normal reniform configuration, it more likely reflects benign reactive change rather than metastatic disease.

ORBIT

Both CT and MR are valuable for imaging of the orbit; each has distinct merits. When evaluating for calcification, such as in retinoblastoma in a child with leukocoria or for bony fracture following trauma, CT is the modality of choice. MR, on the other hand, with its multiplanar capability and superior soft tissue discrimination, has proven to be of tremendous value in orbital imaging. For most orbital abnormalities, including evaluation of the visual pathways, MR is the procedure of choice.

Knowledge of the contents of the various orbital spaces provides insight into the naturally occurring lesions that develop within each area. The retrobulbar space contains both the extraconal and the intraconal spaces, which are separated by the muscle cone or "annulus of Zinn." This muscle cone is formed by the extraocular muscles (superior, inferior, medial, and lateral rectus; superior oblique; and levator palpebrae superior) and a fibrous septum. Together these structures form a cone with its base at the posterior of the globe and its apex at the superior orbital fissure. When identifying an intraconal lesion, an essential issue is whether the lesion arises from the optic nerve sheath complex or is extrinsic to it. The optic nerve sheath complex is composed of the optic nerve and the surrounding perioptic nerve sheath. The optic nerve is an extension of the brain enveloped by CSF and leptomeninges, which form the optic nerve sheath. Therefore, the CSF space that envelops the optic nerve is continuous with the intracranial subarachnoid space. If a lesion arises from the optic nerve sheath complex, the most common lesion is either an optic nerve glioma or optic sheath meningioma.

Optic nerve glioma is the most common tumor of the optic nerve and typically occurs during the first decade of life (Fig. 8.24). There is a high association with neurofibromatosis

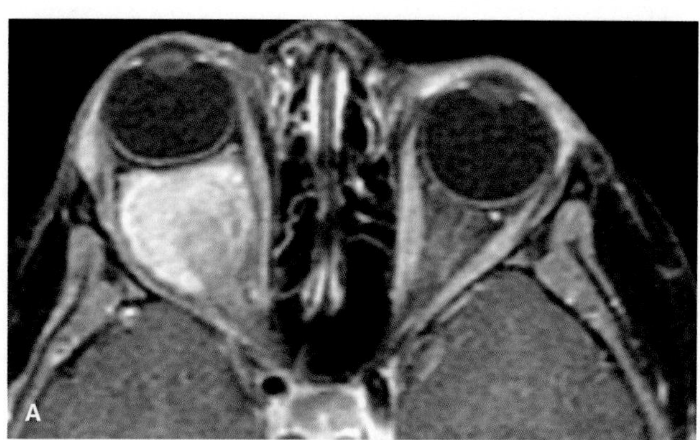

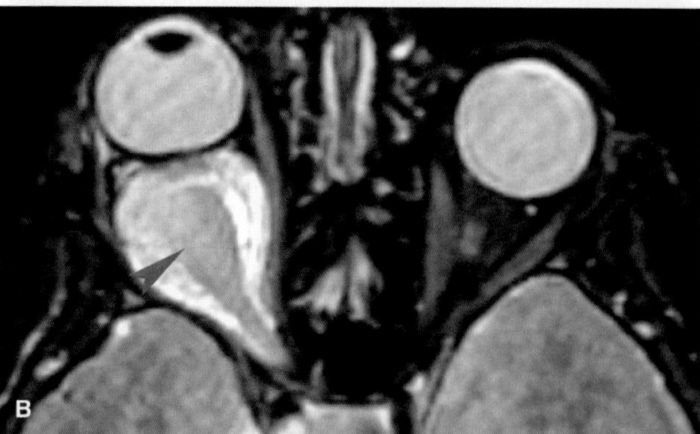

FIGURE 8.24. **Optic Nerve Glioma.** Axial post-gad fat-sat T1WI (**A**) and fat-sat T2WI (**B**) through the orbits. A large contrast enhancing mass involves the right optic nerve. The enlarged optic nerve (*arrowhead*) is visible coursing through markedly thickened optic sheath soft tissue. This soft tissue represents arachnoidal hyperplasia, a finding associated with optic gliomas in patients with neurofibromatosis.

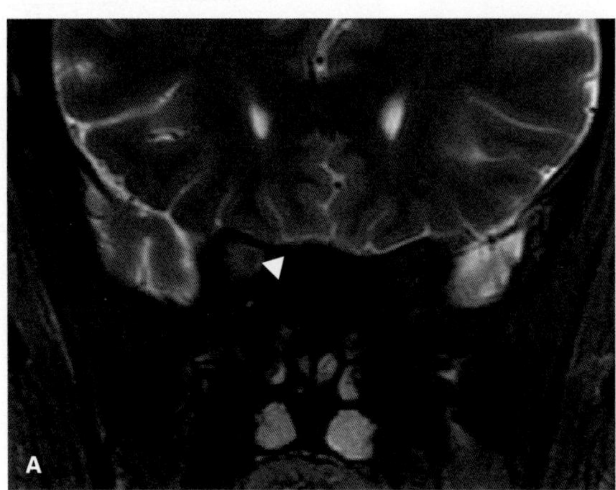

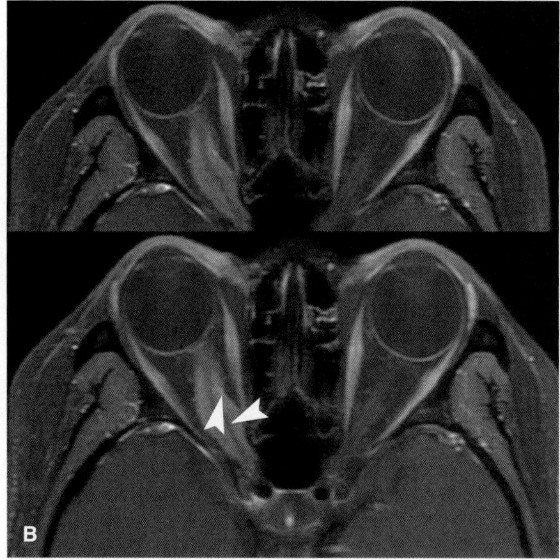

FIGURE 8.25. **Optic Sheath Meningioma. A:** Coronal T2WI. Abnormal enlargement and T2 hyperintensity of the right optic nerve at the level of the orbital apex (*arrow*). **B:** Axial post-gad fat-sat T1WIs through the orbits. "Tram track" enhancement involves the right optic nerve sheath (*arrowhead*) and extends into the optic canal. A somewhat similar pattern may be seen in conditions with infiltration of the optic nerve sheath such as metastatic disease, leukemic infiltrate, and lymphoma.

type 1, particularly when there is bilateral optic nerve involvement. Histologically, these lesions are low-grade pilocytic astrocytomas. The characteristic imaging finding is that of enlargement of the optic nerve sheath complex. The enlarged sheath complex may be tubular, fusiform, or eccentric with kinking. Some optic nerve gliomas have extensive associated thickening of the perioptic meninges. Histologically, this reflects peritumoral-reactive meningeal change, which has been termed "arachnoidal hyperplasia" or "gliomatosis." This finding is often seen in patients with neurofibromatosis.

Optic sheath meningiomas arise from hemangioendothelial cells of the arachnoid layer of the optic nerve sheath. These lesions assume a circular configuration and grow in a linear fashion along the optic nerve. Optic sheath meningiomas demonstrate a characteristic "tram track" pattern of linear contrast enhancement, because the nerve sheath enhances, rather than the nerve itself. MR easily displays any tumor extension along the optic nerve sheath through the orbital apex (Fig. 8.25). In contrast to optic nerve gliomas, meningiomas may invade and grow through the dura, resulting in an irregular and asymmetric appearance. In addition, optic sheath meningiomas may be extensively calcified, whereas optic nerve gliomas rarely have any calcification. In patients with sarcoidosis, leukemia or lymphoma, cellular infiltrates may deposit within the perioptic nerve sheath CSF space. In such cases, contrast enhancement of the perioptic nerve sheath space may mimic the "tram track" appearance of a nerve sheath meningioma. An important differential diagnostic consideration for enhancement of the optic nerve sheath is optic neuritis. In contrast to the conditions just mentioned, which demonstrate enhancement of the optic nerve sheath (i.e., peripheral optic nerve enhancement), optic neuritis demonstrates abnormal T2 hyperintensity and contrast enhancement as a result of inflammation of the optic nerve itself (Fig. 8.26). Optic neuritis presents with an acute visual deficit, often described as "blurring" of vision, and can be the first sign of multiple sclerosis (MS). Approximately 20% of patients with MS initially present with an episode of optic neuritis. In fact, of patients with isolated optic neuritis, approximately 50% eventually are diagnosed with MS.

Vascular Lesions. A variety of vascular lesions may develop in the orbit. The four lesions we will consider include capillary hemangioma, lymphangioma, cavernous hemangioma, and varix. These lesions are readily distinguished by a combination of imaging and clinical findings, including the patient's age (see Table 8.2). *Capillary hemangiomas* develop in infants (younger than 1 year) and are diagnosed within the first weeks of life. Although these lesions may grow rapidly in size, they typically plateau during the first year or two then regress spontaneously. On imaging studies, a capillary hemangioma appears as an infiltrative soft tissue complex, often with multiple vascular flow voids. In contrast, *lymphangiomas* are one of the most common orbital tumors of childhood and occur in an older group of children (3 to 15 years). Lymphangiomas are characterized by their propensity to bleed, and they often contain blood degradation products. An acute hemorrhage may result in marked expansion of the lesion with sudden proptosis (Fig. 8.27). MR reveals a multiloculated, lobular mass with characteristic signal heterogeneity caused by blood degradation products. The older age of presentation, combined with the characteristic heterogeneous signal related to blood products, allows differentiation from the capillary hemangiomas (Fig. 8.28). *Cavernous hemangiomas* are one of the most common orbital masses in adults. In contrast to the other vascular lesions of the orbit, hemangiomas are characterized as a sharply circumscribed, rounded mass (Fig. 8.29). These lesions demonstrate diffuse enhancement, sometimes with a mottled pattern. The venous *varix* is an enormously dilated vein that is characterized by its marked change in size with the Valsalva maneuver.

Superior ophthalmic vein is well visualized on MR studies. Pathology includes thrombosis and enlargement. Thrombosis often occurs in conjunction with cavernous sinus thrombosis and presents as loss of the normal flow void, with signal intensity related to the age of the thrombus. Enlargement of the superior ophthalmic vein may also be seen with cavernous

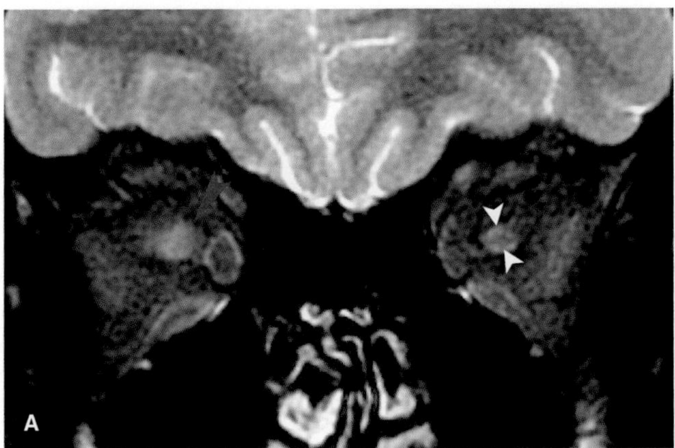

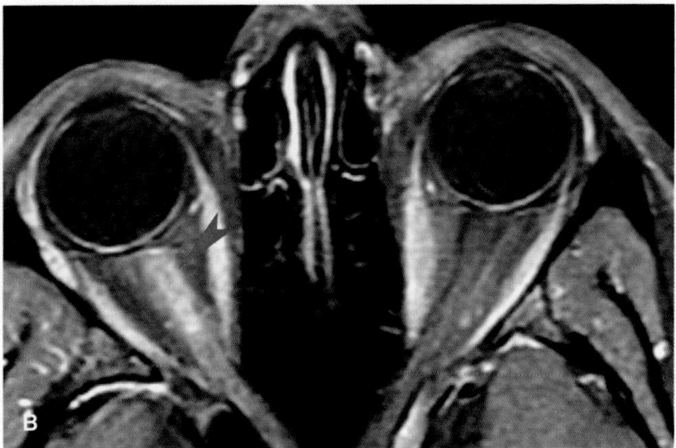

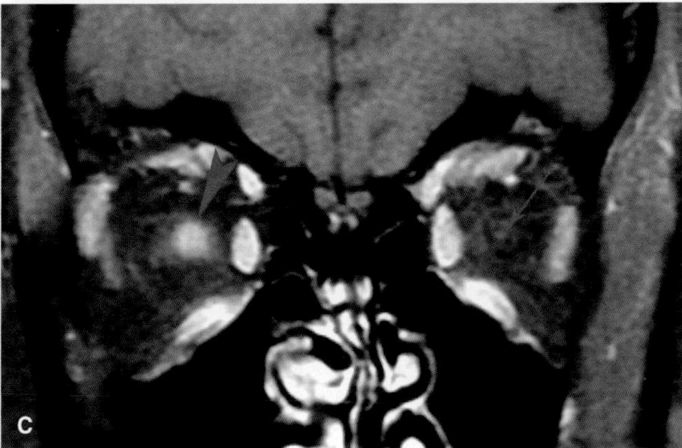

FIGURE 8.26. **Optic Neuritis. A:** Coronal fat-sat T2WI. **B:** Post-gat fat-sat axial. **C:** Post-gad fat-sat coronal T1WI. A 25-year-old woman presented with right-sided visual loss. Abnormal T2 hyperintensity as well as corresponding contrast enhancement are noted involving the right optic nerve (*red arrowheads*) are signs of optic neuritis. Subtle prominence of the left perioptic sheath is a common normal finding (*small white arrowheads*). The normal lack of enhancement of the left optic nerve makes the normal nerve relatively inconspicuous on the post-gad fat-sat T1WI sequences. The dot of slight enhancement (*long arrow*) in the left central nerve on **C**, is in keeping with imaging of the optic disc in the immediate retrobulbar region. Optic neuritis reflects a demyelinating condition often related to multiple sclerosis. Other etiologies include demyelination or inflammation secondary to infections including sinusitis, tuberculosis, and viral agents such as herpes and cytomegalovirus, or as a complication of radiation therapy. Nevertheless, when due to idiopathic demyelination, the condition of optic neuritis often heralds the onset of multiple sclerosis by many years.

carotid fistulas (Fig. 8.30). Cavernous carotid fistulas represent direct or indirect communication between the internal carotid artery and the venous cavernous sinus. These are either spontaneous or posttraumatic, and patients may present with pulsating exophthalmos and bruit.

Pseudotumor and lymphoma are two important orbital lesions that may present with similar imaging findings. Idiopathic inflammatory pseudotumor is a poorly characterized condition that results from an inflammatory lymphocytic infiltrate. This is the most common cause of an intraorbital mass lesion in the adult population. Pseudotumor is often rapidly developing and presents with painful proptosis, chemosis, and ophthalmoplegia. In contrast, lymphoma tends to present with painless proptosis. Lymphoma is the third most common adult orbital mass lesion, following pseudotumor and cavernous hemangioma. On imaging studies, both lymphoma and pseudotumor appear as diffusely infiltrating lesions capable of involving and extending into any retrobulbar structures (Fig. 8.31). Several reports have suggested that T2 shortening of the tumor (dark signal on T2) is suggestive of pseudotumor. Nevertheless, the distinction between these two entities frequently remains very difficult clinically, radiographically, and even histopathologically.

It is reported that a trial dose of steroids may be valuable in differentiating these two entities. Steroids are reported to have a lasting effect, eliminating a pseudotumor lesion. However, the cytolytic effect of steroids on lymphoma may also have a similar but short-lived response that may initially be confounding. In addition, when a diffusely infiltrative mass is encountered in a young child anywhere in the head and neck region, including the orbits, rhabdomyosarcoma should be a consideration.

TABLE 8.2

VASCULAR ORBITAL LESIONS

■ LESION	■ AGE	■ IMAGING FEATURES	■ MORPHOLOGY
Capillary hemangioma	<1 year	Flow voids	Infiltrative lesion
Lymphangioma	3–15 years	Blood products	Multiloculated, lobular mass
Cavernous hemangioma	Adults	Well-circumscribed mass	Rounded mass
Varix	Any age	Dilated vein, may enlarge with Valsalva maneuver	Vascular structure

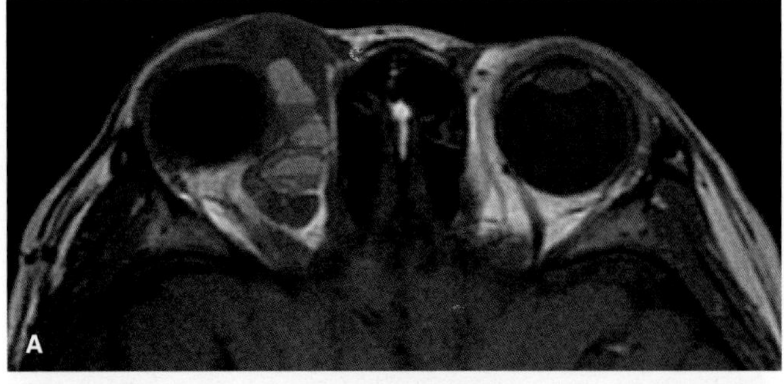

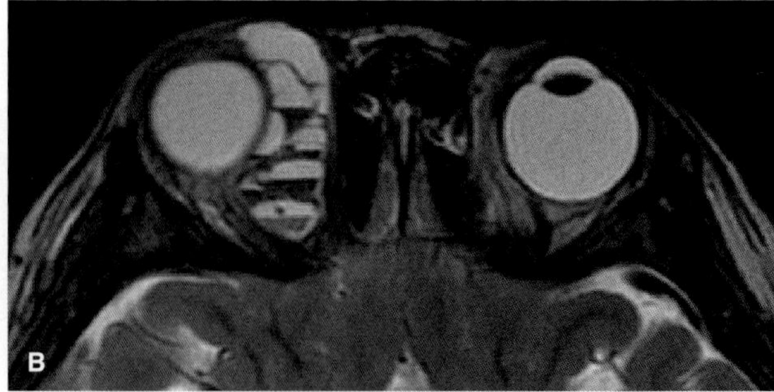

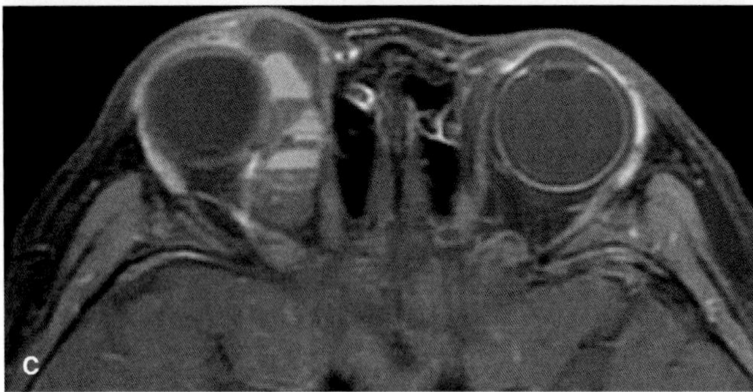

FIGURE 8.27. **Orbital Lymphangioma. A:** Axial T1WI. **B:** Axial T2WI. **C:** Axial Post-gad fat-sat axial T1WI. Imaging reveals a multicystic orbital lesion with numerous fluid–fluid levels (hematocrit effect, i.e., serum layered above red blood cells). Hemorrhage into a lesion is a characteristic feature of lymphangiomas and may be responsible for the rapid development of proptosis.

Thyroid ophthalmopathy (Graves'disease) is a common lesion and is the most frequent cause of unilateral or bilateral proptosis in adults. This condition is the result of an inflammatory infiltration of the orbital muscles and orbital connective tissues. Most patients will have clinical or laboratory evidence of hyperthyroidism, but 10% will not; these are referred to as "euthyroid ophthalmopathy." Imaging findings consist of enlargement of the extraocular muscles with sparing of the tendinous attachments to the globe (Fig. 8.32). This is in contrast to pseudotumor, which typically involves the muscle attachments to the globe. The muscles involved, in decreasing order of frequency, are the *i*nferior, *m*edial, *s*uperior, and *l*ateral rectus (pneumonic "*I'm slow*" reminds one of the order of muscle involvement and the typical orbital symptoms of Graves' disease, namely lid lag and limitation in orbital movement). Eighty percent of patients have bilateral muscle involvement. In some cases of thyroid ophthalmopathy, the extraocular muscles may be normal, and exophthalmos is the result of increased retrobulbar fat.

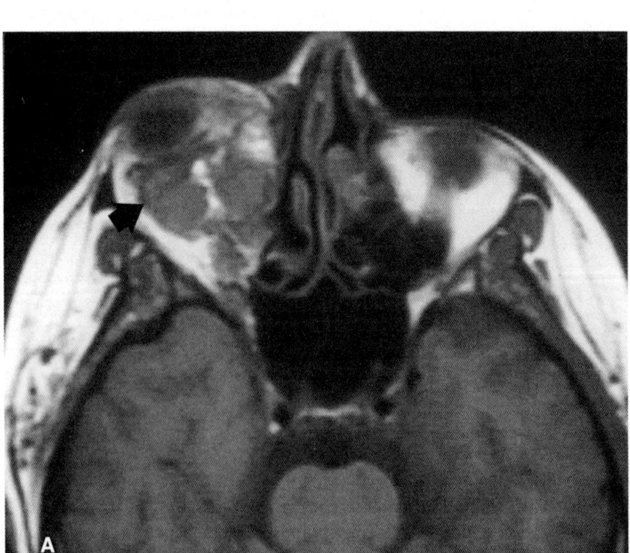

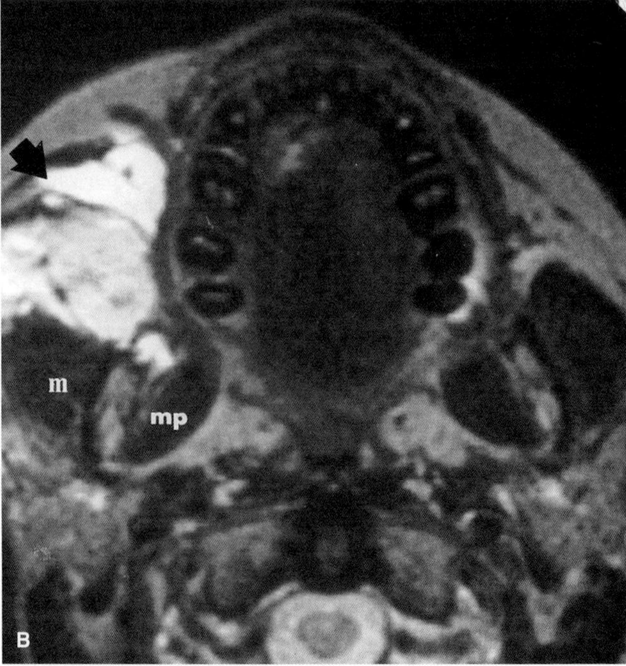

FIGURE 8.28. **Lymphangioma. A:** Axial T1WI through the orbit. **B:** T2WI through the midface. A heterogeneous lesion (*arrows*) extends from the right orbit through the inferior orbital fissure into the masticator space. The heterogeneous signal of this lesion, as well as its tendency to extend across fascial spaces (trans-spatial lesion), is characteristic for lymphangioma. m, masseter muscle; mp, medial pterygoid muscle.

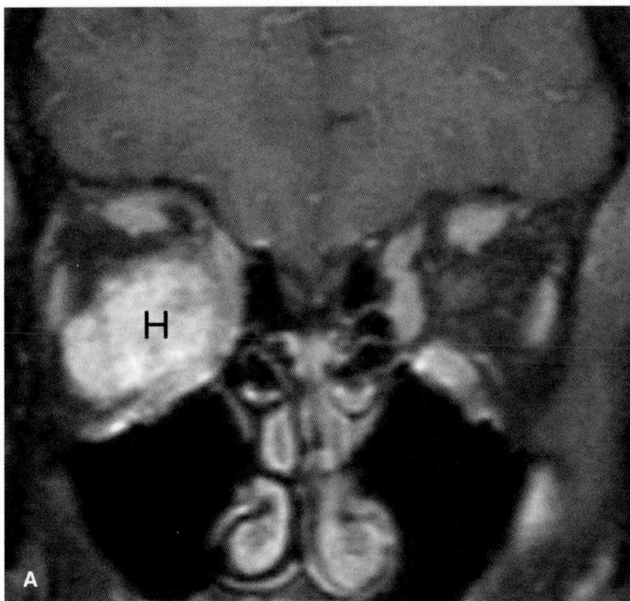

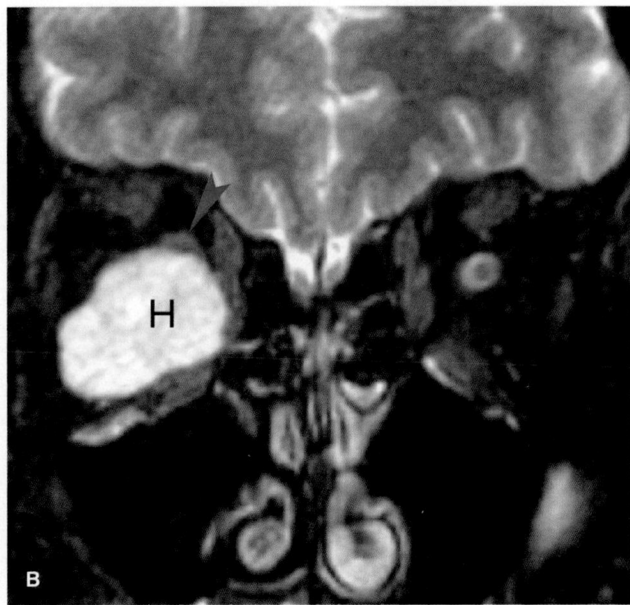

FIGURE 8.29. **Cavernous Hemangioma. A:** Post-gad fat-sat Coronal T1WI. **B:** Fat-sat T2WI through the midorbit. A well-circumscribed retrobulbar mass (*H*) is identified. The optic nerve is clearly separate from the mass (*arrowhead*). The well-circumscribed nature of this mass is characteristic of a cavernous hemangioma, the most common orbital mass in adults.

Lacrimal Gland. The extraconal space primarily contains fat and the lacrimal gland. However, many lesions involving the extraconal space are the result of tumor or inflammation extending from surrounding structures. These may include most of the lesions described earlier, as well as sinus-related inflammation. In contrast, lesions arising from within the extraconal space are primarily lacrimal in origin. Lesions of the lacrimal gland are very nonspecific, but can be divided into inflammatory types (e.g., sarcoidosis, Sjögren syndrome) and neoplastic types. Neoplasms of the lacrimal gland include epithelial and lymphoid tumors. Epithelial tumors are any of the lesions that arise from the salivary glands, such as benign mixed-cell tumor or adenoid cystic carcinoma. Lymphoid tumors include lymphoma and pseudotumor. Although none of these lesions have specific imaging findings, dermoid is one lesion that does have a characteristic finding, consisting of lipid content (Fig. 8.33).

Globe. A variety of lesions may involve the globe, and as usual, clinical history is vital in arriving at a useful differential diagnosis. In the pediatric age group, retinoblastoma is the most common primary ocular malignancy and presents characteristically with leukocoria (white pupillary reflex) and a calcified ocular mass (Fig. 8.34). Other conditions are rare and include developmental abnormalities (persistent hyperplastic primary vitreous tumor and Coats' disease), acquired retinal lesions (retinopathy of prematurity), and infection (primarily endophthalmitis

FIGURE 8.30. **Carotid Cavernous Fistula.** Axial T1WI through the superior orbit. Following a remote head injury, this patient presented with right chemosis. A large flow void is identified within the right cavernous sinus (*straight arrow*). The right superior ophthalmic vein is abnormally dilated (*arrowheads*), but the left vein is normal (*curved arrow*). Dilatation of the superior ophthalmic vein is an important clue to the presence of a carotid cavernous fistula.

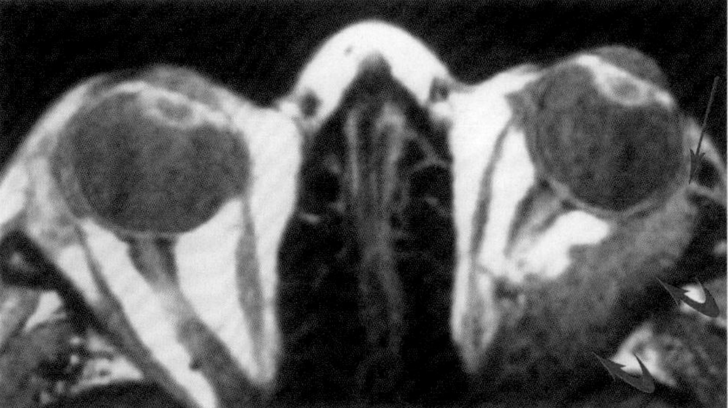

FIGURE 8.31. **Pseudotumor.** Axial T1WI through the orbits. A diffusely infiltrating lesion (*curved arrows*) extends throughout the lateral rectus muscle, including involvement of its tendinous insertion on the globe (*long arrow*). This feature distinguishes pseudotumor from thyroid ophthalmopathy, in which the muscle insertion is spared.

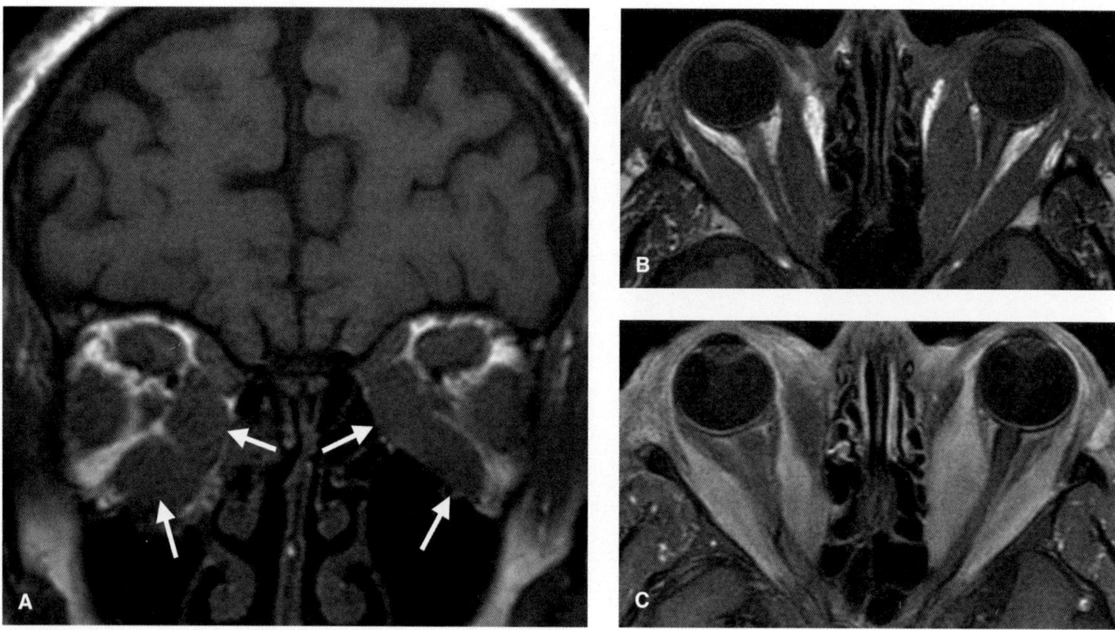

FIGURE 8.32. **Thyroid Ophthalmopathy. A:** Coronal T1WI. **B:** Axial T1WI. **C:** Post-gad fat-sat through the midorbits. Marked extraocular muscle enlargement is identified involving all the muscle bellies, in particular the inferior and medial (*arrows*) rectus muscles. The inferior and medial rectus muscles are the most frequently involved muscles in this disorder. Thyroid ophthalmopathy is the most common cause of proptosis in the adult. Severe muscle hypertrophy may result in orbital apex compression and loss of vision.

secondary to *Toxocara canis*). Note that although retinopathy of prematurity and persistent hyperplastic primary vitreous tumor may be bilateral, Coats' disease and ocular toxocariasis are almost always unilateral. In the adult, common ocular pathology includes retinal and choroidal detachment, uveal melanoma, and metastasis.

CONGENITAL LESIONS

In children, neck masses tend to be benign, including both congenital (thyroglossal duct cysts, branchial cleft cysts, and lymphangiomas/cystic hygromas) and inflammatory

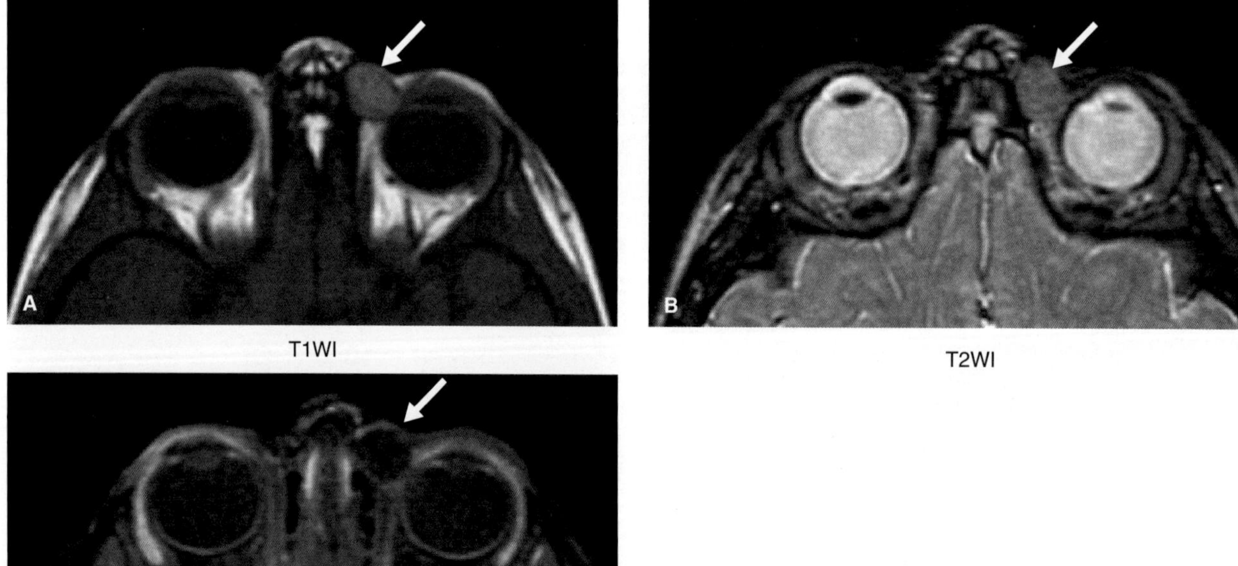

FIGURE 8.33. **Orbital Dermoid. A:** Axial T1WI. **B:** Fat-sat T2WI. **C:** Post-gad fat-sat T1WI through the midorbit. A well-circumscribed mass (*arrow*) is identified in the left medial canthal preseptal space. This lesion reveals intrinsic lipid signal which suppress with fat-sat, characteristic for a dermoid.

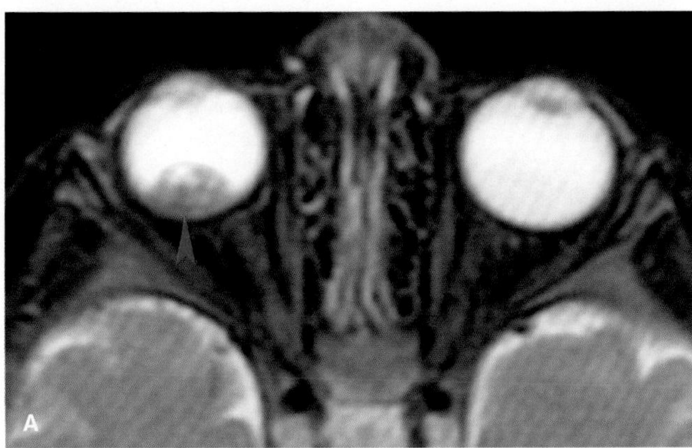

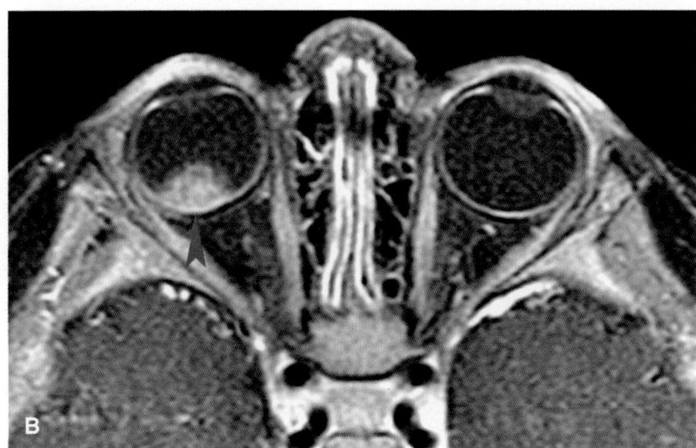

FIGURE 8.34. **Retinoblastoma.** The most common primary ocular malignancy of childhood is retinoblastoma. An 18-month-old infant presented with leukocoria (white pupillary reflex). Axial T2WI (**A**) and post-gad fat-sat T1WI (**B**) reveal an ocular mass confined to the globe without extraocular extension or optic nerve infiltration (*arrowhead* in figure **A** and **B**). MR and CT play an important preoperative role allowing accurate characterization of the full extent of the lesion.

lesions. When malignancy is entertained, the most common lesion in the pediatric age group is lymphoma, followed by rhabdomyosarcoma.

Thyroglossal duct cysts account for about 90% of congenital neck lesions and usually are found in children but may be seen in adults. The thyroglossal duct represents an epithelium-lined tract along which the primordial thyroid gland migrates. This tubular structure originates from the foramen cecum (at the tongue base), extends anterior to the thyrohyoid membrane and strap muscles, and ends at the level of the thyroid isthmus. The duct normally involutes by 8 to 10 weeks of gestation. Because the duct is lined with secretory epithelium, any portion of the thyroglossal duct that fails to involute may give rise to a cyst or sinus tract. In addition, thyroid glandular tissue can arrest anywhere along the course of the thyroglossal duct, giving rise to ectopic thyroid tissue. Seventy-five percent of thyroglossal duct cysts are midline, and most are located at or below the level of the hyoid bone in the region of the thyrohyoid membrane. In fact, thyroglossal duct cysts are the most common midline neck mass.

Surgery is the treatment of choice for these lesions because they may become infected. These lesions tend to recur if incompletely resected. Therefore, sagittal MR is ideal for determining the full extent of the lesion prior to surgery. On CT and MR, these lesions appear as cystic masses with a uniformly thin peripheral rim of capsular enhancement, with occasional septations (Fig. 8.35). Differential diagnostic considerations include necrotic anterior cervical nodes, thrombosed anterior jugular vein, abscess, or obstructed

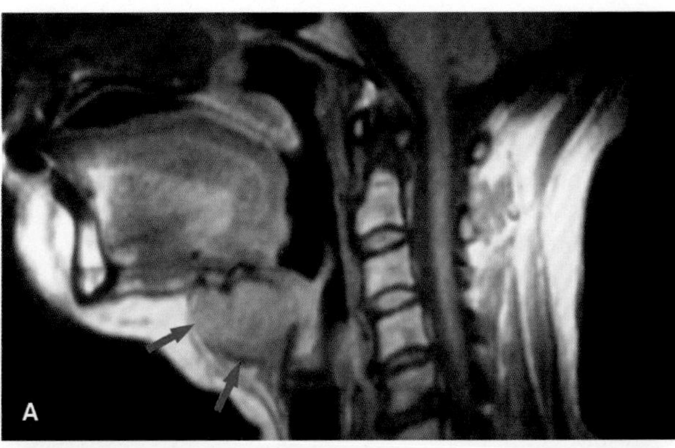

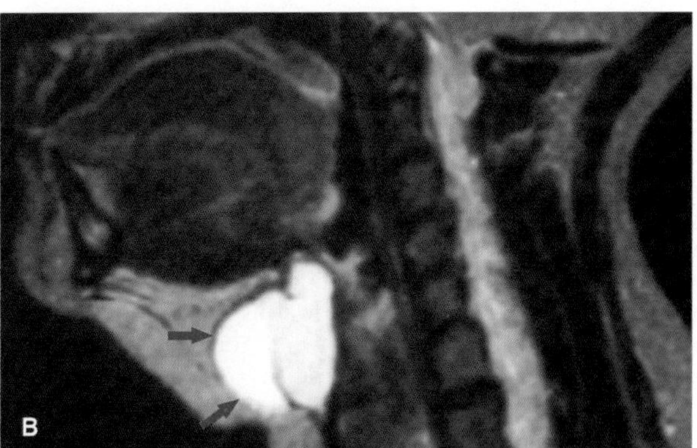

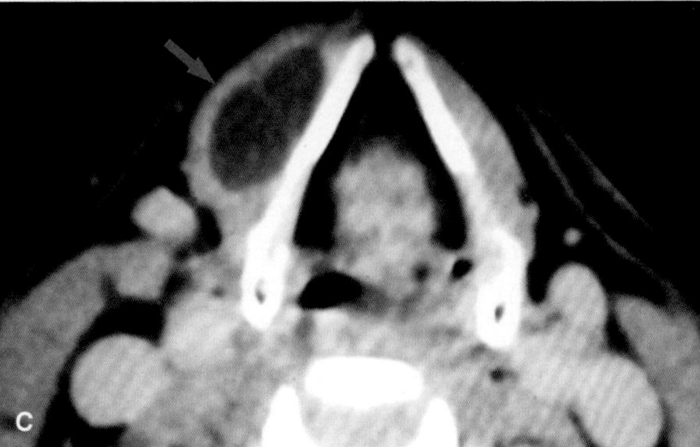

FIGURE 8.35. **Thyroglossal Duct Cyst. A:** Sagittal T1WI. **B:** T2WI. A well-defined, multilobulated cystic mass (*arrows*) is seen below the tongue base. A cystic lesion in this location is highly suggestive of a remnant of the thyroglossal duct. Imaging in the sagittal plane is important in defining the full craniocaudal extent of the lesion. **C:** CT in a different patient. The thyroglossal duct cyst (*arrow*) may be embedded within the strap musculature of the neck. Although most commonly midline, they are off midline in 25% of cases. Differential diagnostic considerations include necrotic anterior cervical node, thrombosed anterior jugular vein, or abscess.

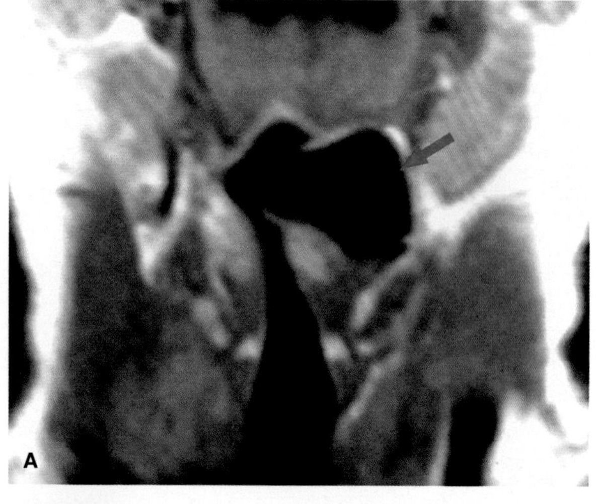

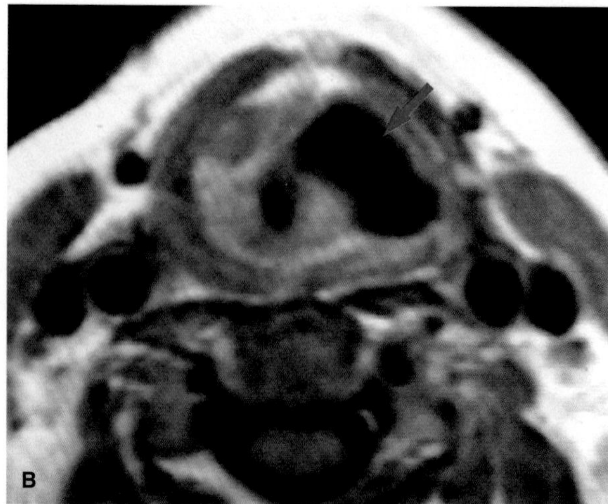

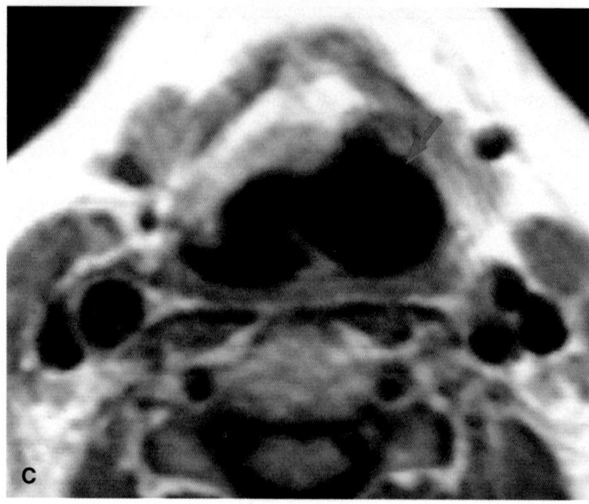

FIGURE 8.36. **Laryngocele.** A trumpet player presented with mild left neck fullness. Coronal (**A**) and axial (**B** and **C**) T1WIs reveal an air-filled mass (*arrows*) associated with the larynx consistent with a laryngocele. These lesions may be fluid filled and mimic a neck abscess or thyroglossal duct cyst. Diagnostic features of the laryngocele are that they communicate with the laryngeal ventricle and are found deep to the strap muscles. In contrast, thyroglossal duct cysts are either superficial or embedded within the strap muscles.

laryngocele. A laryngocele represents an abnormal dilatation of the appendix of the laryngeal ventricle. The laryngeal ventricle separates the false and true cords and anteriorly ends in a blind pouch termed the appendix. The laryngocele develops as a consequence of chronically increased intraglottic pressure, as may be seen in musicians (wind instruments), glass blowers, or excessive coughers. Laryngoceles are classified as internal, external, or mixed, according to their relation to the thyrohyoid membrane. When these lesions are confined to the larynx, they are called internal, but when they protrude above the thyroid cartilage and through the thyrohyoid membrane, they are termed external and typically present as a lateral neck mass near the hyoid bone (Fig. 8.36). Most commonly, laryngoceles have portions that are both in and outside of the thyrohyoid membrane and are called mixed. Laryngoceles that develop without a known predisposing factor should raise the suspicion of an underlying neoplasm obstructing the laryngeal ventricle.

Branchial Cleft Cysts. The structures of the face and neck are derived from the branchial cleft apparatus, which consists of six branchial arches. A branchial cleft cyst, sinus, or fistula may develop if there is failure of the cervical sinus or pouch remnants to regress. Although branchial abnormalities can arise from any of the pouches, the majority (95%) arise from the second branchial cleft. The course of the second branchial cleft begins at the base of the tonsillar fossa and extends between the internal and external carotid arteries. Thus, second branchial cleft cysts are typically found along this pathway, anterior to the middle portion of the sternocleidomastoid muscle and lateral to the internal jugular vein at the level of the carotid bifurcation. The usual clinical presentation is that of a painless neck mass along the anterior border of the sternocleidomastoid muscle, presenting during the first to third decade. These lesions tend to vary in size over time, often enlarging with upper respiratory tract infections.

Branchial cleft cysts are readily identified on CT and MR as well-circumscribed cystic lesions. Wall thickness, irregularity, and enhancement are related to active or prior infections. With MR, the T1W signal characteristics of the cyst may be either hypointense or hyperintense (Fig. 8.37). This signal variability is related to proteinaceous cyst contents, with simple fluid appearing darker on T1, and the presence of proteinaceous contents resulting in T1 shortening, that is, brighter signal on T1WIs. Differential diagnostic considerations include necrotic nodes, abscesses, cystic neural lesions, and thrombosed vessels.

Lymphangiomas are congenital malformations of the lymphatic channels. These lesions are benign and nonencapsulated. Histologically, they are classified as capillary, cavernous, or cystic. Any of these histologic types can be found in a given lesion, but the preponderance of a certain type dictates how the lesion is classified. The capillary lymphangiomas are composed of capillary-size, thin-walled lymphatic channels. In contrast, cavernous lymphangiomas are composed of moderately dilated lymphatics with a fibrous adventitia. Cystic hygromas represent enormously dilated lymphatic channels.

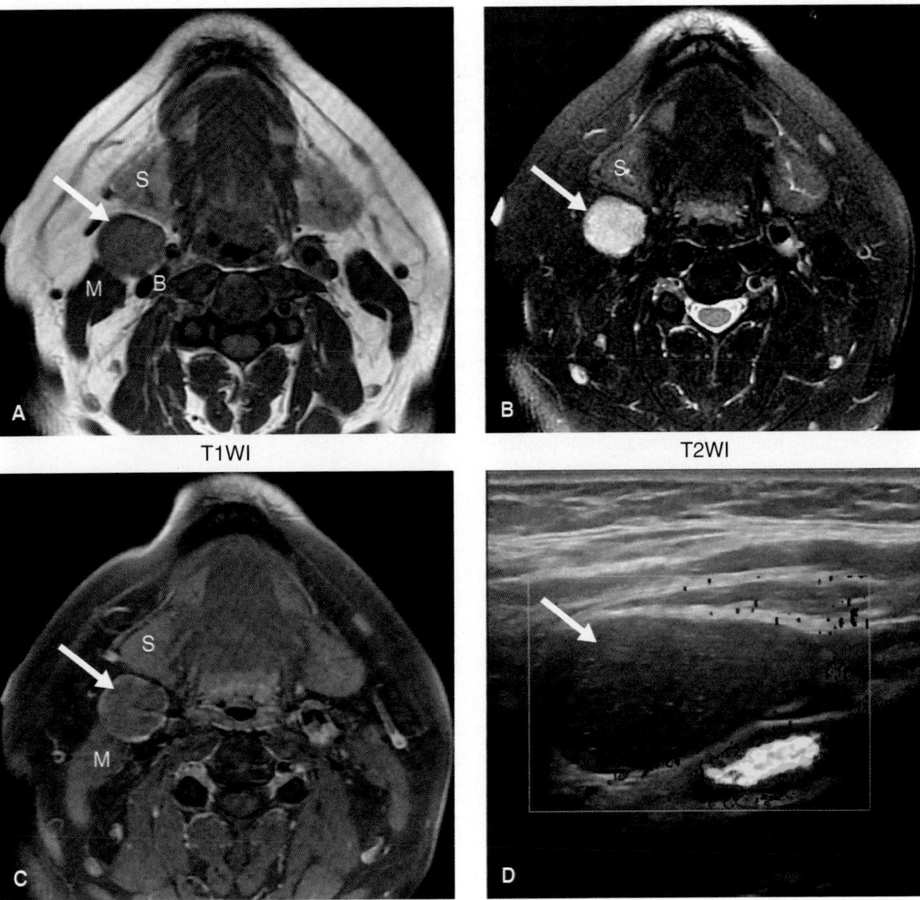

FIGURE 8.37. Branchial Cleft Cyst. Axial T1WI (**A**), T2WI (**B**), T1WI postcontrast (**C**) and ultrasound with doppler (**D**), all obtained through the floor of mouth. A well-rounded, noninfiltrating lesion (*arrow*) is seen anterior to the right sternocleidomastoid muscle (M), which is displaced posteriorly. The submandibular gland (S) is displaced anteriorly. This lesion is at the level of the carotid bifurcation (B). This combination of features is characteristic of a branchial cleft cyst. Branchial cleft cysts may display high signal on the T1WI, the result of T1 shortening effect owing to proteinaceous fluid. Differential diagnostic considerations would include necrotic cervical adenopathy. This especially true in adults, in whom a neck mass is much more likely to be a malignancy rather than a congenital lesion.

The lymphatic system develops from primitive embryonic lymph sacs that are in turn derived from the venous system. If these sacs fail to communicate with the venous system, they dilate as they accumulate lymphatic fluid. Thus, lymphangiomas represent sequestrations of the primitive embryonic lymph sacs. If this defect is localized, the result is an isolated cystic hygroma. However, extensive defects in this lymphovenous communication are incompatible with life

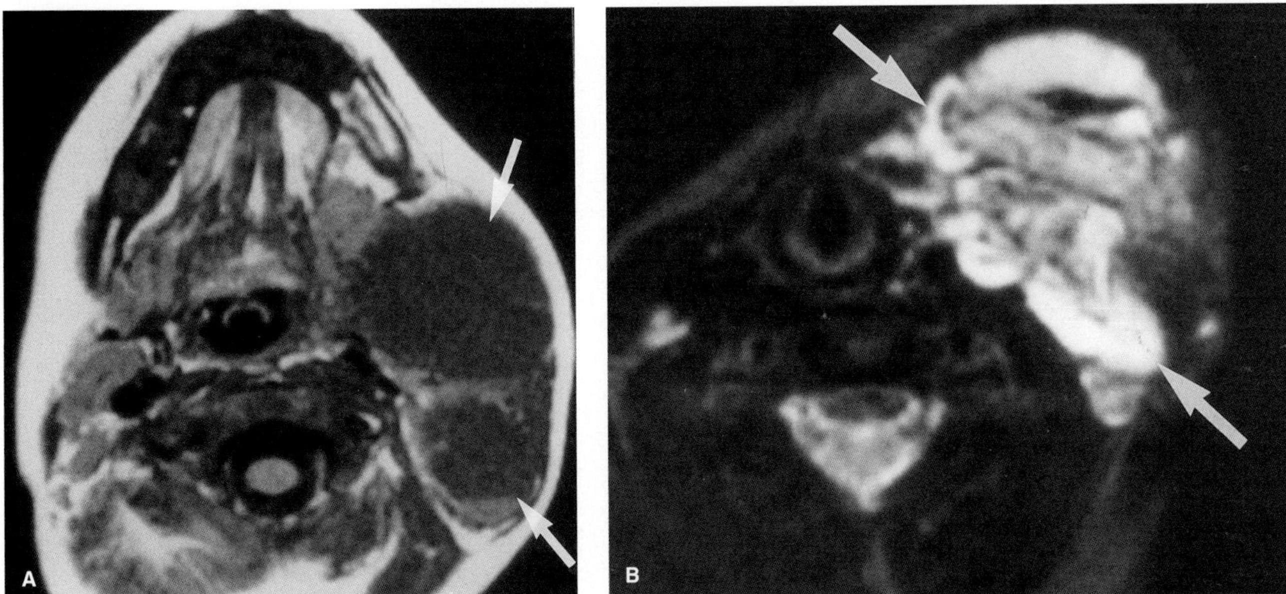

FIGURE 8.38. Cystic Hygroma. A: Axial T1WI at the level of the floor of the mouth. **B:** T2WI at the level of the larynx of a 2-month-old infant. A multiloculated lesion (*arrows*) extends within the soft tissues of the anterior neck. The trans-spatial nature of this lesion and its heterogeneous T2 signal is characteristic of a cystic hygroma or lymphangioma.

and result in fetal hydrops. Various congenital malformation syndromes occur in association with fetal cystic hygromas, including Turner syndrome, fetal alcohol syndrome, Noonan syndrome, and several chromosomal aneuploidies. Most lymphangiomas present by 2 years of age (90%), with 50% presenting at the time of birth. This early presentation reflects that the time of greatest lymphatic development occurs in the first 2 years of life.

Lymphangiomas and cystic hygromas appear as painless compressible neck masses that, if large enough, will transilluminate. The lesions commonly occur in the posterior triangle of the neck. On imaging studies, these lesions are multiloculated cystic masses with septations (Fig. 8.38); they also have a propensity to hemorrhage into themselves. This may result in a dramatic, acute increase in the size of the lesion. On imaging studies, one can expect a hemorrhage-fluid level or heterogeneous signal characteristics associated with blood degradation products. Because these lesions are easily compressible, they tend not to displace adjacent soft tissue structures, and this may prove a helpful differentiating feature from other cystic lesions, such as necrotic lymph nodes.

Suggested Readings

Forghani R, Yu E, Levental M, Som PM, Curtin HD. Imaging evaluation of lymphadenopathy and patterns of lymph node spread in head and neck cancer. *Expert Rev Anticancer Ther* 2015;15(2):207–224.

Glastonbury CM, Harnsberger HR. *Specialty Imaging: Head & Neck Cancer: State of the Art Diagnosis, Staging, and Surveillance*. Salt Lake City, UT: Amirsys; 2012.

Hasso AN. *Diagnostic Imaging of the Head and Neck: MRI with CT & PET Correlations*. Lippincott Williams & Wilkins; 2012.

Koch BL, Hamilton BE, Hudgins PA, Harnsberger HR. *Diagnostic Imaging: Head and Neck*. 3rd ed. Elsevier; 2016.

Plaxton NA, Brandon DC, Corey AS, et al. Characteristics and limitations of FDG PET/CT for imaging of squamous cell carcinoma of the head and neck: a comprehensive review of anatomy, metastatic pathways, and image findings. *AJR Am J Roentgenol* 2015;205(5):W519–W531. https://www.ajronline.org/doi/abs/10.2214/AJR.14.12828

Som PM, Curtin HD, Mancuso AA. Imaging-based nodal classification for evaluation of neck metastatic adenopathy. *AJR Am J Roentgenol* 2000; 174(3):837–844.

Widmann G, Henninger B, Kremser C, Jaschke W. MRI Sequences in head & neck radiology—state of the art. *Rofo* 2017;189(5):413–422. https://pdfs.semanticscholar.org/907b/ea334316fbf574ea0e74e476a0edce52b4ce.pdf

Yousem DM. *Head and Neck Imaging: Case Review Series*. 4th ed. Philadelphia, PA: Elsevier Saunders; 2014.

CHAPTER 9 ■ SPINE IMAGING

ERIK H. L. GAENSLER, DERK D. PURCELL, AND ALYSSA T. WATANABE

This chapter focuses on disorders of the spine, spinal cord, meninges, and paraspinous soft tissues. The first section is divided into sections covering inflammation, infection, neoplasms, vascular diseases, and trauma. The second section focuses on disc degeneration and spinal stenosis. Please refer to the Musculoskeletal section for primary osseous tumors involving the vertebrae (see Chapters 55 and 56) and to Pediatrics for congenital spine anomalies (see Chapter 66).

COMMON CLINICAL SYNDROMES

The clinical syndromes produced by degenerative and nondegenerative diseases can be indistinguishable. Patients with spine disorders present with focal or diffuse back pain, radiculopathy, or myelopathy. Focal back pain without neurologic compromise or fever is not an emergency and is epidemic in our society, with tremendous implications in terms of lost productivity. The most common causes of low back pain are orthopedic, such as muscle and ligament strain, facet joint disease, or discogenic disease that does not compromise the nerve roots. Vertebral metastases or infectious discitis, however, may also cause focal back pain. Since degenerative disease of the spine is far more common than nondegenerative disease, nondegenerative processes may initially be overlooked, with disastrous consequences. Therefore, a good clinical history that specifically addresses any previous cancers, or ongoing fevers and chills, is crucial in raising the suspicion for a nondegenerative process. When history and physical findings are nonspecific, as often is the case, imaging procedures become central to the diagnosis.

In patients with spinal neurologic findings, the history should attempt to distinguish between the clinical syndromes of myelopathy and radiculopathy, as they differ in significant respects, including degree of urgency. Important distinctions between radiculopathy and myelopathy are summarized in Table 9.1.

Myelopathy results from compromise of the spinal cord itself, due to mechanical compression, intrinsic lesions, or inflammatory processes loosely grouped under the term "myelitis." Classic symptoms include bladder and bowel incontinence, spasticity, weakness, and ataxia. With cord compression, a clear motor or sensory spinal cord "level" may develop. Knowing this level is helpful in focusing the imaging examination. The lesion, however, may be several vertebral bodies higher than the apparent dermatomal sensory level, particularly in the thoracic region. Myelopathy often presents without a clear sensory level. In such cases screening of the cord from the cervicomedullary junction to the conus is required.

The spinal cord, like the brain, has limited healing powers. In fact, the spinal cord is less tolerant of injury than the brain. A small mass, such as a 2-cm epidural abscess or hematoma, may permanently damage the cord because of the small diameter of the spinal canal, resulting in permanent paralysis. A similar-sized mass may be asymptomatic within the voluminous calvarium. The "plasticity" of the brain, whereby remaining cortex can assume the function of injured areas through a complex network of redundant neurons, is well documented, particularly in younger patients. The spinal cord, which consists mostly of long linear axonal tracts, demonstrates far less plasticity. After 24 hours of acute severe cord compression, chances of full recovery are significantly diminished. Therefore, acute myelopathy is an emergency, and the radiologist should do everything to facilitate prompt imaging.

Radiculopathy is due to impingement or irritation of the spinal nerves within the spinal canal, lateral recess, neural foramen, or along the extraforaminal course of the nerve. This compromise, typically because of mass effect, results in specific dermatomal sensory deficits and/or muscle group weakness. These are outlined in any neurology or physical diagnosis text and are worth knowing. The most common causes of radiculopathy are disc herniations and spinal stenosis and, in the cervical spine, uncovertebral joint spurring. Of course, malignant and infectious processes compromise spinal nerves, but overall are less common. The peripheral nervous system, unlike the CNS, has significant ability to withstand injury and to regenerate. Therefore, pure radicular symptoms, although at times excruciatingly painful, rarely represent a surgical emergency. Extensive epidural neoplasms and infections may present with mixed myelopathy and radiculopathy. These patients must be imaged with the urgency of a pure cord syndrome.

TABLE 9.1

MYELOPATHY VERSUS RADICULOPATHY

	■ MYELOPATHY	■ RADICULOPATHY
Cause	Spinal cord compromise	Spinal nerve compromise
Typical disease processes	Extramedullary disease: cord compression due to epidural mass effect Cervical spinal stenosis Intramedullary disease: tumor, inflammation, AVMs, SDAVFs	Osteophytic spurring (especially cervical spine) Disc herniations Lumbar spinal stenosis Extramedullary and paraspinous tumors and inflammatory processes compromising nerve roots
Neurologic findings	Ataxia Bowel and bladder incontinence Babinski sign	Weakness and diminished reflexes in specific muscle groups, dermatomal sensory deficits
Accuracy of clinical localization	Often poor; lesion may be several levels higher than anticipated	Usually quite good
Urgency for imaging (of acute presentations)	High–significant deficits may occur if severe cord compression untreated >24 hours.	Low–short delay for conservative treatment usually entails little risk
Preferred imaging modality	MR has no substitute as the initial screening examination	CT, especially with intrathecal contrast is still excellent, particularly in cervical spine

AVMs, arteriovenous malformations; SDAVFs, spinal dural arteriovenous fistulas.

IMAGING METHODS

Conventional radiography of the spine was once the initial test in every spine evaluation, but this is no longer logical or cost effective. Radiographs continue to be useful for ruling out trauma to the vertebral column and other acute screening settings. Plain radiographs and fluoroscopy are indispensable for correct localization in the operating room. Flexion and extension plain films are helpful for assessment of spine stability in spondylolisthesis.

In nondegenerative disease, pay careful attention to the integrity of the pedicles, frequent sites of metastases. Plain radiographs, however, cannot detect early infiltrative changes in the marrow space, which are readily seen on MR.

Myelography. Myelography today is almost always done in conjunction with CT. Indications include complex postoperative cases and patients in whom MR is contraindicated due to incompatible implanted devices. *Ionic contrast agents are absolutely contraindicated for myelography,* as they can result in severe inflammation, seizures, arachnoiditis, and even death. Always personally inspect the vial of contrast you are using, and fill the syringe yourself!

The recommended dosage of nonionic contrast in adults depends on the region to be studied, the size of the patient, and the size of thecal sac. A convenient and conservative rule of thumb in adults is not to exceed 3 g of intrathecal iodine, which works out to 17 mL of 180 mg/mL, 12.5 mL of 240 mg/mL, or 10 mL of 300 mg/mL, three of the standard concentrations.

Myelography begins with a lumbar puncture, with the patient in prone position under fluoroscopy. The preferred puncture site depends on the clinical findings, and usually is the midlumbar region, inferior to the posterior elements of L2 or L3. This injection level will avoid most disc herniations and spinal stenosis, which are usually worse at lower levels, and the conus, which in adults lies between T12/L1 and L1/L2 disc spaces. Take care to place the needle near the midline to reduce the chances of an extra arachnoid injection, or spearing of an exiting nerve. Inject contrast only after spontaneous CSF backflow is established. The complications of poor needle placement include subdural and epidural injection. Examples of these complications are well illustrated in older neuroradiology textbooks and have medicolegal implications. If in doubt where the contrast is going, stop, take frontal and lateral plain films, and examine them carefully. If tumor or infection is suspected, collect adequate CSF for chemistry, cultures, and cytology if this has not already been done. For routine degenerative cases, CSF examination has not proved worthwhile.

C1–C2 punctures are rarely required, and are inherently more dangerous than lumbar injection, as direct injury to the cord or a low-lying posterior inferior cerebellar artery loop can occur. These punctures are best done under lateral fluoroscopy, placing the needle in the posterior third of the spinal canal the between C1 and C2 posterior elements. Classic indications include known blocks caudally, or the need for dense opacification of the cervical and upper thoracic spinal canal for plain films. Today, one of the rare good reasons for a C1–C2 puncture would be complete spine block in the midthoracic region identified by lumbar myelography, with the need to define the upper extent of the block—in a patient with a pacemaker precluding MR. If the pacemaker were not an issue (and some are now MR compatible), MR would be the study of choice. MR is far quicker, more comfortable, and, most importantly, safer for the patient. Even if there is no technical complication with a myelogram, patients with spine block can deteriorate from the subtle fluid and pressure shifts that inevitably accompany needle placement in the subarachnoid space, a syndrome known as "spinal coning." The multiple steps in the evaluation of spine block by plain film myelography followed by CT are shown in Figure 9.1. Contrast this with the simplicity and elegance of MR in a similar case in Figure 9.12. In oncologic cases, MR has the additional benefit of excellent evaluation of the marrow space—not available with CT.

Space-occupying lesions of the spinal canal are categorized according to their location as intramedullary, intradural-extramedullary, and extradural. This classification came from myelography, but works equally well on CT and MR, and is critical for correct differential diagnosis. Intramedullary lesions occur within the spinal cord itself. Extramedullary lesions are by definition outside the cord, but may be either

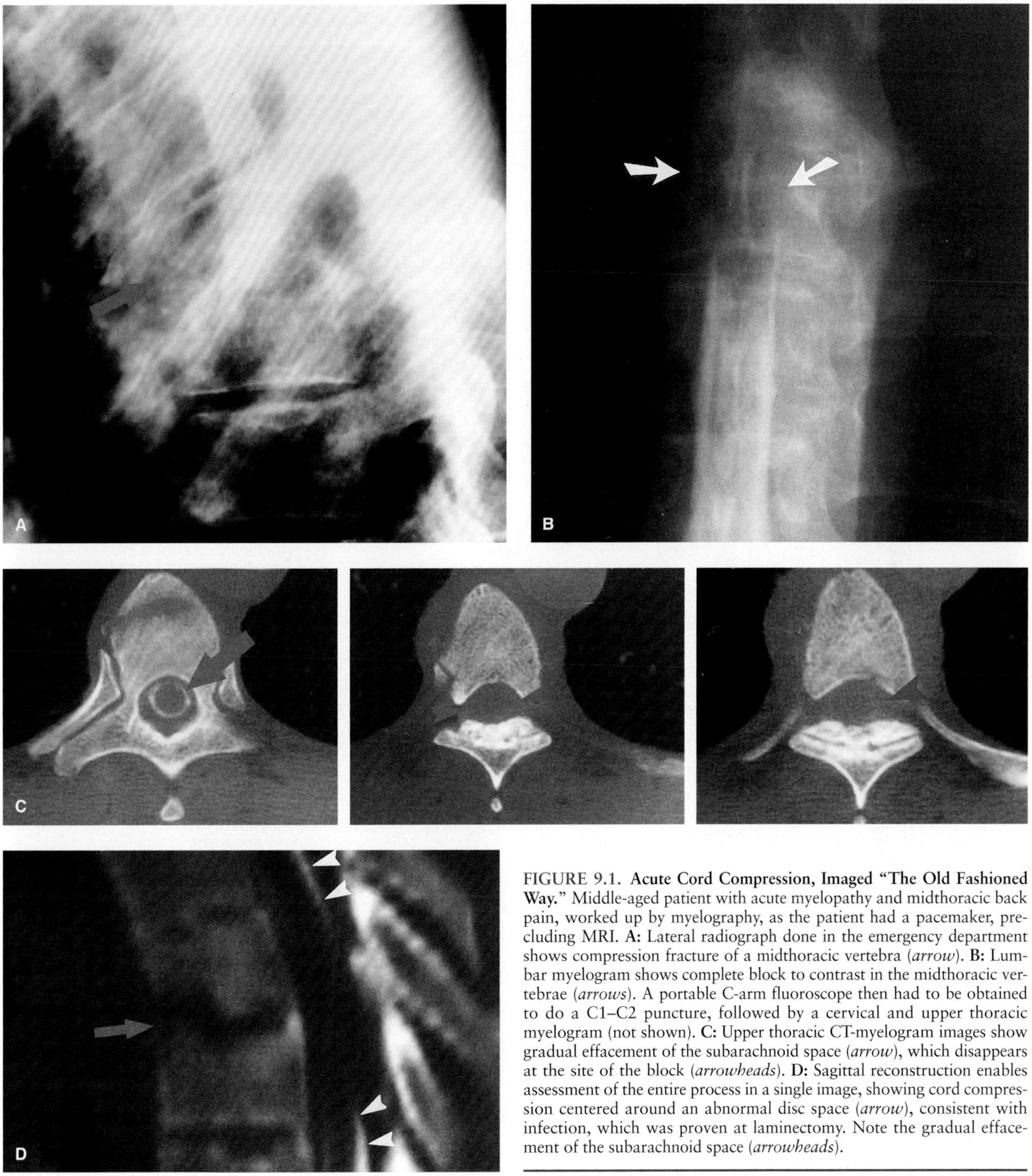

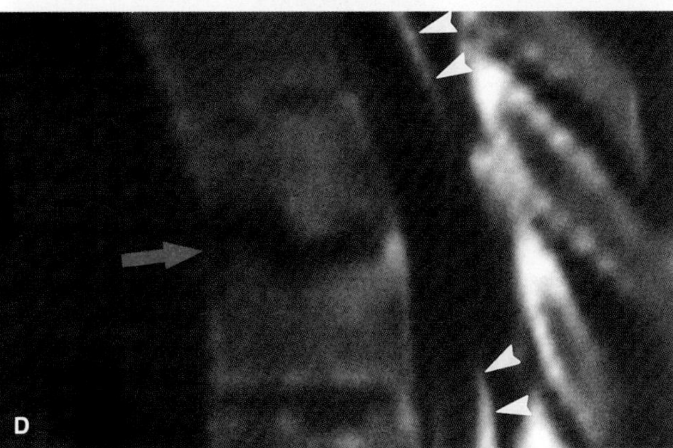

FIGURE 9.1. **Acute Cord Compression, Imaged "The Old Fashioned Way."** Middle-aged patient with acute myelopathy and midthoracic back pain, worked up by myelography, as the patient had a pacemaker, precluding MRI. **A:** Lateral radiograph done in the emergency department shows compression fracture of a midthoracic vertebra (*arrow*). **B:** Lumbar myelogram shows complete block to contrast in the midthoracic vertebrae (*arrows*). A portable C-arm fluoroscope then had to be obtained to do a C1–C2 puncture, followed by a cervical and upper thoracic myelogram (not shown). **C:** Upper thoracic CT-myelogram images show gradual effacement of the subarachnoid space (*arrow*), which disappears at the site of the block (*arrowheads*). **D:** Sagittal reconstruction enables assessment of the entire process in a single image, showing cord compression centered around an abnormal disc space (*arrow*), consistent with infection, which was proven at laminectomy. Note the gradual effacement of the subarachnoid space (*arrowheads*).

intra- or extradural. Please refer to Table 9.2 for a summary of the radiologic appearance and differential diagnosis for each lesion location is outlined in Table 9.2.

Computed Tomography and MRI. CT has largely been replaced by MR for most screening examinations of the spine, except for acute trauma. Low-dose CT myelography remains useful in cases where the limits of the thecal sac or nerve root sleeves need to be precisely defined, such as in complex postoperative states, as discussed in the Degenerative section at the end of this chapter. The key to MR's success has been its superior soft tissue contrast (including the ability to evaluate the marrow compartment), multiplanar capabilities, noninvasiveness, and high sensitivity to gadolinium enhancement.

MR scanning techniques for the spine continue to improve, and with the wide variety of imaging systems available, it makes little sense to recommend specific protocols in a general text.

Gadolinium is essential in the evaluation of infection and intrathecal metastases, but may obscure vertebral metastases by making them isointense with surrounding marrow fat. Also, it is difficult to evaluate hemorrhage on postcontrast images. Always obtain a precontrast T1 "scout" image to avoid these latter two pitfalls.

TABLE 9.2

DIFFERENTIAL DIAGNOSIS OF SPINAL LESIONS BY LOCATION

LOCATION AND IMAGING APPEARANCE

A. INTRADURAL INTRAMEDULLARY

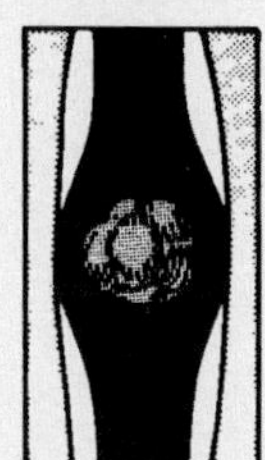

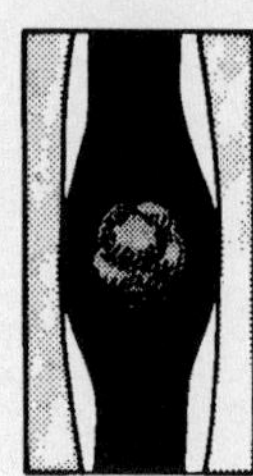

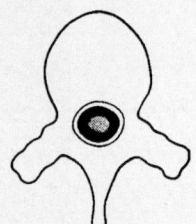

AP Lateral Axial

Cord appears widened in all views. The CSF space appears thinned on all sides in all views.

DIFFERENTIAL DIAGNOSIS

Ependymoma
Astrocytoma
Hemangioblastoma
Lipoma/(Epi)dermoid
Syringohydromyelia
Intramedullary AVM
Rare site: met/abscess

B. INTRADURAL EXTRAMEDULLARY

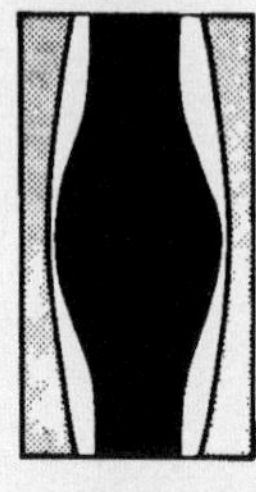

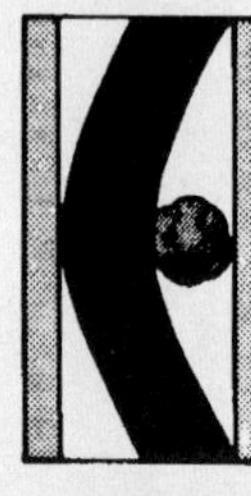

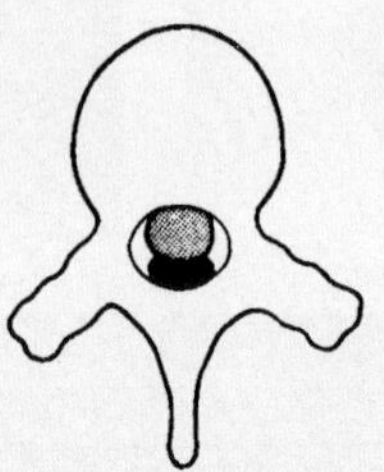

AP Lateral Axial

The contrast/CSF forms acute angles with the mass (which may have a dural attachment—"marble on the carpet"). This results in a "meniscus" around the mass and a widened contrast column between the cord and the mass on one side, with effacement of the CSF on the other.

DIFFERENTIAL DIAGNOSIS

Meningioma
Schwannoma/neurinoma
Neurofibroma
Hemangiopericytoma
Lipoma/(Epi)dermoid
Arachnoid cyst/adhesion
Drop/leptomeningeal met
Veins (extramedullary AVM)

C. EXTRADURAL

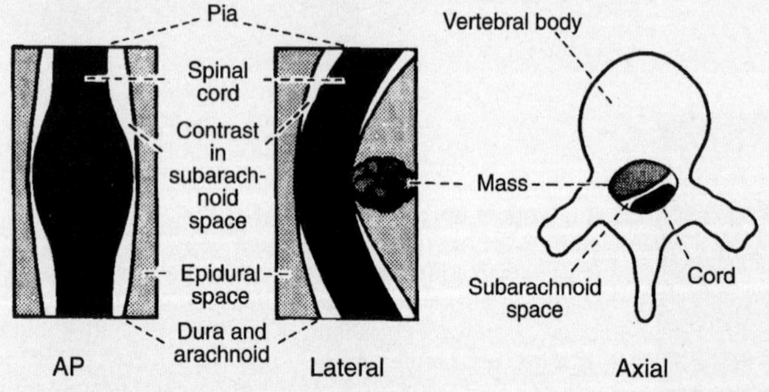

The dura and the sac will be displaced together, away from the mass. The CSF angles around the mass will be obtuse with a "marble under the carpet" appearance. The cord may be widened in one plane by pressure from the mass, with contrast material thinned on both sides of the cord.

DIFFERENTIAL DIAGNOSIS

Degenerative
- Herniated disc
- Synovial cyst
- Osteophyte
- Rheumatoid pannus

Nondegenerative
- Metastasis
- Abscess
- Hematoma
- Primary tumor expansion or invasion
- Epidural lipomatosis

[a]Adapted with permission from Latchaw RE, ed. *MR and CT of the Head, Neck, and Spine.* 2nd ed. St. Louis, MO: Mosby; 1991.
AP, anteroposterior; AVM, arteriovenous malformation; met, metastasis.

Diffusion imaging can help distinguish between vertebral body metastases and compression fractures, as tumor areas show diffusion restriction as compared with fracture zones (see Fig. 9.10). There is promise for diffusion, perfusion, and spectroscopy techniques for intramedullary disease, as the spinal cord represents a "brain" in miniature. Research in this area, however, has lagged work in the brain for two reasons. The small size of the spinal cord makes MR sampling more difficult, and intramedullary lesions are rarer than brain lesions. Spinal cord stroke demonstrates diffusion restriction. Diffusion tensor imaging shows promise in evaluating the long axonal tracts of the cord in conditions such as multiple sclerosis.

Spinal angiography is technically demanding, dangerous in untrained hands, and difficult to interpret. There is no reliable spinal "circle of Willis" allowing collateral flow from multiple sources, although some variable interconnected vascular arcades exist. Catheter-induced complications therefore can have tragic consequences. Excellent texts exist on spinal angiography, but this art is the province of interventional neuroradiologists, who can both diagnose and often treat spinal arteriovenous malformations (AVMs)—the main indication for spinal angiography. Both CT and MR angiography now demonstrate the spinal vasculature with increasing success (Figs. 9.34–9.37).

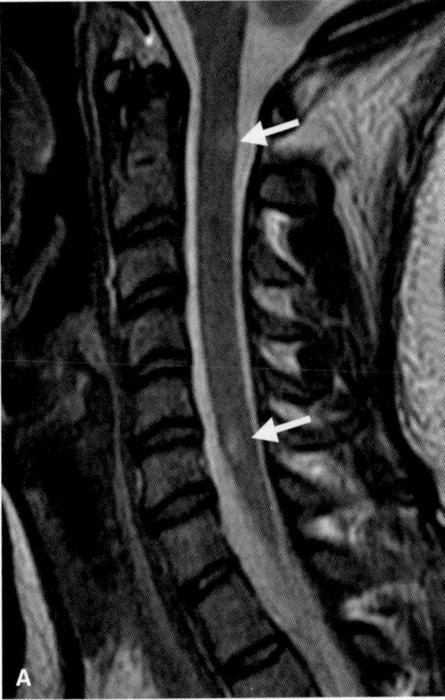

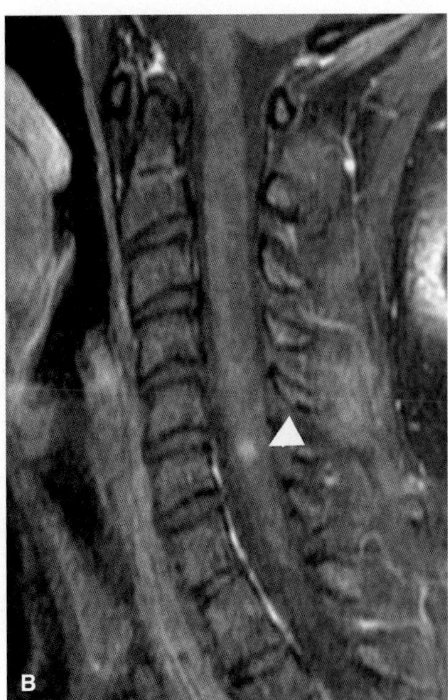

FIGURE 9.2. **Multiple Sclerosis.** Sagittal T2 (**A**) and T1 postcontrast (**B**) images. Multifocal demyelinating plaques (*arrows*) in the cervical cord on the sagittal image. Note how the lesion at C6 (*arrowhead*) enhances, suggesting active inflammation/demyelination. The multiplicity of lesions in the cord (and there were more in the brain) helps exclude a primary spinal cord neoplasm from the differential diagnosis.

Nuclear medicine bone scans are unique in their ability to screen the entire skeleton for metastases in one sitting. Bone scans are highly sensitive but quite nonspecific, as both degenerative and nondegenerative processes will show increased uptake. When such patients are referred for MR, it is critical to be aware of the bone scan findings in order to protocol the examination appropriately. Bone and PET scans are discussed further in the nuclear medicine chapters.

INFLAMMATION

Inflammatory diseases may cause myelopathy, principally through direct involvement of the spinal cord. The mechanism of many of these disorders is not fully understood, and they are sometimes lumped under the term "myelitis." Myelitis may be focal or diffuse. When both clinical and pathologic findings pinpoint a distinct spinal level, the term "transverse myelitis" may be used. Transverse myelitis is not really a specific disease, but rather a category of diseases. Few agree on exactly what processes should be lumped under umbrella term. In my opinion, it is better to describe the imaging findings carefully, and give a differential diagnosis, than to invoke such nonspecific terms in MR reports.

Multiple sclerosis (MS) is the most common spinal cord "inflammatory" disorder, and by far the most frequent cause of intramedullary lesions seen on MR. The epidemiology and pathophysiology of MS are reviewed in detail in Chapter 7. Multiple sclerosis of the brain and spinal cord are similar in terms of patient profile, with the hallmark of the disease being multiple neurologic deficits separated both anatomically and temporally. While imaging can be helpful, the diagnosis ultimately rests on clinical grounds. When spinal MS predominates, it tends to follow a progressive clinical course, as opposed to the relapsing/remitting pattern more characteristic with brain involvement. Many MS patients have mixed presentations, with both brain and spinal cord involvement. Spinal cord disease is isolated in less than 20% of cases. Two-thirds of spinal MS lesions occur in the cervical region.

The best screening protocols include sagittal T2-weighted or inversion recovery sequences, where MS plaques appear as areas of increased signal intensity. As in the brain, plaque enhancement correlates with acute lesion activity (Fig. 9.2). Since the white matter is on the "outside" of the cord, MS plaques tend to be peripheral. Differentiation of a solitary plaque from a glial tumor may be difficult, although MS plaques typically are under two vertebral segments in length, and involve less than half the cross-sectional area of the cord. When a mysterious bright intramedullary lesion is seen on T2-weighted image (T2WI) as in Figure 9.2, the next step should be MR of the brain to search for concomitant MS plaques. The brain and spinal cord are composed of the same tissue types, are physically connected, and share the CSF. A good general rule is when presented with any diffuse spinal process, either intramedullary or leptomeningeal, to look "upstairs," because the same process may also be involving the brain and its coverings.

Devic disease, or neuromyelitis optica (NMO), is an autoimmune disorder affecting the spinal cord and optic nerves. The spinal cord lesions are longer than in MS, and the brain is often spared. There is now a specific test for the NMO IgG antibody, which targets the Aquaporin 4 protein in astrocytes. Treatment differs from MS, and NMO should be mentioned in cases of acute myelitis and optic neuritis.

Lupus Erythematosus. Other CNS inflammatory processes are seen in both the brain and spinal cord. A classic example is systemic lupus erythematosus (SLE), where a necrotizing arteritis leads to cord ischemia and injury. Antibodies may also damage neuronal elements directly. The spinal cord will show diffuse areas of increased signal intensity with cord swelling on T2WI. SLE "lesions" have less well-defined margins than the discrete plaques of MS and may involve the cord over 4 to 5 vertebral body segments. Lupus of the cord may show dramatic improvement on MR after corticosteroids. Multiple sclerosis plaques, in contrast, represent areas of focal myelin destruction, and although the symptoms improve with corticosteroids, the MR findings may improve less dramatically.

Rheumatoid arthritis (RA) is another "collagen-vascular" disease that can compromise the spinal cord, although the mechanisms are different. Focal inflammatory change termed "pannus" destroys the transverse ligament of C1, allowing the odontoid to slide posteriorly relative to C1. This leads to cord compression, particularly in flexion (Fig. 9.3). Therefore, the neurologic injury in RA is due to atlantoaxial (A-A) instability

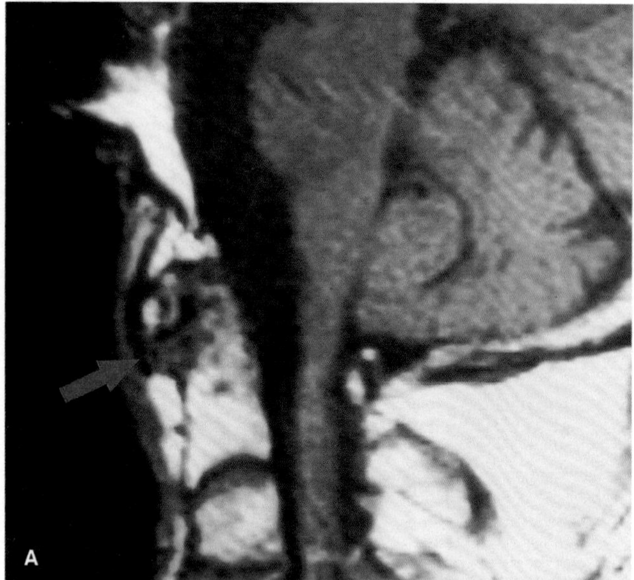

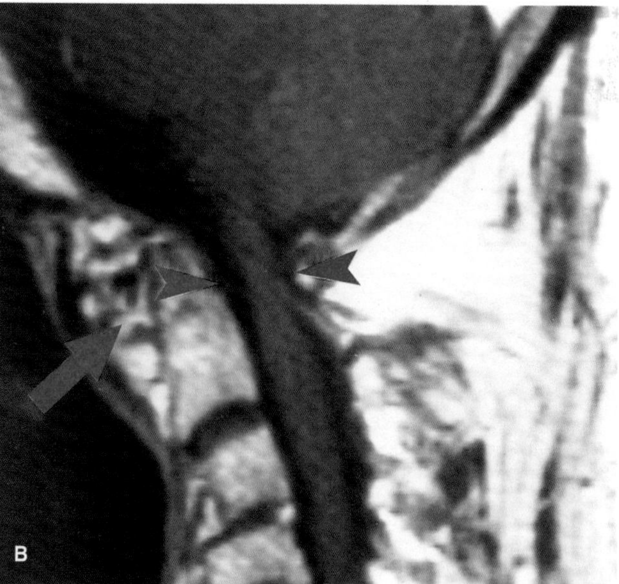

FIGURE 9.3. Rheumatoid Arthritis. A: This elderly patient had myelopathy due to atlantoaxial instability secondary to pannus (*arrow*), which has destroyed the transverse ligament of C1. In extension, no cord impingement is seen. **B:** In flexion, the dens has borderline mass effect on the cord (*arrowheads*). The pannus enhances vigorously with contrast (*arrow*).

rather a primary intramedullary lesion. The instability in time leads to myelomalacia. Sixty percent of RA patients have cervical spine findings, and frank A-A instability is seen in 5%. Patients with spinal RA typically have involvement in their hands and elsewhere. This is a useful discriminator, as a soft tissue mass at the C1–C2 articulation with instability does not necessarily imply RA. A fibrous pseudotumor may occur in the same location with os odontoideum, and can develop in response to any chronically unstable spinal anatomy, including an ununited Type I dens fracture.

Ankylosing spondylitis (AS) shows the classic "bamboo spine," due to extensive bridging of syndesmophytes across multiple vertebral bodies. Without the flexibility of the disc spaces, the rigid AS spine is prone to fracture (*arrow*) with even mild trauma (Fig. 9.4).

Acute viral illnesses are associated with myelitis in a number of ways, either directly or by autoimmune inflammatory change. Herpes zoster is invisible to imaging when latent, but cord swelling and enhancement have been reported with acute "shingles" outbreaks, appearing at spinal levels corresponding to the dermatologic outbreak. Measles provokes an autoimmune reaction that can damage the cord, which has been studied experimentally as a model for MS, and is termed subacute sclerosing panencephalitis. Acute

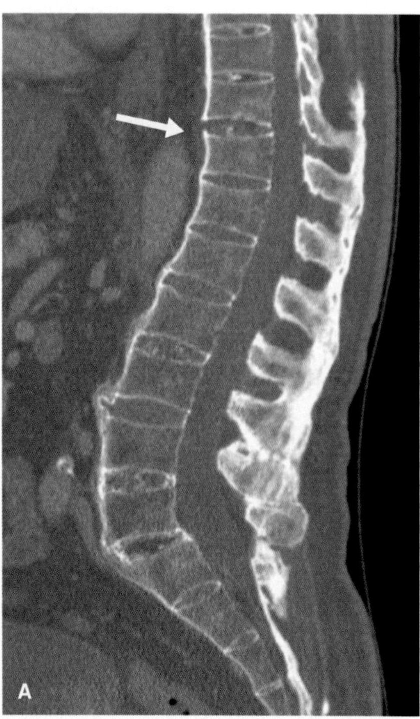

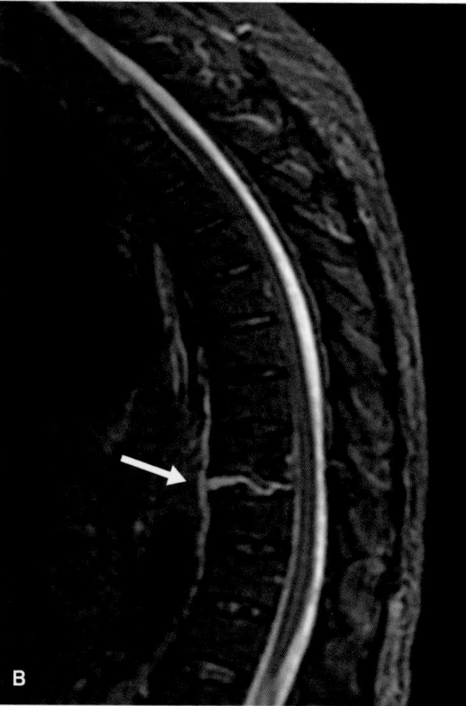

FIGURE 9.4. Ankylosing Spondylitis (AS) With Pseudoarthrosis. A: Sagittal CT reconstruction shows the classic "bamboo spine" of AS, due to extensive bridging of syndesmophytes across multiple vertebral bodies. Without the flexibility of the disc spaces, the very rigid AS spine is prone to fracture of syndesmophytes (*arrow*) with even mild trauma. **B:** Sagittal T2WI MRI centered in the thoracic region demonstrates edema at the fracture site (*arrow*). AS fractures can be associated with instability, and occasionally epidural hematomas, which can lead to paralysis. A low index threshold for imaging is therefore warranted in AS patients with posttraumatic back pain.

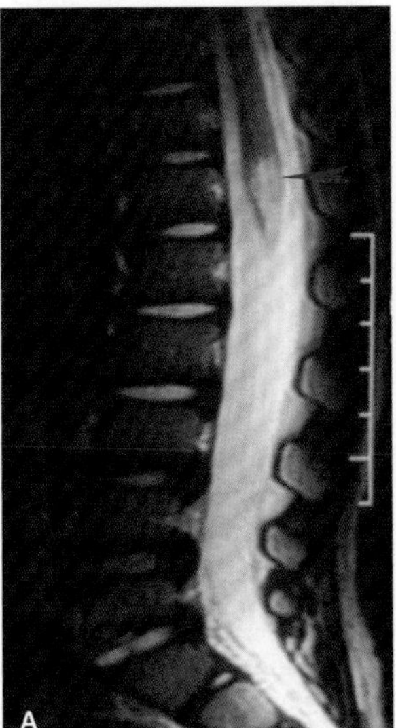
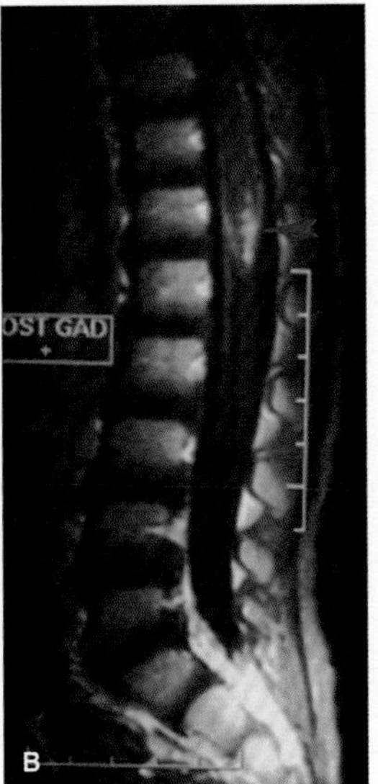

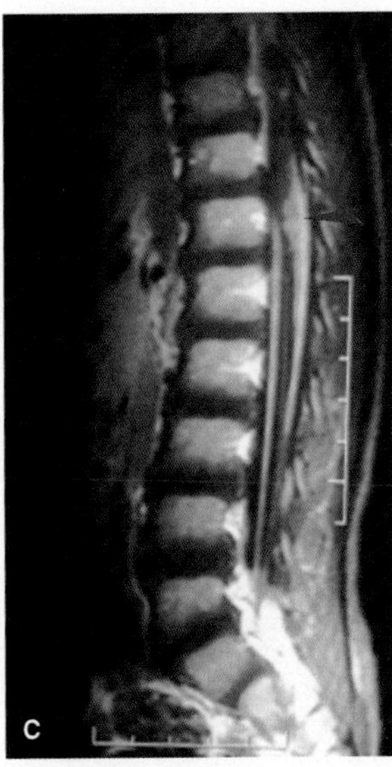
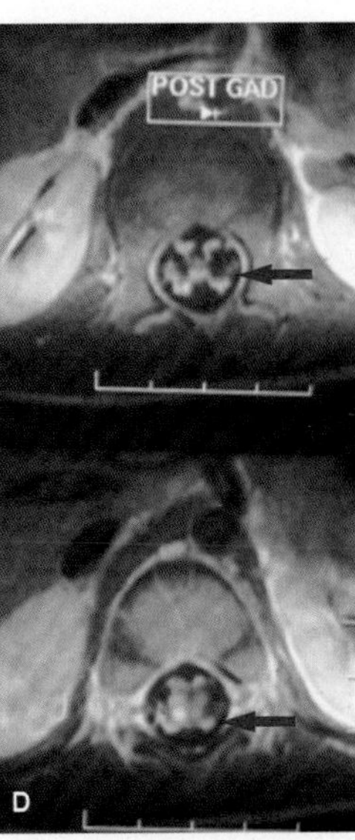

FIGURE 9.5. Guillain–Barré or Acute Inflammatory Demyelinating Polyradiculopathy. This "potty-trained" 3-year-old suffered acute ataxia and loss of bowel control after a diarrheal illness. **A:** T2WI shows edema (*arrowhead*) of the conus medullaris. Sagittal (**B, C**) and axial (**D**) T1-weighted postcontrast images show intense enhancement of the conus (*arrowheads*) and spinal nerves (*arrows*). The patient recovered fully in 6 to 8 weeks.

disseminated encephalomyelitis or ADEM (see Chapter 7) is a monophasic postviral syndrome, which also affects spinal cord as its name, "encephalo*myelitis*," suggests.

Patients with acute viral myelitis typically have sudden high fevers, followed within 4 weeks by rapid onset of motor, sensory, and usually autonomic dysfunction, sometimes referable to a specific spinal cord level. The imaging findings typically are a focal area of cord swelling with high signal on T2WI, with variable enhancement. It is difficult not to draw comparisons with Guillain–Barré syndrome (aka acute inflammatory polyradiculoneuropathy—unfortunately the modern name is more difficult than the classic eponym!). By whatever name, this is a progressive ascending motor weakness that affects more than one limb, but involves peripheral nerves rather than the spinal cord. Guillain–Barré has been seen (very rarely!) after vaccinations, and evolves over a maximum of 4 weeks. Often the spinal nerves enhance (Fig. 9.5). This finding is nonspecific, can be seen in infections and neoplasms involving the CSF pathways, and is even present occasionally in disc disease.

Neurosarcoidosis. Inflammatory conditions involving pia and arachnoid have a similar differential diagnosis whether they involve cerebral or spinal leptomeninges. A classic example is neurosarcoidosis, which can present as diffuse leptomeningeal granulomatous nodules, which typically enhance (Fig. 9.6).

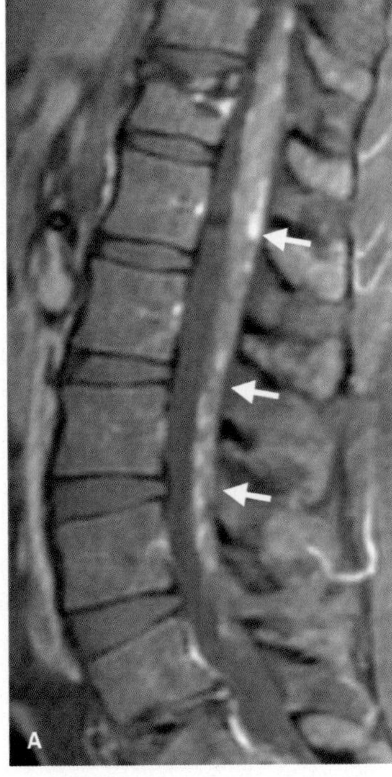
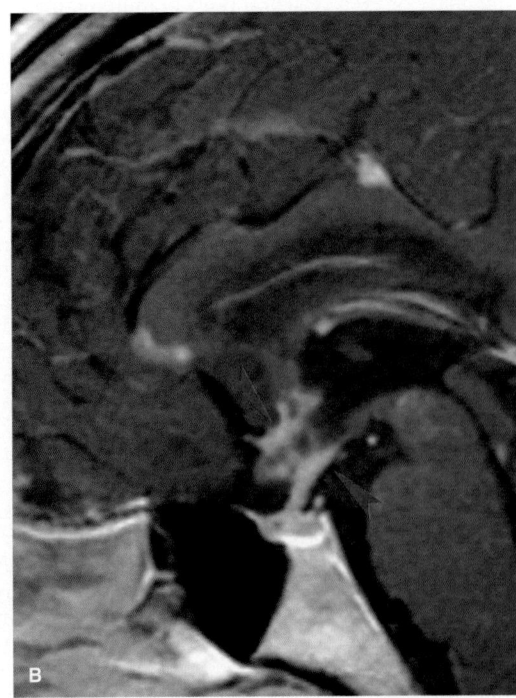

FIGURE 9.6. Neurosarcoidosis. A: Nodular enhancement is evident along the conus and cauda equina nerve roots (*arrows*). **B:** A concomitant scan of the brain reveals leptomeningeal enhancement of the hypothalamus and pituitary stalk (*arrowheads*). Morphology and distribution are characteristics of neurosarcoidosis.

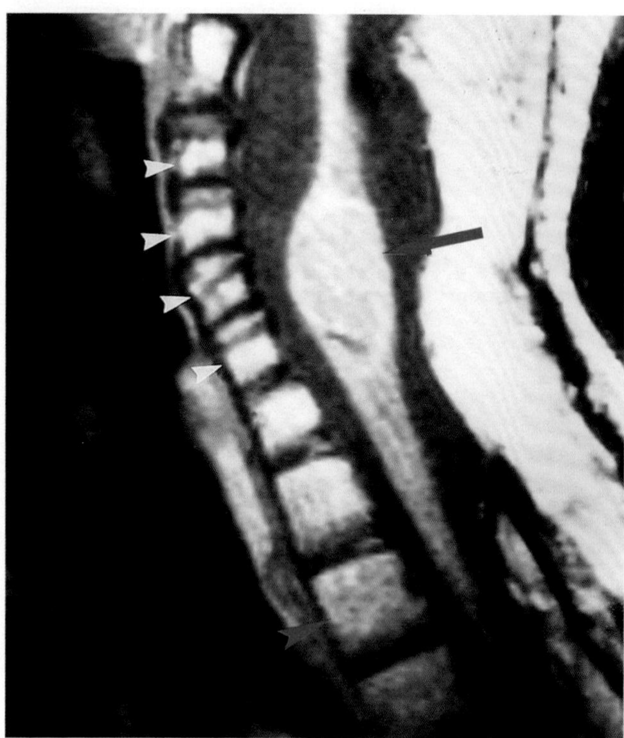

FIGURE 9.7. Radiation (XRT) Effect. This child underwent laminectomy and radiation for an intramedullary astrocytoma (*arrow*). The vertebrae within the XRT field (*white arrowheads*) appear small when compared to those outside the field (*red arrowhead*). The epiphyseal plates of vertebrae, like any other rapidly dividing tissue, are highly sensitive to radiation injury, and suffered growth retardation. Note also the bright post-XRT appearance of the cervical vertebrae, where fat has replaced the radiation-damaged hematopoietic marrow.

This appearance is similar to carcinomatous (see Fig. 9.27) and mycobacterial meningitis, and the distinction must be made on clinical grounds. Sarcoid can also present with intramedullary or even vertebral body granulomatous changes.

Arachnoiditis. The most common causes of arachnoiditis are iatrogenic, including inflammation after spine surgery, spinal anesthesia, or spine "injection" procedures such as epidural nerve blocks. In arachnoiditis, the normally free-layering lumbar roots become adherent to each other, or to the peripheral wall of the thecal sac, giving the sac a "bald" appearance on.

Radiation myelitis is similar to radiation injury to the brain (see Chapter 5). Peak incidence occurs roughly 6 to 12 months after initial treatment, with affected areas demonstrating increased signal intensity on T2WI, with variable enhancement. In the spine, the normal erythropoietic marrow is destroyed and replaced by fat, making the vertebrae bright on T1WI (Fig. 9.28). In growing children, the vertebrae may show arrested growth due to radiation injury to the epiphyses (Fig. 9.7).

The remaining list of "inflammatory" conditions of the spinal cord is long and parallels the differential considerations in the brain. Chemotherapy and other toxins, radiation therapy, metabolic disorders, electrical burns, and lightning are physical factors that can injure the cord. Much of the damage that occurs in spinal cord trauma is not due to the mechanical forces, but the inflammatory reaction that follows. Deficiencies in vitamins such as B_{12} and folate, while not strictly inflammatory, can cause degeneration of the posterior columns.

INFECTION

Infections involving the spine can be classified according to the causative organism, or by anatomic location. Both approaches are useful. Certain infections, such as pediatric pyogenic meningitis, are so dramatic in their presentation that there is little need for imaging, with emergent lumbar puncture and CSF analysis being the cornerstone of diagnosis. Other processes, such as fungal osteomyelitis in the immunocompromised cancer patient, can be difficult to distinguish from metastatic infiltration or mild compression fracture. Evaluation of the pathologic vertebral body is a constant challenge, and the many "rules of thumb" sprinkled throughout this chapter are summarized in Table 9.3.

Pyogenic Infections

Staphylococcus aureus is the most common cause of spine infection in adults, followed by gram-negative bacteria, particularly *Escherichia coli, Pseudomonas,* and *Klebsiella. Salmonella* is associated with sickle cell disease. The vertebrae are seeded hematogenously in most cases, resulting in osteomyelitis that then spreads to the disc space and adjacent vertebral body. The organism seeds via the arterial route, although bacteria may reach the lower spine through Batson venous plexus. Exceptions are children with dermal sinus tracts, or immediate postoperative patients, where a direct portal for infection exists.

Osteomyelitis/Discitis. In adults, the disc itself has a relatively poor blood supply, so primary infection is rare. In children, however, arteries penetrate the growing disc, providing access for primary hematogenous primary infection. Once these vessels have involuted, the most common spinal site of "seeding" is the vertebral body, particularly near the end plates, which have the richest blood supply. Vertebral osteomyelitis then develops (Fig. 9.8), with loss of marrow signal on T1WI and irregularity of the end plates.

As pyogenic infection breaks through the end plate into the disc, discitis ensues, with inevitable infection of the adjacent vertebral body. This creates an osteomyelitis/discitis complex that has been termed "pyogenic spondylodiscitis" (Fig. 9.9). This pattern is suspicious for infection, and unusual with neoplasms (Table 9.3). It can be difficult, though, to distinguish between degenerative endplate changes and early infection. The "Claw Sign" on diffusion-weighted images has been proposed a useful discriminating sign (Fig. 9.10).

Epidural Abscess. Many epidural infections do not have the well-encapsulated "liquid" collections we associate with abscesses elsewhere in the body, and technically are better termed "epidural phlegmon." Epidural infections spread craniocaudally, extending as many as three to four interspaces away from any vertebral abnormality (Fig. 9.11). Such a distant extension is unusual with epidural tumor from metastatic neoplasms (Table 9.3). Epidural abscesses have little room to expand axially, given the confines of the spinal canal, and can quickly lead to cord compression. The epidural space can be seeded hematogenously, but more often is involved by direct extension from the spinal column (Fig. 9.12).

Meningitis typically is due to direct hematogenous seeding of the CSF, rather than contiguous spread of adjacent vertebral infection, unless there is a disruption of the leptomeninges on a congenital or acquired basis. Postcontrast MR is the most sensitive imaging examination for meningitis in both the brain and the spine, as discussed in Chapter 6. It should never be a substitute for lumbar puncture, however, in excluding meningitis.

Spinal cord abscesses are rare, and usually the result of direct seeding of the cord from overwhelming sepsis. Spinal cord pyogenic abscesses, not surprisingly, appear similar to those in the brain: bright centrally with a dark rim on T2WI, with rim enhancement (Fig. 9.13).

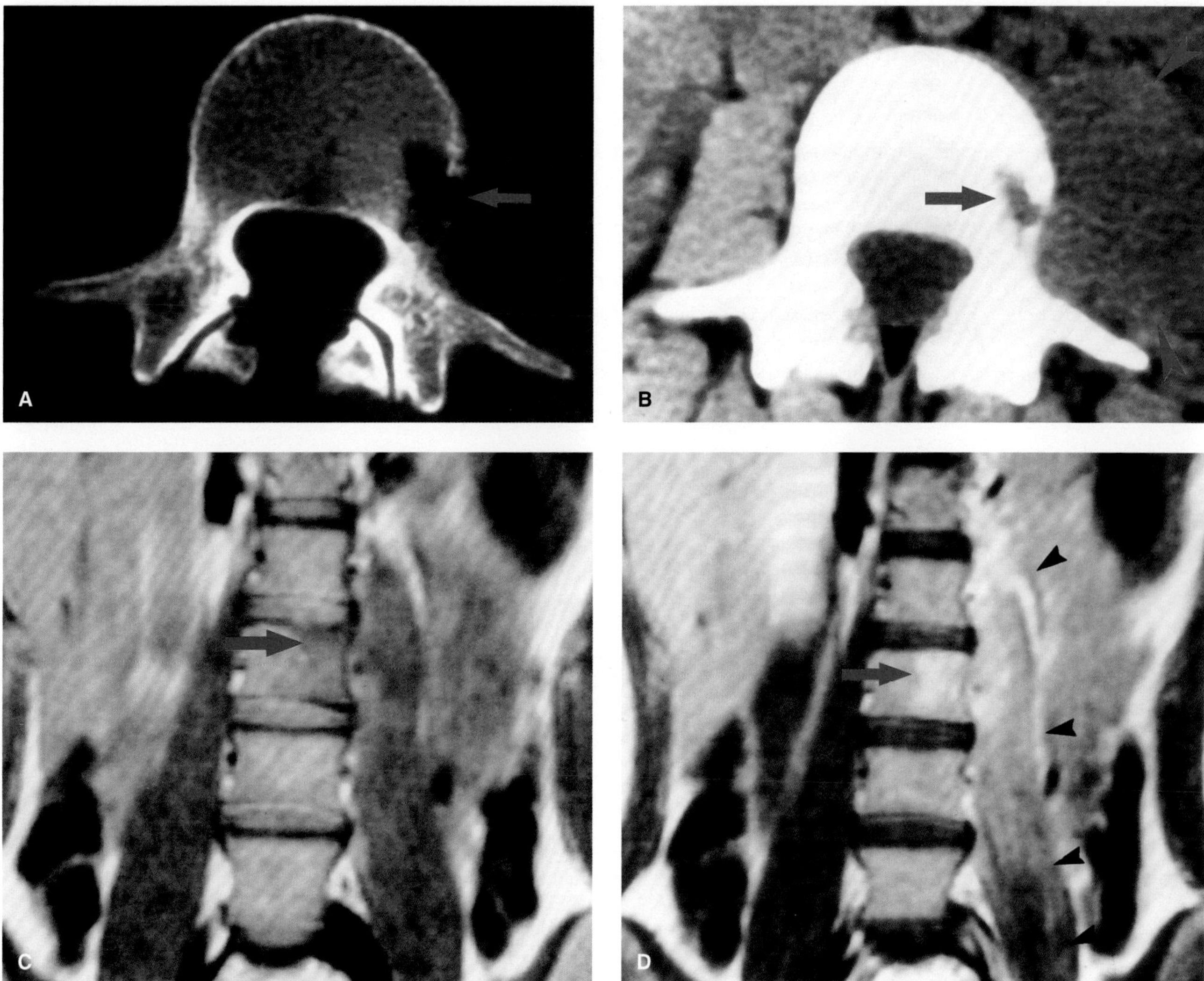

FIGURE 9.8. **Early Osteomyelitis Without Significant Discitis.** This young athlete developed back pain, and a slightly elevated sedimentation rate, with negative blood cultures and negative conventional radiographs, and a bone scan showing increased uptake at L3. A CT, shown with bone windows (**A**) and soft tissue windows (**B**), reveals a destructive process within the vertebral body (*arrows*), which extends into the enlarged left psoas muscle (*arrowheads*). **C:** The unenhanced T1WI in coronal plane shows decreased signal intensity (*arrow*) within the left-sided marrow space of L3, consistent with edema. **D:** Postcontrast T1WI shows marked enhancement within the affected portion of L3 (*arrow*) and the left psoas (*arrowheads*), which is enlarged and enhances all the way into the pelvis. This pattern would be unusual for a tumor. Biopsy yielded *Staphylococcus aureus.* The discs appear spared, which is atypical for *S. aureus.* Note how well the coronal plane shows both the spine and paraspinous tissues over a large area. The coronal plane is very effective in imaging of paraspinous processes.

Conventional radiographs cannot identify a spinal infection unless some disc or bone destruction has occurred, which may take 4 to 8 weeks, with the earliest sign being erosion of the vertebral end plates. Since older patients often have significant loss of vertebral body and disc height because of degenerative processes, evaluation of plain films in the setting of suspected infection is difficult, even after months of symptoms. Late in the infectious course, the end plates may become sclerotic bone as healing occurs, sometimes leading to fusion across the obliterated disc space. Radionuclide bone scans can turn positive in infection far sooner than plain films, but suffer from the same ambiguity: degenerative and nondegenerative processes can look the same. Indium-labeled white cell studies and gallium scans are more specific for infection, but relatively insensitive for small foci of vertebral osteomyelitis. The DWI "Claw Sign" shown in Figure 9.10 is useful is such situations, but in doubt, do a CT-guided aspiration!

Nonpyogenic Infections

Tuberculosis of the spine, or Pott's disease, causes slow collapse of one or usually more vertebral bodies, spreading underneath the longitudinal ligaments (Fig. 9.14). The result is an acute kyphotic or "gibbus" deformity. This angulation, coupled with epidural granulation tissue and bony fragments, can lead to cord compression. Unlike pyogenic infections, the discs can be preserved (see earlier) (see Table 9.3). In late-stage spinal tuberculosis, large paraspinal abscesses without severe pain, frank pus, or fever occur, leading to the expression "cold abscess" (Fig. 9.14D and E). As with other extrapulmonary tuberculosis, the chest film may be unrevealing, with the source being a primary lung lesion that is clinically silent.

Fungal infections can be particularly difficult to differentiate from malignant processes, with the classic problem being

TABLE 9.3

IMAGING EVALUATION OF THE PATHOLOGICALLY COLLAPSED VERTEBRAL BODY

■ CRITERIA	■ INFECTION	■ NEOPLASM	■ OSTEOPOROSIS
Number of vertebrae affected, and pattern	Single vertebral involvement rare Usually at least two vertebrae around an affected disc (pyogenic) or intact disc with subligamentous spread (tuberculosis or fungus)	Isolated or noncontiguous involvement common	Typically several of vertebra show loss of height, to varying degrees
Portions of vertebra affected	Destruction greatest at end plates Posterior elements relatively spared Abnormal marrow signal centered around disc in osteomyelitis/discitis complex	Irregular vertebral body involvement Pedicles typically affected Entire vertebra often infiltrated	Anterior "wedge" deformity of the vertebral body Posterior elements spared Portions of vertebral body retain normal marrow even with acute compression fracture
Marrow signal	Decreased on T1WI Increased on T2WI Normal diffusion Abnormal marrow signal centered around disc in osteomyelitis/discitis complex	Decreased on T1WI Increased on T2WI Restricted diffusion due to "marrow packing" Entire vertebral body usually infiltrated with pathologic compression fracture	T1WI and T2WI normal (unless acute fx.) Diffusion may be increased at the fracture plane Portions of vertebral body retain normal marrow even with acute compression fracture
Disc integrity	Pyogenic: disc involved and enhances Nonpyogenic: disc may be spared	Discs typically spared (prostate cancer an exception)	Discs spared
Epidural component (if present)	Granulation tissue (best seen post-gadolinium) extends several levels above and below the affected vertebrae	Focal mass usually only at level of affected vertebra(e) Lymphoma an exception, with more extensive epidural mass	Rare, unless acute fracture with hematoma, or retropulsion of fragments
Caveats	Discogenic vertebral sclerosis can mimic the osteomyelitis complex on T1-weighted images (but not on enhanced scans)	Gadolinium enhancement may obscure metastases, by reducing their conspicuity relative to fat	Acute compression fractures show marrow edema, and can be difficult to distinguish from pathologic fracture (although posterior elements are usually spared) A follow-up scan in 2–6 months helps make the distinction

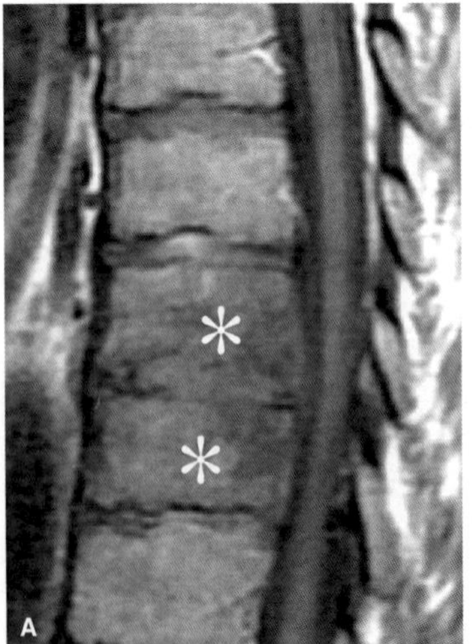

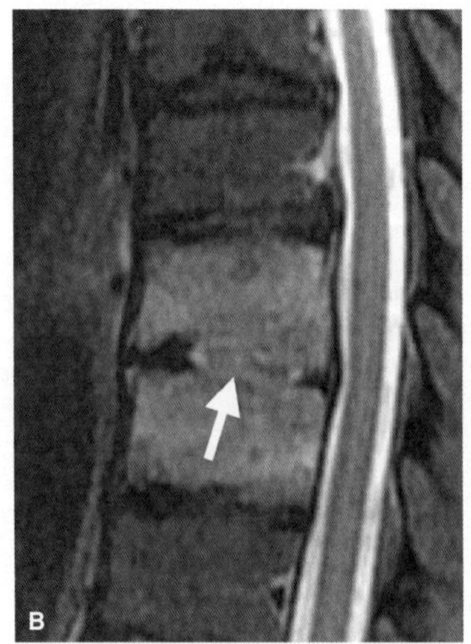

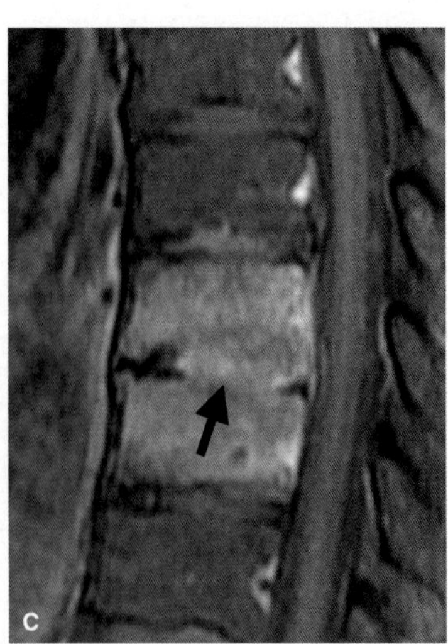

FIGURE 9.9. Pyogenic Spondylodiscitis. A: Sagittal T1-weighted image shows decreased signal intensity in a pair of vertebral bodies (*asterisks*) centered around an abnormal disc. **B:** Sagittal T2-weighted image with fat saturation demonstrates abnormal marrow hyperintensity (edema) and focal hyperintensity in the disc space (*white arrow*). **C:** On the sagittal T1-weighted postcontrast image, the disc enhances intensely (*arrow*), confirming discitis. This "osteomyelitis/discitis complex" is classic for pyogenic infection and virtually rules out neoplasm.

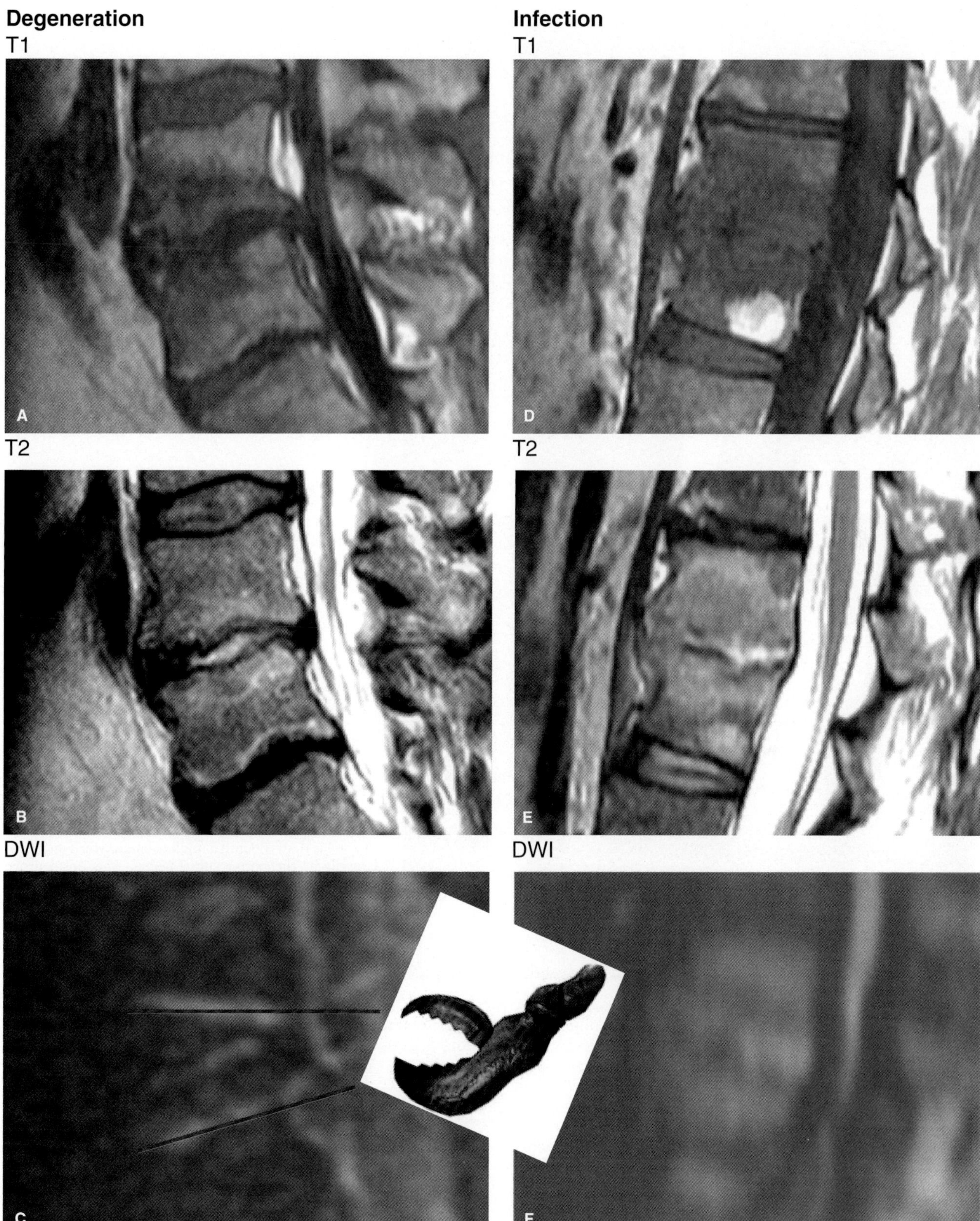

FIGURE 9.10. **Degenerative Endplate Changes Versus Infection: Value of DWI and the "Claw Sign."** The left patient shows degenerative Modic type I vertebral body endplate changes. Marrow edema from chronic micro-trauma is low in signal on T1WI (top-**A**) and becomes bright on T2WI (mid-**B**). On DWI images (lower-**C**) there are paired well defined bands of high signal (*red lines*) several millimeters from the endplate. These bands (*red lines*) resemble a "claw," and represent increased intracellular water at the healing osseous border zone. The right column shows a patient with acute infection. Again, "mirror image" paired abnormal zones spread out from the endplates, showing low signal on T1WI (top-**D**). They become bright on T2WI (mid-**E**). On DWI (lower-**F**), however there is no claw sign, as the infection does not have a chronic hypocellular to hypercellular zone of transition. (Courtesy of Patel KB, Poplawski MM, Pawha PS, Naidich TP, Tanenbaum LN. Diffusion-weighted MRI "claw sign" improves differentiation of infectious from degenerative Modic Type 1 signal changes of the spine. *AJNR Am J Neuroradiol* 2014;35:1647–1652.)

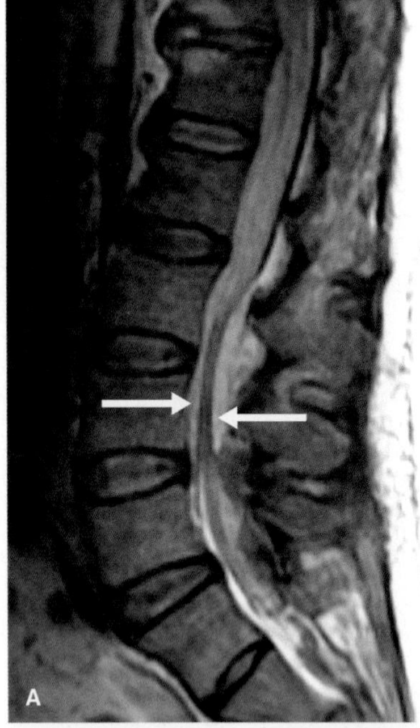

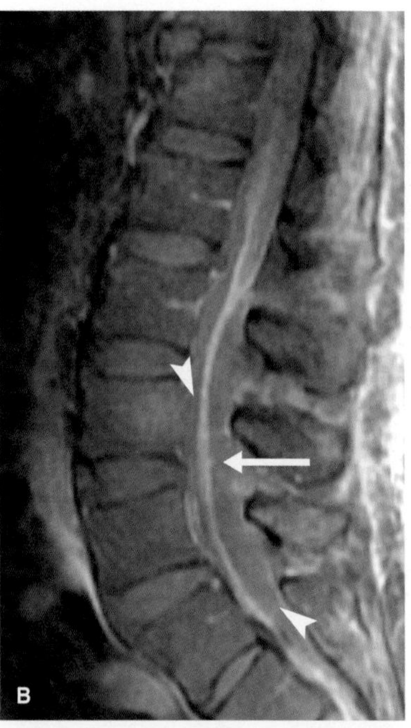

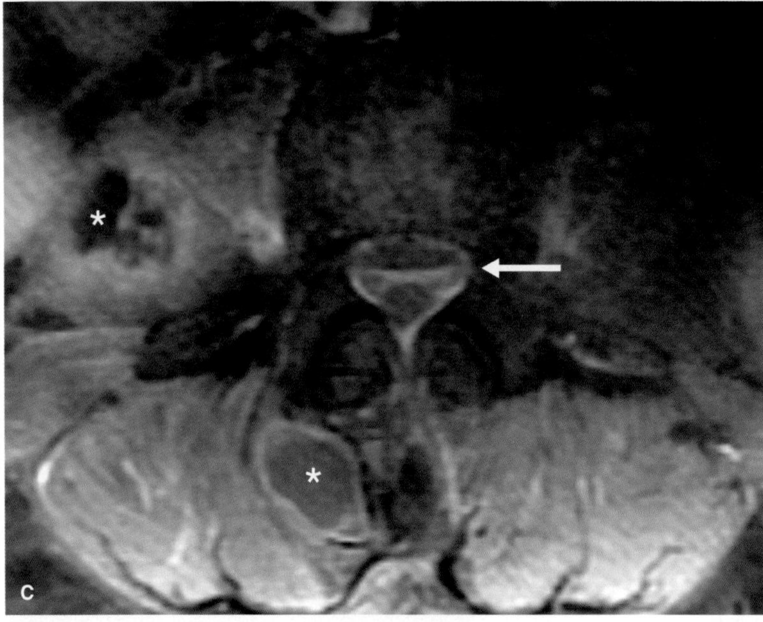

FIGURE 9.11. **Lumbar Epidural Abscess. A:** T2WI sagittal. The lumbar thecal sac is displaced centrally into a ribbon-like structure (*arrows*). **B:** Postcontrast these inwardly displaced dural margins of enhance with contrast (*arrow*). All the intraspinal material compressing the thecal sac (*arrowheads*) is epidural abscess. Typically this requires surgical drainage. **C:** The thecal sac (*arrow*) is flattened into a midline band, which anchored laterally by the exiting spinal nerves. This postcontrast image also demonstrates two right-sided paraspinous abscesses (*asterisks*) that can be safely targeted for catheter drainage and cultures. The earlier the cultures are obtained (preferably prior to antibiotics), the more likely they will be positive.

Candida and *Aspergillus* in the oncology patient mimicking metastatic tumor. Coccidioidomycosis and blastomycosis have specific endemic areas, but with widespread travel, geographic borders have less meaning. Coccidioidomycosis is common in the southwestern United States, and blastomycosis in the southeast. Both are common in Africa and South America, with some variation in strains. Another distinction is that coccidioidomycosis, like tuberculosis, spares the discs, whereas blastomycosis, like actinomycosis, can destroy the discs and the ribs. *Cryptococcus,* usually associated with meningitis, also affects the vertebrae, with well-defined osteolytic changes.

Viruses can affect the cord either primarily or by reactive change (see Inflammatory section above). Poliomyelitis destroys the anterior horns cells directly, as shown in Figure 9.15. Myelopathy is seen in AIDS patients, with vacuolar changes in the spinal cord. This appears to be a direct effect of the HIV virus itself, rather than concomitant infections, or a postinfectious syndrome. The role of MR in AIDS myelopathy is more to exclude other treatable conditions, such as unsuspected cord compression, than to make a highly specific diagnosis.

NEOPLASMS

MR is unique in its ability to detect nonexpansile tumors of the spinal cord, and is the only reliable noninvasive method for detection of tumors within the spinal canal that do not affect bone. When formulating the differential diagnosis for a spinal tumor, it is important to establish the location of the lesion as intramedullary, intradural-extramedullary, or extradural, as shown in Table 9.2. Having determined the "compartment," consider the patient's age when ranking the lesions occurring in that compartment in order of likelihood. In children, 38% of symptomatic spinal canal masses are developmental. Meningiomas constitute a 25% of all intraspinal lesions in adults, but are rare in children.

These figures exclude vertebral metastases, which are the most common neoplasms involving the adult spine. Vertebral

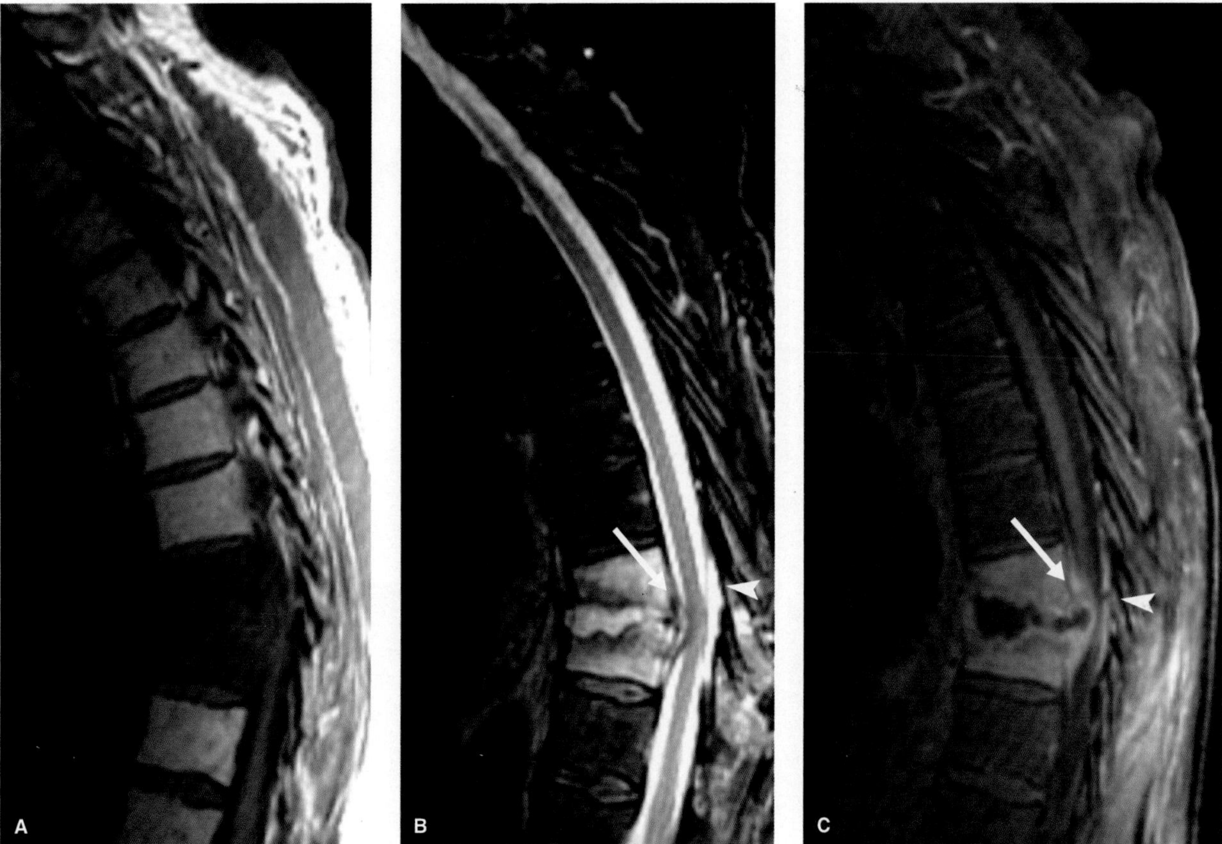

FIGURE 9.12. Impending Cord Compression due to Late Discitis With Epidural Abscess. A: T1WI sagittal image shows complete marrow infiltration of two adjacent vertebral bodies with effacement of the intervening disc, classic for infection. **B:** STIR. Abnormal soft tissue in both the ventral (*arrow*) and dorsal (*arrowhead*) epidural space is beginning to compress the cord. **C:** Postgadolinium T1 with fat saturation shows marked enhancement surrounding the infected disc, which is undergoing lysis. When the organism is not known, CT-guided aspiration is best done before antibiotics, particularly if conservative therapy is planned. Antibiotics will significantly decrease the chances of a definitive culture.

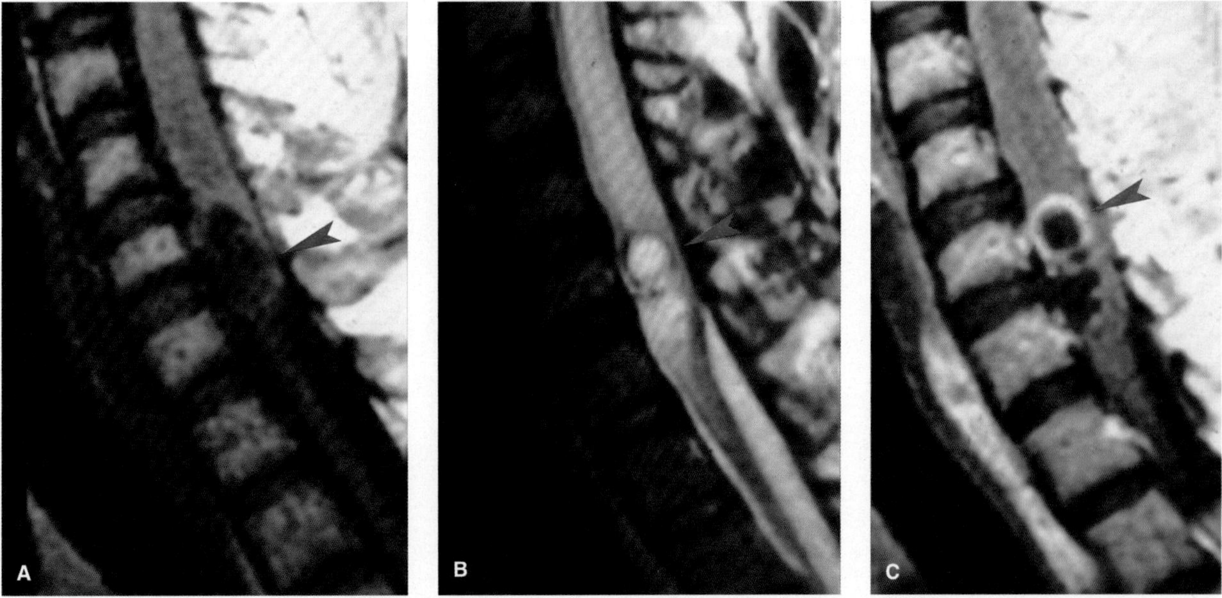

FIGURE 9.13. Spinal Cord Abscess. Sagittal TI-weighted (**A**), T2-weighted (**B**), and T1-weighted postcontrast (**C**) images through the cervical spine show an intramedullary lesion at C6. Note that all the classic features of an abscess in the brain are present, including swelling, edema, a dark rim on T2WI, and rim enhancement. The very long superior extent of the edema on **B** is likely due to CSF flowing through the spinal cord as a result of complete spine block, an interesting condition known as the "presyrinx" state. For further discussion of this entity, see Fischbein NJ, Dillon WP, Cobbs C, Weinstein PR. The "presyrinx" state: a reversible myelopathic condition that may precede syringomyelia. *AJNR Am J Neuroradiol* 1999;20:7–20. (Case Courtesy of Dr. German Zamora, Quito, Ecuador.)

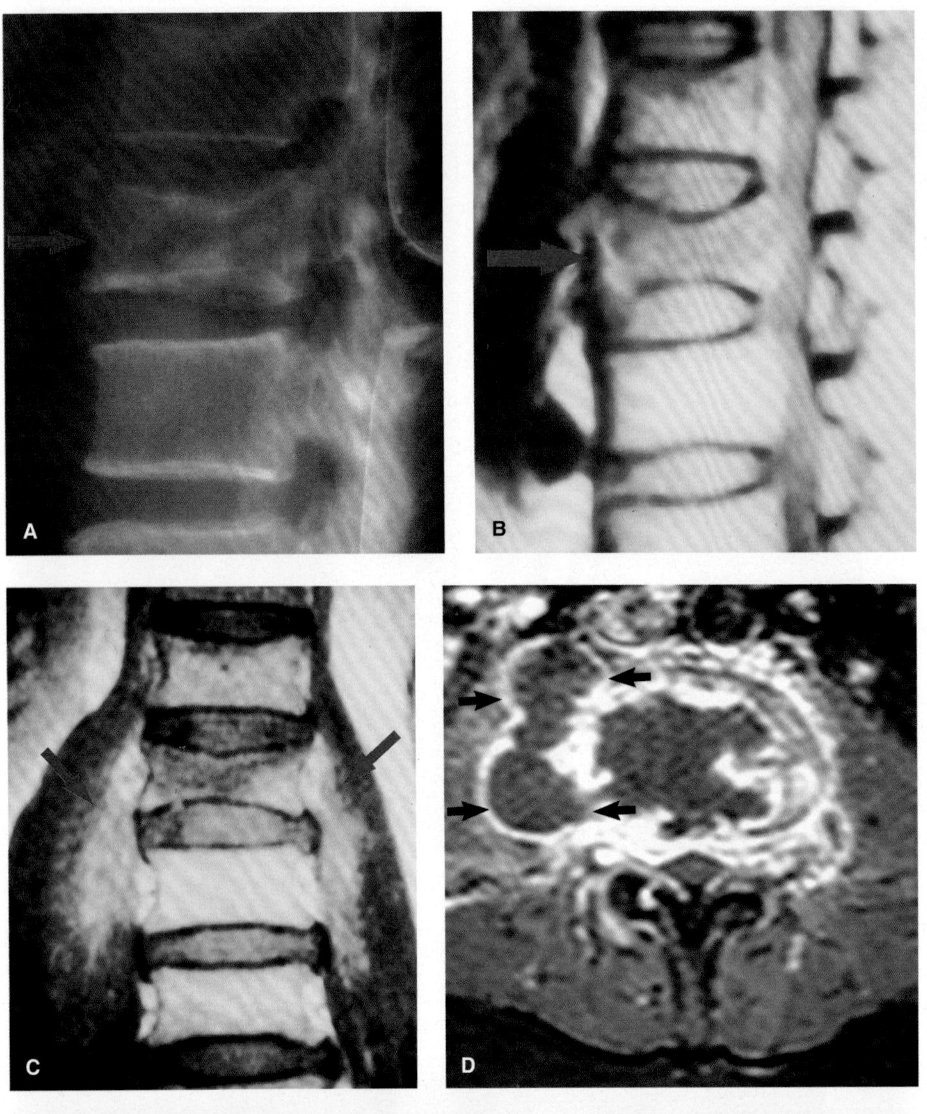

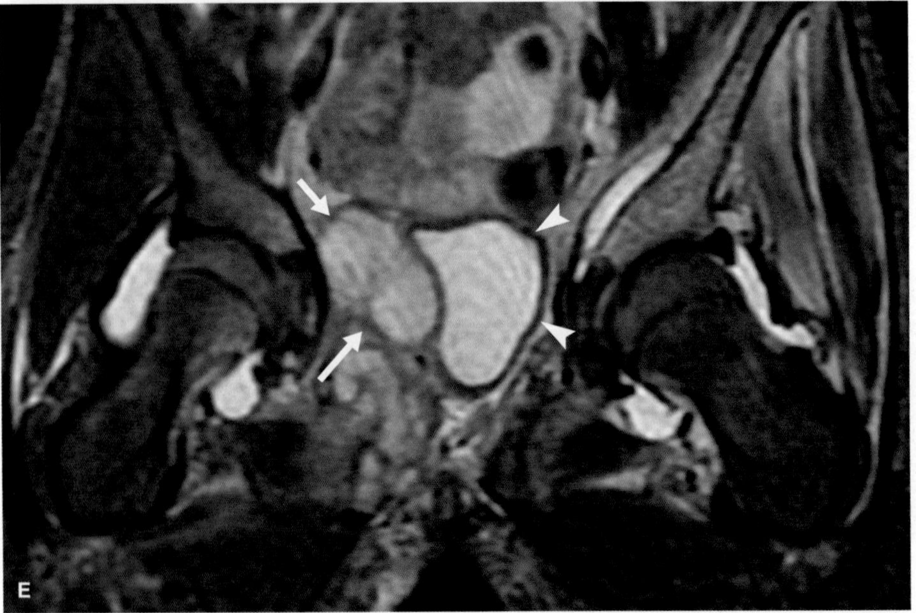

FIGURE 9.14. Tuberculous Osteomyelitis of the Spine (Pott's Disease) and "Cold Abscesses." **A:** Conventional radiograph shows loss of height of L2 (*arrow*), with subtle sclerotic changes. **B:** Enhanced T1WI show abnormal marrow throughout L2 (*arrow*), consistent with a pathologic fracture, making neoplasm or infection prime suspects. Acute compression fractures usually show anterior "wedging," and chronic compression fractures have normal marrow. **C:** Coronal-enhanced images reveal bilateral psoas infiltration (*arrows*), but normal discs, consistent with a nonpyogenic infection such as tuberculosis. Contrast this with the disc involvement seen in Figure 9.9. Metastatic tumor rarely infiltrates the psoas in such a diffuse fashion. **D:** Another patient with more chronic spinal tuberculosis shows a "cold abscess" in the right psoas muscle (*arrows*). **E:** Spread can occur even more diffusely, as shown in this patient with cold abscesses (*arrows*) displacing the bladder (*arrowheads*). (Case courtesy of Dr. Stephen Swanson, Arusha, Tanzania.)

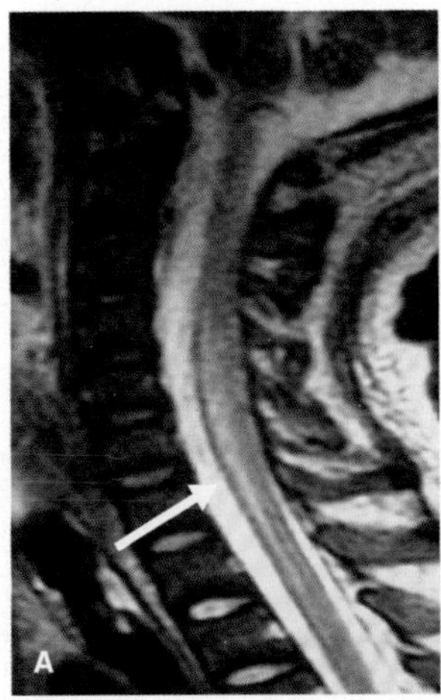

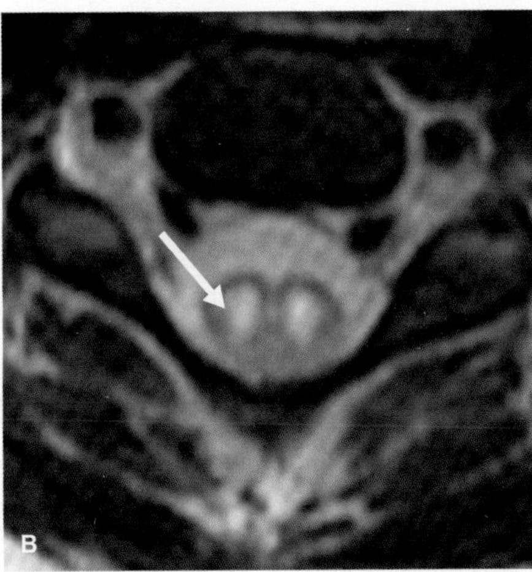

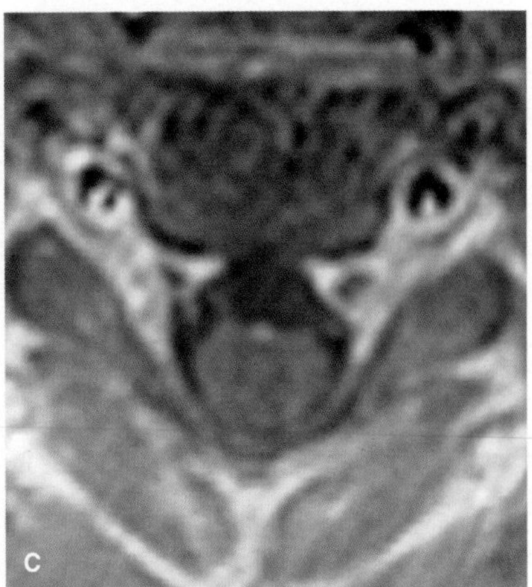

FIGURE 9.15. Poliomyelitis. This patient was admitted with low-grade fever and progressive flaccid weakness of the lower extremities. T2WI sagittal (**A**) and axial (**B**) images show high signal involving the anterior horn cells (*arrows*), without significant enhancement (**C**). Amyotrophic lateral sclerosis (ALS) has similar findings, as the anterior horn cells are also the locus of injury in ALS. (Courtesy of Dr. Rakesh Gupta, Lucknow, India.)

metastases often are found incidentally when evaluating known cancer patients for distant spread. MR is an excellent tool for evaluating these osseous metastases. Signal alterations from tumor infiltration within the normal bright marrow fat on T1WI usually precede any bone changes detectable on plain film or CT (Fig. 9.25). Technetium bone scanning, however, remains the most cost-effective tool for whole body screening. PET is so widely used in oncology today that many vertebral metastases are initially detected on these studies.

Intramedullary Masses

Astrocytomas and ependymomas are the two most common primary intramedullary tumors, but the distinction between them is difficult to make on imaging grounds alone. Both are expansile, low in signal intensity on T1WI, bright on T2WI, with variable enhancement. Both have an increased incidence in neurofibromatosis. Some guidelines, based on involvement of the entire cord diameter and longer cord segments (favors astrocytoma) and presence of cysts and hemorrhage (favors ependymoma), have been proposed to distinguish between the two types of tumors. In any single case, however, they are rarely a substitute for biopsy. Gadolinium contrast is useful to identify the tumor nidus, as well as spread of tumor along CSF pathways.

Ependymomas are the most common spinal cord tumor in adults. They can be divided into the cellular (intramedullary) and myxopapillary (filum terminale) types. Spinal ependymomas are genetically and epidemiologically different from

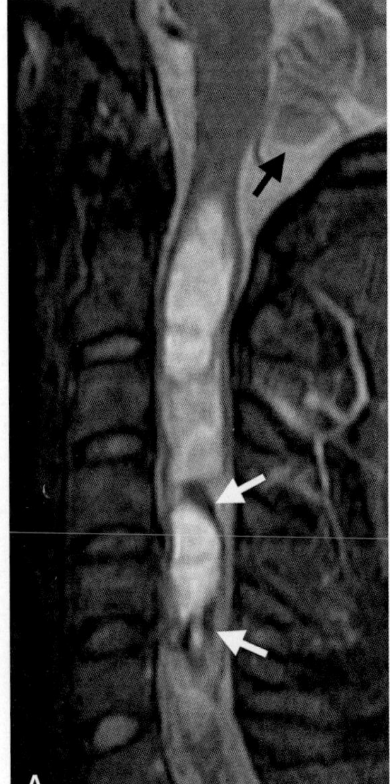

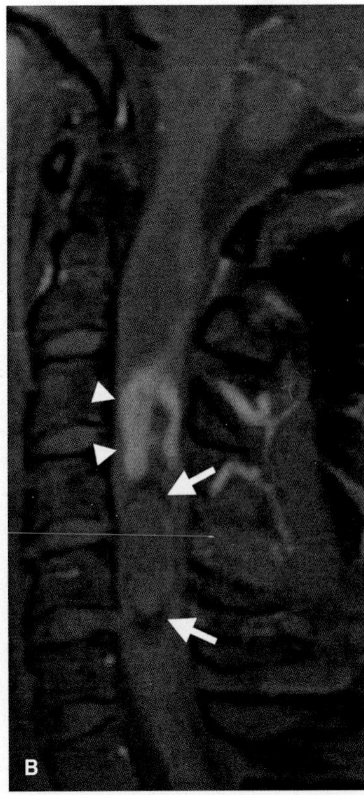

FIGURE 9.16. Ependymoma. A: T2WI shows an expansile, cystic lesion cavity (*white arrows*) within the cervical cord, but the cerebellar tonsils (*black arrow*) are normal in position, so this cannot be a Chiari I (contrast with Fig. 10.26). **B:** Postcontrast image shows an enhancing component (*arrowheads*) at the mid portion of the intramedullary cavity. Irregular hypointensity in the lower portion of the cavity (*arrows*) suggests hemorrhage, a common finding in spinal ependymomas.

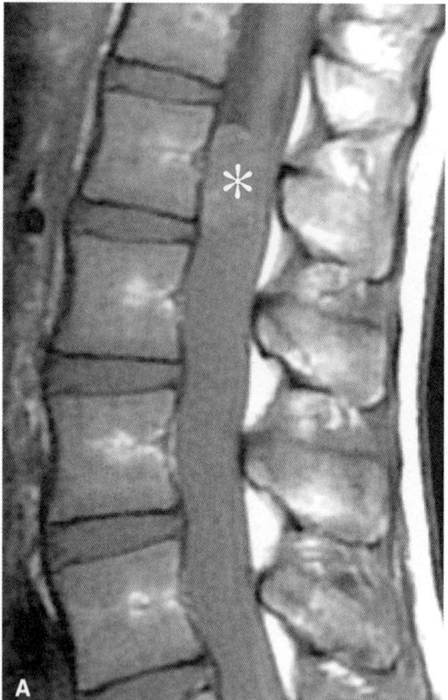

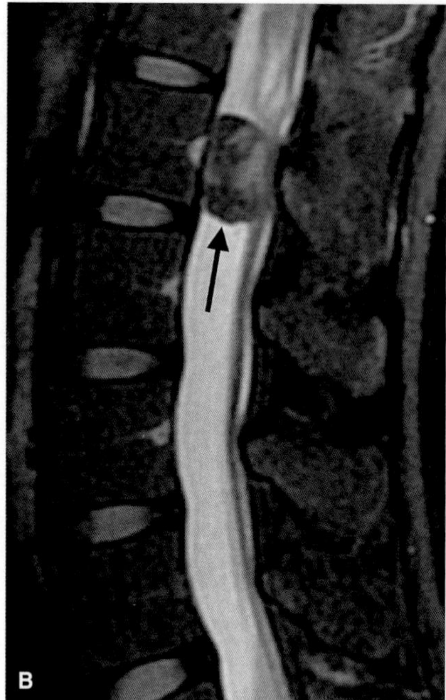

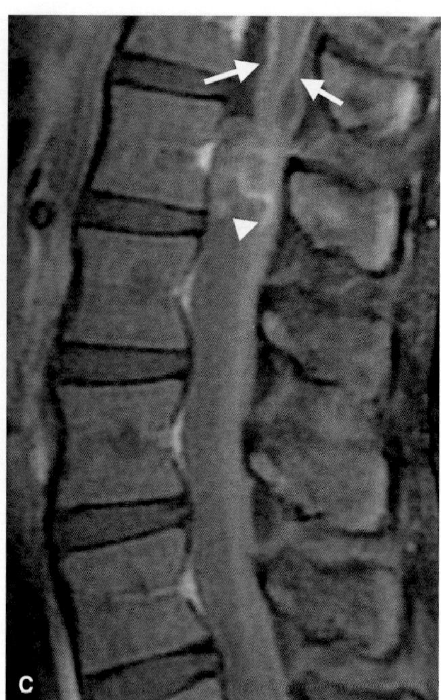

FIGURE 9.17. **Myxopapillary Ependymoma of the Filum Terminale. A:** This patient presented with lower extremity radicular complaints. T1-weighted sagittal image shows an isointense extramedullary mass abutting the conus (*asterisk*). **B:** Sagittal fat-suppressed T2-weighted image demonstrates a low signal mass (*black arrow*). **C:** The mass enhances heterogeneously, with leptomeningeal enhancement of the adjacent conus (*arrows*) and cauda equina nerve root (*arrowhead*).

intracranial types. Peak incidence is in the fourth decade, with a male predominance. These slow-growing neoplasms arise from ependymal cells lining the central canal of the cord, or ependymal cell rests along the filum. Histologically, ependymomas are usually benign, but when intramedullary a complete curative excision may be impossible. Associated hemorrhage can be seen, especially on MR, and cystic areas are common (Fig. 9.16). Filum terminale ependymomas are also known as myxopapillary ependymomas dye to their unique histology. A reasonably specific diagnosis can be made on imaging because of their location adjacent to the conus (Fig. 9.17). Complete resection of myxopapillary ependymomas is possible, as they are typically well encapsulated.

Astrocytoma. Most (75%) astrocytomas occur in the cervical and upper to midthoracic cord, and presentation in the conus is rarer than with ependymomas. Fusiform cord widening, hyperintensity on T2WI, and contrast enhancement often extend over several vertebral body segments (Fig. 9.18). They generally have a lower histologic grade than astrocytomas in the brain. As in the brain, there is considerable histologic variability. Subtypes such as protoplasmic astrocytoma can

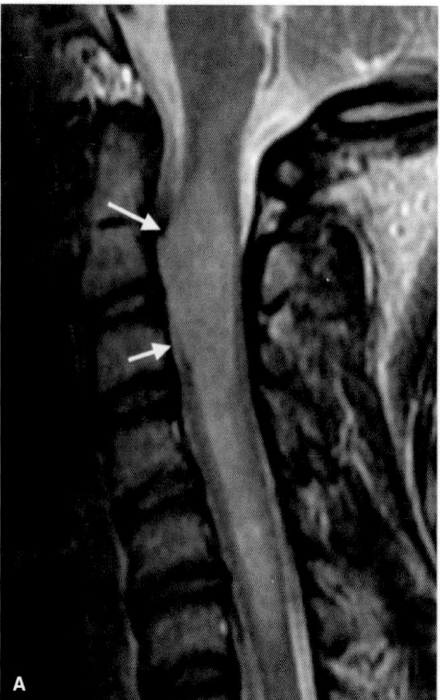

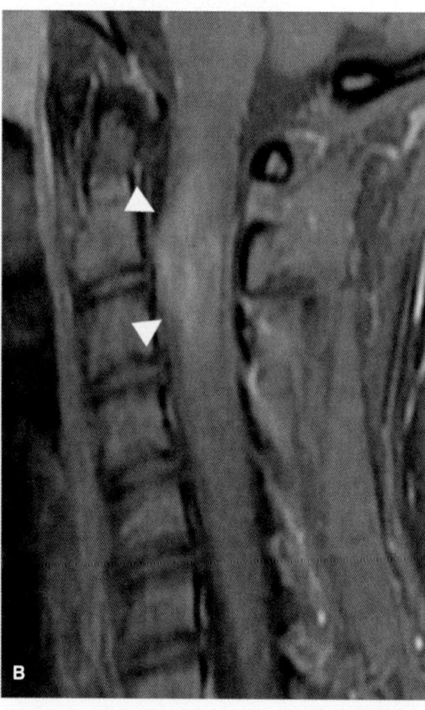

FIGURE 9.18. **Astrocytoma. A:** Sagittal T2-weighted image shows an infiltrative, expansile mass in the upper cervical cord (*arrows*). **B:** Sagittal contrast-enhanced T1-weighted image with fat saturation demonstrates ill-defined enhancement (*arrowheads*).

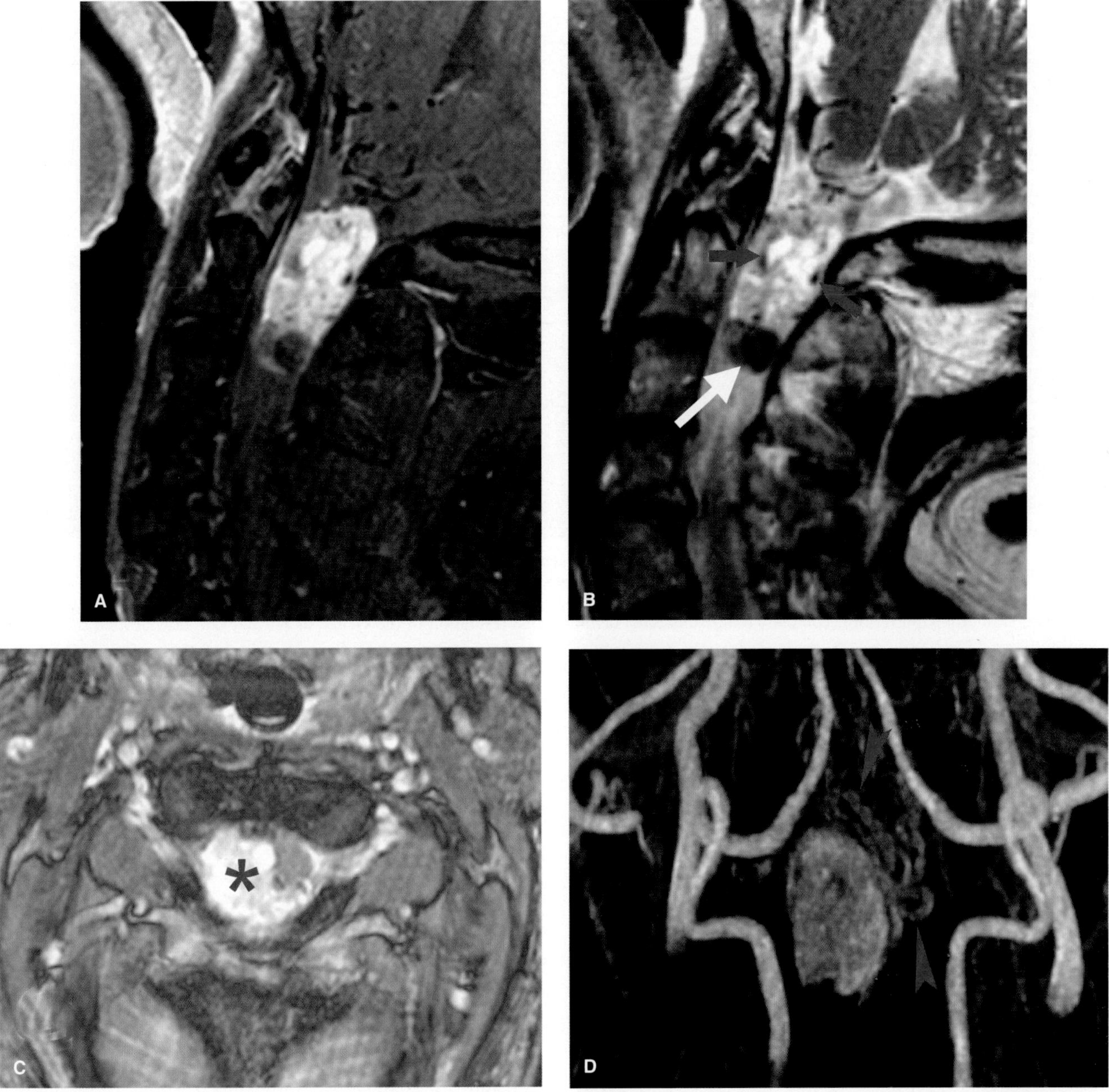

FIGURE 9.19. **Hemangioblastoma. A:** Sagittal contrast-enhanced T1WI shows a large, avidly enhancing intraspinal mass in the upper cervical canal. **B:** Sagittal T2W1 shows a large hypointense focus inferiorly, compatible with intratumoral hemorrhage (*white arrow*). Serpiginous T2 hypointense structures (*red arrows*) represent flow void in this hypervascular mass. **C:** Axial GRE image demonstrates lateral displacement and compression of the cord by the extramedullary mass (*asterisk*). **D:** Coronal MIP reconstruction from a contrast-enhanced MRA demonstrates large feeding vessels (*arrowheads*) adjacent to the hypervascular mass.

involve the spinal cord over a considerable length. Astrocytomas are the most common spinal cord tumor in children, with peak incidence in the third decade, younger than for ependymomas. They may be exophytic, and at times may even appear largely extramedullary. Brainstem gliomas will sometimes extend through the medulla into the upper cervical spine cord. Figure 9.7 shows an expansile cervical cord astrocytoma post laminectomy and radiation.

Hemangioblastomas occur in the spine as well as the posterior fossa. Both types have a high association with von Hippel–Lindau syndrome (see pediatric chapters). These rare tumors, with their characteristic densely enhancing nidus, represent 2% of intraspinal neoplasms. Forty percent are extramedullary and 20% are multiple. The nidus shows vascular hypertrophy (Fig. 9.19) and may be mistaken for an AVM. Intramedullary AVMs, however, typically do not show a related cyst, cord expansion or a non–vascular-enhancing nodule (compare Figs. 9.19 and 9.34).

Syringohydromyelia. Hydromyelia refers to dilation of the central canal of the spinal cord, which is lined by ependyma. Syringomyelia, on the other hand, is a cavity outside the central canal lined by glial cells. Distinction between these two conditions is difficult on high-resolution imaging studies, given that the lining of the cavity cannot be examined histologically. The generic term covering either, "syringohydromyelia," is a bit of a tongue twister, and the abbreviated "syrinx" is often used for both conditions. The etiology of a syrinx can be developmental, such as in the Arnold–Chiari malformations (see Chapter 66). Trauma and tumors, however, can also lead to a syrinx.

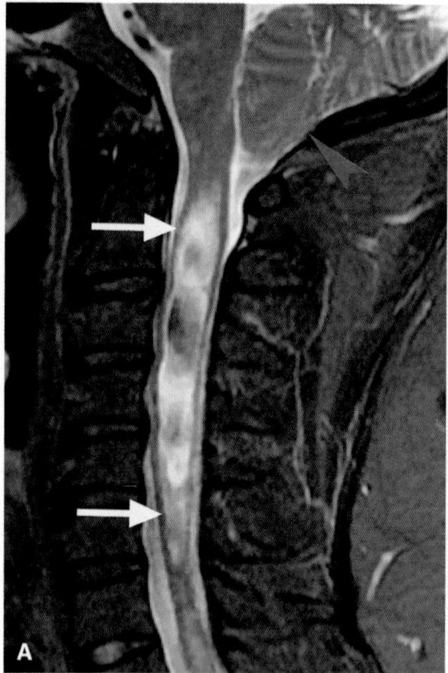

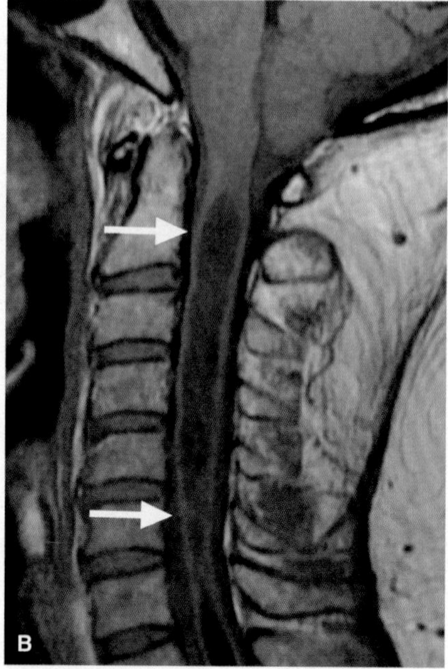

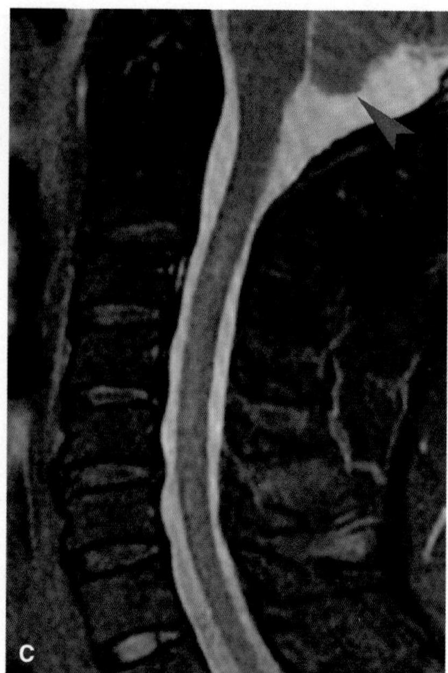

FIGURE 9.20. **Syrinx. A:** T2WI. **B:** T1WI. This intramedullary lesion (*arrows*) shows the classic features of a benign syrinx. The margins of the intramedullary cavity are sharp and the intramedullary contents follow CSF signals on all sequences (patchy hypointensity on T2WI is related to flow). The cause of the syrinx, the low cerebellar tonsils of the Chiari malformation (*arrowhead*), is also seen. **C:** T2WI obtained following suboccipital craniotomy/posterior decompression (*arrowheads*) demonstrated resolution of the syrinx, as normal CSF flow around the cord has been restored.

A syrinx cavity should have very well-defined margins, and its contents should follow CSF signal intensity. Always suspect tumor as a cause of unexplained syrinx. Unless definite benign etiology is apparent, such as prior history of cord contusion or the low cerebellar tonsils of a Chiari I (Fig. 9.20), give gadolinium to search for a tumor nidus. If the "syrinx" borders are indistinct and the signal is brighter than CSF on T1WI and darker than CSF on T2WI, you may be dealing with severe central cord edema, or "presyrinx," which is related to obstruction of CSF flow (Fig. 9.13).

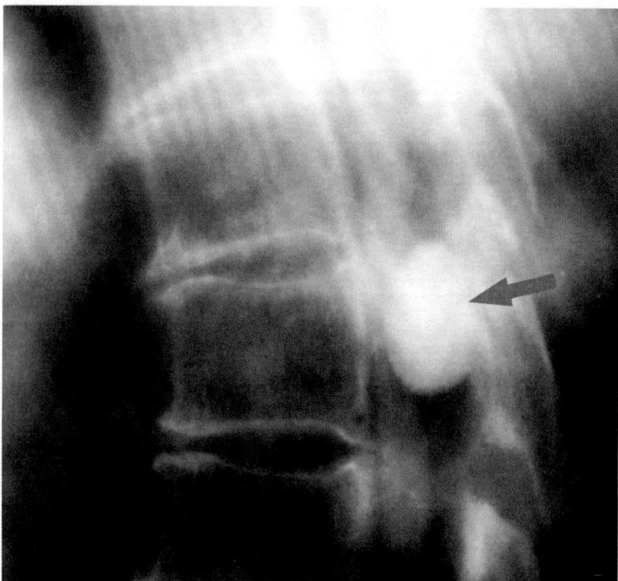

FIGURE 9.21. **Spinal Meningioma.** This intradural but extramedullary mass at T1 is causing chronic severe cord compression. The patient was myelopathic, but remained ambulatory. If an acute lesion such as a vertebral fracture, epidural hematoma, or abscess caused this degree of compression, the patient would likely be paraplegic. The spinal cord is much more tolerant of chronic than acute compression.

Intradural-Extramedullary Masses

Meningioma is the most common intradural tumor in the thoracic region and represents roughly 25% of all adult intraspinal tumors (Fig. 9.21). Most (80%) occur in women, with an average age of 45. Multiple meningiomas raise the question of neurofibromatosis. The usual location is extramedullary-intradural, although there can be an extradural component. CT and MR characteristics are similar to that of intracranial meningiomas, with vigorous enhancement and broad dural bases (Fig. 9.22A and B). The main differential consideration is usually schwannoma, which often will extend out through a neural foramen, and lacks a broad dural base. Schwannomas are less well vascularized than meningiomas, so may undergo cystic necrosis, and often extend out the neural foramina (Fig. 9.22C and D).

Nerve sheath tumors include schwannomas (also known as neurinomas, neurilemmoma, neuroma) and neurofibromas. "Schwannoma" is the preferred term because pathologically these tumors are composed of Schwann cells. They are the most common intraspinal mass, comprising 29% of the total. Schwannomas usually originate from the dorsal sensory nerve roots, but remain extrinsic to the nerve, causing symptoms by mass effect. Most are solitary and sporadic, with a peak presentation in the fifth decade. As MR use for unrelated back pain increases, however, more schwannomas are discovered incidentally in younger patients (Fig. 9.23). Extension into the neural foramen is a frequent finding, especially in the cervical and thoracic regions. Part of the tumor will be intraspinal, and part will be extraspinal, with the waist at the often-expanded

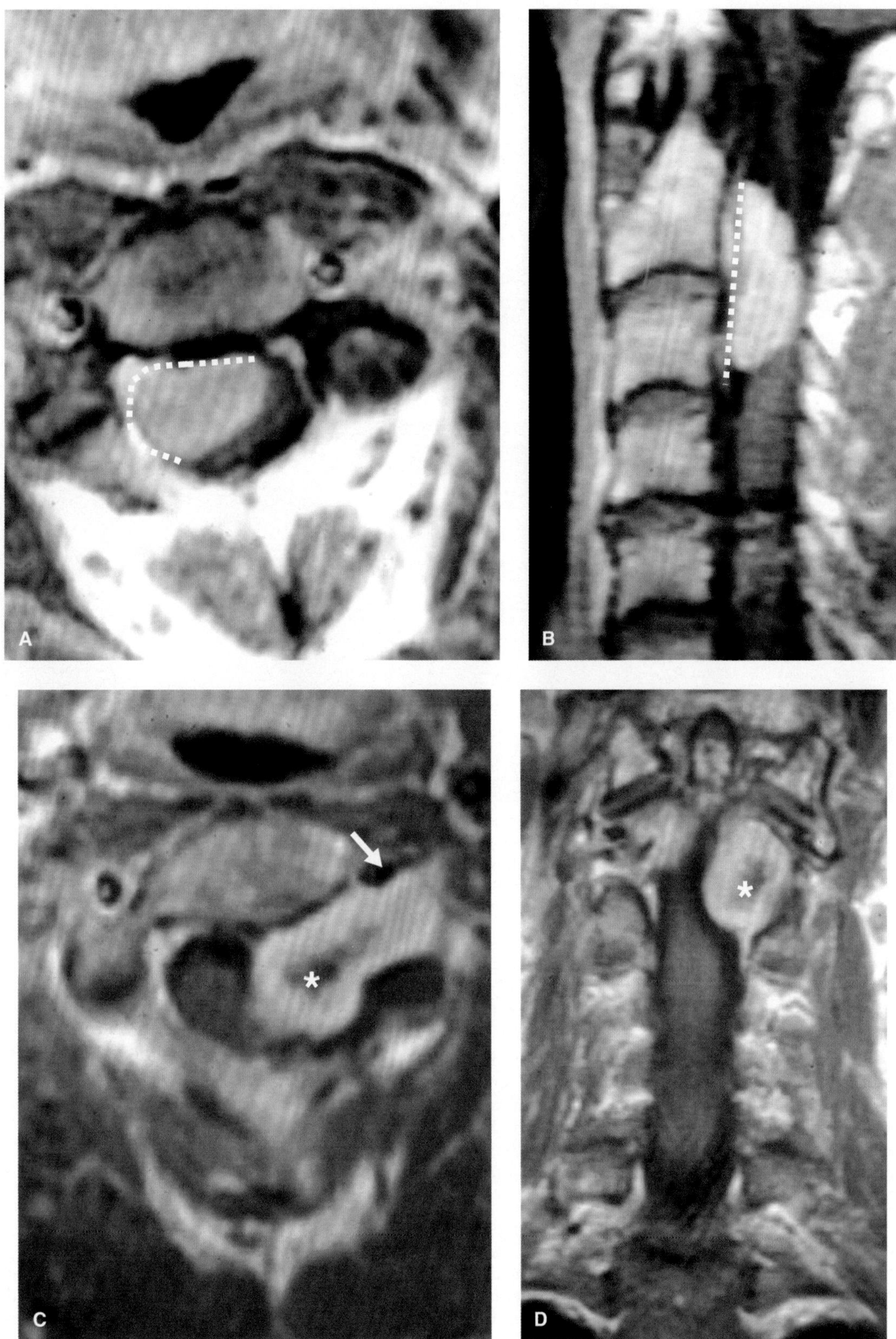

FIGURE 9.22. **Spinal Meningioma Versus Schwannoma. A, B:** Meningiomas have a broad dural base (*dotted lines*), enhance homogeneously due to their excellent blood supply, and do not extend out the neural foramina. **C, D:** Schwannomas do not have a dural base, and thus their blood supply is tenuous. As a result, they often undergo central cystic necrosis (*asterisk*). Often they extend along their parent nerves out neural foramina (*arrow*). The spinal and intracranial presentation of these two tumors is similar. (Please see Chapter 5 for a further discussion of each.) What would your diagnosis be if this lesion was "transplanted to the cerebellopontine angle?" *If you squint a bit, image C looks like a vestibular schwannoma extending into the internal auditory canal, within a miniature posterior fossa!* (Compare to Fig. 5.16 B).

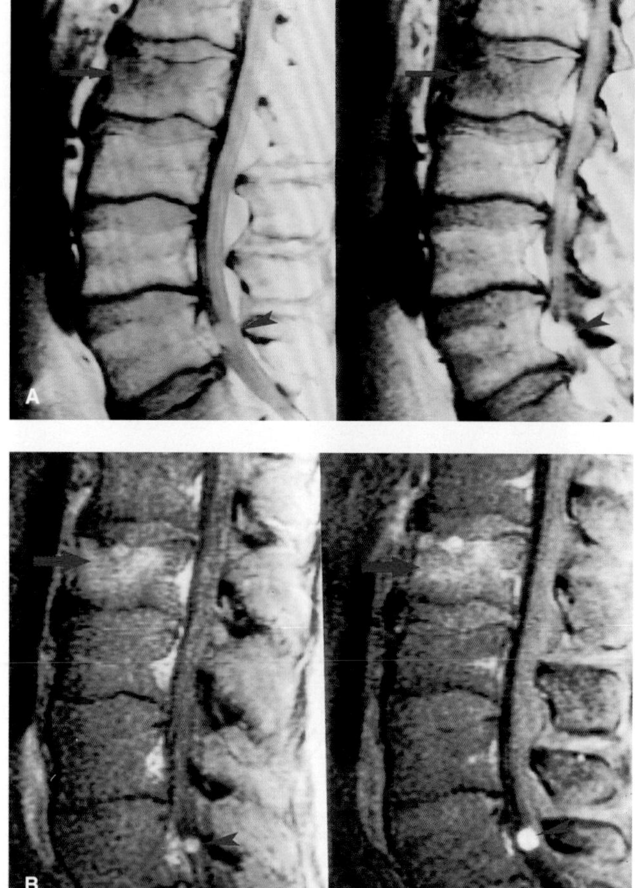

FIGURE 9.23. **Small Incidental Lumbar Schwannoma. A:** This patient had acute focal back pain after an accident, resulting in an acute compression fracture of the superior aspect of L2, which shows marrow edema (*arrow*). A small intraspinal mass was also noted at L5 (*arrowheads*). **B:** This lesion enhanced with contrast (*arrowheads*). Schwannomas of the cauda equina can undergo cystic degeneration as they grow, and if large enough become symptomatic. Note enhancement of the L2 compression fracture (*arrows*) on this fat saturation postcontrast image.

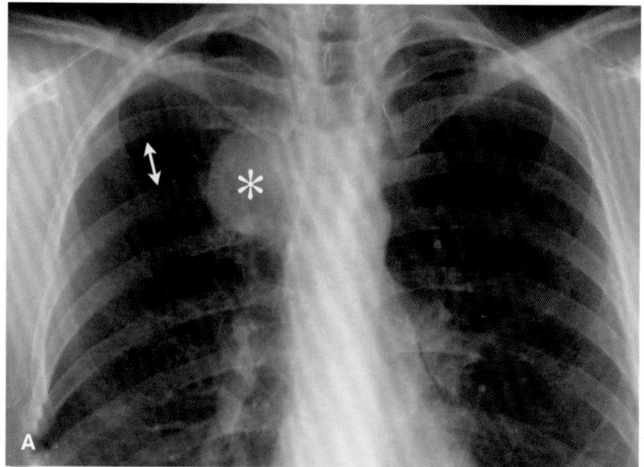

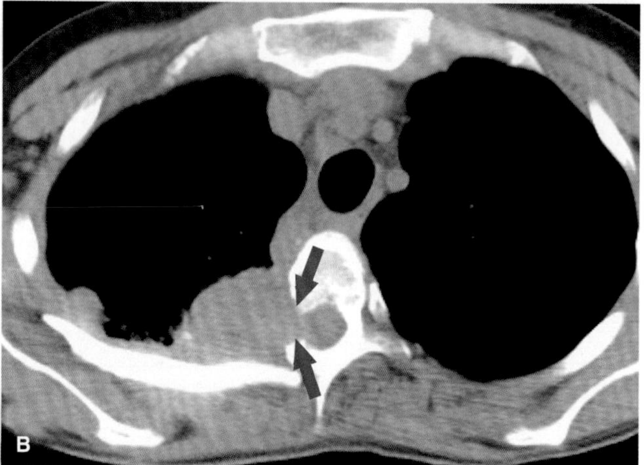

FIGURE 9.24. **Large Thoracic Schwannoma. A:** Anteroposterior chest radiograph shows a posterior mediastinal mass (*asterisk*) with splaying of the ribs (*double-sided arrow*). **B:** Axial CT. Posterior mediastinal mass widens the neural foramen in a "dumbbell" pattern (*arrows*).

bony neural foramen, giving the classic "dumbbell" appearance (Fig. 9.24). In the lumbar region, schwannomas tend to remain within the dural sac (Fig. 9.23). Spinal neurofibromas are associated with neurofibromatosis (NF) type I, and its chromosome 17 abnormalities. These patients may also have dural ectasia and rib abnormalities. Please see Chapter 66 for further discussion.

Intrathecal (Drop) Metastases. The classic cause of spinal intradural-extramedullary metastases is subarachnoid seeding of primary CNS neoplasms, typically medulloblastomas, ependymomas, and germ cell tumors. Tumor cells exfoliate into the CSF and "drop" down into the spinal canal, implant on the pia, and grow into small nodules, giving rise to the term "drop metastases." Non-CNS tumors, such as breast and lung carcinoma and lymphoma also seed the subarachnoid space. Leukemia, which will be discussed later, probably has the highest rate of infiltration of the meninges of any non-CNS tumor. Leptomeningeal metastases can cause considerable inflammation, and patients can present with signs of meningeal irritation, leading to the term "carcinomatous meningitis."

Leptomeningeal metastases classically appear as multiple intradural nodules, usually adherent to the pial reflections, best seen after gadolinium (Fig. 9.27). The differential diagnosis of thickened leptomeninges includes carcinomatous and infectious meningitis, postinfectious states such as Guillain–Barré (Fig. 9.5), granulomatous diseases (Fig. 9.6), and inflammatory arachnoiditis in the postoperative patient. In the immunocompromised patient in particular, diffuse leptomeningeal enhancement requires CSF analysis to distinguish between tumor and infection.

Extradural Masses

Metastases. Neoplasm is the second most common cause of extradural mass, after disc herniations and other degenerative processes. Primary vertebral tumors such as chordomas, giant cell tumors, hemangiomas, and sarcomas are discussed in the "Musculoskeletal" section (see Chapters 55, 56 and 60), and must be kept in the differential diagnosis. The most common extradural neoplasms, however, are metastases of solid tumors such as breast, lung, and prostate carcinoma. Most metastases, like infection, reach the vertebrae via arterial seeding, although prostate carcinoma may preferentially ascend to the lumbar region via Batson venous plexus. The vertebral marrow space, like the liver and the lungs, "filters" a great deal of blood, and provides fertile ground for metastatic deposits.

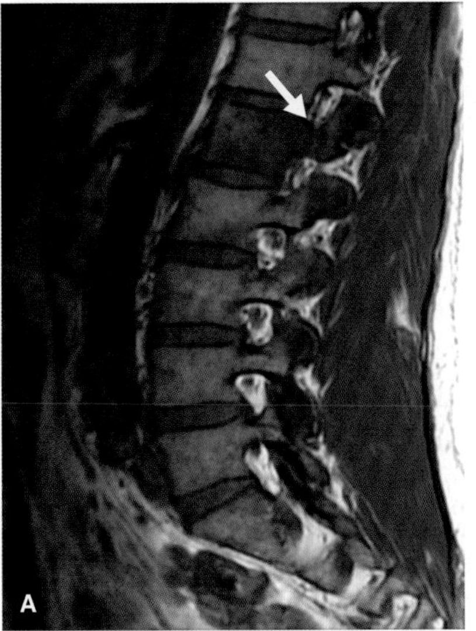
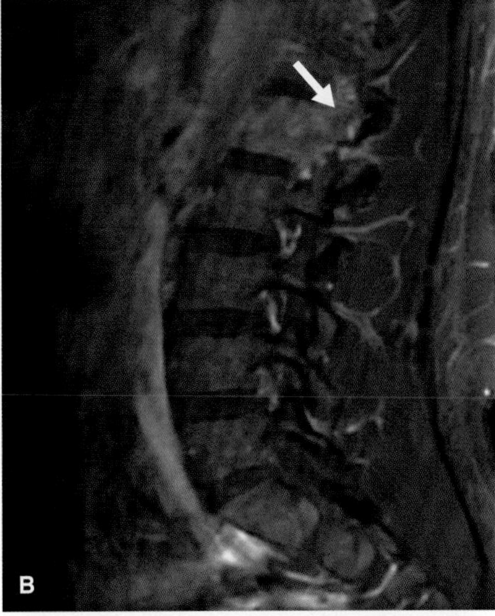
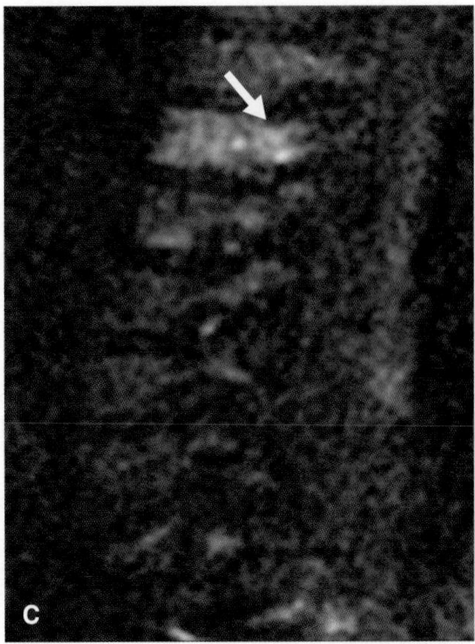

FIGURE 9.25. **Early Vertebral Metastatic Disease. A:** The L1 pedicle (*arrows* throughout) shows low signal on T1WI. The normal fatty marrow, bright on T1, has been replaced by tumor cells, which have higher water content. **B:** STIR images reflect this higher water content due to T2 effects. **C:** DWI is bright due to the greater restriction of water movement in the tightly packed tumor cells.

As these deposits grow, they replace normal marrow, which contains considerable fat, and is bright on T1WI (Figs. 9.27–9.29). Metastases appear as low signal areas on T1WI, becoming high signal on T2WI and STIR, because of their higher water content as compared with fat. Prostate cancer and other densely sclerotic metastases can be somewhat confusing on MR, unless one appreciates that areas of intensely sclerotic bone may be dark on all sequences (Fig. 9.28). Unenhanced T1WI followed and STIR are the mainstay of vertebral body evaluation (Fig. 9.29). Postgadolinium T1 images should be done with fat saturation, as enhancement of metastases can cause them to blend in with normal marrow in conventional T1WI.

Diffusion-weighted imaging (DWI) of the spine is increasing as scanners advance. Metastases will be bright on DWI due to the restriction of water within the infiltrating tumor cells (Fig. 9.26). This effect does not occur with osteoporotic fractures, where extra cellular water may be increased, but not intracellular water. Unfortunately, infiltrated vertebrae can show areas of both tumor (↓ADC) and "pathologic" fracture (↑ADC), confusing the picture.

Once tumor has infiltrated the vertebra, it can spread to the epidural space. Epidural tumor and pathologic compression fractures can lead to myelopathy from mass effect on the spinal cord. A constellation of signs (summarized in Table 9.3) help determine whether a compression fracture is caused by infection, tumor, or is secondary to osteoporosis/trauma (Figs. 9.23 and 9.38–9.39). In general, metastases differ from pyogenic infection in that they involve the vertebrae diffusely

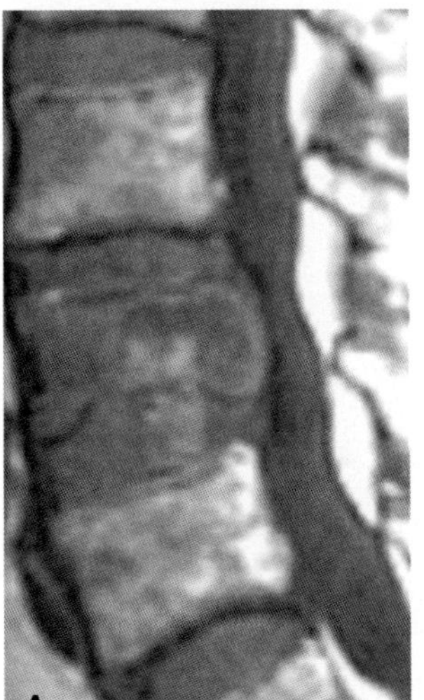
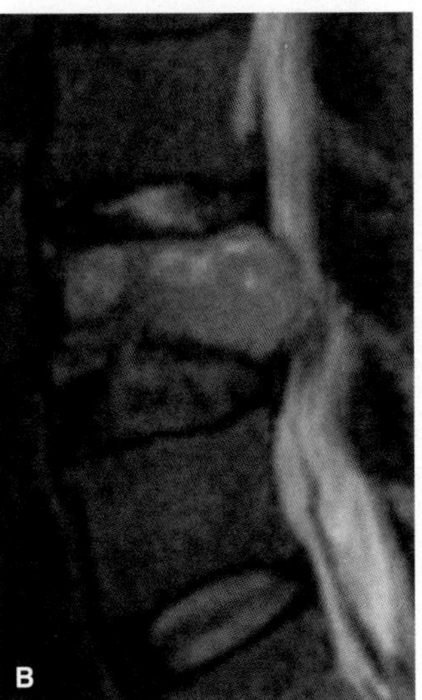
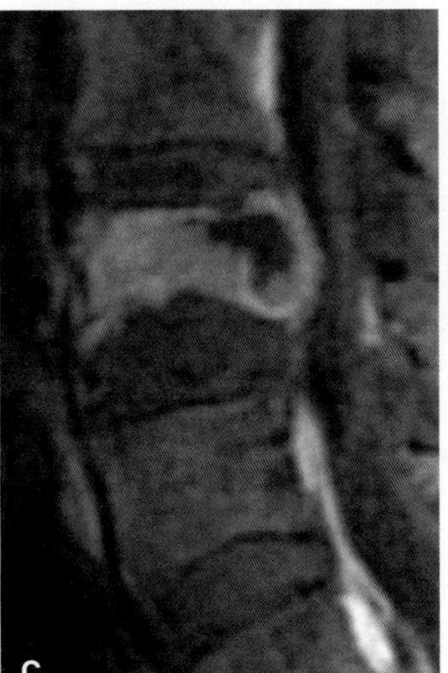
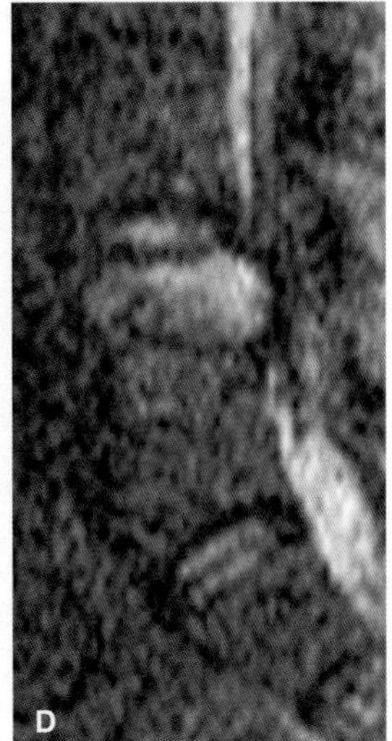

FIGURE 9.26. **Late Vertebral Metastatic Disease. A:** T1WI shows complete infiltration of the marrow of L4, with moderate retropulsion of the posterior portion of the vertebra into the spinal canal. **B:** T2WI shows increased signal, as expected. **C:** Diffuse enhancement after gadolinium. **D:** Diffusion-weighted image shows increased signal. This is due to restricted diffusion of water, which is predominantly intracellular, within the tumor cells packing the marrow space.

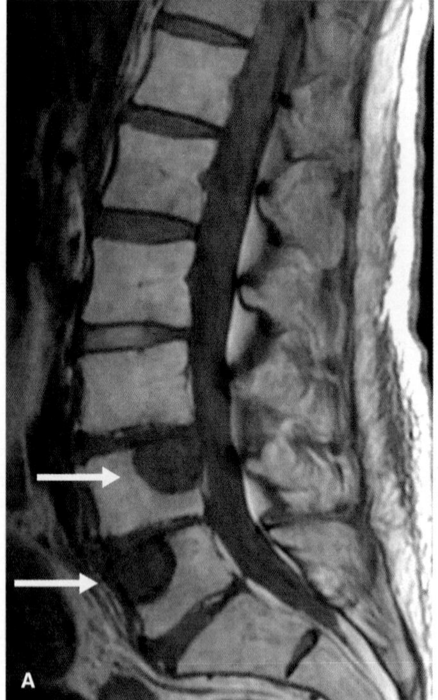

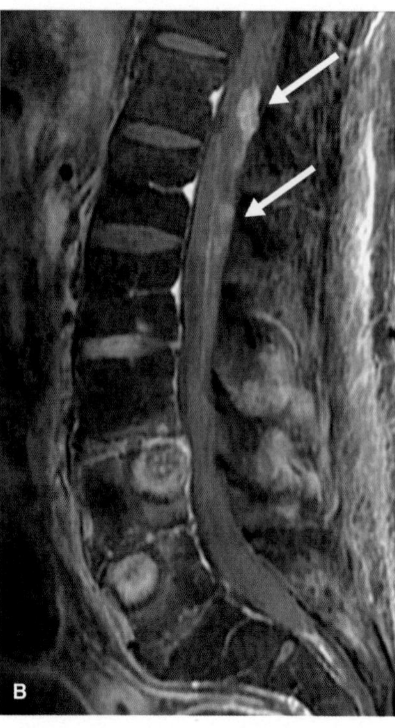

FIGURE 9.27. **Vertebral and Leptomeningeal Metastases From Breast Cancer.** **A:** Large rounded areas of marrow replacement (*arrows*) on T1WI are seen in L4 and L5. **B:** Postgadolinium T1WI images show additional leptomeningeal metastases adherent to the nerves of the cauda equina (*arrows*). These can be overlooked if contrast is not used in oncology patients. Primary brain tumors with leptomeningeal spread (see Fig. 5.15, image F) can present with pial-enhancing lesions in the spine. These are called "drop" metastases, as the tumor cells literally descend along the spinal CSF axis. Medulloblastoma patients are at a particularly high risk for this type of spinal spread.

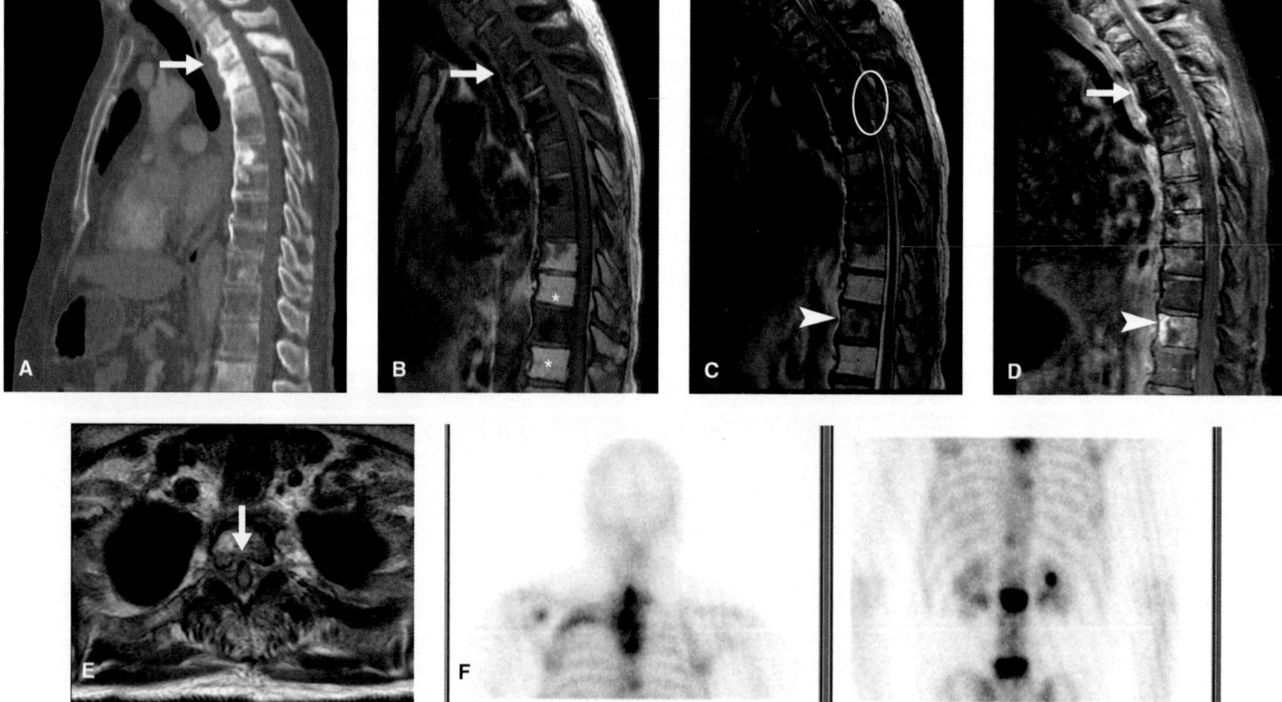

FIGURE 9.28. **Prostate Cancer Metastases.** **A:** Sagittal CT reconstruction shows dense sclerotic areas (*arrow*) in the upper thoracic spine, typical for advanced prostate cancer spread. Most other types of metastases appear lytic on CT. **B, C:** These sclerotic areas represent such dense reactive bone that they appear dark on both T1WI (**B**) and T2WI (**C**), as little marrow fat or water remains (*arrows*.) Note the bright fatty postradiation appearance of the marrow on several lower thoracic vertebrae (*asterisks*). **C:** "Presclerotic" areas of tumor infiltration have a classic bright T2WI appearance for metastases (*arrowhead*). **D:** Sclerotic areas do not enhance (*arrow*), as few vessels are present compared to most metastases, which tend to be hypervascular. Areas of invasion that have not yet become sclerotic do enhance (*arrowhead*). **E:** Epidural tumor is displacing the cord medially (*arrow*) as it fills the lateral portions of the spinal canal. The damaged cord now shows increased signal on T2WI consistent with myelomalacia (see *circled area* on **C**). **F:** Nuclear medicine bone scan demonstrates the sclerotic lesions best, and remain the most efficient way to evaluate lesion burden to the entire skeleton in a single examination. See Chapter 72 for a detailed discussion on this technique.

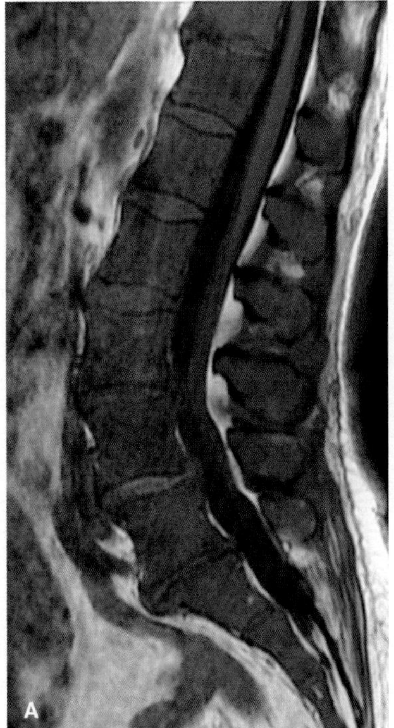

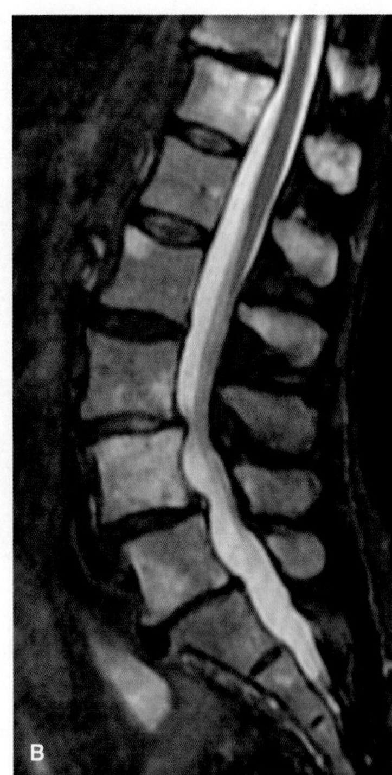

FIGURE 9.29. **Acute Leukemia. A:** The vertebrae are uniformly dark on T1WI, as leukemic cells have completely replaced the normal erythropoietic marrow and fat. A good rule of thumb is that the vertebrae should not be lower in signal than the discs on T1WI. **B:** STIR images show bright marrow due to the increased water content leukemic cells. Myelofibrosis has a similar appearance on T1WI, but would remain dark on STIR due to the acellular fibrosis. (Courtesy Dr. Annie Lai, Berkeley, CA.)

but noncontiguously, sparing the discs. Involvement of the pedicles (Fig. 9.25), lamina, and posterior elements (Fig. 9.30) is another nearly sure sign of neoplasm.

Direct Extension of Paraspinous Tumor. "Round cell tumors" such as lymphoma in adults and neuroblastoma in children can "stealthily" involve the spinal canal, infiltrating through the neural foramina (Fig. 9.31). When CT is used for following lymphoma in the chest and abdomen, subtle involvement of the spinal canal can easily be missed. MR should be used evaluate any lymphoma patient with back pain.

Hematologic malignancies affecting the spine include leukemia, myeloma, and lymphoma. Leukemias change the appearance of the vertebrae in a characteristic fashion: diffuse, even replacement of the marrow with tumor (Fig. 9.29). Solid leukemic infiltrates, or chloromas, can involve the epidural space and cause cord compression.

Multiple myeloma can present as a diffuse and homogeneous low signal in the spine on T1WI, but more typically shows multiple focal defects. Solitary plasmacytomas (Fig. 9.30) are in the differential diagnosis for vertebral plana (totally collapsed

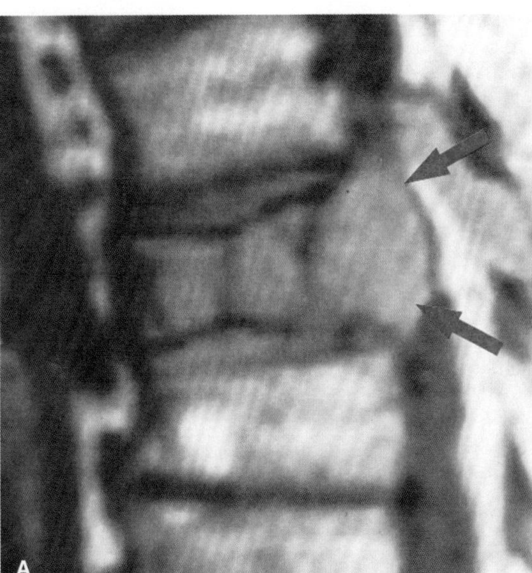

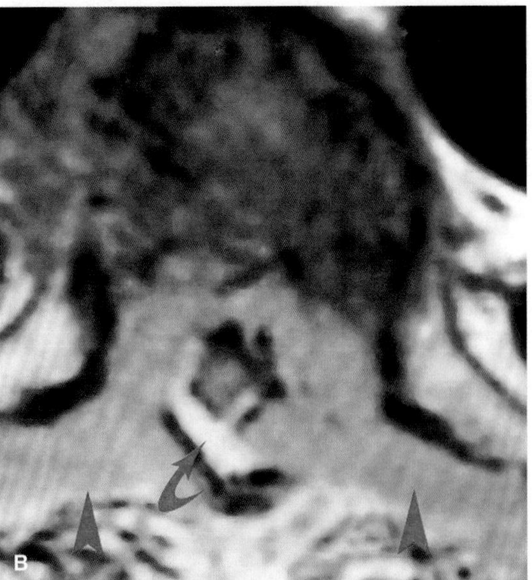

FIGURE 9.30. **Plasmocytoma.** Sagittal (**A**) and axial (**B**) MR images show several features associated with neoplastic infiltration in a midthoracic vertebra. The affected vertebra is completely involved, the discs are spared, and the epidural mass (*arrows*) is limited to the level of affected vertebra. The pedicles and lamina are infiltrated and expanded (*arrowheads*) and the epidural fat (*curved arrow*) is displaced rather than infiltrated. None of these signs alone confirms a neoplastic process, but taken together they are highly suggestive of tumor.

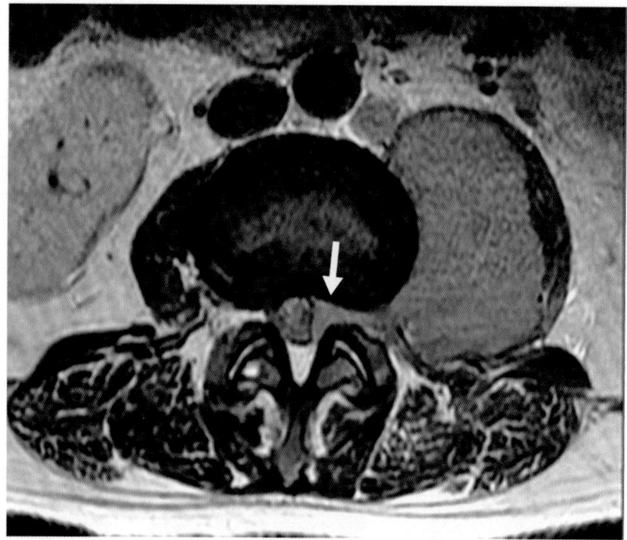

FIGURE 9.31. **Lymphoma Infiltrating the Spinal Canal.** The intraspinal component (*arrow*) of this nodal mass displacing the psoas was missed on a CT. Anytime a patient with lymphoma or other paraspinous tumor presents with back pain, MR is the study of choice. Other paraspinous tumors can infiltrate the spinal canal in a similar fashion, including apical lung (pancoast) tumors, and retroperitoneal and mediastinal carcinomas and sarcomas.

vertebral body), along with eosinophilic granuloma, leukemia, and severe osteoporosis. Technetium bone scans may miss myeloma lesions, which are often relatively "indolent" metabolically. This has made MR spine "screening" of myeloma patients a useful practice.

VASCULAR DISEASES

Spinal Cord Infarction. Vascular diseases of the spine and spinal cord can be divided into cord infarctions and vascular malformations. Spinal "strokes" are quite rare compared with cerebrovascular accidents. The classic scenario is a patient who becomes paralyzed after major thoracic surgery, such as repair of a thoracic aortic aneurysm. Another iatrogenic cause of spinal stroke is spinal epidural steroid injections that inadvertently enter the vasculature supplying the spinal cord.

The affected segments of the cord will appear bright on T2WI and DWI, similar to a brain infarct, followed by the development of myelomalacia. The spinal gray matter in an infarct will be affected a greater degree than the white matter, as is the case in strokes within the brain (Fig. 9.32). Obviously, when a patient in the recovery room after aortic surgery is paraplegic, it does not require great insight to consider a cord infarct. More subtle, however, are cases where atherosclerotic disease or severe degenerative disease leads to thromboembolic cord infarctions. Infarction of the cord must be considered in the differential of any unexplained myelopathy. Acute damage to the cord from viral illness has a similar appearance to stroke, as the gray matter is affected (Fig. 9.15).

Cavernous malformations of the spinal cord resemble "cavernomas" of the brain (Fig. 4.39). They are more dangerous in the spinal cord due to the lack of plasticity, and even a small hemorrhage can be devastating (Fig. 9.33).

Spinal AVM. Spinal stroke can be related to spinal AVM. These lesions are an area of growing interest for two reasons. First, advances in interventional neuroradiology and microsurgery have improved understanding and treatment of these lesions. Second, MR has allowed widespread screening of patients with unexplained myelopathy, leading to the discovery of more patients with spinal AVMs (Fig. 9.37).

AVM is used as a generic term to cover any abnormal vascular complex, which necessarily violates a number of rather complicated spinal AVM classification systems, where true AVMs represent a specific subtype. For a deeper discussion, please refer to the excellent article by Rosenblum. For a first pass at this topic, it is worth going back to the initial question one should ask about any spinal lesion: is the location intramedullary, intradural-extramedullary, or extradural? While an oversimplification, this approach provides a good initial analysis of spinal AVMs.

Intramedullary AVMs have a congenital "nidus" of abnormal vessels within the cord substance, which cause symptoms by hemorrhage or ischemia because of steal phenomenon. They are congenital lesions that can grow as vessels dilate, and typically present in young patients with hemorrhage, leading to acute paraparesis. Some are high flow, with visible signal voids within the cord substance (Fig. 9.34).

Extramedullary AVMs are located in the pia or the dura. When in the dura, they can be as far lateral from the cord as the nerve root sleeves. The classic lesion is the spinal dural arteriovenous fistula (SDAVF), a direct connection between an artery and vein without an intervening nidus of congenitally abnormal vasculature. The direct arterial inflow into the local venous system through the fistula, undamped by the resistance of a capillary bed, raises pressure within the coronal venous plexus draining the spinal cord, which is valveless (Fig. 9.35).

SDAVFs cause symptoms through venous hypertension and congestion of the cord with edema. This edema can be detected on MR as increased signal on T2WI, typically within the conus (Fig. 9.36), which sometimes enhances. The reason for cord enhancement in SDAVFs is not fully understood, but probably results from breakdown of the blood–brain barrier because of either chronic infarction or some sort of capillary leak phenomenon secondary to venous hypertension. These lesions are felt to be acquired rather than congenital, similar to dural AV fistulas in the brain. The key is not to misdiagnose this lesion as tumor, which can lead to a biopsy attempt that ends in disaster due to bleeding.

TRAUMA

In the acute trauma patient, the spine must be evaluated immediately to rule out fractures. Please refer to the Musculoskeletal section for a detailed discussion. Unstable fractures can compromise the diameter of the spinal canal, leading to cord compression and paralysis. Plain films historically have been the first choice in the emergency department, as they can be obtained quickly and inexpensively, without significant interruption of other resuscitation efforts. Recent data show that conventional radiography remains perfectly adequate in low-risk cases.

After severe trauma, however, a modern helical CT of the cervical spine (or the entire spine) takes just a few extra second beyond the mandatory head CT. Subtle lesions, such as fractures of the foramen transversaria (which house the vertebral artery) can be missed on plain films. When complex spine fractures are seen on plain films, CT studies are very helpful to define the relationship of the bone fragments.

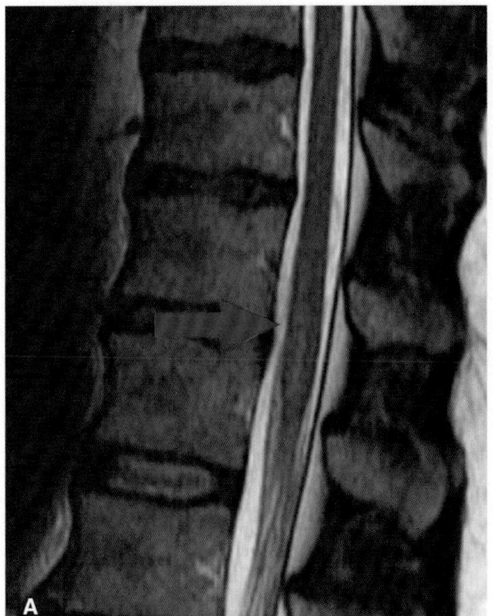

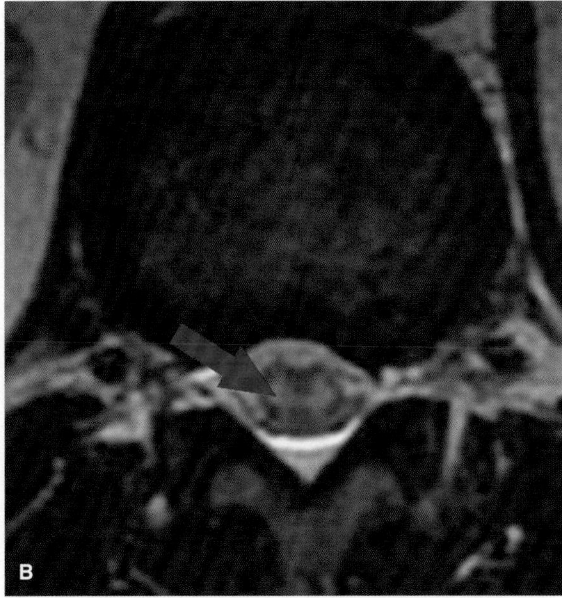

FIGURE 9.32. **Spinal Stroke. A:** Sagittal MR. **B:** Axial MR. This patient developed almost immediate paraplegia after injection of epidural steroids near the thoracolumbar junction. Presumably, these entered the arteries supplying the conus, causing infarction. Note that the high signal on these T2WI images is within the central cord, affecting the gray matter. This is the opposite pattern of spinal MS, where the white matter is preferentially affected.

Acute osteoporotic compression fractures are typically due to minor trauma to weakened vertebrae. This population may benefit from vertebroplasty and other "vertebral augmentation" procedures. Patients with acute compression fractures with marrow edema (Figs. 9.23 and 9.38C and D) are candidates for these stabilizing injections of bone cement, although they remain controversial. Such procedures are not indicated in chronic healed compression fractures (Fig. 9.38A and B), as they are already stable.

Some discussion is needed concerning the immediate and delayed consequences of vertebral trauma to the spinal cord and spinal nerves, which cannot properly be evaluated on plain films or with noncontrast CT. These include cord contusion, epidural hematoma (and their sequelae, such as myelomalacia and syringohydromyelia), and nerve root avulsion.

Cord Contusion. The spinal cord, like the brain, lies suspended in a bath of CSF, contained by arachnoid membranes, dura and bone. The cord, again like the brain, is subject to significant impact against its surrounding bony suit of armor during abrupt acceleration and deceleration. In the brain, contusions appear at the site of a blow and 180 degrees opposite, in the classic coup–contrecoup pattern. Certain bony sites, such as the plenum sphenoidale, tend to traumatize the adjacent brain because of their irregular contour. In the spine, contusions usually occur at sites of fractures, secondary to bony impingement and cord compression (Fig. 9.39).

Spinal cord contusions may occur in the absence of spinal fractures, because of hyperflexion or hyperextension, resulting in myelopathy. The presence of cord hemorrhage has been established as a poor prognostic factor in spinal cord injury patients evaluated by MR. Therefore, T2* or gradient-echo

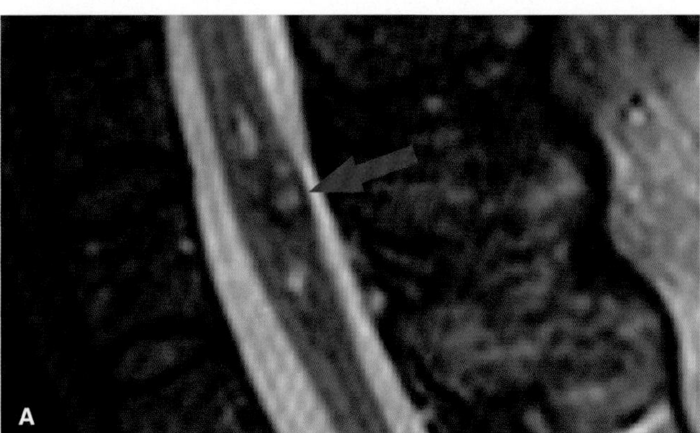

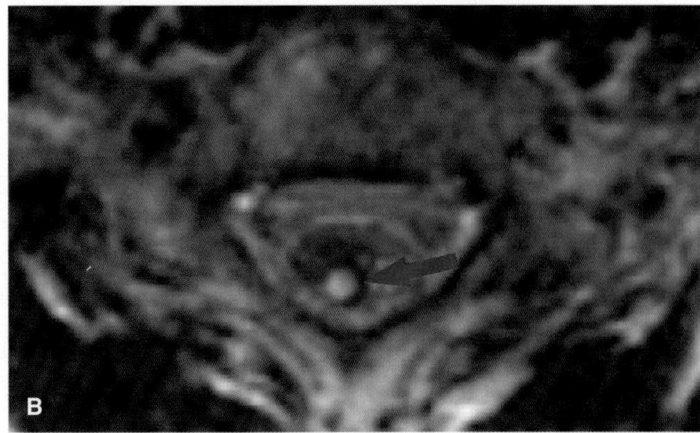

FIGURE 9.33. **Cavernous Malformation.** Sagittal (**A**) and axial (**B**) MR images show an intramedullary lesion with mixed signal intensity. Rounded focus with increased central signal and hemosiderin rim was present on all sequences (*arrow*). No abnormal vessels were seen on MR or angiography, consistent with an occult vascular malformation, which was confirmed surgically.

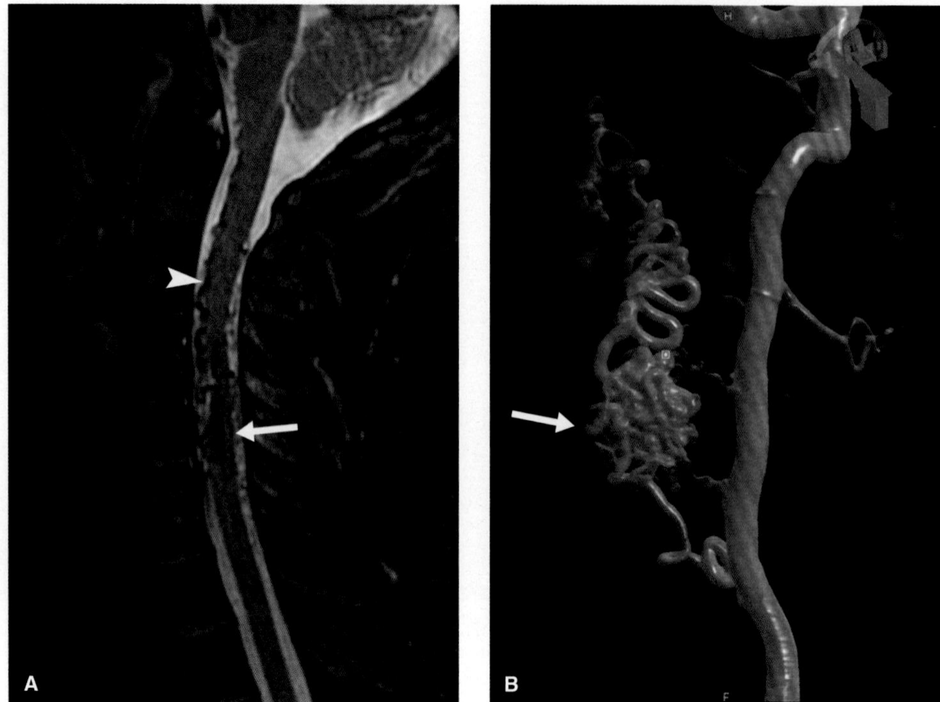

FIGURE 9.34. **Intramedullary Arteriovenous Malformation.** Sagittal T2WI (**A**) image shows multiple serpentine signal voids (*arrow*) within the cervical spinal cord, consistent with an intramedullary arteriovenous malformation. A long draining vessel is also noted in the subarachnoid space (*arrowhead*). **B**: Spinal angiogram injecting the vertebral artery confirms the MR findings, and better demonstrates the nidus of the AVM (*arrow*).

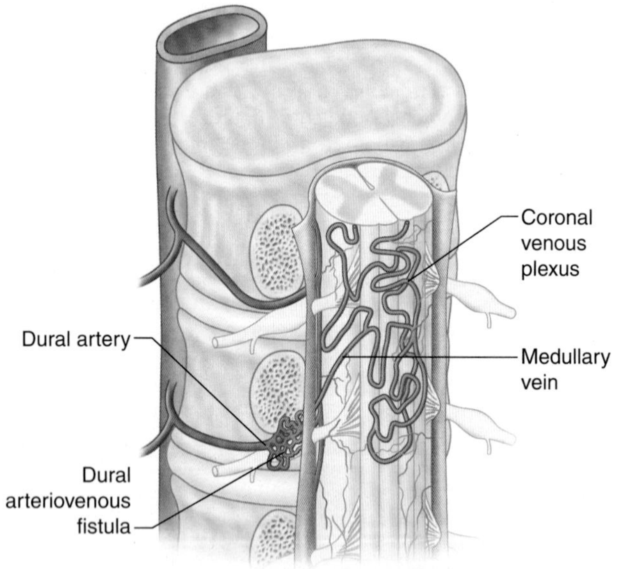

FIGURE 9.35. **Anatomy of a Spinal Dural Arteriovenous Fistula.** The fistula is an abnormal direct connection between an artery and a vein in the dura of the nerve root sleeve. The fistula results in reversal of flow in the draining vein (*arrow*), which in turn feeds the coronal venous plexus with arterial blood under high pressure. The coronal venous plexus dilates, becoming visible to imaging studies, and the cord has difficulty draining its blood because of this fistula-induced venous hypertension and becomes edematous and bright on T2WI (see Fig. 9.36A). (From Rosenblum B, Oldfield EH, Doppman JL, Di Chiro G. Spinal arteriovenous malformations: a comparison of dural arteriovenous fistulas and intradural AVMs in 81 patients. *J Neurosurg* 1987;67:795–802.)

images are a critical portion of any MR protocol for spine trauma. If the spinal cord is injured, myelomalacia results. An area of myelomalacia can enlarge, particularly if adhesions disturb CSF flow, and evolve into a posttraumatic syrinx. The expanding syrinx can cause further neurologic deficit, and require shunting.

Epidural Hematoma. As in the head, extra-axial or, more appropriately, "extramedullary" hematomas can follow trauma, with certain important distinctions. Subdural hematomas are rare in the spine, while epidural hematomas are far more common. The reverse is true in the calvarium, as discussed in Chapter 3.

This distinction can be explained by differences in venous anatomy between the skull and the spine. Most posttraumatic bleeding is venous. In the bony calvarium, the dura is functionally the periosteum, with no potential space between the dura and skull for low-pressure venous blood to accumulate. It takes bleeding under arterial pressure to create an epidural hematoma, by stripping the dura away from the inner table. In the spine, the dura is separated from the bone by epidural fat. In the ventral spinal canal, the epidural space also contains a rich plexus of veins, which drains the vertebral bodies. Trauma, with or without vertebral fracture, can tear these veins, resulting in an epidural hematoma. These hematomas grow with time, leading to cord compression in the setting of normal plain films. CT occasionally detects epidural hematomas in the lumbar spine, if there is sufficient fat to provide contrast. An epidural hematoma in the cervical or thoracic spine usually will be missed unless intrathecal contrast is given. MR therefore is the study of choice, given its ability to image the contents of the spinal canal noninvasively and depict blood-breakdown products (Fig. 9.40).

Nerve Root Avulsion. So far we have focused on the effect of trauma on the spinal cord. Epidural hematomas and

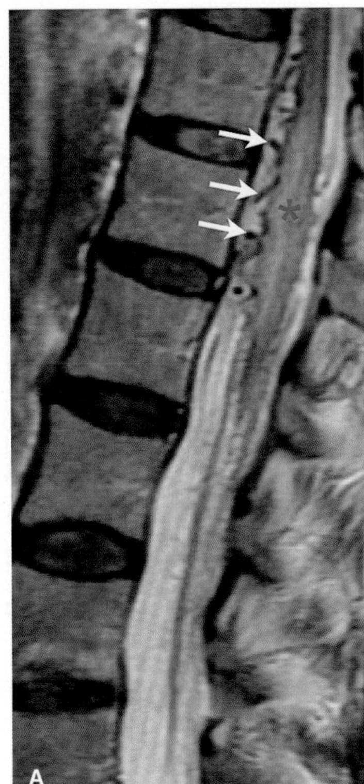

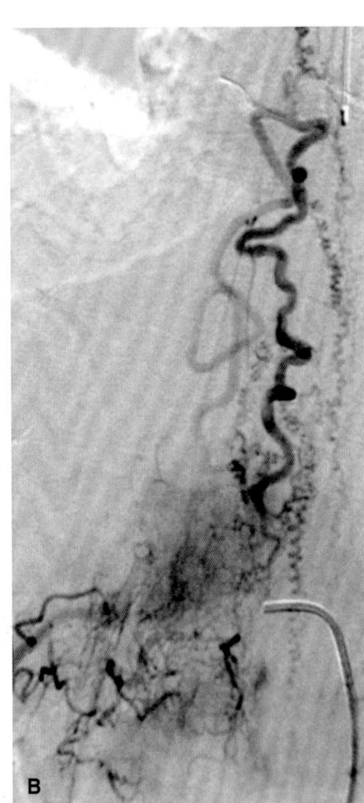

FIGURE 9.36. **Spinal Dural Arteriovenous Fistula. A:** This patient had progressive myelopathy, and the T2-weighted series showed increased signal in the conus (*asterisk*), consistent with edema. Numerous serpiginous flow voids surround the conus (*arrows*). **B:** Spinal angiogram demonstrates dilation of the entire coronal venous plexus.

contusions can also affect nerve roots, and result in radicular complaints. Trauma can cause the spinal nerves to avulse from their connection to the cord. The most common site for root avulsion is the cervical spine, probably because of its wide range of motion during accidents. The nerves supplying the brachial plexus and upper extremities are typically affected, with obvious neurologic deficits. Birth trauma, typically traction on the shoulder, is one of the classic causes of nerve root avulsion at the cervicothoracic junction. This can result in an Erb palsy on the affected side—the shoulder will be adducted and internally rotated, the elbow extended and pronated, and the wrist flexed, all due to injury to the C5, C6, and C7 roots

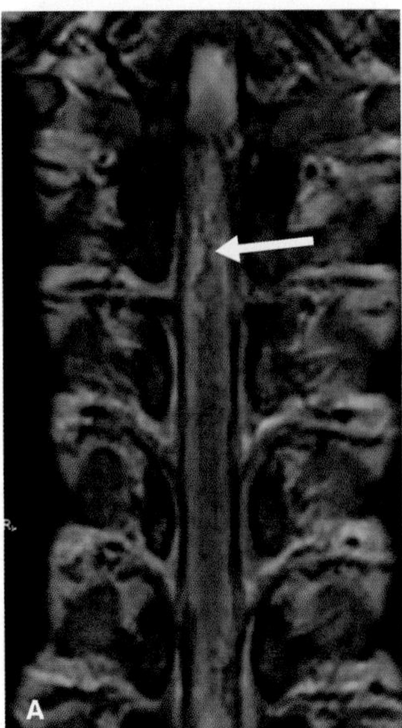

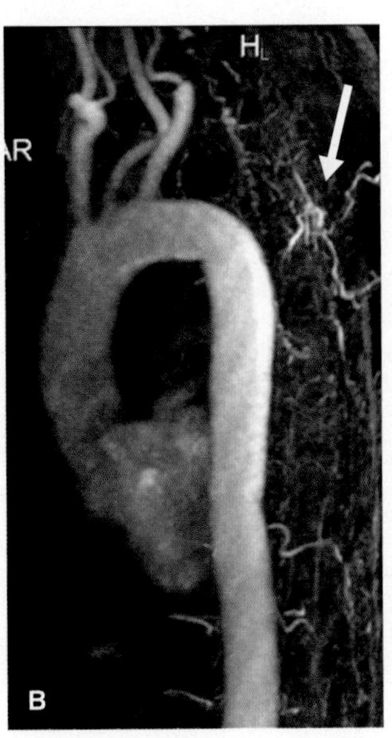

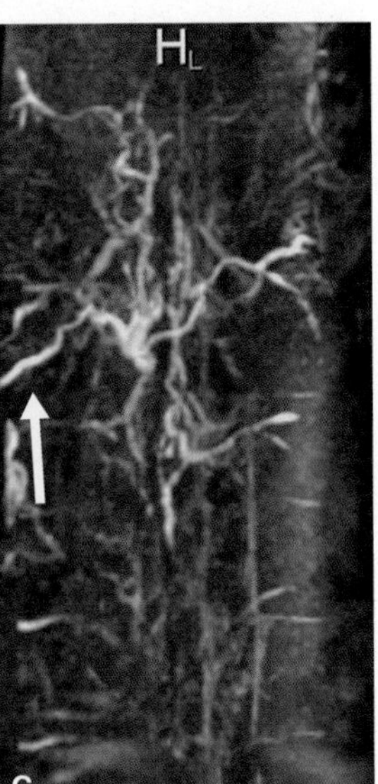

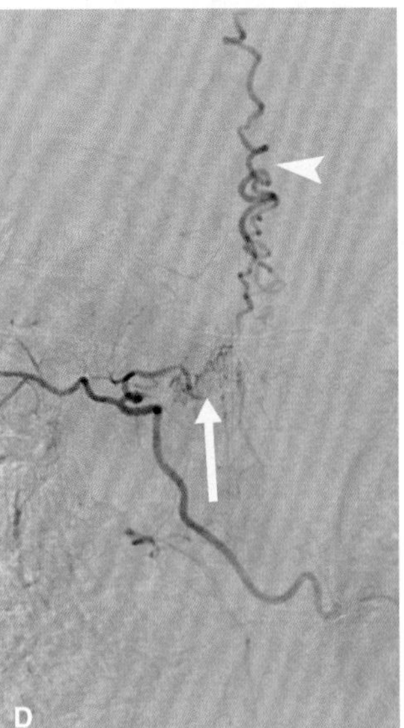

FIGURE 9.37. **Spinal Dural Arteriovenous Fistula (SDAVF). A:** T2 coronal images confirm dilated vessels (*arrow*) dorsal to the spinal cord, initially seen on sagittal scans (not shown). **B:** Postcontrast MRA image demonstrates posterior enlarged vessels over the spine (*arrow*). **C:** The largest vessel, likely the arterial feeder of the SDAVF, is on the right (*arrow*). **D:** Catheter angiogram of right-sided spinal artery at the corresponding thoracic segment confirms the fistula (*arrow*) and engorged draining vein in the subarachnoid space (*arrowhead*). Unlike a true AVM (Fig 9.34) there is no nidus, as this represents a direct shut between artery and a vein. Obliteration of the SDAVF by either surgery or embolization treats the resultant venous hypertension of the cord, which can lead to severe myelopathy. (Case courtesy of Drs. Jonathan Breslau and Bahram Varjavand, Sacramento, CA.)

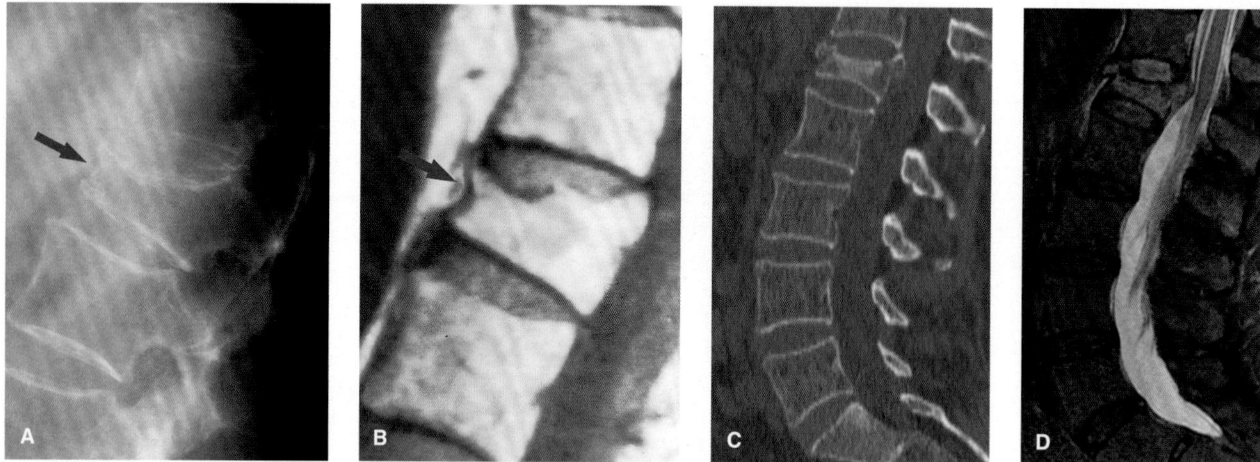

FIGURE 9.38. **Benign Compression Fractures, Chronic and Acute. A:** Conventional radiograph shows a compression fracture of L1 (*arrow*). The vertebral body shows a classic wedge deformity, with greater loss of height anteriorly than posteriorly, with intact pedicles on the anteroposterior view (not shown). This configuration is suggestive of a benign compression fracture. **B:** T1 sagittal MR shows normal marrow signal in the affected vertebrae (*arrow*), confirming a benign cause of the compression fracture, such as osteoporosis. **C:** Sagittal CT reconstruction shows a similar L1 compression the day it occurred, with the fracture planes visible. **D:** STIR image does show homogeneous marrow edema, but a normal marrow fat appearance returned within a year.

(see the Pediatric section). The clinical diagnosis can be confirmed by MR or CT myelography. Typically, CSF will leak out into the epidural space through the tear in the arachnoid and dura from the missing nerve, as can be seen in Figure 9.41. The thoracic spinal nerves (other than T1) and nerves of the lumbar cauda equina rarely undergo avulsion. Given the small field of view needed, thin highly T2-weighted (1 to 2 mm) axial images give excellent detail, and can be reconstructed into "MR-myelograms," much like MR angiograms. MR neurograms are another valuable tool in evaluating both the brachial and lumbar plexus.

While MR is often not practical in the acute setting, it has become a superb noninvasive tool for evaluating the neurologic complications of trauma. MR has increased our understanding of spinal cord injury, and facilitates prediction of long-term outcome.

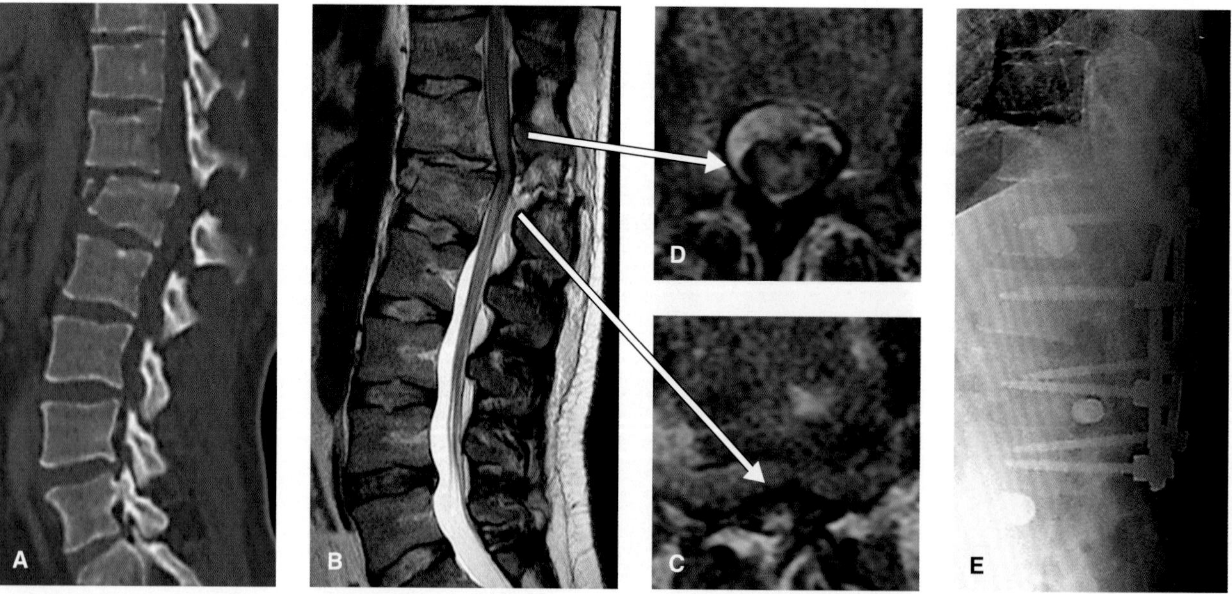

FIGURE 9.39. **Vertebral Fracture With Spinal Cord Contusion.** A 29-year-old male after a mountaineering accident, presenting with profound leg weakness. **A:** CT demonstrates a compression fracture of L1, with retropulsion of L1 into the spinal canal, and distraction of the posterior elements, with instability. **B, C:** T2WI MRI shows compression of the conus. GRE images (not shown) fortunately did not demonstrate hemorrhage into the cord, a poor prognostic sign. **D:** Cord edema extends above the level of the compression, possibly due to ischemia or venous obstruction. **E:** Emergency decompression with internal fixation was performed. With aggressive rehabilitation work, this patient was ambulatory 6 months later. (Courtesy L. Patterson, San Francisco, CA.)

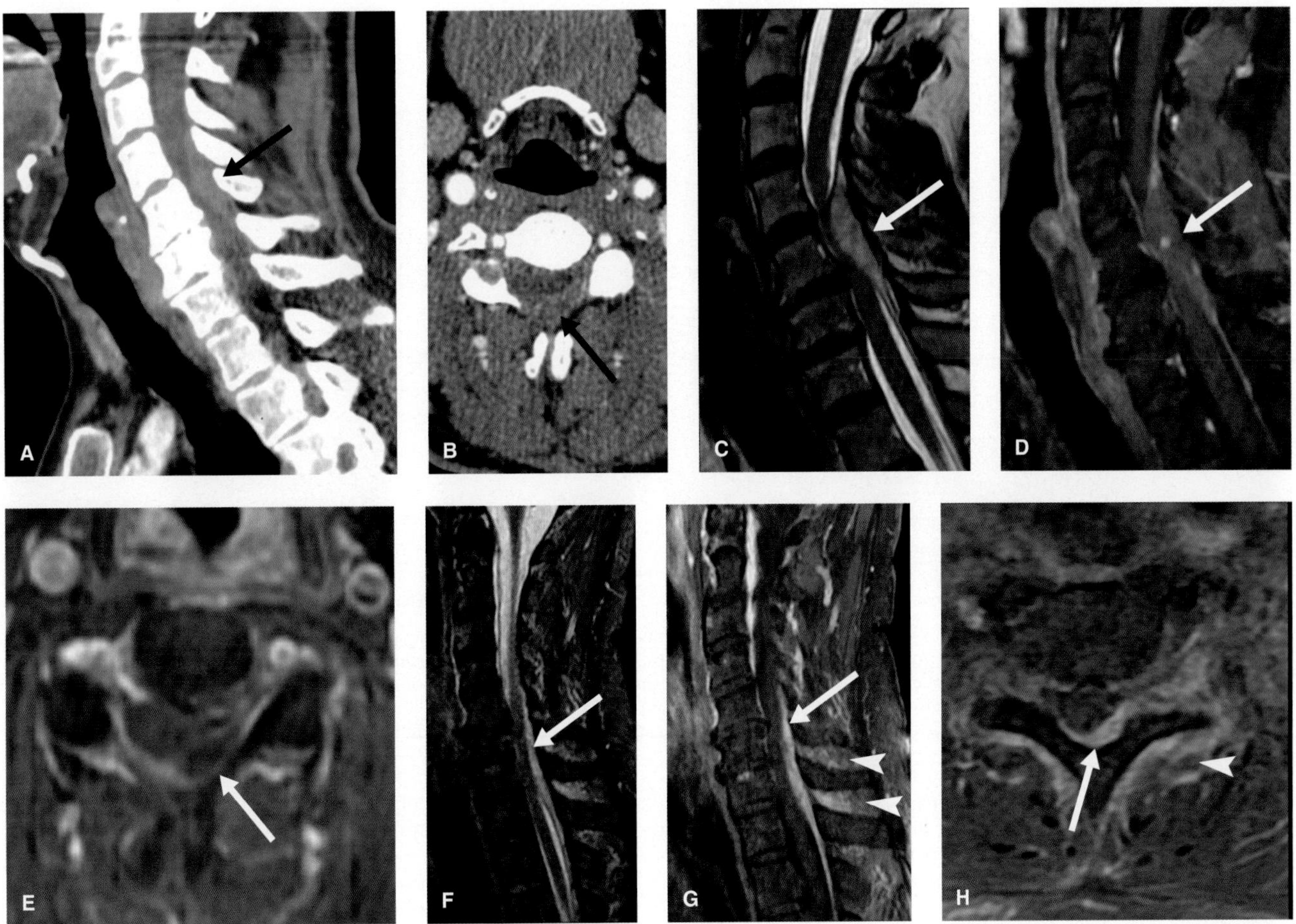

FIGURE 9.40. **Epidural Hematoma (A–E) Versus Epidural Abscess (F–H).** Sagittal (**A**) and axial (**B**) CT images show a slightly hyperdense left-sided posterior epidural collection at C5 (*arrows*), with mass effect on the spinal cord. This is a rare case where CT is positive for an epidural collection, due to the acuteness of the blood in what proved to be a hematoma. T2WI MRI (**C**) shows an intermediate signal epidural mass (*arrow*) with some low signal consistent with early deoxyhemoglobin. Postcontrast T1WI sagittal (**D**) and axial (**E**) images show no significant enhancement of the hematoma (*arrows*). **F:** Epidural abscess shown in a similar location shows high signal on T2WI, as well as significant enhancement (*arrows*, **G**, **H**). The *arrowheads* in images **G** and **H** point to additional enhancement in the posterior paraspinous soft tissues, classic for spreading infection. Note the absence of this type of paraspinous enhancement on images **D** and **E** in the epidural hematoma case.

DEGENERATIVE DISEASES OF THE SPINE

Imaging Methods

Imaging the spine for disc disease and stenosis is done primarily with MRI. CT and CT myelography are useful in patients with MR contraindications or extensive metallic hardware. MR provides more information and a more complete anatomic depiction than CT. For example, MR can determine whether a disc is degenerated by showing loss of signal on T2WIs. MR also shows if annular fibers of the disc are disrupted by noting high signal on the T2WIs (Fig. 9.42). These disc defects have been termed "annular fissures" in the lumbar nomenclature, but surgeons often use the term "high-intensity zone" or HIZ. The HIZ has been associated with internal disc derangement (IDD). IDD may be a cause of axial back pain, and surgeons may perform discectomy with spinal fusion for treatment of IDD.

CT best shows calcified structures, such as osteophytes, bony foraminal stenosis, and ossification of ligaments. Ossification of the posterior longitudinal ligament (OPLL) may be mistaken for disc herniation on MR, is exquisitely depicted on CT (Fig. 9.43).

Sagittal T1WI, T2WI, and T2 fat suppression (such as STIR) are acquired in the sagittal plane on most spine studies. Axial T2WI is used in thoracic and lumbar imaging. Axial gradient echo imaging for the cervical spine has the advantage of providing thinner slices. DWI may be useful to distinguish degenerative disease from infection, as has been described above (see Fig. 9.10—the "Claw Sign"). Contrast is reserved for postoperative cases, or patients where there is additional concern for neoplasm or infection.

Disc Disease

A "Lumbar Disc Nomenclature" multispecialty consensus document was published in 2001 and updated in 2014, addressing the desperate need for clarity and standardization in spine imaging reports (Fig. 9.44). It is critical the radiologist use correct terminology describing disc pathology. Our reports may have legal as well as medical implications!

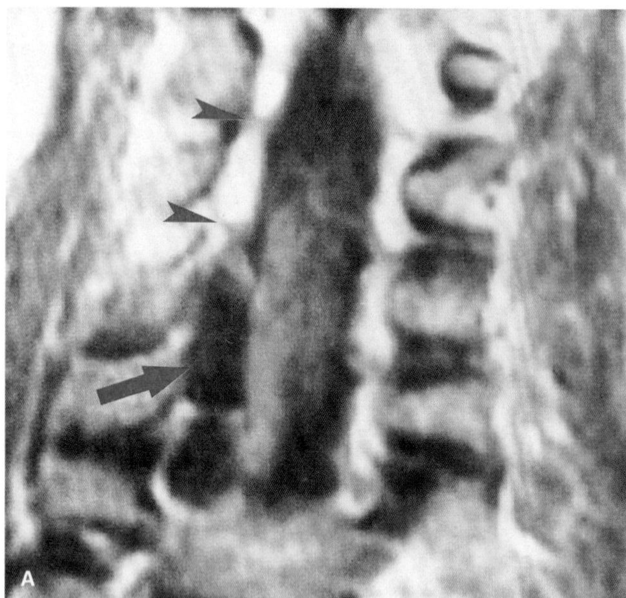

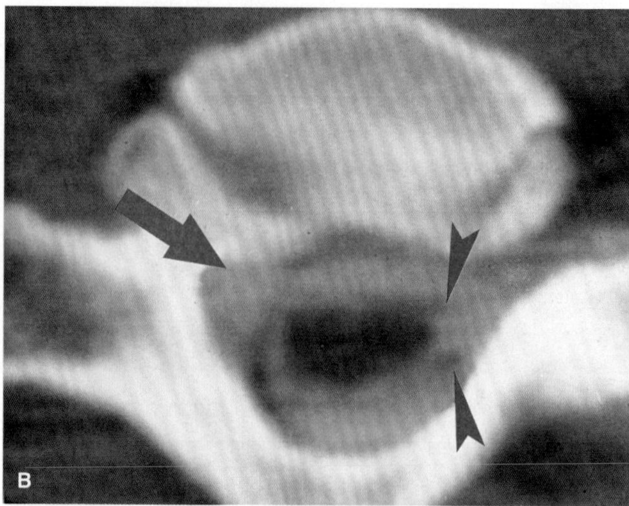

FIGURE 9.41. **Nerve Root Avulsion. A:** Coronal T1WI shows a low signal collection in the right epidural space in the midcervical spine (*arrow*), consistent with CSF that has leaked through avulsed nerve root sleeves. Intact spinal nerves (*arrowheads*) are seen in the upper cervical canal bilaterally traversing through the normal epidural fat. **B:** A CT myelogram confirms the absence of the right-sided nerve roots and the CSF leak (*arrow*). Note the normal roots on the left outlined by myelographic contrast (*arrowheads*).

Disc herniation is defined as a localized or focal displacement of disc material involving less than 25% (90 degrees) of the periphery of the disc, as viewed in the axial plane. Disc herniations are further subcategorized as a protrusion or extrusion based on the shape of the herniation. Up to 50% of the asymptomatic population have disc herniations; hence, just seeing a disc herniation does not necessarily mean it is clinically significant. In fact, many public health experts feel MRI of the lumbar spine is overused, arguing that it identifies too much incidental pathology, to the detriment of patients—and our health care budget!

Always report if a herniation is compressing a nerve root or creating stenosis, in order to help clinicians determine the relevance of the finding. Not all disc herniations require surgery,

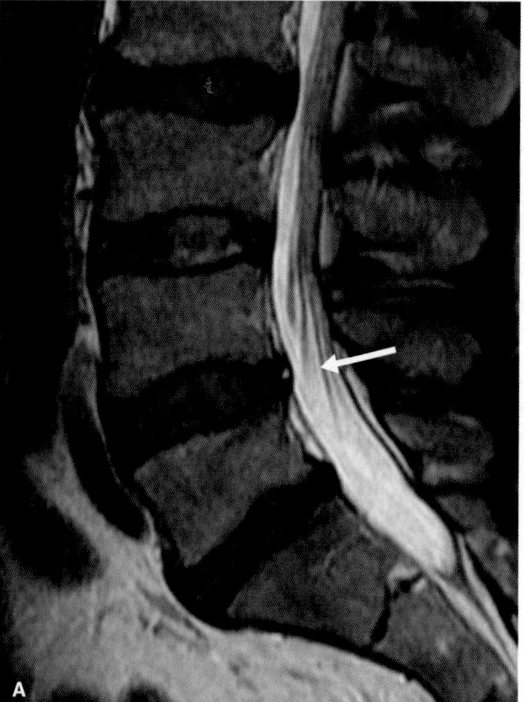

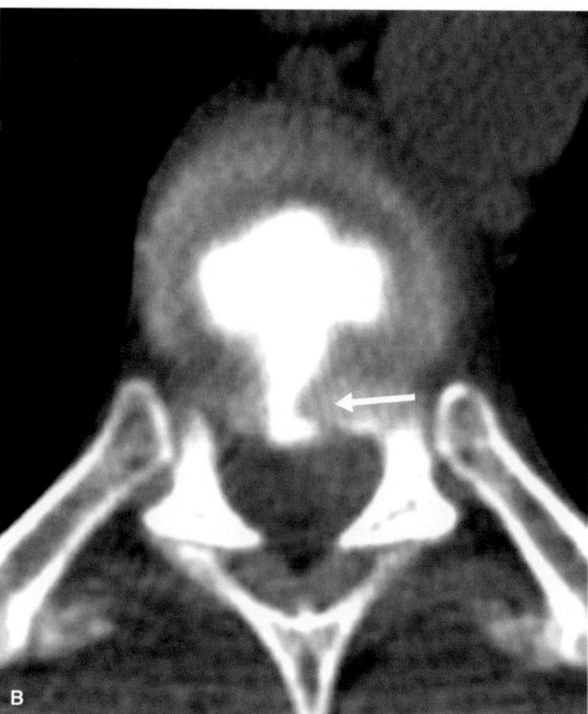

FIGURE 9.42. **Posterior Annular Fissure. A:** The sagittal T2WI shows the lumbar discs to be abnormally low in signal, indicating disc degeneration. The annular fissure is high signal (*arrow*), and thus also known as a "high-intensity zone" (HIZ). **B:** An axial CT discogram showing example of an opacified radial fissure (*arrow*).

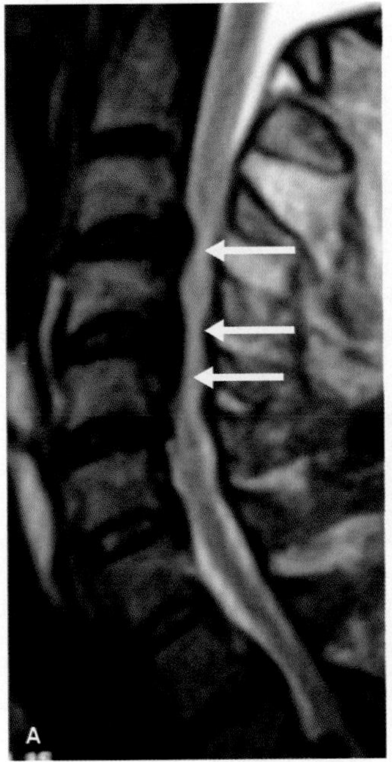

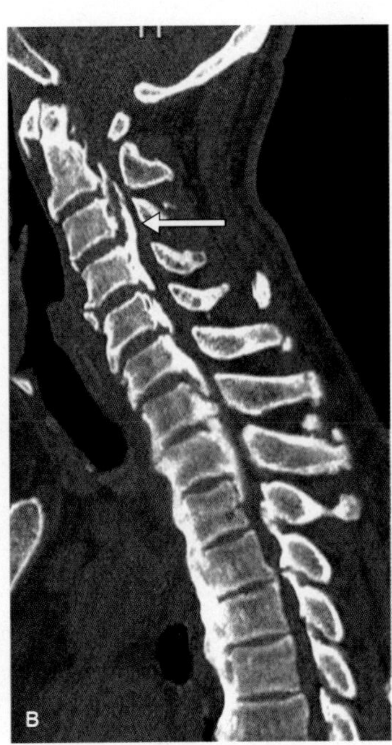

FIGURE 9.43. Ossification of the Posterior Longitudinal Ligament (OPLL). A: Sagittal T2WI image shows confluent wavy low signal intensity within the thickened posterior longitudinal ligament (*arrows*), which could be mistaken for multiple disc extrusions. **B:** Sagittal CT in another patient shows OPLL with better clarity.

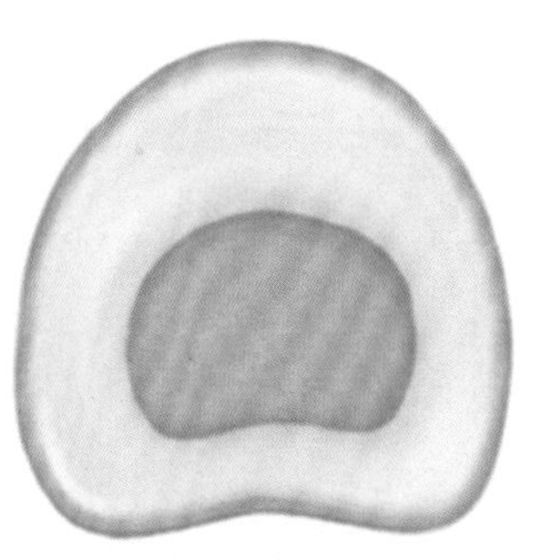

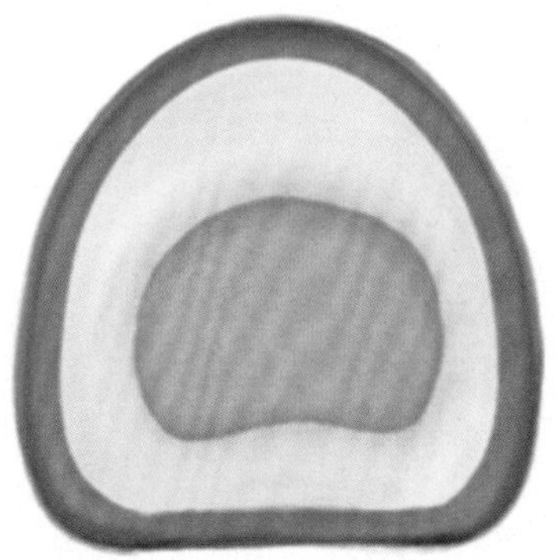

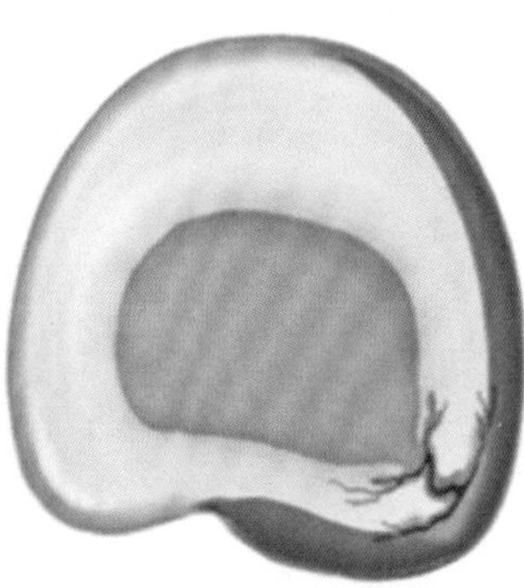

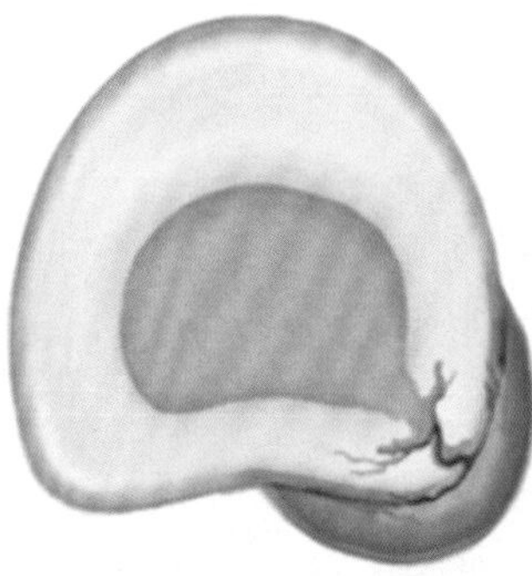

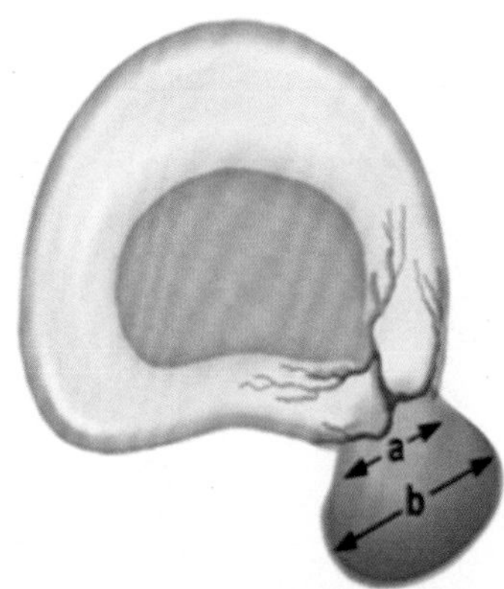

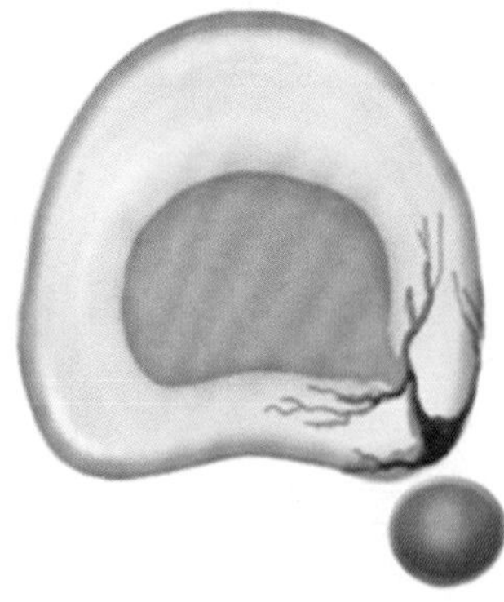

FIGURE 9.44. Summary of Disc nomenclature Based on 2014 Consensus Document. Fardon DF, Williams, AL, Dohring EJ, et al. Lumbar Disc Nomenclature: Version 2.0: Recommendations of the Combined Task Forces of the North American Spine Society, the American Society of Spine Radiology, and the American Society of Neuroradiology. *Spine J* 2014;14(11):2525–2545.

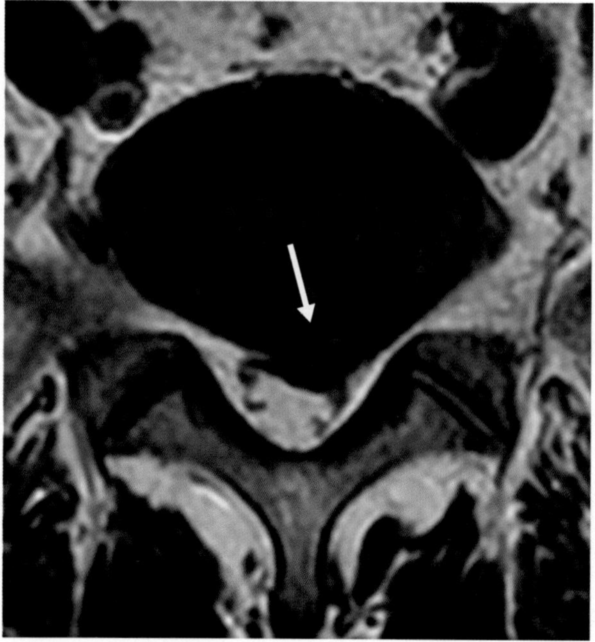

FIGURE 9.45. **Disc Protrusion.** Axial MR image shows left central L4–L5 disc protrusion (*arrow*). Because it is displacing the traversing left L5 nerve root, it could cause symptoms.

and many disc herniations can resorb over time. A disc simultaneously may have more than one herniation. The lexicon described in the lumbar disc nomenclature document is also useful when reporting cervical and thoracic disc disease.

Disc Bulge. A "bulge" involves greater than 25% of the circumference of the disc, and may result from disc degeneration, ligamentous laxity, or bony remodeling. A disc bulge, by definition, is not a disc herniation. Mild disc bulging at L5–S1 <2 mm is considered a normal variant.

Disc Protrusion. A protrusion is defined as displaced disc material extending beyond less than 25% of the disc space, with the greatest measure in any plane being less than the measure of the base (Fig. 9.45). A protrusion has a broad base at its origin, and does not extend above or below the level of the disc in the sagittal plane.

Disc Extrusion. An extrusion is defined as a herniation where the greatest measure of the herniated material is greater than the base at the site of origin. Any disc herniation extending above or below the disc space level should be called an extrusion (Fig. 9.46). The presence of an extrusion, by definition, implies that there is an annular disruption. Extrusions are subclassified as sequestrations if the displaced disc material has lost continuity with the parent disc (Fig. 9.47). The term *migration* signifies displacement of the herniated disc material away from the site of the extrusion. A sequestration can migrate either cephalad or caudally, with about equal

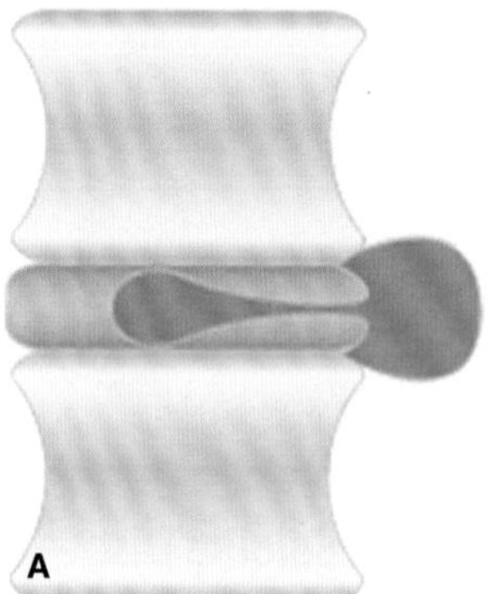

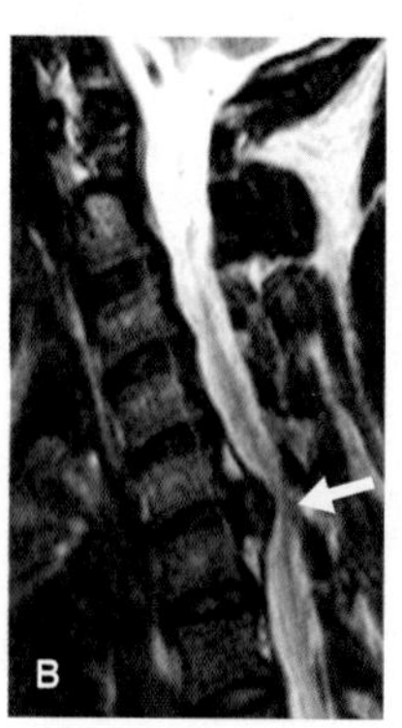

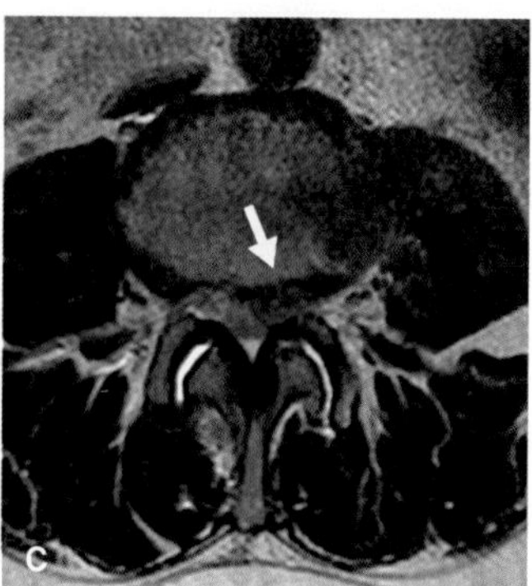

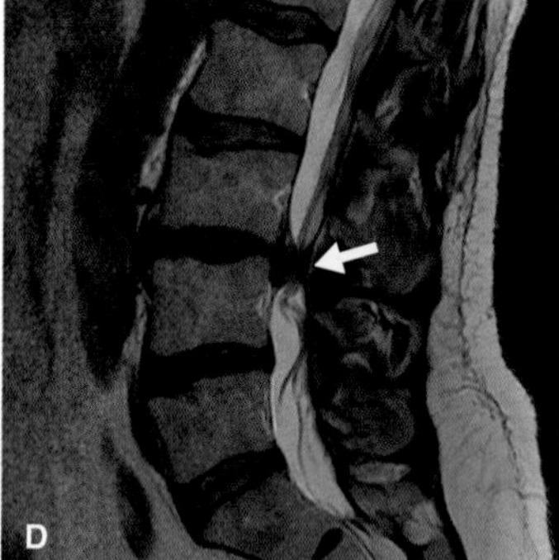

FIGURE 9.46. **Extrusion. A:** Diagram of extrusion (http://radsource.us/spine-nomenclature/). **B:** Sagittal T2-weighted cervical MRI shows an extrusion which is broader at the apex than its base and extends above and below the disc space level. This extrusion is seen elevating the posterior longitudinal ligament (*arrow*). **C, D:** Lumbar disc extrusion (*arrows*.)

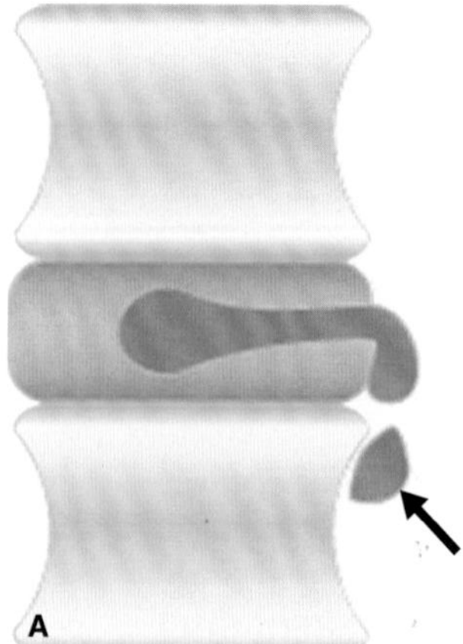

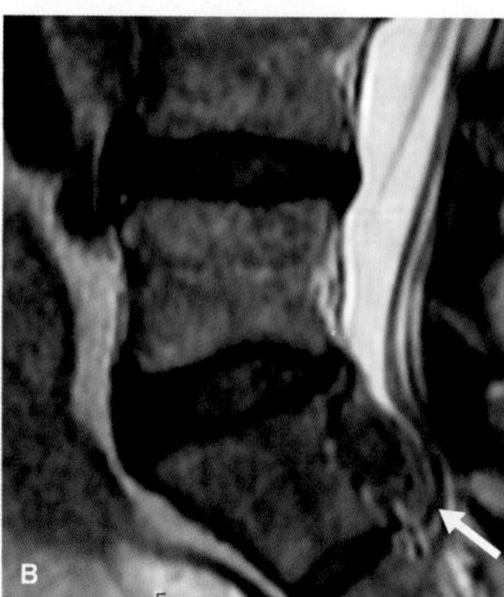

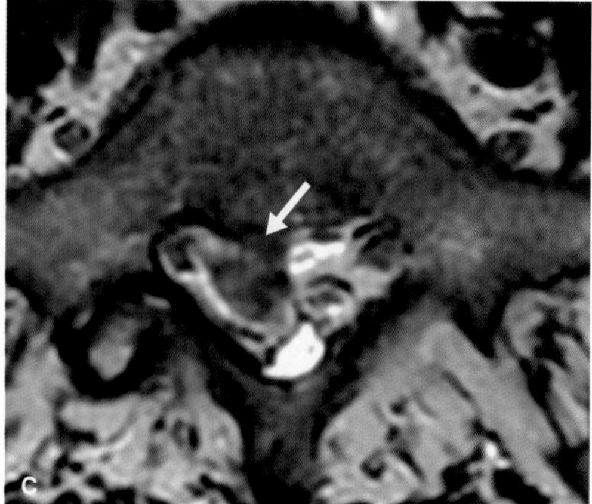

FIGURE 9.47 Sequestration With Caudal Migration. A: Diagram (http://radsource.us/spine-nomenclature/). **B, C:** A fragment of extruded disc material (sequestration) which has separated from the parent disc and has migrated into the right S1 lateral recess (*arrows*). It is seen medial to the S1 root and displacing S2 root, and has mass effect on both.

likelihood. Missing a sequestration can be a cause of failed back surgery. At the very least, the presence of a sequestration means the surgeon must explore more cephalad or caudal in order to remove the free fragment.

Disc Herniation Location

In the axial plane, location of a disc herniation includes central, subarticular, foraminal, extraforaminal, and anterior (Fig. 9.48). The terms right central or left central should replace the use of the term "paracentral" according to the latest nomenclature, but this term is still widely used. The term far lateral is sometimes used synonymously with extraforaminal. Extraforaminal herniations, although not common (<5% of cases) are frequently overlooked, and are a known source of failed back surgery. Because they affect the already exited root, they can mimic symptoms of a disc protrusion from one level more cephalad. For example, in a patient who has multilevel disc disease and symptoms referable to the L3–L4 disc, the disc protrusion may be compressing the traversing L4 nerve root. A lateral or far lateral disc at L4–L5, however, could compress the L4 nerve root and cause the exact same symptoms (Fig. 9.49). If not reported correctly, surgery might be performed at the L3–L4 disc, which is the wrong level! Notifying the surgeon that the disc is lateral to the neural foramen is critical, because the standard surgical approach through the lamina will not allow removal of a far lateral disc.

Herniated discs in the craniocaudal direction through a gap in the vertebral body endplate are referred to as intravertebral herniations or "Schmorl nodes."

SPINAL STENOSIS

Spinal stenosis is encroachment of the bony or soft tissue structures of the spine on one or more of the neural elements, with resulting symptoms. Classically it is divided into congenital and acquired types; however, even the most severe forms of congenital stenosis do not cause symptoms unless a there is component of acquired stenosis (usually degenerative disease of the facets and the discs). A more useful classification of stenosis is on an anatomic basis: central canal, lateral recess and neural foramen. As with disc disease, imaging findings must be matched with clinical findings. Patients can have severe stenosis severe on MRI yet be completely asymptomatic! Incidental stenosis is often seen when screening elderly patients for spinal metastases.

Central Canal Stenosis. Although measurements are tempting when diagnosing central canal stenosis, a subjective assessment as to whether the stenosis (usually in an anteroposterior direction) is mild, moderate, or severe is usually all that is necessary for evaluating the central canal. Absence of any visible CSF within the thecal sac implies severe stenosis, and would probably mean a complete block if a myelogram was performed. An AP spinal canal measurement of 10 mm or greater is considered to be within normal limits in most published articles.

The most common cause of central canal stenosis is degenerative disease of the facets, with bony arthritis that encroaches

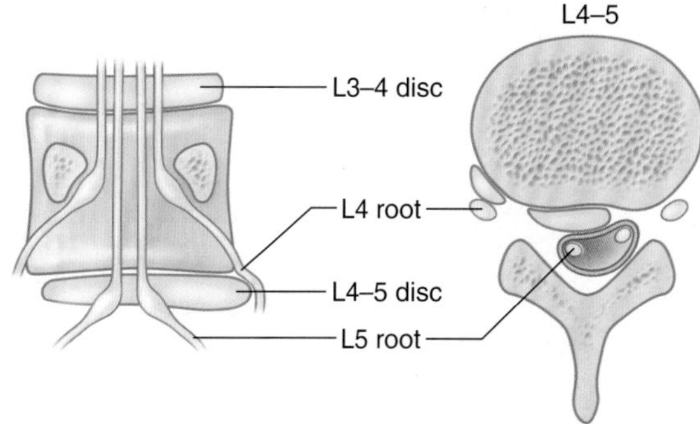

FIGURE 9.49. Schematic of Lateral Disc. This schematic illustrates how a posterior L4–L5 disc protrusion affects the L5 nerve root, yet a lateral L4–L5 disc affects the L4 root.

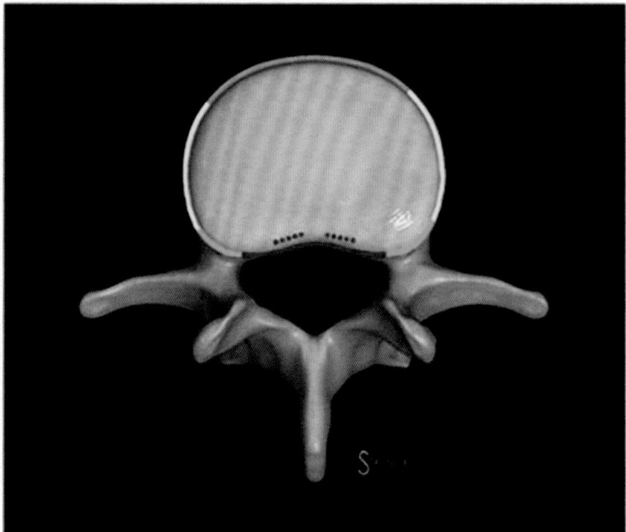

FIGURE 9.48. Zone Map Describing Location of Disc Herniations. Central or right/left central (*red*), subarticular (*blue*), foraminal (*green*), extraforaminal or far lateral (*yellow*) or anterior (*gray*). (From http://radsource.us/spine-nomenclature/)

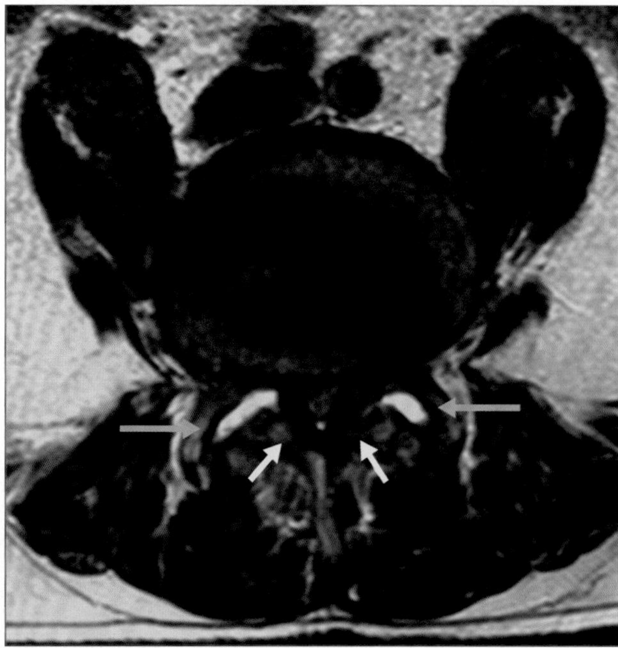

FIGURE 9.50. Spinal Stenosis. An axial T2WI demonstrates severe central canal stenosis with no cerebrospinal fluid seen in the thecal sac. There is a disc bulge, buckling of the ligamentum flavum (*short yellow arrows*) and bilateral facet arthritis with facet effusions (*blue arrows*).

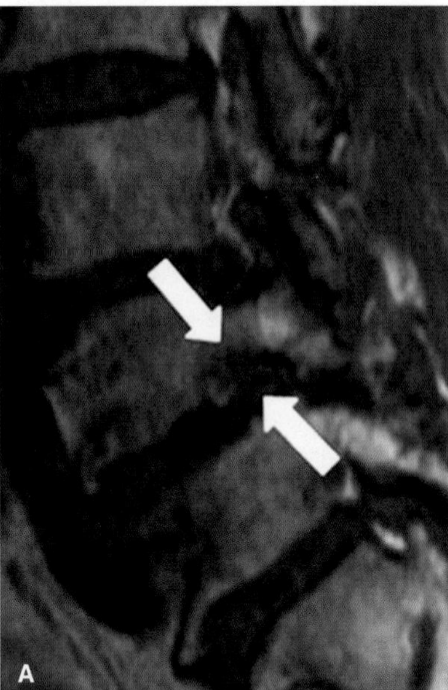
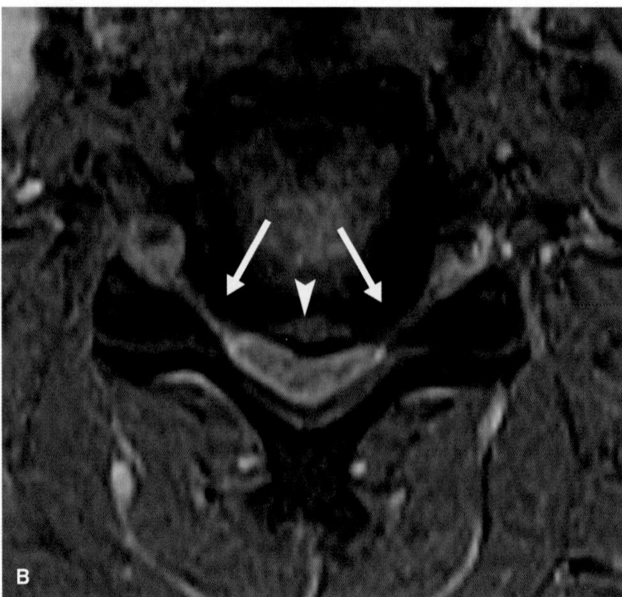

FIGURE 9.51. **Severe Neural Foraminal Stenosis. A:** Sagittal T1WI lumbar MRI shows obliteration of perineural fat and visible nerve root compression. *Arrows* indicate the flattening of the exiting L4 root in the L4–L5 foramen. **B:** Axial cervical gradient echo MRI shows foraminal stenosis due to uncovertebral joint spurring (*arrows*). The patient also has central stenosis due to a disc protrusion (*arrowhead*).

on the central canal. This is also the most common cause of lateral recess stenosis. When the facets undergo degenerative joint disease (DJD), they often have some slippage, which results in buckling of the ligamentum flavum. This is a common cause of central canal stenosis (Fig. 9.50). Frequently disc bulging exacerbates the central canal stenosis.

Neural Foramen Stenosis. DJD of the facets is the most common cause of neuroforaminal stenosis; however, encroachment on the nerve root in the neural foramen can be seen from a lateral disc herniation and spondylolisthesis (Figs. 9.49, 9.51A and 9.52). The lumbar neuroforamina are seen on axial images, just cephalad to the disc space level. The disc space lies at the inferior portion of the neural foramen, and the exiting nerve root lies in the superior or cephalad portion of the neural foramen.

In the cervical spine, the uncovertebral joints (which help stabilize the vertebrae) develop degenerative spurs that narrow the foramina anteromedially (Fig. 9.51B). These joints and their corresponding spurs are not present in the thoracic or lumbar spine.

Lateral Recess Stenosis. The lateral recesses are the bony canals in which the nerve roots lie after they leave the thecal sac and before they enter the neural foramen. Arthritic spurs of the superior articular facet from DJD are the most common cause of encroachment on the lateral recesses. As with the neural foramen, a disc herniation or bulge also can cause nerve root impingement.

Spondylolysis and Spondylolisthesis. Defects in the bony pars interarticularis (spondylolysis) are found in up to 10%

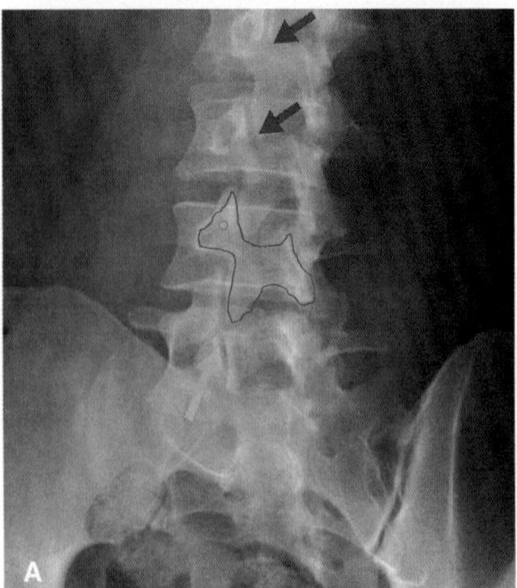
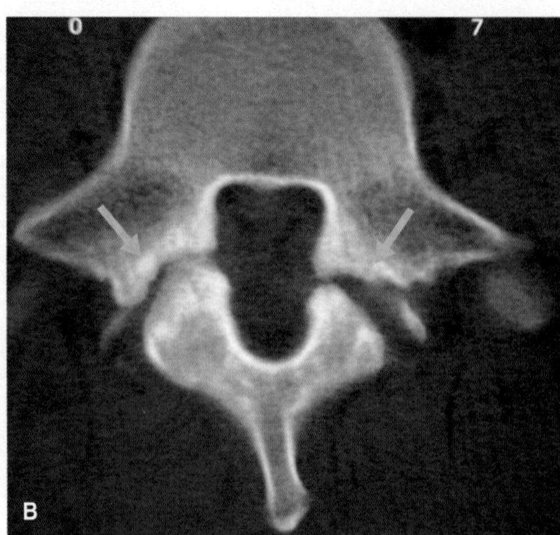
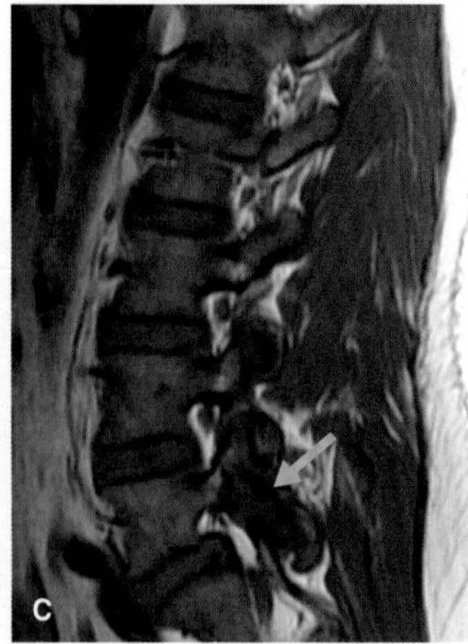

FIGURE 9.52. **Spondylolysis. A:** Oblique x-ray shows a bony defect (*blue arrow*) in the L5 pars interarticularis, also known as the neck of the "Scotty Dog," fractured in this case. A companion intact "Scotty dog" is outlined (to help your imagination) at the L4 level in red, with an intact neck, and a blue eye drawn in! *Red arrows* show intact pars interarticularis at L2 and L3. **B:** An axial CT scan image shows the discontinuity in the bony laminae bilaterally (*arrows*), which indicates the pars fracture. **C:** Sagittal MRI in another patient shows the more subtle appearance of the pars defect.

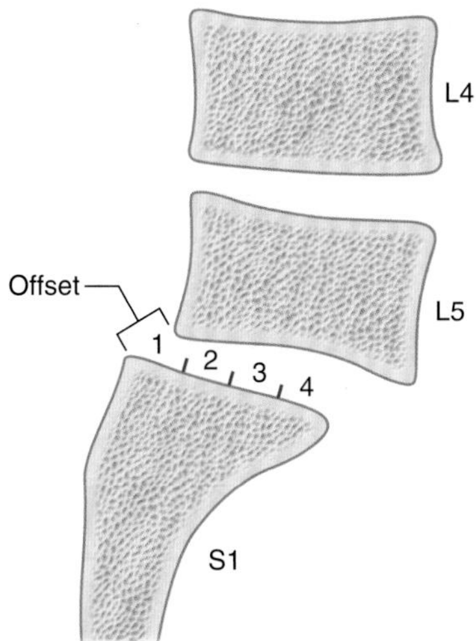

FIGURE 9.53. **Spondylolisthesis Grading Scale.** This schematic shows the grading scale used to gauge the degree of spondylolisthesis. This example would be a Grade I spondylolisthesis because the posterior edge of the slipped L5 vertebral body lies above the first quadrant of the S1 vertebral body.

of asymptomatic individuals, and can be seen on oblique plain films (Fig. 9.52A). They can be a source of low back pain and instability. Prior to disc surgery or other back surgeries, the identification of any spondylolysis is imperative. Failure to note and evaluate spondylolysis is a known source of failed back surgery.

CT is superior to MR imaging at identifying spondylolysis. Spondylolysis is identified on the axial images through the midvertebral body as a break in the normally intact bony ring of the lamina (Fig. 9.52B). Although MR will show spondylolysis defects, these defects can sometimes be very difficult to see (Fig. 9.52C).

Spondylolisthesis (forward displacement of one vertebral body on a lower one) occurs from either slippage of two vertebral bodies following bilateral spondylolysis, or from DJD of the facets with slippage of the facets. If spondylolisthesis is severe, it may result in central canal stenosis, but typically neural foraminal stenosis occurs first. It is most common at L4–L5 and L5–S1 levels.

The Meyerding grading scale is widely used to describe the degree of spondylolisthesis. The more caudal vertebral body is divided into fourths, and the posterior corner of the more cephalad vertebral body is marked at the position where it has slipped forward. If it has slipped forward only into the first quarter of the more caudal vertebral body, it is a Grade I spondylolisthesis (Fig. 9.53). The classification can be summarized as follows: Grade I: 0% to 25%; Grade II: 25% to 50%; Grade III: 50% to 75%; Grade IV: 75% to 100%; and Grade V: greater than 100% (Fig. 9.53).

POSTOPERATIVE CHANGES

Unfortunately, failed back surgery is common. Causes are inadequate surgery (including missed sequestration or lateral disc), failure of a fusion, infection, and development of adjacent level disc disease. CT is useful in evaluating spinal fusions. The signs of pseudarthrosis (failed fusion) on CT may include the presence of a lucent halo around an interbody cage signifying lack of bony incorporation and subsidence of a cage into the vertebral body through a weakness of the

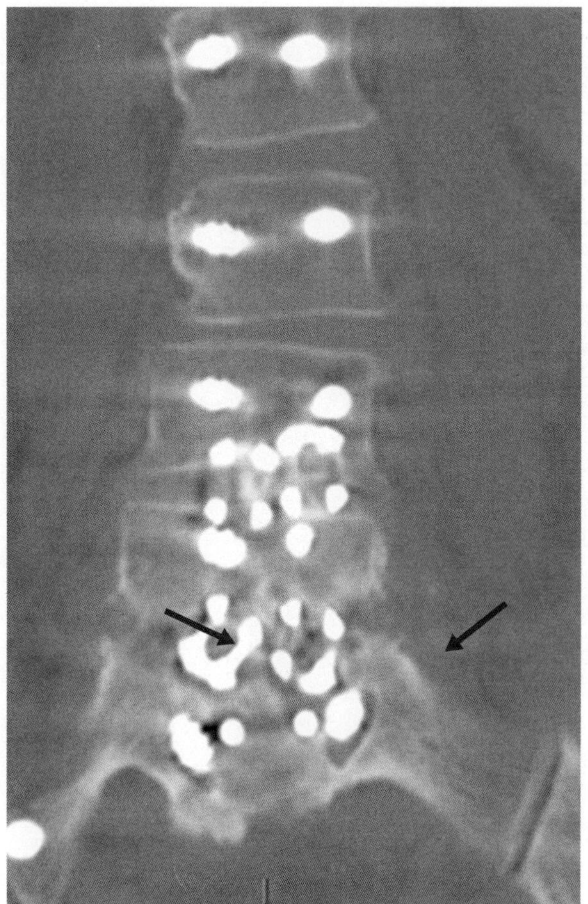

FIGURE 9.54. **Pseudarthrosis.** Coronal CT shows subsidence of cages into the vertebral bodies and lucencies around hardware.

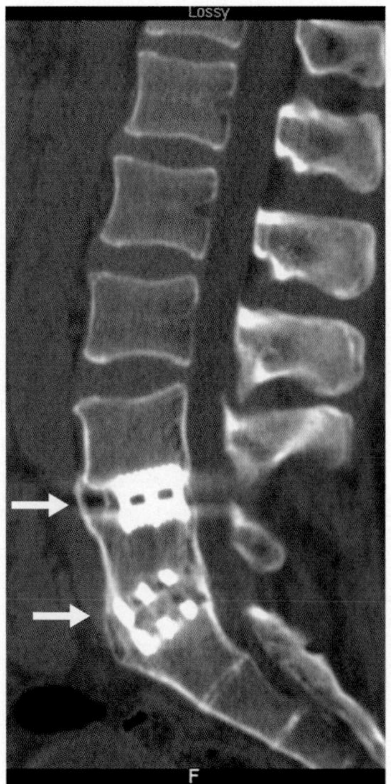

FIGURE 9.55. Sagittal CT shows solid fusion with bone bridging (*arrows*) and incorporation of interbody cages.

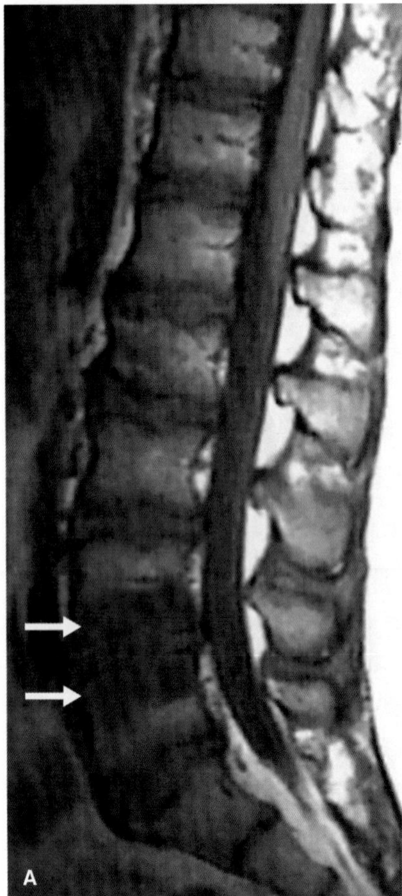

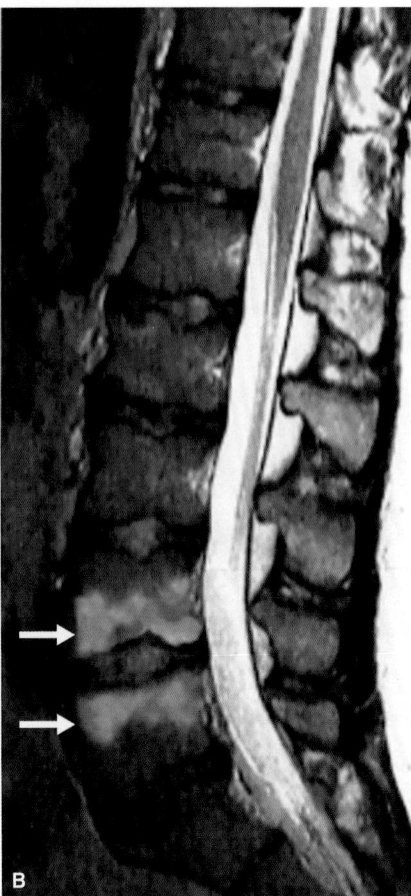

FIGURE 9.56. **Modic Type I Fibrovascular Marrow Changes.** (**A**) Sagittal T1-weighted image in a patient with degenerative disc disease at L4–L5 shows bands of low signal parallel to the end plates (*arrows*). (**B**) These bands become bright on sagittal T2WI (*arrows*). This represents fibrovascular granulation tissue, which may enhance postcontrast. Infection should be considered if bright fluid signal is seen in the disc. For a discussion of the DWI appearance of Modic Type I changes, see Figure 9.10.

endplate (Fig. 9.54). Lucency or pullback of pedicle screws may indicate loose or infected hardware. CT is also helpful in demonstrating incorporation of posterior bone graft material and osseous fusion of facet joints. Bony bridging across the disc space is a CT sign of successful anterior fusion (Fig. 9.55). Fatty marrow ingrowth across the fused disc level is an MRI finding of intact fusion. MR with contrast may be helpful in distinguishing recurrent disc herniation from scar tissue in the setting of discectomy. Many centers have omitted the routine use of gadolinium in the postoperative spine, with the exception of infection.

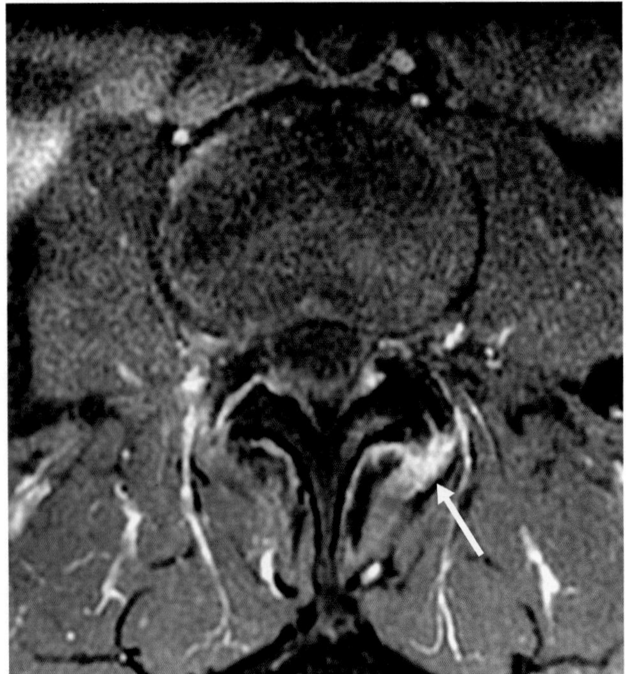

FIGURE 9.57. **Facet Synovitis.** Perifacet enhancement (*arrow*) is best seen on postcontrast T1-weighted fat-suppression imaging.

Bony Abnormalities

Fibrovascular Endplate Marrow Changes. Parallel bands of abnormal signal adjacent to the vertebral body end plates are often seen in association with degenerative disc disease. Please see Table 9.4 for a summary of the Modic Classification, named after the author who first described these changes, and their pathologic correlates.

TABLE 9.4

MODIC TYPE I–III ENDPLATE MARROW CHANGES

- Type I: dark on T1—bright on T2
  - Fibrovascular ingrowth (increased fluid)
- Type II: bright on T1—dark on T2
  - Fatty change (chronic irritation)
- Type III: dark on T1—dark on T2
  - Sclerotic change (end stage)

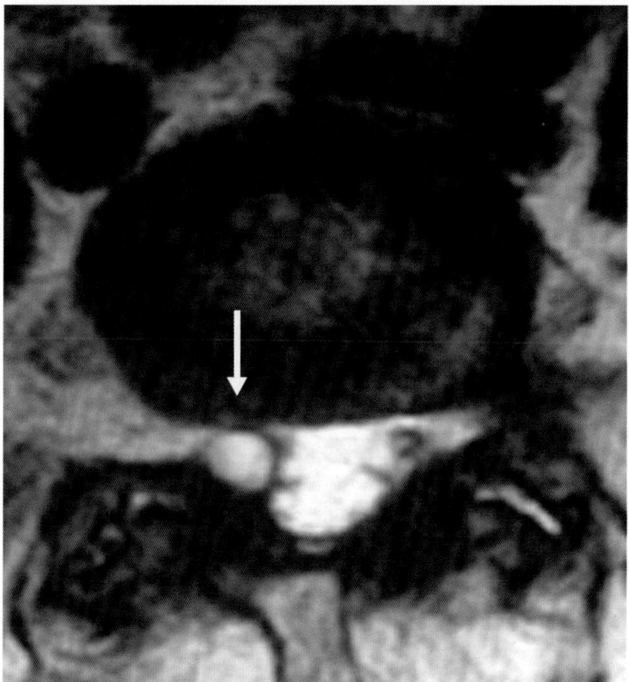

FIGURE 9.58. Typical appearance of intraspinal synovial cyst (*arrow*) projecting into the lateral recess and arising from adjacent degenerated facet joint. The cyst is displacing the traversing nerve root medially.

Modic Type I changes are subcortical low signal bands parallel to the end plates on T1WI, which become bright on T2WI (Fig. 9.56). This usually represents an inflammatory response to degenerative disc disease, but can also be a sign of infection. DWI can be useful to make the distinction between Modic Type I change and infection (Fig. 9.10), as can contrast administration.

Modic Type II changes, the most common appearance, are paired high signal bands on T1WI that remain bright on T2WI. These represent fatty marrow conversion of the previously inflamed bone.

Modic Type III changes are parallel bands of low signal adjacent to the end plates on both T1WI and T2WI. Type III changes represent end-stage bony sclerosis, which can also be seen on plain films. The endplates regions are dark as there is little water or fat within the dense sclerotic bone, not unlike sclerotic prostate cancer metastases (Fig. 9.28).

If you are familiar with acute and chronic appearance of degenerative diseases of joints (such as the knee), there is a clear parallel; repetitive microscopic bone injuries progress from edema, to fatty replacement, and then to bony sclerosis over time.

Facet Disease. Facet disease is a common and often unrecognized source of back pain. Facet synovitis may be associated with facet effusions (Fig. 9.50). Perifacet enhancement can be seen on postcontrast T1-weighted fat-suppression imaging (Fig. 9.57). Facet syndromes can be treated with radiofrequency facet denervation of the medial branches of the sinuvertebral nerves, which supply the facet joints. Another complication of facet disease is the development of synovial cysts. This is most commonly seen in the lumbar spine, but may also occur in the cervical spine (Fig. 9.58). Synovial cysts can potentially be treated with a minimally invasive image-guided injection into the adjacent facet joint or directly into the cyst, which may result in cyst rupture in up to one-third of cases.

Suggested Readings

Aghakhani N, Parker F, David P, et al. Curable cause of paraplegia: spinal dural arteriovenous fistulae. *Stroke* 2008;39:2756–2759.

Atlas S, ed. *Magnetic Resonance Imaging of the Brain and Spine*. 5th ed. Philadelphia, PA: Lippincott Williams & Wilkins; 2016.

Berquist TH. Imaging of the postoperative spine. *Radiol Clin North Am* 2006; 44:407–418.

Birnbaum J, Petri M, Thompson R, Izbudak I, Kerr D. Distinct subtypes of myelitis in systemic lupus erythematosus. *Arthritis Rheum* 2009;60: 3378–3387.

Bley TA, Duffek CC, François CJ, et al. Presurgical localization of the artery of Adamkiewicz with real time resolved 3.0-T MR angiography. *Radiology* 2010;255:873–881.

Cuénod CA, Laredo JD, Chevret S, et al. Acute vertebral collapse due to osteoporosis or malignancy: appearance on unenhanced and gadolinium-enhanced MR images. *Radiology* 1996;199:541–549.

DeSanto J, Ross JS. Spine infection/inflammation. *Radiol Clin North Am* 2011; 49:105–127.

Fardon DF, Williams, AL, Dohring EJ, et al. Lumbar Disc Nomenclature: Version 2.0: Recommendations of the Combined Task Forces of the North American Spine Society, the American Society of Spine Radiology, and the American Society of Neuroradiology. *Spine J* 2014;14(11):2525–2545.

Friedman DP, Flanders AE. Enhancement of gray matter in anterior spinal infarction. *AJNR Am J Neuroradiol* 1992;13:983–985.

Hong SH, Choy JY, Lee JW, Kim NR, Choi JA, Kang HS. MR imaging of the spine: infection or imitation? *Radiographics* 2009;29:599–612.

Jain AK. Tuberculosis of the spine: a fresh look at an old disease. *J Bone Joint Surg Br* 2010;92:905–913.

Koeller KK, Rosenblum RS, Morrison AL. Neoplasms of the spinal cord and filum terminale: radiologic–pathologic correlation. *Radiographics* 2000; 20:1721–1749.

Krings T, Lasjaunias PL, Hans FJ, et al. Imaging in spinal vascular disease. *Neuroimaging Clin N Am* 2007;17:57–72.

Ledermann HP, Schweitzer ME, Morrison WB, Carrino JA. MR imaging findings in spinal infections: rules or myths? *Radiology* 2003;228:506–514.

Looby S, Flanders A. Spine trauma. *Radiol Clin North Am* 2011;49:129–163.

Miyanji F, Furlan JC, Aarabi B, Arnold PM, Fehlings MG. Acute cervical traumatic spinal cord injury: MR imaging findings correlated with neurologic outcomes—prospective study with 100 consecutive patients. *Radiology* 2007;243:820–827.

Modic MT, Steinberg PM, Ross JS, Masaryk TJ, Carter JR. Degenerative disk disease: assessment of changes in vertebral body marrow with MR imaging. *Radiology*. 1988;166 (1): 193–199.

Mulkey SB, Glaiser CM, El-Nabbout B, et al. Nerve root enhancement in spinal MRI in pediatric Guillain Barré syndrome. *Pediatric Neurol* 2010;43: 263–269.

Nguyen GK, Clark R. Adequacy of plain radiography in the diagnosis of cervical spine injuries. *Emerg Radiol* 2005;11:158–161.

Patel KB, Poplawski MM, Pawha PS, Naidich TP, Tanenbaum LN. Diffusion-weighted MRI "claw sign" improves differentiation of infectious from degenerative Modic type 1 signal changes of the spine. *AJNR Am J Neuroradiol* 2014: 35:1647–1652

Poonawalla AH, Hou P, Nelson FA, Wolinsky JS, Narayana PA. Cervical spinal cord lesions in multiple sclerosis: T1-weighted inversion-recovery MR imaging with phase sensitive reconstruction. *Radiology* 2008;246:258–264.

Quencer RM, Post MJ. Spinal cord lesions in patients with AIDS. *Neuroimaging Clin N Am* 1997;7:359–373.

Raya JG, Dietrich O, Reiser MF, Baur-Melnyk A. Methods and applications of diffusion imaging of vertebral bone marrow. *J Magn Reson Imaging* 2006;24:1207–1220.

Reijnierse M, Dijkmans BA, Hansen B, et al. Neurologic dysfunction in patients with rheumatoid arthritis of the cervical spine. Predictive value of clinical, radiographic and MR imaging parameters. *Eur Radiol* 2001;11:467–473.

Rosenblum B, Oldfield EH, Doppman JL, Di Chiro G. Spinal arteriovenous malformations: a comparison of dural arteriovenous fistulas and intradural AVMs in 81 patients. *J Neurosurg* 1987;67:795–802.

Ross JS, Moore KR. *Diagnostic Imaging: Spine*. Salt Lake City, UT: Elsevier; 2016.

Wang PY, Shen WC, Jan JS. Serial MRI changes in radiation myelopathy. *Neuroradiology* 1995;37:374–377.

Wnuk NM, Alkasab TK, Rosenthal DI. Magnetic resonance imaging of the lumbar spine: determining clinical impact and potential harm from overuse. *Spine J*. 2018. pii: S1529-9430(18)30159-1. doi: 10.1016/j.spinee.2018.04.005.

Yoshikawa T, Hayashi N, Yamamoto S, et al. Brachial plexus injury: clinical manifestations, conventional imaging findings, and the latest imaging techniques. *Radiographics* 2006;26:S133–S143 (published online).

SECTION III

CHEST

SECTION EDITOR: Jeffrey S. Klein

CHAPTER 10 ■ METHODS OF EXAMINATION, NORMAL ANATOMY, AND RADIOGRAPHIC FINDINGS OF CHEST DISEASE

JUDY K. TAM AND JEFFREY S. KLEIN

A variety of imaging techniques are available to the radiologist for the evaluation of chest disease. The decision regarding which imaging procedures to perform depends upon many factors, the most important of which are patient age, the availability of various modalities, and the type of information sought. Conventional radiographs of the chest still constitute the most common diagnostic imaging study performed in most radiology departments. The volume of chest CT examinations has dramatically increased in the past 5 to 10 years given its widespread availability and an expanding list of indications for chest CT, including the evaluation of acute aortic disease, trauma evaluation, solitary pulmonary nodule assessment, diagnosis of pulmonary embolism, lung cancer screening, and characterization and monitoring of diffuse lung disease.

IMAGING MODALITIES

Conventional Chest Radiography. Posteroanterior (PA) and lateral chest radiographs are the mainstays of thoracic imaging. Conventional radiographs should be performed as the initial imaging study in most patients with suspected thoracic disease. These radiographs are obtained in most radiology departments on a dedicated chest unit capable of obtaining radiographs with a focus-to-film distance of 6 feet, a high kilovoltage potential (140-kVp) technique, a grid to reduce scatter, and a phototimer to control the length of exposure.

The recognition of proper radiographic technique on frontal radiographs involves assessment of four basic features: *penetration, rotation, inspiration,* and *motion*. Proper penetration is present when there is faint visualization of the thoracic intervertebral disk spaces and discrete branching vessels can be identified through the cardiac shadow and the diaphragm. Rotation is assessed by noting the relationship between a vertical line drawn midway between the medial cortical margins of the clavicular heads and one drawn vertically through the spinous processes of the thoracic vertebrae. Superimposition of these lines (the former in the midline anteriorly and the latter in the midline posteriorly) indicates a properly positioned, nonrotated patient. An appropriate deep inspiration in a normal individual is present when the apex of the right hemidiaphragm is visible below the 10th posterior rib. The cardiac margin, diaphragm, and pulmonary vessels should be sharply marginated in a completely still patient who has suspended respiration during the radiographic exposure (Fig. 10.1).

Portable Radiography. Portable anteroposterior (AP) radiographs are obtained when patients cannot be easily or safely mobilized. Portable radiographs help monitor a patient's cardiopulmonary status; assess the position of monitoring and life support tubes, lines, and catheters; and detect complications related to the use of these devices.

There are technical and patient-related compromises as well as inherent physiologic changes with portable bedside radiography. The maximal kilovoltage potential of portable units requires longer exposures to penetrate cardiomediastinal structures, which results in greater motion artifact. Because critically ill patients are difficult to position for portable radiographs, the patients are often rotated. Inaccuracies in directing the x-ray beam perpendicular to the patient lead to kyphotic or lordotic radiographs. The short focus-to-film distance (typically 40 in) and AP technique result in magnification of intrathoracic structures. On an AP radiograph, the apparent cardiac diameter increases by 15% to 20%, bringing the upper limit of normal for the cardiothoracic ratio from 50% on a PA

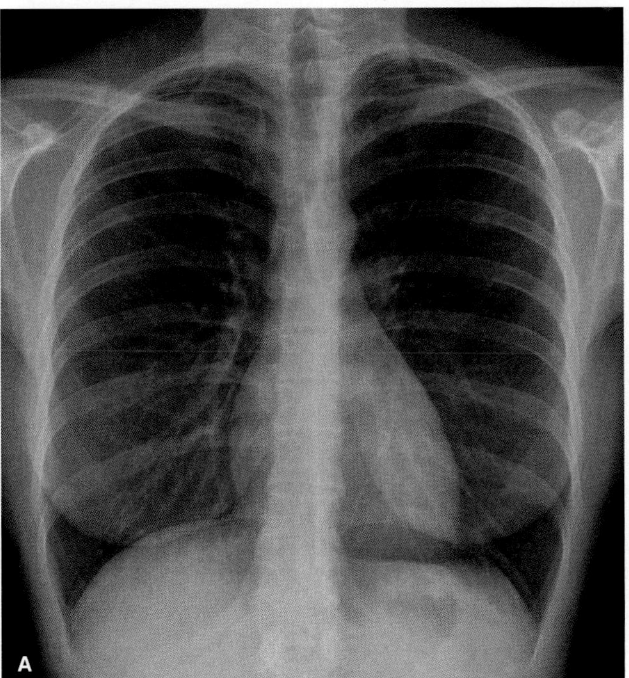

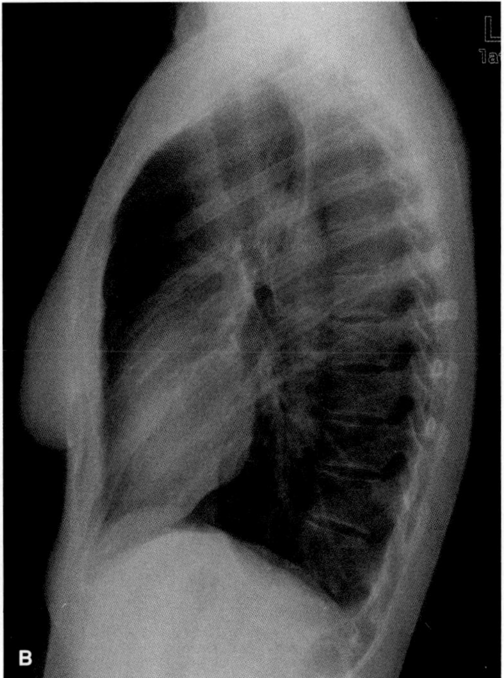

FIGURE 10.1. Normal frontal (**A**) and left lateral (**B**) chest radiographs.

radiograph to 57% on an AP radiograph. Physiologically, the supine position of patients elevates the diaphragm, thus compressing the lower lobes and decreasing lung volumes.

In the supine patient, the normal gravitational effect evens blood flow between upper and lower zones making assessment of pulmonary venous hypertension difficult. Widening of the upper mediastinum or "vascular pedicle" is due to an increase in systemic venous return to the heart. The gravitational layering of free-flowing fluid may hide small effusions. Similarly, a pneumothorax may be difficult to detect because free intrapleural air rises to a nondependent position producing subtle anteromedial or inferior radiolucency.

Digital (Computed) Radiography. The main advantages of digital chest radiography are increased dose efficiency and more consistent image quality. Contrast levels and windows can be adjusted to enhance visualization of various regions in the chest or compensate partly for suboptimal exposure. Although digital images have poorer spatial resolution than their analog counterparts, the benefits of being able to adjust the contrast levels and windows and the availability to view the image on any computer monitor through a PACS (picture archiving and communication system) have resulted in the widespread use of digital chest radiology.

Dual-energy subtraction (DES) chest radiography and *digital tomosynthesis (DTS)* of the chest are advanced radiographic techniques. In the most common form of DES, two sequential exposures at 60 keV and 120 keV are obtained in rapid sequence to produce three frontal images: a standard PA image, a bone-subtracted soft-tissue image, and a bone image (Fig. 10.2). Advantages include improved visualization of lung nodules, detection of calcification within granulomas, visualizing bone islands or healing rib fractures (Fig. 10.3), and enhanced visualization of indwelling lines and catheters.

In DTS of the chest, an x-ray tube moving in a vertical arc exposes a stand-mounted flat panel detector in a single 10- to 12-second breath hold. A series of 50 to 60 frontal tomograms each 5 mm thick are produced using filtered back projection. Uses of DTS of the chest include precise localization of opacities seen on standard two-view radiography, improved detection of nodules (Fig. 10.4), improved visualization of foreign bodies and hardware, and improved detection and characterization of parenchymal disease including airways and interstitial lung disease.

Special Techniques. A *lateral decubitus* radiograph is obtained with a horizontal x-ray beam while the patient lies in the decubitus position. It is used to detect small pleural effusions or to determine whether a pleural effusion on the decubitus side is free flowing (Fig. 10.5). A lateral decubitus radiograph is also used to detect a pneumothorax on the nondependent side. As little as 5 mL of fluid or 15 mL of air can be demonstrated on decubitus radiography.

An *expiratory radiograph* obtained at residual volume (end of maximal expiration) can detect focal or diffuse air trapping and may help in the detection of a small pneumothorax. On expiratory radiography, the volume of air in the pleural space remains stable, whereas the volume of air in the lung parenchyma decreases. Because the lung is also displaced away from the chest wall, the visceral pleural line becomes more visible.

Chest fluoroscopy is used mainly to assess for diaphragmatic paralysis. The "sniff test," in which the patient undergoes chest fluoroscopy while standing and breathes quickly and deeply through the nose, shows paradoxical upward diaphragmatic movement in patients with diaphragmatic paralysis.

Computed Tomography (CT) and High-Resolution Computed Tomography (HRCT). There are several techniques available for acquiring chest CT examinations. Chest CTs are most often acquired in a spiral mode, whereby acquisition occurs continuously while the patient steadily moves through the gantry on the CT scan table, producing a single large volume scan. For HRCT, primarily in younger patients for serial evaluation of diffuse lung disease, an axial mode with thin sections (i.e., ≤1.5 mm thickness) acquired at evenly spaced

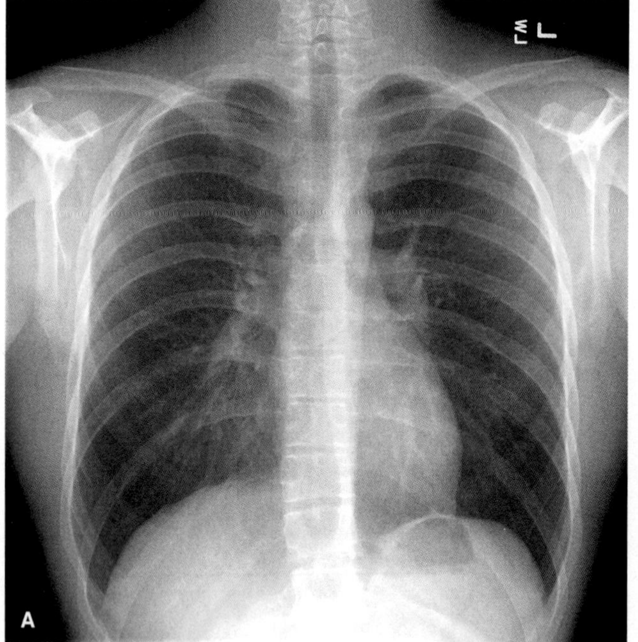

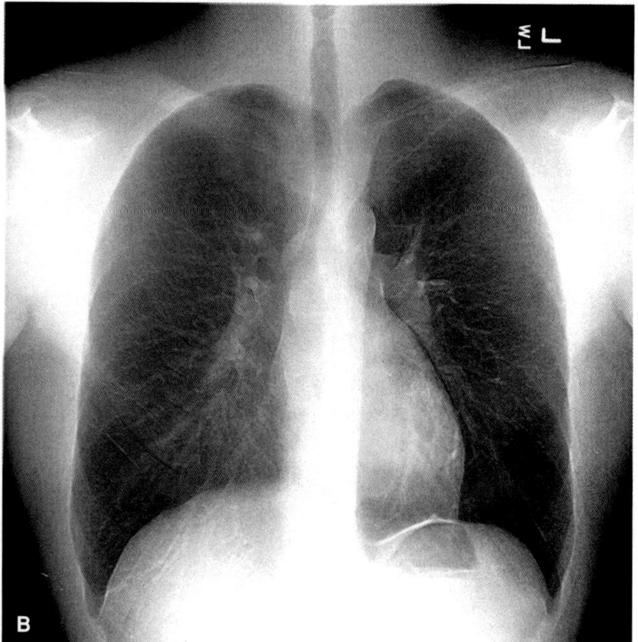

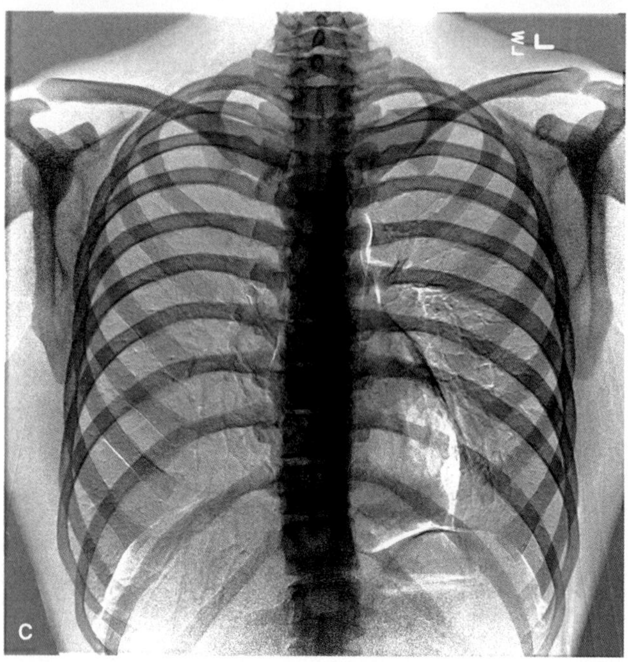

FIGURE 10.2. Dual-Exposure Dual-Energy Frontal Chest Radiographs. A: Chest image obtained at 120 keV. **B:** Soft tissue image. **C:** Bone image.

intervals from lung apices to bases is utilized. Most CT scanners use a multidetector array with 256 to 320 detectors which provides contiguous thin sections of the entire lung in a single breath-hold acquisition. Scans without contrast are usually performed for evaluation or follow-up of parenchymal disease, solitary nodules, and airways disease, whereas intravenous contrast is administered for mediastinal mass evaluation, cancer staging, systemic or pulmonary arterial evaluation, and cardiac studies.

The field of view for image reconstruction is determined by measuring the widest transverse diameter, as seen on the CT scout view. An edge-enhancing computer reconstruction ("sharp" or "lung") algorithm improves the spatial resolution of parenchymal structures and is used for most types of thoracic CT scans. A 512 × 512 matrix size is typically used for image reconstruction. Routine chest CT studies are reconstructed in the axial plane using 2.5- to 3.0-mm slice thickness. Thin-section axial and both sagittal and coronal reconstructions are sent to a PACS workstation for interpretation. Routine settings for CT display of mediastinal structures are WW (window width) = 400 and WL (window level) = 40 and for the lungs are WW = 1,500 and WL = –700.

Expiratory CT scans are useful for the detection of air trapping in patients with airways disease or to assess for the presence of tracheobronchomalacia. Normal and abnormal HRCT findings are reviewed in Chapter 16.

The major advantages of CT are its superior contrast resolution and cross-sectional display format. Superior contrast resolution allows for the differentiation of calcium, soft tissue, and fat within lung nodules or mediastinal structures. Intravenous contrast enhancement improves contrast within structures or masses, as well as within blood vessels (e.g.,

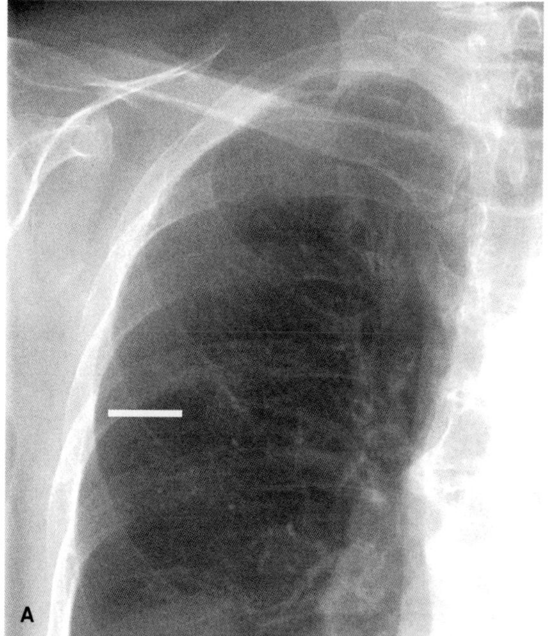

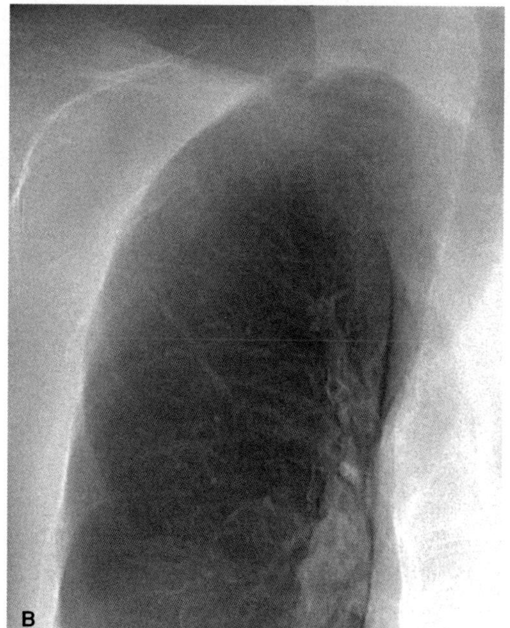

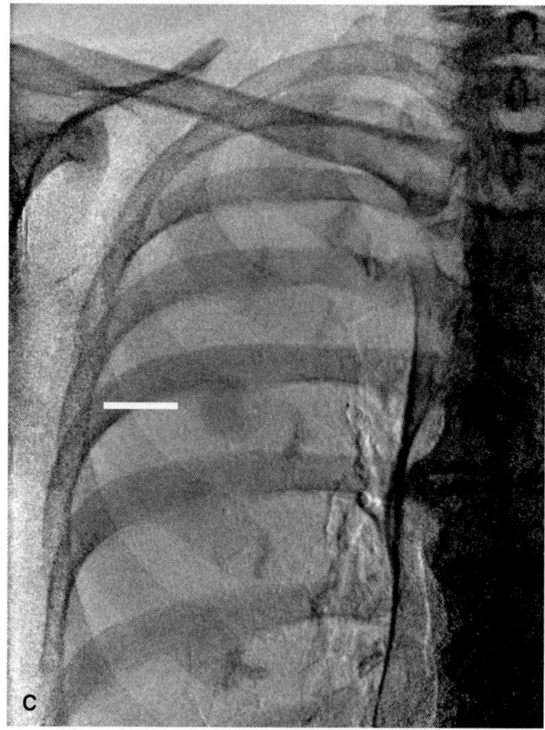

FIGURE 10.3. **Dual-Energy Chest Radiography for Evaluation of a Focal Density. A:** Coned-down view of a frontal chest radiograph shows a focal opacity (*arrow*) overlying the right upper lung. **B:** The soft tissue image with the bone subtracted shows no abnormality. **C:** The bone image shows that the density reflects a healing right anterior 3rd rib fracture (*arrow*).

pulmonary emboli, aortic dissection). The cross-sectional display eliminates the superimposition of structures and allows visualization of parenchymal nodules as small as 1 mm.

The clinical indications for chest CT vary among institutions. The indications for thoracic CT (excluding cardiac indications) are shown in Table 10.1.

Magnetic Resonance Imaging (MRI). As MRI usage expands, studies must be tailored to the individual patient. Morphologic studies usually require only spin echo T1W and T2W sequences in the axial plane. Coronal and sagittal planes are used in selected cases. Mass evaluation may benefit from fat-suppressed sequences and from gadolinium-enhanced sequences. Angiographic acquisitions are often performed with ECG-gated T1W–3D gadolinium-enhanced MR angiography. Respiratory motion is minimized by performing rapid single breath-hold acquisitions or by using respiratory compensation techniques. The latest generation of multichannel scanners with parallel imaging and faster gradients show promise in evaluation of embolic disease without the radiation exposure of CT.

The major advantages of MR are the superior contrast resolution between tumor and fat, the ability to characterize tissues based on T1 and T2 relaxation times, the ability to scan in direct or oblique sagittal and coronal planes, and the lack of need for intravenous iodinated contrast. The ability to obtain images along the long axis of the aorta and cine-MR techniques have made MR the primary modality for imaging of

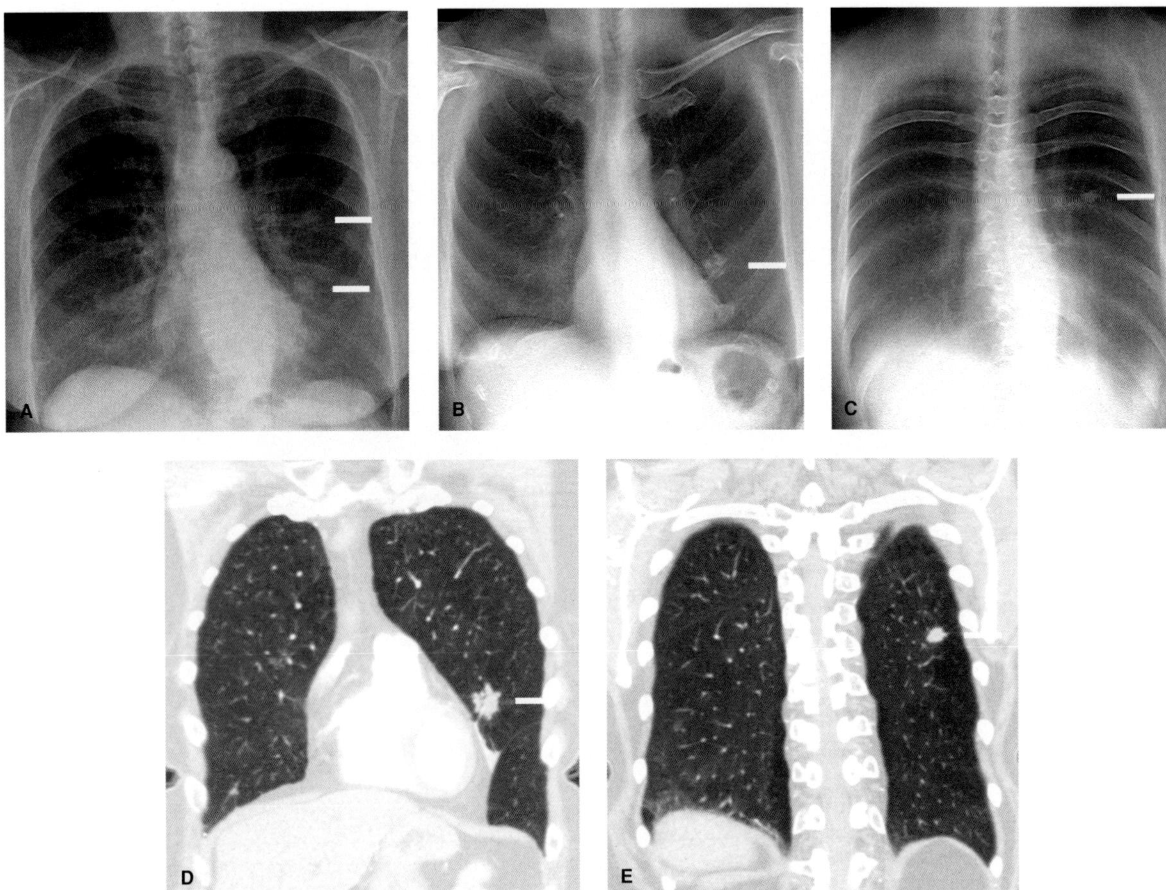

FIGURE 10.4. **Digital Tomosynthesis of the Chest (DTS) for Localization of Lung Nodules.** **A:** Frontal chest radiograph in a 72-year-old woman shows two nodular opacities in the left lung (*arrows*). **B:** Digital tomogram through the anterior chest shows a lobulated nodule in the lingula (*arrow*). **C:** Digital tomogram through the posterior chest shows a second smaller nodule in the superior segment of the left lower lobe (*arrow*). **D, E:** Coronal CT scans confirm the larger lobulated and spiculated lingular nodule (*arrow* in D) and smaller superior segment left lower lobe nodule (*arrow* in E). Biopsy of both lesions showed non–small cell carcinoma.

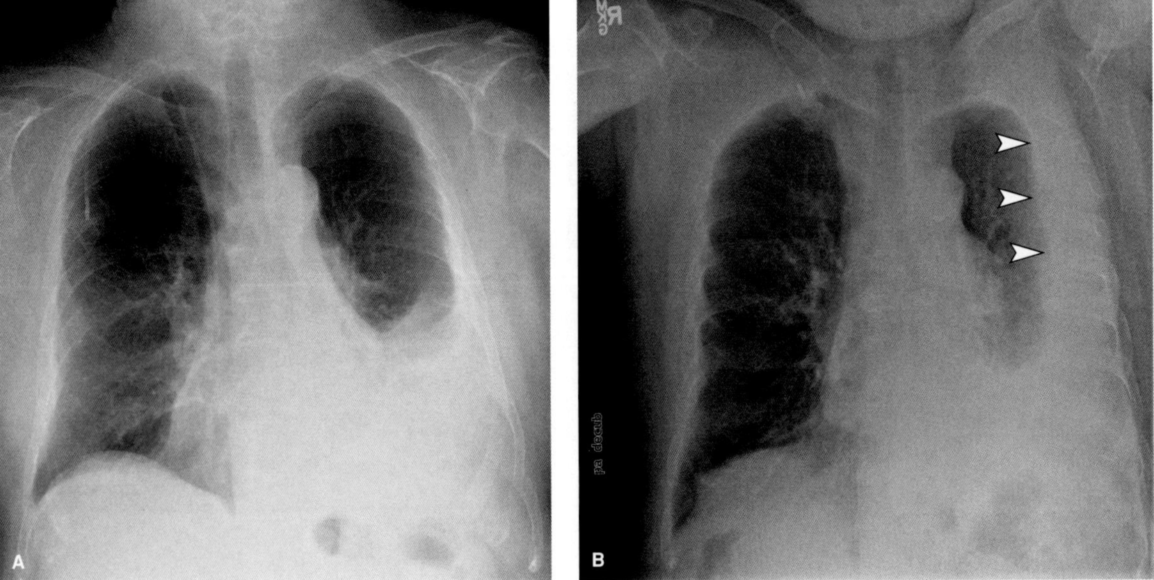

FIGURE 10.5. **Decubitus Radiography for Detecting Free-Flowing Pleural Effusion.** **A:** Upright chest radiograph demonstrates a moderate-sized left pleural effusion. **B:** Left lateral decubitus radiograph shows layering of fluid dependently (*arrowheads*) confirming a free-flowing effusion.

TABLE 10.1

COMMON INDICATIONS FOR CHEST CT

■ INDICATION	■ DETAILS
Evaluation of an abnormality identified on conventional radiography	Solitary pulmonary nodule or mass Localization and characterization of a hilar or mediastinal mass
Staging of lung cancer	Assessment of extent of the primary tumor and the relationship of the tumor to the pleura, chest wall, airways, and mediastinum Detection of hilar and mediastinal lymph node enlargement
Detection of thoracic involvement by malignancy	Extrathoracic malignancies with a propensity to involve the chest (lymphoma; breast, colon, and renal cell carcinoma; melanoma)
Evaluation of complex pleural disease	Detection of empyema Assessment for primary/metastatic pleural malignancy
Detection of pulmonary embolism	CT pulmonary angiography with high injection rate, thin collimation, and precise contrast bolus timing
Detection of lung disease in a patient with pulmonary symptoms and abnormal pulmonary function studies with normal chest radiography	Emphysema Extrinsic allergic alveolitis Small airways disease Immunocompromised patient
Evaluation of patients with chronic diffuse infiltrative lung disease for initial characterization and follow-up	Cystic fibrosis Sarcoidosis Chronic interstitial lung disease Langerhans cell histiocytosis
Lung cancer screening	Current/former smokers 55–75 with 30 pack-year history
Assessment of acute aortic abnormality	Aortic dissection and variants
Evaluation of blunt or penetrating chest injury	Traumatic aortic injury Tracheobronchial injury Esophageal rupture Complex chest wall injuries (flail chest)
Detection of lung involvement in a patient with systemic disease	Rheumatoid arthritis Scleroderma Sarcoidosis

most congenital and acquired thoracic vascular disorders. The characterization of tissues by their T1 and T2 relaxation times allows for the diagnosis of fluid-filled cysts, hemorrhage, and hematoma.

The major disadvantages of thoracic MR are limited spatial resolution, the inability to detect calcium, and difficulties in imaging the pulmonary parenchyma. MR is also more time consuming and expensive than CT. These factors, along with the ability of CT to provide superior or equivalent information in most situations, have limited the use of thoracic MR for most noncardiovascular thoracic disorders. The primary indications for thoracic MR are listed in Table 10.2.

Positron Emission Tomography (PET). PET utilizing fluorodeoxyglucose (FDG) is an imaging modality based on the metabolic activity of neoplastic and inflammatory tissues and is complementary to the anatomic information provided by chest radiography and CT. The role of PET in the chest is mostly for assessment of indeterminate solitary pulmonary nodules, staging of lung cancer, and for baseline assessment and follow-up of lymphoma.

TABLE 10.2

NONCARDIOVASCULAR INDICATIONS FOR MR OF THE THORAX

Assessment of pleural and chest wall masses
Evaluation of mediastinal, cardiovascular, and chest wall invasion by lung tumors
Distinguishing thymic hyperplasia from thymoma
Evaluation of mediastinal masses

Sonography. Transthoracic sonography is commonly used for the detection, characterization, and sampling of pleural, peripheral parenchymal, and mediastinal lesions. The aspiration of small pleural effusions visualized on real-time sonography is preferable to blind thoracentesis. Similarly, sampling of visible pleural masses in patients with malignant effusions can diminish the number of negative pleural biopsies. The aspiration of pleural-based masses and abscesses can be safely performed by ultrasound-guided needle placement into the lesion through the point of contact between the mass and pleura. Large anterior mediastinal masses that have a broad area of contact with the parasternal chest wall may be biopsied without transgressing the lung.

Real-time sonography can also confirm phrenic nerve paralysis without the use of ionizing radiation. It easily detects subpulmonic and subphrenic fluid collections, which may cause diaphragmatic elevation. In the emergency room and critical care settings, thoracic sonography is used to detect pneumothorax and to guide central venous catheterization.

Ventilation/Perfusion Lung Scanning. Ventilation/perfusion (V/Q) lung scintigraphy (see Chapter 72B) is used for the diagnosis of acute pulmonary embolism in select patients and in screening of patients with pulmonary arterial hypertension for the possibility of chronic thromboembolic pulmonary hypertension. Quantitative VQ scanning can be useful in the preoperative planning of lung resection, bullectomy, lung volume reduction surgery for emphysema, and lung transplantation.

Diagnostic pulmonary angiography is performed when CT pulmonary angiography is suboptimal or equivocal. It may also be performed immediately preceding transcatheter interventions for embolization of arteriovenous malformations or thrombolysis of large central pulmonary emboli. Thoracic aortography for traumatic aortic injury and acute nontraumatic aortic disease has also been largely replaced by CT. Evaluation of massive hemoptysis is assessed and treated by bronchial and systemic arteriography and transcatheter embolization.

Transthoracic needle biopsy guided by CT, fluoroscopy, or US is a diagnostic technique utilized in selected patients with pulmonary, pleural, or mediastinal lesions.

CT-guided ablation of lung tumors utilizing radiofrequency ablation, microwave ablation, or cryotherapy is used in the treatment of selected patients with unresectable stage 1 lung cancer and oligometastatic disease to the lungs.

Percutaneous catheter drainage of intrathoracic air or fluid collections, performed by imaging-guided placement of catheters or tubes, is used for the treatment of empyema, pneumothorax, hemothorax, malignant pleural effusion, and other intrathoracic fluid collections. Transcatheter drainage of infected pleural fluid collections is discussed under Management of Pleural Effusion in Chapter 17.

NORMAL CHEST ANATOMY

Tracheobronchial Tree (Fig. 10.6). The trachea is a hollow cylinder composed of a series of C-shaped cartilaginous rings. A flat band of muscle and connective tissue called the *posterior tracheal membrane* completes the rings posteriorly. The tracheal mucosa consists of pseudostratified ciliated columnar epithelium which contains scattered neuroendocrine (APUD) cells. The submucosa contains cartilage, smooth muscle, and seromucous glands.

The trachea is approximately 12 cm long in adults, with an upper limit of normal coronal tracheal diameter of 25 mm in men and 21 mm in women. In cross section, the trachea is oval or horseshoe shaped, with a coronal-to-sagittal diameter ratio of ≥0.6:1.0. A narrowing of the coronal diameter producing a coronal/sagittal ratio of <0.6 is termed a *saber-sheath trachea* and is seen in patients with chronic obstructive pulmonary disease.

On chest radiography, the trachea is seen as a vertically oriented cylindrical lucency extending from the cricoid cartilage superiorly to the main bronchi inferiorly. A slight tracheal deviation to the right after entering the thorax can be a normal radiographic finding. The interface of the right upper lobe (RUL) with the right lateral tracheal wall is called the *right paratracheal stripe* (Fig. 10.6A,B). This stripe should be uniformly smooth and should not exceed 4 mm in width. Thickening or nodularity reflects disease in any of the component tissues. The left lateral wall of the trachea is surrounded by mediastinal vessels and fat and is not normally visible radiographically. The posterior trachea is visualized on the lateral chest (Fig. 10.6C). The tracheoesophageal stripe, which represents the combined thickness of the tracheal and esophageal walls and intervening fat, is visualized when there is air in the upper esophagus. This stripe measures less than 5 mm; thickening is most commonly seen with esophageal carcinoma.

The bronchial system exhibits a branching pattern of asymmetric dichotomy. The daughter bronchi of a parent bronchus vary in diameter, length, and the number of divisions. The main bronchi arise from the trachea at the carina, with the right bronchus forming a more obtuse angle with the long axis of the trachea. The right main bronchus (mean length = 2.2 cm) is considerably shorter than the left main bronchus (mean length = 5 cm) (Fig. 10.6D). The tracheal and main, lobar, and segmental bronchial anatomy are easily seen on multiplanar CT (Fig. 10.6E–O). Bronchi on end can be seen as a ring shadow on chest radiographs. Bronchi gradually lose their cartilaginous support at generations 12 to 15 and these 1- to 3-mm airways are called *bronchioles.* Bronchioles bearing alveoli on their walls are termed *respiratory bronchioles.* Respiratory bronchioles divide into alveolar ducts and alveolar sacs. The airway just before the first respiratory bronchiole is the *terminal bronchiole* and is the smallest bronchiole without respiratory exchange structures. There are approximately 21 to 25 generations between the trachea and the alveoli.

Lobar and Segmental Anatomy (Fig. 10.7). The lungs are divided by the *interlobar fissures,* which are invaginations of the visceral pleura. The minor fissure is only present on the right side and separates the middle from the RUL. The right major (oblique) fissure separates the lower lobe from the upper lobe superiorly and from the middle lobe inferiorly. The RUL bronchus and its artery branch into three segmental branches: anterior, apical, and posterior. The middle lobe bronchus arises from the intermediate bronchus and divides into medial and lateral segmental branches; its blood supply is typically from a branch of the proximal right interlobar pulmonary artery. The right lower lobe (RLL) is supplied by the RLL bronchus and is subdivided into a superior segment and four basal segments: anterior, lateral, posterior, and medial. The blood supply to the RLL is via the RLL pulmonary artery.

The left lung is divided into upper and lower lobes by the left major (oblique) fissure. The left upper lobe (LUL) is analogous to the combined right upper and middle lobes. The LUL is subdivided into four segments: anterior, apicoposterior, and the superior and inferior lingular segments. Arterial supply to the anterior and apicoposterior segments parallels the bronchi and is via branches of the upper division of the left main pulmonary artery. The superior and inferior lingular arteries arise as proximal branches of the left interlobar pulmonary artery, analogous to the middle lobe blood supply. The left lower lobe (LLL) has a superior segment and three basal segments: anteromedial, lateral, and posterior and its blood supply is via the LLL pulmonary artery.

Respiratory Portion of Lung. The *respiratory bronchioles* contain a few alveoli along their walls and give rise to the gas-exchanging units of the lung: the *alveolar ducts* and the *alveolar sacs.* Two types of epithelial cells (pneumocytes) line the pulmonary alveolus. Type 1 pneumocytes are flattened squamous cells covering 95% of the alveolar surface area and are invisible by light microscopy. These cells are incapable of mitosis or repair. The rarer type 2 pneumocytes are cuboidal cells, are visible under light microscopy, and are capable of mitosis. Type 2 pneumocytes are the source of new type 1 pneumocytes and provide a mechanism for repair following alveolar damage. These cells are also thought to be the source of alveolar surfactant, a phospholipid that lowers the surface tension of alveolar walls and prevents alveolar collapse at low lung volumes.

Pulmonary subsegmental anatomy is discussed in Chapter 15, along with the thin-section CT description of these anatomic structures.

Fissures. The interlobar pulmonary fissures represent invaginations of the visceral pleura deep into the substance of the lung (Fig. 10.7). These fissures may completely or incompletely separate the lobes from one another. An incomplete fissure has important consequences regarding interlobar spread of parenchymal consolidation, collateral air drift in patients with lobar bronchial obstruction, and the appearance of pleural effusion in the supine patient. The normal fissures are well delineated on CT (Fig. 10.8A–D).

In most individuals, there are two interlobar fissures on the right and one on the left. The fissures are complete laterally and incomplete medially, with fusion of adjacent lobes. The right and left major fissures are fused in 40% to 70% of individuals, while the *minor fissure* is incomplete in the majority of individuals.

The major and minor fissures are best visualized on lateral radiographs. Variable portions of the major fissures are seen as obliquely oriented, thin white lines coursing anteroinferiorly from posterior to anterior. The left major fissure usually begins more superiorly and has a slightly more vertical course than the right major fissure. At their points of contact with the diaphragm or chest wall, the fissures often have a triangular

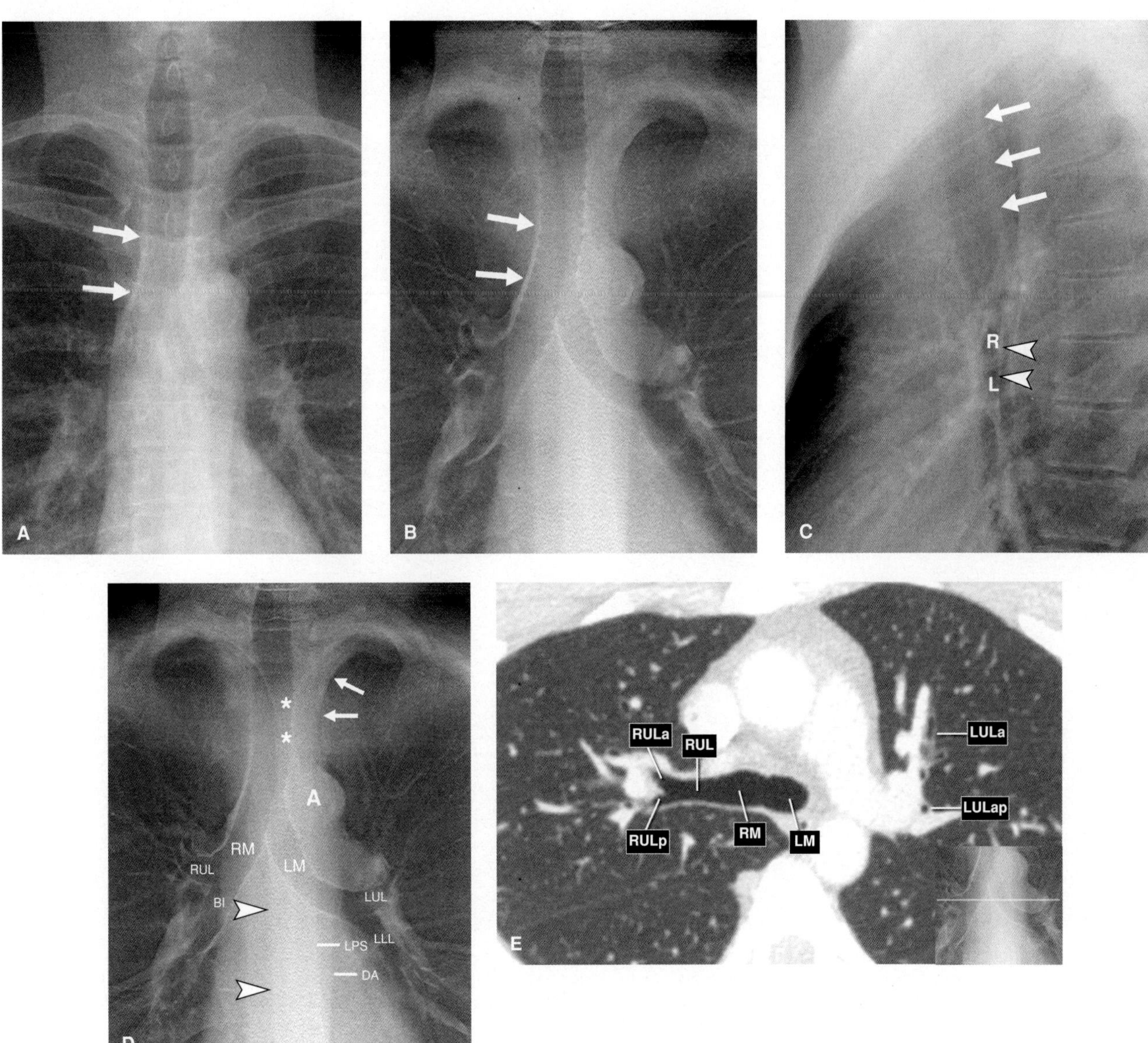

FIGURE 10.6. **Tracheobronchial Tree Anatomy on Radiography and CT. A:** Frontal view of the trachea. Coned-down view of a frontal chest radiograph shows the right paratracheal stripe (*arrows*), composed of the right lateral tracheal wall, a small amount of mediastinal fat, paratracheal lymph nodes, and the visceral and parietal pleural layers of the right upper lobe. **B:** Coned-down frontal tomogram through the trachea shows normal tracheal rings and the right paratracheal stripe (*arrows*). **C:** Coned-down left lateral view of the trachea shows the posterior tracheoesophageal stripe (*arrows*), representing the combined posterior tracheal membrane and anterior wall of the esophagus. The posterior wall of the bronchus intermedius (*arrowheads*), also called the intermediate stem line, is visible on lateral radiographs as it crosses the end-on view of the left upper lobe bronchus (*L*). The end-on right upper lobe bronchus (*R*) is also visible. **D:** Coned-down frontal tomogram through the central airways slightly posterior to Figure 10.6B delineates the main and lobar bronchi. Note the normal posterior junction line (*asterisks*) extending superiorly from the aortic knob (*A*), left subclavian artery interface (*arrows*), and upper portion of the azygoesophageal recess (*arrowheads*), left paraspinal interface (LPS), DA, descending aorta. RM, right main; LM, left main; RUL, right upper lobe; BI, bronchus intermedius; LUL, left upper lobe; LLL, left lower lobe. **E:** Bronchial anatomy on CT. Coned-down axial CT at the level of the main bronchi. RM, right main; RUL, right upper lobe; RULa, right upper lobe anterior segment; RULp, right upper lobe posterior segment; LM, left main; LULa, left upper lobe anterior segment; LULap, left upper lobe apicoposterior segment. Inset, axial level of scan. (*continued*)

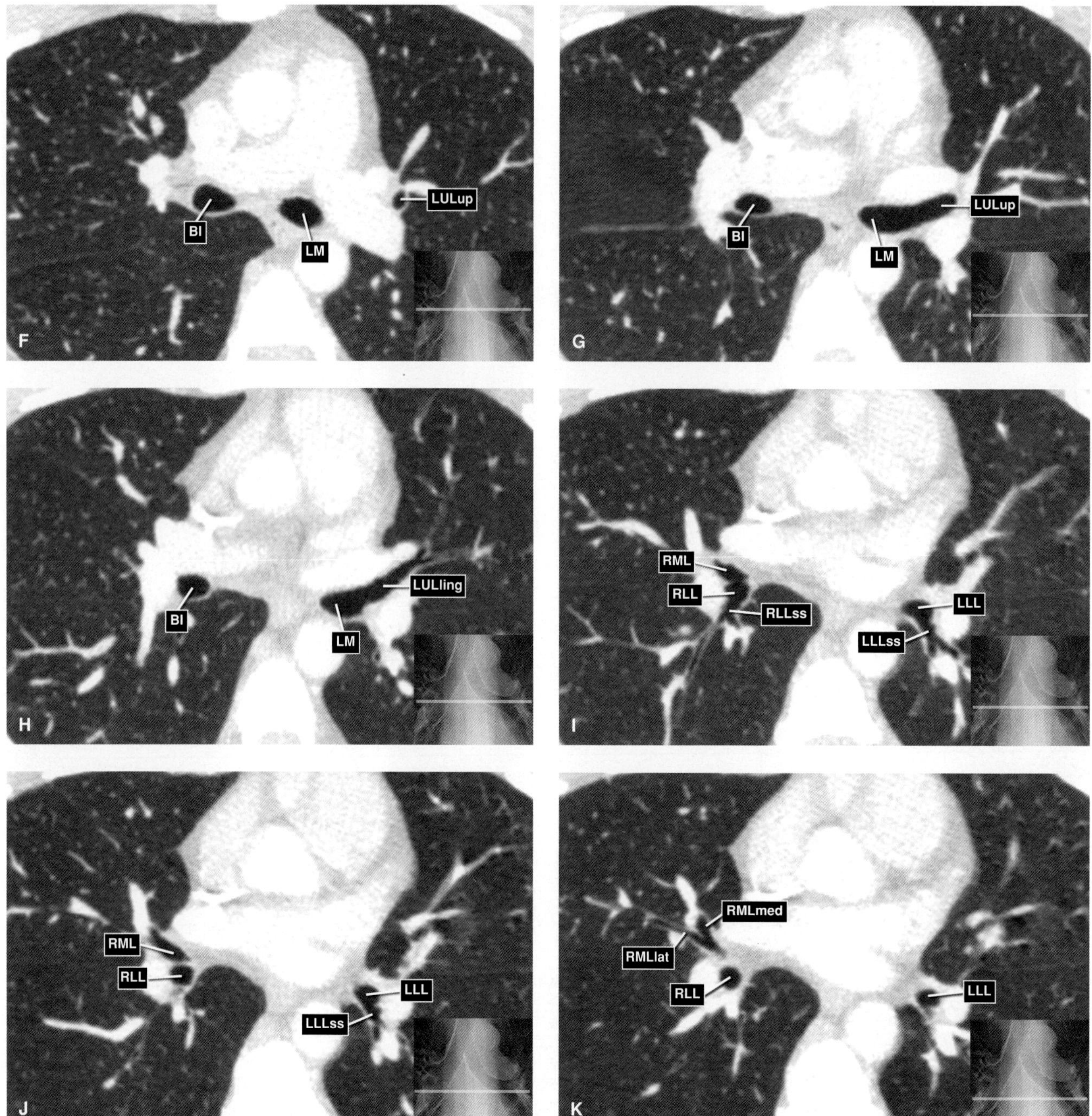

FIGURE 10.6. (*Continued*) **F:** Bronchial anatomy. Coned-down axial CT at the level of the bronchus intermedius. BI, bronchus intermedius; LM, left main; LULup, upper division of left upper lobe (combined anterior and apicoposterior segments). Inset, axial level of scan. **G:** Bronchial anatomy, level of left upper lobe upper division bronchus. BI, bronchus intermedius; LM, left main; LULup, upper division of left upper lobe (combined anterior and apicoposterior segmental bronchi). Inset, axial level of scan. **H:** Bronchial anatomy, level of left upper lobe bronchus, lingular division. Coned-down axial CT. BI, bronchus intermedius; LM, left main; LULling, left upper lobe lingular division. Inset, axial level of scan. **I:** Bronchial anatomy, level of origin of right middle lobe bronchus. Coned-down axial CT. RML, right middle lobe; RLLss, right lower lobe superior segment; LLLss, left lower lobe superior segment; LLL, left lower lobe; RLL, right lower lobe. Inset, axial level of scan. **J:** Bronchial anatomy, level of right middle lobe bronchial origin. Coned-down axial CT. RML, right middle lobe; RLL, right lower lobe; LLL, left lower lobe; LLLss, left lower lobe superior segment. Inset, axial level of scan. **K:** Bronchial anatomy, level of middle and lower lobe bronchi. Coned-down axial CT. RMLmed, right middle lobe medial segment; RMLlat, right middle lobe lateral segment; RLL, right lower lobe; LLL, left lower lobe. Inset, axial level of scan.

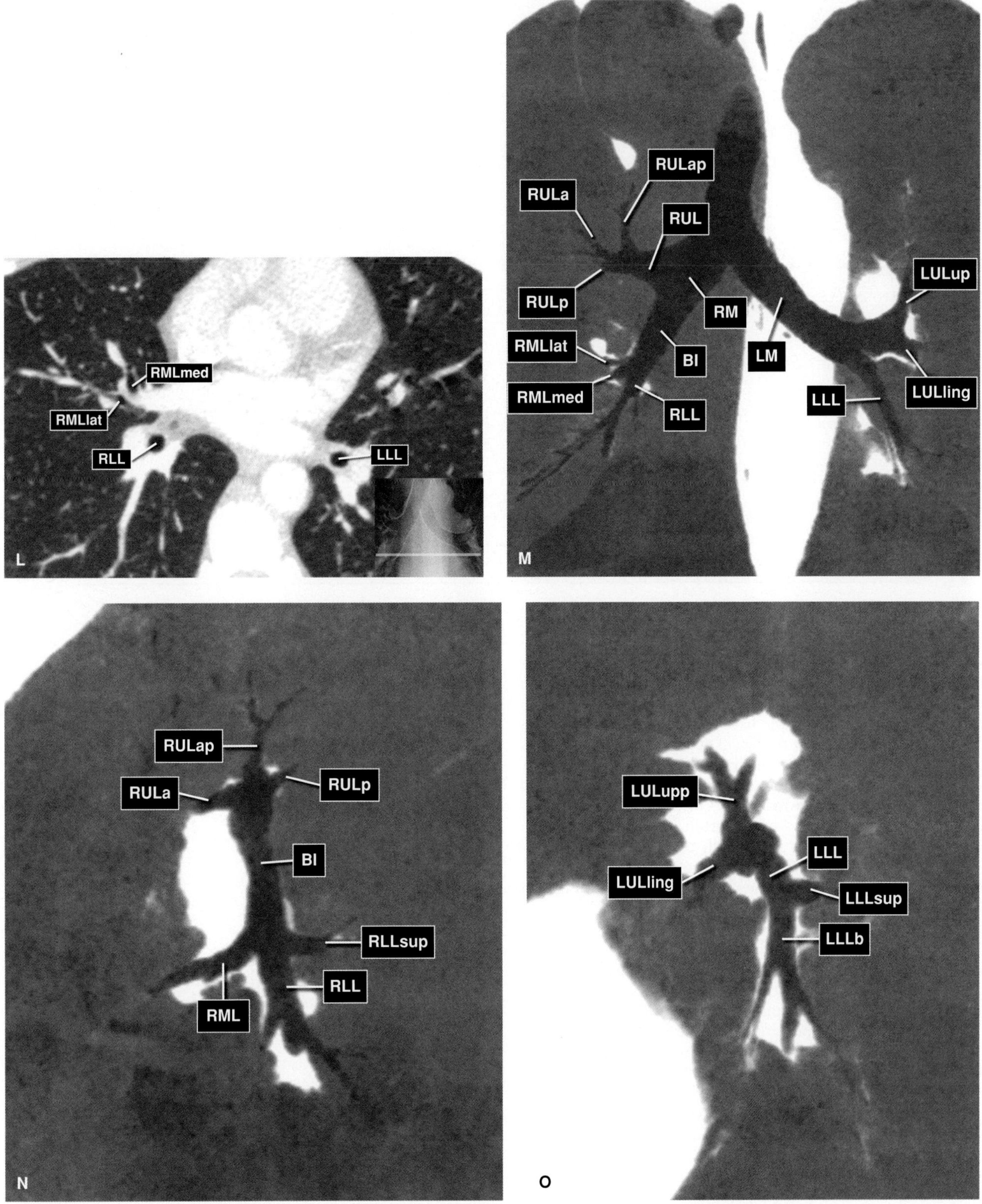

FIGURE 10.6. (*Continued*) **L:** Bronchial anatomy, level of lower lobe bronchi. Coned-down axial CT. RMLmed, right middle lobe medial segment; RMLlat, right middle lobe lateral segment; RLL, right lower lobe; LLL, left lower lobe. Inset, axial level of scan. **M:** Tracheobronchial anatomy. Coronal minIP CT through airways. RM, right main bronchus; RUL, right upper lobe; RULap, right upper lobe apical; RULa, right upper lobe anterior; RULp, right upper lobe posterior; BI, bronchus intermedius; RMLmed, right middle lobe medial segment; RMLlat, right middle lobe lateral segment; RLL, right lower lobe; LM, left main bronchus; LULup, left upper lobe upper division; LULling, LUL lingular segment; LLL, left lower lobe. **N:** Right hilar bronchial anatomy. Sagittal minIP CT through right hilum. RULa, right upper lobe anterior; RULap, right upper lobe apical; RULp, right upper lobe posterior; BI, bronchus intermedius; RML, right middle lobe; RLLsup, right lower lobe superior segment; RLL, right lower lobe. **O:** Left hilar bronchial anatomy. Sagittal minIP CT through left hilum. LULupp, left upper lobe upper division; LULling, left upper lobe lingular; LLL, left lower lobe; LLLsup, left lower lobe superior segment; LLLb, left lower lobe basal trunk.

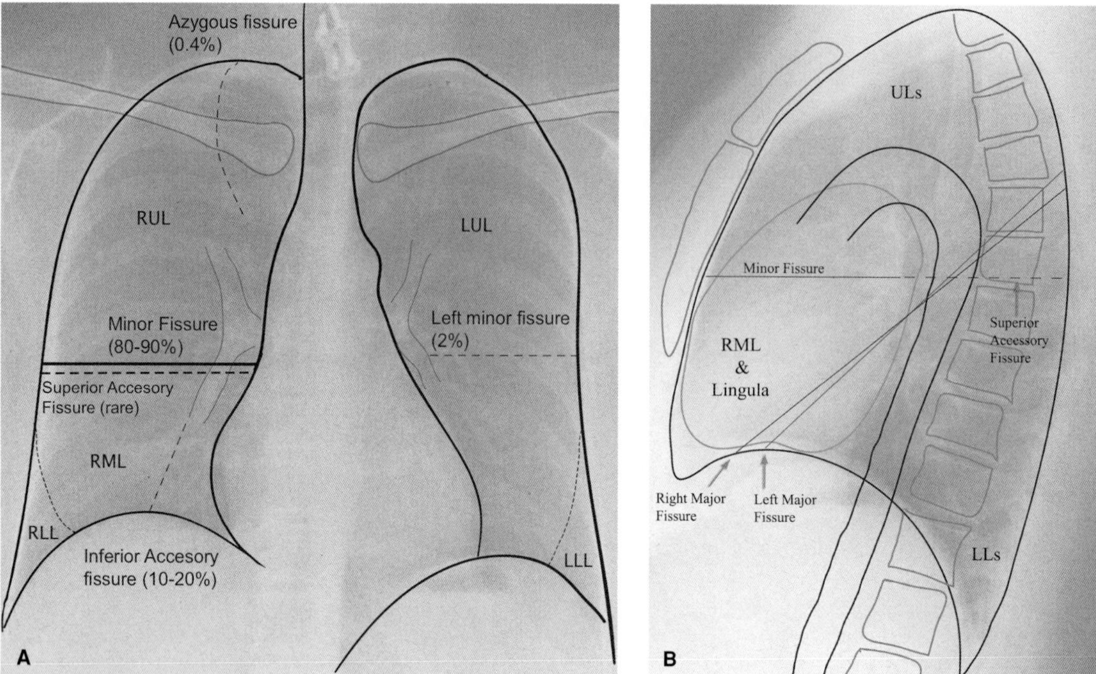

FIGURE 10.7. **Normal Lobar and Fissural Anatomy. A:** Frontal view. **B:** Lateral view. RUL, right upper lobe; LUL, left upper lobe; RML, right middle lobe; RLL, right lower lobe; LLL, left lower lobe; ULs, upper lobes; LLs, lower lobes.

configuration, with the apex of the triangle pointing toward the fissure. Although the major fissures are not normally visualized on frontal radiographs because of their oblique course relative to the x-ray beam, extrapleural fat invaginating into the superolateral aspect of the fissure can create a visible curvilinear edge in the upper thorax. The minor fissure projects at the level of the right fourth rib and is seen as a thin horizontally oriented undulating line on frontal radiographs in approximately 50% of individuals. On a lateral radiograph, the minor fissure is often seen as a thin curvilinear line with a convex superior margin. As a result of the undulating contour of the minor fissure, the posterior aspect of the minor fissure may extend posterior to the right major fissure on lateral radiographs.

The *inferior accessory fissure* (Fig. 10.7A) is the most common accessory fissure and is found in approximately 10% to 20% of individuals. It separates the medial basal from the remaining basal segments of the lower lobe and is often incomplete. It may be seen on frontal radiographs as a thin curvilinear line extending superiorly from the medial third of the hemidiaphragm toward the lower hilum. The inferior accessory fissure is responsible for the juxtaphrenic peak described in upper lobe volume loss. A small triangle of extrapleural fat, seen at its point of insertion on the diaphragm, helps identify the inferior accessory fissure. An inferior accessory fissure can be seen on CT as a curvilinear line extending anterolaterally from just in front of the inferior pulmonary ligament toward the major fissure.

The *azygos fissure* is seen in 0.5% of individuals (Fig. 10.8E). It is composed of four layers of pleura (two visceral, two parietal) and represents an invagination of the right apical pleura by the azygos vein, which has incompletely migrated to its normal position at the right tracheobronchial angle. The azygos fissure appears as a vertical curvilinear line, convex laterally, which extends inferiorly from the lung apex and ends in a teardrop, which is the azygos vein.

The *superior accessory fissure* (Fig. 10.7A) separates the superior segment from the basal segments of the lower lobe. On the right side, it is distinguished from the minor fissure by its posterior location on lateral radiography or CT.

The *left minor fissure* is an uncommon normal variant that separates the lingula from the remaining portions of the upper lobe and is seen occasionally on CT (Fig. 10.8F).

Ligaments. The *inferior pulmonary ligament* is a sheet of connective tissue that extends from the hilum inferiorly toward the hemidiaphragm. It is comprised of fused visceral and parietal pleural layers and tethers the lower lobe to the mediastinum alongside the esophagus. The ligament contains the inferior pulmonary vein and lymph nodes. The inferior pulmonary ligament is sometimes seen on CT scans through the lower thorax as a small, laterally directed beak of mediastinal pleura adjacent to the esophagus (Fig. 10.9). The tethering effect of this ligament on the lower lobe accounts for the medial location and triangular appearance of lower lobe collapse.

The *intersegmental septum* (Fig. 10.9) is a linear structure seen on CT near the inferior pulmonary ligament extending into the lung from the mediastinal pleura.

The *pericardiophrenic ligament* is a triangular density extending toward the lung that is seen along the posterior aspect of the right heart border on lung windows on chest CT (Fig. 10.9). It represents a reflection of pleura over the inferior portion of the phrenic nerve and pericardiophrenic vessels. It is distinguished from the intersegmental septum by its more anterior location and by its characteristic ramifications as branches of the nerve and vessel reflect over the hemidiaphragm.

Pulmonary Arteries. The pulmonary artery is an elastic artery that arises from the right ventricle. The left pulmonary artery is a direct continuation of the main pulmonary artery. The right pulmonary artery branches just below the carina. Within the left hilum, the left pulmonary artery envelopes the upper margin of the left main bronchus and then divides into the upper and lower lobe arteries. The arch formed by the LLL artery over the left hilar bronchi (i.e., the bronchus is hyparterial) is seen on lateral radiography (Fig. 10.10). The right main pulmonary

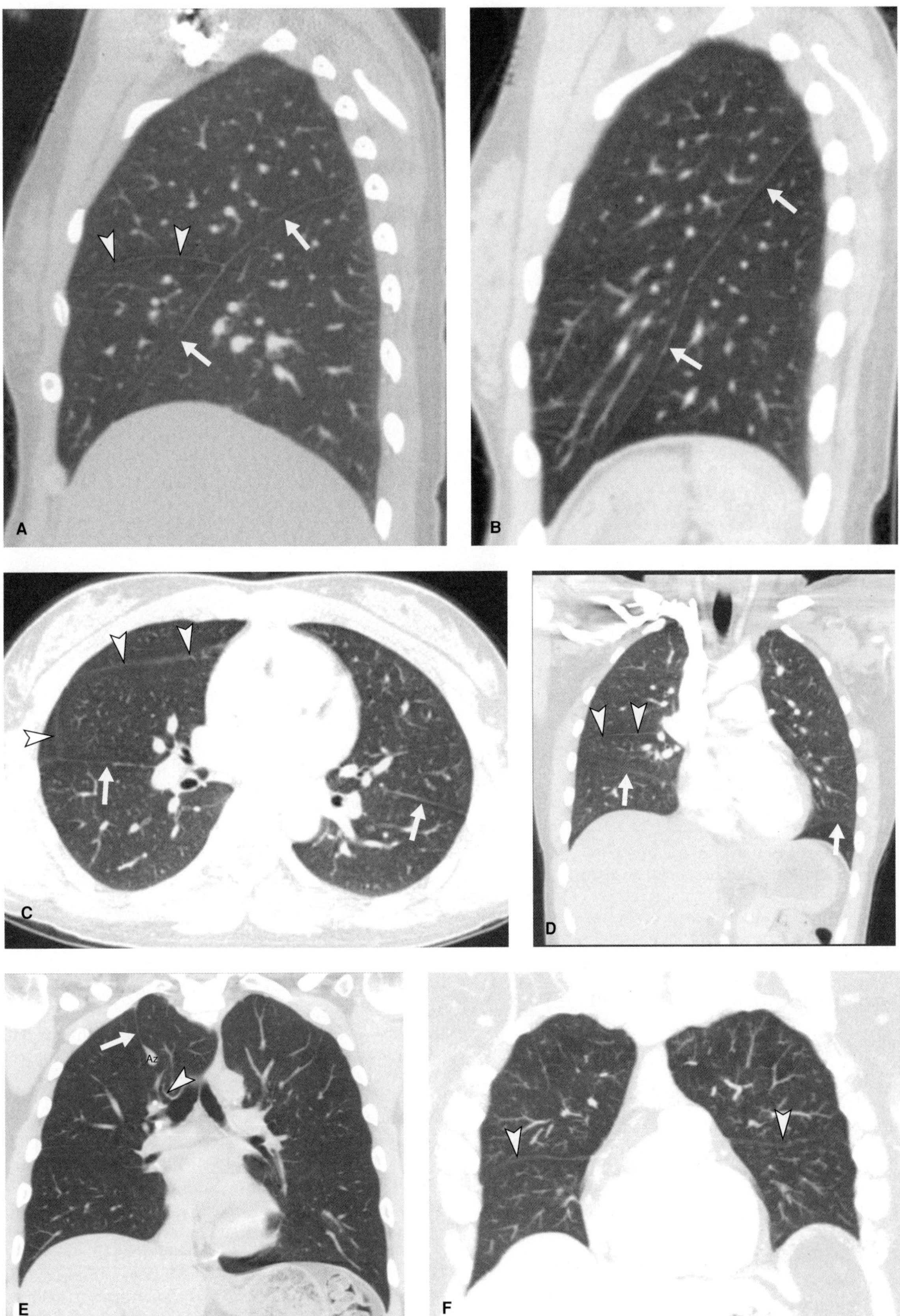

FIGURE 10.8. Fissural Anatomy on CT. A: Sagittal CT through the right lung shows major (*arrows*) and minor (*arrowheads*) fissures. **B:** Sagittal CT through the left lung shows the left major fissure. **C:** Axial CT shows the major fissures as thin lines (*solid arrows*). The minor fissure (*arrowheads*) is indistinct owing to its dome shape and oblique orientation. **D:** Coronal CT shows both major (*arrows*) and minor (*arrowheads*) fissures. **E:** Coronal CT in a different patient shows an azygos fissure (*arrow*) with the azygos vein (Az) situated inferiorly within the fissure. Note anomalous apical segmental bronchus arising from the right main bronchus (*arrowhead*). **F:** Coronal MIP CT in another patient shows bilateral minor fissures (*arrowheads*).

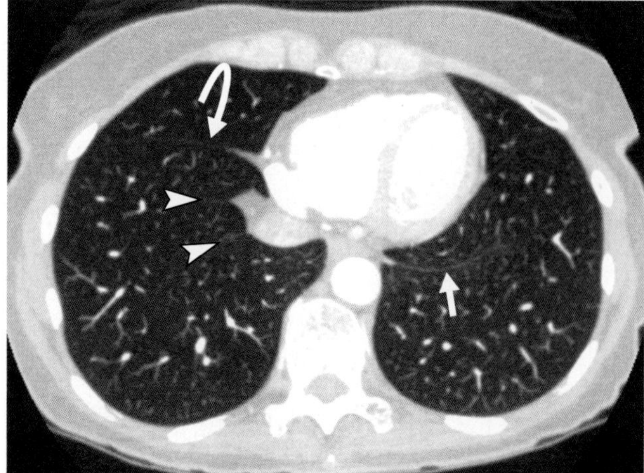

FIGURE 10.9. **Intersegmental Septum and Pericardiophrenic Ligaments.** Axial contrast-enhanced CT scan through the lung bases at lung windows demonstrates a thin curvilinear line (*straight arrow*) extending laterally from the lateral margin of the esophagus into the left lower lobe. This represents the intersegmental septum extending laterally from the inferior pulmonary ligament which lies within the mediastinum. On the right, two linear opacities (*arrowheads*) extending from the fat surrounding the inferior vena cava represent branches of the right pericardiophrenic ligament containing branches of the right phrenic nerve and pericardiophrenic vessels. More anteriorly on the right, the major fissure (*curved arrow*) is seen with mediastinal fat extending into its medial aspect.

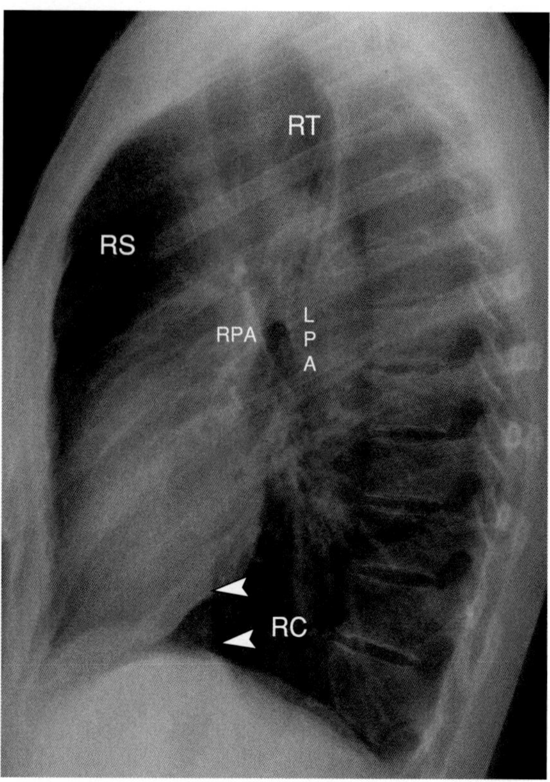

FIGURE 10.10. **Lateral Chest Radiographic Anatomy.** Same patient as Figure 10.1. The right pulmonary artery (RPA) is seen as an oval opacity anterior to the bronchi, while the left pulmonary artery (LPA) arches posteriorly over the left main/upper lobe bronchial confluence. The three normal clear spaces are well depicted. The retrosternal space (RS) is demarcated anteriorly by the posterior margin of the sternum and posteriorly by the heart and ascending aorta and accounts for the anterior junction line seen on frontal radiography. The retrotracheal triangle (RT) is marginated by the posterior wall of the trachea anteriorly, the spine posteriorly, and the aortic arch inferiorly. The retrocardiac space (RC) is demarcated anteriorly by the posterior margin of the heart and the inferior vena cava (*arrowheads*) and by the thoracic spine posteriorly.

artery courses laterally and anterior to the right main bronchus. The right main pulmonary artery divides within the pericardium into the truncus anterior and interlobar arteries. The right interlobar artery courses anterolateral to the bronchus (i.e., the bronchus is eparterial). At the same level that the bronchi lose their cartilage and become bronchioles, the elastic arteries lose their elastic lamina and become muscular arteries.

Bronchial arteries are the primary nutrient vessels of the lung, supplying blood to the bronchial walls to the level of the terminal bronchioles. Mediastinal structures including the trachea, middle third of the esophagus, visceral pleura, mediastinal lymph nodes, vagus nerve, pericardium, and thymus receive a variable amount of blood supply from the bronchial circulation.

The bronchial arteries usually arise from the proximal descending thoracic aorta at the level of the carina and show significant variability. Most commonly, there is one right-sided and two left-sided arteries. The right bronchial artery usually arises from the posterolateral wall of the aorta with an intercostal artery as an intercostobronchial trunk. The left bronchial arteries arise individually from the anterolateral aorta or, rarely, from an intercostal artery. Approximately two-thirds of the blood from the bronchial arterial system returns to the pulmonary venous system via the bronchial veins, with the remaining blood draining via the azygos or hemiazygos systems.

Pulmonary veins arise within the interlobular septa from the alveolar and visceral pleural capillaries. The veins travel in connective tissue envelopes that are separate from the bronchoarterial trunks. The pulmonary veins, which vary in number from three to eight, drain into the left atrium.

Pulmonary lymphatics help clear fluid and particulate matter from the pulmonary interstitium. There are two major lymphatic pathways in the lung and pleura. The visceral pleural lymphatics, which reside in the vascular (innermost) layer of the visceral pleura, form a network over the surface of the lung that roughly parallels the margins of the secondary pulmonary lobules. These peripheral lymphatics penetrate the lung to course centrally within interlobular septa, along with the pulmonary veins, toward the hilum. The parenchymal lymphatics originate in proximity to the alveolar septa ("juxta-alveolar lymphatics") and course centrally with the bronchoarterial bundle. The perivenous and bronchoarterial lymphatics communicate via obliquely oriented lymphatics located within the central regions of the lung. These perivenous lymphatics and their surrounding connective tissue, when distended by fluid, account for the radiographic appearance of Kerley A lines.

Pulmonary interstitium is the scaffolding of the lung and provides support for the airways and pulmonary vessels (Fig. 10.11). It begins within the hilum and extends peripherally to the visceral pleura. The *axial interstitium* extends from the mediastinum and envelopes the bronchovascular bundles. The axial fiber system continues distally as the *centrilobular interstitium* along with the arterioles, capillaries, and bronchioles to provide support for the air-exchanging portions of the lung. The *subpleural interstitium* and interlobular septa are parts of the *peripheral interstitium,* which divides secondary pulmonary lobules. The pulmonary veins and lymphatics lie within the peripheral interstitium. The *intralobular*

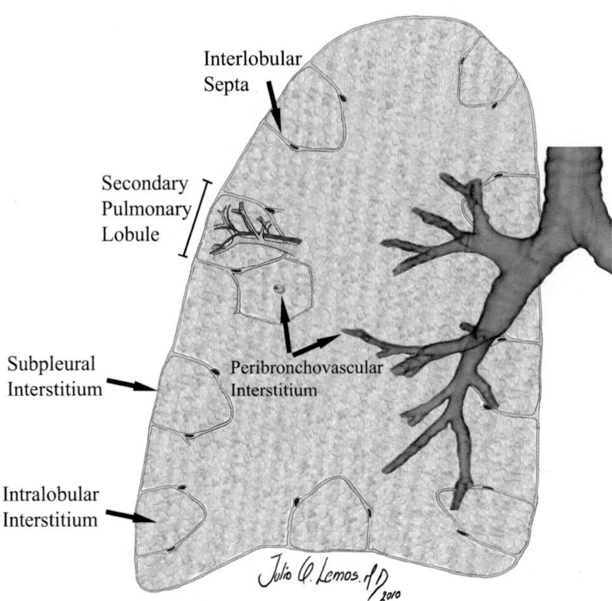

FIGURE 10.11. Diagram of the Pulmonary Interstitium.

interstitium is a thin network of fibers that bridges the gap between the centrilobular and peripheral compartments.

Edema involving the axial interstitium is recognized radiographically as peribronchial cuffing. While pathologic involvement of the intralobular interstitium is difficult to discern radiographically, thickening of portions of this interstitium are occasionally seen as intralobular lines on thin-section CT. Edema of the peripheral and subpleural interstitium accounts for Kerley B lines (or interlobular [septal] lines on thin-section CT) and "thickened" fissures on chest radiographs.

Frontal Chest Radiograph

A knowledge of the normal anatomy depicted on frontal chest radiography is key to detecting and localizing pathologic conditions and to avoid mistaking normal structures for pathologic findings.

Soft tissues of the chest wall consist of the skin, subcutaneous fat, and muscles. The lateral edges of the sternocleidomastoid muscles are readily visible in most patients. The visualization of normal fat in the supraclavicular fossae and the companion shadows of skin and subcutaneous fat paralleling the clavicles help exclude mass, adenopathy, or edema in this region. The inferolateral edge of the pectoralis major muscle is normally seen curving toward the axilla. Both breast shadows should be evaluated routinely to detect evidence of prior mastectomy or distorting mass. The soft tissues lateral to the bony thorax should be smooth, symmetric, and homogeneous in density.

Bones. The thoracic spine, ribs and costal cartilages, clavicles, and scapulae are routinely visible on frontal chest radiography. The thoracic vertebral bodies should be vertically aligned, with visualization of the endplates, pedicles, and spinous processes. Twelve pairs of symmetric ribs should be seen; the upper ribs have smooth superior and inferior cortical margins, while the middle and lower ribs have flanged inferior cortices where the intercostal neurovascular bundles run. Cervical ribs are identified in approximately 2% of individuals and may be associated with symptoms of thoracic outlet syndrome. Costal cartilage calcification is seen in a majority of adults, increases in prevalence with advancing age, and can add multiple shadows to the PA view. Men typically show calcification at the upper and lower margins, while the majority of women develop central cartilaginous calcification (Fig. 17.24).

Lung–Lung Interfaces. A familiarity with the normal mediastinal interfaces is key to the interpretation of the frontal chest radiograph. On frontal radiography, the lung–lung interfaces relate directly to spaces in three regions as seen on lateral radiography: the retrosternal space, the retrotracheal space, and the retrocardiac space (Fig. 10.10).

The retrosternal space reflects contact of the anterosuperior aspect of the upper lobes. This is seen on frontal radiography as the *anterior junction line*, which is a thin vertical line that overlies the thoracic spine (Fig. 10.12A,B). The anterior junction anatomy is an inferior extension of the upper lobe reflections off the innominate veins. The innominate veins produce an inverted V-shaped retromanubrial opacity.

A second potential lung–lung interface is seen on the lateral chest radiograph as the *retrotracheal space or Raider triangle,* a radiolucent region representing contact of the posterosuperior portions of the upper lobes. On lateral chest radiographs, it is bordered anteriorly by the posterior wall of the trachea, inferiorly by the aortic arch, and posteriorly by the thoracic spine. If this space is large, a posterior junction line may be seen on frontal radiography (Fig. 10.12C,D and Table 10.3).

The third potential lung–lung interface occurs in the *retrocardiac space*, located between the posterior border of the heart/IVC and the thoracic spine (Fig. 10.10). If that space is large, the azygoesophageal recess of the RLL may abut the preaortic recess of the LLL to produce an inferior *posterior junction line* on frontal radiographs.

Lung–Mediastinal Interfaces (Table 10.4). The lung–mediastinal interfaces are seen as sharp edges where the lung and adjacent pleura reflect off of various mediastinal structures. The right lateral margin of the superior vena cava is commonly seen as a straight or slightly concave interface with the RUL extending from the level of the clavicle to the superior margin of the right atrium (Fig. 10.13). Prominence or convexity of the caval interface may represent caval dilatation or lateral displacement by a dilated or tortuous aortic arch or other mediastinal mass.

Along the right upper mediastinum, the RUL contacts the right lateral tracheal wall in a majority of individuals. This produces the right paratracheal stripe (Fig. 10.6A,B). The thickness of this line, measured above the level of the azygos vein, should not exceed 4 mm. Thickening or nodularity of the paratracheal stripe is seen in abnormalities of the tissues comprising the stripe, including tracheal tumors, paratracheal lymph node enlargement, and right pleural effusion.

The arch of the azygos vein is seen on frontal radiographs as an oval structure in the right tracheobronchial angle. Supine positioning or performance of the Müller maneuver (forced inspiration against a closed glottis) will increase azygos venous diameter. In general, a diameter of >10 mm on a PA radiograph should raise the possibility of mass, adenopathy, or dilatation of the azygos vein. A dilated azygos vein may be seen with right heart failure, obstruction of venous return to the heart, or a congenital venous anomaly such as azygos continuation of the inferior vena cava. An increase in diameter of the azygos vein from prior comparable radiographs is more important than the absolute measurement.

The *azygoesophageal recess* interface is a vertically oriented interface overlying the thoracic spine (Figs. 10.6D, 10.12C, and 10.13). While normally straight or concave in contour, the middle third of the interface may have a slight rightward convexity at the level of the confluence of the right pulmonary veins with the left atrium. Left atrial dilatation will enlarge and laterally displace this interface, producing a double-density interface composed of the right lateral borders of

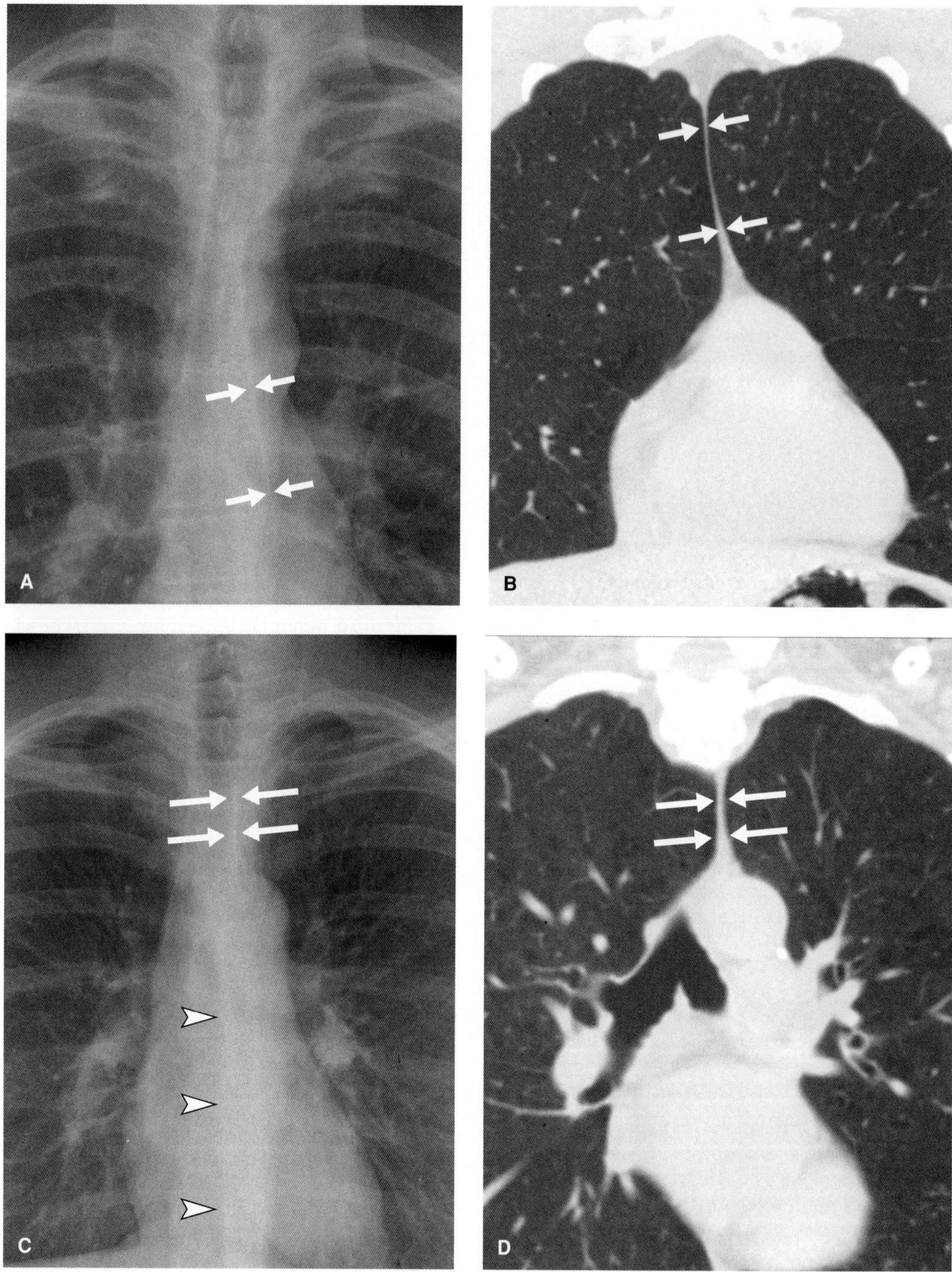

FIGURE 10.12. Anterior and Posterior Junction Lines. A: Coned-down view of frontal radiograph demonstrates a normal anterior junction line (*arrows*). **B:** Coronal CT at lung windows through the anterior thorax in another patient shows the anterior junction line. **C:** Coned-down view of frontal radiograph shows a posterior junction line (*arrows*). The azygoesophageal recess interface (*arrowheads*) is also well delineated. **D:** Coronal CT at lung windows in the same patient shows the posterior junction line (*arrows*) extending superiorly from the aortic arch.

both the right and the left atria. Convexity of the upper third of the interface suggests subcarinal lymph node enlargement or a mass. Convexity of the inferior third may be due to a sliding hiatal hernia, tortuous descending aorta, or enlarged paraesophageal lymph nodes. When air is present in the distal portion of the esophagus and the azygoesophageal recess interfaces with the right lateral wall of the esophagus, a line (the right inferior esophagopleural stripe) rather than an edge is seen.

The *right paraspinal interface* is a straight, vertical interface extending the length of the right hemithorax and represents contact of the right lung with a small amount of tissue lateral to the thoracic spine. It is inconsistently visualized; a focal convexity of this interface suggests spinal or paraspinal disease.

The right heart projects slightly to the right of the lateral margin of the thoracic spine on a normal PA radiograph (Fig. 10.13) and represents the lateral margin of the right

TABLE 10.3

ANTERIOR AND POSTERIOR JUNCTION LINES

■ LINE	■ FEATURES
Anterior junction line	Obliquely oriented from right superior to left inferior Extends from upper sternum to base of heart
Posterior junction line	Vertically oriented in the midline Extends from upper thoracic spine to level of azygos and aortic arches

atrium. The right atrium creates a smooth convex interface with the medial segment of the middle lobe. Individuals with pectus excavatum have a leftward cardiac displacement and therefore this interface may be absent, simulating middle lobe opacification. In patients with right atrial dilatation, this interface may extend well into the right lung.

The right lateral border of the inferior vena cava may be seen at the level of the right hemidiaphragm as a concave lateral interface. The inferior vena caval interface is best visualized on lateral radiographs (Fig. 10.10) and is absent in patients with azygos continuation of the inferior vena cava.

In the uppermost portion of the left mediastinum, one or more interfaces may be recognized above the aortic arch. The interface most often visualized is the subclavian artery (Figs. 10.6D and 10.13). It is unusual for the LUL to interface with the left lateral wall of the trachea to form the left paratracheal stripe because of the intervening subclavian artery and adjacent fat.

The transverse portion of the aortic arch ("aortic knob") creates a convex indentation on the left lung in normal individuals (Fig. 10.13). As the aorta elongates and dilates with age, this interface projects more laterally, and lung may be seen to encircle a greater circumference of the knob.

The left superior intercostal vein may be seen in approximately 5% of individuals on frontal radiographs as a rounded or triangular opacity that focally indents the lung immediately superolateral to the aortic knob. This density, termed

TABLE 10.4

NORMAL LUNG–MEDIASTINAL INTERFACES

Right-sided	Right paraesophageal interface Superior vena cava/right paratracheal stripe Anterior arch of the azygos vein Right paraspinal interface Azygoesophageal recess Lateral margin of right atrium Confluence of right pulmonary veins (right border of left atrium) Right atrium Lateral margin of inferior vena cava
Left-sided	Lateral margin of left subclavian artery Transverse aortic arch Left superior intercostal vein ("aortic nipple") Aortopulmonary window interface Lateral margin of main pulmonary artery Preaortic recess Left paraspinal interface Left atrial appendage Left ventricle Epipericardial fat pad

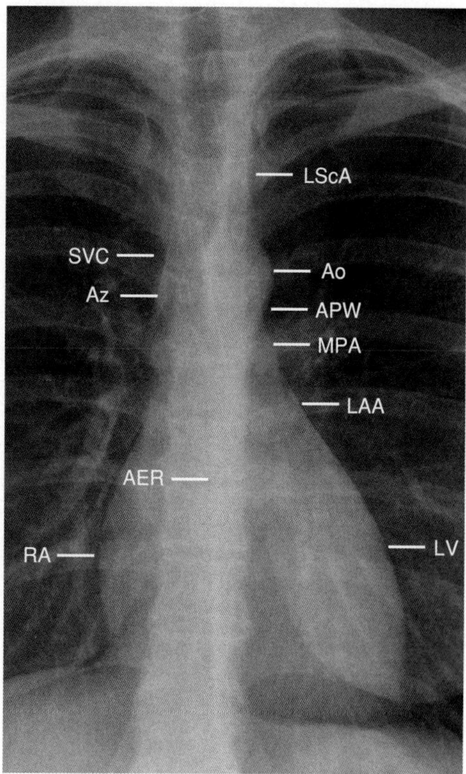

FIGURE 10.13. **Normal Lung–Mediastinal Interfaces.** Coned-down frontal radiograph. On the right (from superior to inferior): SVC, superior vena cava; Az, azygos vein; RA, right atrium. On the left (from superior to inferior): LScA, left subclavian artery; Ao, aortic knob; APW, aortopulmonary window interface; MPA, main pulmonary artery; LAa, left atrial appendage; LV, left ventricle. Also shown is the azygoesophageal recess interface (AER).

the "aortic nipple" (Fig. 10.14), represents the superior intercostal vein as it arches anteriorly from its paraspinal position around the aortic arch to drain into the posterior aspect of the left brachiocephalic vein. When seen, it normally measures <5 mm but may enlarge with elevation of right atrial pressure or with congenital or acquired obstruction of venous return to the right heart.

Immediately inferior to the aortic arch, the LUL contacts the mediastinum to produce the *aortopulmonary window* interface (Fig. 10.13). This interface is usually straight or concave toward the lung; the latter appearance is seen with a tortuous aorta, emphysema, or congenital absence of the left pericardium. A convex lateral interface should suggest mass or lymph node enlargement in the aortopulmonary window.

Immediately inferior to the aortopulmonary window interface is the left lateral border of the main pulmonary artery (Fig. 10.13). The interface of this structure may be convex, straight, or concave toward the lung. Enlargement of the main pulmonary artery is seen as an idiopathic condition in young women, as a result of poststenotic dilatation in valvular pulmonic stenosis or in conditions where there is increased flow or pressure in the pulmonary arterial system, such as left-to-right intracardiac shunts.

The *preaortic recess interface*, seen in a small percentage of normal individuals as a reflection of the LLL with the esophagus anterior to the descending aorta, extends vertically from the undersurface of the aortic knob a variable distance toward the diaphragm. It is usually etched in black (negative Mach effect).

The *left paraspinal interface* (Fig. 10.6D) represents the reflection of the left lung off the paraspinal soft tissues, which

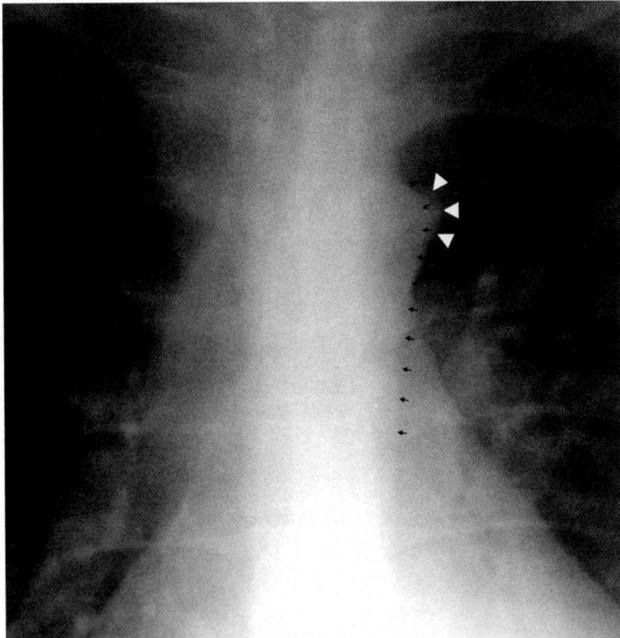

FIGURE 10.14. **Aortic Nipple.** Coned-down frontal chest radiograph shows the contour of the "aortic nipple" formed by the left superior intercostal vein (*white arrowheads*). The *small black arrows* denote the contour of the aortic knob and proximal descending aorta.

largely consist of fat but also contain the sympathetic chain, proximal intercostal vessels, intercostal lymph nodes, and hemiazygos and accessory hemiazygos veins. The left paraspinal interface, in contrast to the right paraspinal interface, is etched in white (positive Mach effect) and can be seen in the majority of individuals. Large vertebral osteophytes, neurogenic tumors, paravertebral hematoma, paraspinal abscess, lipomatosis, and medial pleural effusion can cause lateral displacement of this interface.

The left atrial appendage forms a concave interface immediately below the main pulmonary artery (Fig. 10.13). Straightening or convexity of this interface is seen in patients with left atrial enlargement.

The left ventricle comprises most of the left heart border. A gentle convex margin with the lingula is normal (Fig. 10.13). Abnormalities of the left ventricular contour will be discussed in Section 5 (Cardiac Radiology).

Fat adjacent to the cardiac apex may create a focal convexity or simply obscure the cardiac contour in the cardiophrenic angles. This epipericardial fat is typically unilateral or more prominent on the left (Fig. 10.15) and is most often seen in obese patients and those on corticosteroids. A typical appearance of the fat pad on the lateral radiograph is usually diagnostic (Fig. 10.15B).

The Lungs (Fig. 10.1). The density of the lungs as seen radiographically is attributable solely to the presence of the pulmonary vasculature and enveloping interstitial structures. The arteries are solid cylinders branching along with the bronchi, with both demonstrating a gradual decrease in caliber as they divide. Bronchi smaller than subsegmental bronchi are not visible radiographically. The pulmonary veins can often be traced horizontally to the left atrium, whereas the arteries can be followed to the hila, which are more cephalad than the left atrium. The effects of gravity explain the larger diameter of lower lobe vessels in an upright patient and the equal caliber of upper versus lower lobe vessels in the supine patient. The opacity of the lungs increases inferiorly in women as a result of overlying breast tissue and in men with prominent pectoralis muscles. The opacity of the lung is increased by processes that thicken the interstitium or fill the airspaces. Any process associated with diminished blood flow to the lung or destruction of parenchymal structures results in decreased lung density.

Diaphragm. The diaphragm is the major inspiratory muscle. It originates along multiple costal margins and inserts into the membranous dome. The right hemidiaphragm overlies the liver, and the left hemidiaphragm overlies the stomach and spleen. On frontal radiographs obtained on deep inspiration, the apex of the right hemidiaphragm typically lies at the level of the sixth anterior rib, approximately ½ interspace above the apex of the left hemidiaphragm (Fig. 10.1). A scalloped appearance to the hemidiaphragm is not uncommon. Focal bulges in the diaphragmatic contour are usually a result of acquired diaphragmatic eventration (thinning).

Upper Abdomen. Portions of the liver, spleen, and gastric fundus are routinely visualized on frontal chest radiography. Free intraperitoneal air is seen as a curvilinear lucency beneath the diaphragm on upright chest radiographs. Abnormalities of abdominal situs may be identified by noting the location and appearance of the liver, stomach, and spleen. Enlargement of the liver may cause right diaphragmatic elevation. Intrahepatic air may be seen within the biliary tree, portal vein, or a hepatic abscess. Calcified hepatic lesions or calcified gallstones may be seen in the right upper abdomen. A mass arising within the gastric fundus can occasionally be seen as a soft tissue opacity protruding into a gas-filled gastric lumen. Splenomegaly may be identified by noting a soft tissue mass in the left upper quadrant that displaces the stomach bubble anteromedially and the splenic flexure of the colon inferiorly.

Lateral Chest Radiograph

The lateral chest radiograph is a challenge because of summation of structures in the right and left hemithoraces (Fig. 10.1B). However, knowledge of normal lateral radiographic anatomy can greatly aid in detection and localization of parenchymal and cardiomediastinal processes.

Soft Tissues. Air outlining the anterior axillary folds may render the anterior edges of these skin folds visible overlying the superior aspect of the thorax. The edges are seen as bilateral opacities that are concave anteriorly and can be followed through the level of the thoracic inlet to merge with the soft tissues of the arms.

Bones. The anterior margins of the scapulae project as oblique straight edges overlying the superior and posterior aspects of the thorax, often over the retrotracheal triangle. The anterior and posterior cortical margins of the thoracic vertebral bodies should be aligned forming a gradual kyphosis.

Lung Interfaces. The retrotracheal (or Raider) triangle is bordered by the posterior border of the trachea/esophagus, the anterior border of the spine, and the top of the aortic arch (Fig. 10.10). Masses and airspace disease near the apices, retrotracheal masses (e.g., aberrant subclavian artery or posterior thyroid goiter), or esophageal masses may produce an abnormal opacity in this region.

The superior margin of the aortic arch is seen as a curvilinear opacity projecting posterosuperior to the combined hilar shadow. The descending thoracic aorta is variably seen as a distinct vertically oriented tubular opacity overlying the anterior margin of the thoracic spine; the greater its tortuosity, the more readily evident it is radiographically as it is outlined by the LLL. Rarely, the superior margin of the arch of the azygos vein is visible projecting over the lower aspect of the aortic arch.

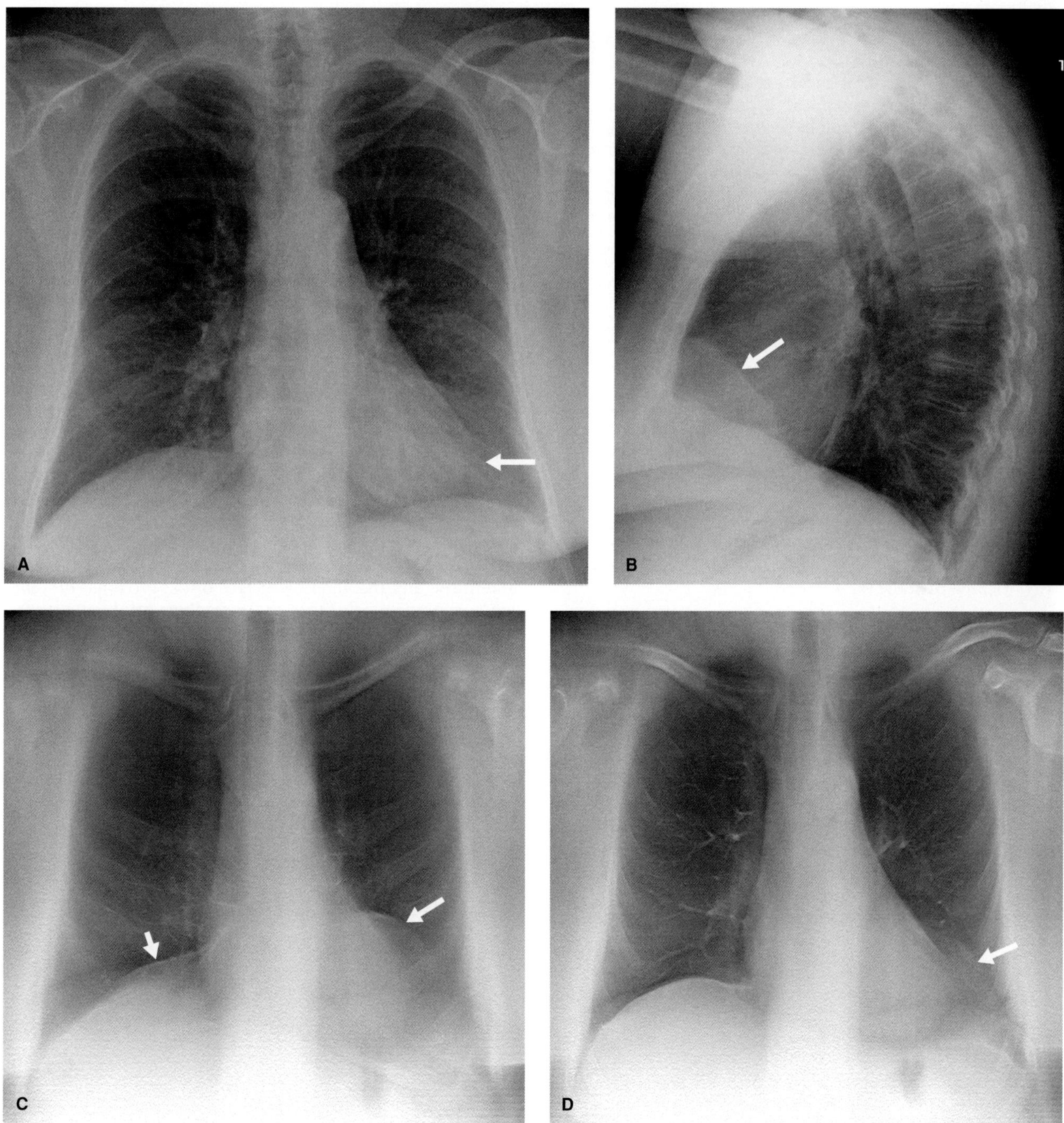

FIGURE 10.15. **Normal Epipericardial Fat Pads. A, B:** Frontal (**A**) and lateral (**B**) chest radiographs show an indistinct left cardiac apex (*arrow* in **A**) due to epipericardial fat seen as the cardiac incisura on lateral radiograph (*arrow* in **B**). **C, D:** Frontal tomograms through the anterior chest demonstrate the right (*short arrow* in **C**) and left (*long arrows* in **C** and **D**) epipericardial fat pads.

The appearance of the retrosternal space depends upon the shape of the sternum and the amount of anterior mediastinal fat. On well-penetrated lateral radiographs, the body of the sternum is readily visible (Fig. 10.1B). A thin retrosternal stripe from a small amount of fat immediately behind the body of the sternum is usually seen. Sternal fracture, infection, tumor, or prior sternotomy can distort or thicken this stripe. Enlargement of internal mammary arteries (as seen in coarctation of the aorta) or enlarged internal thoracic lymph nodes can produce a mass projecting between the concavities of the costal cartilages. Inferiorly, the left lung may be excluded from contacting the anteromedial chest wall by a round or triangular opacity, which represents the cardiac apex and adjacent epipericardial fat. This impression on the anterior surface of the lingula has been termed the *cardiac incisura* and should not be mistaken for a mass (Fig. 10.15B). CT is helpful in equivocal cases. A mass within the anterior (prevascular) mediastinum will create an abnormal opacity in the retrosternal space.

The anterior pericardial reflection can be identified separately from the myocardium on lateral radiographs in 20% of subjects. This thin line represents the pericardial layers between the epicardial and pericardial fat. Nodularity or thickness >2 mm (the "pericardial stripe sign") suggests disease or effusion.

The posterior aspect of the inferior vena cava is visible in a majority of individuals as a concave posterior or straight edge that is visible at the posteroinferior cardiac margin, just above the diaphragm (Figs. 10.1B and 10.10).

The hemidiaphragms appear as parallel dome-shaped structures on lateral radiographs (Figs. 10.1B and 10.10). The posterior portion lies at a more inferior level than the anterior portion, creating a deep posterior costophrenic sulcus and a shallow anterior sulcus. There are several ways to distinguish the right from the left hemidiaphragm on the lateral view. The right hemidiaphragm is typically higher than the left. The anterior left hemidiaphragm is obscured (silhouetted) by the heart, whereas the right hemidiaphragm is seen along its entire AP course. On a well-positioned left lateral chest radiograph, with the right side of the thorax farther from the recording device than the left, the right anterior and posterior costophrenic sulci should project beyond the corresponding left-sided sulci as a result of x-ray beam divergence. Identification of the right and left posterior costophrenic sulci allows identification of the corresponding hemidiaphragms. The presence of air in the stomach or splenic flexure projecting above one hemidiaphragm and below another identifies the more cephalad diaphragm as the left. Occasionally, when both major fissures are visualized, following a major fissure to its point of contact with the diaphragm allows identification of that hemidiaphragm because the left major fissure is more vertically oriented than the right.

Anatomy of the Normal Mediastinum

The mediastinum is a narrow, vertically oriented space that resides between the medial parietal pleural layers of the lungs. It contains central cardiovascular and tracheobronchial structures, the esophagus, fat, and lymph nodes (Fig. 10.16). For the purposes of localizing mediastinal lesions, the mediastinum is most easily divided into three compartments based upon cross-sectional imaging, which is invariably used to localize and characterize these lesions. Within each compartment are readily identifiable structures and a number of spaces in free communication with one another (Table 10.5). The structures and spaces in each compartment and their normal appearance are reviewed here.

Anterior (Prevascular) Mediastinum. The anterior (prevascular) mediastinal compartment includes all structures behind the sternum and anterior to the heart and great vessels, including the internal thoracic lymph nodes, thymus, and the brachiocephalic veins (Fig. 10.17A,B).

The thymus is a triangular or bilobed structure that is largest at puberty and then undergoes gradual fatty involution. In most individuals over the age of 35, the thymus is predominantly fatty, with little or no intermixed glandular (soft tissue) component. The interface of the retrosternal space with the anterior portion of the right and left lungs may be visualized on lateral chest radiographs (see the section "Lateral Chest Radiograph"). The prevascular space generally retains the triangular configuration of the involuted thymus. Normal lymph nodes may be visible on CT within the fat of the prevascular space. Beginning at the level of the aortic arch in most individuals, the anterior portion of the prevascular space tapers to form a thin, vertically oriented linear density that represents the anterior junction line (Fig. 10.12B).

Middle (Visceral) Mediastinum. The middle (visceral) mediastinal compartment extends from the thoracic inlet superiorly to the diaphragm inferiorly and includes the pericardium and its contents, the aortic arch and proximal great arteries, descending thoracic aorta, the central pulmonary arteries and veins, the trachea and main bronchi, the esophagus and thoracic duct, the superior and inferior vena cava, and lymph nodes (Fig. 10.17C–H). Its anterior margin parallels the heart, ascending aorta, and main pulmonary artery, and its margin posteriorly extends to a vertical line parallel through the thoracic vertebrae 1 cm posterior to their anterior margins. The hila may be considered as lateral extensions of the middle mediastinal compartment. The phrenic and vagus nerves are not visible on CT scans but run together in the space between the subclavian arteries and brachiocephalic veins. The recurrent laryngeal nerves lie on each side within the tracheoesophageal groove.

Four middle mediastinal spaces surrounding the trachea and carina can be distinguished (Fig. 10.17B,C). The *right paratracheal space* contains lymph nodes and a small amount of fat. This space extends from the thoracic inlet superiorly to the azygos vein inferiorly. The *pretracheal space* is located between the trachea and the ascending aorta and is contiguous with the precarinal space inferiorly. It contains fat, lymph nodes, and the retroaortic portion of the superior pericardial recess and is the anatomic route used during routine transcervical mediastinoscopy. To the left of the trachea is the *aortopulmonary window*. The borders of the aortopulmonary window are the aortic arch superiorly; the left pulmonary artery inferiorly; the distal trachea, left main bronchus, and esophagus medially; the mediastinal pleural surface of the LUL laterally; the posterior surface of the ascending aorta anteriorly; and the anterior surface of the proximal descending aorta posteriorly. This space contains fat, lymph nodes, the ligamentum arteriosum, and the left recurrent laryngeal nerve. The subcarinal space is outlined posteriorly by the azygoesophageal recess and anteriorly by the posterior aspect of the right pulmonary artery.

The main pulmonary artery can be followed inferiorly to the outflow tract of the right ventricle (Fig. 10.17E). At this level, the right and left atrial appendages and the top of the left atrium may be seen. Also at this level, the right superior pulmonary vein lies anterior to the middle lobe bronchus,

TABLE 10.5

CONTENTS OF THE MEDIASTINUM

■ COMPARTMENT	■ CONTENTS
Anterior (prevascular) mediastinum	Thymus Left brachiocephalic vein Fat Germ cell rests Lymph nodes
Middle (visceral) mediastinum	Heart and pericardium Ascending, transverse, and descending thoracic aorta Main and proximal right and left pulmonary arteries Confluence of pulmonary veins Superior and inferior vena cava Trachea and main bronchi Esophagus Lymph nodes and fat within mediastinal spaces Azygos and hemiazygos veins Thoracic duct
Posterior (paravertebral) mediastinum	Thoracic spine Sympathetic ganglia and intercostal nerves Fat Lymph nodes

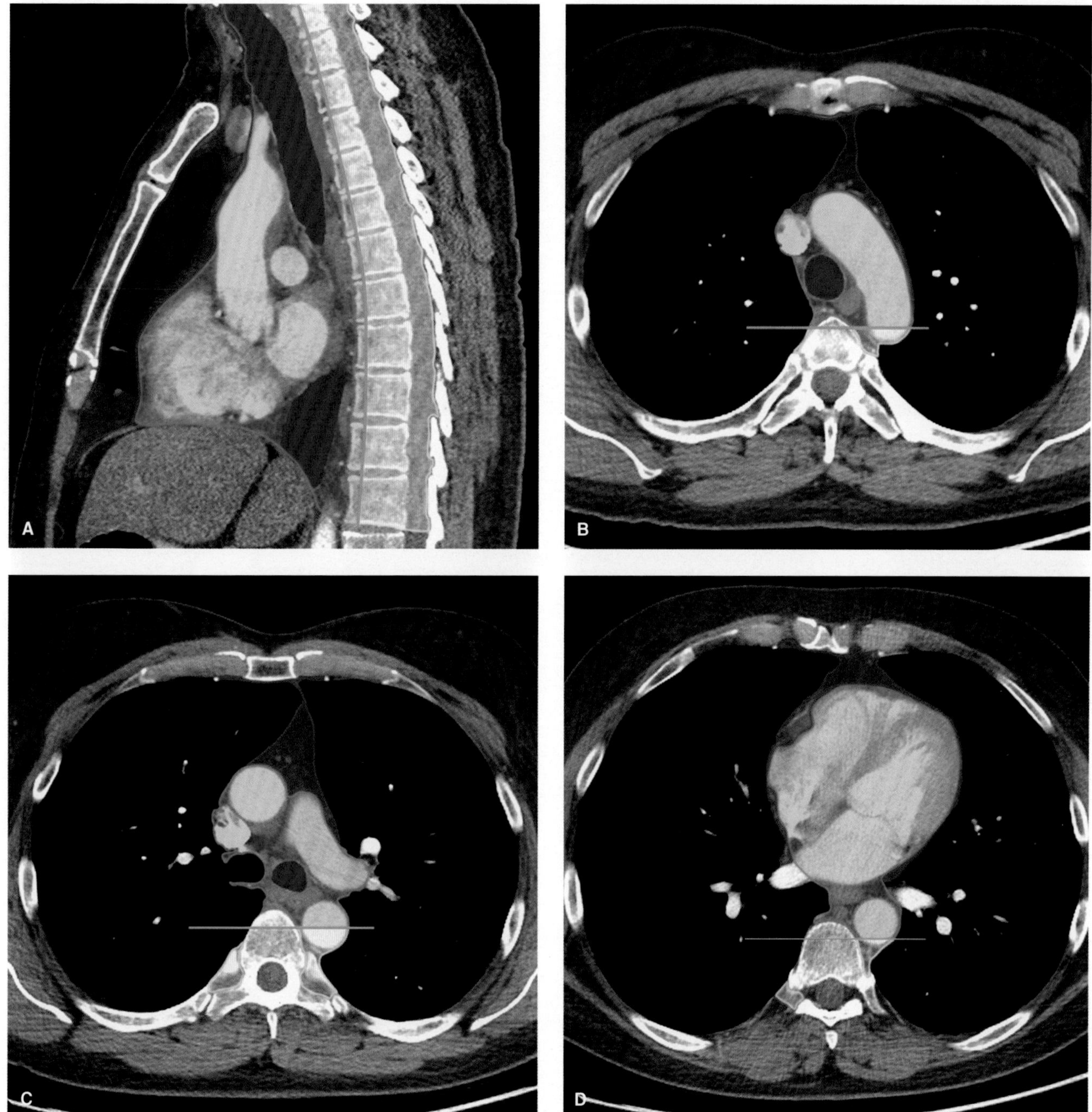

FIGURE 10.16. **Mediastinal Compartments as Defined by the International Thymic Malignancy Interest Group (ITMIG). A:** Midline sagittal contrast CT. **B:** Contrast-enhanced axial CT scan at level of aortic arch. **C:** Contrast-enhanced axial CT scan at level of left pulmonary artery. **D:** Contrast-enhanced axial CT scan at level of left atrium. Prevascular (*purple*), visceral (*blue*), and paravertebral (*yellow*) compartments. *Green line*, boundary between visceral and paravertebral mediastinal compartments. (Reprinted with permission from Carter BW, Benveniste MF, Madan R, et al. ITMIG classification of mediastinal compartments and multidisciplinary approach to mediastinal masses. *Radiographics* 2017;37(2):417; Figure 1.)

which in turn lies immediately anterior to the RLL bronchus. Inferiorly, the right atrium, right ventricle, and left ventricle are identified (Fig. 10.17F–H).

Nodal Stations. The International Association for the Study of Lung Cancer (IASLC) created a standard classification scheme for mediastinal lymph nodes (Fig. 13.19) to provide greater uniformity in the evaluation of nodal disease in patients with lung cancer and other malignancies.

Posterior (Paravertebral) Mediastinum. The posterior (paravertebral) mediastinal compartment lies behind the visceral mediastinum and includes the spine and paravertebral soft tissues including the thoracic duct, azygos and hemiazygos veins, sympathetic chain, proximal intercostal vessels and nerves, and lymph nodes and fat. The azygos and hemiazygos veins lie on the right and left sides, respectively, posterolateral to the descending aorta within a fat-containing space that also contains the thoracic duct, the sympathetic chains (normally not visible), and small lymph nodes (Fig. 10.17E–G,I). Inferiorly, this space is continuous with the retrocrural space and laterally with the paraspinal space, which contains the intercostal arteries, veins, and lymph nodes.

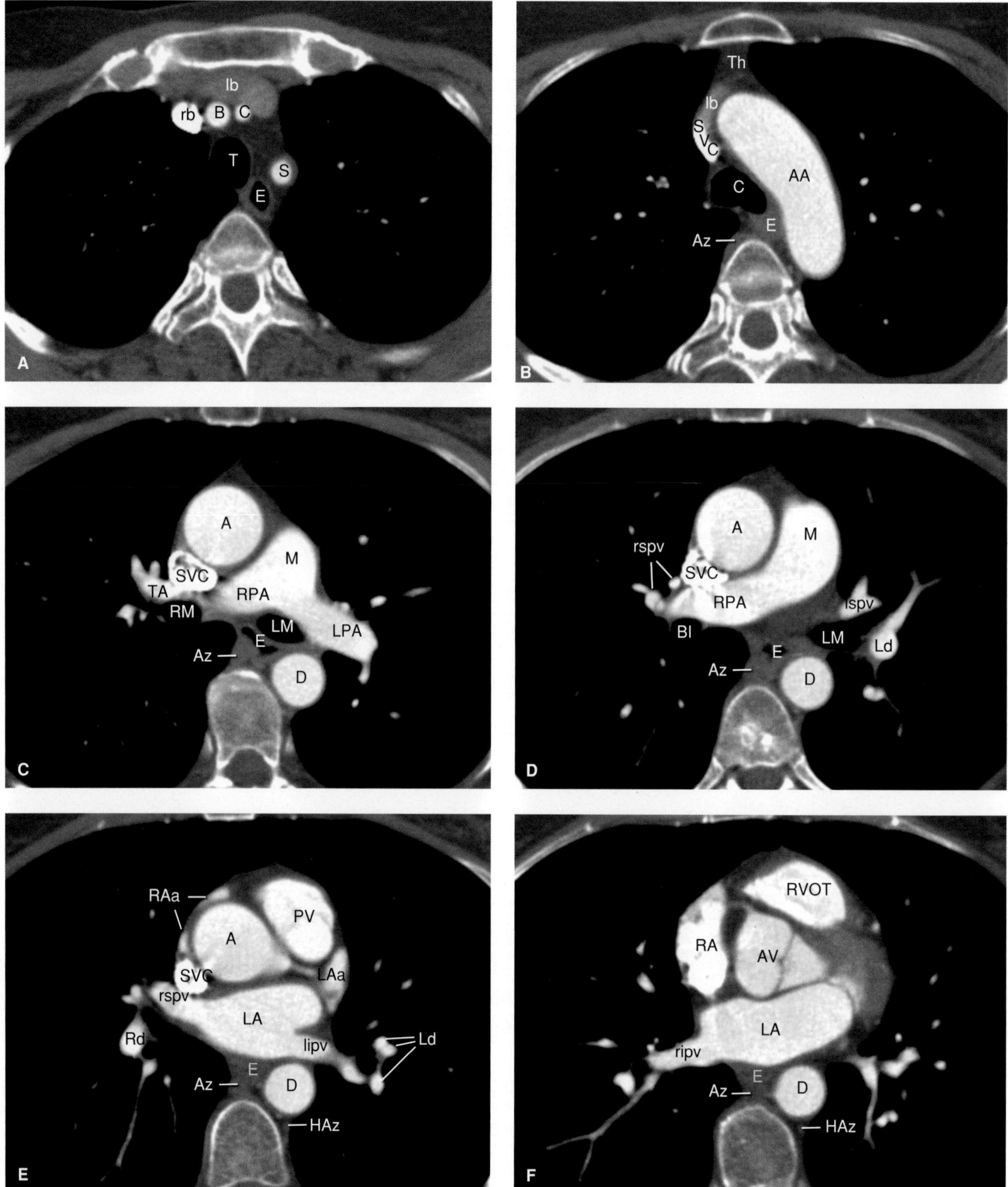

FIGURE 10.17. **Normal Mediastinal Anatomy on Coned-Down Axial CT. A: Supra-aortic level.** rb, right brachiocephalic vein; lb, left brachiocephalic vein; B, brachiocephalic artery; C, common carotid artery; S, left subclavian artery; T, trachea; E, esophagus. **B: Aortic arch level.** Th, thymus with fatty involution; lb, left brachiocephalic vein; SVC, superior vena cava; AA, aortic arch; C, tracheal carina; E, esophagus; Az, azygos vein. **C: Main and left pulmonary artery level.** SVC, superior vena cava; A, ascending aorta; D, descending aorta; M, main pulmonary artery; LPA, left pulmonary artery; RPA, right pulmonary artery; TA, truncus anterior branch of right pulmonary artery; RM, right main bronchus; LM, left main bronchus; E, esophagus; Az, azygos vein. **D: Right pulmonary artery level.** A, ascending aorta; SVC, superior vena cava; M, main pulmonary artery; RPA, right pulmonary artery; rspv, branches of right superior pulmonary vein; lspv, left superior pulmonary vein; BI, bronchus intermedius; LM, left main bronchus; Ld, left descending pulmonary artery; E, esophagus; Az, azygos vein; D, descending aorta. **E: Level of left atrium.** RAa, right atrial appendage; SVC, superior vena cava; A, ascending aorta; PV, pulmonic valve; LAa, left atrial appendage; LA, left atrium; rspv, right superior pulmonary vein; lipv, left inferior pulmonary vein; Rd, right lower lobe pulmonary artery; Ld, basal segmental branches of left lower lobe pulmonary artery; D, descending aorta; E, esophagus; Az, azygos vein; Haz, hemiazygos vein. **F: Level of aortic valve.** RA, right atrium; RVOT, right ventricular outflow tract; AV, aortic valve; ripv, right inferior pulmonary vein; LA, left atrium; D, descending aorta; E, esophagus; Az, azygos vein; HAz, hemiazygos vein.

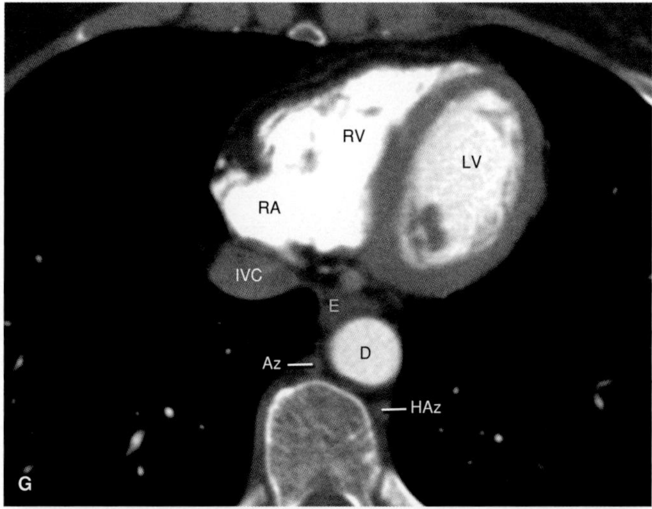

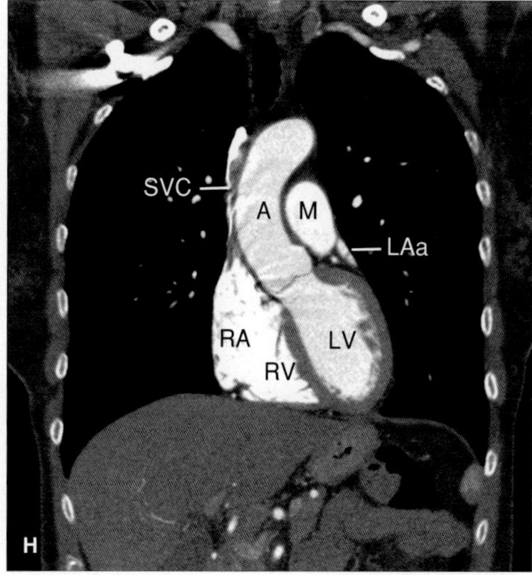

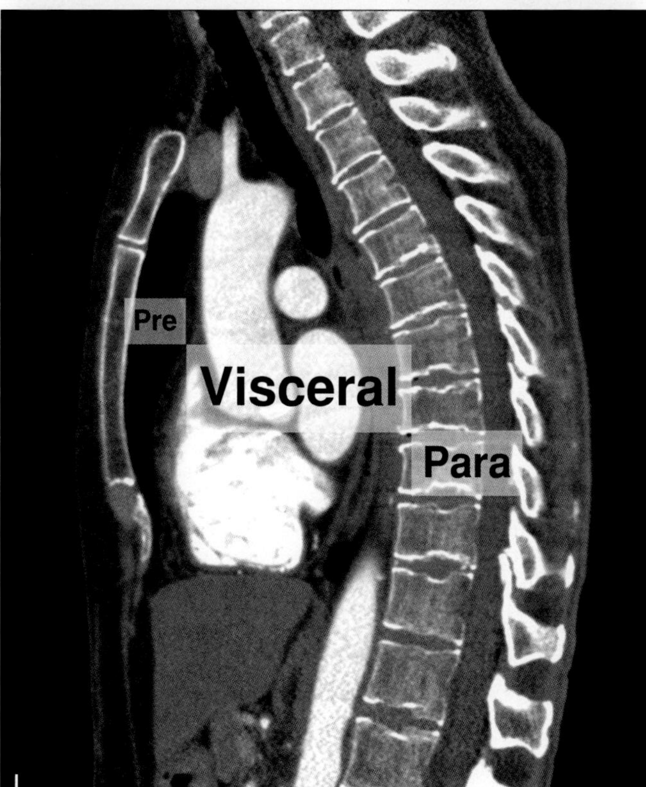

FIGURE 10.17. (*Continued*) **G: Level of the ventricles.** RA, right atrium; RV, right ventricle; LV, left ventricle; IVC, inferior vena cava; D, descending aorta; E, esophagus; Az, azygos vein; HAz, hemiazygos vein. **H: Normal coronal mediastinal anatomy.** SVC, superior vena cava; RA, right atrium; RV, right ventricle; A, ascending aorta; M, main pulmonary artery; LAa, left atrial appendage; LV, left ventricle. **I: Normal sagittal mediastinal anatomy.** The components of the prevascular (Pre), visceral (Visceral), and paravertebral (Para) mediastinal compartments are well demonstrated.

Normal Hilar Anatomy

Frontal View. The hilum represents the junction of the lung with the mediastinum and is composed of upper lobe pulmonary veins and branches of the pulmonary artery and corresponding bronchi (Fig. 10.18). These are all enveloped by small amounts of fat, with intermixed lymph nodes. On frontal radiographs, the right and left pulmonary arteries comprise the predominant portion of the hilar opacity. While the hilum is also composed of the superior pulmonary veins, lobar bronchi, bronchopulmonary lymph nodes, and a small amount of fat, these structures contribute little to the overall hilar density. In over 90% of normal individuals, the left hilar shadow is higher than the right. This is because the left pulmonary artery, which comprises the predominant portion of the left hilar shadow, ascends over the left main and upper lobe bronchus, whereas the right pulmonary artery lies inferior to the RUL bronchus. In the remainder of individuals, the right and left hila lie at the same level. A right hilum which is higher than the left suggests volume loss in either the RUL or the LLL.

The shape of the right hilum on frontal radiographs has been likened to a sideways V, with the opening pointing rightward (Fig. 10.18A). The upper portion of the V is composed primarily of the truncus anterior and the posterior division of the right superior pulmonary vein. The right interlobar artery forms the lower half of the V, as it descends lateral to the bronchus intermedius. The right inferior pulmonary vein crosses the lower right hilar shadow but does not contribute to its opacity.

Left Lateral View. On a true lateral radiograph, the right and left hilar shadows are not completely superimposed and comprise a combination of the right and left pulmonary arteries

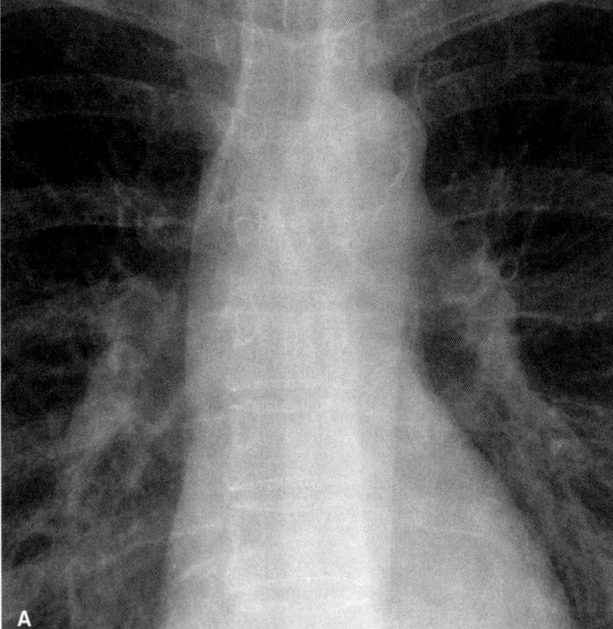

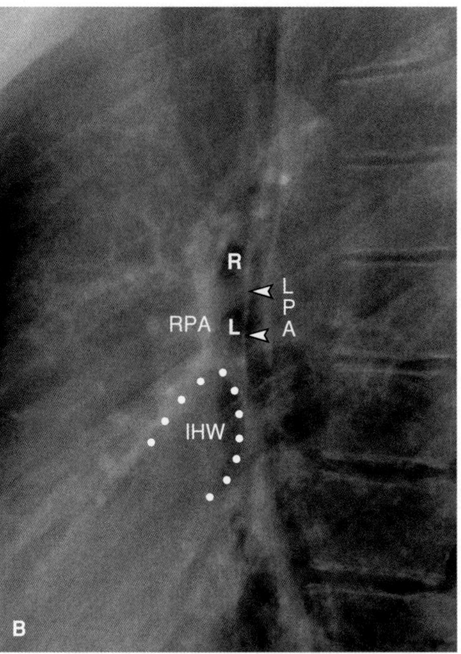

FIGURE 10.18. **Normal Frontal and Lateral Hilar Anatomy. A:** Coned-down frontal radiograph. Note that the left hilum is slightly higher than the right. **B:** Coned-down lateral radiograph. Same patient as Figure 10.6C. RPA, right pulmonary artery; LPA, left pulmonary artery; R, right upper lobe bronchus; L, left main/upper lobe bronchial confluence; *arrowheads*, posterior wall of bronchus intermedius (intermediate stem line); IHW, inferior hilar window (denoted by *dotted area*).

and the superior pulmonary veins (Figs. 10.6C and 10.18B). The anterior aspect of the hilar shadow is composed of the transverse portion of the right pulmonary artery, which produces an oval opacity projecting immediately anterior to the bronchus intermedius. The confluence of the right superior pulmonary veins overlaps the lower portion of the right pulmonary artery and contributes to its opacity. Superiorly and posteriorly, the comma-shaped left pulmonary artery passes above and behind the round or oval lucency representing the horizontally oriented LUL bronchus summating on a portion of the left main bronchus and then descends behind the LLL bronchus (Fig. 10.18B). The confluence of left superior pulmonary veins, which lies behind the level of the right superior pulmonary vein, creates an opacity that occupies the posteroinferior aspect of the composite hilar shadow. The avascular aspect of the composite hilar shadow, inferior to the shadow of the right pulmonary artery and veins and anterior to the descending left pulmonary artery and left superior vein, is called the *inferior hilar window* (Fig. 10.18B). This region is roughly triangular in shape, with its apex at the junction of the LUL and LLL bronchi and its base directed anteriorly and inferiorly. The RML and lingular veins cross the inferior hilar window, but because of their small size, they do not contribute significant opacity to this area.

The RUL bronchus is seen on lateral radiographs in approximately 50% of individuals as an end on, round lucency at the upper margin of the composite hilar shadow. The posterior wall of the bronchus intermedius is a thin vertical line, less than 2 mm thick, extending inferiorly from the posterior aspect of the RUL bronchus (Fig. 10.18B). This line, termed the intermediate stem line, is seen in 95% of patients and extends inferiorly to bisect the end-on lucency of the left main/LUL bronchus on a lateral radiograph. This structure is visible because air within the intermediate bronchus anteriorly and lung within the azygoesophageal recess posteriorly outlines its posterior wall. Thickening or nodularity of this line is seen in bronchogenic carcinoma, pulmonary edema, or enlargement of azygoesophageal recess lymph nodes.

The LUL bronchus is seen on lateral radiographs in 75% of individuals and lies approximately 4 cm inferior to the RUL bronchus. This bronchus is visualized with greater frequency than the RUL bronchus because it is outlined by the left pulmonary artery and other mediastinal structures, while the RUL bronchus is contacted only by the right main pulmonary artery anteroinferiorly and the azygos arch superiorly. The projection of the intermediate stem line over the LUL bronchus also helps identify this bronchus. Below the oval lucency of the LUL bronchus, the basal trunk of the LLL bronchus can sometimes be identified, with its anterior wall visible as a white line, outlined by air in the bronchial lumen and air in the lung.

Pleural Anatomy

The pleura is a serosal membrane that envelopes the lung and lines the costal surface, diaphragm, and mediastinum. It is composed of two layers (visceral and parietal) that join at the hilum. Blood supply to the parietal pleura is via the systemic circulation, while the visceral pleura is supplied by the pulmonary circulation. The parietal pleura is contiguous with the chest wall and diaphragm and therefore extends deep posteriorly into the costophrenic sulci, while the visceral pleura is adherent to the surface of the lung. The pleural space is a potential space between the two pleural layers and normally contains a small amount of fluid (<5 mL) that reduces friction during breathing.

The normal costal, diaphragmatic, and mediastinal pleura is not visible on conventional radiography or CT. On thin-section CT, a 1- to 2-mm stripe may be seen lining the intercostal spaces between adjacent ribs (Fig. 10.19). This "intercostal stripe" represents the combination of the two pleural layers, the endothoracic fascia, extrapleural fat, and the innermost intercostal muscle (Fig. 10.20). Internal to the ribs, the normal pleura is not seen and the inner cortex of rib appears to contact the lung. The presence of soft tissue between the inner

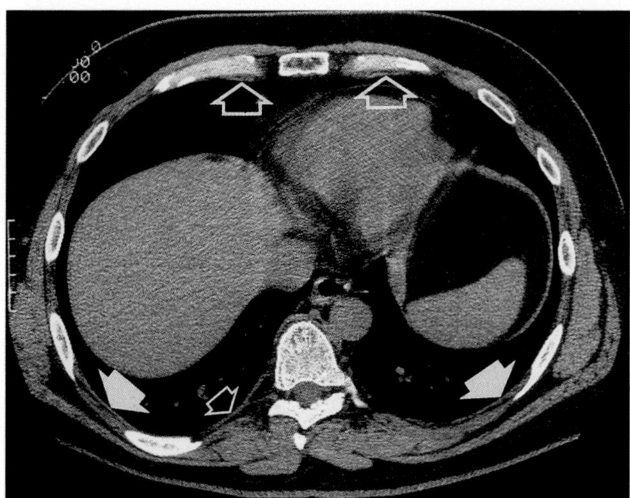

FIGURE 10.19. **HRCT of the Pleura.** HRCT scan through the lung bases demonstrates normal intercostal stripes (*solid arrows*) that are separated from the intercostal muscles by a layer of fat. An intercostal vein (*small open arrow*) is seen in the paravertebral region. Anteriorly, the transverse thoracic muscles (*large open arrows*) line the parasternal pleural surface.

rib and the lung, best appreciated on thin-section CT studies, indicates pleural thickening. The innermost intercostal muscle is anatomically absent in the paravertebral area, and if a thin line is visible between the lung and paravertebral fat or rib, it represents a combination of the two pleural surfaces and the endothoracic fascia.

Chest Wall Anatomy

The radiographic anatomy of the soft tissues and bony structures of the chest wall were discussed in the section on the normal frontal radiograph. CT provides detailed anatomic information about the normal chest wall and axillae. A detailed knowledge of normal cross-sectional chest wall and axillary anatomy is key to accurate localization and characterization of disease processes. Chest wall anatomy as seen on CT at six representative levels is shown in Figure 10.21.

Diaphragmatic Anatomy

The diaphragm is composed of striated muscles and a large central tendon separating the thoracic and abdominal cavities. The diaphragmatic muscle arises from the posterior aspect of the xiphoid process and anterolaterally, laterally, and posterolaterally from the 6th to 12th costal cartilages and ribs. The diaphragmatic crura originate from the upper lumbar vertebrae and course to the posterior aspect of the central tendon. The diaphragm has three normal openings and two potential gaps. The *aortic hiatus* lies in the midline, immediately behind the diaphragmatic crura and anterior to the 12th thoracic vertebral body (Fig. 10.22A). The aorta, thoracic duct, and azygos and hemiazygos veins traverse this opening. The *esophageal hiatus* usually lies slightly to the left of midline, cephalad to the aortic hiatus, and transmits the esophagus and vagus nerves (Fig. 10.22B). The caval foramen contains the inferior vena cava and pierces the central tendon of the diaphragm at the level of the eighth thoracic intervertebral disk space (Fig. 10.22C). The foramina of Morgagni are triangular gaps in the muscles of the anteromedial diaphragm. This cleft is normally occupied by fat and the internal mammary vessels and is a site of potential intrathoracic herniation of abdominal contents. The foramina of Bochdalek are defects in the closure of the posterolateral diaphragm at the junction of the pleuroperitoneal membrane with the transverse septum. Hernias through the foramina of Morgagni and Bochdalek are discussed in Chapter 17.

On CT scans, the domes of the diaphragms are rounded interfaces on either side of the chest at the level of the base of the heart. In some patients, the diaphragm has an undulating or nodular appearance due to contraction of the slips of the diaphragmatic muscles. This appearance is seen with increasing frequency in older patients and is more common on the left than the right. Posteriorly, the superior aspects of the diaphragmatic crura are seen. The crura are curvilinear soft tissue structures that arise from the upper two to three lumbar vertebrae. Their associated esophageal and aortic openings within the bundles of the crura are well visualized on CT (Fig. 10.22). The inferior aspects of the diaphragmatic crura within the upper abdomen may have a rounded appearance in the axial plane and should not be mistaken for enlarged retrocrural lymph nodes.

RADIOGRAPHIC FINDINGS IN CHEST DISEASE

Parenchymal lung disease on chest radiographs can be divided into those processes that produce an abnormal increase in the density of the lung (opacity) and those that produce an abnormal decrease in lung density (lucency). The normal density of the lungs is a result of the relative proportion of air to soft tissue (blood or parenchyma) in a ratio of 11 to 1. Processes that increase the relative amount of soft tissue cause a significant

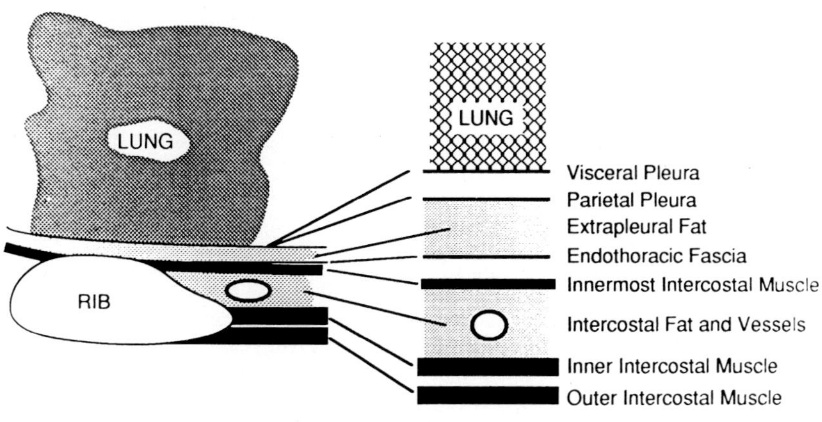

FIGURE 10.20. **Normal Pleural and Chest Wall Anatomy.** The visceral pleura is 0.1 to 0.2 mm thick and is composed of a single layer of mesothelial cells and its associated fibroelastic fascia, called the subpleural interstitium, that is part of the peripheral interstitial network. The parietal pleura is 0.1 mm thick and is composed of a single layer of mesothelial cells lining a loose connective tissue layer containing systemic capillaries, lymphatic vessels, and sensory nerves. Outside the parietal pleura is the fibroelastic endothoracic fascia, which is separated from the pleura by a thin layer of extrapleural fat. The endothoracic fascia lines the ribs and intercostal muscles.

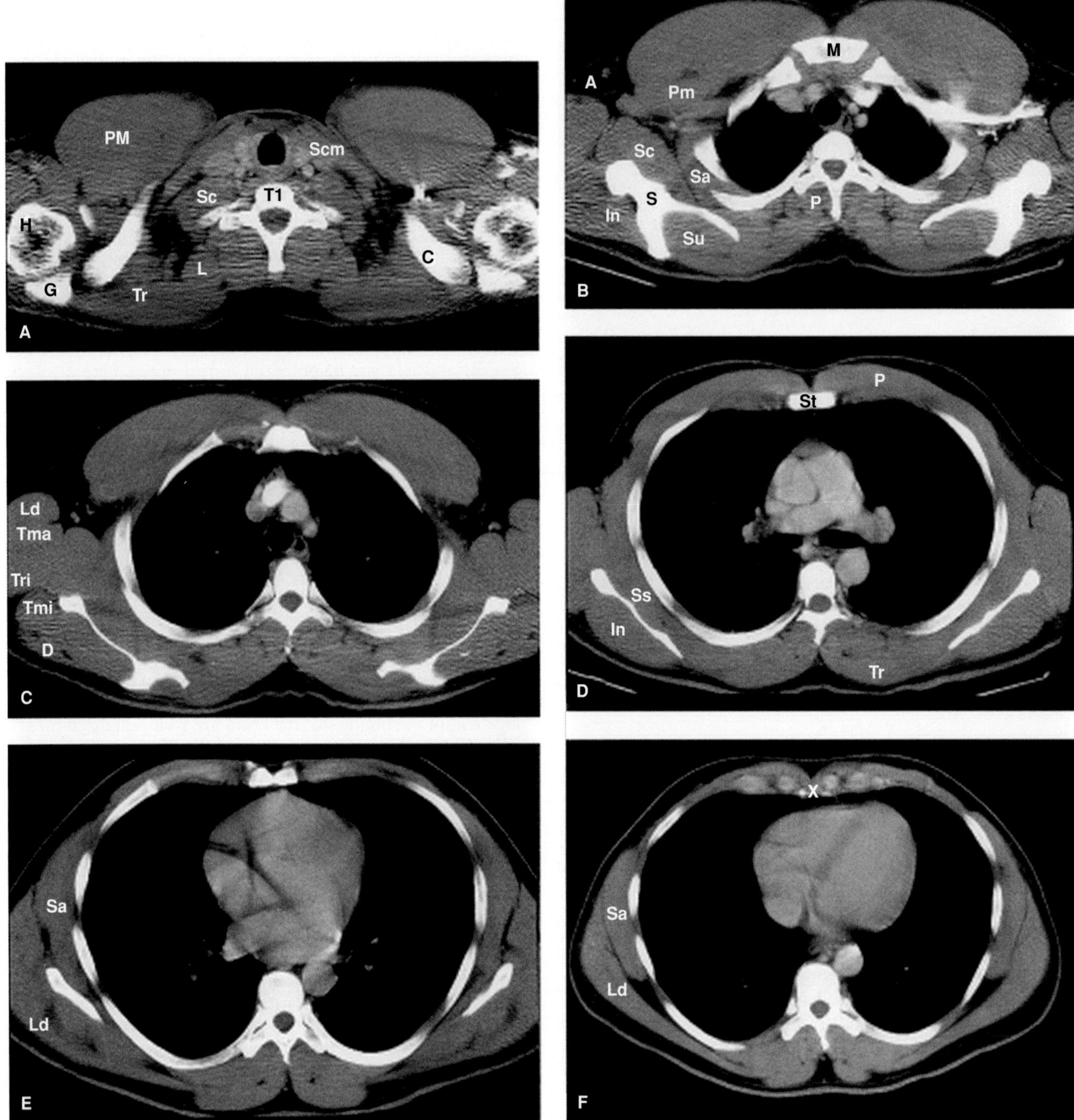

FIGURE 10.21. **Normal Chest Wall Anatomy on CT. A: Level of the thoracic inlet.** PM, pectoralis major muscle; Tr, trapezius muscle; L, levator scapulae muscle; Sc, scalene muscle; Scm, sternocleidomastoid muscle; H, humeral head; G, glenoid; C, distal clavicle; T1, first thoracic vertebral body. **B: Level of the axillary vessels.** Pm, pectoralis minor muscle; Sa, serratus anterior muscle; Su, supraspinatus muscle; In, infraspinatus muscle; Ss, subscapularis muscle; P, paraspinal muscles; M, manubrium of the sternum; S, body of the scapula; A, axilla with normal lymph nodes. **C: Level of the sternomanubrial joint.** Ld, latissimus dorsi muscle; Tma, teres major muscle; Tri, long head of the triceps muscle; Tmi, teres minor muscle; D, deltoid muscle. **D: Level of the body of the sternum.** P, pectoralis muscles; Ss, subscapularis muscle; In, infraspinatus muscle; Tr, trapezius muscle; St, body of the sternum. **E: Level of tip of scapula.** Ld, latissimus dorsi muscle; Sa, serratus anterior muscle. **F: Level of the xiphoid process.** Ld, latissimus dorsi muscle; Sa, serratus anterior muscle; X, xiphoid process of the sternum.

decrease in this ratio and are more easily discernible than diffuse processes which destroy blood vessels and parenchyma and cause little change in this ratio, thereby producing only small decreases in overall lung density. CT, by virtue of its superior contrast resolution, is significantly more sensitive than radiography in demonstrating subtle decreases in overall radiographic density of the lungs.

Abnormal pulmonary opacities may be classified into airspace opacities, opacity resulting from atelectasis, interstitial opacities, nodular or mass-like opacities, and branching

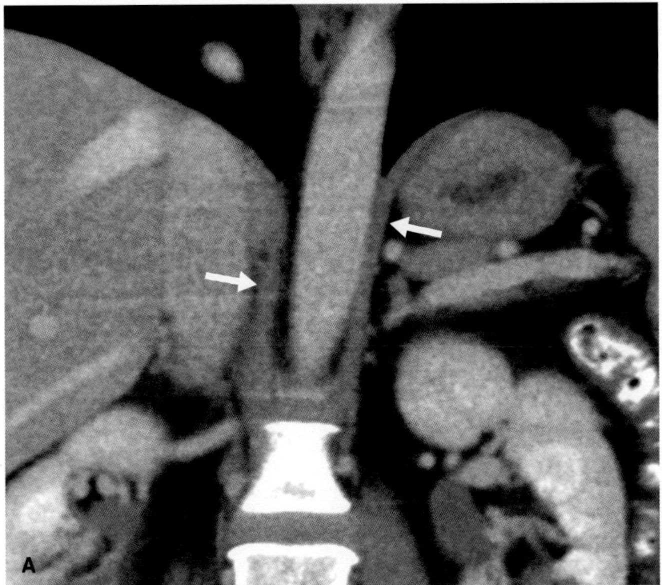

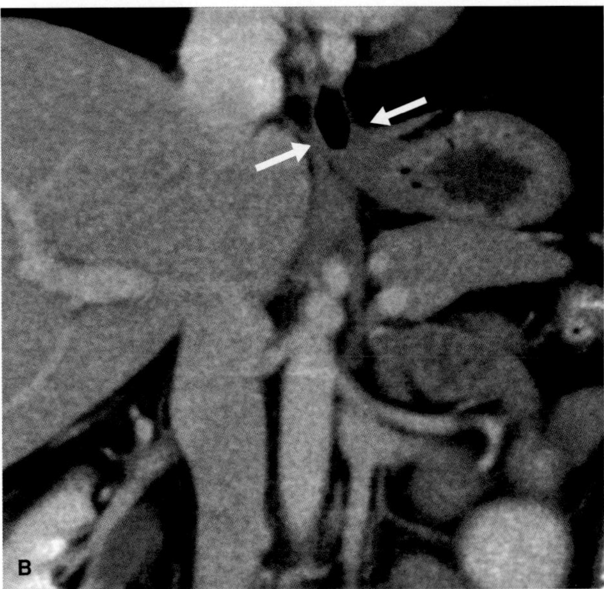

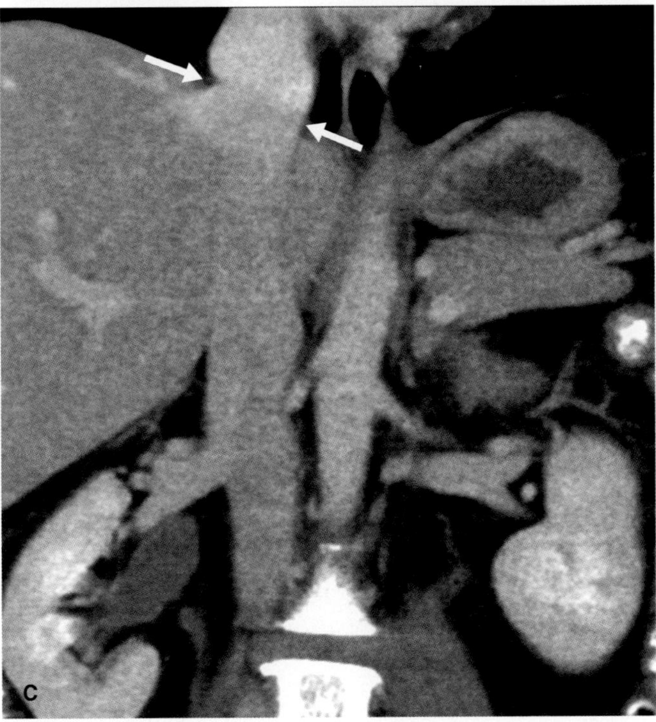

FIGURE 10.22. **Normal Diaphragmatic Hiatuses on CT. A:** Coned-down coronal contrast-enhanced CT through the posterior aspect of the upper abdomen shows the aortic hiatus situated between the diaphragmatic crura (*arrows*). **B:** Coned-down coronal contrast-enhanced CT anterior to (**A**) shows the esophageal hiatus (*arrows*). **C:** Coned-down coronal contrast-enhanced CT anterior to (**B**) shows the caval hiatus (*arrows*).

opacities (Table 10.6). These patterns have been shown to accurately represent pulmonary pathologic processes in correlative radiographic–pathologic studies and are a practical means of generating a meaningful differential diagnosis.

Pulmonary Opacity

Airspace Disease. Radiographic findings of airspace disease are listed in Table 10.7. Airspace opacities occur when air within the terminal airspaces of the lung is replaced by material of soft tissue density, such as blood, transudate, exudate, or neoplastic cells. A segmental distribution of disease may be seen in a process such as pneumococcal pneumonia, which begins in the terminal airspaces and spreads to other airspaces via interalveolar channels (pores of Kohn) and channels bridging preterminal bronchioles with alveoli (canals of Lambert). Initially, the opacity is poorly marginated because the airspace-filling process extends in an irregular fashion to involve adjacent airspaces, creating an irregular interface with the x-ray beam. Airspace nodules, which are typically poorly marginated, round opacities, 6 to 8 mm in diameter, may be seen at the leading edge of an airspace-filling process. These nodules represent filling of acini or other sublobular structures and are most often seen in diffuse alveolar pulmonary edema and transbronchial spread of cavitary tuberculosis.

A characteristic of airspace-filling processes is the tendency of airspace shadows to coalesce as they extend through the lung. When the airspaces are rendered opaque by the presence of intra-alveolar cellular material and fluid, the normally aerated bronchi become visible as branching tubular lucencies

TABLE 10.6

PATTERNS OF PULMONARY OPACITY

■ TYPE		■ EXAMPLE
Airspace (alveolar) filling		Pneumococcal pneumonia Pulmonary edema
Atelectasis	Lobar Subsegmental	Endobronchial neoplasm Linear atelectasis
Interstitial opacities	Reticular Reticulonodular Linear	Idiopathic pulmonary fibrosis Sarcoidosis Interstitial pulmonary edema
Nodular	Miliary (<2 mm) Micronodule (2–7 mm) Nodule(s) (7–30 mm)	Miliary tuberculosis Acute hypersensitivity pneumonitis Granulomatous diseases Lung cancer Hamartoma Metastases
	Mass (>30 mm)	Lung cancer Abscess
Tubular/branching		Mucocele

called *air bronchograms* (Fig. 10.23). Rarely, severe interstitial disease encroaching upon the airspaces may produce an air bronchogram; this is most typically seen in "alveolar" sarcoid. When the airspace-filling process extends to the interlobar fissure, it is seen as a sharply marginated lobar opacity.

A pattern of parenchymal opacity that reliably represents an airspace-filling process is the "bat's wing" or "butterfly" pattern of disease. In this pattern, dense airspace opacities occupy the central regions of lung and abruptly terminate as they extend laterally before reaching the peripheral portions of the lung. This distribution of disease appears almost exclusively in patients with pulmonary edema. Another feature of airspace-filling processes is the tendency to rapidly change over time. The development or resolution of parenchymal opacities within hours usually indicates an airspace-filling process; prominent exceptions include atelectasis and interstitial pulmonary edema. The differential diagnosis of diffuse confluent airspace opacities is reviewed in Table 10.8.

The CT findings of airspace disease are similar to those described on chest radiography. These are: (1) lobar, segmental, and/or lobular distribution of disease; (2) poorly marginated opacities that tend to coalesce; (3) airspace nodules; and (4) air bronchograms. A lobar or segmental distribution of disease is easily appreciated on cross-sectional imaging. CT can show individually opacified lobules, termed a "patchwork quilt" appearance. This pattern is classically seen in bronchopneumonia (Fig. 10.24) but is also present in other airspace processes. Coalescence of opacities, commonly seen in pulmonary edema and pneumonia, is best assessed on serial CT studies. When diseases cause only airspace filling, airspace nodules are present and the interlobular septa are normal or obscured. On thin-section CT, these nodules are usually seen within the peribronchiolar (centrilobular) region of the pulmonary lobule. Air bronchograms or bronchiolograms are usually better appreciated on thin-section CT than on radiographs owing to the superior contrast resolution and

TABLE 10.7

RADIOGRAPHIC CHARACTERISTICS OF AIRSPACE DISEASE

Lobar or segmental distribution
Poorly marginated
Airspace nodules
Tendency to coalesce
Air bronchograms
Bat's wing (butterfly) distribution
Rapid change over time

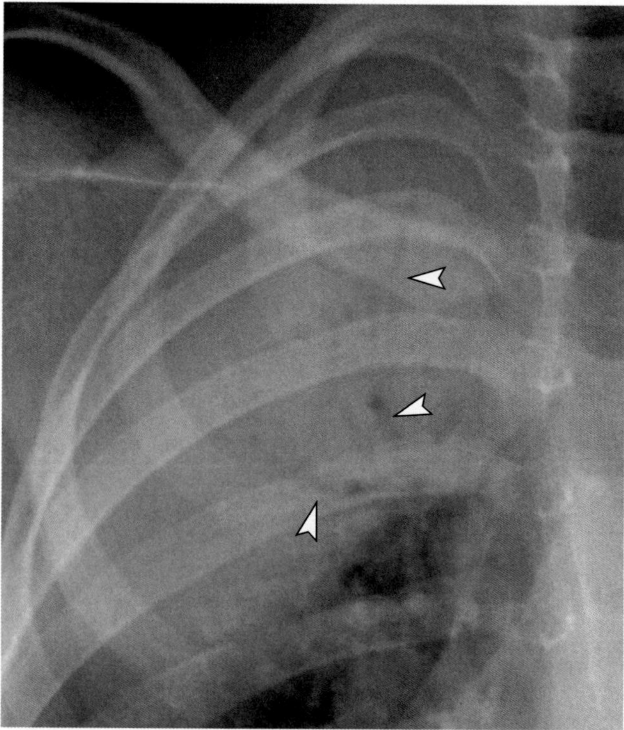

FIGURE 10.23. **Air Bronchograms in Air Space Disease.** Coned-down frontal radiograph in a 4-year-old with lobar pneumonia shows right upper lobe airspace opacification with branching tubular lucencies (*arrowheads*) reflecting air bronchograms.

TABLE 10.8

DIFFUSE CONFLUENT AIRSPACE OPACITY

■ TYPE	■ EXAMPLE
Pulmonary edema	Cardiogenic Fluid overload/renal failure Increased capillary permeability (see Table 12.2)
Inflammatory	Acute hypersensitivity pneumonitis Acute eosinophilic pneumonia Acute lupus pneumonitis
Pneumonia	*Pneumocystis jiroveci* Gram-negative bacteria Viral (influenza) Fungi Histoplasmosis Aspergillosis
Hemorrhage	See Table 12.3
Neoplasm	Adenocarcinoma (mucinous) Lymphoma
Alveolar proteinosis	Acute silica inhalation Lymphoma Leukemia AIDS

the cross-sectional nature of CT. This is particularly true in those regions of the lung where bronchi course in the transverse plane (anterior segments of upper lobes, middle lobe and lingula, and superior segments of the lower lobes).

Atelectasis reflects loss of lung volume and is usually but not invariably associated with an increase in radiographic density. There are five basic mechanisms of atelectasis (Table 10.9).

TABLE 10.9

TYPES OF PULMONARY ATELECTASIS

■ TYPE	■ EXAMPLE
Obstructive (resorptive)	Lung cancer (endobronchial)
Passive (relaxation)	Pleural effusion Pneumothorax
Compressive	Bulla
Cicatricial	Postprimary tuberculosis Radiation fibrosis
Adhesive	Respiratory distress syndrome of the newborn

Obstructive or *resorptive atelectasis* is the most common form of atelectasis and is secondary to complete endobronchial obstruction of a lobar bronchus with resorption of gas distally. Complete obstruction of a central bronchus may not produce atelectasis if collateral airflow to the obstructed lung (via pores of Kohn, canals of Lambert, or incomplete interlobar fissures) allows the lung to remain inflated. An obstructed lobe or lung containing a high partial pressure of oxygen, as may be seen in patients receiving supplemental oxygen, will collapse more rapidly (sometimes within minutes) than does lung containing ambient air due to the rapid absorption of oxygen from the alveolar spaces into the alveolar capillaries. Lung cancer, mucus plugs, foreign bodies, and malpositioned endotracheal tubes are the most common causes of endobronchial obstruction and secondary resorptive atelectasis.

Passive or *relaxation atelectasis* results from the mass effect of pleural air or fluid on the underlying lung, as the lung recoils inward when dissociated from the chest wall. The degree of atelectasis depends on the size of the pleural collection and the compliance of the lung and visceral pleura.

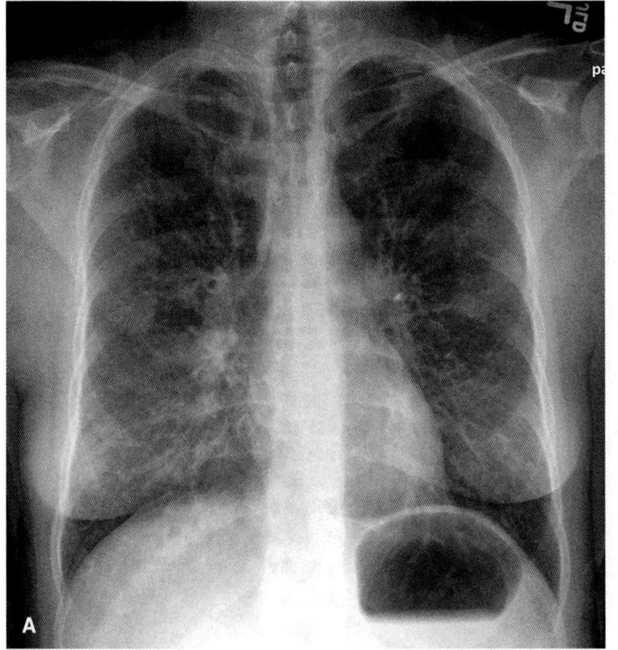

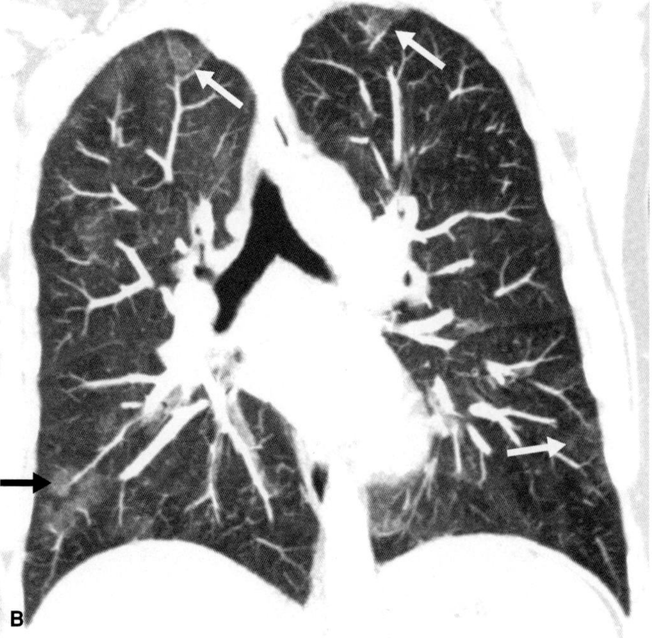

FIGURE 10.24. **Lobular Air Space Disease in Bronchopneumonia. A:** Frontal chest radiograph in a 47-year-old female with bronchopneumonia shows bilateral patchy airspace opacities. **B, C:** Coronal CT scan through the carina (**B**) and posterior lungs (**C**) shows multifocal lobular ground-glass opacities (*arrows*). (*continued*)

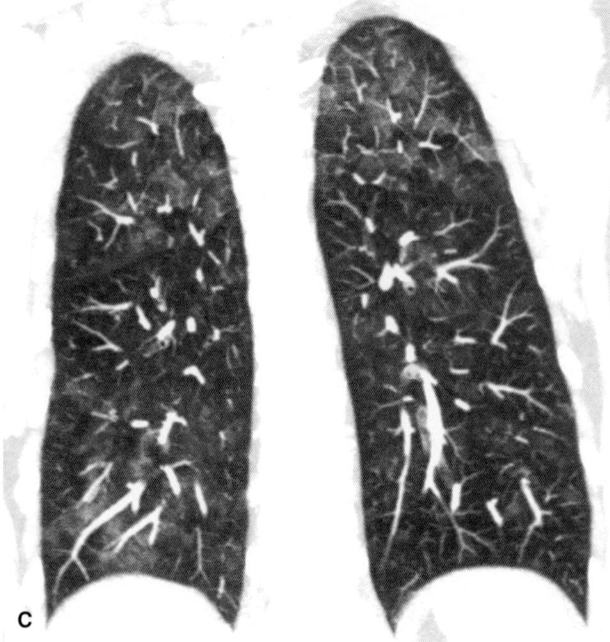

FIGURE 10.24. (*Continued*)

A large pleural or chest wall mass or elevated diaphragm can also produce passive atelectasis.

Compressive atelectasis is a form of passive atelectasis in which an intrapulmonary mass compresses adjacent lung parenchyma. Common causes include bullae, lung abscesses, and large tumors.

Processes resulting in parenchymal fibrosis reduce alveolar volume and produce *cicatricial atelectasis*. Localized cicatricial atelectasis is most often seen in association with chronic upper lobe fibronodular tuberculosis. The radiographic appearance is that of severe lobar volume loss with scarring, bronchiectasis, and compensatory hyperinflation of the adjacent lung. Diffuse cicatricial atelectasis is seen in interstitial fibrosis of any etiology. An overall increase in lung density, with reticular opacities and diminished lung volumes, is characteristic of this condition.

TABLE 10.10

RADIOGRAPHIC SIGNS IN LOBAR ATELECTASIS

■ DIRECT SIGNS	■ INDIRECT SIGNS
Displacement of interlobar fissure	Bronchovascular crowding
Increased density of atelectatic lung	Ipsilateral diaphragm elevation Ipsilateral tracheal/cardiac/mediastinal shift Hilar elevation (upper lobe atelectasis) or depression (lower lobe atelectasis) Compensatory hyperinflation of other lobe(s) Shifting granuloma Ipsilateral small hemithorax Ipsilateral rib space narrowing

Adhesive atelectasis occurs in association with surfactant deficiency. Type 2 pneumocytes, which produce surfactant, may be injured as a result of general anesthesia, ischemia, or radiation. Surfactant deficiency causes increased alveolar surface tension and results in diffuse alveolar collapse and volume loss. Radiographs typically show decreased lung volume and an increase in density.

Lobar Atelectasis. The only direct radiographic finding of lobar atelectasis is the displacement of an interlobar fissure (Table 10.10). There are several indirect findings of atelectasis, most of which reflect attempts to compensate for the volume loss (Table 10.10 and Fig. 10.25). Diminished aeration results in increased density in the affected portion of the lung and bronchovascular crowding. Ipsilateral shift of the trachea, heart, or mediastinum and hilar structures is a common finding in lobar atelectasis. Shift of the entire mediastinum is typical of

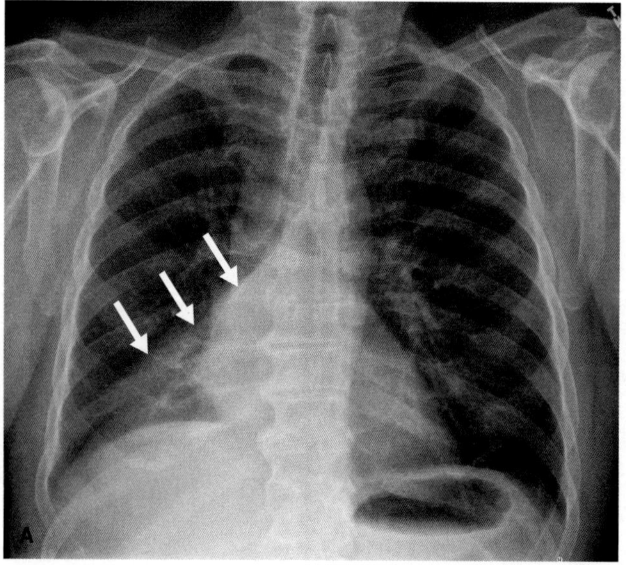

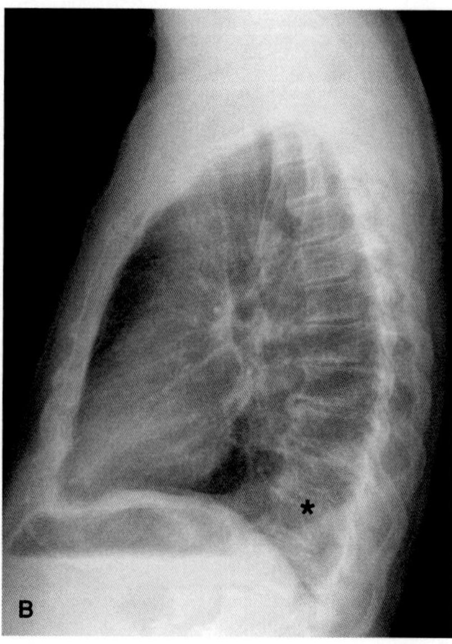

FIGURE 10.25. **Right Lower Lobe Atelectasis.** Frontal chest radiograph (**A**) in a patient with right lower lobe atelectasis shows a homogeneous triangular opacity in the right lower lung that obscures the medial right hemidiaphragm. *Arrows*, displaced right major fissure. On the lateral radiograph (**B**), there is opacity overlying the lower spine (*asterisk*) and the posterior right diaphragm is obscured.

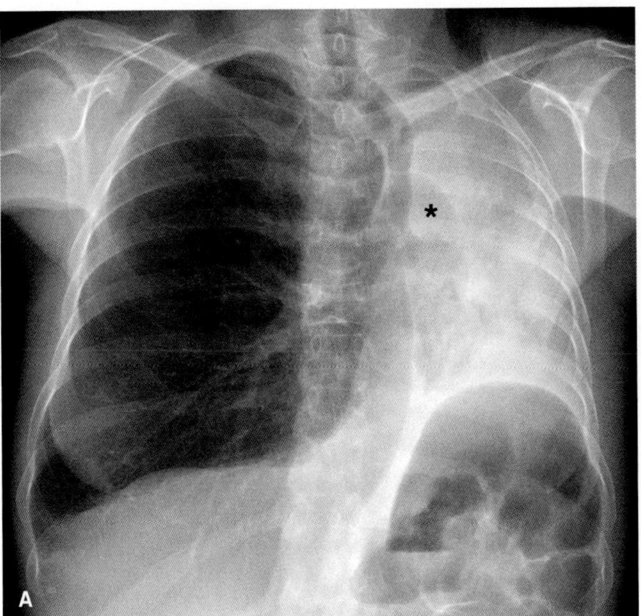

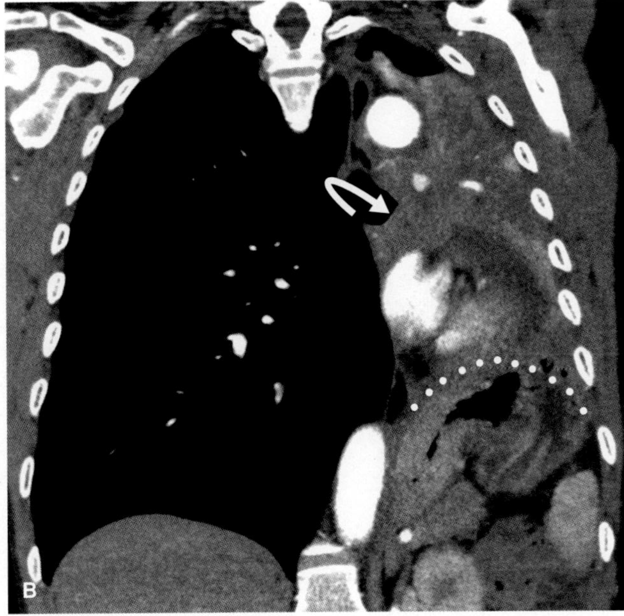

FIGURE 10.26. **Atelectasis of the Entire Lung. A:** Frontal chest radiograph in a 62-year-old man with shortness of breath and hemoptysis demonstrates complete left lung atelectasis. Note marked leftward mediastinal shift with overinflation of the anterior right upper lobe (*asterisk*) and elevation of the left diaphragm. **B:** Contrast-enhanced coronal CT shows virtually complete left lung atelectasis with leftward mediastinal shift and an elevated left hemidiaphragm (*dotted line*). A mass (*curved arrow*) is seen obstructing the left main bronchus as the cause of the atelectasis. Bronchoscopy revealed an obstructing squamous cell carcinoma.

collapse of an entire lung (Fig. 10.26). Compensatory hyperinflation, which represents an attempt by the remaining normal lung to partially fill the space lost by the atelectatic lung, usually develops with chronic volume loss and is not seen in acute collapse. It is seen as increased lucency of lung with attenuation of pulmonary vascular markings. In complete lung or upper lobe atelectasis, the contralateral upper lobe may herniate across the midline bowing the anterior junction line toward the affected side (Fig. 10.26). A characteristic but seldom seen plain radiographic finding of compensatory hyperinflation is the "shifting granuloma," in which a pre-existing granuloma in an adjacent aerated lung changes position as it moves toward the collapsed lobe. In atelectasis of a lung, a decrease in size of the hemithorax with approximation of the ribs may be seen. The absence of air bronchograms helps distinguish resorptive lobar atelectasis from lobar pneumonia, particularly if the atelectatic lobe is only slightly diminished in volume. A triangular configuration with the apex at the pulmonary hilum is common to all types of lobar atelectasis. The fissure bordering the collapsed lobe typically assumes a concave configuration. Complete lobar atelectasis can be difficult to detect on frontal and lateral radiographs but is easily appreciated on CT.

Segmental Atelectasis. Atelectasis of one or several segments of a lobe may be difficult to visualize on plain radiographs. The appearance ranges from a thin linear opacity to a wedge-shaped opacity that does not abut an interlobar fissure. Segmental atelectasis is better appreciated on CT.

Subsegmental (Platelike) Atelectasis. Bandlike linear opacities representing linear atelectasis are commonly associated with low lung volumes. This is seen in patients with pleuritic chest pain, postoperative patients, or patients with massive hepatosplenomegaly or ascites. Subsegmental atelectasis tends to occur at the lung bases. The linear shadows are 2 to 10 cm in length and are typically oriented perpendicular to the costal pleura (Fig. 10.27). Pathologically, these areas of linear collapse are deep to invaginations of visceral pleura formed by incomplete fissures or scars.

Rounded Atelectasis. This uncommon form of atelectasis, typically affecting the lower lobe, is most closely associated with asbestos-related pleural disease but may be seen in any condition associated with an exudative (proteinaceous) pleural effusion. Pleural adhesions which form in the resolving phase of a pleural effusion can cause the adjacent lung to roll up into a ball as it re-expands. Rounded atelectasis is often found along the inferior and posterior costal pleural surfaces adjacent to an area of pleural fibrosis or plaque formation. Conventional radiographs reveal a well-defined, 2- to 7-cm pleural-based mass adjacent to an area of pleural thickening in the lower posterior lung. The identification of a curvilinear bronchovascular bundle or "comet tail" entering the anterior inferior margin of the mass, as seen on lateral radiographs, is characteristic. The round or wedge-shaped mass forms an acute angle with the pleura adjacent to an area of pleural thickening, usually in the inferior and posterior thorax. Posterior displacement of the major fissure as a sign of atelectasis is best appreciated on sagittal CT reformations (Fig. 10.28). The atelectatic lung can be seen to enhance following intravenous contrast administration. When the characteristic CT findings are seen in a patient with a known history of pleural disease, the appearance is diagnostic and no further evaluation is necessary.

Right Upper Lobe Atelectasis (Fig. 10.29A,B). In RUL atelectasis, the lung collapses superiorly and medially, with superomedial displacement of the minor fissure and anteromedial displacement of the upper half of the major fissure, producing a right upper paramediastinal density on frontal radiographs, which can obliterate the normal right paratracheal stripe and azygos vein. A central convex mass will prevent part of the usual fissure concavity. This appearance produces the S sign of Golden (Fig. 13.13B). The trachea is deviated toward the right, and the right hilum and hemidiaphragm are elevated. "Tenting" or "peaking" of the right hemidiaphragm is occasionally seen and represents fat within the inferior aspect of a stretched inferior accessory fissure. Compensatory hyperinflation of the

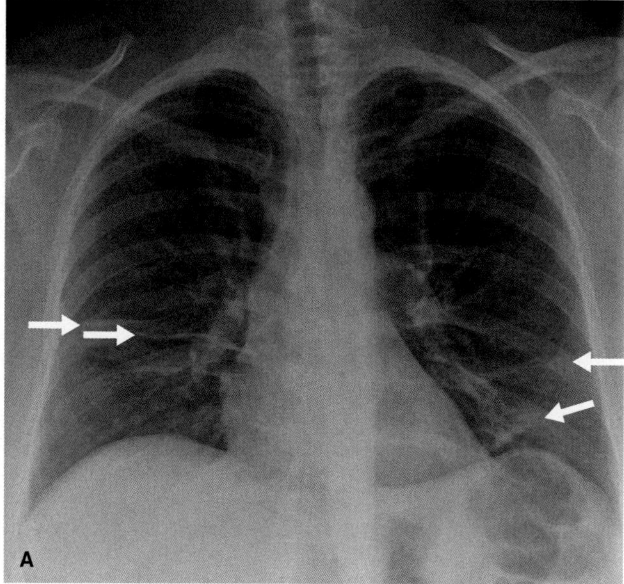

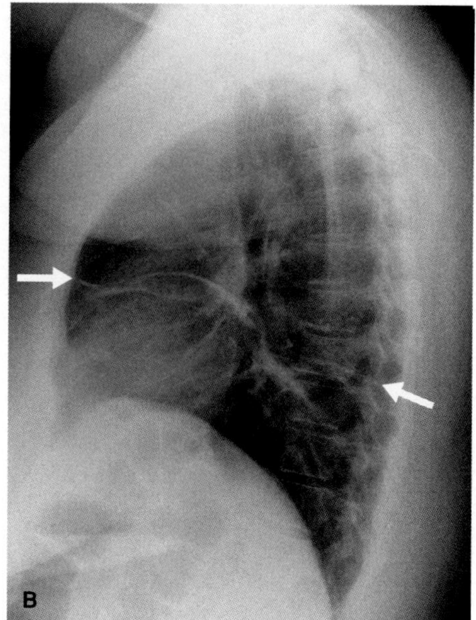

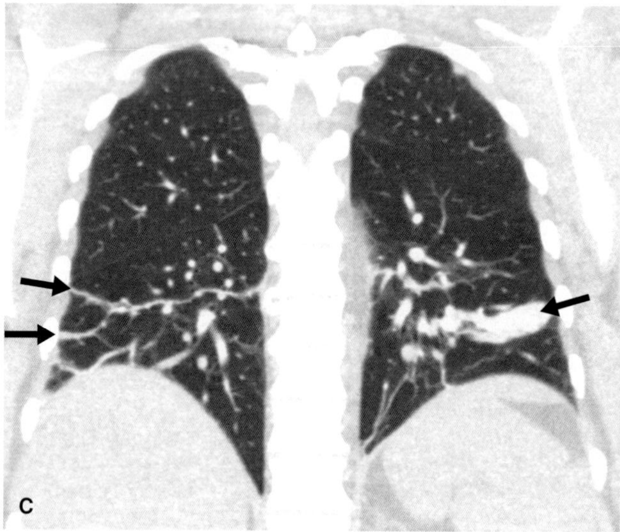

FIGURE 10.27. Subsegmental (Platelike) Atelectasis. A, B: Frontal (**A**) and lateral (**B**) chest radiographs and coronal CT scan (**C**) in a man with abdominal pain shows diminished lung volumes and bilateral lower zone coarse linear opacities (*arrows*) parallel to the diaphragms and perpendicular to the costal pleura, representing areas of subsegmental atelectasis.

middle and lower lobes may be seen in chronic atelectasis, and the LUL may herniate across the midline anteriorly toward the right. Scarring from tuberculosis, endobronchial tumor, and mucus plugging are common causes of RUL atelectasis.

Left upper lobe atelectasis (Fig. 10.29C,D) has a different appearance from RUL atelectasis because of the absence of a minor fissure. The LUL collapses anteriorly, maintaining a broad area of contact with the anterior costal pleural surface. The major fissure shifts anteriorly and is seen marginating a long, narrow band of increased opacity paralleling the anterior chest wall on lateral radiographs. Diagnosis on frontal radiographs may be difficult. There is subtle increased opacity in the left upper thorax, which can obliterate the aortic knob, AP window, and left upper cardiac margin. The apex of the left hemithorax remains lucent as a result of hyperinflation of the superior segment of the LLL. Leftward tracheal displacement, left hilar and left diaphragmatic elevation, and leftward bulging of the anterior junction line from an overinflated RUL are additional clues to the diagnosis. An uncommon finding on the frontal radiograph in LUL atelectasis is a crescent of air ("Luftsichel") along the left upper mediastinum, which represents a portion of the overinflated superior segment of the LLL interposed between the aortic arch medially and the collapsed upper lobe laterally (Fig. 10.29C). Postinflammatory cicatrization and endobronchial tumor are the most common causes of LUL atelectasis.

Middle lobe atelectasis (Fig. 10.29E,F) displaces the minor fissure posteroinferiorly and the major fissure anterosuperiorly. Because of the minimal thickness of the collapsed middle lobe and the oblique orientation of the inferiorly displaced minor fissure, the detection of middle lobe atelectasis on frontal radiographs is difficult. The only finding on frontal radiographs may be a vague density over the right lower lung, with obscuration of the right heart margin. The lateral radiograph shows a typical triangular density, with its apex at the hilum.

Right Lower Lobe Atelectasis (Fig. 10.25). The RLL collapses toward the lower mediastinum owing to the tethering effect of the pulmonary ligament. This results in inferior displacement of the upper half of the major fissure and posterior displacement of the lower half, producing a triangular opacity in the right lower paravertebral space that obscures the medial right hemidiaphragm on frontal radiographs. The lateral margin of this triangular opacity is formed by the displaced major fissure. The right interlobar pulmonary artery is obscured within the collapsed lower lobe, a finding that helps distinguish the triangular opacity of RLL atelectasis from a medial pleural effusion, which tends to displace the interlobar artery laterally

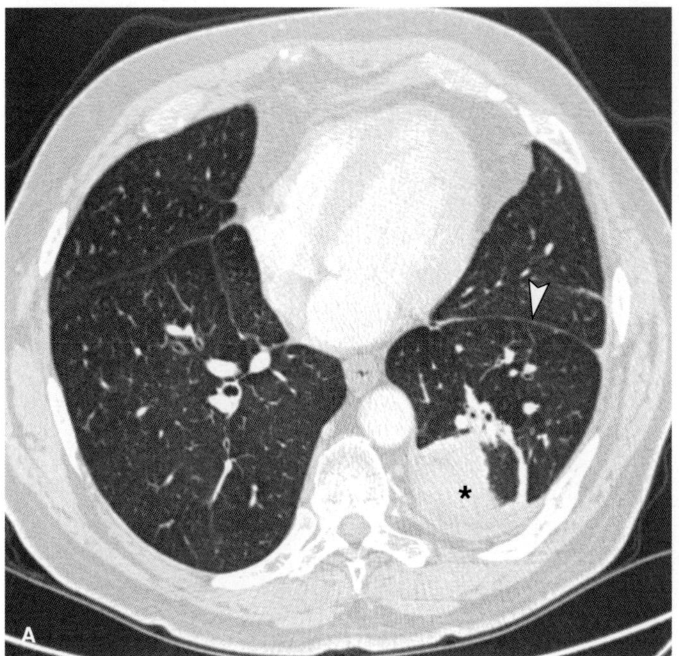

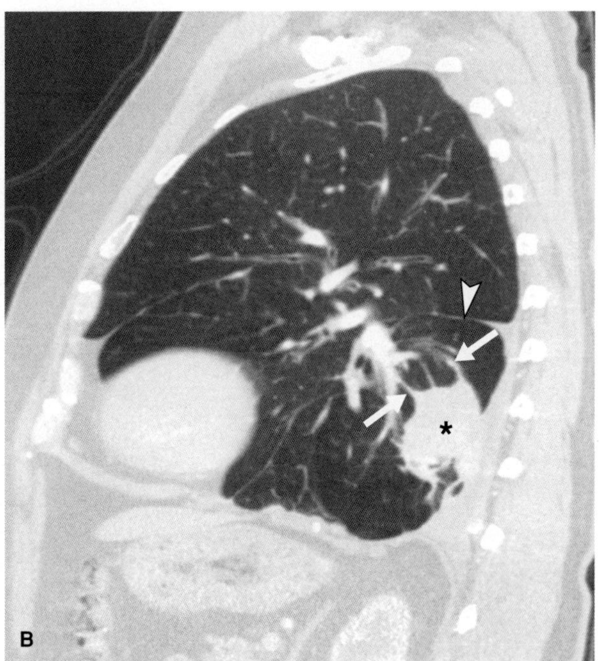

FIGURE 10.28. **Rounded Atelectasis. A, B:** Contrast-enhanced axial (**A**) and left sagittal CT scan (**B**) at lung windows in a patient with left lower lobe rounded atelectasis shows a pleural-based mass (*asterisk*) in the posteroinferior left lower lobe associated with pleural thickening. Note the vessels coursing into the mass (*arrows* in **B**) and the associated volume loss as evidenced by posterior and inferior displacement of the left major fissure (*arrowheads* in A and **B**).

rather than obscure it. The right hemidiaphragm may be elevated. On lateral radiographs, a vague triangular opacity with its apex at the hilum and its base over the posterior portion of the right hemidiaphragm and posterior costophrenic sulcus may be seen. Mucus plugs, foreign bodies, and endobronchial tumors are the most common causes of RLL atelectasis.

Combined middle and right lower lobe atelectasis may be seen with obstruction of the bronchus intermedius by a mucus plug or tumor. The appearance on the frontal radiograph is characteristic, with a homogeneous triangular opacity sharply marginated superiorly by the depressed minor fissure and obscuration of both the right heart border and the right hemidiaphragm (Fig. 10.29G,H). Cardiac and mediastinal shift toward the right is common.

Left lower lobe atelectasis (Fig. 10.29I) is similar in appearance to atelectasis of the RLL. A triangular opacity in the left

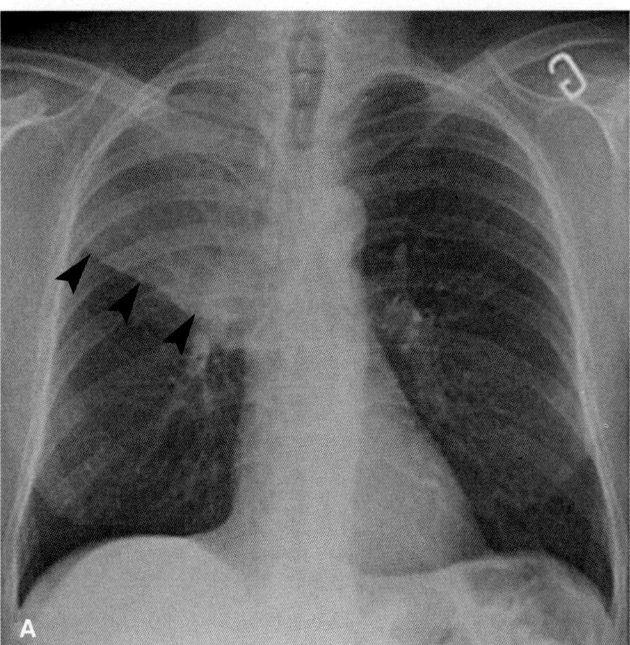

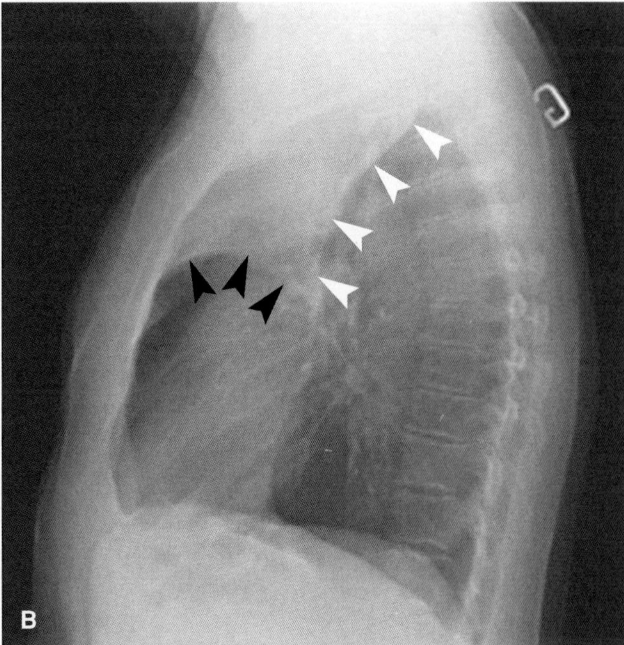

FIGURE 10.29. **Lobar Atelectasis. A, B:** Right upper lobe atelectasis. Frontal (**A**) chest radiograph shows opacification of the right upper lobe with superior displacement of the minor fissure (*arrowheads*). Lateral (**B**) radiograph demonstrates anterior displacement of the major fissure (*arrows*) and superior displacement of the minor fissure (*arrowheads*). (*continued*)

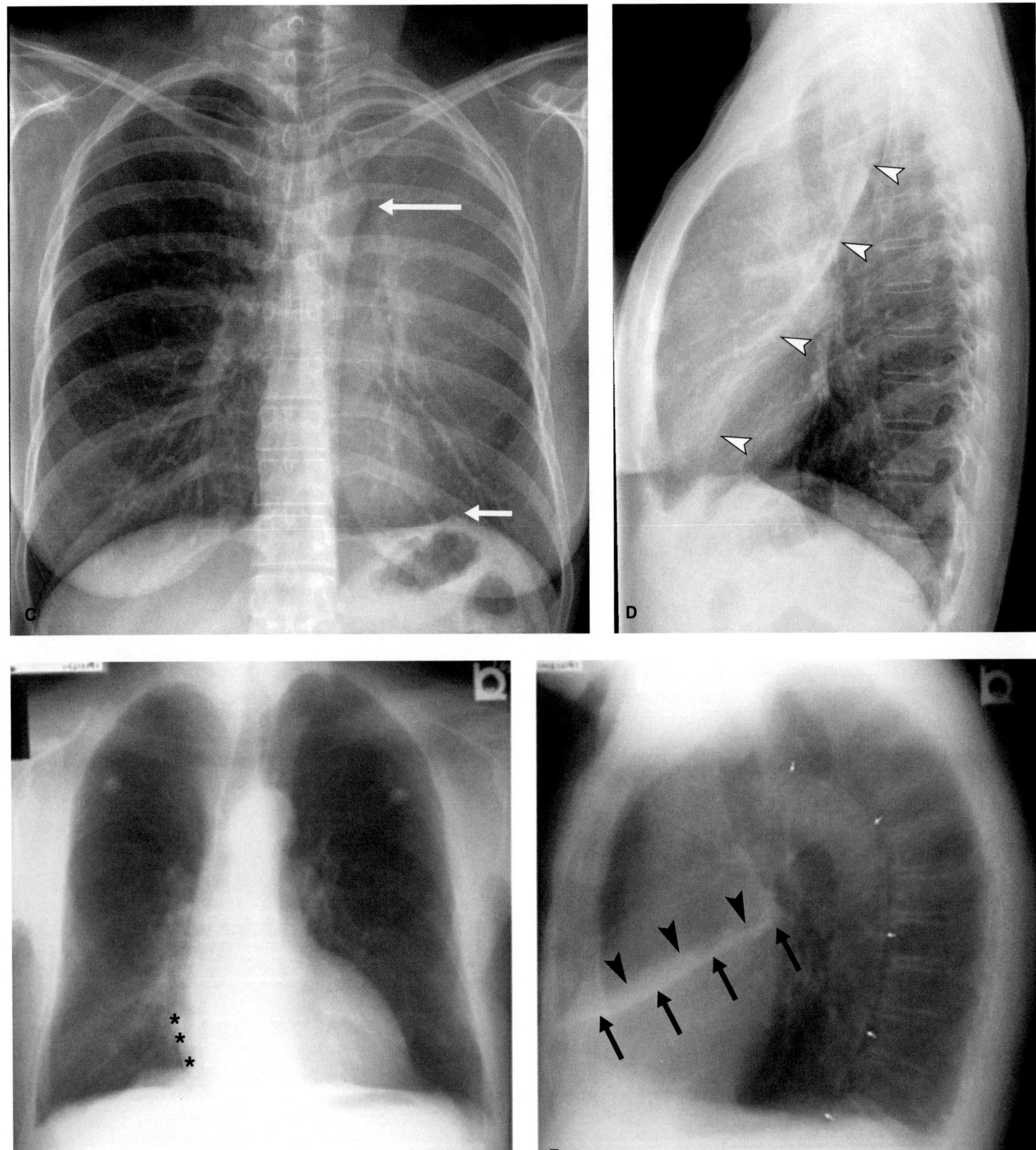

FIGURE 10.29. (*Continued*) **C,D:** Left upper lobe atelectasis. Frontal (**C**) and lateral (**D**) chest radiographs in a patient shows left upper lung opacity obscuring the left mediastinal interfaces. On the frontal (**C**) radiograph, there is a subtle left juxtaphrenic peak (*short arrow*) representing an inferior accessory fissure tenting the left hemidiaphragm as a result of left upper lobe volume loss. A lucency (*long arrow*) outlining the aortic knob represents compensatory hyperinflation of the superior segment of the left lower lobe (*luftsichel sign*). The lateral (**D**) radiograph shows the anteriorly displaced left major fissure (*arrowheads*) outlining the opacified, atelectatic left upper lobe. **E,F:** Right middle lobe atelectasis. On the frontal (**E**) radiograph, the right midcardiac border has an obscured contour (*asterick*). The lateral (**F**) radiograph shows the atelectatic middle lobe outlined by the inferiorly displaced minor fissure (*arrowheads*) and anterior and superiorly displaced major fissure (*arrows*).

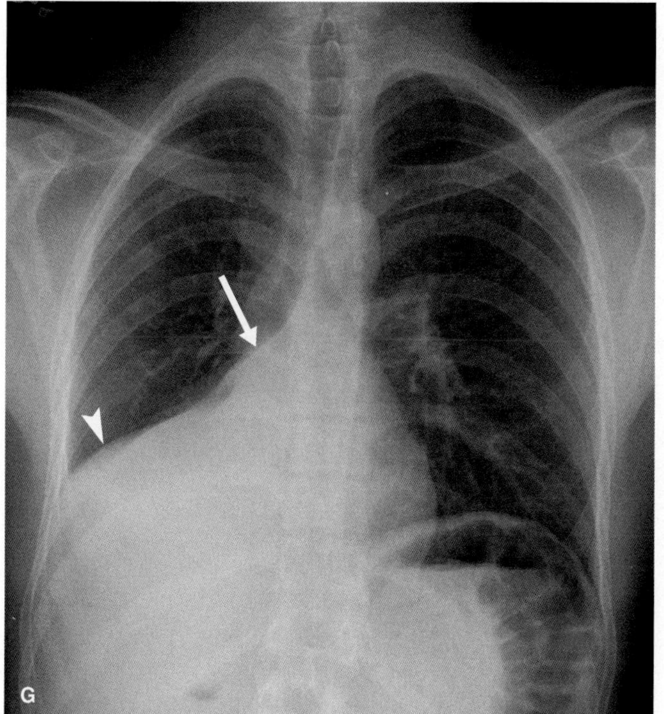

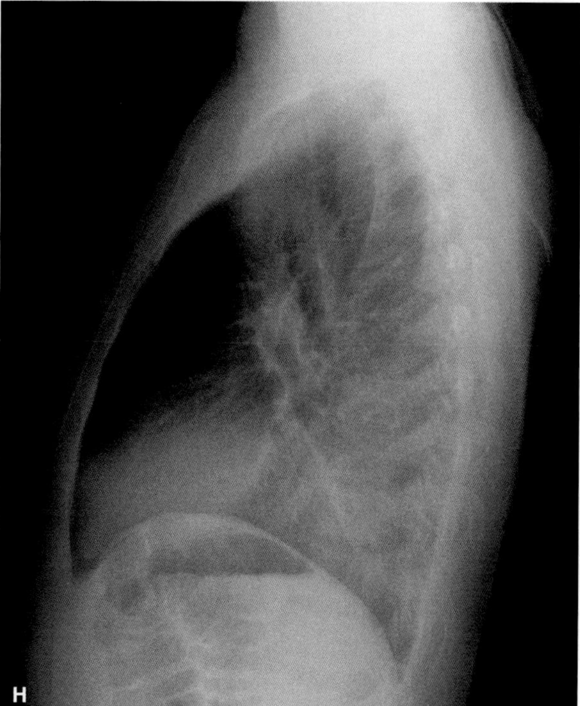

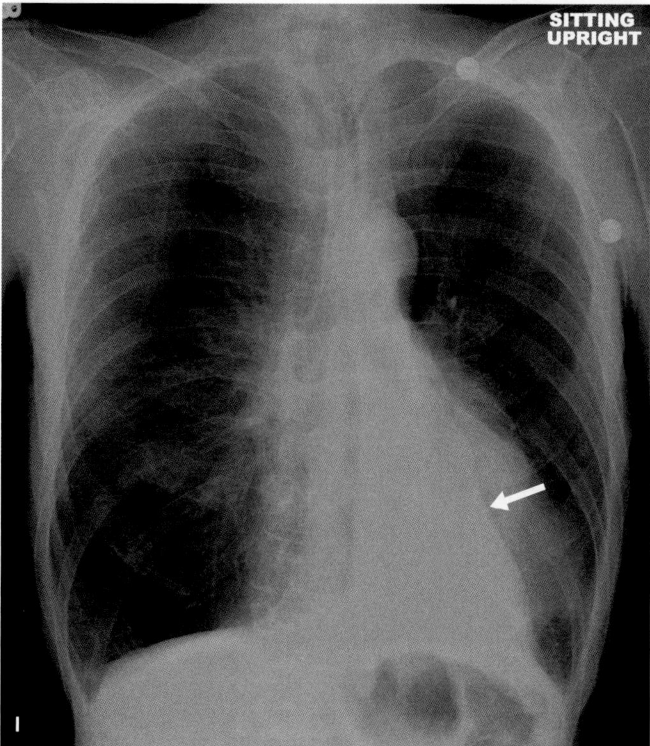

FIGURE 10.29. (*Continued*) G, H: Right middle and lower lobe atelectasis. Frontal (G) and lateral (H) chest radiographs in a 14-year old male with asthma show complete middle and right lower lobe atelectasis. On the frontal (G) view, the displaced major (*arrow*) and minor (*arrowhead*) fissures are visible. Note obscuration of the right heart border and right hemidiaphragm by the opacified, atelectatic lobes. I: Left lower lobe atelectasis. Upright frontal radiograph in a patient with severe ephysema and left lower lobe atelectasis due to an obstructing lung cancer shows an opacified left lower lobe obscuring the left hemidiaphragm. Note leftward mediastinal shift and displacement of the left major fissure (*arrow*) outlining the atelectatic lobe.

lower paramediastinal region, with loss of the medial retrocardiac diaphragmatic outline, is seen on frontal radiographs. In addition, the left hilum is displaced inferiorly and the interlobar artery is obscured. The diaphragm may be elevated and the heart shifted toward the left. Compensatory hyperinflation of the LUL may be seen. The LLL commonly is atelectatic in postoperative patients who have undergone cardiac surgery.

Atelectasis of an entire lung is most often seen with obstructing masses in the main bronchus or by a malpositioned endotracheal tube. Air bronchograms are absent. The trachea and heart are shifted toward the side of atelectasis, with herniation of the contralateral anteromedial lung across the midline, causing widening of the retrosternal space on lateral radiographs and bulging of the anterior junction line toward the ipsilateral side on frontal radiographs (Fig. 10.26). The ipsilateral chest wall may show approximation of the ribs. Left lung atelectasis may be recognized by noting superior displacement of the gastric air bubble or splenic flexure of the colon due to ipsilateral diaphragmatic elevation.

Interstitial Disease. Interstitial opacities are produced by processes that thicken the interstitial compartments of the

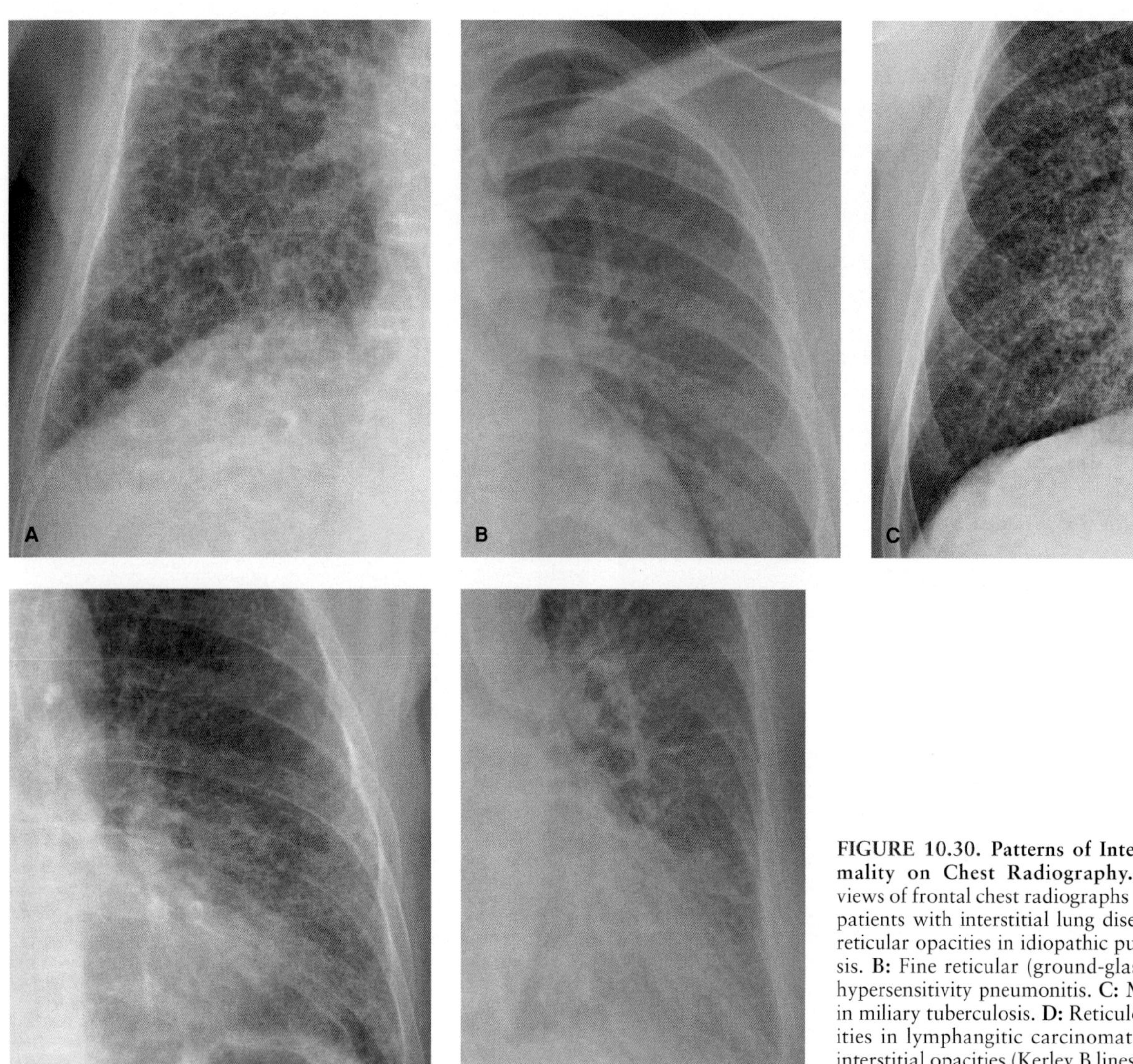

FIGURE 10.30. Patterns of Interstitial Abnormality on Chest Radiography. Coned-down views of frontal chest radiographs in five different patients with interstitial lung disease. **A:** Coarse reticular opacities in idiopathic pulmonary fibrosis. **B:** Fine reticular (ground-glass) opacities in hypersensitivity pneumonitis. **C:** Miliary nodules in miliary tuberculosis. **D:** Reticulonodular opacities in lymphangitic carcinomatosis. **E:** Linear interstitial opacities (Kerley B lines) in pulmonary edema.

lung. Water, blood, tumor, cells, fibrous tissue, or any combination of these may render the interstitial space visible on radiographs. Radiographic patterns of interstitial disease are divided into reticular/ground-glass, reticulonodular, nodular, and linear patterns on plain radiographs (Fig. 10.30 and Table 10.11). The predominant interstitial pattern of opacity produced depends on the nature of the underlying disease and the portion of the interstitium affected.

Reticular pattern refers to a network of curvilinear opacities that usually involves the lungs diffusely. The subdivision of reticular opacities into fine, medium, and coarse opacities refers to the size of the lucent spaces created by these intersecting curvilinear opacities (Fig. 10.30A). A fine reticular pattern, also known as "ground-glass" opacity, is seen in processes that line or thicken the parenchymal interstitium of the lung to produce a fine network of lines with intervening lucent spaces on the order of 1 to 2 mm in diameter (ground-glass opacity can also reflect airspace disease when the alveolar material incompletely fills the airspaces) (Fig. 10.30B). Diseases that commonly produce this appearance include interstitial pulmonary edema and usual interstitial pneumonitis. Medium reticulation, also termed honeycombing, refers to reticular interstitial opacities where the intervening spaces are 3 to 10 mm in diameter. This pattern is most commonly seen in pulmonary fibrosis involving the parenchymal and peripheral interstitial spaces. Coarse reticular opacities with spaces greater than 1 cm in diameter are seen most commonly in diseases that produce cystic spaces as a result of parenchymal destruction. The most common interstitial diseases associated with coarse reticulation are usual interstitial pneumonia, sarcoidosis, and Langerhans cell histiocytosis of the lung.

Nodular opacities represent small round lesions within the pulmonary interstitium. In contrast to airspace nodules, interstitial nodules are homogeneous and sharply defined, as their margins are surrounded by normally aerated lung. Unlike airspace nodules which tend to be uniform in diameter (approximately 8 mm), interstitial nodular opacities can be subdivided based on size into miliary nodules (<2 mm), micronodules (2 to 7 mm), nodules (7 to 30 mm), or masses (>30 mm). A micronodular or miliary pattern is seen predominantly in granulomatous processes (e.g., miliary tuberculosis or histoplasmosis) (Fig. 10.30C), hematogenous pulmonary metastases (most commonly thyroid and renal cell carcinoma), and pneumoconioses (silicosis). Nodules and masses are most often seen in metastatic disease to the lung.

Reticulonodular opacities may be produced by the overlap of numerous reticular opacities or by the presence of both nodular and reticular opacities. Although this appearance appears to

TABLE 10.11

PATTERNS OF INTERSTITIAL PULMONARY OPACITY

■ PATTERN	■ ETIOLOGY	■ EXAMPLE
Linear	Interstitial edema	
	Neoplastic	Lymphangitic carcinomatosis
	Infection	Mycoplasma
		Viral
	Idiopathic	Amyloidosis (alveolar septal form)
Reticular: acute	Interstitial edema	
	Infection	Viral
		Mycoplasma
		Pneumocystis jiroveci
Reticular: chronic	Postinfectious scarring	Tuberculosis (postprimary)
		Histoplasmosis (chronic)
		Coccidioidomycosis (chronic)
	Collagen vascular disease	Rheumatoid lung
		Scleroderma
		Dermatomyositis/polymyositis
		Ankylosing spondylitis
		Mixed connective tissue disease
	Granulomatous disease	Sarcoidosis
		Langerhans cell histiocytosis
	Lymphoproliferative	Lymphocytic interstitial pneumonitis
	Inhalational	Asbestosis
		Silicosis and coal worker's pneumoconiosis
		Hypersensitivity pneumonitis (chronic)
		Chronic aspiration
	Drug reaction	Nitrofurantoin
		Chemotherapeutic agents
		Amiodarone
	Radiation pneumonitis (chronic)	
	Idiopathic	Idiopathic pulmonary fibrosis
		Nonspecific interstitial pneumonitis
		Lymphangioleiomyomatosis
		Neurofibromatosis
Nodular	Infection	Mycobacterial
		Fungal
		Varicella (healed)
	Inhalational diseases	Silicosis and coal worker's pneumoconiosis
		Berylliosis
		Siderosis
		Heavy metal dust
		Talcosis
		Hypersensitivity pneumonitis
	Granulomatous disease	Sarcoidosis
		Langerhans cell histiocytosis (early)
	Neoplastic	Metastatic disease
		Lymphomatoid granulomatosis
	Idiopathic	Pulmonary alveolar microlithiasis
		Amyloidosis (parenchymal nodular form)
		Pleuropulmonary fibroelastosis (upper lobe)

be frequent on radiographs, only a few diseases actually show reticulonodular involvement on pathology specimens. Silicosis, sarcoidosis, and lymphangitic carcinomatosis (Fig. 10.30D) are diseases that may give rise to true reticulonodular opacities.

Linear patterns of interstitial opacities are seen in processes that thicken the axial (bronchovascular) or peripheral interstitium of the lung. Because the axial interstitium surrounds the bronchovascular structures, thickening of this compartment produces parallel linear opacities radiating from the hila when visualized in length or peribronchial "cuffs" when viewed end on. This pattern of interstitial disease may be impossible to distinguish from airways diseases, such as bronchiectasis and asthma, which primarily thicken the walls of airways. Thickening of the peripheral interstitium of the lung produces linear opacities that are either 2- to 6-cm long lines which are <1 mm thick and are obliquely oriented, coursing through the substance of the lung toward the hila (Kerley A lines) or shorter (1- to 2-cm) thin lines that are peripheral and course

TABLE 10.12

CAUSES OF PULMONARY LUCENCY

■ DISTRIBUTION			■ EXAMPLE
Localized			Cavity Cyst Bulla Bleb Pneumatocele
Unilateral	Technical factors		Grid cutoff Patient rotation
	Extrapulmonary	Chest wall/soft tissue	Absent pectoralis muscle (Poland syndrome) Mastectomy
		Pleural disease	Contralateral pleural effusion/thickening Pneumothorax
	Pulmonary	Diminished blood flow	Hypoplastic lung/pulmonary artery Pulmonary embolism Mediastinal/hilar tumor Fibrosing mediastinitis Lobar atelectasis/resection
		Diminished pulmonary blood flow and hyperinflation	Swyer–James syndrome Endobronchial tumor/foreign body (check-valve effect)
Bilateral	Technical factors		Overpenetrated radiograph
	Extrapulmonary		Bilateral mastectomies
	Pulmonary	Diminished pulmonary blood flow	Congenital heart disease Chronic thromboembolic pulmonary hypertension
		Diminished pulmonary blood flow and hyperinflation	Asthma Emphysema

perpendicular to and contact the pleural surface (Kerley B lines) (Fig. 10.30E). Kerley A lines correspond to thickening of connective tissue sheets within the lung, which contain lymphatic communications between the perivenous and bronchoarterial lymphatics, while Kerley B lines represent thickened peripheral subpleural interlobular septa (Fig. 12.1). A linear pattern of disease is seen in pulmonary edema, lymphangitic carcinomatosis, and acute viral or atypical bacterial pneumonia. The thin-section CT findings of interstitial lung disease are reviewed in Chapter 15.

Pulmonary nodule refers to a discrete round opacity within the lung measuring less than 3 cm in diameter, whereas a round opacity greater than 3 cm in diameter is termed a *pulmonary mass.* A solitary pulmonary nodule presents a common diagnostic dilemma and is discussed in Chapter 13.

Mucoid Impaction. Branching tubular opacities that are distinguished from normal vascular shadows invariably represent mucus-filled, dilated bronchi and are termed *bronchoceles, mucoceles,* or *mucoid impaction.* Their appearance has been likened to that of a gloved finger or the shape of the letters V or Y, depending upon the length of airway and number of branches involved. When the bronchoceles occur in a central perihilar location, they may be the result of: (1) nonobstructive bronchiectasis such as in cystic fibrosis or allergic bronchopulmonary aspergillosis, (2) postobstructive bronchiectasis distal to an endobronchial tumor, or (3) a congenitally atretic bronchus (Fig. 16.2). A typical location—immediately distal to the expected location of the apical segmental bronchus and a hyperlucent segment or lobe distal to the bronchocele owing to collateral air drift—should suggest the diagnosis of a congenitally atretic bronchus.

Pulmonary Lucency

Abnormal lucency of the lung may be localized or diffuse (Table 10.12). Focal radiolucent lesions of the lung include cavities, cysts, bullae, blebs, and pneumatoceles (Fig. 10.31). These lesions are usually recognized by identification of the wall of the lucent lesion.

Cavities form when a pulmonary mass undergoes necrosis and communicates with an airway, leading to gas within its center. The wall of a cavity is, by definition, greater than 1 mm thick and is usually irregular or lobulated. Lung abscess and necrotic neoplasm are the most common cavitary pulmonary lesions (Fig. 10.31A). A *bulla* is a gas collection within the pulmonary parenchyma that is >1 cm in diameter and has a thin wall <1 mm thick. It represents a focal area of parenchymal destruction (emphysema) and may contain fibrous strands, residual blood vessels, or alveolar septa (Fig. 10.31B). An *air cyst* is any well-circumscribed intrapulmonary gas collection with a smooth, thin wall >1 mm thick. While some of these lesions have a true epithelial lining and are therefore true cysts (i.e., a bronchogenic cyst that communicates with a bronchus), most are likely postinflammatory or posttraumatic lesions. A *bleb* is a collection of gas <1 cm in size within the layers of the visceral pleura, usually found in the lung apex (Fig. 10.31C). These small gas collections are indistinguishable from paraseptal emphysema. Rupture of an apical bleb can lead to spontaneous pneumothorax. *Pneumatoceles* are thin-walled, gas-containing structures that represent distended airspaces distal to a check-valve obstruction of a bronchus or bronchiole, most commonly secondary to staphylococcal pneumonia (Fig. 10.31D), or result from pulmonary laceration following blunt or penetrating trauma. These lesions

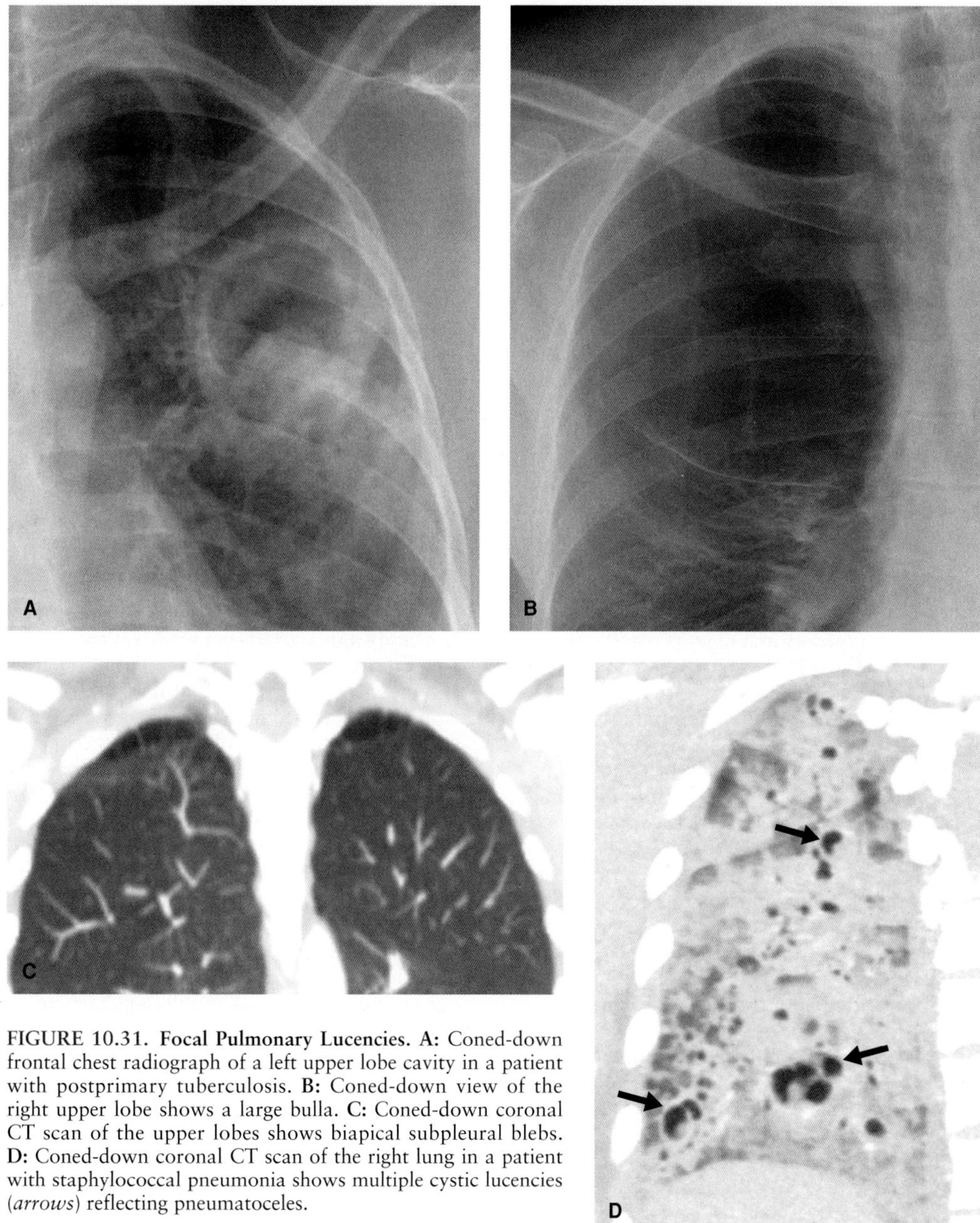

FIGURE 10.31. **Focal Pulmonary Lucencies. A:** Coned-down frontal chest radiograph of a left upper lobe cavity in a patient with postprimary tuberculosis. **B:** Coned-down view of the right upper lobe shows a large bulla. **C:** Coned-down coronal CT scan of the upper lobes shows biapical subpleural blebs. **D:** Coned-down coronal CT scan of the right lung in a patient with staphylococcal pneumonia shows multiple cystic lucencies (*arrows*) reflecting pneumatoceles.

generally resolve within 4 to 6 months. *Bronchiectatic cysts* are usually multiple, round, thin-walled lucencies found in clusters in the lower lobes and represent saccular dilatations of airways in varicose or cystic bronchiectasis.

Unilateral pulmonary hyperlucency must be distinguished from differences in lung density resulting from technical factors or overlying soft tissue abnormalities. Congenital absence of the pectoralis muscle (Poland syndrome) (Fig. 17.18) or mastectomy can produce apparent hyperlucency.

True unilateral hyperlucent lung is a result of decreased blood flow to the lung. Diminished blood flow may result from a primary vascular abnormality, shunting of blood away from a lung that traps air, or a combination of the two. Hypoplasia of the right or left pulmonary artery produces an ipsilateral lung that is hyperlucent and diminished in size. A similar appearance may be produced by lobar resection or atelectasis, where the remaining lobe or lung hyperinflates to accommodate the hemithorax, thereby attenuating pulmonary vessels and producing hyperlucency. Pulmonary arterial obstruction may be secondary to extrinsic compression or invasion by a hilar mass or to pulmonary embolism. A check-valve effect from an endobronchial tumor or foreign body can produce air trapping, resulting in shunting of blood and unilateral hyperlucency. The Swyer–James syndrome or unilateral hyperlucent lung syndrome is a condition that follows adenoviral infection during infancy (Fig. 16.23). An asymmetric obliterative bronchiolitis with severe air trapping on expiration and secondary unilateral pulmonary artery hypoplasia produces the hyperlucency in this condition. Emphysema, if asymmetric, can produce a hyperlucent lung; this is most common with severe bullous disease.

Bilateral hyperlucent lungs may be simulated by an overpenetrated radiograph or by a thin patient. True bilateral hyperlucent lungs are the result of diminished pulmonary blood flow. This may be the result of congenital pulmonary stenosis, most commonly associated with tetralogy of Fallot, or secondary to an acquired obstruction of the pulmonary circulation, as in pulmonary arterial hypertension or chronic thromboembolic disease. Pulmonary emphysema results in hyperinflation with air trapping on expiration, destruction of the pulmonary microvasculature, and attenuation of lobar and segmental vessels, thereby producing bilateral hyperlucency. Asthma produces transient air trapping and diffuse bilateral vascular attenuation, resulting in both hyperinflation and hyperlucency.

Mediastinal Masses

Mediastinal masses are recognized on frontal radiographs as a soft tissue density that causes obliteration or displacement of the mediastinal contours or interfaces. The lung–mass interface typically is well defined laterally, where it is convex with the adjacent lung and creates obtuse angles with the lung at its superior and inferior margins (Fig. 11.4). This latter characteristic is diagnostic of an extrapulmonary lesion, whether mediastinal or pleural. Lateral displacement of the trachea or heart may be seen with large mediastinal masses, sometimes first recognized by displacement of an indwelling endotracheal tube, nasogastric tube, or intravascular catheter.

Virtually every patient with a mediastinal mass will undergo further workup with CT or MR. US is usually limited to the evaluation of vascular masses and for real-time imaging guidance during transthoracic needle biopsy.

The vascular origin of a mediastinal mass is readily apparent on contrast-enhanced CT, MR, and, occasionally, transthoracic or transesophageal US. The recognition of fat within a mediastinal mass on CT or MR limits the differential diagnosis to a small number of entities, including diaphragmatic hernia, lipoma, teratoma, epicardial fat, and thymolipoma. A fat–fluid level is virtually diagnostic of a mature teratoma. Although calcification is occasionally detected radiographically within mediastinal masses, CT is considerably more sensitive and provides more specific characterization of the calcification. Coarse calcification within an anterior mediastinal mass should suggest the diagnosis of a teratoma (especially if a tooth is seen) or thymoma. Curvilinear rim-like calcification should suggest a cyst or an aneurysm. Conversely, the presence of calcification within an untreated mediastinal mass virtually excludes the diagnosis of lymphoma.

Frontal and lateral chest radiographs help localize a mediastinal mass to the anterior (prevascular), middle (visceral), or posterior (paravertebral) mediastinal compartments (Chapter 11). For instance, if the contours of a lesion are outlined by air and seen above the clavicles, then the lesion must be in the posterior mediastinum. Conversely, if the contours of a lesion are lost at the thoracic inlet level, it must be in the anterior mediastinum. CT and MR provide more precise information regarding structures involved by the mediastinal mass, help narrow the differential diagnosis, and help guide appropriate diagnostic procedures.

Mediastinal Widening

Mediastinal widening is described as an increase in the transverse diameter of the mediastinum on frontal chest radiographs (Fig. 11.30). True mediastinal disease is often difficult to distinguish from technical factors causing mediastinal widening, such as AP technique, supine positioning, and rotation. Mediastinal lipomatosis is the most common cause of uniform mediastinal widening on frontal radiographs. Clues to the presence of mediastinal disease include increasing mediastinal width compared to prior frontal radiographs, mass effect on adjacent mediastinal structures (tracheal deviation or displacement of an indwelling nasogastric tube or central venous catheter), increased density of the mediastinum, and obscuration of the normal mediastinal contours such as the aortic knob and right paratracheal stripe. While normal measurements have been developed for mediastinal width, there is such great individual variability that absolute measurements are not useful.

Pneumomediastinum and Pneumopericardium

The diagnosis of *pneumomediastinum* is usually made on conventional radiographs. Small amounts of extraluminal air appear as linear or curvilinear lucencies lining anatomic structures within the mediastinal contours (Fig. 11.31). Larger collections may be seen outlining the cardiac silhouette, mediastinal vessels, tracheobronchial tree, or esophagus. The most common finding is air outlining the left heart border, where a curvilinear lucency representing pneumomediastinum is paralleled by a thin curvilinear opacity representing the combined thickness of the visceral and parietal pleura of the lingula. Another sign of pneumomediastinum is the "continuous diaphragm" sign (Fig. 11.31A), in which air dissects between the pericardium and central diaphragm allowing visualization of the central portion of the diaphragm in contiguity with the right and left hemidiaphragms, each of which is outlined by air in the lower lobes, respectively. While this sign is fairly specific for pneumomediastinum, pneumopericardium may produce a similar finding. Small amounts of mediastinal air are often more easily appreciated on the lateral radiograph, with air outlining the aortic root or main or central pulmonary arteries.

There are three entities that may mimic some of the radiographic findings of pneumomediastinum. These entities have significantly different etiologies and therapeutic implications: pneumopericardium, medial pneumothorax, and Mach bands. Air in the pericardial sac typically surrounds the heart and is limited superiorly by the normal pericardial reflections around the proximal ascending aorta and main pulmonary artery. Pneumopericardium in an adult is often seen in the early postoperative period following pericardiotomy for cardiac surgery but can also develop in patients with alveolar rupture due to mechanical ventilation or as the result of trauma (Fig. 10.32). Air within the pericardium rises to a nondependent position on decubitus positioning, unlike mediastinal air, which is not mobile.

The differentiation of pneumomediastinum from a medial pneumothorax is also aided by decubitus radiographs as pleural air will rise nondependently along the lateral pleural space. In contrast to pneumothorax, pneumomediastinum may outline intramediastinal structures (pulmonary artery, trachea) and is often bilateral. However, the distinction between pneumomediastinum and medial pneumothorax may be impossible, and the two conditions often coexist. Paramediastinal lucent bands created by Mach effect are easily distinguished from pneumomediastinum. The lateral margin of lucent Mach bands consists of lung parenchyma, as opposed to the thin pleural line seen with mediastinal air. These bands represent an optical illusion (caused by a retinal reinforcement response) that disappears when the interface between mediastinal soft tissues and lung is covered.

Hilar Disease

Frontal radiographic findings of enlarged hilar lymph nodes, a dilated pulmonary artery, or a hilar mass include hilar enlargement, increased hilar density, a lobulated hilar contour, and distortion of central bronchi. An abnormal hilum is most easily appreciated by comparison with the contralateral hilum and by review of prior chest radiographs (Figs. 11.32 and 11.33). CT will often show a left hilar mass that is not evident on routine radiographs. On the right, the normally sharp right hilar angle, formed by the intersection of the lower lateral aspect of the right superior pulmonary vein with the

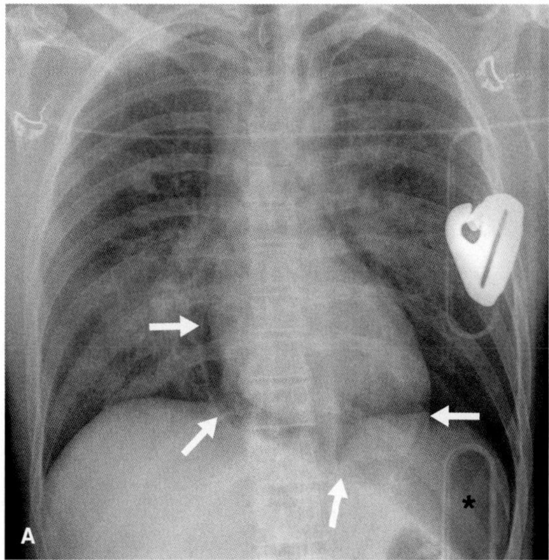

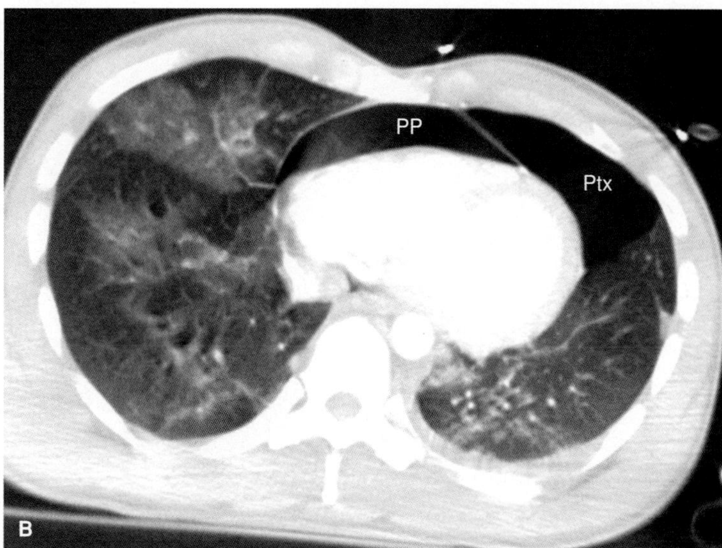

FIGURE 10.32. **Pneumopericardium. A:** Supine portable chest radiograph in a patient who sustained blunt chest trauma shows abnormal lucency (*arrows*) outlining the cardiac silhouette. There is a left basilar pneumothorax seen as an abnormal lucency in the left lower chest/upper abdomen (*asterisk*). The patchy bilateral airspace opacities reflect contusions. **B:** Axial contrast-enhanced CT scan through the heart shows pneumopericardium (*PP*) and a left pneumothorax (*Ptx*).

upper lateral aspect of the right interlobar pulmonary artery, is often distorted or obscured by a hilar mass. An increase in density of the hilar shadow is seen with a hilar mass that lies primarily anterior or posterior to the normal hilar vascular shadows. In such patients, the enlarged hilar nodes will produce an increase in density on frontal views and a lobulated appearance when viewed in profile on a lateral radiograph.

When an abnormally dense hilum is noted, the relationship between the vessels and the density must be assessed. A density through which the normal hilar vessels can be seen constitutes a "hilum overlay" sign, which indicates a mass superimposed on the hilum (Figs. 11.5 and 11.10). Conversely, vascular structures that converge only as far as the lateral margin of the increased hilar density indicate enlargement of intrahilar vascular structures (the "hilum convergence" sign). Lateral radiograph or CT will clarify the abnormality. In patients with small lung volumes or exaggerated kyphosis, a mass in the lower right hilum on frontal radiographs may be simulated by the end-on projection of a horizontally oriented right interlobar artery. Comparison with prior radiographs will usually resolve the matter, with CT reserved for equivocal cases.

Tumors involving the lobar bronchi or bronchus intermedius may produce luminal narrowing of the bronchi and enlargement of the hilar shadow (Fig. 11.15). Occasionally, an endobronchial mass produces an abrupt cutoff of the bronchus radiographically.

Right or left hilar enlargement from pulmonary artery dilatation is caused by increased flow or increased pressure in the pulmonary arterial circulation (Fig. 11.37). Pulmonary artery dilatation is usually assessed by measuring the right interlobar pulmonary artery on frontal radiographs. The upper limit of normal for the transverse diameter of the proximal right interlobar artery, as measured on a PA radiograph at a level immediately lateral to the proximal portion of the bronchus intermedius, is 17 mm in men and 15 mm in women.

The lateral radiograph can confirm the presence of hilar abnormality seen on frontal radiography and may demonstrate a mass when the frontal radiograph is normal. Hilar masses that lie predominantly anterior or posterior to the hilar vessels are best visualized on the lateral view. Because the lateral radiograph is a composite of both hilar shadows, the cumulative density of bilateral hilar masses may produce a significant increase in the normal density of the composite shadow, which is more easily appreciated on a lateral than on a frontal view. The lateral radiographic findings of a hilar mass are an abnormal size of or a lobulated contour to the normal vascular shadows, the presence of soft tissue in a region that is normally radiolucent, an increase in density of the composite hilar shadow, and abnormalities of the central bronchi. An increase in the size and density of the composite hilar shadow is best appreciated by comparison with prior radiographs, as is usually seen with bilateral hilar lymph node enlargement from sarcoidosis. Hilar lymph node enlargement produces lobulation of the normally smooth outlines of the right and left main pulmonary arteries. There are additional findings unique to the lateral radiograph that suggest the presence of a hilar mass and may allow lateralization of the hilar abnormality. Because the RUL bronchus is visualized on the lateral radiograph in only a minority of individuals, visualization of the RUL bronchial lumen, particularly if it was invisible on a prior lateral radiograph, may reflect mass or adenopathy in the upper right hilum. A lobulated posterior wall of the bronchus intermedius, or a thickness >3 mm, indicates an abnormality of the bronchus (bronchitis or bronchogenic carcinoma), thickening of the axial interstitium (pulmonary edema or lymphangitic carcinomatosis), or enlargement of lymph nodes in the posterior aspect of the lower right hilum.

The normal anatomy of the inferior hilar window was reviewed earlier in this chapter. The identification of a soft tissue mass >1 cm in diameter within this radiolucent region is an indication of unilateral or bilateral hilar mass. Occasionally, the silhouetting of the anterior wall of the LLL bronchus, recognized as a concave anterior curvilinear structure contiguous with the anterior aspect of the LUL bronchus, allows lateralization of a mass to the left lower hilum. The added opacity of a mass within the normally radiolucent inferior hilar window produces an oval opacity to the composite hilar shadow on lateral radiographs (Fig. 10.33).

CT is the most sensitive imaging modality in detecting and localizing enlarged hilar lymph nodes and masses. Although contrast enhancement is rarely necessary to assess mediastinal nodes, it simplifies identification of enlarged vascular structures or nonenhancing hilar nodes (defined as nodes that exceed 10 mm in short-axis diameter) or masses. On axial or

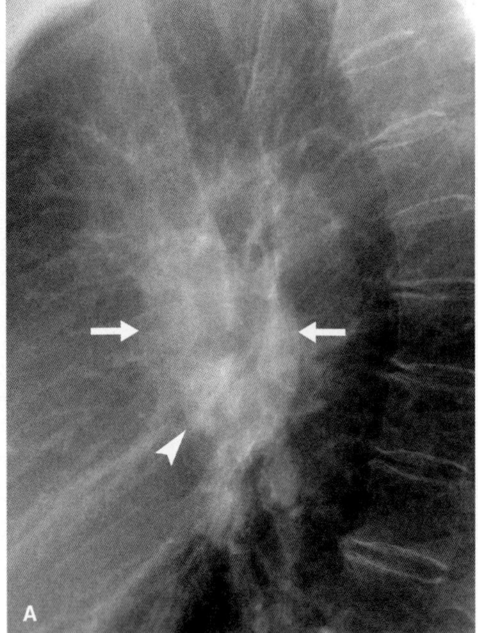

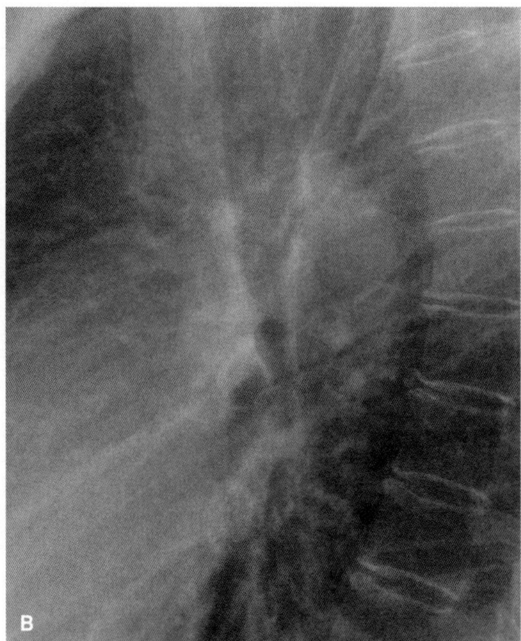

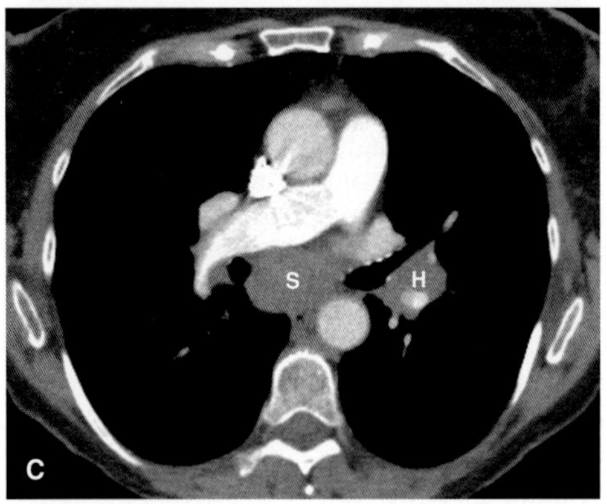

FIGURE 10.33. **Hilar Lymph Node Enlargement on Lateral Radiography. A:** Coned-down lateral radiography in a patient with hilar and mediastinal lymph node enlargement from sarcoidosis shows an oval opacity (*arrows*) overlying the hila. There is filling in of the inferior hilar window (*arrowhead*). **B:** Coned-down view of a prior lateral chest radiograph in the same patient shows normal hilar anatomy. **C:** Contrast-enhanced axial CT through the hila shows subcarinal (*S*) and left hilar (*H*) lymph node enlargement accounting for the opacity seen on lateral radiography.

coronal T2-weighted MR, hilar masses are round masses of low or intermediate signal intensity, in distinction to the signal void of flowing blood within the hilar vessels or of air in the bronchi. Displacement or distortion of the hilar vessels provides indirect evidence of hilar disease. Tumor invasion of a branch of the pulmonary artery or vein within the hilum produces a filling defect within the vessel on contrast-enhanced CT or intraluminal signal on MR. The density characteristics of hilar masses on CT can help provide important information for differential diagnosis. For example, a round, cystic hilar mass with imperceptible walls in an asymptomatic young person is typical of a bronchogenic cyst.

Enlarged hilar lymph nodes can be detected by CT without the use of intravenous contrast. A detailed knowledge of the normal hilar vascular and bronchial anatomy, as seen on CT, is necessary for the identification of subtle hilar contour abnormalities. In those portions of the hilum where lung directly contacts a wall of a bronchus, thickening or lobulation of the normal thin linear shadow of the bronchial wall indicates hilar abnormality. Lymph node enlargement in these regions is obscured on frontal radiographs by the overlying cardiac and hilar vascular shadows. CT is more sensitive than conventional radiographs or MR for the detection of masses within lobar or proximal segmental bronchi. If an endobronchial mass is associated with a large extraluminal component, it produces a radiographically visible hilar soft tissue mass and obstructive atelectasis.

Enlarged hilar lymph nodes may have different appearances on CT. Enlargement of discrete lymph nodes, most commonly seen in sarcoidosis, appears as multiple distinct round masses (Fig. 11.36B). When tumor or an inflammatory process extends through the nodal capsule to involve contiguous nodes, a single large mass of confluent lymph nodes is produced that may be difficult to distinguish from a primary hilar bronchogenic carcinoma. This latter appearance is most often seen in hilar nodal metastases from small cell carcinoma of the lung or lymphoma (Fig. 11.15). The CT density of enlarged hilar or enlarged mediastinal lymph nodes can provide clues to the diagnosis (see Table 11.4).

An abnormally small hilum indicates a diminution in the size of the right or left pulmonary artery.

Pleural Effusion

The radiographic appearance of pleural effusions depends on multiple factors, including the amount of fluid present, the patient's position during the radiographic examination, and the presence or absence of adhesions between the visceral and parietal pleura. Small amounts of pleural fluid initially collect between the lower lobe and diaphragm in a subpulmonic location. As the amount of pleural fluid increases, it spills into the posterior and lateral costophrenic sulci. A moderate amount of pleural fluid (>175 mL) in the erect patient has a

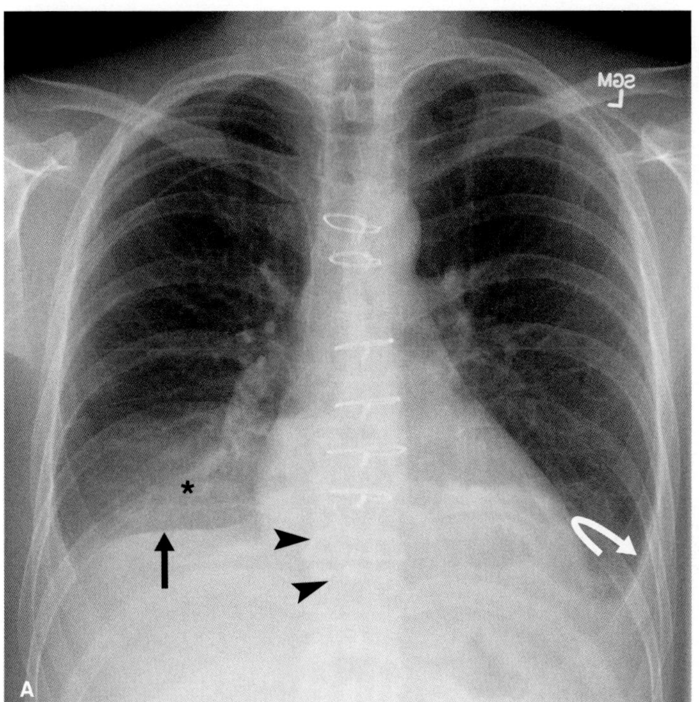

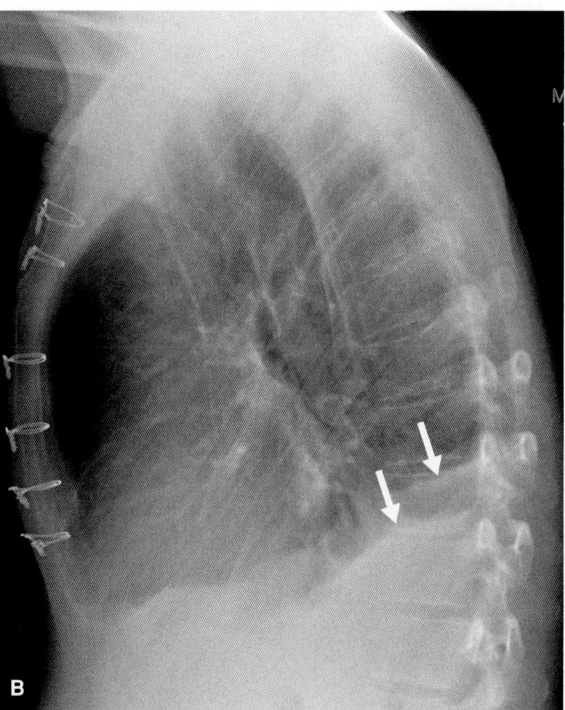

FIGURE 10.34. **Pleural Effusions on Upright Chest Radiography. A:** Frontal chest radiograph in a patient status post coronary artery bypass graft surgery shows a right pleural effusion that is partly subpulmonic (*arrow*) and a left effusion seen as a typical lateral meniscus (*curved arrow*). Note the hazy opacity overlying the right lower lung (*asterisk*) reflecting posteriorly situated fluid seen en face. **B:** Lateral radiograph shows effusions blunting both posterior costophrenic sulci (*arrows*).

characteristic appearance on the frontal radiograph, with a homogeneous lower zone opacity seen in the lateral costophrenic sulcus with a concave interface toward the lung. This concave margin, known as a *pleural meniscus,* appears higher laterally than medially on frontal radiographs because the lateral aspect of the effusion, which surrounds the costal surface of the lung, is tangent to the frontal x-ray beam. Similarly, the meniscus of pleural fluid on lateral radiographs peaks anteriorly and posteriorly (Fig. 10.34).

In patients with suspected pleural effusion, a lateral decubitus film with the affected side down is the most sensitive technique to detect small amounts of fluid. With this technique, as small as 5 mL of pleural fluid may be seen layering between the lung and lateral chest wall. While a moderate-size, free-flowing collection should be obvious on upright radiographs, a large pleural effusion can cause passive atelectasis of the entire lung, producing an opaque hemithorax. It may be difficult to distinguish the latter condition from collapse of an entire lung. A massive pleural effusion should produce mass effect resulting in contralateral mediastinal shift, whereas a collapsed lung without pleural effusion will demonstrate volume loss and result in mediastinal shift toward the opaque side. In some patients, CT or US may be necessary to distinguish pleural fluid from collapsed lung.

CT is sensitive in detecting free pleural fluid. On axial scans, pleural fluid layers posteriorly with a characteristic meniscoid appearance and has a CT attenuation value of 0 to 20 HU. Small effusions may be difficult to differentiate from pleural thickening, fibrosis, or dependent atelectasis, and decubitus scans are useful in making this distinction.

US is particularly useful in detecting free-flowing pleural effusions, which are usually seen as anechoic collections at the base of the pleural space surrounding atelectatic lung.

Pleural fluid may become loculated between the pleural layers to produce an appearance indistinguishable from that of a pleural mass. Fluid loculated within the costal pleural layers appears as a vertically oriented elliptical opacity with a broad area of contact with the chest wall, producing a sharp, convex interface with the lung when viewed in tangent. CT is commonly utilized to detect and localize loculated pleural fluid collections. The characteristic finding is a sharply marginated lenticular mass of fluid attenuation conforming to the concavity of the chest wall that forms obtuse angles at its edges and compresses and displaces the subjacent lung (Fig. 17.2). Multiple loculated pleural fluid collections can mimic pleural metastases or malignant mesothelioma radiographically. CT or US can confirm the fluid characteristics of these pleural "masses."

Pleural fluid may extend into the interlobar fissures, producing characteristic findings. Free fluid within the minor fissure is usually seen as smooth, symmetric thickening on a frontal radiograph. Fluid within the major fissure is normally not visible on frontal radiographs, as the fissures are viewed en face. An exception is fluid extending into the lateral aspect of an incomplete major fissure, which produces a curvilinear density extending from the inferolateral to the superomedial aspect of the lung. Fluid loculated between the leaves of visceral pleura within an interlobar fissure results in an elliptic opacity oriented along the length of the fissure (Fig. 17.7). These loculated collections of pleural fluid are termed "pseudotumors" and are most often seen within the minor fissure on frontal radiographs in patients with congestive heart failure. The tendency for these opacities to disappear rapidly with diuresis has led to the term "vanishing lung tumor." Although a characteristic appearance on plain radiographs is usually sufficient for diagnosis, the CT demonstration of a localized fluid collection in the expected location of the major or minor fissure is confirmatory.

An uncommon appearance of pleural effusion is seen when fluid accumulates between the lower lobe and diaphragm and is termed a *subpulmonic* effusion. While small amounts of pleural fluid normally accumulate in this location, it is

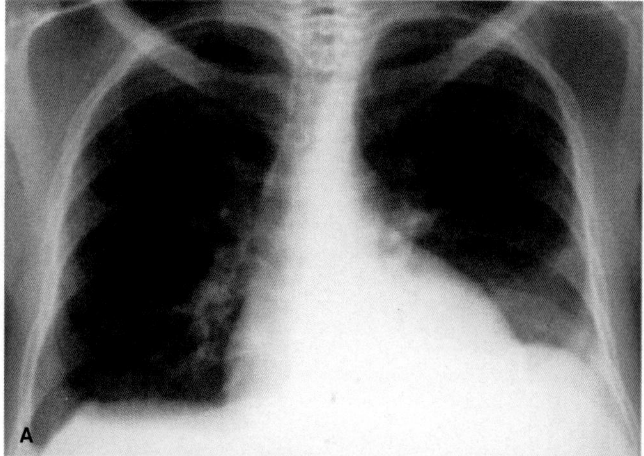

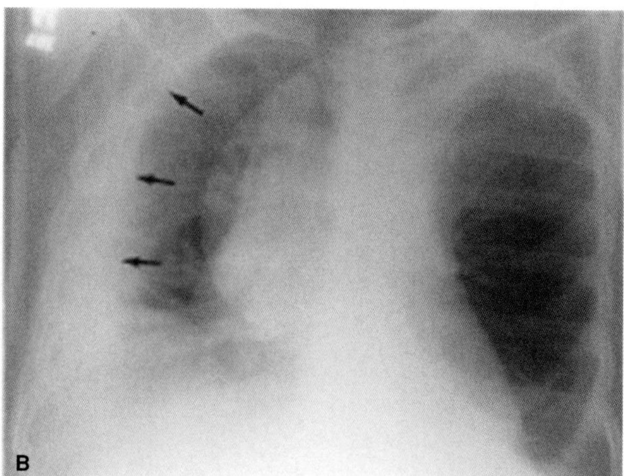

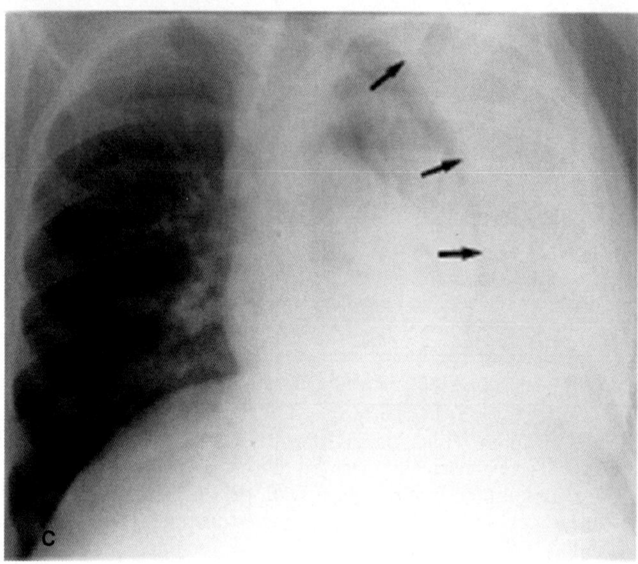

FIGURE 10.35. **Bilateral Subpulmonic Pleural Effusions. A:** An upright posteroanterior radiograph in a 41-year-old woman with ascites demonstrates apparent elevation of both hemidiaphragms. Right (**B**) and left (**C**) decubitus films demonstrate dependent layering of the subpulmonic pleural fluid (*arrows*).

uncommon for larger effusions to remain subpulmonic without spilling into the posterior and lateral costophrenic sulci. A subpulmonic effusion may be difficult to appreciate on upright chest radiographs because the fluid collection mimics an elevated hemidiaphragm. Clues to its presence on frontal radiographs include apparent and new elevation of the diaphragm, lateral peaking of the hemidiaphragm that is accentuated on expiration, a minor fissure that is close to the diaphragm (right-sided effusions), and an increased separation of the gastric air bubble from the base of the lung (left-sided effusions). Despite the atypical subpulmonic accumulation of fluid with the patient upright, the effusion will layer dependently on lateral decubitus radiographs (Fig. 10.35).

The radiographic detection of pleural effusion in the supine patient can be difficult because fluid accumulates in a dependent location posteriorly. The most common finding is a hazy opacification of the affected hemithorax with obscuration of the hemidiaphragm and blunting of the lateral costophrenic angle. Fluid extending over the apex of the lung may produce a soft tissue cap with a concave interface inferiorly, while medial fluid may cause an apparent mediastinal widening.

Pneumothorax

The classic radiographic finding of a pneumothorax on upright chest films is visualization of the visceral pleura as a thin curvilinear line that parallels the chest wall, separating the partially collapsed lung centrally from pleural air peripherally (Fig. 10.36). An expiratory radiograph may aid in the detection of a small pneumothorax by increasing the volume of intrapleural air relative to lung, thereby displacing the visceral pleural reflection away from the chest wall and by exaggerating the differences in density of pneumothorax (black) to lung (gray) at the end of expiration.

The detection of a pneumothorax is difficult when chest films are obtained in the supine position. Approximately 30% of pneumothoraces imaged on supine radiographs are undetected. Because critically ill patients, especially those in the ICU, are at risk of a pneumothorax from iatrogenic trauma or barotrauma, the recognition of a pneumothorax on a supine film is particularly important. In a supine patient, the most nondependent portion of the pleural space is anterior or anteromedial. Small pneumothoraces will initially collect in these regions and will fail to produce a visible pleural line. The affected hemithorax may appear hyperlucent. Anteromedial air may sharpen the borders of mediastinal soft tissue structures, resulting in improved visualization of the cardiac margin and aortic knob. The lateral costophrenic sulcus may appear abnormally deep and hyperlucent, a finding known as the "deep sulcus" sign (Fig. 10.37). Visualization of the anterior costophrenic sulcus owing to air anteriorly and inferiorly produces the "double diaphragm" sign, as the dome and anterior portions of the diaphragm are outlined by lung and pleural air, respectively. When an anterior pneumothorax is suspected on a supine radiograph, an upright film, lateral

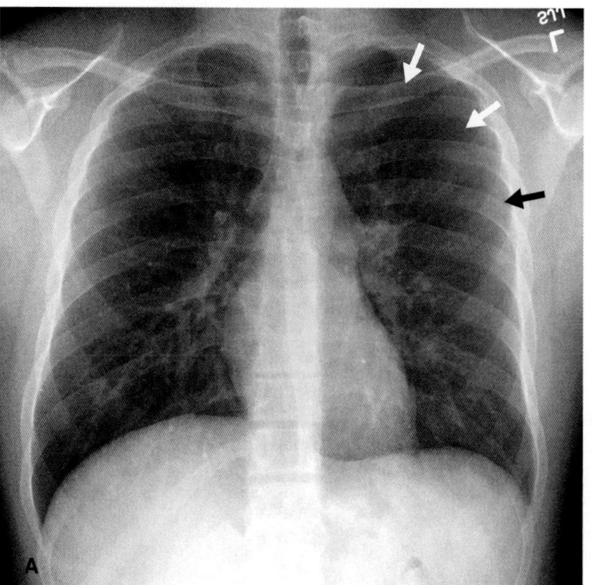

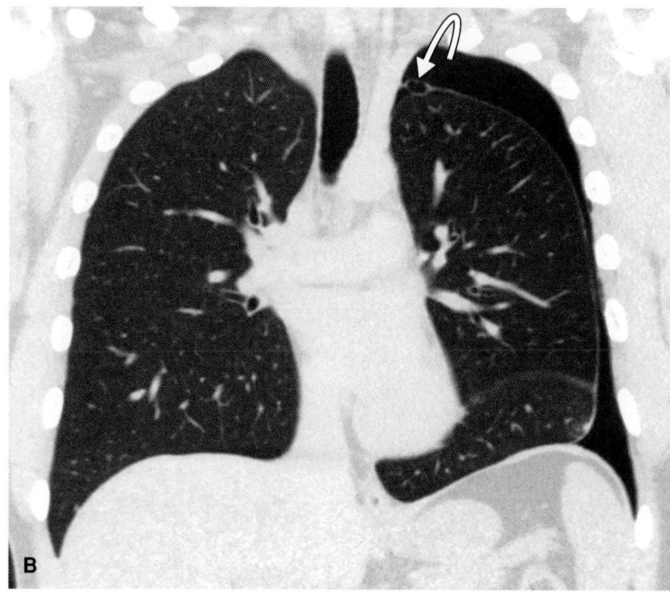

FIGURE 10.36. **Pneumothorax on Radiography and CT. A:** Upright frontal chest radiograph in a 28-year-old man shows a left pneumothorax with a visible visceral pleural line (*arrows*). **B:** Coronal CT scan shows the left pneumothorax and a left apical bleb (*curved arrow*) that is likely responsible for the spontaneous pneumothorax.

decubitus film with the affected side up, ultrasound, or CT scan should be obtained

Subpulmonic pneumothoraces are rare. Radiographically, a localized area of hyperlucency is seen inferiorly, with the visceral pleural line paralleling the hemidiaphragm. Loculated pneumothoraces develop as the result of adhesions between visceral and parietal pleura and may be found anywhere in the pleural space. CT is often necessary for diagnosis.

Several entities produce a curvilinear line or interface or hyperlucency on chest radiographs and must be distinguished from a pneumothorax. Skin folds resulting from the compression of redundant skin by the portable radiographic cassette can produce a curvilinear interface that simulates the visceral pleural line. A skin fold produces an edge or interface with atmospheric air (Fig. 10.38). The interface produced by a skin fold rarely continues over the lung apex and is often seen to

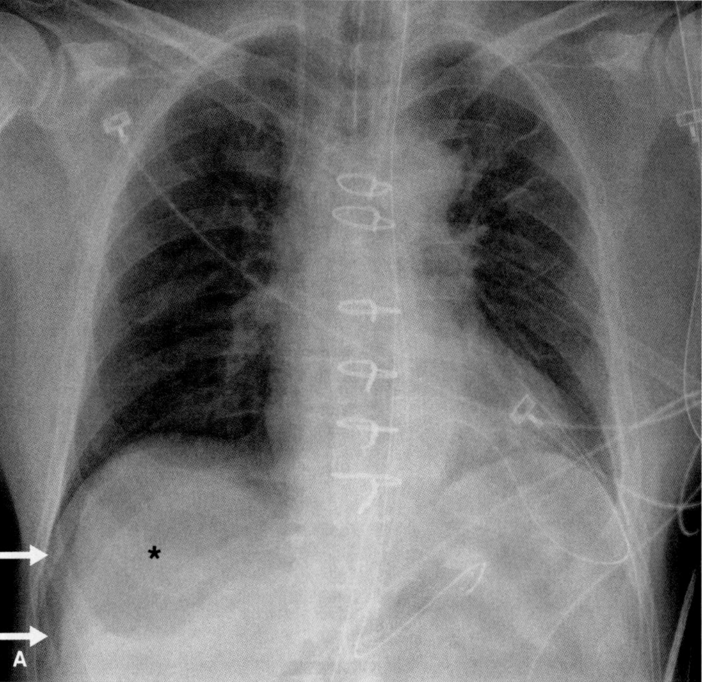

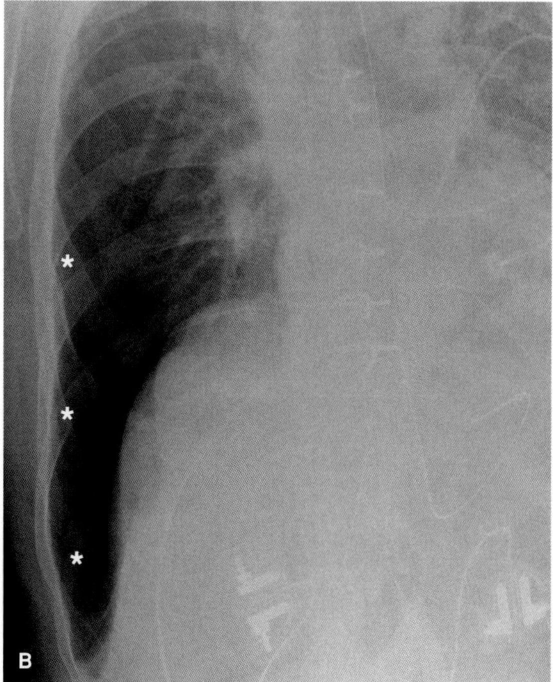

FIGURE 10.37. **Pneumothorax in Supine Patient. A:** Portable chest radiograph in a supine patient status post right-sided central line placement shows abnormal lucency over the right upper abdomen (*asterisk*) and an apparent deep right lateral costophrenic sulcus ("deep sulcus" sign) (*arrows*). **B:** A coned-down cross-table left lateral decubitus radiograph of the right side shows a large right pneumothorax (*asterisks*).

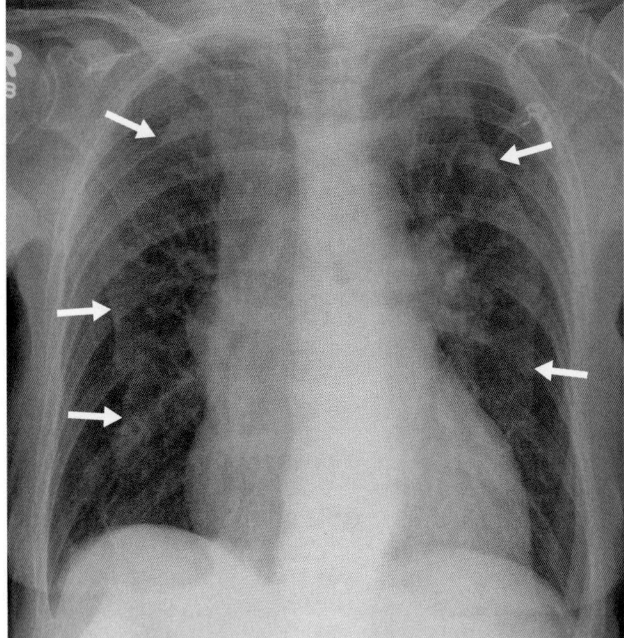

FIGURE 10.38. **Skin Folds Simulating Pneumothorax.** A portable chest radiograph shows bilateral curvilinear densities overlying both lungs (*arrows*) reflecting skin folds outlined by air. Skin folds are often bilateral, appear as edges rather than the thin curvilinear line of the visceral pleura, and do not extend over the lung apex.

extend beyond the chest wall. Pulmonary vascular opacities may be followed peripheral to the skin fold interface. Bullae may simulate pneumothorax by producing localized or unilateral hyperlucency. They are marginated by thin curvilinear walls that are concave rather than convex to the chest wall. The distinction of pneumothorax from bullous disease may be difficult but is usually evident by the clinical presentation. However, since this distinction has important therapeutic implications, certain patients may require CT.

Portable bedside ultrasound is useful for detecting a pneumothorax in the emergency or critical care setting. In normal patients, the lung is seen to slide at the interface with the pleura. This sliding is absent when a pneumothorax is present.

Localized Pleural Thickening

Localized pleural thickening is seen as a flat, smooth, slightly raised soft tissue opacity extending over one or two intercostal spaces that displaces the lung from the innermost cortical margin of the ribs when viewed in tangent. Localized pleural thickening viewed en face is usually undetectable radiographically because the lesion does not significantly attenuate the x-ray beam and does not present a raised edge that can be recognized as a distinct opacity. An exception is the presence of pleural calcification, which can usually be recognized as discrete thin linear or curvilinear calcific densities paralleling the inner surface of the ribs when viewed end-on or as geographic areas of increased density with round or lobulated borders when viewed en face (Fig. 17.16). Focal areas of pleural fibrosis are best appreciated on CT scans, where they are easily distinguished from deposits of subpleural fat by their density.

An additional radiographic finding that mimics the appearance of focal pleural thickening is the apical cap. This is a curvilinear subpleural opacity, <5 mm thick, occasionally calcified, with a smooth concave inferior margin which represents nonspecific fibrosis of the apical lung and adjacent visceral pleura (Fig. 10.39). While it is usually bilateral and symmetric, slight asymmetry in thickness is common. Any growth of the opacity, significant asymmetry, inferior convexity of the opacity, rib destruction, or symptoms should prompt a CT or MR examination to exclude an apical neoplasm (Pancoast or superior sulcus tumor) (Fig. 13.14).

Diffuse Pleural Thickening

Fibrothorax appears as a thin, smooth band of soft tissue with a sharp internal margin seen immediately beneath and parallel to the inner margin of the ribs and intercostal spaces. It is usually

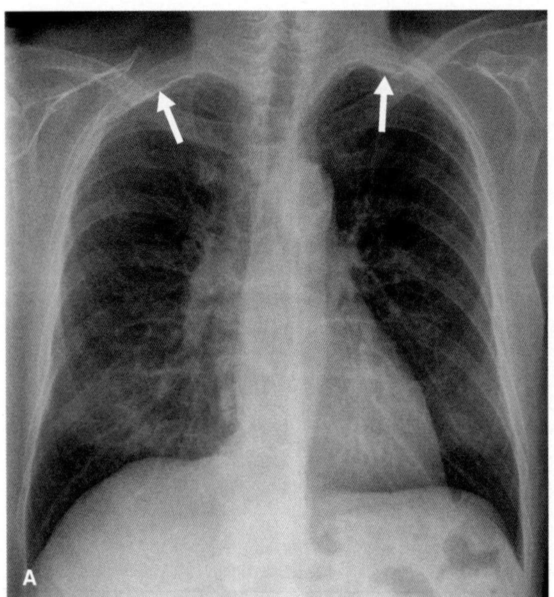

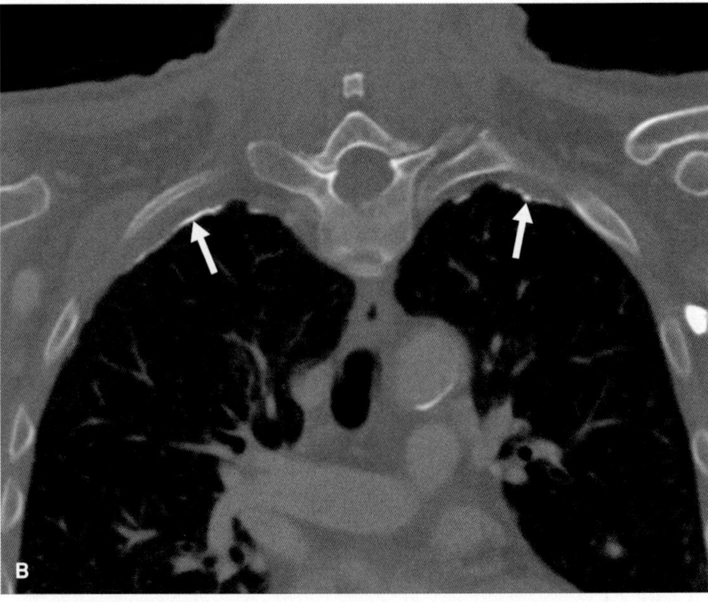

FIGURE 10.39. **Apical Cap Reflecting Fibrosis. A:** Frontal chest radiograph shows bilateral curvilinear calcified apical opacities (*arrows*). **B:** Coned-down contrast-enhanced coronal CT at lung windows shows the calcified apical caps (*arrows*) reflecting subpleural fibrosis.

unilateral and extends over large areas of the dependent (posterior and inferior) portions of the pleural space. Anterior or posterior costal pleural thickening creates a veil-like opacity without sharp margins when viewed en face on frontal radiographs. Blunting of the lateral costophrenic sulcus may be seen on frontal radiographs (Fig. 17.15), while sparing of the posterior costophrenic sulcus and an absence of layering fluid on decubitus positioning help distinguish pleural fibrosis from a small effusion. Fibrothorax tends to spare the interlobar fissures and mediastinal pleura. CT and HRCT are more sensitive than conventional radiographs in detecting pleural thickening. The diminished volume of the affected hemithorax seen with extensive fibrothorax is more easily appreciated on axial CT images than on frontal radiographs (Fig. 17.12). CT provides an unimpeded view of the underlying lung in patients with diffuse pleural thickening, allowing detection of associated interstitial pulmonary fibrosis. This is important in evaluating patients with suspected asbestosis and in assessing the extent of pulmonary disease in patients being considered for pleurectomy.

Pleural and Extrapleural Lesions

The shape and margins of a peripheral opacity on conventional radiographs help define the opacity as parenchymal, pleural, or extrapleural. Pleural masses form obtuse angles with the adjacent normal pleura, in distinction to peripheral lung lesions which usually contact the normal pleura at acute angles. Pleural and extrapleural masses are usually vertically oriented elliptic opacities. Pleural lesions tend to have smooth, well-defined margins as they compress normal lung. These sharp, smooth margins are best appreciated on radiographic projections, with the x-ray beam tangent to the interface between the mass and the lung (Fig. 17.14). A mass sharply outlined by lung on one view but poorly marginated on the orthogonal view should suggest a pleural or extrapleural process. In contrast, intraparenchymal lesions are surrounded by air and will have similar margins on both views. Pleural lesions, unlike parenchymal lesions, do not change position with respiratory motion. Lung disease is often confined to a lobe, while pleural disease may extend across fissures. Pedunculated pleural lesions such as localized fibrous tumors are rare but can present with radiographic features of either pleural or parenchymal lesions.

Despite the aforementioned features, the distinction of pleural from peripheral parenchymal lesions may be difficult. This distinction has important diagnostic implications; parenchymal processes are best evaluated by examination of expectorated sputum or by bronchoscopy, whereas pleural lesions will require thoracentesis or pleural biopsy. CT is often used to help distinguish between pleural and parenchymal disease. A peripheral lesion that is completely surrounded by lung on CT is intraparenchymal, with the exception being the rare pleural lesion arising within an interlobar fissure. Peripheral lung masses generally have irregular margins and may contain air bronchograms. Those parenchymal lesions that contact the pleura will form acute angles with the chest wall. The CT appearance of pleural and extrapleural or chest wall lesions are similar. Both pleural and extrapleural lesions are sharply defined and form obtuse angles with the chest wall; rib destruction or subcutaneous mass is the only finding that localizes an extrapulmonary lesion to the chest wall (Fig. 17.22). When a peripheral parenchymal lesion invades the pleura, determining the origin of the mass may be impossible. CT can further characterize peripheral lesions by their density; a smooth fatty mass is almost certainly a pleural lipoma (Fig. 17.13), whereas a homogeneous pleural or extrapleural soft tissue mass is most likely a localized fibrous tumor of pleura or neurogenic tumor (Figs. 11.24 and 17.14). The signal intensity on MR images may be useful in the characterization of focal pleural masses. Loculated fluid collections will show homogeneous low signal on T1 and high signal on T2. Lipomas demonstrate homogeneous high signal intensity on T1 and low signal on fat-suppressed T1. Localized fibrous tumors of pleura are typically of intermediate signal intensity on T1 and high signal intensity on T2, respectively, due to the high cellularity of these tumors.

Chest Wall Lesions

Chest wall lesions become evident radiographically when (1) they extend into the thorax and become outlined by displaced lung, (2) there is bone displacement or destruction by the mass, or (3) they protrude externally from the skin surface to be outlined by air in the atmosphere. CT, MR, and US are all useful in assessing the characteristics of chest wall lesions. While CT and MR are most useful in determining the extent of intrathoracic involvement by chest wall lesions, US is the least expensive and simplest method of characterizing the nature of palpable chest wall masses. The radiographic findings of chest wall lesions involving specific bony or soft tissue components of the chest wall are detailed in the section on chest wall disease in Chapter 17.

Diaphragmatic Abnormalities

Radiographic findings of diaphragmatic disorders include elevation and depression of the diaphragm and abnormalities of diaphragmatic contour. The diagnostic considerations of diaphragmatic disease are reviewed in Chapter 17.

Suggested Readings

Chou SH, Kicska GA, Pipavath SN, Reddy GP. Digital tomosynthesis of the chest: current and emerging applications. *Radiographics* 2014;34(2):359–372.

Gibbs JM, Chandrasekhar CA, Ferguson EC, Oldham SA. Lines and stripes: where did they go?—from conventional radiography to CT. *Radiographics* 2007; 27(1):33–48.

Heitzman R. *The Mediastinum: Radiologic Correlations with Anatomy and Pathology*. Berlin: Springer-Verlag; 1988:311–349.

Im JG, Webb WR, Rosen A, Gamsu G. Costal pleura: appearances at high-resolution CT. *Radiology* 1989;171:125–131.

Kuhlman JE, Collins J, Brooks GN, Yandow DR, Broderick LS. Dual-energy subtraction chest radiography: what to look for beyond calcified nodules. *Radiographics* 2006;26:79–92.

Müller NL, Webb WR. Radiographic imaging of the pulmonary hila. *Invest Radiol* 1985;20:661–671.

Nason LK, Walker CM, McNeeley MF, Burivong W, Fligner CL, Godwin JD. Imaging of the diaphragm: anatomy and function. *Radiographics* 2012; 32(2):E51–E70.

Proto AV, Speckman JM. The left lateral radiograph of the chest. Part 1. *Med Radiogr Photogr* 1979;55:29–74.

Proto AV, Speckman JM. The left lateral radiograph of the chest. *Med Radiogr Photogr* 1980;56:38–64.

Schaefer-Prokop C, Neitzel U, Venema HW, Uffmann M, Prokop M. Digital chest radiography: an update on modern technology, dose containment and control of image quality. *Eur Radiol* 2008;18(9):1818–1830.

Wilkinson GA, Fraser RG. Roentgenography of the chest. *Appl Radiol* 1975; 4:41–53.

CHAPTER 11 ■ MEDIASTINUM AND HILA

JEFFREY S. KLEIN

This chapter will review the radiologic approach to mediastinal masses, diffuse mediastinal disease, and hilar abnormalities.

MEDIASTINAL MASSES

Localized mediastinal abnormalities are common diagnostic challenges for the radiologist. Patients with mediastinal masses tend to present in one of three ways: (1) with symptoms related to local mass effect or invasion of adjacent mediastinal structures (e.g., stridor in a patient with thyroid goiter); (2) as the result of a search for mediastinal abnormality in a patient with a predisposing condition (e.g., a patient with myasthenia gravis and concern for thymoma); or (3) as an incidental finding on chest radiography or CT. Occasionally, a mediastinal mass is discovered in the course of an evaluation for known malignancy (e.g., a patient with non-Hodgkin lymphoma [NHL]). Contrast-enhanced multidetector row CT (MDCT) is the primary cross-sectional modality used to evaluate mediastinal masses. MR is typically reserved for specific problem solving and is most useful for: (1) assessing lesions in patients who cannot receive iodinated contrast; (2) likely vascular lesions; (3) confirming the cystic nature of lesions that have high attenuation due to proteinacious contents; and (4) distinguishing thymic hyperplasia from thymic neoplasms. PET is used to confirm increased metabolic activity in suspected malignancy, to assess response of mediastinal tumors to therapy, particularly lymphoma, and to distinguish residual or recurrent tumor from fibrosis (Table 11.1).

For the purposes of the following discussion, the mediastinum is divided into three compartments: anterior (prevascular), middle (visceral), and posterior (paravertebral) compartments, as described in Chapter 10.

Anterior (Prevascular) Mediastinal Masses (Table 11.2)

Vascular Structures. Perhaps the most common thoracic inlet mass is seen in older patients as tortuous arterial structures, in particular the confluence of the right brachiocephalic and right subclavian arteries or left subclavian artery bulging laterally into the upper lobe to produce a thoracic inlet mass (Fig. 11.1). Since the "mass" is situated anteriorly in the thoracic inlet, its lateral border above the clavicle is indistinct, whereas masses that are posterior or paravertebral in location are sharply outlined by apical lung which extends higher posteriorly than anteriorly. This finding is termed the "thoracic inlet" or "cervicothoracic" sign, and helps localize thoracic inlet masses, thereby suggesting the etiology of such lesions. Tortuous arterial structures may be identified by the presence of atherosclerotic calcification, and can often be seen on a lateral chest radiograph as a "mass" projecting posterior to the tracheal air column which is sharply outlined posteriorly. In contrast to other masses in the thoracic inlet, a tortuous vessel is usually associated with tracheal deviation toward the side of the mass, whereas most goiters and other inlet masses displace the trachea contralaterally.

An uncommon vascular cause of an anterior mediastinal or prevascular mass is an aneurysm arising from the right sinus of Valsalva or an ascending aortic aneurysm extending anteriorly. Sinus of Valsalva aneurysms are typically seen incidentally on cardiac CT or MR and not detected radiographically. A prevascular mass arising from the ascending aorta as seen on lateral chest radiography that contains curvilinear calcification should suggest an ascending aortic aneurysm or foregut cyst as potential causes.

Thyroid Masses. In a small percentage of patients with a cervical thyroid goiter, a thyroid carcinoma, or an enlarged gland from thyroiditis, extension of the thyroid through the thoracic inlet into the superior mediastinum may occur. These lesions are usually discovered as incidental findings on chest radiography; a minority of patients will present with complaints of dyspnea or dysphagia as a result of tracheal or esophageal compression respectively. Thyroid goiters, either uninodular or multinodular, arise from the lower pole of the thyroid or thyroid isthmus and can enter the superior mediastinum anterior to the trachea (80% of cases) or to the right and posterolateral to the trachea (20% of cases). In a very small minority of patients with intrathoracic goiter, the connection of the intrathoracic component of the goiter to the cervical gland is a thin fibrous band or is absent and therefore not obvious on cross-sectional imaging.

On chest radiography, an anterosuperior mediastinal mass typically deviates the trachea contralaterally and either posteriorly (anterior masses) or anteriorly (posterior masses). Coarse, clumped calcifications are common in thyroid goiters. Radioiodine studies should be performed as the initial imaging procedure, although false-negative results do occur. CT usually shows characteristic findings: (1) well-defined margins;

TABLE 11.1

UTILITY OF IMAGING MODALITIES IN EVALUATION OF MEDIASTINAL MASSES

MODALITY	UTILITY	LIMITATIONS
Conventional radiography	▪ Ready availability ▪ Low radiation dose ▪ Global assessment of chest ▪ Compartmentalization of mass	
Multi-detector CT	▪ High contrast resolution ▪ Ready availability ▪ Detection of calcification ▪ Superior spatial resolution to MR	Ionizing radiation Iodinated contrast
Magnetic resonance imaging	▪ Iodinated contrast contraindicated ▪ Vascular lesions ▪ Confirms cysts (foregut, pericardial) ▪ Thymic mass vs. hyperplasia	Inability to detect Ca^{++} Lower spatial resolution than CT
FDG-PET	▪ Measures metabolic activity ▪ Distinguishes necrosis/fibrosis from viable tumor ▪ Global assessment of regional/distant metastases ▪ Assess treatment response	

TABLE 11.2

ANTERIOR (PREVASCULAR) MEDIASTINAL MASSES

Common	
Vascular	▪ Tortuous/dilated brachiocephalic/ right subclavian artery
Thyroid	▪ Colloid nodule ▪ Goiter
Parathyroid	▪ Adenoma
Lymphatic	▪ Lymphoma • Hodgkin • Non-Hodgkin ▪ Metastatic disease
Thymic	▪ Thymoma ▪ Thymic hyperplasia
Germ cell neoplasm	▪ Teratoma (benign)
Mesenchymal tumors	▪ Lipoma
Uncommon	
Vascular	▪ Ascending aortic aneurysm ▪ Sinus of Valsalva aneurysm
Thyroid	▪ Carcinoma
Parathyroid	▪ Hyperplasia ▪ Carcinoma
Lymphatic	▪ Lymphangioma ▪ Inflammatory
Thymic	▪ Thymic cyst ▪ Thymolipoma ▪ Thymic neuroendocrine tumor (carcinoid) ▪ Thymic carcinoma
Germ cell neoplasm	▪ Teratoma (malignant) ▪ Seminoma ▪ Endodermal sinus tumor ▪ Embryonal cell carcinoma ▪ Choriocarcinoma
Mesenchymal tumors	▪ Leiomyoma ▪ Fibroma ▪ Hemangioma ▪ Hamartoma

(2) continuity of the mass with the cervical thyroid; (3) coarse calcifications; (4) cystic or necrotic areas; (5) baseline high CT attenuation (because of intrinsic iodine content); and (6) intense enhancement (>25 H) as a result of the hypervascularity of most thyroid masses and prolonged enhancement (resulting from active uptake of iodine from contrast media) following intravenous contrast administration (Fig. 11.2). MR is useful in depicting the longitudinal extension of thyroid goiters without the use of intravenous contrast.

Parathyroid Masses. In approximately 2% of patients, the parathyroid glands fail to separate from the thymus in the neck and descend with the gland into the anterosuperior mediastinum. These glands can be found near the thoracic inlet in or about the thymus. This becomes important in the small percentage of patients with persistent clinical and biochemical evidence of hyperparathyroidism following routine neck exploration and parathyroidectomy. Most of these ectopic parathyroid lesions are small (<3 cm) adenomas; rarely, they represent hyperplastic glands or parathyroid carcinoma. When US fails to localize a lesion in the neck, CT, MR, or technetium[99] sestamibi (Tc-99m-sestamibi) scanning may be useful in detecting mediastinal lesions (Fig. 11.3).

Lymphangiomas. These uncommon masses are tumors comprised of dilated lymphatic channels. The cystic or cavernous form (cystic hygroma) is most commonly discovered in infancy and is often associated with chromosomal abnormalities, including Turner syndrome and trisomies 13, 18, and 21. In infants, these lesions tend to extend from the neck into the anterior mediastinum; less commonly they may arise primarily within the anterior mediastinum in older patients.

Thymomas (Thymic Epithelial Neoplasms). Thymoma is the second most common primary mediastinal neoplasms in adults after lymphoma. These lesions are neoplasms that arise from thymic epithelium with varying numbers of intermixed lymphocytes. Thymic epithelial neoplasms are divided into *thymomas*, in which the neoplastic component reflects thymic epithelial cells, and *thymic carcinomas*, in which the epithelial component shows signs of overt atypia. The World Health

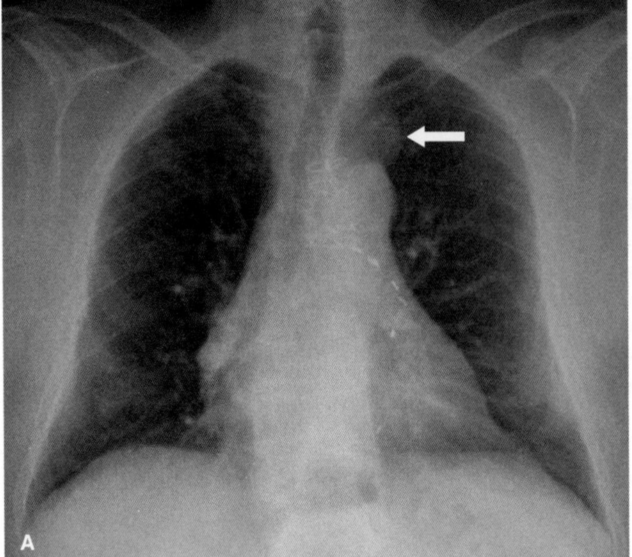

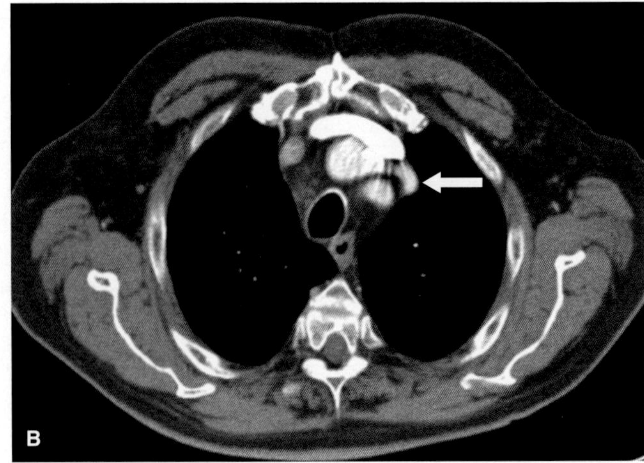

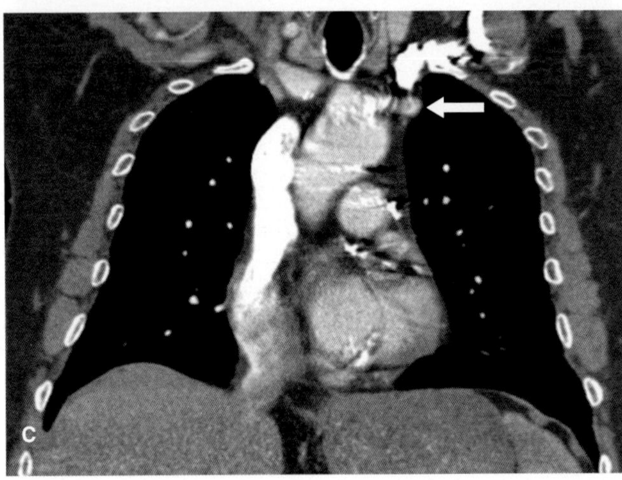

FIGURE 11.1. Tortuous Left Common Carotid Artery Producing Superior Mediastinal "Mass." A: Chest radiograph demonstrates a left superior mediastinal mass (*arrow*). **B** and **C:** Axial (**B**) and coronal (**C**) contrast-enhanced scans show a tortuous left common carotid artery arising from the aortic arch (*arrows* in **B** and **C**) as producing the "mass."

Organization classifies these neoplasms based upon the morphology of the epithelial component and the ratio of epithelial cells to lymphocytes. The classification system divides these neoplasms into types A, AB, B1, B2, B3, and C, with a spectrum of histologic changes ranging from the classic encapsulated thymoma (A), which has a favorable prognosis, to thymic carcinoma (C), which generally carries a poor prognosis. For the staging of thymic epithelial neoplasms, the International Thymic Malignancy Interest Group (ITMIG) has developed a detailed classification system based on TNM descriptors.

The average age at diagnosis of thymoma is 45 to 50; these lesions are rare in patients under the age of 20. While most often associated with myasthenia gravis, thymoma has been associated with other paraneoplastic syndromes such as pure red cell aplasia and hypogammaglobulinemia. Of patients with myasthenia gravis, 10% to 15% have a thymoma, while a larger percentage of patients with thymoma (30% to 50%) have or will develop myasthenia. Autoimmune diseases that have been associated with thymoma include Grave disease and lupus.

On chest radiography, thymomas are seen as round or oval, smooth or lobulated soft tissue masses arising near the origin of the great vessels at the base of the heart. CT is best for characterizing thymomas and detecting local invasion preoperatively (Fig. 11.4). As a result of their firm consistency, thymomas characteristically maintain their shape where they contact the sternum anteriorly and heart and great vessels posteriorly. Compared to type A tumors, higher-grade thymomas, particularly types B3 and C, tend to show larger size, more irregular margins, heterogeneous enhancement, regions of necrosis, mediastinal nodal metastases, and calcification. Invasion of tumor through the thymic capsule is present in 33% to 50% of patients (Fig. 11.5). In the majority of these patients, microscopic capsular invasion cannot be determined on CT or MR. Local invasion of mediastinal pleura, pericardium, lung, chest wall, diaphragm, and great vessels occurs in decreasing order of frequency in a minority of patients. Contiguity of a thymoma with the adjacent chest wall or mediastinal structures cannot be used as reliable evidence of invasion of these structures. Drop metastases to dependent portions of the pleural space are a recognized route of spread of thymoma that has invaded the pleura. Extrathoracic metastases are rare, although transdiaphragmatic spread of a pleural tumor into the retroperitoneum has been described. For these reasons, it is important to image the entire thorax and upper abdomen in any patient with suspected invasive disease.

In patients with myasthenia gravis who are being evaluated for thymoma, CT can demonstrate tumors that are not visible on conventional radiography. However, very small thymic tumors may not be distinguishable from a normal or hyperplastic gland with CT, particularly in younger patients with a large amount of residual thymic tissue.

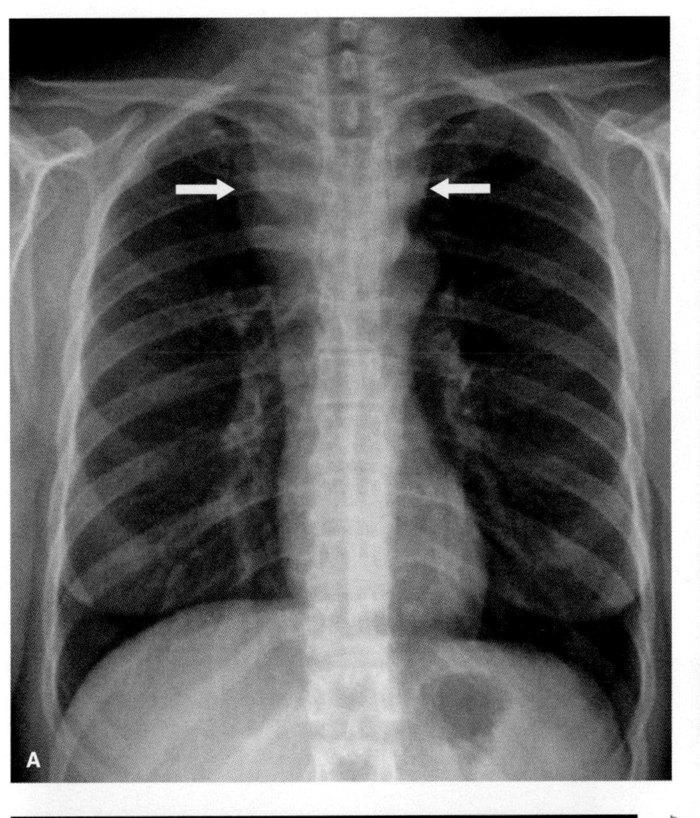

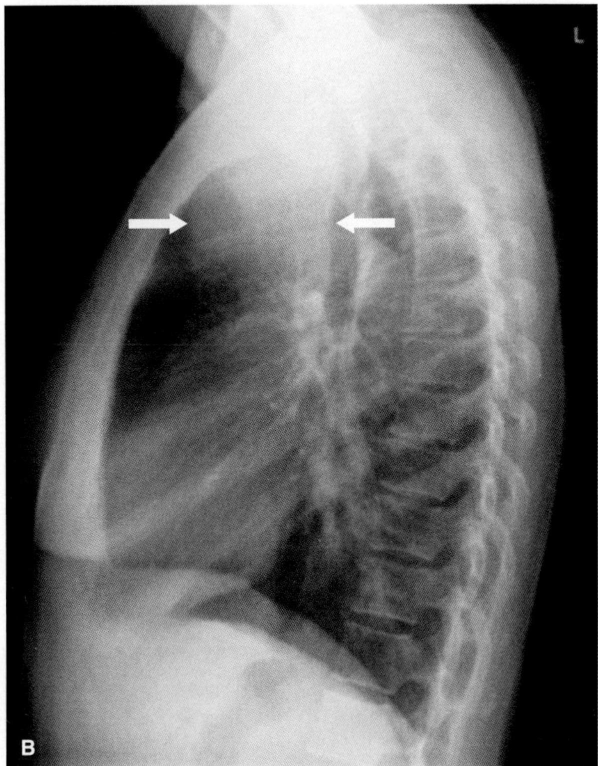

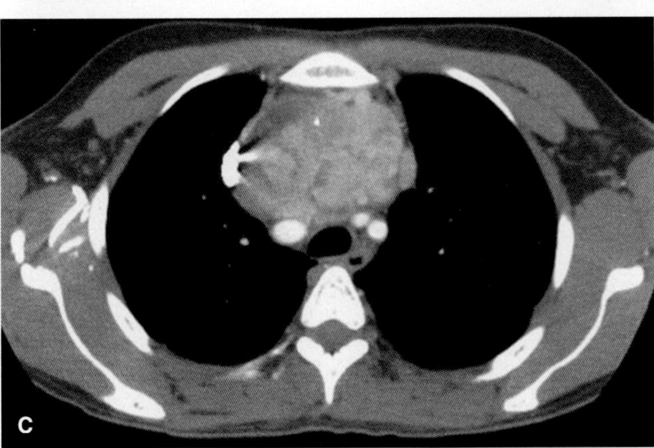

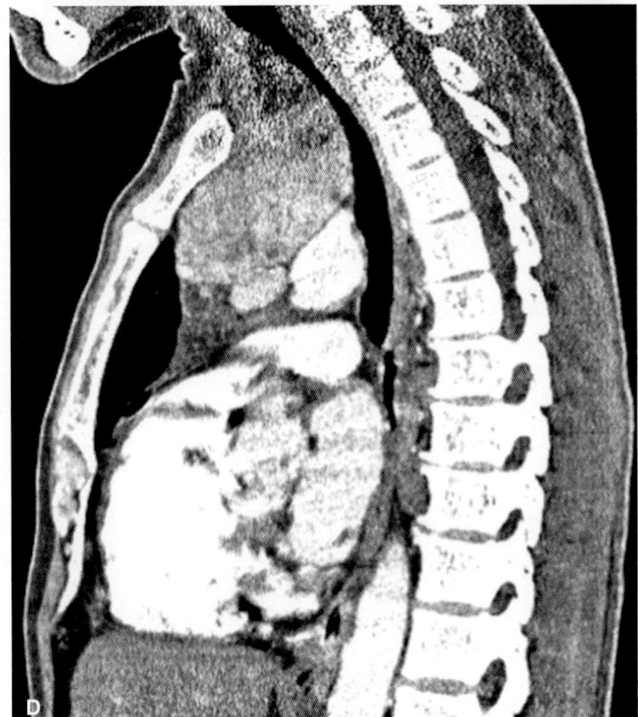

FIGURE 11.2. **Thyroid Goiter.** Frontal (**A**) and lateral (**B**) radiographs show a lobulated anterior and superior mediastinal mass (*arrows*). **C:** Axial contrast-enhanced CT at the level of the manubrium shows a mixed attenuation mass with foci of calcification and regions of low attenuation anterior to the trachea and great vessels. **D:** Sagittal-reformatted midline scan shows the mass extending from the thoracic inlet into the anterior mediastinum.

Thymic cysts may be congenital or acquired. Congenital unilocular thymic cysts are rare lesions that represent remnants of the thymopharyngeal duct and contain thin or gelatinous fluid. They are characterized histologically by an epithelial lining, with thymic tissue in the cyst wall, which distinguishes thymic cysts histologically from other congenital cystic lesions within the anterior mediastinum. Acquired multilocular thymic cysts are postinflammatory in nature and have been associated with AIDS, prior radiation or surgery, and autoimmune conditions such as Sjögren syndrome, myasthenia gravis, and aplastic anemia; in these latter conditions, clinical and radiologic distinction of multilocular thymic cyst from cystic thymoma may be difficult; in fact, the two conditions can coexist. Large cysts will be evident as masses on conventional radiography, and CT or MR will demonstrate the cystic nature of the lesion. If the distinction between a true thymic cyst, cystic degeneration of a thymoma or lymphoma, germ cell neoplasm, or lymphangioma is impossible

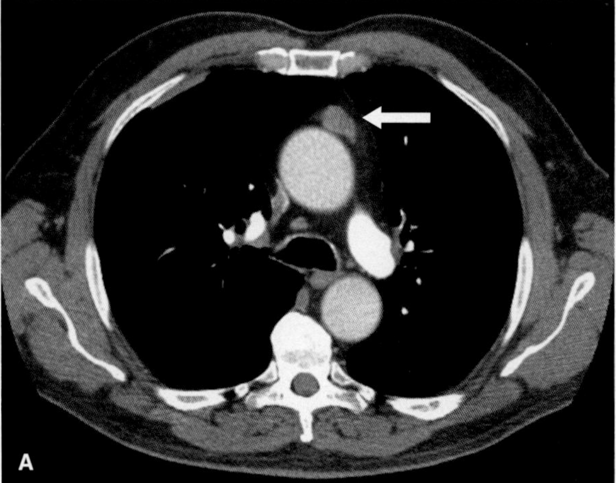

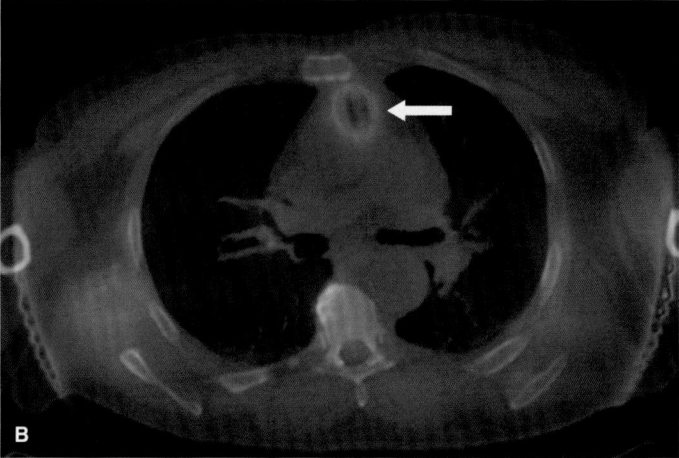

FIGURE 11.3. **Parathyroid Adenoma.** **A:** Axial contrast-enhanced CT through the upper chest in a 60-year-old male with hypercalcemia demonstrates a preaortic nodule (*arrow*). **B:** Fused SPECT-CT Tc-99m-sestamibi shows increased activity within the lesion (*arrow*). Surgical exploration confirmed an ectopic parathyroid adenoma.

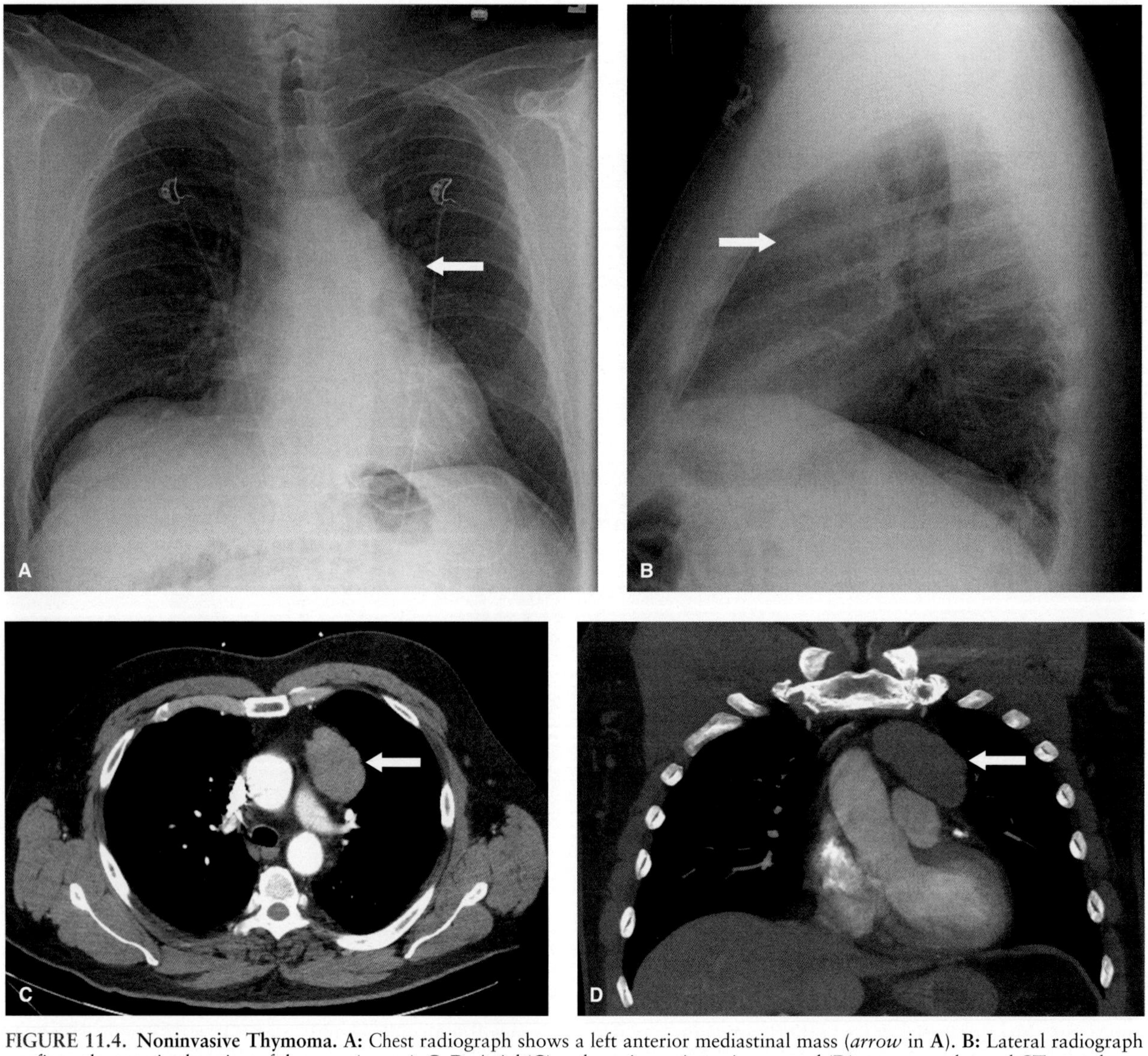

FIGURE 11.4. **Noninvasive Thymoma.** **A:** Chest radiograph shows a left anterior mediastinal mass (*arrow* in **A**). **B:** Lateral radiograph confirms the anterior location of the mass (*arrow*). **C, D:** Axial (**C**) and maximum intensity coronal (**D**) contrast-enhanced CT scan shows a lobulated left anterior mediastinal mass (*arrows* in **C, D**). Surgical resection revealed a noninvasive thymoma.

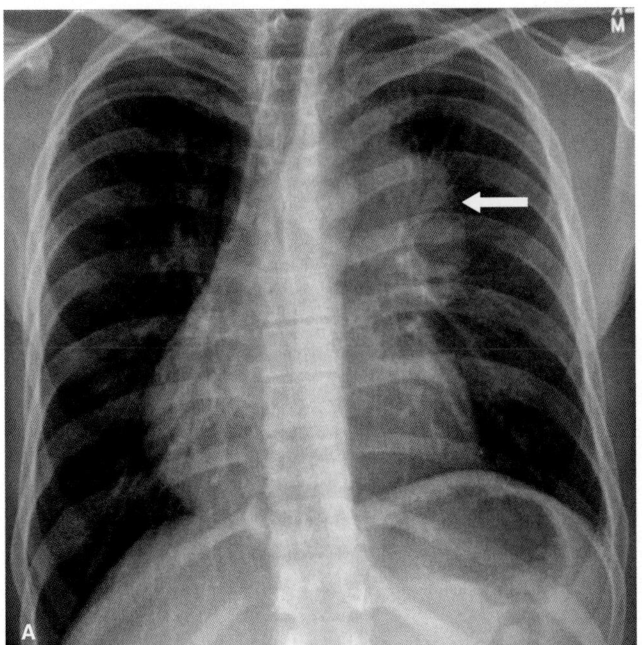

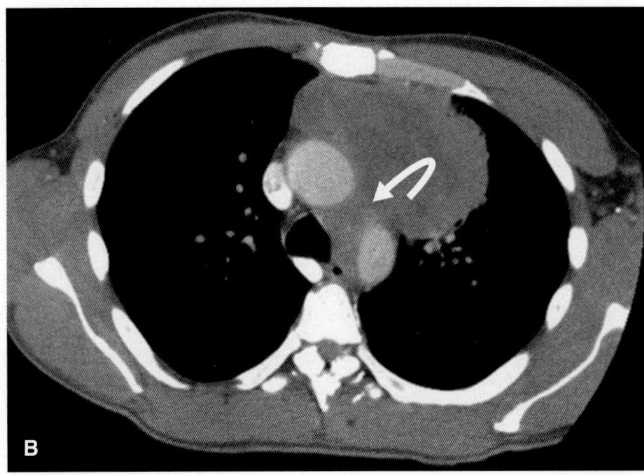

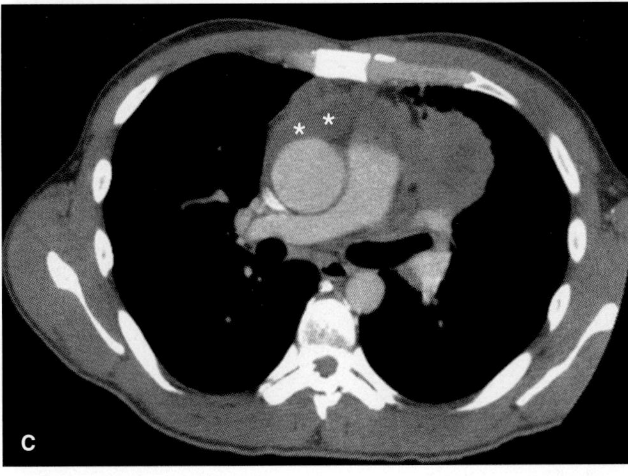

FIGURE 11.5. **Invasive Thymoma. A:** Posteroanterior chest radiograph reveals a left mediastinal mass (*arrow*) with an irregular lateral border. **B:** CT confirms a solid left anterior mediastinal mass (*arrow*) with foci of necrosis. Note soft tissue infiltration of the aortopulmonary window (*curved arrow*) indicating mediastinal invasion. **C:** Axial scan more inferiorly shows broad mediastinal contact by the tumor with associated pericardial effusion (*asterisks*). Mediastinal and pericardial invasion were confirmed at surgery.

on clinical and radiologic grounds, the lesion should be biopsied or resected.

Thymolipoma is a rare, benign thymic neoplasm that consists primarily of fat with intermixed rests of normal thymic tissue. These masses are asymptomatic and therefore are typically large when first detected. Chest radiographs show a large anterior mediastinal mass that, because of its pliable nature, tends to envelope the heart and diaphragm. CT demonstrates a fatty mass with interspersed soft tissue densities. Resection is curative.

Thymic Carcinoid. Neuroendocrine tumors of the thymus are rare malignant neoplasms believed to arise from thymic cells of neural crest origin (amine precursor uptake and decarboxylation [APUD] or Kulchitsky cells). The most common histologic type is carcinoid tumor, which, as with similar lesions arising within the bronchi, ranges in differentiation and behavior from typical carcinoid to atypical carcinoid to small cell carcinoma. Approximately 40% of patients have Cushing syndrome as a result of adrenocorticotropic hormone secretion by the tumor. These patients tend to have smaller lesions at the time of diagnosis since they present early with signs of corticosteroid excess. The carcinoid syndrome associated with thymic carcinoid is uncommon. This lesion is indistinguishable from thymoma on plain radiographs and CT scans.

Thymic Hyperplasia is defined as enlargement of a thymus that is normal on gross and histologic examination. This rare entity occurs primarily in children as a rebound effect in response to an antecedent stress, discontinuation of chemotherapy, or treatment of hypercortisolism. An association with Grave disease has also been noted. The term *thymic hyperplasia* has been used incorrectly to describe the histologic findings of lymphoid follicular hyperplasia of the thymus, found in 60% of patients with myasthenia gravis. In contrast to most cases of true thymic hyperplasia, lymphoid hyperplasia does not produce thymic enlargement. Most patients with thymic hyperplasia have normal sized or diffusely enlarged glands on CT (Fig. 11.6); occasionally thymic hyperplasia will present as a mass that is radiographically indistinguishable from thymoma. Most cases can be resolved by noting a decrease in size on follow-up studies, thereby obviating the need for biopsy. Chemical shift MR with in- and out-of-phase sequences can distinguish hyperplasia, which shows signal decrease on out-of-phase chemical shift imaging due to the presence of microscopic fat within hyperplastic tissue, from thymic neoplasms that do not decrease in signal intensity.

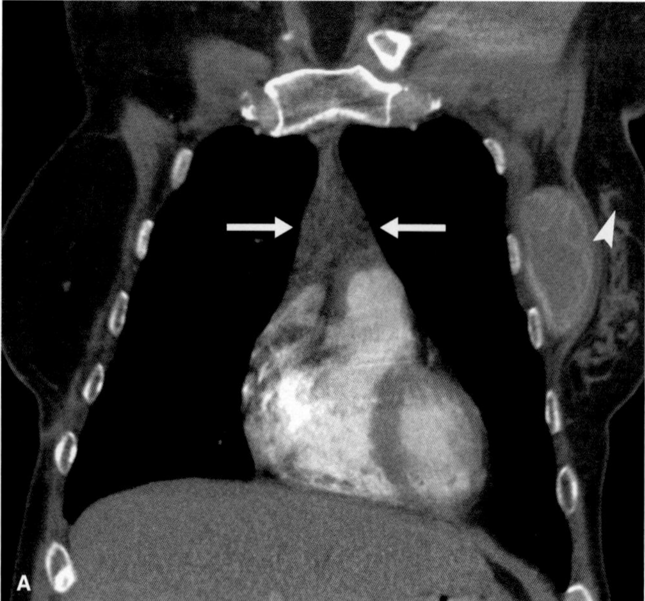

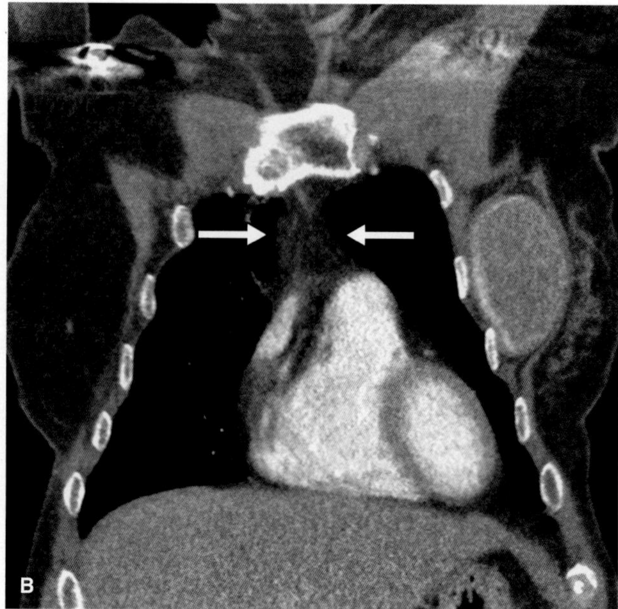

FIGURE 11.6. **Thymic Hyperplasia. A:** Coronal contrast-enhanced CT through the anterior mediastinum in a 55-year-old woman who recently completed chemotherapy for left breast cancer shows a diffusely enlarged thymus (*arrows*) with predominantly soft tissue attenuation. Note left breast prosthesis (*arrowhead*). **B:** Coronal CT scan years later following completion of chemotherapy shows a decrease in size of the thymus (*arrows*) with almost uniform fat attenuation.

Thymic Lymphoma. The thymus is involved in 40% to 50% of patients with the nodular sclerosing subtype of Hodgkin disease. Its radiographic appearance is indistinguishable from that of other solid neoplasms arising within the thymus. The presence of lymph node enlargement in other portions of the mediastinum or anterior chest wall involvement should suggest the diagnosis.

Lymphoma. Hodgkin disease or NHL is the most common primary mediastinal neoplasm in adults. Hodgkin disease involves the thorax in 85% of patients at the time of presentation. The majority (90%) of patients with intrathoracic involvement have mediastinal lymph node enlargement; this most commonly involves the anterior mediastinal and hilar nodal groups. The anterior mediastinum is the most frequent site of a localized nodal mass in patients with Hodgkin disease, particularly those with the nodular sclerosing type (Fig. 11.7). Isolated enlargement of mediastinal or hilar nodes outside the anterior mediastinum should suggest an alternative diagnosis. Only 25% of patients with Hodgkin lymphoma have disease limited to the mediastinum at the time of diagnosis. NHL involves the thorax in approximately 40% of patients at presentation. In contrast to Hodgkin disease, only 50% of patients with NHL and intrathoracic disease have mediastinal nodal involvement, and only 10% of NHL patients have disease that is limited to the mediastinum. Of the various subtypes of NHL that present with mediastinal masses, lymphoblastic lymphoma and diffuse large B-cell lymphoma are the most common (Fig. 11.8). Lymphoma involving a single mediastinal or hilar nodal group is much more common in NHL than in Hodgkin disease. NHL most commonly involves middle mediastinal and hilar lymph nodes; juxtaphrenic and posterior mediastinal nodal involvement is uncommon but is seen almost exclusively in NHL. Patterns of pulmonary parenchymal involvement in lymphoma are discussed in Chapter 13.

While Hodgkin disease spreads in a fairly predictable pattern from one nodal group to an adjacent group, NHL is felt to be a multifocal disorder in which patterns of involvement are unpredictable. Localized intrathoracic Hodgkin disease is usually treated with radiation therapy, with 90% response rates. More widespread Hodgkin disease and NHL are treated with chemotherapy, with better response rates for Hodgkin disease than for NHL.

On conventional radiography, lymphoma involving the anterior mediastinum is indistinguishable from thymoma or germ cell neoplasm and presents as a lobulated mass projecting to one or both sides of the mediastinum (Fig. 11.7). Calcification in untreated lymphoma is extremely uncommon, and its presence within an anterior mediastinal mass should suggest another diagnosis. Involvement of other lymph node stations in the mediastinum, hila, neck, or axilla makes lymphoma more likely. An enlarged spleen displacing the gastric air bubble medially, seen in the upper abdominal portion of the frontal chest radiograph, provides an additional clue to the diagnosis.

MDCT is performed in virtually all patients with lymphoma. The advantages of chest CT include the ability to better characterize and localize masses seen on chest radiographs; detection of subradiographic sites of involvement that can alter disease staging, prognosis, and therapy; guidance for transthoracic or open biopsy; the ability to monitor response to therapy; and detection of relapse. The appearance of nodal involvement in lymphoma varies; most commonly, discrete enlarged solid lymph nodes or conglomerate masses of nodes are seen (Fig. 11.7C). Parenchymal involvement is usually the result of direct extranodal extension of a tumor from hilar nodes along the bronchovascular lymphatics; this is better appreciated on CT than on chest radiography. Likewise, a tumor extending from the mediastinum to the pericardium, subpleural space, and chest wall is best appreciated on CT or MR. On MR, untreated lymphoma appears as a mass of uniform low signal intensity on T1WIs and uniform high signal intensity or intermixed areas of low and high signal intensity on T2WIs. The areas of low signal intensity on T2WIs of untreated patients may be a result of foci of fibrotic tissue in nodular sclerosing Hodgkin disease.

Patients with successfully treated mediastinal Hodgkin disease often have residual soft tissue density in the affected

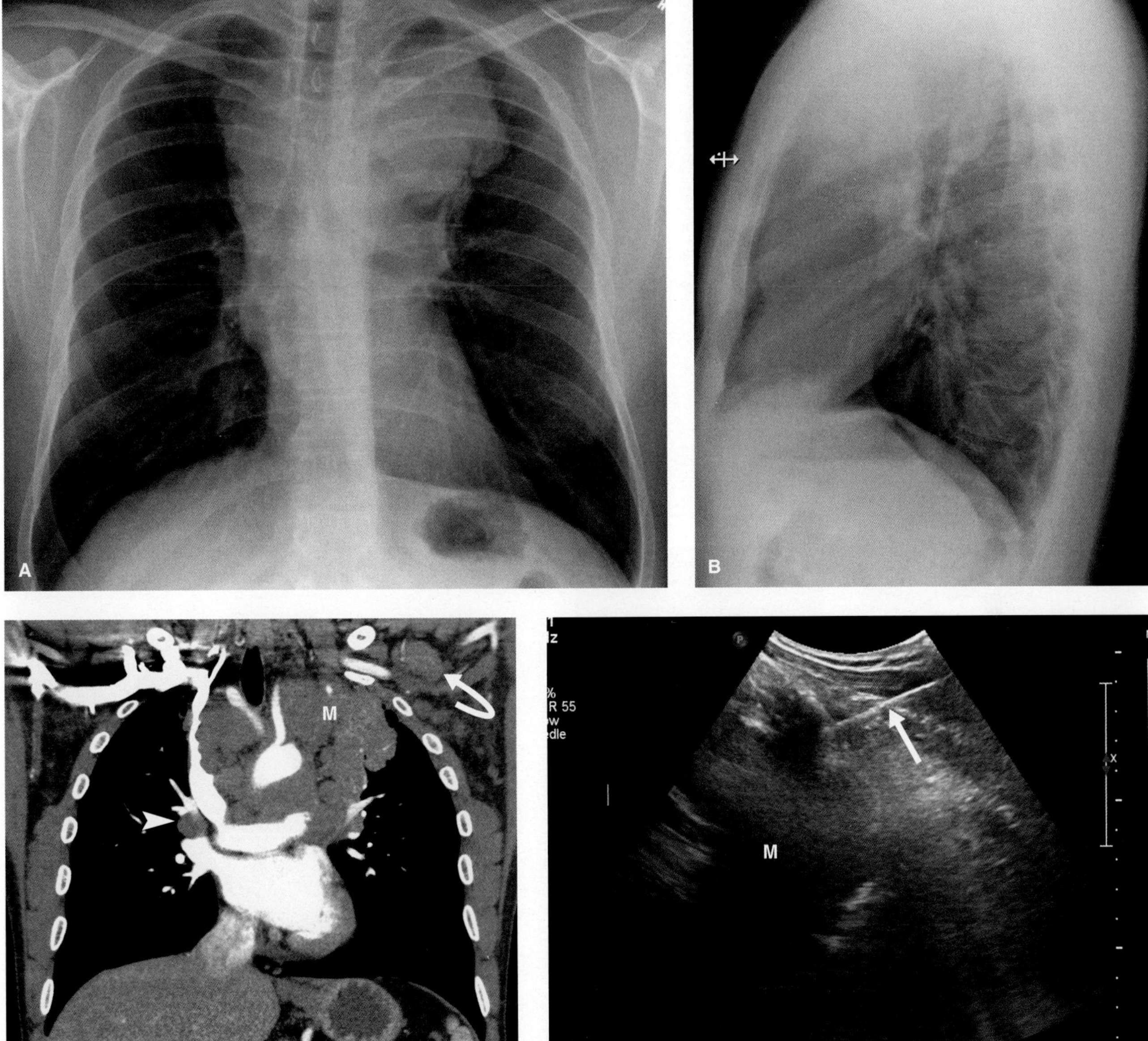

FIGURE 11.7. **Hodgkin Lymphoma. A, B:** Posteroanterior (**A**) and lateral (**B**) chest radiographs in a 35-year-old man shows a large, lobulated anterior and superior mediastinal mass. **C:** Coronal contrast-enhanced CT at the level of the aortic arch shows a large superior mediastinal mass (M) encompassing the arch and great vessels. Note enlarged right hilar (*arrowhead*) and left axillary (*curved arrow*) lymph nodes. **D:** Ultrasound-guided core needle biopsy shows the mass (M) with biopsy needle (*arrow*) at edge of lesion. Core biopsy demonstrated nodular sclerosing subtype of Hodgkin disease.

mediastinal compartments, with dystrophic calcification commonly seen within treated nodes (Fig. 11.9). CT and fluorodeoxyglucose (FDG)-PET are used to monitor the response of lymphoma to therapy. While CT can accurately assess tumor regression and detect relapse within nodal groups outside the treated region, the ability to distinguish residual tumor from sterilized fibrotic masses is limited. Residual soft tissue masses have been reported in up to 50% of patients, most commonly with nodular sclerosing Hodgkin disease, and are more common when the pretreatment mass is large. Some patients with residual masses on CT or MR will have tumor recurrence within 6 to 12 months after the completion of therapy. In general, the appearance of high signal intensity regions on T2WIs more than 6 months after treatment should suggest recurrence. FDG-PET is clearly superior to CT or MR in distinguishing recurrent tumor from fibrosis in both Hodgkin disease and NHL.

Germ Cell Neoplasms, which include teratoma, seminoma, choriocarcinoma, endodermal sinus tumor, and embryonal cell carcinoma, arise from collections of primitive germ cells that arrest in the anterior mediastinum on their journey to the gonads during embryologic development. Since they are histologically indistinguishable from germ cell tumors arising in the testes and ovaries, the diagnosis of a primary malignant mediastinal germ cell neoplasm requires exclusion of a primary gonadal tumor as a source of mediastinal metastases. A key in distinguishing primary from metastatic mediastinal germ cell neoplasm is the presence of retroperitoneal lymph node involvement in metastatic gonadal tumors.

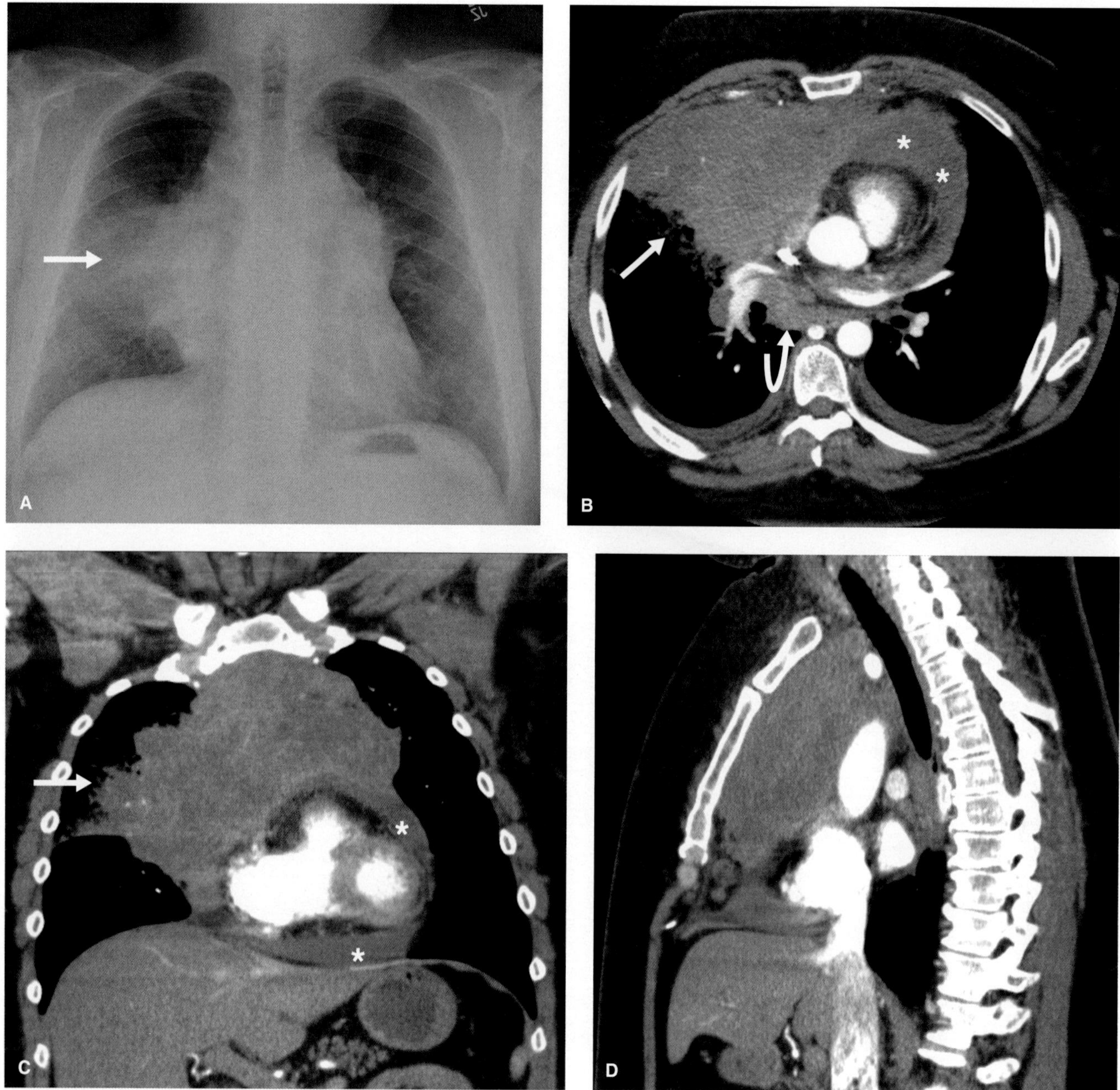

FIGURE 11.8. **Non-Hodgkin Lymphoma, Diffuse Large B-Cell Type. A:** Chest radiograph shows a mediastinal mass extending into the right perihilar lung (*arrow*). **B, C, D:** Axial (**B**), coronal (**C**), and sagittal (**D**) contrast-enhanced CT scan shows a large anterior mediastinal mass with mixed attenuation extending into the right upper lobe (*arrows* in **B** and **C**) with associated right hilar and subcarinal lymph node enlargement (*curved arrows*) small pleural effusions and a pericardial effusion (*asterisks* in **B** and **C**). Core needle biopsy showed diffuse large B-cell lymphoma.

The most common benign mediastinal germ cell neoplasm is teratoma, comprising 60% to 70% of mediastinal germ cell neoplasms. Teratomas may be cystic or solid. Cystic or mature teratoma is the most common type of teratoma seen in the mediastinum; these lesions commonly contain tissues of ectodermal, mesodermal, and endodermal origin. Solid germ cell tumors are usually malignant, with seminoma comprising 25% to 50% of such lesions. Most germ cell neoplasms are detected in patients 20 to 40 years of age. While benign tumors have a slight female preponderance (female/male, 60%/40%), malignant tumors are seen almost exclusively in males.

Radiographically, these tumors have an appearance similar to thymoma. While the majority are located in the anterior mediastinum, up to 10% are found in the posterior mediastinum. Benign lesions are often round or oval and smooth in contour; an irregular, lobulated, or ill-defined margin suggests malignancy. Calcification is present in 33% to 50% of tumors but is nonspecific unless in the form of a tooth. On CT, benign teratomas are usually cystic and may contain soft tissue, bone, teeth, fat, or, rarely, fat-fluid levels (Fig. 11.10). Malignant teratoma, seminoma, choriocarcinoma, and endodermal sinus (yolk sac) tumors are malignant lesions seen primarily in young men. Seminoma is the most common malignant germ cell neoplasm, accounting for 30% of these tumors. The radiographic findings are nonspecific. CT typically shows a large lobulated soft tissue mass that may contain areas of

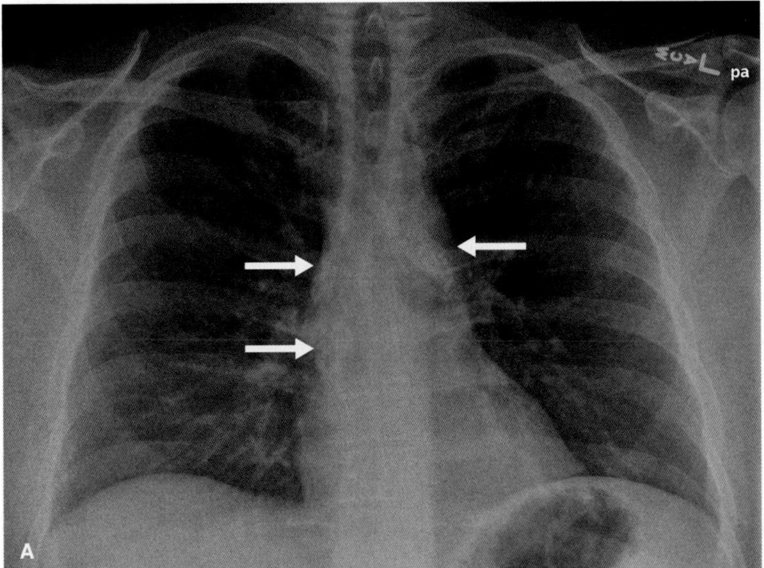

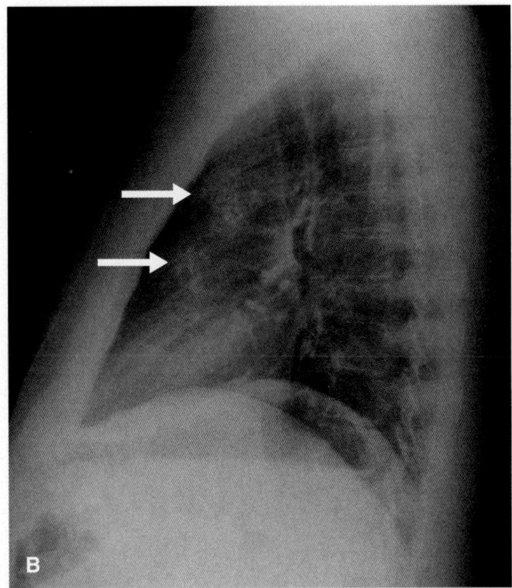

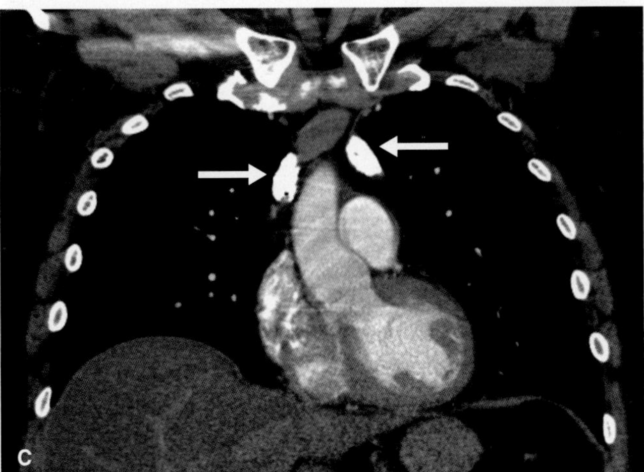

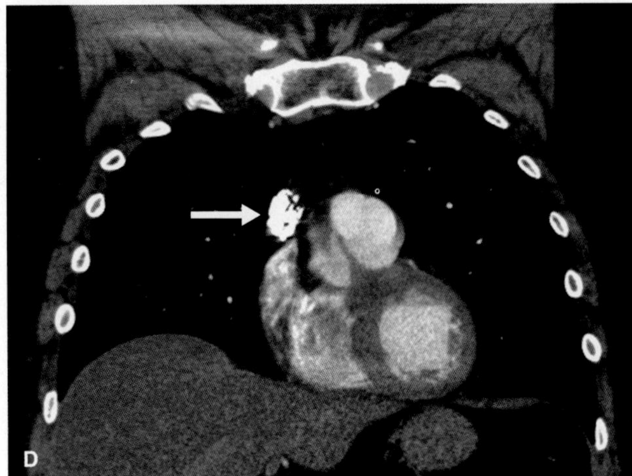

FIGURE 11.9. **Treated Hodgkin Lymphoma With Residual Calcified Nodes. A, B:** Chest radiographs in frontal (**A**) and lateral (**B**) projections demonstrate coarse anterior and superior mediastinal calcification (*arrows*). **C, D:** Contrast-enhanced coronal CT scans through the anterior mediastinum (**C, D**) show multiple calcified nodes (*arrows*) reflecting treated tumor.

hemorrhage, calcification, or necrosis (Fig. 11.11). Elevated serum levels of human chorionic gonadotropin (beta-HCG) or alpha-fetoprotein (alpha-FP) are helpful in the diagnosis of suspected malignant mediastinal germ cell neoplasm, while clinical or CT evidence of gynecomastia is an additional clue to diagnosis.

Mesenchymal Tumors. Benign and malignant tumors arising from the fibrous, fatty, muscular, or vascular tissues of the mediastinum may present as mediastinal masses, most commonly in the anterior mediastinum. Lipomas can occur in any location in the mediastinum but are most often anterior. The diagnosis is made by recognition of a well-defined mass of uniform fatty attenuation (under −50 HU). The presence of soft tissue elements should raise the possibility of a thymolipoma or liposarcoma (Fig. 11.12); the latter may show evidence of invasion of adjacent structures at the time of diagnosis. Fat within a mature teratoma or transdiaphragmatic herniation of omental fat is usually easily distinguished from a lipoma.

Hemangiomas are benign tumors composed of vascular channels and may be associated with the syndrome of hereditary hemorrhagic telangiectasia. A pathognomonic sign on chest radiographs is the recognition of phleboliths within a smooth or lobulated soft tissue mass. Angiosarcomas are rare malignant vascular neoplasms that are indistinguishable from other invasive neoplasms arising within the anterior mediastinum.

Leiomyomas are rare benign neoplasms that arise from smooth muscles within the mediastinum. Similarly, fibromas and hamartomas (tumors that contain more than one mesenchymal element) can rarely present as anterior mediastinal masses.

Middle (Visceral) Mediastinal Masses (Table 11.3)

Lymphatic/Lymph Node Enlargement and Masses. Most middle mediastinal lymph node masses are malignant, representing metastases from lung cancer, extrathoracic malignancy, or lymphoma. Benign causes of middle mediastinal lymph node enlargement include foregut cysts, vascular anomalies or

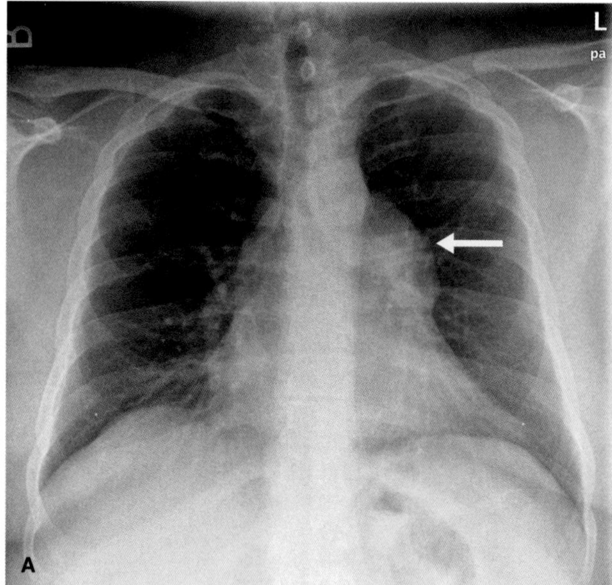

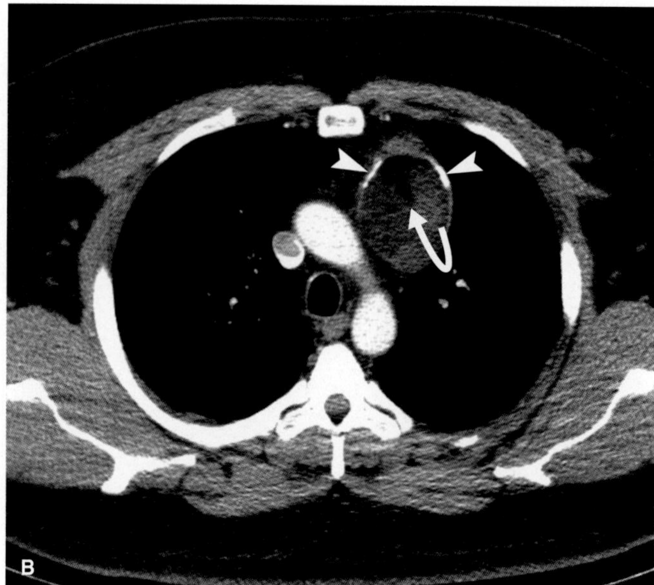

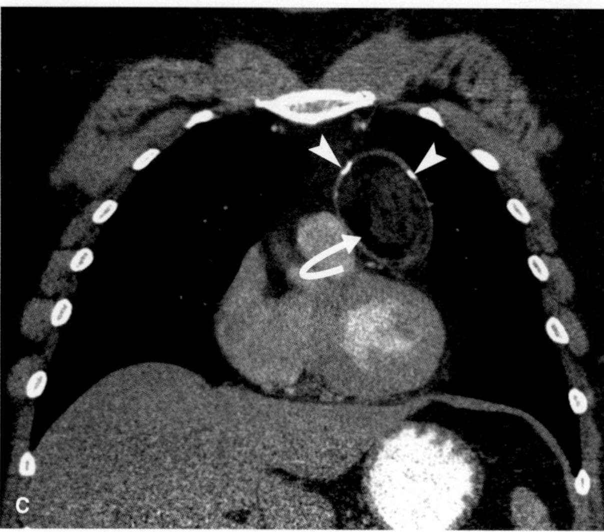

FIGURE 11.10. **Mature Teratoma. A:** Frontal chest radiograph in a 42-year-old man shows a left mediastinal mass (*arrow*). **B, C:** Axial (**B**) and coronal-reformatted (**C**) contrast-enhanced CT in a reveals a rounded anterior mediastinal mass with peripheral calcification (*arrowheads* in **B** and **C**) containing fat (*curved arrow* in **B** and **C**) and soft tissue elements. Surgical resection confirmed a mature teratoma.

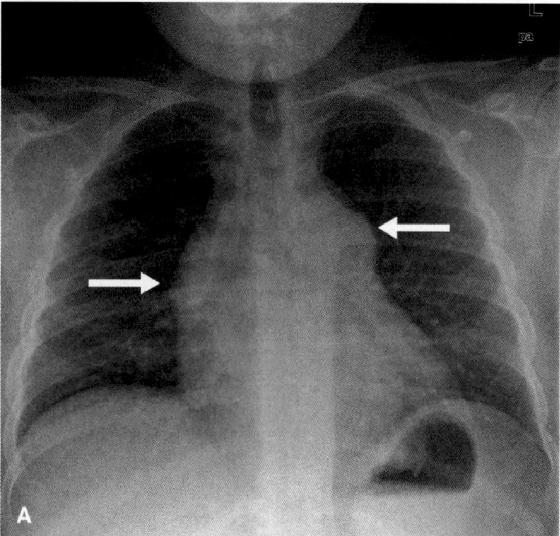

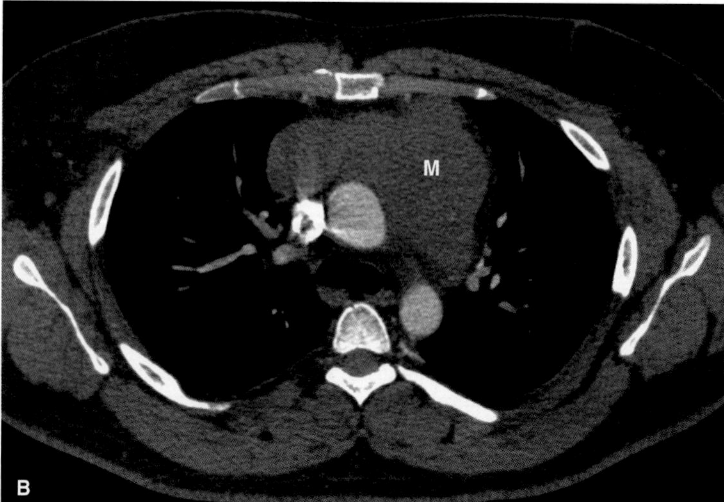

FIGURE 11.11. **Malignant Nonseminomatous Germ Cell Tumor. A:** Posteroanterior chest radiograph in a 30-year-old man reveals a mediastinal mass (*arrows*). **B:** Axial contrast-enhanced CT demonstrates a lobulated anterior mediastinal soft tissue mass (M). CT-guided biopsy showed a nonseminomatous tumor with mixed yolk sac and embryonal elements.

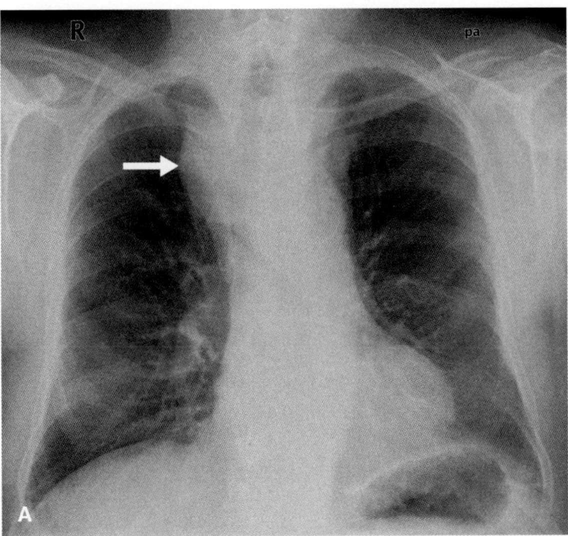

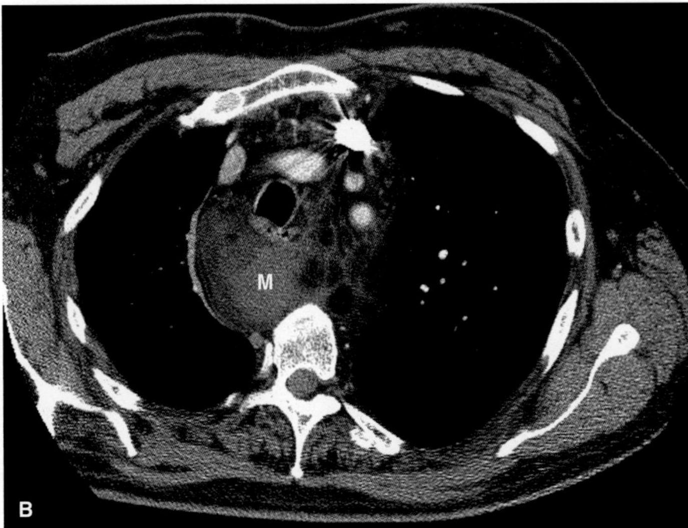

FIGURE 11.12. Liposarcoma of Mediastinum. A: Frontal chest radiograph in an 83-year old man with dysphagia shows a superior mediastinal mass (*arrow*). **B:** Contrast-enhanced axial CT shows a mixed attenuation mass (M) with fatty and soft tissue elements infiltrating the mediastinum. CT-guided biopsy showed a liposarcoma confirmed at surgery.

aneurysms (Fig. 11.13), sarcoidosis, mycobacterial and fungal infection, and angiofollicular lymph node hyperplasia (Castleman disease).

On conventional radiography, several findings suggest that a middle mediastinal mass represents lymph node enlargement. The presence of multiple bilateral mediastinal masses that distort the lung/mediastinal interface is relatively specific for lymph node enlargement. Occasionally, calcification can be detected within enlarged lymph nodes on plain radiographs; CT is more sensitive in detecting nodal calcification and its distribution within lymph nodes.

One of the prime indications for performing thoracic CT is to detect the presence of enlarged mediastinal lymph nodes. CT is most often obtained to confirm an abnormal chest radiographic finding or to evaluate a patient with suspected mediastinal disease despite normal radiographs (a patient with a suspicious solitary pulmonary nodule or with cervical Hodgkin disease). MDCT allows for the recognition of abnormally enlarged lymph nodes that would not be evident on chest radiography. In general, abnormal lymph nodes are seen as round or oval soft tissue masses that measure >1.0 cm in their short-axis diameter. Although CT is unable to distinguish between benign inflammatory nodes and those involved by malignancy based upon size criteria alone, CT can provide useful information about the internal density of the nodes (Table 11.4). A standardized classification system for hilar and mediastinal lymph nodes is the International Association for the Study of Lung Cancer (IASLC) lymph node map, which is used with the eighth edition of the TNM classification system for lung cancer. This lymph node classification system, based upon the Mountain-Dressler American Thoracic Society lymph node map, groups intrathoracic lymph nodes into stations

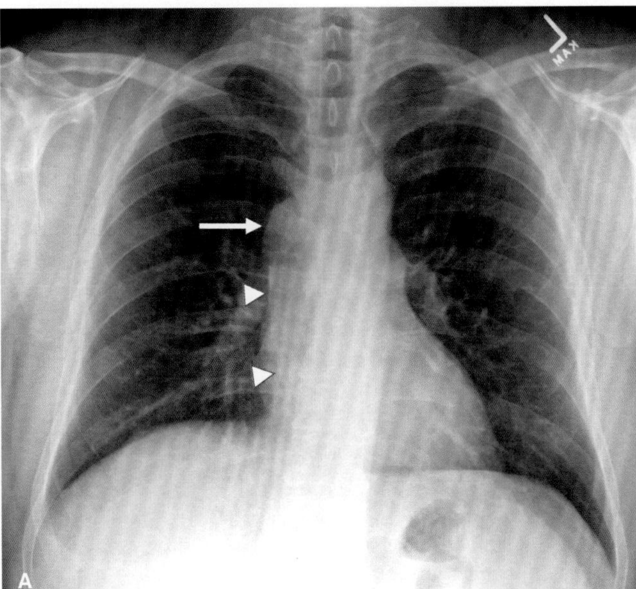

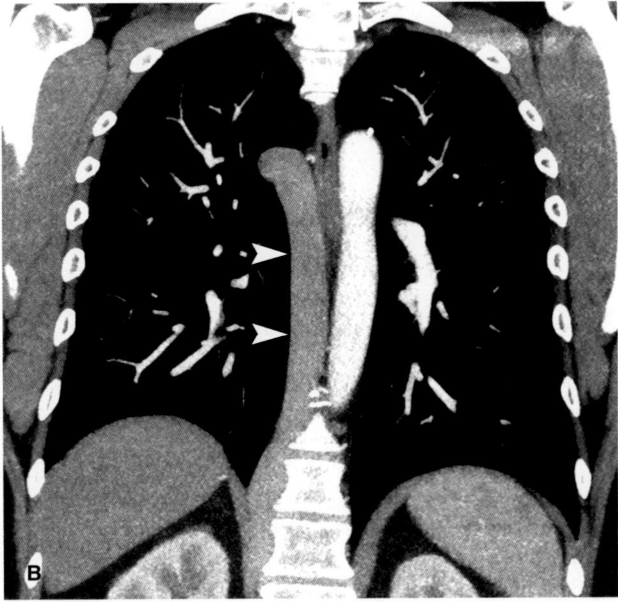

FIGURE 11.13. Azygos Continuation of the Inferior Vena Cava (IVC) as Right Paratracheal Mass. A: Frontal chest radiograph in an asymptomatic 40-year-old man demonstrates a right paratracheal mass (*arrow*), contiguous with a vertically oriented tubular opacity (*arrowheads*). **B:** Coronal contrast-enhanced CT shows a dilated azygos vein (*arrowheads*). The intrahepatic IVC (not shown) was absent; no other anomalies were identified.

TABLE 11.3

MIDDLE (VISCERAL) MEDIASTINAL MASSES

Lymphatic	Malignancy	▪ Primary intrathoracic malignancy • Non–small cell carcinoma • Small cell carcinoma • Primary pulmonary lymphoma • Carcinoid tumor • Extrathoracic malignancy with nodal spread ▪ Head and neck CA ▪ Breast CA ▪ Genitourinary (renal cell, seminoma) ▪ Melanoma ▪ Systemic malignancy • Lymphoma • Leukemia (T cell) • Kaposi sarcoma
	Inflammatory	▪ Infection • Mycobacterial ▪ Tuberculosis • Fungal ▪ Histoplasmosis ▪ Coccidioidomycosis ▪ Blastomycosis • Viral ▪ Measles ▪ Mononucleosis ▪ Granulomatous • Sarcoidosis ▪ Other • Castleman disease
Cyst		▪ Foregut cyst • Bronchogenic cyst • Enteric cyst • Neurenteric cyst ▪ Mesothelial cyst • Pericardial cyst
Tracheal/central bronchial malignancy		▪ Carcinoid tumor ▪ Salivary gland tumor • Mucoepidermoid CA • Adenoid cystic CA ▪ Bronchogenic carcinoma • Squamous cell carcinoma • Small cell carcinoma
Vascular		▪ Thoracic aortic aneurysm ▪ Double aortic arch ▪ Dilated azygos vein ▪ Dilated main pulmonary artery ▪ Esophageal varices
Esophageal		▪ Neoplasms • Leiomyoma • GIST • Carcinoma ▪ Diverticula ▪ Hiatal hernia

TABLE 11.4

CT DENSITY OF MEDIASTINAL/HILAR LYMPH NODES

▪ DENSITY	▪ PATTERN	▪ CONDITION
Calcification	Central or punctate	▪ Mycobacterial ▪ Fungal ▪ Amyloidosis ▪ Sarcoidosis ▪ Silicosis ▪ Mycobacterial infection ▪ Treated lymphoma
	Peripheral (EGGSHELL)	
	Complete	
Hypervascular		▪ Carcinoid tumor ▪ Small cell carcinoma ▪ Metastases • Renal cell carcinoma • Thyroid carcinoma ▪ Castleman disease
Necrosis		▪ Infection • Mycobacterial • Fungal • Whipple disease (Tropheryma whipplei) ▪ Metastases • Squamous cell carcinoma • Seminoma • Lymphoma

and correlates with easily identifiable CT and anatomic landmarks. The IASLC lymph node mapping system can be found in Chapter 13, Figure 13.19.

In addition to the detection and characterization of enlarged mediastinal nodes, CT can help guide diagnostic nodal tissue sampling. This is usually most helpful in the setting of suspected bronchogenic carcinoma, where accurate staging of mediastinal nodal disease is important for prognostic purposes and treatment planning. The detection of enlarged lymph nodes on CT may suggest biopsy via endobronchial ultrasound (EBUS), endoscopic ultrasound (EUS), or mediastinoscopy.

As mentioned above, mediastinal lymph node enlargement is common in Hodgkin disease and NHL. Lymphoma accounts for 20% of all mediastinal neoplasms in adults, and most patients with intrathoracic lymphoma have concomitant extrathoracic disease. In most patients, the nodal enlargement is bilateral but asymmetric (Fig. 11.14). Nodular sclerosing Hodgkin disease commonly results in lymph node enlargement, predominantly within the anterior mediastinum and thymus. Isolated posterior nodal enlargement is usually seen only in patients with NHL.

Leukemia, particularly the T-lymphocytic varieties, can cause intrathoracic lymph node enlargement. The lymph node enlargement is usually confined to the middle mediastinal and hilar nodes.

The most common source of metastases to middle mediastinal nodes is lung cancer. In the majority of patients, symptoms or radiographic findings suggest the presence of a primary tumor in the lung. In a small percentage of patients, particularly those with small cell carcinoma, the primary carcinoma may be inconspicuous or invisible on conventional radiography, with nodal metastases being the only visible abnormality

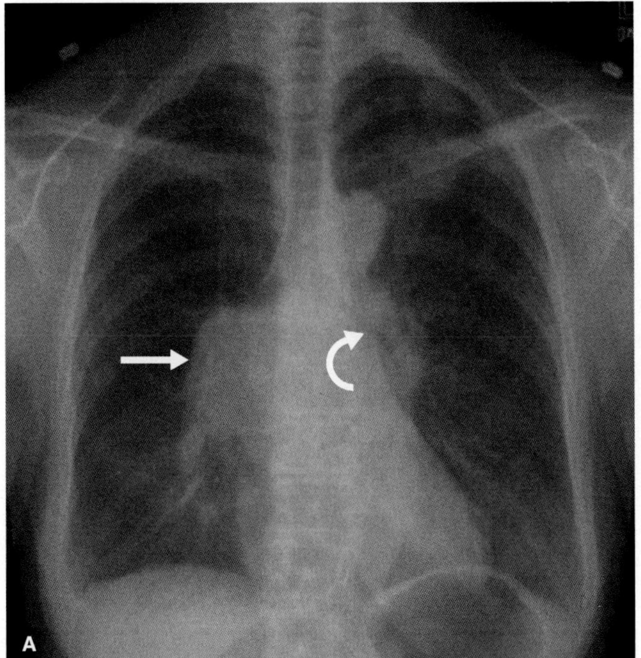

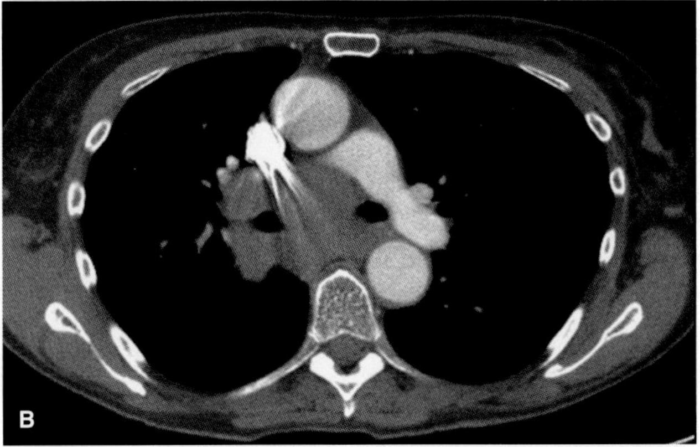

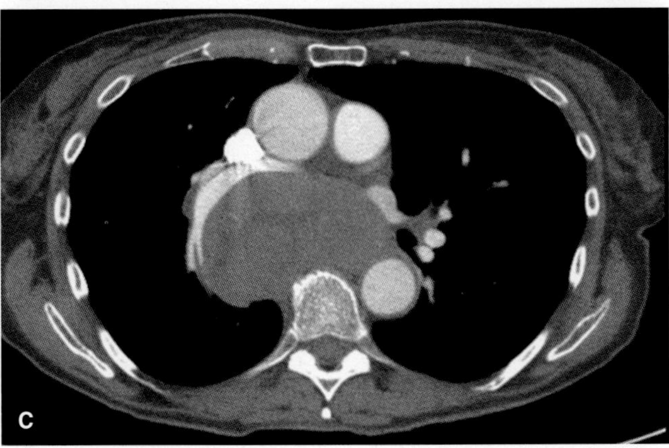

FIGURE 11.14. **Right Hilar/Middle Mediastinal Mass due to Non-Hodgkin Lymphoma. A:** Chest radiograph shows a right hilar and subcarinal mass (*arrow*). Note splaying of the carina and narrowing of the left main bronchus (*curved arrow*). The density overlying the left upper lobe is an artifact. **B** and **C:** Axial contrast-enhanced CT scans show a right hilar and subcarinal soft tissue mass. CT-guided core biopsy of the subcarinal component revealed non-Hodgkin lymphoma.

(Fig. 11.15). Lymph node enlargement is often unilateral on the side of the visible pulmonary or hilar abnormality (Fig. 13.20A). Paratracheal and aorticopulmonary nodes are most commonly involved. Since the accuracy of CT in predicting the presence or absence of mediastinal lymph node metastases is approximately 60% to 70%, PET-CT should be performed in virtually all patients with lung cancer for accurate staging. A more thorough discussion of mediastinal nodal involvement in lung cancer may be found in Chapter 13.

Lymph node metastases from extrathoracic malignancies can result in mediastinal node enlargement, either with or without concomitant pulmonary metastases. These mediastinal nodal metastases may result from inferior extension of neck masses (thyroid carcinoma, head and neck tumors); extension along lymphatic channels from below the diaphragm (testicular or renal cell carcinoma, gastrointestinal malignancies); or hematogenous extension (breast carcinoma, melanoma, Kaposi sarcoma).

Mediastinal lymph node enlargement is very common in patients with sarcoidosis, occurring in 60% to 90% of patients at some stage of their disease. Nodal enlargement is typically bilateral and symmetric and involves the hila as well as the mediastinum; this usually allows for differentiation of sarcoidosis from lymphoma and metastatic disease. In sarcoidosis, the enlarged nodes produce a lobulated appearance on chest radiographs and CT, because the enlarged nodes do not coalesce. This is in contrast to lymphoma and nodal metastases, in which the intranodal tumor extends through the nodal capsule to form conglomerate-enlarged nodal masses. Right and left paratracheal lymph nodes are typically involved; anterior or posterior mediastinal nodal enlargement has been described with greater frequency recently, probably as a result of the improved sensitivity of CT as compared to radiography for detecting nodal enlargement in these regions.

A variety of infections, most commonly histoplasmosis, coccidioidomycosis, blastomycosis, and tuberculosis can cause mediastinal nodal enlargement (Fig. 11.16). Typically these patients have parenchymal opacities on chest radiographs, but isolated lymph node enlargement may be seen in primary tuberculosis, particularly in children and young adults. Bacterial infections such as anthrax, bubonic plague, and tularemia are uncommon causes of lymph node enlargement. Typically, there will be signs and symptoms of acute infection, and chest radiographs will show evidence of pneumonia. Bacterial lung abscesses also may be associated with reactive lymph node enlargement. Hilar and mediastinal lymph nodes may be enlarged in patients with measles, pneumonia, and infectious mononucleosis.

Angiofollicular or giant lymph node hyperplasia, known as *Castleman disease (CD)* is a lymphoproliferative disorder characterized by enlargement of hilar and mediastinal lymph

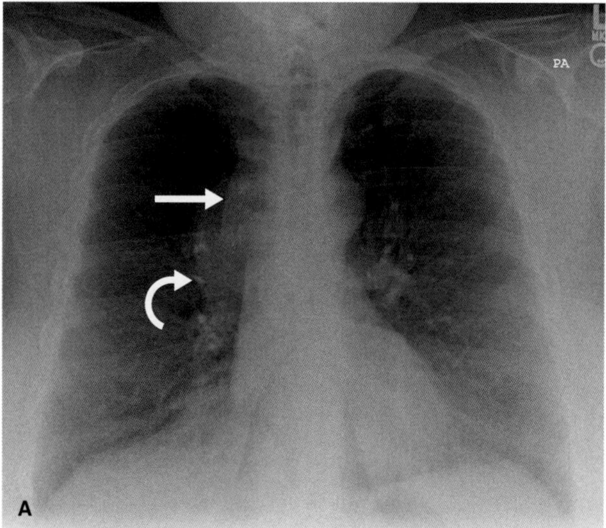

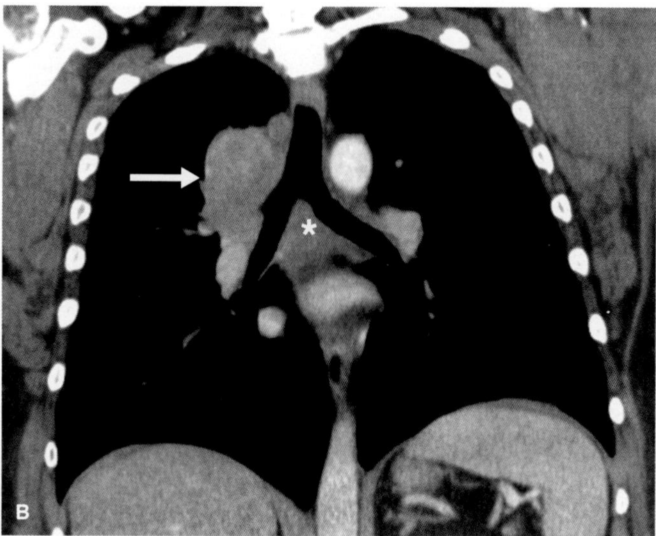

FIGURE 11.15. **Middle Mediastinal/Hilar Lymph Node Enlargement From Small Cell Carcinoma of Lung. A:** Frontal chest radiograph in a 46-year-old man with small cell carcinoma of lung shows right paratracheal (*straight arrow*) and right hilar (*curved arrow*) lymph node enlargement. **B:** Coronal contrast-enhanced CT scan at the level of the tracheal carina shows a lobulated right paratracheal and right hilar soft mass (*straight arrow*) with associated subcarinal lymph node enlargement (*asterisk*).

nodes, predominantly in the middle and posterior mediastinal compartments. The disease can be localized (unicentric or one lymph node group) producing a single group of enlarged lymph nodes or multicentric involving multiple lymph node groups and organs containing lymphatic tissue. The unicentric form of CD has an excellent prognosis whereas multicentric disease is most often associated with HIV and human herpesvirus 8 (HHV-8) infection and has a more variable clinical course. In the more common hyaline vascular subtype, the disease presents as an asymptomatic mediastinal soft tissue mass. The less common plasma cell subtype is associated with multicentric disease and is often associated with systemic symptoms. Histologically, there is replacement of normal nodal architecture with multiple germinal centers and multiple small vessels with hyalinized walls that course perpendicularly toward the germinal centers to give a characteristic "lollipop" appearance on light microscopy. The vascular nature of these masses accounts for the intense enhancement seen on contrast-enhanced CT. Calcification within these masses has been described. Unicentric lesions are cured by resection, whereas multicentric disease associated with HHV-8 infection is treated by rituximab and HHV-8 negative disease with siltuximab.

FIGURE 11.16. **Tuberculous Lymph Node Enlargement.** Coronal contrast-enhanced CT at the level of the tracheal carina in a child with primary tuberculosis demonstrates enlarged bilateral hilar and subcarinal lymph nodes with necrosis. Specimens obtained by bronchoscopy revealed *Mycobacterium tuberculosis*.

Foregut and Mesothelial Cysts are common mediastinal lesions that typically present as asymptomatic masses on routine chest radiographs in young adults. CT and MR show findings characteristic of the cystic nature of these lesions.

Bronchogenic cysts result from anomalous budding of the tracheobronchial tree during embryologic development. To be characterized as bronchogenic in origin, the wall of the cyst must be lined by a respiratory epithelium with pseudostratified columnar cells and contain seromucous glands; some may contain cartilage and smooth muscle within their walls. It is often difficult to distinguish between bronchogenic and enteric cysts based on their location and pathologic appearance; the term *foregut cyst* has been used to describe those lesions that cannot be specifically characterized. The majority of bronchogenic cysts (80% to 90%) arise within the mediastinum in the vicinity of the tracheal carina. Most mediastinal lesions are asymptomatic; occasionally, compression of the tracheobronchial tree or esophagus may produce dyspnea, wheezing, or dysphagia. Rarely, mediastinal cysts become secondarily infected after communication with the airway or esophagus, or they cause symptomatic compression after rapid enlargement following hemorrhage. Bronchogenic cysts are seen as soft tissue masses in the subcarinal or right paratracheal space on frontal chest radiographs; less common sites of involvement include the hilum, posterior mediastinum, and periesophageal region. They appear as a single smooth, round, or elliptic mass; a minority are lobulated in contour. MDCT is the method of choice for the diagnosis of a mediastinal cyst. If a well-defined, thin-walled mass of fluid density (0 to 10 H) is seen that fails to enhance following intravenous contrast administration, it can be assumed to represent a benign cyst (Fig. 11.17). High CT attenuation (>40 H) suggesting a solid

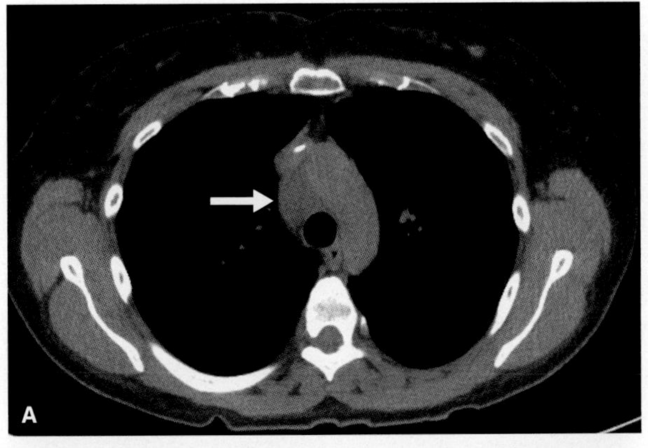

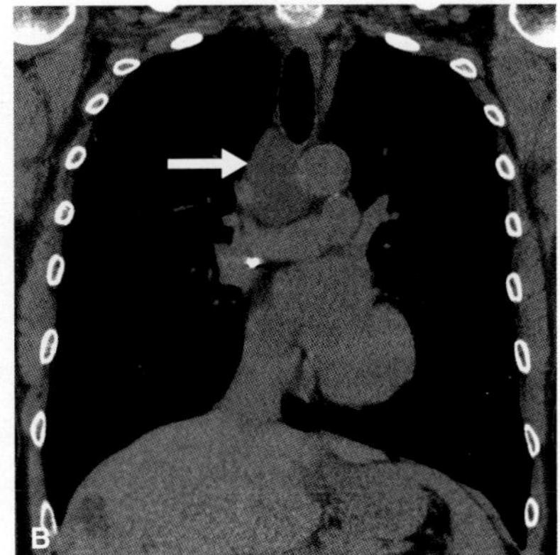

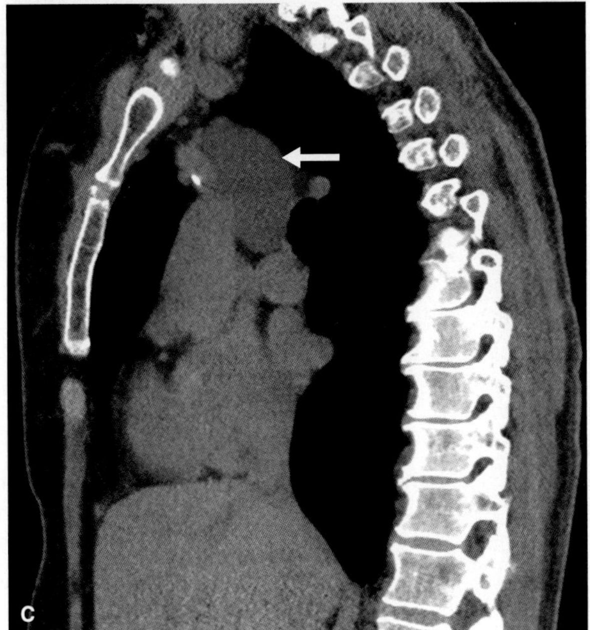

FIGURE 11.17. **Bronchogenic Cyst.** Axial (**A**), coronal (**B**) and sagittal (**C**) unenhanced (**A**) CT scans in a 38-year-old man demonstrate a smooth, oval-shaped low-attenuation right paratracheal mass (*arrows*) consistent with a bronchogenic cyst.

mass can be seen when the cyst is filled with mucoid material, milk of calcium, or blood. Calcification of the cyst wall has been described but is uncommon. MR shows characteristic low signal intensity on T1WIs and high signal intensity on T2WIs. The presence of proteinaceous material within the cyst will shorten T1 relaxation times, yielding high signal intensity on T1WIs; no change in signal will be seen on postcontrast MR studies. While resection is required for definitive diagnosis, most patients with characteristic imaging features who are asymptomatic are managed nonsurgically. Both transbronchoscopic and percutaneous needle aspiration and drainage have been described for diagnosis and treatment of these lesions.

Pericardial cysts arise from the parietal pericardium and contain clear serous fluid surrounded by a layer of mesothelial cells. Most often, they arise in the anterior cardiophrenic angle, with right-sided lesions being twice as common as left-sided lesions; approximately 20% arise more superiorly within the mediastinum. These lesions usually present as incidental asymptomatic round or oval masses in the cardiophrenic angle (Fig. 11.18). Their pliable nature can be demonstrated with a change in patient position. CT typically shows a unilocular cystic mass adjacent to the heart; MR or US via a subxiphoid approach shows findings characteristic of a simple cyst. As with bronchogenic cysts, there have been reports of cysts with high attenuation on CT that on resection are found to be filled with proteinaceous or mucoid material. The differential diagnosis for cardiophrenic angle masses includes pericardial cyst, an enlarged

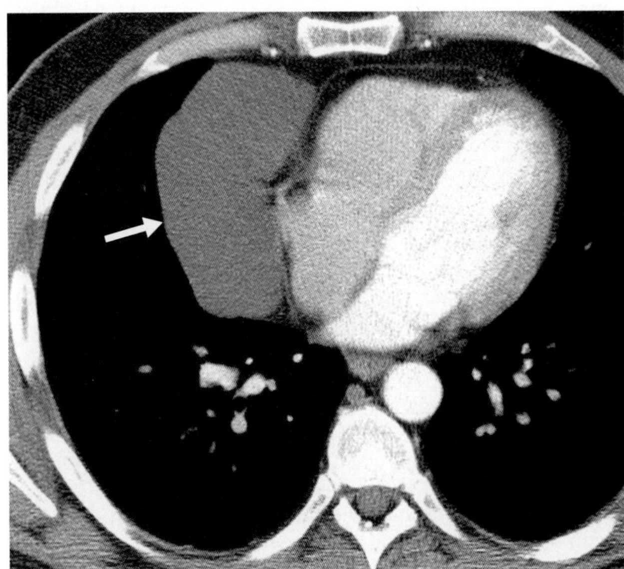

FIGURE 11.18. **Pericardial Cyst.** Enhanced CT scan through heart shows a smooth, sharply marginated, low-attenuation mass (*arrow*) in the right cardiophrenic angle, consistent with a pericardial cyst.

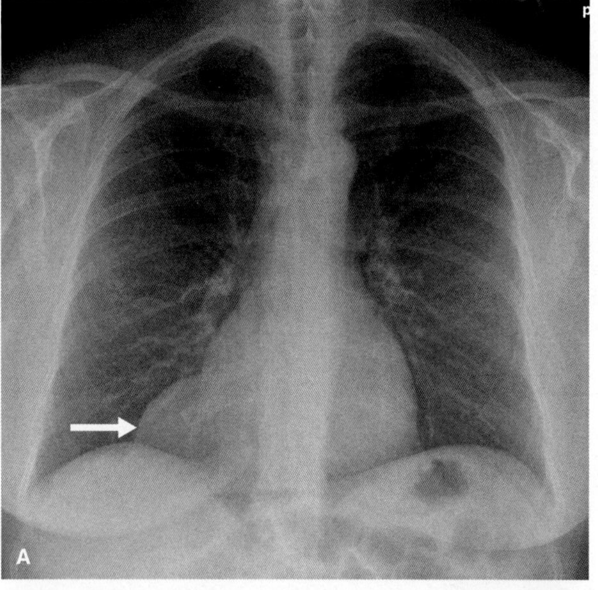

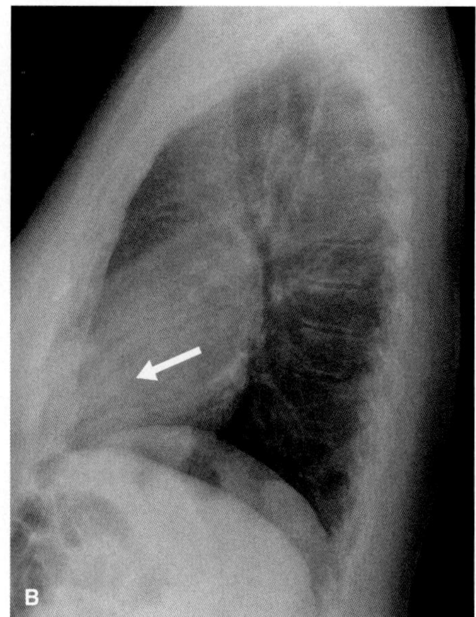

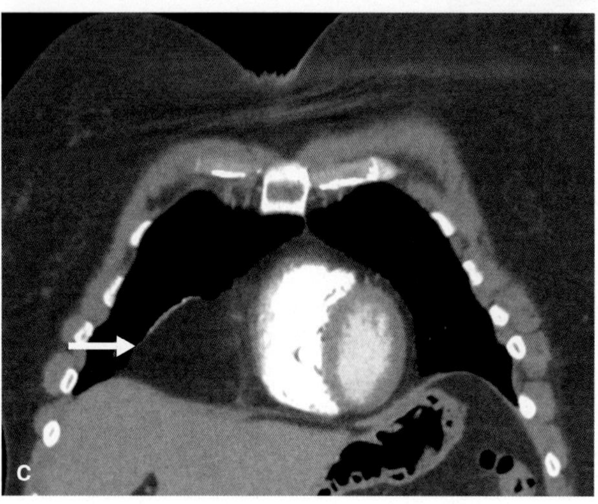

FIGURE 11.19. **Enlarged Epipericardial Fat Pad as Cardiophrenic Angle Mass. A, B:** Frontal (**A**) and lateral (**B**) chest radiographs show a right cardiophrenic angle mass (*arrows*). **C:** Coronal contrast-enhanced CT through the anterior chest shows a uniform attenuation fatty mass (*arrow*) reflecting an enlarged epipericardial fat pad.

epipericardial fat pad (Fig. 11.19), enlarged juxtaphrenic lymph nodes, and diaphragmatic hernias (discussed in Chapter 17).

Tracheal and Central Bronchial Masses commonly produce upper airway symptoms with obstructive pneumonitis and atelectasis and rarely present as asymptomatic mediastinal masses. Occasionally, central airway masses present as radiographic abnormalities when they distort the tracheal air column or mediastinal contour. These masses are discussed in Chapter 15.

Esophageal Lesions. Lesions in the middle or distal third of the esophagus may present as visceral mediastinal masses. Common presenting symptoms include dysphagia and aspiration pneumonia, although many patients are asymptomatic.

The majority of esophageal neoplasms, excluding lesions that arise at the esophagogastric junction, are squamous cell carcinomas. Unlike benign neoplasms of the posterior mediastinum, these lesions, when seen on chest radiographs, are rarely asymptomatic. Typically these patients have a history of dysphagia and significant weight loss. Difficulty in detecting asymptomatic lesions and the absence of a serosa account for the advanced stage of most esophageal carcinoma at presentation and a 5-year survival rate of less than 20%. Patients with esophageal carcinoma may have abnormal radiographic findings which may include abnormal convexity of the azygoesophageal recess, mediastinal widening from the tumor itself or associated esophageal dilatation (distal tumors), thickening of the tracheoesophageal stripe (proximal tumors), and tracheal deviation or narrowing. The diagnosis is usually made on barium esophagram and confirmed by endoscopic biopsy. CT scanning has proved accurate for staging esophageal carcinoma: findings include an intraluminal mass; thickening of the esophageal wall; loss of fat planes between the esophagus and adjacent mediastinal structures (usually the trachea, with upper esophageal lesions, and the descending aorta, with lower esophageal lesions); and evidence of nodal and distant metastases.

Several benign esophageal neoplasms, including leiomyoma and gastrointestinal stromal tumors (GISTs) can present as smooth, solitary mediastinal masses projecting laterally from the posterior mediastinum on frontal chest radiographs. They generally involve the lower third of the esophagus from the level of the subcarinal space to the esophageal hiatus. Initial evaluation is with barium esophagram, which shows a smooth, broad-based mass forming obtuse margins with the esophageal wall. CT demonstrates a smooth, well-defined soft tissue mass adjacent to the esophagus that enhances with intravenous contrast. The smooth nature of these tumors and the absence of esophageal dilatation above the mass helps distinguish benign tumors from carcinoma.

Pulsion diverticula arising at the cervicothoracic esophageal junction or distal esophagus are false diverticula representing mucosal outpouchings through defects in the muscular layer of the esophagus. A large proximal pulsion diverticulum (Zenker) may extend through the thoracic inlet and appear as a retro-esophageal superior mediastinal mass containing an air–fluid level on upright chest radiographs. A distal pulsion diverticulum appears as a juxtadiaphragmatic mass with an air–fluid level projecting to the right of midline. Barium esophagram is diagnostic.

A dilated esophagus resulting from functional (achalasia, scleroderma) or anatomic (stricture, carcinoma) obstruction may produce a mass that courses vertically over the length of the mediastinum, projecting toward the right side on frontal chest radiographs (Fig. 11.20). An air–fluid level on upright films is usually present. A completely air-filled, dilated esophagus appears as a thin curvilinear line along the medial right thorax, because the right lateral wall of the esophagus is outlined by intraluminal air medially and the right lung laterally. An esophagram or CT will confirm the diagnosis of a dilated esophagus; determination of the cause of obstruction often requires endoscopy or occasionally esophageal manometry.

Esophageal varices may produce a round or lobulated retrocardiac mass in patients with portal hypertension. The diagnosis is usually made by endoscopic recognition of submucosal varices involving the distal esophagus. The varices are readily recognized on contrast CT, MR, or portal venography.

A common cause of a mass in the inferior visceral mediastinum is a hiatal hernia. This results from a separation of the superior margins of the diaphragmatic crura and stretching of the phrenoesophageal ligament. The stomach is by far the most common structure in the hernia sac (Fig. 11.21); the gastric cardia (sliding hernia) or fundus (paraesophageal hernia)

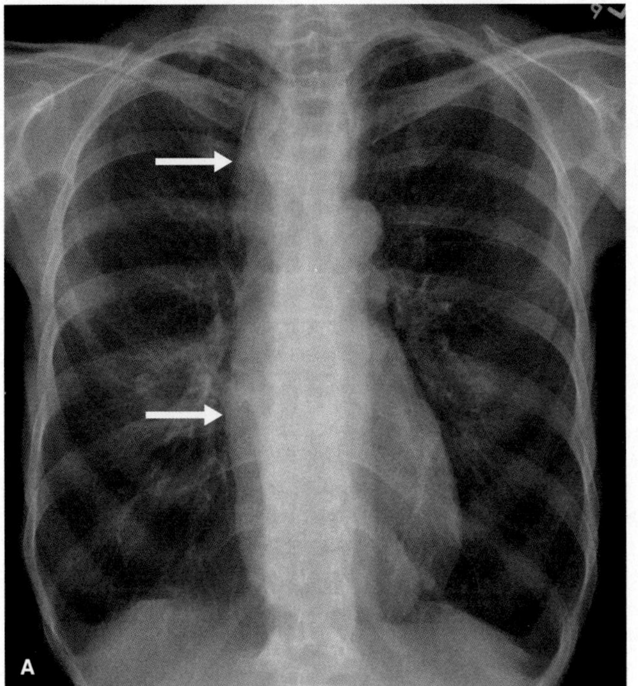

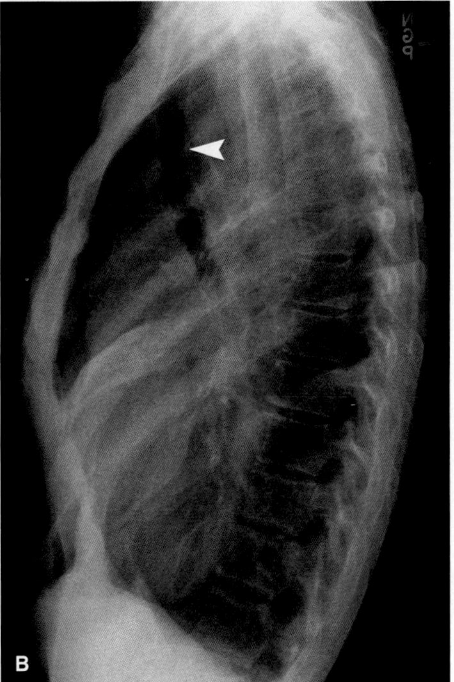

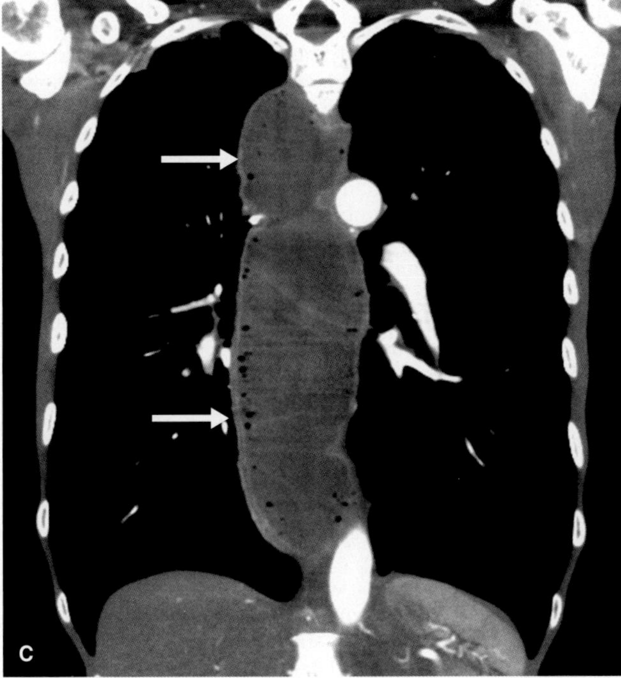

FIGURE 11.20. **Achalasia. A, B:** Frontal (**A**) and lateral (**B**) chest radiographs in a 52-year-old man with achalasia demonstrate a vertically oriented right mediastinal mass (*arrows* in A) that deviates the trachea anteriorly (*arrowhead* in **B**). **C:** Contrast-enhanced coronal CT through the posterior chest shows a dilated esophagus containing ingested material (*arrows*).

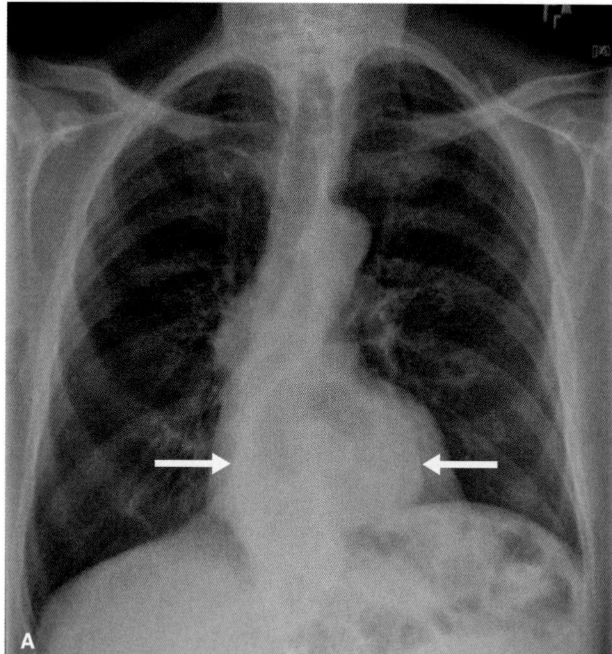

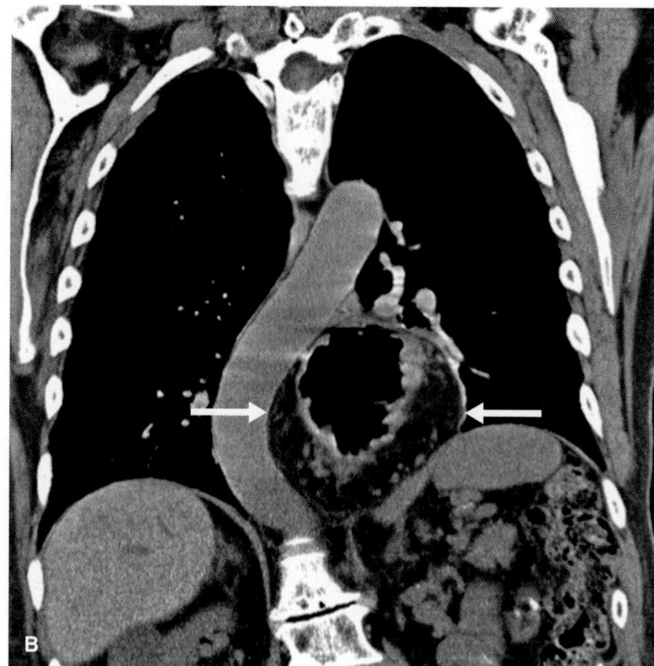

FIGURE 11.21. **Hiatal Hernia. A:** Chest radiograph shows a retrocardiac mass containing air (*arrows*). **B:** Coronal CT scan at the level of the descending aorta shows a hiatal hernia (*arrows*).

may be involved. Rarely, omental fat, ascitic fluid, or a pancreatic pseudocyst herniates through the esophageal hiatus into the mediastinum (Fig. 11.22). The characteristic location at the esophageal hiatus and the presence of a rounded density containing an air or air–fluid level on upright films are diagnostic. Barium esophagram or CT will confirm the diagnosis.

Enteric/Neurenteric Cysts. Enteric cysts are fluid-filled masses lined by enteric epithelium. Esophageal cysts usually arise intramurally or immediately adjacent to the esophagus (Fig. 11.23). When an enteric cyst has a persistent communication with the spinal canal (canal of Kovalevsky) and is associated with congenital defects of the thoracic spine (anterior spina bifida, hemivertebrae, or butterfly vertebrae), it is termed a *neurenteric cyst*. CT or MR can confirm the cystic nature of these masses. If the cyst communicates with the GI tract, it may contain air or an air–fluid level or opacify with contrast during an upper GI series.

Diaphragmatic Hernias, which may present as paracardiac masses, are discussed in Chapter 17.

Vascular Lesions. Congenital or acquired anomalies of the heart and great vessels are common middle mediastinal masses and are discussed in the sections on Pediatric and Cardiac Radiology.

Neurogenic Lesions. Rarely, a neurofibroma arising from the phrenic nerve may present as a middle mediastinal juxtacardiac mass.

Posterior (Paravertebral) Mediastinal Masses (Table 11.5)

Neurogenic Tumors. Posterior mediastinal masses arising from neural elements are classified by their tissue of origin. Three groups have been recognized: (1) tumors arising from intercostal nerves (schwannoma, neurofibroma); (2) sympathetic ganglia (ganglioneuroma, ganglioneuroblastoma, and neuroblastoma); and (3) paraganglionic cells (paraganglionoma). Tumors in each of these three groups may be benign or malignant neoplasms (6). Although neurogenic tumors can occur at any age, they are most common in young patients. Neuroblastoma and ganglioneuroma are most common in children, whereas schwannoma and neurofibroma affect adults more frequently.

Histologically, both schwannoma and neurofibroma are comprised of spindle cells that arise from the Schwann cell. While neurofibroma is an encapsulated tumor that contains interspersed neurons, schwannoma is not encapsulated and contains no neuronal elements. Both tumors are more common in patients with neurofibromatosis. Multiple lesions in the mediastinum, particularly bilateral apicoposterior masses, are virtually diagnostic of neurofibromatosis. A small percentage of schwannomas (10%) are locally invasive (malignant schwannoma).

Radiographically, intercostal nerve tumors appear as round or oval paravertebral soft tissue masses. CT shows a smooth or lobulated paraspinal soft tissue mass, which may erode the adjacent vertebral body or rib (Fig. 11.24). CT demonstration of tumor extension from the paravertebral space into the spinal canal via an enlarged intervertebral foramen is characteristic of a "dumbbell" neurofibroma. MR is the modality of choice for imaging a suspected neurofibroma. In addition to the occasional demonstration of both intra- and extra-spinal canal components, MR of neurofibromas shows typical high signal intensity on T2WIs and often enhances following gadolinium administration.

Tumors that arise from the sympathetic ganglia represent a continuum from the histologically benign ganglioneuroma found in adolescents and young adults to the highly malignant neuroblastoma seen almost exclusively in children under the age of 5. These tumors generally present as elongated, vertically oriented paravertebral soft tissue masses with a broad area of contact with the posterior mediastinum (Fig. 11.25). These findings may help distinguish these lesions from schwannomas or neurofibromas, which usually maintain an acute angle with the vertebral column and posterior mediastinum and therefore tend to show sharp superior and inferior margins on lateral chest radiographs. Large masses may erode vertebral bodies

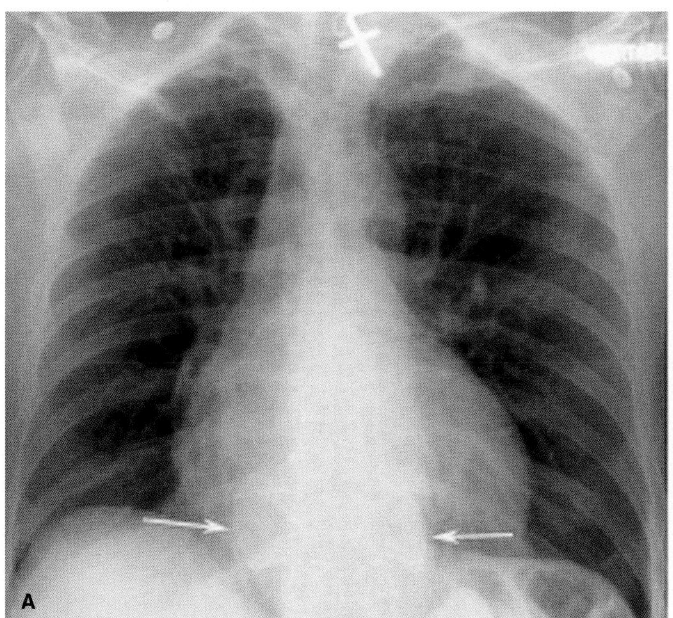

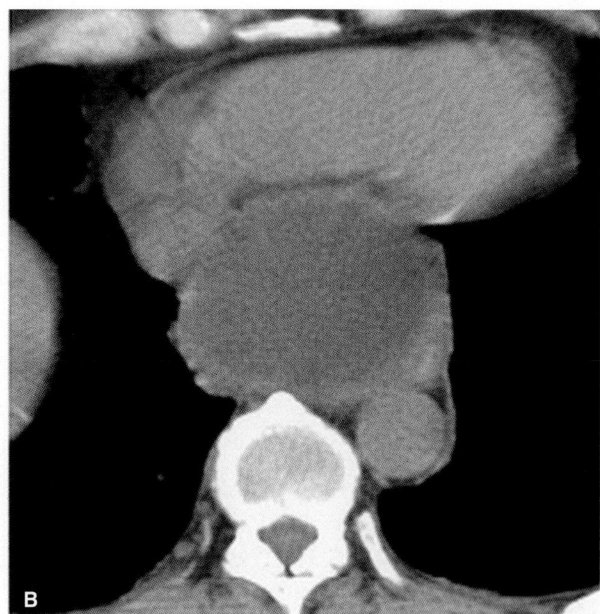

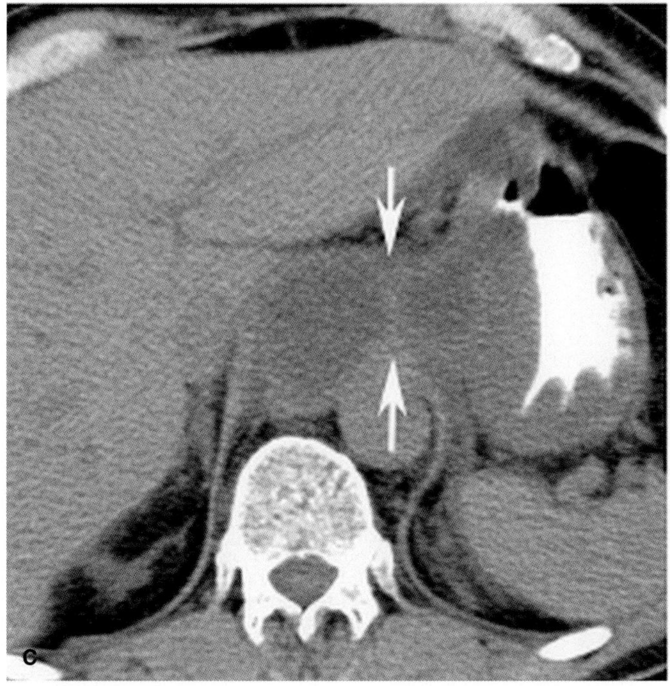

FIGURE 11.22. **Pancreatic Pseudocyst as Mediastinal Mass. A:** Portable chest radiograph in a 62-year-old man with an episode of severe pancreatitis 7 months earlier shows a retrocardiac mass (*arrows*). **B:** Unenhanced axial CT through the lower chest shows a thick-walled cystic mediastinal mass. **C:** Axial scan through the upper abdomen shows communication of the abdominal and thoracic components of the pseudocyst (*arrows*) through the esophageal hiatus.

or ribs. Calcification, seen in up to 25% of cases, is a helpful diagnostic feature of these tumors but does not help distinguish benign from malignant neoplasms. Because these tumors often produce catecholamines, urinary levels of vanillylmandelic acid or metanephrines, which are byproducts of catecholamine metabolism, may be elevated. Prognosis depends upon the histologic features of the tumor and the patient's age and extent of disease at the time of diagnosis.

Mediastinal paragangliomas are tumors that arise from neural crest or chromaffin cells that lie in proximity to the thoracolumbar sympathetic ganglia of the autonomic nervous system. The posterior mediastinum is the site of fewer than 25% of mediastinal paragangliomas, with the majority arising in the anterior or middle mediastinum. Radiographically, these tumors are indistinguishable from other neurogenic tumors. However, most patients have hypertension and biochemical evidence of excess catecholamine production. CT and angiography demonstrates a hypervascular mass. I-123 metaiodobenzylguanidine (MIBG), Ga-68 DOTA (DOTATATE) PET-CT, or F-18-FDG PET-CT can be used to confirm the diagnosis.

Vertebral Abnormalities. A variety of conditions that affect the thoracic spine may manifest as posterior mediastinal masses. These lesions typically produce lateral deviation of the paraspinal reflection on frontal radiographs. Often, the bony origin of these lesions is not obvious on initial examination, making distinction from neurogenic tumors and other posterior mediastinal masses difficult.

Neoplastic, infectious, metabolic, traumatic, or degenerative processes of the thoracic spine may produce a paraspinal mass by one of four mechanisms: (1) expansion of vertebral body or posterior elements (multiple myeloma, aneurysmal

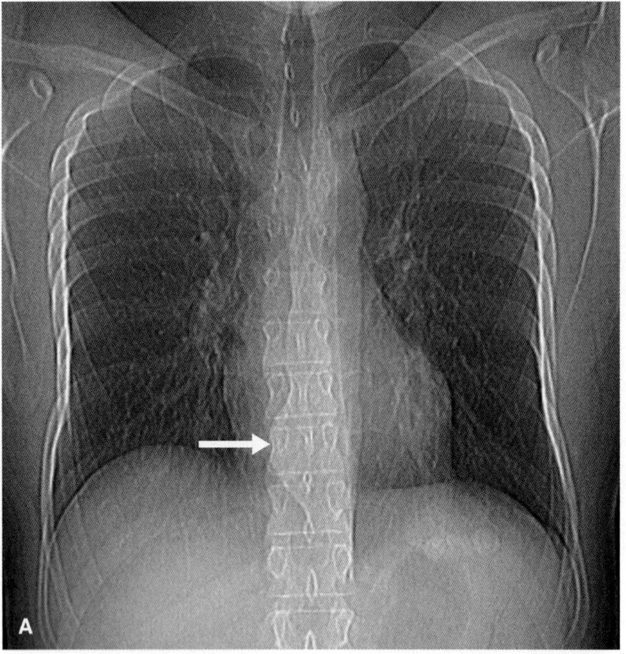

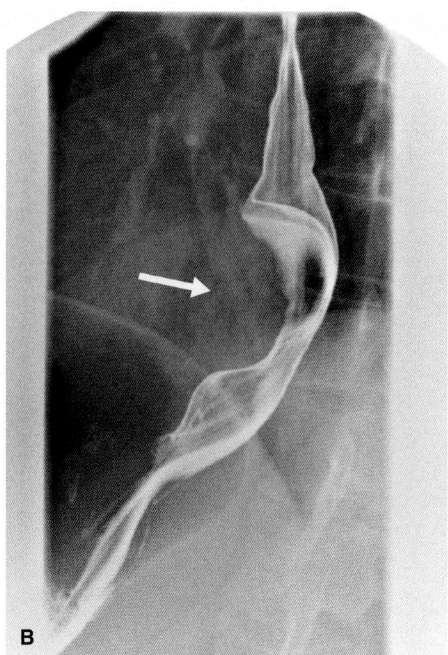

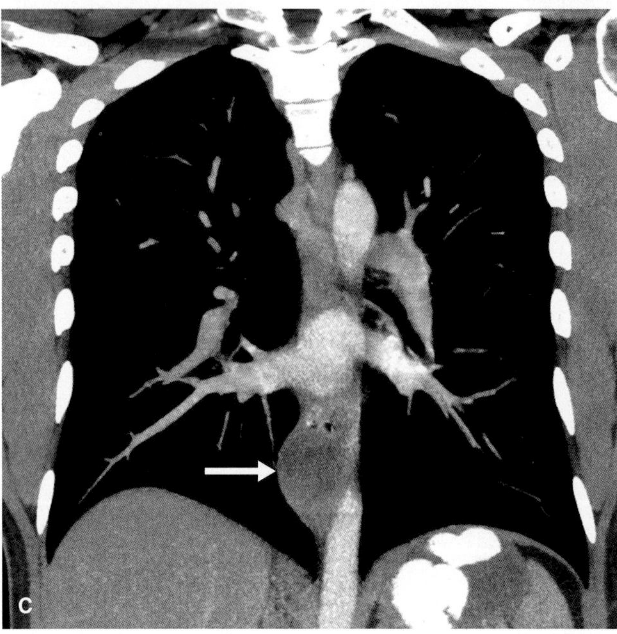

FIGURE 11.23. Esophageal Duplication Cyst. **A:** Frontal scout view from CT in a 31-year-old man with odynophagia shows a mass (*arrow*) deforming the lower azygoesophageal recess. **B:** Barium esophagram in right posterior oblique projection shows a submusocal distal esophageal mass (*arrow*). **C:** Coronal contrast-enhanced CT demonstrates a low-attenuation mass (*arrow*). Surgery confirmed an esophageal duplication cyst.

bone cyst); (2) extraosseous extension of infection, tumor, or marrow elements (infectious spondylitis (Fig. 11.26), metastatic carcinoma, extramedullary hematopoiesis, respectively); (3) pathologic fracture and paraspinal hematoma formation (any destructive neoplastic or inflammatory process, trauma); or (4) protrusion of degenerative osteophytes. Neoplastic processes are usually easily identified by expansion and destruction of vertebral bodies, with sparing of intervertebral disks. Bronchogenic, breast, or renal cell carcinoma are the most common primary sites of thoracic spinal metastases. Infectious spondylitis is distinguished from neoplastic processes by the presence of a paravertebral mass centered at the point of maximal bone destruction. In patients with a paravertebral abscess secondary to tuberculosis or bacterial infection, narrowing of the adjacent disk space and destruction of vertebral end-plates are important clues to the diagnosis. Extramedullary hematopoiesis is seen almost exclusively in conditions associated with ineffective production or excessive destruction of erythrocytes, such as thalassemia major, congenital spherocytosis, and sickle cell anemia. It is recognized by noting expansion of the medullary space and cyst formation within long bones, ribs, and vertebral bodies, with associated lobulated paraspinal soft tissue masses. These masses, which represent hyperplastic bone marrow that has extruded from the vertebral bodies and posterior ribs, are typically seen in the lower thoracic and upper lumbar region. Traumatic injuries to the thoracic spine are usually obvious from the patient's history and recognition of spine fracture on radiographic and CT studies of the spine. Degenerative disk disease may produce a localized paraspinal mass on frontal radiographs. Well-penetrated films will show the characteristic inferolaterally projecting osteophytes at the level of the mass, which are most commonly right sided because of the inhibitory

TABLE 11.5

POSTERIOR (PARAVERTEBRAL) MEDIASTINAL MASSES

Neurogenic	▪ Intercostal nerve • Schwannoma • Neurofibroma • Neurofibrosarcoma ▪ Sympathetic ganglia • Ganglioneuroma • Ganglioneuroblastoma • Neuroblastoma ▪ Paraganglioma
Vertebral	▪ Trauma • Paraspinal hematoma ▪ Infection • Paraspinal abscess ▪ Staphylococcus ▪ Tuberculosis ▪ Neoplasm • Metastatic disease • Myeloma • Lymphoma ▪ Degenerative • Osteophytosis ▪ Other • Extramedullary hematopoiesis
Vascular	▪ Thoracic aortic aneurysm ▪ Double aortic arch ▪ Dilated azygos vein ▪ Dilated main pulmonary artery ▪ Esophageal varices
Cyst	▪ Lateral thoracic meningocele

effect of the pulsating descending aorta on left-sided osteophyte formation.

Lateral Thoracic Meningoceles represent an anomalous herniation of the spinal meninges through an intervertebral foramen, resulting in a paravertebral soft tissue mass. Most meningoceles are discovered in middle-aged patients as asymptomatic masses. They are slightly more common on the right, and are multiple in 10% of cases. There is a high association between lateral thoracic meningoceles and neurofibromatosis. A meningocele is the most common posterior mediastinal mass in patients with neurofibromatosis; conversely, approximately two-thirds of patients with meningoceles have neurofibromatosis. Chest radiographs typically reveal a round, well-defined paraspinal mass that is indistinguishable from a neurofibroma. Additional clues to the diagnosis include rib erosion, enlargement of the adjacent neural foramen, vertebral anomalies, or kyphoscoliosis. When a lateral meningocele is associated with kyphoscoliosis, it is usually found at the apex of the scoliotic curve on the convex side. MR demonstration of a herniated subarachnoid space is the diagnostic technique of choice; conventional or CT myelography, which demonstrates filling of the meningocele with contrast, is reserved for equivocal cases.

Rarely, malignant lymph node enlargement may produce a recognizable paraspinal mass. This is most often seen in NHL, metastatic lung cancer, and seminoma; other mediastinal or extrathoracic sites of involvement are invariably present.

Despite the advances in detection and characterization of mediastinal masses with cross-sectional imaging, most patients will require tissue sampling for definitive diagnosis. However, the radiologist can use the information provided by CT or MR to help limit the differential diagnosis and thereby guide the appropriate evaluation and treatment. In a large percentage of cases, when tissue sampling is required, it can be accomplished by CT- or US-guided transthoracic biopsy.

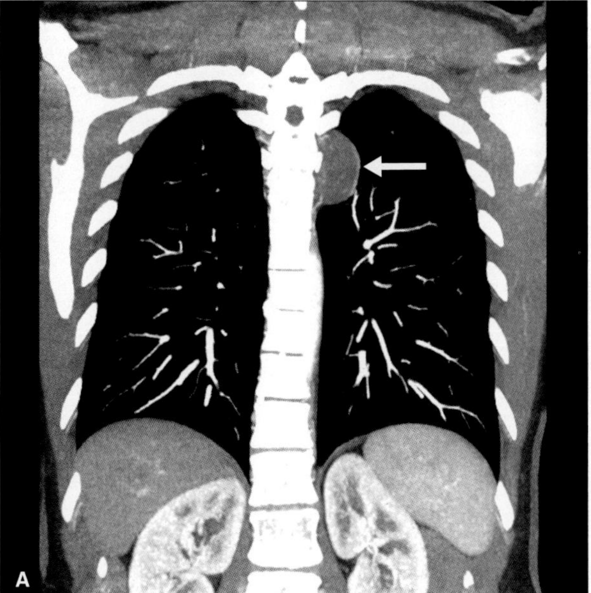

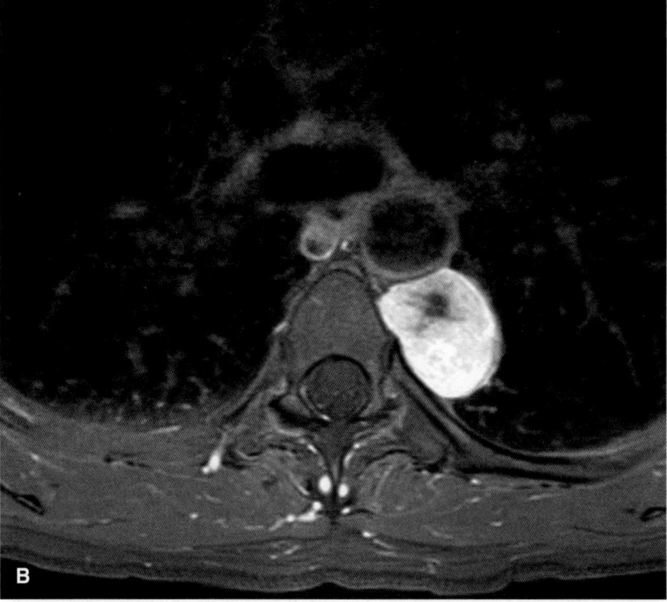

FIGURE 11.24. **Schwannoma. A:** Contrast-enhanced coronal maximum intensity projection CT in an asymptomatic 39-year-old woman demonstrates a left upper paravertebral soft tissue mass (*arrow*). **B:** Axial T1-weighted fat saturated post contrast MR shows enhancement of the lesion. CT-guided biopsy confirmed a schwannoma.

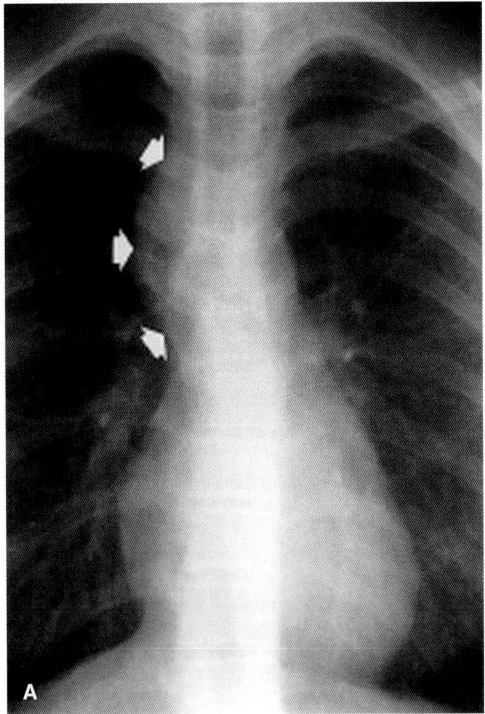

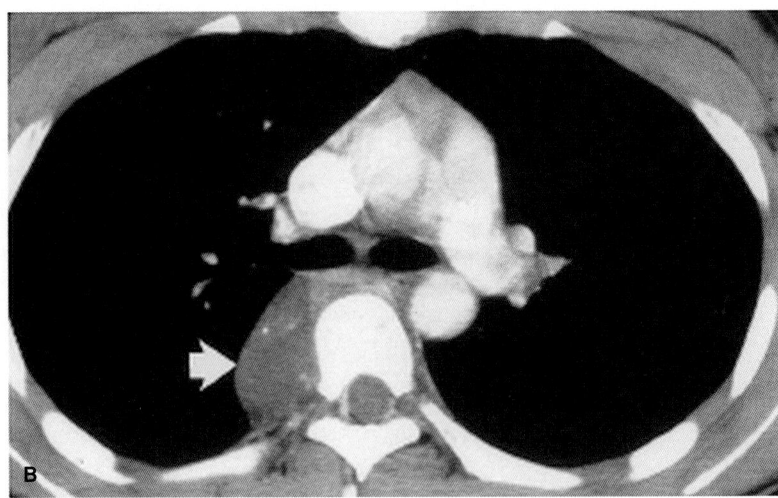

FIGURE 11.25. **Ganglioneuroma. A:** Posteroanterior radiograph in a 15-year-old female reveals an oval, vertically oriented, right-sided mediastinal mass (*arrows*). **B:** Contrast-enhanced CT shows a low-attenuation posterior mediastinal mass (*arrow*) with calcification. This was surgically proven to be ganglioneuroma.

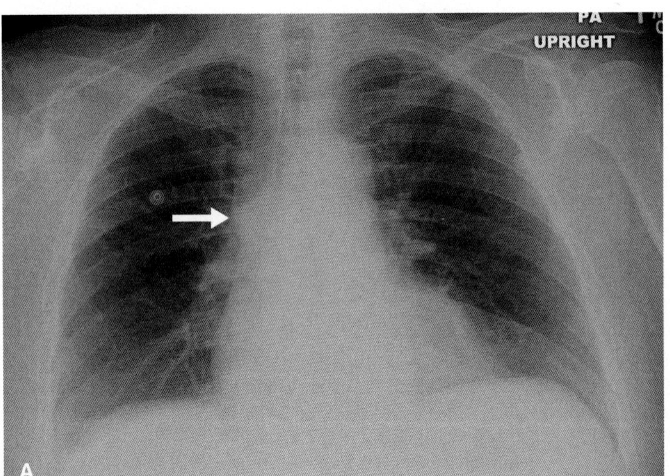

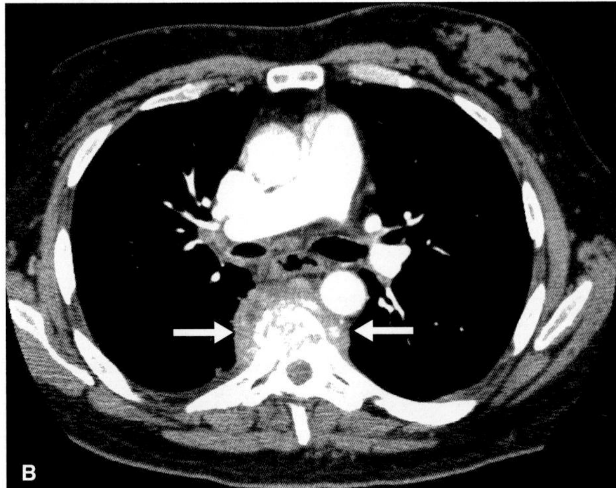

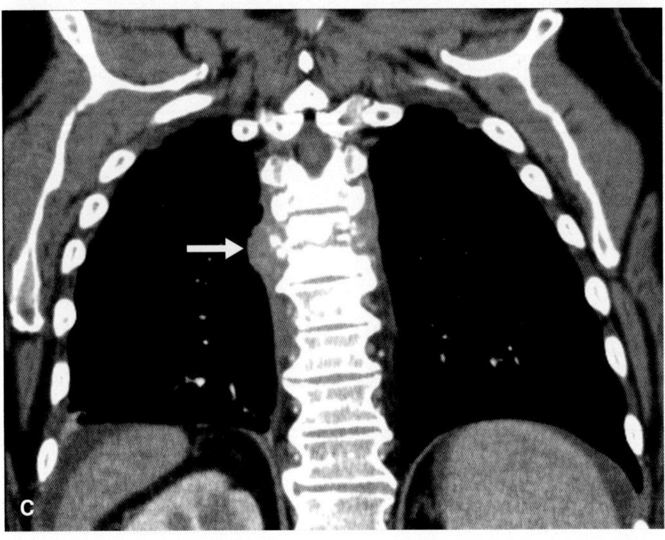

FIGURE 11.26. **Discitis/Osteomyelitis of Thoracic Spine as Paravertebral Mass. A:** Frontal chest radiograph in a 53-year-old man with cirrhosis, fever, and back pain shows a subtle right mediastinal mass (*arrow*). **B, C:** Axial (**B**) and coronal (**C**) contrast-enhanced CT shows disc space narrowing and vertebral end-plate destruction with a paravertebral inflammatory mass (*arrows*). Biopsy showed staphylococcal infection.

DIFFUSE MEDIASTINAL DISEASE (TABLE 11.6)

Mediastinal Infection is an uncommon condition that may be divided into acute and chronic forms based upon etiology, clinical features, and radiologic findings. The distinction between acute and chronic infection is important because there are considerable differences in treatment and prognosis.

Acute mediastinitis is caused by bacterial infection that most often develops following esophageal perforation or is a complication of cardiothoracic or esophageal surgery. Esophageal perforation may complicate esophageal instrumentation (e.g., endoscopy, biopsy, dilatation, or stent placement); penetrating chest trauma; esophageal carcinoma; foreign body or corrosive ingestion; or vomiting. Spontaneous esophageal perforation following prolonged vomiting is termed *Boerhaave syndrome*. In this condition, a vertical tear occurs along the left posterolateral wall of the distal esophagus, just above the esophagogastric junction, leading to signs and symptoms of acute mediastinitis. Less commonly, acute mediastinitis may develop from mediastinal extension of infection in the neck, retropharyngeal space, lungs, pleural space, pericardium, or spine.

The clinical presentation of acute mediastinitis is usually dramatic and is characterized by severe retrosternal chest pain, fever, chills, and dysphagia, often accompanied by evidence of septic shock. Physical examination may reveal findings associated with pneumomediastinum, with subcutaneous emphysema in the neck and an apical, systolic crunching sound on chest auscultation (Hamman sign).

The most common chest radiographic findings are widening of the superior mediastinum in 66% of patients and pleural effusion in 50% of patients. Specific findings such as mediastinal air or air–fluid levels are less common. When mediastinitis occurs in association with Boerhaave syndrome, pneumoperitoneum and left hydropneumothorax may also be seen.

When esophageal perforation is suspected, an esophagram or CT with oral contrast should be performed to detect leakage of contrast into the mediastinum and to localize the exact site of perforation. In a patient who is not at risk for aspiration, a water-soluble contrast agent is administered initially. Once gross contrast extravasation has been excluded, barium is then given for superior radiographic detail. The sensitivity of the esophagram for detecting contrast leakage is highest when the study is obtained within 24 hours of the perforation.

MDCT is the radiologic study of choice for the diagnosis of acute mediastinitis. CT findings include extraluminal gas, bulging of the mediastinal contours, and focal or diffuse soft tissue infiltration of mediastinal fat. Localized fluid collections suggest focal abscess formation (Fig. 11.27). Associated findings include mediastinal venous thrombosis, pneumothorax, pleural effusion or empyema, subphrenic abscess, and vertebral osteomyelitis.

While the clinical and radiographic diagnosis of mediastinitis is often straightforward, it may be difficult in postoperative patients who have undergone recent median sternotomy. In these patients, infiltration of mediastinal fat and focal air or fluid collections may be normal findings on postoperative CT scans performed days to weeks following the removal of intraoperatively placed mediastinal drains. In such patients, the progression of findings on follow-up CT scans will correctly identify the majority of those with postoperative mediastinal infection.

The prognosis for patients with acute mediastinitis varies with the underlying etiology and the extent of mediastinal involvement at the time of diagnosis. Esophageal perforation is associated with the poorest outcome, with a mortality approaching 50%. A delay in diagnosis and treatment of the mediastinal infection of greater than 24 hours is associated with a significant increase in overall morbidity and mortality.

In addition to its sensitivity in the diagnosis of mediastinitis, CT can be used to guide treatment and predict outcome. Those patients with evidence of extensive mediastinal infection, seen on CT as diffuse infiltration of the mediastinal fat without evidence of abscess formation, have a mortality approaching 50%. In contrast, patients with discrete mediastinal abscesses that are amenable to surgical or percutaneous drainage, or with small localized abscesses that are amenable to antibiotic therapy alone, have a more favorable prognosis. In addition, patients with mediastinal abscesses and contiguous empyema or subphrenic abscess may respond favorably to drainage of these extramediastinal collections.

TABLE 11.6

DIFFUSE MEDIASTINAL WIDENING

Smooth	▪ Mediastinal lipomatosis ▪ Malignancy • Lymphoma • Small cell carcinoma • Metastatic disease ▪ Mediastinal hemorrhage • Arterial • Traumatic aortic/arch vessel laceration • Ruptured aortic aneurysm • Venous • Superior vena cava/right atrial injury ▪ Mediastinitis • Acute bacterial • Chronic (sclerosing) • Histoplasmosis • Other ▪ Dilated esophagus • Achalasia • Scleroderma • Stricture • Distal esophageal malignancy
Lobulated	▪ Lymph node enlargement (see Table 11.3) ▪ Malignancy • Small cell carcinoma • Metastatic disease ▪ Vascular • Tortuous great vessels ▪ Superior vena cava thrombosis ▪ Neurofibromatosis

Chronic Fibrosing (Sclerosing) Mediastinitis. The hallmarks of chronic fibrosing mediastinitis are chronic inflammatory changes and mediastinal fibrosis. The most common cause of this rare condition is granulomatous infection, usually secondary to *Histoplasma capsulatum*. Infection by other fungi including blastomycosis and aspergillosis, tuberculosis, radiation therapy, sarcoidosis and drugs (methysergide) are less common causes. Idiopathic mediastinal fibrosis, which is probably an autoimmune process, is related to fibrosis in other regions, including the retroperitoneum, intraorbital fat, and thyroid gland.

Several theories have been advanced to explain the pathogenesis of fibrosing mediastinitis owing to histoplasmosis. The most widely accepted theory suggests that affected patients develop an idiosyncratic hypersensitivity response to a fungal antigen released from ruptured mediastinal granulomas resulting in a fibroinflammatory reaction.

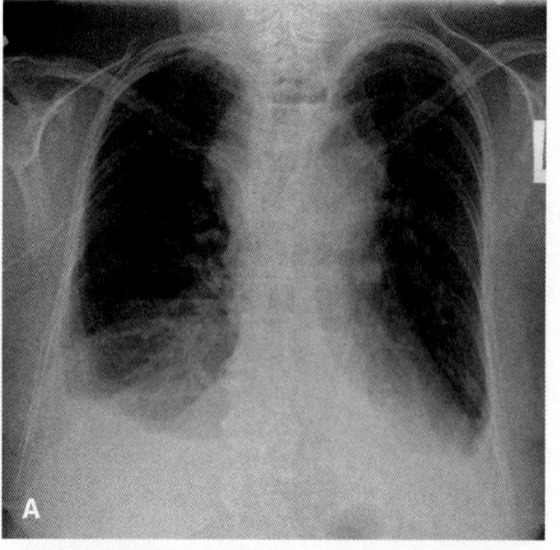

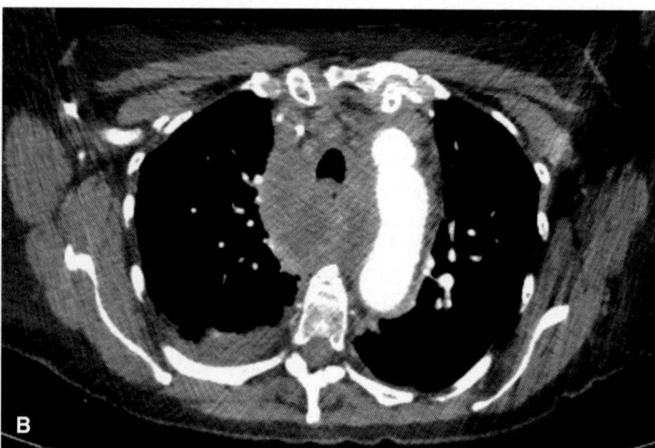

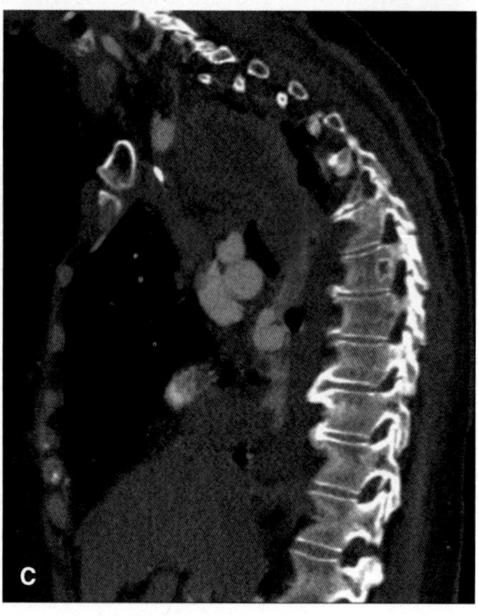

FIGURE 11.27. **Acute Mediastinitis From Esophageal Perforation.** **A:** Frontal chest radiograph in a 67-year-old female with a documented upper esophageal perforation from a foreign body shows a widened upper mediastinum with bilateral pleural effusions. **B, C:** Contrast-enhanced axial (**B**) and sagittal (**C**) CT scans show mixed fluid and soft tissue attenuation material within the upper mediastinum surrounding the esophagus representing bacterial mediastinitis.

Clinically, this condition occurs in adults and presents with a variety of symptoms, depending upon the extent of fibrosis and the mediastinal structures compromised by the fibrotic process. The superior vena cava (SVC) is the most commonly affected structure, with involvement in over 75% of symptomatic patients. The SVC syndrome manifests with headache, epistaxis, cyanosis, jugular venous distention, and edema of the face, neck, and upper extremities. The most serious and potentially fatal manifestation of fibrosing mediastinitis is obstruction of the central pulmonary veins, which produces pulmonary edema that may mimic severe mitral stenosis. Patients with involvement of the tracheobronchial tree may have cough, dyspnea, wheezing, hemoptysis, and obstructive pneumonitis. Dysphagia or hematemesis can be seen with esophageal involvement. Less commonly, pulmonary arterial hypertension and cor pulmonale can develop from narrowing of the pulmonary arteries. Rarely constrictive pericarditis can develop.

The most common finding noted on chest radiographs is asymmetric lobulated widening of the upper mediastinum, most often on the right. When the process is secondary to granulomatous infection, enlarged calcified lymph nodes may be seen. Narrowing of the tracheobronchial tree may be evident. The sequelae of vascular involvement may be seen, including oligemia from pulmonary arterial compression or venous hypertension and pulmonary edema from involvement of the central pulmonary veins. Postobstructive atelectasis or consolidation may also be seen.

MDCT is the modality of choice for the diagnosis and assessment of chronic sclerosing mediastinitis. Enlarged lymph nodes with calcification are the most common finding (Fig. 11.28). The fibrotic infiltration of the mediastinal fat that is characteristic of this condition is seen as abnormal soft tissue density replacing the normal mediastinal fat with obliteration of the normal mediastinal interfaces. MDCT delineates the degree of involvement of the mediastinal vessels, trachea, and central bronchi. In patients with significant SVC involvement, collateral venous channels within the mediastinum and chest wall are well demonstrated.

A definitive diagnosis of chronic fibrosing mediastinitis and the establishment of the underlying etiology are difficult. Skin tests for histoplasmosis and tuberculosis may add additional information but are usually not helpful. The precise diagnosis, and more important the distinction from infiltrating malignancy, may require biopsy, but in most cases typical imaging findings provide a confident presumptive diagnosis. In those patients with noncalcified mediastinal or hilar masses that lack ancillary findings of histoplasmosis such as lung, hepatic, or splenic calcifications, biopsy may be necessary to establish a diagnosis.

Mediastinal Hemorrhage. Injury to mediastinal vessels resulting from blunt or penetrating thoracic trauma is the most common cause of mediastinal hemorrhage. Blunt chest trauma most often occurs in the setting of a motor vehicle accident, when rapid deceleration and thoracic cage compression produce shearing effects at the aortic isthmus. Iatrogenic trauma, usually from attempts at central line placement, can also cause mediastinal hemorrhage. Spontaneous hemorrhage

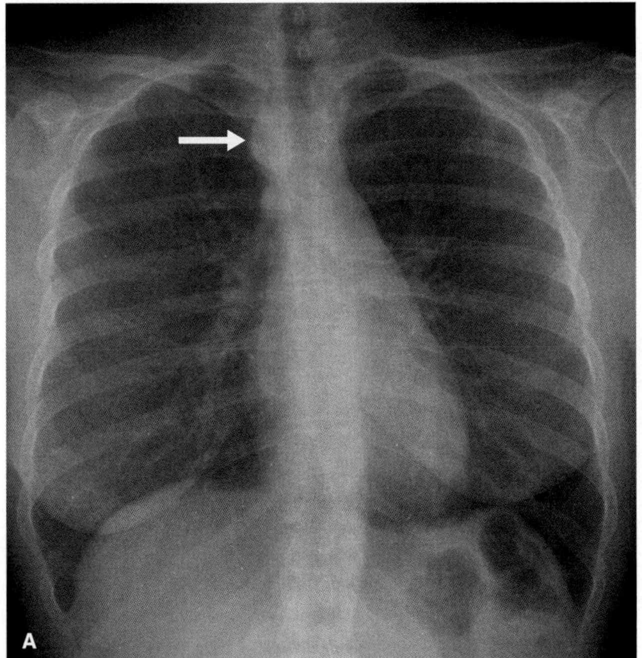

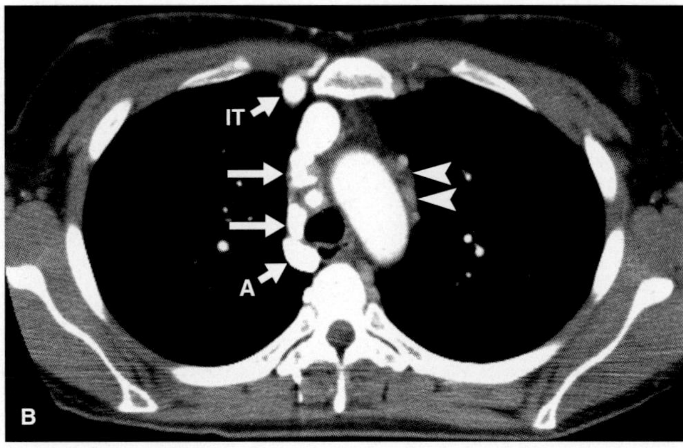

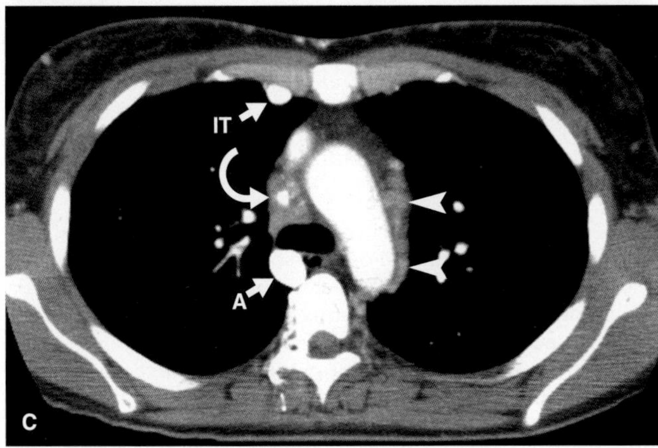

FIGURE 11.28. **Fibrosing Mediastinitis From Histoplasmosis.** **A:** Posteroanterior chest radiograph in an asymptomatic 33-year-old woman shows calcifications in the right paratracheal region (*arrow*). **B, C:** Axial contrast-enhanced CT scan at the level of the aortic arch demonstrates calcified right paratracheal nodes (*arrows* in **B**) with calcified thrombosis of the superior vena cava (*curved arrow* in **C**) and dilated right internal thoracic (IT), azygos (A), and subcutaneous venous collaterals. Note lobulated dilatation of the unenhanced left superior intercostal vein (*arrowheads* in **C**) along the aortic arch representing additional mediastinal venous collaterals.

may develop in patients with a coagulopathy, or with aortic rupture from aneurysm or dissection. Chronic hemodialysis, radiation vasculitis, and bleeding into a mediastinal mass are rare causes of mediastinal hemorrhage.

In the nontraumatic setting, the signs and symptoms of mediastinal hemorrhage are often mild or absent. The patient may complain of retrosternal chest pain radiating toward the back. Rarely, SVC compression may result in the SVC syndrome. Extension of blood from the mediastinum superiorly into the retropharyngeal space may result in neck stiffness, odynophagia, or stridor.

The main radiographic finding in mediastinal hemorrhage of any cause is a focal or diffuse widening of the mediastinum that obscures the normal mediastinal contours. In mediastinal hemorrhage, the mediastinum develops a flat or slightly convex outward contour, unlike the round, lobulated, or irregular contour seen with enlarged lymph nodes or a localized mediastinal mass. Blood extending from the mediastinum into the pleural or extrapleural space produces a free-flowing effusion or a loculated extrapleural collection, respectively. Rarely, extension of blood into the lungs via the bronchovascular interstitium produces interstitial opacities that mimic pulmonary edema. Serial radiographs may show rapid changes in mediastinal or pleural fluid collections in patients with persistent hemorrhage. CT demonstrates abnormal soft tissue within the mediastinum that obliterates the normal interfaces between the mediastinal fat, the vessels, and the airways (Fig. 11.29). Freshly clotted blood is high in attenuation and is usually easily appreciated on CT. CT is also superior to radiography in demonstrating the extramediastinal extent of hemorrhage and is useful in demonstrating associated thoracic injuries in patients following blunt chest trauma.

Mediastinal Lipomatosis is a benign, asymptomatic condition characterized by excessive deposition of fat in the mediastinum. Predisposing conditions include obesity, Cushing disease, and corticosteroid therapy. However, this entity is unassociated with identifiable conditions in approximately 50% of patients.

The common finding on conventional radiography is smooth, symmetric widening of the superior mediastinum. If the amount of fat deposition is marked, the mediastinum widening may show lobulated margins. The trachea remains midline in position in patients with mediastinal lipomatosis, whereas mediastinal tumor infiltration or mediastinal hemorrhage usually cause tracheal deviation or narrowing. Fat may also accumulate in the paraspinal regions, chest wall, and cardiophrenic angles; the latter produces enlargement of the epipericardial fat pads that is a clue to the proper diagnosis.

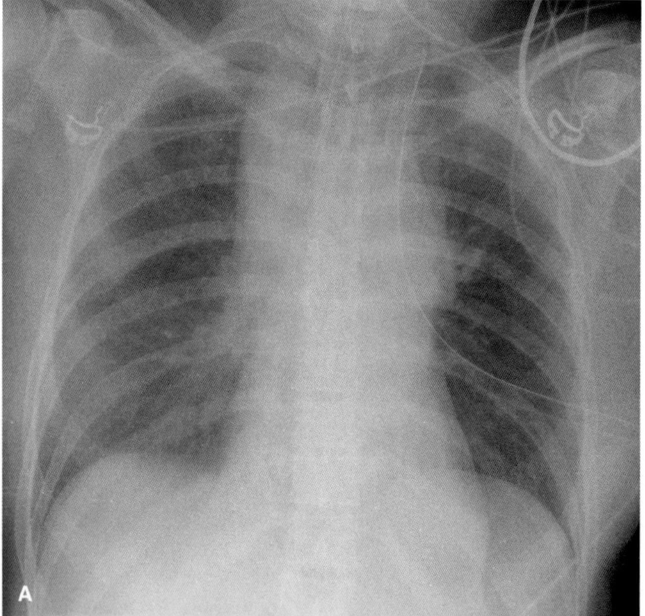

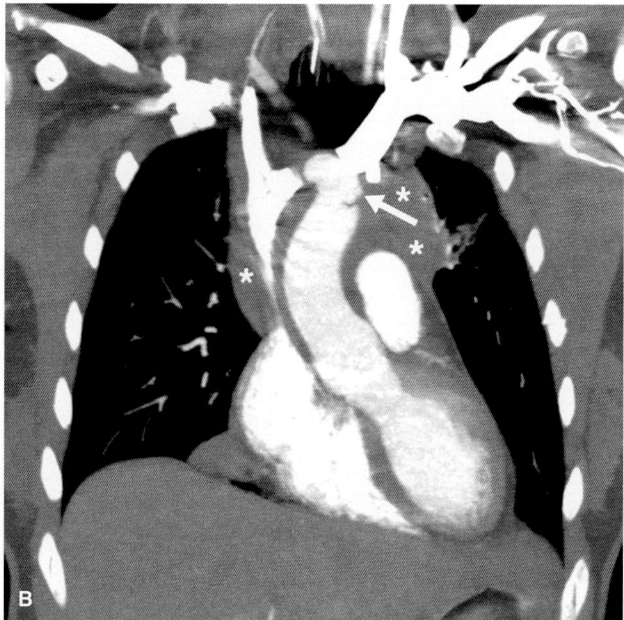

FIGURE 11.29. **Mediastinal Hematoma From Traumatic Aortic Injury. A:** Portable chest radiograph in a 38-year-old woman involved in a motor vehicle accident demonstrates a widened mediastinum. **B:** Coronal maximum intensity projection CT aortogram demonstrates a traumatic pseudoaneurysm of the aortic arch (*arrow*) with extensive mediastinal hematoma (*asterisks*).

CT provides a definitive diagnosis by demonstrating abundant, homogeneous, unencapsulated fat that bulges the mediastinal contours (Fig. 11.30). Displacement or compression of mediastinal structures, particularly the trachea, is typically absent. Heterogeneity within the fat suggests other primary or superimposed conditions, such as neoplastic infiltration, infection, hemorrhage, or fibrosis.

Malignancy. Malignant involvement of the mediastinum is typically seen as discrete masses or lymph node enlargement. Rarely, diffuse soft tissue infiltration of the mediastinal fat may occur, either alone or in association with focal lesions. Plain radiographs are nonspecific, usually demonstrating mediastinal widening. CT shows soft tissue infiltration of the normal mediastinal fat and obliteration of the normal tissue planes. This pattern is most common with extracapsular spread of lymphoma or small cell carcinoma of the lung. The latter disease has a high propensity to invade mediastinal structures and therefore may present with symptoms of airway obstruction or SVC syndrome.

Pneumomediastinum is the presence of extraluminal gas within the mediastinum. Possible sources of such gas include the lungs, trachea, central bronchi, esophagus, external trauma including surgery and penetrating injury, and extension of gas from the neck or abdomen (Table 11.7).

Air from the lungs is the most common source of pneumomediastinum. The mechanism of pneumomediastinum formation involves a sudden rise in intrathoracic and intra-alveolar pressure that leads to alveolar rupture. The extra-alveolar air first collects within the bronchovascular interstitium and then dissects centrally to the hilum and mediastinum (the Macklin

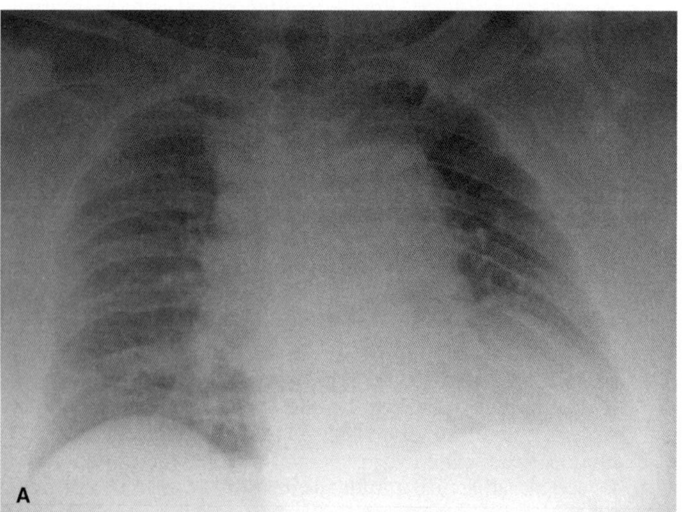

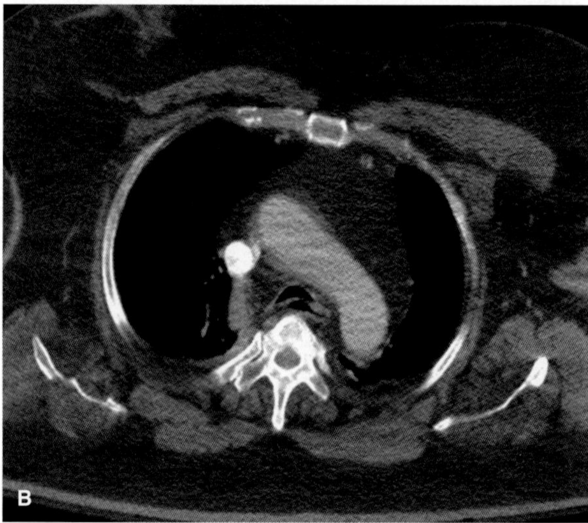

FIGURE 11.30. **Mediastinal Lipomatosis. A:** Frontal chest radiograph in a 54-year-old man shows a widened mediastinum. **B:** Axial contrast-enhanced CT at the level of the aortic arch shows abundant mediastinal fat accounting for the mediastinal widening on radiography.

TABLE 11.7

CAUSES OF PNEUMOMEDIASTINUM

Intrathoracic	▪ Alveolar • Valsalva maneuver • Positive pressure ventilation ▪ Tracheobronchial tree • Bronchial stump dehiscence • Tracheobronchial injury ▪ Esophagus • Boerhaave syndrome • Traumatic esophageal injury ▪ Endoscopic interventions • Carcinoma with fistula ▪ Infection with fistula formation • Histoplasmosis • Tuberculosis
Extrathoracic	▪ Recent sternotomy ▪ Pneumoperitoneum/ pneumoretroperitoneum ▪ Subcutaneous emphysema in neck ▪ Penetrating injury ▪ Laryngeal injury

effect). Less commonly, the air may dissect peripherally toward the subpleural interstitium and rupture through the visceral pleura to produce a pneumothorax.

Pneumomediastinum most commonly complicates mechanical ventilation in patients with ARDS, because the combination of positive pressure ventilation and noncompliant lungs predisposes to alveolar rupture. Spontaneous pneumomediastinum can occur with deep inspiratory or Valsalva maneuvers during strenuous exercise, childbirth, weightlifting, and inhalation of drugs such as marijuana, nitrous oxide, and crack cocaine. Patients with asthma are prone to pneumomediastinum; this is related to the airways obstruction that characterizes this disease (Fig. 11.31). Prolonged vomiting from any cause may lead to intrathoracic pressures that are sufficiently high to produce pneumomediastinum. In patients with diabetic ketoacidosis, pneumomediastinum may result from the deep inspirations associated with Kussmaul breathing as patients attempt to correct the underlying acidosis. Blunt chest trauma can result in pneumomediastinum as a result of an abrupt increase in intra-alveolar pressure and shearing forces affecting the alveolar walls.

Pneumomediastinum arising from the tracheobronchial tree or esophagus usually is a result of traumatic disruption of these structures. The marked shearing forces that develop with blunt trauma may lead to fracture of the trachea or mainstem bronchi. Penetrating trauma to the tracheobronchial tree is usually iatrogenic and may follow endotracheal intubation, bronchoscopy, or tracheostomy. Rarely, neoplasms or inflammatory lesions (e.g., tuberculosis) may erode through the tracheal wall and into the peritracheal fat. Esophageal rupture is most often spontaneous, usually in the setting of severe, prolonged vomiting (Boerhaave syndrome). In addition to pneumomediastinum, a left hydropneumothorax and pneumoperitoneum may be present in this condition. Spontaneous esophageal rupture may occur during childbirth, during a severe asthmatic episode, or with blunt chest trauma. Endoscopic procedures, stent placement, esophageal dilatation, corrosive ingestion, and carcinoma may lead to esophageal perforation. Mediastinal gas may be produced by bacterial organisms in acute mediastinitis.

Air within the soft tissues of the neck from penetrating trauma or laryngeal fracture may lead to pneumomediastinum by extending inferiorly through the retropharyngeal and prevertebral spaces, or along the sheaths of the great vessels. Deep space infections in the neck can spread along the same fascial planes and lead to mediastinitis. The term *Ludwig angina* describes the substernal chest pain caused by the intramediastinal extension of such infections. Rarely, pneumomediastinum develops as air dissects superiorly from the retroperitoneum through the aortic hiatus or from the peritoneal cavity along the internal mammary vascular sheaths.

The symptoms associated with pneumomediastinum vary with the underlying etiology, extent of mediastinal air, and presence of mediastinitis. Mediastinal air without infection is generally asymptomatic and does not require treatment. In some patients with spontaneous pneumomediastinum, there may be substernal, pleuritic-type chest pain of sudden onset that can be related to a specific inciting incident, such as vomiting or the Valsalva maneuver. Dyspnea may be present. In adults, mediastinal air under pressure usually escapes into the neck, producing crepitus over the neck, supraclavicular regions, and chest wall. Rarely, mediastinal air under pressure may produce a tension pneumomediastinum in which the clinical findings are those of cardiac tamponade. Patients with mediastinitis and pneumomediastinum are usually seriously ill with chest pain, high fevers, dyspnea, and signs of sepsis. The radiographic findings of pneumomediastinum are reviewed in Chapter 10.

THE HILA

Unilateral Hilar Enlargement/Increased Density (Table 11.8)

An abnormal hilum as seen radiographically can appear as enlargement, increased density, or both. Increased density can occasionally result from a parenchymal abnormality superimposed on the hilum on frontal radiography, and while the lateral radiograph is most helpful in this regard, CT will often be necessary to localize the abnormality to the hilum. Comparison with the contralateral hilum and review of prior radiographs are most helpful in detecting hilar abnormality.

Malignancy. A hilar mass usually represents bronchogenic carcinoma or confluent lymph node metastases (Fig. 11.32). Unilateral hilar enlargement may be the presenting radiographic feature of squamous cell carcinoma, where the hilar mass represents the extraluminal extension of an endobronchial tumor from its origin within a central (i.e., lobar or proximal segmental) bronchus. Concomitant hilar lymph node involvement may contribute to hilar enlargement in some of these patients. Approximately 20% of patients with squamous cell carcinoma have a hilar mass on chest radiograph. In contrast, patients with adenocarcinoma and large cell carcinoma more commonly present with a peripheral pulmonary nodule or mass. In many patients, the hilar mass may be obscured by adjacent atelectasis or obstructive pneumonitis.

Unilateral hilar enlargement resulting from metastatic lymph node involvement is most often seen in small cell carcinoma (Fig. 11.15). The propensity of this tumor for early invasion of the bronchial submucosa and peribronchial lymphatics accounts for the high incidence of widespread hematogenous and hilar and mediastinal lymph node metastases at the time of diagnosis. Plain film evidence of enlarged hilar lymph nodes resulting from metastases from adenocarcinoma of lung or large cell carcinoma are seen in only 10% to 15% of patients. CT is more sensitive than radiography for detecting enlarged hilar nodes and should be performed in all patients to guide further staging procedures and for proper preoperative or treatment planning.

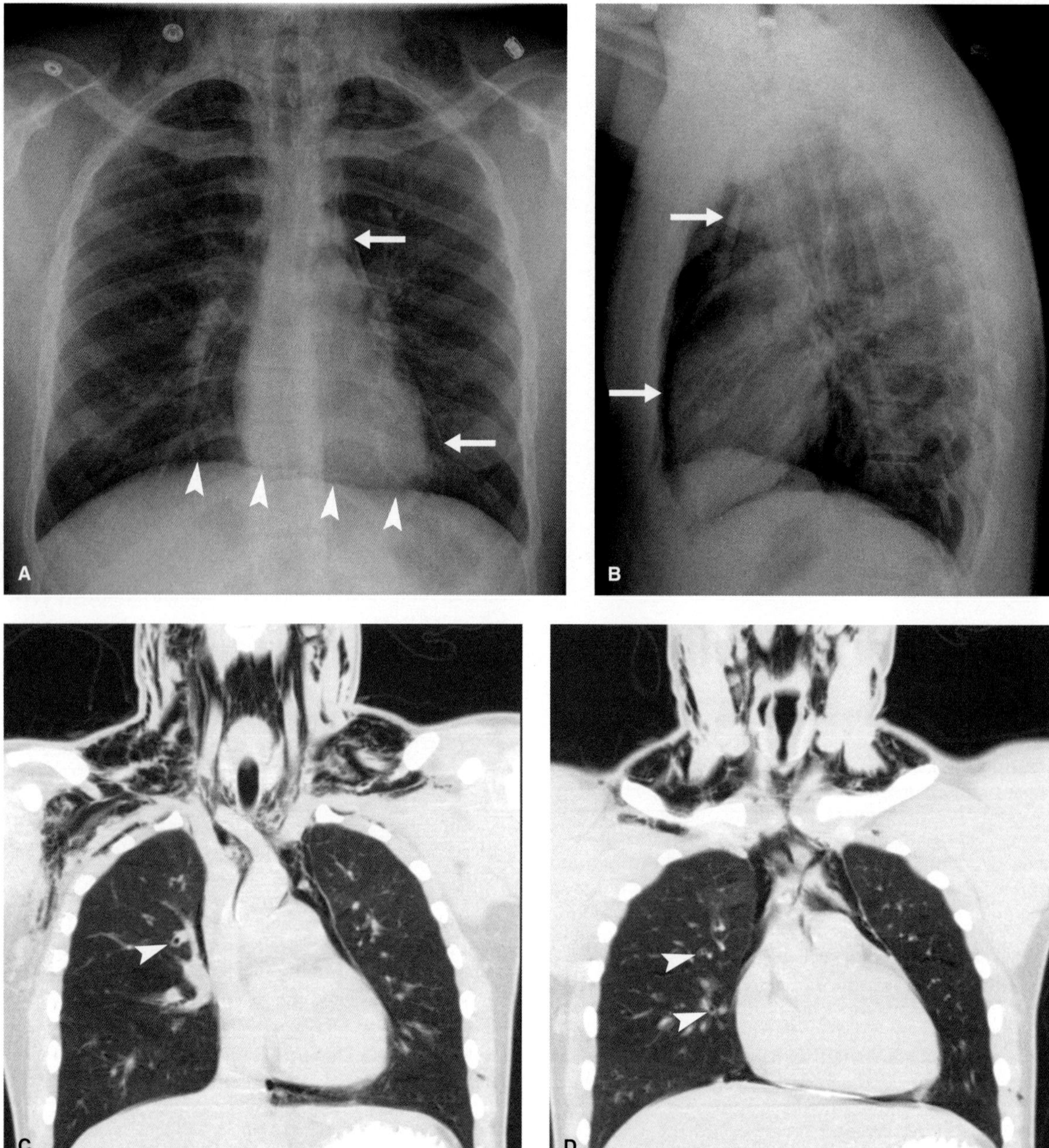

FIGURE 11.31. **Pneumomediastinum.** A, B: Frontal (A) and lateral (B) chest radiographs in a patient with an acute asthma exacerbation shows perihilar bronchial cuffing (*arrow*) and pneumomediastinum extending into the neck producing subcutaneous emphysema. Note the ability to see the diaphragm as a continuous interface ("continuous diaphragm" sign) (*arrowheads*). C, D: Coronal CT scans at the level of the ascending aorta show airways thickening (*arrow*) and confirms pneumomediastinum extending into the neck.

Metastases to hilar and mediastinal lymph nodes from extrathoracic malignancies are uncommon, occurring in approximately 2% of patients. The malignancies that are most often associated with intrathoracic nodal metastases are genitourinary (renal and testicular); head and neck (skin, larynx, and thyroid); breast; and melanoma (Fig. 11.33). In renal cell carcinoma and seminoma, lymphatic spread of tumor to retroperitoneal nodes and up the thoracic duct to the posterior mediastinum is the mode of spread to thoracic nodes. Although there is no direct communication between the thoracic duct and anterior mediastinal lymph nodes, reflux of tumor emboli through incompetent valves may allow tumor spread to hilar, paratracheal, and intraparenchymal lymphatics. Head and neck tumors reach the mediastinum via lymphatic spread from cervical lymph nodes. Intrathoracic nodal metastases from breast carcinoma are often seen late in the course of disease, often years after the initial diagnosis. Malignant melanoma is the extrathoracic neoplasm with the highest incidence of intrathoracic nodal metastases; patients with nodal disease will almost invariably have radiographic evidence of parenchymal metastases.

Although 75% of patients presenting with Hodgkin lymphoma have evidence of intrathoracic lymph node enlargement, isolated unilateral hilar lymph node enlargement is uncommon. The thoracic manifestations in NHL differ in primary pulmonary lymphoma versus lymphoma that primarily

TABLE 11.8

UNILATERAL HILAR ENLARGEMENT

Lymph node enlargement	Malignancy	■ Bronchogenic carcinoma ■ Lymph node metastases • Bronchogenic carcinoma • Head and neck CA • Breast carcinoma • Melanoma • Genitourinary malignancy ■ Renal cell carcinoma ■ Testicular malignancy ■ Lymphoma
	Infection	■ Mycobacterial infection • TB • Nontuberculous (MAI) ■ Fungal infection • Histoplasmosis • Coccidioidomycosis • Blastomycosis ■ Bacterial • Lung abscess • Plague • Tularemia ■ Viral infection • Measles • Mononucleosis
Vascular	Pulmonary artery dilation	■ Valvular pulmonic stenosis (left) ■ Pulmonary artery aneurysm • Behçet's • Hughes–Stovin ■ Pulmonary artery thromboembolism
Cyst	Foregut	Bronchogenic cyst

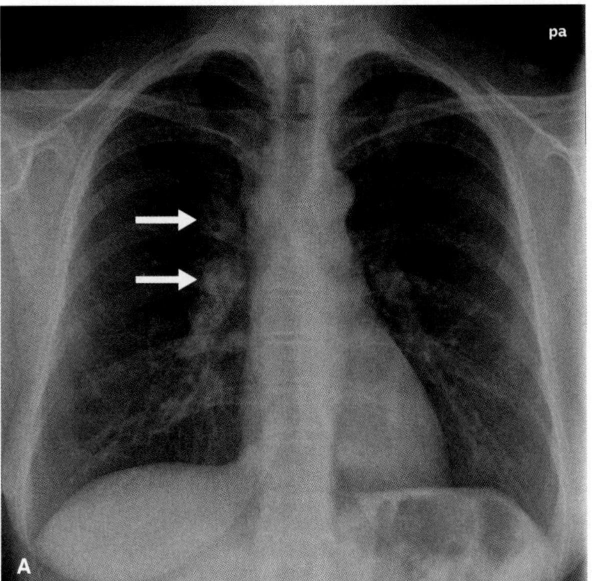

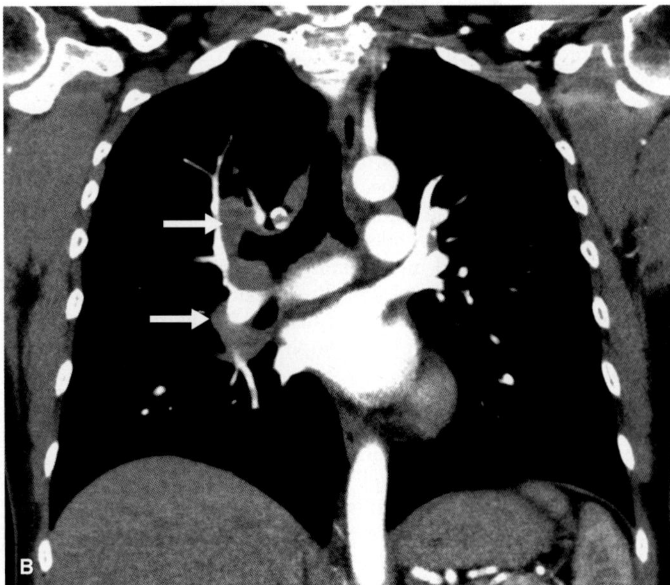

FIGURE 11.32. **Bronchogenic Carcinoma as Enlarged Hilar Lymph Nodes. A:** Frontal chest radiograph in a 49-year-old woman with chest tightness shows an enlarged right hilum (*arrows*). **B:** Coronal contrast-enhanced CT through the right hilum shows a enlarged right hilar lymph nodes (*arrows*). Bronchoscopic biopsy revealed non–small cell carcinoma.

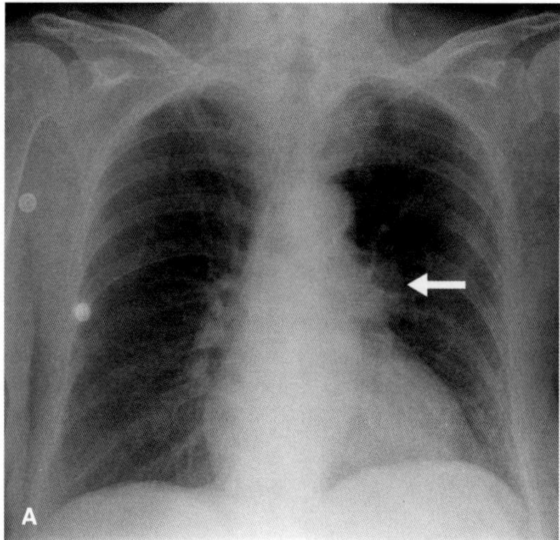

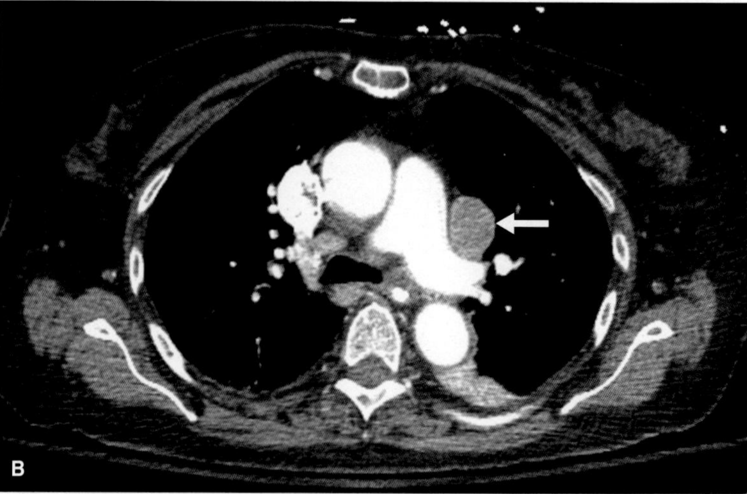

FIGURE 11.33. **Hilar Nodal Metastases From Ovarian Carcinoma. A:** Frontal chest radiograph in an 83-year-old woman with ovarian carcinoma shows a left hilar mass (*arrow*). **B:** Axial contrast-enhanced CT shows an enlarged left hilar lymph node (*arrow*) reflecting metastatic disease.

involves extrathoracic sites with secondary pulmonary involvement. Thoracic involvement in primary pulmonary lymphoma is largely limited to parenchymal and pleural disease, whereas secondary pulmonary lymphoma generally manifests as intrathoracic lymph node enlargement, with 35% showing hilar or middle mediastinal lymph node enlargement (Fig. 11.14).

Infection. Unilateral hilar or mediastinal lymph node enlargement is a characteristic feature in primary pulmonary tuberculosis (see Fig. 14.8) in distinction to postprimary tuberculosis; an exception is the severely immunocompromised patient with AIDS. Isolated lymph node enlargement as a manifestation of primary tuberculosis is more common in children than in adults. There is almost always concomitant parenchymal disease in immunocompetent patients with lymph node enlargement. Fungal infections such as histoplasmosis and coccidioidomycosis may present with hilar lymph node enlargement, typically associated with patchy or lobar airspace opacification in the ipsilateral lung (see Fig. 14.17). A variety of bacterial infections have been associated with unilateral hilar lymph node enlargement, including plague, tularemia, and anaerobic lung abscess. A characteristic finding in patients with pneumonic plague is the detection on unenhanced CT of increased attenuation within hilar and mediastinal nodes that drain regions of parenchymal involvement owing to intranodal hemorrhage. Tularemia (*Francisella tularensis*) causes parenchymal consolidation in association with hilar lymph node enlargement and pleural effusion.

The viral infections most commonly associated with hilar lymph node enlargement are infectious mononucleosis and measles pneumonia. The thorax is infrequently involved in mononucleosis, but hilar lymph node enlargement is the most common manifestation of intrathoracic disease. Lymph node enlargement may accompany the reticular interstitial opacities of typical measles pneumonia, or it may be associated with nodular, segmental, or lobar opacities and pleural effusion in atypical measles pneumonia.

Pulmonary Artery Enlargement. Although unilateral hilar enlargement is most often the result of a mass or enlarged lymph nodes, abnormal enlargement of the right or left pulmonary artery may cause hilar enlargement (Fig. 11.34). Vascular disorders that produce unilateral pulmonary artery enlargement include poststenotic dilatation of the left pulmonary artery from valvular or postvalvular pulmonic stenosis (Fig. 11.35), pulmonary artery aneurysms, and distention of the pulmonary artery by bland or tumor thrombus. Patients with congenital valvular pulmonic stenosis may develop poststenotic dilatation or aneurysms of the main and left pulmonary arteries from the jet effect of blood upon these vessels. Rarely, stenoses resulting from pulmonary artery vasculitis, congenital rubella, or Williams syndrome may lead to poststenotic dilatation of a pulmonary artery. Aneurysms of the central pulmonary arteries are usually associated with congenital heart disease, such as pulmonic stenosis and left-to-right shunts from ventricular septal defect and patent ductus arteriosus. Rare vasculitides such as Behçet disease and Hughes–Stovins syndrome may present with pulmonary artery aneurysms. A large pulmonary embolus lodging in the proximal portion of a pulmonary artery may cause proximal dilatation. Obviously, these patients are symptomatic and will show characteristic findings on perfusion lung scan or CT pulmonary angiography.

Bronchogenic Cyst is an uncommon cause of a hilar mass. CT and MR will show a round, smooth, thin-walled cyst, usually found in an asymptomatic young adult. Because the hilum is an unusual location for a bronchogenic cyst, and distinction from a necrotic tumor or lymph node mass cannot be made radiographically, these lesions should be biopsied or removed.

Bilateral Hilar Enlargement

Bilateral hilar enlargement is the result of enlargement of hilar lymph nodes or the central pulmonary arteries (Table 11.9).

Enlarged Lymph Nodes

Malignancy. The malignancies producing bilateral hilar lymph node enlargement are similar to those producing unilateral enlargement. In distinction to unilateral nodal enlargement, metastases are uncommon causes of bilateral hilar nodal enlargement. The most frequent solid tumors producing bilateral hilar disease are small cell carcinoma of the lung, lymphoma, and malignant melanoma.

Bilateral hilar lymph node involvement by lymphoma is more common in Hodgkin disease than NHL. Hilar involvement is virtually never seen without concomitant anterior

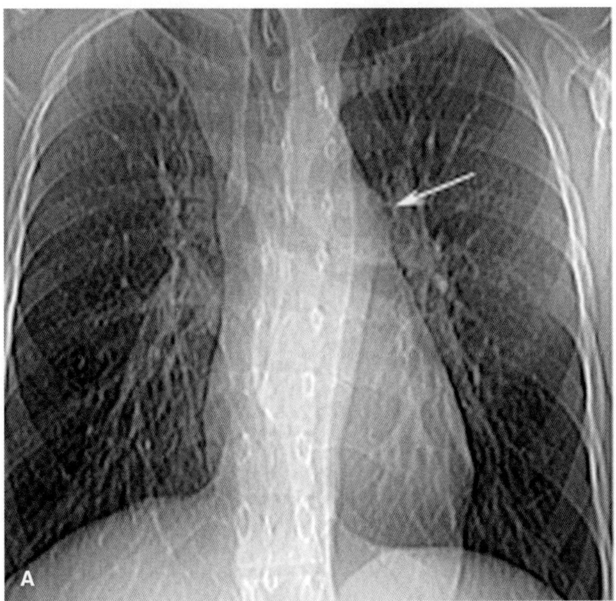

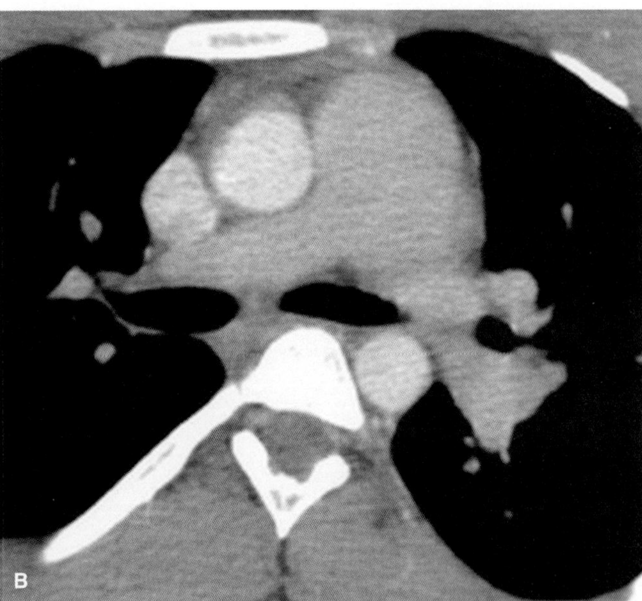

FIGURE 11.34. **Unilateral Hilar Enlargement From Idiopathic Dilatation of the Pulmonary Artery. A:** Scout view from chest CT shows abnormal convexity in the region of the main pulmonary artery (*arrow*). Note thoracic scoliosis. **B:** Enhanced CT scan shows dilated main pulmonary artery with normal right and left pulmonary arteries. Physical examination and echocardiogram showed no evidence of pulmonic valve disease.

mediastinal nodal enlargement in Hodgkin disease, whereas NHL may produce isolated hilar disease.

The most common chest radiographic manifestation of leukemic involvement of the thorax is hilar and mediastinal lymph node enlargement; it is seen in up to 25% of patients. Lymph node enlargement is much more common in the lymphocytic than the myelogenous form, particularly in chronic lymphocytic leukemia.

Infection. Mediastinal and hilar lymph node enlargement from infection is most often seen in tuberculous and fungal infection with histoplasmosis and coccidioidomycosis. In these diseases, the lymph node enlargement may be unilateral or bilateral. With bilateral disease, the enlargement is asymmetric in distinction to sarcoidosis, which is typically symmetric. Bacterial infection from *Bacillus anthracis* (anthrax) and *Yersinia pestis* (plague) may produce bilateral hilar lymph node enlargement. In anthrax infection, the lymph node enlargement is often associated with patchy airspace opacities in the lower lobes. The bubonic form of plague may produce marked hilar and mediastinal adenopathy without pneumonia. Recurrent bacterial infection complicating cystic fibrosis is often associated with bilateral hilar lymph node enlargement, and distinction from pulmonary artery enlargement from pulmonary hypertension may be difficult radiographically.

Sarcoidosis is associated with bilateral hilar lymph node enlargement in 80% of patients. Most of these patients have concomitant paratracheal lymph node enlargement, and nearly half have concomitant radiographic parenchymal disease. The pattern

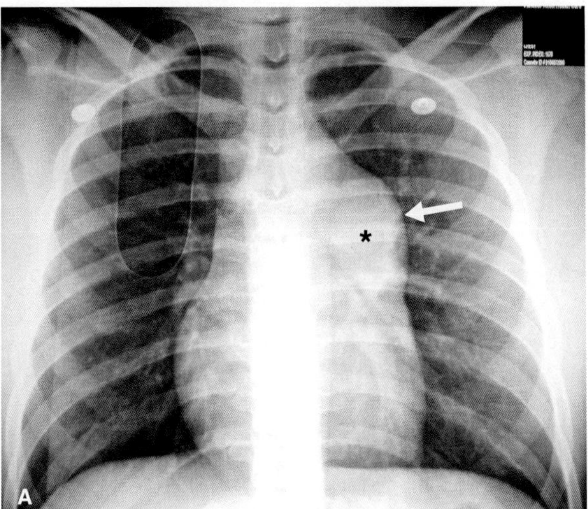

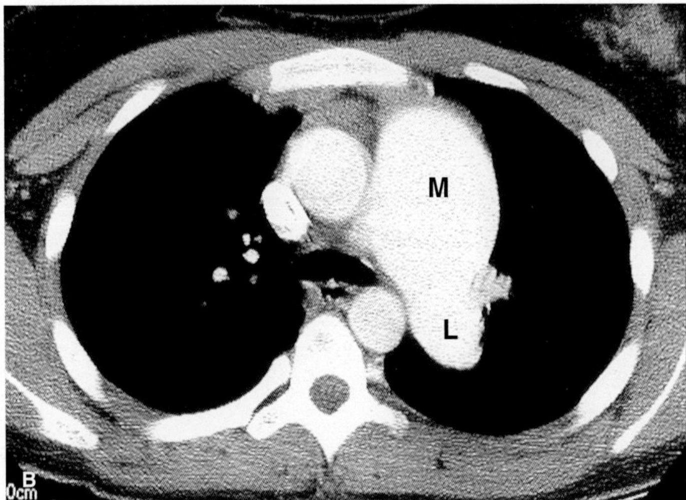

FIGURE 11.35. **Left Hilar Enlargement in Valvular Pulmonic Stenosis. A:** Chest radiograph shows a middle mediastinal mass (*arrow* in [**A**]) with left hilar enlargement (*asterisk* in [**A**]). **B:** Axial contrast-enhanced CT shows marked main (M) and left (L) pulmonary arterial dilatation as a result of valvular pulmonic stenosis.

TABLE 11.9

BILATERAL HILAR ENLARGEMENT

Lymph node enlargement	Malignancy	■ Primary intrathoracic malignancy • Non–small cell carcinoma • Small cell carcinoma • Primary pulmonary lymphoma • Carcinoid tumor • Extrathoracic malignancy with nodal spread • Head and neck CA • Breast CA • Genitourinary (renal cell, seminoma) • Melanoma ■ Systemic malignancy • Lymphoma • Leukemia (T cell)
	Infection	■ Tuberculosis ■ Fungal infection • Histoplasmosis ■ Viral infection • Measles • Mononucleosis
	Granulomatous	■ Sarcoidosis ■ Berylliosis
	Inhalational	■ Silicosis
Vascular	Pulmonary artery dilation	■ Pulmonary arterial HTN ■ Increased pulmonary blood flow • Left-to-right shunt • Pulmonary venous HTN • Anemia

of lymph node involvement in sarcoidosis has been termed the 1-2-3 sign, with 1 = right paratracheal, 2 = right hilar, and 3 = left hilar lymph node enlargement (Fig. 11.36). The enlarged nodes produce symmetric, lobulated hilar masses on plain film, since the enlarged nodes remain separate. In 20% of patients, the involved lymph nodes will calcify; usually the calcifications are punctate in appearance, but occasionally peripheral "eggshell" calcification is seen. In some patients, the involved nodes can be seen to enhance after contrast administration on CT. In the majority of patients, the enlarged nodes resolve within 2 years of discovery; in a small percentage, the nodes remain enlarged for many years.

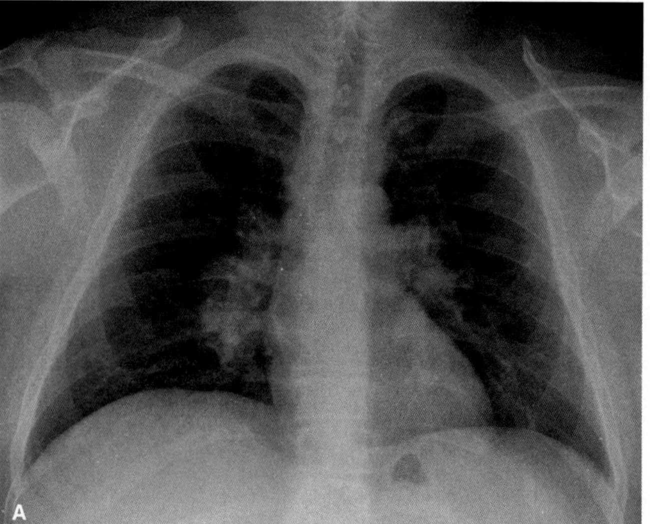

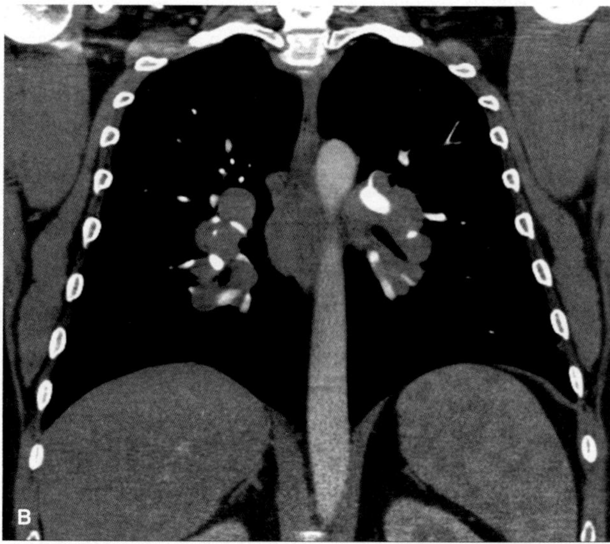

FIGURE 11.36. **Bilateral Hilar Lymph Node Enlargement in Sarcoidosis. A:** Posteroanterior radiograph in a 46-year-old man with sarcoidosis reveals bilateral hilar lymph node enlargement with subtle upper and mid-lung reticulonodular opacities. **B:** Contrast-enhanced coronal CT at the level of the carina shows bilateral hilar lymph node enlargement.

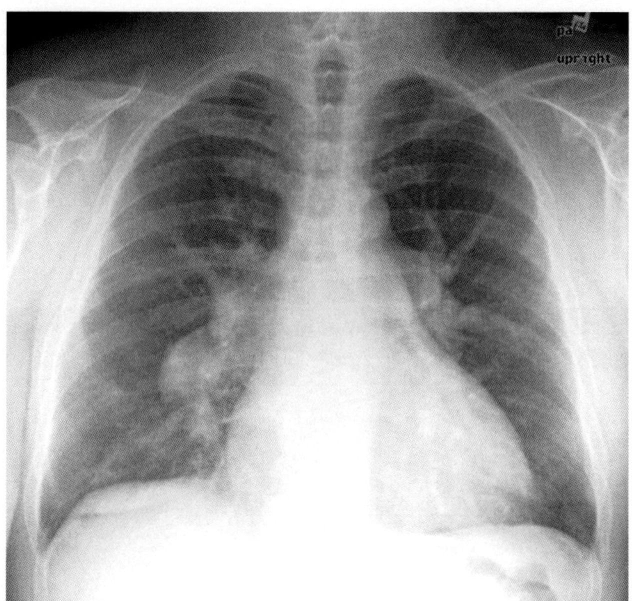

FIGURE 11.37. Bilateral Hilar Enlargement in Pulmonary Arterial Hypertension. Frontal chest radiograph shows marked central pulmonary arterial dilatation with attenuation of peripheral vasculature ("pruning") in a patient with severe pulmonary arterial hypertension due to COPD.

Berylliosis and Silicosis. The hilar and mediastinal lymph node enlargement of chronic berylliosis is radiographically indistinguishable from that of sarcoidosis. Similarly, silicosis can produce hilar and mediastinal lymph node enlargement; eggshell calcification of hilar nodes is highly suggestive of this entity, although peripheral nodal calcification may also be seen with sarcoidosis, histoplasmosis, or amyloidosis.

Enlarged Pulmonary Arteries

Bilateral pulmonary artery enlargement is seen with increased flow or increased resistance in the pulmonary circulation (Fig. 11.37). The conditions associated with bilateral pulmonary arterial enlargement are reviewed in Chapter 12.

Small Hila

Bilaterally small hila (Table 11.10) can be seen in some adults with severe pulmonary overinflation from emphysema or in those with diminished pulmonary blood flow due to congenital pulmonary outflow obstruction (tetralogy of Fallot, Ebstein anomaly) or rarely fibrosing mediastinitis.

The most common causes of a small hilum are atelectasis and resection of a portion of lung, which leave a small residual hilar artery supplying the remaining lobe or lobes. Hypoplasia of the pulmonary artery, often with associated abnormalities of the ipsilateral lung (hypogenetic lung syndrome, Swyer–James syndrome) (see Fig. 16.23), is another cause of a small hilum. Less commonly, invasion of the proximal pulmonary artery by mediastinal tumor, or obstruction of the pulmonary artery due to fibrosing mediastinitis, can produce a diminutive hilum. In any patient in whom a small hilum is a new radiographic finding, a CT scan should be performed to assess the mediastinum for central obstructing lesions. The left hilum can appear small in patients in whom the hilar shadow is obscured by the upper left heart margin or by fat in the region of the aortopulmonic interface. In these cases, the lateral radiograph will usually show a left pulmonary artery of normal size.

TABLE 11.10

SMALL HILUM/HILA

Unilateral	Congenital	▪ Absence or hypoplasia of the pulmonary artery ▪ Pulmonary agenesis, aplasia, hypoplasia ▪ Congenital pulmonary venolobar (Scimitar) syndrome (hypogenetic lung)
	Acquired	▪ Constrictive bronchiolitis (Swyer–James syndrome) ▪ Lobar atelectasis ▪ Lobar resection ▪ Pulmonary artery narrowing • Fibrosing mediastinitis
Bilateral		▪ Emphysema ▪ Decreased pulmonary blood flow • Fibrosing mediastinitis • Tetralogy of Fallot • Valvular pulmonic stenosis • Ebstein anomaly

Suggested Readings

Carter BW, Benveniste MF, Madan R, et al. IASLC/ITMIG staging system and lymph node map for thymic epithelial neoplasms. *Radiographics* 2017;37(3):758–776.

Carter BW, Benveniste MF, Madan R, et al. ITMIG classification of mediastinal compartments and multidisciplinary approach to mediastinal masses. *Radiographics* 2017;37(2):413–436.

El-Sherief AH, Lau CT, Wu CC, et al. International association for the study of lung cancer (IASLC) lymph node map: radiologic review with CT illustration. *Radiographics* 2014;34(6):1680–1691.

Inaoka T, Takahashi K, Mineta M, et al. Thymic hyperplasia and thymus gland tumors: differentiation with chemical shift MR imaging. *Radiology* 2007;243(3):869–876.

Katabathina VS, Restrepo CS, Martinez-Jimenez S, Riascos RF. Nonvascular, nontraumatic mediastinal emergencies in adults: a comprehensive review of imaging findings. *Radiographics* 2011;31(4):1141–60.

Kligerman SJ, Auerbach A, Franks TJ, Galvin JR. Castleman disease of the thorax: clinical, radiologic, and pathologic correlation: from the radiologic pathology archives. *Radiographics* 2016;36:1309-1332.

McAdams HP, Kirejczyk WM, Rosado-de-Christenson ML, Matsumoto S. Bronchogenic cyst: imaging features with clinical and histopathologic correlation. *Radiology* 2000;217(2):441–446.

McLoud TC, Kalisher L, Stark P, Greene R. Intrathoracic lymph node metastases from extrathoracic neoplasm. *AJR Am J Roentgenol* 1978;131(3):403-407.

McNeeley MF, Chung JH, Bhalla S, Godwin JD. Imaging of granulomatous fibrosing mediastinitis. *AJR Am J Roentgenol* 2012;199(2):319–327.

Webb WR. Chapter 3. The pulmonary hila. In: Webb WR, Higgins CB, eds. *Thoracic Imaging. Pulmonary and Cardiovascular Radiology*. Philadelphia, PA: Wolters Kluwer; 2017:78–105.

Webb WR. Chapter 6: Lymphoma and lymphoproliferative disease. In: Webb WR, Higgins CB, eds. *Thoracic Imaging. Pulmonary and Cardiovascular Radiology*. Philadelphia, PA: Wolters Kluwer; 2017:179–201.

Whitten CR, Khan S, Munneke GJ, Grubnic S. A diagnostic approach to mediastinal abnormalities. *Radiographics* 2007;27(3):657–671.

CHAPTER 12 ■ PULMONARY VASCULAR DISEASE

CURTIS E. GREEN AND JEFFREY S. KLEIN

PULMONARY EDEMA

Basic Principles. Under normal conditions, the interstitial space of the lung is kept dry by pulmonary lymphatics located within the axial and peripheral interstitium of the lung. The lymphatics drain the small amounts of transudated fluid that enters the interstitial spaces as an ultrafiltrate of plasma. Because there are no lymphatic structures immediately within the alveolar walls (parenchymal interstitium), filtered interstitial fluid is drawn to the lymphatics by a pressure gradient from the alveolar interstitium to the axial and peripheral interstitium. When the rate of fluid accumulation in the interstitium exceeds the lymphatic drainage capabilities of the lung, fluid accumulates first within the interstitial space. As the amount of extravascular fluid increases, fluid accumulates in the corners of the alveolar spaces. Progressive fluid accumulation eventually produces flooding of the alveolar spaces, resulting in airspace pulmonary edema. While interstitial edema may leave the gas-exchanging properties of the lung unaffected, flooding of the alveolar spaces leads to impaired oxygen and carbon dioxide exchange.

Excess fluid accumulation in the lung is caused by one of three basic mechanisms. The most common mechanism involves a change in the normal Starling forces that govern fluid movement in the lung. Because normal fluid movement is determined by the differences in hydrostatic and oncotic pressure between the pulmonary capillaries and surrounding alveolar interstitium, an imbalance in these forces may lead to pulmonary edema. This imbalance of forces is most commonly the result of increased capillary hydrostatic pressure (hydrostatic pulmonary edema) and less commonly diminished plasma oncotic or interstitial hydrostatic pressure. A second mechanism is obstruction or absence of the normal pulmonary lymphatics, which leads to the excess accumulation of interstitial fluid. Thirdly, a wide variety of disorders can injure the epithelium of the capillaries and alveoli, causing an increase in capillary permeability that allows protein-rich fluid to escape from the capillaries into the pulmonary interstitium.

Imaging findings in pulmonary edema result from both the interstitial and the airspace components and depend to some extent on the cause of the edema, as will be discussed later. The radiographic appearance of interstitial pulmonary edema results from thickening of the components of the interstitial spaces by fluid. Thickening of the axial interstitium results in the loss of definition of the intrapulmonary vascular shadows and thickening of the peribronchovascular interstitium causing peribronchial cuffing and tram tracking. Edema within alveolar septa produces ground-glass opacity initially in only the dependent lung zones and then throughout the lungs, most severe in the dependent zones. Involvement of peripheral and subpleural interstitial structures produces Kerley lines and subpleural edema. Kerley A and B lines represent thickening of central connective tissue septa and peripheral interlobular septa, respectively (Fig. 12.1). Subpleural edema is the accumulation of fluid within the innermost (interstitial) layer of the visceral pleura and is best seen on lateral radiographs as smooth thickening of the interlobar fissures. The radiographic changes of interstitial pulmonary edema may progress to those of airspace edema or, if successfully treated, resolve within 12 to 24 hours.

Airspace pulmonary edema develops when fluid in the interstitial spaces extends into the alveoli. The upright chest radiograph typically shows bilaterally symmetric airspace opacities predominately in the mid and lower lung zones. Airspace nodules and the findings of interstitial edema (Kerley B lines and subpleural edema) are usually present peripherally. As with interstitial edema, the airspace opacities of alveolar edema may change rapidly, often within hours. The differential diagnosis of diffuse airspace opacities has been reviewed (see Table 10.9). Thin-section CT can be useful for identification and assessment of pulmonary edema as the findings of thickening of subpleural, septal, and bronchovascular structures are fairly specific. Mild parenchymal edema produces a ground-glass pattern around the hila (Fig. 12.2). Early alveolar edema is seen as centrilobular airspace nodules surrounding the arteries within the lobular core, whereas severe alveolar edema produces dense perihilar airspace opacification.

Hydrostatic pulmonary edema (normal capillary permeability) is the most common form of pulmonary edema. It is usually caused by an elevation in the pulmonary venous pressure (pulmonary venous hypertension [PVH]). The classic cause of PVH is left ventricular systolic failure, but renal failure and a variety of cardiac and noncardiac abnormalities have the same physiology. Decreased capillary oncotic pressure, such as present in patients with hypoalbuminemia secondary to the nephrotic syndrome or liver failure, can cause findings identical to those in patients with elevated hydrostatic pressure.

The *causes of PVH* may be divided into four major categories: obstruction to left ventricular inflow, left ventricular systolic dysfunction (LV failure), mitral valve regurgitation, and systemic or pulmonary volume overload. The classic cause of obstruction to left ventricular inflow is mitral stenosis, but

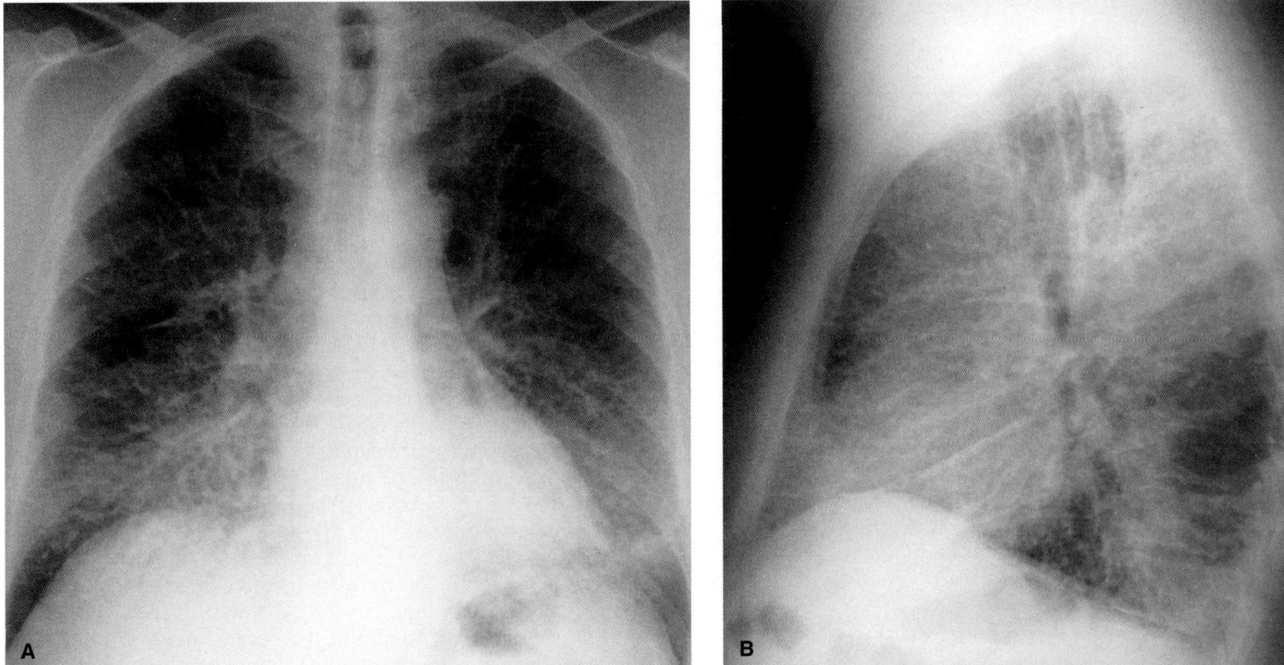

FIGURE 12.1. **Interstitial Pulmonary Edema Caused by Cardiac Disease.** Posteroanterior (**A**) and lateral (**B**) chest films in a 65-year-old man with an anterior wall myocardial infarction showing hydrostatic interstitial edema as evidenced by prominent upper lobe vessels (redistribution of pulmonary blood flow), indistinct lower lung zone pulmonary vessels, peripheral linear opacities (thickened interlobular septa or Kerley B lines), and thickened fissures (subpleural edema) resulting from acute left ventricular failure. Note the absence of cardiomegaly.

poor left ventricular compliance (diastolic dysfunction), such as caused by hypertrophy or chronic ischemic subendocardial fibrosis, is more common. Mimickers of mitral stenosis such as left atrial myxomas are rare. Obstruction of the central pulmonary veins from tumor, fibrosing mediastinitis, or pulmonary vein thrombosis may also be associated with the radiographic findings of PVH. Common causes of LV failure include ischemic heart disease, aortic valve stenosis and regurgitation, and nonischemic cardiomyopathy (Table 12.1). Severe mitral valve regurgitation can cause PVH directly by elevating left atrial pressure or secondarily by causing LV failure. Acute pulmonary volume overload is relatively common and most frequently due to iatrogenic overhydration. Acute postinfarction ventricular septal defect is a rare cause. Patients with acute or chronic renal failure may develop pulmonary edema because of increased pulmonary capillary hydrostatic

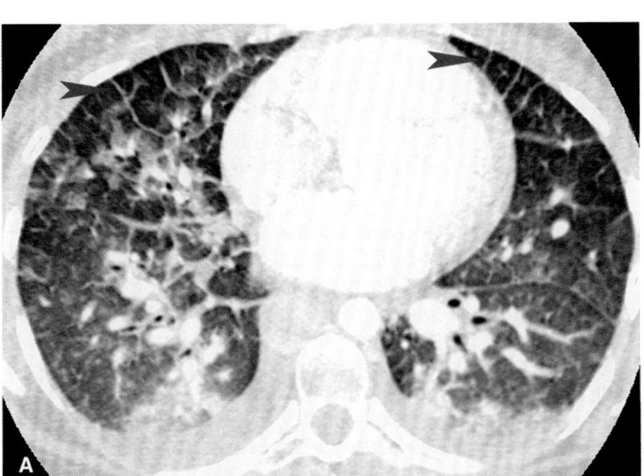

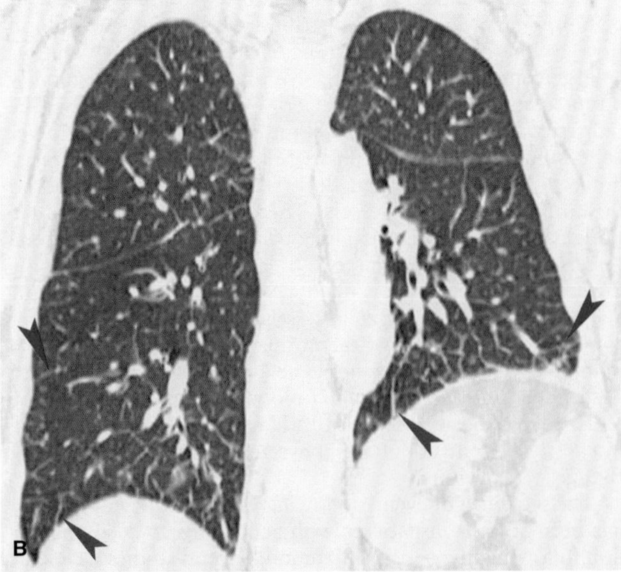

FIGURE 12.2. **Thin-Section CT of Hydrostatic Interstitial Pulmonary Edema. A:** Axial scan in a 28-year-old woman with postpartum cardiomyopathy showing thickening of the interlobular septal (*arrowheads*) and bronchovascular bundles with dependent patchy ground-glass and airspace opacities and bilateral pleural effusions. **B:** Coronal reconstruction in a different patient with hydrostatic interstitial edema. Thickened septal lines (*arrowheads*) and bronchovascular bundles and scattered ground-glass opacities are present, but there is no airspace consolidation.

TABLE 12.1

CAUSES OF PULMONARY VENOUS HYPERTENSION AND PULMONARY EDEMA

Left ventricular systolic dysfunction	Ischemic heart disease Left ventricular outflow obstruction (aortic stenosis, hypertension, coarctation, hypertrophic obstructive cardiomyopathy) Aortic stenosis Hypoplastic left heart syndrome
Obstruction to left ventricular inflow	Mitral valve stenosis Decreased left ventricular compliance (hypertrophy, pericardial constriction or tamponade, restrictive cardiomyopathy) Left atrial tumors Cor triatriatum and supravalvular mitral ring
Mitral regurgitation	Endocarditis Papillary muscle rupture or dysfunction Ruptured chordae Mitral prolapse
Systemic or pulmonary volume overload	Overhydration Renal failure Ventricular septal rupture
Pulmonary venous obstruction	
Central pulmonary veins	Fibrosing mediastinitis Pulmonary vein stenosis (tumor invasion, postcardiac ablation or surgery) Pulmonary venous thrombosis
Intrapulmonary veins	Pulmonary venoocclusive disease

pressure caused by a combination of hypervolemia and LV dysfunction.

The classic radiographic findings of PVH are enlargement of pulmonary veins and redistribution of pulmonary blood flow to the nondependent lung zones. Pulmonary venous enlargement is seen as progressive dilatation of horizontally oriented pulmonary veins on serial chest radiographs. The redistribution of pulmonary blood flow results from lower zone pulmonary venous constriction causing increased resistance to lower zone blood flow, with resultant preferential flow into upper lobe vessels. Therefore, with PVH in the upright patient with normal lung parenchyma, the upper zone vessels are frequently as large as or larger in diameter than the lower zone vessels. This is the opposite of the normal appearance, in which the lower zone vessels are larger than the upper zone vessels as a result of the normal gravitational effects on pulmonary blood flow. It should be noted that in patients with basilar lung disease, pulmonary blood flow may appear to be redistributed in the absence of PVH and with upper lobe lung disease (e.g., centrilobular emphysema) distribution may not change.

The sequence of events following the development of PVH has been studied in patients with acute cardiac decompensation following myocardial infarction. Several studies have correlated the radiographic findings of PVH in the erect patient with measurements of pulmonary capillary wedge pressure (PCWP) using flow-directed balloon occlusion (e.g., Swan–Ganz) catheters. When PCWP is normal (8 to 12 mm Hg), the chest radiograph is normal. Mild elevation of PCWP (12 to 18 mm Hg) produces constriction of lower lobe vessels and enlargement of upper lobe vessels. Progressive elevation of PCWP (19 to 25 mm Hg) leads to the findings of interstitial pulmonary edema: loss of vascular definition, peribronchial cuffing, and Kerley lines (Fig. 12.1). PCWP above 25 mm Hg produces alveolar filling with radiographic findings of bilateral airspace opacities in the perihilar and lower lung zones.

Atypical Radiographic Appearances of PVH. Several conditions may give rise to atypical radiographic appearances of PVH. Because the distribution of edema is affected by gravity, it is not surprising that edema fluid accumulates posteriorly or unilaterally in patients maintaining a prolonged supine or decubitus position, respectively. The diagnosis of unilateral edema is suggested by typical radiographic and clinical findings of pulmonary edema in one lung that resolve rapidly or redistribute with changes in patient positioning. Another cause of asymmetric or unilateral pulmonary edema is an interruption in the blood supply to one lung. This may be seen in pulmonary artery hypoplasia or in an acquired obstruction to pulmonary arterial blood flow such as central pulmonary embolism (PE) or extrinsic compression of the pulmonary artery from tumor or fibrosis. In these conditions, the lung with diminished pulmonary blood flow is "protected" from the transudation of fluid and the development of pulmonary edema. Bronchogenic carcinoma, lymphoma, or other causes of unilateral lymph node enlargement can impede normal lymphatic drainage and predispose to unilateral pulmonary edema. Similarly, unilateral pulmonary venous obstruction from tumor or fibrosing mediastinitis will predispose to edema on the affected side. Unilateral pulmonary edema may develop in the lung that is reexpanded by the rapid evacuation of a large pleural fluid collection or pneumothorax. This is known as *reexpansion pulmonary edema* and is discussed in a subsequent section.

Alveolar pulmonary edema localized to the right upper lung may be seen in patients with severe mitral regurgitation, likely as a result of preferential regurgitant flow of blood into the right upper lobe pulmonary vein across the superiorly and posteriorly oriented mitral valve. Affected patients will usually have typical radiographic findings of interstitial edema elsewhere in the lungs (Fig. 12.3).

Patients with pulmonary emphysema frequently have unusual appearances of alveolar edema. Areas of bullae, most commonly in the apical portions of the lungs, are spared from the development of alveolar edema because the pulmonary blood flow to these regions has already been obliterated by the emphysematous process. These emphysematous regions within adjacent areas of airspace opacification can simulate cavity formation and may be difficult to distinguish radiographically from necrotizing pneumonia or pneumatocele formation. Comparison with previous radiographs and correlation with the clinical course will aid in the proper diagnosis.

Increased Capillary Permeability Edema. Rapidly progressive respiratory compromise caused by leakage of protein-rich edema fluid into the lung, resulting from damage to the pulmonary microcirculation, may develop as a complication of a variety of systemic conditions. When respiratory failure develops as a result of this condition and is associated with increased lung stiffness (noncompliance) it is termed *acute lung injury* or when severe *acute respiratory distress syndrome* (ARDS). The edema associated with this syndrome is called *lung injury* or *increased capillary permeability edema,* as compared to the normal alveolar capillary permeability of hydrostatic edema. Many pulmonary and nonpulmonary disorders have been associated with increased permeability edema (Table 12.2); the most common are shock, severe trauma, burns, sepsis, narcotic overdose, and pancreatitis. Although the precise pathogenesis of capillary permeability edema has

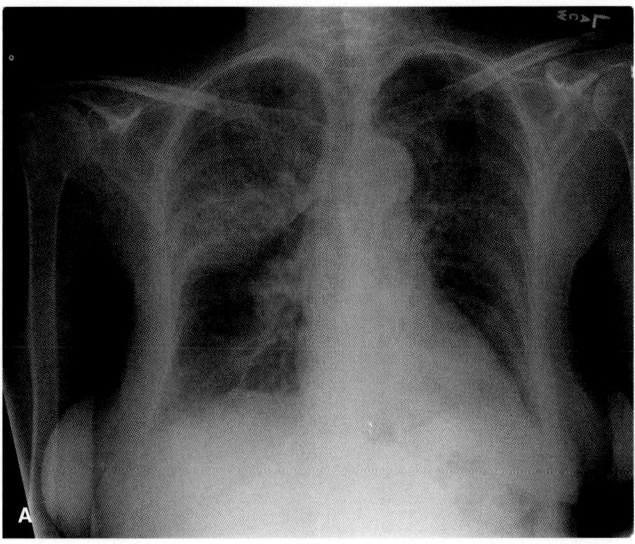

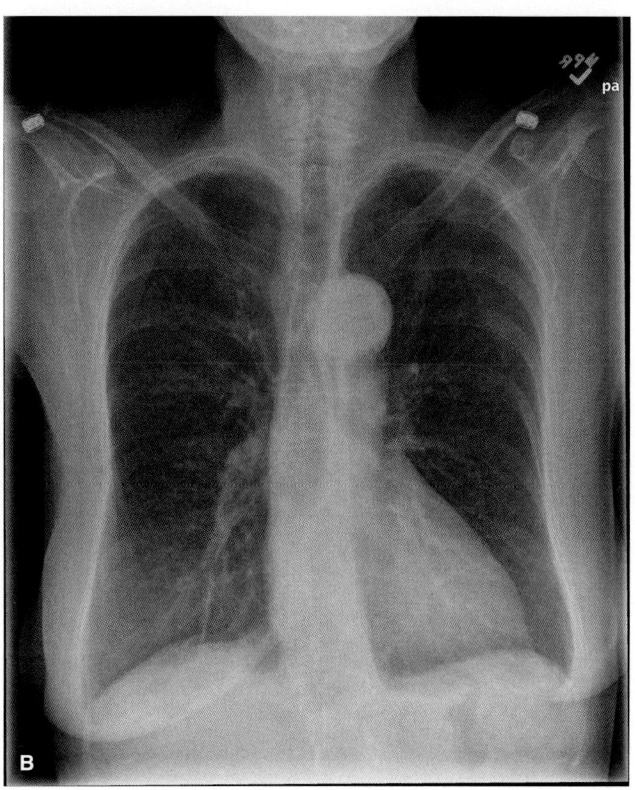

FIGURE 12.3. **Right Upper Lobe Edema in Acute Severe Mitral Valve Regurgitation. A:** Frontal chest radiograph at presentation demonstrates severe edema in the upper portion of the right lung with mild edema elsewhere. **B:** Radiograph obtained 2 days later demonstrates resolution of edema.

yet to be completely elucidated, current evidence suggests that recruitment and activation of neutrophils in the lung with release of enzymes and oxygen radicals are key factors in the development of capillary endothelial damage.

TABLE 12.2

ETIOLOGIES OF INCREASED PERMEABILITY PULMONARY EDEMA

Septicemia	Gram-negative bacteria
Shock	
Major surgery	
Burns	
Acute pancreatitis	
Disseminated intravascular coagulation	
Drugs	Narcotics Heroin Crack cocaine Aspirin
Inhalation of noxious fumes	Nitrogen dioxide (silo-filler's disease) Hydrocarbons Smoke Chlorine Phosgene
Aspiration of fluid	Fresh or salt water near drowning Gastric fluid aspiration (Mendelson syndrome)
Fat embolism	
Amniotic fluid embolism	

The pathologic changes associated with ARDS are those of diffuse alveolar damage and are common to all patients regardless of the underlying etiology. Within 12 to 24 hours following the initial insult (stage 1 or exudative ARDS), damage to capillary endothelium produces engorged capillaries and proteinaceous interstitial edema. Within the first week (stage 2 or proliferative ARDS), the injury to type 1 pneumocytes leads to the flooding of alveoli with edema fluid and proteinaceous and cellular debris, which form hyaline membranes lining the distal airways and alveoli. In stage 3 (fibrotic) ARDS, occurring 10 to 14 days following the initial insult, type 2 pneumocytes proliferate in an attempt to reline the denuded alveolar surfaces, and fibroblastic tissue proliferates within the airspaces. This fibroblastic tissue may resolve and leave minimal scarring or, particularly in those with severe disease and long-standing oxygen requirements, result in extensive interstitial fibrosis.

Radiographically, ARDS follows a predictable pattern. Chest radiographs become abnormal by 12 to 24 hours following the onset of dyspnea and demonstrate patchy peripheral airspace opacities (Fig. 12.4). CT scans show diffuse ground-glass and airspace opacities. Interlobular septal thickening is usually minimal or absent (Fig. 12.5). These opacities coalesce over the next several days to produce confluent bilateral airspace opacities with air bronchograms. Radiographic improvement in the opacities may be seen within the first week, but this is often caused by the effects of increasing positive pressure ventilation rather than true histologic improvement. After 1 week, the airspace opacities gradually give way to a coarse reticulonodular pattern that may resolve over the course of several months or remain unchanged, in which case the pattern represents irreversible pulmonary fibrosis (i.e., honeycombing). Pneumonia complicating ARDS is difficult to diagnose radiographically, but it should be suspected when a focal area of airspace opacification or a significant pleural effusion develops during the course of the disease. Likewise, the superimposition of LV failure may be impossible to recognize but is suggested by rapid clinical and radiographic

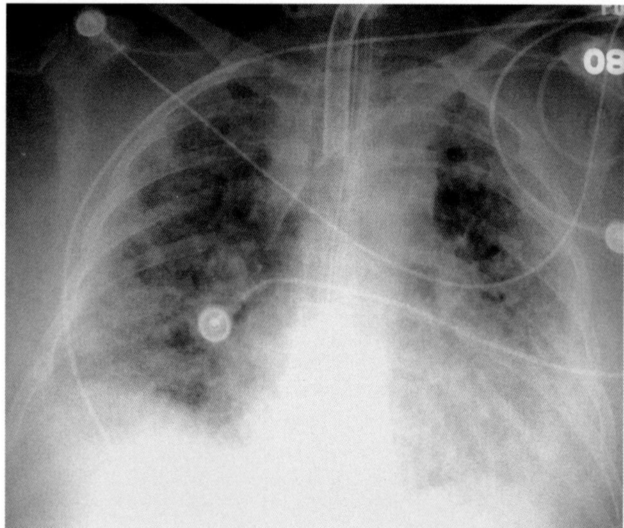

FIGURE 12.4. **Increased Permeability (Lung Injury) Edema in Acute Respiratory Distress Syndrome.** Portable chest radiograph in a 46-year-old woman with severe pancreatitis and respiratory failure reveals bilateral airspace opacification with a somewhat peripheral distribution, representing diffuse alveolar damage and permeability edema.

deterioration associated with changes in measured PCWP and edema fluid protein content. Pneumomediastinum and pneumothorax may result as a complication of positive pressure ventilation to noncompliant lungs and should be sought on portable chest radiographs.

Radiographic Distinction of Hydrostatic From Increased Capillary Permeability Edema. Beyond identifying the presence of pulmonary edema, the ability to distinguish between types of pulmonary edema has significant diagnostic and therapeutic importance. Milne et al. have described the chest radiographic findings that can be used to distinguish cardiac and overhydration edema from increased capillary permeability edema. In pulmonary edema associated with chronic cardiac failure, the heart is usually enlarged and displays an inverted (redistributed) pulmonary blood flow pattern. The distribution of edema is even from central to peripheral over the lower lung zones. The vascular pedicle, which represents the mediastinal width at the level of the superior vena cava and left subclavian artery, is widened (>53 mm on posteroanterior radiograph), reflecting increased circulating blood volume. Lung volumes are diminished because of decreased pulmonary compliance from edema. Peribronchial cuffing/Kerley lines and pleural effusions represent interstitial and intrapleural transudation of fluid respectively. These findings may be difficult to interpret, however. Furthermore, cardiac size per se is not particularly useful in distinguishing cardiac-related edema from other causes of hydrostatic and capillary leak edema for the following reasons: many patients with heart failure will not have radiographically evident cardiac enlargement; many patients with cardiac enlargement are not in failure; and enlargement of the cardiac silhouette may be caused by pericardial fluid, mediastinal fat, and poor lung expansion. Cardiomegaly is the best considered evidence of a chronic condition rather than an indicator of a specific problem.

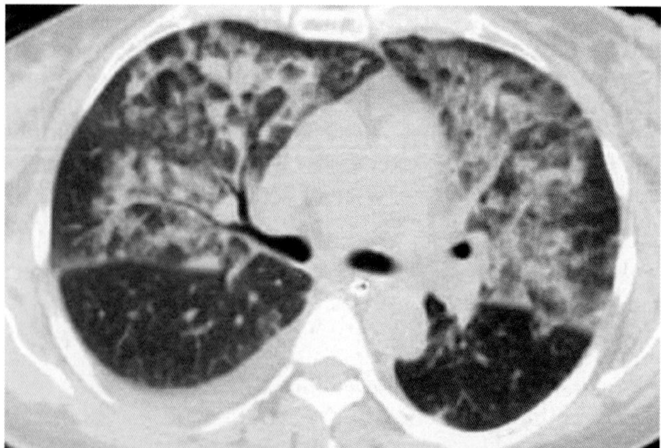

FIGURE 12.5. **Thin-Section CT of Lung Injury Edema.** Geographic, nondependent ground-glass and airspace opacities are present, but interlobular septal thickening is mostly absent.

Capillary permeability edema can sometimes be distinguished from hydrostatic edema by the following: a nondependent or peripheral distribution of edema, an absence of other signs of hydrostatic edema such as interlobular septal thickening and subpleural edema, and, most importantly, a lack of short-term change. It should be noted that some factors may render radiographic distinction of types of pulmonary edema difficult. Radiographs of supine patients will make evaluation of pulmonary blood flow distribution and vascular pedicle width difficult. The presence of severe alveolar edema will obscure underlying vascular markings. Many patients with capillary permeability edema will be overhydrated in attempts to maintain circulating blood volume, producing complex radiographic findings. Finally, most intubated patients will suffer from more than one problem.

Neurogenic pulmonary edema following head trauma, seizure, or increased intracranial pressure is a complex phenomenon that appears to involve both hydrostatic and increased permeability mechanisms. Massive sympathetic discharge from the brain in these conditions produces systemic vasoconstriction and increased venous return, with resultant increase in LV diastolic pressure and hydrostatic pulmonary edema. The presence of protein-rich edema fluid and normal PCWP in some patients suggests that increased permeability may be a contributing factor.

High-altitude pulmonary edema develops in certain individuals after rapid ascent to altitudes above 3,500 m. Edema typically develops within 48 to 72 hours of ascent and appears to reflect a varied individual response to hypoxemia, in which scattered areas of pulmonary arterial spasm result in transient pulmonary arterial hypertension (PAH). This produces an increase in high-pressure blood flow to uninvolved areas, resulting in damage to the capillary endothelium and increased permeability edema, typically with a patchy distribution. Resolution usually occurs within 24 to 48 hours after the administration of supplemental oxygen or a return to sea level.

Reexpansion Pulmonary Edema. Rapid reexpansion of a collapsed lung following evacuation of a large pneumothorax or pleural effusion present for >48 hours may result in the development of unilateral pulmonary edema. Risk factors include young age and prolonged duration of lung collapse. Recent evidence points toward a hydrostatic mechanism for the development of reexpansion edema. Gradual reexpansion of the lung by slow removal of pleural air or fluid over a 24- to 48-hour period and administration of supplemental oxygen will help limit the incidence and severity of this complication.

Acute Upper Airway Obstruction. Pulmonary edema may be seen during or immediately after treatment of acute upper airway obstruction. The proposed mechanism involves the creation of markedly negative intrathoracic pressure by attempts to inspire against an extrathoracic airway obstruction, producing

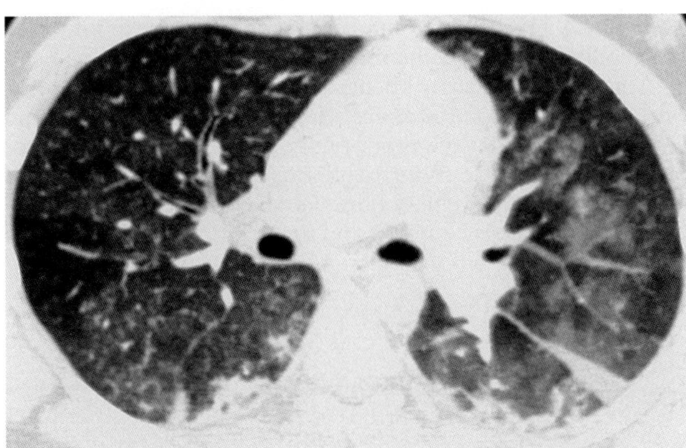

FIGURE 12.6. **Fat Embolism Producing Permeability Edema.** CT in an 18-year-old man with dyspnea and hypoxemia 48 hours after intramedullary rod placement for a femoral fracture shows asymmetric ground-glass and airspace opacities with small left pleural effusion.

decreased interstitial hydrostatic pressure thereby promoting transudation of fluid into the lung. There are no distinguishing radiographic features.

Amniotic Fluid Embolism. A severe and often fatal form of pulmonary edema may develop in a pregnant woman when amniotic fluid gains access to the systemic circulation during labor. There is an association of this entity with fetal distress and demise, because the mucin within fetal meconium plays a key role in the pathogenesis of this disorder. Embolic obstruction of the pulmonary vasculature by mucin and fetal squames within the amniotic fluid leads to sudden PAH and cor pulmonale with decreased cardiac output and pulmonary edema. An anaphylactoid reaction and disseminated intravascular coagulopathy (DIC) from factors within the amniotic fluid contribute to vascular collapse. Radiographically, there are typically bilateral confluent airspace opacities indistinguishable from pulmonary edema of other etiologies. In severe cases, there may be enlargement of the central pulmonary arteries and right heart as a manifestation of cor pulmonale. The diagnosis can be confirmed by identification of fetal squames and mucin in blood samples obtained from indwelling pulmonary artery catheters.

Fat Embolism. The embolization of marrow fat to the lung is a common complication occurring 24 to 72 hours after the fracture of a long bone such as the femur. Within the lung, the fat is hydrolyzed to its component fatty acids, causing increased pulmonary capillary permeability and hemorrhagic pulmonary edema. Radiographically and on CT, confluent ground-glass and airspace opacities are seen (Fig. 12.6). The diagnosis is made by recognizing findings of systemic fat embolism (petechial rash, CNS depression) and pulmonary changes in the appropriate time period following trauma. Most patients have a mild course with minimal respiratory compromise, whereas a minority will develop progressive respiratory failure leading to death.

PULMONARY HEMORRHAGE AND VASCULITIS

Hemorrhage or hemorrhagic edema of the lung can result from trauma, bleeding diathesis, infections (invasive aspergillosis, mucormycosis, *Pseudomonas,* influenza), drugs (penicillamine), PE, fat embolism, ARDS, and autoimmune diseases (Table 12.3). The autoimmune diseases associated with pulmonary hemorrhage include Goodpasture syndrome, idiopathic pulmonary hemorrhage, granulomatosis with polyangiitis, systemic lupus erythematosus, rheumatoid arthritis, and polyarteritis nodosa.

TABLE 12.3

CAUSES OF PULMONARY HEMORRHAGE

Spontaneous	Thrombocytopenia Hemophilia Anticoagulant therapy
Trauma	Pulmonary contusion
Embolic disease	Pulmonary embolism Fat embolism
Vasculitis	Autoimmune Goodpasture syndrome Idiopathic pulmonary hemorrhage Table 12.5. Antineutrophil cytoplasmic antibody (ANCA)-associated vasculitides Infectious Gram-negative bacteria Influenza Aspergillosis Mucormycosis
Drugs	Penicillamine

Goodpasture syndrome is an autoimmune disease characterized by damage to the alveolar and renal glomerular basement membranes by a cytotoxic antibody. The antibody is directed primarily against renal glomerular basement membrane and cross reacts with alveolar basement membrane to produce the renal injury and pulmonary hemorrhage characteristic of this disorder. Young adult men are most commonly affected and present with cough, hemoptysis, dyspnea, and fatigue. The pulmonary complaints usually precede clinical evidence of renal failure. Chest radiographs show bilateral coalescent airspace opacities that are radiographically indistinguishable from those of pulmonary edema (Fig. 12.7). CT scans demonstrate

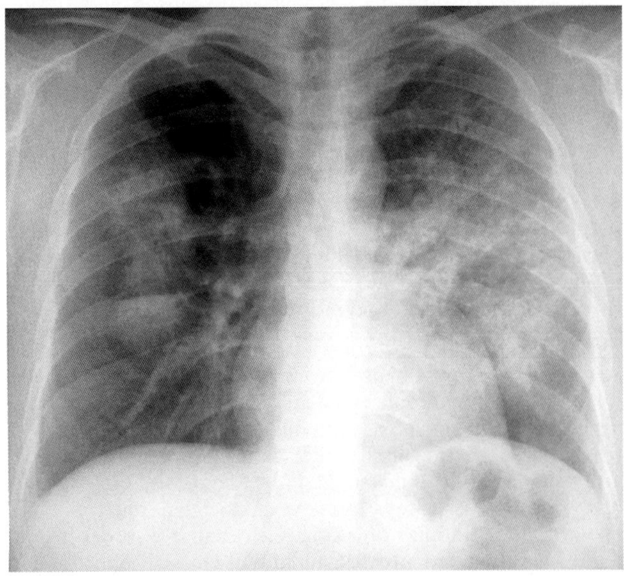

FIGURE 12.7. Frontal chest radiograph in a patient with Goodpasture syndrome shows asymmetric bilateral airspace disease representing intra-alveolar blood.

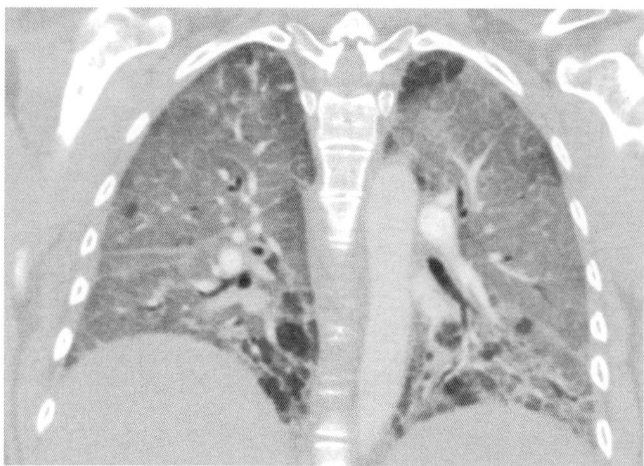

FIGURE 12.8. CT of Pulmonary Hemorrhage. Coronal CT through the posterior lungs in a patient with pulmonary hemorrhage shows extensive bilateral ground-glass opacities with associated interlobular septal thickening, producing a "crazy-paving" pattern on CT.

ground-glass and airspace opacities without interlobular septal thickening acutely. Within several days, the airspace opacities resolve, giving rise to reticular opacities in the same distribution owing to resorption of blood products into the pulmonary interstitium. This results in the so-called crazy paving pattern (Fig. 12.8). Complete radiographic resolution is seen within 2 weeks, except in those with recurrent episodes of hemorrhage, in whom the reticular opacities persist and represent pulmonary fibrosis. The diagnosis is made by immunofluorescent studies of renal or lung tissue, which show a smooth wavy line of fluorescent staining along the basement membrane. The overall prognosis is poor, although the use of immunosuppressive drugs and plasmapheresis has improved survival.

Idiopathic Pulmonary Hemorrhage. The pulmonary manifestations of idiopathic pulmonary hemorrhage are clinically and radiographically indistinguishable from those of Goodpasture syndrome. In distinction to Goodpasture syndrome, this disorder is most common in children, with an equal sex distribution. The diagnosis is one of exclusion and is suggested when pulmonary hemorrhage and anemia are found in a patient with normal renal function and urinalysis and an absence of antiglomerular basement membrane antibodies.

Other Vasculitides. Granulomatosis with polyangiitis, systemic lupus erythematosus, rheumatoid arthritis, and polyarteritis nodosa are autoimmune disorders associated with a systemic immune complex vasculitis. The development of pulmonary hemorrhage in these diseases is secondary to small vessel pulmonary arteritis and capillaritis, which results in spontaneous hemorrhage. The pulmonary manifestations of these diseases are discussed in subsequent sections.

Differentiation of pulmonary hemorrhage from pulmonary edema or pneumonia may be difficult, particularly because many causes of pulmonary edema and pneumonia may have a significant hemorrhagic component. The rapid development of airspace opacities associated with a dropping hematocrit and hemoptysis should suggest the diagnosis. Hemoptysis, however, is not always present. Associated renal disease, hematuria, or findings of a collagen vascular disorder or systemic vasculitis may provide additional clues. The distinction of pulmonary hemorrhage from pneumonia is made by the absence of fever or purulent sputum and the finding of a normal or elevated carbon monoxide–diffusing capacity. This latter determination is directly related to the volume of gas exchanging intravascular and extravascular intrapulmonary red blood cells and is therefore elevated in pulmonary hemorrhage or hemorrhagic edema but decreased in pneumonia. The presence of hemosiderin-laden macrophages in sputum, bronchoalveolar lavage fluid, or tissue specimens is evidence of chronic or recurrent intrapulmonary hemorrhage. A rapid radiographic improvement of the airspace opacities in pulmonary hemorrhage is common and may aid in diagnosis.

PULMONARY EMBOLISM

PE is a common cause of acute chest symptoms. While it is associated with significant morbidity and mortality, treatment with anticoagulation can significantly reduce the likelihood of recurrent emboli that might result in chronic thromboembolic pulmonary hypertension (CTPH) or death. Since anticoagulation has associated morbidity, particularly in elderly and debilitated patients, an accurate determination of the presence or absence of PE is necessary.

The radiologist plays a central role in the diagnostic evaluation of the patient with suspected PE. This section will briefly review the aspects of patient evaluation not related to imaging and then detail the various imaging modalities available to the radiologist.

Clinical and Laboratory Findings. The majority of patients with PE have a variety of nonspecific symptoms, including dyspnea (84%), pleuritic chest pain (74%), anxiety (59%), and cough (53%), and in some patients asymptomatic embolization can occur. Physical examination may reveal tachypnea (respiratory rate >16/min), rales, and a prominent pulmonary component of the second heart sound.

The main laboratory test obtained in patients with suspected PE is a plasma D-dimer level. D-dimer is a degradation product of fibrin and is a very sensitive indicator of the presence of venous thrombosis. Enzyme-linked immunosorbent assay D-dimer measurements have a sensitivity for deep venous thrombosis (DVT) of 98% to 100%, and therefore a normal value will effectively exclude the possibility of DVT and PE, particularly when the clinical probability for PE is low.

Radiologic Evaluation. A number of imaging techniques can be employed in the evaluation of the patient with suspected PE. These include the chest radiograph, ventilation/perfusion (V/Q) lung scintigraphy, CT angiography, and conventional pulmonary angiography. Noninvasive methods of imaging DVTs include compression and Doppler US of the legs, lower extremity indirect CT venography (CTV), and magnetic resonance venography of the extremities and pelvis. The relatively noninvasive nature and high accuracy of these techniques to diagnose DVT and an increasing familiarity with their performance and interpretation among radiologists have led to their widespread use in the workup of PE. The American College of Radiology has developed appropriateness guidelines for utilization of imaging studies in evaluation of patients with suspected PE.

Chest radiography is the first examination obtained in all patients with suspected PE and has an ACR appropriateness rating of 9 in all clinical scenarios. Although the majority of patients with PE will have abnormal radiographs, a significant percentage of patients will have normal chest radiographs. The radiographic findings include cardiac, pulmonary arterial, parenchymal, pleural, and diaphragmatic changes.

Cardiac enlargement, or more precisely right heart enlargement, is an uncommon finding seen with massive or extensive PE producing cor pulmonale. Enlargement of the central pulmonary arteries from PAH may also be seen but is more commonly a late sequela of chronic thromboembolic disease. The most common radiographic findings in PE without infarction are peripheral airspace opacities and linear atelectasis. Localized peripheral oligemia with or without distended proximal vessels (Westermark sign) is exceedingly rare. The airspace opacification represents localized pulmonary hemorrhage produced by bronchial and pulmonary venous collateral flow to the obstructed region and is seen with peripheral but not central emboli. Volume loss in the lower lung from adhesive atelectasis caused by ischemic injury to type 2 pneumocytes and secondary surfactant deficiency may produce diaphragmatic elevation and the development of linear atelectasis.

Less than 10% of all PEs result in lung infarction. Collateral bronchial arterial and retrograde pulmonary venous flow prevent infarction in most patients. The distinction between embolism with and without infarction is usually impossible radiographically and is of limited importance, as treatment is identical. Infarction from embolism occurs with greater frequency in patients with underlying heart failure because of their limited collateral bronchial arterial flow to the ischemic region. In PEs with infarction, the cardiac, pulmonary arterial, and peripheral vascular changes are indistinguishable from those seen in embolism without infarction.

Radiographic features that suggest infarction include the presence of a pleural effusion and the development of a pleura-based wedge-shaped opacity (Hampton hump). This opacity, typically found in the posterior or lateral costophrenic sulcus of the lung, is wedge shaped, homogeneous, and lacks an air bronchogram. The blunted apex of the wedge points toward the occluded feeding vessel, whereas the base is against the pleural surface (Fig. 12.9). It is often obscured by surrounding areas of hemorrhage in the early phases following infarction, but becomes more obvious with time as the peripheral areas of hemorrhage resolve. A distinction between PE with and without infarction is usually made by noting changes in the radiographic opacities with time. In embolism without infarction, the airspace opacities should resolve completely within 7 to 10 days, whereas infarcts resolve over the course of several weeks or months and usually leave a residual linear parenchymal scar and/or localized pleural thickening.

None of the aforementioned radiographic findings, either alone or in combination, are useful in making a firm diagnosis of PE. Conversely, a completely normal radiograph may be seen in up to 40% of patients with emboli. The prime utility of the chest radiograph in the evaluation of PE is to identify conditions that mimic PE clinically, such as pneumonia or pneumothorax, and as an aid to the interpretation of the ventilation/perfusion lung scan.

Ventilation/Perfusion (V/Q) Lung Scintigraphy. The IV administration of macroaggregated albumin radiolabeled with technetium (Tc-99m) has long been used to assess the patency of the pulmonary circulation. The sensitivity of this technique allows for the confident exclusion of PE when a technically adequate perfusion scan is normal. The addition of ventilation scanning increases the specificity of an abnormal perfusion scan and is always performed in conjunction with the perfusion scan when possible.

V/Q scanning is no longer commonly used, however, in the evaluation of the patient with suspected PE for a number of reasons including the low likelihood of either a normal or high-probability study—a result that clinicians can confidently rely upon to guide treatment decisions; significant inter-observer variability in the interpretation of V/Q studies; and the high accuracy of CT angiography in detecting pulmonary emboli. The ACR gives V/Q scanning an appropriateness score of 7 in a patient with high pretest probability, but only 2 with low pretest probability or negative D-dimer. Because the radiation dose to the breast is less with V/Q scanning than with CT angiography, the combined American Thoracic Society/Society for Thoracic Radiology Task Force now recommends it as the first imaging study in pregnant women with a normal chest radiograph. The same consideration could apply to young individuals with high pretest probability, normal chest radiographs, and no history of chronic pulmonary disease (ACR score = 7). It is also an option in patients with severe risk of adverse reaction to contrast material.

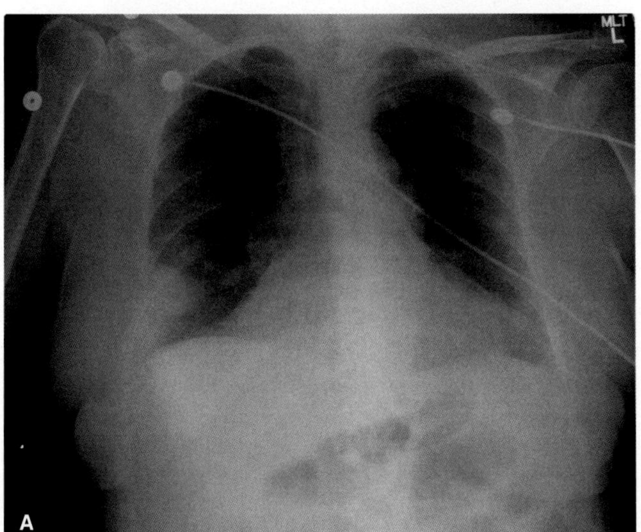

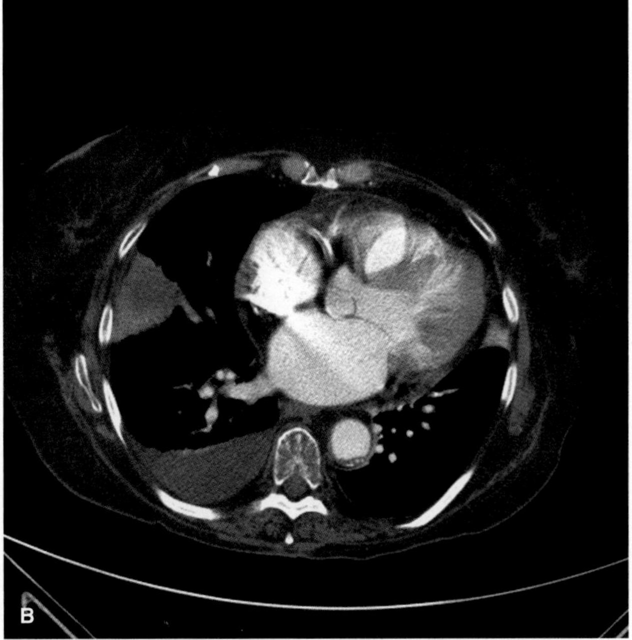

FIGURE 12.9. **Pulmonary Infarct Secondary to Acute Pulmonary Embolism. A:** Frontal chest radiograph shows a wedge-shaped area of consolidation in the periphery of the right lung. **B:** Axial CT shows wedge-shaped, pleural-based consolidation with central hypoattenuation consistent with early necrosis.

CT Pulmonary Angiography. CT angiography of the pulmonary arteries (CTPA) using MDCT is currently the recommended study for detection of PE (ACR score of 9 in patients with high pretest probability, 5 in patients with low pretest probability, and 7 in pregnant patients). Not only is accuracy high for detection of pulmonary emboli, but a negative study has a high negative predictive value for near-term pulmonary thromboembolic events.

Contiguous or overlapping 1- to 2-mm scans through the entire thorax during injection of 80 to 120 mL of 300 to 350 mg I(iodine)/mL nonionic contrast injected through an 18-gauge or larger IV catheter at 5 mL/s allow routine dense opacification of second- and third-order subsegmental pulmonary arteries. Scanning during expiratory phase of respiration has been shown to decrease the number of inadequate scans although makes evaluation of the pulmonary parenchyma more difficult. Scans must be interpreted on workstations in a paging or cine mode to allow efficient review and accurate interpretation of the large data sets produced by the current 64- to 256-channel MDCT scanners.

Acute emboli are recognized as intraluminal filling defects (Fig. 12.10) or nonopacified vessels with a convex filling toward the proximal lumen. Secondary findings that can be seen on CT include peripheral oligemia (Westermark sign), pleura-based wedge-shaped consolidation reflecting peripheral hemorrhage or infarct, linear atelectasis, and pleural effusion. The detection of a high-attenuation thrombus in the pulmonary arteries on unenhanced CT in patients with PE has been rarely described. Chronic emboli should be suggested when the filling defect is adherent to the vessel wall rather than in the center of the lumen or when a web is present (Fig. 12.11). Common diagnostic pitfalls in the detection of PE on CTPA include motion artifact, streak artifact from dense contrast or catheters, partial volume averaging of obliquely oriented vessels, prominent hilar lymphoid tissue, poorly opacified pulmonary veins, mucus-filled bronchi, and regional areas of increased pulmonary arterial resistance from consolidation or atelectasis, all of which can simulate intraluminal arterial filling defects.

At present MDCT is widely considered the first-line diagnostic modality for the evaluation of suspected PE. Confident detection of a discrete intraluminal filling defect is highly specific for PE. Conversely, multiple studies have shown that the negative predictive value of a good quality CTPA for PE is greater than 95%.

Although the ability to detect small emboli has improved significantly with MDCT, the main limitation of CTPA remains the reliable detection of small (subsegmental) emboli, although the frequency and clinical significance of such emboli are subjects of significant debate. In addition to the detection of emboli, up to two-thirds of patients with acute chest symptoms who are studied with CTPA to exclude PE have an alternative diagnosis suggested by findings detected on CT, something not possible with techniques such as perfusion scintigraphy, MR angiography, and conventional angiography that only assess the pulmonary vasculature.

Pulmonary angiography was traditionally considered to be the gold standard in the diagnosis of PE, but has been almost

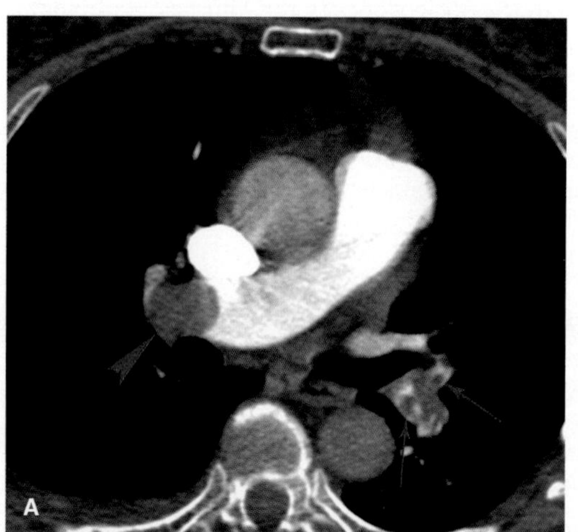

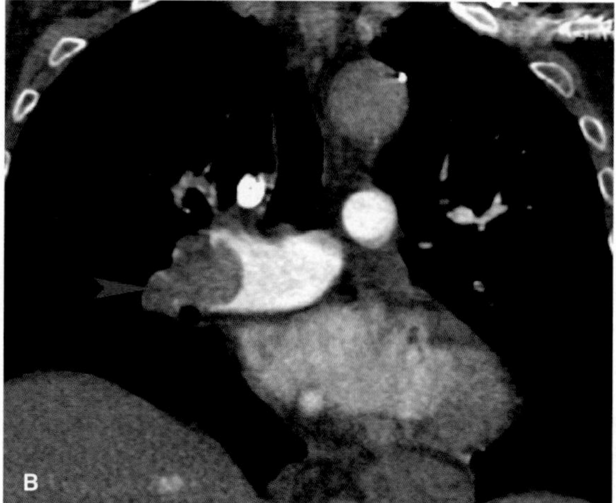

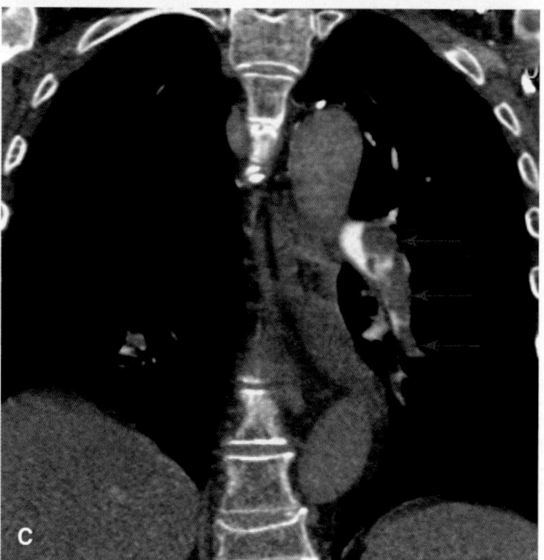

FIGURE 12.10. **Pulmonary Embolism on CT Angiography.** Axial (**A** and **B**) and coronal (**C**) reconstructed images from a CT pulmonary angiogram show nearly occlusive thrombus in the right main pulmonary artery (*arrowheads*) and the left lower lobe pulmonary artery and its branches (*arrows*).

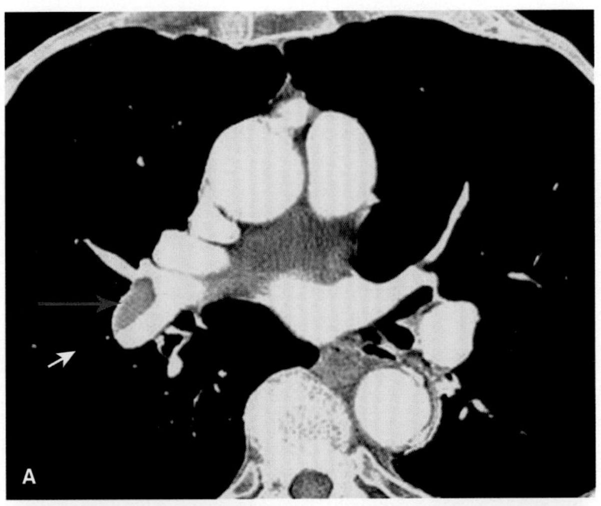

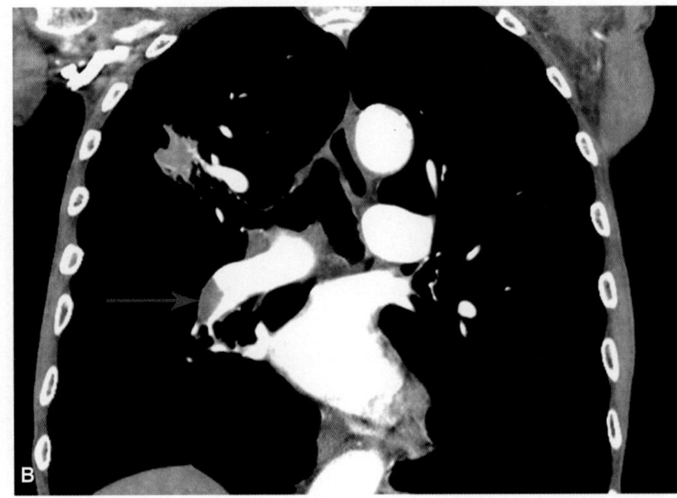

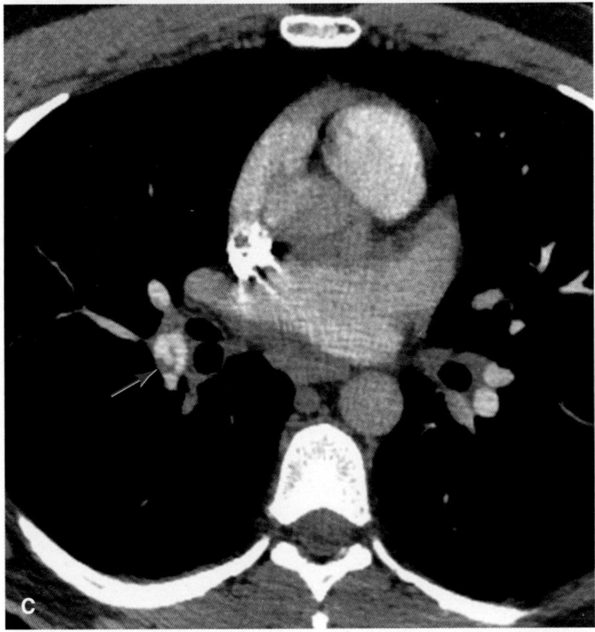

FIGURE 12.11. Chronic Pulmonary Emboli. CT pulmonary angiogram in axial (**A**) and coronal (**B**) planes demonstrate a large filling defect (*arrows*) adherent to the anterolateral wall of the pulmonary artery to the right lower lobe. (**C**) Axial scan in a different patient demonstrates a linear defect in the right interlobar artery (*arrow*).

entirely supplanted by CTA. Digital subtraction angiography is the technique selectively used when a definitive diagnosis of PE or DVT cannot be achieved by less invasive means. This study, which requires right heart and pulmonary arterial catheterization with selective injection of nonionic contrast, can be performed safely in a majority of patients. The accuracy of pulmonary arteriography in the diagnosis of PE is high. On the basis of clinical follow-up of patients with negative studies, the sensitivity of pulmonary angiography is 98% to 99%, although as with CTPA, the accuracy for the detection of subsegmental PE is closer to 66%.

PE is diagnosed on pulmonary angiography when an intraluminal filling defect or the trailing end of an occluding thrombus is outlined by contrast. Secondary signs, including a prolonged arterial phase, diminished peripheral perfusion, and delay in the venous phase, are nonspecific and are not used to diagnose PE. Once a thrombus is unequivocally identified, the study is terminated. The only exception would be a patient who is considered a candidate for surgical thrombectomy or thrombolytic therapy, where precise knowledge of the laterality, location, and extent of the thrombus is required.

Noninvasive Imaging for DVT. The use of noninvasive techniques for the diagnosis of DVT is an important component of the evaluation of pulmonary thromboembolic disease (see Chapter 34), as 90% of PEs arise from the lower extremities and because the treatment for proximal (i.e., above-the-knee) DVT is identical to that for proven PE. A confident diagnosis of proximal DVT can provide an endpoint in the evaluation of thromboembolic disease.

When performed by skilled personnel, compression US has a sensitivity of 90% to 95% and a specificity of 95% to 98% for the diagnosis of acute DVT when compared to contrast venography.

Indirect CTV, typically performed after contrast injection has been administered for CTPA, has been used to allow detection of thigh and pelvic DVT. Axial or helical scans performed from the popliteal fossa to the diaphragm obtained approximately 3 minutes after the initiation of contrast injection for CTPA have been shown in preliminary studies to have a high accuracy in the detection of proximal lower extremity and pelvic DVT. The addition of CTV to CTPA can provide incremental information for the diagnosis of venous thromboembolic disease, particularly when a proximal DVT is detected

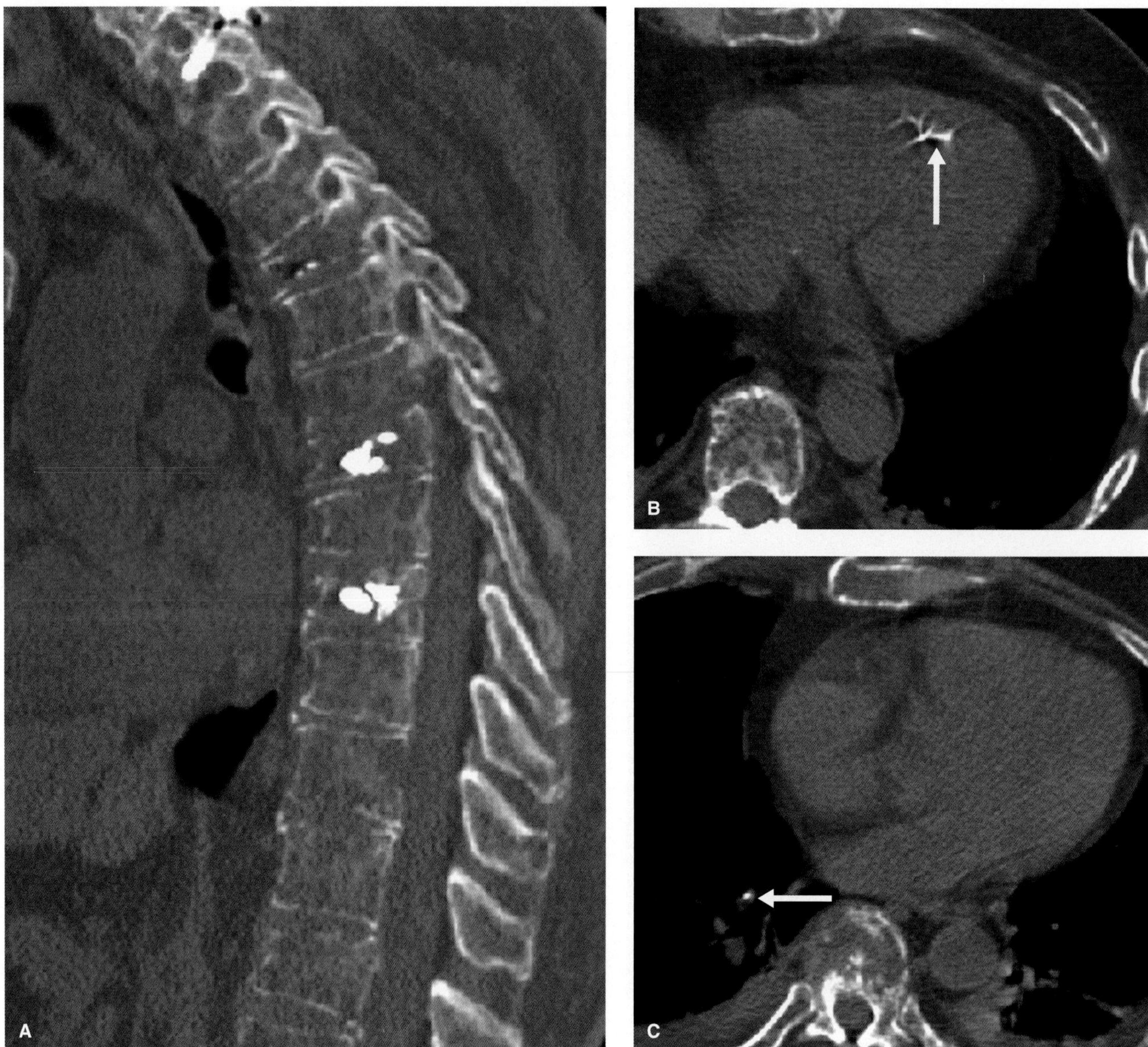

FIGURE 12.12. Embolized Methyl Methacrylate Following Vertebroplasty. A: Sagittal reconstruction through the thoracic spine shows severe osteoporosis, multilevel vertebral height loss and bone cement in three vertebral bodies. **B:** Noncontrast scan at the level of the ventricles shows bone cement in the right ventricular apex (*arrow*). **C:** Scan at a slightly lower level shows cement in a branch of the posterobasal segment artery (*arrow*).

in a patient with a poor-quality, equivocal, or negative CTPA study. MR venography and radionuclide scintigraphy can be used to detect DVT, but these are not used routinely in clinical practice for this purpose.

Nonthrombotic pulmonary embolism can rarely occur. The most commonly described conditions are: (1) air embolism, usually as a result of air within a venous catheter or air injected during contrast-enhanced CT; (2) macroscopic fat embolism following long bone fracture, with pulmonary embolization of marrow elements; (3) methylmethacrylate embolization complicating vertebroplasty (Fig. 12.12); and (4) radioactive seed implant embolization from prostate brachytherapy.

Pulmonary tumor emboli can develop in a small percentage of patients with malignancies such as renal cell carcinoma, breast cancer, hepatocellular carcinoma, and GI malignancy. These tumor emboli may lead to significant respiratory symptoms because of occlusion of small vessels. Imaging features are uncommon but include central pulmonary arterial dilation and enlarged, nodular peripheral pulmonary artery branches on thin-section CT (Fig. 12.13).

PULMONARY ARTERIAL HYPERTENSION

PAH is defined as a systolic pressure in the pulmonary artery exceeding 30 mm Hg either measured directly by right heart catheterization or as estimated by echocardiography. The diagnosis of PAH is usually evident from the clinical history, physical findings, and appearance on chest radiographs. The typical radiographic findings of PAH are enlarged main and hilar pulmonary arteries that taper rapidly toward the lung periphery (Fig. 12.14). Associated enlargement of the RV, seen on lateral radiographs as prominence of the anterosuperior cardiac

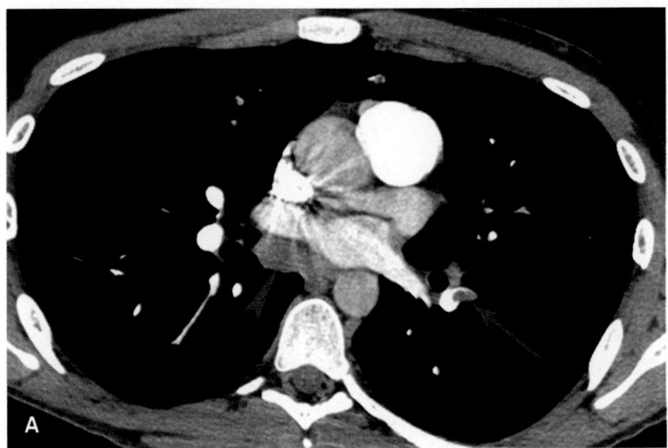

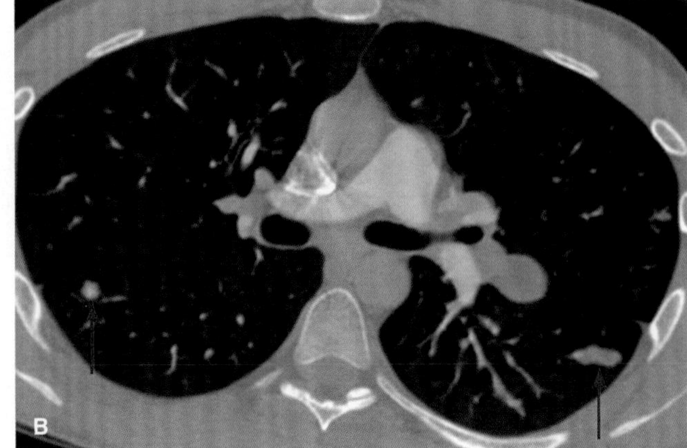

FIGURE 12.13. Pulmonary Tumor Emboli From Metastatic Renal Cell Carcinoma. A: Axial CT image shows a filling defect (*arrow*) representing a tumor embolus in the artery to the anteromedial basal segment artery of the left lower lobe. An enlarged subcarinal lymph node (*arrowhead*) is also present. **B:** Round and ovoid metastases (*arrows*) to the lung are present in the superior segments.

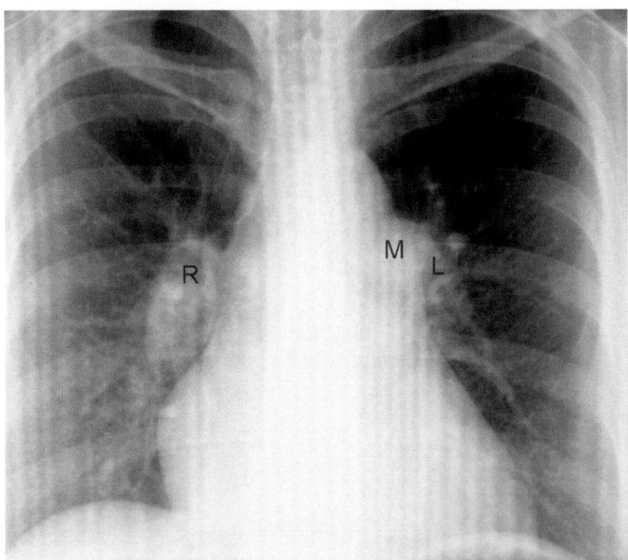

FIGURE 12.14. Pulmonary Arterial Hypertension. Posteroanterior chest radiograph in a 29-year-old woman with idiopathic pulmonary hypertension shows enlarged main (M), right (R), and left (L) pulmonary arteries with diminutive peripheral vessels.

margin with obliteration of the retrosternal airspace, is an additional clue to the diagnosis. Occasionally, hypertension-induced atherosclerotic lesions in the large elastic pulmonary arteries can produce mural calcification on radiography or CT, a rare finding that is relatively specific for PAH. A useful measurement for enlargement of the central pulmonary arteries, usually indicating PAH in the absence of a left-to-right shunt, is a transverse diameter of the proximal interlobar pulmonary artery on posteroanterior chest radiograph that exceeds 16 mm. CT measurement of the main pulmonary artery is even more useful. In patients younger than 50 years, a ratio of the diameter of the main pulmonary artery (measured at the level of the main right pulmonary artery) to the transverse diameter of the ascending aorta at the same level greater than 1 strongly correlates with a mean pulmonary artery pressure greater than 20 mm Hg. Because the aorta normally enlarges with advancing age, in patients older than 50 years, a maximum transverse measurement of the main pulmonary artery greater than 29 mm correlates better (Fig. 12.15). All of this assumes that the patient does not have pulmonary overcirculation, in which case the peripheral vessels will also be enlarged. Flattening or bowing of the interventricular septum toward the LV indicates RV hypertension. A normal measurement of the main or right interlobar pulmonary artery does not exclude PAH, as patients with mild or even moderate elevation of pulmonary artery pressure may have normal-sized

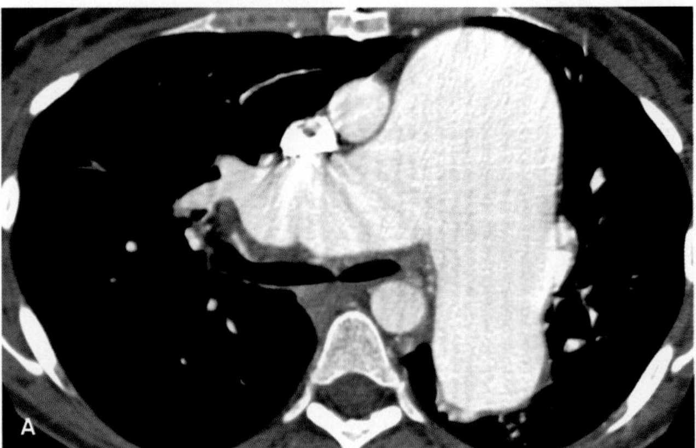

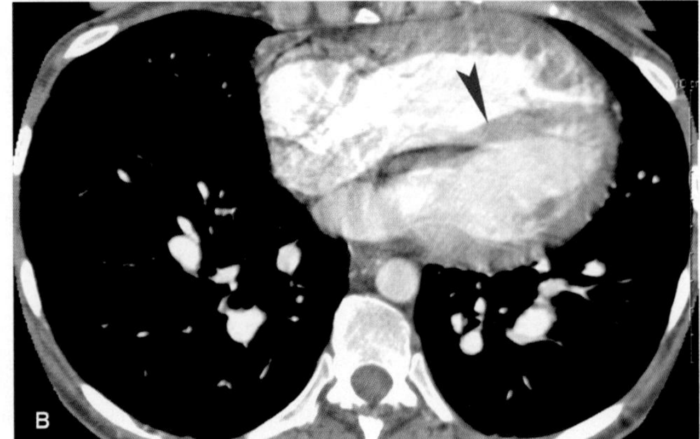

FIGURE 12.15. Pulmonary Arterial Hypertension. Axial CT scans through at the level of the main pulmonary arteries (**A**) and the ventricles (**B**) show marked enlargement of the pulmonary trunk and both main pulmonary arteries. Flattening of the interventricular septum (*arrowhead*) indicates high right ventricular pressure.

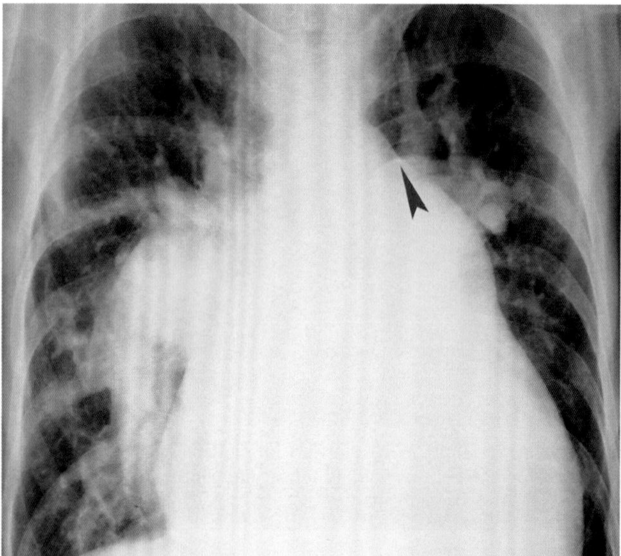

FIGURE 12.16. **Acquired Eisenmenger Syndrome.** A frontal radiograph of a 56-year-old man with an atrial septal defect shows massive enlargement of the central pulmonary arteries and heart with "pruning" of the peripheral vessels and calcium in the left pulmonary artery (*arrowhead*) consistent with high pulmonary arterial resistance.

arteries. Those patients with long-standing PAH will develop RV hypertrophy, with eventual RV dilatation and right heart failure (cor pulmonale). MR may also demonstrate intraluminal signal during the early diastolic phase of the cardiac cycle, a finding indicative of turbulent flow caused by the increased vascular resistance that is sometimes seen with marked elevation of pulmonary artery pressure.

In addition to PAH, enlargement of the central pulmonary arteries may be seen in conditions associated with increased flow through the pulmonary circulation. This occurs in patients with a high cardiac output, such as anemia, those

TABLE 12.4

CAUSES OF PULMONARY ARTERIAL HYPERTENSION

Chronic pulmonary venous hypertension

Lung disease/chronic hypoxemia
  Emphysema/chronic bronchitis
  Cystic lung disease
    Langerhans cell histiocytosis
    Lymphangioleiomyomatosis
  Cystic fibrosis
  Interstitial fibrosis
    Usual interstitial pneumonitis
    Sarcoidosis
    Radiation fibrosis (rare)
  Small airways disease

Constrictive bronchiolitis

Chronic hypoventilation
  Obesity and obstructive sleep apnea
  Chest wall deformity (kyphoscoliosis)

Idiopathic (primary) pulmonary hypertension
Eisenmenger syndrome

Pulmonary vasculitis (plexogenic pulmonary arteriopathy)
  Connective tissue diseases (scleroderma, lupus, mixed connective tissue disease)
  ANCA-positive vasculitis (see Table 12.5)
  HIV infection

Drugs (fenfluramine, dexfenfluramine, "fen-phen")
Chronic pulmonary thromboembolic disease

ANCA-positive vasculitis
  Granulomatosis with polyangiitis
  Eosinophilic granulomatosis with polyangiitis (Churg–Strauss syndrome)
  Microscopic polyangiitis
  Drug-induced vasculitis

ANCA, antineutrophil cytoplasmic antibody.

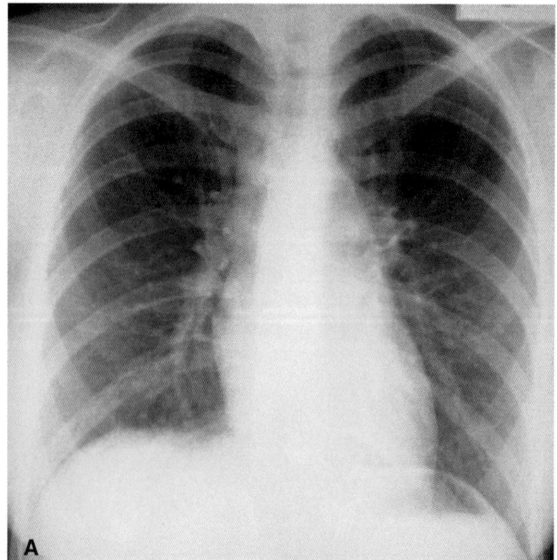

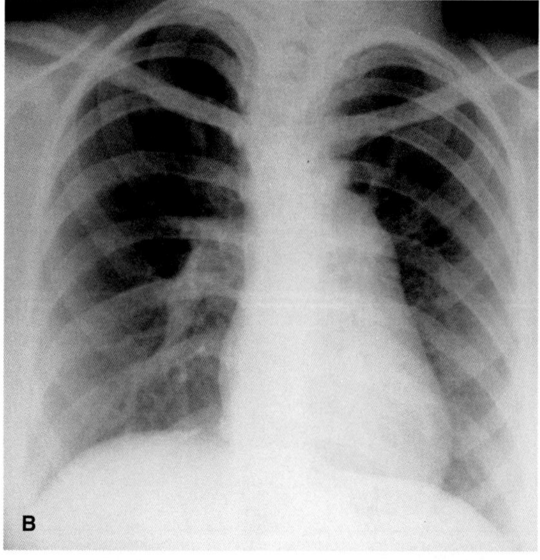

FIGURE 12.17. **Congenital Eisenmenger Syndrome. A:** Frontal chest radiograph in a 19-year-old woman with complete atrioventricular canal. The chest radiograph is normal except for mild prominence of the pulmonary trunk, which could be normal for a patient this age. The history of cyanosis since early childhood strongly suggests congenitally elevated pulmonary arterial resistance. Pulmonary artery pressure was suprasystemic. **B:** Frontal radiograph in a 16-year-old girl with a ventricular septal defect shows an enlarged pulmonary trunk and slightly prominent right pulmonary artery.

TABLE 12.5

ANTINEUTROPHIL CYTOPLASMIC ANTIBODY (ANCA)-ASSOCIATED VASCULITIDES

Antineutrophil cytoplasmic antibody (ANCA) positive vasculitis
Granulomatosis with polyangiitis
Eosinophilic granulomatosis with polyangiitis (Churg–Strauss syndrome)
Microscopic polyangiitis
Drug-induced vasculitis

with thyrotoxicosis, or those with left-to-right shunts. The latter includes atrial and ventricular septal defects, patent ductus arteriosus, and partial anomalous pulmonary venous return. Early in the course of left-to-right shunts, the pulmonary artery pressure is normal or slightly elevated, because pulmonary vascular resistance drops to compensate for the increased flow. In these patients, there is enlargement of both central and peripheral pulmonary arteries, producing "shunt vascularity" on chest radiographs. If uncorrected, some of these individuals will develop muscular hypertrophy of the pulmonary arterioles with medial hyperplasia and intimal fibrosis causing an increase in pulmonary vascular resistance (Eisenmenger syndrome). These patients have typically very large hearts owing to long-standing overcirculation with superimposed pulmonary hypertension (Fig. 12.16). Many patients with Eisenmenger physiology have high pulmonary resistance and are cyanotic since early childhood. They typically present with relatively unimpressive chest radiographs with a normal heart size and slightly enlarged pulmonary trunk (Fig. 12.17).

An increase in resistance to pulmonary blood flow is the most common cause of PAH (Table 12.4). The most common causes are parenchymal lung disease and obesity hypoventilation syndrome. Other causes include severe chest wall deformity, diffuse pleural fibrosis, recurrent PE, pulmonary vasculitis (e.g., lupus and scleroderma), and idiopathic (primary) pulmonary hypertension. Chronic elevation of pulmonary venous pressure can also result in PAH. This is most commonly the result of mitral stenosis, although any impedance to pulmonary venous return to the left heart can produce venous hypertension. Less common entities in this group include left atrial tumor, cor triatriatum, pulmonary

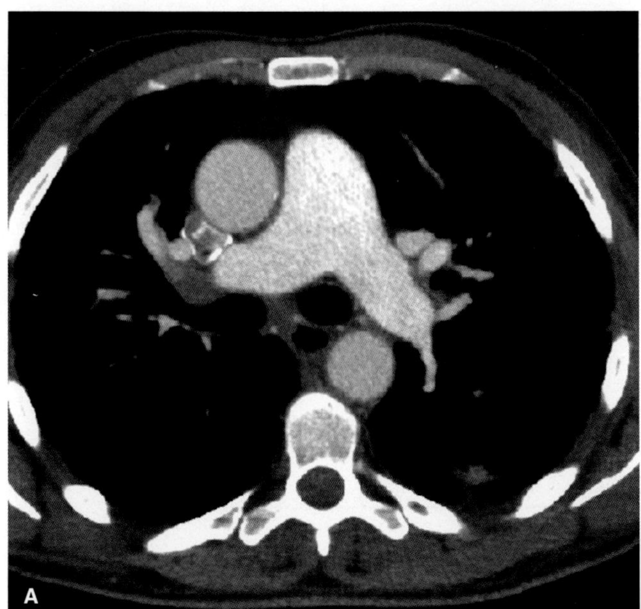

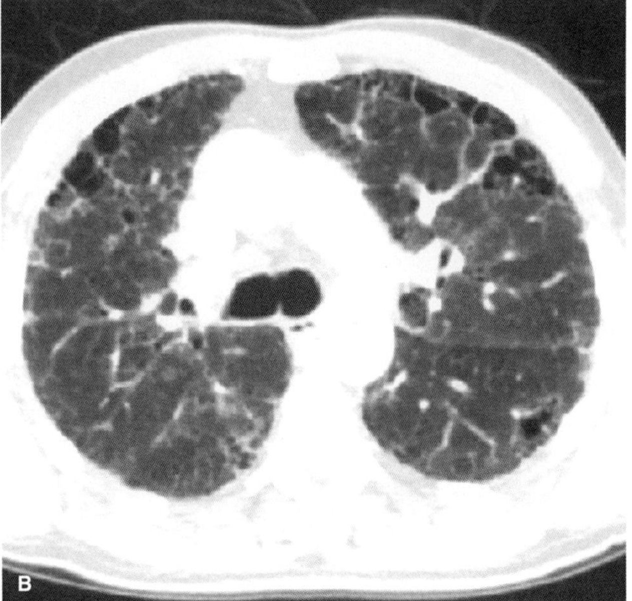

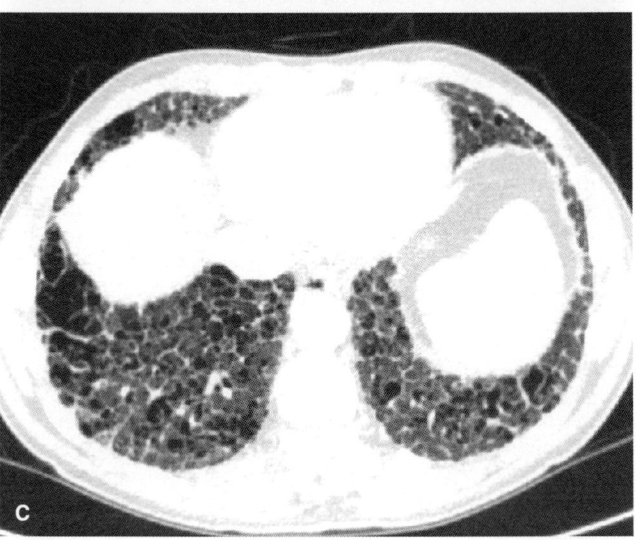

FIGURE 12.18. **Pulmonary Arterial Hypertension in a Patient With Somewhat Atypical Appearing Usual Interstitial Pneumonia. A:** Contrast-enhanced CT at the level of the main pulmonary artery demonstrates enlargement of the pulmonary trunk and right and left main pulmonary arteries. Scans at the level of the carina (**B**) and lung bases (**C**) show widespread interstitial thickening, ground-glass opacities, and early honeycomb cyst formation with a basilar predominance.

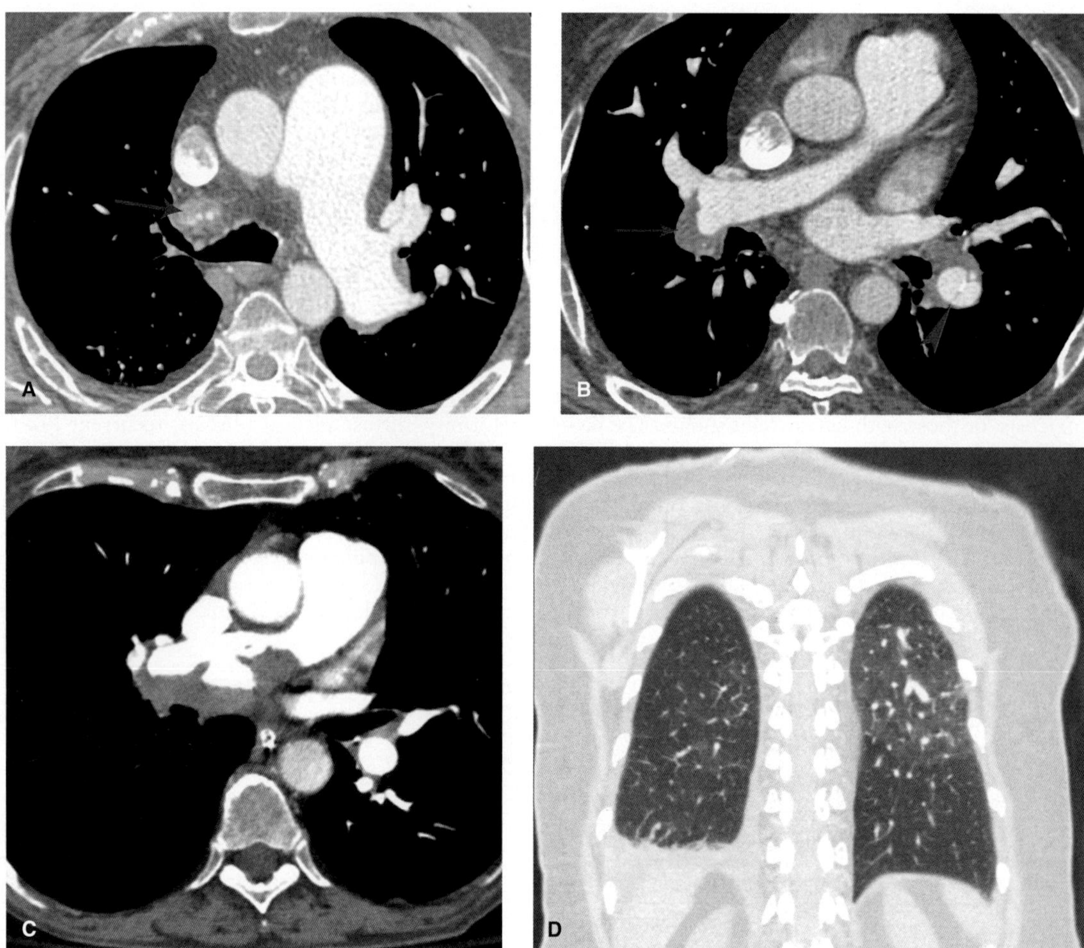

FIGURE 12.19. Chronic Thromboembolic Pulmonary Hypertension (CTEPH). A: Enhanced CT scan at the level of the main pulmonary artery shows dilated main and left pulmonary arteries, with thrombosis of the truncus anterior branch of the right pulmonary artery (*arrow*). **B:** At the level of the hila, there is an eccentric filling defect (*arrow*) in the right interlobar artery and a web-like filling defect (*arrowhead*) containing calcification in the left interlobar artery. These findings are characteristic of chronic unresolved emboli. **C:** Different patient with CTEPH. Axial scan at the level of the central pulmonary arteries demonstrates extensive chronic clot in the right main pulmonary artery and an enlarged pulmonary trunk. **D:** Coronal reconstruction through the posterior lungs in a third patient demonstrates a large area of decreased perfusion in the lower portion of the lung with engorgement of vessels in the upper portion of the lung.

vein stenosis or occlusion, and pulmonary venoocclusive disease (PVOD). Chronic LV failure rarely, if ever, results in PAH owing to relatively short chronicity. An important clue to the presence of mitral stenosis is enlargement of the LA and appendage. Unfortunately, the pulmonary trunk may be enlarged in patients with LV failure from ischemic heart disease owing to concomitant emphysema.

Parenchymal lung disease, particularly emphysema and diffuse interstitial fibrosis, are common causes of PAH. The mechanisms by which these disorders produce increased vascular resistance include chronic hypoxemia and reflex vasoconstriction and the development of irreversible changes in pulmonary arteriolar caliber, with widespread obliteration of the pulmonary vascular bed. The radiographic findings of emphysema and interstitial fibrosis are usually evident radiographically by the time PAH has developed (Fig. 12.18).

Chronic hypoxemia from alveolar hypoventilation is the likely mechanism for PAH that complicates pleural fibrosis, kyphoscoliosis, and the obesity hypoventilation syndrome. Pleural thickening and kyphoscoliosis are readily evident radiographically. The obesity hypoventilation (obstructive sleep apnea) syndrome is usually associated with marked truncal obesity and lungs that are diminished in volume (mostly owing to diaphragmatic elevation) but are normal in appearance.

Disorders of the pulmonary arteries that produce PAH include chronic PEs, vasculitis, and pulmonary arteriopathy resulting from long-standing increased pulmonary blood flow from left-to-right shunt. Occlusion of lobar and segmental vessels producing PAH can result from failure of pulmonary thromboemboli to lyse or completely recanalize (Fig. 12.19). Rarely, pulmonary vasculitis resulting from diseases such as rheumatoid lung disease or Takayasu arteritis produces obliteration of the pulmonary vasculature and leads to PAH.

CT angiographic findings of CTPH correlate with conventional angiographic findings and include focal stenoses, bandlike or weblike filling defects, and eccentric wall thickening (Figs. 12.11 and 12.19). Lung windows in patients with CTPH classically demonstrate a pattern of mosaic attenuation, with the hyperlucent regions demonstrating attenuated vascular markings (mosaic oligemia) as compared to areas of increased attenuation that result from hyperemia from intact pulmonary artery branches.

Idiopathic or primary pulmonary hypertension encompasses diseases of the pulmonary arterioles and venules that are not attributable to other etiologies and have characteristic histologic findings. *Plexogenic pulmonary arteriopathy, recurrent microscopic PE,* and *PVOD* are the three diseases that

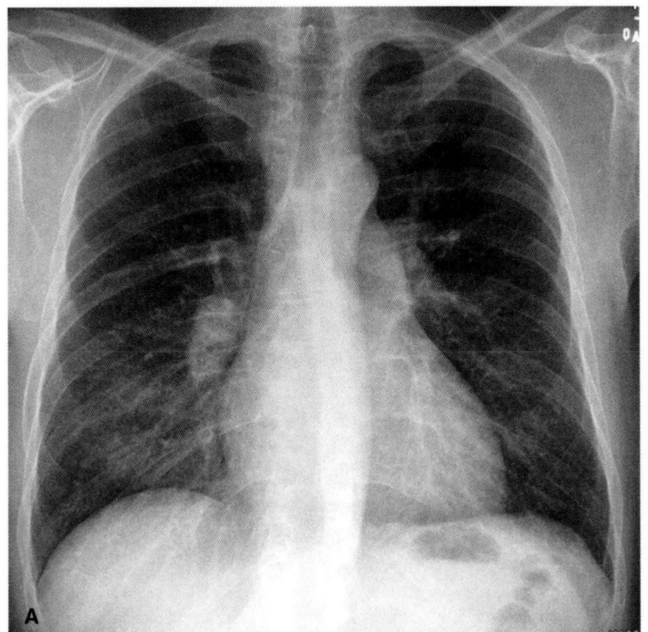

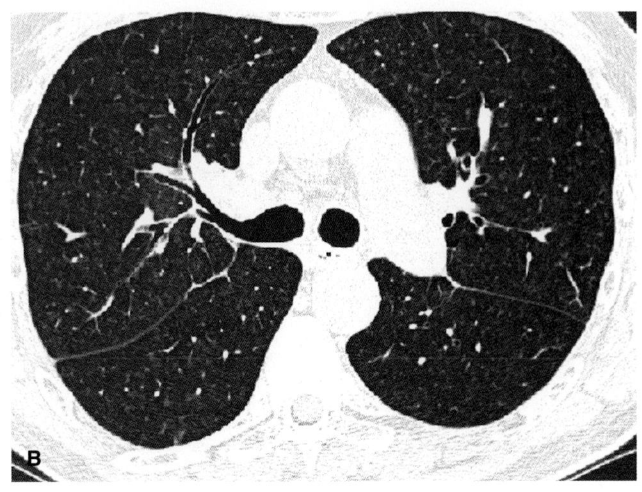

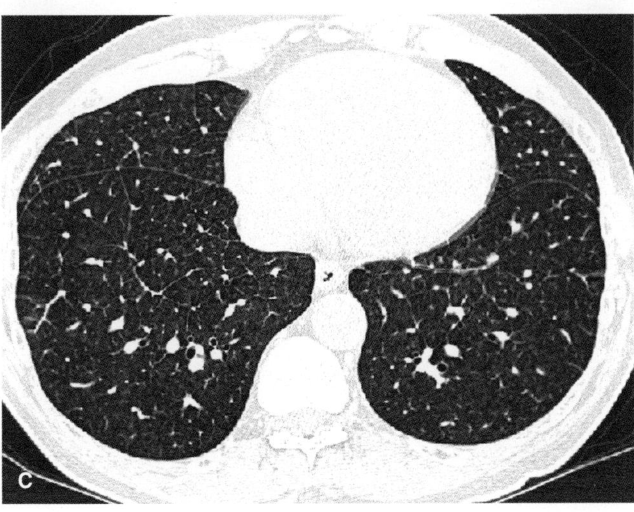

FIGURE 12.20. **Pulmonary Venoocclusive Disease. A:** Frontal chest radiograph shows enlargement of the central pulmonary arteries, normal size to small peripheral vessels and Kerley B-lines in the bases. Axial thin-section CT scans at the carina (**B**) and mid-heart (**C**) levels demonstrate diffuse centrilobular ground-glass nodules and interlobular septal thickening.

comprise this category. Plexogenic pulmonary arteriopathy is a disease among young women in whom medial hypertrophy and intimal fibrosis obliterate the muscular arteries. Dilated vascular channels within the periphery of the obliterated vessel produce the plexogenic lesions seen on biopsy in virtually all patients with this disease. Progressive dyspnea and fatigue develop with characteristic physical findings of PAH and cor pulmonale. In plexogenic pulmonary arteriopathy, pulmonary perfusion scans typically show normal perfusion or small, nonsegmental peripheral perfusion defects, allowing distinction from large-vessel thromboembolic disease. Microembolic disease is clinically and radiographically indistinguishable from plexogenic arteriopathy. In this entity, plexogenic lesions within arterioles are absent. Perfusion scans are more likely to show small perfusion defects in this disorder. The presence of small microemboli histologically is not a distinguishing feature, because in situ thrombosis within diseased arterioles can have a similar appearance.

In PVOD (Fig. 12.20), the obliteration of small intrapulmonary venules results in interstitial pulmonary edema. A condition related to PVOD is *pulmonary capillary hemangiomatosis* (PCH), which is characterized by the proliferation of capillaries throughout the pulmonary interstitium, resulting in venular obstruction. The transmission of increased pressure to the arterial side leads to medial hypertrophy and obliteration of vessel lumina with resultant arterial hypertension. Risk factors for PVOD/PCH include administration of chemotherapeutic agents, exposure to organic solvents, and systemic sclerosis. An autosomal recessive familial form due to an EIF2AK4 mutation has also been identified.

The diagnosis of PVOD/PCH and its distinction from idiopathic PH is important as the clinical course of PVOD/PCH tends to be more aggressive and patients with PVOD/PCH treated with vasodilator therapy for PH are at risk for life-threatening pulmonary edema. Chest radiographs often show interstitial or airspace pulmonary edema with a normal heart size. Perfusion lung scanning is usually normal or shows small peripheral nonsegmental defects. The combination of pulmonary edema with a normal heart size, absent findings for PVH, normal PCWP, and the insidious onset of dyspnea should suggest this diagnosis rather than left heart failure, mitral valve disease, or large vessel pulmonary venous occlusion. Thin-section CT features of PVOD and PCH are those of PVH and include interlobular septal thickening, centrilobular nodular ground-glass opacities, and pleural effusions. A definitive diagnosis can only be made by characteristic findings on open lung biopsy. The prognosis is universally poor, with most patients succumbing to their disease within 2 years of diagnosis.

Suggested Readings

https://acsearch.acr.org/docs/69404/EvidenceTable

Buckner CB, Walker CW, Purnell GL. Pulmonary embolism: chest radiographic abnormalities. *J Thorac Imaging* 1989;4:23–27.

Frazier AA, Rosado-de-Christenson ML, Galvin JR, Fleming MV. Pulmonary angiitis and granulomatosis: radiologic-pathologic correlation. *Radiographics* 1998;18:687–710.

Gosselin MV, Rassner UA, Thieszen SL, Phillips J, Oki A. Contrast dynamics during CT pulmonary angiogram: analysis of an inspiration associated artifact. *J Thorac Imaging* 2004;19(3):1–7.

Hansell DM. Small-vessel diseases of the lung: CT-pathologic correlates. *Radiology* 2002;225:639–653.

Ketai LH, Godwin D. A new view of pulmonary edema and acute respiratory distress syndrome. *J Thorac Imaging* 1998;13:147–171.

Leung AN, Bull TM, Jaeschke R, et al. An official American Thoracic Society/Society of Thoracic Radiology clinical practice guideline: evaluation of suspected pulmonary embolism in pregnancy. *Am J Respir Crit Care Med* 2011;184:1200–1208.

Milne EN, Pistolesi M, Miniati M, Giuntini C. The radiologic distinction of cardiogenic and noncardiogenic edema. *AJR Am J Roentgenol* 1985;144:879–894.

Ng CS, Wells AU, Padley SP. A CT sign of chronic pulmonary arterial hypertension: the ratio of the main pulmonary artery to aortic diameter. *J Thorac Imaging* 1999;14:270–278.

Pistolesi M, Miniati M, Milne ENC, Giuntini C. The chest roentgenogram in pulmonary edema. *Clin Chest Med* 1985;6:315–344.

Primack SL, Miller RR, Müller NL. Diffuse pulmonary hemorrhage: clinical, pathologic and imaging features. *AJR Am J Roentgenol* 1995;164:295–300.

Remy-Jardin M, Pistolesi M, Goodman LR, et al. Management of suspected acute pulmonary embolism in the era of CT angiography: a statement from the Fleischner Society. *Radiology* 2007;245(2):315–329.

Stein PD, Athanasoulis C, Alavi A, et al. Complications and validity of pulmonary angiography in acute pulmonary embolism. *Circulation* 1992;85:462–468.

The PIOPED investigators. Value of the ventilation/perfusion scan in acute pulmonary embolism: results of the prospective investigation of pulmonary embolism diagnosis (PIOPED). *JAMA* 1990;263:2753–2759.

Tillie-Leblond I, Mastora I, Radenne F, et al. Risk of pulmonary embolism after a negative spiral CT angiogram in patients with pulmonary disease: 1-year clinical follow-up study. *Radiology* 2002;223:461–467.

CHAPTER 13 ■ PULMONARY NEOPLASMS AND NEOPLASTIC-LIKE CONDITIONS

JEFFREY S. KLEIN

THE SOLITARY PULMONARY NODULE

The radiologic evaluation of a solitary pulmonary nodule (SPN) remains one of the most common and most difficult diagnostic dilemmas in thoracic radiology (Table 13.1). The prevalence of SPNs has increased as a result of the growing use of multidetector CT and the use of low-dose CT screening for lung cancer. Before embarking on a detailed diagnostic evaluation of an SPN, one must determine whether a focal opacity seen on chest radiography is real or artifactual. When a focal opacity is detected radiographically, efforts should be made to ascertain if it is truly intrathoracic, which should begin with a careful review of a lateral radiograph to localize the opacity. Densities seen on only a single view may reflect artifacts, skin, chest wall or pleural lesions, or true intrapulmonary nodules. Occasionally, physical examination can reveal a skin lesion that accounts for the opacity. Chest fluoroscopy can be useful to help localize an opacity seen on only a single radiographic projection and can identify the opacity as within the chest wall or alternatively in the lung. If available, dual-energy chest radiography with review of the bone image can be used as a problem solving tool to identify calcified lesions such as healed rib fractures or bone islands, calcified granulomas of lung, or calcified pleural plaques that may produce a nodular opacity on frontal radiographs. Chest tomosynthesis likewise can provide coronal tomographic images that localize a focal density to the chest wall or lungs. A limited chest CT obtained without intravenous contrast focused on the area in question can definitively delineate the location and nature of a nodular radiographic opacity.

Comparison chest radiographs, when available, should be reviewed to determine if nodular opacities were evident previously. An opacity completely stable in size for more than 2 years is considered benign and obviates further evaluation. If there is any concern that a nodule previously seen has enlarged, a chest CT should be obtained for further characterization.

Once a new or enlarging SPN has been identified, the radiologist should initiate an investigation to determine whether the nodule has features that are definitely benign, highly suspicious for malignancy, or lacks clear benign or malignant features and is therefore indeterminate.

Clinical Factors. Before considering the radiologic features used to characterize a lung nodule, there are several important clinical factors to be considered. In a patient under the age of 35, particularly a nonsmoker without a history of malignancy, an SPN is invariably a granuloma, hamartoma, or an inflammatory lesion. These nodules can be followed with conventional radiography to confirm their benign nature. Patients over the age of 35, particularly those who are current or recent cigarette smokers, have a significant incidence of malignant SPNs. SPNs in a patient over 35 years of age should never be followed radiographically without tissue confirmation unless a benign pattern of calcification or the presence of intralesional fat is identified on radiographs or thin-section CT or there has been radiographically documented lack of growth over a minimum of 2 years. A history of cigarette smoking, prior lung or head and neck cancer, or asbestos exposure raises the likelihood for malignancy in a patient with an SPN. Alternatively, if the patient is from an area where histoplasmosis or tuberculosis is endemic, the likelihood of a granuloma is greater; in such patients, a conservative approach may be warranted. Finally, the finding of an SPN in a patient with an extrathoracic malignancy raises the possibility of a solitary pulmonary metastasis. An SPN that arises more than 2 years after the diagnosis of an extrathoracic malignancy and proves to be malignant is almost always a primary lung tumor rather than a metastasis; breast carcinoma and melanoma are notable exceptions to this rule.

Growth Pattern. Pulmonary malignancies grow at a relatively predictable rate. The growth rate of an SPN is usually expressed as the *doubling time* or the time it takes for a nodule to double its volume. For a sphere, this corresponds to a 26% increase in diameter. Although some benign lesions (mostly hamartomas and histoplasmomas) may exhibit a growth rate similar to that of malignant lesions, the absence of growth or an extraordinarily slow or rapid rate of growth of a solid nodule is reliable evidence that an SPN is benign. Studies have shown that lung cancer presenting as a solid SPN has a doubling time of approximately 180 days. Therefore, a doubling time of less than 1 month or greater than 2 years reliably characterizes a solid lesion as benign. Infectious lesions and rapidly growing metastases from choriocarcinoma, seminoma, or osteogenic sarcoma comprise the majority of rapidly growing solitary nodules, while lack of growth or a doubling time exceeding 2 years is seen in hamartomas and histoplasmomas. However, some malignancies such as some well-differentiated adenocarcinomas (i.e., adenocarcinoma in situ [AIS] and minimally invasive adenocarcinoma [MIA]) and carcinoid tumors may have a doubling time of greater than 2 years, particularly if the nodule is subsolid (i.e., ground glass or mixed soft tissue/ground glass) in attenuation.

In patients with clinical and imaging characteristics suggesting an indeterminate SPN, particularly lesions ≤8 mm in

TABLE 13.1

DIFFERENTIAL DIAGNOSIS OF A SOLITARY PULMONARY NODULE

■ ETIOLOGY			
Neoplasm	Benign		Hamartoma Sclerosing pneumocytoma Inflammatory myofibroblastic tumor
	Malignant	Primary	Carcinoid tumor Bronchogenic carcinoma Lymphoma (non-Hodgkin)
		Metastatic	Carcinoma Sarcoma
Infection	Bacterial		Abscess Round pneumonia Nocardiosis
	Fungal		Histoplasmoma Coccidioidoma Blastomyces
	Mycobacterial		Tuberculoma
	Parasitic		Amebic abscess Echinococcal cyst Paragonimiasis Dirofilariasis
Connective tissue disease			Granulomatosis with polyangiitis Rheumatoid nodule
Vascular			Hematoma Infarct Pulmonary artery aneurysm Arteriovenous malformation
Airway		Congenital	Bronchogenic cyst Mucocele Infected bulla Traumatic lung cyst
Miscellaneous			Amyloidoma

diameter, thin-section CT analysis of nodule volume appears to provide a noninvasive method of assessing nodule growth and determining which lesions require biopsy or resection. This technique is more accurate than cross-sectional measurements in determining nodule volume and distinguishing between growing malignant SPNs and stable benign lesions. If a decision is made to simply follow an SPN radiologically, either because of a high likelihood of benignity or because the patient cannot tolerate or refuses an invasive diagnostic procedure, the lesion should be followed by thin-section CT.

Size. Although size does not reliably discriminate benign from malignant SPNs, the larger the lesion, the greater the likelihood of malignancy. Masses exceeding 4 cm in diameter are usually malignant. However, the converse does not hold true; many pulmonary malignancies are less than 2 cm in diameter at the time of diagnosis, particularly if detected by screening chest CT. Nodules <6 mm in diameter have a less than 1% likelihood of malignancy even in high-risk patients, and, therefore, most radiologists will not recommend evaluation of such lesions unless there is a very high clinical likelihood of malignancy.

Margin (Border, Edge) Characteristics. The appearance of the margin (i.e., border or edge) of an SPN is a helpful sign in determining the nature of the lesion. The edge characteristics are best evaluated on thin-section CT, as this technique is considerably more accurate than plain radiographs. The margins of an SPN may be sharp or ill defined. A round, smooth nodule is most likely a granuloma or hamartoma, although a rare primary pulmonary malignancy such as a carcinoid tumor, adenocarcinoma, or a solitary metastasis may have a perfectly smooth margin. A notched or lobulated margin may be seen in hamartomas but malignant lesions including carcinoid tumors and some lung cancers will have a lobulated border. Pathologic examination has shown that the lobulated edge of a malignant nodule represents mounds of tumor extending into the adjacent lung. A spiculated margin is highly suspicious for malignancy (Fig. 13.1). The term *corona radiata* has been used to describe this appearance, in which linear densities radiate from the edge of a nodule into the adjacent lung. Pathologically, these linear radiations represent reoriented connective tissue (interlobular) septa drawn into the tumor by the cicatrizing (scarring) nature of many malignant lung tumors (Fig. 13.1C). Tumor extension from the nodule or fibrosis and edema of these connective tissue septa may thicken these linear densities. However, it has been shown that spiculation is not specific for malignancy, as benign processes that produce cicatrization can have an identical appearance. Benign lesions that have a spiculated border include lipoid pneumonia, organizing pneumonia, tuberculomas, and the mass lesions of progressive massive fibrosis in complicated silicosis. A peripherally situated pulmonary nodule may contact the costal pleura or interlobar fissure via a linear opacity known as a "pleural tail" (Fig. 13.2), which reflects pleural retraction associated with

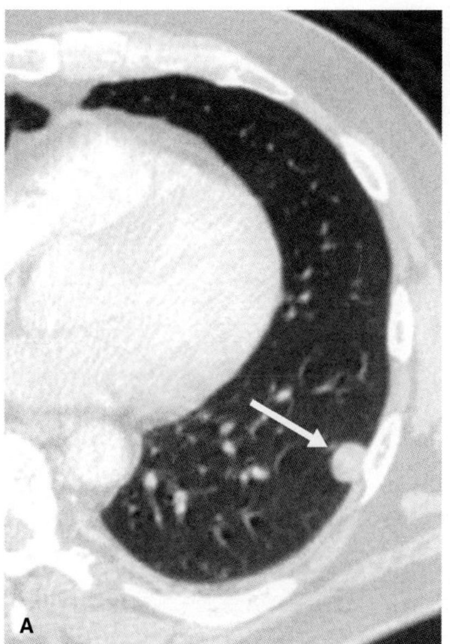

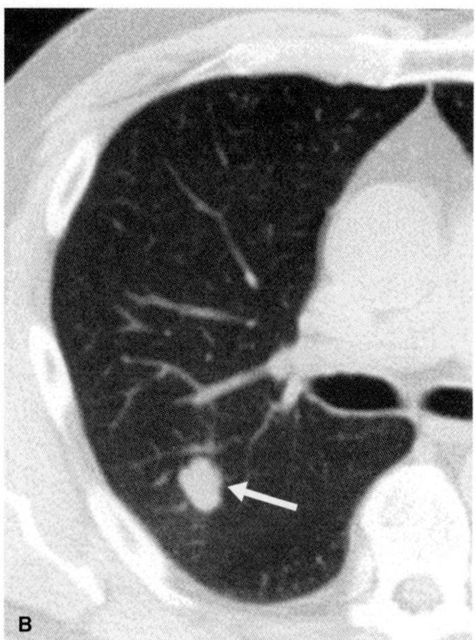

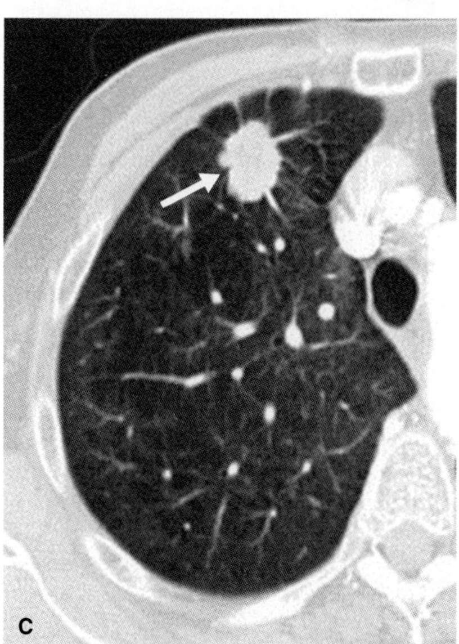

FIGURE 13.1. Edge or Marginal Characteristics of Solitary Pulmonary Nodules as Demonstrated on CT. A: Smooth borders in a granuloma. **B:** Lobulated contour of a hamartoma. **C:** Spiculated border in lung cancer.

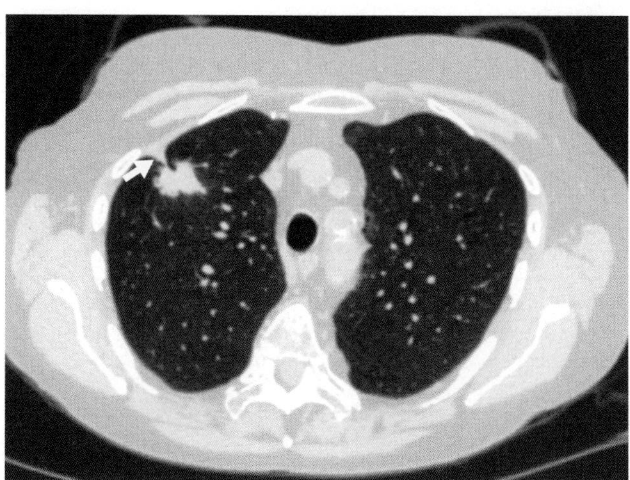

FIGURE 13.2. Pleural Tail Associated With Lung Adenocarcinoma. Axial CT through a spiculated right upper lobe adenocarcinoma shows a triangular density (*arrow*) extending from the lesion to the anterolateral costal pleural surface reflecting a pleural tail.

fibrosis related to the lesion and is not specific for malignancy. As with the corona radiata, the recognition of this line, while suggestive of malignancy (particularly adenocarcinoma), is not specific and may be seen in peripheral granulomas. An SPN with an ill-defined margin may be benign or malignant, with benign nodules usually reflecting a resolving inflammatory process.

There are additional characteristics of the border of an SPN that help identify the nature of the lesion. The presence of small "satellite" nodules around the periphery of a dominant nodule is strongly suggestive of benign disease, particularly granulomatous infection. The identification of feeding and draining vessels emanating from the hilar aspect of an SPN is pathognomonic of a pulmonary arteriovenous malformation (AVM) (Fig. 13.3). A posttraumatic pulmonary artery pseudoaneurysm will show marked contrast enhancement and contiguity with the feeding artery on CT. The presence of a halo of ground-glass opacity encircling an SPN in an immunocompromised, neutropenic patient should suggest the diagnosis of invasive fungal infection. Finally, a nodule or mass adjacent to an area of pleural thickening with a "comet tail" of bronchi and vessels entering the hilar aspect of the

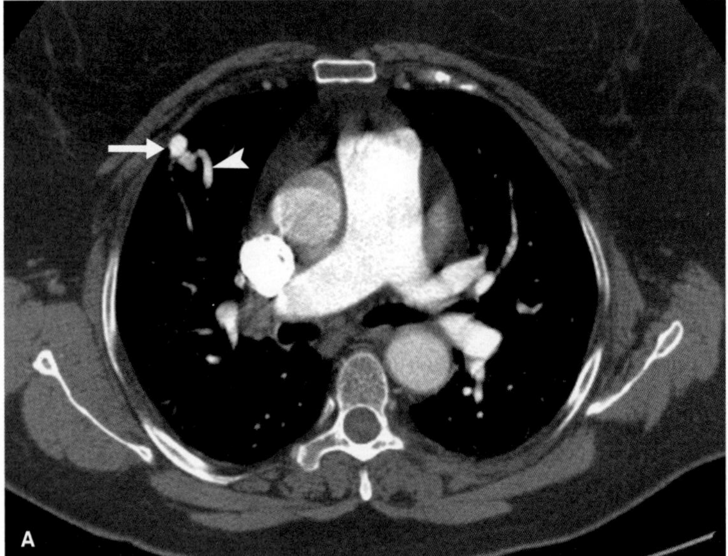

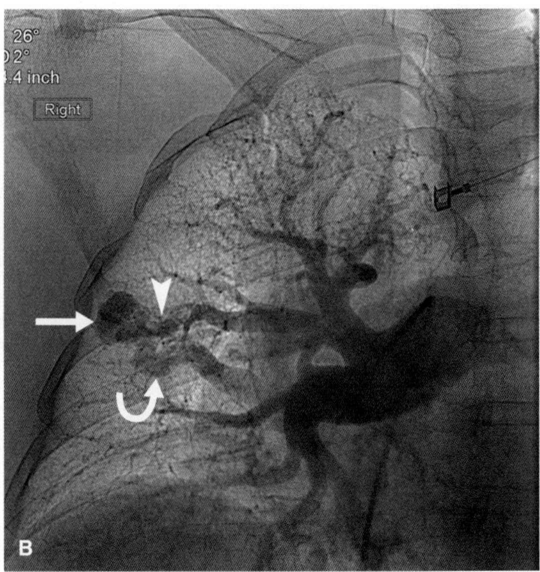

FIGURE 13.3. **Arteriovenous Malformation. A:** Contrast-enhanced axial CT shows a densely enhancing pleural nodule (*arrow*) with a feeding vessel (*arrowhead*). **B:** Digital subtraction right pulmonary angiogram in the left anterior oblique projection shows the lobulated malformation (*arrow*) with a feeding artery (*arrowhead*) and large draining vein (*curved arrow*) confirming the arteriovenous malformation.

mass and associated lobar volume loss is characteristic of rounded atelectasis.

Density. The density of an SPN is probably the single most important factor in characterizing the lesion as benign or indeterminate. In general, lesions that are calcified are benign. There are five patterns of calcification that when present in a solid nodule that is smooth or lobulated reliably indicates benignity. These patterns can be identified on conventional radiography but thin-section CT is often necessary to detect and characterize the calcification. *Complete, central, or peripheral rim-like calcification* within an SPN is specific for a healed granuloma from tuberculosis or histoplasmosis. *Concentric* or *laminated calcification* indicates a granuloma and allows confident exclusion of neoplasm. *Popcorn calcification* within a nodule is diagnostic of a pulmonary hamartoma in which the cartilaginous component has calcified.

It is important to remember that calcification within an SPN is synonymous with a benign lesion only if the calcification follows one of the five patterns of benign calcification (Fig. 13.4). Approximately 10% of malignant nodules contain calcification on CT. A bronchogenic carcinoma that arises in an area of previous granulomatous infection may engulf a preexisting calcified granuloma as it enlarges. In this situation, the calcification will be eccentric in the nodule, allowing distinction from a centrally calcified granuloma. Malignant pulmonary neoplasms occasionally demonstrate small or microscopic foci of calcification, particularly adenocarcinomas that produce mucin or psammoma bodies. The rare solitary pulmonary metastasis from osteosarcoma or chondrosarcoma may contain calcium, but the diagnosis in these patients will usually be obvious clinically.

The identification of fat within an SPN is diagnostic of a pulmonary hamartoma (Fig. 13.5). A discussion of the radiographic and CT features of a pulmonary hamartoma can be found in the section "Lesions Presenting as SPNs."

With the routine use of thin-section MDCT, we know that many SPNs are not completely solid in attenuation and contain nonsolid (i.e., ground-glass or cystic) components. These subsolid lesions, which can be pure ground glass or mixed solid and ground glass in attenuation, are particularly important when seen on low-dose CT lung screening in high-risk patients, as data from lung cancer screening trials have shown that the majority of subsolid nodules that persist beyond 3 months reflect adenocarcinoma. Conversely, the majority of pure ground-glass attenuation nodules are benign. Ground-glass nodules <6 mm in diameter almost invariably reflect atypical adenomatous hyperplasia (AAH) or focal fibrosis. While pure ground-glass nodules >6 mm may reflect malignancy, the minority that are malignant represent indolent lepidic-predominant adenocarcinoma with an excellent prognosis. Subsolid nodules reflecting adenocarcinoma are discussed under Adenocarcinoma in the section on Lung Cancer.

Recently, it has been recognized that some lung cancers can present on CT as cystic lesions with wall thickening or nodularity (Fig. 13.6). The majority of these lesions prove to be adenocarcinoma. The mechanism of the development of the cystic airspaces is unknown. Any cystic lesion that on follow-up develops wall thickening (in the absence of infection or trauma) or mural nodularity is suspicious and may require biopsy or resection for diagnosis.

It is important to remember that not all SPNs can be reliably characterized by their internal attenuation characteristics. A lesion with a diameter greater than 3 cm (termed a "mass"), those showing lobulated or spiculated margins, and thick-walled cavitary lesions have a high likelihood of malignancy regardless of internal density and almost invariably require tissue diagnosis when detected. Likewise, the demonstration of an air bronchogram or bubbly lucencies within an SPN is highly suspicious for adenocarcinoma (Fig. 13.7).

Contrast-Enhanced CT. Several studies have demonstrated the utility of dynamic, contrast-enhanced CT in the evaluation of SPNs, with virtually all malignant lesions demonstrating an increase in attenuation of greater than 15 H after contrast administration (Fig. 13.8). Therefore, lack of significant (i.e., >15 H) enhancement of a solid nodule 6 to 30 mm in diameter following intravenous iodinated contrast administration effectively excludes malignancy (sensitivity = 98%).

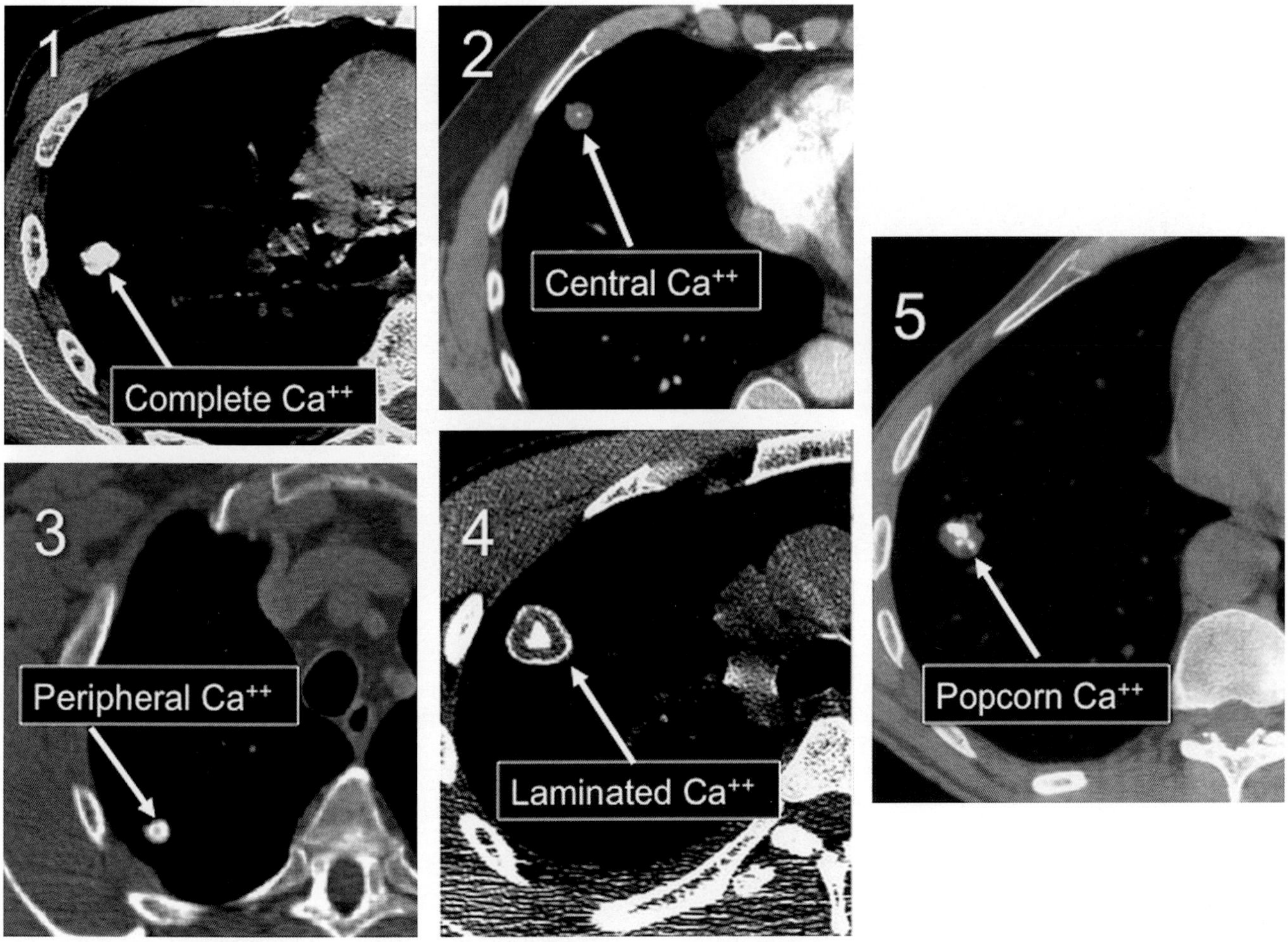

FIGURE 13.4. **Patterns of Benign Calcification in Solitary Pulmonary Nodules.** Ca^{++}, calcification.

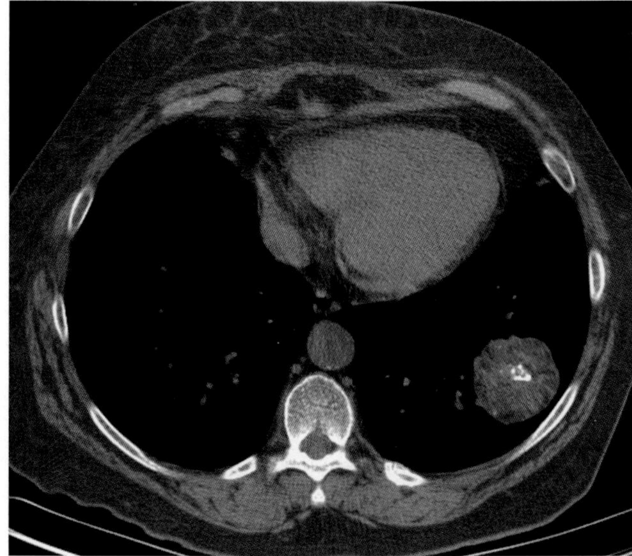

FIGURE 13.5. **Fat in Pulmonary Hamartoma.** Unenhanced CT scan through a left lower lobe mass shows peripheral foci of fat with soft tissue density and coarse calcification, findings diagnostic of a hamartoma.

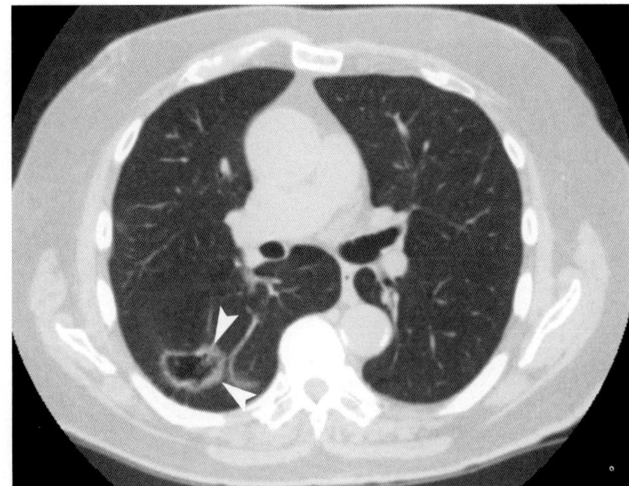

FIGURE 13.6. **Cystic Adenocarcinoma.** Axial CT scan through the mid lungs shows a cystic lesion in the superior segment of the right lower lobe with ill-defined thickening along its medial wall (*arrowheads*). CT core biopsy showed adenocarcinoma, confirmed at surgical resection.

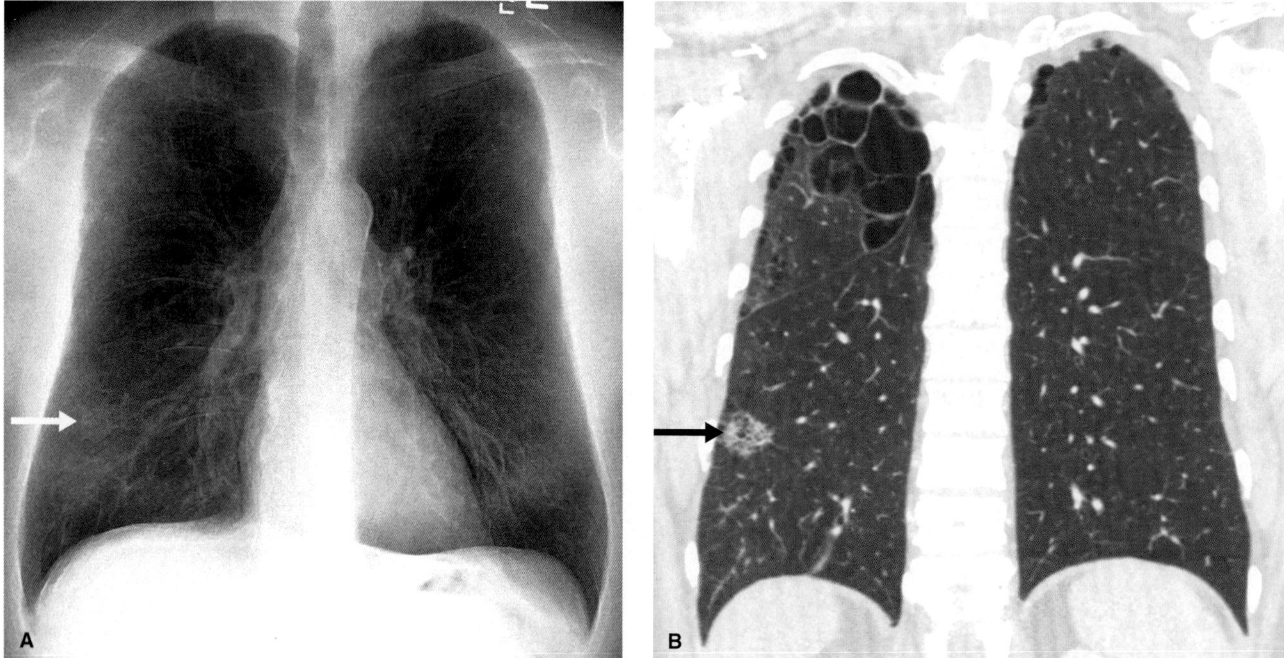

FIGURE 13.7. **Cystic ("Bubbly") Lucencies in Adenocarcinoma. A:** Soft tissue image from a dual energy chest radiograph shows a vague nodular density overlying the lower right lung. **B:** Coronal CT through the posterior lungs shows an irregular subsolid right lower lobe nodule (*arrow*) containing small cystic lucencies. Biopsy revealed adenocarcinoma.

PET. PET using fluorine-18-labeled fluorodeoxyglucose (FDG) has shown a high accuracy in the distinction between benign and malignant SPNs (Fig. 13.9). For lesions >8 mm in diameter, the sensitivity of FDG-PET/CT is 97%, with a specificity of 85%; the relatively lower specificity reflects inflammatory lesions such as active granulomas that are FDG avid. False-negative PET studies are seen in patients with lesions <10 mm in diameter and low metabolically active malignancies such as carcinoid tumor and preinvasive or MIA.

Management Decisions. Recommendations from the Fleischner Society for the follow-up of incidentally detected solid and subsolid lung nodules were recently updated and provide guidelines for the frequency and length of follow-up (Tables 13.2 and 13.3). For the management of lung nodules detected on

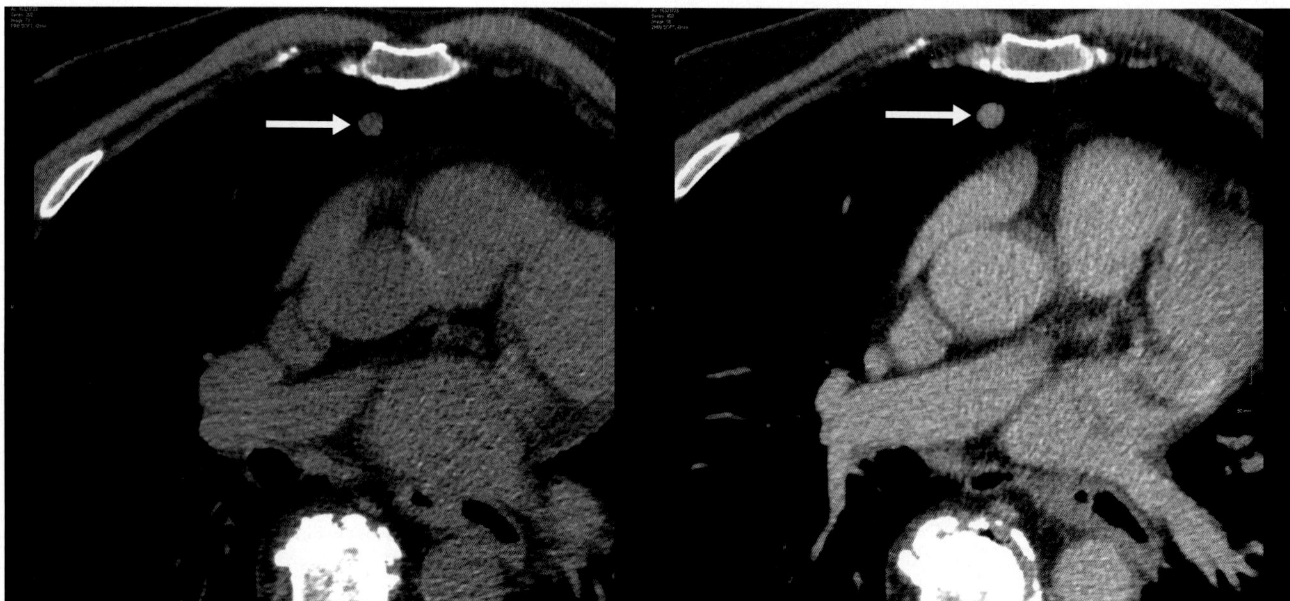

FIGURE 13.8. **CT Nodule Enhancement Study.** Paired coned-down contrast-enhanced axial CT scans targeted to a right upper lobe nodule (*arrow*) in an 80-year-old man shows a smoothly marginated nodule at baseline (*left*) found to enhance 50 Hounsfield units 2 minutes after intravenous contrast administration (*right*). CT-guided biopsy showed a carcinoid tumor.

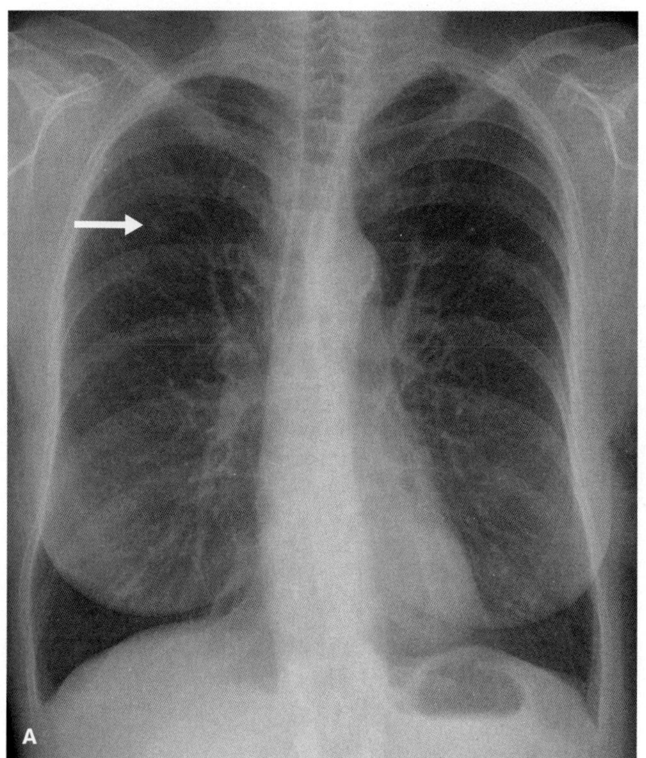

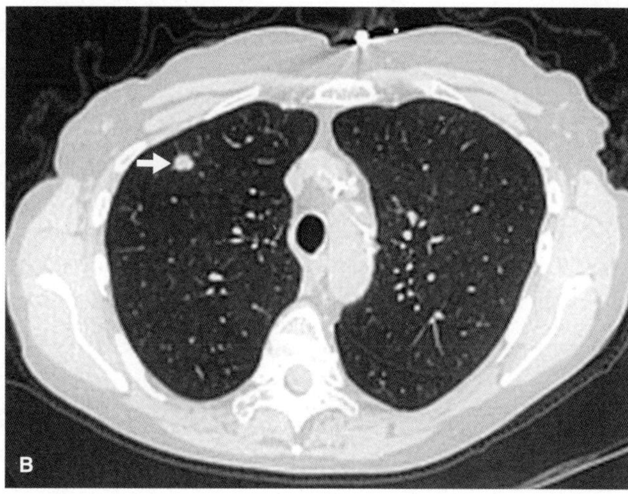

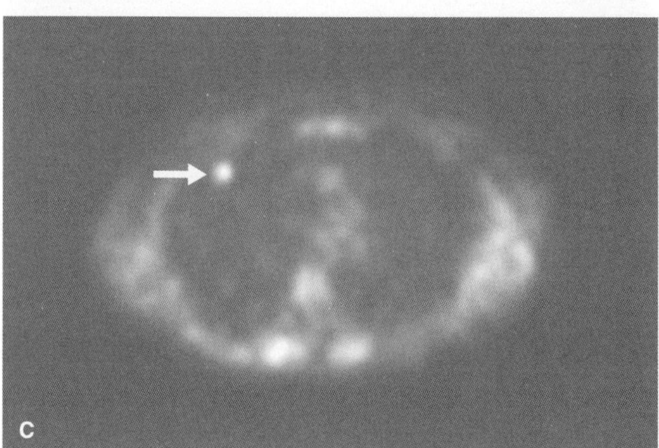

FIGURE 13.9. PET for Evaluation of Solitary Pulmonary Nodule. A: Frontal chest radiograph shows a small right upper lobe nodule (*arrow*). B: Axial CT through the upper lobes confirms the presence of a 9-mm diameter irregular nodule in the right upper lobe (*arrow*). C: Axial PET shows increased FDG uptake within the nodule (*arrow*). Biopsy showed adenocarcinoma.

TABLE 13.2

FLEISCHNER SOCIETY 2017 GUIDELINES FOR THE MANAGEMENT OF SMALL INCIDENTAL SOLID LUNG NODULES ON CT

■ NODULE SIZE (VOLUME)	■ LOW-RISK PATIENT	■ HIGH-RISK PATIENT
<6 mm (<100 mm^3)	No follow-up needed	Optional follow-up @ 12 months
6–8 mm (100–250 mm^3)	CT @ 6–12 months Consider @ 18–24 months	Follow-up CT @ 6–12 months, then @ 18–24 months
>8 mm (>250 mm^3)	Consider CT @ 3 months, PET/CT, or biopsy	Consider CT @ 3 months, PET/CT, or biopsy

MacMahon H, Naidich DP, Goo JM, et al. Guidelines for management of incidental pulmonary nodules detected on CT images: from the Fleischner Society 2017. *Radiology* 2017;284(1):228–243.

TABLE 13.3

FLEISCHNER SOCIETY GUIDELINES FOR MANAGEMENT OF SUBSOLID LUNG NODULES

■ SOLITARY NODULE	■ MANAGEMENT	■ COMMENTS
Subsolid <6 mm (<100 mm^3)	No follow-up needed	F/U @ 2 and 4 years if suspicious
Ground glass ≥6 mm (>100 mm^3)	CT @ 6–12 months then every 2 years × 5 years	If solid component or growth, consider resection
Part-solid nodule ≥6 mm (>100 mm^3)	F/U CT @ 3–6 months If stable and solid component <6 mm, annual CT × 5 years	Persistent part-solid nodules highly suspicious PET-CT for solid component >6 mm

MacMahon H, Naidich DP, Goo JM, et al. Guidelines for management of incidental pulmonary nodules detected on CT images: from the Fleischner Society 2017. *Radiology* 2017;284(1):228–243.

low-dose screening CT in high-risk patients, the American College of Radiology has developed the Lung-RADS™ system used by ACR-accredited screening programs which provides a structured series of recommendations for the reporting and management of screening-detected SPNs (Table 13.4).

When measuring a solid or subsolid nodule on CT at baseline or follow-up, the average diameter of two measurements (the largest diameter and a second perpendicular to the largest) in any of the axial, sagittal, or coronal planes rounded to the nearest millimeter obtained should be recorded for lesions <10 mm in diameter; for lesions ≥10 mm, bidimensional measurements should be given. For subsolid lesions with a solid component, a single largest diameter of the solid component should also be measured.

Patients with indeterminate SPNs should have either FDG-PET, CT follow-up, or undergo transthoracic biopsy or resection. When the lesion is very likely to be malignant, it is reasonable to forgo biopsy and proceed directly to thoracoscopy or thoracotomy for resection. However, there are several reasons to perform a preoperative biopsy on an indeterminate SPN. The primary reason to biopsy an indeterminate SPN is to make the diagnosis of a benign lesion, thereby avoiding an unnecessary thoracoscopy or thoracotomy. This would most benefit the patient with a reasonable likelihood of having a benign lesion. Factors suggesting benignity include: age under 35, nonsmoker, patient from an area endemic for tuberculosis or histoplasmosis, nodule <2 cm with smooth margins, recent symptoms of a lower respiratory infection, and a doubling time of less than 30 days or greater than 2 years. The other major indication for the biopsy of an indeterminate but suspicious SPN is a patient with limited pulmonary reserve who is a poor surgical candidate for pulmonary resection. In these patients, a biopsy can provide a diagnosis and guide nonoperative therapy. Because most SPNs are peripherally situated in the lung, transthoracic needle biopsy (TNB) is the procedure of choice for tissue sampling. Peripheral lesions requiring biopsy that are too small for successful TNB (i.e., lesions ≤5 mm in diameter) can be sampled with video-assisted thoracoscopic surgery (VATS). Patients with SPNs that are centrally situated with a large bronchus entering the lesion should undergo transbronchoscopic biopsy.

A solid SPN that is judged to be benign based on patient age, growth rate, the presence of benign calcification, or those with a specific benign diagnosis provided by TNB should be followed with radiographs or CT for a minimum of 2 years to confirm their benign nature. The radiographic follow-up consists of frontal and lateral chest radiographs if the lesions are radiographically apparent or thin-section CT at 6-month intervals for 1 year and then at 2 years.

Lesions Presenting as SPNs

The differential diagnosis of an SPN is shown in Table 13.2. In addition to lung cancer (particularly adenocarcinoma), granulomas (e.g., tuberculosis and histoplasmosis) and other infections such as nocardiosis and dirofilaria, there are a number of entities that may produce an SPN. Many of these entities are discussed elsewhere in the text.

Carcinoid Tumors. While carcinoid tumors may present as SPNs (Fig. 13.8), the majority (80%) are central endobronchial lesions that present with wheezing, atelectasis, or obstructive pneumonitis. A detailed discussion of carcinoid tumors can be found in the section on malignant pulmonary neoplasms.

Pulmonary hamartoma reflects a benign neoplasm composed of an abnormal arrangement of the mesenchymal and epithelial elements found in normal lung. Histologically, the mesenchymal component is comprised of cartilage surrounded by fibromyxoid tissue with variable amounts of fat, smooth muscle, and entrapped bronchial epithelium outlining the lobules; calcification and ossification are seen in 30%. These tumors are seen most commonly in the fourth and fifth decades of life. Approximately 90% of hamartomas arise within the pulmonary parenchyma, accounting for approximately 5% of all SPNs.

These lesions usually present as smooth or lobulated SPNs on chest radiography. While the diagnosis is often suggested on plain radiographs, CT is obtained in most patients. A confident diagnosis of hamartoma can be made when HRCT shows a nodule or mass demonstrating a smooth or lobulated border and containing focal fat (Figs. 13.1B and 13.5). Calcification, when present, is in the form of multiple clumps of calcium dispersed throughout the lesion ("popcorn" calcification) (Figs. 13.4 and 13.5). As a rule, hamartomas that contain calcium also contain fat. While hamartomas tend to grow slowly, the presence of characteristic thin-section CT findings allows for observation alone. Rapid growth, pulmonary symptoms, or very large lesions usually warrant tissue sampling.

Non-Hodgkin Lymphoma. Primary pulmonary lymphoma arising from the bronchus-associated lymphoid tissue ([BALT] which arises from the mucosa-associated lymphoid tissue [MALT] found along the bronchi) are low-grade B-cell lymphomas that present in adults in their 50s. The most common radiographic finding is an SPN (Fig. 13.10) or focal airspace opacity. The diagnosis is made by immunohistochemistry and flow cytometry of resected specimens or of aspirated cells obtained by TNB.

Sclerosing Pneumocytoma (Hemangioma). This benign epithelial tumor is classified as an adenoma and typically affects

TABLE 13.4

LUNG-RADS™ REPORTING AND DATA SYSTEM OF THE AMERICAN COLLEGE OF RADIOLOGY FOR LOW-DOSE CT SCREENING EXAMS

LUNG-RADS™ VERSION 1.0 ASSESSMENT CATEGORIES RELEASE DATE: APRIL 28, 2014						
CATEGORY	CATEGORY DESCRIPTOR	CATEGORY	FINDINGS	MANAGEMENT	PROBABILITY OF MALIGNANCY (%)	ESTIMATED POPULATION PREVALENCE (%)
Incomplete	—	0	Prior chest CT examination(s) being located for comparison Part or all of lungs cannot be evaluated	Additional lung cancer screening CT images and/or comparison to prior chest CT examinations is needed	N/A	1
Negative	No nodules and definitely benign nodules	1	No lung nodules Nodule(s) with specific calcifications: complete, central, popcorn, concentric rings and fat-containing nodules	Continue annual screening with low-dose CT (LDCT) in 12 months	<1	90
Benign appearance or behavior	Nodules with a very low likelihood of becoming a clinically active cancer due to size or lack of growth	2	Solid nodule(s): <6 mm New <4 mm Part-solid nodule(s): <6 mm total diameter on baseline screening Non-solid nodule(s) (GGN): <20 mm OR ≥20 mm and unchanged or slowly growing Category 3 or 4 nodules unchanged for ≥3 months			
Probably benign	Probably benign finding(s)—short-term follow-up suggested; includes nodules with a low likelihood of becoming a clinically active cancer	3	Solid nodule(s): ≥6 to <8 mm at baseline OR new 4 mm to <6 mm Part-solid nodule(s) ≥6 mm total diameter with solid component <6 mm OR new <6 mm total diameter Non-solid nodule(s) (GGN) ≥20 mm on baseline CT or new	6-month LDCT	1–2	5

(*continued*)

TABLE 13.4

LUNG-RADS™ REPORTING AND DATA SYSTEM OF THE AMERICAN COLLEGE OF RADIOLOGY FOR LOW-DOSE CT SCREENING EXAMS (*Continued*)

LUNG-RADS™ VERSION 1.0 ASSESSMENT CATEGORIES RELEASE DATE: APRIL 28, 2014						
CATEGORY	**CATEGORY DESCRIPTOR**	**CATEGORY**	**FINDINGS**	**MANAGEMENT**	**PROBABILITY OF MALIGNANCY (%)**	**ESTIMATED POPULATION PREVALENCE (%)**
Suspicious	Findings for which additional diagnostic testing and/or tissue sampling is recommended	4A	Solid nodule(s): ≥8 to <15 mm at baseline OR growing <8 mm OR new 6 to <8 mm Part-solid nodule(s): ≥6 mm with solid component ≥6 mm to <8 mm OR with a new or growing <4-mm solid component Endobronchial nodule	3-month LDCT; PET/CT may be used when there is a ≥8-mm solid component.	5–15	2
		4B	Solid nodule(s) ≥15 mm OR new or growing and ≥8 mm Part-solid nodule(s) with: a solid component ≥8 mm OR a new or growing ≥4-mm solid component	Chest CT with or without contrast, PET/CT and/or tissue sampling depending on the probability of malignancy and comorbidities. PET/CT may be used when there is a ≥8-mm solid component.	>15	2
		4X	Category 3 or 4 nodules with additional features or imaging findings that increases the suspicion of malignancy			
Other	Clinically significant or potentially clinically significant findings (non-lung cancer)	S	Modifier—may add on to category 0–4 coding	As appropriate to the specific finding	N/A	10
Prior lung cancer	Modifier for patients with a prior diagnosis of lung cancer who return to screening	C	Modifier—may add on to category 0–4 coding			

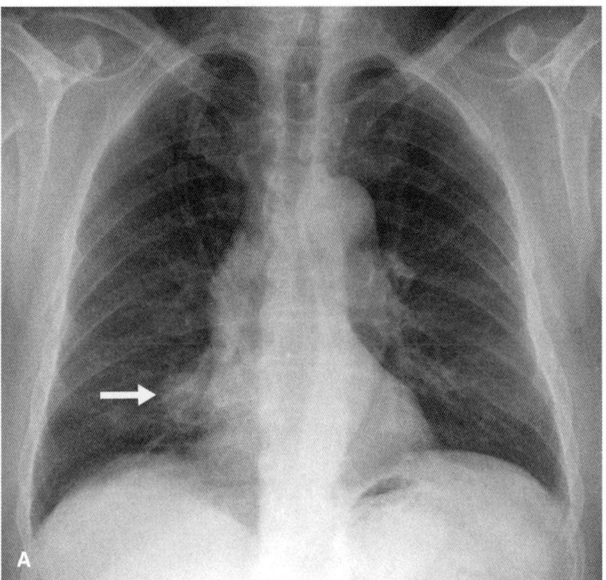

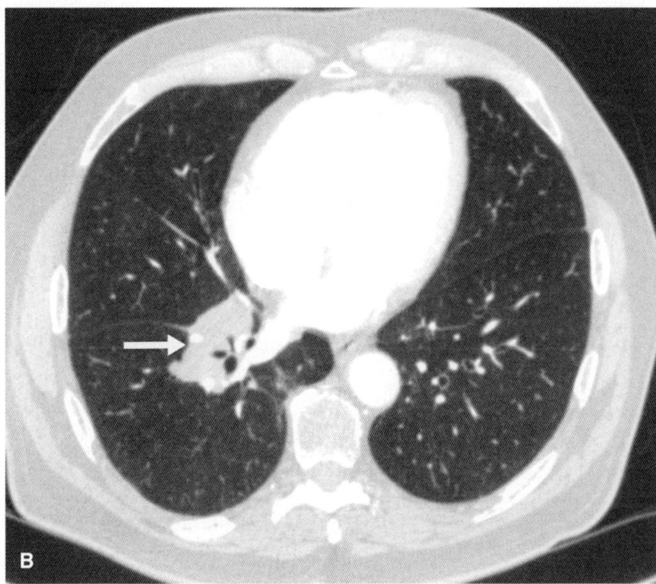

FIGURE 13.10. Non-Hodgkin's Lymphoma as a Solitary Pulmonary Mass. A: Frontal chest radiograph shows a medial right lower lobe mass (*arrow*). **B:** Axial CT shows the mass (*arrow*) within the medial middle and right lower lobes with patent bronchi extending through the proximal part of the lesion. Bronchoscopic biopsy showed non-Hodgkin lymphoma.

females and presents as a solitary, smoothly marginated juxtapleural nodule that enhances densely due to its vascular nature. The lesion may contain foci of low attenuation and may be calcified on thin-section CT analysis.

Inflammatory myofibroblastic tumor (plasma cell granuloma, inflammatory pseudotumor) of lung is characterized histologically by myofibroblasts which are spindle cells admixed with chronic inflammation—containing plasma cells. These lesions present as smoothly marginated SPNs in children and young adults.

Lipoid Pneumonia. The inadvertent aspiration of mineral oils ingested by elderly patients to treat constipation may produce a localized pulmonary lesion. Patients with gastroesophageal reflux or disordered swallowing mechanisms are at particular risk. Radiographically, a focal area of airspace opacification or a solid mass may be seen in the lower lobes. A spiculated appearance to the edge of the mass is not uncommon, as the oil may produce a chronic inflammatory reaction in the surrounding lung that leads to fibrosis. While CT can demonstrate fat within the lesion, most patients with the mass-like form of this entity require resection for definitive diagnosis.

Bronchogenic Cyst. Fluid-filled cystic lesions of the lung may produce an SPN. Intrapulmonary bronchogenic cysts are uncommon causes of SPNs; 90% of these lesions are found in the middle mediastinum. The characteristic finding is a sharply marginated cyst on CT in a young patient, although distinction from an infected bulla, echinococcal cyst, mucocele, or thin-walled lung abscess may be impossible. Superinfection of a lung bulla may produce an SPN or mass. In such patients, the radiographic or CT appearance of an intraparenchymal air–fluid level within a thin-walled localized air collection (usually in an upper lobe) with typical bullous changes in other portions of lung usually allows for the proper diagnosis.

Focal Organizing Pneumonia. Occasionally, patients who have a resolving pneumonia or even those with a focal mass-like form of cryptogenic organizing pneumonia will have an SPN detected on radiography or CT. These lesions often show irregular and indistinct margins and may be FDG avid on PET,

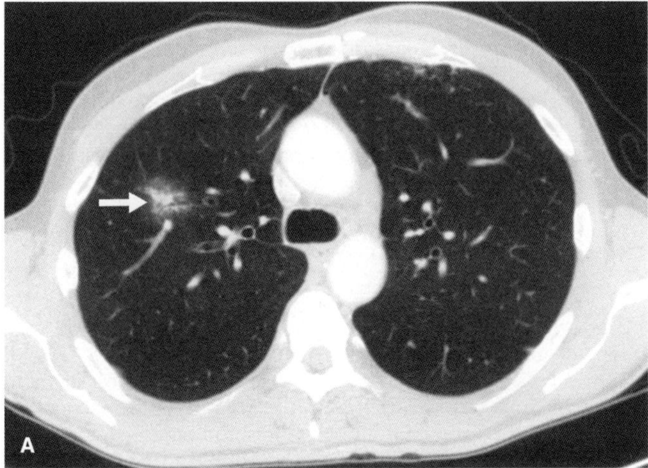

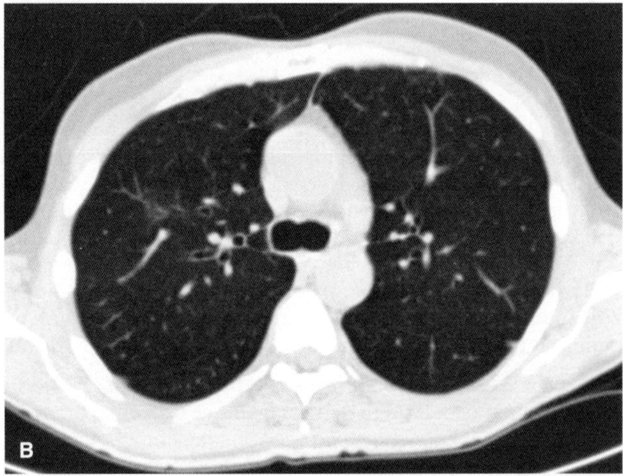

FIGURE 13.11. Focal Organizing Pneumonia as Subsolid Lesion. A: Axial CT at the level of the carina shows a subsolid lesion in the right upper lobe (*arrow*). **B:** Repeat Axial CT 8 weeks later show almost complete resolution of the lesion, consistent with a resolving inflammatory process.

TABLE 13.5

WORLD HEALTH ORGANIZATION CLASSIFICATION OF PRIMARY LUNG TUMORS

Epithelial	Adenocarcinoma Squamous cell carcinoma Neuroendocrine tumors Large cell carcinoma Salivary gland tumors Papillomas Adenomas Adenosquamous carcinoma Sarcomatoid carcinoma	 Mucoepidermoid carcinoma Adenoid cystic carcinoma Sclerosing pneumocytoma Pleuropulmonary blastoma
Mesenchymal	Hamartoma Chondroma Inflammatory myofibroblastic tumor Pleuropulmonary blastoma	
Lymphohistiocytic	Mucosa-associated lymphoid tumors (MALToma) Diffuse large cell lymphoma Lymphomatoid granulomatosis	
Tumors of ectopic origin	Germ cell tumors Melanoma Intrapulmonary thymoma	

Adapted from Travis WD, Brambilla E, Nicholson AG, et al. The 2015 World Health Organization classification of lung tumors: impact of genetic, clinical and radiologic advances since the 2004 classification. *J Thorac Oncol* 2015;10(9):1243–1260.

thereby showing a significant overlap of findings with those of lung cancer (Fig. 13.11). Sometimes a history of recent lower respiratory tract infection will be present. Radiologic follow-up, perhaps after empiric antibiotic therapy, will allow distinction from malignancy in most patients, although a minority will require surgical resection for definitive diagnosis.

Hematoma/Traumatic Lung Cyst. Blunt or penetrating chest trauma can result in the formation of traumatic lung cysts or hematomas, seen as round opacities often containing air or an air/fluid level.

LUNG TUMORS

In 2015, the World Health Organization updated its classification of lung tumors (Table 13.5). While epithelial neoplasms comprise the majority of malignant lung tumors, there are also mesenchymal and lymphohistiocytic malignancies that may arise within the lung.

Lung Cancer

Lung cancer is a malignant epithelial neoplasm that arises within the pulmonary parenchyma. It remains the leading cause of death from malignancy in the United States and most industrialized countries for both men and women. Although survival rates for lung cancer are poor, radiology plays a central role in diagnosis and management. This section will review the key pathologic, epidemiologic, and radiologic features of lung cancer with an emphasis on the radiologic staging of this disease.

Cytologic and Pathologic Features. Bronchogenic carcinoma is a malignant neoplasm that arises from the bronchial or alveolar epithelium. Ninety-nine percent of malignant epithelial neoplasms of the lungs arise from the bronchi or lungs, while fewer than 0.5% arise from the trachea. Bronchogenic carcinoma is divided into four main histologic subtypes based on their gross and microscopic features: adenocarcinoma, squamous cell carcinoma, small cell carcinoma, and large cell carcinoma (Table 13.6, Fig. 13.12).

Adenocarcinoma is the most common type of lung cancer, accounting for approximately 43% of all lung carcinomas. It has the weakest association with smoking and is the most common subtype of lung cancer in nonsmokers. Whereas these tumors most often develop in the upper lobes as SPNs, they are found in the central portions of the lungs in about one-fourth of cases. Adenocarcinomas arise from bronchiolar or alveolar epithelium and have an irregular or spiculated appearance where they invade adjacent lung producing an irregularly marginated pulmonary nodule or mass on imaging (Fig. 13.12A,B). Fibrosis in and about the tumor is common. Histologically, adenocarcinomas demonstrate gland formation and mucin production.

While most adenocarcinomas are seen on thin-section CT as lobulated or spiculated solid SPNs, it is common to see ground-glass or cystic components within these lesions. The presence of ground glass in an adenocarcinoma presenting as an SPN represents lepidic growth of tumor cells along the alveolar walls, whereas the solid (soft tissue) component reflects invasive tumor. The histologic appearance of preinvasive, minimally invasive, and invasive adenocarcinoma of the lung correlates well with thin-section CT features, which in turn correlates with prognosis. Table 13.7 reviews the classification of premalignant lesions (i.e., AAH), preinvasive malignant adenocarcinoma (AIS), MIA, and invasive adenocarcinoma correlated with the expected thin-section CT features.

Squamous cell carcinoma is the second most common subtype of lung cancer accounting for approximately 23% of all cases. This tumor arises centrally within a lobar or segmental bronchus. Grossly, these tumors are polypoid masses that grow into the bronchial lumen while simultaneously invading the bronchial wall. The central location and endobronchial component of the tumor account for the presenting symptoms of cough and hemoptysis and for the common radiographic findings of a hilar mass with or without obstructive

TABLE 13.6

COMMON SUBTYPES OF LUNG CARCINOMA

■ TYPE	■ % OF LUNG CARCINOMA	■ IMAGING FEATURES	■ TREATMENT
Adenocarcinoma	43	Peripheral nodule Peripheral mass	I–II = surgery III–IV = XRT/chemo
Squamous cell carcinoma	23	Hilar mass Necrotic/cavitary lung mass Atelectasis	I–II = surgery III–IV = XRT/chemo
Small cell carcinoma	13	Hilar mass Mediastinal mass	Chemotherapy
Other (large cell, carcinoid)	21	Lung mass Endobronchial mass	Variable

pneumonitis or atelectasis. Central necrosis is common in large tumors; cavitation may be seen if communication has occurred between the central portion of the mass and the bronchial lumen (Fig. 13.12C). Histologically, squamous cell carcinoma is characterized by invasion of the bronchial wall by nests of malignant cells with abundant cytoplasm. The microscopic identification of keratin pearls and intercellular bridges, seen in well-differentiated lesions, is specific for this tumor.

Small cell carcinoma, a type of neuroendocrine tumor of the lung, accounts for 13% of bronchogenic carcinomas and arises centrally within the main or lobar bronchi. These tumors are the most malignant neoplasms arising from bronchial neuroendocrine (Kulchitsky) cells and are alternatively referred to as Kulchitsky cell cancers or KCC-3. Typical carcinoid tumors (KCC-1) represent the least malignant type, with atypical carcinoid tumors (KCC-2) intermediate in aggressiveness. Small cell carcinomas exhibit a small endobronchial component

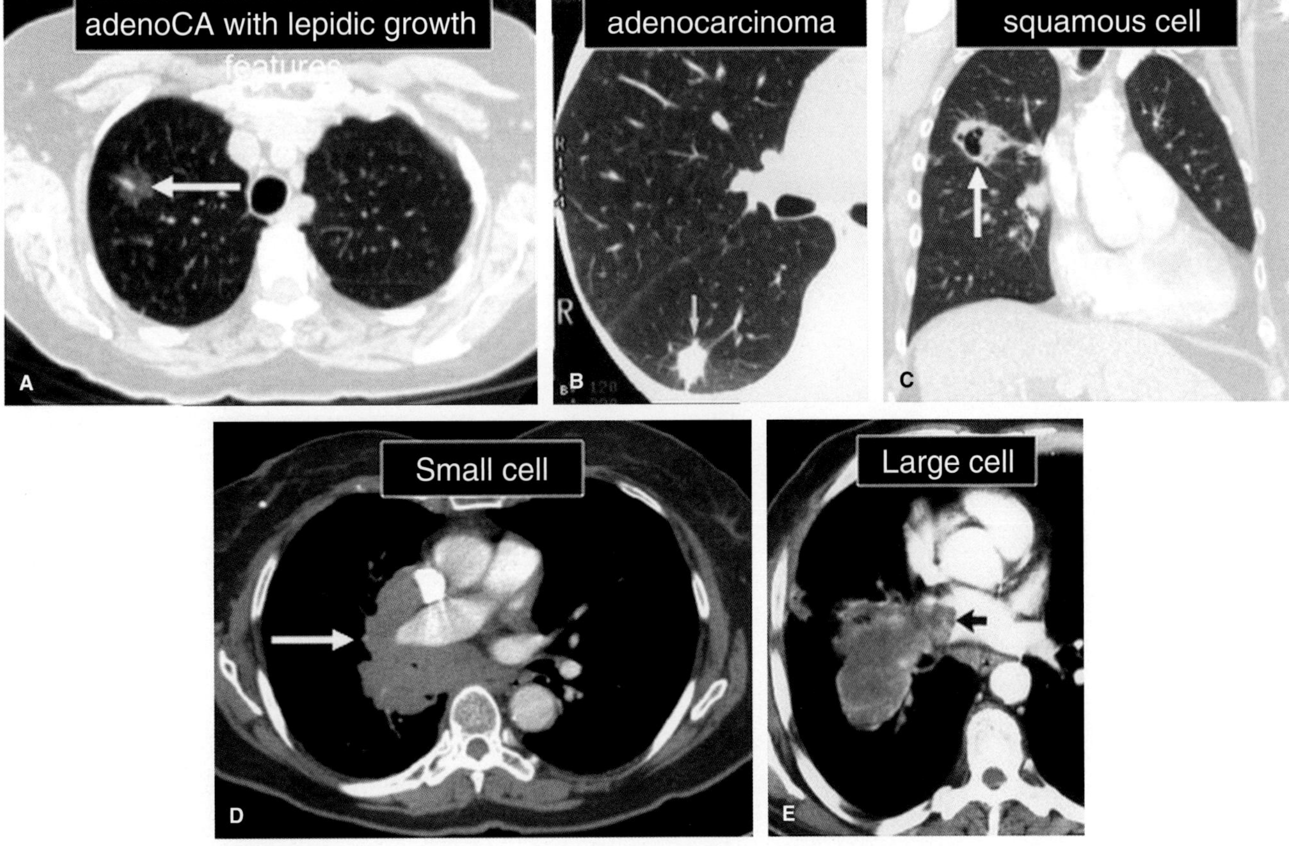

FIGURE 13.12. **Typical CT Appearances of the Subtypes of Bronchogenic Carcinoma. A:** Subsolid (mixed solid/ground-glass attenuation) solitary nodule. **B:** Spiculated peripheral SPN. **C:** Cavitary mass. **D:** Large right hilar mass. **E:** Large mass with left atrial invasion (*arrow*).

TABLE 13.7

CLASSIFICATION OF PREMALIGNANT LESIONS AND ADENOCARCINOMA OF LUNG

■ SUBTYPE	■ IMAGING CHARACTERISTICS	■ EXAMPLE
Atypical adenomatous hyperplasia	Ground-glass nodule <5 mm diameter	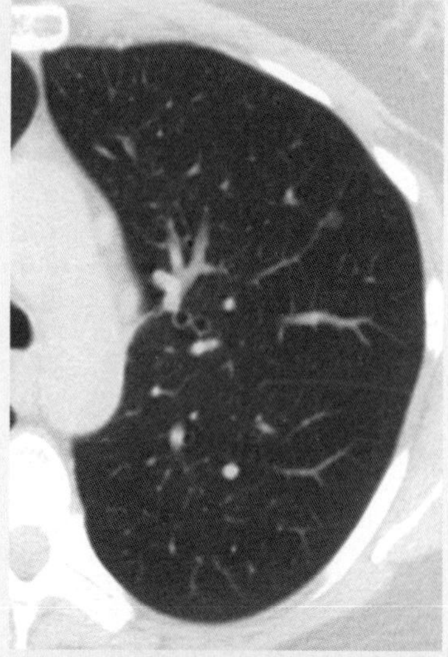
Adenocarcinoma in situ	Ground-glass nodule <30 mm +/– small soft tissue/cystic elements	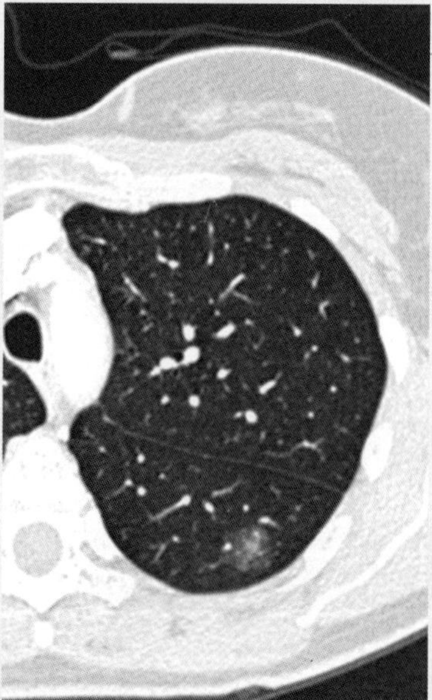
Minimally invasive adenocarcinoma	Ground-glass nodule <30 mm with soft tissue nodule <5 mm	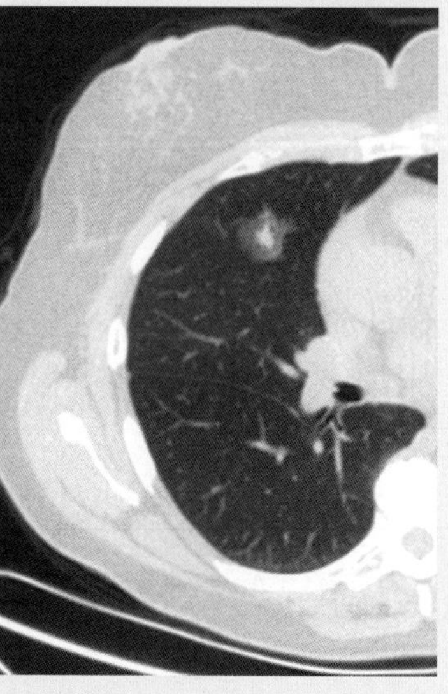

TABLE 13.7

CLASSIFICATION OF PREMALIGNANT LESIONS AND ADENOCARCINOMA OF LUNG (*Continued*)

■ SUBTYPE	■ IMAGING CHARACTERISTICS	■ EXAMPLE
Lepidic-predominant adenocarcinoma	Subsolid nodule/mass with soft tissue nodule >5 mm	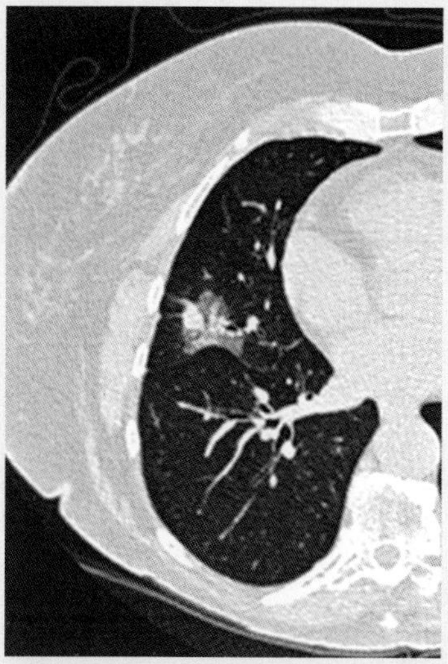
Invasive adenocarcinoma (micropapillary, papillary, acinar, lepidic, solid, invasive mucinous)	Solid nodule/mass	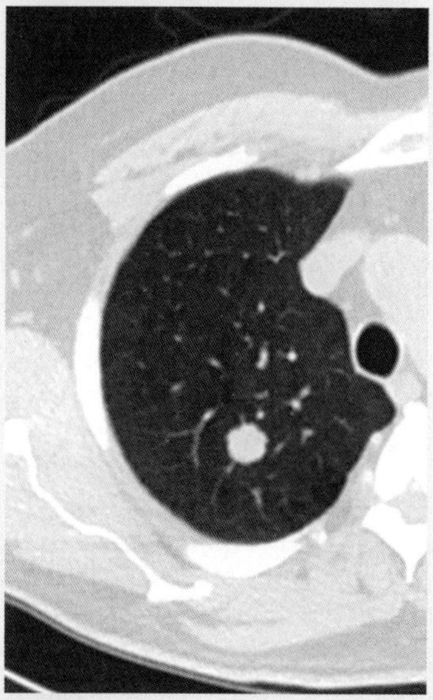
	Focal/multifocal airspace consolidation	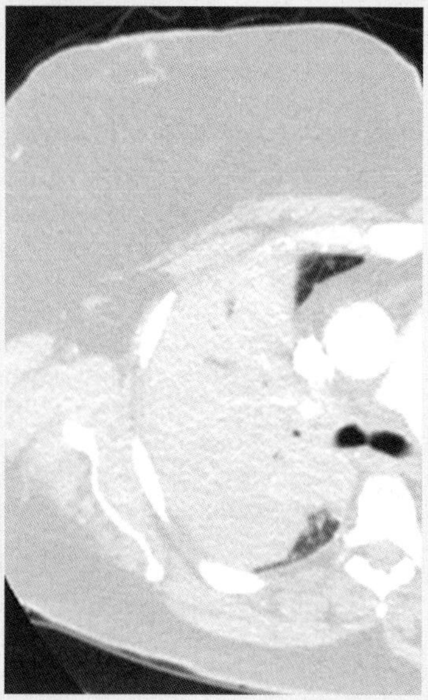

(*continued*)

TABLE 13.7

CLASSIFICATION OF PREMALIGNANT LESIONS AND ADENOCARCINOMA OF LUNG (*Continued*)

■ SUBTYPE	■ IMAGING CHARACTERISTICS	■ EXAMPLE
	Diffuse nodular opacities	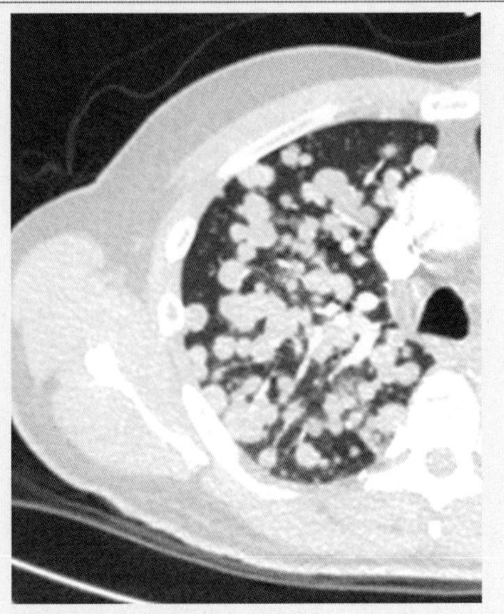

invading the bronchial wall and peribronchial tissues early in the course of disease. This produces a hilar or mediastinal mass with extrinsic bronchial compression and obstruction. Invasion of the submucosal and peribronchial lymphatics leads to local lymph node enlargement (Fig. 13.12D) and hematogenous dissemination, which are almost invariable at the time of presentation. Microscopically, these malignant cells are tightly clustered with nuclei molded together because of the scant amount of cytoplasm. This lesion is distinguished from carcinoid tumor histologically by the presence of mitoses. Electron microscopy and immunocytochemistry demonstrate the presence of intracytoplasmic neurosecretory granules.

Large cell neuroendocrine tumors are uncommon high-grade neuroendocrine tumors (the other is small cell carcinoma) that present as lung nodules or masses indistinguishable from other types of lung cancer.

Large cell carcinoma is occasionally diagnosed when a non–small cell lung cancer lacks the histologic characteristics of squamous cell carcinoma or adenocarcinoma. Histologic features include large cells with abundant cytoplasm and prominent nucleoli. This tumor tends to arise peripherally as a solitary mass and is often large at the time of presentation (Fig. 13.12E).

Epidemiology. The majority of patients with lung cancer are cigarette smokers who are over 40 years of age. Men are most commonly affected, although the percentage of female lung cancer patients has risen steadily in parallel with the increased prevalence of heavy cigarette smoking among women.

In addition to cigarette smoke, well-recognized risk factors for the development of lung cancer include chronic obstructive pulmonary disease (COPD), emphysema, asbestos exposure, previous Hodgkin lymphoma, radon exposure, and diffuse interstitial or localized lung fibrosis. Cigarette smoke is by far the leading cause of lung cancer, with approximately 87% of cases attributed to smoking. The relationship between cigarette smoke and lung cancer is irrefutable, with the intensity of smoking (number of pack-years) showing the greatest positive correlation with development rates of malignancy. Lung cancer is uncommon in nonsmokers, and cigarette smoking is associated with a 10- to 30-fold increase in the incidence of lung cancer as compared to nonsmokers. Cessation of smoking decreases the risk of developing lung cancer, with the greatest decline found in those with the longest smoking cessation interval. Carcinogens in cigarette smoke produce cellular atypia and squamous metaplasia of the bronchiolar epithelium that may precede malignant transformation. Small cell carcinoma and squamous cell carcinoma are the two histologic subtypes, with the strongest association with cigarette smoking in men, while cigarette smoking in women is associated with an increased incidence of all histologic subtypes.

Asbestos exposure is associated with an increased incidence of bronchogenic carcinoma, malignant pleural mesothelioma, laryngeal carcinoma, and esophagogastric carcinoma. Lung cancer may follow prolonged exposure (usually 20 years or greater in duration) from the mining or processing of asbestos fibers. A long latency period from the initial asbestos exposure, generally 35 years or longer, is necessary for the development of lung cancer. While asbestos exposure alone is associated with a fourfold increase in the incidence of lung cancer, concomitant cigarette smoking, perhaps by acting as a cocarcinogen, is associated with a 40- to 50-fold increase in the incidence as compared to the nonexposed, nonsmoking individual.

Patients previously treated for mediastinal Hodgkin disease with radiation, chemotherapy, or a combination of the two have an eightfold increase in lung cancer beginning 10 years after treatment. Exposure to inhaled radioactive material, particularly radon, is associated with the development of small cell carcinoma of lung 20 years or more after the exposure.

Diffuse interstitial fibrosis in patients with usual interstitial pneumonitis due to scleroderma, rheumatoid lung disease, or idiopathic pulmonary fibrosis has been associated with an increased incidence of bronchogenic carcinoma, particularly adenocarcinoma. Rarely a lung cancer will develop in a region of parenchymal scarring or granuloma formation such as can be seen in patients with prior tuberculosis.

Radiographic Findings. The radiographic findings in lung cancer depend on the subtype of cancer and the stage of disease at the time of diagnosis. The two most common findings are an SPN (size between 2 mm and 3 cm) or lung mass (3 cm or larger in size) and a hilar mass with or without bronchial obstruction. All cell types can present with a pulmonary nodule. Because squamous and small cell carcinoma arise from the central bronchi, the majority of these types of bronchogenic carcinoma produce a hilar mass (Fig. 13.12C,D). The hilar mass represents either the extraluminal portion of the bronchial tumor or hilar lymph node enlargement from metastatic disease. Extension of the hilar lesion into the mediastinum or the presence of mediastinal nodal metastases can produce a smooth or lobulated mediastinal mass. Marked mediastinal nodal enlargement producing a lobulated mediastinal contour is characteristic of small cell carcinoma. Extensive replacement of the mediastinal fat by either primary tumor or extracapsular nodal extension may produce diffuse mediastinal widening with loss of the mediastinal fat planes and compression or invasion of the trachea or central bronchi, esophagus, and mediastinal vascular structures, as seen on contrast-enhanced CT.

Obstruction of the bronchial lumen by the endobronchial component of a tumor can result in several different radiographic findings. The most common finding is resorptive atelectasis or obstructive pneumonitis of the lung distal to the obstructing lesion. Resorptive atelectasis is recognized by the classic findings of lobar or whole lung collapse, whereas obstructive pneumonitis results in minimal or no atelectasis or occasionally an increase in the volume of the affected portion of the lung. An abnormal increase in lobar or whole lung volume is recognized radiographically by a bulging interlobar fissure marginating the obstructed lobe or by mediastinal shift, respectively, and is termed "drowned lung." Occasionally, the mass producing the lobar atelectasis creates a central convexity in the normally concave contour of the collapsed lobe, producing the S sign of Golden (Fig. 13.13). Most commonly, the opacity of the obstructed lung obscures the underlying central lesion. The lung with obstructive pneumonitis is not infected but rather shows a chronic inflammatory infiltrate and alveolar filling with lipid-laden macrophages; the latter finding accounts for the descriptive terms "golden" or "endogenous lipoid pneumonia."

Additional radiographic features of atelectasis that should suggest obstruction by tumor include obliteration of the main or proximal lobar bronchial air column, hilar mass, combined middle and lower lobe atelectasis, and atelectasis or opacification that persists beyond 3 to 4 weeks. CT confirms the presence of lobar atelectasis and may demonstrate mucus bronchograms within the lung distal to the obstructing lesion. The central mass is readily distinguished from vascular structures,

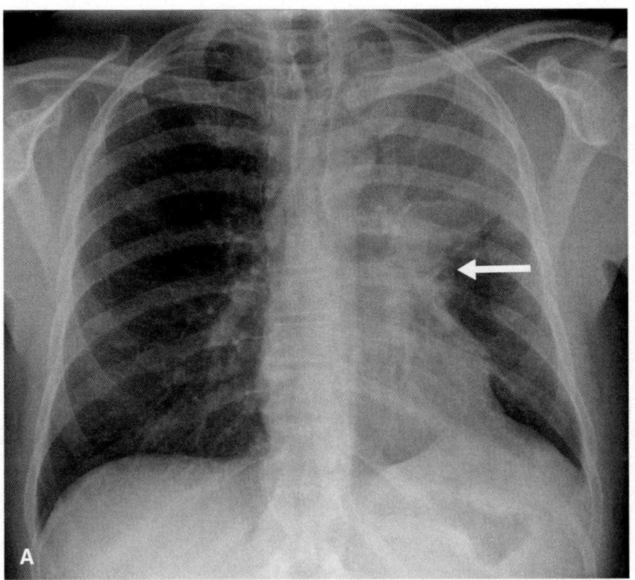

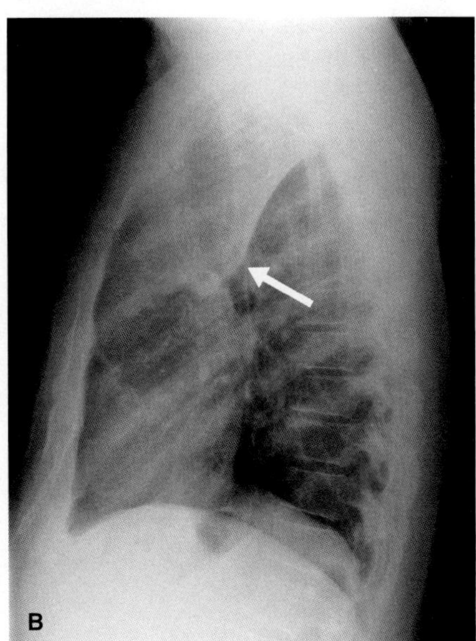

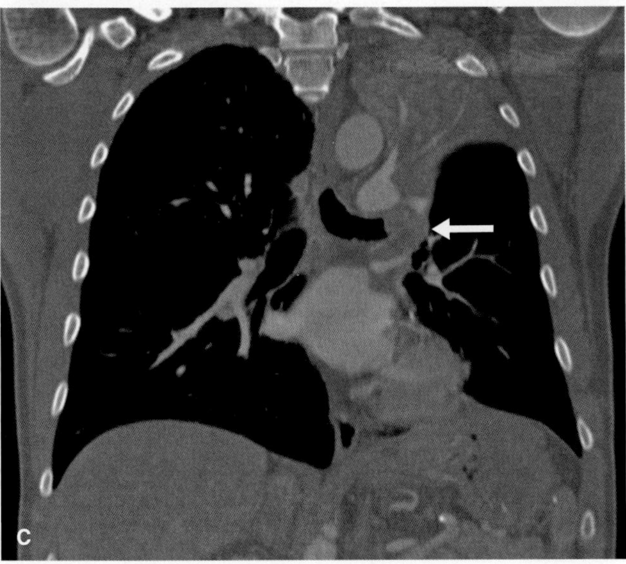

FIGURE 13.13. Hilar Mass due to Squamous Cell Carcinoma. A, B: Frontal (**A**) and lateral (**B**) chest radiographs in a 58-year-old male smoker with hemoptysis shows left upper lobe atelectasis. Note hilar convexity reflecting the obstructing mass (*arrow*). **C:** Coronal contrast-enhanced CT scan shows a left hilar mass (*arrow*) occluding the left upper lobe bronchus. Note the absence of air bronchograms within the atelectatic lung.

with narrowing or occlusion of the bronchial lumen best seen on images viewed at lung windows. The central tumor is usually distinguished from atelectatic lung by the contrast between the perfused but nonventilated enhancing lung and the low-attenuation, poorly enhancing central mass. An uncommon manifestation of bronchial obstruction by lung cancer is the development of mucoid impaction (mucocele). This represents mucus within the dilated segmental bronchi distal to the obstructing neoplasm. The appearance has been likened to a gloved hand, with the dilated bronchi representing the fingers of the glove. Radiographic visualization of the mucocele requires collateral ventilation to the obstructed lobe or segment.

Tumors that arise from the bronchiolar or alveolar epithelium—namely, adenocarcinoma and large cell carcinoma—commonly produce an SPN or mass on chest radiography. The radiographic evaluation of the SPN, in particular the size, growth rate, shape, margins, and internal density, has been reviewed in detail earlier in this chapter. A notched, lobulated, or spiculated margin to the nodule is common in lung cancer (Fig. 13.2). The radially spiculated appearance of a peripheral nodule has been termed "corona radiata." While it was initially thought to be pathognomonic for malignancy, the finding of a corona radiata is nonspecific and can be seen in granulomas or organizing pneumonia. The edge characteristics of an SPN are best appreciated on thin-section (i.e., ≤1.5 mm) CT images through the lesion.

Cavitation of solitary malignant nodules is uncommon but is most often seen in squamous cell carcinomas (Fig 13.12C). The walls of cavitating neoplasms tend to be thicker and more nodular than those of cavitary inflammatory lesions. The presence of air bronchograms or bubbly lucencies within a nodule or mass (Fig. 13.7) or mixed solid/ground-glass attenuation is highly suggestive of an adenocarcinoma (Fig. 13.12A, Table 13.7). Eccentric calcification within nodules may represent dystrophic calcification of necrotic regions, granulomas engulfed by an enlarging tumor, or calcification of mucin or psammoma bodies secreted by tumor cells in adenocarcinomas.

The size and growth pattern of an SPN are important characteristics. Masses ≥3 cm in diameter seen in adults over 35 years of age have a high incidence of malignancy. The volume doubling time (equivalent to a 26% increase in diameter) for a malignant nodule usually ranges from 1 month (some squamous cell and large cell carcinomas) to nearly 5 years (preinvasive or minimally invasive adenocarcinoma).

Pancoast (superior sulcus) tumor is a peripheral neoplasm arising in that portion of the lung apex indented superiorly by the subclavian artery. Although they can be of any cell type, the majority of these lesions are squamous cell carcinomas or adenocarcinomas. The presenting symptoms are related to invasion of adjacent structures, with arm pain and muscular atrophy attributable to brachial plexus involvement, Horner syndrome from involvement of the sympathetic chain, and shoulder pain from chest wall invasion (Fig. 13.14). The chest

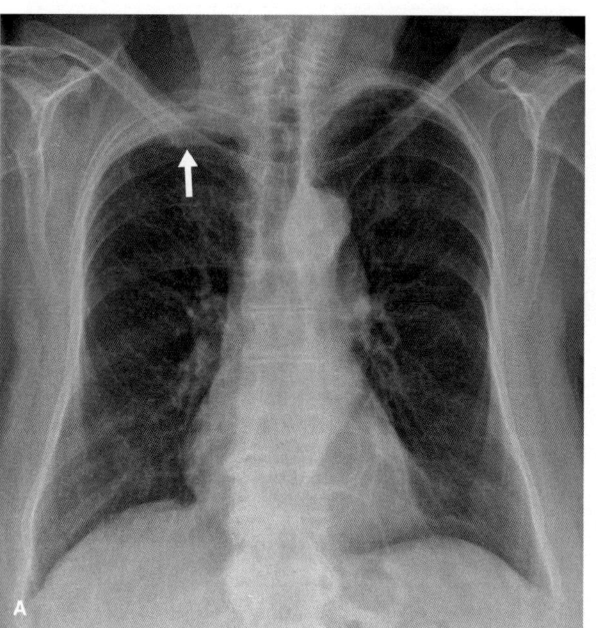

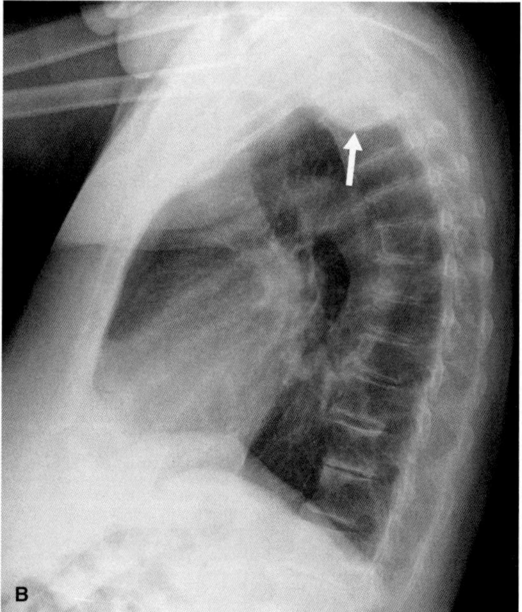

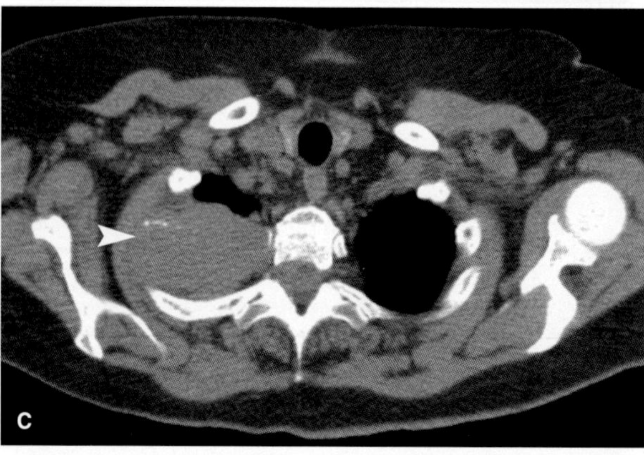

FIGURE 13.14. Superior Sulcus (Pancoast) Tumor. **A, B:** Frontal (**A**) and lateral (**B**) radiographs in a 79-year-old woman with right chest pain shows a right apical mass (*arrow*). **C:** Axial CT scan shows a right apical soft tissue mass with destruction of the lateral right second rib (*arrowhead*). Diagnosis was non–small cell carcinoma.

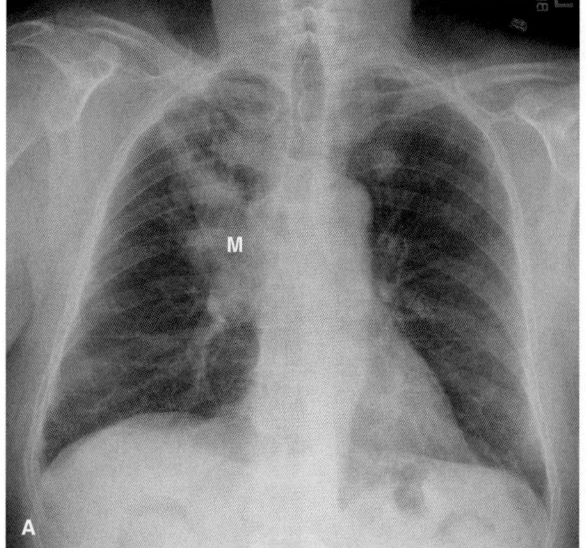

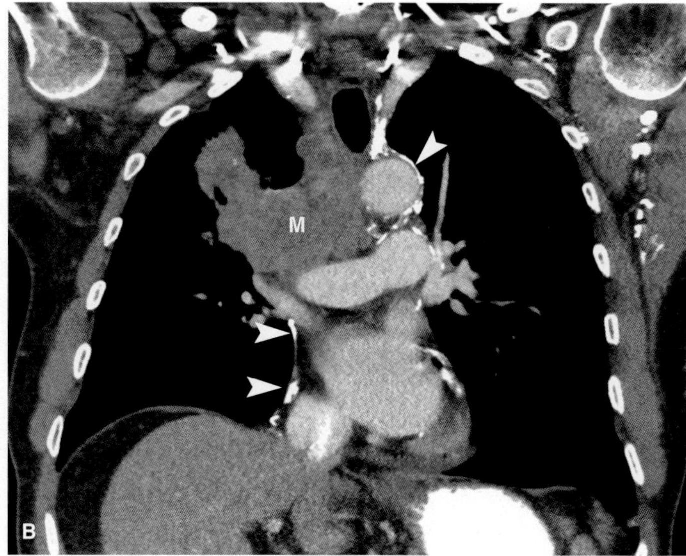

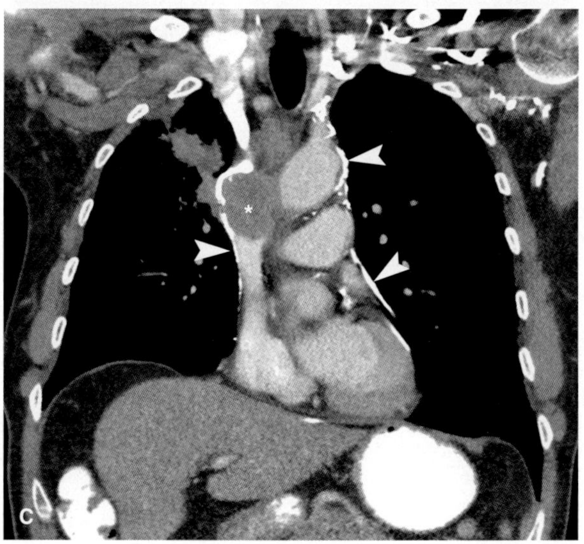

FIGURE 13.15. Superior Vena Cava Syndrome in Non–Small Cell Carcinoma. A: Frontal chest radiograph in a 73-year-old man with facial swelling shows a right hilar and mediastinal mass (*M*) involving the right upper lobe. **B, C:** Coronal contrast-enhanced CT shows a large right upper lobe and hilar mass (*M*) with invasion of the superior vena cava (*asterisk* in **C**). Note the associated dilated mediastinal venous collaterals including the right and left pericardiophrenic veins (*arrowheads* in **B** and **C**).

radiographic finding of an apical density may be mistaken for a pleuroparenchymal fibrous cap, which is a common finding in older individuals. Apical soft tissue thickening exceeding 5 mm, asymmetric thickness of biapical opacities exceeding 5 mm, enlargement on serial radiographs, or evidence of rib destruction should prompt further evaluation with CT or MR. The presence of a mass with an inferior convex margin toward the lung and/or the presence of rib or vertebral body destruction are uncommon plain film findings. CT demonstrates the apical region to better advantage and is best for determining the extent of chest wall and vertebral invasion. Coronal and sagittal MR is useful for determining the relationship of the mass to the subclavian artery, brachial plexus, and spinal canal.

Airspace opacification caused by lung cancer is an uncommon radiographic finding in the absence of an obstructing endobronchial lesion. Mucinous adenocarcinoma may produce airspace opacification as malignant cells grow along the pre-existing parenchymal lattice while producing large amounts of mucus. The diffuse form may present as lobar or multilobar airspace opacification or as diffuse bilateral airspace nodules (Table 13.7). These latter appearances may be indistinguishable from pneumonia or edema, although the clinical findings, chronicity of the process, and cytologic examination of sputum and bronchoscopy specimens should provide the correct diagnosis. The production of copious amounts of watery mucus by these tumors is termed bronchorrhea and may be seen in affected patients.

Superior vena cava (SVC) syndrome results from obstruction of the SVC from compression or invasion by mediastinal tumor, particularly small cell carcinoma or lymphoma. Lung cancer is the most common cause of SVC syndrome (Fig. 13.15).

A malignant pleural effusion is an exudative fluid collection in a patient with proven malignancy that shows malignant cytology on thoracentesis or tumor on pleural biopsy. The detection of a malignant pleural effusion has been upstaged in the most recent lung cancer staging classification to M1a or stage IVa lung cancer because of a worse prognosis relative to the presence of nodal metastases. Although the presence of a pleural effusion in patients with bronchogenic carcinoma is associated with a poor prognosis, it is not synonymous with malignant pleural involvement because central lymphatic obstruction and postobstructive infection can produce benign effusions in patients with malignancy. Smooth or lobulated pleural thickening or a discrete pleural mass suggests malignant pleural involvement. Contrast-enhanced CT may demonstrate pleural thickening or mass with associated pleural fluid on plain radiographs (Fig. 13.16). The utility of CT in the diagnosis of pleural and chest wall invasion is discussed in the section on lung cancer staging. Chest wall invasion is detected radiographically by the presence of an extrathoracic soft

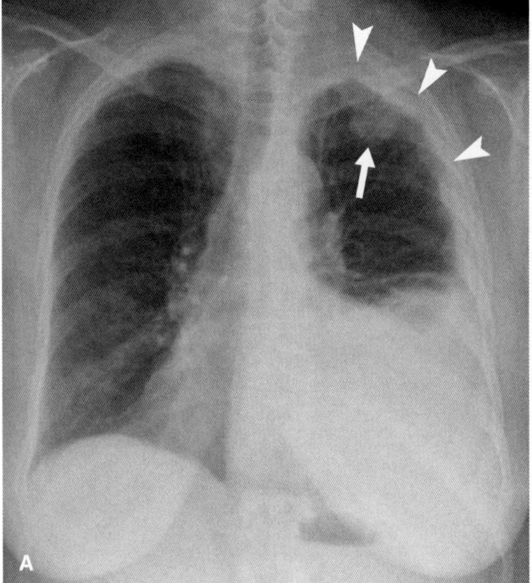

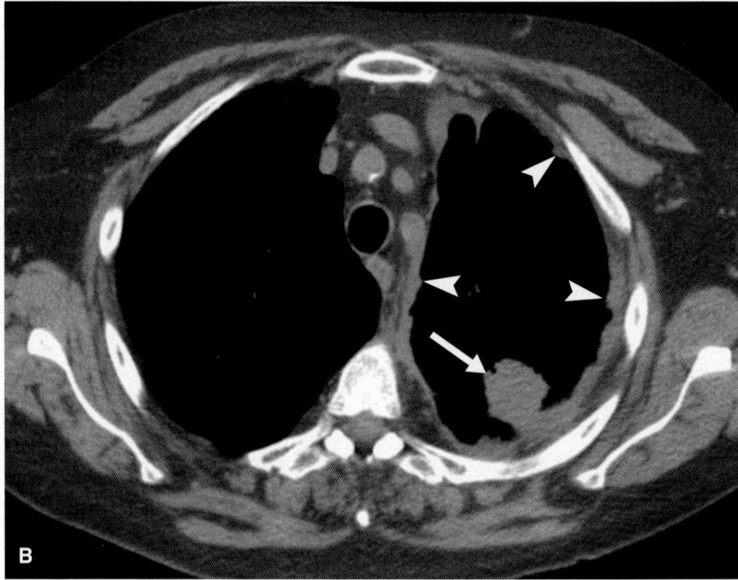

FIGURE 13.16. **Malignant Pleural Involvement in Bronchogenic Carcinoma. A:** Frontal chest radiograph shows a left apical lesion (*arrow*) with a moderate left pleural effusion and associated lobulated left pleural thickening (*arrowheads*). **B:** Non–contrast-enhanced CT through the upper lobes reveals an irregular left upper lobe lesion (*arrow*) with circumferential irregular left pleural thickening (*arrowheads*). Analysis of pleural fluid cytology revealed adenocarcinoma.

tissue mass or rib destruction. CT is more sensitive in detecting subtle bone destruction, while MR is better for detecting invasion of chest wall fat or muscle, particularly in superior sulcus tumors. Diaphragmatic elevation and paralysis may be seen with malignant invasion of the phrenic nerve. Progressive enlargement of the cardiac silhouette may be seen in patients with a malignant pericardial effusion; echocardiography and pericardiocentesis are diagnostic.

Lymphangitic carcinomatosis (LC) represents invasion of the lymphatic channels of the lung by tumor. Invasion of lymphatics or neoplastic involvement of the hilar and mediastinal nodes leads to retrograde (centrifugal) lymphatic flow with dilatation of lymphatic channels, interstitial deposits of tumor, and fibrosis. Radiographically, the typical findings are linear and reticulonodular opacities with peribronchial cuffing and subpleural edema or pleural effusion. In lung cancer, invasion and obstruction of lymphatics at the site of tumor may produce a segmental or lobar distribution of opacities. Lymphangitic spread to hilar and mediastinal lymph nodes produces unilateral lymph node enlargement with interstitial opacities, while hematogenous dissemination of tumor to the pulmonary capillaries with secondary lymphatic invasion leads to bilateral interstitial abnormalities. Unilateral or asymmetric involvement of the lungs by lymphangitic tumor suggests lung cancer rather than an extrapulmonary site (Fig. 13.17). CT best demonstrates the characteristic smooth or beaded thickening of the interlobular septa and bronchovascular interstitium.

While prevention of lung cancer is the best and most cost-effective solution to the problem of lung cancer mortality, this is not achievable as long as the addictive habit of cigarette smoking is not entirely eliminated. Early detection and treatment can improve survival rates from this deadly disease. Screening with periodic chest radiographs in high-risk patients has not been shown to be effective because chest radiographs only detect lesions exceeding 1 cm in diameter. The results of the largest randomized study using CT for lung cancer screening, the National Lung Screening Trial (NLST), has shown that low-dose MDCT can reduce lung cancer mortality and as a result low-dose CT screening is now widely performed in the United States for eligible high-risk patients (i.e., ages 55 to 75 with a 30-pack-year history of cigarette smoking).

Diagnostic Evaluation. Efforts to diagnose lung cancer should also attempt to stage the patient whenever possible so that management decisions, particularly regarding resectability, can be made expeditiously. Cytologic examination of sputum or bronchoalveolar lavage fluid is simple and inexpensive and is most useful in central tumors. Bronchoscopy with endobronchial biopsy is useful for the visualization and biopsy of main or lobar bronchial lesions, with endobronchial ultrasound (EBUS)-guided needle biopsy used to sample subcarinal masses. Endoscopic ultrasound (EUS) is useful in mediastinal nodal sampling of periesophageal lymph nodes in patients with lung cancer. CT- or fluoroscopic-guided transthoracic biopsy of peripheral masses can establish a diagnosis in over 90% of patients with lung cancer. FDG-PET scans may complement CT and decrease the need for more invasive staging procedures.

CT is obtained in all patients with possible lung cancer for diagnostic and staging evaluation and to guide efforts at tissue sampling. The detection of distal lesions in the adrenal gland, liver, or bones with biopsy of accessible lesions can provide both diagnostic and staging information. The relationship of the tumor to the central airways determines the utility of transbronchoscopic endobronchial or endotracheal biopsy, while the detection of large subcarinal nodes can direct transcarinal biopsy using EBUS guidance. The pleura may be evaluated for thickening, masses, or effusions, suggesting that thoracentesis or closed pleural biopsy is the appropriate initial diagnostic procedure. Thoracotomy with resection of a peripheral lesion is appropriate for suspicious solitary lesions lacking clinical or CT evidence of unresectable nodal, mediastinal, pleural, or extrathoracic metastases. In some cases, patients with peripheral lesions may benefit from more limited surgery using VATS. Radiology may occasionally play a role in VATS by guiding placement of localizing needles and wires preoperatively using CT or intraoperative sonographic guidance.

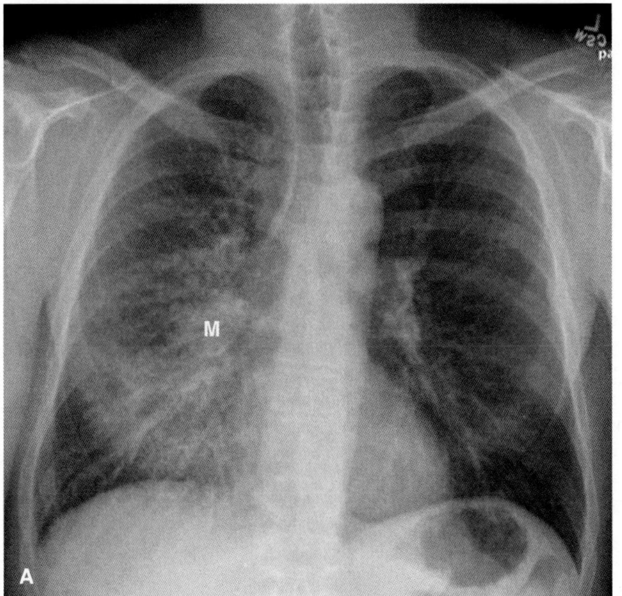

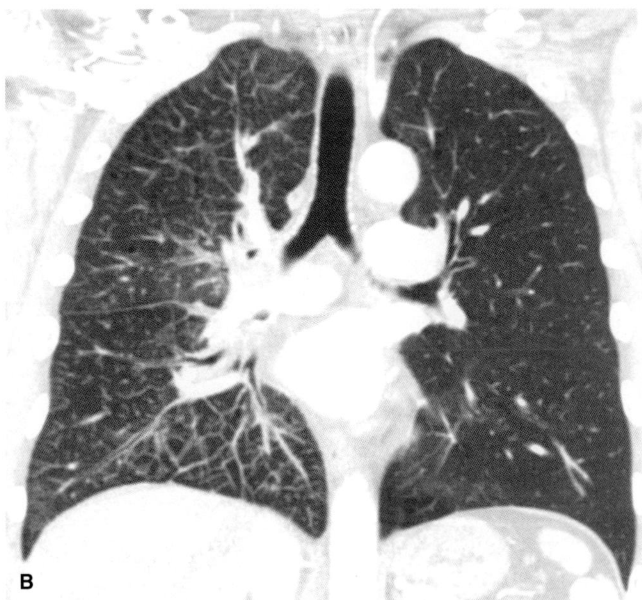

FIGURE 13.17. Lymphangitic Carcinomatosis From Lung Cancer. A: Chest radiograph in a 57-year-old female with cough shows unilateral right-sided linear interstitial opacities associated with a right hilar mass (*M*). **B:** Coronal CT through the level of the hila shows smooth thickening of the interlobular septa representing lymphangitic carcinomatosis.

FDG-PET/CT scans have been shown to have a very high sensitivity and moderately high specificity in detecting malignant tumors. Because malignant tumors have a higher rate of glucose metabolism than most benign processes, increased FDG uptake is suggestive of malignancy. The current threshold for lung cancer detection appears to be a lesion size of ≥8 mm. FDG-PET/CT is the most accurate noninvasive imaging method of detecting lymph node metastases in patients with lung cancer, although most patients with enlarged lymph nodes will undergo endoscopic or mediastinoscopic lymph node biopsy if surgical resection is being considered.

Radiologic Staging of Lung Cancer. The primary role of the radiologist in imaging the patient with lung cancer is to determine the anatomic extent or stage of the tumor. This has prognostic importance, helps determine treatment options, and is useful for investigators assessing the effectiveness of treatments applied to patients with a similar extent of disease. The staging of lung cancer is based on the extent of the primary tumor (T), the presence of nodal involvement (N), and evidence of distant metastases (M). Using this TNM classification, lung cancer is divided into four stages. This scheme was modified in 2017, representing the 8th edition of the TNM staging system (Table 13.8). In patients with small cell carcinoma, which is almost invariably not a surgically curable disease, patients have been traditionally divided into two groups: those with disease limited to one hemithorax (limited disease) and those with contralateral lung or extrathoracic spread (extensive disease). However, the new edition of the TNM lung cancer staging system applies to the staging of both non–small cell and small cell lung cancer as well as typical and atypical carcinoid tumors.

The major distinction in lung cancer staging is the division of patients with stage I or II (potentially resectable) from those with stage III and IV (usually unresectable) disease (Table 13.9). Stage IIIa disease represents T1–T2N2 disease (i.e., tumor <5 cm with ipsilateral mediastinal nodal involvement), a T3 lesion with ipsilateral N1 nodal disease, or a T4 lesion associated with no nodal (N0) or ipsilateral hilar nodal involvement (N1). Stage IIIb disease represents T1–T2N3 disease (contralateral hilar, mediastinal, scalene, or supraclavicular nodal involvement) or T3–T4N2 disease. Stage IV disease reflects contralateral lung, pleural/pericardial, or distant metastatic spread of disease.

Primary Tumor (T). The new TNM classification has further subdivided the T designation of the primary tumor to better reflect survival statistics based on the longest diameter of the tumor and improvements in surgical resection of patients with multiple nodules in the same lobe or lung. There is now subdivision of tumors by I-cm increments into T1a (0 to 1 cm), T1b (1 to 2 cm), and T1c (2 to 3 cm). Similarly, T2 tumors (those >3 m in diameter) are divided by 1-cm increments into T2a (3 to 4 cm) and T2b (4 to 5 cm). Now included in the T2 designation are tumors involving a main bronchus and those associated with atelectasis of an entire lung, tumor characteristics that were formerly T3 designations (Table 13.7). T3 lesions are those >5 cm in diameter or that invade the parietal pleura or pericardium, chest wall, or phrenic nerve or the presence of multiple nodules in the same lobe. T4 lesions are >7 cm, those that invade a structure that cannot be resected, or the presence of multiple nodules in different lobes of the same lung.

Chest Wall Invasion. Tumors invading the chest wall (including the superior pulmonary sulcus), diaphragm, mediastinal pleura, pericardium, or proximal main bronchus are classified as T3 lesions. In patients with superior sulcus tumors, vertebral body or mediastinal invasion or involvement of the brachial plexus or subclavian artery above the lung apex precludes surgical resection. Lower-grade superior sulcus tumors can be treated by local irradiation followed by en bloc resection of the tumor and chest wall with reasonable survival rates.

Rib destruction or presence of an extrathoracic soft tissue mass are the only plain film findings specific for chest wall invasion; pleural thickening adjacent to a lung mass is nonspecific and need not indicate chest wall invasion. The CT diagnosis of chest wall invasion can be difficult, although CT should be obtained if this is suspected. CT findings suggestive

TABLE 13.8

TNM CLASSIFICATION OF LUNG CANCER—EIGHTH EDITION

T (primary tumor)		
T0		No primary tumor
	T_{IS}	Carcinoma in situ
T1		Tumor <3 cm
	T1a (mi)	Minimally invasive adenocarcinoma (MIA)
	T1a	Tumor ≤1 cm
	T1b	Tumor >1 cm–≤2 cm
	T1c	Tumor >2 cm–≤3 cm
T2		Tumor >3 cm–≤5 cm
	T2a	Tumor invades visceral pleura
	T2a	Tumor involves main bronchus/atelectasis to hilum
	T2a	Tumor >3 cm–≤4 cm
	T2b	Tumor >4 cm–≤5 cm
T3		Tumor >5 cm–≤7 cm
		Tumor invades chest wall/pericardium/phrenic nerve
		Separate tumor nodule(s), same lobe
T4		Tumor >7 cm
		Tumor invades trachea/carina/esophagus/mediastinum/diaphragm/heart/great vessels/recurrent laryngeal nerve/spine
		Separate tumor nodule(s), separate lobe, ipsilateral
N (lymph nodes)		
N_X		Lymph node metastases cannot be assessed
N0		No lymph node metastases
	N1	Ipsilateral hilar/peribronchial/intrapulmonary lymph node(s)
N1	N1a	Single station N1 involvement
	N1b	Multiple station N1 involvement
N2	N2	Ipsilateral mediastinal/subcarinal lymph node(s)
	N2a1	Single station N2 involvement without N1 involvement
	N2a2	Single station N2 involvement with N1 involvement
	N2b	Multiple station N2 involvement
N3		Contralateral hilar/mediastinal or scalene/supraclavicular lymph node involvement
M (metastatic disease)		
M0		No distant metastases
M1	M1a	Malignant pleural/pericardial effusion/nodules
	M1a	Separate tumor nodule, contralateral
	M1b	Single extrathoracic metastasis
	M1c	Multiple extrathoracic metastases/one or more organs

Adapted from Detterbeck FC, Boffa DJ, Kim AW, Tanoue LT. The eighth edition lung cancer stage classification. *Chest* 2017;151(1):193–203.

of chest wall invasion are obtuse angles at the point of contact of the tumor and pleura, >3 cm of contact between tumor and pleura, pleural thickening adjacent to the mass, and infiltration of extrapleural fat. Extrathoracic extension of the mass or rib destruction is a specific but insensitive CT finding for chest wall invasion (Fig. 13.14B).

MR is equal to CT in its ability to diagnose chest wall invasion. Coronal MR images are useful in superior sulcus tumors to determine chest wall, brachial plexus, or subclavian artery involvement.

Mediastinal Invasion. Tumor invasion of the mediastinum with involvement of the heart, great vessels, trachea, carina, esophagus, diaphragm, or recurrent laryngeal nerve (T4 tumor) precludes resection. Localized invasion of the pericardium (T3 tumor) does not prevent resection. Mediastinal pleural invasion is difficult to assess preoperatively and has no significant impact on survival aside from other tumor characteristics, and so it has been eliminated from the T classification in the new staging system.

On conventional radiographs, a mediastinal mass, mediastinal widening, or diaphragmatic elevation (from phrenic nerve involvement) suggests invasion. As with the diagnosis of chest wall invasion, CT demonstration of tumor mass in contiguity with the mediastinal pleura or thickening of the mediastinal pleura does not necessarily indicate mediastinal extension or unresectability. However, a significant mediastinal mass that is contiguous with a lung tumor, compresses mediastinal vessels or esophagus, or replaces mediastinal fat strongly suggests this diagnosis. Unless there are definitive CT findings demonstrating mediastinal invasion by the primary tumor, simply describing the tumor as contiguous with the mediastinum is sufficient and does not typically alter the surgical approach to potentially resectable patients.

Central Airway Involvement. Tumors that involve a main bronchus (T2 tumors) are resectable regardless of their distance from the carina. Although tracheal or carinal involvement (T4 tumor) can be treated by carinal resection with end-to-side anastomosis of the remaining bronchus to the tracheal stump ("sleeve pneumonectomy"), most surgeons would consider this unresectable. Although radiographs can occasionally demonstrate a mass within the main bronchus or trachea, CT is more accurate in assessing the relationship of the mass to the trachea and tracheal carina (Fig. 13.18). However, CT is known to underestimate the mucosal or submucosal extent of tumor as seen bronchoscopically. Therefore, any patient with a central lesion should undergo bronchoscopy to determine the proximal extent of the tumor unless CT shows obvious carinal or tracheal invasion.

Multiple Tumor Nodules in the Same Lobe. The current staging system for non–small cell lung cancer classifies cases of satellite tumor nodules in the same lobe as the primary tumor as T3 disease, based on prognosis. In the absence of mediastinal nodal (N2) disease and distant metastases, most patients with multiple nodules in the same lobe with adequate pulmonary reserve will undergo attempt at curative resection.

Pleural/Pericardial Effusion. Malignant pleural or pericardial thickening, nodularity, or effusion is M1a disease and precludes curative resection. In a patient with lung cancer, pleural effusion can occur for a variety of reasons including pleural invasion, obstructive pneumonia, and lymphatic or pulmonary venous obstruction by tumor. Although the presence of effusion associated with lung cancer indicates a poor prognosis, only those patients with tumor cells in the pleural fluid or on pleural biopsy are considered unresectable. Other patients with effusion are considered to have "resectable" lesions despite their poor prognosis. Usually conventional radiographs, including decubitus films, are sufficient

TABLE 13.9

STAGING GROUPS FOR EIGHTH EDITION OF TNM CLASSIFICATION OF LUNG CANCER WITH 5-YEAR SURVIVAL DATA BY STAGE

STAGE		T	N	M	5-YEAR SURVIVAL (CLINICAL STAGING) (%)
I	1A1	T1a (mi)	N0	M0	92
		T1a			
	1A2	T1b	N0	M0	83
	1A3	T1c	N0	M0	77
	1B	T2a	N0	M0	68
II	IIA	T2b	N0	M0	60
	IIB	T1a-c	N1	M0	53
		T2a	N1	M0	
		T2b	N1	M0	
III	IIIA	T1a-c	N2	M0	36
		T2a-b	N2	M0	
		T3	N1	M0	
		T4	N0	M0	
		T4	N1	M0	
	IIIB	T1a-c	N3	M0	26
		T2a-b	N3	M0	
		T3	N2	M0	
		T4	N2	M0	
	IIIC	T3	N3		13
		T4	N3	M0	
IV	IVA	Any T	Any N	M1a	10
		Any T	Any N	M1b	
	IVB	Any T	Any N	M1c	0

to diagnosis a pleural effusion. Thoracentesis with cytologic examination and/or pleural biopsy is necessary for definitive diagnosis of malignant pleural involvement. Pleural thickening >1 cm, lobulated pleural thickening, or circumferential pleural thickening (i.e., involvement of the mediastinal pleura) on CT strongly suggests pleural invasion (Fig. 13.16B). While PET can be useful in characterizing pleural effusions in patients with lung cancer as malignant, caution is advised in patients who have undergone prior pleurodesis, as inflammation from intrapleural talc administration can be FDG avid on PET.

Lymph Node Metastases (N) (Fig. 13.19). While selected patients with ipsilateral mediastinal or subcarinal node (N2) metastases are considered potentially resectable, most patients with N2 nodal disease based on preoperative imaging or nodal biopsy have a poor prognosis and are usually offered

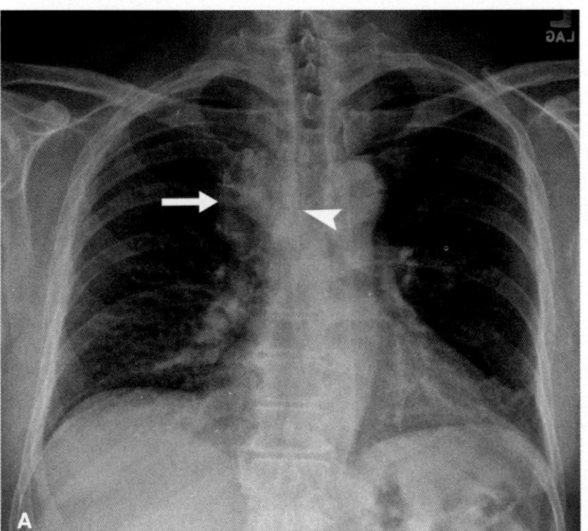

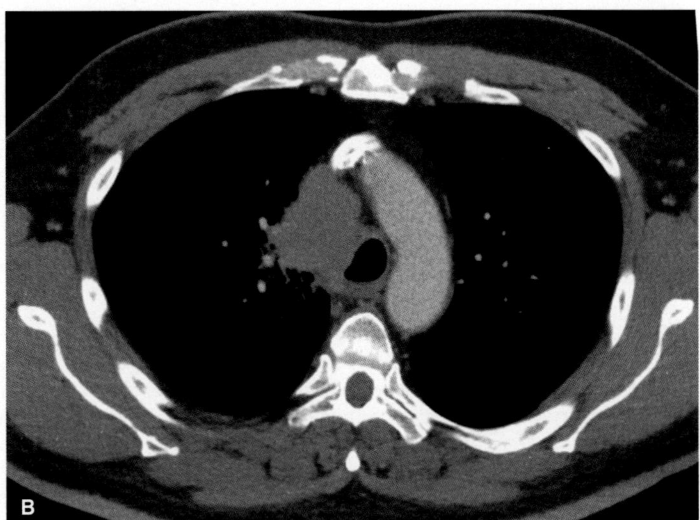

FIGURE 13.18. Tracheal Involvement by Non–Small Cell Carcinoma. A: Frontal chest radiograph shows a right paratracheal mass (*arrow*) with indistinctness of the right lower lateral tracheal wall (*arrowhead*). **B:** Axial contrast-enhanced CT through the level of the distal trachea shows a soft tissue mass involving the trachea with a large extraluminal component. Bronchoscopy shows invasion of the right tracheal wall by tumor. Biopsy revealed non–small cell carcinoma.

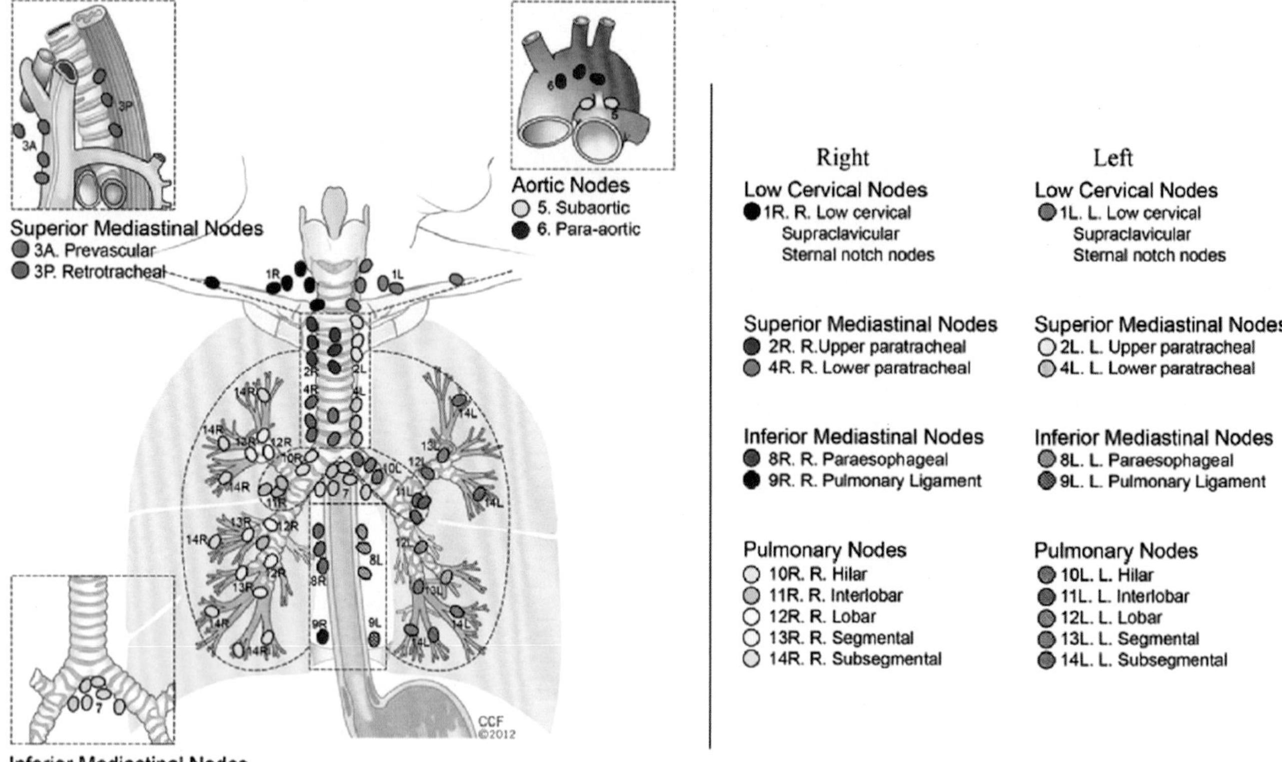

FIGURE 13.19. **Proposed IASLC Nodal Zones for Lung Cancer Staging.** (From El-Sherief AH, Lau CT, Wu CC, Drake RL, Abbott GF, Rice TW. International Association for the Study of Lung Cancer (IASLC) lymph node map: radiologic review with CT illustration. *Radiographics* 2014;34(6):1680–1691.)

neoadjuvant therapy. Those patients with pathologic N2 disease from nonbulky intracapsular nodal metastases limited to one mediastinal nodal station that are detected microscopically following surgical resection have a better survival and, therefore, resection may be appropriate. Contralateral hilar/mediastinal or supraclavicular nodal (N3) disease is unresectable (Fig. 13.20). An addition to the nodal classification system is the subclassification of the nodal involvement into single or multiple nodal stations within the N1 and N2 regions, and the presence of N2 (mediastinal) nodal involvement without N1 involvement, termed skip nodal metastases.

The detection of a large mediastinal mass on chest radiograph in a patient with lung cancer requires mediastinoscopic or transthoracic biopsy confirmation of tumor invasion before deeming the patient unresectable. A normal chest radiograph or the suggestion of hilar or mediastinal lymph node enlargement should prompt a chest CT to assess the status of the lymph nodes. No single measurement allows completely accurate distinction of normal from malignant nodes. This is because malignant involvement does not always enlarge the lymph node (producing false-negative findings and reducing sensitivity), while enlarged nodes in patients with lung cancer may represent reactive hyperplasia rather than tumor replacement (producing false-positive findings and reducing specificity). If a small nodal diameter (5 mm) is used as the dividing point between benign and malignant, sensitivity will be excellent but specificity will be low. However, choosing a large nodal diameter (2 cm) increases specificity but decreases sensitivity. Radiologists should use a short-axis nodal diameter of 1 cm, as this value achieves the best compromise of sensitivity and specificity.

CT is relatively inaccurate in determining the nodal status of the patient with lung cancer. Both sensitivity and specificity for nodal metastases, when a short-axis diameter of 1 cm or greater is used as abnormal, are approximately 60% to 65% on a patient-by-patient basis and, may be, even lower when looking at individual nodal stations. Although CT cannot be considered accurate enough to determine with certainty whether or not mediastinal lymph nodes are involved by tumor, it can provide information of value in guiding invasive staging procedures such as EBUS-guided biopsy, mediastinoscopy, EUS-guided biopsy, and transthoracic or open biopsy. As discussed earlier, integrated PET-CT provides superior accuracy in nodal staging of lung cancer.

In select institutions, mediastinoscopy and endobronchial/endoscopic techniques complement CT in the nodal staging of lung cancer. Most patients with lung cancer who have PET-positive and/or enlarged mediastinal nodes on CT that are accessible to mediastinoscopy (i.e., pretracheal, anterior subcarinal, and right tracheobronchial nodes), EBUS (pretracheal, paratracheal, subcarinal, hilar and interlobar nodes), or EUS (subcarinal, paraesophageal, inferior pulmonary ligament) should have nodal sampling. The decision of whether patients with negative PET or CT studies for nodal enlargement should undergo empiric nodal sampling remains controversial. Patients with borderline pulmonary function benefit most from preoperative nodal sampling because a positive mediastinoscopic biopsy almost certainly precludes any attempt at resection.

Metastatic Disease (M). Each patient with proven lung cancer should be carefully evaluated for the presence of distant metastases (M1). Unequivocal evidence of metastases can obviate an unnecessary thoracotomy. Common sites of extrathoracic spread in patients with lung cancer include lymph

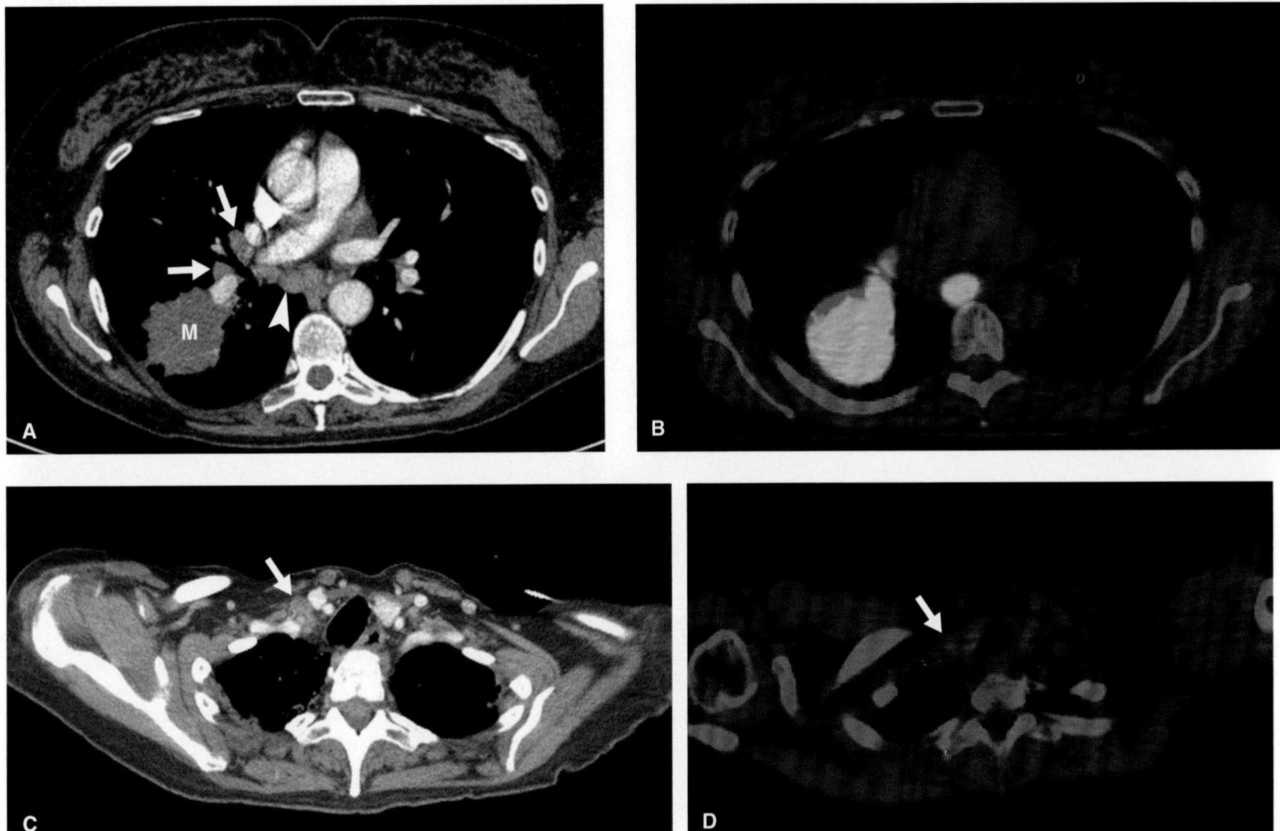

FIGURE 13.20. Lymph Node Metastases in Bronchogenic Carcinoma. A: Contrast-enhanced axial CT through the mid lungs demonstrates a right lower lobe mass (*M*) with enlarged right hilar–interlobar (*small arrows*) (N1 disease) and subcarinal (*arrowhead*) (N2 disease) nodes. **B:** Fused axial PET-CT at the same level shows marked increased FDG activity in the mass and nodes. **C:** Scan at the lung apices shows an enlarged right supraclavicular node (*arrow*) (N3 disease). **D:** Fused axial PET-CT at the same level shows increased FDG activity in the supraclavicular node (*arrow*). Ultrasound-guided biopsy of the supraclavicular node showed metastatic adenocarcinoma.

nodes, liver, adrenal gland, bone, and brain. Metastases to the other lung, although intrathoracic, are also considered M1 disease. Involvement of these sites probably represents hematogenous spread of tumor from the lung.

The designation of metastatic disease has been further subclassified in the new lung cancer staging system into patients without metastatic disease (M0), those with malignant pleural or pericardial disease or a contralateral lung metastasis (M1a), those with a single site of extrathoracic metastatic disease (M1b), and those with multiple extrathoracic metastases in one or more organs (M1c).

CT of the chest and upper abdomen is part of the initial evaluation in virtually all patients evaluated for bronchogenic carcinoma. This is adequate for assessing the liver, spleen, adrenal glands, and upper abdominal lymph nodes for evidence of metastases. US or MR may be used to distinguish soft tissue hepatic masses from incidental cysts. Whole-body FDG-PET imaging is used to detect bone metastases. Conventional radiographs or CT are obtained to assess specific foci of abnormally increased radionuclide uptake or to evaluate localized bone pain.

Imaging of the brain with MR is routinely performed for lung cancer staging, except in patients with stage IA lung cancer and no clinical evidence of brain metastases.

Approximately 60% to 65% of patients with small cell carcinoma have metastatic disease at the time of diagnosis. Because it is likely that all patients with small cell carcinoma have gross or microscopic metastatic disease at presentation, these patients are generally not candidates for curative surgical resection. However, accurate staging of these patients for extrathoracic involvement determines prognosis and allows for proper assessment of response to chemotherapy. An additional reason for extrathoracic staging of small cell carcinoma is the ability to manage localized bone or soft tissue involvement with radiation or resection.

Adrenal lesions are seen in approximately 10% of patients undergoing staging CT examinations for bronchogenic carcinoma. However, approximately 5% of normal individuals are known to have benign adrenocortical adenomas. In fact, isolated adrenal masses in patients with non–small cell bronchogenic carcinoma are twice as likely to be adenomas than metastases. In some patients, the adrenal nodule or mass may be the only extrathoracic site of abnormality, making accurate diagnosis of the adrenal lesion crucial in determining staging and management.

Methods used to distinguish adenomas from malignant (primary or metastatic) adrenal lesions include CT, chemical-shift MR, FDG-PET, and fine-needle aspiration biopsy. The combined ability of unenhanced CT to detect lipid-rich adenomas (≤10 H) and delayed enhanced CT to detect lipid-poor adenomas (≥60% relative washout at 15 minutes) has been utilized with high accuracy to distinguish between adenomas and malignant adrenal lesions. Chemical shift MR is occasionally used to characterize adrenal lesions. PET has a sensitivity approaching 100% for detecting adrenal metastases (Fig. 13.21), such that a negative study effectively

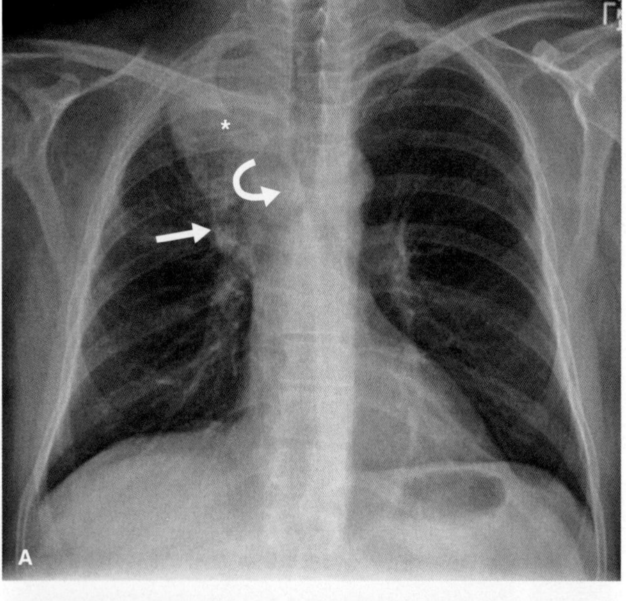

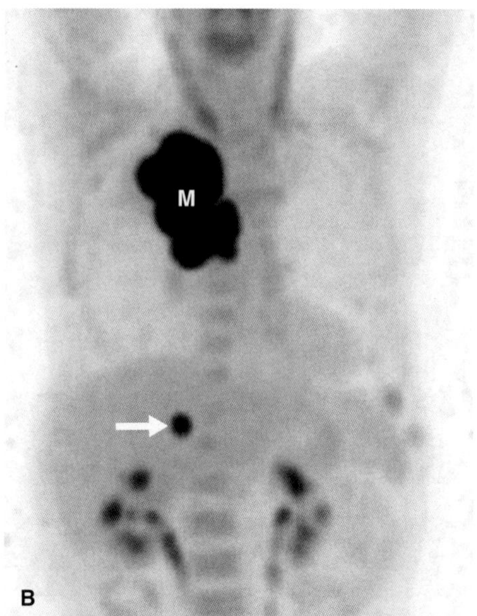

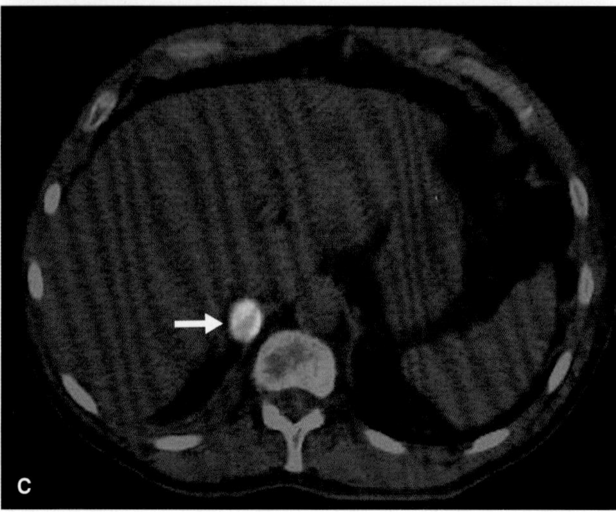

FIGURE 13.21. Adrenal Metastasis From Bronchogenic Carcinoma. A: Frontal chest radiograph shows right upper lobe atelectasis (*asterisk*) and a right hilar mass (*arrow*) with narrowing of the distal trachea/right main bronchus (*curved arrow*). **B:** Coronal maximum intensity projection image from a PET shows marked increased radiotracer activity in the mass (*arrow*) which replaces the right upper lobe. There is a focus of increased activity in the right upper abdomen (*arrow*). **C:** Fused axial image from PET-CT shows the focal uptake within the right adrenal gland (*arrow*).

excludes this possibility. However, adenomas can be FDG avid and produce false-positive studies; therefore, isolated, FDG-positive adrenal lesions may require biopsy for definitive characterization.

NONEPITHELIAL LUNG TUMORS AND TUMOR-LIKE CONDITIONS

Lymphoma. Parenchymal involvement in Hodgkin disease is two to three times more common than in non-Hodgkin lymphoma. Most cases of primary pulmonary non-Hodgkin lymphoma arise from the BALT and represent low-grade B-cell lymphomas. These BALT lymphomas are also termed extranodal marginal zone lymphomas (MZL) and have been associated with autoimmune diseases, in particular Sjögren syndrome and rheumatoid arthritis. Less common forms of pulmonary lymphoma include diffuse large B-cell lymphoma.

Parenchymal abnormalities in Hodgkin lymphoma usually produce linear and coarse reticulonodular opacities that extend directly into the lung from enlarged hilar lymph nodes. Extensive areas of parenchymal involvement can produce mass-like opacities and areas of airspace opacification. Atelectasis in Hodgkin disease is rarely caused by extrinsic nodal compression of the bronchi but rather develops from an obstructing endobronchial tumor. Extension into the subpleural lymphatics may produce subpleural plaques or masses that are visible only by CT. While parenchymal involvement in Hodgkin disease does not occur in the absence of hilar and mediastinal nodal disease (excluding patients who have undergone mediastinal irradiation), non-Hodgkin lymphoma may involve the parenchyma without concomitant nodal disease in up to 50%. The parenchymal involvement most often appears as nodules/masses (Fig. 13.22) or airspace opacities; the latter may simulate lobar pneumonia. Coarse reticulonodular or tree-in-bud opacities are uncommon; rarely, a nodule or mass is the sole manifestation of intrathoracic disease.

Lymphomatoid granulomatosis presents a T cell–rich primary pulmonary B-cell lymphoma associated with Epstein–Barr virus (EBV) infection. Central nervous system and skin involvement are seen in up to 50% of affected patients. Histologically, there are multiple round nodules containing lymphocytes that infiltrate small- and medium-sized arteries resulting in necrosis. Radiographically, there are multiple nodular opacities with a lower lobe predilection. Cavitation as a result of vascular invasion is common. Overall prognosis is poor and is

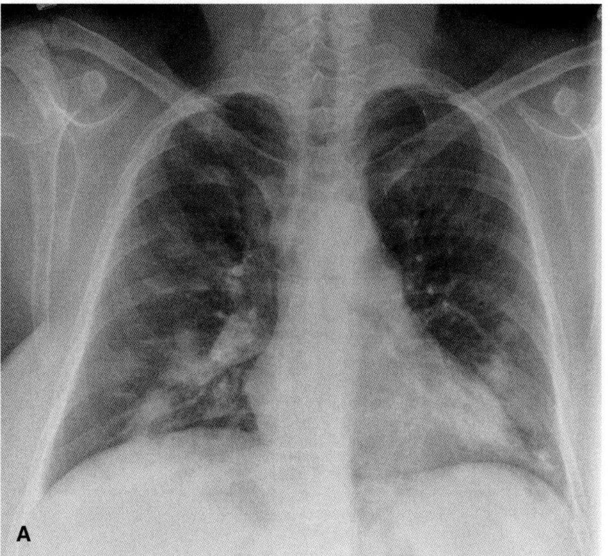

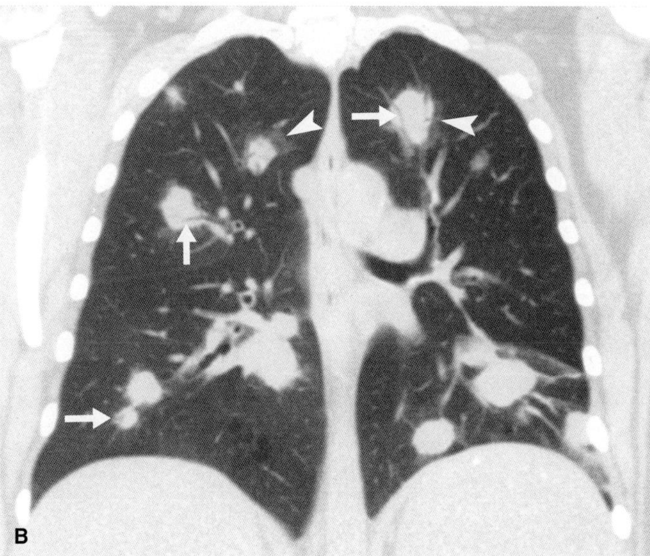

FIGURE 13.22. T-Cell Lymphoma Involving Lungs. A: Frontal chest radiograph in a 57-year-old woman shows multiple bilateral pulmonary nodules. **B:** Coronal CT through the posterior lungs shows multiple nodules. Note patent bronchi (*arrows*) and adjacent ground-glass opacities (*arrowheads*) associated with several of the nodules.

graded from 1 (good prognosis) to 3 (poor prognosis) based on the number of malignant B lymphocytes containing EBV RNA per high-powered field.

Follicular Bronchiolitis, Lymphocytic Interstitial Pneumonitis (LIP), and Nodular Lymphoid Hyperplasia. Follicular bronchiolitis and lymphoid interstitial pneumonitis are related inflammatory conditions associated with autoimmune and immunologic diseases including Sjögren syndrome, rheumatoid arthritis, and myasthenia gravis and immunocompromised states including common variable immunodeficiency and HIV infection. Affected patients have cough and dyspnea and a history of frequent respiratory infections. Patients with follicular bronchiolitis, most often seen associated with rheumatoid arthritis, have small, ill-defined centrilobular nodules representing lymphoid hyperplasia around small bronchi and bronchioles. LIP, a predominantly interstitial disease seen almost exclusively in patients with Sjögren syndrome and children with HIV infection (where it is associated with EBV infection), produces a lower lobe reticulonodular and linear pattern of disease radiographically, often with intermixed areas of airspace opacification. CT findings include diffuse ground-glass opacity, poorly defined centrilobular nodules, interlobular septal thickening, and thin-walled cysts (Fig. 13.23); lymph node enlargement may be an associated finding. Nodular lymphoid hyperplasia is likely a form of LIP in which one or several nodules or masses reflecting reactive lymphoid hyperplasia around small airways are seen.

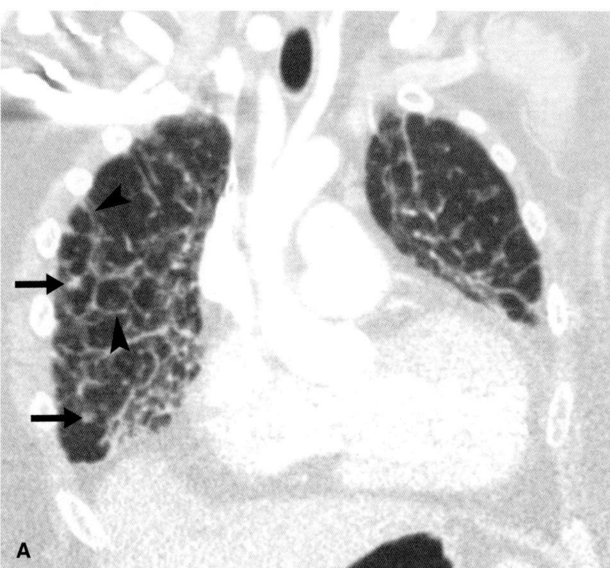

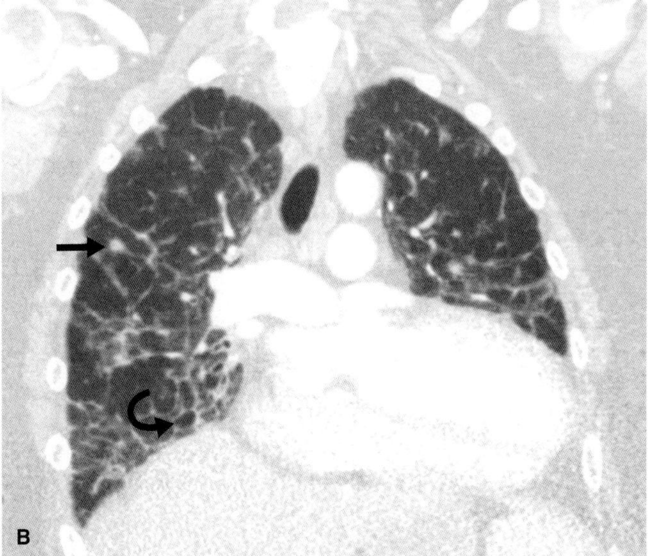

FIGURE 13.23. Lymphocytic Interstitial Pneumonitis in Common Variable Immunodeficiency. Coronal reformatted CT scans at lung windows through the anterior (**A**) and mid (**B**) lungs in a patient with immunodeficiency show ill-defined centrilobular nodules (*arrows* in **A**), reticular opacities (*arrowheads* in **A**), and cystic lesions (*curved arrow* in **B**) indicative of lymphocytic interstitial pneumonitis.

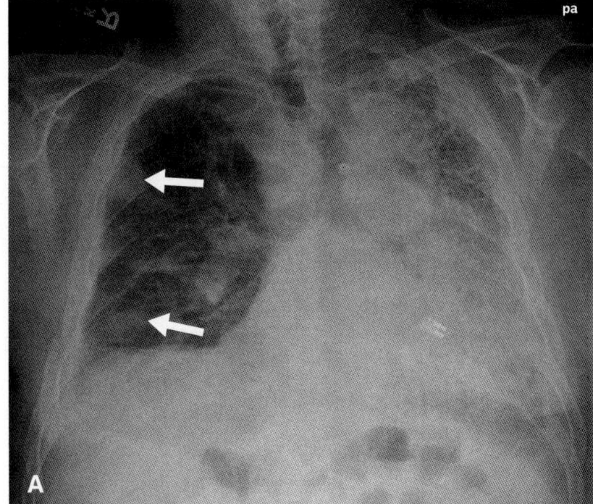

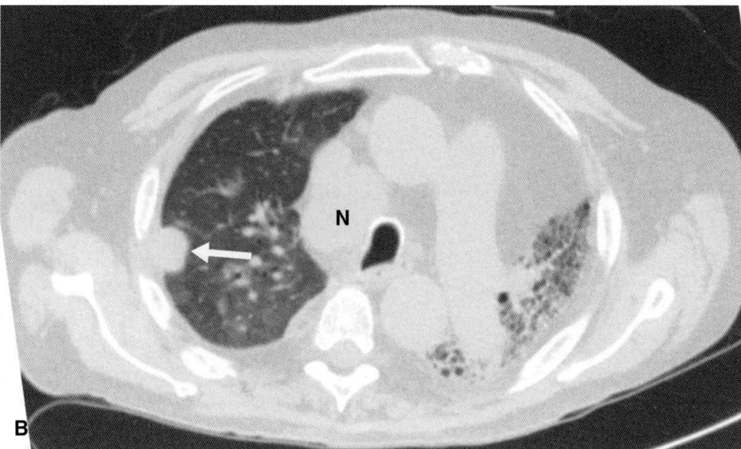

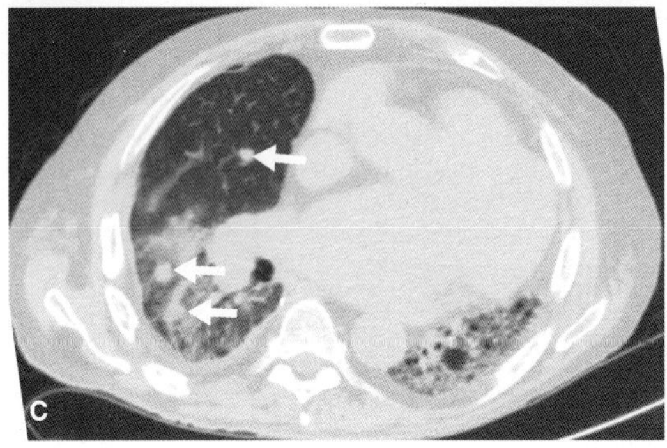

FIGURE 13.24. **Posttransplant Lymphoproliferative Disorder. A:** Frontal chest radiograph in a patient s/p right lung transplantation for idiopathic pulmonary fibrosis shows right lung nodules (*arrows*). **B, C:** Axial CT scans show multiple right lung nodules (*arrows* in **B** and **C**) and ground-glass opacities in the right lung. Note markedly enlarged right paratracheal lymph node (*N* in **B**). Biopsy revealed lymphoma.

Posttransplant lymphoproliferative disorder represents a spectrum of entities ranging from benign polyclonal lymphoid proliferation to aggressive non-Hodgkin lymphoma that develop in a small percentage of transplant patients, with lung transplant recipients most commonly affected. Infection with EBV is responsible for most cases. The disease often presents with extranodal disease, with the lung commonly involved. The most common imaging finding is that of solitary or multiple sharply marginated lung nodules or masses (Fig. 13.24). Treatment varies but for indolent forms of disease, reduction in immunosuppression is effective.

Leukemia. While leukemic involvement of the lung is found in approximately one-third of patients at autopsy, clinical or radiographic evidence of parenchymal infiltration is uncommon during life. The majority of pulmonary disease in leukemic patients is caused by pneumonia complicating immunosuppression, edema from cardiac disease, or hemorrhage owing to thrombocytopenia. Parenchymal involvement in leukemia usually takes the form of interstitial infiltration by leukemic cells, with resultant peribronchial cuffing and reticulonodular opacities on chest radiography. Focal accumulation of leukemic cells can produce a chloroma and the radiographic appearance of an SPN. An unusual pulmonary manifestation of leukemia is *pulmonary leukostasis*, which is seen in acute leukemia or those in blast crisis in whom the peripheral white blood cell count exceeds 100,000 to 200,000/cm^3. In this condition, the white cell blasts clump within the pulmonary microvasculature to produce dyspnea. Approximately half of affected patients have normal radiographs, while the remainder demonstrate a diffuse reticulonodular pattern of disease.

Kaposi sarcoma (KS) of the lung is most often seen in AIDS patients or transplant recipients and is associated with infection by human herpesvirus 8 (HHV-8). Pulmonary involvement typically follows skin, oropharyngeal, and/or visceral involvement. The histologic features are characteristic: clusters of spindle cells with numerous mitotic figures are separated by thin-walled vascular channels containing red blood cells. The tumor involves the tracheobronchial mucosa and the peribronchovascular, alveolar, and subpleural interstitium of the lung. KS produces small-to-medium, poorly marginated nodular and coarse linear opacities that extend from the hilum into the mid- and lower lung. CT shows the typical peribronchovascular location of the opacities and may demonstrate air bronchograms traversing mass-like areas of confluent disease. The mass-like opacities often parallel the long axis of the bronchovascular structures and have been described as "flame-shaped." A bloody pleural effusion is present in up to 50% of patients; this is attributed to lesions within the subpleural interstitium of the lung. Hilar and mediastinal lymph node enlargement is found in 20% of patients. Important diagnostic features of pulmonary KS are the slow rate of progression of disease (usually over many months) and the absence of fever or pulmonary symptoms despite extensive parenchymal disease.

The diagnosis of pulmonary KS is usually made indirectly by the visualization of typical endobronchial lesions in a patient with characteristic chest radiographic and CT findings.

Pulmonary blastoma is a rare malignant tumor affecting children and young adults. The tumors are comprised of both mesenchymal and epithelial elements of lungs, the latter simulating the appearance of fetal lungs at 10 to 16 weeks' gestation. Pulmonary blastomas are difficult to distinguish histologically from carcinosarcomas. These tumors tend to be extremely large at presentation (Fig. 13.25). Diagnosis is made by resection of the lesion. The prognosis is poor because many lesions have metastasized by the time of diagnosis.

Diffuse idiopathic pulmonary neuroendocrine cell hyperplasia (DIPNECH) is a preneoplastic proliferation of neuroendocrine cells found in the mucosa of small airways. Affected patients are middle-aged women that present either with

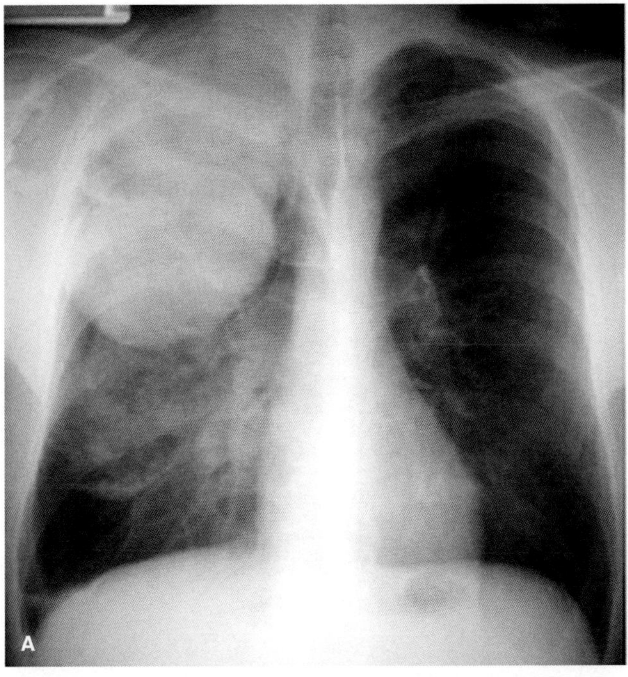

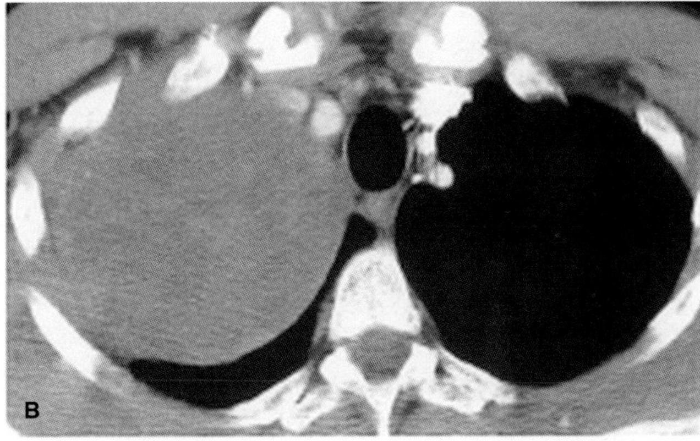

FIGURE 13.25. **Pulmonary Blastoma. A:** Posteroanterior radiograph in a 29-year-old man with hemoptysis shows a large right upper lobe mass. **B:** Enhanced CT shows a large mass that occupies much of the right upper lobe. Pathologic examination of the pneumonectomy specimen revealed pulmonary blastoma.

asymptomatic small lung nodules that simulate metastatic disease or with symptoms of cough, dyspnea, and wheezing diagnosed as COPD or asthma. In these latter patients, there are histologic findings of neuroendocrine cell hyperplasia and constrictive bronchiolitis with pulmonary functional evidence of airway obstruction. Mosaic lung attenuation and air trapping are typically seen on inspiratory and expiratory CT, respectively. Nodules <5 mm in diameter represent carcinoid tumorlets, while larger nodules represent typical carcinoid tumors (see Fig. 16.22).

TRACHEAL AND BRONCHIAL MASSES

Tracheal Neoplasms. Intratracheal masses may be divided into neoplastic and nonneoplastic masses. Primary tracheal tumors are rare; however, 90% of all primary tracheal tumors in adults are malignant. The majority of primary tracheal malignancies arise from tracheal epithelium or mucous glands (90%); the remainder arise from the mesenchymal elements of the tracheal wall (10%). Squamous cell carcinoma is the most common primary tracheal malignancy, accounting for at least 50% of all malignant tracheal neoplasms (Fig. 13.26). These tumors affect middle-aged male smokers and are associated with laryngeal, bronchogenic, or esophageal malignancies in up to 25% of cases. The majority arise in the distal trachea within 3 to 4 cm of the tracheal carina, with the cervical trachea the next most common site. Cough, hemoptysis, dyspnea, and wheezing are common presenting symptoms. Patients may be mistakenly treated for asthma before the correct diagnosis is made. Adenoid cystic carcinoma is a malignant neoplasm that arises from the tracheal salivary glands and accounts for 40% of primary tracheal malignancies. This neoplasm tends to involve the posterolateral wall of the distal two-thirds of the trachea (Fig. 13.27) or main or lobar bronchi.

The diagnosis of a primary tracheal malignancy is rarely made prospectively on chest radiographs, although well-penetrated radiographs can demonstrate distortion of the tracheal air column by a mass. CT typically shows a lobulated or irregular soft tissue mass that eccentrically narrows the tracheal lumen and has a variable extraluminal component (Fig. 13.27). Masses >2 cm in diameter are likely to be malignant, while those <2 cm are more likely benign. Calcification is uncommon. Resectability of these lesions depends on the length of tracheal involvement and the extent of mediastinal invasion at the time of diagnosis. CT is particularly well suited for determining mediastinal involvement and is the modality of choice for imaging tracheal neoplasms. The prognosis in patients with squamous cell carcinoma is poor, as up to 50% of patients have mediastinal extension of tumor at the time of diagnosis. While adenoid cystic carcinoma has a better prognosis, these slow-growing lesions are locally invasive with a tendency toward late recurrence and metastases.

A variety of other lesions comprise the remainder of primary tracheal malignancies and include mucoepidermoid carcinoma, carcinoid tumor, adenocarcinoma, lymphoma, small cell carcinoma, leiomyosarcoma, fibrosarcoma, and chondrosarcoma. Chondrosarcoma arises from tracheal cartilage and is identified by the presence of calcified chondroid matrix within the tumor. The trachea may be secondarily involved by malignancy either by direct invasion or by hematogenous spread. Laryngeal carcinoma may extend below the vocal cords to involve the cervical trachea. There is also a tendency for tumor to recur at the tracheostomy site in patients who have undergone total laryngectomies for carcinoma. Papillary and follicular carcinomas are the most common types of thyroid malignancy to invade the trachea. Squamous cell carcinoma of the upper third of the esophagus can invade the posterior tracheal wall and may produce a tracheoesophageal fistula. Lung cancer may involve the trachea by direct proximal extension from central bronchi, by extranodal spread of tumor from metastatic pretracheal or paratracheal lymph nodes, or by direct invasion of large right upper lobe tumors (Fig. 13.18). CT is best at demonstrating tumor invasion of the tracheal wall and the extent of intraluminal mass. The extrathoracic primary tumors that are most often associated with hematogenous endotracheal metastases are carcinomas of the breast, kidney, and colon and melanoma. These lesions may appear on CT as irregular thickening of the tracheal wall or as well-defined, localized nodules or masses that are indistinguishable from benign tracheal tumors.

Chondroma, fibroma, squamous cell papilloma, hemangioma, and granular cell tumors are the most common benign

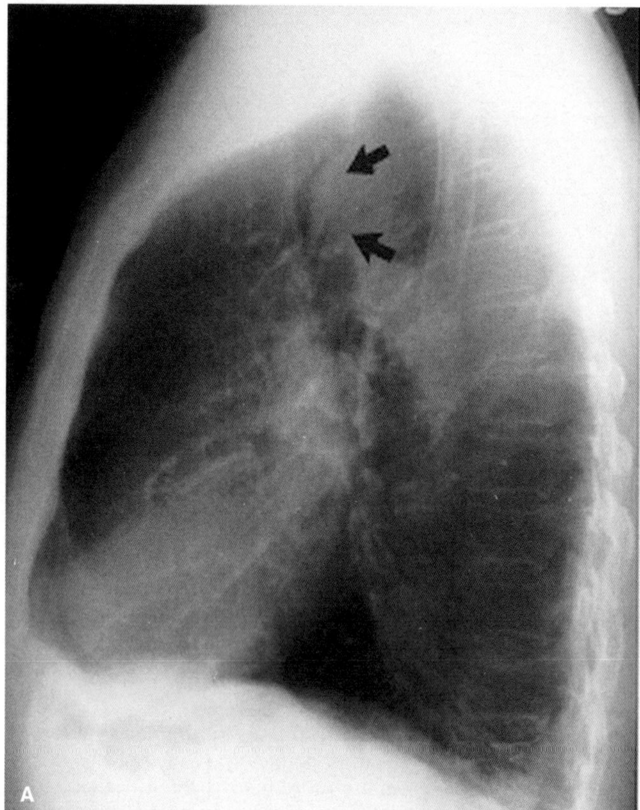

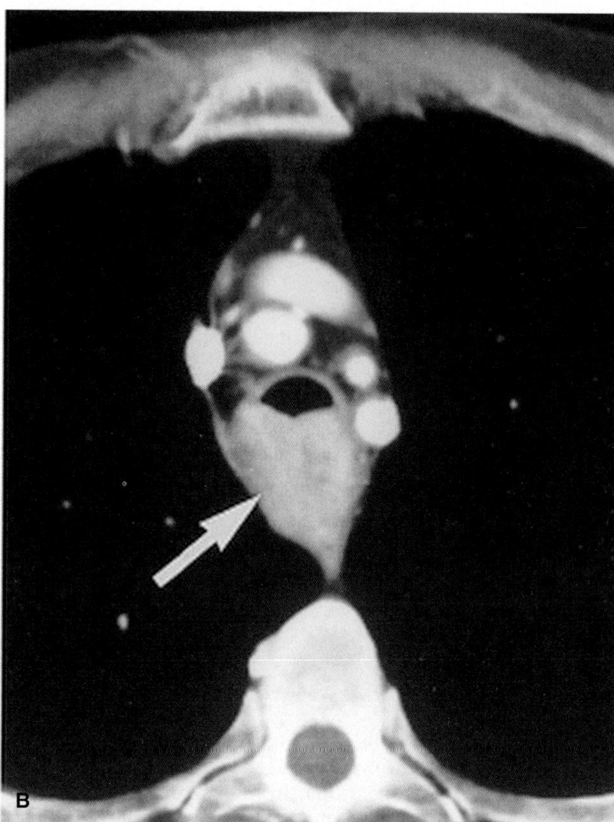

FIGURE 13.26. Squamous Cell Carcinoma of the Trachea. A: Lateral chest radiograph in a 68-year-old man shows a mass in the midtrachea (*black arrows*). **B:** CT scan demonstrates an enhancing mass (*arrow*) in the posterior trachea with narrowing of the tracheal lumen. Bronchoscopic biopsy showed squamous cell carcinoma.

tracheal tumors in adults. A *chondroma* arises from the tracheal cartilage and produces a well-circumscribed endoluminal mass. CT may demonstrate stippled cartilaginous calcification within the mass. *Fibromas* are sessile or pedunculated fibrous masses arising in the cervical trachea. *Squamous cell papilloma* is a mucosal lesion caused by infection with human papilloma virus. This disease typically produces multiple laryngeal masses in children born to women with venereal warts (condylomata acuminata). The trachea, bronchi, and lungs may become involved over time. These lesions usually regress by adolescence and, therefore, are uncommon causes of a solitary tracheal lesion in adults. *Hemangiomas* are seen in the cervical trachea almost exclusively in infants and young children; they appear as focal masses on CT. *Granular cell tumor* is a neoplasm that arises from neural elements in the tracheal or bronchial wall. These lesions usually involve the cervical trachea or main bronchi but can arise in smaller bronchi (Fig. 13.28). CT shows a broad-based or pedunculated soft tissue mass that may invade the tracheal wall. This neoplasm has a tendency toward local recurrence.

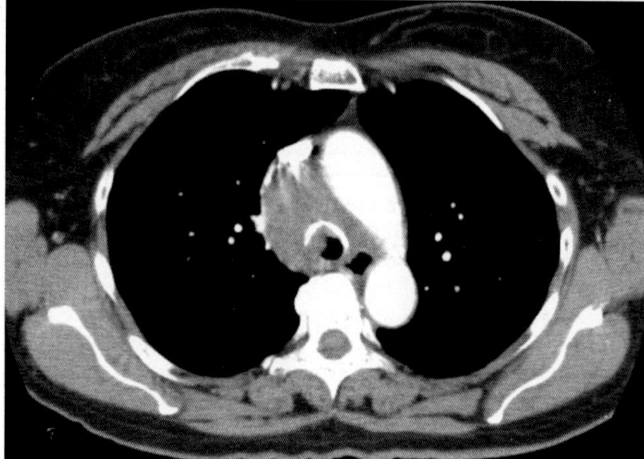

FIGURE 13.27. Adenoid Cystic Carcinoma of Trachea. Axial CT scan through the distal trachea shows an intratracheal mass irregularly narrowing the tracheal lumen with a large extraluminal/mediastinal component. Bronchoscopic biopsy showed adenoid cystic carcinoma.

Nonneoplastic intratracheal masses from ectopic intratracheal thyroid or thymic tissue have been reported and are radiographically indistinguishable from intratracheal neoplasms. Intratracheal thyroid is seen in women with extratracheal goiters. The intratracheal tissue is likewise goitrous and most commonly found in the posterolateral wall of the cervical trachea, although any portion of the trachea may be involved. Mucus may appear as intratracheal masses in patients with excess sputum production or diminished clearance mechanisms. They are typically low-attenuation masses on CT that change position or disappear after an effective cough.

Primary malignant neoplasms of the central bronchi include lung cancer, carcinoid tumor, and salivary gland tumors (adenoid cystic carcinoma, mucoepidermoid carcinoma, and pleomorphic adenoma). Carcinoid and salivary gland tumors account for approximately 2% of all tracheobronchial neoplasms; 90% of these lesions arise in a bronchus or the lung, while the remainder arise within the trachea. Carcinoid tumor accounts for nearly 90%, adenoid cystic carcinoma 8%, and mucoepidermoid 2% of these lesions. However, adenoid cystic

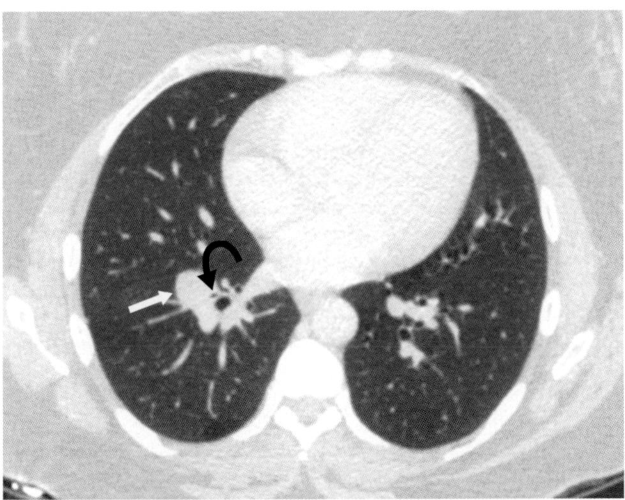

FIGURE 13.28. **Granular Cell Tumor of Lung.** CT scan at lung windows through the lower lobes shows a smoothly bordered mass (*arrow*) that narrows the anterior basal segmental bronchus (*curved arrow*). Surgical lobectomy revealed a granular cell tumor arising from the segmental bronchus.

carcinoma accounts for 90% and carcinoid 10% of all malignant tracheal neoplasms excluding lung cancer.

Carcinoid tumors arise from neuroendocrine (amine precursor uptake and decarboxylation or Kulchitsky) cells within the airways. There is a spectrum of histologic differentiation and malignant behavior in tumors of Kulchitsky cell origin ranging from the low-grade malignant-typical carcinoid to atypical carcinoid to the highly malignant small cell carcinoma. Eighty percent of bronchial carcinoid tumors arise within the central bronchi, and patients present with cough, dyspnea, wheezing, recurrent episodes of atelectasis or pneumonia, or hemoptysis (Fig. 13.29). The hemoptysis may be massive and is attributable to the highly vascular nature of these lesions. The average age at diagnosis is 50. Histologically, these tumors show sheets or trabeculae of uniform cells separated by a fibrovascular stroma. The cells may contain intracytoplasmic inclusions; immunohistochemistry will reveal a variety of neuroendocrine products including serotonin, vasoactive intestinal polypeptide, adrenocorticotropic hormone, and antidiuretic hormone. Carcinoid syndrome is seen in fewer than 3% of cases.

Radiologically, central bronchial carcinoids present with atelectasis or pneumonia secondary to large airway obstruction. A hyperlucent lobe or lung of diminished volume may result from incomplete obstruction or collateral airflow with reflex hypoxic vasoconstriction; this finding is also rarely seen in lung cancer. Carcinoid tumors arising within the lung appear as well-defined smooth or lobulated nodules or masses. Calcification or ossification is seen in 10% of pathologic specimens but is rarely visualized radiographically. CT is ideally suited to demonstrate the relationship of the mass to the central airways. The typical appearance on CT is a smooth or lobulated soft tissue mass within a main or lobar bronchus (Fig. 13.29). The presence of a small intraluminal and large extraluminal soft tissue component has given rise to the descriptive term "iceberg tumor." Atypical carcinoids tend to have more irregular margins and inhomogeneous contrast enhancement and are much more likely to be associated with hilar and mediastinal lymph node metastases. In some cases, the presence of small punctate peripheral calcifications or marked contrast enhancement on CT may allow distinction from lung cancer. Indium-labeled octreotide nuclear imaging has proven useful in the staging of carcinoid tumors, particularly the preoperative assessment of nodal or distant metastases. Given the relatively high false negative rate of FDG-PET for typical carcinoid tumors, octreotide scanning for TNM staging should be considered in all patients with known or suspected carcinoid tumor.

The prognosis for patients with typical bronchial carcinoid is excellent with a 5-year survival rate of 90%. Regional lymph node metastases, seen in approximately 5% of operative specimens,

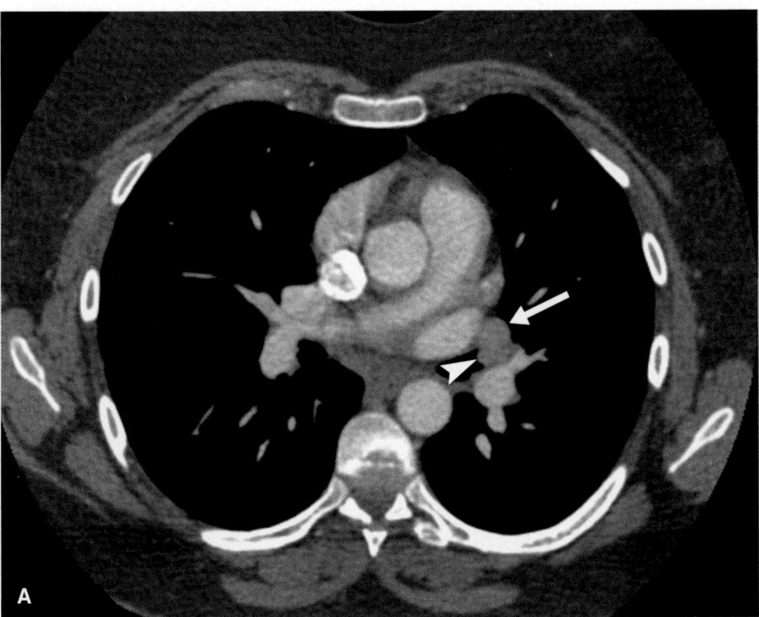

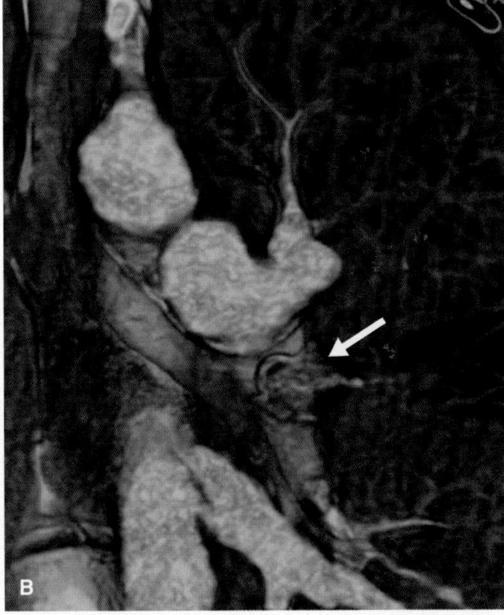

FIGURE 13.29. **Carcinoid Tumor, Left Upper Lobe Bronchus. A:** Contrast-enhanced axial CT through the mid chest shows a lobulated soft tissue mass (*arrow*) in the left hilum with an endoluminal component in the left upper lobe bronchus (*arrowhead*). **B:** Coronal volume-rendered CT reconstruction through the left hilum shows the mass (*arrow*) within the left upper lobe bronchus. Bronchoscopic biopsy revealed typical carcinoid tumor.

lower the 5-year survival rate to 70%. Atypical carcinoids are associated with metastases in up to 70% of cases, although these may appear many years after discovery of the primary tumor. The 5-year survival rate in these patients is less than 50%.

Pulmonary hamartoma is a benign neoplasm comprised of disorganized epithelial and mesenchymal elements normally found in the bronchus or lung. Histologically, these lesions contain cartilage surrounded by fibrous connective tissue, with variable amounts of fat, smooth muscle, and seromucous glands; calcification and ossification are seen in 30% of cases. Ninety percent of these lesions arise within the pulmonary parenchyma as nodules or masses (Figs. 13.1B and 13.5); fewer than 10% are endobronchial. Endobronchial hamartomas are usually pedunculated lesions with fatty centers covered by fibrous tissue that contain little cartilage. Patients are usually diagnosed in the fifth decade. Central bronchial hamartomas present with cough or upper airway obstruction. CT shows a soft tissue mass that is usually indistinguishable from a bronchial carcinoid.

METASTATIC DISEASE TO THE THORAX

The spread of extrapulmonary neoplasm to the lung may occur by direct invasion of the pulmonary parenchyma or as a result of hematogenous dissemination, with the latter mechanism much more common. Uncommonly, a tumor can disseminate throughout the lungs via the tracheobronchial tree as in laryngotracheal papillomatosis and some cases of mucinous adenocarcinoma. Transpleural spread of tumor can be seen in cases of invasive thymoma.

Direct invasion of the lung may occur with mediastinal, pleural, or chest wall malignancies. The most common mediastinal malignancies to invade the lung are esophageal carcinoma, lymphoma, and malignant germ cell tumors or any malignancy metastasizing to mediastinal or hilar lymph nodes. Malignant mesothelioma and metastases to the pleura or chest wall can extend through the pleura to invade the adjacent lung.

Hematogenous metastases to the lung may be seen with any tumor that gains access to the SVC, inferior vena cava, or thoracic duct because the pulmonary artery is the final common pathway for these channels. Although only a minority of tumor emboli survive within the pulmonary interstitium, those that do produce one of two morphologic and radiographic appearances: pulmonary nodules or LC.

Pulmonary nodules are the most common manifestation of hematogenous metastases to the lung. They are most commonly seen in carcinomas of the lung, breast, kidney, thyroid, colon, uterus, and head and neck. Although most patients have multiple nodules, metastases can present as SPNs. SPNs caused by metastases are typically smooth in contour, while primary bronchogenic tumors tend to be lobulated or spiculated. The likelihood that an SPN represents a solitary metastasis in a patient with a synchronous extrathoracic malignancy is slightly less than 50%, while SPNs in patients with prior malignancy are almost always primary lung cancer or a granuloma. However, the site of the primary tumor may affect the likelihood that an SPN is a metastasis. Carcinoma of the rectosigmoid colon, osteogenic sarcoma, renal cell carcinoma, breast cancer, and melanoma are more likely to result in solitary pulmonary metastasis. It should be cautioned that what may appear as a solitary metastasis on plain radiographs may be only one of multiple pulmonary nodules as shown by chest CT.

Nodular pulmonary metastases are usually smooth or lobulated lesions that are found in greater numbers in the peripheral portions of the lower lobes because of the greater pulmonary blood flow to these regions. However, metastatic nodules can be ill-defined, thereby simulating inflammatory lesions. CT is the modality of choice for the evaluation of pulmonary metastases (Fig. 13.30). There are no characteristic features of nodular metastases that allow distinction among different primary neoplasms. Similarly, the distinction between metastases and granulomas is usually impossible. The demonstration of calcification within multiple pulmonary nodules in the absence of a history of a primary bone-forming neoplasm such as osteogenic sarcoma or chondrosarcoma is diagnostic of granulomatous disease. Although primary mucinous adenocarcinomas of the colon and ovary may rarely produce calcification within pulmonary metastases, these microscopic calcifications are usually too small to be detected even on CT. Additionally, in patients with miliary nodular opacities, the presence of one or more larger nodules interspersed with uniformly sized miliary nodules is highly suggestive of metastases from melanoma or carcinoma of the lung, thyroid, or kidney.

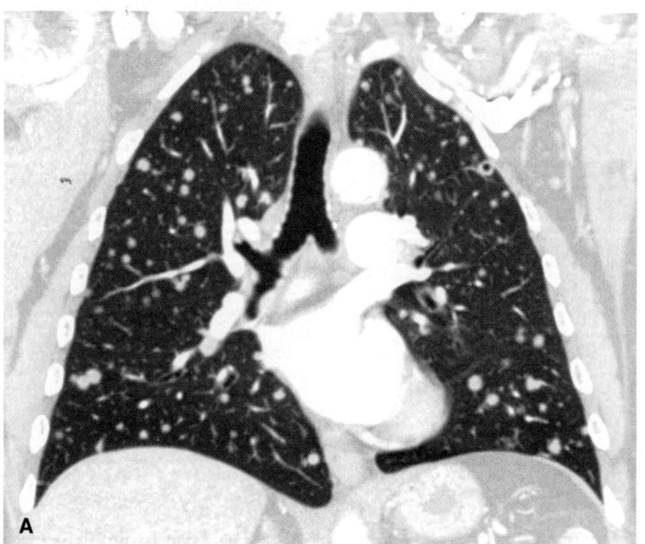

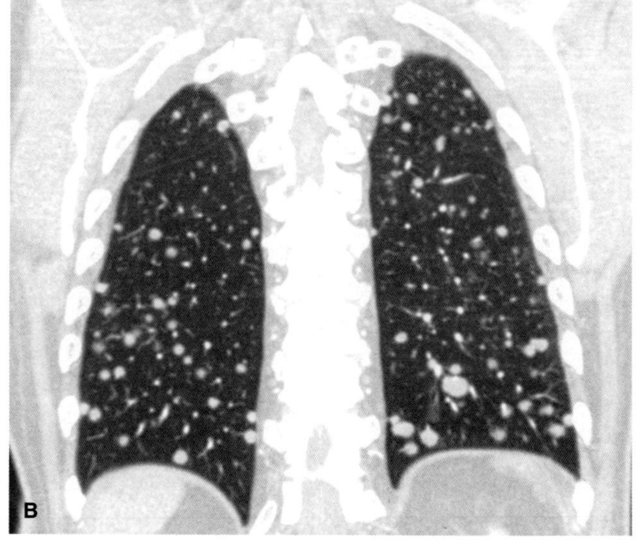

FIGURE 13.30. **Nodular Pulmonary Metastases. A, B:** Coronal CT scans through the mid (**A**) and posterior (**B**) lungs show innumerable bilateral smooth pulmonary nodules reflecting hematogenous metastases from melanoma.

The diagnosis of nodular pulmonary metastases is usually presumptive based on the demonstration of multiple pulmonary nodules in a patient with a known malignancy with a propensity for lung metastases. In some patients, particularly those with SPNs and no evidence of additional sites of metastases or those with a history of a prior localized malignancy, a biopsy of the nodule should be performed. In selected patients, resection of a solitary pulmonary metastasis or several peripheral metastases may be undertaken. CT is the best imaging modality to follow the response of metastases to chemotherapy, with resolution or stability of nodules indicating a positive response.

Lymphangitic Carcinomatosis (LC). While direct parenchymal lymphatic invasion and obstruction of hilar and mediastinal lymph nodes by bronchogenic carcinoma is the most common cause of unilateral LC, extrapulmonary malignancies may invade pulmonary lymphatics after hematogenous dissemination to both lungs to produce interstitial deposits of tumor. In LC, the tumor cells invade the lymphatics within the peribronchovascular and peripheral interstitium resulting in lymphatic dilatation, interstitial edema, and fibrosis. The most common extrathoracic malignancies to produce LC are carcinomas of the breast, stomach, pancreas, and prostate. Occasionally, LC will present in a patient without a known primary malignancy. Most patients with LC have slowly progressive dyspnea and a nonproductive cough.

The chest radiographic findings in LC complicating extrathoracic malignancy correlate with the involvement of the peribronchovascular and peripheral interstitium seen pathologically. Peribronchial cuffing and linear opacities, particularly Kerley B lines, are characteristically seen. Coarse reticulonodular opacities may also be present. Concomitant hilar and mediastinal lymph node enlargement need not be present.

The predominant CT findings in LC are thickening of interlobular septa and the subpleural interstitium (Fig. 13.17). While nodular thickening of the septa, reflecting tumor nodules, is characteristic of LC, it is seen in only a minority of patients. The thickened septal lines do not distort the pulmonary lobule, a feature that helps distinguish LC from interstitial fibrosis, which characteristically distorts the normal lobular shape. Visibility of the intralobular bronchioles or prominence of the centrilobular vessel is frequently seen, as is thickening of the peribronchovascular interstitium within the central (parahilar) portions of the lung. The findings may be unilateral or even limited to one lobe, particularly when LC occurs secondary to bronchogenic carcinoma. Because most patients with LC have pathologic involvement of the peribronchovascular interstitium, the diagnosis is best made by transbronchial biopsy. In a patient with the appropriate history, the CT appearance of lymphangitic spread may be specific enough to obviate the need for transbronchial biopsy. Occasionally, the HRCT study will demonstrate the typical findings of LC when conventional radiographs are normal or equivocal.

Pulmonary Arterial Tumor Emboli. Rarely, extrathoracic tumors can invade the systemic venous circulation and embolize to the lung as macroscopic tumor emboli that then grow within the pulmonary arterial vasculature. Examples include hepatocellular carcinoma and renal cell carcinoma that can invade the hepatic veins and renal veins, respectively, gaining access to the right heart and pulmonary vasculature. Macroscopic tumor emboli appear as tubular or branching intravascular lesions that often expand the lumen of the involved artery (Fig. 12.11). Peripheral pulmonary arterial tumor emboli can result in pulmonary infarction.

Suggested Readings

Aquino SL. Imaging of metastatic disease to the thorax. *Radiol Clin North Am* 2005;43(3):481–495.

Bankier AA, MacMahon H, Goo JM, Rubin GD, Schaefer-Prokop CM, Naidich DP. Recommendations for measuring pulmonary nodules at CT: a statement from the Fleischner Society. *Radiology* 2017;285(2):584–600.

Detterbeck FC, Boffa DJ, Kim AW, Tanoue LT. The eighth edition lung cancer stage classification. *Chest* 2017;151(1):193–203.

Goldstraw P, Chansky K, Crowley J, et al. The IASLC lung cancer staging project: proposals for revision of the TNM stage groupings in the forthcoming (eighth) edition of the TNM classification for lung cancer. *J Thorac Oncol* 2016; 11(1):39–51.

Kim SK, Allen-Auerbach M, Goldin J, et al. Accuracy of PET/CT in characterization of solitary pulmonary lesions. *J Nucl Med* 2007;48(2):214–220.

Kligerman S, Digumarthy S. Staging of non-small cell lung cancer using integrated PET/CT. *AJR Am J Roentgenol* 2009;193(5):1203–1211.

Lung-RADS. American College of Radiology. https://www.acr.org/-/media/ACR/Files/RADS/Lung-RADS/LungRADSAssessmentCategories.pdf

MacMahon H, Naidich DP, Goo JM, et al. Guidelines for management of incidental pulmonary nodules detected on CT images: from the Fleischner Society 2017. *Radiology* 2017;284(1):228–243.

Ngo AVH, Walker CM, Chung JH, et al. Tumors and tumorlike conditions of the large airways. *AJR Am J Roentgenol* 2013;201(2):301–313.

Sirajuddin A, Raparia K, Lewis VA, et al. Primary pulmonary lymphoid lesions: radiologic and pathologic findings. *RadioGraphics* 2016;36(1):53–70.

Song JW, Oh YM, Shim TS, Kim WS, Ryu JS, Choi CM. Efficacy comparison between (18)F-FDG PET/CT and bone scintigraphy in detecting bony metastases of non-small-cell lung cancer. *Lung Cancer* 2009;65(3):333–338.

Swensen SJ, Viggiano RW, Midthun DE, et al. Lung nodule enhancement at CT: multicenter study. *Radiology* 2000;214(1):73–80.

Travis WD, Brambilla E, Nicholson AG, et al. The 2015 World Health Organization classification of lung tumors: impact of genetic, clinical and radiologic advances since the 2004 classification. *J Thorac Oncol* 2015;10(9):1243–1260.

Truong MT, Ko JP, Rossi SE, et al. Update in the evaluation of the solitary pulmonary nodule. *RadioGraphics* 2014;34(6):1658–1679.

Wu C, Klein JS. Lung cancer: radiologic manifestations and diagnosis. Chapter 24. In: Chung, Wu NL, eds. *Imaging of the Chest*. Philadelphia, PA: WB Saunders; 2017.

CHAPTER 14 ■ PULMONARY INFECTION

JEFFREY S. KLEIN

INFECTION IN THE NORMAL HOST

The bronchopulmonary system is open to the atmosphere and therefore is relatively accessible to airborne microorganisms. Multiple host defense mechanisms exist at the level of the pharynx, trachea, and central bronchi. When these mechanisms fail, pathogenic organisms can penetrate to the small distal bronchi and the pulmonary parenchyma. Once the invading organisms penetrate the parenchyma, there is activation of both the cellular and humoral immune systems. This response may manifest clinically and radiographically as pneumonia, and in a normal host will often lead to eradication or at least suppression of the infecting organisms. If the immune response is impaired, a lower respiratory tract infection may lead to a very severe illness and often death, despite appropriate antibiotic therapy.

Mechanisms of Disease and Radiographic Patterns. Microorganisms responsible for producing pneumonia enter the lung and cause infection by three potential routes: via the tracheobronchial tree, via the pulmonary vasculature, or via direct spread from infection in the mediastinum, chest wall, or upper abdomen.

Infection via the tracheobronchial tree is generally secondary to inhalation or aspiration of infectious microorganisms and can be divided into three subtypes based on gross pathologic appearance and radiographic patterns: lobar pneumonia, lobular or bronchopneumonia, and atypical pneumonia. As will be discussed in later sections, certain organisms will typically produce one of these three patterns, although there is considerable overlap.

Lobar pneumonia is typical of pneumococcal pulmonary infection. In this pattern of disease, the inflammatory exudate begins within the distal airspaces. The inflammatory process spreads via the pores of Kohn and canals of Lambert to produce nonsegmental consolidation. If untreated, the inflammation may eventually involve an entire lobe (Fig. 14.1). Because the airways are usually spared, air bronchograms are common and significant volume loss is unusual.

Bronchopneumonia is the most common pattern of disease and is most typical of staphylococcal pneumonia. In the early stages of bronchopneumonia, the inflammation is centered primarily in and around lobular bronchi. As the inflammation progresses, exudative fluid extends peripherally along the bronchus to involve the entire pulmonary lobule. Radiographically, multifocal opacities that are roughly lobular in configuration produce a "patchwork quilt" appearance because of the interspersion of normal and diseased lobules (Fig. 14.1B). While bronchopneumonia is the most common cause of multifocal patchy airspace opacities, there is a broad list of differential diagnostic considerations. Exudate within the bronchi accounts for the absence of air bronchograms in bronchopneumonia. With coalescence of affected areas, the pattern may resemble lobar pneumonia.

In atypical pneumonia, most often the result of viral and mycoplasma pulmonary infection, there is inflammatory thickening of bronchiolar and alveolar walls and the pulmonary interstitium. This results in a radiographic pattern of small airways thickening and irregular linear and nodular opacities which reflect a combination of small airways, alveolar and peripheral interstitial disease. Air bronchograms are absent because the alveolar spaces remain aerated. Segmental and subsegmental atelectasis from small airways obstruction is common.

The spread of infection to the lung via the pulmonary vasculature usually occurs in the setting of systemic sepsis. The pattern of parenchymal involvement is patchy and bilateral. The lung bases are most severely involved, because blood flow is greatest in the dependent portions of the lungs. Pulmonary infection from direct spread usually results in a localized parenchymal process adjacent to an extrapulmonary source of infection. If an organism causes extensive parenchymal necrosis, abscess formation may result.

Bacterial Pneumonia

Community-acquired bacterial pneumonia accounts for between 500,000 and 1 million hospitalizations in the United States annually, and is most often due to infection by *Streptococcus pneumoniae, Mycoplasma pneumoniae, Chlamydia pneumoniae,* and *Legionella pneumophila.* Table 14.1 lists the most common organisms responsible for bacterial pneumonia and typical radiographic and thin-section CT findings in affected patients.

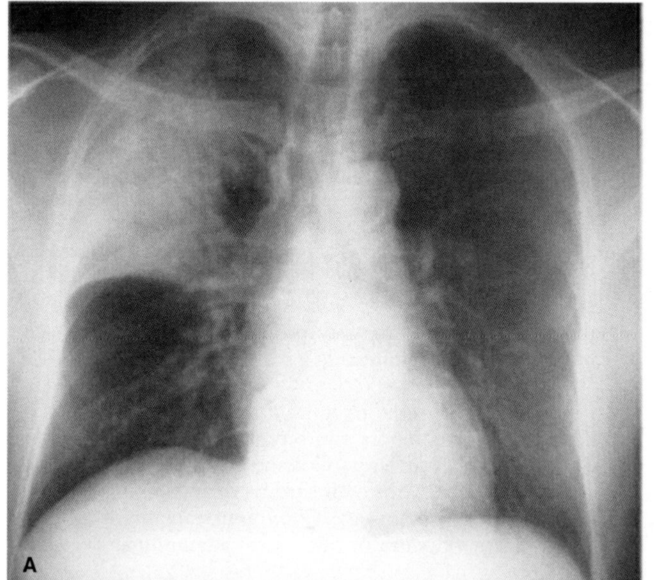

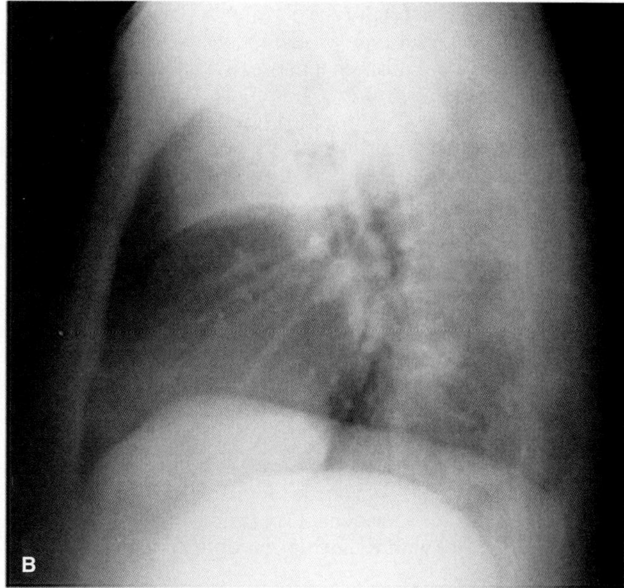

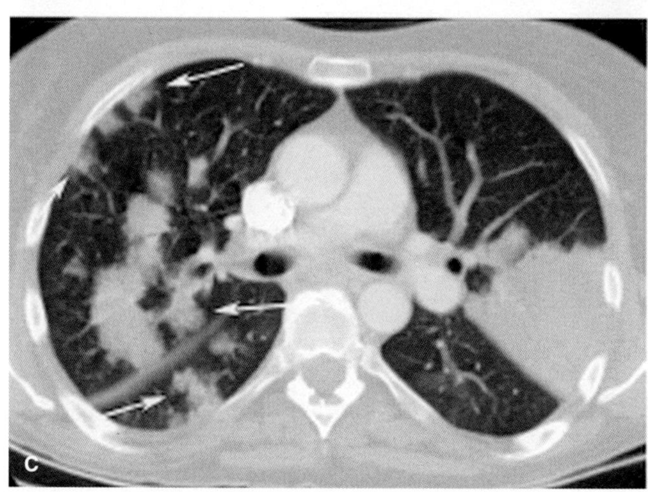

FIGURE 14.1. Pneumococcal Pneumonia. A, B: Frontal (**A**) and lateral (**B**) radiographs in a 57-year-old man with fever, chills, and productive cough demonstrate airspace opacification in the right upper lobe with air bronchograms. Sputum culture was positive for *Streptococcus pneumoniae*. **C:** CT scan in another patient with pneumococcal pneumonia shows dense multifocal segmental airspace opacification in the upper lobes. Note the lobular pattern of opacity in the right upper lobe and superior segment of the right lower lobe (*arrows*), reflecting regions of bronchopneumonia.

TABLE 14.1

ORGANISMS CAUSING BACTERIAL PNEUMONIA AND IMAGING PATTERNS

■ ORGANISMS	■ PATTERNS OF DISEASE	■ ASSOCIATED FINDINGS
■ *Streptococcus pneumoniae* ■ *Legionella pneumophila* ■ *Klebsiella pneumoniae* ■ *Haemophilus influenzae*	■ **Lobar/sublobar consolidation** ■ Air bronchograms	■ Round pneumonia ■ Bulging fissure (Klebsiella) ■ Pleural effusion (Klebsiella)
■ *Staphylococcus aureus* ■ *Pseudomonas aeruginosa* ■ *Escherichia coli* ■ *Anaerobic bacteria* ■ *Actinomyces israelii*	■ **Lobular/patchy consolidation** ■ Absence of air bronchograms ■ Bronchial wall thickening	■ Effusion/empyema ■ Cavitation/abscess ■ Pneumatoceles ■ Chest wall involvement (Actinomyces)
■ *Mycoplasma pneumoniae* ■ *Chlamydia pneumoniae*	■ **Ill-defined nodular/patchy opacities** ■ Reticular opacities ■ Bronchial wall thickening	
■ *Nocardia asteroides*	■ **Nodules/masses** ■ Consolidation (mass-like)	■ Cavitation ■ Crazy paving (with alveolar proteinosis)

Gram-Positive Bacteria

Streptococcus pneumoniae (pneumococcus). S. pneumoniae is a gram-positive organism that may cause infection in healthy individuals but is much more commonly seen in the elderly, alcoholics, and other compromised hosts. It is the most commonly isolated bacteria in patients with pneumonia who require hospitalization. Patients with sickle cell disease or who have undergone splenectomy are at particular risk for severe pneumococcal pneumonia.

Pneumococcal pneumonia tends to begin in the lower lobes or the posterior segments of the upper lobes. Initially there is involvement of the terminal airways, but rather than remaining localized to this site, there is rapid development of an airspace inflammatory exudate. The spread of infection to contiguous airspaces via interalveolar connections accounts for the nonsegmental distribution and homogeneity of the resultant consolidation.

The typical radiographic appearance of acute pneumococcal pneumonia is lobar consolidation (Fig. 14.1A,B). Air bronchograms are usually evident. Cavitation in pneumococcal pneumonia is rare, with the exception of infections caused by serotype 3. Uncomplicated parapneumonic effusion or empyema may be seen in up to 50% of patients. With appropriate therapy, complete clearing may be seen in 10 to 14 days. In older patients or those with underlying disease, complete resolution may take 12 to 16 weeks.

Patients with pneumococcal pneumonia occasionally present with atypical radiographic patterns of disease. Patchy lobular opacities similar to those seen with bronchopneumonia (Fig. 14.1C) or rarely, a reticulonodular pattern may be seen. In some patients, the atypical appearance may relate to the presence of pre-existing lung disease (e.g., emphysema), partial treatment, or an impaired immune response. In children and young adults, pneumococcal pneumonia may present as a spherical opacity ("round pneumonia") simulating a parenchymal mass (Fig. 14.2).

Staphylococcus aureus pneumonia is an important cause of nosocomial pneumonia, and typically affects debilitated patients. It may also develop following hematogenous spread to the lungs in patients with endocarditis or indwelling catheters and intravenous drug users. Community-acquired infection may complicate influenza or other viral pneumonias.

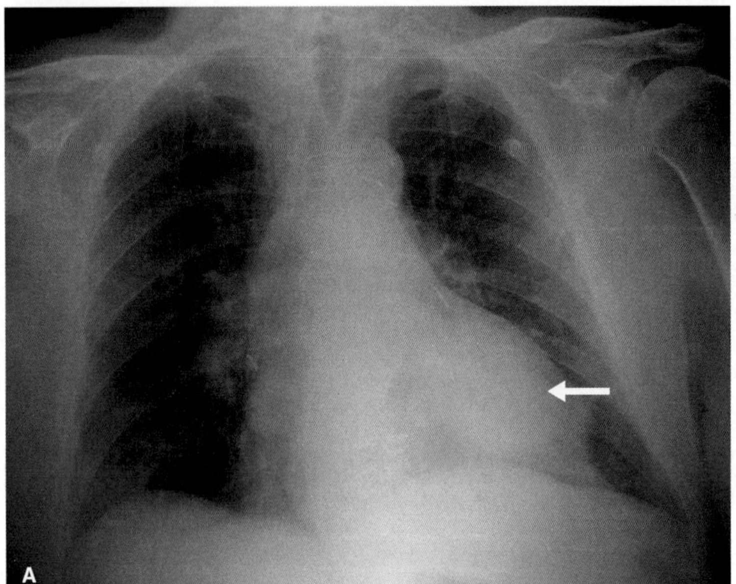

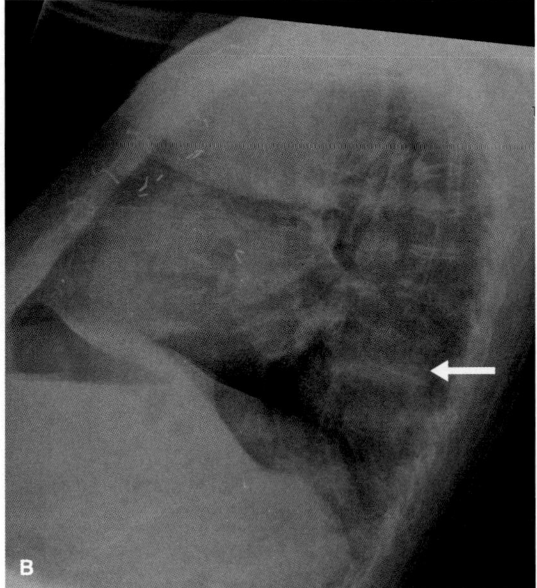

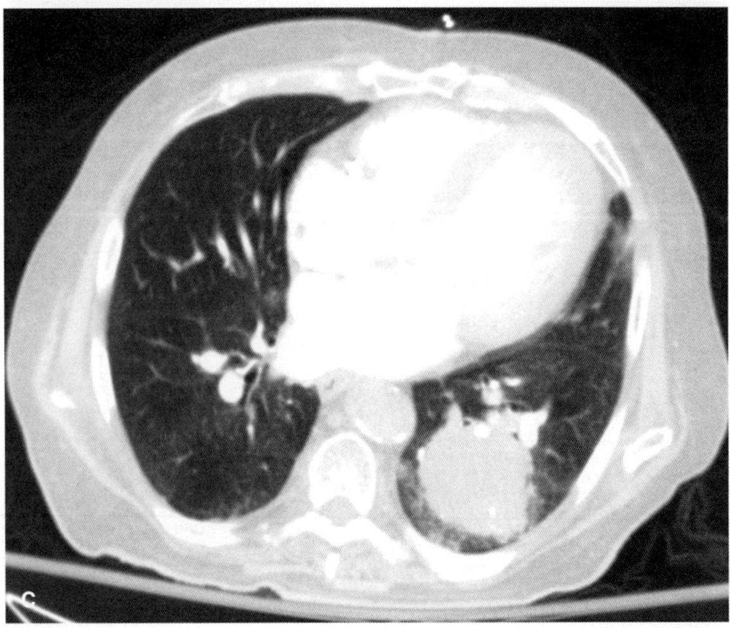

FIGURE 14.2. **Round Pneumonia. A, B:** Frontal (**A**) and lateral (**B**) chest radiographs in a 76-year-old man with cough and fever demonstrates a left lower lobe mass (*arrows*). **C:** Axial CT scan shows the left lower lobe mass with ill-defined margins. Blood cultures revealed pneumococcal infection.

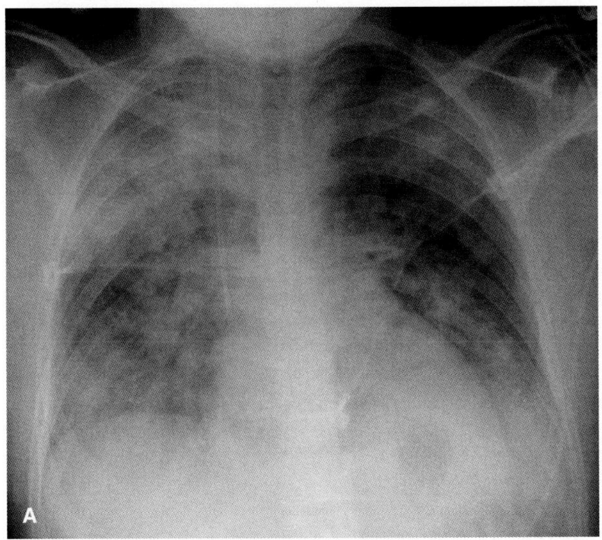

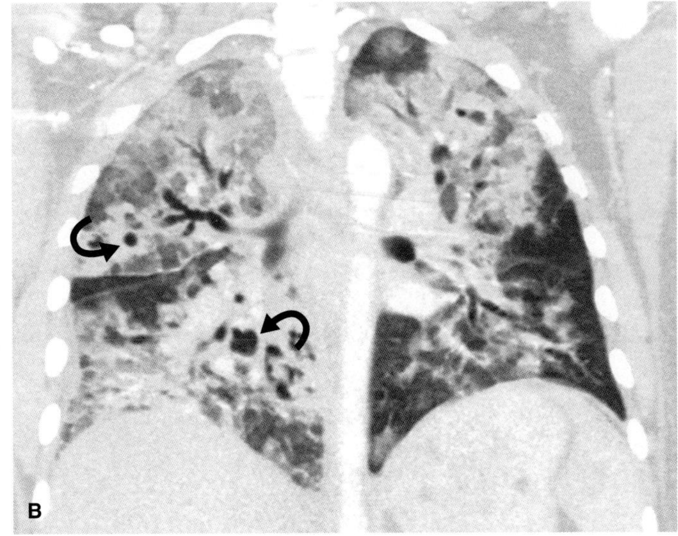

FIGURE 14.3. ***Staphylococcus aureus* Pneumonia. A:** Frontal chest radiograph in a patient with Staphylococcal pneumonia demonstrates multifocal airspace opacification. **B:** Contrast-enhanced coronal CT through the mid-lungs shows multifocal airspace and ground-glass opacification. The presence of pneumatoceles (*curved arrows*) is consistent with staphylococcal pulmonary infection.

S. aureus typically produces a bronchopneumonia and appears radiographically as patchy opacities. In severe cases, the opacities may become confluent to produce lobar opacification. Because the inflammatory exudate fills the airways, air bronchograms are rarely seen. In adults, the process is often bilateral and may be complicated by abscess formation in 15% to 30% of patients. In patients who develop pulmonary infection from hematogenous seeding, multiple bilateral poorly defined nodular opacities develop that eventually become more sharply defined and cavitate. Pneumatocele formation occurs in 15% to 30% of patients and may lead to pneumothorax. Pneumatoceles may be distinguished from abscesses by their thin walls, rapid change in size, and tendency to develop during the late phase of infection (Fig. 14.3). Pleural effusion is common, seen in 30% to 50% of patients, and can rapidly result in empyema.

Gram-Negative Bacteria. Gram-negative bacteria are increasingly important causes of pneumonia in hospitalized patients, accounting for over 50% of nosocomial pulmonary infections. While gram-negative organisms may be isolated from only a small percentage of healthy individuals, the isolation rate in hospitalized and severely ill patients ranges from 40% to 75%. The organisms most often responsible for pneumonia include members of the Enterobacteriaceae family (*Klebsiella pneumoniae*, *Escherichia coli*, *Proteus mirabilis*, *Serratia marcescens*); *Pseudomonas aeruginosa*; *Haemophilus influenzae*; and *L. pneumophila*.

The radiographic appearance of gram-negative bacterial pneumonia varies from small ill-defined nodules to patchy areas of opacification that may become confluent and resemble lobar pneumonia. Involvement is usually bilateral and multifocal, and the lower lobes are most frequently affected. Abscess formation and cavitation are relatively common. Parapneumonic effusion is common and is often complicated by empyema formation.

Klebsiella pneumoniae. *Klebsiella* pneumonia occurs predominantly in older alcoholic men and debilitated hospitalized patients. Radiographically it appears as a homogeneous lobar opacification containing air bronchograms. Three features, when present, can help distinguish it radiographically from pneumococcal pneumonia: (1) the volume of the involved lobe may be increased by the exuberant inflammatory exudate, producing a bulging interlobar fissure; (2) an abscess may develop, with cavity formation, which is uncommon in pneumococcal pneumonia; and (3) the incidence of pleural effusion and empyema is higher. Pulmonary gangrene may be seen but is uncommon.

Haemophilus influenzae. In adults, *H. influenzae* infection is most common in patients with chronic obstructive pulmonary disease (COPD), alcoholism, diabetes mellitus, and those with an anatomic or functional splenectomy. It most often causes bronchitis, although it may extend to produce bilateral lower lobe bronchopneumonia.

Pseudomonas aeruginosa pneumonia most often affects debilitated patients, particularly those requiring mechanical ventilation. There is a high mortality rate associated with the disease. The radiographic pattern of parenchymal involvement depends upon the method by which the organisms reach the lung. Patchy opacities with abscess formation, which mimic staphylococcal pneumonia, are common when the infection reaches the lung via the tracheobronchial tree. Diffuse, bilateral, ill-defined nodular opacities usually reflect hematogenous dissemination. Pleural effusions are common and are usually small.

Legionella pneumophila. Legionnaires disease is caused by infection with *L. pneumophila,* a gram-negative bacillus commonly found in air conditioning and humidifier systems. This infection tends to affect older men. Community-acquired infection is seen in patients with COPD or malignancy, while nosocomial infection primarily affects immunocompromised patients or those with renal failure or malignancy.

The characteristic radiographic pattern is airspace opacification, which is initially peripheral and sublobar. In some patients, the airspace opacities appear as a round pneumonia. The infection progresses to lobar (Fig. 14.4) or multilobar involvement despite the initiation of antibiotic therapy. At the peak of disease, the parenchymal involvement is usually bilateral. Pleural effusions are seen in approximately 30% of patients. Cavitation is not seen except in the immunocompromised patients. The radiographic resolution of pneumonia is often prolonged and may lag behind symptomatic improvement.

Anaerobic Bacterial Infection. The majority of anaerobic lung infections arise from aspiration of infected oropharyngeal contents. Approximately 25% of patients give a history of

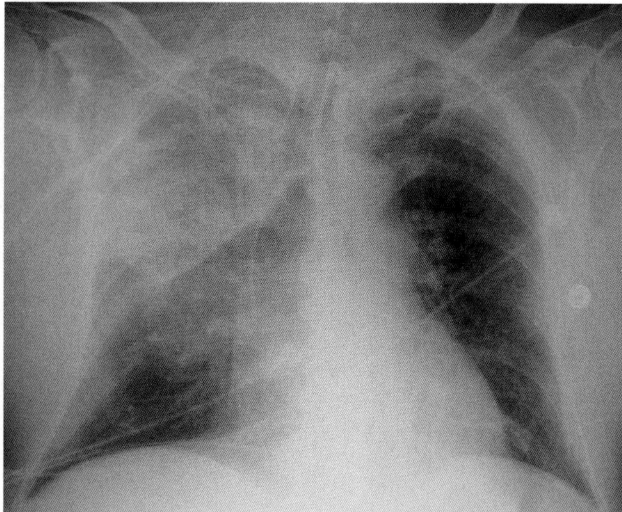

FIGURE 14.4. ***Legionella pneumophila* Pneumonia.** Portable chest radiograph in a 53-year-old renal transplant recipient on mechanical ventilation demonstrates dense right upper lobe and superior segment right lower lobe airspace opacification. Bronchoscopy showed *Legionella pneumophila* pneumonia.

impaired consciousness, and many are alcoholic. The most common organisms responsible are the gram-negative bacilli *Bacteroides* and *Fusobacterium*, although the majority of pulmonary infections are polymicrobial. All anaerobic pulmonary infections produce a similar radiographic appearance. The distribution of parenchymal opacities reflects the gravitational flow of aspirated material. When aspiration occurs in the supine position, it is the posterior segments of the upper lobes and superior segments of the lower lobes that are predominantly involved, whereas aspiration in the erect position leads to involvement of basal segments of the lower lobes. The typical radiographic appearance is peripheral lobular and segmental airspace opacities. Cavitation within areas of consolidation is relatively common, and discrete lung abscesses may be seen in up to 50% of patients (Fig. 14.5). Hilar and/or mediastinal lymph node enlargement may be seen in those with lung abscesses. Empyema, with or without bronchopleural fistula formation, is a common complication and is seen in up to 50% of patients.

Atypical Bacterial Infections

Actinomycosis. *A. israelii* is an anaerobic gram-positive filamentous bacterium that is a normal inhabitant of the human oropharynx. It causes disease when it gains access to devitalized or infected tissues that facilitate its growth. Actinomycosis most commonly follows dental extractions, manifesting as mandibular osteomyelitis or a soft tissue abscess. The lungs may be infected by aspiration of infectious oral debris or, less commonly, by direct extension from the primary site of disease.

The radiographic pattern of actinomycosis is often indistinguishable from that of nocardiosis. Findings consist of nonsegmental airspace opacities in the periphery of the lower lobes. In some cases, the infection manifests as a localized mass-like opacity that mimics lung cancer (Fig. 14.6). If therapy is not instituted, a lung abscess may develop. Thoracic actinomycosis is characterized by its ability to spread to contiguous tissues without regard for normal anatomic barriers. Extension into the pleural space can cause empyema, while chest wall involvement is characterized by osteomyelitis of the ribs and chest wall abscess. Involvement of the ribs is seen as wavy periosteal reaction or lytic rib destruction. If the pleuropulmonary disease becomes chronic, extensive fibrosis may be seen. Rarely, the disease is disseminated and a miliary pattern is seen.

Mycoplasma displays both bacterial and viral characteristics and are considered as a separate group. They are probably the most common atypical pneumonia and account for 10% to 15% of all community-acquired pneumonia. Affected patients usually have a subacute illness of 2 to 3 weeks' duration. Symptoms include fever, nonproductive cough, headache, and malaise. Unusual physical findings include bullous myringitis and rash.

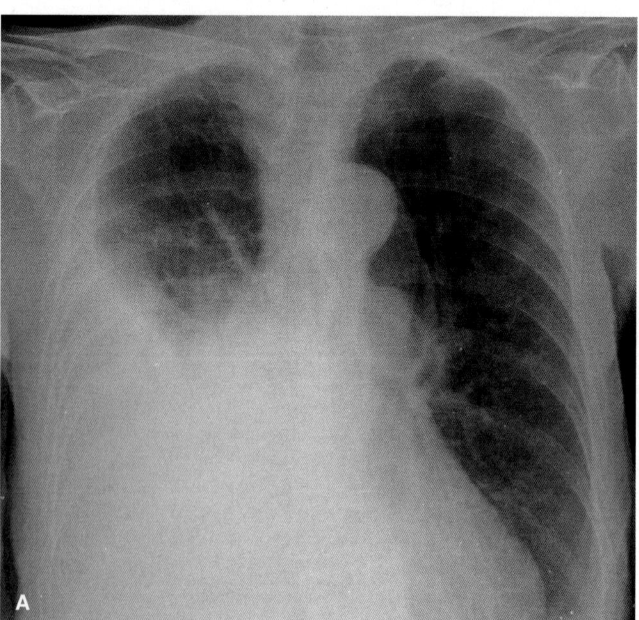

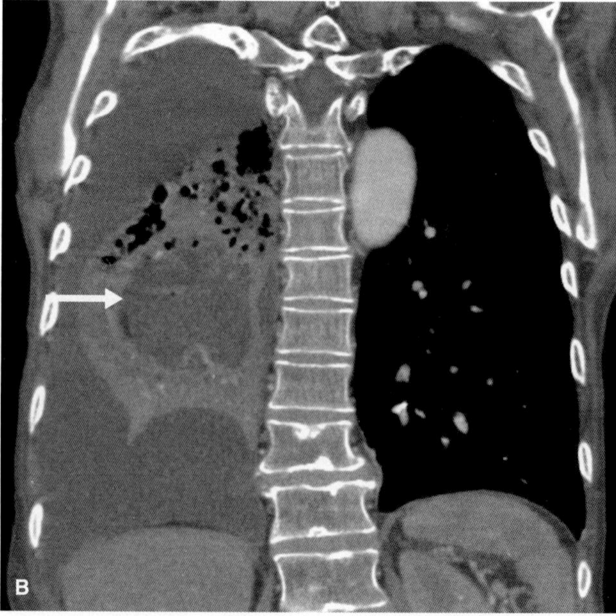

FIGURE 14.5. **Necrotizing Anaerobic Pneumonia With Abscess Formation and Parapneumonic Effusion. A:** Frontal chest radiograph in a 58-year-old man with fever and progressive shortness of breath shows a large right pleural effusion. **B:** Contrast-enhanced coronal CT scan shows a consolidated and atelectatic right lung containing a large abscess (*arrow*) and associated parapneumonic effusion. Anaerobic organisms were recovered from sputum cultures.

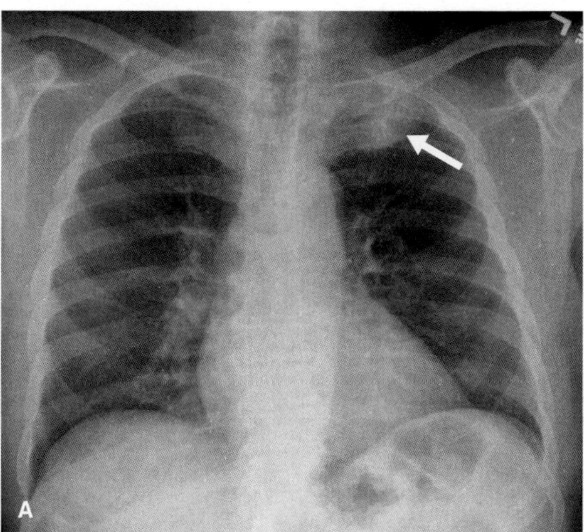

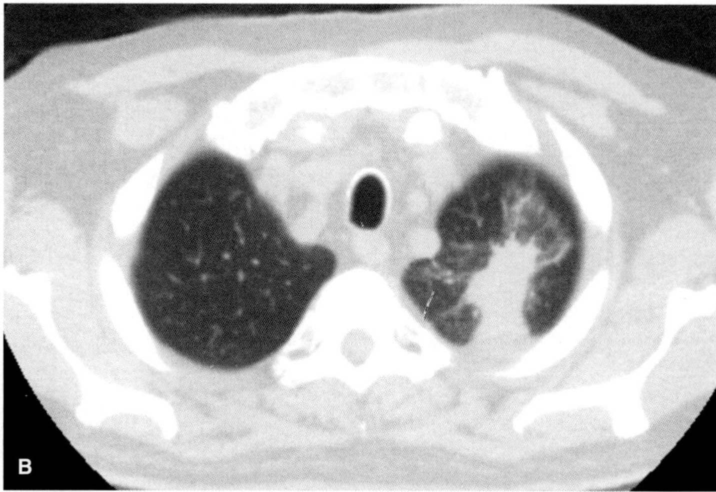

FIGURE 14.6. *Actinomyces* **Pulmonary Infection. A:** Frontal chest radiograph shows a vague opacity projecting over the left first rib (*arrow*). **B:** Axial CT through the upper lungs shows an irregular mass with adjacent ground glass that extends posteriorly to create a broad area of contact with the pleural surface. CT-guided transthoracic biopsy revealed *Actinomyces israelii* infection.

In the early stages of infection, interstitial inflammation leads to a fine reticular pattern on the chest radiograph. This may progress to patchy segmental ground-glass or airspace opacities (Fig. 14.7), which may coalesce to produce lobar consolidation. CT of mycoplasma pneumonia usually appears as patchy airspace opacities with a tree-in-bud appearance that reflects infectious bronchiolitis. The process is often unilateral and tends to involve the lower lobes. Pleural effusion may be seen in the consolidative form of disease and occurs most commonly in children. Lymph node enlargement is uncommon but may be seen in children. Radiographic resolution may require 4 to 6 weeks.

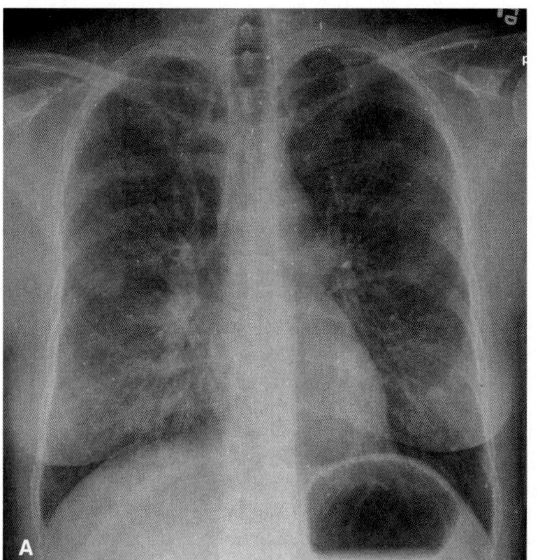

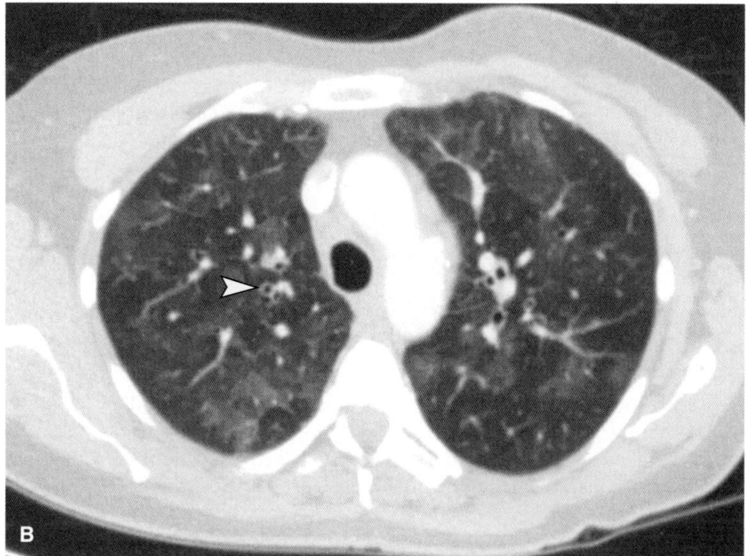

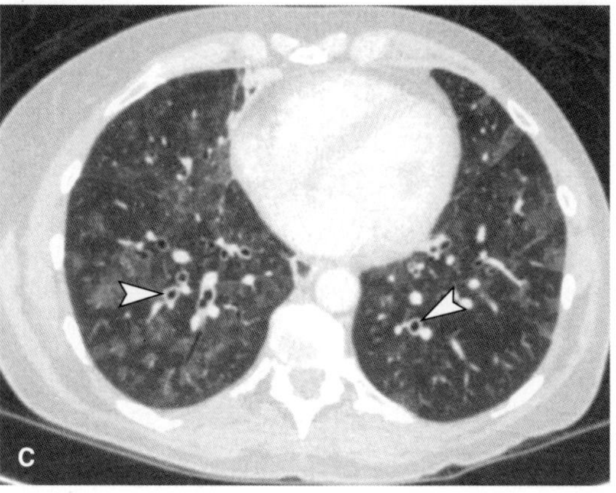

FIGURE 14.7. ***Mycoplasma*** **Pneumonia. A:** Frontal chest radiograph in a 42-year-old woman with *Mycoplasma* pneumonia demonstrates diffuse fine reticular opacities. **B, C:** Axial CT through the upper (**B**) and lower (**C**) lungs shows centrilobular and lobular areas of ground-glass opacity with associated bronchial wall thickening (*arrowheads*).

Mycobacterial Infections

Mycobacterium tuberculosis is an aerobic acid-fast bacillus. Two principal forms of tuberculous pulmonary disease are recognized clinically and radiographically: primary tuberculosis (TB) and postprimary or "reactivation" disease. The inflammatory response to *Mycobacterium tuberculosis* differs from the normal response to bacterial organisms in that it involves cell-mediated immunity (delayed hypersensitivity). Initially, droplet nuclei laden with bacilli are inhaled and implanted in a subpleural location. In most patients, the bacilli are phagocytized and killed by alveolar macrophages. If the bacilli overcome the immune response of the host, an inflammatory focus is established. The macrophages are then transformed into epithelioid cells, which aggregate to form granulomas. The granulomas are usually well formed by 1 to 3 weeks, coinciding with the development of delayed hypersensitivity. The granulomas typically demonstrate central caseous necrosis, thereby distinguishing them from the granulomas seen in sarcoidosis. Inflammation and enlargement of draining hilar and mediastinal lymph nodes is common in primary disease, particularly in children and immunocompromised patients.

In primary infection, the parenchymal disease and adenopathy may completely resolve, or there may be a residual focus of scarring or calcification. In some situations, usually in infants under the age of 1 year, local parenchymal disease progresses and is termed *progressive primary TB*. More commonly, the disease will be contained by the granulomatous response and recur years later (reactivation or postprimary TB) in the setting of weakened host defenses from aging, alcoholism, diabetes, cancer, or HIV infection. Postprimary TB develops under the influence of hypersensitivity, with caseous necrosis seen histologically.

Primary TB has classically been a disease of childhood, although the incidence of primary disease has increased with the HIV disease. Most patients with primary TB are asymptomatic and have no radiographic sequelae of infection. In some patients a Ranke complex, consisting of a calcified parenchymal focus (the Ghon lesion) and nodal calcification, is seen. If the patient is symptomatic, a nonspecific focal pneumonitis occurs and is seen as small, ill-defined areas of segmental or lobar opacification (Fig. 14.8). The parenchymal consolidation may mimic a bacterial pneumonia, but the clinical and radiographic course is much more indolent. Cavitation is relatively uncommon in the immunocompetent patient. The pulmonary focus may resolve completely or persist as a Ghon lesion or a Ranke complex. *Tuberculomas* are discrete nodular opacities that may develop in primary TB but are much more common in postprimary disease. Unilateral pleural effusion is seen in 20% of cases and is usually associated with parenchymal disease. In the absence of positive pleural fluid stain or culture, the presumptive diagnosis of a tuberculous pleural effusion is made by demonstrating granulomas on parietal pleural biopsy or detecting elevated adenosine deaminase levels in pleural fluid samples. If a tuberculous empyema develops, it may break through the parietal pleura to form an extrapleural collection (empyema necessitatis). Unilateral hilar or mediastinal lymph node enlargement is common, particularly in children, and may be the sole radiographic manifestation of infection. The detection of necrotic lymph node enlargement in a patient with TB suggests active disease (see Fig. 11.16). Bilateral hilar or mediastinal lymph node enlargement may be seen, but this is uncommon and is almost invariably asymmetric in distinction to lymph node enlargement in sarcoidosis. During the primary tuberculous infection, there is hematogenous dissemination of the organism to regions with a high partial pressure of oxygen; these include the lung apices, renal medullae, and bone marrow. These microscopic foci are clinically silent and serve as a source of reactivation disease.

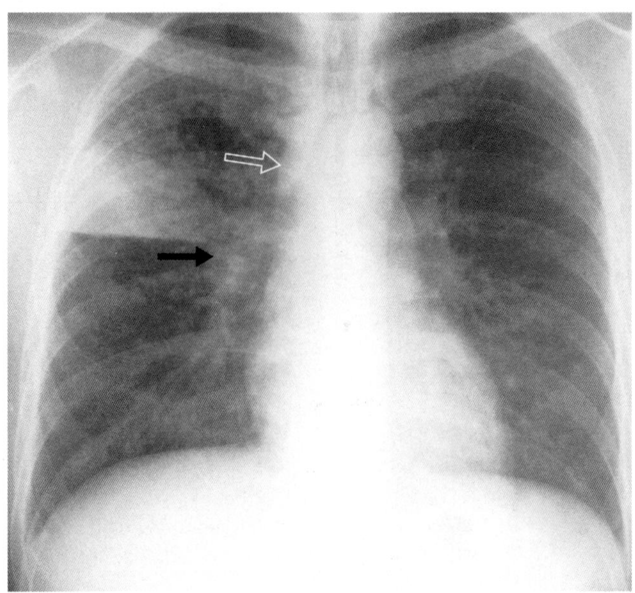

FIGURE 14.8. **Primary Tuberculosis.** A frontal chest radiograph in a 32-year-old homeless man shows airspace disease within the anterior segment of the right upper lobe, with right hilar (*solid arrow*) and paratracheal (*open arrow*) lymph node enlargement. Sputum stains and cultures revealed *Mycobacterium tuberculosis*.

Postprimary TB usually reflects reactivation of previous quiescent disease, but in 30% to 40% actually reflects recently acquired infection. Affected patients often present with cough and constitutional symptoms, including chills, night sweats, and weight loss. Reactivation tends to occur in the apical and posterior segments of the upper lobes and the superior segments of the lower lobes. Ill-defined patchy and nodular opacities are commonly seen. Cavitation is an important radiographic feature of postprimary infection and usually indicates active and transmissible disease (Fig. 14.9). The cavitary focus may lead to transbronchial spread of organisms and result in a multifocal bronchopneumonia. Erosion of a cavitary focus into a branch of the pulmonary artery can produce an aneurysm (Rasmussen aneurysm) and cause hemoptysis. With appropriate antimicrobial treatment, the disease is usually controlled by a granulomatous response. Parenchymal healing is associated with fibrosis, bronchiectasis, and volume loss (cicatrizing atelectasis) in the upper lobes.

There are several late complications of pulmonary TB. Interstitial fibrosis can cause pulmonary insufficiency and secondary pulmonary arterial hypertension. Hemoptysis may be secondary to bronchiectasis, mycetoma formation in an old tuberculous cavity, or erosion of a calcified peribronchial lymph node (broncholith) into a bronchus. Bronchostenosis is a result of healed endobronchial TB.

Miliary TB may complicate either primary or reactivation disease. It results from hematogenous dissemination of tubercle bacilli and produces diffuse bilateral 2- to 3-mm pulmonary nodules (Fig. 14.10). Miliary disease is associated with a high mortality and requires prompt therapy.

Atypical Mycobacterial Infection. There are several nontuberculous mycobacteria that may cause pulmonary disease. The most common organisms responsible for pulmonary disease are *Mycobacterium avium-intracellulare* (MAI) or *Mycobacterium kansasii*. Disease in nonimmunocompromised patients typically affects patients with underlying lung disease including COPD and bronchiectasis. The radiographic features of the most common form of pulmonary MAI infection are often indistinguishable from those of reactivation TB,

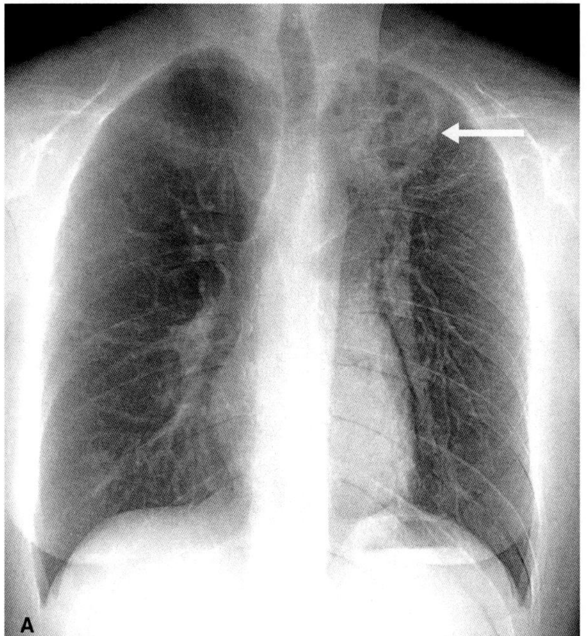

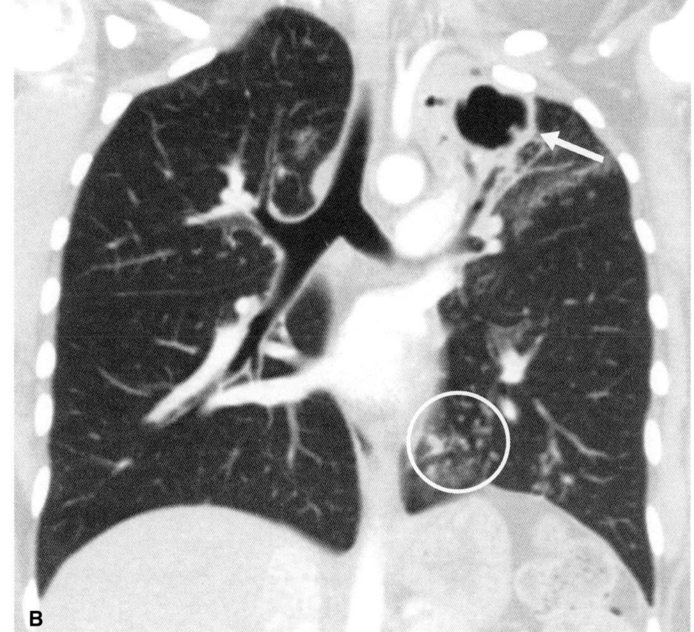

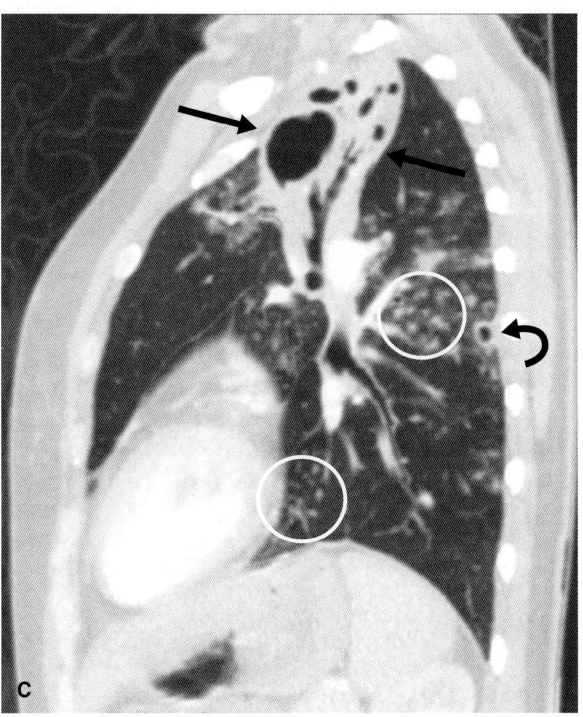

FIGURE 14.9. **Postprimary (Reactivation) Tuberculosis. A:** Frontal dual-energy subtraction chest radiograph in a 46-year-old woman shows left apical cavitary disease (*arrow*) with associated left upper lobe volume loss. **B, C:** Contrast-enhanced coronal (**B**) and sagittal (**C**) CT scans show the left upper lobe consolidation (*arrows*) with dependent tree-in-bud opacities (*circles*) reflecting endobronchial spread of disease. Note additional superior segment left lower lobe cavity (*curved arrow* in **C**). Sputum cultures were positive for *Mycobacterium tuberculosis*.

with chronic fibrocavitary opacities involving the upper lobes (Fig. 14.11). While cavitation is common, pleural effusion, lymph node enlargement, and miliary spread are distinctly unusual. A second pattern of disease with MAI in middle-aged and elderly women presents with small centrilobular nodules and bronchiectasis, often in a middle lobe and lingular distribution (Fig. 14.12). A third form of disease reflects a hypersensitivity reaction to inhaled MAI in hot water systems and has been termed "hot-tub lung" to reflect one of the more common causes of this condition. The imaging characteristics are those of hypersensitivity pneumonitis with centrilobular ground-glass nodules and ground-glass opacities, indistinguishable from subacute hypersensitivity pneumonitis from other inhaled organic antigens.

MAI infection in the setting of AIDS is discussed in the section "Infection in the Immunocompromised Host."

Although the disease caused by nontuberculous mycobacteria tends to be more indolent than that seen with *M. tuberculosis*, it is often difficult to treat effectively. Standard treatment for pulmonary MAI is a combination of three antibiotics for a minimum of one year.

Table 14.2 reviews the common imaging features of MTB and atypical mycobacterial infection.

Viral Pneumonia

Viruses are a major cause of upper respiratory tract and airways infection, although pneumonia is relatively uncommon. The diagnosis of viral pneumonia is often one of exclusion. Chest radiographic features are nonspecific and usually demonstrate a pattern of bronchopneumonia or reticulonodular opacities.

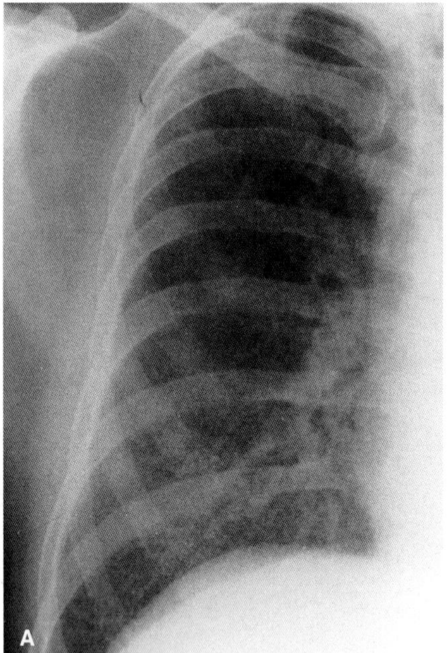

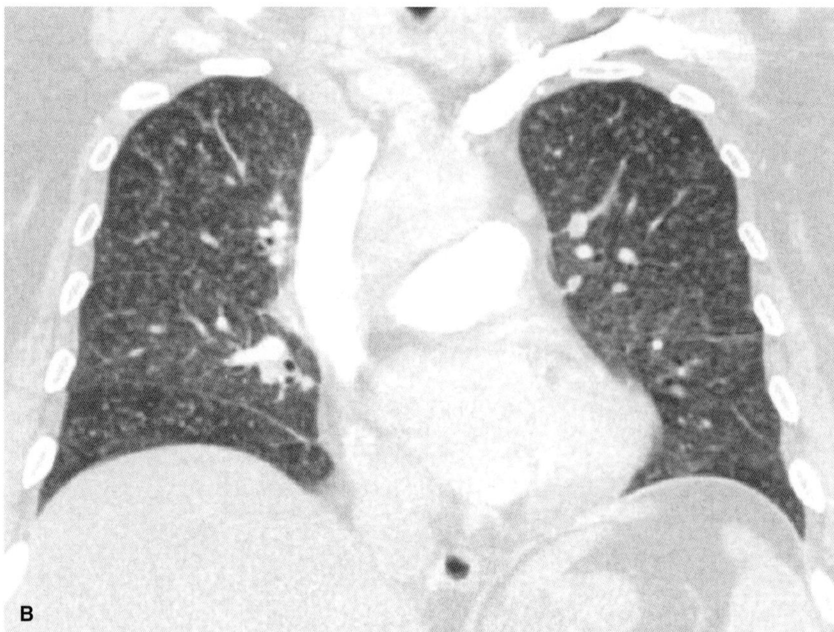

FIGURE 14.10. **Miliary Tuberculosis. A:** Coned-down view of a frontal radiograph demonstrates innumerable micronodular opacities characteristic of micronodular (miliary) interstitial disease. Transbronchial biopsy demonstrated caseating granulomas containing acid-fast bacilli. **B:** Coronal reformation at lung windows of a CT scan in another patient with proven miliary tuberculosis shows innumerable randomly distributed small lung nodules.

Resolution is usually complete, but permanent sequelae may be seen including bronchiectasis, constrictive bronchiolitis (which may produce a unilateral hyperlucent lung or Swyer–James syndrome), and pulmonary fibrosis.

Influenza. In adults, the most common cause of viral pneumonia is influenza. Outbreaks of influenza can occur in pandemics, epidemics, or sporadically. In most patients the disease is confined to the upper respiratory tract, but in elderly persons, those with underlying cardiopulmonary disease or immunocompromise, and in pregnant women, a severe hemorrhagic pneumonia may develop. In adults with influenza pneumonia, there is often bilateral lower lobe patchy airspace opacification. CT shows ground-glass or airspace opacities with centrilobular nodules (Fig. 14.13). Bacterial superinfection with *Streptococcus* or *Staphylococcus* organisms contributes to a fulminating course that may result in death. The development of lobar consolidation, pleural effusion, or cavitation suggests bacterial superinfection.

Respiratory syncytial virus and parainfluenza virus are common causes of epidemic viral pneumonia in children. When seen in adults, the disease is usually in the setting of a debilitated or immunocompromised patient (Fig. 14.14). Findings are similar to other viral pneumonias: patchy airspace opacities, bronchial wall thickening (particularly in RSV pneumonia) and centrilobular nodules and tree-in-bud opacities.

Varicella zoster, which causes chickenpox and shingles, may produce a severe pneumonia in adults. Patients on immunosuppressive therapy or with lymphoma are at greatest risk. Chest radiographs characteristically show diffuse bilateral ill-defined nodular opacities 5 to 10 mm in diameter. These opacities usually resolve completely, although in some patients they involute and calcify to produce innumerable small (2 to 3 mm) calcified nodules (Fig. 14.15).

Adenovirus is a frequent cause of upper and occasionally lower respiratory tract infection. Hyperinflation and bronchopneumonia accompanied by lobar atelectasis are the most frequent radiographic manifestations of adenovirus pneumonia; however, adenovirus in children may present as lobar or segmental consolidation.

The most common causes of viral pneumonia and typical imaging findings are shown in Table 14.3.

Fungal Pneumonia

Fungal infections are now seen with increased frequency because of an increase in the incidence of disease caused by pathogenic fungi in healthy hosts and the emergence of opportunistic species in immunocompromised hosts. Fungi can cause pulmonary disease by several mechanisms. Some fungi, including *Histoplasma capsulatum, Coccidioides immitis*, and *Blastomyces dermatitidis,* are endemic fungi and most commonly infect normal hosts. Other fungi, most notably *Aspergillus, Candida*, *Cryptococcus*, and *Mucormycosis* (*zygomycosis*), are opportunistic pathogens in immunocompromised individuals. In all cases, the fungi elicit a necrotizing granulomatous reaction. The high mortality of untreated invasive infection and the availability of effective antifungal therapy with triazoles (fluconazole, intraconazole, voriconazole, and posaconazole), lipid-based amphotericin B and the endocardins (e.g., caspofungin) has made the early and accurate diagnosis of fungal infection imperative. A number of serologic assays (complement fixation, immunodiffusion) and histologic methods are available for the accurate diagnosis of fungal infection.

Histoplasmosis. *H. capsulatum* is endemic to certain areas of North America, most notably the Ohio, Mississippi, and St. Lawrence river valleys and Mexico. The overwhelming majority (95% to 99%) of infections by *H. capsulatum* are asymptomatic. A routine chest film demonstrating multiple well-defined calcified nodules less than 1 cm in size, with or without calcified hilar or mediastinal lymph nodes, may be the only indication of prior infection.

Acute histoplasmosis most often presents with the abrupt onset of flu-like symptoms. The chest radiograph in such patients may be normal or may show nonspecific changes,

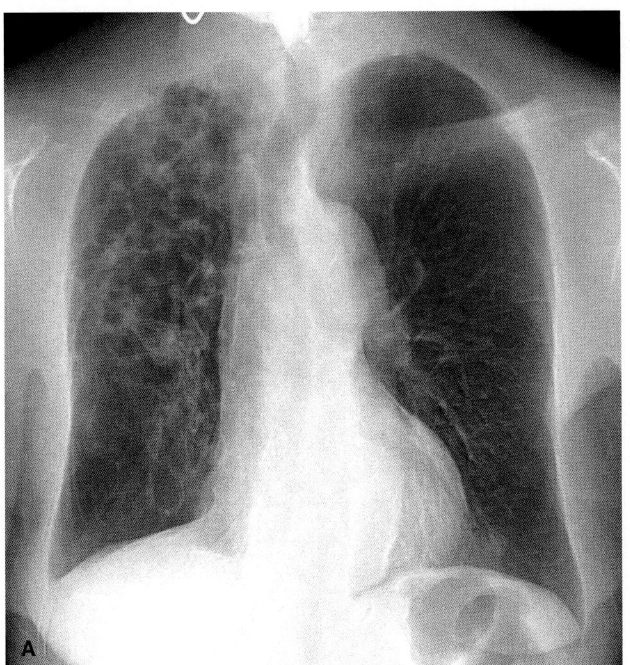

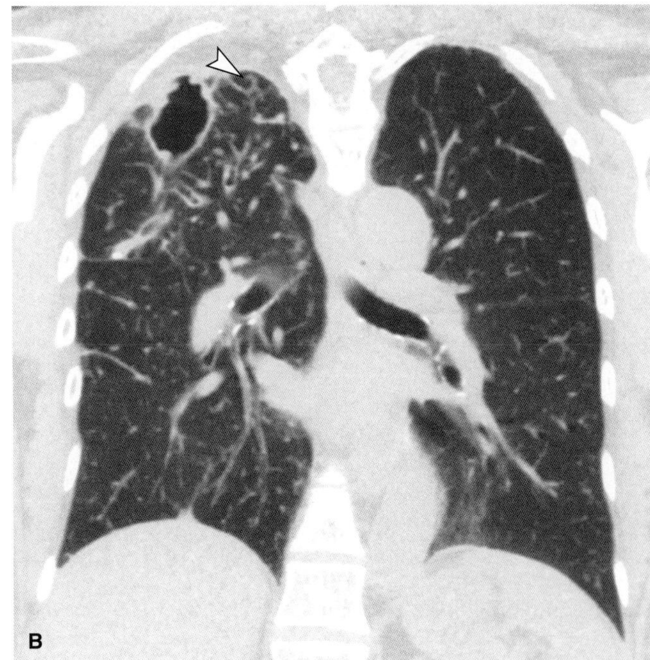

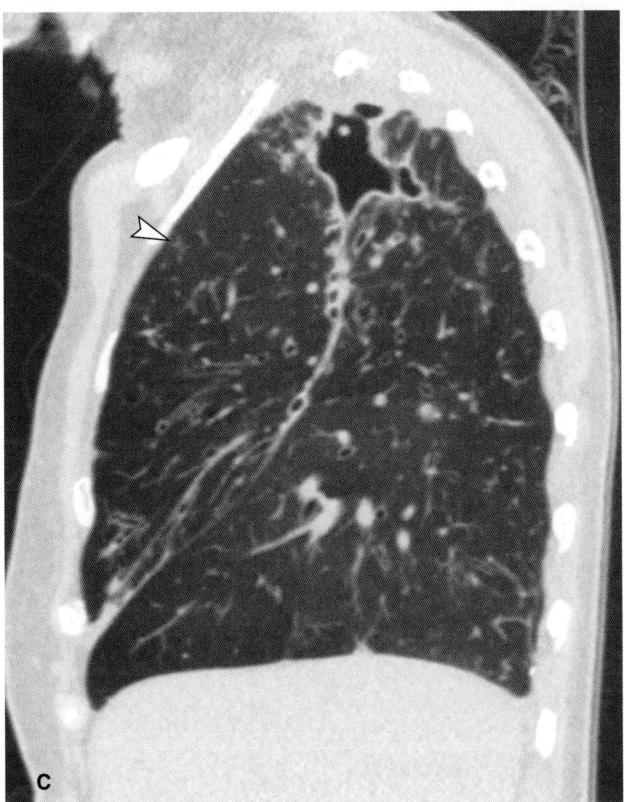

FIGURE 14.11. ***Mycobacterium avium-intracellulare* (MAI) Infection-Fibrocavitary Form. A:** Frontal dual-energy subtraction chest radiograph in a 62-year-old woman with MAI infection demonstrates right upper lobe volume loss with multiple cavities. **B, C:** Coronal (**B**) and sagittal (**C**) CT scans reveal an irregular right apical cavity with right lung cylindrical bronchiectasis, small nodules, and tree-in-bud opacities (*arrowheads*). Note the similarity in appearance to postprimary tuberculosis.

including subsegmental airspace opacities with or without associated hilar lymph node enlargement (Fig. 14.16). The inhalation of a large inoculum of organisms can produce widespread, fairly discrete nodular opacities 3 to 4 mm in diameter with hilar adenopathy. Alternatively, acute histoplasmosis may result in a solitary nodule <3 cm in diameter, termed a *histoplasmoma*. Histoplasmomas are most common in the lower lobes and frequently calcify.

H. capsulatum can also cause chronic pulmonary disease, usually in patients with underlying emphysema. Unilateral or bilateral upper lobe cicatrizing atelectasis with marked hilar retraction may mimic the radiographic findings seen in postprimary TB. Similarly, chronic upper lobe fibrocavitary disease may be seen. Involvement of the mediastinum by chronic granulomatous inflammation may lead to fibrosing mediastinitis, while endobronchial disease can produce bronchostenosis.

Asymptomatic blood-borne dissemination of *H. capsulatum* is common, as judged by the frequency of calcified splenic granulomas in residents of endemic areas. Clinically apparent disseminated histoplasmosis, however, is extremely rare and is usually seen in infants or immunocompromised adults. The chest film most commonly shows widespread 2- to 3-mm nodules that

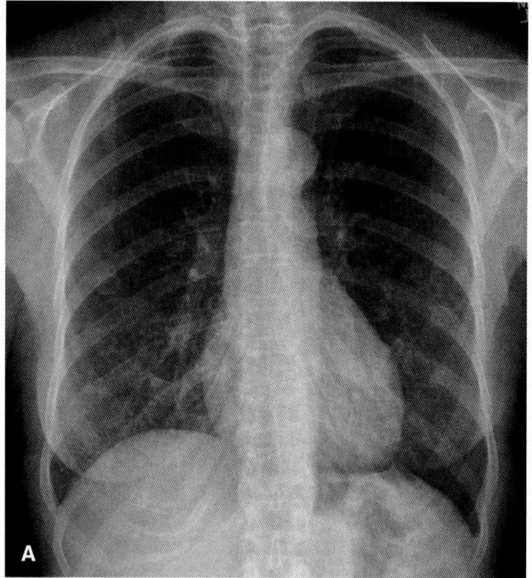

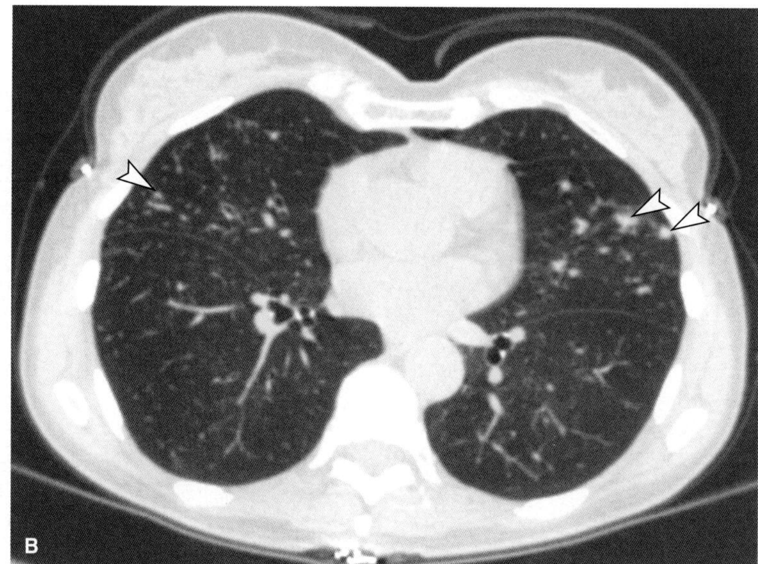

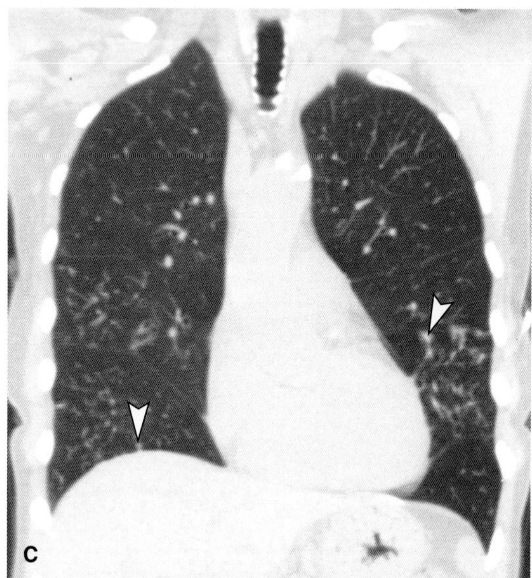

FIGURE 14.12. ***Mycobacterium avium-intracellulare* (MAI) Infection-Nodular Bronchiectatic Form. A:** Frontal chest radiograph in a 54-year-old woman with MAI infection shows mid and lower zone reticulonodular opacities. **B, C:** Axial (**B**) and coronal (**C**) CT scans show middle lobe, lingular and right lower lobe cylindrical bronchiectasis, tree-in-bud opacities, and nodules (*arrowheads* in **B** and **C**).

TABLE 14.2

FEATURES OF MTB AND ATYPICAL MYCOBACTERIAL INFECTION

ORGANISMS	DISEASE FORM	IMAGING FINDINGS
Mycobacterium tuberculosis	Primary	▪ Mediastinal/hilar lymph node enlargement (necrotic) ▪ Segmental/lobar consolidation ▪ Pleural effusion ▪ Miliary opacities
	Postprimary	▪ Consolidation with cavitation ▪ Centrillobular nodules/tree-in-bud opacities
	Inactive (previous) disease	▪ Calcified nodules +/– lymph nodes ▪ Fibronodular changes in upper lungs
Nontuberculous (atypical) mycobacteria	Fibrocavitary	▪ Single/multiple cavities ▪ Centrilobular nodules ▪ Tree-in-bud opacities
	Nodular bronchiectatic	▪ Cylindrical bronchiectasis (esp ML/lingula) ▪ Centrilobular nodules ▪ Patchy consolidation
	Allergic ("hot-tub lung")	▪ Centrilobular ground-glass nodules ▪ Ground-glass opacity ▪ Air trapping (expiratory CT)

ML, middle lobe.

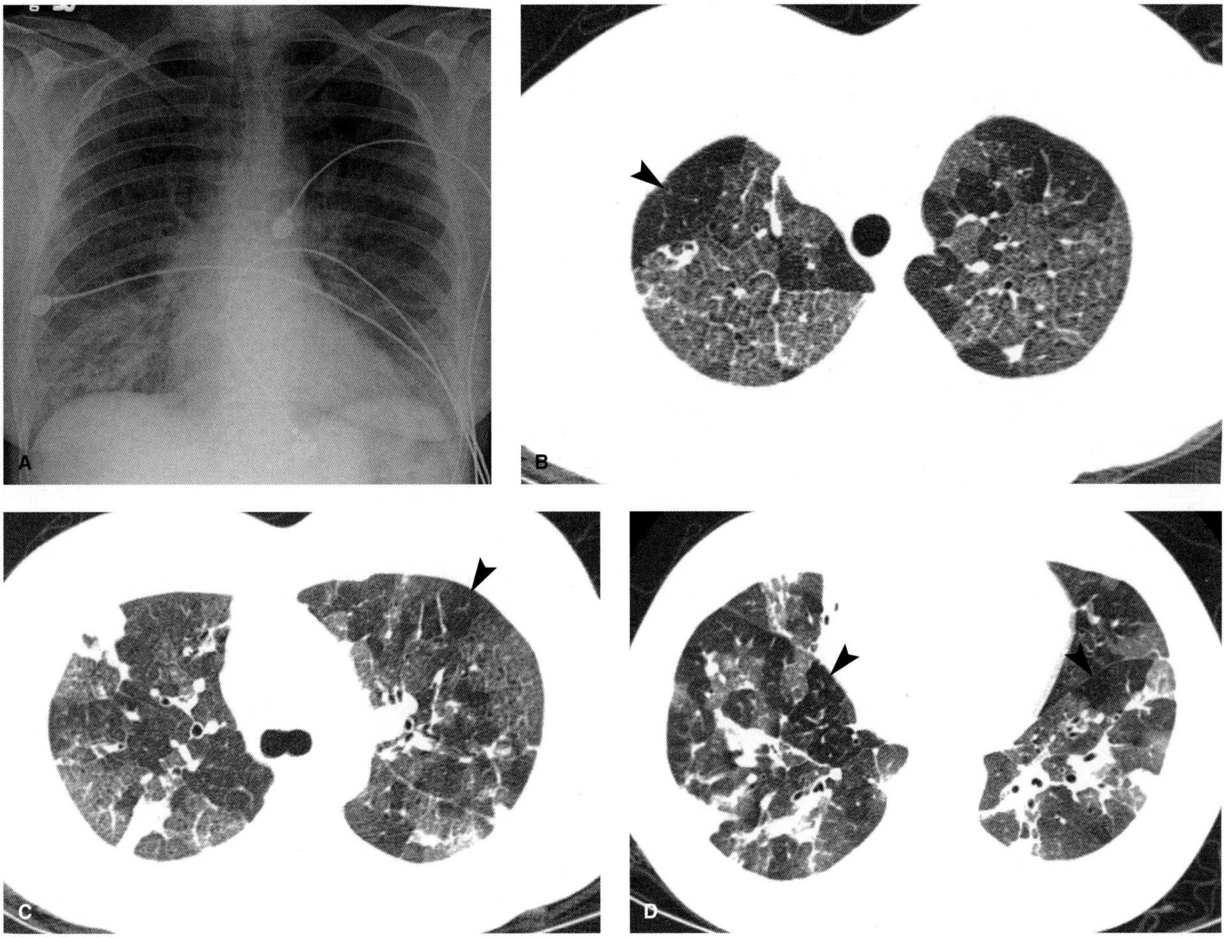

FIGURE 14.13. *Influenza* **Pneumonia. A:** Frontal chest radiograph in a 42-year-old woman with *Influenza* pneumonia shows bilateral fine reticular opacities with right lower lobe airspace opacification. **B–D:** Axial CT scans through the upper (**B**), mid (**C**) and lower (**D**) lungs show bronchial wall thickening, geographic ground-glass opacities with intra-and interlobular septal thickening ("crazy-paving"), and scattered lobular airspace opacification. There are lobular and subsegmental areas of hyperlucency (*arrowheads* in **B–D**) reflecting small airways disease with secondary air trapping.

are indistinguishable from those of miliary TB, though reticular opacities and patchy areas of consolidations may also be seen.

Coccidioidomycosis. C. immitis is endemic to the southwestern United States and the San Joaquin Valley of California. There are three types of clinical and radiographic coccidioidal pulmonary infection: acute, chronic, and disseminated coccidioidomycosis. Acute coccidioidomycosis develops in 40% of infected adults. These patients develop a self-limiting viral-type illness, which is referred to as "valley fever" when associated

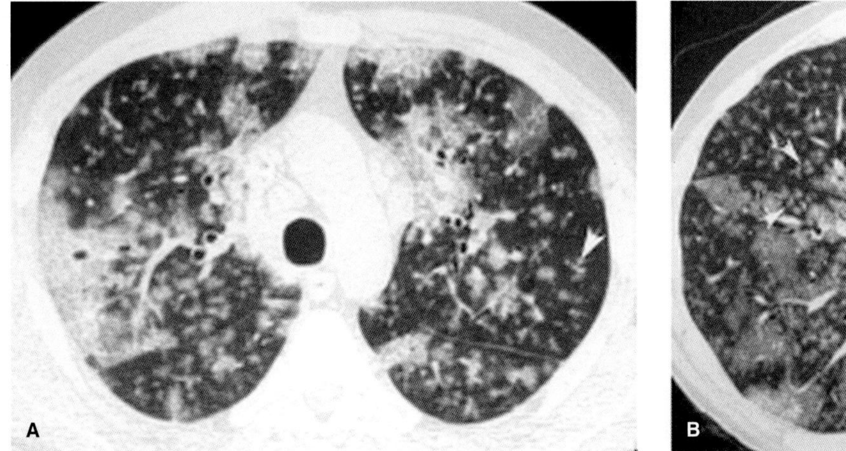

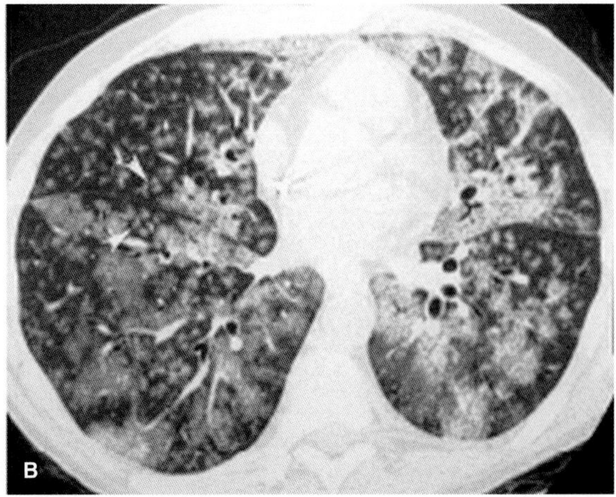

FIGURE 14.14. *Parainfluenza* **Virus Pneumonia. A, B:** CT through upper lungs (**A**) and mid-lungs (**B**) in a patient with acute myelogenous leukemia (AML) shows striking bronchopneumonia and bronchiolitis (*arrowheads*). *Parainfluenza* virus was isolated from bronchoalveolar lavage fluid.

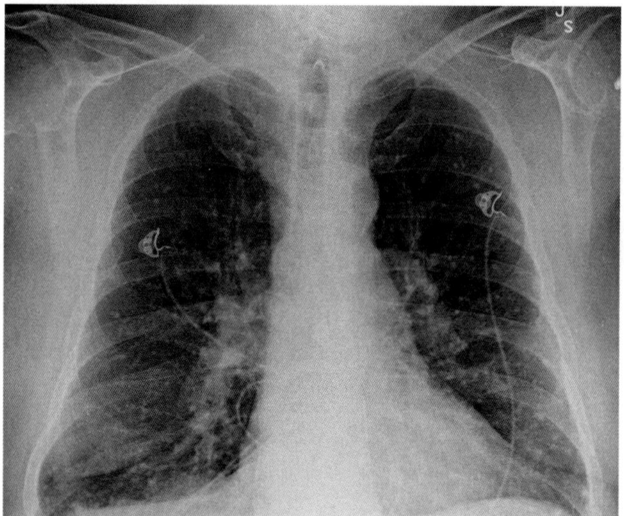

FIGURE 14.15. **Healed *Varicella* Pneumonia.** Frontal chest radiograph in a patient with a history of *Varicella* pneumonia shows innumerable scattered calcified nodules.

with erythema nodosum and arthralgias. The chest radiograph may be normal or show focal or multifocal airspace or nodular opacities (Fig. 14.17) that resolve over several months. Hilar and mediastinal lymph node enlargement and pleural effusion may be seen with parenchymal disease.

Disseminated (miliary) coccidioidomycosis is relatively rare and usually affects immunocompromised patients and non-Caucasians. The typical appearance is that of miliary lung nodules often superimposed upon the changes of acute infection (i.e., nodules/consolidation).

Patients whose symptoms or radiographic abnormalities persist beyond 6 weeks are considered to have chronic coccidioidomycosis. The radiographic features of chronic *persistent* disease include coccidioidal nodules or masses (coccidioidomas) and persistent areas of consolidation. Coccidioidal nodules are areas of round pneumonia, usually located in the subpleural regions of the upper lobes. These nodules tend to cavitate rapidly and produce characteristic thin-walled cavities. In chronic *progressive* disease, upper lobe fibrocavitary disease similar to postprimary TB and histoplasmosis is seen.

Blastomycosis. North American blastomycosis, caused by *B. dermatitidis,* is a chronic systemic disease primarily affecting the lungs and skin. Its geographic distribution overlaps that of histoplasmosis but extends farther to the east and north. The pulmonary infection is often asymptomatic. Symptomatic infection resembles that of an acute bacterial pneumonia. The radiographic findings in pulmonary blastomycosis are nonspecific. The most common manifestation of disease is homogeneous nonsegmental airspace opacification with a propensity for the upper lobes. A less common presentation is single or multiple masses (Fig. 14.18), which cavitate in 15% of cases. Pulmonary masses tend to occur in patients with prolonged symptoms (>1 month) and may mimic lung cancer. Pleural effusion and lymph node enlargement are uncommon. A disseminated miliary form may be seen in immunocompromised hosts.

Aspergillus species are responsible for a spectrum of pulmonary diseases in humans. This includes aspergilloma or mycetoma formation within preexisting cavities, semi-invasive (chronic necrotizing) aspergillosis in patients with mildly impaired immunity, invasive pulmonary aspergillosis in the neutropenic lymphoma or leukemia patient, and allergic bronchopulmonary aspergillosis in the hyperimmune patient.

An aspergilloma (mycetoma, fungus ball) is a ball of hyphae, mucus, and cellular debris that colonizes a pre-existing bulla or a parenchymal cavity created by some other pathogen or destructive process such as post-primary TB. Invasion into adjacent lung parenchyma does not occur unless host defense mechanisms are compromised. The mycetoma is usually asymptomatic, but may cause hemoptysis, which may be massive (>350 mL/24 h). An aspergilloma is seen as a solid round mass within an upper lobe cavity, with an "air crescent" separating the mycetoma from the cavity wall (Fig. 14.19). Progressive apical pleural thickening adjacent to a cavity is a common radiographic finding and should prompt a search for a complicating mycetoma. Semi-invasive and invasive aspergillosis are discussed later in this chapter, while allergic bronchopulmonary aspergillosis, which is primarily a large airways process, is reviewed in Chapter 16.

The clinical types of pulmonary fungal infection and associated imaging patterns are summarized in Table 14.4.

TABLE 14.3

VIRAL PULMONARY INFECTION—COMMON ORGANISMS AND PATTERNS OF DISEASE

■ ORGANISMS	■ PATTERNS OF DISEASE	■ ASSOCIATED FINDINGS
CMV	■ **Ground-glass opacities** ■ Reticulonodular opacities ■ Patchy airspace opacities ■ Nodules (uncommon)	
Influenza	■ **Lobular/patchy consolidation** ■ Absence of air bronchograms ■ Bronchial wall thickening	■ **Bacterial** superinfection
Varicella-zoster	■ **Centrilobular nodular opacities** ■ Confluent airspace opacities	■ Small calcified nodules (chronic)
RSV	■ **Centrilobular nodules** ■ **Airspace opacities** ■ Ground-glass opacities ■ Bronchial wall thickening	
Adenovirus	■ **Lobular/patchy consolidation** ■ **Ground-glass opacities**	■ Unilateral hyperlucent lung (Swyer–James) syndrome (chronic)

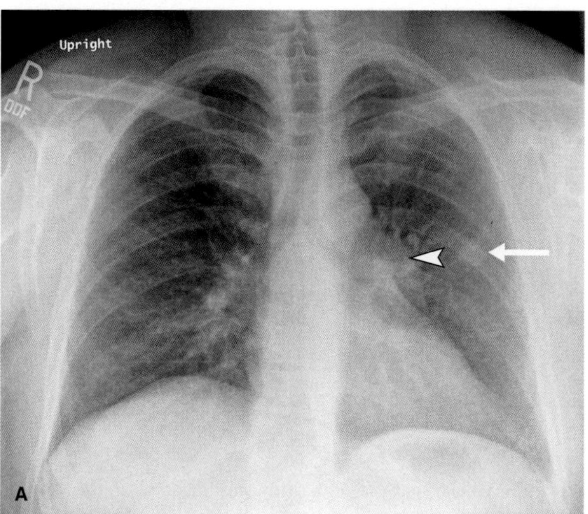

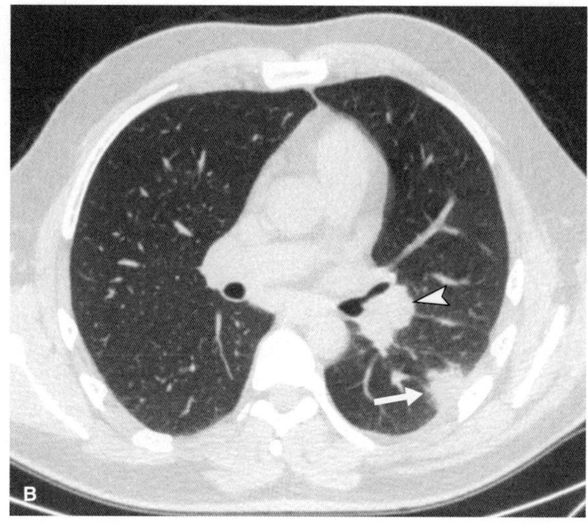

FIGURE 14.16. **Acute Histoplasmosis. A:** Frontal chest radiograph in a 38-year-old man with histoplasmosis shows a left mid-lung nodule (*arrow*) with associated left hilar enlargement (*arrowhead*). **B:** Axial CT shows an irregular superior segment left lower lobe nodule (*arrow*) with ill-defined margins and an enlarged left hilum (*arrowhead*) reflecting lymph node enlargement.

Parasitic Infection

Parasitic infections (Table 14.5) of the lung are relatively uncommon in the United States. However, increased travel to countries where parasites are endemic, the immigration of people from these regions to the United States, and growing numbers of immunocompromised patients require a familiarity with these infections. In general, parasitic diseases of the thorax are manifested by either a direct invasion of lungs and pleura or, less commonly, a hypersensitivity reaction.

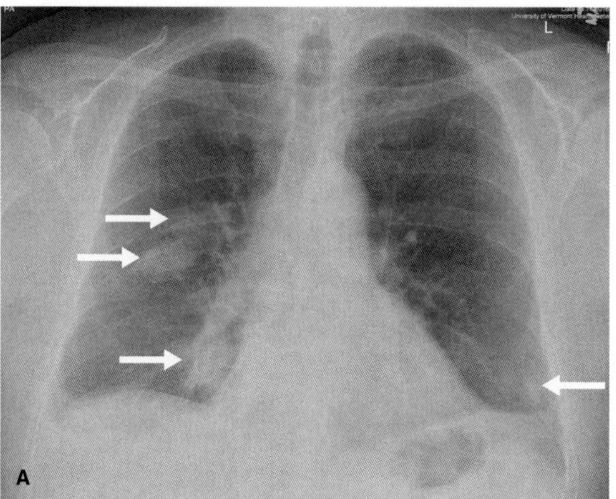

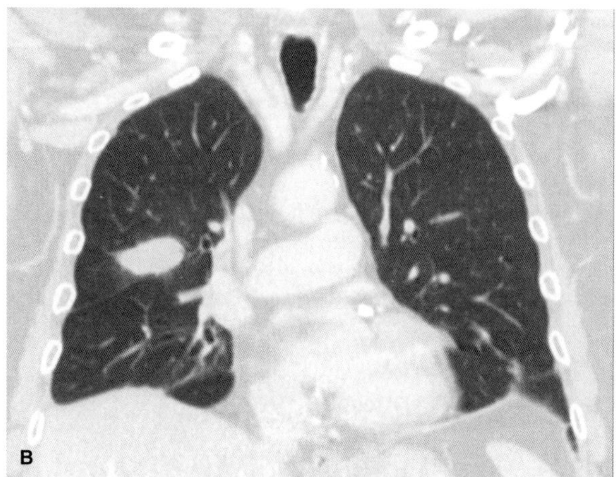

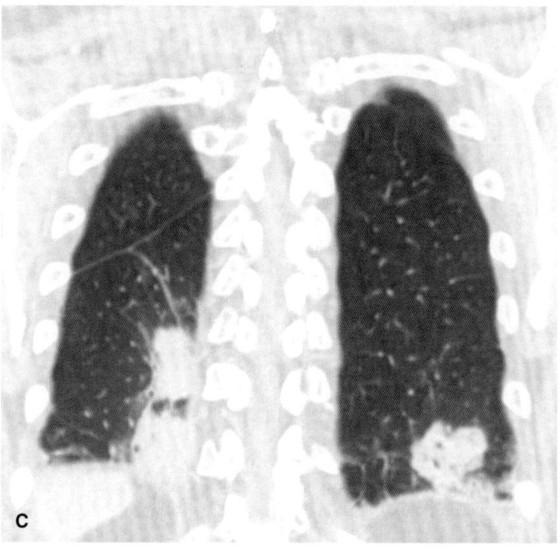

FIGURE 14.17. **Primary *Coccidioides* Infection. A:** Frontal radiograph in a 54-year-old man with a clinical diagnosis of Valley fever shows multiple right mid and lower lung and left basilar nodules (*arrows*). **B, C:** Coronal CT scans through the middle (**B**) and posterior lungs (**C**) confirms multiple bilateral nodules and masses. Several nodules contain patent bronchi. CT-guided transthoracic biopsy of the peripheral lung lesion revealed coccidioidomycosis.

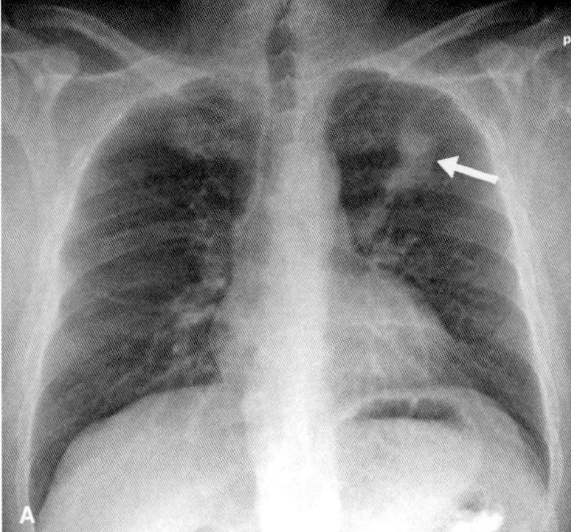

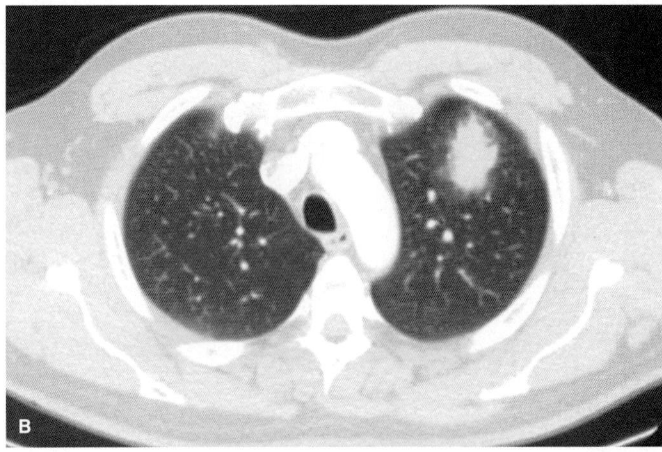

FIGURE 14.18. ***Blastomyces dermatitidis*** **Infection. A:** Chest radiograph in a 39-year-old male shows an ill-defined mass in the left upper lobe (*arrow*). **B:** CT scan through the upper lobes demonstrates an irregular left upper lobe mass with surrounding ground-glass opacity. Biopsy revealed *Blastomyces dermatitidis* infection.

Amebiasis. Symptomatic infection with *Entamoeba histolytica* is usually confined to the GI tract and liver. If the infection remains confined to the subphrenic space, a right pleural effusion and basilar atelectasis may result from local diaphragmatic inflammation. The most common method of pleuropulmonary involvement by amebiasis is by the direct intrathoracic extension of infection from a hepatic abscess. This transdiaphragmatic spread of organisms may extend into the right pleural space to produce an empyema or may involve the right lower lobe to produce an amebic pneumonia or lung abscess.

Hydatid Disease (Echinococcosis) of the Lung. Echinococcus granulosus is the cause of most cases of human hydatid disease. The disease is endemic in sheep-raising areas and is relatively uncommon in the United States. Dogs, coyotes, and wolves are the usual definitive hosts, with sheep, goats, and cattle acting as intermediate hosts. When a human becomes an accidental intermediate host, disease may result. The larval organisms travel to the liver and lungs and, if they survive host defenses, encyst and gradually enlarge. Pulmonary echinococcal cysts are composed of three layers: an exocyst (chitinous layer), which is a protective membrane; an inner endocyst, which produces the "daughter cysts"; and a surrounding capsule of compressed, fibrotic lung known as the pericyst.

Pulmonary echinococcal cysts characteristically present as well-circumscribed, spherical soft tissue masses. In distinction to hepatic cysts, lung cysts do not have calcified walls. The cysts range in size from 1 to 20 cm, with a predilection for the lower lobes and the right side. While most cysts remain asymptomatic, patients may present when the cyst develops a communication with the bronchial tree. If the pericyst ruptures, a thin crescent of air will be seen around the periphery of the cyst, producing the "meniscus" or "crescent" sign. If the cyst itself ruptures, the contents of the cyst are expelled into the airways, producing an air–fluid level. On occasion, the cyst wall may be seen crumpled and floating within an uncollapsed pericyst, producing the pathognomonic "sign of the camalote" or "water lily" sign. Rarely, a cyst will rupture into the pleural space, producing a large pleural effusion.

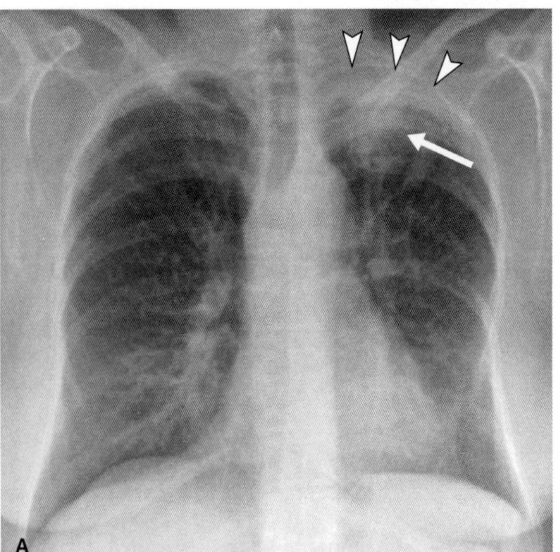

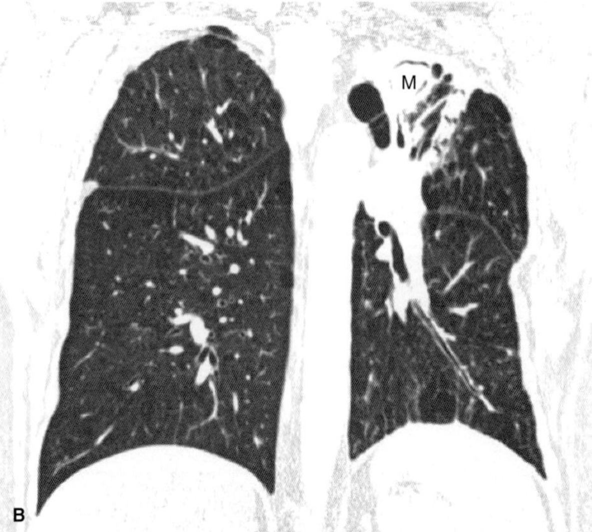

FIGURE 14.19. **Aspergilloma. A:** Chest radiograph in a 67-year-old woman with hemoptysis reveals left upper lobe volume loss, a left upper lobe mass (*arrow*) with associated apical pleural thickening (*arrowheads*). Note changes from prior left thoracotomy for bullectomy. **B:** Coronal reformatted CT scan reveals left apical scarring and a mass (M) within a bulla. There are emphysematous changes bilaterally.

TABLE 14.4

FUNGAL PULMONARY INFECTIONS: ORGANISMS AND TYPICAL IMAGING FINDINGS

ORGANISMS	FORM OF DISEASE	ASSOCIATED FINDINGS
Histoplasma capsulatum	▪ Acute	▪ Segmental consolidation ▪ Nodule/mass ▪ Hilar lymph node enlargement
	▪ Disseminated	▪ Miliary nodules
	▪ Chronic	▪ Upper lobe cicatrizing atelectasis ▪ Fibrocavitary disease
	▪ Chronic mediastinal	▪ Fibrotic mediastinal/hilar mass w/Ca^{++}
Coccidioides immitis	▪ Acute	▪ Focal/multifocal airspace/nodular opacities ▪ Lymph node enlargement ▪ Pleural effusion ▪ Diffuse small nodules (heavy exposure)
	▪ Disseminated	▪ Miliary nodules
	▪ Chronic persistent	▪ Nodules/consolidation (+/– cavitation)
	▪ Chronic progressive	▪ Fibrocavitary disease
Blastomyces dermatitidis	▪ Acute	▪ Focal airspace consolidation ▪ Single/multiple nodules/masses
	▪ Disseminated	▪ Miliary nodules
Aspergillus fumigatus	▪ Invasive	▪ Nodule/mass/focal consolidation with halo +/– cavitation
	▪ Semi-invasive	▪ Upper lobe mass/consolidation (associated with emphysema/fibrosis) ▪ Adjacent pleural thickening
	▪ Saprophytic	▪ Nodule/mass in cyst/cavity/bulla (+/– mobile) ▪ Adjacent pleural thickening
	▪ Allergic	▪ Mucoid impaction (+/– high attenuation) within proximal varicose bronchiectasis
Cryptococcus neoformans	▪ Acute	▪ Single/multiple nodules ▪ Focal nonsegmental consolidation
	▪ Disseminated	▪ Miliary nodules
Candida albicans	▪ Hematogenous	▪ Random/miliary nodules
	▪ Aspiration	▪ Lower lobe centrilobular nodules/tee-in-bud ▪ Lobular consolidation
Pneumocystis jiroveci	▪ Acute	▪ Diffuse ground-glass opacity ▪ Airspace consolidation ▪ Pneumatocele formation

Paragonimiasis results from infection with the lung fluke *Paragonimus westermani*. The organism is found predominantly in eastern Asia and is usually acquired by eating raw crabs or snails. Infestation of the lung may be asymptomatic, or a patient may present with cough, hemoptysis, dyspnea, and fever. In 20% of affected patients, the chest radiograph is normal. The most common radiographic finding is multiple cysts with variable wall thickness. These cystic opacities may become confluent and are often associated with focal atelectasis and subsegmental consolidation. Dense linear opacities representing the burrows of the organisms may be identified. Because the flukes penetrate the pleura, effusions are common and may be massive.

Schistosomiasis. Human schistosomiasis is caused by three blood flukes: *Schistosoma mansoni*, *Schistosoma japonicum*, and *Schistosoma haematobium*. It is one of the most important parasitic infestations of humans worldwide, although it is rarely acquired in the United States. The life cycle of the fluke is complex, with human infestation acquired through contact with infested water. The larvae penetrate the skin or oropharyngeal mucosa and travel via the venous circulation to the pulmonary capillaries. As the larvae pass through the lungs, an acute allergic response may develop, presenting radiographically as transient airspace opacities (eosinophilic pneumonia) that resolve spontaneously. The larvae then pass through the pulmonary capillaries into the systemic circulation. *S. japonicum* and *S. mansoni* eventually migrate to the mesenteric venules, while *S. haematobium* migrates to bladder venules. The mature flukes produce ova, which may embolize to the lungs, where they implant in and around small pulmonary arterioles. The organism induces granulomatous inflammation and fibrosis, which leads to an obliterative arteriolitis, resulting in pulmonary hypertension and cor pulmonale. Radiographically, a diffuse fine reticular pattern is most commonly seen in association with dilatation of the central pulmonary arteries. Small nodular opacities resembling miliary TB may be seen as granulomata forming around ova.

Dirofilariasis. The nematode *Dirofilaria immitis* (dog heartworm) can be transmitted from infected dogs to humans by mosquitoes. Pulmonary involvement appears as an

TABLE 14.5

PARASITIC PULMONARY INFECTIONS IN HUMANS AND IMAGING FINDINGS

■ DISEASE	■ ORGANISMS	■ IMAGING FINDINGS
Amebiasis	▪ *Entamoeba histolytica*	▪ Right lower lobe pneumonia/abscess ▪ Right pleural effusion/empyema
Hydatid disease	▪ *Echinococcus granulosus* ▪ *Echinococcus multilocularis*	▪ Lower lobe cysts (right) ▪ Air crescent sign ▪ Air–fluid level ▪ "Camalote"/"water lily" sign
Paragonimiasis	▪ *Paragonimus westermani*	▪ Cyst/cysts with cavitation ▪ Pleural effusion
Schistosomiasis	▪ *Schistosoma mansoni* ▪ *Schistosoma japonicum* ▪ *Schistosoma haematobium*	▪ Acute • Lobular air space opacities ▪ Chronic • Reticular opacities • Pulmonary arterial hypertension • Miliary nodules
Dirofilariasis	▪ *Dirofilaria immitis*	▪ Subpleural solitary pulmonary nodule

asymptomatic subpleural solitary pulmonary nodule that represents an inflammatory reaction surrounding a dead worm that has embolized from a peripheral vein to lodge in a peripheral pulmonary artery branch. The diagnosis is made on resection of the nodule.

Toxoplasmosis. Toxoplasma infection is reviewed in the section "Infection in the Immunocompromised Host."

COMPLICATIONS OF PULMONARY INFECTION

There are a number of acute and chronic complications of pulmonary infection that may produce characteristic radiologic findings and therefore are important to be aware (Table 14.6).

Parapneumonic Effusion. Pleural effusions associated with underlying pneumonia, termed parapneumonic effusions, are the most common complication of pneumonia, seen in up to 50% of patients (Fig. 14.5). Complicated parapneumonic effusions and empyemas represent a spectrum from exudative effusions with low pH and elevated LDH and protein in the former to frank pus with loculations in the latter. A detailed discussion of the imaging features of parapneumonic effusions can be found in Chapter 17.

Chest Wall Involvement. Uncommonly, a peripheral pulmonary infection will extend through the pleural membranes to invade the chest wall. When an empyema collection extends to create an infected subcutaneous collection in the chest wall it is termed *empyema necessitatis.* The organisms most often associated with this rare complication of pulmonary infection include TB, *A. israelii*, nocardiosis, fungus, and staphylococcal infection.

Lung abscess is most often the result of aspiration of mouth anaerobes with or without aerobes, and is seen 10 to 14 days following aspiration. Patients at greatest risk for lung abscess formation include poor dental hygiene and conditions that predispose to aspiration such as alcoholism, seizures, altered consciousness, and drug overdose. Some lung abscesses develop as an embolic complication of septic thrombophlebitis or tricuspid endocarditis. Abscesses appear as nodules or masses typically with central necrosis with or without air–fluid levels, and develop in the gravity dependent portions of the lungs (posterior upper lobes, superior segment, and subpleural regions of the lower lobes (Figs. 14.5 and 14.20).

Pulmonary gangrene is a rare complication of severe pulmonary infection when a portion of lung is sloughed. This rare complication occurs when there is thrombosis of pulmonary vessels as a result of the infection. It can be seen in severe

TABLE 14.6

COMPLICATIONS OF PULMONARY INFECTION

	■ SITE OF COMPLICATION			
	■ LUNG/AIRWAYS	■ PLEURA/CHEST WALL	■ VASCULAR	■ MEDIASTINUM
Acute	Abscess Gangrene Pneumatocele	Parapneumonic effusion/ empyema	Mycotic aneurysm	
Chronic	Bronchiectasis Swyer–James syndrome Broncholithiasis Bronchial stenosis Interstitial fibrosis	Empyema necessitatis		Fibrosing mediastinitis

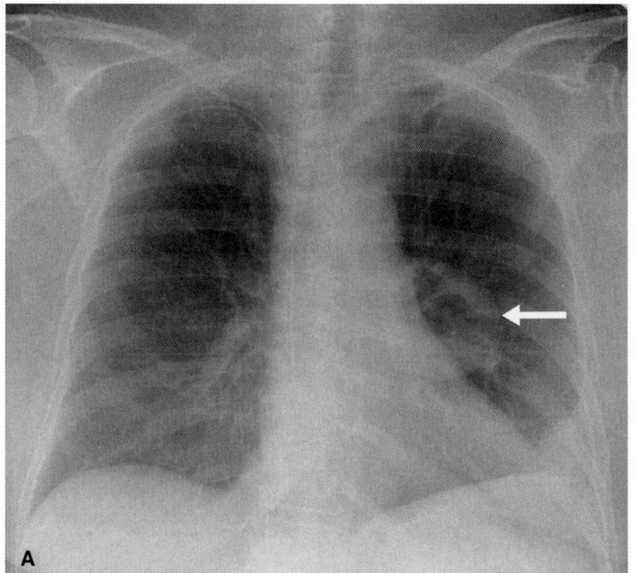

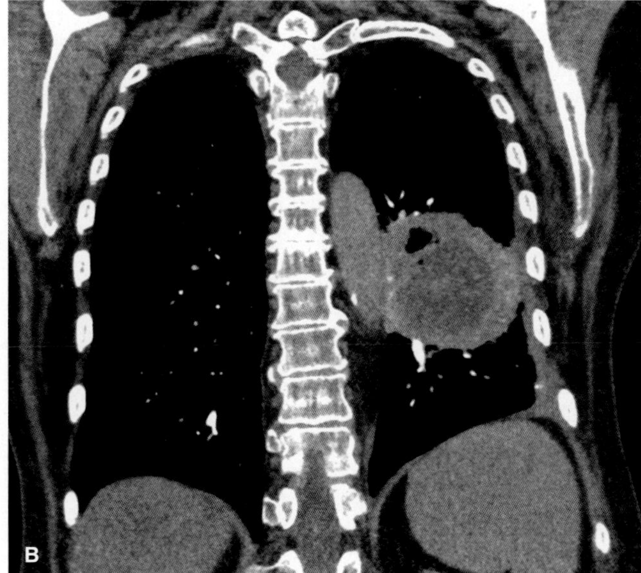

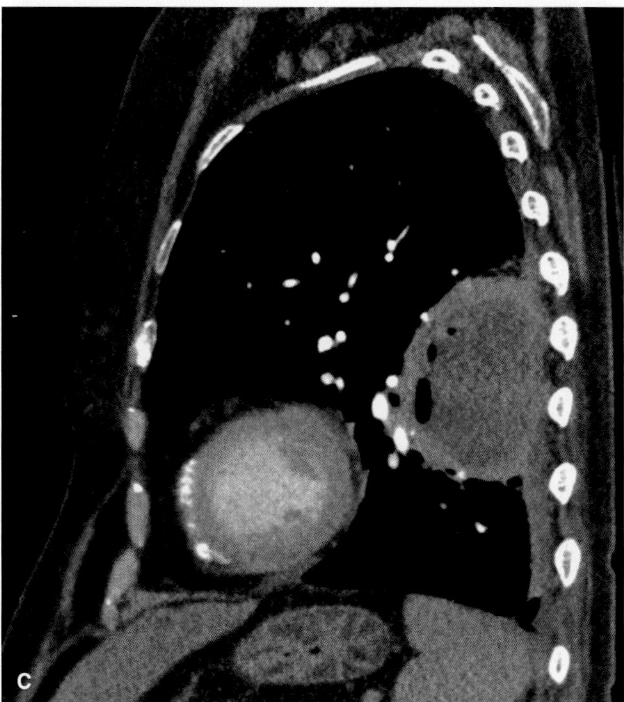

FIGURE 14.20. Lung Abscess. A: Frontal chest radiograph in a 38-year-old man with a 2-month history of fever and purulent sputum shows a cavitary lesion (*arrow*) in the superior segment of the left lower lobe. **B, C:** Contrast-enhanced coronal (**B**) and sagittal (**C**) CT shows a thick-walled lesion containing air and fluid reflecting a lung abscess. Note adjacent posterior pleural thickening related to the abscess.

bacterial pneumonia but is more closely associated with invasive pulmonary fungal infection. Imaging findings include a nodule or mass within a cavity with a crescent of air surrounding the sloughed portion of the lung. Treatment can be medical or surgical.

Mycotic aneurysm is a rare complication of pulmonary infection or infective endocarditis. While a lung nodule or mass adjacent to a hilar vessel in a patient with endocarditis or pneumonia should suggest the diagnosis, contrast CT is the definitive diagnostic procedure as it demonstrates the relationship of the mass with the pulmonary arterial vasculature.

Bronchiectasis. While postinfectious bronchiectasis is now less common in industrialized nations, pulmonary infection due to viral pneumonia, atypical mycobacteria, bacterial infection, and fungal infection may result in localized bronchiectasis. Bronchiectasis is reviewed in more detail in Chapter 16.

Swyer–James syndrome is an uncommon postinfectious form of constrictive bronchiolitis that typically results from a severe viral or mycoplasma infection in infancy or childhood. Typical radiologic findings include a hyperlucent lung with normal or small volume, attenuated vasculature, expiratory air trapping, and occasionally proximal bronchiectasis (see Fig. 16.23).

Bronchial Stenosis. This is a rare complication of infection and when seen is most often associated with endobronchial TB or fungal infections such as histoplasmosis.

Broncholithiasis. This condition reflects the presence of an endobronchial calcified nodule, most often seen as a result of erosion of a calcified peribronchial lymph node resulting from histoplasmosis or TB. Imaging findings include the identification of an endobronchial calcified nodule, often with distal atelectasis, bronchiectasis, or mucoid impaction (see Fig. 16.10). Thin-section CT is the diagnostic imaging modality of choice.

Fibrosing Mediastinitis (Sclerosing Mediastinitis). A rare condition that produces mediastinal fibrosis can develop in a small subset of patients with prior *Histoplasma* infection, perhaps as an immunologic reaction to fungal antigens. Other fungal infections, autoimmune disorders, drugs, and fibroinflammatory diseases have been associated with fibrosing mediastinitis. Pathologically dense fibrous tissue is seen to infiltrate the mediastinum. Clinically this condition presents with signs and symptoms related to obstruction of central airways, vessels, or of the esophagus. Radiologically there is mediastinal widening with calcifications visible. A focal mediastinal mass can also be seen. CT typically demonstrates either a localized calcified right paratracheal or subcarinal mass, or soft tissue infiltration of the middle mediastinum with compression or obliteration of structures (see Fig. 11.28). Secondary pulmonary parenchymal changes are the result of central airway and vascular compromise.

INFECTION IN THE IMMUNOCOMPROMISED HOST

Immunocompromise is defined as a decrease in the normal host defense mechanisms that fight infection. Immunocompromised patients include those with HIV infection, underlying hematologic malignancy, and individuals receiving chemotherapeutic and immunosuppressive therapy, particularly organ transplant recipients. The types of pulmonary infection seen in the immunocompromised patient depend on the specific defect(s) in host defense mechanisms. While the majority of pulmonary complications in immunocompromised patients are infectious in nature, noninfectious complications of disease can account for up to 25% of lung disease in this population. The accurate identification of the predominant radiographic pattern of abnormality in the immunocompromised patient helps limit the differential diagnostic considerations (Tables 14.7 and 14.8). With the advent of highly active antiretroviral therapy (HAART) and effective prophylaxis, the incidence of opportunistic infection in HIV/AIDS has decreased dramatically. Bacterial respiratory infections now account for most pulmonary infections in individuals living with HIV in the developed world.

TABLE 14.7

RADIOLOGIC PATTERNS OF PULMONARY DISEASE AND ETIOLOGIES IN HIV INFECTION

■ PATTERN	■ COMMON ETIOLOGIES
Focal lung disease	■ Bacterial infection ■ Fungal infection ■ Mycobacterial infection ■ Non-Hodgkin lymphoma ■ Bronchogenic carcinoma
Diffuse lung disease	■ PJP ■ CMV pneumonia ■ Lymphocytic interstitial pneumonitis
Nodules	■ Non-Hodgkin lymphoma ■ Mycobacterial infection ■ Fungal infection ■ Septic emboli (IVDA)
Lymph node enlargement	■ Mycobacterial infection ■ Fungal infection ■ Non-Hodgkin lymphoma ■ Bronchogenic carcinoma
Pleural effusion	■ Parapneumonic effusion/empyema ■ Mycobacterial infection ■ Fungal infection ■ Non-Hodgkin lymphoma

TABLE 14.8

PULMONARY INFECTIONS IN HEMATOPOIETIC STEM CELL TRANSPLANT RECIPIENTS

■ PHASE	■ TIME	■ COMMON INFECTIONS
Pre-engraftment	0–30 days	■ Aspergillosis ■ Bacterial infection ■ RSV pneumonia
Early post-transplantation	30–100 days	■ Cytomegalovirus ■ *Pneumocystis jiroveci* ■ Aspergillosis
Late post-transplantation	>100 days	■ Bacterial ■ Aspergillosis ■ Viral • Adenovirus • RSV • *Varicella zoster* • *Parainfluenza*

Bacterial Pneumonia. Bacteria are the most common cause of pneumonia in immunocompromised hosts. In HIV-infected patients, bacterial pneumonia may occur early in the course of infection and has an incidence six times that seen in the normal population. Recurrent bacterial pneumonia is categorized as an AIDS-defining illness for patients with HIV infection. The most common organisms causing pneumonia in HIV patients are *S. pneumoniae, H. influenzae, S. aureus, E. coli,* and *P. aeruginosa*. Uncommon causes of bacterial pneumonia in the AIDS population include *Nocardia asteroides*, *Rhodococcus equi*, *Bartonella henselae,* and *Bartonella quintana* (bacillary angiomatosis). In the non-HIV immunocompromised patient, *S. aureus* and gram-negative aerobes including *Klebsiella, Proteus, E. coli, Pseudomonas, Enterobacter,* and *Serratia* are the most common bacterial pathogens. Bacterial pneumonia is characterized by focal segmental or lobar airspace opacities. Cavitation is more frequent in the immunocompromised population than in normal individuals and may occur as multiple microabscesses. Multilobar involvement and diffuse pneumonia may occur and are distinctly unusual in normal individuals. Pleural effusions and empyema are uncommon.

Renal transplant recipients and patients on high-dose corticosteroids are at increased risk of pneumonia caused by *L. pneumophila* and *Legionella micdadei* (Pittsburgh agent). *L. pneumophila* causes multilobar focal areas of consolidation (Fig. 14.4), sometimes with cavitation and pleural effusion. The Pittsburgh agent causes a characteristic appearance of multiple, well-circumscribed, centrally cavitating nodules.

Nocardia is a gram-positive, branching, filamentous bacillus that is weakly acid fast. *N. asteroides* is the most important cause of pulmonary disease. It is usually an opportunistic infection in patients on immunosuppressive therapy, those with lymphoma or leukemia, and patients with alveolar proteinosis. The most frequent radiographic presentation is a homogeneous, nonsegmental airspace opacity or a mass. Cavitation is frequent (Fig. 14.21). Infection may extend into the pleural space and chest wall to produce empyema and osteomyelitis, respectively. Hilar lymph nodes may be enlarged. Treatment is with sulfonamides.

Tuberculosis. The incidence of TB has increased considerably since the onset of the AIDS epidemic. Most cases are caused

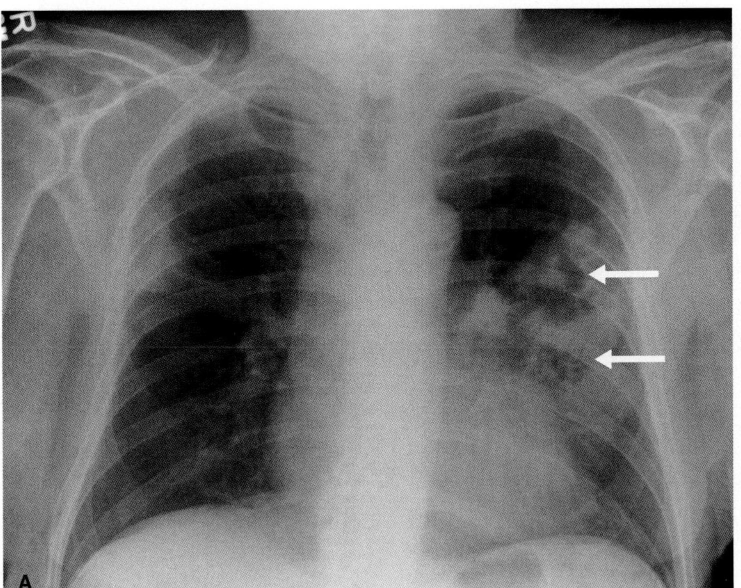

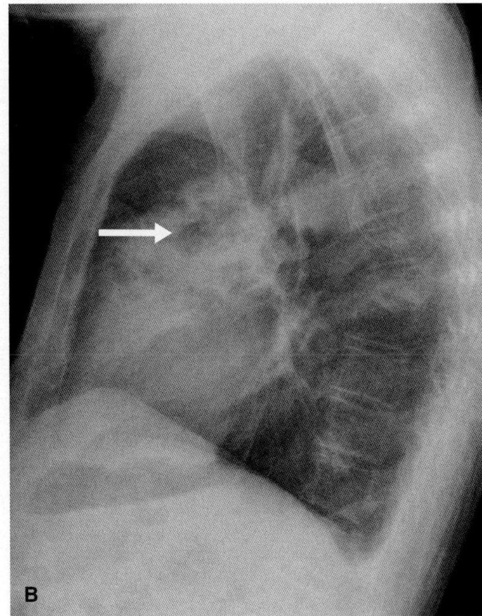

FIGURE 14.21. **Nocardia Pneumonia. A, B:** Frontal (**A**) and lateral (**B**) chest radiographs in a 34-year-old man with *Nocardia asteroides* pneumonia shows bilateral airspace opacification with areas of cavitation within the left upper lobe (*arrows* in **A** and **B**).

by reactivation of previously acquired disease. The diagnosis of TB in immunocompromised hosts is complicated because skin reactivity and sputum analysis are less sensitive in immunocompromised hosts and the yield of bronchoalveolar lavage is decreased in this patient population. The chest radiographic findings depend on the stage of HIV infection and the degree of immune dysfunction, which can be estimated by the CD4 count. In the early stages of AIDS (CD4+ >200 cells/mm^3), a postprimary pattern of upper lobe fibrocavitary disease indistinguishable from that seen in the immunocompetent patient is most common. Later in the course of AIDS (CD4+ 50 to 200 cells/mm^3), the radiographic features most often associated with primary disease are seen and include lobar consolidation, mediastinal and hilar lymphadenopathy, and pleural effusion. Rim-enhancing nodes with central necrosis on CT scans are a characteristic finding and should strongly suggest TB in a patient with AIDS. In advanced AIDS (CD4 <50 cells/mm^3), the radiographic findings are atypical and are characterized by diffuse reticular or nodular (miliary) opacities.

Mycobacterium avium-intracellulare (MAI) infection is the most common nontuberculous mycobacterial infection in AIDS patients. The disease primarily affects the GI tract, but disseminated disease can involve the chest. Lymphadenopathy is the major radiographic manifestation, but nonspecific focal airspace opacity or diffuse nodular opacities may be seen. Infection by *M. kansasii* may produce a pattern identical to that of postprimary TB.

Viral pneumonia other than CMV is uncommon in AIDS but can be seen in other immunocompromised patients (Fig. 14.14).

Cytomegalovirus is a common cause of viral pneumonia in patients with impaired cell-mediated immunity, specifically renal transplant recipients and lymphoma. It is an uncommon cause of pneumonia in the AIDS population. Chest radiographs and CT show diffuse bilateral ground-glass opacity or nodular opacities (Fig. 14.22).

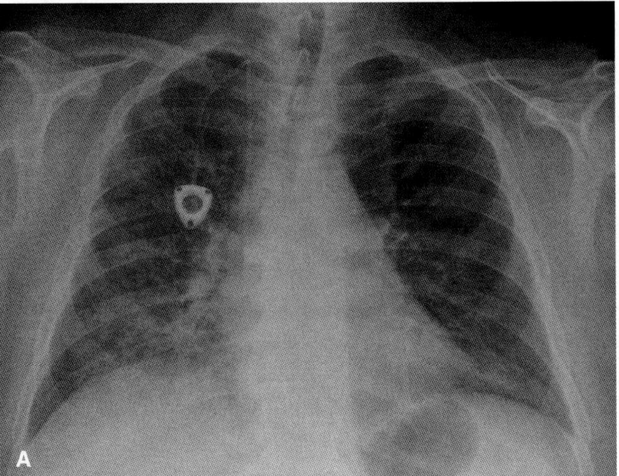

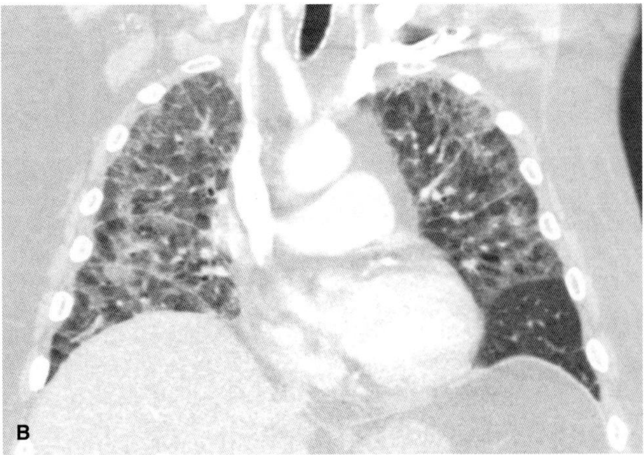

FIGURE 14.22. ***CMV* pneumonia. A:** Frontal chest radiograph in a 43-year-old bone marrow transplant recipient shows bilateral asymmetric reticulonodular opacities. **B:** Contrast-enhanced coronal CT scan through the mid-lungs shows bilateral ground-glass opacities with minimal interlobular septal thickening. Transbronchial lung biopsy revealed *CMV* infection.

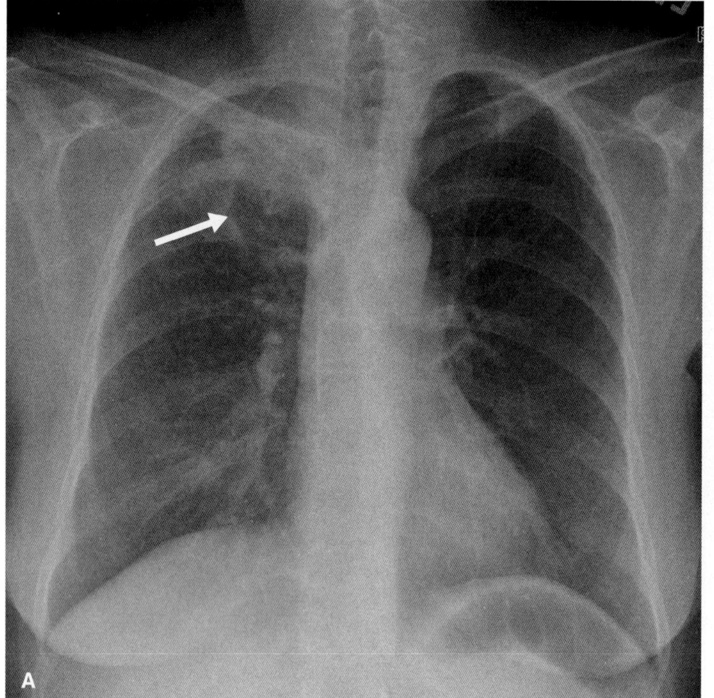

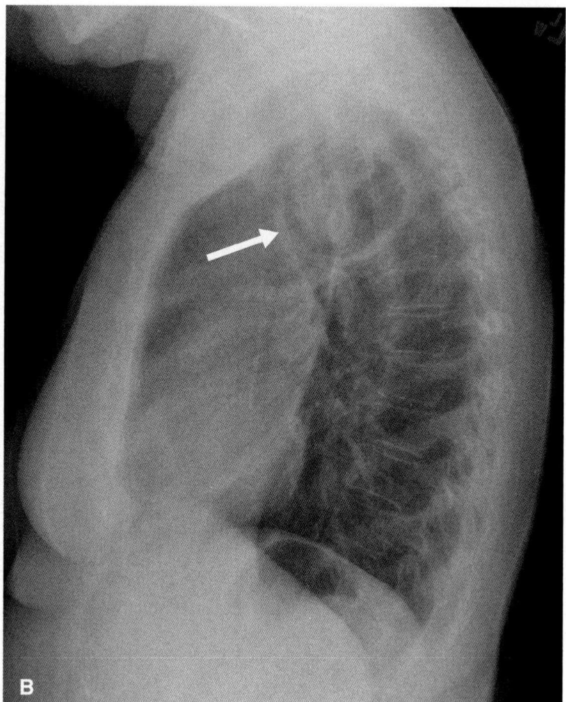

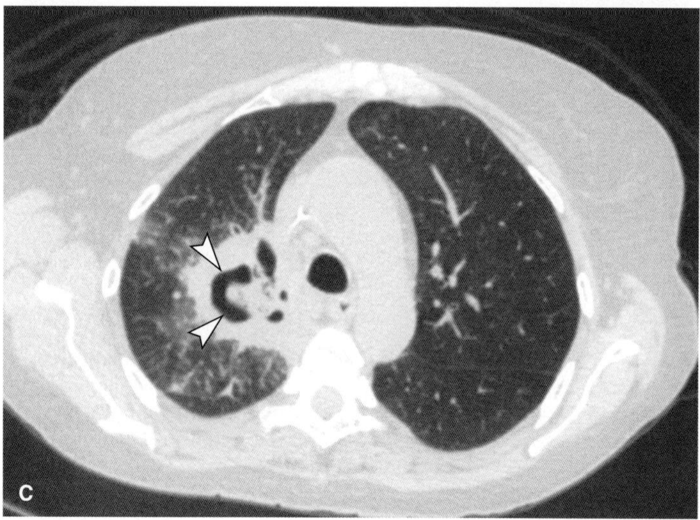

FIGURE 14.23. **Invasive Aspergillosis. A, B:** Posteroanterior (**A**) and lateral (**B**) radiographs in a hematopoietic stem cell transplant recipient with a history of non-Hodgkin lymphoma demonstrates a large right upper lobe cavity (*arrow*) with adjacent consolidation. **C:** Axial CT scan through the upper lobes shows a right upper lobe cavitary mass with adjacent ground-glass opacity. Note the crescentic air within the lesion (*arrowheads*).

Aspergillosis. Invasive aspergillus infection usually occurs in severely immunocompromised patients with neutropenia, most commonly those with leukemia or those receiving chemotherapy or corticosteroids. It occurs less frequently in AIDS patients, usually in the terminal stages of disease. The radiographic manifestations range from large nodular opacities to diffuse parenchymal consolidation (Fig. 14.23). The organism tends to invade blood vessels, causing infarction. Much of the observed opacity represents hemorrhage and edema. If pleural effusion develops, it usually indicates empyema. Cavitation, in the form of an air crescent, is not usually evident on chest films early in the course of disease, but it characteristically develops when the patient's complement of circulating neutrophils returns to a normal level (Fig. 14.23C). CT is useful for the early diagnosis of invasive aspergillosis. The demonstration of a zone of relative decreased attenuation surrounding a dense, mass-like opacity has been termed the "CT halo sign" and is relatively specific for invasive aspergillosis in a neutropenic patient. The halo represents a region of edema and hemorrhage where an air crescent will develop, separating the region of infected, necrotic lung from normal parenchyma.

Semi-invasive aspergillosis is an unusual form of *Aspergillus* pulmonary infection seen in patients with mild degrees of immunosuppression. The organism invades previously diseased lung tissue, producing slowly progressive airspace opacification or chronic cavitary disease.

Coccidioidomycosis in AIDS and other immunocompromised hosts is usually manifested by disseminated infection rather than the localized granulomatous disease seen in normal hosts. Pulmonary involvement is usually diffuse and produces miliary nodules, diffuse nodules, or reticulonodular opacities. Hilar and mediastinal lymphadenopathy and pleural effusions are uncommon.

Cryptococcosis. Cryptococcus neoformans is a budding yeast commonly found in soil and bird droppings. *Cryptococcus* is the most common cause of fungal infection in the AIDS population but can affect any immunocompromised patient. In some patients, particularly those with AIDS, the organism disseminates from its portal of entry in the lung to involve the CNS, bones, and mucocutaneous tissues. Meningitis is the most serious consequence of infection. There are several

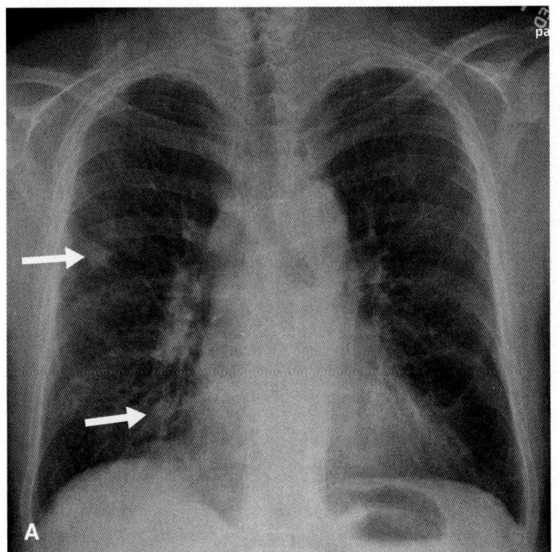

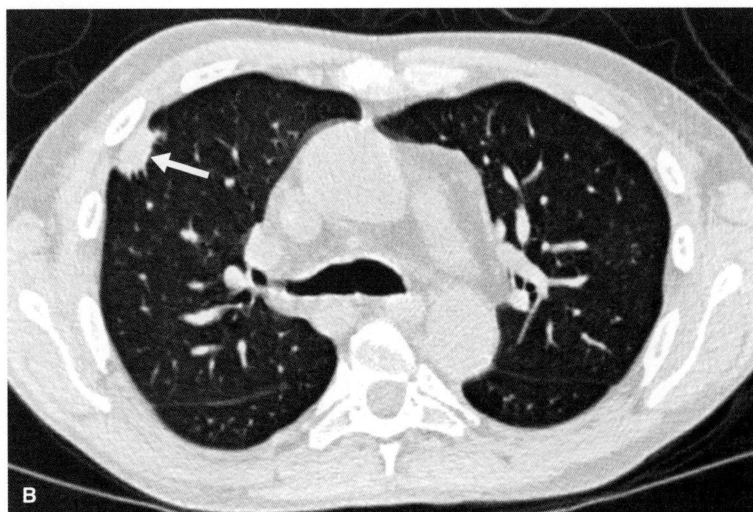

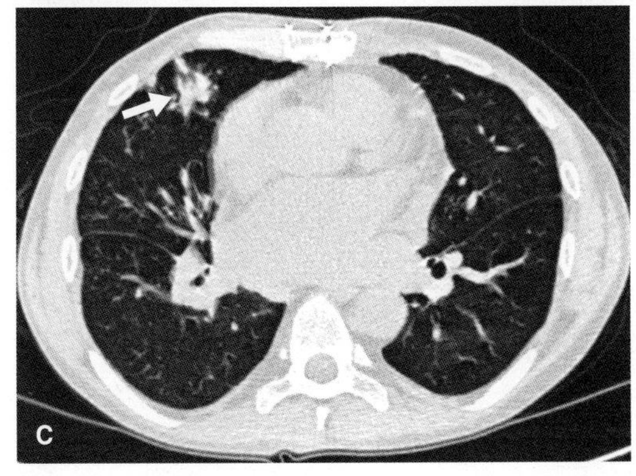

FIGURE 14.24. ***Cryptococcus*** **in Lung Transplant Recipient. A:** Frontal chest radiograph in a 35-year-old bilateral single lung transplant recipient shows several right lung nodules (*arrows*). **B, C:** Axial CT scans through the upper (**B**) and mid-lungs (**C**) show upper and middle lobe nodules (*arrows*). Stains and culture of a transthoracic needle biopsy aspirate showed cryptococcal infection.

chest radiographic patterns of disease: single or multiple nodules or masses (mimicking lung cancer) (Fig. 14.24), single or multiple patchy airspace opacities, and multiple small nodules (mimicking miliary TB). Cavitation, lymph node enlargement, and pleural effusion are more commonly seen in AIDS patients than in normal hosts.

Candidiasis. *Candida albicans* is an unusual cause of pneumonia in the immunocompromised patient. Patients with severe neutropenia caused by lymphoma or leukemia in the late stages of disease are most susceptible. The diagnosis is often difficult because *Candida* is a common colonizer in immunocompromised patients and its presence is often associated with other opportunistic infections. Chest radiographs in patients with *Candida* pneumonia show diffuse, bilateral, nonsegmental airspace or interstitial opacities. Miliary nodules may be seen, but cavitation, adenopathy, and pleural effusion are uncommon features.

Mucormycosis (zygomycosis) is a rare cause of pneumonia in immunocompromised patients with lymphoma, leukemia, or diabetes. Pulmonary infection is commonly accompanied by paranasal sinus infection, which may extend to involve the brain or meninges. Chest radiographic appearances include a solitary nodule (Fig. 14.25) or mass or focal airspace opacity, which may cavitate. Pleural effusion is uncommon.

Pneumocystis jiroveci Pneumonia. *P. jiroveci* (PJP) is a fungus commonly found in human lungs, although clinically significant pneumonia is seen only in immunocompromised individuals. PJP is most common in AIDS patients, usually in the late stages of HIV infection (CD4 <200 cells/mm^3). With the advent of HAART, the incidence of PJP has decreased significantly in the developed world. PJP still occurs in patients with HIV infection who are undiagnosed, not taking or responding to HAART, and those failing or not taking prophylaxis with trimethoprim sulfamethoxazole. Despite HAART and prophylaxis, PJP remains the most common AIDS-defining opportunistic infection. Organ transplant recipients on immunosuppressive drugs (particularly corticosteroids) and patients with lymphoreticular malignancies are also at increased risk for PJP.

The chest radiograph may be normal in the early phase of disease. In such patients, thin-section CT of the lung may provide evidence of subradiographic disease. As the disease progresses, a fine reticular or ground-glass pattern develops, particularly in the parahilar regions (Fig. 14.26). Progressive disease leads to confluent symmetric airspace opacification. Thin-walled cysts or pneumatoceles may develop during the course of disease and are responsible for an increased incidence of spontaneous pneumothorax complicating PJP. Pleural effusion or lymph node enlargement is distinctly uncommon (<5%) and should suggest an alternative or additional diagnosis. The diagnosis of PJP in AIDS is made by histopathologic demonstration of organisms from induced sputum or bronchoscopic specimens.

Toxoplasmosis. *Toxoplasma gondii* is an obligate intracellular protozoan whose definitive host is the cat. Humans acquire the organism by ingestion of material contaminated by oocyst-containing stool. It has been estimated that toxoplasmosis exists in a chronic asymptomatic form in 50% of the population of the United States. Disease can be recognized in four clinicopathologic forms: congenital, ocular, lymphatic, and generalized. Pulmonary involvement is usually seen in the generalized form of the disease, which affects immunocompromised hosts, including those with AIDS, organ transplant recipients, and patients with leukemia or lymphoma.

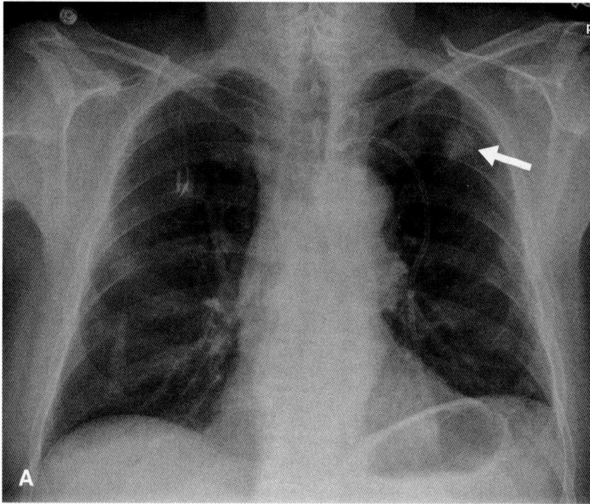

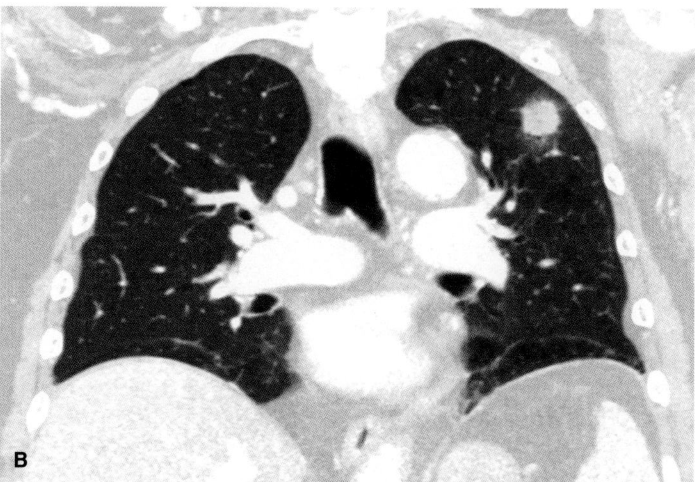

FIGURE 14.25. ***Mucormycosis*** **Infection in Bone Marrow Transplant Recipient. A:** Frontal chest radiograph in a patient with biopsy-proven mucormycosis shows a well-defined left upper lobe nodule (*arrow*). **B:** Contrast-enhanced coronal CT scan shows a left upper lobe nodule with irregular, somewhat indistinct margins with minimal surrounding ground glass.

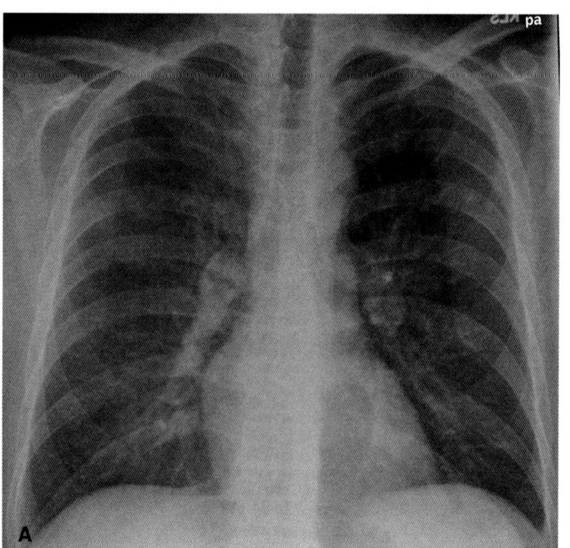

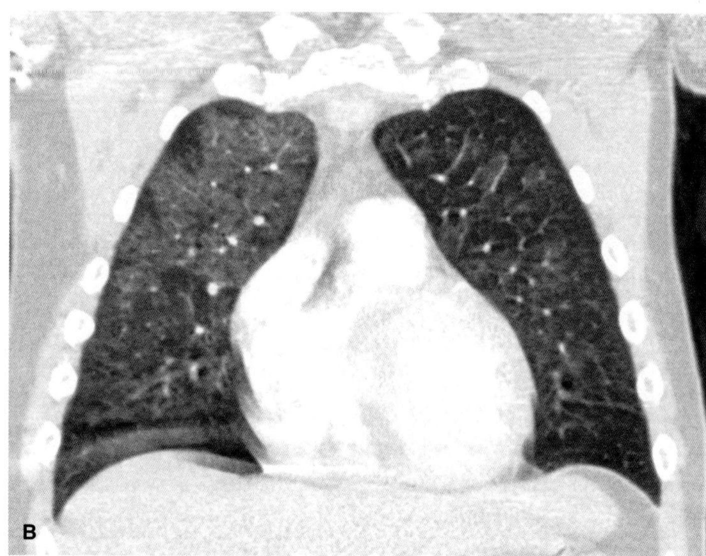

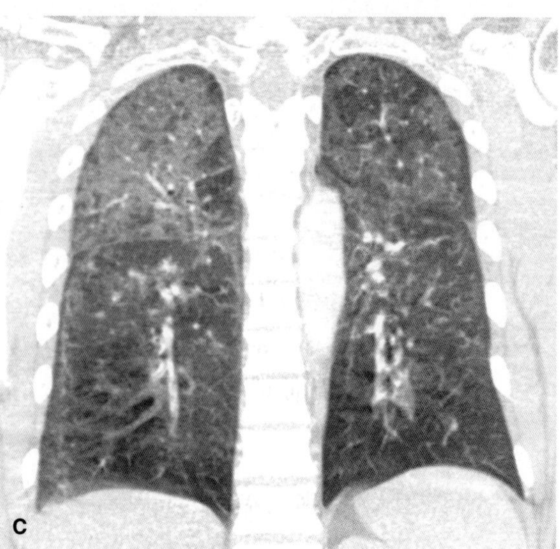

FIGURE 14.26. ***Pneumocystis jiroveci*** **Pneumonia (PJP). A:** Frontal chest radiograph in an HIV-positive patient with *Pneumocystis* pneumonia shows fine reticular opacities. **B, C:** Coronal CT scans through the anterior (**B**) and posterior lungs (**C**) show bilateral ground-glass opacities.

The radiographic findings in pulmonary toxoplasmosis include diffuse reticular opacities that resemble those of acute viral pneumonia. Less commonly, airspace opacities with air bronchograms may be seen. Hilar and mediastinal lymph node enlargement is common, while pleural effusion is rare. With generalized disease, most often seen in patients with AIDS, diffuse bilateral small nodular opacities may be seen.

Hematopoietic stem cell transplant (HSCT) recipients have a high (40% to 60%) incidence of pulmonary complications. Because of the predictable course of immune suppression, a timeline of expected pulmonary complications can be constructed to help narrow the differential diagnosis for radiographic abnormalities in patients following HSCT. The time following HSCT can be divided into three phases: the neutropenic phase, the early phase, and the late phase. The neutropenic phase lasts for the first 30 days approximately, followed by the early phase (from 30 to 100 days), and finally the late phase (more than 100 days post-HSCT). Complications can be infectious or noninfectious; the most common infections develop according to the time of presentation after transplantation as detailed in Table 14.6.

Suggested Readings

Ahuja J, Kanne JP. Thoracic infections in immunocompromised patients. *Radiol Clin North Am* 2014;52:121–136.

Bartlett JG, Finegold SM. Anaerobic infections of the lung and pleural space. *Am Rev Respir Dis* 1974;110:56–77.

Brecher CW, Aviram G, Boiselle PM. CT and radiography of bacterial respiratory infections in AIDS patients. *AJR Am J Roentgenol* 2003;180:1203–1209.

Cheon JE, Im JG, Kim MY, Lee JS, Choi GM, Yeon KM. Thoracic actinomycosis: CT findings. *Radiology* 1998;209(1):229–233.

Chong S, Lee KS, Yi CA, Chung MJ, Kim TS, Han J. Pulmonary fungal infection: imaging findings in immunocompetent and immunocompromised patients. *Eur J Radiol* 2006;59:371–383.

Franquet T. Imaging of pulmonary viral pneumonia. *Radiology* 2011;260: 18–39.

Jude CM, Nayak NB, Patel MK, Deshmukh M, Batra P. Pulmonary coccidioidomycosis: pictorial review of chest radiographic and CT findings. *Radiographics* 2014;34:912–925.

Martinez S, McAdams HP, Batchu CS. The many faces of pulmonary nontuberculous mycobacterial infection. *AJR Am J Roentgenol* 2007;189: 177–186.

Martinez S, Restrepo CS, Carrillo JA, et al. Thoracic manifestations of tropical parasitic infections: a pictorial review. *Radiographics* 2005;25:135–155.

Morris A, Lundgren JD, Masur H, et al. Current epidemiology of Pneumocystis pneumonia. *Emerg Infect Dis* 2004;10:1713–1720.

Nachiappan AC, Rahbar K, Shi X, et al. Pulmonary tuberculosis: role of radiology in diagnosis and management. *Radiographics* 2017;37:52–72.

Oh YW, Effmann EL, Godwin JD. Pulmonary infections in immunocompromised hosts: the importance of correlating the conventional radiologic appearance with the clinical setting. *Radiology* 2000;217:647–656.

Reittner P, Muller NL, Heyneman L, et al. Mycoplasma pneumoniae pneumonia. Radiographic and high-resolution CT features in 28 patients. *AJR Am J Roentgenol* 2000;174:37–41.

Rossi SE, McAdams HP, Rosado-de-Christensen ML, Franks TJ, Galvin JR. Fibrosing mediastinitis. *Radiographics* 2001;21:737–757.

Sharma S, Maycher B, Eschun G. Radiological imaging in pneumonia: recent innovations. *Curr Opin Pulm Med* 2007;13:159–169.

Tarver RD, Teague SD, Heitkamp DE, Conces DJ, Jr. Radiology of community-acquired pneumonia. *Radiol Clin North Am* 2005;43:497–512.

Vilar J, Domingo ML, Soto C, Cogollos J. Radiology of bacterial pneumonia. *Eur J Radiol* 2004;51(2):102–113.

CHAPTER 15 ■ DIFFUSE LUNG DISEASE

CURTIS E. GREEN AND JEFFREY S. KLEIN

Diffuse lung disease represents a broad spectrum of disorders that primarily affect the pulmonary interstitium (Table 15.1). These diseases present in a variety of manners, most typically with symptoms of progressive dyspnea. Some patients, however, present with minimal or no symptoms and interstitial lung disease is discovered either incidentally or during radiologic screening for interstitial disease associated with collagen vascular disease. Restrictive lung disease and hypoxemia on pulmonary function tests are characteristically present. The radiographic findings produced by interstitial disease are reviewed in Chapter 10. Thin-section CT has revolutionized the diagnosis of interstitial lung disease, and its role in the evaluation of interstitial disease is detailed in this chapter.

THIN-SECTION CT OF THE PULMONARY INTERSTITIUM

Normal Anatomy. Thin-section CT provides the most direct radiographic method for assessment of the pulmonary interstitium. The general utility of thin-section CT in the evaluation of chronic interstitial lung disease is outlined in Table 15.2. The pulmonary interstitium is the scaffolding of the lung, providing support for the airways, gas-exchanging units, and vascular structures. It is a continuous network of connective tissue fibers that begins at the lung hilum and extends peripherally to the visceral pleura (see Fig. 10.11). The central interstitial compartment extending from the mediastinum peripherally and enveloping the bronchovascular bundles is termed the *axial* or *bronchovascular interstitium*. The axial interstitium is contiguous with the interstitium surrounding the small centrilobular arteriole and bronchiole within the secondary pulmonary lobule, where it is called the *centrilobular interstitium*. The most peripheral component of the interstitium is the *subpleural* or *peripheral interstitium*, which lies between the visceral pleura and the lung surface. Invaginations of the subpleural interstitium into the lung parenchyma form the borders of the secondary pulmonary lobules and represent the interlobular septa. Extending between the centrilobular interstitium within the lobular core and the interlobular septal/subpleural interstitium in the lobular periphery is a fine network of connective tissue fibers that support the alveolar spaces called the *intralobular, parenchymal,* or *alveolar interstitium.*

The secondary pulmonary lobule is defined as that subsegment of lung supplied by three to five terminal bronchioles and separated from adjacent secondary lobules by intervening connective tissue (interlobular septa) (Fig. 15.1). Each terminal bronchiole further subdivides into respiratory bronchioles, alveolar ducts, alveolar sacs, and alveoli. The unit of lung subtended from a single terminal bronchiole is called a *pulmonary acinus*. The centrilobular artery and preterminal bronchiole are located in the center of the secondary lobule. Pulmonary veins and lymphatics run at the margins of lobules within the interlobular septa, with lymphatics and connective tissue found within the contiguous subpleural interstitium. The secondary pulmonary lobule is typically polyhedral in shape, with each side ranging from 1.0 to 2.5 cm in length. The interlobular septa are most prominent over the periphery of the lung, where they are readily seen on CT. At the

TABLE 15.1

ACRONYMS FOR DIFFUSE LUNG DISEASES

■ ABBREVIATION	■ DISEASE
AFOP	Acute fibrinous and organizing pneumonia
AIP	Acute interstitial pneumonia
COP	Cryptogenic organizing pneumonia
CPFE	Combined pulmonary fibrosis and emphysema
CWP	Coal worker's pneumoconiosis
DIP	Desquamative interstitial pneumonia
IIP	Idiopathic interstitial pneumonia
IPAF	Interstitial pneumonia with autoimmune features
IPF	Idiopathic pulmonary fibrosis
LIP	Lymphocytic interstitial pneumonitis
LAM	Lymphangioleiomyomatosis
LCH	Langerhans cell histiocytosis
NSIP	Nonspecific interstitial pneumonia
OP	Organizing pneumonia
PAP	Pulmonary alveolar proteinosis
PMF	Progressive massive fibrosis
PPFE	Pleuroparenchymal fibroelastosis
RB-ILD	Respiratory bronchiolitis–associated interstitial lung disease
SLE	Systemic lupus erythematosus
TS	Tuberous sclerosis
UIP	Usual interstitial pneumonia

surface of the lung, these septa are short structures that course perpendicular to the pleural surface and completely separate adjacent lobules. Within the parahilar portions of the lung, the interlobular septa are longer and more obliquely oriented and incompletely marginate the secondary lobules.

Normal Thin-Section CT Findings. Thin-section CT can demonstrate much of the normal anatomy of the secondary pulmonary lobule. Interlobular septa are normally 0.1 mm thick and can be seen in the lung periphery, particularly along the superior and inferior pleural surfaces (Fig. 15.2). Centrilobular arteries (1 mm in diameter) are V- or Y-shaped structures on thin-section CT seen within 5 to 10 mm of the pleural surface. Normal intralobular (0.7 mm) and acinar (0.3 to 0.5 mm) arteries are commonly seen. Normal airways are visible only to within 3 cm of the pleura. The centrilobular bronchiole, with a diameter of 1 mm and a wall thickness of 0.15 mm, is not normally visible on thin-section CT. Pulmonary veins (0.5 cm) are occasionally seen as linear or dot-like structures within 1 to 2 cm of the pleura and, when visible, indicate the locations of interlobular septa. The peribronchovascular, centrilobular, and intralobular interstitial compartments are not normally visible on thin-section CT.

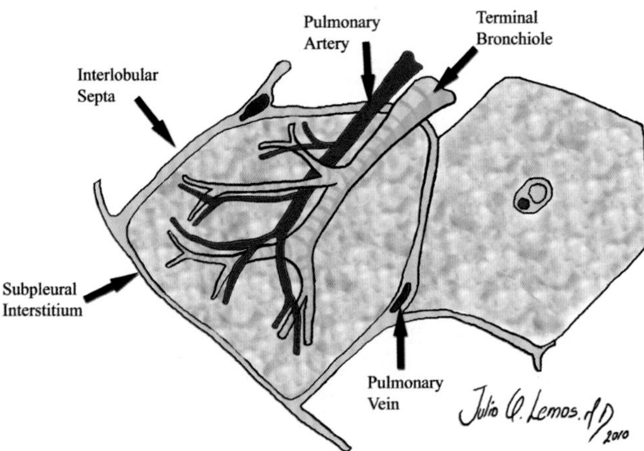

FIGURE 15.1. Diagram of the Normal Secondary Pulmonary Lobule.

TABLE 15.2

UTILITY OF THIN-SECTION CT IN THE EVALUATION OF CHRONIC INTERSTITIAL LUNG DISEASE

1. Detection of clinically suspected parenchymal abnormality when the chest radiograph is normal or shows questionable abnormality
2. Characterization of diffuse parenchymal abnormalities
3. Determining likelihood of usual interstitial pneumonitis/idiopathic pulmonary fibrosis
4. Biopsy planning:
   - Determination of route for biopsy, that is, transbronchial, open lung, or bronchoalveolar lavage
   - Targeting biopsy to area(s) of active disease, avoiding areas of end-stage fibrosis
5. Monitoring of response to therapy or progression of disease
6. Detecting complications associated with diffuse lung disease or its treatment
   - Infection
   - Malignancy
   - Drug toxicity

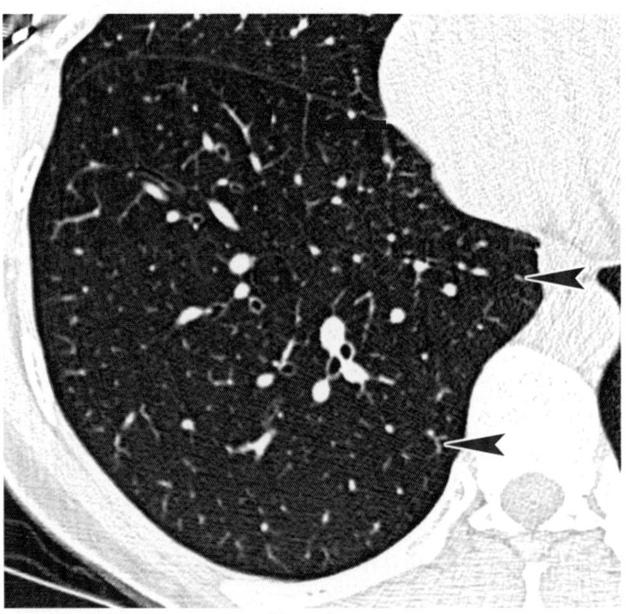

FIGURE 15.2. Thin-Section CT of Normal Lobular Anatomy. Normal interlobular septum (*arrow*) and centrilobular arteries (*arrowheads*) are clearly visible.

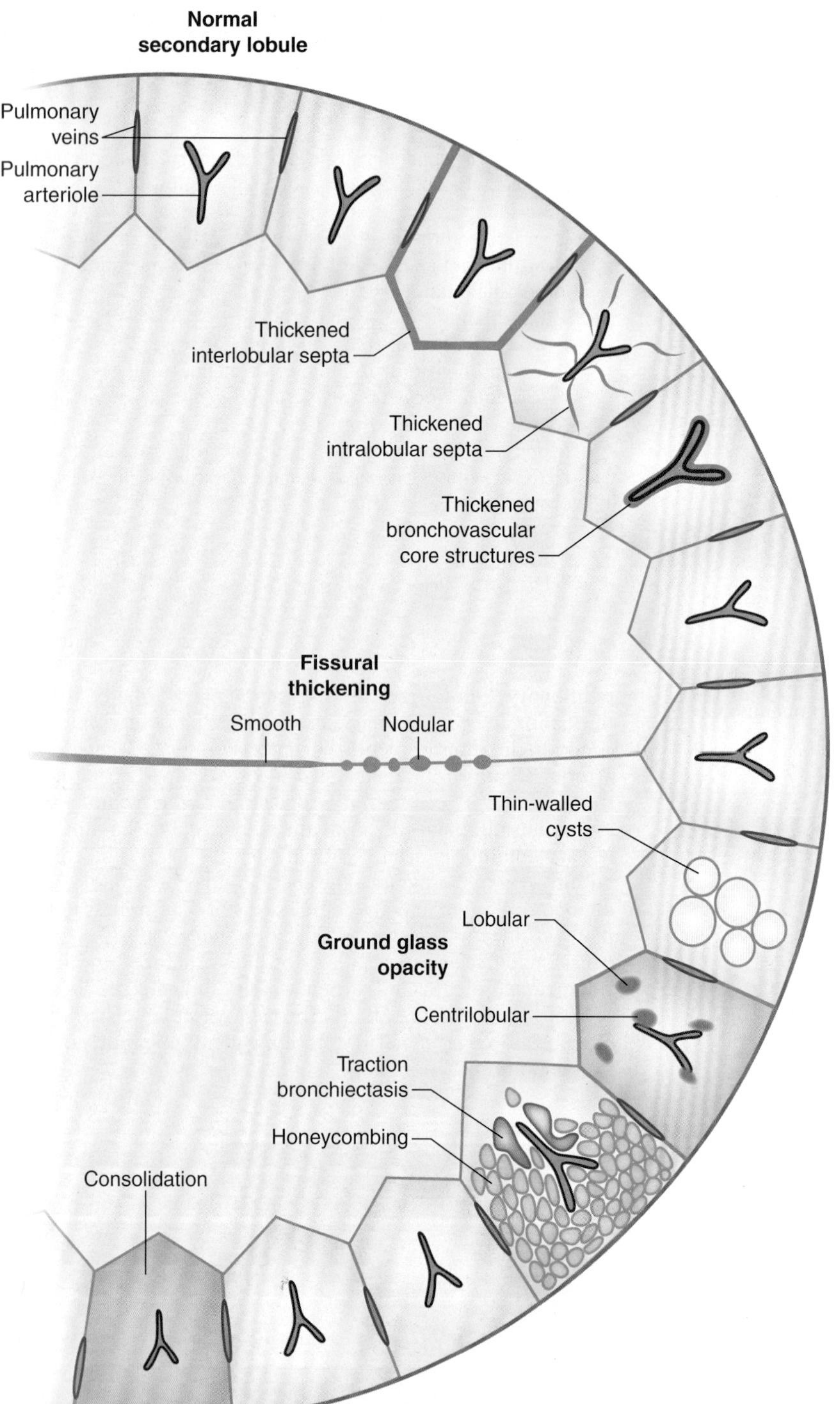

FIGURE 15.3. Thin-Section CT Findings in Interstitial Lung Disease. (Reprinted with permission from *The Radiologist*, Baltimore, MD: Lippincott Williams & Wilkins; 1998.)

Thin-Section CT Signs of Disease

The signs of interstitial lung disease on thin-section CT are illustrated in Fig. 15.3, and their differential diagnosis is listed in Table 15.3.

Interlobular (Septal) Lines. Septal thickening is most often seen as thin, short, 1- to 2-cm lines oriented perpendicular to and intersecting the costal pleura. These lines are best visualized in the subpleural and juxtadiaphragmatic regions of the lung, where they outline the anterior and posterior margins of secondary lobules. In the central regions of the lung, the thickened septa can completely envelope lobules to produce polygonal structures. Although septa can be seen in normal individuals, these lines are thicker (>1 mm) and more numerous in patients with diseases primarily affecting the interlobular interstitium, such as interstitial pulmonary edema, idiopathic pulmonary fibrosis (IPF), and lymphangitic carcinomatosis (Fig. 15.4). Interlobular lines on thin-section CT are the equivalent of Kerley B lines seen in the inferolateral portions of the lungs on frontal radiographs. Within the central regions of the lung, long (2 to 6 cm) linear opacities representing obliquely oriented connective tissue septa are the equivalent of radiographic Kerley A lines.

TABLE 15.3

DIFFERENTIAL DIAGNOSTIC RCT FEATURES IN INTERSTITIAL LUNG DISEASE

■ CT FINDING	■ DIFFERENTIAL DIAGNOSIS	■ CT FINDING	■ DIFFERENTIAL DIAGNOSIS
Interlobular (septal) lines	Interstitial edema Lymphangitic carcinomatosis Sarcoidosis UIP	Irregular lung interfaces	Pulmonary edema UIP Sarcoidosis
Intralobular lines	UIP Alveolar proteinosis Hypersensitivity pneumonitis (chronic)	Micronodules, random distribution	Miliary tuberculosis or histoplasmosis Hematogenous metastases Silicosis/coal worker's pneumoconiosis (CWP) EG
"Thickened" fissures	Pulmonary edema Sarcoidosis Lymphangitic carcinomatosis	Micronodules, perilymphatic distribution	Sarcoidosis Lymphangitic carcinomatosis Silicosis/CWP
Peribronchovascular interstitial thickening	Pulmonary edema (smooth) Sarcoidosis (nodular) Lymphangitic carcinomatosis (smooth or nodular)	Ground-glass opacities	UIP Desquamative interstitial pneumonia Acute interstitial pneumonia (AIP) Hypersensitivity pneumonitis
Centrilobular nodules	Hypersensitivity pneumonitis OP/COP RB-ILD		OP/COP RB-ILD Hemorrhage *Pneumocystis jiroveci* pneumonia Cytomegalovirus pneumonia Alveolar proteinosis
Subpleural lines	Asbestosis IPF	Architectural distortion Traction bronchiectasis	UIP Sarcoidosis
Parenchymal bands	UIP Sarcoidosis	Conglomerate mass	Silicosis/CWP Sarcoidosis Silicosis
Honeycombing	UIP Hypersensitivity pneumonitis (chronic) Sarcoidosis	Consolidation	CWP Radiation fibrosis BOOP/COP Sarcoidosis
Thin-walled cysts	Langerhans cell histiocytosis Lymphangioleiomyomatosis Tuberous sclerosis		AIP UIP

Intralobular Lines. In some patients, a lattice of fine lines is seen within the central portion of the pulmonary lobule radiating out toward the thickened lobular borders to produce a "spoke-and-wheel" or "spider web" appearance. These lines are not normally visible on thin-section CT and represent thickening of the intralobular or parenchymal interstitium. Thickened intralobular lines usually result from fibrosis and are most commonly seen in IPF and other causes of usual interstitial pneumonitis (UIP). Thickened intralobular lines can also be seen in other infiltrative diseases such as pulmonary alveolar proteinosis (PAP).

"Thickened" Fissures. The apparent thickening of interlobar fissures in patients with interstitial lung disease is usually a direct extension of the thickening of interlobular septa to involve the subpleural interstitium of the lung. While such a process normally involves all pleural surfaces equally, the "thickening" is usually best appreciated on the fissures, where two layers of visceral pleura—and therefore two layers of subpleural interstitium—are seen outlined on either side by aerated lung. The fissural thickening can be smooth or nodular. Smooth fissural thickening is virtually indistinguishable from a small amount of pleural fluid within the fissure and is most commonly seen with pulmonary edema. Nodular fissural thickening is commonly seen in sarcoidosis and lymphangitic carcinomatosis (Fig. 15.4), where the nodules lie within the subpleural lymphatics.

Thickened bronchovascular structures of the lung result from thickening of the peribronchovascular interstitium. This produces apparent enlargement of perihilar vascular structures and thickening of bronchial walls, which are the thin-section CT equivalent of peribronchial cuffing and tram tracking seen radiographically. Pulmonary edema causes smooth thickening of the peribronchovascular interstitium whereas sarcoidosis causes nodular thickening (Fig. 15.5A). Lymphangitic carcinomatosis can result in either smooth or irregular peribronchovascular thickening (Fig. 15.6).

Centrilobular (Lobular Core) Abnormalities. Thickening of the axial interstitium within the lobular core produces an abnormal prominence of the "dot-like" or branching centrilobular arteriole. Diseases that commonly produce this appearance include pulmonary edema, lymphangitic carcinomatosis, and UIP. The centrilobular bronchiole is not normally seen on

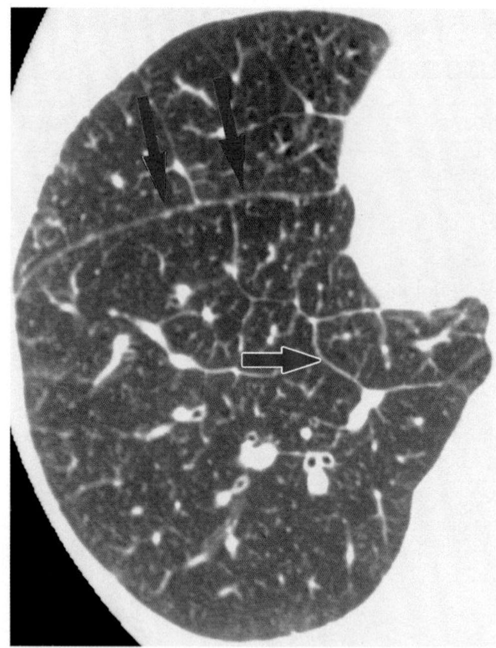

FIGURE 15.4. **Interlobular (Septal) Lines in Lymphangitic Carcinomatosis.** A thin-section CT scan through the upper lobes in a patient with lymphangitic carcinomatosis shows thickened interlobular septa (*small arrow*). Note the presence of nodular fissural thickening (*large arrows*), another common finding in this entity.

thin-section CT but may be rendered visible as a result of luminal dilatation or thickening of the centrilobular interstitium. Small airways disease can produce centrilobular bronchiolar abnormalities, which are seen on thin-section CT as fluid-filled dilated branching Y-shaped structures that produce a "tree-in-bud" appearance. Ill-defined centrilobular nodules represent disease of the bronchiole and adjacent parenchyma and are

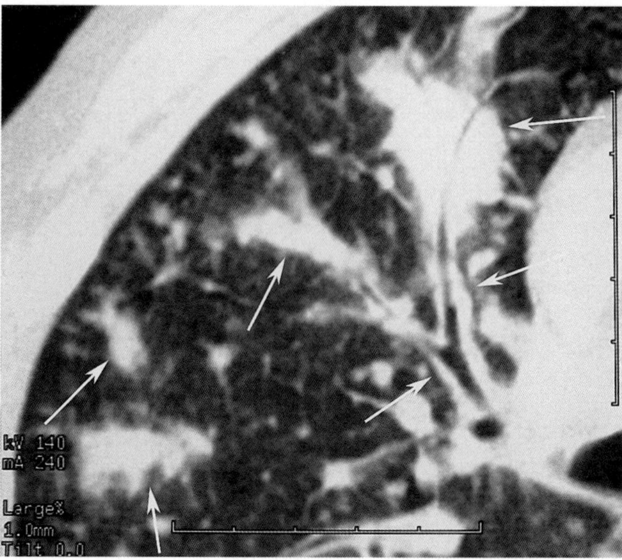

FIGURE 15.6. **Thickened Bronchovascular Structures in Lymphangitic Carcinomatosis.** In a patient with lymphangitic carcinomatosis, a thin-section CT shows both smooth and nodular thickening of the bronchovascular structures (*arrows*) that represent lymphatic tumor surrounding the axial interstitium.

commonly present in subacute hypersensitivity pneumonitis (Fig. 15.7), cryptogenic organizing pneumonia (COP), respiratory bronchiolitis–associated interstitial lung disease (RB-ILD) as well as other disorders.

Subpleural Lines. These 5- to 10-cm-long curvilinear opacities are found within 1 cm of the pleura and parallel the chest wall. They are most frequent in the posterior portions of the lower lobes and remain unchanged on prone scans. They probably represent an early phase of lung fibrosis and should be distinguished from a similar line that is seen as a result

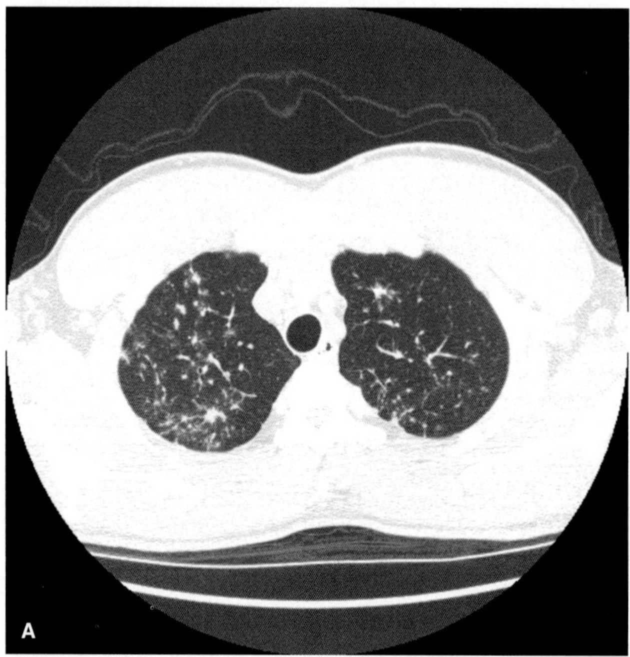

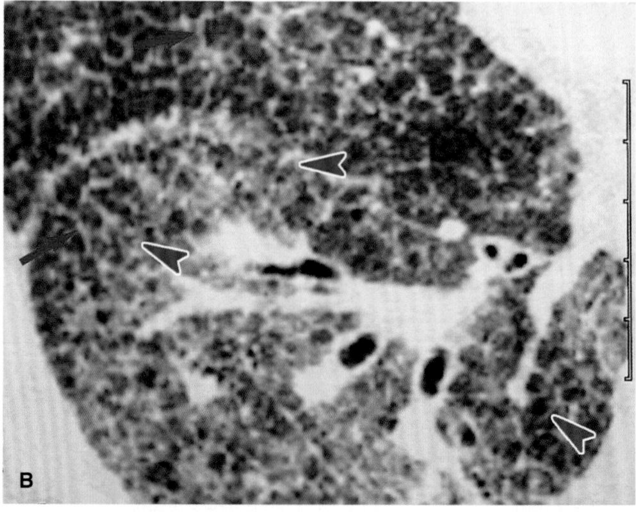

FIGURE 15.5. **Interstitial Thickening. A:** Thin-section CT in a patient with sarcoidosis shows nodular interstitial thickening and scattered irregular nodules. **B:** A targeted thin-section CT through the right lower lobe in a patient with UIP shows thickening of intralobular (*long arrows*) and interlobular (*arrowheads*) lines associated with ground-glass opacity.

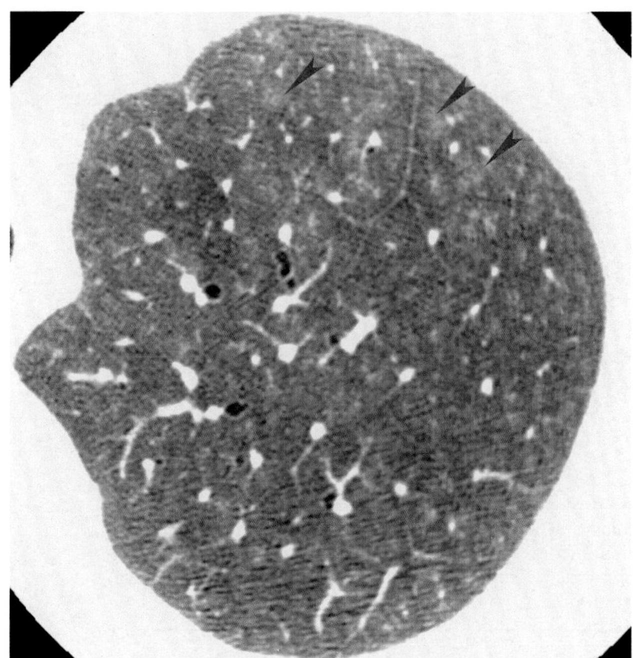

FIGURE 15.7. **Centrilobular Ground-Glass Nodules in Subacute Hypersensitivity Pneumonitis.** Thin-section CT shows the typical poorly defined centrilobular nodules (*arrowheads*) of subacute hypersensitivity pneumonitis.

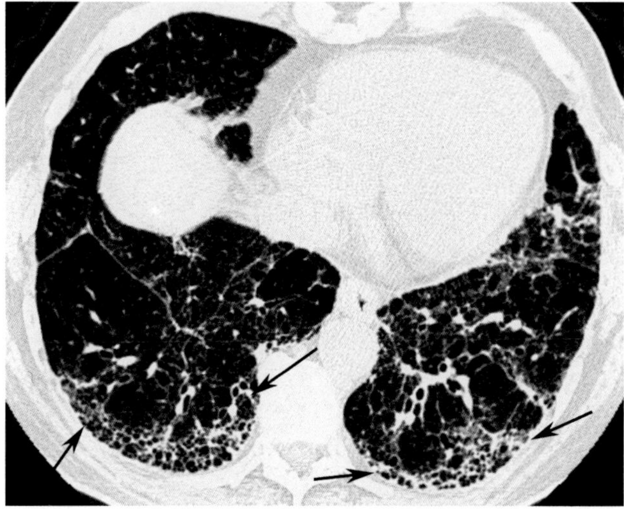

FIGURE 15.8. **Honeycomb Lung in Usual Interstitial Pneumonia.** Thin-section CT in a patient with IPF shows peripheral honeycombing (*arrows*) resulting from end-stage pulmonary fibrosis.

of atelectasis in the dependent portion of the lungs in normal individuals. Subpleural lines are most often seen in patients with asbestosis and, less commonly, IPF.

Parenchymal bands are nontapering linear opacities, 2 to 5 cm in length, that extend from the lung to contact the pleural surface. These fibrotic bands can be distinguished from vessels and thickened septa by their length, thickness, course, absence of branching, and their association with regional parenchymal distortion. Parenchymal bands are frequently seen in asbestosis, IPF, and sarcoidosis.

Honeycomb cysts are small (6 to 10 mm) cystic spaces with thick (1 to 3 mm) walls, most often present in the posterior subpleural regions of the lower lobes, and result from end-stage pulmonary fibrosis from a variety of etiologies. Pathologically, the cysts are lined by bronchiolar epithelium and are the result of bronchiolectasis. Most patients show additional signs of interstitial disease, including thickened interlobular and intralobular lines, parenchymal bands, irregularity of lung interfaces, and areas of ground-glass opacity. Honeycombing is frequently seen in UIP (Fig. 15.8) and chronic hypersensitivity pneumonitis, and occasionally in sarcoidosis.

Thin-walled cysts are a common manifestation of late stages of Langerhans cell histiocytosis of lung (LCH), also referred to as eosinophilic granulomatosis, and lymphangioleiomyomatosis (LAM). These cysts are slightly larger in diameter (10 mm) and have thinner walls than honeycomb cysts. Honeycomb cysts usually have shared walls, while the cysts of LCH and

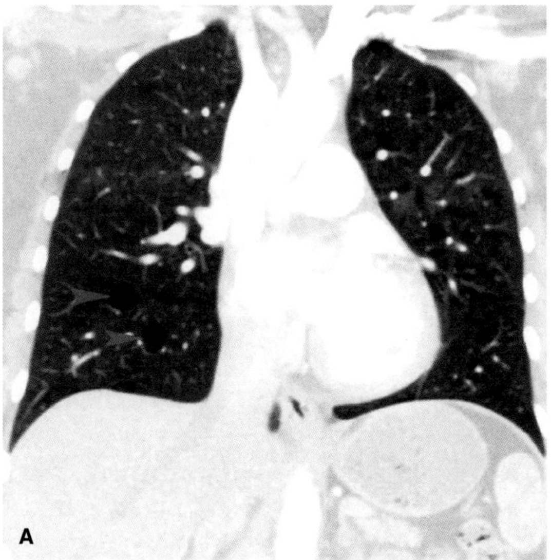

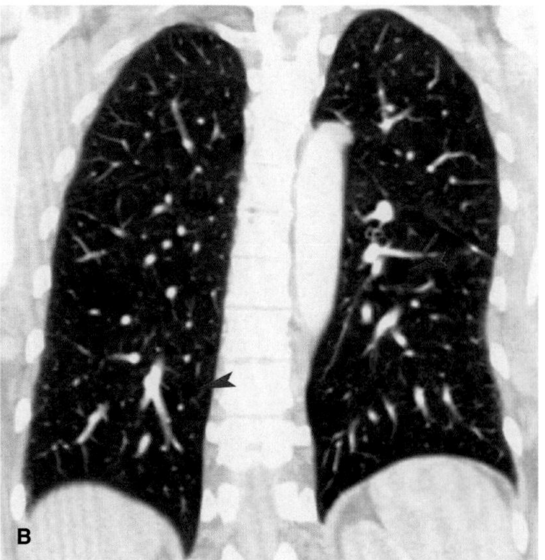

FIGURE 15.9. **Thin-Walled Cysts in Lymphangioleiomyomatosis (LAM). A, B:** Coronal reconstructions of a thin-section CT of a patient with LAM show multiple, thin-walled cysts (*arrowheads*). Although variably sized, the cysts are fairly uniform in shape.

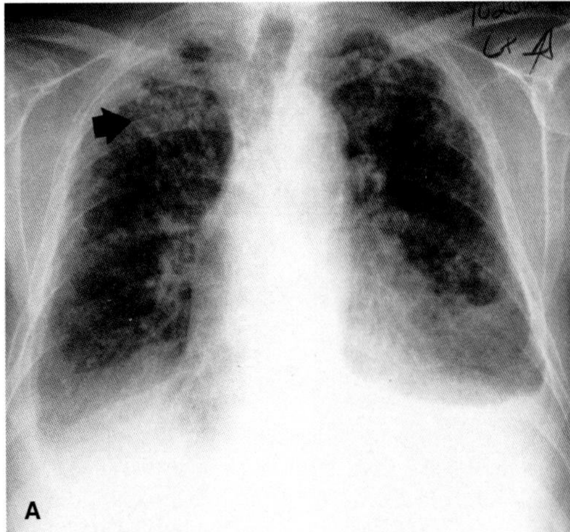

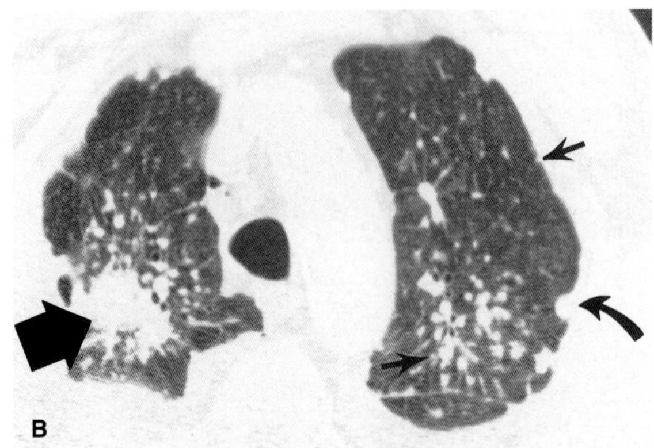

FIGURE 15.10. **Nodules and a Conglomerate Mass in Silicosis. A:** Posteroanterior radiograph of a 79-year-old patient with silicosis shows diffuse nodules as well as a conglomerate mass in the right upper lobe (*arrow*). **B:** Thin-section CT scan through the upper lobes shows peribronchovascular and subpleural micronodules (*small arrows*), larger nodules (*curved arrow*), and a conglomerate mass representing progressive massive fibrosis in the right upper lobe (*large arrow*). The pleural effusions are caused by concomitant congestive heart failure.

LAM do not. The cysts of LCH and LAM are usually evenly distributed from central to peripheral portions of the upper lobes (Fig. 15.9), with or without lower lobe involvement, while honeycombing tends to occur in the subpleural regions of the lower lobes. Normal lung may be found in the intervening spaces between the cysts of LCH and LAM. Honeycombing uniformly destroys lung and produces distortion of lung interfaces and traction bronchiectasis, features not typically found in either LCH or LAM.

Irregularity of Lung Interfaces. A common thin-section CT sign of interstitial disease, irregularity of the normally smooth interface between the bronchovascular bundles and the surrounding lung, reflects edema, or fibrosis or infiltration of the axial interstitium by granulomas or tumor. Similarly, irregularity of the interface between fissures or pleural surfaces and adjacent lung indicates peripheral interstitial disease. UIP (Fig. 15.5B) and sarcoidosis are the most common causes of irregular lung interfaces.

Micronodules. These 1- to 3-mm, sharply marginated, round opacities seen on thin-section CT represent conglomerates of granulomas or tumor cells within the interstitium. These are most often seen in sarcoidosis, LCH, silicosis (Fig. 15.10), miliary tuberculosis (TB) or histoplasmosis, metastatic adenocarcinoma, and lymphangitic carcinomatosis. They may be seen along the central bronchovascular structures (sarcoidosis, LCH); within interlobular septa or subpleural interstitium (sarcoidosis, lymphangitic carcinomatosis, silicosis); or within the substance of the pulmonary lobules (metastatic adenocarcinoma, miliary granulomatous infection). Nodules predominating in the peribronchovascular, interlobular, and subpleural regions—those portions of the interstitium where the lymphatics lie—are said to have a "perilymphatic" distribution.

Ground-Glass Opacity. Ground-glass opacity is defined as an area of increased attenuation (on thin-section CT) within which the normal parenchymal structures are visible. Multifocal areas of ground-glass opacity can sometimes be identified in patients with diffuse interstitial lung disease. These regions often respect lobular borders and do not demonstrate air bronchograms. They result from abnormalities below the resolution of the CT scan and are most often produced by thickening of the alveolar septa, with or without the lining of the alveolar spaces, by inflammatory exudate or fluid. Diseases commonly associated with this appearance include desquamative interstitial pneumonia (DIP), *Pneumocystis jiroveci* pneumonia, acute hypersensitivity pneumonitis (Fig. 15.11), nonspecific interstitial pneumonia (NSIP), and interstitial pulmonary edema. The ground-glass densities are occasionally confined to the immediate centrilobular regions of the pulmonary lobules, where they appear as fuzzy nodular densities that outline the normally invisible centrilobular bronchiole (Fig. 15.7). This reflects involvement of the peribronchovascular interstitium and surrounding alveoli by an inflammatory process and is seen in hypersensitivity pneumonitis, COP, and panbronchiolitis. The presence of ground-glass opacities is important because it often implies an active inflammatory process or edema that is reversible and warrants aggressive treatment. Ground-glass abnormality associated with a predominant pattern of honeycombing indicates microscopic pulmonary fibrosis, however.

Architectural Distortion and Traction Bronchiectasis. Processes that result in extensive parenchymal fibrosis can distort the normal architecture of the lung, creating irregularities of the lung-mediastinal, lung-pleural, and lung-vascular interfaces. Parenchymal distortion is often better appreciated on thin-section CT than on plain radiographs. Sarcoidosis and

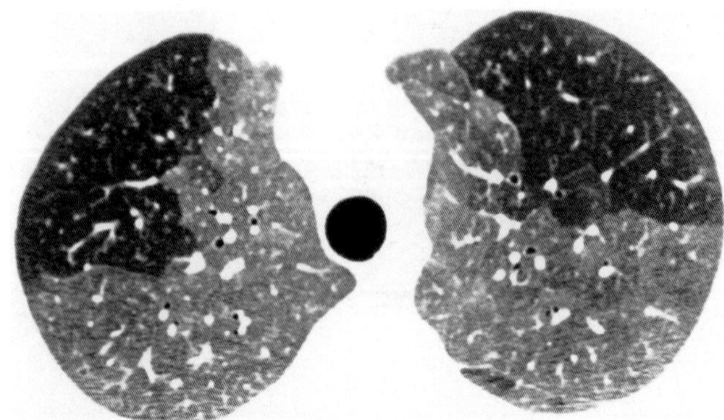

FIGURE 15.11. **Ground-Glass Opacity in Acute Hypersensitivity Pneumonitis.** A thin-section CT through the upper lobes shows widespread ground-glass opacity in a patient with hypersensitivity pneumonitis. Note that the pulmonary vessels are still visible within the areas of abnormality.

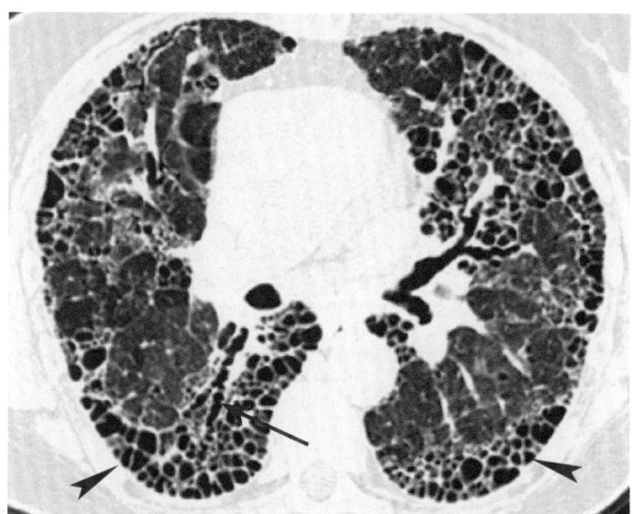

FIGURE 15.12. **Architectural Distortion and Traction Bronchiectasis in Usual Interstitial Pneumonia.** Thin-section CT through the lower lobes shows extensive peripheral honeycombing (*blue arrowheads*), traction bronchiectasis (*red arrow*), and architectural distortion.

UIP (Fig. 15.12) are the diseases most commonly associated with architectural distortion.

A finding commonly associated with architectural distortion is *traction bronchiectasis*, in which fibrosis causes traction on the walls of bronchi, resulting in irregular dilatation. While this usually involves segmental and subsegmental bronchi, it can also be seen at the intralobular level, where traction bronchiolectasis contributes to honeycombing. Traction bronchiectasis is most commonly seen in UIP (Fig. 15.12), but is also common in fibrotic sarcoidosis and radiation fibrosis.

Conglomerate Masses. In some patients with extensive pulmonary fibrosis, masses of fibrotic tissue develop in the parahilar regions of the upper lobes, often associated with peripheral bullae. On CT, these masses are seen to contain crowded vessels and dilated bronchi. They are most often seen in patients with end-stage sarcoidosis but can occur in complicated silicosis with progressive massive fibrosis (PMF) (Fig. 15.10) or radiation fibrosis following treatment of Hodgkin lymphoma or lung cancer. A similar finding is seen rarely in intravenous drug users when a granulomatous fibrosis results as a response to intravenous talc or starch mixed with narcotics.

Consolidation refers to increased lung density that obscures underlying blood vessels; air bronchograms are commonly present. This finding can be seen with any airspace-filling process (Fig. 15.13) but occasionally occurs in interstitial diseases such as UIP and sarcoidosis.

CHRONIC INTERSTITIAL LUNG DISEASE

Chronic interstitial lung disease usually results from diffuse inflammatory processes that primarily affect the axial and parenchymal interstitium of the lung. A wide variety of disease processes can result in diffuse damage to the pulmonary interstitium. Careful evaluation of all available radiologic studies and correlation with clinical findings and laboratory data are essential to the accurate diagnosis of chronic interstitial lung disease (Table 15.4). However, the majority of patients with interstitial lung disease will require histologic examination of lung tissue for definitive diagnosis.

Chronic Interstitial Pulmonary Edema

Chronic elevation of pulmonary venous pressure may lead to increased interstitial markings on plain radiographs. The interstitial thickening is caused by distention of pulmonary lymphatics and chronic interstitial edema and is seen most commonly in patients with long-standing mitral stenosis or LV failure. Radiographically, peribronchial cuffing, tram tracking, poor definition of vascular markings, and linear or reticular opacities may be seen. Redistribution of blood flow to the upper lobes, a manifestation of pulmonary venous hypertension, and prominence of the fissures caused by subpleural edema and fibrosis are concomitant findings. Honeycombing is not a feature of chronic pulmonary venous hypertension; its presence in a patient with cardiac disease should suggest another cause of pulmonary fibrosis (e.g., amiodarone lung toxicity).

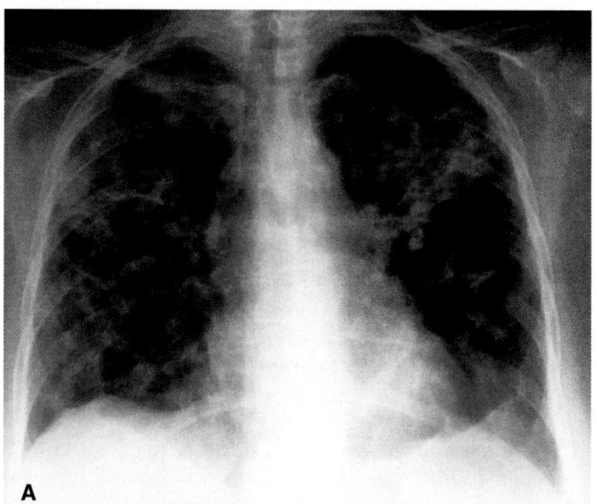

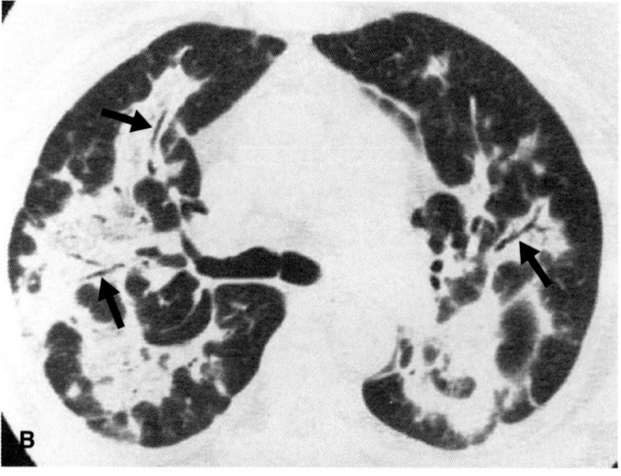

FIGURE 15.13. **Consolidation in Cryptogenic Organizing Pneumonia (COP). A:** Posteroanterior radiograph in a 53-year-old patient with fever, dyspnea, and a dry cough shows patchy consolidation and diminished lung volumes. **B:** Thin-section CT scan shows multifocal areas of consolidation in a peribronchial distribution. Note air bronchograms with mild bronchial dilatation (*arrows*) within the consolidated areas. An open-lung biopsy showed COP.

TABLE 15.4

DIFFERENTIAL DIAGNOSTIC FEATURES IN CHRONIC INTERSTITIAL LUNG DISEASE

■ FINDING	■ DIFFERENTIAL DIAGNOSIS

Upper zone distribution	Tuberculosis (postprimary)
	Chronic fungal infection
	  Histoplasmosis
	  Coccidioidomycosis
	Sarcoidosis
	Langerhans cell histiocytosis
	Silicosis
	Ankylosing spondylitis
	Hypersensitivity pneumonitis (chronic)
	Radiation fibrosis from treatment of head and neck malignancy

Lower zone distribution	Idiopathic pulmonary fibrosis Asbestosis Rheumatoid lung Scleroderma Neurofibromatosis Dermatomyositis/polymyositis Chronic aspiration
Normal or increased lung volumes	Sarcoidosis Langerhans cell histiocytosis Lymphangioleiomyomatosis Tuberous sclerosis Interstitial disease superimposed on emphysema
Honeycombing	Idiopathic pulmonary fibrosis Sarcoidosis Eosinophilic granuloma Rheumatoid lung Scleroderma Pneumoconiosis Hypersensitivity pneumonitis Chronic aspiration Radiation fibrosis

Miliary nodules	Tuberculosis
	Fungi
	  Histoplasmosis
	  Coccidioidomycosis
	  Cryptococcosis
	Silicosis
	Metastases
	  Thyroid carcinoma
	  Renal cell carcinoma
	  Bronchogenic carcinoma
	  Melanoma
	  Choriocarcinoma
	Sarcoidosis
	Langerhans cell histiocytosis

Hilar/mediastinal lymph node enlargement	Sarcoidosis Lymphangitic carcinomatosis Lymphoma Hematogenous metastases Tuberculosis Fungal infection Silicosis
Pleural disease	Asbestosis (plaques) Lymphangitic carcinomatosis (effusion) Rheumatoid lung disease (effusion/thickening) Lymphangioleiomyomatosis (chylous effusion)

Abnormalities of soft tissues and bony thorax	Skin nodules
	  Neurofibromatosis
	Subcutaneous calcifications
	  Dermatomyositis
	  Scleroderma
	Erosion of distal clavicles
	  Rheumatoid lung
	  Scleroderma
	Rib lesions
	Ribbon ribs/erosion of inferior rib margins
	  Neurofibromatosis
	Erosion of superior margins
	  Rheumatoid lung
	  Scleroderma
	Kyphoscoliosis
	  Neurofibromatosis
	Lytic bone lesions
	  Metastases
	  Langerhans cell histiocytosis

Connective Tissue Disease

These disorders are associated with immunologically mediated inflammation and damage to connective tissues throughout the body. The most common thoracic manifestations of this group of heterogeneous disorders are vasculitis and interstitial fibrosis, although the pleura, chest wall, diaphragm, and heart may also be affected.

Rheumatoid Lung Disease (Table 15.5). Rheumatoid arthritis produces a chronic arthritis of peripheral joints. Extra-articular manifestations are seen in up to 75% of patients. In contrast to the disease as a whole, which is more common in women, pulmonary involvement is more common in men. The pleuropulmonary manifestations of rheumatoid disease typically follow the onset of joint disease and tend to be seen in patients with high serum rheumatoid factor titers and eosinophilia, but in up to 15% of patients, pleuropulmonary involvement precedes the joint disease.

The most common radiographic manifestation of parenchymal lung involvement is an interstitial pneumonitis and fibrosis, which histologically is a form of UIP. This begins

TABLE 15.5

MANIFESTATIONS OF RHEUMATOID DISEASE IN THE CHEST

■ MANIFESTATION	■ RADIOGRAPHIC FINDINGS
Serositis	
Pleuritis	Pleural effusion, thickening
Pericarditis	Pericardial effusion
Interstitial pneumonitis (UIP, NSIP)	Pulmonary fibrosis (basilar predominance)
Organizing pneumonia	Patchy peribronchovascular and subpleural consolidation
Necrobiotic nodules	Multiple peripheral cavitating nodules
Caplan syndrome	Multiple peripheral cavitating nodules
Bronchiolitis obliterans	Hyperinflation
Pulmonary arteritis	Pulmonary arterial hypertension and right heart enlargement Pulmonary hemorrhage

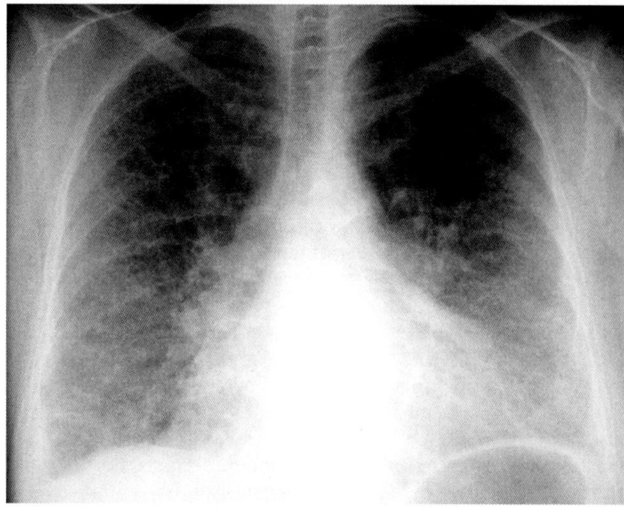

FIGURE 15.14. Honeycombing in Rheumatoid Lung. Posteroanterior radiograph in a patient with end-stage rheumatoid lung disease demonstrates a medium reticular opacity caused by honeycomb cysts. Note the predominant peripheral distribution of disease. Bilateral pleural effusions and cardiac enlargement caused by pericardial effusion are also evident.

as an alveolitis (inflammation of the alveolar interstitium) that is seen radiographically as fine reticular or ground-glass opacities with a lower zone predominance. There is gradual progression to end-stage pulmonary fibrosis with the development of a basilar medium or coarse reticular or reticulonodular pattern (honeycombing) (Fig. 15.14). Thin-section CT is more sensitive in detecting the earliest parenchymal changes than conventional radiographs and is also more sensitive in depicting the development of interstitial fibrosis (Fig. 15.15). Predominant upper lobe fibrosis, cavitation, and bulla formation are rare. This less common pattern of lung involvement is indistinguishable from that seen with ankylosing spondylitis and must be distinguished from postprimary fibrocavitary TB by acid-fast staining of sputum.

Less common parenchymal manifestations of rheumatoid disease are lung nodules (Fig. 15.15) and changes attributable to organizing pneumonia. Necrobiotic (rheumatoid) nodules in the lung can produce peripheral well-defined nodular opacities on chest radiographs that are histologically indistinguishable from the subcutaneous rheumatoid nodules seen on the extensor surfaces of the elbows and knees in these patients. The lung nodules commonly evolve into thick-walled cavities, which tend to wax and wane in parallel with the flares of arthritis. Similar nodules may develop in the lungs of coal miners and silica or asbestos workers with rheumatoid arthritis as a hypersensitivity response to inhaled dust particles (Caplan syndrome). Caplan syndrome is usually indistinguishable radiographically from the necrobiotic nodules of simple rheumatoid disease, although the presence of the associated characteristic small nodular or irregular parenchymal opacities of simple pneumoconiosis helps make this distinction. Organizing pneumonia (OP) and bronchiolitis obliterans (constrictive bronchiolitis) are also associated with rheumatoid disease. The clinical, functional, and

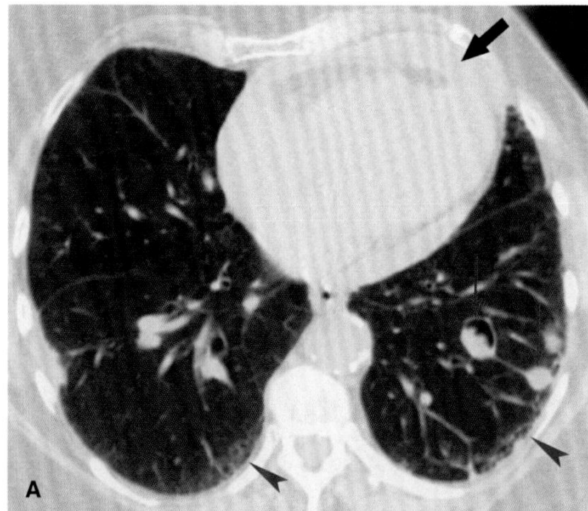

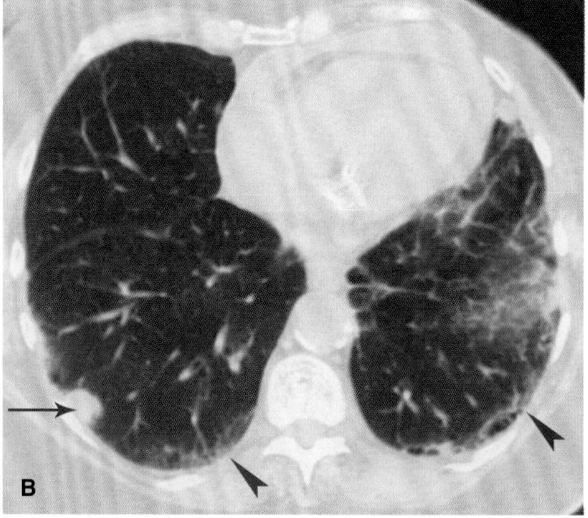

FIGURE 15.15. Rheumatoid Lung Disease and Rheumatoid Nodules. Thin-section axial CT scans through the lung bases in a patient with rheumatoid arthritis asymmetric subpleural reticulation (*blue arrow heads*) reflecting interstitial pneumonitis. Note cavitating and solid bilateral rheumatoid nodules (*red arrows* in **A** and **B**) and pericardial effusion (*black arrow*), additional findings seen in patients with rheumatoid chest disease.

radiographic findings are similar to those of OP or bronchiolitis obliterans associated with systemic lupus erythematosus (SLE), drugs, or viral infection.

Pleuritis is the most common thoracic manifestation of rheumatoid disease and is found in 20% of patients. As with pulmonary involvement, there is a male predilection for pleural disease. Pleural effusions are exudative and have a characteristically low glucose concentration.

Enlargement of the central pulmonary arteries and right heart dilatation may be seen on chest radiographs in patients with pulmonary arterial hypertension. This is an uncommon manifestation of rheumatoid disease that usually develops secondary to diffuse interstitial fibrosis. Rarely, the pulmonary arteries are involved as a part of the systemic vasculitis seen in extra-articular rheumatoid disease. There are no parenchymal abnormalities associated with rheumatoid pulmonary arteritis.

Abnormalities that may be seen in the chest wall of individuals with rheumatoid arthritis include tapered erosion of the distal clavicles, rotator cuff atrophy with a high-riding humeral head, bilateral symmetric glenohumeral joint space narrowing with or without superimposed degenerative joint disease, and superior rib notching or erosion.

Systemic Lupus Erythematosus. This disease of young and middle-aged women typically involves inflammation of multiple organs mediated by auto-antibodies and circulating immune complexes. The thorax is commonly affected and may be the initial site of involvement. The thoracic disease is often limited to the pleura and pericardium, although the lung, heart, diaphragm, and intercostal muscles are involved in as many as one-third of patients. In the pleura and pericardium, a fibrinous serositis produces painful exudative pleural and pericardial effusions. Radiographically, the pleural effusions are small or moderate in size and can be unilateral or bilateral. The effusions usually resolve with corticosteroid therapy. Pleural fibrosis results in diffuse pleural thickening and is present in the majority of patients with long-standing disease.

Pulmonary involvement may take the form of acute lupus pneumonitis or chronic interstitial disease. Acute lupus pneumonitis is characterized by rapid onset of fever, dyspnea, and hypoxemia, and may require mechanical ventilation. These patients have pathologic changes that are indistinguishable from those seen in ARDS, with diffuse alveolar damage (DAD) producing an exudative intra-alveolar edema with hyaline membrane formation. Radiographically, rapidly coalescent bilateral airspace opacities are seen, while the typical thin-section CT finding is one of ground-glass opacity (Fig. 15.16). These findings are difficult to distinguish from those seen in diffuse alveolar hemorrhage associated with pulmonary vasculitis, severe pneumonia related to immunosuppressive therapy,

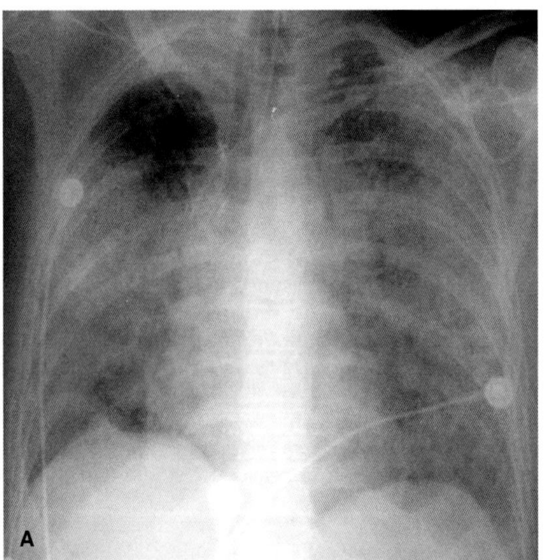

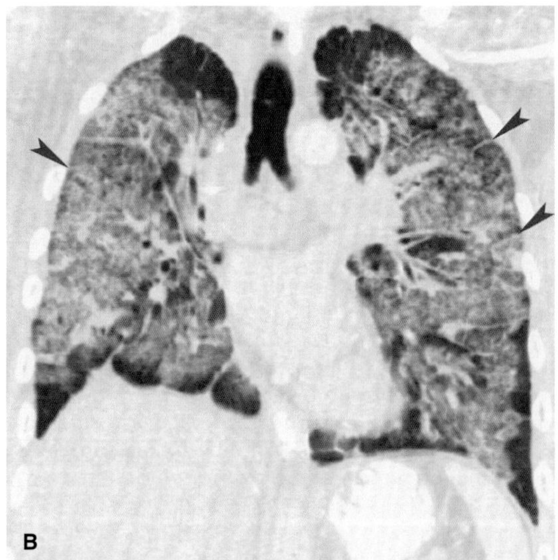

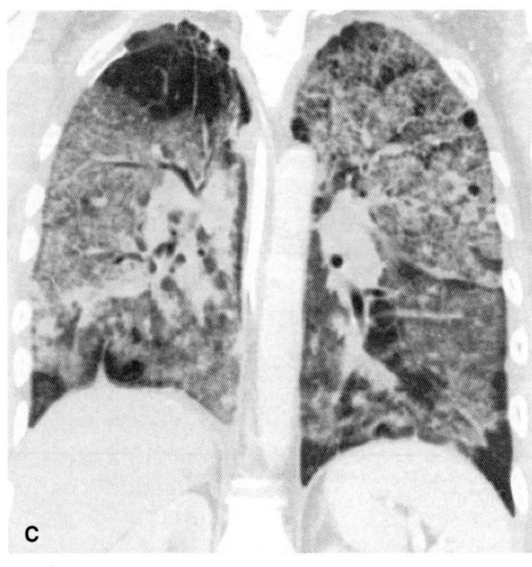

FIGURE 15.16. **Acute Lupus Pneumonitis.** Frontal chest radiograph (**A**) in a 45-year-old woman with lupus and acute respiratory failure shows diffuse bilateral airspace and ground-glass opacities. Coronal CT through the mid (**B**) and posterior (**C**) thorax shows bilateral ground-glass opacities with foci of consolidation and associated interlobular septal thickening (*arrows*); findings seen in diffuse alveolar damage.

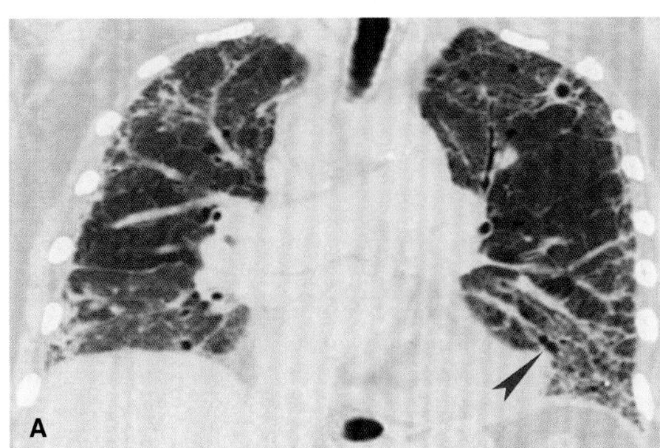

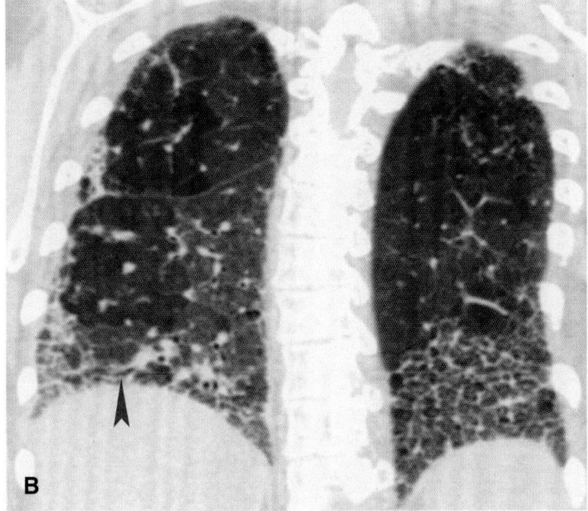

FIGURE 15.17. **Scleroderma With Fibrotic Nonspecific Interstitial Pneumonitis (NSIP).** CT with coronal reformations through the mid (**A**) and posterior (**B**) thorax in a patient with biopsy-proven NSIP complicating scleroderma shows bilateral lower lobe predominant peripheral reticulation and ground-glass opacities, with traction bronchiectasis (*arrowheads*) and minimal honeycomb cyst formation.

or pulmonary edema secondary to renal failure. The diagnosis of acute lupus pneumonitis is made by excluding pneumonia and pulmonary edema and by noting an improvement following the initiation of immunosuppressive therapy.

Radiographic evidence of UIP is distinctly uncommon in SLE, but fibrosis is said to be present pathologically in one-third of patients. When seen radiographically, the pattern is one of basilar reticular opacities that are indistinguishable from those seen in rheumatoid lung disease or scleroderma. Therefore, the presence of severe interstitial fibrosis in a patient with clinical features of SLE should prompt consideration of the diagnosis of an overlap syndrome (mixed connective tissue disease). As with rheumatoid lung disease and scleroderma, thin-section CT is the most sensitive technique for demonstrating early interstitial disease.

Additional chest radiographic findings in SLE include elevation of the hemidiaphragms with decreased lung volumes and resultant basilar areas of linear atelectasis. Diaphragmatic elevation is present in as many as 20% of patients and is the result of diaphragmatic weakness from a primary myopathy unrelated to corticosteroid therapy. Rarely, the central pulmonary arteries are enlarged from pulmonary arterial hypertension secondary to pulmonary vasculitis. Pulmonary embolism with or without infarction may produce peripheral parenchymal opacities and results from deep venous thrombosis that develops in the presence of a circulating lupus anticoagulant. OP has been described in patients with SLE but is indistinguishable clinically and radiographically from lupus pneumonitis, because both conditions produce parenchymal opacities that are responsive to steroids. Superior rib erosions may be present and are indistinguishable from similar findings in rheumatoid arthritis or scleroderma.

Scleroderma (progressive systemic sclerosis) produces inflammation and fibrosis of the skin, esophagus, musculoskeletal system, heart, lungs, and kidneys in young and middle-aged women. The etiology and pathogenesis are unknown. The lungs are involved pathologically in nearly 90% of patients, although only 25% of patients have respiratory symptoms or radiographic evidence of pulmonary involvement. Pulmonary function testing is more sensitive than conventional radiography in the diagnosis of lung disease and shows the typical diminished lung volumes, preserved flow rates, and low diffusing capacity of interstitial pulmonary fibrosis. Pathologically, the parenchymal changes are those of interstitial fibrosis with a pattern of NSIP. Severe pulmonary involvement is reflected radiographically as a coarse reticular or reticulonodular pattern involving the subpleural regions of the lower lobes. The most common thin-section CT findings are ground-glass opacities, reticulation, and eventually traction bronchiectasis in a lower zone, subpleural distribution (Fig. 15.17). Thin-section CT is more sensitive than the chest radiograph in detecting and evaluating interstitial disease. Progressive loss of lung volume is seen with advancing pulmonary fibrosis. The development of large (1 to 5 cm) subpleural lower lobe cysts may lead to spontaneous pneumothorax.

Pulmonary arterial hypertension with enlarged central pulmonary arteries and RV dilatation is seen in up to 50% of patients with scleroderma and may be seen in the absence of interstitial fibrosis. In these patients, thickening and obliteration of small muscular pulmonary arteries and arterioles are responsible for the development of pulmonary arterial hypertension. Pleural effusions are significantly less common in scleroderma than in rheumatoid disease or SLE and may be a helpful distinguishing feature. Pleural thickening is more often attributable to extension of pulmonary interstitial fibrosis into the interstitial layer of the pleura than to pleuritis.

Several additional chest radiographic findings may be seen in patients with scleroderma. Eggshell calcification of mediastinal lymph nodes has been reported, although it is more common in silicosis and sarcoidosis. A dilated air-filled esophagus may be identified on the upright chest radiograph and is a manifestation of esophageal dysmotility from smooth muscle atrophy and fibrosis. An air–fluid level within a dilated esophagus suggests secondary distal esophageal stricture formation from chronic reflux esophagitis. Functional or anatomic esophageal obstruction may result in aspiration with the development of lower lobe pneumonia. Because patients with scleroderma are at a greater risk for developing lung cancer, particularly bronchioloalveolar cell carcinoma, the appearance of a mass or persistent airspace opacity should raise this possibility. Patients with the subcutaneous calcification, Raynaud phenomenon, esophageal dysmotility, sclerodactyly, and telangiectasia (CREST) syndrome, a variant of scleroderma, may have radiographically visible calcifications within the subcutaneous tissues of the chest wall. Superior rib notching or erosion may also be seen.

Dermatomyositis and polymyositis involve autoimmune inflammation and destruction of skeletal muscle, producing

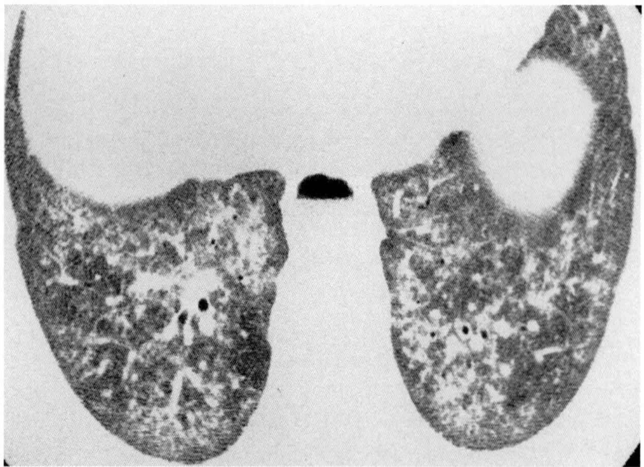

FIGURE 15.18. Polymyositis. Thin-section CT through the lung bases shows reticulation and ill-defined centrilobular nodules, likely reflecting interstitial pneumonitis and organizing pneumonia, respectively in a patient with polymyositis.

proximal muscle pain and weakness (polymyositis) and occasionally associated with a skin rash (dermatomyositis). The thoracic manifestations of these diseases include respiratory and pharyngeal muscle weakness. Interstitial pneumonitis is seen in 5% to 10% of patients and is indistinguishable from that associated with rheumatoid lung disease, SLE, scleroderma, or IPF. A fine reticular interstitial pattern in acute disease leads to a chronic, coarse reticular or reticulonodular process that is predominantly basilar in distribution. Most patients with polymyositis and interstitial lung disease have clinical manifestations of rheumatoid arthritis or scleroderma, and these patients tend to respond favorably to corticosteroids. As with scleroderma, the early parenchymal changes may be subradiographic but can be demonstrated on thin-section CT studies through the lower lobes. Airspace consolidation and ground-glass opacity represent organizing pneumonia and DAD, respectively (Fig. 15.18). Additional chest radiographic findings in polymyositis reflect the involvement of skeletal muscle. Small lung volumes with diaphragmatic elevation and basilar linear atelectasis are secondary to diaphragmatic and intercostal muscle involvement. Pharyngeal and upper esophageal muscle weaknesses predispose to aspiration pneumonia. The chest radiograph should be examined carefully for lung masses because bronchogenic carcinoma accounts for a significant percentage of the malignancies seen with a higher-than-normal frequency in patients with dermatomyositis or polymyositis.

Sjögren Syndrome. This autoimmune disorder of middle-aged women is characterized by the sicca syndrome (dry eyes [keratoconjunctivitis sicca], dry mouth [xerostomia], and dry nose [xerorhinia]) which results from lymphocytic infiltration of the lacrimal, salivary, and mucous glands, respectively. Most patients with the sicca syndrome have associated manifestations of other collagen vascular diseases, such as rheumatoid arthritis, scleroderma, or SLE.

The chest is involved in approximately one-third of patients with Sjögren syndrome with or without associated collagen vascular disease. The most common manifestation is interstitial fibrosis, which is indistinguishable from that seen with other collagen vascular disorders. Involvement of tracheobronchial mucous glands leads to thickened sputum with mucus plugging and recurrent bronchitis, bronchiectasis, atelectasis, and pneumonia. Thin-section CT demonstrates both interstitial opacities and the presence of small airways involvement with bronchiolectasis and a "tree-in-bud" appearance. Pleuritis and pleural effusion are less common.

Patients with Sjögren syndrome are at increased risk for developing lymphocytic interstitial pneumonitis (LIP) and non-Hodgkin pulmonary lymphoma. The radiographic appearance of LIP is lower lobe coarse reticular or reticulonodular opacities that are indistinguishable from interstitial fibrosis. Thin-section CT shows ground-glass opacity with scattered, thin-walled cysts. The development of lymphoma in these patients should be suspected when nodular or alveolar opacities develop in the lung in association with mediastinal lymph node enlargement.

Ankylosing Spondylitis. Approximately 1% to 2% of individuals with ankylosing spondylitis develop pulmonary disease in the form of upper lobe pulmonary fibrosis. The fibrotic changes are commonly associated with the development of bullae and cavities, which are prone to mycetoma formation with *Aspergillus*. The diagnosis should be suspected in a young to middle-aged man with characteristic spine changes (kyphosis and spinal ankylosis) who has abnormally increased lung volumes and upper lobe fibrobullous disease, the latter of which simulates postprimary fibrocavitary TB.

Overlap Syndromes and Mixed Connective Tissue Disease. Some patients with collagen vascular disease have features of more than one of the recognized syndromes discussed above. These patients are classified as having an overlap syndrome with thoracic manifestations characteristic of the other disorders. Patients with a distinct form of overlap syndrome, called *mixed connective tissue disease*, have clinical features of SLE, scleroderma and polymyositis, and have serum antibodies to extractable nuclear antigen. The thoracic manifestations of mixed connective tissue disease include UIP, pulmonary arterial hypertension caused by plexogenic pulmonary arteriopathy, and pleural effusion and thickening from a fibrinous pleuritis like that found in patients with SLE.

Interstitial Pneumonia With Autoimmune Features. The development of interstitial fibrosis is a relatively common occurrence in patients with an established autoimmune disorder such as rheumatoid arthritis, scleroderma, mixed connective tissue disease, and systemic lupus. There is a group of patients, however, in whom interstitial pneumonia is the first and perhaps only clinical manifestation of autoimmune disease, but who do not meet criteria for a specific autoimmune disorder. These individuals have suggestive but inconclusive clinical or laboratory evidence of an underlying autoimmune disorder. In the past, this category has been given a number of names including undifferentiated connective tissue disease-associated ILD, lung-dominant connective tissue disease and autoimmune-featured ILD.

Idiopathic Chronic Interstitial Pneumonias

The idiopathic interstitial pneumonias (IIPs) are characterized by an inflammatory process in the lung that can result in pulmonary fibrosis. In 2013, a joint task force of the American Thoracic Society and European Respiratory Society updated the classification of the idiopathic pneumonias and regrouped them into five categories (Table 15.6): chronic fibrosing IIP, smoking-related IIP, acute or subacute IIP, rare IIP, and unclassifiable IIP. These disorders are most accurately characterized by their histologic appearance. Unfortunately, confusion arises when clinical terms are used interchangeably with the aforementioned histologic terms in describing these disorders. When possible (when the histology is known), it is most accurate to use the histologic term to describe a particular disorder, while reserving clinical terms such as *IPF* or *rheumatoid lung* for interstitial disease associated with specific clinical diseases for which histology is unavailable.

TABLE 15.6

ATS/ERS CLASSIFICATION OF IDIOPATHIC INTERSTITIAL PNEUMONIAS

Chronic fibrotic IIP	Idiopathic pulmonary fibrosis Nonspecific interstitial pneumonia
Smoking-related IIP	Respiratory bronchiolitis–associated interstitial lung disease Desquamative interstitial pneumonia
Acute or subacute IIP	Bronchiolitis obliterans–organizing pneumonia/cryptogenic organizing pneumonia Acute interstitial pneumonia Acute exacerbation of IIP
Rare IIP	Lymphocytic interstitial pneumonia Idiopathic pleuroparenchymal fibroelastosis
Unclassifiable IIP	

Chronic Fibrosing Idiopathic Interstitial Pneumonias

Usual Interstitial Pneumonia. UIP is the most common of the IIPs and is the pattern associated with IPF. It is likely the result of repetitive injury to the lung. The initial response in the lung is inflammation, which is followed by repair and eventually fibrosis. The pathologic abnormalities seen in UIP represent a spectrum of findings, characterized in the early stage of disease by marked proliferation of macrophages in the alveolar airspaces associated with a mild and uniform thickening of the interstitium by mononuclear cells. Late in the course of disease, the pathologic findings are characterized by thickening of the alveolar interstitium by mononuclear inflammatory cells and fibrous tissue. A distinguishing histologic feature of UIP is that different stages of the disease are seen simultaneously within different portions of the lung (temporal heterogeneity).

Patients with UIP typically present in the fifth to seventh decades, with a slight male preponderance. Presenting symptoms include progressive dyspnea or a nonproductive cough. Pulmonary function tests show restrictive disease and a decreased diffusing capacity of the lungs for carbon monoxide (DLCO). Most cases of UIP are idiopathic, but up to 30% of patients with UIP have an associated collagen vascular or immunologic disorder. This is most often rheumatoid arthritis, but it can also be SLE, scleroderma, or dermatomyositis/polymyositis. The criteria for the CT diagnosis of UIP as recommended by the Fleischner Society are listed in Table 15.7.

The radiographic manifestations of UIP parallel the pathologic changes. The earliest radiographic changes are basilar fine to medium reticular opacities or ground-glass densities (Fig. 15.19A). As the disease progresses, a coarse reticular or reticulonodular pattern is seen, which almost invariably leads to the formation of honeycomb cysts (3 to 10 mm in diameter) and progressive loss of lung volume (Figs. 15.8 and 15.12). Extensive pulmonary fibrosis may be associated with findings of pulmonary arterial hypertension. Upper lobe bullae may be seen and predispose to the development of spontaneous pneumothorax. Hilar lymph node enlargement and pleural effusions have been described but are rare and should suggest an alternative diagnosis.

Thin-section CT findings in UIP differ with the stage of the disease and vary from one lung region to another. As fibrosis develops, findings include irregular septal or subpleural thickening (in contrast to the smooth septal thickening seen with edema or lymphangitic spread of carcinoma), intralobular lines, irregular interfaces, honeycombing, and traction bronchiectasis (Figs. 15.12 and 15.19B). The changes are typically most severe in the peripheral and basal portions of the lungs, which can be helpful in differential diagnosis. Mildly enlarged mediastinal lymph nodes are often seen.

In most patients with IPF, the disease progresses inexorably, with an overall mean survival of <5 years. Previously, there was no effective treatment for IPF, but two new drugs, nintedanib and pirfenidone, have been approved by the FDA. Neither is curative, but both appear to slow progression of disease by inhibiting scar formation. There is an increased incidence of lung cancer in patients with IPF, with adenocarcinoma the most common histologic subtype. For this reason,

TABLE 15.7

CT CRITERIA FOR DIAGNOSIS OF USUAL INTERSTITIAL PNEUMONIA/IDIOPATHIC PULMONARY FIBROSIS

	■ TYPICAL UIP CT PATTERN	■ PROBABLE CT UIP PATTERN	■ CT PATTERN INDETERMINATE FOR UIP	■ CT FEATURES MOST CONSISTENT WITH NON-IPF DIAGNOSIS
Distribution	Basal predominant (occasionally diffuse), and subpleural predominant; distribution is often heterogeneous	Basal and subpleural predominant; distribution is often heterogeneous	Variable or diffuse	Upper or mid-lung predominant fibrosis; peribronchovascular predominance with subpleural sparing
Features	Honeycombing; reticular pattern with peripheral traction bronchiectasis or bronchiolectasis; absence of features to suggest an alternative diagnosis	Reticular pattern with peripheral traction bronchiectasis or bronchiolectasis; honeycombing is absent; absence of features to suggest an alternative diagnosis	Evidence of fibrosis with some inconspicuous features suggestive of non-UIP pattern	Any of the following: predominant consolidation, extensive pure ground-glass opacity (without acute exacerbation). Extensive mosaic attenuation with extensive sharply defined lobular air trapping on expiration, diffuse nodules or cysts

From Lynch DA, Sverzellati N, Travis WD, et al. Diagnostic criteria for idiopathic pulmonary fibrosis: a Fleischner Society White Paper. *Lancet Respir Med* 2018;6(2):138–153.

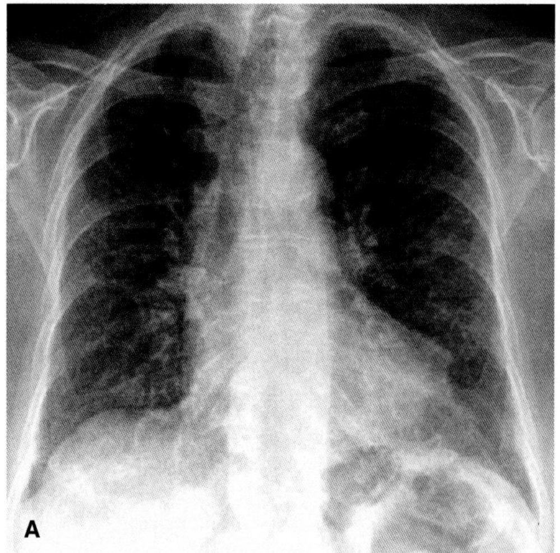

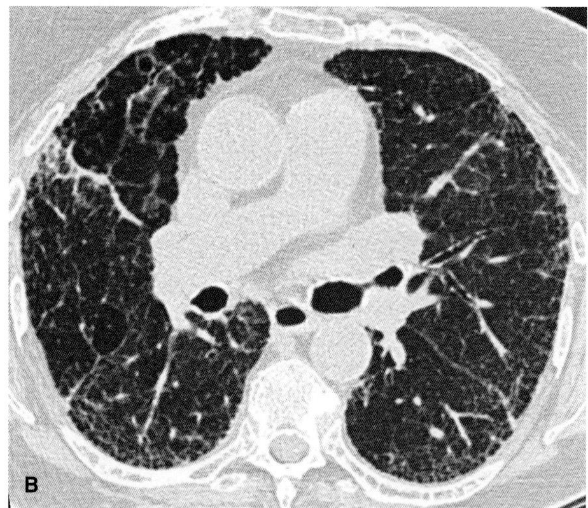

FIGURE 15.19. **Usual Interstitial Pneumonia (UIP). A:** Posteroanterior radiograph in a patient with UIP demonstrates bilateral coarse reticular opacities. **B:** A thin-section CT through the mid-lungs shows peripheral reticulation.

it is probably not advisable to follow these patients with traditional HRCT technique (thin sections every centimeter) as the majority of the lung is not imaged and cancers may not be detected in a timely manner.

Nonspecific Interstitial Pneumonitis. NSIP is a recently introduced term used to describe interstitial pneumonias that cannot be otherwise classified as UIP, AIP, COP, RB-ILD, or DIP. Many cases of NSIP are seen in association with collagen vascular disease or as drug reactions. The pathologic changes are temporally homogeneous, as compared to UIP, which is typically heterogeneous. Pathologists generally divide NSIP into cellular and fibrotic forms of disease, with correlative findings on thin-section CT. Those with cellular NSIP show areas of ground-glass and consolidation on thin-section CT in a peripheral and lower zone distribution (Fig. 15.20). Bronchial dilatation and linear opacities are more typical of the fibrotic form of NSIP (Fig. 15.17), but in distinction to UIP, honeycombing is rare. While cellular NSIP is usually responsive to steroids, fibrotic NSIP has a poor prognosis, similar to that of UIP.

Smoking-Related Idiopathic Interstitial Pneumonias

Respiratory Bronchiolitis–Associated Interstitial Lung Disease. RB-ILD is a disorder seen only in cigarette smokers and characterized by inflammation within and around the respiratory bronchioles. The histology of RB-ILD overlaps with that of DIP, and some authors have suggested that RB-ILD is an early form of DIP. Patients with RB-ILD are typically young, heavy smokers with mild cough and dyspnea. Pulmonary function tests show restrictive or mixed restrictive–obstructive patterns. Symptoms respond to smoking cessation or steroid therapy, and there is no progression to end-stage fibrosis.

The chest radiograph is normal in up to 21% of cases of RB-ILD, but diffuse linear and nodular opacities and basilar atelectasis are often seen. The most common thin-section CT findings are scattered ground-glass opacities and small centrilobular nodules, often with an upper lobe-predominant distribution (Fig. 15.21). Linear opacities are rare and honeycombing is not seen. Emphysema is often a concomitant finding.

Desquamative Interstitial Pneumonia. DIP is a disorder characterized by the accumulation of macrophages within alveolar spaces. Ninety percent of patients with DIP are cigarette smokers.

The typical radiographic findings in DIP are basilar reticular opacities with normal or minimally diminished lung volumes. Ground-glass opacities are seen in only 33% of cases, while honeycombing is rare. Up to 22% of patients have a normal chest radiograph. Thin-section CT shows ground-glass opacities, most often within the peripheral aspects of the bases (Fig. 15.22). Irregular linear opacities, honeycombing, and traction bronchiectasis can be seen but are much less common than in UIP. Ground-glass abnormalities often improve or completely resolve with corticosteroid therapy.

Acute or Subacute Idiopathic Interstitial Pneumonias

Organizing Pneumonia/Cryptogenic Organizing Pneumonia. OP refers to a disorder characterized by the widespread deposition of granulation tissue (fibroblasts, collagen, and capillaries) within peribronchiolar airspaces and bronchioles. Most cases of organizing pneumonia are idiopathic and properly referred to as COP. A number of conditions have been associated with this disorder in which case it is usually referred to as OP. These include viral infection (influenza, adenovirus, and measles); toxic fume inhalation (sulfur dioxide and chlorine); collagen vascular disease (rheumatoid arthritis and SLE); organ transplantation (bone marrow, lung, and heart–lung); drug reactions; and chronic aspiration.

Patients with COP often have a subacute illness, with several months' history of nonproductive cough and dyspnea. The physical examination may reveal rales or wheezes. Pulmonary function tests usually show a restrictive pattern of disease with diminished lung volumes and normal to increased flow rates. The DLCO is significantly decreased. Pathologically, a mononuclear cell exudate in the bronchioles and surrounding alveoli organizes to form intrabronchiolar and intra-alveolar granulation tissue. A characteristic of this disease is the uniformity of the histologic changes and the absence of parenchymal distortion and fibrosis; these features help distinguish COP from UIP, which can have similar clinical, functional, and radiographic features.

Radiographs in patients with COP reveal patchy bilateral airspace or ground-glass opacities (Fig. 15.13A), with

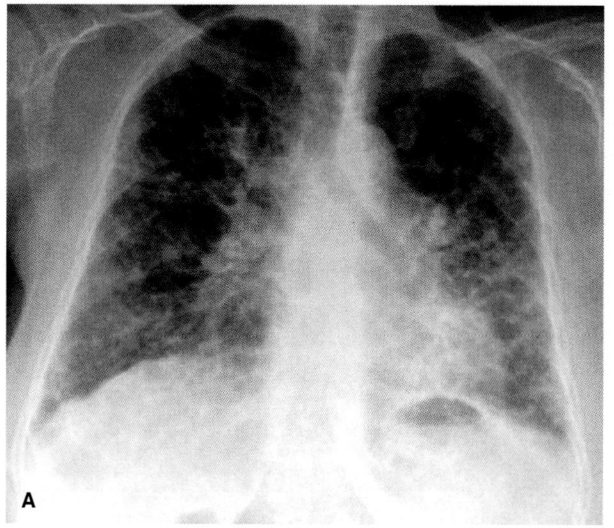

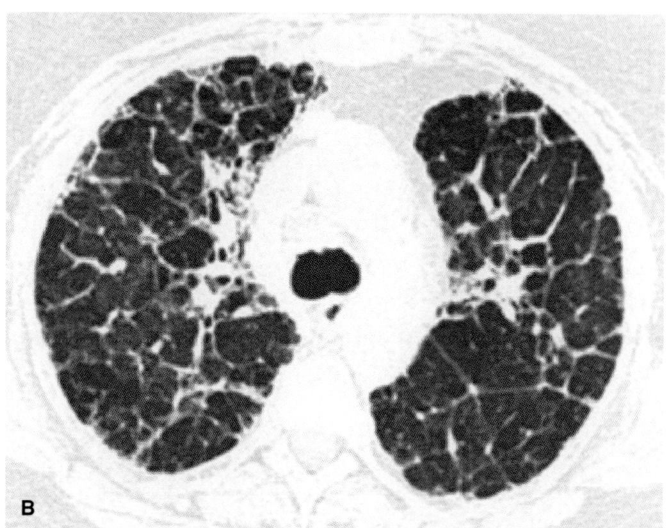

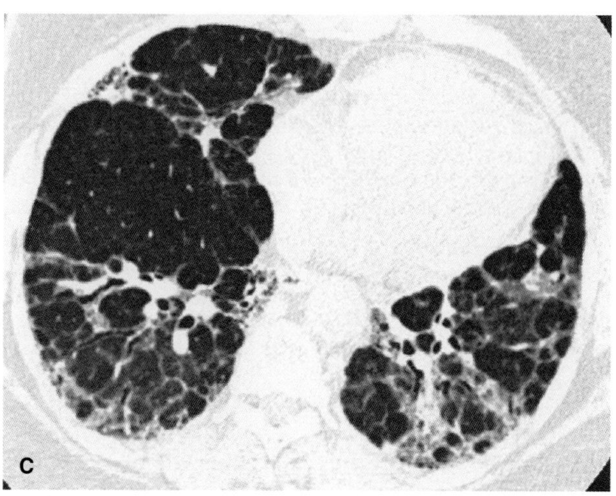

FIGURE 15.20. **Nonspecific Interstitial Pneumonia (NSIP). A:** Frontal chest radiograph demonstrates coarse interstitial markings throughout both lungs. **B:** Thin-section CT scans at the level of the carina demonstrate thickened interlobular septa with medial upper lobe traction bronchiectasis. **C:** Thin-section CT through the lung bases shows traction bronchiectasis, minimal honeycombing, and ground-glass opacities. Open-lung biopsy demonstrated NSIP.

scattered nodular opacities in some patients. The most common thin-section CT findings are patchy consolidation or ground-glass opacity with either a subpleural or peribronchial pattern of distribution (Fig. 15.13B). More recently, a thin-section CT finding of patchy ground-glass opacities surrounded by crescentic regions of more dense consolidation, termed the so-called "reversed halo" sign, has been described in patients with COP that while not specific should suggest the diagnosis (Fig. 15.23). Small ill-defined peribronchial nodules are seen less commonly. Bronchiectasis and bronchial wall thickening are commonly seen in the involved areas of lung.

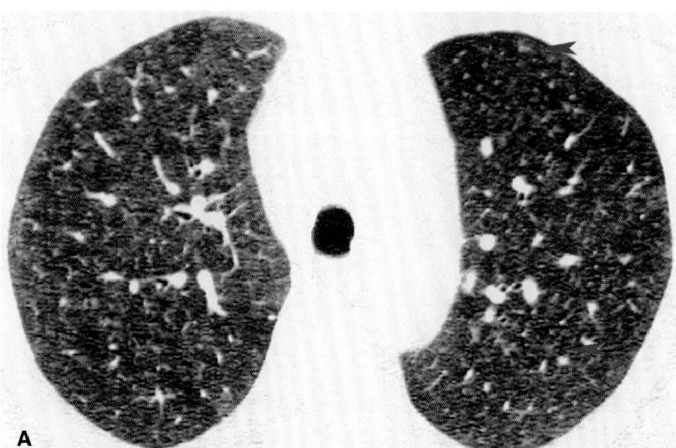

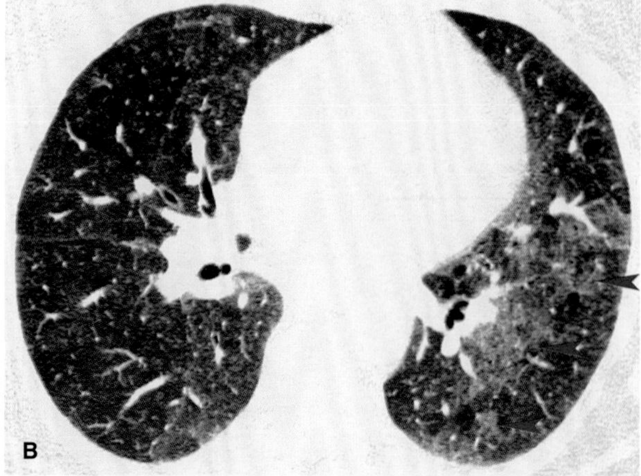

FIGURE 15.21. **Respiratory Bronchiolitis–Associated Interstitial Lung Disease (RB-ILD).** Thin-section CT scans through the upper lobes (**A**) and lower lobes (**B**) in a patient with biopsy-proven RB-ILD demonstrate bilateral centrilobular (*arrowheads*) and geographic regions of ground-glass opacity.

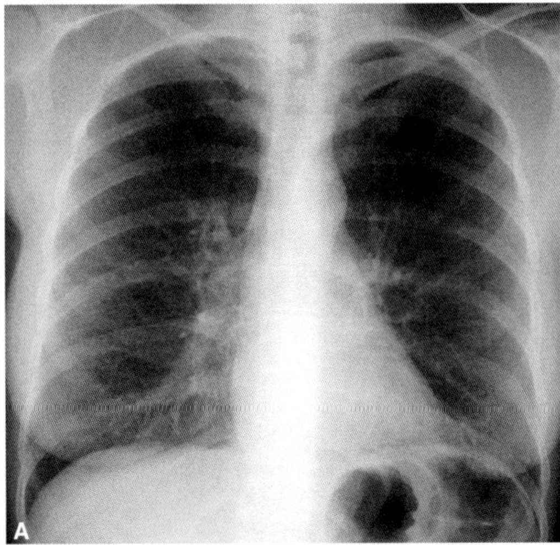

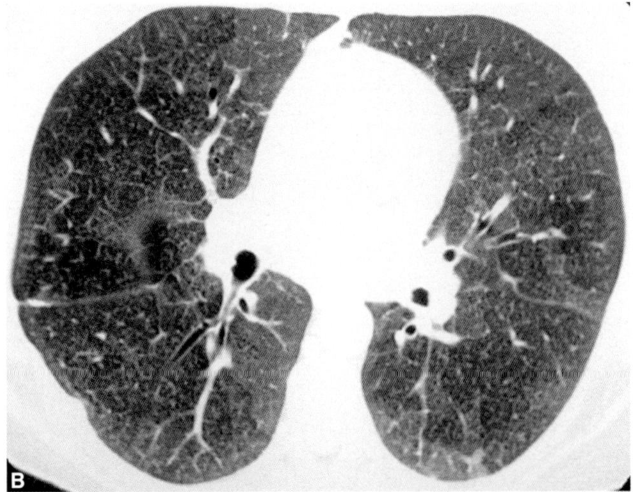

FIGURE 15.22. Desquamative Interstitial Pneumonia (DIP). Chest radiograph (**A**) and thin-section CT (**B**) show fine reticular or ground-glass opacities in a smoker with DIP.

The diagnosis of COP is made by recognizing the characteristic CT findings or based on the histologic changes on open-lung biopsy.

Acute Interstitial Pneumonia. Also known as the Hamman–Rich syndrome, AIP is an acute, aggressive form of idiopathic interstitial pneumonitis and fibrosis. Patients with AIP typically present with a brief history of cough, fever, and dyspnea that progress rapidly to severe hypoxemia and respiratory failure requiring mechanical ventilation. The pathologic manifestations of AIP are those of ARDS, and the disease has been termed *idiopathic ARDS*. The histologic findings are those of DAD with minimal mature collagen deposition. A characteristic of the process is that it is diffuse and temporally homogeneous. Chest radiographs and thin-section CT scans show findings of ARDS, with diffuse ground-glass opacity and consolidation with air bronchograms (Fig. 15.24). On CT, there is often a gradient of increasing density from anterior to posterior lung. Linear opacities, honeycombing, and traction bronchiectasis are uncommon. As in other forms of ARDS, the mortality rate ranges from 60% to 90%. Fibrosis can develop but tends to stabilize and does not progress beyond the recovery phase.

Acute Exacerbation of Interstitial Pneumonia. Acute worsening of chronic interstitial pneumonia (also referred to as accelerated phase of interstitial pneumonia) results from DAD, can result in acute respiratory failure, and occurs most commonly in patients with IPF. CT demonstrates extensive and usually rapidly progressive ground glass and sometimes consolidation superimposed on the underlying fibrosis (Fig. 15.25). Acute exacerbation should be considered in any patient with IPF who presents with acute respiratory failure and new parenchymal opacities, but it is important to first exclude more common causes of pulmonary opacities such as infection and hydrostatic pulmonary edema before making the diagnosis.

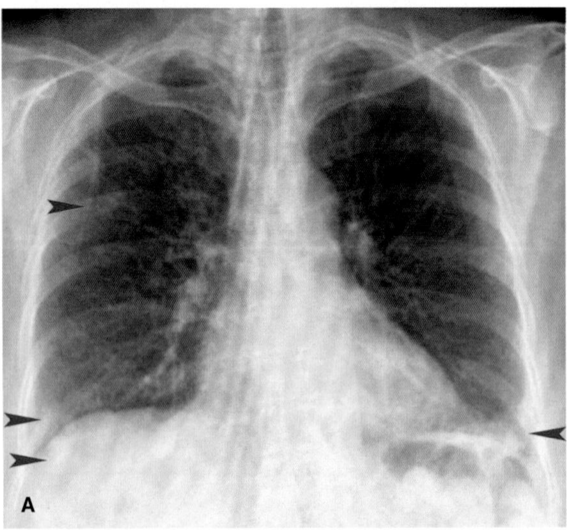

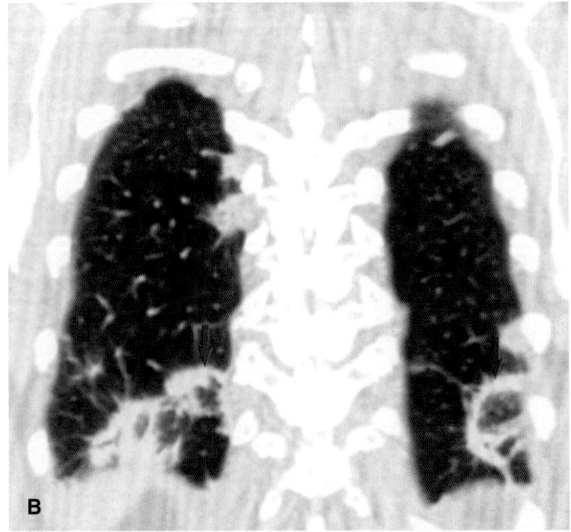

FIGURE 15.23. "Reversed Halo" Sign in Cryptogenic Organizing Pneumonia (COP). Frontal chest radiograph (**A**) in a 53-year-old woman with dry cough and shortness of breath shows ill-defined densities in the peripheral right lung and both lung bases (*arrowheads*). CT with coronal reformation (**B**) shows bilateral, lower zone predominant peripheral mass-like opacities, several of which demonstrate dense peripheral consolidation or a reversed halo sign (*arrows*). Diagnosis was by open-lung biopsy.

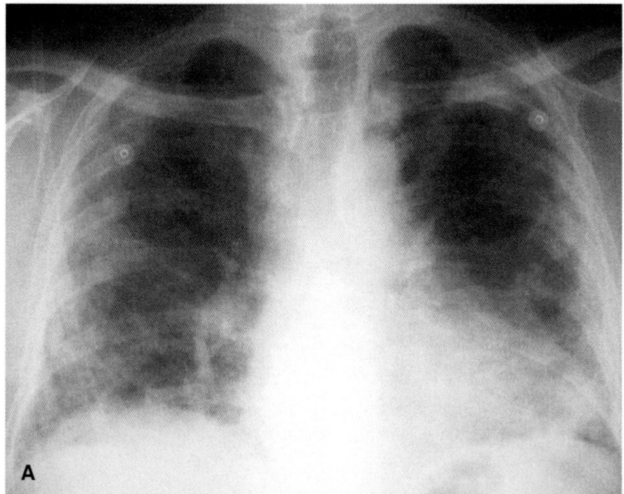

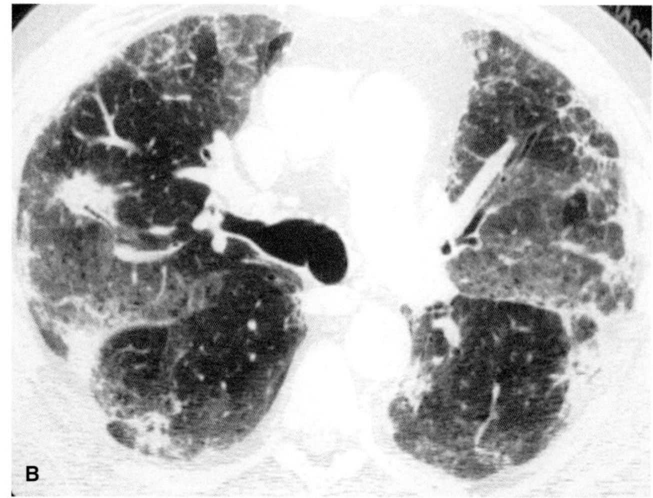

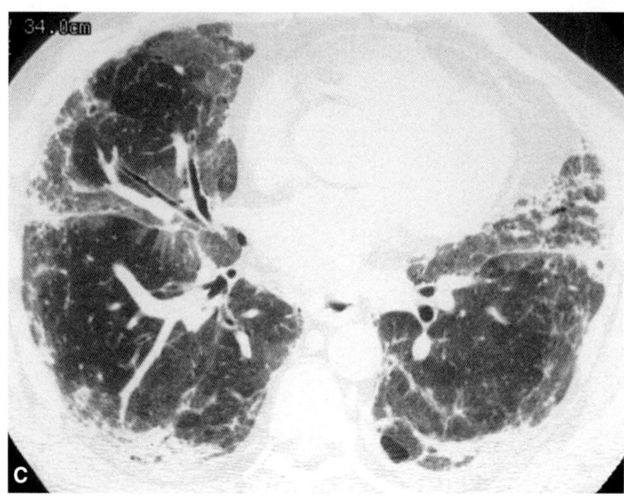

FIGURE 15.24. **Acute Interstitial Pneumonia (Hamman–Rich Syndrome).** Frontal radiograph (**A**) in a patient with biopsy-proven acute interstitial pneumonia demonstrates peripheral airspace and ground-glass opacity. CT scans through the upper lobe bronchus (**B**) and lower lungs (**C**) show predominantly peripheral ground-glass and reticular opacities with scattered airspace opacities.

Rare Idiopathic Interstitial Pneumonias

Lymphocytic interstitial pneumonia is discussed in Chapter 13 (Pulmonary Neoplasms).

Pleuroparenchymal fibroelastosis (PPFE) is a rare, potentially fatal disease characterized by elastic tissue-rich fibrosis involving the pleura and adjacent lung parenchyma. While most cases are idiopathic, patients who have received radiation or chemotherapy, and bone marrow and lung transplant recipients may be at particular risk. Typically, the upper lung zones are most severely involved. CT scans demonstrate (Fig. 15.26) irregular pleural thickening, upper lobe volume loss, architectural distortion, and traction bronchiectasis. Mid- and lower zone involvement is relatively common, but tends to look more like NSIP. On occasion, PPFE can be mimicked by sarcoidosis, ankylosing spondylitis-associated fibrosis, and chronic hypersensitivity pneumonitis; although with the occasional exception of chronic hypersensitivity pneumonitis, these do not usually have as extensive pleural involvement.

Unclassifiable Idiopathic Interstitial Pneumonia

In some cases of IIP, the clinical, pathologic, and imaging findings do not allow for a specific diagnosis. A common cause of this is the unavailability of histopathology because of the high risk of open-lung biopsy. It is common to find a CT pattern of probable or definite UIP in these patients. Regardless of whether a definitive diagnosis is made, those patients with fibrosis have a poor prognosis. Management may be guided by disease behavior.

Other Chronic Interstitial Lung Diseases

Neurofibromatosis (NF) is an autosomal-dominant neurocutaneous syndrome, which is divided into two types: type 1, or von Recklinghausen disease, and type 2. The classic manifestations of NF1 are cutaneous café-au-lait spots and neurofibromas of cutaneous and subcutaneous peripheral nerves and nerve roots. In addition, there is often involvement of the skeletal, vascular, and pulmonary systems. The condition is also associated with a variety of neoplasms, including meningiomas, optic gliomas, neurofibrosarcomas, and pheochromocytomas.

There are several thoracic manifestations of NF1. Cutaneous and subcutaneous neurofibromas may be seen along the chest wall or projecting over the lungs. The spine may show a kyphoscoliosis, with scalloping of the posterior aspect of the vertebral bodies caused by dural ectasia. "Ribbon rib" deformities and rib notching may be seen. Mediastinal masses in patients with NF1 include neurofibromas, lateral thoracic meningoceles, and extra-adrenal pheochromocytomas.

Parenchymal lung disease is seen in approximately 20% of patients with NF1. The findings include diffuse interstitial fibrosis and bulla formation. The interstitial fibrosis is predominantly lower zonal and bilaterally symmetric. Bullae usually develop

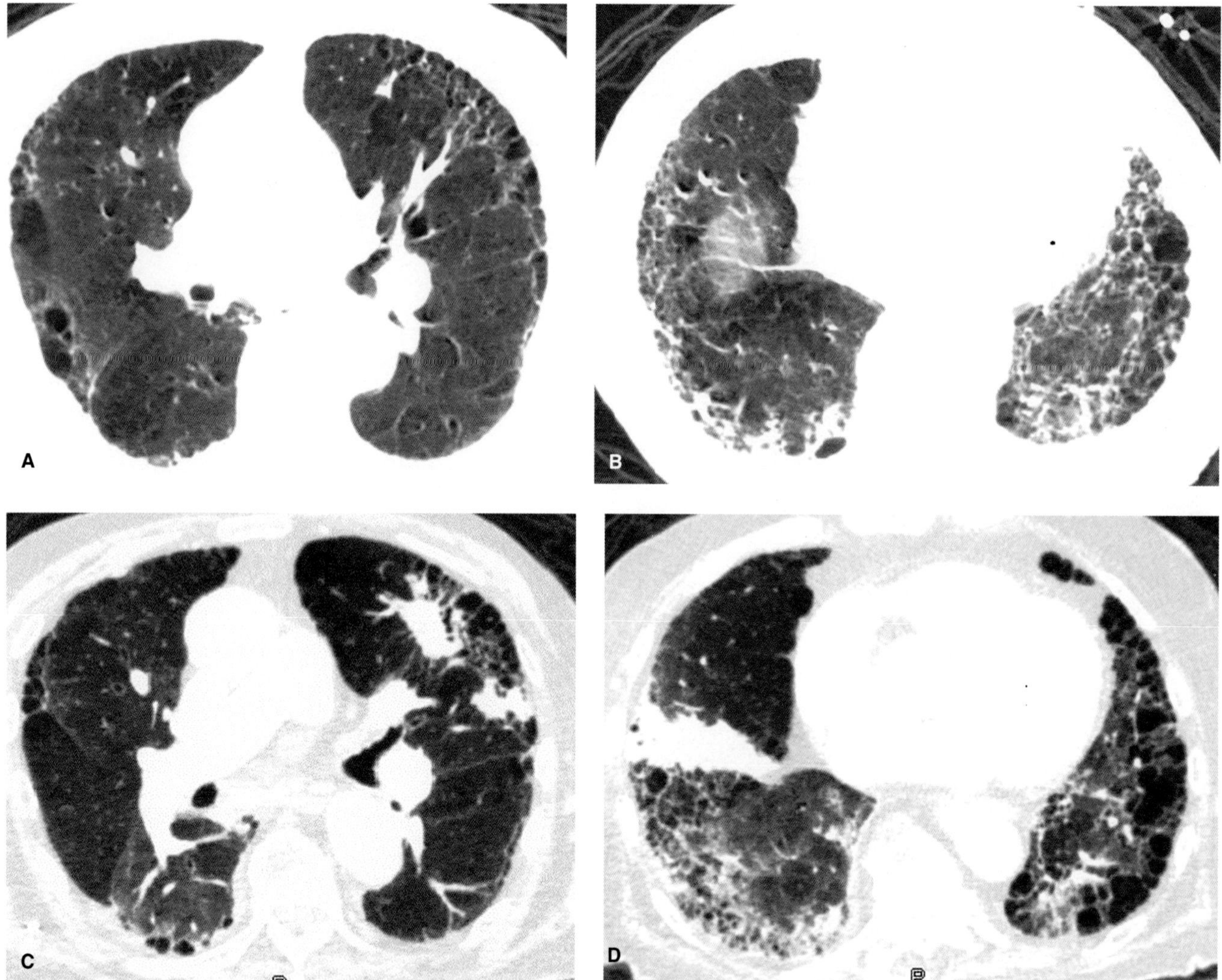

FIGURE 15.25. **Acute Exacerbation of Interstitial Lung Disease. A, B:** Axial CT scans at the mid-lung and base from 2012 demonstrate interstitial thickening, architectural distortion, and honeycomb cysts in a patient with IPF and rapid respiratory decompensation. **C, D:** CT scan performed in 2015 demonstrates worsening of fibrosis and new areas of consolidation in both lungs. The appearance is indistinguishable from pneumonia, but there was no clinical or bronchoscopic evidence of infection.

in the upper zones, with asymmetric involvement of the lungs. Pulmonary symptoms are usually minimal or absent, with pulmonary function tests showing a mixed obstructive/restrictive pattern. A small number of patients will develop respiratory failure caused by pulmonary fibrosis, with secondary development of pulmonary arterial hypertension and cor pulmonale.

Tuberous Sclerosis (TS). TS is an autosomal-dominant neurocutaneous syndrome with variable expression. The classical clinical triad of TS is seizures, mental retardation, and adenoma sebaceum. Additional manifestations include intracranial calcifications, cerebral cortical and periventricular hamartomas, renal angiomyolipomas, cardiac rhabdomyomas, retinal phakomas, and sclerotic bone lesions.

Pulmonary involvement in TS is rare and is seen in approximately 1% of cases. Patients with pulmonary TS tend to be older and have a lower incidence of seizures and mental retardation. The pulmonary involvement is indistinguishable clinically, pathologically, and radiographically from that seen in LAM. Pathologically, there is smooth muscle proliferation in the peribronchovascular and parenchymal interstitium of the lung. Small adenomatoid nodules measuring several millimeters in diameter may be seen scattered throughout the lungs.

Radiographically, there are symmetric bilateral reticular or reticulonodular opacities. In the later stages of disease, a pattern of coarse reticular or small cystic opacities may be seen. The cysts are uniform in size and <1 cm in diameter. Thin-section CT is best at depicting the presence of thin-walled pulmonary cysts and can help detect associated extrapulmonary abnormalities, including renal angiomyolipomas and periventricular tubers. A helpful feature in distinguishing TS from other chronic interstitial lung diseases is the normal to increased lung volumes in patients with TS caused by small airways obstruction and expiratory air trapping. In distinction to LCH and sarcoidosis, which have a predominant upper zone distribution of disease, pulmonary TS tends to affect the entire lung uniformly. Pneumothorax is common and results from the rupture of a subpleural cyst. Pleural effusions are uncommon. The pulmonary involvement often leads to pulmonary arterial hypertension and cor pulmonale, which are associated with high mortality.

Lymphangioleiomyomatosis. LAM is an uncommon condition that is seen exclusively in women. The average age at diagnosis is 43 years. Although LAM shares many features with pulmonary TS, it is not an inherited condition and lacks the extrapulmonary features of TS.

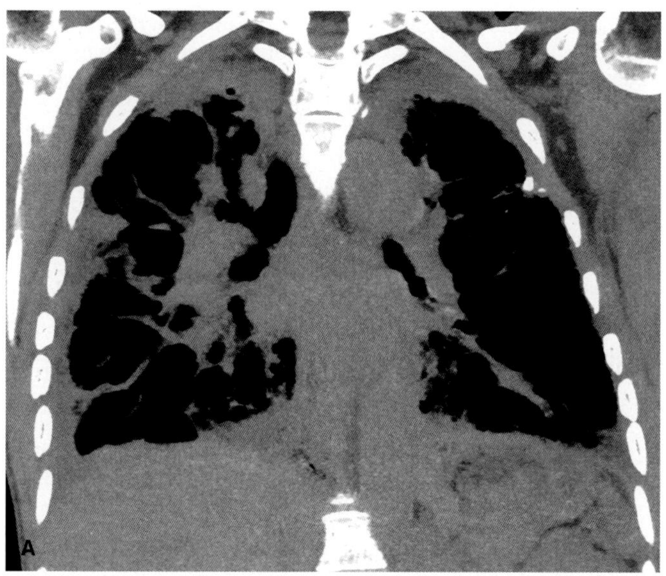

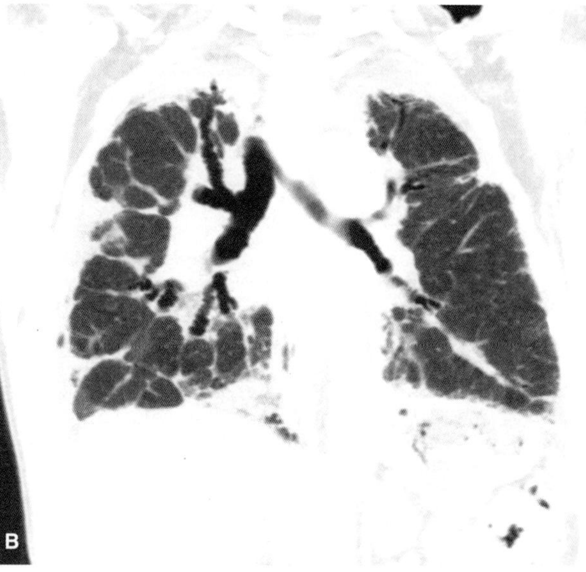

FIGURE 15.26. **Idiopathic Pleuroparenchymal Fibroelastosis.** Coronal CT reconstructions in mediastinal (**A**) and lung (**B**) windows demonstrate extensive pleural thickening and adjacent consolidation involving the periphery of the right lung and left apex with bronchiectasis and upper lobe volume loss.

On gross pathologic examination, patients with advanced LAM show replacement of the normal lung architecture by cysts. These cysts, which range from 0.2 to 2.0 cm in diameter, are separated by thickened interstitium containing numerous interlacing bundles of smooth muscle. Smooth muscle proliferation is also seen within the walls of pulmonary veins, bronchioles, and lymphatics. The smooth muscle proliferation within lymphatic channels causes lymphatic obstruction and dilatation that may lead to the development of chylothorax, chyloperitoneum, or chylopericardium. Similarly, smooth muscle proliferation within mediastinal and retroperitoneal lymph nodes may result in nodal enlargement. The perilymphatic smooth muscle proliferation and nodal enlargement help distinguish LAM pathologically from the pulmonary involvement of TS.

The patient with LAM is typically a woman of childbearing age who presents with progressive dyspnea or a spontaneous pneumothorax. Hemoptysis may be seen in some patients, presumably related to pulmonary venous obstruction by the smooth muscle proliferation.

The chest radiograph may be normal early in the disease. Eventually, symmetric bilateral fine reticular or reticulonodular opacities are seen. The late radiographic pattern is one of cysts and honeycombing; the cysts tend to have thinner walls than those seen with IPF or NF (Fig. 15.9). As in TS, the lung volumes are typically normal or increased. Large, recurrent chylous pleural effusions may be unilateral or bilateral. Spontaneous pneumothorax is also a common finding and may be bilateral.

Thin-section CT demonstrates thin-walled cysts distributed throughout the lungs (Figs. 15.9 and 15.27B). In less severely involved areas, the intervening lung is normal. Interlobular septal thickening is generally mild or absent. Although thin-walled cysts are seen in a variety of other diseases, the thin-section CT findings in a patient with a characteristic

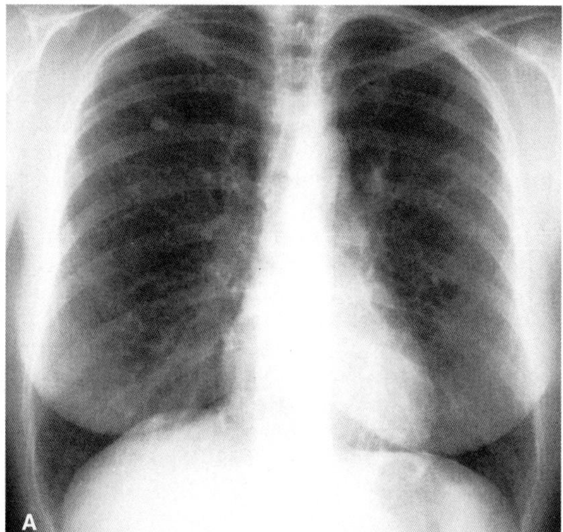

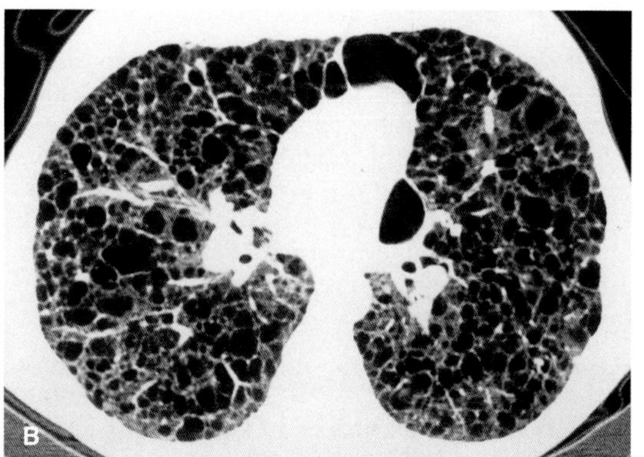

FIGURE 15.27. **Lymphangioleiomyomatosis (LAM). A:** Posteroanterior radiograph in a 36-year-old patient with LAM shows diffuse coarse reticular opacities with normal lung volumes. **B:** Thin-section CT in another patient with LAM shows almost complete replacement of the parenchyma by thin-walled cysts.

history (a woman with dyspnea, spontaneous pneumothorax, and chylous pleural effusions) are diagnostic.

The prognosis of patients with symptomatic LAM is poor, with approximately 70% of patients dying within 5 years. In some patients, the administration of antiprogesterone agents such as tamoxifen may slow the progression of disease.

Alveolar Septal Amyloidosis. Amyloidosis encompasses a group of diseases characterized by the extracellular deposition of insoluble fibrillary proteins termed *amyloid*. Amyloid represents a number of proteins that are distinctive biochemically but similar physically, in that their polypeptide chains form β-pleated sheets. Amyloidosis has traditionally been classified into four forms: (1) primary, in which there is no associated chronic disease or in which there is an underlying plasma cell disorder; (2) secondary, in which an underlying chronic abnormality such as TB is present; (3) familial, which is very uncommon and usually localized to nervous tissue; and (4) senile, which affects many organs in patients over 70. More recently, a classification scheme has been developed that is based on the specific protein comprising amyloid. In this scheme, the most important forms are amyloid L (AL), usually seen with plasma cell dyscrasias and associated with the deposition of immunoglobulin light chains, and amyloid A (AA), which occurs in patients with chronic inflammatory diseases such as familial Mediterranean fever and certain neoplasms including multiple myeloma, lymphoma, and leukemia.

There are three major patterns of amyloid deposition within the lungs and airways: tracheobronchial, nodular parenchymal, and diffuse parenchymal (alveolar septal). In most cases, these patterns occur independently but can overlap.

In alveolar septal amyloidosis, the amyloid is deposited in the parenchymal interstitium and within the media of small blood vessels. Within the alveolar septa, amyloid deposits are located between the endothelial cells lining the septal capillaries and the alveolar epithelium; inflammatory cells are typically absent.

This process is usually seen in older patients who have symptoms of chronic progressive dyspnea. Recurrent hemoptysis may also be seen as a result of medial dissection of the involved pulmonary arteries. Radiographically, patients with parenchymal alveolar septal disease show evidence of interstitial disease, with fine reticular or reticulonodular opacities that may become more coarse and confluent over time. Thin-section CT demonstrates interlobular septal thickening, reticulation, and micronodules. Fibrosis and lymph node enlargement are uncommon. The radiographic appearance simulates that seen in silicosis or sarcoidosis.

The diagnosis is made on lung biopsy by the identification of amorphous eosinophilic material thickening the alveolar septa that appears apple green in color when stained with Congo red and viewed under polarized light. There is no effective treatment.

Chronic Aspiration Pneumonia. Patients who repeatedly aspirate may develop chronic interstitial abnormalities on chest radiographs. With repeated episodes of aspiration over months to years, a residuum of irregular reticular interstitial opacities may persist, probably representing peribronchial scarring. A reticulonodular pattern may be seen as the result of granulomas forming around food particles. These chronic interstitial abnormalities can be observed between episodes of acute aspiration pneumonitis.

INHALATIONAL DISEASE

Pneumoconiosis

The term *pneumoconiosis* is used to describe the nonneoplastic reaction of the lungs to inhaled inorganic dust particles. The inorganic dust pneumoconioses result from the inhalation and retention of asbestos, silica, or coal particles within the lung. With time, the accumulation of these particles leads to two types of pathologic reactions that may be seen alone or in combination: fibrosis, which may be focal and nodular or diffuse and reticular; and the aggregation of particle-laden macrophages. Organic dust inhalational syndromes, which are discussed at the end of this section, are not associated with the retention and accumulation of particles within the lungs. Instead, the organic dusts induce a hypersensitivity reaction known as hypersensitivity pneumonitis or extrinsic allergic alveolitis.

Asbestosis. *Asbestos* is the generic term for a group of fibrous silicates that are resistant to heat and various chemical insults. Asbestos is divided into two major subgroups: the serpentines and the amphiboles. The serpentines are curly, flexible, and smooth; the only commercially important serpentine is chrysotile. The amphiboles have straight, needlelike fibers; this subgroup includes crocidolite and amosite. The different types of asbestos fibers vary in their potential to cause disease, with the amphiboles having a greater fibrogenic and carcinogenic potential than the serpentines. At present, >90% of the asbestos used in the United States is chrysotile.

Asbestos inhalation may cause disease of the pleura, parenchyma, airways, and lymph nodes. Pleural disease is the most common of these and usually manifests as parietal pleural plaques. Other pleural manifestations include pleural effusion, localized visceral pleural fibrosis, diffuse pleural fibrosis, and mesothelioma. The pleural manifestations of asbestos exposure are discussed in more detail in Chapter 17. The pulmonary parenchymal manifestations of asbestos inhalation include interstitial fibrosis (asbestosis), rounded atelectasis, and bronchogenic carcinoma.

Asbestosis is defined as a diffuse parenchymal interstitial fibrosis caused by the inhalation of asbestos fibers. The development of asbestosis depends on both the length and severity of exposure, and clinical manifestations are usually not apparent for 20 to 40 years following initial exposure. Pathologically, a large number of "asbestos bodies" will be seen in lung tissue. This characteristic structure consists of a core transparent asbestos fiber surrounded by a coat of iron and protein. Asbestos bodies are usually found within interstitial fibrous tissue or airspaces and only rarely in pleural plaques. The number of asbestos bodies and fibers per gram of digested lung tissue is roughly proportional to the degree of occupational exposure and the severity of interstitial fibrosis. On gross examination of affected lungs, fibrosis is most prominent in the subpleural regions of the lower lobes. Microscopically, the appearance varies from a slight increase in interstitial collagen to complete obliteration of normal architecture and formation of thick fibrous parenchymal bands and cystic spaces (honeycombing).

The majority of patients with asbestos-related pleuropulmonary disease are asymptomatic. Patients beyond the early stages of interstitial fibrosis will often experience shortness of breath and a restrictive pattern on pulmonary function tests. These patients are also at risk of developing asbestos-associated neoplasia, particularly bronchogenic carcinoma and pleural mesothelioma, and require close clinical follow-up.

The radiographic findings in asbestosis occur in two forms: small and large opacities. Small opacities may be reticular, nodular, or a combination of the two. The changes produced on chest radiographs are divided into three stages. The earliest finding is a fine reticulation, predominantly in the lower lung zones, which is a manifestation of early interstitial pneumonitis and fibrosis. With time, the small irregular opacities become more prominent, creating a coarse reticular pattern of disease. In later stages, the reticular opacities may extend

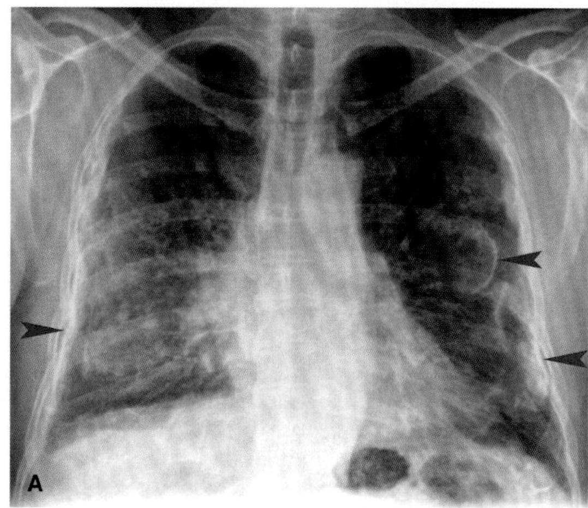

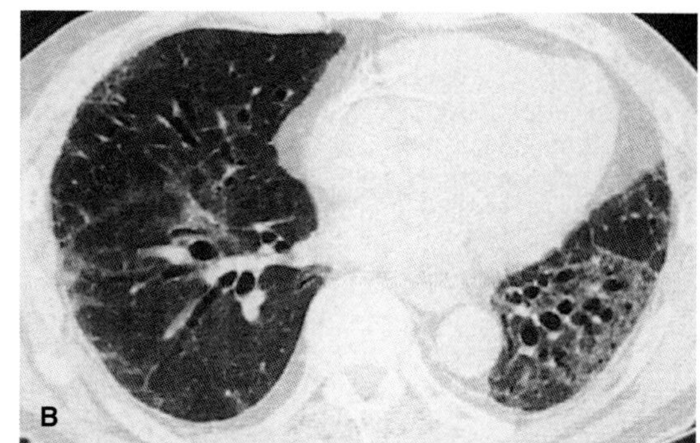

FIGURE 15.28. **Asbestosis. A:** Frontal chest radiograph shows course basilar interstitial markings and calcified pleural plaques (*arrowheads*). **B:** Thin-section CT through the lung bases shows left lower lobe honeycombing, peripheral ground-glass opacities, and traction bronchiectasis bilaterally.

into the mid- and upper lung zones, with progressive obscuration of the cardiac and diaphragmatic margins and progressive diminution of lung volumes. Large opacities, that is, those measuring greater than 1 cm in diameter, are invariably associated with widespread interstitial fibrosis and pleural plaques. These large opacities show lower zone predominance and may be well-defined or ill-defined and multiple.

Thin-section CT is a sensitive means of detecting both the pleural and parenchymal changes associated with clinical asbestosis. Interlobular septal thickening is the most common thin-section CT finding in asbestos-exposed individuals. Intralobular septal thickening and small centrilobular "dot-like" opacities, the latter caused by peribronchiolar fibrosis, are also common. Many cases will progress to honeycombing. The thin-section CT findings are those of UIP (Figs. 15.12 and 15.19), but patients with asbestosis may also have pleural disease, which may help to distinguish between these two entities (Fig. 15.28). Additionally, ground-glass opacity is relatively uncommon in asbestosis compared with IPF and other forms of UIP.

Identification of intrafissural plaques, especially if they contain calcification, is also possible with thin-section CT. Characteristic CT features of focal lung masses in asbestos-exposed individuals may allow for conservative management of these lesions. For example, a wedge-shaped or round mass adjacent to focal pleural thickening, with evidence of lobar volume loss and a "comet tail" bronchovascular bundle coursing into it, can be confidently diagnosed as rounded atelectasis by thin-section CT, obviating biopsy.

Silicosis. Silica is an abundant mineral composed of regularly arranged molecules of silicon dioxide. It is ubiquitous in the earth's crust and exposure to a high concentration may lead to pathologic and radiologic changes. Occupations associated with such levels of exposure include mining, quarrying, foundry work, ceramic work, and sandblasting. Two distinct histopathologic reactions to inhaled silica are *silicotic nodules* and *silicoproteinosis*.

Silicotic nodules measure from 1 to 10 mm in diameter and are made up of dense concentric lamellae of collagen. They are typically most numerous in the upper lobes and parahilar regions of lung; calcification or ossification of the nodules is common. Coalescence of these nodules produces areas of PMF. PMF may occupy an entire lobe, with areas of emphysema often present adjacent to these masses. Focal necrosis is common within the central portions of these large conglomerate lesions and is often the result of ischemia or superinfection by TB or anaerobic bacteria. Exposure of 10 to 20 years is usually required for the radiographic changes of fibrotic silicosis to develop. The classic radiographic appearance is multiple well-defined nodules ranging from 1 to 10 mm in diameter. These tend to be diffuse with an upper zone predominance of nodules and calcify in approximately 20% of cases. A reticular pattern of disease may be seen preceding or associating with the nodular pattern and is sometimes the earliest radiographic finding. This pattern of reticulonodular opacities is often referred to as "simple" silicosis, in contrast to the large conglomerate opacities that characterize "complicated" silicosis (Fig. 15.10). These conglomerate opacities represent areas of PMF and most commonly develop in the peripheral portions of the upper and mid-lung zones. The opacities tend to migrate toward the hila, leaving areas of emphysema between the pleural surface and the areas of progressive fibrosis. These conglomerate areas may cavitate, often in association with superimposed tuberculous infection. Hilar lymph node enlargement may be seen at any stage, and these hilar nodes often demonstrate peripheral "eggshell" calcification. Clinically, the diagnosis of fibrotic silicosis is based on identification of a diffuse reticular, nodular, or reticulonodular pattern on the chest radiograph in a patient with an appropriate exposure history. Patients may be asymptomatic for many years, but may worsen functionally in conjunction with progression of the radiographic changes. The pulmonary fibrosis and associated restrictive functional impairment of silicosis may progress even after the individual is removed from the offending environment.

Silicoproteinosis usually occurs in individuals exposed to very high concentrations of silica. It is characterized by filling of alveolar spaces with lipoproteinaceous material similar to that seen in idiopathic alveolar proteinosis. There is little collagen deposition associated with this reaction and the well-defined collagenous nodule is not typically seen. Acute silicoproteinosis presents radiographically with diffuse airspace disease and is indistinguishable in appearance from idiopathic alveolar proteinosis. As do patients with fibrotic silicosis, those with acute silicoproteinosis have an increased susceptibility to TB. They are also predisposed to superinfection with *Nocardia*, which may produce mass-like consolidation and chest wall involvement.

Coal Worker's Pneumoconiosis. The inhalation of large amounts of carbon-containing inorganic material may lead to significant pulmonary disease. The exposure levels required to cause this disease occur almost exclusively in the workplace. Since the most common occupation producing this entity is coal mining, the resultant disease is termed coal worker's pneumoconiosis (CWP).

CWP has two characteristic pathologic findings: the coal dust macule and PMF. The coal dust macule results from the deposit of carbonaceous material within the lung. Coal dust macules are round or stellate nodules ranging in size from 1 to 5 mm. They are composed of pigment-laden macrophages with minimal or absent collagen formation. They are found within the interstitium adjacent to respiratory bronchioles, and are scattered throughout the lungs with a predilection for the apices. The coal dust macule or nodule is the hallmark of simple CWP and is generally not associated with functional impairment. In fact, radiographic abnormalities may be absent in simple CWP. Complicated CWP is characterized by the presence of PMF. PMF is defined as nodular or mass-like lesions exceeding 2 to 3 cm in diameter that are composed of irregular fibrosis and pigment. PMF is most common in the posterior segments of the upper lobes and superior segments of the lower lobes. The conglomerate masses may cross interlobar fissures. Central cavitation is common and is most often a result of infarction from obliteration of pulmonary vessels by the fibrotic masses. Occasionally, superinfection of the masses by TB or fungus accounts for central necrosis and cavitation. The mass lesions of complicated CWP are similar to those seen in complicated silicosis. It should be noted that despite their name, the lesions of PMF may not progress with time and are not necessarily massive in size.

Patients with CWP usually present with respiratory difficulties only when PMF has developed, as those with simple pneumoconiosis are generally asymptomatic. In complicated CWP, there is progressive dyspnea which may lead to cor pulmonale. Because many coal workers also smoke cigarettes, the development of centrilobular emphysema and chronic bronchitis may complicate the clinical picture.

Radiographically, "simple" CWP presents typically as upper zone reticulonodular or small nodular opacities. A purely reticular pattern may also be seen, especially in the early stages of the process. The nodules range from 1 to 5 mm in diameter and correspond to conglomerates of coal dust macules seen pathologically. The lesions are indistinguishable radiographically from the nodules of simple silicosis. In as many as 10% of coal miners, some of these nodules will calcify centrally. This is in distinction to the diffuse calcification of silicotic nodules. The nodular opacities of simple CWP do not progress after coal dust exposure has ceased. The lesions of complicated pneumoconiosis (PMF) range in size from 2 cm to an entire lobe and are seen in the upper portion of the lungs. PMF usually begins peripherally as a mass with a smooth, well-defined lateral border and an ill-defined medial border. PMF gradually "migrates" toward the hilum, creating a zone of emphysema between the opacities and the chest wall. These lesions may mimic primary carcinoma, particularly if a background of nodular opacities is not appreciated. The PMF seen with CWP may develop years after exposure to coal dust has ceased and may progress in the absence of further exposure.

Certain complicating factors may alter the radiographic appearance of CWP. TB is relatively common in patients with CWP and may produce central cavitation in some patients with PMF. Caplan syndrome or "rheumatoid pneumoconiosis," seen in coal workers with rheumatoid arthritis, is characterized radiographically by nodular opacities 0.5 to 5 cm in diameter that develop rapidly and tend to appear in crops. The nodules are more sharply defined and seen more peripherally than the masses of PMF. These lesions are not specific for CWP and may be seen in patients with silicosis or asbestosis.

Miscellaneous Pneumoconioses. A variety of inorganic dusts other than asbestos, silica, and coal dust can cause pleuropulmonary disease but are far less common. Chronic berylliosis produces a reaction that mimics sarcoidosis and is discussed in the section "Granulomatous Diseases." Aluminum workers may develop disabling pulmonary fibrosis after years of exposure to aluminum dust, usually from bauxite mining. Radiographic changes include fine to coarse reticular or reticulonodular opacities distributed throughout the lungs, along with greatly diminished lung volumes and marked pleural thickening. Apical bullae may be seen, which produce spontaneous pneumothoraces. Hard metal pneumoconiosis, formerly called giant cell interstitial pneumonitis, may result from exposure to cobalt and tungsten alloys and can cause interstitial pneumonitis with varying degrees of fibrosis. The chest radiograph demonstrates a reticulonodular pattern that may be very coarse and, if advanced, may be associated with small cystic shadows. Lymph node enlargement may be seen.

Hypersensitivity Pneumonitis

Hypersensitivity pneumonitis or *extrinsic allergic alveolitis* is an immunologic pulmonary disorder associated with the inhalation of one of the antigenic organic dusts. These dusts must be of small particle size to penetrate into the alveolar spaces and incite a host inflammatory response. A wide variety of etiologic agents have been implicated, including many thermophilic bacteria, true fungi, and various animal proteins. Some of the more common disease entities include farmer's lung (exposure to moldy hay); humidifier lung (exposure to water reservoirs contaminated by thermophilic bacteria); and bird fancier's lung (exposure to avian proteins in feathers and excreta).

The development of hypersensitivity pneumonitis depends upon the size, number, and immunogenicity of the inhaled organic particles, and the immune response of the host. Two forms of the disease are distinguished by their clinical presentation and immunopathogenesis. Acute disease develops 4 to 6 hours following exposure to the inciting antigen and is mediated by a type 3 (immune complex) reaction. Typical symptoms include cough, dyspnea, and fever. Chronic disease is often insidious and commonly results in interstitial pulmonary fibrosis. Patients with chronic disease often have malaise, chronic cough, and progressive dyspnea. This form of disease appears to be mediated by a type 4 (cell-mediated) immune reaction.

The histopathologic features of the different types of hypersensitivity pneumonitis are usually indistinguishable, except in rare situations where antigenic material can be identified in the pathologic preparations. The pathologic features are dependent on the intensity of exposure to the allergen and on the stage of disease when tissue biopsy is obtained. Early findings include capillary congestion and inflammation within alveolar septae. In later stages of acute disease, bronchiolitis and alveolitis with granuloma formation are present. With repeated antigenic exposure, there is a progressive increase in interstitial fibrosis, which is initially patchy in distribution but may progress to diffuse interstitial fibrosis.

The radiographic changes of hypersensitivity pneumonitis parallel the pathologic findings. The chest radiograph may be normal early in the acute stage of disease. Within hours, fine nodular or ground-glass opacities develop, most often in the lower lobes; progressive airspace opacification may simulate pulmonary edema. Within hours to days, the opacities resolve and the chest radiograph becomes normal. With continued or repeated exposures, the chest radiograph will remain abnormal between acute episodes. The chronic changes appear as diffuse coarse reticular or reticulonodular opacities in the

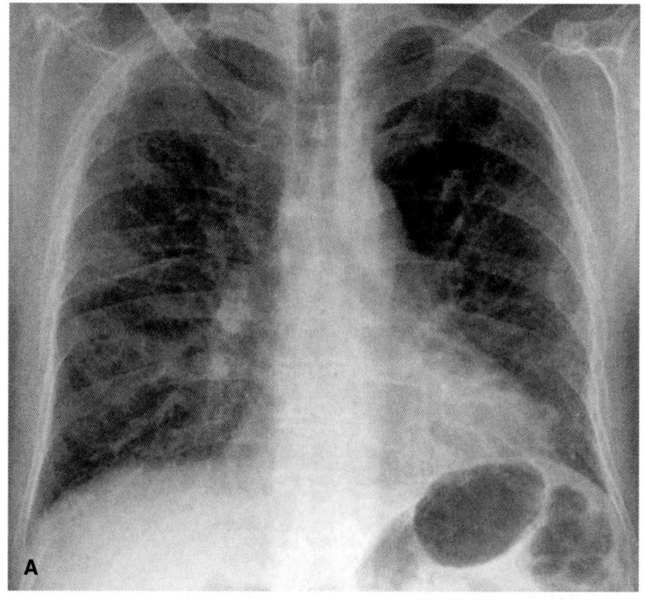

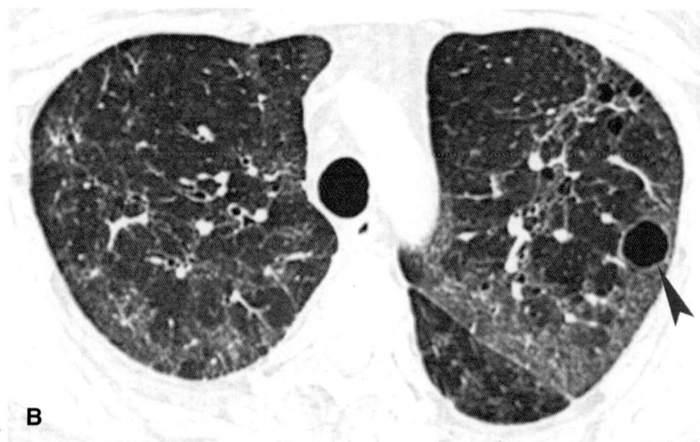

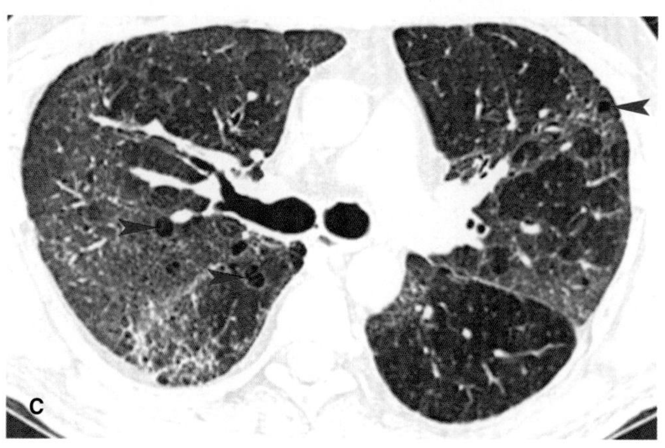

FIGURE 15.29. **Chronic Hypersensitivity Pneumonitis.** Chest radiograph (**A**) in a farmer with chronic progressive dyspnea shows bilateral reticular opacities without zonal predilection. Axial CT scans through the upper (**B**) and mid-lungs (**C**) show bilateral areas of reticulation and ground-glass opacity. Note the presence of cysts (*arrowheads*), which have been described in hypersensitivity pneumonitis and likely reflect overdistending regions of lung distal to small airway involvement.

mid-lung and upper lung zones; a honeycomb pattern with loss of lung volume may be seen. The diagnosis of hypersensitivity pneumonitis should be considered when repeated episodes of rapidly changing ground-glass or airspace opacification are seen in a patient with underlying coarse interstitial lung disease. Hilar or mediastinal lymph node enlargement and pleural effusion are uncommon findings in patients with hypersensitivity pneumonitis.

Thin-section CT may be very helpful in the diagnosis of hypersensitivity pneumonitis, particularly in the subacute phase, when chest radiographs may be normal or quite nonspecific. The most common findings in the acute phase of disease are airspace opacities. The subacute phase is characterized by patchy areas of ground-glass opacity and poorly defined ("fuzzy") centrilobular nodules (Figs. 15.7 and 15.11). These findings may be superimposed on one another and both show a predilection in the mid- and lower lung zones. In the chronic phase of the disease, findings are those of fibrosis: interlobular and intralobular interstitial thickening, honeycombing, and traction bronchiectasis (Fig. 15.29). Distribution of disease is varied, but sometimes there is relative sparing of the costophrenic angles, which may help to distinguish hypersensitivity pneumonitis from UIP.

The diagnosis of hypersensitivity pneumonitis is made by eliciting a history that suggests a temporal relationship between the patient's symptoms and certain exposures. The intermittent exposure of susceptible persons to high concentrations of antigen leads to recurrent episodes that typically begin 4 to 6 hours following exposure. The symptoms usually persist for 12 hours and then resolve spontaneously if the exposure has been terminated. Repeated exposure to the inciting antigen will result in acute exacerbations, with typical symptoms and radiographic findings. Chronic disease is more difficult to diagnose and develops when there is a continuous low level of exposure to the antigen. The prognosis for patients whose disease is recognized at an early stage is good if the offending agent can be removed from the patient's environment. In the more insidious chronic form of disease, the diagnosis is often delayed and considerable interstitial fibrosis may be present at the time of diagnosis. These patients generally suffer from chronic respiratory insufficiency.

GRANULOMATOUS DISEASES

Sarcoidosis

Sarcoidosis is a multisystem granulomatous disease of unknown etiology characterized histologically by noncaseating granulomas that may progress to fibrosis. The disease is seen more commonly in blacks than whites and is rare in Asians. Black women are at particular risk for this disease. Most patients are 20 to 40 years of age at the time of diagnosis; however, because patients with this disease are often asymptomatic, many cases are never identified.

Although numerous theories have been proposed, the etiology of sarcoidosis is unknown. Whatever the etiologic agent, the underlying pathogenesis involves activation of pulmonary macrophages that, in turn, recruit mononuclear cells to the pulmonary interstitium, leading to the formation of granulomas. The activated macrophages also stimulate proliferation of T-helper lymphocytes in the lung, which induces an overactivity of B lymphocytes, resulting in the hypergammaglobulinemia characteristically seen in this disease. The excess number of T-helper lymphocytes in the lung may be detected in bronchoalveolar lavage (BAL) fluid of patients with sarcoidosis and is helpful in the differential diagnosis of this condition.

The pathologic changes of sarcoidosis follow a fairly predictable pattern. The earliest changes involve the pulmonary interstitium, with the development of a nonspecific lymphocytic and histiocytic infiltrate. This progresses to the formation of microscopic granulomas. The granulomas contain palisading epithelioid histiocytes with intermixed multinucleated giant cells and, in contrast to tuberculous granulomas, are typically noncaseating. The giant cells in the granulomas may contain dark-staining lamellated structures within their cytoplasm called Schaumann bodies, which are characteristic of sarcoidosis. The granulomas are found most commonly within the axial (peribronchovascular) and peripheral or subpleural interstitium of the lung, but may involve the parenchymal (alveolar) interstitium and airway mucosa; the airway lesions may be visualized bronchoscopically. Involvement of the axial interstitium of the lung accounts for the high (approximately 90%) diagnostic yield of blind transbronchial biopsy in sarcoidosis, since this technique usually provides samples of the bronchial wall, the surrounding axial interstitium, and adjacent airspaces. The small granulomas usually resolve after months or years. In some patients, the microscopic granulomas coalesce to form larger nodules. Rarely, these nodules grow to form large, well-defined masses or poorly marginated opacities that contain air bronchograms and simulate an airspace-filling process. In this "alveolar" form of sarcoidosis, the airspaces are not filled with material but are compressed and obliterated by the exuberant granuloma formation within the surrounding interstitium.

In 20% of patients, fibrous tissue is deposited at the periphery of the granulomas and eventually grows inward to replace the granulomas, resulting in interstitial fibrosis. The fibrosis tends to progress over time, with the development of broad bands of fibrous tissue extending from the hilar regions toward the lung apices, producing hilar elevation and distortion of the hilar vessels and upper mediastinum. Masses of fibrous tissue may develop in the parahilar regions of the upper lobes, with peripheral areas of emphysema or cyst formation. These cysts predispose a patient to spontaneous pneumothoraces and provide a site for mycetoma formation.

Lymph node involvement in sarcoidosis is characterized by replacement of the normal nodal architecture with granulomas that are indistinguishable from those found in the pulmonary parenchyma. As with parenchymal involvement, these may regress, coalesce, or undergo fibrosis.

The clinical presentation of sarcoidosis may be dominated by pulmonary or extrapulmonary manifestations of the disease, but a considerable percentage of patients are asymptomatic and are identified by incidental findings on chest radiographs. Pulmonary symptoms are present in 25% of patients and include dyspnea and a nonproductive cough. Common extrapulmonary findings include fever, malaise, uveitis, and erythema nodosum. In a minority of patients, involvement of the liver, heart, kidneys, or CNS may dominate the clinical picture.

Common laboratory findings in sarcoidosis include hypercalcemia, hypergammaglobulinemia, and elevated serum angiotensin-converting enzyme levels. Cutaneous anergy to purified protein derivative (PPD) tuberculin skin test reflects an abnormality of delayed hypersensitivity found in these patients. Pulmonary function tests vary from normal in those with minimal or no parenchymal disease to a severe restrictive pattern with low diffusing capacity in patients with end-stage pulmonary fibrosis.

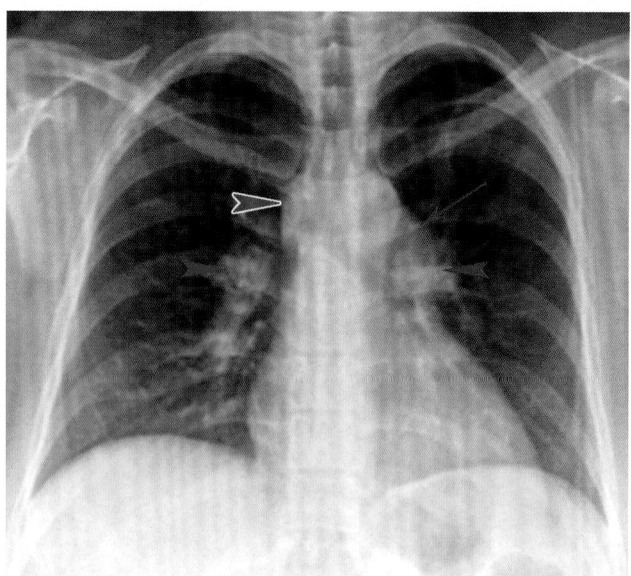

FIGURE 15.30. **Sarcoidosis.** Posteroanterior radiograph in an asymptomatic 26 year old shows enlargement of right paratracheal (*blue arrowhead*), bilateral hilar (*red arrowheads*), and aortopulmonary window (*arrow*) lymph nodes, characteristic of sarcoidosis.

Lymph Node Enlargement. Enlargement of mediastinal and hilar lymph nodes is found in 80% of patients with sarcoidosis and is associated with radiographically normal lungs in slightly more than half of these patients. The classic appearance on chest radiographs is the combination of right paratracheal and bilateral symmetric hilar lymph node enlargement (Fig. 15.30). The symmetric enlargement is a key feature that allows distinction from malignancy and TB, conditions that usually produce unilateral or asymmetric lymph node enlargement. Left paratracheal lymph node enlargement is common, as determined by CT, although enlargement of these nodes is usually not appreciated on radiographs because the region is obscured by the aorta and great vessels on frontal radiographs. The enlarged nodes tend to have a lobulated contour because the individual nodes remain discrete. Mediastinal (paratracheal) lymph node enlargement without concomitant hilar enlargement is uncommon and should suggest lymphoma or metastatic disease. Similarly, unilateral hilar nodal enlargement is unusual, seen in only 5% of individuals. CT has shown that in involvement of anterior mediastinal, posterior mediastinal, subcarinal, and aortopulmonary lymph nodes occurs with greater frequency than was previously thought, based on the radiographic appearance.

The enlarged lymph nodes regress within 2 years in 75% of affected patients. A small percentage of patients will have persistent lymph node enlargement for years. The development of parenchymal opacities concomitant with the resolution of lymph node enlargement is a helpful feature in differentiating sarcoidosis from lymphoma, in which enlarged lymph nodes do not regress when parenchymal abnormalities develop. Calcification of involved lymph nodes is seen in up to 20% of patients and may involve only the periphery of the node ("eggshell" calcification).

Lung Disease. The lung is involved radiographically in only 40% to 50% of patients with sarcoidosis, despite the nearly

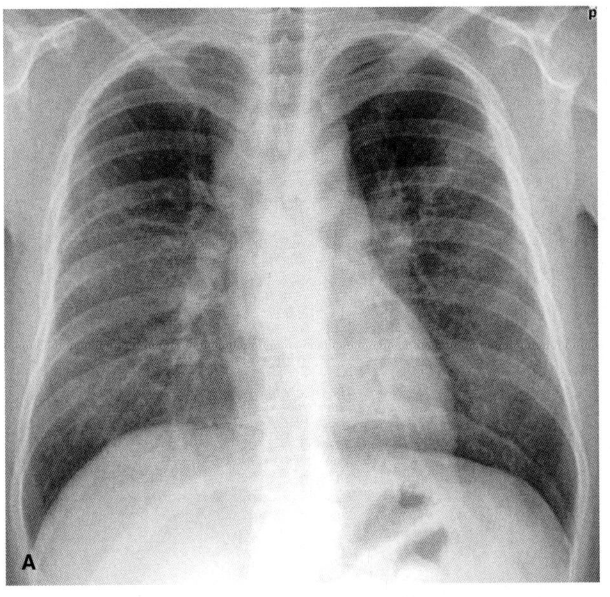

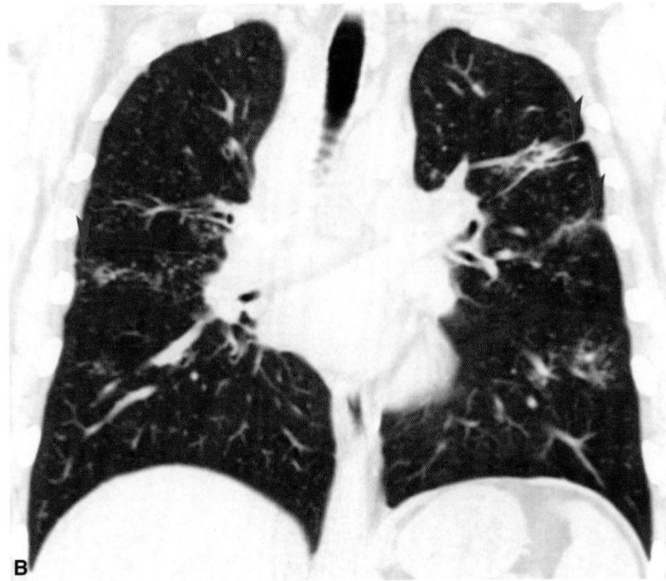

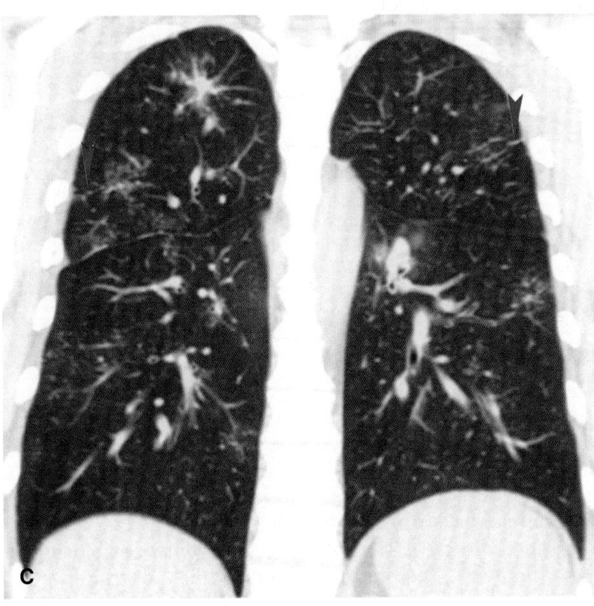

FIGURE 15.31. **Sarcoidosis With Reticulonodular Opacities.** Frontal radiograph (**A**) in a patient with sarcoidosis shows bilateral predominantly mid-zone reticulonodular opacities in association with bilateral hilar and paratracheal lymph node enlargement. CT scans with coronal reformations through the mid (**B**) and posterior (**C**) lungs shows patchy areas of clustered micronodules with some admixed reticulation (*arrowheads*) in the upper and mid-lungs.

90% yield from transbronchial biopsy of the lung. The most common parenchymal abnormality is that bilateral symmetric reticulonodular opacities show a predilection for the mid- and upper lung zones (Fig. 15.31). The reticulonodular opacities represent the combination of granulomas and fibrosis. CT shows that most nodules lie predominantly in a peribronchovascular and subpleural location (Fig. 15.32A). The appearance of reticulonodular opacities never precedes the enlargement of hilar and mediastinal lymph nodes. The earliest parenchymal finding is a diffuse micronodular pattern, identical in appearance to miliary TB, which represents the superimposition of microscopic granulomas (Fig. 15.32B). This pattern, which is rarely identified radiographically, may precede the development of hilar lymph node enlargement.

In approximately 10% of patients, the coalescence of granulomas produces one of two unusual radiographic manifestations of parenchymal sarcoidosis. Exuberant interstitial granulomas can obliterate adjacent airspaces, producing poorly defined airspace opacities that may contain air bronchograms. In some cases, intra-alveolar inflammation and granulomas contribute to the alveolar pattern of disease. These airspace opacities are primarily seen in the peripheral portions of the mid-lung zone, thereby simulating eosinophilic pneumonia and cryptogenic organizing radiographically. The presence of reticulonodular opacities elsewhere in the lung or concomitant symmetric hilar and mediastinal lymph node enlargement, best seen on CT and thin-section CT, provides important clues to the diagnosis.

Nodular or mass-like sarcoidosis develops in a manner similar to alveolar disease. These masses can be quite large and typically have a sharp margin. Air bronchograms are often demonstrated on CT and thin-section CT (Fig. 15.32C); cavitation is extremely rare.

Pulmonary fibrosis develops in 20% of patients with long-standing parenchymal involvement. The chest radiograph shows coarse linear opacities extending obliquely from the hila toward the upper and mid-lung zones. There is considerable distortion and elevation of the hila, with scalloping of the lung-mediastinal interface. Occasionally, conglomerate masses of fibrosis form in the upper perihilar regions that simulate the PMF of complicated silicosis. On CT, these masses contain air bronchograms with traction bronchiectasis. Distortion and obstruction of the airways from fibrosis can lead to secondary air trapping, with resultant alveolar septal

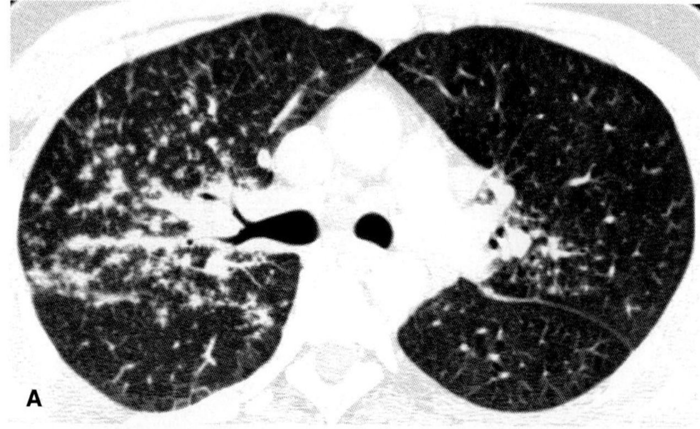

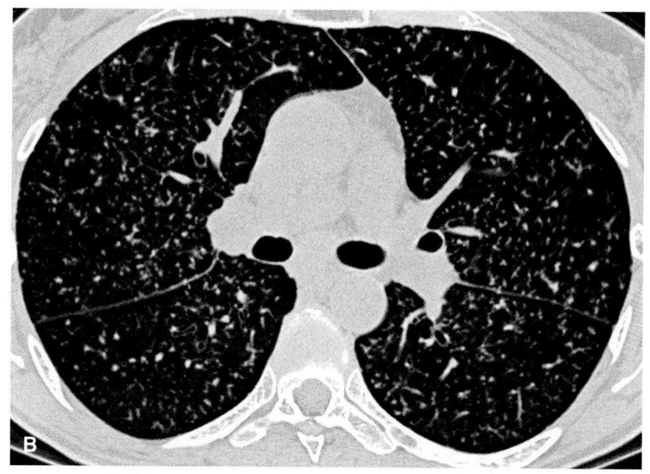

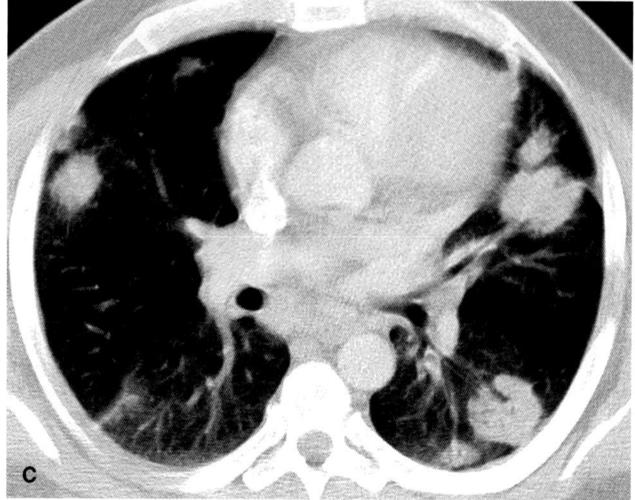

FIGURE 15.32. **CT Appearances of Pulmonary Sarcoidosis.** Sarcoidosis in three different patients showing (**A**) typical perilymphatic nodules, (**B**) miliary nodules, and (**C**) mass-like opacities. The latter two appearances are uncommon.

disruption and cicatricial emphysema or bullae formation (Fig. 15.33). An increase in radiographic lung volumes may accompany these cystic changes, a finding that is characteristic of bullous sarcoidosis. Mycetomas can develop within the cysts and lead to massive hemoptysis from erosion into bronchial arteries. Cysts may also rupture into the pleural space and produce spontaneous pneumothoraces.

Pleural Changes. Pleural thickening or effusion occurs in approximately 7% of patients with sarcoidosis and is the result of granulomatous inflammation of the visceral and parietal pleura. Aggregation of nodules along the pleural surface can cause pleural pseudoplaques.

Miscellaneous Findings. Endobronchial granulomas can result in fibrosis of the bronchial wall and bronchial stenosis with air trapping. Pulmonary arterial hypertension is an uncommon finding and is usually secondary to long-standing pulmonary fibrosis.

Thin-Section CT Findings. Thin-section CT is clearly more sensitive than chest radiographs in detecting the parenchymal abnormalities of sarcoidosis. A variety of thin-section CT findings has been described in this disease, which represent both the granulomatous and fibrotic responses seen histologically (Figs. 15.31B and 15.32). The most frequent finding is the presence of interstitial nodules, 3 to 10 mm in diameter, seen as nodular thickening of the peribronchoarterial (axial) interstitium and interlobular septa or as subpleural nodules. The nodules correlate closely with the coalescing noncaseating granulomas seen microscopically on tissue specimens. Septal thickening, thickening of bronchovascular bundles, architectural distortion, lung cysts, honeycombing, and central conglomerate masses with crowded, ectatic bronchi are findings indicative of fibrosis from long-standing disease. Segmental or mass-like airspace opacities, termed "alveolar" sarcoid, usually indicate the presence of active disease and resolve with corticosteroid therapy. Likewise, the finding of patchy areas of ground-glass density has been shown to correlate with increased uptake on gallium scans and may be indicative of an active alveolitis. Several recent papers have showed good correlation between conventional CT and thin-section CT findings and pulmonary function tests.

Radiographic Staging of Sarcoidosis. The chest radiographic manifestations of sarcoidosis have been divided into five stages (Table 15.8). These stages generally parallel the course of disease and are useful for prognostic purposes. Stage 1 disease is associated with a 75% rate of resolution, whereas only 30% of patients with stage 2 and 10% of patients with stage 3 disease resolve.

The diagnosis of sarcoidosis is usually based on the histologic demonstration of noncaseating granulomas involving multiple organs. Tissue is most often obtained by bronchoscopically guided transbronchial biopsy, which provides a diagnosis in up to 90% of patients. Biopsy of organs likely to be involved in this disease, such as the liver and scalene lymph nodes, will provide a diagnosis in a majority of patients. Percutaneous needle biopsy can provide diagnostic tissue specimens in those with mass-like pulmonary lesions. In certain situations, the diagnosis of sarcoidosis is made on a constellation of chest radiographic findings and characteristic eye or skin changes.

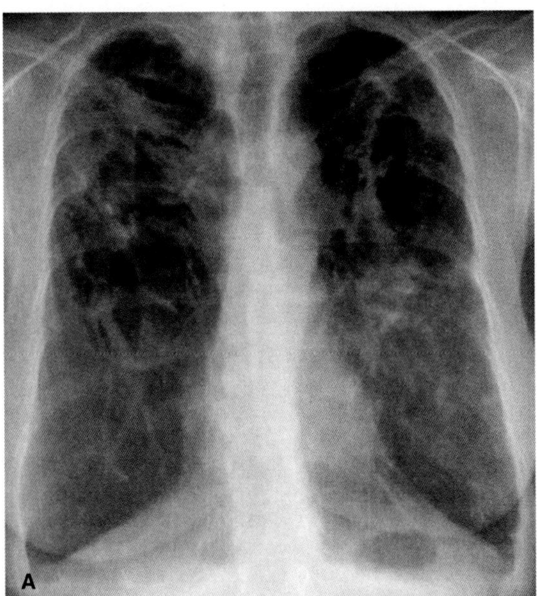
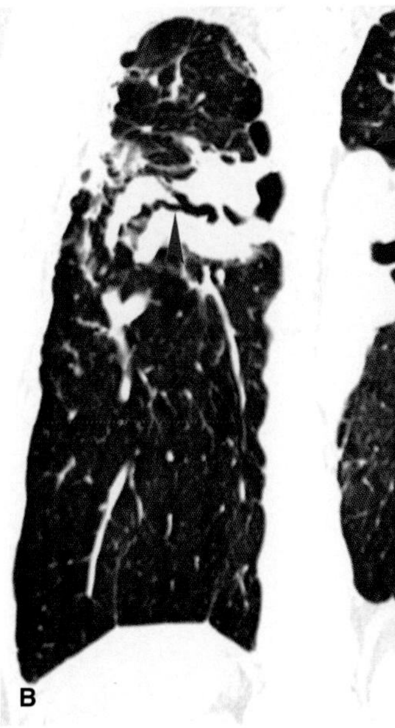
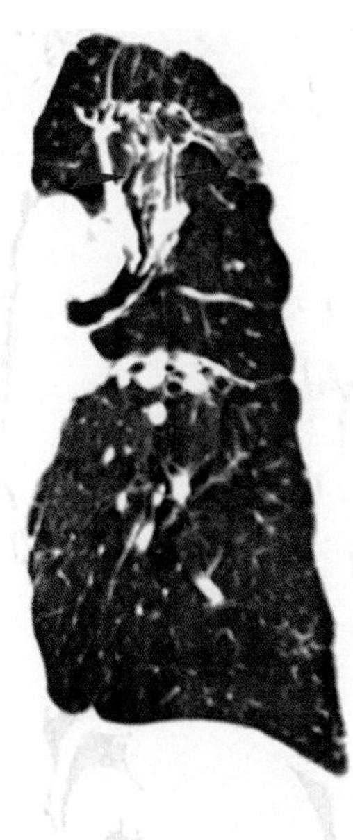

FIGURE 15.33. **Stage IV (Fibrotic) Sarcoidosis.** In a 65-year-old woman with a 25-year history of sarcoidosis, frontal chest radiograph (**A**) shows coarse reticular opacities with marked elevation and distortion of the hila and mediastinal reflections. CT scan with coronal reformation (**B**) shows parahilar fibrosis with traction bronchiectasis (*arrowheads*). Note the relative absence of nodules in this stage of disease.

Berylliosis

Although berylliosis is actually an inhalational lung disease, it is discussed here because of the clinical, pathologic, and radiographic similarities to sarcoidosis. This uncommon disease produces noncaseating granulomas in multiple organs, with primary lung involvement. The radiographic features of berylliosis are indistinguishable from those of sarcoidosis. Hilar and mediastinal lymph node enlargement and bilateral reticulonodular opacities are the most common findings. Progression to end-stage interstitial fibrosis with honeycombing or upper lobe bullous disease may occur, with the latter predisposing the patient to aspergilloma formation and spontaneous pneumothoraces.

Langerhans Cell Histiocytosis of Lung

The entity of LCH includes several disorders with similar pathologic features that differ in age at the time of diagnosis, mode of presentation, specific organs involved, and prognosis. The form of this disease affecting adults presents with predominant involvement of lung and bones. The disease most commonly affects young adults and has no sex predilection.

TABLE 15.8

RADIOGRAPHIC STAGING OF SARCOIDOSIS

■ STAGE	■ RADIOGRAPHIC FINDINGS
0	Normal chest radiograph
1	Bilateral hilar lymph node enlargement
2	Bilateral hilar lymph node enlargement and parenchymal disease
3	Parenchymal disease only
4	Pulmonary fibrosis

There is a very high association between pulmonary involvement and cigarette smoking.

Pathologically, LCH of lung demonstrates multiple small nodules, which are found predominantly in the axial interstitial tissues of the upper and mid-lung zones around small bronchioles. The nodules are granulomas composed predominantly of cells with eosinophilic cytoplasm known as Langerhans cells. They are normally found in the skin, where they act as antigen-processing cells, and appear to proliferate in the lung and other organs in response to an unidentified antigenic stimulus. In some patients, the nodular phase of disease may be preceded by an exudative phase, with filling of the alveolar spaces with a cellular exudate containing the Langerhans cells. The small peribronchiolar nodules may coalesce to form larger nodules, which may cavitate, or they may extend to infiltrate the alveolar septa and induce an interstitial inflammatory reaction. The nodules may resolve completely, but in most patients, the central portions of the nodules undergo fibrosis, producing a stellate nodular lesion that is characteristic of pulmonary LCH histologically. In the late stages, characteristic findings include fibrosis and the development of small, uniform, thin-walled cysts. Larger peripheral cysts or bullae may develop in the apical regions, presumably as a result of bronchiolar obstruction by fibrosis, with distal air trapping.

Pulmonary symptoms are present in two-thirds of patients with LCH of lung at presentation. Cough and the gradual onset of dyspnea are the most common complaints. Pleuritic chest pain may indicate the development of a spontaneous pneumothorax from rupture of a subpleural cyst. Pulmonary function tests reflect the fibrosis and cystic changes seen in this disorder, with characteristic restrictive and obstructive patterns of disease and a diminished diffusing capacity.

The radiographic findings in LCH of the lung usually follow a predictable pattern. Although the earliest changes in LCH of the lung are associated with filling of alveoli, the radiographic demonstration of airspace opacities is uncommon. The earliest findings are small to medium nodular opacities that tend to have an upper and mid-lung zone distribution (Fig. 15.34). In some cases, the nodules coalesce to form larger nodules or masses, which rarely cavitate. The

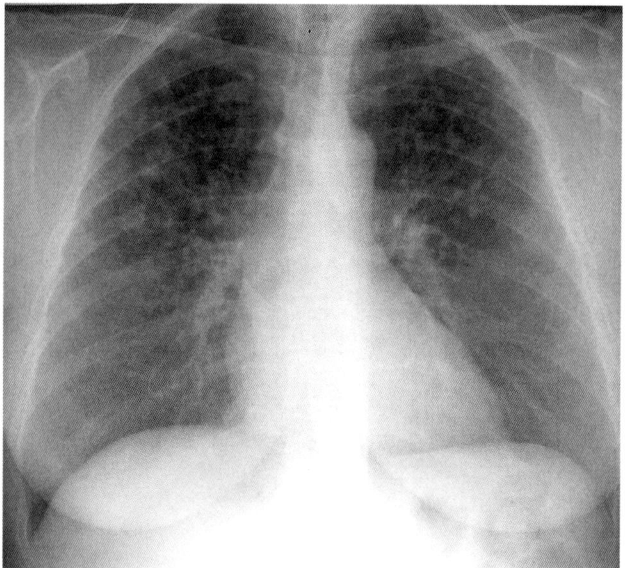

FIGURE 15.34. **Langerhans Cell Histiocytosis (LCH) of Lung.** Posteroanterior radiograph in a 52-year-old woman with LCH shows a nodular pattern with a middle and upper zone predominance.

nodular pattern may resolve completely or be replaced by a predominantly reticulonodular or reticular pattern that represents the fibrotic phase of the disease. Late stages of the disease are characterized by a coarse reticular pattern with intermixed thin-walled cysts. These cysts account for the relative preservation or increase in lung volumes typical of LCH, which is a distinguishing feature of this disease. Hilar or mediastinal lymph node enlargement is distinctly uncommon, a feature that helps distinguish LCH from sarcoidosis. Pneumothorax from rupture of a cyst or bulla is the presenting finding or develops during the course of disease in up to 25% of patients. Pleural effusion in the absence of a pneumothorax is rare. Extrapulmonary manifestations include well-defined lytic rib or vertebral lesions.

The parenchymal changes of LCH of the lung are best demonstrated on thin-section CT. Thin-section CT in patients with a relatively short duration of symptoms (<6 months) shows well-defined interstitial nodules of varying size, sometimes with cavitation, and cyst formation in the upper lungs. More long-standing disease is characterized by larger cysts (Fig. 15.35) and honeycombing. Nodules and thick-walled cysts can transform into thin-walled cysts, suggesting that the sequence of evolution of LCH lesions is as follows: nodule →cavitated nodule→thick-walled cyst→thin-walled cyst.

Features which help distinguish LCH of lung from emphysema are the presence of nodules (with or without cavitation) and thin-walled cysts in LCH that lack a constant relationship to the centrilobular core structures. The thin-section CT distinction of LCH from LAM in a woman is more difficult; an upper zone distribution and the presence of nodules favor LCH. Nodules in LAM also tend to be more uniform in shape, whereas nodules in LCH can be bizarre appearing.

The diagnosis of LCH of lung is made by noting the characteristic stellate nodular lesions with Langerhans cells on open-lung biopsy specimens. The treatment for symptomatic patients is corticosteroid therapy, although more than half of the patients with lung disease stabilize or improve spontaneously.

Granulomatosis With Polyangiitis

Granulomatosis with polyangiitis (GPA), formerly referred to as Wegener granulomatosis, is a systemic autoimmune disorder characterized pathologically by a necrotizing granulomatous vasculitis involving the upper and lower respiratory tracts and kidneys. The characteristic lesions in the lungs are discrete nodules or masses of granulomatous inflammation with central necrosis and cavitation. The lesions involve pulmonary vessels, accounting for the high incidence of central necrosis and for the occasional presentation with pulmonary hemorrhage. Mucosal and submucosal lesions may be present in the tracheobronchial tree and are seen almost exclusively in women.

Most patients with GPA are middle-aged, with a slight male predominance. The respiratory tract is affected in 100% of patients, with symptoms usually dominated by sinus and nasal mucosal involvement. Pulmonary involvement may be asymptomatic or manifested by cough, dyspnea, or chest pain. Presentation with pulmonary hemorrhage and hemoptysis may

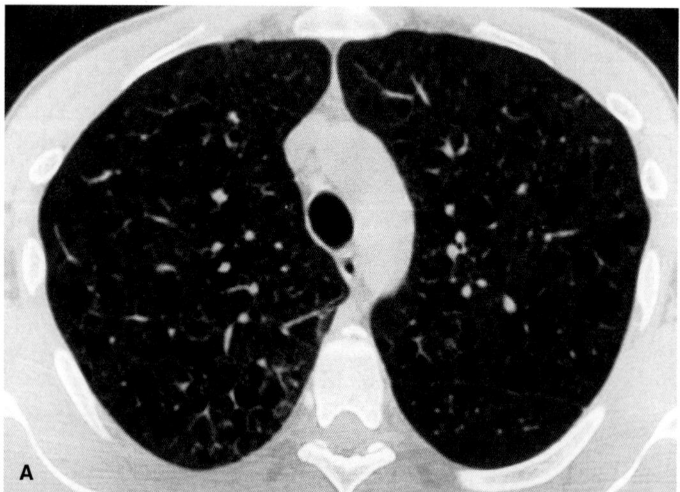

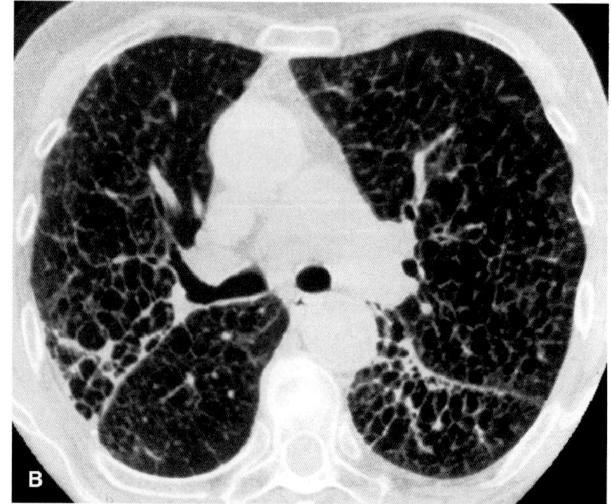

FIGURE 15.35. **Langerhans Cell Histiocytosis on Thin-Section CT. A:** Thin-section CT in a 39-year-old smoker with Langerhans cell histiocytosis shows multiple cysts with thin but well-defined walls. **B:** In another patient with LCH, the cysts are more extensive, with little normal intervening parenchyma. Note the irregular shape of many of these cysts.

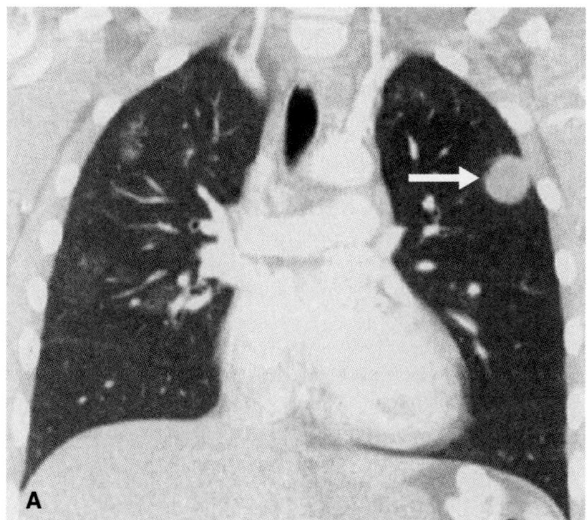

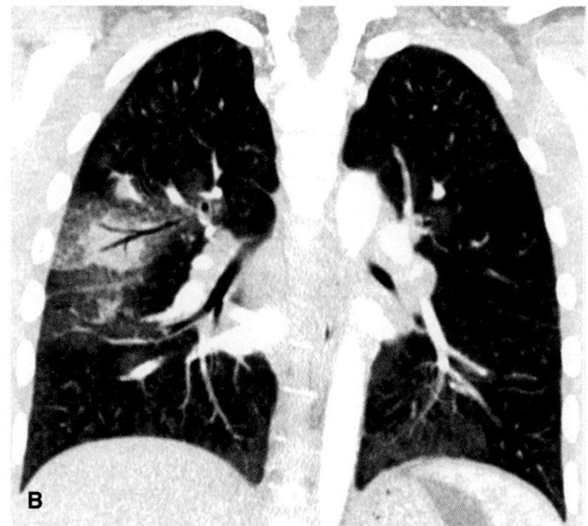

FIGURE 15.36. **Granulomatosis With Polyangiitis. A, B:** Coronal CT reconstructions through the mid (**A**) and posterior (**B**) lungs in a patient with GPA show a left upper lobe nodule (*arrow* in **A**) and ground-glass opacity in the right upper and left lower lobes.

mimic other pulmonary–renal syndromes such as Goodpasture syndrome and idiopathic pulmonary hemorrhage. Renal involvement usually follows involvement of the respiratory tract and is seen in almost 90% of patients.

The characteristic chest radiographic features of lung involvement in GPA are multiple sharply marginated nodules or masses (Fig. 15.36A); solitary lesions are seen in up to one-third of patients. Irregular, thick-walled cavitary lesions are seen in 50% of patients during the course of disease. Localized or diffuse areas of airspace opacification can represent hemorrhage or pneumonia, the latter often a result of complicating *Staphylococcus aureus* infection. Tracheal or bronchial lesions may be present and are usually best appreciated on CT, where they appear as calcified mucosal or submucosal deposits which produce irregular narrowing of the airway lumen. The airway lesions are usually not associated with parenchymal disease, but endobronchial lesions may produce distal atelectasis. Pleural effusion from pleural involvement is not uncommon. Pneumothorax may result from rupture of a cavitary lesion into the pleural space. Lymph node enlargement is not seen in this disease.

The diagnosis of GPA is be made by biopsy of involved tissues, usually nasal mucosa or lung, showing granulomatous inflammation and vasculitis that are characteristic of this disease. The pathologic changes in the kidneys are often nonspecific, and therefore renal biopsy is often nondiagnostic. This disease usually responds dramatically to cyclophosphamide (Cytoxan) therapy. Some patients with disease limited to the chest respond to oral co-trimoxazole (Bactrim). Untreated patients invariably die of renal failure or, less commonly, progressive respiratory disease. High serologic titers for the presence of antineutrophil cytoplasmic antibody are specific for the diagnosis of GPA, although a negative test does not exclude the diagnosis, particularly in patients with limited or inactive disease.

EOSINOPHILIC LUNG DISEASE

This term refers to a heterogeneous group of allergic diseases characterized by excess eosinophils in the lung and occasionally blood. Fraser and Pare have classified these diseases into three groups: idiopathic, those of known etiology, and those associated with autoimmune or collagen vascular disorders (Table 15.9).

Idiopathic Eosinophilic Lung Disease

The idiopathic disorders associated with eosinophilic lung disease include simple pulmonary eosinophilia, chronic eosinophilic pneumonia, and hypereosinophilic syndrome.

Simple pulmonary eosinophilia, also known as Löffler syndrome, is a transient pulmonary process characterized pathologically by pulmonary infiltration with an eosinophilic exudate. Most patients have a history of allergy, most commonly asthma. The characteristic radiographic findings are

TABLE 15.9

EOSINOPHILIC LUNG DISEASE

Idiopathic	Simple pulmonary eosinophilia (Löffler syndrome) Acute eosinophilic pneumonia Chronic eosinophilic pneumonia Hypereosinophilic syndrome
Known etiology	Drugs Antibiotics Penicillins Nitrofurantoin Nonsteroidal anti-inflammatory agents Aspirin Chemotherapeutic agents Bleomycin Methotrexate Parasites Filaria *Strongyloides* *Ascaris* Hookworm
Autoimmune disease	Granulomatosis with polyangiitis Sarcoidosis Rheumatoid lung disease Polyarteritis nodosa Allergic angiitis and granulomatosis (Churg–Strauss syndrome)

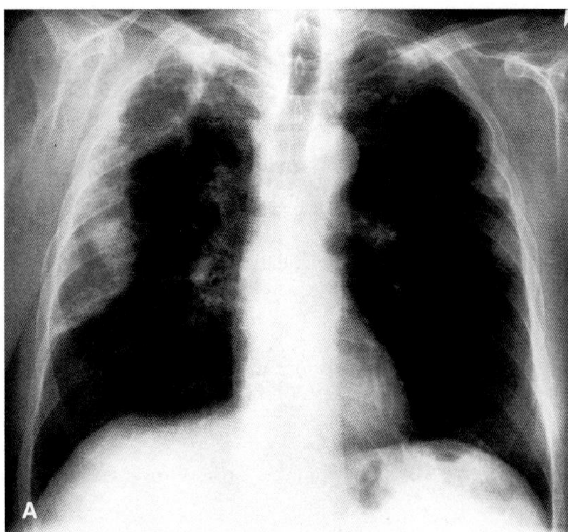

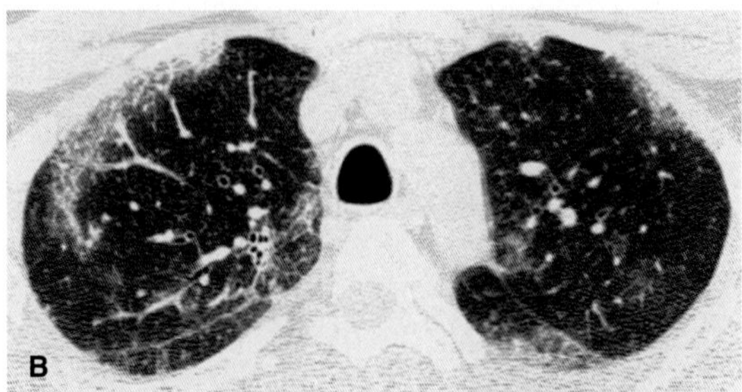

FIGURE 15.37. Eosinophilic Pneumonia. A: In a 38-year-old man with asthma, shortness of breath, and peripheral eosinophilia, a frontal chest film demonstrates bilateral peripheral airspace opacities. The patient's symptoms and the radiographic findings improved rapidly following initiation of corticosteroid therapy. **B:** CT scan in a different patient with eosinophilic pneumonia shows peripheral ground-glass opacity with reticulation in the upper lungs.

peripheral, homogeneous, ill-defined areas of airspace opacities that may parallel the chest wall (Fig. 15.37); this latter feature is best appreciated on CT. The opacities in Löffler syndrome have been described as fleeting, because there is a tendency for rapid clearing in one area with new involvement in other areas. A dry cough, dyspnea, and peripheral blood eosinophilia are common but are not invariably present. The diagnosis is based on the combination of pulmonary symptoms, blood eosinophilia, and characteristic radiographic findings. Most patients having a self-limiting illness that resolves spontaneously within 4 weeks.

Acute eosinophilic pneumonia is an idiopathic condition characterized by severe dyspnea and hypoxia lasting <5 days and >25% eosinophils on pulmonary lavage. Progression is rapid as is resolution after steroid therapy. CT abnormalities consist of patchy ground glass and interlobular septal thickening.

Chronic Eosinophilic Pneumonia. Patients with symptoms and radiographic abnormalities that last longer than 1 month are considered to have chronic eosinophilic pneumonia. The clinical and radiographic features are similar to those of Löffler syndrome, although there is a distinct predilection for women. Patients are usually symptomatic with fever, malaise, and dyspnea. The pulmonary symptoms and radiographic opacities respond dramatically to corticosteroid therapy and improve within 4 to 7 days, although relapse upon discontinuation of treatment is common.

Hypereosinophilic syndrome is a systemic disorder with a male predominance that is characterized by multiple organ damage from eosinophilic infiltration of tissues. Blood eosinophilia is prolonged and marked in this condition. The major chest radiographic findings are associated with cardiac involvement causing congestive heart failure: cardiomegaly, pulmonary edema, and pleural effusions. Pulmonary parenchymal infiltration with eosinophils may produce interstitial or airspace opacities.

Eosinophilic Lung Disease of Identifiable Etiology

Pulmonary eosinophilia of known etiology includes drug- and parasite-induced eosinophilic lung disease. Drugs associated with pulmonary eosinophilia include nitrofurantoin and penicillin. The parasitic infections most commonly responsible are filaria and the roundworms *Ascaris lumbricoides* and *Strongyloides stercoralis*. These parasites may produce pulmonary eosinophilia as they migrate through the alveolar capillaries and into the alveoli during their tour of the body. These disorders are usually indistinguishable clinically and radiographically from Löffler syndrome.

Eosinophilic Lung Disease Associated With Autoimmune Diseases

A number of autoimmune disorders are associated with eosinophilic pulmonary infiltrates. These include GPA, sarcoidosis, rheumatoid lung disease, polyarteritis nodosa, and allergic angiitis and granulomatosis. The first three disorders have a variety of thoracic manifestations and are discussed elsewhere. The predominant chest radiographic finding in polyarteritis nodosa is hemorrhage caused by a vasculitis involving the bronchial arterial circulation. This condition is discussed in Chapter 12. Allergic angiitis and granulomatosis (Churg–Strauss syndrome) is a multisystem disorder in which asthma, blood eosinophilia, necrotizing vasculitis, and extravascular granulomas are invariable features. Pulmonary involvement, as seen radiographically or pathologically, is indistinguishable from chronic eosinophilic pneumonia.

DRUG-INDUCED LUNG DISEASE

Drugs can induce a variety of adverse effects in the chest. The majority of cases of drug-induced chest disease are iatrogenic, although accidental or intentional drug overdoses may also result in severe pulmonary disease. The clinical and imaging findings are often difficult to distinguish from infection, pulmonary edema, or a pulmonary manifestation of the disease being treated. The major histiologic principal patterns of drug-induced lung damage are DAD, UIP, NSIP, bronchiolitis obliterans–organizing pneumonia (BOOP), eosinophilic lung disease, and pulmonary hemorrhage (Table 15.10). DAD, eosinophilic lung disease, and pulmonary hemorrhage are usually the result of an acute lung insult. UIP, NSIP, and BOOP are more commonly due to chronic toxicity.

TABLE 15.10

HISTOLOGIC PATTERNS IN DRUG-INDUCED LUNG TOXICITY

■ HISTOLOGY	■ COMMON CAUSES
DAD	cyclophosphamide bleomycin carmustine (BCNU) gold salts mitomycin melphalan
UIP	cyclophosphamide bleomycin methotrexate
NSIP	carmustine amiodarone methotrexate gold salts chlorambucil
Eosinophilic pneumonia	pencillamine sulfasalazine nitrofurantoin NSAIDs para-aminosalicylic acid
BOOP	bleomycin gold salts cyclophosphamide methotrexate amiodarone nitrofurantoin penicillamine sulfasalazine rituximab nivolumab pembrolizumab
Hemorrhage	anticoagulants amphotericin B cyclophosphamide mitomycin

DAD most commonly results from an acute insult to the lungs resulting in damage to type II pneumocytes and the alveolar endothelium. The initial manifestation is pulmonary edema, frequently in a geographic or nondependent distribution without much-associated pleural fluid or interlobular septal thickening. After discontinuation of the offending drug, it may resolve, stabilize, or progress to fibrosis frequently in a UIP pattern (Fig. 15.38). Drugs that commonly cause DAD include chemotherapeutic agents (busulfan, bleomycin, BCNU, and cyclophosphamide), gold salts, mitomycin, and melphalan. Opiates can also cause acute pulmonary edema.

UIP can be the result of DAD or occur as a result of chronic drug toxicity. The drugs most commonly implicated in this form of lung disease are amiodarone, nitrofurantoin (Fig. 15.39), and the chemotherapeutic agents cyclophosphamide, bleomycin, and methotrexate. Radiographically, patients present with bilateral, predominantly lower lobe, coarse reticular and linear opacities with diminished lung volumes. In patients undergoing chemotherapy for malignancy, the findings are difficult to distinguish from those of lymphangitic carcinomatosis, pulmonary hemorrhage, or opportunistic pneumonia. Pulmonary edema is the major differential diagnosis in patients receiving amiodarone therapy. The diagnosis can usually be made by excluding one of these other processes or thin-section CT.

NSIP (also referred to as chronic interstitial pneumonia when known to result from drug toxicity) is most commonly encountered with amiodarone, methotrexate, and BCNU therapy. Gold salts and chlorambucil are less common causes.

OP is a relatively common result of pulmonary drug toxicity and usually responds well to cessation of therapy and steroids. A large number of drugs have been reported to cause OP, most commonly bleomycin, cyclophosphamide, methotrexate, and gold salts; and less commonly amiodarone, nitrofurantoin, penicillamine, and sulfasalazine. Biologic agents including the TNF-α monoclonal antibody rituximab, used in non-Hodgkin lymphoma and rheumatoid arthritis, have been shown to rarely produce organizing pneumonia with associated interstitial pneumonitis (Fig. 15.40).

Eosinophilic pneumonia results from a hypersensitivity response to a metabolite of the drug combined with an endogenous protein. Antibody production directed against this hapten-protein complex leads to antibody-mediated immediate or immune complex hypersensitivity reactions. It is usually associated with

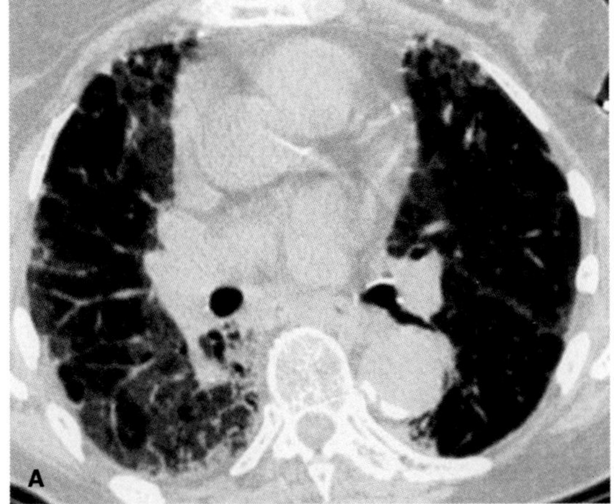

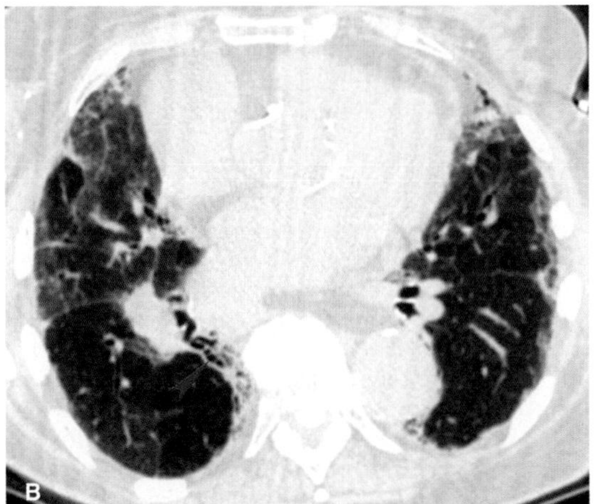

FIGURE 15.38. **Usual Interstitial Pneumonia (UIP) From Nitrofurantoin Administration.** Axial CT scans through the mid and lower lungs in an elderly woman receiving nitrofurantoin prophylaxis for recurrent urinary tract infections show bilateral subpleural reticulation with traction bronchiectasis (*arrowhead*) consistent with UIP.

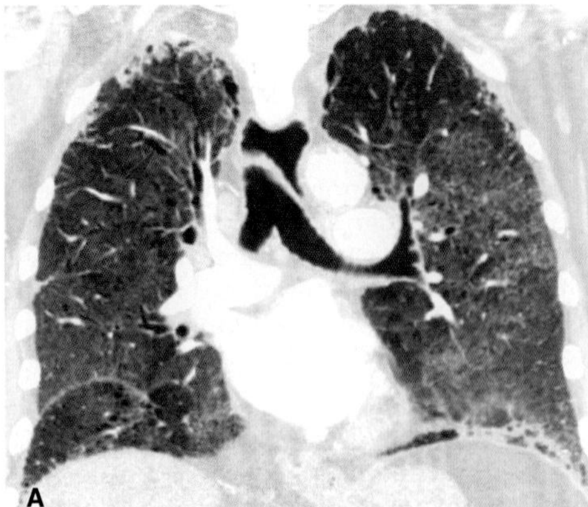

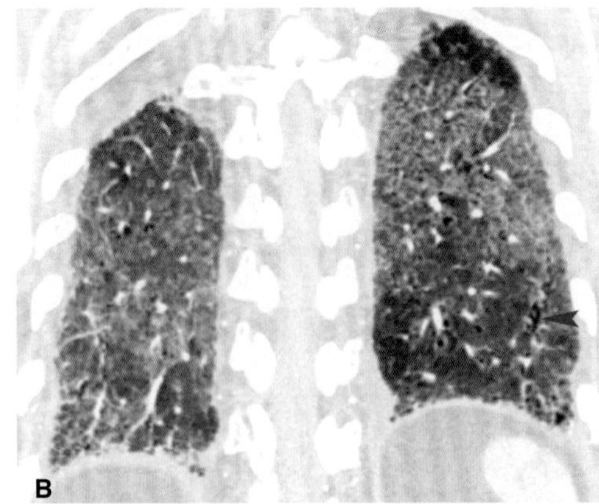

FIGURE 15.39. **Cytoxan-Induced Diffuse Alveolar Damage.** Coronal CT scans through the mid- (**A**) and posterior (**B**) lungs in a patient with biopsy-proven mixed proliferative and organizing diffuse alveolar damage from cytoxan show bilateral ground-glass and reticular opacities, with foci of traction bronchiectasis (*arrowheads*).

fever, skin rash, and blood eosinophilia. Radiographically, fleeting peripheral patchy airspace opacities develop hours to days after the initiation of drug therapy. The opacities often respond to corticosteroid therapy. Penicillin and sulfonamide antibiotics are the drugs most often associated with hypersensitivity reactions.

Pulmonary hemorrhage may be caused by drug-induced pulmonary vasculitis, complicate anticoagulation therapy, or result from drug-induced thrombocytopenia. Penicillamine therapy has been associated with pulmonary hemorrhage in patients with rheumatoid arthritis, but the mechanism is unknown. Affected individuals typically have hemoptysis and a falling hematocrit associated with the rapid development of diffuse bilateral airspace opacities. The diagnosis of hemorrhage is usually confirmed by bloody fluid return on BAL. Lavage also shows an increased percentage of alveolar macrophages containing hemosiderin. The opacities of diffuse pulmonary hemorrhage resolve completely without residual scarring unless accompanied by pulmonary infarction which may leave pleural and parenchymal scars.

Other Manifestations. Pulmonary nodules are an uncommon manifestation of chronic lung injury from bleomycin or cyclophosphamide, and in this situation, they are radiographically indistinguishable from pulmonary metastases.

A number of drugs, most commonly procainamide, hydralazine, and isoniazid, have been associated with a lupus-like syndrome that is often indistinguishable from SLE. Pleural and pericardial effusions are common. Basilar interstitial disease has been described but is uncommon.

Obliterative bronchiolitis is a small-airways inflammatory process that results in granulation tissue within bronchioles causing air trapping which can be severe enough to result in respiratory insufficiency. It can result from a variety of insults including aspiration, organ transplantation, viral infection, collagen vascular disease; and drugs, especially penicillamine, and is described in more detail in Chapter 16.

A chronic granulomatous vasculitis may develop as a response to particulate substances such as talc or starch mixed with illicit intravenous drugs. This can lead to obliteration of the pulmonary vasculature, producing pulmonary hypertension and RV failure. Radiographically, the lungs may show an interstitial pattern of disease, with enlargement of the central pulmonary arteries and right heart. The radiographs may rarely show central conglomerate masses that are indistinguishable from PMF of silicosis or end-stage sarcoidosis.

Enlargement of the hilar and mediastinal lymph nodes on chest radiographs is an uncommon manifestation of drug toxicity. Dilantin and methotrexate are the main drugs associated with this rare complication. The lymphadenopathy is usually part of a systemic hypersensitivity reaction and regresses with removal of the offending agent.

Specific Agents (Table 15.11)

Nitrofurantoin is an oral antibiotic used widely in the treatment of urinary tract infections. There are two distinct patterns of nitrofurantoin-associated pulmonary reaction: acute and chronic. The acute form, seen in approximately 90% of cases, most likely represents a hypersensitivity reaction. The chest radiograph demonstrates interstitial or mixed alveolar/interstitial infiltrates with a basal predominance, often accompanied by small pleural effusions. The chronic form occurs after weeks to years of continuous therapy and is probably caused by direct toxic damage. Interstitial pneumonitis and fibrosis indistinguishable from IPF are seen pathologically (Fig. 15.38).

Bleomycin is a cytotoxic antibiotic used in the treatment of lymphoma, squamous cell carcinoma, and testicular cancer. Bleomycin-induced lung disease is related to the cumulative dosage of the drug. Free oxygen radicals within the lung are felt to play a major role in the lung injury and account for the deleterious effects of supplemental oxygen administration in patients with bleomycin toxicity. The typical radiographic pattern is that of bilateral lower lobe reticular opacities. A minority of patients will demonstrate acute patchy or confluent airspace opacities as a result of a hypersensitivity reaction to the drug or DAD. The reticular or airspace opacities tend to have a basal predominance. Solitary or multiple pulmonary nodules constitute an unusual radiographic appearance of bleomycin lung toxicity that is indistinguishable radiographically from pulmonary metastases, but the lesions generally disappear following cessation of the drug.

Alkylating Agents. Drugs such as busulfan, which is used in the treatment of myeloproliferative disorders, and cyclophosphamide (Cytoxan), used widely in the treatment of malignancies and autoimmune disease, cause clinically recognizable pulmonary toxicity in 1% to 4% of patients. Pathologic findings include organizing intra-alveolar exudate, fibrosis, and

TABLE 15.11

SPECIFIC DRUG TOXICITIES

■ DRUG	■ PRIMARY PATHOLOGY	■ TREATMENT	■ INCIDENCE	■ PROGNOSIS
cyclophosphamide	DAD NSIP BOOP	d/c drug	Common	Good
carmustine	DAD NSIP	d/c drug	20–50%	Good
bleomycin	DAD NSIP BOOP	d/c drug	3–5%	Poor
amiodarone	NSIP BOOP Pleural effusions	d/c drug	5–10%	Good
gold salts	DAD and NSIP BOOP	d/c drug	1%	Good
methotrexate	NSIP HSP BOOP	None	5–10%	Good
nitrofurantoin	NSIP	d/c		Good
nivolumab	BOOP	d/c	5%	Good

the presence of large atypical type 2 pneumocytes. Radiographically, a diffuse reticular pattern with basal predominance is seen; airspace opacities may be present and are more common with busulfan than cyclophosphamide.

Cytosine Arabinoside (Ara-C) is an antimetabolic agent generally used to treat acute leukemia. Pulmonary toxicity develops in 15% to 30% of treated patients within 30 days of administration and is manifested as pulmonary edema resulting from increased capillary permeability.

Methotrexate is an antimetabolite used for the treatment of malignancies and autoimmune diseases such as rheumatoid arthritis and psoriasis. In contrast to bleomycin and the alkylating agents, methotrexate usually causes reversible pulmonary disease caused by a hypersensitivity reaction rather than direct

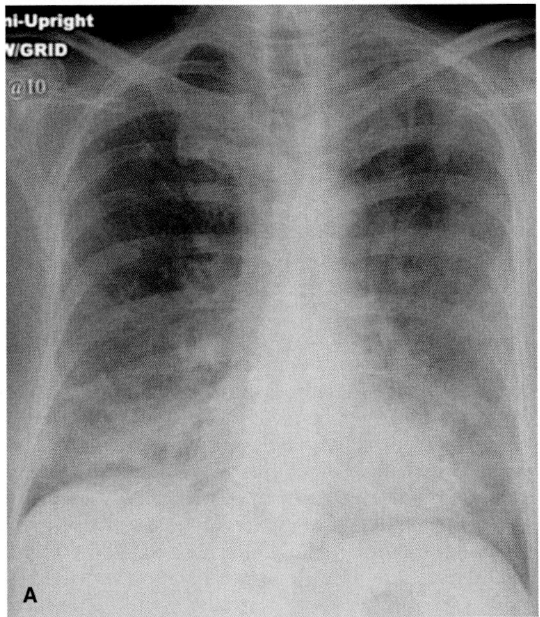

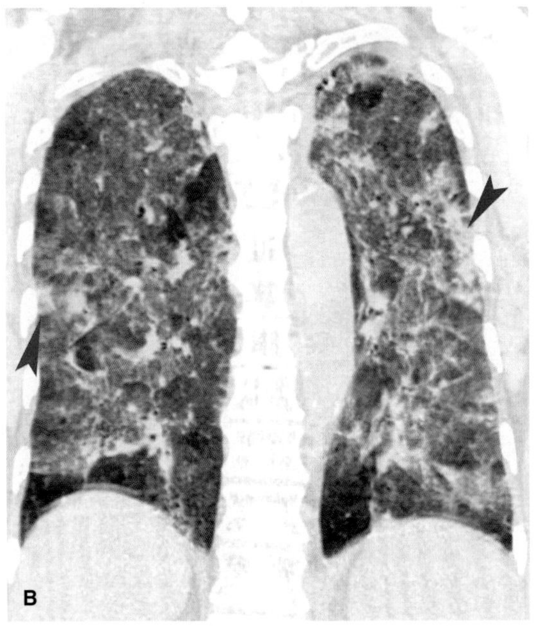

FIGURE 15.40. **Rituximab-Induced Diffuse Lung Disease.** Chest radiograph (**A**) in a patient receiving rituximab to prevent renal transplant rejection shows a diffuse bilateral pattern of ground-glass and basilar airspace opacification. CT with coronal reformation (**B**) shows a mixed pattern of ground-glass and patchy airspace opacities (*arrowheads*) and minimal reticulation. Open-lung biopsy showed a mixed pattern of organizing pneumonia and interstitial pneumonitis. The patient responded to discontinuation of the rituximab and corticosteroid administration.

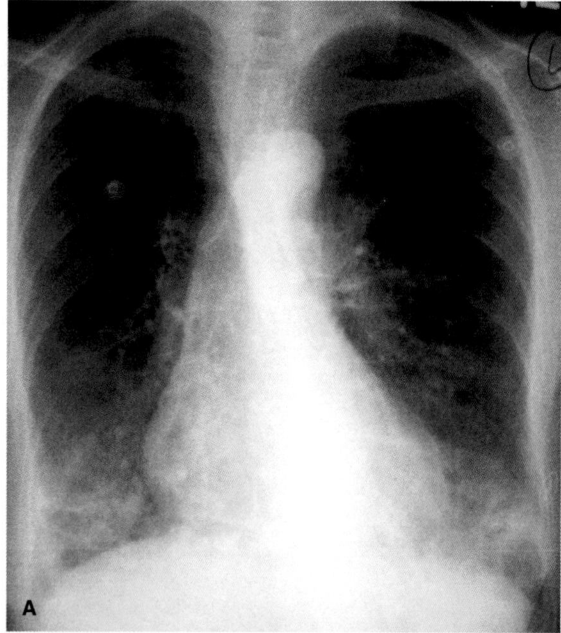

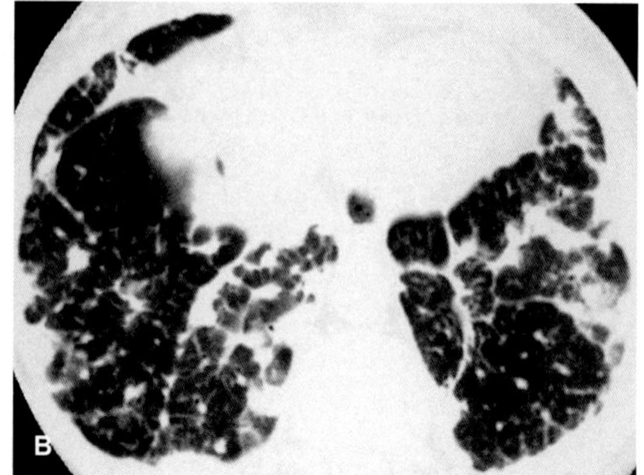

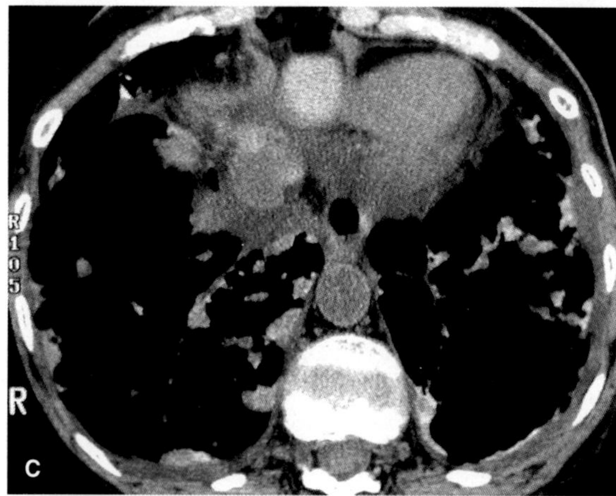

FIGURE 15.41. **Amiodarone Lung Toxicity.** Frontal chest radiograph (**A**) in a 64-year-old patient who experienced progressive shortness of breath while receiving amiodarone for ventricular tachycardia shows cardiomegaly, basilar coarse interstitial opacities, and small pleural effusions. Thin-section unenhanced CT scan through the lung bases at lung windows (**B**) shows coarse reticular and nodular opacities, which were high attenuation at mediastinal windows (**C**), consistent with amiodarone lung toxicity.

toxic damage to the lung. DAD leading to restrictive lung disease is seen in approximately 10% of cases, however, and appears radiographically as a diffuse reticular pattern.

Amiodarone, an antiarrhythmic agent, is an important cause of drug-induced pulmonary damage, affecting approximately 5% of individuals on chronic therapy. Amiodarone is concentrated in the lung and has a long tissue half-life. The exact mechanism of lung damage is unknown but relates to the accumulation of phospholipids, which disturb metabolic functions in the lung. Pathologically, there is inflammation and fibrosis of the alveolar septae, with an accumulation of lipid-laden alveolar macrophages and hyperplasia of type 2 pneumocytes.

Pulmonary toxicity begins months to years after the initiation of therapy. Patients typically present with dyspnea or a nonproductive cough, which may be difficult to distinguish from congestive heart failure or pneumonia. The chest film typically shows airspace and reticular opacities. CT findings show significant overlap with findings of pulmonary edema—which is common in these patients—with reticulation and, ground-glass and airspace opacities. Findings of fibrosis and high attenuation within parenchymal abnormalities should strongly suggest amiodarone toxicity (Fig. 15.41). Amiodarone should be withdrawn or the dose diminished at the earliest sign of toxicity because the drug has an extraordinarily long half-life (approximately 90 days). The cessation of amiodarone at an early stage of toxicity, with occasional use of corticosteroids, usually provides relief.

MISCELLANEOUS DISORDERS

Pulmonary alveolar proteinosis is a rare disease in which the lipoproteinaceous material surfactant deposits in abnormal amounts within the airspaces of the lung. Idiopathic PAP has a predilection for males in their 20s to 40s, although the disease has been reported in children. In adults, PAP has been seen in patients with acute silicoproteinosis and immunocompromised patients with lymphoma, leukemia, or AIDS. These conditions are associated with an acquired defect of alveolar macrophages that causes them to fail to phagocytize surfactant, resulting in the accumulation of surfactant within the alveolar spaces. Pathologically, the alveoli are filled with a lipoproteinaceous material that stains deep pink with periodic acid–Schiff. The interstitium is usually not involved, but some patients may have chronic interstitial inflammation and fibrosis.

Patients with PAP are often asymptomatic, although some complain of progressive dyspnea and a nonproductive cough. The absence of orthopnea is an important clinical feature

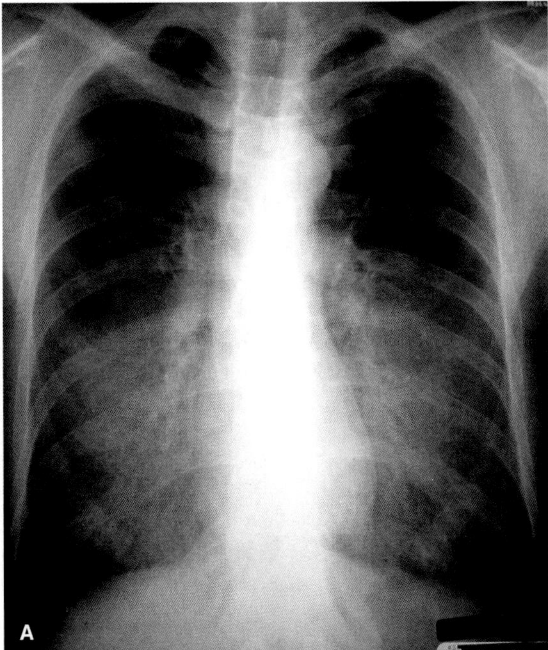

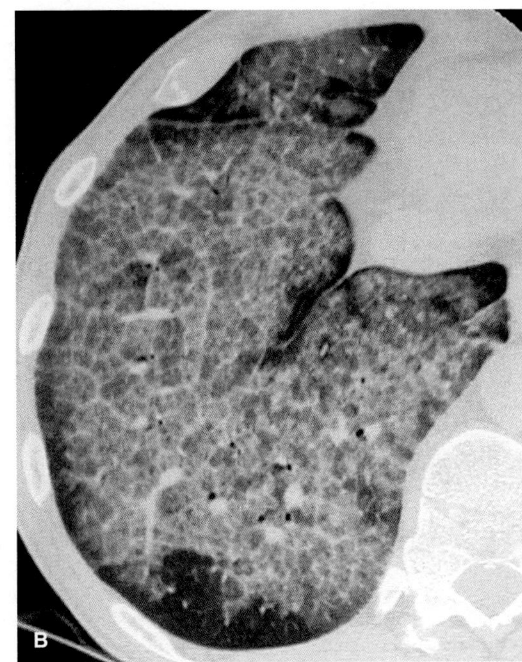

FIGURE 15.42. Pulmonary Alveolar Proteinosis (PAP). A: Frontal chest radiograph in a 34-year-old man with PAP demonstrates subtle bilateral ground-glass opacities. **B:** A CT scan viewed at the lung windows shows a mixed pattern of ground-glass attenuation superimposed on thickened interlobular and intralobular lines, which has been termed "crazy paving" and is characteristic of this disorder.

distinguishing PAP from pulmonary edema secondary to congestive heart failure.

The typical radiographic finding in alveolar proteinosis is bilateral symmetric perihilar airspace opacification, which is indistinguishable in appearance from pulmonary edema (Fig. 15.42). Airspace nodules are commonly seen at the periphery of the confluent opacities. Cardiomegaly, pleural effusions, and evidence of pulmonary venous hypertension are notably absent. Thin-section CT scans typically show geographic ground-glass opacities superimposed upon thickened interlobular and intralobular septa, a pattern that has been described as "crazy paving." While crazy paving in the proper clinical setting is characteristic of this disease, a number of other conditions can produce this pattern on thin-section CT, most commonly pulmonary edema (particularly permeability edema), atypical pneumonia and pulmonary hemorrhage, and rarely, bronchoalveolar cell carcinoma.

Patients with PAP are particularly prone to superinfection of the lung with *Nocardia, Aspergillus, Cryptococcus,* and atypical mycobacteria. The factors responsible for this may include macrophage dysfunction and the favorable culture medium of intra-alveolar lipoproteinaceous material. Infection by one of these organisms should be suspected in any patient with PAP who develops symptoms of pneumonia or radiographic findings of focal parenchymal opacification or cavitation and pleural effusion. CT helps in the early detection of opportunistic infection, because pneumonia or abscess formation may be obscured by the underlying process on conventional radiographs.

Prior to the advent of BAL, one-third of patients died from respiratory failure or opportunistic infections, while the remaining two-thirds either stabilized or resolved spontaneously. Repeated BAL with saline has significantly reduced the mortality from this disease. The duration of treatment with BAL varies; some patients require repetitive long-term therapy, while others resolve after a single treatment. Recently, the recognition that patients with PAP have deficient levels of granulocyte-macrophage colony-stimulating factor (GM-CSF) in alveolar macrophages has led to therapy with GM-CSF, which is an alternative to lung lavage for treatment of this disease.

Alveolar microlithiasis is a rare disorder characterized by the deposition of minute calculi within the alveolar spaces. While alveolar microlithiasis can affect individuals of any age without sex predilection, there is a very high incidence of this disease in siblings. The underlying abnormality responsible for the formation of these calculi, known as calcospherites, is unknown. These are small calculi, measuring less than 1 mm in diameter, which are composed of calcium phosphate. Pathologically, these calculi are found within normal alveoli; interstitial fibrosis may develop in long-standing disease. The radiographic findings are specific: confluent bilateral dense micronodular opacities that, because of their high intrinsic density, produce the so-called "black pleura sign" at their interface with the chest wall. Apical bullous disease is common and may lead to spontaneous pneumothorax. The diagnosis is made by a history of alveolar microlithiasis in a sibling of an affected individual in combination with typical radiographic findings. Biopsy is usually unnecessary. The majority of patients are asymptomatic at presentation despite the marked radiographic abnormalities, a feature that is characteristic of this disorder. Most patients develop progressive respiratory insufficiency, although some remain stable for years. There is no effective treatment.

Diffuse pulmonary ossification is an uncommon condition characterized by the formation of bone within the lung parenchyma. The nodular form of this disease is seen in severe, chronic untreated mitral stenosis, while more irregular ossification is seen in chronic inflammatory conditions such as amyloidosis and UIP. The condition is appreciated as nodular or linear areas of high attenuation on thin-section CT. Other conditions that can produce high-attenuation material in the lung parenchyma include pulmonary calcification in secondary hyperparathyroidism, in which there is an upper lobe predilection, and amiodarone lung toxicity, in which the deposition of an iodinated metabolite of amiodarone accumulates in the lung, liver, and thyroid.

Acute fibrinous and organizing pneumonia refers to a pattern of lung injury characterized by organizing pneumonia and fibrin within the alveolar space that does not meet strict histopathologic criteria for DAD or organizing pneumonia. Many causes have been suggested including toxic fume inhalation, drug toxicity, autoimmune disease, and infection. The clinical course may be fulminant resulting in death, or subacute with eventual recovery. In the fulminant form, the imaging findings are indistinguishable from DAD, and in the subacute form from OP.

Combined pulmonary fibrosis and emphysema syndrome (CPFE) is a clinical syndrome resulting from the coexistence of emphysema and pulmonary fibrosis, whether both secondary to smoking or of different etiologies. Most patients with fibrosis and emphysema will have symptoms predominantly due to one or the other. In some patients, however, the combination of the physiologic effects of emphysema (increased lung volume and compliance with reduced maximal expiratory flow) and pulmonary fibrosis (decreased lung volume and compliance with maintenance of expiratory flow) results in relatively normal spirometric measurements, but severely impaired gas exchange. Thin-section CT plays an important role in identifying these patients as clinical and laboratory assessment may fail to recognize the combination of abnormalities. The distinction is important clinically as the prognosis is different than in patients with fibrosis or emphysema alone. The CT findings are the same regardless of whether the patient has CPFE syndrome or not, with upper zone centrilobular emphysema and basilar fibrosis (most frequently in a UIP pattern). In some cases it is difficult to assess the relative extent of each as there can be overlap in the appearance of emphysema, especially the paraseptal variety, and honeycomb cysts.

References and Suggested Readings

Aylwin ACB, Gishen P, Copley SJ. Imaging appearance of thoracic amyloidosis. *J Thorac Imaging* 2005;20(1):41–46.

Fischer A, Antoniou KM, Brown KK, et al. An official European Respiratory Society/American Thoracic Society research statement: interstitial pneumonia with autoimmune features. *Eur Respir J* 2015;46(4):976–987.

Frankel SK, Cool CD, Lynch DA, Brown KK. Idiopathic pleuroparenchymal fibroelastosis: description of a novel clinicopathologic entity. *Chest* 2004;126(6):2007–2013.

Holbert JM, Costello P, Li W, Hoffman RM, Rogers RM. CT features of pulmonary alveolar proteinosis. *AJR Am J Roentgenol* 2001;176(5):1287–1294.

Jankowich MD, Rounds SIS. Combined pulmonary fibrosis and emphysema syndrome: a review. *Chest* 2012;141(1):222–231.

Johkoh T, Müller NL, Akira M, et al. Eosinophilic lung diseases: diagnostic accuracy of thin-section CT in 111 patients. *Radiographics* 2000;216(3):773–780.

Kazerooni EA. High-resolution CT of the lungs. *AJR Am J Roentgenol* 2001;177(3): 501–519.

Kim KI, Kim CW, Lee MK, et al. Imaging of occupational lung disease. *Radiographics* 2001;21(6):1371–1391.

Kim EA, Lee KS, Johkoh T, et al. Interstitial lung diseases associated with collagen vascular diseases: radiologic and histopathologic findings. *Radiographics* 2002;22(Suppl 1):S151–S165.

Kligerman SJ, Franks TJ, Galvin JR. From the radiologic pathology archives: organization and fibrosis as a response to lung injury in diffuse alveolar damage, organizing pneumonia, and acute fibrinous and organizing pneumonia. *Radiographics* 2013;33(7):1951–1975.

Koyama T, Ueda H, Togashi K, Umeoka S, Kataoka M, Nagai S. Radiologic manifestations of sarcoidosis in various organs. *Radiographics* 2004;24(1): 87–104.

Lynch DA, Rose CS, Way D, King TE. Hypersensitivity pneumonitis: sensitivity of high-resolution CT in a population-based study. *AJR Am J Roentgenol* 1992;159(3):469–472.

Lynch DA, Sverzellati N, Travis WD, et al. Diagnostic criteria for idiopathic pulmonary fibrosis: a Fleischner Society White Paper. *Lancet Respir Med* 2018; 6(2):138–153.

Mayberry JP, Primack SL, Muller NL. Thoracic manifestations of systemic autoimmune diseases: radiographic and high-resolution CT findings. *Radiographics* 2000;20(6):1623–1635.

Pallisa E, Sanz P, Roman A, Majo J, Andreu J, Caceres J. Lymphangiomyomatosis: pulmonary and abdominal findings with pathologic correlation. *Radiographics* 2002;22(Suppl 1):S185–S198.

Pandit-Bhalla M, Diethelm L, Ovella T, Sloop GD, Valentine VG. Idiopathic interstitial pneumonias: an update. *J Thorac Imaging* 2003;18(1):1–13.

Reddy TL, Tominaga M, Hansell DM, et al. Pleuroparenchymal fibroelastosis: a spectrum of histopathological and imaging phenotypes. *Eur Respir J* 2012:40(2):377–385.

Rossi SE, Erasmus JJ, McAdams HP. Pulmonary drug toxicity: radiologic and pathologic manifestations. *Radiographics* 2000;20(5):1245–1259.

Sundar KM, Gosselin MV, Chung H, Cahill BC. Pulmonary Langerhans cell histiocytosis: emerging concepts on pathobiology, radiology, and clinical evolution of disease. *Chest* 2003;123(5):1673–1683.

Sverzellati N, Lynch DA, Hansell DM, et al. American Thoracic Society-European Respiratory Society classification of the idiopathic interstitial pneumonias: advances in knowledge since 2002. *Radiographics* 2015;35(7): 1849–1872.

CHAPTER 16 ■ AIRWAYS DISEASE AND EMPHYSEMA

VIVEK KALIA AND JEFFREY S. KLEIN

INTRODUCTION

Airways disease describes a broad spectrum of congenital and acquired conditions that may be asymptomatic but more commonly produce symptoms of shortness of breath or cough. The imaging of airways disease is important to understand as affected patients will usually be referred for imaging early in the course of their evaluation. This chapter will review the radiographic and CT findings associated with diseases of the large airways (i.e., trachea, central bronchi, and bronchi) and small airways diseases.

TRACHEA AND CENTRAL BRONCHI

Congenital Tracheal and Bronchial Anomalies

Tracheal agenesis, cartilaginous abnormalities of the trachea, tracheal webs and stenosis, tracheoesophageal fistulas, and vascular rings and slings present as breathing and feeding difficulties in the neonatal and infancy period. These are uncommon congenital lesions that are discussed in Chapter 67.

Tracheal bronchus, or bronchus suis, so called because it is the normal pattern of tracheal branching in pigs, consists of an accessory bronchus to all or a portion of the right upper lobe that arises from the right lateral tracheal wall within 2 cm of the tracheal carina (Fig. 16.1). It most often supplies the apical segment of the right upper lobe. While it is usually an incidental finding on chest CT in 0.5% to 1.0% of the population, there is an association with congenital tracheal stenosis. Most patients are asymptomatic, though resultant retained secretions may produce expiratory stridor and/or recurrent infections.

Bronchial Atresia. This is characterized by atresia of a segmental or subsegmental bronchus with a normal distal airway. The patent airway distal to the atretic segment often fills with mucus (i.e., bronchocele) and the distal lung parenchyma becomes hyperinflated due to air trapping. Patients are usually asymptomatic but may present with recurrent infections. CT often shows a geographic hyperlucent segment of lung parenchyma, frequently in the upper lobes, and associated with a hyperdense tubular structure (the bronchocele) (Fig. 16.2).

Bronchial Branching Anomalies. Congenital branching anomalies of the bronchi are common asymptomatic findings on chest CT and reflect either *displaced* bronchi (the bronchus arises from an abnormal location) or *supernumerary* bronchi (where a bronchus supplies a portion of lung in addition to the normal bronchus).

Focal Tracheal Disease

Focal disorders of the trachea may produce narrowing or dilatation of the tracheal lumen (Table 16.1). They may be characterized as benign neoplasms (such as papilloma and carcinoid), malignant neoplasms (such as squamous cell carcinoma and adenoid cystic carcinoma), and nonneoplastic conditions (such as tuberculosis [TB], postintubation stenosis, and foreign body).

Focal tracheal dilatation is caused by congenital or acquired abnormalities of the elastic membrane or cartilaginous rings of the trachea. Localized tracheal dilatation may be seen with tracheoceles, with acquired tracheomalacia related to prolonged endotracheal intubation, or as a result of tracheal traction from severe unilateral upper lobe parenchymal scarring. Tracheoceles, also known as paratracheal air cysts, may be congenital or acquired. The most common tracheocele represents a true tracheal diverticulum due to herniation of the tracheal air column through a weakened posterior tracheal membrane. These lesions occur almost exclusively in the cervical trachea because the pressure gradient from the extrathoracic trachea to the atmosphere with the Valsalva maneuver favors their formation in this region. Tracheoceles are usually asymptomatic and are easily recognized on CT as circular lucencies along the right posterolateral trachea at the thoracic inlet.

Extrinsic Mass Effect. The most common cause of extrinsic mass effect on the trachea is a tortuous or dilated aortic arch or brachiocephalic artery, typically seen as rightward deviation of the distal trachea in older individuals. An intrathoracic goiter or a large paratracheal lymph node mass is an additional cause of extrinsic tracheal mass effect. Extrinsic mass effect can also be seen with congenital vascular anomalies, such as

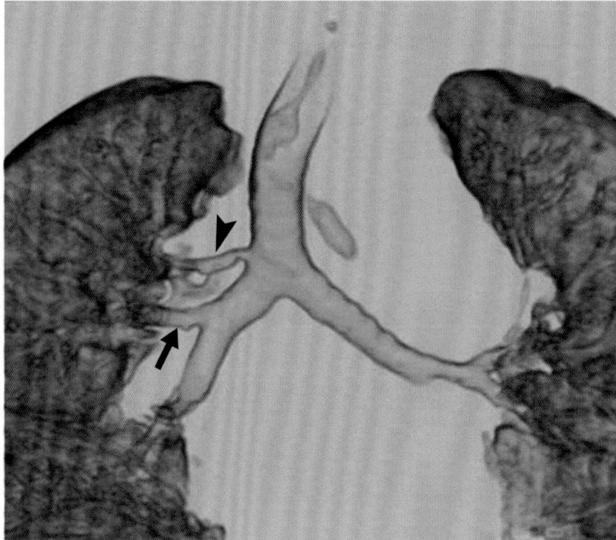

FIGURE 16.1. **Tracheal Bronchus.** Shaded surface rendering of a helical CT dataset reveals an anomalous bronchus (*arrowhead*) supplying a portion of the right upper lobe arising from the right lateral tracheal wall above the tracheal carina. Note the right upper lobe bronchus (*arrow*).

an aberrant left pulmonary artery (PA) and aortic ring, or with a large mediastinal bronchogenic cyst. Because the tracheal cartilage provides resiliency, extrinsic masses tend to displace the trachea without narrowing its lumen. Traction deformity of the trachea is generally seen in cicatrizing processes that asymmetrically affect the lung apices, most commonly postprimary TB, histoplasmosis, and radiation fibrosis. Occasionally, the distal trachea is narrowed in patients with sclerosing mediastinitis, although this disorder more commonly affects the central bronchi.

Focal Tracheal Stenosis. Focal tracheal or central (main and proximal lobar) bronchial narrowing may result from inflammatory disorders that affect the tracheal or central bronchial walls. Cartilaginous damage or the development of granulation tissue and fibrosis from a tracheostomy or at the site of a previously inflated endotracheal tube balloon cuff can lead to focal tracheal narrowing (Fig. 16.3). Tracheal stenosis has a typical hourglass deformity on frontal radiography. Those patients with tracheomalacia from cartilage damage may manifest narrowing only during phases of the respiratory cycle when extratracheal pressure exceeds intratracheal pressure. Therefore, patients with extrathoracic tracheomalacia, most often at the site of a prior tracheostomy, demonstrate tracheal narrowing on inspiration, whereas patients with intrathoracic tracheomalacia, usually from prior endotracheal intubation, have tracheal narrowing on expiration. Postintubation stenosis is rare with the low-pressure, high-volume endotracheal tube cuffs in current use. Granulomatosis with polyangiitis (GPA) can produce a necrotizing granulomatous inflammation of the trachea and central bronchi, leading to focal cervical tracheal narrowing or, in advanced disease, narrowing of the entire length of the trachea. The diagnosis of tracheal involvement by GPA is made by the radiographic demonstration of tracheal narrowing in association with upper airway and renal involvement and characteristic findings on biopsy.

A number of infectious processes may result in tracheal or bronchial inflammation and stenosis. Endotracheal and endobronchial tuberculoses are usually associated with cavitary TB, where the production of large volumes of infected sputum predisposes to tracheal and central bronchial infections. Upper tracheal inflammation and stenosis may result from histoplasmosis and coccidioidomycosis. Invasive tracheobronchitis from aspergillosis, candidiasis, and mucormycosis has been described in immunocompromised patients. Tracheal scleroma is a chronic granulomatous disorder caused by infection with *Klebsiella rhinoscleromatis*. This disease is uncommon in the United States and is seen most commonly in people of lower socioeconomic status in Central and South America and Eastern Europe.

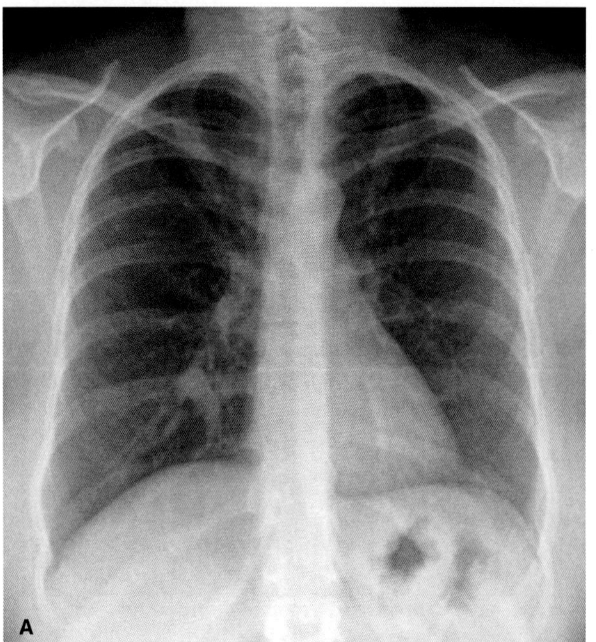

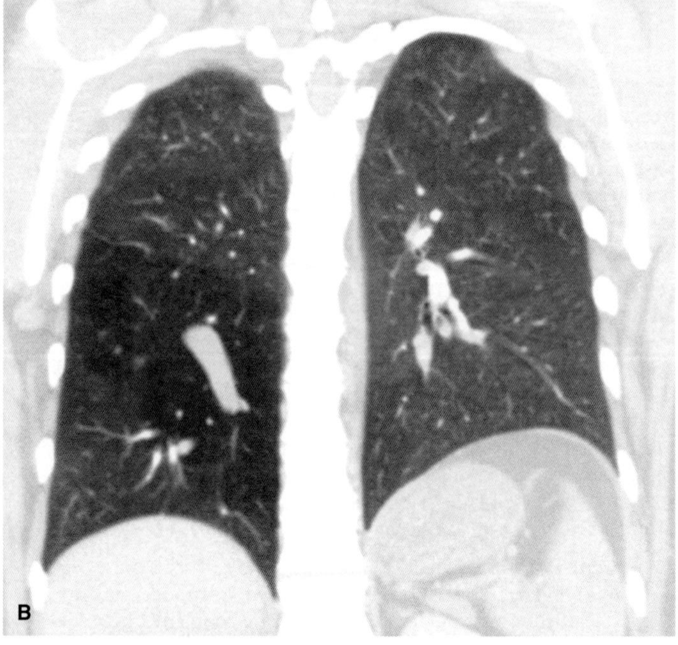

FIGURE 16.2. **Bronchial Atresia. A:** Frontal chest radiograph in an asymptomatic patient shows a curvilinear opacity in the medial right lower lung. **B:** Coronal CT through the posterior lungs shows a tubular opacity in the right lower lobe representing a dilated, mucus-filled bronchus surrounded by hyperlucent lung. Note that the dilated bronchus is larger in diameter than the normal vessels in the lungs.

TABLE 16.1

CAUSES OF FOCAL TRACHEAL DISEASE

Narrowing	Extrinsic
	  Thyroid goiter
	  Paratracheal lymph node mass
	  Asymmetric or unilateral upper lobe fibrosis
	    Tuberculosis
	    Histoplasmosis
	Intrinsic
	  Tracheomalacia
	    Endotracheal tube cuff
	    Tracheostomy site
	  Granulomatosis with polyangiitis
	  Sarcoidosis
	  Infection
	    Tuberculosis
	    Fungus
	    Histoplasmosis
	    Coccidioidomycosis
	    Aspergillosis
	    Scleroma

Masses	Neoplasm
	  Malignant
	    Primary
	      Squamous cell carcinoma
	      Adenoid cystic carcinoma (cylindroma)
	    Metastatic
	      Direct invasion
	        Laryngeal carcinoma
	        Thyroid carcinoma
	        Esophageal carcinoma
	        Bronchogenic carcinoma
	      Hematogenous (endobronchial)
	        Breast carcinoma
	        Renal cell carcinoma
	        Colon carcinoma
	        Melanoma
	  Benign
	    Chondroma
	    Fibroma
	    Squamous cell papilloma
	    Hemangioma
	    Granular cell myoblastoma
	Nonneoplastic
	  Ectopic thyroid or thymus
	  Mucus

Dilatation	Tracheoceles Tracheomalacia Upper lobe fibrosis

Tracheal and bronchial masses are mostly neoplasms and are discussed in Chapter 13.

Diffuse Tracheal Disease

Diffuse disorders of the trachea manifest as either narrowing or dilatation of the tracheal lumen. Diffuse tracheal narrowing may be seen with saber-sheath trachea, amyloidosis, tracheobronchopathia osteochondroplastica, relapsing polychondritis, GPA, or tracheal scleroma (Table 16.2). The latter two conditions may cause diffuse tracheal narrowing, but more commonly the involvement is limited to the cervical trachea.

TABLE 16.2

CAUSES OF DIFFUSE TRACHEAL DISEASE

Tracheal narrowing	Congenital tracheal stenosis (complete cartilage rings) Saber-sheath trachea Amyloidosis Tracheobronchopathia osteochondroplastica Relapsing polychondritis Granulomatosis with polyangiitis Tracheal scleroma
Tracheal dilatation	Tracheobronchomegaly (Mounier–Kuhn syndrome) Tracheomalacia Pulmonary fibrosis

Diffuse Tracheal Narrowing

Congenital tracheal stenosis is a rare condition in which there is incomplete septation of the cartilage rings, producing a long segment tracheal narrowing or "napkin ring" trachea. This anomaly is often associated with other congenital cardiovascular anomalies, in particular anomalous origin of the left PA from the right PA ("PA sling").

Saber-sheath trachea is a fixed deformity of the intrathoracic trachea in which the coronal diameter is diminished to less than two-thirds of the sagittal diameter. The tracheal wall is uniformly thickened, and calcification of the cartilaginous rings is present in most cases. This entity most commonly affects older men with chronic obstructive pulmonary disease (COPD). The tracheal narrowing likely reflects the chronic transmission of increased intrapleural pressure seen in obstructive lung disease and tracheal injury from chronic cough. The characteristic findings are apparent on frontal radiographs and CT (Fig. 16.4).

Amyloidosis is characterized by the deposition of a fibrillar protein–polysaccharide complex in various organs. It may involve the airways as part of localized or systemic disease. Submucosal deposits in the tracheobronchial tree are more commonly a manifestation of localized disease and may be associated with nodular or alveolar septal deposits in the lungs. Mass-like circumferential deposits that irregularly narrow the tracheal lumen are best demonstrated on CT and can result in recurrent atelectasis and pneumonia. Calcification of these deposits occurs in only 10% of cases. The diagnosis is made by the presence of typical protein–polysaccharide deposits demonstrated following Congo red staining of tracheal or bronchial wall biopsy specimens. This typically demonstrates apple-green birefringence when viewed under polarized light (Fig. 16.5).

Tracheobronchopathia osteochondroplastica is a rare disorder characterized by the presence of multiple submucosal osseous and cartilaginous deposits within the trachea and central bronchi of elderly men. The lesions arise as enchondromas from the tracheal and bronchial cartilage, and then project internally to produce nodular submucosal deposits that irregularly narrow the tracheal lumen and have a characteristic appearance and feel on bronchoscopy. The diagnosis is generally made on bronchoscopy and CT, where calcified plaques can be seen involving the anterior and lateral walls of the trachea. Sparing of the membranous posterior wall of the trachea, which lacks cartilage, is a helpful feature that distinguishes this entity from tracheobronchial amyloid (Fig. 16.6). While usually asymptomatic, patients may have recurrent infection related to bronchial obstruction by the masses.

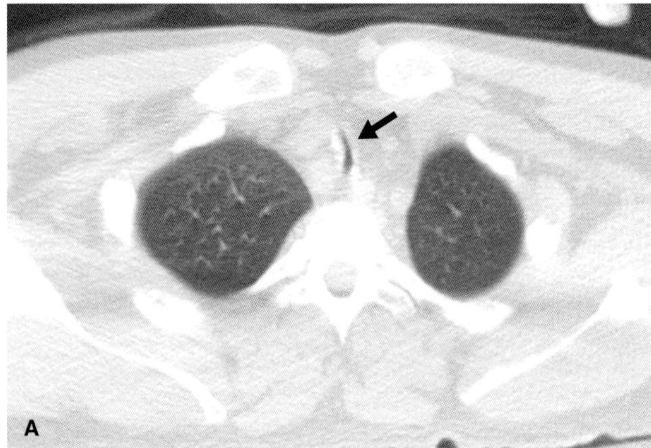
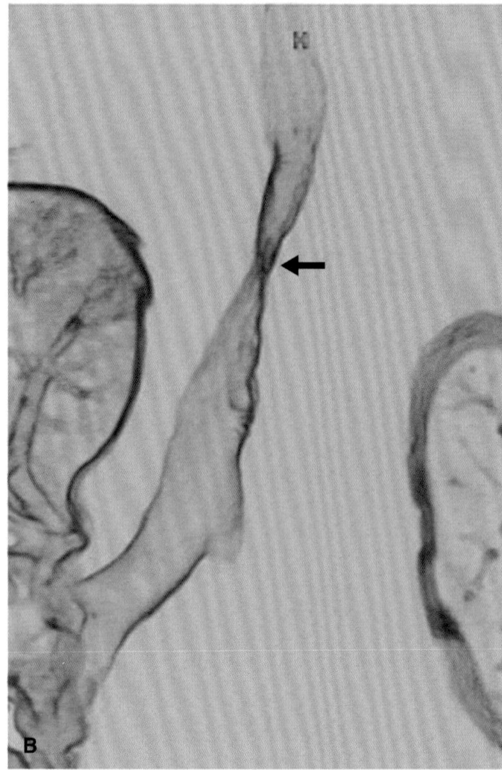

FIGURE 16.3. **Tracheal Stenosis From Prior Intubation.** Axial CT scan at lung windows through the upper trachea (**A**) and shaded surface rendering from helical CT scan (**B**) show marked narrowing (*arrows*) of the trachea in the coronal plane because of prior intubation with resultant stenosis.

Relapsing polychondritis is a systemic autoimmune disorder that commonly affects the cartilage of the earlobes, nose, larynx, tracheobronchial tree, joints, and large elastic arteries. Early in the disease, tracheal wall inflammation associated with cartilage destruction leads to an abnormally compliant and dilated trachea. Later in the disease, fibrosis leads to diffuse fixed narrowing of the tracheal lumen. Respiratory complications secondary to involvement of the upper airway cartilage account for nearly 50% of all deaths from this condition. The diagnosis is made by noting recurrent inflammation at two or more cartilaginous sites, most commonly the pinnae of the ear (producing cauliflower ears) and the bridge of the

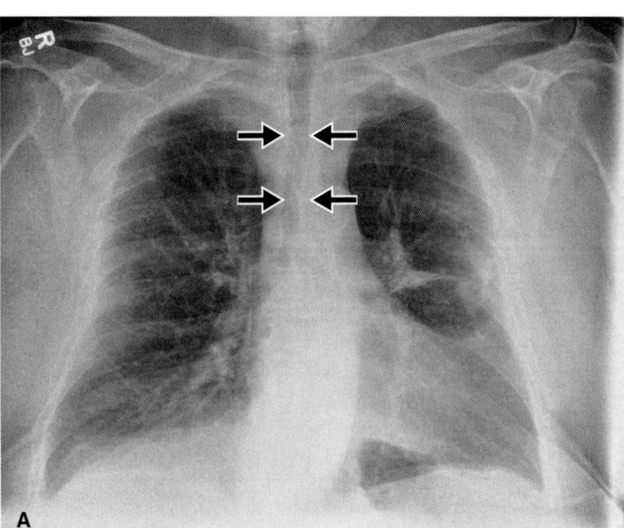
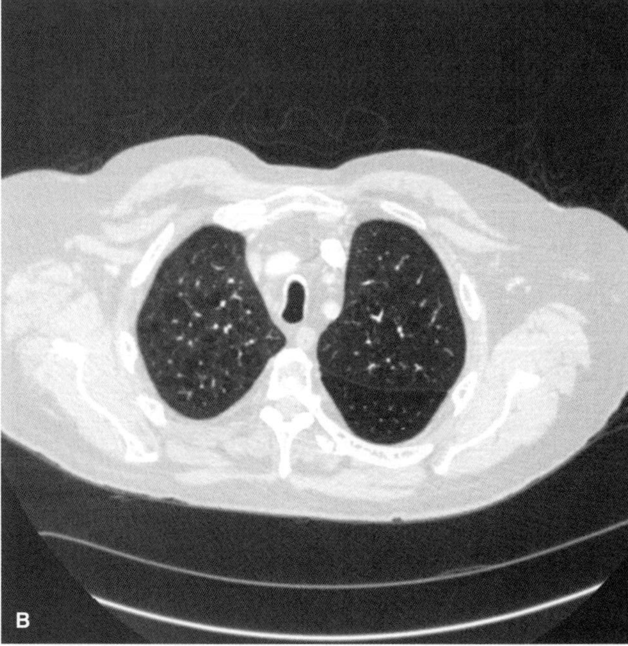

FIGURE 16.4. **Saber-Sheath Trachea. A:** Frontal chest radiograph in a 76-year-old man with COPD demonstrates uniform narrowing of the intrathoracic trachea (*arrows*). **B:** Axial CT through the upper lungs shows the typical saber-sheath configuration of the trachea, with sagittal narrowing and coronal elongation. Note the presence of upper lobe emphysema, a common associated finding.

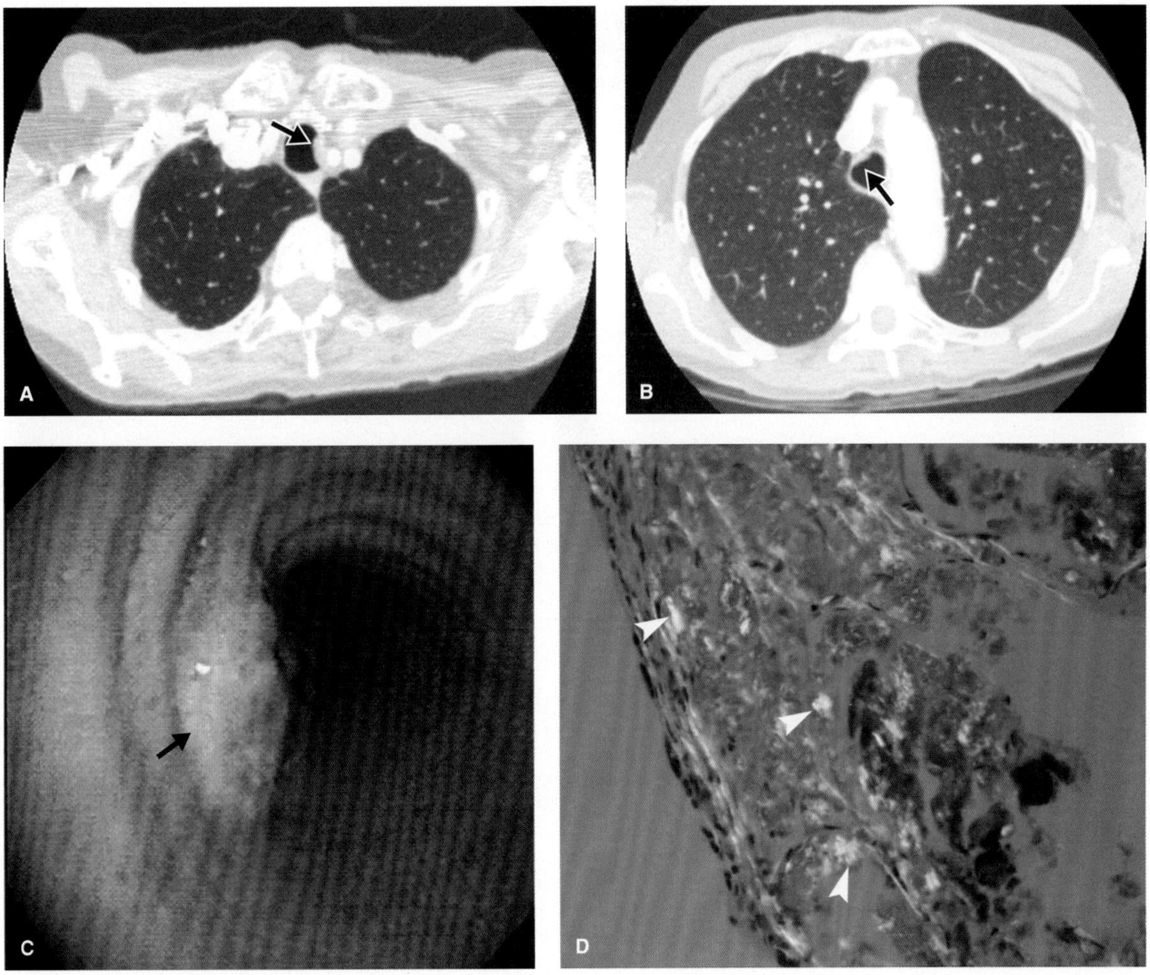

FIGURE 16.5. Amyloidosis of the Trachea. CT scans at lung windows through the upper (**A**) and lower (**B**) trachea demonstrate broad-based nodular lesions (*arrows*) along the tracheal wall. **C:** Image from fiber-optic bronchoscopy shows a raised yellowish lesion (*arrow*) along the left lateral proximal tracheal wall. **D:** Photomicrograph obtained under polarized light following Congo red staining of the endobronchial biopsy specimen shows typical apple-green birefringent crystals (*arrowheads*) characteristic of amyloid deposits.

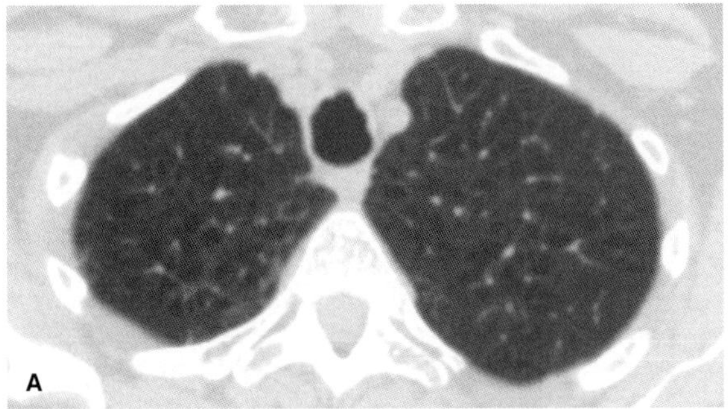

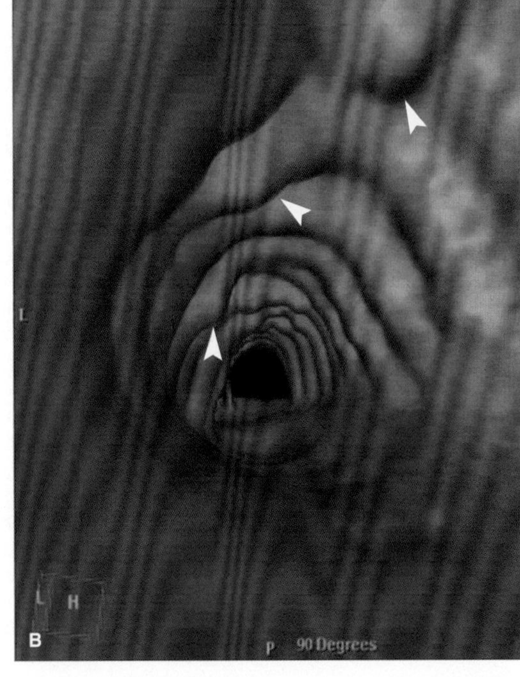

FIGURE 16.6. Tracheobronchopathia Osteochondroplastica. A, B: Axial CT scan through the upper trachea (**A**) and endoluminal rendering of the trachea (**B**) demonstrate nodular protrusions (*arrowheads* in **B**) extending from the cartilaginous rings of the tracheal wall.

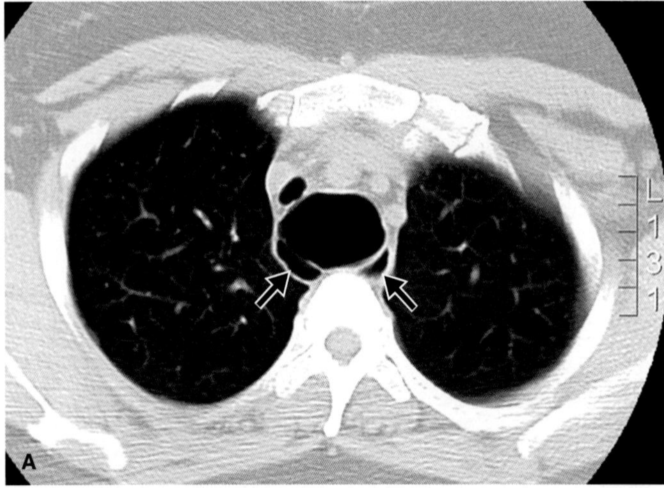

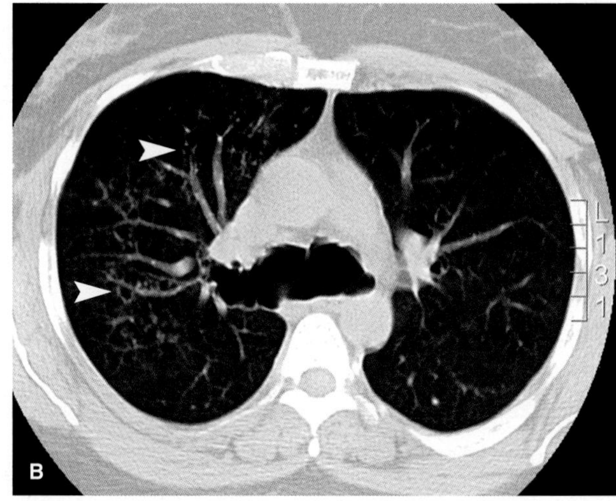

FIGURE 16.7. **Tracheobronchomegaly (Mounier–Kuhn Syndrome).** CT scans at lung windows at the level of the trachea (**A**) and carina (**B**) show marked tracheal and main bronchial dilatation in a patient with Mounier–Kuhn syndrome. Note the presence of characteristic diverticula along the central airways (*arrows*) and concomitant varicose bronchiectasis within the right upper lobe (*arrowheads*). (Case courtesy of Matthew Brewer MD, Milwaukee, WI.)

nose (producing a saddle nose deformity). Radiographs and CT show diffuse smooth thickening of the wall of the trachea and central bronchi, with narrowing of the lumen.

Diffuse Tracheal Dilatation

Tracheobronchomegaly (Mounier–Kuhn syndrome) is a congenital disorder of the elastic and smooth muscle components of the tracheal wall. An association with Ehlers–Danlos syndrome, a congenital defect in collagen synthesis, and cutis laxa, a congenital defect in elastic tissue, has been reported. The disease is found almost exclusively in men under the age of 50. Abnormal compliance of the trachea and central bronchi leads to central bronchial collapse during coughing. The airways obstruction impairs mucociliary clearance, predisposing the patient to recurrent episodes of pneumonia and bronchiectasis. Symptoms are indistinguishable from those associated with chronic bronchitis and bronchiectasis. On frontal radiographs, the trachea and central bronchi measure greater than 3.0 and 2.5 cm, respectively, in coronal diameter. The trachea has a corrugated appearance caused by the herniation of tracheal mucosa and submucosa between the tracheal cartilages (Fig. 16.7). The lungs are typically hyperinflated and may demonstrate bullae.

Tracheobronchomalacia (TBM) with diffuse tracheal and central bronchial dilatation may result from a congenital or acquired defect of tracheal cartilage causing softness of the tracheal cartilage rings and a tendency for airway collapse. Congenital disorders most often associated with TBM include relapsing polychondritis, Ehlers–Danlos syndrome, and mucopolysaccharidosis. Acquired TBM is more common than the congenital form and is most often associated with COPD. TBM may also result from prolonged intubation, prior tracheostomy, and extrinsic tracheal compression by mediastinal masses and vascular anomalies. Symptoms and radiographic findings are similar to those of tracheobronchomegaly—cough, dyspnea, wheezing, and recurrent respiratory infection.

The imaging hallmark of tracheomalacia is excessive airway collapse on expiration, seen best on dynamic expiratory CT using a low-dose CT acquisition performed during a forced expiratory maneuver. A reduction in the cross-sectional area of the trachea exceeding 50% on the expiratory CT, particularly if there is a crescentic "frown-like" configuration to the trachea in cross section, should suggest the diagnosis (Fig. 16.8), although this sign is not specific, as a significant percentage of normal patients will show dynamic airway collapse on expiratory CT. An additional clue to the presence of TBM is the recognition of a "lunate"-shaped trachea, in which the coronal diameter of the trachea exceeds the sagittal diameter on axial CT obtained at normal inspiration.

In some patients with long-standing interstitial pulmonary fibrosis, diffuse tracheal dilatation may be seen. The etiology of the tracheal dilatation may relate to long-standing elevation in transpulmonary pressures caused by diminished lung compliance or to chronic coughing.

Tracheal and Bronchial Injury

Injury to the trachea or main bronchi is most often seen with blunt chest trauma from a deceleration-type injury. Concomitant aortic laceration, great vessel injury, or rib (particularly an upper anterior rib), sternum, scapula, or vertebral fracture is the rule and may dominate the clinical picture. The mechanism of injury is forceful compression of the central tracheobronchial tree against the thoracic spine during impact. The fractures generally involve the proximal main bronchi (80%) or distal trachea (15%) within 2 cm of the tracheal carina; the peripheral bronchi are involved in 5% of cases. Horizontal laceration or transection parallel to the tracheobronchial cartilage is the most common form of injury.

The diagnosis of tracheobronchial injury is often first suggested on early posttrauma chest radiographs by the presence of pneumothorax and pneumomediastinum, particularly in a patient not receiving mechanical ventilation (Fig. 16.9A). Typically, the pneumothorax fails to respond to chest tube drainage owing to a large air leak at the site of airway injury. The subtended lung remains collapsed against the lateral chest wall ("fallen lung" sign) (Fig. 16.9B). An aberrant endotracheal tube or an overdistended balloon cuff is a further clue to the presence of an unsuspected tracheobronchial disruption. As many as one-third of tracheobronchial injuries have a delayed diagnosis; these patients may present with a collapsed lung or pneumonia secondary to bronchial stenosis. Definitive diagnosis is by bronchoscopy. MDCT with three-dimensional reconstruction and shaded surface displays may be useful in patients who develop bronchial occlusion or stenosis because of a delay in diagnosis.

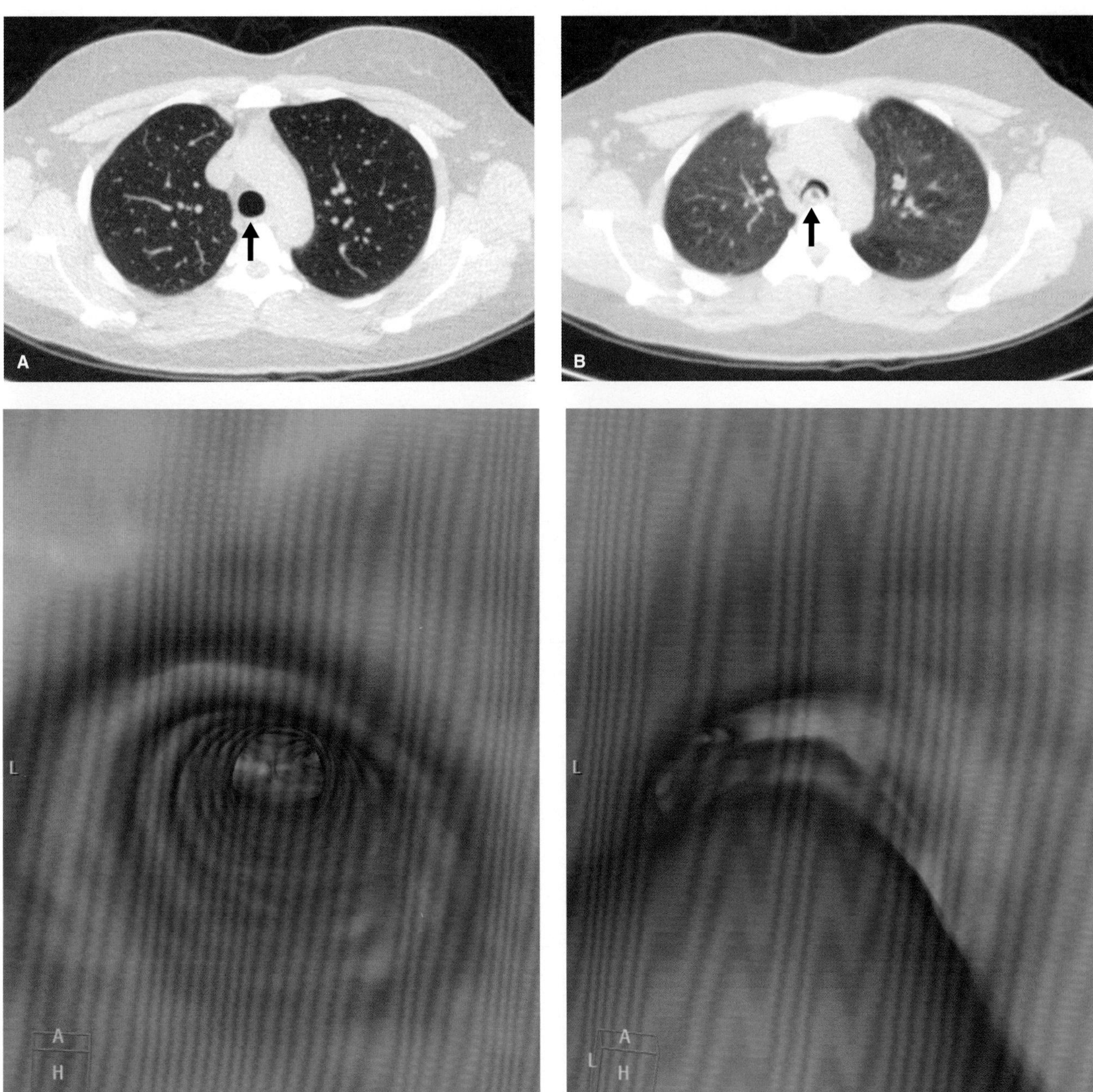

FIGURE 16.8. **Tracheobronchomalacia in Ehlers–Danlos Syndrome.** Paired inspiratory (**A**) and low-dose expiratory (**B**) CT scans through the mid trachea (*arrows*) at lung windows show a normal rounded configuration of the trachea on inspiration with marked collapse during dynamic expiratory CT with a "frown-like" configuration with buckling of the posterior tracheal membrane. **C, D:** Paired endotracheal renderings at inspiration (**C**) and expiration (**D**) show collapse of the posterior tracheal membrane with marked luminal narrowing.

Penetrating tracheal injuries usually involve the cervical trachea and result from gunshot or stab wounds to the neck. Injury to the intrathoracic trachea is usually associated with fatal penetrating cardiovascular injury.

Broncholithiasis

Broncholithiasis, the presence of calcified material within the tracheobronchial tree, develops from erosion of a calcified peribronchial lymph node into the bronchial lumen (Fig. 16.10). Most calcified lymph nodes result from granulomatous lymph node inflammation caused by histoplasmosis or TB. Broncholiths may occlude the airway and lead to bronchiectasis, obstructive atelectasis, or pneumonia. Patients are often asymptomatic but may have cough productive of stones or calcified material (lithoptysis). Hemoptysis may develop from erosion of the broncholith into a bronchial vessel.

CHRONIC OBSTRUCTIVE PULMONARY DISEASE

The diseases known collectively as COPD include asthma, chronic bronchitis, bronchiectasis, and emphysema. The

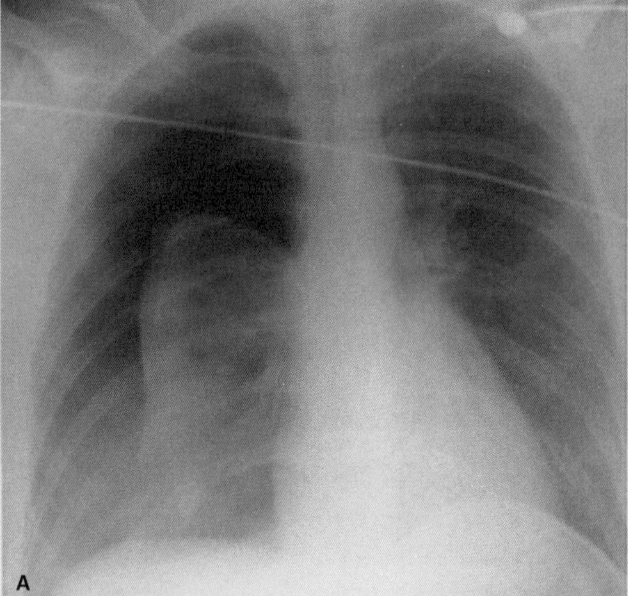

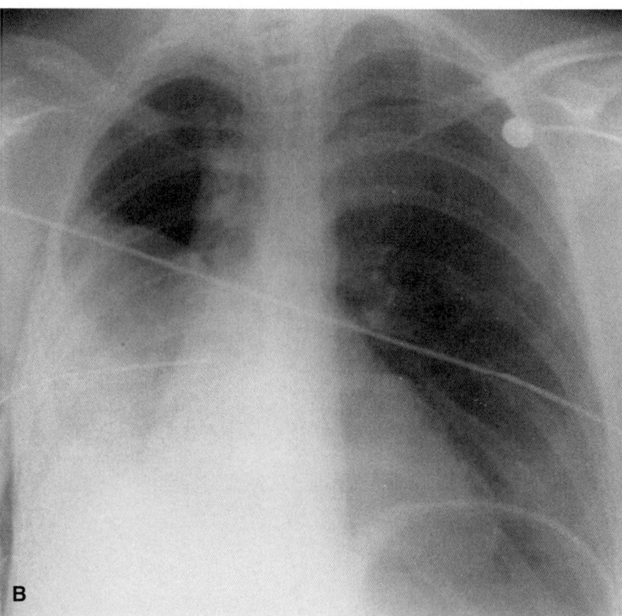

FIGURE 16.9. Injury of the Right Main Bronchus. A: An upright chest film shows a broken right clavicle with a large right pneumothorax and pneumomediastinum in a 24-year-old woman struck by a car. **B:** A film obtained following chest tube placement shows a persistent pneumothorax. A large air leak was noted from the tube. Bronchoscopy revealed complete disruption of the right main bronchus, which was confirmed at thoracotomy.

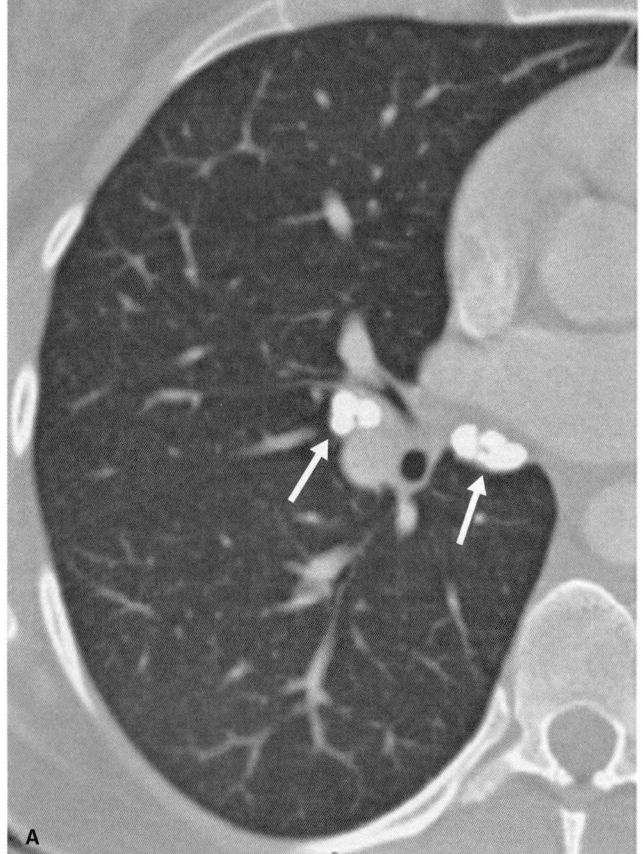

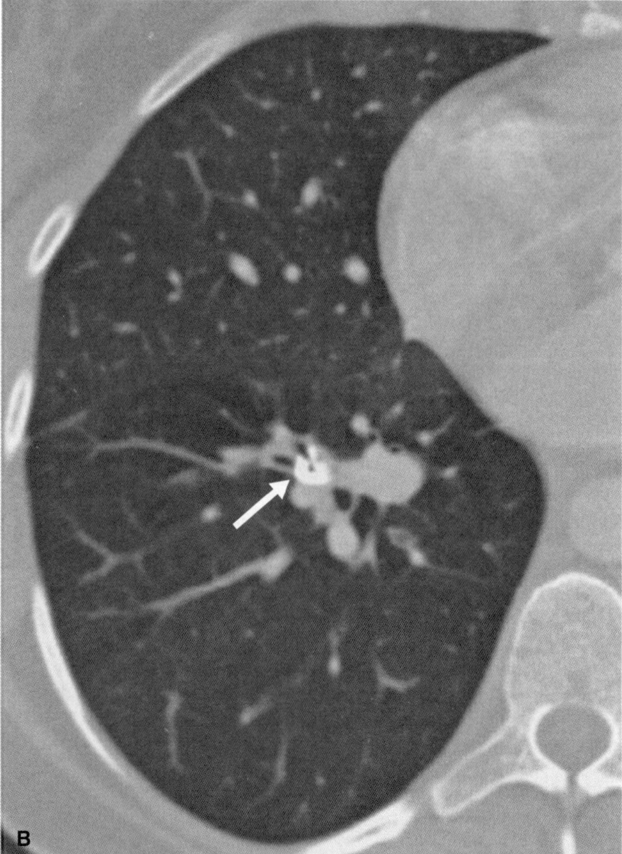

FIGURE 16.10. Broncholithiasis. Targeted reconstruction of the right lung from a CT in a 33-year-old woman with hemoptysis at the level of the middle lobe bronchus (**A**) and proximal basal segmental right lower lobe bronchi (**B**) show calcified lymph nodes (*arrows*) in the right hilum and azygoesophageal recess (*arrows* in **A**) with a calcified node within the anterior basal segmental bronchus (*arrow* in **B**).

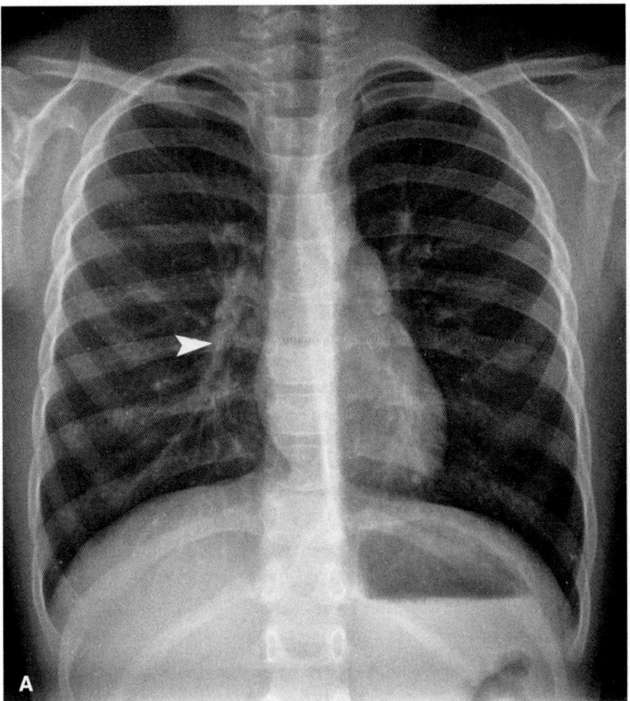

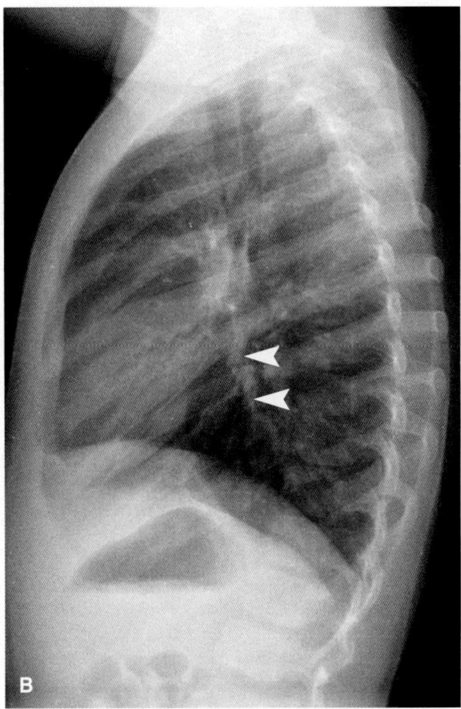

FIGURE 16.11. **Asthma. A, B:** Frontal (**A**) and lateral (**B**) chest radiographs in a child with an acute asthma exacerbation shows perihilar bronchial cuffing (*arrowheads*) and bronchial wall thickening in the lower lobes (*arrowheads* in **B**).

common pathophysiology in this group of diseases is obstruction to expiratory airflow.

Asthma and Chronic Bronchitis

Asthma is an airways disorder characterized by the rapid onset of bronchial narrowing with spontaneous resolution or improvement as a result of therapy. A wide variety of inciting factors and agents has been identified. Many patients have an allergic history and develop episodic bronchial constriction from excessive production of immunoglobulin E following exposure to antigenic stimuli. This results in bronchial smooth muscle contraction, bronchial wall inflammation, and excessive mucus production. These responses narrow the bronchial lumen and produce symptoms of coughing, wheezing, and dyspnea.

The radiographic findings in uncomplicated asthma are primarily the result of diffuse airways narrowing. Hyperinflation producing increased lung volume, flattening or inversion of the diaphragm, attenuation of the peripheral vascular markings, and prominence of the retrosternal airspace is the result of expiratory air trapping. Bronchial wall inflammation and thickening appear radiographically as peribronchial cuffing and "tram tracking." In some patients, the hila are prominent from transient pulmonary arterial hypertension caused by hypoxic vasoconstriction.

There are several reasons to obtain a chest radiograph in patients with asthma. Tracheal and central bronchial narrowing from extrinsic or intrinsic lesions may produce dyspnea and wheezing that may be mistaken for asthma. Bacterial pneumonia may induce airway hyperreactivity and present as an acute asthmatic attack. Complications of asthma may be detected on chest radiographs obtained during and following the asthmatic episode. Mucus plugs can cause bronchial obstruction and resorptive atelectasis; pneumonia can develop in these collapsed regions. Expiratory airflow obstruction with resultant alveolar rupture and dissection of air medially may produce pneumomediastinum (Fig. 16.11). If the extra-alveolar air dissects peripherally to the subpleural space to form subpleural blebs, pneumothorax may result. Both pneumomediastinum and pneumothorax may be exacerbated in ventilated patients receiving high–positive-pressure ventilation.

Chronic bronchitis is a clinical and not a radiographic diagnosis. It is defined as the excess production and expectoration of sputum that occurs on most days for at least 3 consecutive months in at least 2 consecutive years. The majority of individuals with chronic bronchitis are cigarette smokers. Morphologically, the lower lobe bronchi are most often affected, with thickening of their walls from mucous gland hyperplasia. Fifty percent of patients with a history of chronic bronchitis have normal chest radiographs. Some patients show peribronchial cuffing or tram tracks when the thick-walled and mildly dilated bronchi are viewed end on or in length, respectively. Other patients have a "dirty chest," in which the peripheral lung markings are accentuated. This radiographic appearance lacks a definite pathologic correlate but may represent thickened airway walls, smoking-related small airways disease (i.e., respiratory bronchiolitis), or prominent PAs from pulmonary arterial hypertension complicating associated centrilobular emphysema. CT in patients with chronic bronchitis may show bronchial wall thickening and mucus plugging (Fig. 16.12).

Bronchiectasis

Bronchiectasis is defined as an abnormal permanent dilatation of bronchi. This is distinguished from transient bronchial dilatation that can be seen within areas of airspace consolidation in patients with pneumonia. Morphologically, bronchiectasis is divided into three groups: cylindrical, varicose, and cystic (saccular). Cylindrical bronchiectasis is characterized by mild diffuse dilatation of the bronchi. Varicose bronchiectasis is cystic bronchial dilatation interrupted by focal areas of narrowing, an appearance that has been likened to a string of

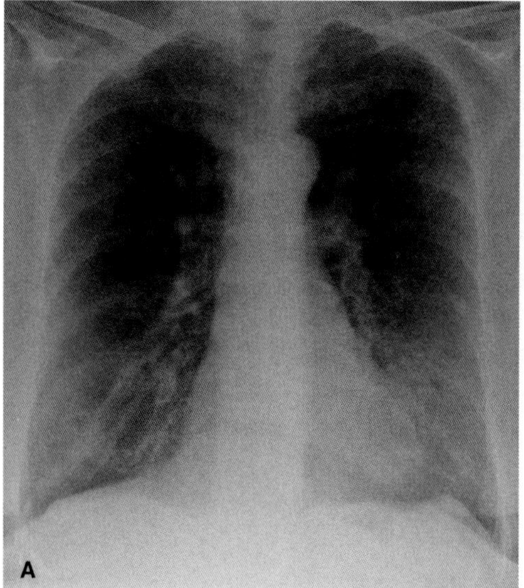

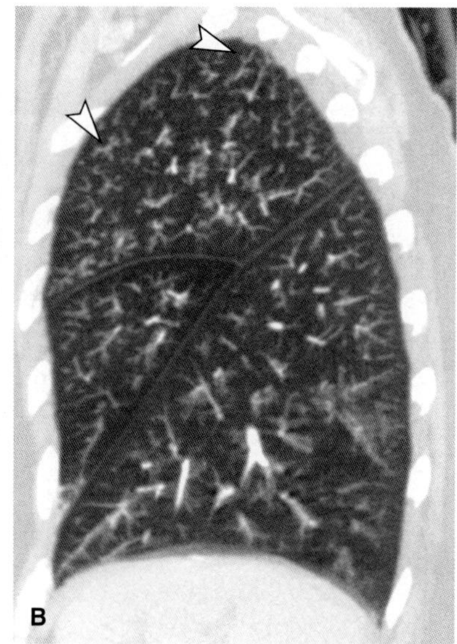

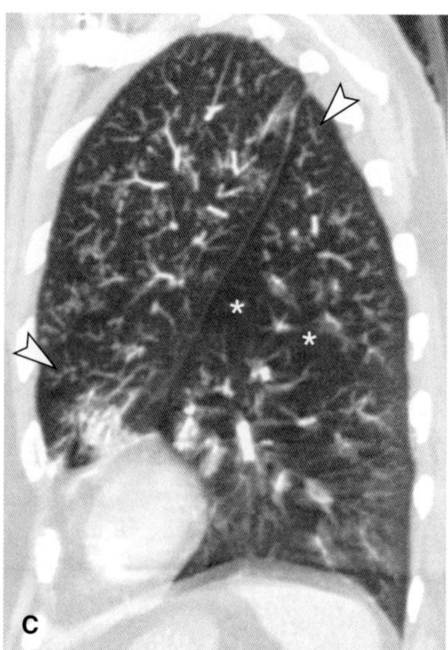

FIGURE 16.12. **"Dirty Chest" of Chronic Bronchitis. A:** Frontal chest radiograph in a patient with a history of chronic bronchitis and chronic obstructive pulmonary disease shows hyperinflation with increased parenchymal markings. **B, C:** Sagittal maximum intensity projection CT scans through the right (**B**) and left (**C**) lungs show upper lobe predominant centrilobular tree-in-bud opacities (*arrowheads*) and mosaic attenuation (*asterisks* in **C**), the latter likely due to air trapping.

pearls. Cystic bronchiectasis is seen as clusters of bronchi with marked localized saccular dilatation. Bronchiectasis may be localized or generalized. Localized bronchiectasis is most commonly a result of prior infection, whereas generalized bronchiectasis is seen in patients with cystic fibrosis (CF). Patients usually have a history of chronic sputum production and recurrent lower respiratory infections. Hemoptysis associated with enlargement of bronchial arteries is common and may be massive and life threatening.

The chest radiographic findings of bronchiectasis are typically nonspecific. Scarring, volume loss, and loss of the sharp definition of the normal bronchovascular markings are present in the affected regions. Parallel linear shadows representing the walls of cylindrically dilated bronchi seen in length may be visualized. Cystic bronchiectasis has a characteristic appearance of multiple peripheral thin-walled cysts, with or without air–fluid levels that tend to cluster together in the distribution of a bronchovascular bundle. The findings tend to be peripheral in most cases of localized bronchiectasis; central bronchiectasis is seen only in allergic bronchopulmonary aspergillosis (ABPA), cystic fibrosis, bronchial atresia, or acquired central bronchial obstruction.

CT is the most sensitive imaging technique in the diagnosis of bronchiectasis. The CT appearance of bronchiectasis depends on the site of involvement and the type of bronchiectasis. In the upper and lower lobes, all bronchi are imaged in cross section, and their luminal diameter can be directly compared to that of the accompanying PAs. Cylindrical bronchiectasis in these regions appears as multiple dilated thick-walled circular lucencies, with the adjoining smaller artery giving each dilated bronchus the appearance of a "signet ring" (Fig. 16.13). In the mid-lung, where the bronchi course horizontally, the appearance is that of parallel linear opacities ("tram tracks"). Mucoid impaction within dilated upper or lower lobe bronchi may be mistaken for lung nodules unless one observes the vertical nature of the opacity on sequential axial images. In the mid-lung regions, impacted bronchi sectioned in length are recognized as branching, fingerlike opacities. Cystic bronchiectasis in any region is easily recognized as clusters of rounded lucencies, often containing air–fluid levels; this appearance has been likened to a cluster of grapes. Varicose bronchiectasis cannot be differentiated from cylindrical bronchiectasis unless sectioned longitudinally in the mid-lung regions, where the pattern of dilatation simulates the contour of a caterpillar. The detection of varicose bronchiectasis, along with the classically described "finger-in-glove" appearance of mucoid impaction, in an asthmatic patient should suggest the diagnosis of ABPA.

Bronchiectasis is caused by a variety of disorders, all of which predispose the bronchi to chronic inflammation, with resultant cartilage damage and dilatation (Table 16.3).

Cystic fibrosis is a hereditary disease in young whites characterized in the lung by the production of abnormally thick, tenacious mucus. The thick mucus plugs the small airways and leads to bronchial obstruction and infection. A vicious cycle of recurrent infection, most often with *Pseudomonas aeruginosa* or *Staphylococcus aureus*, eventually causes severe bronchiectasis. The bronchiectasis is associated with functional airways obstruction and dyspnea. Hemoptysis, sometimes massive, may complicate the bronchiectasis and may require treatment by transcatheter bronchial artery embolization. Chest radiographs in affected patients show hyperinflation due to air trapping and predominantly upper lobe bronchiectasis that tends to be more extensive than non-CF bronchiectasis. CT delineates the severity and extent of bronchiectasis and shows associated small airways disease seen as tree-in-bud opacities and mosaic attenuation due to air trapping (Fig. 16.13). Distal atelectasis and obstructive pneumonitis are common findings. The pulmonary hila may be prominent from enlarged lymph nodes caused by chronic infection or from vascular dilatation associated with pulmonary arterial hypertension. The diagnosis rests on a positive family history and a sweat test showing an abnormally high concentration of chloride. Improvements in antibiotic therapy and pulmonary physiotherapy have increased long-term survival, but the overall prognosis remains poor, with most patients succumbing to respiratory insufficiency in young adulthood. Management includes antibiotics to prevent infection, mucolytics (such as dornase alfa) and chest physiotherapy to thin, loosen, and expel mucus. More recently, patients with at least one G551D mutation in the

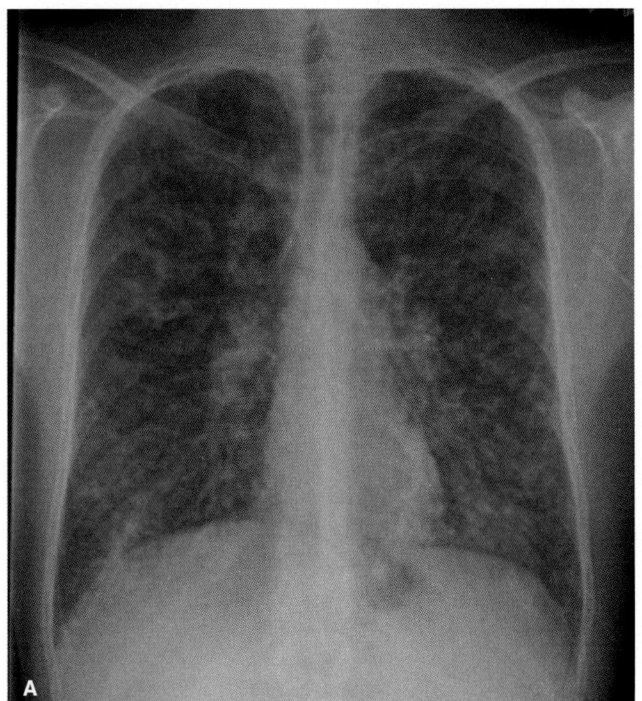

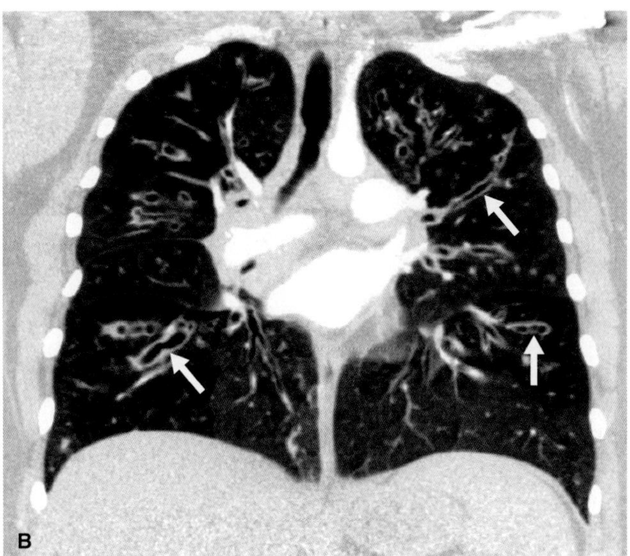

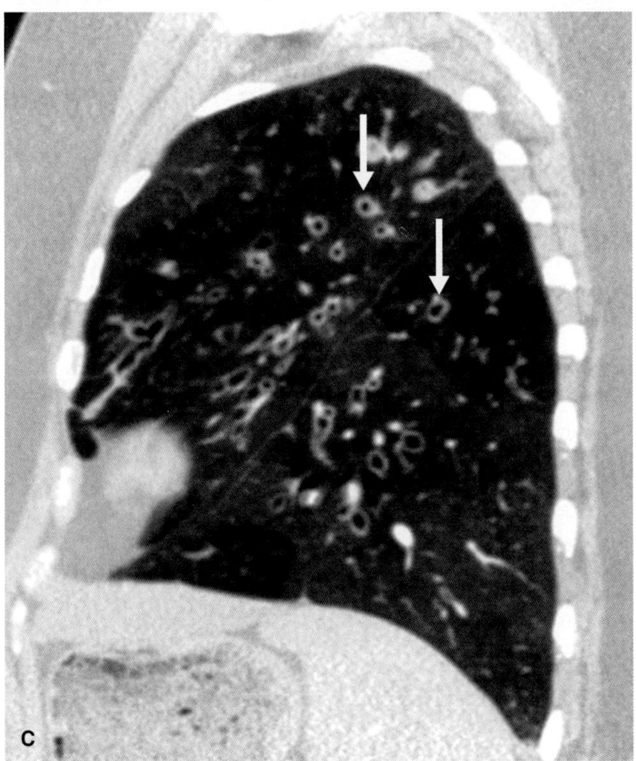

FIGURE 16.13. **Bronchiectasis in Cystic Fibrosis. A:** Chest radiograph in a patient with cystic fibrosis. The lungs are hyperinflated with multiple linear and tubular branching opacities. Note the bilateral hilar enlargement as a result of pulmonary arterial hypertension and reactive lymph node enlargement. **B:** Coronal reformatted CT scan through the trachea shows bilateral cylindrical bronchiectasis (*arrows*) and mosaic attenuation due to airways disease. **C:** Sagittal reformation through the left lung shows the left lung cylindrical bronchiectasis in cross section as "signet rings" (*arrows*).

cystic fibrosis transmembrane conductance regulator (CFTR) gene can be treated with ivacaftor, which potentiates chloride transport and leads to improvements in respiratory symptoms and lung function.

Primary ciliary dyskinesia, also known as ***dysmotile cilia syndrome***, is a disorder in which the epithelial cilial motion is abnormal and ineffective. A variety of structural cilial abnormalities may be found, the most common of which is an absence of the outer dynein arms of the peripheral microtubules of the cilia. The abnormality may result in rhinitis, sinusitis, bronchiectasis, dysmotile spermatozoa and sterility, situs inversus, and dextrocardia. The triad of sinusitis, situs inversus, and bronchiectasis is known as Kartagener syndrome. Chest radiographs show diffuse bronchiectasis and hyperinflation; situs inversus is seen in approximately 50% of patients. The diagnosis is made on the basis of the clinical and radiographic findings along with studies of cilial anatomy and motion on samples obtained from nasal biopsy.

Postinfectious Bronchiectasis. Severe childhood pneumonia, usually a sequela of infection with adenovirus, measles, or pertussis, may cause severe bronchial damage and recurrent infection with resultant bronchiectasis. In some patients,

TABLE 16.3

SPECIFIC CAUSES OF BRONCHIECTASIS

Localized	Tuberculous scarring, upper lobes (postprimary disease)
	Bronchial disease
	Extrinsic compression
	Enlarged hilar nodes
	Bronchial stenosis/occlusion
	Bronchial atresia
	Tuberculosis
	Sarcoidosis
	Prior bronchial injury
	Endobronchial mass
	Carcinoid tumor
	Bronchogenic carcinoma
	Foreign body
Diffuse	Cystic fibrosis
	Primary ciliary dyskinesia/dysmotile cilia syndrome
	Congenital immunodeficiency
	Inflammatory bowel disease (ulcerative colitis)
	Postinfectious
	Adenovirus (Swyer–James syndrome)
	Measles
	Pertussis
	Chronic aspiration
	Allergic bronchopulmonary aspergillosis
	Pulmonary fibrosis (traction bronchiectasis)
	α-1-antitrypsin deficiency

childhood bronchitis and bronchiolitis are associated with obstructive airways disease and an underdeveloped lung, the latter known as Swyer–James syndrome (see "Small Airways Disease" section).

Allergic bronchopulmonary aspergillosis represents a hypersensitivity reaction to *Aspergillus* antigens and is characterized clinically by asthma, blood eosinophilia, bronchiectasis with mucus plugging, and circulating antibodies to *Aspergillus* antigen. An immediate (type 1) hypersensitivity reaction to *Aspergillus* antigen accounts for acute episodes of wheezing and dyspnea, while an immune complex-mediated (type 3) hypersensitivity within the lobar bronchi leads to bronchial wall inflammation and proximal bronchiectasis. Affected patients invariably have an allergic history, and ABPA is often associated with known asthma or cystic fibrosis. Patients with this disorder have recurrent episodes of cough, wheezing, and expectoration of mucus plugs. The chest radiograph shows proximal, predominantly upper lobe bronchiectasis; consolidation due to associated eosinophilic pneumonia is seen in the majority of patients during the acute phase of the disease. The dilated bronchi may be seen as dilated air-filled tubules or as broadly branching opacities characteristic of mucoid impaction within the dilated bronchi. CT is helpful in characterizing the opacities as dilated bronchi (Fig. 16.14). The detection of central varicose bronchiectasis with normal peripheral bronchi in a susceptible patient should suggest the diagnosis. Corticosteroids are the treatment of choice.

Bronchial Obstruction. Bronchiectasis can develop distal to an endobronchial obstruction caused by neoplasm, atresia, or stenosis. Slow-growing central bronchogenic neoplasms that have a large endoluminal component (e.g., carcinoid tumor) may obstruct the distal bronchi and produce bronchiectasis with mucus plugging (mucoceles). Similarly, bronchial atresia or bronchostenosis from trauma or chronic bronchial infection (e.g., endobronchial TB) can lead to distal bronchial dilatation. The radiographic recognition of mucocele formation in patients with endobronchial obstruction is dependent on adequate collateral ventilation to the lung supplied by the obstructed airway. Unfortunately, in most patients, collapse of lung around the dilated mucus-filled bronchus precludes diagnosis on plain radiographs. CT will show the central airway obstruction and dilated mucus bronchograms and can help guide bronchoscopic examination and biopsy.

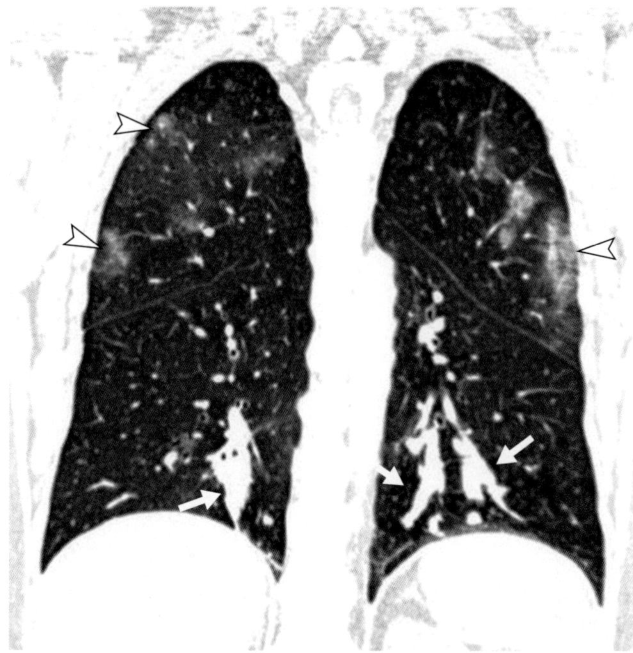

FIGURE 16.14. Allergic Bronchopulmonary Aspergillosis (ABPA). Coronal reformatted CT scan through the posterior chest at lung windows in a patient with ABPA shows bilateral lower lobe mucoid impaction (*arrows*) and patchy upper lobe ground-glass opacities (*arrowheads*).

Peribronchial Fibrosis. *Traction bronchiectasis* is a term used to describe the effect of severe pulmonary fibrosis on the peripheral airways. Airways that traverse regions of parenchymal fibrosis and honeycombing often become irregularly dilated as their walls are retracted by the fibrotic process. This occurs most commonly in the upper lobes in patients with long-standing TB and in the subpleural regions of the lower lobes in patients with idiopathic pulmonary fibrosis. Because the accompanying fibrosis precludes visualization of the dilated bronchi radiographically, traction bronchiectasis is best appreciated on thin-section CT studies of the lung.

Emphysema

Definition and Subtypes. Emphysema is a pathologic diagnosis that is defined as an abnormal, permanent enlargement of the airspaces distal to the terminal bronchiole, accompanied by destruction of alveolar walls, and without obvious fibrosis. The pathologic classification of emphysema is based on the portion of the secondary pulmonary lobule affected. *Centrilobular emphysema* is the most common and is characterized by airspace distention in the central portion of the lobule, with sparing of the more distal portions of the lobule. This form of emphysema affects the upper lobes to a greater extent than the lower lobes (Fig. 16.15). *Panlobular emphysema* results in

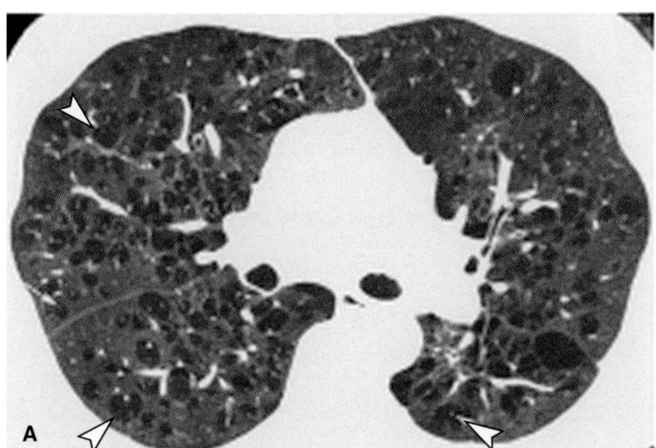

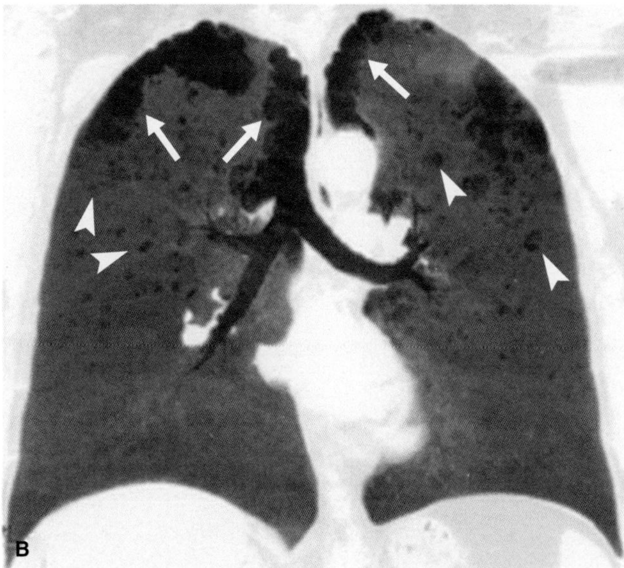

FIGURE 16.15. **Centrilobular and Paraseptal Emphysema on CT. A:** CT scan through the mid lungs in a patient with centrilobular emphysema shows discrete lucencies (*arrowheads*) lacking perceptible walls and containing centrilobular artery branches. **B:** In another patient with both centrilobular and paraseptal emphysema, a coronal minimum intensity reconstruction CT shows subpleural lucencies, reflecting paraseptal emphysema (*arrows*) with associated centrilobular emphysema (*arrowheads*).

uniform distention of the airspaces throughout the substance of the lobule, from the central respiratory bronchioles to the peripheral alveolar sacs and alveoli. In contrast to centrilobular emphysema, this form has a predilection for the lower lobes (Fig. 16.16). *Paraseptal emphysema* is seen as selective distention of peripheral airspaces adjacent to interlobular septa, with sparing of the centrilobular region. This form of emphysema is most often seen in the immediate subpleural regions of the upper lobes (Fig. 16.15). Paraseptal emphysema may coalesce to form apical bullae; rupture of these bullae into the pleural space may give rise to spontaneous pneumothoraces. *Paracicatricial* or *irregular emphysema* refers to destruction of lung tissue associated with fibrosis that bears no consistent relationship to a given portion of the lobule. It is most often seen in association with old granulomatous inflammation (Fig. 16.17).

Etiology and Pathogenesis. The most common etiologic factor for the development of emphysema is cigarette smoking. This is associated predominantly with centrilobular emphysema but may be a contributing factor in the development of panlobular emphysema. The pathogenesis of centrilobular emphysema is complex and has not been completely elucidated. Cigarette smoke leads to excess neutrophil deposition in the lung. This results in the release of proteases (e.g., elastase) and antiprotease inhibitors, which in turn leads to destruction of alveolar septa. Inflammation and obstruction of small airways likely contributes to distal airspace distention and alveolar septal disruption. The association between deficiency of the serum protein α-1-antitrypsin (α-1-antiprotease inhibitor) and the development of panlobular emphysema is well established. This disease is inherited as an autosomal recessive trait. Individuals who are homozygous for two of either of the recessive genes S or Z (ZZ or SS genotype) develop panlobular emphysema by middle age. Heterozygotes (one normal [M] allele and one Z or S allele) have a slightly increased incidence of emphysema. Cigarette smoking, by producing excess antiprotease inhibitors, can accelerate the development of emphysema in patients with the ZZ, SS, and heterozygotic genotypes.

Clinical Findings and Functional Abnormalities. Because a definitive diagnosis of emphysema requires tissue, the diagnosis during life is based on a combination of clinical, functional, and radiographic findings. The vast majority of patients with emphysema are long-term cigarette smokers. Symptoms associated with emphysema include dyspnea and a productive cough; the latter is attributed to chronic bronchitis, which often accompanies centrilobular emphysema. The functional hallmarks of emphysema are decreased airflow and diffusing capacity. Expiratory airflow obstruction is expressed as a decrease in the volume of air expired in the first second of a forced expiratory maneuver from total lung capacity (FEV_1) and a decrease in the ratio of FEV_1 to the total volume of air expired during a forced expiratory maneuver (FEV_1/FVC). Airflow obstruction is secondary to increased airways resistance and decreased driving pressure (i.e., elastic recoil). In patients with moderate to severe emphysema, the predominant factor limiting expiratory airflow is the decreased elastic recoil that results from parenchymal destruction. Airflow obstruction, however, is not invariably present in patients with mild emphysema. Diffusing capacity, measured by the diffusion of carbon monoxide from the alveoli into the bloodstream during a single breath hold ($DL_{CO}SB$), assesses the integrity and surface area of the alveolocapillary membrane. The diffusing capacity in emphysema is decreased because the volume of pulmonary parenchyma available for gas exchange is diminished. The severity of the emphysema correlates well with the $DL_{CO}SB$. Although an abnormal diffusing capacity is more sensitive than abnormal spirometry in diagnosing emphysema, it is nonspecific. Since $DL_{CO}SB$ depends on both the surface area available for gas diffusion and the number and hemoglobin content of red blood cells within the pulmonary capillaries, any process affecting these factors can alter the measurement of $DL_{CO}SB$. For example, a decreased $DL_{CO}SB$ can be seen in any disease that diminishes the volume of pulmonary capillaries available for gas diffusion (e.g., pulmonary embolism); interferes with gas exchange across the alveolocapillary membrane (e.g., interstitial pulmonary fibrosis), or produces airway obstruction, thereby diminishing the gas-exchanging airspaces (i.e., cystic fibrosis).

Radiologic Evaluation. Frontal and lateral chest radiographs are the initial radiographic examinations obtained in patients with suspected emphysema. The plain radiographic

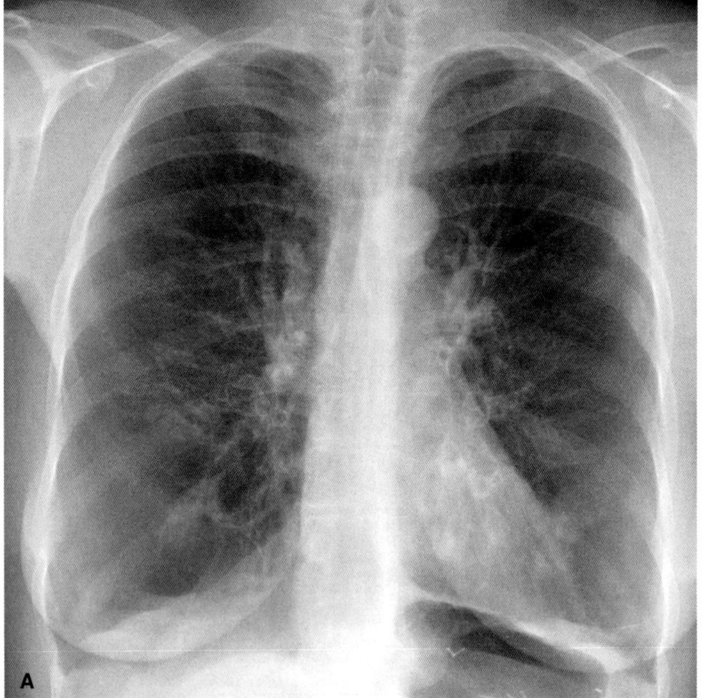

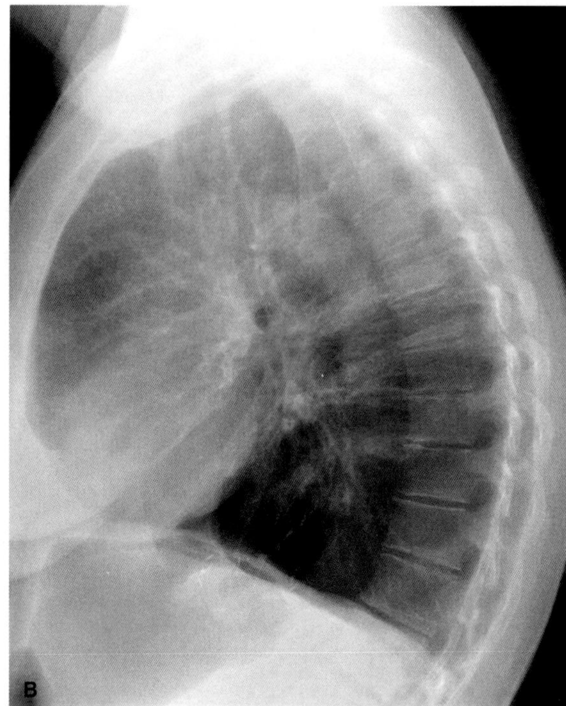

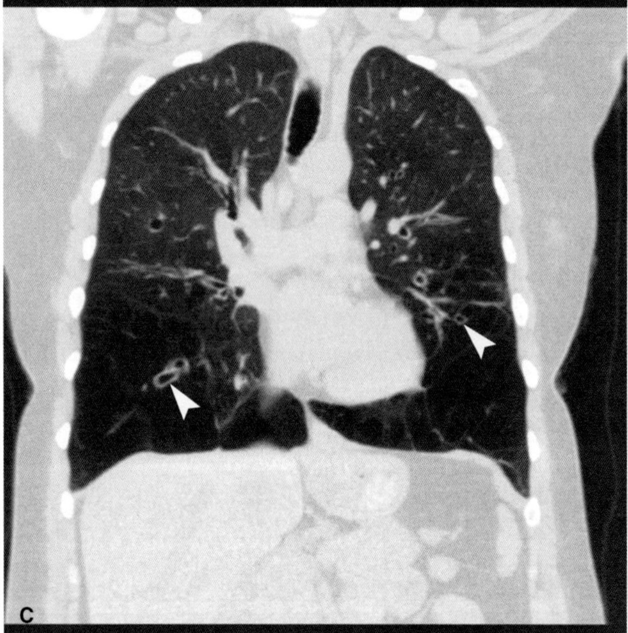

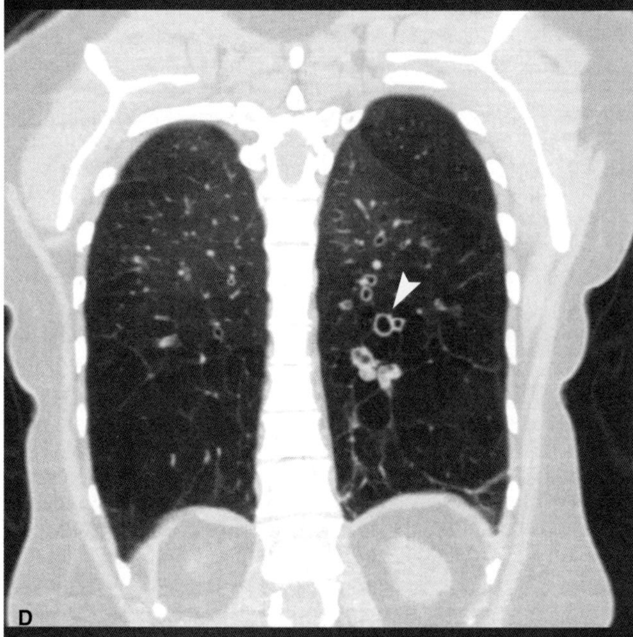

FIGURE 16.16. **Panlobular Emphysema Associated With Alpha-1-Antitrypsin Deficiency. A, B:** Frontal (**A**) and lateral (**B**) chest radiographs in a 63-year-old woman with known alpha-1-antitrypsin deficiency show hyperinflated lungs with marked bibasilar hyperlucency. **C, D:** Coronal CT scans through the mid and posterior lungs show uniform destruction of secondary pulmonary lobules. Note the presence of bronchiectasis (*arrowheads*), another common finding in patients with alpha-1-antitrypsin deficiency.

findings of emphysema are listed in Table 16.4. Hyperinflation is the most important plain radiographic finding and reflects the loss of lung elastic recoil. It is the radiographic equivalent of an abnormally increased total lung capacity. The abnormal increase in lung volumes is best detected by noting inferior displacement and flattening of the normally convex superior hemidiaphragms, right or obtuse angles to the normally acute-angled costophrenic sulci, and an increase in anteroposterior chest diameter (best appreciated by noting an increase in the depth of the retrosternal clear space) (Fig. 16.18). Absent or attenuated peripheral vascular markings are caused by parenchymal destruction and obliteration of peripheral pulmonary arteries traversing emphysematous areas. When the characteristic thin walls of bullae are seen marginating the peripheral avascular regions, emphysema can be diagnosed with certainty. Increased radiolucency of the lungs on radiographs resulting from pulmonary hyperinflation and attenuation of peripheral vascular markings is difficult to detect because it is subject to various patient and technical factors and therefore is an inaccurate indicator of the presence

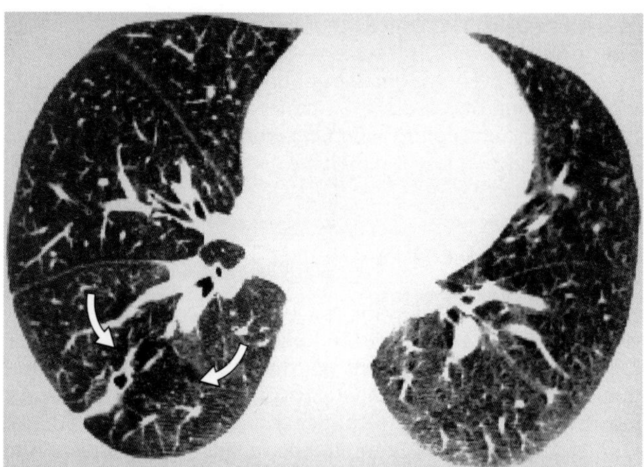

FIGURE 16.17. **Paracicatricial Emphysema.** HRCT scan in a patient with focal right lower lobe postinflammatory scarring and bronchiectasis shows focal hyperlucency (*arrows*) representing paracicatricial emphysema.

of emphysema. It is well recognized that many patients with severe centrilobular emphysema have minimal or no hyperinflation on chest radiographs, and they tend to show increased lung markings rather than peripheral vascular attenuation. In such patients, the increased markings may reflect the presence of smoking-related small airways disease (e.g., respiratory bronchiolitis-associated interstitial lung disease [RB-ILD]). The effects of emphysema and chronic hypoxemia on the right side of the heart may be appreciated as enlargement of the central pulmonary arteries and right ventricle in those with complicating pulmonary arterial hypertension and cor pulmonale.

TABLE 16.4

RADIOGRAPHIC FINDINGS IN PULMONARY EMPHYSEMA

■ FINDING	■ EXPLANATION
Diffuse hyperlucency (panlobular)	Destruction of pulmonary capillary bed and alveolar septa
Flattening and depression of the hemidiaphragms; increased retrosternal airspace (panlobular > centrilobular)	Hyperinflation caused by loss of elastic recoil of lung
Bulla	Thin-walled region of confluent (panlobular > centrilobular) emphysematous destruction
Enlarged central PAs; right heart enlargement (centrilobular)	Loss of pulmonary capillary bed; associated chronic hypoxemia causes increased pulmonary vascular resistance
Increased peripheral vascular markings (centrilobular)	Small airways disease Increased pulmonary vascularity

The use of the term *COPD* to describe patients with the radiographic findings of emphysema is inaccurate and should be discouraged. COPD is a functional diagnosis, whereas chest radiography depicts anatomy only. In fact, patients with radiographic findings of hyperinflation and vascular attenuation, while they invariably have emphysema morphologically, may

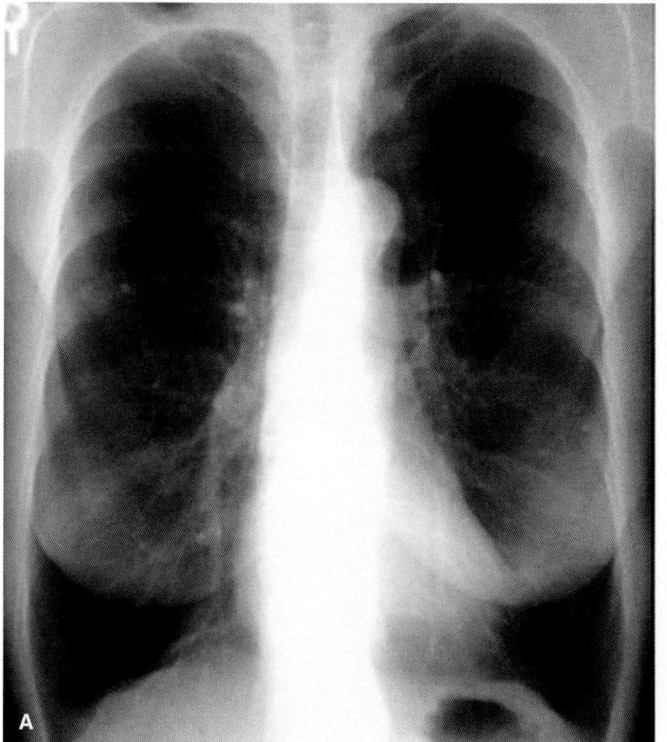

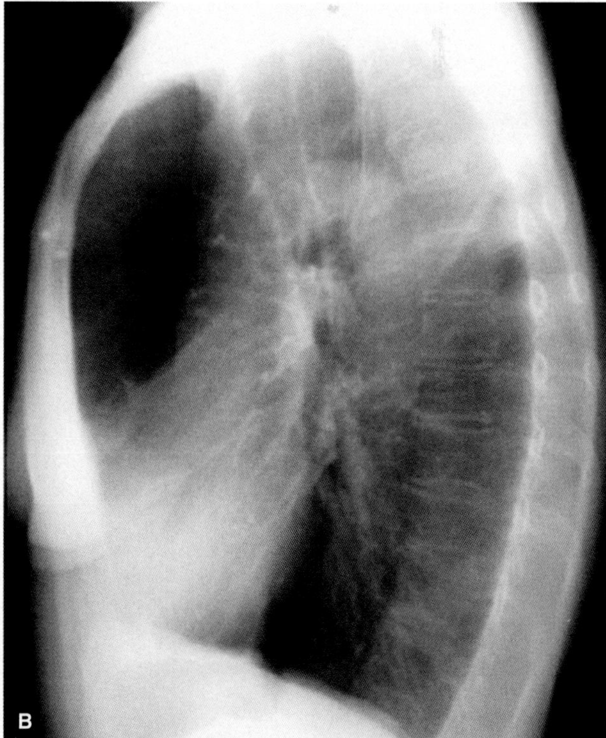

FIGURE 16.18. **Chest Radiographs in Emphysema.** Posteroanterior (**A**) and lateral (**B**) chest radiographs in a 62-year-old woman with emphysema show hyperinflation with hyperlucency, upper lobe vascular attenuation, flattening of the diaphragms, and an increased retrosternal airspace, reflecting severe emphysema.

rarely lack functional evidence of airflow obstruction and therefore do not have COPD.

Widespread, extensive emphysema may be accurately diagnosed on chest radiographs, but mild disease is often not evident radiographically. CT provides a confident diagnosis of emphysema in the absence of chest radiographic findings of hyperinflation or parenchymal abnormalities. CT is ideally suited to the diagnosis of emphysema because of its cross-sectional nature and high contrast resolution. Thin-section CT (<1.5 mm slice thickness) provides better characterization of centrilobular emphysema than thicker (3 to 5 mm) collimation. CT is useful for assessing the distribution of emphysema, particularly in patients considered for lung volume reduction surgery (LVRS). Centrilobular emphysema on thin-section CT scan is seen as discrete, well-defined areas of low attenuation lacking definable walls adjacent to the core centrilobular structures within secondary pulmonary lobules (Fig. 16.15). Thin-section CT can detect mild centrilobular emphysema imperceptible on chest radiography and not discernable on 5-mm thick scans because of partial volume averaging of small emphysematous areas within the thickness of the scan section. Minimum-intensity projection (minIP) imaging, in which the lowest voxel within a slab of 1-mm CT images is displayed, is the most accurate method of quantifying emphysema (Fig. 16.15B).

Treatment of Emphysema. Advances in operative techniques now provide surgical options and endobronchial intervention for the treatment of emphysema. LVRS is a method of relieving patient dyspnea by resecting severely emphysematous regions of lung and improving respiratory mechanics. This technique, specifically benefits those with mostly upper lobe emphysema and low exercise capacity prior to surgery. An alternative surgical technique available to treat patients with emphysema, particularly younger patients with α-1-antitrypsin deficiency, is single- or double-lung transplantation. Augmentation therapy for patients with moderate severity disease due to α-1-antitrypsin involves intravenous infusion of pooled plasma protein concentrate to increase blood and tissue levels of α-1-antitrypsin and reduce the rate of decline in lung function. The bronchoscopic placement of one-way endobronchial valves that prevent air entry but allow air egress from emphysematous lung that lacks collateral ventilation via incomplete fissures can reduce lung volumes, improve lung function, and relieve dyspnea in select patients.

BULLOUS LUNG DISEASE

Bullae are thin-walled cystic spaces that exceed 1 cm in diameter and are found within the lung parenchyma (Fig. 16.19). Bullae most often represent confluent areas of emphysematous lung and may be seen as part of generalized emphysema. However, in a minority of patients, bullae are not associated with emphysema. For example, the increased lung weight and chronically elevated transpleural pressure in patients with lower lobe interstitial pulmonary fibrosis predispose to bullae formation. Bullae may also be seen in diseases that cause chronic upper lobe fibrosis, such as sarcoidosis, pulmonary Langerhans cell histiocytosis, and ankylosing spondylitis. In these diseases, chronic bronchiolar obstruction leads to distal airspace distention, alveolar septal disruption, and the development of bullae. A rare cause of lung cysts or bullae is Birt–Hogg–Dubé syndrome, which is an autosomal dominant disorder characterized by skin fibrofolliculomas, malignant renal tumors, and thin-walled lung cysts, the latter predisposing to spontaneous pneumothorax.

Primary bullous disease (Table 16.5) is a group of disorders in which bullae are isolated lesions without intervening areas of emphysema or interstitial lung disease. Primary bullous lung disease may be familial and has been found in association with Marfan or Ehlers–Danlos syndrome, IV drug use, HIV infection, and vanishing lung syndrome, which is an accelerated form of paraseptal emphysema seen in young adult men (Fig. 16.19). Most patients are asymptomatic unless large bullae compress normal parenchyma and cause compressive

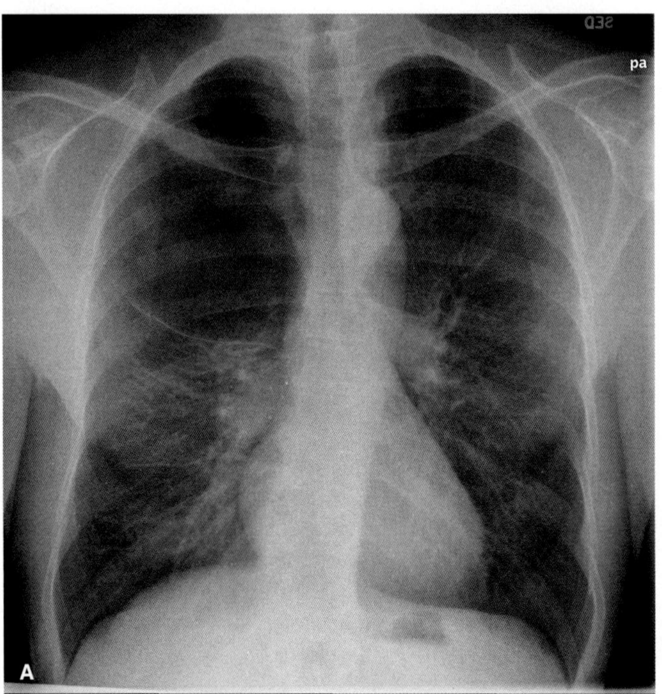

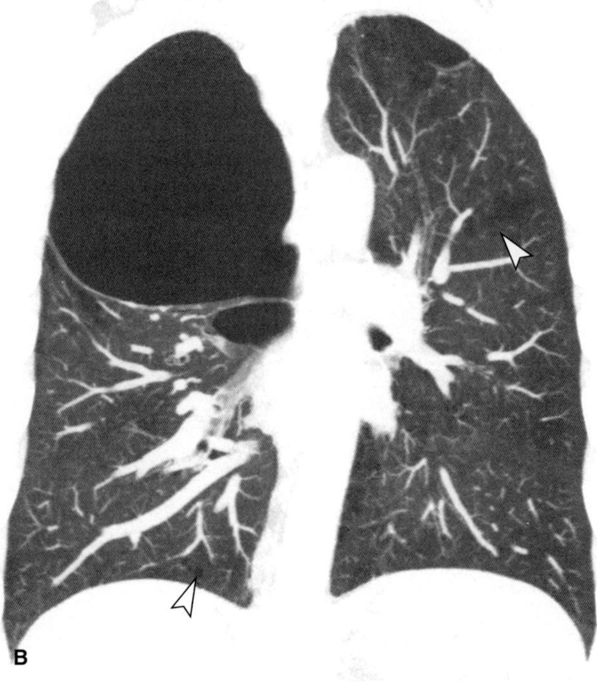

FIGURE 16.19. **Bullous Lung Disease. A:** Frontal chest radiograph in a 27-year-old man shows a large right upper lobe bulla. **B:** Coronal CT through the mid lungs shows a large bulla with additional smaller bullae bilaterally (*arrowheads*).

TABLE 16.5

CAUSES OF PRIMARY BULLOUS LUNG DISEASE

Familial
Vanishing lung disease
Marfan syndrome
Ehlers–Danlos syndrome
IV drug use
HIV infection
Birt–Hogg–Dubé syndrome

atelectasis and dyspnea. Radiographically, isolated bullae have an upper lobe distribution and appear as rounded, thin-walled lucencies of varying size. These lesions can become huge as a result of air trapping and cause depression of the ipsilateral lung and hemidiaphragm and may even produce contralateral mediastinal shift. CT is useful in evaluating the extent of bullous disease and the amount of compressed pulmonary tissue.

Spontaneous pneumothorax occurs when a subpleural bulla ruptures into the pleural space. These patients may be difficult to manage; persistent air leaks lead to prolonged and often unsuccessful closed-tube drainage of the pleural space and reexpansion of the lung. When a bulla becomes secondarily infected, chest radiographs or CT will demonstrate an air–fluid level within the bulla that resolves over several weeks with the administration of antibiotics. A cancer may rarely develop within the wall of a bulla. Symptomatic patients and those with enlarging bullae should be considered for bullectomy. Radioisotopic lung perfusion studies may be performed preoperatively to assess the amount of perfused and potentially functional lung parenchyma compressed by the bullae.

SMALL AIRWAYS DISEASE

The small airways are defined as non–cartilage-bearing bronchioles with a luminal diameter <2 mm. Small airway abnormalities are not discernable radiographically but are commonly detected on thin-section CT. As the definitive diagnosis of small airways disease usually requires open lung biopsy, and physiologic tests are not particularly accurate for diagnosis, imaging is an important component of patient evaluation. While many patients with small airways abnormalities are asymptomatic, a number of disorders primarily affecting the small airways that present as cough, wheezing, or shortness of breath can be diagnosed on CT. This section will review the spectrum of inflammatory and fibrotic conditions that may manifest as small airways disease.

CT in Small Airways Disease. Thin-section CT is a sensitive indicator of the presence of small airways disease. The CT findings of small airways disease include both direct and indirect findings. The direct CT signs of small airways disease include centrilobular nodules, seen as sharply defined or ground-glass attenuation nodules situated within 5 mm of the costal pleural surface, and centrilobular tree-in-bud opacities which are branching Y- or V-shaped tubular opacities. Pathologically, these tree-in-bud opacities reflect dilated and mucus-filled preterminal bronchioles or peribronchiolar inflammation and fibrosis.

The indirect CT signs of small airways disease include proximal bronchial dilatation, most often seen in patients with chronic obliterative small airways disease (i.e., constrictive bronchiolitis), and hyperlucent regions due to expiratory air trapping. Those portions of lung most severely affected by small airways disease are poorly ventilated and perfused and appear relatively hyperlucent relative to normal lung, producing a pattern of mosaic attenuation. A mosaic attenuation appearance on CT can also be seen in patients with primary pulmonary vascular disease, most typically chronic

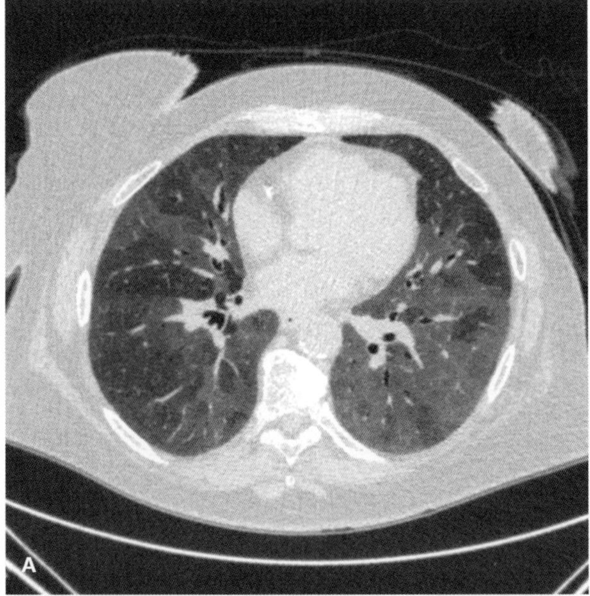

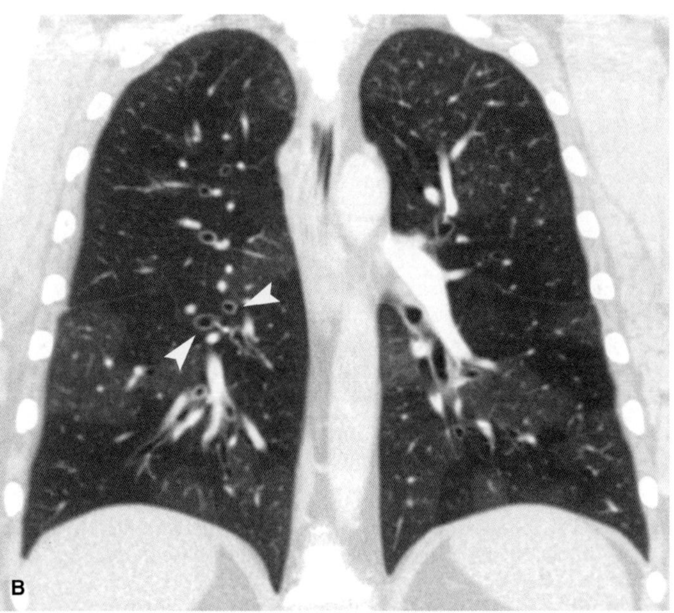

FIGURE 16.20. **Mosaic Attenuation due to Ground-Glass Infiltrative Disease Versus Mosaic Perfusion From Small Airways Disease. A:** Axial CT through the lower lungs in a patient with *Pneumocystis jiroveci* pneumonia demonstrates bilateral ground-glass opacity with spared regions. Note the normal airways and uniform caliber of vessels within involved and uninvolved regions. **B:** Coronal CT through the posterior lungs in a patient with constrictive bronchiolitis shows regions of abnormal decreased attenuation due to air trapping. The presence of mild bronchial dilatation in the right perihilar lung (*arrowheads*) and small size of vessels within lucent regions help confirm mosaic attenuation due to mosaic perfusion from airways disease and associated decreased perfusion of involved regions.

TABLE 16.6

CLINICAL AND IMAGING FEATURES OF SMALL AIRWAYS DISEASE

ENTITY	ASSOCIATED CONDITIONS	CT FINDINGS
Infectious bronchiolitis	Viral/atypical/mycobacterial infection	Tree-in-bud opacities
Diffuse panbronchiolitis	None	Tree-in-bud opacities, bronchial dilatation/thickening
Respiratory bronchiolitis-associated interstitial lung disease	Cigarette smoking	Centrilobular and geographic ground-glass opacities
Hypersensitivity pneumonitis (subacute)	Inhaled organic antigen	Centrilobular ground-glass nodules, air trapping on expiratory scans
Follicular bronchiolitis	Rheumatoid arthritis, Sjögren syndrome	Centrilobular ground-glass nodules
Constrictive bronchiolitis	Transplant patients, drug reactions, inhalation injury, postinfectious, inflammatory bowel disease	Mosaic attenuation with air trapping on expiratory scans, bronchial dilatation (late)
Diffuse idiopathic pulmonary neuroendocrine cell hyperplasia (DIPNECH)	Carcinoid tumor	Mosaic attenuation with air trapping on expiratory scans, bronchial thickening, nodule(s)

thromboembolic pulmonary hypertension, and in infiltrative processes such as *Pneumocystis jiroveci* pneumonia and desquamative interstitial pneumonitis that produce geographic ground-glass opacification. The use of both inspiratory and expiratory CT can help distinguish between mosaic attenuation due to airways or vascular disease (termed mosaic perfusion) and mosaic attenuation due to infiltrative disorders. In patients with mosaic perfusion due to small airways disease, expiratory CT demonstrates attenuated vessels within more lucent regions of lung indicating that the lucency is the result of decreased perfusion, whereas vessel size is uniform between regions of normal lung and ground-glass infiltration (Fig. 16.20).

Bronchiolitis, or small airways disease, refers to an inflammation of the small airways (Table 16.6). Pathologically, bronchiolitis is histologically classified as either cellular/proliferative or constrictive/obliterative subtype. Centrilobular bronchioles located at the center of the secondary pulmonary lobule are not normally visible, only visible when abnormal. *Infectious bronchiolitis* is often a disease of young children caused by respiratory syncytial virus or adenovirus and produces respiratory distress and radiographic hyperinflation that are indistinguishable from asthma. However, there is an increasing recognition of infectious bronchiolitis in adults caused by a variety of microorganisms (Fig. 16.21). A specific but uncommon cause of bronchiolitis is *diffuse* or *Asian panbronchiolitis*, which is associated with sinus disease and results in progressive pulmonary symptoms of airways disease, including cough and sputum production. Bronchiolar and peribronchial inflammation is commonly a result of heavy cigarette smoking. This latter disease is termed *RB-ILD*, and it presents with signs and symptoms of interstitial lung disease. RB-ILD is reviewed in Chapter 15. Bronchiolitis is also a prominent feature of patients with subacute hypersensitivity pneumonitis, which is also reviewed in Chapter 15. A mononuclear cell-infiltrative bronchiolitis can be seen in patients with inflammatory bowel disease, *Follicular bronchiolitis* reflects a form of diffuse lymphoid hyperplasia of peribronchiolar lymphoid follicles of unclear clinical significance seen in patients with rheumatoid arthritis or Sjögren syndrome. Thin-section CT shows ill-defined centrilobular ground-glass nodules and occasional bronchial dilatation.

Constrictive bronchiolitis, also known as *bronchiolitis obliterans,* is a subacute disease characterized pathologically by a mononuclear cell inflammatory process within the walls of respiratory bronchioles that leads to the formation of granulation tissue, which plugs small airways. This results in dyspnea and functional airways obstruction. This disorder may be idiopathic or secondary to viral infection, toxic fume inhalation (e.g., silo-filler's disease), drug reaction (e.g., penicillamine), collagen vascular disorders (e.g., rheumatoid arthritis), organ transplantation, or chronic aspiration. Lung, heart–lung, and bone marrow transplant patients (Fig. 16.20B) are at particularly risk. Constrictive bronchiolitis in the adult may be the result of an early childhood lower respiratory infection with adenovirus, measles, or mycoplasma, in which case it is known as unilateral hyperlucent lung or Swyer–James syndrome. In Swyer–James syndrome, the bronchiolitis causes diffuse small airways obliteration, air trapping, and destruction

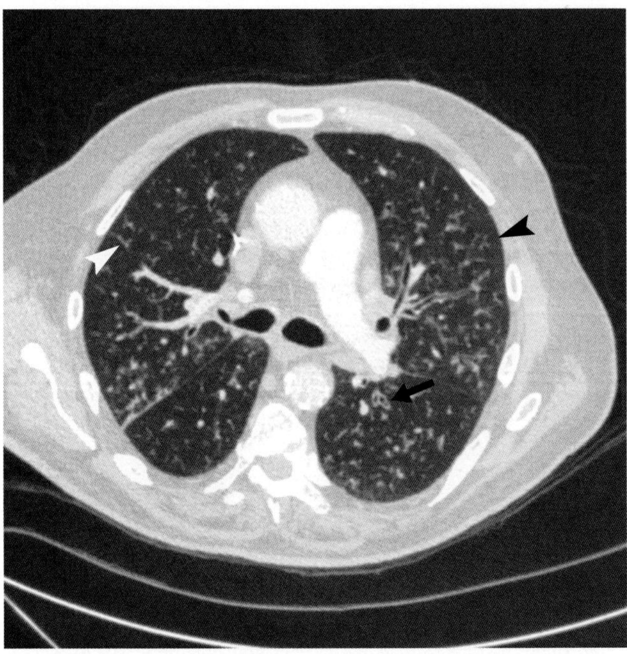

FIGURE 16.21. Infectious Bronchiolitis With Tree-in-Bud Opacities. Axial CT through the mid lungs in a patient with mycoplasma pneumonia shows centrilobular tree-in-bud opacities (*arrowheads*) and thickened bronchi (*arrows*).

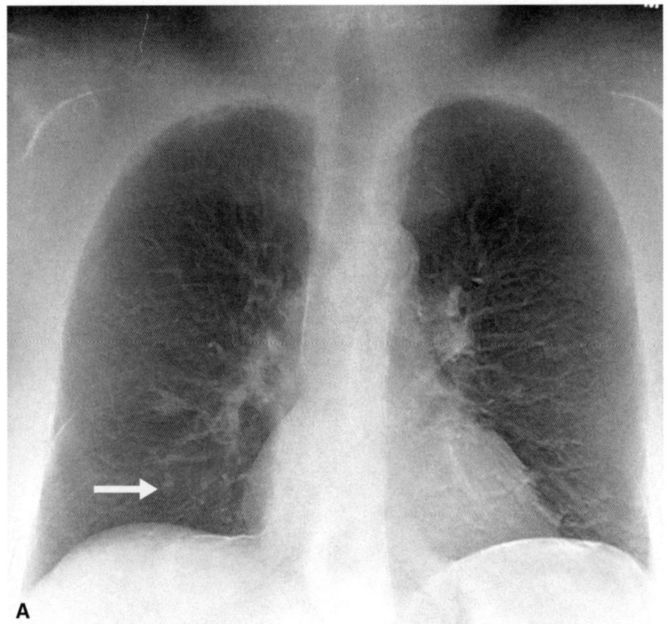

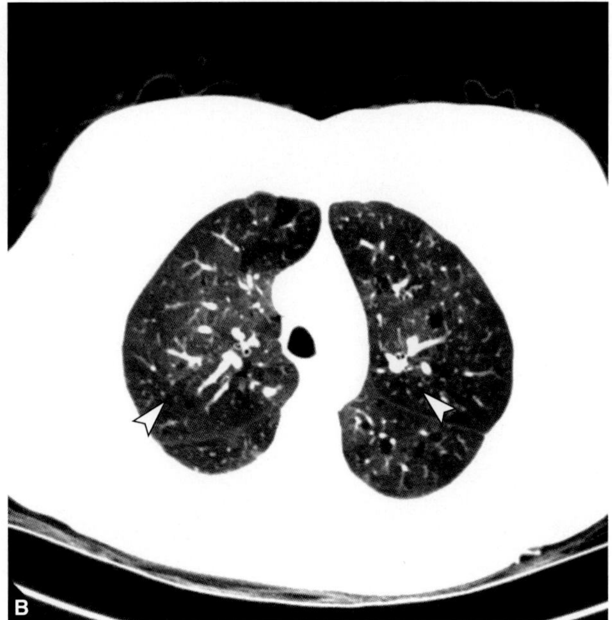

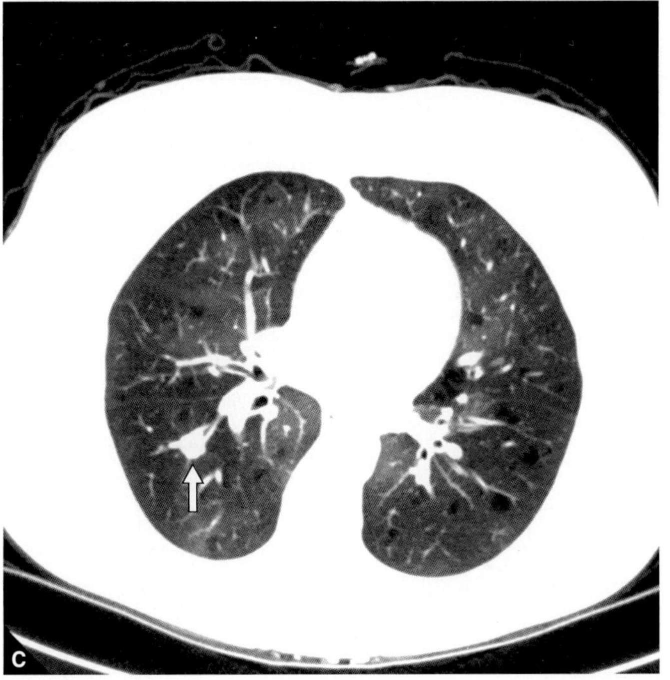

FIGURE 16.22. **Diffuse Idiopathic Pulmonary Neuroendocrine Cell Hyperplasia (DIPNECH). A:** Dual-energy subtraction frontal chest radiograph in a 53-year-old woman with a long history of asthma shows a nodule in the right lower lung (*arrow*). **B:** Axial CT through the upper lungs (**B**) shows marked mosaic perfusion. There are multiple small nodules (*arrowheads*). **C:** Axial CT at the level of the nodule seen radiographically shows that a right lower lobe nodule that lies along a bronchovascular bundle (*arrow*). CT-guided biopsy of the right lower lobe nodule revealed a typical carcinoid tumor. Subsequent surgical biopsy of another nodule revealed carcinoid tumorlet.

of alveolar walls and emphysema owing to overdistention of peripheral airspaces. Because postinfectious bronchiolitis obliterans affects the lungs asymmetrically and usually occurs during a period of lung growth and development, the affected lung is typically small and hyperlucent and the ipsilateral PA is hypoplastic. Most patients with the Swyer–James syndrome are asymptomatic, whereas some patients complain of dyspnea or recurrent lower respiratory tract infections. A rare form of constrictive bronchiolitis, termed diffuse idiopathic pulmonary neuroendocrine cell hyperplasia (DIPNECH), is seen in middle-aged women who demonstrate severe airflow limitation and thin-section CT findings of air trapping with bronchial thickening and dilatation in association with one or multiple small nodules representing neuroendocrine cell tumorlets or, if the nodules are >5-mm diameter, carcinoid tumors (Fig. 16.22).

The chest radiograph in patients with pure constrictive bronchiolitis may be normal despite the presence of severe dyspnea and functional evidence of airflow obstruction. The most common radiographic abnormality in this disorder is diffuse reticulonodular opacities with associated hyperinflation. Central bronchiectasis has been described particularly in those with constrictive bronchiolitis that developed as a complication of heart–lung transplantation. In patients with Swyer–James syndrome, the affected lung is normal or small in volume, and marked unilateral air trapping is seen on fluoroscopy or expiratory films. The air trapping is caused by bronchiolar obstruction with collateral air drift to the distal airspaces on inspiration that cannot escape on expiration. The ipsilateral hilum is small and the pulmonary vasculature is reduced, accounting for the hyperlucency seen radiographically and on CT (Fig. 16.23). Perfusion lung scanning shows

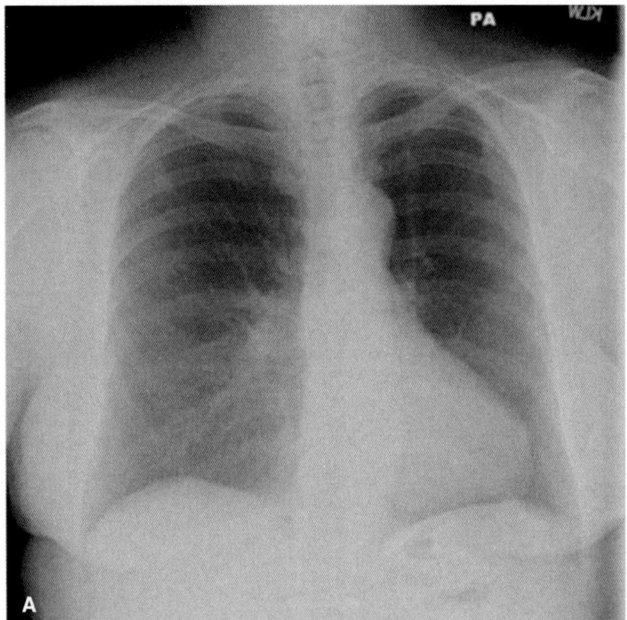

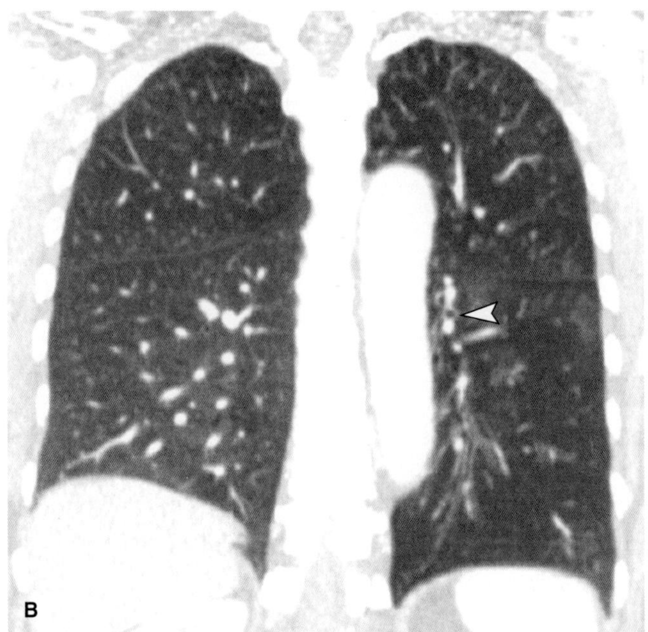

FIGURE 16.23. **Unilateral Hyperlucent Lung (Swyer–James) Syndrome. A:** Chest radiograph shows subtle decrease in left lung volume with a small left hilum and attenuated vascularity. **B:** Coronal reformatted CT scan through the level of the descending aorta at lung windows shows left lung hyperlucency with mild central bronchial dilatation and thickening (*arrowhead*).

decreased perfusion of the affected lung, while the ventilation study shows decreased ventilation with markedly delayed radioisotope washout. This latter finding helps distinguish the Swyer–James syndrome from primary central PA occlusion or hypoplastic lung, conditions in which ventilation is maintained.

Suggested Readings

Barnes D, Gutiérrez Chacoff J, Benegas M, et al. Central airway pathology: clinic features, CT findings with pathologic and virtual endoscopy correlation. *Insights Imaging* 2017;8(2):255–270.

Berniker AV, Henry TS. Imaging of small airways diseases. *Radiol Clin North Am* 2016;54(6):1165–1181.

Carden KA, Boiselle PM, Waltz DA, Ernst A. Tracheomalacia and tracheobronchomalacia in children and adults: an in-depth review. *Chest* 2005;127(3):984–1005.

Chung JH, Kanne JP, Gilman MD. CT of diffuse tracheal diseases. *AJR Am J Roentgenol* 2011;196(3):W240–W246.

Foster WL Jr, Gimenez EI, Roubidoux MA, et al. The emphysemas: radiologic-pathologic correlations. *Radiographics* 1993;13(2):311–328.

Hansell DM. Small airways diseases: detection and insights with computed tomography. *Eur Respir J* 2001;17(6):1294–1313.

Hansell DM, Bankier AA, MacMahon H, McLoud TC, Müller NL, Remy J. Fleischner Society: glossary of terms for thoracic imaging. *Radiology* 2008; 246(3):697–722.

Lynch DA. Imaging of small airways disease and chronic obstructive pulmonary disease. *Clin Chest Med* 2008;29(1):165–179.

Marom EM, Goodman PC, McAdams HP. Focal abnormalities of the trachea and main bronchi. *AJR Am J Roentgenol* 2001;176(3):707–711.

Milliron B, Henry TS, Veeraraghavan S, Little BP. Bronchiectasis: mechanisms and imaging clues of associated common and uncommon diseases. *Radiographics* 2015;35(4):1011–1030.

Rice A, Nicholson AG. The pathologist's approach to small airways disease. *Histopathology* 2009;54(1):117–133.

Semple T, Calder A, Owens CM, Padley S. Current and future approaches to large airways imaging in adults and children. *Clin Radiol* 2017;72(5):356–374.

Stagnaro N, Rizzo F, Torre M, Cittadini G, Magnano G. Multimodality imaging of pediatric airways disease: indication and technique. *Radiol Med* 2017;122(6):419–429.

Washko GR. Diagnostic imaging in COPD. *Semin Respir Crit Care Med* 2010; 31(3):276–285.

CHAPTER 17 ■ PLEURA, CHEST WALL, DIAPHRAGM, AND MISCELLANEOUS CHEST DISORDERS

JEFFREY S. KLEIN

PLEURA

Anatomy, Physiology, and Pathophysiology

The pleura is a serous membrane subdivided into visceral pleura, which covers the lung and forms the interlobar fissures, and parietal pleura, which lines the mediastinum, diaphragm, and thoracic cage. Both the visceral and parietal pleurae consist of a single layer of mesothelial cells and their basement membrane, and a dense sheet of irregular connective tissue with varying ratios of collagen to elastin. The potential space between the visceral and parietal pleura is the pleural space. The parietal and visceral pleurae meet at the hila, and form a thin double-layered fold at the medial lung base inferior to the inferior pulmonary veins termed the pulmonary ligament. A small amount of fluid totaling 2 to 5 mL is normally present in the pleural space to serve as a lubricant that allows smooth gliding of the visceral pleura along the parietal pleura during breathing. The volume of fluid within the pleural space is the result of a dynamic equilibrium between formation and resorption. The formation of pleural fluid follows Starling law and depends upon hydrostatic and oncotic forces in both the systemic capillaries of the parietal pleura and the pleural space. Under normal conditions, pleural fluid is formed by filtration from systemic capillaries in the parietal pleura and resorbed via the parietal pleural lymphatics (Fig. 17.1).

The radiologically detectable manifestations of pleural diseases are limited and include effusion, thickening, and calcification.

Pleural Effusion

Pleural effusions form when an imbalance occurs between formation and reabsorption (Table 17.1). Pleural effusions may be classified by their gross appearance (bloody, chylous, purulent, serous), the underlying disease process (Table 17.2), or by the pathophysiology of abnormal pleural fluid formation (i.e., transudative vs. exudative) (Tables 17.1). This latter differentiation is made by measuring the protein, lactic acid dehydrogenase (LDH), and glucose concentration of the pleural fluid obtained by thoracentesis (Table 17.3).

Specific Causes of Pleural Effusion

Congestive Heart Failure. Congestive heart failure is the most common condition to produce a transudative pleural effusion. The effusions are typically bilateral and larger on the right. An isolated right effusion is twice as common as an isolated left effusion.

Parapneumonic Effusion and Empyema. A parapneumonic effusion is defined as an effusion associated with pneumonia. Peripheral parenchymal infection produces an exudative pleural effusion by causing visceral pleural inflammation that increases pleural capillary permeability. Inflammatory thickening of the pleural membranes with lymphatic obstruction may also be a contributing factor. Empyema results when the parenchymal infection extends into the pleural space. Parenchymal infections that typically result in empyema formation are bacterial pneumonia, septic emboli, and lung abscess, whereas fungal, viral, and parasitic infections are uncommon causes. Less commonly, infection may extend into the pleural space from the spine, mediastinum, and chest wall.

Forty percent of bacterial pneumonias have an associated pleural effusion. *Staphylococcus aureus* and gram-negative pneumonias are the most common cause of parapneumonic effusion and empyema. The natural history of parapneumonic effusions may be divided into three stages. Stage I is an exudative stage; visceral pleural inflammation causes increased capillary permeability and pleural fluid accumulation. Most of these sterile exudative effusions resolve with appropriate antibiotic therapy. A stage II parapneumonic effusion is a fibrinopurulent pleural fluid collection containing bacteria

TABLE 17.1

PATHOPHYSIOLOGY OF ABNORMAL PLEURAL FLUID FORMATION

■ MECHANISM	■ DISEASE ENTITY	■ TRANSUDATE/EXUDATE
Increased interstitial fluid production	CHF, parapneumonic effusion, permeability pulmonary edema, lung transplantation	Transudate
Increased hydrostatic pressure	LV or RV failure, SVC syndrome, pericardial tamponade	Transudate
Increased capillary permeability		Exudate
Decreased capillary oncotic pressure	Low protein states	Transudate
Impaired fluid resorption	Malignancy	Exudate
Elevated systemic venous pressure		Transudate

and neutrophils. Fibrin deposition on the visceral and parietal pleura impairs fluid resorption and produces loculations. If the infection is not treated, the loculations will impair attempts at closed pleural fluid drainage. A stage III parapneumonic effusion develops 2 to 3 weeks after initial pleural fluid formation and is characterized by the ingrowth of fibroblasts over the pleura, which produces pleural fibrosis and entraps the lung. Dystrophic calcification of the pleura may develop following resolution of the pleural infection. Tuberculous pleural effusion or empyema resulting from the rupture of subpleural caseating granulomas may complicate pulmonary infection or occur as the primary manifestation of disease. Effusions in tuberculosis (TB) are more common in young adults with pulmonary disease and in HIV-positive individuals with severe immunodeficiency. The pleural fluid is characteristically straw colored, with greater than 70% lymphocytes and a low glucose concentration.

Radiographically, empyema most often appears as a loculated pleural fluid collection. On CT, it is elliptic in shape and is seen most often within the posterior (costal pleura) and inferior (subpulmonic) pleural space. The collection conforms to and maintains a broad area of contact with the chest wall (Fig. 17.2). The distinction of empyema from peripheral lung abscess has important therapeutic implications; empyemas require external drainage, whereas lung abscesses usually respond to postural drainage and antibiotic therapy. Contrast-enhanced chest CT is most useful in making this distinction (Table 17.4). Detection of an empyema may be difficult when there is extensive parenchymal consolidation. In these cases, CT and US are useful in detecting parapneumonic fluid collections and guiding diagnostic thoracentesis and pleural drainage. Findings on CT that are fairly specific for the presence of

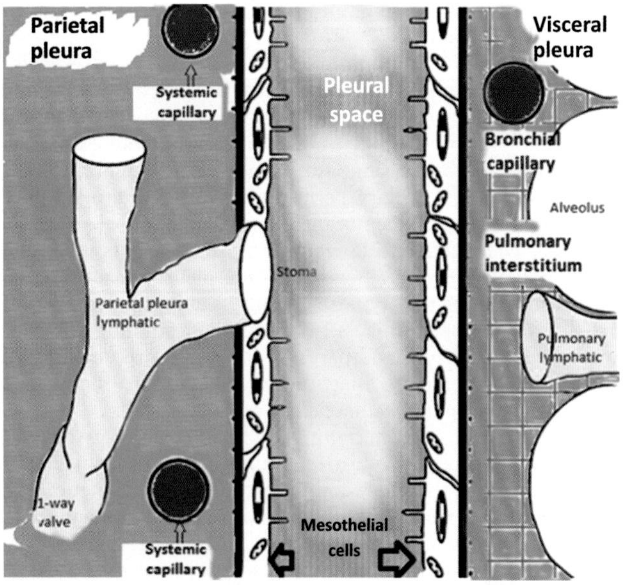

FIGURE 17.1. Normal Pleural Fluid Physiology. (Diagram modified from Miserocchi G. Physiology and pathophysiology of pleural fluid turnover. *Eur Respir J* 1997;10(1):219–225, with permission.)

TABLE 17.2

ETIOLOGY OF PLEURAL EFFUSIONS

■ DISEASE CATEGORY	■ ENTITY
Infection	Bacterial Fungal Viral Mycobacterial Parasitic
Cardiovascular	Congestive heart failure Constrictive pericarditis Superior vena cava obstruction Post-myocardial infarction or pericardiotomy (Dressler) syndrome Pulmonary infarction
Neoplastic	Lung cancer Metastatic disease Lymphoma Chest wall/pleural neoplasm
Collagen vascular	Systemic lupus erythematosus Rheumatoid arthritis
Inhalational	Asbestos-related pleural effusion
Trauma	Blunt or penetrating trauma ▪ Hemothorax ▪ Chylothorax Esophageal rupture
Abdominal disease	Pancreatitis Subphrenic abscess Cirrhosis (hepatic hydrothorax) Ascites (any cause)
Miscellaneous	Drugs Myxedema Ovarian tumors (Meigs syndrome)

TABLE 17.3

CHEMICAL CHARACTERISTICS OF TRANSUDATIVE VERSUS EXUDATIVE EFFUSIONS

Transudate	Exudate
TP_{fluid}/TP_{serum} <0.5	TP_{fluid}/TP_{serum} >0.5
LDH_{fluid}/LDH_{serum} <0.6	LDH_{fluid}/LDH_{serum} >0.6
LDH_{fluid} <200 IU/L	LDH_{fluid} >200 IU/L
Specific gravity <1.016	Specific gravity >1.016
Diseases:	**Diseases:**
Cardiogenic	Infection
Hypoproteinemic	Infarction
Myxedematous	Neoplasm
Cirrhotic (hepatic hydrothorax)	Inflammation (serositis)
Nephrotic syndrome	

an exudative pleural effusion include thickening and enhancement of the parietal pleura, the presence of loculations, and the detection of discrete soft tissue lesions along the parietal pleura outlined by low-attenuation pleural fluid. Hemorrhagic effusions can occasionally be recognized on CT by their intrinsic high attenuation or the presence of a fluid–fluid level caused by dependent cellular blood elements.

Neoplasms. Pleural effusion may be seen with benign or malignant intrathoracic tumors. The tumors most commonly associated with pleural effusion are, in order of frequency, lung carcinoma, breast carcinoma, pelvic tumors, gastric carcinoma, and lymphoma. Pleural fluid may result from pleural involvement by tumor or from lymphatic obstruction anywhere from the parietal pleura to the mediastinal nodes. The effusions are exudative and may be bloody.

Demonstration of malignant cells on cytologic examination of pleural fluid obtained at thoracentesis is necessary for

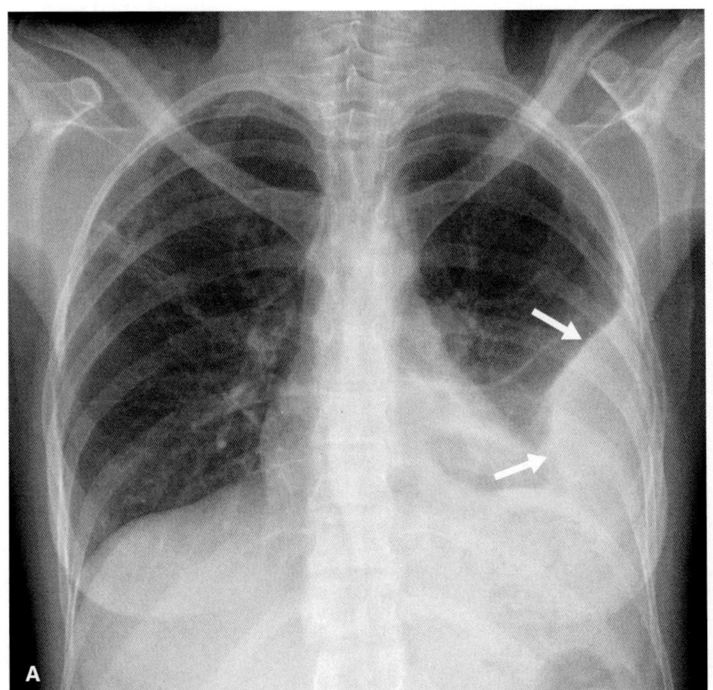

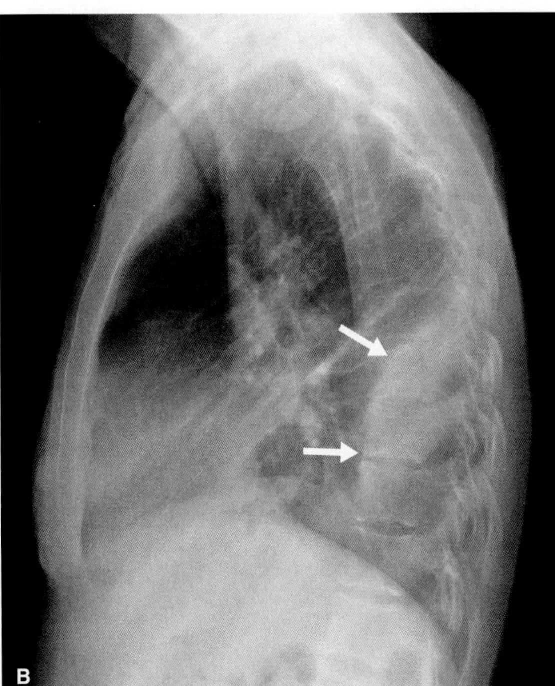

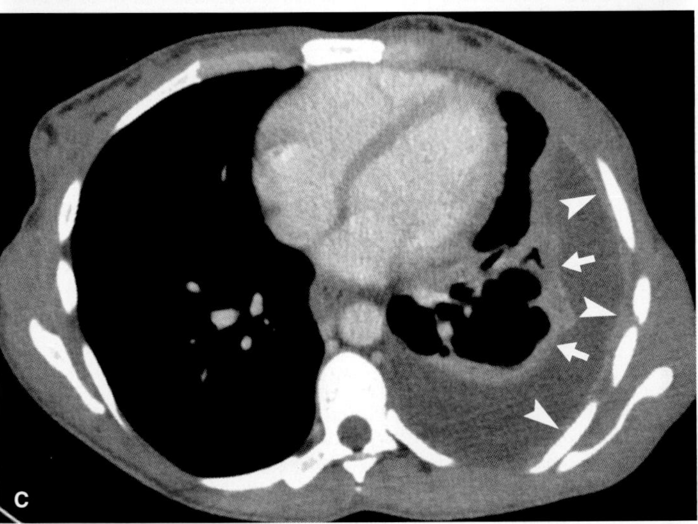

FIGURE 17.2. Empyema on Radiography and CT. A, B: Frontal (**A**) and lateral (**B**) chest radiographs in a 37-year-old woman with empyema show a loculated left lateral and posterior pleural fluid collection (*arrows*). **C:** Contrast-enhanced axial CT shows a left pleural fluid collection with enhancing parietal (*arrowheads*) and visceral (*short arrows*) pleural surfaces characteristic of an empyema. The patient subsequently underwent successful image-guided catheter drainage with resolution of the collection.

TABLE 17.4

EMPYEMA VERSUS LUNG ABSCESS ON CT

■ FEATURE	■ EMPYEMA	■ ABSCESS
Shape	Oval, oriented longitudinally	Round
Margin	Thin, smooth ("split pleura" sign)	Thick, irregular
Angle with chest wall	Obtuse	Acute
Effect on lung	Compression	Consumption
Treatment	External drainage	Antibiotics, postural drainage

the diagnosis of a malignant effusion. Image-guided closed or thoracoscopic biopsy is reserved for patients with negative cytologic examination. Clues to the presence of a malignant pleural effusion include smooth or nodular pleural thickening, mediastinal or hilar lymph node enlargement or mass, and solitary or multiple parenchymal nodules. CT is useful in demonstrating pleural masses or underlying parenchymal lesions in those with large effusions (Fig. 17.3).

Trauma. Blunt or penetrating trauma to the chest, including iatrogenic trauma from thoracotomy, thoracostomy, or placement of central venous catheters, may result in a hemothorax. Hemothorax results from laceration of vessels within the lung, mediastinum, chest wall, or diaphragm. Intrapleural blood coagulates rapidly, and septations form early. In some individuals, pleural motion causes defibrination, which lyses the clotted blood. In the acute setting, pleural fluid of high CT attenuation (>80 H) may be seen (Fig. 17.4); associated rib fractures or subcutaneous emphysema should suggest the diagnosis. An acute hemothorax is treated with thoracostomy tube drainage, while thoracotomy is generally reserved for persistent bleeding or hypotension.

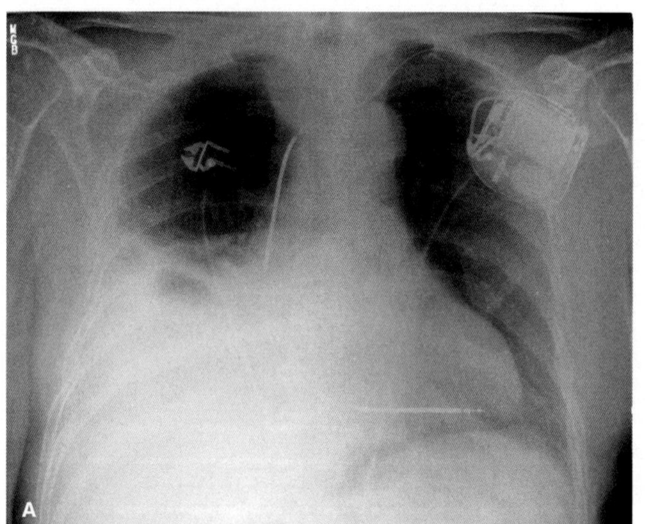

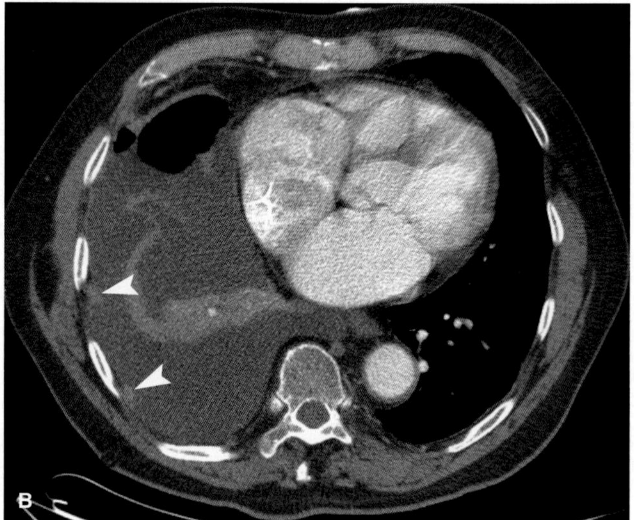

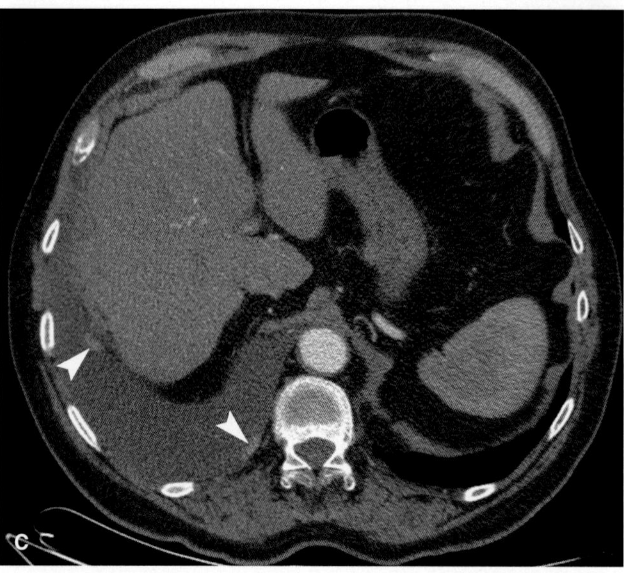

FIGURE 17.3. **Malignant Pleural Effusion: CT Diagnosis. A:** Frontal chest radiograph in a 69-year-old man with a history of renal cell carcinoma shows a moderate right pleural effusion. **B, C:** Contrast-enhanced axial CT scans at the level of the left atrium (**B**) and upper abdomen (**C**) show parietal pleural nodules (*arrowheads*) reflecting tumor implants associated with the pleural effusion. Pleural fluid cytology confirmed metastatic pleural disease.

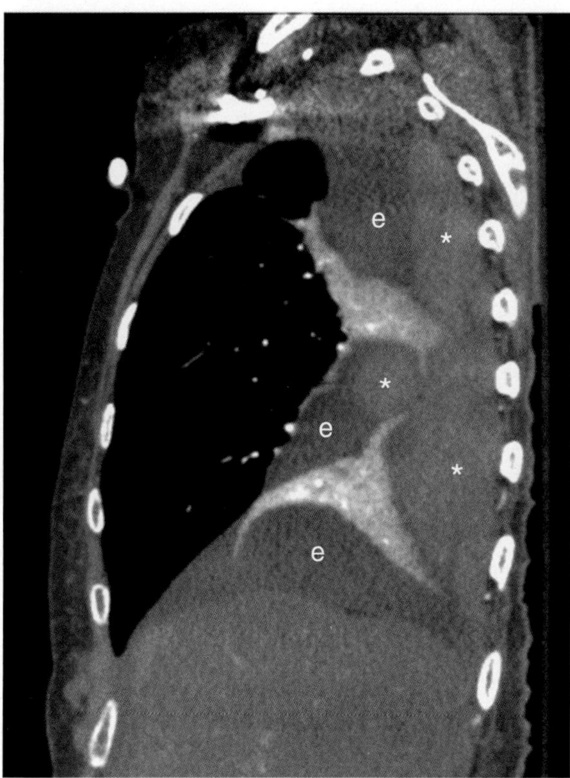

FIGURE 17.4. **Hemothorax.** Contrast-enhanced sagittal CT through the right hemithorax in a patient who has sustained blunt chest trauma with a right rib fracture shows a pleural effusion (e) containing dependent high-attenuation material (*asterisks*) representing clotted blood in a traumatic hemothorax.

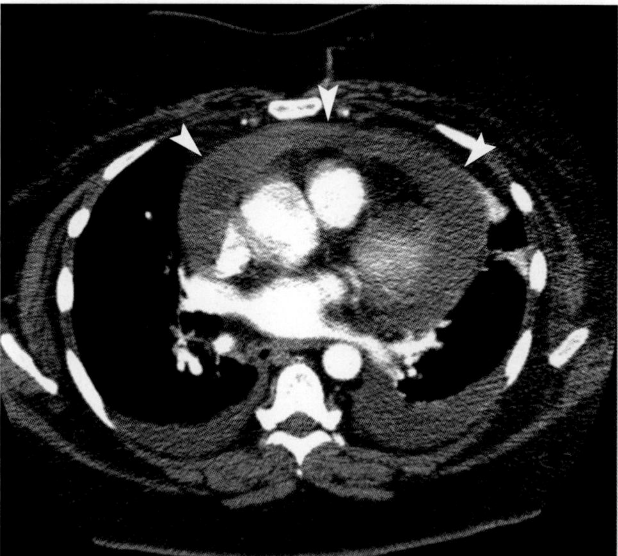

FIGURE 17.5. **Serositis With Pleural and Pericardial Effusions.** Axial CT scan in a 54-year-old patient with lupus erythematosus shows bilateral pleural and a pericardial effusion. Note subtle thickening and enhancement of the pericardium (*arrowheads*) indicating the presence of pericarditis.

Esophageal perforation from prolonged vomiting (Boerhaave syndrome) or as a complication of esophageal dilatation may produce a pleural effusion, most commonly on the left side. Elevated salivary amylase levels and low pH within pleural fluid in a patient clinically suspected to have esophageal perforation is diagnostic.

Extravascular placement of a central line can result in a hydrothorax when intravenous solution is inadvertently infused into the pleural or extrapleural space.

Collagen Vascular and Autoimmune Disease. Systemic lupus erythematosus has a reported incidence of pleural effusions ranging from 33% to 74% (Fig. 17.5). These exudative effusions are a result of pleural inflammation; patients often present with pleuritic chest pain. Cardiomegaly is a common associated radiographic finding and may be caused by pericardial effusion, hypertension, renal failure, or lupus-associated endocarditis or myocarditis. Pleural effusion is the most common intrathoracic manifestation of rheumatoid arthritis and is most frequently seen in male patients following the onset of joint disease.

The effusions occur independent of pulmonary parenchymal involvement but may develop following intrapleural rupture of peripheral rheumatoid nodules. The effusions of rheumatoid arthritis are exudative, with lymphocytosis, low glucose concentration, and low pH (<7.2). Rheumatoid effusions may persist unchanged for years. Autoimmune syndromes producing pleural and pericardial effusions have been described following myocardial infarction (Dressler syndrome) or cardiac surgery (postpericardiotomy syndrome). Both are characterized by fever, pleuritis, pneumonitis, and pericarditis developing within days to weeks of the precipitating event. The radiographic findings include enlargement of the cardiac silhouette, pleural effusions, and parenchymal airspace opacities. A serosanguinous exudative pleural effusion is seen in over 80% of patients. Treatment with nonsteroidal anti-inflammatory drugs usually results in symptomatic and radiographic improvement.

Abdominal Disease. Radioisotope studies have demonstrated that peritoneal fluid may enter the pleural space via transdiaphragmatic lymphatic channels or through defects in the diaphragm. The lymphatic channels are larger on the right side, accounting for the higher incidence of right-sided effusions associated with ascites or liver failure (hepatic hydrothorax).

Pancreatitis. Acute or chronic pancreatitis can cause pleural effusions that are most often left sided because of the proximity of the pancreatic tail to the left hemidiaphragm. The effusion associated with acute pancreatitis is typically exudative and may be bloody. Pleural effusion from chronic pancreatitis may cause pleuritic chest pain and shortness of breath. Rupture of the pancreatic duct can lead to a pancreaticopleural fistula. A high amylase concentration in the pleural fluid should suggest the pancreas as the etiology of the effusion, although elevated amylase may be seen in pleural effusions caused by malignancy or esophageal perforation.

Subphrenic Abscess. Subphrenic abscess complicating abdominal surgery or perforation of a hollow viscus can cause diaphragmatic paresis, basilar atelectasis, and pleural effusion. Patients with a pleural effusion associated with upper abdominal pain, fever, and leukocytosis should have CT or US examination and when applicable, percutaneous catheter drainage of the abscess.

Pelvic Tumors. An association between benign pleural effusions and pelvic tumors has long been recognized. First described with ovarian fibroma (Meigs syndrome), a number of pelvic and abdominal tumors, including pancreatic and ovarian malignancy, lymphoma, and uterine leiomyomas, have been found to cause pleural effusion. The effusions in Meigs syndrome are usually transudative and resolve after removal of the pelvic tumor.

Chylothorax. Chylothorax is a pleural collection containing triglycerides in the form of chylomicrons resulting from extravasation of thoracic duct contents secondary to

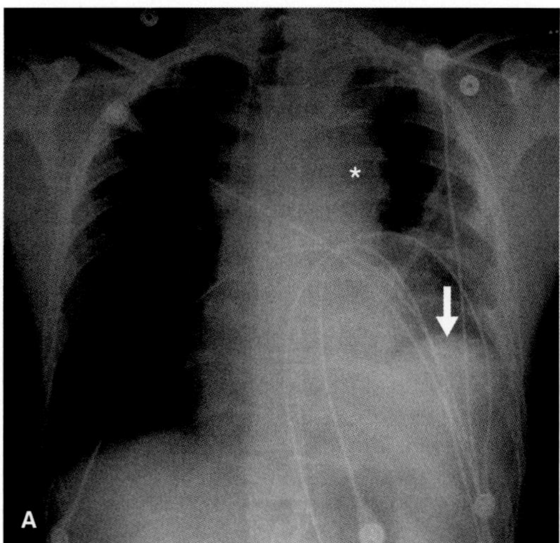

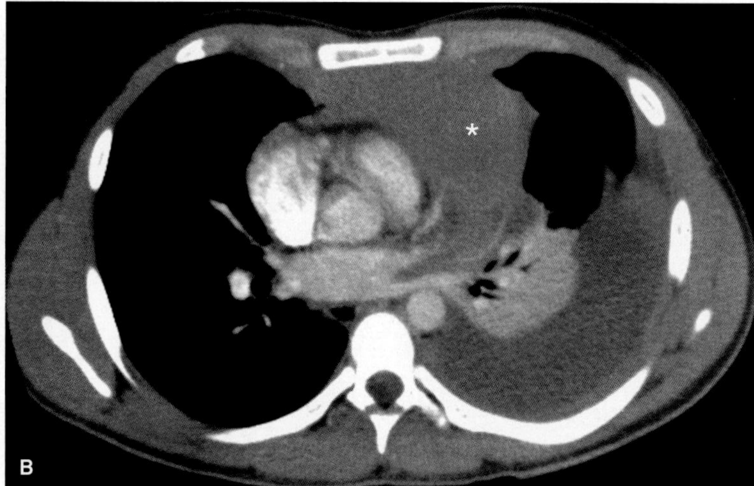

FIGURE 17.6. Chylous Pleural Effusions Caused by Lymphoma. A: Frontal chest radiograph in a 34-year-old man with non-Hodgkin lymphoma shows a mediastinal mass (*asterisk*) with a subpulmonic left pleural effusion (*arrow*). **B:** Contrast-enhanced axial CT through the mid-chest shows an anterior mediastinal mass (*asterisk*) with a left pleural effusion and passive left lower lobe atelectasis. Left thoracentesis revealed a milky effusion found to be chylous based on elevated pleural fluid triglyceride levels.

malignancy, iatrogenic trauma, or TB (Fig. 17.6). The thoracic duct originates from the cisterna chyli at the level of the first lumbar vertebra and ascends along the right paravertebral space, entering the thorax via the aortic hiatus. As it ascends, the duct crosses from right to left at the level of the sixth thoracic vertebra to lie alongside the upper esophagus. A knowledge of this anatomy is useful as disruption of the upper duct caused by direct trauma or obstruction with rupture produces a left chylothorax, while injury to the lower intrathoracic duct produces a right chylothorax. At the level of the left subclavian artery, the duct arches anteriorly to empty into the confluence of the left internal jugular and subclavian veins. The radiographic appearance is indistinguishable on conventional radiographs and CT from other causes of free-flowing effusions. The diagnosis is confirmed by triglyceride levels exceeding 110 mg/dL in the pleural fluid.

Pulmonary Embolism. Infarction complicating pulmonary embolism is a well-recognized cause of pleural effusion. The effusion may be associated with elevation of the ipsilateral diaphragm and peripheral wedge-shaped opacities (Hampton hump). The pleural effusion is typically a small, unilateral, serosanguineous exudate.

Drugs. Drugs may cause pleural effusions as a result of pleural inflammation (methysergide) or by producing a lupus-like syndrome (phenytoin, isoniazid, hydralazine, procainamide). Nitrofurantoin has been associated with an immunologic reaction that causes pleuropulmonary disease with eosinophilia.

Management of Pleural Effusion. Transudative pleural effusions are managed by treatment of the underlying disorder, because the pleura is intrinsically normal in these diseases. Management of parapneumonic effusions is best guided by evaluation of the likelihood that the effusion, if not drained, would result in prolonged hospitalization, pleural fibrosis with resultant respiratory impairment, local spread of infection, or death. This likelihood is based on the anatomy, bacteriology, and chemistry (i.e., ABCs) of the fluid collection (Table 17.5). In general, larger, loculated collections with positive gram

TABLE 17.5

PARAPNEUMONIC EFFUSION: ANATOMY, BACTERIOLOGY, AND CHEMISTRY

Categorizing Outcome					
Pleural space Anatomy	Pleural fluid Bacteriology	Pleural fluid Chemistry	Category	Risk of poor outcome	Drainage
A_0 = free-flowing effusion <10 mm	B_x = culture and Gram stain unknown	C_x = pH unknown	1	Very low	No
A_1 = small to moderate free-flowing effusion >10 mm and <½ hemithorax	B_0 = negative culture and Gram stain	C_0 = pH >7.20	2	Low	No
A_2 = large free-flowing (>½ hemithorax), loculated, or thickened parietal pleura	B_1 = positive culture or Gram stain	C_1 = pH <7.20	3	Moderate	Yes
	B_2 = Pus		4	High	Yes

Colice GL, Curtis A, Deslauriers J, et al. Medical and surgical treatment of parapneumonic effusions: an evidence-based guideline. *Chest* 2000;118(4):1158–1171.

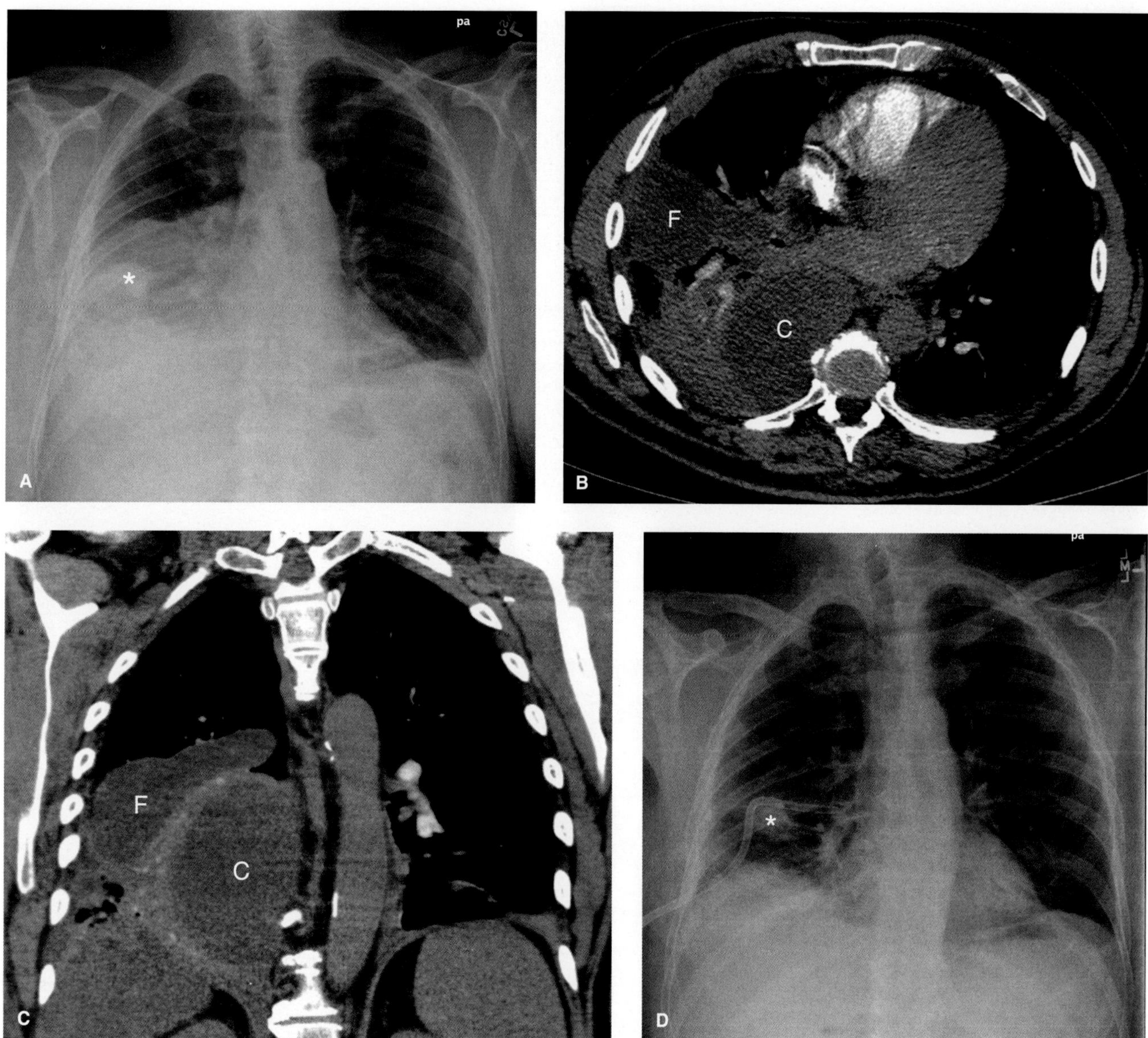

FIGURE 17.7. **CT-Guided Percutaneous Empyema Drainage Using Fibrinolytics. A:** Frontal chest radiograph in a 64-year-old man with cough and fever shows abnormal opacity over the right lower lung consistent with a pleural effusion with a loculated intrafissural component (*asterisk*). **B, C:** Contrast-enhanced axial (**B**) and coronal (**C**) CT scans demonstrate a multiloculated right pleural fluid collections with locules in the major fissure (F) and in the lower posteromedial costal pleural space (C). **D:** Frontal chest radiograph following image-guided transcatheter drainage with intrapleural fibrinolytic therapy shows the drainage catheter with marked radiographic improvement, with only a minor fissural component remaining (*asterisk*).

stains or cultures and pH <7.20 are associated with a moderate to high risk for poor outcome as detailed above and should be drained if possible. The choice of drainage procedure depends on various factors, including patient age and underlying condition, length of illness, and access to image-guided therapy and thoracoscopy. Although intrapleural fibrinolytic therapy using tissue plasminogen activator with concomitant DNAse will help a certain subset of patients with complex parapneumonic effusions (Fig. 17.7), some will require open pleural drainage by video-assisted thoracoscopic surgery (VATS) or thoracotomy with decortication. In contrast, malignant pleural effusions most often require closed drainage and pleural sclerosis, with talc being the current agent of choice. Trials of other pleurodesis agents have not shown superiority while being marred by higher cost. It is notable that talc pleurodesis can cause FDG-PET positive nodularity that is a source of false-negative PET evaluations. Some patients may benefit from VATS drainage and sclerosis. Select patients can be managed as outpatients with indwelling silastic catheters (e.g., PleurX™ catheter, CareFusion Corp, San Diego, CA), which allow intermittent patient-directed drainage of fluid. Patients with chylothorax secondary to lymphoma or TB require therapy directed at the underlying cause. Those patients with chylothorax due to traumatic thoracic duct disruption often require surgical ligation of the duct, although image-guided thoracic duct embolization can be performed successfully in select patients.

Patients with pleural effusions from trauma, pulmonary embolism, autoimmune disorders, and drug reactions often require no specific therapy. Exceptions include the postcardiac injury patients (Dressler syndrome), who are treated with nonsteroidal anti-inflammatory agents, and patients with

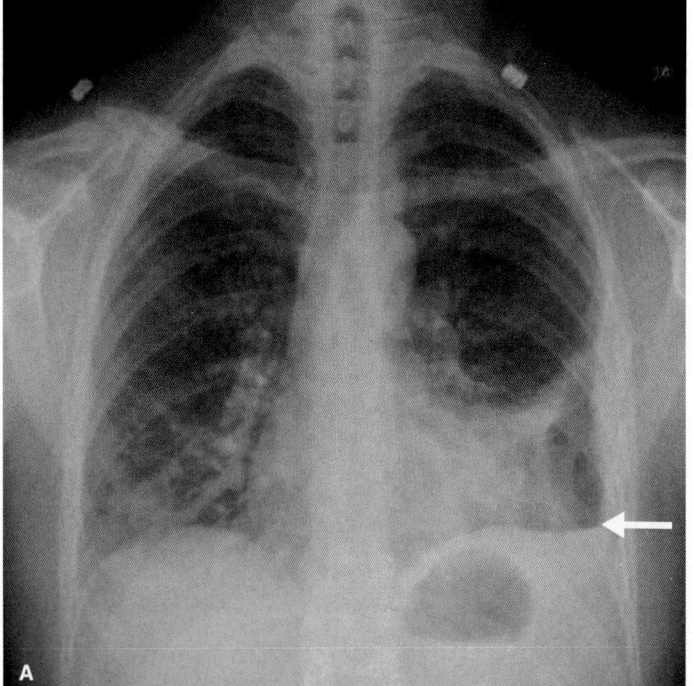

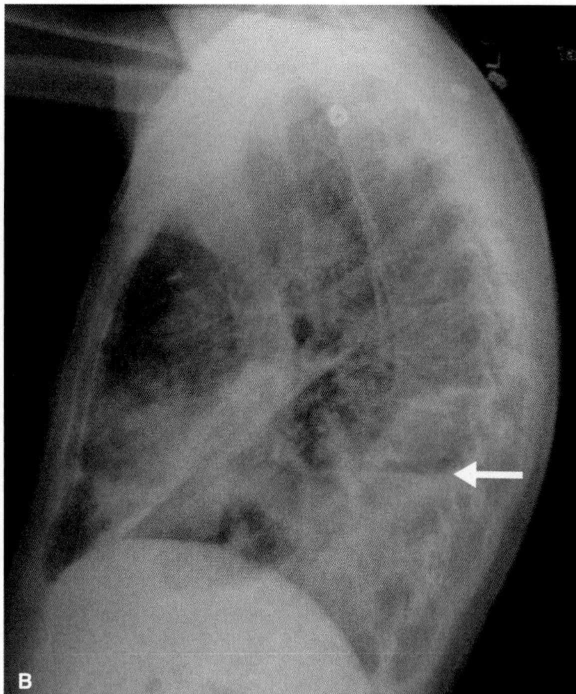

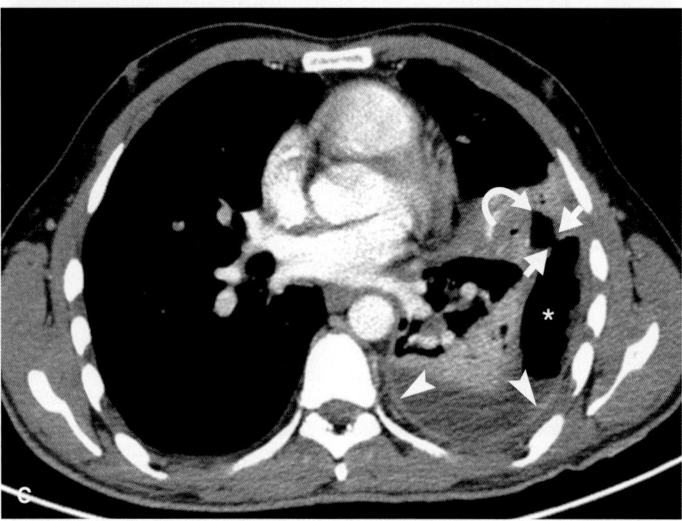

FIGURE 17.8. Bronchopleural Fistula and Empyema Complicating Pneumonia. Frontal (**A**) and lateral (**B**) radiographs demonstrate bilateral lower lobe and lingular consolidation, with a left lower loculated hydropneumothorax (*arrows*). **C:** Contrast-enhanced axial CT shows lingular and left lower lobe airspace opacification with a cavitation in the lingula (*curved arrow*) associated with a bronchopleural fistula (*short arrows*). A loculated pleural air and fluid collection is present (*asterisk*) with enhancement of the parietal pleura (*arrowheads*).

large hemothoraces that require large bore tube drainage to prevent pleural fibrosis and lung entrapment.

Bronchopleural Fistula

A bronchopleural fistula is a communication between the lung and the pleural space that often originates from a peripheral airway. A bronchopleural fistula from a bronchus typically results in an empyema, while an air leak from peripheral airspaces may cause an intractable pneumothorax without associated infection. Bronchopleural fistulas often develop from dehiscence of a bronchial stump following lobectomy or pneumonectomy, or as the result of a necrotizing pulmonary infection. Presenting symptoms include fever, cough, and dyspnea; large air leaks may be noted in patients with pleural drains. Radiographically, a bronchopleural fistula presents as a loculated intrapleural air and fluid collection. An air–fluid level in the postpneumonectomy space should suggest the diagnosis. CT is useful in evaluating patients with suspected bronchopleural fistula and empyema (Fig. 17.8), as it can distinguish a hydropneumothorax from a peripheral lung abscess and occasionally demonstrate the actual fistulous communication.

Following pneumonectomy, the residual space gradually fills with fluid and appears radiographically as an opaque hemithorax with ipsilateral mediastinal shift. The radiographic findings suggesting bronchopleural fistula formation complicating pneumonectomy are described in the previous section. CT and MR are useful in evaluating the postpneumonectomy space for evidence of tumor recurrence, and may help in the diagnosis of postoperative bronchopleural fistula and empyema.

Pneumothorax

Pneumothorax results from air entering the pleural space and may be traumatic or spontaneous (Table 17.6). Spontaneous pneumothorax is further subdivided into a primary form,

TABLE 17.6

ETIOLOGY OF PNEUMOTHORAX

Spontaneous	Primary (idiopathic)	Subpleural bleb
	Secondary	Obstructive airways disease
		■ COPD/emphysema
		■ Asthma
		■ Cystic fibrosis
		Infection
		■ Cavitating pneumonia
		■ Lung abscess/septic embolus
		■ Pneumatocele
		Obstructive airways disease
		■ COPD/emphysema
		■ Asthma
		■ Cystic fibrosis
		Infection
		■ Cavitating pneumonia
		■ Lung abscess/septic embolus
		■ Pneumatocele
		Neoplasm
		■ Lung cancer (peripheral)
		■ Metastases (cavitary)
		Cystic lung disease
		■ Langerhan cell histiocytosis
		■ Sarcoidosis (stage IV)
		■ Lymphangioleiomyomatosis
		■ Tuberous sclerosis
		■ Birt–Hogg–Dube syndrome
		Collagen vascular disease
		■ Marfan syndrome
		■ Ehlers–Danlos disease
		■ Cutis laxa
		Catamenial pneumothorax
Traumatic	Iatrogenic	Thoracic/abdominal surgery
		Percutaneous interventions
		■ Lung/pleural biopsy
		■ Thoracentesis
		■ Pleural drainage
		Central lung/pacemaker placement
		Mechanical ventilation
		Esophageal biopsy/dilatation
		Transbronchial lung biopsy
	Noniatrogenic	Penetrating trauma
		■ Gunshot wound
		■ Stab wound
		Blunt trauma
		■ Tracheobronchial injury
		■ Esophageal rupture
		■ Rib fracture

which has no identifiable etiology, and a secondary form, which is associated with underlying parenchymal lung disease. Patients with a pneumothorax typically present with the sudden onset of dyspnea and pleuritic chest pain.

Radiographically, pneumothorax on upright radiography is recognized by crescentic nondependent lucency that parallels the chest wall and displaces the visceral pleural line centrally. In a supine patient, such as in the ER or ICU setting, a pneumothorax can be undetectable as air in the pleural space rises nondependently and creates indiscernible increased lucency over the lower thorax and upper abdomen (Fig. 17.9). Signs of pneumothorax on supine radiography include a hyperlucent upper abdomen (particularly on the right over the normally dense liver), the "deep sulcus" sign, the "double diaphragm" sign, the epicardial fat pad sign (for left pneumothorax), and an unusually sharp heart border. In patients with pre-existing pleural adhesions, a pneumothorax can present as a loculated lucency within the pleural space including the interlobar fissures.

On CT, pneumothorax is identified by nondependent lucency over the lower anterior thorax. It is not uncommon in trauma patients to detect a small basilar pneumothorax overlying the lower chest that is not evident radiographically.

Traumatic Pneumothorax. Trauma is the most common cause of pneumothorax. Penetrating injuries can produce pneumothorax by introducing air from the atmosphere into the pleural space or by laceration of the visceral pleura, resulting in an air leak from the lung. Gunshot and knife wounds to the chest and

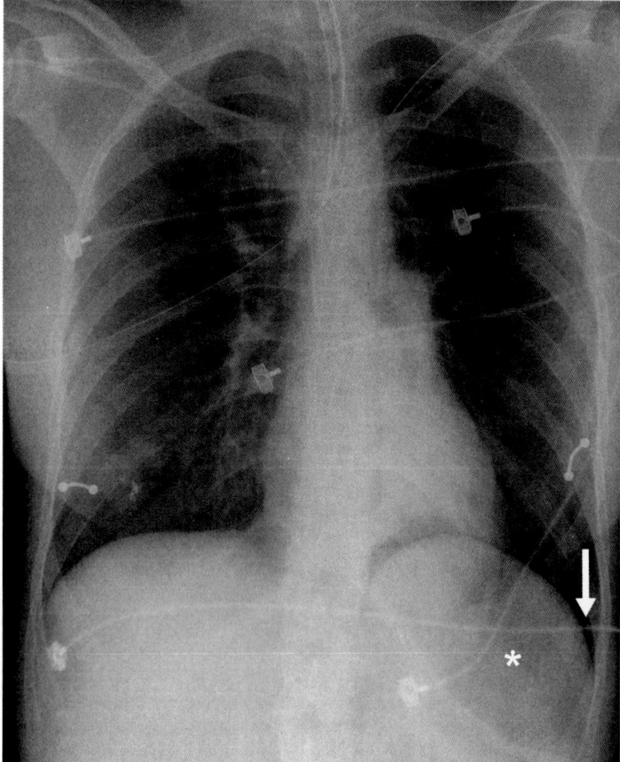

FIGURE 17.9. **Pneumothorax in Supine Patient.** Supine portable chest radiograph of a 27-year-old woman following attempted left subclavian venous catheterization showing abnormal lucency over the left upper abdomen (*asterisk*) with a deep left lateral costophrenic sulcus (*arrow*) representing a pneumothorax.

upper abdomen, central line placement, thoracentesis, transbronchial biopsy, and transthoracic needle biopsy are common penetrating injuries that cause traumatic pneumothorax. Blunt chest trauma may cause pneumothorax by two different mechanisms: (1) an acute increase in intrathoracic pressure results in extra alveolar interstitial air because of alveolar disruption, which tracks peripherally and ruptures into the pleural space; and (2) laceration of the tracheobronchial tree can produce a pneumothorax with a large bronchopleural fistula. In patients with rib fractures, the free edge of the fractured ribs can project inward to lacerate the lung and cause pneumothorax.

Primary Spontaneous Pneumothorax. This most often occurs in young or middle-aged men. A familial incidence and a propensity for tall, thin individuals have been noted. Affected patients may have blebs or bullae in the lung apices that are responsible for the development of recurrent pneumothoraces. Treatment of the initial episode is with closed tube drainage, with thoracoscopic bullectomy reserved for recurrent episodes or persistent air leak.

Secondary Spontaneous Pneumothorax. Multiple entities have been associated with secondary spontaneous pneumothorax. Chronic obstructive pulmonary disease is the most common predisposing condition. Acute obstruction to expiration from bronchoconstriction (asthma) or the performance of the Valsalva maneuver (crack cocaine or marijuana smoking, transvaginal childbirth) may cause spontaneous pneumothorax. Pneumothorax may complicate cystic fibrosis (Fig. 17.10) or the cystic lung changes in diseases such as sarcoidosis, Langerhan cell histiocytosis of lung, lymphangioleiomyomatosis, and idiopathic pulmonary fibrosis with subpleural honeycomb cyst formation. Necrotizing pneumonia or lung abscess caused by gram-negative or anaerobic bacteria, TB, or *Pneumocystis jiroveci* pneumonia can lead to pneumothorax, particularly in the mechanically ventilated patient. Metastases to the lung are an infrequent cause of pneumothorax and rarely are a presenting feature of disease. In these cases, pneumothorax develops when necrotic subpleural metastases rupture into the pleural space.

Sarcomas, particularly osteogenic sarcoma, lymphoma, and germ cell malignancies, are the most common malignancies to produce spontaneous pneumothorax. Marfan syndrome is the most common connective tissue disease producing pneumothorax; it usually results from the rupture of apical bullae. Other connective tissue diseases that can produce pneumothorax are Ehlers–Danlos syndrome and cutis laxa.

Mechanically ventilated patients are particularly at risk for pneumothorax because of the administration of positive pressure, underlying emphysema, complicating necrotizing pneumonia, and frequent line placements and other invasive procedures. Not uncommonly, patients with ARDS on mechanical ventilation develop small peripheral cystic airspaces which can rupture into the pleural space. When these are seen to develop on serial chest radiographs, impending pneumothorax can be suggested.

A particularly rare type of recurrent pneumothorax that occurs with menstruation is catamenial pneumothorax. This condition affects women in their fourth decade and is most likely caused by the cyclical necrosis of pleural endometrial implants, which creates an air leak between the lung and pleura. Rarely, air entering the peritoneal cavity during menstruation gains access to the pleural cavity via diaphragmatic defects. The predilection for right-sided pneumothoraces in this disorder indicates a key role for right-sided diaphragmatic defects. The pneumothoraces tend to be small and resolve spontaneously. Catamenial pneumothorax is managed by inducing amenorrhea.

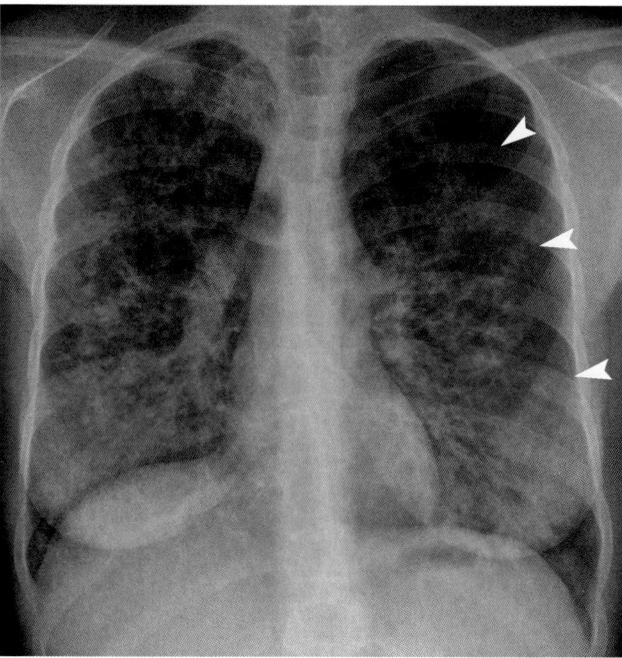

FIGURE 17.10. **Spontaneous Pneumothorax Complicating Cystic Fibrosis.** Upright frontal chest radiograph in a 27-year-old woman with acute exacerbation of cystic fibrosis demonstrates coarse reticular opacities and a left pneumothorax. Note the visceral pleural line (*arrowheads*) outlined by pleural air.

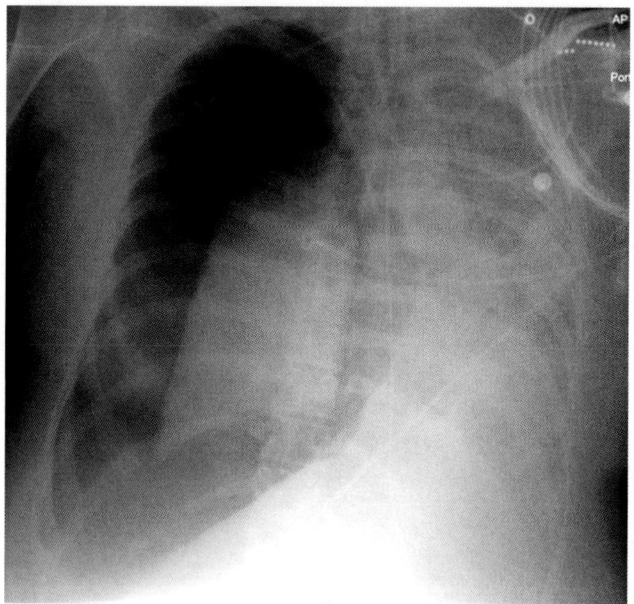

FIGURE 17.11. **Tension Pneumothorax.** Portable radiograph in a 27-year-old woman with ARDS complicating pneumonia demonstrates a large right pneumothorax with enlargement of the right hemithorax, marked diaphragmatic depression, and contralateral mediastinal shift.

Tension pneumothorax is a critical condition that most often results from iatrogenic trauma in mechanically ventilated patients. Tension pneumothorax results from a check-valve pleural defect that allows air to enter but not exit the pleural space. This leads to a pleural air collection that has a pressure exceeding atmospheric pressure during at least a portion of the respiratory cycle, causing complete collapse of the underlying lung and impairing venous return to the heart. Clinically, patients present with tachypnea, tachycardia, cyanosis, and hypotension. Radiographically, the involved hemithorax is expanded and hyperlucent, with a medially retracted lung, ipsilateral diaphragmatic depression or inversion, and contralateral mediastinal shift (Fig. 17.11). It is important to remember that contralateral mediastinal shift from pneumothorax does not invariably indicate tension, since an imbalance in the degree of negative intrapleural pressure can produce shift in the absence of tension. Therefore, tension pneumothorax remains a clinical diagnosis. Immediate evacuation of the pleural space should be performed with a needle, catheter, or large-bore thoracostomy tube.

Focal Pleural Disease

Focal pleural disease may be divided into localized pleural thickening, pleural calcification, or pleural mass (Table 17.7).

Localized pleural thickening from fibrosis is usually the end result of peripheral parenchymal and pleural inflammatory disease, with pneumonia as the most common cause. Additional causes include pulmonary embolism with infarction, asbestos exposure, trauma, prior chemical pleurodesis, and drug-related pleural disease.

Pleural calcification is most often unilateral and involves the visceral pleura. It is usually the result of prior hemothorax or empyema (e.g., TB), although pleural fibrosis from any cause may calcify. Asbestos exposure can cause bilateral calcified parietal pleural plaques. Visceral pleural calcifications from pleural hemorrhage or infection are indistinguishable radiographically. Initially, the calcification is punctate, but it often progresses to become sheet-like. CT is particularly useful in characterizing pleural calcification (Fig. 17.12). The presence of fluid within calcified pleural layers seen on CT suggests an active empyema and is most often seen in patients with prior TB. The use of CT in the evaluation of asbestos-related focal pleural disease and calcification is discussed in a subsequent section.

Pleural Mass. Focal pleural masses are usually benign neoplasms such as lipomas; loculated pleural fluid can mimic a pleural mass radiographically. Thoracic lipomas may arise in the chest wall or subpleural fat. Homogeneous fat attenuation on CT scan (–30 to –100 H) is diagnostic (Fig. 17.13). *Localized fibrous tumors of pleura* (LFTP) are uncommon pleural tumors. While most often benign, approximately 15% will recur locally after resection. These lesions appear as well-defined, spherical or oblong masses that arise from subpleural mesenchymal cells and are benign in approximately 80% of cases. These tumors are occasionally attached to the pleura by a narrow pedicle, a finding that is virtually pathognomonic and accounts for changes in intrapleural location occasionally seen with changes in patient positioning. CT usually shows a smoothly marginated, pleura-based soft tissue mass with either uniform soft tissue attenuation or inhomogeneous enhancement caused by areas of necrosis (Fig. 17.14). An association between LFTP and hypertrophic pulmonary

TABLE 17.7

FOCAL PLEURAL DISEASE

■ FINDING	■ ENTITY	
Mimics of focal pleural thickening	Apical cap Companion shadow of ribs Subpleural fat deposition	
Focal pleural thickening	Pneumonia Pulmonary infarct Trauma Asbestos-related pleural plaques (bilateral)	
Calcification	Visceral ■ Hemothorax ■ Empyema Parietal ■ Asbestos-related pleural plaques (bilateral)	
Pleural/extrapleural mass	Neoplasm	Benign ■ Localized fibrous tumor ■ Lipoma ■ Neurofibroma Malignant ■ Metastasis ■ Mesothelioma ■ Myeloma
	Other	Hematoma Loculated pleural effusion Healed rib fracture Splenosis

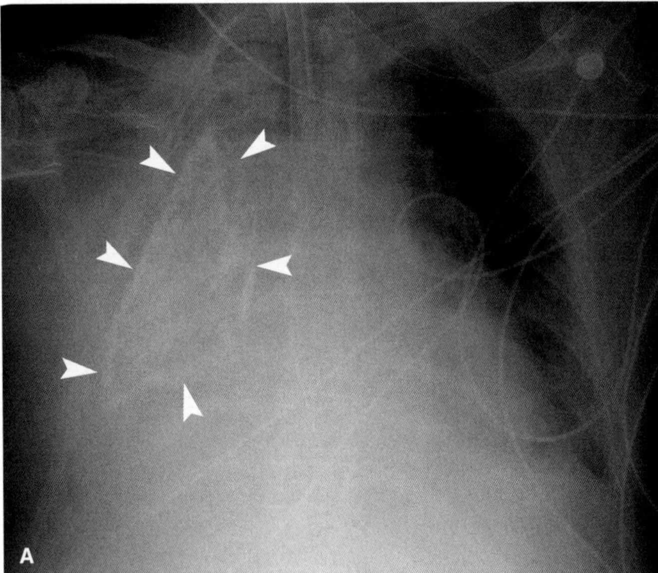

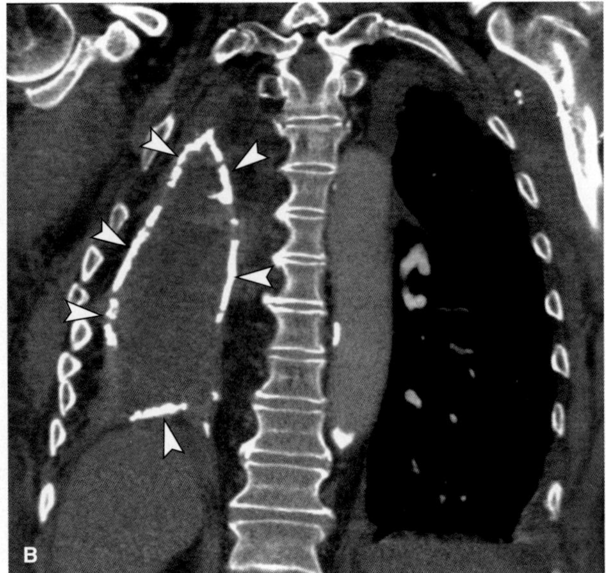

FIGURE 17.12. **Pleural Calcification Following Thoracotomy. A:** Frontal portable chest radiograph in a 74-year-old man with prior right thoracotomy and pneumonectomy shows a small opacified right hemithorax and dense peripheral calcification (*arrowheads*). **B:** Coronal CT scan shows a thick rind of pleural calcification (*arrowheads*) within a contracted right hemithorax.

osteoarthropathy and hypoglycemia is recognized. Unlike malignant mesothelioma, there is no association between LFTP and asbestos exposure.

Diffuse Pleural Disease

Diffuse pleural disease usually represents diffuse pleural fibrosis (fibrothorax), pleural malignancy, or multiloculated pleural effusion (Table 17.8).

Fibrothorax (diffuse pleural fibrosis) is defined as pleural thickening extending over more than one-fourth of the costal pleural surface. Fibrothorax most commonly results from the resolution of an exudative pleural effusion (including asbestos-related effusions), empyema, or hemothorax. The fibrothorax can encompass the entire lung and produce a trapped lung. Affected patients may develop a chronic pleural effusion due to abnormally low intrapleural pressures that recurs following thoracentesis (Fig. 17.15). When this causes a restrictive ventilatory defect, pleurectomy (decortication) may be necessary to restore function to the underlying lung.

Pleural Malignancy. Metastatic disease to the pleura commonly causes irregular or nodular pleural thickening, usually in association with a pleural effusion. The malignant tumors with a propensity to metastasize to the pleura include adenocarcinomas of the lung, breast, ovary, kidney, and GI tract. Malignant mesothelioma is seen almost exclusively in asbestos-exposed individuals.

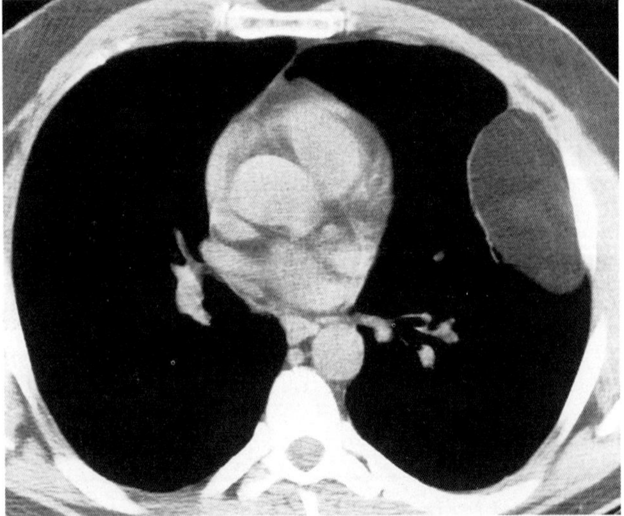

FIGURE 17.13. **Pleural Lipoma.** CT scan in a patient with an asymptomatic mass discovered as an incidental chest radiographic finding shows a left anterolateral pleura-based mass with homogeneous fatty attenuation representing a lipoma.

TABLE 17.8

DIFFUSE PLEURAL DISEASE

■ FINDING	■ ENTITY
Smooth pleural thickening	Pleural fibrosis ▪ Hemothorax ▪ Prior empyema ▪ Serositis ▪ Prior pleurodesis Pleural effusion (supine radiographs) Extrapleural fat deposition
Lobulated/nodular	Malignancy ▪ Primary Mesothelioma ▪ Metastatic disease Adenocarcinoma (lung, breast, ovary, renal, GI) Thymoma (invasive) Lymphoma Effusion ▪ Empyema ▪ Prior pleural adhesions

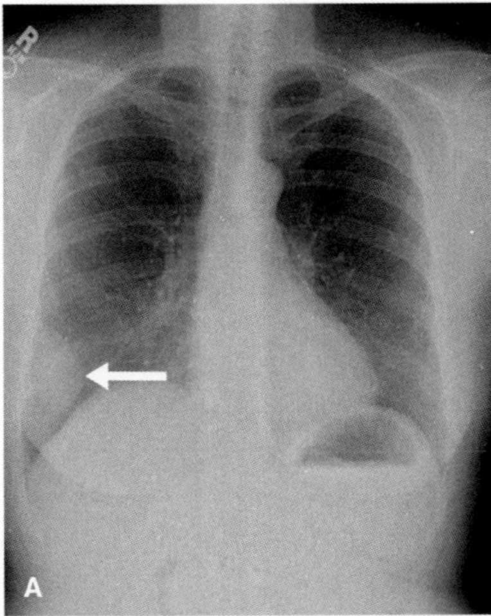

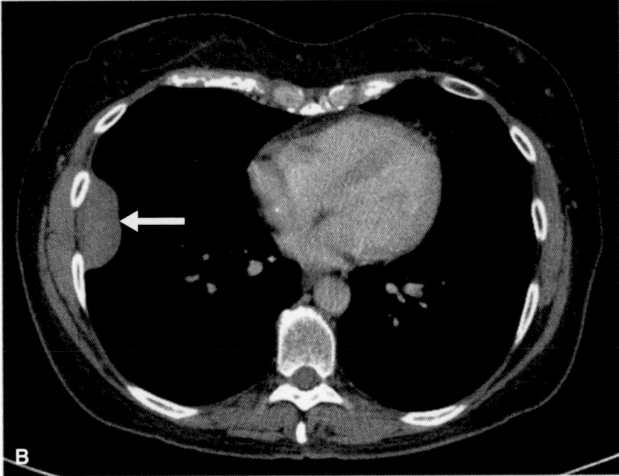

FIGURE 17.14. Localized Fibrous Tumor of Pleura. A: Chest radiograph in a 47-year-old woman shows a smooth intrathoracic mass in the lower right lateral chest with obtuse superior and inferior margins. **B:** Contrast-enhanced axial CT scan shows a sharply defined soft tissue mass (*arrow*) with tapered obtuse margins, along the right lateral costal pleural surface, typical of a pleural mass. Note the absence of chest wall involvement. Biopsy confirmed a localized fibrous tumor of pleura.

Malignant pleural disease is most often caused by one of four conditions: metastatic adenocarcinoma (see Fig. 13.16), invasive thymoma or thymic carcinoma, mesothelioma, and rarely lymphoma. Pleural malignancy presents radiographically as multiple discrete pleural masses or nodular pleural thickening, although the pleural lesions are often obscured by an associated malignant pleural effusion. Contrast-enhanced CT can distinguish solid pleural masses from loculated pleural fluid and can show discrete pleural masses or thickening in patients with large effusions. In contrast to benign pleural thickening, malignant pleural disease is more likely when the pleural thickening on CT is circumferential and nodular, greater than 1 cm in thickness, and/or involves the mediastinal pleura. Mesothelioma is radiographically indistinguishable from metastatic pleural disease and will be discussed in the next section. Chest wall invasion by pleural tumor, seen as rib destruction or soft tissue infiltration of the subcutaneous fat and musculature, is better appreciated on CT or MR than on plain films. The diagnosis of malignant pleural disease is made by cytologic examination of fluid obtained at thoracentesis, closed or thoracoscopically guided pleural biopsy, or by thoracotomy.

Asbestos-Related Pleural Disease

Prolonged exposure to the inorganic silicate mineral fibers generically known as asbestos can result in a variety of pleural

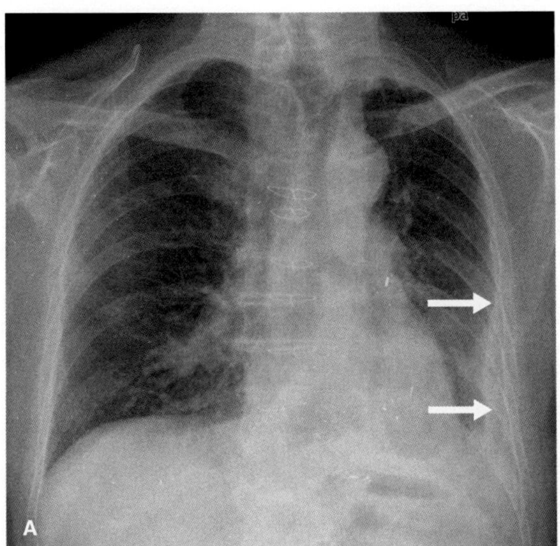

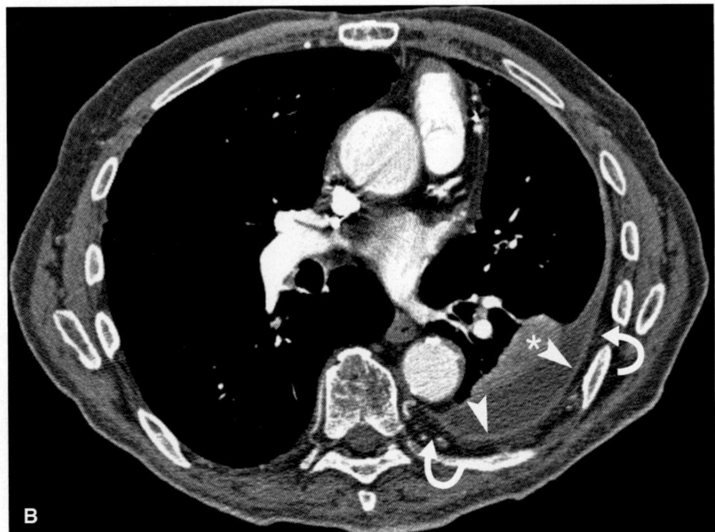

FIGURE 17.15. Diffuse Pleural Fibrosis With Lung Entrapment. A: Frontal chest radiograph in a patient with a history of prior coronary artery bypass graft surgery shows marked volume loss in the left hemithorax with left lower lateral pleural thickening (*arrows*). **B:** Contrast-enhanced axial CT scan (**B**) through the mid-chest shows volume loss in the left hemithorax with smooth thickening of the left costal parietal pleural surface (*arrowheads*) and hypertrophy of the extrapleural fat (*curved arrows*). There is associated rounded atelectasis within the left lower lobe (*asterisk*). The pleural effusion is due to trapped lung with associated highly negative intrapleural pressure. Note sparing of the mediastinal pleural surface, typical of benign pleural disease.

and pulmonary disorders. Benign pleural disease is the most common thoracic manifestation of asbestos inhalation and includes pleural plaques, pleural effusions, and diffuse pleural fibrosis. Malignant asbestos-related pleural disease manifests as malignant mesothelioma.

Benign Asbestos-Related Pleural Disease

Pleural plaques are the most common benign manifestation of asbestos inhalation. These plaques develop 20 to 30 years after the initial asbestos exposure and are more frequent with increasing length and severity of exposure to the fibers. Asbestos plaques are found on the parietal pleura, most commonly over the diaphragm and lower posterolateral chest wall. The mediastinal pleural surface and costophrenic sulci are characteristically spared. The plaques are discrete, bilateral, slightly raised (2 to 10 mm thick) foci of pleural thickening that are pearly white and shiny in gross appearance. Histologically, the plaques are comprised of dense bands of collagen. Punctate or linear calcification within the plaques is common and is more frequent as the plaques enlarge. Asbestos bodies (short, straight asbestos fibers coated with iron and protein that microscopically look like small dumbbells) are not seen within the plaques. Visceral pleural plaques, seen as discrete flat regions of pleural thickening within the major fissures on CT, are most commonly associated with interstitial fibrosis. Most patients with isolated asbestos-related pleural plaques are asymptomatic.

When viewed en face, calcified plaques appear as geographic areas of opacity that have been likened to a holly leaf (Fig. 17.16). CT is extremely sensitive in detecting calcified and noncalcified pleural plaques in asbestos-exposed individuals and can distinguish pleural plaques and diffuse pleural fibrosis from subpleural fat deposits that may mimic pleural disease on conventional radiography. Although plaques are invariably bilateral on gross examination of the pleural space in affected individuals, it is not unusual to see unilateral plaques (most often left sided) on radiography or CT.

Pleural effusion occurs 10 to 20 years after the initial exposure to asbestos and is the earliest manifestation of asbestos-related pleural disease. The development of asbestos-related effusion appears to be dose related. The effusions are usually small, unilateral or bilateral, and exudative and may be bloody. The diagnosis of a benign asbestos-related pleural effusion is one of exclusion and, in addition to a history of exposure, requires the exclusion of TB or pleural malignancy (i.e., mesothelioma or metastatic adenocarcinoma). A long latency period between the initial exposure and the development of pleural effusion (>20 years) should prompt a diagnostic evaluation for malignant mesothelioma. While most asbestos-related pleural effusions resolve spontaneously, up to one-third recur and some patients develop diffuse pleural fibrosis.

Diffuse pleural thickening or fibrosis may follow asbestos-related pleural effusion or result from the confluence of pleural plaques. Diffuse asbestos pleural thickening is defined as smooth, flat pleural thickening extending over one-fourth of the costal pleural surface. In distinction to pleural plaques, which affect the parietal pleura alone, diffuse pleural fibrosis involves both the parietal and visceral pleura. Radiographically, diffuse pleural thickening is seen as a smooth thickening of the pleura involving the lower thorax with blunting of the costophrenic sulci (Fig. 17.16). CT is useful in determining the extent of pleural thickening, involvement of the interlobar fissures, and to detect underlying fibrotic or emphysematous lung disease. Diffuse pleural fibrosis can result in symptomatic restrictive lung disease.

Malignant Asbestos-Related Pleural Disease

Malignant mesothelioma is a rare malignant pleural neoplasm associated with asbestos exposure. Unlike other pleural and parenchymal manifestations of asbestos, it does not appear to be a dose-related phenomenon. Mesothelioma most often occurs 30 to 40 years after the initial exposure. Although the incidence increases with heavy exposure, malignant mesothelioma may also develop after minimal exposure and contrasts with the linear relationship between the development of benign asbestos pleural disease and the dose of asbestos exposure. Crocidolite is the fiber type most often implicated in the development of malignant mesothelioma, although chrysotile likely accounts for the majority of asbestos-related mesotheliomas,

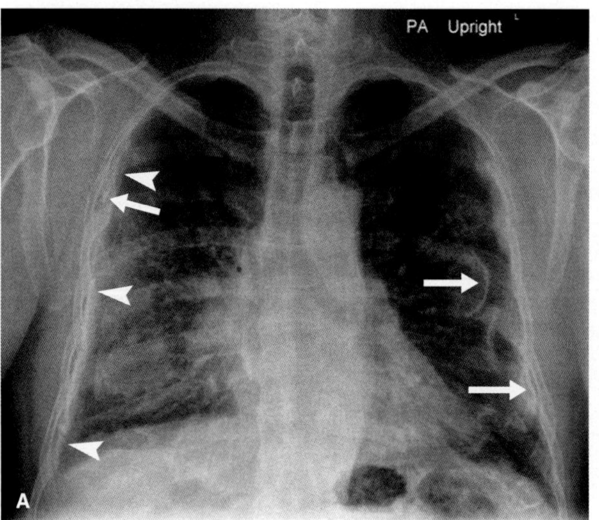

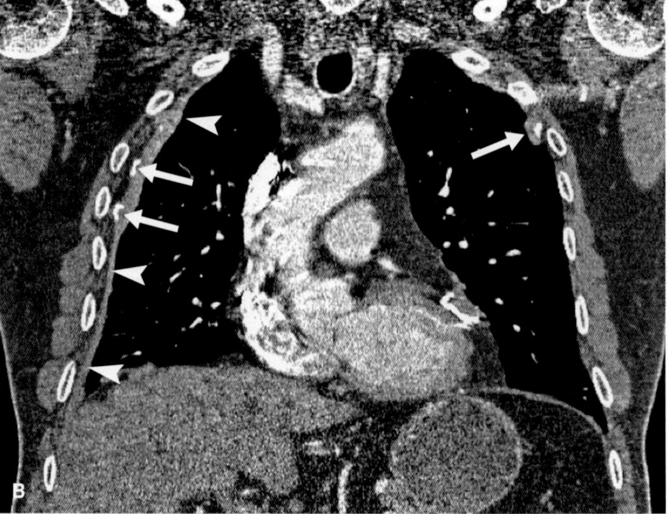

FIGURE 17.16. **Calcified Pleural Plaques and Diffuse Pleural Fibrosis in Asbestos-Related Pleural Disease.** Frontal chest radiograph (**A**) shows bilateral calcified plaques (*arrows*) and more diffuse thickening along the right lateral pleural surface (*arrowheads*). Coronal CT at the level of the ascending aorta (**B**) confirms the presence of bilateral pleural plaques (*arrows*) and also shows thickening along the right lateral pleural surface (*arrowheads*). Note the subtle decrease in volume of the right hemithorax, best evidenced by narrowing of the intercostal spaces. The absence of mediastinal pleural involvement is typical for benign pleural processes.

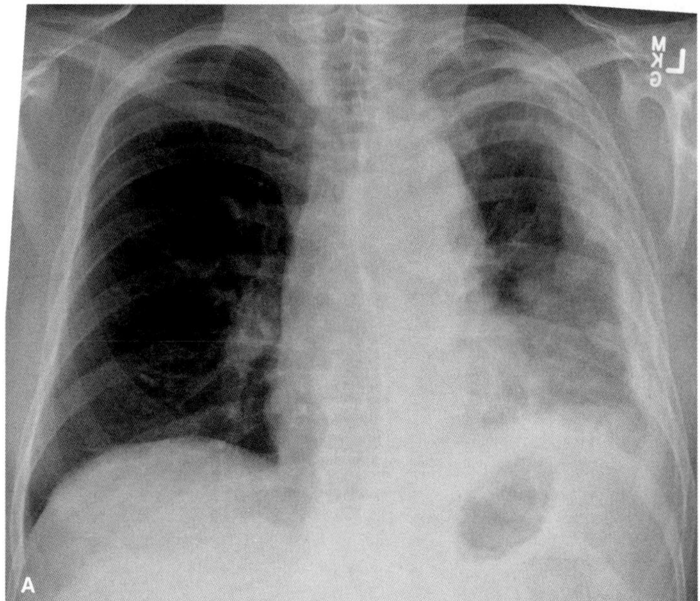

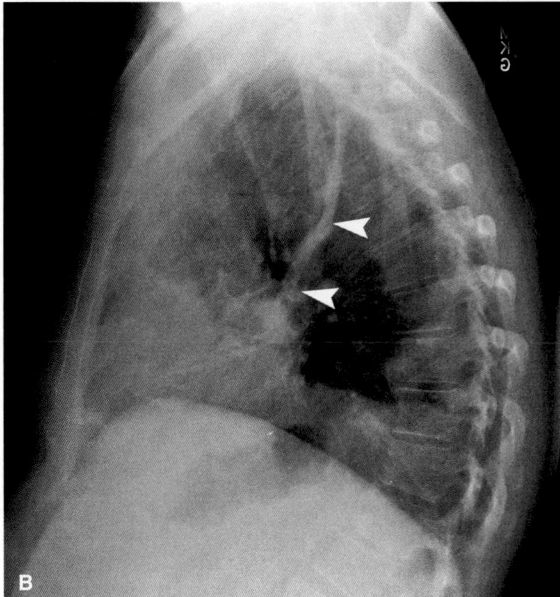

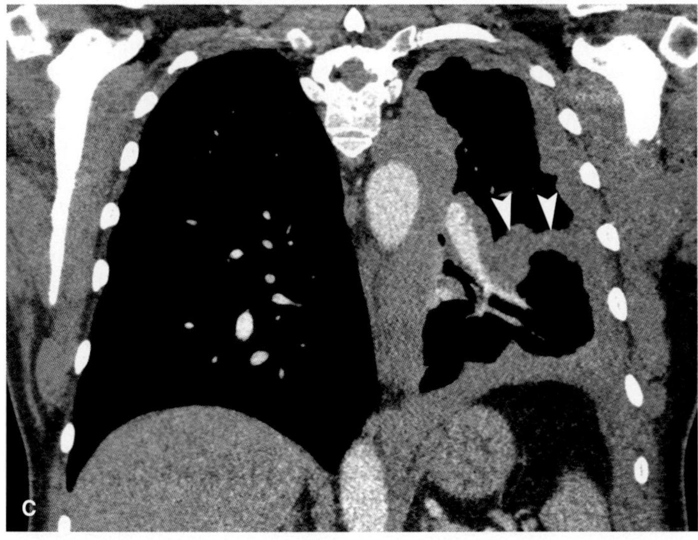

FIGURE 17.17. **Mesothelioma. A, B:** Frontal (**A**) and lateral (**B**) chest radiographs show nodular circumferential left pleural thickening and volume loss in the left hemithorax. Note thickening of the left major fissure on the lateral radiograph (*arrowheads* in **B**). **C:** Contrast-enhanced coronal CT at the level of the proximal descending aorta shows circumferential nodular left pleural thickening with extension into the major fissure (*arrowheads*). CT-guided biopsy confirmed an epithelial subtype of mesothelioma.

because it is the most widely used form of asbestos. Pathologically, mesothelioma is divided into epithelial, sarcomatous, and mixed types, with the epithelial form the most common and associated with a better prognosis than the sarcomatous and mixed subtypes.

Mesothelioma typically grows by contiguous spread from the pleural space into the lung, chest wall, mediastinum, and diaphragm; distant metastases are not uncommon. It most often appears radiographically as thick (>1 cm) and nodular diffuse pleural thickening. Calcification or, rarely, ossification is seen in 20% of tumors, although calcified pleural plaques may be seen in uninvolved areas of the pleura. A pleural effusion is often present, which, if large, may obscure the pleural tumor. Malignant involvement of the mediastinal pleural surface may prevent contralateral mediastinal shift despite extensive pleural tumor volume and effusion, a finding that may help distinguish mesothelioma from metastatic disease. CT is the imaging modality of choice in the evaluation of malignant mesothelioma and depicts the extent of pleural involvement and invasion of the chest wall and mediastinum (Fig. 17.17). Diaphragmatic invasion by tumor, best assessed by MR or CT, is important only in those patients otherwise considered for resection. Adenopathy is seen in the ipsilateral hilum and mediastinum in approximately 50% of patients. While the radiologic findings may be highly suggestive of mesothelioma, metastatic pleural malignancy can have a similar appearance, so histologic confirmation is necessary.

The diagnosis of malignant mesothelioma is made histologically and often requires the use of special stains. The epithelial type of malignant mesothelioma may be indistinguishable from adenocarcinoma on light microscopy. Staging of mesothelioma is by the TNM classification system. Stage I or II disease reflects tumor limited to the ipsilateral pleural, lung, or diaphragm without nodal or distant spread. While surgical resection by pleurectomy or extrapleural pneumonectomy may benefit selected patients with stage I or II disease and good pulmonary reserve, the median survival from the time of diagnosis in all patients with mesothelioma is only 12 to 21 months.

CHEST WALL

Disorders of the soft tissues or bony structures of the chest wall may come to attention because of local symptoms or physical findings, during evaluation of pulmonary or pleural

TABLE 17.9

CHEST WALL LESIONS

Neoplasms	Cutaneous/ subcutaneous	Mole Nevus Wart Neurofibroma
	Rib	Chondrosarcoma Osteosarcoma Metastasis
	Soft tissues	Primitive neuroectodermal (Askin) tumor Fibrosarcoma Liposarcoma Melanoma Metastasis
Infection		Staphylococcus Tuberculosis
Trauma		Hematoma

disease, or as an incidental finding on radiographic or CT studies (Table 17.9).

Soft Tissues

Congenital absence of the pectoralis muscle results in hyperlucency of the affected hemithorax on frontal radiographs. *Poland syndrome* is an autosomal recessive disorder characterized by unilateral absence of the sternocostal head of the pectoralis major, ipsilateral syndactyly, and rib anomalies (Fig. 17.18). There may be associated aplasia of the ipsilateral breast. Patients who have had a mastectomy will also show unilateral hyperlucency. In those who have undergone a modified radical mastectomy, the horizontally oriented inferior edge of the hypertrophied pectoralis minor muscle may be identified on frontal radiographs.

A variety of skin lesions such as moles, nevi, warts, neurofibromas, and accessory nipples may produce a nodular opacity on frontal radiographs that mimics a solitary pulmonary nodule. Examination of the skin surface should be performed in any patient with a new nodular opacity seen on chest radiography, and repeat radiographs obtained with a radiopaque marker over the skin lesion will confirm the nature of the opacity and avoid unnecessary follow-up radiographs and chest CT. Chest wall abscesses may present as localized, painful, fluctuant subcutaneous masses. *Staphylococcus* and *Mycobacterium tuberculosis* are the most common organisms responsible. The diagnosis is usually obvious clinically. Chest radiographs demonstrate a poorly defined opacity on the frontal radiograph when the abscess involves the anterior or posterior chest wall. CT shows a localized fluid collection with an enhancing wall and is used to determine the location and extent of the collection prior to drainage.

Soft tissue neoplasms of the chest wall are rare. They are most often detected clinically as a mass protruding from the chest wall and appear as nonspecific extrathoracic soft tissue masses on chest radiographs. The most common benign neoplasm of the chest wall is a lipoma. Lipomas may be intrathoracic or extrathoracic, or they may project partially within and outside the thorax (dumbbell lipoma). CT shows a sharply circumscribed mass of fatty density, while MR shows characteristic high and intermediate signal intensity on T1WIs and T2WIs, respectively.

Fibrosarcomas and liposarcomas are the most common primary malignant soft tissue neoplasms of the chest wall in adults. Malignant tumors often present with symptoms of localized chest wall pain and a visible, palpable mass. Patients who have received chest wall radiation are at particular risk for developing sarcomas. Radiographically, these soft tissue masses are often associated with bony destruction.

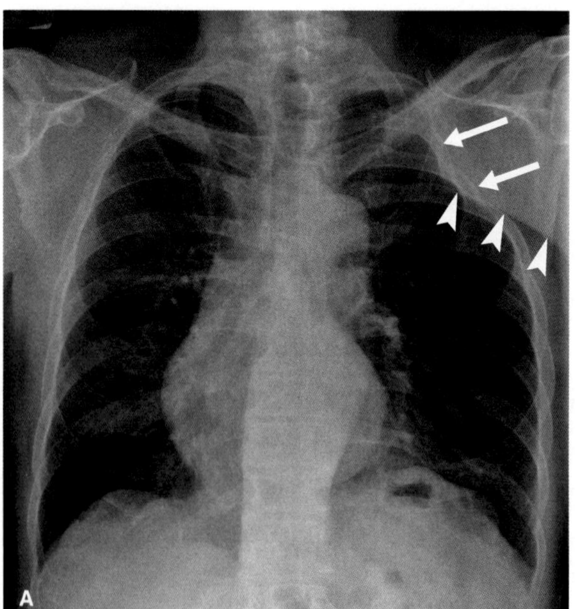

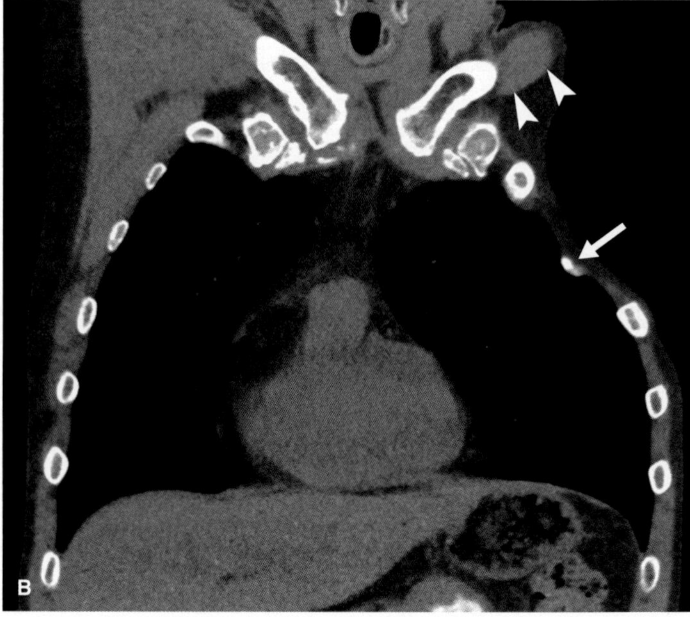

FIGURE 17.18. Poland Syndrome. A: Frontal chest radiograph in a patient with Poland syndrome shows hypoplastic left 3rd and 4th ribs (*arrows*) and hyperlucency of the left hemithorax due to absence of the left pectoralis major muscle. Note the hypertrophied left pectoralis minor muscle outlined by air (*arrowheads*). **B:** Coronal CT through the anterior chest shows a hypoplastic left 3rd rib (*arrow*) and absence of the left pectoralis major muscle with intact left pectoralis minor muscle (*arrowheads*).

CT best depicts the bone destruction and intrathoracic component of tumor, while MR shows the extent of tumor and delineates tumor from surrounding muscle and subcutaneous fat. A rare malignant neoplasm arising from the chest wall of children and young adults is the Askin tumor, which arises from primitive neuroectodermal rests in the chest wall. These small round blue-cell tumors are histologically similar to Ewing sarcoma of bone, present as chest wall or pleural masses, and are very aggressive with a high mortality rate.

The Bony Thorax

Congenital Anomalies (Table 17.10). The most common congenital anomalies of the ribs are bony fusion and bifid ribs, neither of which have clinical significance. Intrathoracic ribs are extremely rare congenital anomalies where an accessory rib arises from a vertebral body or the posterior surface of a rib and extends inferolaterally into the thorax, usually on the right side (Fig. 17.19). Osteogenesis imperfecta and neurofibromatosis may be associated with thin, wavy, "ribbon" ribs. A relatively common congenital anomaly is the cervical rib, which arises from the seventh cervical vertebral body. Cervical ribs are usually asymptomatic, although in a minority of individuals with the thoracic outlet syndrome, the rib or associated fibrous bands can compress the subclavian artery, producing secondary ischemic symptoms, or compress the subclavian vein and brachial plexus, producing pain, weakness, and swelling of the upper extremity and potentially subclavian vein thrombosis (Paget von Schroetter syndrome). Decompression of the space by surgical resection of the cervical rib can relieve the symptoms in selected patients.

Rib notching is seen in a variety of pathologic conditions. Inferior rib notching is much more common than superior rib notching and is caused by enlargement of one or more of the structures that lie in the subcostal grooves (intercostal nerve, artery, or vein). The notching predominantly affects the posterior aspects of the ribs bilaterally and may be narrow, wide, deep, or shallow.

The most common cause of bilateral inferior rib notching is coarctation of the aorta distal to the origin of the left subclavian artery. In this condition, blood circumvents the aortic obstruction and reaches the descending aorta via the subclavian, internal mammary, and intercostal arteries. The increased blood flow in the intercostal arteries produces tortuosity and dilatation of these vessels, which erodes the inferior margins of the adjacent ribs. Other causes of aortic obstruction that can lead to inferior rib notching include aortic thrombosis and Takayasu arteritis. Congenital heart diseases associated with decreased pulmonary blood flow may be associated with rib notching as the intercostal arteries enlarge in an attempt to supply collateral blood flow to the oligemic lungs. Superior vena caval obstruction can cause increased flow through intercostal veins and thereby result in rib notching. Multiple intercostal neurofibromas in neurofibromatosis type 1 are the most common nonvascular cause of inferior rib notching. Associated findings of neurofibromatosis include ribbon ribs, thoracic kyphoscoliosis, and scalloping of the posterior aspect of the vertebral bodies due to dural ectasia.

Superior rib notching is much less common than inferior rib notching. The pathogenesis of superior rib notching is unknown, although a disturbance of osteoblastic and osteoclastic activity and the stress effect of the intercostal muscles are proposed mechanisms. Paralysis is the most common condition associated with superior rib notching. Other etiologies include rheumatoid arthritis, systemic lupus erythematosus, and rarely, marked tortuosity of the intercostal arteries from severe, long-standing aortic obstruction.

TABLE 17.10

RIB LESIONS

Congenital	Fusion anomalies
	Cervical rib
	Ribbon ribs
	Rib notching
	  Inferior
	    Coarctation of the aorta
	    Tetralogy of Fallot
	    Superior vena cava obstruction
	    Blalock–Taussig shunt (unilateral right)
	    Neurofibromatosis
	  Superior
	    Paralysis
	    Collagen vascular disease
	      Rheumatoid arthritis
	      Systemic lupus erythematosus

Trauma	Healing rib fracture
Nonneoplastic tumors	Fibrous dysplasia Eosinophilic granuloma Brown tumor

Neoplasms	Benign
	  Osteochondroma
	  Enchondroma
	  Osteoblastoma
	Malignant
	  Primary
	    Chondrosarcoma
	    Osteogenic sarcoma
	    Fibrosarcoma
	  Metastatic
	    Multiple myeloma
	    Metastases
	    Breast carcinoma
	    Bronchogenic carcinoma
	    Renal cell carcinoma
	    Prostate carcinoma

Osteomyelitis	*Staphylococcus aureus* Tuberculosis Actinomycosis Nocardiosis

Trauma. Rib and costal cartilage fractures may result from blunt or penetrating trauma to a normal rib cage or from minimal trauma to abnormal ribs, such as those affected by metastases. An acute rib fracture is seen as a thin vertical lucency; malalignment of the superior and inferior cortices of the rib may occasionally be the only radiographic finding. The tendency to affect the posterolateral aspects of the ribs explains the utility of obtaining ipsilateral posterior oblique radiographs for suspected fracture, because this projection best displays the fracture line. In any patient with an acute rib fracture, a careful search should be made for associated pneumothorax, hemothorax, and pulmonary contusion or laceration. Since the first three ribs are well protected by the clavicles, scapulae, and shoulder girdles, fracture of these ribs

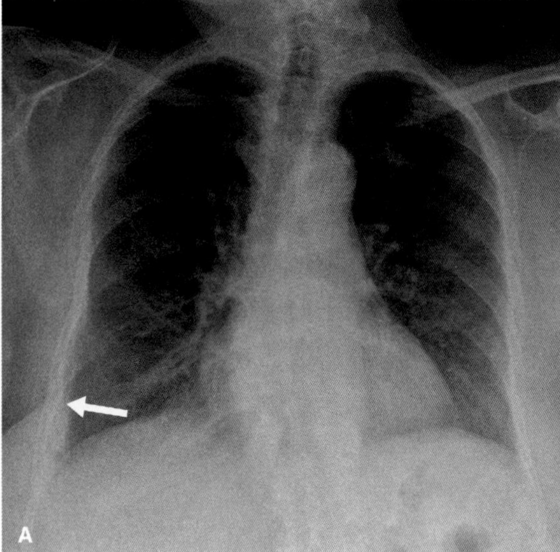

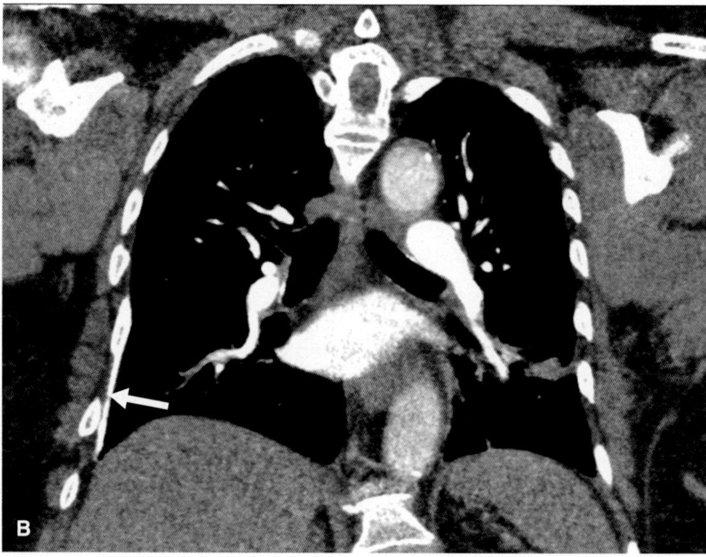

FIGURE 17.19. **Intrathoracic Rib. A:** Frontal chest radiograph in an asymptomatic female shows a linear opacity in the right lower lateral chest (*arrow*). **B:** Contrast-enhanced coronal CT through the mid-chest shows the opacity represents an intrathoracic rib (*arrow*) extending inferiorly from the lateral right 6th rib (*arrow*).

indicates severe trauma and should prompt a careful evaluation for associated great vessel and visceral injury. Fractures of the 10th, 11th, or 12th ribs may be associated with injury to the liver or spleen. Severe blunt trauma to the rib cage, in which multiple contiguous ribs are fractured in more than one place, is termed a "flail chest." This results in a free segment of the chest wall that moves paradoxically inward on inspiration and outward on expiration. These posttraumatic chest wall injuries are best evaluated with CT and the use of surface renderings that best depict the extent of injury and are helpful for preoperative planning of repair (Fig. 17.20). Healing rib fractures will demonstrate callus formation, which may be exuberant in patients receiving corticosteroids. Multiple contiguous healed rib fractures, particularly if bilateral, should suggest chronic alcoholism or a prior motor vehicle accident. Bilateral symmetric anterolateral fractures should suggest injury from chest compression during cardiopulmonary resuscitation efforts.

Nonneoplastic Lesions. The ribs are the most common site of involvement by monostotic fibrous dysplasia (Fig. 17.21). The typical appearance is an expansile lesion in the posterior aspect of the rib with a lucent or ground-glass density; rarely, the lesion is sclerotic. Multiple rib involvement from polyostotic fibrous dysplasia can result in severe restrictive pulmonary disease. Langerhan cell histiocytosis can cause lytic lesions in patients under age 30. These are usually solitary lytic lesions, which can be expansile but do not have sclerotic margins; this latter feature helps distinguish these lesions from fibrous dysplasia. Brown tumors from hyperparathyroidism can also produce lytic rib lesions.

Neoplasms. Primary osteochondral neoplasms or metastatic disease can involve the ribs. Osteochondromas are the most common benign neoplasm of ribs, followed in relative frequency by enchondromas and osteoblastomas. Primary malignant neoplasms of the ribs in adults are uncommon. Chondrosarcoma is the most common primary rib malignancy, with osteogenic sarcoma and fibrosarcoma less common. Rib involvement from multiple myeloma or metastatic carcinoma can produce solitary or multiple lytic lesions and is much more common than primary tumors. Myeloma can also cause permeative bone destruction that is indistinguishable from severe osteoporosis; an associated soft tissue mass is a clue to the diagnosis (Fig. 17.22). The diagnosis of myeloma is made by identification of a monoclonal spike on serum protein electrophoresis and typical findings of abnormal aggregates of plasma cells on bone marrow biopsy. The most common metastatic lesions to ribs are from lung and breast cancer, which produce multiple lytic lesions when dissemination is hematogenous or localized rib destruction when invasion is by contiguous spread. Expansile lytic rib metastases are seen most commonly from renal cell and thyroid carcinoma. Sclerotic rib metastases are most commonly seen in breast and prostate carcinoma, although lung cancer and carcinoid tumors can produce blastic metastases (Fig. 17.23).

Infection. Chest wall infection and osteomyelitis of the ribs usually develop from contiguous spread from the lung, pleural space, and vertebral column. Less commonly, infection complicates penetrating chest trauma or spreads to the ribs hematogenously. Pleuropulmonary infections that may traverse the pleural space and produce a chest wall infection include TB, fungus, actinomycosis, and nocardiosis. Radiographs may demonstrate bone destruction, periostitis, and subcutaneous emphysema; bone scans can detect subradiographic bone involvement. CT can demonstrate bone destruction, soft tissue swelling, and abscesses within the chest wall. In addition, CT may show involvement of the adjacent pleural space, lung, sternum, or vertebral column.

Costal Cartilages. Ossification of the costal cartilages is a normal finding on frontal chest radiographs in adults. Female costal cartilage ossification involves the central portion of the cartilage, extending from the rib toward the sternum in the shape of a solitary finger, while male costal cartilage ossification involves the peripheral portion of the cartilage and has the appearance of two fingers ("peace" sign). These typical patterns of male and female costal cartilage ossification are seen in 70% of patients (Fig. 17.24) and do not apply to the first rib.

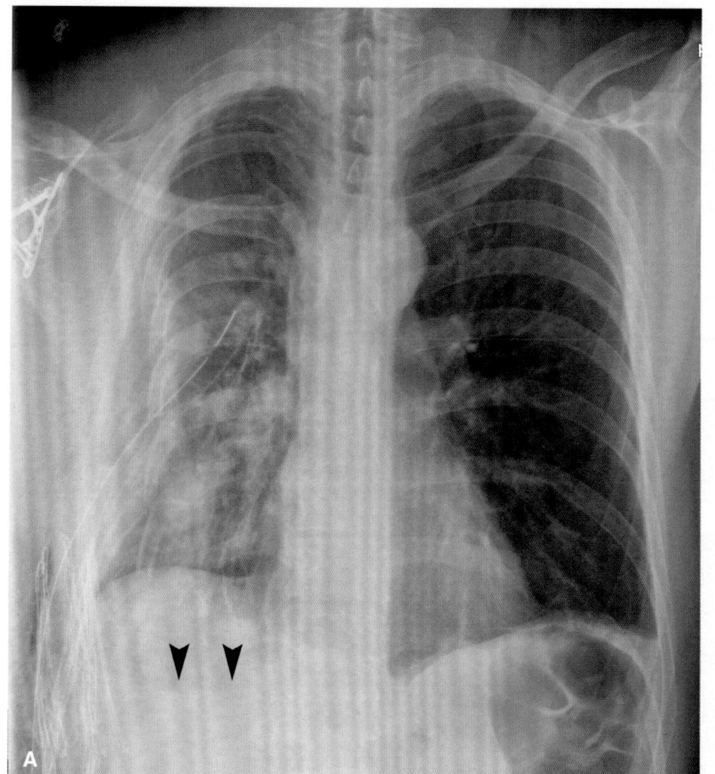

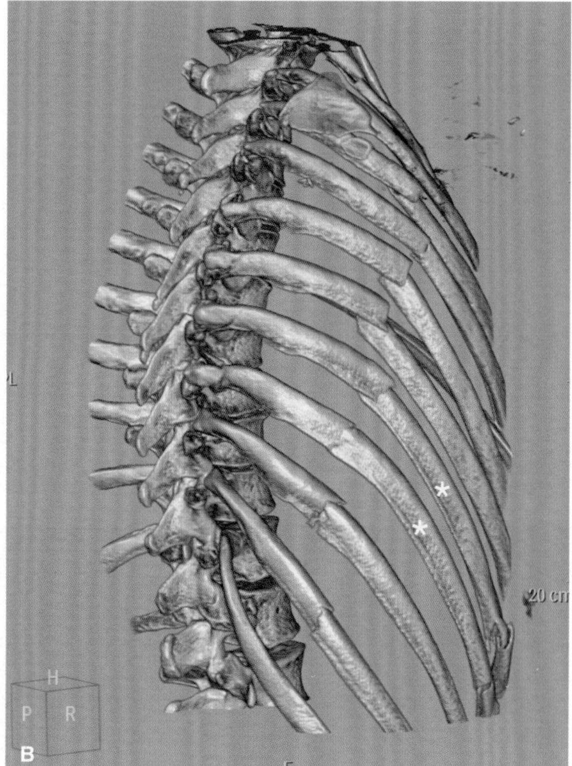

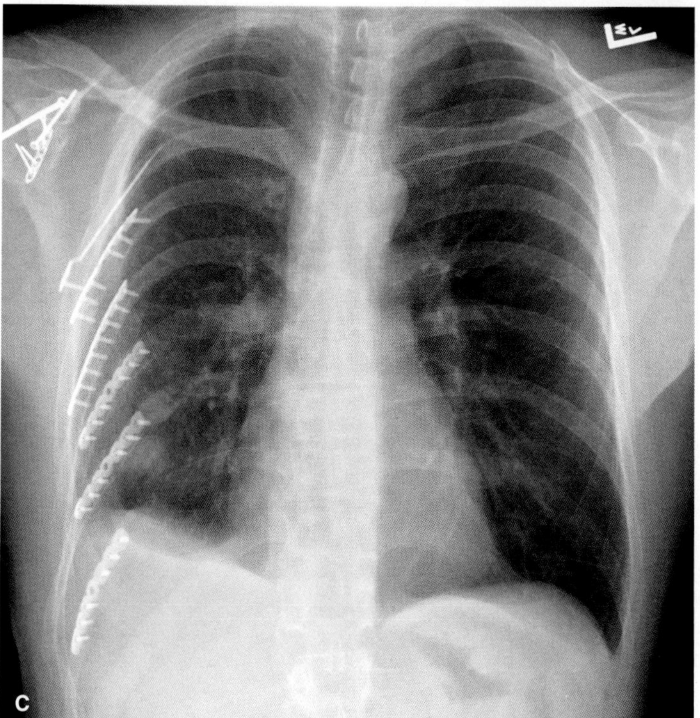

FIGURE 17.20. **Flail Chest. A:** Upright frontal chest radiograph in a 38-year-old man who sustained blunt chest trauma several weeks previously shows multiple displaced right rib fractures. There is a right hydropneumothorax (*arrowheads* = air–fluid level) despite the presence of a right thoracostomy tube. Note repair of associated right scapular fracture. **B:** Surface-rendered CT from a right posterior oblique projection with the scapula removed shows multiple displaced right rib fractures. There are at least two contiguous ribs with two fractures each (*asterisks*), meeting the definition of a flail segment. **C:** Frontal radiograph following surgical repair of the flail chest shows fixation plates and pins transfixing the rib fractures with improvement in fracture fragment alignment.

Scapula. Scapular abnormalities that are visible on frontal radiographs include congenital, posttraumatic, and neoplastic lesions. Scapular fractures may result from direct trauma to the upper back and shoulder or from impaction of the humeral head into the glenoid. A winged scapula is identified when the scapula is superiorly displaced from its normal position and the inferior portion is posteriorly displaced from the chest wall. This causes foreshortening of its appearance on the frontal radiograph and a "mass" on radiography where the protruding scapula is outlined by atmospheric air (Fig. 17.25). This deformity typically results from disruption of innervation by the long thoracic nerve to the serratus anterior muscle that helps maintain scapular contact with the chest wall. Metastatic disease to the scapula is recognized by the presence of lytic destructive lesions; lung and breast cancer are the most commonly associated primary malignancies.

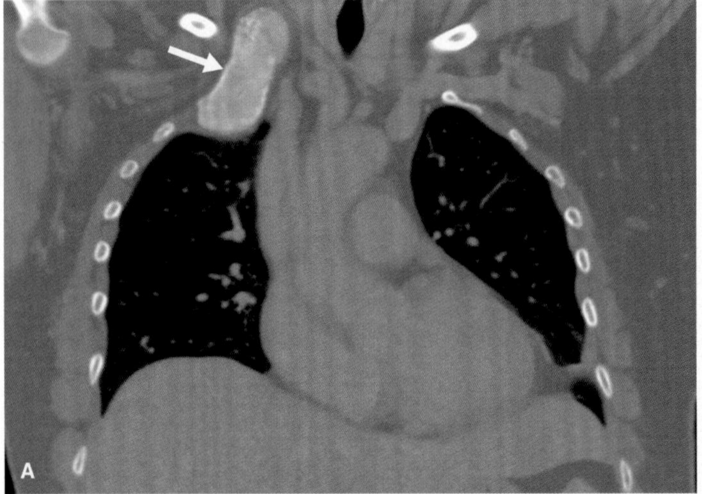
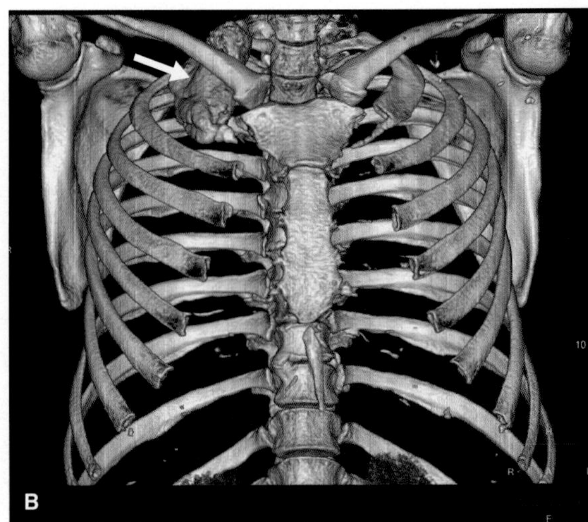
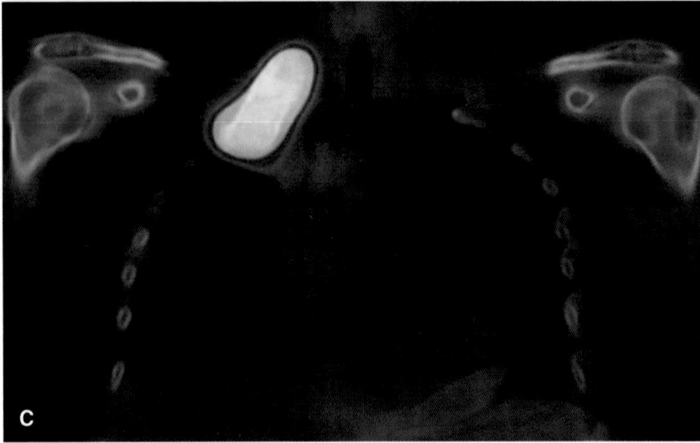

FIGURE 17.21. **Fibrous Dysplasia. A, B:** Contrast-enhanced coronal (**A**) and frontal projection surface-rendered CT (**B**) in a 34-year-old male with a palpable right supraclavicular mass shows a dense mass (*arrow*) replacing the right first rib and extending into the right supraclavicular space. **C:** Fused FDG PET-CT shows marked increased activity within the mass. Surgical resection revealed fibrous dysplasia.

Clavicle. A variety of diseases can affect the clavicle in adults. The distal third of the clavicle is commonly fractured in blunt trauma. Rheumatoid arthritis and hyperparathyroidism can produce erosion of the distal clavicles. The distal clavicle is sharply defined in rheumatoid arthritis and tapers to a point, whereas in hyperparathyroidism it is often indistinct and irregular. Additional findings in rheumatoid arthritis include narrowing of the glenohumeral joint and a high riding humeral head caused by rotator cuff atrophy. Primary malignant neoplasms of the clavicle include Ewing or osteogenic sarcoma. Metastases to the clavicle are usually associated with lesions in other portions of the bony thorax. Osteomyelitis of

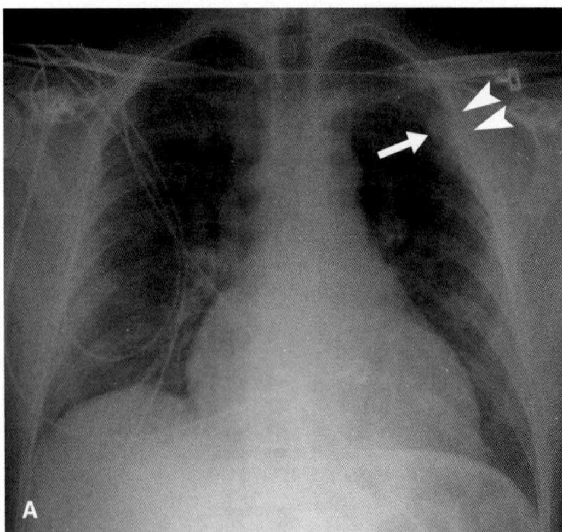
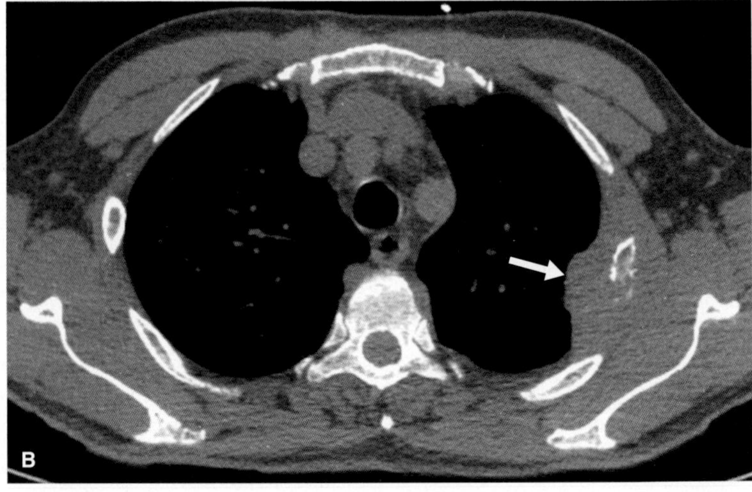

FIGURE 17.22. **Myeloma Producing a Chest Wall Mass. A:** Frontal chest radiograph in a 67-year-old man with a history of myeloma shows an extrapulmonary mass in the left upper chest (*arrow*) with destruction of the left 3rd rib laterally (*arrowheads*). **B:** Axial CT shows a mass (*arrow*) in the left lateral chest wall with associated rib destruction. Biopsy showed myeloma.

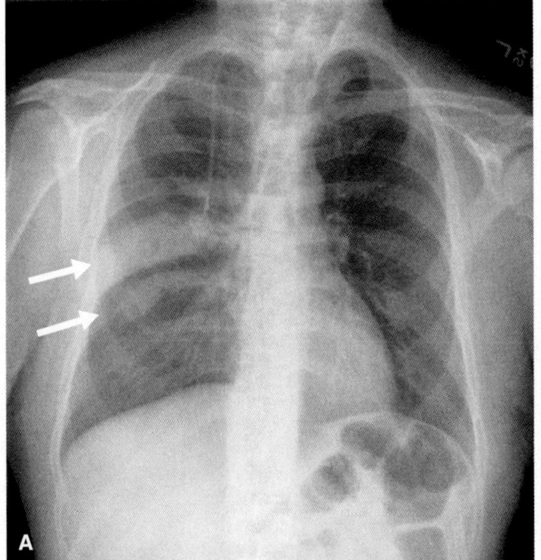

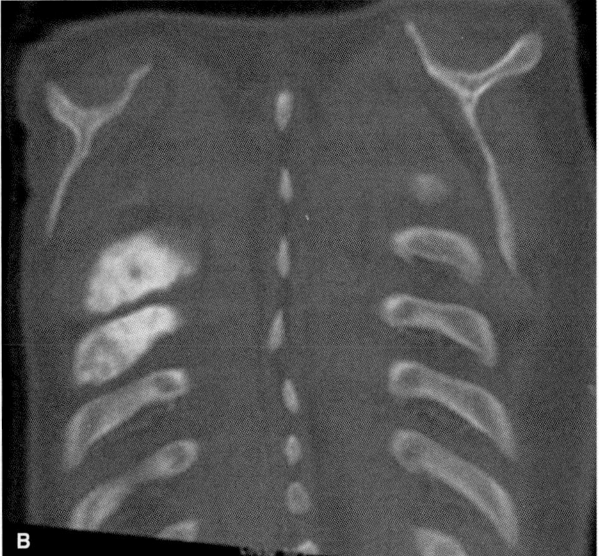

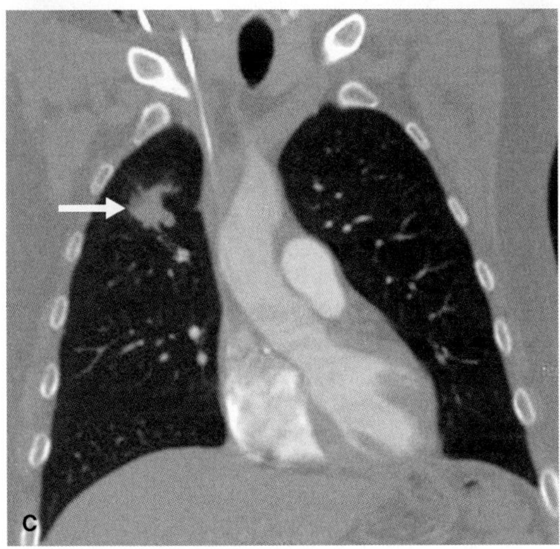

FIGURE 17.23. **Blastic Bone Metastases From Lung Cancer.** Chest radiograph (**A**) shows sclerotic, expansile changes in two contiguous right posterior ribs (*arrows*) and the mid-thoracic spine. Coronal-reformatted CT (**B**) through the posterior chest wall shows blastic changes in the two contiguous ribs. Coronal-reformatted CT (**C**) through the ascending aorta shows a spiculated right upper lobe nodule (*arrow*) reflecting the patient's primary non–small-cell lung cancer.

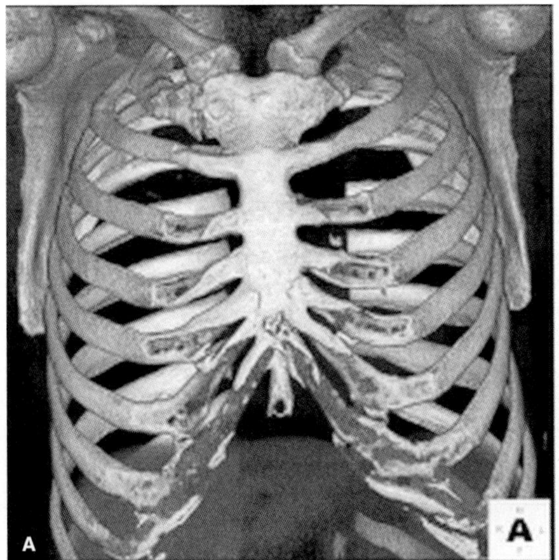

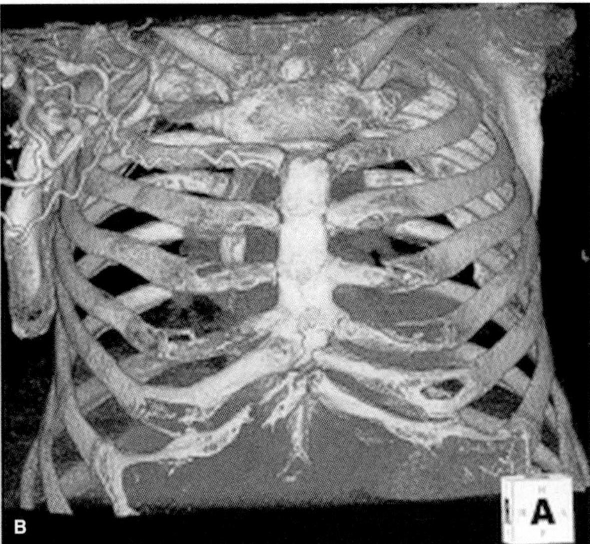

FIGURE 17.24. **Normal Ossification Patterns in Men and Women.** Shaded-surface three-dimensional reconstructions of the anterior chest wall show typical ossification patterns of costal cartilages in a woman (**A**) and a man (**B**).

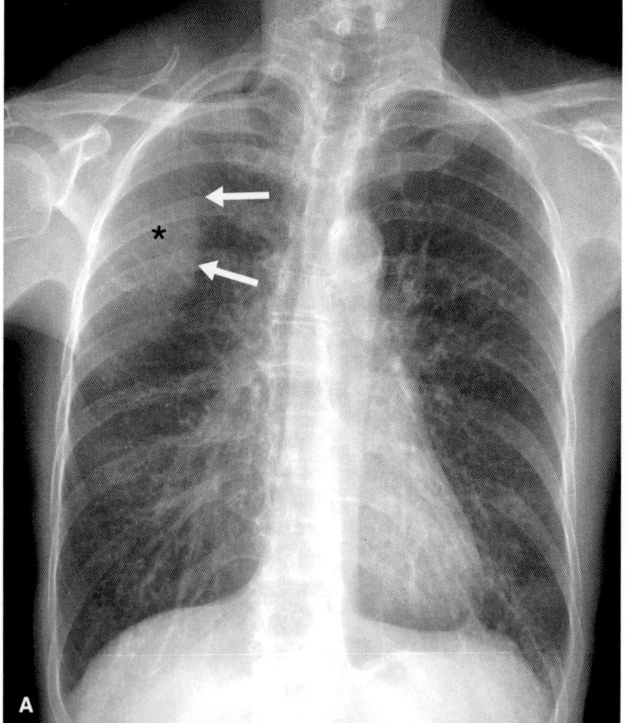

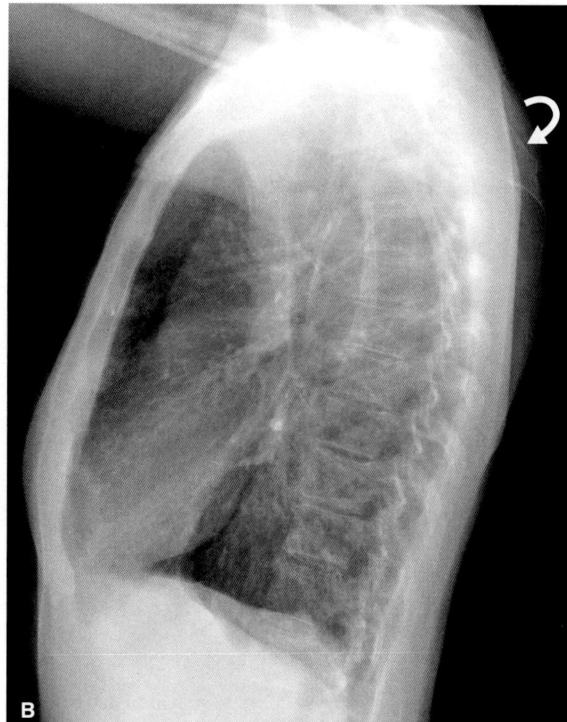

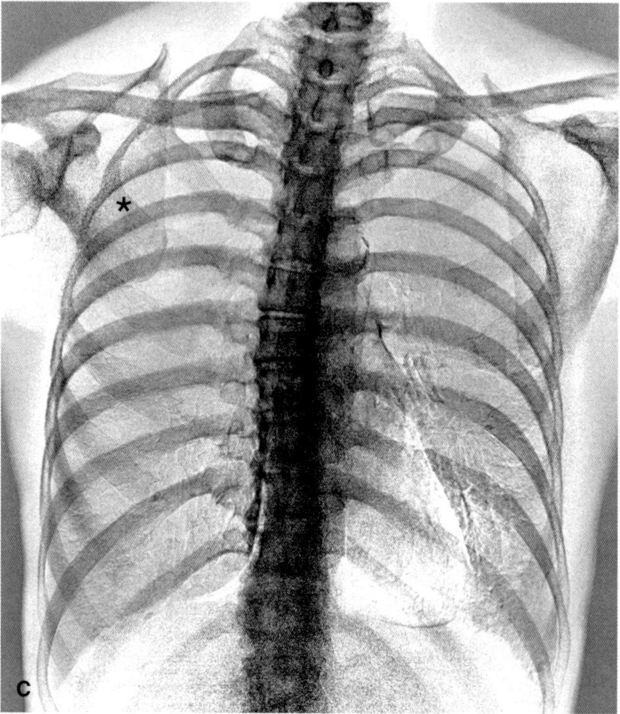

FIGURE 17.25. **Winged Scapula. A:** Frontal chest radiograph in an asymptomatic man shows an opacity (*asterisk*) with a sharp medial border (*arrows*) and indistinct lateral border over the right upper chest. **B:** Lateral chest radiograph shows a scapula protruding from the posterior chest wall (*curved arrow*). **C:** Bone image from dual energy chest radiograph shows the right scapula (*asterisk*) has a foreshortened appearance consistent with a winged scapula.

the clavicle is uncommon and is most often seen in intravenous drug users. Paget disease can involve the clavicle, but there is often concomitant pelvic bone and calvarial involvement.

Thoracic Spine. Numerous thoracic spine abnormalities are visible on chest radiographs. Congenital anomalies, including hemivertebrae, butterfly vertebra, spina bifida, and scoliosis, can be seen on well-penetrated frontal radiographs. Vertebral compression fractures caused by trauma, osteoporosis, or metastases are best seen on lateral radiographs and may produce an exaggerated kyphosis. Large bridging osteophytes may mimic a paraspinal mass on frontal radiographs or a pulmonary nodule on lateral films. Vertebral osteomyelitis is seen as destruction of vertebral bodies and intervertebral discs, often associated with a paraspinal abscess. Chronic anemia in patients with thalassemia major or sickle cell disease may result in prevertebral or paravertebral masses of extramedullary hematopoiesis, which represent herniated hyperplastic bone marrow. Sickle cell anemia produces a characteristic appearance of H-shaped or "Lincoln log"

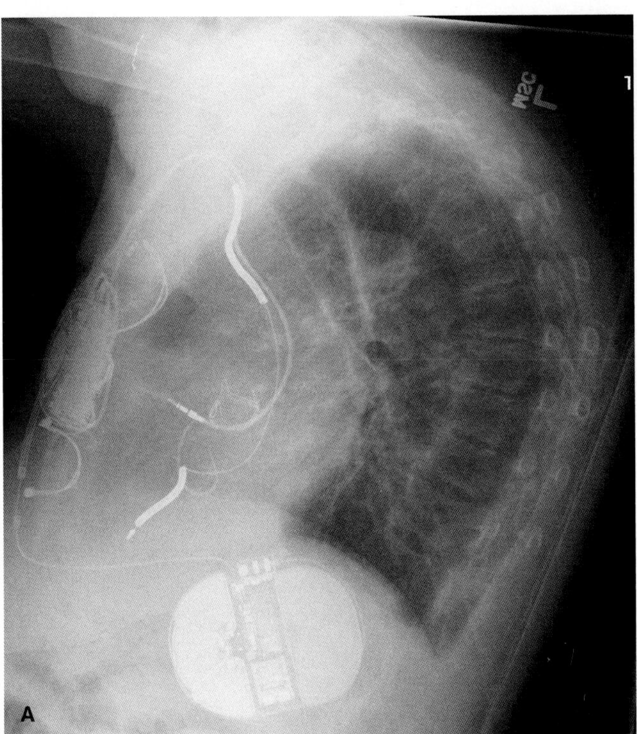
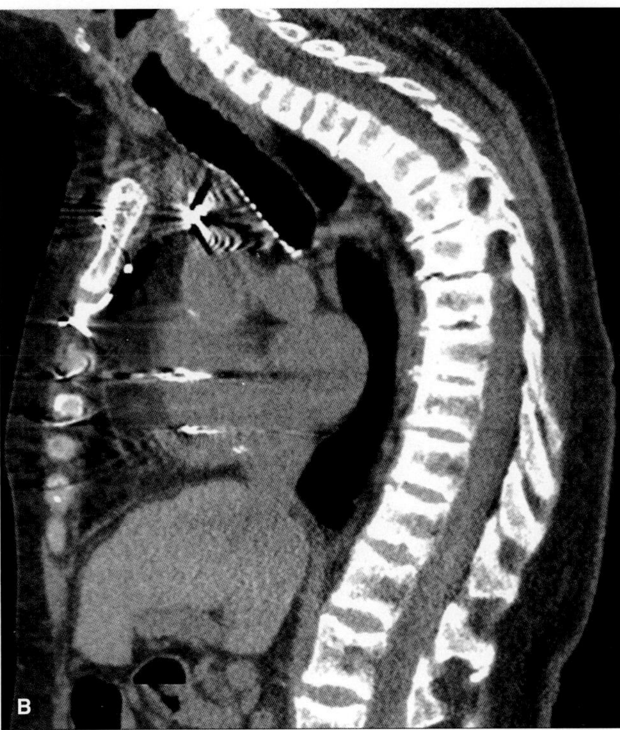

FIGURE 17.26. **Rugger Jersey Spine. A:** Lateral chest radiograph in a 87-year-old man with chronic renal failure shows end-plate sclerosis throughout the thoracic spine. **B:** Midline sagittal CT shows the typical changes of a rugger-jersey spine.

vertebrae on lateral chest radiographs that is pathognomonic of this disease. Similarly, a "rugger jersey" appearance to the thoracic spine on lateral chest films suggests renal osteosclerosis (Fig. 17.26).

Sternum. Developmental sternal deformities include pectus excavatum (funnel chest), pectus carinatum (pigeon breast), and abnormal segmentation. In pectus excavatum, the sternum is inwardly depressed and the ribs protrude anterior to the sternum. It often has an autosomal dominant pattern of inheritance but may occur sporadically. Pectus excavatum is commonly associated with congenital connective tissue disorders, such as Marfan syndrome, Poland syndrome, osteogenesis imperfecta, and congenital scoliosis. Most patients are asymptomatic. A clinically insignificant systolic murmur can result from compression of the right ventricular outflow tract, although some patients with pectus deformities and systolic murmurs have mitral valve prolapse. Pectus excavatum has a characteristic appearance on frontal chest radiograph. The heart is displaced to the left and the combination of the depressed soft tissues of the anterior chest wall and the vertically oriented anterior ribs results in loss of the right heart border. The findings on frontal radiographs may be mistakenly attributed to middle lobe opacification from pneumonia or atelectasis. The typical inward depression of the midsternum and lower sternum is seen on lateral chest radiographs (Fig. 17.27). CT helps define the deformity and in severe cases is used for preoperative planning of surgical correction.

Pectus carinatum is an outward bowing of the sternum that may be congenital or acquired. The congenital form is seen more commonly in boys and in families with a history of chest wall deformities or scoliosis. Congenital atrial or ventricular septal defects and severe childhood asthma account for the majority of the acquired cases of pectus carinatum. Affected patients are asymptomatic. The characteristic outward bowing of the sternum with deepening of the retrosternal airspace is seen on lateral radiographs (Fig. 17.28).

Severe blunt trauma to the chest, most often associated with deceleration injury from a motor vehicle accident, can result in fracture or dislocation of the sternum. Sternal body fracture and sternomanubrial dislocation are associated with a 25% to 45% mortality rate from concomitant injuries to the aorta, diaphragm, heart, tracheobronchial tree, and lung. Sternal films or lateral radiographs will show the fracture and often demonstrate a retrosternal hematoma; CT may be useful in those patients with normal plain films and a high suspicion of sternal injury.

A prior median sternotomy is the most common sternal abnormality seen on conventional radiography and chest CT. Circular wires encompassing the sternum are seen spaced along its length within the interspaces between costal cartilages. The vertical lucency representing the sternotomy may heal, but in many patients bony union does not occur. In the early postoperative period, a retrosternal hematoma may be seen, which normally resolves within the first several weeks. The radiologist plays a key role in the evaluation of possible sternal wound infection. Radiographic evidence of bony destruction and air in the sternal incision appearing weeks after sternotomy are specific but insensitive findings for osteomyelitis. Bone scans are not particularly useful, as there will be increased radionuclide uptake for months following sternotomy. CT is the modality of choice in the evaluation of sternal wound infection. The CT findings of sternal osteomyelitis include bone destruction, peristernal soft tissue mass, enhancing fluid collection, and gas. The extent of infection, specifically associated mediastinitis, can also be determined.

DIAPHRAGM

Unilateral Diaphragmatic Elevation. The differential diagnosis of unilateral diaphragmatic elevation is listed in Table 17.11. Eventration of the diaphragm is a result of congenital absence, underdevelopment, or atrophy of diaphragmatic

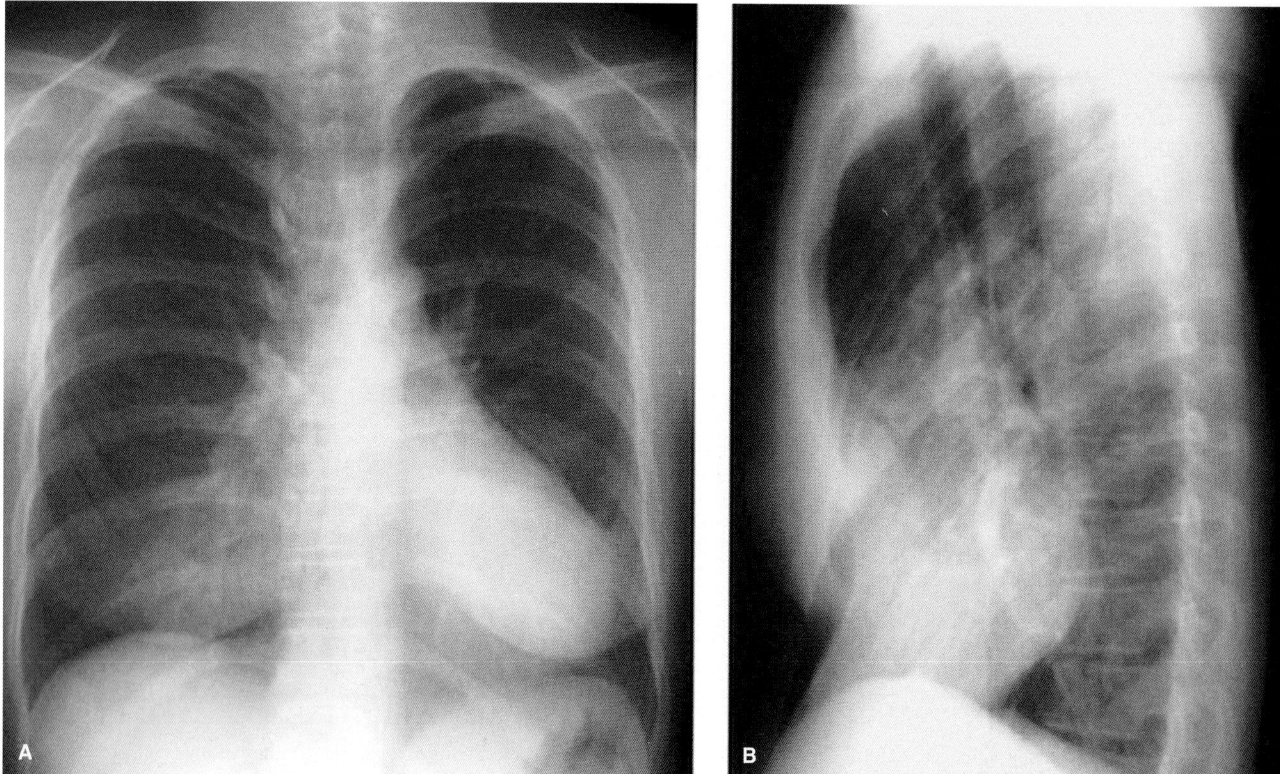

FIGURE 17.27. **Pectus Excavatum. A, B:** Frontal (**A**) and lateral (**B**) chest radiographs show changes of pectus excavatum. Note the apparent middle lobe opacity on the frontal radiograph that is typical of this condition.

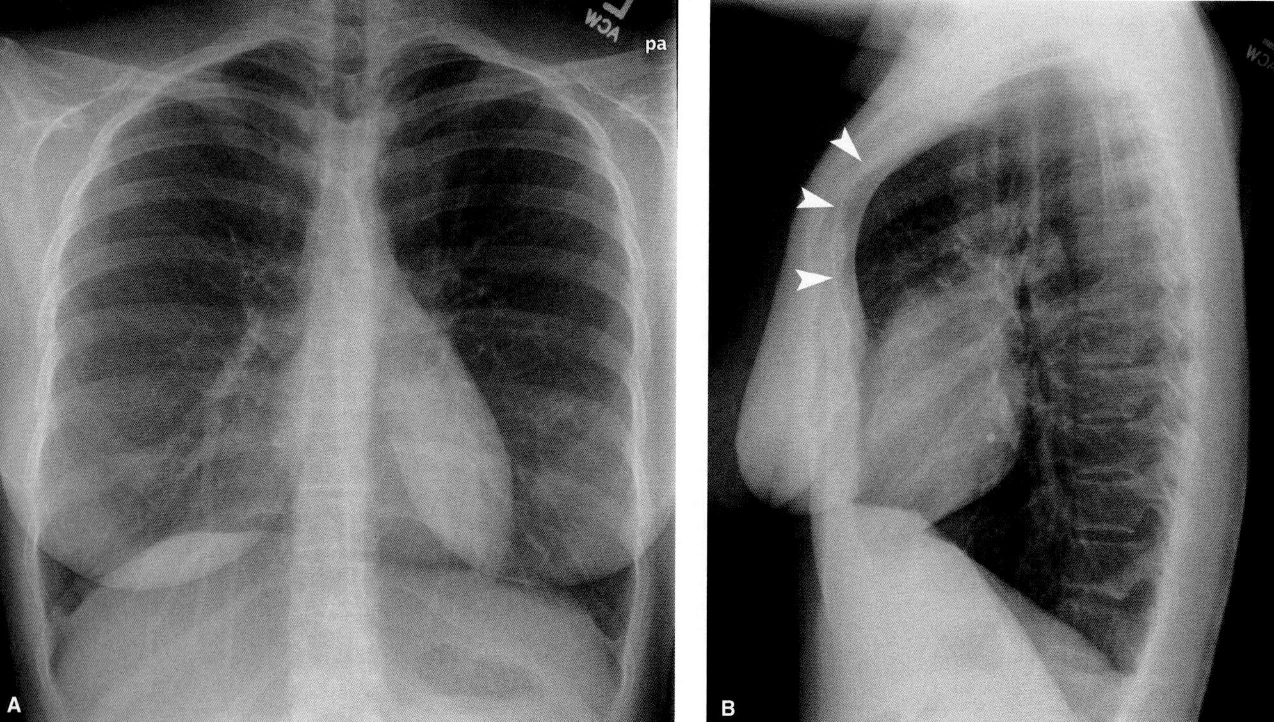

FIGURE 17.28. **Pectus Carinatum. A, B:** Frontal (**A**) and lateral (**B**) chest radiographs in an asymptomatic woman showed the typical anterior bowing of the sternum on lateral radiography (*arrowheads*) reflecting a pectus carinatum deformity.

TABLE 17.11

UNILATERAL DIAPHRAGMATIC ELEVATION

Eventration	
Diminished lung volume	Congenital Hypoplastic lung Acquired Lobar/lung atelectasis Pulmonary resection
Paralysis	Idiopathic Iatrogenic phrenic nerve injury Phrenic crush (tuberculosis) Intraoperative Malignant invasion of phrenic nerve Bronchogenic carcinoma Inflammation of diaphragmatic muscle Pleuritis Lower lobe pneumonia Subphrenic abscess
Upper abdominal mass	Hepatomegaly or liver mass Splenomegaly Gastric/colonic distention Ascites (usually bilateral) Diaphragmatic hernia[a] Subpulmonic pleural effusion[a]

[a]Apparent diaphragmatic elevation.

musculature. This produces a localized elevation of the hemidiaphragm on frontal radiographs in older individuals (Fig. 17.29), which on the right is indistinguishable from the rare foramen of Morgagni hernia. Complete diaphragmatic eventration is indistinguishable radiographically from diaphragmatic paralysis.

Unilateral diaphragmatic paralysis may be caused by surgical injury or neoplastic involvement of the phrenic nerve, which affects the right and left hemidiaphragms with equal frequency. Idiopathic phrenic nerve dysfunction resulting from a viral neuritis is a common cause of diaphragmatic paralysis in male patients and is usually right sided. A positive fluoroscopic or ultrasonographic sniff test (paradoxical superior movement of the diaphragm with sniffing, a result of the effects of negative intrathoracic pressure on a flaccid diaphragm during inspiration) is diagnostic. Chronic loss of lung volume, particularly from collapse or resection of the lower lobe, results in diaphragmatic elevation. This is also a common sequela of chronic cicatrizing atelectasis of the upper lobe from TB.

An enlarged liver or hepatic mass can produce right hemidiaphragmatic elevation by direct pressure on the undersurface of the hemidiaphragm. Similarly, an enlarged spleen, gas-distended stomach, or enlarged splenic flexure can produce an elevated left hemidiaphragm. Irritation of the superior surface of the hemidiaphragm by a pleural or pleura-based parenchymal process (e.g., infarct, pneumonia) or of the undersurface of the diaphragm by a subphrenic abscess, hepatitis, or cholecystitis may cause the diaphragm to become flaccid, leading to elevation. A subpulmonic effusion may simulate an elevated hemidiaphragm.

Bilateral diaphragmatic elevation that is not effort related may be caused by a neuromuscular disturbance or intrathoracic or intra-abdominal disease. Radiographically, the

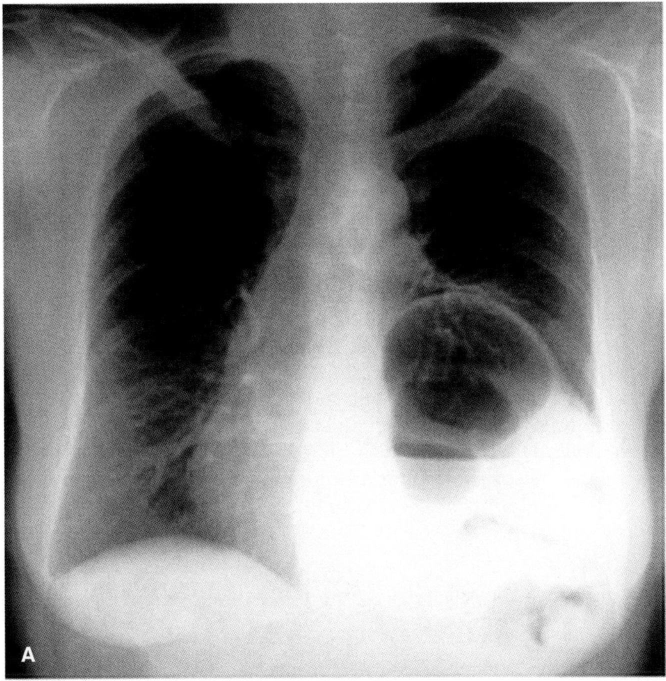

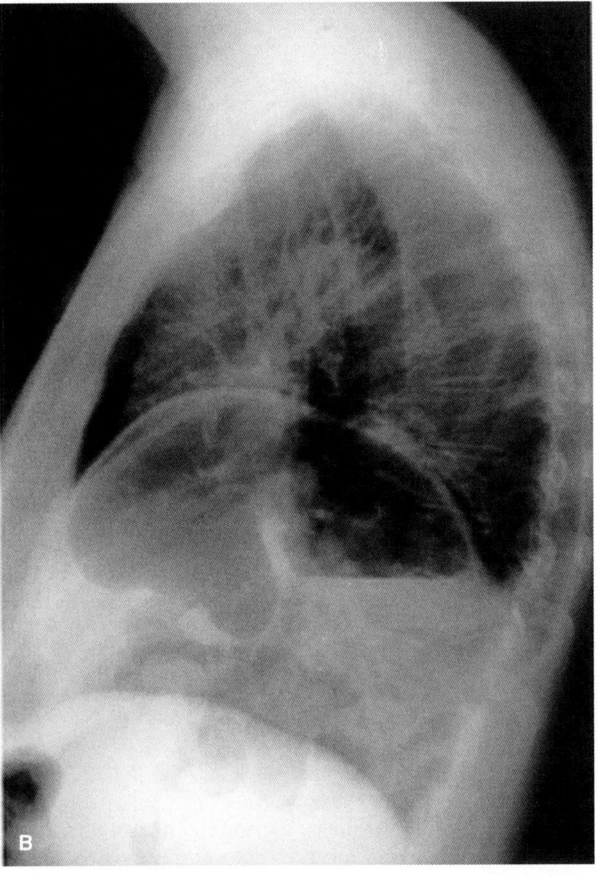

FIGURE 17.29. **Eventration of the Diaphragm.** Posteroanterior (**A**) and lateral (**B**) chest radiographs in an asymptomatic 61-year-old woman reveal marked elevation of the left hemidiaphragm representing diaphragmatic eventration.

diaphragms are elevated on both frontal and lateral views. Bibasilar linear atelectasis or passive lobar or segmental lower lobe atelectasis may be seen. Bilateral phrenic nerve disruption or intrinsic diaphragmatic muscular disease will produce bilateral diaphragmatic paralysis and elevation. Common disorders include cervical cord injury, multiple sclerosis, and the myopathy associated with systemic lupus erythematosus. In these patients, fluoroscopic or real-time US imaging of the diaphragms demonstrates a positive sniff test.

Lung restriction caused by interstitial fibrosis, bilateral pleural fibrosis, or chest wall disease (most commonly from obesity) can produce bilateral diaphragmatic elevation. An increase in intra-abdominal volume, most often from ascites, hepatosplenomegaly, or pregnancy, can restrict diaphragmatic motion. These conditions may be distinguished from bilateral paralysis by observation of normal but diminished inferior excursion of the diaphragms on fluoroscopy, US, or inspiratory/expiratory radiographs.

Diaphragmatic Depression. Depression and flattening of one hemidiaphragm is seen with unilateral overinflation of a lung, usually as a compensatory mechanism when the contralateral lung is small or as a result of a large ipsilateral pneumothorax (Fig. 17.11). Distinction between these two entities is usually possible by the clinical history and by characteristic findings in those with pneumothorax. A tension pneumothorax may cause inversion of the hemidiaphragm. Bilateral diaphragmatic depression is either a permanent finding—a result of abnormally increased lung compliance in patients with emphysema—or a transient finding in those with asthma and expiratory air trapping.

Diaphragmatic Hernias. There are three types of nontraumatic diaphragmatic hernias. The most common is the *esophageal hiatal hernia*, which represents herniation of a portion of the stomach through the esophageal hiatus. These are usually seen as incidental asymptomatic masses on chest radiographs, although some patients may have symptoms of gastroesophageal reflux or, rarely, severe pain from strangulation of the herniated stomach. Hiatal hernias are seen projecting behind the heart on frontal chest radiographs in the immediate supradiaphragmatic region of the posterior mediastinum. An air–fluid level may be seen in the hernia. An esophagram is confirmatory. CT shows widening of the esophageal hiatus and depicts the contents of the hernia sac, which often include stomach, omental fat, and, rarely, ascitic fluid.

Bochdalek Hernia. The foramen of Bochdalek is a defect in the hemidiaphragm at the site of the embryonic pleuroperitoneal canal. Large hernias through the Bochdalek foramen present in the neonatal period with hypoplasia of the ipsilateral lung and respiratory distress. In adults, small hernias through this foramen are common and are predominantly seen on the left side, presumably because of the protective effect of the liver, which prevents herniation of right infradiaphragmatic fat through the right foramen of Bochdalek. The hernia typically appears as a posterolateral mass above the left hemidiaphragm, although it can occur anywhere along the posterior diaphragmatic surface (Fig. 17.30). CT shows the diaphragmatic defect with herniation of retroperitoneal fat, omentum, spleen, or kidney.

Morgagni Hernia. A defect in the parasternal portion of the diaphragm, the foramen of Morgagni, is the least common type of diaphragmatic hernia. A Morgagni hernia is invariably right sided and appears as an asymptomatic cardiophrenic angle mass (Fig. 17.31). The diagnosis is made by noting herniation of omental fat, liver, or transverse colon through the paracardiac portion of the right hemidiaphragm on CT scans through the lung bases. The presence of omental vessels within a fatty paracardiac mass is diagnostic (Fig. 17.31C). Coronal CT can demonstrate the diaphragmatic defect, distinguishing this entity from partial eventration of the hemidiaphragm.

Traumatic Hernia. Traumatic herniation of abdominal contents through a tear or rupture of the central or posterior aspect of the hemidiaphragm may follow blunt thoracoabdominal trauma or penetrating injury. The left side is affected in more than 90% of cases because the liver dissipates the traumatic forces and protects the right hemidiaphragm from injury. Radiographically, the diagnosis should be suspected when the left hemidiaphragmatic contour is indistinct or elevated or when gas-filled loops of bowel or stomach are seen in the left lower thorax following severe trauma. Early diagnosis is often difficult because associated thoracic and abdominal injuries may obscure the clinical and radiographic findings. The diagnosis is often made after the traumatic episode, with symptoms caused by intestinal obstruction with strangulation (pain, vomiting, fever), compression of the left lung (cough, dyspnea, chest pain), or as an incidental finding, particularly if only fat and no viscus has herniated through the defect (Fig. 17.32). In addition to the stomach, the small intestine, colon, omentum, spleen, kidney, fat, and the left lobe of the liver can also herniate through the defect. The diagnosis is usually made by CT demonstrating bowel herniating into the thorax through a constricting diaphragmatic defect. The resultant narrowing or "waist" of the herniated intestine as it traverses the diaphragmatic defect differentiates a hernia from simple diaphragmatic elevation. Coronal and sagittal CT reconstructions can characterize the herniated tissues and detect associated visceral injuries (Fig. 17.32B,C). In addition to the detection of intrathoracic herniation of abdominal contents, CT can usually depict the diaphragmatic defect, even in the absence of visceral herniation. Other CT findings suggestive of traumatic diaphragmatic injury include thickening or retraction of the diaphragm away from the traumatic injury, a narrowing or waist of the diaphragm on the herniated viscus ("collar" or "waist" sign) (Fig. 17.32C) and contact between the posterior ribs and the liver (right-sided injury) or stomach (left-sided injury), termed the "dependent viscera" sign.

Diaphragmatic Tumors. Primary diaphragmatic tumors are extremely rare, with an equal incidence of benign and malignant lesions. Benign lesions include lipomas, fibromas, schwannomas, neurofibromas, and leiomyomas. Echinococcal cysts and extralobar sequestrations may be found within the diaphragm. Fibrosarcomas are the most common primary malignant diaphragmatic lesion. Radiographically, they appear as focal extrapulmonary masses obscuring all or part of the hemidiaphragm and are indistinguishable from masses arising within the diaphragmatic pleura. CT may show the origin of the mass, although the relationship of the mass to the diaphragm is best appreciated on coronal MR or transabdominal US. Direct invasion of the diaphragm by lower lobe lung cancer, mesothelioma, or a subphrenic neoplasm is much more common than primary diaphragmatic malignancy.

CONGENITAL LUNG DISEASE IN ADULTS

Bronchogenic cysts represent anomalous outpouchings of the primitive foregut that no longer communicate with the tracheobronchial tree. They are commonly present as asymptomatic mediastinal masses of water attenuation and are in Chapter 11.

Congenital pulmonary airway malformation (CPAM) and congenital lobar overinflation (emphysema) are discussed in Chapter 67.

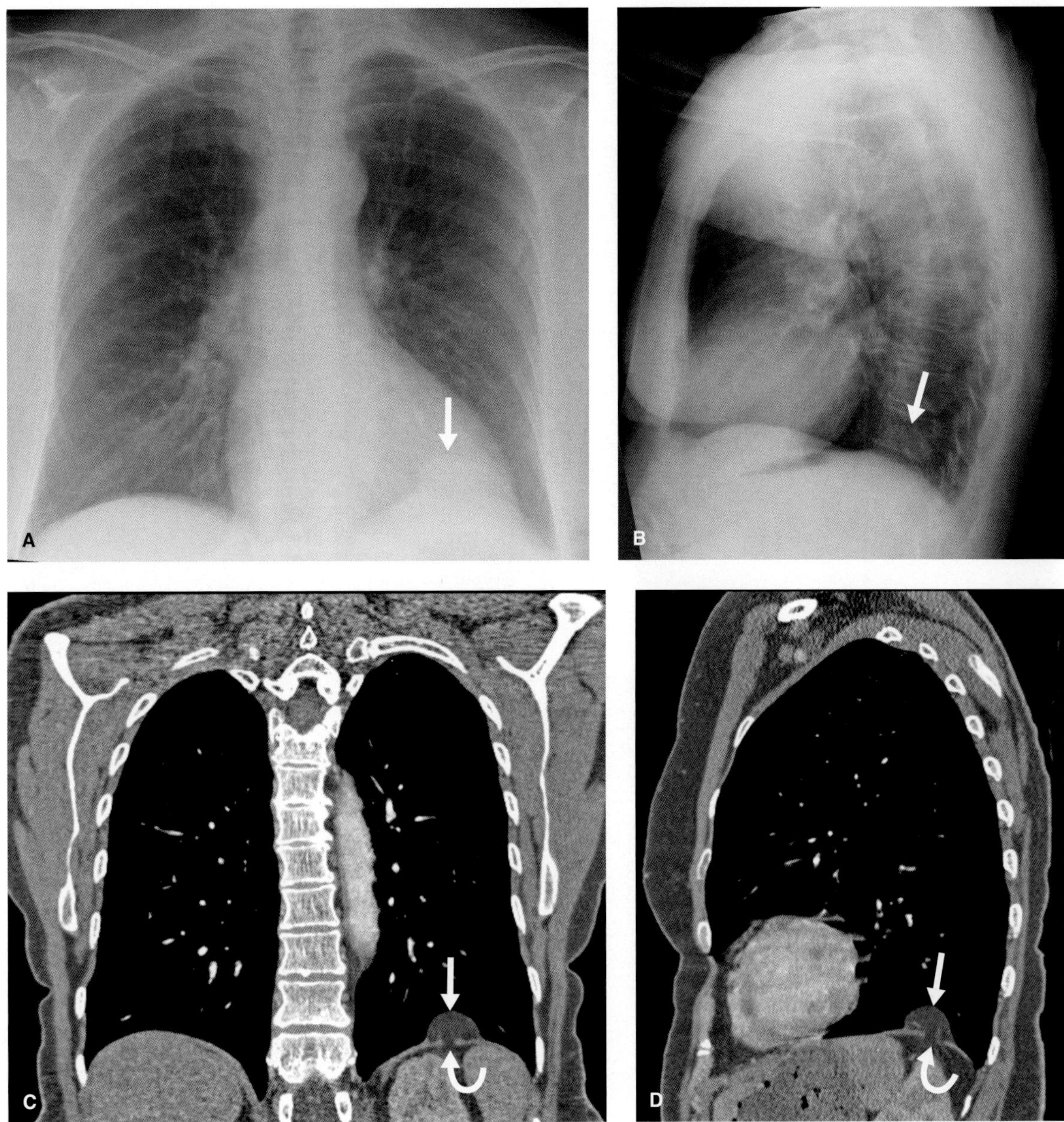

FIGURE 17.30. **Foramen of Bochdalek Hernia. A, B:** Frontal (**A**) and lateral (**B**) chest radiographs in an asymptomatic 62-year-old woman show a mass (*arrow* in **A,B**) arising from the posterior left hemidiaphragm. **C, D:** Coronal (**C**) and sagittal CT scans through the diaphragm shows fat (*arrow* in **C,D**) herniating through the foramen of Bochdalek (*curved arrow* in **C,D**).

Bronchial atresia is discussed in Chapters 16 and 67.

Bronchopulmonary sequestration is a congenital abnormality resulting from the independent development of a portion of the tracheobronchial tree that is isolated from the normal lung and maintains its fetal systemic arterial supply. Grossly, the sequestered lung is cystic and bronchiectatic. These patients most often present with recurrent pneumonia from recurrent infection in the sequestered lung, although some (mostly extralobar sequestrations) are discovered as asymptomatic posterior mediastinal or diaphragmatic masses.

Pulmonary sequestration is divided into intralobar and extralobar forms. *Intralobar sequestration* is contained within the visceral pleura of the normal lung. *Extralobar sequestration* is enclosed by its own visceral pleural envelope and may be found adjacent to the normal lung or within or below the diaphragm. Most patients with intralobar sequestration present with pneumonia. Extralobar sequestration is usually asymptomatic and is seen as an incidental finding in a neonate with other severe congenital anomalies. Intralobar sequestration is more common than the extralobar type, by a ratio of 3 to 1. Both forms are found in the lower lobes, but extralobar sequestration is predominantly left sided (90%), whereas one-third of intralobar sequestrations are right sided. A major differentiating feature between the two types is the arterial supply to and venous drainage from the sequestered lung. An intralobar sequestration is supplied by a single large artery that arises from the infradiaphragmatic aorta and enters the sequestered lung via the pulmonary ligament. The venous drainage is typically via the pulmonary veins, although systemic venous drainage can occur. In contrast, an extralobar sequestration receives several small branches from systemic and occasionally pulmonary arteries, with venous drainage into the systemic venous system (inferior vena cava, azygos, or hemiazygos veins).

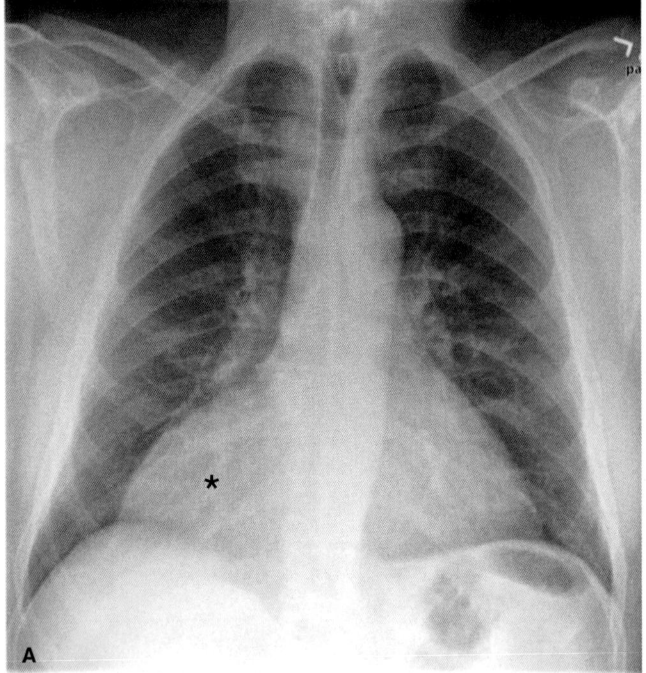

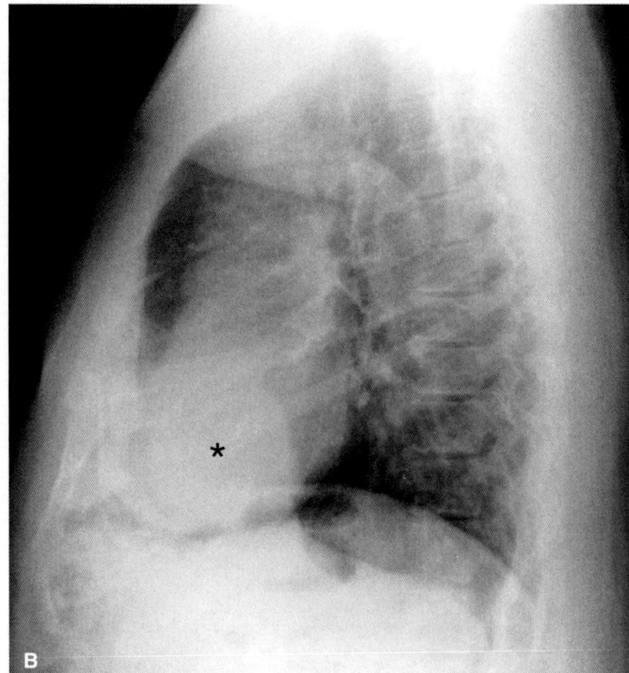

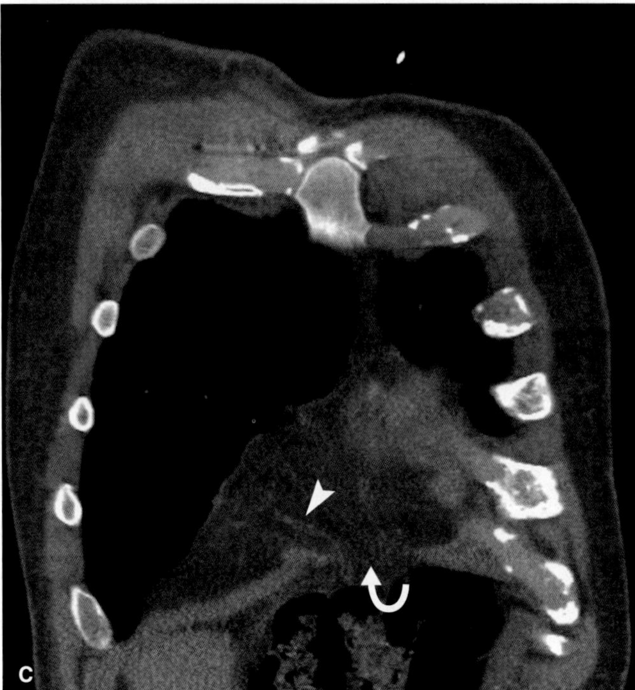

FIGURE 17.31. **Foramen of Morgagni Hernia.** Frontal (**A**) and lateral (**B**) chest radiographs in a 60-year-old woman reveal a large mass in the right cardiophrenic angle (*asterisk*). **C:** Coronal CT scan at the level of the anterior diaphragm shows a fatty paracardiac mass containing omental vessels (*arrowhead*). The defect in the medial diaphragm is visible (*curved arrow*).

Sequestration appears as a solid posterior mediastinal mass or as a solitary or multicystic air collection. Air–fluid levels are seen when infection has produced communication of the sequestered lung with the normal tracheobronchial tree. The definitive diagnosis is made by the demonstration of abnormal systemic arterial supply to the abnormal lung, which is usually accomplished by CT angiography (Fig. 17.33). Catheter angiography is usually reserved for preoperative patients in whom precise demonstration of the origin and number of the systemic feeders is necessary.

Hypoplastic lung is a developmental anomaly resulting in a small lung. This entity is discussed in Chapter 67.

Hypogenetic lung syndrome/scimitar syndrome, a variant of the hypoplastic lung, is characterized by an underdeveloped right lung with abnormal venous drainage of the lung to the inferior vena cava just above or below the right hemidiaphragm or eventration, dextroposition of the heart, and herniation of left lung anteriorly into the right hemithorax. This entity is discussed in Chapter 67.

Arteriovenous Malformation. Pulmonary arteriovenous malformations (AVMs) are abnormal vascular masses in which a focal collection of congenitally weakened capillaries dilates to become a tortuous complex of vessels fed by a

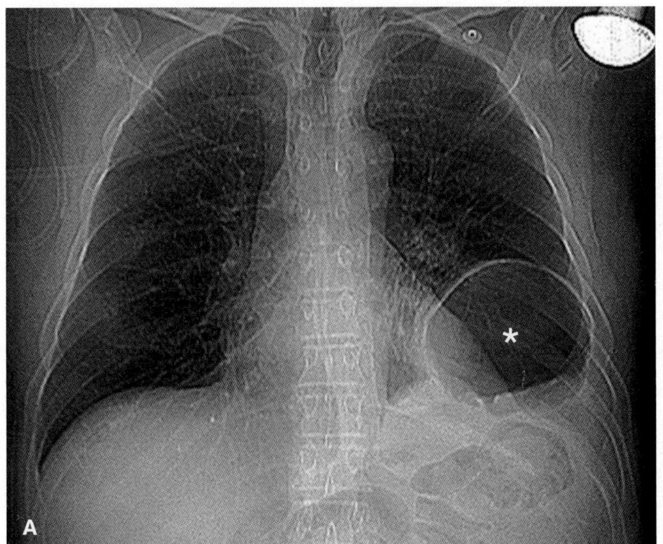

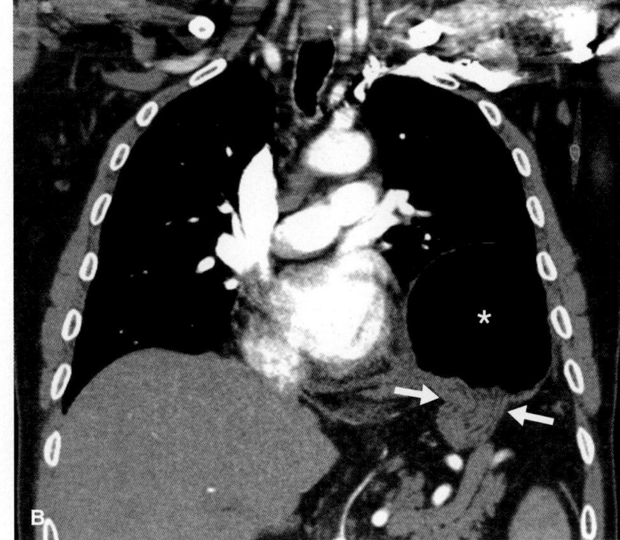

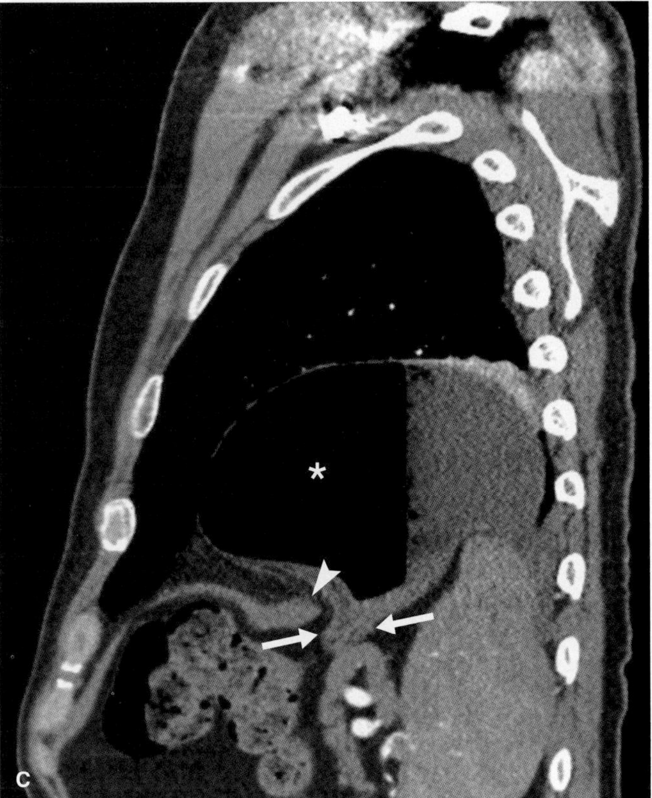

FIGURE 17.32. **Traumatic Diaphragmatic Hernia. A:** Scout radiograph in a patient with prior blunt chest trauma shows an abnormal lucency (*asterisk*) in the left lower chest. **B, C:** Contrast-enhanced coronal (**B**) and sagittal (**C**) CT scans show the stomach (*asterisk*) herniating through a diaphragmatic defect that produces a waist-like narrowing on the herniated stomach (*arrows* in **B** and **C**). Note anterior edge of injured diaphragm (*arrowhead* in **C**).

single pulmonary artery and drained by a single pulmonary vein. Most pulmonary AVMs do not come to attention until early adulthood. They are detected either incidentally, as part of a screening evaluation in patients with hereditary hemorrhagic telangiectasia (Osler–Weber–Rendu disease), a condition that is present in approximately 80% of all patients with pulmonary AVMs, or because of a variety of symptoms. The most common pulmonary symptoms are hemoptysis and dyspnea, the latter attributable to hypoxia caused by the intrapulmonary right-to-left shunt. Nonpulmonary symptoms most often relate to CNS disease. Stroke may occur from paradoxical right-to-left cerebral emboli or from thrombosis resulting from secondary polycythemia caused by chronic hypoxemia. Brain abscess may develop from paradoxical septic emboli.

The chest radiograph of a pulmonary AVM usually shows a solitary pulmonary nodule, most often located in the subpleural portions of the lower lobes. Approximately one-third of patients have multiple lesions. The lesion is often lobulated and has feeding and draining vessels emanating from the mass and extending toward the hilum. The morphology of the lesions is best demonstrated on CT. The feeding and draining vessels can be demonstrated by CT or MR (Fig. 13.3). Angiography is reserved for preoperative evaluation and for patients undergoing therapeutic transcatheter embolization with spring coils, which is the treatment of choice for patients with multiple AVMs.

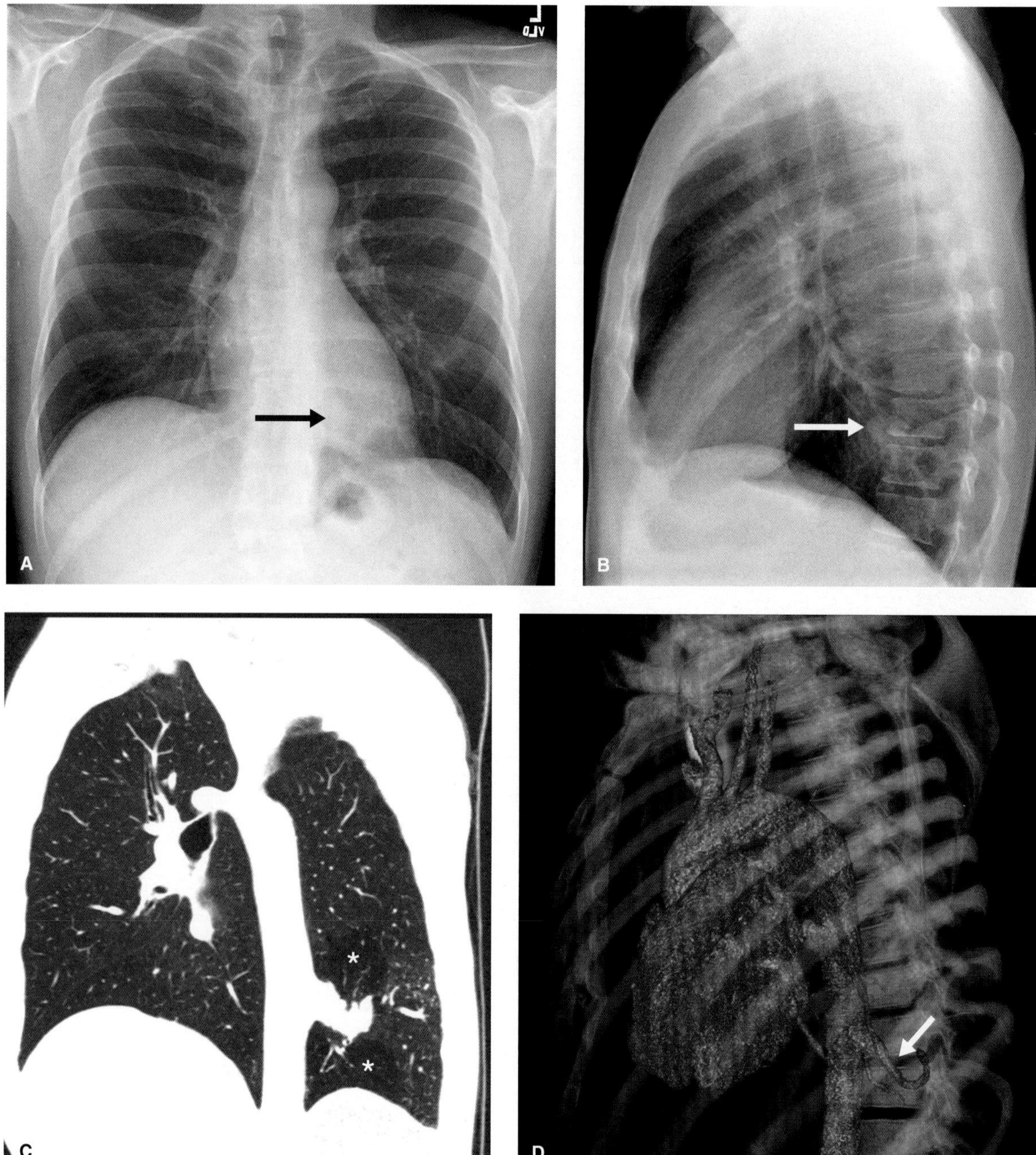

FIGURE 17.33. **Intralobar Pulmonary Sequestration. A, B:** Frontal (**A**) and lateral (**B**) chest radiographs in a 28-year-old man with a history of prior pneumonia show an abnormal opacity in the medial left lower lobe (*arrow*). **C:** Oblique coronal CT shows abnormally lucent lung within the left lower lobe (*asterisks*) with an opacity extending into the abnormal lung from the descending aorta. **D:** Oblique sagittal shaded surface rendering from a CT aortogram shows that the curvilinear opacity reflects a artery arising from the descending aorta (*arrow*), diagnostic of systemic arterial supply to a left lower lobe pulmonary sequestration.

TRAUMATIC LUNG DISEASE

Pulmonary contusion usually follows blunt chest trauma and typically develops adjacent to the site of impact or at distant sites due to shear injury. Blood and edema fluid fill the alveoli of the lung within the first 12 hours after trauma, producing scattered areas of airspace opacification that may rapidly become confluent and may be difficult to distinguish from aspiration pneumonia (Fig. 17.34). Patients may have shortness of breath and hemoptysis; blood can usually be suctioned from the endotracheal tube. The typical radiographic course is stabilization of opacities by 24 hours and improvement within 2 to 7 days. Progressive opacities seen more than 48 hours after trauma should raise the suspicion of aspiration pneumonia or developing ARDS.

Pulmonary Laceration, Traumatic Lung Cyst, and Pulmonary Hematoma. Pulmonary laceration is a common sequela of penetrating or blunt chest trauma. In the latter situation, it represents a shearing injury to the substance of the lung. The elastic properties of the lung quickly transform the linear laceration into a rounded air cyst. These cysts may be

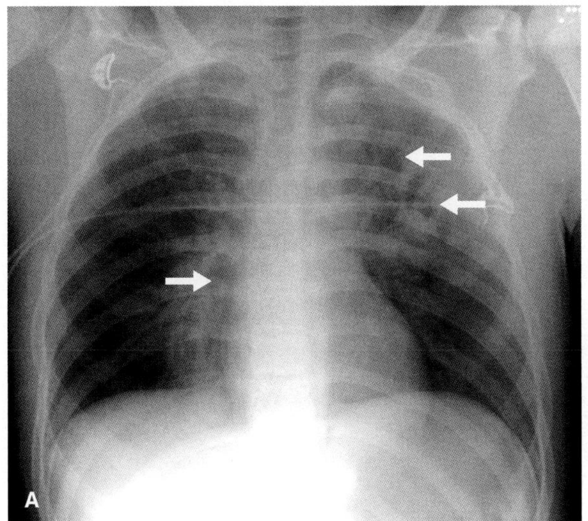

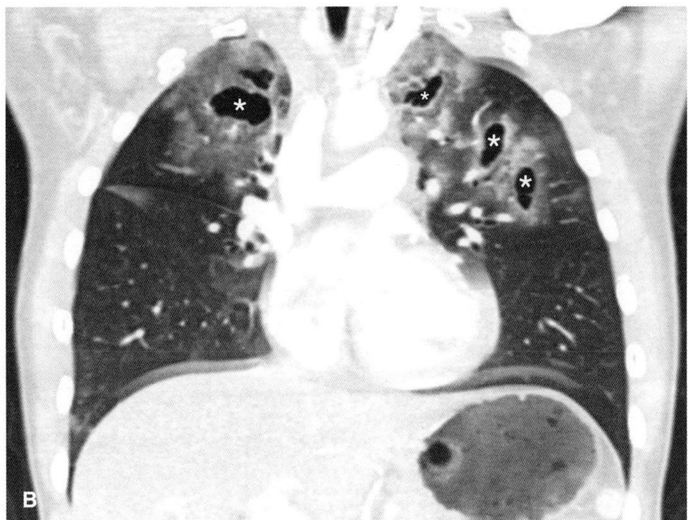

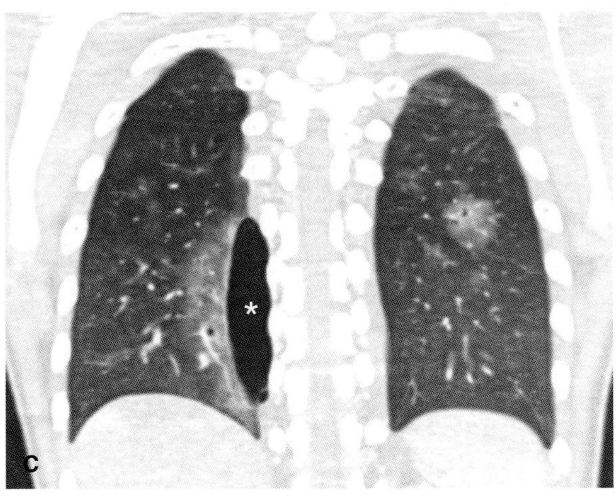

FIGURE 17.34. **Pulmonary Contusions and Traumatic Lung Cysts. A:** Portable chest radiograph in a patient involved in a motor vehicle accident shows medial right lung and left upper lobe airspace opacification. Subtle lucencies are visible within the opacified areas (*arrows*). **B, C:** Coronal CT scans through the mid- (**B**) and posterior (**C**) thorax show bilateral upper lobe and medial right lower lobe ground-glass and airspace opacifications with thin-walled lucencies (*asterisks*), reflecting lung contusions and traumatic lung cysts, respectively. There is an associated left 1st rib fracture and apical pleural fluid collection.

filled with varied amounts of blood as a result of laceration of pulmonary capillaries; those that are completely filled with blood are more appropriately termed *pulmonary hematomas*. On radiographs and CT, these cysts appear as rounded lucencies that may contain air or an air–fluid level (Fig. 17.34). Initially, these cysts are often obscured by the adjacent contused lung, only to be recognized after resorption of the blood. The cysts tend to shrink gradually over a period of weeks to months. The term *traumatic lung cyst* or *pneumatocele* can be used for these lesions; the latter term is also used to describe air cysts that result from a check-valve overdistention of the distal lung, as seen in certain types of pneumonia.

ASPIRATION

Aspiration in the adult can involve the aspiration of solid or liquid materials or of a foreign body. Aspiration of a tooth can occur after head trauma or following traumatic intubation. Foreign-body aspiration in adults is uncommon but should be considered in any patient with cough, wheezing, or nonresolving atelectasis or pneumonia or lobar/lung hyperinflation, particularly if accompanied by an endobronchial abnormality on CT.

Aspiration pneumonia and *pneumonitis* are terms used to describe the different pulmonary inflammatory responses to aspirated material. As was discussed in the chapter on infection, aspiration pneumonia describes a mixed anaerobic infection resulting from the aspiration of infected oropharyngeal contents. The aspiration of oropharyngeal or gastric secretions may also occur in a "pure" form uncomplicated by infection, producing aspiration pneumonitis.

Aspiration of oropharyngeal or gastric secretions, with or without food particles, is not an uncommon event. It is seen in debilitated patients with chronic diseases, in patients with tracheal or gastric tubes, in unconscious patients, and in those who have suffered strokes, seizures, or trauma. More chronic and less easily recognizable forms of aspiration may occur in patients with anatomic abnormalities of the upper GI tract (Zenker diverticulum, esophageal stricture) or functional disorders (gastroesophageal reflux, neuromuscular dysfunction).

Gastric fluid is highly irritating to the lungs and often stimulates explosive coughing and associated deep inspirations, leading to widespread distribution of the fluid throughout both lungs and into the peripheral airspaces. The hydrochloric acid contained in gastric fluid causes direct damage to both the bronchiolar lining and the alveolar wall. The severity of the resultant pneumonitis depends upon several factors: it is increased with a pH of the aspirated fluid <2.5, large volume of aspirated fluid, large particulate matter in the aspirated fluid, and young age. The massive aspiration of gastric contents is known as Mendelson syndrome. When the aspirate includes particulate material, the particles are distributed by gravity and may incite a granulomatous foreign body–type reaction.

Three basic radiographic patterns of aspiration pneumonitis have been observed: (1) extensive bilateral airspace opacification; (2) diffuse but discrete airspace nodular opacities; and

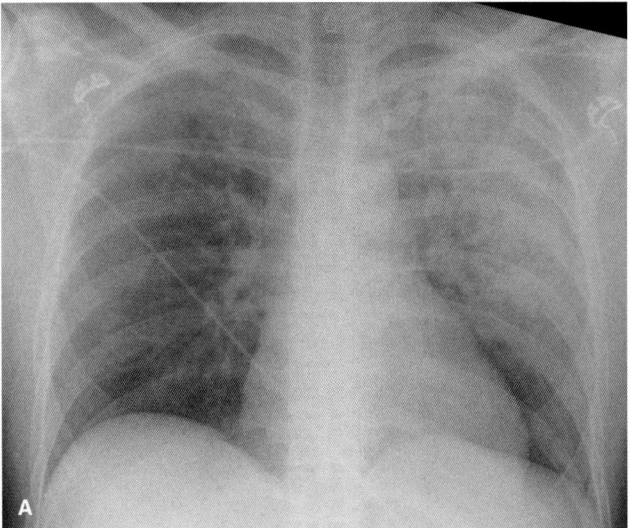

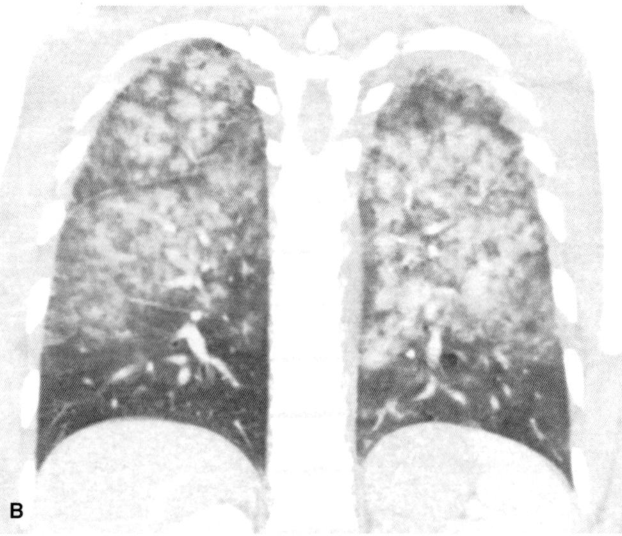

FIGURE 17.35. **Aspiration Bronchiolitis/Pneumonitis. A:** Portable frontal chest radiograph in a patient with a witnessed aspiration event demonstrates dense left upper lobe and patchy right upper lobe airspace opacification. **B:** Coronal CT scan through the posterior chest shows a bilateral dependent centrilobular and lobular airspace opacification reflecting aspiration bronchiolitis and bronchopneumonia.

(3) irregular parenchymal opacities that are not obviously airspace filling in nature. Parenchymal involvement is most often bilateral, with a predilection for the basal and perihilar regions (Fig. 17.35). When a significant amount of admixed food is present, the opacities are usually posterior and segmental. Atelectasis is often present, presumably airway obstruction caused by food particles. The radiographic appearance may worsen over the first few days but then demonstrates rapid improvement. A worsening of the radiographic appearance at this stage suggests development of a complicating infection, ARDS, or superimposed pulmonary embolism.

Chronic Aspiration Pneumonitis. Patients who repeatedly aspirate may develop chronic interstitial abnormalities on chest radiographs. With repeated episodes of aspiration over months to years, irregular reticular interstitial opacities may persist, probably representing peribronchial scarring. A reticulonodular pattern may be seen, caused by granulomas forming around food particles. These chronic interstitial abnormalities can be observed in between episodes of acute aspiration pneumonitis.

Exogenous Lipoid Pneumonia. Multifocal areas of consolidation or masses can result from the aspiration of lipid material and are classically seen in older patients with swallowing disorders or gastroesophageal reflux who ingest mineral oil as a laxative or inhale oily nose drops. When solitary, the lesion can mimic lung cancer. CT findings of fat attenuation with a compatible clinical history are diagnostic of this entity (Fig. 17.36).

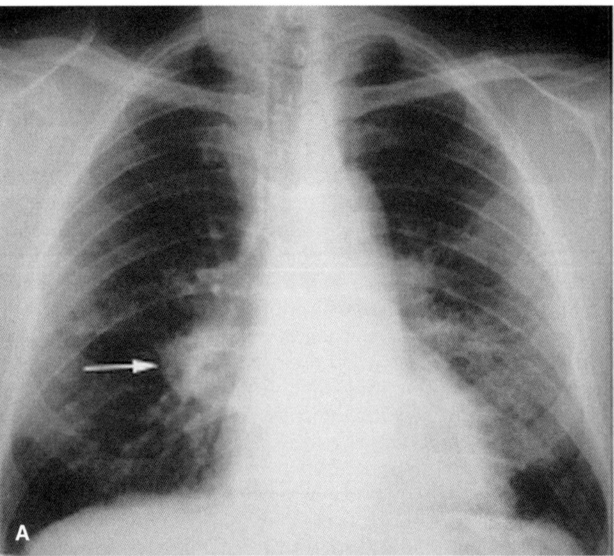

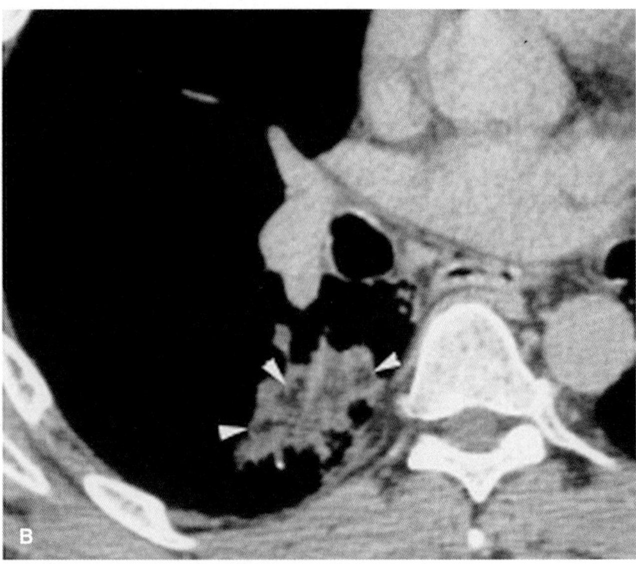

FIGURE 17.36. **Exogenous Lipoid Pneumonia. A:** Frontal chest radiograph in a 77-year-old man who used mineral oil as a laxative shows a superior segment right lower lobe mass (*arrow*) with associated lower lung interstitial changes present for 3 years. Coned-down axial CT through the right lower lobe (**B**) shows fat attenuation within the mass (*arrowheads*), indicative of lipoid pneumonia.

RADIATION-INDUCED LUNG DISEASE

Radiation-induced lung injury is most often seen in three clinical situations: patients treated for unresectable lung cancer, the treatment of mediastinal lymphoma or thymoma, and patients treated for stage I to stage IIIa breast cancer. The pulmonary effects of external irradiation depend on several variables. The volume of lung treated will affect the incidence of radiation injury; the greater the volume irradiated, the more likely that radiation injury will occur. Most radiation treatment is limited to less than one-third to one-half of the lung, as an equivalent dose administered to an entire lung or both lungs would cause serious lung injury. The total dose and the method of fractionation will affect the incidence of radiation injury. Doses under 20 Gy rarely produce lung injury, while doses exceeding 30 Gy, particularly if administered to a significant portion of the lungs, have a significant incidence of radiation pneumonitis. Administration of a single large dose is more deleterious than fractionation of a similar total dose over the course of several weeks. There is variation in the susceptibility to radiation among individuals; a given dose may cause pneumonitis in one patient whereas another remains unaffected. The concomitant use of chemotherapeutic agents (particularly bleomycin) or the withdrawal of corticosteroid therapy may accentuate the deleterious effects of radiation. The mechanism of radiation-induced lung injury is not completely understood,

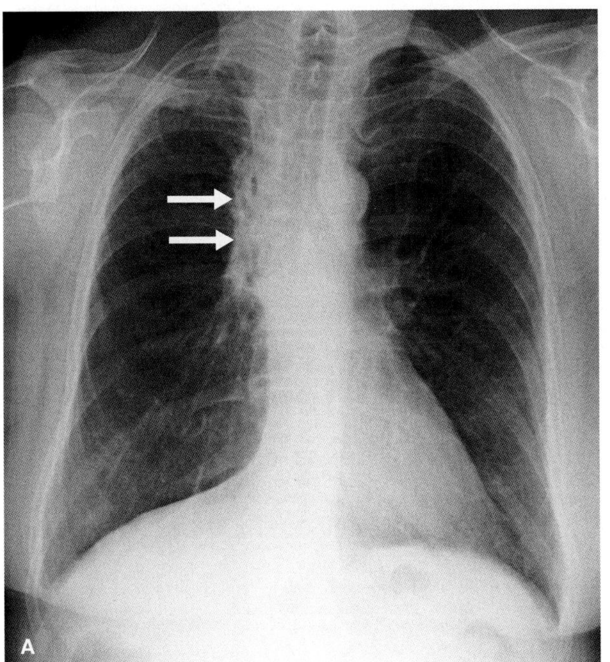

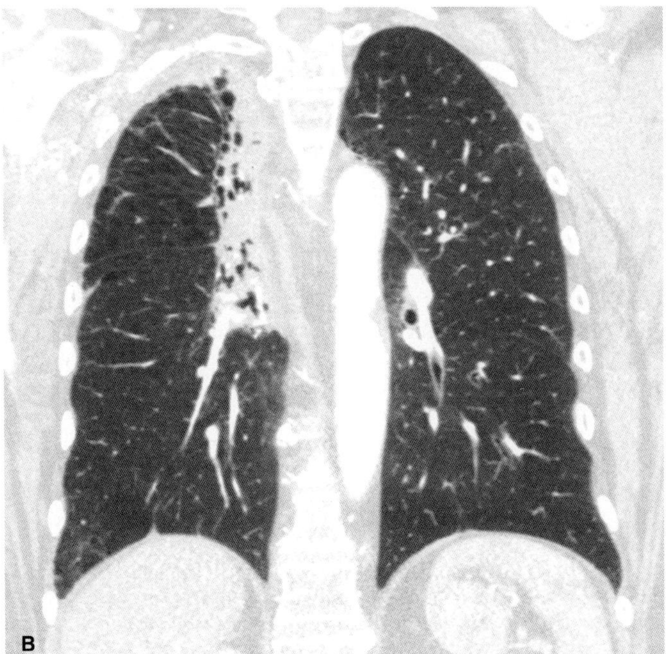

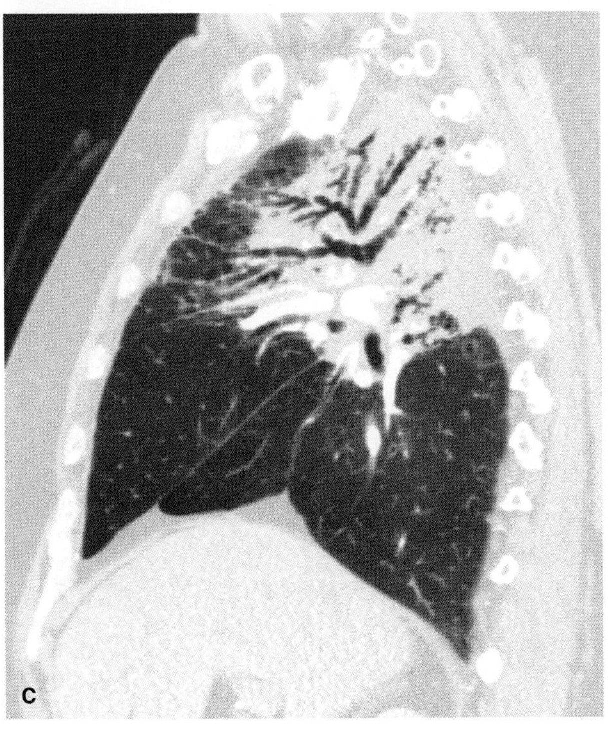

FIGURE 17.37. **Radiation Fibrosis. A:** Frontal chest radiograph in a woman previously irradiated for unresectable non–small-cell carcinoma shows a sharply demarcated right paramediastinal opacity (*arrows*) with right hilar elevation. **B, C:** Coronal (**B**) and sagittal CT (**C**) scans show dense, sharply defined right paravertebral airspace opacification containing dilated bronchi representing radiation fibrosis.

but the acute effects involve injury to capillary endothelial and pulmonary epithelial cells that line the alveoli. This diffuse alveolar damage produces a cellular, proteinaceous intra-alveolar exudate and hyaline membranes that is indistinguishable histologically from ARDS. These changes develop 4 to 12 weeks following the completion of therapy. Whereas most patients with acute radiation pneumonitis are asymptomatic, dyspnea and a nonproductive cough may be present.

Radiographically, a sharply marginated, localized area of airspace opacification is seen that does not conform to lobar or segmental anatomic boundaries and directly corresponds to the radiation port. Adhesive atelectasis of the involved portion of lung is common because the radiation produces a loss of surfactant by damaging type 2 pneumocytes. The pneumonitis may resolve completely with or without the administration of corticosteroids, or it may progress to pulmonary fibrosis. Pulmonary fibrosis corresponds histologically to a reparative phase, with regeneration of type 2 pneumocytes, reorganization of the parenchyma, ingrowth of granulation tissue, and eventually interstitial fibrosis. Fibrosis appears as coarse linear opacities or occasionally as a homogeneous parenchymal opacity with severe cicatrizing atelectasis of the involved portion of the lung. The sharp margination of the parenchymal fibrotic changes may be difficult to appreciate on plain radiographs but is usually obvious on CT or MR studies. Fibrotic tissue is characteristically low signal on T2W MR sequences, a finding that is helpful in distinguishing fibrosis from recurrent tumor, which typically produces high signal on T2WIs. The parenchymal changes are usually stable by 1 year following radiation therapy. Pleural thickening caused by fibrosis is a common finding. Small pleural and pericardial effusions are also common.

The diagnosis of radiation pneumonitis is usually made by excluding infection or malignancy as a cause of the patient's symptoms and by the presence of typical radiographic findings following a course of radiation therapy to the chest. This distinction may require bronchoalveolar lavage and transbronchial biopsy. An increased number of lymphocytes in the bronchoalveolar lavage fluid and an absence of malignant cells confirm the diagnosis. The demonstration of airspace opacification on CT that conforms to a known portal of radiation is usually sufficient for the diagnosis (Fig. 17.37). Treatment is generally supportive, with severe cases requiring corticosteroid therapy.

Suggested Readings

Baumann MH, Strange C, Heffner JE, et al; AACP Pneumothorax Consensus Group. Management of spontaneous pneumothorax. An American College of Chest Physicians Delphi Consensus Statement. *Chest* 2001;119(2):590–602.

Colice GL, Curtis A, Deslauriers J, et al. Medical and surgical treatment of parapneumonic effusions: an evidence-based guideline. *Chest* 2000; 118(4):1158–1171.

Desir A, Ghaye B. CT of blunt diaphragmatic rupture. *Radiographics* 2012; 32(2):477–498.

Guttentag AR, Salwen JK. Keep your eyes on the ribs: The spectrum of normal variants and diseases that involve the ribs. *Radiographics* 1999;19(5):1125–1142.

Kaewlai R, Avery LL, Asrani AV, Novelline RA. Multidetector CT of blunt thoracic trauma. *Radiographics* 2008;28(6):1555–1570.

Kim M, Lee KY, Lee KW, Bae KT. MDCT evaluation of foreign bodies and liquid aspiration pneumonia in adults. *AJR Am J Roentgenol* 2008;190(4):907–915.

Larici AR, del Ciello A, Maggi F, et al. Lung abnormalities at multimodality imaging after radiation therapy for non-small cell lung cancer. *Radiographics* 2011;31(3):771–789.

Leung AN, Muller NL, Miller RR. CT in the differential diagnosis of diffuse pleural disease. *AJR Am J Roentgenol* 1990;154(3):487–492.

Light RW (ed). *Chapter 2. Physiology of the pleural space.* In: *Pleural Diseases*. 6th ed. Philadelphia, PA: Lippincott Williams & Wilkins; 2013.

Miserocchi G. Physiology and pathophysiology of pleural fluid turnover. *Eur Respir J* 1997;10(1):219–225.

Nam SJ, Kim S, Lim BJ, et al. Imaging of primary chest wall tumors with radiologic-pathologic correlation. *Radiographics* 2011;31(3):749–770.

Nason LK, Walker CM, McNeeley MF, Burivong W, Fligner CL, Godwin JD. Imaging of the diaphragm: anatomy and function. *Radiographics* 2012;32(2):E51–E70.

Nickell LT Jr, Lichtenberger JP 3rd, Khorashadi L, Abbott GF, Carter BW. Multimodality imaging for characterization, classification, and staging of malignant pleural mesothelioma. *Radiographics* 2014;34(6):1692–1706.

Peterman TA, Brothers SK. Pleural effusions in congestive heart failure and in pericardial disease. *N Engl J Med* 1983;309(5):313.

Qureshi NR, Gleeson FV. Imaging of pleural disease. *Clin Chest Med* 2006; 27(2):193–213.

Talbot BS, Gange CP Jr, Chaturvedi A, Klionsky N, Hobbs SK, Chaturvedi A. Traumatic rib injury: patterns, imaging pitfalls, complications, and treatment. *Radiographics* 2017;37(2):628–651.

SECTION IV

BREAST RADIOLOGY

SECTION EDITOR: Brandi T. Nicholson

CHAPTER 18 ■ NORMAL ANATOMY AND HISTOPATHOLOGY

CARRIE M. ROCHMAN, JONATHAN V. NGUYEN, AND BRANDI T. NICHOLSON

OVERVIEW

A thorough understanding of the normal anatomy and imaging appearance of the breast is important. When we have a good reference for what normal looks like, we are more likely to detect something that is abnormal. In addition, normal structures can mimic pathology. Identifying the spectrum of appearance of normal structures will improve cancer detection and also help reduce unnecessary biopsies and follow-up. To understand normal breast anatomy, we will proceed from superficial to deep (Fig. 18.1).

SKIN

The skin of the breast is uniformly thin measuring 2 to 3 mm in thickness. When the skin of the breast becomes thickened, it may indicate underlying pathology. Invasive breast cancers can cause overlying focal skin thickening and/or skin retraction. Inflammatory breast cancer can cause a more diffuse pattern of skin thickening or *peau d'orange* involving the entire breast. Unilateral skin thickening is commonly seen after radiation therapy to the breast. Diffuse bilateral skin thickening can be seen in systemic disorders (heart failure, renal failure, etc.) that cause fluid overload or edema. Skin thickness is best evaluated on mammography when the area of concern is tangential to the x-ray beam. Skin thickness is easily seen with ultrasound or MRI (Fig. 18.2).

There are multiple structures that normally reside in the skin. Hair follicles, sebaceous glands, and sweat glands all occur within the dermis of the breast. Blocked pores can result in the formation of epidermoid cysts, which are also sometimes referred to as sebaceous cysts. Most commonly these cysts contain keratin. They may become superinfected. The palpable lump may cause a woman to seek medical attention or the mass may be seen on screening mammography. The location of the structure in the skin is an indication to its benign etiology. The skin can often be seen wrapping around the structure with a "claw sign." A thin tract to the overlying skin surface may also be visible. On physical examination, a prominent pore or "black head" is often present (Fig. 18.3).

Skin lesions can also cause a pseudo mass on mammography. A raised skin lesion will often demonstrate radiolucency surrounding the mass which represents air trapped during breast compression. Air can also be seen trapped within crevices of a skin lesion. We have our technologists place a metallic BB at the site of prominent skin lesions to avoid unnecessary work ups. Sometimes multiple skin lesions can be a sign of a systemic process such as neurofibromatosis (Fig. 18.4).

NIPPLE–AREOLAR COMPLEX

The nipple–areolar complex (NAC) is usually located at the 4th intercostal space in a nonpendulous breast. The areola consists of pigmented skin, rings of smooth muscle, and specialized apocrine glands called Montgomery glands. These Montgomery glands open to the skin surface at the Morgagni tubercles which are 1- to 2-mm raised bumps around the periphery of the areola. There are approximately 10 to 15 ductal openings on the surface of each nipple. The major milk ducts converge to form a lactiferous sinus which then extends to the surface of the nipple. Because the duct epithelium extends to the surface of the nipple, breast cancer can involve the NAC.

There is normal variation in the appearance of the nipple. Nipples may be retracted or inverted. A slit-like cleft in the nipple may be present (Fig. 18.5). Nipple inversion or retraction is most often benign when the appearance of the nipples is bilateral, symmetric, and long standing. When new or asymmetric nipple inversion or retraction is present, it may be due to an underlying malignancy (Fig. 18.6). It is important to position a patient with the nipple in profile on at least one of the mammographic views to evaluate for nipple inversion or retraction. Nipple in profile view is also important to ensure that the nipple does not obscure a subareolar mass. A nipple shadow can also simulate a pseudo mass (Fig. 18.7). When in doubt a skin marker such as a BB can be placed to mark the location of the nipple.

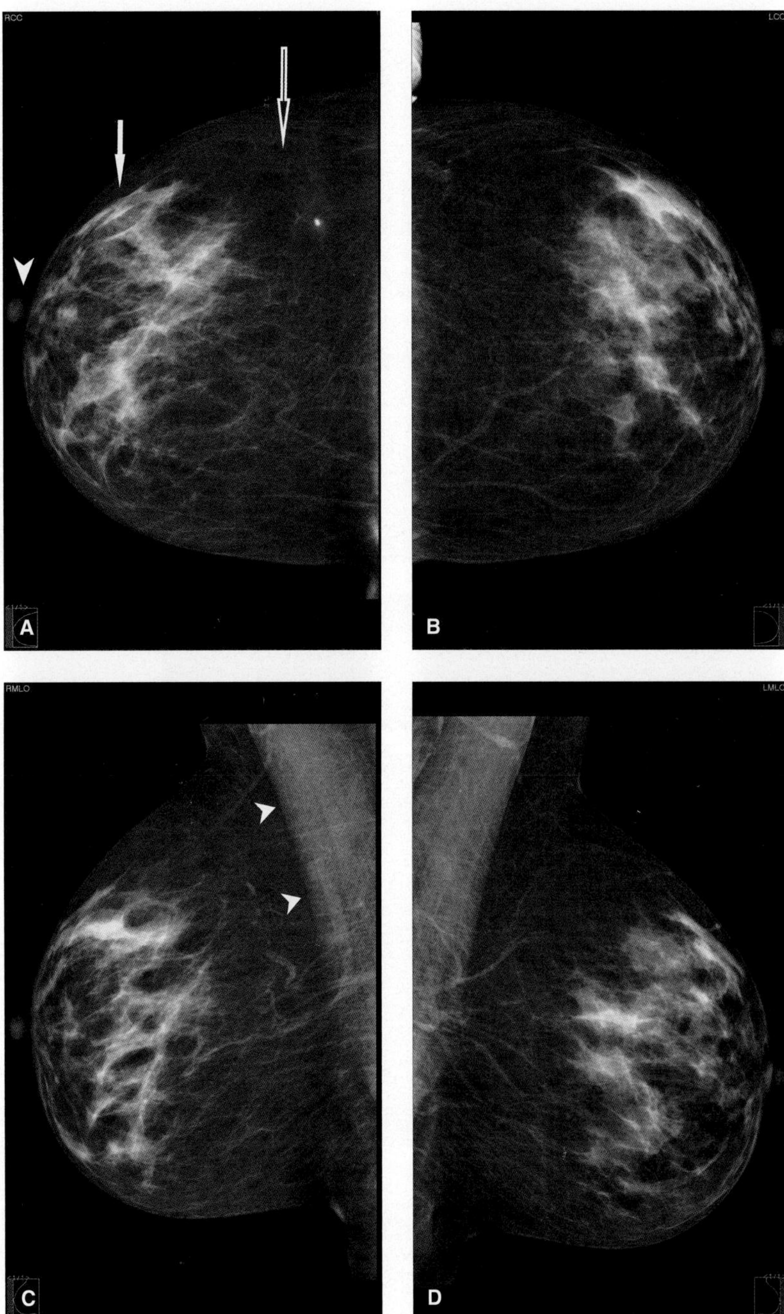

FIGURE 18.1. **Normal Mammogram. A:** Right cranial caudal (RCC) view showing normal appearance of the nipple (*arrowhead*), normal fibroglandular breast tissue (*solid arrow*), and normal fatty tissue (*open arrow*). **B:** Left cranial caudal (LCC) view. **C:** Right mediolateral oblique (RMLO) view. Pectoralis major muscle can be seen on MLO view (*arrowheads*). **D:** Left mediolateral oblique (LMLO) view.

Posterior acoustic shadowing is often seen when evaluating the nipple with ultrasound due to abundant fibrous tissue. Maintaining good contact of the US transducer with the skin can also be challenging. Liberal usage of ultrasound gel is helpful to prevent artifacts due to poor contact. It is also useful to angle to ultrasound probe from multiple planes around the nipple to image retro areolar structures (Fig. 18.8).

Nipple enhancement is commonly seen on MRI after the administration of IV contrast. Normal nipple enhancement is symmetric, thin, and continuous with persistent kinetics. Asymmetric, thick, or nodular enhancement may be the result of an underlying malignancy (Fig. 18.9).

Paget disease of the NAC is characterized by malignant cells in the epidermis of the nipple. It is most commonly seen with ductal carcinoma in situ (DCIS). Patients may present with erythema, scaly, or eczema-like changes. When a patient presents with these signs and symptoms, diagnostic evaluation is necessary to search for underlying calcifications or a mass. If imaging is negative, a referral to a breast surgeon or dermatologist is necessary for possible skin biopsy or additional evaluation with MRI.

The NAC contains abundant sensory innervation. Adequate anesthesia is required when performing breast interventions around the NAC.

SUBCUTANEOUS TISSUE

The breast tissue lies between the facial planes of the superficial pectoral fascia and the deep pectoral fascia. Interspersed and connecting the facial layers are the Cooper suspensory ligaments (Fig. 18.10). The Cooper ligaments create an internal framework or scaffolding that supports the breast. Cooper ligaments are easily seen with mammography and MRI.

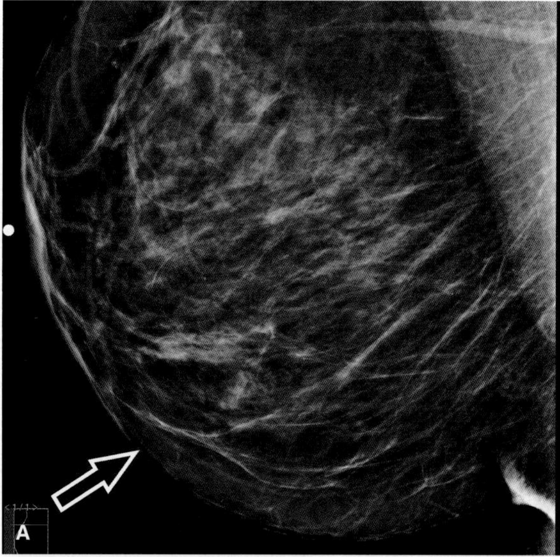

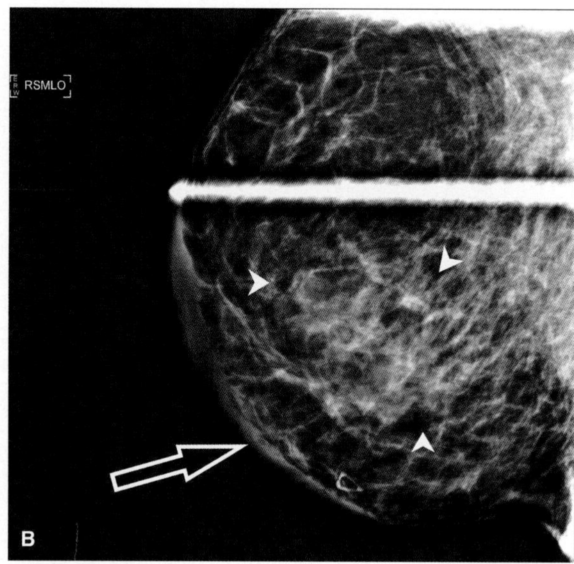

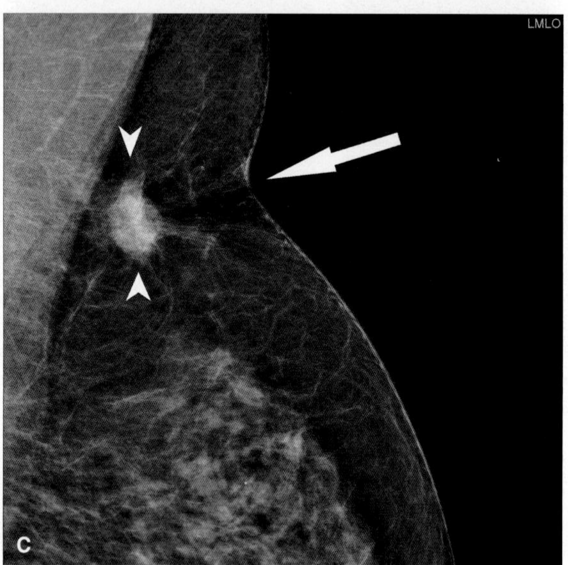

FIGURE 18.2. **Comparison of Skin Thickness. A:** Normal skin thickness on asymptomatic screening mammogram (*open arrow*). **B:** Image from the same patient 2 years later shows diffuse skin thickening (*open arrow*) due to inflammatory breast cancer. There is a large mass present (*arrowheads*) which is an invasive ductal carcinoma. **C:** Different patient with skin retraction (*solid arrow*) due to underlying invasive ductal carcinoma (*arrowheads*).

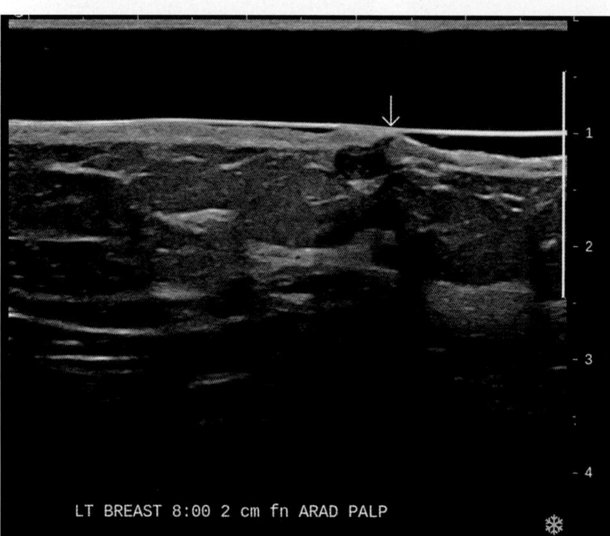

FIGURE 18.3. **Sebaceous Cyst.** Ultrasound image shows a superficial oval mass in the skin. A dermal tract is seen extending to the skin surface (*arrow*) which is characteristic.

Normally, they have a scalloped appearance with undulating curves that can resemble the waves of the ocean. Straightening or distortion of the normal architecture of the Cooper ligaments can be an important sign of malignancy (Fig. 18.11). Thickening of the ligaments can be seen with both malignancy or with edema. When thickening of the skin and Cooper ligaments seen, careful imaging evaluation and clinical evaluation is needed to determine if underlying breast cancer is present. The imaging appearance can be similar to infectious mastitis which is more commonly seen in lactating patients. Thickening of the Cooper ligaments can also cause retraction of the nipple or overlying skin. This feature can also be a clue to an underlying breast cancer.

Adipose tissue is present in variable quantity in the breast. The amount of fat in the breast is related to both age and body mass index. Obese women tend to have a large amount of fat in their breasts. Very thin women have very little fat. After menopause, the stoma of the breast becomes more fatty.

Fat causes low attenuation of x-rays, so it appears dark gray on mammography, which is distinctly different from fibroglandular tissue or masses. Mammograms are helpful to determine when fat is present in a mass such as a lipoma or hamartoma. On ultrasound, fat is a medium gray. Some masses can appear similar. Assessment of compressibility is a useful technique to

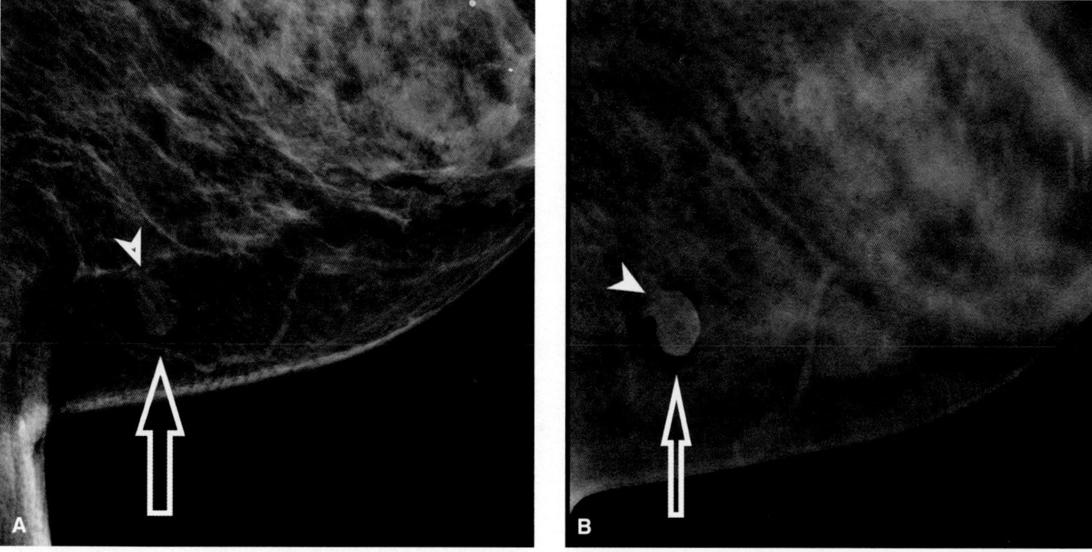

FIGURE 18.4. Nevus Simulating a Mass. Oval circumscribed mass is seen with a surrounding dark halo due to air gap around the nevus (*open arrow*). The halo is absent at the site of attachment to the skin (*arrowhead*). Nevus can be seen on both (**A**) two-dimensional digital mammography and (**B**) digital breast tomosynthesis (DBT).

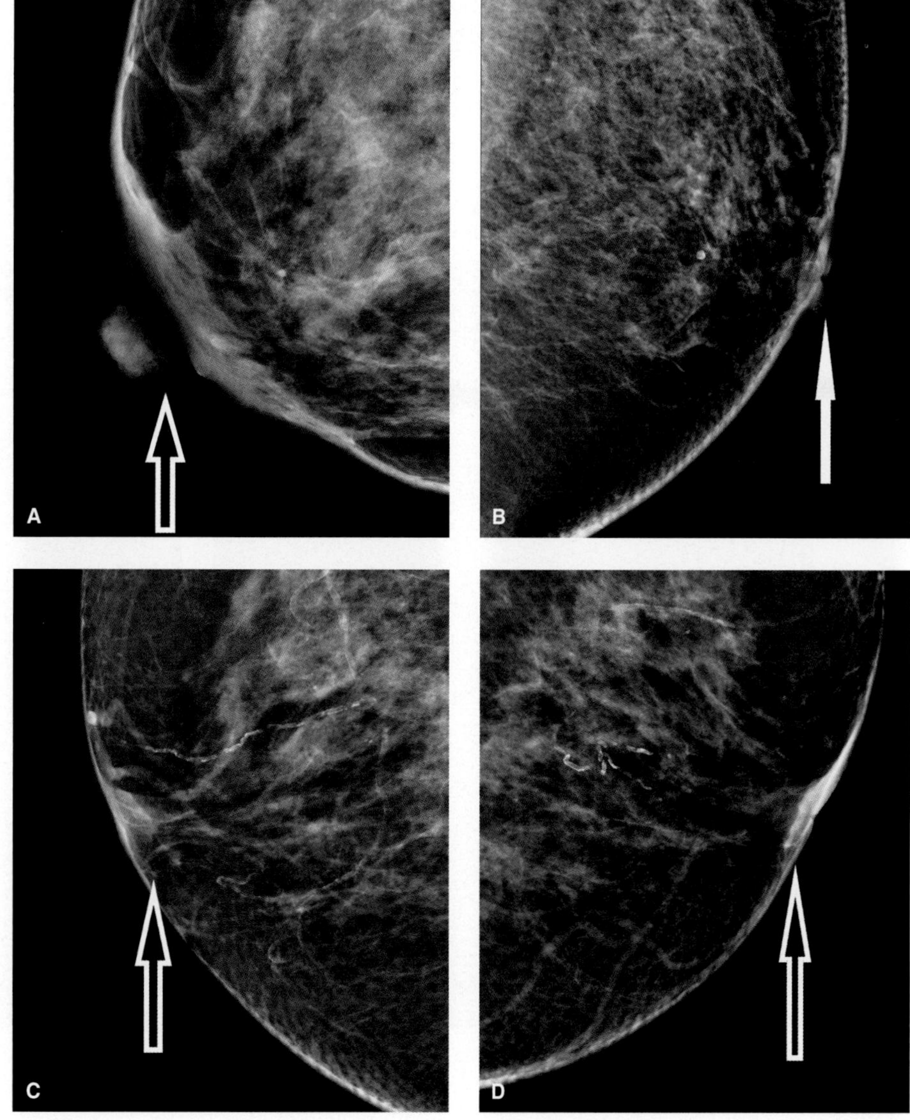

FIGURE 18.5. Normal Appearance of the Nipple. A: Most common, normal appearance of the nipple (*open arrows*). **B:** Normal nipple with cleft (*arrows*). **C, D:** Bilateral nipple inversion (*open arrows*). Nipple inversion is often benign when this appearance is bilateral, symmetric, and long standing.

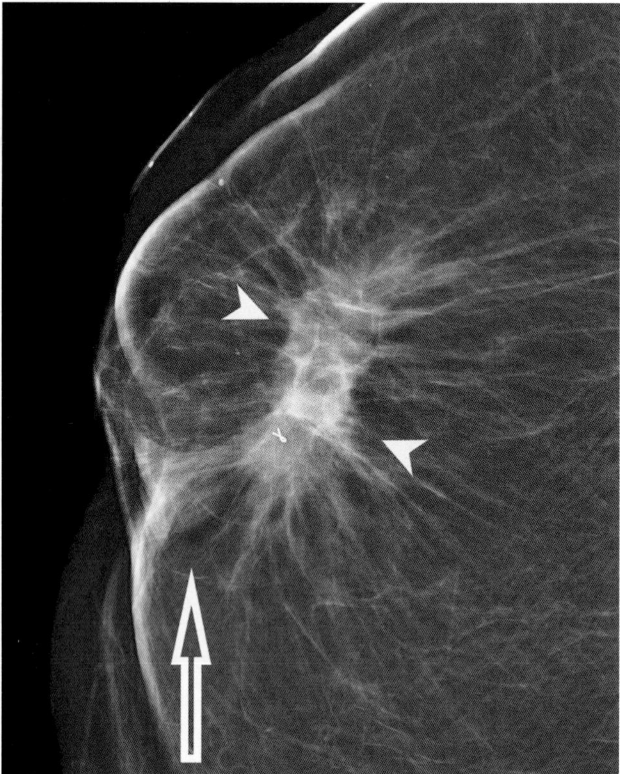

FIGURE 18.6. **Pathologic Nipple Retraction.** Retracted nipple (*open arrow*) due to underlying high-density spiculated mass which is a known invasive breast cancer (*arrowheads*).

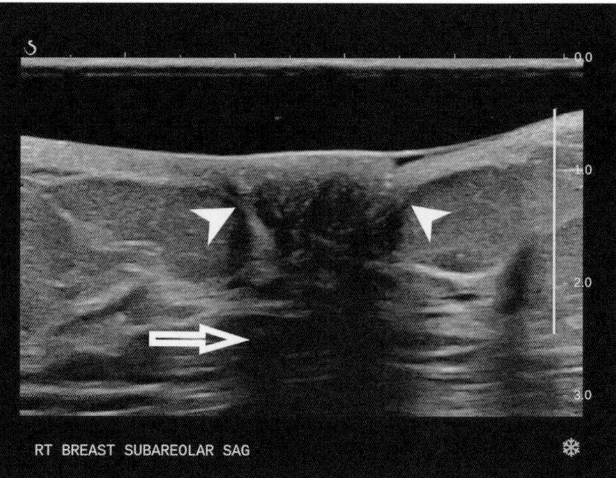

FIGURE 18.8. **Nipple on Ultrasound.** Normal appearance of the nipple on ultrasound (*arrowheads*). Prominent shadowing is often seen posterior to the nipple due to ultrasound beam attenuation (*open arrow*).

determine if a mass is a fat lobule versus an isoechoic mass. Fat is the most compressible structure in the breast. The AP dimension of a fat lobule will decrease by 30% or more if compressed with the ultrasound transducer (Fig. 18.12).

MILK DUCTS AND LOBULES

The glandular tissue of the breast is composed of the lobules and milk ducts. These structures are formed by the epithelium

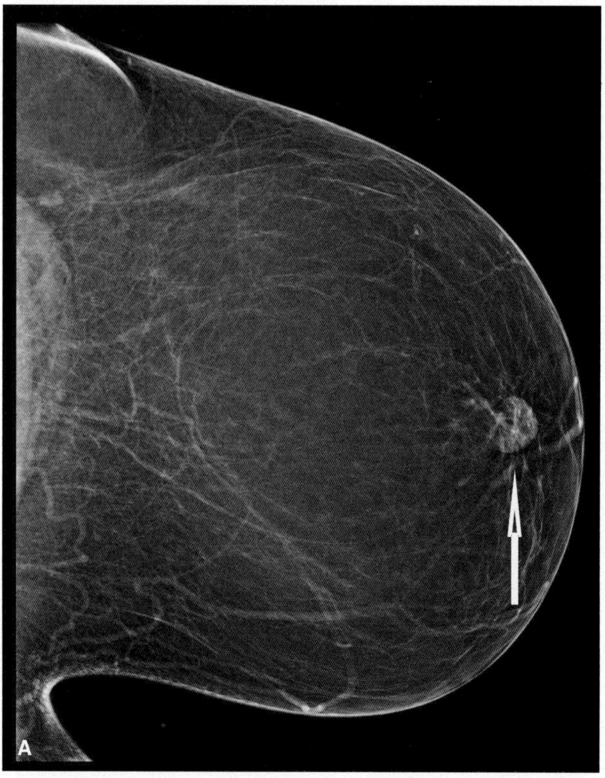

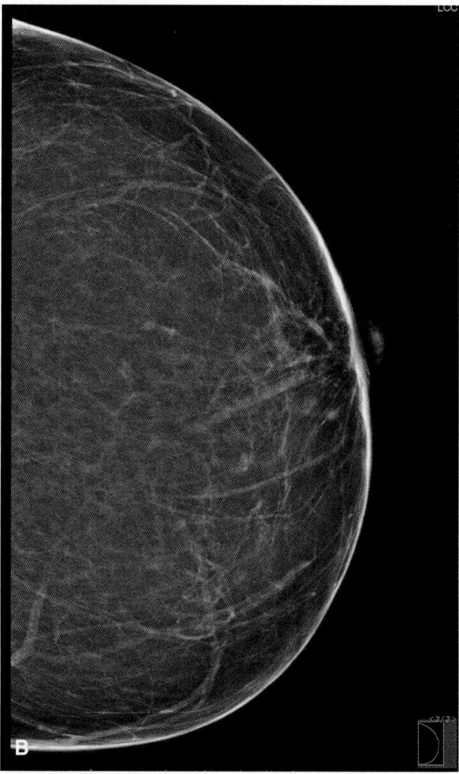

FIGURE 18.7. **Nipple Simulating a Mass. A:** If the nipple is not imaged in profile, it can simulate a breast mass (*open arrow*). **B:** Repeat imaging with nipple in profile confirms that no breast mass is present.

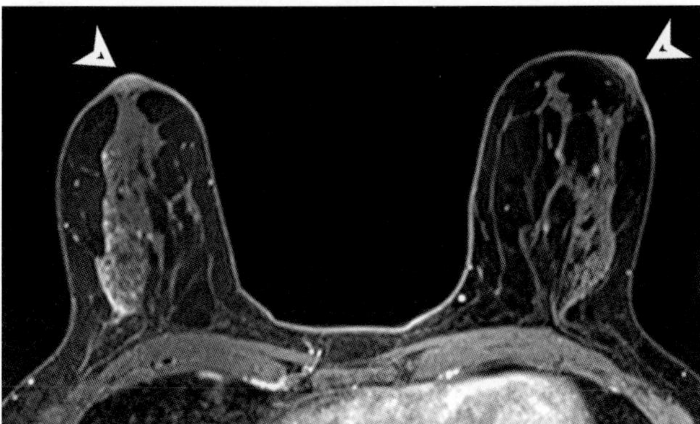

FIGURE 18.9. **Nipples on MRI.** Normal appearance of the nipples on MRI (*arrowheads*).

that invaginates during embryology. These structures are important, because the majority of breast cancers arise from either the ducts or the lobules. Thus, most breast cancers are adenocarcinomas, arising from epithelium.

The ductal system of the breast is arranged like the branches of a tree (Fig. 18.13). There are approximately 10 to 15 milk ducts that extend to the surface of the nipple with a reported range between 5 and 20. Behind each nipple orifice, there is a slightly dilated portion known as the lactiferous sinus. This is believed to be an important reservoir for milk during lactation and breast feeding. The milk ducts then continue to branch as they extend posteriorly to drain a lobe of the breast. Some ductal systems are quite small, and only extend a few centimeters. Others are quite large and may occupy almost an entire quadrant.

A ductal system is best demonstrated on galactography (Fig. 18.14). During galactography, a single duct orifice on the nipple is cannulated with a small probe. A small amount of iodinated contrast material is injected into the duct and mammogram views are performed. Most ductal carcinomas begin in a single ductal system. Suspicious microcalcifications that are linear or segmental may be conforming to the shape of a ductal system. These distributions are the most worrisome for DCIS (Fig. 18.15).

Each ductal system drains a lobe of the breast. Within each lobe there are 20 to 40 lobules. Within each lobule, there are 10 to 100 alveoli. The alveoli are the smallest functional units responsible for milk production. The terminal duct lobular unit (TDLU) is made up of the terminal duct and the lobule that it drains. It is an important structural and functional unit of the breast. The TDLU gives rise to numerous pathologies and is the site where most ductal and lobular carcinomas are thought to arise (Fig. 18.16).

If the acini become dilated, they form cysts. Cysts and fibrocystic changes are very common, seen in 30% to 50% of women. Fortunately, cysts and fibrocystic changes do not increase breast cancer risk. But, they are commonly encountered in breast imaging and can lead to mammography screening recalls to determine if a suspicious mass is solid or cystic. Fortunately ultrasound is a reliable tool to determine if a mass is solid, cystic, or complex (both solid and cystic).

STROMA

The lobules and milk ducts are interspersed with fat and fibrous stroma. Together this is call fibroglandular tissue. The amount of fat relative to the amount of fibroglandular tissue can vary. When this is measured on mammography, it is called *breast density*. Breast density is important, because it can mask a cancer on mammography. Mammograms have reduced sensitivity in dense tissue. Breast density is also an independent risk factor for breast cancer.

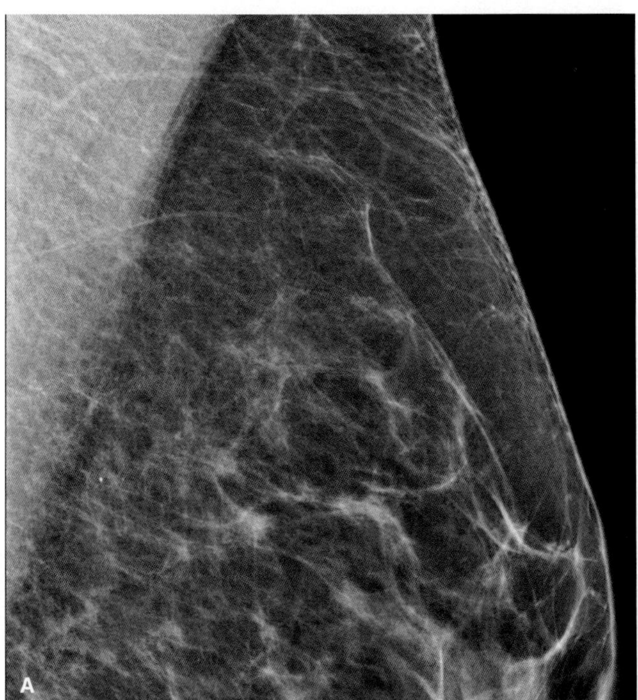

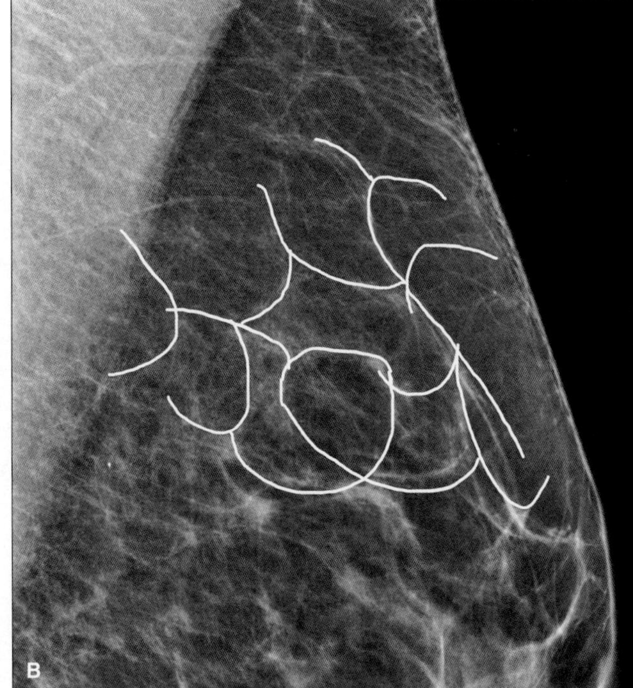

FIGURE 18.10. **Cooper Ligaments. A:** Normal Cooper ligaments are seen as fine, thin curved lines on mammography. **B:** Normal Cooper ligaments are outlined with *white line*.

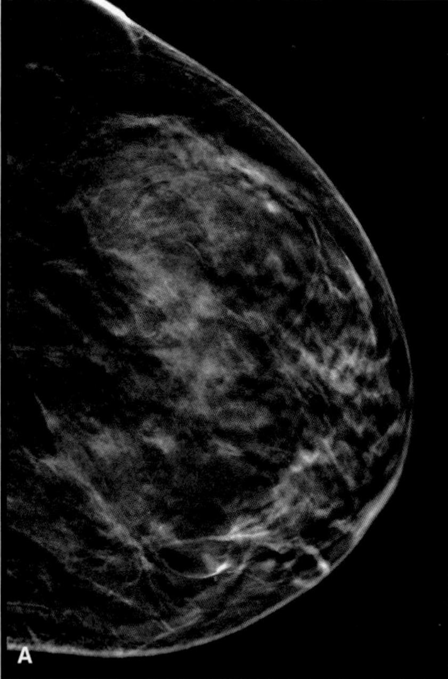

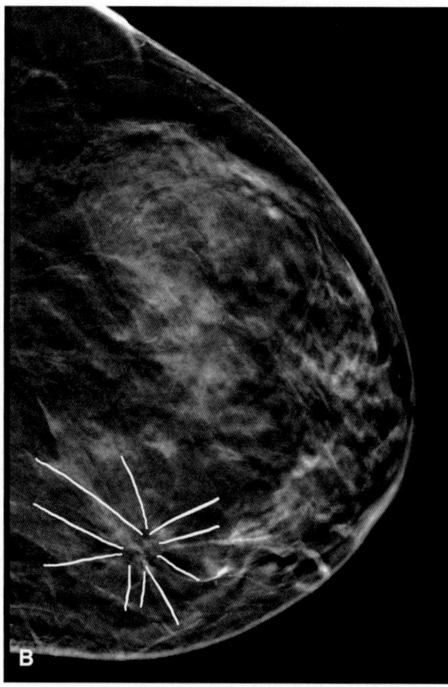

FIGURE 18.11. Straightening of Cooper Ligaments. A: Straightening of Cooper ligaments can be seen. This is also known as architectural distortion. **B:** Abnormal straight Cooper ligaments are outlined with *white line*.

In most women, the majority of fibroglandular tissue is in the upper outer quadrants. There is usually less breast tissue in the lower inner quadrant and in the retromammary fat. Beware of something that develops in these areas (Fig. 18.17). It is also important to carefully examine the fat–glandular interface to detect invasive breast cancers (Fig. 18.18). A breast mass can cause focal outward bulge or focal retraction (Fig. 18.19).

The breasts may be symmetric or asymmetric in size. Asymmetric breast size is almost always normal in the absence of clinical symptoms or mammographic abnormalities (Fig. 18.20). However, a "shrinking breast" may be a sign of a large invasive lobular carcinoma (ILC). With ILC, the breast becomes less compressible as the tumor infiltrates through the breast. Because the breast does not compress as much, it looks smaller, or "shrinking," when compared to prior mammograms (Fig. 18.21).

CHEST WALL

The chest wall includes the muscles and ribs deep to each breast. The pectoralis muscles of the chest wall lie immediately deep to the breast. Pectoralis major is seen on the mediolateral oblique (MLO) view of the mammogram and is an important landmark when assessing image quality and positioning (see Chapter 19). Pectoralis can also be seen (Fig. 18.22). The muscles of the chest wall are covered by a layer of fascia and have a different innervation than the breast. Care must be taken to avoid the chest wall muscles during percutaneous

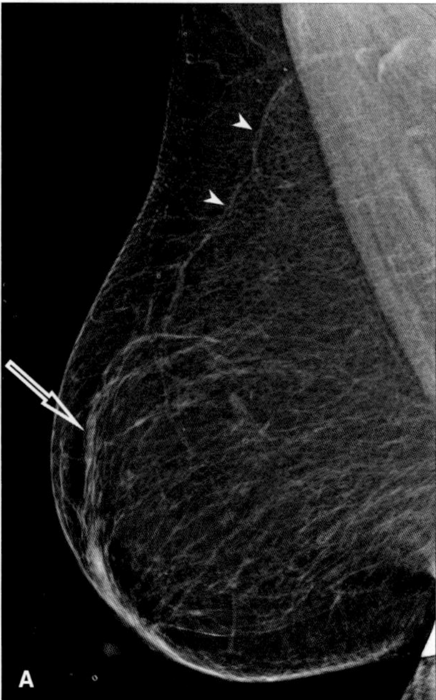

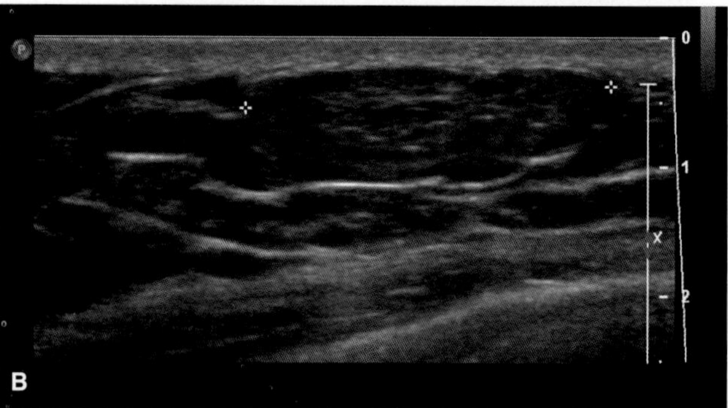

FIGURE 18.12. Fat on Mammography and Ultrasound. A: Fat on mammography is dark gray due to minimal x-ray beam attenuation. The scant fibroglandular tissue (*open arrow*), Copper ligaments, and blood vessels (*arrowheads*) are easily seen. **B:** Fat lobule on ultrasound.

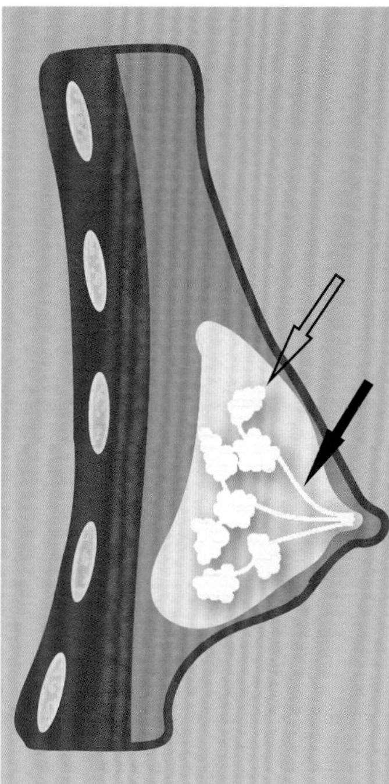

FIGURE 18.13. **Cartoon of Ductal and Lobular Anatomy.** Numerous ducts are seen converging at the nipple (*solid arrow*). Lobules are the functional unit of the breast and site of milk formation (*open arrow*).

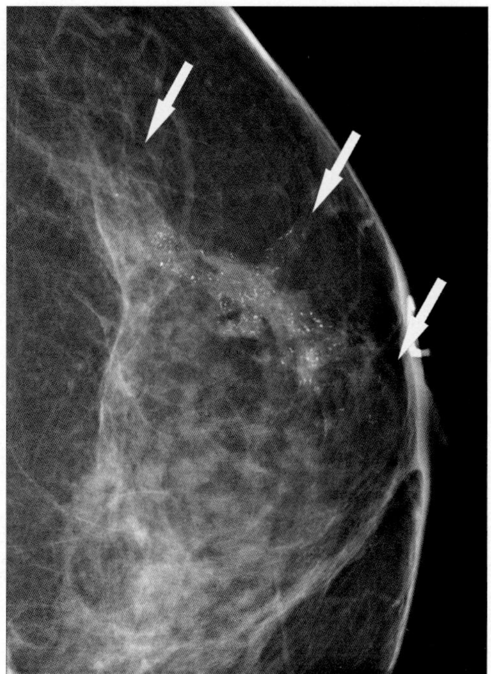

FIGURE 18.15. **DCIS in Segmental Distribution.** Fine pleomorphic calcifications are seen extending from the nipple in a segmental distribution that follows the ductal anatomy (*arrows*). This is highly suspicious for malignancy. Biopsy showed high-grade DCIS.

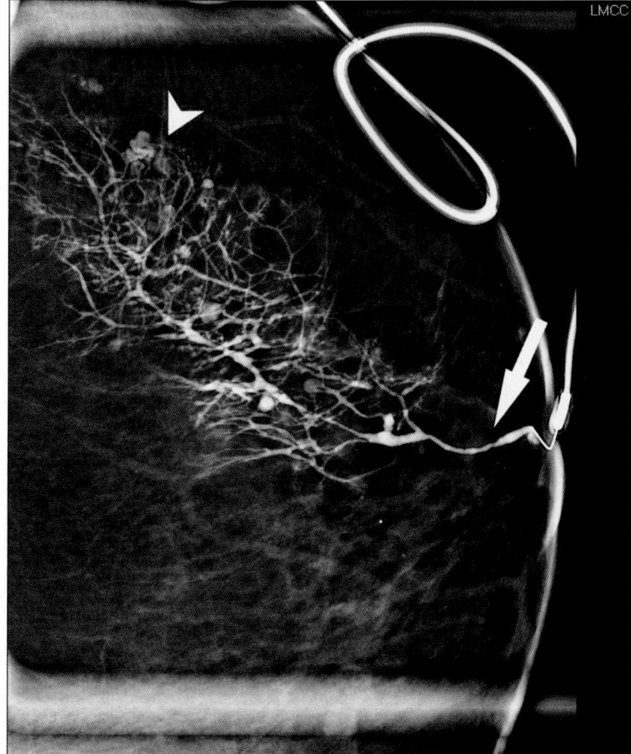

FIGURE 18.14. **Normal Galactogram.** Administration of iodinated contrast material into a single duct demonstrates the normal milk duct seen directly behind the nipple (*solid arrow*). Numerous branches of the ductal system are seen. There is contrast extending into the lobules (*arrowhead*), some of which are mildly distended into tiny cysts.

interventions or biopsy. Muscle invasion from breast cancer is an important prognostic feature. Muscle invasion may be suspected when a breast mass is fixed or not freely mobile. The presence of muscle invasion is best seen with MRI (see Chapter 22). Loss of the fat plane is occasionally seen on mammography. However, because the mass is fixed to the chest wall, it is often difficult to image. Evaluation of muscle invasion is limited on ultrasound due to posterior acoustic shadowing caused by many breast cancers which obscures detail of the underlying muscle.

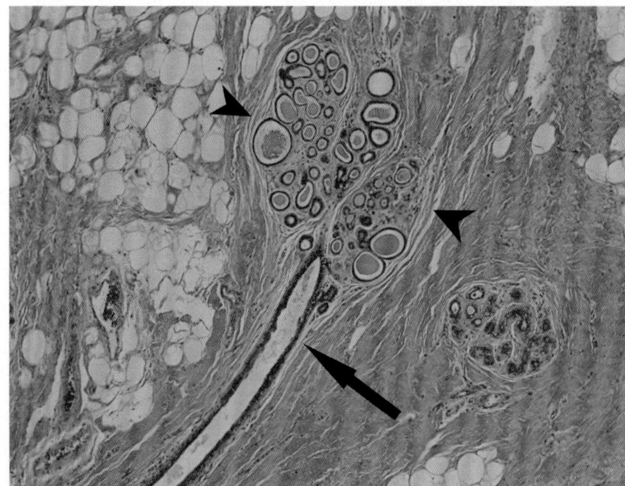

FIGURE 18.16. **Histopathology of Normal TDLU.** H&E stain of normal breast tissue reveals the elongated tubular terminal duct (*arrow*) and the lobular unit (*arrowheads*). (Histopathology slide provided by Dr. Kristen Atkins.)

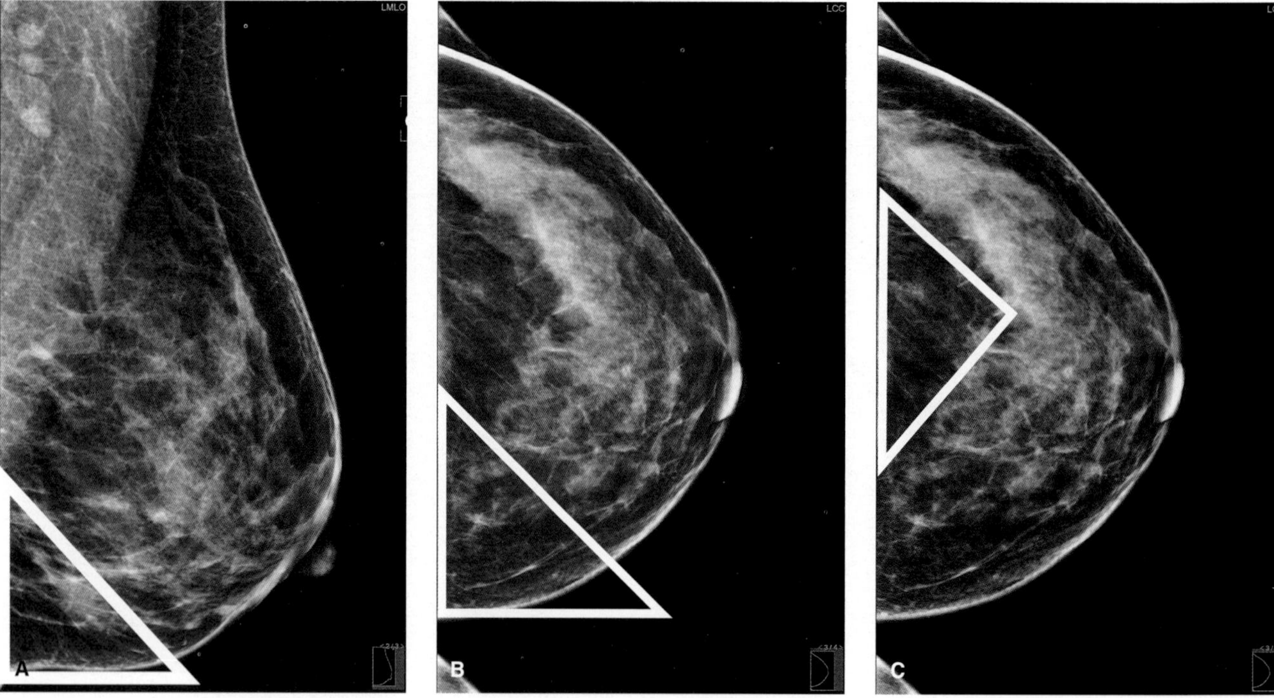

FIGURE 18.17. **Lower Inner Quadrant and Retromammary Fat.** There is usually less breast tissue in the (**A**) lower, (**B**) inner quadrant, and (**C**) retromammary fat. Beware of masses or asymmetries that develop in these locations.

MALE BREAST

The male breast anatomy is similar to that of a prepubescent girl. It is composed of a NAC and rudimentary milk ducts. Genetically and hormonally normal males do not develop lobules and thus do not develop pathologies that arise from the lobules. Men can develop breast cancer, but it is almost always invasive ductal carcinoma (IDC) or DCIS. The male breast can also develop hypertrophic changes called gynecomastia. This is usually related to estrogen or medication-induced stimulation (see Chapter 20).

LYMPHATICS

Lymphatic drainage of the breast is important because it is the most common method of spread for breast cancers. Lymph node metastasis is one of the strongest prognostic features for patients with breast cancer. Survival decreases with increasing numbers of metastatic lymph nodes.

A normal axillary lymph node is oval, circumscribed, and contains a fatty hilum. They have a "reniform" or kidney-like shape (Fig. 18.23). Normal nodes have a broad range of long- and short-axis lengths. In a study performed by Deurloo et al.,

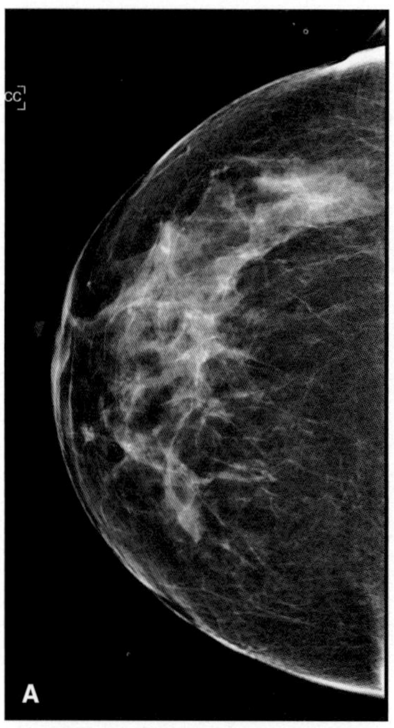

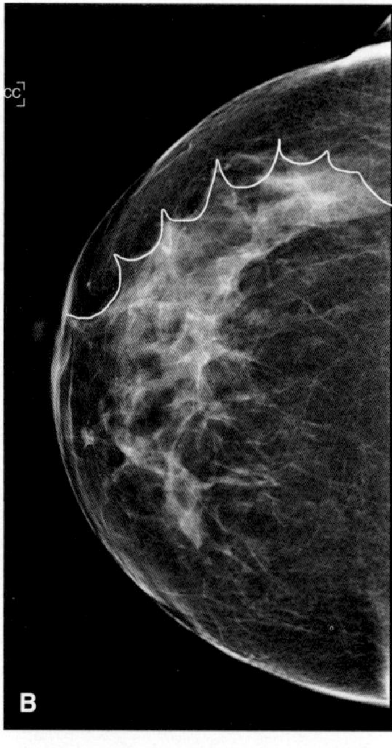

FIGURE 18.18. **Normal Fat–Glandular Interface. A:** The interface of the glandular tissue and fat normally has a scalloped appearance with gentle curving lines. **B:** Fat–glandular interface is outlined in *white*.

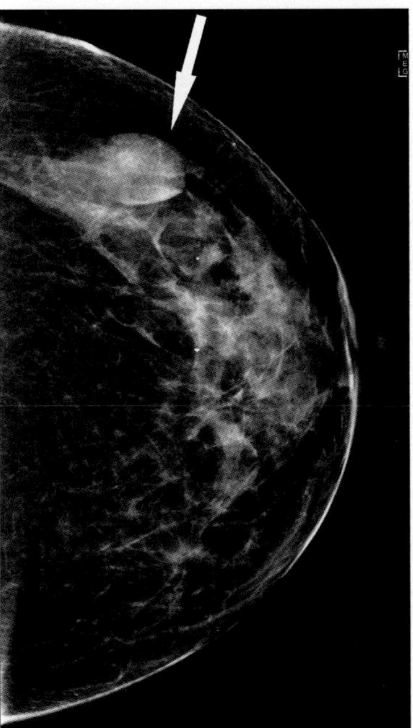

FIGURE 18.19. **Mass Causing Outward Bulge at Fat–Glandular Interface.** The normal fat–glandular interface is distorted by a mass that is causing a focal outward convex bulge (*arrow*).

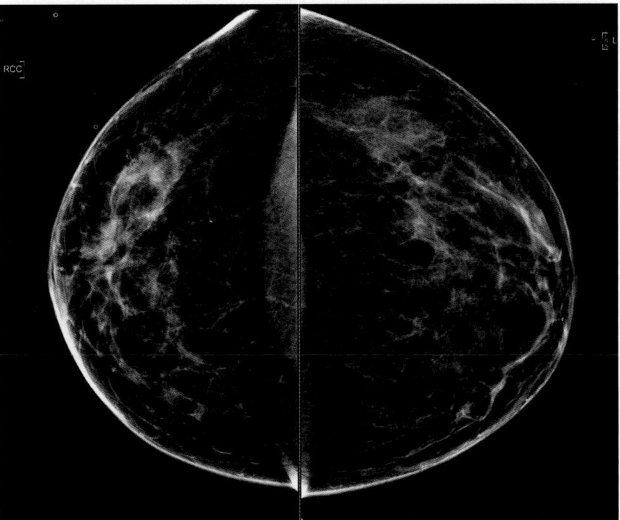

FIGURE 18.21. **Shrinking Breast.** Bilateral CC views showing asymmetric breast size. The right breast is smaller than the left. On prior mammograms (not shown) breasts were symmetric in size. There is also increased density on the right and architectural distortion. Biopsy revealed invasive lobular carcinoma.

the morphology and cortical thickness were found to be the strongest predictors of metastasis. We use 2.3 mm as the maximum cortical thickness for a normal node in a patient *with* breast cancer. The normal cortical thickness of an axillary lymph node in women *without* breast cancer can be up to 3 mm. It is also important to look at other features of the nodes such as loss of the fatty hilum. Focal cortical thickening can also be a sign of metastasis. The afferent lymphatic channels first pass through the *cortex* of a node. Thus, the immediate subcortical region is often the first place that a metastasis is deposited. Be suspicious of a ball-like projection from the cortex of a node. An indistinct or irregular margin of a node can be a sign of extra capsular extension of the metastasis into the surrounding fat (Fig. 18.24).

Majority of the vascular supply to a lymph node is through the hilum. The feeding artery enters the hilum and the draining vein exits through the hilum. Cancer causes neoangiogenesis. Lymph node metastasis can cause abundant *extra hilar blood flow*, or multiple feeding vessels around a node that do not pass through the hilum.

Change over time is also very important when evaluating lymph nodes, regardless of the absolute size or morphology. If a node is unchanged over many years (in the absence of treatments that prevent cancer growth such as chemotherapy),

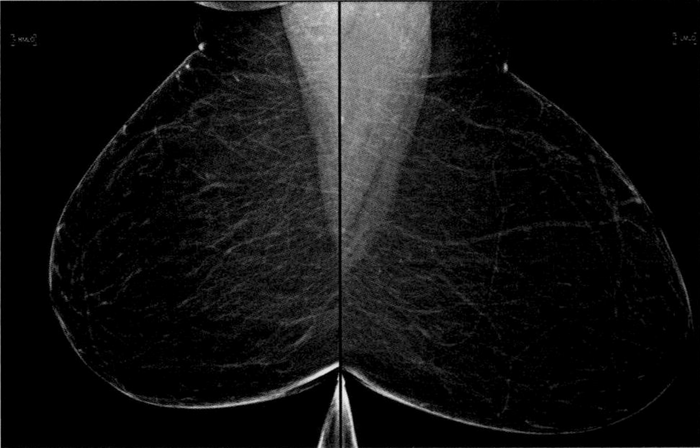

FIGURE 18.20. **Asymmetric Breast Size.** Bilateral MLO views showing asymmetric breast size. The right breast is smaller than the left. Asymmetric breast size is common. It is a benign finding when it is long standing and not associated with other signs of malignancy.

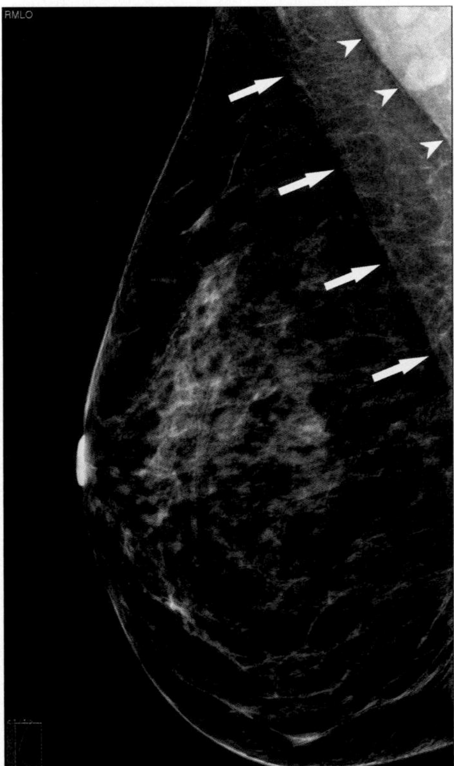

FIGURE 18.22. **Pectoralis Major and Minor.** MLO mammogram shows pectoralis major muscle (*arrows*) and pectoralis minor muscle (*arrowheads*).

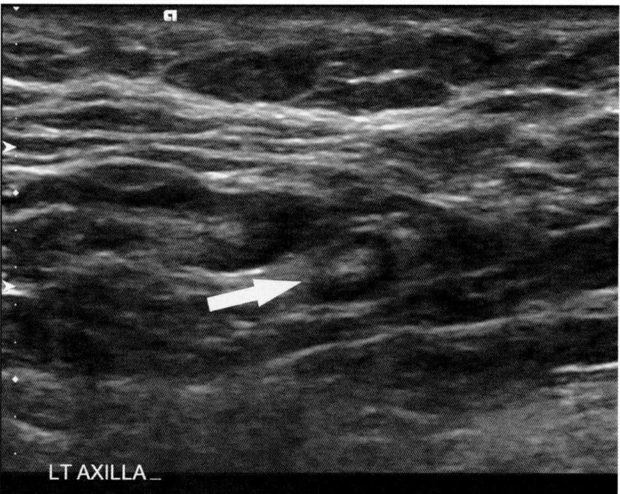

FIGURE 18.23. **Normal Lymph Node** (*arrow*). Gray scale ultrasound image of the axilla shows a normal appearing lymph node. Note the reniform shape, uniform thin cortex, circumscribed margin, and normal echogenic fatty hilum.

TABLE 18.1

SUSPICIOUS LYMPH NODE FEATURES

Cortical thickness >2.3 mm
Loss of fatty hilum
Focal cortical thickening
Indistinct margin
Increased extra hilar blood flow
Increasing size over time

it is likely benign. A node that has increased in size or has new suspicious features is worrisome. Keep in mind that it is normal for nodes to fluctuate slightly in response to infection or inflammation. If a patient has a clinical explanation for enlarged nodes (recent flu shot, eczema flair, etc.), it is reasonable to perform a short term follow-up to ensure that the nodes return to normal size (Table 18.1).

There are numerous lymphatic channels that course throughout the breast and locations of draining lymph nodes (Table 18.2). There is a large lymphatic plexus under the NAC that is called the subareolar or Sappey plexus. Periductal lymphatic vessels lie adjacent to the duct wall. Lymphatic drainage moves from superficial to deep, and from the breast to the axilla and internal mammary (IM) chain. About 75% to 97% of the lymphatic drainage of the breast is to the lymph nodes in the axilla. Less than 10% of lymphatic drainage is to the IM chain. The first lymph node encountered is called the *sentinel lymph node*. This node can be identified at the time of surgery by using mapping techniques that involve injection of a blue dye and/or a radioisotope (^{99m}Tc-sulfur colloid). These substances are then traceable to the sentinel node. Less than one-quarter of the lymphatic drainage of the breast is to the IM nodes which extend along a vertical parasternal plane adjacent to the IM artery and vein. These nodes are seen in the intercostal spaces adjacent to the sternum.

The axillary nodes are divided into three levels (Fig. 18.25). *Level I* nodes are lateral to the pectoralis minor muscle. *Level II* nodes are posterior to pec minor. *Level III* nodes are medial to pec minor. Level III nodes are sometimes called infra clavicular nodes. When nodes are located between the pectoralis major and pectoralis minor muscles, they are called *Rotter nodes*. The level I nodes are most easily identified and removed during axillary lymph node dissection. Thus, it is important to alert your surgical colleague if there are abnormal nodes present in the other locations deep to the muscles.

It is common to see several axillary lymph nodes on routine MLO mammography views (Fig. 18.26). The number of nodes seen is largely dependent on the positioning technique of the mammography technologist. Because the nodes reside in the pocket of fat just posterior to the pectoralis muscle, they may slip out from under the compression paddle. If nodes are present on a mammogram, you should evaluate their size and morphology. If nodes are not present mammographically, they cannot be assessed. If a node is seen on the current examination, but was not included on the priors, it is likely due to positioning and should not be viewed as new or suspicious if the size and morphology are otherwise normal.

Enlarging or abnormal axillary nodes require further investigation. Both malignant and benign infectious or inflammatory etiologies can lead to enlarged lymph nodes. Adenopathy can be bilateral or unilateral which can help

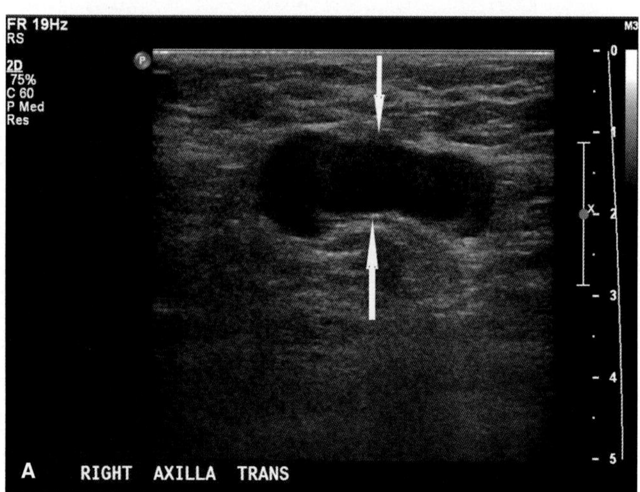

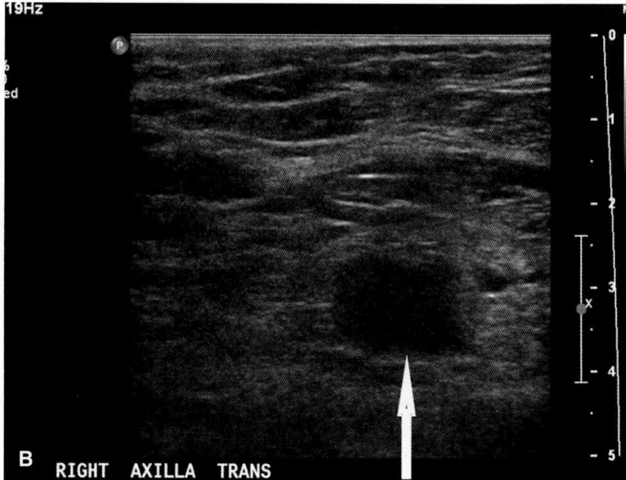

FIGURE 18.24. **Suspicious Lymph Nodes on Ultrasound.** Ultrasound images showing (**A**) diffuse cortical thickening (*arrows*) and (**B**) indistinct margin and loss of normal fatty hilum (*arrows*).

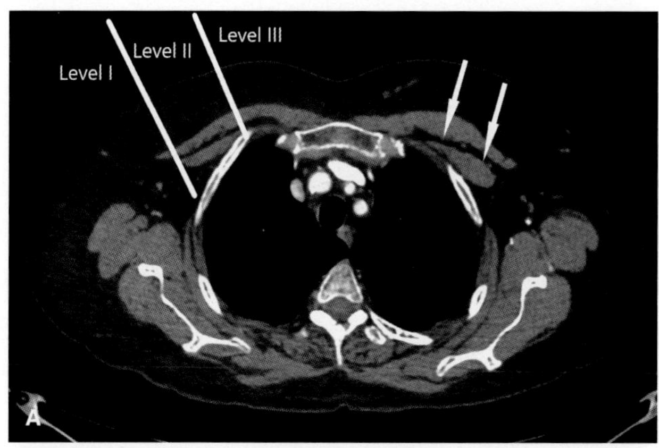

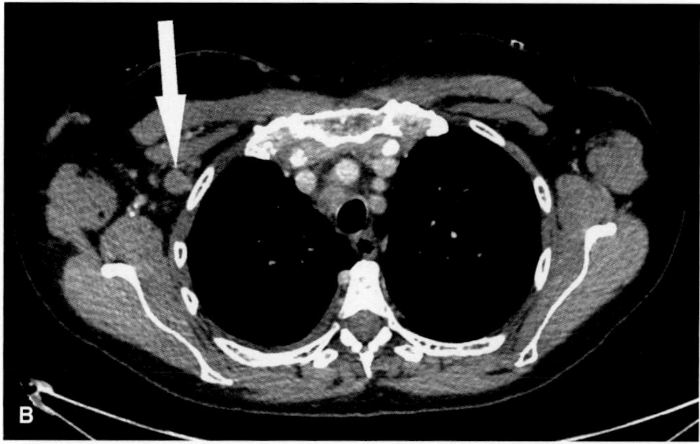

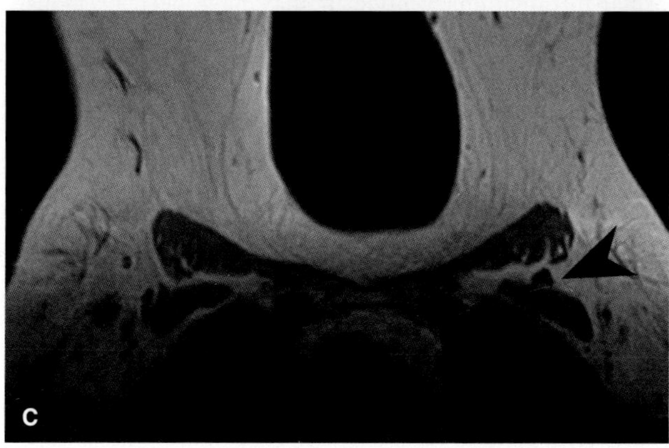

FIGURE 18.25. **Lymph Node Levels of the Axilla. A:** Axial CT scan of the chest. Axillary lymph nodes are divided into three levels. Level I nodes are lateral to the pectoralis minor muscle (*arrows*). Level II nodes are deep to pectoralis minor. Level III nodes are medial to pectoralis minor. **B:** Enlarged level II lymph node (*arrow*) in a patient with a known ipsilateral breast cancer (not shown). Mediastinal adenopathy is also present. **C:** Lymph nodes that are located between the pectoralis major and minor are called Rotter nodes (*arrowhead*).

narrow the differential diagnosis. It is important to remember that unilateral axillary adenopathy may be due to breast cancer, even if the mammogram is normal since some breast cancers are mammographically occult. To diagnostically evaluate the axillary lymph nodes, a targeted ultrasound is most commonly performed. Other cross-sectional imaging such as CT scan or MRI can also be useful.

We routinely image axillary lymph nodes in the setting of a new breast cancer diagnosis or in the setting of a highly suspicious (BI-RADS 5) breast mass that has not yet undergone biopsy. The axilla is imaged routinely as this received the majority of lymphatic drainage. The IM nodes are imaged when there is a cancer in the medial half of the breast. Lymphatic drainage to the IM nodes is more likely when the primary tumor is in the medial breast.

Lymph nodes can also be found *in* the breast and are called *intramammary nodes* (Fig. 18.27). Intramammary nodes are most often a normal incidental finding. They are almost always found in the fat, usually adjacent to a vessel. Intramammary nodes do not occur in the fibroglandular breast tissue. This distinction can be difficult when a patient is extremely thin, with little subcutaneous fat. Intramammary nodes are similar in appearance to nodes elsewhere. They are oval, circumscribed, and fat containing. The anatomy of an intramammary node is easily evaluated with digital breast tomosynthesis. Targeted ultrasound can also be performed if a suspected intramammary node is seen mammographically. The presence or absence of intramammary nodes does not fluctuate. Thus, a **new** mass should not be classified as a

TABLE 18.2

LYMPH NODE LOCATIONS

Axilla	Level I Level II Level III Rotter's
Internal Mammary Chain	
Supraclavicular	
Intramammary	

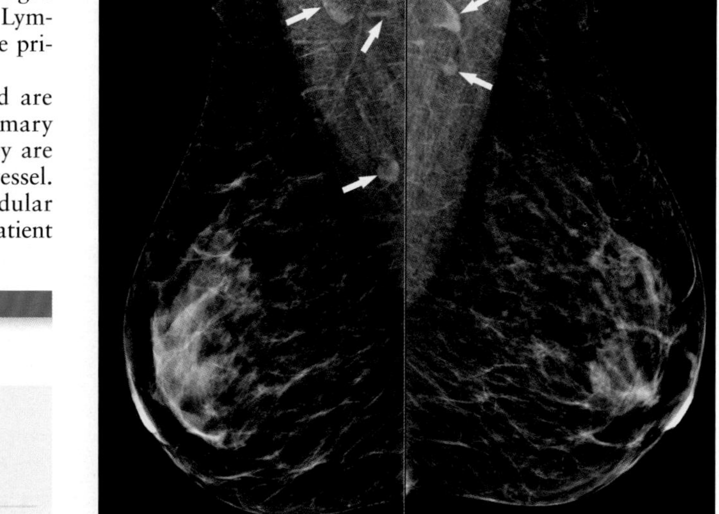

FIGURE 18.26. **Lymph Nodes on MLO Mammogram.** Lymph nodes (*arrows*) are commonly seen on MLO mammographic views.

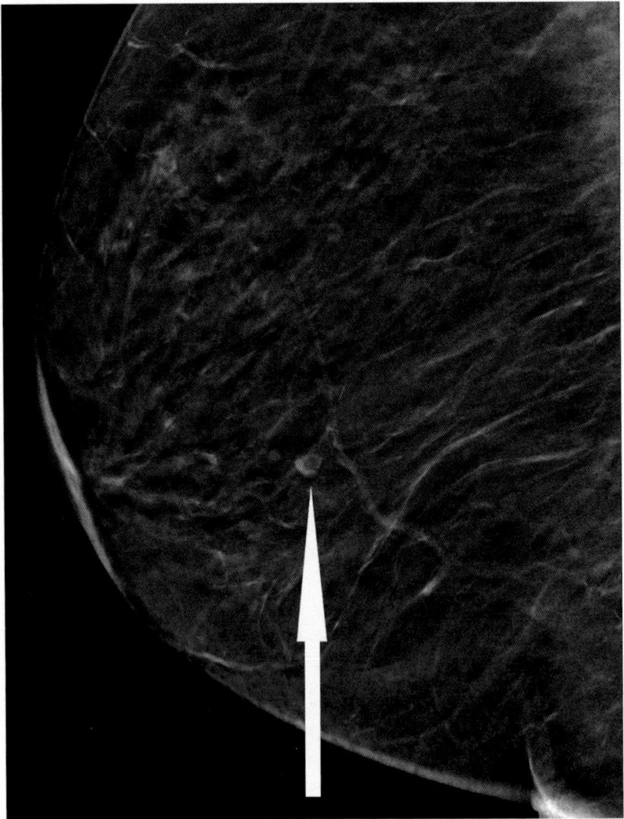

FIGURE 18.27. **Normal Intramammary Node.** Normal intramammary lymph nodes (*arrow*) are often seen. Nodes are located in the fat, often near a blood vessel. A fatty hilum is often visible as seen on this image with digital breast tomosynthesis (DBT).

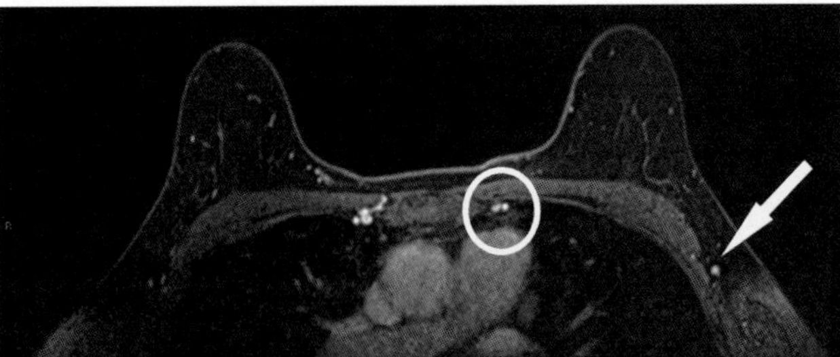

FIGURE 18.28. **Blood Supply Seen on MRI.** Blood supply to the breast is primarily from the internal mammary artery and vein (*circle*) and the lateral thoracic artery and vein (*arrow*).

normal intramammary node. It may have been previously obscured or not included on the films.

BLOOD SUPPLY

Knowledge of the blood supply to the breast is helpful to avoid damage to a large vessel during a biopsy. Blood supply also affects the pattern of normal physiologic background enhancement during MRI. The blood supply to the breast is from the IM artery that supplies the medial and central parts of the breast and the lateral thoracic artery which supplies the upper and outer portions of the breast. Minor contributions to arterial flow are also made by the pectoral branch of the thoracoacromial artery and branches from the intercostal arteries (Fig. 18.28).

Major venous drainage of the breast parallels the arterial supply. Superficial veins on the breast can become enlarged and quite noticeable during pregnancy and lactation. Thrombophlebitis of a superficial vein is called Mondor disease. It has many etiologies including prior surgery, trauma, dehydration, pregnancy, or other thrombogenic conditions. Patients usually present with a tender palpable cord and a linear area of skin erythema (Fig. 18.29).

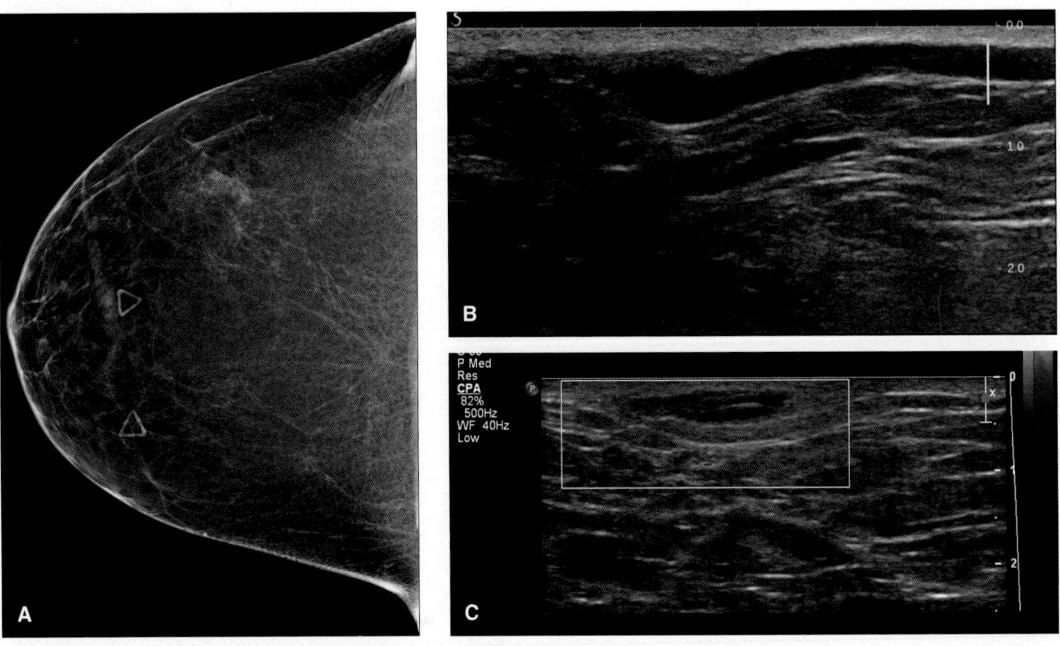

FIGURE 18.29. **Mondor Thrombophlebitis. A:** CC mammogram shows a palpable tube-like structure marked with the *triangles*. **B:** Gray scale ultrasound shows a superficial tubular structure with low level echoes compatible with a thrombosed superficial vein. **C:** There is no detectable flow on Doppler imaging due to thrombosis.

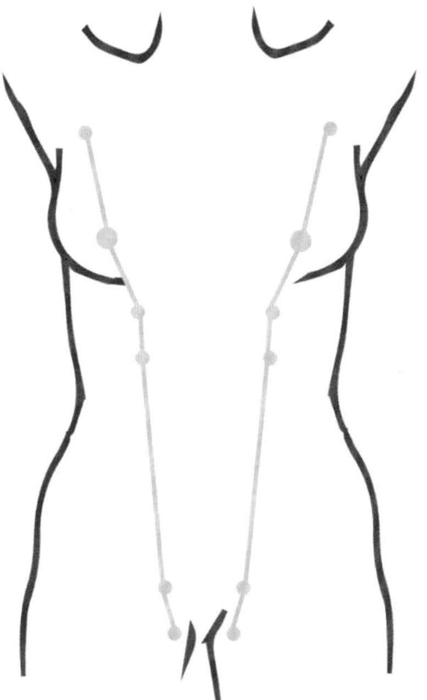

FIGURE 18.30. **Milk Streak.** Development of the milk streak occurs during embryology (*tan lines*). Incomplete regression of the milk streak can lead to the formation of accessory nipples or breast tissue at these locations.

EMBRYOLOGY AND DEVELOPMENT

The human breast changes throughout a woman's lifetime. Breast development begins during the 5th week of development and is the same for both males and females. The ventral ectoderm folds inward to form two symmetric lines known as the "milk streak." The milk streak extends from the axilla to the groin (Fig. 18.30). Over the thorax, this line continues to thicken to form a ridge. The remainder of the line begins to regress. Incomplete regression of the milk streak can lead to the formation of accessory nipples or breast tissue. Accessory breast tissue is most common in the axilla, seen in 2% to 6% of women. This accessory breast tissue can undergo normal physiologic changes and even produce milk during lactation. Importantly, cancers can also develop in accessory breast tissue. It is also common for women to have an accessory nipple present. Accessory nipples are often small, pigmented, and can be mistaken for a nevus.

The presence of accessory nipples is called *polythelia*. The presence of accessory breast tissue is termed *polymastia*. Congenital absence of the breast is termed *amastia*. When a nipple is present without underlying breast tissue, it is known as *amazia* (Table 18.3). Congenital anomalies of the breast can coexist with abnormal development of other structures. Poland syndrome was first described in 1841 and is the association of absence of the pectoral muscle, chest wall deformity, breast anomalies, and symbrachydactyly, with hypoplasia of the middle phalanges and central skin webbing (Fig. 18.31).

TABLE 18.3

DEVELOPMENTAL ANOMALIES OF THE BREAST

Polythelia	Presence of accessory nipples
Polymastia	Presence of accessory breast tissue
Amastia	Congenital absence of the breast
Amazia	Nipple is present without underlying breast tissue

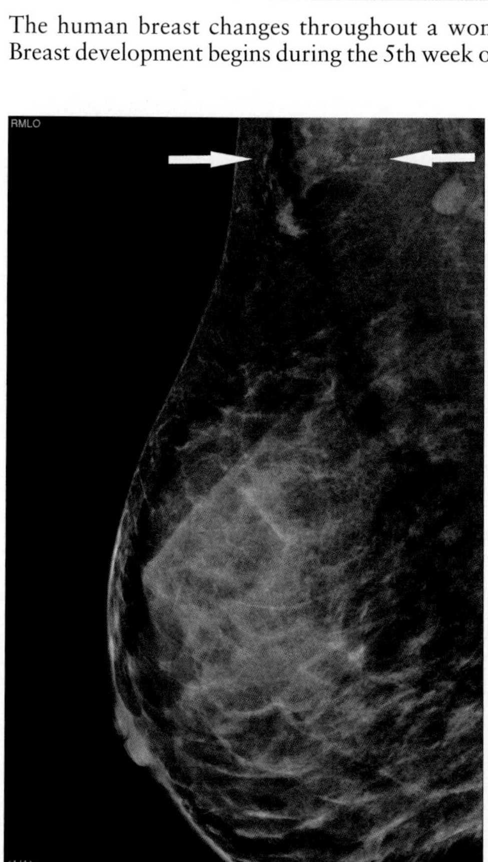

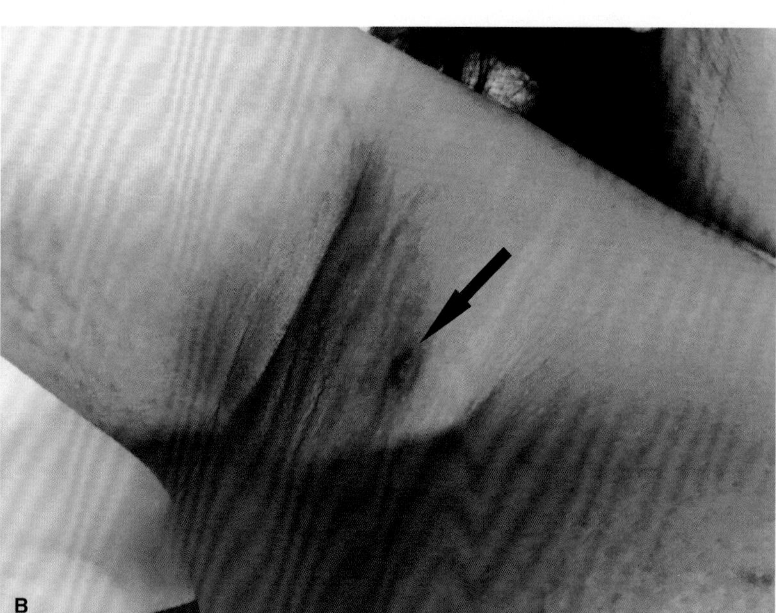

FIGURE 18.31. **Accessory Breast Tissue in the Axilla. A:** Right MLO mammogram showing accessory breast tissue in the axilla (*arrows*). **B:** Photograph of the axilla showing an accessory nipple (*black arrow*).

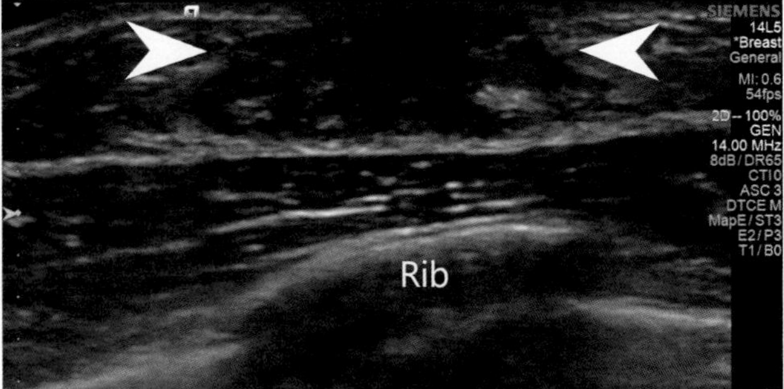

FIGURE 18.32. **Breast Bud on Ultrasound.** Normal breast bud in a 7-year-old girl with a tender palpable subareolar lump. Breast bud is often hypoechoic and extends directly posterior to the nipple. This must not be mistaken for a mass. Trauma from biopsy can interfere with normal breast development.

Breast development continues throughout fetal development with budding and branching of the epithelium to form ducts. After birth, the male breast remains rudimentary, consisting only of ductal structures and not lobules. The female breast continues to develop during puberty. Development of the milk ducts is predominantly under the effects of estrogen. The TDLUs and lobules begin to form in later adolescence and in the early 20s under both estrogen and progesterone stimulation. The lobules will be the site of milk production during pregnancy and lactation.

Breast development is termed *thelarche*. In young girls, the first sign of breast development is a nickel size lump directly behind the nipple called the *breast bud*. A breast bud can be tender and palpable, and may present for diagnostic evaluation. It may initially be asymmetric. It is extremely important NOT to biopsy the breast bud. Iatrogenic trauma to the breast bud can halt further development and leave the patient with a subsequent marked deformity and underdevelopment of the breast (Fig. 18.32).

CHANGES OVER TIME: PREGNANCY, LACTATION, AND MENOPAUSE

Important changes occur in the breast during pregnancy and lactation which will change the normal imaging appearance of the breast. During pregnancy, there is accelerated development of the lobules under the influence of progesterone. The effects are most pronounced in the second and third trimesters. There is an increase in the number of acini and an increase in the intralobular stroma. Fibroglandular elements occupy a greater percentage of the breast relative to fat. Mammographic breast density markedly increases. In the late third trimester, the acini begin to secrete colostrum and then milk which will also increase the breast density. If a lactating woman presents for imaging evaluation we ask that she breast feed or pump immediately prior to the examination to minimize the amount of fluid present (Fig. 18.33).

Pregnancy and lactation also change the appearance of the breast tissue on both ultrasound and MRI. On ultrasound, the fibroglandular tissue becomes more hypoechoic. Dilated, fluid-filled milk ducts can also be seen. On MRI, there is marked enhancement of the background parenchyma. Screening breast MRI is not routinely performed in women that are pregnant because it is not known how gadolinium contrast agent will affect a fetus.

There is normal involution of the breast tissue with menopause and declining circulating estrogen and progesterone. The fibroglandular tissue becomes more fatty replaced. Because the risk of breast cancer continues to increase with advancing age, a new or developing mass or asymmetry in a postmenopausal woman should be viewed suspiciously. There may be a transient increase in fibroglandular tissue in postmenopausal women using hormone replacement therapy (HRT). However, the use of HRT has declined over the past decade due to association with increased breast cancer risk.

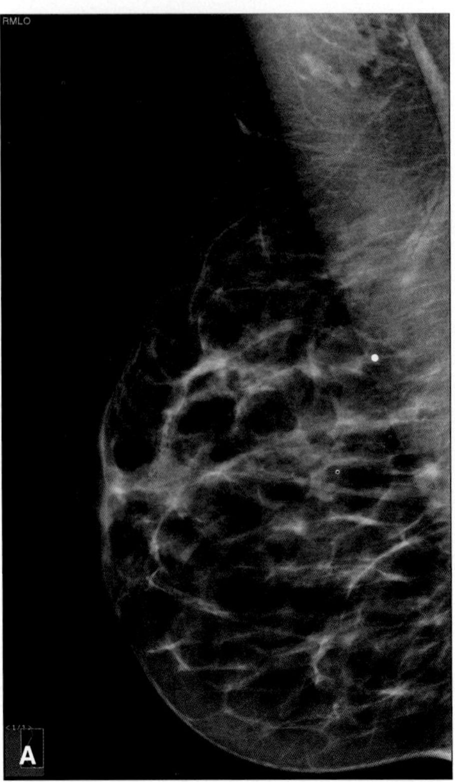

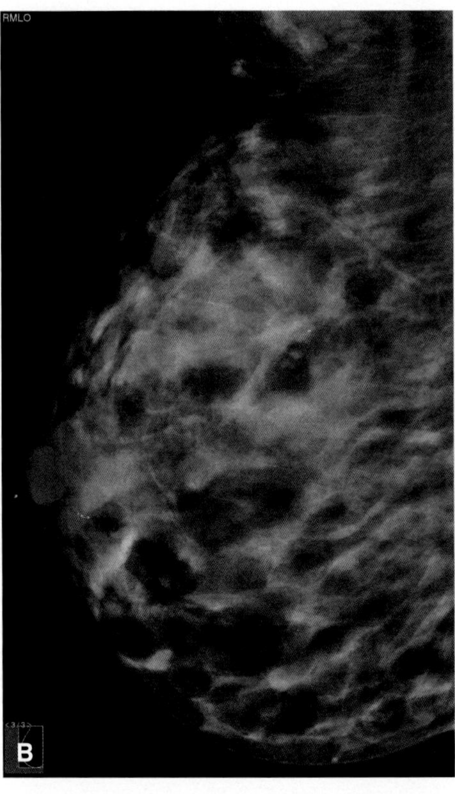

FIGURE 18.33. **Lactational Changes. A:** Normal MLO mammogram before pregnancy. **B:** Normal MLO mammogram in the same patient while lactating. There is marked increase in the fibroglandular tissue and breast density.

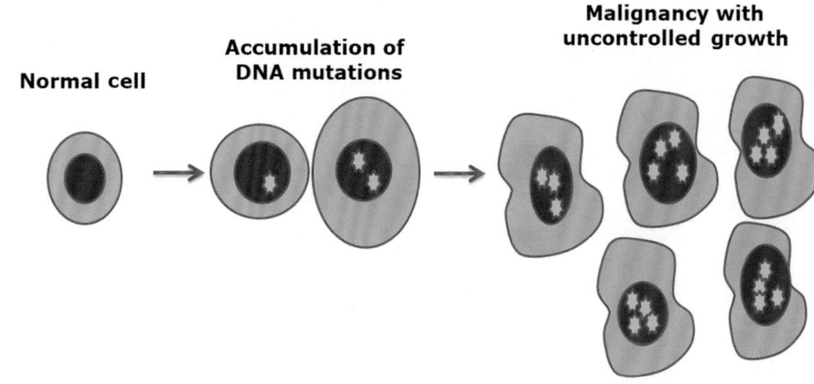

FIGURE 18.34. Cartoon representation of DNA mutations in the cell nucleus leading to uncontrolled cell growth of malignancy.

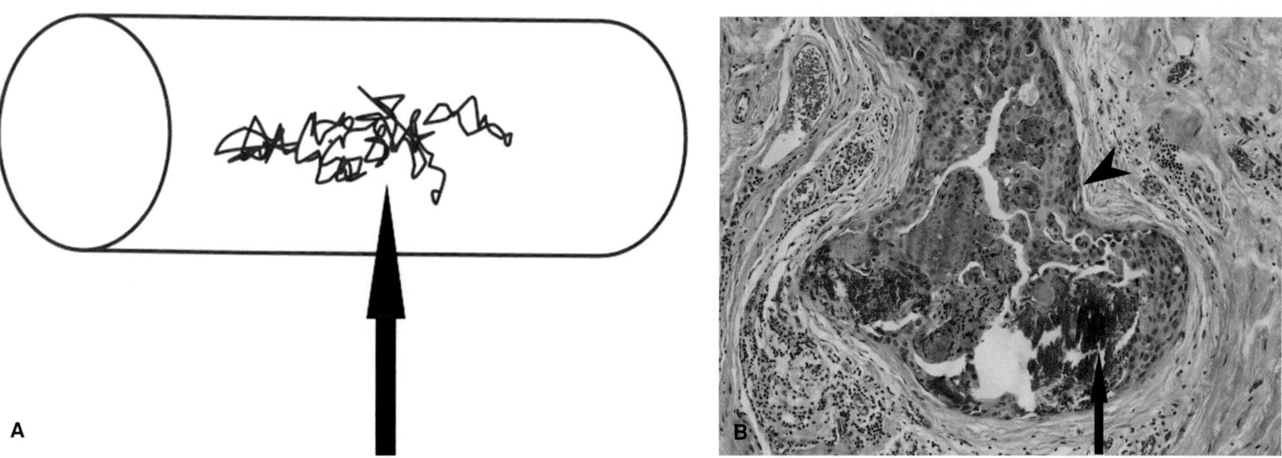

FIGURE 18.35. **DCIS. A:** Cartoon drawing of a milk duct containing calcifications of DCIS (*arrow*). **B:** Histopathology of DCIS. H&E stain showing distended duct (*arrowhead*) lumen filled with abnormal cells of DCIS. There is necrosis and calcification present (*arrow*). The calcifications are detectable on mammography. (Histopathology slide provided by Dr. Kristen Atkins.)

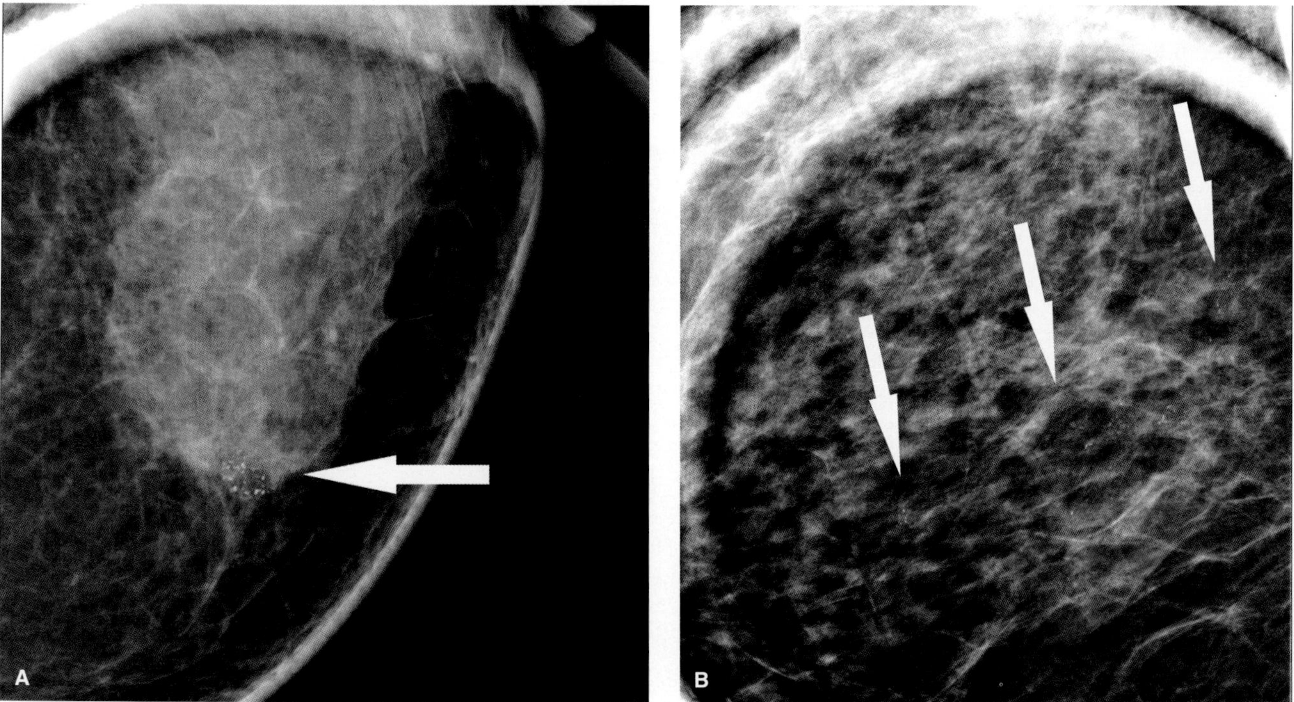

FIGURE 18.36. **Mammographic Appearance of DCIS.** Spot magnification mammograms. **A:** A group of fine pleomorphic calcifications (*arrow*). Biopsy showed high-grade DCIS. **B:** Segmental fine pleomorphic calcifications following the distribution of the milk duct (*arrows*). Biopsy showed high-grade DCIS.

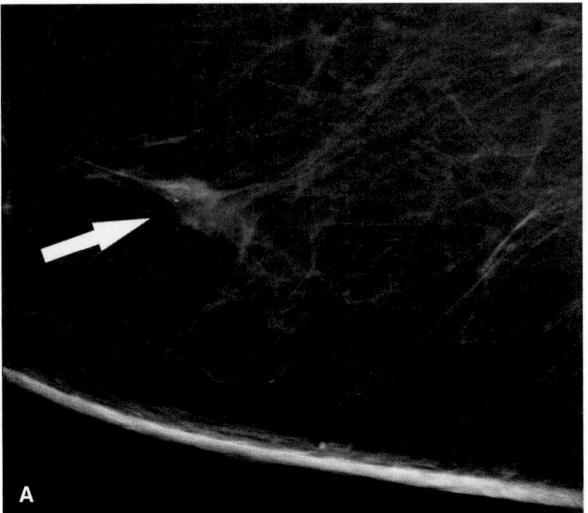

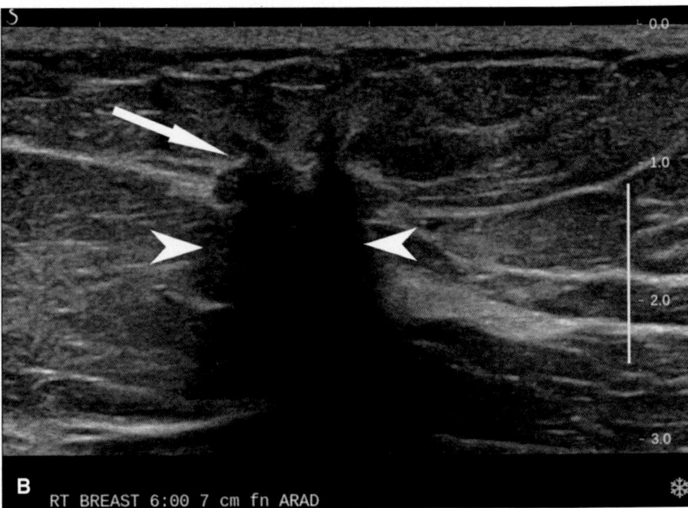

FIGURE 18.37. **Mammographic and Ultrasound Appearance of Invasive Ductal Carcinoma. A:** ML spot magnification view shows an irregularly shaped, high-density mass with spiculated margin and fine pleomorphic calcifications. **B:** Gray scale ultrasound shows the same mass (*arrow*) with the irregular shape and speculated margin. Mass also exhibits posterior acoustic shadowing (*arrowheads*). Imaging appearance is highly suggestive of malignancy.

PATHOPHYSIOLOGY OF BREAST CANCER

Breast cancer is the most common nondermatologic malignancy in women and the second most common cause of cancer deaths (American Cancer Society). Most breast cancers arise from the epithelium of the milk ducts and the lobules. Thus, majority of breast cancers are adenocarcinomas. Cancers arise after the accumulation of DNA mutations that result in uncontrolled cell growth (Fig. 18.34). Most breast cancers arise from ductal cells in the TDLU. There is a spectrum in the histopathologic appearance of breast disease that progresses from usual ductal hyperplasia, atypical ductal hyperplasia, DCIS, and IDC. Malignant cells of DCIS are confined to the milk duct. It has not broken through the basement membrane and thus, by definition, has no potential for metastatic spread (Fig. 18.35). However, DCIS, is categorized as "breast cancer" because of the likelihood of transformation to invasive disease. DCIS classically appears as calcifications on mammography or nonmass enhancement on MRI. The distribution of DCIS often follows the anatomy of a milk duct or ductal system (Fig. 18.36).

IDC is the most common form of breast cancer. It begins in the milk duct and spreads beyond the basement membrane to invade the stroma. It classically presents as a breast mass that can be seen with mammography, ultrasound, and MRI (Fig. 18.37). IDC has the potential to spread to the lymph nodes and metastasize throughout the body.

Less commonly, breast cancer may arise from cells of the lobules which is termed ILC. The cancer cells of ILC lack e-cadherin. Thus, the cells do not "stick" together, but rather form a web of infiltrative cells. ILC is classically more challenging to detect with imaging. ILC can present as a breast mass,

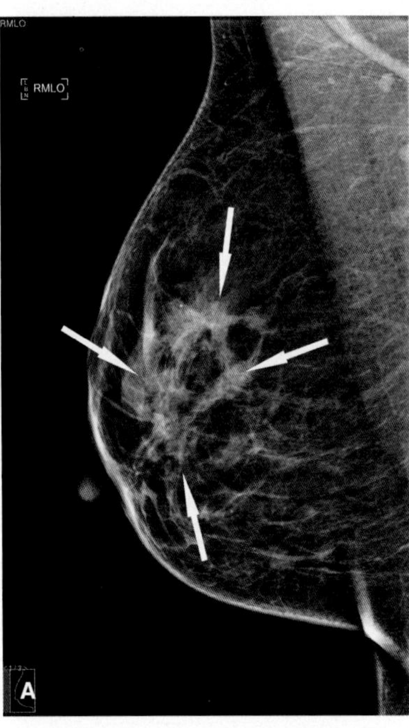

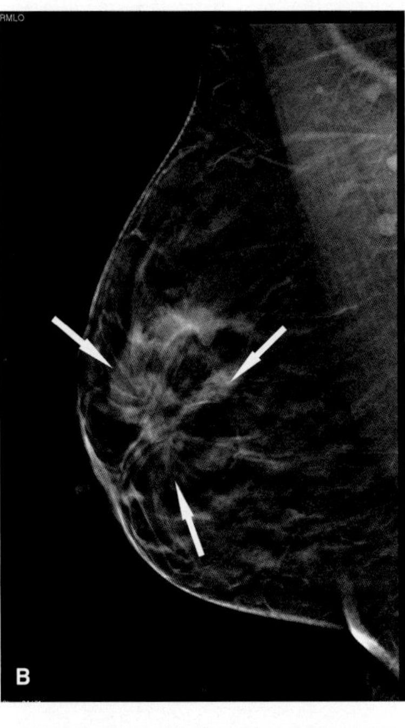

FIGURE 18.38. **Mammographic Appearance of Invasive Lobular Carcinoma. A:** Two-dimensional digital mammography and (**B**) digital breast tomosynthesis (DBT) reveal a large area of architectural distortion (*arrows*). Biopsy showed invasive lobular carcinoma.

an asymmetry, or architectural distortion (Fig. 18.38). The use of imaging techniques such as digital breast tomosynthesis and MRI has increased our ability to detect ILC. In contrast to DCIS, lobular carcinoma in situ (LCIS) is *not* considered breast cancer. It is a high-risk lesion that increases breast cancer risk.

Suggested Readings

American Cancer Society. Breast Cancer Statistics 2017. cancer.org/BreastCancerStats2017.

American College of Radiology. *American College of Radiology Manual on Contrast Media. Version 10.3*. Reston, VA: ACR Committee on Drugs and Contrast Media; 2017.

Beals RK, Crawford S. Congenital absence of the pectoral muscles. *Clin Orthop Relat Res* 1976;119:166–171.

Cao MM, Hoyt AC, Bassett LW. Mammographic signs of systemic disease. *Radiographics* 2011;31(4):1085–1100.

Chlebowski RT, Stefanick, ML, Anderson GA. Breast cancer in postmenopausal women after hormone therapy. *JAMA* 2011;305(5):466–467.

DeFilippis EM, Arleo EK. The ABCs of accessory breast tissue: basic information every radiologist should know. *AJR Am J Roentgenol* 2014;202(5):1157–1162.

Deurloo EE, Tanis PJ, Gilhuijs KG, et al. Reduction in the number of sentinel lymph node procedures by preoperative ultrasonography of the axilla in breast cancer. *Eur J of Cancer* 2003;39(8):1068–1073.

Harvey JA, Nicholson BT, Cohen MA. Finding early invasive breast cancers: a practical approach. *Radiology* 2008;248(1):61–76.

Hultborn KA, Larsen LG, Raghnult I. The lymph drainage from the breast to the axillary and parasternal lymph nodes: studied with the aid of colloidal AU198. *Acta Radiol* 1955;43(1):52–64.

McTiernan A, Martin CF, Peck JD, et al. Estrogen-plus-progestin use and mammographic density in postmenopausal women: Women's Health Initiative randomized trial. *J Natl Cancer Inst* 2005;97(18):1366–1376.

Nicholson BT, Harvey JA, Cohen MA. Nipple-areolar complex: normal anatomy and benign and malignant processes. *Radiographics* 2009;29(2):509–523.

Osborne MP, Boolbol SK. Breast anatomy and development. In: Harris JR, Lippman ME, Morrow M, Osborne CK, eds. *Breast Diseases*. 5th ed. Philadelphia, PA: Wolters Kluwer Health; 2014.

Santen R, Mansel R. Benign breast disorders. *N Engl J Med* 2005;353(3):275–285.

Stavros AT. *Breast Ultrasound*. Philadelphia, PA: Lippincott Williams & Wilkins; 2004.

CHAPTER 19 ■ IMAGING THE SCREENING PATIENT

JONATHAN V. NGUYEN, CARRIE M. ROCHMAN, AND BRANDI T. NICHOLSON

INTRODUCTION

Breast imaging is essential in the evaluation of the breast to aid in the detection of early breast cancer in asymptomatic women and to evaluate clinical breast symptoms. Breast imaging encompasses mammography, ultrasound, magnetic resonance imaging (MRI), and some functional imaging modalities. Mammography is the primary imaging modality used for breast cancer screening.

SCREENING FOR BREAST CANCER

Support for Screening

Breast cancer survival is influenced by the size of the tumor and the lymph node status at the time of diagnosis. Small tumors with negative axillary lymph nodes have survival rates well above 90%. Such cancers are detected far more often with screening mammography than with physical examination. Several randomized controlled trials have proven the efficacy of screening mammography in reducing breast cancer mortality from the identification of lower-stage malignancies.

In 1963, the Health Insurance Plan of New York (HIP) invited 31,000 women aged 40 to 64 years to participate in four annual screenings for breast cancer by mammography and physical examination. This study group was compared with a control group of women who received routine medical care. Nine years after beginning the study, there was a 29% reduction in breast cancer mortality in the group receiving annual screening.

Multiple trials of mammographic screening were begun in the late 1970s and early 1980s. They were population based, meaning that all women living within a specific geographical area who were within the age range under study were included in the trial. Breast cancer mortality was compared between women invited to screening and those not invited (controls). When the data from all centers were combined, the reduction in breast cancer mortality among women aged 40 to 74 years was 24% in the group invited to mammographic screening.

The actual benefit of screening mammography for women of all ages is likely to exceed that which has been demonstrated by the randomized clinical trials. Breast cancer mortality data on all women invited for screening, regardless of whether they actually underwent mammography, were used in calculating the reduction of mortality attributable to screening. Compliance rates for obtaining mammography among trial invitees ranged from 61% to 89%. The technology used for mammography has improved greatly since the time that the trials began, resulting in earlier detection of breast cancer. Recent evaluations of the impact of mammographic screening in the community setting (service screening) have shown breast cancer mortality reductions of up to 50% among screened women; however, it is difficult to determine the contribution of screening relative to that of improvements in therapy in lowering the death rate from breast cancer.

The goal of screening asymptomatic women is to find breast cancer in its earliest stages when treatment has the highest chance for survival. In a well-established screening program, over 50% of cancers will be minimal; minimal cancers are defined as those that are noninvasive or invasive but less than 1 cm in size with negative nodes. Over 80% of breast cancer discovered by screening mammography should be node negative.

Screening Guidelines

There is controversy over the age at which mammographic screening should begin and also the frequency of such screening. Traditionally, the recommendation for screening mammography was to start annual screening at age 40 and continue until there is less than 10 years of life expectancy.

In 2009, the U.S. Preventive Services Task Force (USPSTF) withdrew its support for mammographic screening for women in their 40s and recommended that women aged 50 to 74 years be screened biennially, which they reaffirmed in their 2016 recommendation statement. The USPSTF concluded that the benefit gained from screening was not high enough to offset the downsides of screening (false-positive results, anxiety, and possible overdiagnosis and overtreatment). They chose to use a 15% reduction in mortality in their meta-analysis even though mortality reductions of up to 44% have been reported with screening in this age group. Observational studies have shown that women aged 40 to 49 years were more likely to have late-stage cancers diagnosed if they were screened at 2-year intervals when compared with a 1-year screening interval. Other studies of cancers that occur between screens have shown that a greater proportion of breast cancers grow faster in younger women than in older women. It is for this reason that the American College of Radiology and the Society of Breast Imaging at this time continue to recommend annual mammographic screening for women at age 40 and older. The American Cancer Society (ACS) recommends starting annual screening at age 45, with an option to transition to biennial screening at age 55. Although it is clear both that mammographic screening can reduce breast cancer mortality for women in their 40s and that annual mammographic screening is more effective in reducing breast cancer deaths for women in this age group, economic considerations and more research into individual patient factors may favor modifications in screening strategies.

Women potentially at high risk for development of breast cancer should seek expert advice regarding the age at which screening should begin, the periodicity of mammography, and the possible addition of other screening modalities. A risk assessment should be performed. Factors known to increase a woman's risk include the following: (1) A personal history of breast or ovarian cancer. (2) Laboratory evidence that the woman is a carrier of the BRCA1 or BRCA2 genetic mutation. These mutations confer an estimated risk of up to 80% for development of breast cancer by age 70. (3) Having a mother, sister, or daughter with breast cancer. (4) Atypical ductal hyperplasia (ADH) or lobular neoplasia diagnosed on a previous breast biopsy. (5) A history of chest irradiation received between the ages of 10 and 30 years. Women who are at high risk (lifetime risk for breast cancer of greater than 20%) should undergo annual screening MR in addition to mammographic screening. This is further elaborated on in Chapter 22. In addition, it would be appropriate to start screening with mammography as early as ages 25 to 30 in these women. Screening with US can be considered in high-risk women who cannot undergo MR screening.

When adopting a screening policy, the physician must remember that all women are at risk for developing breast cancer. The ACS estimates that one woman in every eight will develop the disease during her lifetime. The majority of women who contract breast cancer will not have histories that place them at higher risk.

TECHNICAL FACTORS IN SCREENING

Mammography Physics

Because both high contrast and high spatial resolution are needed for optimal mammography, standard radiographic equipment cannot be used for this examination. Mammography must be performed on a unit dedicated to this purpose. Mammographic equipment and technique differ from standard radiography in several ways. The anode material that is used to generate the x-rays in most dedicated film screen mammography units is molybdenum. This allows the production of lower-energy x-rays, which in turn produces greater contrast between soft tissue structures. The structures of the breast do not differ greatly in their inherent contrast, so these low-kilovolt photons are extremely important in producing a high-contrast image. Some units also have rhodium anodes that can be used to increase the contrast in more dense breasts, while keeping radiation dose and time of exposure low. Full-field digital mammography (FFDM) units often use tungsten anodes, which are more efficient, have better longevity, and can yield lower radiation doses than molybdenum anodes. The image processing possible with digital mammography allows high-quality mammograms utilizing tungsten anodes. The radiologist must be able to discern tiny microcalcifications on mammograms; some of these calcifications may be 0.1 mm or less in size. The small focal spot size used in mammography units and high-resolution digital radiographic detectors or high-resolution, single intensifying screens used with single emulsion film contribute to the creation of images with high resolution.

Compression. All mammographic units are equipped with compression paddles that squeeze the breast against the image receptor or film holder. Good compression of the breast is essential to high-quality mammography for several reasons. Compression spreads overlapping breast structures so that true masses can be differentiated from summation shadows that occur because of overlapping soft tissues. The breast is immobilized during compression so motion unsharpness or blurring due to patient movement is minimized. Geometric unsharpness, caused by the finite focal spot dimension, is minimized by bringing the breast structures closer to the film. Compression renders the breast nearly uniform in thickness so that the film density of tissues near the nipple will be similar to those near the chest wall. Radiation dose can be reduced by good compression; a thinner breast requires fewer photons for penetration.

Unfortunately, some women find breast compression uncomfortable. However, most can tolerate it once the benefits of compression are explained. During routine mammography, the breast is compressed for just a few seconds while each film is taken. Many units are equipped with automated compression devices so the technologist can release the tension immediately after the film is exposed.

Other factors important to consider in the production of high-quality mammograms include the x-ray generator, beam filtration, whether or not a grid is used, film-intensifying screen combinations, and the film-processing system. All of these factors are interrelated and must be optimized to produce technically acceptable films of the breast.

FFDM. FFDM units have been commercially available since 2000 and now account for the majority of mammography units in the United States. FFDM uses an electronic system for image capture and display. It has higher contrast resolution and better dynamic range than film screen mammography. Spatial resolution is lower with FFDM, but its greater contrast resolution still makes high-quality images possible. The radiation dose from FFDM is comparable to that of film screen mammography in smaller breasts; it may be lower in larger breasts. Advantages of FFDM over film screen mammography include a higher speed of image acquisition and thus increased throughput of patients, the ability to perform image processing (which may lead to fewer repeat films due to optimization of brightness and contrast), other image processing algorithms (which may result in increased conspicuity of certain features including microcalcifications, integration of computer-aided detection, and diagnosis software programs), electronic storage thus eliminating lost films and the need for film storage, and the possibility of teleradiology.

The Digital Mammographic Imaging Screening Trial, a multicenter trial that enrolled more than 49,000 women in the United States and Canada, found no significant differences in the sensitivity of FFDM compared to film screen mammography for all women enrolled. However, FFDM performed significantly better than film screen mammography in premenopausal and perimenopausal women, in women younger than 50 years, and in women with dense breasts. These findings along with the technical advantages of FFDM have resulted in the steady replacement of film screen mammography with FFDM for breast cancer detection and diagnosis.

Radiation Risk

An increased susceptibility to breast cancer has been documented among women exposed to high doses of radiation (1 to 20 Gy). The survivors of the atomic bomb explosions in Japan, patients undergoing radiation therapy, and sanatoria patients undergoing multiple chest fluoroscopies for monitoring of tuberculosis therapy are all groups having an increased incidence of breast cancer. Such data raised questions about the risk incurred from the low doses of radiation received during screening mammography.

A controlled study of the effects of low doses of radiation such as those received during mammography would require large numbers of women in both the study and control groups. Close to 100 million patients in each group would be required in order to provide statistically significant data. Clearly, this would not be practical or possible. As such, estimates or risk have been hypothesized by extrapolation from data obtained at higher doses using a linear dose–response model.

Follow-up data from the Japanese atomic bomb survivors have shown progressively decreasing radiation risk with increased age at exposure. Women exposed in their youth and teens suffered the highest increase in risk. No increased risk was demonstrable for women aged 40 years or older at exposure. Studies of the other populations sustaining significant breast radiation exposure have also supported a diminished risk with advancing age at exposure. Estimated lifetime risk of breast cancer death from a single mammogram in the age group from 40 to 49 years is approximately 2 in 1 million. In women aged 50 to 59 years, this risk is reduced to less than 1 in 1 million; progressive reductions in risk are seen at older ages. These theoretical risks should be weighed against the risk of dying from spontaneous breast cancer, which would be approximately 700 per million in women aged 40 to 49 years and 1,000 per million in women aged 50 to 59 years. Based on projection models, routine screening mammography is not associated with an increased radiation-induced mortality.

The American College of Radiology recommends that the average glandular dose delivered by a single mammographic view should not exceed 3 mGy, although most mammographic views are approximately 2 mGy. To put radiation dose from mammography in perspective, the average effective dose from a standard two-view mammogram is 0.44 mSv, while the effective dose from natural background radiation in the United States is 3 mSv per year.

Positioning of Screening Mammography

Mammography can be performed with the patient seated or standing. Most screening practices prefer the standing position because it allows faster throughput and is less cumbersome for the technologist to achieve proper positioning. Patients are able to lean into the unit to a greater degree when standing, thus allowing more of the posterior breast tissues to be imaged.

In the United States, two views of each breast are generally taken for screening mammography. In some European countries, a single mediolateral oblique (MLO) view is taken for screening examinations, but studies have shown that one-view examinations miss 20% to 25% of breast cancers. Moreover single-view mammography would lead to an excessive number of patients being called back for additional views. The standard views for screening mammography are the MLO view and the craniocaudal (CC) view.

MLO View. The MLO view, when properly positioned, depicts the greatest amount of breast tissue. To perform an MLO view, the x-ray tube and image receptor, which are fixed with respect to one another, are moved to an angle that parallels the orientation of the patient's pectoralis major muscle. The technologist is given flexibility in choosing the angle so that the greatest amount of breast tissue possible can be imaged. The angle is generally between 40 and 60 degrees from the horizontal.

The patient is asked to relax her arm and chest muscles and to lean into the machine. The breast is placed on the image receptor and compression is applied from the superomedial direction, the same direction from which the x-rays will be generated. The breast must be pulled anteriorly and spread in a superior–inferior direction as much as possible to minimize overlapping structures and to maximize the amount of tissue imaged. The nipple should be in profile. Compression must be applied (Fig. 19.1). By convention, in the MLO view, a marker indicating the side (left or right) and type of view is placed near the axillary tissues of the breast.

CC View. For the CC view, the unit is placed in the vertical position so that the x-ray tube is perpendicular to the floor. Photons will travel from the anode located superior to the breast to the image receptor underneath the breast. The breast is placed on the image receptor, pulled anteriorly, and spread horizontally before the compression plate is applied to the superior skin surface (Fig. 19.2). The nipple should again be in profile. The chest wall should rest against the image receptor. The markers indicating the side imaged and type of view should be placed near the skin close to the lateral aspect of the breast. By convention, when displaying the CC view, the lateral breast is positioned at the superior aspect of the image.

Supplemental Views. Certain supplemental views may need to be required to visualize the breast tissue completely or optimally. An anterior compression view, typically on an MLO, can be performed to better evaluate the anterior breast parenchyma in large breasts. An exaggerated craniocaudal lateral (XCCL) view can be performed to visualize the lateral posterior breast tissue on the CC projection (Fig. 19.3). Similarly, a cleavage view can be performed to visualize medial breast tissue in the CC projection.

Image Quality

High image quality is necessary to optimize sensitivity and specificity of screening mammography. The technologist plays a key role in the positioning of the patient to produce the best images for interpretation. The technologist also should identify any technical issues and repeat any mammographic view during a screening examination, so that the patient does not need to return for repeat images on a separate date.

MLO. A properly positioned MLO mammogram should show the pectoralis major muscle down to the level of a line drawn perpendicular to the muscle through the nipple (posterior nipple line). The nipple should be in profile so that the subareolar area can be adequately evaluated. The

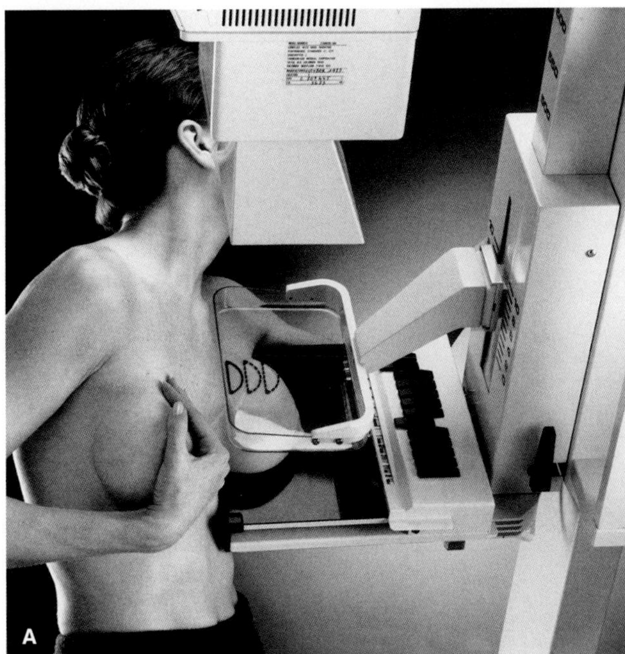

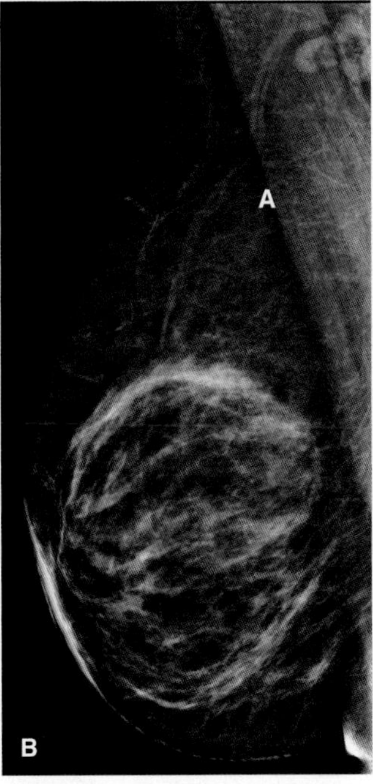

FIGURE 19.1. **Mediolateral Oblique (MLO) View. A:** Patient positioning for an MLO View. (Courtesy of General Electric Medical Systems, Milwaukee, WI.) **B:** Mammogram of MLO projection.

inframammary fold should be visible to ensure that the inferior portion of the breast has been imaged (Fig. 19.4).

CC. When evaluating a CC mammogram, optimal positioning can be assured when pectoralis muscle is seen centrally on the film and the nipple is in profile (Fig. 19.5). An alternative method of assuring appropriate visualization of posterior tissues is to measure the distance from the nipple to the edge of the film through the central axis of the breast; this distance should be within 1 cm of the length of the posterior nipple line as seen on the MLO view.

Artifacts. There are several mammographic artifacts that the technologist and radiologist should be able to identify that may obscure or be confused with a true breast abnormality. Motion artifact is one of the most common artifacts that can limit image quality. Patient motion causes blur, which can obscure detail of normal structures and abnormalities, particularly microcalcifications (Fig. 19.6). To limit motion, the technologist should instruct the patient to remain still or hold their breath during imaging. Increasing compression can also aid in reducing the effect of patient motion on image quality.

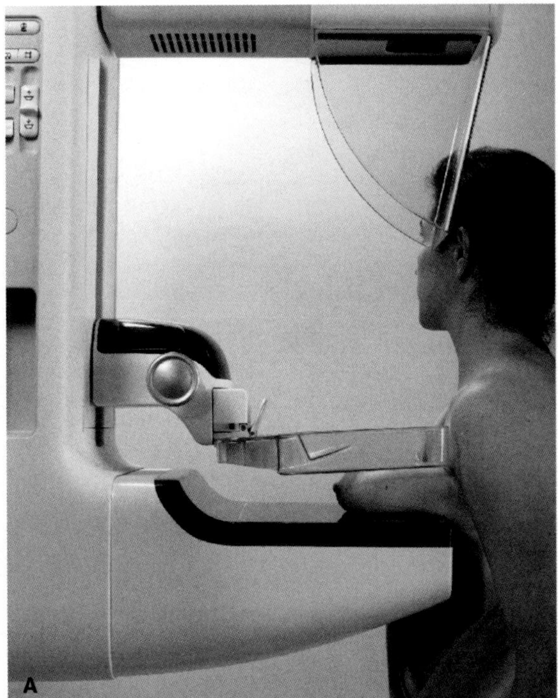

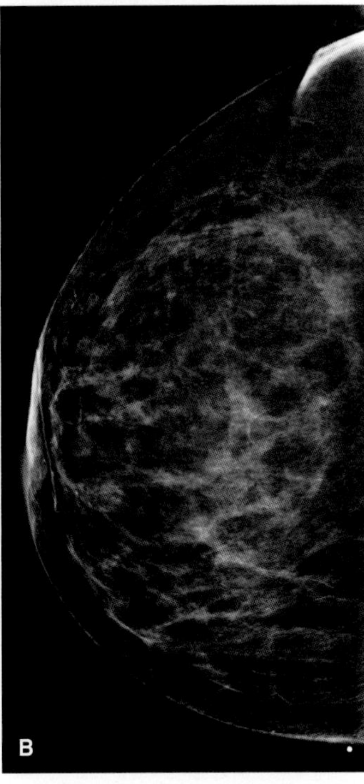

FIGURE 19.2. **Craniocaudal (CC) View. A:** Patient positioning for the CC View. (Courtesy of Hologic Inc, Bedford, MA.) **B:** Mammogram of CC projection.

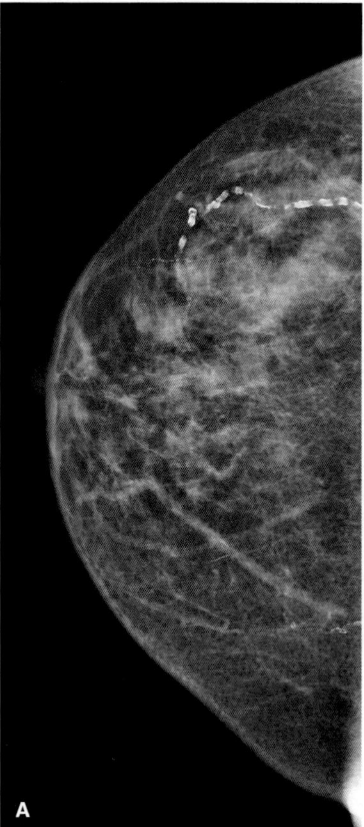

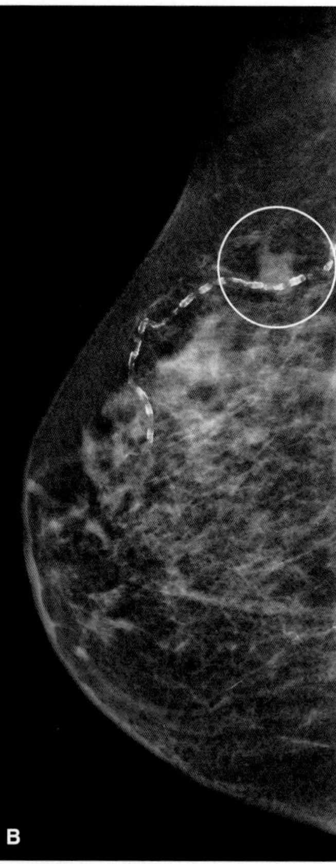

FIGURE 19.3. **Exaggerated Craniocaudal Lateral (XCCL) View. A:** Right craniocaudal view does not fully include lateral breast tissue. **B:** Right XCCL identifies a mass in the lateral breast tissue (*arrow*). Biopsy of this mass demonstrated invasive ductal carcinoma.

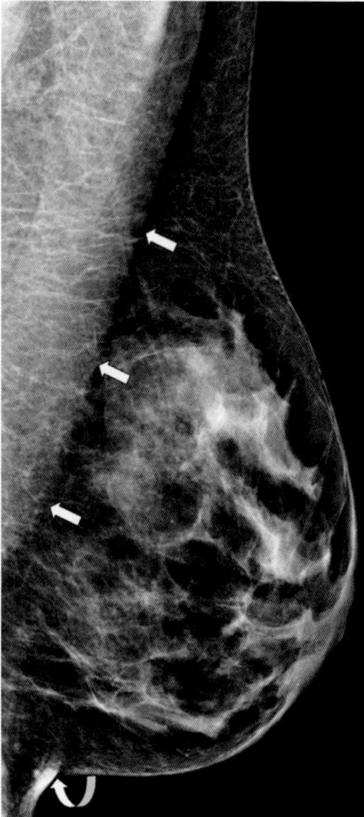

FIGURE 19.4. **MLO Positioning.** Normal mediolateral oblique view of left breast. The pectoralis muscle (*arrows*) is seen from the axilla to below the level of the posterior nipple line. The inframammary fold (*curved arrow*) is well seen and the nipple is in profile.

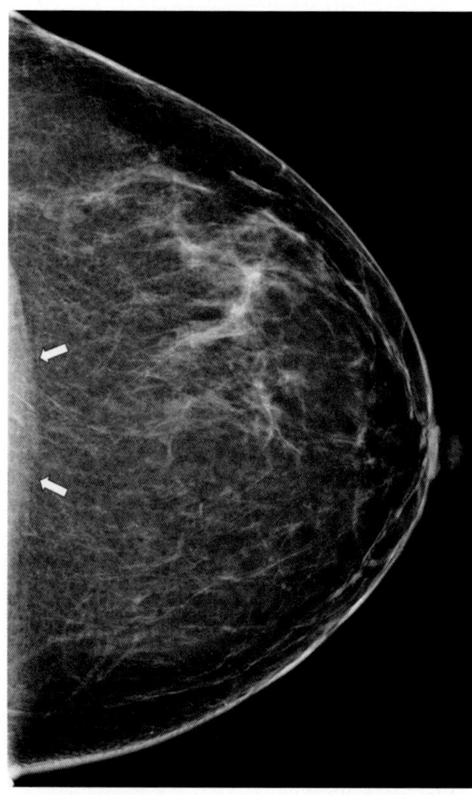

FIGURE 19.5. **CC Positioning.** Normal craniocaudal view of the left breast. Note that the nipple is in profile and the pectoralis muscle (*arrows*) is seen posteriorly indicating optimal visualization of breast tissue.

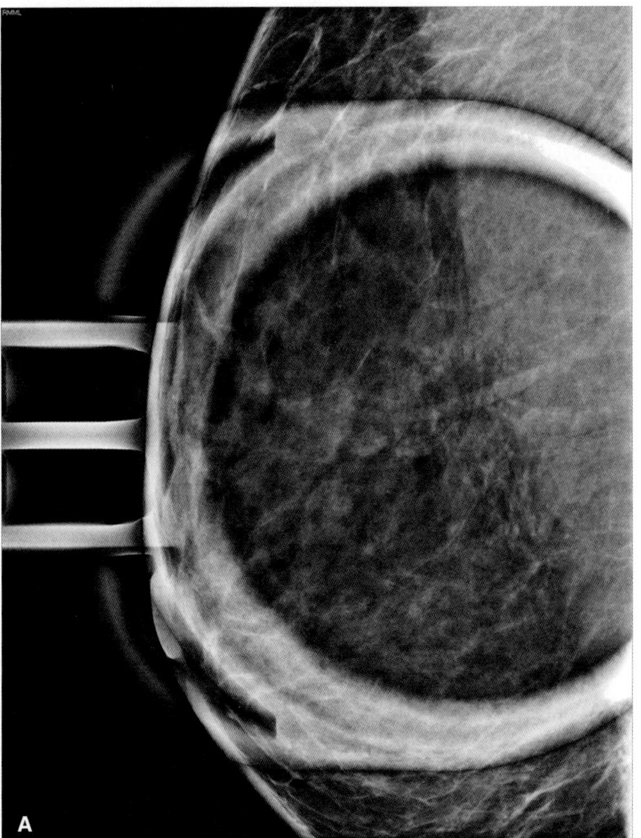

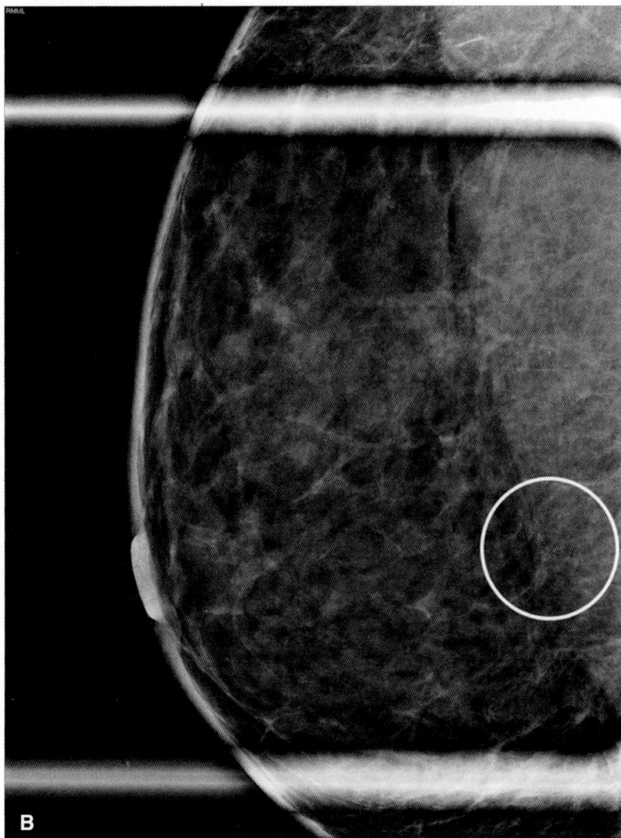

FIGURE 19.6. **Blur. A:** Magnification mediolateral view with blur. **B:** Repeat magnification ML view without blur allows easier identification of the suspicious group of amorphous calcifications (*circle*). Ductal carcinoma in situ was found on biopsy.

Patients should also be reminded prior to mammography to avoid antiperspirant and skin creams. Typically, these cause radiopaque densities on the skin and could be mistaken for microcalcifications within the breast (Fig. 19.7). If the technologist recognizes this artifact, they should attempt to clean the skin before repeating the mammogram. Hardware or processing errors can also create artifacts on the mammographic image, including ghosting, grid lines, dead pixels, edge processing, and pixel dropout, which the radiologist should recognize and usually recommend repeat imaging.

BREAST IMPLANTS

Approximately 2 million women have breast implants in the United States. Women with reconstructed breasts without native breast tissue after mastectomy do not require screening mammography. Women with implants for breast augmentation should undergo screening mammography. The presence of implants can make screening mammography more difficult, with one prospective study demonstrating lower sensitivity of mammography in women with breast implants. The standard CC and MLO projections with the implant included are performed to maximize the amount of breast tissue included. To optimize sensitivity and visualization in the anterior breast parenchyma, which is usually compressed by the implant, two additional implant-displaced (ID) views are also performed with the implant displaced back against the chest wall with the breast tissue pulled forward (Fig. 19.8). In total, four mammographic views are performed per breast, compared to the usual two views per breast.

Implant Types

Implants are commonly characterized by both their material and location. The two most widely used materials in implants are silicone and saline. Silicone implants appear uniformly hyperdense on mammography. Saline implants are less dense than silicone, where the x-ray beam is able to penetrate the filling material. Unlike in silicone-filled implants, the radial folds and implant valve are typically visible in a saline-filled implant due to the lower density. There are also dual-lumen implants, consisting of both saline and silicone lumens, but are utilized less commonly. Regardless of the material, after the implant is placed in the breast, the body normally generates a fibrous capsule around the implant. The fibrous capsule plays an important role in the description of rupture. Implants are also described by their location: subglandular or subpectoral. Subpectoral implants are less associated with capsular contracture than subglandular implants. Capsular contracture is a clinical diagnosis where there is abnormal constriction of the fibrous capsule on the implant, and clinically the patient states the implant feels abnormally spherical and firm.

Implant Rupture

Mammograms can help detect implant-related complications, including rupture. When saline implants rupture, there is rapid decompression and clinically the diagnosis is obvious. On mammography, the saline implant will be decompressed and retracted against the chest wall (Fig. 19.9A). For silicone

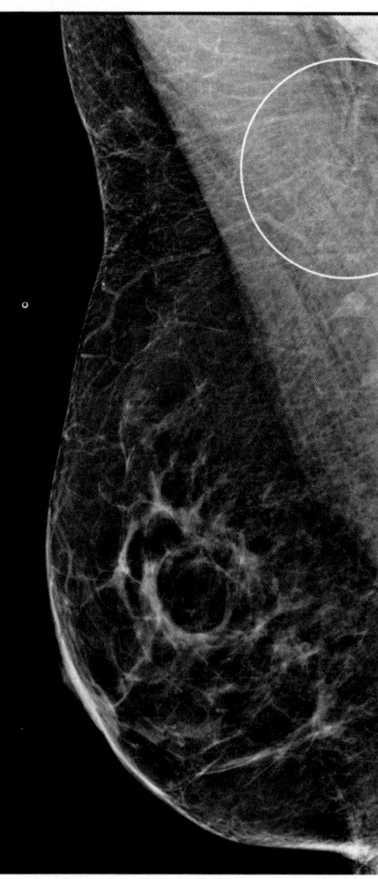

FIGURE 19.7. **Deodorant.** Deodorant is seen in the right axilla overlying the pectoralis muscle (*circle*). Many deodorants, powders, and ointments contain radiopaque components, which may simulate calcifications.

implants, evaluation of implant rupture is more difficult given the density of the silicone filling. The presence of a contour bulge or obvious radiopaque silicone extending away from the implant suggests intra- or extracapsular rupture (Fig. 19.9B). However, MR imaging has been shown to be the most sensitive imaging study to evaluate for silicone implant rupture. MR evaluation of implants will be covered further in Chapter 21.

TOMOSYNTHESIS

Digital breast tomosynthesis (DBT), also referred to as three-dimensional (3D) mammography, allows the breast to be viewed in a 3D format as multiple thin-slice images spanning the entire breast. The patient is positioned exactly the same as standard digital mammography during DBT. The difference is during the image acquisition; the x-ray tube pivots in an arc while the patient and the breast remain stationary. The tomosynthesis images are reconstructed from the projection images, similar to computed tomography. The tomosynthesis images consist of multiple thin (usually 1-mm) "slices" of the breast after reconstruction. The images can either then be analyzed by the radiologist by scrolling through the slice images manually or displayed as a cine loop, where the images are automatically scrolled through like a movie clip.

The advantages behind DBT in the interpretation of mammograms are twofold. In the screening population, interpretation relies heavily on the detection of masses, asymmetries, and architectural distortion. Overlying fibroglandular tissue has a masking effect on the detection of these lesions, which is why sensitivity decreases with increasing breast density. Through the use of thin slices through areas of fibroglandular tissue, the reader has an increased chance of detecting the cancer (Fig. 19.10). Alternately, superimposition of normal fibroglandular tissue is commonly mistaken as a mass or asymmetry, which subsequently resolves with additional diagnostic imaging (which would be classified as a false positive). The addition of

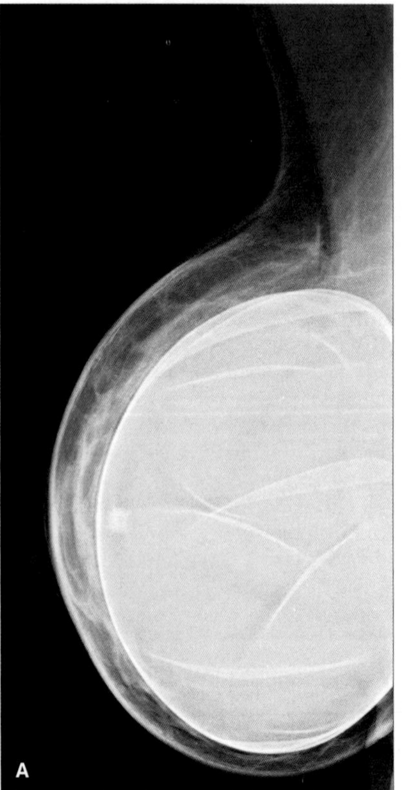

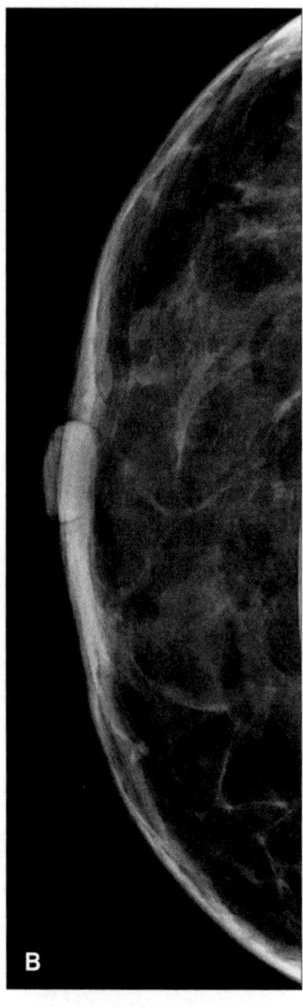

FIGURE 19.8. **Implant Displaced (ID) View.** Right craniocaudal views of a patient with a right breast implant. **A:** Full craniocaudal mammogram views all breast parenchyma and implant. **B:** Implant-displaced view demonstrates increased visualization and evaluation of the anterior breast parenchyma.

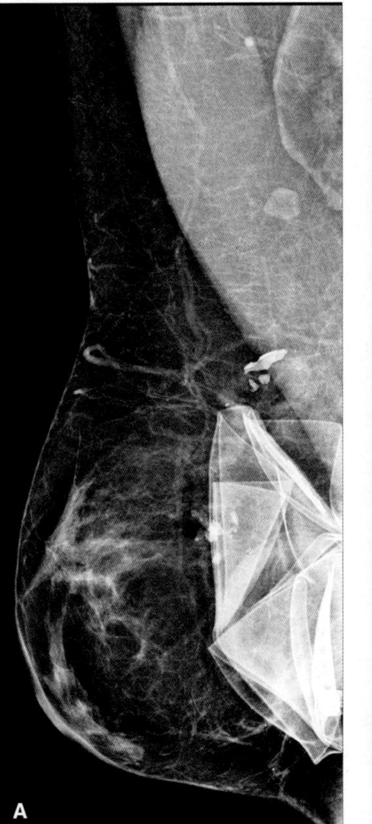

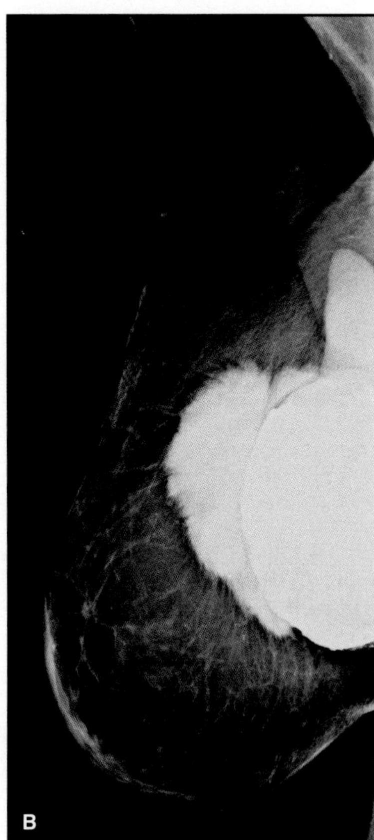

FIGURE 19.9. **Implant Rupture. A:** Right mediolateral oblique view demonstrates a deflated subglandular saline implant. Dystrophic calcifications of the fibrous capsule are also noted. **B:** Right mediolateral oblique view demonstrates hyperdense material extending anteriorly and superiorly from the subglandular silicone implant, consistent with extracapsular rupture.

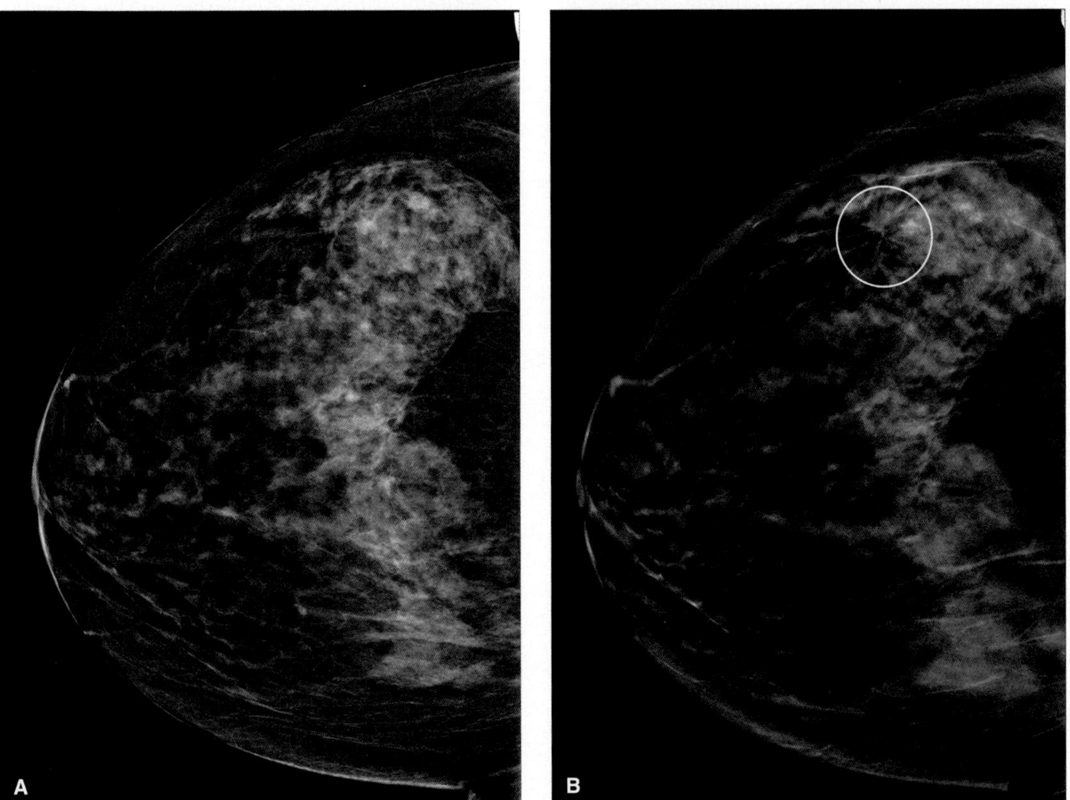

FIGURE 19.10. **Tomosynthesis. A:** Right CC view. **B:** Right CC tomosynthesis slice. The area of architectural distortion in the lateral breast is much more conspicuous on the tomosynthesis image (*circle*). Further workup and biopsy revealed invasive ductal carcinoma.

DBT to digital mammography would aid the radiologist in differentiating true masses from superimposing breast tissue.

Studies have confirmed that DBT has advantage over FFDM with improved overall accuracy in the screening population. The Oslo Tomosynthesis Screening Trial comparing FFDM with combined DBT and FFDM demonstrated a 27% increase in cancer detection rate and a 15% reduction in false-positive interpretations of screening mammography. Several other studies have demonstrated similar statistically significant increases in sensitivity and reduction in false-positive rates with the addition of DBT to FFDM in both the screening and diagnostic setting.

One consideration with DBT is patient dose. The tomosynthesis images are interpreted alongside a two-dimensional (2D) image, which was traditionally obtained with a standard digital mammogram image. Obtaining a 2D image and tomosynthesis images resulted in about a 38% increase in radiation dose per view. In 2013, the FDA approved the use of the first synthetic 2D image, which generates a 2D image from the DBT image acquisition data. The implementation of creating synthetic 2D, in place of obtaining separate 2D image, eliminates the additional radiation for patients undergoing DBT, with radiation doses on par with standard 2D FFDM images.

INTERPRETING THE MAMMOGRAM

Maximizing Your Interpretation

Classic mammographic signs of malignancy are spiculated masses or pleomorphic clusters of microcalcifications; however, only about 40% of all breast carcinoma presents in these ways. In the remainder of cases, more indeterminate findings for malignancy are present. Breast cancer can present as masses, architectural distortion, asymmetries, or calcifications. There are several characteristics of each finding that are more suspicious for malignancy than others. The radiologist must look at each mammogram with great care, so that false-negative diagnoses are minimized.

In most practices, patients are asked to complete a brief history form that includes questions relevant to breast health and cancer risk. This first allows the technologist to appropriately identify which patients should be set up for diagnostic evaluation prior to imaging. Also, knowledge of the patient's history prior to image interpretation is helpful for the radiologist to ensure findings associated with prior surgical scars, posttraumatic changes, or hormone replacement are appropriately interpreted.

Viewing conditions are extremely important for optimal interpretation. The room must be darkened. Computer workstations should be used for FFDM interpretation with high-resolution monitors and magnification capability. If films are being interpreted, all adjacent view box light should be blocked out. Dedicated mammography film alternators and view boxes can do this automatically. If standard view boxes or alternators are used, exposed blackened film can be cut to mask out unwanted light.

As mentioned previously, a screening mammogram consists of two views of each breast: the CC and the MLO views. A reasonable approach to viewing mammograms is discussed below; however radiologists will develop their own individual processes for reviewing studies. Whatever protocol a radiologist chooses should be consistent and thorough to optimize efficiency and cancer detection.

First, confirm that the name and other patient identifiers are correct (i.e., you are reading the correct study) and that the images are of adequate quality. As mentioned previously, images must have good contrast, compression, positioning, and lack of blur or other artifacts. An overview screen with the entire current study compared with prior studies is helpful to check for obvious abnormalities and changes from the previous studies. Next, examine each CC view to look for imaging findings suggestive of disease in the breast parenchymal pattern, such as masses or asymmetries. View the image at full resolution or a magnifying glass to maximize visualization of calcifications and architectural distortion. All visible breast parenchyma should be scanned systematically to ensure that all parts of the breast have been examined. Compare the left and right CC views, side by side, to identify more subtle asymmetries. If tomosynthesis views were obtained, they should be analyzed next. The process is then repeated for the MLO views and any additional views that may have been obtained as part of the study.

If a finding is identified, compare with the prior mammograms to assess whether the finding is new, growing, or stable by using as many prior studies as possible. Typically, findings that have been stable for 2 years are considered benign. Any suspicious mammographic change in the finding should warrant further workup with diagnostic imaging. For masses or asymmetries, a suspicious change could include increase in size, increase in density, or development of more suspicious margins. For calcifications, an increase in number or extent is considered a suspicious change. Keep in mind that malignant masses or calcifications that are unchanged in appearance for up to 4.5 years have been reported. Although such a long period of stability is unusual, these reports emphasize the need for highly suspicious–appearing lesions or calcifications to undergo biopsy regardless of their apparent lack of change in size on serial films. Such lesions may have been overlooked or misinterpreted on a previous study.

The importance of comparing current mammograms with previous films cannot be overstated. Comparison with previous films will allow detection of subtle changes, in turn suggesting the need for further evaluation of such areas at an earlier time than might be possible if no comparison had been made (Fig. 19.11). Benign breast lesions may appear new when compared to priors or enlarge over time, and interval mammographic changes are commonly due to benign etiologies, but such changes should be fully evaluated through the use of diagnostic evaluation from the screening setting.

Interpreting mammograms is primarily pattern recognition as radiologists try to detect signs of malignancy from normal breast parenchyma. As radiologists gain more experience interpreting mammograms, the better they perform. One study examined the influence of volume of screening mammograms interpreted to performance outcomes in the United States. They found that higher-volume readers demonstrate lower false-positive rates (screening mammograms that were falsely interpreted as abnormal) and similar cancer detection rates than radiologists with lower annual volumes. The U.S. Food and Drug Administration requires radiologists who interpret mammograms to have read at least 960 mammograms within the last 2 years.

Breast Density

The breast is composed of radiopaque breast parenchyma and radiolucent fatty elements. The relative amount of tissue density to fat is classified into four mammographic density categories by the Breast Imaging Reporting and Data System (BI-RADS) lexicon. In the 4th edition of BI-RADS released in 2003, the four density categories were split by quartiles as follows: almost entirely fatty (<25%), scattered fibroglandular densities (25% to 50%), heterogeneously dense (50% to 75%),

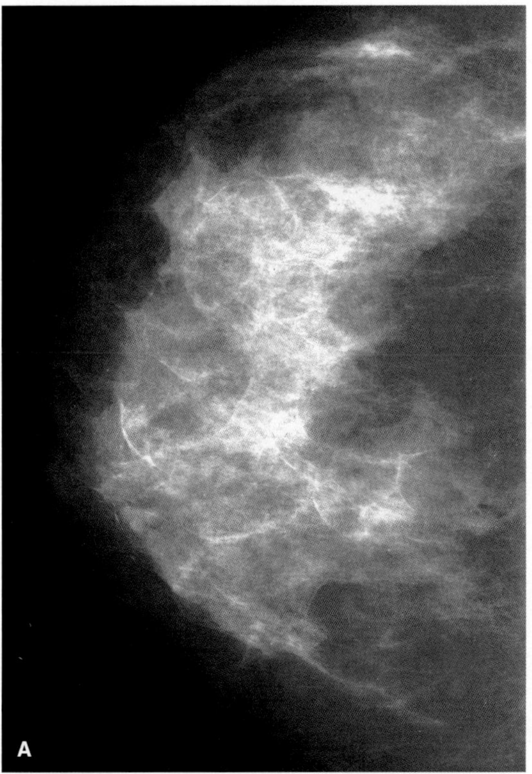

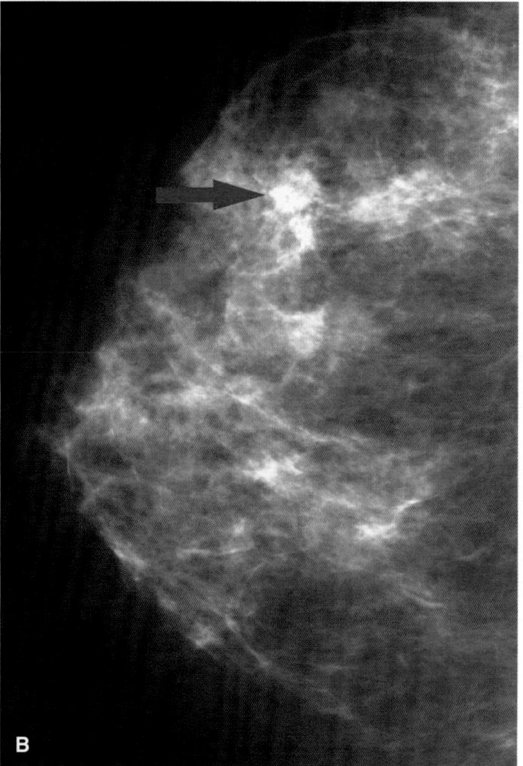

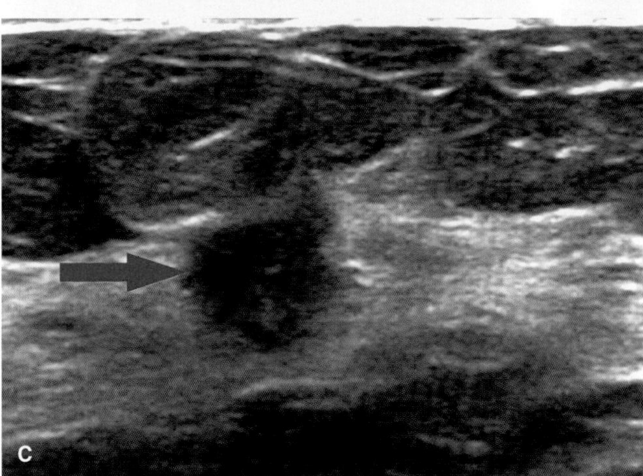

FIGURE 19.11. Infiltrating Ductal Carcinoma. **A:** Craniocaudal mammogram shows dense mammary parenchyma but no evidence of malignancy. **B:** Mammogram 1 year later shows development of a subtle new mass (*arrow*). **C:** US shows an irregular, solid mass (*arrow*) with indistinct margins. Biopsy demonstrated an infiltrating duct carcinoma.

and extremely dense (>75%). The 5th edition of BI-RADS released in 2014 updated the density categories in an effort to have radiologists account for masking effect when categorizing breast density (Fig. 19.12). The density categories in the 5th edition of BI-RADS are listed as: BI-RADS a—the breasts are almost entirely fatty; BI-RADS b—there are scattered areas of fibroglandular density; BI-RADS c—the breasts are heterogeneously dense, which may obscure small masses; and BI-RADS d—the breasts are extremely dense, which lowers the sensitivity of mammography. The distribution of tissue density as gathered by the Breast Cancer Surveillance Consortium (BCSC) from 934,098 negative screening mammograms obtained from 1994 to 2008 can be seen on Figure 19.13. Most breast density categorization are performed subjectively by the radiologists. Several automated breast density assessment softwares are currently available that can help improve reliability.

Increased breast density has shown to decrease sensitivity of mammograms in the detection of malignancy due to masking effect. Mammography is based on the detection of cancers due to their inherent contrast difference with the adjacent structures, with the most contrast difference with fat density. With increasing breast density, overlapping radiopaque dense breast tissue may obscure underlying cancers. In a study performed by Carney, the sensitivity of mammography in fatty breasts was 88%, compared to 62% in extremely dense breasts.

Another reason breast density is important is that breast density is an independent risk factor for breast cancer. The increased risk in breast cancer is likely due to the fact that breast cancers typically arise from epithelial cells, which is found in the glandular breast parenchyma. Higher breast density means more glandular tissue, which means more epithelial cells that may turn into malignancy. McCormack performed a meta-analysis of research studies examining the relationship of breast density and cancer risk and demonstrated relative risks in the incidence of breast cancer of heterogeneously dense and extremely dense patients at 2.92 and 4.64, respectively.

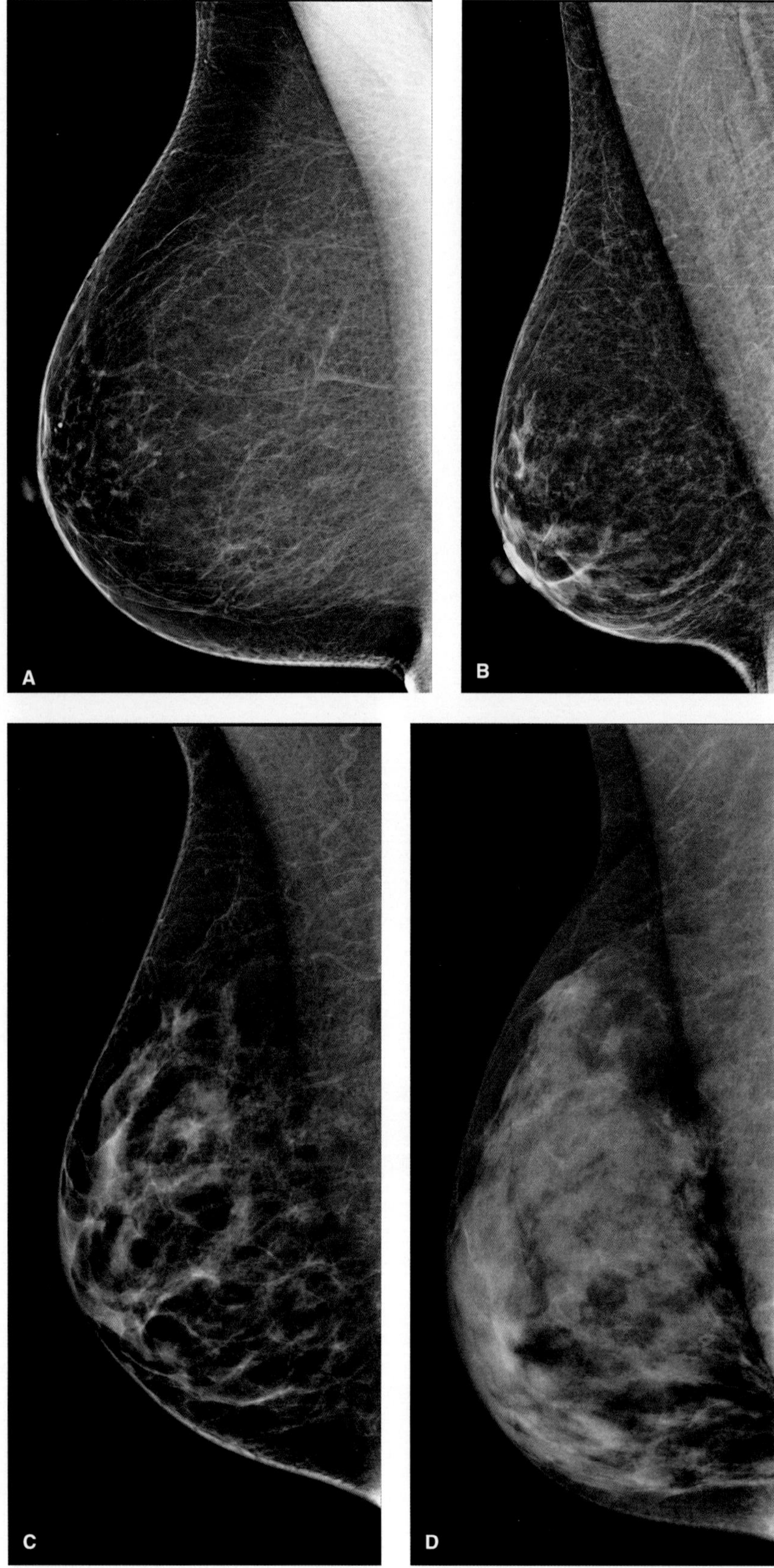

FIGURE 19.12. **Breast Density in the MLO Projections.** A: Fatty. B: Scattered fibroglandular tissue. C: Heterogeneously dense. D: Extremely dense.

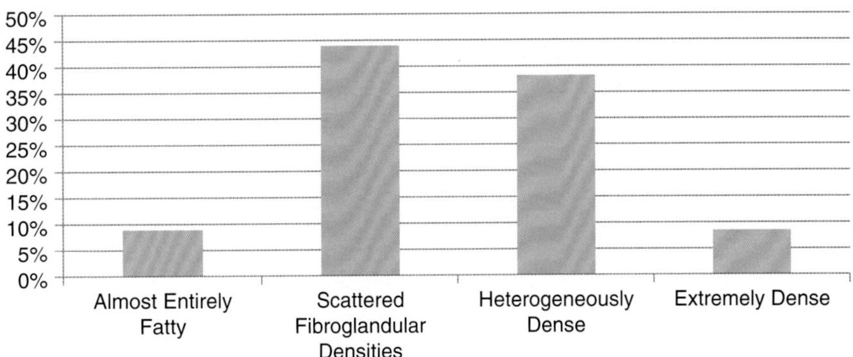

FIGURE 19.13. Distribution of Tissue Densities.

Because of these factors, several states have passed breast density notification legislation mandating that women who are categorized as BI-RADS c (heterogeneously dense) or BI-RADS d (extremely dense) are notified. As of 2018, currently 35 states have mandatory breast density notification laws in effect and several others are working on introducing their own. The legislation varies from state to state but most generally inform the woman that mammography may be less sensitive due to their breast density and that they should discuss adjunct screening modalities with their primary care physician.

THE USE OF OTHER IMAGING MODALITIES FOR BREAST CANCER SCREENING

Mammography is the only imaging modality that has been proven to reduce breast cancer mortality when used to screen asymptomatic women. However, the overall sensitivity of mammography varies across the population and can be as low as 42% in women with dense breasts. Because of this fact, other imaging modalities have been developed as a supplement to traditional digital mammography in the screening population. MR is being used for breast cancer screening in conjunction with mammography in high-risk women. Screening ultrasound is currently being used as a supplemental tool for women with dense breasts. Several functional images have also shown promise for the same population.

Screening Breast Ultrasound

Several single-institution studies have shown that whole breast screening US can detect small nonpalpable invasive cancers not seen mammographically in women with heterogeneously dense or extremely dense breasts. A multi-institution trial of screening breast US as an adjunct to mammography in high-risk women reported an incremental cancer detection rate of 4.2/1,000 women screened with both modalities as compared to mammography alone; however, false positives were also increased substantially when US was used. Several follow-up studies have confirmed an additional cancer detection rate of 3 per 1,000 examinations in women with dense breasts.

Studies comparing mammography, breast US, and breast MR for screening in high-risk women have shown that supplemental screening with US adds no benefit when these women are appropriately screened with mammography and breast MR. US screening may, however, be useful in high-risk women in whom MR is contraindicated or cannot be tolerated. In addition to high false-positive rates, there are challenges to the incorporation of US as a screening modality. US is highly dependent on the operator and on the equipment and technique used for scanning. It is also a time consuming, labor-intensive examination, which should be performed by a radiologist or technologist trained in the technique.

Automated breast ultrasound units have been developed, which uncouples image acquisition from interpretation. The advantages of automated breast over handheld sonography include minimizing operator dependence, improved consistency and reproducibility, and do not require physician time for image acquisition. Disadvantages include more shadowing artifacts and possible lack of coverage for axillary and lateral regions of large breasts. Recent studies examining automated breast ultrasound have shown similar additional cancer yield rates of approximately 3 per 1,000 examinations.

Functional Imaging

Mammography and ultrasound are considered structural imaging, where the radiologist is trying to interpret physical changes within the breast. Functional imaging aims to analyze the physiologic activity within the breast. Functional imaging modalities have the benefit of increased sensitivity over structural imaging studies. MRI with contrast capitalizes on the detection of blood flow to cancers through intravenous contrast, which enhances the lesion. In regards to screening for breast cancer, MRI is currently only recommended as a supplement to mammography in high-risk women. Breast MRI will be discussed separately in Chapter 21.

Contrast-enhanced spectral mammography (CESM) has been developed to also aid in the detection of increased blood flow associated with breast cancer, without the high expense, long lengths of examination, and limited availability concerns of MRI. To obtain the images, the patient is first administered intravenous iodinated contrast, then placed in compression, similar to the standard mammographic views. However, during each image acquisition, the mammographic unit obtains two images: a low-energy image and a high-energy image. The low-energy image appears similar to a standard 2D image. The high-energy image is processed to highlight the iodine-enhanced portions of the breast and suppress the background breast tissue. The high-energy image allows the radiologist to see areas of abnormal enhancement (Fig. 19.14). Early research studies have demonstrated CESM to perform with similar sensitivity in cancer detection to MRI, with both demonstrating improved detection over standard mammography.

Breast-specific gamma imaging (BSGI) employs the use of technetium-99m sestamibi to detect malignancy. The modality takes advantage of the fact that sestamibi demonstrates increased uptake in breast cancer. Like the previously mentioned examinations in this section because this modality is functional, rather than anatomic, breast density of the patient does not affect the sensitivity of the examination. One study

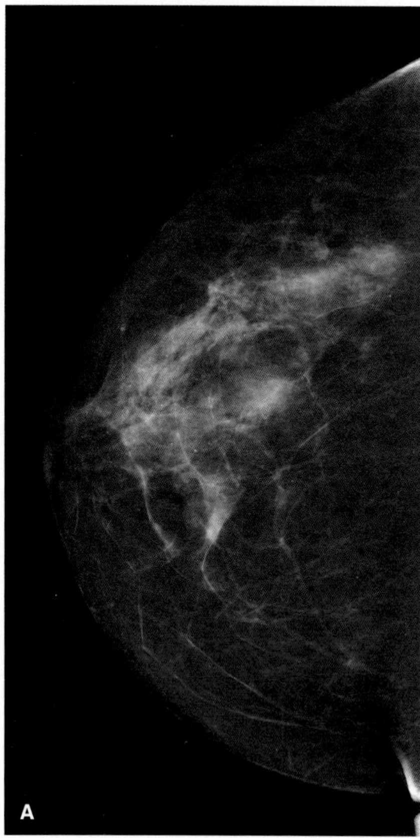

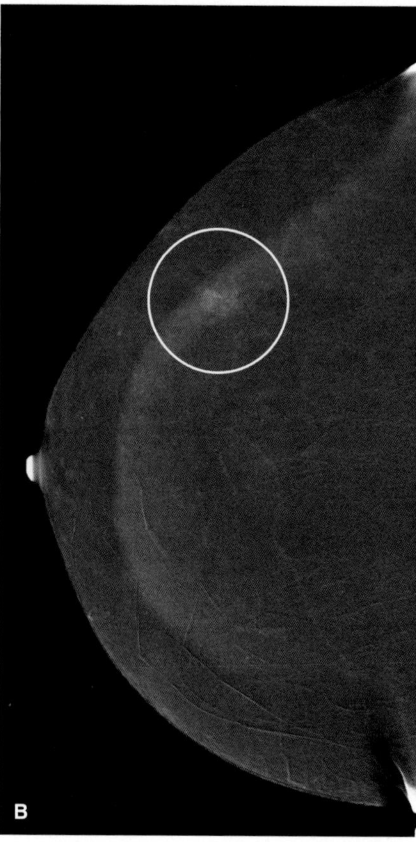

FIGURE 19.14. **Contrast-Enhanced Spectral Mammography (CESM). A:** Right CC view. **B:** Right CC CESM image. Area of enhancement in the lateral view correlates with a tubular carcinoma (*circle*).

by Brem demonstrated a sensitivity of 96.4% and a specificity of 59.5%. The big disadvantage with BSGI includes its high relative radiation level. Hendrick noted that the radiation dose of a single BSGI was comparable to a lifetime annual screening mammography. Ongoing research is currently being performed to increase the sensitivity of the detectors to allow for lower administered doses of technetium-99m sestamibi.

CONCLUSION

Screening mammography continues to be the single best test for early detection of breast cancer in order to reduce breast cancer mortality. However, it is likely that in the coming years a more individualized approach based on risk and other factors will be used in breast cancer screening, involving personalized screening strategies and supplemental imaging modalities.

Suggested Readings

Are you dense? Available from http://www.areyoudenseadvocacy.org/dense/ Updated 2018. Accessed April 5, 2018.

American Cancer Society. Breast Cancer Facts & Figures 2017–2018. Atlanta, GA: American Cancer Society, Inc. 2017. https://www.cancer.org/content/dam/cancer-org/research/cancer-facts-and-statistics/breast-cancer-facts-and-figures/breast-cancer-facts-and-figures-2017-2018.pdf. Accessed June 22, 2018.

American College of Radiology. ACR appropriateness criteria. Available from https://www.acr.org/Quality-Safety/Appropriateness-Criteria Updated 2017. Accessed 9/28, 2017.

Ayyala RS, Chorlton M, Behrman RH, Kornguth PJ, Slanetz PJ. Digital mammographic artifacts on full-field systems: what are they and how do I fix them? *Radiographics* 2008;28(7):1999–2008.

Berg WA, Blume JD, Cormack JB, et al. Combined screening with ultrasound and mammography vs mammography alone in women at elevated risk of breast cancer. *JAMA* 2008;299(18):2151–2163.

Brem RF, Floerke AC, Rapelyea JA, Teal C, Kelly T, Mathur V. Breast-specific gamma imaging as an adjunct imaging modality for the diagnosis of breast cancer. *Radiology* 2008;247(3):651–657.

Brem RF, Lenihan MJ, Lieberman J, Torrente J. Screening breast ultrasound: past, present, and future. *AJR Am J Roentgenol* 2015;204(2):234–240.

Buist DS, Anderson ML, Haneuse SJ, et al. Influence of annual interpretive volume on screening mammography performance in the United States. *Radiology* 2011;259(1):72–84.

Carney PA, Miglioretti DL, Yankaskas BC, et al. Individual and combined effects of age, breast density, and hormone replacement therapy use on the accuracy of screening mammography. *Ann Intern Med* 2003;138(3):168–175.

Chiarelli AM, Edwards SA, Prummel MV, et al. Digital compared with screen-film mammography: performance measures in concurrent cohorts within an organized breast screening program. *Radiology* 2013;268(3):684–693.

Ciatto S, Houssami N, Bernardi D, et al. Integration of 3D digital mammography with tomosynthesis for population breast-cancer screening (STORM): a prospective comparison study. *Lancet Oncol* 2013;14(7):583–589.

Curpen BN, Sickles EA, Sollitto RA, Ominsky SH, Galvin HB, Frankel SD. The comparative value of mammographic screening for women 40–49 years old versus women 50–64 years old. *AJR Am J Roentgenol* 1995;164(5):1099–1103.

D'Orsi C, Sickles E, Mendelson E, Morris E, et al. *ACR BI-RADS® Atlas: Breast Imaging Reporting and Data System*. 5th ed. Reston, VA: American College of Radiology; 2013.

Elkin EB, Hudis C, Begg CB, Schrag D. The effect of changes in tumor size on breast carcinoma survival in the U.S.: 1975–1999. *Cancer* 2005;104(6):1149–1157.

Fallenberg EM, Schmitzberger FF, Amer H, et al. Contrast-enhanced spectral mammography vs. mammography and MRI—clinical performance in a multi-reader evaluation. *Eur Radiol* 2017;27(7):2752–2764.

Feig SA, Ehrlich SM. Estimation of radiation risk from screening mammography: recent trends and comparison with expected benefits. *Radiology* 1990;174(3 Pt 1):638–647.

Gennaro G, Bernardi D, Houssami N. Radiation dose with digital breast tomosynthesis compared to digital mammography: per-view analysis. *Eur Radiol* 2018;28(2):573–581.

Helvie MA, Chan HP, Adler DD, Boyd PG. Breast thickness in routine mammograms: effect on image quality and radiation dose. *AJR Am J Roentgenol* 1994;163(6):1371–1374.

Hendrick RE. Radiation doses and cancer risks from breast imaging studies. *Radiology* 2010;257(1):246–253.

Hendrick RE, Smith RA, Rutledge JH 3rd, Smart CR. Benefit of screening mammography in women aged 40-49: a new meta-analysis of randomized controlled trials. *J Natl Cancer Inst Monogr* 1997;(22):87–92.

Hooley RJ, Greenberg KL, Stackhouse RM, Geisel JL, Butler RS, Philpotts LE. Screening US in patients with mammographically dense breasts: initial experience with Connecticut Public Act 09-41. *Radiology* 2012;265(1):59–69.

Kelly KM, Dean J, Comulada WS, Lee SJ. Breast cancer detection using automated whole breast ultrasound and mammography in radiographically dense breasts. *Eur Radiol* 2010;20(3):734–742.

Kerlikowske K, Grady D, Barclay J, Sickles EA, Ernster V. Effect of age, breast density, and family history on the sensitivity of first screening mammography. *JAMA* 1996;276(1):33–38.

Kerlikowske K, Zhu W, Hubbard RA, et al; Breast Cancer Surveillance Consortium. Outcomes of screening mammography by frequency, breast density, and postmenopausal hormone therapy. *JAMA Intern Med* 2013;173(9):807–816.

Lee-Felker SA, Tekchandani L, Thomas M, et al. Newly diagnosed breast cancer: comparison of contrast-enhanced spectral mammography and breast MR imaging in the evaluation of extent of disease. *Radiology* 2017;285(2):389–400.

Linver MN, Paster SB. Mammography outcomes in a practice setting by age: prognostic factors, sensitivity, and positive biopsy rate. *J Natl Cancer Inst Monogr* 1997;(22):113–117.

McCormack VA, dos Santos Silva I. Breast density and parenchymal patterns as markers of breast cancer risk: a meta-analysis. *Cancer Epidemiol Biomarkers Prev* 2006;15(6):1159–1169.

Miglioretti DL, Rutter CM, Geller BM, et al. Effect of breast augmentation on the accuracy of mammography and cancer characteristics. *JAMA* 2004; 291(4):442–450.

Nystrom L, Rutqvist LE, Wall S, et al. Breast cancer screening with mammography: overview of Swedish randomised trials. *Lancet* 1993;341(8851):973–978.

Oeffinger KC, Fontham ET, Etzioni R, et al. Breast cancer screening for women at average risk: 2015 guideline update from the American Cancer Society. *JAMA* 2015;314(15):1599–1614.

Paci E, Duffy SW, Giorgi D, et al. Quantification of the effect of mammographic screening on fatal breast cancers: The Florence Programme 1990-96. *Br J Cancer* 2002;87(1):65–69.

Pisano ED, Gatsonis C, Hendrick E, et al. Diagnostic performance of digital versus film mammography for breast-cancer screening. *N Engl J Med* 2005;353(17):1773–1783.

Saslow D, Boetes C, Burke W, et al. American Cancer Society guidelines for breast screening with MRI as an adjunct to mammography. *CA Cancer J Clin* 2007;57(2):75–89.

Scaranelo AM, Marques AF, Smialowski EB, Lederman HM. Evaluation of the rupture of silicone breast implants by mammography, ultrasonography and magnetic resonance imaging in asymptomatic patients: correlation with surgical findings. *Sao Paulo Med J* 2004;122(2):41–47.

Shapiro S. Evidence on screening for breast cancer from a randomized trial. *Cancer* 1977;39(6 Suppl):2772–2782.

Siu AL; U.S. Preventive Services Task Force. Screening for breast cancer: U.S. Preventive Services Task Force recommendation statement. *Ann Intern Med* 2016;164(4):279–296.

Skaane P, Bandos AI, Gullien R, et al. Comparison of digital mammography alone and digital mammography plus tomosynthesis in a population-based screening program. *Radiology* 2013;267(1):47–56.

Tabar L, Fagerberg CJ, Gad A, et al. Reduction in mortality from breast cancer after mass screening with mammography. Randomised trial from the Breast Cancer Screening Working Group of the Swedish National Board of Health and Welfare. *Lancet* 1985;1(8433):829–832.

Tabar L, Vitak B, Chen HH, Yen MF, Duffy SW, Smith RA. Beyond randomized controlled trials: organized mammographic screening substantially reduces breast carcinoma mortality. *Cancer* 2001;91(9):1724–1731.

US Preventive Services Task Force. Screening for breast cancer: U.S. Preventive Services Task Force recommendation statement. *Ann Intern Med* 2009; 151(10):716–726, W-236.

Vyborny CJ, Schmidt RA. Mammography as a radiographic examination: an overview. *Radiographics* 1989;9(4):723–764.

Wald NJ, Murphy P, Major P, Parkes C, Townsend J, Frost C. UKCCCR multicentre randomised controlled trial of one and two view mammography in breast cancer screening. *BMJ* 1995;311(7014):1189–1193.

Weigert J, Steenbergen S. The Connecticut experiment: the role of ultrasound in the screening of women with dense breasts. *Breast J* 2012;18(6): 517–522.

White E, Miglioretti DL, Yankaskas BC, et al. Biennial versus annual mammography and the risk of late-stage breast cancer. *J Natl Cancer Inst* 2004; 96(24):1832–1839.

Yaffe MJ. AAPM tutorial. Physics of mammography: image recording process. *Radiographics* 1990;10(2):341–363.

Zuley ML, Bandos AI, Ganott MA, et al. Digital breast tomosynthesis versus supplemental diagnostic mammographic views for evaluation of noncalcified breast lesions. *Radiology* 2013;266(1):89–95.

CHAPTER 20 ■ IMAGING THE DIAGNOSTIC PATIENT

JONATHAN V. NGUYEN, CARRIE M. ROCHMAN, AND BRANDI T. NICHOLSON

INTRODUCTION

While screening mammography is performed on asymptomatic women to hopefully identify early-stage breast cancer, diagnostic examinations are used to work up abnormal screening mammograms and to evaluate patients with clinical symptoms. Due to the nature of the patient population diagnostic examinations have higher abnormal interpretation rates, higher positive predictive values, and higher cancer detection rates, which can be about 10 times more prevalent than in the screening population. The distinction between screening and diagnostic examination is important as diagnostic examinations usually require specifically targeted imaging with mammography and/or sonography.

DIAGNOSTIC MAMMOGRAPHY

Diagnostic mammography is done in women who have had a recent abnormal screening mammogram, who have a current sign or symptom of malignancy, are being followed for a probably benign finding, or have a personal history of breast cancer. Diagnostic mammogram views can include the traditional full views, like craniocaudal (CC) and mediolateral oblique (MLO), as well as other specific views to best evaluate the area of concern or needing follow-up (Table 20.1).

Spot Compression Views

Spot compression mammographic views are used to evaluate equivocal findings seen on full-field mammographic views. Spot compression involves a smaller compression paddle than the one used for full-field views, which apply compression to a specific area within the breast. Spot compression views are essential in the diagnostic workup for masses, architectural distortion, and asymmetries. Compression has several benefits for mammography: decreases breast thickness to improve contrast, reduces blurriness of the image, and displaces glandular tissue. The last characterstic is an important aspect in diagnostic imaging. Typically, glandular tissue is soft and mobile, which is easily displaced with spot compression views. It can be common for superimposition of normal glandular tissue to mimic a mass or asymmetry, which can resolve with spot compression views. In contrast, breast cancers tend to be firm and not easily compressible due to the desmoplastic response initiated by some tumors resulting in less displacement on spot compression views. Therefore, spot compression views allow better visualization and characterization of mammographic masses. Any indeterminate mammographic finding that persists after spot compression views should further be evaluated with ultrasound.

Magnification Views

Microcalcifications are commonly seen on mammographic images and typically represent a benign process. Most of the microcalcifications recommended for biopsy result in benign pathology (70% to 80%). However, they can also be a sign of underlying malignancy, most commonly ductal carcinoma in situ. Proper evaluation and characterization during diagnostic evaluation is important to increase the positive predictive value for a biopsy of calcifications.

When microcalcifications are being evaluated, typically magnification views in the CC and true lateral (either ML or LM) projections are performed. A lateral projection is used for magnification views over the MLO projection to evaluate for milk of calcium and for better localization. Magnification views are of higher resolution than full-field views, which allows more accurate assessment of the morphology of microcalcifications and the borders of masses, when present.

When evaluating calcifications, first verify and try to localize them within the breast, to ensure they are not within the skin or artifact. Tangential views can be performed if there is suspicion for dermal calcifications (Fig. 20.1). Then assess if they can be classified as a specific benign morphology, and be given a Breast Imaging Reporting and Data System (BI-RADS)

TABLE 20.1

DIAGNOSTIC MAMMOGRAPHIC VIEWS

■ VIEW	■ ABBREVIATION	■ PURPOSE
90-degree lateral	ML (mediolateral) or LM (lateromedial)	Localizing lesion seen in one view Demonstrate milk of calcium due to its gravity dependency
Spot compression	SC	Determine whether lesion is real or is a summation shadow
Spot compression with magnification	M	Better definition of margins of masses and morphology of calcifications
Exaggerated craniocaudal	XCCL	Show lesions in outer aspect of breast and axillary tail not seen on CC view
Cleavage view	CV	Show lesions deep in posteromedial breast not seen in CC view
Tangential	TAN	Verify skin lesions Show palpable lesions obscured by dense tissue
Rolled views	CCRM (rolled medial) or CCRL (rolled lateral)	Verify true lesions Determine location of lesion seen in one view by seeing how location changes
Lateromedial oblique	LMO	Improved visualization of superomedial tissue Improved tissue visualization and comfort for women with pectus excavatum, recent sternotomy, prominent pacemaker

2: benign finding assessment. One classic example is milk of calcium, where calcium deposits within cysts can be seen layering on the magnification ML view (Fig. 20.2). The morphology, distribution, and comparison to priors are all essential in proper characterization of calcifications. If the calcifications are indeterminate (Fig. 20.3), a stereotactic biopsy should be performed, which will be covered in Chapter 23.

True Lateral and Rolled CC Views

Asymmetries, mammographic findings that do not conform to a radiosense mass and that are only viewed in one project, on a mammographic examination can be hard to interpret. Most of these findings end up to be superimposition of breast tissues; however the other possibility is a true breast lesion that is either obscured or not included in the image in the other projection. These one-view findings can be evaluated with true lateral and rolled CC views when digital breast tomosynthesis (DBT) is not available. If the one-view finding is seen only in the MLO projection, acquisition of a mediolateral (ML) or lateromedial (LM) view can either help to resolve

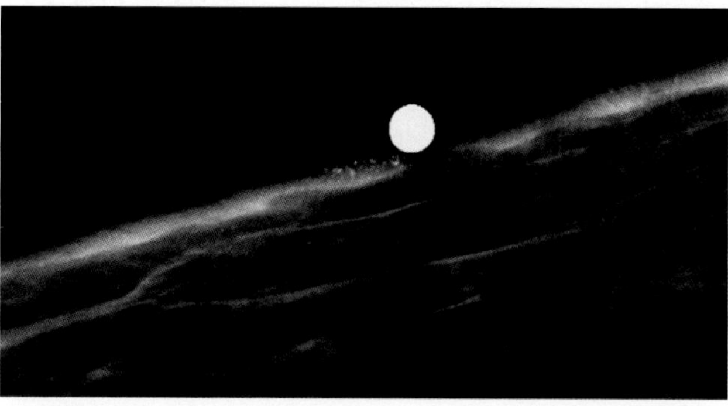

FIGURE 20.1. **Skin Calcifications.** Tangential view showing calcifications to be in the skin. A radiopaque marker had been placed on the skin at the site of the calcifications. This was done to facilitate positioning for the tangential view.

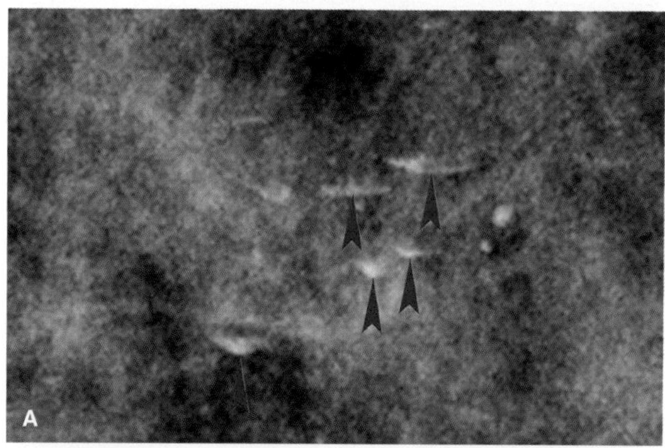

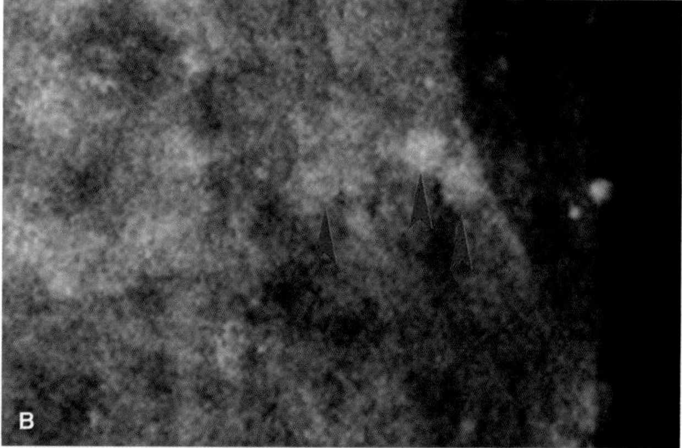

FIGURE 20.2. **Milk of Calcium in Breast Cysts. A:** Magnification of a 90-degree lateral mammogram showing milk of calcium or layering calcifications (*arrowheads*). **B:** Craniocaudal magnification view of the same area showing smudged, rounded calcifications (*arrowheads*). This change in configuration between views is typical of sedimented calcium. The calcium is layering in the bottom of microcysts and so it appears as a line or meniscus when viewed from the side in the lateral projection. When viewed from the top, these calcifications simply appear smudged and rounded.

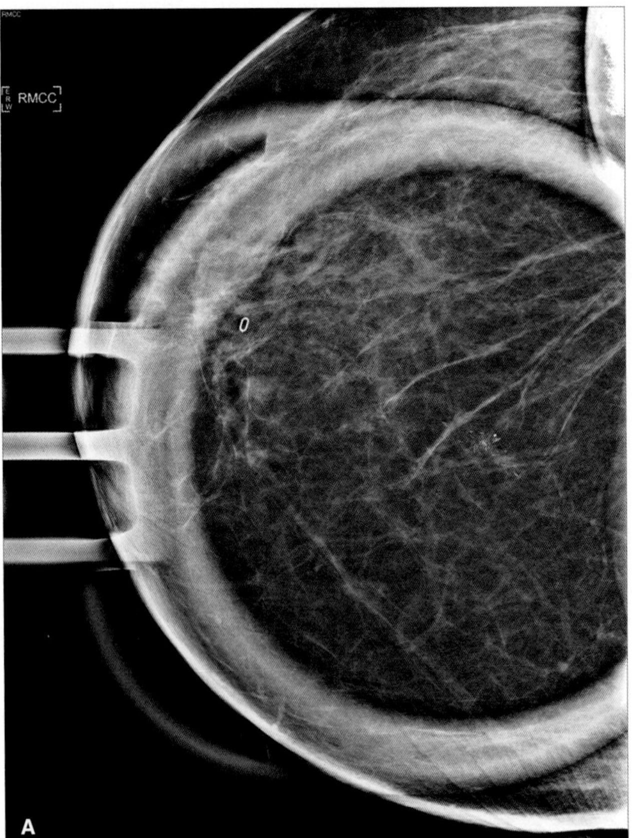

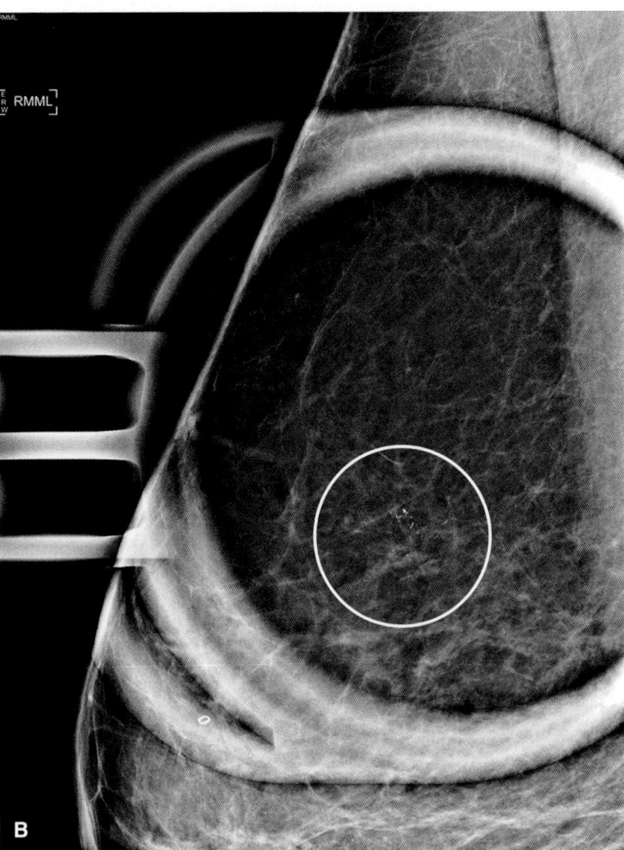

FIGURE 20.3. Suspicious Calcifications. A: Right magnification CC view. **B:** Right magnification ML view. A group of fine pleomorphic calcifications are identified (*circle*). Patient has history of prior benign biopsy marked by clip more anteriorly. Biopsy of the calcifications revealed ductal carcinoma in situ.

superimposition or aid in localization, if a true breast lesion is present. Lateral lesions will appear more inferior on the true lateral view compared to the MLO view, while medial lesions will appear more superior on the true lateral view compared to the MLO view. If the one-view finding is seen only in the CC projection, rolled CC views can be obtained. Rolled CC views are obtained by rolling the superior breast either medially (CC rolled medial) or laterally (CC rolled lateral) before the breast is compressed in the CC projection. These rolled CC views can also resolve or localize findings. For example, superior lesions will project more lateral on the rolled CC lateral (CCRL) image, while the inverse is true for inferior lesions. Spot compression views can also help resolve asymmetries as superimposition of breast tissue.

Tomosynthesis

Tomosynthesis in the diagnostic setting has been shown to perform comparable or superior to conventional diagnostic mammography. One study demonstrated improved efficiency with tomosynthesis in the diagnostic setting, with decreased amount of additional images needed compared to traditional 2D mammography. Due to its improved ability to differentiate superimposition versus true breast lesions, along with improved characterization of masses, tomosynthesis is increasingly being used in the diagnostic setting in lieu of 2D mammographic views; to evaluate masses, asymmetries, and architectural distortion (Fig. 20.4). Tomosynthesis can be done in full or spot compression views as needed. For highly suspicious lesions, tomosynthesis can also improve evaluation of extent, due to its increased sensitivity in the detection of masses. Tomosynthesis also has a great role in resolving whether a one-view asymmetry represents a true breast lesion or summation of normal breast structures.

Ultrasound

High-resolution ultrasound is an important tool in the diagnostic setting. Ultrasound consists of using mechanical/sound waves that travel through the body. As the pulse wave interacts with objects, there is echo generation, which the ultrasound probe can detect and uses to generate an image. The advantages of ultrasound are that it is less limited by breast density than mammography, is widely available, has no radiation, and sensitive in the detection of masses. The big disadvantages of ultrasound are that it is operator dependent, and has difficulty detecting calcifications and some forms of architectural distortion, which can both be signs of malignancy. Therefore, ultrasound is usually done alongside mammographic evaluation.

A limitation of mammography is differentiating cystic from solid masses. Ultrasound is useful for differentiating if a mammographic mass is solid or cystic. On ultrasound, simple cysts have a specific appearance; they are circumscribed, anechoic masses, usually with posterior acoustic enhancement (Fig. 20.5). For solid masses, ultrasound can additionally help to characterize margins and other imaging features that are suggestive of benign or malignant etiology. A common benign breast mass is a fibroadenoma. Fibroadenomas typically appear circumscribed, oval, and homogeneously

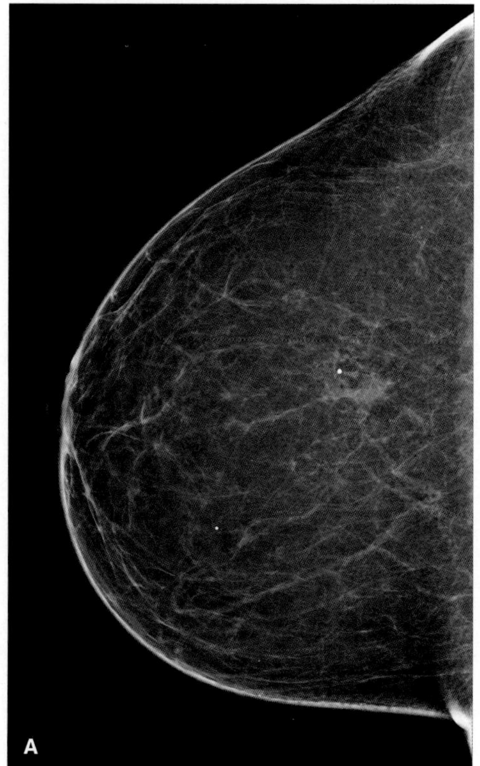

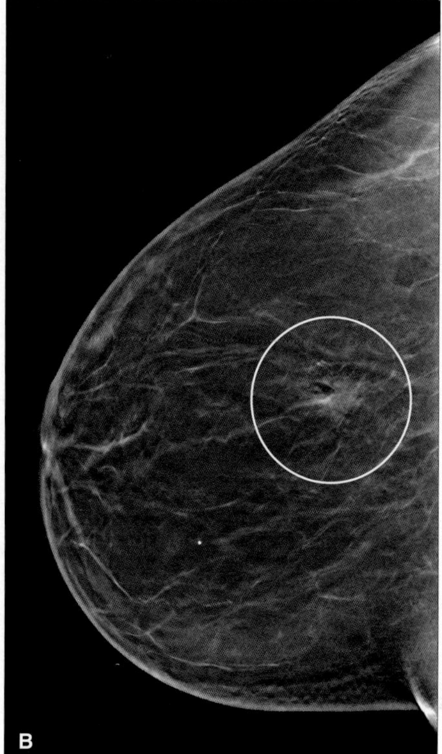

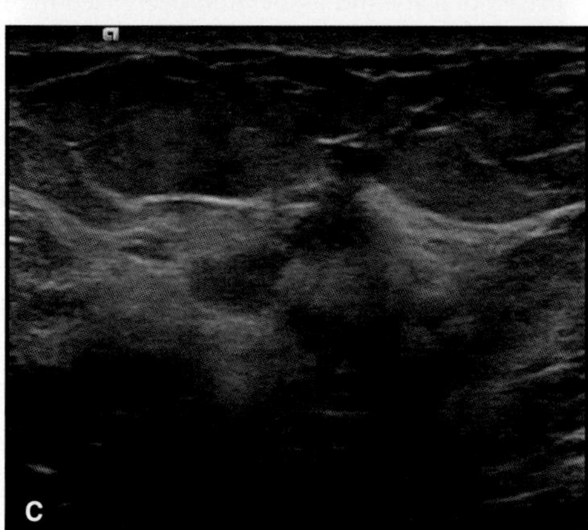

FIGURE 20.4. **Tomosynthesis in Diagnostic Examination.** **A:** Screening right CC identifies a developing asymmetry in the posterior aspect. **B:** Tomosynthesis allows better visualization and characterization. The finding now appears as an irregular-shaped mass with indistinct margins (*circle*). **C:** Ultrasound confirms an irregular-shaped mass. Biopsy revealed IDC.

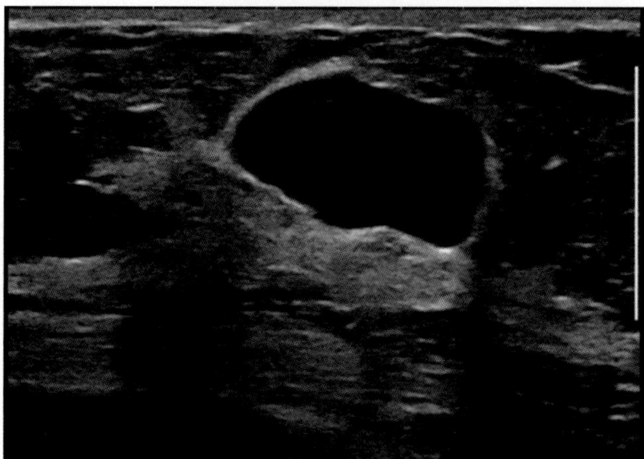

FIGURE 20.5. **Simple Cyst.** The classic sonographic appearance of a simple cyst is an anechoic circumscribed oval or round mass with posterior acoustic enhancement.

hypoechoic and these masses can be given a BI-RADS 3: probably benign impression on baseline examinations (Fig. 20.6). If a specific benign finding, such as a simple cyst or lymph node, is not identified, and the finding does not demonstrate benign features on ultrasound, then a biopsy is typically warranted (BI-RADS 4: suspicious finding or BI-RADS 5: highly suspicious for malignancy, depending on level of concern for cancer). If a lesion is identified under ultrasound, an ultrasound-guided biopsy can be performed, which will be covered separately in Chapter 23.

EVALUATION OF THE SYMPTOMATIC PATIENT

Patients with signs or symptoms of breast disease are not appropriate for a screening examination. Instead, these patients are seen for a diagnostic study with the imaging workup tailored to the specific situation. The American College of Radiology has created expert panels involving subspecialists to develop

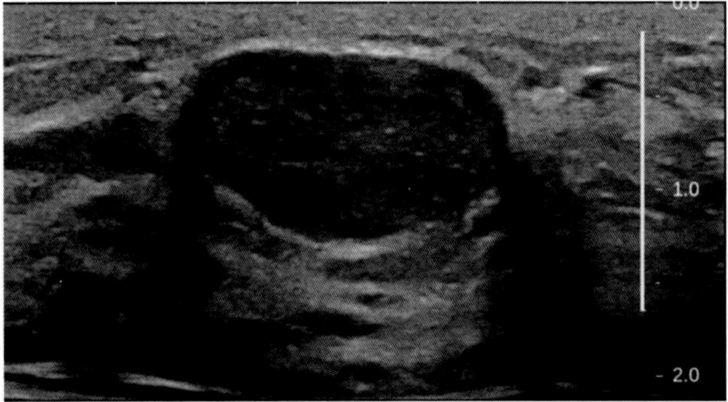

FIGURE 20.6. **Fibroadenoma.** Solid mass with benign appearing features. Oval in shape, circumscribed margins, homogeneously hypoechoic. Biopsy was performed at the patient's request and confirmed fibroadenoma.

appropriateness criteria, which are recommendations on initial imaging and workup of various clinical symptoms based on current evidence-based best practice, for different clinical scenarios. Within breast imaging, specific details of the symptom, age of patient, risk for breast cancer, and relative radiation levels of the imaging modalities all factor into what would be the appropriate workup for a patient.

Palpable Breast Mass

Palpable breast masses in women are frequent breast complaints seeking medical advice. Determining a true breast mass from normal structures on physical examination can be difficult and takes proper technique and experience. Few patients presenting for diagnostic evaluation with palpable abnormalities were discovered to have breast cancer. Common benign palpable findings in patients include cysts, fibroadenomas, or normal breast structures. Research has shown that cancers presenting as palpable abnormalities, tend to be more aggressive and have a poorer diagnosis than screen-detected cancers.

Because of the association of palpable breast mass and malignancy, imaging evaluation is necessary in most patients presenting with a palpable complaint. The initial imaging modality recommended differs, typically based on age, and is listed in Table 20.2. Mammography is indicated for women of appropriate age for routine screening, which is typically 40 years of age. Starting with mammography for ages 30 to 39 years could be considered, particularly if they are considered high risk for the development of breast cancer. Some palpable findings can be deemed specific benign, based on the mammogram images, such as fat-containing masses. When a patient has a finding suspicious for malignancy, having a complete mammogram examination can help to determine extent of disease and evaluate the asymptomatic contralateral breast. Also, comparison with priors can be helpful in the interpretation of the mammogram. A radiopaque marker is typically placed over the site of the palpable mass to aid the radiologist in the interpretation of the clinical symptom. Spot compression views should also be performed of the palpable abnormality. The radiologist should examine the area around the radiopaque marker for masses or asymmetries that would explain the patient's symptoms. A study performed by Faulk, demonstrated a 9% increase in cancer detection with spot compression views in the workup of patients presenting with a palpable breast mass. DBT can be used in place of digital mammography with equivalent or improved performance. DBT can aid with the lesion characterization, particularly where obscuring breast parenchyma is present.

TABLE 20.2

INITIAL IMAGING RECOMMENDATION FOR A PALPABLE BREAST MASS

■ AGE	■ INITIAL IMAGING RECOMMENDATION
<30 years	Ultrasound
30–39 years	Mammography or ultrasound
≥40 years	Mammography

Whether the mammogram is negative or identified a mass, ultrasound is generally performed next in the evaluation of a palpable finding. Ultrasound is able to identify lesions that are mammographically occult and also characterize mammographic findings. When an ultrasound identifies a solid or complex solid or cystic mass an ultrasound-guided biopsy is warranted (Fig. 20.7).

In women with a recent normal screening mammogram, who are under the typical screening age (some use 30 years, others 35 or 40 years of age as the cut-off for when to begin with ultrasound over mammography), or are pregnant, ultrasound is recommended as the initial test. Ultrasound is preferred in young and pregnant women because of the relative radiation risk from mammography and their typically higher breast density and associated decreased mammographic sensitivity. If the ultrasound identifies a suspicious finding, a mammogram should be performed to evaluate for extent of disease.

The use of both mammographic and ultrasound imaging in the evaluation of palpable abnormalities is effective in ruling out malignancy. Studies have shown at least a 97% negative predictive value with combined negative or normal mammographic and ultrasound examinations. However, a biopsy may still be warranted if the clinical examination finding is deemed suspicious despite normal imaging.

Breast Pain

Breast pain, also referred to as mastalgia or mastodynia, is a commonly reported breast symptom. One study discovered that around 70% of women experience some breast pain or tenderness within their lifetime. Breast pain is the second most common breast symptom that women seek medical advice for and can be severe enough to have effect on quality of life. The cause of breast pain is not incompletely understood, and many theories have been presented, including hormonal factors, fluid–electrolyte balance, and inflammation from physiologic processes within the breast, such as fibrocystic changes or duct ectasia. However, no study has fully identified the etiology of mastalgia for patients, as it is likely multifactorial. Fortunately, breast pain is very rarely associated with malignancy.

Mastalgia can be divided into cyclic and noncyclic breast pain. Cyclic breast pain is defined by intermittent breast pain that spikes during the luteal phase, right before the menses, and is thought to be primarily hormonal in etiology due to its relationship to the menstrual cycle. Usually, the pain or tenderness is also associated with swelling in the breasts. The pain can be either unilateral or bilateral. Usually, no imaging evaluation of cyclic breast is necessary, as the likelihood of malignancy is low.

Noncyclical breast pain tends to be unilateral and more focal than cyclical breast pain. Similar to cyclical breast pain, noncyclical breast pain has a low likelihood of malignancy. Dujim examined 987 women presenting for diagnostic examination with breast pain compared to 987 screening patients.

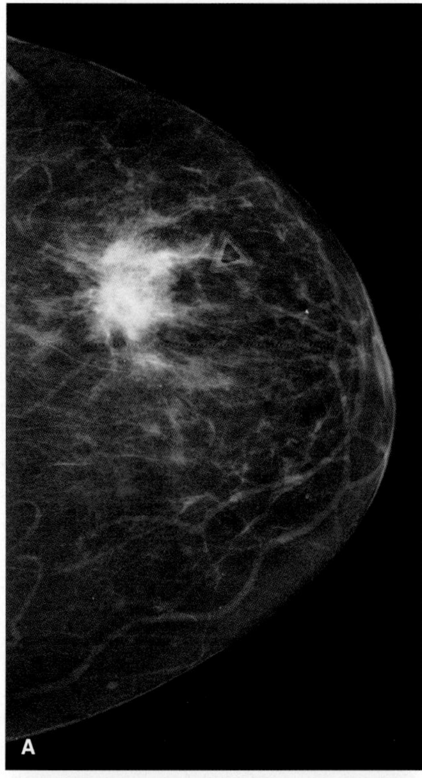

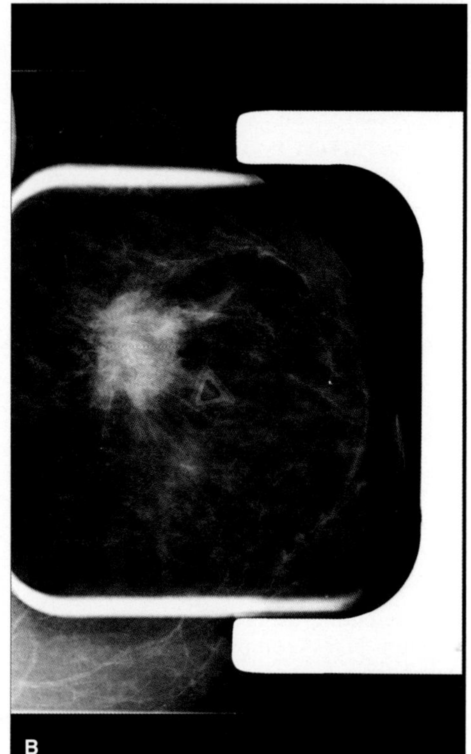

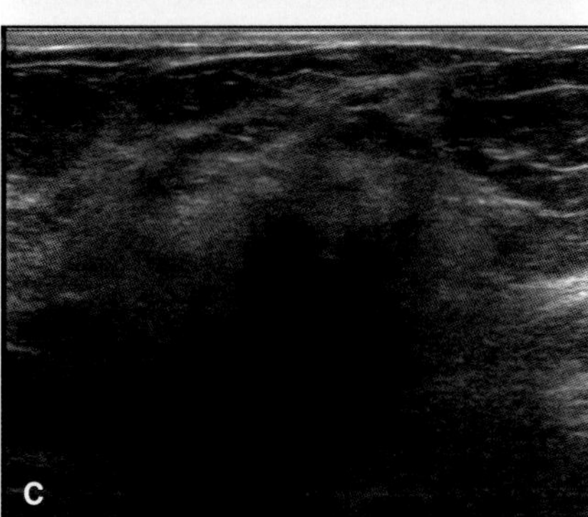

FIGURE 20.7. **Workup of a Palpable Mass. A:** Patient presents with palpable mass. Triangle marker is placed on the skin by the technologist to communicate to the radiologist the area of clinical concern. An irregularly shaped hyperdense mass with speculated margins is identified. **B:** Spot compression view. The mass persists on spot compression views. **C:** US of the finding shows an irregular hypoechoic solid mass with indistinct margins. Biopsy demonstrated infiltrating duct carcinoma.

In the population with breast pain, the study demonstrated no difference in breast cancer incidence between the painful breast and the contralateral nonpainful breast. Also, the cancer incidence between the diagnostic population and the screening population had no significant difference.

Imaging still has some role in the evaluation of noncyclical pain, despite its very low yield in cancer detection. Mastitis or abscesses are benign treatable etiologies that can be identified by imaging. Also, negative imaging may offer some reassurance to patients, who may be concerned that their pain is a representation of malignancy. If imaging evaluation is performed for noncyclical breast pain, usually mammography is performed for women older than 40 years of age. Ultrasound is the initial examination for women younger than 30 years of age. Between 30 and 39 years of age, either mammography or ultrasound may be appropriate for initial evaluation.

Nipple Discharge

Nipple discharge is the third common breast complaint, after a palpable mass and breast pain. The nipple discharge should first be categorized as pathologic, meaning it could be a result of underlying breast malignancy, or physiologic, which is a result of normal bodily functions. Pathologic nipple discharge presents as serous or bloody in color, spontaneous, unilateral, and arising from a single duct. Physiologic nipple discharge can be green, yellow, or milky in color, nonspontaneous (only presents with expression), bilateral, and usually arises from multiple ducts. Several studies have demonstrated that physiologic nipple discharge is not associated with increased identification or development of breast cancer. Because of this fact, physiologic nipple discharge does not warrant nonstandard imaging evaluation outside of screening. For pathologic nipple discharge, intraductal papilloma is the most common etiology accounting for 35% to 56% of cases. However, an underlying malignancy is identified in 5% to 23% of cases.

The standard of care for the initial evaluation for women presenting with pathologic nipple discharge is dependent on age, similar to the recommendations for a palpable mass (Table 20.3). On mammography, careful attention should be made to any suspicious masses or calcifications on the symptomatic side. If mammography is negative, an ultrasound is generally performed. The retroareolar region is usually evaluated as most lesions causing nipple discharge are near the nipple, rather than deep in the breast (Fig. 20.8). If mammography

TABLE 20.3

INITIAL IMAGING RECOMMENDATION FOR PATHOLOGIC NIPPLE DISCHARGE

■ AGE	■ INITIAL IMAGING RECOMMENDATION
<30 years	Ultrasound
30–39 years	Mammography or ultrasound
≥40 years	Mammography

and ultrasound are negative, both galactography (also known as ductography) and breast MR imaging, which will be covered in subsequent chapters, have been demonstrated to be useful in the evaluation of pathologic nipple discharge.

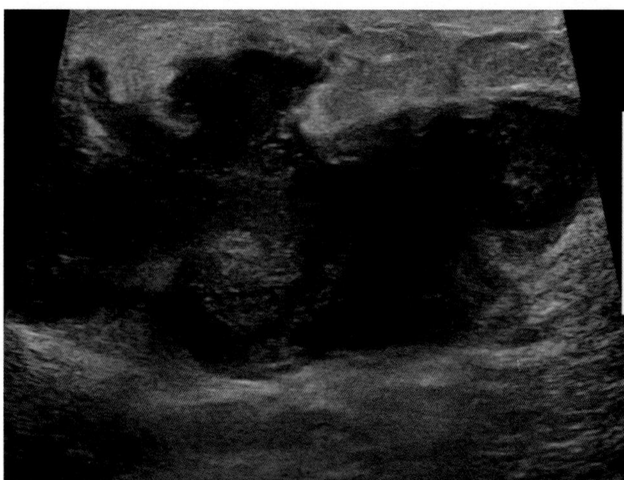

FIGURE 20.9. **Abscess.** Ultrasound of a tender erythematous left breast revealed an abscess, which typically appears as a hypoechoic irregularly shaped collection.

Inflammation of the Breast

Breast inflammation, presenting as breast erythema and swelling, is a less common breast complaint, but warrants imaging evaluation when there is concern for abscess. Infection mastitis and breast abscesses typically occur in younger women. Mastitis is a common complication for breast feeding women, and typically caused by *Staphylococcus aureus*. Ultrasound is typically the modality of choice for initial evaluation, as these patients are usually presenting with pain and cannot tolerate the compression of mammography. On ultrasound, mastitis is characterized by an area of heterogeneously altered echotexture from the edema within the parenchyma, skin thickening, and increased vascularity. An abscess typically presents as a palpable mass with overlying erythema and appears sonographically as an irregular, indistinct, heterogeneously hypoechoic collection, sometimes with multiple loculations (Fig. 20.9). If an abscess is identified, an ultrasound-guided drainage can be performed to obtain fluid for analysis, as well as aid in resolution.

One important mimic of infection mastitis that a radiologist should be aware of is inflammatory breast cancer (IBC). If the patient is older and antibiotics do not provide complete

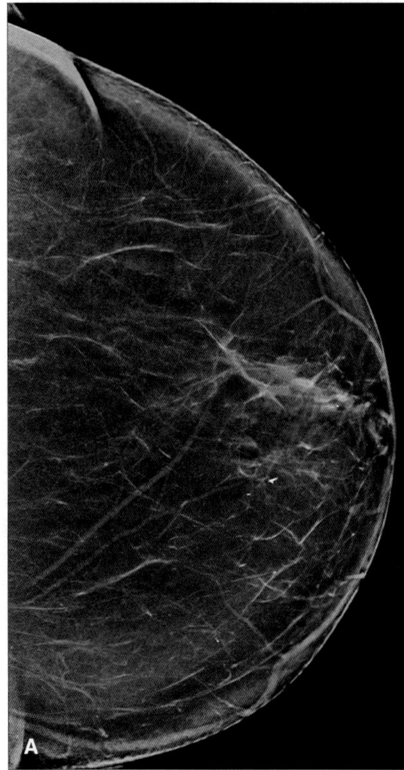

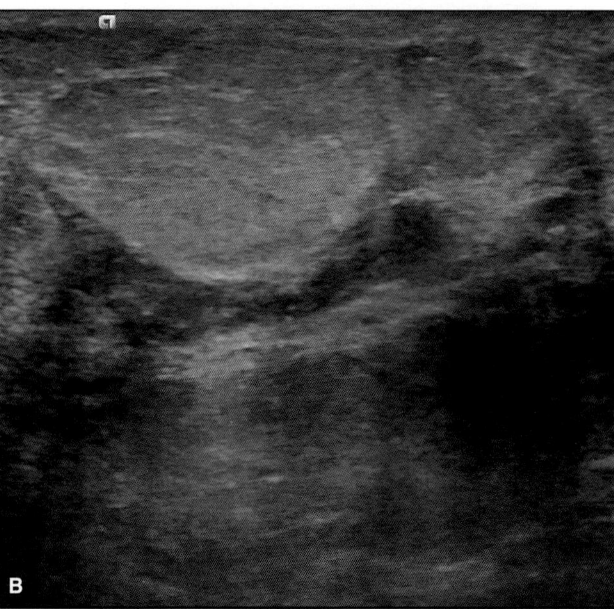

FIGURE 20.8. **Workup of a Patient With Pathologic Left Nipple Discharge. A:** Mammography demonstrates focal asymmetry in the left subareolar region. **B:** Ultrasound demonstrates an intraductal mass correlating with the mammographic finding. Biopsy revealed DCIS.

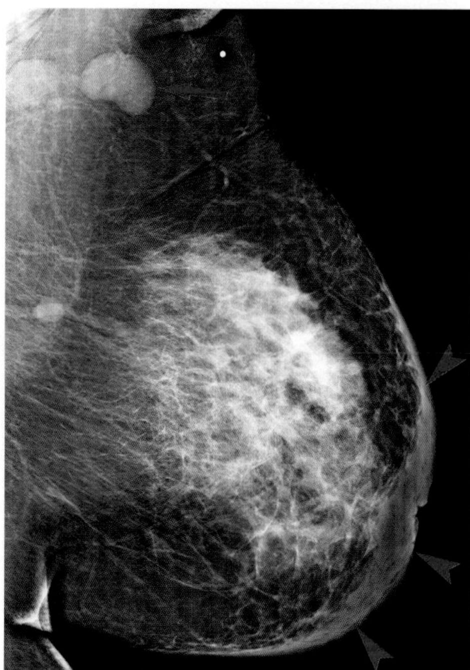

FIGURE 20.10. **Inflammatory Carcinoma.** Mediolateral oblique view demonstrates a diffuse increase in parenchymal density, along with skin thickening (*arrowheads*). An enlarged, dense lymph node (*arrow*) is seen in the axilla. The lymph node was palpable and was marked with a radiopaque skin marker. Pathology confirmed malignant adenopathy.

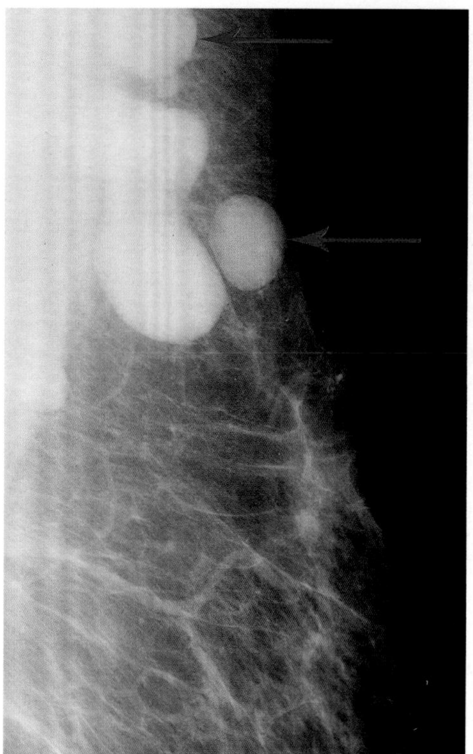

FIGURE 20.11. **Lymphoma.** Hodgkin disease involves the axillary lymph nodes. The nodes are homogeneous, dense, and enlarged (*arrows*).

resolution within 1 to 2 weeks, IBC should be a consideration. Inflammatory carcinoma is a rare subtype of breast cancer accounting for 2% to 5% of all breast cancers. Patients present with breast erythema, swelling, and tenderness, sometimes with a rapid onset. They may see skin changes known was *peau d'orange*, where there is small dimpling in the skin, like the outside of an orange. IBC is a clinical diagnosis, but a skin punch biopsy can sometimes be diagnostic to confirm the diagnosis.

On mammography, IBC can create imaging findings of diffuse breast enlargement, diffuse increased density, skin thickening, and enlarged axillary lymph nodes (Fig. 20.10). Ultrasound may be used if there is an identifiable mass on mammography as a way to obtain a target for ultrasound-guided biopsy. IBC behaves aggressively and around 20% to 40% of patients will have distant metastases on diagnosis. Breast MRI imaging and body imaging staging cross-sectional studies with computed tomography (CT) may be used needed to provide additional staging information.

Paget Disease

If a patient presents with itching, eczema, or ulceration of the nipple, Paget disease should be a consideration. Paget disease is characterized pathologically as invasion of the epidermis of the nipple by malignant cells. Surgical biopsy is the diagnostic standard for the diagnosis of Paget disease within the nipple. However, imaging plays an important role as it is estimated that 90% of women have an underlying malignancy deeper in the breast. Complete mammographic evaluation should be the first imaging test performed for initial evaluation to identify signs of malignancy; however, it can be negative in many cases. Ultrasound and MRI imaging can also be useful in identifying underlying disease and evaluating extent for surgical planning. Breast MR has the best accuracy at finding an underlying malignancy.

Axillary Adenopathy

Axillary lymph nodes are frequently visualized on the MLO mammogram. Normally, they have lucent centers or notches resulting from fat in the hilum. Fatty infiltration of the nodes themselves can cause lucent enlargement and replacement and is benign.

Mammographically, pathologic axillary nodes appear homogeneously dense and enlarged. A variety of processes can result in replacement of normal nodal architecture. Malignant involvement of axillary nodes can be the result of primary breast cancer, metastatic disease, lymphoma, or leukemia (Fig. 20.11). Axillary nodes can also become pathologically enlarged because of inflammation. Patients with rheumatoid arthritis, systemic lupus erythematosus, scleroderma, and psoriasis may have axillary adenopathy. These diseases more often give bilateral adenopathy, along with lymphoma and leukemia, whereas unilateral axillary adenopathy is more concerning for metastatic breast or skin cancer. Some inflammatory processes can give unilateral adenopathy, such as a recent inoculation or a cat scratch in the ipsilateral arm (Table 20.4).

TABLE 20.4

DIFFERENTIAL OF AXILLARY ADENOPATHY

■ UNILATERAL	■ BILATERAL
Ipsilateral infection	Systemic infections, such as HIV
Metastasis from ipsilateral breast cancer	Systemic granulomatous/ autoimmune diseases
Metastasis from melanoma from ipsilateral side	Lymphoma/leukemia

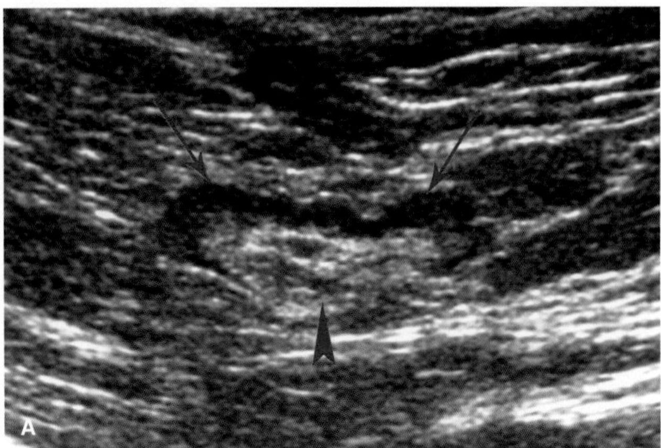

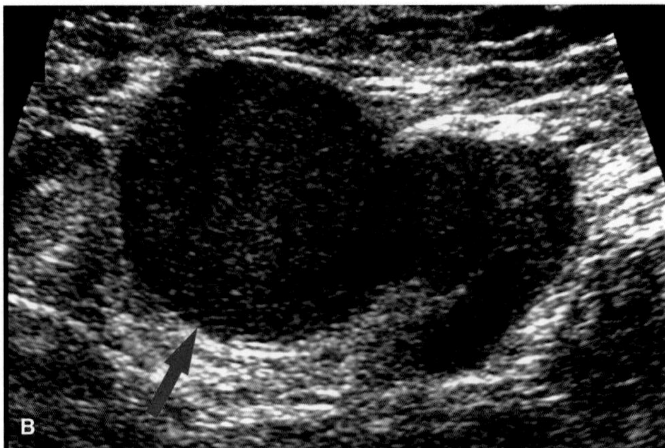

FIGURE 20.12. **Axillary Lymph Nodes. A:** US image of a normal axillary lymph node. The cortex is diffusely thin (*arrows*), while the hilum (*arrowhead*) is hyperechoic due to fat cells with areas of hyperechoic reflective interfaces from vessels and trabeculae. **B:** A 40-year-old woman with a new diagnosis of locally advanced right breast invasive ductal carcinoma. US of the right axilla showed enlarged hypoechoic lymph nodes (*arrow*) indicative of metastatic disease.

Coarse calcifications in axillary nodes may reflect granulomatous disease. Gold deposits, seen in patients being treated for rheumatoid arthritis, are occasionally seen in axillary nodes and may be confused with calcifications.

Ultrasound can be used to assess the axillary nodes at the time of a new diagnosis of breast cancer. Benign or normal lymph nodes have a hyperechoic hilum with a thin hypoechoic cortical rim. The upper limit of normal cortical thickness ranges in the literature from 2.3 to 3 mm. Metastatic deposits in the node create focal hypoechoic cortical thickening or at times complete replacement of the lymph node (resulting in absence of the fatty hilum) (Fig. 20.12). If any suspicious nodes are identified, they can be biopsied under ultrasound guidance to determine the etiology of nodal enlargement.

THE MALE BREAST

A normal male breast appears on mammography as a mound of subcutaneous fat without glandular tissue (Fig. 20.13). Gynecomastia is the most common indication for imaging a male breast. Gynecomastia is a benign proliferation of ductal and stromal tissue in men. Many causes of gynecomastia have been discovered (Table 20.5) and gynecomastia can manifest at any age, depending on the etiology. Men typically present with a palpable mass or tender thickening in the subareolar location.

The initial imaging evaluation of a palpable mass in a male depends on the patient's age (Table 20.6). Because gynecomastia has such a typical and specific benign appearance on mammography, the ACR recommends mammography as the initial imaging modality for any male greater than or equal to 25 years of age. Gynecomastia generally appears as a triangular or flame-shaped area of subareolar glandular tissue

TABLE 20.5

ETIOLOGIES OF GYNECOMASTIA

Idiopathic
Drugs (including anabolic steroids, leuprolide acetate, thiazide diuretics, cimetidine, tricyclic antidepressants, estrogen, spironolactone, digitalis, and marijuana)
Cirrhosis
Hypogonadism
Hormone-secreting neoplasms
Hyperthyroidism
Chronic renal disease

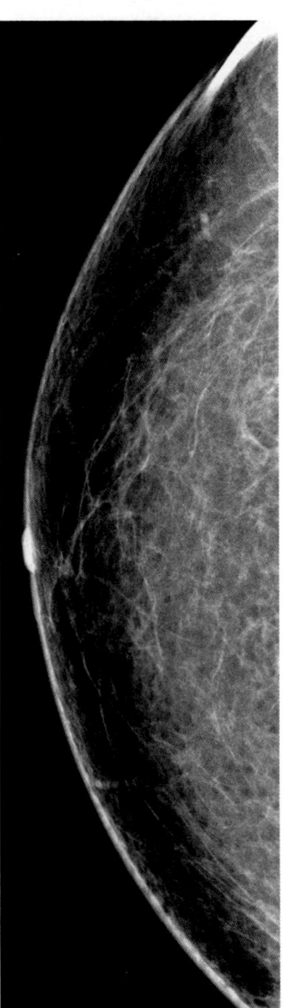

FIGURE 20.13. **Male Breast.** Relatively normal male breast, which is a mound of subcutaneous fat. Note the lack of glandular tissue.

TABLE 20.6

INITIAL IMAGING RECOMMENDATION FOR PALPABLE MALE BREAST MASS

■ AGE	■ INITIAL IMAGING RECOMMENDATION
<25 years	Ultrasound
≥25 years	Mammography

that points toward the nipple with fat interspersed within the parenchymal elements (Fig. 20.14). Gynecomastia can be unilateral or bilateral. When bilateral, it is most frequently asymmetric. The three patterns of gynecomastia include nodular, dendritic, and diffuse glandular.

Breast cancer in men is rare, making up 1% of all breast cancers and with an incidence of approximately 1 per 100,000 men. Risk factors include BRCA 1 or BRCA 2 mutation, Klinefelter syndrome, family history, and history of chest radiation. Breast cancer images are similar in men as in women. Male breast cancer typically presents as a mass with suspicious features since men almost always get invasive ductal carcinoma (IDC) due to the development differences in their breasts compared to women (see chapter 19). IDC accounts for about 80% of the breast cancer types in men (Fig. 20.15).

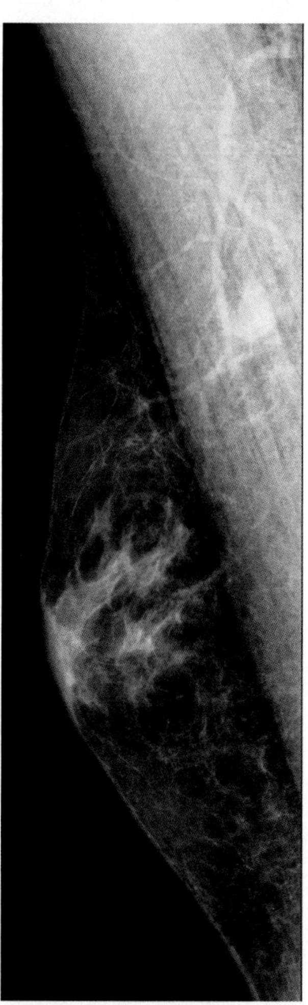

FIGURE 20.14. **Gynecomastia.** Mediolateral oblique view of a male with dendritic gynecomastia. Glandular tissue is seen in the subareolar area. This tissue gradually intersperses with the fat and does not appear as a mass.

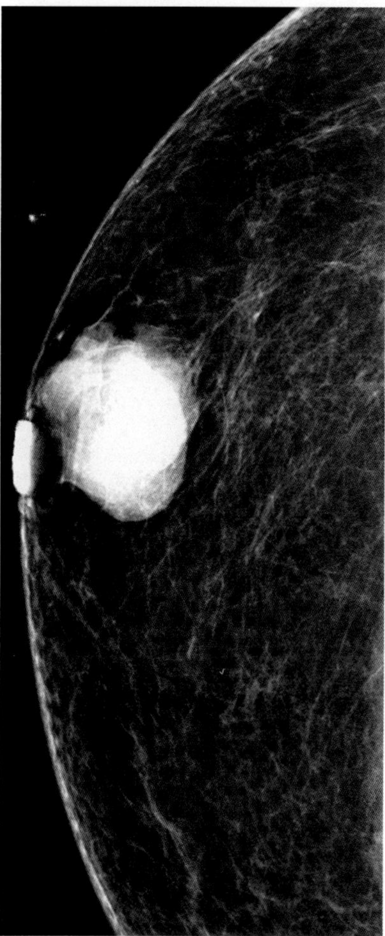

FIGURE 20.15. **Male Breast Cancer.** Mediolateral oblique view of the breast in a male. The mass has a defined interface with the surrounding fat.

ASSESSMENT AND RECOMMENDATION

The role of diagnostic examinations is to assign a final BI-RADS assessment to help guide management. Any imaging, either mammographic or sonographic, that would aid in the evaluation of a finding or symptom, should be performed before a decision on management is given. In essence, each BI-RADS assessment is associated with a management recommendation (Table 20.7).

The BI-RADS 0: incomplete assessment is given to abnormal findings on screening mammograms that require additional imaging. In general, the BI-RADS 0: incomplete assessment should rarely be given in the diagnostic setting. Ideally all imaging is completed while the patient is present, to minimize return visits and anxiety. In addition the role of the diagnostic examination is to fully characterize the lesion into a final assessment category. However, if the patient is unable to complete imaging evaluation, then a BI-RADS 0: incomplete assessment would be appropriate. BI-RADS 0: incomplete assessment can also be used when prior imaging from an outside institution is not available at the time of diagnostic

TABLE 20.7

BI-RADS ASSESSMENTS AND RECOMMENDATIONS

■ BI-RADS ASSESSMENT	■ RECOMMENDATION
BI-RADS 0	Needs additional imaging evaluation and/or prior images for comparison
BI-RADS 1	Routine screening
BI-RADS 2	Routine screening
BI-RADS 3	Short term follow-up
BI-RADS 4	Tissue diagnosis
BI-RADS 5	Tissue diagnosis
BI-RADS 6	Appropriate action should be taken

evaluation or other information is needed prior to confidently determining the final category.

If the diagnostic evaluation reveals an imaging finding as (BI-RADS 1: negative) or as specific benign finding (BI-RADS 2: benign), than the patient can return to routine screening. One caveat in patients presenting with a highly suspicious clinical symptom is that tissue diagnosis may still be warranted in the setting of BI-RADS 1: negative or BI-RADS 2: benign results.

BI-RADS 3: probably benign assessment should be given to findings that have a less than 2% chance to represent malignancy. A landmark study performed by Sickles, confirmed that three finding types identified on initial evaluation fit this criterion (Table 20.8). If priors are available and a finding is new, then it would not be appropriate to give a BI-RADS 3: probably benign assessment, despite the presence of probably benign imaging features. In this scenario, a BI-RADS 4: suspicious assessment should be used and biopsy recommended.

If the diagnostic evaluation yields a concerning finding, BI-RADS 4: suspicious assessment is used and tissue sampling is recommended. If the finding is highly suspicious (>95% chance) of malignancy based on imaging features, than a BI-RADS 5: highly suggestive of malignancy is given. For these lesions, the radiologist should perform imaging during the diagnostic examination for staging. Tissue sampling is recommended for BI-RADS 5: highly suggestive of malignancy findings.

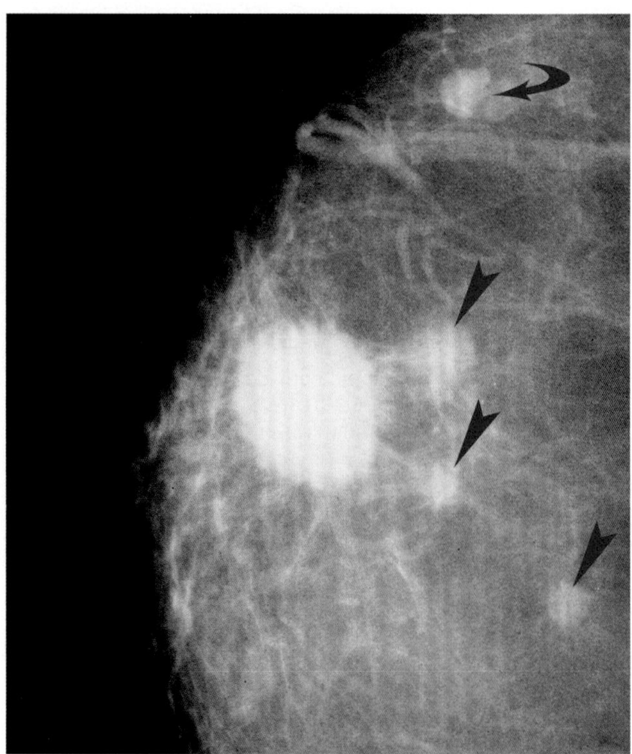

FIGURE 20.16. Multifocal Carcinoma. Craniocaudal view. The largest mass was palpable. The others were discovered by mammography (*arrowheads*). The more well-defined nodule (*curved arrow*) probably represented an intramammary lymph node.

BREAST CANCER STAGING

Staging plays an essential role in the prognosis and treatment of patients diagnosed with breast cancer. The American Joint Committee of Cancer (AJCC) developed a tumor-node-metastasis (TNM) staging system that allows the clinician to assign a stage to the patient. The radiologists role is to help provide this information to the clinician.

Tumor (T) stage is based on tumor size and extent. When evaluating masses, the maximum measurement is recorded regardless of imaging modality. Involvement of the skin, nipple, and chest wall are also important descriptors that impact the T stage. When a BI-RADS 5: highly suspicious of malignancy lesion is present, the remainder of the breast should be evaluated for extent or multifocal disease, as this will affect the surgical plan (Fig. 20.16). The contralateral breast should also be evaluated to ensure the patient does not have bilateral cancer. Women with history of breast cancer are at a slightly increased risk for a contralateral breast cancer, compared to women with no breast cancer history. MR imaging is the most sensitive test for staging breast cancer, often additional sites of cancer that are mammographically occult. This will be further covered in Chapter 22.

TABLE 20.8

FINDINGS APPROPRIATE TO BE GIVEN BI-RADS 3 ASSESSMENT ON INITIAL IMAGING

Group of round calcifications
Oval, circumscribed mass
Focal asymmetry

Lymph node (N) stage has strong implications to the treatment plan of the patient, as well as prognosis. Lymph node stage can be assessed both clinically or with imaging. Ultrasound is superior to mammography in evaluating the axillary node status. As mentioned previously, lymph nodes are assessed primarily by their size and morphology to determine if they are normal or abnormal. Enlarged nodes, even in cancer patients, are not always secondary to metastatic disease, so tissue sampling either by image-guided biopsy or surgical biopsy is often performed. Surgical management of the axilla is a controversial issue and ever adapting to balance survival rates and recurrence risk. The role of the radiologist is to document the imaging findings to assist the surgeon and oncologist in their decision making.

Metastatic disease (M) stage, like lymph node status, plays a large role in the treatment plan of the patient. Distal staging imaging is not needed in most newly diagnosed breast cancer patients. Body imaging may be ordered by the referring clinician when there is a higher likelihood for metastatic disease, usually in patients with locally advanced breast cancer at presentation or in patients who have recurred.

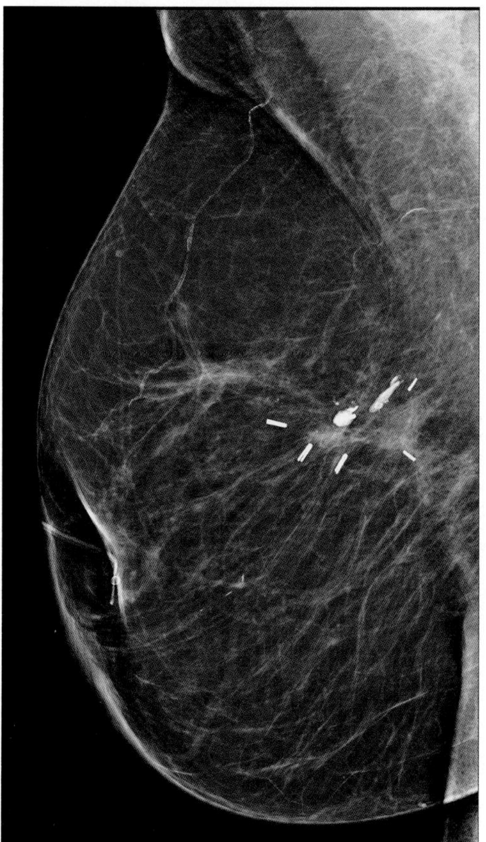

FIGURE 20.17. **Postoperative Scar.** Postoperative scar demonstrates focal asymmetry with architectural distortion and dystrophic calcifications

POSTOPERATIVE SURVEILLANCE

The recurrence rate for patients undergoing optimal treatment, with either mastectomy or breast conservation therapy, for breast cancer is 1% to 2% a year, although the risk increases with positive node status and positive surgical margins. Patients who undergo mastectomy for surgical treatment do not require subsequent ipsilateral screening mammography, as the mastectomy theoretically removes all of the breast tissue. However, any palpable abnormality on the mastectomy side should be assessed with ultrasound to evaluate for possible recurrence.

Annual mammography, with either 2D or DBT, should still be performed for women who underwent breast conservation therapy to detect any evidence of recurrence. Although no strict guidelines exist for posttreatment surveillance, some institutions perform these mammograms in the diagnostic setting. One advantage is that the radiologist can perform additional pictures, such as magnification views of the lumpectomy bed, if they believe it would aid in the detection of local recurrence.

Imaging findings of the postoperative breast depend on how recent the surgery was performed. Mass-like postoperative fluid collections are common within the first year of surgery. The lumpectomy site is commonly associated with scar formation and dystrophic or fat necrosis calcifications instead of a mass (Fig. 20.17). The scar formation appears mammographically as architectural distortion, which either stabilizes or diminishes in conspicuity over the years. Any calcifications that develop within the lumpectomy site should be examined closely. Breast edema and skin thickening are common findings if the patient receives radiation treatment. Evidence of recurrence include enlarging masses, developing asymmetries, or new or increasing suspicious calcifications within or adjacent to the lumpectomy bed. These findings should be evaluated with diagnostic imaging and biopsied if the findings are indeterminate (Fig. 20.18).

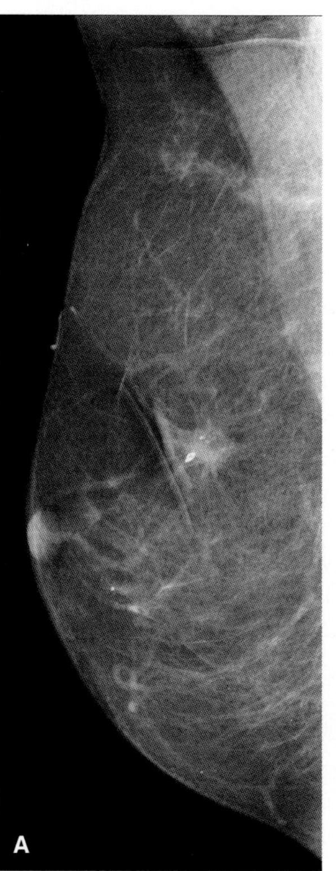

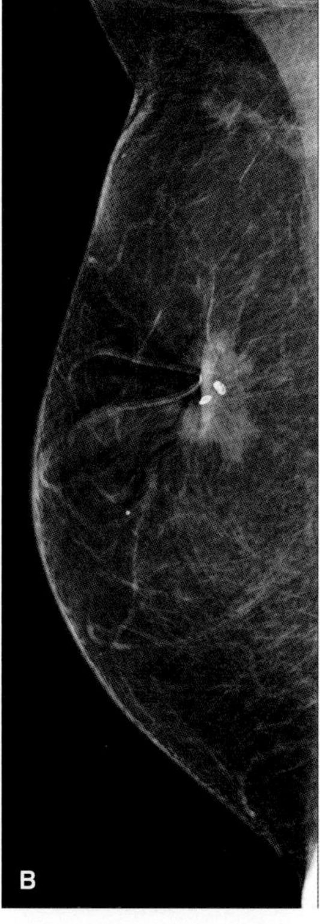

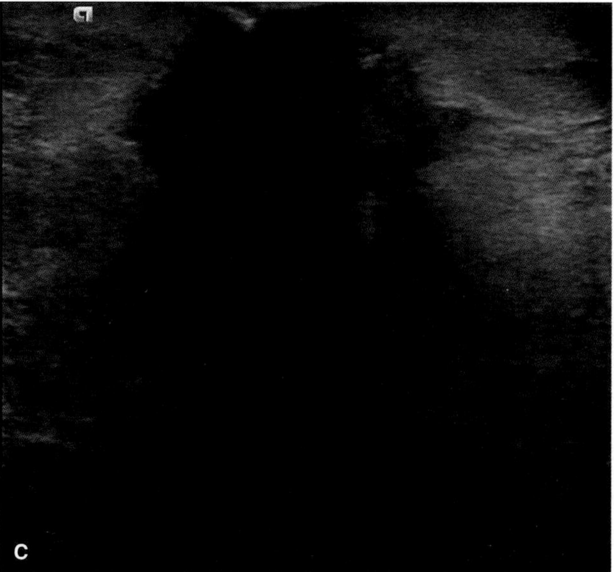

FIGURE 20.18. **Local Recurrence. A:** RMLO two years prior for comparison. **B:** RMLO current examination demonstrates an enlarging mass at the lumpectomy site. Biopsy revealed recurrent IDC. **C:** Ultrasound demonstrates an irregular spiculated mass correlating with the mammographic finding. Biopsy revealed IDC.

CONCLUSION

Diagnostic imaging is used to work up symptomatic patients or those with abnormal screening mammograms. Diagnostic breast imaging is essential in separating benign findings that have no chance of malignancy from suspicious lesions, which will then need to undergo a biopsy to determine if malignant. Appropriate imaging and recommendations will maximize the sensitivity for detecting malignancy and specificity to avoid unnecessary procedures.

Suggested Readings

Ader DN, Browne MW. Prevalence and impact of cyclic mastalgia in a United States clinic-based sample. *Am J Obstet Gynecol* 1997;177(1):126–132.

American College of Radiology. ACR appropriateness criteria. https://www.acr.org/Quality-Safety/Appropriateness-Criteria. Updated 2017.

Bahl M, Baker JA, Greenup RA, Ghate SV. Diagnostic value of ultrasound in female patients with nipple discharge. *AJR Am J Roentgenol* 2015;205(1):203–208.

Barton MB, Elmore JG, Fletcher SW. Breast symptoms among women enrolled in a health maintenance organization: frequency, evaluation, and outcome. *Ann Intern Med* 1999;130(8):651–657.

Berger N, Luparia A, Di Leo G, et al. Diagnostic performance of MRI versus galactography in women with pathologic nipple discharge: a systematic review and meta-analysis. *AJR Am J Roentgenol* 2017;209(2):465–471.

Berkowitz JE, Gatewood OM, Gayler BW. Equivocal mammographic findings: evaluation with spot compression. *Radiology* 1989;171(2):369–371.

Brandt KR, Craig DA, Hoskins TL, et al. Can digital breast tomosynthesis replace conventional diagnostic mammography views for screening recalls without calcifications? A comparison study in a simulated clinical setting. *AJR Am J Roentgenol* 2013;200(2):291–298.

Chansakul T, Lai KC, Slanetz PJ. The postconservation breast: part 1, expected imaging findings. *AJR Am J Roentgenol* 2012;198(2):321–330. doi: 10.2214/AJR.10.7298.

Chansakul T, Lai KC, Slanetz PJ. The postconservation breast: part 2, imaging findings of tumor recurrence and other long-term sequelae. *AJR Am J Roentgenol* 2012;198(2):331–343.

Clarke M, Collins R, Darby S, et al; Early Breast Cancer Trialists' Collaborative Group (EBCTCG). Effects of radiotherapy and of differences in the extent of surgery for early breast cancer on local recurrence and 15-year survival: An overview of the randomised trials. *Lancet* 2005;366(9503):2087–2106.

Dennis MA, Parker SH, Klaus AJ, Stavros AT, Kaske TI, Clark SB. Breast biopsy avoidance: the value of normal mammograms and normal sonograms in the setting of a palpable lump. *Radiology* 2001;219(1):186–191.

D'Orsi CJ, Sickles EA, Mendelson EB, et al. *ACR BI-RADS Atlas: Breast Imaging Reporting and Data System.* Reston, VA: American College of Radiology; 2013.

Duijm LE, Guit GL, Hendriks JH, Zaat JO, Mali WP. Value of breast imaging in women with painful breasts: observational follow up study. *BMJ* 1998;317(7171):1492–1495.

Ecanow JS, Abe H, Newstead GM, Ecanow DB, Jeske JM. Axillary staging of breast cancer: what the radiologist should know. *Radiographics* 2013;33(6):1589–1612.

Faulk RM, Sickles EA. Efficacy of spot compression-magnification and tangential views in mammographic evaluation of palpable breast masses. *Radiology* 1992;185(1):87–90.

Giess CS, Frost EP, Birdwell RL. Interpreting one-view mammographic findings: minimizing callbacks while maximizing cancer detection. *Radiographics* 2014;34(4):928–940.

Goksel HA, Yagmurdur MC, Demirhan B, et al. Management strategies for patients with nipple discharge. *Langenbecks Arch Surg* 2005;390(1):52–58.

Hooley RJ, Scoutt LM, Philpotts LE. Breast ultrasonography: state of the art. *Radiology* 2013;268(3):642–659.

Howard MB, Battaglia T, Prout M, Freund K. The effect of imaging on the clinical management of breast pain. *J Gen Intern Med* 2012;27(7):817–824.

Lee SC, Jain PA, Jethwa SC, Tripathy D, Yamashita MW. Radiologist's role in breast cancer staging: providing key information for clinicians. *Radiographics* 2014;34(2):330–342.

Liberman L, Morris EA, Dershaw DD, Abramson AF, Tan LK. MR imaging of the ipsilateral breast in women with percutaneously proven breast cancer. *AJR Am J Roentgenol* 2003;180(4):901–910.

Lim HS, Jeong SJ, Lee JS, et al. Paget disease of the breast: Mammographic, US, and MR imaging findings with pathologic correlation. *Radiographics* 2011;31(7):1973–1987.

Margolis NE, Morley C, Lotfi P, et al. Update on imaging of the postsurgical breast. *Radiographics* 2014;34(3):642–660.

Moy L, Slanetz PJ, Moore R, et al. Specificity of mammography and US in the evaluation of a palpable abnormality: retrospective review. *Radiology* 2002;225(1):176–181.

Newman LA, Sahin AA, Cunningham JE, et al. A case-control study of unilateral and bilateral breast carcinoma patients. *Cancer* 2001;91(10):1845–1853.

Nguyen C, Kettler MD, Swirsky ME, et al. Male breast disease: pictorial review with radiologic-pathologic correlation. *Radiographics* 2013;33(3):763–779.

Peppard HR, Nicholson BE, Rochman CM, Merchant JK, Mayo RC 3rd, Harvey JA. Digital breast tomosynthesis in the diagnostic setting: indications and clinical applications. *Radiographics* 2015;35(4):975–990.

Sickles EA. Breast calcifications: mammographic evaluation. *Radiology* 1986;160(2):289–293.

Sickles EA. Periodic mammographic follow-up of probably benign lesions: results in 3,184 consecutive cases. *Radiology* 1991;179(2):463–468.

Sickles EA, Miglioretti DL, Ballard-Barbash R, et al. Performance benchmarks for diagnostic mammography. *Radiology* 2005;235(3):775–790.

Siegel RL, Miller KD, Jemal A. Cancer statistics, 2017. *CA Cancer J Clin* 2017;67(1):7–30.

Smith RL, Pruthi S, Fitzpatrick LA. Evaluation and management of breast pain. *Mayo Clin Proc* 2004;79(3):353–372.

Stavros AT, Thickman D, Rapp CL, Dennis MA, Parker SH, Sisney GA. Solid breast nodules: use of sonography to distinguish between benign and malignant lesions. *Radiology* 1995;196(1):123–134.

Ulitzsch D, Nyman MK, Carlson RA. Breast abscess in lactating women: US-guided treatment. *Radiology* 2004;232(3):904–909.

Yeh ED, Jacene HA, Bellon JR, et al. What radiologists need to know about diagnosis and treatment of inflammatory breast cancer: A multidisciplinary approach. *Radiographics* 2013;33(7):2003–2017.

Zuley ML, Bandos AI, Ganott MA, et al. Digital breast tomosynthesis versus supplemental diagnostic mammographic views for evaluation of noncalcified breast lesions. *Radiology* 2013;266(1):89–95.

CHAPTER 21 ■ BREAST IMAGING REPORTING AND DATA SYSTEM

CARRIE M. ROCHMAN, JONATHAN V. NGUYEN AND BRANDI T. NICHOLSON

INTRODUCTION

The Breast Imaging Reporting and Data System (BI-RADS®) was created by the American College of Radiology (ACR) to standardize mammography practice and reporting. It is intended to improve communication through breast imaging reports and standardize recommendations and management of breast lesions. BI-RADS was created in response to substantial problems with inconsistent quality and radiation doses in facilities performing mammography in the late 1980s. This coincided with the Mammography Quality Standards Act (MQSA) which was enacted by the United States Congress in 1992 to regulate the quality of care in mammography "to ensure that all women have access to quality mammography for the detection of breast cancer in its earliest, most treatable stages."

There are several components of the BI-RADS atlas including sections devoted to breast imaging lexicon, reporting system, and guidance for each of the modalities used in breast imaging (mammography, ultrasound, and magnetic resonance imaging [MRI]). There are also sections of the atlas devoted to follow-up and outcome monitoring and a data dictionary of terms (Table 21.1). BI-RADS helps radiologists to describe findings, apply appropriate assessment and recommendations, audit their breast imaging practice to ensure maintenance of quality standards, and improve patient care. As breast imaging changes and evolves, so does BI-RADS which is currently in its fifth edition, published in 2013.

The lexicon is the largest component of the BI-RADS atlas. The terms and recommended reporting format are meant to standardize the radiology report to make reports meaningful and unambiguous to the nonradiologist. The descriptors used in the lexicon are evidence based, to help categorize a finding and its likelihood of malignancy. Using the lexicon can help the radiologist determine the risk of malignancy associated with a finding. The breast imaging lexicon is organized by modality: mammography, ultrasound, and MRI.

MAMMOGRAPHY LEXICON

Breast Composition

Breast composition, or breast density, refers to the amount of fibroglandular tissue in the breast relative to the amount of fat. Interestingly, it has nothing to do with perceived "lumpiness" or "dense tissue" on physical examination. Breast density is assessed on mammography. Fibroglandular tissue attenuates x-rays more than fat. Thus, dense breast tissue appears white on a mammogram. X-rays pass more easily through fat, so fat appears dark gray. Breast composition is classified as (a) the breasts are almost entirely fatty; (b) there are scattered areas of fibroglandular density; (c) the breasts are heterogeneously dense, which may obscure small masses; and (d) the breasts are extremely dense, which lowers the sensitivity of mammography (Fig. 21.1; Table 21.2). The assessment of breast composition should be based on the densest area. The location of the dense tissue can also be included in the report (e.g., retroareolar, upper outer quadrant, etc.) to communicate with the referring physician where sensitivity is limited. Breast composition and impact on masking malignancy and breast cancer risk are discussed further in Chapter 19.

Masses

A breast mass is defined as a three-dimensional (3D) structure that occupies space in the breast. It can be seen on two different mammographic projections and has outward convex margins.

There are benign and malignant etiologies for breast masses. Careful characterization and assessment are important to ensure that you do not miss a cancer or perform unnecessary workup or biopsy benign masses. If a breast cancer presents as a mass, it is most often an invasive cancer, so accurate characterization and assessment are critical to avoid delay in diagnosis.

TABLE 21.1

ACR BI-RADS® ATLAS SECTIONS

Mammography (lexicon, reporting, and guidance)
Ultrasound (lexicon, reporting, and guidance)
Magnetic resonance imaging (lexicon, reporting, and guidance)
Follow-up and outcome monitoring
Data dictionary

TABLE 21.2

BI-RADS® BREAST COMPOSITION CATEGORIES

a. The breasts are almost entirely fatty.
b. There are scattered areas of fibroglandular density.
c. The breasts are heterogeneously dense, which may obscure small masses.
d. The breasts are extremely dense, which lowers the sensitivity of mammography.

TABLE 21.3

BI-RADS® MASS DESCRIPTORS: MAMMOGRAPHY

Shape	Oval Round Irregular
Margin	Circumscribed Obscured Microlobulated Indistinct Spiculated
Density	High density Equal density Low density Fat containing

On mammography, masses are characterized by their shape, margin, and density (Table 21.3). Shape may be oval, round, or irregular. An **oval** mass has a shape similar to an egg (Fig. 21.2). One axis is longer than the others. A **round** mass looks like a sphere or a ball (Fig. 21.3). An **irregular** mass is neither round nor oval. With an irregular mass, there can be small projections that extend from the dominant portion of the mass (Fig. 21.4). A mass with an irregular shape is more likely to be assessed as BI-RADS 4: Suspicious or BI-RADS 5: Highly Suspicious for Malignancy compared to those that are oval or round.

Margin describes the border or edge of a mass at the interface with the surrounding tissue. Margin may be classified as circumscribed, obscured, indistinct, microlobulated, or spiculated. A **circumscribed** margin is a well-defined, smooth interface between the mass and the surrounding tissue (Fig. 21.5). You could take a pencil and draw a thin line at the margin of the mass. Many benign processes have a circumscribed margin such as cysts, fibroadenomas, and intramammary lymph nodes. But, be aware that some cancers can also have circumscribed margins. Phyllodes tumors and invasive ductal carcinomas (IDCs) such as high-grade IDC, medullary, mucinous, and papillary subtypes of IDC can appear circumscribed. If more than 25% of the margin is not well seen due to overlapping fibroglandular tissue, it is considered **obscured** (Fig. 21.6). This is less frequent with the increased use of digital breast tomosynthesis (DBT). An **indistinct** margin has a very vague interface between the mass and the surrounding tissue (Fig. 21.7). The margin often looks "fuzzy." In older versions of BI-RADS, this was also termed ill-defined. A **microlobulated** margin has several small bumps along the surface (Fig. 21.8). This margin is often seen with benign clustered microcysts, but can also be a worrisome sign of malignancy when associated with a solid mass. A **spiculated** margin has straight lines extending out from the mass (Fig. 21.9). The spiculations are often due to a desmoplastic reaction surrounding the tumor. A mass with a spiculated margin is assessed as BI-RADS 5: Highly Suggestive of Malignancy in almost all cases. It is important to distinguish a spiculated mass from architectural distortion (AD). AD is also characterized by straight lines, but lacks a 3D structure

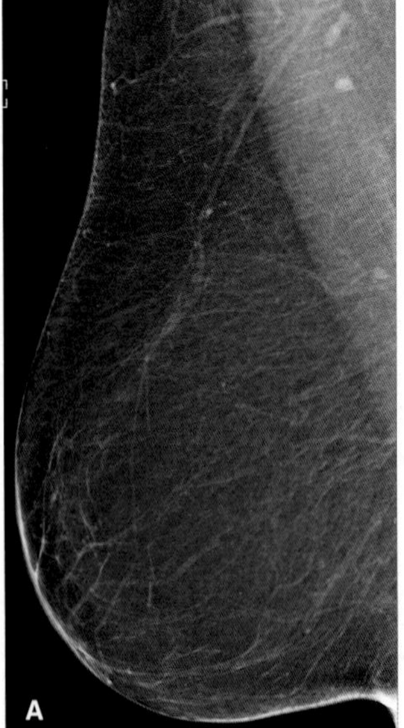

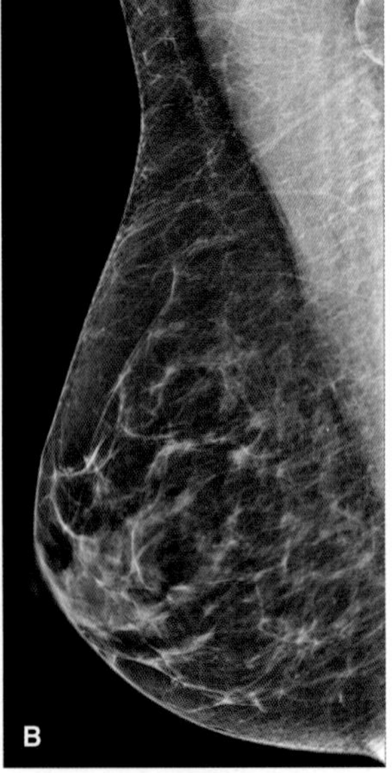

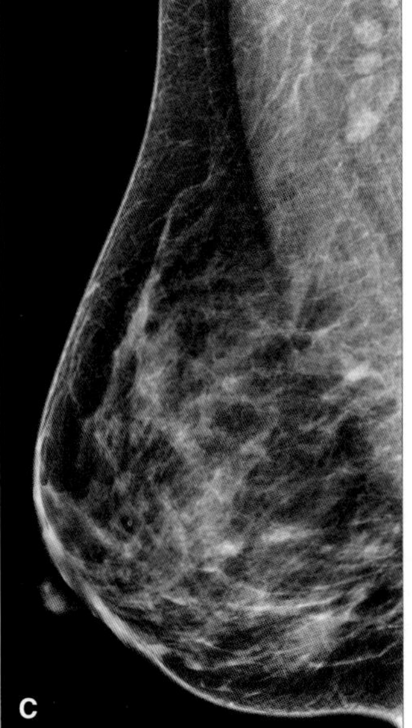

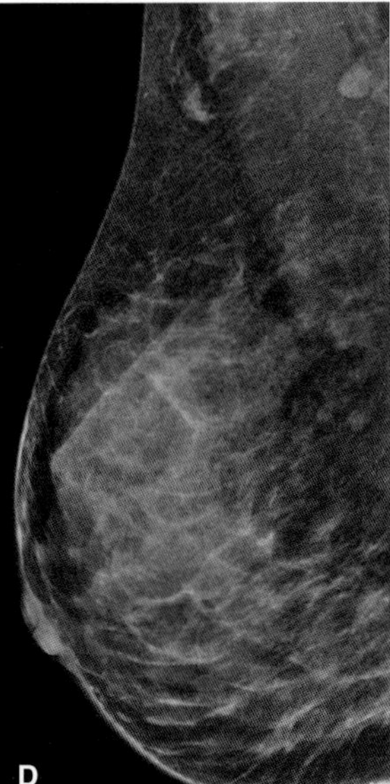

FIGURE 21.1. **Breast Density Categories. A:** The breasts are almost entirely fatty. **B:** There are scattered areas of fibroglandular density. **C:** The breasts are heterogeneously dense, which may obscure small masses. **D:** The breasts are extremely dense, which lowers the sensitivity of mammography.

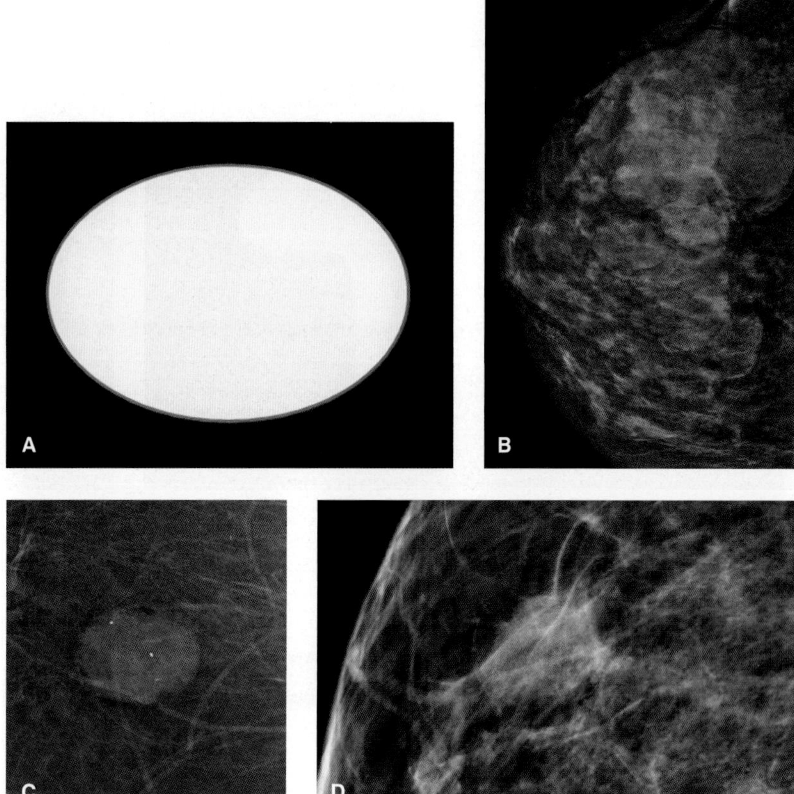

FIGURE 21.2. **Oval Shape on Mammography.** **A:** Oval shape is similar to an ellipse or egg. **B:** Multiple oval circumscribed masses on mammography. Ultrasound showed multiple simple cysts. **C:** Oval circumscribed mass. Biopsy showed fibroadenoma. **D:** Oval mass with obscured margin. Biopsy showed high grade invasive ductal carcinoma (IDC).

and outward convex margins (Fig. 21.10). When describing the margin of a mass, you should always choose the most worrisome feature. For example, if the majority of a mass is circumscribed, but a portion is indistinct, the mass should be characterized as indistinct (Fig. 21.11).

The density of a mass refers to x-ray attenuation relative to the fibroglandular tissue. Invasive breast cancers are often composed of densely packed cells and fibrosis that are theorized to attenuate x-rays more than the surrounding tissue. Thus, they often appear as high density (or more white) on a mammogram or as a high-density mass. Density is characterized as fat containing, low density, equal density, or high density. A **fat-containing** mass has an area that is as dark gray as a fat lobule (Fig. 21.12). When a mass is oval circumscribed and fat containing, it is almost always benign. Circumscribed fat-containing masses include lipomas, oil cysts, galactoceles, lymph nodes, and hamartomas. Keep in mind that not *all* fat-containing masses are benign. A cancer can engulf or trap fat as it grows. These cancers usually have a suspicious shape or margin (Fig. 21.13). A **low-density** mass is less white than the surrounding tissue (Fig. 21.14). Low density is commonly seen with cysts and is often a more benign feature. However, when a cancer is growing in an infiltrative pattern through the fat, it can appear as a low-density mass. An **equal-density**

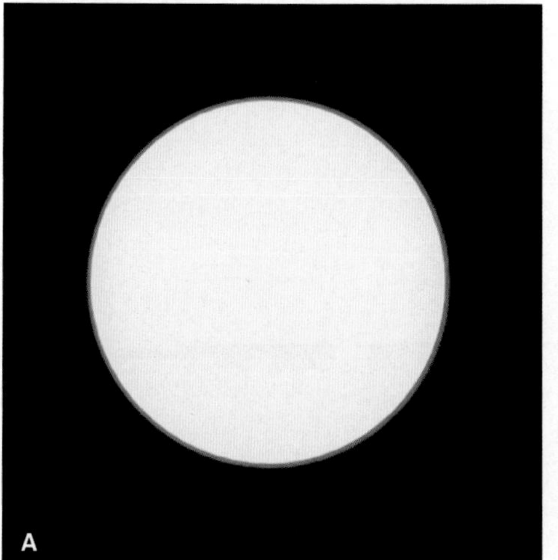

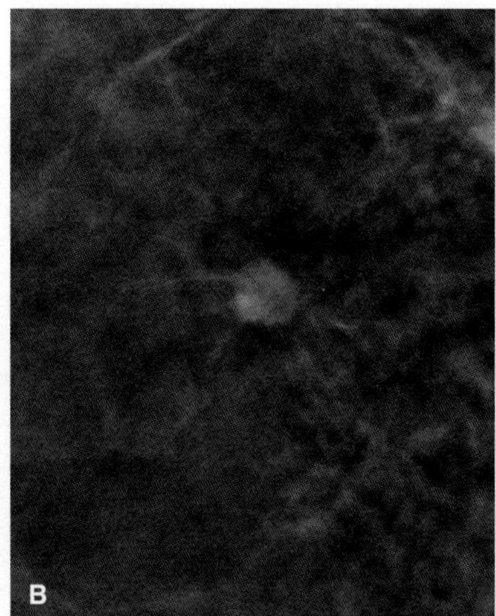

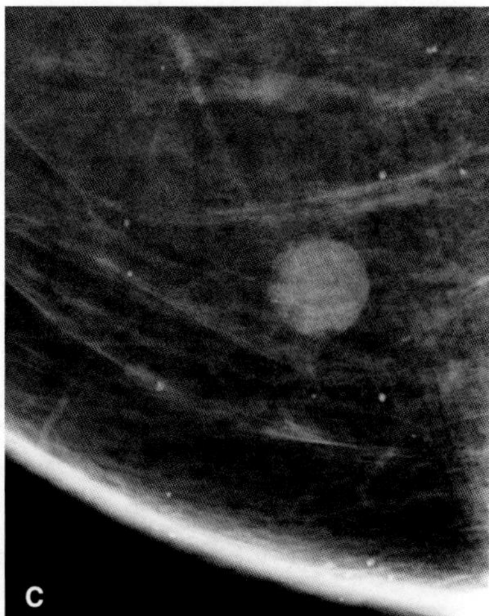

FIGURE 21.3. **Round Shape on Mammography.** **A:** Round shape should resemble a ball or sphere. **B:** Round spiculated mass. Biopsy showed invasive ductal carcinoma (IDC). **C:** Round circumscribed mass. Ultrasound showed an epidermal inclusion cyst.

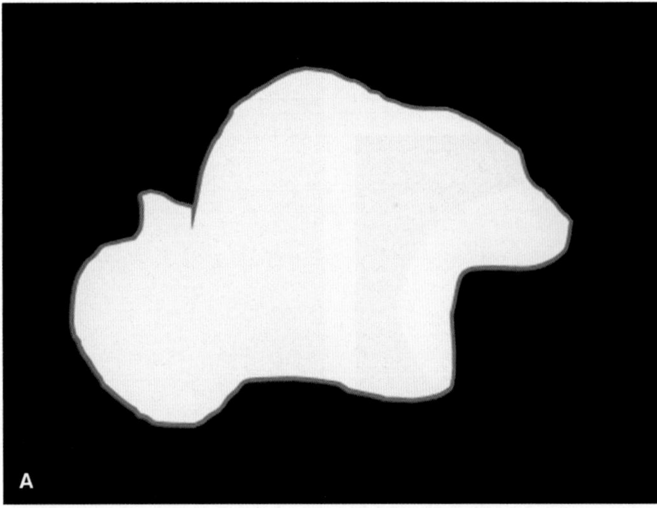

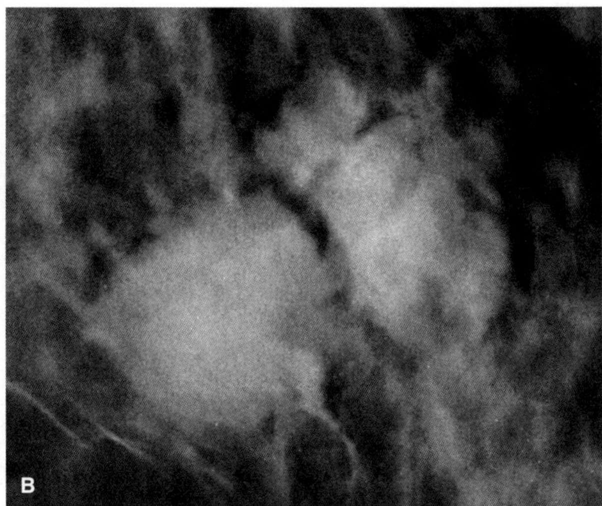

FIGURE 21.4. **Irregular Shape on Mammography. A:** Irregular shape is neither round nor oval. **B:** Irregular mass on digital breast tomosynthesis (DBT). Biopsy showed invasive ductal carcinoma (IDC).

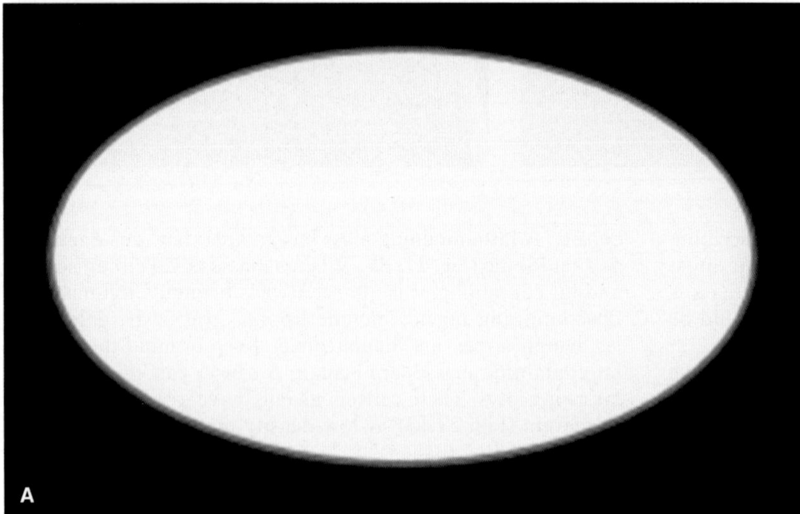

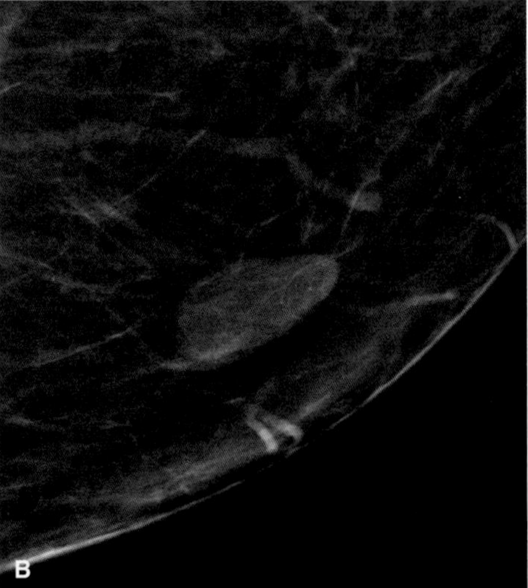

FIGURE 21.5. **Circumscribed Margin on Mammography. A:** Circumscribed margin is well defined, smooth interface. **B:** Circumscribed mass that was stable for many years mammographically. Mass is a probable fibroadenoma.

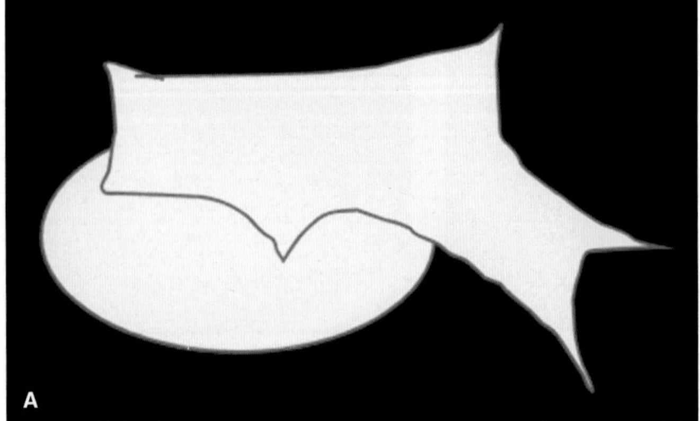

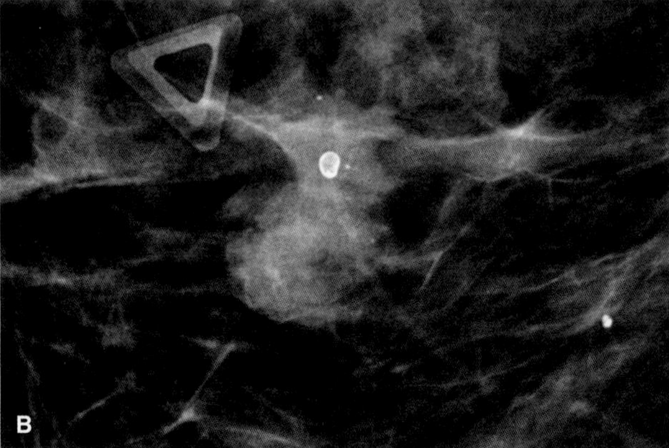

FIGURE 21.6. **Obscured Margin on Mammography. A:** More than 25% of the margin is not seen due to overlapping tissue. **B:** Obscured mass on mammography. The triangle marker signifies that the mass is palpable. Biopsy showed invasive ductal carcinoma (IDC).

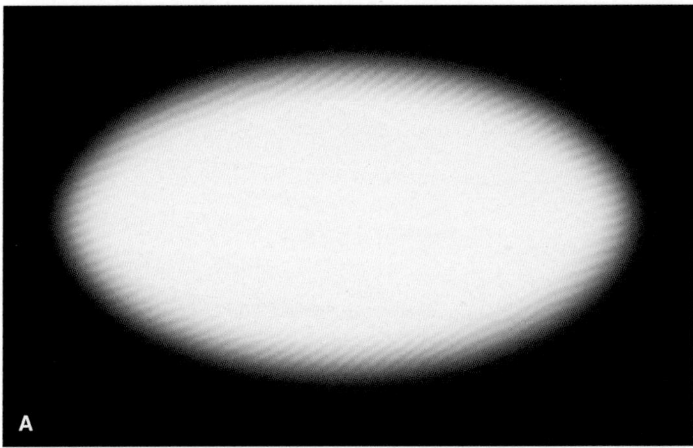
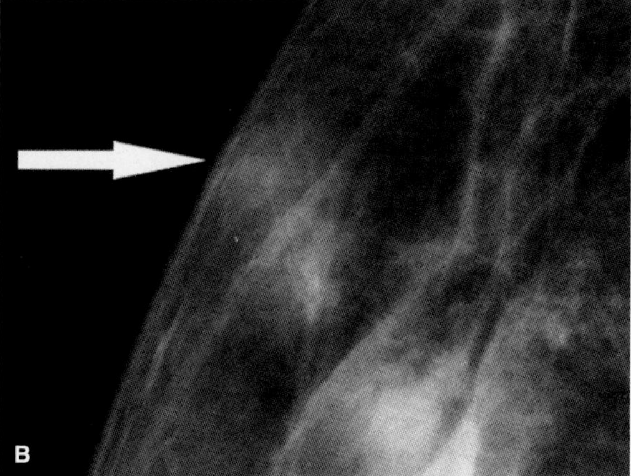

FIGURE 21.7. **Indistinct Margin on Mammography. A:** Vague or fuzzy interface between the mass and the surrounding tissue. **B:** Indistinct mass on mammography (*arrow*). Biopsy showed fat necrosis.

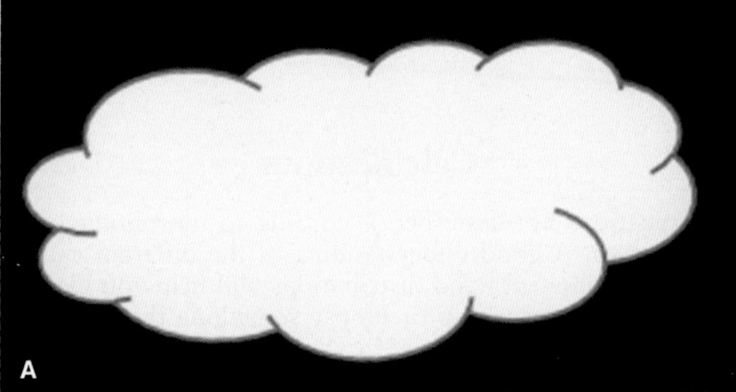

FIGURE 21.8. **Microlobulated Margin on Mammography. A:** A microlobulated margin has several small bumps along the surface. **B:** Microlobulated mass on DBT. Mass was mixed solid and cystic on ultrasound (not shown). Biopsy revealed fibrocystic changes.

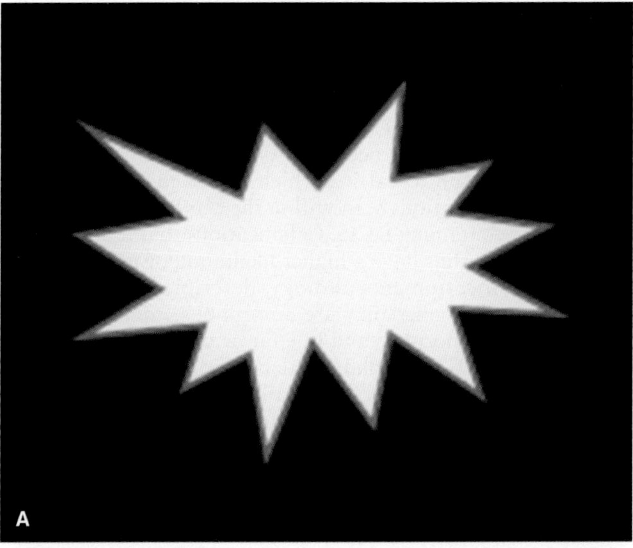
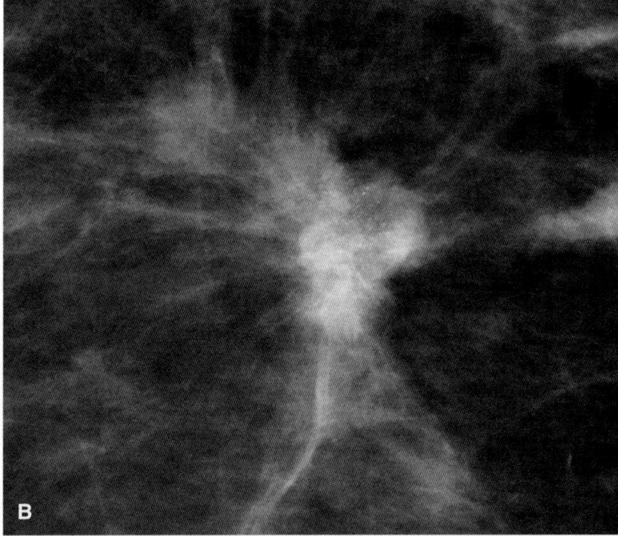

FIGURE 21.9. **Spiculated Margin on Mammography. A:** Spiculated margin has straight lines extending out from the mass. **B:** Spiculated mass on mammography. There are associated fine pleomorphic calcifications. Appearance is highly suggestive of malignancy. Biopsy showed invasive ductal carcinoma (IDC).

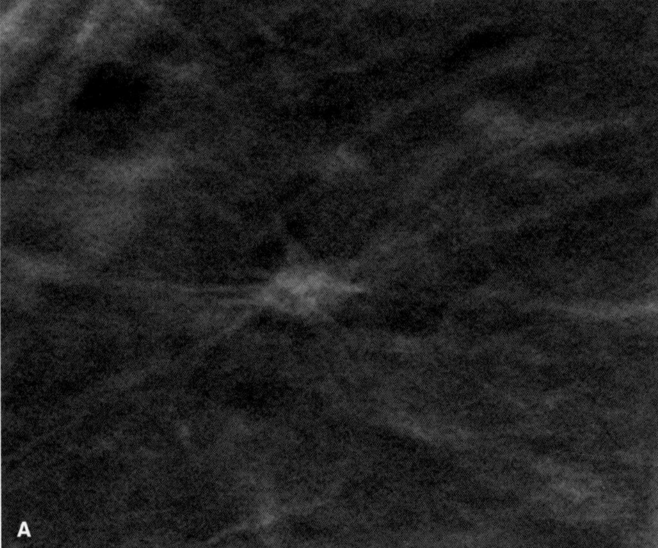

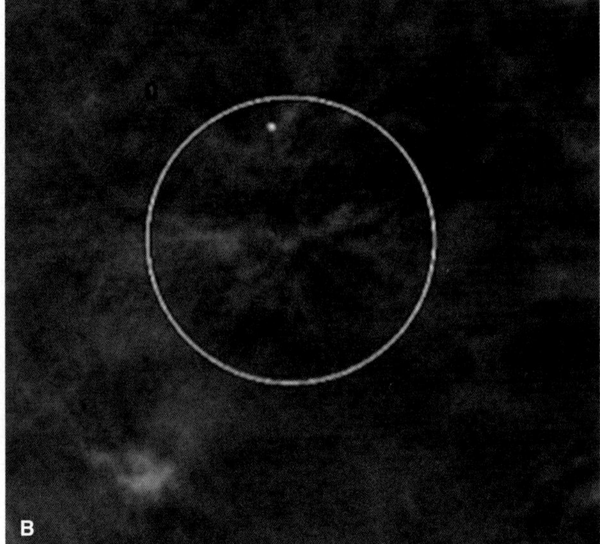

FIGURE 21.10. **Spiculated Mass Versus Architectural Distortion. A:** Spiculated mass. Mass has a three-dimensional shape and outward convex margins. Biopsy showed invasive lobular carcinoma (ILC). **B:** Architectural distortion seen on DBT with multiple straight lines radiating from a central point. There is no underlying mass. Biopsy showed radial scar.

mass has an x-ray attenuation similar to the surrounding tissue (Fig. 21.15). This is seen with both benign and malignant masses. A **high-density** mass is whiter than the surrounding tissue and is the most worrisome of the mass–density categories. Many invasive cancers are high density (Fig. 21.16).

A thorough analysis and categorization of the shape, margin, and density of all masses seen mammographically is imperative to determine the likelihood of malignancy. A combination of features helps guide assessment and recommendation.

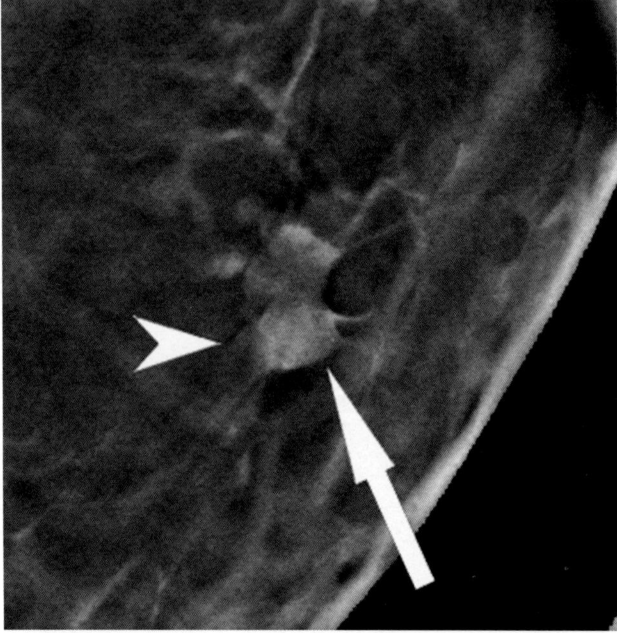

FIGURE 21.11. **Margin With Mixed Features.** Breast mass on DBT with margin that is partly circumscribed (*arrow*) and partly indistinct (*arrowhead*). The mass is most correctly described by the "worst" feature—indistinct. Pathology at biopsy and surgical excision showed papilloma with atypia.

Calcifications

Calcifications are described according to morphology and distribution. A good understanding of the different calcification morphologies and distributions will help you identify cancer, but not work up or biopsy something that is clearly benign (like a calcified artery!). Digital mammography offers high spatial resolution, around 0.1 mm/pixel. Because of this, we can detect microcalcifications in the tissue, which is an important feature of many breast cancers.

Pathologic microcalcifications are often associated with necrotic tumor debris. This is most commonly seen with ductal carcinoma in situ (DCIS). By definition, an "in situ" cancer has not crossed the basement membrane. Cells of DCIS fill the milk but do not invade the adjacent stroma. DCIS does not have direct access to the vascular system. Nutrients can only diffuse across the cell layers as they multiply. The cancerous cells at the center of a duct, furthest from the basement membrane and furthest from the vasculature, cannot get enough nutrients from diffusion alone. The tumor cells in the center of the duct die or become necrotic. As these necrotic cells accumulate, they begin to calcify, which results in a thin layer of "casting" calcifications seen within the center of the lumen of a milk duct containing DCIS. Calcifications that follow a ductal distribution thus have a higher likelihood of malignancy.

The calcification morphology descriptors that can be associated with malignancy are amorphous, coarse heterogeneous, fine pleomorphic, and fine linear or fine linear branching (Table 21.4). **Amorphous** calcifications can be the most difficult to identify. They are small and fuzzy in appearance (Fig. 21.17). It is often difficult to count an exact number of amorphous calcifications. The differential diagnosis of amorphous calcifications includes DCIS (often low grade), high-risk lesions (atypical ductal hyperplasia, atypical lobular hyperplasia, and lobular carcinoma in situ), fibrocystic changes, and sclerosing adenosis. **Coarse heterogeneous** calcifications are larger, between 0.5 and 1 mm (Fig. 21.18). The differential diagnosis includes DCIS (often high grade), degenerating fibroadenoma or papilloma, fibrocystic changes, or fat necrosis. **Fine pleomorphic calcifications** are usually <0.5 mm in size and have a variety of sizes and shapes (Fig. 21.19).

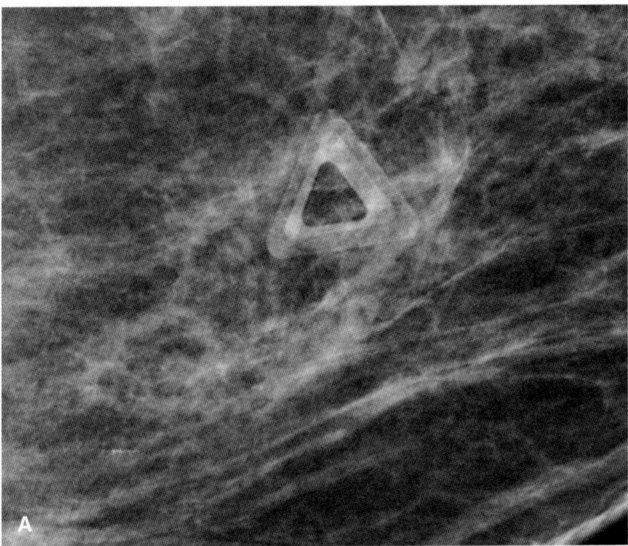

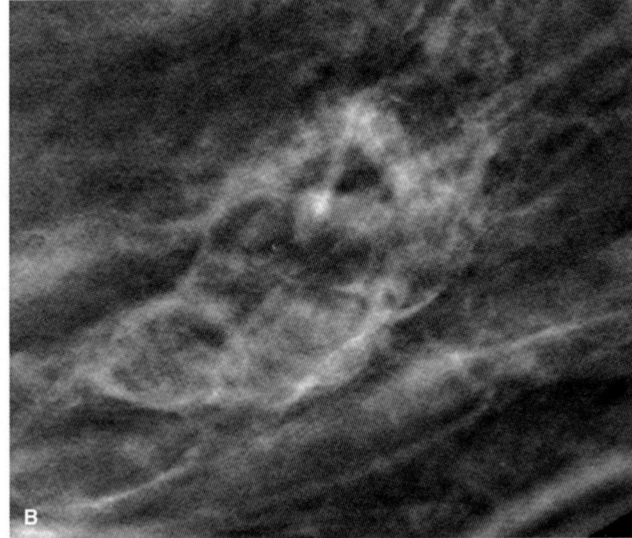

FIGURE 21.12. **Fat-Containing Mass. A:** Fat-containing mass on mammography. **B:** Fat-containing mass on DBT. Patient had a history of trauma and bruising at this location. The triangle marker indicates that the mass is palpable. Appearance is compatible with fat necrosis.

The differential diagnosis is similar to coarse heterogeneous calcifications but the likelihood of malignancy is higher for fine pleomorphic at about 30%. **Fine linear or fine linear branching** calcifications are thin and linear. Their appearance is similar to a ductal system or branches of a tree. You may see calcifications that look like a "Y" or a "V" that suggest their location within the branches of a milk duct. This group of calcifications has the highest likelihood of malignancy of all the calcification morphology descriptors at about 70% and almost always requires biopsy (Fig. 21.20).

In addition to morphology, accurate description of the distribution of calcifications can help determine the likelihood of malignancy (Table 21.5). **Diffuse** calcifications are scattered randomly throughout the breast and have the lowest correlation with malignancy (Fig. 21.21). **Regional** calcifications occupy a large area that is more than one ductal system (Fig. 21.22). **Grouped** calcifications occupy a small area, usually within 2 cm (Fig. 21.23). **Linear** calcifications are arranged in a line, which is suggestive of location within a milk duct (Fig. 21.24). This can be seen with DCIS, since it often starts in a single duct. *Segmental* calcifications are wedge shaped with the broad base closer to the chest wall and tapering toward the nipple (Fig. 21.25). These calcifications span more than half the distance from the chest wall to the nipple. The distribution

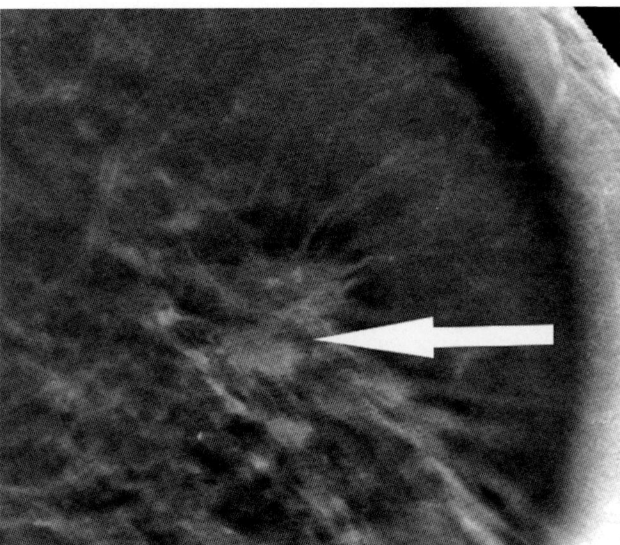

FIGURE 21.13. **Cancer-Engulfing Fat.** There is low attenuation fat within this irregular spiculated mass (*arrow*). Biopsy showed invasive ductal carcinoma (IDC).

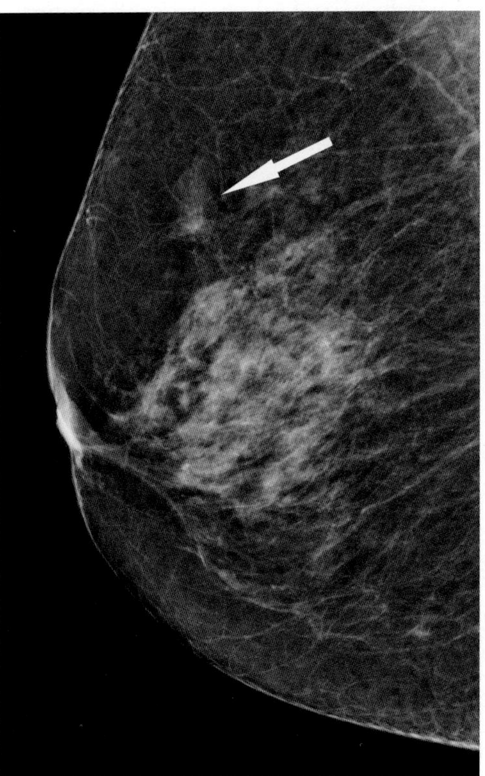

FIGURE 21.14. **Low-Density Mass.** Low-density mass seen on mammogram (*arrow*). Ultrasound revealed a simple cyst.

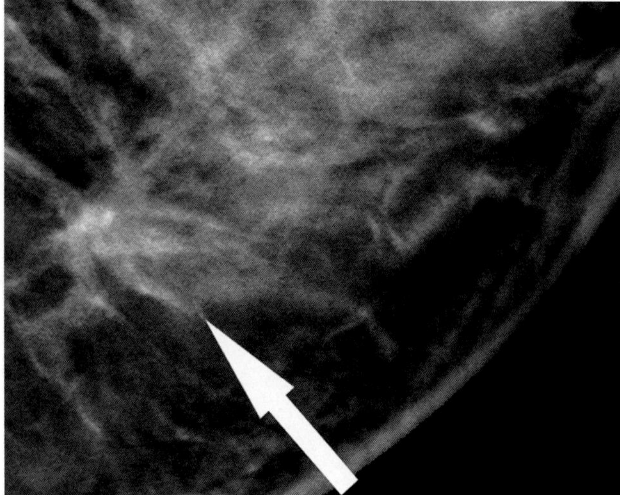

FIGURE 21.15. **Equal-Density Mass.** Irregular spiculated mass is seen (*arrow*). It is equal in density or similar in attenuation to the surrounding tissue. Biopsy showed invasive lobular carcinoma (ILC).

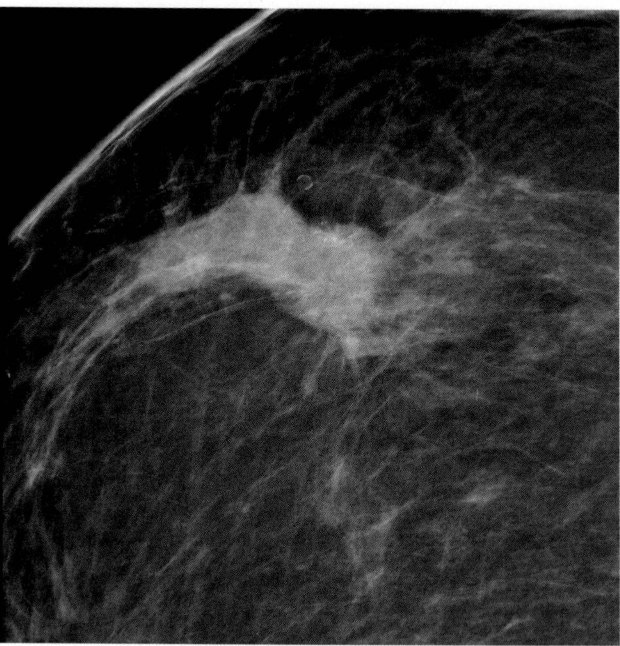

FIGURE 21.16. **High-Density Mass.** Irregular, speculated, high-density mass. The mass is whiter than the surrounding breast tissue. Biopsy showed invasive ductal carcinoma (IDC).

can resemble a triangle and correspond to an entire ductal system and all of its branches. This distribution is often a worrisome finding, with the likelihood of malignancy around 62%.

There are also many benign breast calcifications. Some form of calcification is frequently seen on mammograms. Many benign calcifications have a very specific benign appearance and do not require additional imaging evaluation or biopsy. The typically benign calcifications are skin, vascular, coarse or "popcorn-like," large rod-like, round, rim, dystrophic, milk of calcium, and suture (Table 21.6). **Skin** calcifications are usually lucent centered and multiple in number. They are usually superficial on one of the mammographic views. Special views such as a tangential view can help confirm their location in the skin (Fig. 21.26). They are common in the inframammary fold, cleavage, and areola. They can also be seen in scars. **Vascular** calcifications are in the walls of arteries. They often have a "tram-track" appearance of two double lines. They follow the path of the arterial supply to the breast. They are often wider at the posterior aspect of the

TABLE 21.4

BI-RADS® CALCIFICATION MORPHOLOGY DESCRIPTORS AND LIKELIHOOD OF MALIGNANCY

■ SUSPICIOUS MORPHOLOGY	■ LIKELIHOOD OF MALIGNANCY
Amorphous	21%
Coarse heterogeneous	13%
Fine pleomorphic	29%
Fine linear or fine linear branching	70%

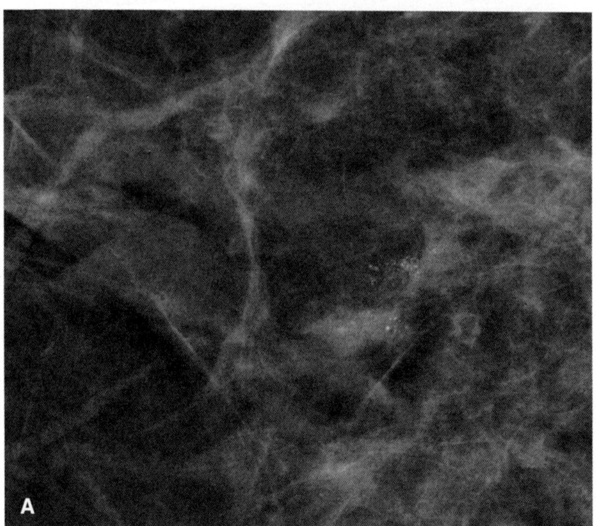

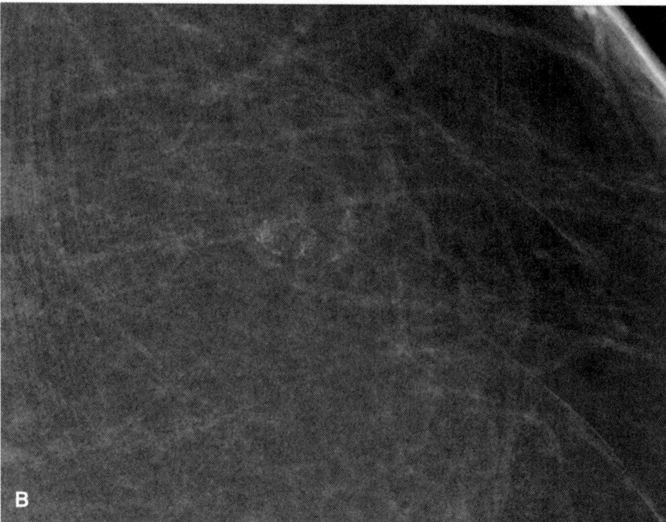

FIGURE 21.17. **Amorphous Calcifications. A:** Numerous small and fuzzy calcifications are present. They are difficult to count. Biopsy showed fibrocystic changes. **B:** Biopsy showed atypical ductal hyperplasia.

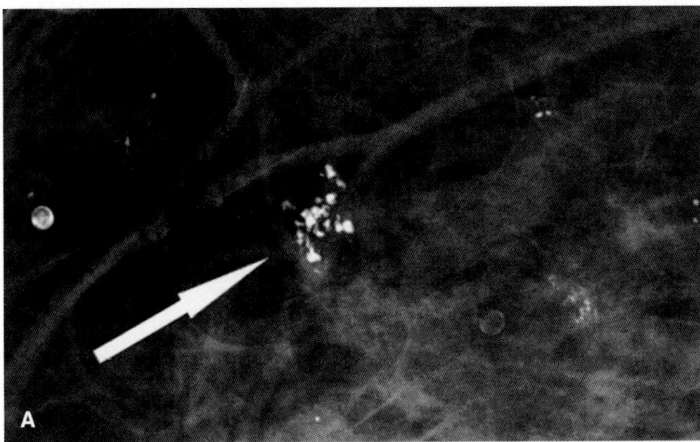

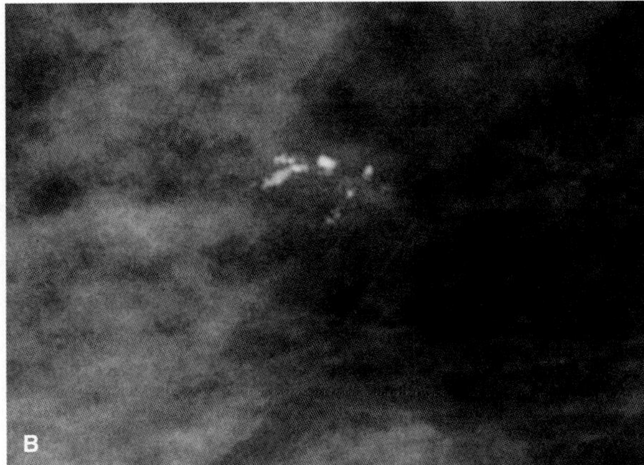

FIGURE 21.18. **Coarse Heterogeneous Calcifications. A:** This group of coarse heterogeneous calcifications (*arrow*) was stable mammographically for many years and likely represents a degenerated fibroadenoma. **B:** Coarse heterogeneous calcifications in a different patient. Biopsy showed high-grade DCIS.

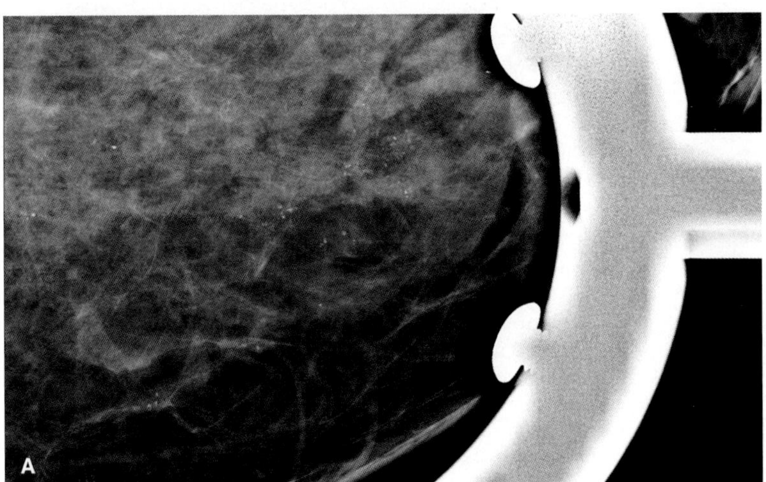

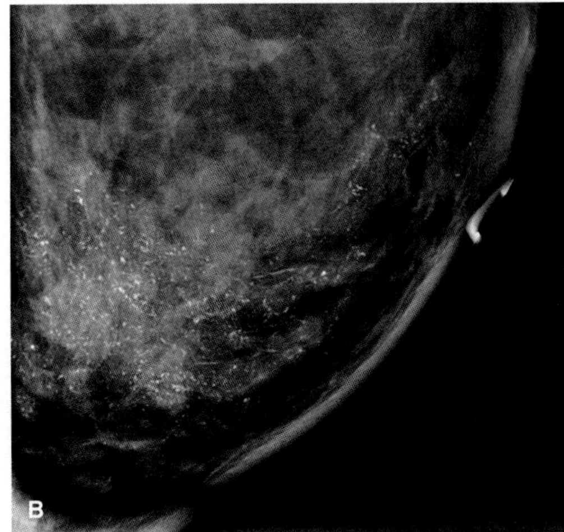

FIGURE 21.19. **Fine Pleomorphic Calcifications. A:** Fine pleomorphic calcifications. Biopsy showed high-grade DCIS. **B:** Segmental fine pleomorphic calcifications. Biopsy showed high-grade DCIS. Surgical pathology after mastectomy showed DCIS and multiple areas of invasive ductal carcinoma (IDC).

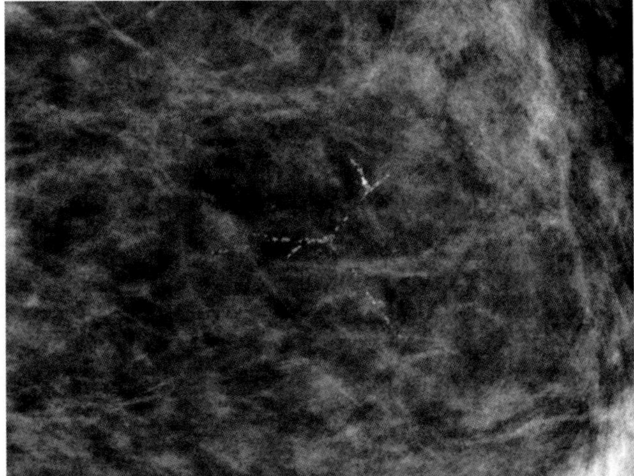

FIGURE 21.20. **Fine Linear or Fine Linear Branching Calcifications.** Fine linear or fine linear branching calcifications. Note the "V" and "Y" shapes where the calcifications are filling the branching ducts. Biopsy showed high-grade DCIS.

breast and become narrower as they branch toward the nipple. DBT or magnification views can help identify if a tube is associated with the calcifications. Vascular calcifications are different from the casting calcifications of DCIS. Vascular calcifications are in the wall of the tube (artery), not in the center of the tube (milk duct) as seen in DCIS (Fig. 21.27). **Coarse or**

TABLE 21.5

BI-RADS® CALCIFICATION DISTRIBUTION DESCRIPTORS AND LIKELIHOOD OF MALIGNANCY

■ DISTRIBUTION	■ LIKELIHOOD OF MALIGNANCY
Diffuse	0%
Regional	26%
Grouped	31%
Linear	60%
Segmental	62%

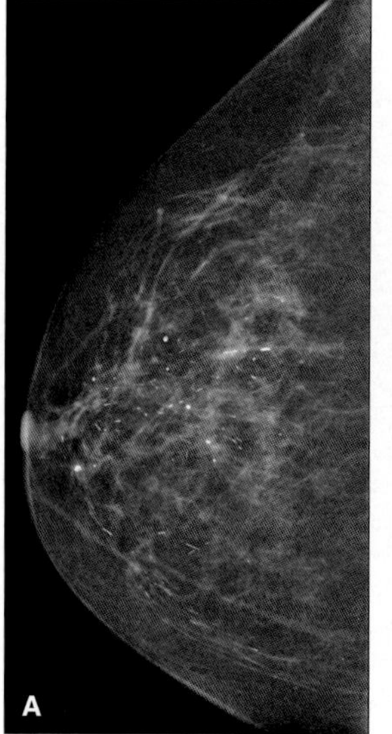

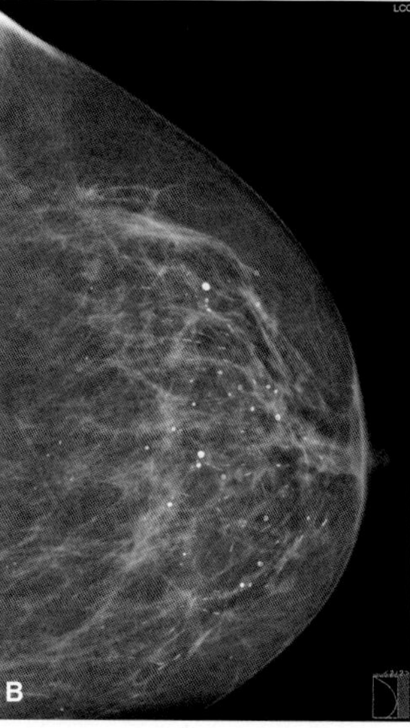

FIGURE 21.21. **Diffuse Calcifications. A:** Right CC and (**B**) left CC mammograms show bilateral diffuse large rod-like and rim calcifications. Appearance is compatible with benign secretory calcifications and calcified oil cysts. Diffuse bilateral distribution is frequently a benign finding.

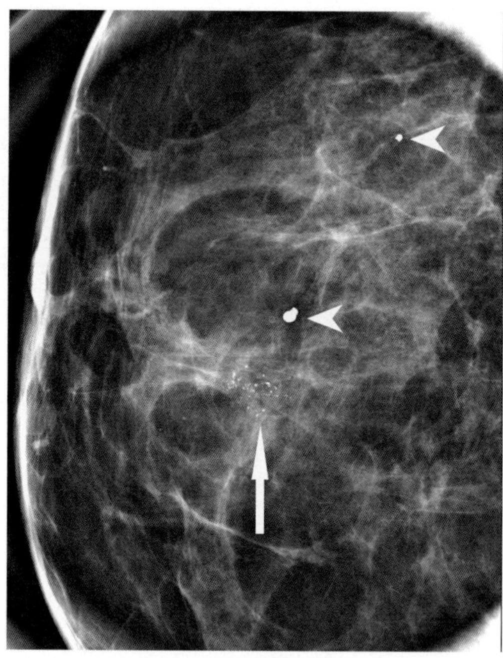

FIGURE 21.23. **Grouped Calcifications.** Grouped fine pleomorphic calcifications (*arrow*). Biopsy showed high-grade DCIS. There are incidental benign dystrophic calcifications (*arrowheads*).

"popcorn-like" calcifications are large, around 2 to 3 mm in size. As their name implies, they look like a piece of popcorn. They can be seen with an oval, circumscribed mass which is an involuting or degenerating fibroadenoma (Fig. 21.28). **Large rod-like** calcifications are benign calcifications of the duct. Branching pattern is common. They are smooth and cigar shaped. They are most often diffuse, bilateral, and seen almost exclusively in postmenopausal women. Large rod-like calcifications are also called secretory calcifications (Fig. 21.29). **Round** calcifications can be benign or malignant. They look like smooth round circles. They are often numerous and identical in appearance. Distribution of these calcifications is key. Diffuse or regional round calcifications are benign. Grouped round calcifications that have a low likelihood of malignancy are followed mammographically under BI-RADS 3 protocol (see Chapter 20). Round calcifications that are linear, segmental, new, increasing, or near a known cancer are suspicious (Fig. 21.30).

Milk of calcium refers to calcium that has precipitated out of the fluid within a cyst. They look like fuzzy puddles when viewed from the top down on the craniocaudal (CC) view. They can be indistinct and hard to see on CC views. When viewed from the side on medial-lateral or lateral-medial (ML or LM) view, they form a tiny curvilinear meniscus or teacup. It is important to note that these calcifications change shape on different mammographic projections (Fig. 21.31).

There are several typically benign calcifications associated with prior trauma or surgery. **Rim** calcifications are usually round or oval calcifications with a lucent center. Appearance resembles an eggshell. They are most often calcification of the wall of an oil cyst or fat necrosis (Fig. 21.32). **Dystrophic** calcifications may also have a lucent center but are more irregular in shape (Fig. 21.33). They are also the result of prior trauma, surgery, or radiation. **Suture** calcifications are deposited around suture material. They have the shape and

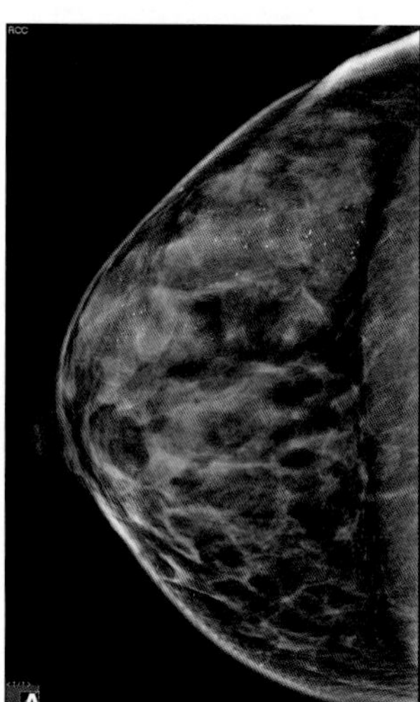

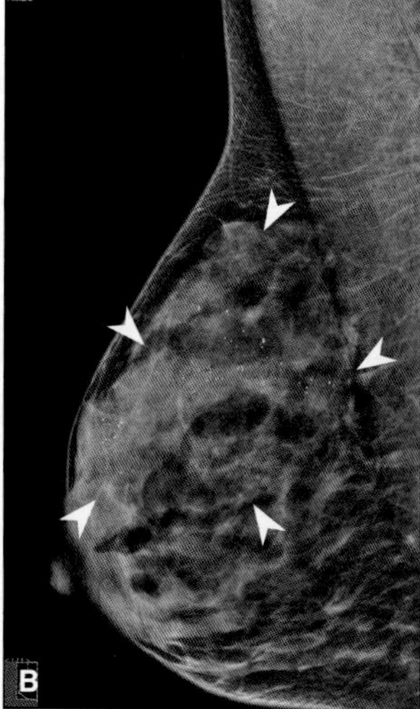

FIGURE 21.22. **Regional Calcifications.** Round calcifications are seen occupying an entire quadrant (*arrowheads*) seen on (**A**) CC view and (**B**) MLO view. Biopsy showed fibrocystic changes.

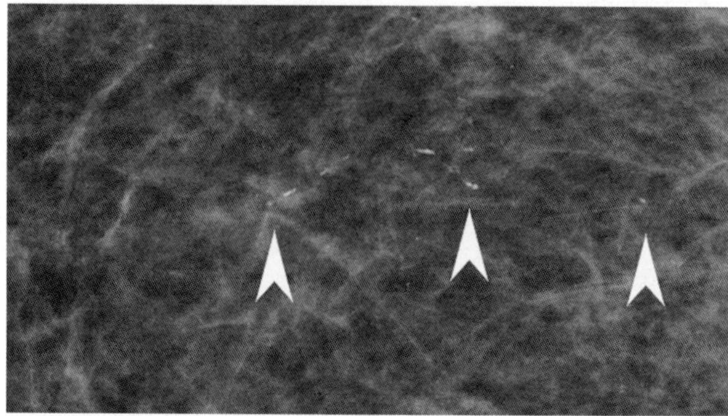

FIGURE 21.24. **Linear Calcifications.** Fine linear branching calcifications are seen in a linear distribution (*arrowheads*). Biopsy revealed high-grade DCIS.

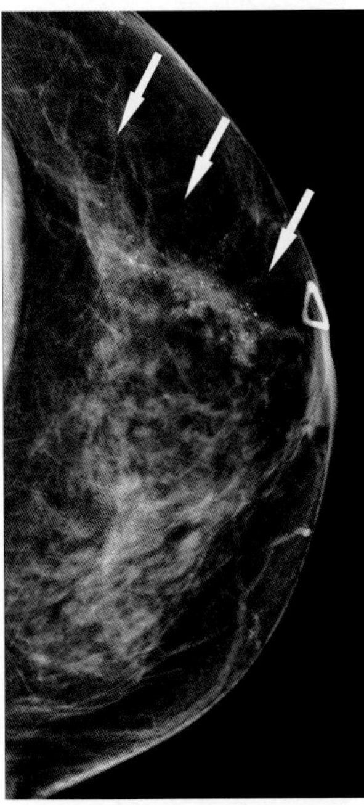

FIGURE 21.25. **Segmental Calcifications.** Fine pleomorphic calcifications involving the entire ductal system from the chest wall to the nipple (*arrows*). Biopsy showed high-grade DCIS. A triangle marker is on the skin which indicates that a palpable lump is also present.

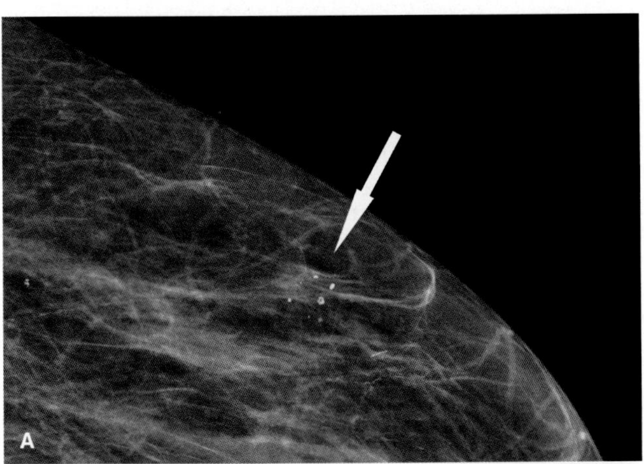

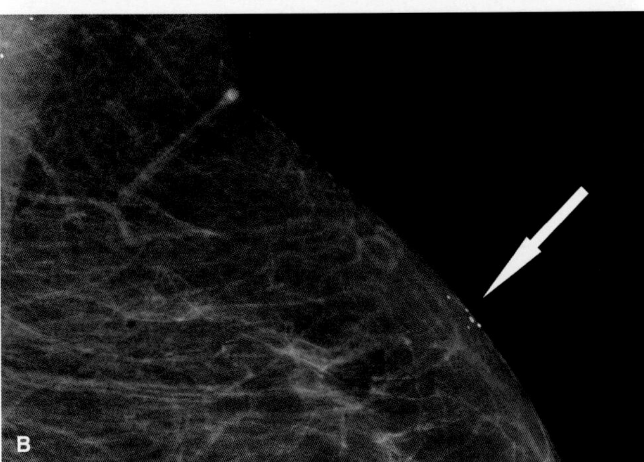

FIGURE 21.26. **Skin Calcifications. A:** CC view showing a group of round and lucent-centered calcifications (*arrow*). **B:** MLO view confirms the location of the calcifications in the skin (*arrow*).

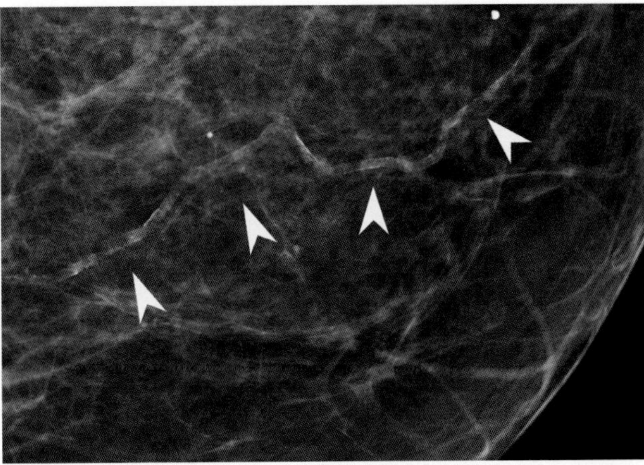

FIGURE 21.27. **Vascular Calcifications.** Calcifications with a "tram-track" appearance (*arrowheads*) are compatible with vascular calcifications.

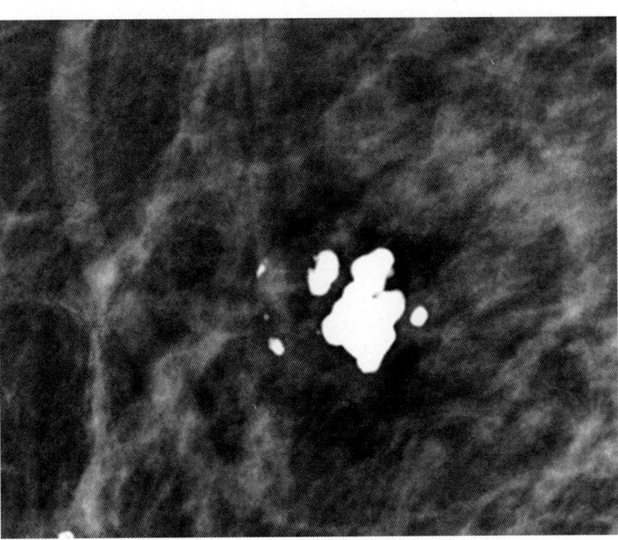

FIGURE 21.28. **Coarse or "Popcorn-Like" Calcifications.** Popcorn-like calcifications are commonly seen in degenerated fibroadenomas. The calcifications are specific and benign. They require no further workup or intervention.

TABLE 21.6

BI-RADS® TYPICALLY BENIGN CALCIFICATIONS

Skin
Vascular
Coarse or "popcorn-like"
Large rod-like
Round
Rim
Dystrophic
Milk of calcium

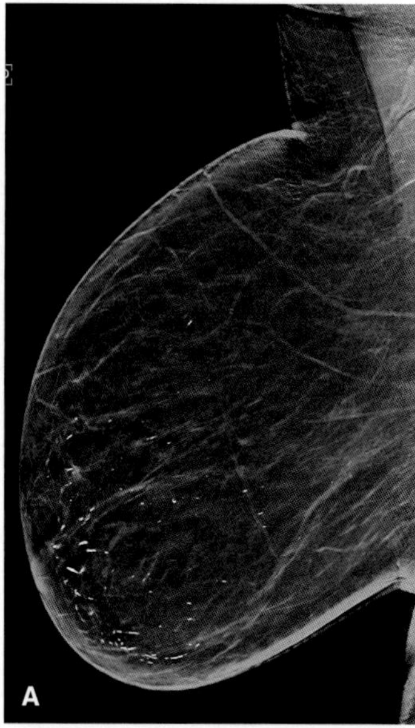

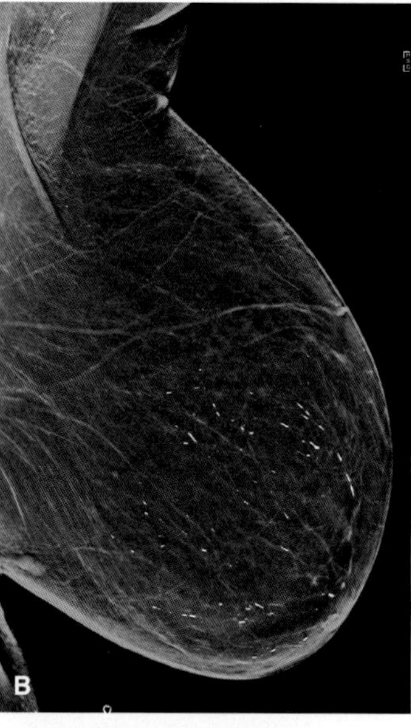

FIGURE 21.29. **Large Rod-Like Calcifications. A:** Right MLO and (**B**) left MLO synthetic 2D views show bilateral diffuse large rod-like calcifications. Appearance is compatible with benign secretory calcifications.

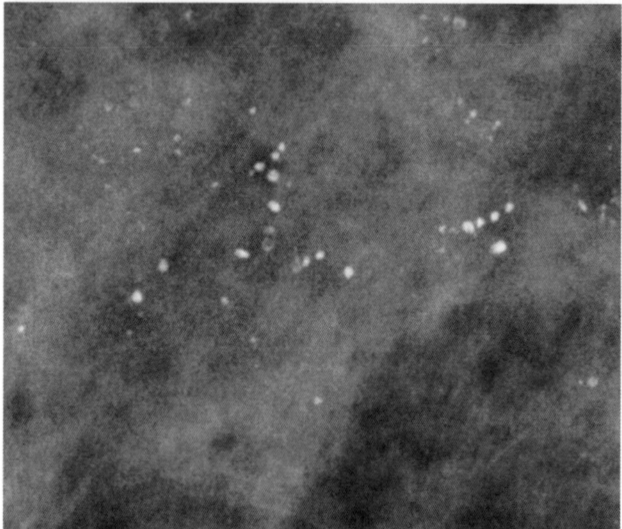

FIGURE 21.30. **Round Calcifications.** Round calcifications. Biopsy showed fibrocystic changes.

appearance of suture material with loops and knots. Patients will always have a history of surgery.

Architectural Distortion

Normal breast tissue consists of undulating intermixed fat lobules and fibroglandular tissue. Normally the lines that mark the interface of tissue and fat are soft, respectful, and similar to waves in an ocean. The thin Cooper ligaments are also visible mammographically and have a similar appearance. When a fibrosing process is present, these lines become straight and the normal architecture is distorted. On mammography, this looks like straight lines, often radiating from a central point. The adjacent parenchyma may look retracted or "pulled in." There is no definite mass present with pure architectural distortion (AD). If there are straight lines radiating from a mass, it should be described as a spiculated mass. If there is no definite mass present, straight lines indicate AD (Fig. 21.34).

There are both benign and malignant etiologies for AD. Prior surgery, trauma, fibrosis, fibrocystic changes, or a radial

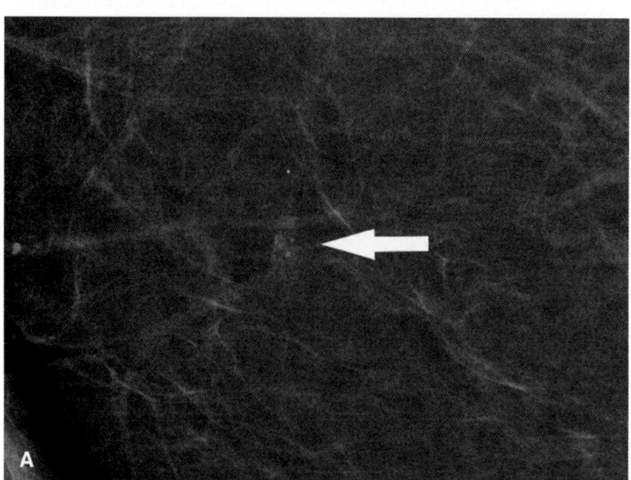

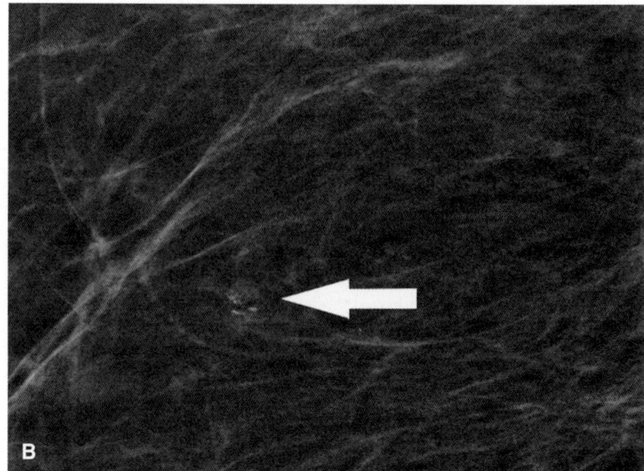

FIGURE 21.31. **Milk of Calcium. A:** A small group of calcifications that are smudgy and amorphous on CC view (*arrow*). **B:** Calcifications "layer" and resemble teacups on the ML view (*arrow*).

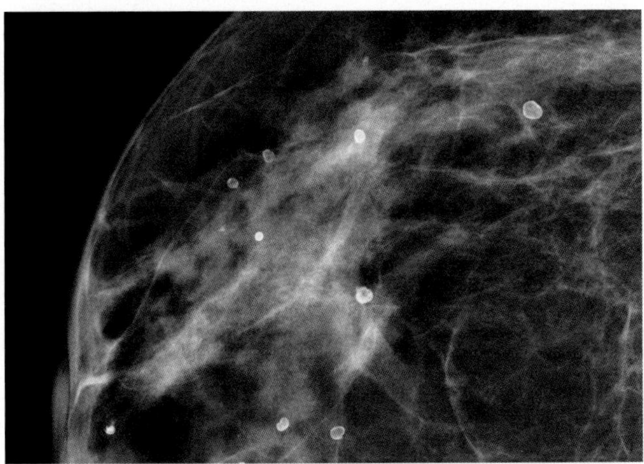

FIGURE 21.32. **Rim Calcifications.** Benign rim or eggshell calcifications. These are commonly seen with fat necrosis and calcified oil cysts.

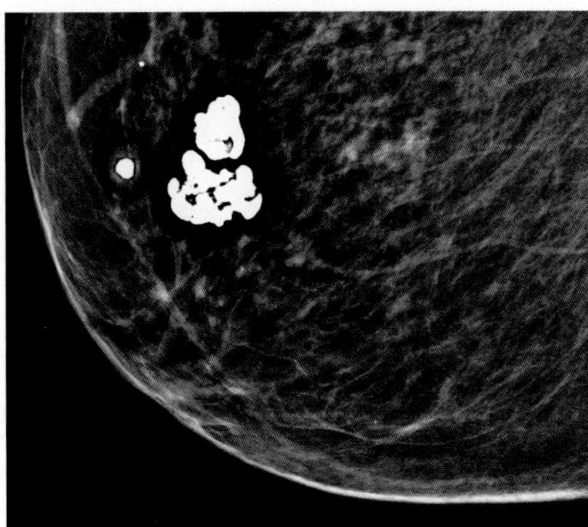

FIGURE 21.33. **Dystrophic Calcifications.** Large smooth calcifications with lucent center. Dystrophic calcifications can be seen with prior trauma, surgery, or radiation.

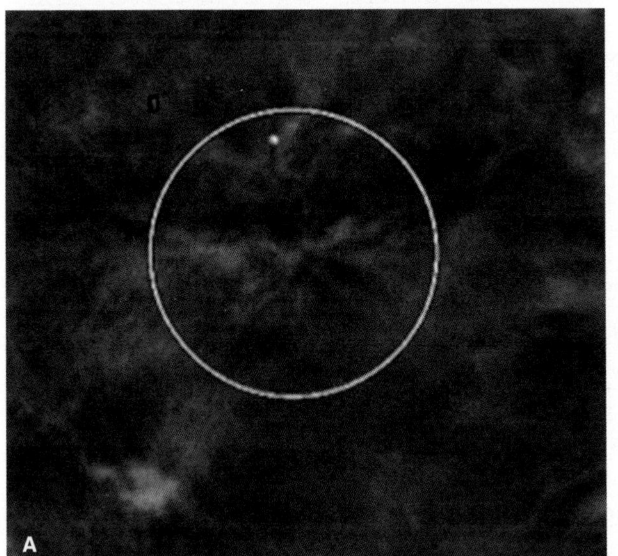

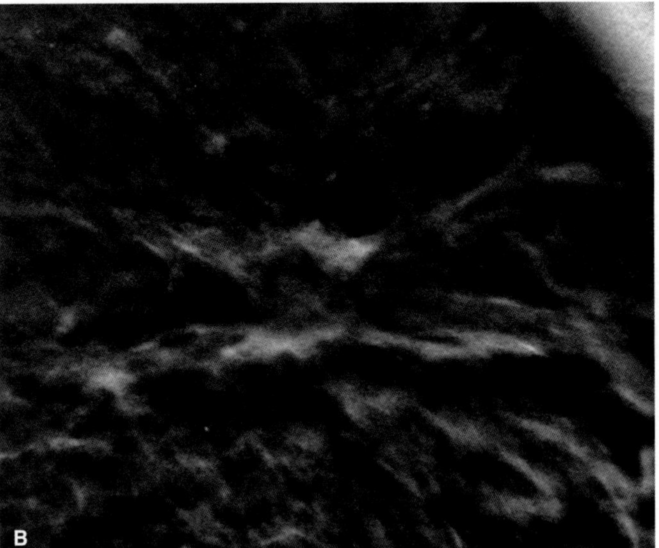

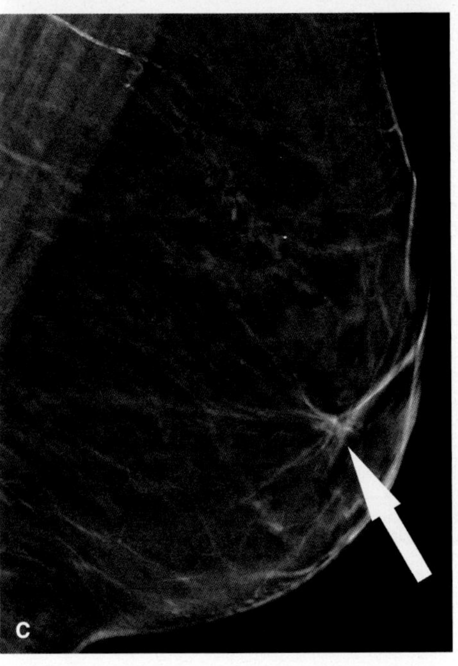

FIGURE 21.34. **Architectural Distortion. A:** Circle surrounds multiple straight lines of architectural distortion. Biopsy showed radial scar. **B:** Architectural distortion seen on DBT. Biopsy showed invasive ductal carcinoma (IDC). **C:** Architectural distortion seen on DBT due to a surgical scar (*arrow*).

TABLE 21.7

CAUSES OF ARCHITECTURAL DISTORTION

Invasive breast cancer—ILC and IDC
Prior surgery
Radial scar
Fibrocystic changes
Fibrosis

scar can cause AD (Table 21.7). However, it can also be seen with cancer. Without a history of prior surgery to explain AD, biopsy is necessary. AD can be seen with both IDC and invasive lobular carcinoma (ILC). AD is a classic appearance of ILC which may present without a visible mass.

AD can be difficult to detect mammographically. Luckily, it is more easily seen with DBT. This has led to increased cancer detection, with the greatest impact in scattered and heterogeneous breast density categories. AD exhibits a high positive predictive value (PPV) for malignancy (60% to 83%) at diagnostic 2D mammography.

Asymmetries

As the name implies, an asymmetry is seen in only one breast, different from the other side. An asymmetry resembles a clump of normal fibroglandular tissue often with interspersed fat. It is not a mass (does not have a definable 3D shape or outward convex margins). An asymmetry often represents summation of normal structures but can occasionally be seen with malignancy. Asymmetries are subdivided into four groups: asymmetry, global asymmetry, focal asymmetry, and developing asymmetry (Table 21.8).

An **asymmetry** is seen only on one mammographic view. It often represents superimposition of normal structures (Fig. 21.35). A **global asymmetry** is large, involving more than one quadrant. In the absence of other suspicious findings (e.g., calcifications, AD, nipple retraction, or a palpable mass), it is most often a benign variant or normal anatomy (Fig. 21.36). A **focal asymmetry** is seen on two mammographic views and is smaller than a quadrant (Fig. 21.37). A **developing asymmetry** is the most suspicious type of asymmetry. It is new or larger when compared to priors (Fig. 21.38). It has the highest association with malignancy—with a PPV of approximately 12.8% at screening and 26.7% at diagnostic mammography. When seen on screening, it should always be evaluated with diagnostic mammography to determine the underlying cause. If there is no specific benign cause identified for a developing asymmetry (trauma, underlying cyst, etc.), biopsy should be performed.

Associated Features

As you can see from the lexicon, breast cancer can present as a mass, calcifications, AD, or asymmetry. It is also important to recognize that these findings can occur alone or together, which is important to recognize. It is important to also describe findings that are seen together such as calcifications adjacent to a mass. A combination of suspicious findings will increase the likelihood of malignancy.

Skin retraction, nipple retraction, skin thickening, trabecular thickening, and axillary adenopathy are also important signs of malignancy (Table 21.9). Sometimes it is the associated feature that you first recognize as a sign of something abnormal. These associated findings should be viewed suspiciously with a search to determine the underlying cause (Fig. 21.39).

TABLE 21.8

BI-RADS® ASYMMETRIES

Asymmetry (seen on one view)
Focal asymmetry (seen on two views)
Global asymmetry
Developing asymmetry

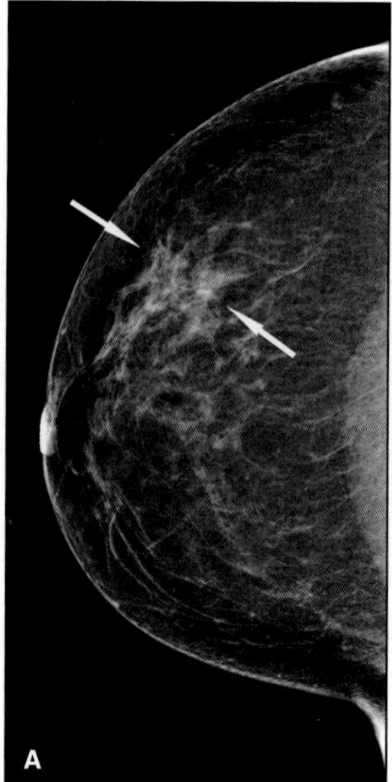

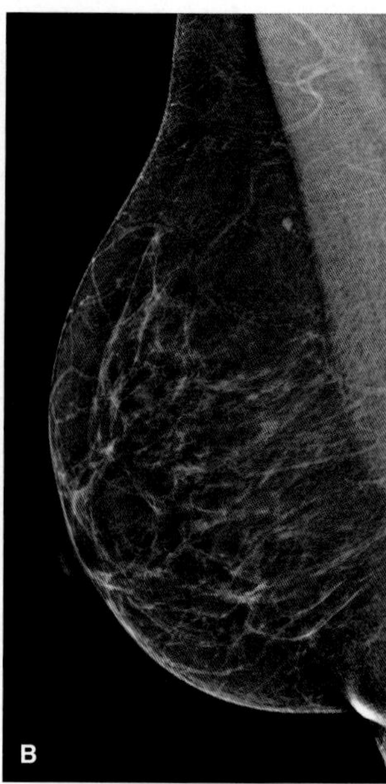

FIGURE 21.35. **Asymmetry. A:** Asymmetric tissue is seen on the CC view only (*arrows*). **B:** There is no corresponding finding on MLO. Diagnostic evaluation with tomosynthesis and ultrasound revealed normal-appearing breast tissue.

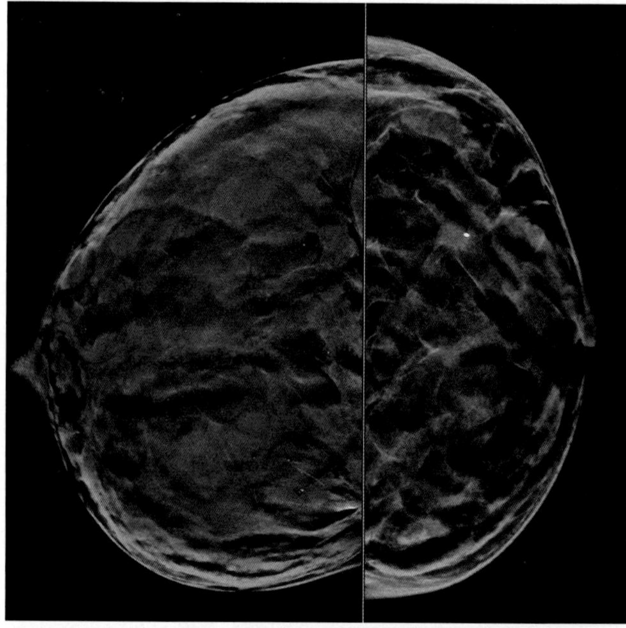

FIGURE 21.36. **Global Asymmetry.** Bilateral CC views from a lactating patient show asymmetric tissue on the right. She is only breastfeeding on the right, which is the likely etiology of the asymmetry.

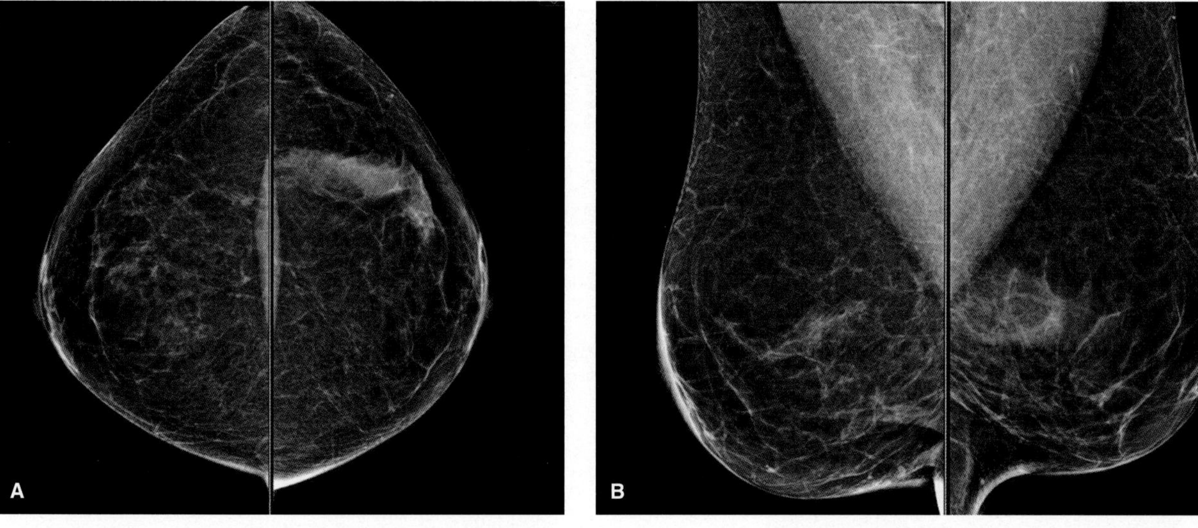

FIGURE 21.37. **Focal Asymmetry. A:** Bilateral CC views and (**B**) bilateral MLO views showing a focal asymmetry in the left breast.

TABLE 21.9

BI-RADS® ASSOCIATED FEATURES

Skin retraction
Nipple retraction
Skin thickening
Trabecular thickening
Axillary adenopathy
Architectural distortion
Calcifications

ULTRASOUND LEXICON

There is a separate BI-RADS lexicon for ultrasound imaging of the breast. Masses are described on ultrasound according to their shape, margin, orientation, echo pattern, and posterior features. As with mammography, accurate characterization of breast masses on ultrasound will guide assessment, recommendation, and improve cancer detection (Table 21.10).

The shape descriptors are the same as those on mammography: *oval, round,* and *irregular* (Fig. 21.40). Margin is classified as circumscribed or not circumscribed. A **circumscribed**

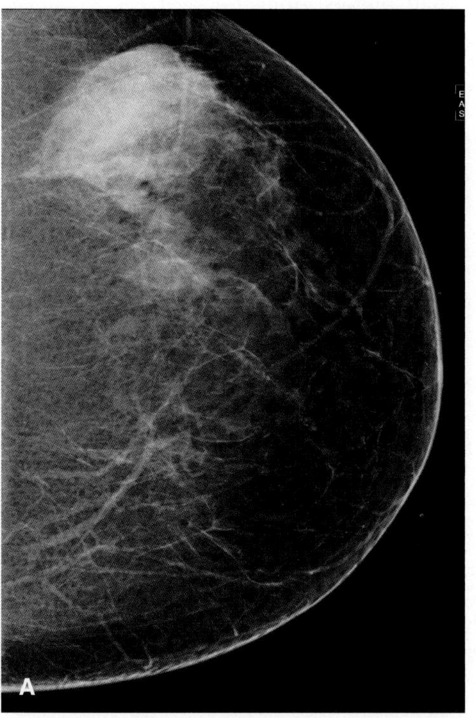

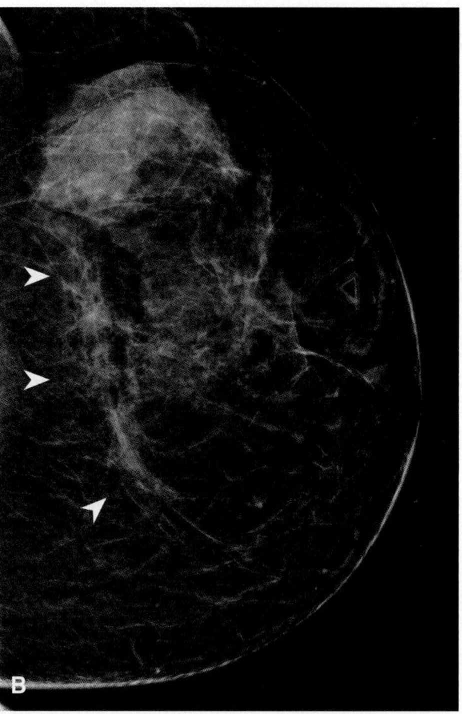

FIGURE 21.38. **Developing Asymmetry. A:** Left CC view from 2 years prior. **B:** Current left CC view showing a developing asymmetry (*arrowheads*). This finding was also palpable, which is marked with a triangle. Biopsy showed invasive ductal carcinoma with lobular features.

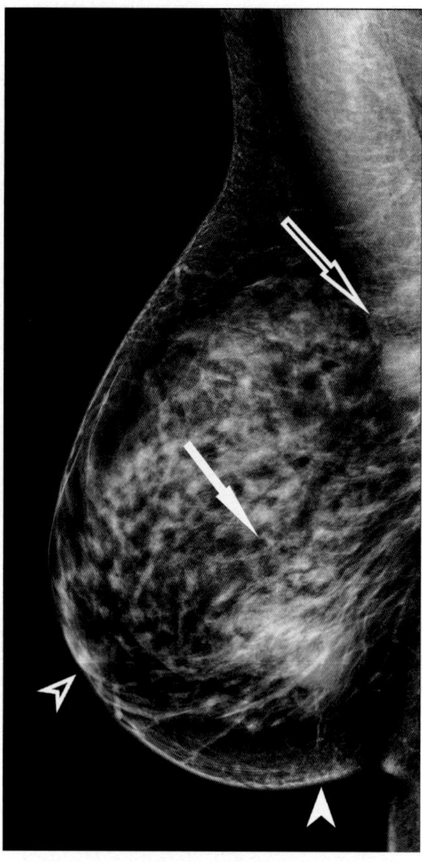

FIGURE 21.39. **Associated Features of Malignancy.** There is an irregular-shaped high-density mass with indistinct margin present (*solid arrow*). Biopsy showed invasive ductal carcinoma. Also note the adenopathy in the low axilla (*open arrow*), skin thickening (*solid arrowhead*), and nipple retraction (*open arrowhead*). The combination of the mass plus the associated features increases the level of suspicion for malignancy.

TABLE 21.10

BI-RADS® MASS DESCRIPTORS: ULTRASOUND

Shape	Oval Round Irregular
Margin	Circumscribed Indistinct Angular Microlobulated Spiculated
Echo pattern	Anechoic Hyperechoic Complex cystic and solid Hypoechoic Isoechoic Heterogeneous
Orientation	Parallel Not parallel
Posterior features	No posterior features Enhancement Shadowing Combined pattern

margin is a well-defined, smooth interface between the mass and the surrounding tissue. The not-circumscribed margins include indistinct, angular, microlobulated, and spiculated (Fig. 21.41). The definition of circumscribed, indistinct, microlobulated, and spiculated margins is similar to mammography. An **indistinct** margin has a very vague interface between the mass and the surrounding tissue. The margin often looks "fuzzy." A **microlobulated** margin has several small bumps along the surface. A **spiculated** margin has straight lines extending out from the mass. **Angular** margin is

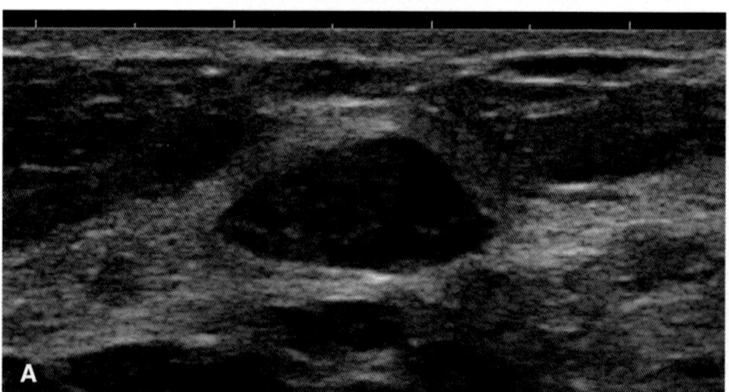

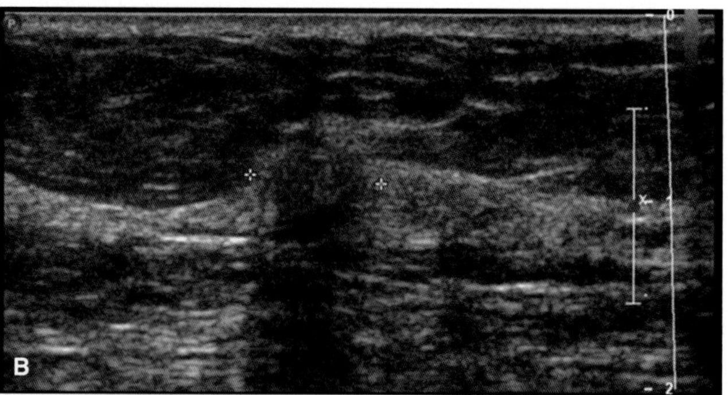

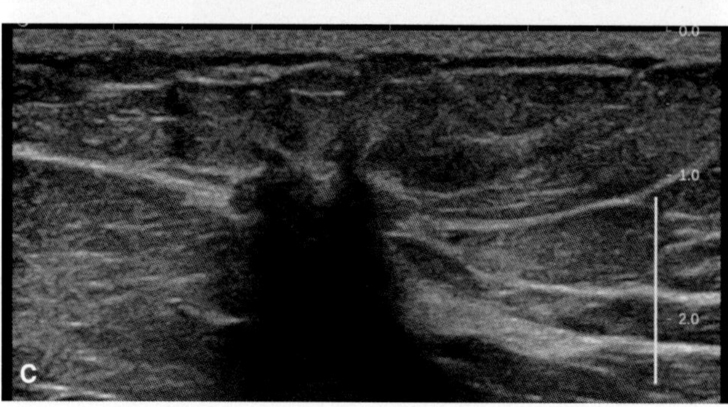

FIGURE 21.40. **Ultrasound Shape.** Multiple grayscale ultrasound images from different patients. **A:** Oval mass. **B:** Round mass. **C:** Irregular mass.

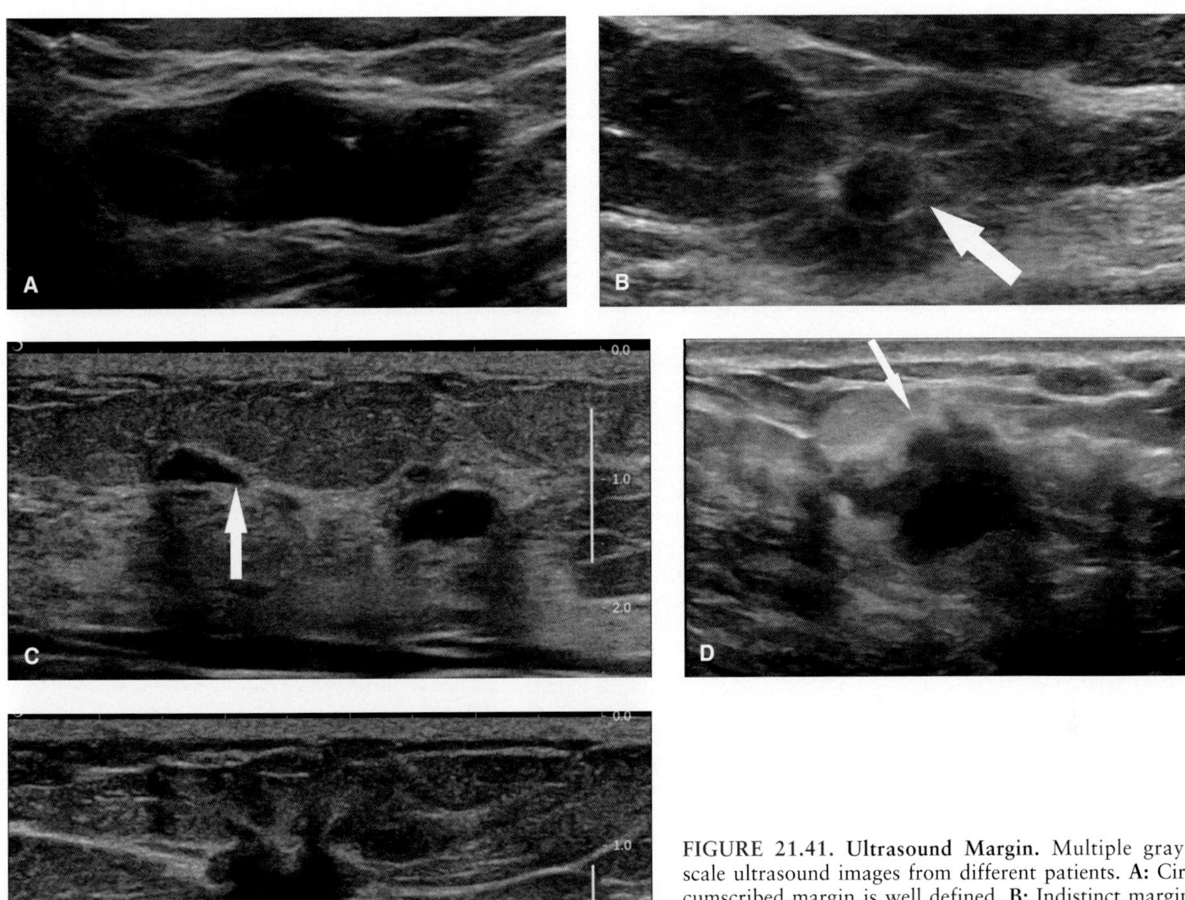

FIGURE 21.41. **Ultrasound Margin.** Multiple grayscale ultrasound images from different patients. **A:** Circumscribed margin is well defined. **B:** Indistinct margin has a very vague interface (*arrow*). **C:** Angular margin is forming acute angles or tail-like extensions (*arrow*). **D:** Microlobulated margin has several small bumps along the surface (*arrow*). **E:** Spiculated margin has straight lines extending out from the mass.

unique to ultrasound. The edges of the mass are forming acute angles or tail-like extensions. This can signify extension of the mass from a milk duct.

The echo pattern of a mass refers to the echogenicity of the internal contents. If no sound waves are reflected, the mass is **anechoic** or completely black inside. This is common in fluid-containing structures such as a simple cyst. A **hyperechoic** mass is more echogenic or "white" than the fat. A **hypoechoic** mass is less echogenic or darker than fat. An **isoechoic** mass is the same as the fat around it. These masses may be difficult to identify. A **complex cystic and solid** mass contains both fluid components in addition to solid material. A **heterogeneous** mass has mixed features (Fig. 21.42).

The orientation of a mass relative to the chest wall and the posterior features deep to a mass are also important. Normal fibroglandular tissue and many benign findings (such as cysts and fibroadenomas) are most often parallel to the chest wall. A mass that is antiparallel (or taller than wide) is often suspicious for invasive breast cancer (Fig. 21.43). Posterior features describe the appearance of the tissue deep to a mass. Posterior features are described as: **no posterior features, enhancement, shadowing,** or **combined pattern.** Structures with a high water content (such as cysts or necrotic tumors) often exhibit posterior acoustic enhancement. Invasive breast cancers, dense fibrosis, and large calcifications cause posterior acoustic shadowing due to attenuation of the ultrasound beam (Fig. 21.44).

Ultrasound is very good at demonstrating the fluid content within a finding. There are several cystic breast masses (Fig. 21.45; Table 21.11). If a mass is completely anechoic with a thin imperceptible wall, it may be classified as a **simple cyst.** Numerous adjacent tiny cysts (1 to 3 mm in size) are termed **clustered microcysts.** Simple cysts and clustered microcysts are benign. A **complicated cyst** has diffuse low-level echoes present. These may be indistinguishable from a hypoechoic solid mass and prompt aspiration or biopsy. A **complex cystic and solid mass** has both solid- and fluid-containing spaces. This cystic mass has the highest association with malignancy. A complex cystic and solid mass may also represent an abscess, hematoma, fat necrosis, or postsurgical collection. Correlation with clinical history is important to determine if a patient has a history of infectious symptoms or recent trauma or surgery.

Associated features may also be seen on ultrasound such as AD, duct changes, skin thickening or retraction, edema, and vascularity. Modern, high-frequency transducers may also detect calcifications in or around a mass as well as calcifications in a duct. Elastography is a tool designed to assess the "stiffness" of tissue. Since many cancers are made of densely packed malignant cells, they may exhibit firm or *hard* elastography assessment. Elastography may also be assessed as *intermediate* or *soft.*

Ultrasound is also used to image lymph nodes in the axilla as they are not always seen on mammographic views. See

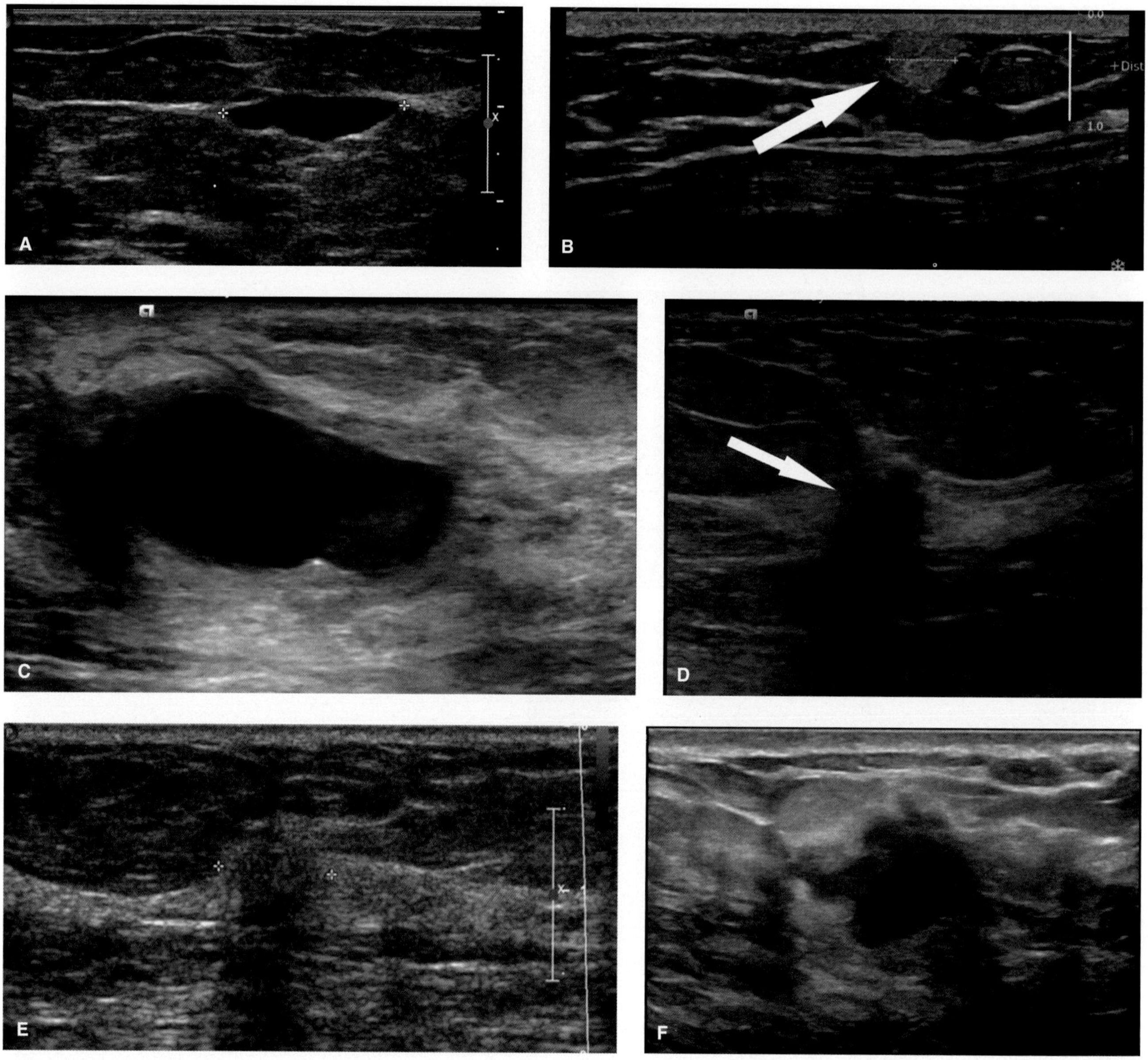

FIGURE 21.42. **Ultrasound Echo Pattern.** Multiple grayscale ultrasound images from different patients. **A:** Anechoic mass compatible with a simple cyst. **B:** Echogenic mass compatible with fat necrosis (*arrow*). Margin has straight lines extending out from the mass. This finding was associated with an entirely fat-containing mass on mammography (not shown). **C:** Complex cystic and solid mass. Finding underwent cyst aspiration and completely resolved. **D:** Hypoechoic mass (*arrow*). Biopsy showed invasive ductal carcinoma. **E:** Isoechoic mass that is similar to the adjacent fat. Mass is conspicuous due to posterior shadowing. **F:** Heterogeneous internal echo pattern.

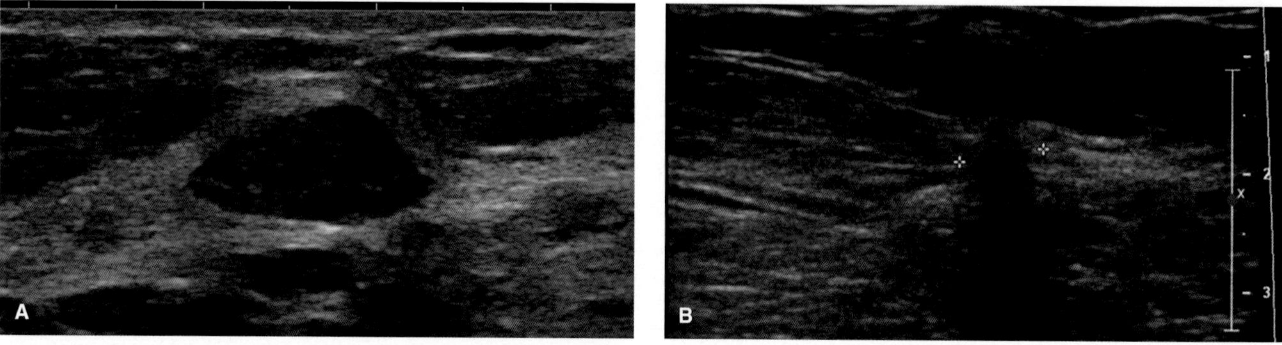

FIGURE 21.43. **Orientation. A:** Parallel. Mass is parallel to the chest wall. Imaging appearance is most suggestive of a fibroadenoma. **B:** Not parallel. Mass is taller than wide. Biopsy showed invasive ductal carcinoma (IDC).

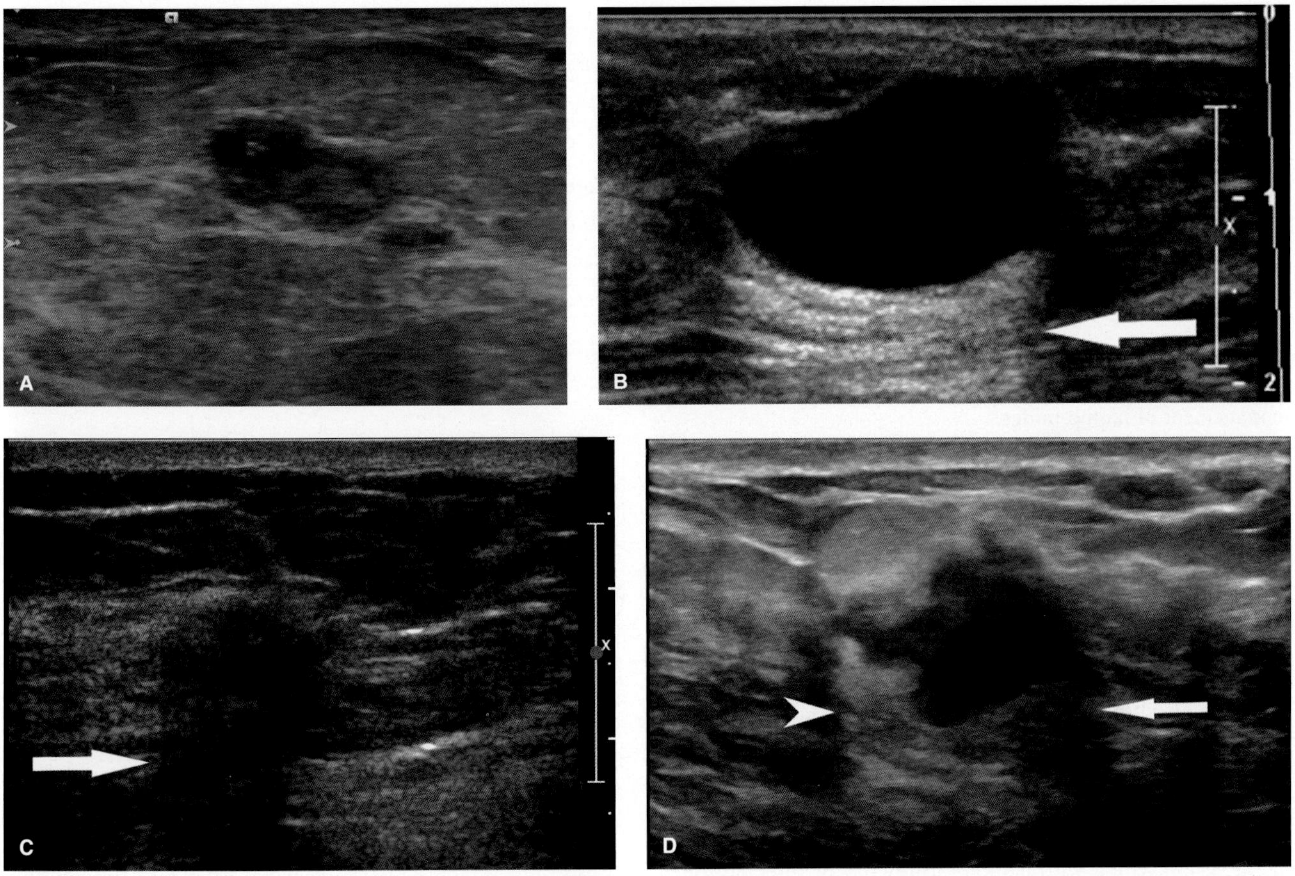

FIGURE 21.44. **Posterior Features. A:** No posterior features. **B:** Enhancement (*arrow*). **C:** Shadowing (*arrow*). **D:** Mixed features with areas of posterior acoustic enhancement (*arrowhead*) and shadowing (*arrow*).

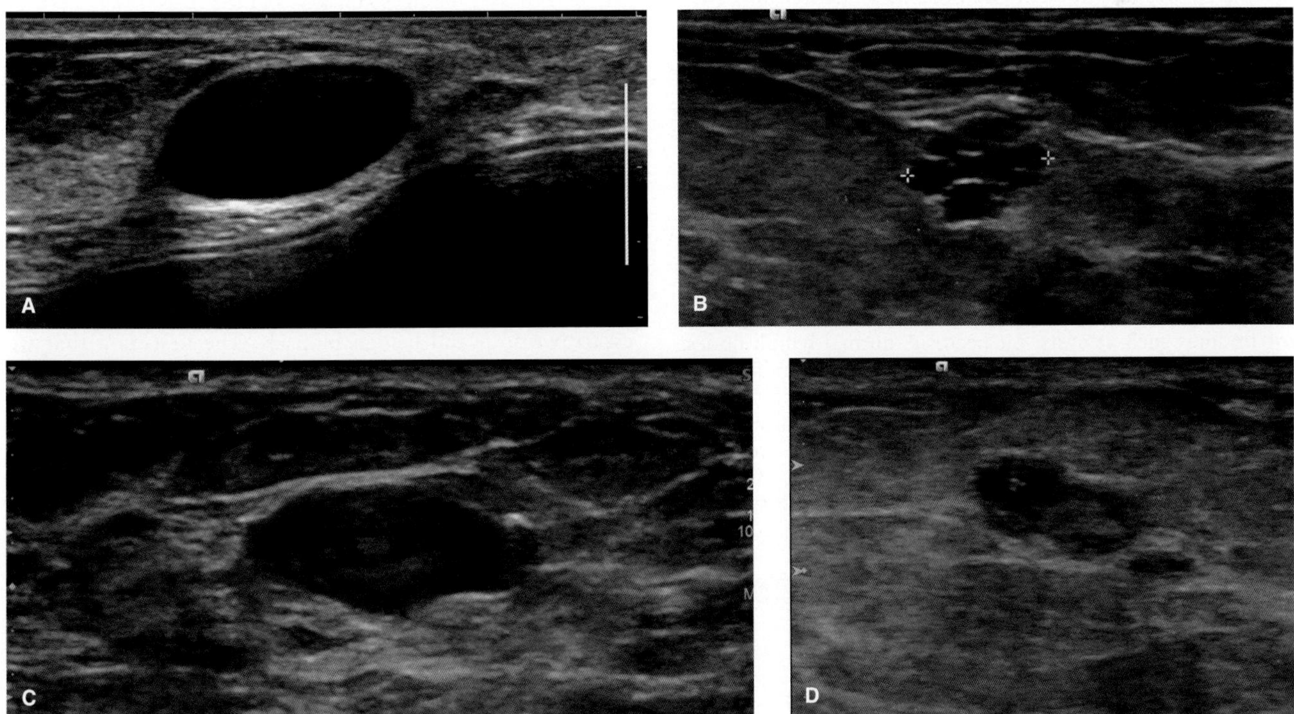

FIGURE 21.45. **Cystic Breast Masses on Ultrasound. A:** Simple cyst. **B:** Clustered microcysts. **C:** Complicated cyst with diffuse low-level internal echoes. **D:** Complex solid and cystic mass.

TABLE 21.11

CYSTIC BREAST MASSES ON ULTRASOUND

Simple cyst	Benign
Clustered microcysts	Benign
Complicated cyst	Benign cyst with debris, rarely malignancy
Complex solid and cystic mass	Benign cyst with debris, abscess, hematoma, papilloma, malignancy

Chapters 18 and 20 for further discussion of evaluation and management of lymph nodes.

MRI LEXICON

BI-RADS atlas also provides lexicon and guidance for MRI, which will be discussed in detail in Chapter 22.

REPORTING

BI-RADS also provides guidance for reporting. Clear communication to referring providers is improved with a consistent, standardized report. We typically begin each breast imaging report with the patient's history. This includes age, gender, and reason for the examination. We also include family and surgical history, if known. It is important to describe the location of the lesion which will facilitate follow-up or intervention. Careful understanding of lesion location will also help correlate findings between different imaging modalities. For every lesion it is important to include laterality, clock face, depth, and distance from the nipple (Table 21.12).

In the Impression section of the report, all lesions are given an assessment category and recommendation. BI-RADS Assessment Categories are numbered 0 to 6 (Table 21.13). Assessment **Category 0** is used when a finding needs additional evaluation or when prior films are needed for comparison. This is most commonly used when a lesion is detected at screening mammography. Additional mammographic views or perhaps an ultrasound is needed to further assess the finding and determine the likelihood of malignancy. Assessment **Category 1** is a negative examination. Only the normal structures of the breast are present. There are no suspicious findings that require intervention or attention on follow-up. Assessment **Category 2** is a benign finding. There is a lesion present, but it has a specific benign appearance. This is commonly used for findings such as cysts, fat necrosis, normal lymph nodes, etc. Assessment **Category 3** is a probably benign finding. The likelihood of malignancy is low, <2%. Findings in Assessment Category 3 usually undergo short interval follow-up for a total of 2 years (see Chapter 20). Assessment **Category 4** is for findings that have a likelihood of malignancy between 2% and 95%. This is a very broad range! Category 4 can be further subdivided based on the likelihood of malignancy into Categories 4A (2% to 10%), 4B (10% to 50%), and 4C (50% to 95%). Assessment **Category 5** is for lesions with a very high likelihood of malignancy (>95%). This category is used for classic appearance of cancers. Examples of BI-RADS Assessment Category 5 findings include irregular, spiculated, high-density masses or segmental fine linear branching calcifications. Assessment **Category 6** is a known or biopsy-proven malignancy.

TABLE 21.12

LOCATION OF A LESION

Laterality (right or left)
Quadrant and clock face
Depth
Distance from the nipple

TABLE 21.13

BI-RADS® ASSESSMENT CATEGORIES

Category 0	Incomplete—need additional imaging evaluation and/or prior films for comparison
Category 1	Negative
Category 2	Benign
Category 3	Probably benign
Category 4	Suspicious
Category 5	Highly suggestive of malignancy
Category 6	Known biopsy-proven malignancy

FOLLOW-UP AND OUTCOME MONITORING

In addition to the lexicon discussed earlier in the chapter, BI-RADS is also a quality assurance tool. It provides guidance to help radiologists assess their performance and identify potential areas of improvement.

Statistical Terms

Under MQSA, data are collected at all facilities performing breast imaging to create a clinically relevant medical audit. This audit allows interpreting physicians to assess their performance and the performance of their facility. Well-established benchmarks are published for comparison. Although it may seem like a daunting task, collecting this data helps radiologists identify areas of deficiency and create appropriate plans for quality improvement.

First, we must know what data to collect and how they are used. The goal of breast imaging is to identify breast cancer at the earliest most treatable stage, while minimizing unnecessary workup and benign biopsies. The first data that we must collect are the overall number of studies performed for each modality. This is important, because the benchmarks are different for screening mammography, diagnostic mammography, screening ultrasound, and MRI. A **screening examination** (mammogram, ultrasound, or MRI) is performed on an asymptomatic woman. She does not have any current breast complaints, abnormal physical examination, or known abnormal imaging findings. We are deciding if she is normal or if there is an unsuspected underlying malignancy. A **diagnostic examination** (mammogram, ultrasound, or MRI) is performed if the patient has a clinical sign or symptom of breast cancer, unresolved abnormal breast imaging such as a recent abnormal screening examination, or she is undergoing short-term surveillance due to recent biopsy or surgery that requires follow-up.

Next, we classify our breast imaging results. In screening, a screening recall is given BI-RADS 0 assessment and is considered a **positive examination.** In diagnostic imaging, a request for tissue diagnosis, BI-RADS 4 or 5 assessment, is considered a positive examination. A **negative examination** is BI-RADS 1 or 2 in screening and BI-RADS 1, 2, or 3 in diagnostic imaging. (Please note that BI-RADS 3 should not be used for screening mammography.) An examination can be classified as **true positive (TP)** if there is a tissue diagnosis of breast cancer (DCIS or invasive breast cancer) within 1 year after a positive examination. An examination can be classified as **true negative (TN)** if there is NO known tissue diagnosis of breast cancer within 1 year after a negative examination. An examination can be classified as **false negative (FN)** if there is a known tissue diagnosis of breast cancer within 1 year after a negative examination. An examination can be classified as **false positive (FP)** if there is NO known tissue diagnosis of breast cancer within 1 year after a positive examination. If you add these numbers (TP + TN + FN + FP), this should equal the total number of examinations performed at your facility. We then use these numbers to calculate our sensitivity TP/(TP + FN), specificity TN/(TN + FP), cancer detection rate per 1,000 patients imaged, recall rate, abnormal interpretation rate, and PPV. PPV is a very important benchmark. It is defined as the percentage of diagnostic examinations that result in a tissue diagnosis of breast cancer within 1 year. PPV = TP/(TP + FP). PPV is further subdivided into three definitions. PPV_1 is used for positive results at screening. PPV_2 is used for positive results at diagnostic examinations for which tissue diagnosis or biopsy is recommended. PPV_3 is the percentage of biopsies performed that result in a cancer diagnosis. This is also known as the positive biopsy rate.

This data collection can seem very intimidating. But in the era of electronic medical records and breast reporting software, it is becoming more efficient and reliable.

Medical Audit

The basic clinically relevant audit is fairly easy to perform if the above data are collected. Once an audit is performed, comparison to national benchmarks is essential to assess performance and identify areas in need of improvement. Benchmarks are set through scholarly articles and by the Breast Cancer Surveillance Consortium (BCSC). Radiologists can also participate in the National Mammography Database (NMD) in which they upload their audit data and compare their performance to national standards.

Because there are multiple sources for benchmarks, the standards can vary. For example, in BI-RADS, Carney et al. suggest that the minimally acceptable performance for cancer detection in screening mammography is ≥2.5 cancers per 1,000 screening examinations. Please note that this is much lower than the benchmark set by the BCSC at 4.7 cancers per 1,000 women screened. An acceptable recall rate for screening mammography is between 5% and 12%. Most breast imagers aim for a recall rate <10%. With the increased use of DBT, which has fewer false positives, recall rates are continuing to decline.

Increased data collected and metrics compared can continue to help radiologists improve performance. Of the data collected, a concerted effort to review false-negative examinations is imperative. This can help individual radiologists and their colleagues avoid delay in diagnosis. Audits should be performed at least once every 12 months. The data does rely on volume, so audits and identification of trends are less reliable for practices with a very small number of cases.

Suggested Readings

Alshafeiy TI, Nguyen JV, Rochman CM, Nicholson BT, Patrie JT, Harvey JA. Outcome of architectural distortion detected only at breast tomosynthesis versus 2D mammography. *Radiology* 2018:288(1):38–46.

Andersson I, Ikeda DM, Zackrisson S, et al. Breast tomosynthesis and digital mammography: a comparison of breast cancer visibility and BIRADS classification in a population of cancers with subtle mammographic findings. *Eur Radiol* 2008;18:2817–2825.

Bahl M, Baker JA, Kinsey EN, Ghate SV. Architectural distortion on mammography: correlation with pathologic outcomes and predictors of malignancy. *AJR Am J Roentgenol* 2015;205(6):1339–1345.

Bent CK, Bassett LW, D'Orsi CJ, Sayre JW. The positive predictive value of BI-RADS microcalcification descriptors and final assessment categories. *AJR Am J Roentgenol* 2010;194(5):1378–1383.

Berg WA, Arnoldus CL, Teferra E, Bhargavan M. Biopsy of amorphous breast calcifications: pathologic outcome and yield at stereotactic biopsy. *Radiology* 2001;221:495–503.

Berg WA, Campassi CI, Ioffe OB. Cystic lesions of the breast: sonographic-pathologic correlation. *Radiology* 2003;227:183–191.

Burnside ES, Ochsner JE, Fowler KJ, et al. Use of microcalcification descriptors in BI-RADS® 4th edition to stratify risk of malignancy. *Radiology* 2007;242:388–395.

Burnside ES, Sickles EA, Bassett LW, et al. The ACR BI-RADS® experience: learning from history. *J Am Coll Radiol* 2009;6(12):851–860.

Carney PA, Sickles EA, Monsees BS, et al. Identifying minimally acceptable interpretive performance criteria for screening mammography. *Radiology* 2010;255(2):354–361.

Chang YW, Kwon KH, Goo DE, Choi DL, Lee HK, Yang SB. Sonographic differentiation of benign and malignant cystic lesions of the breast. *J Ultrasound Med* 2007;26:47–53.

Conway BJ, McCrohan JL, Rueter FG, Suleiman OH. Mammography in the eighties. *Radiology* 1990;177:335–339.

D'Orsi CJ, Getty DJ, Swets JA, Pickett RM, Seltzer SE, McNeil BJ. Reading and decision aids for improved accuracy and standardization of mammographic diagnosis. *Radiology* 1992;184:619–622.

D'Orsi CJ, Sickles EA, Mendelson EB, Morris EA, eds. ACR BI-RADS® Atlas, Breast Imaging Reporting and Data System. 5th ed. Reston, VA: American College of Radiology; 2013.

Galkin BM, Feig SA, Muir HD. The technical quality of mammography in centers participating in a regional breast cancer awareness program. *Radiographics* 1988;8:133–145.

Haas BM, Kalra V, Geisel J, Raghu M, Durand M, Philpotts LE. Comparison of tomosynthesis plus digital mammography and digital mammography alone for breast cancer screening. *Radiology* 2013;269:694–700.

Kaas R, Kroger R, Hendriks JH, et al. The significance of circumscribed malignant mammographic masses in the surveillance of BRCA 1/2 gene mutation carriers. *Eur Radiol* 2004;14:1647–1653.

Karssemeijer N, Frieling JT, Hendriks JH. Spatial resolution in digital mammography. *Invest Radiol* 1993;28:413–419.

Lacquement MA, Mitchell D, Hollingsworth AB. Positive predictive value of the Breast Imaging Reporting and Data System. *J Am Coll Surg* 1999; 189(1):34–40.

Lazarus E, Mainiero MB, Schepps B, Koelliker SL, Livingston LS. BI-RADS lexicon for US and mammography: interobserver variability and positive predictive value. *Radiology* 2006;239:385–391.

Leung JW, Sickles EA. Developing asymmetry identified on mammography: correlation with imaging outcome and pathologic findings. *AJR Am J Roentgenol* 2007;188(3):667–675.

Liberman L, Abramson AF, Squires FB, Glassman JR, Morris EA, Dershaw DD. The breast imaging reporting and data system: positive predictive value of mammographic features and final assessment categories. *AJR Am J Roentgenol* 1998;171(1):35–40.

McLelland R. Mammography 1984: challenge to radiology. *AJR Am J Roentgenol* 1984;143:1–4.

Mendelson EB, Berg WA, Merritt CR. Toward a standardized breast ultrasound lexicon, BI-RADS: ultrasound. *Semin Roentgenol* 2001;36:217–225.

Schrading S, Kuhl CK. Mammographic, US, and MR imaging phenotypes of familial breast cancer. *Radiology* 2008;246:58–70.

Sickles EA. Nonpalpable, circumscribed, noncalcified solid breast masses: likelihood of malignancy based on lesion size and age of patient. *Radiology* 1994;192:439–442.

Sickles EA. Findings at mammographic screening on only one standard projection: outcomes analysis. *Radiology* 1998;208(2):471–475.

Skaane P, Bandos AI, Gullien R, et al. Comparison of digital mammography alone and digital mammography plus tomosynthesis in a population-based screening program. *Radiology* 2013;267:47–56.

Stavros AT, Thickman D, Rapp CL, Dennis MA, Parker SH, Sisney GA. Solid breast nodules: use of sonography to distinguish between benign and malignant lesions. *Radiology* 1995;196:123–134.

U.S. Food and Drug Administration. About Mammography Quality Standards Act (MQSA). Available from https://www.fda.gov/Radiation-EmittingProducts/MammographyQualityStandardsActandProgram/AbouttheMammographyProgram/default.htm. Accessed December 2017.

Wang Y, Ikeda DM, Narasimhan B, et al. Estrogen receptor-negative invasive breast cancer: imaging features of tumors with and without human epidermal growth factor receptor type 2 overexpression. *Radiology* 2008; 246:367–375.

Woods RW, Sisney GS, Salkowski LR, Shinki K, Lin Y, Burnside ES. The mammographic density of a mass is a significant predictor of breast cancer. *Radiology* 2011;258(2):417–425.

CHAPTER 22 ■ BREAST MAGNETIC RESONANCE IMAGING

BRANDI T. NICHOLSON, CARRIE M. ROCHMAN, AND JONATHAN V. NGUYEN

INTRODUCTION TO MRI

Although mammography is the most cost-effective way to screen for breast cancer and has reduced breast cancer deaths by 20% to 35% in women who screen, it remains limited in its ability to detect all breast cancers due to breast density, age, tumor type, and risk factors. Its limited sensitivity results in 10% to 30% of breast cancers missed on digital mammography. Tomosynthesis (DBT) has improved mammographic sensitivity but is still unable to visualize as many cancers as contrast-enhanced magnetic resonance (ce-MR) imaging of the breast.

Initial investigation of breast MR imaging started in the early 1980s, but at that time it was of limited benefit due to the lack of contrast. However, in 1985, gadolinium diethylenetriaminepentaacetic acid (DTPA) became available which made ce-MR imaging promising as a breast imaging tool. The benefits of ce-MR are that it has high spatial and soft tissue resolution and lacks ionizing radiation. ce-MR is the most sensitive test currently available for detecting breast cancer with a cancer detection rate (CDR) of up to 18/1,000.

INDICATIONS

The current uses of breast MR imaging are listed in Table 22.1.

Screening

High-Risk Screening. The American Cancer Society (ACS) guidelines recommend ce-MR as an adjunct to clinical breast examinations and annual mammography for women at risk for hereditary breast cancer, untested first-degree relatives of women with BRCA mutations, and any patient with a family history predictive of a lifetime cancer risk of at least 20%. The American College of Radiology (ACR) appropriateness criteria state that ce-MR is "usually appropriate" for women considered high risk. Their definition of high risk is similar to those of the ACS: women with a BRCA gene mutation and their untested first-degree relatives, women with a history of chest irradiation between 10 to 30 years of age, women with 20% or greater lifetime risk of breast cancer. Table 22.2 shows the appropriateness scale used by the ACR. This recommendation was based on a review of at least six prospective, nonrandomized studies of high-risk women, which reported significantly higher sensitivity for MR (77% to 100%) compared with mammography only (25% to 40%) or mammography plus ultrasound (US) ± clinical breast examinations (49% to 67%), despite substantial differences in patient populations and MR technique. Table 22.3 lists the sensitivity, specificity, negative predictive value (NPV) and positive predictive value (PPV) for breast MR. The sensitivity of breast MR holds true for both invasive and in situ disease, and unlike mammography, the sensitivity of MR is not impacted by breast density. Figure 22.1 shows a ce-MR screening detected invasive ductal carcinoma (IDC).

The ACS most recently updated their recommendations in July 2017 and continues to state "women who are at high risk for breast cancer based on certain factors should get an MRI and a mammogram every year." Breast MR continues to find additional cancers over mammography on subsequent/yearly examinations in high-risk women, so is recommended to be done annually. Figure 22.2 shows an annual screening MR diagnosing a new invasive ductal cancer not seen on the prior year MR examination. The ACR appropriateness criteria also state that ce-MR "may be appropriate" for women

TABLE 22.1

INDICATIONS FOR CONTRAST-ENHANCED BREAST MAGNETIC RESONANCE (CE-MR) IMAGING OF THE BREAST

Breast cancer screening of high-risk patients
Preoperative staging of breast cancer
Postoperative evaluation in women with positive margins after lumpectomy
Monitoring response to neoadjuvant chemotherapy
Detection of mammographically occult malignancy in patients with axillary nodal metastasis
Workup of nipple discharge (*selectively*)
Evaluation of silicone implants

of intermediate risk: women with a personal history of breast cancer, lobular neoplasia, atypical ductal hyperplasia, or 15% to 20% lifetime risk of breast cancer. These women are included on a case-by-case basis in annual breast MR imaging screening due to their slightly elevated risk.

Personal History of Breast Cancer. Having a personal history of breast cancer is not a strong recommendation to screen with MR but does fall into the intermediate risk and "may be appropriate" category per the ACR. However, because ce-MR is so sensitive, it does find more cancers than mammography alone, specifically more DCIS and small invasive cancers not yet involving lymph nodes, in all patient populations. MR imaging can also distinguish scar and fibrosis from recurrence in women status post breast conservation therapy (BCT) and can be helpful in patients with concerning mammogram or clinical examination. Figure 22.3 shows the benefit of ce-MR in a woman with a history of cancer and limited mammograms. The patient in Figure 22.3 had a history of bilateral breast cancer with benign mammographic postsurgical changes bilaterally on mammography. The MR reveals extensive disease in the left breast and no enhancement in the right breast.

Extent of Disease

Preoperative Staging. BCT is a common treatment for women with breast cancer. It includes surgery plus radiation and has been shown to have equal survival, for early stage cancers, as mastectomy. The rates of local recurrence after BCT range from 3% to 19% at 10 years. Local recurrence is defined as reappearance of cancer in the ipsilateral breast or on the ipsilateral chest wall and regional recurrence is defined as tumor in the regional lymph nodes (ipsilateral axillary, supraclavicular, infraclavicular, and/or internal mammary nodes). Figure 22.4 shows a patient with a history of left breast cancer who now has regional recurrence in an abnormal left internal mammary node. Breast MR best demonstrates internal mammary node disease compared to mammography (not visible) and US.

Cancers at greater than 2 cm from the index lesion are unlikely to be removed by a typical lumpectomy, may be too far away to be detected on the margin by pathology, and can contribute to in-breast recurrences. MR imaging can detect additional sites of disease not visible on mammography and/or US at a rate of 10%, specifically incidental findings greater than 2 cm from the known cancer. Figure 22.5 shows a second site of ipsilateral invasive disease in a different quadrant of the primary disease detected on cancer staging MR. Women with multicentric (disease in more than one quadrant of the breast) disease are typically not able to undergo BCT.

There are subsets of women who may benefit more than others by preoperative breast MR. This would include women who should otherwise be getting breast MR for high-risk screening, premenopausal women, those who have dense breast tissue, and those with invasive lobular carcinoma (ILC). The patient in Figure 22.3 had mammographically occult ILC detected on ce-MR. A different patient shown in Figure 22.6 has dense breast tissue. She presented with a palpable finding and was found to have ILC. On staging MR, additional foci concerning for more extensive disease were present. The patient went on to mastectomy confirming the extent of disease shown on her MR. MR imaging is the most accurate study for determining tumor size when correlated with histopathology.

The impact of breast MR on surgical planning is variable. A meta-analysis of 12 studies found that MR benefitted some patients by finding additional sites of proven, true positive (TP),

TABLE 22.3

SENSITIVITY, SPECIFICITY, NEGATIVE PREDICTIVE VALUE (NPV), AND POSITIVE PREDICTIVE VALUE (PPV) OF BREAST CE-MR IMAGING

Sensitivity	77–100
Specificity	30–97
NPV	99
PPV	25

Numbers are rounded %.

TABLE 22.2

AMERICAN COLLEGE OF RADIOLOGY (ACR) APPROPRIATENESS CRITERIA, RATING SCALE. THE APPROPRIATENESS IS RATED ON AN ORDINAL SCALE THAT USES INTEGERS FROM 1 TO 9 GROUPED INTO THREE CATEGORIES

■ RATING	■ APPROPRIATENESS	■ BENEFIT
1, 2, or 3	"Usually not appropriate"	Harms of doing the procedure or treatment outweigh the benefits
4, 5, or 6	"May be appropriate"	Risks and benefits are equivocal or unclear
7, 8, or 9	"Usually appropriate"	Benefits of doing a procedure or treatment outweigh the harms or risks

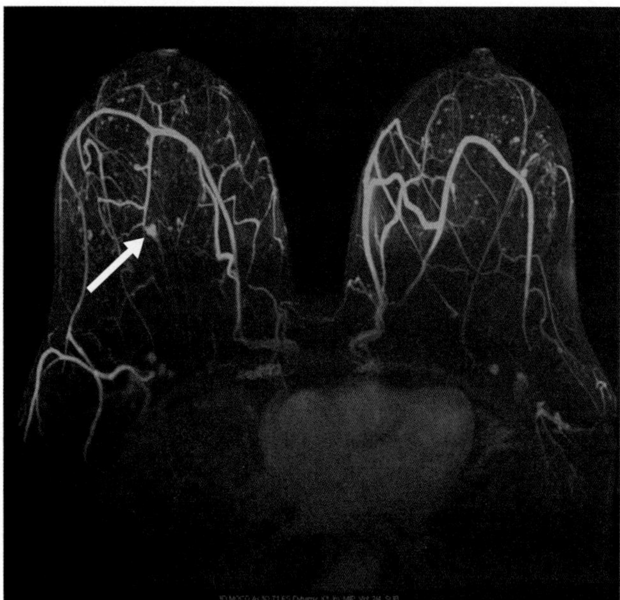

FIGURE 22.1. **Screening Breast ce-MR Detected Invasive Ductal Cancer.** High-risk screening postcontrast axial maximum intensity projection (MIP) breast MR demonstrating a mammographically occult (not shown) small round mass with irregular margins and homogeneous enhancement (*arrow*) in the right breast.

disease. This resulted in mastectomy or larger lumpectomy instead of smaller lumpectomy due to additional significant disease. In less but still an important percent of women, MR can unfortunately overestimate lesion size, multicentricity, and contralateral involvement, which results in unnecessary mastectomies and larger lumpectomies, due to false positive (FP) findings.

Specific to ILC, the second most common type of invasive breast cancer, it is more common to have a more diffuse and infiltrative growth pattern compared to IDC. This makes it more often missed or underestimated on mammography, like in Figure 22.3. In these patients, preoperative breast MR has been shown to alter management in nearly a third, as in Figure 22.6. Overall, breast MR finds contralateral, otherwise occult, malignancy in 3% to 6% of women regardless of their primary malignancy histology. Figure 22.7 shows an MR in a patient who underwent staging MR for a known left IDC. The MR revealed a suspicious mass in the right breast that was found to represent DCIS.

Extramammary Disease on MR. MR imaging can also visualize structures outside the breast parenchyma. This includes the axilla, dome of the liver, mediastinum, and bones of the ribcage and sternum. Extramammary findings are seen in about one-third of breast MR examinations with about 20% of those proving to be malignant, and as one might suspect, these findings are more likely to be malignant in women undergoing breast MR for cancer staging. The most common sites for breast cancer to metastasis are the bone, lung, brain, liver, and lymph nodes (in descending order) (see Fig. 22.8 for examples). All but the brain can be seen on a routine breast MR imaging. When present findings are more likely to be malignant in the bone, lung, and lymph nodes. In contrast, lesions in the liver are much more likely to be benign (95%) as in Figure 22.8C and D. Pleural effusions are also common, seen in nearly 90% of healthy women undergoing screening MR, and are typically benign in the screening population. MR is also able to demonstrate direct extension of a tumor into the muscle better than either mammography or US. Muscle invasion is suspected when there is enhancement of the muscle; loss of the fat plane or muscle edema does *not* correlate with invasion. Figure 22.9 shows two patients with muscle edema; however, only the patient with enhancement in the muscle had extension of tumor into the muscle histologically.

Post Lumpectomy With Positive Margins. MR can be beneficial in women who did not undergo preoperative MR but are found to have positive margins on lumpectomy. MR can see and localize additional disease in up to 80% of these women.

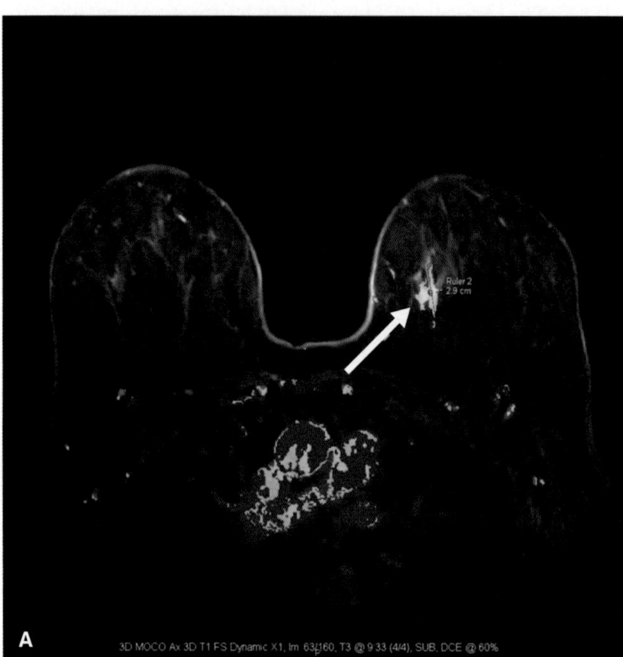

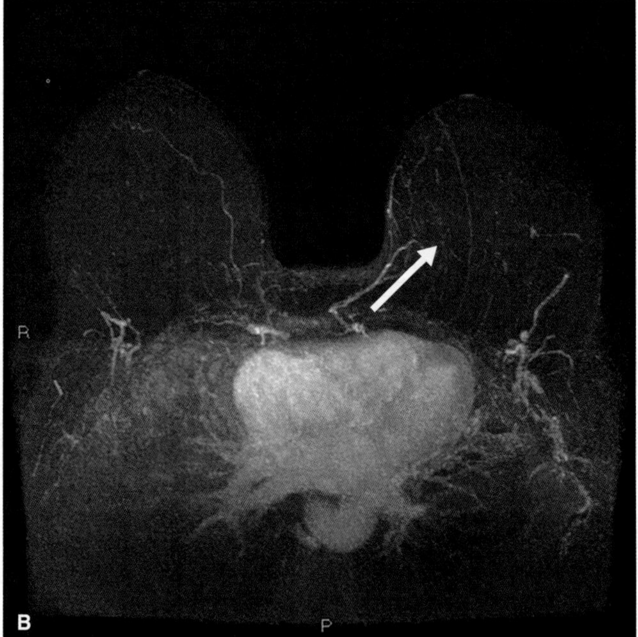

FIGURE 22.2. **Annual Screening Breast ce-MR With a New Invasive Ductal Cancer. A:** Current postcontrast axial T1W with FS subtracted breast MR with superimposed computer-aided detection, with an irregular, heterogeneously enhancing mass with irregular margins (*arrow*) in the left breast. **B:** On the 1-year prior examination, no suspicious enhancement is present (*arrow*) in this area.

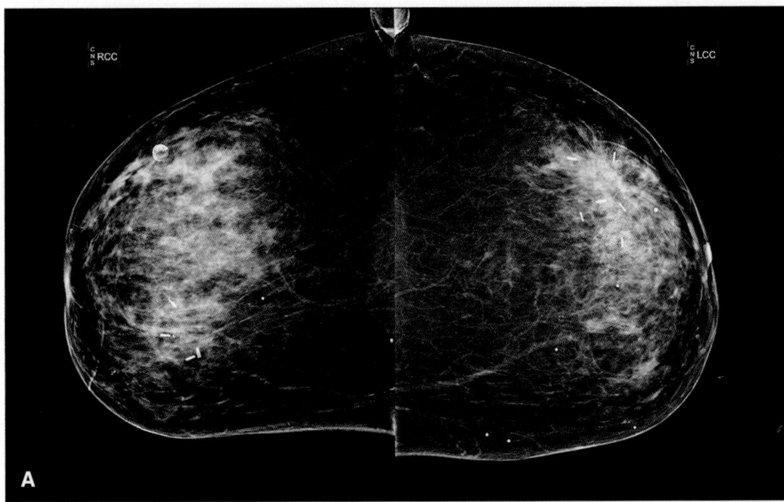

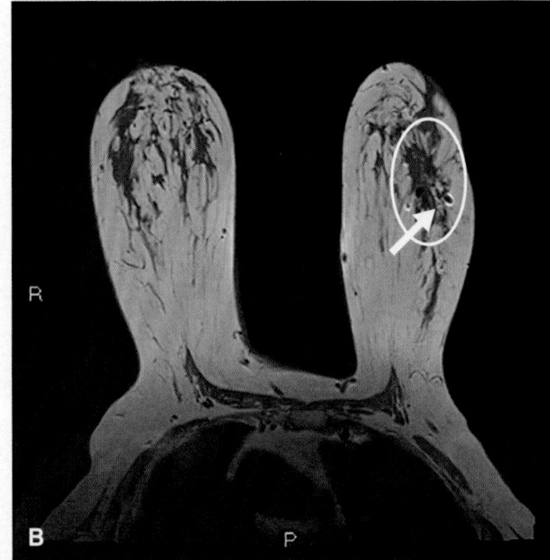

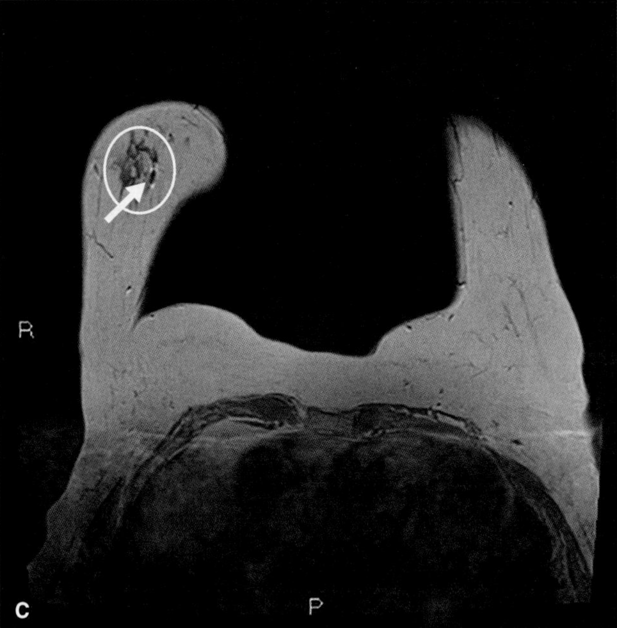

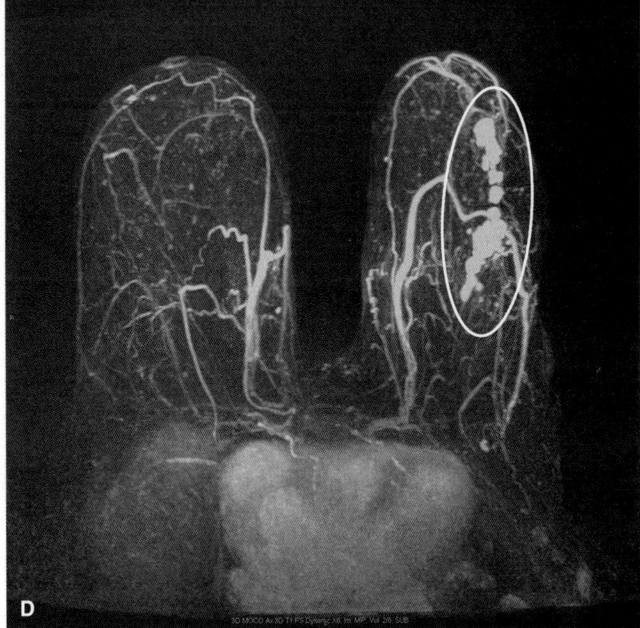

FIGURE 22.3. **ce-MR Imaging in Patient Status Post Bilateral Lumpectomy. A:** Bilateral mammogram (craniocaudal views of each breast) showing bilateral lumpectomy scars (surgical clips). **B, C:** T1W non-FS axial breast MR images at appropriate levels to demonstrate the distortion (*circles*) and susceptibility artifact from clips (*arrows*) in the left (**B**) and right (**C**) breasts. **D:** Postcontrast axial MIP image showing highly suspicious segmental nonmass enhancement at the left lumpectomy bed (*circle*) proven to be recurrent invasive lobular carcinoma and no suspicious enhancement at the right lumpectomy bed.

Postsurgical inflammation and infection can create FP results on MR imaging. Imaging between days 28 and 35 after surgery has been found most sensitive and specific compared to more sooner. Women also better tolerate the MR the further out from surgery due to pain.

Neoadjuvant Monitoring. Neoadjuvant chemotherapy is most often used in women with locally advanced breast cancer in an effort to shrink tumor burden; however, more women are becoming candidates for neoadjuvant chemotherapy. The goal of neoadjuvant chemotherapy is no longer only to enable or lessen surgery but to also improve cure rates and is therefore being used more often. In 2012, ce-MR was shown to be superior to clinical examination at all time points for assessing response to therapy. The addition of functional imaging such as diffusion-weighted imaging (DWI), magnetic resonance spectroscopy (MRS), and other advanced MR technology to the routine breast MR examination may offer prognostic indicators of early response to therapy. Early data on DWI and MRS are promising. However, performing MRS and DWI are challenging and these technical difficulties may prove difficult to overcome.

Metastatic Disease With Suspected Breast Primary

Although it is an uncommon initial presenting symptom for women with breast cancer (<1% of patients), historically women with metastatic axillary disease suspected to be from a breast cancer would have undergone total mastectomy with axillary node dissection. This scenario is now an indication for performing preoperative breast MR. In these women, MR

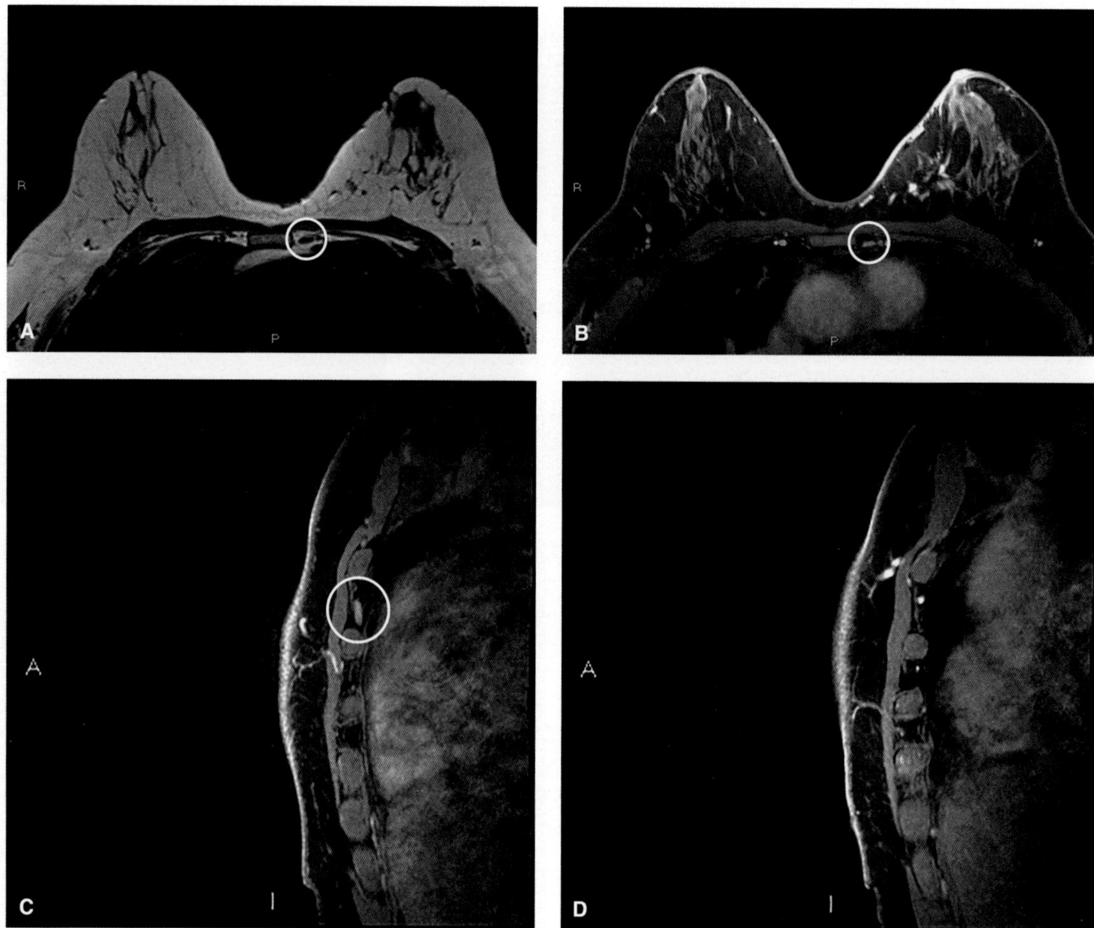

FIGURE 22.4. **Internal Mammary Node on Breast MR. A:** Axial T1W non-FS image shows an abnormal internal mammary node on the left (*circle*). **B:** This node enhances (*circle*) on the axial postcontrast T1W with FS image. **C:** Sagittal sequences can often demonstrate the internal mammary nodes the best, as seen on the sagittal postcontrast T1W with FS image (*circle*). **D:** The contralateral side on sagittal postcontrast T1W with FS image has no suspicious nodes present.

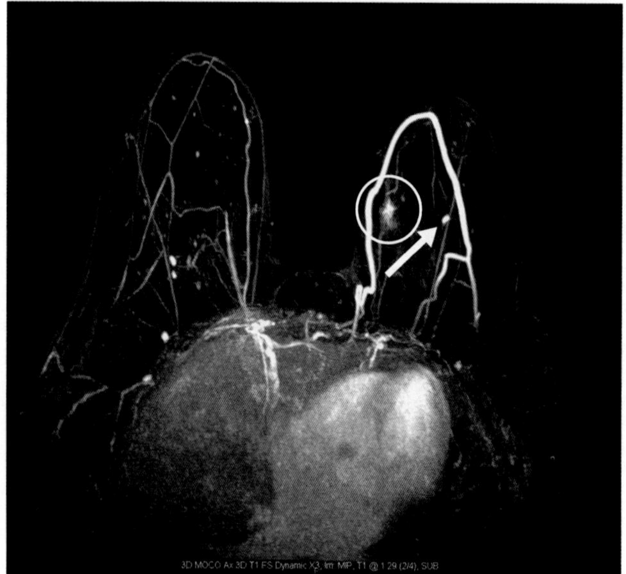

FIGURE 22.5. **Multicentric Breast Cancer Detected on Breast MR.** Postcontrast MIP image shows the known cancer as an irregular enhancing mass in the medial breast (*circle*). The mammographically occult (not shown) ipsilateral mass is oval, circumscribed, and homogeneously enhancing (*arrow*). The two findings are in different quadrants.

is able to find two-thirds of the primary breast cancers, and once the tumors are identified, radiologists are able to find them 80% of the time on US, the so-called "second-look" or "targeted" US. Given the specificity of MR and the possibility of benign processes in these patients, a preoperative biopsy should be done to confirm that the MR finding represents malignancy. Figure 22.10 shows a woman with a recent screening mammogram demonstrating a metastatic axillary node. The breast MR was ultimately needed to identify her primary breast cancer which was later found on "second-look" US.

Nipple Discharge

Discharge represents about 10% of all breast symptoms, third to breast pain and breast masses. Suspicious discharge includes spontaneous, unilateral, single duct, serous, or sanguineous discharge. Most of the time, this is due to a benign papilloma, but it can also be secondary to malignancy in up to 10% to 15% of cases. Mammography is commonly normal in this patient population, and therefore, galactography is commonly done for the preoperative workup in these women (Chapter 23). Given the high sensitivity of ce-MR to detect both invasive and in situ breast cancer and its sensitivity to detect papillomas, it makes sense to consider MR in the evaluation of these women. Although

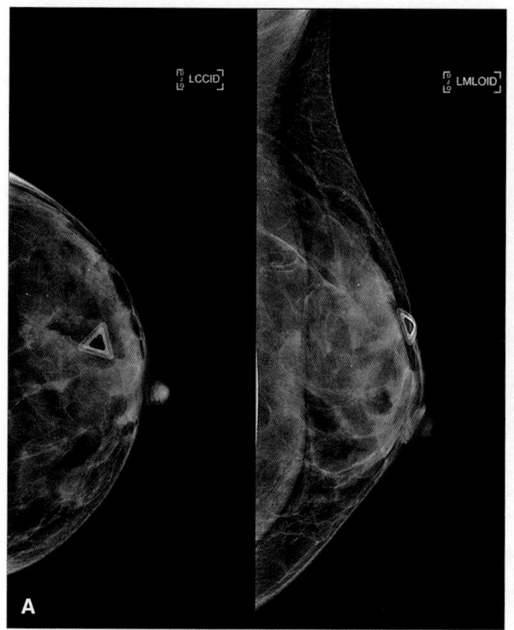

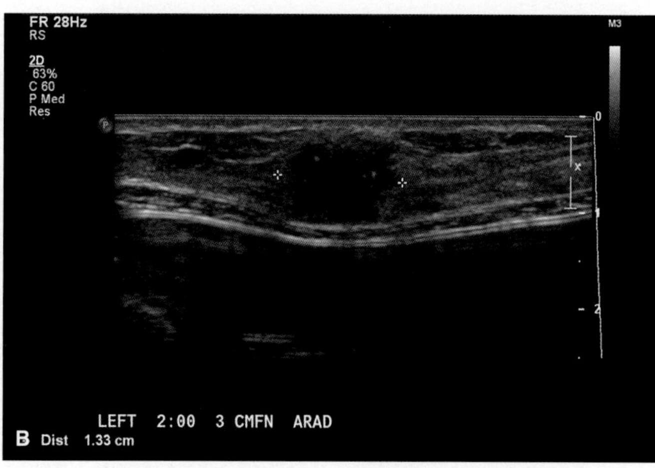

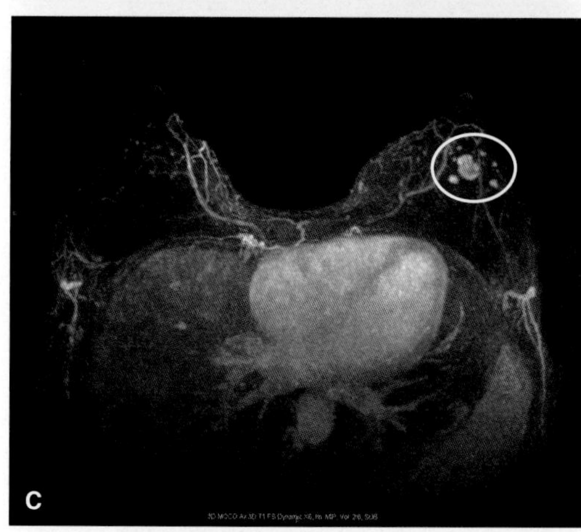

FIGURE 22.6. **Invasive Lobular Carcinoma (ILC) on Breast MR.** A 48-year-old woman presents with a palpable lump. Her mammogram (**A**) shows dense breast tissue obscuring her palpable mass (under *triangle*). **B:** Breast US demonstrates a 13-mm round, indistinct, hypoechoic mass (*calipers*). This mass underwent US-guided core needle biopsy and was found to be an ILC. **C:** Breast MR was done due to breast density and histology. The contrast-enhanced axial MIP shows the primary tumor surrounded by several suspicious enhancing foci asymmetric (*circle*) from the normal right breast. Mastectomy confirmed extensive disease.

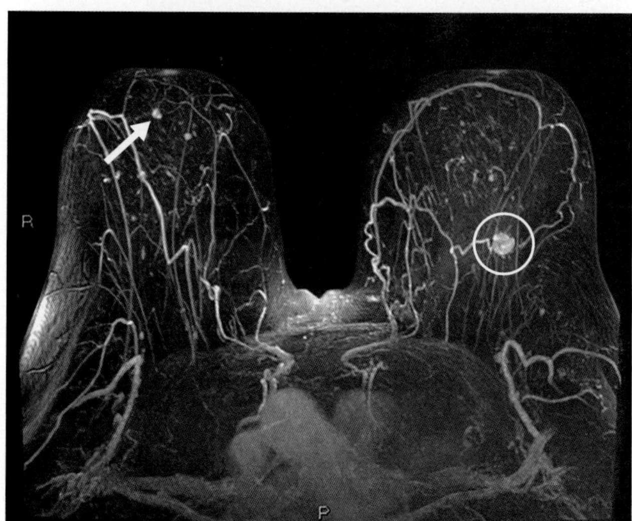

FIGURE 22.7. **Contralateral Mammographically Occult Disease on Breast MR.** Contrast-enhanced axial MIP image shows a round, irregular, heterogeneously enhancing mass (*circle*) which is the known left invasive ductal carcinoma. In the contralateral breast, there is a small focus in the anterior third (*arrow*) found to be DCIS on core needle biopsy.

nipple discharge is not a listed indication for breast MR, it is used in a case-by-case basis with good results. Women who may benefit from MR for discharge include those in whom the galactogram failed, who are otherwise considered high risk for breast cancer, or who have other suspicious findings on imaging or physical examination concerning for malignancy. Figure 22.11 shows how a breast MR can help in the workup for women with nipple discharge, especially when galactogram has failed. A small papilloma was found on her MR.

Biopsy Planning

A normal MR does not exclude malignancy; as sensitive as it is, it is not perfect. For this reason, a breast MR is not part of the typical prebiopsy workup in patients who have a finding on conventional (mammogram and US). The sensitivity of MR to detect cancer when conventional imaging is abnormal is near 90% (90.9% for invasive disease and 73% for DCIS) with a reasonable specificity of about 70%. However, a negative MR is not good enough to allow us to avoid a biopsy. Rarely, MR can assist us in localizing single-view mammographic findings that are not amenable to stereotactic or DBT-guided biopsy; fortunately, this is uncommon.

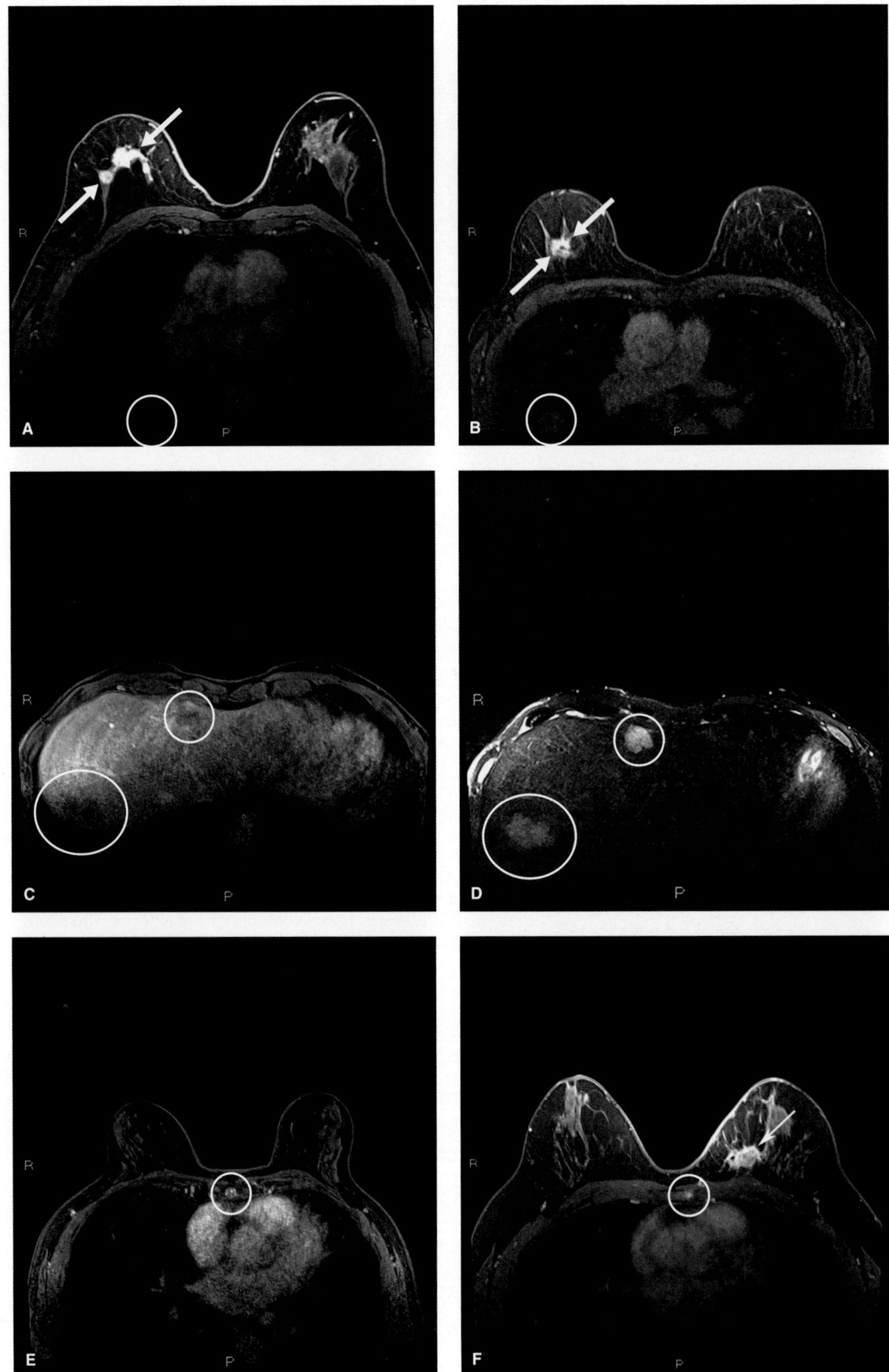

FIGURE 22.8. **Incidental Findings on Breast MR. A, B:** Two patients with current invasive breast cancer in the right breast (*arrows*) who had incidental lung masses detected on staging breast MR (*circles*). Workup was done for both patients with PET-CT and biopsy; one was proven benign (**A**) and the other primary lung cancer (**B**). **C, D:** Patient undergoing staging breast MR for advanced breast cancer with numerous abnormal metastatic nodes (not shown) revealing multiple liver masses (*circles*). The masses were heterogeneously enhancing on postcontrast T1W with FS (**C**) and hyperintense on T2W images (**D**). Workup with liver protocol MR (not shown) demonstrated benign hemangiomas. Liver lesions are so common that they are more likely benign even in cancer patients. **E, F:** Two patients with incidental enhancing sternal masses (*circles*) on postcontrast T1W with FS (**E**) and postcontrast T1W with FS and subtraction images (**F**). The first patient was imaged for high-risk screening and the sternal mass was stable in retrospect for many years and deemed benign. The second patient had a concurrent breast cancer (**F**, *arrow*) in the left breast with numerous metastatic nodes (not shown). The sternal mass underwent biopsy and was found to be metastatic disease.

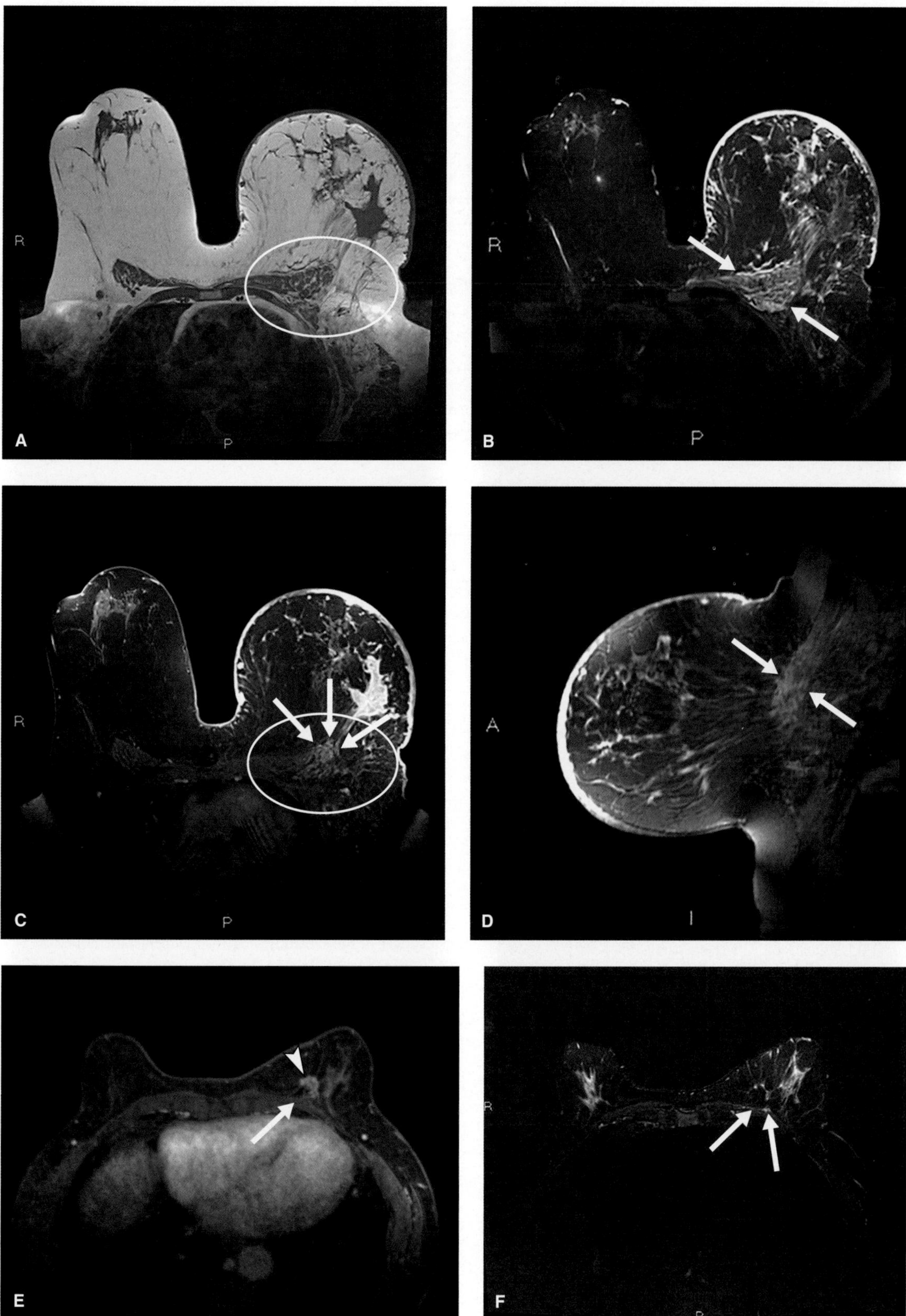

FIGURE 22.9. Using MR Imaging to Determine Tumor Extension Into the Pectoralis Muscle. **A–D:** Multiple MR images on a patient with advanced invasive breast cancer. **A:** T1W non-FS axial MR image showing muscle location (*circle*) with surrounding thickening of the Cooper ligaments and skin from edema. **B:** Same level on T2W with FS axial MR image. Increased T2 signal consistent with edema is present in the pectoralis muscle (*arrows*) and throughout the breast and skin. **C:** Postcontrast T1W with FS axial MR at the same level shows enhancement (*arrows*) in the muscle (*circle*) confirmed to correlate with chest wall invasion histologically. **D:** Sagittal postcontrast T1W with FS again shows the muscle enhancement (*arrows*). **E, F:** A second patient with a smaller invasive breast cancer (E, *arrowhead*) close to the muscle with increased T2 signal from edema on T2W with FS axial MR (F, *arrows*) without enhancement (E, *arrow*) in the muscle. Patient did not have muscle extension on lumpectomy.

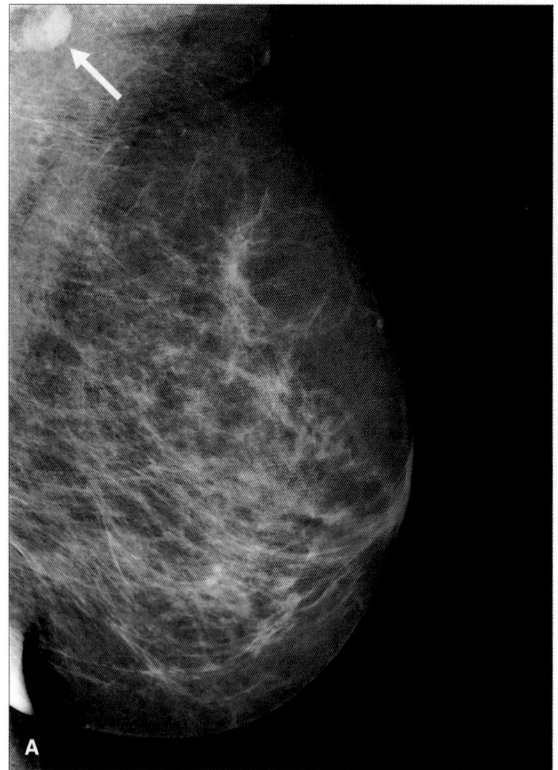

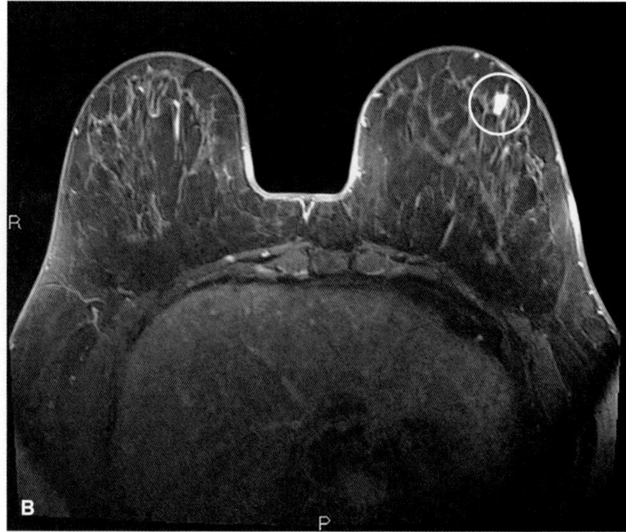

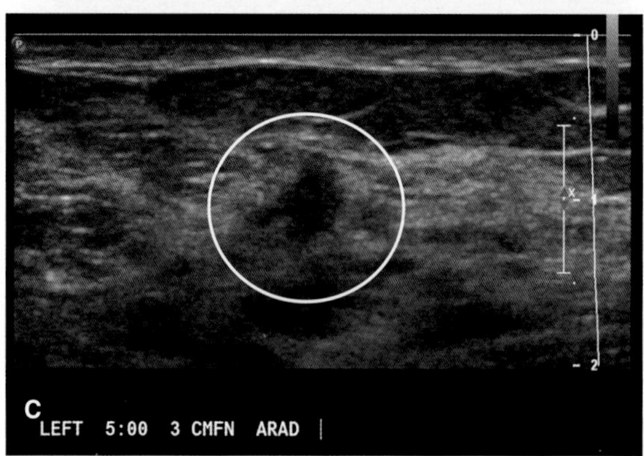

FIGURE 22.10. **Metastatic Axillary Lymph Node Involvement With Unknown Primary. A:** Screening mammogram showing new left axillary adenopathy (*arrow*). Initial breast US did not find a primary (not shown). Core biopsy of the node confirmed breast origin. **B:** Contrast-enhanced breast MR demonstrated an enhancing mass in the lower outer quadrant (*circle*). **C:** Targeted or second-look US was able to find the primary mass at 5:00 (*circle*) which was confirmed to be an invasive breast cancer of the same histology as the metastatic node.

Implant Evaluation

Implant Rupture. Breast MR is useful in the setting of evaluating the integrity of silicone breast implants as it is the imaging test with the highest sensitivity and specificity for implant rupture, making it the most accurate study. It has a reported sensitivity of 72% to 94% and specificity of 85% to 100%, compared to about 25% sensitivity and 85% specificity for mammography and US. It should be noted that the diagnosis of *saline* implant rupture does not require MR; it can be diagnosed clinically by rapid breast shrinking and can be seen as a collapsed or absent implant on mammography or US (see Fig. 19.9A in Chapter 19 for the mammographic appearance of saline rupture).

There are two types of silicone implant ruptures: intracapsular (more common) and extracapsular (see Fig. 19.9B in Chapter 19 for the mammographic appearance of silicone rupture). The integrity of the fibrous capsule determines which rupture type is present. Figure 22.12 shows the two types of implant rupture and the fibrous capsule on breast MR. In intracapsular rupture, the fibrous capsule remains intact and the characteristic imaging finding is called the "linguine sign." This is shown in Figure 22.12A and B. The linguine appearance comes from the collapsed implant membrane (dark signal) layering dependently in the silicone (bright on T2W images). When extracapsular rupture is present, silicone signal is seen outside the dark fibrous capsule. Figure 22.12C and D shows extracapsular rupture. In evaluation of silicone implants, MR technique is done to suppress or emphasize the signal from water, fat, or silicone, making silicone visible beyond the capsule. Silicone can be seen in the breast parenchyma as well as the lymph nodes. MR evaluation for implant rupture does not require contrast administration.

Peri-Implant Fluid Collections. In addition to rupture, breast MR can be used to image women with peri-implant fluid collections. Fluid can be present due to infection or breast implant–associated anaplastic large cell lymphoma (BIA-ALCL). Infection is usually diagnosed clinically with US used as needed to direct therapy including aspiration. Infection after implant reconstruction is common with about 6% of women with implants developing an infection at some point. Breast MR is *un*commonly performed in this clinical setting. ALCL is a type of non-Hodgkin lymphoma, is rare, and appears to be associated more commonly with textured implants. The first

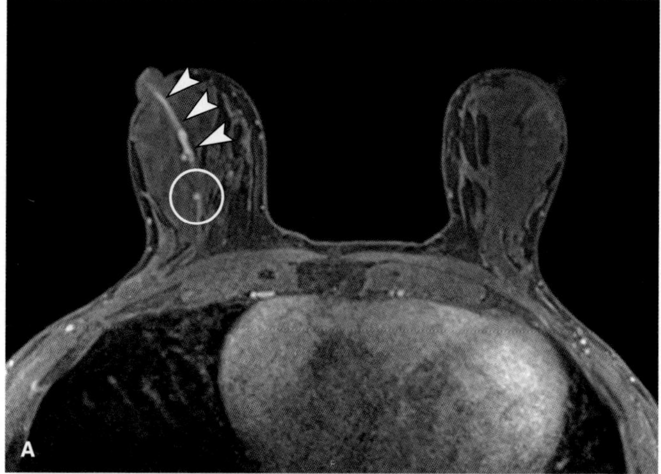

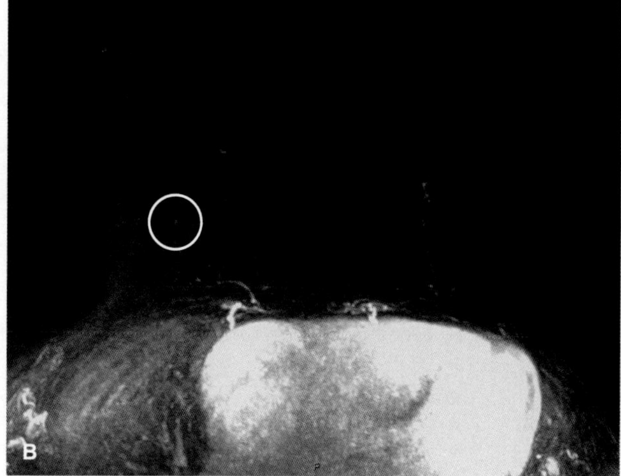

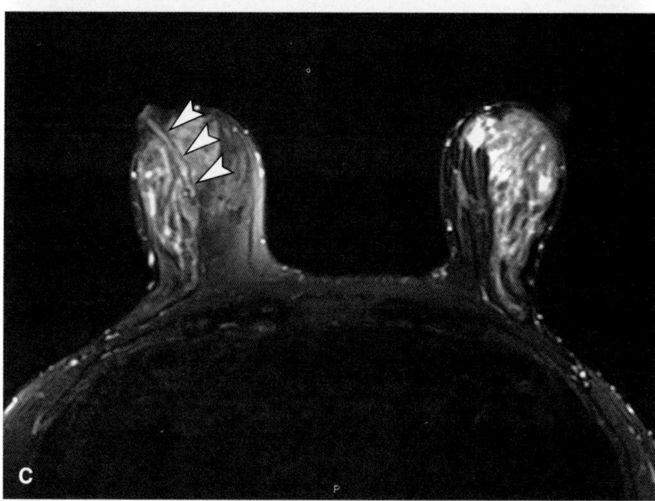

FIGURE 22.11. **MR in a Patient With Nipple Discharge Who Failed Galactogram. A:** Postcontrast T1W with FS axial MR image showing an enhancing focus in the central right breast (*circle*) as well as a dilated hyperintense duct on T1W duct (*arrowheads*). **B:** Postcontrast MIP shows only enhancement in the focus (*circle*); there is a lack of enhancement in the dilated duct. **C:** T2W with FS axial MR again shows the dilated iso- to slightly hyperintense duct on T2 (*arrowheads*). The signal in the duct is consistent with blood. This patient was found to have a small papilloma occult on mammogram (not shown) at MR-guided biopsy.

case was reported in 2007. The absolute risk of developing ALCL is reported to be extremely low between 0.1 and 0.3 per 100,000 patients per year in women with implants. Most patients present well after the implant was placed with breast swelling secondary to fluid (with or without a mass) around the implant. Aspiration of the fluid or biopsy of a mass if present allows for confirmation of ALCL versus infection. In ALCL, women with fluid only have a better prognosis than those with a mass. Treatment is implant removal. The need for radiation and/or chemotherapy in these patients is less well understood. Figure 22.13 shows a patient with a peri-implant fluid collection that was ultimately diagnosed as BIA-ALCL.

TECHNIQUE

Imaging Parameters

The ACR practice parameters for the performance of ce-MR imaging were revised in 2013 and amended in 2014. Table 22.4 lists the performance guidelines by technical factor. For a facility to be accredited for breast MR, they have to follow the ACR guidelines, but specific protocols will vary across institutions. In addition, for ACR accreditation, they must be able to do mammographic correlation, breast US, and MR imaging–guided procedures or have a relationship with a facility that can provide those services for them.

MR imaging equipment specifications and performance must also meet all state and federal requirements. Patients are scanned in the prone position with the breasts hanging into a dedicated breast coil. Body coils should not be used for breast MR examinations. The breast should be imaged in axial or sagittal planes or a combination of the two. Core pulse sequences when evaluating the breast for cancer include a three-plane localizer, T1W images, T2W images with fat saturation (FS), three-dimensional FS gradient echo series precontrast administration, and typically 3 or more postcontrast acquisitions. Table 22.5 shows what information is gained from the various sequences. It is recommended to use fat saturation to maximize the contrast between enhancing cancers and breast fat, which is bright on MR imaging. Subtraction is also done to accentuate the enhancing abnormalities on the study.

Cancers enhance differently than background glandular tissue due to more permeable vessels that result in more rapid early enhancement and more rapid washout of contrast. A breast MR protocol includes several time points which allows us the ability to not only assess an area as enhancing but also its kinetics over time. The first postcontrast time point is at about 90 seconds, the best time to detect breast cancer given its more rapid enhancement compared to the parenchyma. Sequential time points are acquired based on individual protocols with the delayed time point typically at 4 to 5 minutes.

Kinetics

There are three kinetic curves defined in the BI-RADS Atlas. They are classified based on the degree of early enhancement (slow,

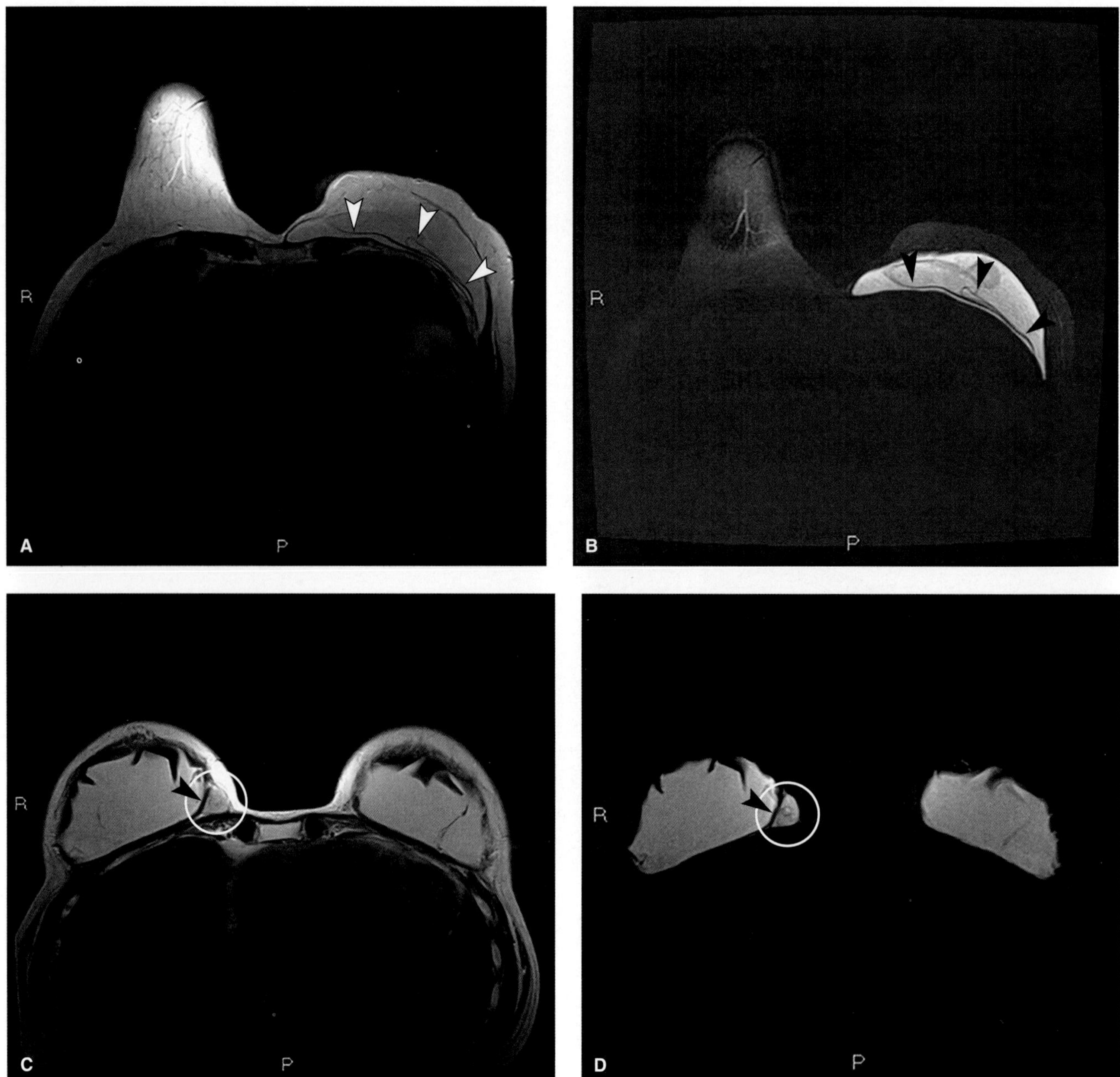

FIGURE 22.12. **MR of Silicone Implant Rupture. A, B:** Axial silicone sequences showing the linguine sign in the posterior–inferior aspect of the left implant (*arrowheads*). The linguine sign is secondary to the collapsed implant membrane layering dependently in the silicone. The silicone remains within the fibrous capsule in an intracapsular rupture. **C, D:** Axial silicone sequences in a second patient who has extracapsular rupture. There is silicone signal (*circle*) outside the dark fibrous capsule (*black arrowhead*).

medium, and fast) and the delayed change in enhancement after the peak (persistent, plateau, and washout). Figure 22.14 shows the kinetic curves as described in the ACR BI-RADS Atlas. The definition of fast initial is >100% increase in signal intensity within the first 2 minutes, medium as 50% to 100% increase, and slow as <50% increase. For the delayed phase, persistent is >10% increase in signal over time, plateau as no significant change from the peak, and washout as >10% decrease in signal from peak. The most concerning curve is the one with fast initial and washout delayed kinetics. However, kinetics performs poorly overall for predicting malignancy except in masses with washout delayed kinetics. Morphology should be used over kinetics to determine if biopsy or follow-up is appropriate. Computer-aided diagnosis (CAD) software is used to aid interpretation of breast MR imaging. The software helps to provide the kinetic information in an objective fashion. The CAD software color codes the findings if they reach a threshold initial enhancement, often set at 50% to 60%. The color selected is based on the delayed curve. Figure 22.3 shows a mass that colors predominately yellow due to a plateau enhancement curve. Figure 22.15 shows all three enhancement kinetics. The patient in Figure 22.15C and D is the same as in Figure 22.5.

Artifacts

Most common artifacts on breast MR relate to patient factors and attempts at fat saturation. Patient factors include positioning, motion, and metallic artifacts. Technical factors include things like selection of field of view and anatomic coverage,

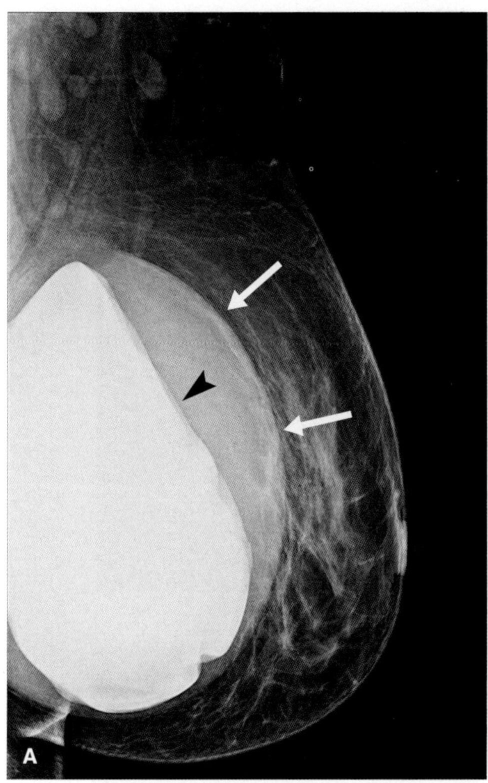

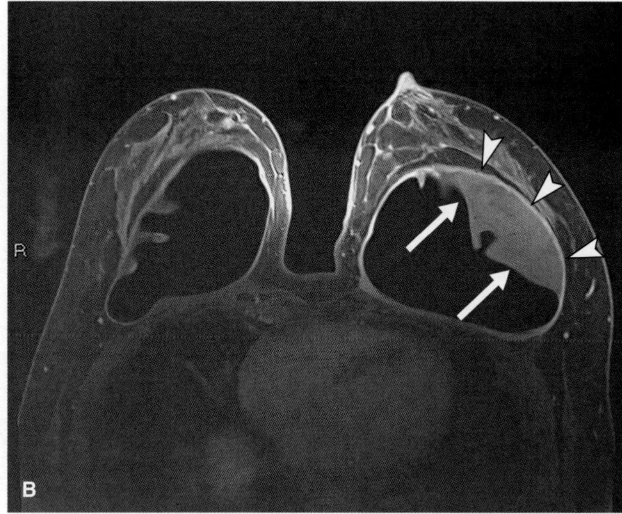

FIGURE 22.13. **Breast Implant-Associated Anaplastic Large Cell Lymphoma. A:** The patient presented on a mammography with a peri-implant fluid collection (*arrows*) with mass effect on the underlying silicone implant (*arrowhead*). US confirmed fluid density (not shown). **B:** A contrast-enhanced breast MR was done to evaluate for a mass and extent of disease. It showed a complex fluid collection (between *arrowheads* and *arrows*) surrounding the implant (*arrows*) with minimal enhancement at the edge of the fluid (*arrowheads*).

the coil type, issues with fat saturation, and various artifacts. To minimize patient factors, each breast should be positioned symmetrically, centered in the coil and avoid touching the coil elements. Poor positioning can compress parts of the breast, limit comparison of right to left, and create high signal (where breast touches the coil) artifacts. Technical factors impact the

TABLE 22.4

ACR TECHNICAL GUIDELINES FOR THE PERFORMANCE OF BREAST MR IMAGING

■ TECHNICAL FACTOR	■ GUIDELINES
Field strength	1.5-T magnet has traditionally been considered a minimum technical requirement because of the relationship between field strength and resolution
Slice thickness	3 mm or less
In-plane resolution	1 mm or less
Fat suppression	Chemical fat suppression and/or image subtraction
Imaging both breasts	Simultaneous bilateral imaging with a dedicated breast coil
Contrast	Gadolinium contrast as a bolus with a standard dose of 0.1 mmol/kg followed by a saline flush of at least 10 mL
Scan time	Kinetic information should be reported based on enhancement data determined at specified intervals separated by 4 minutes or less

TABLE 22.5

INFORMATION GAINED FROM MR IMAGING SEQUENCES

■ SEQUENCE	■ INFORMATION
T1W images	Differentiation of adipose tissue from glandular tissue
T2W fat-suppressed images	Identification of fluid-filled structures such as cysts
Dynamic images	Morphology and enhancement kinetics

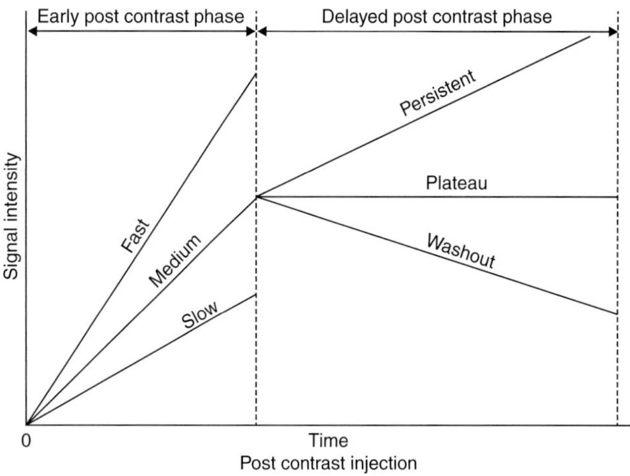

FIGURE 22.14. **Breast MR Kinetic Curves.**

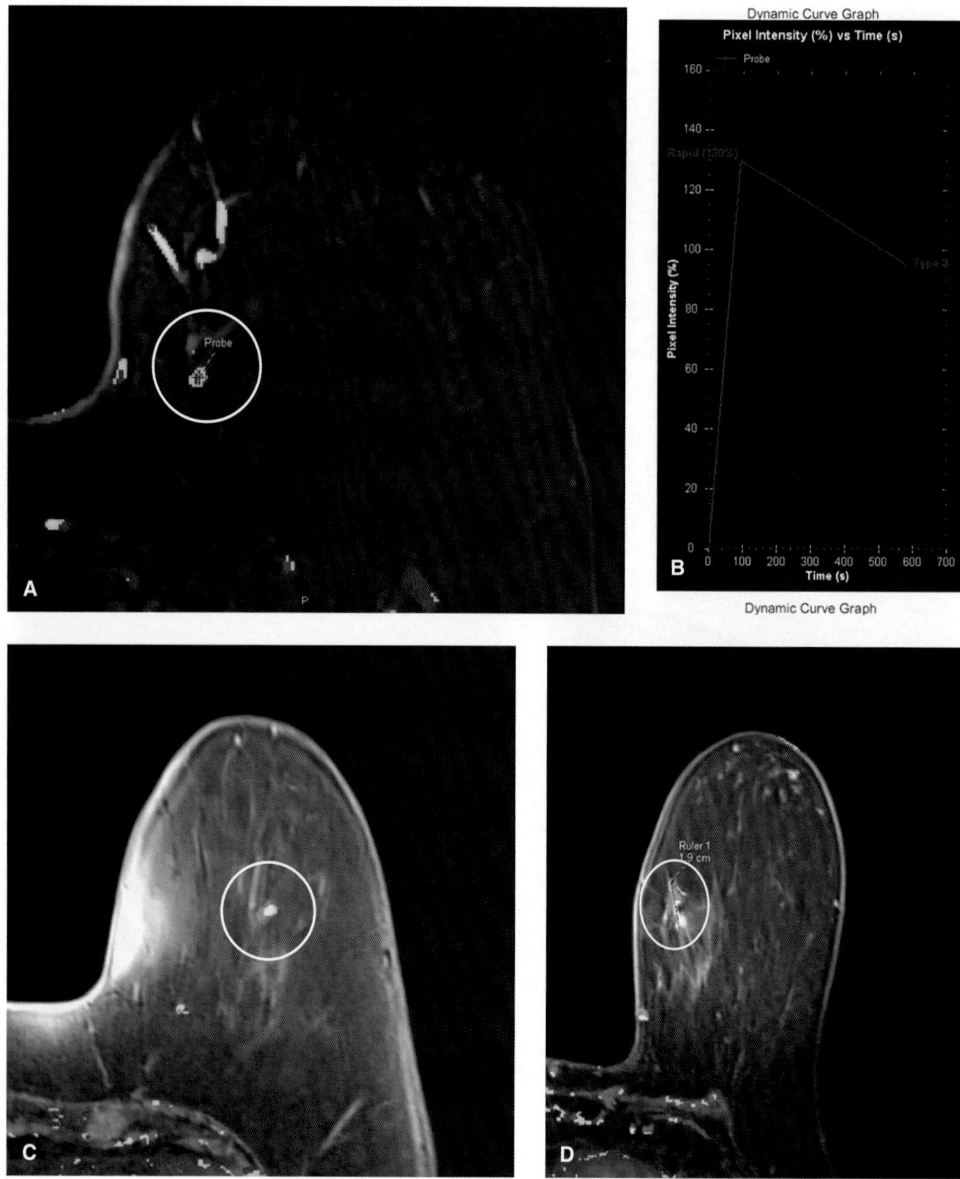

FIGURE 22.15. **Enhancement Curves on Dynamic Breast MR. A, B:** Small round, irregular, homogeneously enhancing mass with a fast initial and washout delayed enhancement curve (*circle*, **A**). **C, D:** The patient from Figure 22.5 had two sites of cancer. The smaller additional mass (**C**, *circle*) had plateau kinetics and is therefore colored yellow and the larger primary mass (**D**, *oval*) had persistent kinetics and is color-coded blue (*curves* not shown).

image quality and if not done well can create artifacts on the image. For breast MR, the FOV should adequately include both breasts and the low axilla which typically is from the level of the clavicle to just inferior to the inframammary fold. If the technologist fails to use the breast coil and images with the body coil, the image will be grainy.

One of the key technical factors in breast MR is fat saturation. To do chemical fat saturation, the MR unit applies a pulse at a frequency of 3.5 ppm (224 Hz at 1.5 T) below the water peak. This can be challenging in a patient who is predominately fatty or one that lacks fat (extreme fibroglandular tissue). When the peak is incorrectly applied, fat remains bright obscuring detection of bright cancers. Other common artifacts are from motion of blood flow, respiratory movement, and patient motion. These are detected along the phase-encoding direction. For this reason, the phase-encoding direction for breast MR is set left to right on axial images and superior to inferior on sagittal sequences to minimize its impact on the study. Figure 22.16 shows some common artifacts on breast MR, including patient motion, failed fat saturation, and chemical shift artifact.

INTERPRETATION

The first edition of the BI-RADS Atlas was released in 1993 and included lexicon related to mammography only. Work on MR breast lexicon began in 1997. Testing and review of the lexicon took 6 years with the BI-RADS—MR imaging first appearing in the BI-RADS Atlas, 4th edition, in 2003. The 5th edition of BI-RADS was released in 2013 and included recommendations related to report content (i.e., clinical history, comparison to prior examinations, and protocol description) as well as lexicon vocabulary, specifically to MR imaging lexicon.

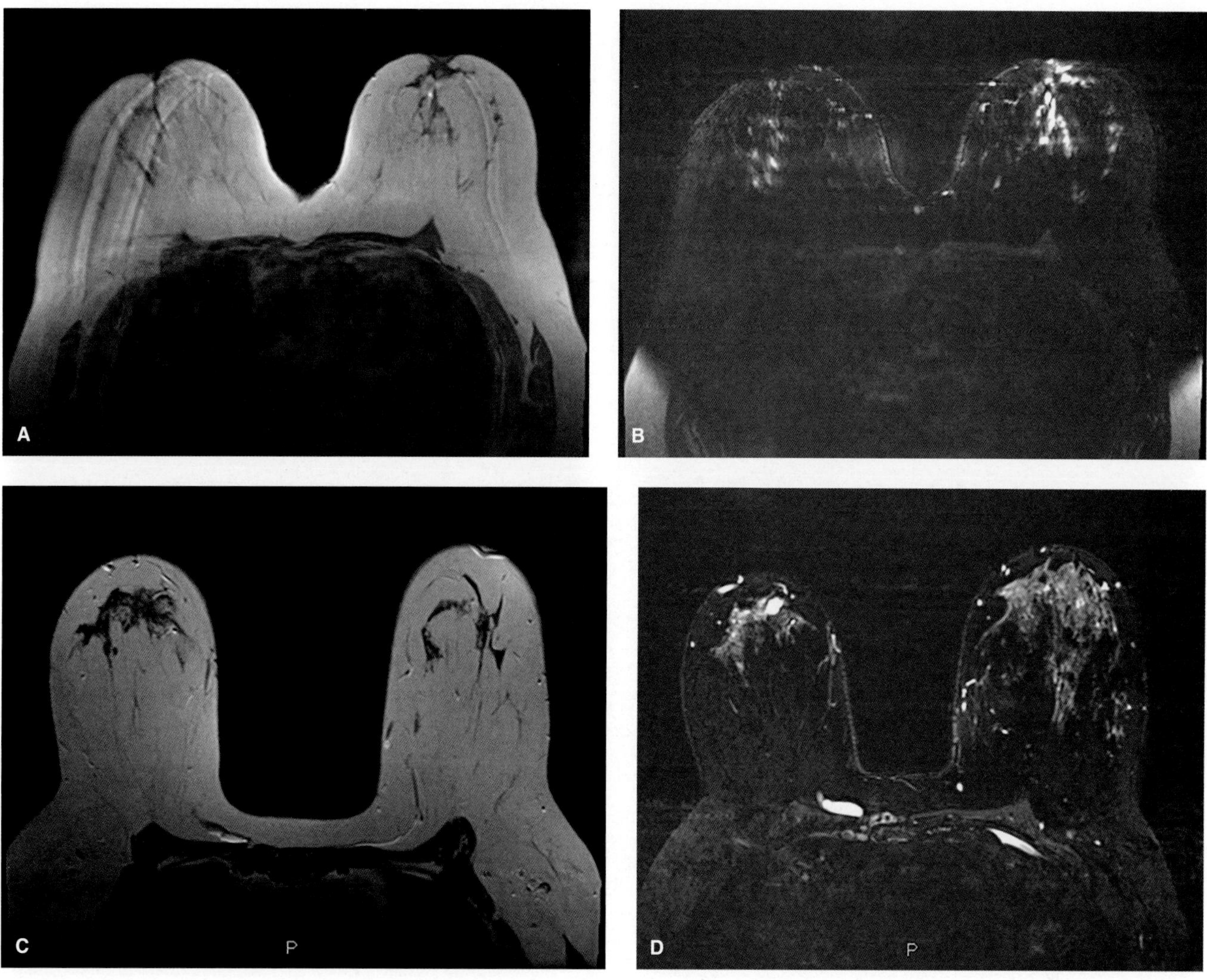

FIGURE 22.16. **Common Artifacts on Breast MR. A, B:** Patient motion creating repetitive bands on the T1W without FS image (**A**) and motion blurring on the T2W with FS image (**B**). **C–F:** A different patient who had an initial breast MR for cancer staging where FS failed and the study required repeating. **C, D:** Initial and repeat axial T2W without (**C**) and with (**D**) successful FS images. *(continued)*

Background Parenchymal Enhancement and Fibroglandular Tissue

Background Parenchymal Enhancement. As directed by the atlas, MR reports should include a description of background parenchymal enhancement (BPE) or the normal enhancement of a patient's fibroglandular tissue (see Table 22.6). Figure 22.17 shows examples of each of the BPE levels. This is assessed at the first postcontrast image which, as described in the technique section, occurs at approximately 90 seconds.

A higher degree of BPE affects the abnormal interpretation rate and is more common in younger women (50 years and younger). Luckily, no effect is observed on breast MR PPV, CDR, sensitivity, or specificity related to BPE. However, greater BPE has been shown to be associated with a higher probability of developing breast cancer. Specifically, women with mild, moderate, and marked BPE can be up to nine times more likely to develop breast cancer.

BPE is affected by hormone levels. In general, there is less BPE in the postmenopausal patient and during the second week of the menstrual cycle in premenopausal women. The least amount of BPE is observed during the proliferative phase (days 3 to 7) and the highest during the secretory phase (days 21 to 27). Therefore, screening breast MR should be performed during first half of the menstrual cycle (days 3 to 14). The effect of the menstrual cycle on BPE may differ based on the patient's breast density. In women who do not have regular cycles, serum progesterone levels can be used to time the examination. For cancer staging, MR imaging studies are usually done without consideration of a patient's cycle to facilitate expedited clinical decision making.

Fibroglandular Tissue. Along with the amount of BPE, reports are to comment on the amount of fibroglandular tissue present, similar to breast density on mammography. Table 22.7 lists the categories of fibroglandular tissue and Figure 22.18 shows examples on MR. It is interesting to note that the degree of BPE does not depend on the amount of fibroglandular tissue and can be present at various levels regardless of time in menstrual cycle or menopausal status.

Findings

The three finding types we describe based on the atlas lexicon are a focus, a mass, or an area of nonmass enhancement (NME). Table 22.8 lists the lexicon related to the three finding types.

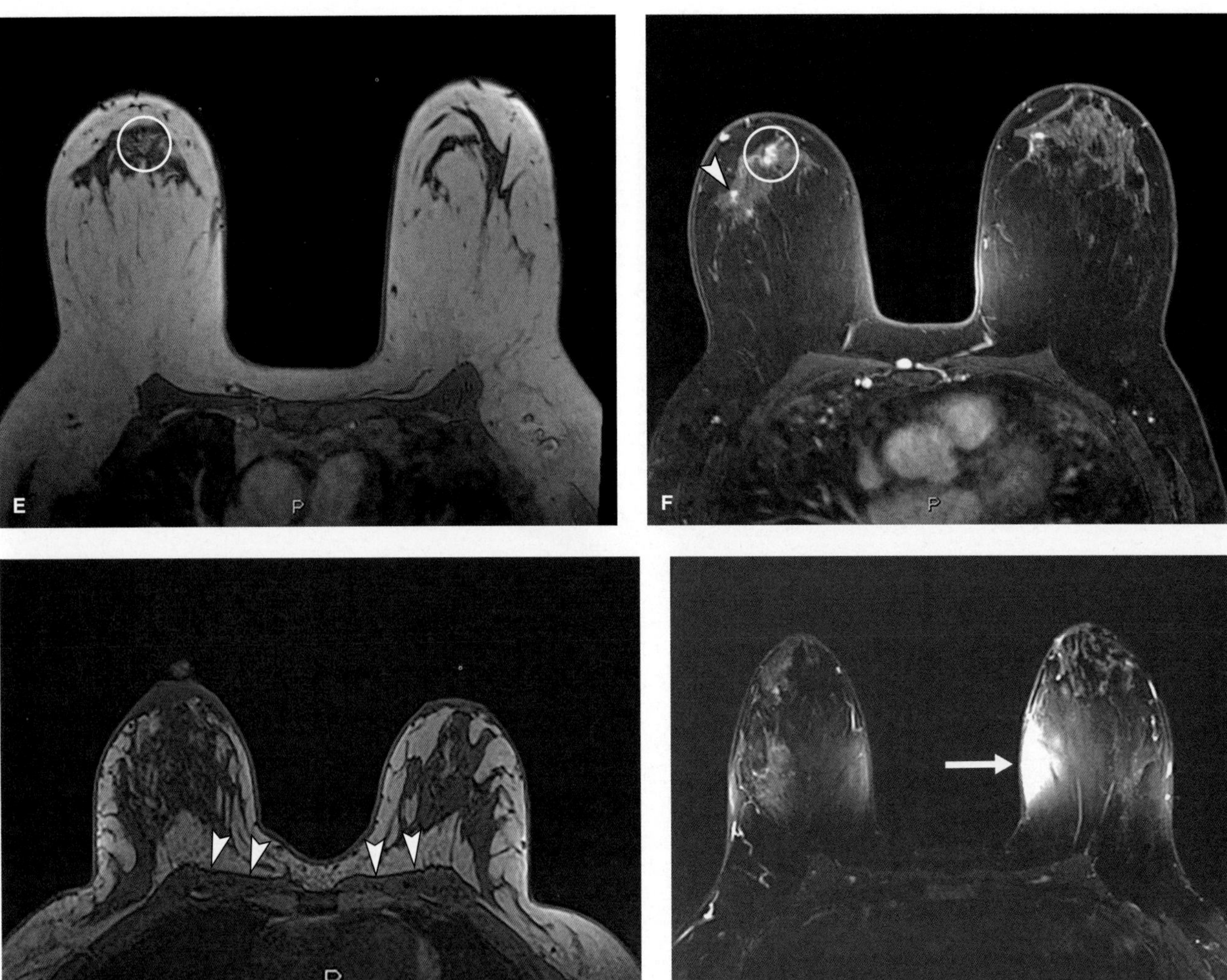

FIGURE 22.16. (*Continued*) **E, F:** Initial and repeat axial postcontrast T1W without (**E**) and with (**F**) successful FS images. The breast tissue is hyperintense without FS on the first sequence (**E**) which obscures easy detection of the bright, secondary to enhancement, cancer (*circles*) in the right anterior breast. In addition to the known cancer, having FS makes detection of the additional foci of disease posterolateral (*arrowhead*) possible. **G:** Chemical shift artifact degrading the axial T1W without FS image. This artifact occurs at the fat–fluid interfaces due to spatial misregistration secondary to the 224-Hz frequency shift between the tissues and creates a dark band at the interface. This happens on all images with a fat–fluid interface but can be minimized with proper technique. **H:** Flair (*arrow*) happens when the tissue is too close to the coil. Bright areas are created on the image, as on this axial T2W with FS image.

Focus. A focus is defined as a unique punctate enhancing dot, usually <5 mm, that lacks features of a mass (see Fig. 22.19). Shape, margin, distribution, or internal enhancement are *not* used to further characterize a focus; so if you *are* able to assess these features, then the finding is more appropriately categorized as a mass. When there are multiple bilateral foci, it is considered benign and categorized as part of the patient's BPE and not described separately as a finding. The patient in Figure 22.17B would be an example of this imaging appearance. A focus can be present due to both malignant and benign histologies. Table 22.9 lists the differential diagnosis for a focus. Features that are more typical of malignancy include a dominant or single focus, one that does not have features suggestive of a lymph node (no fatty hilum), a change from prior examination, or associated suspicious kinetics (washout delayed pattern). If a focus is hyperintense on T2WI, it is more likely benign, especially if it also is felt to be stable and have a fatty hilum or persistent delayed kinetics. The overall rate of malignancy for a focus is low at about 3%, but if the focus is new and/or hypointensity on T2WI foci, the rate for malignancy can be as high as 30%.

TABLE 22.6

BACKGROUND PARENCHYMAL ENHANCEMENT CATEGORIES

Minimal
Mild
Moderate
Marked

Mass. To be called a mass, the finding needs to be 3-dimensional with convex outward margins. For masses, we describe their shape, margin, and internal enhancement characteristics. Since nearly all histologies could present as a mass on MR, we use the lexicon terms to help to stratify if a mass is more likely benign or malignant. For example, irregular is the most concerning for malignancy of the three shapes.

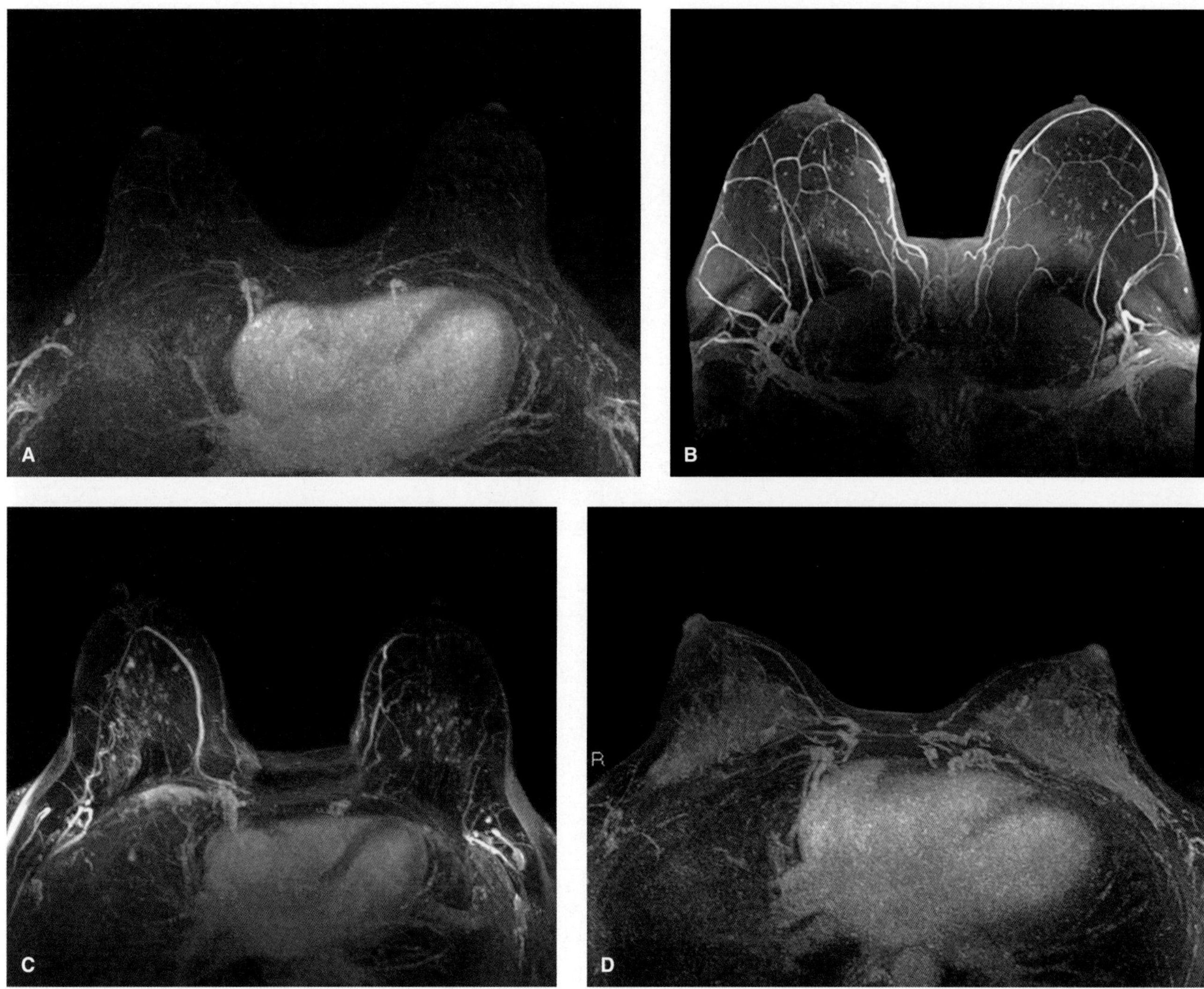

FIGURE 22.17. **Background Parenchymal Enhancement Levels on Breast MR. A:** Minimal. **B:** Mild. **C:** Moderate. **D:** Marked.

Figure 22.5 showed a nice example of an irregular malignant mass. The two noncircumscribed margins, spiculated and irregular, are more concerning for malignancy than a circumscribed margin. Figure 22.20 shows the contrast of a highly concerning spiculated mass and a more benign-appearing circumscribed mass. Of the internal enhancement patterns rim is the most concerning. Therefor a round, spiculated, rim-enhancing mass would be highly concerning for malignancy.

MR can also help us predict the subtype of cancer. A lower-grade IDC will more likely have irregular or spiculated margins, whereas a circumscribed mass with rim enhancement is more often a high-grade, sometimes triple negative, IDC and is at higher risk of lymph node involvement.

There are some imaging features that are specific for benign findings. The two most common benign breast masses are fibroadenomas and cysts. A fibroadenoma will classically be oval, circumscribed, hyperintense on T2W images with nonenhancing dark internal septations as shown in Figure 22.21, whereas a cyst, also oval, circumscribed, and hyperintense on T2W images, will lack any internal enhancement.

Nonmass Enhancement. NME is defined as enhancement that is not a mass nor a focus and stands out compared to BPE. The distribution and internal enhancement pattern are the terms used in describing NME, much like the distribution and morphology are for calcifications. There are six options for distribution with regional, multiple regions, and diffuse being suggestive of benign processes, the most common cause being fibrocystic changes. It is important to note that multicentric cancer can overlap with benign appearances. In contrast, segmental distribution has a high PPV for malignancy (34.5%). In internal enhancement patterns, clustered ring is most concerning for malignancy (36.7% PPV), followed by clumped internal enhancement (27.5% PPV). NME in a patient with a known ipsilateral cancer, of older age or that is extensive, has also been shown to have a higher PPV for malignancy

TABLE 22.7

FIBROGLANDULAR TISSUE CATEGORIES

Almost entirely fatty
Scattered fibroglandular tissue
Heterogeneous fibroglandular tissue
Extreme fibroglandular tissue

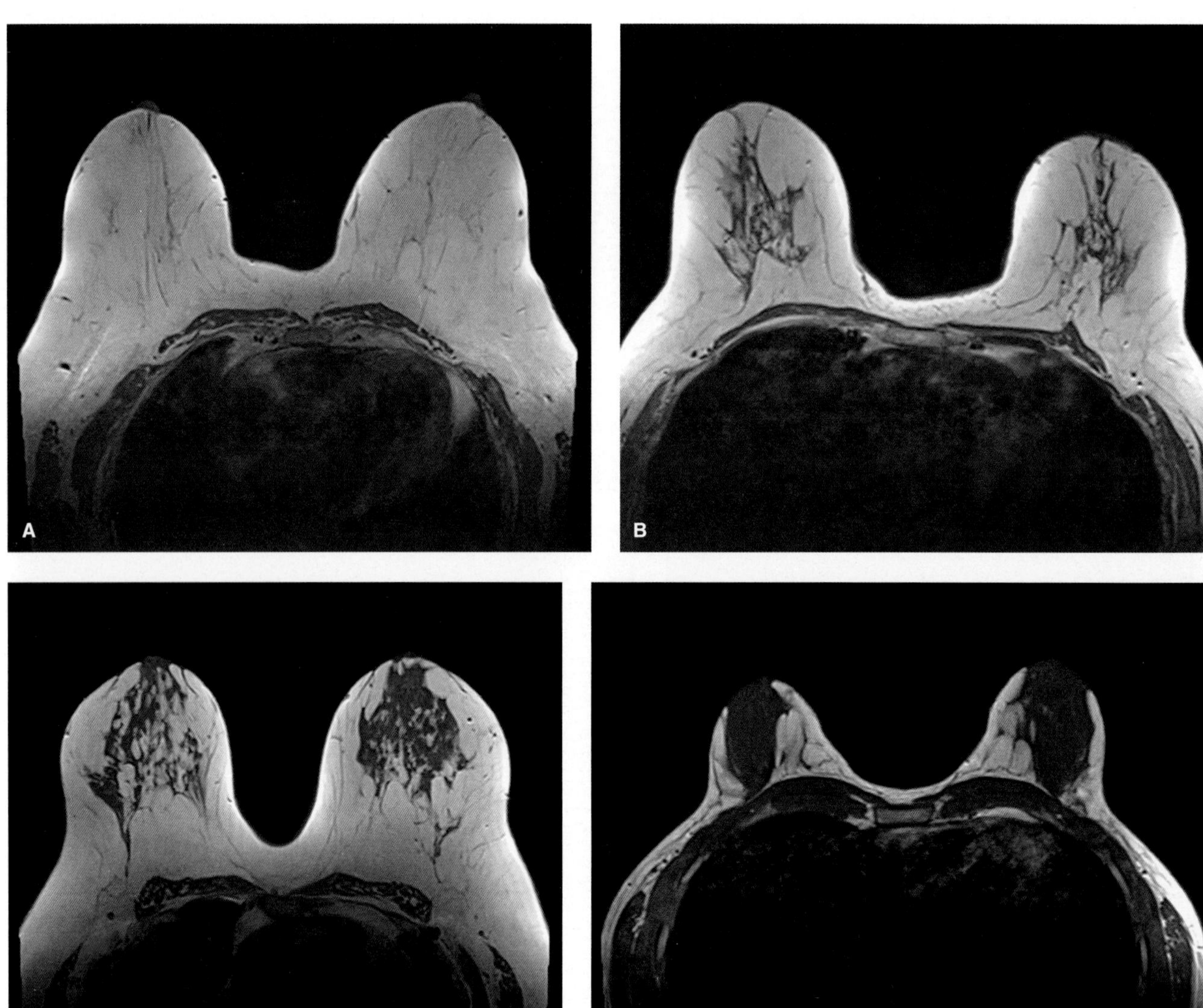

FIGURE 22.18. **Amount of Fibroglandular Tissue on Breast MR. A:** Almost entirely fatty. **B:** Scattered fibroglandular tissue. **C:** Heterogeneous fibroglandular tissue. **D:** Extreme fibroglandular tissue.

compared to other patients. The most common malignancy to present as NME is DCIS. All three patients in Figure 22.22 were found to have DCIS. Table 22.10 lists the differential diagnosis of NME.

WORKUP OF ABNORMAL MRI

When there is an abnormality (BI-RADS 4: suspicious finding or BI-RADS 5: highly suspicious finding) on breast MR, a patient can undergo an MR-guided biopsy or evaluation with mammography and/or US to find a correlate. Overall, masses seen on MR are more likely found with conventional imaging (mammogram and/or US) than NME. NME is found about half as often as masses (30% compared to 60% on average). For all findings, increasing size, more suspicious imaging features (BI-RADS 5 > BI-RADS 4), rim enhancement (mass), and clumped enhancement (NME) are more likely to have an US correlate. When a landmark is nearby (such as a surgical scar or cyst), the ability to find a correlate is also improved. In addition to US, DBT and contrast-enhanced mammography (a mammogram examination with intravenous contrast administration) can be used to find correlates for biopsy planning. About 1/8 cases of US-guided biopsies of initial MR finding that were deemed benign concordant at initial radiology–pathology review were found to not correspond with the MR finding on follow-up. Confirmation of biopsy target and follow-up are vital to the success of image-guided biopsies.

RISKS OF MRI

A good quality of breast MR is that there is no radiation exposure to the patient. However, contrast exposure may not be without some risk to patients. In 1997, nephrogenic systemic fibrosis (NSF) was first described in the United States and has since been linked to gadolinium-based contrast agents. NSF is a multisystemic fibrosing disease that primarily affects the skin but can progress to internal organ involvement. Death is rare but has been reported. Patients with severe renal impairment who undergo a ce-MR are at most risk for NSF; for this reason, breast ce-MR is not usually performed in women with GFR <30. In addition to the risk of NSF, there is evidence that gadolinium is retained by the body with deposition in the

TABLE 22.8

BREAST MRI LEXICON LIST OF FINDINGS AND TERMS

■ FINDINGS	■ TERMS	
Focus		
Masses	Shape	Oval[b] Round[a] Irregular[a]
	Margin	Circumscribed[b] Irregular[a] Spiculated[a]
	Internal enhancement characteristics	Homogeneous[b] Heterogeneous[a] Rim enhancement[a] Dark internal septations[b]
Nonmass enhancement (NME)	Distribution	Focal Linear Segmental[b] Regional[a] Multiple regions[a] Diffuse[a]
	Internal enhancement patterns	Homogeneous Heterogeneous Clumped[b] Clustered ring[b]

[a]Terms more often associated with malignancy.
[b]Terms more often associated with benign findings.

bone and brain. Deposition of linear gadolinium agents in the brain appears to be dose dependent but not associated with any neurologic symptoms and is unrelated to renal function. Table 22.11 lists the various breast MR contrast agents and whether they are linear or macrocyclic. Early data suggest that macrocyclic ionic gadolinium agents may not deposit in the brain and may therefore be safer for use.

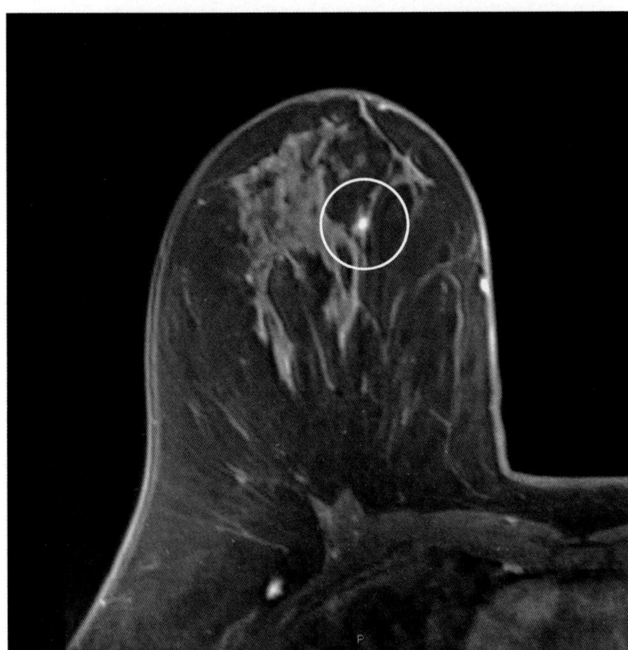

FIGURE 22.19. **Focus on Breast MR.** The focus (*circle*) is too small to characterize and therefore does not meet criteria for a mass or nonmass enhancement.

TABLE 22.9

DIFFERENTIAL DIAGNOSIS OF A FOCUS ON BREAST MRI

Intramammary lymph node
Papilloma
Small fibroadenoma
Fibrocystic changes
Usual ductal hyperplasia
Atypical ductal hyperplasia
Invasive ductal carcinoma
Ductal carcinoma in situ

Ha et al. (2014); Ha and Comstock (2014).

Further investigation into this phenomenon is important in the high-risk women population since many of these patients will be recommended for annual breast MR over 40+ years. MultiHance (gadobenate dimeglumine) and Magnevist (gadopentetate dimeglumine) are common breast contrast agents and are both linear ionic with label warnings regarding NSF. Many institutions are moving toward Gadavist (gadobutrol) and Dotarem (gadoterate meglumine) since they are macrocyclic agents. Data on all agents show reasonable sensitivity for detecting breast cancer, some slightly improved over others.

FUTURE OF MR IMAGING

Breast MR imaging in high-risk women has a CDR of up to 18/1,000 additional cancers over mammography and in average-risk women 15.5/1,000 additional cancers. Unfortunately, MR is a high-cost imaging modality with limited availability. Research looking at ways to shorten the protocol and reduce the reading time is ongoing. Shorter table time and quicker read times would reduce cost and allow for more widespread use of MR imaging for screening purposes. Kuhl has evaluated an abbreviated MR protocol that includes only the pre- and postcontrast sequences and a maximum intensity projection (MIP) sequence. Her group found they maintained the sensitivity of MR (CDR of 18/1,000) with an acquisition time of 10 minutes and a reading time of less than 1 minute.

TABLE 22.10

DIFFERENTIAL DIAGNOSIS OF NME ON BREAST MRI

Fibrocystic changes
Inflammatory benign lesions
Usual ductal hyperplasia
Atypical ductal hyperplasia
Invasive lobular carcinoma
Ductal carcinoma in situ

Milosevic et al. (2017).

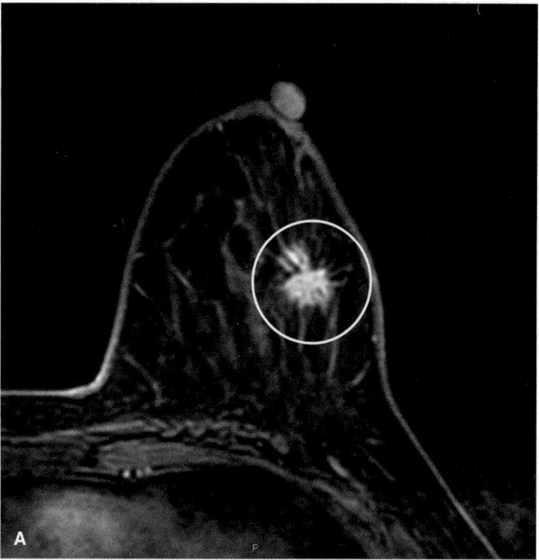

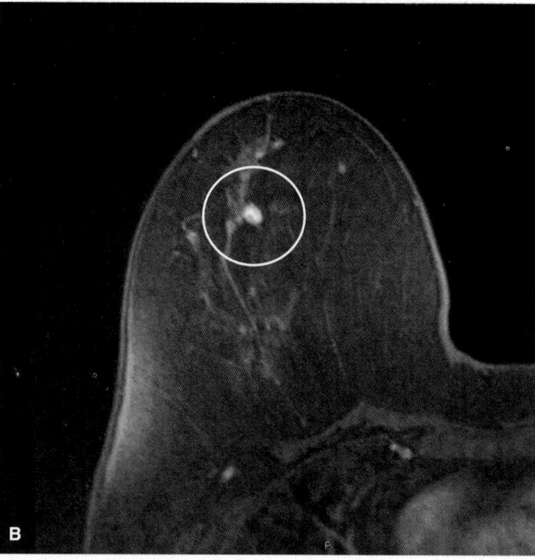

FIGURE 22.20. **Mass Margins on Breast MR.** Comparison of a highly suspicious spiculated margin mass (**A**, *circle*) to one that has a benign circumscribed margin (**B**, *circle*). Although the circumscribed mass has more benign features, if it is new or enlarging, it should undergo biopsy, as some cancers can mimic benign lesions.

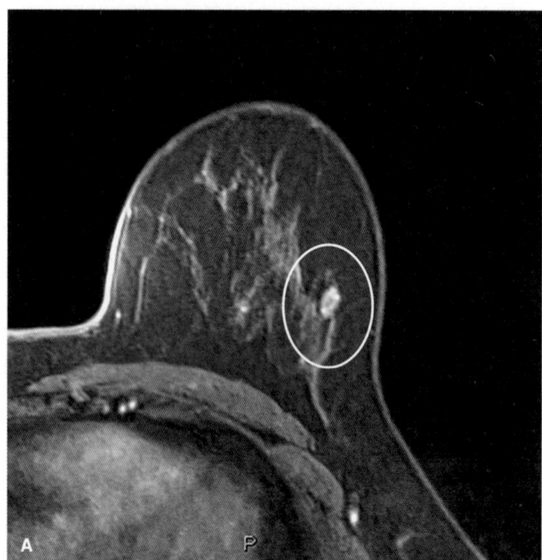

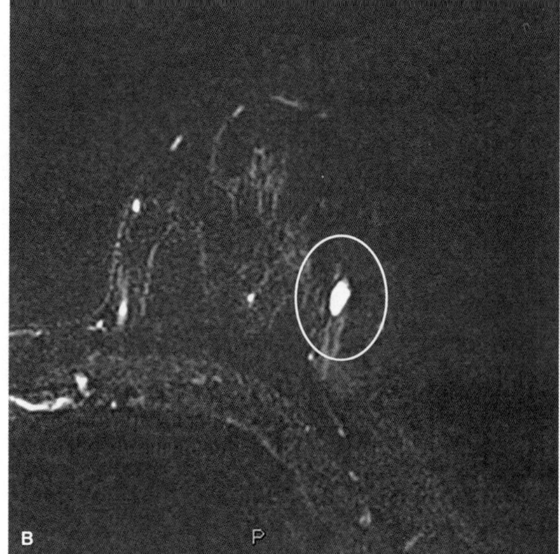

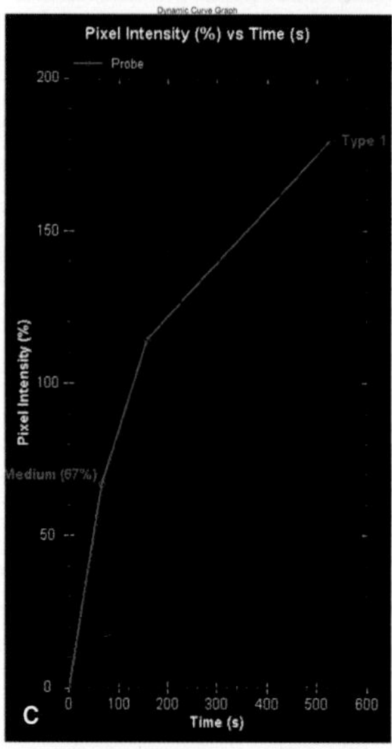

FIGURE 22.21. **Fibroadenoma on Breast MR.** A fibroadenoma is most often an enhancing oval (**A**, *oval*), circumscribed, hyperintense on T2W images (**B**, *oval*) mass with nonenhancing dark internal septations (dark areas within mass in **A**) with benign kinetics (**C**).

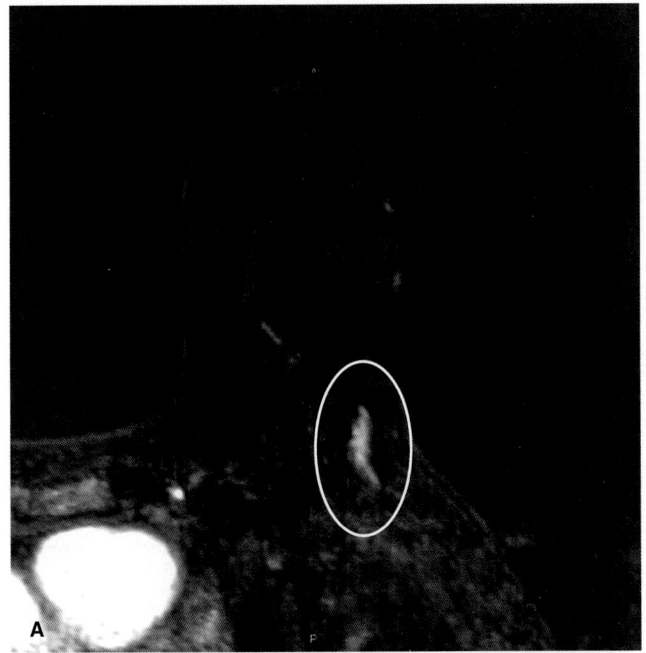

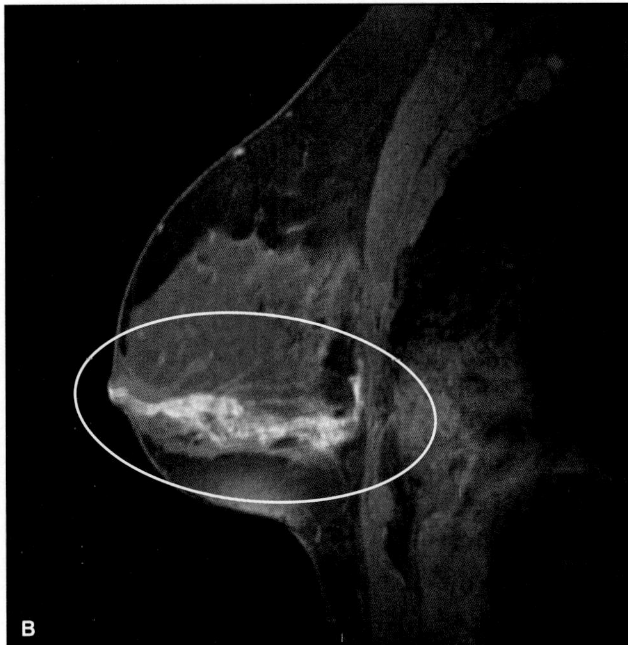

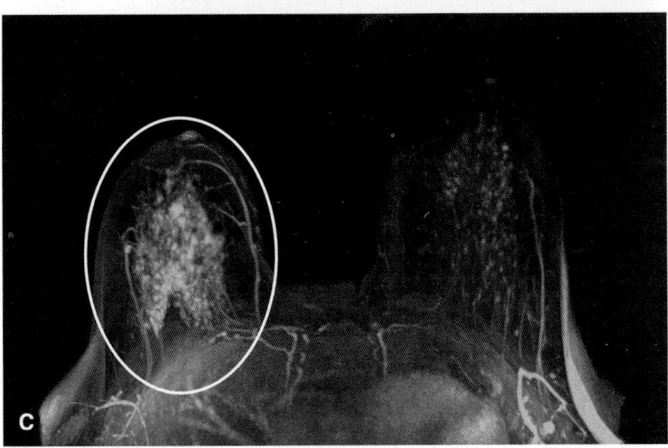

FIGURE 22.22. **NME on Breast MR.** All of the following areas of NME underwent biopsy and were found to be ductal carcinoma in situ (DCIS). **A:** Linear, conforming to the expected ductal distribution. **B:** Segmental, involving a segment of the breast. **C:** Regional, involving more than one ductal system. Regional is more often benign; however, was from extensive DCIS in this case.

Benefits of an abbreviated protocol include additional time slots for imaging, improved compliance and less patient motion, reduced image storage, and lessened physician fatigue. Potential limitations of this protocol are the inability to confidently determine whether a lesion is benign fat containing (no T1W non-FS images), decreased confidence in being able to declare a finding as specific benign (no T2W images), loss of kinetic information (no delayed time points), and a need to occasionally recall women for a full ce-MR imaging study.

TABLE 22.11

BREAST MR CONTRAST AGENTS AND TYPE

■ BRAND NAME	■ AGENT	■ STRUCTURE
Dotarem	Gadoterate meglumine	Macrocyclic
Gadavist	Gadobutrol	Macrocyclic
MultiHance	Gadobenate dimeglumine	Linear
OptiMARK	Gadoversetamide	Linear
Omniscan	Gadodiamide	Linear
ProHance	Gadoteridol	Macrocyclic
Magnevist	Gadopentetate dimeglumine	Linear

Other groups are looking at abbreviated protocols that include the T2W images or two postcontrast time points. A trial comparing an abbreviated breast MR (including a T2W image) against DBT in women with dense breasts is ongoing in 2017 and will add to our understanding of its application for screening women with average risk and dense breasts.

CONCLUSION

Breast MR is the most sensitive study to evaluate for breast cancer. It has many uses including, but not limited to, screening of high-risk women, preoperative staging of breast cancer, and implant evaluation. It requires the administration of gadolinium when done to evaluate for breast cancer which may not be without some risk. Future studies will look at the issues related to repetitive doses of gadolinium. Given the high sensitivity of breast MR, there is an interest in reducing the cost so that more women can benefit. It is likely that in the near future an abbreviated protocol will allow more widespread use of MR as a screening tool.

Suggested Readings

Agarwal K, Sharma U, Sah RG, et al. Pre-operative assessment of residual disease in locally advanced breast cancer patients: a sequential study by quantitative diffusion weighted MRI as a function of therapy. *Magn Reson Imaging* 2017;42:88–94.

Alduk AM, Brcic I, Podolski P, Prutki M. Correlation of MRI features and pathohistological prognostic factors in invasive ductal breast carcinoma. *Acta Clin Belg* 2017;72(5):306–312.

Amano Y, Aoki R, Kumita S, Kumazaki T. Silicone-selective multishot echo-planar imaging for rapid MRI survey of breast implants. *Eur Radiol* 2007;17(7):1875–1878.

American Cancer Society. Breast cancer early detection and diagnosis. Available from https://www.cancer.org/cancer/breast-cancer/screening-tests-and-early-detection/american-cancer-society-recommendations-for-the-early-detection-of-breast-cancer.html Accessed September 8, 2017.

American College of Radiology. *ACR BI-RADS Atlas Breast Imaging and Reporting Data System*. 5th ed. Reston, VA: American College of Radiology; 2013.

American College of Radiology (ACR). Breast magnetic resonance imaging (MRI) accreditation program requirements. Available from https://www.acr.org/~/media/ACRAccreditation/Documents/Breast-MRI/Requirements.pdf Accessed September 14, 2017.

American College of Radiology (ACR). Diagnostic radiology: magnetic resonance imaging (MRI) practice parameters and technical standards. ACR practice parameter for the performance of contrast-enhanced magnetic resonance imaging (MRI) of the breast. Available from https://www.acr.org/~/media/ACR/Documents/PGTS/guidelines/MRI_Breast.pdf Accessed September 8, 2017.

Badan GM, Roveda DJ, Paito S, et al. Ductal carcinoma in situ of the breast: evaluation of main presentations on magnetic resonance imaging compared with findings on mammogram and histology. *Rev Assoc Med Bras (1992)* 2016;62(5):421–427.

Ballesio L, Maggi C, Savelli S, et al. Role of breast magnetic resonance imaging (MRI) in patients with unilateral nipple discharge: preliminary study. *Radiol Med* 2008;113(2):249–264.

Baur A, Bahrs SD, Speck S, et al. Breast MRI of pure ductal carcinoma in situ: sensitivity of diagnosis and influence of lesion characteristics. *Eur J Radiol* 2013;82(10):1731–1737.

Berg WA, Gutierrez L, NessAiver MS, et al. Diagnostic accuracy of mammography, clinical examination, US, and MR imaging in preoperative assessment of breast cancer. *Radiology* 2004;233(3):830–849.

Bird RE, Wallace TW, Yankaskas BC. Analysis of cancers missed at screening mammography. *Radiology* 1992;184(3):613–617.

Bolan PJ, Kim E, Herman BA, et al. MR spectroscopy of breast cancer for assessing early treatment response: results from the ACRIN 6657 MRS trial. *J Magn Reson Imaging* 2017;46(1):290–302.

Braun M, Polcher M, Schrading S, et al. Influence of preoperative MRI on the surgical management of patients with operable breast cancer. *Breast Cancer Res Treat* 2008;111(1):179–187.

Brennan S, Liberman L, Dershaw DD, Morris E. Breast MRI screening of women with a personal history of breast cancer. *AJR Am J Roentgenol* 2010;195(2):510–516.

Chang YW, Kwon KH, Choi DL, et al. Magnetic resonance imaging of breast cancer and correlation with prognostic factors. *Acta Radiol* 2009;50(9):990–998.

Chikarmane SA, Michaels AY, Giess CS. Revisiting nonmass enhancement in breast MRI: analysis of outcomes and follow-up using the updated BI-RADS atlas. *AJR Am J Roentgenol* 2017;209(5):1178–1184.

Cho N, Im SA, Kang KW, et al. Early prediction of response to neoadjuvant chemotherapy in breast cancer patients: comparison of single-voxel (1) H-magnetic resonance spectroscopy and (18)F-fluorodeoxyglucose positron emission tomography. *Eur Radiol* 2016;26(7):2279–2290.

Ciatto S, Houssami N, Bernardi D, et al. Integration of 3D digital mammography with tomosynthesis for population breast-cancer screening (STORM): a prospective comparison study. *Lancet Oncol* 2013;14(7):583–589.

Clauser P, Carbonaro LA, Pancot M, et al. Additional findings at preoperative breast MRI: the value of second-look digital breast tomosynthesis. *Eur Radiol* 2015;25(10):2830–2839.

Clemens MW, Nava MB, Rocco N, Miranda RN. Understanding rare adverse sequelae of breast implants: anaplastic large-cell lymphoma, late seromas, and double capsules. *Gland Surg* 2017;6(2):169–184.

Cohen JB, Carroll C, Tenenbaum MM, Myckatyn TM. Breast implant-associated infections: the role of the National Surgical Quality Improvement Program and the local microbiome. *Plast Reconstr Surg* 2015;136(5):921–929.

Daniel BL, Gardner RW, Birdwell RL, Nowels KW, Johnson D. Magnetic resonance imaging of intraductal papilloma of the breast. *Magn Reson Imaging* 2003;21(8):887–892.

Dao TH, Rahmouni A, Campana F, Laurent M, Asselain B, Fourquet A. Tumor recurrence versus fibrosis in the irradiated breast: differentiation with dynamic gadolinium-enhanced MR imaging. *Radiology* 1993;187(3):751–755.

Dash N, Lupetin AR, Daffner RH, Deeb ZL, Sefczek RJ, Schapiro RL. Magnetic resonance imaging in the diagnosis of breast disease. *AJR Am J Roentgenol* 1986;146(1):119–125.

de Almeida JR, Gomes AB, Barros TP, Fahel PE, Rocha Mde S. Predictive performance of BI-RADS magnetic resonance imaging descriptors in the context of suspicious (category 4) findings. *Radiol Bras* 2016;49(3):137–143.

Debald M, Abramian A, Nemes L, et al. Who may benefit from preoperative breast MRI? A single-center analysis of 1102 consecutive patients with primary breast cancer. *Breast Cancer Res Treat* 2015;153(3):531–537.

de Bresser J, de Vos B, van der Ent F, Hulsewe K. Breast MRI in clinically and mammographically occult breast cancer presenting with an axillary metastasis: a systematic review. *Eur J Surg Oncol* 2010;36(2):114–119.

de Jong D, Vasmel WL, de Boer JP, et al. Anaplastic large-cell lymphoma in women with breast implants. *JAMA* 2008;300(17):2030–2035.

Delille JP, Slanetz PJ, Yeh ED, Kopans DB, Garrido L. Physiologic changes in breast magnetic resonance imaging during the menstrual cycle: perfusion imaging, signal enhancement, and influence of the T1 relaxation time of breast tissue. *Breast J* 2005;11(4):236–241.

DeMartini WB, Liu F, Peacock S, Eby PR, Gutierrez RL, Lehman CD. Background parenchymal enhancement on breast MRI: impact on diagnostic performance. *AJR Am J Roentgenol* 2012;198(4):W373–W380.

Dontchos BN, Rahbar H, Partridge SC, et al. Are qualitative assessments of background parenchymal enhancement, amount of fibroglandular tissue on MR images, and mammographic density associated with breast cancer risk? *Radiology* 2015;276(2):371–380.

El Yousef SJ, Duchesneau RH, Alfidi RJ, Haaga JR, Bryan PJ, LiPuma JP. Magnetic resonance imaging of the breast. Work in progress. *Radiology* 1984;150(3):761–766.

Feig S. Cost-effectiveness of mammography, MRI, and ultrasonography for breast cancer screening. *Radiol Clin North Am* 2010;48(5):879–891.

Fortunato L, Sorrento JJ, Golub RA, Cantu R. Occult breast cancer. A case report and review of the literature. *N Y State J Med* 1992;92(12):555–557.

Frei KA, Kinkel K, Bonel HM, Lu Y, Esserman LJ, Hylton NM. MR imaging of the breast in patients with positive margins after lumpectomy: influence of the time interval between lumpectomy and MR imaging. *AJR Am J Roentgenol* 2000;175(6):1577–1584.

Gao Y, Ibidapo O, Toth HK, Moy L. Delineating extramammary findings at breast MR imaging. *Radiographics* 2017;37(1):10–31.

Gorczyca DP, DeBruhl ND, Mund DF, Bassett LW. Linguine sign at MR imaging: does it represent the collapsed silicone implant shell? *Radiology* 1994;191(2):576–577.

Ha R, Comstock CE. Breast magnetic resonance imaging: management of an enhancing focus. *Radiol Clin North Am* 2014;52(3):585–589.

Ha R, Sung J, Lee C, Comstock C, Wynn R, Morris E. Characteristics and outcome of enhancing foci followed on breast MRI with management implications. *Clin Radiol* 2014;69(7):715–720.

Hambly NM, Liberman L, Dershaw DD, Brennan S, Morris EA. Background parenchymal enhancement on baseline screening breast MRI: impact on biopsy rate and short-interval follow-up. *AJR Am J Roentgenol*. 2011;196(1):218–224.

Harvey SC, Di Carlo PA, Lee B, Obadina E, Sippo D, Mullen L. An abbreviated protocol for high-risk screening breast MRI saves time and resources. *J Am Coll Radiol* 2016;13(11S):R74–R80.

Harvey JA, Hendrick RE, Coll JM, Nicholson BT, Burkholder BT, Cohen MA. Breast MR imaging artifacts: how to recognize and fix them. *Radiographics* 2007;27(Suppl 1):S131–S145.

Hennigs A, Riedel F, Marme F, et al. Changes in chemotherapy usage and outcome of early breast cancer patients in the last decade. *Breast Cancer Res Treat* 2016;160(3):491–499.

Houssami N, Ciatto S, Macaskill P, et al. Accuracy and surgical impact of magnetic resonance imaging in breast cancer staging: systematic review and meta-analysis in detection of multifocal and multicentric cancer. *J Clin Oncol* 2008;26(19):3248–3258.

Houssami N, Hayes DF. Review of preoperative magnetic resonance imaging (MRI) in breast cancer: should MRI be performed on all women with newly diagnosed, early stage breast cancer? *CA Cancer J Clin* 2009;59(5):290–302.

Igarashi T, Ashida H, Morikawa K, Motohashi K, Fukuda K. Use of BI-RADS-MRI descriptors for differentiation between mucinous carcinoma and fibroadenoma. *Eur J Radiol* 2016;85(6):1092–1098.

Ikeda DM. Progress report from the American College of Radiology Breast MR Imaging Lexicon Committee. *Magn Reson Imaging Clin N Am* 2001;9(2):295–302.

Jatoi I, Proschan MA. Randomized trials of breast-conserving therapy versus mastectomy for primary breast cancer: a pooled analysis of updated results. *Am J Clin Oncol* 2005;28(3):289–294.

Kajihara M, Goto M, Hirayama Y, et al. Effect of the menstrual cycle on background parenchymal enhancement in breast MR imaging. *Magn Reson Med Sci* 2013;12(1):39–45.

Kang SS, Ko EY, Han BK, Shin JH, Hahn SY, Ko ES. Background parenchymal enhancement on breast MRI: influence of menstrual cycle and breast composition. *J Magn Reson Imaging* 2014;39(3):526–534.

Kazama T, Nakamura S, Doi O, Suzuki K, Hirose M, Ito H. Prospective evaluation of pectoralis muscle invasion of breast cancer by MR imaging. *Breast Cancer* 2005;12(4):312–316.

Keech JA Jr, Creech BJ. Anaplastic T-cell lymphoma in proximity to a saline-filled breast implant. *Plast Reconstr Surg* 1997;100(2):554–555.

King V, Gu Y, Kaplan JB, Brooks JD, Pike MC, Morris EA. Impact of menopausal status on background parenchymal enhancement and fibroglandular tissue on breast MRI. *Eur Radiol* 2012;22(12):2641–2647.

Kramer SC, Rieber A, Gorich J, et al. Diagnosis of papillomas of the breast: value of magnetic resonance mammography in comparison with galactography. *Eur Radiol* 2000;10(11):1733–1736.

Kriege M, Brekelmans CT, Boetes C, et al. Efficacy of MRI and mammography for breast-cancer screening in women with a familial or genetic predisposition. *N Engl J Med* 2004;351(5):427–437.

Kriege M, Brekelmans CT, Boetes C, et al. Differences between first and subsequent rounds of the MRISC breast cancer screening program for women with a familial or genetic predisposition. *Cancer* 2006;106(11):2318–2326.

Kucher C, Steere J, Elenitsas R, Siegel DL, Xu X. Nephrogenic fibrosing dermopathy/nephrogenic systemic fibrosis with diaphragmatic involvement in a patient with respiratory failure. *J Am Acad Dermatol* 2006;54(2 Suppl):S31–S34.

Kuhl CK, Schrading S, Leutner CC, et al. Mammography, breast ultrasound, and magnetic resonance imaging for surveillance of women at high familial risk for breast cancer. *J Clin Oncol* 2005;23(33):8469–8476.

Kuhl CK, Schrading S, Strobel K, Schild HH, Hilgers RD, Bieling HB. Abbreviated breast magnetic resonance imaging (MRI): first postcontrast subtracted images and maximum-intensity projection-a novel approach to breast cancer screening with MRI. *J Clin Oncol* 2014;32(22):2304–2310.

Lee JY, Park JE, Kim HS, et al. Up to 52 administrations of macrocyclic ionic MR contrast agent are not associated with intracranial gadolinium deposition: multifactorial analysis in 385 patients. *PLoS One* 2017;12(8):e0183916.

Lehman CD, Gatsonis C, Kuhl CK, et al. MRI evaluation of the contralateral breast in women with recently diagnosed breast cancer. *N Engl J Med* 2007;356(13):1295–1303.

Lehman CD, Isaacs C, Schnall MD, et al. Cancer yield of mammography, MR, and US in high-risk women: prospective multi-institution breast cancer screening study. *Radiology* 2007;244(2):381–388.

Liberman L, Morris EA, Dershaw DD, Abramson AF, Tan LK. MR imaging of the ipsilateral breast in women with percutaneously proven breast cancer. *AJR Am J Roentgenol* 2003;180(4):901–910.

Lubina N, Schedelbeck U, Roth A, et al. 3.0 tesla breast magnetic resonance imaging in patients with nipple discharge when mammography and ultrasound fail. *Eur Radiol* 2015;25(5):1285–1293.

Machida Y, Shimauchi A, Kuroki Y, et al. Single focus on breast magnetic resonance imaging: diagnosis based on kinetic pattern and patient age. *Acta Radiol* 2017;58(6):652–659.

Mahoney MC, Gatsonis C, Hanna L, DeMartini WB, Lehman C. Positive predictive value of BI-RADS MR imaging. *Radiology* 2012;264(1):51–58.

Manganaro L, D'Ambrosio I, Gigli S, et al. Breast MRI in patients with unilateral bloody and serous-bloody nipple discharge: a comparison with galactography. *Biomed Res Int* 2015;2015:806368.

Mann RM, Hoogeveen YL, Blickman JG, Boetes C. MRI compared to conventional diagnostic work-up in the detection and evaluation of invasive lobular carcinoma of the breast: a review of existing literature. *Breast Cancer Res Treat* 2008;107(1):1–14.

Mann RM, Loo CE, Wobbes T, et al. The impact of preoperative breast MRI on the re-excision rate in invasive lobular carcinoma of the breast. *Breast Cancer Res Treat* 2010;119(2):415–422.

McDonald RJ, McDonald JS, Kallmes DF, et al. Intracranial gadolinium deposition after contrast-enhanced MR imaging. *Radiology* 2015;275(3):772–782.

Meissnitzer M, Dershaw DD, Lee CH, Morris EA. Targeted ultrasound of the breast in women with abnormal MRI findings for whom biopsy has been recommended. *AJR Am J Roentgenol* 2009;193(4):1025–1029.

Milosevic ZC, Nadrljanski MM, Milovanovic ZM, Gusic NZ, Vucicevic SS, Radulovic OS. Breast dynamic contrast enhanced MRI: fibrocystic changes presenting as a non-mass enhancement mimicking malignancy. *Radiol Oncol* 2017;51(2):130–136.

Morris EA. Review of breast MRI: indications and limitations. *Semin Roentgenol* 2001;36(3):226–237.

Moschetta M, Telegrafo M, Rella L, Stabile Ianora AA, Angelelli G. Let's go out of the breast: prevalence of extra-mammary findings and their characterization on breast MRI. *Eur J Radiol* 2014;83(6):930–934.

Nelson HD, Fu R, Cantor A, Pappas M, Daeges M, Humphrey L. Effectiveness of breast cancer screening: systematic review and meta-analysis to update the 2009 U.S. Preventive Services Task Force recommendation. *Ann Intern Med* 2016;164(4):244–255.

Newburg AR, Chhor CM, Young Lin LL, et al. Magnetic resonance imaging-directed ultrasound imaging of non-mass enhancement in the breast: outcomes and frequency of malignancy. *J Ultrasound Med* 2017;36(3):493–504.

Nguyen J, Nicholson BT, Patrie JT, Harvey JA. Incidental pleural effusions detected on screening breast MRI. *AJR Am J Roentgenol* 2012;199(1):W142–W145.

O'Neill AC, Zhong T, Hofer SOP. Implications of breast implant-associated anaplastic large cell lymphoma (BIA-ALCL) for breast cancer reconstruction: an update for surgical oncologists. *Ann Surg Oncol* 2017;24(11):3174–3179.

Pengel KE, Loo CE, Wesseling J, Pijnappel RM, Rutgers EJ, Gilhuijs KG. Avoiding preoperative breast MRI when conventional imaging is sufficient to stage patients eligible for breast conserving therapy. *Eur J Radiol* 2014;83(2):273–278.

Piper ML, Roussel LO, Koltz PF, et al. Characterizing infections in prosthetic breast reconstruction: a validity assessment of national health databases. *J Plast Reconstr Aesthet Surg* 2017;70(10):1345–1353.

Prince MR, Zhang H, Morris M, et al. Incidence of nephrogenic systemic fibrosis at two large medical centers. *Radiology* 2008;248(3):807–816.

Sanyal S, Marckmann P, Scherer S, Abraham JL. Multiorgan gadolinium (Gd) deposition and fibrosis in a patient with nephrogenic systemic fibrosis–an autopsy-based review. *Nephrol Dial Transplant* 2011;26(11):3616–3626.

Sardanelli F, Newstead GM, Putz B, et al. Gadobutrol-enhanced magnetic resonance imaging of the breast in the preoperative setting: results of 2 prospective international multicenter phase III studies. *Invest Radiol* 2016;51(7):454–461.

Saslow D, Boetes C, Burke W, et al. American cancer society guidelines for breast screening with MRI as an adjunct to mammography. *CA Cancer J Clin* 2007;57(2):75–89.

Scaranelo AM, Marques AF, Smialowski EB, Lederman HM. Evaluation of the rupture of silicone breast implants by mammography, ultrasonography and magnetic resonance imaging in asymptomatic patients: correlation with surgical findings. *Sao Paulo Med J* 2004;122(2):41–47.

Schnall MD, Blume J, Bluemke DA, et al. MRI detection of distinct incidental cancer in women with primary breast cancer studied in IBMC 6883. *J Surg Oncol* 2005;92(1):32–38.

Shah AT, Jankharia BB. Imaging of common breast implants and implant-related complications: a pictorial essay. *Indian J Radiol Imaging* 2016;26(2): 216–225.

Smith RA, Duffy SW, Gabe R, Tabar L, Yen AM, Chen TH. The randomized trials of breast cancer screening: what have we learned? *Radiol Clin North Am* 2004;42(5):793–806.

Soderstrom CE, Harms SE, Farrell RS Jr, Pruneda JM, Flamig DP. Detection with MR imaging of residual tumor in the breast soon after surgery. *AJR Am J Roentgenol* 1997;168(2):485–488.

Tabar L, Yen MF, Vitak B, Chen HH, Smith RA, Duffy SW. Mammography service screening and mortality in breast cancer patients: 20-year follow-up before and after introduction of screening. *Lancet* 2003;361(9367):1405–1410.

Van Zee KJ, Ortega Perez G, Minnard E, Cohen MA. Preoperative galactography increases the diagnostic yield of major duct excision for nipple discharge. *Cancer* 1998;82(10):1874–1880.

Varadarajan R, Edge SB, Yu J, Watroba N, Janarthanan BR. Prognosis of occult breast carcinoma presenting as isolated axillary nodal metastasis. *Oncology* 2006;71(5–6):456–459.

Warner E, Plewes DB, Hill KA, et al. Surveillance of BRCA1 and BRCA2 mutation carriers with magnetic resonance imaging, ultrasound, mammography, and clinical breast examination. *JAMA*. 2004;292(11):1317–1325.

Warner E, Plewes DB, Shumak RS, et al. Comparison of breast magnetic resonance imaging, mammography, and ultrasound for surveillance of women at high risk for hereditary breast cancer. *J Clin Oncol* 2001;19(15):3524–3531.

Wasif N, Garreau J, Terando A, Kirsch D, Mund DF, Giuliano AE. MRI versus ultrasonography and mammography for preoperative assessment of breast cancer. *Am Surg* 2009;75(10):970–975.

Wiener JI, Chako AC, Merten CW, Gross S, Coffey EL, Stein HL. Breast and axillary tissue MR imaging: correlation of signal intensities and relaxation times with pathologic findings. *Radiology* 1986;160(2):299–305.

Yang XP, Han YD, Ye JJ, et al. Comparison of gadobenate dimeglumine and gadopentetate dimeglumine for breast MRI screening: a meta-analysis. *Asian Pac J Cancer Prev* 2014;15(12):5089–5095.

Yeatman TJ, Cantor AB, Smith TJ, et al. Tumor biology of infiltrating lobular carcinoma. Implications for management. *Ann Surg* 1995;222(4):549–559; discussion 559–561.

Yilmaz R, Bender O, Celik Yabul F, Dursun M, Tunaci M, Acunas G. Diagnosis of nipple discharge: value of magnetic resonance imaging and ultrasonography in comparison with ductoscopy. *Balkan Med J* 2017;34(2):119–126.

Yitta S, Joe BN, Wisner DJ, Price ER, Hylton NM. Recognizing artifacts and optimizing breast MRI at 1.5 and 3 T. *AJR Am J Roentgenol* 2013;200(6): W673–W682.

CHAPTER 23 ■ IMAGE-GUIDED BREAST PROCEDURES

BRANDI T. NICHOLSON, CARRIE M. ROCHMAN, AND JONATHAN V. NGUYEN

INTRODUCTION TO BREAST BIOPSIES

Suspicious imaging findings require histologic or cytologic examination for definitive diagnosis. Historically, women underwent surgical excision for suspicious breast findings. However, the current standard of care is to perform percutaneous image-guided procedures and now the majority, >80% of over 1.6 million, of biopsies are done with image guidance. Stereotactic-guided biopsies were the first to be developed in the late 1980s. Since then image guidance for procedures has continued to improve and can be done using mammographic, stereotactic, tomosynthesis (DBT), ultrasound (US), or magnetic resonance (MR) imaging and has the same accuracy of surgical biopsy. In addition, image-guided biopsy is less invasive, has minimal to no scarring, and can be performed quickly compared to surgical biopsy. It also allows most women to avoid surgery (±80% of results will be benign) or to plan for neoadjuvant treatments in the setting of malignancy and decrease the number of necessary surgeries during their treatment. When image-guided procedures cannot be done, patients continue to be referred for localization and surgical excision. Localization and excision is also done for image-guided procedures with discordant, high-risk or malignant results.

BREAST BIOPSY

Indications

Indications for core biopsy are similar to those for surgical biopsy. A complete diagnostic examination must be done before biopsy is recommended. A lesion assessed at diagnostic as BI-RADS 4: suspicious finding or BI-RADS 5: highly suspicious finding should be recommended for sampling. For a BI-RADS 3: probably benign finding, short interval follow-up is the recommendation of choice. However, there are times when a biopsy should be performed as is listed in Table 23.1. Technical difficulties such as inadequate visualization of the lesion, breast thickness, or location of the finding may occasionally preclude the use of an image-guided biopsy. In these instances the patient is referred to a breast surgeon for surgical biopsy.

Needle Types

There are several needle types used in image-guided breast biopsies. These include small (typically 22- to 25-gauge) needles for fine-needle aspiration (FNA) and larger (hollow 9- to 12-gauge) needles for core needle biopsy (CNB).

Fine-Needle Aspiration. FNA was first reported in 1930 and remains an inexpensive, safe and relatively accurate method for obtaining histology. A limitation of FNA is that it requires the pathologist to have special expertise and is associated with more false positives (FP) and false negatives (FN) compared to CNB.

Core Needle Biopsy. CNB was introduced in the 1990s and can be done with a spring-loaded needle or a vacuum-assisted device and is the preferred method over FNA due to its improved sensitivity (84% to 88% compared to 72% to 77%). Both methods demonstrate similar specificity of 94% to 98%. An additional advantage to CNB over FNA is that it obtains more tissue allowing for a more easy ability to grade tumors and evaluate receptor status. However, CNB is more costly and more invasive than FNA.

For CNB, either a 14-gauge automated biopsy gun or a 9- to 12-gauge vacuum-assisted needle is used. The standard 14-gauge gun works by a spring action mechanism that fires the needle through the lesion. The inner cannula containing the tissue notch is projected through the lesion first and then the cutting cannula is fired over it so that a small core of tissue is retained within the specimen notch. With the vacuum-assisted devices, suction is used to bring the tissue into the specimen notch of the needle, which is then cut by an inner rotating cannula. Vacuum-assisted devices generally require only a single needle pass to obtain multiple specimens, whereas standard core biopsy requires multiple passes, one for each specimen. The vacuum-assisted needle offers improved ability to adequately sample microcalcifications when compared with the standard biopsy gun. Calcifications can be subject to the most risk of upgrade to malignancy after a benign or high-risk CNB

TABLE 23.1

INDICATIONS FOR IMAGE-GUIDED BIOPSY

BI-RADS 3: probably benign finding[a]	Follow-up not possible On transplant list or otherwise immunocompromised Known ipsilateral breast cancer Patient preference
BI-RADS 4: suspicious finding	
BI-RADS 5: highly suspicious finding	

[a]Short interval follow-up is the recommendation of choice.

result. With vacuum-assisted needle biopsy there is a larger volume of tissue obtained which is associated with decreased upgrade rates compared with the smaller gauge automated devices. The vacuum-assisted needles are the device of choice for stereotactic-, DBT-, and MR-guided procedures. They are also occasionally used in US-guided biopsies when small (5 mm or less in diameter) findings are being sampled.

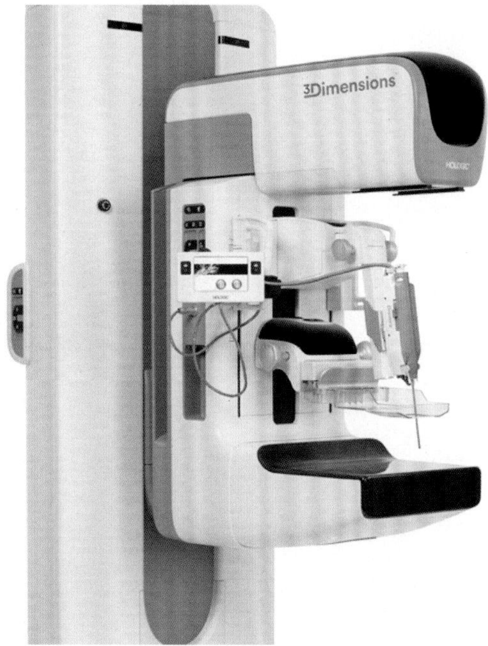

FIGURE 23.2. **Add-on Stereotactic Biopsy Unit.** The biopsy device attaches to a mammography unit allowing for multifunctionality of the mammography suite. (Courtesy of Hologic Inc, Bedford, MA.)

Guidance

Core biopsies can be guided by stereotactic, DBT, US, or MR imaging. MR and DBT-guided procedures have increased in utilization as the technology develops and becomes more widely available. All methods are highly accurate with reported success rates of ≥98%. When determining the method of guidance one first considers which method the lesion is best seen and is most accessible, and second on consideration of patient comfort. For example, if the finding is only visible on a DBT study that will be the guidance used. If the finding is also visible with US, then US is usually selected as it is comfortable for patients and quick to perform. If a patient has more than one finding and histology results will affect management decisions, more than one biopsy is done.

Stereotactic Biopsy. Currently, there are two types of stereotactic units available as shown in Figures 23.1 and 23.2. The first is a prone-dedicated unit and the second an add-on unit. Prone tables have the advantage of the patient positioned lying down which can minimize patient motion and vasovagal reactions. However, there can be limited access to the chest wall or far posterior or lateral findings and women can find it uncomfortable due to body habitus, mobility issues, and neck/shoulder discomfort. Prone tables also limit utilization of the room to only one purpose. In contrast, the add-on unit attaches to a standard mammography machine and allows utilization of the room for routine imaging between procedures. The patient can be positioned either sitting or lying down and is often more comfortable compared to the prone position. There are different lesion locations that can be difficult to access with the add-on unit, so each method has its limitations.

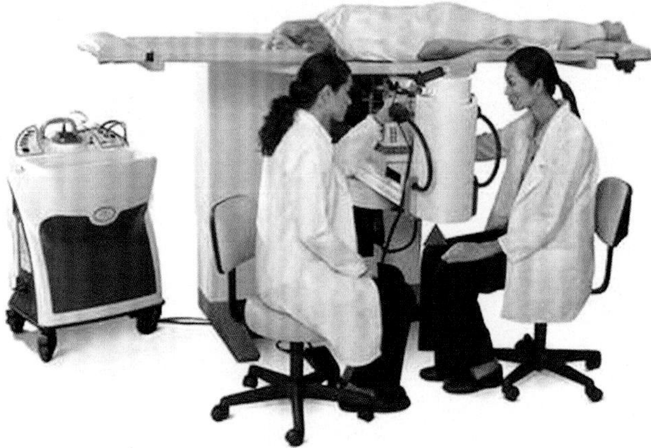

FIGURE 23.1. **Dedicated Stereotactic Biopsy Unit.** The x-ray tube (*red arrowhead*) moves independent of the compressed breast so stereo images can be obtained. The needle guide is adjusted so that the biopsy needle (*red arrow*) will be centered in the lesion. (Courtesy of Hologic Inc, Bedford, MA.)

The most common findings sampled using stereotactic-guidance are calcifications. Figure 23.3 shows BI-RADS 4 calcifications and the imaging steps of a stereotactic biopsy. Occasionally, other findings like a mass, an asymmetry, or architectural distortion is only or best seen mammographically and will be referred for stereotactic biopsy as well like in Figure 23.4. A 9- to 12-gauge vacuum-assisted needle is used for these types of biopsies.

During a stereotactic biopsy the x-ray tube head moves independent of the compressed breast. The target for biopsy is centered in the aperture while the breast is in compression. The initial image is taken straight on to confirm it is centered. Then two images each at 15-degree oblique from center are obtained. Calculation of the amount of deviation of the lesion in these two oblique views allows the exact determination of the depth of the lesion. The needle guide is adjusted for exact positioning of the needle in three dimensions to the center of the lesion. After the injection of local anesthetic, a small skin incision is made to permit needle entry into the breast. Positioning of the needle is verified with stereotactic views and biopsies are taken. Inadequate breast thickness, usually around 30 mm or less, may lead to an unsuccessful biopsy due to technical limitations of the biopsy device and needle. Women with thin breast tissue in compression may not be able to undergo a stereotactic biopsy and will be sent for primary surgical excision.

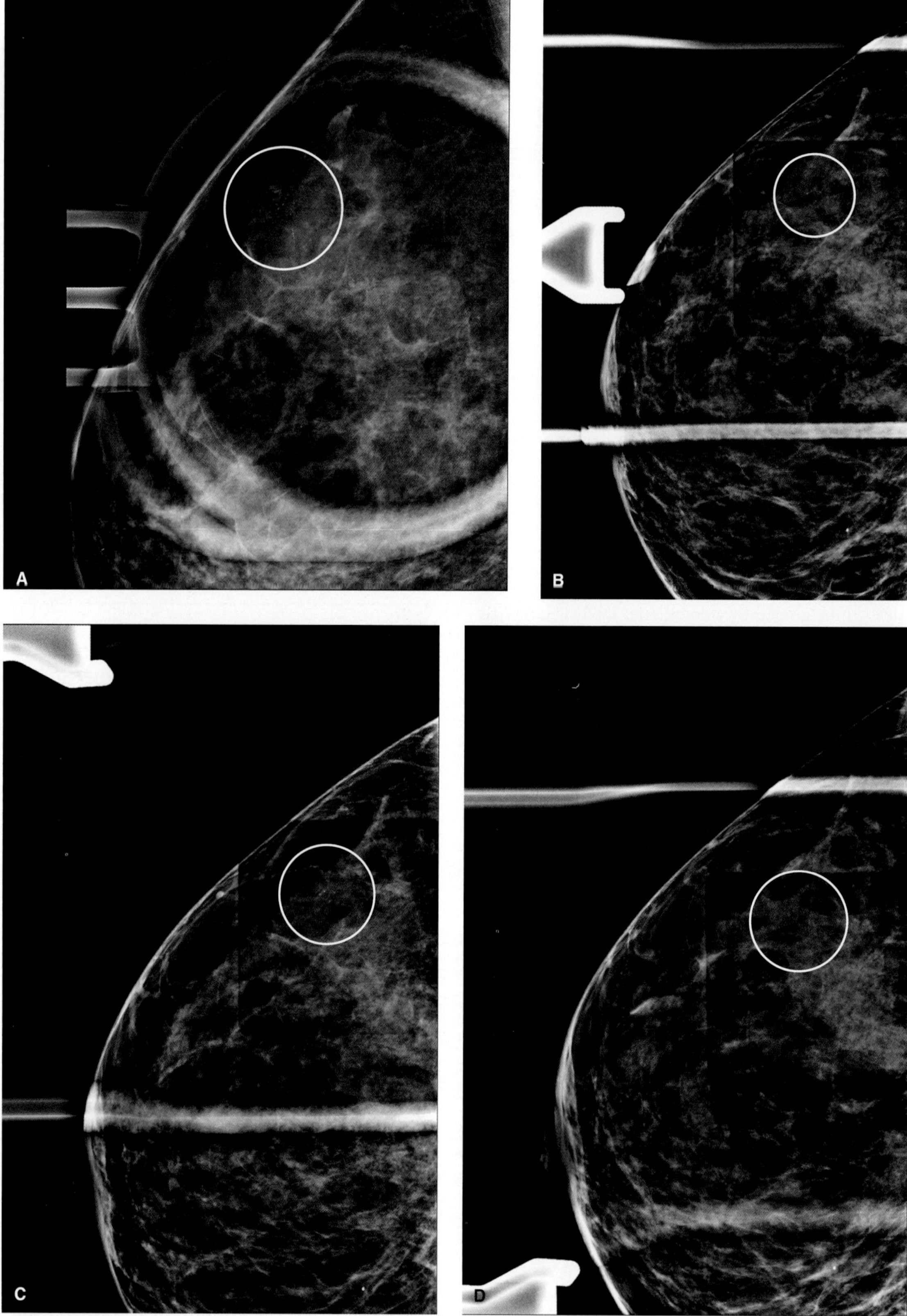

FIGURE 23.3. **Stereotactic Biopsy Steps. A:** Left magnification view showing BI-RADS 4 grouped fine pleomorphic calcifications recommended for biopsy (*circle*). **B:** The scout image with the calcifications well positioned in the opening of the compression paddle (*circle*). **C, D:** Two oblique views are taken 15° off-center and the target is identified for the software (*circles*).

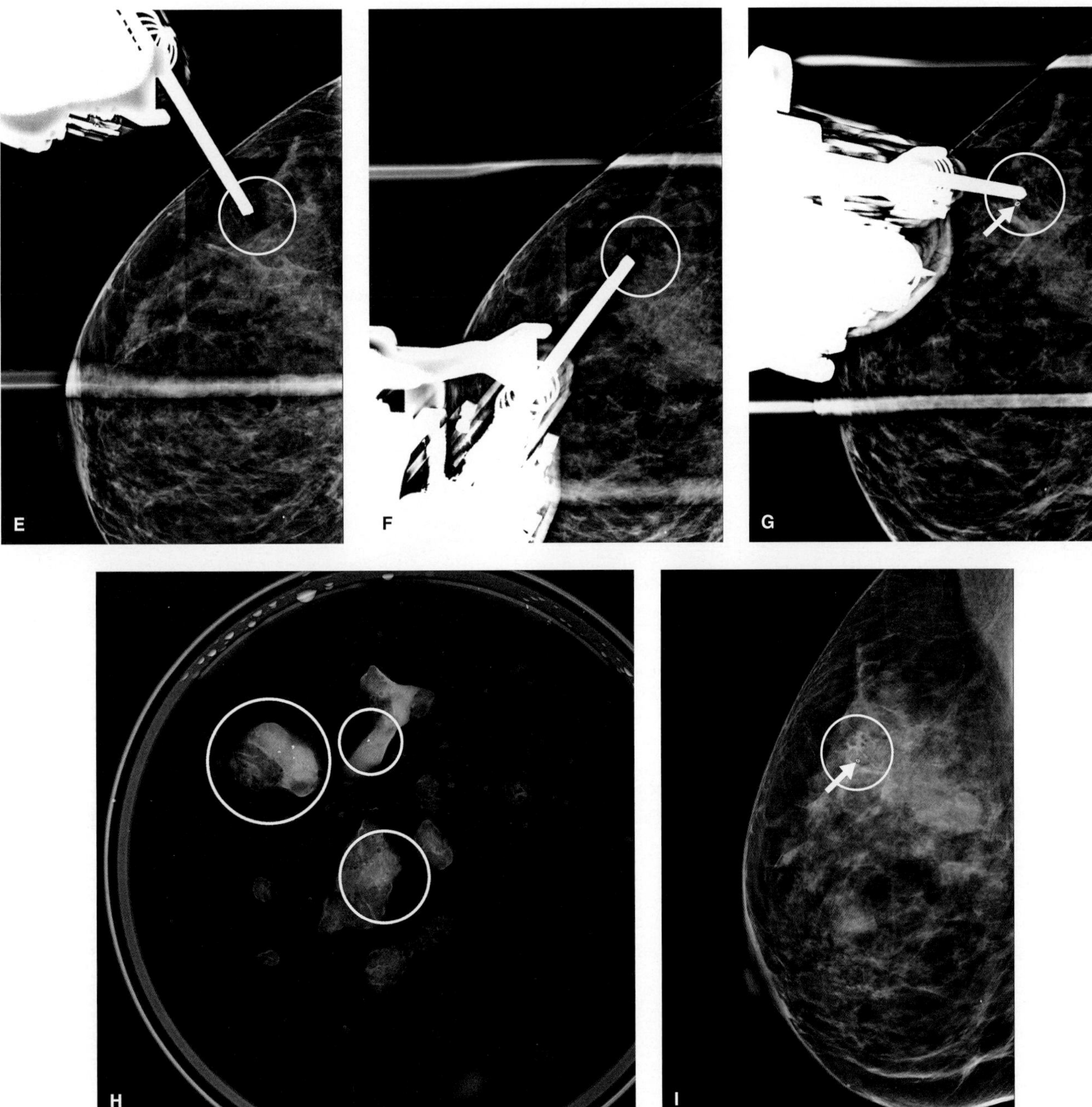

FIGURE 23.3. (*Continued*) **E, F:** After the skin is prepped and the tissue is anesthetized the needle is placed with the leading edge or tip at the target (*circles*) and two additional oblique views are taken to confirm positioning. The needle is then advanced and sampling is performed. **G:** After sampling is complete a biopsy marker is placed at the biopsy site (*arrow*). Biopsy site changes can also be appreciated with decrease in calcifications (*circle*). **H:** The specimen radiograph confirms calcifications were obtained at the time of biopsy (*circles*). **I:** The final step of the procedure is to obtain a two-view postbiopsy mammogram, ML view shown, to see the biopsy marker related to the target. The *arrow* points to the marker in the expected location compared to (**A**) and a decrease in number of calcifications (*circle*). Biopsy result was ductal carcinoma in situ, concordant.

After sampling is complete, a radiograph is taken of the tissue samples, this is called a specimen radiograph as demonstrated in Figure 23.3H. This allows confirmation that the intended target has been removed. Confirming that calcifications are present in the tissue being sent to pathology improves the accuracy of the procedure. The same process can be done for masses and asymmetries where you are looking to confirm that dense tissue is present in the sample instead of only fat. Figure 23.4B shows density within one of the samples in a stereotactic biopsy done for a mass. If there is an inadequate sample, additional tissue can be taken before removal of the needle.

Once the sampling is complete, a marker can and should be placed at the biopsy site. Markers are designed such that they can be placed through the vacuum-assisted open bore needle. A postbiopsy mammogram will demonstrate the metallic marker. Figure 23.3I shows a postclip mammogram with the marker in the expected location.

Tomosynthesis Biopsy. Some findings are only visible on or are more conspicuous with tomosynthesis. A common imaging finding where this would be true is an area of architectural distortion seen only on slices from a DBT examination as in Figure 23.5. For this or other like findings

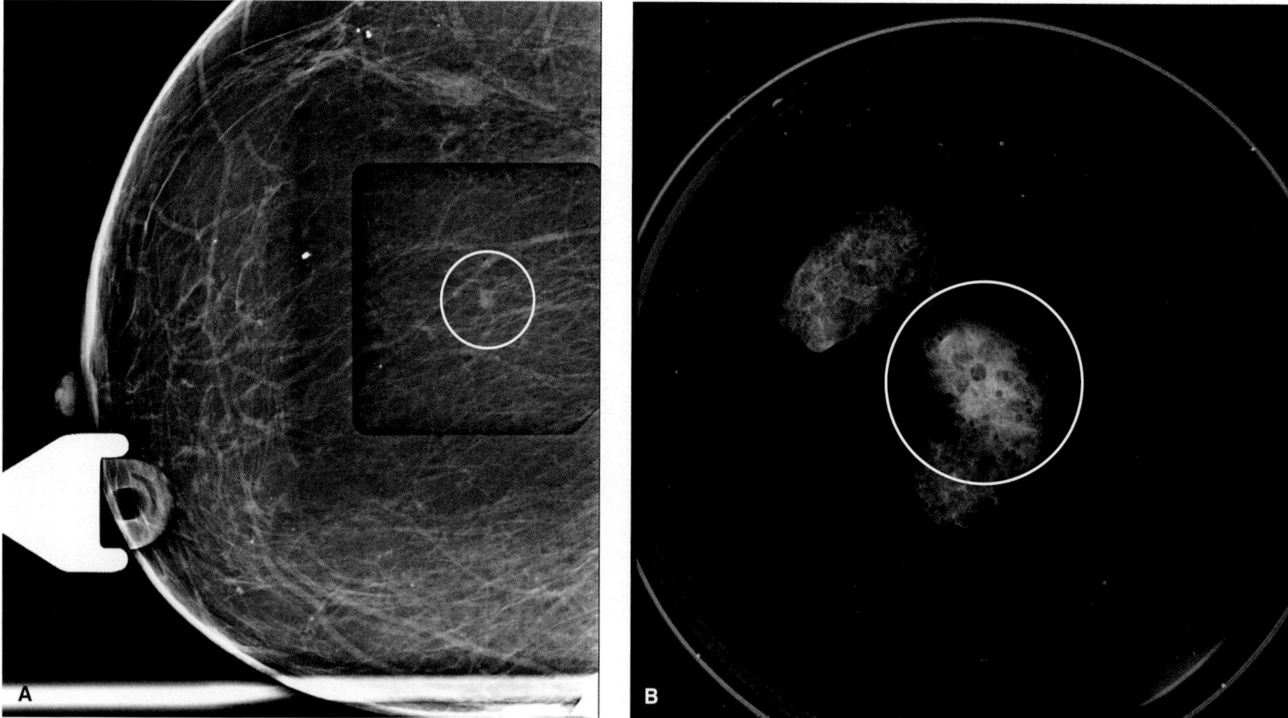

FIGURE 23.4. **Stereotactic Biopsy for Mass. A:** Scout image showing the target (*circle*). A small mass that could not be seen with ultrasound (not shown) and underwent stereotactic biopsy. **B:** A specimen radiograph can confirm targeting when dense tissue is present instead of only fat (*circle*). Pathology result was invasive ductal carcinoma, concordant.

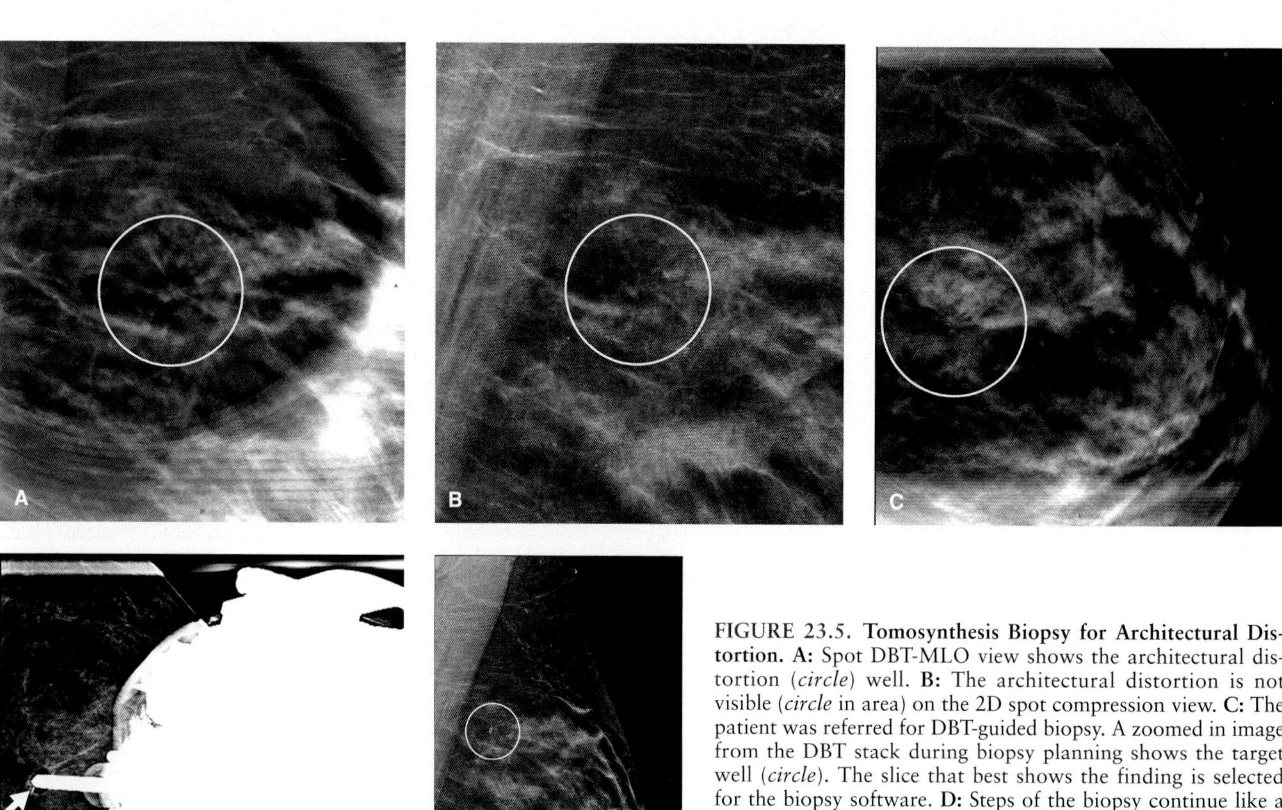

FIGURE 23.5. **Tomosynthesis Biopsy for Architectural Distortion. A:** Spot DBT-MLO view shows the architectural distortion (*circle*) well. **B:** The architectural distortion is not visible (*circle* in area) on the 2D spot compression view. **C:** The patient was referred for DBT-guided biopsy. A zoomed in image from the DBT stack during biopsy planning shows the target well (*circle*). The slice that best shows the finding is selected for the biopsy software. **D:** Steps of the biopsy continue like a stereotactic biopsy with the final step being placement of the marker (*arrow*). **E:** The postbiopsy mammogram can be done using DBT or 2D. The full MLO, in this case the synthesized two-dimensional view from the DBT stack, shows the marker (*circle*) in the expected location. Pathology result was radial scar, concordant.

DBT is the only guidance that may allow for successful image-guided CNB. DBT-guided biopsies were not initially available when DBT imaging began and procedures were done as best as possible using landmarks with stereotactic-guidance or were sent for primary surgical excision with localization. The development of DBT capable biopsy units has allowed image-guided biopsies of less conspicuous findings without sending patients to surgery primarily. In 2013, Schrading et al. published their initial results of DBT-guided biopsies and found that it performed superior to stereotactic guidance. There are several units available and they include both prone and add-on devices. The same 9- to 12-gauge vacuum-assisted needle is used for DBT-guided biopsies as in stereotactic-guidance. Many steps of a DBT-guided procedure are similar to stereotactic-guidance (see Fig. 23.5). The breast is placed into compression, the target is centered in the aperture, and imaging is done for targeting. Unlike the stereotactic where two obliques are taken, in

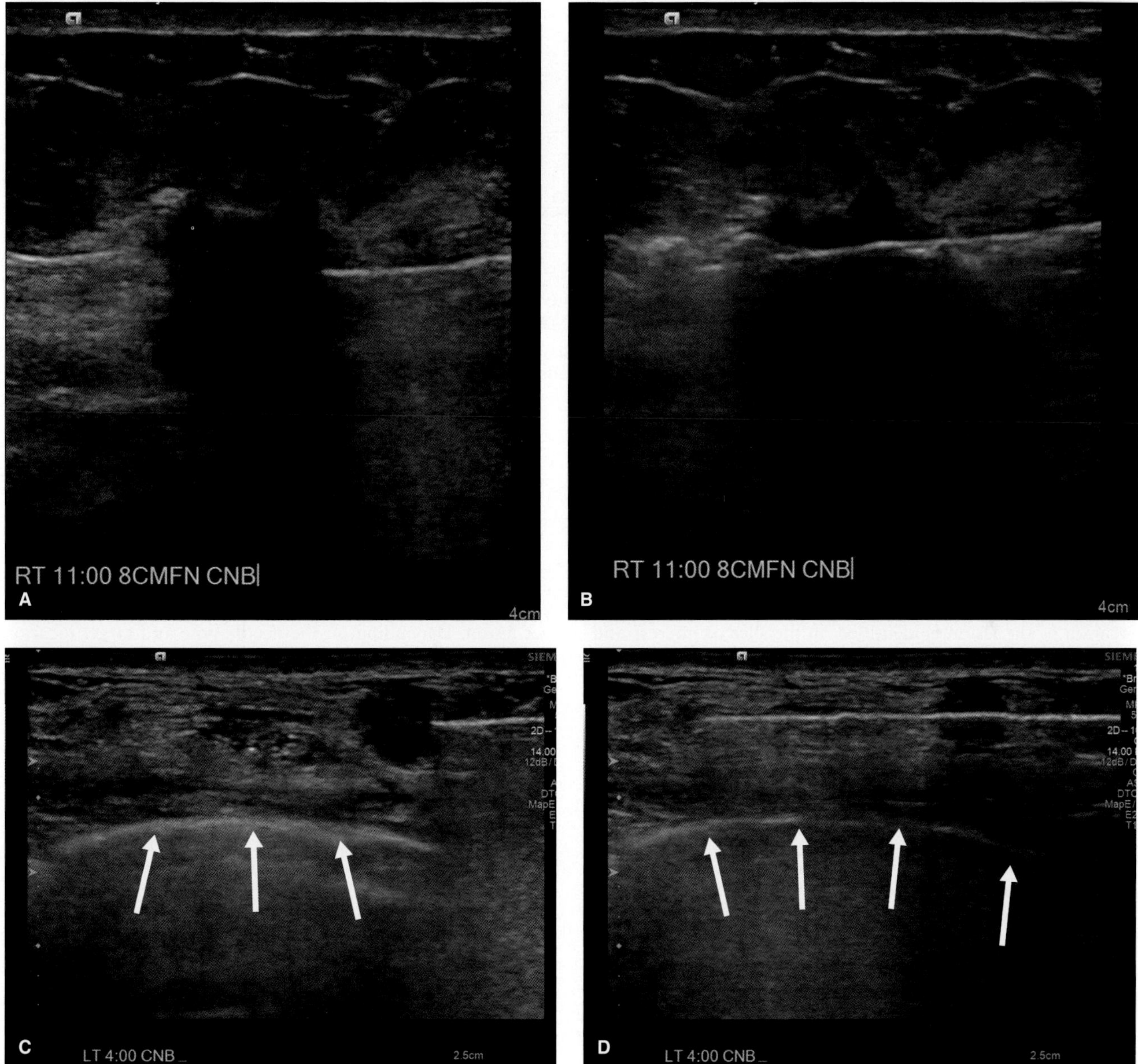

FIGURE 23.6. **Ultrasound Biopsy of Mass. A, B:** Large, irregular, indistinct, and hypoechoic mass in a large breast undergoing ultrasound-guided core needle biopsy. **A:** The 14-gauge throw needle is positioned at the leading edge of the mass before the sample is taken. **B:** Postfire image shows the needle through the mass in a parallel approach. Pathology result was invasive ductal carcinoma, concordant. **C, D:** A smaller mass in a thinner breast can undergo successful and safe core biopsy. **C:** The 14-gauge throw needle is positioned at the leading edge of the mass as in the first case. Maintaining needle visualization and a parallel approach becomes more important in a thin breast. **D:** The postfire image shows the needle through the mass and safely traversing the tissue away from the chest wall. Pathology result was invasive ductal carcinoma, concordant.

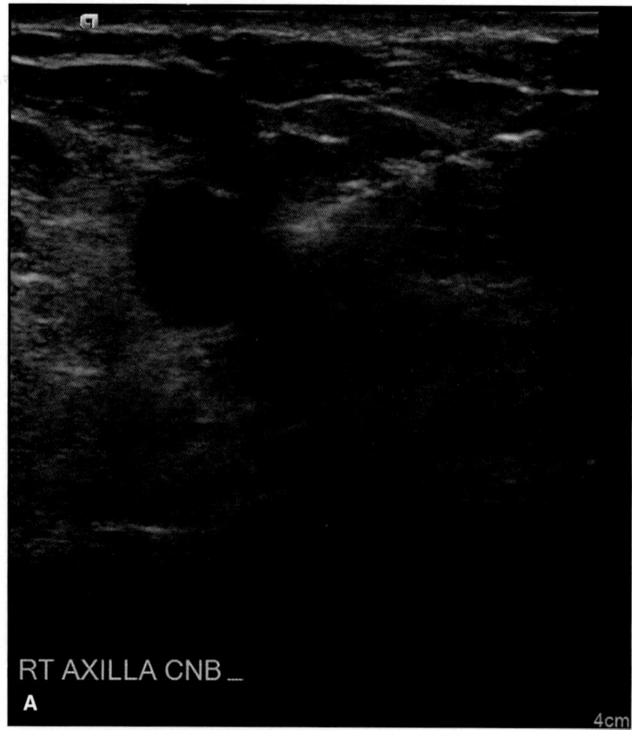

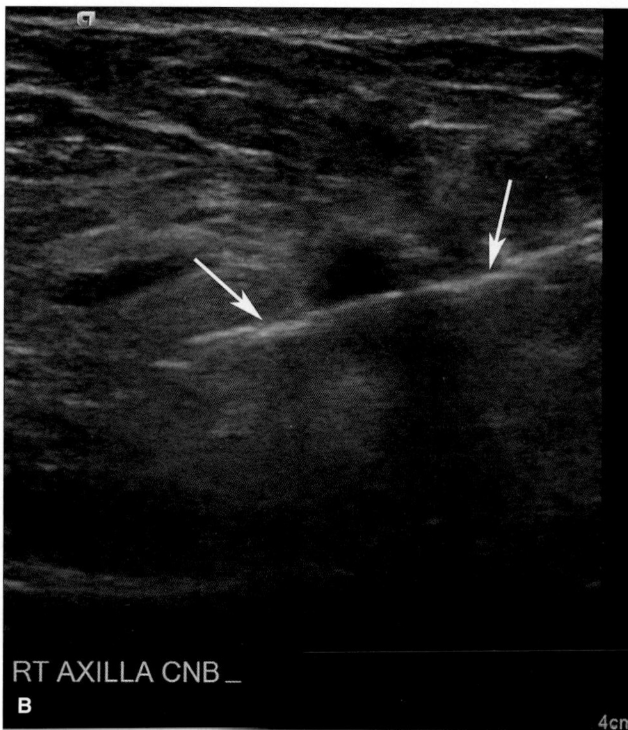

FIGURE 23.7. **Ultrasound Biopsy of Axillary Node. A, B:** The approach for an axillary node biopsy is at an angle. **A:** The needle is positioned at the leading edge of the node before the inner trocar is advanced through the node. **B:** The inner trocar can be seen exposed after advancement within the node (*arrows* at each edge of the visible trocar). When the needle is fired the trocar is covered but the needle tip does not advance making it safe for the axilla. Pathology result was metastatic node, concordant.

DBT-guided procedures the x-ray tube head moves in an arc over the breast and a tomosynthesis stack is obtained. The location of the lesion is identified on the slice of interest and the depth is directly calculated. The procedure continues as for a stereotactic biopsy as above concluding with obtaining a specimen radiograph and marker placement. Compared to stereotactic-guided, DBT biopsies tend to be faster to perform with fewer exposures taken during the procedure and no increase in complications. Inadequate breast thickness can impact the success of DBT biopsies as in stereotactic guidance.

Ultrasound Biopsy. US-guided biopsy was first described by Parker et al. (1993) and was shown to be fast, accurate, and without significant complications. This paved the way for widespread use of US guidance for breast biopsies and it is currently the method of choice for lesions that are well seen with US. Adequate sonographic visualization of the lesion is essential if core biopsy is to be performed with US guidance which means that the most common lesions sampled are masses and axillary lymph nodes. Both 14-gauge automated biopsy needles and larger gauge vacuum-assisted needles can be utilized. In general, US-guided procedures are preferred over other methods because they are more comfortable for women, allow for real-time visualization of the needle throughout the procedure, are less expensive, and take less time to perform. Specifically, US-guided CNB has been found to be up to 56% and 30% less expensive compared to surgical and stereotactic biopsy, respectively.

For US-guided CNB local anesthetic is used at the skin entrance site. A small incision is made in the skin to allow entrance of the needle into the breast. Anesthetic is also placed along the expected needle path and around the target lesion. Depending on the needle type and target location the approach may be parallel to the chest wall (breast masses undergoing automated CNB shown in Fig. 23.6) or at an angle (axillary node with a spring-loaded semi-automated needle shown in Fig. 23.7). The goal is to ensure sampling of the target lesion without risk to the patient. Most women can successfully undergo an US-guided biopsy regardless of breast thickness.

In addition, FNA or aspiration of fluid-filled masses can be done with US guidance. FNA is done with small needles (22- to 25-gauge). Local anesthetic is used at the skin and along the needle path. The needle is then advanced into the finding and under real-time visualization the sample is obtained. A skin incision is not necessary. If a cytopathologist or pathologist is present during the FNA they can do a preliminary review. If the sample is inconclusive then the procedure can be converted to CNB with an improvement in sensitivity.

In settings where the finding is an indeterminate mass, solid versus cystic finding, an aspiration can be attempted before consideration of a CNB. Figure 23.8 shows an aspiration without resolution of the finding for which a CNB was then performed. If a finding can be proven fluid filled by a successful aspiration a CNB can be avoided. In addition, women will request aspiration of simple cysts (BI-RADS 2: benign finding) secondary to pain. The procedure steps are the same for aspirations as for in an FNA and shown in Figure 23.9.

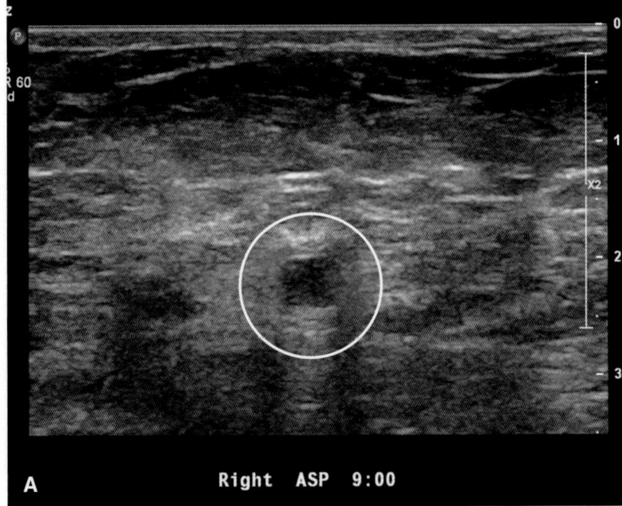

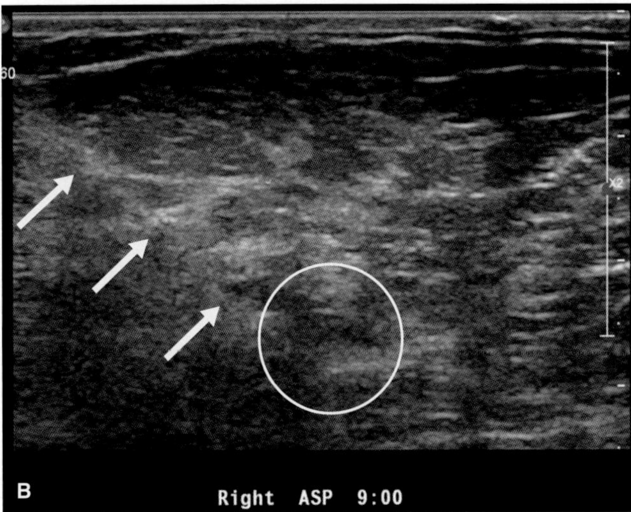

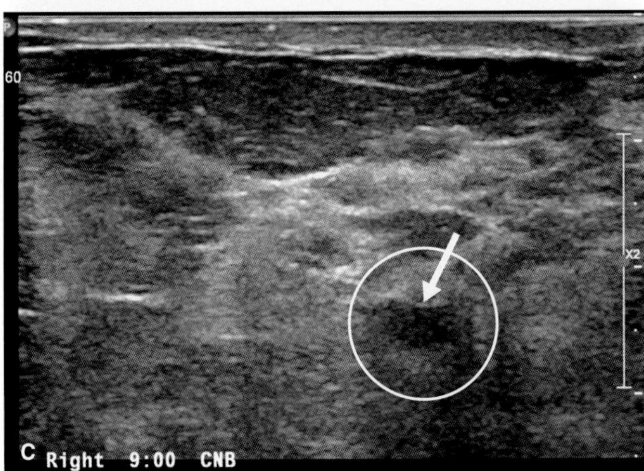

FIGURE 23.8. **Failed Aspiration of Indeterminate Mass. A:** Ultrasound shows a round, circumscribed, hypoechoic indeterminate mass (*circle*). **B:** During aspiration the 22-gauge spinal needle can be seen traversing the tissue (*arrows*) into the mass (*circle*) at an angle. **C:** The postaspiration ultrasound image demonstrates incomplete resolution of the finding (*circle*). The *arrow* shows the flatter contour postaspiration. The patient was then set up for a core needle biopsy, images not shown. Pathology result was benign and concordant.

Magnetic Resonance Imaging Biopsy. With the increased use of contrast-enhanced MR (ce-MR) imaging to screen high-risk women and stage women newly diagnosed with breast cancer there are more MR only BI-RADS 4 and BI-RADS 5 findings. With this came the need to develop methods to localize and sample these imaging findings. MR-guided localizations began in the mid 1990s and demonstrated that it was possible to obtain tissue with reasonable accuracy and positive predictive value. However, it was desired to be able to perform a CNB so surgery could be avoided in most patients. Some of the earliest reports of MR-guided biopsies were in the late 1990s. Now, CNB done with MR guidance is common place in facilities doing high-volume breast MR imaging.

Figure 23.10 shows a patient with linear nonmass enhancement and the imaging steps of the MR-guided biopsy. To perform an MR-guided biopsy physicians use dedicated grid systems that are designed to specifically fit on the breast coil. These grid systems communicate with one of several MR-guidance software programs that aid in the targeting of the enhancing breast lesion. In order to visualize the MR findings during the biopsy, contrast is given to ensure appropriate targeting. The procedure needs to be performed in a timely manner such that the contrast has not washed out of the target before sampling has occurred. In addition, women must remain still during all the imaging and the biopsy portion to ensure accurate targeting. The patient is imaged at intervals during the procedure and intermittently removed from the magnet so additional steps of the biopsy can be performed.

Like other procedures, local anesthetic is given at the skin entrance site and along the needle path. A skin nick is required to allow access of the biopsy needle and a large bore vacuum-assisted MR-compatible biopsy needle is used.

Some women have claustrophobia and will require anti-anxiolytics for this procedure, something that is relatively uncommon in non–MR image-guided breast procedures. There are unfortunately some MR findings that can be difficult or impossible to biopsy due to their far posterior or medial location or related to the patient's breast thickness. These are similar limitations as seen in stereotactic and DBT-guided biopsies. In women with excessively thin breasts one can consider direct image-guided localization or placement of a biopsy marker under MR guidance followed by localization using mammographic guidance (see below "Localization" section) as alternatives to sampling.

Biopsy Markers

Biopsy markers should be placed after image-guided biopsies for several reasons. They provide confirmation that the intended target has been sampled and they aid in future

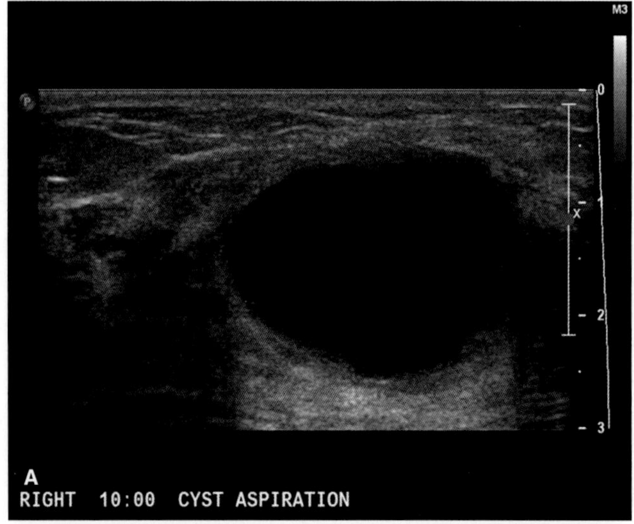

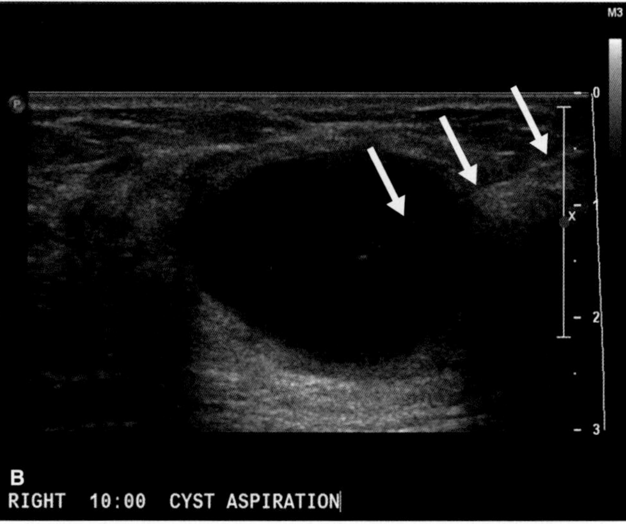

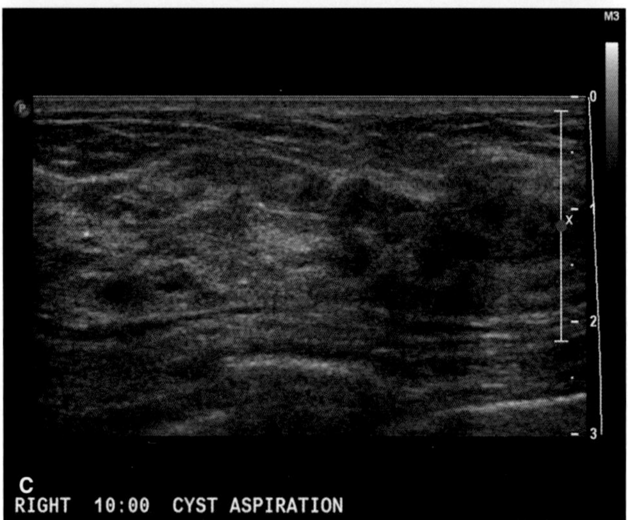

FIGURE 23.9. **Simple Cyst Aspiration. A:** Ultrasound shows a large painful simple cyst. **B:** During aspiration the 22-gauge spinal needle can be seen traversing the tissue (*arrows*) into the cyst at an angle. **C:** Complete resolution of the cyst is confirmed on the postaspiration image.

localization (limiting the amount of tissue that needs to be removed to accurately get the target). Markers come in a variety of shapes and can help differentiate biopsy sites when more than one biopsy has been done.

Confirmation of Targeting. Confirmation of targeting is necessary for all biopsies. The typical outcomes are shown in Figures 23.3, 23.5, and 23.10 where the markers are in their expected locations. Figure 23.11 is an example of the marker

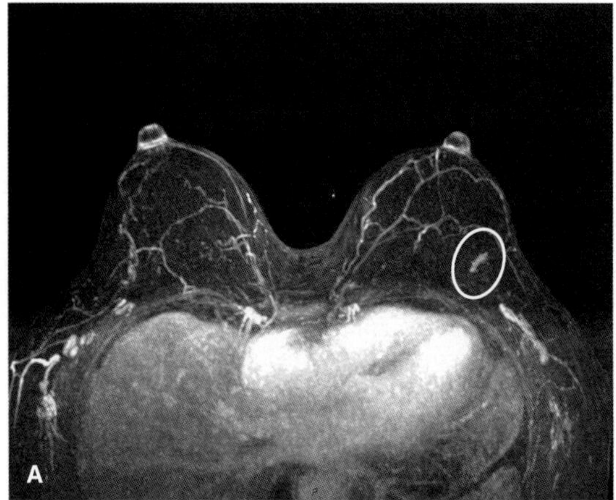

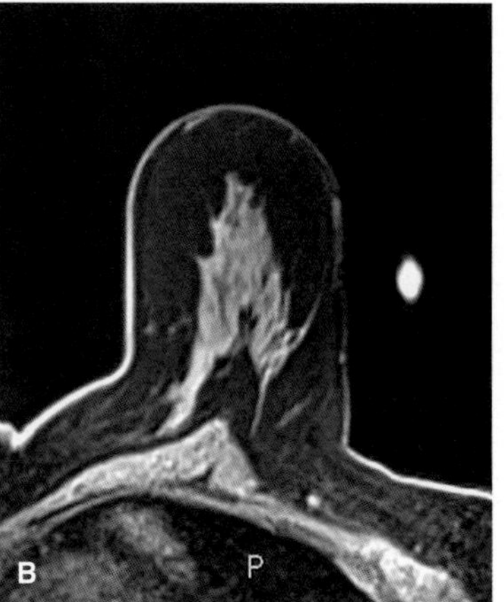

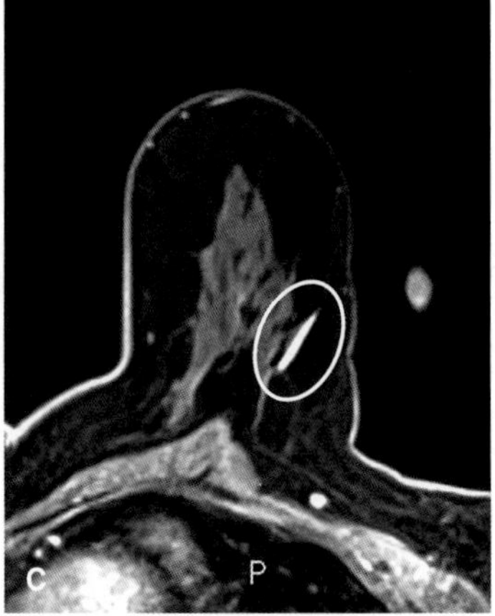

FIGURE 23.10. **MRI Biopsy. A:** Maximum intensity projection of ce-MRI showing linear NME in the posterior lateral left breast (*oval*). **B:** The patient is positioned prone in the scanner with her breast in the compression grid. Before contrast is given imaging is done to confirm adequate thickness, target is accessible within the grid, and MRI technical factors are optimized. **C:** Contrast is then given to identify the target for biopsy (*oval*).

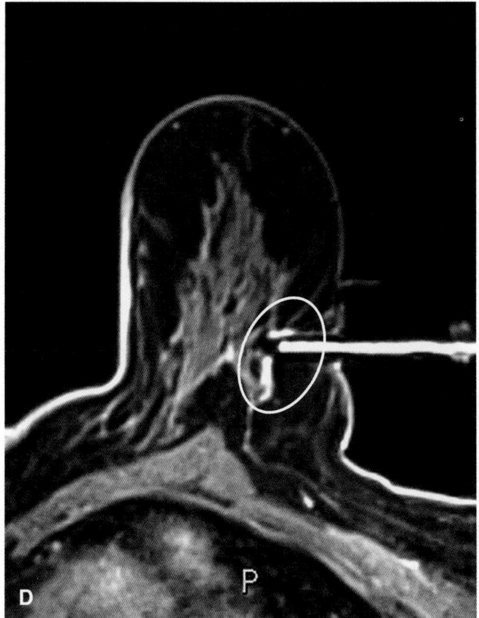

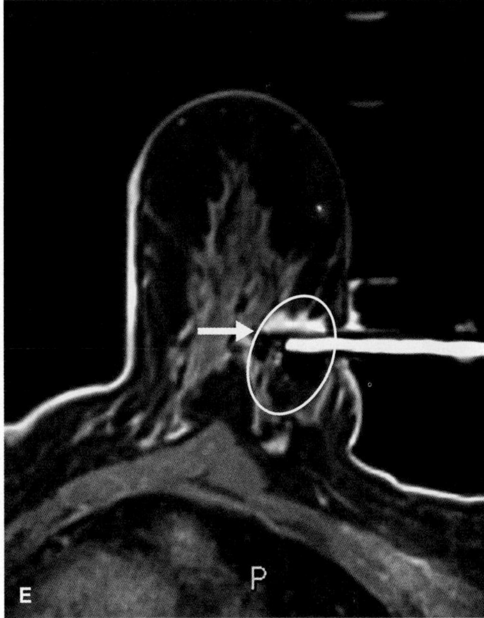

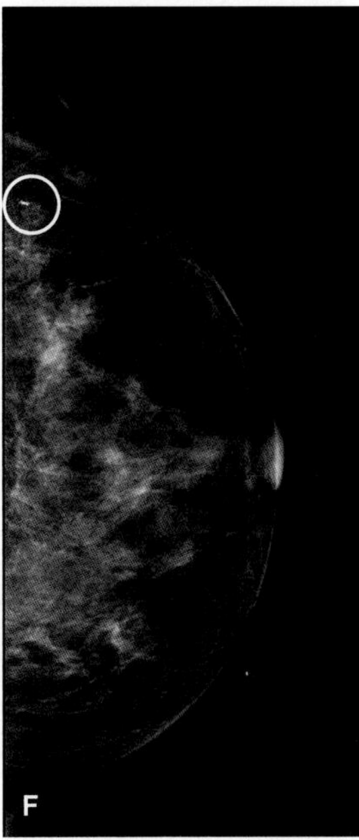

FIGURE 23.10. (*Continued*) **D:** After the skin is prepped and the tissue is anesthetized a gadolinium-filled introducer is placed into the breast with the tip in the target (*oval*). **E:** The gadolinium-filled introducer is replaced with the biopsy needle and sampling is done. After sampling the introducer is placed back into the breast and a final image is done to confirm biopsy site changes where expected. The oval shows the biopsy site changes in good location and the *arrow* shows the air–fluid level from normal postbiopsy bleeding (remember the patient is prone so air is "below" the fluid). **F:** As in all biopsies a marker is placed and a postbiopsy two-view mammogram is done. The CC projection is shown with the marker in the expected location, posterior lateral left breast near the tissue fat interface (*circle*). Pathology result is atypical ductal hyperplasia, concordant.

being off. In these settings, the patient should be notified of the discrepancy and plans for a repeat biopsy, typically with another modality or with a change in position, or for surgical excision if appropriate. In all cases, all tissue should be sent for pathology review.

Future Localization. Localizations done when a marker has been placed have been shown to be associated with higher negative margin rates in cancer patients. Occasionally, the entire mammographic finding is removed during sampling and the marker is the only imaging finding useful for localization. One may think that if the imaging finding is gone after biopsy that there is no residual pathology, however studies have confirmed that removal of the imaging finding does not correlate with an absence of residual tumor.

One should consider placing a marker in aspiration of a cyst when fluid is sent for cytologic evaluation. Fluid is sent when it is bloody or there is a concern for a solid component. The cyst may resolve completely with the procedure and results may dictate a need for surgery. If the cyst does not recur before surgery, the marker can then be used for localization. Biopsy markers are not routinely placed at the time of benign simple cyst aspirations.

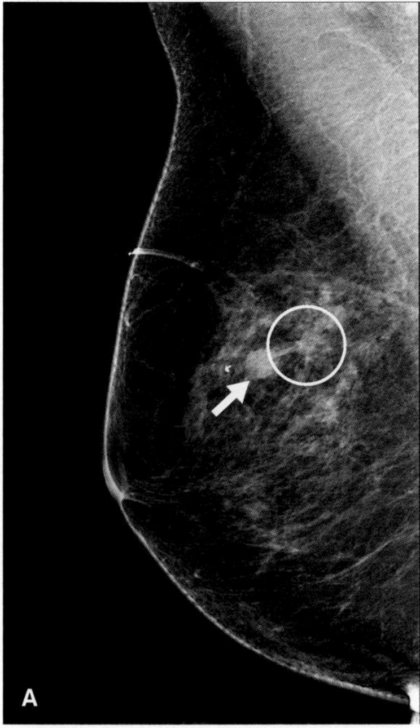
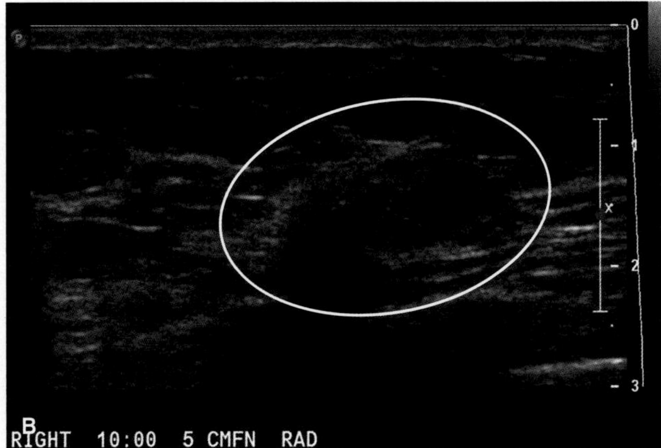

FIGURE 23.11. **Malpositioned Clip. A:** MLO mammogram showing an asymmetry with distortion (*circle*) posterior to a round mass (*dashed arrow*) and remote biopsy clip. **B:** Targeted ultrasound showed a mass (*oval*) felt to correlate with the mammographic finding. This mass underwent ultrasound-guided biopsy, images not shown, with marker placement. (*continued*)

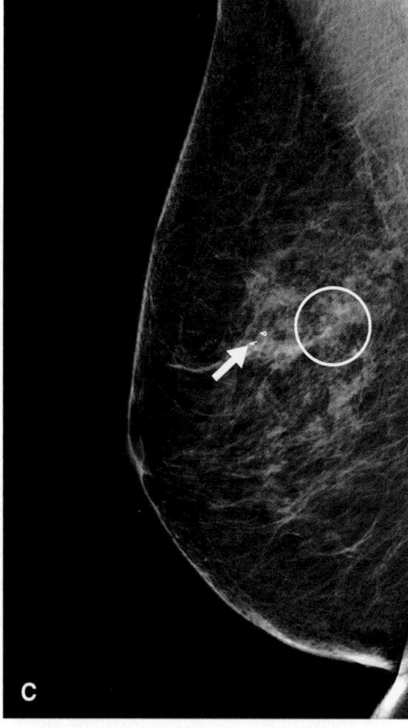

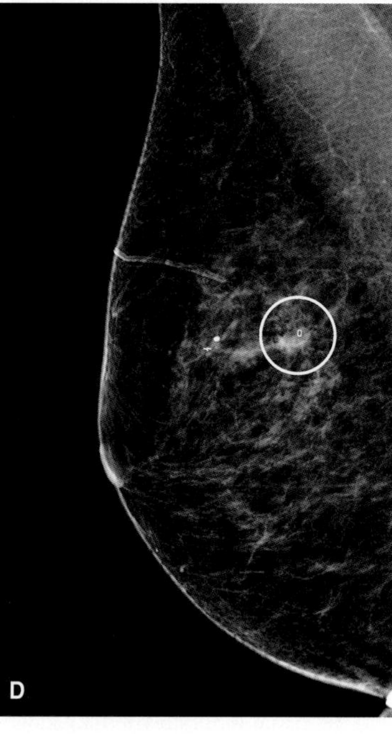

FIGURE 23.11. (*Continued*) **C:** Postbiopsy mammogram revealed the marker was malpositioned anterior to the target (*arrow*). *Circle* shows the expected location. The patient then underwent stereotactic-guided biopsy, images not shown, with marker placement. **D:** Postbiopsy mammogram now shows the marker in good location (*circle*). Pathology result of the stereotactic biopsy was invasive lobular carcinoma, concordant. The ultrasound biopsy result was benign.

Even large lesions require marker placement. If the finding is malignant the patient may undergo neoadjuvant chemotherapy and the mass may shrink such that it is not visible after treatment. The marker can allow for successful image-guidance localization and lumpectomy as in Figure 23.12. Again, surgery remains indicated in this scenario as absence of residual imaging finding does not exclude residual tumor. Without a biopsy marker the patient would potentially need mastectomy when the tumor is no longer visible.

Complications

Overall, image-guided breast biopsies are safe. Complications are uncommon and listed in Table 23.2. Most women have minimal bleeding during a core biopsy which is controlled with manual compression postprocedure. Clinically significant bleeding occurs in a small number of patients, less than 1% with use of 14-gauge needles. Bleeding risk has been found to be similar even with larger gauge or vacuum-assisted biopsy devices. Risk of bleeding can be increased in women using anticoagulation medications and these medications are ideally held for procedures. Although, if the medication cannot be stopped studies have found that the biopsy can still be safe to perform with only slight increase risk of bleeding. Infection is reported to occur in less than 1% of patients as well. Pneumothorax is a very rare complication of image-guided breast biopsy. This is minimized and should not occur with careful planning, direct image guidance, and safe approaches to sample the target (i.e., a parallel approach in US-guided CNB, see Figure 23.6).

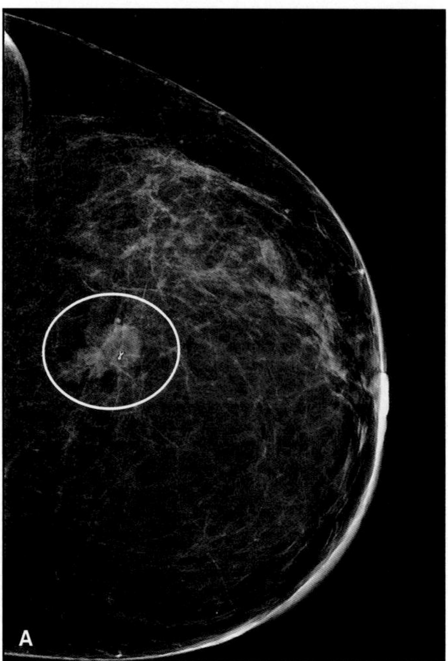

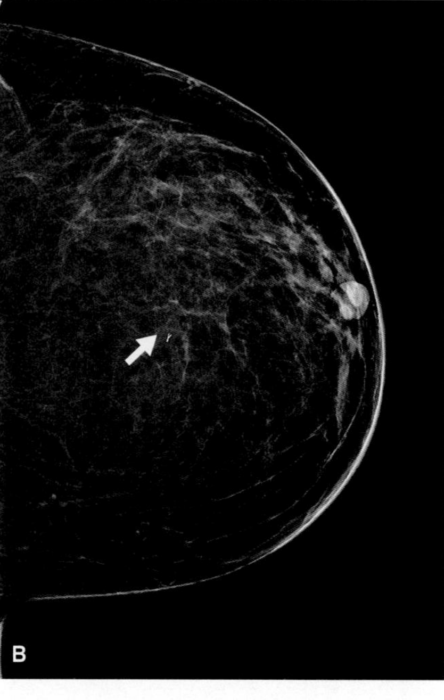

FIGURE 23.12. **Neoadjuvant Chemotherapy. A:** Postbiopsy mammogram shows the biopsy marker well positioned within a conspicuous large mass (*oval*). **B:** After neoadjuvant chemotherapy the mass is barely visible but the marker (*arrow*) can be used to localize for surgery, allowing for breast conservation treatment.

TABLE 23.2

COMPLICATIONS OF IMAGE-GUIDED BIOPSIES

Hemorrhage
Infection
Pneumothorax (rare)

Radiology–Pathology Concordance

The accuracy of image-guided CNB in diagnosing breast carcinoma approaches that of surgical biopsy with reported sensitivities of 85% to 100% and specificities of 96% to 100%. In order to achieve such high sensitivities and specificities, it is essential that the mammographic, US, and MR appearances of the lesion be correlated with the pathologic diagnosis. If there is discordance between results and imaging, repeat core biopsy or excisional biopsy should be performed, as in Figure 23.13. In cases where atypical ductal hyperplasia (ADH) is diagnosed by core biopsy, excisional biopsy should be performed due to

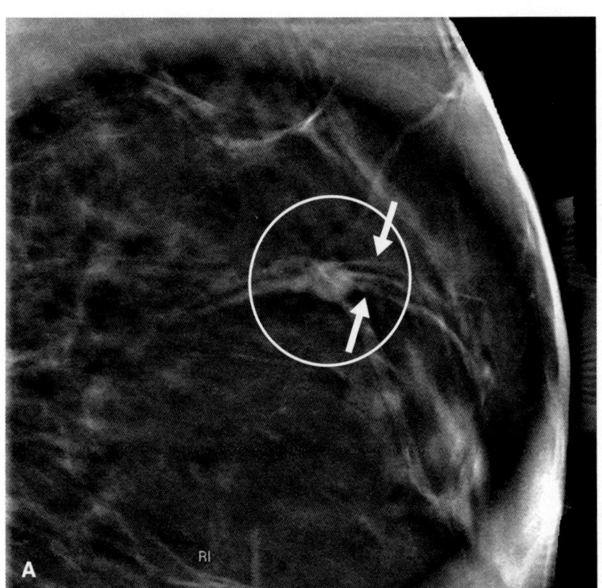

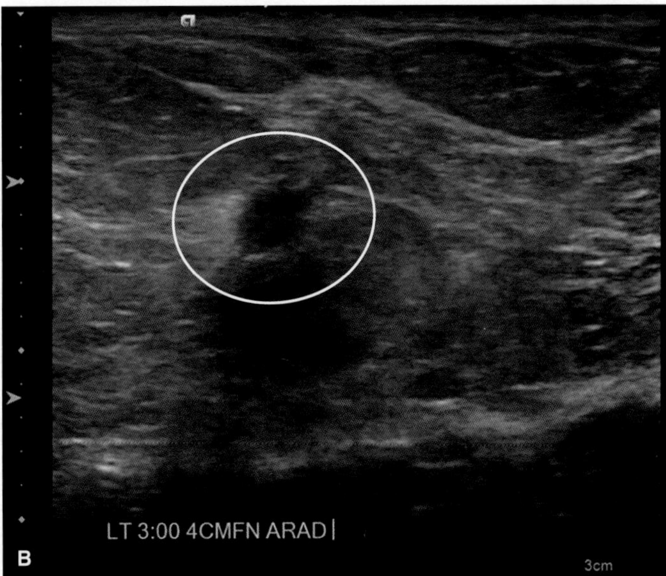

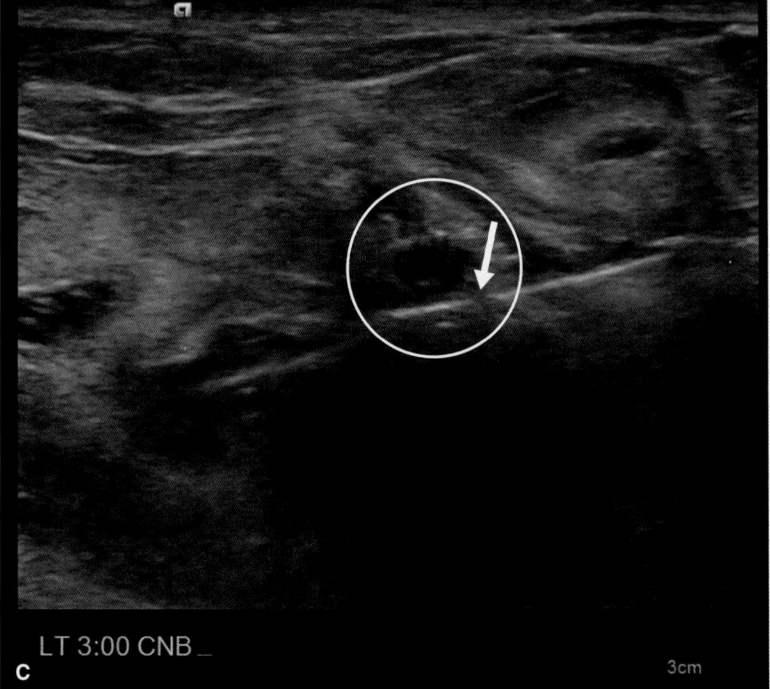

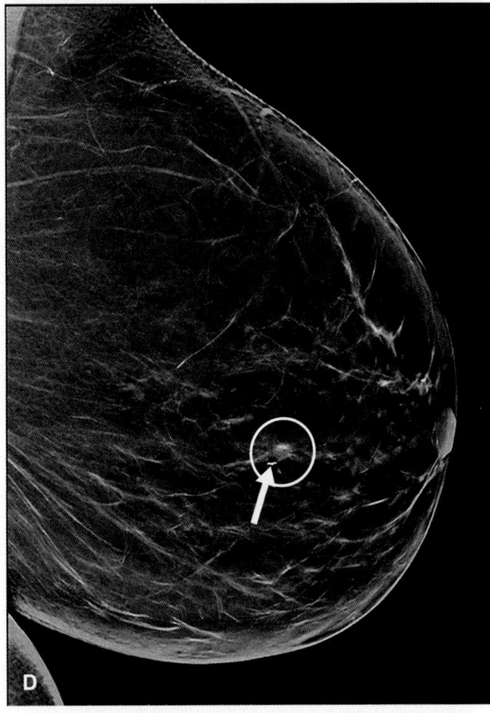

FIGURE 23.13. Benign Discordant Biopsy. A: BI-RADS 5: highly suspicious finding (*circle*) due to round shape with spiculated margins (between *arrows*). **B:** Ultrasound demonstrated the mass (*circle*). **C:** The patient underwent an US-guided CNB where in retrospect the needle path (*arrow*) is under the mass (*circle*). **D:** Postbiopsy ML shows the marker (*arrow*) next to the mass (*circle*). Pathology result was benign fibrofatty tissue, discordant. (*continued*)

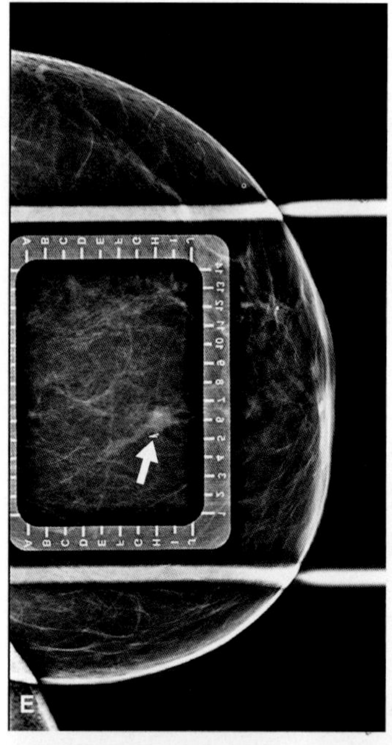

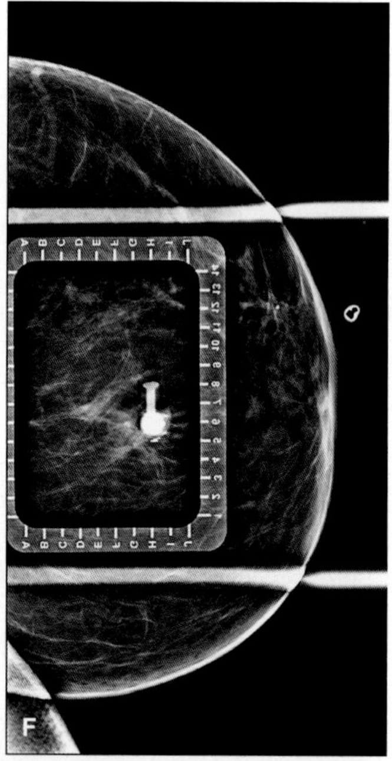

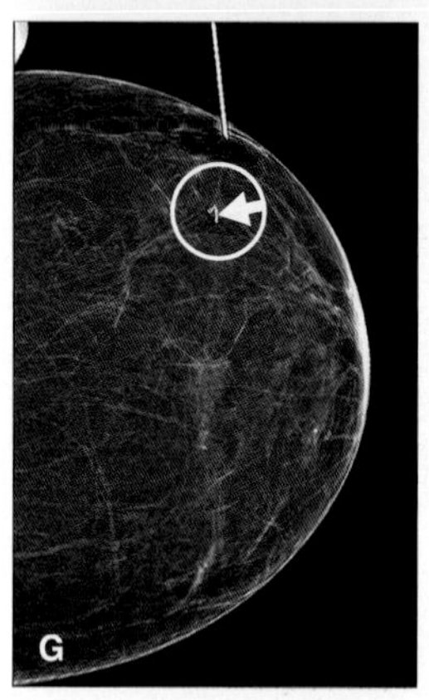

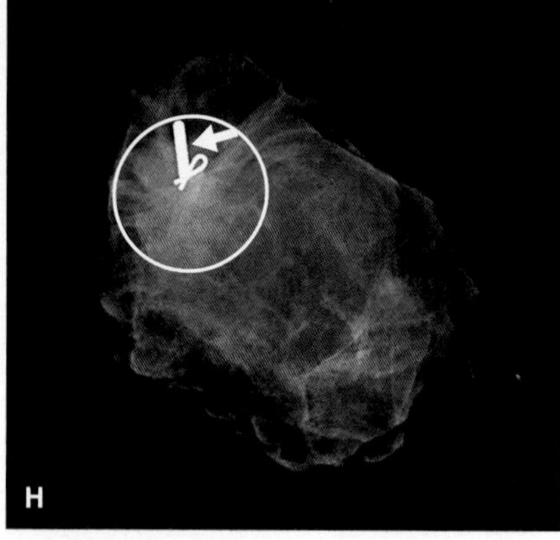

FIGURE 23.13. (*Continued*) **E:** The patient was set up for localization and excision. The planning localization LM image shows the biopsy marker (*arrow*) in the fat adjacent to the mass. The mass lies at H-6. **F:** The introducer for the radioseed goes through the mass at H-6. **G:** CC view obtained at 90 degrees from the prior view allows placement of the radioseed (*arrow*) into the mass (*circle*). **H:** Excisional specimen radiograph shows the mass (*circle*), clip (*ribbon shape*), and radioseed (*arrow*) were successfully removed. Pathology result was invasive ductal carcinoma, concordant.

a reported upgrade rate of 15% to 30% of ADH on CNB to carcinoma at excision. Postcore biopsy management of papillary lesions, mucin-containing lesions, lobular neoplasia (including lobular carcinoma in situ and atypical lobular hyperplasia), and radial scars remains controversial.

Follow-Up After Benign Biopsy

There is no consensus on follow-up after benign image-guided biopsy. The success of image-guided biopsies hinges on the ability to trust a negative result. The FN rate of image-guided CNB is about 1.5%. Many of the FN biopsies are recognized at the time of the procedure or when the histology results show discordance with the imaging finding during radiology–pathology review. However, to ensure the remaining potential FN cases are discovered imaging follow-up is necessary. Some institutions will do a 6-month follow-up after a benign biopsy, others 1 year. Studies have shown that there is no difference in the ability to detect the FN biopsies at either 6 or 12 months. A safe approach is to do a 6-month follow-up for nonspecific benign results and a 12-month follow-up when specific benign results are obtained.

TABLE 23.3

INDICATIONS FOR SURGICAL EXCISION

Needle biopsy results	Malignant Benign discordant Atypia
Unsuccessful image-guided biopsy	Tissue too thin to perform needle biopsy Location inaccessible Patient factors
Patient preference	

LOCALIZATION

Indications

Localizations have been done successfully since the 1970s. There are several indications for recommending and performing image-guided localization as listed in Table 23.3.

The classic example of a discordant result necessitating surgical excision is when benign results are obtained in the setting of a BI-RADS 5 lesion, like demonstrated in Figure 23.13. There are some benign histology results that are excised due to their risk of being upgraded to malignancy at excision. ADH is the most common of these and is associated with the

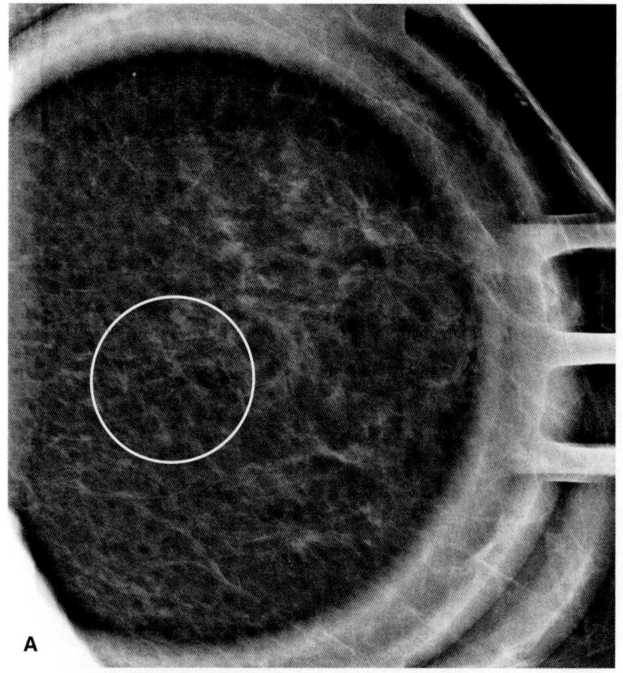

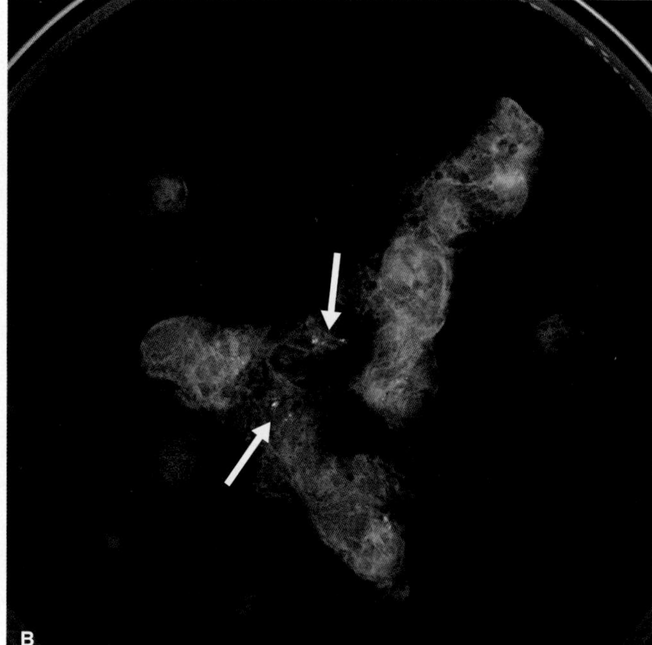

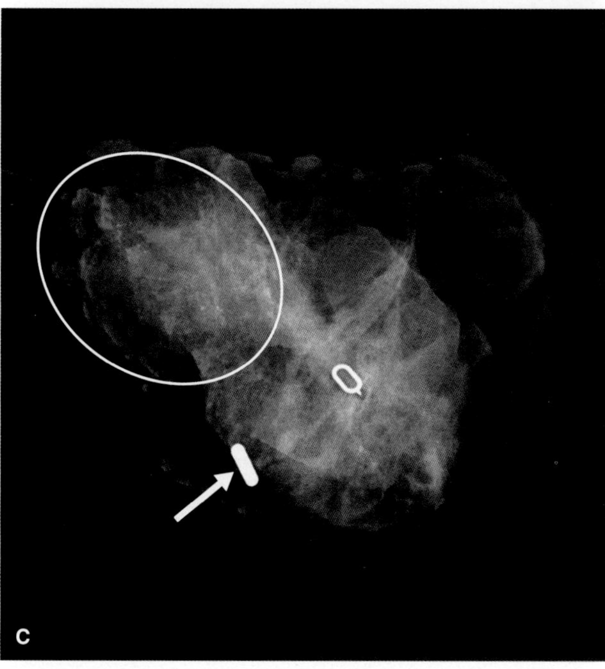

FIGURE 23.14. **Atypical Ductal Hyperplasia. A:** Magnification view shows BI-RADS 4: suspicious grouped fine pleomorphic calcifications (*circle*) recommended for stereotactic biopsy. **B:** Biopsy was done with numerous calcifications obtained (*arrows* on representative calcifications). Pathology result was atypical ductal hyperplasia, concordant. **C:** Surgical excision was recommended and radioseed localization was performed. The surgical specimen shows additional calcifications (*oval*) and both the radioseed (*arrow*) and biopsy marker (*circle* shape) were retrieved. Pathology result was ductal carcinoma in situ, concordant.

highest upgrade rates of all the high-risk lesions. ADH has an unacceptably high upgrade rate to either DCIS or invasive carcinoma regardless of imaging finding, needle gauge, or number of samples. Figure 23.14 shows an example of calcifications upgraded to DCIS at excision.

Localization Devices

Needle-Wire Systems. Localizations are generally performed using needle-wire systems, which allow placement of a wire through an introducing needle that has been positioned in the breast at the site of the abnormality. The commercially available wires differ mainly in the configuration of the anchoring end. Figure 23.15 shows several needle-wire types. Needle-wire system requires the localization be done on the same day as the surgery. They are inexpensive, done with any modality of image guidance (included MR), and are the most common method for localization worldwide. Positive margin rates with needle-wire localization have been reported to be as high as 45% to 57% with reexcision rates of 20% to 70%. The limitation regarding scheduling and the undesirably high-positive margins and reexcision rates have encouraged the development of other tools.

Non-Wire Localizations. Newer methods include radioseed localization (RSL), radar localization, radiofrequency identification (RFID), and magnetic tracers. Each of these newer methods have pros and cons. A significant positive for patients is the ability to place the tracer in advance of the surgery.

Radioseed Localization. RSL is a done using a seed filled with low-activity iodine 125 (I-125) and was first described in

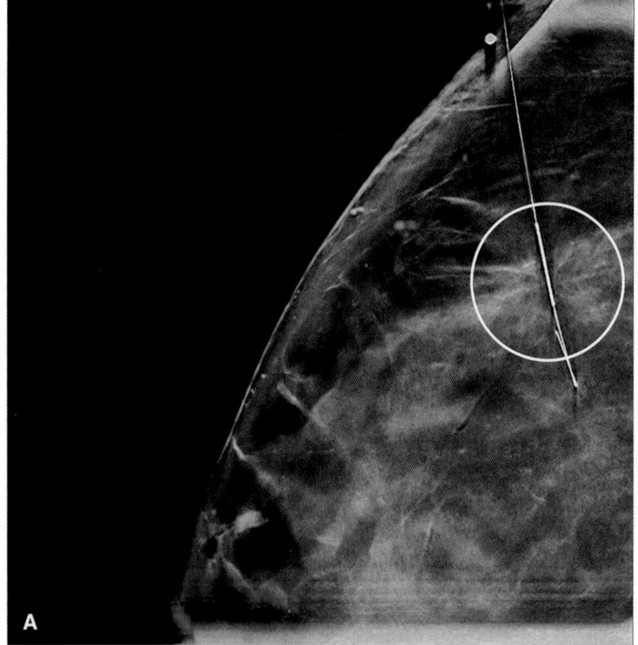

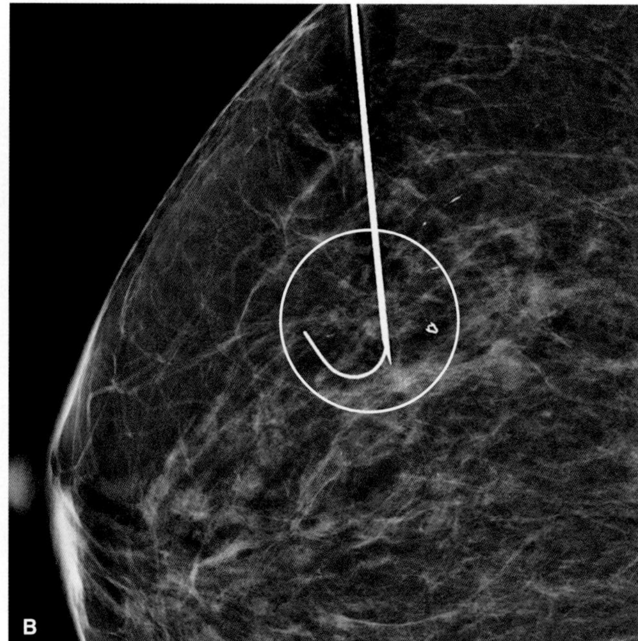

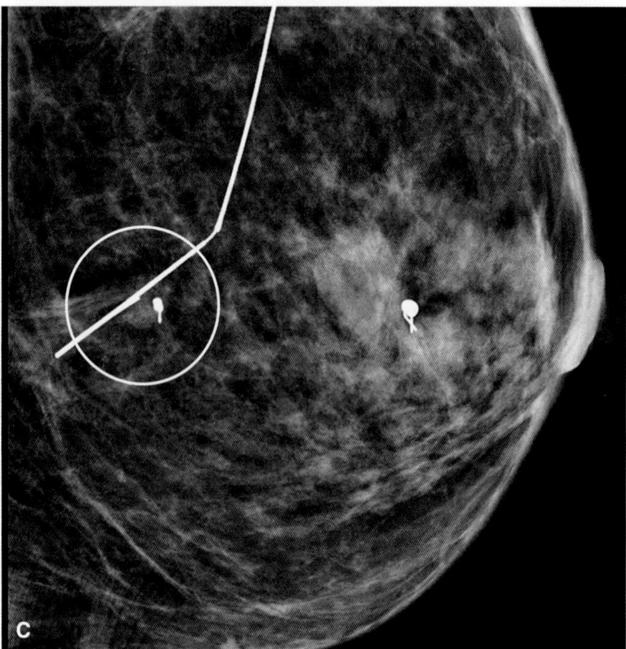

FIGURE 23.15. **Needle-Wire Types. Mammographic Appearance of Three Needle-Wire Combinations. A:** Kopans spring-hookwire. The stiffener (thickened part of wire) is placed through the target (*circle*). **B:** Homer J-wire. The hook is formed just past the target (*circle*). **C:** The hookwire. The thickened portion of the wire (last 25 mm of the wire) is positioned through the target (*circle*). In all cases the goal is to go through the target with the tip beyond the lesion.

2001. Localizations done with I-125 seeds have been found to have lower positive margin and reexcision rates compared to needle-wire localizations. The I-125 radioseeds can be placed using mammographic (including mammographic, stereotactic, or DBT) and US guidance. The half-life of I-125 is 60 days which allows for placement up to 5 days before surgery creating flexibility in scheduling. Using radioseeds are safe as long as safety precautions are followed. Figures 23.13 and 23.14 show RSLs. However, instituting RSL can take months due to state and federal mandates related to radioactivity which limits its widespread use.

Radar Localization. The SAVI SCOUT (Cianna Medical, Aliso Viejo, California) reflector uses infrared (IR) light for localization and was first approved for use by the FDA in 2014. The SAVI SCOUT measures 12 mm, has two antennas, and is stimulated to emit electromagnetic waves by IR light given off by the handpiece used by the surgeon. Figure 23.16 shows an example of a SAVI SCOUT localization. It can be placed up to 30 days ahead of surgery allowing for even more flexibility of scheduling. The surgeon is directed by both an auditory and numeric signal on the handpiece. Early studies show a reexcision rate comparable to both RSL and needle-wire localization.

Radiofrequency Identification. RFID is the size of a grain of rice and is a tiny microchip that stores a unique identification number and has an antenna that responds to interrogation by the reader. RFID has FDA approval for placement into humans and are undergoing early evaluation for their use in localization of breast lesions. They function via an RFID reader which sends a signal to the implanted tag's antenna which then sends a response signal back to the reader allowing localization with a display on an LCD screen and an audio signal. An RFID is safe to

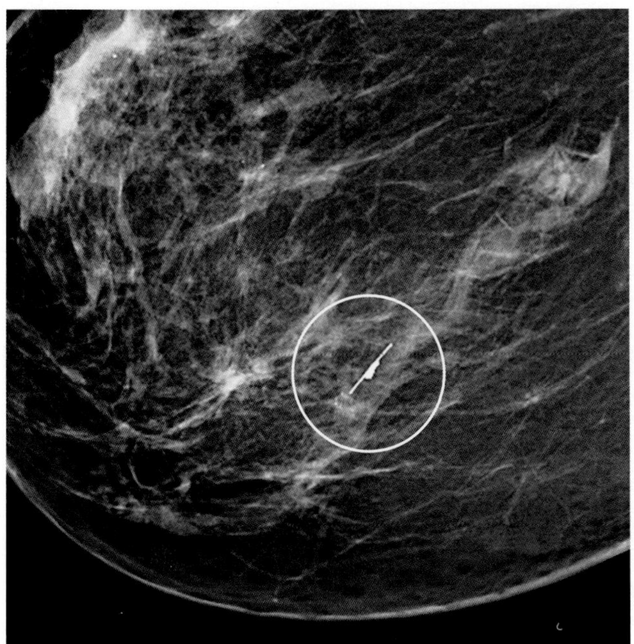

FIGURE 23.16. **SAVI SCOUT.** Mammographic image of a SAVI SCOUT (*circle*) surgical guidance which uses electromagnetic waves.

image with MR, however has an artifact that would make it not ideal to place before obtaining a diagnostic MR. RFID remains too new a technology to have much data about its success.

Magnetic Tracers. The Magseed system (Endomagnetics, Austin, Texas) was approved by the FDA in 2016. Like the SAVI SCOUT it can be placed up to 30 days before surgery. It measures only 1 mm × 5 mm, is magnetic, and detected by the Sentimag probe held by the surgeon. Special OR equipment is needed as ferromagnetic instruments interfere with the magnet. Given this is the newest method there is not yet enough data about its utility in breast localization.

Guidance

Mammographic Localization. Mammographic guidance is the most common image-guidance utilized for localization. Most mammographic units are equipped with a compression paddle that contains one large hole marked on the edge with a grid that is used to help localize the finding. The patient is usually seated during imaging and the lesion or biopsy marker to be localized is located centered within the opening in the compression plate. The skin surface closest to the lesion should be used for needle placement. For example, if the lesion is located at 12 o'clock position, a craniocaudal approach should be used. A single mammographic image is taken showing the paddle and its reference grid as well as the imaging finding. Shadows of crosshairs are projected on the skin to allow for correct access such that the needle inserted parallel to the x-ray beam will traverse the target. Local anesthetic is given in the skin and along the needle path before the needle is placed. Once the needle (with wire) is positioned through the target the position is confirmed by a second image. If the needle position is satisfactory, the patient, with needle in place, is carefully removed from the mammography unit so that the tube can be rotated 90 degrees. The patient is then repositioned in the unit and compressed along an axis parallel to the needle. A film is taken to assess the depth of the needle tip with respect to the lesion. The needle must be beyond

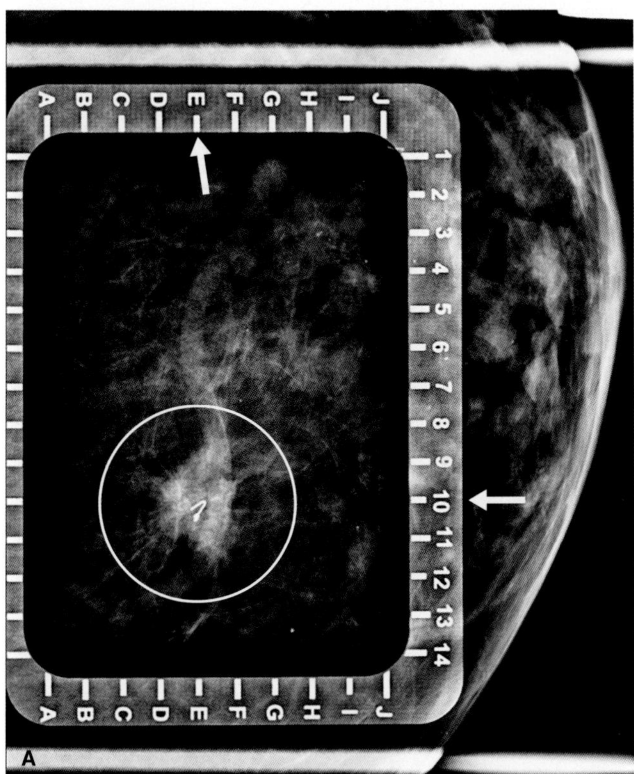

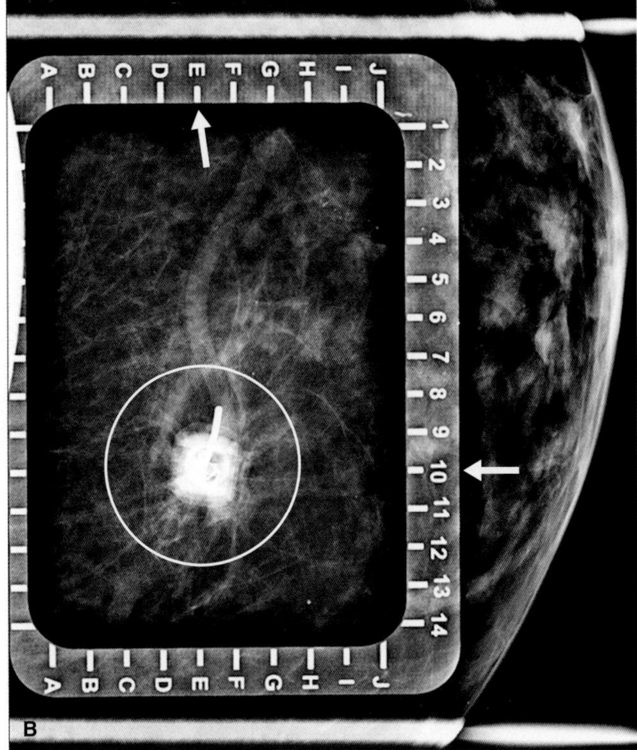

FIGURE 23.17. **Mammographic-Guided Needle-Wire Localization. A:** Scout image with the patient in compression using the localization paddle. The mass with biopsy marker (*circle*) are positioned at E-10 (*arrows*). **B:** The needle is advanced into the breast through the mass (*circle*) at E-10 (*arrows*). Crosshairs are projected on the skin to aid in entering at the correct location (not shown). (*continued*)

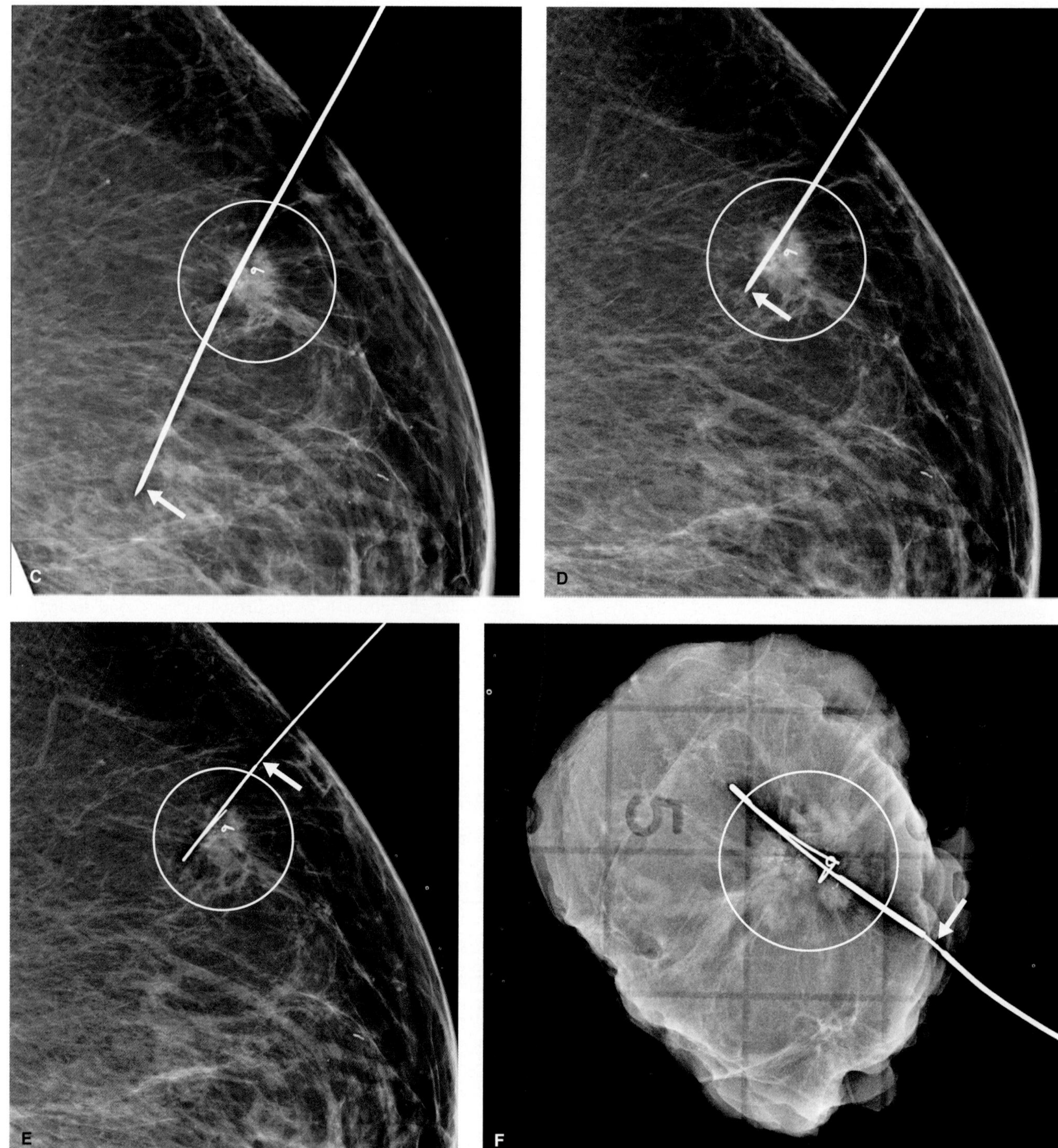

FIGURE 23.17. (*Continued*) **C:** Once the needle is placed, compression is released and an image at 90 degrees from the initial view is taken where the needle should be seen traversing the mass (*circle*) with the tip (*arrow*) beyond the target. **D:** The needle is pulled back such that the tip (*arrow*) lies past the mass (*circle*). The wire is pinned at this location and the needle removed. **E:** The final image shows the hookwire through the mass (*circle*) with the tip beyond the target and the transition (thin portion at the *arrow*) at the leading edge of the target. **F:** Surgical specimen radiograph confirms removal of the wire and the mass (*circle*). In addition to the mass the biopsy marker and associated calcifications can be seen. The transition (*arrow*) remains at the leading edge of the mass. Pathology result was invasive ductal carcinoma with ductal carcinoma in situ, concordant.

the lesion in order to proceed. This assures a fixed relationship between the needle and the lesion. Optimally, the tip of the needle for a wire localization should be 1 to 2 cm beyond the lesion with the wire through the target. Once the depth of the needle tip is satisfactory, the wire (which is in the needle) can be left behind as the needle is withdrawn. Figure 23.17 shows the imaging steps for a mammographic-guided needle-wire localization. The patient is then sent to the operating room for surgical excision.

Bracketed localization is advocated for nonpalpable lesions over 2 cm in size or in cases where the surgeon requests additional guidance. More than one localization wire is placed to demarcate the extent of the lesion. This technique is particularly helpful for areas of microcalcifications over 2 cm in

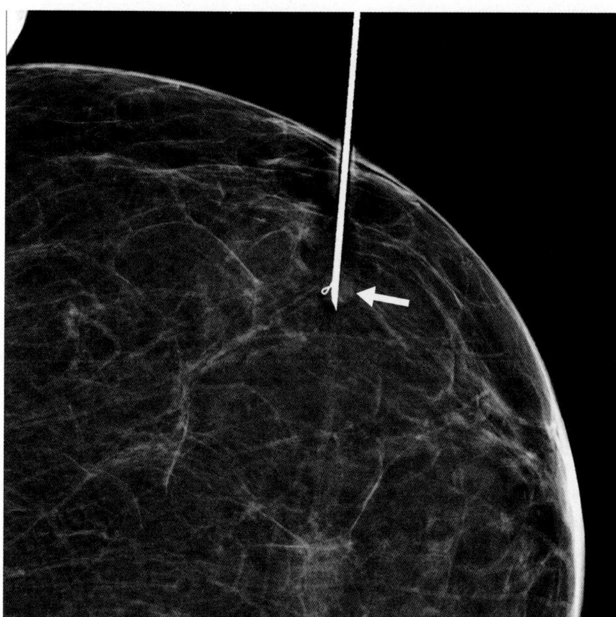

FIGURE 23.18. **Radioseed Placement.** Last image taken before deployment of radioseed from Figure 23.13 with the tip in the mass (*arrow*). The radioseed was well positioned in the mass in Figure 23.13G.

diameter; it promotes complete removal of such lesions. All localizations should be planned with the input of the surgeon performing the excision.

Mammographic localization with any of the other methods (Radioseed, SAVI SCOUT, RFID, or Magseed) is similar to the above described steps. However, instead of placing the tip of the needle 1 to 2 cm beyond the lesion, the tip of the needle is positioned such that the device will be within or immediately adjacent to the target when deployed. Figure 23.18 shows the needle tip in the mass before deployment of the radioseed placed in Figure 23.13.

Ultrasound Localization. For findings that are visible with US, it is the preferred localization method as it is fast, safe, comfortable for patients, and may be more accurate. The steps for localization are similar as those for biopsy and aspiration. Upon visualization of the target the shortest distance from the skin which allows the needle to approach the target at a slight obliquely is selected. Local anesthetic is placed in the skin and along the needle path to the target. For needle-wire localizations the needle is advanced through the target until the tip is seen beyond the lesion at about 1 cm. The needle is then removed while the wire is left behind, pinned such that the tip remains beyond the finding. Figure 23.19 shows the wire related to the mass in an US-guided placement. If one of the other devices are being used the goal is to deploy the localization marker within or immediately adjacent to the target. This typically means the tip of the needle should be at the desired final location of the localization device. Upon localization with US guidance the patient should have a two-view mammogram to confirm location of the wire or other devices. There are some newer biopsy markers that are designed to be visible on US which has increased the number of lesions that can be localized with US.

Magnetic Resonance Localization. There are some findings that will need MR-guided localization. This includes findings that were sampled with MR guidance but have a malpositioned biopsy marker that cannot be used to guide a mammographic localization. It also includes lesions that were not amenable to MR-guided biopsy. The same grid system that is used for MR-guided core biopsy is used for localization. Contrast is given as breast MR findings are either only or best seen with contrast enhancement. Software is used to guide the position of the MR-compatible needle wire to the correct location. The needle wire is placed along the plane of compression into the target. Unlike mammographic guidance, there is no repositioning of the patient. This can result in less exact positioning of the wire. A two-view mammogram is done with the wire in place following removal of the needle to give the surgeon reference of the wire position in the breast.

In MR localizations it is especially important to do careful radiology–pathology review of the final surgical pathology to ensure the desired target was removed. X-ray specimen radiography, described below, may not identify the lesion in these patients. Discordant cases should undergo postoperative MR to ensure the finding has been removed.

Specimen Radiograph

Once the surgical excision has been performed, the excised tissue should be sent for x-ray. Figures 23.13 to 23.15 and 23.17

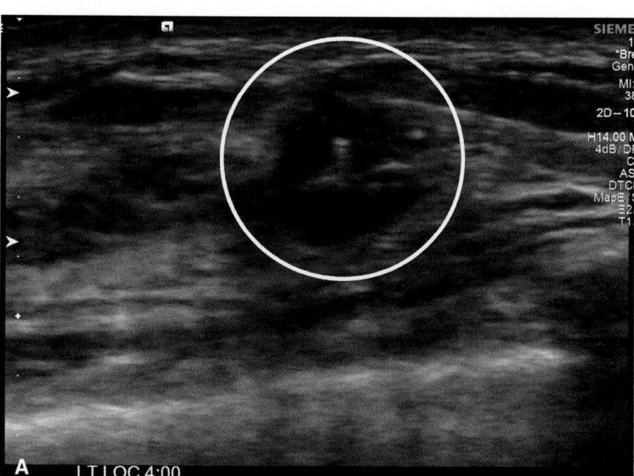

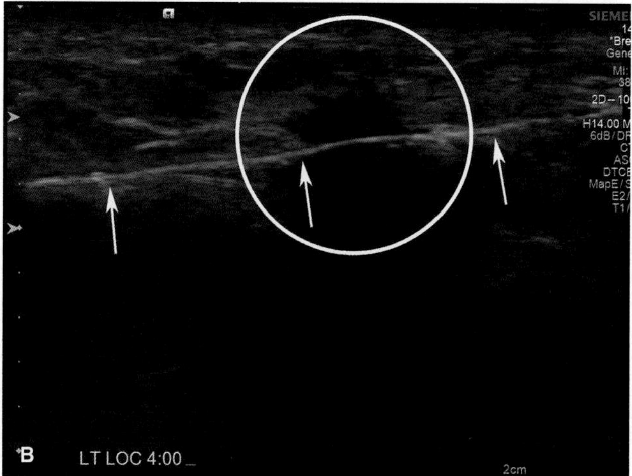

FIGURE 23.19. **Ultrasound-Guided Needle-Wire Localization. A:** Ultrasound image of the target mass (*circle*). **B:** Ultrasound image of the hookwire (*arrows*, post removal of the needle) through the mass (*circle*). The postprocedure mammogram is shown in Figure 23.15C.

contain surgical specimen radiographs. Specimens assure that the mammographic abnormality and/or the biopsy marker has been removed. It is also important to communicate where the finding lies compared to the tissue edge. Additional tissue can be removed as directed by the location of the finding in the specimen radiograph potentially improving rate of negative margins. The x-ray also confirms removal of the entire wire and the other localization tools (Radioseed, SAVI SCOUT, RFID, and Magseed). Imaging and handheld detector information is used in combination to document removal of the newer devices. In a small number of cases (1% to 6.7%), localization will fail and the lesion or clip will not be removed. Issues leading to a higher fail rate include placing the wire >5 mm from the intended target, having more than one lesion, a small breast, calcifications as the target, a small specimen, and small lesions. In most of these cases, the localization will have to be repeated.

GALACTOGRAPHY

Suspicious nipple discharge is an uncommon complaint, occurring in about 5% to 10% of women. In 10% to 15% of these women it is due to breast cancer, the rest of the causes are benign with the most common etiology representing a papilloma. Table 23.4 lists the differential diagnosis for suspicious nipple discharge. Galactography is indicated for women with spontaneous, unilateral, single duct clear, or bloody nipple discharge. Often their conventional imagings (mammography and US) are normal. Performing a galactogram allows for visualization of the cause in most women which in turn can direct surgery. Directed surgery has an increased likelihood of finding pathology compared to a blind retroareolar excision. The procedure involves injecting less than 1 cc of iodinated contrast material into the offending duct using a 30-gauge

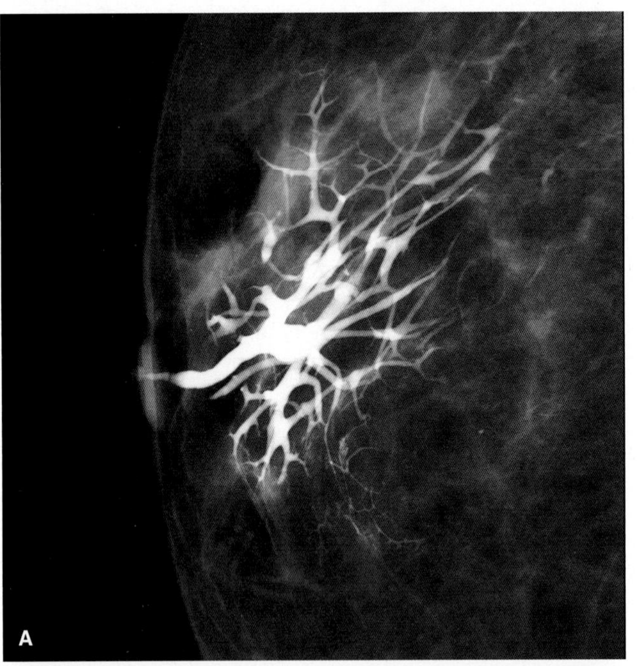

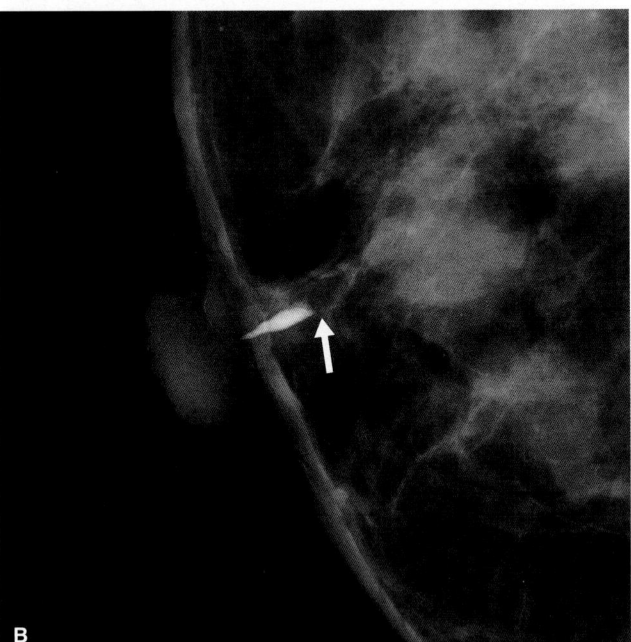

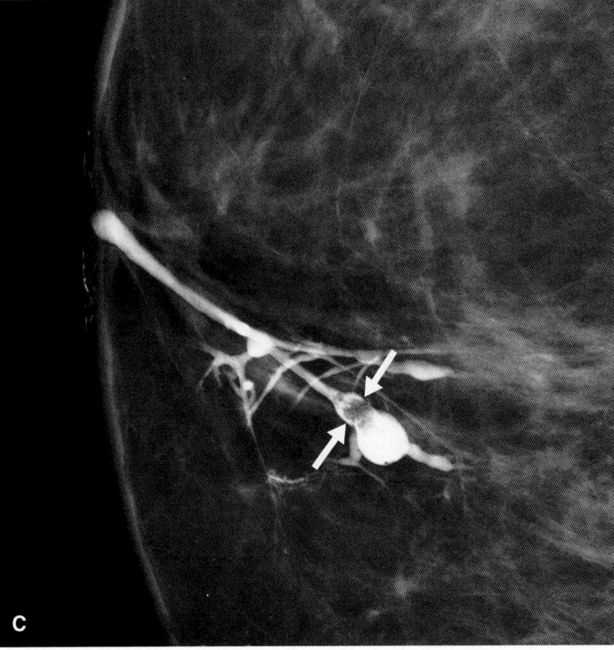

FIGURE 23.20. Galactogram. A: Normal ductal system. **B:** Abrupt termination of duct (*arrow*) consistent with an intraductal mass. Excision pathology result was papilloma. **C:** Filling defect in a side branch (*between arrows*). Excision pathology result was papilloma.

TABLE 23.4

DIFFERENTIAL DIAGNOSIS FOR SUSPICIOUS NIPPLE DISCHARGE

Ductal carcinoma in situ
Papilloma
Duct ectasia
Mastitis
Fibrocystic changes

blunt tip catheter. Topical analgesic can be placed onto the nipple areolar complex but is not necessary to do the procedure. After the duct is filled with contrast multiple images are taken to look for intraductal masses as evidenced by filling defects within the opacified duct. Figure 23.20 shows three galactogram findings, including normal. In some patients a biopsy marker is placed using mammographic-guidance at the location of the filling defect as was done in Figure 23.21 for one of the patients in Figure 23.20. The steps for placing the marker are similar to performing mammographic needle-wire localization. The marker allows for easier targeting on a separate day without the need to repeat the galactogram.

Galactography can be unsuccessful for several reasons; these include a failure to elicit discharge, failure to cannulate the duct, extravasation of contrast material through the duct wall, or imaging of the incorrect ductal system. Contraindications to galactography include an allergy to iodinated contrast material; premedication can be given if needed. MR is receiving increased use for preoperative evaluation of suspicious nipple discharge as an alternative to ductography and has now been shown in many studies to be equal to or more sensitive. Figure 23.22 shows a patient who underwent galactography for suspicious nipple discharge that later benefited from preoperative breast MRI.

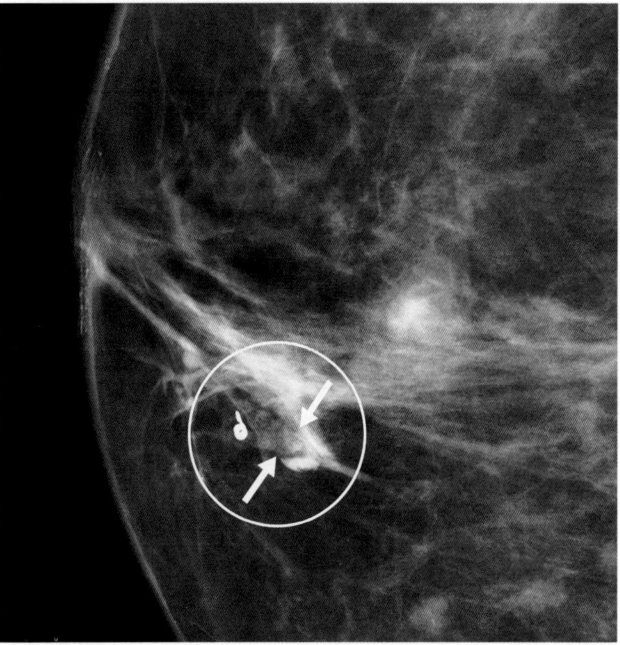

FIGURE 23.21. Galactogram With Clip. Single mammogram image after clip placement (*circle*) at the site of filling defect (*between arrows*) seen on Figure 23.20C.

CONCLUSION

Image-guided biopsies are safe, reliable, and the preferred method for obtaining tissue diagnosis for imaging findings. With most findings being secondary to benign histology, a CNB can avoid surgery in the majority of women. The FN

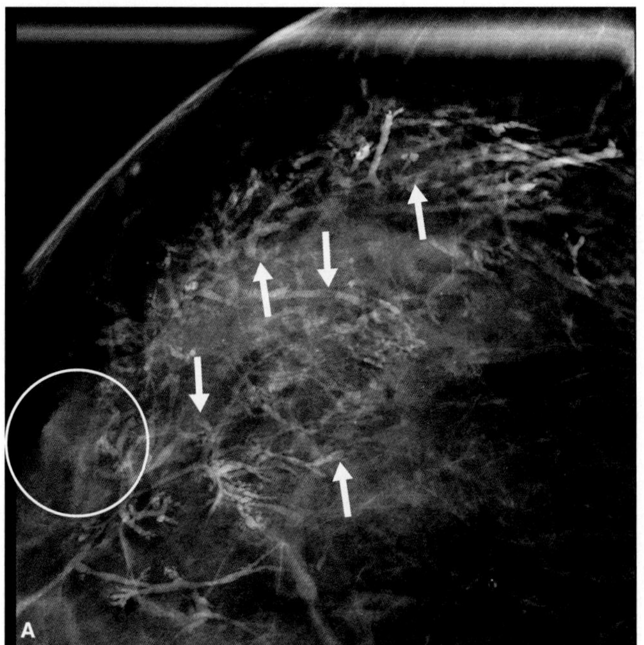

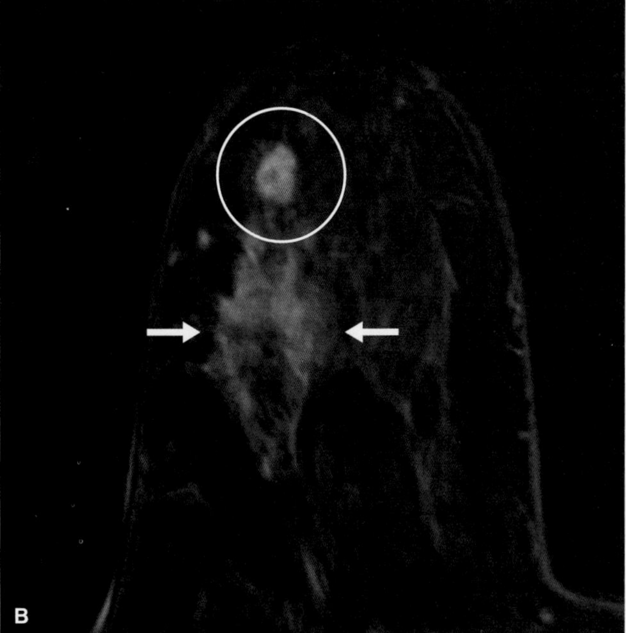

FIGURE 23.22. Galactogram with US and MRI. Patient presented with suspicious nipple discharge and underwent a galactogram (**A**) demonstrating numerous filling defects and irregularity of the ductal system (*arrows*). Mass effect can be seen from what is later found to be a mass (*circle*). **B:** MRI was done due to the worrisome appearance on galactogram. MRI shows a discrete round, irregular, homogeneously enhancing mass (*circle*) with associated segmental nonmass enhancement (*between arrows*) that correlates with the abnormal ducts on galactogram. (*continued*)

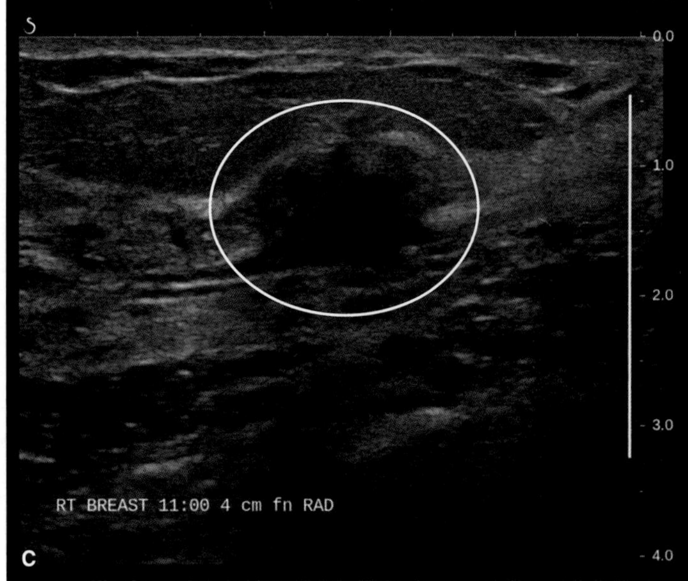

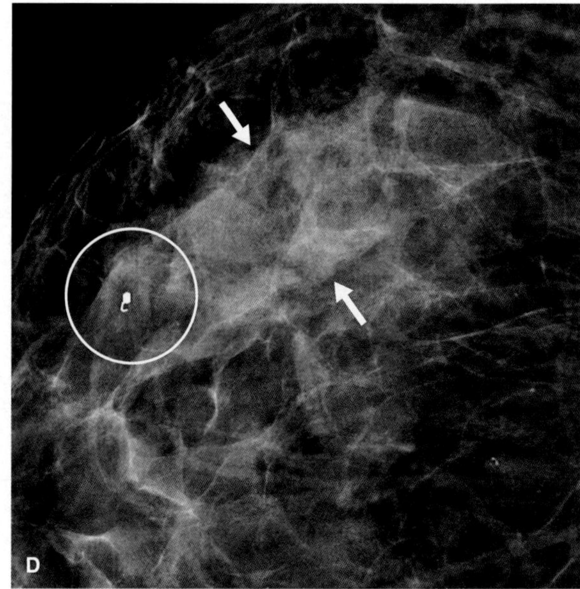

FIGURE 23.22. (*Continued*) **C:** Targeted US shows the BI-RADS 5: highly suspicious mass (*circle*) and US-guided CNB was performed, not shown. **D:** Postbiopsy mammogram shows the mass location (*circle* with biopsy marker) and its relationship to the prior galactogram abnormality and NME on MRI (*between arrows*). Pathology result of the mass was invasive ductal carcinoma. The patient later underwent mastectomy for widespread associated ductal carcinoma in situ.

rate of biopsies is low enough to be an acceptable method to exclude malignancy when careful radiology–pathology concordance is done as well as imaging follow-up when benign. When surgery is needed image-guided localization can be done to facilitate removal of the appropriate imaging finding.

Suggested Readings

Bassett L, Winchester DP, Caplan RB, et al. Stereotactic core-needle biopsy of the breast: a report of the Joint Task Force of the American College of Radiology, American College of Surgeons, and College of American Pathologists. *CA Cancer J Clin* 1997;47(3):171–190.

Berger N, Luparia A, Di Leo G, et al. Diagnostic performance of MRI versus galactography in women with pathologic nipple discharge: a systematic review and meta-analysis. *AJR Am J Roentgenol* 2017;209(2):465–471.

Bourke AG, Taylor DB, Westcott E, Hobbs M, Saunders C. Iodine-125 seeds to guide removal of impalpable breast lesions: radio-guided occult lesion localization—a pilot study. *ANZ J Surg* 2016;87(11):E178–E182.

Brancato B, Crocetti E, Bianchi S, et al. Accuracy of needle biopsy of breast lesions visible on ultrasound: audit of fine needle versus core needle biopsy in 3233 consecutive samplings with ascertained outcomes. *Breast* 2012;21(4):449–454.

Britton PD, Sonoda LI, Yamamoto AK, Koo B, Soh E, Goud A. Breast surgical specimen radiographs: how reliable are they?. *Eur J Radiol.* 2011; 79(2):245–249. http://re5qy4sb7x.search.serialssolutions.com/?url_ver=Z39.88-2004&rft_val_fmt=info:ofi/fmt:kev:mtx:journal&rfr_id=info:sid/Ovid:medl&rft.genre=article&rft_id=info:doi/10.1016%2Fj.ejrad.2010.02.012&rft_id=info:pmid/20303687&rft.issn=0720-048X&rft.volume=79&rft.issue=2&rft.spage=245&rft.pages=245-9&rft.date=2011&rft.jtitle=European+Journal+of+Radiology&rft.atitle=Breast+-surgical+specimen+radiographs%3A+how+reliable+are+they%3F.&rft.aulast=Britton.

Chetlen AL, Kasales C, Mack J, Schetter S, Zhu J. Hematoma formation during breast core needle biopsy in women taking antithrombotic therapy. *AJR Am J Roentgenol* 2013;201(1):215–222.

Cox CE, Russell S, Prowler V, et al. A prospective, single arm, multi-site, clinical evaluation of a nonradioactive surgical guidance technology for the location of nonpalpable breast lesions during excision. *Ann Surg Oncol* 2016;23(10):3168–3174.

Dauphine C, Reicher JJ, Reicher MA, Gondusky C, Khalkhali I, Kim M. A prospective clinical study to evaluate the safety and performance of wireless localization of nonpalpable breast lesions using radiofrequency identification technology. *AJR Am J Roentgenol* 2015;204(6):W720–W723.

Diamantis A, Magiorkinis E, Koutselini H. Fine-needle aspiration (FNA) biopsy: historical aspects. *Folia Histochem Cytobiol* 2009;47(2):191–197.

Elvecrog EL, Lechner MC, Nelson MT. Nonpalpable breast lesions: correlation of stereotaxic large-core needle biopsy and surgical biopsy results. *Radiology* 1993;188(2):453–455.

Fischer U, Kopka L, Grabbe E. Magnetic resonance guided localization and biopsy of suspicious breast lesions. *Top Magn Reson Imaging* 1998;9(1):44–59.

Follacchio GA, Monteleone F, Meggiorini ML, et al. Radio-localization of non-palpable breast lesions under ultrasonographic guidance: current status and future perspectives. *Curr Radiopharm* 2017;10(3):178–183.

Frank HA, Hall FM, Steer ML. Preoperative localization of nonpalpable breast lesions demonstrated by mammography. *N Engl J Med* 1976;295(5):259–260.

Gisvold JJ, Goellner JR, Grant CS, et al. Breast biopsy: a comparative study of stereotaxically guided core and excisional techniques. *AJR Am J Roentgenol.* 1994;162(4):815–820.

Graham RA, Homer MJ, Sigler CJ, et al. The efficacy of specimen radiography in evaluating the surgical margins of impalpable breast carcinoma. *AJR Am J Roentgenol* 1994;162(1):33–36.

Gray RJ, Salud C, Nguyen K, et al. Randomized prospective evaluation of a novel technique for biopsy or lumpectomy of nonpalpable breast lesions: radioactive seed versus wire localization. *Ann Surg Oncol* 2001;8(9):711–715.

Ha D, Dialani V, Mehta TS, Keefe W, Iuanow E, Slanetz PJ. Mucocele-like lesions in the breast diagnosed with percutaneous biopsy: is surgical excision necessary? *AJR Am J Roentgenol* 2015;204(1):204–210.

Hartmann LC, Degnim AC, Santen RJ, Dupont WD, Ghosh K. Atypical hyperplasia of the breast—risk assessment and management options. *N Engl J Med* 2015;372(1):78–89.

Harvey J, March D. *Making the diagnosis: A practical guide to breast imaging.* 1st ed. Philadelphia, PA: Saunders; 2013:584.

Hughes JH, Mason MC, Gray RJ, et al. A multi-site validation trial of radioactive seed localization as an alternative to wire localization. *Breast J* 2008;14(2):153–157.

Jackman RJ, Burbank F, Parker SH, et al. Stereotactic breast biopsy of nonpalpable lesions: Determinants of ductal carcinoma in situ underestimation rates. *Radiology* 2001;218(2):497–502.

Jeffries DO, Dossett LA, Jorns JM. Localization for breast surgery: the next generation. *Arch Pathol Lab Med* 2017;141(10):1324–1329.

Khan S, Diaz A, Archer KJ, et al. Papillary lesions of the breast: To excise or observe? *Breast J* 2017. doi: 10.1111/tbj.12907.

Kohler J, Krause B, Grunwald S, et al. Ultrasound and mammography guided wire marking of non-palpable breast lesions: analysis of 741 cases. *Ultraschall Med* 2007;28(3):283–290.

Kuhl CK, Elevelt A, Leutner CC, Gieseke J, Pakos E, Schild HH. Interventional breast MR imaging: clinical use of a stereotactic localization and biopsy device. *Radiology* 1997;204(3):667–675.

Lee CH, Philpotts LE, Horvath LJ, Tocino I. Follow-up of breast lesions diagnosed as benign with stereotactic core-needle biopsy: frequency of mammographic change and false-negative rate. *Radiology* 1999;212(1):189–194.

Levin DC, Parker L, Schwartz GF, Rao VM. Percutaneous needle vs surgical breast biopsy: previous allegations of overuse of surgery are in error. *J Am Coll Radiol* 2012;9(2):137–140.

Liberman L. Centennial dissertation. Percutaneous imaging-guided core breast biopsy: state of the art at the millennium. *AJR Am J Roentgenol* 2000;174(5):1191–1199.

Liberman L, Evans WP, 3rd, Dershaw DD, et al. Radiography of microcalcifications in stereotaxic mammary core biopsy specimens. *Radiology* 1994;190(1):223–225.

Liberman L, Feng TL, Dershaw DD, Morris EA, Abramson AF. US-guided core breast biopsy: use and cost-effectiveness. *Radiology* 1998;208(3):717–723.

Mahoney MC, Newell MS. Breast intervention: how I do it. *Radiology* 2013;268(1):12–24.

Mango VL, Wynn RT, Feldman S, et al. Beyond wires and seeds: reflector-guided breast lesion localization and excision. *Radiology* 2017;284(2):365–371.

Menes TS, Rosenberg R, Balch S, Jaffer S, Kerlikowske K, Miglioretti DL. Upgrade of high-risk breast lesions detected on mammography in the breast cancer surveillance consortium. *Am J Surg* 2014;207(1):24–31.

Meyer JE, Smith DN, DiPiro PJ, et al. Stereotactic breast biopsy of clustered microcalcifications with a directional, vacuum-assisted device. *Radiology* 1997;204(2):575–576.

Nassar A. Core needle biopsy versus fine needle aspiration biopsy in breast—a historical perspective and opportunities in the modern era. *Diagn Cytopathol* 2011;39(5):380–388.

Nicholson BT, Harvey JA, Patrie JT, Mugler JP, 3rd. 3D-MR ductography and contrast-enhanced MR mammography in patients with suspicious nipple discharge; a feasibility study. *Breast J* 2015;21(4):352–362.

Nurko J, Mancino AT, Whitacre E, Edwards MJ. Surgical benefits conveyed by biopsy site marking system using ultrasound localization. *Am J Surg* 2005; 190(4):618-622.

Orel SG, Schnall MD, Newman RW, Powell CM, Torosian MH, Rosato EF. MR imaging-guided localization and biopsy of breast lesions: initial experience. *Radiology* 1994;193(1):97–102.

Parker SH, Burbank F, Jackman RJ, et al. Percutaneous large-core breast biopsy: a multi-institutional study. *Radiology* 1994;193(2):359–364.

Parker SH, Jobe WE, Dennis MA, et al. US-guided automated large-core breast biopsy. *Radiology* 1993;187(2):507–511.

Parker SH, Lovin JD, Jobe WE, Burke BJ, Hopper KD, Yakes WF. Nonpalpable breast lesions: stereotactic automated large-core biopsies. *Radiology* 1991;180(2):403–407.

Penco S, Rizzo S, Bozzini AC, et al. Stereotactic vacuum-assisted breast biopsy is not a therapeutic procedure even when all mammographically found calcifications are removed: analysis of 4,086 procedures. *AJR Am J Roentgenol* 2010;195(5):1255–1260.

Philpotts LE, Hooley RJ, Lee CH. Comparison of automated versus vacuum-assisted biopsy methods for sonographically guided core biopsy of the breast. *AJR Am J Roentgenol* 2003;180(2):347–351.

Quinn SF, Demlow T, Dunkley B. Temno biopsy needle: Evaluation of efficacy and safety in 165 biopsy procedures. *AJR Am J Roentgenol* 1992;158(3):641–643.

Reicher JJ, Reicher MA, Thomas M, Petcavich R. Radiofrequency identification tags for preoperative tumor localization: proof of concept. *AJR Am J Roentgenol* 2008;191(5):1359–1365.

Sakamoto N, Ogawa Y, Tsunoda Y, Fukuma E. Evaluation of the sonographic visibility and sonographic appearance of the breast biopsy marker (UltraClip®) placed in phantoms and patients. *Breast Cancer* 2017;24(4):585–592.

Salkowski LR, Fowler AM, Burnside ES, Sisney GA. Utility of 6-month follow-up imaging after a concordant benign breast biopsy result. *Radiology* 2011;258(2):380–387.

Schrading S, Distelmaier M, Dirrichs T, et al. Digital breast tomosynthesis-guided vacuum-assisted breast biopsy: initial experiences and comparison with prone stereotactic vacuum-assisted biopsy. *Radiology* 2015;274(3):654–662.

Seow JH, Phillips M, Taylor D. Sonographic visibility of breast tissue markers: a tissue phantom comparison study. *Australas J Ultrasound Med* 2012;15(4):149–157.

Shetty MK. Presurgical localization of breast abnormalities: an overview and analysis of 202 cases. *Indian J Surg Oncol* 2010;1(4):278–283.

Smith DN, Rosenfield Darling ML, Meyer JE, et al. The utility of ultrasonographically guided large-core needle biopsy: results from 500 consecutive breast biopsies. *J Ultrasound Med* 2001;20(1):43–49.

Thomassin-Naggara I, Lalonde L, David J, Darai E, Uzan S, Trop I. A plea for the biopsy marker: how, why and why not clipping after breast biopsy? *Breast Cancer Res Treat* 2012;132(3):881–893.

van la Parra RF, Kuerer HM. Selective elimination of breast cancer surgery in exceptional responders: historical perspective and current trials. *Breast Cancer Res* 2016;18(1):8.

Van Zee KJ, Ortega Perez G, Minnard E, Cohen MA. Preoperative galactography increases the diagnostic yield of major duct excision for nipple discharge. *Cancer* 1998;82(10):1874–1880.

Wang M, He X, Chang Y, Sun G, Thabane L. A sensitivity and specificity comparison of fine needle aspiration cytology and core needle biopsy in evaluation of suspicious breast lesions: a systematic review and meta-analysis. *Breast* 2017;31:157–166.

Wang J, Simsir A, Mercado C, Cangiarella J. Can core biopsy reliably diagnose mucinous lesions of the breast? *Am J Clin Pathol* 2007;127(1):124–127.

SECTION V

CARDIAC RADIOLOGY

SECTION EDITOR: Seth Kligerman

CHAPTER 24 ■ INTRODUCTION TO CARDIAC ANATOMY, PHYSIOLOGY, AND IMAGING TECHNIQUES

KATE HANNEMAN AND SETH KLIGERMAN

INTRODUCTION

Basic knowledge of cardiac anatomy and physiology is essential to selecting an appropriate cardiac imaging technique for a particular clinical indication and for accurate interpretation of cardiac imaging studies. This chapter will review cardiac anatomy, physiology, and imaging techniques.

CARDIAC ANATOMY

The four-chambered heart lies primarily in the left hemithorax, termed *levoposition* (Fig. 24.1). The cardiac apex is normally located to the left of midline (*levocardia*). *Dextrocardia* indicates that the apex of the heart is to the right of midline. *Dextroposition* means that the heart is displaced to the right lying primarily in the right hemithorax; however, there is no anatomic alteration in the heart itself.

Situs Solitus. Normal anatomic positioning is termed *situs solitus*. With respect to cardiac anatomy, this means that the morphologic right atrium (RA) is on the right and the morphologic left atrium (LA) in on the left. Right-sided organs include a trilobed lung (with eparterial bronchus) in the chest and the liver in the abdomen. Left-sided organs include a bilobed lung (with hyparterial bronchus) in the chest and the spleen in the abdomen.

Situs Abnormalities. *Situs inversus totalis* means that all major organs are reversed or mirrored from their normal positions. With respect to cardiac anatomy, the morphologic RA is on the left and the morphologic LA is on the right. Although there is a slightly increased risk of congenital heart disease (CHD), in most cases situs inversus is discovered incidentally. Kartagener syndrome is a combination of situs inversus with dextrocardia, bronchiectasis, and sinusitis (Fig. 24.2). *Situs ambiguous* is associated with a higher incidence of complex CHD, and means that there are components of situs solitus and situs inversus in the same person. In the setting of CHD, isomerism is a situation where some paired structures on opposite sides of the body are symmetrical mirror images of each other. Left isomerism is associated with polysplenia. Each lung contains only two lobes and hyparterial bronchi. The incidence of CHD is increased, most commonly atrial septal defects (ASDs) or anomalous pulmonary venous return. Right isomerism is associated with asplenia. There are bilateral minor fissures and three lobes in each lung. Associated cardiac anomalies are usually more complex and severe than in left isomerism.

Right Atrium. The right border of the cardiac silhouette is formed primarily of the RA (Figs. 24.1 and 24.3). The RA receives systemic venous return from the superior vena cava (SVC), inferior vena cava (IVC), and coronary sinus. The RA is divided into two portions. The smooth posterior wall develops from the sinus venosus, with the SVC and IVC in continuity posteriorly (Fig. 24.4). The trabeculated anterior wall is derived from the embryonic RA. The RA appendage extends superiorly and medially from the SVC opening. The RA appendage is triangular or pyramidal shaped with a broad base and contains thick, coarse, pectinate muscles extending toward the atrioventricular (AV) valve. The crista terminalis is a smooth, thickened muscular ridge that runs from the mouth of the SVC and fades inferiorly to the mouth of the IVC. It divides the two portions of the atrium and corresponds to an external sulcus terminalis. The medial or posterior wall of the RA is the interatrial septum, which contains a smooth, central, dimpled area called the fossa ovalis. Inflow from the SVC, IVC, and coronary sinus enters the smooth posterior portion of the RA. The SVC has a free opening, whereas the IVC is partially guarded by a thin eustachian valve, which

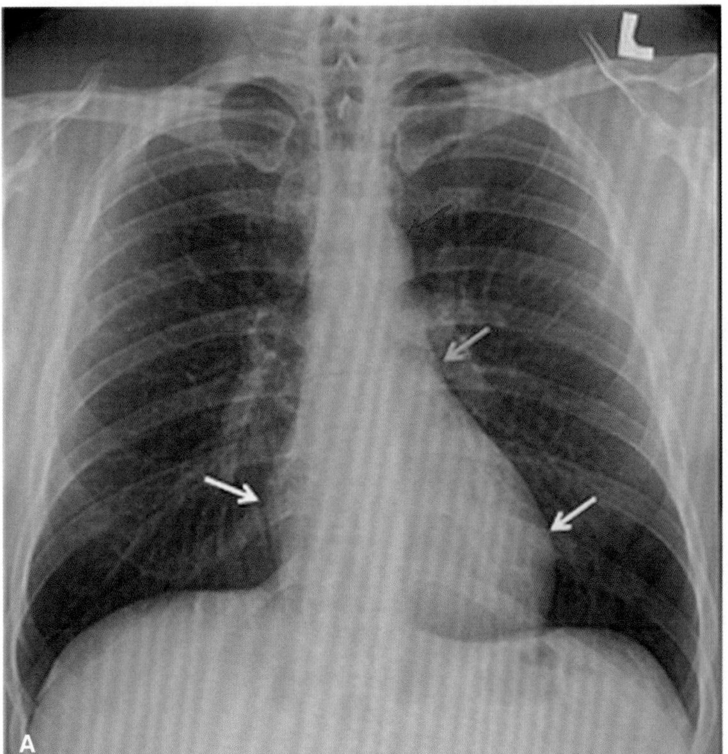

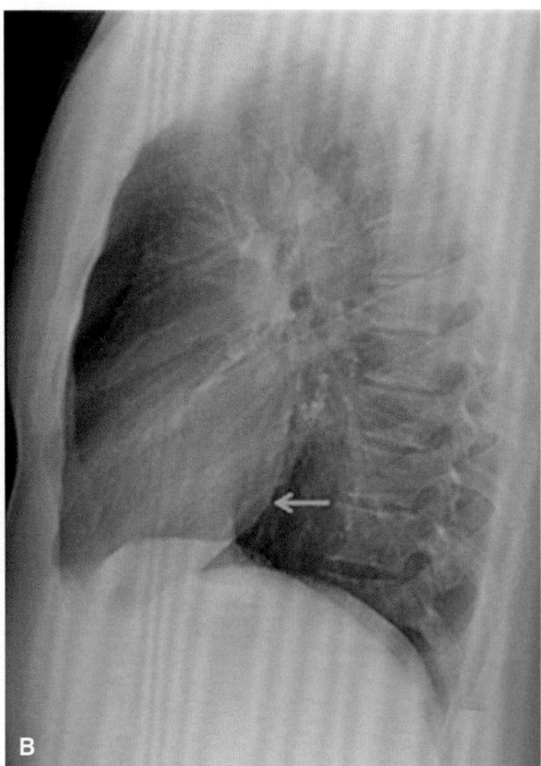

FIGURE 24.1. **Normal Chest Radiograph. A:** Normal posterior–anterior chest radiograph demonstrates situs solitus, levocardia, and normal heart size. The left ventricle (LV) (*yellow arrow*) is border forming on the left. The right atrium (RA) (*white arrow*) is border forming on the right. The aortic arch (*red arrow*) is of normal contour, and the pulmonary artery (PA) (*blue arrow*) is concave. **B:** Normal lateral chest radiograph. The inferior vena cava (IVC) intersection with the LV can be evaluated (*green arrow*).

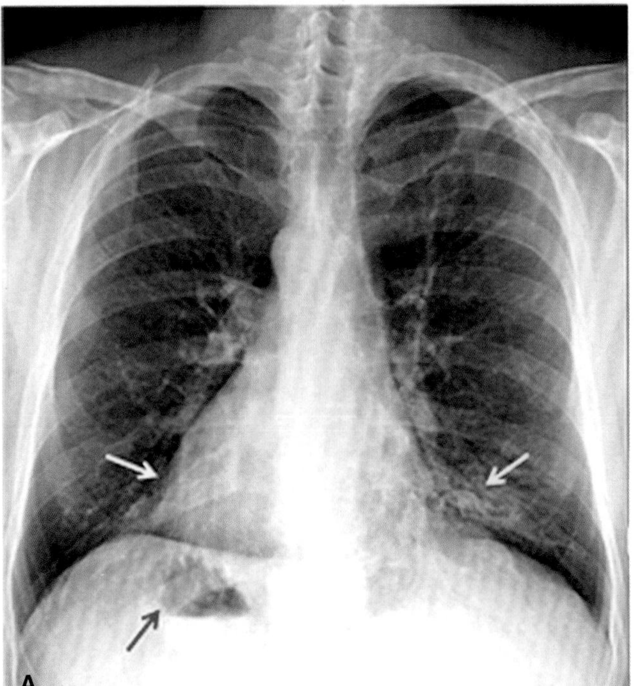

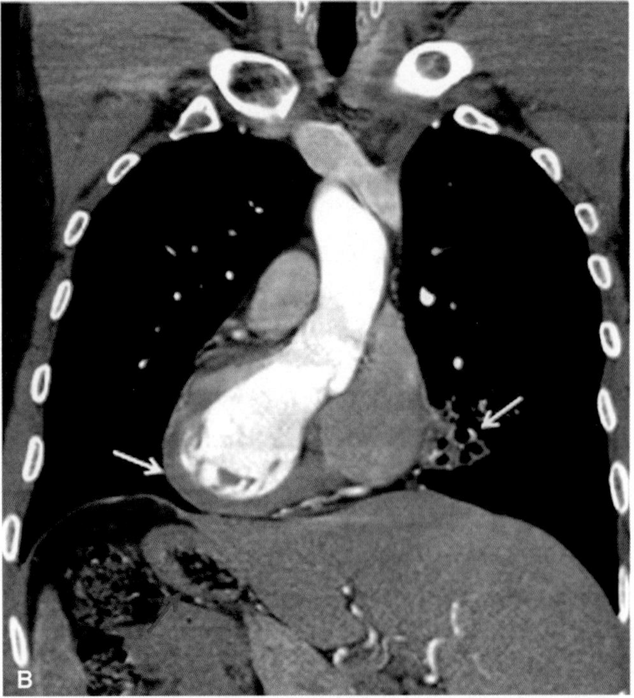

FIGURE 24.2. **Kartagener Syndrome With Situs Inversus. A:** Posterior–anterior chest radiograph. **B:** Coronal contrast-enhanced CT of chest. The cardiac apex is on the right in keeping with dextrocardia (*white arrows*). The stomach is also on the right (*red arrows*). There is bronchiectasis particularly in the left middle and lower lobes (*yellow arrows*).

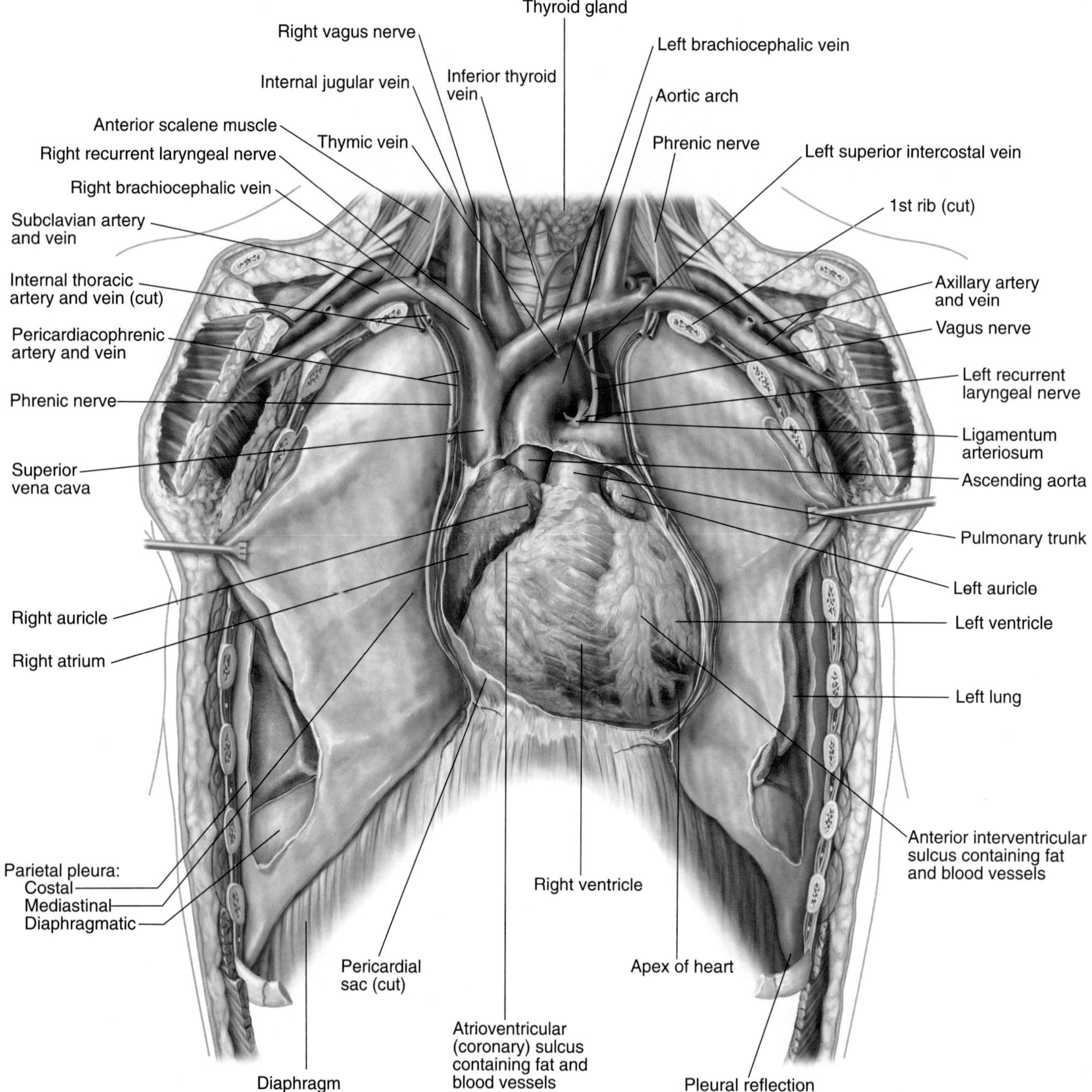

FIGURE 24.3. **Cardiothoracic Anatomy: Frontal View of the Heart After Cutaway of the Chest Wall, Pleural Surfaces, and Pericardial Surface.** Note the relationship of the RA, RV, left atrial appendage, and LV to the great vessels. (Reproduced with permission from Tank PW, Gest TR, and Burkel W. *Atlas of Anatomy*. Philadelphia, PA: Wolters Kluwer/Lippincott Williams & Wilkins; 2009.)

is occasionally absent or perforated. The coronary sinus enters the RA anterior and medial to the IVC. Its opening is guarded by the thebesian valve between the orifice of the IVC and the tricuspid valve.

Right Ventricle. The right ventricle (RV) is the most anterior chamber and abuts the sternum (Fig. 24.1). The tricuspid AV valve separates the RV from its upstream atria (usually the RA). The RV is divided into a posterior or inferior portion (inflow or sinus portion), which is heavily trabeculated, and a less-trabeculated anterior or superior portion (outflow tract or pulmonary conus) (Figs. 24.4 and 24.5). The two portions of the RV are divided by the crista supraventricularis, which courses between the pulmonary valve and the tricuspid valve. The moderator band (also known as the septomarginal band) is a muscular band that extends from the base of the anterior papillary muscle to the interventricular septum. It carries part of the right bundle branch of the conduction system and is a consistent feature of the RV. The infundibulum (conus arteriosus) is the smooth cephalic portion of the RV that leads to the pulmonary trunk. Morphologically, the RV is distinguished from the left ventricle (LV) by having coarser trabeculae (particularly at the apex), a moderator band, a muscular

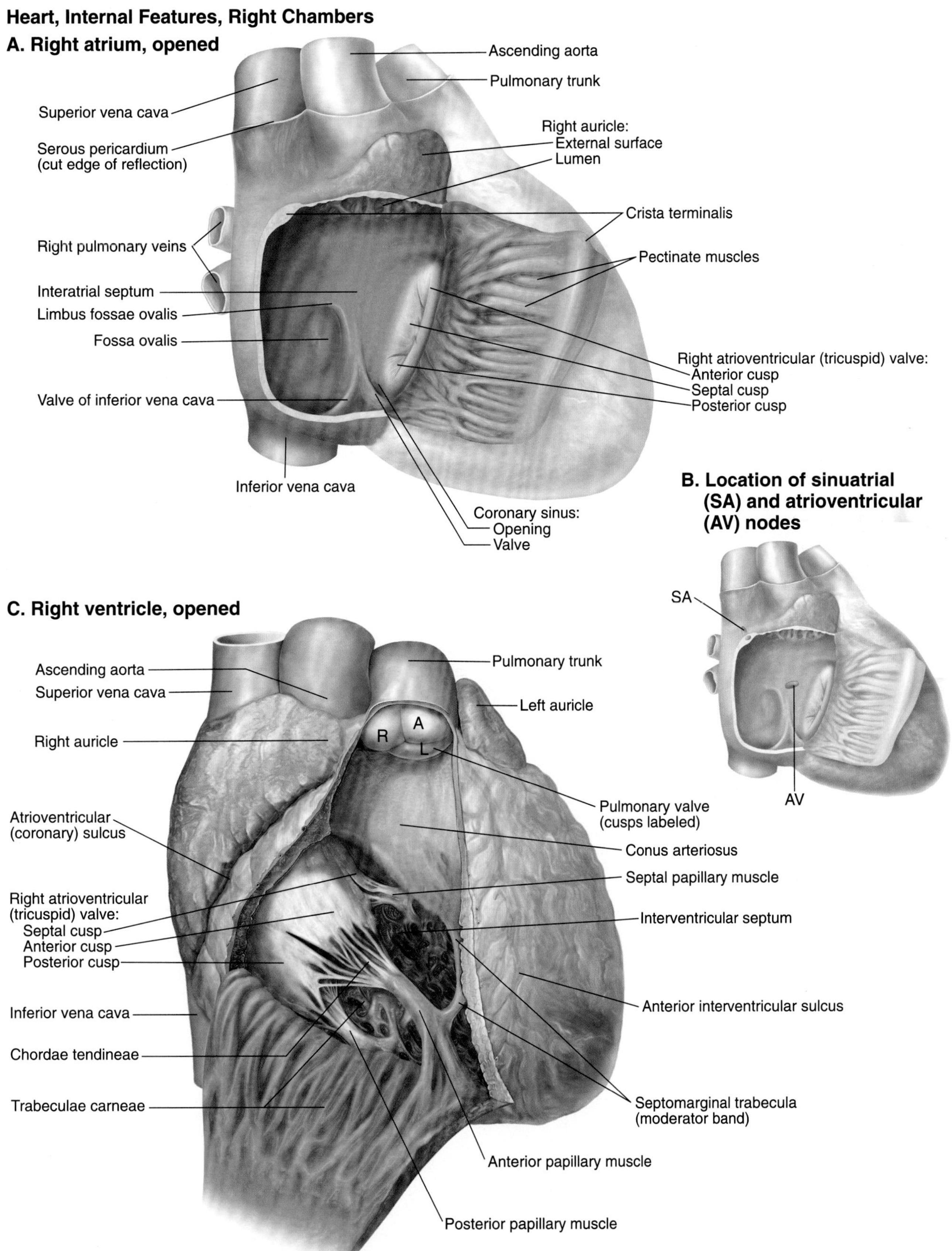

FIGURE 24.4. **Cutaway Views of the RA and RV.** (Reproduced with permission from Tank PW, Gest TR, and Burkel W. *Atlas of Anatomy*. Philadelphia, PA: Wolters Kluwer/Lippincott Williams & Wilkins; 2009.)

Sectional View of the Heart

A. Plane of section

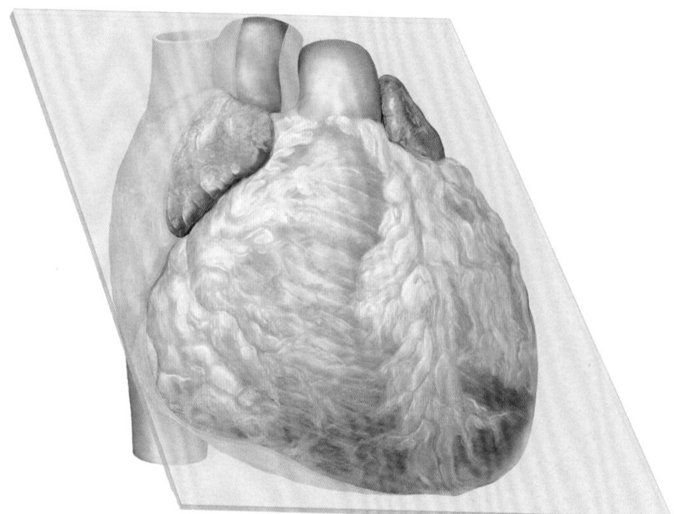

B. Section through the heart showing the posteroinferior portion

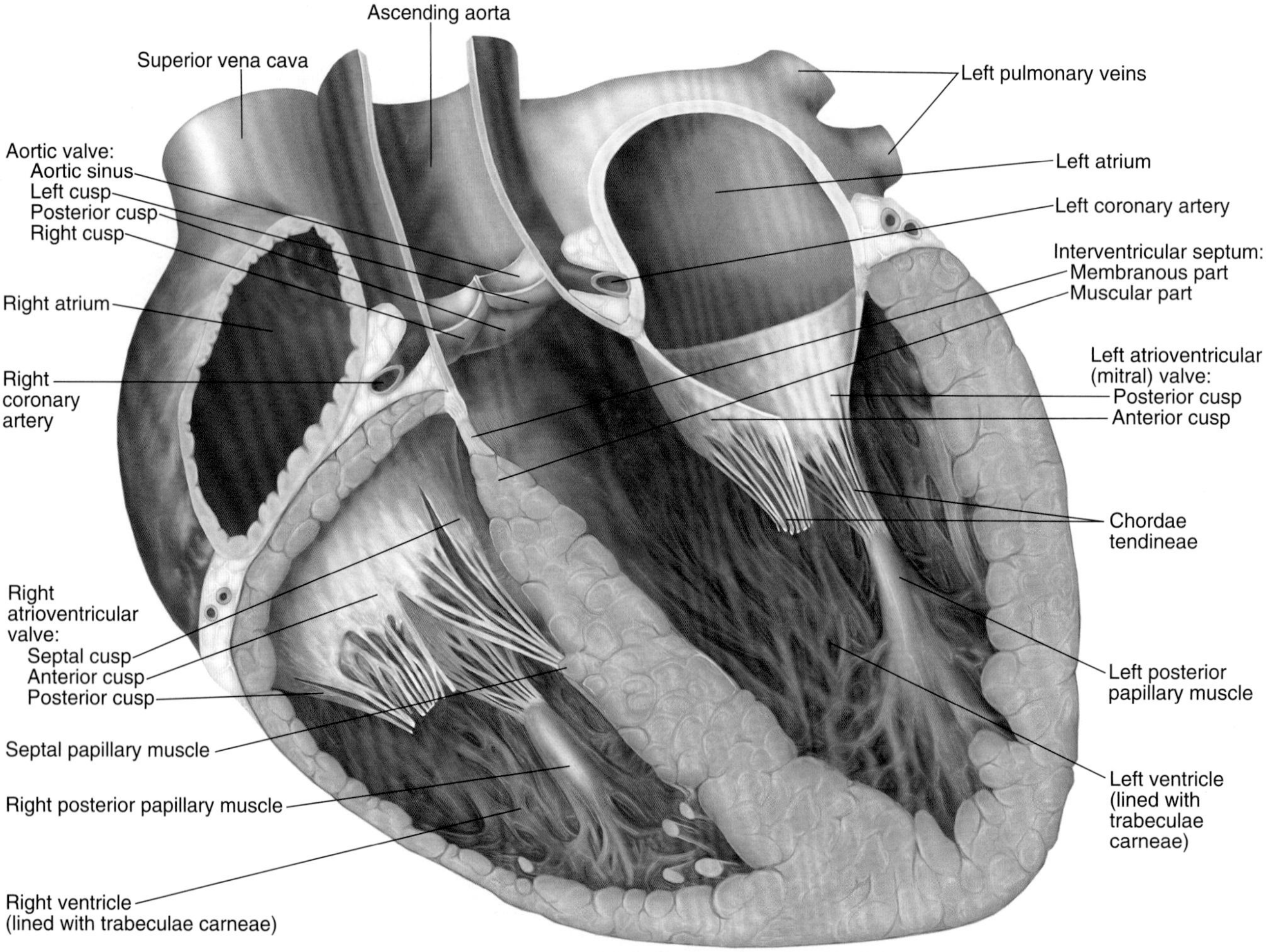

FIGURE 24.5. **Bisection Through the Long Axis of the Heart.** (Reproduced with permission from Tank PW, Gest TR, and Burkel W. *Atlas of Anatomy*. Philadelphia, PA: Wolters Kluwer/Lippincott Williams & Wilkins; 2009.)

infundibulum, apical displacement of the right AV valve, and lack of fibrous continuity between its inlet and outflow valves. The RV has a much thinner wall compared with the LV as it normally operates at much lower pressures. Desaturated blood from the right heart circulates through the lungs via the pulmonary arteries.

Pulmonary Arteries. The muscular pulmonary conus extends to the tricuspid pulmonary valve, with the pulmonary trunk extending superiorly and to the left. The left PA extends posteriorly, coursing over the top of the left main stem bronchus, then descending posteriorly. The right PA extends horizontally to the right, bifurcates within the pericardial sac, and exits the right hilum as the truncus anterior (which supplies the right upper lobe) and the interlobar artery (which supplies the right middle and lower lobes). The left main stem bronchus is hyparterial, meaning that it lies below the PA. The right bronchus is eparterial, meaning that it lies next to the right PA.

Pulmonary Veins. The pulmonary veins connect to the LA, transferring oxygenated blood from the lungs back to the heart. Typically there are two pulmonary veins on each side, superior and inferior. Normal variants include direct drainage from the right middle lobe into the LA. Occasionally a portion of the pulmonary venous return will be to the right heart or SVC, termed partial anomalous pulmonary venous return (PAPVR). PAPVR from the right lung is twice as common as PAPVR from the left lung. The most common form of PAPVR is one in which a right upper pulmonary vein (typically draining the right upper and middle lobes) connects to the RA or the SVC. This form is often associated with a sinus venosus ASD. Total anomalous pulmonary venous return (TAPVR) is a rare congenital malformation in which all four pulmonary veins drain into systemic veins, usually the SVC or IVC, or drain directly into the RA. An ASD is required for survival prior to repair.

Left Atrium. The LA is subcarinal and midline, and is the most superior and posterior cardiac chamber (Fig. 24.6). The smooth walls of the LA are nestled between the right and left bronchi, and its posterior wall abuts the anterior wall of the esophagus. The left atrial appendage is long, slender, and finger like, and projects superiorly and to the left. The pectinate muscles are fewer and smaller compared with the RA, and are confined to the inner surface of the LA appendage. The pulmonary veins enter the posterior part of the LA with the left-sided veins located more superior than the right-sided veins. The LA is relatively smooth walled on its internal aspect. The coronary sinus runs behind the LA, from posterosuperior to anteroinferior.

Left Ventricle. The mitral valve separates the LV from its upstream atria (usually the LA). The anterior leaflet of the mitral valve lies near the interventricular septum and extends to the posterior (noncoronary) cusp of the aortic valve (Figs. 24.5 and 24.6). The smaller posterior mitral leaflet lies posteriorly and to the left. There are two papillary muscles which attach to the mitral valve via chordae tendineae, anterolateral and posteromedial. The chordae tendineae are strong fibrous cords. The inflow portion of the LV is posterior to the anterior leaflet of the mitral valve. The outflow portion of the LV is anterior and superior to the anterior mitral leaflet. The interventricular septum has a high membranous portion that is contiguous with the aortic root. The more muscular inferior portion of the septum extends to the left ventricular apex. The walls of the LV are much thicker compared with the RV. The LV is separated from the RV by the interventricular septum which is concave, bulging into the RV. The LV inflow and outflow tracts are relatively smooth and the apex is lined by fine trabeculae.

Aorta. The LV outflow tract leads to the aortic root through the aortic valve which is typically tricuspid, composed of right, left, and posterior (or noncoronary) cusps. The sinuses of Valsalva are the reservoirs created by the closure of the aortic valve and from which the right and left coronary arteries arise. The aortic arch gives rise to the right brachiocephalic artery, left common carotid artery, and left subclavian artery. The descending aorta typically descends to the left of midline.

Coronary Arteries. The right coronary artery arises from the right coronary cusp and the left main coronary artery arises from the left coronary cusp. Coronary anatomy will be detailed in Chapter 25.

Ligamentum Arteriosum. The ligamentum arteriosum arises from the superior, proximal left PA, and crosses through the aorticopulmonary window to the inferior aspect of the distal aortic arch. The ligamentum arteriosum is the remnant of the ductus arteriosus, which closes functionally in the first 24 hours of life, and closes anatomically by 10 days of life.

Conduction System. The sinoatrial (SA) node consists of specialized neuromuscular tissue that measures approximately 5 to 20 mm and is located on the anterior endocardial surface of the RA just above the SVC and right atrial appendage junction, near the crista terminalis. Electrical propagation spreads to both atria via Purkinje-like fibers and is recorded as the P wave on an electrocardiogram (ECG). The AV node is a 2- × 5-mm region of neuromuscular tissue on the endocardial surface, along the right side of the interatrial septum, just inferior to the ostium of the coronary sinus. The impulse is collected and delayed approximately 0.7 second in the AV node before passing into the bundle of His. The bundle of His is a 20-mm-long tract which extends down the right side of the membranous interventricular septum. The bundle of His bifurcates into right and left bundles before arborizing through the two ventricles via the Purkinje system. The interventricular septum activates from superior to inferior, with the anterior or septal RV being the first to activate and the posterior or basal LV being the last to activate.

CARDIAC PHYSIOLOGY

The cardiac cycle is a series of pressure changes that take place within the heart, resulting in movement of blood through different chambers of the heart and the body. The contraction of the atria precedes that of the ventricles. The cardiac cycle is divided into ventricular diastole and systole. Diastole represents ventricular filling, and systole represents ventricular contraction and ejection. Systole and diastole occur in both the right and left heart, although with different pressures. Diastole begins with closing of the aortic and pulmonic valves and ends with closing of the mitral and tricuspid valves, encompassing isovolumic ventricular relaxation and ventricular filling. Isovolumic relaxation is the period immediately after ventricular contraction when the aortic and pulmonic valves have closed, but the AV valves have not yet opened. After the ventricle fills and transitions to contraction, the pressure gradient will eventually exceed that of the aorta and main pulmonary artery and will close the AV valves. AV valve closure is the source of the first heart sound, denoted as S1. Systole begins when the AV valves close and concludes with closure of the aortic and pulmonic valve, encompassing isovolumic ventricular contraction and ventricular ejection. The time between closing of the AV valves and opening of the aortic and pulmonic valves is the period of isovolumic contraction. Eventually, the pressure within the ventricle exceeds the

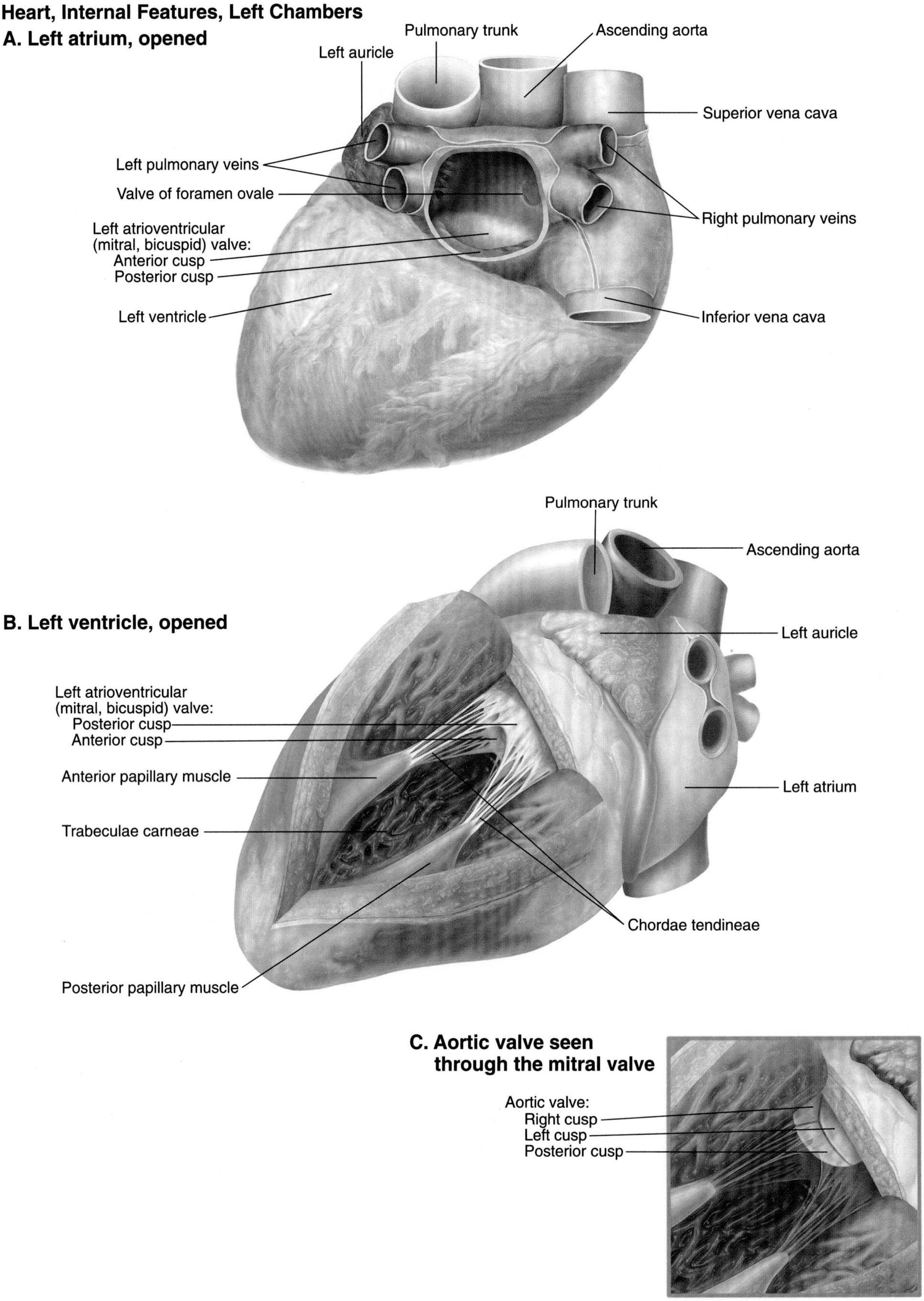

Heart, Internal Features, Left Chambers

A. Left atrium, opened

Pulmonary trunk
Ascending aorta
Left auricle
Superior vena cava
Left pulmonary veins
Valve of foramen ovale
Left atrioventricular (mitral, bicuspid) valve:
Anterior cusp
Posterior cusp
Right pulmonary veins
Left ventricle
Inferior vena cava

B. Left ventricle, opened

Pulmonary trunk
Ascending aorta
Left auricle
Left atrioventricular (mitral, bicuspid) valve:
Posterior cusp
Anterior cusp
Anterior papillary muscle
Left atrium
Trabeculae carneae
Chordae tendineae
Posterior papillary muscle

C. Aortic valve seen through the mitral valve

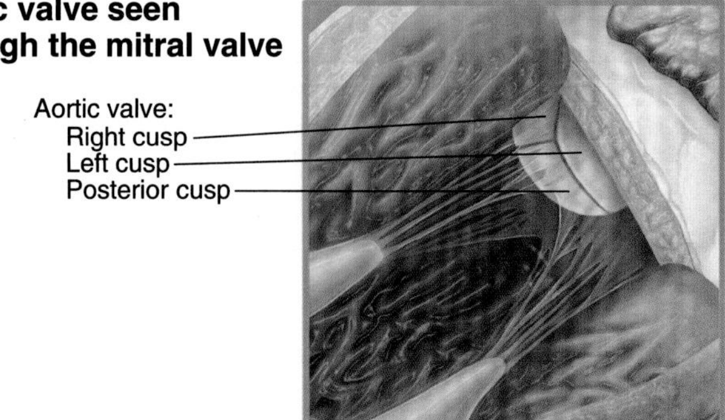

FIGURE 24.6. **Cutaway Views of the LV and LA.** (Reproduced with permission from Tank PW, Gest TR, and Burkel W. *Atlas of Anatomy*. Philadelphia, PA: Wolters Kluwer/Lippincott Williams & Wilkins; 2009.)

pressure in the aorta and main pulmonary artery, and the aortic and pulmonic valves open, marking the beginning of ventricular ejection. The aortic and pulmonic valve closure is the source of the second heart sound, denoted as S2.

IMAGING TECHNIQUES

Chest Radiography

Depending on the clinical indication, a chest radiograph may be the first imaging modality a patient with cardiac pathology undergoes. Chest radiography techniques include posterior–anterior (PA) and anterior–posterior (AP) frontal projections and lateral projection.

Frontal Projection. The right border of the cardiac silhouette is formed primarily by the RA, with the SVC entering superiorly and the IVC often seen at its lower margin (Fig. 24.1). The left border of the heart is created primarily by the LV and LA appendages. The pulmonary artery, aortopulmonary window, and aortic arch extend superiorly.

Lateral Projection. The RV is border forming anteriorly adjacent to the sternum, with its outflow tract extending superiorly and posteriorly. The LA is border forming in the high posterior, subcarinal region. The LV is border forming inferiorly and posteriorly.

Global cardiac size can be evaluated on chest radiography using the cardiothoracic ratio (CTR). The CTR is assessed as the ratio of maximal horizontal cardiac diameter to maximal horizontal thoracic diameter (measured from the inner edge of ribs/pleura). A normal CTR on a PA radiograph is less than 0.5. A CTR greater than 0.5 on a PA radiograph is suggestive of cardiomegaly, although not chamber specific.

Left atrial enlargement can be directly visualized on a frontal chest radiograph using the double density sign (Fig. 24.7). This occurs when the right side of the LA indents the adjacent lung and forms its own distinct silhouette. LA enlargement can be confirmed by an oblique measurement greater than 7 cm, measured from the inferior midpoint of left main bronchus to the right border of the LA. Enlargement of the left atrial appendage appears as an extra convexity inferior to the main pulmonary artery. On the lateral view, the LA is the most posterior chamber and when enlarged will encroach on or overlie the spine. Indirect signs of LA enlargement include splaying of the carina (with an increase in the tracheal bifurcation angle to over 90 degrees), posterior displacement of the left mainstem bronchus on the lateral radiograph, and superior displacement of the left mainstem bronchus on the frontal radiograph.

Right atrial enlargement is more difficult to evaluate on chest radiography compared with LA enlargement. Nonspecific findings of RA enlargement include increased convexity along the right heart border (Fig. 24.8).

Left ventricular enlargement results in displacement of the left heart border and apex leftward, inferiorly, or posteriorly. Rounding of the cardiac apex can also be seen. LV enlargement can be evaluated using the Hoffman–Rigler sign, which is considered positive if the distance between the LV border and the posterior border of IVC exceeds 1.8 cm, measured at a level 2 cm above the intersection of the diaphragm and IVC on a lateral radiograph (Fig. 24.9).

Right ventricular enlargement is not as easily detected as LV enlargement. RV enlargement should be considered in the setting of a large CTR if the Hoffman–Rigler sign is negative for LV enlargement. Other signs of RV enlargement include uplifted cardiac apex on the frontal radiograph and filling of

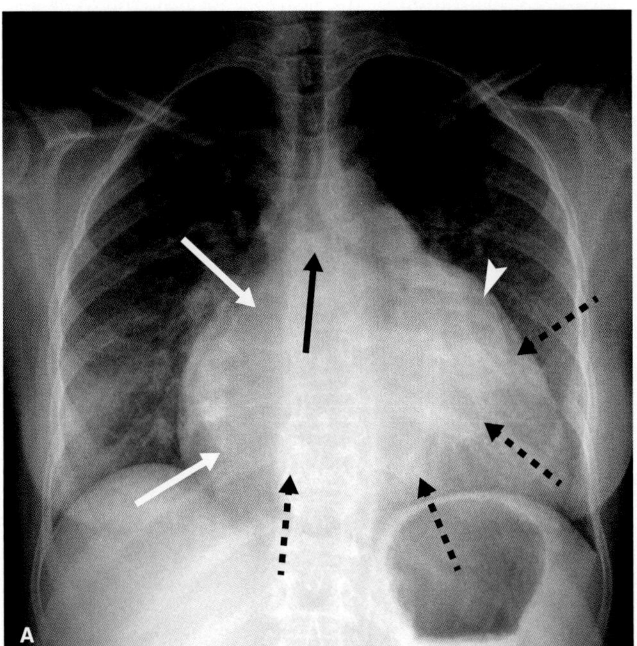

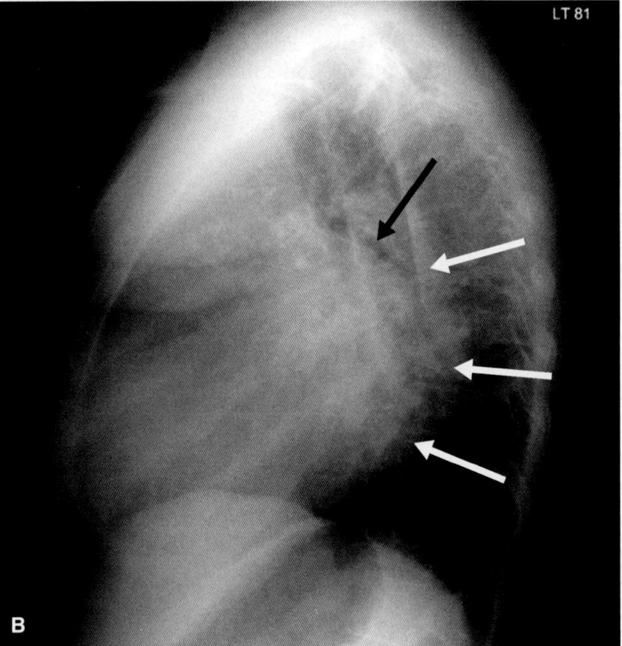

FIGURE 24.7. **Left Atrial Enlargement. A:** Posterior–anterior chest radiograph in a patient with severe mitral stenosis shows the classic findings of left atrial (LA) enlargement including a double density along the right heart border (*white arrows*), splaying of the carina (*black arrow*), and enlargement of the LA appendage (*white arrowhead*). The LA is so large that it appears like a large posterior mediastinal mass (*black-dotted arrows*). **B:** On the lateral view, the LA is the most posterior chamber and when enlarged encroaches on or overlies the spine (*white arrows*). In addition, there is posterior displacement of the left mainstem bronchus (*black arrow*).

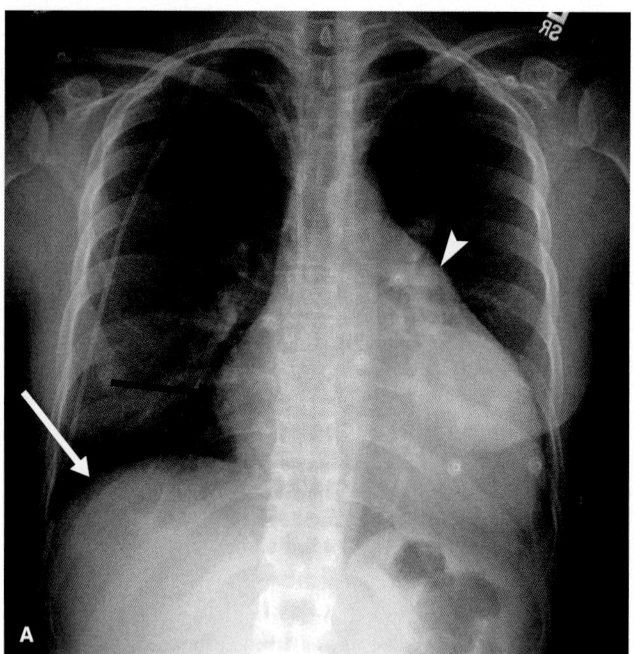

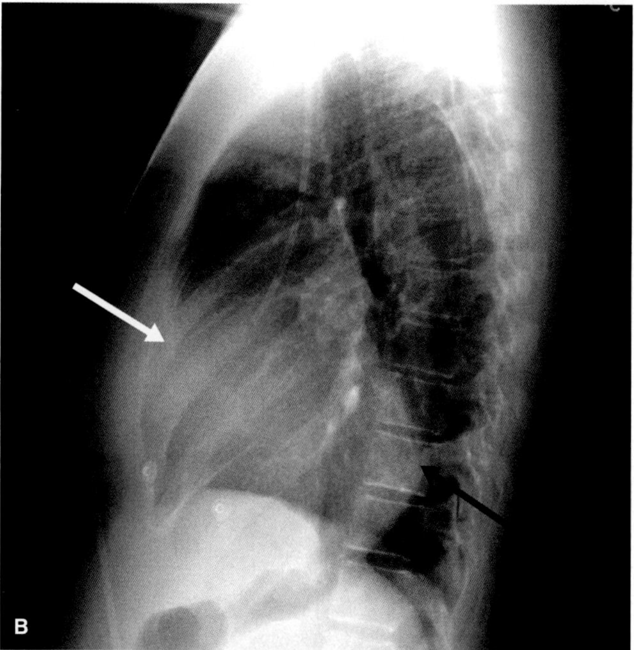

FIGURE 24.8. **Right Atrial and Right Ventricular Dilation in a 35-Year-Old Woman With Pulmonary Arterial Hypertension and Severe Tricuspid Regurgitation. A:** PA radiograph shows increased convexity to the right of the spine (*black arrow*). The left heart border has a more rounded contour than normal (*white arrow*) due to posterior displacement of the heart from right ventricular dilation. The pulmonary artery is enlarged (*white arrowhead*). **B:** Lateral radiograph shows increased soft tissue attenuation in the retrosternal space (*white arrow*). In addition, there is increased density overlying the spine, which is usually a sign of left atrial enlargement (*black arrow*). However, the right heart was so dilated in this case that the right atrium became the most posterior cardiac chamber. There are no signs of left atrial enlargement such as double density along the right heart border, splaying of the carina, enlargement of the left atrial appendage, or posterior displacement of the left mainstem bronchus.

the retrosternal air space (more than one-third of the sternal length) on the lateral radiograph (Fig. 24.8).

Echocardiography

Echocardiography is widely available and is routinely used in the diagnosis, evaluation, and follow-up of patients with cardiac disease. Echocardiography is useful in assessing the cardiac chamber size and function. Ventricular function can be evaluated using M-mode, two-dimensional (2D), and three-dimensional (3D) echocardiography. In addition to allowing visualization of the heart, echocardiography is also useful in the assessment and quantification of blood flow using techniques such as pulsed- or continuous-wave Doppler. These techniques can be used to evaluate for abnormal

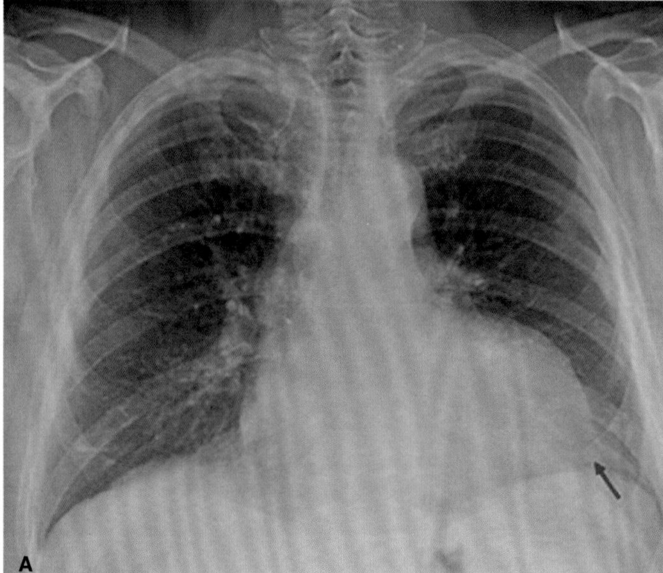

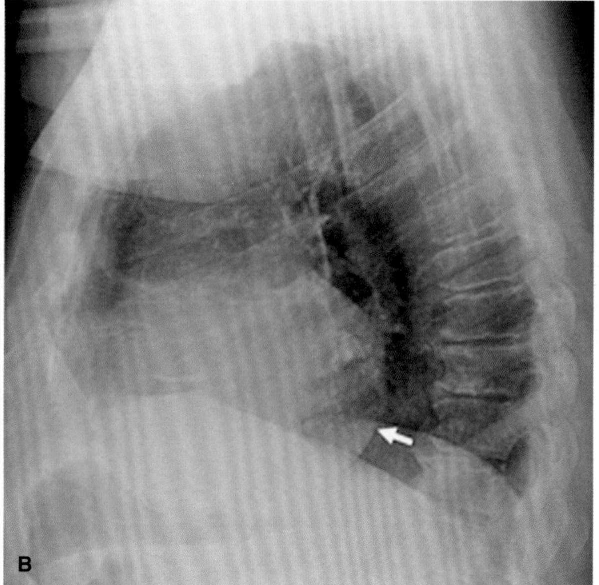

FIGURE 24.9. **Left Ventricular Enlargement. A:** Posterior–anterior chest radiograph demonstrates prominence of the LV with the apex pointing downward (*red arrow*). **B:** Lateral chest radiograph demonstrates the posterior margin of the LV (*white arrow*) projecting behind the IVC. The cardiothoracic ratio is >0.5 and the Hoffman–Rigler sign is positive.

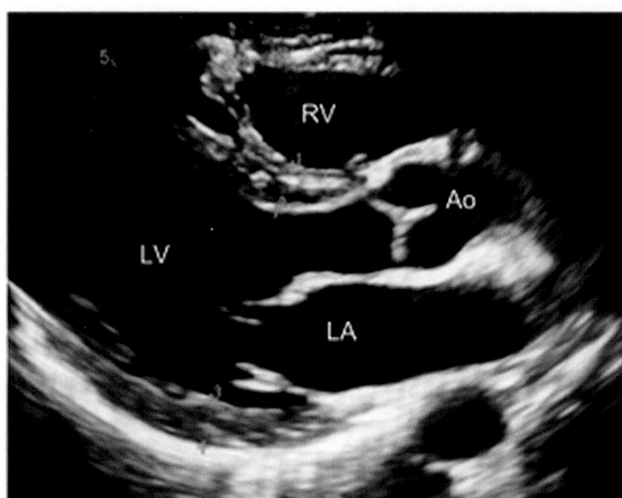

FIGURE 24.10. Echocardiography Parasternal Long-Axis View. Transthoracic parasternal long-axis image in diastole is obtained with the patient in left lateral decubitus position and demonstrates the *LA*, *LV*, aortic root (*Ao*), and a portion of the *RV*, in addition to the mitral and aortic valves.

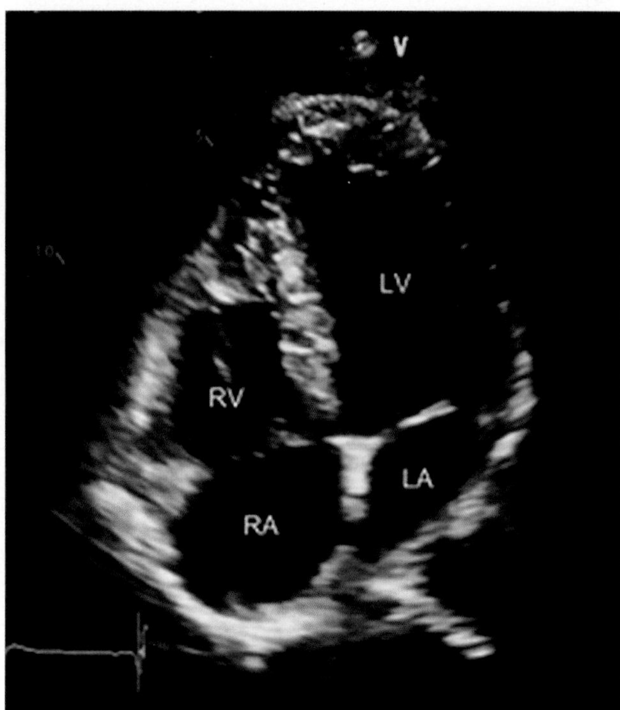

FIGURE 24.11. Echocardiography Apical Four-Chamber View. Transthoracic apical four-chamber view is obtained with the patient supine with left arm abducted and demonstrates the *LA*, *LV*, *RA*, and *RV* in addition to the mitral and tricuspid valves.

communications between the left- and right-sided cardiac chambers, valve regurgitation, and tissue motion. Speckle tracking echocardiography allows for assessment of myocardial contraction and deformation.

Transthoracic echocardiography (TTE) is the most common type of echocardiography, in which the ultrasound probe is placed on the chest or abdomen to obtain still images or movie clips of the heart. The main TTE windows—which refer to the physical location of the transducer—are suprasternal, parasternal, apical, and subcostal (subxiphoid). Echocardiography views refer to the image plane as it relates to the axis of the heart. Standard views in the parasternal window include long-axis view (useful to evaluate the size and contractility of the ventricles and to assess the morphology and function of the mitral and aortic valves) and short-axis view (Fig. 24.10). Standard views in the apical window include four-chamber view (useful for visualization of all four cardiac chambers including the apex, assessment of ejection fraction using the Simpson method, and assessment of mitral inflow), five-chamber view (which includes the aortic valve and is useful for assessment of aortic stenosis), and two- and three-chamber views (Fig. 24.11). Subcostal views include four-chamber, short-axis, and IVC views (which allow for estimation of a patient's volume status).

Transesophageal echocardiography (TEE) is a less common way to perform echocardiography, in which a specialized probe containing an ultrasound transducer at its tip is passed into the patient's esophagus. TEE is advantageous in certain circumstances as many cardiovascular structures can be imaged more clearly using this technique. The posterior aspect of the heart is directly anterior to the esophagus, reducing the attenuation of the ultrasound signal. TEE is useful in imaging the LA and left atrial appendage when thrombus or clot is suspected. Disadvantages of TEE include the fact that this is a more invasive test and requires sedation.

Nuclear Imaging

Nuclear medicine uses small amounts of radioactive materials called radiotracers to image the heart noninvasively. There are several different nuclear medicine imaging techniques that provide unique information regarding cardiac function, blood flow, and myocardial inflammation.

Radionuclide ventriculography is a noninvasive study, which provides information on cardiac function. Evaluation of cardiac function with radionuclide ventriculography is accurate, although exposure to radiation is a disadvantage compared with other imaging modalities.

Myocardial perfusion imaging (MPI) is one of the most widely used nuclear cardiology techniques. Myocardial perfusion images are typically obtained at both rest and stress. Stress can be achieved using exercise (typically walking on a treadmill or riding a stationary bicycle) or using a pharmacologic agent to vasodilate the coronary arteries (most commonly adenosine, dipyridamole, or regadenoson) or to increase myocardial contraction and heart rate (such as dobutamine). A small amount of radiopharmaceutical such as technetium (^{99m}Tc) sestamibi is injected at both rest and stress. Images of the heart are then acquired using a single-photon emission computed tomography (SPECT) camera which detects the radiation released by the tracer. If there is coronary artery narrowing resulting in stress-induced myocardial ischemia, a decrease in blood flow to the affected area of myocardium will be detected at stress but not at rest (unmatched defect). Areas of myocardium that are scarred in the setting of an infarct will have a defect at both rest and stress (matched defect).

Positron emission tomography (PET) is most commonly used in oncology; however, it is also used to provide information about the blood supply and metabolic activity of the heart. Intravenous radiotracers used in PET perfusion imaging include Rubidium-82, Nitrogen-13 ammonia, and Oxygen-15 water with images typically acquired at both stress and rest, similar to MPI. Intravenous injection of ^{18}F-fluorodeoxyglucose (^{18}F-FDG) in combination with myocardial glucose suppression

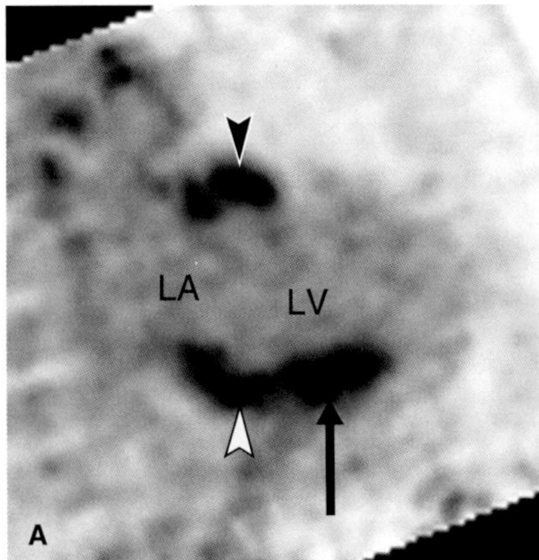

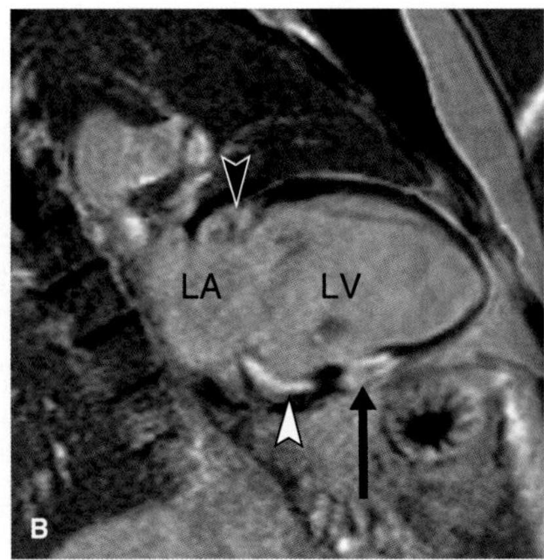

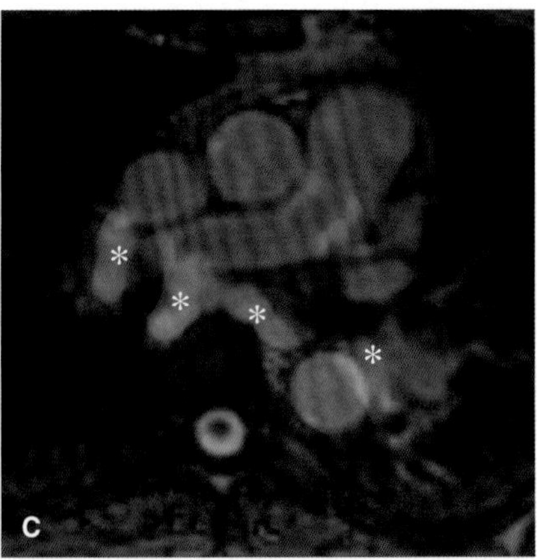

FIGURE 24.12. **Positron Emission Tomography. A:** ^{18}F-fluorodeoxyglucose (^{18}F-FDG) PET image reconstructed in a two-chamber view in a patient with cardiac sarcoidosis shows intense uptake in the inferior wall (*white arrowhead*) and anterior wall (*black arrowhead*) at the base and in the inferior wall at the midcavity level (*black arrow*). **B:** Corresponding image from an MRI shows corresponding foci midmyocardial, subepicardial, and transmural delayed enhancement due to inflammation and fibrosis. **C:** Fused image from PET and MRI examinations shows intense FDG uptake in mediastinal and hilar lymphadenopathy (*) which is bilateral and symmetric. LV, left ventricle; LA, left atrium.

(typically achieved by having patients fast or eat a low-carbohydrate diet for several hours prior to the study) can be used to evaluate for inflammation in patients with known or suspected cardiac sarcoidosis (Fig. 24.12).

Cardiac CT

Cardiac CT has an important role in the evaluation of coronary and cardiac anatomy. Modern multidetector CT scanners acquire high-resolution 3D datasets of the heart. Suppression of motion artifacts due to the beating heart is achieved by synchronizing data acquisition or reconstruction with the patient's ECG. Several different cardiac synchronization methods are available.

Prospective ECG-triggering synchronizes the x-ray exposure to specific portions of the cardiac cycle, allowing for reduced radiation dose. Axial images are only acquired during a specified portion of the cardiac cycle, starting at a predetermined delay from the R wave, for example, 70% to 80% of the R–R interval. The interval that the patient is scanned can be increased (e.g., to 60% to 80% of the R–R interval) or decreased (e.g., to 73% to 78% of the R–R interval) depending on the choice of the operator, leading to a respective increase or decrease in the radiation dose. During the remainder of the cardiac cycle, the CT tube current is turned off and therefore no radiation is delivered. The number of axial scans required to complete the study depends on both the superior-to-inferior length of the region to be scanned and the number of detector rows of the scanner. For instance, a 64-detector row CT scanner with a detector width of 0.625 mm acquires a 4-cm axial slab with each rotation. Therefore, if the total superior-to-inferior length of the heart is 16 cm, it would require four axial scans to complete the study (Fig. 24.13). However, a CT scanner with 256 detector rows and a detector width

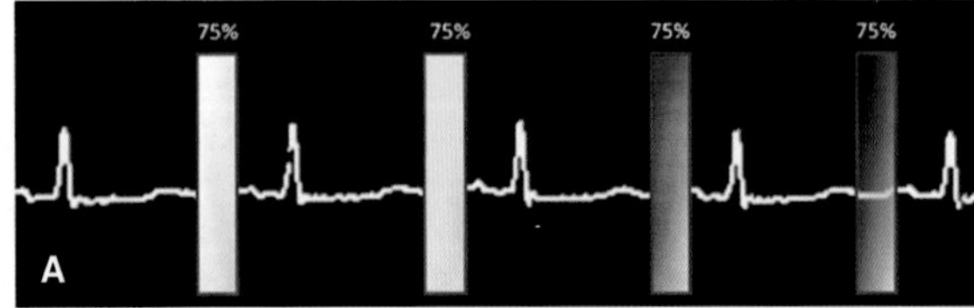

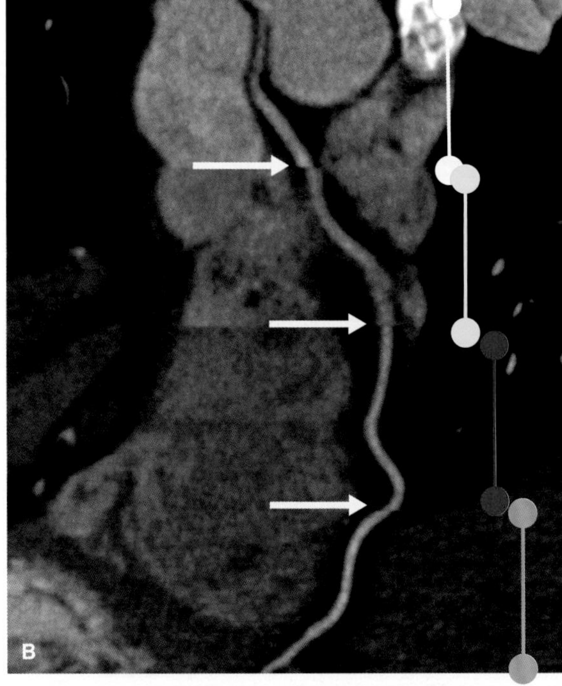

FIGURE 24.13. **Prospective Gating With Multiple Axial Acquisitions. A:** Using a prospective ECG-triggered technique, axial images are only acquired over a prespecified portion of the cardiac cycle (*colored boxes*). In this example, they are obtained during 75% of the R–R interval, during end diastole before the atrial contraction. With most scanners, multiple sequential axial images are required with this technique to scan the entire heart. After each axial acquisition, the scanner turns off, the table moves to the next portion of the heart, and then the next axial acquisition is obtained at the same percentage of the R–R interval. This axial "step-and-shoot" acquisition continues until the entire preselected anatomy is scanned. **B:** Example of an axial "step-and-shoot" acquisition using a 64-slice scanner. Each axial slice scans a 4-cm slab of the heart requiring a total of four axial scans to cover the entire heart. The axial images are spliced together creating the edge artifact along different slabs (*white arrows*), which is most conspicuous along the course of the right coronary artery.

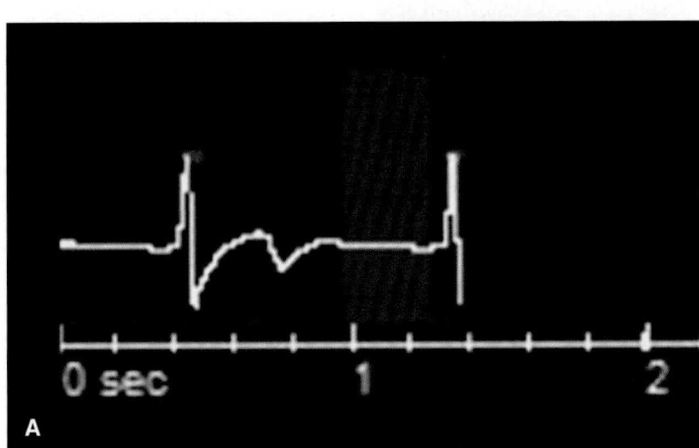

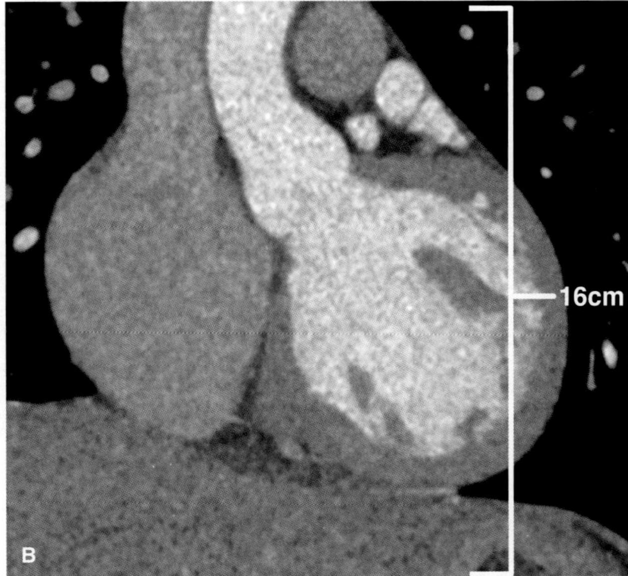

FIGURE 24.14. **Prospective Gating With a Single Axial Acquisition. A:** Using a prospective ECG-triggered technique, axial images are only acquired over a prespecified portion of the cardiac cycle (*navy box*, in this case targeting diastole). With many scanners, this would require multiple axial acquisitions, as seen in Figure 24.13 above. However, with certain CT scanners that have a large number of detector rows, the entire heart, as seen in (**B**), can be imaged during a single axial rotation. Currently, two different vendors have scanners that can cover up to 16 cm with a single axial rotation.

of 0.625 mm would only require a single axial rotation to cover the entire area (Fig. 24.14). When multiple axial slices are required, the scanner turns off between axial acquisitions, the table moves to the next region of the heart, and the scanner turns back on during the preselected portion of the cardiac cycle. This pattern of scanning has thus been termed "step-and-shoot." Another method of prospective scanning is the use of dual-source technology to allow for very fast, high-pitch, prospectively triggered helical scans. Using this high–temporal resolution technique, the entire heart is imaged during a single diastolic phase during a single heartbeat allowing for very-low-dose imaging (Fig. 24.15). With any form of prospective acquisition, images are only acquired during a portion of the R–R interval. Therefore, reconstructions in phases outside that interval are not possible and function cannot be assessed.

Retrospective ECG gating most commonly uses a low-pitch scan to acquire redundant CT data. Images are acquired throughout entire cardiac cycle over multiple continuous heartbeats with simultaneous ECG recording (Fig. 24.16). The desired cardiac phase is selected retrospectively, providing flexibility to reconstruct images at multiple cardiac phases. More recently, large detector row scanners with 16 cm of coverage can cover the entire heart in a single axial rotation. With this technology, a retrospective scan can be performed by an

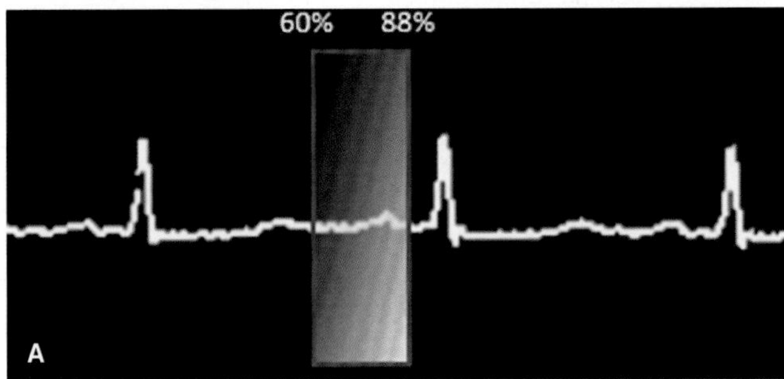

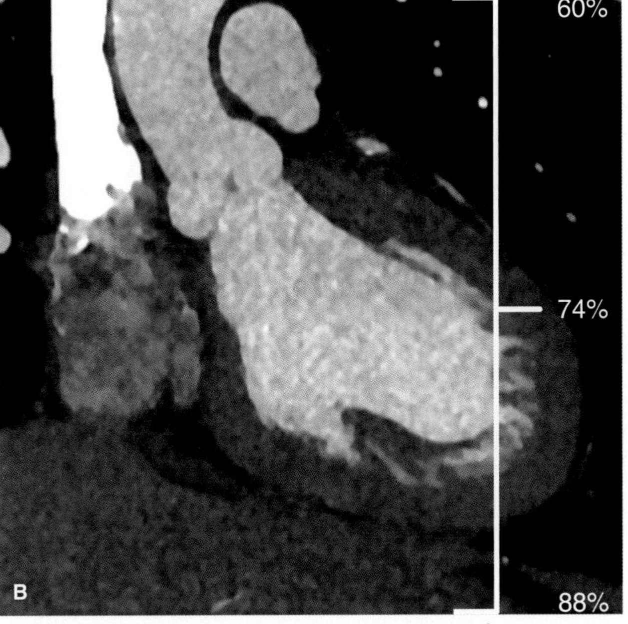

FIGURE 24.15. **Prospective Gating Using a High-Pitch Helical Technique. A:** While most vendors have scanners that perform prospective gating using an axial acquisition, one vendor uses two offset x-ray cameras coupled with a rapid table movement and high temporal resolution to create a high-pitch helical scan. In most instances, the entire scan is obtained during one diastolic portion of one heartbeat. Because the scan is helical, different slices are obtained at different portions of the R–R interval. For instance, in this example (**B**), which is acquired from superior to inferior, the top slices are obtained at 60% of the R–R interval. This percentage increases as the scan moves inferiorly so the most inferior slices are obtained at 88% of the R–R interval.

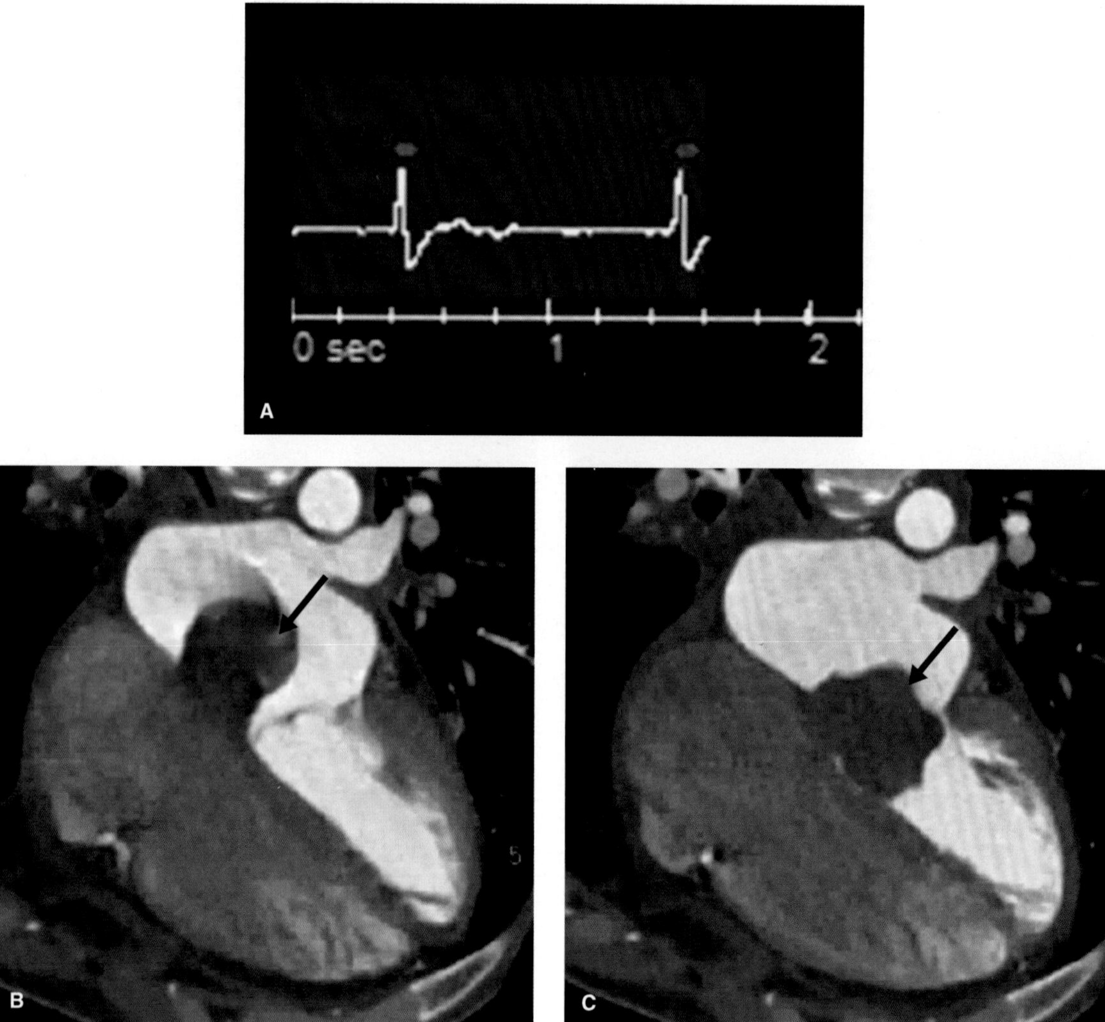

FIGURE 24.16. **A:** Using a retrospective ECG-gating technique without ECG dose modulation, images are acquired throughout the cardiac cycle using full tube current (*navy box*). This allows for retrospective selection and reconstruction of any desired cardiac phase(s) without any decrease in image quality at the cost of higher dose. With most scanners, these scans are obtained helically. **B, C:** Images from a cardiac CTA obtained during systole (**B**) and diastole (**C**) in a patient with a left atrial myxoma (*black arrows*) show low image noise creating high image quality throughout the cardiac cycle.

axial acquisition that occurs during the entire cardiac cycle. Retrospective ECG gating has the advantage of allowing for quantification of cardiac volumes and function. In addition, it is also helpful in patients with arrhythmias as the scan can be edited to remove data from irregular beats, such as in a premature ventricular contraction. However, this extra data comes at the cost of a higher radiation dose. This dose may be reduced with the use of ECG modulation of the tube current with concentration of the highest dose at a desired prespecified cardiac phase. Using dose modulation, images are still acquired throughout the entire cardiac cycle; however, a lower dose is applied over most of the cardiac cycle with full dose only over a shorter portion (typically diastole) (Fig. 24.17). While reduced dose phases can be used to assess cardiac function, they should not be used to evaluate for coronary artery disease.

Coronary artery calcium score (CACS) CT is a valuable imaging technique used to quantify coronary artery calcification. A low-dose ECG-gated nonenhanced CT is acquired through the heart (Fig. 24.18). CACS is a well-established test for risk-stratifying asymptomatic patients and is an independent predictor of long-term prognosis. The Agatston CACS is calculated based on a weighted density score given to the highest attenuation value multiplied by area of the calcification speck. Please refer to Chapter 25 for further details on calcium scoring.

Coronary CT angiography (CTA) is widely performed to assess the coronary arteries accurately and noninvasively (Fig. 24.19). Rapid technologic developments have led to improved spatial and temporal resolution. For example, expansion of multislice CT systems to 320-slice systems has allowed for acquisition of whole-heart coverage in one gantry rotation. Dual-energy CT can remove or reduce the depiction of coronary calcification to improve intraluminal evaluation of calcified vessels and provide detailed analysis of coronary plaque composition by decreasing beam hardening and enabling material decomposition.

Coronary CTA has high diagnostic accuracy for CAD compared to catheter angiography. Several professional societies have issued guidelines, expert consensus documents, and appropriateness criteria for coronary CTA. The clinical utility of coronary CTA in the setting of suspected stable CAD has been investigated in several large prospective trials, which

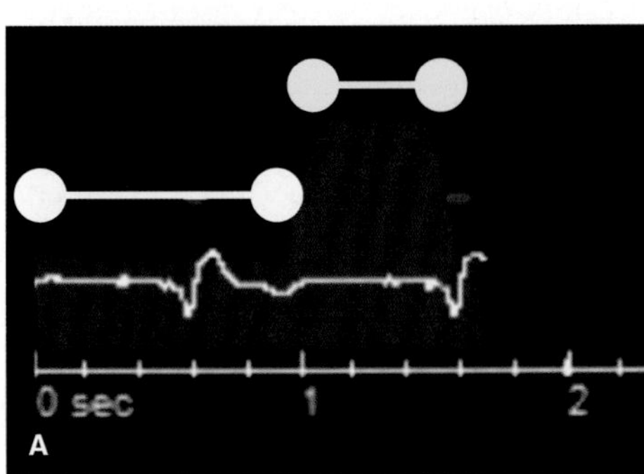

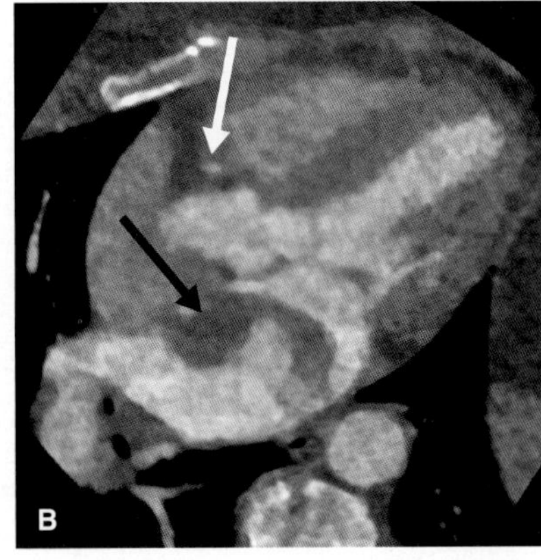

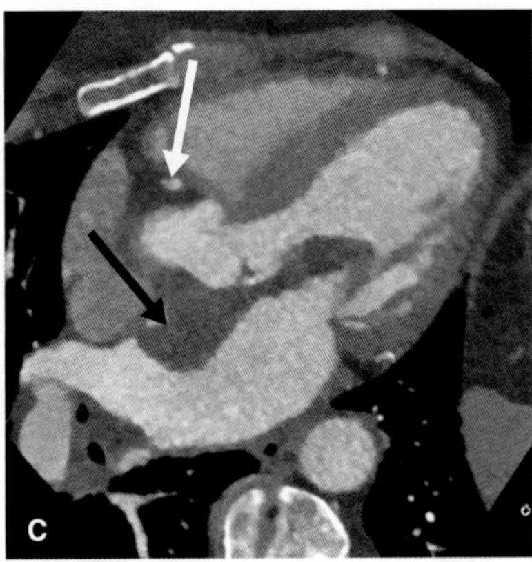

FIGURE 24.17. **A:** Using retrospective gating with ECG-based modulation of the tube current, images are acquired over the entire cardiac cycle. However full current (mA) is only delivered over a prespecified portion of the cardiac cycle (*yellow line*) and the remainder of the cardiac cycle receives a lower amount of current (*white line*). **B:** Images from a retrospectively gated CTA using ECG dose modulation in a patient with a left atrial myxoma show the effect of ECG dose modulation. With most scanners, these scans are obtained helically. During systole, when the mA is lowered, the images appear grainier due to increased noise. This can limit detailed evaluation of smaller structures, such as the right coronary artery (*white arrow*). However, the larger LA myxoma (*black arrow*) is still well visualized. **C:** During end diastole, when ECG dose modulation is off and the mA is maximized, the image has an overall better image quality due to decreased noise. Both the RCA (*white arrow*) and myxoma (*black arrow*) can be well visualized.

have demonstrated that coronary CTA is clinically useful as an alternative to or in addition to functional testing. Several large randomized trials have compared coronary CTA to the current standard of care in patients with acute chest pain, demonstrating the safety of a negative coronary CTA to identify patients for discharge from the emergency department. Coronary CTA is not recommended for cardiovascular risk assessment in asymptomatic adults. Please refer to Chapter 25 for further information of coronary CTA.

FIGURE 24.18. **Coronary Artery Calcium Score CT.** A low-dose ECG-gated nonenhanced CT is acquired through the heart allowing for visualization and quantification of coronary calcium (*red arrow*).

Cardiac MRI

Cardiac magnetic resonance imaging (MRI) is considered the reference standard for the assessment of cardiac structure and function. Cardiac MRI is a noninvasive imaging technique that does not expose the patient to ionizing radiation. Gadolinium-based contrast agents are frequently used in cardiac MRI. Using older gadolinium-based contrast agents, patients with impaired renal function demonstrated a risk of developing nephrogenic systemic fibrosis (NSF), which is predominantly associated with the administration of gadolinium-based

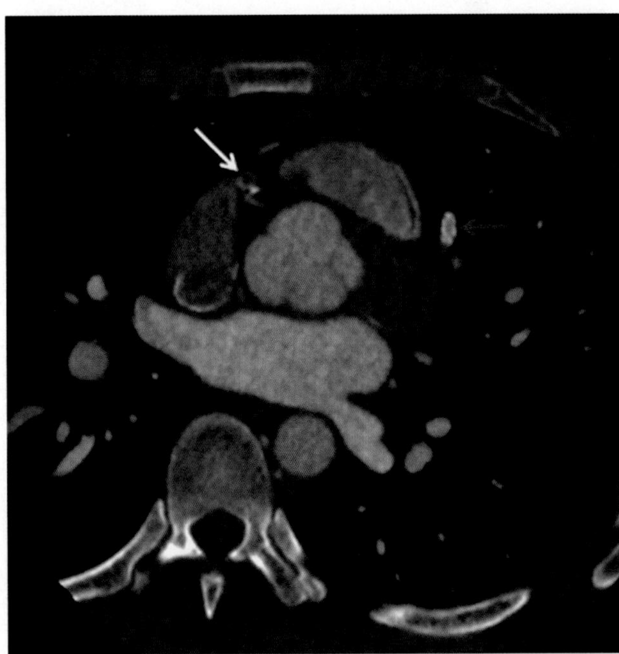

FIGURE 24.19. **Coronary CT Angiography.** Axial coronary CTA image demonstrates chronic total occlusion (CTO) of the proximal right coronary artery (*white arrow*) and a patent stent in the proximal left anterior descending coronary artery (*red arrow*).

contrast agents with linear structure. However, due to the improved safety profile of newer type II gadolinium agents, which are the ones most commonly used in cardiac MRI, the American College of Radiology (ACR) recently changed its guidelines. The new guidelines state that the assessment of renal function in any patient receiving a single dose of a type II agent is optional given the exceedingly low or possibly nonexistent risk of developing NSF. Nonetheless, any gadolinium agent should only be administered if deemed necessary by a supervising radiologist. Gadolinium deposition in the brain has been detected following repeated administration of gadolinium-based contrast agents, although no adverse clinical effects have been demonstrated to date.

Cardiac MRI contraindications previously included implanted devices, such as pacemakers and implantable cardioverter defibrillators (ICDs), given concerns that magnetic fields and radiofrequency energy could interact with and cause malfunction of the device or permanent damage to the device, leads, or heart at the lead–tissue interface. Multiple MRI-conditional cardiovascular implantable electronic devices (CIED) are now available. Very low rates of complications or clinically significant device parameter changes have been reported following MRI in patients with these devices. A recent expert consensus statement on MRI in patients with CIEDs has been published with recommendations and protocols for patients with conditional and nonconditional CIEDs. These guidelines state that it is reasonable for a patient with an MRI nonconditional CIED system to undergo MRI if there are no fractured, epicardial, or abandoned leads, MRI is the best test for the condition, and there is an institutional protocol and a designated responsible MRI physician and CIED physician.

Cardiac MRI indications include assessment of cardiac size and function, myocardial ischemia and viability, cardiomyopathies, myocarditis, iron overload, valvular disease, vascular diseases, and CHD. Cardiac MRI studies typically involve acquisition of a set of sequences that are tailored to the specific clinical indication, with studies typically lasting between 45 and 90 minutes in duration. The study begins with acquisition of localizers to assist with image planning. Conventional MRI techniques are adapted for cardiac imaging using ECG gating and high–temporal resolution sequences.

Cardiac imaging planes are typically used in cardiac MRI, as opposed to the standard body imaging planes (axial, coronal, and sagittal). Cardiac imaging planes include short-axis, two-chamber, three-chamber, and four-chamber planes (Fig. 24.20).

Cine imaging of the heart is typically achieved by acquiring a set of retrospectively gated balanced steady-state free precession (bSSFP) images in standard cardiac imaging planes (Fig. 24.20). Cine bSSFP has good temporal resolution and intrinsic image contrast due to the relatively high T2:T1 ratio of blood compared to myocardium. bSSFP techniques are produced by emitting an excitation radiofrequency pulse with short repetition time (TR) followed by gradient refocusing, and are less vulnerable to T2* effects compared with gradient recalled echo (GRE) imaging. Cine images are often obtained with ECG-triggered segmented imaging, in which the cardiac cycle is divided into multiple segments. Each image is composed of information gathered over multiple heartbeats. This approach requires multiple breath-holds to acquire a complete set of cardiac images. More recently, free-breathing and 3D volumetric cine acquisitions have been described which

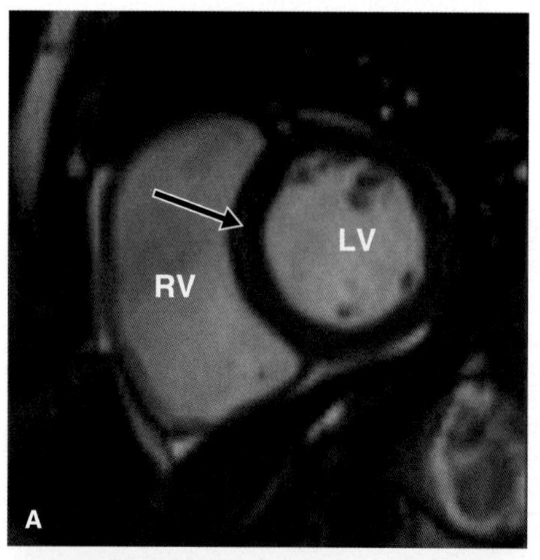

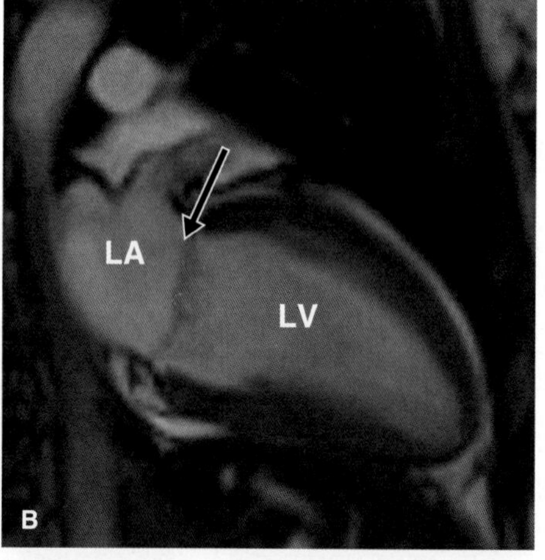

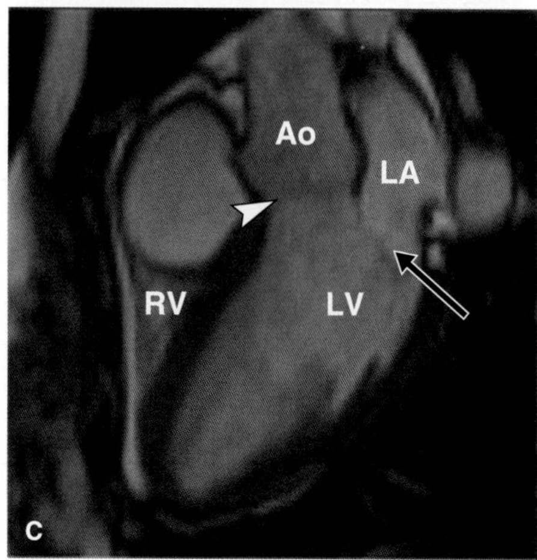

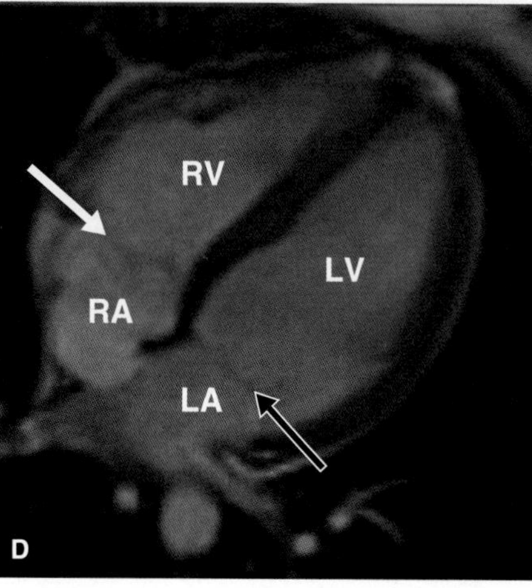

FIGURE 24.20. **Cardiac MRI Imaging Planes.** Cardiac MRI balanced steady-state free precession (bSSFP) images in standard cardiac imaging planes. **A:** Short-axis image demonstrates the left ventricle (*LV*) and right ventricle (*RV*) separated by the interventricular septum (*black arrow*). **B:** Two-chamber image demonstrates the left atrium (*LA*) and left ventricle (*LV*), which are separated by the mitral valve (*black arrow*). **C:** Three-chamber image demonstrates the *LA*, *LV*, and aortic root (*Ao*) as well as the mitral (*black arrow*) and aortic (*white arrowhead*) valves. **D:** Four-chamber image demonstrates the *LV*, *RV*, *LA*, and right atrium (*RA*) as well as the mitral (*red arrow*) and tricuspid (*white arrow*) valves.

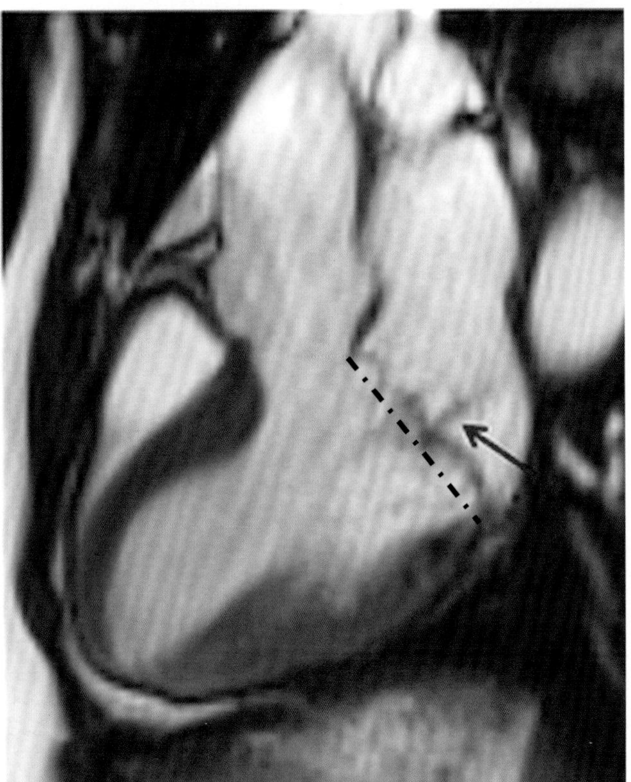

FIGURE 24.21. **Mitral Regurgitation.** Cardiac MRI three-chamber bSSFP image demonstrates moderate mitral regurgitation, which is visualized qualitatively as signal dephasing (*red arrow*). In systole, the mitral valve leaflets extend posterior to the mitral valve plane (*dotted black line*) consistent with mitral valve prolapse.

eliminate or minimize the need for breath holding and result in much shorter acquisition times. 3D cine imaging also eliminates the need for images to be acquired in multiple planes, thereby reducing planning and scan time.

A short-axis stack of images covering both ventricles from the base to apex is usually acquired. Quantification of ventricular end-diastolic and end-systolic volumes, ejection fraction, stroke volume, cardiac output, and myocardial mass can be achieved by contouring endocardial and epicardial borders at end-diastole and end-systole using cardiac postprocessing software according to standardized guidelines. Turbulent flow causes signal dephasing, allowing valvular disease (including regurgitation) to be assessed qualitatively (Fig. 24.21). Atrial size can evaluated visually or by assessing cross-sectional areas or volumes.

Phase contrast MRI is a technique that allows for reliable quantification of regurgitant and shunt flow volumes, visualization of time-resolved flow patterns, and assessment of wall shear stress and turbulence. Common indications for phase contrast imaging include valvular disease and CHD. Phase contrast imaging is traditionally acquired as a 2D slice prescribed in an oblique plane perpendicular through the vessel of interest using gated phase contrast sequences sensitized to through-plane velocity. The typical acquisition is a time-resolved or multiphase 2D GRE sequence. Two sets of raw image data are acquired with a difference in the gradient first moment, from which both velocity and magnitude images are reconstructed (Fig. 24.22). 2D phase contrast acquisitions can be acquired in breath-hold or free breathing, usually with a segmented acquisition. An important parameter in acquiring phase contrast imaging is the velocity encoding value, or VENC. Typically the VENC is set to be slightly greater than the largest velocities expected. A low VENC results in higher-phase signal-to-noise ratio. However, unwanted flow–related aliasing occurs if too low a value of VENC is selected.

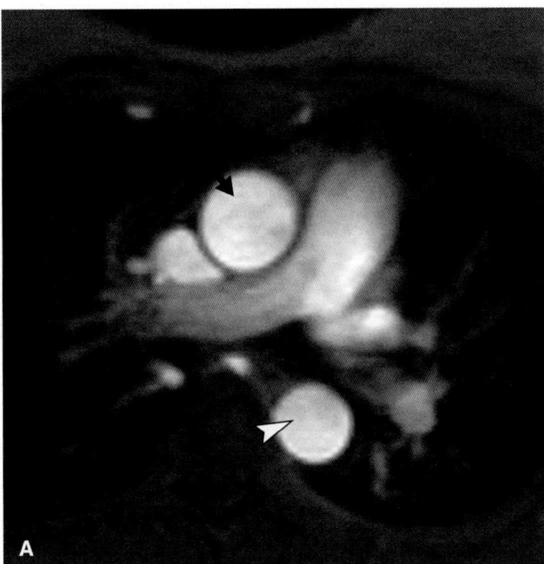

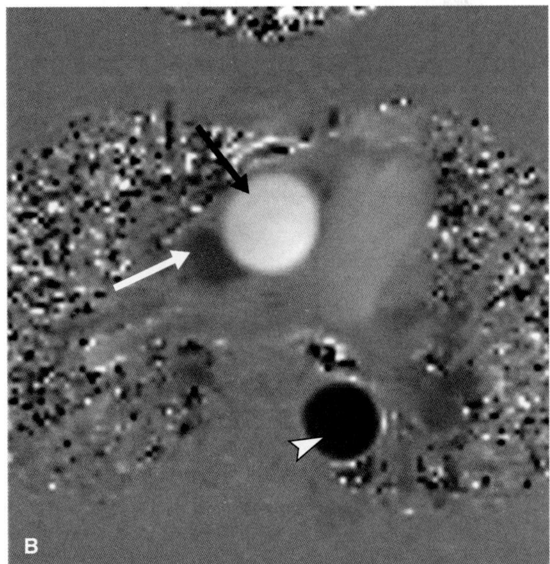

FIGURE 24.22. **Phase Contrast MRI. 2D** Phase contrast images were acquired orthogonal to the ascending (*black arrow*) and descending (*white arrowhead*) thoracic aorta at the level of the main pulmonary artery. **A:** The magnitude image provides anatomic information without specifying direction of flow. **B:** The phase image allows for quantification of the velocity of blood flow. Blood flowing superiorly, such as that in the ascending aorta (*black arrow*), appears as bright signal whereas blood flowing inferiorly, such as in the descending thoracic aorta (*white arrowhead*), appears dark in signal. While the blood in the superior vena cava (SVC, *white arrow*) also flows inferiorly, the signal in the SVC is not as dark as that of the descending thoracic aorta because the velocity of flow in the SVC is much less than that of the aorta.

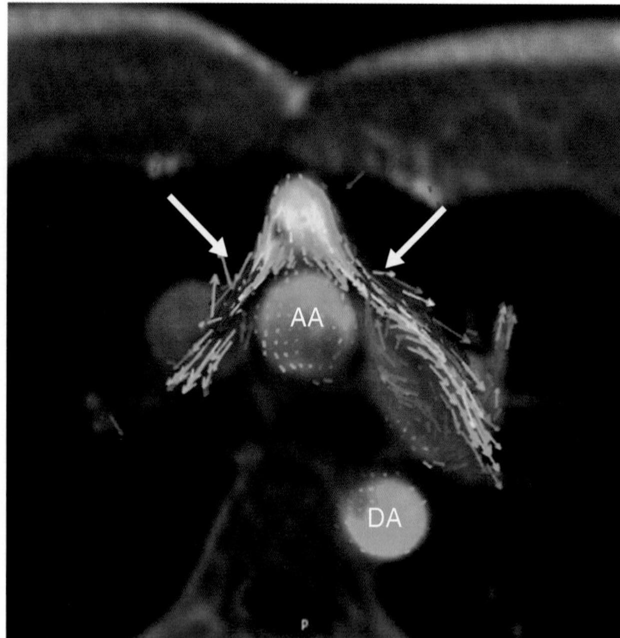

FIGURE 24.23. **4D Flow Phase Contrast MRI.** Axial oblique image from a 4D flow phase contrast MRI in a patient with complete transposition of the great arteries status post arterial switch surgery and Lecompte maneuver, shows areas of increased velocities in the proximal left and right pulmonary arteries (*white arrows*). These vessels are narrowed as they extend around the ascending aorta, which is a common late complication following arterial switch procedure. An advantage of 4D flow is that many different imaging planes can be reformatted at the time of analysis, without restrictions to predefined imaging planes. AA, ascending aorta; DA, descending thoracic aorta.

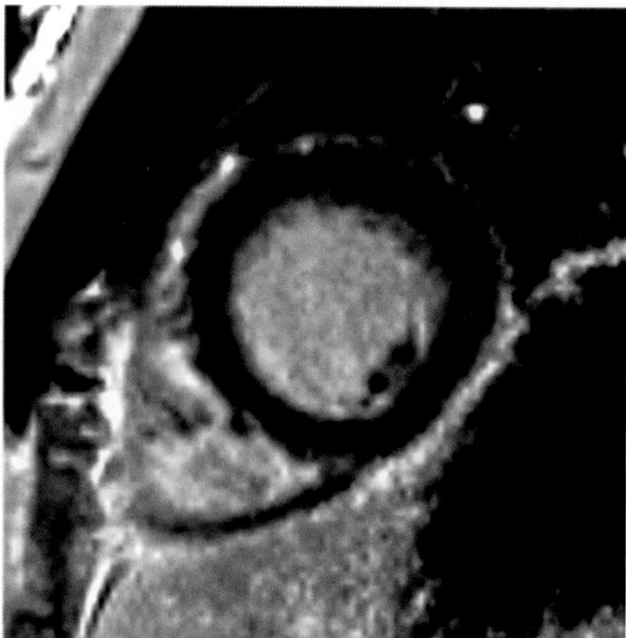

FIGURE 24.24. **Late Gadolinium Enhancement Cardiac MRI.** Short-axis late gadolinium-enhanced image in a healthy volunteer demonstrates normal nulling of the myocardium, which appears black.

More recently, ECG-synchronized 3D phase contrast MRI using three-directional velocity encoding, or four-dimensional (4D) flow MRI, has been described and is now routinely used in many centers. 4D-flow MRI consists of a volumetric time-resolved acquisition that is gated to the cardiac cycle, providing a time-varying vector field of blood flow in addition to anatomic images. An advantage of 4D flow is that many different imaging planes can be reformatted at the time of analysis, without restrictions to predefined imaging planes (Fig. 24.23). For both 2D and 4D phase contrast approaches, background error must be removed using postprocessing algorithms. The most common approach is to measure the phase in the static background tissue surrounding the flow, and then use these measurements to estimate the phase correction throughout the image.

Late gadolinium enhancement (LGE) imaging is a reproducible method for assessing infarct and macroscopic or replacement fibrosis, with prognostic value in patients with ischemic and nonischemic cardiomyopathies. The presence, extent, and pattern of delayed enhancement are helpful in diagnosing and monitoring patients with cardiomyopathies.

LGE imaging is typically acquired 10 to 20 minutes after administration of 0.1 to 0.2 mmol/kg gadolinium-based contrast agent. Gadolinium is paramagnetic and therefore reduces T1 time. Gadolinium-based contrast agents distribute in the extracellular space and under normal circumstances do not enter myocardial cells. In certain pathologic conditions, the volume of distribution of contrast is increased due to expansion of the extracellular space (such as collagen deposition in the setting of fibrosis) or myocardial cell membrane disruption (such as infarction), leading to enhancement on LGE images. Normal myocardium will appear black (Fig. 24.24). Areas of infarct and fibrosis with higher gadolinium concentration and consequently shorter T1 and faster recovery will appear bright (Figs. 24.12 and 24.25). The blood pool typically has bright signal as well due to the presence of gadolinium in the blood.

The most commonly used sequences for LGE imaging are inversion recovery (IR) or phase-sensitive inversion recovery (PSIR) using ECG-gated, segmented FLASH readout. With IR sequences, an adequate inversion time (TI) must be selected to null the signal from normal myocardium and provide the best tissue contrast between infarct/fibrosis and normal myocardial

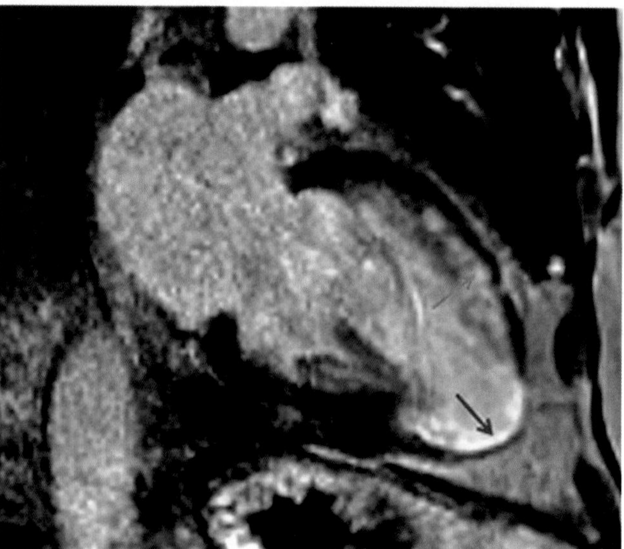

FIGURE 24.25. **Myocardial Infarct on Late Gadolinium Enhancement Cardiac MRI.** Two-chamber late gadolinium–enhanced (LGE) image demonstrates subendocardial hyperintensity at the mid-to-apical anterior wall (*orange arrow*) and transmural enhancement at the apex (*red arrow*) in keeping with an infarct.

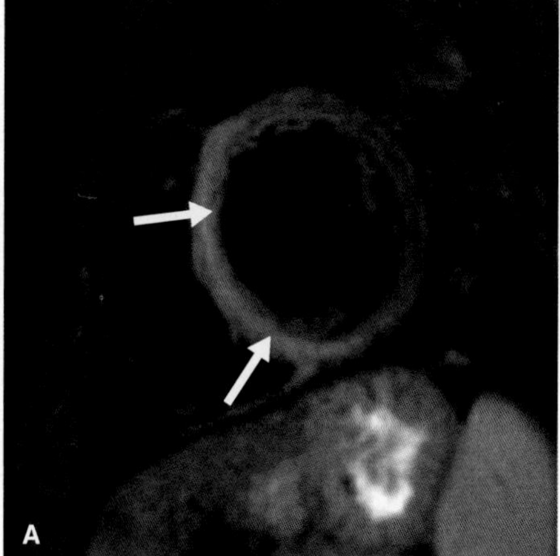

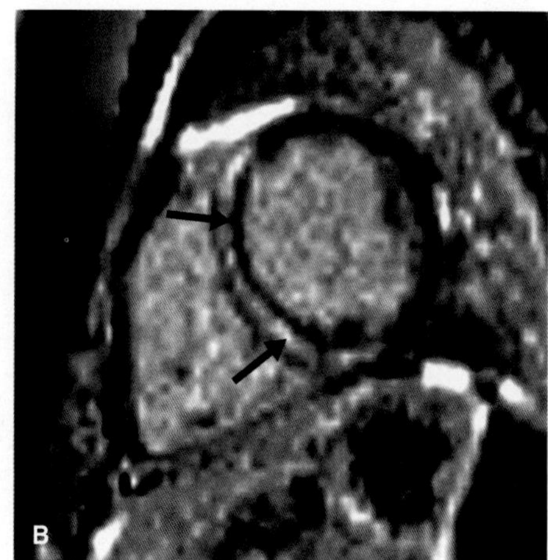

FIGURE 24.26. **Myocarditis. A:** Short-axis T2-weighted black-blood cardiac MRI demonstrates linear midwall hyperintensity (*white arrows*) in the interventricular septum in a patient with viral myocarditis. **B:** Late gadolinium–enhanced image demonstrates corresponding enhancement in the interventricular septum (*black arrows*).

tissue. Optimal TI varies depending on several factors including cardiac output and contrast kinetics. The TI can be determined by trial and error or by using a Look–Locker sequence that acquires a series of images with variable TI during one breath-hold. PSIR techniques partially overcome the limitation of appropriate TI selection. More recently, the use of IR or PSIR with single-shot steady-state free precession (SSFP) has been used for rapid multislice coverage or in cases where patients have arrhythmias or difficulty breath holding.

Cardiac tissue characterization has also been described using multiple noncontrast techniques including T2-weighted imaging, T2* imaging, T1-weighted imaging with and without fat suppression, and diffusion-weighted imaging (DWI). These techniques are useful both for myocardial tissue characterization as well as tumor assessment.

T2-weighted imaging is used for the assessment of myocardial edema and inflammation, such as in the setting of acute infarction, myocarditis, stress cardiomyopathy, and cardiac sarcoidosis. Similar to LGE, the extent and pattern of signal abnormality are helpful in distinguishing between different underlying etiologies. In general, the long T2 relaxation times of water-bound protons result in high signal intensity of edematous tissue on T2-weighted imaging (Fig. 24.26). Standard myocardial T2-weighted imaging typically utilizes turbo spin–echo (TSE) readouts with or without fat saturation pulses, combined with dark-blood preparation. More recently, T2-weighted, SSFP-based sequences have been described. Limitations of T2-weighted imaging include an incomplete dark-blood preparation resulting in a bright-rim blood artifact adjacent to the endocardium.

T2 imaging* is used for assessment of myocardial iron, most commonly in the setting of transfusion-dependent anemias such as β-thalassemia major. Intracellular iron results in shortening of the MRI relaxation parameter T2* due to magnetic field inhomogeneity. Myocardial T2* can be quantified reproducibly and has been shown to correlate inversely with iron deposition. T2* techniques include gradient-echo imaging with multiple breath-holds, multiecho gradient-echo imaging with a single breath-hold (Fig. 24.27), and black-blood imaging using a double IR sequence with acquisition of multiecho T2* images in late diastole. Myocardial T2* is commonly assessed using a midventricular slice by sampling a region of interest in the interventricular septum. Liver T2* can also be quantified as the short-axis slices of the myocardium often include portions of the liver in the field of view.

Parametric mapping techniques allow for quantification of myocardial tissue based on changes in T1, T2, and T2* relaxation times and extracellular volume (ECV). T1 and T2 are intrinsic magnetic properties of tissue that represent longitudinal and transverse recovery times of hydrogen atoms after excitation, respectively. Each tissue has its own characteristic range of T1 and T2 values, which may be altered in disease. T2* is always less than or equal to T2 and results primarily from inhomogeneities in the main magnetic field. Parametric mapping allows for quantification, potentially standardizing cardiac MRI measurements of myocardial tissue properties.

T1 maps can be produced of noncontrast (or native) myocardial T1 values or postcontrast myocardial T1 values. The combination of pre- and postcontrast T1 mapping allows for calculation of the myocardial partition coefficient, lambda, with subsequent derivation of ECV by adjustment for the contrast distribution volume using hematocrit. A benefit of native T1 mapping over LGE techniques is that administration of contrast is not required.

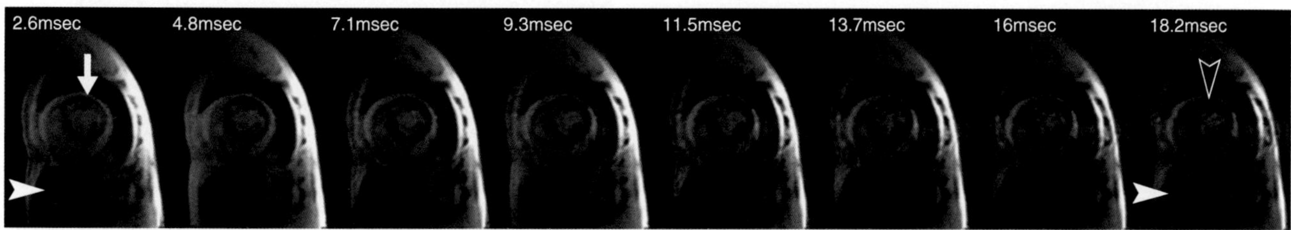

FIGURE 24.27. **T2* Imaging With MRI.** Short-axis multiecho gradient echo sequence obtained through the left ventricular midcavity shows rapid degradation of myocardial signal at increasing echo times from 2.6 ms (*white arrow*) to 18.2 ms (*black arrowhead*). This is secondary to the increased myocardial iron deposition in this patient with hemochromatosis. Short-axis imaging also allows for liver T2* quantification (*white arrowhead*) which is usually involved in most cases of hemochromatosis.

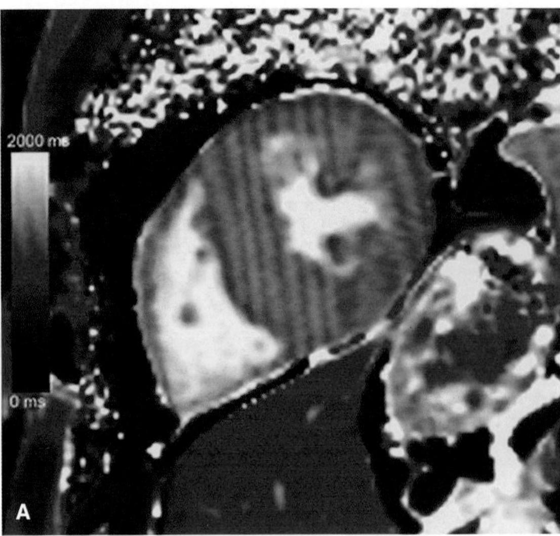

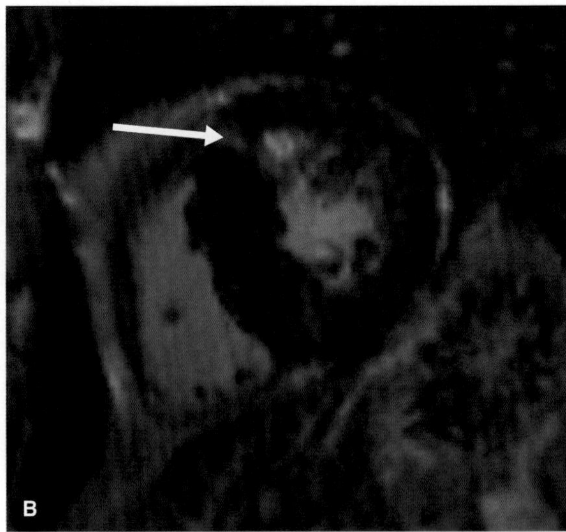

FIGURE 24.28. **Hypertrophic Cardiomyopathy. A:** Short-axis noncontrast cardiac MRI T1 map in a patient with asymmetric septal hypertrophic cardiomyopathy (HCM). Noncontrast T1 values at the interventricular septum (1,320 ms at 3T) are elevated above the normal reference range in keeping with fibrosis. **B:** Late gadolinium–enhanced image demonstrates fibrosis at the anterior right ventricular insertion point (*white arrow*) and hypertrophied anterior septum.

Noncontrast myocardial T1 values are elevated, postcontrast T1 values are reduced, and ECV values are elevated when the extracellular space is expanded, such as in the setting of myocardial fibrosis (Fig. 24.28). Elevated noncontrast T1 and ECV values have also been described in the setting of cardiac amyloid infiltration and myocardial edema. On the other hand, noncontrast T1 values are reduced in several conditions including iron overload, fat infiltration, Fabry disease, and hemorrhage.

Multiple different T1 mapping techniques are currently available, including modified Look–Locker inversion recovery (MOLLI), shortened MOLLI sequence (ShMOLLI), saturation recovery single-shot acquisition (SASHA), and saturation pulse prepared heart-rate-independent inversion recovery (SAPPHIRE) techniques. IR techniques have been shown to underestimate native myocardial T1, whereas saturation recovery techniques yield higher accuracy but lower precision. T1 values vary based on other factors including magnetic field strength, with significantly higher noncontrast T1 values at 3T compared to 1.5T. Therefore, absolute T1 measurements must be interpreted based on the specific technique employed.

T2 maps can be generated by obtaining a series of images to calculate a T2 decay curve, from which myocardial T2 relaxation times can be directly determined. T2 values are elevated in myocardial edema, including acute infarction, myocarditis, stress cardiomyopathy, and sarcoidosis (Fig. 24.29). Several different T2 mapping techniques have been described. In general, a T2 preparation pulse is applied to impart T2 signal contrast, and a subsequent readout is performed by using an SSFP or fast low-angle shot (FLASH) sequence. SSFP-based

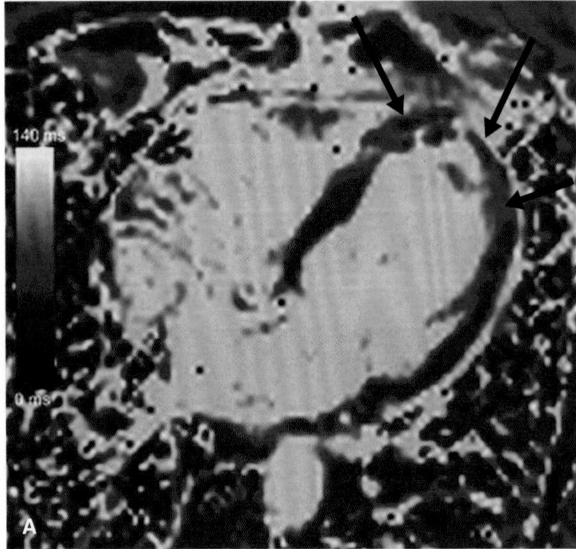

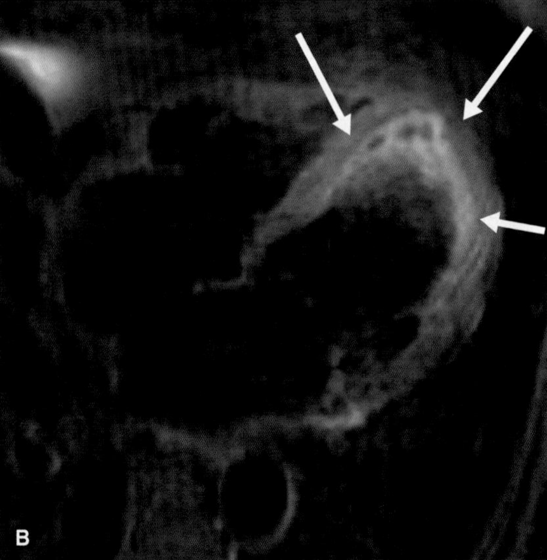

FIGURE 24.29. **Stress Cardiomyopathy. A:** Four-chamber cardiac MRI T2 map in a patient with stress (Takotsubo) cardiomyopathy. T2 values are elevated at the apex (70 ms, *black arrows*) above the normal reference range in keeping with edema. **B:** Four-chamber cardiac MRI black-blood T2-weighted image demonstrates corresponding hyperintensity at the apex (*white arrows*) due to edema.

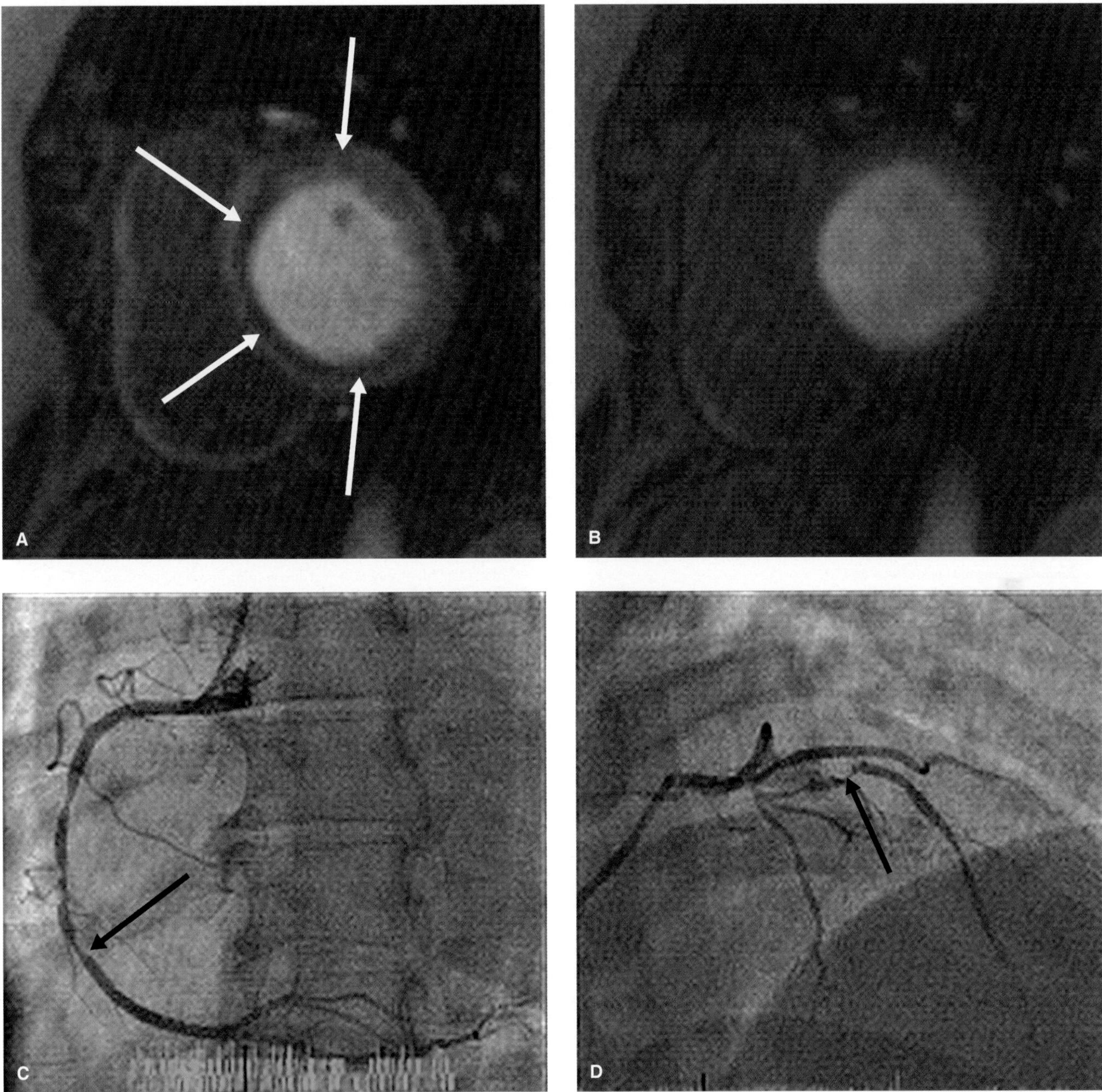

FIGURE 24.30. **Stress Perfusion Cardiac MRI and Catheter Coronary Angiography. A:** Short-axis stress perfusion cardiac MRI image demonstrates subendocardial hypoperfusion (low signal intensity) at the anterior wall, anterior septum, inferior septum, and inferior wall (*white arrows*). **B:** Short-axis rest perfusion cardiac MRI image demonstrates no rest perfusion defect. There was no evidence of late gadolinium enhancement to suggest the presence of infarct or fibrosis (not shown). **C:** Coronary catheter angiography image demonstrates several areas of severe (>70%) stenosis in the proximal and mid right coronary artery (*black arrow*). **D:** Coronary catheter angiography image demonstrates several areas of severe (>70%) stenosis in the left anterior descending and right coronary arteries (*black arrow*).

T2-mapping may slightly overestimate T2 values, but offers more signal-to-noise and less image artifacts.

Cardiac MRI perfusion imaging can be used to characterize coronary flow reserve and myocardial perfusion under rest and stress conditions. Perfusion is typically assessed using first-pass imaging, where contrast enhancement during the first pass of a contrast agent bolus through the cardiac chambers and the myocardium is evaluated and measured. Cardiac MRI perfusion studies primarily rely on the use of T1-weighted techniques, with multiple images acquired every heartbeat for a duration of approximately 60 heartbeats, covering a precontrast phase, the first pass of the contrast agent, and recirculation of contrast. The acquisition is too long for a single breath-hold and motion-correction algorithms can be applied during postprocessing (Fig. 24.30).

Suggested Readings

Achenbach S, Marwan M, Schepis T, et al. High-pitch spiral acquisition: a new scan mode for coronary CT angiography. *J Cardiovasc Comput Tomogr* 2009;3:117–121.

ACR Committee on Drugs and Contrast Media. ACR manual on contrast media. Available from https://www.acr.org/-/media/ACR/Files/Clinical-Resources/Contrast_Media.pdf. 2017.

Agatston AS, Janowitz WR, Hildner FJ, Zusmer NR, Viamonte MJ, Detrano R. Quantification of coronary artery calcium using ultrafast computed tomography. *J Am Coll Cardiol* 1990;15:827–832.

Baksi AJ, Pennell DJ. T1 mapping in heart failure: from technique to prognosis, toward altering outcome. *Circ Cardiovasc Imaging* 2013;6:861–863.

Blanke P, Bulla S, Baumann T, et al. Thoracic aorta: prospective electrocardiographically triggered CT angiography with dual-source CT—feasibility, image quality, and dose reduction. *Radiology* 2010;255:207–217.

Budoff MJ, Shaw LJ, Liu ST, et al. Long-term prognosis associated with coronary calcification: observations from a registry of 25,253 patients. *J Am Coll Cardiol* 2007;49:1860–1870.

Burt JR, Zimmerman SL, Kamel IR, Halushka M, Bluemke DA. Myocardial T1 mapping: techniques and potential applications. *RadioGraphics* 2014; 34:377–395.

Carpenter JP, He T, Kirk P, et al. On T2* magnetic resonance and cardiac iron. *Circulation* 2011;123:1519–1528.

Chareonthaitawee P, Beanlands RS, Chen W, et al. Joint SNMMI-ASNC expert consensus document on the role of (18)F-FDG PET/CT in cardiac sarcoid detection and therapy monitoring. *J Nucl Med* 2017;58:1341–1353.

Coelho-Filho OR, Rickers C, Kwong RY, Jerosch-Herold M. MR myocardial perfusion imaging. *Radiology* 2013;266:701–715.

Dass S, Suttie JJ, Piechnik SK, et al. Myocardial tissue characterization using magnetic resonance noncontrast t1 mapping in hypertrophic and dilated cardiomyopathy. *Circ Cardiovasc Imaging* 2012;5:726–733.

Doltra A, Amundsen BH, Gebker R, Fleck E, Kelle S. Emerging concepts for myocardial late gadolinium enhancement MRI. *Current Cardiology Reviews* 2013;9:185–190.

Douglas PS, Hoffmann U, Patel MR, et al. Outcomes of anatomical versus functional testing for coronary artery disease. *N Engl J Med* 2015;372:1291–1300.

Dvorak RA, Brown RK, Corbett JR. Interpretation of SPECT/CT myocardial perfusion images: common artifacts and quality control techniques. *RadioGraphics* 2011;31:2041–2057.

Eitel I, Friedrich MG. T2-weighted cardiovascular magnetic resonance in acute cardiac disease. *J Cardiovasc Magn Reson* 2011;13:13.

Flett AS, Hayward MP, Ashworth MT, et al. Equilibrium contrast cardiovascular magnetic resonance for the measurement of diffuse myocardial fibrosis: preliminary validation in humans. *Circulation* 2010;122:138–144.

Germain P, El Ghannudi S, Jeung MY, et al. Native T1 mapping of the heart—a pictorial review. *Clin Med Insights Cardiol* 2014;8:1–11.

Gimbel JR, Bello D, Schmitt M, et al. Randomized trial of pacemaker and lead system for safe scanning at 1.5 Tesla. *Heart Rhythm* 2013;10:685–691.

Giri S, Chung YC, Merchant A, et al. T2 quantification for improved detection of myocardial edema. *J Cardiovasc Magn Reson* 2009;11:56.

Gold MR, Sommer T, Schwitter J, et al. Full-body MRI in patients with an implantable cardioverter-defibrillator: primary results of a randomized study. *J Am Coll Cardiol* 2015;65:2581–2588.

Gulani V, Calamante F, Shellock FG, Kanal E, Reeder SB. Gadolinium deposition in the brain: summary of evidence and recommendations. *Lancet Neurol* 2017;16:564–570.

He T, Gatehouse PD, Kirk P, et al. Black-blood T2* technique for myocardial iron measurement in thalassemia. *J Magn Reson Imaging* 2007;25:1205–1209.

Heidary S, Patel H, Chung J, et al. Quantitative tissue characterization of infarct core and border zone in patients with ischemic cardiomyopathy by magnetic resonance is associated with future cardiovascular events. *J Am Coll Cardiol* 2010;55:2762–2768.

Higgins CB, Reinke RT, Jones NE, Broderick T. Left atrial dimension on the frontal thoracic radiograph: a method for assessing left atrial enlargement. *AJR Am J Roentgenol* 1978;130:251–255.

Ho SY, Cabrera JA, Sanchez-Quintana D. Left atrial anatomy revisited. *Circ Arrhythm Electrophysiol* 2012;5:220–228.

Hoffman RB, Rigler LG. Evaluation of left ventricular enlargement in the lateral projection of the chest. *Radiology* 1965;85:93–100.

Hoffmann U, Truong QA, Schoenfeld DA, et al. Coronary CT angiography versus standard evaluation in acute chest pain. *N Engl J Med* 2012;367:299–308.

Huang TY, Liu YJ, Stemmer A, Poncelet BP. T2 measurement of the human myocardium using a T2-prepared transient-state TrueFISP sequence. *Magn Reson Med* 2007;57:960–966.

Indik JH, Gimbel JR, Abe H, et al. 2017 HRS expert consensus statement on magnetic resonance imaging and radiation exposure in patients with cardiovascular implantable electronic devices. *Heart Rhythm* 2017;14:e97–e153.

Kellman P, Arai AE. Cardiac imaging techniques for physicians: late enhancement. *J Magn Reson Imaging* 2012;36:529–542.

Kronenberg MW, Parrish MD, Jenkins DW Jr, Sandler MP, Friesinger GC. Accuracy of radionuclide ventriculography for estimation of left ventricular volume changes and end-systolic pressure-volume relations. *J Am Coll Cardiol* 1985;6:1064–1072.

Kuruvilla S, Adenaw N, Katwal AB, Lipinski MJ, Kramer CM, Salerno M. Late gadolinium enhancement on cardiac magnetic resonance predicts adverse cardiovascular outcomes in nonischemic cardiomyopathy: a systematic review and meta-analysis. *Circ Cardiovasc Imaging* 2014;7:250–258.

Langman DA, Goldberg IB, Finn JP, Ennis DB. Pacemaker lead tip heating in abandoned and pacemaker-attached leads at 1.5 Tesla MRI. *J Magn Reson Imaging* 2011;33:426–431.

Lin SL, Hsu TL, Liou JY, et al. Usefulness of transesophageal echocardiography for the detection of left atrial thrombi in patients with rheumatic heart disease. *Echocardiography* 1992;9:161–168.

Litt HI, Gatsonis C, Snyder B, et al. CT angiography for safe discharge of patients with possible acute coronary syndromes. *N Engl J Med* 2012;366:1393–1403.

Malik SB, Chen N, Parker RA 3rd, Hsu JY. Transthoracic echocardiography: pitfalls and limitations as delineated at cardiac CT and MR imaging. *RadioGraphics* 2017;37:383–406.

Miller JM, Rochitte CE, Dewey M, et al. Diagnostic performance of coronary angiography by 64-row CT. *N Engl J Med* 2008;359:2324–2336.

Nayak KS, Nielsen JF, Bernstein MA, et al. Cardiovascular magnetic resonance phase contrast imaging. *J Cardiovasc Magn Reson* 2015;17:71.

Paul JF, Abada HT. Strategies for reduction of radiation dose in cardiac multislice CT. *Eur Radiol* 2007;17:2028–2037.

Pedersen SF, Thrysøe SA, Robich MP, et al. Assessment of intramyocardial hemorrhage by T1-weighted cardiovascular magnetic resonance in reperfused acute myocardial infarction. *J Cardiovasc Magn Reson* 2012;14:1–8.

Petersen SE, Aung N, Sanghvi MM, et al. Reference ranges for cardiac structure and function using cardiovascular magnetic resonance (CMR) in Caucasians from the UK Biobank population cohort. *J Cardiovasc Magn Reson* 2017;19:18.

Pica S, Sado DM, Maestrini V, et al. Reproducibility of native myocardial T1 mapping in the assessment of Fabry disease and its role in early detection of cardiac involvement by cardiovascular magnetic resonance. *J Cardiovasc Magn Reson* 2014;16:99.

Puntmann VO, Isted A, Hinojar R, Foote L, Carr-White G, Nagel E. T1 and T2 mapping in recognition of early cardiac involvement in systemic sarcoidosis. *Radiology* 2017;285:63–72.

Roujol S, Weingartner S, Foppa M, et al. Accuracy, precision, and reproducibility of four T1 mapping sequences: a head-to-head comparison of MOLLI, ShMOLLI, SASHA, and SAPPHIRE. *Radiology* 2014;272:683–689.

Sado DM, Maestrini V, Piechnik SK, et al. Noncontrast myocardial T1 mapping using cardiovascular magnetic resonance for iron overload. *J Magn Reson Imaging* 2015;41:1505–1511.

Sadowski EA, Bennett LK, Chan MR, et al. Nephrogenic systemic fibrosis: risk factors and incidence estimation. *Radiology* 2007;243:148–157.

Schindler TH, Schelbert HR, Quercioli A, Dilsizian V. Cardiac PET imaging for the detection and monitoring of coronary artery disease and microvascular health. *JACC Cardiovasc Imaging* 2010;3:623–640.

Schulz-Menger J, Bluemke DA, Bremerich J, et al. Standardized image interpretation and post processing in cardiovascular magnetic resonance: Society for Cardiovascular Magnetic Resonance (SCMR) board of trustees task force on standardized post processing. *J Cardiovasc Magn Reson* 2013;15:35.

SCOT-HEART Investigators. CT coronary angiography in patients with suspected angina due to coronary heart disease (SCOT-HEART): an open-label, parallel-group, multicentre trial. *Lancet* 2015;385:2383–2391.

Sheehan F, Redington A. The right ventricle: anatomy, physiology and clinical imaging. *Heart* 2008;94:1510–1515.

Simonetti OP, Finn JP, White RD, Laub G, Henry DA. "Black blood" T2-weighted inversion-recovery MR imaging of the heart. *Radiology* 1996; 199:49–57.

Spieker M, Haberkorn S, Gastl M, et al. Abnormal T2 mapping cardiovascular magnetic resonance correlates with adverse clinical outcome in patients with suspected acute myocarditis. *J Cardiovasc Magn Reson* 2017;19:38.

Sun Z, Lin C, Davidson R, Dong C, Liao Y. Diagnostic value of 64-slice CT angiography in coronary artery disease: a systematic review. *Eur J Radiol* 2008;67:78–84.

Usman M, Ruijsink B, Nazir MS, Cruz G, Prieto C. Free breathing whole-heart 3D CINE MRI with self-gated Cartesian trajectory. *Magn Reson Imaging* 2017;38:129–137.

Vasanawala SS, Hanneman K, Alley MT, Hsiao A. Congenital heart disease assessment with 4D flow MRI. *J Magn Reson Imaging* 2015;42(4):870–886.

Wassmuth R, Prothmann M, Utz W, et al. Variability and homogeneity of cardiovascular magnetic resonance myocardial T2-mapping in volunteers compared to patients with edema. *J Cardiovasc Magn Reson* 2013;15:27–27.

Xue H, Kellman P, Larocca G, Arai AE, Hansen MS. High spatial and temporal resolution retrospective cine cardiovascular magnetic resonance from shortened free breathing real-time acquisitions. *J Cardiovasc Magn Reson* 2013;15:102.

CHAPTER 25 ■ CORONARY ARTERY ANOMALIES AND DISEASE

SETH KLIGERMAN

Noninvasive imaging of the coronary arteries can be obtained through various modalities including ultrasound (echocardiography), CT, and MRI. While echocardiography is a useful tool to rapidly assess systolic and diastolic myocardial function and complications of myocardial infarct, its ability to directly assess the coronary arteries is limited. Due to its excellent spatial resolution as low as 0.5 mm and temporal resolution as low as 66 ms, cardiac CTA has become the primary tool to directly visualize the anatomy as well as congenital and acquired anomalies of the coronary arteries. While cardiac MRI can be used to assess the coronary arteries, its strength lies in its ability to assess for myocardial damage after infarction and to guide therapy.

CORONARY ARTERY ANATOMY

The coronary arteries course through the epicardial fat to supply oxygenated blood to the myocardium. Coronary artery anatomy is highly variable, and the size and distribution of the coronary arteries vary from person to person. Given this, it is important to distinguish normal variant anatomy from congenital abnormalities. It is also imperative to distinguish between benign congenital anomalies and ones that can compromise myocardial blood flow with subsequent myocardial ischemia, infarction, or sudden cardiac death.

Left Main Coronary Artery

The coronary arteries arise from the sinuses of Valsalva, which are three anatomic outpouchings in the ascending aorta. The left main coronary artery and right coronary artery (RCA) arise from the left and right sinuses, respectively (Fig. 25.1). No coronary artery should arise from the noncoronary sinus, which is directed posteriorly toward the interatrial septum.

After its origin from the left sinus of Valsalva, the left main coronary artery courses laterally to the left before dividing. It is usually the largest coronary artery but is of variable length. In most people, the left main coronary artery bifurcates into an anteriorly directed left anterior descending coronary artery (LAD) and a posteriorly directed left circumflex coronary artery (LCx) (Fig. 25.2). In approximately 20% to 30% of patients, the left main coronary artery trifurcates with a ramus intermedius branch arising between the LAD and LCx (Fig. 25.3).

Left Anterior Descending Coronary Artery

The LAD is usually a large vessel that runs along the anterior surface of the left ventricle (LV) (Fig. 25.4). The LAD can be of variable length but usually wraps around the left ventricular apex before terminating. The LAD is divided into three portions, proximal, mid, and distal (Fig. 25.5). The proximal

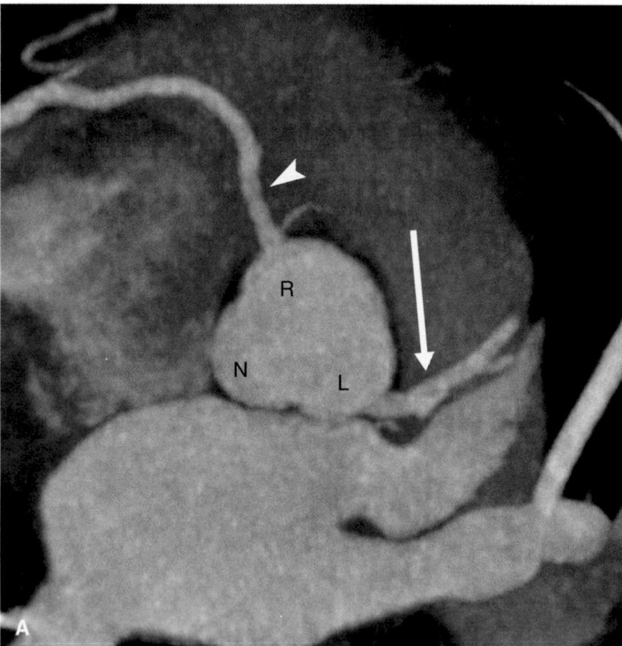

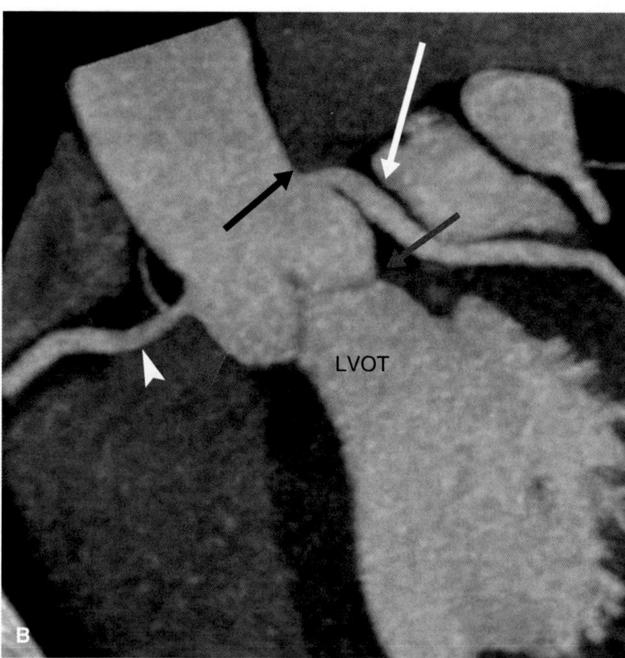

FIGURE 25.1. **Normal Coronary Ostial Anatomy. A:** A 7-mm thick MIP image transverse to the aortic sinus from a coronary CTA shows the left (*L*), right (*R*), and noncoronary (*N*) sinuses. The left main coronary artery (*white arrow*) and right coronary artery (*white arrowhead*) arise normally from the left and right coronary sinuses, respectively. **B:** Coronal oblique 5-mm thick MIP image through the left ventricular outflow tract (*LVOT*) shows that the ostia for the left main (*white arrow*) and right (*white arrowhead*) coronary arteries originate from the aortic root between the level of the sinuses of Valsalva (*red arrowhead*) and sinotubular junction (*black arrow*). The aortic valve leaflets attach at the annulus (*red arrow*) which separates the LVOT from the aortic root.

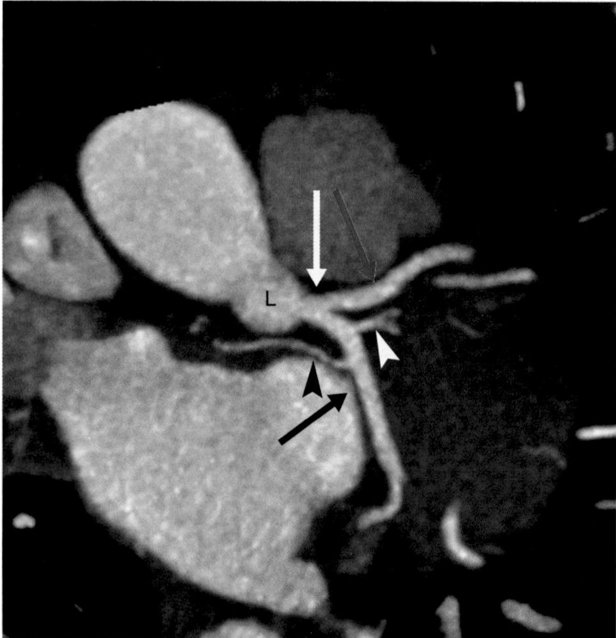

FIGURE 25.2. **Normal Anatomy of the Left Main Coronary Artery.** Double oblique multiplanar reformat shows the left main coronary artery (*white arrow*) arises from the left sinus of Valsalva (*L*). In this patient, the left main is only 4 mm long before bifurcating into left anterior descending (LAD, *red arrow*) and left circumflex (LCx) coronary arteries (*black arrow*). The sinoatrial (SA) nodal branch artery arises from the left circumflex (*black arrowhead*) which occurs in about one-third of patients. An early first obtuse marginal branch is also seen (*white arrowhead*). The left main coronary artery can vary in length from a few millimeters to a few centimeters.

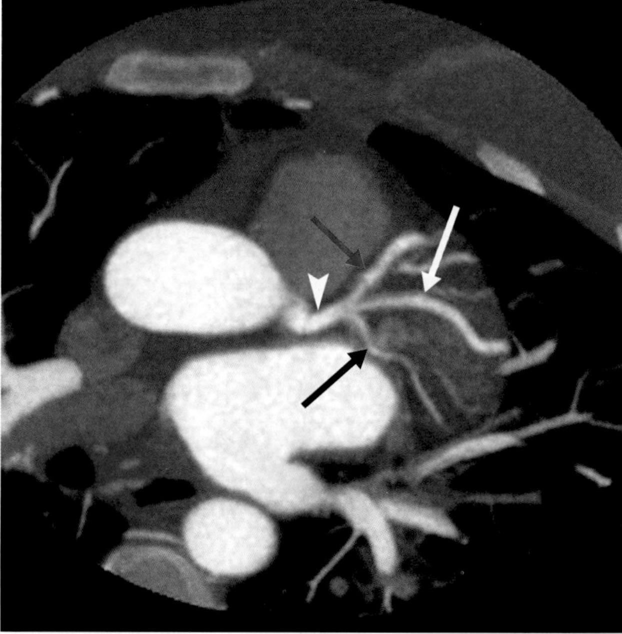

FIGURE 25.3. **Ramus Intermedius.** Axial oblique 4-mm thick MIP image through the left main coronary artery (*white arrowhead*) shows that the vessel trifurcates into the left anterior descending (*red arrow*), left circumflex (*black arrow*), and ramus intermedius branches (*white arrow*). A ramus intermedius is present in 20–30% of the population and may be a diminutive vessel, or as in this case, a large caliber vessel.

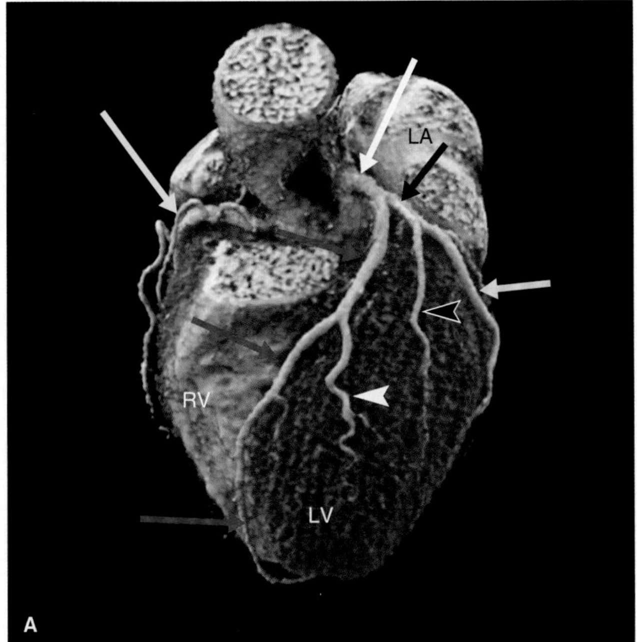

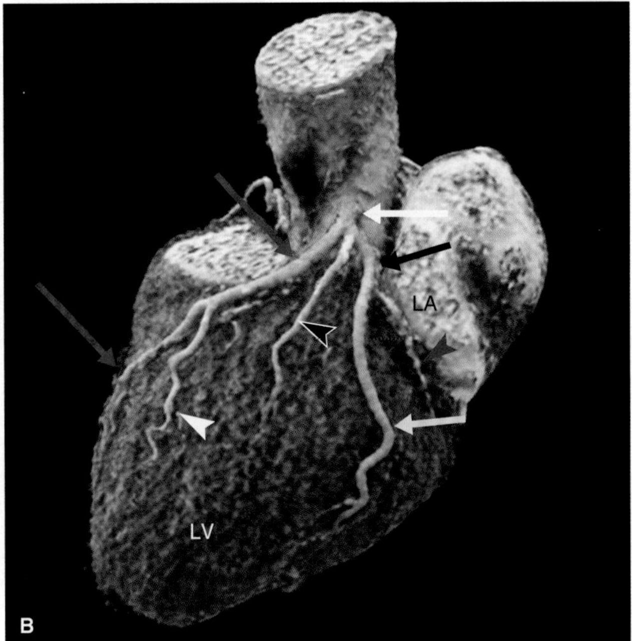

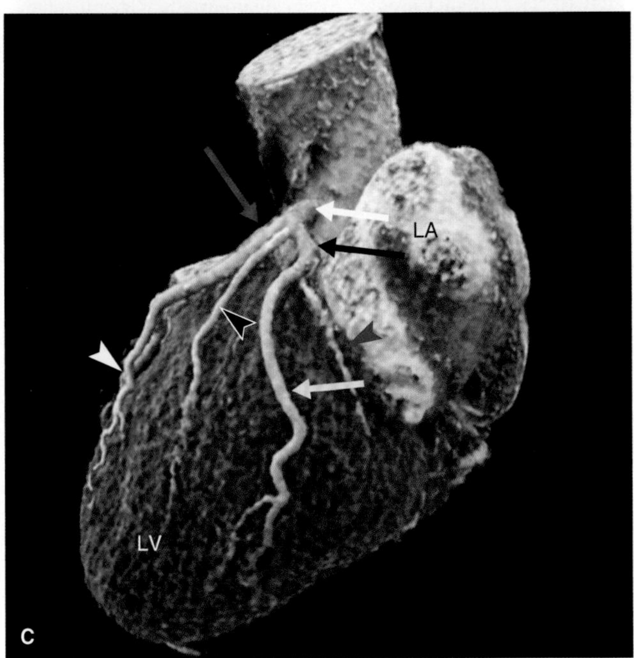

FIGURE 25.4. **Left Anterior Descending (LAD) and Left Circumflex (LCx) Coronary Artery Anatomy.** Volume-rendered images of the heart from a coronary CTA in (**A**) anterior, (**B**) anterolateral, and (**C**) lateral projections show the left main coronary artery arising from the left sinus of Valsalva (*white arrows*). The LAD (*red arrows*) courses in the anterior interventricular groove between the right ventricle (*RV*) and left ventricle (*LV*). Diagonal branches (*white arrowheads*) arise from the lateral aspect of the LAD to supply portions of the anterolateral LV. The left circumflex (*black arrows*) has a more posterolateral course between the LV and left atrium (*LA*). Two obtuse marginal (OM) arteries, a smaller first (*black arrowheads*) and a larger second (*pink arrows*), arise from the left circumflex to supply portions of the anterolateral and inferolateral surface of the LV, respectively. After the second OM, the LCx the distal LCx is small in caliber (*red arrowheads*), a common finding in a right-dominant anatomy. On the anterior view (**A**), the right coronary artery (RCA, *yellow arrow*) arises from the right sunus if Valsalva.

LAD extends from its origin to the ostium of the first large septal branch or diagonal branch, whichever arises first. The mid-LAD extends from end of the proximal LAD to one-half the distance to the LV apex, and the distal LAD is defined as the end of the mid-LAD to its termination.

The LAD gives rise to both septal branches and diagonal branches (Figs. 25.4 and 25.6). While smaller than the LAD itself, the diagonal and septal branches are needed to supply oxygenated blood to the anterolateral and anteroseptal LV myocardium, respectively. Numerous small septal branches arise from the inferomedial aspect of the LAD and dive into the anterior portion of the interventricular septum. The diagonal branches arise from the lateral aspect of the LAD and course over the anterolateral aspect of the LV. Although the number varies, most patients have between two and four diagonals.

Left Circumflex Coronary Artery

At the bifurcations of the left main, the LCx courses posterolaterally between the LV and left atrium (Fig. 25.2). The LCx gives rise to obtuse marginal (OM) vessels that supply oxygenated blood to the inferolateral aspect of the LV (Fig. 25.4). Blood supply to the anterolateral aspect of the LV at the base and mid-cavity level can occur via the OM or diagonal vessels, depending on the patient's anatomy. The size and number of OM branches vary, but most patients have at least two visible OM vessels. Once the LCx reaches the inferolateral aspect of the left atrioventricular (AV) groove and begins to wrap around the inferior aspect of the LV, it is usually a diminutive vessel since most people are right dominant. However, in patients who have left or codominant circulation (representing approximately 10%

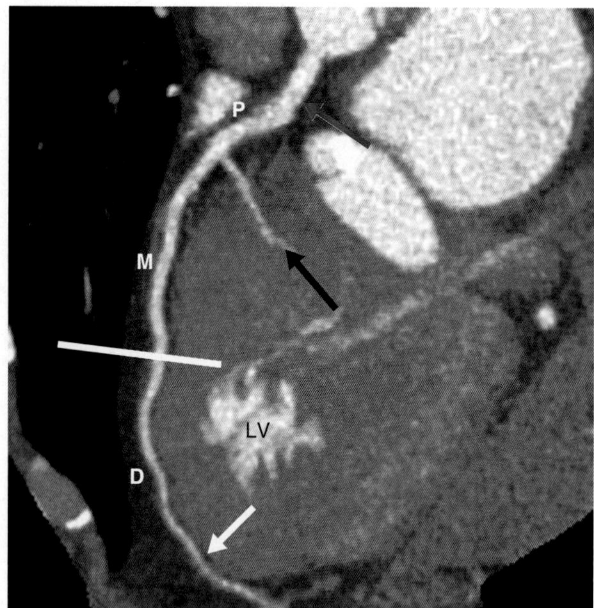

FIGURE 25.5. **Left Anterior Descending (LAD) Coronary Artery Segmentation.** Curved MPR of LAD (*red arrow*) shows the vessel coursing over the anterior wall of the left ventricle (*LV*). The proximal LAD extends from the origin of the LAD to the ostium of the first large septal (*black arrow*) or diagonal vessel, whichever arises first. To divide the mid and distal LAD, a line is drawn at the mid-way point (*white line*) between the end of the proximal LAD (*white arrow*) and LV apex (*white arrow*). The mid-LAD (*M*) extends from the end of the proximal LAD (*P*) to this line and the distal LAD (*D*) is defined as the end of the mid-LAD to the termination of the LAD. The LCx is not visualized in this plane.

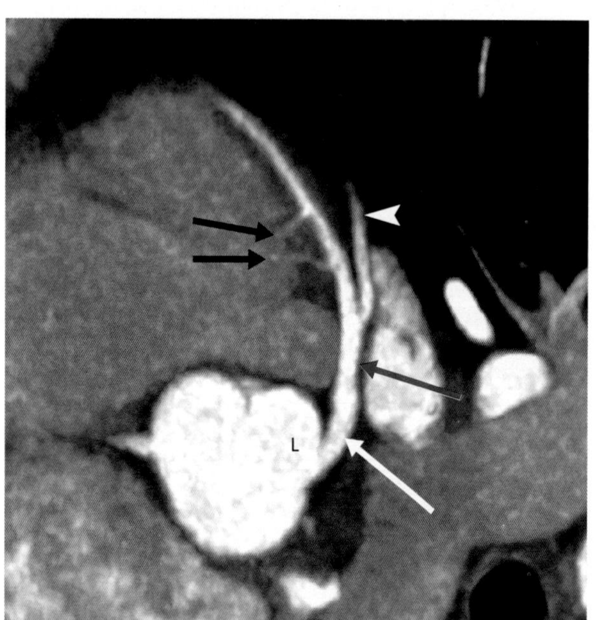

FIGURE 25.6. **Septal and Diagonal Branches of the Left Anterior Descending (LAD) Coronary Artery.** Double oblique 3-mm thick MIP image shows the left main coronary artery (*white arrow*) arising from the left sinus of Valsalva (*L*). The left main bifurcates into the LAD (*red arrow*) and LCx (not seen). The branches of the LAD that extend laterally to supply portions of the anterolateral wall of the left ventricle are called diagonal branches (*white arrowhead*). The septal branches (*black arrows*) are more numerous but small in size. They supply the anteroseptal portion of the left ventricle.

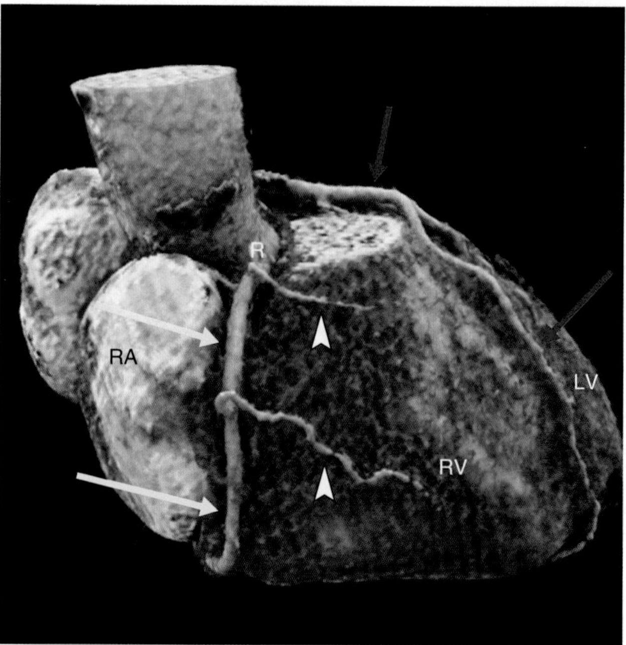

FIGURE 25.7. **Right Coronary Artery Anatomy.** Right lateral volume-rendered image from a coronary CTA shows the right coronary artery (RCA, *yellow arrows*) arising from the right sinus of Valsalva (*R*). The RCA courses in the right atrioventricular groove between the right atrium (*RA*) and right ventricle (*RV*). Acute marginal branches (*white arrowheads*) arise anteriorly and supply to the anterior free wall of the RV. The LAD (*red arrows*) can be seen coursing over the anterior wall of the left ventricle (*LV*).

and 20% of the population, respectively), the distal LCx will be larger in size (Fig. 25.7).

Ramus Intermedius

In approximately 20% to 30% of patients, the left main coronary artery will trifurcate into the LAD, LCx, and a middle branch called the ramus intermedius or intermediate branch (Fig. 25.3). This branch can vary in size and distribution; in some patients, it courses anterolaterally in a distribution similar to a diagonal branch, while in other cases it courses more posteriorly in a distribution similar to an OM branch.

Right Coronary Artery

The RCA arises from the anterior-facing right sinus of Valsalva (Figs. 25.1 and 25.7). Since approximately 70% of patients are right dominant, the RCA is a large vessel that courses anteriorly in the right AV groove and gives rise to the posterior descending artery (PDA) and posterior left ventricular (PLV) branches (Figs. 25.7 and 25.8). The RCA is divided into three territories (Fig. 25.9). The proximal RCA is defined as the ostium of the RCA to one-half the distance to the acute margin of the heart. The mid-RCA is defined as the end of the proximal RCA to the acute margin of the heart, and the distal RCA is defined as the end of the mid-RCA to the origin of the PDA.

As the RCA courses in the right AV groove, acute marginal branches arise from the RCA and course anteriorly and extend to the anterior surface of the right ventricle (Fig. 25.7). In right-dominant patients, the distal RCA will divide into two branches along the undersurface of the heart, the PDA and PLV (Fig. 25.8).

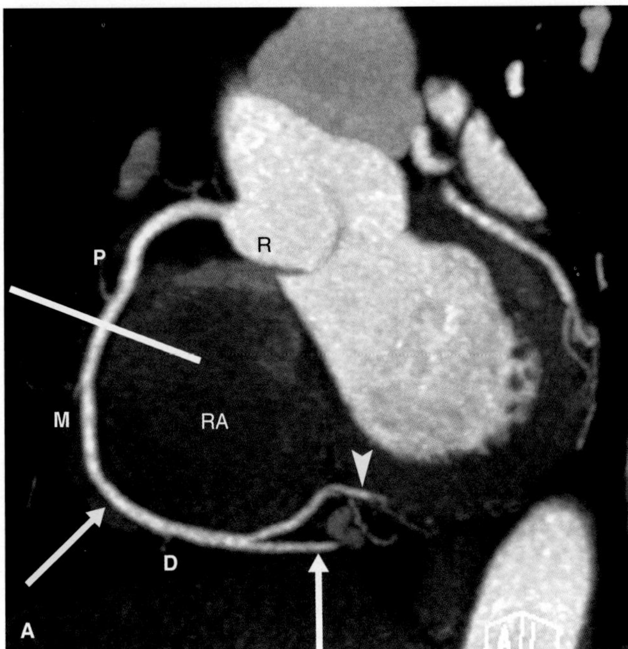

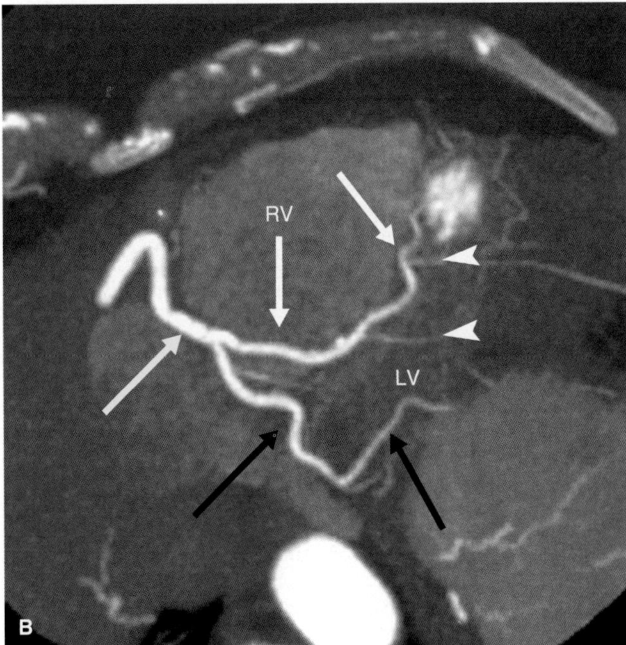

FIGURE 25.8. Right Coronary Artery (RCA) Anatomy. A: "C-view" of RCA as it courses in the right atrioventricular groove between the right atrium (*RA*) and right ventricle (not visualized in this plane) shows its division into three territories. The proximal RCA (*P*) is defined as the ostium from the right sinus (*R*) to one-half the distance (*white line*) to the acute margin, or angle, of the heart (*yellow arrow*). The mid-RCA (*M*) is defined as the end of the proximal RCA to the acute margin of the heart. The distal RCA (*D*) is defined as the end of the mid-RCA to the origin of the posterior descending artery (PDA, *white arrow*). The posterior left ventricular branch (PLV, *yellow arrowhead*) courses over the PDA. **B:** Distal RCA anatomy (*yellow arrow*) is often best seen on an inferior view of the heart. The distal RCA divides into the PDA (*white arrows*) and the PLV (*black arrows*). The PDA courses in the inferior interventricular groove between the inferior surface of the left ventricle (*LV*) and right ventricle (*RV*) and gives rise to small septal branches that supply the inferoseptal segments (*white arrowheads*). The PLV (*black arrow*) supplies the inferior and inferolateral portions of the left ventricular base. The size and extent of the PDA and PLV greatly vary depending on dominance and size of the LAD and LCx, both of which were relatively small in this patient. This patient is right heart dominant with a single PDA arising from the RCA, as seen in 70% of the population.

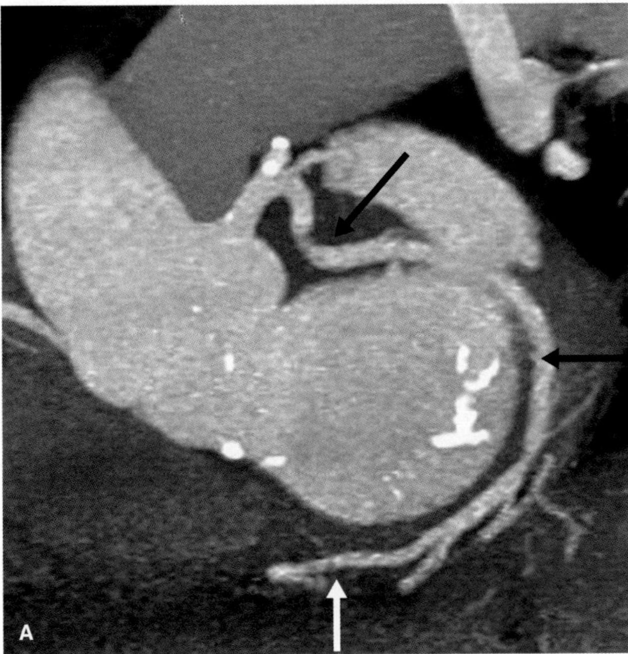

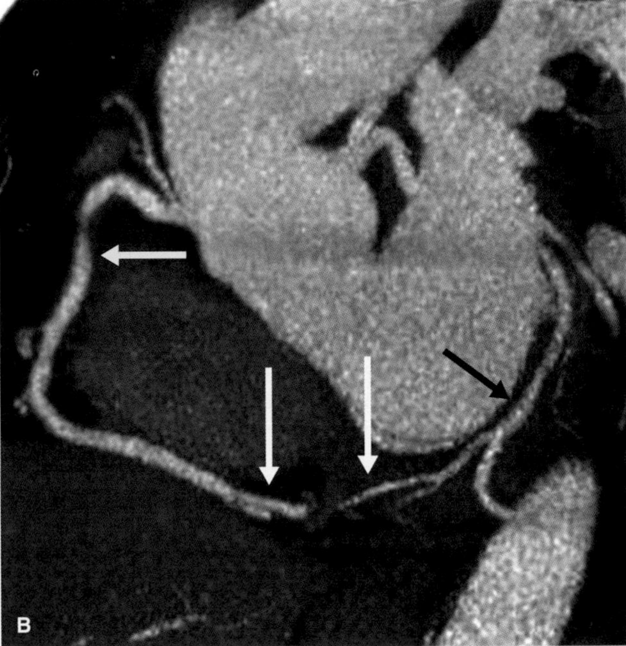

FIGURE 25.9. Left Dominance and Codominance. A: Coronal oblique MIP image shows a large LCx (*black arrows*) giving rise to the PDA (*white arrow*) denoting a left-dominant system. The RCA, which is not visualized, was small in size. **B:** Coronal oblique MIP in another patient shows two PDAs (*white arrows*), one arising from the RCA (*yellow arrow*) and the other arising from the LCx (*black arrow*) consistent with a codominant system.

Posterior Descending Artery

In the majority of patients, the PDA arises from the RCA and thus they are considered right dominant (Fig. 25.8). In approximately 10% of patients, the PDA arises from the left circumflex, and the patient is considered left dominant (Fig. 25.9A). In the remainder of patients, both the RCA and LCx give rise to a PDA branch, and these patients are often considered balanced or codominant (Fig. 25.9B).

Whichever vessel gives rise to the PDA, the vessel courses in the posterior interventricular sulcus to supply the inferior wall of the LV (Fig. 25.8). Like the LAD, the PDA gives rise to septal branches that supply the inferolateral aspect of the left ventricular septum. The PDA is of variable size and length. In patients with a smaller LAD, the PDA tends to be a larger artery and vice versa (Fig. 25.8).

Posterior Left Ventricular Branch

Arising from the distal RCA, the posterior left ventricular branch (PLV), also called the PLB, course laterally and extends along the posterior AV groove between the inferior aspect of the left atrium and LV (Fig. 25.8). It is of variable size and length. Depending on the patient's anatomy, in right-dominant patients either the PLV or LCx can supply the inferolateral wall at the base of the heart.

Conus Branch

The conus branch is usually the first branch of the RCA, although it can have a separate origin from the right coronary sinus in 17% to 50% of patients (Fig. 25.10). The conus branch extends anteriorly to supply blood to the right ventricular outflow tract (RVOT) or conus. In some instances, the conus acts as a collateral pathway for blood flow to the LAD, and this circuit is often referred to as the arterial circle of Vieussens.

Sinoatrial Nodal Branch

The sinoatrial (SA) nodal branch is a small vessel that most often originates from the RCA (Fig. 25.14) but arises from the LCx in about one-third of patients (Fig. 25.2). Less commonly, the SA branch can arise from the left main coronary artery, directly from the aorta (Fig. 25.11), or there may be two SA arteries supplied by both the LCx and RCA. Depending on its origin, the SA nodal branch courses posteriorly (RCA origin) or medially (LCx origin) and terminates in the region of the SA node located along the posterior aspect of where the superior vena cava enters the right atrium. It is important not to mistake this normal vessel for an anomalous coronary artery.

Atrioventricular Nodal Branch

In most patients, the AV nodal branch arises from the very distal "U-shaped" aspect of the distal RCA as it courses superior to the PDA. It is a small vessel that courses superiorly toward the posterior annulus of the mitral valve (Fig. 25.12).

CORONARY ARTERY ANOMALIES

Occurring in between 0.5% and 1.5% of the population, coronary artery anomalies are frequently encountered on cardiac CT. While many of these anomalies have little clinical

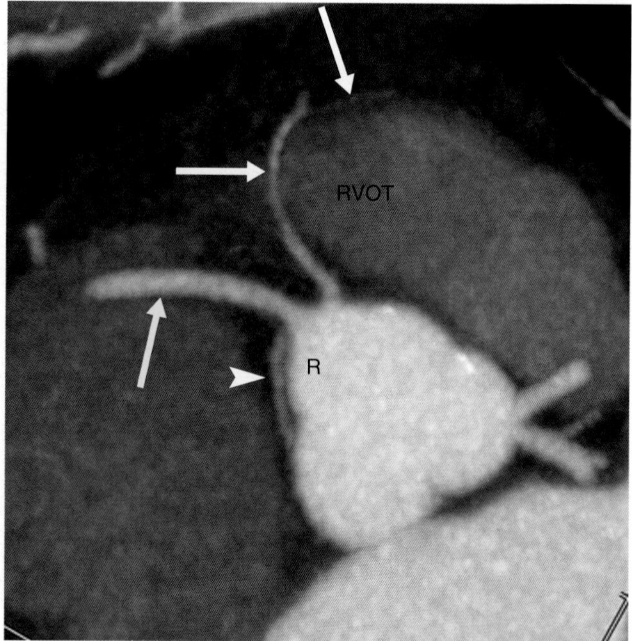

FIGURE 25.10. Anatomy of the Conus Artery. Axial oblique MIP image shows the RCA (*yellow arrow*) arising from the right sinus of Valsalva (*R*). The conus branch (*white arrows*) usually is the first vessel to arise from the very proximal RCA; however, in this case, it arises directly from the right aortic sinus which is a common benign anatomic variant. The conus courses superiorly and anteriorly to supply the right ventricular outflow tract (*RVOT*) and is an important pathway for collateralization. The sinoatrial nodal branch (*white arrowhead*) arises from the proximal RCA and is partially visualized as it courses posteriorly.

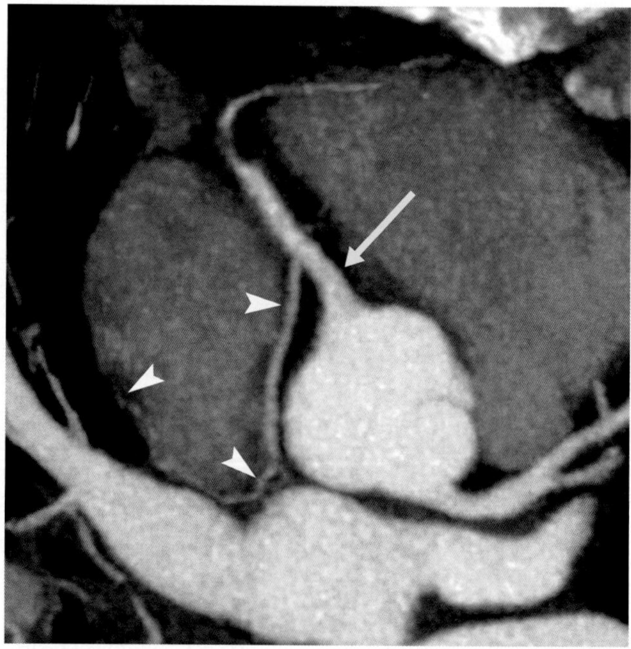

FIGURE 25.11. Sinoatrial (SA) Nodal Branch Anatomy. Curved multiplanar reformat image shows the SA branch (*white arrowheads*) arising from the proximal RCA (*yellow arrow*) and coursing posteriorly to end between left atrium (LA) and superior portion of the right atrium. The SA branch most commonly arises from the RCA but can originate from the LCx (Fig. 25.2). In rare instances, both the RCA and LCx give rise to separate SA nodal branches.

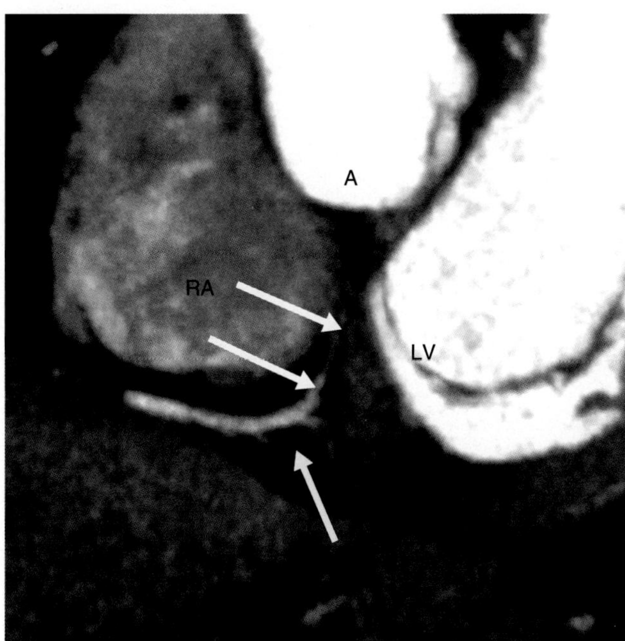

FIGURE 25.12. **Atrioventricular (AV) Nodal Branch Anatomy.** Coronal oblique MPR image shows the AV nodal branch (*white arrows*) arising from the distal right coronary artery *(yellow arrow)*. The AV nodal branch extends superiorly between the right atrium (*RA*) and left ventricle (*LV*) toward the aortic root (*A*).

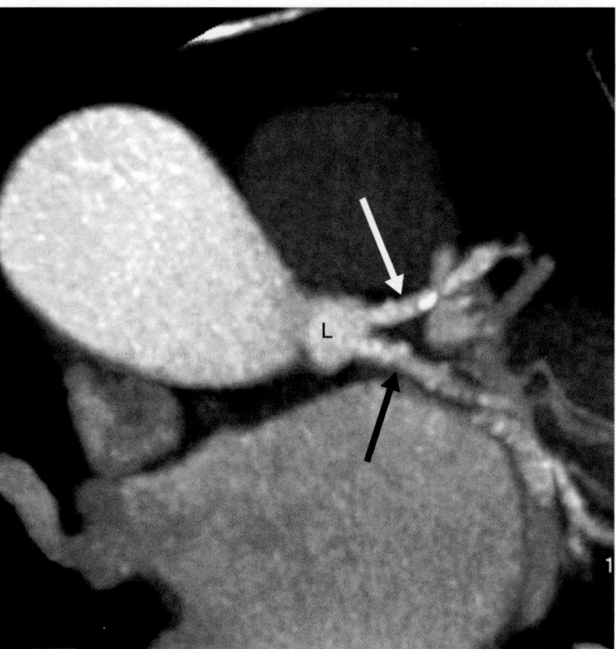

FIGURE 25.13. **Absent Left Main Coronary Artery.** Axial oblique image from a coronary CTA shows complete absence of the left main coronary artery. The left anterior descending (*white arrow*) and left circumflex (*black arrow*) coronary arteries arise directly from the left sinus of Valsalva (*L*). This is a rare but benign congenital variant.

significance, anomalous coronary anatomy can lead to sudden cardiac death. Some of these anomalies can lead to symptoms and thus be the reason for the study; however, they are often clinically silent and are frequently an incidental finding. It is also important to remember that although anomalous coronary anatomy is best visualized with electrocardiography (ECG)-gated CT angiography, the improved temporal resolution of modern scanners often allows for a basic assessment of coronary artery origins and course on nongated thoracic CT scans.

There are many ways to subdivide these anomalies. One of the more commonly used methods is to divide them based on anomalous origin, course, and termination. No matter how one chooses to classify these anomalies, it is important to recognize that even though many of the anomalies are benign, others can lead to a reduction in coronary blood flow and major adverse cardiac events (MACEs).

ABNORMALITIES IN ORIGIN

There are numerous congenital coronary artery anomalies associated with an anomalous origin. While it may be an isolated finding, in some instances, such as in patients with a single coronary artery, multiple anomalies or origin and course may coexist. These anomalies include absence of the left main coronary artery, anomalous location of the coronary ostium outside the aortic root, and anomalous origin of the coronary ostium from the incorrect sinus.

Abnormalities in Origin, Benign

Absence of the Left Main Coronary Artery. Absence of the left main coronary artery is a benign variant that occurs in approximately 0.4% to 2% of the population. In this situation, the LAD and LCx have independent origins from the left sinus of Valsalva (Fig. 25.13).

Anomalous Origin of the Coronary Arteries Outside of the Aortic Root. In certain instances, the coronary arteries may arise from a location outside of the sinuses. While some of these anomalies may be potentially malignant, as discussed later, many are benign. A high origin of a coronary artery occurs when its ostium is located 1 cm or greater above the sinotubular junction. This most commonly affects the RCA (Fig. 25.14). Although this origin is benign, its location could lead to accidental injury during surgical manipulation of the ascending aorta.

Retroaortic. In a retroaortic course, the anomalous coronary artery arises from the opposite sinus and courses posteriorly between the aorta and left atrium. This most commonly occurs when the LCx or left main coronary artery arises from the right sinus of Valsalva, either directly from the aorta or from the proximal RCA (Fig. 25.15A). In rare instances, the RCA can arise from the left sinus with a retroaortic course (Fig. 25.15B). While these are benign anomalies, they can be inadvertently injured during aortic valve or annular surgery.

Anterior to Pulmonary Outflow Tract (Prepulmonic or Precardiac). A prepulmonic course occurs when an anomalous coronary artery courses anterior to the RVOT (Fig. 25.16). Most commonly, this abnormality involves the LAD or left main coronary artery. This prepulmonic vessel often arises directly from the proximal RCA in the setting of a single coronary artery (Fig. 25.17). If the LAD has a prepulmonic course, the LCx may have a retroaortic course or can arise directly from the left sinus. In addition, the anomaly may be accompanied by a small anomalous septal branch arising from the right cusp to supply the basilar septum. Less commonly, the RCA may have a prepulmonic course, usually in the setting of a single left coronary artery.

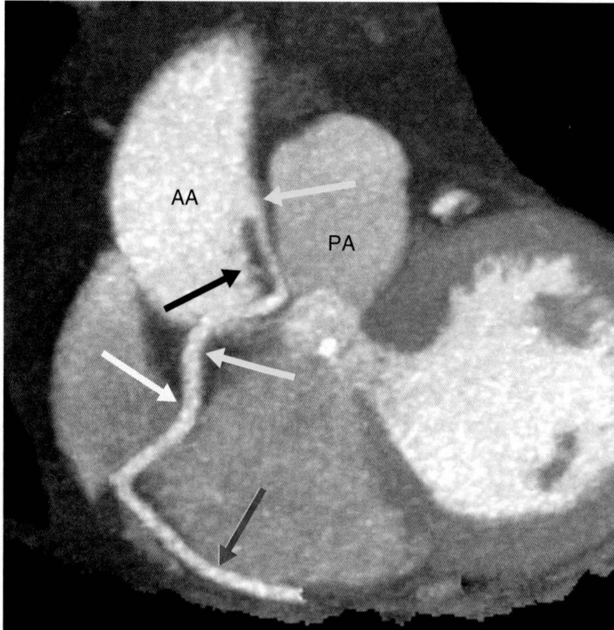

FIGURE 25.14. High Origin of the Right Coronary Artery (RCA). Sagittal oblique MIP image shows the RCA (*yellow arrows*) arising from the ascending aorta (*AA*) and coursing inferiorly between the aorta and pulmonary artery (*PA*) before entering the AV groove (*white arrow*). A high origin, which is a benign anomaly, occurs when a coronary artery ostium is located greater than 1 cm above the sinotubular junction (*black arrow*). This most commonly affects the RCA.

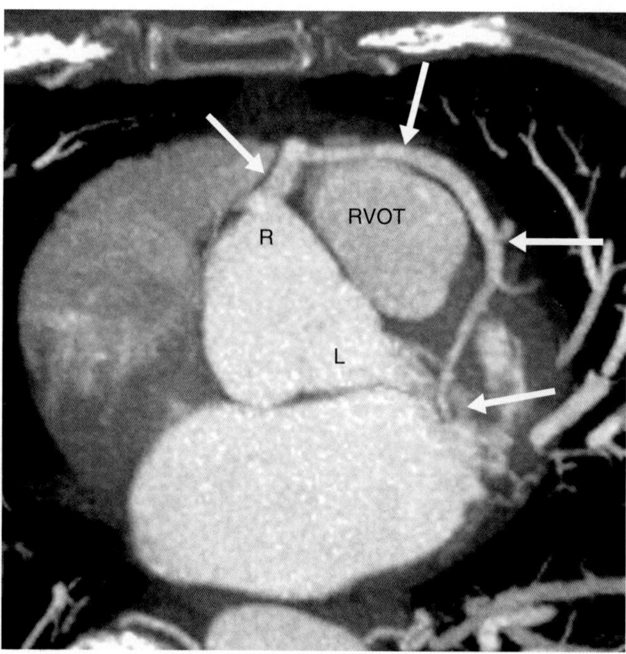

FIGURE 25.16. Prepulmonic Course. Axial oblique image from a coronary CTA shows that the left main coronary artery (*white arrows*) arises from the right sinus of Valsalva (*R*) and courses anteriorly around the right ventricular outflow tract (*RVOT*), consistent with a prepulmonic or precardiac course. No coronary artery arises from the left sinus of Valsalva (*L*). This is a benign anomaly.

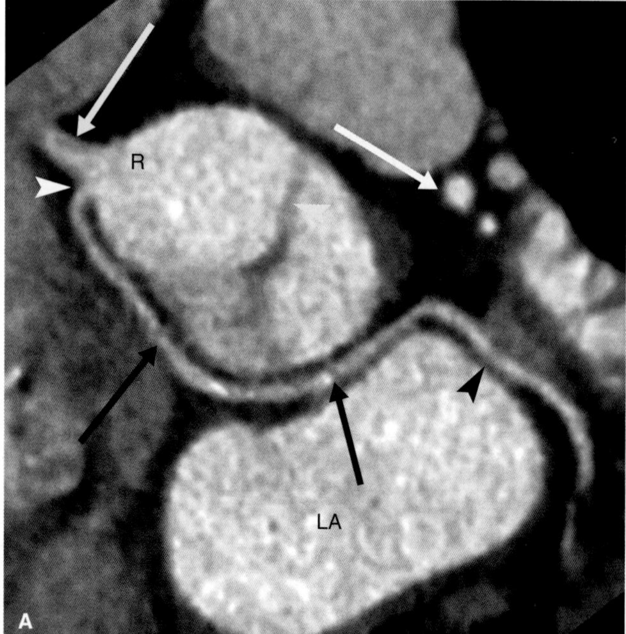

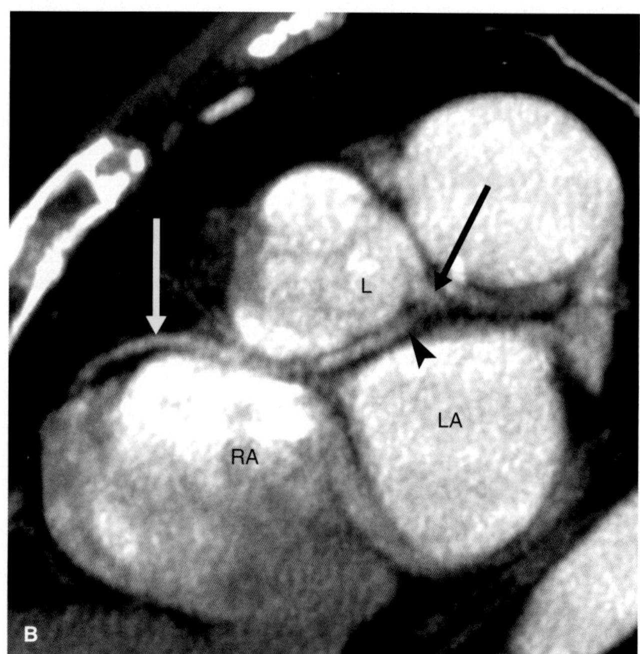

FIGURE 25.15. Retroaortic Course. A: Axial oblique image through the aortic root from a coronary CTA in a 47-year-old man shows that the origin of the LCx (*white arrowhead*) is from the right coronary sinus (*R*). The LCx then courses posteriorly (*black arrows*) between the aortic root and left atrium (*LA*) before entering its normal territory (*black arrowheads*). The LCx has a separate ostium from the RCA (*yellow arrow*). The LAD (*white arrow*) originated from the left coronary sinus. Incidental note is made of a bicuspid aortic valve (*yellow arrowhead*). **B:** Sagittal oblique image from a coronary CTA in a 9-year-old child shows ostium of the RCA (*black arrow*) arising from the left sinus (*L*) and coursing posteriorly between the left atrium and aortic root (*black arrowhead*) before entering the right atrioventricular groove (*yellow arrow*). While the LCx anomaly is not uncommon, a retroaortic course of the RCA is extremely rare. Both are benign courses.

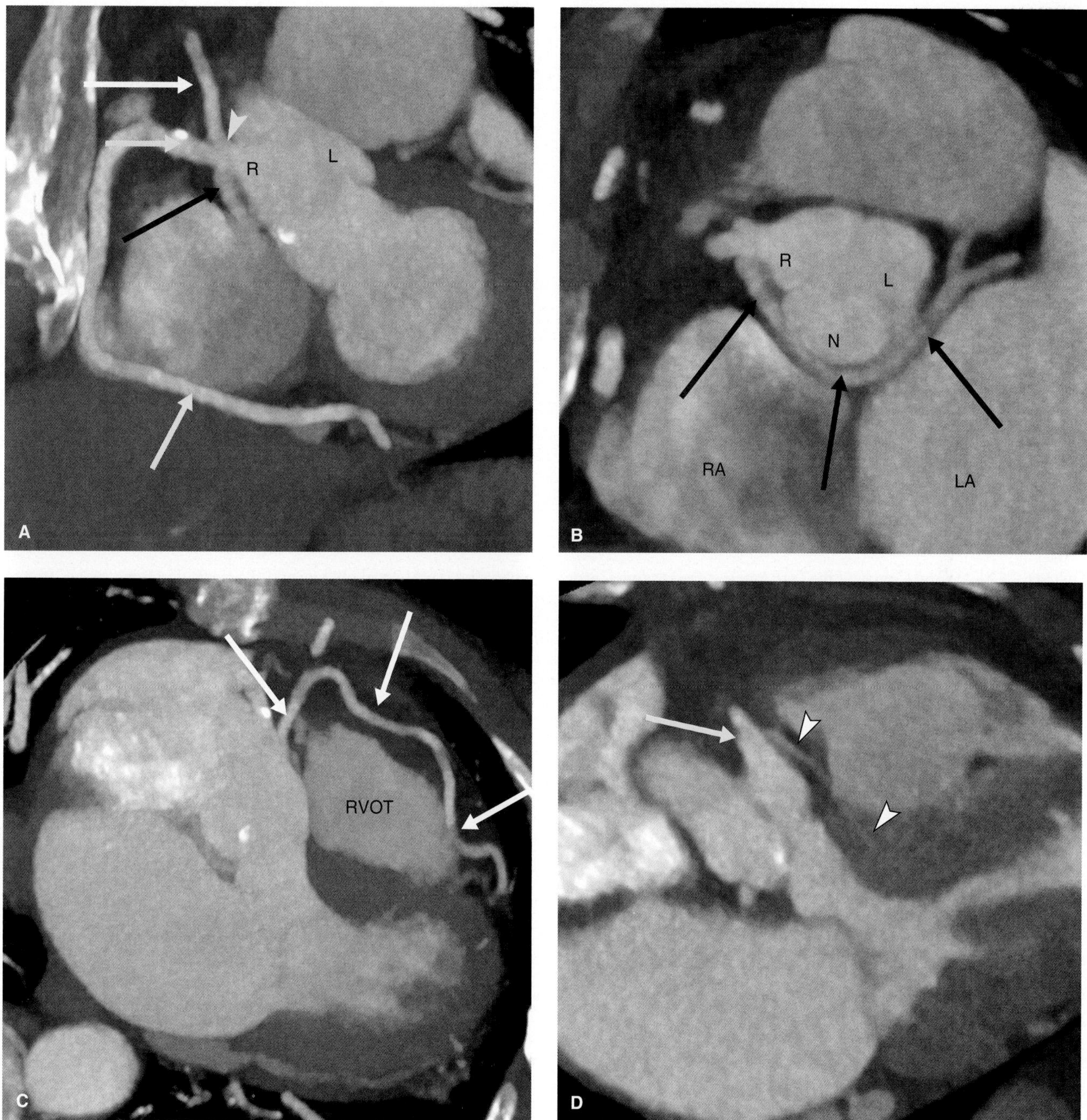

FIGURE 25.17. Incidental Discovery of a Single Right Coronary Artery in a 54-Year-Old Woman With Atypical Chest Pain. A: C-view of the RCA shows a single right coronary artery (*yellow arrowhead*) arising from the right sinus (*R*) and trifurcating into the RCA (*yellow arrows*), with large branches extending both superiorly (*white arrow*) and inferiorly (*black arrow*). Except for mild atherosclerotic disease, the RCA is otherwise normal. No coronary artery arises from the left sinus (*L*). **B:** Coronal oblique MIP shows that the inferiorly directed artery in **A** (*black arrow*) represents a retroaortic LCx (*black arrows*) coursing posteriorly between the right atrium (*RA*), left atrium (*LA*), and noncoronary sinus (*N*). **C:** Axial oblique MIP image shows that the superiorly directed artery in A (*white arrow*) is a prepulmonic LAD (*white arrows*) which courses around the right ventricular outflow tract (*RVOT*). **D:** In addition to these three larger vessels, axial oblique MIP shows a very small anomalous septal branch (*white arrowheads*) originating from the proximal RCA (*yellow arrow*) to supply basilar septum. In this instance of a single coronary artery, all of the anomalous courses are benign. However, there are numerous configurations of single coronary arteries which can have both benign and potentially malignant configurations.

Septal (Intramyocardial) Course. A septal course usually involves the LAD arising from the right coronary sinus (Figs. 25.17D and 25.18). It is important to recognize the inferomedial course of the vessel that dives into the proximal aspect of the left ventricular septum as this distinguishes this benign course from the potentially malignant interarterial course discussed below. Although it can rarely be associated with myocardial ischemia, in most instances it is benign.

Noncoronary Sinus. Origin from the noncoronary sinus is an extremely rare anomaly. This can occur with the RCA or left

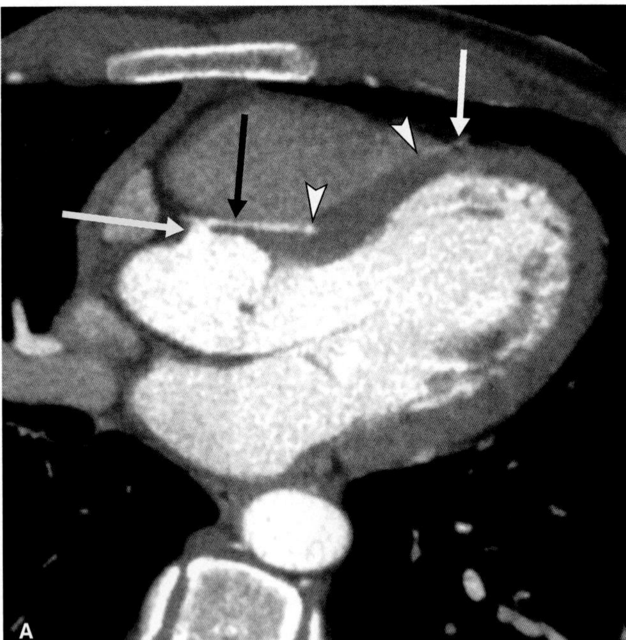

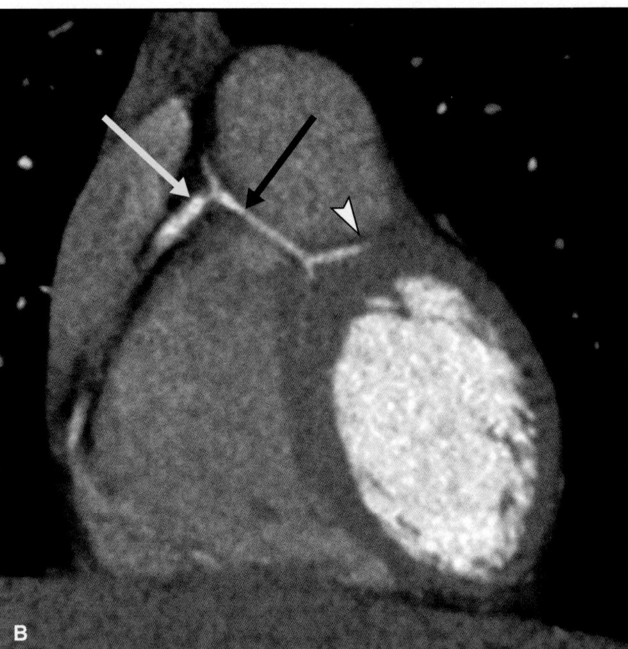

FIGURE 25.18. Septal Course of the Left Anterior Descending Coronary Artery (LAD). A: Axial oblique and (**B**) coronal oblique images from a coronary CTA show the LAD arising from the proximal RCA (*yellow arrows*) and coursing inferiorly and medially (*black arrows*) before diving into the interventricular septum (*white arrowheads*). The proximal and mid LAD (*white arrowheads*) run in the wall of the left ventricle consistent with a long-segment myocardial bridge. The distal LAD (*white arrow*) reenters its normal location in the epicardial fat. This benign course needs to be delineated from the potentially malignant interarterial course where the coronary artery crosses directly between the main pulmonary artery and aorta and does not have the inferiorly directed course as seen in this case.

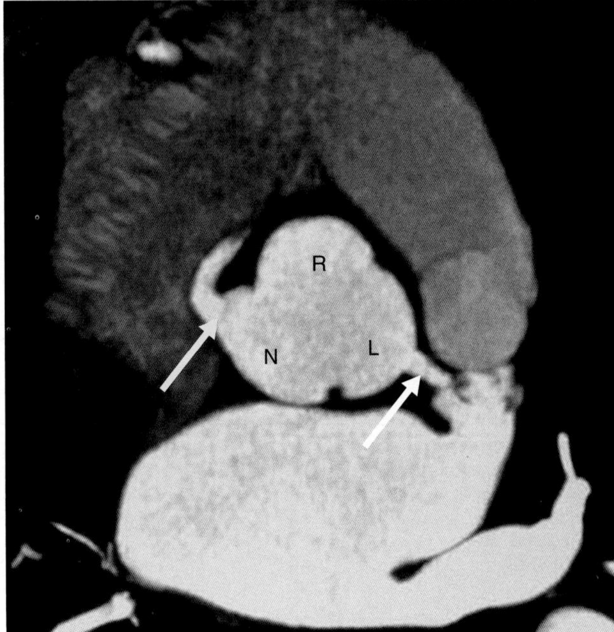

FIGURE 25.19. Maximum-intensity projection image through the sinuses of Valsalva in a 43-year-old woman with atypical chest pain shows the RCA (*yellow arrow*) arising from the noncoronary sinus (*N*). The left main (*white arrow*) arises from the left sinus (*L*). No coronary artery arises from the right sinus (*R*). A coronary artery arising from the noncoronary sinus is an extremely rare anomaly. (Courtesy of Jacobo Kirsch, MD.)

main coronary artery (Fig. 25.19). Although there is little information on this anomaly given its rarity, it is often considered a benign anomaly.

Abnormalities in Origin, Possibly Malignant

Interarterial Course. With an interarterial course, a coronary artery arises from the opposite sinus and courses medially between the aorta and pulmonary artery. This can involve the RCA (Fig. 25.20), left main (Fig. 25.21), or LAD. Unlike the retroaortic or septal course, an interarterial course, especially when involving the left main or LAD, can lead to myocardial ischemia, infarction, and sudden cardiac death. The cause of this is believed to be multifactorial. When the artery courses medially, it can experience extrinsic compression between the aorta and pulmonary artery. Compression can worsen during exercise due to physiologic dilation of the aorta and pulmonary artery at a time when myocardial oxygen demand increases. Proximal compression can also occur as the vessel passes through the aortic wall, which is termed an *intramural course*. The intramural course can be of various lengths and is often identified on imaging by soft tissue attenuation surrounding the proximal coronary artery. As it courses through the wall of the aorta, the narrowed vessel has an ovoid shape with an increased height/width ratio (Figs. 25.20 and 25.21). In addition, the coronary artery ostium is often dysplastic and "slit like," further reducing blood flow into the vessel. Lastly, the proximal vessel can have a tangential course with an acute angulation that leads to a further reduction in blood flow.

An interarterial course of the RCA is more common than those involving the left system. In patients with an interarterial RCA, a higher incidence of symptoms and adverse cardiac events has been reported in those with a more superior course

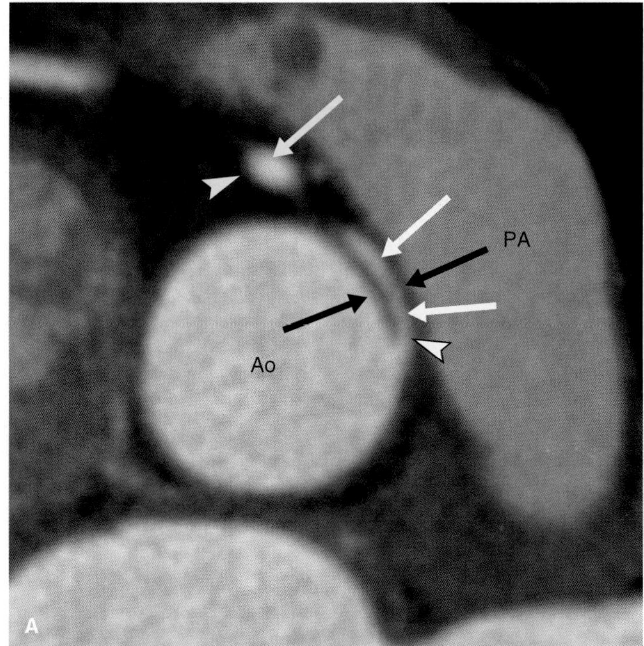

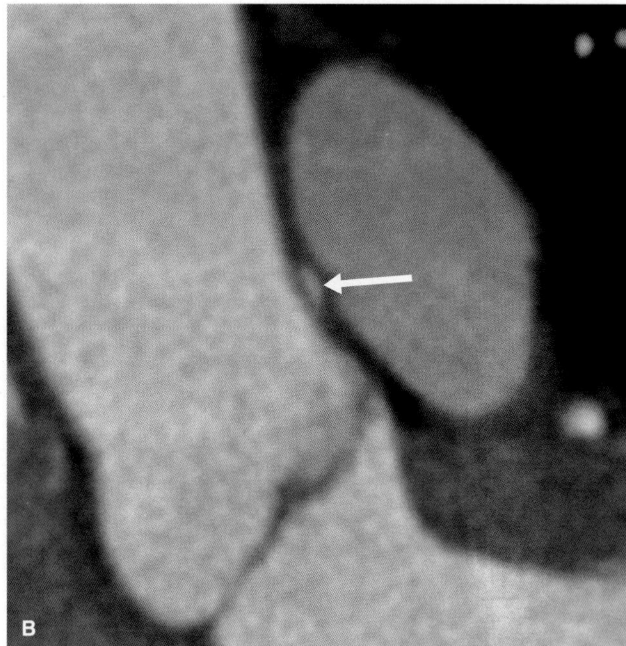

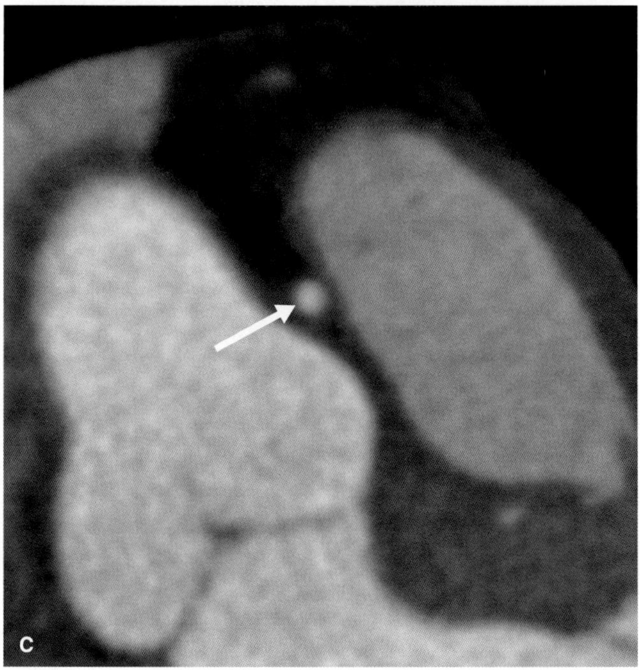

FIGURE 25.20. **Incidental Finding of an Interarterial Course of the Right Coronary Artery (RCA) in a 56-Year-Old Man. A:** Axial oblique image from a coronary CTA shows the proximal RCA (*white arrows*), which arises just above the left coronary sinus, coursing between the aorta (*Ao*) and pulmonary artery (*PA*). The proximal vessel is narrowed and surrounded by soft tissue attenuation (*black arrows*), whereas the RCA 2 cm distal (*yellow arrow*) is normal in size and surrounded by epicardial fat (*yellow arrowhead*). The soft tissue attenuation represents the intramural portion of the artery where it courses in the wall of the aorta. In addition, whereas coronary arteries should have a relatively straight course from its ostium, this interarterial RCA takes a near-90-degree turn rightward just distal to its ostium (*white arrowhead*) creating an acute angulation. **B:** Sagittal oblique image through the proximal RCA (*white arrow*) shows marked narrowing and an abnormal ovoid configuration of the vessel which is taller than it is wide. **C:** Sagittal oblique image a few centimeters distal to the RCA ostium shows a normal rounded appearance to the RCA (*white arrow*) where the height and width are equal. The findings in **A** and **B** are diagnostic on an interarterial course. An interarterial course of the RCA can be an incidental finding or can lead to ischemia.

of the interarterial vessel (between the aorta and pulmonary artery) as compared to those with a more inferior course (between the aorta and right ventricular outflow tract). However, in most patients, an interarterial course of the RCA is an incidental finding which does not cause ischemia. When an interarterial course of an RCA is identified, surgical correction is recommended if the patient has chest pain, ischemia, syncope, presyncope, or LV dysfunction in the appropriate vascular territory. Asymptomatic adults often undergo a stress test to determine whether there is inducible ischemia in the affected vascular distribution. If ischemia is absent on stress testing, many currently favor no intervention. However, practices vary depending on the patient's age and the specific institution.

Compared to the RCA, an interarterial course of the LAD or left main has a higher association with myocardial ischemia and sudden cardiac death. Surgical correction is recommended in most cases even if the finding is incidental. This can occur via various techniques including unroofing, reimplantation, or bypass.

Anomalous Origin of the Left Main Coronary Artery From the Pulmonary Artery. Anomalous origin of the left main coronary artery from the pulmonary artery (ALCAPA), or Bland–Garland–White syndrome, is a rare congenital anomaly with an estimated incidence of 1/300,000 live births. In utero, admixture of blood and high pulmonary pressures allow for adequate perfusion of the left main coronary artery. In the neonatal period, pulmonary pressures remain high enough to allow for adequate perfusion of the left main coronary artery with pulmonary arterial blood. However, during the first few months of life, pulmonary artery pressures begin to decrease. Once this occurs, the timing of symptoms depends on the presence or

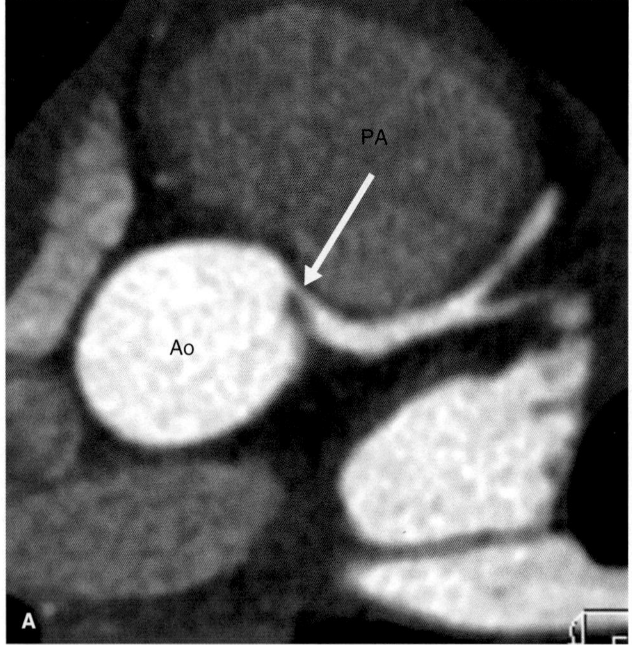

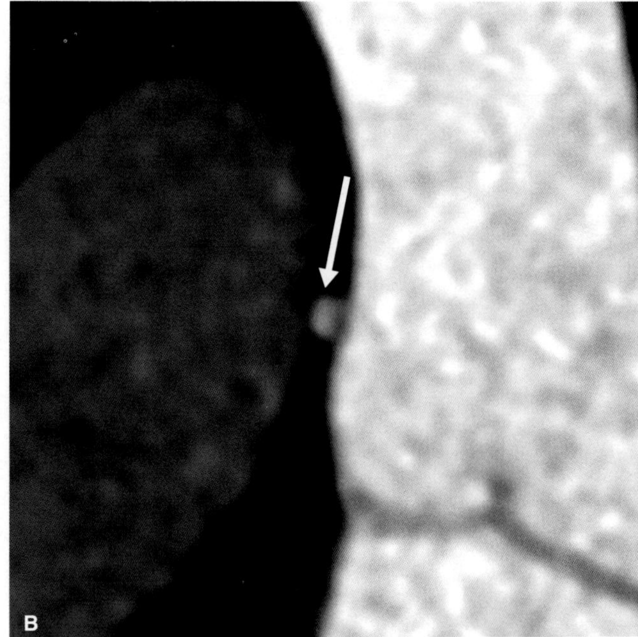

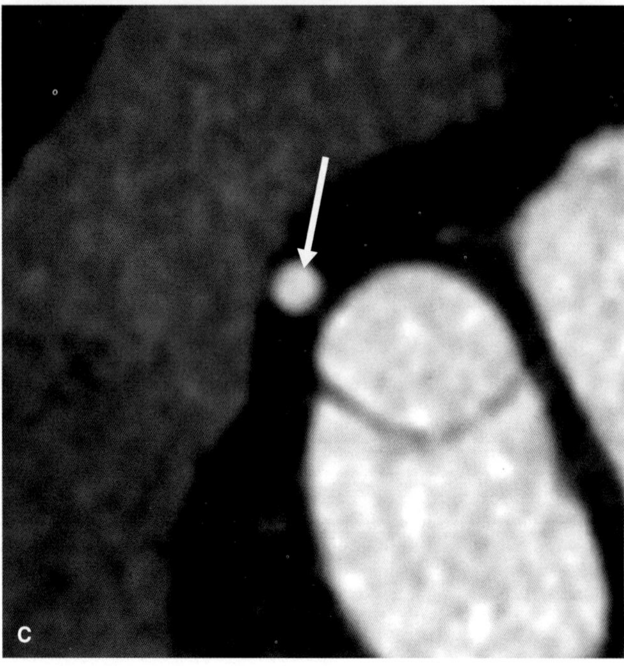

FIGURE 25.21. Interarterial Course of the Left Main Coronary Artery in a 14-Year-Old Boy Who Presented to the Emergency Department after Cardiac Arrest while Playing Basketball. A: Axial oblique image from a coronary CTA shows the left main coronary artery (*white arrow*), which arises above the right coronary sinus, coursing between the aorta (*Ao*) and pulmonary artery (*PA*). The proximal vessel is severely narrowed. **B:** Sagittal oblique image through the proximal left main near the ostium shows severe narrowing of the LM (*white arrow*), which has an ovoid shape as it courses between the aorta and pulmonary artery. The vessel measures 2 × 1 mm in diameter. **C:** Sagittal oblique image 1 cm distal to the ostium; the LM has a more normal rounded shape and size (*white arrow*), measuring 4 × 4 mm. A 5-mm intramural course of the proximal left main was confirmed at surgery. Interarterial course of the left main or LAD is less common than that of the RCA but has a much high incidence of sudden cardiac death.

absence of collaterals. In the absence of adequate collaterals, the decrease in pulmonary pressures leads to inadequate blood flow from the PA into the left main coronary artery. This can lead to myocardial ischemia, infarct, and cardiac death in 90% of infants in the first year of life (Fig. 25.22). However, if robust RCA collaterals are present, high pressure systemic blood from the RCA will flow retrograde into the left main distribution and ultimately into the main pulmonary artery due to lower pulmonary pressures. This retrograde blood flow from the RCA to the left main and into the main pulmonary artery creates a physiologic state akin to a fistula (Fig. 25.23). Due to preferential flow into the lower-pressure PA and not the microcirculation, capillary hypoperfusion may lead to chronic subendocardial ischemia. Patients with this pattern of ALCAPA often present in their third or fourth decade of life with subacute symptoms such as angina, dyspnea, palpitations, and fatigue. While some patients with ALCAPA may be asymptomatically discovered in their eighth decade of life, ventricular arrhythmia and sudden death are still common in this population.

Single Coronary Artery. With a single coronary artery, all coronary artery branches arise from a single vessel which can have various benign or potentially malignant anomalous courses (Fig. 25.17). A single RCA is more common than left.

Ostial Atresia. Ostial atresia is an extremely rare abnormality where the ostium of the RCA or left main does not develop (Fig. 25.24). It more commonly affects the left main coronary artery ostium than the RCA ostium. While the ostium is atretic, just distal to the atretic segment normal coronary artery anatomy is present. This anomaly is often associated with sudden cardiac death in newborns but patients can survive into adulthood if collateral pathways between the opposite coronary circulation exist.

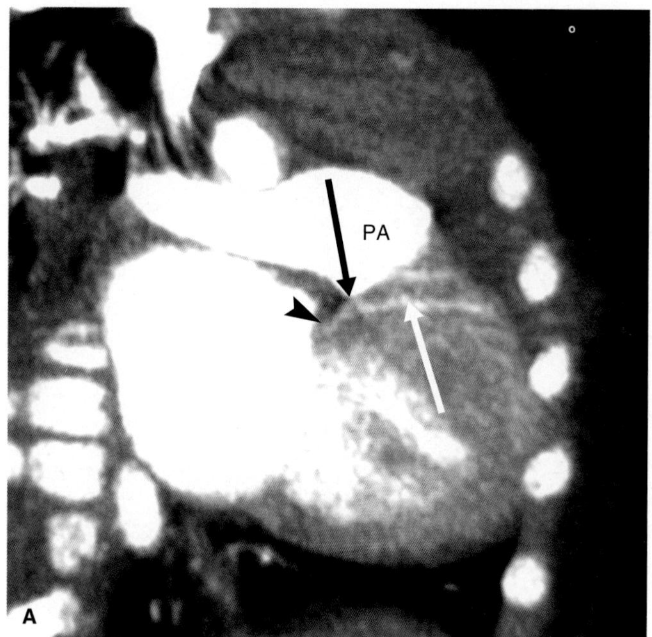

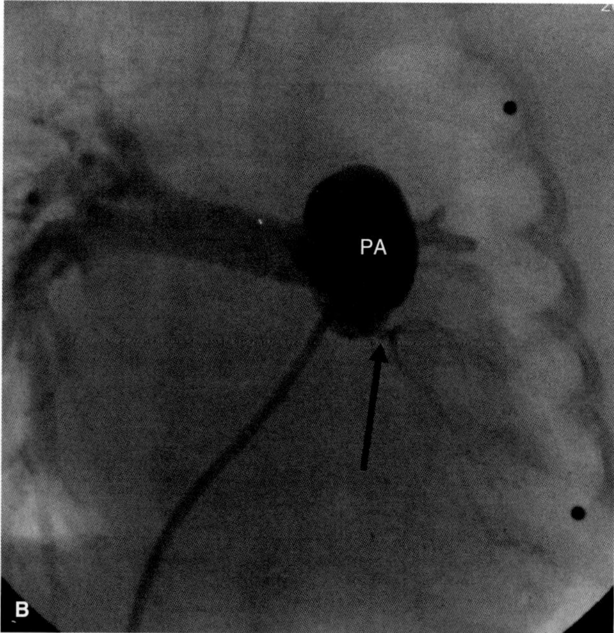

FIGURE 25.22. **Anomalous Origin of the Left Main Coronary Artery From the Pulmonary Artery (ALCAPA) in an 8-Week-Old Infant With Poor Feeding, Lethargy, and Irritability. A:** Sagittal oblique image from a CTA shows the left main coronary artery (*black arrow*) arising from the pulmonary artery (*PA*) with subsequent bifurcation into the LAD (*white arrow*) and LCx (*black arrowhead*). **B:** Anterior image from catheter angiography confirms the presence of ALCAPA with the left main (*black arrow*) arising from the PA.

ABNORMALITIES IN COURSE

Myocardial Bridging

An intramyocardial course of a coronary artery, or **myocardial bridging**, is a common incidental finding and has been reported in up to 58% of patients undergoing coronary CTA and in up to 86% of autopsies. Bridging most often involves the mid-LAD where a band of myocardial tissue extends around the vessel (Fig. 25.25). The depth and length of the bridged segment can vary significantly from a few millimeters to a few centimeters. While the vessel is compressed during systole, this rarely leads to symptoms as the coronary

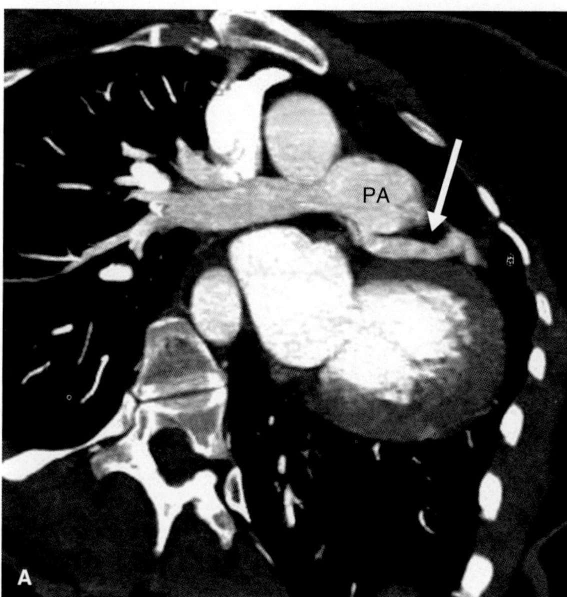

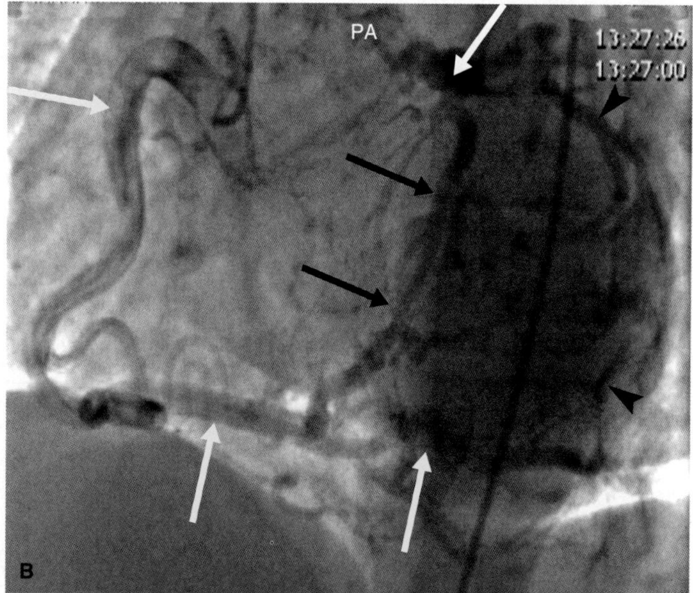

FIGURE 25.23. **Anomalous Origin of the Left Main Coronary Artery From the Pulmonary Artery (ALCAPA) in a 50-Year-Old Woman With Chest Pain. A:** Coronal oblique image of the left main coronary artery from a gated CTA of the chest shows a dilated left main coronary artery (*white arrow*) arising from the pulmonary artery (*PA*), consistent with ALCAPA. **B:** Coronary angiogram with a right coronary artery (RCA) injection shows a diffusely dilated RCA and associated branches (*yellow arrows*). Flow from these dilated vessels fills the left circumflex (*black arrowheads*), left anterior descending (*black arrows*), and left main (*white arrow*) via retrograde flow. The blood then drains into the pulmonary artery (*PA*) creating a large fistula. Due to the presence of collateral circulation, the patient was able to survive into adulthood with this congenital abnormality.

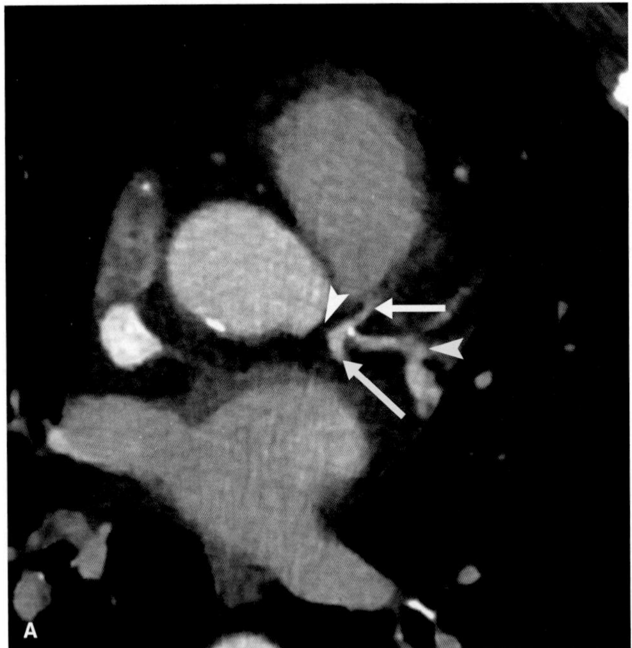

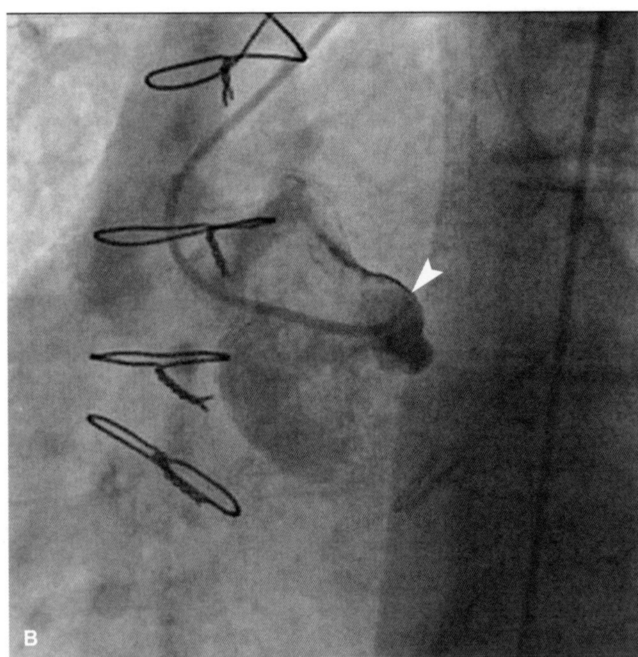

FIGURE 25.24. **Ostial Atresia in a 51-Year-Old Woman. A:** Axial oblique MPR through the expected location of the left main coronary artery shows complete absence of the vessel (*white arrowhead*). The left main distal to the atresia can be seen trifurcating into the LAD (*white arrow*), ramus intermedius (*yellow arrowhead*), and LCx (*yellow arrow*). The patient underwent coronary artery bypass surgery when she was 15 for surgically proven left main ostial atresia. **B:** Still image from a coronary angiogram with injection in the expected location of the left main ostium shows no hint of ostial development (*white arrowhead*).

arteries fill during diastole. Although the vast majority of myocardial bridges are an incidental finding on coronary CTA, myocardial bridges can lead to angina and ischemia through various mechanisms including phasic systolic vessel compression, persistent diastolic lumen diameter reduction, increased blood flow velocities, retrograde systolic flow, and reduced coronary flow reserve. In addition, there is an increased incidence of coronary artery atherosclerotic disease

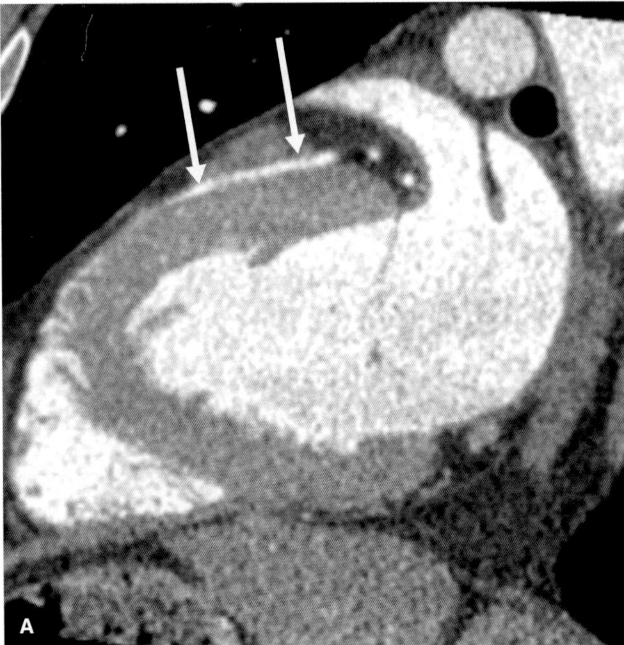

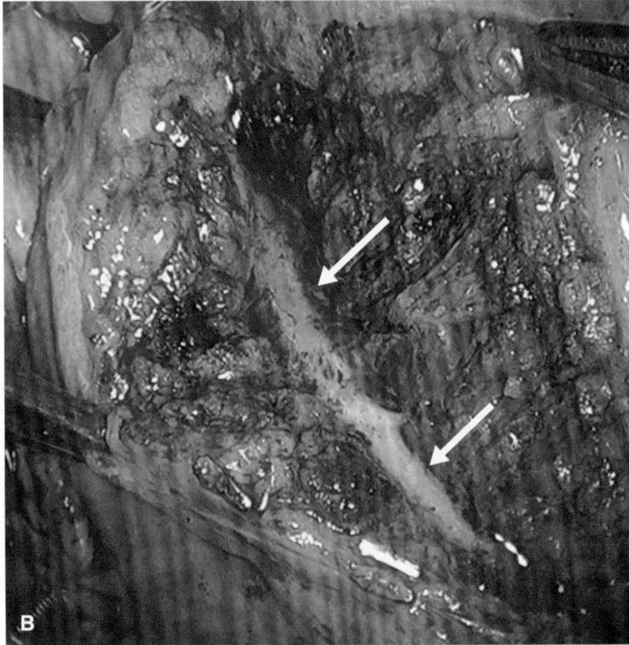

FIGURE 25.25. **Myocardial Bridging in a 22-Year-Old Man With Repeated Visits to the Emergency Department for Chest Pain. A:** Sagittal oblique image from a coronary CTA shows the mid-LAD diving into the left ventricular myocardium (*white arrows*), consistent with a 38-mm myocardial bridge which measured 8 mm in depth. No other abnormalities were found, and stress imaging showed no abnormality. Although this is a common incidental finding and of little clinical significance in the majority of patients, due to his repeated symptoms and lack of other explanation for pain, the patient elected to undergo surgery. **B:** Surgical image during myotomy shows the mid-LAD surrounded by myocardium (*white arrow*). Two months after surgery, the patient returned to the emergency department with chest pain similar to that experienced prior to surgery.

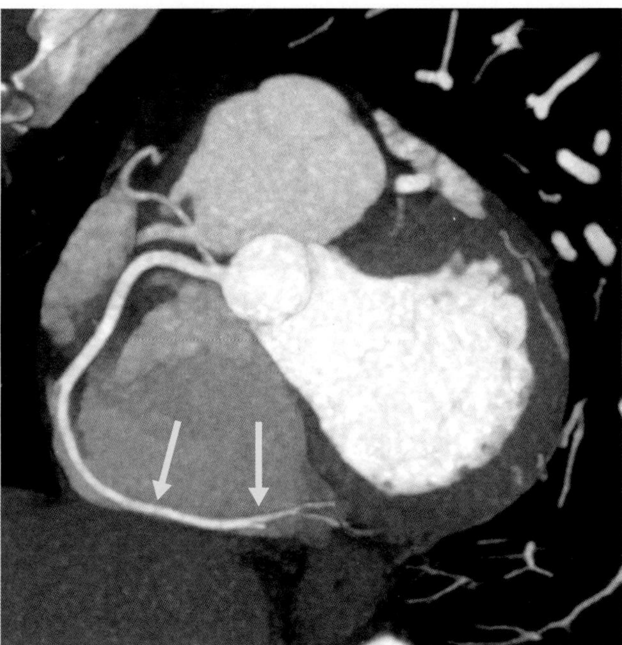

FIGURE 25.26. **Intracavitary Course of the RCA in a 40-Year-Old Man Presenting to the Emergency Department With Chest Pain.** C-view of the RCA (*yellow arrows*) shows the distal RCA coursing within the right atrium. This is a benign course, although the vessel could be theoretically injured during various forms of intervention.

proximal to the bridge, although the bridged segment is typically free of disease. Although there are no definitive imaging findings to distinguish between incidental and symptomatic bridges, deep bridges are more likely to be symptomatic.

Intracavitary Course

Compared to myocardial bridging, an intracavitary course of the coronary artery, where the vessel dives into a cardiac chamber, is relatively rare. In most reported instances, this involves the RCA extending into the right atrium (Fig. 25.26). In one large autopsy series of 331 patients, this abnormal course was seen in 1.8%. However, in a retrospective review of over 9,284 coronary CTAs, the anomaly was seen in only 0.15% of the studies. This anomalous course should not cause any symptoms in relation to compression, but the vessel could be inadvertently injured during right heart cannulation, instrumentation, ablation therapy, or even central line placement.

Split (Double) Coronary Artery

A split or double coronary artery is an extremely rare anomaly. In most instances, there is one coronary artery arising from the sinus of Valsalva, which then divides in its proximal portion into two parallel coronary arteries that mirror their courses. Since in most cases there is a single ostium, many have preferred to use the term "split" to describe this anomaly (Fig. 25.27A). In rarer instances, there is a true "double" or duplicate coronary artery where each has an independent origin from the aortic sinus with near-parallel courses (Fig. 25.27B). In general, this is a benign anomaly.

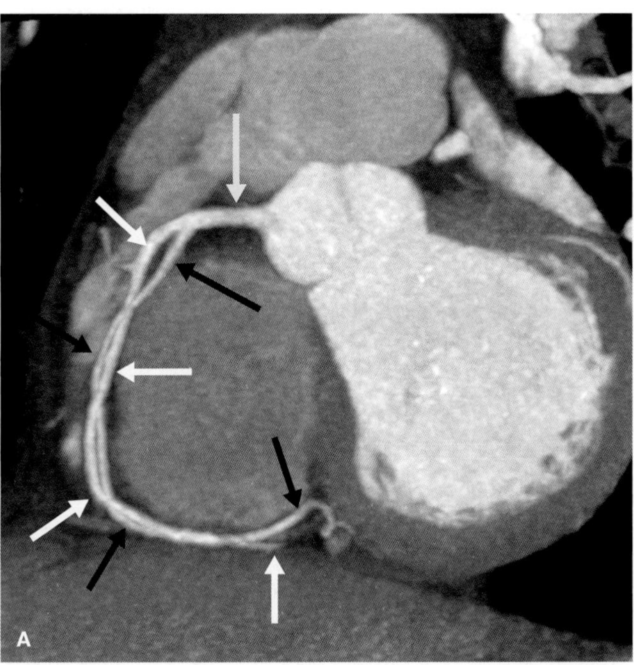

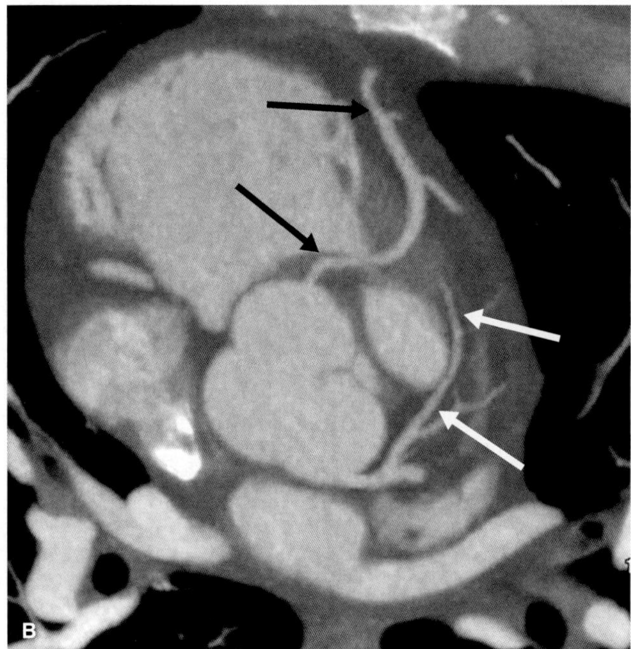

FIGURE 25.27. **Incidental Findings of Extranumerary Coronary Arteries in Two Patients Presenting to the Emergency Department With Chest Pain. A:** A 6-mm MIP C-view of the RCA in a 38-year-old man shows a single RCA proximally (*yellow arrow*), although a few centimeters distal to its origin, the vessel splits in two. The larger vessel (*white arrows*) gives rise to various acute marginal (AM) branches and continues distally as the PDA. The smaller vessel (*black arrows*) does not give rise to any AM branches and continues as the PLV. **B:** Dual left anterior descending (LAD) coronary artery in a 30-year-old man. Axial oblique MIP shows two LAD vessels. The first is a smaller LAD arising from the left main coronary artery which supplies the proximal LAD territory (*white arrows*). The second is a larger LAD arising from the right coronary sinus and supplying the mid and distal LAD territory through a septal course (*black arrows*). These are both benign anomalies.

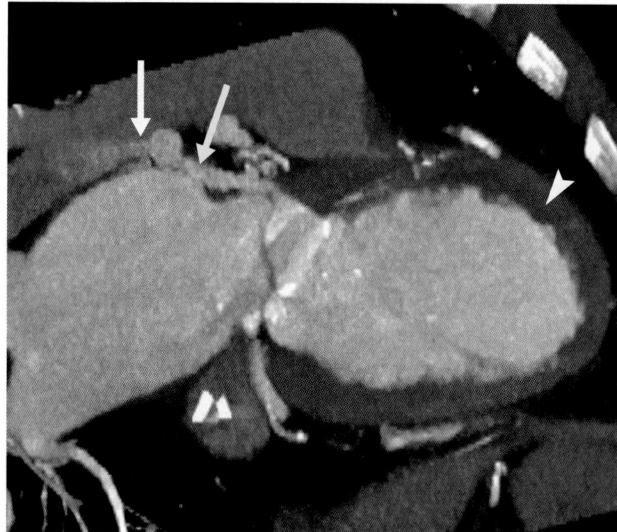

FIGURE 25.28. **Coronary Artery Fistula.** Sagittal oblique multiplanar reformat from a retrospectively gated coronary CTA showed diffuse tortuosity and dilation of the LCx (*yellow arrow*), a portion of which drains into the left pulmonary artery (*white arrow*). The LAD territory shows subendocardial hypoperfusion (*white arrowhead*).

ABNORMALITIES IN TERMINATION

Coronary Fistula

Coronary artery fistulas may be acquired but are most often congenital. Fistulas can involve either the left or right coronary systems, and the literature varies on which distribution is most common. No matter which coronary artery is involved, drainage is most commonly to the right side (from the coronary sinus to the pulmonary artery) and physiologically acts like a left-to-right shunt. In nearly all cases, the involved coronary artery is markedly dilated and tortuous and such a finding on CT should lead to suspicion of a fistula (Fig. 25.28; Video 25.1). Although a fistula can be incidentally found, patients often present with congestive heart failure due to long-standing shunt, ischemia due to a steal phenomenon (preferential flow of blood through lower-pressure fistula instead of through higher-pressure capillary bed), or endocarditis.

CORONARY ARTERY DISEASE

Coronary artery disease (CAD) is the leading cause of mortality of both men and women in the western world. One of the most common indications for coronary CTA is for the assessment of CAD. The excellent spatial resolution of coronary CTA allows for evaluation of coronary artery stenosis, remodeling, and characterization of coronary plaque. Just as important, a normal coronary CTA examination can exclude CAD as the cause of a patient's symptoms.

Although there are multiple indications for coronary CTA, one of its main uses is in patients with nonacute chest pain and a low to intermediate pretest probability of having severe obstructive coronary disease. The use of coronary CTA in patients with a high probability of having obstructive CAD is questionable. More recently, the use of coronary CTA in select patients with acute chest pain has become more widely adopted. However, as discussed in more detail below, this test should not be performed in patients having acute coronary syndrome (ACS) with ST elevation or elevated troponin levels.

Coronary Artery Calcification

While coronary artery CTA is not recommended for screening, noncontrast evaluation of the coronary artery calcification (CAC) in asymptomatic patients is recommended in specific populations. This includes low-risk patients with a family history of premature coronary heart disease (male first-degree relative <55 years or female first-degree relative <65 years) and patients with intermediate-risk factors (10-year risk of coronary heart disease of 10% to 20%) and no history of CAD. In addition, asymptomatic adults ≥40 years of age with diabetes can also undergo screening. Per the U.S. Preventative Task Force, screening CAC should not be obtained in low-risk patients (<10% 10-year risk of coronary heart disease). In addition, as CAC is a screening study, it should not be performed in patients who have previously had a MACE.

In the appropriate patient population, coronary artery calcium scoring (CACS) has been a well-validated marker for cardiovascular risk and can provide incremental value to other population-based data, such as the Framingham Risk Score (FRS). Higher CACS is indicative of a greater likelihood of cardiovascular death. Compared to individuals with a 0 CACS, the hazard ratio for having a major coronary event was 3.89, 7.08, and 6.84 in patients with a 1 to 100, 101 to 300, and >300 CACS, respectively. In patients with extremely high scores (Agatston score >1,000), the relative risk was 10.8. A 0 CACS is also of important prognostic value as those without coronary calcium are unlikely to develop a MACE. In a review of 25,903 asymptomatic subjects without coronary calcium, less than 1% had a cardiac event during a 51-month follow-up period.

Currently, CACS is performed using prospective ECG gating with data reconstructed at a 2.5-mm slice thickness. A tube potential of 120 kV is still recommended for CACS as this kV was used for the initial Agatston scoring method, and lowering the kV (70 kV, 80 kV, or 100 kV) would increase the calcium score due to blooming artifact. While older research studies report a radiation dose of around 1.5 mSv for a CACS, modern scanners can perform this at a fraction of this dose.

Once the CACS scan is reconstructed, various software packages automatically highlight areas along the coronary artery territories with an attenuation greater than 130 HU (Fig. 25.29). These areas are then manually selected or rejected by the radiologist or technologist to calculate an Agatston score which takes into account both the size and highest density of the plaque. By entering the Agatston score into a CACS calculator, the patient's score can be compared to those of the same age, gender, and ethnicity. While asymptomatic patients may undergo CACS for screening, many institutions perform CACS as part of their routine protocol for patients undergoing contrast-enhanced coronary CTA.

Coronary Plaque and Remodeling

An advantage of coronary CTA is its ability to characterize coronary atherosclerotic plaque. In general, coronary plaques can be characterized by their composition, pattern of remodeling, and degree of luminal narrowing.

Coronary artery plaques, or fibroatheromas, are classified as calcified, noncalcified, or mixed. While CAC can be either intimal or medial in location, intimal calcifications are the calcifications related to atherosclerotic disease. Intimal calcifications, which occur due to an osteoblastic-like factor released from intimal vascular smooth muscles cells, are associated with hypertension, dyslipidemia, cigarette smoking, and other proinflammatory conditions. The noncalcified portion

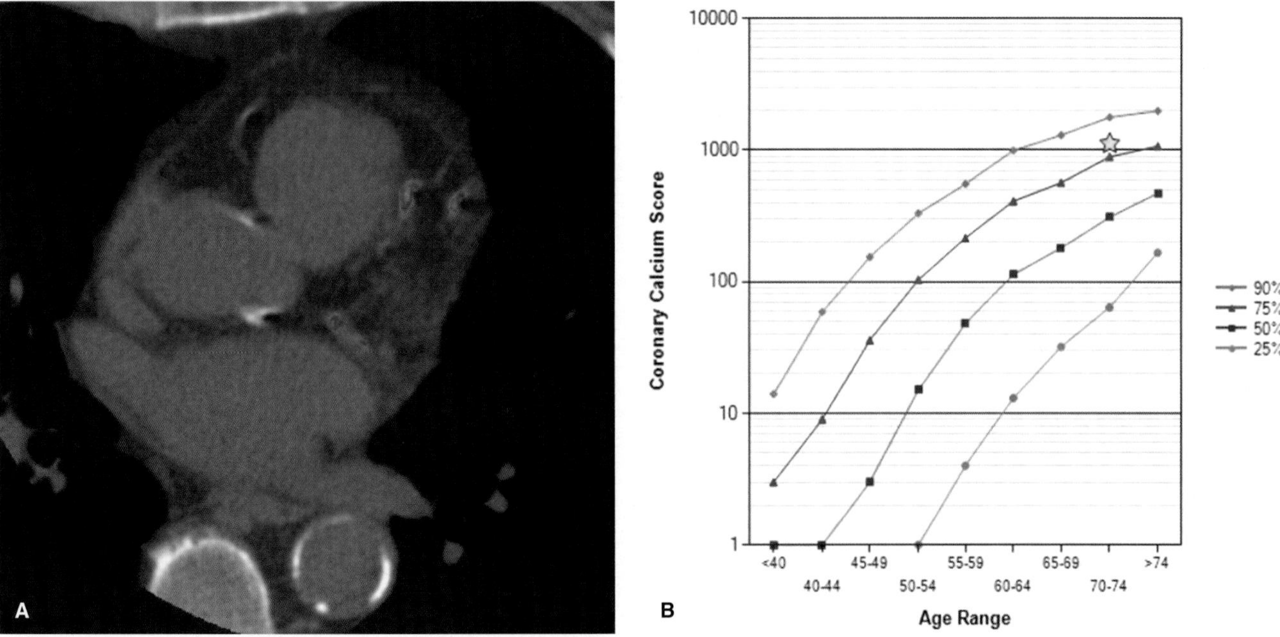

FIGURE 25.29. **Calcium Scoring for Prediction of Future Cardiac Events.** A 73-year-old asymptomatic man with a history of hypertension, smoking, and hyperlipidemia undergoes a calcium score CT. **A:** Axial image from a calcium score CT shows areas of atherosclerotic disease in the LAD distribution and LCx distribution marked as red and blue, respectively. **B:** The patient's total calcium score via the Agatston method was 1,121 which places the patient in the 83rd percentile for patients of the same age, gender, and ethnicity who are free of clinical cardiovascular disease and diabetes.

of a plaque is comprised of two main components within the intima, a fibrous cap which overlies a lipid-rich necrotic core.

Pathologically, plaques can be classified as stable or vulnerable. Atherosclerotic plaques are more vulnerable to rupture with a thinner fibrous cap and larger underlying necrotic core. When the fibrous cap ruptures, the highly thrombogenic necrotic core enters the coronary artery lumen to cause an acute thrombotic event. Plaque rupture is the leading cause of MACEs, and the severity of event will vary depending on the degree of luminal thrombosis. Plaque erosions can also lead to major cardiac events and occur when a portion of the coronary artery endothelium sloughs off. As the endothelium provides a nonthrombogenic surface, the loss of the endothelial layers can precipitate thrombosis formation in the region of the absent endothelium. Since plaque erosion is less common and no current noninvasive imaging techniques are available to predict this process, it will not be discussed.

Imaging manifestations on coronary CTA to help to identify vulnerable plaques include positive remodeling and low-attenuation plaques. Positive remodeling refers to outward growth or expansion of both the coronary artery and associated plaque (Fig. 25.30). The causes of positive remodeling are complex, but it is primarily caused by medial and adventitial inflammation which weakens the underlying framework of the coronary artery and causes its outward expansion. In addition to the medial and adventitial inflammation, intimal inflammation causes thinning of the fibrous cap. As the vessel expands outward, the inflamed and thinned fibrous cap is stretched making it more prone to rupture. In the presence of a large necrotic core, tension and inflammation of the fibrous cap increase making the plaque more vulnerable to rupture. It is important to remember that positive remodeling (outward growth) and negative remodeling (inward growth, stenosis) usually occur together. In cases where positive remodeling is the predominant growth pattern, luminal narrowing may be only mild to moderate, and therefore, the patients will remain asymptomatic. It is also important to remember that positive remodeling can lead to a visual overestimation of stenosis.

The attenuation of the noncalcified plaque can also be assessed to identify vulnerable lesions. In general, a high-attenuation plaque tends to correspond to a fibroatheroma with a larger and thicker fibrous cap and thus has a smaller likelihood of rupture. On the other hand, a low-attenuation plaque, defined as a plaque with attenuation value <30 HU, corresponds to a plaque with a larger lipid-rich necrotic core and thus has a higher propensity to rupture (Fig. 25.30). While either the presence of positive remodeling or low-attenuation plaque on coronary CTA increases the risk of a future acute coronary event, the presence of both findings dramatically increases the risk. In a study by Motoyama et al. assessing plaque characteristics associated with subsequent development of an acute coronary event in 1,059 patients, 22.5% of patients with both findings develop an acute event compared to 3.7% with one finding and 0.5% with neither positive remodeling nor low-attenuation plaque.

An additional coronary CTA finding that may be indicative of a thin-cap atheromatous vulnerable plaque is termed the "napkin-ring" sign (Fig. 25.31). This is visualized as a rim of high attenuation surrounding an area of low attenuation representing the inflamed fibrous cap surrounding the necrotic lipid core, and its presence can be an independent predictor of a future acute coronary event. The presence of these imaging findings should be mentioned in the coronary CTA report, as they may lead to changes in patient therapy.

Coronary Stenosis. Negative remodeling, or inward growth of a plaque, causes coronary artery stenosis. This stenosis can occur rapidly in the setting of an acute coronary thrombosis or plaque rupture. However, in many instances, stenosis occurs slowly due to continued growth of a stable plaque.

As CT technology has continued to improve, there has been increasing sensitivity and negative predictive value for morphologic evaluation of the coronary arteries in comparison to catheter-based angiography. More recent multicenter trials using 64-slice CT have demonstrated even greater efficacy for morphologic evaluation. A 2008 meta-analysis of

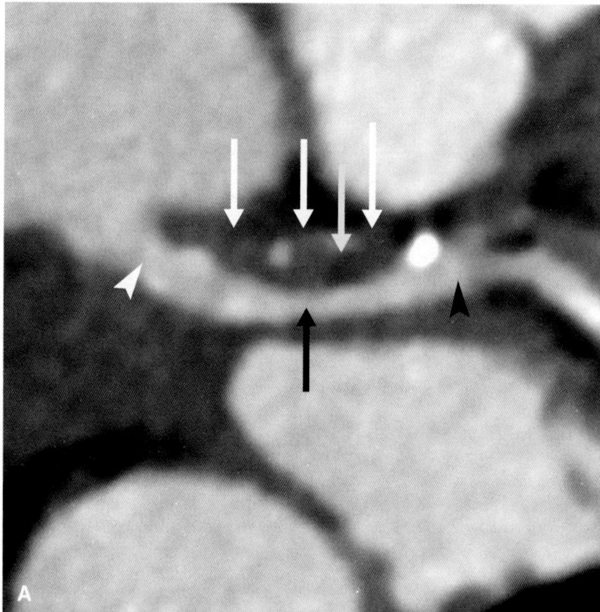

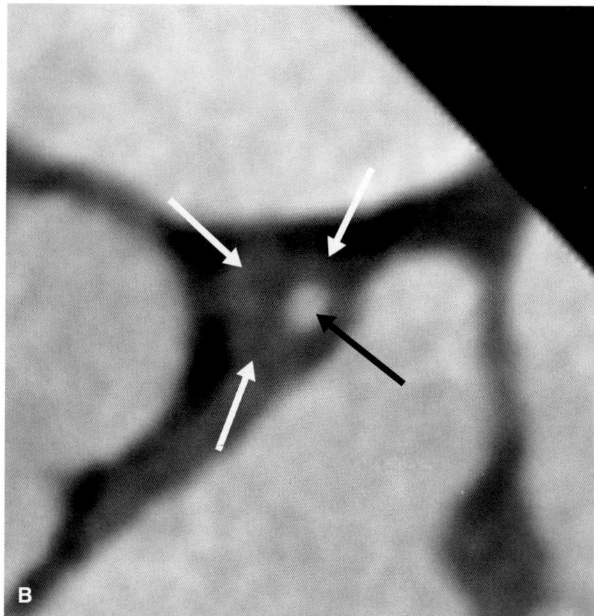

FIGURE 25.30. **Positive Remodeling in a 55-Year-Old Man With Atypical Chest Pain. A, B:** Axial oblique (**A**) and transverse (**B**) images of the left main coronary artery (LM) show exuberant mixed, but predominantly noncalcified, plaque which partially wraps around the vessel (*white arrows*). The plaque leads to outward growth of the vessel, termed positive remodeling. Within the positive remodeling, there is a focus of low-density plaque measuring 10 HU (*yellow arrow*). The presence of both these findings suggests a "vulnerable plaque" with a greater likelihood to rupture and potentially cause an acute myocardial event. Including the plaque, the maximum transverse diameter of the vessel measured in **B** was 8 mm, whereas the proximal and distal LM have a maximal diameter of 6 mm and 4 mm, respectively. This illustrates the outward growth (positive remodeling) of the vessel. The luminal diameters of the proximal (*white arrowhead*, **A**), mid (*black arrow*, **A, B**), and distal (*black arrowhead*, **A**) LM are 5 mm, 3 mm, and 4 mm, respectively, consistent with a 33.3% stenosis. While the positive remodeling is a predominant feature, there is usually a concomitant component of negative remodeling (stenosis) as well.

64-slice coronary CTA among 1,296 patients in 28 studies showed a pooled sensitivity of 98%, specificity of 89%, positive predictive value (PPV) of 93%, and negative predictive value of 100% in comparison with catheter angiography. A more recent meta-analysis using dual-source CT technology demonstrated similarly excellent results even in the setting of higher heart rates. The most recently published multisociety appropriateness guidelines for coronary CTA consider stable symptomatic patients at low to intermediate risk for coronary events suitable for this test.

When reviewing a coronary CTA, it is imperative to use both multiplanar reformatted (MPR) reconstructions and axial images to assess the degree of stenosis. While maximum-intensity projection or volume-rendered images can supplement the use of MPRs, they should not be used for primary diagnosis. Multiple vendors offer software tools beyond MPRs

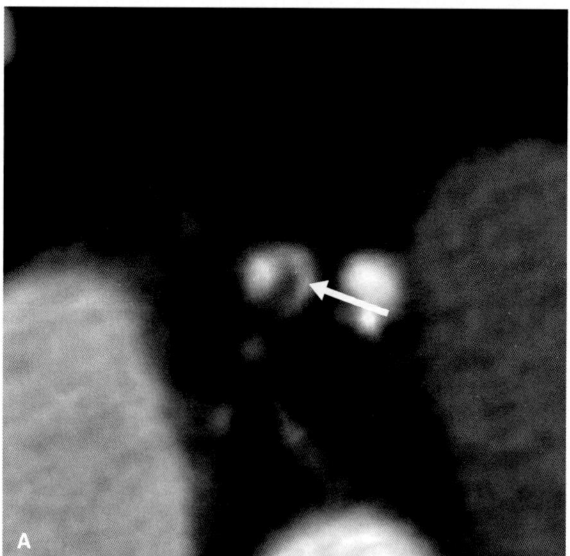

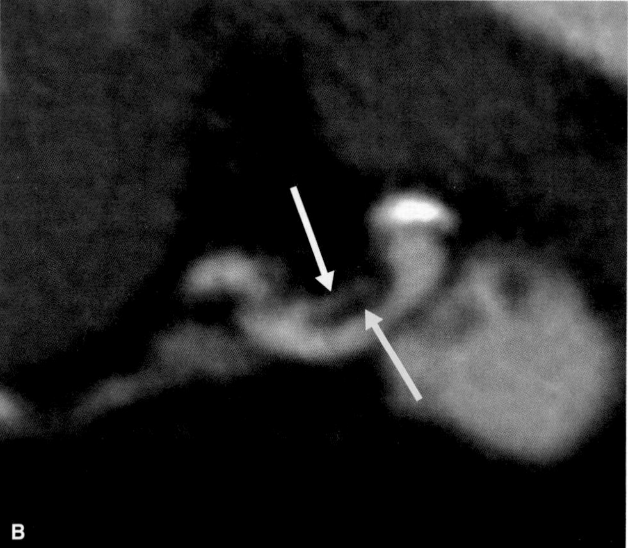

FIGURE 25.31. **Napkin-Ring Sign.** Transverse (**A**) and longitudinal (**B**) images through the mid-LCx show positive remodeling with only a mild stenosis. The positive remodeling demonstrates a few areas of low attenuation plaque (*yellow arrow*). In addition, there is fine linear enhancement along the periphery of the noncalcified plaque, creating a "napkin-ring" sign (*white arrows*, **A, B**). This is another finding suggestive of a "vulnerable plaque."

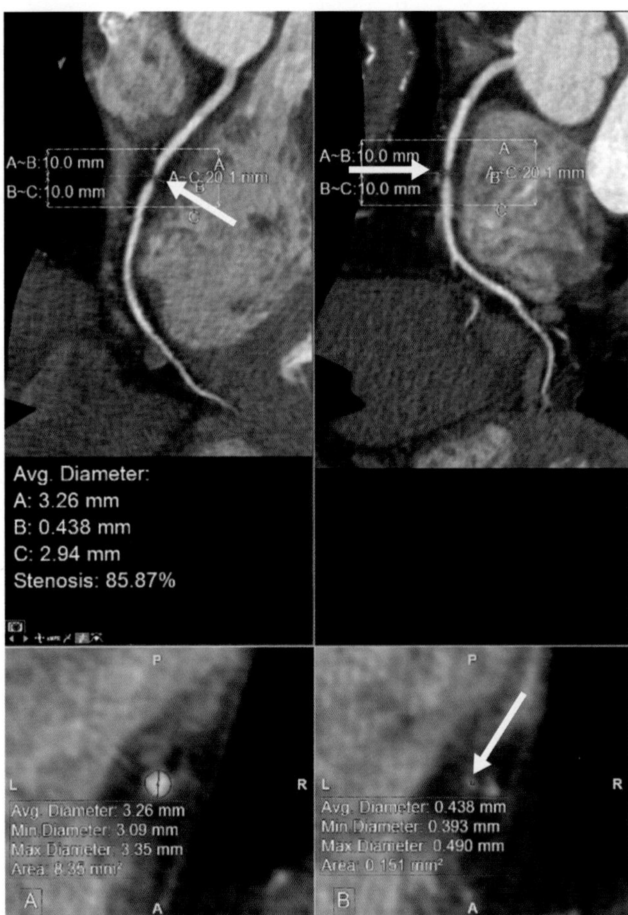

FIGURE 25.32. **Semi-Automated Stenosis Measurement in a 70-Year-Old Man With a Severe Stenosis in the LCx.** Curved MPR images through the LCx show a focal area of noncalcified plaque leading to a stenosis (*white arrows*). The diameter 1 cm proximal and distal to the stenosis measures 3.3 mm and 2.9 cm, respectively, for a mean diameter of 3.1 cm. The diameter in the areas of stenosis measures 0.44 mm. This corresponds to an 86% stenosis.

which can perform semiautomated stenosis calculations, assess plaque morphology, measure total plaque volume, and create curved MPR images of each vessel (Fig. 25.32).

For all vessels except the left main coronary artery, where a stenosis >50% is considered severe, coronary stenosis is quantified as absent (0%), minimal (1% to 24%), mild (25% to 49%), moderate (50% to 69%), severe (70% to 99%), and occlusive (100%) (Fig. 25.33). In patients with stable chest pain, a coronary artery etiology is highly unlikely in those with absent, minimal, or mild stenosis. Although a 70% or greater stenosis is considered severe, a stenosis ≥50% can potentially lead to hemodynamic compromise and therefore may be significant. Therefore, the presence of a moderate stenosis may require functional assessment with exercise ECG, exercise or pharmacologic nuclear stress testing, or stress echocardiography. In patients with a severe stenosis, functional assessment or an invasive catheter angiography should be considered.

In addition to evaluation of anatomic stenosis, the myocardium should be closely evaluated to assess for subendocardial myocardial perfusion defects (Fig. 25.34). In the presence of a significant stenosis, this usually represents an area of myocardial ischemia or infarct. If a retrospective ECG-gated coronary CTA is performed, at least 10 phases should be reconstructed at uniform intervals to allow for assessment of biventricular function which can be quantified using various software tools. Even with the use of ECG mA modulation, functional data can still be obtained throughout the cardiac cycle. This can be useful to evaluate for regional wall motion abnormalities associated with myocardial ischemia or infarct (Fig. 25.35).

While the negative predictive value of coronary CTA for assessment of coronary stenosis is excellent, the PPV is less optimal. One of the main reasons for this is the presence of moderate and even severe stenosis which is not hemodynamically significant, as determined by functional imaging or invasive catheter angiography. Cardiac CT stress imaging and CT fractional flow reserve (CT-FFR) are two newer techniques that can help provide physiologic data which can further increase the PPV of coronary CTA.

In myocardial perfusion CT, images of the heart and coronary arteries are obtained during the early portion of first-pass circulation, when iodinated contrast is predominantly intravascular. Akin to nuclear medicine stress testing, this is often done both at rest and during pharmacologic stress. A single acquisition, where the heart is scanned once during rest and once during stress, or a dynamic acquisition, where the heart is scanned multiple times during both stress and rest, can be performed. While the dynamic acquisition provides more detailed perfusion data, the radiation dose will be higher albeit similar in range to a ^{99m}Tc and less than a ^{201}Tl and dual-isotope SPECT for viability assessment. Stress and rest attenuation maps of the myocardium can be generated to determine if a coronary stenosis seen on CTA correlates with myocardial hypoperfusion. Similar to MRI stress testing, which is discussed in more detail below, myocardial ischemia on first-pass perfusion will manifest as regional subendocardial hypoperfusion corresponding to a specific vascular territory during stress that should improve or resolve during rest. Infarcted tissue should show persistent perfusion defect(s) during rest imaging. Iodinated contrast will concentrate in infarcted tissue and can be visualized by obtaining a third scan 5 to 10 minutes after the last contrast administration. Although delayed-enhancement CT shows high accuracy for the detection of infarcted tissue, it often underestimates the degree of infarct size when compared to MRI.

The second method is CT-FFR. The concept of CT-FFR is derived from invasive coronary angiography where the differences in pressure across a stenosis are directly measured. An FFR measurement of 1 means that there is no change in pressure across a stenosis, whereas an FFR of 0.7 means that the pressure distal to the stenosis is only 70% of that proximal to the stenosis. In general, a FFR of 0.8 or lower is considered hemodynamically significant. With CT-FFR, the data from a standard coronary CTA undergo computational fluid dynamic modeling and deep machine-based learning algorithms. This allows for both anatomic and hemodynamic information to be obtained from a single acquisition. Multiple studies have shown that the use of CT-FFR in conjunction with coronary CTA improves accuracy and specificity (Fig. 25.36). This can change treatment strategy and avoid unnecessary invasive testing, especially in those with anatomically moderate stenosis.

Coronary CTA in the Setting of Acute Chest Pain. ACS includes myocardial infarction with ST elevation (STEMI), myocardial infarct without ST elevation (NSTEMI), and unstable angina. In patients with acute chest pain and ECG changes or elevated cardiac troponin levels, the first line of therapy is thrombolysis and revascularization. Except in very rare exceptions, noninvasive imaging should not be performed in patients with ACS. However, coronary CTA is an excellent tool to assess patients presenting to the ED with acute chest pain, a low to intermediate risk of CAD, and a negative troponin level. In general, a coronary etiology of the chest pain is unlikely in patients without a significant stenosis on coronary CTA. Multiple prospective trials have been performed to compare the use of coronary CTA to standard

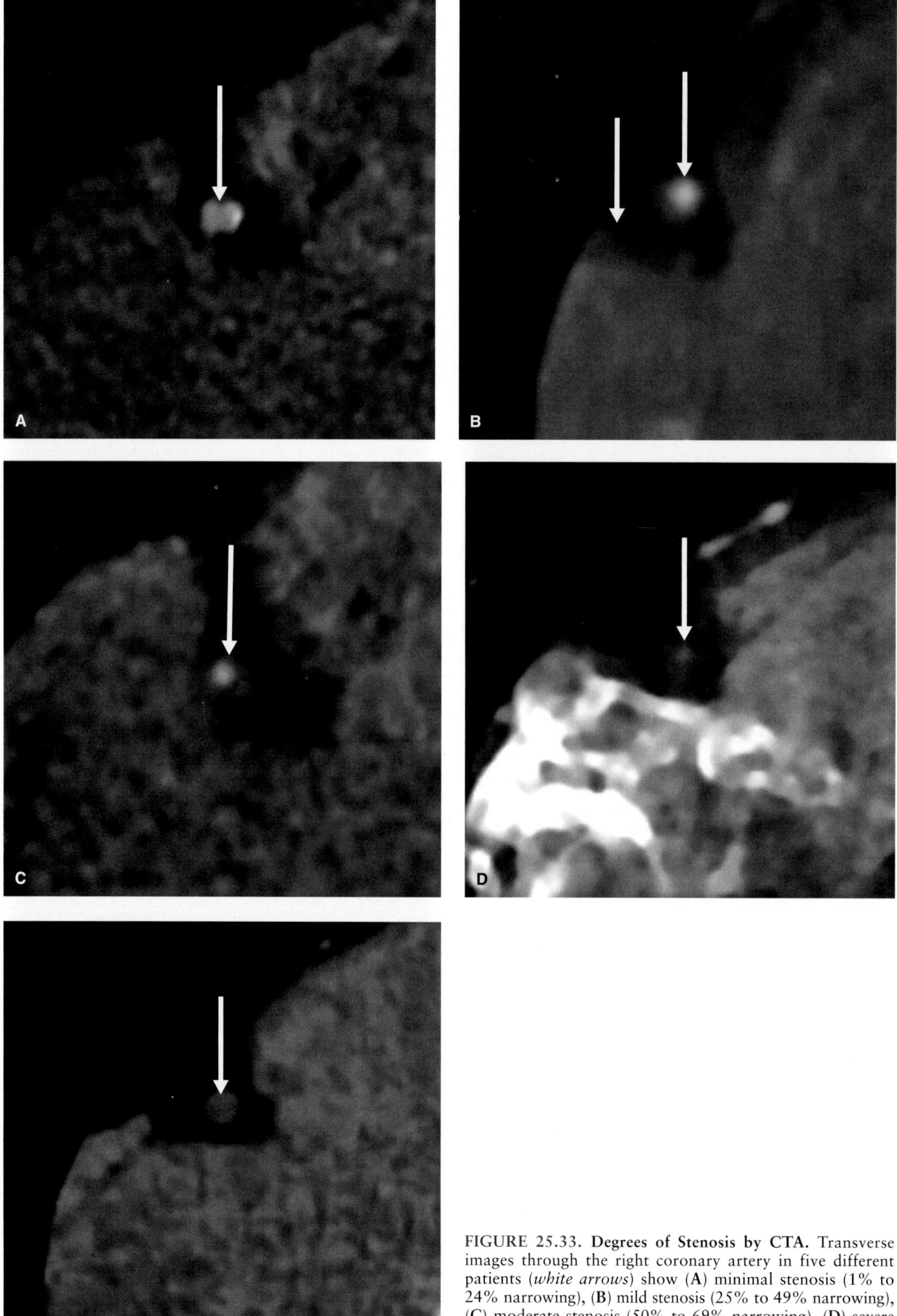

FIGURE 25.33. **Degrees of Stenosis by CTA.** Transverse images through the right coronary artery in five different patients (*white arrows*) show (**A**) minimal stenosis (1% to 24% narrowing), (**B**) mild stenosis (25% to 49% narrowing), (**C**) moderate stenosis (50% to 69% narrowing), (**D**) severe stenosis (70% to 99% narrowing), and (**E**) occlusion (100% stenosis).

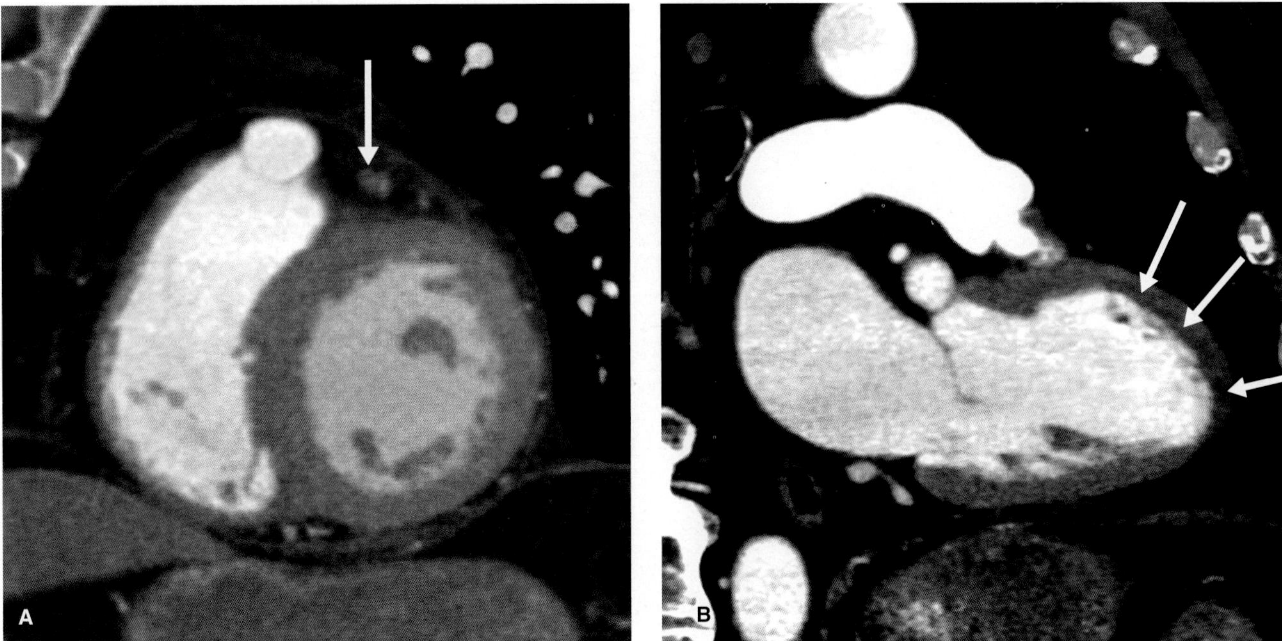

FIGURE 25.34. **Subendocardial Hypoperfusion in a 60-Year-Old Woman With Chest Pain. A:** Short-axis image through the mid-cavity of the left ventricle shows a severe stenosis of the LAD (*white arrow*). **B:** Two-chamber image demonstrates subendocardial hypoperfusion in the LAD distribution (*white arrows*). On CT, the hypoperfused myocardium could represent ischemic or infarcted tissue.

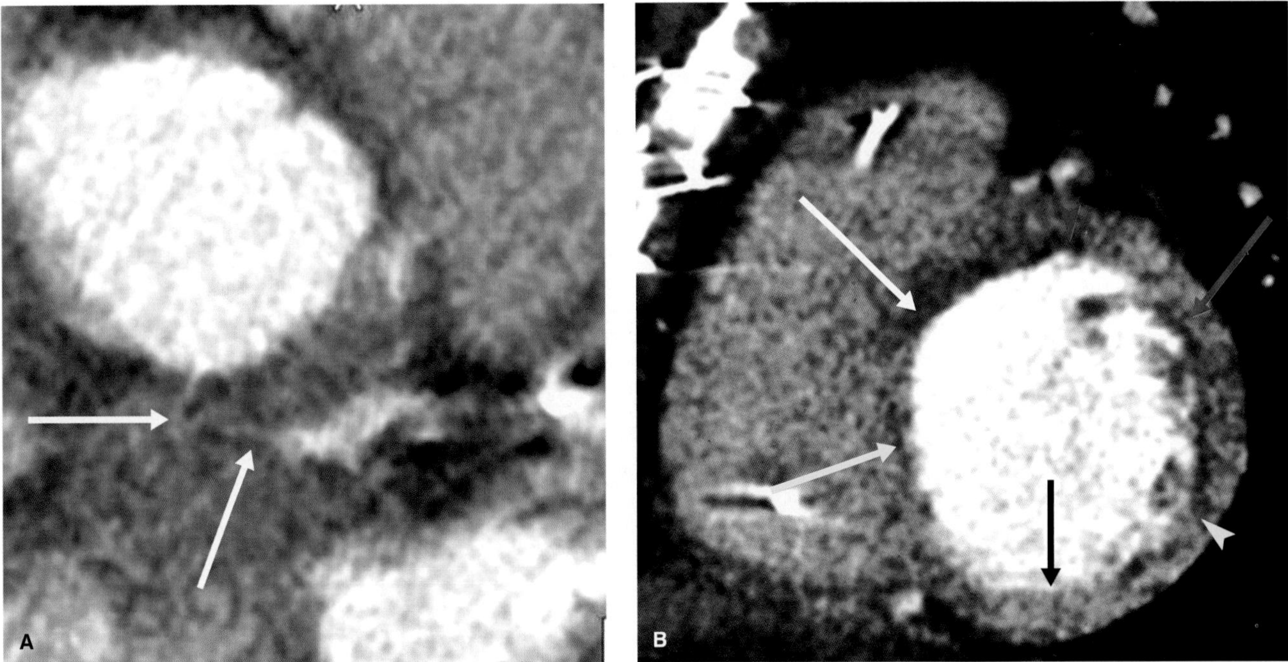

FIGURE 25.35. **Left Main Coronary Artery Territory Myocardial Infarct in a 60-Year-Old Man in Disseminated Intravascular Coagulation (DIC), Platelet Count of 2,950/mL, Troponin I of 57.7 ng/mL, and a Heart Rate of 122 bpm. A:** Axial oblique image from a retrospectively gated coronary CTA shows near-complete occlusion of the LM (*white arrows*). **B:** Short-axis image through the base shows subendocardial hypoperfusion involving the anteroseptal (*white arrow*), anterior (*red arrowhead*), anterolateral (*red arrow*), and portions of the inferolateral (*yellow arrowhead*) and inferoseptal (*yellow arrow*) segments. These findings are consistent with infarcts in both the LAD and LCx distributions. The inferior segment (*black arrow*) and portion of the inferolateral and inferoseptal segment are supplied by the RCA which was normal.

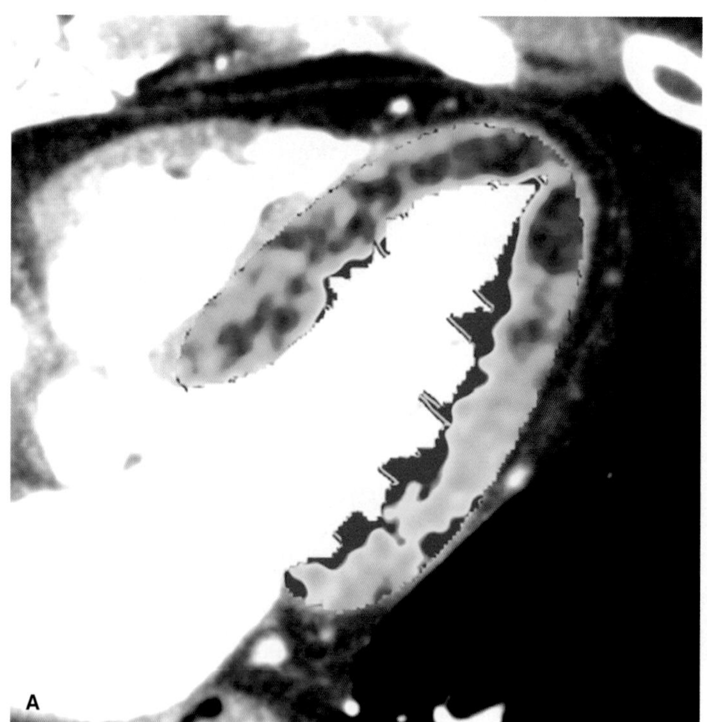

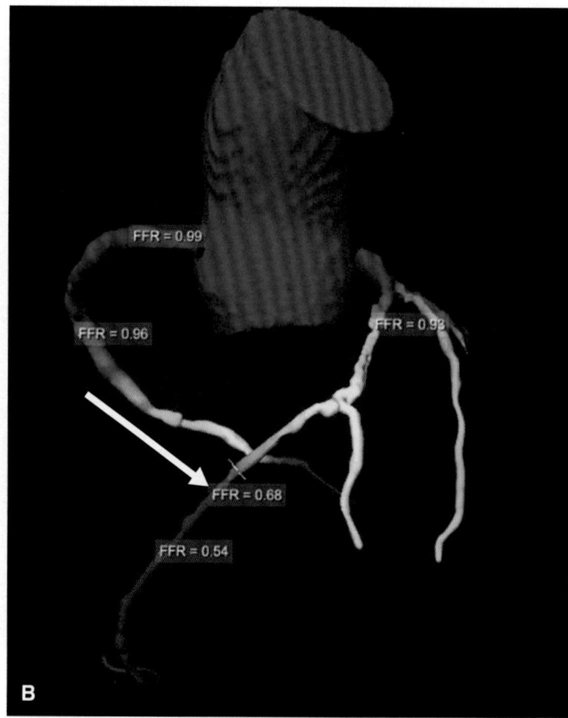

FIGURE 25.36. **Myocardial Perfusion Imaging and CT-FFR in a 75-Year-Old Man With Episodic Chest Pain. A:** Four-chamber image from a stress perfusion CT shows hypoperfusion (*blue pixels*) in the septum and apex consistent with LAD territory ischemia. The rest perfusion study was normal. **B:** CT-FFR image from the same patient shows significantly reduced flow in the mid and distal LAD (*white arrow*), with CT-FFR values less than 0.8. Flow in the LCx and RCA territories is normal. The patient underwent stenting of his LAD. (Images courtesy of Joseph Schoepf, MD.)

of care therapy, such as functional stress test, in the emergency department setting. Each showed that coronary CTA, compared to the standard of care, allows for earlier discharge without a significant difference in adverse cardiac events. Similar to patients with stable chest pain, those with a moderate stenosis may still have hemodynamic compromise and may need to undergo functional testing or invasive coronary angiography (Fig. 25.37).

MRI IN CORONARY ARTERY DISEASE

MR Imaging of the Coronary Arteries

While coronary CTA is the primary noninvasive technique for evaluating the coronary arteries, coronary MR angiography (cMRA) has demonstrated value as a potential alternative technique. Coronary MRA has some distinct advantages as studies can be performed without intravenous contrast and patients are not exposed to ionizing radiation. However, compared to coronary CTA, cMRA is limited due to its reduced spatial resolution, longer exam times, and operator dependency. Although there are advocates for using this technology in the assessment of CAD, cMRA is not currently used for the assessment of CAD in most institutions. Coronary MRA is accepted as a tool to assess for anomalous coronary arteries and coronary artery aneurysms, especially in the pediatric population or those with severe contrast allergies (Fig. 25.38). At 1.5 T, cMRA is performed using a whole-heart, free-breathing, 3D steady–state free precession (SSFP) sequence. Blood appears bright on SSFP sequences due its inherent T2/T1 weighting, obviating the need for contrast. At 3 T, gadolinium contrast agents are recommended due to the different sequences used.

MR Assessment of the Myocardium in Coronary Artery Disease

MRI is one of the strongest tools in the noninvasive evaluation of cardiomyopathies. It is considered the gold standard for evaluating cardiac function and can differentiate between ischemic and nonischemic etiologies of myocardial injury and dysfunction. The below section will concentrate on the use of cardiac MRI for ischemic cardiomyopathies, as its use in the assessment of nonischemic cardiomyopathies is presented in a different chapter.

When a patient undergoes a cardiac MRI with a known or suspected ischemic cardiomyopathy, the radiologist has four main goals: confirm (or refute) the suspected diagnosis, evaluate cardiac function and morphology, assess for myocardial viability, and look for any complications. Functional evaluation is performed using an SSFP sequence at 1.5 T and either a GRE of SSFP sequence at 3 T. To acquire a single slice along a prespecified cardiac plane, an expiratory breath-held, retrospectively gated, segmented sequence is obtained over multiple heart beats. Depending on the patient-related factors, such as heart rate, rhythm, and breath-hold ability, as well as technical factors, such as use of parallel imaging, k-space filling techniques, and TR optimization, this breath hold can last between 5 and 12 seconds. Although protocols vary by institution, in most instances, a single SSFP (or GRE) cine sequence is obtained in the two-, three-, and four-chamber planes. However, the mainstay for functional evaluation is the short-axis plane. Using a 6- to 8-mm slice thickness, sometimes with a 2-mm gap between slices, a short-axis stack of cine SSFP (or GRE) sequences are obtained through the entire cardiac axis from the mitral valve plane to the cardiac apex.

When placed in a cine viewer, SSFP imaging allows detailed assessment of wall motion and thickness. Due to the territorial

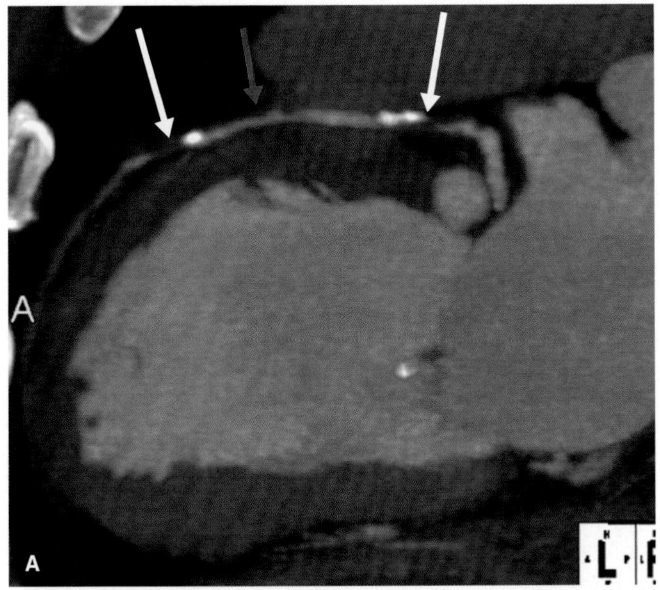

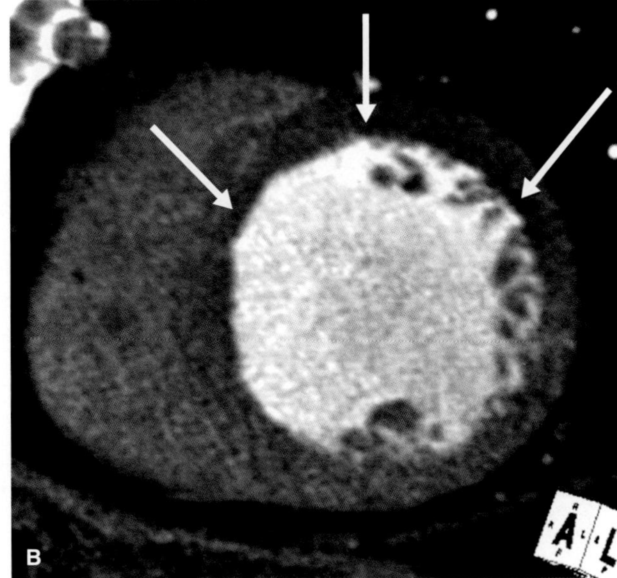

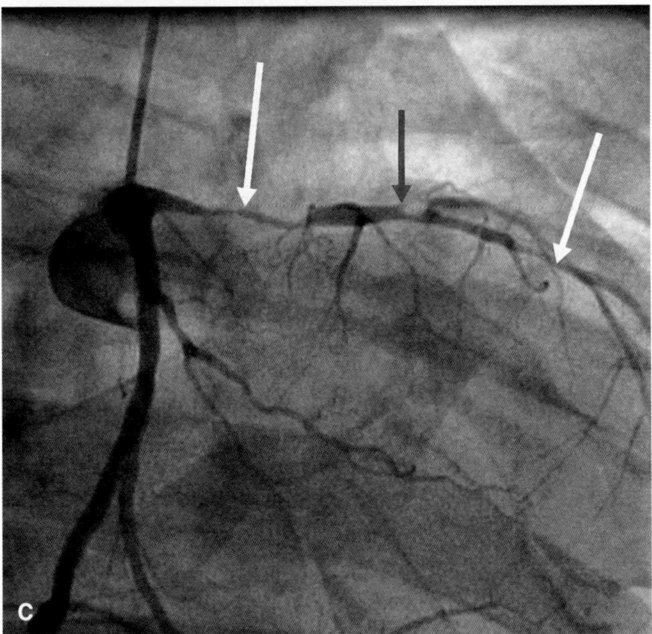

FIGURE 25.37. **Coronary CTA in a 46-Year-Old Man With a History of Smoking and Hypercholesterolemia Who Presented to the Emergency Department With Mild Chest Pain and Normal Troponin Levels. A:** Longitudinal image through the LAD shows multiple areas of calcified and mixed plaque leading to two long-segment areas of severe stenosis (*white arrows*) and a focal area of severe stenosis in between (*red arrow*). There were only areas of mild plaque and stenosis in the LCx and RCA distributions. **B:** Short-axis image through LV base shows subendocardial hypoperfusion in the LAD distribution (*white arrows*). **C:** Right anterior oblique image from subsequent cardiac catheterization shows two long-segment areas of severe stenosis (*white arrows*) and more focal severe stenosis (*red arrow*) corresponding to findings on CTA.

distribution of the coronary arteries, myocardial infarct or ischemia will manifest as a wall motion abnormality localized to a specific vascular territory (Figs. 25.39 to 25.41). Depending on the severity of injury, the wall motion can be described as hypokinetic (reduced contractility), akinetic (no contractility), or dyskinetic (paradoxical movement). This distribution of motion abnormality due to infarct can significantly vary given the heterogeneity of coronary artery distribution and location of obstruction. In most patients, the anterior and anteroseptal segments at the base and mid-cavity levels are supplied by the LAD and its branches (Fig. 25.39). Portions of the anterolateral segments can be supplied by diagonal branches from the LAD depending on a patient's anatomy. The LCx and its OM branches will often supply the inferolateral segment but can also supply portions of the anterolateral and/or inferior segments depending on size and dominance (Fig. 25.40). At the apical level, in many patients, the anterior, lateral, and septal segments are supplied by the LAD distribution and the inferior segment is supplied by the PDA. The cardiac apex (segment 17) is usually supplied by the LAD. If the left main is involved, myocardium in both the LAD and LCx distributions will be affected. If a patient is right dominant, the RCA and its PDA and PLV branches will supply the inferoseptal, inferior, and possibly portions of the inferolateral segments at the base and mid-cavity levels, depending on the size and extent of the PLV branch (Figs. 25.41 and 25.42). Wall motion abnormalities corresponding to one of these vascular distributions is a good clue that the underlying etiology is coronary in origin. Even in multivessel disease where wall motion abnormalities may involve multiple territories, the degree of dysfunction and extent of myocardial injury often varies between territories allowing for diagnosis.

Other signs of myocardial injury due to infarct depend on the acuity of the injury. In the setting of a recent MI, there may be increased subendocardial signal intensity in the myocardium on T2-weighted sequences secondary to myocardial edema. These T2-weighted sequences are usually performed using a double inversion recovery, "black blood," preparation used to null the signal in the blood pool or a triple inversion recovery preparation to null both the signal in blood

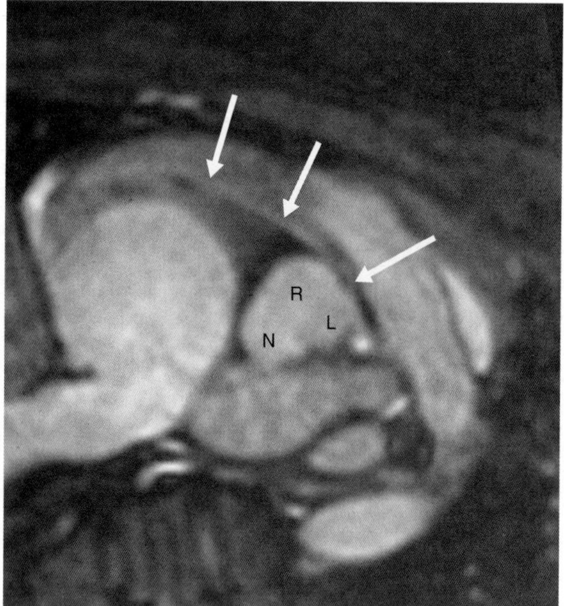

FIGURE 25.38. A 3D SSFP MRA of the coronary arteries in a 15-year-old boy with chest pain and an abnormal echocardiogram show an interarterial course of the RCA which is narrowed proximally (*white arrows*). Although there are advocates for using coronary MRA to assess for atherosclerotic coronary artery disease, most institutions use cMRA to assess for anomalous coronary arteries and coronary artery aneurysms, especially in the pediatric population or those with severe contrast allergies (*R, L, N* = right, left, and noncoronary sinuses, respectively).

and fat (Fig. 25.41; Video 25.4). It should also be mentioned that myocardial edema can sometimes be seen on an SSFP sequence due to its T2/T1 weighting (Fig. 25.42). Microvascular obstruction (MO), another sign of an acute or subacute infarct, is discussed below.

As the myocardium remodels after an infarct, the affected segments can become thinned depending on the severity of injury. This thinning is often associated with worsening function as the affected segments may become akinetic or dyskinetic (Figs. 25.39, Videos 25.2 and 25.3; 25.40 and 25.42). While myocardial thinning often suggests scarring, it does not necessarily indicate nonviable myocardium, which is assessed using delayed enhancement imaging.

First-pass myocardial perfusion imaging is performed during the administration of intravenous gadolinium, which is a contrast medium that shortens T1 relaxation. In areas of ischemia and infarct, subendocardial predominant hypoperfusion is often seen corresponding to the region(s) of wall motion abnormality identified in cine imaging (Fig. 25.41).

Ten to 15 minutes after the injection of gadolinium, delayed images are usually acquired. Although gadolinium is an extracellular agent, it can accumulate in areas where there has been acute myocyte injury secondary to cell membrane disruption seen in acute or subacute infarct (Figs. 25.41 and 25.42) or it can accumulate in areas with an increased interstitial space, such as in an area of scarring as seen in chronic infarct (Figs. 25.39 and 25.40). This retained gadolinium leads to T1 shortening in the affected areas. To highlight the effects of gadolinium, the delayed enhancement sequences are performed at a set inversion time which is used to null the signal of the normal myocardium. As myocardial injury from an infarct starts in the subendocardial region of the ventricle and extends outward, subendocardial late gadolinium enhancement corresponding to a coronary artery segmental territory is indicative of myocardial infarction. The extent of LGE is directly related to the likelihood of successful revascularization with bypass grafting or percutaneous coronary intervention. Subendocardial enhancement measuring <50% of the regional myocardial thickness is associated with functional recovery after revascularization (Fig. 25.41), while areas of >50% transmural LGE extent are much less likely to respond to revascularization (Figs. 25.39, 25.40, and 25.42). If the infarct involves the entire thickness of the myocardium, it is called a transmural infarct. Large transmural infarcts, especially those in the LAD distribution, are more likely to cause left ventricular aneurysms (Fig. 25.39). Due to alterations of blood flow, anterior left ventricular aneurysms have a propensity to develop thrombus which can subsequently embolize.

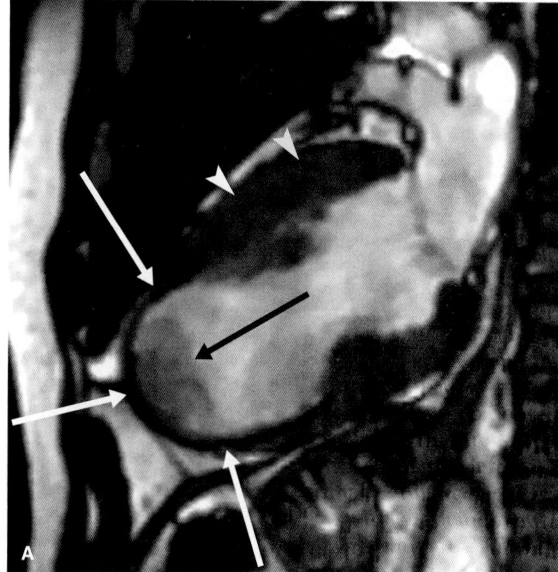

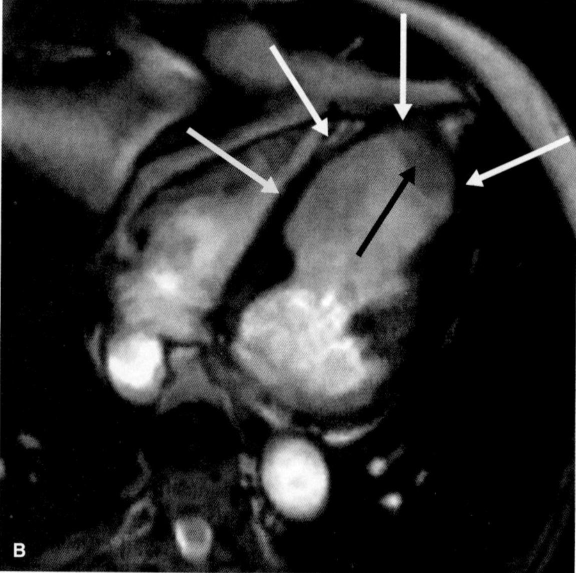

FIGURE 25.39. **Transmural LAD Territory Infarct With Apical Aneurysm and Thrombus in a 77-Year-Old Man. A, B:** 2-chamber (**A**) and 4-chamber (**B**) images from a cine SSFP sequences demonstrate thinning of all the apical segments of the left ventricle (*white arrows*) which were also dyskinetic. The anteroseptal segment at the mid-cavity level was also thinned and akinetic (*yellow arrow*). The anterior segments at the mid-cavity level (*white arrowhead*, **A**) and base (*yellow arrowhead*) were hypokinetic. There is a low-signal mass in the left ventricular apex consistent with a thrombus (*black arrows*).

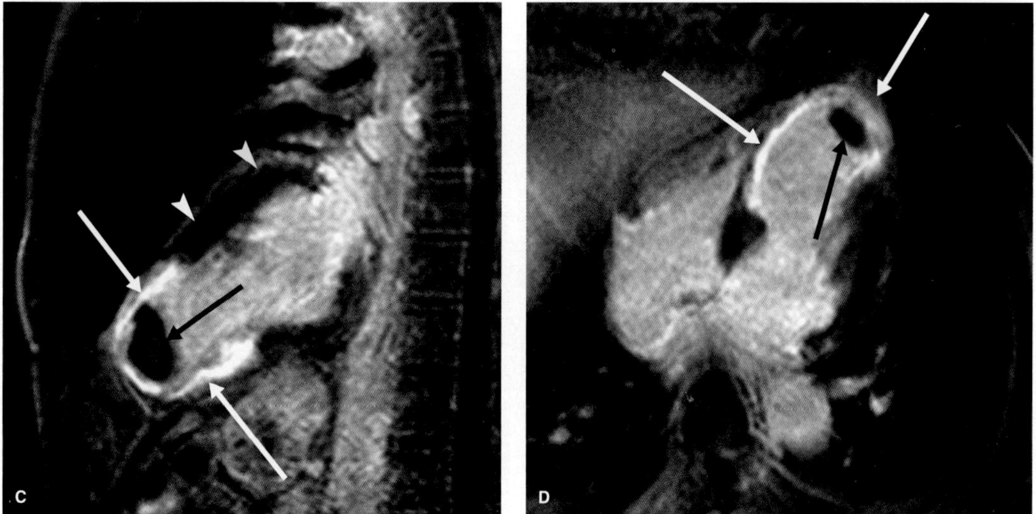

FIGURE 25.39. (*Continued*) **C, D:** 2-chamber (**C**) and 4-chamber (**D**) gadolinium delayed enhancement images shows transmural enhancement of the dyskinetic to akinetic segments (*white arrows*) consistent with non-viable myocardium. However, the hypokinetic anterior segments at the mid-cavity (*white arrowhead*) and base (*yellow arrowhead*) show no enhancement and could improve function with revascularization. The apical thrombus (*black arrows*) is devoid of signal.

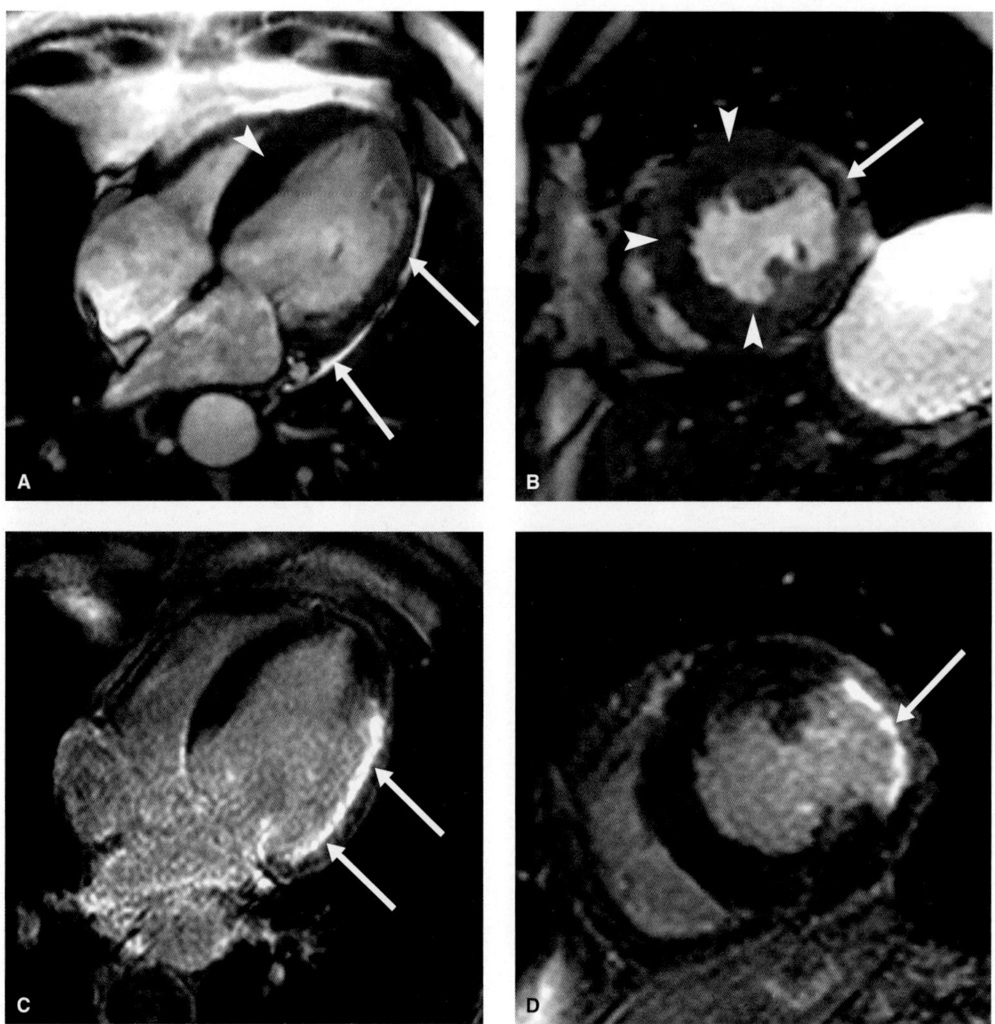

FIGURE 25.40. **Left Circumflex Territory Infarct (LCx) in a 67-Year-Old Patient With History of Myocardial Infarction. A, B:** 4-chamber (**A**) and mid-cavity short axis (**B**) images from SSFP cine sequences show thinning of the anterolateral segments and portions of the inferolateral segments of the left ventricle at the base and mid-cavity levels (*white arrows*). These segments were also akinetic. **C, D:** 4-chamber (**C**) and mid-cavity short-axis (**D**) LGE images show transmural enhancement in the akinetic segments (*white arrows*) consistent with non-viable myocardium. Although this territory could potentially be supplied by a large diagonal branch from the LAD, cardiac catheterization confirmed a proximal LCx occlusion in this right coronary artery dominant patient.

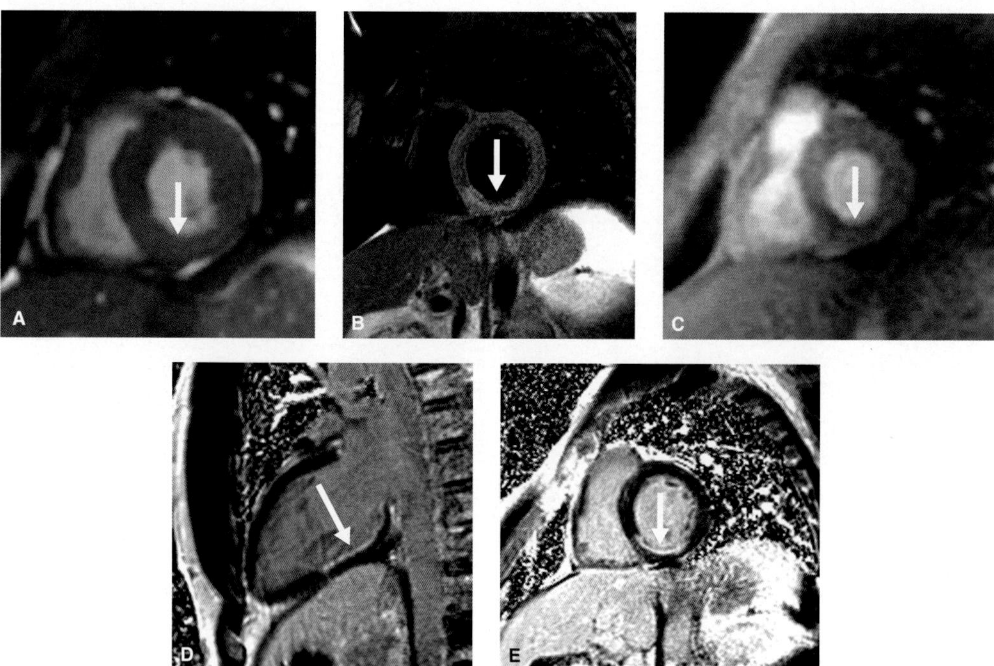

FIGURE 25.41. **Subacute Myocardial Infarct in the RCA Distribution in a Patient With Right Coronary Artery Dominance but a Relatively Small Posterior Left Ventricular Branch. A:** Short axis image through the base of the left ventricle from a cine SSFP sequence shows mild thinning of the inferior segment which was hypokinetic (*white arrow*). **B:** T2-weighted triple inversion recovery image through the base shows subendocardial high signal due to edema from recent infarct (*white arrow*). **C:** Short-axis perfusion image at the base shows subendocardial hypoperfusion which can be seen with ischemia or infarct (*white arrow*). **D, E:** Short-axis (**D**) and two-chamber (E) LGE images show thin subendocardial delayed enhancement (*white arrows*) involving the inferior segment at the base and mid-cavity level consistent with infarct. Given that the enhancement is less than 50% of the myocardial thickness, the underlying myocardium is considered viable, and the patient is likely to recover function after reperfusion.

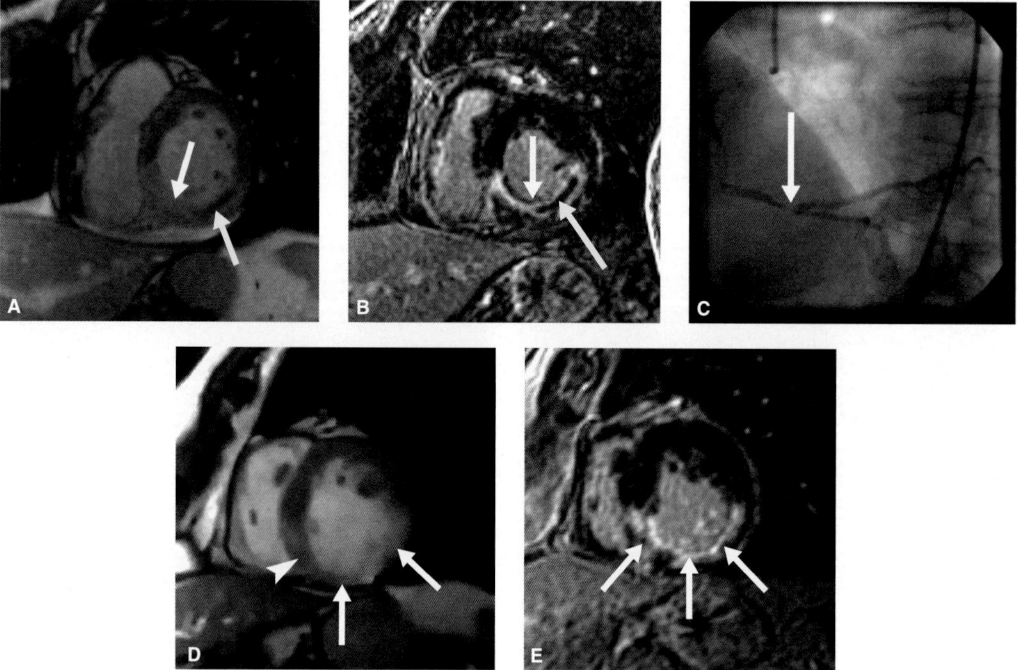

FIGURE 25.42. **Subacute Myocardial Infarct in the RCA Distribution in a Patient With Right Coronary Artery Dominance and a Large Posterior Lateral Ventricular Branch. A:** Short axis image from a SSFP cine sequence at the mid-cavity level obtained after intravenous contrast injection shows severe edema and early enhancement of the inferoseptal, inferior, and inferolateral segments (*white arrows*). An areas of low signal within these segments represents a focus of microvascular obstruction (MVO, *yellow arrow*). **B:** Short axis LGE image at the same level shows near transmural infarct (*white arrow*) with a large focus of MVO (*yellow arrow*). **C:** Right anterior oblique image from a cardiac catheterization performed one week earlier shows the severe stenosis in the distal RCA (*white arrow*). The PLV is a large branch which explain the extent of injury to the inferolateral segment. **D:** Image from a cine SSFP sequence 6 months later at the same level as (**A**) shows thinning the inferior and inferolateral segments (*white arrows*) which were akinetic. Although the inferoseptal segment appears thicker, it was also akinetic (*white arrowhead*). **E:** Short axis LGE image 6-months later at the same level as (**C**) shows thinning and near transmural enhancement of the affected segments (*white arrow*) with associated functional decline consistent with abnormal left ventricular remodeling. The MVO has resolved.

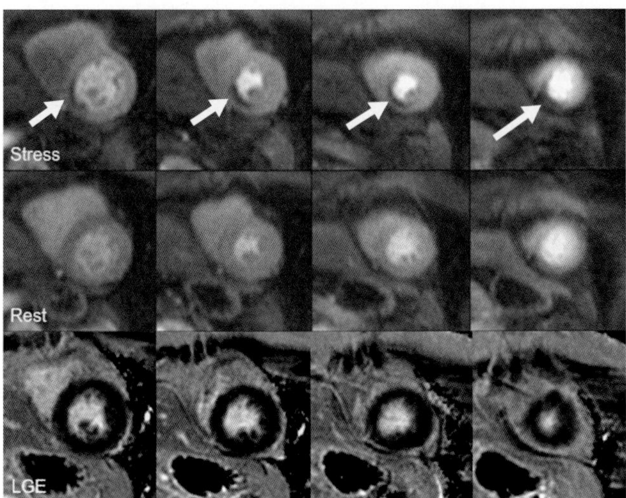

FIGURE 25.43. **Cardiac MRI Stress Test.** Stress imaging (first row) shows hypoperfusion of the inferior segments from the base to the apex (*white arrows*) which resolves on rest imaging (middle row). Delayed-enhancement imaging demonstrates no evidence of infarct. Subsequent cardiac catheterization showed a severe PDA stenosis requiring stent placement.

Microvascular obstruction (MO) is a specific form of myocardial reperfusion injury that occurs after therapy for an acute MI. The cause of MO is multifactorial and is thought to be caused by the release of cytotoxic mediators that cause local vasoconstriction, capillary endothelial swelling, myocardial edema, hemorrhage, and microembolization of atherosclerotic debris. The exact timing of MO is unclear, but it occurs nearly immediately after reperfusion, can increase in size and extent up to 48 hours after injury, and can be seen up to 1 month after reperfusion. Given severity of the injury, gadolinium cannot diffuse into the areas of MO. Therefore, on LGE imaging, the areas of MO appear as dark, nonenhanced areas surrounded by enhancing infarct (Fig. 25.42). When present, MO is an indicator of severe myocardial injury that often leads to adverse left ventricular remodeling and is an independent predictor of worse patient outcomes.

MRI in the Assessment of Ischemia. Stress MR imaging using SSFP and perfusion imaging can be used to distinguish ischemia from prior myocardial infarction. Rest followed by stress MR imaging is often performed using pharmacologic agents such as adenosine because of the challenges of introducing MR-compatible equipment into the MR imaging suite to perform physiologic stress testing. Similar to other imaging-based stress techniques, segmental, subendocardial hypoperfusion on stress imaging which returns to normal on rest imaging suggests myocardial ischemia (Fig. 25.43). Since LGE is performed, stress MRI can also assess for areas of scarring from infarct. Although not as widely used, recent studies of stress MR imaging demonstrate sensitivity of 0.82 to 0.92 and specificity of 0.75 to 0.94, suggesting that stress MR imaging is as good as conventional approaches of stress imaging.

TREATMENT OF CORONARY ARTERY DISEASE

Coronary Stents

Compared to coronary angioplasty alone, coronary stents create a larger residual diameter and reduce the rate of restenosis. In-stent restenosis occurs in up to 35% of patients with bare-metal stents and up to 10% of patients with drug-eluting stents. In addition to restenosis, stent thrombosis, sometimes fatal, can occur.

Coronary CTA can be used to evaluate for stent occlusion and restenosis (Fig. 25.44). In general, stents ≥3 mm in diameter are more likely to be evaluable. However, evaluation can

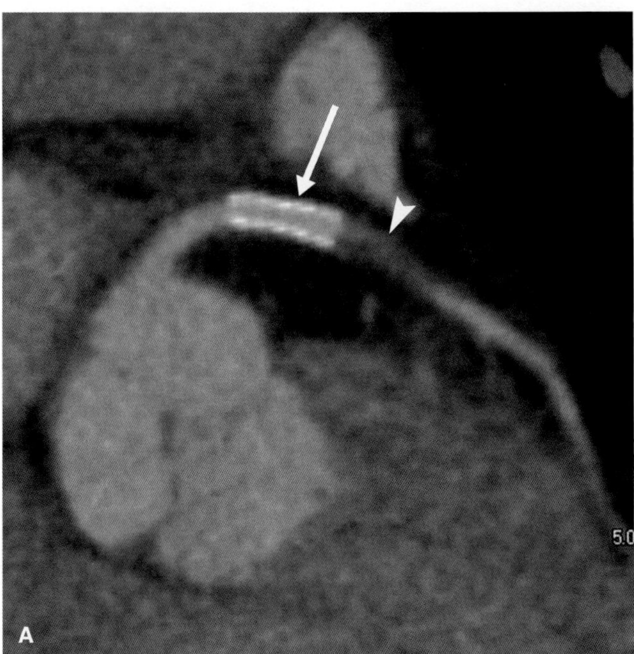

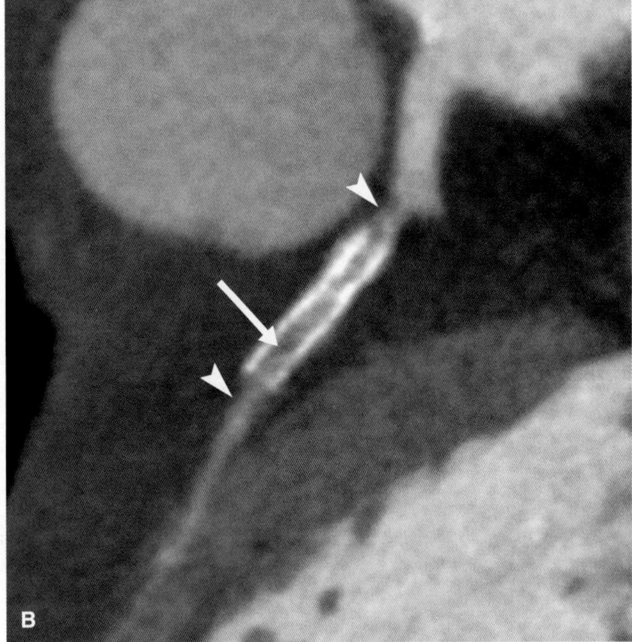

FIGURE 25.44. **Stent Evaluation Using Coronary CTA. A:** Curved MPR image through the LAD in a 59-year-old woman with chest pain shows a patent stent (*white arrow*) with no in-stent restenosis. However, there is a severe stenosis distal to the stent (*white arrowhead*). **B:** Curved MPR through the LAD in a 66-year-old man demonstrates an area of hypoattenuation in the distal aspect of the stent due to in-stent restenosis (*white arrow*). In addition, there are moderate stenoses in the LAD proximal and distal to the stent (*white arrowheads*). While the negative predictive value for CTA in assessing in-stent restenosis is high, the positive predictive value is low.

be difficult given the metal artifact created by the struts of the stent. In one large meta-analysis using 64-slice CT, the overall NPV of CT was high at 97% but the PPV was very low at 53%. In general, thin-slice image reconstruction with a sharp kernel, small field of view, and use of wide windows is recommended to optimize stent visualization. Low-kV imaging, which will often reduce contrast dose and increase the attenuation of contrast, will increase the metallic artifact associated with stents.

Coronary Artery Bypass Grafts

Since its introduction in 1962, coronary artery bypass grafting (CABG) has remained the definitive treatment for advanced CAD. Patency of the coronary grafts is critical for long-term survival and depends on the type of graft that is used. In the VA Cooperative Study, internal mammary grafts had a patency rate of 85% after 10 years, as compared to 61% for saphenous vein grafts (SVG). ECG-gated CTA is an excellent tool for assessing the patency of coronary artery bypass grafts. Since internal mammary artery grafts originate from the subclavian artery, it is important to perform an ECG-gated evaluation of the entire chest. In most instances, the left internal mammary artery (LIMA) is used due to its proximity to the left ventricular apex. This vessel is dissected from the parasternal region and anastomosed to the LAD due to its higher patency rate (Fig. 25.45). Due to its high patency rate, the LIMA graft usually appears as a well-opacified, small-caliber vessel coursing inferiorly through the anterior mediastinum and eventually into the epicardial fat where it will anastomose with the distal LAD. Although stenosis is most common near the distal anastomosis, it can occur anywhere along the vessel.

SVG are harvested from the legs and attached as a free graft to the ascending aorta and coronary artery distal to the site of obstruction. A rightward-directed SVG usually is directed toward the RCA distribution and will anastomose with the PDA. Leftward-directed SVG can anastomose with various vessels including the LAD, diagonal, OM, and LCx arteries (Fig. 25.46). While an SVG can supply a single vessel, in some instances a sequential or "jump graft" will be used where a single vein is anastomosed to multiple adjacent vessels, such as a diagonal and OM vessel. When evaluating a SVG, it is important to evaluate the entire graft for patency and signs of opacification distal to the graft, which suggests graft patency. When an SVG does thrombose, all that may be visible is a small vascular outpouching from the ascending aorta, a finding that is sometimes referred to as the "nubbin sign" (Fig. 25.46).

It is also important to evaluate for complications such as SVG aneurysm (SVGA) (Fig. 25.47). Aneurysms of saphenous venous grafts after coronary artery bypass are not uncommon, but the exact incidence is unknown. Nearly 70% of SVGA occur more than 10 years after initial CABG, while approximately 10% occur within the first 5 years. The size widely varies, but in case reports, the average SVGA exceeded 6 cm in diameter and SVG-to-RCA distribution grafts are most common. The pathophysiology leading to SVGA is primarily due to accelerated atherosclerosis. While most cases are asymptomatic, SVGAs can become symptomatic due to thrombosis, rupture, fistulization with adjacent structures, or compression of adjacent structures. Both surgical and percutaneous approaches have been used to treat aneurysms with variable success.

Pseudoaneurysms of either internal mammary or saphenous vein bypass grafts are a rare complication. They most commonly occur due to graft breakdown and dehiscence (Fig. 25.48). Compared to SVGAs, they tend to occur at the proximal or distal anastomotic sites and within the first weeks to months after surgery. Treatment is usually surgical.

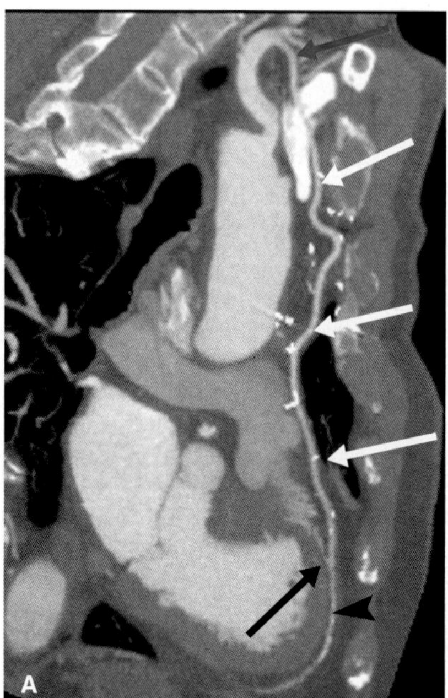

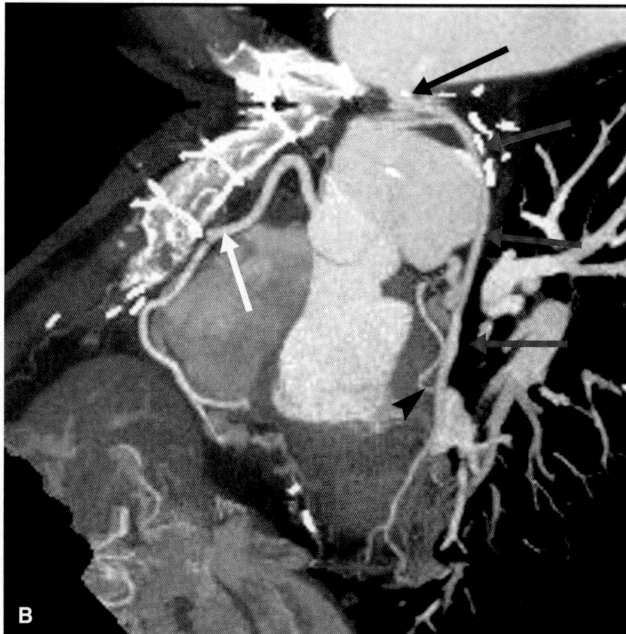

FIGURE 25.45. **Bypass Graft Assessment in a 60-Year-Old Man Status Post Coronary Artery Bypass. A:** Curved parasagittal maximum-intensity projection (MIP) image from a gated CTA of the chest shows a patent left internal mammary artery (LIMA) bypass graft (*white arrows*) arising from the left subclavian artery (*red arrow*) and anastomosing with the distal LAD (*black arrow*). There is good opacification of the LAD distal to the anastomosis (*black arrowhead*). **B:** Curved MIP shows a patent saphenous vein graft (*red arrows*) arising from the aorta (*black arrow*) and anastomosing with the second obtuse marginal artery (*black arrowhead*). The RCA (*white arrow*) is without significant disease. ECG-gated CTA of the thorax is an excellent tool for assessing the patency of coronary artery bypass grafts.

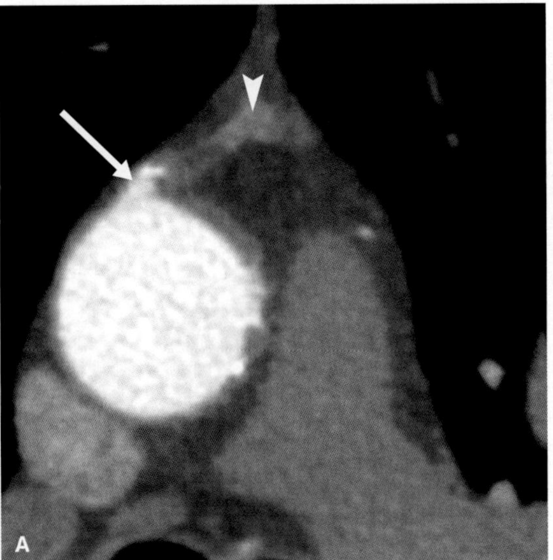

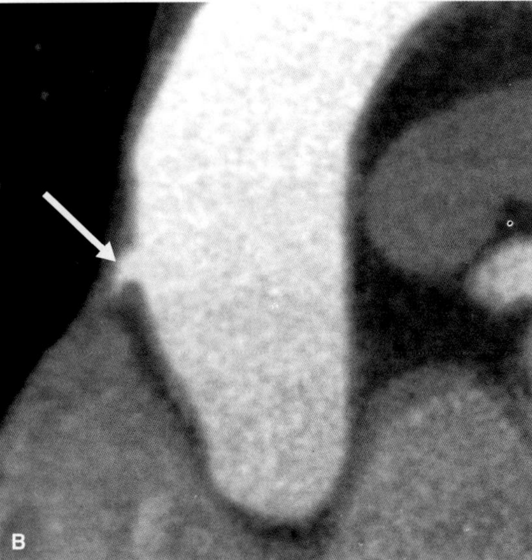

FIGURE 25.46. **Saphenous Vein Graft (SVG) Occlusions on Coronary CTA in a 64-Year-Old Woman With a History of CABG. A:** Axial oblique image through the ascending aorta shows a small outpouching from the aorta (*white arrow*) with a subtle thrombosed saphenous vein to diagonal bypass graft (*white arrowhead*). **B:** The patient's saphenous vein to posterior descending artery bypass graft (*white arrow*) was also thrombosed. The appearance of these small outpouchings from the aorta has been referred to as the "nubbin sign."

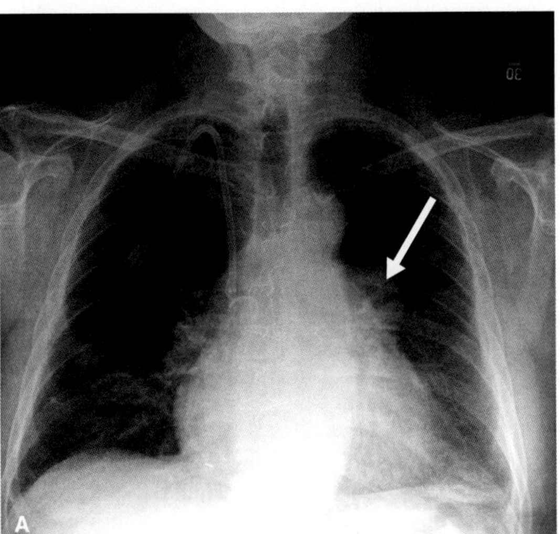

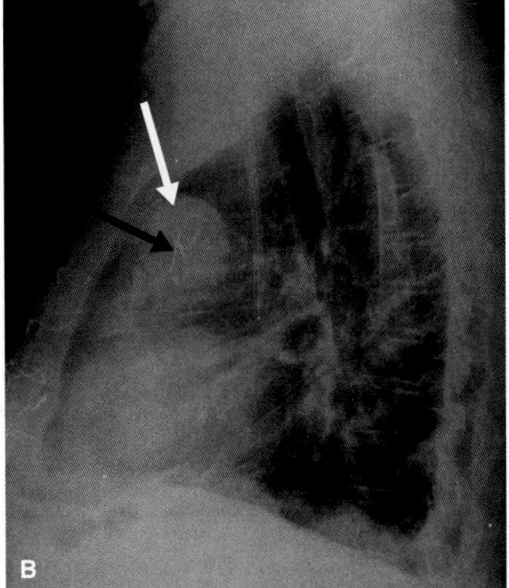

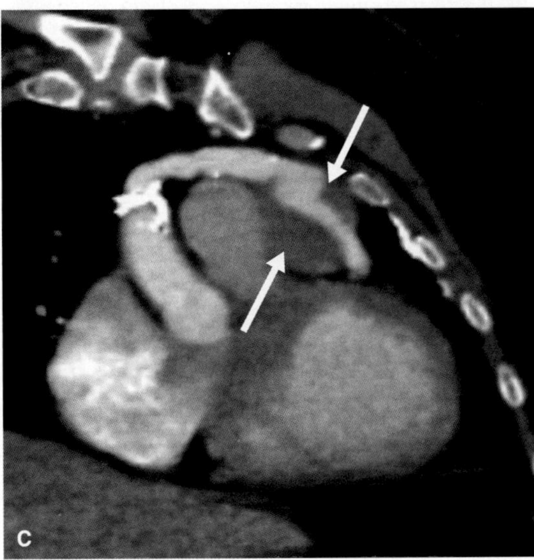

FIGURE 25.47. **Incidental Findings of a Saphenous Vein Graft Aneurysm (SVGA) in a 77-Year-Old Man. A:** Posterioranterior and (**B**) lateral chest radiographs showed a well-rounded mass in the anterior mediastinum (*white arrows*). Given the location and adjacent coronary artery bypass clips (*black arrow*, **B**), the finding is concerning for a bypass graft aneurysm. **C:** Coronary oblique MPR image from a gated CTA shows the SVGA (*white arrows*). SVGA is a late complication after CABG.

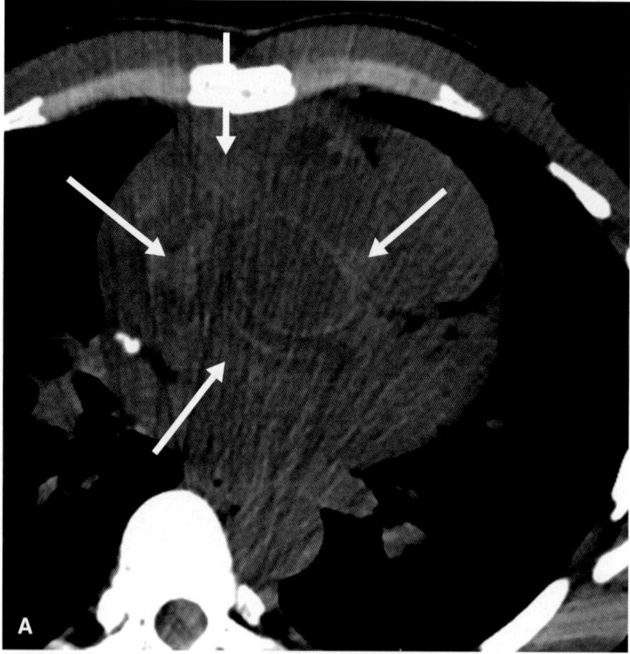

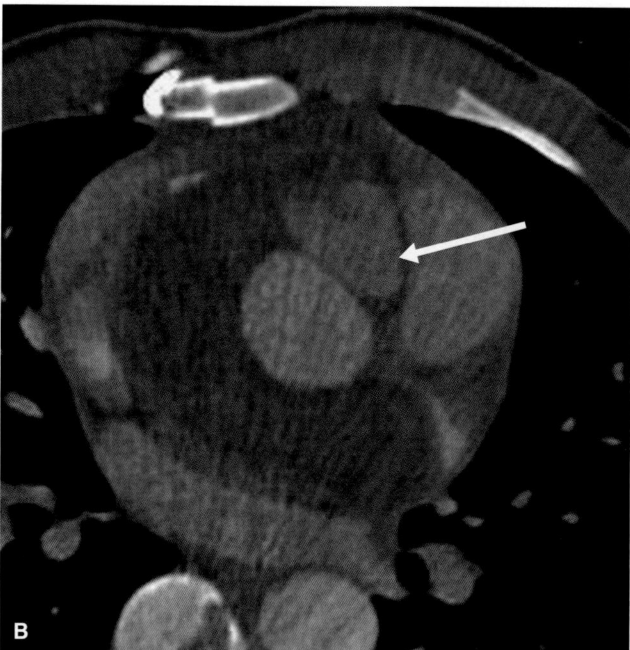

FIGURE 25.48. **Saphenous Venous Graft Pseudoaneurysm in a 40-Year-Old Man With Worsening Chest Pain 2 Days After Surgery. A:** Axial noncontrast image from a gated CTA shows heterogeneous fluid collection surrounding the aortic root with areas of high attenuation suggestive of blood products (*white arrows*). **B:** Axial image at the same level after administration of contrast shows contrast extravasation near the right sinus of Valsalva (*white arrow*). The patient underwent redo sternotomy which showed that the RCA saphenous venous graft had dehisced from its aortic anastomosis. Bypass graft pseudoaneurysms are uncommon and usually occur at the anastomotic sites.

CORONARY ARTERY ANEURYSM AND PSEUDOANEURYSM

Coronary artery aneurysm is defined as a segment of the coronary artery that measures more than 1.5 times the adjacent normal coronary artery. Of all of the different etiologies of coronary artery aneurysms, atherosclerotic disease is the most common, accounting for approximately 50% of coronary artery aneurysms diagnosed in adults (Fig. 25.49). The exact incidence is unknown as many atherosclerotic coronary artery aneurysms (ACAA) are detected incidentally.

The most common cause of aneurysms in the pediatric population is Kawasaki disease (KD), which is a systemic small- and medium-vessel vasculitis which occurs in infants and young children (Fig. 25.49). It is the leading cause of acquired childhood heart disease in the United States, and coronary artery aneurysms are a major cause of morbidity in this population. Smaller coronary artery aneurysms may decrease in size or resolve in patients with KD, but giant aneurysms (>8 mm) do not regress and can lead to myocardial infarct or death due to rupture or stenosis/thrombosis. In addition to atherosclerosis and KD, there are many additional causes of coronary artery aneurysms including other vasculitides, connective tissue disease, inflammatory conditions, and fistulas.

Coronary artery pseudoaneurysms are rare and usually iatrogenic due to coronary catheterization (Fig. 25.50). They can also occur from infection, trauma, or even be idiopathic. Due to their risk of rupture, treatments include stenting, coil embolization, or surgical repair with or without bypass grafting.

CORONARY ARTERY DISSECTION

There are three main causes of coronary artery dissection. The most common cause is percutaneous interventions such as angioplasty, where coronary dissections occur in less than 1% of cases. In most cases, these dissections are limited and can be successfully treated with stent placement. Retrograde extension into the aorta can occur but is uncommon.

Type A aortic dissections involve the ascending aorta and can extend into the aortic root. When the aortic root is involved, obstruction of coronary blood flow can occur via two mechanisms. First, the intimal flap can directly cover the ostium of a coronary artery. Second, the dissection can extend from the aorta into the coronary artery (Fig. 25.51). Both causes can lead to coronary occlusion. When there is suspicion for a type A dissection, ECG gating should be used so the aortic root and coronary arteries can be evaluated in detail.

Spontaneous coronary artery dissections (SCAD) are the third main cause of coronary dissection. This process usually affects younger women and although considered rare, in one institution, SCAD was the cause of MI in 24% of women less than 50 years of age undergoing cardiac catheterization. The occurrence of SCAD is most commonly associated with pregnant or postpartum patients and in patients undergoing intense exercise (Fig. 25.52). However, other etiologies include fibromuscular dysplasia, connective tissue disorders, systemic inflammatory conditions, hormonal therapy, and even intense emotional stress. Almost all patients present with ACS, and treatment depends on the extent of the dissection and can range from conservative therapy to CABG.

MECHANICAL COMPLICATIONS OF MYOCARDIAL INFARCTION

Left ventricular free wall rupture, ventricular septal rupture (VSR), and papillary muscle rupture are three catastrophic mechanical complications after acute myocardial infarction. Although timing can vary, these entities usually occur within the

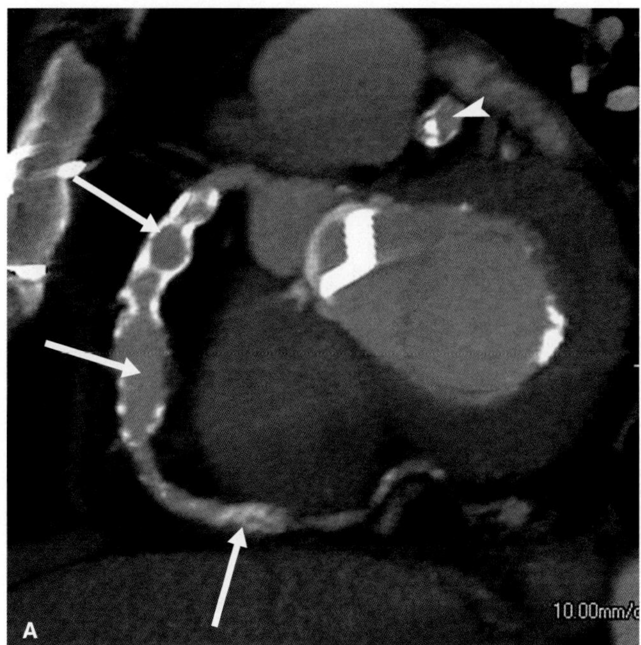

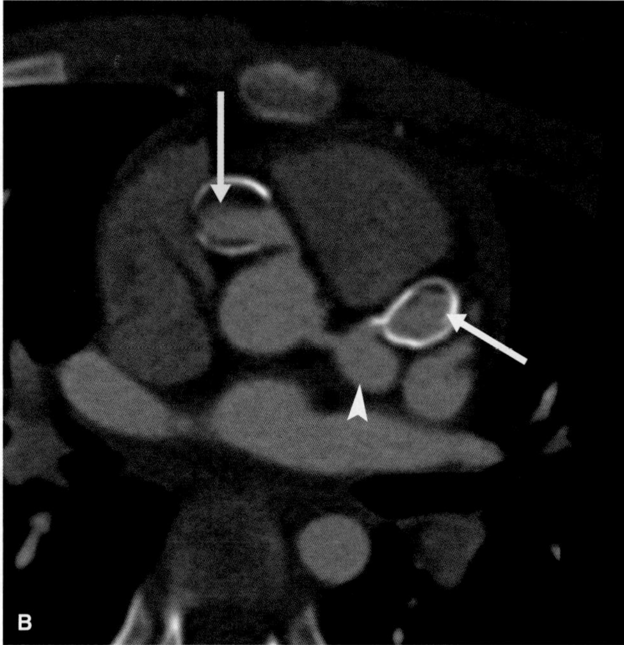

FIGURE 25.49. Coronary Artery Aneurysms. A: Sagittal oblique MPR image through the RCA in an 81-year-old man shows extensive atherosclerotic disease with multiple RCA aneurysms (*white arrows*). The partially visualized LAD is also aneurysmal (*white arrowhead*). **B:** Axial oblique image in a 5-year-old girl with a history of Kawasaki disease shows large aneurysms of the proximal LAD (*white arrow*), LCx (*white arrowhead*), and RCA (*yellow arrow*). Atherosclerotic disease is the most common cause of coronary artery aneurysms in adults, while Kawasaki disease is the most common cause in children.

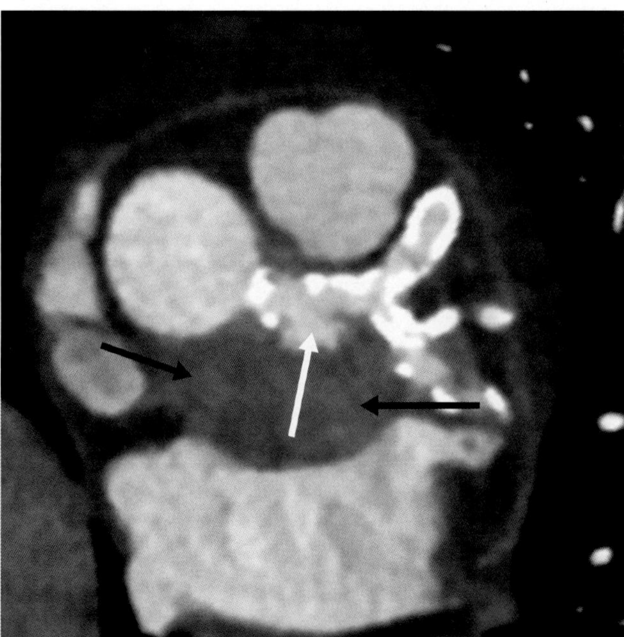

FIGURE 25.50. Axial oblique MPR in a 68-year-old man with diffusely aneurysmal and calcified coronary arteries shows a defect in the posterior wall of the left main coronary artery (LM, *white arrow*) with surrounding hematoma (*black arrows*). The patient had undergone cardiac catheterization the day prior, and the injury was thought to be iatrogenic. However, a large hole in the LM was confirmed during surgery which required repair.

first week after infarction and may be lethal if not quickly recognized and treated. These entities may be lethal if not quickly recognized and treatment usually involves surgical repair.

A left ventricular pseudoaneurysm, also referred to as left ventricular free wall rupture, occurs when there is a tear through the myocardium which is contained by adjacent pericardium or scar tissue (Fig. 25.53). Myocardial infarct is the most common cause, but other etiologies include cardiac surgery, trauma, and infection. Although many patients die immediately after the rupture, a patient can survive if the rupture is contained. It is important to differentiate true aneurysms and pseudoaneurysm due to different treatments and outcomes. Although most pseudoaneurysms involve the inferior and inferolateral walls and most true aneurysms occur in the anterior walls, both pathologies can occur in both regions and thus location alone does not make the diagnosis. In general, true aneurysms have a broad neck (Fig. 25.54). Pseudoaneurysms usually have a narrow neck that has a diameter less than 50% of that of the maximal diameter of the distal outpouching.

Although quite rare, a VSR occurs in 0.17% to 0.31% of patients 1 to 5 days after an acute MI. Septal rupture can develop after transmural infarct and leads to a left-to-right shunt which can lead to complete hemodynamic collapse (Fig. 25.55). Even with surgical intervention, overall operative mortality is 42.9%.

While the left ventricular anteromedial papillary muscle has a dual blood supply, the posteromedial papillary muscle of the LV is usually supplied only by the PDA. Therefore, the posteromedial papillary muscle is 6 to 12 times more likely to rupture after MI. Rupture usually occurs 2 to 7 days after an acute MI, and if left untreated, up to 50% of patients can die within 24 hours and 94% at 2 months. If this muscle ruptures, the posterior leaflet of the mitral valve becomes incompetent causing severe mitral regurgitation which is often directed rightward, more notably toward the right superior pulmonary vein (RSPV). As pressures in the RSPV increase, there is decreased pulmonary venous return causing asymmetric right-sided edema, which is most pronounced in the right upper lung (Fig. 25.56).

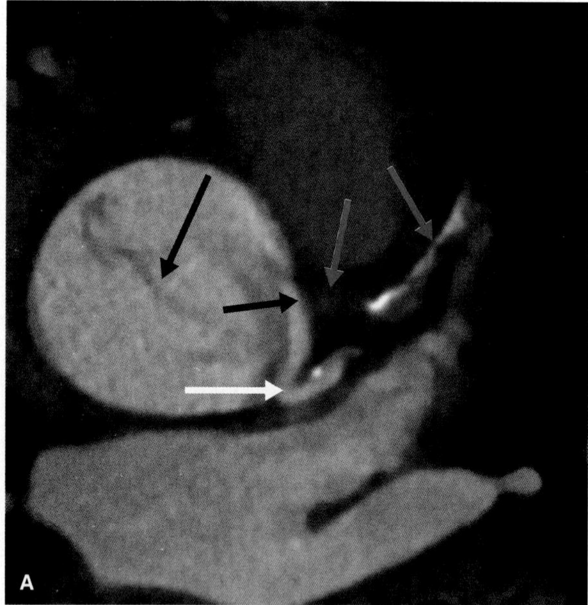

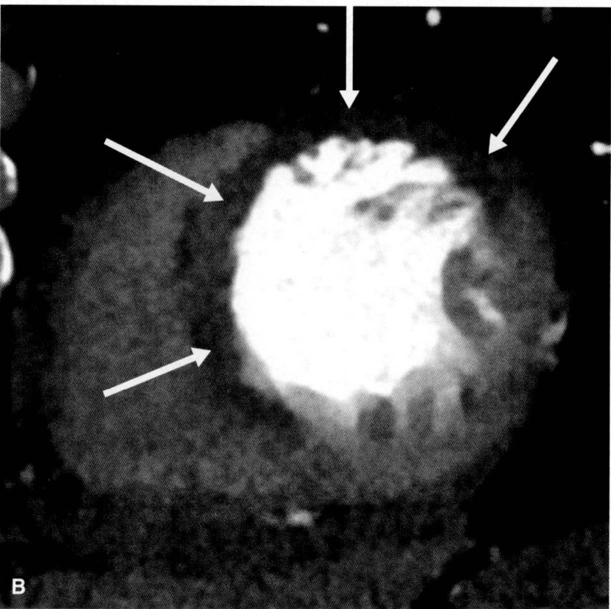

FIGURE 25.51. **Type A Aortic Dissection Extending Into the LAD in a 55-Year-Old Man With Hypertension. A:** Axial oblique image through the aortic root shows the type A dissection. The dissection flap (*black arrows*) extended into and occluded the left anterior descending coronary artery (*red arrows*). Fortunately for the patient, he had an uncommon coronary artery variant where the LAD and LCx have separate ostia from the left sinus of Valsalva (absent left main). Because of this, the LCx remained patent (*white arrow*). **B:** Short-axis image through the base of the heart shows transmural infarction of the anterior, anteroseptal, and inferoseptal segments due to LAD occlusion (*white arrows*). The LCx and RCA territories show normal perfusion.

ADDITIONAL CONSIDERATIONS

As modern scanners continue to improve their spatial and temporal resolution, aspects of cardiac pathology can be assessed on nearly any routine chest or abdomen CT (Fig. 25.57). While ECG gating is necessary to assess the coronary arteries in detail, in many instances, the coronary ostia can be visualized on routine scans, even those that are performed without intravenous contrast. Similarly, myocardial perfusion defects or other sequelae of infarct, such as fatty metaplasia or calcification of the myocardium, left ventricular aneurysm, and thrombus are often visible. Therefore, routine evaluation of the heart should be added to one's search pattern as part of the assessment on any chest or abdomen CT.

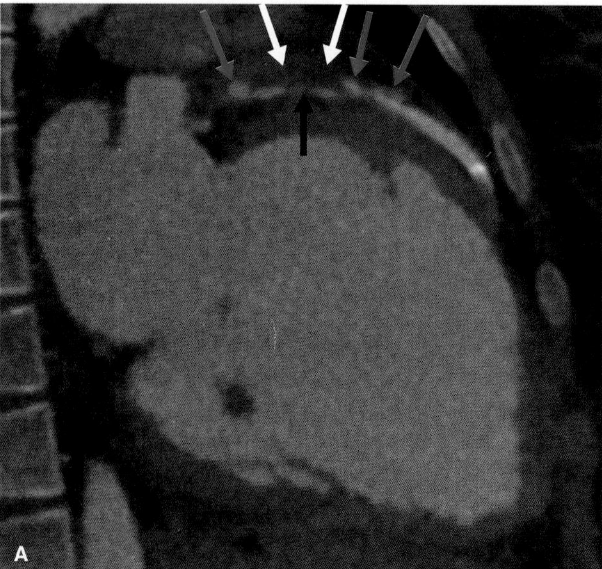

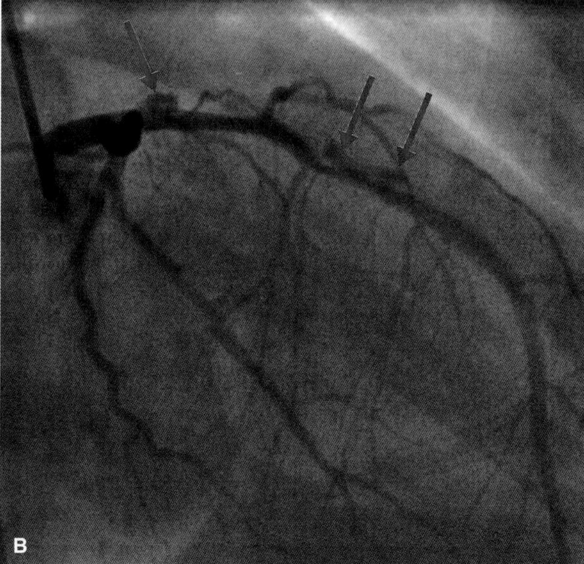

FIGURE 25.52. **A 24-Year-Old Woman With a History of Spontaneous Coronary Artery Dissection (SCAD) With Subsequent Stenting After Giving Birth to Her Second Child. A:** Longitudinal image through the proximal LAD shows soft tissue attenuation surrounding the vessel corresponding to the thrombosed false lumen (*white arrows*) which compresses true lumen (*black arrow*). There are a few areas of contrast outpouchings that represent persistent filling of the false lumen (*red arrows*). The left ventricle is severely dilated and the patient's ejection fraction was 31%. **B:** Right anterior oblique image from a coronary catheterization shows areas of persistent filling of the false lumen (*red arrows*) corresponding to the findings on CTA.

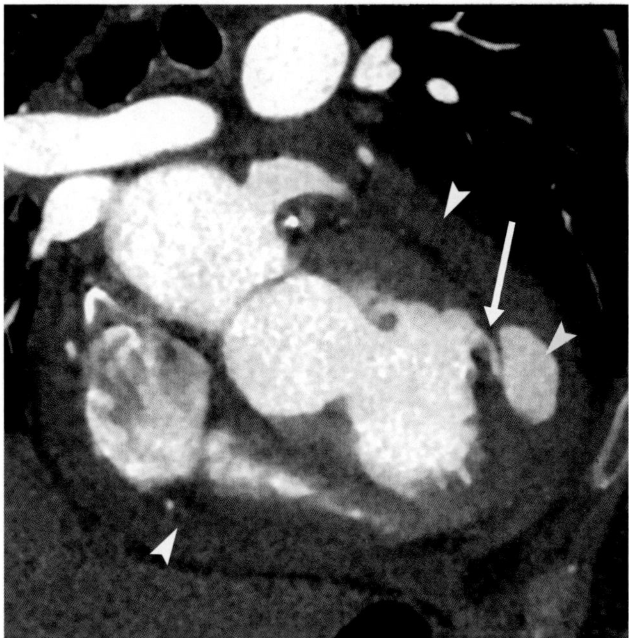

FIGURE 25.53. **Retrospectively Gated Coronary CTA in a 61-Year-Old Man With Recent LAD Territory Infarct.** Coronal oblique reformat shows the narrow-necked tear through the left ventricular myocardium (*white arrow*) with distal pseudoaneurysm (*yellow arrowhead*) and surrounding hemopericardium (*white arrowheads*). Pseudoaneurysm formation represents a myocardial rupture contained by surrounding pericardium or scarring. Although most common in the inferior segments, they can occur anteriorly as well.

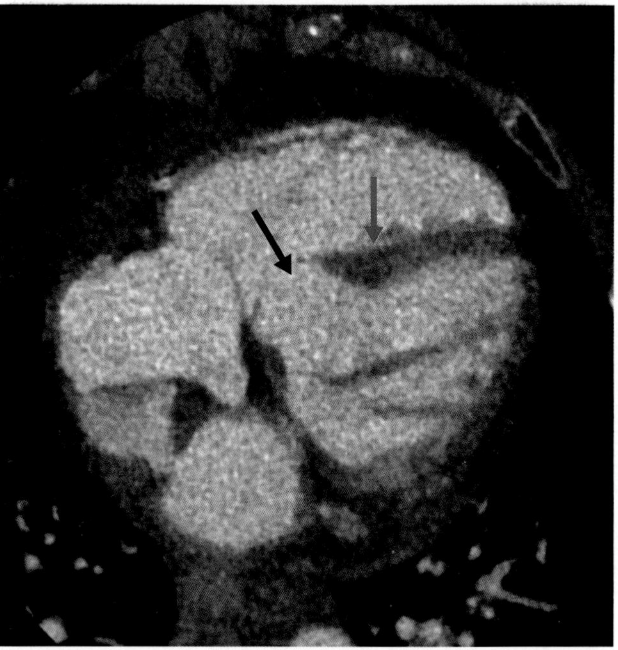

FIGURE 25.55. Four-chamber image from a cardiac CTA in a 78-year-old woman who developed worsening shortness of breath 4 days after LAD territory infarct shows a large defect in the anteroseptal segment at the base (*black arrow*) consistent with a postinfarct ventricular septal rupture. The edges of the myocardium adjacent to the rupture are hypoattenuating due to the infarct (*red arrow*). The patient died 1 day later.

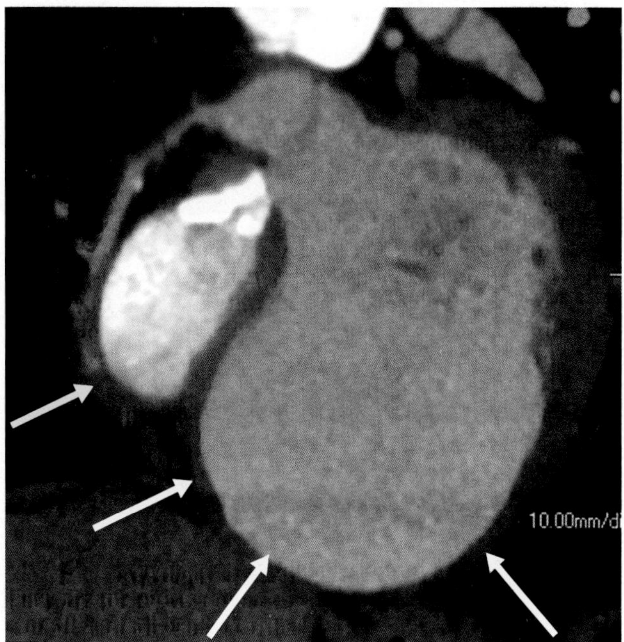

FIGURE 25.54. Coronal oblique image through the base of the heart in a 61-year-old man shows a large wide-mouthed true aneurysm of the inferior wall which is surrounded by thin myocardium (*white arrows*). The RCA is chronically occluded (*yellow arrow*). Due to its large size, the patient underwent surgery with mesh repair of the inferior wall. Pathology confirmed the imaging diagnosis of an aneurysm. Although aneurysms are more common in the anterior segments, they can occur inferiorly as well.

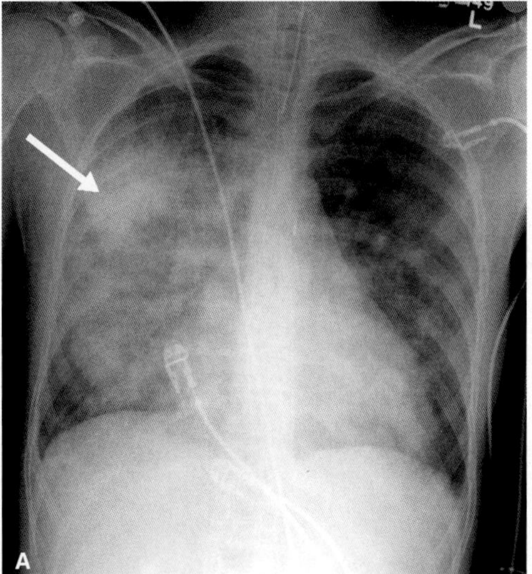

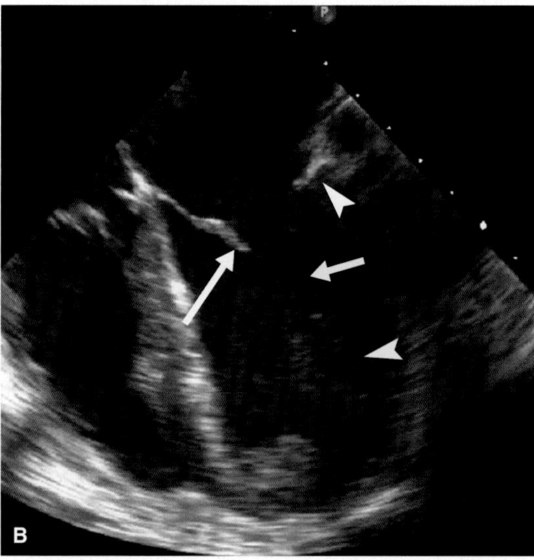

FIGURE 25.56. **A:** AP radiograph in a 49-year-old woman with severely worsening dyspnea 7 days after RCA territory infarct shows asymmetric edema most notably in the right upper lung (*white arrow*). **B:** Four-chamber view from a bedside echocardiogram shows a flair posterior leaflet (*white arrow*) leading to severe acute mitral regurgitation. The anterior leaflet (*white arrow*) is still attached to its chordae (*yellow arrow*) and papillary muscle (*yellow arrowhead*). The rightward and superior direction of the jet causes this characteristic finding. The patient underwent emergent surgery to repair the valve.

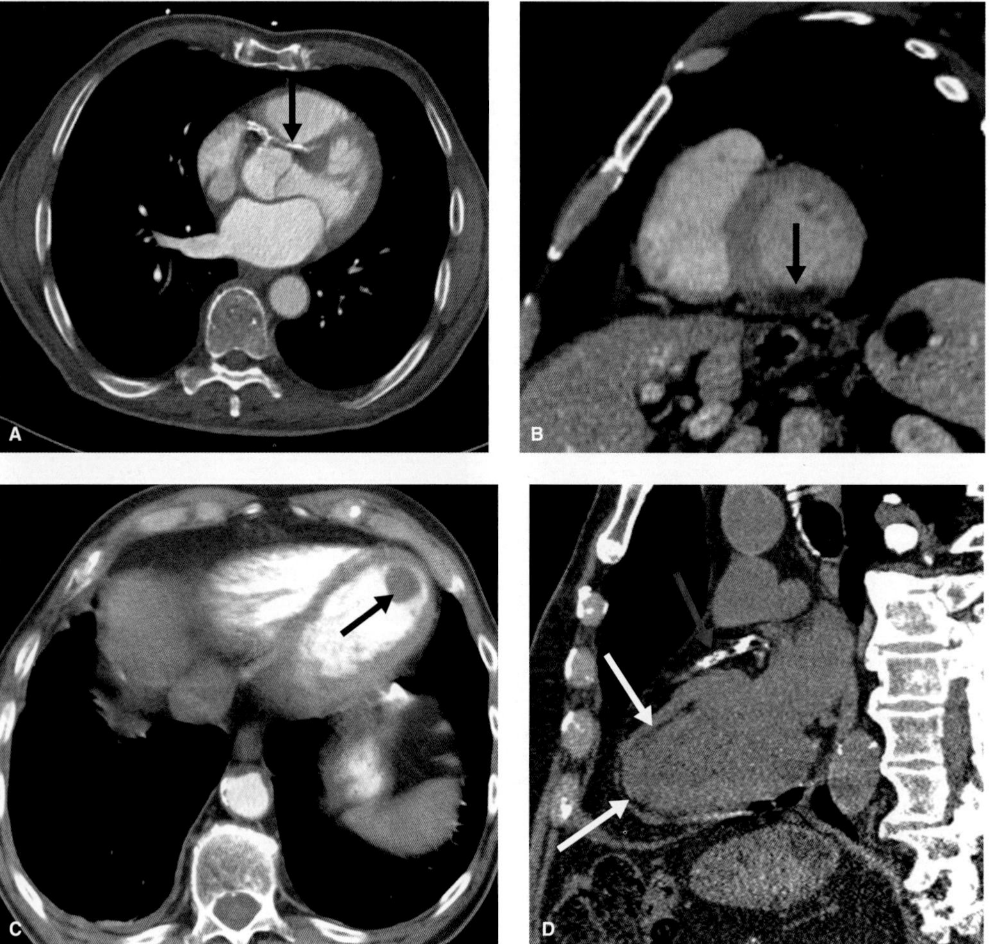

FIGURE 25.57. **Cardiac Findings on Nongated CT Examinations. A:** Axial image from a contrast-enhanced CT of the chest in a 71 year old shows an anomalous septal course of the left anterior descending coronary artery (*black arrow*). **B:** Short-axis reconstruction from a routine chest CT in a 59-year-old man shows subendocardial hypoperfusion in the inferior wall (*black arrow*). The patient had an acute MI 2 days prior. **C:** Axial image from an abdominal CT in a 63-year-old woman shows a left ventricular apical aneurysm with a 2-cm thrombus (*black arrow*). The finding was unknown to the primary team. **D:** Sagittal oblique MPR in an 85-year-old woman shows extensive calcification in the LAD territory (*red arrow*) with subendocardial fatty metaplasia of the associated myocardium due to old infarct (*white arrows*). Fatty metaplasia is a common finding and can be visualized with or without contrast.

Suggested Readings

Abdel-Aty H, Zagrosek A, Schulz-Menger J, et al. Delayed enhancement and T2-weighted cardiovascular magnetic resonance imaging differentiate acute from chronic myocardial infarction. *Circulation* 2004;109(20):2411–2416.

Achenbach S, Giesler T, Ropers D, et al. Detection of coronary artery stenoses by contrast-enhanced, retrospectively electrocardiographically-gated, multislice spiral computed tomography. *Circulation* 2001;103(21):2535–2538.

Alford WC Jr, Stoney WS, Burrus GR, Frist RA, Thomas CS Jr. Recognition and operative management of patients with arteriosclerotic coronary artery aneurysms. *Ann Thorac Surg* 1976;22(4):317–321.

Angelini P. Coronary artery anomalies: an entity in search of an identity. *Circulation* 2007;115(10):1296–1305.

Arnaoutakis GJ, Zhao Y, George TJ, Sciortino CM, McCarthy PM, Conte JV. Surgical repair of ventricular septal defect after myocardial infarction: outcomes from the Society of Thoracic Surgeons National Database. *Ann Thorac Surg* 2012;94(2):436–443; discussion 443–444.

Bastarrika G, Lee YS, Huda W, Ruzsics B, Costello P, Schoepf UJ. CT of coronary artery disease. *Radiology* 2009;253(2):317–338.

Bazzocchi G, Romagnoli A, Sperandio M, Simonetti G. Evaluation with 64-slice CT of the prevalence of coronary artery variants and congenital anomalies: a retrospective study of 3,236 patients. *Radiol Med* 2011;116(5):675–689.

Bourassa MG, Butnaru A, Lesperance J, Tardif JC. Symptomatic myocardial bridges: overview of ischemic mechanisms and current diagnostic and treatment strategies. *J Am Coll Cardiol* 2003;41(3):351–359.

Budoff MJ, Dowe D, Jollis JG, et al. Diagnostic performance of 64-multidetector row coronary computed tomographic angiography for evaluation of coronary artery stenosis in individuals without known coronary artery disease: results from the prospective multicenter ACCURACY (Assessment by Coronary Computed Tomographic Angiography of Individuals Undergoing Invasive Coronary Angiography) trial. *J Am Coll Cardiol* 2008;52(21):1724–1732.

Burke AP, Kolodgie FD, Farb A, Weber D, Virmani R. Morphological predictors of arterial remodeling in coronary atherosclerosis. *Circulation* 2002;105(3):297–303.

Cademartiri F, La Grutta L, Malago R, et al. Prevalence of anatomical variants and coronary anomalies in 543 consecutive patients studied with 64-slice CT coronary angiography. *Eur Radiol* 2008;18(4):781–791.

Chen YF, Chien TM, Chen CW, Lin CC, Lee CS. Double right coronary artery or split right coronary artery? *Int J Cardiol* 2012;154(3):243–245.

Coelho-Filho OR, Rickers C, Kwong RY, Jerosch-Herold M. MR myocardial perfusion imaging. *Radiology* 2013;266(3):701–715.

Cook CM, Petraco R, Shun-Shin MJ, et al. Diagnostic accuracy of computed tomography-derived fractional flow reserve: a systematic review. *JAMA Cardiol* 2017;2(7):803–810.

Cowles RA, Berdon WE. Bland-White-Garland syndrome of anomalous left coronary artery arising from the pulmonary artery (ALCAPA): a historical review. *Pediatr Radiol* 2007;37(9):890–895.

Cury RC, Abbara S, Achenbach S, et al. CAD-RADS: Coronary Artery Disease – Reporting and Data System. An expert consensus document of the Society of Cardiovascular Computed Tomography (SCCT), the American College of Radiology (ACR) and the North American Society for Cardiovascular Imaging (NASCI). Endorsed by the American College of Cardiology. *J Am Coll Radiol* 2016;13(12 Pt A):1458–1466. e9.

Daoud AS, Pankin D, Tulgan H, Florentin RA. Aneurysms of the coronary artery. Report of ten cases and review of literature. *Am J Cardiol* 1963;11:228–237.

Dash D. Complications of coronary intervention: abrupt closure, dissection, perforation. *Heart Asia* 2013;5(1):61–65.

de Agustin JA, Marcos-Alberca P, Hernandez-Antolin R, et al. Collateral circulation from the conus coronary artery to the anterior descending coronary artery: assessment using multislice coronary computed tomography. *Rev Esp Cardiol* 2010;63(3):347–351.

Detrano R, Guerci AD, Carr JJ, et al. Coronary calcium as a predictor of coronary events in four racial or ethnic groups. *N Engl J Med* 2008;358(13):1336–1345.

Dodge JT Jr, Brown BG, Bolson EL, Dodge HT. Lumen diameter of normal human coronary arteries. Influence of age, sex, anatomic variation, and left ventricular hypertrophy or dilation. *Circulation* 1992;86(1):232–246.

Duarte R, Cisneros S, Fernandez G, et al. Kawasaki disease: a review with emphasis on cardiovascular complications. *Insights Imaging* 2010;1(4):223–231.

Eckart RE, Scoville SL, Campbell CL, et al. Sudden death in young adults: a 25-year review of autopsies in military recruits. *Ann Intern Med* 2004;141(11):829–834.

Erol C, Seker M. The prevalence of coronary artery variations on coronary computed tomography angiography. *Acta Radiol* 2012;53(3):278–284.

Farb A, Burke AP, Tang AL, et al. Coronary plaque erosion without rupture into a lipid core. A frequent cause of coronary thrombosis in sudden coronary death. *Circulation* 1996;93(7):1354–1363.

Ferencik M, Ropers D, Abbara S, et al. Diagnostic accuracy of image postprocessing methods for the detection of coronary artery stenoses by using multidetector CT. *Radiology* 2007;243(3):696–702.

Fischman DL, Leon MB, Baim DS, et al. A randomized comparison of coronary-stent placement and balloon angioplasty in the treatment of coronary artery disease. Stent Restenosis Study Investigators. *N Engl J Med* 1994;331(8):496–501.

Frances C, Romero A, Grady D. Left ventricular pseudoaneurysm. *J Am Coll Cardiol* 1998;32(3):557–561.

Frazier AA, Qureshi F, Read KM, Gilkeson RC, Poston RS, White CS. Coronary artery bypass grafts: assessment with multidetector CT in the early and late postoperative settings. *Radiographics* 2005;25(4):881–896.

Friedman BM, Dunn MI. Postinfarction ventricular aneurysms. *Clin Cardiol* 1995;18(9):505–511.

Galli A, Lombardi F. Postinfarct left ventricular remodelling: a prevailing cause of heart failure. *Cardiol Res Pract* 2016;2016:2579832.

Garcia MJ, Lessick J, Hoffmann MH; CATSCAN Study Investigators. Accuracy of 16-row multidetector computed tomography for the assessment of coronary artery stenosis. *JAMA* 2006;296(4):403–411.

Goetti R, Feuchtner G, Stolzmann P, et al. Delayed enhancement imaging of myocardial viability: low-dose high-pitch CT versus MRI. *Eur Radiol* 2011;21(10):2091–2099.

Goldman S, Zadina K, Moritz T, et al. Long-term patency of saphenous vein and left internal mammary artery grafts after coronary artery bypass surgery: results from a Department of Veterans Affairs Cooperative Study. *J Am Coll Cardiol* 2004;44(11):2149–2156.

Goldstein JA, Chinnaiyan KM, Abidov A, et al. The CT-STAT (Coronary Computed Tomographic Angiography for Systematic Triage of Acute Chest Pain Patients to Treatment) trial. *J Am Coll Cardiol* 2011;58(14):1414–1422.

Greenland P, Bonow RO, Brundage BH, et al. ACCF/AHA 2007 clinical expert consensus document on coronary artery calcium scoring by computed tomography in global cardiovascular risk assessment and in evaluation of patients with chest pain: a report of the American College of Cardiology Foundation Clinical Expert Consensus Task Force (ACCF/AHA Writing Committee to Update the 2000 Expert Consensus Document on Electron Beam Computed Tomography) developed in collaboration with the Society of Atherosclerosis Imaging and Prevention and the Society of Cardiovascular Computed Tomography. *J Am Coll Cardiol* 2007;49(3):378–402.

Hamirani YS, Wong A, Kramer CM, Salerno M. Effect of microvascular obstruction and intramyocardial hemorrhage by CMR on LV remodeling and outcomes after myocardial infarction: a systematic review and meta-analysis. *JACC Cardiovasc Imaging* 2014;7(9):940–952.

Harris PJ, Behar VS, Conley MJ, et al. The prognostic significance of 50% coronary stenosis in medically treated patients with coronary artery disease. *Circulation* 1980;62(2):240–248.

Hecht HS, Budoff MJ, Berman DS, Ehrlich J, Rumberger JA. Coronary artery calcium scanning: clinical paradigms for cardiac risk assessment and treatment. *Am Heart J* 2006;151(6):1139–1146.

Hobbs RE, Millit HD, Raghavan PV, Moodie DS, Sheldon WC. Coronary artery fistulae: a 10-year review. *Cleve Clin Q* 1982;49(4):191–197.

Hoffmann U, Truong QA, Schoenfeld DA, et al. Coronary CT angiography versus standard evaluation in acute chest pain. *N Engl J Med* 2012;367(4):299–308.

Holmes DR Jr, Leon MB, Moses JW, et al. Analysis of 1-year clinical outcomes in the SIRIUS trial: a randomized trial of a sirolimus-eluting stent versus a standard stent in patients at high risk for coronary restenosis. *Circulation* 2004;109(5):634–640.

Hulten EA, Blankstein R. Pseudoaneurysms of the heart. *Circulation* 2012;125(15):1920–1925.

Hwang JH, Ko SM, Roh HG, et al. Myocardial bridging of the left anterior descending coronary artery: depiction rate and morphologic features by dual-source CT coronary angiography. *Korean J Radiol* 2010;11(5):514–521.

Iemura J, Oku H, Shirotani H. Right coronary artery pseudoaneurysm after blunt injury to the chest. *Heart* 1996;76(1):86.

Ilia R, Rosenshtein G, Weinstein J, Cafri C, Abu-Ful A, Gueron M. Left anterior descending artery length in left and right coronary artery dominance. *Coron Artery Dis* 2001;12(1):77–78.

Javadi MS, Lautamaki R, Merrill J, et al. Definition of vascular territories on myocardial perfusion images by integration with true coronary anatomy: a hybrid PET/CT analysis. *J Nucl Med* 2010;51(2):198–203.

Jeudy J, White CS, Kligerman SJ, et al. Spectrum of coronary artery aneurysms: from the radiologic pathology archives. *Radiographics* 2018;38(1):11–36.

Jones BM, Kapadia SR, Smedira NG, et al. Ventricular septal rupture complicating acute myocardial infarction: a contemporary review. *Eur Heart J* 2014;35(31):2060–2068.

Joshi SD, Joshi SS, Athavale SA. Origins of the coronary arteries and their significance. *Clinics (Sao Paulo)* 2010;65(1):79–84.

Kanza RE, Allard C, Berube M. Cardiac findings on non-gated chest computed tomography: a clinical and pictorial review. *Eur J Radiol* 2016;85(2):435–451.

Kar S, Webel RR. Diagnosis and treatment of spontaneous coronary artery pseudoaneurysm: rare anomaly with potentially significant clinical implications. *Catheter Cardiovasc Interv* 2017;90(4):589–597.

Kashiwagi M, Tanaka A, Kitabata H, et al. Feasibility of noninvasive assessment of thin-cap fibroatheroma by multidetector computed tomography. *JACC Cardiovasc Imaging* 2009;2(12):1412–1419.

Kim PJ, Hur G, Kim SY, et al. Frequency of myocardial bridges and dynamic compression of epicardial coronary arteries: a comparison between computed tomography and invasive coronary angiography. *Circulation* 2009;119(10):1408–1416.

Kim SY, Seo JB, Do KH, et al. Coronary artery anomalies: classification and ECG-gated multi-detector row CT findings with angiographic correlation. *Radiographics* 2006;26(2):317–333; discussion 333–334.

Kim RJ, Wu E, Rafael A, et al. The use of contrast-enhanced magnetic resonance imaging to identify reversible myocardial dysfunction. *N Engl J Med* 2000;343(20):1445–1453.

Kishi S, Giannopoulos AA, Tang A, et al. Fractional flow reserve estimated at coronary CT angiography in intermediate lesions: comparison of diagnostic accuracy of different methods to determine coronary flow distribution. *Radiology* 2018;287(1):76–84.

Kitagawa T, Yamamoto H, Horiguchi J, et al. Characterization of noncalcified coronary plaques and identification of culprit lesions in patients with acute coronary syndrome by 64-slice computed tomography. *JACC Cardiovasc Imaging* 2009;2(2):153–160.

Knaapen M, Koch AH, Koch C, et al. Prevalence of left and balanced coronary arterial dominance decreases with increasing age of patients at autopsy. A postmortem coronary angiograms study. *Cardiovasc Pathol* 2013;22(1): 49–53.

Kosar P, Ergun E, Ozturk C, Kosar U. Anatomic variations and anomalies of the coronary arteries: 64-slice CT angiographic appearance. *Diagn Interv Radiol* 2009;15(4):275–283.

Krasuski RA, Magyar D, Hart S, et al. Long-term outcome and impact of surgery on adults with coronary arteries originating from the opposite coronary cusp. *Circulation* 2011;123(2):154–162.

Krishnan B, Cross C, Dykoski R, et al. Intra-atrial right coronary artery and its ablation implications. *JACC Clin Electrophysiol* 2017;3(9):1037–1045.

Kumar A, Beohar N, Arumana JM, et al. CMR imaging of edema in myocardial infarction using cine balanced steady-state free precession. *JACC Cardiovasc Imaging* 2011;4(12):1265–1273.

Kumbhani DJ, Ingelmo CP, Schoenhagen P, Curtin RJ, Flamm SD, Desai MY. Meta-analysis of diagnostic efficacy of 64-slice computed tomography in the evaluation of coronary in-stent restenosis. *Am J Cardiol* 2009;103(12): 1675–1681.

Kutty RS, Jones N, Moorjani N. Mechanical complications of acute myocardial infarction. *Cardiol Clin* 2013;31(4):519–531, vii–viii.

Le Breton H, Pavin D, Langanay T, et al. Aneurysms and pseudoaneurysms of saphenous vein coronary artery bypass grafts. *Heart* 1998;79(5):505–508.

Lee BY. Anomalous right coronary artery from the left coronary sinus with an interarterial course: is it really dangerous? *Korean Circ J* 2009;39(5): 175–179.

Lee HJ, Hong YJ, Kim HY, et al. Anomalous origin of the right coronary artery from the left coronary sinus with an interarterial course: subtypes and clinical importance. *Radiology* 2012;262(1):101–108.

Lempel JK, Jeudy J, Kligerman SJ, White CS. The nubbin sign. *J Thorac Imaging* 2013;28(3):W42.

Litt HI, Gatsonis C, Snyder B, et al. CT angiography for safe discharge of patients with possible acute coronary syndromes. *N Engl J Med* 2012; 366(15):1393–1403.

Lowe JE, Oldham HN Jr, Sabiston DC Jr. Surgical management of congenital coronary artery fistulas. *Ann Surg* 1981;194(4):373–380.

Madhavan MV, Tarigopula M, Mintz GS, Maehara A, Stone GW, Genereux P. Coronary artery calcification: pathogenesis and prognostic implications. *J Am Coll Cardiol* 2014;63(17):1703–1714.

Malagutti P, Nieman K, Meijboom WB, et al. Use of 64-slice CT in symptomatic patients after coronary bypass surgery: evaluation of grafts and coronary arteries. *Eur Heart J* 2007;28(15):1879–1885.

Mandal S, Tadros SS, Soni S, Madan S. Single coronary artery anomaly: classification and evaluation using multidetector computed tomography and magnetic resonance angiography. *Pediatr Cardiol* 2014;35(3):441–449.

Masci PG, Bogaert J. Post myocardial infarction of the left ventricle: the course ahead seen by cardiac MRI. *Cardiovasc Diagn Ther* 2012;2(2):113–127.

Miller JA, Anavekar NS, El Yaman MM, Burkhart HM, Miller AJ, Julsrud PR. Computed tomographic angiography identification of intramural segments in anomalous coronary arteries with interarterial course. *Int J Cardiovasc Imaging* 2012;28(6):1525–1532.

Miller JM, Rochitte CE, Dewey M, et al. Diagnostic performance of coronary angiography by 64-row CT. *N Engl J Med* 2008;359(22):2324–2336.

Min JK, Leipsic J, Pencina MJ, et al. Diagnostic accuracy of fractional flow reserve from anatomic CT angiography. *JAMA* 2012;308(12):1237–1245.

Mohara J, Konishi H, Kato M, Misawa Y, Kamisawa O, Fuse K. Saphenous vein graft pseudoaneurysm rupture after coronary artery bypass grafting. *Ann Thorac Surg* 1998;65(3):831–832.

Mohlenkamp S, Hort W, Ge J, Erbel R. Update on myocardial bridging. *Circulation* 2002;106(20):2616–2622.

Motoyama S, Kondo T, Sarai M, et al. Multislice computed tomographic characteristics of coronary lesions in acute coronary syndromes. *J Am Coll Cardiol* 2007;50(4):319–326.

Motoyama S, Sarai M, Harigaya H, et al. Computed tomographic angiography characteristics of atherosclerotic plaques subsequently resulting in acute coronary syndrome. *J Am Coll Cardiol* 2009;54(1):49–57.

Mowatt G, Cook JA, Hillis GS, et al. 64-Slice computed tomography angiography in the diagnosis and assessment of coronary artery disease: systematic review and meta-analysis. *Heart* 2008;94(11):1386–1393.

Musiani A, Cernigliaro C, Sansa M, Maselli D, De Gasperis C. Left main coronary artery atresia: literature review and therapeutical considerations. *Eur J Cardiothorac Surg* 1997;11(3):505–514.

Narula J, Achenbach S. Napkin-ring necrotic cores: defining circumferential extent of necrotic cores in unstable plaques. *JACC Cardiovasc Imaging* 2009;2(12):1436–1438.

Opolski MP, Pregowski J, Kruk M, et al. The prevalence and characteristics of intra-atrial right coronary artery anomaly in 9,284 patients referred for coronary computed tomography angiography. *Eur J Radiol* 2014;83(7): 1129–1134.

Pejkovic B, Krajnc I, Anderhuber F, Kosutic D. Anatomical aspects of the arterial blood supply to the sinoatrial and atrioventricular nodes of the human heart. *J Int Med Res* 2008;36(4):691–698.

Pena E, Nguyen ET, Merchant N, Dennie C. ALCAPA syndrome: not just a pediatric disease. *Radiographics* 2009;29(2):553–565.

Polacek P, Kralove H. Relation of myocardial bridges and loops on the coronary arteries to coronary occulsions. *Am Heart J* 1961;61:44–52.

Raff GL, Abidov A, Achenbach S, et al. SCCT guidelines for the interpretation and reporting of coronary computed tomographic angiography. *J Cardiovasc Comput Tomogr* 2009;3(2):122–136.

Ramirez FD, Hibbert B, Simard T, et al. Natural history and management of aortocoronary saphenous vein graft aneurysms: a systematic review of published cases. *Circulation* 2012;126(18):2248–2256.

Renapurkar R, Desai MY, Curtin RJ. Intracavitary course of the right coronary artery: an increasingly recognized anomaly by coronary computed tomography angiography. *J Thorac Imaging* 2010;25(3):W77–W78.

Ropers D, Pohle FK, Kuettner A, et al. Diagnostic accuracy of noninvasive coronary angiography in patients after bypass surgery using 64-slice spiral computed tomography with 330-ms gantry rotation. *Circulation* 2006;114(22): 2334–2341; quiz 2334.

Rossi A, Merkus D, Klotz E, Mollet N, de Feyter PJ, Krestin GP. Stress myocardial perfusion: imaging with multidetector CT. *Radiology* 2014;270(1):25–46.

Said SA, van der Werf T. Dutch survey of coronary artery fistulas in adults: congenital solitary fistulas. *Int J Cardiol* 2006;106(3):323–332.

Sakuma H. Coronary CT versus MR angiography: the role of MR angiography. *Radiology* 2011;258(2):340–349.

Salavati A, Radmanesh F, Heidari K, Dwamena BA, Kelly AM, Cronin P. Dual-source computed tomography angiography for diagnosis and assessment of coronary artery disease: systematic review and meta-analysis. *J Cardiovasc Comput Tomogr* 2012;6(2):78–90.

Saremi F, Goodman G, Wilcox A, Salibian R, Vorobiof G. Coronary artery ostial atresia: diagnosis of conotruncal anastomotic collateral rings using CT angiography. *JACC Cardiovasc Imaging* 2011;4(12):1320–1323.

Sari I, Kizilkan N, Sucu M, et al. Double right coronary artery: report of two cases and review of the literature. *Int J Cardiol* 2008;130(2):e74–e77.

Sarwar A, Shaw LJ, Shapiro MD, et al. Diagnostic and prognostic value of absence of coronary artery calcification. *JACC Cardiovasc Imaging* 2009;2(6):675–688.

Saw J, Aymong E, Sedlak T, et al. Spontaneous coronary artery dissection: association with predisposing arteriopathies and precipitating stressors and cardiovascular outcomes. *Circ Cardiovasc Interv* 2014;7(5):645–655.

Serruys PW, de Jaegere P, Kiemeneij F, et al. A comparison of balloon-expandable-stent implantation with balloon angioplasty in patients with coronary artery disease. Benestent Study Group. *N Engl J Med* 1994;331(8):489–495.

Shah DJ, Kim HW, James O, et al. Prevalence of regional myocardial thinning and relationship with myocardial scarring in patients with coronary artery disease. *JAMA* 2013;309(9):909–918.

Shen WF, Tribouilloy C, Mirode A, Dufosse H, Lesbre JP. Left ventricular aneurysm and prognosis in patients with first acute transmural anterior myocardial infarction and isolated left anterior descending artery disease. *Eur Heart J* 1992;13(1):39–44.

Stone GW, Moses JW, Ellis SG, et al. Safety and efficacy of sirolimus- and paclitaxel-eluting coronary stents. *N Engl J Med* 2007;356(10):998–1008.

Syed M, Lesch M. Coronary artery aneurysm: a review. *Prog Cardiovasc Dis* 1997; 40(1):77–84.

Taylor AJ, Cerqueira M, Hodgson JM, et al. ACCF/SCCT/ACR/AHA/ASE/ ASNC/NASCI/SCAI/SCMR 2010 appropriate use criteria for cardiac computed tomography. A Report of the American College of Cardiology Foundation Appropriate Use Criteria Task Force, the Society of Cardiovascular Computed Tomography, the American College of Radiology, the American Heart Association, the American Society of Echocardiography, the American Society of Nuclear Cardiology, the North American Society for Cardiovascular Imaging, the Society for Cardiovascular Angiography and Interventions, and the Society for Cardiovascular Magnetic Resonance. *Circulation* 2010;122(21):e525–e555.

Tesche C, De Cecco CN, Albrecht MH, et al. Coronary CT angiography-derived fractional flow reserve. *Radiology* 2017;285(1):17–33.

Topaz O, DiSciascio G, Cowley MJ, et al. Absent left main coronary artery: angiographic findings in 83 patients with separate ostia of the left anterior descending and circumflex arteries at the left aortic sinus. *Am Heart J* 1991;122(2):447–452.

Tunick PA, Slater J, Kronzon I, Glassman E. Discrete atherosclerotic coronary artery aneurysms: a study of 20 patients. *J Am Coll Cardiol* 1990;15(2): 279–282.

Varga-Szemes A, Meinel FG, De Cecco CN, Fuller SR, Bayer RR, 2nd, Schoepf UJ. CT myocardial perfusion imaging. *AJR Am J Roentgenol* 2015;204(3): 487–497.

Veltman CE, de Graaf FR, Schuijf JD, et al. Prognostic value of coronary vessel dominance in relation to significant coronary artery disease determined with non-invasive computed tomography coronary angiography. *Eur Heart J* 2012;33(11):1367–1377.

Virmani R, Burke AP, Farb A. Plaque rupture and plaque erosion. *Thromb Haemost* 1999;82 Suppl 1:1–3.

Virmani R, Burke AP, Farb A, Kolodgie FD. Pathology of the vulnerable plaque. *J Am Coll Cardiol* 2006;47(8 Suppl):C13–C18.

Virmani R, Burke AP, Kolodgie FD, Farb A. Vulnerable plaque: the pathology of unstable coronary lesions. *J Interv Cardiol* 2002;15(6):439–446.

Virmani R, Burke AP, Kolodgie FD, Farb A. Pathology of the thin-cap fibroatheroma: a type of vulnerable plaque. *J Interv Cardiol* 2003;16(3):267–272.

Vliegenthart R, Henzler T, Moscariello A, et al. CT of coronary heart disease: part 1, CT of myocardial infarction, ischemia, and viability. *AJR Am J Roentgenol* 2012;198(3):531–547.

Warnes CA, Williams RG, Bashore TM, et al. ACC/AHA 2008 guidelines for the management of adults with congenital heart disease: a report of the American College of Cardiology/American Heart Association Task Force on Practice Guidelines (writing committee to develop guidelines on the management of adults with congenital heart disease). *Circulation* 2008;118(23):e714–e833.

Weustink AC, Nieman K, Pugliese F, et al. Diagnostic accuracy of computed tomography angiography in patients after bypass grafting: comparison with invasive coronary angiography. *JACC Cardiovasc Imaging* 2009;2(7):816–824.

Yamagishi M, Terashima M, Awano K, et al. Morphology of vulnerable coronary plaque: insights from follow-up of patients examined by intravascular ultrasound before an acute coronary syndrome. *J Am Coll Cardiol* 2000; 35(1):106–111.

Yamamoto H, Kitagawa T, Ohashi N, et al. Noncalcified atherosclerotic lesions with vulnerable characteristics detected by coronary CT angiography and future coronary events. *J Cardiovasc Comput Tomogr* 2013;7(3): 192–199.

Yamanaka O, Hobbs RE. Coronary artery anomalies in 126,595 patients undergoing coronary arteriography. *Cathet Cardiovasc Diagn* 1990;21(1):28–40.

Yau JM, Singh R, Halpern EJ, Fischman D. Anomalous origin of the left coronary artery from the pulmonary artery in adults: a comprehensive review of 151 adult cases and a new diagnosis in a 53-year-old woman. *Clin Cardiol* 2011;34(4):204–210.

Yoshida S, Sakuma K, Ueda O. Acute mitral regurgitation due to total rupture in the anterior papillary muscle after acute myocardial infarction successfully treated by emergency surgery. *Jpn J Thorac Cardiovasc Surg* 2003;51(5):208–210.

Zarins CK, Taylor CA, Min JK. Computed fractional flow reserve (FFTCT) derived from coronary CT angiography. *J Cardiovasc Transl Res* 2013;6(5): 708–714.

Zeina AR, Odeh M, Blinder J, Rosenschein U, Barmeir E. Myocardial bridge: evaluation on MDCT. *AJR Am J Roentgenol* 2007;188(4):1069–1073.

Zenooz NA, Habibi R, Mammen L, Finn JP, Gilkeson RC. Coronary artery fistulas: CT findings. *Radiographics* 2009;29(3):781–789.

CHAPTER 26 ■ CARDIAC MASSES

JAY S. LEB AND SETH KLIGERMAN

INTRODUCTION

Cardiac masses are a relatively uncommon entity which can be classified as either a tumor or tumorlike condition. The prevalence of cardiac tumors is low, estimated at 0.002% to 0.03% on autopsy series. In fact, many of the cardiac lesions detected are usually tumorlike lesions, with thrombus representing most cases. Cardiac tumors can be further classified as primary or secondary, with secondary tumors due to metastatic disease being 20 to 40 times more common than primary cardiac tumors (Fig. 26.1). While the classification of theses lesions into benign or malignant entities is an important prognostic factor, any cardiac tumor or tumorlike condition can cause significant morbidity or mortality by causing embolic, arrhythmogenic, or obstructive manifestations. Advances in cardiac imaging, particularly cross-sectional imaging, have significantly expanded the role of imaging in the evaluation of these lesions.

IMAGING TECHNIQUES AND PROTOCOLS

Cardiac masses are often detected incidentally on routine echocardiography or computed tomography (CT) studies, performed for other reasons. With the increasing temporal resolution of conventional CT, there are an increasing number of incidental cardiac lesions detected on routine chest and abdominal imaging. Once discovered, localization of the lesion is the first important diagnostic step. Knowing the location of the lesion alone can aid in narrowing the differential diagnosis (Figs. 26.2 and 26.3). Many times, reported cardiac lesions either reflect normal structures or are related to extracardiac lesions from the adjacent structures, including the pericardium, mediastinum, or lungs. Visualization of the epicardium and/or pericardium can be helpful in distinguishing intra- versus extracardiac lesions. Localizing the epicenter of the lesion within the heart will aid in the diagnosis of cardiac masses. Detecting calcification, fat, or fibrous tissue within the lesion will help narrow the diagnosis. Imaging features can also aid in determining if the lesion has benign or malignant features (Table 26.1). Of course, one of the most crucial questions to answer is whether the lesion is a mass or a thrombus.

Echocardiography

Several imaging modalities are available to evaluate cardiac masses, each with different advantages and disadvantages. Transthoracic echocardiography remains the first-line imaging technique used to evaluate cardiac masses, as it is widely available, readily performed, and relatively inexpensive. It provides excellent real-time imaging to evaluate heart morphology, and ventricular and valvular function. However, the poor soft tissue contrast of echocardiography and its restricted acoustic windows limit its ability to completely characterize cardiac masses. Echocardiographic evaluation of the adjacent extracardiac structures is also limited and the extent of local involvement is not always assessed. In addition, large infiltrative extracardiac masses may be misinterpreted as primarily intracardiac in location due to the narrow field of view. While transesophageal echocardiography is superior in its available acoustic windows, it remains limited by its restricted fields of view and soft tissue contrast.

Cross-Sectional Imaging

With recent advances in techniques, cross-sectional imaging with cardiac CT and cardiac magnetic resonance imaging (CMR) is increasingly relied on for further evaluation of suspected cardiac lesions. ECG gating, the ability to time the imaging acquisition to the patient's electrocardiogram, limits motion artifact and can help provide functional analysis.

Cardiac CT. ECG-gated cardiac CT—with high spatial resolution, multiplanar image reconstruction capabilities, and fast acquisition times—allows for the accurate detection and localization of cardiac masses. Although the ability of CT to characterize tissue is not as good as MRI, CT is excellent in detecting the presence of fat, fluid, and calcification within lesions. Retrospective ECG gating, where the heart is imaged throughout the cardiac cycle, may be helpful to demonstrate movement of the mass during the cardiac cycle. Disadvantages of cardiac CT include decreased temporal resolution, exposure to ionizing radiation, and inferior soft tissue contrast as compared with MRI. The need for intravenous contrast limits CT availability in patients with renal failure or prior contrast allergy.

Intravenous, nonionic contrast is an important component in the CT evaluation of cardiac lesions. If the location

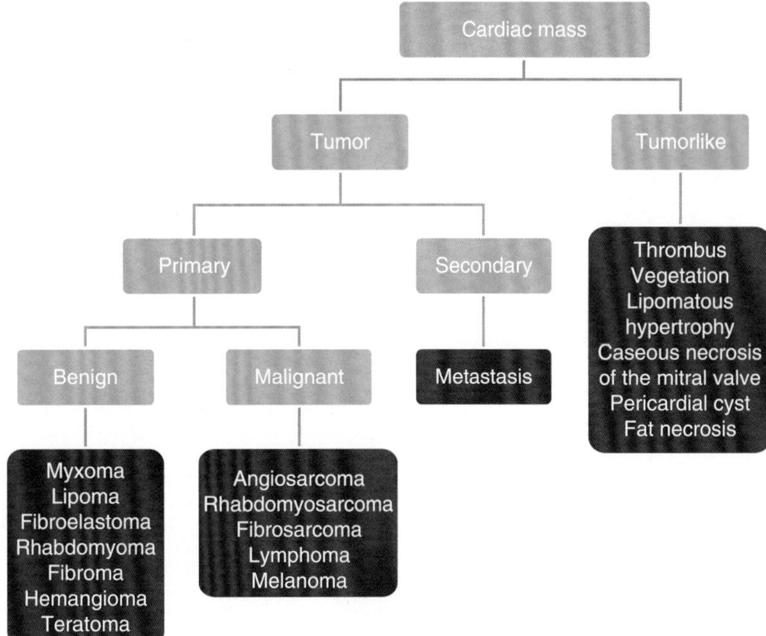

FIGURE 26.1. Overview of Cardiac Mass Subtypes.

of the lesion in question is known, the contrast timing can be tailored to opacify the region of interest by using either bolus tracking or timing-bolus techniques. Bolus tracking is performed by placing a region of interest in a specific area (depending on what needs to be opacified for the examination) and serial images are obtained, with subsequent triggering of the scan when the density within the region of interest exceeds a designated threshold value. Timing-bolus technique utilizes a preliminary scan using a small quantity of contrast (10 to 20 mL), and the transit time for the time for the contrast to peak (TTP) in the region of interest is calculated. Otherwise, a larger volume of contrast should be administered to ensure adequate opacification of all chambers. Delayed-phase imaging may be helpful in assessing tumor enhancement or to

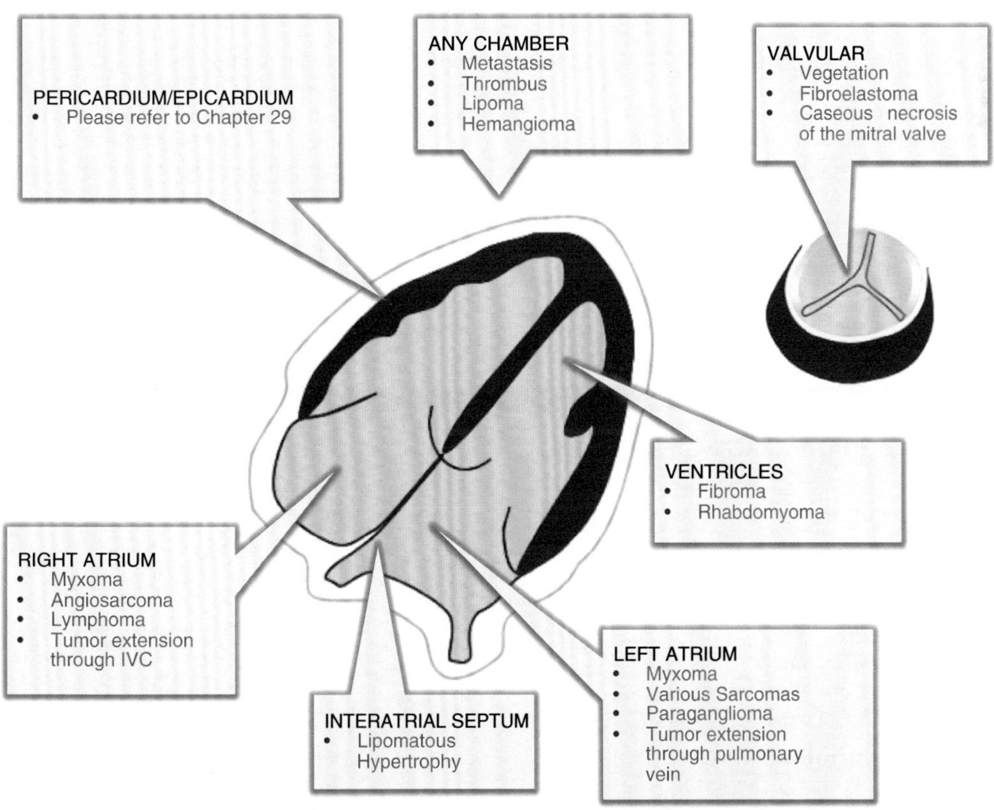

FIGURE 26.2. Schematic Depiction of the Typical Location of Common Cardiac Masses.

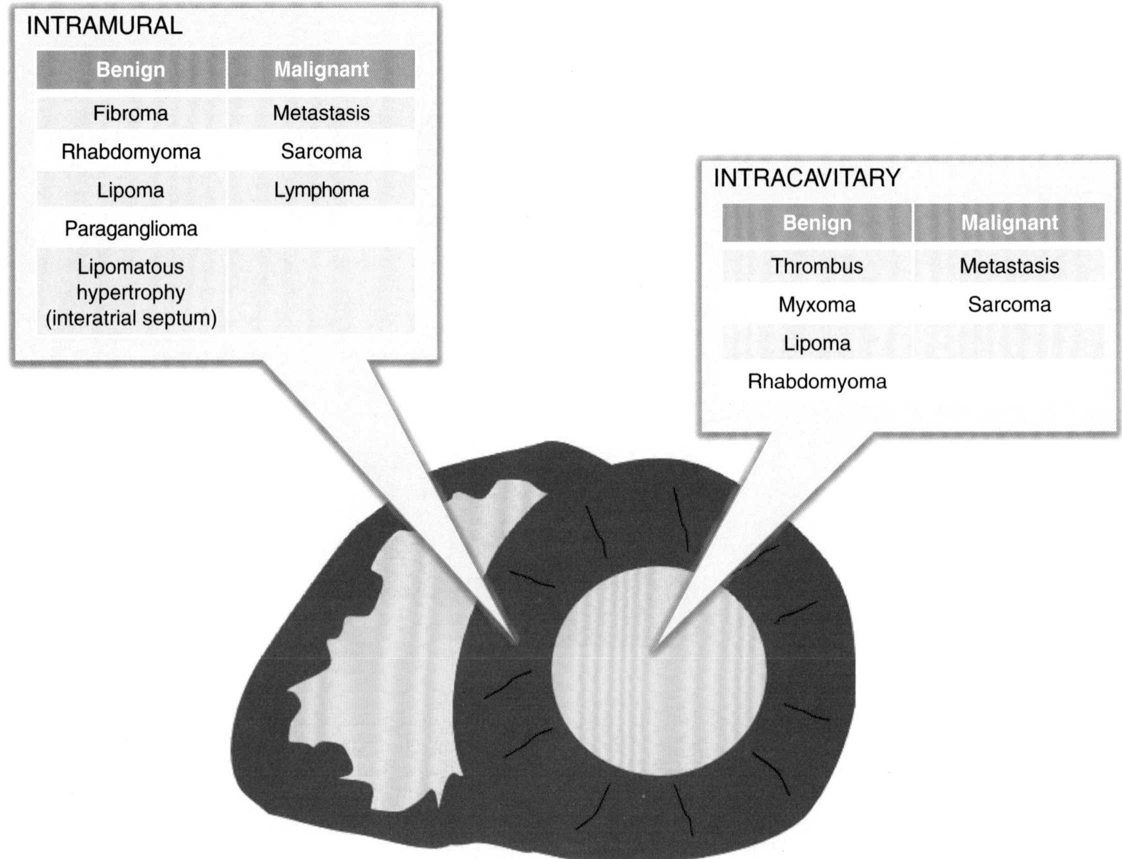

INTRAMURAL
Benign
Malignant
Fibroma
Metastasis
Rhabdomyoma
Sarcoma
Lipoma
Lymphoma
Paraganglioma
Lipomatous hypertrophy (interatrial septum)
INTRACAVITARY
Benign
Malignant
Thrombus
Metastasis
Myxoma
Sarcoma
Lipoma
Rhabdomyoma

FIGURE 26.3. **Schematic Depiction of Common Cardiac Masses and Their Location With Relation to the Myocardium.**

improve opacification of the right atrium, IVC, or left atrial appendage.

Cardiac MRI. Cardiac MRI is currently the modality of choice in evaluating cardiac masses. It is noninvasive, offers multiplanar imaging, unrestricted fields of view, and provides excellent soft tissue contrast. Gradient echo cine imaging allows for excellent localization of the mass and simultaneously allows for functional analysis. T1- and T2-weighted imaging (T1W and T2W) provides valuable anatomic definition and tissue characterization. However, definitive differentiation between benign and malignant lesions based on these signal characteristics alone are difficult due to the wide overlap of many tumors, as most tumors demonstrate low to intermediate signal on T1W imaging and high signal on the T2W imaging. Fat-saturation techniques are routinely used to evaluate for the presence of fat. Postcontrast T1–based perfusion and late gadolinium enhancement (LGE) images are key sequences to evaluate for lesion vascularity and enhancement (Table 26.2).

The cardiac MR protocol is tailored to detect the lesion, evaluate its morphology, and define its tissue components. Scout images and nontargeted axial images of the chest are

TABLE 26.1

BENIGN VERSUS MALIGNANT IMAGING FEATURES

■ FEATURES	■ BENIGN	■ MALIGNANT
Size	■ Small, <5 cm	■ Large, >5 cm
Number of lesions	■ Single	■ Multiple
Location	■ Left sided	■ Right sided
Margins	■ Smooth ■ Well-defined borders ■ No extension through tissue planes	■ Irregular ■ Ill-defined borders ■ Direct invasion through tissue planes
Pericardium	■ No involvement	■ Hemorrhagic pericardial effusion ■ Pericardial invasion or multiple nodular masses
Tissue characteristics	■ Homogeneous ■ Absent to minimal early enhancement. ■ Variable delayed enhancement	■ Heterogeneous due to hemorrhage and necrosis ■ Prominent early enhancement. ■ Variable delayed enhancement

TABLE 26.2

SUMMARY AND EXPLANATION OF THE CARDIAC MR SEQUENCES UTILIZED IN THE DETECTION AND EVALUATION OF CARDIAC MASSES

■ SEQUENCES	■ DESCRIPTION	■ UTILITY
3D scout images and transaxial images	■ Either SSFP or FSE ■ Large field of view ■ Covers the entire thorax	■ Overview of anatomy ■ Visualization of large lesions involving the mediastinum/lungs
Cine SSFP	■ Performed in the standard two-chamber, four-chamber, and stacked short-axis views ■ Can also be performed in planes to optimally visualize the lesion	■ Confirmation/localization of the lesion ■ Assesses lesion size, mobility, effect on the myocardial function, and valvular structures
T1W +/– fat saturation	■ T1W black blood double IR FSE images; triple IR used to null fat	■ T1 tissue characterization ■ Assesses for fat components, hemorrhage, or necrosis
T2W +/– fat saturation	■ T2W black blood double IR FSE images; triple IR used to null fat	■ T2 tissue characterization ■ Assesses for edema or necrosis
Myocardial tagging (optional)	■ Different tagging sequence techniques can be utilized	■ Evaluates for the presence of infiltration into the myocardium or pericardium ■ Detection of a noncontractile intramyocardial mass
Perfusion imaging	■ During the administration of gadolinium (0.1–0.2 mmol/kg) ■ Dynamic FLASH imaging	■ Assesses lesion vascularity and distinguishes from myocardium or thrombus
Early postcontrast T1W	■ 3D volumetric breath-hold T1 fat-saturated or T1W double IR FSE images	■ Assesses lesion enhancement and distinguishes from myocardium or thrombus
Late gadolinium enhancement	■ 10 minutes after contrast injection ■ Segmented double inversion recovery FSE sequence ■ Inversion time (typically 200–300 ms) set to achieve appropriate nulling of the normal myocardium, determined via a TI scout or Look–Locker sequence	■ Assesses lesion enhancement and distinguishes from myocardium or thrombus ■ Can also perform imaging at an inversion time of 600 ms to aid in distinguishing thrombus versus mass

first utilized to help locate the lesion and plan subsequent targeted imaging. Steady-state free precession (SSFP) cine images are then performed and prescribed based on the location of the mass. In general, the entire mass should be evaluated in at least one plane to ensure accurate characterization. After the mass is localized, T1W and T2W sequences should be obtained through the lesion prior to contrast administration to characterize the tissue types. In lesions localized near or within the pericardium, myocardial tissue tagging—a dynamic tagged sequence—can aid in the detection of myocardial infiltration or adhesions. In addition, tagging sequences can help detect the presence of a noncontractile intramyocardial mass, such as a rhabdomyoma, or differentiate a true mass versus asymmetric focal hypertrophic cardiomyopathy.

After localization and basic tissue characterization, postcontrast imaging following the intravenous administration of gadolinium-based contrast is a key component to the MR evaluation. The tumor should be imaged during first-pass perfusion to allow for detection of early arterial enhancement. Afterward, T1-postcontrast imaging should be performed in the same plane as the T1W precontrast images to allow for accurate comparison. LGE images are performed 10 to 15 minutes after the administration of contrast, which is useful to detect late gadolinium enhancement of the mass or surrounding myocardial enhancement due to the mass. The LGE characteristics may help differentiate thrombus or other benign lesions from the malignant ones which typically demonstrate increasingly greater enhancement. Utilizing longer inversion recovery times (such as 600 ms) can distinguish a thrombus from a tumor.

While an excellent tool for cardiac mass evaluation, MRI does have its limitations. First off, MRI examinations require a patient to lie supine in a relatively enclosed tube for a prolonged period, often greater than 1 hour. Sedation may be necessary for patients with severe claustrophobia or those who cannot follow instructions. This can prolong imaging time due to the need to perform multiaverage sequences. In addition, small masses may not be detected on MRI due to its relatively decreased spatial resolution compared to other modalities such as CT (Table 26.3).

BENIGN CARDIAC TUMORS

Myxoma. Myxomas are benign lesions of endocardial origin. They are the most common primary cardiac tumor and represent 50% of all benign cardiac masses and 25% of all primary cardiac tumors. They usually occur in the fourth to seventh decades of life and approximately 60% of affected patients are female. Myxomas arise from undifferentiated and totipotent mesenchymal stem cell and have a gelatinous composition described as an acid mucopolysaccharide–rich stroma. Greater than 90% of cases are sporadic and usually solitary. However, cardiac myxomas can be seen in patients with the Carney complex, which is an autosomal dominant disorder characterized by an increased risk of tumors including cardiac and

TABLE 26.3

SUMMARY OF CARDIAC MASS IMAGING FEATURES ON CT AND MRI

CARDIAC LESION	LOCATION	CT FEATURES	T1W	T2W	PERFUSION/T1W+	LGE	OTHER
Myxoma	Left atrium, interatrial septum attached to the fossa ovalis	Hypodense lesion	Isointense	Hyperintense areas	Mild	Heterogeneous	Lobular, at times on a stalk
Lipoma	Endocardial, intramyocardial, or epicardial in or around any chamber	Homogenous lesion with fat density	Hyperintense	Hyperintense	Absent	Absent	Suppresses on fat suppression images
Papillary fibroelastoma	Valve leaflets, most commonly the aortic	Small mobile homogenous lesion	Hypo/ Isointense	Iso/hyperintense	Absent	Variable but usually moderate	Unlike vegetation, will not typically cause valvular destruction
Rhabdomyoma	Ventricles, intramyocardial or intracavitary	Smooth nodules in the myocardium	Isointense	Iso/hyperintense	Absent/mild	Absent/minimal	Frequently multifocal
Fibroma	Ventricles, intramyocardial	Homogenous low attenuation mass	Isointense	Hypointense	Absent	Intense	No enhancement on perfusion imaging due to avascularity
Hemangioma	Any chamber, intracavitary	Heterogeneous lesion, may have calcification	Iso/hyperintense	Hyperintense	Intense	Intense	Hypervascular on perfusion
Paraganglioma	Left atrium, the atrial roof or posterior wall	Well defined lesion with intense enhancement	Hypo/isointense	Hyperintense	Intense	Intense	Light bulb bright on T2W
Metastasis	Endocardial, intramyocardial, or epicardial in or around any chamber	Infiltrative lesion	Variable, commonly hypointense	Hyperintense	Variable (mild to intense)	Heterogeneous	Melanoma will be high on T1W and low on T2W
Angiosarcoma	Right atrium/ventricle	Hemorrhagic lesion	Heterogeneous	hyperintense	Intense	Heterogenous	May have pericardial involvement with a hemorrhagic effusion
Other sarcomas	Left atrium	Usually hypodense	Hypo/isointense	Hyperintense	Moderate/intense	Heterogeneous/ homogenous	Can extend into the pulmonary veins
Lymphoma	Anywhere but classically near right AV groove	Infiltrating lesion, low/ isoattenuating to the myocardium	Hypo/isointense	Iso/hyperintense	Absent/mild	Variable, at times none	Infiltrative tumor which grows along framework of heart
Thrombus	Any chamber	Homogenous lesion	Hypointense	Hypointense	Absent	Absent	Nulls at longer inversion time, around 600 msec
Lipomatous hypertrophy of the interatrial septum	Interatrial septum, always spares the fossa ovalis	Homogenous lesion with fat density	Hyperintense	Hyperintense	Absent	Absent	Suppresses on fat suppression images, barbell in shape

cutaneous myxomas. Other Carney complex associations include hyperpigmented skin lesions, endocrinopathy, and extracardiac neoplasms such as breast fibroadenomas, melanotic schwannomas, or pituitary adenomas. In cases where myxomas are multifocal, extra-atrial, or recurrent, association with the Carney complex should be suspected.

There is a varied clinical presentation in patients with a cardiac myxoma, depending on the lesion location, size, and its effect on cardiac function. The triad of intracardiac obstruction, embolization of tumor, and constitutional symptoms is classically described. Since the majority of tumors occur in the left atrium, symptoms are commonly related to mitral valve obstruction and include dyspnea and orthopnea from pulmonary edema (Fig. 26.4b). Right atrial tumors can present with findings of tricuspid valve obstruction, including peripheral edema and syncope.

As demonstrated on imaging, myxomas are commonly intracavitary with 75% to 80% of myxomas found in the left atrium, with the majority arising from the interatrial septum near the fossa ovalis. A minority of cases may arise from the chamber walls or valve surfaces. Larger tumors may obstruct or prolapse through the mitral valve. Ten to twenty percent of tumors occur in the right atrium. Myxomas originating in the ventricular chamber or atrioventricular valves are rare. Most cardiac myxomas are well-defined lesions which are ovoid or round in shape (Fig. 26.4A). They may be pedunculated on a discrete stalk or have a broad stalk or base of attachment with the pedunculated lesions having an increased chance of prolapsing and obstructing the adjacent atrioventricular valve. While the majority of myxomas are smooth or lobulated, there is a subset of villous or papillary myxomas which has multiple fragile, villous extensions, increasing the risk for embolization. Embolization is of much greater concern for left atrial masses due to the downstream systemic circulation (Fig. 26.4B).

Aside from lesion detection and localization, imaging will aid in lesion characterization. On echocardiography, myxomas may be homogeneous or heterogeneous, with hyperechoic areas representing focal calcification and hypoechoic regions relating to cystic, necrotic, or hemorrhagic components. In general, echocardiography is an excellent tool to visualize the myxoma's effect on surrounding structures, including valvular obstruction. On CT, myxomas are usually hypodense masses attached to the interatrial septum in the region of the fossa ovalis and may enhance heterogeneously with contrast administration. CT is an excellent tool for detection of calcification, which is visible in approximately 10% of cases. On MRI, myxomas classically demonstrate isointense signal on T1W images and hyperintense signal on T2W images. However, because myxomas have varying components within them, including hemorrhagic, myxomatous, cystic, fibrous, and/or necrotic tissue, many are heterogeneous in signal. The lesion is usually hyperintense to myocardium on bright-blood SSFP sequences and will enhance following the administration of gadolinium-based contrast agents (Fig. 26.4A,B). For most cases of cardiac myxomas, the key imaging feature in the diagnosis remains its location and relationship with the interatrial septum. When in this characteristic location, there is little else in the differential diagnosis. When in an atypical location, the differential diagnosis can include a variety of tumors including benign tumors such as fibroelastomas, hemangiomas, and malignancies such as metastases.

Lipoma. Intracardiac lipomas are benign lesions which constitute approximately 10% of all primary cardiac tumors. Lipomas consist of encapsulated mature adipose cells which are commonly well defined, round or oval in shape, and broad-based. The majority of cases arise from the epicardial surface and extend outward into the pericardial space. However, lipomas

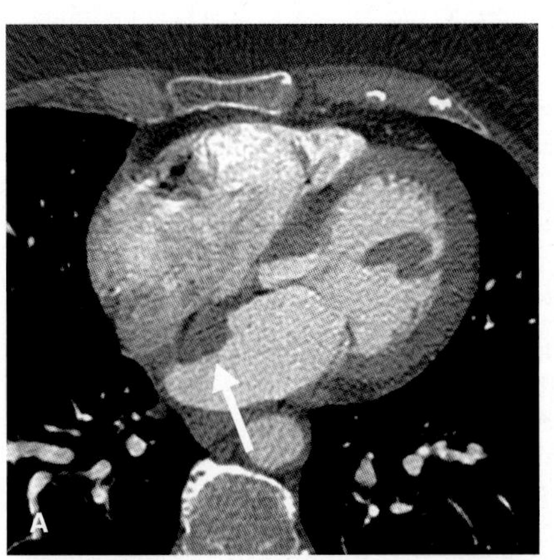

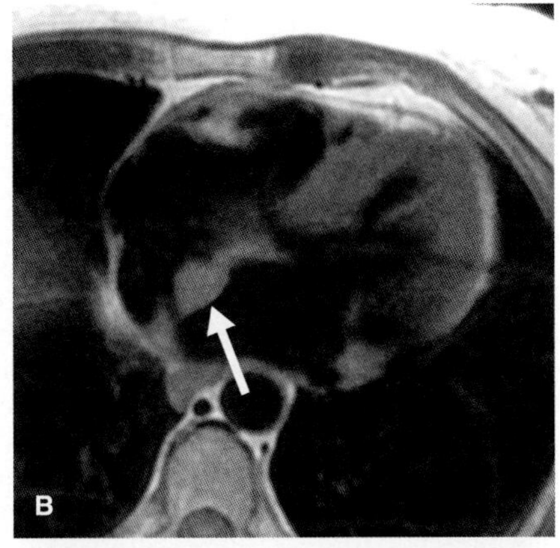

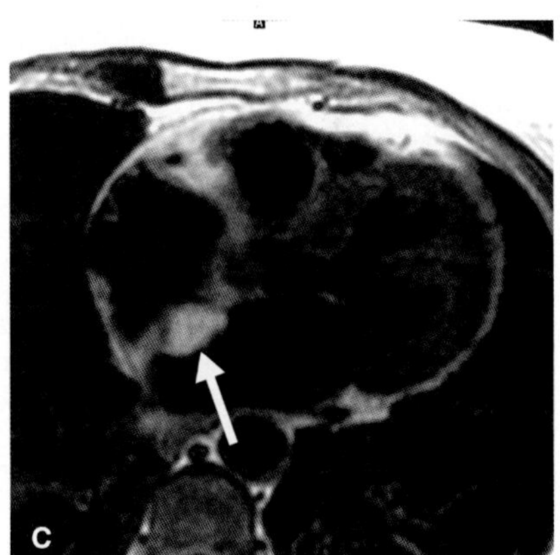

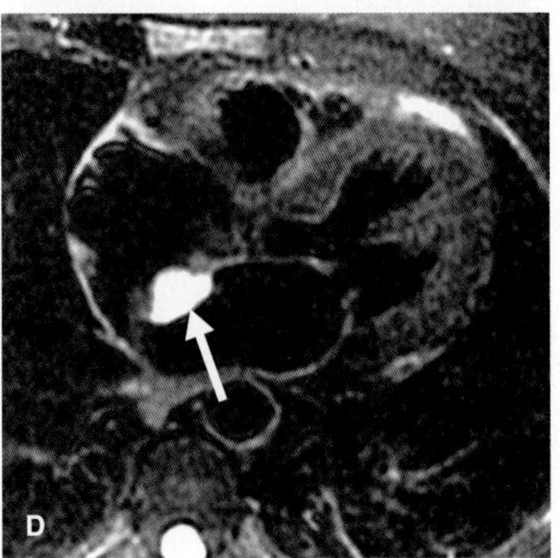

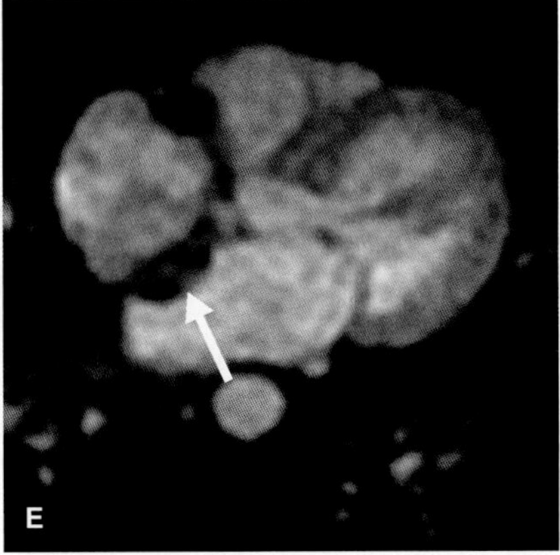

FIGURE 26.4a. **Cardiac Myxoma.** Axial postcontrast CT (**A**) demonstrates a broad-based hypodense mass (*arrow*) extending from the interatrial septum into the left atrium. It demonstrates isointense signal on T1W images (**B**), hyperintense signal on T2W images without (**C**) and with fat saturation (**D**), and heterogeneous enhancement on early postcontrast T1W imaging (**E**). After surgical removal, pathology was consistent with an atrial myxoma. (*continued*)

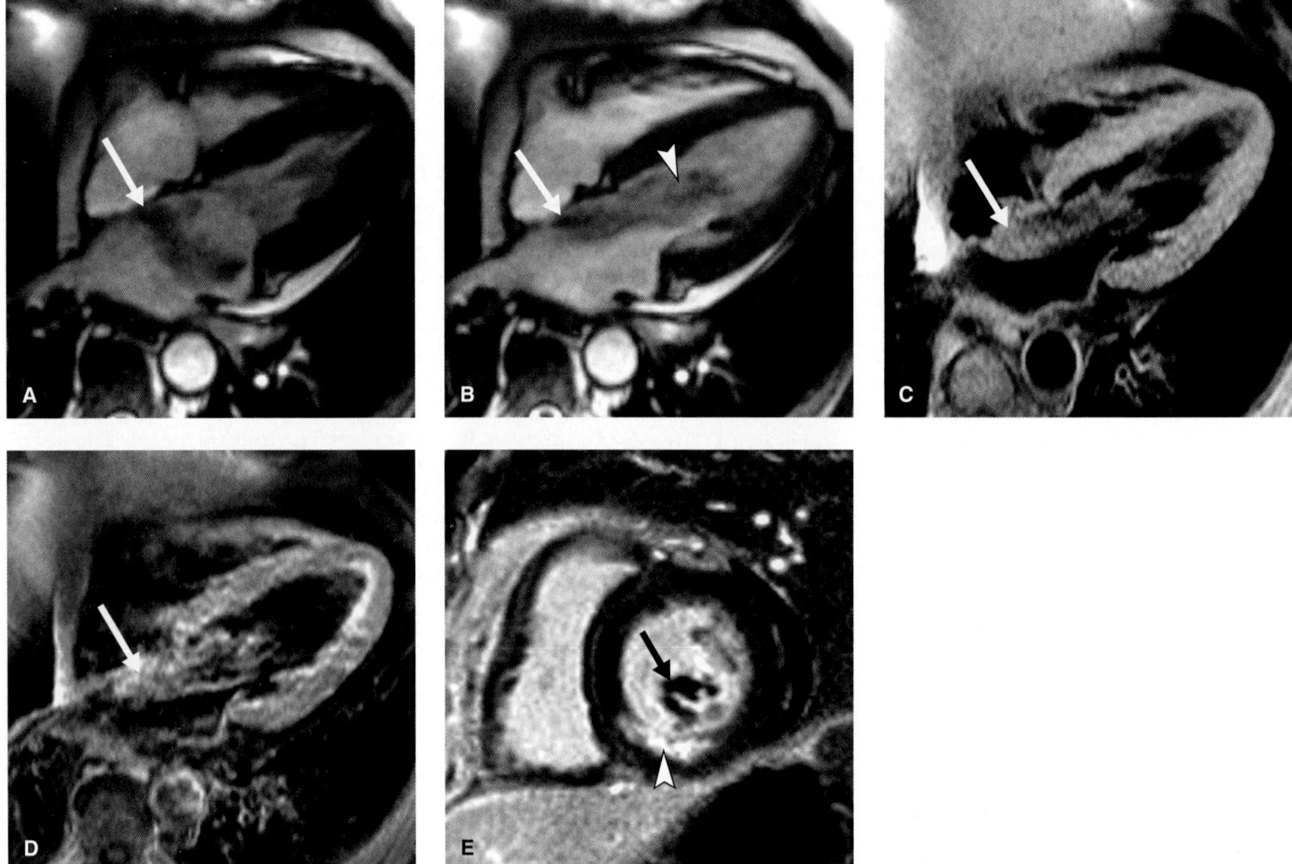

FIGURE 26.4b. (*Continued*) Villous cardiac myxoma with embolization into the right coronary artery in a 40-year-old woman. 4-chamber SSFP images obtained during systole (**A**) and diastole (**B**) shows a large left atrial mass attached to the region of the fossa ovalis (*white arrows*). The edges of the mass are ill-defined. During diastole, the mass prolapses through the mitral valve into the left ventricle (*white arrowhead,* **B**). On T1 weighted precontrast image (**C**), the mass is predominantly isointense to hypointense in signal compared to the myocardium. The mass shows heterogenous enhancement on T1W post-contrast imaging (**D**) which ranged from hypointense to hyperintense (*white arrow,* **D**) to myocardium. Delayed enhancement image (**E**) shows subendocardial infarct in the inferior wall due to RCA territory infarct (*white arrowhead*). Portions of the tumor can be seen in the left ventricle (*black arrow*). Myxoma tumor thrombus was removed from the RCA during cardiac catheterization and confirmed pathologically.

can also arise from the endocardium and pericardium. Most cases are asymptomatic and often discovered incidentally; however, larger lesions can cause obstruction to flow or impinge on ventricular wall motion when located in the pericardial space.

On CT, lipomas are homogeneous, well-defined lesions demonstrating density within the fatty range measuring less than −50 HU. On MRI, lipomas will follow fat signal on all sequences, decrease in signal with fat-suppression techniques, and will not demonstrate enhancement. The presence of a chemical shift/"India ink" artifact at the interface between the lipoma and the surrounding tissue on SSFP sequences is another characteristic finding (Fig. 26.5). While both cardiac lipomas and lipomatous hypertrophy of the interatrial septum will demonstrate identical signal characteristics, the location of the lesion within the interatrial septum with sparing of the fossa ovalis will allow differentiation of lipomatous hypertrophy from a true lipoma.

Papillary Fibroelastoma. Papillary fibroelastomas are benign endocardial–based lesions which constitute approximately 10% of all primary cardiac tumors. Fibroelastomas contain avascular dense connective tissue covered in a single layer of endothelium. They are generally small in size, measuring less than 1 to 1.5 cm on average. Pathologically, they have multiple papillary frond-like projections which are attached by a stalk-like projection to the valvular endocardium. Their appearance on gross pathologic examination has been compared to a sea anemone. Ninety percent of fibroelastomas occur on cardiac valves and they account for 75% of all valvular neoplasms. However, as they can occur on any endocardial surface, they should remain in the differential diagnosis when an endocardial-based mass is present. Most occur on the aortic and mitral valves and are usually located on the aortic side of the aortic valve and the atrial side of the atrioventricular valves, away from the free edge of the leaflet. No known familial cases of papillary fibroelastomas have been reported and they are usually solitary. Most cases of papillary fibroelastoma are asymptomatic and discovered incidentally; however, due to their friable nature and propensity for thrombus formation on their surface, there is an association with transient ischemic attacks and strokes.

Echocardiography is usually the best modality to detect and evaluate papillary fibroelastomas. The excellent temporal resolution of ultrasound allows for detection of these small, highly mobile lesions which are attached to the valve leaflets. Fibroelastomas will appear as homogeneous soft tissue attenuation lesions on ECG-gated CT, which can be used for presurgical planning (Fig. 26.6). On MRI, the lesions will demonstrate intermediate signal on T1W images and hyperintense signal on T2W images. Cine SSFP MR sequences may demonstrate turbulent flow surrounding the low signal mass. While there may be mild enhancement on T1W postcontrast imaging, fibroelastomas often show intense enhancement on delayed enhancement sequences obtained 10 minutes after the administration of intravenous contrast due to the presence of

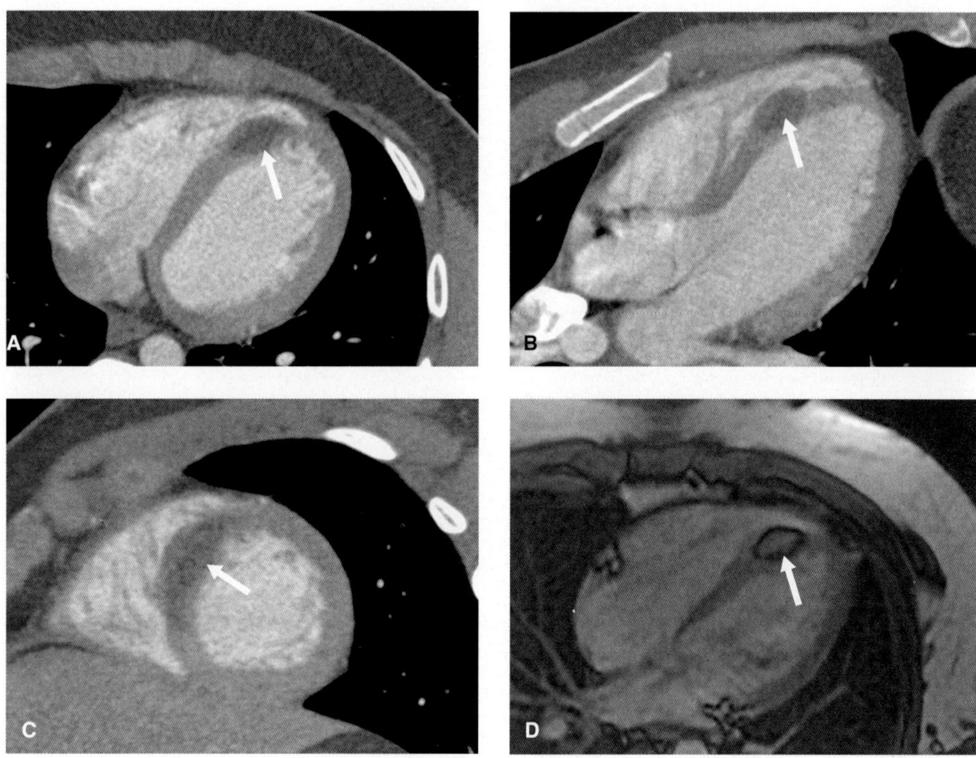

FIGURE 26.5. **Cardiac Lipoma.** Axial CT image (**A**) with multiplanar reconstructions in the three-chamber (**B**) and short-axis (**C**) views demonstrates a hypodense intramural mass (*arrow*) in the apical interventricular septal segment. Axial SSFP MR image (**D**) demonstrates peripheral "India ink" artifact (*arrow*) indicating the presence of a fat-containing lesion. These findings are most consistent with an intramyocardial lipoma.

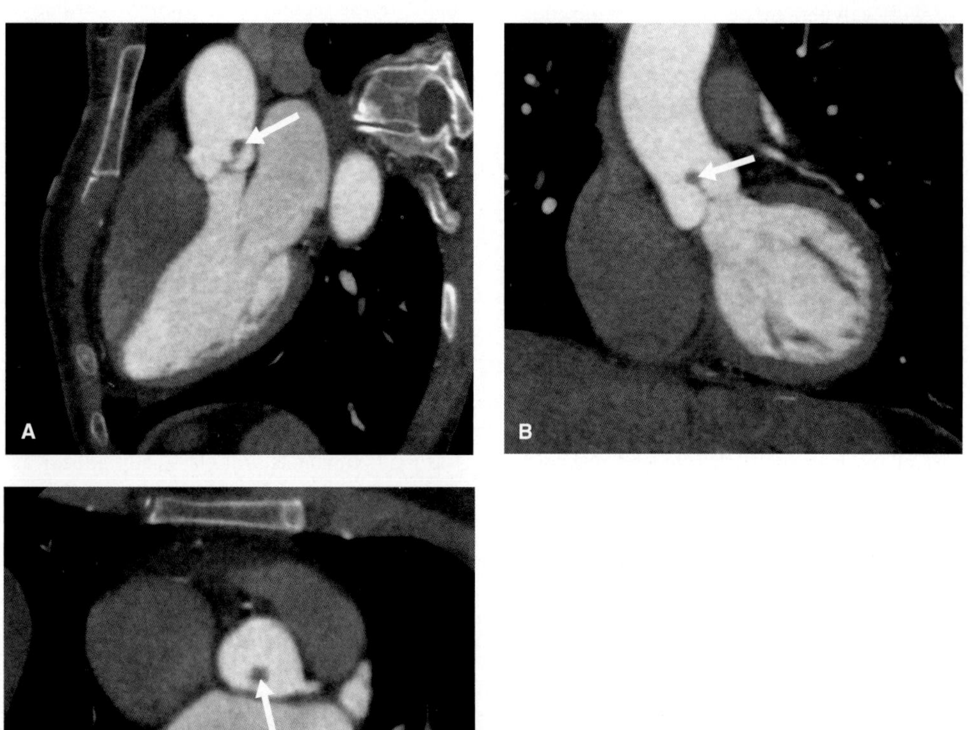

FIGURE 26.6. **Valvular Papillary Fibroelastoma.** Multiplanar CT images in the three-chamber (**A**), LVOT (**B**), and aortic valve (**C**) views demonstrate a pedunculated mass (*arrow*) arising from the commissure between the left and right aortic valve leaflets. Pathology was consistent with a papillary fibroelastoma.

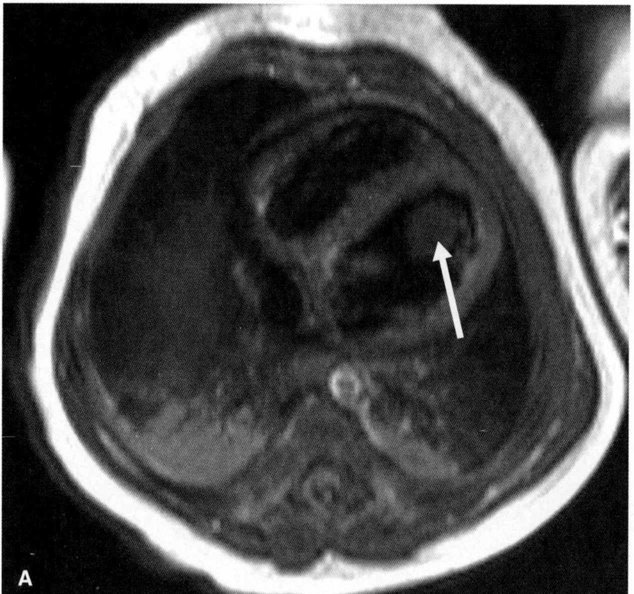

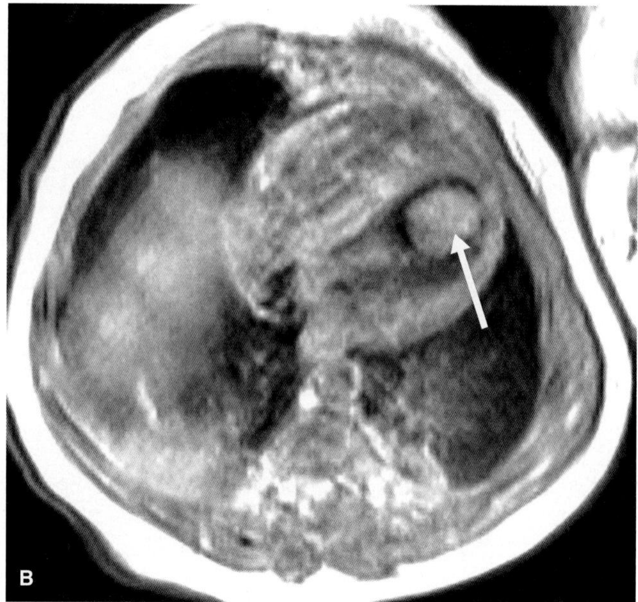

FIGURE 26.7. **Cardiac Rhabdomyoma.** Axial CMR T1W imaging (**A**) demonstrates a hypointense intracavitary mass (*arrow*) which demonstrates mild hyperintense signal (*arrow*) on the T2W sequences (**B**) in a newborn with known tuberous sclerosis.

fibrous tissue. The presence of delayed gadolinium enhancement is a key feature in distinguishing a fibroelastoma from a vegetation, which is the main differential diagnosis for a valvular mass. In general, while inflamed tissue surrounding a vegetation may enhance on delayed imaging, enhancement within a vegetation is usually mild or absent. In addition, as vegetations represent infected thrombi, there is often destruction of the associated valve with valvular or perivalvular regurgitation, which is absent with fibroelastoma. Lastly, patients with infective endocarditis are often febrile, septic, and the lungs may demonstrate subpleural cavitary nodules due to septic emboli. These findings are absent in fibroelastomas.

Rhabdomyoma. Cardiac rhabdomyomas are benign congenital tumors which are the most common primary tumors in infants and children. They account for 50% to 75% of pediatric cardiac tumors, equally affecting males and females. Rhabdomyomas are hamartomas of altered enlarged cardiac myocytes which arise as small intramural nodules in the ventricular myocardium, measuring between 1 and 3 cm on average. While these tumors may be solitary and occur in isolation, 50% of cases are seen in patients with tuberous sclerosis and are usually multiple. The presence of multiple cardiac rhabdomyomas has a 95% association with tuberous sclerosis, and almost all patients with this genetic disorder will have cardiac rhabdomyomas in infancy. The majority of cases are asymptomatic and many of the tumors will regress with age, usually before the age of 4. Occasionally, rhabdomyomas can cause in utero arrhythmias, or protrude into the ventricular chamber causing obstruction, heart failure, and intrauterine demise.

Most rhabdomyomas are detected on pre- or postnatal echocardiograms, seen as solid hyperechoic masses either within the ventricular myocardium or intracavitary and attached to the myocardium. Given that their attenuation is similar to normal myocardium, rhabdomyomas may be difficult to detect on CT but can appear as smooth, intramyocardial nodules. On MRI, they are isointense to normal myocardium on T1W images, mildly hyperintense on T2W images, and will demonstrate minimal to no hyperenhancement after administration of contrast (Fig. 26.7). The differential for a cardiac mass in a neonate or infant includes rhabdomyoma, fibroma, teratoma, and rhabdomyosarcoma. Rhabdomyomas can be differentiated by their multiplicity, homogeneous soft tissue signal, hyperintense signal on T2W sequences (as opposed to cardiac fibromas), and minimal to no enhancement.

Fibroma. Cardiac fibromas are benign fibrous hamartomas which are the second most common cardiac tumors in infants and children. About one-third of cases are found in infants before the age of 1, while 15% of cardiac fibromas are found in adolescents and adults. They are nonencapsulated fibrous tumors composed of neoplastic fibroblasts and abundant collagen. Fibromas are typically solitary, intramural tumors measuring between 2 and 7 cm. It may be a discrete mass or focal wall thickening, mimicking focal hypertrophy. The left ventricular wall or interventricular septum are common locations, with rarer cases found in the right atrium or ventricle. These tumors have an association with Gorlin syndrome (also termed basal cell nevus syndrome), an autosomal dominant syndrome of basal cell carcinoma, odontogenic keratocysts, and other neoplasms. One-half to two-thirds of the cardiac fibromas are symptomatic with a range of symptoms including chest pain, heart failure, arrhythmias, syncope, or sudden cardiac death.

On CT, fibromas will classically appear as a well-defined, homogeneous low attenuation mass located within the left ventricular myocardium. Coarse calcifications are present in 15% to 20% of cases and are often located centrally. After contrast, fibromas demonstrate mild enhancement on CT. On MRI, fibromas are usually isointense to the adjacent myocardium on T1W MR sequences, and hypointense on the T2W images due to their fibrous components. While fibromas are avascular and will show no enhancement during perfusion imaging, they will classically show intense enhancement with late gadolinium imaging due to their large amount of collagen creating an expanded extracellular space for contrast to pool into (Fig. 26.8). The differential diagnosis for an intramural myocardial lesion includes metastatic disease, rhabdomyoma (particularly in children), hemangioma, rhabdomyosarcoma, and focal hypertrophic cardiomyopathy which can mimic a mass. However, the combination of hypointense signal on the T2W

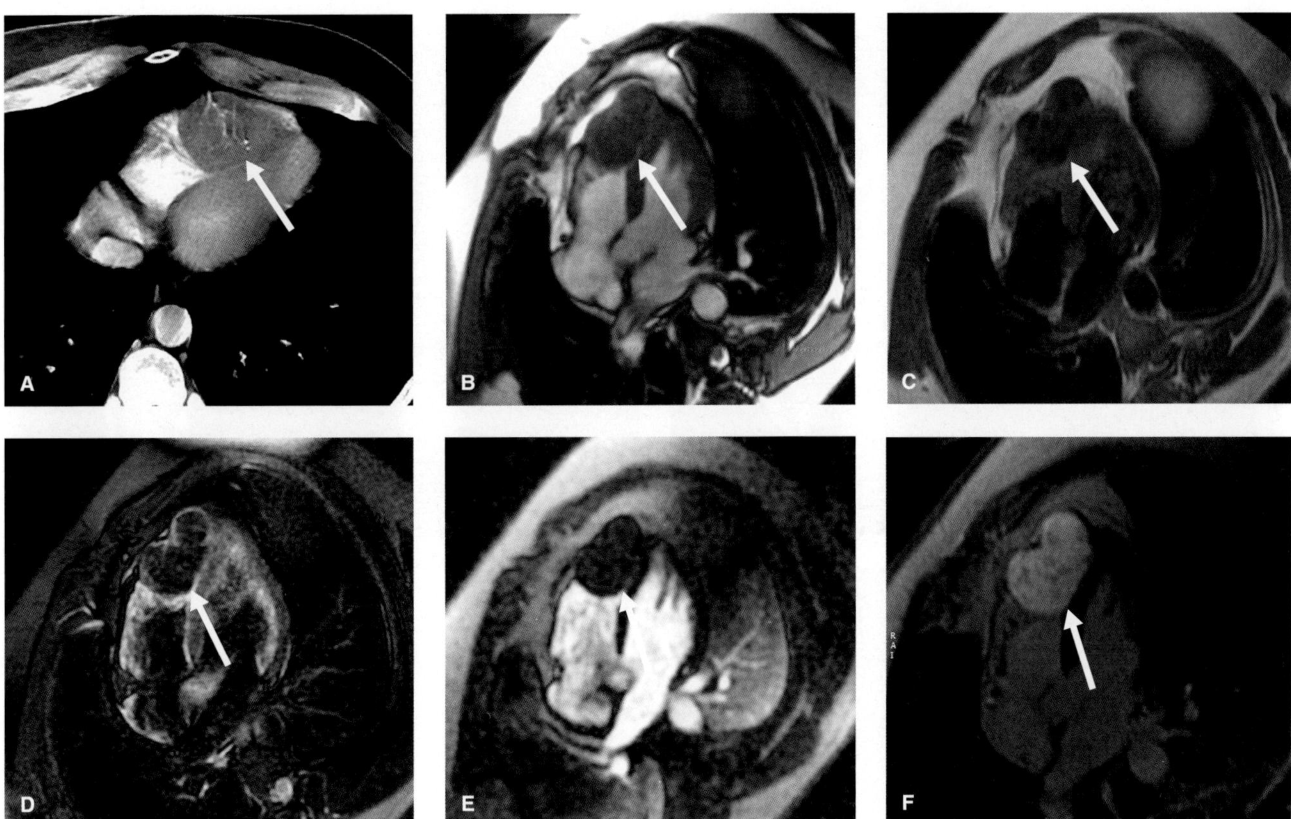

FIGURE 26.8. **Cardiac Fibroma.** Axial nongated postcontrast CT (**A**) demonstrates a large mass within the right ventricular apex (*arrow*) with several calcified foci. It demonstrates hypointense signal on T1W images (**B**), hypointense signal on T2W images (**C**) without and with fat saturation (**D**), lack of contrast enhancement during perfusion (**E**) indicating avascularity, and hyperintense homogeneous enhancement on LGE imaging (**F**). The diagnosis of cardiac fibroma was confirmed after surgical removal.

sequences and intense LGE is very uncommon in any other entity aside for a fibroma.

Hemangioma. Cardiac hemangiomas are rare tumors that account for 5% to 10% of all primary benign cardiac tumors. They are composed of vascular endothelial cells and can be arteriovenous, capillary, or cavernous in type. Fifty percent of cases are made up of the arteriovenous type, which is made up of dysplastic arterial and venous structures. Hemangiomas can be located in any part of the heart with 75% of cases being intramural. Intracavitary tumors are usually smaller and can be connected to the endocardium by a short stalk. Cardiac hemangiomas are commonly asymptomatic, although patients may present with dyspnea on exertion. There is an association with Kasabach–Merritt syndrome, which is characterized by multiple hemangiomas causing recurrent thrombocytopenia and consumptive coagulopathy.

On cardiac CT, hemangiomas are heterogeneous in density and will exhibit heterogeneous enhancement after contrast administration. Some cases may demonstrate internal calcifications. On MRI, they are heterogeneous and predominately hyperintense on both the T1W and T2W images. On both perfusion and delayed-phase imaging, the arteriovenous and capillary subtypes will demonstrate intense enhancement due to their vascular components, except in the areas of calcification (Fig. 26.9).

Paraganglioma. Cardiac paragangliomas are rare cardiac tumors derived from clustered neuroendocrine cells and are closely related to pheochromocytomas. They typically occur in adults during the third or fourth decades. Like any paraganglioma found within the body, they may produce catecholamines which can cause hypertension or other symptoms attributable to excess catecholamine production. Five percent to 10% of cardiac paragangliomas can be metastatic, with osseous involvement being the most common. Cardiac paragangliomas can be present in patients with the Carney triad, which is made up of extra-adrenal pheochromocytoma, gastrointestinal stromal tumor (GIST), and pulmonary chondroma (this is not to be confused with the Carney complex mentioned regarding cardiac myxomas). They most commonly occur in the left atrial wall, in the location of the normal cardiac paraganglioma cells, typically involving either the left atrial roof or posterior wall. Other reported locations include the interatrial septum or right atrium.

On both CT and MRI, cardiac paragangliomas will commonly show intense enhancement following contrast administration, both on the early- and delayed-phase imaging. Central necrosis and hemorrhage along with scattered internal calcification may be present as well. Paragangliomas are typically hypo- to isointense on T1W imaging and extremely hyperintense on T2W sequences (Fig. 26.10). Focal cardiac abnormal uptake on iodine-123 or iodine-131 metaiodobenzylguanidine (MIBG) scintigraphy is highly specific for cardiac paragangliomas as it is selectively taken up by extra-adrenal paragangliomas.

Other Benign Cardiac Neoplasms. Additional rare benign neoplasms include teratomas, lymphangiomas, and hamartomas. Cardiac teratomas are germ cell tumors made up of several different types of tissue and are like any other teratoma in the body. They are commonly found in infants/children as complex multilocular, heterogeneous cystic masses growing within the pericardial sac, typically on the right side. They are

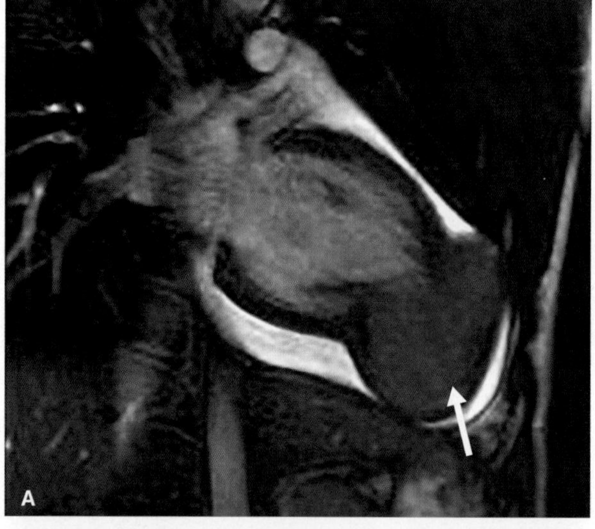

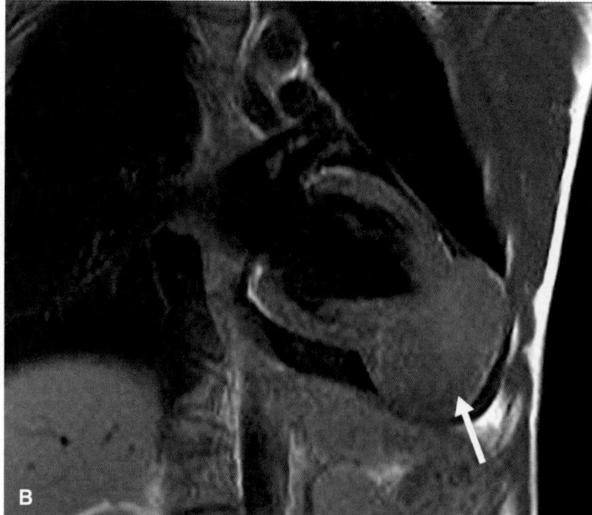

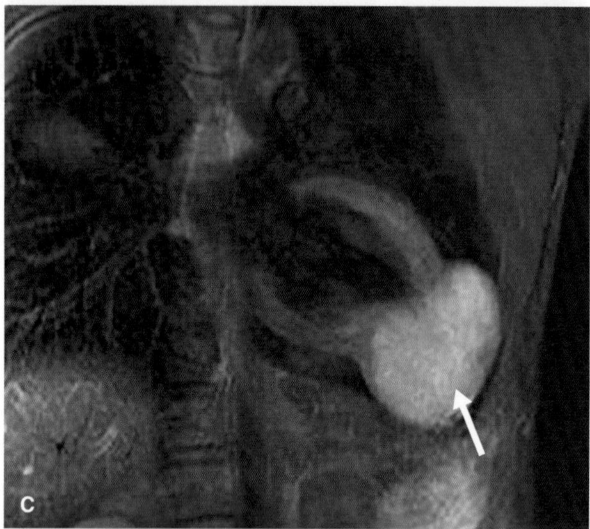

FIGURE 26.9. **Cardiac Hemangioma.** Multiple cardiac MR images in the two-chamber view demonstrate an exophytic large mass (*arrow*) arising from the left ventricular apex which demonstrated iso- to mildly hyperintense signal on the SSFP (**A**) and T1W images (**B**), and intense enhancement on the postcontrast imaging (**C**). Findings were consistent with a hemangioma after surgical removal.

usually large in size and associated with a pericardial effusion. Teratomas will demonstrate calcification and fat and commonly exhibit an attachment to the aorta via a pedicle.

Cardiac lymphangiomas are benign abnormal collections of lymphatic vessels which are rare benign neoplasms, most commonly found in children. They are typically multiloculated cystic lesions within the pericardial space and may be associated with a chylous pericardial effusion. On CT, they appear as well-circumscribed lesions with varying degrees of attenuation values. On MRI, there may be areas of high signal intensity on the T1W images due to proteinaceous material within them. Lymphangiomas will also demonstrate hyperintense signal on T2W images due to their cystic spaces.

Cardiac hamartomas are extremely rare and are composed of hypertrophied disorganized myocytes with interstitial fibrosis. They most commonly occur within the left ventricular myocardium and will demonstrate enhancement on both CT and MRI. On MRI, hamartomas will demonstrate similar signal characteristics to the normal myocardium but will demonstrate avid enhancement on the early and delayed-phase imaging postcontrast administration (Fig. 26.11). Distinguishing hamartomas from the focal form of hypertrophic cardiomyopathy on imaging may be extremely difficult. These two entities will share some histologic features but can be distinguished by the lack of increased vascularity and more diffuse myocardial involvement seen with hypertrophic cardiomyopathy.

MALIGNANT CARDIAC TUMORS

Metastatic Disease

Metastatic disease involving the heart is the most common cardiac mass found in the adult population. It is approximately 20 to 40 times more common than all primary cardiac tumors and is associated with a poor prognosis. Approximately 10% of patients with primary malignancy have cardiac metastatic involvement, although this is often only visible on histopathology. Metastatic disease can involve the heart via a number of pathways including: hematogenous or lymphatic seeding from a tumor at a different site of the body, direct tumor invasion from an adjacent primary within the mediastinum or lungs, or transvenous intracavitary contiguous extension from the inferior vena cava (IVC), superior vena cava (SVC), or pulmonary veins. Lung cancer is the most common metastatic lesion to the heart accounting for 30% to 40% of cases followed by hematologic malignancies, breast cancer, and esophageal cancer. Direct

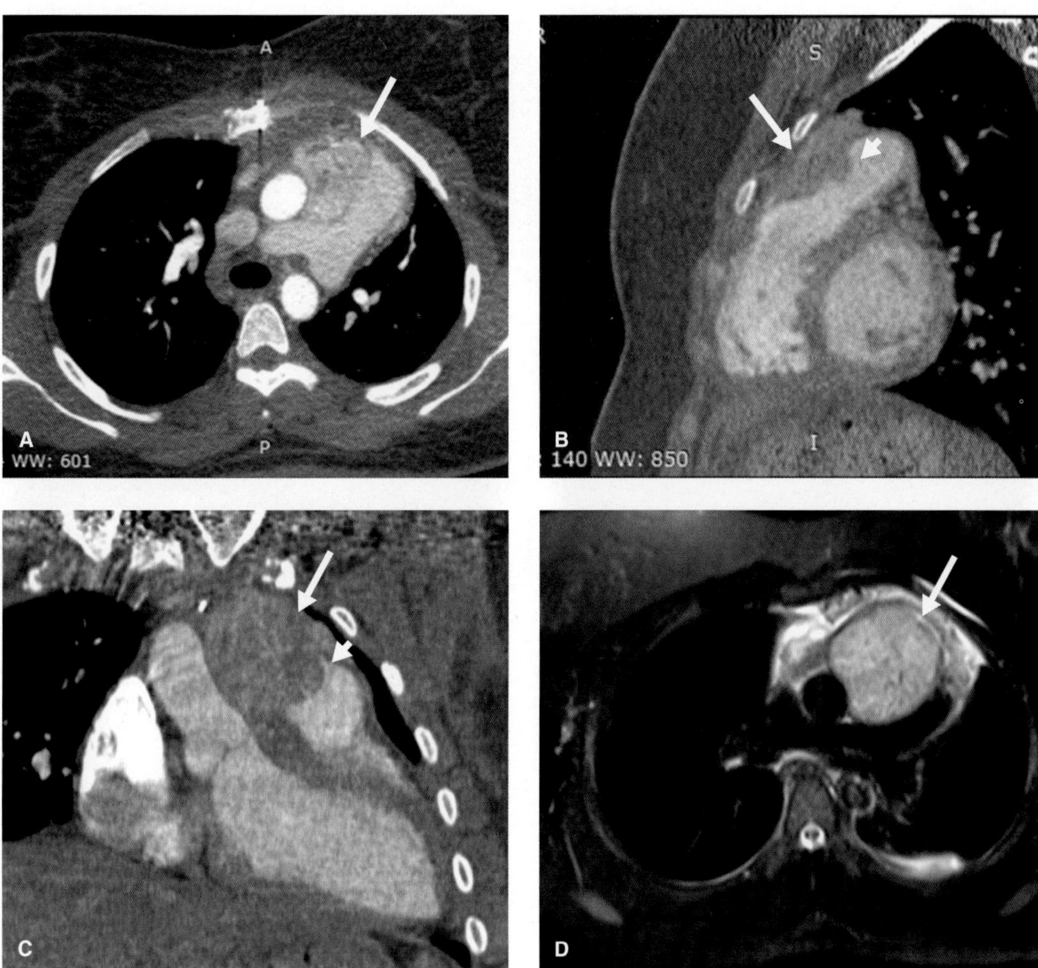

FIGURE 26.10. **Paraganglioma.** Axial postcontrast ECG-gated CT (**A**) demonstrates an avidly enhancing mediastinal mass situated between the ascending aorta and main pulmonary artery (*arrow*). Sagittal (**B**) and coronal (**C**) oblique CT-reconstructed images demonstrate invasion of the mass (*arrow*) into the right ventricular outflow tract (*arrowhead*). The lesion (*arrow*) demonstrates hyperintense signal on T2W fat-saturation MR axial images (**D**). Findings were consistent with a paraganglioma after surgical resection.

invasion or lymphatic extension to the pericardium and epicardium is the most common route of spread and is often accompanied by a malignant pericardial effusion. Melanomas, renal cell carcinomas, and sarcomas are the most common tumors to spread to the heart hematogenously and usually result in intramural involvement. Abdominal and pelvic malignancies can invade the IVC and grow superiorly into the right atrium.

While most cases of cardiac metastasis are clinically silent, symptoms usually manifest due to altered cardiac function, flow obstruction, or involvement of the electrical conduction system related to the location that is involved. Range of symptoms include syncope, left- or right-sided heart failure, arrhythmias, heart block, or significant pericardial effusions that can lead to cardiac tamponade. Obstructive symptoms are commonly seen in transvenous extension of disease, with involvement of the SVC/IVC and right atrium.

When imaging the heart for metastatic disease, the most common findings will include pericardial involvement and/or intracavitary masses. Many cases of cardiac metastatic disease will have an associated malignant pericardial effusion. Echocardiography is the best initial evaluation for pericardial involvement, specifically to evaluate for an effusion, its effect on cardiac function, and assessment for tamponade physiology. While echocardiography may demonstrate pericardial thickening or nodularity, it does not evaluate the entire pericardium and may not detect pericardial deposits. Please refer to Chapter 29 on pericardial disease.

Both CT and MRI will provide a broader anatomic evaluation of the heart in assessing for metastatic disease, as they are able to evaluate the entire heart as well as its surrounding structures. Metastatic involvement of the myocardium will present on CT/MRI as a discrete mass or masses. CT is the best modality to evaluate for lung cancer invasion into the pulmonary veins and is excellent at assessing for invasion of abdominal tumors into the IVC and right atrium. While a routine contrast enhancement CT may detect cardiac metastases, ECG gating should be considered if there is concern for cardiac involvement. The presence of heterogeneous enhancement on CT will help distinguish tumor thrombus from bland thrombus which is a frequent clinical dilemma.

As with primary cardiac masses, CMR will offer superior tissue characterization of cardiac metastatic disease and will provide excellent functional and hemodynamic assessment. In general, metastatic lesions will demonstrate low signal on T1W images and high signal on T2W images. Melanoma or hemorrhagic lesions may demonstrate high signal on the T1W

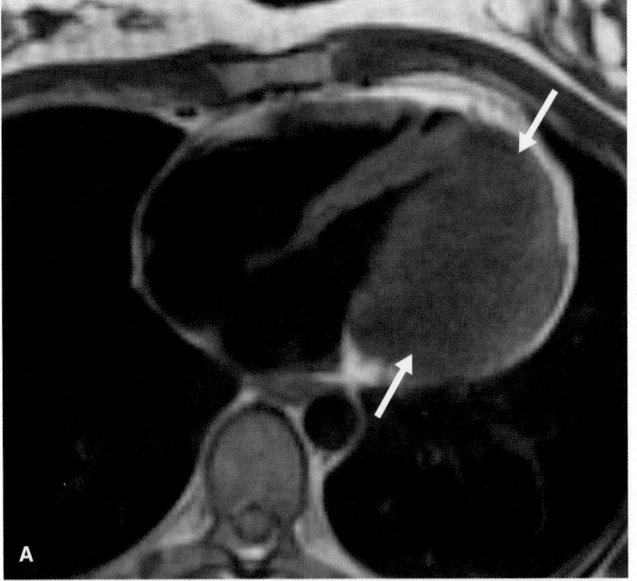

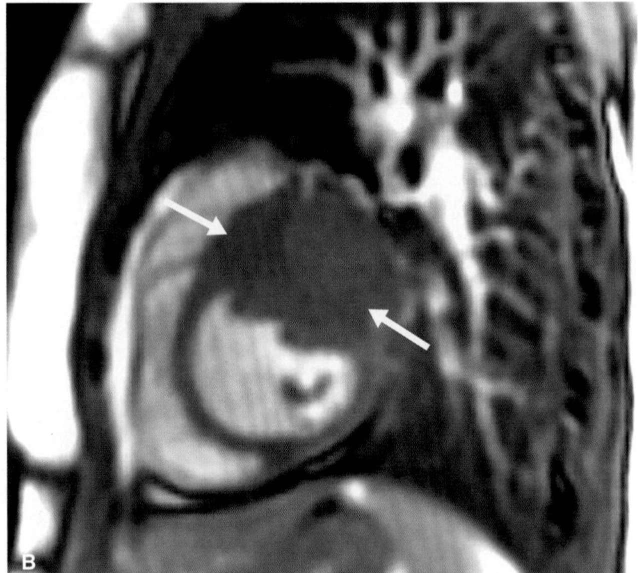

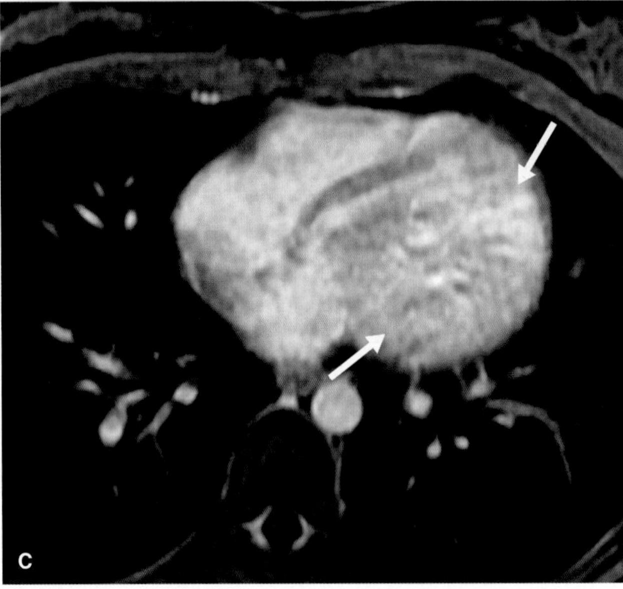

FIGURE 26.11. **Cardiac Hamartoma.** Axial T1W (**A**) and short-axis SSFP (**B**) MR images demonstrate a large intramural isointense lesion (between the *arrows*) in the anterior and anterolateral segments of the left ventricle, which demonstrates diffuse enhancement on the postcontrast axial image (**C**) in a patient with a known recurrent hamartoma.

images as well. These lesions will generally demonstrate heterogeneous enhancement, which may not be clearly detected on postcontrast CT images (Fig. 26.12). Due to its ability to detect subtle metastatic foci, MRI is superior to CT for accurate extent of disease evaluation. In addition, delayed enhancement imaging with a long inversion time (TI = 600) allows for differentiation of tumor from thrombus, as the prolonged inversion time selectively nulls avascular tissue. Therefore, thrombus will be hypointense on the long inversion time images, while enhancing tumor will demonstrate hyperintense signal.

Sarcoma. Primary cardiac sarcomas are neoplastic lesions which arise from the mesenchymal cells within the cardiac muscle. They are the most common primary malignant tumor of the heart, accounting for one-third of cases and include several subtypes (Table 26.4). Angiosarcoma is the most common differentiated cardiac sarcoma, compromising nearly 40% of cases. Undifferentiated sarcomas are the second most common sarcoma involving the heart, making up 25% of cases. Rhabdomyosarcoma is the most common primary cardiac malignancy in childhood and accounts for 4% to 7% of all cardiac sarcomas. Other types of primary cardiac sarcomas include leiomyosarcoma, osteosarcoma, and fibrosarcoma.

Cardiac sarcomas primarily affect adults between the third and fifth decades and are extremely rare in children. They carry a poor prognosis with mean survival ranging from 3 months to 4 years. At presentation, many cases exhibit evidence of metastatic disease, frequently involving the lungs. Dyspnea is the common symptom, with other presentations including chest pain, arrhythmias, tamponade, and/or death.

Typical locations and imaging appearances of cardiac sarcomas vary based on the histologic subtype. They may be intramural with infiltration and thickening of the myocardium and/or intracavitary, and will commonly demonstrate components of hemorrhage and necrosis. Pericardial involvement with a hemorrhagic pericardial effusion and nodular thickening

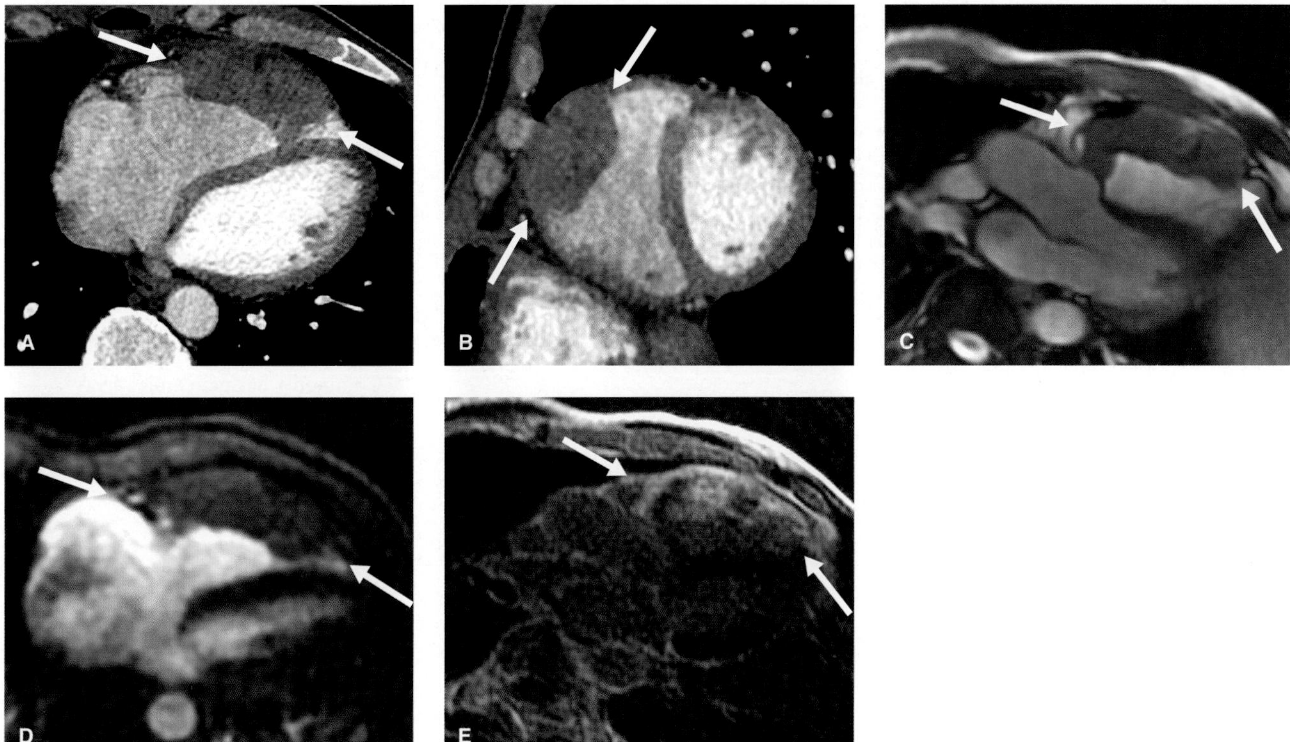

FIGURE 26.12. **Cardiac Metastasis.** Postcontrast nongated CT in the axial (**A**) and short-axis (**B**) planes, in a patient with known metastatic lung cancer, demonstrates an infiltrative mass (between the *arrows*) in the free wall of the right ventricle. It demonstrates hypo- to isointense signal in relation to the myocardium on the SSFP sequence (**C**) and heterogeneous enhancement on the perfusion (**D**) and late gadolinium engagement (**E**) images.

of the pericardium is another common feature. Invasion into the mediastinum or valvular destruction may be present.

Cardiac angiosarcoma is the only cardiac sarcoma that predominately arises in the right atrium in the region of the right atrioventricular groove. While there may be a discrete right atrial mass, tumor can often be seen extending anteriorly along the wall of the right atrium and right ventricle. Encasement of the right coronary artery is a common finding. On both CT and MRI, they appear as heterogeneous soft tissue masses with areas of necrosis. A characteristic finding is intense enhancement within the soft tissue component of the tumor and rapid enhancement on first-pass perfusion (Fig. 26.13). The main differential for an infiltrative mass in the region of the right atrioventricular groove is metastatic disease or lymphoma.

While angiosarcomas predominate in the right atrium and rhabdomyosarcoma have no chamber predilection, the other histologic subtypes of cardiac sarcomas usually occur in the left atrium. They present as large masses that infiltrate along the wall of the left atrium. As they crawl and invade along the left atrial wall, they often invade and obstruct the pulmonary veins and/or the mitral annulus. Although myxomas—which are the most common primary cardiac tumor—also occur in the left atrium, they are not infiltrative and do not invade into the pulmonary veins. In addition, the vast majority of left atrial myxomas occur along the interatrial septum in the region of the fossa ovalis, a finding that is not seen with left atrial sarcomas. Like other aggressive tumors, left atrial sarcomas appear as heterogeneous soft tissue masses, often with areas of necrosis. Enhancement is usually present but is often not as pronounced as with right atrial angiosarcomas. In general, it is often difficult to differentiate between the histologic subtypes of cardiac sarcoma on imaging, although prominent osteoid matrix in a large left atrial mass should raise the suspicion for a cardiac osteosarcoma.

Lymphoma. Primary cardiac lymphoma is defined as lymphoma exclusively involving the heart and/or pericardium. It is usually of the non-Hodgkin B-cell type, most commonly occurring in immunocompromised patients, often related to infection with the Epstein–Barr virus. Others more susceptible to primary cardiac lymphoma include posttransplant patients or those with HIV/AIDS. It is quite rare, making up 1.3% of primary cardiac tumors and only 0.5% of extranodal lymphomas at autopsy. Secondary cardiac lymphoma due to systemic lymphoma involving the heart is more common, with one study showing approximately 30% of patients with lymphoma having cardiac involvement at autopsy. Primary cardiac lymphoma commonly involves the right side of the heart, particularity the right atrium and has a predilection for the right atrioventricular groove similar to angiosarcoma. Most common clinical presentation includes arrhythmias including atrioventricular block, heart failure, dyspnea, or a pericardial effusion.

On cross-sectional imaging, primary cardiac lymphoma will manifest as an ill-defined, infiltrative epicardial or myocardial mass, or multiple masses usually along the right side of the heart, with an associated pericardial effusion. The right atrium is most commonly involved, followed by the

TABLE 26.4

SUMMARY OF CARDIAC SARCOMA SUBTYPES AND THEIR IMAGING FEATURES

■ CARDIAC SARCOMA SUBTYPES	■ MALIGNANT CARDIAC TUMORS (%)	■ COMMON TUMOR LOCATION	■ IMAGING AND OTHER FEATURES
Angiosarcoma	37–40	Right atrium	■ Two morphologic types: 1. Well-defined mass protruding into the right atrium 2. Diffusely infiltrating mass along the right side of the heart ■ Has a propensity for hemorrhage and necrosis ■ Commonly has pericardial invasion and a hemorrhagic pericardial effusion
Undifferentiated sarcoma	24–33	Left atrium	■ May be a discrete mass or an irregular infiltrative lesion ■ Commonly hemorrhagic
Leiomyosarcoma	8–10	Posterior wall of the left atrium or IVC	■ Sessile lobulated hypodense mass on CT ■ May be multifocal ■ May arise or invade into the pulmonary veins
Osteosarcoma	3–9	Left atrium	■ Typically large tumors which are centered in the left atrium, unlike osteosarcoma metastases to the heart ■ Commonly contain large foci of calcification
Rhabdomyosarcoma	4–7	No chamber predilection	■ Most common primary malignant tumor in children, but can affect all ages ■ May be solitary or multifocal intramural masses
Liposarcoma	<1%	Left or right atrium	■ May show foci of fat density on CT ■ On MRI, fat-saturation sequences are not particularly helpful unlike cardiac lipoma or lipomatous hypertrophy of the interatrial septum

right ventricle and then the left-sided chambers. A unique feature of lymphoma is its tendency to extend along the epicardium, encasing adjacent structures including the coronary arteries, aortic root, or pulmonary vessels. In addition, it may diffusely involve the myocardium, masquerading as myocardial hypertrophy or it can demonstrate nodular or lobulated intracavitary components. The lesion will usually be hypo- to isodense to the surrounding myocardium on CT with heterogeneous enhancement, postcontrast administration. CMR best depicts the extent of the myocardial and pericardial involvement due to its better tissue characterization. On MRI, it will demonstrate isointense signal to the myocardium on T1W images, hyperintense signal on T2W images, and variable enhancement postcontrast (Fig. 26.14). Differential diagnosis for an ill-defined infiltrative lesion along the epicardial surface includes metastatic disease or sarcomas. Lymphoma may be distinguished from these entities by their homogeneous signal throughout the lesion. This homogeneous signal in cardiac lymphoma is due to the absence of necrosis or hemorrhage, which causes the variable signal demonstrated in metastatic lesions and sarcoma. When solely within the myocardium, it can be mistaken for hypertrophic cardiomyopathy and when intracavitary, it may be confused for a thrombus or myxoma.

Tumorlike Lesions

Thrombus. Intracardiac thrombus is the most common intracardiac lesion and can involve any cardiac chamber. In the right atrium and right ventricle, thrombi are commonly attached to intravascular catheters/lines or are the sequelae of deep venous thrombosis with subsequent embolization. In atrial fibrillation, thrombus will usually form in the left atrial appendage due to poor blood flow, while in the setting of ventricular dysfunction it will form in akinetic or aneurysmal portions of the ventricle, often in the left ventricular apex.

Differentiating thrombus from other cardiac lesions is a frequent diagnostic question. While postcontrast cardiac CT imaging is an excellent tool for detecting and localizing intracavitary thrombi, it is limited in differentiating thrombus from tumor. Thrombus is hypodense on CT and does not enhance. Given this, thrombus is often best delineated during the portal venous phase of imaging where it appears hypodense to

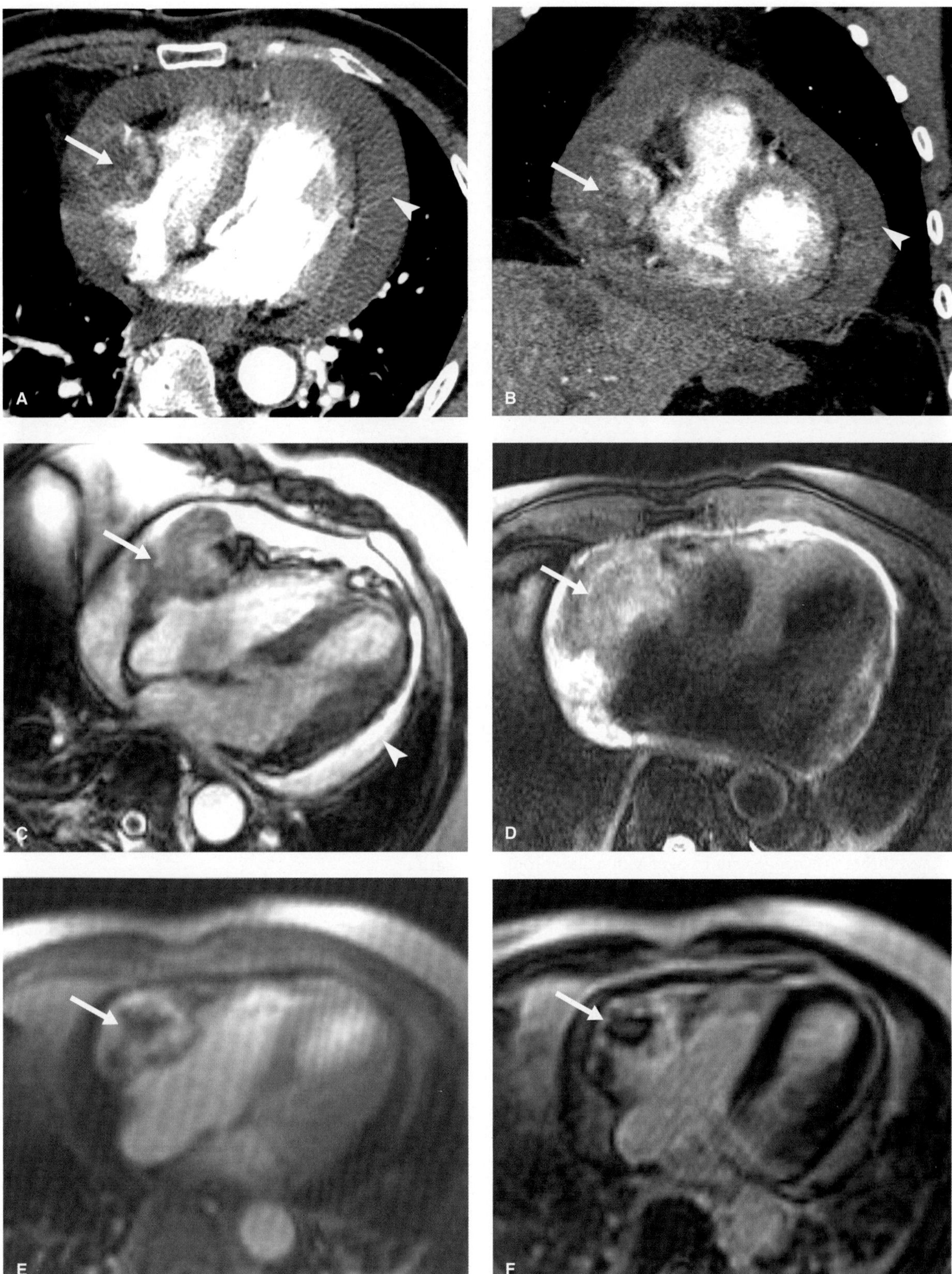

FIGURE 26.13. Cardiac Angiosarcoma. Axial (**A**) and coronal (**B**) postcontrast CT images demonstrate a heterogeneous enhancing mass in the right atrioventricular groove (*arrow*) with a pericardial effusion (*arrowhead*). CMR shows a heterogeneous hyperintense lesion on the SSFP (**C**) and T2W images (**D**) with avid enhancement on both the perfusion (**E**) and LGE (**F**) sequences. The central nonenhancing area within the mass represents necrosis.

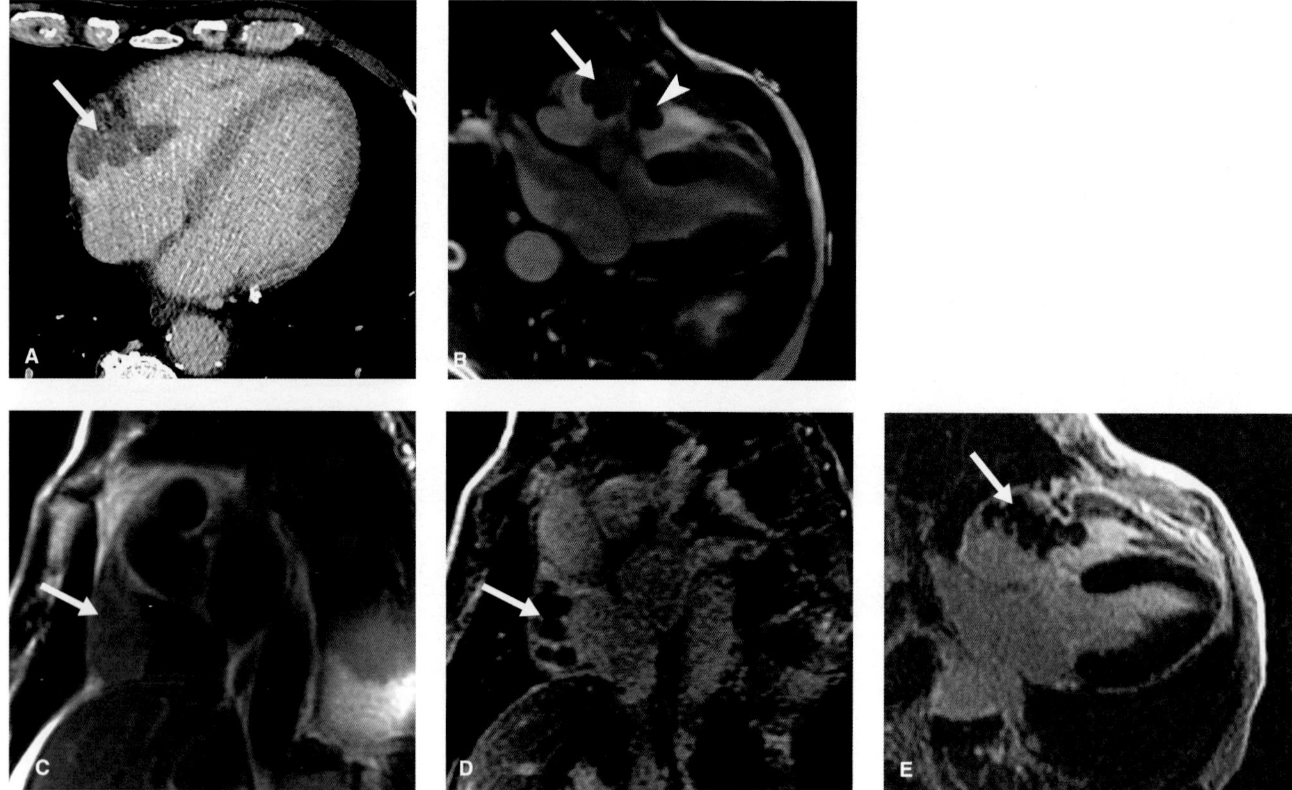

FIGURE 26.14. **Cardiac Lymphoma.** Postcontrast axial CT (**A**) and MR SSFP imaging in the four-chamber view (**B**) demonstrate a multilobulated mass (*arrow*) in the right atrium extending along the lateral aspect into the right ventricle (*arrowhead*). It demonstrates isointense signal on the T2W images and minimal to no enhancement on LGE images. Biopsy results were consistent with B-cell lymphoma.

the normally enhancing myocardium. CMR is the imaging of choice in distinguishing thrombus from tumor. Imaging characteristics of thrombus change with its age, with acute thrombus demonstrating hyperintense signal on T1W and T2W sequences and chronic thrombus demonstrating hypointense signal on both sequences. Subacute thrombus will be hyperintense on T1W images and hypointense on T2W images. Thrombus will characteristically show no contrast uptake on first-pass perfusion or T1W postcontrast images. Importantly, thrombus will demonstrate dark signal on delayed enhancement sequences with a long inversion time of 600 ms (Fig. 26.15) and at times more intermediate signal using a standard inversion time of 300 ms, a finding that is absent in most tumors. One recent study has shown that performing a dedicated TI scout ("Look–Locker") sequence through the mass can distinguish the two entities, as thrombus demonstrated a typical pattern of hyper/isointensity with a short inversion time and hypointensity with long inversion time in 94% of cases, with only 2% of tumors demonstrating the same signal pattern. Of note, chronic organised thrombus may demonstrate peripheral enhancement on late gadolinum enhancement imaging due to fibrous material forming around it.

Lipomatous Hypertrophy of the Interatrial Septum. Lipomatous hypertrophy is a benign process characterized by proliferation of adipose cells within the interatrial septum. It occurs in up to 8% of the population and can be associated with an increased body mass index and large amounts of epicardial fat. The amount of fat usually will increase with age. The fat within the atrial septum is made up of mature unencapsulated adipose tissue resembling brown fat and can be metabolically active on FDG-PET. Most cases are incidentally discovered and are asymptomatic, with very rare cases causing supraventricular arrhythmias and sudden death.

Cross-sectional imaging will demonstrate a dumbbell-shaped fatty mass in the interatrial septum, commonly with asymmetric enlargement of its posterolateral component. The dumbbell shape is created by the sparing of the fossa ovalis. On MRI, the lesion will follow normal fat characteristics with both hyperintense signal on T1W and T2W sequences and loss of signal with fat-suppression techniques (Fig. 26.16). Normal septal thickness measures less than 1 cm, with cases of lipomatous hypertrophy measuring greater than 2 cm. Cases measuring up to 7 cm have been described as well. Cardiac lipoma is the main differential diagnosis and will have a true fibrous capsule. Sparing of the fossa ovalis is a key feature in lipomatous hypertrophy that helps in distinguishing it from other abnormalities.

Vegetations. Valvular vegetations are adherent lesions made up of platelets, fibrin, and inflammatory cells that seed the valvular leaflets, usually in an area of endocardial injury. In infective endocarditis, these lesions are also composed of microorganisms, either bacterial or fungal. Noninfective endocarditis is rare and can be due to nonbacterial thrombotic endocarditis (NBTE) seen in the setting of malignancy or Libman–Sacks endocarditis which occurs in patients with systemic lupus erythematosus (SLE) due to deposition of immune complexes. The vegetations are irregular or rounded in shape, measuring a few millimeters to greater than 1 cm. Differential diagnosis includes papillary fibroelastoma, with infective endocarditis usually leading to leaflet destruction as opposed to papillary fibroelastoma which is a benign entity.

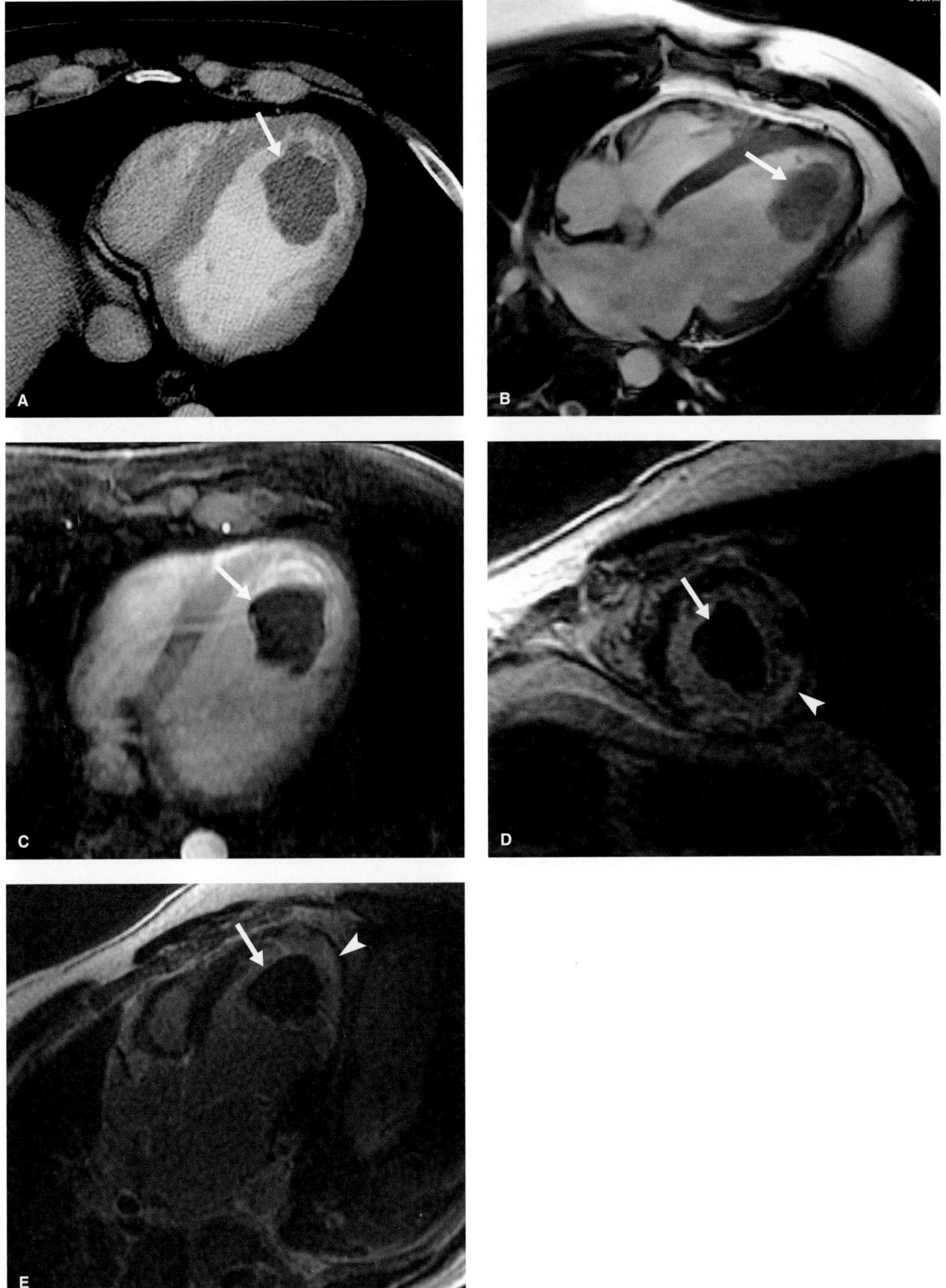

FIGURE 26.15. **Interventricular Thrombus.** Postcontrast nongated axial CT (**A**) and SSFP MR (**B**) images demonstrate a hypodense/hypointense lesion in the apical cavity of the left ventricle (*arrow*). It demonstrates no enhancement on the early post contrast images (**C**) and the LGE images in the short-axis (**D**) and three-chamber (**E**) views, although the left ventricular apical myocardium does demonstrate late gadolinium enhancement (*arrowhead*). Findings are consistent with an apical myocardial infarct and interventricular thrombus.

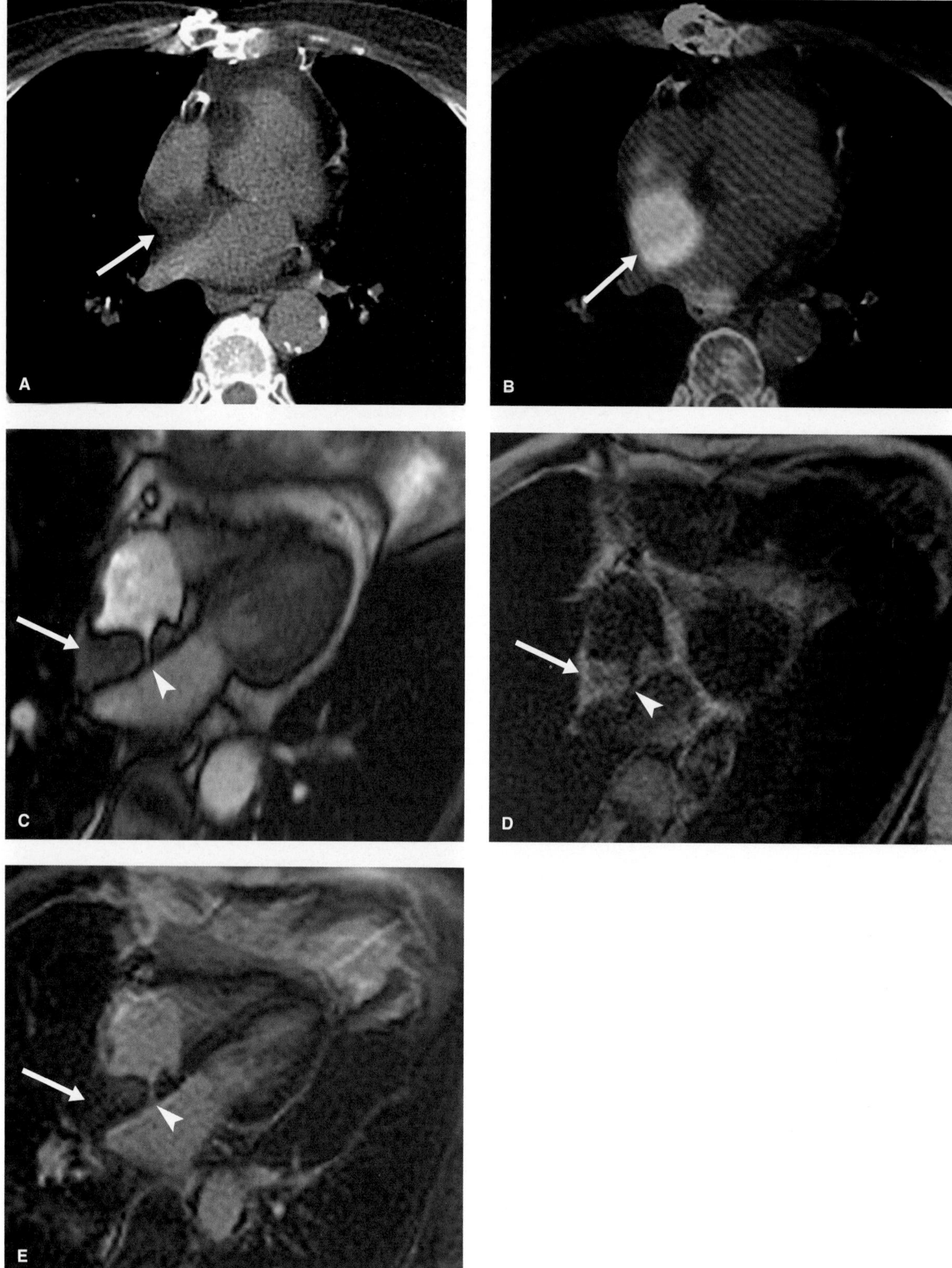

FIGURE 26.16. Lipomatous Hypertrophy of the Interatrial Septum. Axial CT (**A**) demonstrates a low-density lesion in the interatrial septum (*arrow*) which is FDG avid on a PET-CT due to the presence of brown fat (**B**). Follow-up CMR shows a lesion within the interatrial septum on the SSFP (**C**) image, which spares the fossa ovalis (*arrowhead*) and demonstrates hyperintense signal on T1W (**D**) and no LGE (**E**).

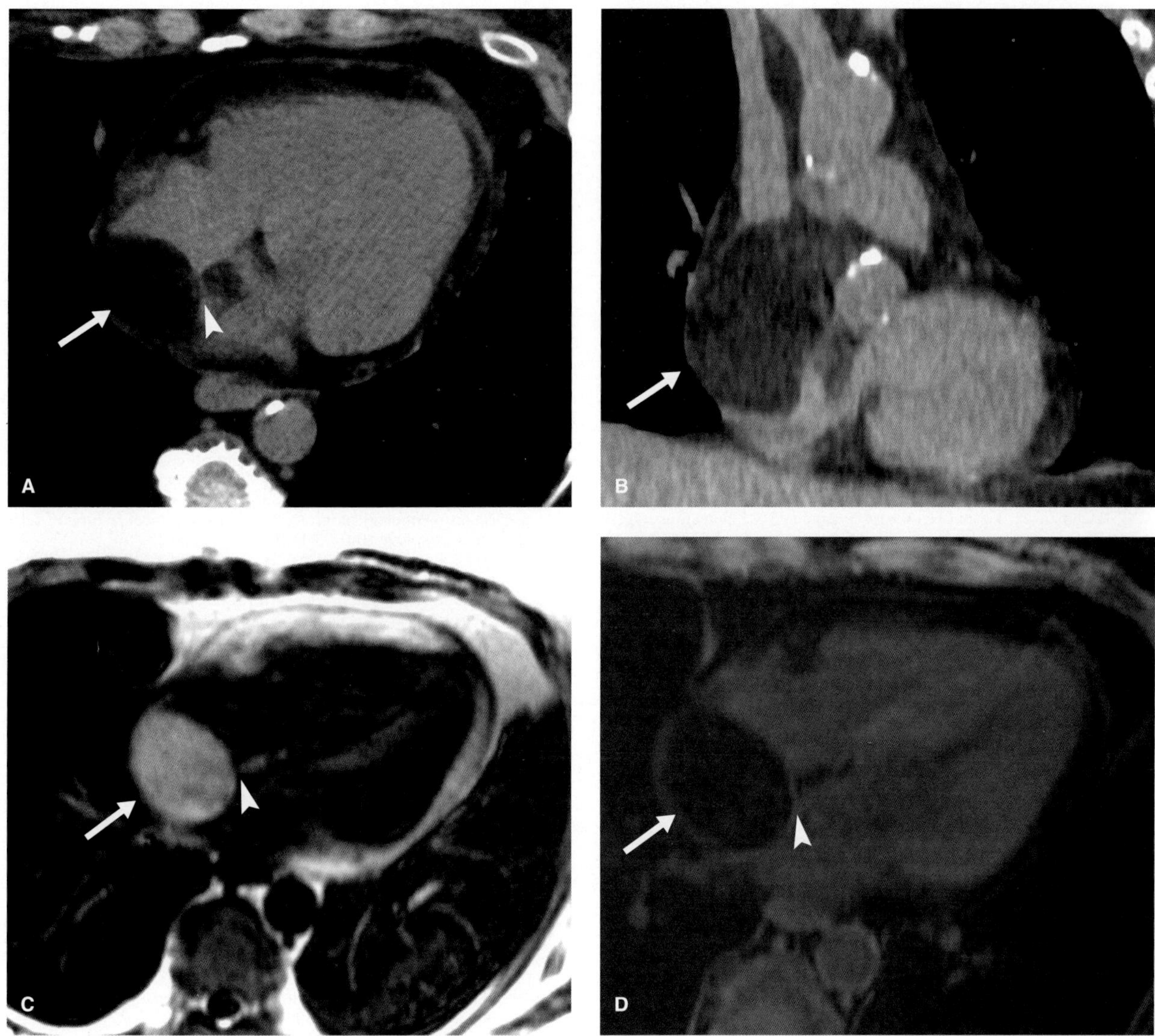

FIGURE 26.17. **Large Lipomatous Hypertrophy of the Interatrial Septum.** Noncontrast CT in the four-chamber (**A**) and coronal oblique (**B**) views demonstrates a large lesion in the interatrial septum measuring fat density (*arrow*), which spares the fossa ovalis (*arrowhead*), in a patient with a known supraventricular tachycardia. The lesion demonstrates homogenous hyperintense signal on the T1W images without fat suppression (**C**) and complete dropout of signal on the T1W images with fat suppression (**D**), consistent with fat.

Normal Anatomic Structures. Several normal anatomic structures may appear as pseudomasses on echocardiography but which are commonly distinguished from true pathology on cross-sectional imaging. The two most common structures are the crista terminalis and the eustachian valve. The crista terminalis is a normal anatomic structure which demarcates the area of embryologic fusion of the primitive right atrium and the sinus venosus. It is a vertically oriented smooth muscle ridge within the right atrium, which extends from the SVC to the IVC. The eustachian valve is a normal ridge of tissue at the junction of the right atrium and IVC, which in utero directed blood flow from the IVC into the fossa ovalis.

Suggested Readings

American College of Radiology. *ACR Manual on Contrast Media. Version 10.3.* Reston, VA: ACR; 2017.

Araoz PA, Mulvagh SL, Tazelaar HD, Julsrud PR, Breen JF. CT and MR imaging of benign primary cardiac neoplasms with echocardiographic correlation. *Radiographics* 2000;20(5):1303–1319.

Asopa S, Patel A, Khan OA, Sharma R, Ohri SK. Non-bacterial thrombotic endocarditis. *Eur J Cardiothorac Surg* 2007;32:696–701.

Bader RS, Chitayat D, Kelly E, et al. Fetal rhabdomyoma: prenatal diagnosis, clinical outcome, and incidence of associated tuberous sclerosis complex. *J Pediatr* 2003;143:620–624.

Becker AE. Primary heart tumors in the pediatric age group: a review of salient pathologic features relevant for clinicians. *Pediatr Cardiol* 2000;21(4): 317–323.

Beghetti M, Gow RM, Haney I, Mawson J, Williams WG, Freedom RM. Pediatric primary benign cardiac tumors: a 15-year review. *Am Heart J* 1997; 134:1107–1114.

Beghetti M, Prieditis M, Rabeyka IM, Mawson J. Images in cardiovascular medicine. Intrapericardial teratoma. *Circulation* 1998;97:1523–1524.

Bergey PD, Axel L. Focal hypertrophic cardiomyopathy simulating a mass: MR tagging for correct diagnosis. *AJR Am J Roentgenol* 2000;174(1): 242–244.

Beroukhim RS, Prakash A, Buechel ER, et al. Characterization of cardiac tumors in children by cardiovascular magnetic resonance imaging: a multicenter experience. *J Am Coll Cardiol* 2011;58:1044–1054.

Buckley O, Madan R, Kwong R, Rybicki FJ, Hunsaker A. Cardiac masses, part 1: imaging strategies and technical considerations. *AJR Am J Roentgenol* 2011a;197(5):W837–W841.

Buckley O, Madan R, Kwong R, Rybicki FJ, Hunsaker A. Cardiac masses, part 2: key imaging features for diagnosis and surgical planning. *AJR Am J Roentgenol* 2011b;197:W842–W851.

Burke AP, Rosado-de-Christenson M, Templeton PA, Virmani R. Cardiac fibroma: clinicopathologic correlates and surgical treatment. *J Thorac Cardiovasc Surg* 1994;108:862–870.

Burke AP, Virmani R. Cardiac myxoma: a clinicopathologic study. *Am J Clin Pathol* 1993;100:671–680.

Burke A, Virmani R. Tumors of the heart and great vessels. In: *Atlas of Tumor Pathology, 3rd Series, Fascicle 16*. Washington, DC: Armed Forces Institute of Pathology; 1996.

Bussani R, De-Giorgio F, Abbate A, Silvestri F. Cardiac metastases. *J Clin Pathol* 2007;60:27–34.

Carson W, Chiu SS. Image in cardiovascular medicine. Eustachian valve mimicking intracardiac mass. *Circulation* 1998;97:2188.

Chiles C, Woodard PK, Gutierrez FR, Link KM. Metastatic involvement of the heart and pericardium: CT and MR imaging. *Radiographics* 2001;21:439–449.

Chun EJ, Choi SI, Jin KN, et al. Hypertrophic cardiomyopathy: assessment with MR imaging and multidetector CT. *Radiographics* 2010;30(5):1309–1328.

Cina SJ, Smialek JE, Burke AP, Virmani R, Hutchins GM. Primary cardiac tumors causing sudden death: a review of the literature. *Am J Forensic Med Pathol* 1996;17:271–281.

Dell'Amore A, Lanzanova G, Silenzi A, Lamarra M. Hamartoma of mature cardiac myocytes: case report and review of the literature. *Heart Lung Circ* 2011;20:336–340.

Edwards FH, Hale D, Cohen A, Thompson L, Pezzella AT, Virmani R. Primary cardiac valve tumors. *Ann Thorac Surg* 1991;52(5):1127–1131.

Fan CM, Fischman AJ, Kwek BH, Abbara S, Aquino SL. Lipomatous hypertrophy of the interatrial septum: increased uptake on FDG PET. *AJR Am J Roentgenol* 2005;184:339–342.

Ghadimi Mahani M, Lu JC, Rigsby CK, Krishnamurthy R, Dorfman AL, Agarwal PP. MRI of pediatric cardiac masses. *AJR Am J Roentgenol* 2014;202:971–981.

Goldberg AD, Blankstein R, Padera RF. Tumors metastatic to the heart. *Circulation* 2013;128:1790–1794.

Gowda RM, Khan IA, Nair CK, Mehta NJ, Vasavada BC, Sacchi TJ. Cardiac papillary fibroelastoma: a comprehensive analysis of 725 cases. *Am Heart J* 2003;146:404–410.

Goyal P, Weinsaft JW. Cardiovascular magnetic resonance imaging for assessment of cardiac thrombus. *Methodist Debakey Cardiovasc J* 2013;9(3):132–136.

Grebenc ML, Rosado de Christenson ML, Burke AP, Green CE, Galvin JR. Primary cardiac and pericardial neoplasms: radiologic-pathologic correlation. *Radiographics* 2000;20:1073–1103.

Grebenc ML, Rosado de Christenson ML, Green CE, Burke AP, Galvin JR. Cardiac myxoma: imaging features in 83 patients. *Radiographics* 2002;22:673–689.

Grizzard JD, Ang GB. Magnetic resonance imaging of pericardial disease and cardiac masses. *Magn Reson Imaging Clin N Am* 2007;15:579–607.

Hamidi M, Moody JS, Weigel TL, Kozak KR. Primary cardiac sarcoma. *Ann Thorac Surg* 2010;90(1):176–181.

Hamilton BH, Francis IR, Gross BH, et al. Intrapericardial paragangliomas (pheochromocytomas): imaging features. *AJR Am J Roentgenol* 1997;168:109–113.

Hananouchi GI, Goff WB 2nd. Cardiac lipoma: six-year follow-up with MRI characteristics, and a review of the literature. *Magn Reson Imaging* 1990;8(6):825–828.

Heyer CM, Kagel T, Lemburg SP, Bauer TT, Nicolas V. Lipomatous hypertrophy of the interatrial septum: a prospective study of incidence, imaging findings, and clinical symptoms. *Chest* 2003;124:2068–2073.

Hoey ET, Mankad K, Puppala S, Gopalan D, Sivananthan MU. MRI and CT appearances of cardiac tumours in adults. *Clin Radiol* 2009;64:1214–1230.

Jeudy J, Kirsch J, Tavora F, et al. From the radiologic pathology archives: cardiac lymphoma: radiologic-pathologic correlation. *Radiographics* 2012;32(5):1369–1380.

Kaji T, Takamatsu H, Noguchi H, et al. Cardiac lymphangioma: case report and review of the literature. *J Pediatr Surg* 2002;37:E32.

Kassop D, Donovan MS, Cheezum MK, et al. Cardiac masses on cardiac CT: a review. *Curr Cardiovasc Imaging Rep* 2014;7:9281.

Lembcke A, Meyer R, Kivelitz D, et al. Images in cardiovascular medicine: papillary fibroelastoma of the aortic valve: appearance in 64-slice spiral computed tomography, magnetic resonance imaging, and echocardiography. *Circulation* 2007;115:e3–e6.

Luna A, Ribes R, Caro P, Vida J, Erasmus JJ. Evaluation of cardiac tumors with magnetic resonance imaging. *Eur Radiol* 2005;15:1446–1455.

McAllister HA Jr. Primary tumors and cysts of the heart and pericardium. *Curr Probl Cardiol* 1979;4(2):1–51.

McCarthy PM, Piehler JM, Schaff HV, et al. The significance of multiple, recurrent, and complex cardiac myxomas. *J Thorac Cardiovasc Surg* 1986;91(3):389–396.

Menon SC, Miller DV, Cabalka AK, Hagler DJ. Hamartomas of mature cardiac myocytes. *Eur J Echocardiogr* 2008;9:835–839.

Mirowitz SA, Gutierrez FR. Fibromuscular elements of the right atrium: pseudomass at MR imaging. *Radiology* 1992;182:231–233

Motwani M, Kidambi A, Herzog BA, Uddin A, Greenwood JP, Plein S. MR imaging of cardiac tumors and masses: a review of methods and clinical applications. *Radiology* 2013;268:26–43.

O'Donnell DH, Abbara S, Chaithiraphan V, et al. Cardiac tumors: optimal cardiac MR sequences and spectrum of imaging appearances. *AJR Am J Roentgenol* 2009;193:377–387.

Parmley LF, Salley RK, Williams JP, Head GB 3rd. The clinical spectrum of cardiac fibroma with diagnostic and surgical considerations: noninvasive imaging enhances management. *Ann Thorac Surg* 1988;45:455–465.

Paydarfar D, Krieger D, Dib N, et al. In vivo magnetic resonance imaging and surgical histopathology of intracardiac masses: distinct features of subacute thrombi. *Cardiology* 2001;95(1):40–47.

Pazos-López P, Pozo E, Siqueira ME, et al. Value of CMR for the differential diagnosis of cardiac masses. *JACC Cardiovasc Imaging* 2014;7:896–905.

Prakash P, Kalra MK, Stone JR, Shepard JA, Digumarthy SR. Imaging findings of pericardial metastasis on chest computed tomography. *J Comput Assist Tomogr* 2010;34:554–558.

Rajiah P, Kanne JP, Kalahasti V, Schoenhagen P. Computed tomography of cardiac and pericardiac masses. *J Cardiovasc Comput Tomogr* 2011;5:16–29.

Reynen K. Cardiac myxomas. *N Engl J Med* 1995;333:1610–1617.

Salanitri JC, Pereles FS. Cardiac lipoma and lipomatous hypertrophy of the interatrial septum: cardiac magnetic resonance imaging findings. *J Comput Assist Tomogr* 2004;28:852–856.

Scheffel H, Baumueller S, Stolzmann P, et al. Atrial myxomas and thrombi: comparison of imaging features on CT. *AJR Am J Roentgenol* 2009;192:639–645.

Seguin JR, Coulon P, Huret C, Grolleau-Roux R, Chaptal PA. Intrapericardial teratoma in infancy: a rare disease. *J Cardiovasc Surg* 1986;27:509–511.

Semionov A, Sayegh K. Multimodality imaging of a cardiac paraganglioma. *Radiol Case Rep* 2016;11:277–281.

Shanmugam G. Primary cardiac sarcoma. *Eur J Cardiothorac Surg* 2006;29:925–932.

Sparrow PJ, Kurian JB, Jones TR, Sivananthan MU. MR imaging of cardiac tumors. *Radiographics* 2005;25(5):1255–1276.

Sun JP, Asher CR, Yang XS, et al. Clinical and echocardiographic characteristics of papillary fibroelastomas: a retrospective and prospective study in 162 patients. *Circulation* 2001;103(22):2687–2693.

Sütsch G, Jenni R, von Segesser L, Schneider J. Heart tumors: incidence, distribution, diagnosis. Exemplified by 20,305 echocardiographies. *Schweiz Med Wochenschr* 1991;121(17):621–629.

Syed IS, Feng D, Harris SR, et al. MR imaging of cardiac masses. *Magn Reson Imaging Clin N Am* 2008;16:137–164.

Tada H, Asazuma K, Ohya E, et al. Images in cardiovascular medicine. Primary cardiac B-cell lymphoma. *Circulation* 1998;97(2):220–221.

Tomasian A, Iv M, Lai C, Jalili M, Krishnam MS. Cardiac hemangioma: features of cardiovascular magnetic resonance. *J Cardiovasc Magn Reson* 2007;9:873–876.

Werdan K, Dietz S, Löffler B, et al. Mechanisms of infective endocarditis: pathogen-host interaction and risk states. *Nat Rev Cardiol* 2014;11(1):35–50.

Zakaria RH, Barsoum NR, El-Basmy AA, El-Kaffas SH. Imaging of pericardial lymphangioma. *Ann Pediatr Cardiol* 2011;4:65–67.

CHAPTER 27 ■ VALVULAR DISEASE

ALBERT HSIAO AND KATE HANNEMAN

VALVE STRUCTURE AND FUNCTION

The four cardiac valves—aortic, mitral, pulmonary, and tricuspid—separate the chambers of the heart and their outflow vessels. The *inlet valves*, mitral and tricuspid, separate the ventricles from their upstream atria. The *outlet valves*, aortic and pulmonary, separate these great vessels from their upstream ventricles. It is worthwhile reflecting briefly on these definitions as they become useful, especially for patients with congenital heart disease (CHD). For example, the aorta may arise from the right ventricle in patients with transposition of the great vessels. To avoid confusion, it is helpful to remember that valves are defined by their downstream chamber or vessel. In the case of transposition, for example, blood passes from the right ventricle, through the *aortic valve* into the aorta.

The primary function of the cardiac valves is to provide minimal resistance to forward flow, while preventing backward regurgitant flow (Fig. 27.1). This is a particularly remarkable feat for the mitral valve, which provides minimal resistance to inflow, while withstanding pressures of over 100 mm Hg during left ventricular systolic contraction. The mitral valve apparatus is comprised of the valve leaflets (anterior and posterior), chordae tendineae, and papillary muscles (Fig. 27.2). The two leaflets are each divided into three scallops, separated by two clefts. The middle scallop is larger than the other two. Surrounding the leaflets is the mitral annulus, which is a continuous fibrous ring that surrounds the leaflets. The mitral annulus is in *fibrous continuity* with the aortic valve. During each systolic contraction, the valve leaflets rapidly coapt to prevent regurgitant flow, which is aided by the contraction of the papillary muscles which maintain tension throughout systole. The chordae tendineae attach the papillary muscles to the leaflets and to the commissural areas between the leaflets, maintaining tension and preventing prolapse of the leaflets into the atrium. Injury to either the anterolateral or posteromedial papillary muscle can cause failure of the mitral valve. The anterolateral papillary muscle is generally supplied by the left anterior descending coronary artery or the left circumflex coronary artery. The posteromedial papillary muscle is generally supplied by the right coronary artery.

The tricuspid valve, which typically separates the right ventricle from the right atrium, is so named because of its three leaflets. The anterior, posterior, and septal leaflets are attached by chordae tendineae to three papillary muscles—anterior, posterior, and septal. Papillary muscles of the right ventricle are more varied in their attachments. The anterior papillary muscle can attach to the anterior leaflet alone, or to both the anterior and septal leaflets. The posterior papillary muscle can attach to the posterior and septal leaflets. The septal papillary muscle can attach to the septal and anterior leaflet. Additional chordae may further support the papillary muscles, connect points on the right ventricular wall, or directly attach the septal leaflet to the right ventricular wall.

The aortic and pulmonary valves are normally each formed by three cusps. The cusps of the aortic valve are named according to the sinuses of Valsalva from which coronary arteries typically arise (Fig. 27.3). The left main coronary artery arises from the left sinus of Valsalva. The right coronary artery arises from the right sinus of Valsalva. The last cusp (typically posterior) is named the noncoronary cusp. The left and right cusps typically abut or "face" the pulmonary valve and are thus referred to as the "facing" sinuses of Valsalva.

The cusps of the pulmonary valve are named by their relationship to the aortic valve and are called the right, left, and

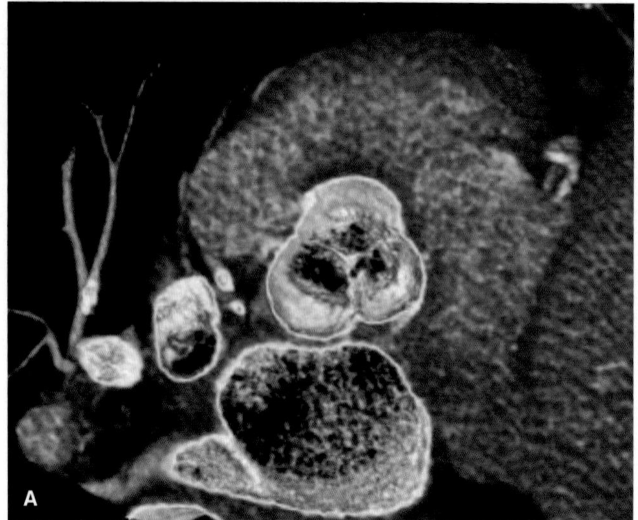

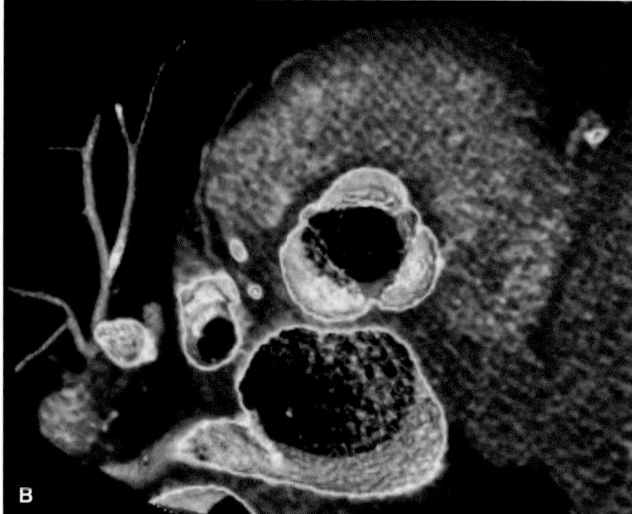

FIGURE 27.1. **3D Reconstruction of a Normal Trileaflet Aortic Valve During Diastole (A) and Systole (B) From Cardiac CT.** During diastole, the leaflets coapt normally to prevent regurgitation of blood into the left ventricle. During systole, the leaflets open widely to allow passage of blood into the aorta.

nonseptal (or anterior) cusps (Fig. 27.4). Similar to the aortic valve, the pulmonary valve opens during ventricular systole. The valve closes at the end of ventricular systole as the pressure in the right ventricle drops.

IMAGING EVALUATION OF VALVE DISEASE

Echocardiography

Echocardiography is the primary modality for evaluation of suspected valve disease, often as a follow-up to a heart murmur detected on physical examination. Due to its widespread accessibility and relatively low cost, echocardiography is the dominant modality for initial evaluation and grading severity of valve disease. Due to their location, the mitral and aortic valves are generally well visualized by transthoracic echocardiography (TTE). When further anatomic detail is required, transesophageal echocardiography (TEE) can be used. Because of their anterior location near the sternum, however, sonographic windows for evaluating the pulmonary and tricuspid valves are limited.

Radiography and CT

Although chest radiography and computed tomography (CT) are not primary modalities used for evaluation of valve disease, secondary signs of valve disease can be present on these examinations. It is important to recognize the typical locations of the valves on radiograph in order to appropriately identify surgical prosthesis, valvular calcification, and chamber

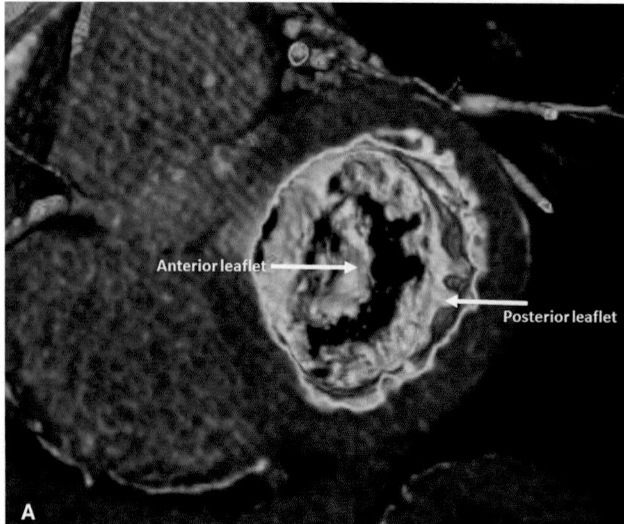

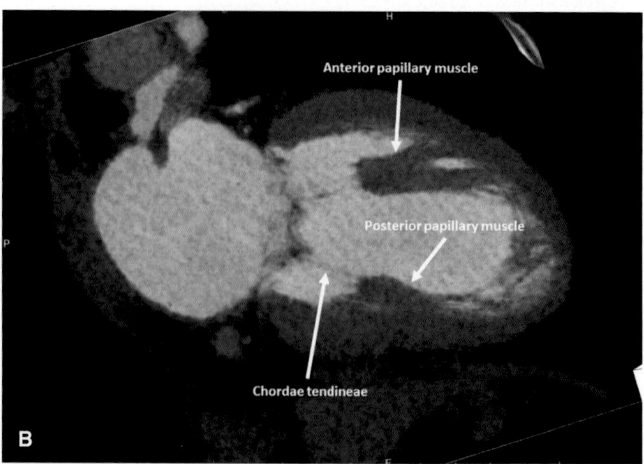

FIGURE 27.2. **3D Reconstruction in Short Axis (A) and Minimum Intensity Projection (MinIP) Image in Long Axis (B) From a Cardiac CT Illustrating the Anatomy of the Mitral Valve.** The anterior leaflet lies medially and the posterior leaflet lies laterally. Each valve is attached to the papillary muscles via thin chordae tendineae.

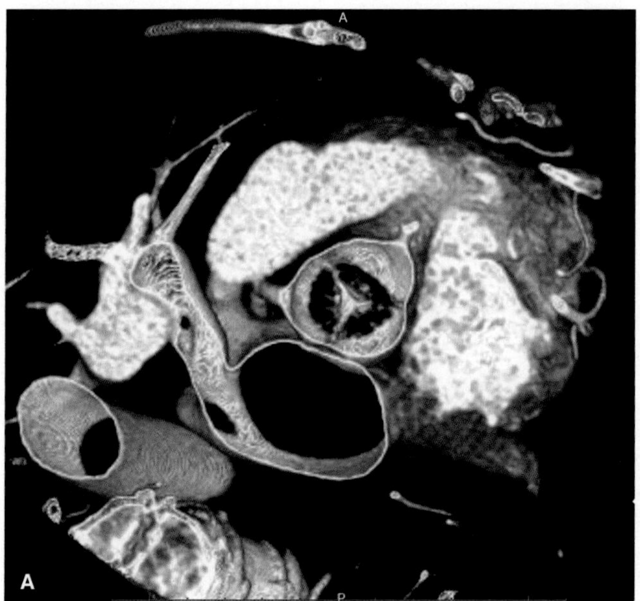

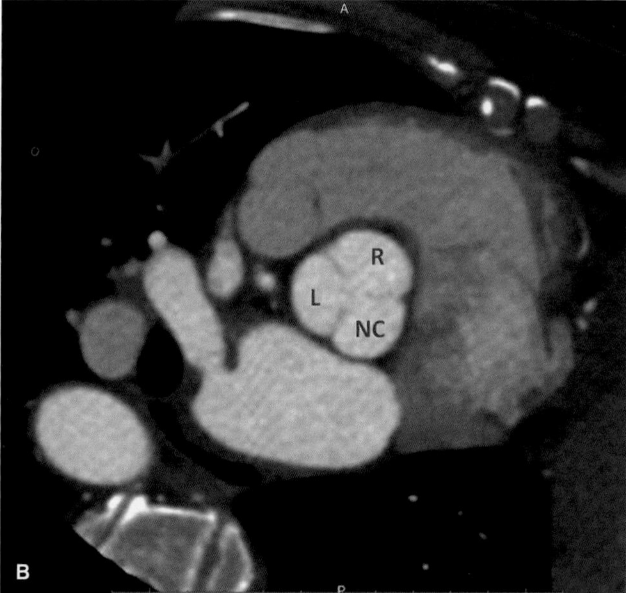

FIGURE 27.3. **3D Reconstruction (A) and Multiplanar Reformat (B) From Cardiac CT at the Sinuses of Valsalva, Viewed From Above.** The coronary arteries arise from the left and right cusps (labeled as *L* and *R*), while the noncoronary cusp abuts the interatrial septum (labeled *NC*).

enlargement (Figs. 27.5 to 27.8). In patients with mitral stenosis (MS), for example, the atrium may be enlarged due to the greater resistance of flow into the left ventricle. In patients with substantial mitral regurgitation, the left ventricle and atrium may both be enlarged due to greater stroke volumes needed to maintain cardiac output and the volume of regurgitant blood passing backward into the atrium.

Mitral annular calcifications (MACs) are a common radiologic finding on chest radiography and CT. It can be seen in up to 35% of elderly patients and can be seen as an "O"- or "C"-shaped dense structure at the expected location of the mitral annulus. On chest CT, the findings are readily localized to the annulus. It is believed to represent chronic degeneration of the fibrous ring of the mitral valve and may be seen in younger patients with renal disease or abnormal calcium metabolism. One rare variant of MAC is known as caseous MAC or caseous calcification of the mitral annulus (CCMA). Because it is infrequent, it can be misdiagnosed as abscess, infection, or tumor. It is often localized to the posterior atrioventricular groove and represents a caseous transformation of the annular ring. The mechanism of liquefaction and caseation is not well understood. Characteristic images from one such patient with caseous MAC are shown in Figure 27.9.

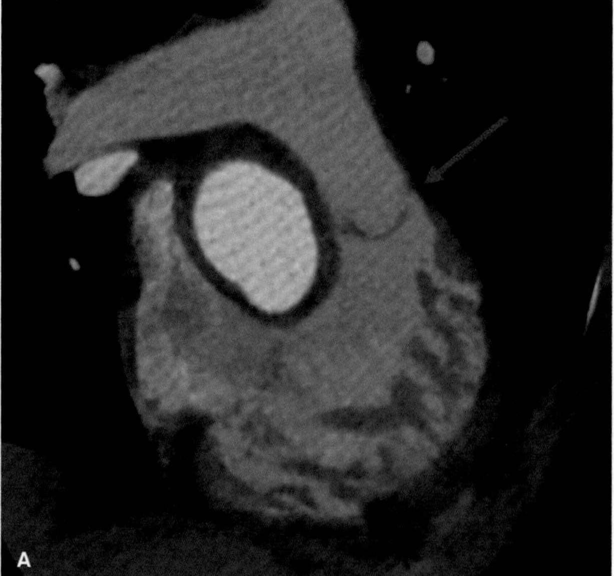

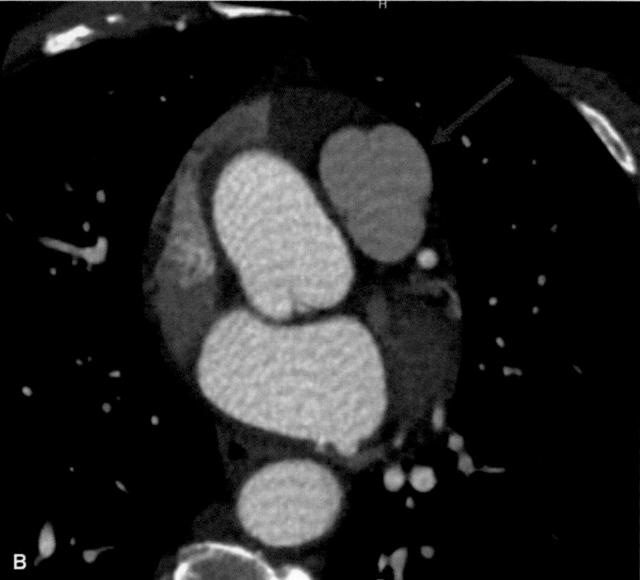

FIGURE 27.4. **Reconstructed 3D images of the pulmonary valve from cardiac CT.** MinIP reformat of the right ventricular outflow tract (**A**) shows the location of the pulmonary valve leaflets. Multiplanar reformat at the level of the pulmonary valve (**B**) shows the three cusps of the pulmonary valve. *Red arrows* highlight the location of the pulmonary valve.

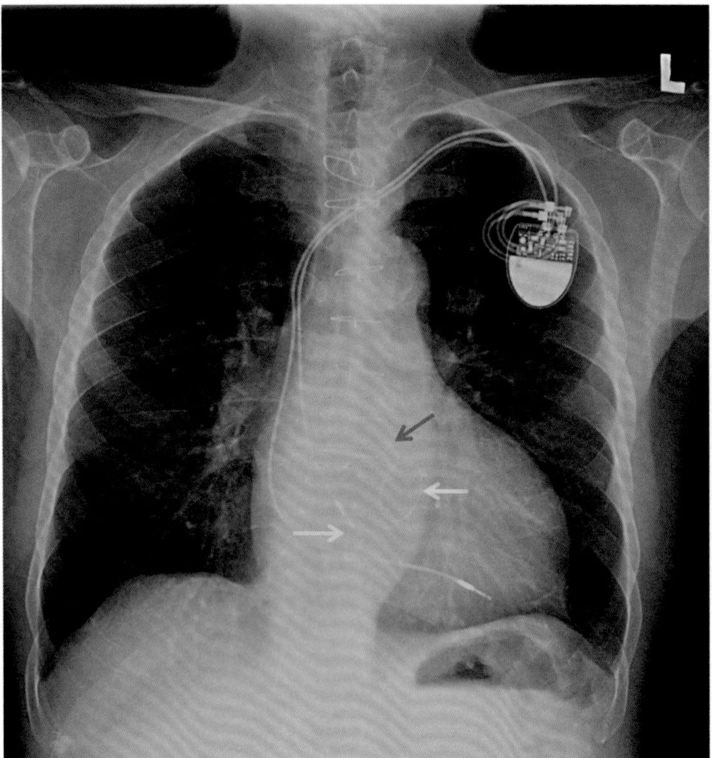

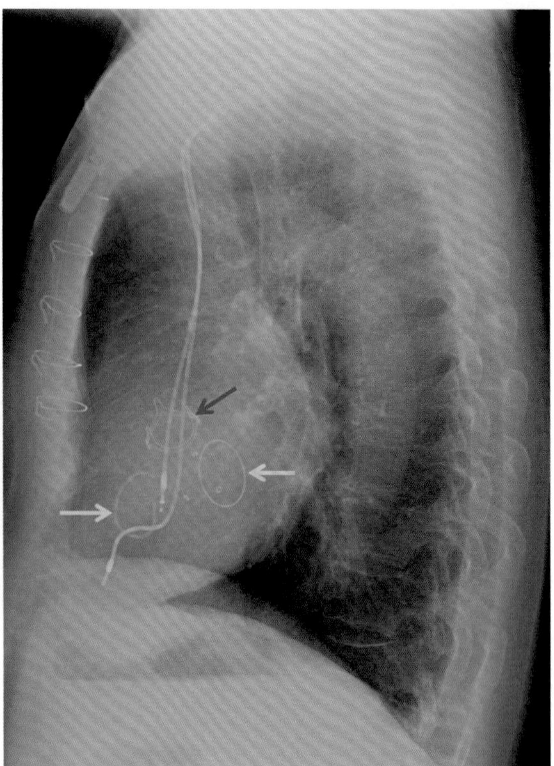

FIGURE 27.5. Frontal and lateral radiographs showing bioprosthetic aortic valve replacement (upper, *red arrow*), mitral valve replacement (right, *orange arrow*), and tricuspid annuloplasty ring (left, *green arrow*).

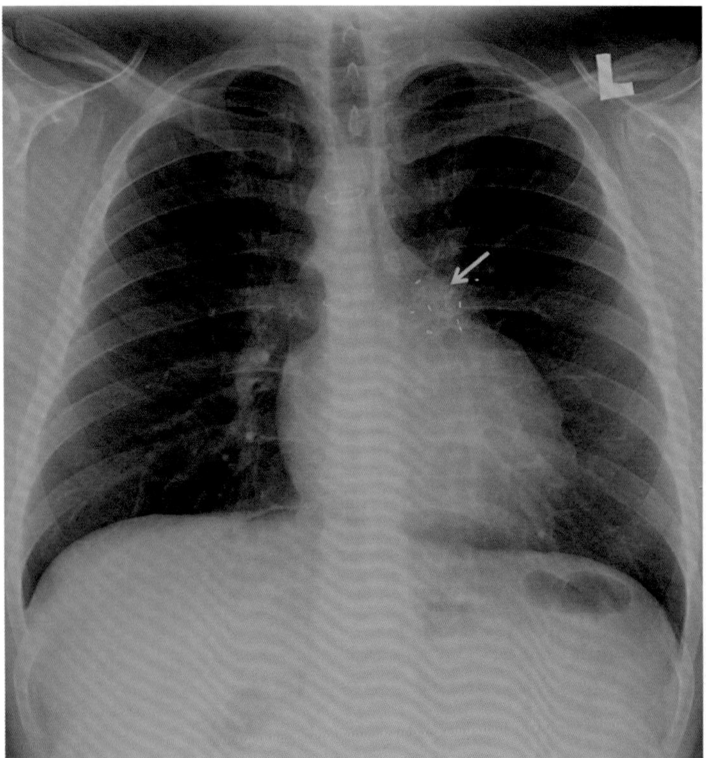

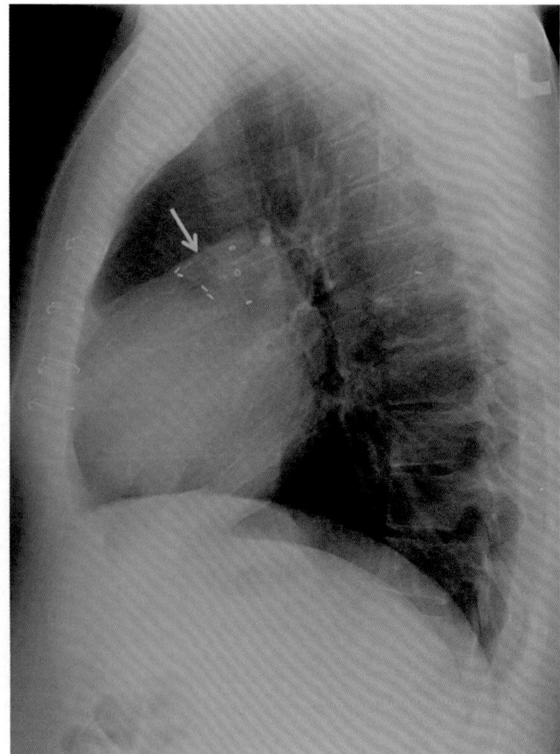

FIGURE 27.6. Frontal and lateral radiographs in a patient with repaired tetralogy of Fallot and right aortic arch showing a bioprosthetic pulmonary valve replacement (*blue arrow*).

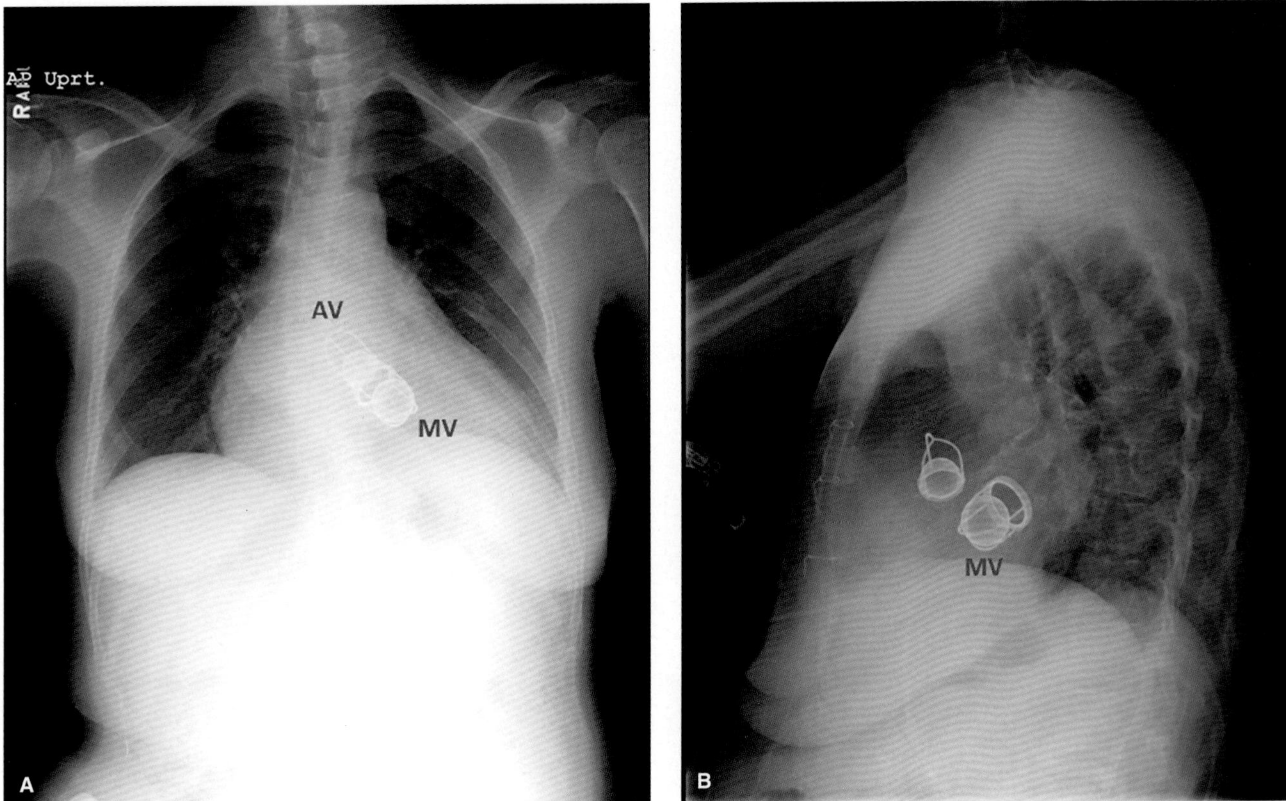

FIGURE 27.7. Frontal and lateral radiographs in a patient with Starr–Edwards caged ball valve prostheses in the mitral and aortic positions.

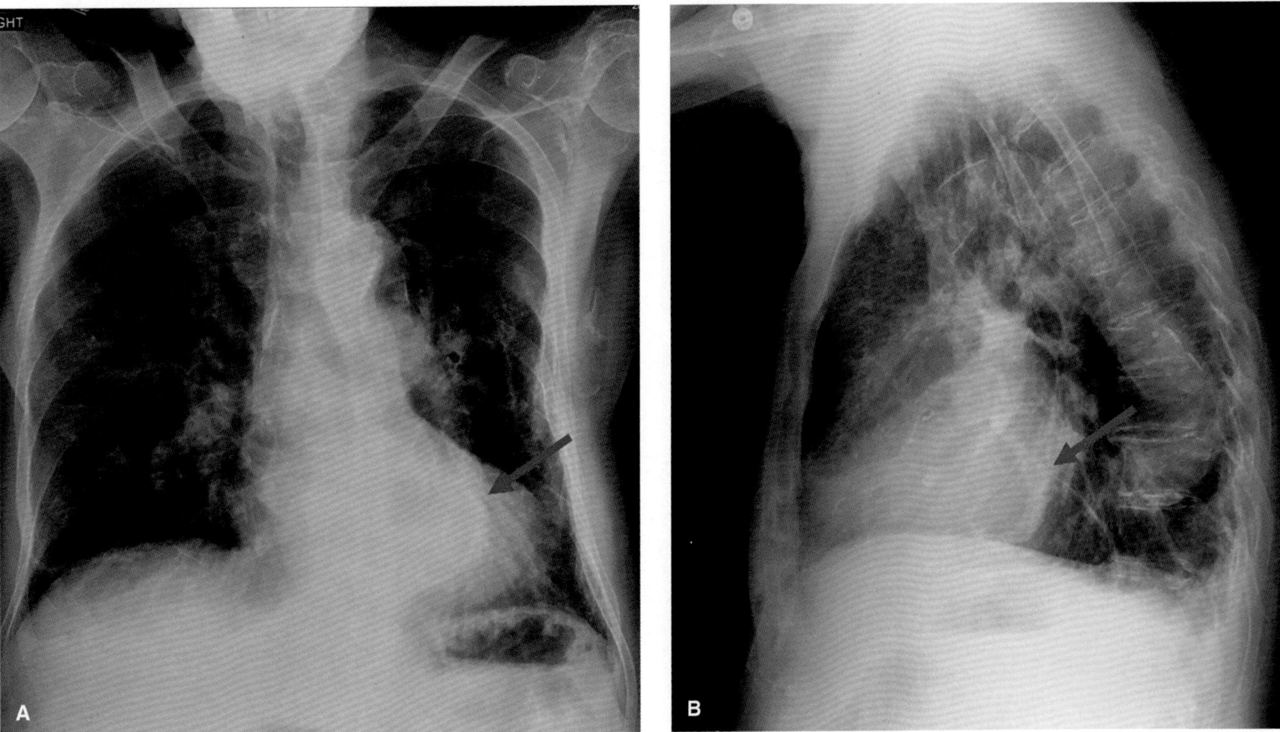

FIGURE 27.8. Radiographs in frontal (**A**) and lateral (**B**) projections and maximum intensity projection (MIP) CT reconstructions in coronal (**C**) and sagittal (**D**) planes from a patient with heavy mitral annular calcifications. *Red arrows* highlight the location of the mitral annular calcification. (*continued*)

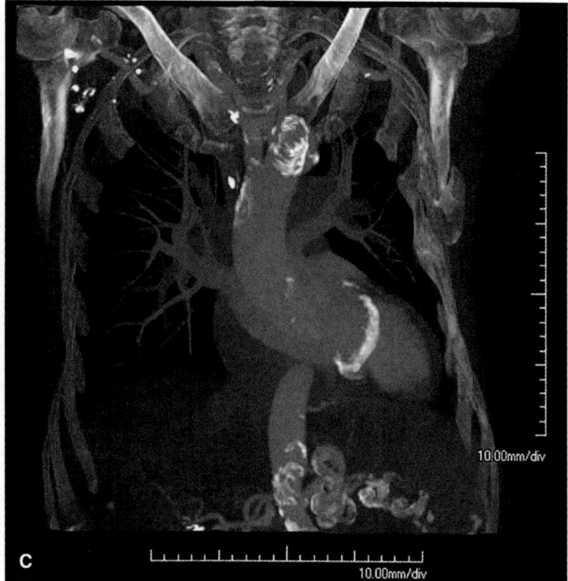

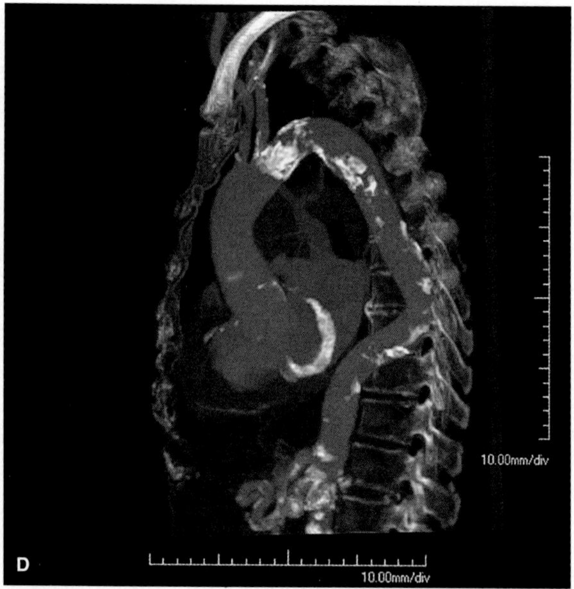

FIGURE 27.8. (*Continued*)

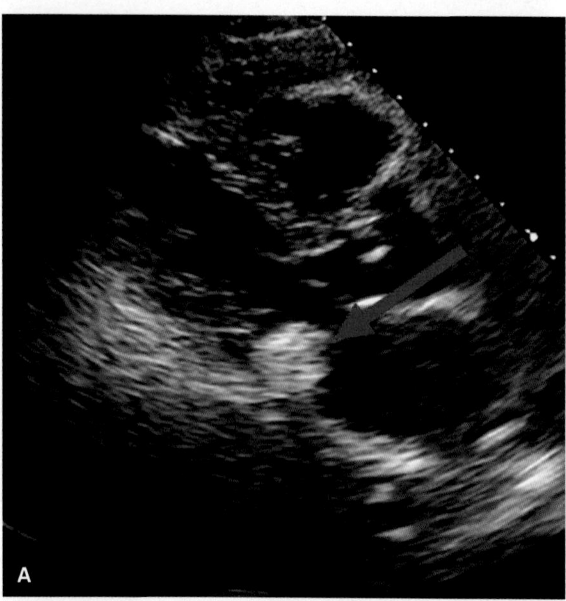

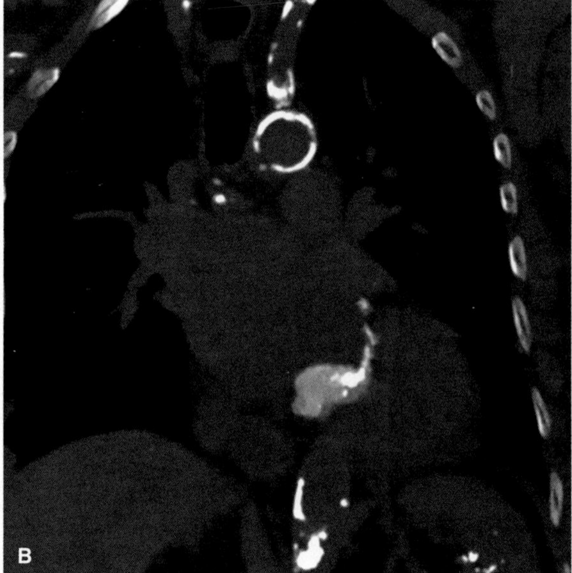

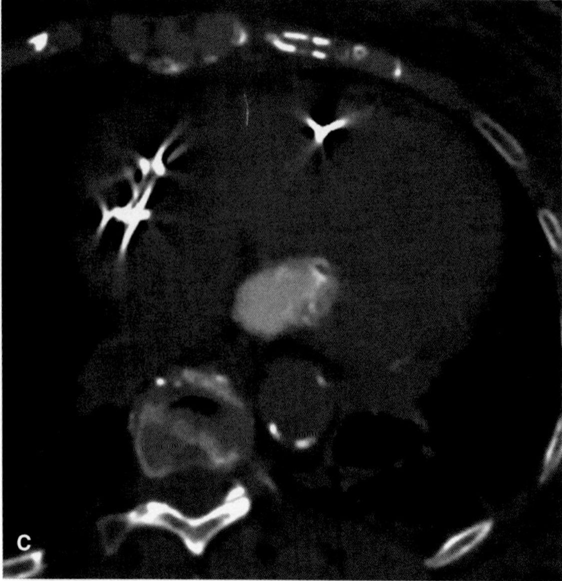

FIGURE 27.9. Images From Transesophageal Echocardiography (**A**) and Computed Tomography in Coronal (**B**) and Axial (**C**) Planes From a Patient With Caseous Mitral Annular Calcifications. Echocardiography shows an echogenic mass centered on the mitral annulus, which is also seen in corresponding CT slices.

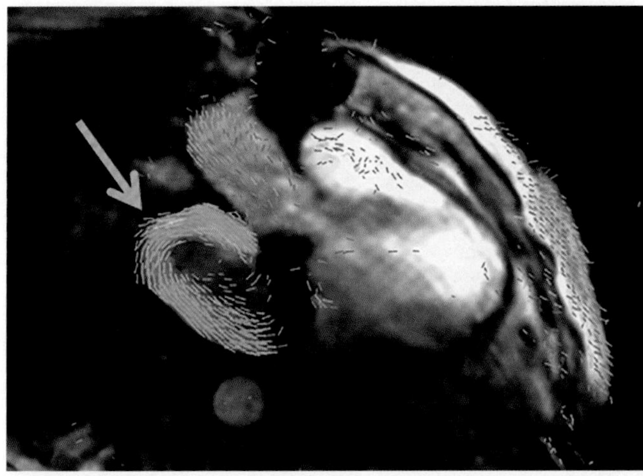

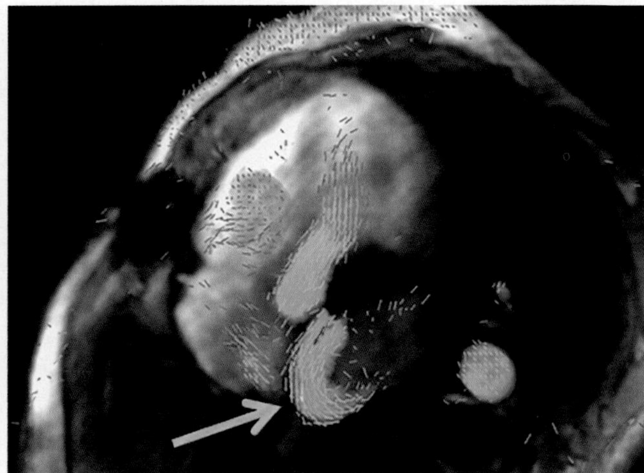

FIGURE 27.10. 4D Flow MRI Images From a Patient With Prior Mitral Valve Repair and Recurrent Severe Mitral Regurgitation. Large *yellow arrows* highlight the regurgitant jet. Note the regurgitant jet wraps around the posterior wall of the left atrium, the so-called "Coanda effect," which is a qualitative feature of severe mitral regurgitation often observed echocardiographically. In this case, regurgitant volume exceeded 60 mL/beat with a regurgitant fraction near 50%, consistent with severe mitral regurgitation.

Cardiac MRI

MRI has become an essential modality for evaluating the valves, especially the pulmonary and tricuspid valves in patients with CHD, as these valves are not well evaluated echocardiographically due to their position. Further, as MRI has become the quantitative gold standard for complete visualization of the heart and measurement of blood flow, its role in quantifying valve function has gradually increased. While echocardiography can readily measure blood velocities with Doppler ultrasound with high temporal resolution, measurement of total blood flow volume is a unique characteristic of MRI. We highlight several uses of MRI for measuring flow velocity and flow volume below.

Phase-Contrast MRI

Phase-contrast MRI is the clinical gold standard for noninvasive measurement of blood flow and is routinely used to quantify the severity of valvular stenosis or regurgitation. It utilizes the understanding that moving protons traveling in the direction of a bipolar magnetic gradient will acquire phase, and this phase can be mapped directly back to the speed of the moving proton (*refer to Cardiac MRI Technique chapter for more details*). Measurements of blood flow are typically performed perpendicular to the direction of blood flow, centered in the vessel or valve of interest. It is known that these measurements can be impaired by the presence of turbulent flow, such as near a stenosis or within an aneurysmal vessel, and thus measurements should be performed where the phase-contrast technique is least affected by patient geometries.

Typically, for valvular stenosis, peak velocities are measured near or just distal to the location of severe stenosis. Mean and peak velocities can then be converted to a pressure gradient according to the modified Bernoulli equation:

$$\Delta P = 4v^2,$$

where ΔP is the pressure gradient across the valve in mm Hg and v is the velocity in m/s.

For example, given a peak velocity of 350 cm/s across a pulmonary valve, the peak pressure gradient is estimated to be 49 mm Hg ($4 \times 3.5 \times 3.5 = 49$).

For valvular regurgitation, two approaches are commonly used: (a) measuring the amount of regurgitant flow below a zero baseline near the valve or vessel of interest, and (b) directly measuring the regurgitant jet during the systolic portions of the cardiac cycle where regurgitation is observed (Figs. 27.10 and 27.11).

Valvular regurgitation is generally quantified with two primary metrics: regurgitant volume (RVol) and regurgitant fraction (RF). First, RVol is defined as the amount of blood flow backward through the valve and is typically defined in units of either liters per minute (L/min) or milliliters per beat (mL/beat). Second, RF is defined as the RVol divided by the forward flow volume. If, for example, a patient has a net cardiac output of 6 L/min, with 8 L/min going forward across an inlet valve during diastole and 2 L/min going backward during systole, the RF is 25% (2 L/min divided by 8 L/min). In the same example, if the heart rate is 50 beats/min, the RVol of 2 L/min can also be described as 40 mL/beat (2,000 mL/min divided by 50 beats/min).

Quantification of Ventricular Stroke Volume

Valvular regurgitation may also be quantified by measuring the differences in stroke volume between the left and right ventricles by either MRI or CT. These measurements are however only applicable to patients with a single regurgitant valve without concomitant shunts (abnormal connections between the left and right heart, such as an anomalous pulmonary vein or atrial septal defect). For example, for a patient with isolated mitral regurgitation, the mitral RVol can be estimated using the difference in stroke volume between the left and right ventricles. If two or more valves are regurgitant, it would be difficult to determine the contribution of each without the use of phase-contrast MRI.

AORTIC VALVE

Congenital Aortic Valve Disease

Bicuspid aortic valve (BAV) is the most common CHD, affecting approximately 1% of adults. In BAV, two of the leaflets of the aortic valve may be partly or completely fused, resulting in a two-cusped (bicuspid) valve rather than the normal three-cusped valve (Figs. 27.12 and 27.13). BAV is associated with aortopathy, with approximately half of these patients demonstrating dilation of the aortic root and proximal ascending

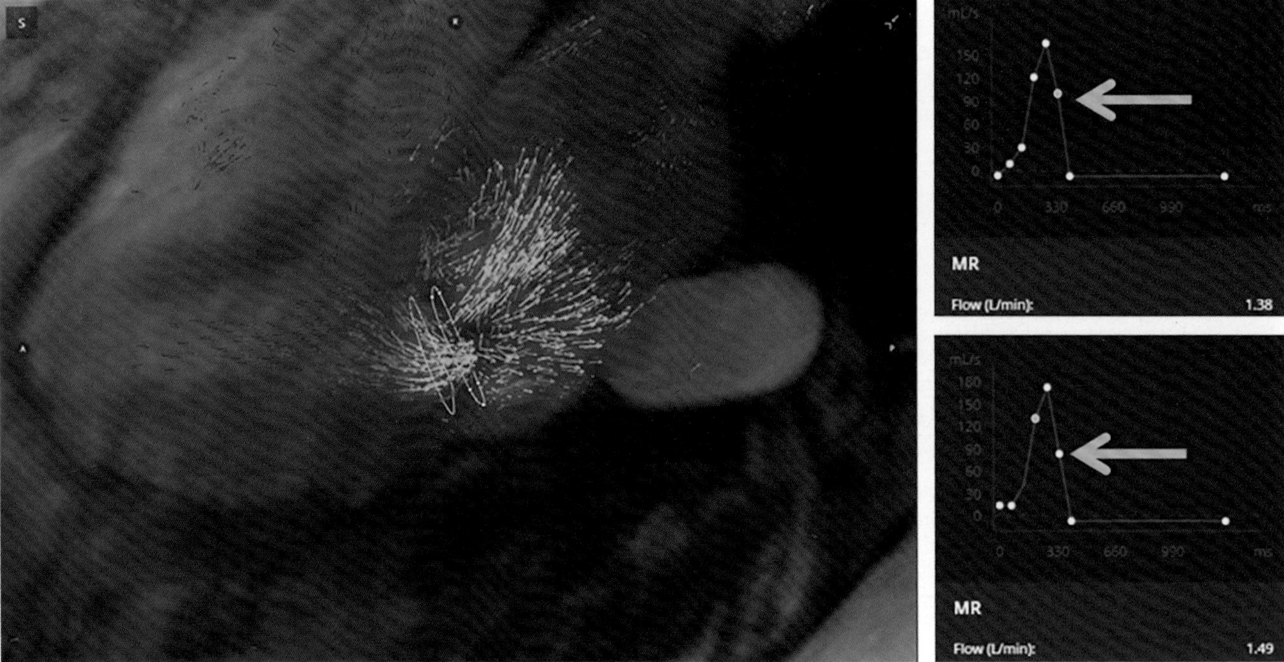

FIGURE 27.11. **4D Flow MRI Images From a Patient With Mitral Regurgitation and a Complex Mitral Regurgitant Jet.** The duration of the regurgitant jet is short-lived, as shown by the flow curves, resulting in a lower total regurgitant volume.

aorta (Fig. 27.14). This dilation is important to identify, as patients are predisposed to complications including aneurysm formation, aortic dissection and rupture. BAV is also associated with aortic coarctation. BAV can also be complicated by aortic stenosis and regurgitation, which can coexist. Cardiac CT and MRI imaging is useful to confirm valve morphology and to evaluate for valvular and aortic complications.

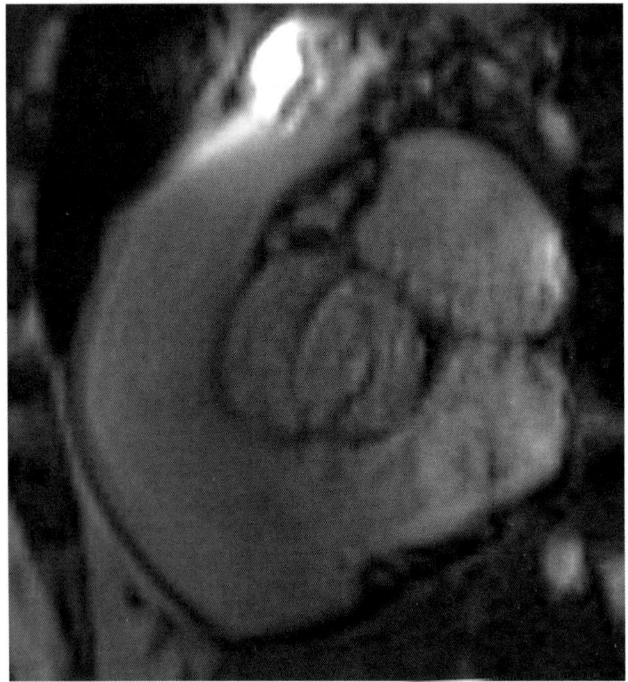

FIGURE 27.12. Oblique MRI image through the aortic root in a patient with bicuspid aortic valve, showing a "fish-mouth" opening of the valve during systole.

Flow acceleration across the aortic valve may also be caused by subaortic membranes that lie within the left ventricular outflow tract (LVOT). Occasionally, these may be too thin to resolve with MRI but can be inferred based on the location of the flow acceleration starting below the level of the aortic valve (Fig. 27.15). Subaortic membrane is the most common type of subaortic stenosis, typically resulting in a murmur. It can occur in isolation or associated with other CHD, including Shone complex.

Acquired Aortic Valve Disease

Acquired aortic valve disease is often caused by degenerative calcification and chronic leaflet deterioration. Less commonly acquired causes of acquired aortic valve disease include prior rheumatic heart disease affecting the aortic valve, radiation-induced heart disease typically more than a decade after mediastinal radiation, and infective endocarditis (IE).

Aortic Stenosis

Aortic stenosis is the most common valve disease, generally occurring among older patients. While BAV can predispose to early development of aortic stenosis, even a normal trileaflet aortic valve may eventually thicken and calcify with age (Fig. 27.16). Clinical management of aortic valve stenosis is guided by clinical stages and estimates of aortic valve area (AVA), primarily performed with echocardiography.

The most reliable echocardiographic measurement of AVA is determined by the *continuity equation*, which states that the blood flow passing through a tube must be equal, measured at any location along that tube, in order to satisfy conservation of mass. To estimate AVA echocardiographically, measurements of blood velocity are measured in the relatively normal LVOT and at the stenotic aortic valve, and a measurement of the LVOT diameter is also obtained. AVAs below 1.5 cm^2 are

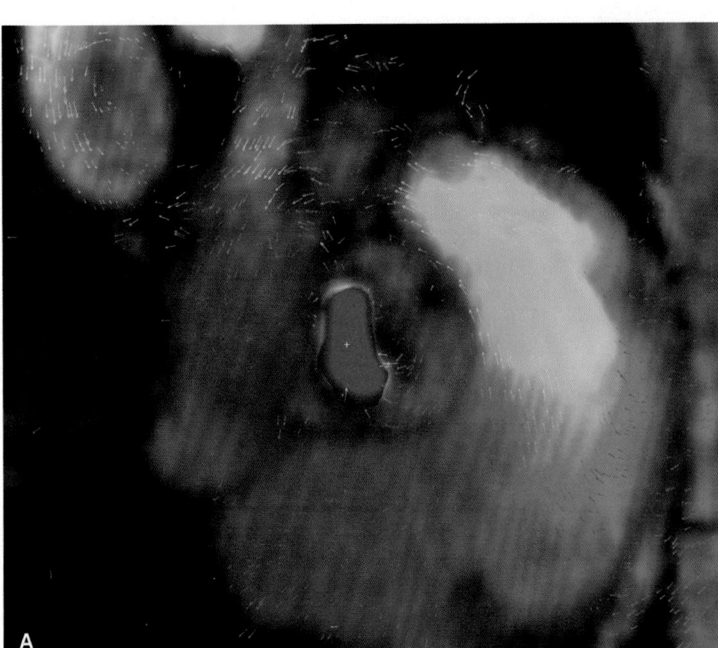

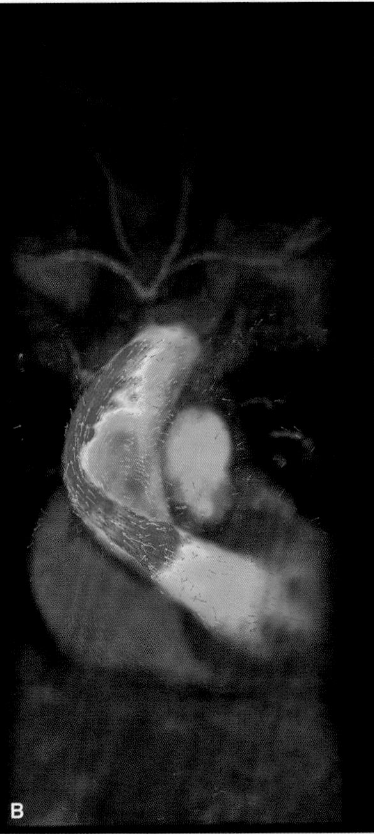

FIGURE 27.13. Cross-Section Through the Aortic Valve (A) and Coronal Plane Through the Aorta (B) From a Patient With Bicuspid Aortic Valve. Note the "fish-mouth" shaped jet of systolic flow through aortic valve resulting in an eccentric jet shearing along the wall of the ascending aorta.

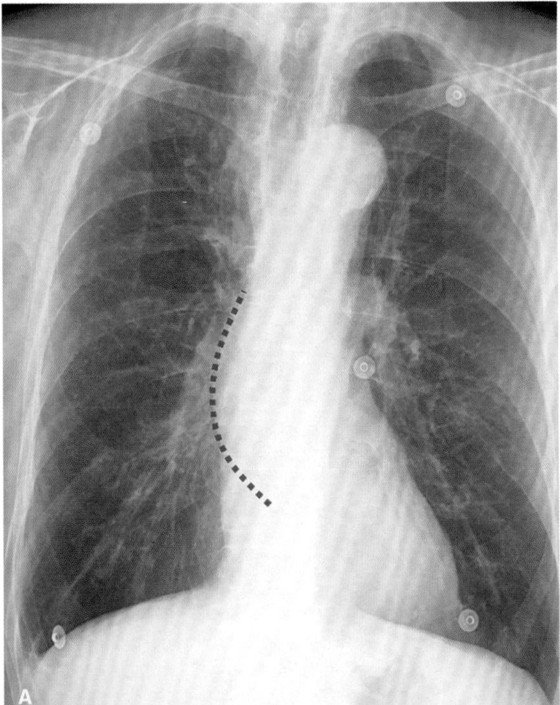

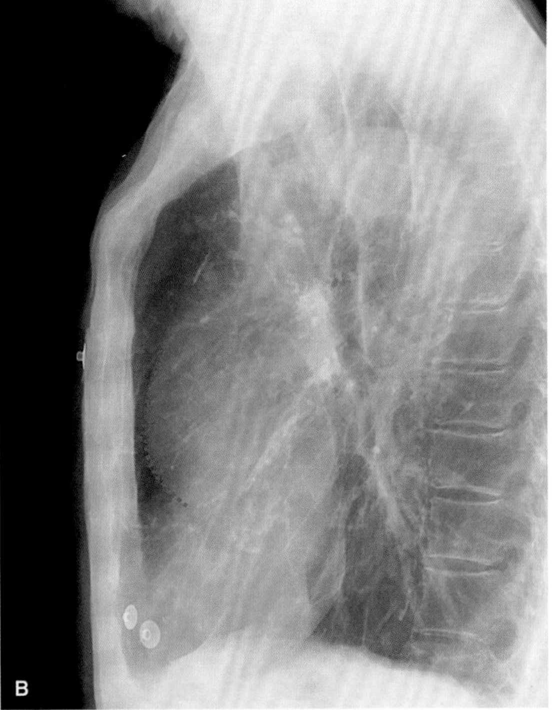

FIGURE 27.14. Ectatic Ascending Aortic Contour in a Patient With Bicuspid Aortic Valve and Aortic Stenosis. Frontal (**A**) and lateral (**B**) radiographs show the ectatic contour of the ascending aorta highlighted by the *red dashed line*. CT (**C**) confirmed the presence of ascending aortic aneurysm. (*continued*)

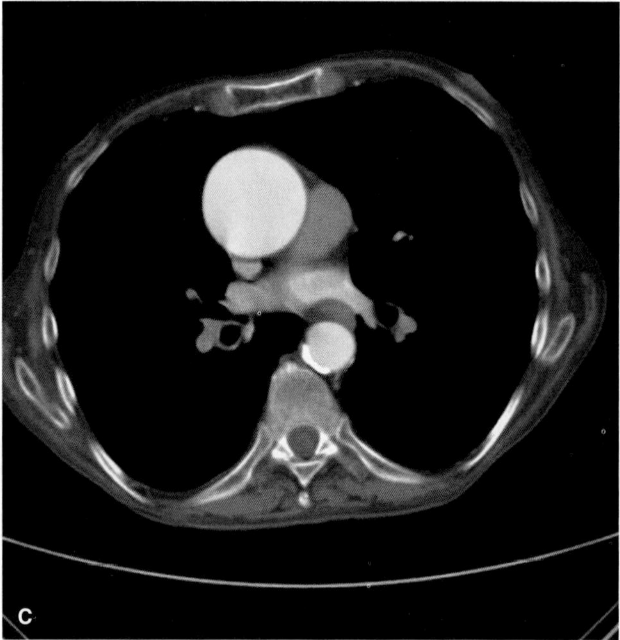

FIGURE 27.14. (*Continued*)

considered moderate, below 1 cm^2 are considered severe, and areas less than 0.5 cm^2 are considered critical. Severe stenosis typically correlates with peak aortic velocities over 4 m/s mean gradients exceeding 40 mm Hg.

Radiographic findings in aortic stenosis are variable and depend on the severity of disease. In the setting of mild aortic stenosis, the chest radiograph is often normal or mild dilation of the ascending aorta may be present. In more severe disease, valvular calcification may be identified along with signs of left ventricular dilation and left heart failure (Figs. 27.16 and 27.17).

When aortic stenosis is sufficiently severe, patients may undergo surgical aortic valve replacement or transcatheter aortic valve replacement (TAVR). The latter approach has made it feasible to treat aortic stenosis in patients who were previously not considered candidates for open surgical repair. The choice of a surgical valve versus TAVR is currently based on multiple clinical factors, including surgical risk, patient preference, and comorbid conditions.

Preprocedure planning for TAVR is now routinely performed with cardiac CT, for measurement of the size of the aortic annulus, evaluation of vascular access, and prediction of projection angles for prosthesis deployment. Accurate measurement of the aortic annulus is essential to choose an appropriately sized device. If the device is sized too small for the aortic annulus, this may result in paravalvular leak, which is associated with greater morbidity and mortality. If the device is sized too large for the aortic annulus, this may result in aortic annular rupture, especially in patients with heavy annular calcifications. Aortic annular rupture is a rare but serious complication and is associated with high rates of perioperative mortality.

The aortic annulus is typically measured in systole in a double oblique plane immediately below the hinge points of the aortic valve cusps. Aortic annular measurements include maximum and minimum diameters, perimeter, and cross-sectional area.

Aortic Regurgitation

Aortic regurgitation is typically graded qualitatively with echocardiography, but when needed for clinical management, RVol and RF can be quantified using MRI. This may be necessary if echocardiographic windows are limited, or when the regurgitant jet is particularly eccentric. In aortic regurgitation, the total left ventricular stroke volume is initially increased through compensatory mechanisms, resulting in dilation and concentric left ventricular hypertrophy. This mechanism eventually fails in the setting of severe or long-standing regurgitation, resulting in heart failure. Left ventricular dilation can be identified on chest radiography when moderate to severe and at earlier stages with cardiac-gated CT and cardiac MRI. Retrospectively gated cardiac CT acquired throughout the cardiac cycle, or cine cardiac

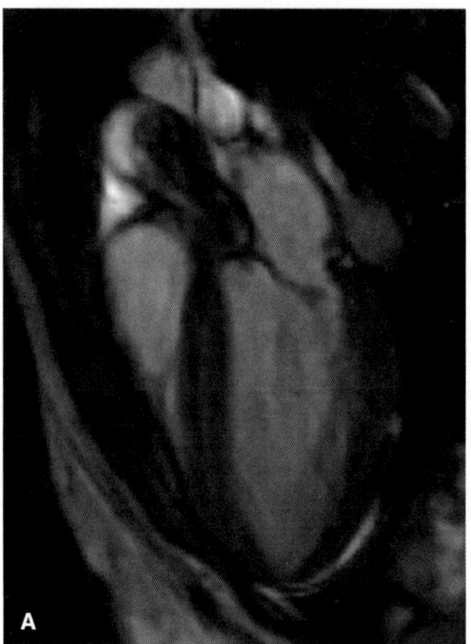

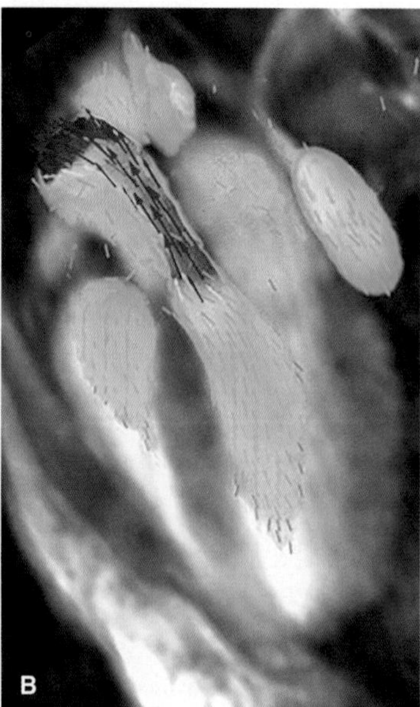

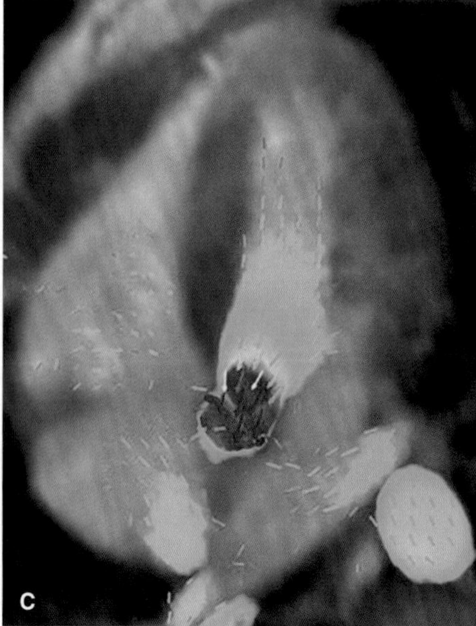

FIGURE 27.15. **Left Ventricular Three-Chamber SSFP (A) and Vector-Overlay 4D Flow (B, C) Images Showing Flow Acceleration Across the Aortic Valve in a Patient With a Subaortic Membrane Prior to Surgical Resection.** Close inspection shows that the flow acceleration begins at a level just below the aortic valve plane, consistent with subaortic membrane, not the aortic valve itself.

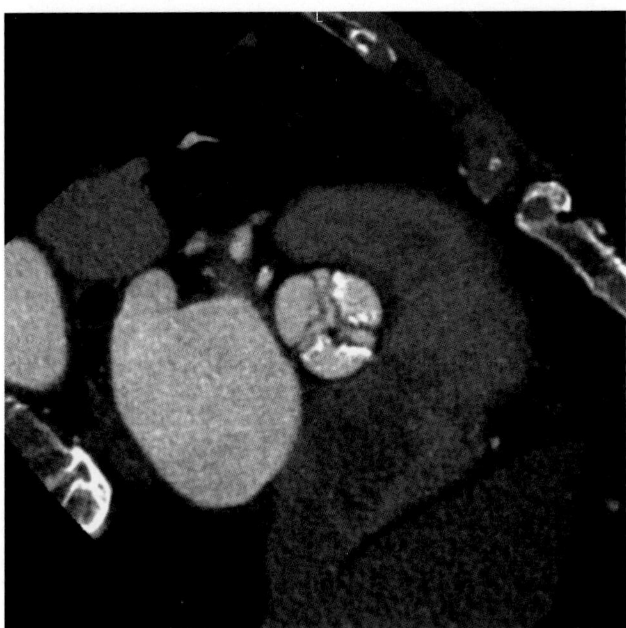

FIGURE 27.16. **Multiplanar Reformat of a Cardiac CT Showing the Aortic Valve During Systole.** Heavily calcified aortic valve leaflets in a patient with severe aortic stenosis show restricted opening of the aortic valve.

MRI acquired in the aortic valve plane, can demonstrate a coaptation defect of the aortic valve (Figs. 27.18 and 27.19).

MITRAL VALVE

Congenital Mitral Valve Disease

Mitral valve prolapse (MVP) is defined as bowing or prolapse of the mitral leaflet of 2 mm or more beyond the annular plane into the left atrium in ventricular systole (Fig. 27.20). MVP is the most common cause of severe nonischemic mitral regurgitation. Patients with MVP are at increased risk for ventricular arrhythmia and sudden death. MVP is caused by rupture or elongation of the chordae tendineae. Both anterior and posterior leaflets can be involved; however, the middle scallop of the posterior leaflet (P2 segment) is the most commonly affected. The prolapsed valve scallop is classified as a billowing leaflet (with bowing of the leaflet body) or flail leaflet (with free leaflet edge prolapse). Associated imaging findings include leaflet thickening. Conditions that are associated with secondary MVP include connective tissue disorders (such as Marfan syndrome) and CHD (such as ostium secundum ASD and aortic coarctation). Echocardiography is typically the first-line imaging investigation in cases of suspected MVP; however, CT and MRI are useful for detailed anatomic and functional evaluation and surgical planning.

Congenital cleft mitral valve can be seen in isolation or in association with other forms of CHD. Mitral cleft is characterized by division of one of the leaflets (typically the anterior leaflet). Cleft mitral valve is associated with progressive mitral regurgitation. In isolated mitral cleft, the cleft is oriented toward the LVOT rather than the inlet septum, as is the case of patients with an endocardial cushion defect (AVSD).

Though relatively uncommon, MS can occur congenitally with hypoplasia of the mitral valve annulus, fusion of the mitral valve commissure, and shortened or thickened chordae tendineae. This can be seen in association with multiple left-sided cardiac anomalies in what is known as Shone complex, including parachute mitral valve (in which all chordae attach to a single papillary muscle) or a supramitral ring. Other associated left-heart congenital abnormalities include aortic coarctation, aortic valve stenosis, and subvalvular aortic stenosis.

Acquired Mitral Valve Disease

MS is more often acquired (most commonly due to rheumatic heart disease) than congenital. MS characteristically results in increased left atrial (LA) pressure, as a compensatory mechanism in order to maintain normal cardiac output. This compensation results in LA enlargement and increased pulmonary venous pressure, eventually leading to pulmonary hypertension. On chest radiography, findings in left atrial enlargement include the double-density sign and elevation of the left main bronchus with splaying of the carina (Fig. 27.21). Echocardiography, CT,

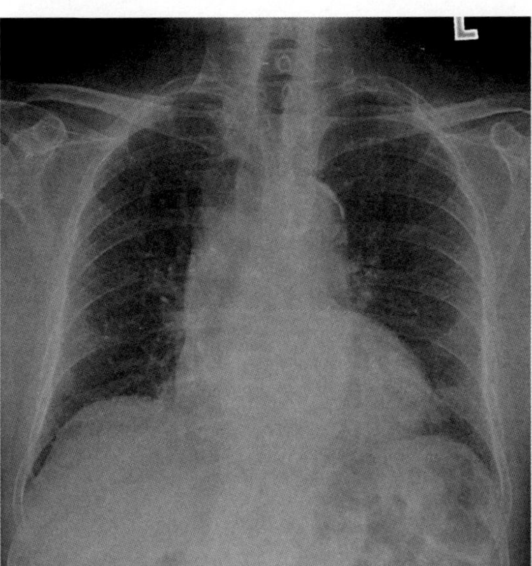

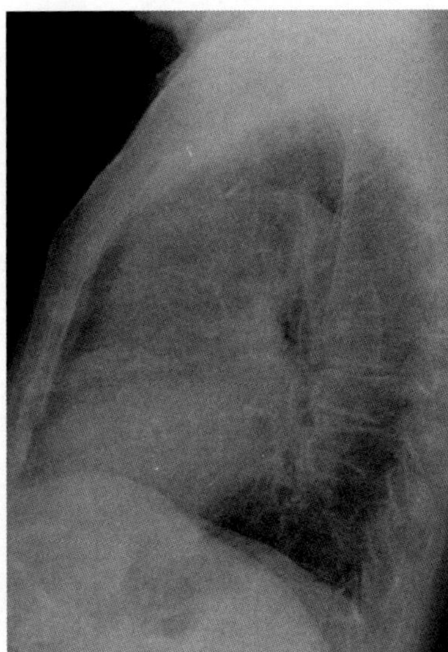

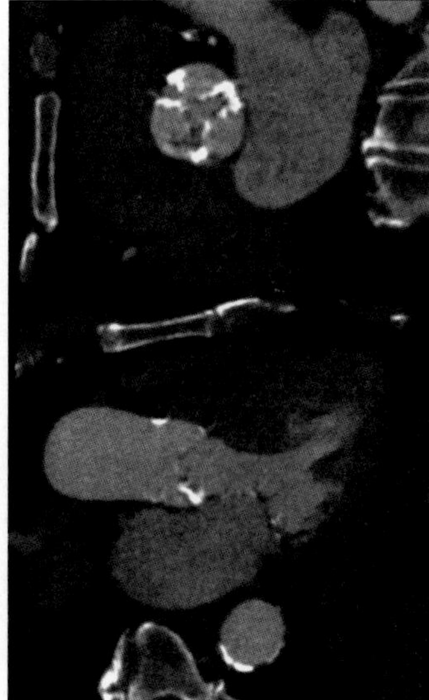

FIGURE 27.17. Frontal and lateral radiographs and cardiac CT images in a patient with severe aortic stenosis and moderate aortic valve calcification (seen on lateral chest radiograph and CT images).

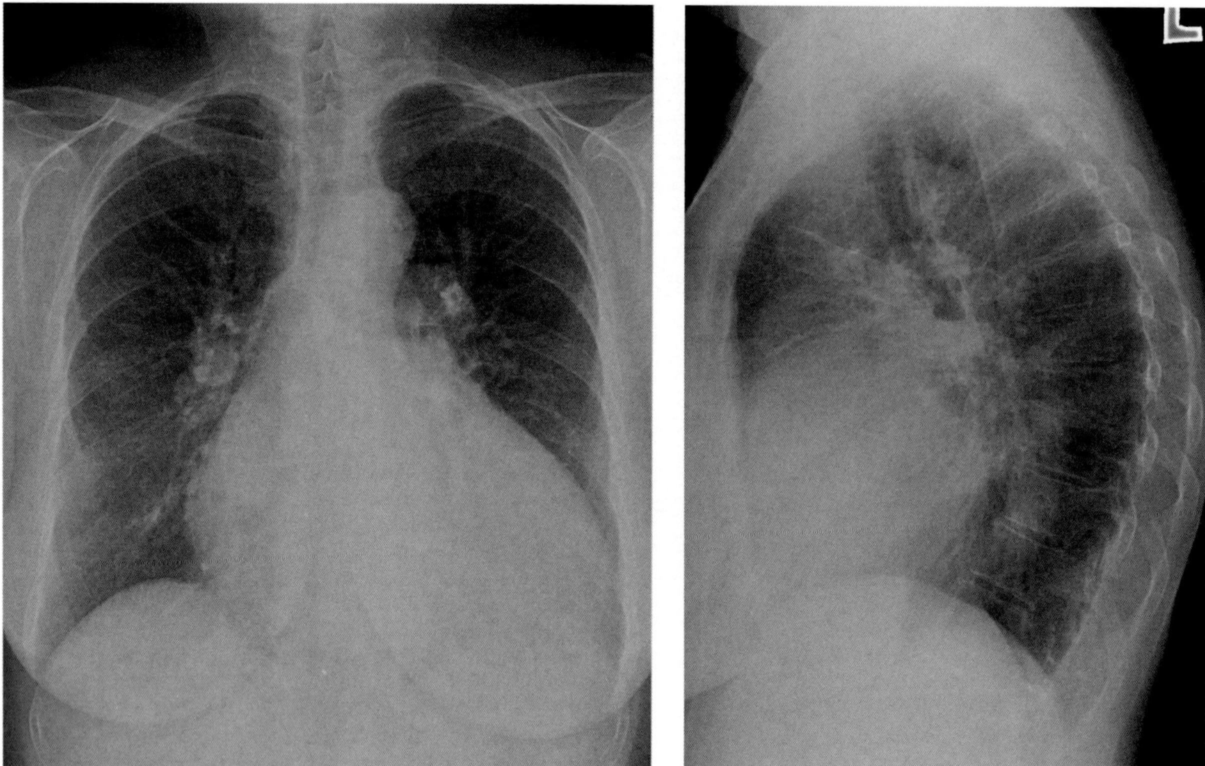

FIGURE 27.18. **Frontal and Lateral Radiographs in a Patient With Severe Aortic Regurgitation.** The left atrium and left ventricle are dilated.

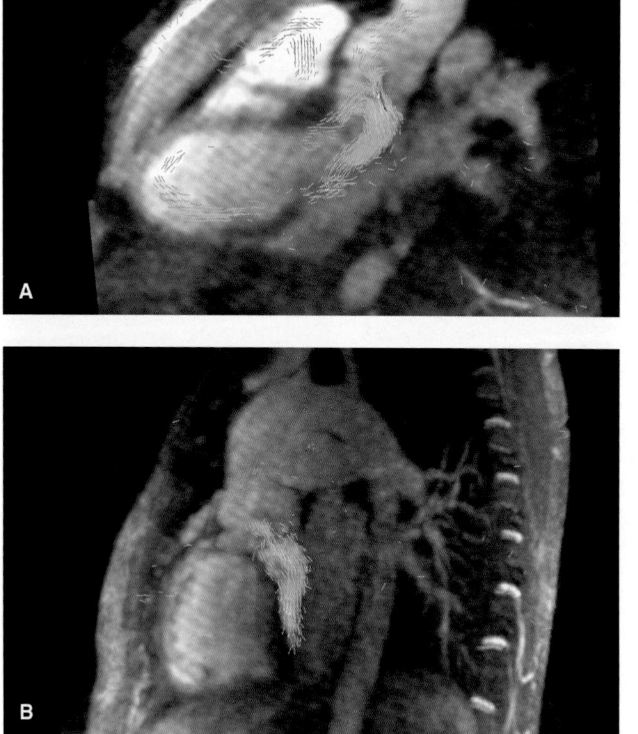

FIGURE 27.19. 4D flow MRI in three-chamber view (**A**) and oblique sagittal aortic view (**B**) showing an eccentric regurgitant jet from the aortic valve.

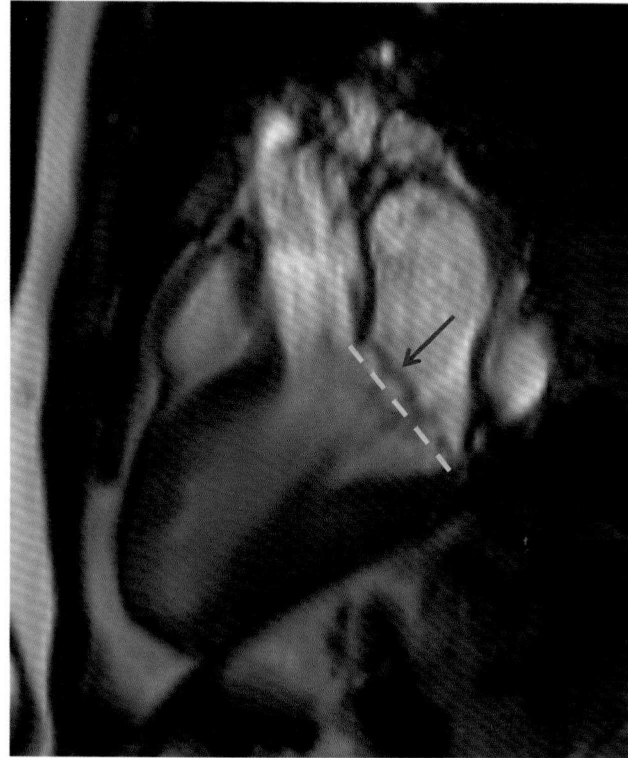

FIGURE 27.20. Cardiac MRI three-chamber SSFP image demonstrates mitral valve prolapse (*red arrow*) by several millimeters beyond the mitral annular plane (*yellow dotted line*).

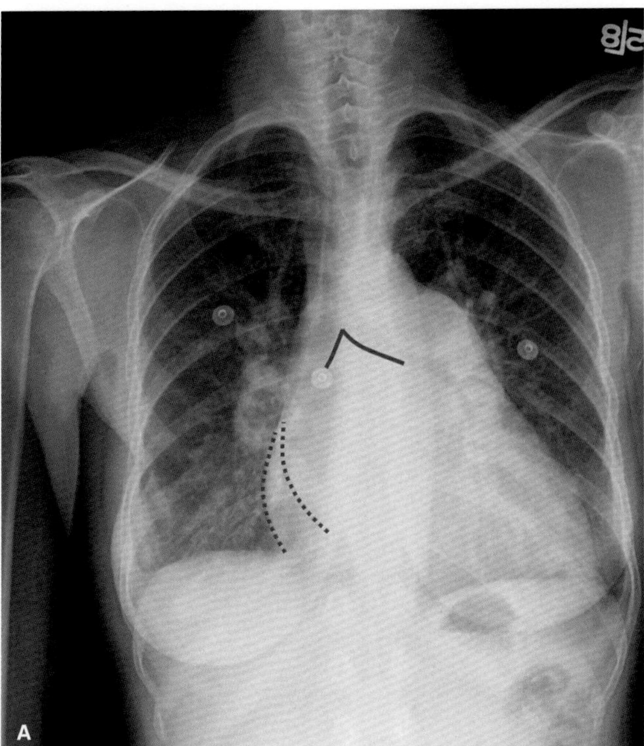

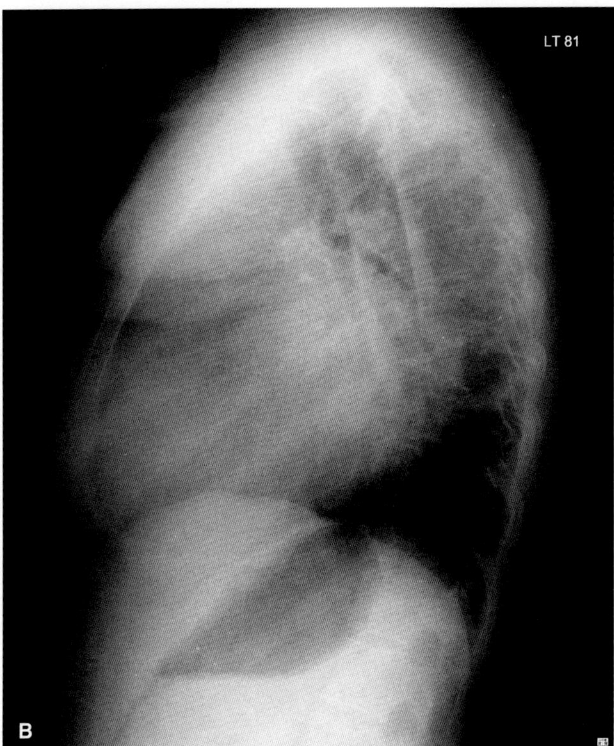

FIGURE 27.21. **PA (A) and Lateral (B) Chest X-Rays in a Patient With Mitral Stenosis.** There is severe left atrial enlargement with posterior bulging of the left atrial contour, double-density along the right heart border (*dotted red lines*), and splaying of the carina (*solid blue lines*). Note the marked enlargement of the pulmonary arteries, presumably from long-standing pulmonary vascular congestion from backup of blood related to mitral stenosis.

and MRI are useful in assessing mitral valve anatomy (leaflet mobility, thickening, and calcification), mitral valve area, and the left ventricle (Figs. 27.22 and 27.23).

Unlike the aortic valve, which lies downstream of a pumping ventricle, the mitral inflow relies on passive relaxation of the left ventricle to draw in blood from the pulmonary venous system. Thus, relatively small pressure gradients can have much more significant hemodynamic consequences. The transmitral gradient, measured by Doppler echocardiography, combined with mitral valve planimetry and pressure half-time, is used as the noninvasive clinical standard for assessing severity of MS. In rough numbers, a mean gradient of greater than 5 mm Hg is considered severe, while a mean gradient of greater than 10 mm Hg is considered very severe. The severity of MS may also be measured invasively by performing simultaneous right and left heart catheterizations to obtain mean pulmonary capillary wedge pressure (PCWP) or transseptal LA pressure and comparing these against left ventricular pressure during diastole.

Ischemic MR is defined as MR caused by changes of left ventricular structure and function related to ischemia (and is covered in greater detail in Chapter 28). Acute ischemic mitral regurgitation is caused by rupture of a papillary muscle occurring during the acute phase of myocardial infarction, and is associated with high mortality. This can sometimes be witnessed radiographically as one of the uncommon causes of asymmetric

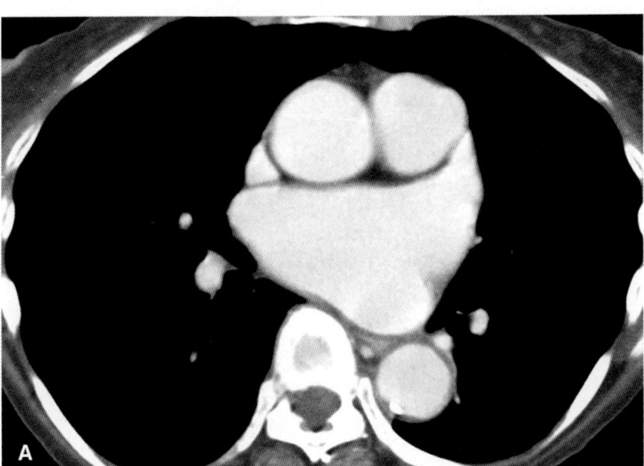

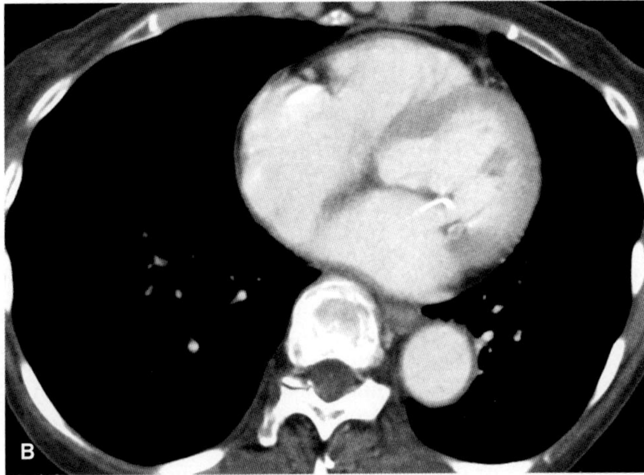

FIGURE 27.22. Enlarged left atrial appendage (**A**) and mitral calcifications (**B**) in a patient with mitral stenosis.

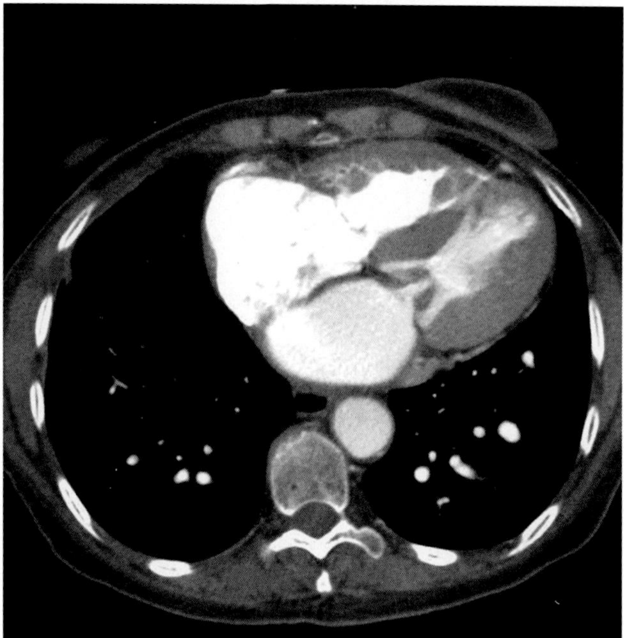

FIGURE 27.23. Thickened mitral valve leaflets in a patient with severe mitral stenosis.

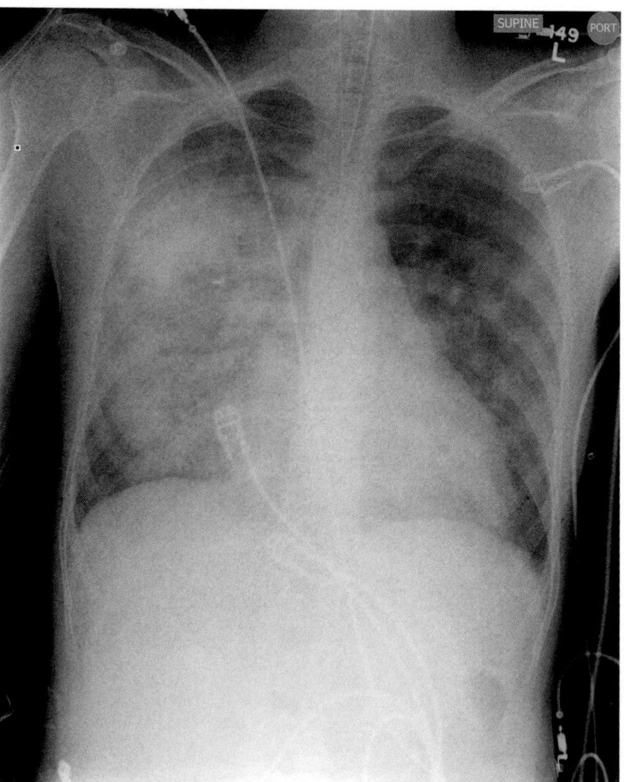

FIGURE 27.24. Chest X-Ray Demonstrating Asymmetric Right Upper Lobe and Right Middle Lobe Pulmonary Edema in a Patient With Acute Mitral Regurgitation. Acute mitral regurgitation is an uncommon but well-known cause of asymmetric pulmonary edema.

pulmonary edema (Fig. 27.24). Chronic ischemic mitral regurgitation occurs more than 2 weeks after infarction with absence of structural mitral valve disease, and is caused by modifications of the geometry and kinetics of the subvalvular apparatus, resulting from abnormalities of regional myocardial contraction. Imaging plays an important role in assessment of LV size, wall motion and function, mitral valve morphology, and the severity of MR.

While we have shown several examples of primary mitral valve regurgitation above, mitral valve regurgitation can also occur *secondarily* as a result of left ventricular failure. As the left ventricle dilates, so does the mitral annulus, which limits the ability of the mitral valve leaflets to properly coapt (Fig. 27.25). This form of mitral regurgitation is known as *secondary mitral regurgitation*. It can be difficult, however, in certain clinical situations to differentiate between primary and secondary mitral regurgitation. This can pose a clinical dilemma as surgical repair is indicated for primary mitral regurgitation, while the benefit of surgery is less certain in secondary regurgitation. Discriminating between primary and secondary mitral regurgitation is further confounded though, as severe primary mitral regurgitation can itself lead to left ventricular dilatation.

TRICUSPID VALVE

Congenital Tricuspid Valve Disease

Ebstein anomaly accounts for less than 1% of CHD but is the most common cause of congenital tricuspid regurgitation. Ebstein anomaly is characterized by variable and abnormal developmental anomaly of the tricuspid valve including apical displacement of the septal and posterior tricuspid valve leaflets, redundancy and fenestration of the anterior tricuspid leaflet, and dilation of the true tricuspid annulus. The right atrium and right ventricle often dilate, and tricuspid regurgitation is common. On frontal chest radiography, the heart may have a globular or box shape (Fig. 27.26). Pulmonary vascularity is either normal or decreased. Cardiac MRI is useful in visualizing the tricuspid valve and leaflet attachments and quantifying biventricular size and function (Figs. 27.27 and 27.28). Apical displacement of the septal leaflet >8 mm/m^2 has been proposed as a cutoff for Ebstein anomaly (rather than absolute displacement >1.5 to 2 cm). In normal human hearts, the septal and posterior leaflets are slightly apically displaced relative to the anterior mitral valve leaflet (<8 mm/m^2).

Tricuspid atresia (TA) is a cyanotic type of CHD characterized by agenesis of the tricuspid valve. There is an obligatory intra-atrial connection through an ASD or patent foramen ovale (PFO) which is necessary for survival. A small ventricular septal defect (VSD) is often also present. The right ventricle is typically small and hypoplastic, while the right atrium is dilated and hypertrophied. TA is associated with right-sided aortic arch and transposition of the great arteries (TGA). Patients with TA without TGA typically have some degree of pulmonary stenosis (PS). Chest radiography may demonstrate decreased pulmonary vascularity and flat or concave main pulmonary artery. Cardiac CT and MRI often depict fatty or muscular separation of the right atrium from the right ventricle.

Tricuspid stenosis is rare and is most often congenital or acquired due to rheumatic heart disease. A characteristic hemodynamic feature of tricuspid stenosis is increased pressure gradient between the right atrium and right ventricle (>5 mm Hg), resulting in venous congestion. The right atrium is usually enlarged.

PULMONARY VALVE

Pulmonary Stenosis

Congenital PS refers to dynamic or fixed anatomic obstruction to blood flow from the RV to the pulmonary arterial vasculature. The level of obstruction can be categorized as

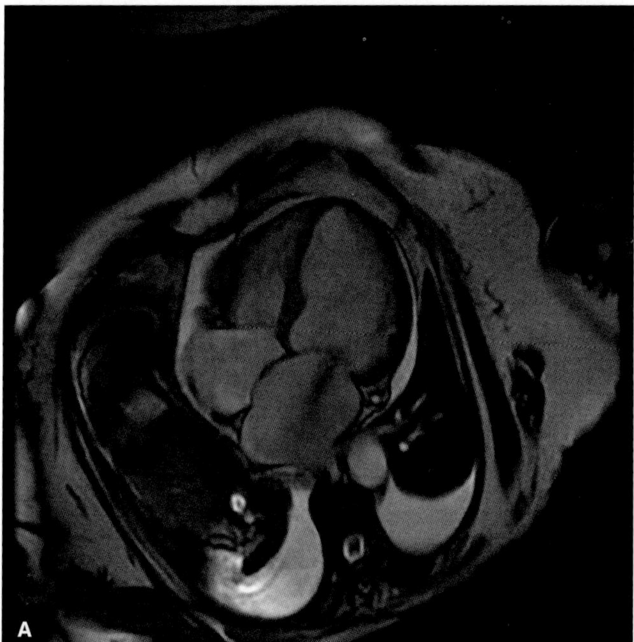

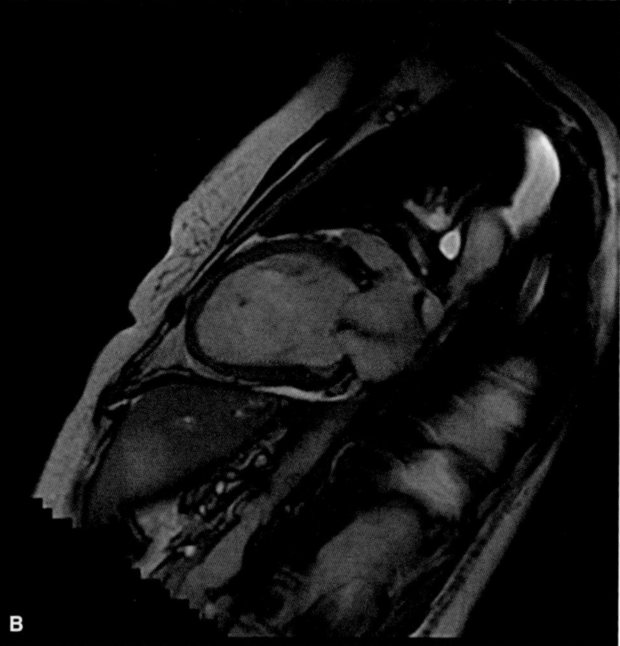

FIGURE 27.25. **Systolic SSFP Images in Four-Chamber (A) and Two-Chamber (B) Views Showing a Central Dephasing Jet Into the Left Atrium due to Secondary Mitral Regurgitation.** In secondary mitral regurgitation, there may not be an underlying defect of the mitral valve but rather a dilation of the left ventricle from cardiomyopathy that causes regurgitation.

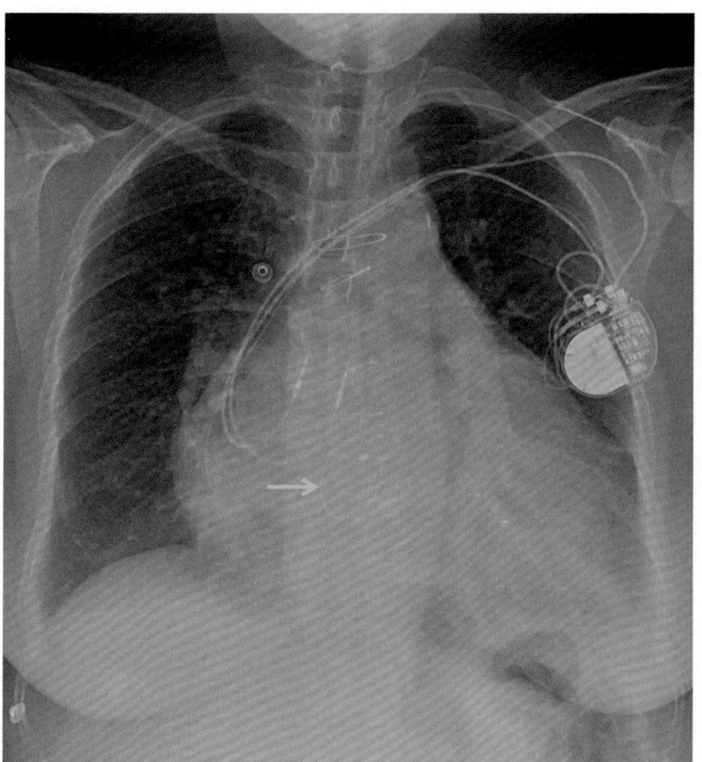

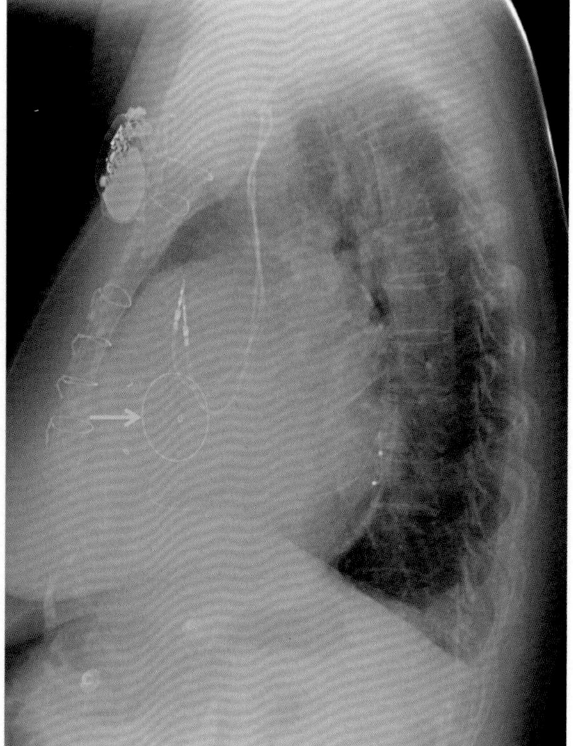

FIGURE 27.26. **Frontal and Lateral Radiographs in a Patient With Ebstein Anomaly and Tricuspid Valve Replacement.** The right atrium and right ventricle are dilated. There is a left chest wall pacemaker generator with two right atrial leads and a coronary sinus lead. *Green arrows* highlight the location of the tricuspid valve.

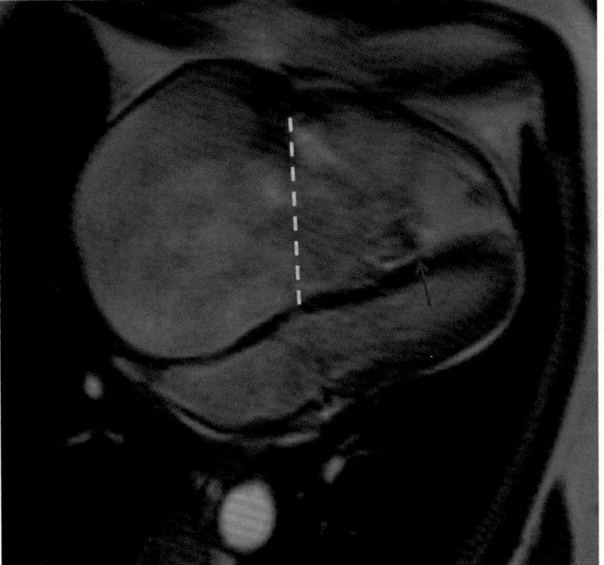

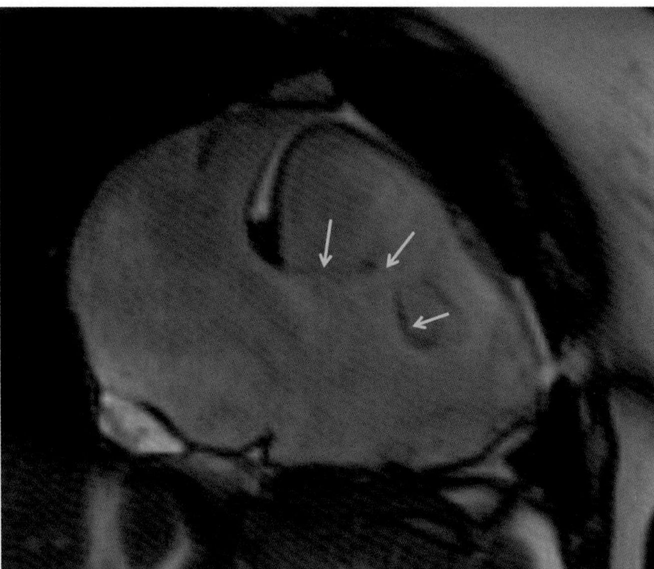

FIGURE 27.27. Cardiac MRI four-chamber and right ventricular two-chamber SSFP images in a patient with Ebstein anomaly demonstrate apical displacement of the septal tricuspid valve leaflet (*red arrow*) in relation to the tricuspid annulus plane (*yellow dotted line*), elongated anterior tricuspid valve leaflet (*green arrows*), and right atrial and right ventricular dilation.

valvular, subvalvular, or supravalvular and can be found in association with more complicated congenital heart defects. Isolated pulmonary valve stenosis accounts for approximately 10% of all CHDs. The valve commissures may be partially fused resulting in a narrow central orifice, often leading to poststenotic dilation of the main pulmonary artery (Fig. 27.29). Alternatively, the valve leaflets may be irregular and thickened without commissural fusion, as is the case in the majority of patients with Noonan syndrome. Subvalvular PS occurs due to narrowing of the infundibular or subinfundibular right ventricular outflow tract (RVOT) and is present in individuals with tetralogy of Fallot (TOF). Double-chambered RV is a rare condition resulting from fibromuscular narrowing of the RVOT with subvalvular right

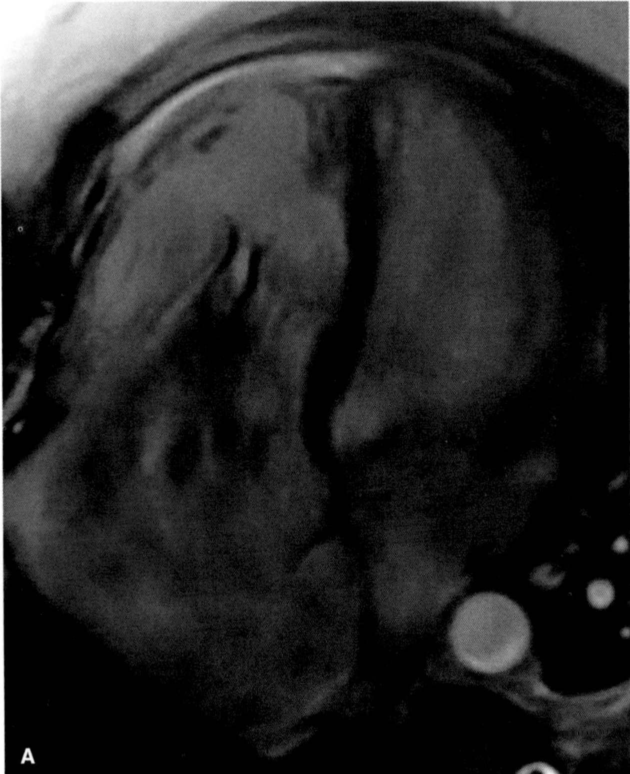

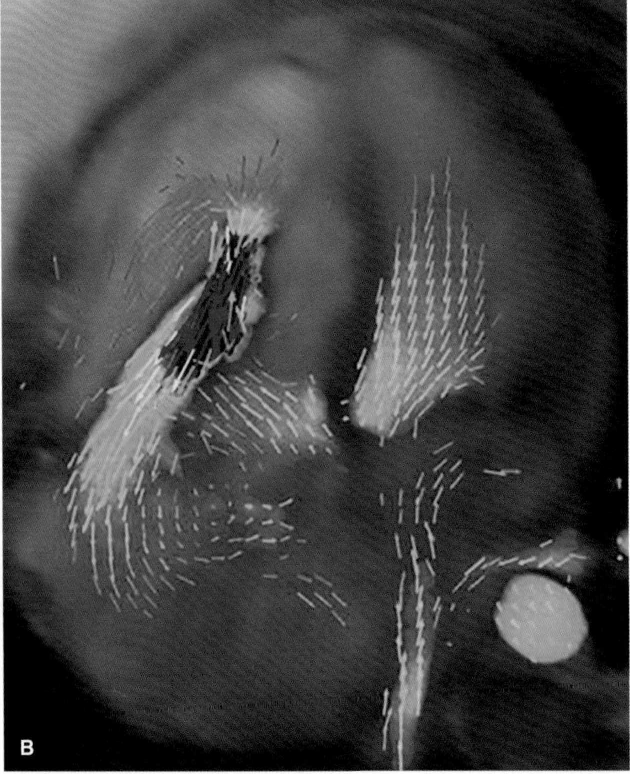

FIGURE 27.28. Four-chamber SSFP (**A**) and vector-overlay 4D flow images in four-chamber (**B**) and right ventricular three-chamber (**C**) views showing apical displacement of the tricuspid valve with severe tricuspid regurgitation during systole.

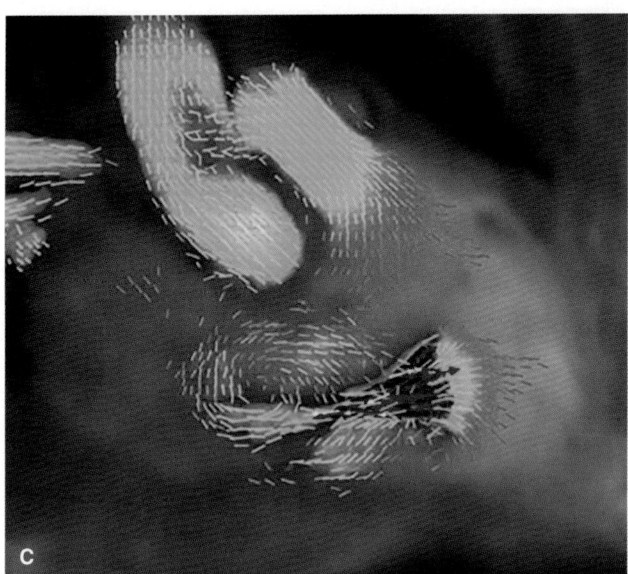

FIGURE 27.28. (*Continued*)

ventricular outflow obstruction. Supravalvular PS can result from obstruction at the level of the main pulmonary artery, at its bifurcation, or more distal branches. Multiple sites of obstruction are common. Approximately 20% of patients with TOF have associated supravalvular PS.

Pulmonary Regurgitation

Patients with congenital PS or TOF often undergo pulmonary valvuloplasty or surgical repair during infancy or early childhood. Such patients are often left with incompetent pulmonary valves. Quantification of pulmonary valve regurgitation and stenosis is commonly performed by MRI for these patients over the course of their lifetime. While initially chronic pulmonary regurgitation was considered less consequential, it has become clear that patients with severe pulmonary regurgitation may eventually dilate their right ventricle and develop right ventricular failure. Unfortunately, the pulmonary valve is not readily visualized echocardiographically due to its position behind the sternum. MRI is therefore commonly used to measure both the severity of pulmonary regurgitation and measure the severity of dilation of the right ventricle to determine the need for surgical or interventional valve replacement (Fig. 27.30).

ACQUIRED DISEASES OF MULTIPLE VALVES

Infective Endocarditis

Valve IE refers to an infection of the valve leaflets as well as prosthetic valves. Intravenous drug users are at increased risk. IE is associated with high morbidity and mortality even with appropriate treatment. Once infection is initiated, the clotting pathway often results in vegetation formation, which often appears as an irregular mobile or fixed mass attached to the low-pressure side of a valve. Fragments of vegetation can break off resulting in pulmonary septic emboli (in the setting of right heart disease) and TIA or stroke (in the setting of left heart disease). Eventually, the valve leaflets may be destroyed leading to valvular regurgitation and heart failure. Echocardiography is useful for diagnosing IE, assessing the severity of disease, and following patients undergoing treatment. Cardiac CT and MRI are useful in identifying and characterizing vegetations, valve destruction, and perivalvular extension. TEE is

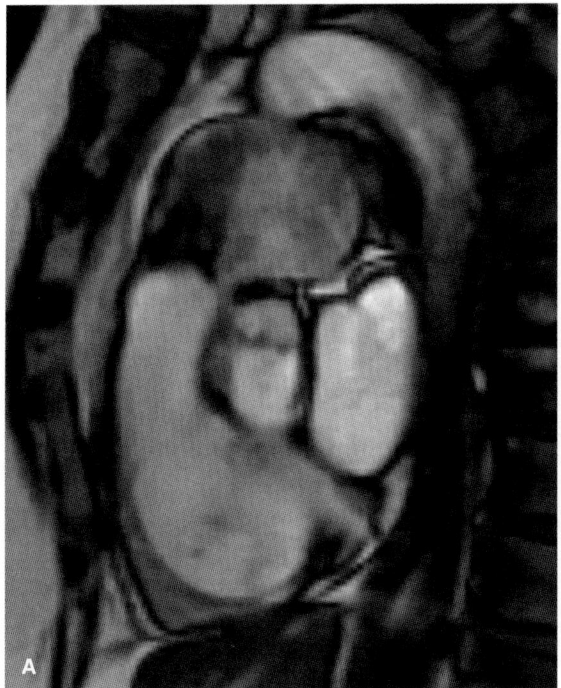

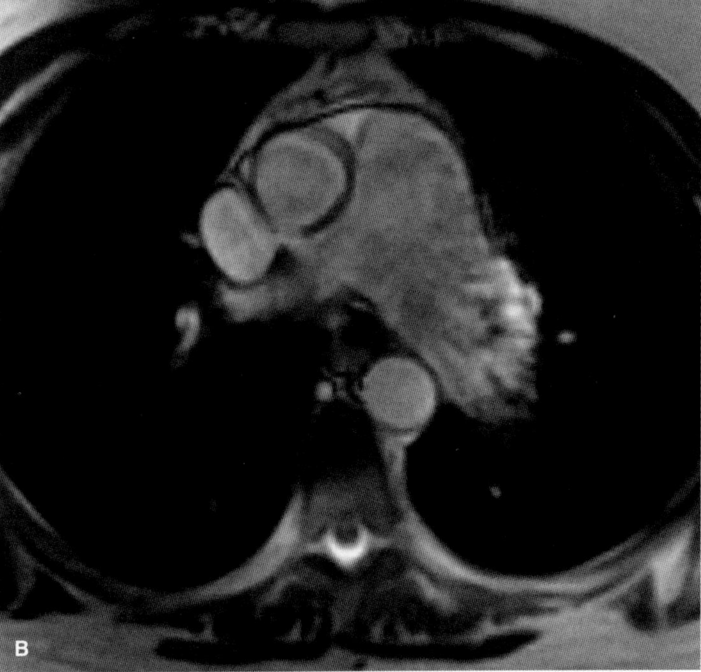

FIGURE 27.29. **SSFP Images of the Pulmonary Outflow Tract (A) and the Main Pulmonary Artery (B) Showing Pulmonary Stenosis with Flow Acceleration begins at the Level of the Pulmonary Valve.** There is associated enlargement of the main and left pulmonary arteries.

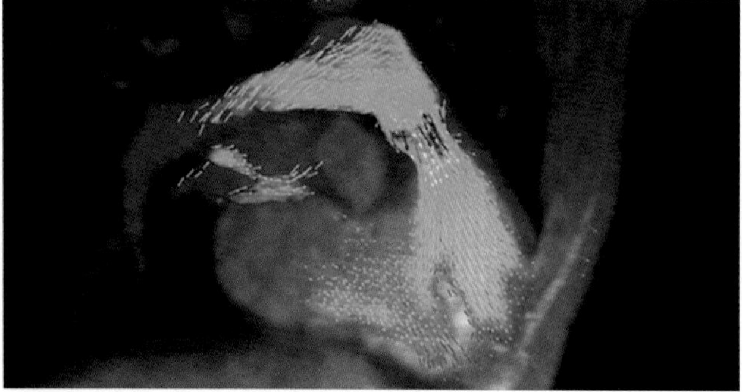

FIGURE 27.30. **Right Ventricular Three-Chamber View From 4D Flow MRI Showing Free (Severe) Pulmonary Regurgitation in a Patient With Repaired Tetralogy of Fallot.** In this patient, right ventricular volume exceeded 160 mL/m^2 and the pulmonary regurgitant fraction measured 48%, which was sufficient to warrant surgical repair.

often superior in detecting small vegetations and valve perforations. However, CT has several advantages including very short image acquisition time, assessment of the perivalvular extent of disease including abscesses, and in prosthetic valve endocarditis where acoustic shadowing decreases the sensitivity of TEE. MRI has an important role in diagnosing cerebral embolic events.

Nonbacterial Endocarditis

Libman–Sacks nonbacterial endocarditis is a common heart-related manifestation in patients with systemic lupus erythematosus (SLE). Small valve vegetations typically affect the ventricular and atrial sides of the mitral valve. Unlike IE, these lesions rarely result in hemodynamically significant valve dysfunction and rarely embolize.

Rheumatic Heart Disease

Rheumatic valve disease refers to valve fibrosis and scarring caused by an autoimmune reaction to infection with group A streptococci, resulting in valve stenosis and/or regurgitation. The highest incidence of rheumatic fever is observed in children in underdeveloped or developing countries where antibiotics are not routinely used for pharyngitis. The most commonly involved valve in rheumatic heart disease is the mitral valve by far, followed by aortic, tricuspid, and pulmonary valves in that order. In most cases, the mitral valve is involved along with one or more other valves (Fig. 27.30). The majority of patients with MS have a history of rheumatic fever. MS is a progressive disease and patients frequently undergo repeat imaging including echocardiography, CT, or MRI. Patients commonly present with shortness of breath and fatigue related to left heart failure. Chronic elevation of LA pressure needed to move blood across the stenotic mitral valve results in atrial dilation and elevated pulmonary pressure. Approximately 30% to 40% of symptomatic patients with MS develop atrial fibrillation.

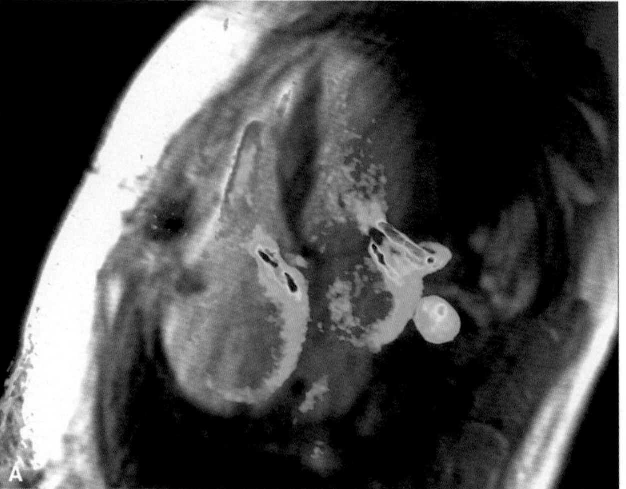

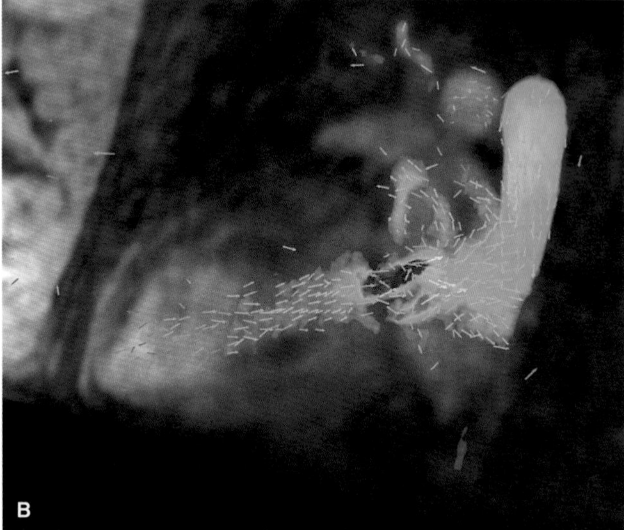

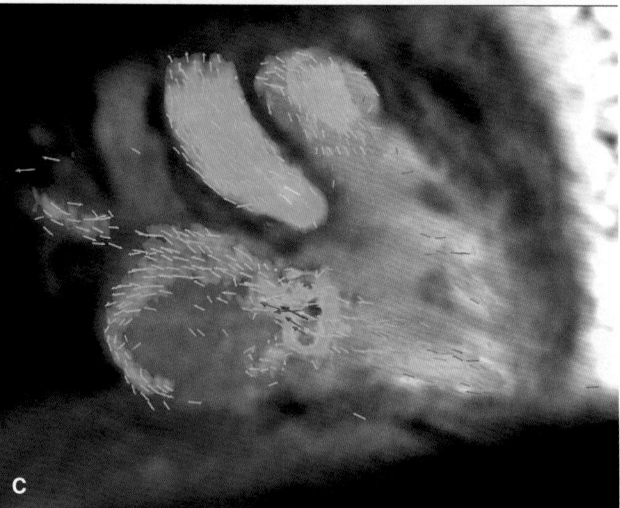

FIGURE 27.31. 4D flow MR images in four-chamber (**A**), left ventricular two-chamber (**B**), and right ventricular three-chamber (**C**) views showing severe mitral and tricuspid regurgitation in a patient with rheumatic heart disease.

Carcinoid Valve Disease

Carcinoid heart disease is a frequent occurrence in patients with carcinoid syndrome. Approximately 30% to 40% of

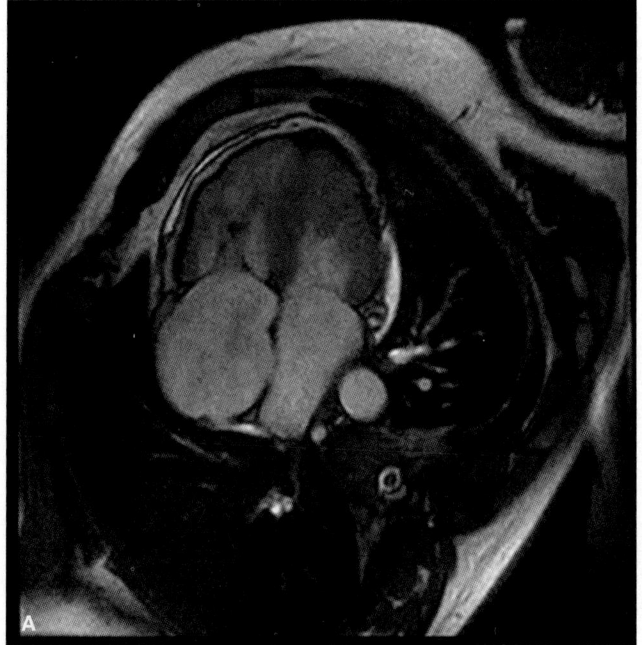

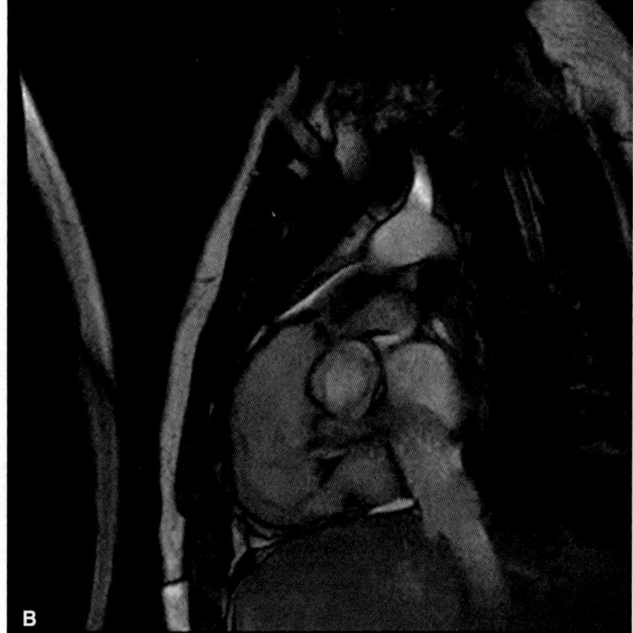

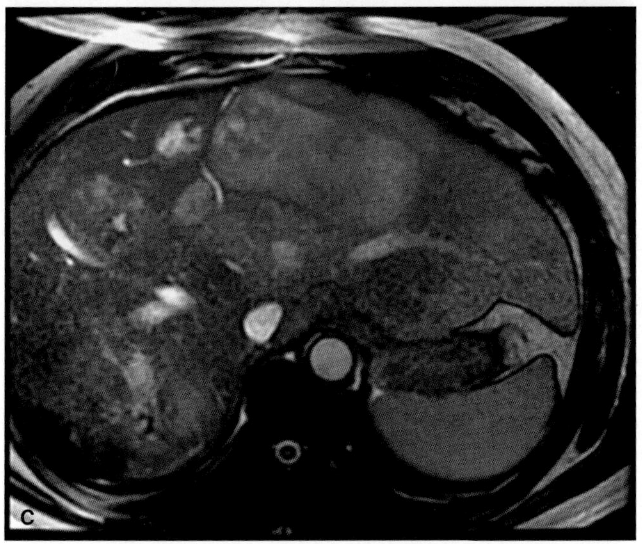

FIGURE 27.32. **SSFP MRI Images in Four-Chamber View (A) and Right Ventricular Outflow Tract View (B) of the Heart and Axial View of the Liver (C) in a Patient With Carcinoid Heart Disease due to Metastatic Neuroendocrine Tumor.** Note the restricted opening of the tricuspid valve during diastole on the four-chamber view. During systole in the right ventricular outflow tract view, pulmonary stenosis and tricuspid regurgitation are evident. Multiple hepatic neuroendocrine metastases in the liver are responsible for the right-sided carcinoid valve disease.

patients with neuroendocrine tumors (most commonly midgut carcinoids) present with carcinoid syndrome, including episodes of flushing, hypotension, diarrhea, and bronchospasm. The vast majority of patients with neuroendocrine metastases to the liver will develop carcinoid syndrome, as the vasoactive substance reaches the systemic circulation via the hepatic vein. Chronic exposure to excessive circulating serotonin is considered an important contributing factor to the development of carcinoid heart disease. Carcinoid heart disease is characterized by the development of plaque-like, fibrous endocardial thickening involving the heart valves (mainly tricuspid and pulmonary). The first-line imaging modality is TTE. Imaging features include thickening of valve leaflets/cusps and subvalvular apparatus, retraction and altered motion of the leaflets/cusps, and valve regurgitation (ranging from mild to severe) (Fig. 27.32). Pulmonary valve involvement may be underappreciated on TTE. Cardiac MRI may be useful to evaluate the pulmonary valve, identify cardiac metastases, and assess right ventricular size and function. Cardiac CT may be helpful in assessment of the degree of structural valvular damage and assessing the degree of calcification, if present.

POSTOPERATIVE COMPLICATIONS FOLLOWING VALVE SURGERY

Postoperative complications following valve surgery include infection, dehiscence, and perivalvular leak. Perivalvular leak has been described after both aortic and mitral valve replacements and occur due to incomplete apposition of the sewing ring to the native annular tissue. Late complications include valve regurgitation, IE, anastomotic dehiscence, pseudoaneurysm and thromboembolic events (Fig. 27.33).

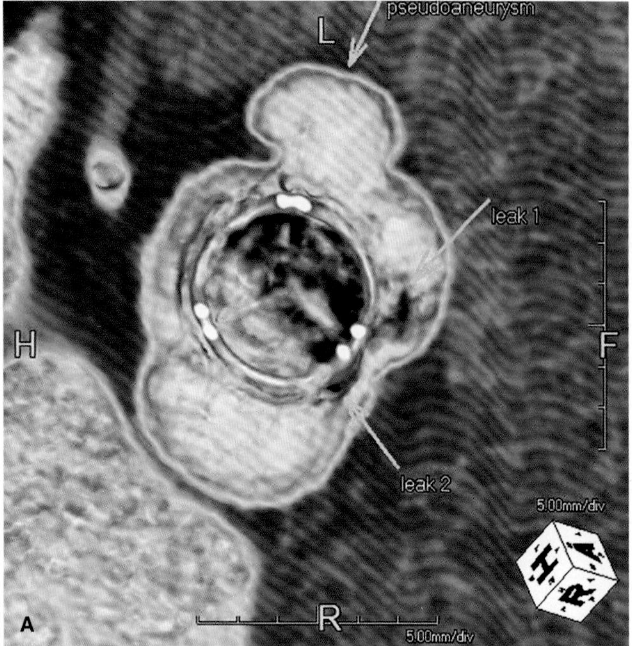

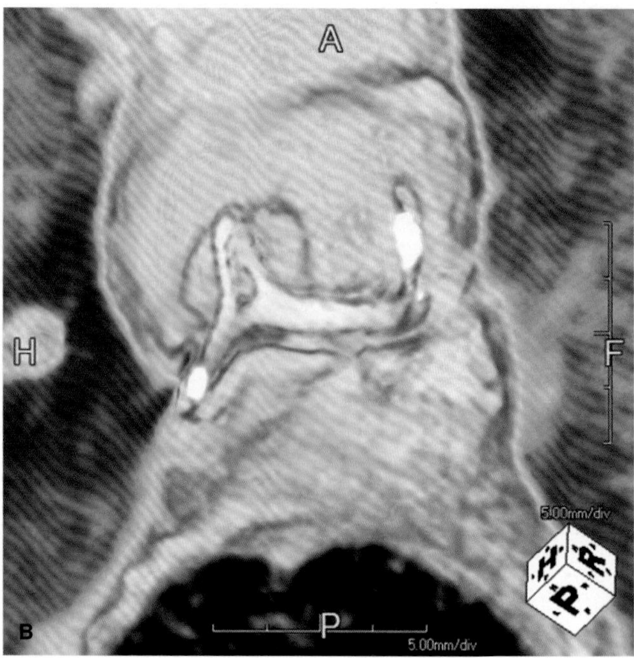

FIGURE 27.33. 3D Reconstructed Images From a Cardiac CTA Showing a Paravalvular Leak and Pseudoaneurysm That Have Developed Around a Bioprosthetic Aortic Valve. *Arrows* highlight the locations of pseudoaneurysm and paravalvular leak. These were presumed to be the result of infection sometime after valve replacement surgery.

Suggested Readings

Attenhofer Jost CH, Connolly HM, Dearani JA, Edwards WD, Danielson GK. Ebstein's anomaly. *Circulation* 2007;115(2):277–285.

Basso C, Perazzolo Marra M, Rizzo S, et al. Arrhythmic mitral valve prolapse and sudden cardiac death. *Circulation* 2015;132(7):556–566.

Baumgartner H, Hung J, Bermejo J, et al; American Society of Echocardiography; European Association of Echocardiography. Echocardiographic assessment of valve stenosis: EAE/ASE recommendations for clinical practice. *J Am Soc Echocardiogr* 2009;22(1):1–23.

Bennett CJ, Maleszewski JJ, Araoz PA. CT and MR imaging of the aortic valve: radiologic-pathologic correlation. *Radiographics* 2012;32(5):1399–1420.

Blanke P, Joseph S, Leipsic J. CT in transcatheter aortic valve replacement. *Radiology* 2013;269(3):650–669.

Bolling SF, Iannettoni MD, Dick M, Rosenthal A, Bove EL. Shone's anomaly: operative results and late outcome. *Ann Thorac Surg* 1990;49(6):887–893.

Cevasco M, Shekar PS. Surgical management of tricuspid stenosis. *Ann Cardiothorac Surg* 2017;6(3):275–282.

Ciarka A, Van de Veire N. Secondary mitral regurgitation: pathophysiology, diagnosis, and treatment. *Heart* 2011;97(12):1012–1023.

Colen TW, Gunn M, Cook E, Dubinsky T. Radiologic manifestations of extra-cardiac complications of infective endocarditis. *Eur Radiol* 2008;18(11):2433–2445.

Davar J, Connolly HM, Caplin ME, et al. Diagnosing and managing carcinoid heart disease in patients with neuroendocrine tumors: an expert statement. *J Am Coll Cardiol* 2017;69(10):1288–1304.

Dhoble A, Chakravarty T, Nakamura M, et al. Outcome of paravalvular leak repair after transcatheter aortic valve replacement with a balloon-expandable prosthesis. *Catheter Cardiovasc Interv* 2017;89(3):462–468.

Elgendy IY, Conti CR. Caseous calcification of the mitral annulus: a review. *Clin Cardiol* 2013;36(10):E27–E31.

Feneis JF, Kyubwa E, Atianzar K, et al. 4D flow MRI quantification of mitral and tricuspid regurgitation: reproducibility and consistency relative to conventional MRI. *J Magn Reson Imaging* 2018. doi: 10.1002/jmri.26040.

Hsiao A, Lustig M, Alley MT, et al. Rapid pediatric cardiac assessment of flow and ventricular volume with compressed sensing parallel imaging volumetric cine phase-contrast MRI. *AJR Am J Roentgenol* 2012;198(3):W250–W259.

Hsiao A, Tariq U, Alley MT, Lustig M, Vasanawala SS. Inlet and outlet valve flow and regurgitant volume may be directly and reliably quantified with accelerated, volumetric phase-contrast MRI. *J Magn Reson Imaging* 2015;41(2):376–385.

Kanwar A, Thaden JJ, Nkomo VT. Management of patients with aortic valve stenosis. *Mayo Clin Proc* 2018;93(4):488–508.

Koo HJ, Yang DH, Oh SY, et al. Demonstration of mitral valve prolapse with CT for planning of mitral valve repair. *Radiographics* 2014;34(6):1537–1552.

Leon MB, Smith CR, Mack M, et al. Transcatheter aortic-valve implantation for aortic stenosis in patients who cannot undergo surgery. *N Engl J Med* 2010;363(17):1597–1607.

Liu J, Frishman WH. Nonbacterial thrombotic endocarditis: pathogenesis, diagnosis, and management. *Cardiol Rev* 2016;24(5):244–247.

Loukas M, Housman B, Blaak C, Kralovic S, Tubbs RS, Anderson RH. Double-chambered right ventricle: a review. *Cardiovasc Pathol* 2013;22(6):417–423.

Maganti K, Rigolin VH, Sarano ME, Bonow RO. Valvular heart disease: diagnosis and management. *Mayo Clin Proc* 2010;85(5):483–500.

Marwick TH, Lancellotti P, Pierard L. Ischaemic mitral regurgitation: mechanisms and diagnosis. *Heart* 2009;95(20):1711–1718.

Murillo H, Restrepo CS, Marmol-Velez JA, et al. Infectious diseases of the heart: pathophysiology, clinical and imaging overview. *Radiographics* 2016;36(4):963–983.

Nishimura RA, Otto CM, Bonow RO, et al. 2017 AHA/ACC Focused Update of the 2014 AHA/ACC Guideline for the Management of Patients With Valvular Heart Disease: A Report of the American College of Cardiology/American Heart Association Task Force on Clinical Practice Guidelines. *Circulation* 2017;135(25):e1159–e1195.

Ordovas KG, Muzzarelli S, Hope MD, et al. Cardiovascular MR imaging after surgical correction of tetralogy of Fallot: approach based on understanding of surgical procedures. *Radiographics* 2013;33(4):1037–1052.

Otto CM, Bonow RO. *Valvular Heart Disease: A Companion to Braunwald's Heart Disease*. 3rd ed. Philadelphia, PA: Elsevier/Saunders; 2015.

Pasic M, Unbehaun A, Buz S, Drew T, Hetzer R. Annular rupture during transcatheter aortic valve replacement: classification, pathophysiology, diagnostics, treatment approaches, and prevention. *JACC Cardiovasc Interv* 2015;8(1):1–9.

Saremi F, Gera A, Ho SY, Hijazi ZM, Sánchez-Quintana D. CT and MR imaging of the pulmonary valve. *Radiographics* 2014;34(1):51–71.

Saremi F, Hassani C, Millan-Nunez V, Sánchez-Quintana D. Imaging evaluation of tricuspid valve: analysis of morphology and function with CT and MRI. *AJR Am J Roentgenol* 2015;204(5):W531–W542.

Schultz CJ, Moelker A, Piazza N, et al. Three dimensional evaluation of the aortic annulus using multislice computer tomography: are manufacturer's guidelines for sizing for percutaneous aortic valve replacement helpful? *Eur Heart J* 2010;31(7):849–856.

Séguéla PE, Houyel L, Acar P. Congenital malformations of the mitral valve. *Arch Cardiovasc Dis* 2011;104(8–9):465–479.

Siegel MJ, Bhalla S, Gutierrez FR, Billadello JB. MDCT of postoperative anatomy and complications in adults with cyanotic heart disease. *Am J Roentgenol* 2005;184(1):241–247.

Sievers HH, Schmidtke C. A classification system for the bicuspid aortic valve from 304 surgical specimens. *J Thorac Cardiovasc Surg* 2007;133(5):1226–1233.

Van Dyck M, Glineur D, de Kerchove L, El Khoury G. Complications after aortic valve repair and valve-sparing procedures. *Ann Cardiothorac Surg* 2013;2(1):130–139.

Vasanawala SS, Hanneman K, Alley MT, Hsiao A. Congenital heart disease assessment with 4D flow MRI. *J Magn Reson Imaging* 2015;42(4):870–886.

Verma S, Siu SC. Aortic dilatation in patients with bicuspid aortic valve. *N Engl J Med* 2014;370(20):1920–1929.

Warnes CA. Bicuspid aortic valve and coarctation: two villains part of a diffuse problem. *Heart* 2003;89(9):965–966.

Wasowicz M, Meineri M, Djaiani G, et al. Early complications and immediate postoperative outcomes of paravalvular leaks after valve replacement surgery. *J Cardiothorac Vasc Anesth* 2011;25(4):610–614.

Webb WR, Higgins CB. *Thoracic Imaging: Pulmonary and Cardiovascular Radiology*. 3rd ed. Lippincott Williams & Wilkins; 2016.

Yalonetsky S, Tobler D, Greutmann M, et al. Cardiac magnetic resonance imaging and the assessment of Ebstein anomaly in adults. *Am J Cardiol* 2011;107(5):767–773.

Zakkar M, Amirak E, Chan KM, Punjabi PP. Rheumatic mitral valve disease: current surgical status. *Prog Cardiovasc Dis* 2009;51(6):478–481.

Zhu D, Bryant R, Heinle J, Nihill MR. Isolated cleft of the mitral valve: clinical spectrum and course. *Tex Heart Inst J* 2009;36:553–556.

CHAPTER 28 ■ NONISCHEMIC CARDIOMYOPATHIES

ELIZABETH WEIHE AND SETH KLIGERMAN

Cardiomyopathies refer to specific diseases of the myocardium, most commonly caused by ischemic heart disease as discussed in Chapter 25. There is however, a wide spectrum of factors unrelated to ischemic heart disease that can lead to cardiomyopathy, including infection, immunologic abnormalities, hemodynamic pathologies, toxic injuries, and genetic factors. This cluster of diverse and sometime rare diseases is referred to as *nonischemic cardiomyopathies*.

Although nonischemic cardiomyopathies have a broad spectrum of causes (Table 28.1), they all have a final common pathway of myocardial injury, which can lead to mechanical and electrical dysfunction and clinical heart failure.

Establishing a diagnosis of nonischemic cardiomyopathy can sometimes be challenging on physical examination, ECG, and echocardiogram, as many of the findings are nonspecific and overlap with ischemic heart disease. Over the last 20 years, cardiac MRI has emerged as a unique and powerful tool that can help establish etiology, evaluate function, and assess extent of disease. Cardiac MRI is now considered the reference standard for assessing chamber size, left ventricular function, and ventricular mass in cardiomyopathies. Tissue characterization techniques, including late gadolinium enhancement, T1 mapping, T2 mapping, T2* mapping, can be utilized to better assess the fibrosis, inflammation, edema, and iron deposition within the heart respectively. However, as cardiac MRI is contraindicated in some patients, ECG-gated cardiac CTA can also serve as a tool to diagnose certain nonischemic cardiomyopathies through detailed evaluation of cardiac function and morphology. Specific imaging features can help determine the underlying etiology of a patient's clinical heart failure and thereby guide management and treatment decision.

This chapter will highlight several of the salient imaging findings associated with various nonischemic cardiomyopathies.

HYPERTROPHIC CARDIOMYOPATHY

Hypertrophic cardiomyopathy (HCM) is an autosomal dominant genetic cardiomyopathy seen in 0.05% to 0.2% of the population and is the leading case of sudden cardiac death in young adults and athletes. Over 900 unique mutations in sarcomere contractile proteins have been identified that lead to early-onset ventricular hypertrophy. This genetic heterogeneity leads to the varied phenotypic expressions seen in patients with HCM.

The imaging hallmark of HCM on cardiac MRI is focal, regional, or diffuse left ventricular hypertrophy with measurements often exceeding 20 mm as measured at end-diastole. The left ventricle is generally not dilated, and the ejection fraction is usually normal or increased, leading to obliteration of the LV cavity during systole. Asymmetric septal involvement is the most common form of HCM, with other variants including apical, symmetric, midventricular, mass-like and noncontiguous HCM (Fig. 28.1).

Histologically, HCM is differentiated from hypertension-related hypertrophy by the presence of myofiber disarray with focal areas of necrosis and subsequent fibrosis, most often seen in the midmyocardium. On late gadolinium-delayed enhancement imaging, this will lead to a classic pattern of hazy midmyocardial enhancement or less frequently as nodular enhancement in the interventricular septum at the RV insertion points (Fig. 28.2). These patterns of enhancement would be atypical for cardiac amyloidosis, as discussed below.

TABLE 28.1

CAUSES OF NONISCHEMIC CARDIOMYOPATHY

Hypertrophic cardiomyopathy
Sarcoidosis
Amyloidosis
Myocarditis
Hemochromatosis
Dilated cardiomyopathy
Stress cardiomyopathy (Takotsubo cardiomyopathy)
Left ventricular noncompaction
Fabry disease
Gaucher disease
Loeffler endocarditis
Mitochondrial abnormalities
Ion channel diseases

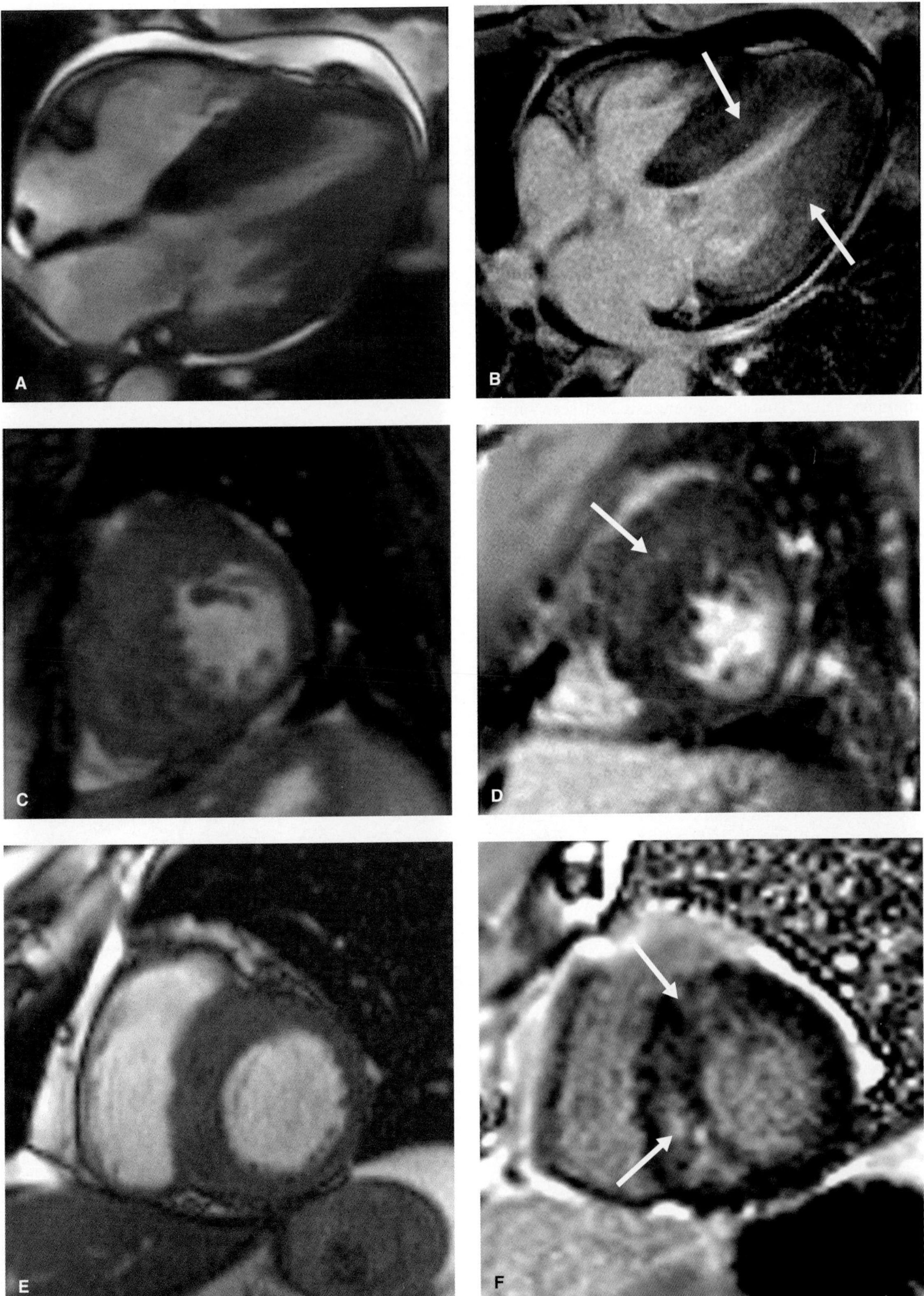

FIGURE 28.1. **Hypertrophic Cardiomyopathy: Focal, Regional, or Diffuse Wall Thickening of the Left Ventricle is the Hallmark of HCM.** Diffuse HCM as seen on four-chamber SSFP view (**A**) involves the entire LV. Corresponding delayed enhancement images show hazy, midmyocardial-delayed enhancement (**B**). Mass-like HCM is seen as irregular focal/regional thickening as seen in the anteroseptal wall on short-axis SSFP view (**C**). Corresponding patchy midmyocardial-delayed enhancement is seen in the region of wall thickening (**D**). Asymmetric septal HCM is the most common variant, most characteristically seen as focal hypertrophy of the anteroseptal and inferoseptal segments at the base of the heart (**E**), again with corresponding patchy foci of midmyocardial-delayed enhancement (**F**).

Delayed enhancement is identified in over 80% of HCM patients and is associated with increased incidence of ventricular tachyarrhythmias, which can lead to sudden cardiac death.

Asymmetric septal HCM is the most common form of HCM, usually involving the anteroseptal segments, most notably at the base of the left ventricle. Approximately 20% to 30% of these patients develop an obstructive form of HCM, sometimes referred to as hypertrophic obstructive cardiomyopathy (HOCM), where narrowing of the left ventricular outflow track (LVOT) by the hypertrophied myocardium causes flow acceleration across the LVOT. This increase in velocity lowers the pressure in the LVOT which causes the mitral valve apparatus to be pulled toward the LVOT during systole. The systolic anterior motion of the mitral valve (SAM) causes further narrowing of the LVOT, worsening obstruction, and has been associated with worse outcomes. Due to the SAM, the mitral leaflets are often pulled open during systole leading to a characteristic mitral regurgitant jet directly posterolaterally toward the left-sided pulmonary veins. This phenomenon is best seen on the three-chamber SSFP cine imaging (Fig. 28.3).

Apical HCM variant is characterized by pronounced ventricular hypertrophy at the LV apex, which leads to the characteristic "spade-like" configuration of the left ventricle on vertical long-axis view of the heart (Fig. 28.4). This HCM variant is associated with hypertension but has an overall better prognosis as it is less commonly associated with sudden cardiac death than septal hypertrophy. However, up to 5 % of all HCMs with left apical involvement develop left apical aneurysms, which increase the risk for thromboembolic disease and the development of clinical heart failure (Fig. 28.5).

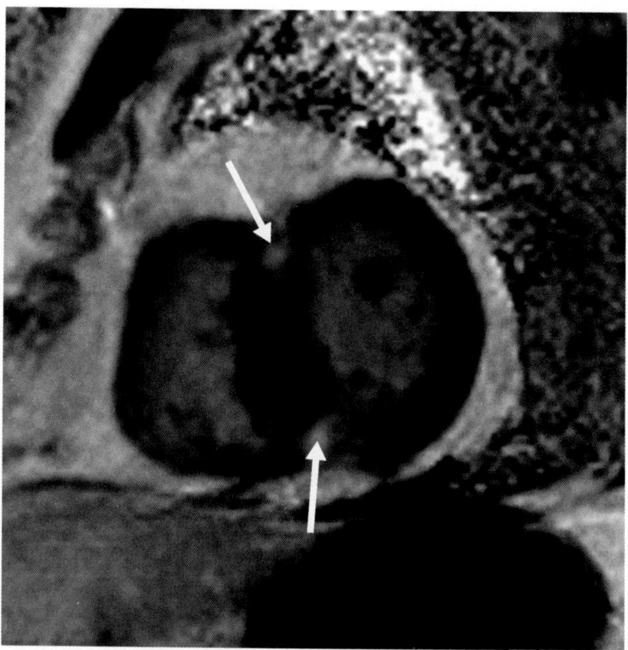

FIGURE 28.2. Short-axis–delayed gadolinium enhancement imaging in a 17-year-old man with hypertrophic cardiomyopathy shows thickening of the anteroseptal and inferoseptal segments with delayed enhancement isolated to the right ventricular insertion points (*arrows*). In HCM, this pattern is much less common than hazy mid-myocardial enhancement.

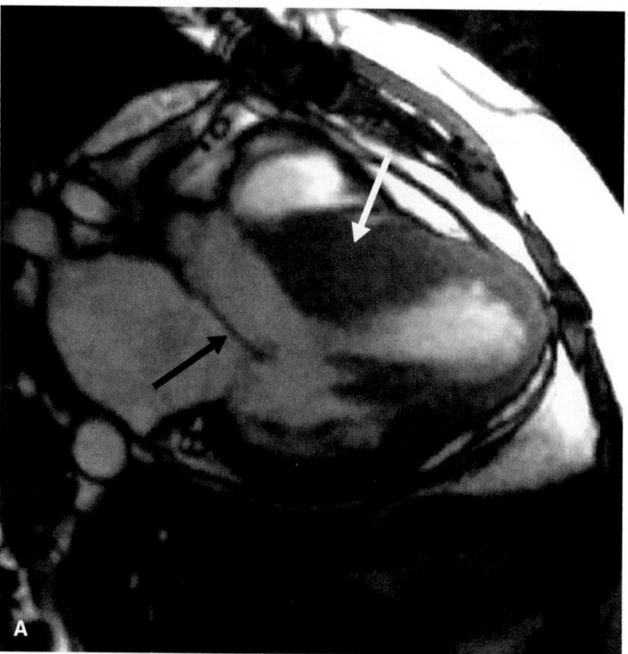

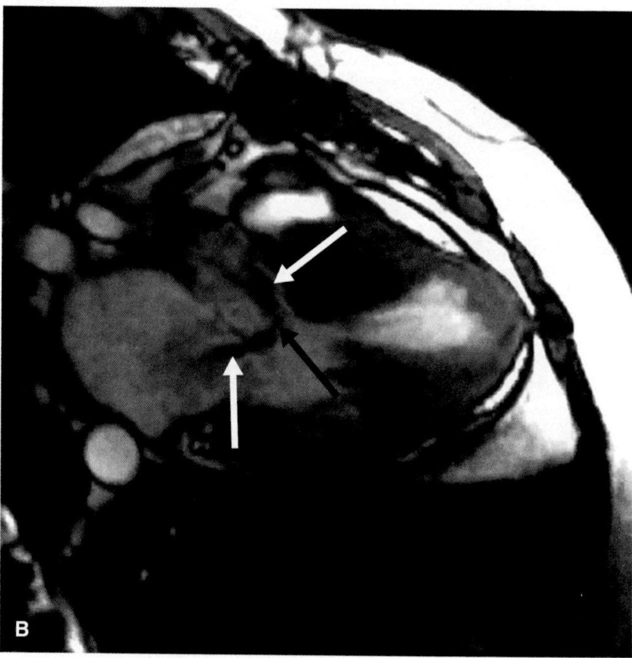

FIGURE 28.3. **Hypertrophic Obstructive Cardiomyopathy (HOCM) in a 48-Year-Old Man. A:** Three-chamber image at the end of diastole shows asymmetric hypertrophy of the basilar septum (*white arrow*). The mitral valve leaflets are closed (*black arrow*), and the aortic valve has yet to open. **B:** Three-chamber image obtained during early systole demonstrates marked narrowing of the left ventricular outflow track (LVOT, *white arrow*) due to two factors. First, the hypertrophied basilar septum contracts and narrows the LVOT. Second, the narrowing increases the velocity of blood across the LVOT, as demarcated by the black dephasing jet (*white arrow*). This increased velocity lowers the pressure in the LVOT. The reduced pressure during systole leads to the anterior leaflet of the mitral valve being sucked toward and narrowing the LVOT (*black arrow*), which is called systolic anterior motion of mitral valve (SAM). In addition, because the SAM causes the mitral valve to be pulled open, a characteristic jet of mitral regurgitation is commonly seen (*red arrow*). LVOT obstruction is a risk factor for cardiovascular death in this patient population.

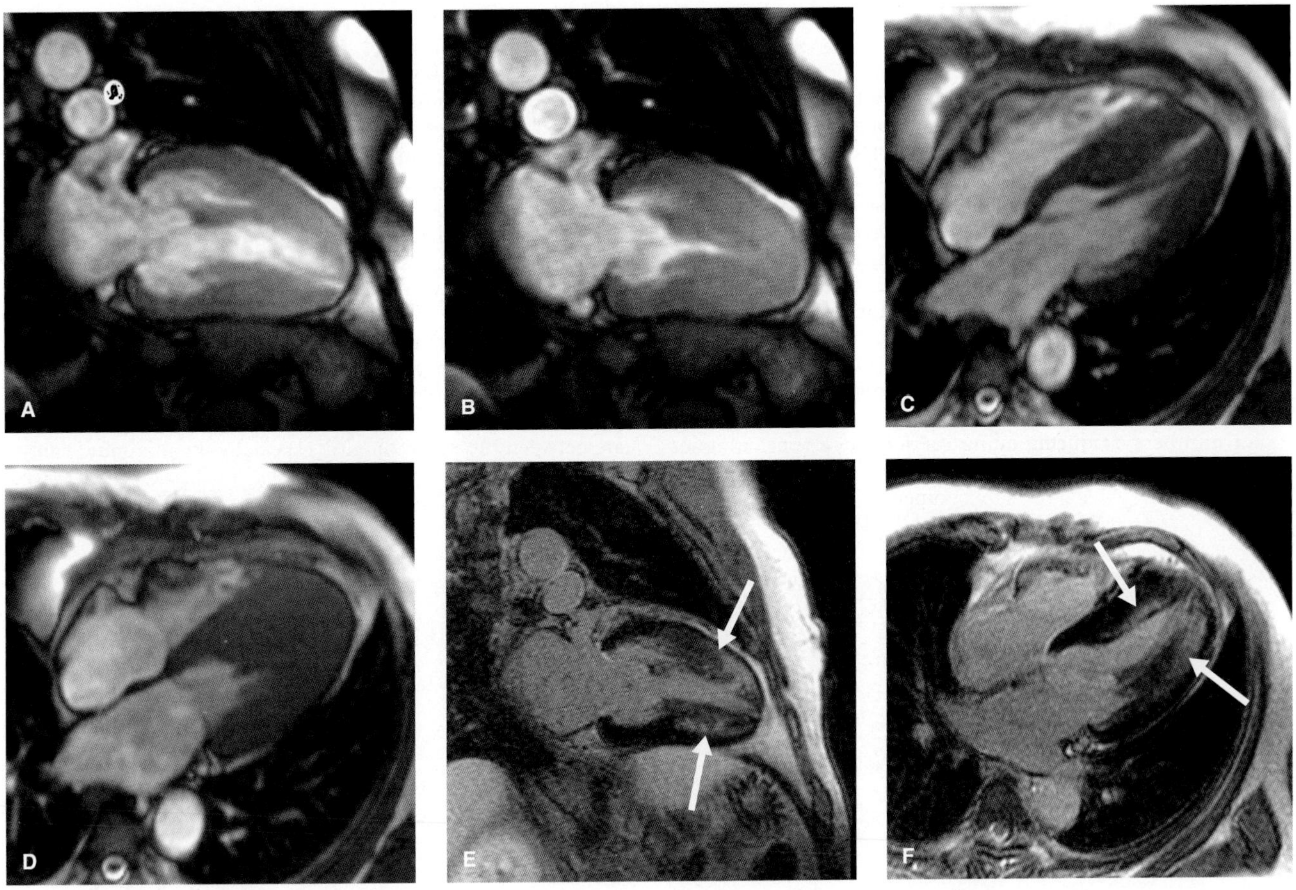

FIGURE 28.4. **Apical Hypertrophic Cardiomyopathy Variant.** Apical HCM variant is characterized by focal thickening of the left ventricular apex, which leads to the "spade-like" configuration of the left ventricle, seen in both two-chamber SSFP imaging (**A, B**) and four-chamber SSPF imaging (**C, D**) during diastole and systole, respectively. **E, F**: Two-chamber (**E**) and four-chamber (**F**) delayed enhancement images show classic hazy, midmyocardial enhancement corresponding to the hypertrophied segments (*arrows*).

In certain instances, HCM may present with diffuse myocardial involvement (Fig 28.1A, B) and may have a morphological appearance nearly identical to some cases of hypertensive heart disease. While the presence of usually severe systemic hypertension and other clinical information can elucidate between etiologies, in some instances patient with HCM can also have hypertension. T1-tissue mapping will usually show higher T1 values in HCM compared to hypertensive disease, but both disease states lead to increased T1 values. The best way to differentiate between the two is the presence of characteristic hazy mid-myocardial delayed enhancement in HCM which will be absent in hypertensive heart disease. If delayed enhancement is absent, differentiation between the two can be quite difficult based on imaging alone.

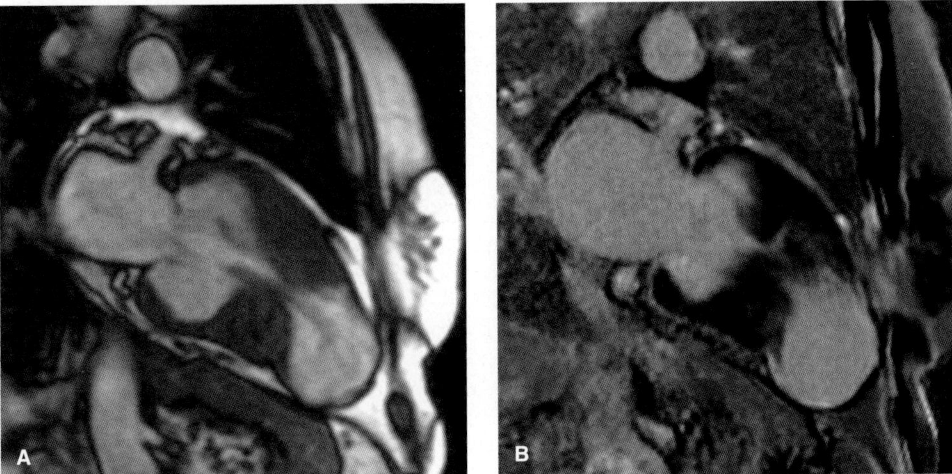

FIGURE 28.5. Two-chamber SSFP (**A**) and delayed enhancement images (**B**) in a man with apical predominant HCM show a large apical aneurysm secondary to increased pressures at the cardiac apex. Delayed enhancement is seen in the thinned left apex. This is a rare finding, occurring in less than 5% of patients with HCM. Compared to patients without apical aneurysm, those with apical aneurysms are at an increased risk of adverse cardiac events.

FABRY DISEASE

Fabry disease is an X-linked disorder which results in the pathologic accumulation of glycosphingolipid within different tissues, including the heart. Clinical and morphologic cardiac manifestations of Fabry disease mimic those of HCM. Compared to HCM, hazy midmyocardial-delayed enhancement is often isolated to the inferolateral segments of the left ventricle despite relatively diffuse hypertrophy (Fig. 28.6).

One of the best ways to differentiate between Fabry disease, HCM, and cardiac amyloidosis, which is discussed below, is through T1-tissue mapping. As detailed in Chapter 24, precontrast T1-tissue mapping maps the native T1 relaxation of myocardium over multiple inversion times using a T1 mapping sequence. Although the exact numbers vary depending on sequence type, magnet strength, and manufacturer, the approximate native T1 values of myocardium at 1.5 T are 950 ± 21 ms and at 3 T are 1,052 ±23 ms. Since fat has a shorter native T1 than myocardium, the lipid accumulation in Fabry disease causes significant shortening of native T1 relaxation with values reported at 853 ± 53 ms at 1.5 T (Fig. 28.6). The other cardiomyopathy with such a low native T1 of myocardium is cardiac iron overload, which has different imaging findings as discussed below.

While Fabry disease causes a reduction in native myocardial T1 values, the myocardial fibrosis and extracellular expansion in HCM and cardiac amyloid lead to an increase in myocardial T1 values. As the degree of fibrosis is usually worse in amyloid than in HCM, patients with amyloid usually have a higher native T1 value of around 1,100 ms at 1.5 T compared to the native T1 value in HCM which is usually around 1,000 ms at 1.5 T. This distinction can help differentiate between these pathologies, especially if gadolinium cannot be used.

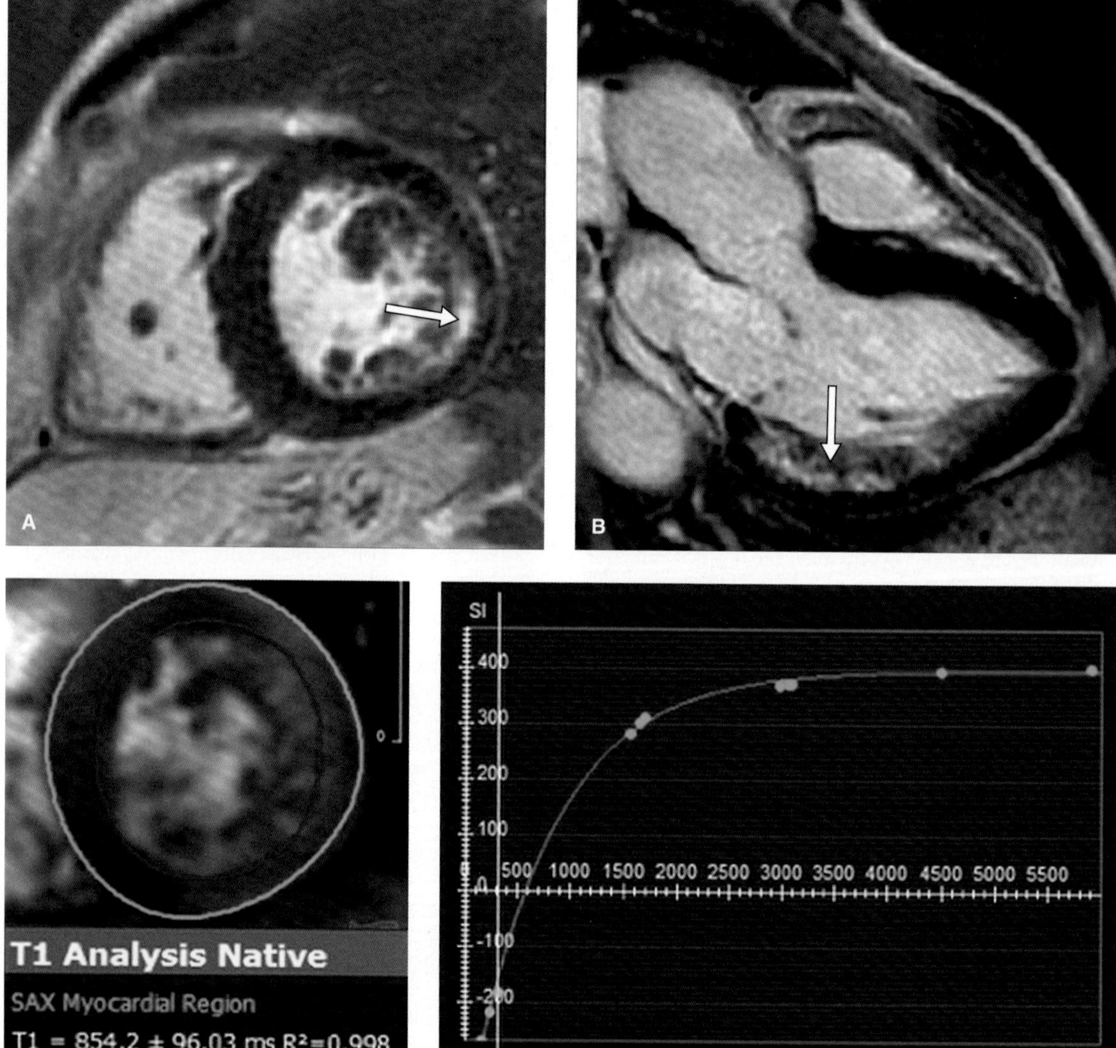

FIGURE 28.6. Fabry Disease. Short-axis (**A**) and three-chamber view (**B**) delayed enhancement imagings show the characteristic midmyocardial-delayed enhancement of the inferolateral left ventricular wall in a patient with known Fabry disease (*arrows*). **C, D:** T1 mapping can be used to help distinguish Fabry disease from HCM. Normal T1 relaxation time of the myocardium at 3 T is around 1,000 ms whereas in this patient with Fabry disease it is 854 ms. Decreased T1 relaxation times in patients with Fabry disease is secondary to intramyocardial lipid deposition within the myocardium, as seen in this patient with Fabry disease with a calculated T1 relaxation timeof 854 ms (**C, D**). T1 values in patient with HCM will be increased.

CARDIAC AMYLOIDOSIS

Cardiac amyloidosis is a restrictive cardiomyopathy that is caused by the random abnormal deposition of extracellular amyloid fibrils within the heart, including within the myocardium, atria, coronary arteries, and valves. This infiltrative process can be caused by a heterogeneous group of disorders with AL amyloidosis being the most common etiology of cardiac amyloidosis. AL amyloidosis is caused by the deposition of fibrils of monoclonal immunoglobulin light chains associated with B-cell dyscrasias such a multiple myeloma. Physiologically, amyloid deposition in the heart leads to thickening of myocardium with impaired myocardial relaxation and diastolic dysfunction. While systolic dysfunction does occur, left ventricular ejection fraction in patients with amyloid is usually only mildly reduced.

Although tissue biopsy is the gold standard for diagnosis as amyloid deposition is established by the presence of apple-green birefringence on polarizing light microscopy, cardiac MRI has become a powerful tool in defining cardiac involvement in cardiac amyloidosis. The imaging hallmark of cardiac amyloidosis is diffuse concentric left ventricular hypertrophy of the myocardium which initially leads to an elevated left ventricular mass index with initial decrease in ventricular volumes. Similar findings can occur in the right ventricle but are less pronounced. Once diastolic and subsequent systolic dysfunction ensues, the ventricular volumes gradually increase in size. Biatrial dilation often is present secondary to increased ventricular pressures from the diastolic dysfunction. Atrial wall thickening can also occur due to amyloid deposition. Pleural and pericardial effusions are also common (Fig. 28.7).

Another clue to the diagnosis of cardiac amyloid is the presence of circumferential subendocardial hypoperfusion on dynamic first pass perfusion sequence obtained during the administration of gadolinium. Approximately 10 minutes after the injection of gadolinium, delayed imaging is obtained to assess for fibrosis. However, in patients with amyloid, the selection of an accurate inversion time to properly null myocardium and assess for scarring can be quite difficult. The deposition of amyloid in the myocardium leads to dramatic expansion of the extracellular space and thus a pronounced increase in the deposition of gadolinium in the myocardium. Due to this, the amount of gadolinium within the myocardium often exceeds or is similar to that in the blood pool. When an inversion scout sequence is obtained, the increased myocardial gadolinium concentration actually causes the myocardial signal to null before or at the same time as the gadolinium in the blood pool. While this can lead to confusion, it is a finding not seen with other cardiomyopathies.

Delayed gadolinium enhancement is most classically described as diffuse subendocardial LV enhancement although sometimes with associated RV and/or atrial wall enhancement. However, linear or patchy foci of enhancement of the subendocardial, midmyocardial, or subepicardial enhancement can also be observed. The constellation of findings of circumferential left ventricular hypertrophy with diffuse subendocardial hypoperfusion and delayed enhancement in the setting of biatrial enlargement, diastolic dysfunction, and abnormal T1 kinetics before (T1-tissue mapping) and after (abnormal myocardial nulling) the administration of contrast can allow one to reliably make the diagnosis of cardiac amyloid on MRI (Figs. 28.7 and 28.8).

LOEFFLER ENDOCARDITIS

Hypereosinophilic syndrome (HES) is defined by peripheral blood eosinophilia which can lead to multiple system dysfunction and damage. The classic cardiac manifestation of HES is known as Loeffler endocarditis. Cardiac involvement begins with eosinophilic infiltration into the endocardium with necrosis, followed by the thrombotic stage where thrombus forms on the damaged endocardium and the later stage where endomyocardial fibrosis and scarring of the chordae tendonae occurs.

Loeffler endocarditis is a restrictive cardiomyopathy which can involve one or both ventricles. On delayed enhancement sequences, a classic circumferential subendocardial pattern of fibrosis is present corresponding to the eosinophilic destruction of this portion of the myocardium. While this pattern can mimic that seen with cardiac amyloidosis, the presence of adherent ventricular thrombi, appearing as areas of low signal of delayed enhancement imaging, helps to differentiate. Over time, this subendocardial fibrosis leads to obliteration of the ventricular cavity and a restrictive cardiomyopathy (Fig. 28.9).

DILATED CARDIOMYOPATHIES

Nonischemic-dilated cardiomyopathies are characterized by cardiac chamber dilation coupled with impaired contractility of the left ventricle or both the left ventricle and right ventricle. Approximately 50% of dilated cardiomyopathies are idiopathic or genetic in origin; however, there are a wide range of secondary etiologies including ischemia, post myocarditis, toxic/metabolic triggers, peripartum cardiomyopathy, drug toxicity, infiltrative disease, and connective tissue disorders. Idiopathic-dilated cardiomyopathies are typically seen in younger patients

Dilated cardiomyopathies all have increased systolic and diastolic volumes with decreased ejection fractions. Ventricular thickness is often mildly thinned to normal and is associated with increased end-diastole volumes, greater than 140 mL for the LV and greater than 150 mL for the RV, indexed to body surface area. SSPF cine imaging is used to assess global or regional ventricular dysfunction and decreased LV and/or RV ejection fractions.

Given the variable histologic appearance seen in nonischemic-dilated cardiomyopathy, delayed gadolinium enhancement is often not seen. If present, it characteristically appears as thin, linear midmyocardial enhancement most often involving the interventricular septum. Studies have shown the presence of delayed enhancement within the midmyocardium is associated with increased mortality and increased number of significant arrhythmic events (Fig. 28.10).

ARRHYTHMOGENIC RIGHT VENTRICULAR CARDIOMYOPATHY

Arrhythmogenic right ventricular cardiomyopathy (ARVC) also referred to as arrhythmogenic right ventricular dysplasia (ARVD). ARVC is usually transmitted with an autosomal dominant pattern, although incomplete penetrance and limited phenotypic expression likely contributes to an underdiagnosis of disease within families. ARVC accounts for 5% of the cases of sudden cardiac death in the patients less than 35 years old, and therefore the diagnosis is aggressively pursued so treatment can be initiated as soon as possible.

The diagnosis of ARVC is made by presence of major and minor criteria defined in 1994 and revised in 2010, where ECG findings, genetic testing, family history, biopsy, and noninvasive imaging all aid in the diagnosis. Although these criteria are very specific, they lack sensitivity particularly in patients with incomplete expression of the disease.

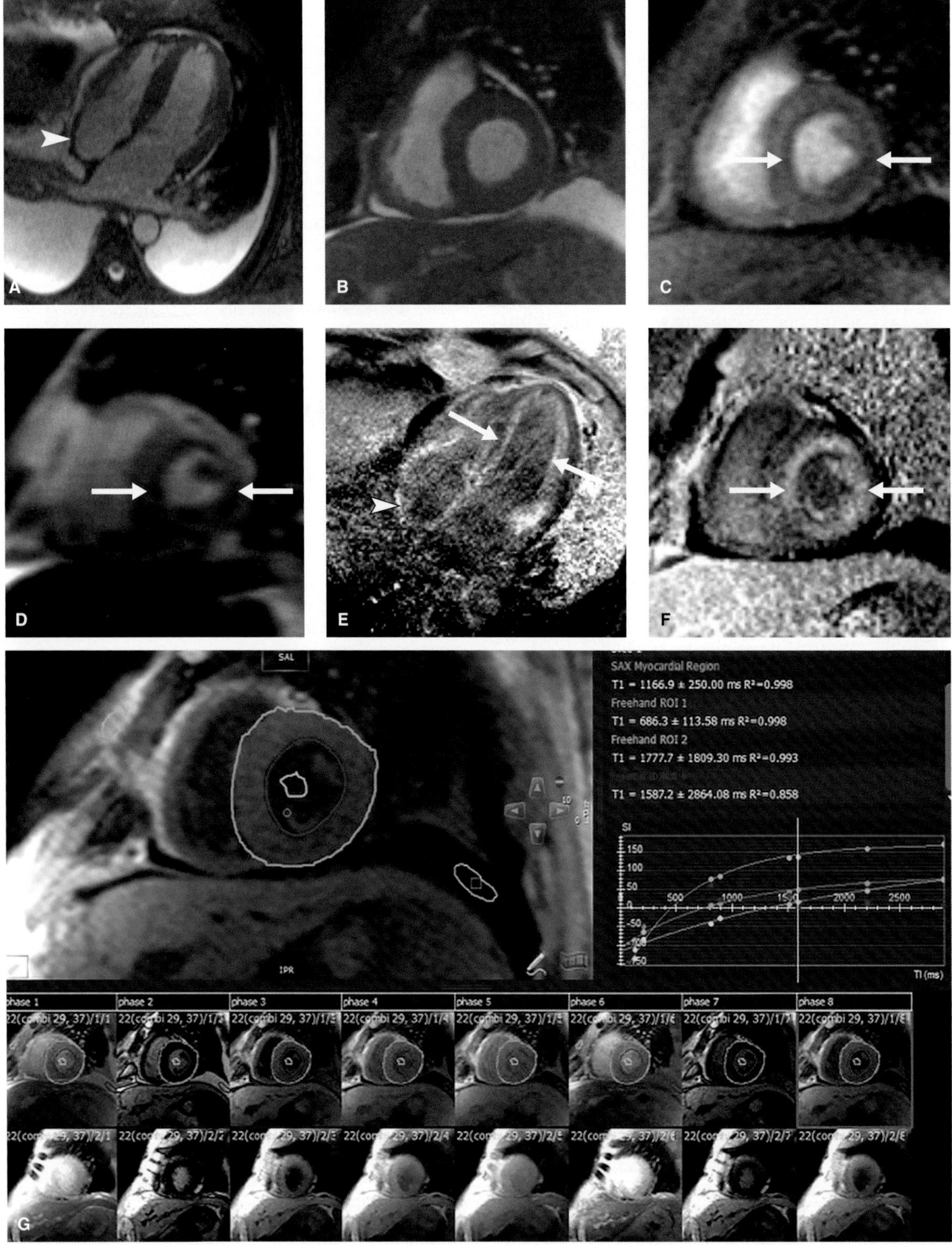

FIGURE 28.7. **Cardiac Amyloidosis in a 60-Year-Old Man With Diastolic Dysfunction. A, B:** Four-chamber (**A**) and short-axis images through the base of the left ventricle (**B**) obtained during diastole show biventricular hypertrophy and biatrial enlargement. In addition, the wall of the right atrium is thickened (**A**, *arrowhead*). Large bilateral pleural effusions are present. **C:** First-pass perfusion image through the same level as (**B**) shows circumferential subendocardial hypoperfusion (*arrows*). **D:** Image from a TI inversion scout sequence obtained at 180 ms shows that the myocardium, especially the subendocardial layer, is nulled (*arrows*). However, the blood pool is still bright and has yet to null. In nearly all other normal and pathologic states, the blood pool will null before the myocardium. **E, F:** Four-chamber (**E**) and short-axis (**F**) LGE images show the classic subendocardial-delayed enhancement pattern (*arrows*). Notice the enhancement of the right atrial wall (**E**, *arrowhead*) due to amyloid deposition corresponding to the areas of thickening seen in (**A**). Mild right ventricular subendocardial LGE is also present. **G:** Precontrast T1 mapping in a patient with known cardiac amyloidosis is calculated by plotting a decay curve of signal intensity of the myocardium at multiple inversion times. Normal T1 relaxation time of the myocardium at 1.5 T is around 950 ms. In this patient with known cardiac amyloidosis, the precontrast T1 relaxation time was 1,167 ms.

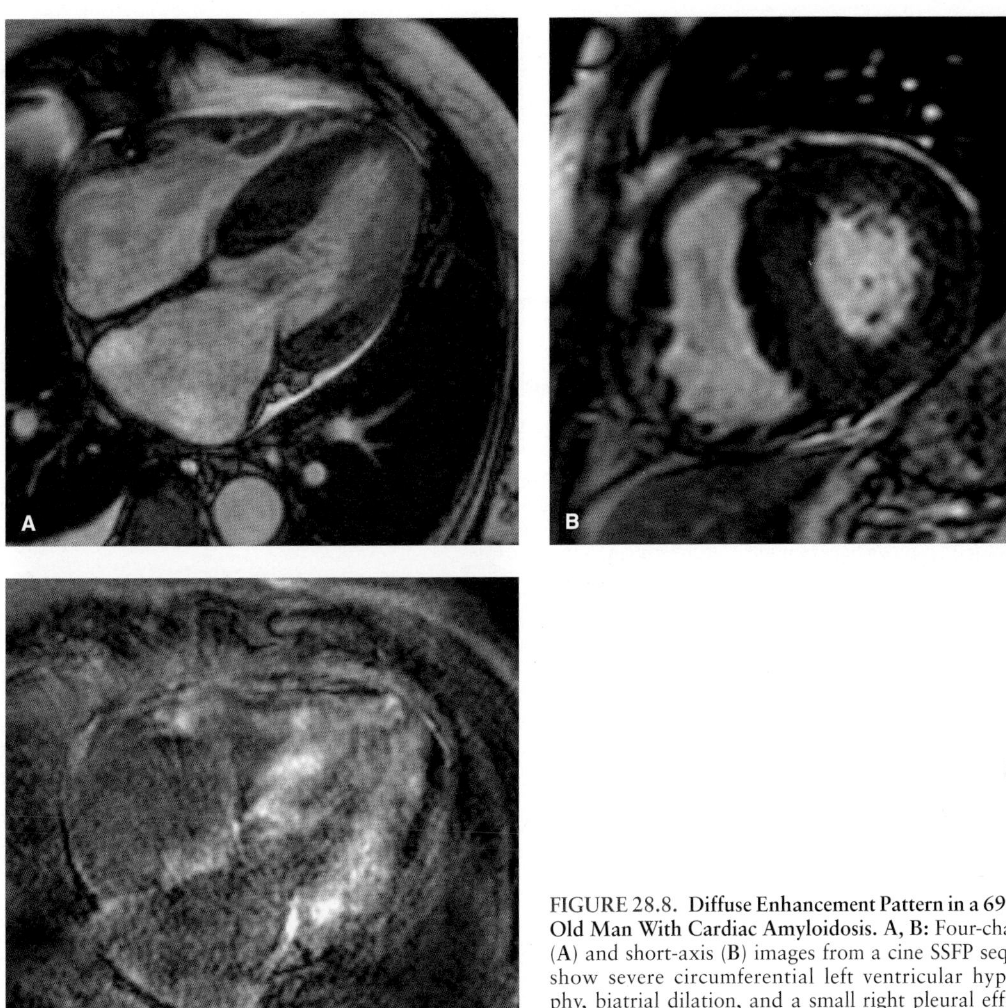

FIGURE 28.8. **Diffuse Enhancement Pattern in a 69-Year-Old Man With Cardiac Amyloidosis. A, B:** Four-chamber (**A**) and short-axis (**B**) images from a cine SSFP sequence show severe circumferential left ventricular hypertrophy, biatrial dilation, and a small right pleural effusion. **C:** Four-chamber–delayed gadolinium enhancement image shows diffuse biventricular and biatrial enhancement. Endomyocardial biopsy confirmed cardiac amyloidosis.

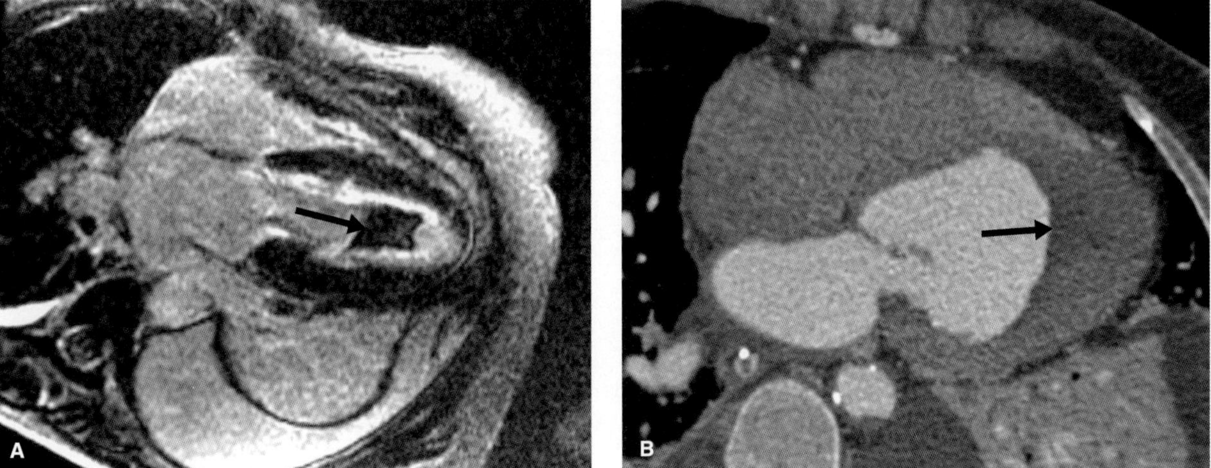

FIGURE 28.9. **Loeffler Endocarditis.** Classic diffuse subendocardial-delayed enhancement of left ventricle is seen in Loeffler endocarditis, with adherent thrombi detected as low-signal intensity on delayed enhancement imaging (**A**, *arrow*). Over time, the subendocardial fibrosis leads to the obliteration of the LV cavity, as seen on the CT scan of a second patient with Loeffler endocarditis (*arrow*), ultimately resulting in a restrictive cardiomyopathy (**B**).

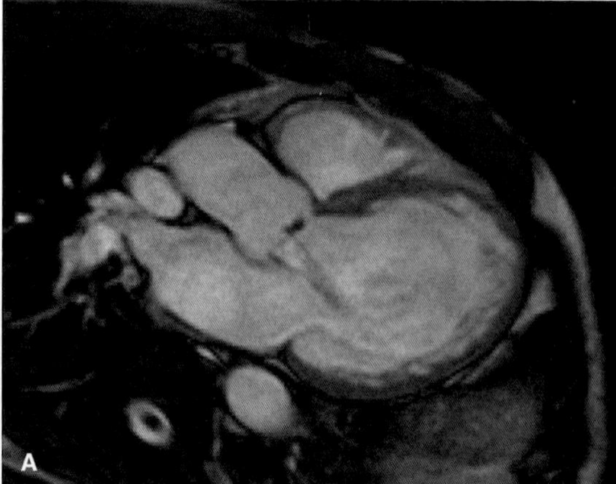

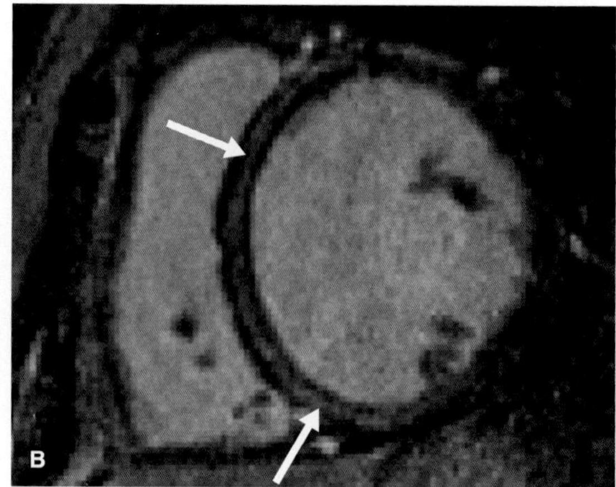

FIGURE 28.10. **Nonischemic-Dilated Cardiomyopathy.** SSFP imaging of the LVOT shows mild dilation of the right left ventricle with normal to mildly thinned left ventricular myocardium (**A**) in a patient with a nonischemic-dilated cardiomyopathy. Delayed enhancement is commonly absent in those with nonischemic-dilated cardiomyopathy. However when present, it is most commonly seen in a linear midmyocardial distribution (**B**, *arrows*).

Cardiac MRI can detect morphologic and functional changes in the right ventricle, including right ventricular dilation, reduced RV ejection fraction, and focal areas of RV dyskinesia leading to small "aneurysms." These findings are often best seen on RVOT and four-chamber SSFP cine imaging. These regional wall motion abnormalities in the right ventricle remain the most reliable features of early ARVC. Fibrofatty replacement of the right ventricular myocardium does occur but is often not seen until later in the course of disease. In addition, it is now recognized that areas of macroscopic fat can be seen in the RV in patients without ARVC. Because of this, the presence of myocardial fat on MRI is not considered a major or minor criterion to make the diagnosis of ARVC. Similarly, while delayed gadolinium enhancement is seen in the right ventricle in 60% to 70% of patients with confirmed ARVC, it is also not considered a criterion for diagnosis by MRI (Fig. 28.11).

Although ARVC/ARVD is classically described as a RV predominant disease, genetic testing and imaging advantage has increased our awareness of the LV dominant and biventricular phenotypes of the disease. In excess of 75% of ARVC have LV involvement in the advance disease. Delayed enhancement of the LV most often involves inferior and lateral LV wall in a subepicardial and midmyocardial distribution.

MYOCARDITIS

Myocarditis is focal inflammation of the myocardium, most commonly triggered by a viral infection and can lead to a new dilated cardiomyopathy in an otherwise healthy patient. Acute myocarditis can present as chest pain, hemodynamic instability, and ischemic-like ECG changes, mimicking acute myocardial infarction. Although the patients are typically

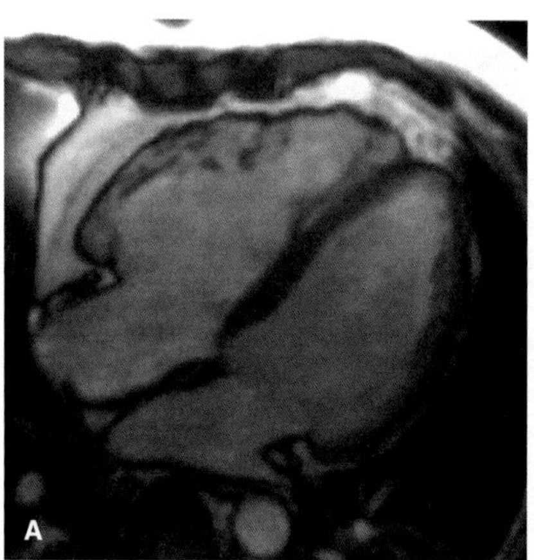

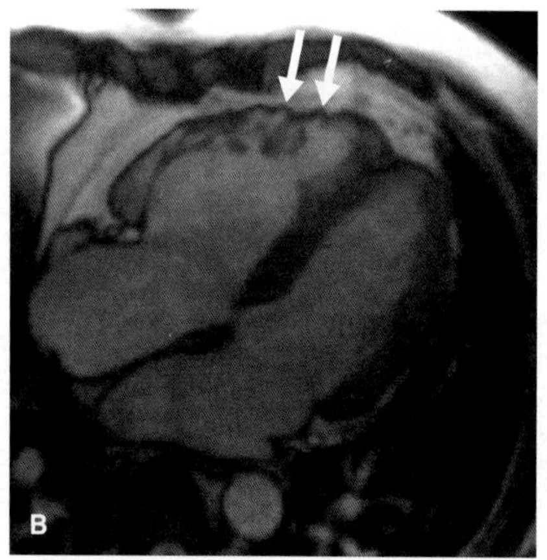

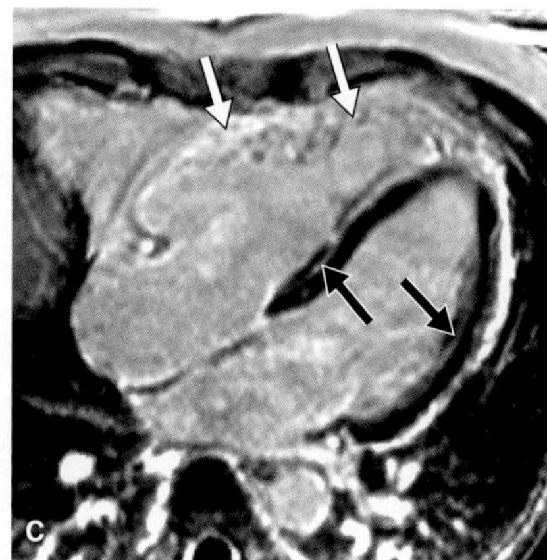

FIGURE 28.11. **Arrhythmogenic Right Ventricular Cardiomyopathy (ARVC) in a 34-Year-Old Woman Revived After an Incidence of Ventricular Fibrillation Arrest. A, B:** Four-chamber SSFP images during diastole (**A**) and systole (**B**) show a dilated RV with a reduced ejection fraction of 32%. The ratio of the patient's RV end-diastolic volume (RV-EDV) to body surface area (BSA) was significantly elevated at 133 mL/m^2. Additionally, there are multiple small dyskinetic foci on the free wall of the best seen on systole (*arrows*, **B**). This constellation of findings would equate to one major criterion in the diagnosis of ARVC. A definitive diagnosis requires the presence of two major, one major and two minor, or four minor criteria which are based on imaging, pathologic, and physiologic abnormalities as well as family history. **C:** In this more advanced case of ARVC, delayed enhancement along the free wall of the right ventricle (*white arrows*) with additional foci of involvement in the interventricular septum (*black arrow*) and lateral aspect of the left ventricle (*black arrow*). While delayed enhancement is commonly seen in cases of ARVC, it is not a criterion for its diagnosis.

younger with fewer coronary risk factors, often times emergent coronary catheterization is performed to exclude ischemic heart disease.

Cardiac MR is often performed in symptomatic patients with a clinical suspicion for myocarditis. In the acute inflammatory phase, T2-weighted images can demonstrate global or regional areas of increased intensity to signify myocardial edema. While myocardial edema can be visually assessed, it can also be quantitatively measured. When the average signal of myocardium is twice that of skeletal muscle as measured on T2-weighted nonfat saturated images, a diagnosis of myocardial edema can be made. In addition, global relative enhancement can be quantified by comparing the ratio of myocardial to skeletal muscle enhancement on precontrast and early postcontrast T1-weighted images. An abnormal global relative enhancement ratio is defined as greater than 3.2:1 and occurs secondary to acute cell membrane rupture which leads to increased intracellular gadolinium deposition. On delayed enhancement imaging, patchy nodular and/or linear enhancement is present in a subepicardial and midmyocardial distribution. It can often involve the right ventricle as well. Subendocardial enhancement is uncommon but can occur. However, it will not correspond to a vascular territory like that seen with infarct. Adjacent pericardial enhancement due to pericardial inflammation can occur allowing one to diagnosis myopericarditis (please refer to Chapter 29). The presence of two of the three above criteria (myocardial edema ratio, global relative enhancement, characteristic delayed enhancement pattern) allow one to reliably make the diagnosis of myocarditis.

While delayed gadolinium enhancement in cases of myocarditis can signify expansion of the extracellular space due to myocardial fibrosis, it can also represent intracellular gadolinium deposition due to myocyte cell membrane disruption. This is an important distinction as fibrosis is permanent while injured myocytes can heal. Therefore, a follow-up cardiac MR a few weeks after diagnosis is recommended as it can differentiate between the two. Delayed enhancement that persists or resolves on follow-up imaging represents areas of fibrosis or repaired myocardium, respectively. This is important as the presence of fibrosis is a predictor of all-cause mortality and cardiac mortality in patients with biopsy-proven viral myocarditis (Fig. 28.12).

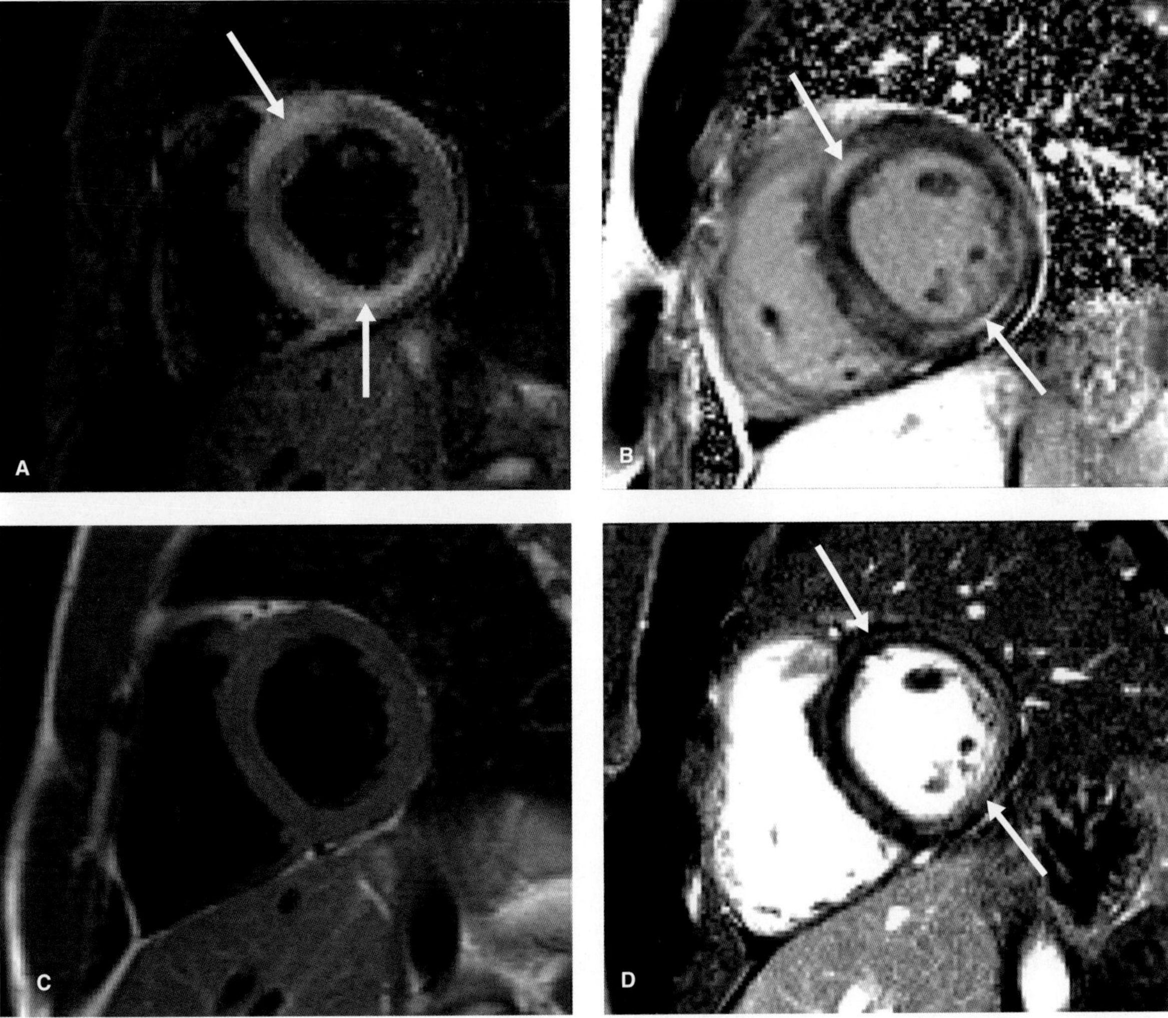

FIGURE 28.12. **Myocarditis in a 17-year-old man with chest pain, elevated troponin levels, and a normal coronary angiogram.** During the acute inflammatory stage myocarditis, increased signal is seen in the anterior, septal, and inferior walls of the left ventricle on this T2W fat saturation image through the mid-cavity of the left ventricle (**A**) signifying edema (*arrows*). Relatively diffuse linear midmyocardial and subepicardial delayed enhancement is present (**B**, *arrows*), compatible with the diagnosis of acute myocarditis. In the acute setting of myocarditis, delayed gadolinium enhancement can be secondary to acute myocyte injury and/or scarring. **C.** Follow up imaging 4 months later reveals resolution of the previously seen edema on T2-weighted imaging. **D.** In addition, there has been a decrease in delayed enhancement. Residual areas of linear midmyocaridal enhancement represent permanent fibrosis (*arrows*).

CARDIAC SARCOIDOSIS

Sarcoidosis is a systemic inflammatory disorder characterized by the deposition of noncaseating nonnecrotic granulomas in the affected organs. On autopsy, 20% to 60% of patients have histologic changes of cardiac sarcoid, but only about 5% of patients have the clinical manifestations associated with cardiac sarcoidosis, which include heart failure, arrhythmias, electrical conduction disorders, or sudden cardiac death. A diagnosis of cardiac sarcoid is confirmed either by the presence of noncaseating granulomas on endomyocardial biopsy or clinical criteria which include abnormalities on the ECG, cardiac echo, cardiac MRI, and radionuclide imaging.

During the inflammatory/early phase of cardiac sarcoid, focal wall thickening can be seen on SSFP or T1-weighted imaging. Edema (best seen with T2-weighted sequences) and regional wall motion abnormalities can occur. Delayed enhancement is extremely variable with biventricular linear and/or nodular lesions occurring predominantly in a subepicardial/midmyocardial distribution. Transmural enhancement can occur but is uncommon. As the disease progresses, increased fibrosis and scarring occurs, resulting in focal wall thinning and additional wall motion abnormalities (Fig. 28.13).

The cardiac MR findings of sarcoidosis can look identical to those of myocarditis, so it is important to correlate with patient's history and to identify other associated findings in the chest such as mediastinal lymphadenopathy or characteristic parenchymal changes. Cardiac sarcoid, especially in its late stages, can mimic ischemic cardiomyopathy with wall thinning and transmural enhancement although the enhancement of sarcoid usually does not correspond to a vascular territory and foci of subepicardial and midmyocardial are often present. In addition, right ventricular–delayed enhancement, relatively uncommon in ischemic cardiomyopathy, usually exists. Finally, cardiac sarcoidosis can present with RV predominant involvement mimicking ARVC (Fig. 28.14). Endomyocardial biopsy may be needed to differentiate.

LEFT VENTRICULAR NONCOMPACTION

Left ventricular noncompaction (LVNC) is a genetically heterogeneous disease seen in both pediatric and adult populations, where the normal morphogenesis of myocardial tissue into compact myocardium is disrupted. This leads to highly trabeculated left ventricular myocardium and ultimately can cause heart failure, arrhythmias, and sudden cardiac death.

MRI allows for optimal visualization of the left ventricular myocardium. Hypertrabeculation spares the septum but often involves the anterolateral, and inferolateral segments at the base and mid-cavity levels and much of the cardiac apex. On cine SSPF imaging, a ratio of greater than 2.3:1 of noncompacted to compacted left ventricular myocardium at end-diastole is suggestive of LVNC. The compacted myocardium in LVNC is often quite thin and systolic function is usually decreased in regions of hypertrabeculation. Delayed enhancement is more commonly detected in older children/adults and is seen both in areas of hypertrabeculation and in the adjacent midmyocardium (Fig. 28.15).

While the diagnosis should be straightforward, debate exists in making the diagnosis in asymptomatic patients, especially in athletes, with normal left ventricular function. In one large study looking at over 1,000 athletes, over 8% of healthy

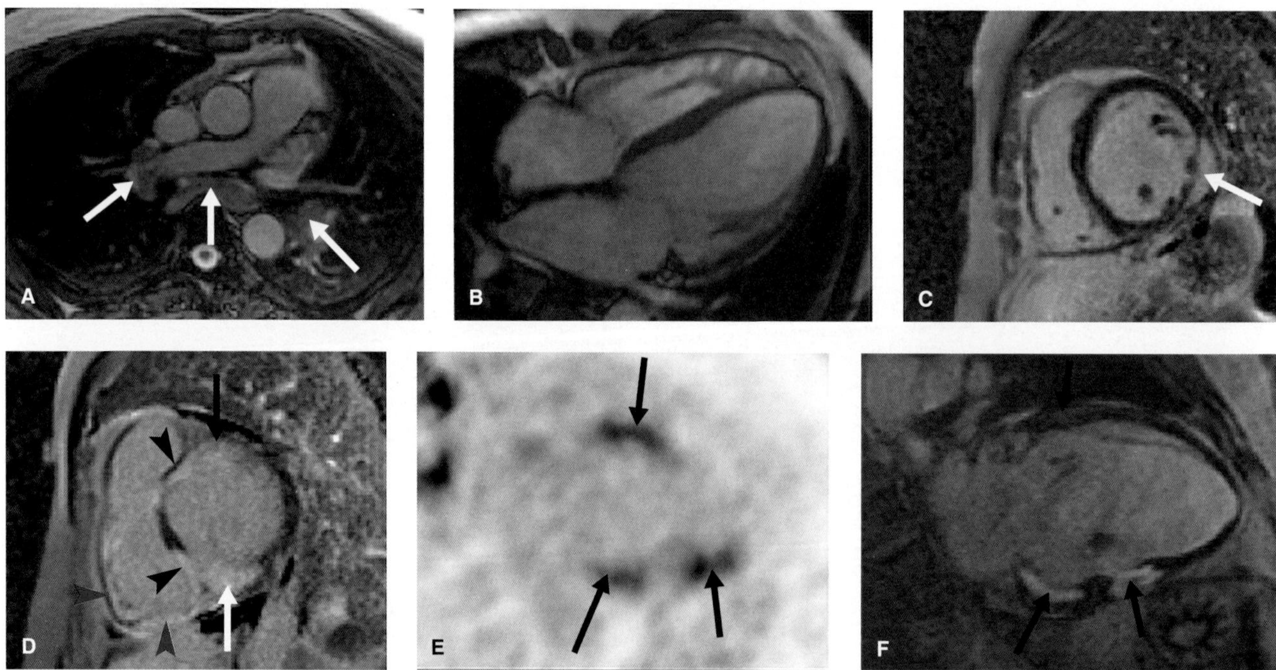

FIGURE 28.13. **Cardiac Sarcoidosis.** Bilateral mediastinal and hilar adenopathy is seen on scout imaging (**A**, *white arrows*) in patient with known sarcoidosis, who was being evaluated for cardiac involvement. On SSFP four-chamber imaging, the left ventricle is mildly dilated (**B**), which is nonspecific but compatible with decreased systolic function as seen on echocardiogram. Corresponding delayed enhancement imaging confirms the diagnosis of cardiac sarcoidosis with nodular midmyocardial delayed enhancement primary involving the inferolateral segment at the mid cavity level (**C**, *white arrow*). At the base (**D**) there is more extensive delayed enhancement in the inferior (*white arrow*), inferoseptal (*white arrowhead*), anteroseptal (*black arrowhead*), and anterior (*black arrow*) segments of the left ventricle which is nearly transmural in some areas. In addition, there is robust-delayed enhancement involving the right ventricle (*red arrowheads*). Cardiac FDG PET scan also be used to diagnose cardiac sarcoid as patchy/focal areas of myocardial uptake are seen along the anterior and inferior left ventricular wall (**E**, *arrows*), which correspond to focal-delayed enhancement seen on two-chamber view of the previous cardiac MRI (**F**, *arrows*).

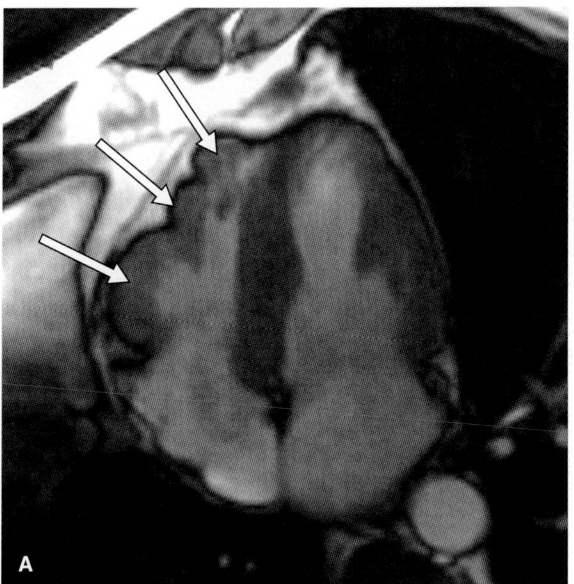

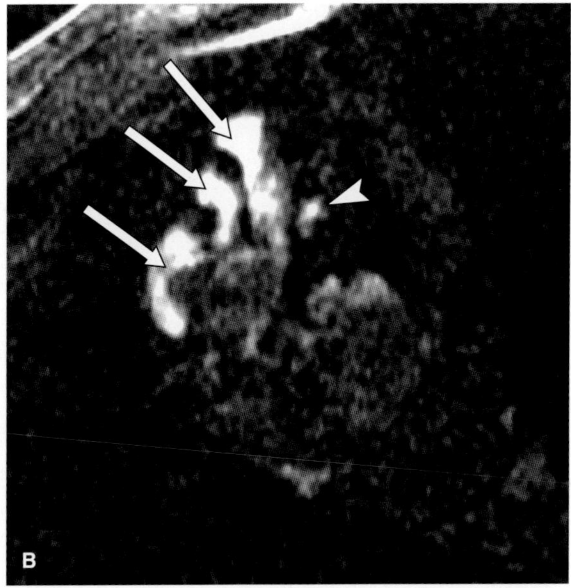

FIGURE 28.14. **Sarcoid Mimicking ARVC in a 48-Year-Old Man. A:** Four-chamber SSFP image obtained during systole shows multiple dyskinetic areas along the RV free wall. The right ventricular ejection fraction and end-diastolic volumes were normal. **B:** Delayed enhancement image obtained at the same level as (**A**) shows intense enhancement in the RV wall (*white arrows*). Additionally, there were areas of delayed enhancement in the left ventricle (*arrowhead*). Biopsy revealed multiple noncaseating granulomas consistent with sarcoidosis.

asymptomatic athletes met the diagnostic criteria for LVNC. However, when athletes with hypertrabeculation were compared to patients with LVNC, those with LVNC demonstrated a significantly increased LV end-diastolic volume and reduced LV ejection fraction (EF: 46.3% vs. 60.3%). Therefore, caution should be made in making the diagnosis in asymptomatic patients with normal ejection fraction and no delayed enhancement.

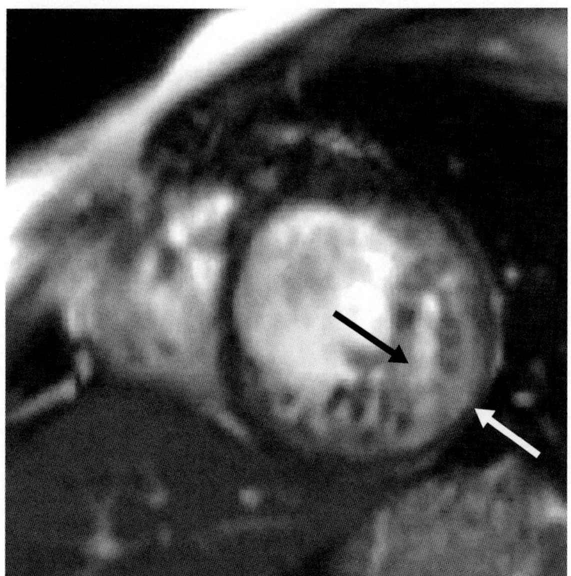

FIGURE 28.15. **Left ventricular noncompaction (LVNC).** Short-axis image in end-diastole at the midcavity level in a 28-year-old woman with LVNC shows hypertrabeculation of the inferolateral left ventricular wall (*black arrow*) with relative thinning of the adjacent compacted myocardium (*white arrow*). The ratio of noncompacted:-compacted myocardium is 4.5:1, much greater than the 2.3:1 ratio used as the cutoff for diagnosis.

STRESS-INDUCED (TAKOTSUBO) CARDIOMYOPATHY

Takotsubo cardiomyopathy, also known as apical ballooning syndrome or "broken heart" syndrome, is stress-induced cardiomyopathy, most frequently seen in postmenopausal women after a severe emotional or physical event. Patients present with acute-onset heart failure and ECG changes mimicking acute coronary syndrome but lack any signs of ischemic heart disease on left heart catheterization. The hallmark of the disease is a transient hypokinesis or akinesis of the mid and apical segments of the left ventricle with hypercontractility of the basilar segments. This ultimately leads to the hallmark configuration of the left ventricle, resembling a *takotsubo,* a Japanese pot used to catch octopi.

SSFP functional imaging shows characteristic ballooning of the left ventricular apex. T2-weighted imaging on cardiac MRI can demonstrate signal abnormality/edema in the regions of wall motion abnormalities and extends across vascular territories. However, the edema often resolves within 2 weeks of symptom onset, which is in contrast to STEMI and myocarditis where it can persist 2 to 3 months after the cardiac event. Typically, no perfusion defects or delayed enhancements are seen in patients with Takotsubo cardiomyopathy, which again also helps differentiate this entity from ischemic heart disease and acute myocarditis (Fig. 28.16).

IRON OVERLOAD CARDIOMYOPATHY

Iron overload cardiomyopathy occurs secondary to iron deposition in the myocardium, either related to genetic disorders of iron metabolism or increased circulating iron related to transfusion. This can lead to either dilated or restrictive phenotypes

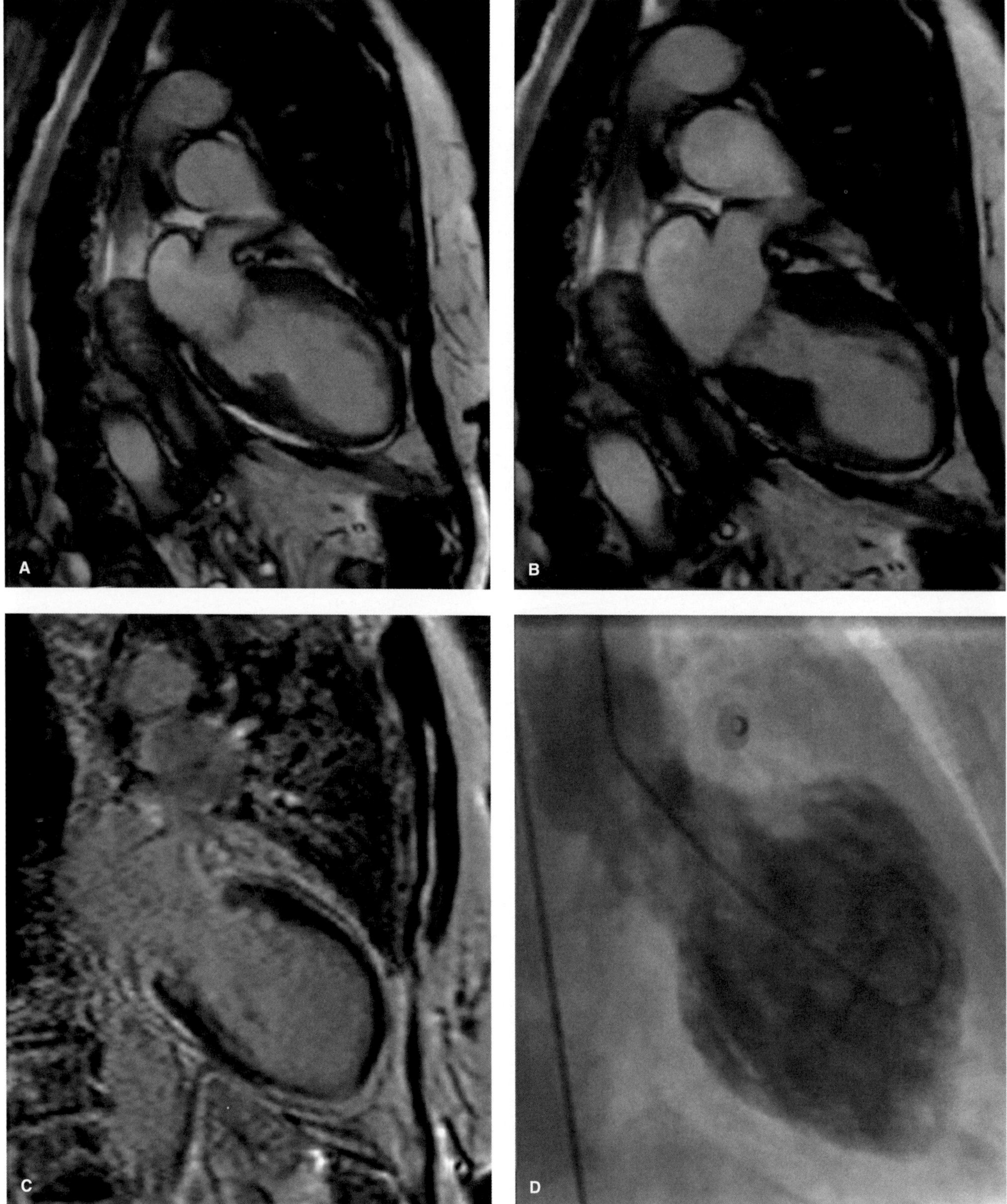

FIGURE 28.16. **Stress-Induced/Takotsubo Cardiomyopathy in a 55-Year-Old Woman Who Accidentally Ran Over Her Dog.** The relative hyperkinesis of the left ventricular base and hypokinesis of the left ventricular mid cavity and apex leads to the characteristic apical ballooning seen between end-diastole (**A**) and end-systole (**B**) on two-chamber SSPF imaging in a patient with Takotsubo cardiomyopathy. No corresponding areas of delayed enhancement are often detected (**C**). Ventriculogram (**D**) performed during cardiac catheterization demonstrates the characteristic appearance of a *takotsubo*, a Japanese octopus pot, at end-systole in the cardiac cycle.

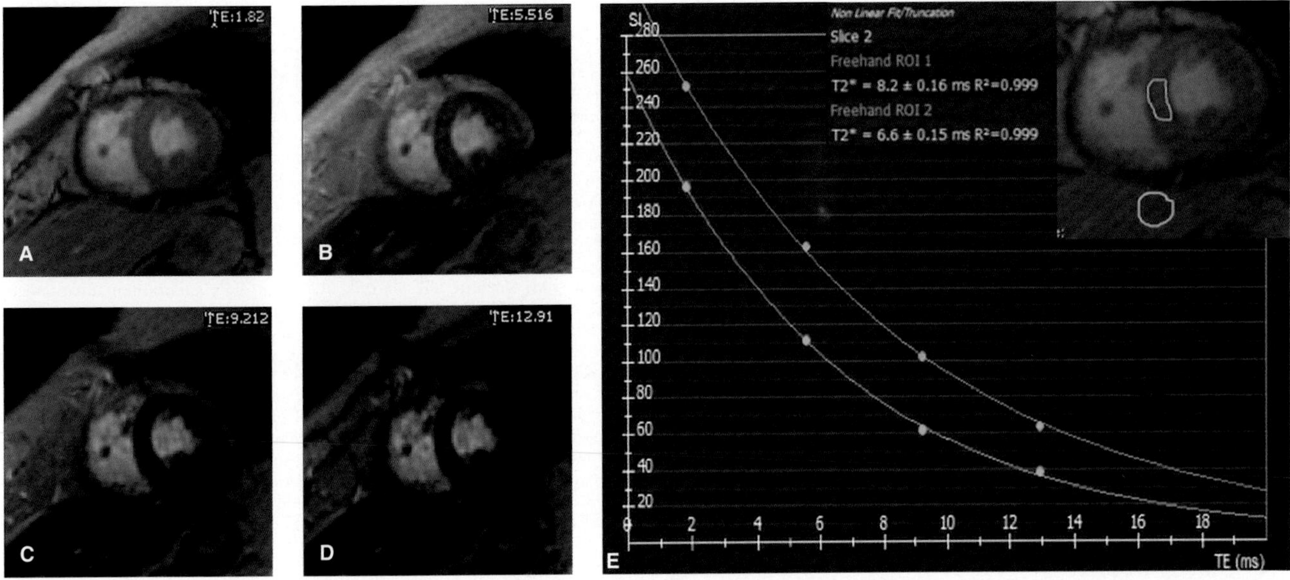

FIGURE 28.17. **Iron Overload Cardiomyopathy.** Gradient echo sequences of a patient with iron overload cardiomyopathy are performed at different echo times (TE) on images. **A–D:** Regions of interest as drawn over the heart and liver at each time point to determine the signal intensity (SI). The inherent decay curve (E) allows for the calculation of the T2* relaxation time. T2* relaxation time of the heart was 8 ms and the liver was 7 ms, signifying severe deposition of iron in both the myocardium and liver in a patient with known primary hemochromatosis.

of iron overload cardiomyopathy, ultimately resulting in clinical heart failure, conduction abnormalities, and pulmonary hypertension.

Cardiac MR T2* mapping can be used for quantitative assessment of iron deposition as iron deposition generates local field inhomogeneities which result in T2* shortening. T2* values >20 ms are considered within normal range (normal mean 40 ms), with T2* values 10 to 20 ms indicating mild to moderate iron loading and T2* values <10 ms indicating severe iron loading, thereby helping risk stratify patients at risk for heart failure and arrhythmias (Fig. 28.17).

Suggested Readings

Alfakih K, Plein S, Thiele H, Jones T, Ridgway JP, Sivananthan MU. Normal human left and right ventricular dimensions for MRI as assessed by turbo gradient echo and steady-state free precession imaging sequences. *J Magn Reson Imaging* 2003;17(3):323–329.

Anderson LJ. Assessment of iron overload with T2* magnetic resonance imaging. *Prog Cardiovasc Dis* 2011;54(3):287–294.

Arbustini E, Weidemann F, Hall JL. Left ventricular noncompaction: a distinct cardiomyopathy or a trait shared by different cardiac diseases? *J Am Coll Cardiol* 2014;64(17):1840–1850.

Assomull RG, Lyne JC, Keenan N, et al. The role of cardiovascular magnetic resonance in patients presenting with chest pain, raised troponin, and unobstructed coronary arteries. *Eur Heart J* 2007;28(10):1242–1249.

Banypersad SM, Moon JC, Whelan C, Hawkins PN, Wechalekar AD. Updates in cardiac amyloidosis: a review. *J Am Heart Assoc* 2012;1(2):e000364.

Belloni E, Cobelli FD, Esposito A, et al. MRI of cardiomyopathy. *AJR Am J Roentgenol* 2008;191(6):1702–1710.

Bluemke DA. MRI of nonischemic cardiomyopathy. *AJR Am J Roentgenol* 2010;195(4):935–940.

Chao BH, Cline-Parhamovich K, Grizzard JD, Smith TJ. Fatal Loeffler's endocarditis due to hypereosinophilic syndrome. *Am J Hematol* 2007;82(10):920–923.

Choudhury L, Mahrholdt H, Wagner A, et al. Myocardial scarring in asymptomatic or mildly symptomatic patients with hypertrophic cardiomyopathy. *J Am Coll Cardiol* 2002;40(12):2156–2164.

Chu WC, Au WY, Lam WW. MRI of cardiac iron overload. *J Magn Reson Imaging* 2012;36(5):1052–1059.

Chun EJ, Choi SI, Jin KN, et al. Hypertrophic cardiomyopathy: assessment with MR imaging and multidetector CT. *Radiographics* 2010;30(5):1309–1328.

Corrado D, Link MS, Calkins H. Arrhythmogenic right ventricular cardiomyopathy. *N Engl J Med* 2017;376(1):61–72.

Cury RC, Abbara S, Sandoval LJ, et al. Images in cardiovascular medicine. Visualization of endomyocardial fibrosis by delayed-enhancement magnetic resonance imaging. *Circulation* 2005;111(9):115–117.

Dabir D, Child N, Kalra A, et al. Reference values for healthy human myocardium using a T1 mapping methodology: results from the International T1 Multicenter cardiovascular magnetic resonance study. *J Cardiovasc Magn Reson* 2014;16:69.

De Cobelli F, Esposito A, Belloni E, et al. Delayed-enhanced cardiac MRI for differentiation of Fabry's disease from symmetric hypertrophic cardiomyopathy. *AJR Am J Roentgenol* 2009;192(3):W97–W102.

Dote K, Sato H, Tateishi H, Uchida T, Ishihara M. Myocardial stunning due to simultaneous multivessel coronary spasms: a review of 5 cases. *J Cardiol* 1991;21(2):203–214.

Elliott P, McKenna WJ. Hypertrophic cardiomyopathy. *Lancet* 2004;363(9424):1881–1891.

Eriksson MJ, Sonnenberg B, Woo A, et al. Long-term outcome in patients with apical hypertrophy cardiomyopathy. *J Am Coll Cardiol* 2002;39(4):638–645.

Felker GM, Thompson RE, Hare JM, et al. Underlying causes and long-term survival in patients with initially unexplained cardiomyopathy. *N Engl J Med* 2000;342(15):1077–1084.

Feng D, Edwards WD, Oh JK, et al. Intracardiac thrombosis and embolism in patients with cardiac amyloidosis. *Circulation* 2007;116(21):2420–2426.

Fernandez-Perez GC, Aguilar-Arjona JA, de la Fuente GT, et al. Takotsubo cardiomyopathy: assessment with cardiac MRI. *AJR Am J Roentgenol* 2010;195(2):W139–W145.

Friedrich MG, Sechtem U, Schultz-Menger J, et al. Cardiovascular magnetic resonance in myocarditis: A JACC White Paper. *J Am Coll Cardiol* 2009;53(17):1475–1487.

Gati S, Chandra N, Bennett RL, et al. Increased left ventricular trabeculation in highly trained athletes: do we need more stringent criteria for the diagnosis of left ventricular non-compaction in athletes? *Heart* 2013;99(6):401–408.

Goitein O, Matetzky S, Beinart R, et al. Acute myocarditis: noninvasive evaluation with cardiac MRI and transthoracic echocardiography. *AJR Am J Roentgenol* 2009;192(1):254–258.

Grün S, Schumm J, Greulich S, et al. Long-term follow up of biopsy-proven viral myocarditis: predictors of mortality and incomplete recovery. *J Am Coll Cardiol* 2012;59(18):1604–1615.

Gulati A, Jabbour A, Ismail TF, et al. Association of fibrosis with mortality and sudden cardiac death in patients with nonischemic dilated cardiomyopathy. *JAMA* 2013;309(9):896–908.

Hansen MW, Merchant N. MRI of hypertrophic cardiomyopathy: part I, MRI appearances. *AJR Am J Roentgenol* 2007;189(6):1335–1343.

Hunold P, Schlosser T, Eggebrecht H, et al. Myocardial late enhancement in contrast-enhanced cardiac MRI: distinction between infarction scar and non-infarction-related disease. *AJR Am J Roentgenol* 2005;184(5):1420–1426.

Ismail TF, Prasad SK, Pennell DJ. Prognostic importance of late gadolinium enhancement cardiovascular magnetic resonance in cardiomyopathy. *Heart* 2012;98(6):438–442.

Jain A, Tandri H, Calkins H, Bluemke DA. Role of cardiovascular magnetic resonance imaging in arrhythmogenic right ventricular dysplasia. *J Cardiovasc Magn Reson* 2008;10:32.

Jassal DS, Nomura CH, Neilan TG, et al. Delayed enhancement cardiac MR imaging in noncompaction of left ventricular myocardium. *J Cardiovasc Magn Reson* 2006;8(3):489–491.

Jeudy J, Burke AP, White CS, Kramer GB, Frazier AA. Cardiac sarcoidosis: the challenge of radiologic-pathologic correlation: from the radiologic pathology archives. *Radiographics* 2015;35(3):657–679.

Kirk P, Roughton M, Porter JB, et al. Cardiac T2* magnetic resonance for prediction of cardiac complications in thalassemia major. *Circulation* 2009;120(20):1961–1968.

Kremastinos DT, Farmakis D. Iron overload cardiomyopathy in clinical practice. *Circulation* 2011;124(20):2253–2263.

Kwong RY, Heydari B, Abbasi S, et al. Characterization of cardiac amyloidosis by atrial late gadolinium enhancement using contrast-enhanced cardiac magnetic resonance imaging and correlation with left atrial conduit and contractile function. *Am J Cardiol* 2015;116(4):622–629.

Laissy JP, Hyafil F, Feldman LJ, et al. Differentiating acute myocardial infarction from myocarditis: diagnostic value of early- and delayed-perfusion cardiac MR imaging. *Radiology* 2005;237(1):75–82.

Maceira AM, Joshi J, Prasad SK, et al. Cardiovascular magnetic resonance in cardiac amyloidosis. *Circulation* 2005;111(2):186–193.

Mahrholdt H, Goedecke C, Wagner A, et al. Cardiovascular magnetic resonance assessment of human myocarditis: a comparison to histology and molecular pathology. *Circulation* 2004;109(10):1250–1258.

Marcus FI, McKenna WJ, Sherrill D et al. Diagnosis of arrhythmogenic right ventricular cardiomyopathy/dysplasia: proposed modification of the Task Force Criteria. *Circulation* 2010;121(13):1533–1541.

Maron BJ. Hypertrophic cardiomyopathy: a systematic review. *JAMA* 2002;287(10):1308–1320.

Moon JC, McKenna WJ, McCrohon JA, Elliott PM, Smith GC, Pennell DJ. Toward clinical risk assessment in hypertrophic cardiomyopathy with gadolinium cardiovascular magnetic resonance. *J Am Coll Cardiol* 2003;41(9):1561–1567.

Moon JC, Mogensen J, Elliott PM, et al. Myocardial late gadolinium enhancement cardiovascular magnetic resonance in hypertrophic cardiomyopathy caused by mutations in troponin I. *Heart* 2005;91(8):1036–1040.

Moon JC, Sachdev B, Elkington AG, et al. Gadolinium enhanced cardiovascular magnetic resonance in Anderson-Fabry disease. Evidence for a disease specific abnormality of the myocardial interstitium. *Eur Heart J* 2003;24(23):2151–2155.

Morita H, Rehm HL, Menesses A, et al. Shared genetic causes of cardiac hypertrophy in children and adults. *N Engl J Med* 2008;358(18):1899–1908.

Murphy DT, Shine SC, Cradock A, Galvin JM, Keelan ET, Murray JG. Cardiac MRI in arrhythmogenic right ventricular cardiomyopathy. *AJR Am J Roentgenol* 2010;194(4):W299–W306.

Oechslin E, Jenni R. Left ventricular noncompaction revisited: a distinct phenotype with genetic heterogeneity? *Eur Heart J* 2011;32(12):1446–1456.

Ordovas KG, Higgins CB. Delayed contrast enhancement on MR images of myocardium: past, present, and future. *Radiology* 2011;261(2):358–374.

Patel AR, Kramer CM. Role of cardiac magnetic resonance in the diagnosis and prognosis of nonischemic cardiomyopathy. *JACC Cardiovasc Imaging* 2017;10(10 Pt A):1180–1193.

Peritz DC, Vaugh A, Ciocca M, Chung EH. Hypertrabeculation vs left ventricular noncompaction on echocardiogram: a reason to restrict athletic participation. *JAMA Intern Med* 2014;174(8):1379–1382.

Petersen SE, Selvanayagam JB, Wiesmann F, et al. Left ventricular non-compaction: insights from cardiovascular magnetic resonance imaging. *J Am Coll Cardiol* 2005;46(1):101–105.

Pica S, Sado DM, Maestrini V, et al. Reproducibility of native myocardial T1 mapping in the assessment of Fabry disease and its role in early detection of cardiac involvement by cardiovascular magnetic resonance. *J Cardiovasc Magn Reson* 2014;16:99.

Puntmann VO, Carr-White G, Jabbour A, et al. T1-mapping and outcome in nonischemic cardiomyopathy: all-cause mortality and heart failure. *JACC Cardiovasc Imaging* 2016;9(1):40–50.

Richardson P, McKenna W, Bristow M, et al. Report of the 1995 World Health Organization/International Society and Federation of Cardiology Task Force on the definition and classification of cardiomyopathies. *Circulation* 1996;93(5):841–842.

Rowin EJ, Maron BJ, Haas TS, et al. Hypertrophic cardiomyopathy with left ventricular apical aneurysm: implications for risk stratifications and management. *J Am Coll Cardiol* 2017;69(7):761–773.

Salanitri GC. Endomyocaridal fibrosis and intracardiac thrombus occurring in idiopathic hypereosinophilic syndrome. *AJR Am J Roentgenol* 2005;184(5):1432–1433.

Salemi VM, Rochitte CE, Shiozaki AA, et al. Late gadolinium enhancement magnetic resonance imaging in the diagnosis and prognosis of endomyocardial fibrosis patients. *Circ Cardiovasc Imaging* 2011;4(3):304–311.

Sen-Chowdhry S, Syrris P, Ward D, Asimaki A, Sevdalis E, McKenna WJ. Clinical and genetic characterization of families with arrhythmogenic right ventricular dysplasia/cardiomyopathy provides novel insights into patterns of disease expression. *Circulation* 2007;115(13):1710–1720.

Tandri H, Castillo E, Ferrari VA, et al. Magnetic resonance imaging of arrhythmogenic right ventricular dysplasia: sensitivity, specificity, and observer variability of fat detection versus functional analysis of the right ventricle. *J Am Coll Cardiol* 2006;48(11):2277–2284.

Tandri H, Friedrich MG, Calkins H, Bluemke DA. MRI of arrhythmogenic right ventricular cardiomyopathy/dysplasia. *J Cardiovasc Magn Reson* 2004;6(2):557–563.

Tavora F, Cresswell N, Li L, Ripple M, Solomon C, Burke A. Comparison of necropsy finding in patients with sarcoidosis dying suddenly from cardiac sarcoidosis versus dying suddenly from other causes. *Am J Cardiol* 2009;104(4):571–577.

Teraoka K, Hirano M, Ookubo H, et al. Delayed contrast enhancement of MRI in hypertrophic cardiomyopathy. *Magn Reson Imaging* 2004;22(2):155–161.

te Riele AS, Tandri H, Bluemke DA. Arrhythmogenic right ventricular cardiomyopathy (ARVC): cardiovascular magnetic resonance update. *J Cardiovasc Magn Reson* 2014;16:50.

van den Boomen M, Slart RHJA, Hulleman EV, et al. Native T1 reference values for nonischemic cardiomyopathies and populations with increased cardiovascular risk: a systemic review and meta-analysis. *J Magn Reson Imaging* 2018;47(4):891–912.

vanden Driesen RI, Slaughter RE, Strugnell WE. MR findings in cardiac amyloidosis. *AJRAm J Roentgenol* 2006;186(6):1682–1685.

Vasaiwala SC, Finn C, Delpriore J, et al. Prospective study of cardiac sarcoid mimicking arrhythmogenic right ventricular dysplasia. *J Cardiovasc Electrophysiol* 2009;20(5):473–476.

Vignaux O, Dhote R, Duboc D, et al. Detection of myocardial involvement in patients with sarcoidosis applying T2-weighted, contrast-enhanced, and cine magnetic resonance imaging: initial results of a prospective study. *J Comput Assist Tomogr* 2002;26(5):762–767.

Vogelsberg H, Mahrholdt H, Deluigi CC, et al. Cardiovascular magnetic resonance in clinically suspected cardiac amyloidosis: noninvasive imaging compared to endomyocardial biopsy. *J Am Coll Cardiol* 2008;51(10):1022–1030.

Wu AH. Management of patients with non-ischemic cardiomyopathy. *Heart* 2007;93(3):403–408.

Yilmaz A, Ferreira V, Klingel K, Kandolf R, Neubauer S, Sechtem U. Role of cardiovascular magnetic resonance imaging (CMR) in the diagnosis of acute and chronic myocarditis. *Heart Fail Rev* 2013;18(6):747–760.

Zuccarino F, Vollmer I, Sanchez G, Navallas M, Pugliese F, Gayete A. Left ventricular noncompaction: imaging findings and diagnostic criteria. *AJR Am J Roentgenol* 2015;204(5):W519–W530.

CHAPTER 29 ■ IMAGING OF THE PERICARDIUM

SETH KLIGERMAN

ANATOMY AND NORMAL APPEARANCE ON IMAGING

The pericardium is a two-layer, fibrous sac that surrounds the heart which is composed of two layers. The innermost layer is the visceral pericardium that lines the epicardial surface of the heart. It is separated from the outermost portion of the myocardium by a layer of epicardial fat which can vary in thickness. The parietal pericardium is composed of two layers. The inner layer of the parietal pericardium and visceral pericardium, both of which are lined by mesothelial cells, form the serous pericardium. These two serous layers are attached and adherent to one another at or near sites of attachments of the great vessels to the heart. The potential space where visceral and parietal serous layers are not attached is the pericardial cavity. The mesothelial cells of both serous layers secrete a small amount of fluid into the pericardial space to lubricate the cavity and therefore the space normally contains 15 to 35 mL of pericardial fluid. This serous pericardium is encased in the outermost layer of the parietal pericardium, the fibrous pericardium. The fibrous pericardium is attached to the mesothelial layer of the parietal pericardium and is composed of various layers of collagen and elastic fibers. Peripheral to those layers lays the epipericardial connective tissue layer containing large bundles of collagen which form parts of the pericardial ligaments which loosely anchor the pericardium to the manubrium, xiphoid process, and central tendon of the diaphragm. Superiorly, the fibrous layer continues over the aortic arch where it blends with the deep cervical fascia.

On chest radiography (CXR), the pericardium usually cannot be visualized. However, certain disease processes, which will be discussed later, can lead to visualization of the pericardium on CXR but this evaluation is limited compared to cross-sectional imaging.

On computed tomography (CT), the pericardium is best visualized anterior to the anterior wall of the right ventricle where it is outlined by both epicardial and mediastinal fat (Figs. 29.1 and 29.2). Although there may be certain areas where it is not well seen, it is present except for rare circumstances. Normally, the pericardium appears as a thin 1 to 2 mm thick curvilinear band of soft tissue surrounding the heart which extends superior to inferiorly from the great vessels to diaphragmatic surface, respectively. A pericardial thickness greater than 4 mm in diameter is considered abnormal. However, since fluid is often found in the pericardial sac, it is important not to confuse an effusion with pericardial thickening although the delineation between the two may be difficult. Fluid in numerous pericardial sinuses and recesses, as discussed below, is common and should not be mistaken for pathology.

On MRI, the parietal pericardium will appear as a low-signal line surrounded by bright epicardial and mediastinal fat on T1- and T2-weighted imaging without fat saturation (Fig. 29.3). On steady state free precession (SSFP) imaging, which is a common sequence in cardiac MRI to evaluate cardiac motion (cine MRI), the pericardium still appears low in signal compared to the adjacent fat. Additional sequences can be used to visualize the pericardium, especially when certain diseases are suspected. Spatial modulation of magnetization (tagging), free-breathing, nongated cine, T1-weighted postcontrast sequences, and delayed enhancement sequences can all be used to assess for various pathologic processes and will be discussed below.

Pericardial Sinuses and Recesses

The portion of the visceral pericardium that covers the vessels is arranged in the form of two short tubes. One encloses the proximal portions of the ascending aorta and pulmonary trunk and is termed the arterial mesocardium. The other encloses the superior (SVC), inferior vena cava (IVC) and the four pulmonary veins and is termed the venous mesocardium. This normal arrangement of the visceral pericardium can lead to outpouchings (recesses) or tunnels (sinuses) which often contain pericardial fluid, even in the absence of a pericardial effusion. These structures occur in specific locations around the heart and they can be categorized depending on whether they arise from the oblique sinus, the transverse sinus, or pericardial cavity proper.

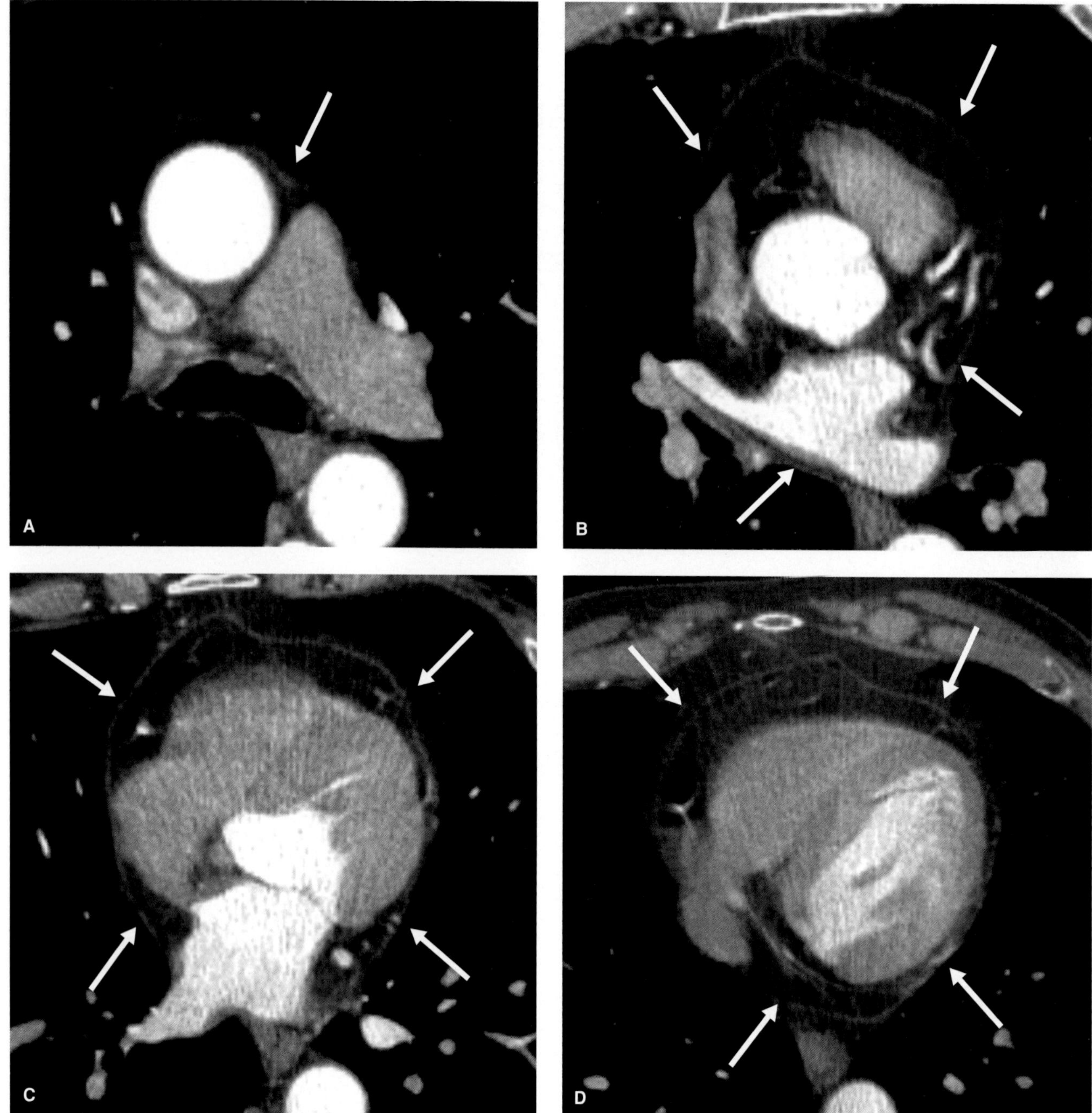

FIGURE 29.1. **A** to **D:** Normal pericardial anatomy on axial CT in a 61-year-old man. Axial images at the level of the (**A**) ascending aorta, (**B**) aortic root, (**C**) left atrium, and (**D**) coronary sinus demonstrates a curvilinear band of soft tissue surrounding the heart from the level of the great vessels to the diaphragm (*arrows*). In this patient, the pericardium is well visualized as it outlined by mediastinal fat and prominent epicardial fat. Although the entire pericardium is often difficult to visualize, it is almost always present. Up to 35 mL of fluid is normally found in the pericardial sac and it is important not to confuse a small amount of physiologic fluid with pericardial thickening.

The oblique sinus is found posterior and superior to the left atrium (Fig. 29.4). The oblique sinus is contiguous with the subcarinal region and forms a posterior pericardial recess. Given its extension into the subcarinal region, it can be mistaken for lymphadenopathy. Similar to all other sinuses and recesses, the fluid will measure simple fluid attenuation and signal on both CT (–10 to 10 HU) and MRI, respectively.

The transverse sinus lies superior to the left atrium, posterior to the aorta and main pulmonary artery, but anterior to the oblique sinus (Fig. 29.4). It communicates with several recesses including the right pulmonic, left pulmonic, superior aortic, and inferior aortic recesses. The left and right pulmonary recesses are usually small in size and form the lateral extents of the transverse sinus. The superior aortic recess extends superiorly along the ascending aorta, has anterior and posterior components, and is often visible on CT. The anterior portion lies anterior to the ascending aorta and pulmonary artery and can vary in shape and extent (Fig. 29.4). The posterior portion can be seen on CT as a crescentic-shaped fluid collection posterior of the ascending aorta. In some instances, this recess can have a prominent superior extension and can be confused for a mediastinal cyst mass leading to unnecessary

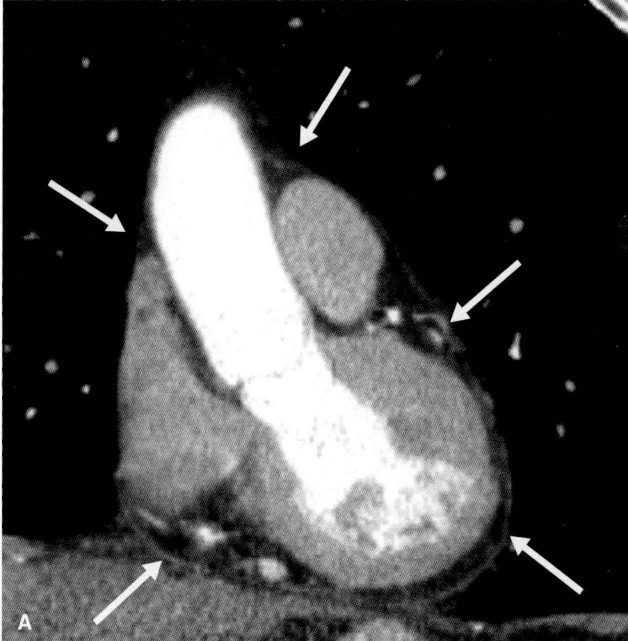

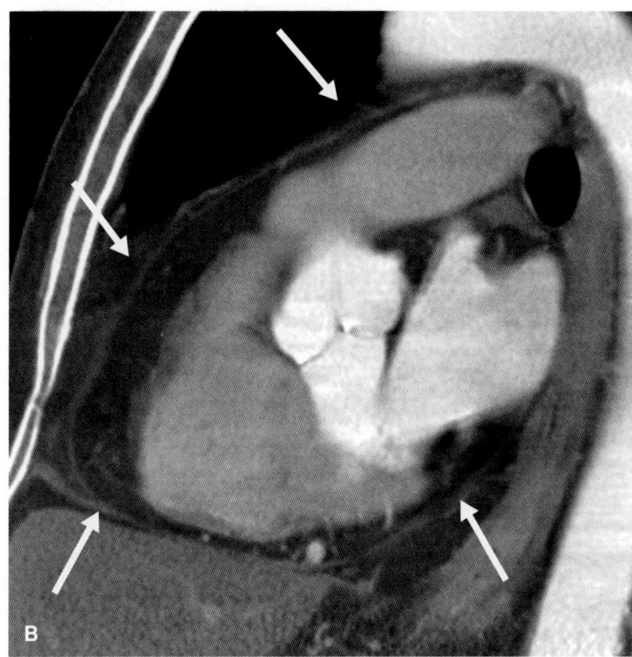

FIGURE 29.2. **A, B:** Normal pericardium on CT. 5-mm thick ray-sum parasagittal image of the thorax (**A**) and coronal oblique multiplanar reconstruction base of the left ventricle (**B**) shows the extent of the pericardium which encloses the heart (*arrows*).

intervention (Fig. 29.5). The inferior aortic recess is often less conspicuous and is located between the right lateral aspect of the ascending aorta and the right atrium with its most inferior extent at the level of the aortic annulus.

In addition to the above, there are three recesses of the pericardial cavity proper. These include the postcaval recess, the left pulmonary vein recess, and right pulmonary vein recess. The postcaval recess is posterior and to the right of the SVC. The left and right pulmonary venous recesses are located between the superior and inferior pulmonary veins on each side. In most instances, there is only a trace amount of fluid in these recesses and they are not visible. However, on occasion, the sleeve around the right inferior pulmonary vein can be filled with fluid and can mimic adenopathy or a tumor (Fig. 29.6). Fluid in the sleeve will often be seen on both sides of the vein and does not narrow the vein. The characteristic location and fluid attenuation can help differentiate this from pathology.

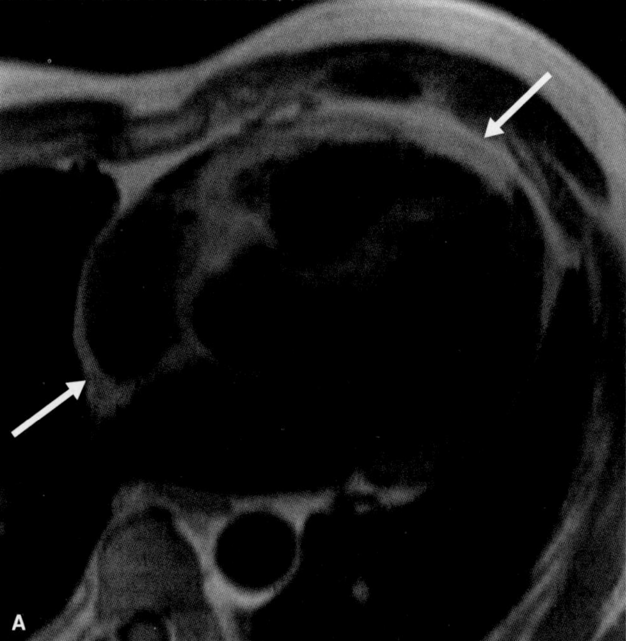

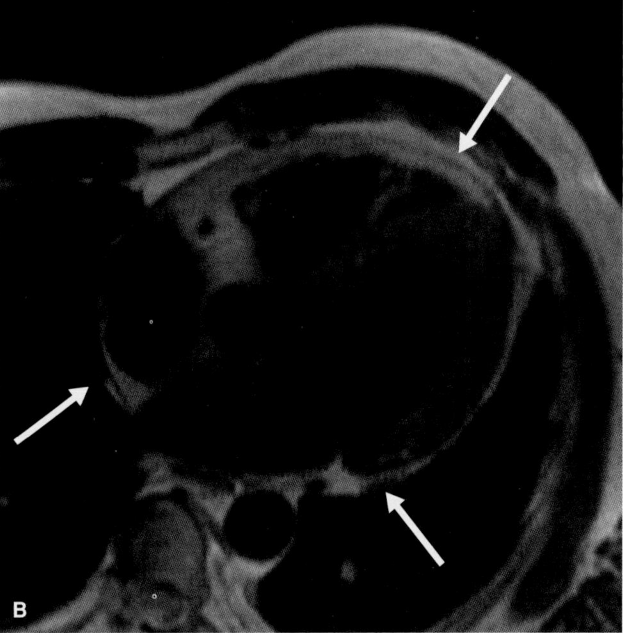

FIGURE 29.3. **A to D:** Normal appearance of pericardium on MRI. Four-chamber T1-weighted (**A**), T2-weighted (**B**), steady-state free precession (**C**), and delayed enhancement (**D**) images in a 38-year-old man with arrhythmogenic right ventricular dysplasia shows a normal pericardium (*arrows*) which is isointense to hypointense to adjacent myocardium on all sequences. Similar to CT, the pericardium is best seen when outlined by hyperintense mediastinal fat and may not be visible in certain areas but is almost always present. (*continued*)

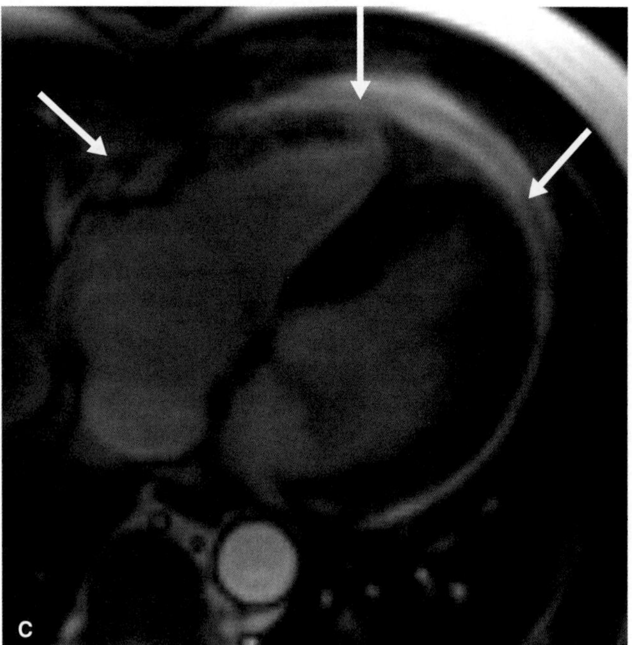

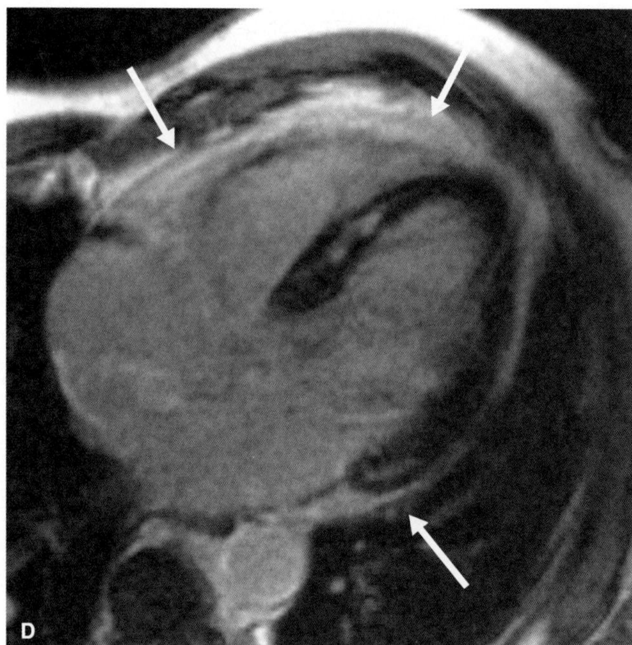

FIGURE 29.3. (*Continued*)

Blood supply to the pericardium is supplied by branches from the thoracic aorta and pericardiophrenic arteries. Venous drainage occurs through *venae pericardiales* which drain to the azygos vein, SVC, or brachiocephalic veins. Innervation predominantly occurs through branches of the phrenic nerve although vagal innervation from the esophageal plexus supplies some of the posterior pericardium. The lymphatic drainage of the pericardium is primarily directed toward the tracheobronchial nodes and less frequently toward the prepericardial lymphatic vessels and nodes.

CONGENITAL ANOMALIES OF THE PERICARDIUM

Pericardial Cyst

Pericardial cysts are uncommon benign congenital lesions occurring in 1 in 100,000 patients. The majority occur at the cardiophrenic angles, on the right greater than the left. A minority occur in other parts of the mediastinum but are

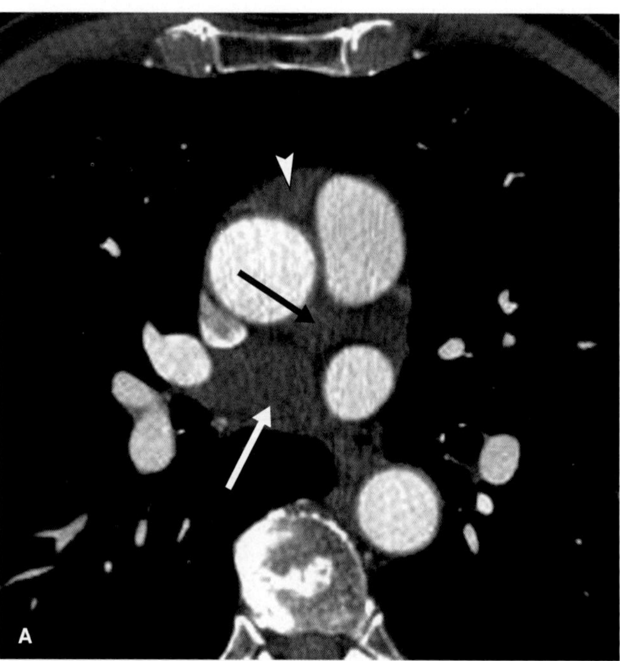

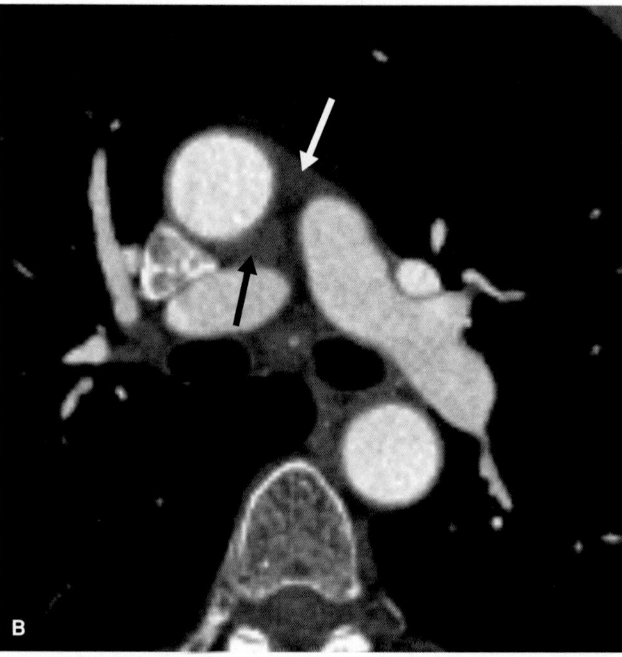

FIGURE 29.4. **A** to **C**: Oblique and transverse sinuses anatomy in a 44-year-old man. **A:** Axial CT image demonstrates a normal amount of fluid in the oblique sinus (*white arrow*), which is located superior to the left atrium. Fluid is also present in the transverse sinus (*black arrow*) which is more anterior. Fluid in the superior aortic recess (*white arrowhead*) communicates with the transverse sinus. **B:** Axial image more superiorly shows fluid in the superior aortic recess, which is divided into anterior (*white arrow*) and posterior portions (*black arrow*).

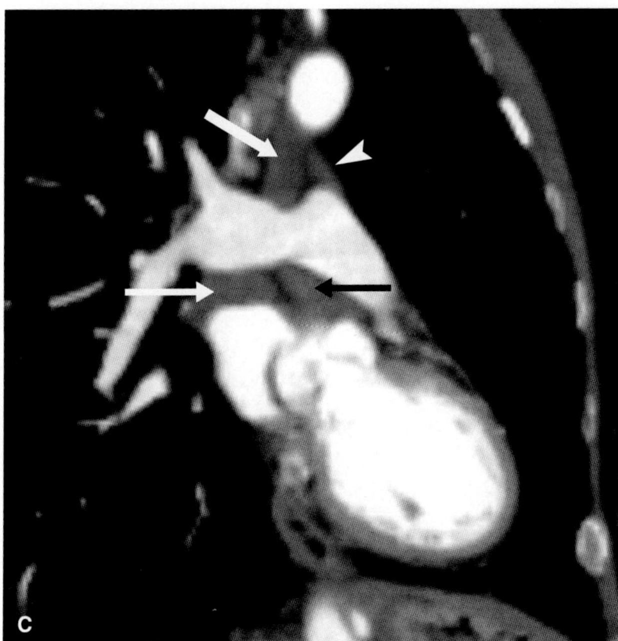

FIGURE 29.4. (*Continued*) **C:** Sagittal oblique image shows that the more posterior oblique sinus (*white arrow*) does not communicate with the more anterior transverse sinus (*black arrow*). Fluid can also be seen in the anterior (*white arrowhead*) and posterior (*fat white arrow*) aspects of the superior aortic recess. Fluid in this location is common and should not be confused with adenopathy or other pathology.

usually attached to the pericardium. Most patients are asymptomatic but up to one-third may present with chest pain, dyspnea or cough, particularly if the cyst compresses adjacent structures.

Imaging features of pericardial cysts are often characteristic. On chest radiography, the cyst typically manifests as a rounded density that contacts the hemidiaphragm and anterior chest wall (Fig. 29.7). On CT, pericardial cysts typically appear as thin-walled, round, or ovoid lesions with internal homogeneous attenuation. While most cysts should measure simple fluid attenuation on CT (–10 HU to 10 HU), pericardial cysts, similar to other mediastinal cysts, can contain proteinaceous material or blood products. This can lead to increased attenuation on CT. However, even if increased, the attenuation should be homogeneous throughout the cyst. If the diagnosis of a cyst cannot be definitively made on CT, MRI can help with the diagnosis (Fig. 29.7). Most cysts in the body will appear high in signal on T2-weighted images and low in signal on T1-weighted images due to the inherent signal characteristics of fluid. However, pericardial and other mediastinal cysts can have variable signal intensity on both T1- and T2-weighted images depending on the degree of proteinaceous material or blood products. Cysts with a moderate or high protein concentration can appear intermediate or high signal on T1-weighted imaging and intermediate or low in signal on T2-weighted imaging, respectively. On both MRI and CT, internal septations should be absent and while the wall of the cyst may enhance, no internal enhancement should be seen. Pericardial cysts can displace or if very large compress surrounding structures but there should be no evidence of invasion. Internal enhancement, heterogeneous signal (MRI) or attenuation (CT), thickened wall, numerous septations, or invasion into surrounding structures should raise the possibility of a cystic tumor, as discussed later in the chapter.

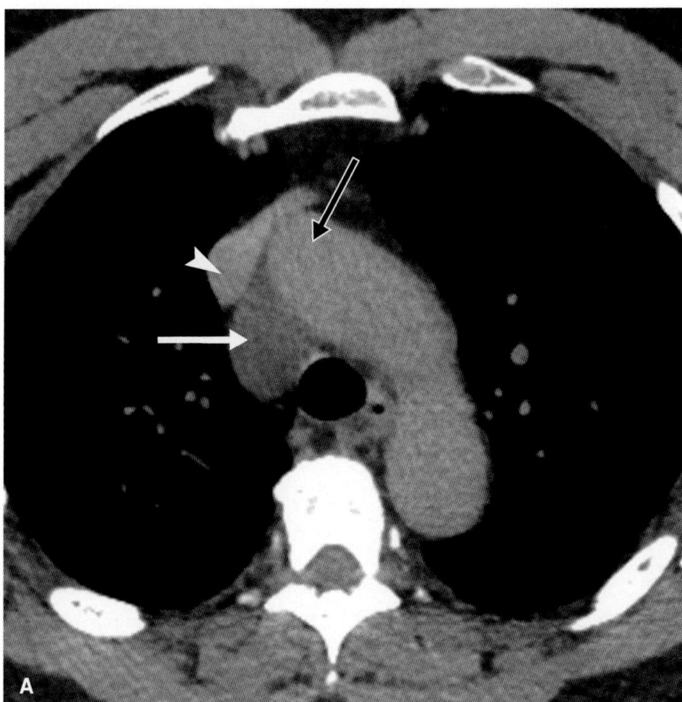

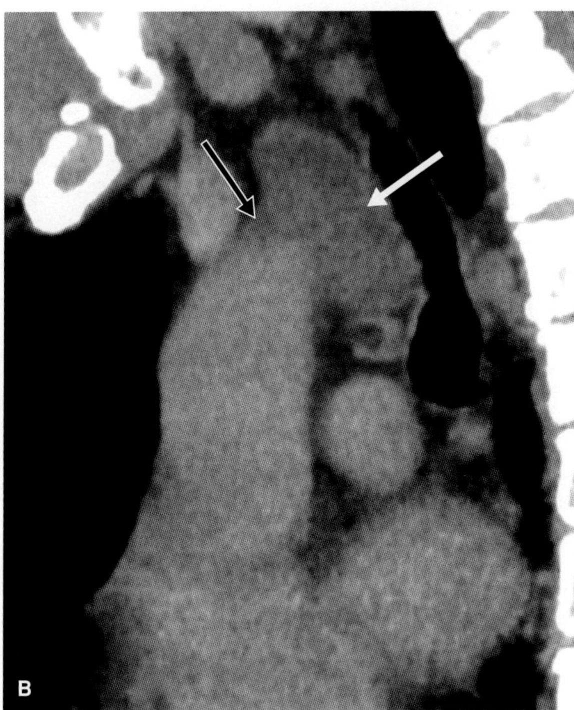

FIGURE 29.5. **A, B:** 42-year-old man with "high-riding" superior pericardial recess mimicking a mediastinal cyst. **A:** Axial image at the level of the aortic arch vessels shows a "cystic mass" in the right paratracheal region (*arrow*) between the proximal aortic arch (*black arrow*) and superior vena cava (*white arrowhead*). **B:** Sagittal image shows that this fluid collection (*white arrow*) communicates with the superior aortic recess (*black arrow*), consistent with a "high-riding superior aortic recess." This anatomic variant can be easily confused with a mediastinal cystic mass which could lead to unnecessary intervention.

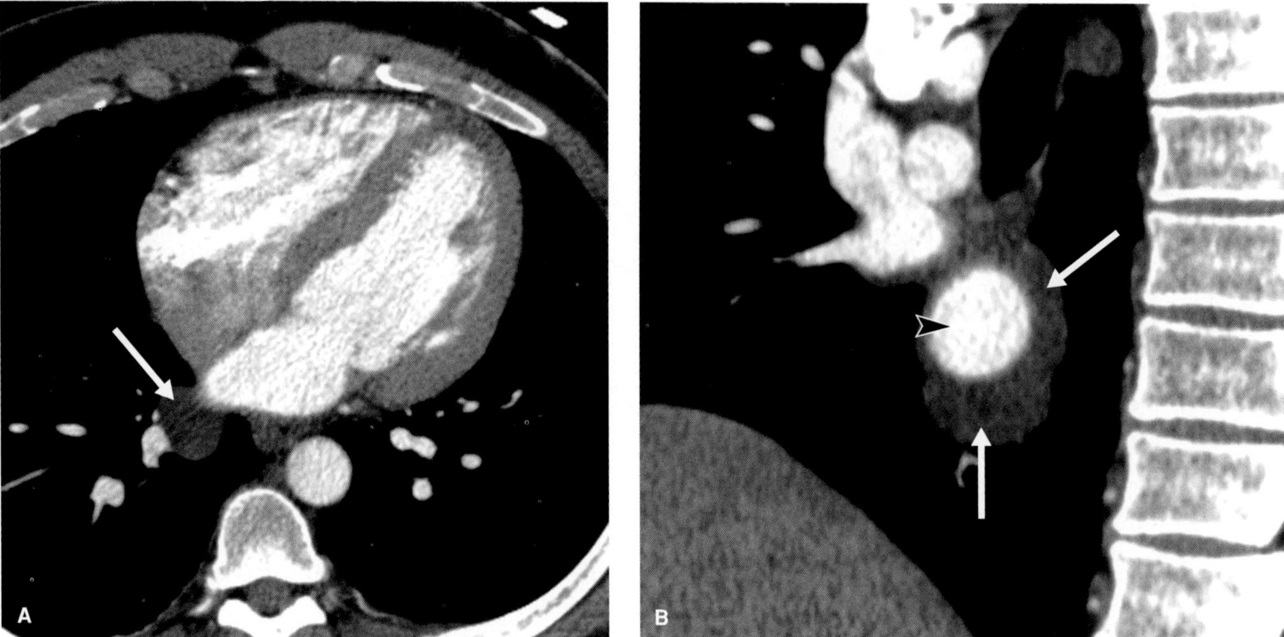

FIGURE 29.6. **A, B:** Axial-oblique (**A**) and sagittal-oblique (**B**) multiplanar reformats shows fluid in a serosal sleeve (*white arrows*) that surrounds the right inferior pulmonary vein (*black arrowhead*, Figure 6B) in a 26-year-old man. This collection has a characteristic appearance of fluid attenuation surrounding but not narrowing the pulmonary vein and should not be confused with a mass or adenopathy.

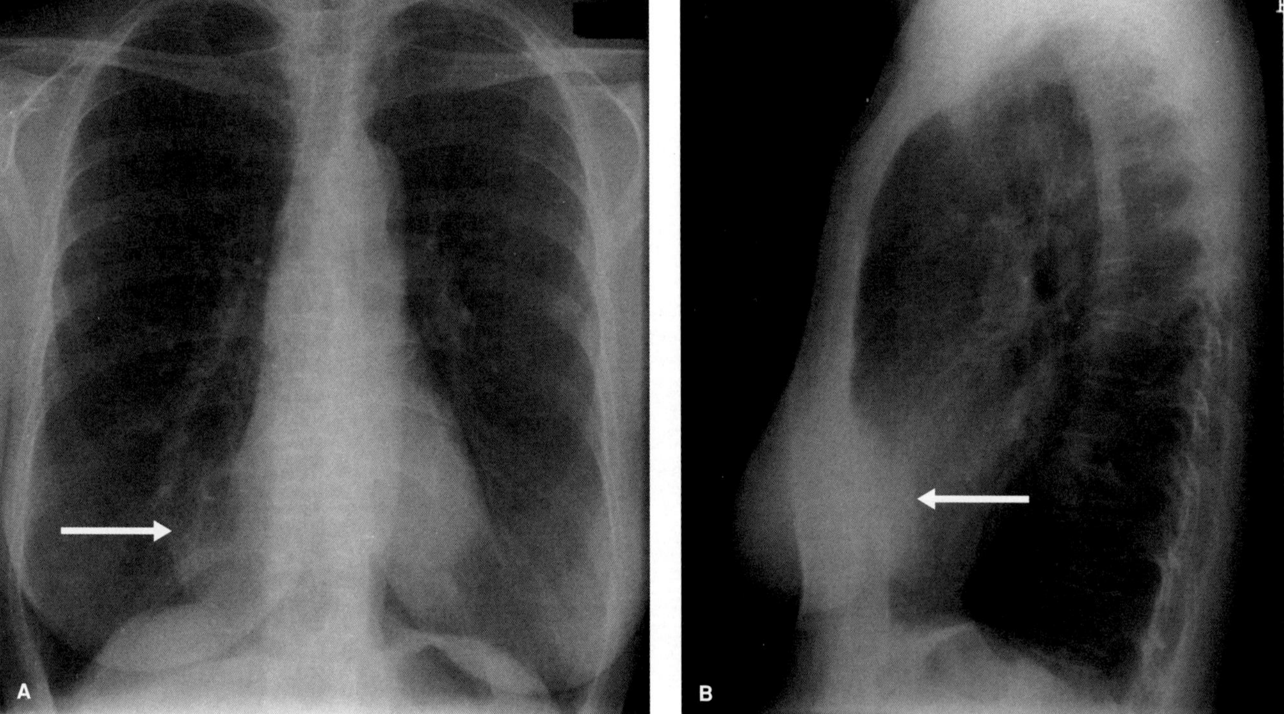

FIGURE 29.7. **A** to **G:** MRI of a pericardial cyst incidentally discovered on a chest radiograph (**A, B**). PA (**A**) and lateral (**B**) radiographs in a 59-year-old woman with a cough shows a smooth, ovoid mass in the right cardiophrenic sulcus (*white arrow*).

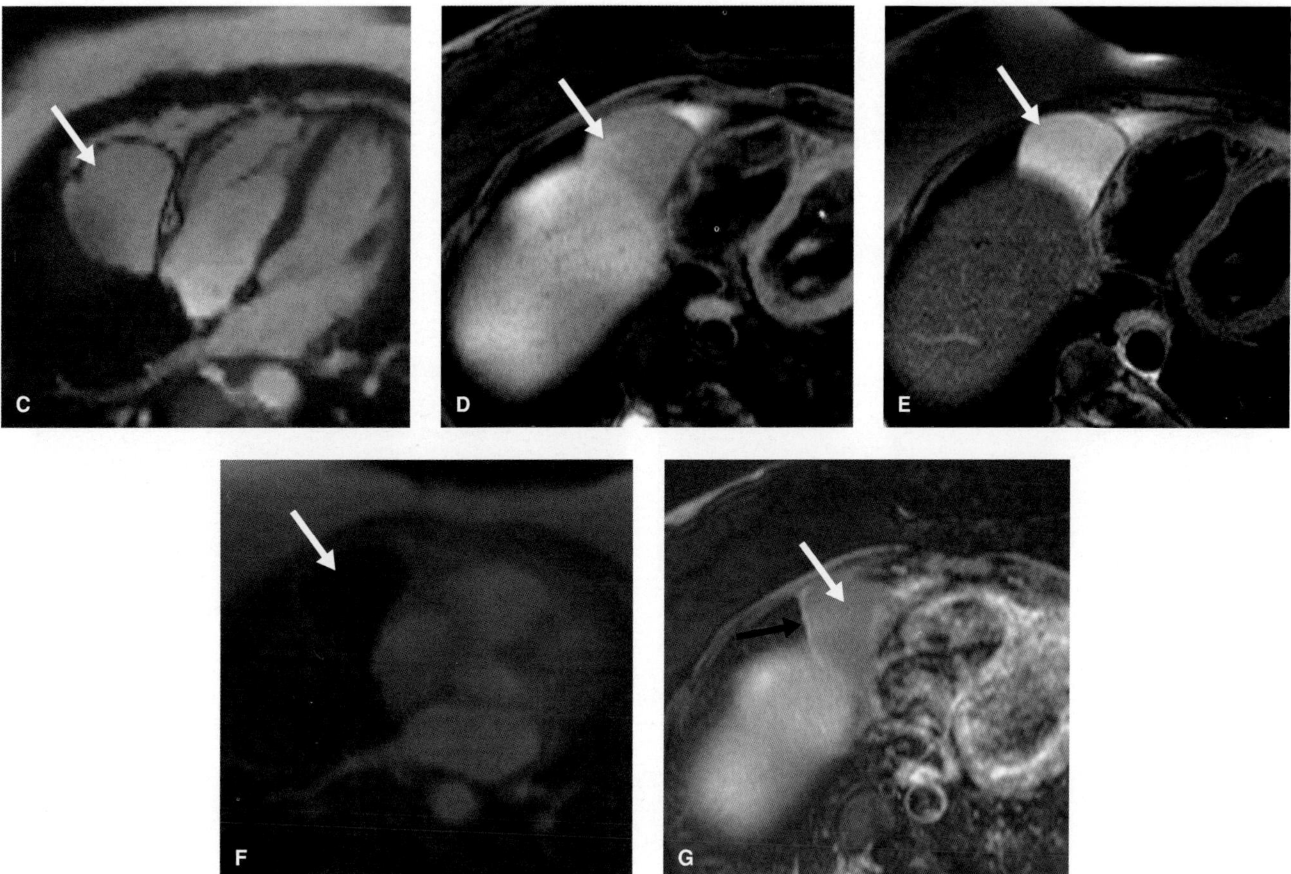

FIGURE 29.7. (*Continued*) **C**: Four-chamber cine SSFP sequence shows homogeneous high signal within the mass which is contiguous with the pericardium (*arrow*). **D**: Axial noncontrast T1-weighted and (E) T2-weighted demonstrates homogeneous isointense (Figure 4D, *white arrow*) and hyperintense signal in the lesion compared to myocardium (Figure 4E, *white arrow*), respectively. **F**: First-pass perfusion imaging shows absence of perfusion in the homogeneously low-signal mass (*arrow*). **G**: T1-weighted sequence after the administration of contrast shows no appreciable internal enhancement of the lesion although there is mild rim enhancement (*black arrow*). Homogeneous signal, a thin smooth rim, lack of perfusion, and lack of enhancement all help to characterize this lesion as a benign cyst. Due to the varying degree of proteinaceous material within any mediastinal cyst, the signal on T1-weighted sequences can range from low (simple fluid) to high (large concentration of protein) and vice-versa on T2-weighted imaging.

Pericardial diverticula often cannot be distinguished from pericardial cysts but can be suspected if there is a direct connection of a cyst-like structure to fluid in the pericardial space. Additionally, since there is a retained connection with the pericardium, fluid within a pericardial diverticulum can change over time (Fig. 29.8). Most pericardial cysts and diverticula do not undergo treatment but symptomatic cysts may require aspiration or surgery.

Pericardial Defect

Absence of the pericardium or pericardial defects are most commonly postsurgical. In rare instances, absence of the pericardium can be congenital abnormality estimated to occur in one in 7,000 to one in 13,000 people. The defects can be partial or complete and are much more common on the left. Most pericardial defects, especially those with complete absence, are asymptomatic and the findings are often incidental. However, in very rare instances, portions of the left atrium can herniate through a partial defect and become incarcerated. This can lead to infarction of portions of the left atrium, most notably the left atrial appendage, with subsequent syncope and sudden death. Although these defects usually occur in isolation, 30% to 50% of patients will have an associated congenital anomaly such as an atrial septal defect, patent ductus arteriosus, bicuspid aortic valve, or pulmonary abnormalities.

Absence of the pericardium can be a difficult diagnosis to make on CXR. Leftward rotation of the heart is present but usually more pronounced in those with complete defects. The best clue on radiograph is the interposition of lung between the main pulmonary artery and transverse aorta on frontal radiographs in patients with complete absence or larger partial defects (Fig. 29.9). If a smaller defect is present over the left atrium, bulging of the left upper heart border can be seen due to left atrial herniation.

The appearance of congenital absence of the pericardium on CT and MRI depends on whether it is partial or complete. In complete and certain partial left-sided defects, there is a leftward rotation of the heart into the left chest, with interposition of the medial portion of the left upper lobe between the aorta and pulmonary artery (Fig. 29.9). If the defect is partial, the heart bulges leftward in the region of the left atrial appendage. The actual defect in partial absence may be difficult to visualize on CT given that portions of the pericardium can be difficult to see in even normal studies. MRI can improve detection of the pericardium. If the left-sided defect is complete, the entire heart is typically displaced to the left and the cardiac apex is positioned posteriorly.

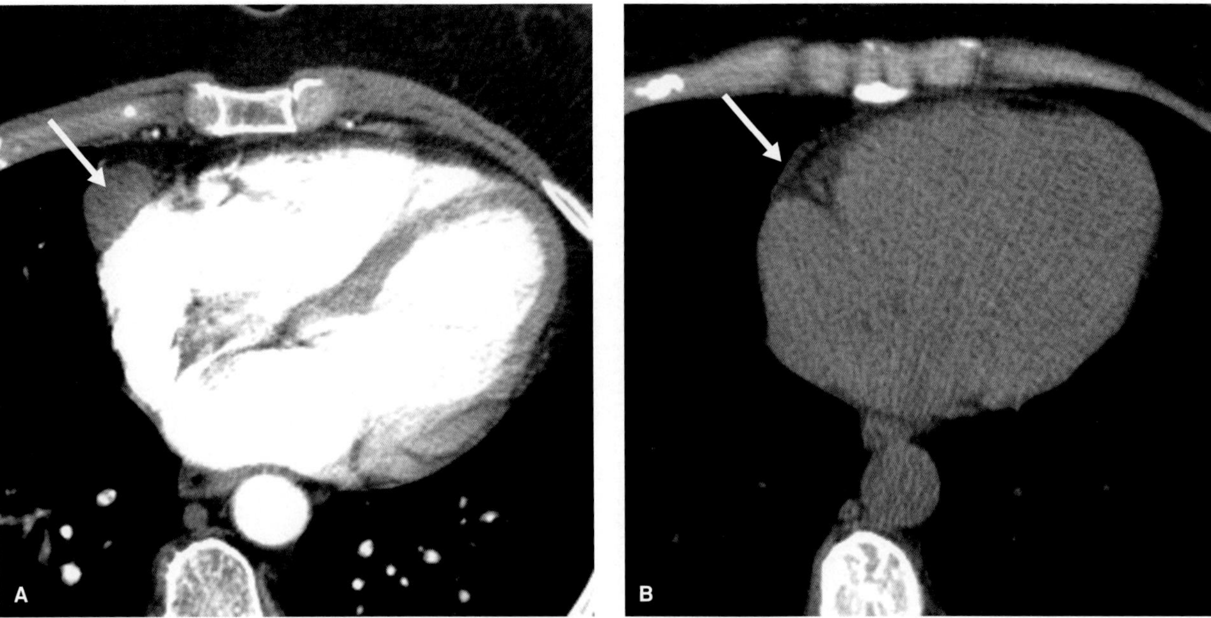

FIGURE 29.8. **A, B:** Pericardial diverticulum in a 66-year-old woman. **A:** Axial contrast-enhanced CT shows a small, ovoid cystic structure contiguous with the pericardium, though to represent a small pericardial cyst (*white arrow*). **B:** Follow-up imaging 6 months later shows that the lesion has disappeared (*white arrow*) confirming that this cystic structure represented a pericardial diverticulum that maintained a connection to the pericardium.

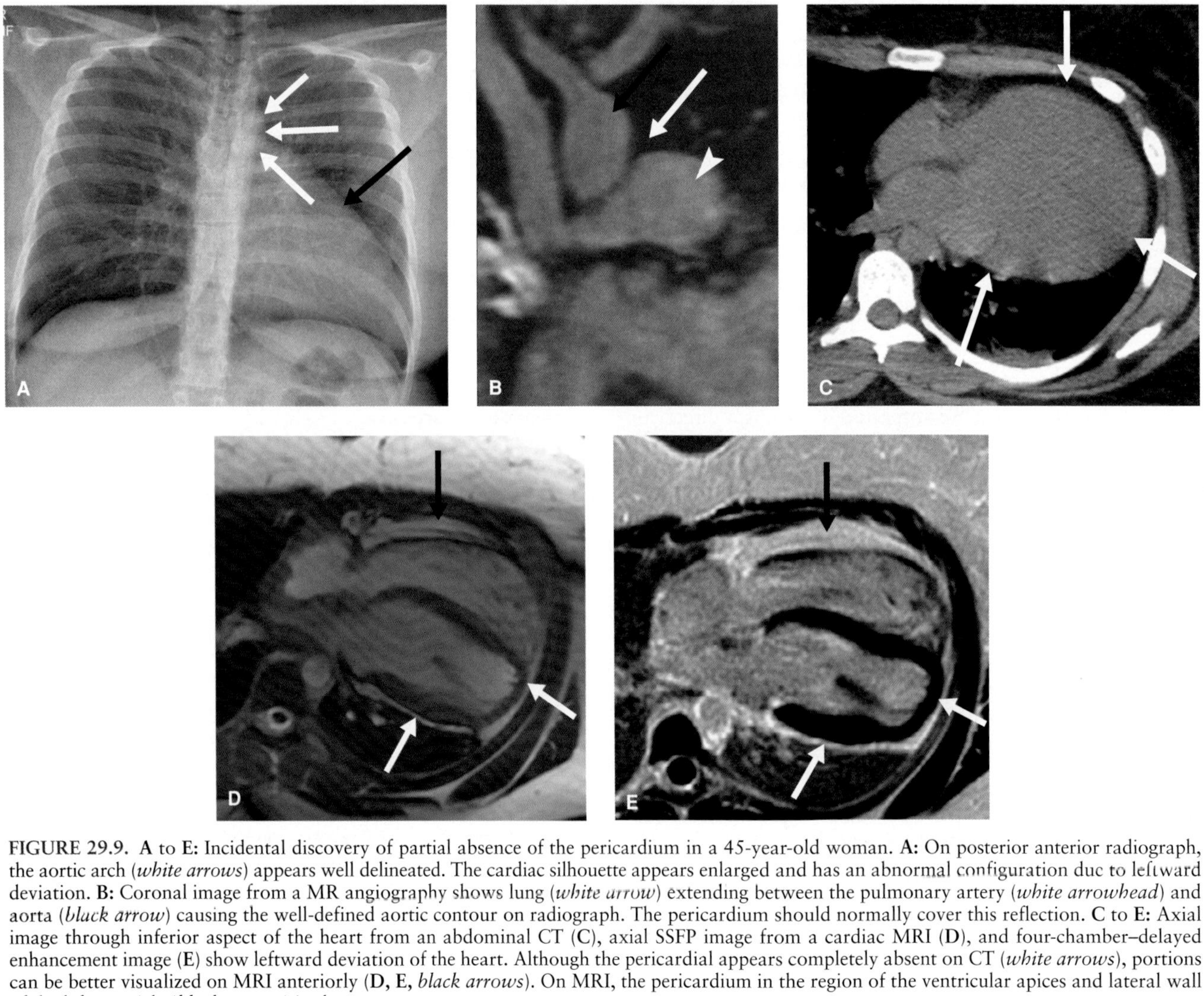

FIGURE 29.9. **A** to **E:** Incidental discovery of partial absence of the pericardium in a 45-year-old woman. **A:** On posterior anterior radiograph, the aortic arch (*white arrows*) appears well delineated. The cardiac silhouette appears enlarged and has an abnormal configuration due to leftward deviation. **B:** Coronal image from a MR angiography shows lung (*white arrow*) extending between the pulmonary artery (*white arrowhead*) and aorta (*black arrow*) causing the well-defined aortic contour on radiograph. The pericardium should normally cover this reflection. **C** to **E:** Axial image through inferior aspect of the heart from an abdominal CT (**C**), axial SSFP image from a cardiac MRI (**D**), and four-chamber–delayed enhancement image (**E**) show leftward deviation of the heart. Although the pericardial appears completely absent on CT (*white arrows*), portions can be better visualized on MRI anteriorly (**D, E,** *black arrows*). On MRI, the pericardium in the region of the ventricular apices and lateral wall of the left ventricle (*black arrows*) is absent.

ACQUIRED PERICARDIAL DISEASES

Pericardial Effusion

Pericardial effusion, the accumulation of fluid in the pericardial space, is a common imaging finding. Depending on the characteristics of the fluid, an effusion can be characterized as transudative, exudative, hemorrhagic, or pyogenic (Fig. 29.10). Transudative effusions are common in processes that lead to an increase in right atrial pressure, such as congestive heart failure and pulmonary hypertension. There are numerous causes of exudative effusions that include infection, inflammation, malignancy, autoimmune disorders, and trauma. Exudative effusions are common in pericarditis as discussed below. Hemopericardium occurs when blood products are present in the pericardium which can occur with trauma or aortic dissection.

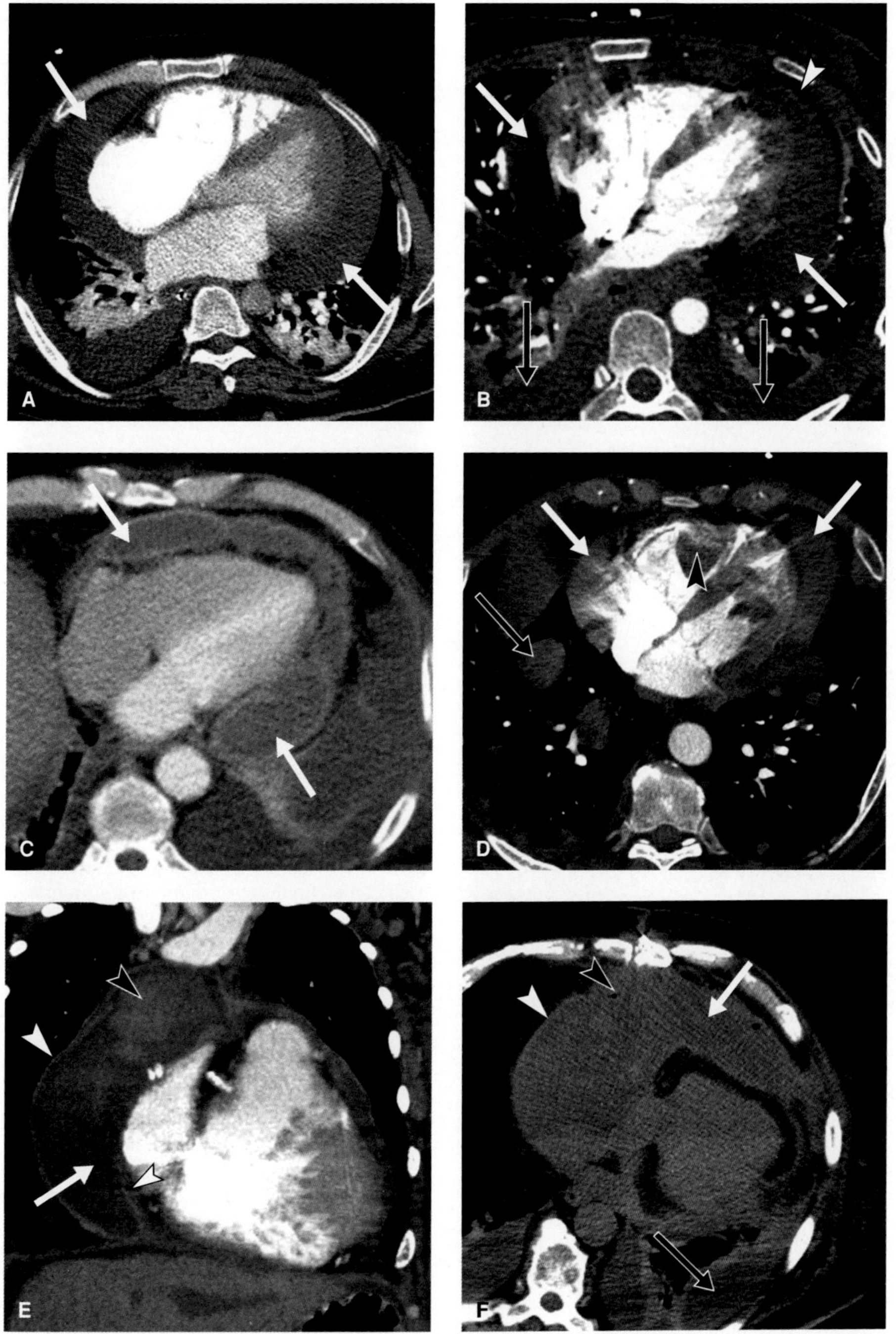

FIGURE 29.10. **A** to **F**: Types of material in pericardial effusions on CT. **A**: Axial CT in a 36-year-old man with nephrotic syndrome demonstrates a large transudative effusion (*white arrow*). The pericardium is not visibly thickened. **B**: Axial CT shows a sterile exudative effusion in a 33-year-old woman with lupus-related pleuritis (*black arrows*) and pericarditis (*white arrows*). Notice the mild pericardial enhancement (*white arrowhead*). **C**: Axial CT in a 27-year-old man with acute tuberculous pericarditis shows a multi-loculated effusion (*white arrows*) with pericardial thickening and enhancement. Draining showed bloody and purulent fluid that grew out acid-fast bacilli. **D**: Moderate-sized malignant pericardial effusion (*white arrows*) on an axial image from a CT scan in 66-year-old man with thyroid cancer. There are associated pulmonary (*black arrow*) and cardiac (*black arrowhead*) metastases. **E**: Coronal CT in a 69-year-old patient status post cardiac surgery shows a heterogeneous pericardial effusion (*white arrow*) with foci of increased attenuation (*black arrowhead*) due to hemopericardium. There is associated pericardial thickening and enhancement (*white arrowhead*). **F**: Pyopericardium in a 50-year-old man status post cardiac surgery with methicillin-resistant *Staphylococcus aureus* (MRSA) infection shows a large heterogeneous pericardial effusion (*white arrow*) with pericardial thickening (*white arrowhead*) and foci of air (*black arrowhead*). There is an associated right-sided empyema (*black arrow*). Frank pus was removed during pericardiocentesis.

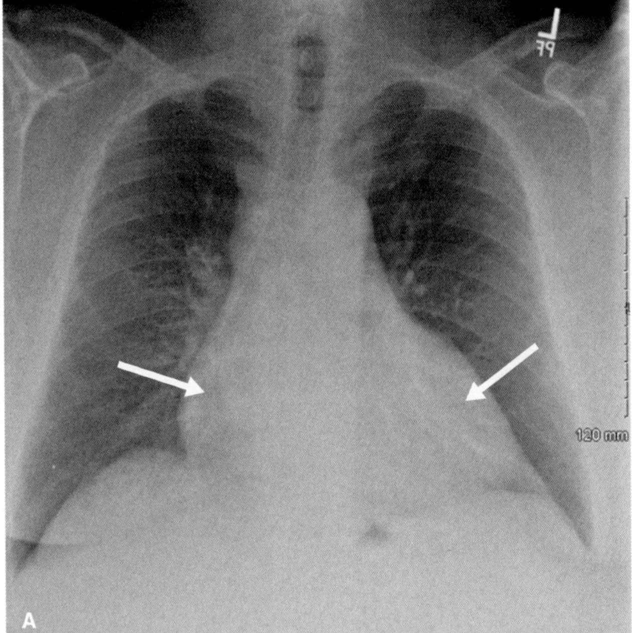

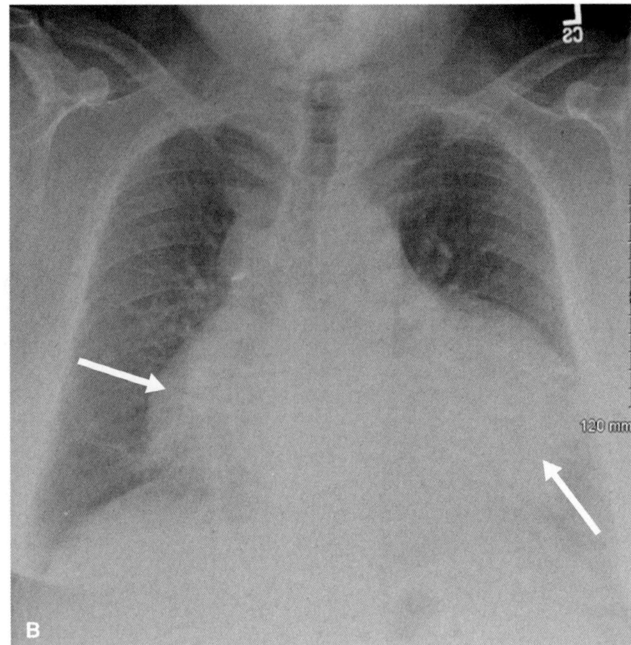

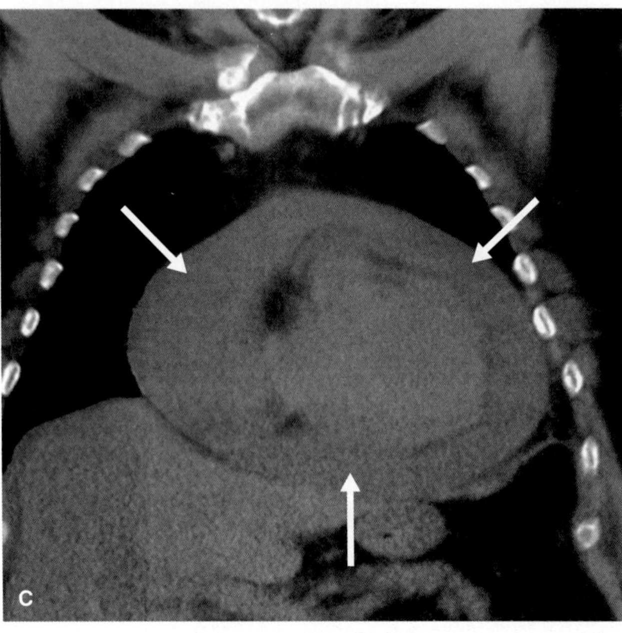

FIGURE 29.11. A to C: Diagnosis of a pericardial effusion on frontal radiograph. A: PA radiograph in a 71-year-old woman who presents to the emergency department with a cough and fever demonstrate a mildly enlarged cardiac silhouette (*white arrows*). B: PA radiograph obtained 3 weeks later due to worsening chest pain and dyspnea shows a dramatic increase in the size of the cardiac silhouette (*white arrows*), which has a globular shape, over a short period of time. These findings should raise the suspicion of a pericardial effusion. C: 10-mm thick coronal ray-sum image from a CT obtained a few hours later shows a circumferential pericardial effusion (*white arrows*). Although there is no pericardial thickening or enhancement, this does not exclude the diagnosis of acute pericarditis. A pericardial drain was placed which revealed serosanguinous fluid. A viral etiology was suspected given the history of recent fever.

In pyopericardium, frank pus fills the pericardial space and carries a high mortality rate. Although most effusions are small and asymptomatic, symptomatology varies depending on the cause of effusion and rapidity of accumulation.

The detection of a pericardial effusion on chest radiography can be difficult. Large effusions can often be suggested if the heart has an enlarged, "water bottle" morphology on a frontal CXR or if there is a rapid increase in the size of the cardiac silhouette over a short period of time (Fig. 29.11). On the lateral radiograph, a fat pad sign suggests the presence of a pericardial effusion and occurs when pericardial fluid is outlined on both sides lower attenuation mediastinal and epicardial fat (Fig. 29.12).

If a clinically significant pericardial effusion is suspected, echocardiography is often used as the initial technique due to its wide availability and ease of use. However, echocardiography has limitations, including a poor acoustic window, difficulty in characterizing the pericardial collection, and difficulty in assessing the thickness of the pericardium. Both CT and MRI can help quantify both the size and tissue characteristics of the effusion and associated pericardium. On CT, an increase in density above that of simple fluid may indicate an exudative or hemorrhagic process, although there is overlap. As discussed below in greater detail, patients with active pericardial inflammation or infection will often demonstrate pericardial enhancement after the administration of intravenous contrast (Fig. 29.10B, C, E, F). The presence of pericardial nodularity or other signs of malignancy should raise the concern for a malignant pericardial effusion (Fig. 29.10D). In patients with a history of trauma, surgery, or aortic dissection, high-density fluid suggests hemopericardium (Fig. 29.10E).

MRI is also a valuable tool to help characterize a pericardial effusion. Most effusions are high in signal on T2-weighted and SSFP sequences, even if the effusion is complex in nature. On T1-weighted sequences, simple transudative effusions typically display homogeneous low-signal intensity and do

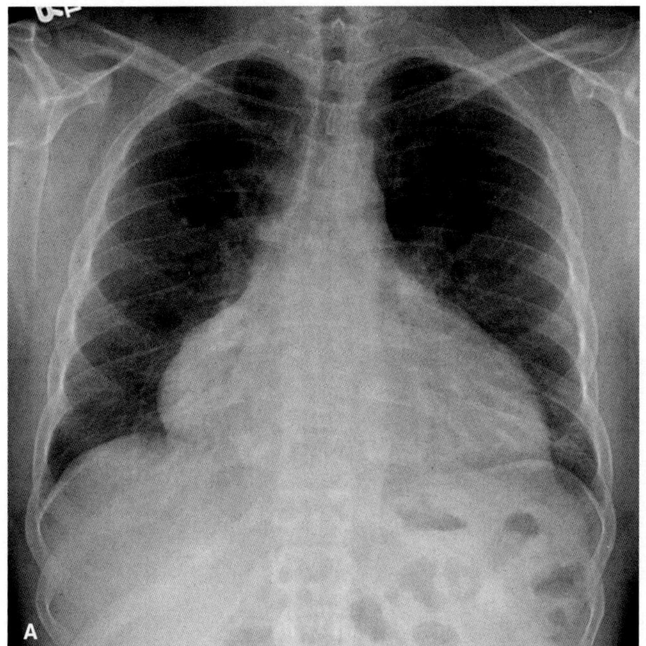

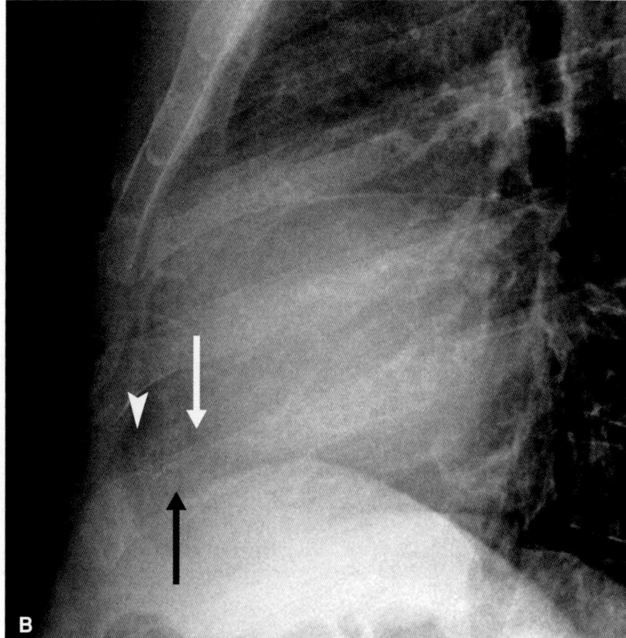

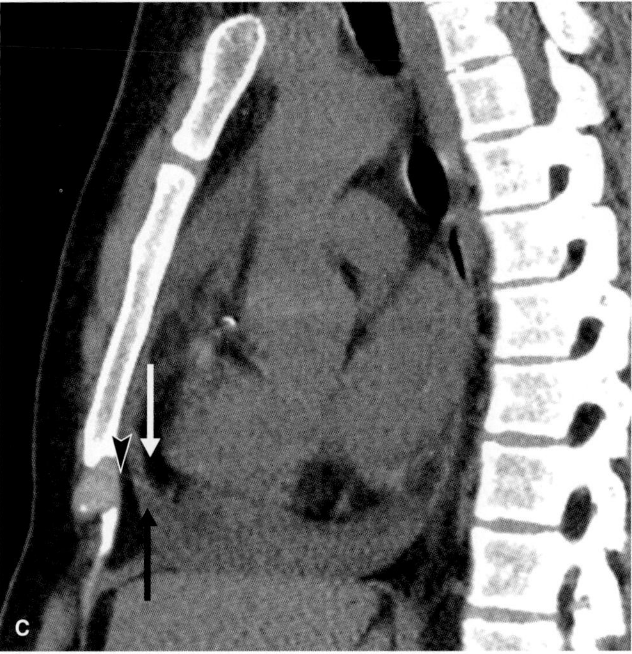

FIGURE 29.12. A to **C:** Fat pad sign on a lateral radiograph in a 38-year-old man with shortness of breath. **A:** PA radiograph shows a globular appearing cardiac contour. There are no associated findings of fluid overload. **B:** Coned-down view of the heart on the lateral radiograph shows higher attenuation fluid (*black arrow*) outlined by epicardial fat centrally (*white arrow*) and mediastinal fat peripherally (*white arrowhead*). **C:** Corresponding CT shows the pericardial effusion (*black arrow*) outlined by epicardial (*white arrow*) and mediastinal (*black arrowhead*) fat which correlates with the findings on lateral radiograph.

not enhance (Fig. 29.13). However, in cases of a moderate or large pericardial effusion, areas of increased signal can occur on T1-weighted sequences due to the nonlinear motion of the pericardial fluid. However, this finding will not be present on T2-weighted and SSFP sequences which can help differentiate this artifact from an exudative or hemorrhagic effusion which will have abnormal signal intensity on all sequences.

On delayed enhancement imaging, the appearance of a pericardial effusion will differ depending on whether the images are reconstructed using a magnitude or phase sensitive inversion technique (PSIR). In essence delayed imaging using a magnitude reconstruction represents an absolute value of longitudinal magnetization while PSIR preserves its polarity. In delayed enhancement imaging, an inversion prepulse is given and the timing of the sequence is set to when the recovering longitudinal magnetization of the myocardium returns to 0 (or is nulled) which causes the myocardium to appear black. With magnitude imaging, tissues that both relax faster (voxels containing gadolinium or fat) or slower (voxels containing water) will both appear bright in signal. Therefore, it can be difficult to differentiate epicardial fat from pericardial fluid using magnitude imaging (Fig. 29.13D). However, PSIR preserves the information about the polarity of the longitudinal relaxation so voxels that relax slower than myocardium, such as those containing water, are ascribed darker signals. Voxels that relax faster than myocardium, such as those with fat and gadolinium, appear as bright pixels. Therefore, using the PSIR reconstruction, pericardial fluid will appear very dark while epicardial fat will appear bright (Fig. 29.13E). This is a useful tool that not only allows differentiation between tissues but also elucidate pathology such as in the case of pericardial thickening or adjacent myocardial inflammation.

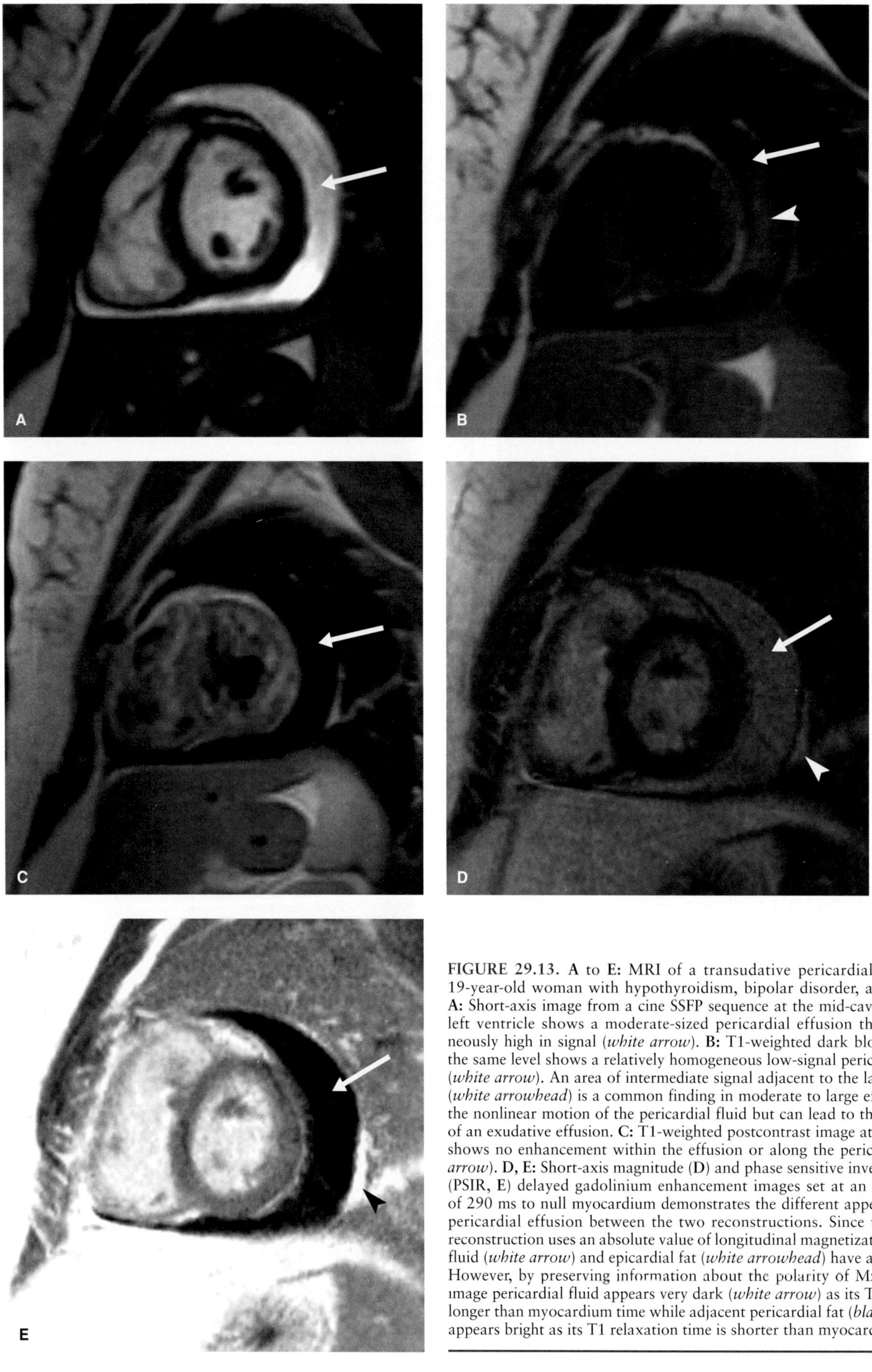

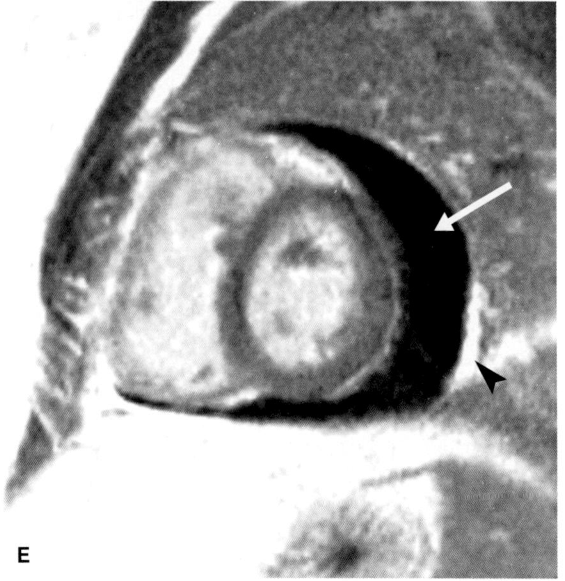

FIGURE 29.13. **A** to **E:** MRI of a transudative pericardial effusion in a 19-year-old woman with hypothyroidism, bipolar disorder, and chest pain. **A:** Short-axis image from a cine SSFP sequence at the mid-cavity level of the left ventricle shows a moderate-sized pericardial effusion that is homogeneously high in signal (*white arrow*). **B:** T1-weighted dark blood imaging at the same level shows a relatively homogeneous low-signal pericardial effusion (*white arrow*). An area of intermediate signal adjacent to the lateral segments (*white arrowhead*) is a common finding in moderate to large effusions due to the nonlinear motion of the pericardial fluid but can lead to the misdiagnosis of an exudative effusion. **C:** T1-weighted postcontrast image at the same level shows no enhancement within the effusion or along the pericardium (*white arrow*). **D, E:** Short-axis magnitude (**D**) and phase sensitive inversion recovery (PSIR, **E**) delayed gadolinium enhancement images set at an inversion time of 290 ms to null myocardium demonstrates the different appearances of the pericardial effusion between the two reconstructions. Since the magnitude reconstruction uses an absolute value of longitudinal magnetization (Mz), both fluid (*white arrow*) and epicardial fat (*white arrowhead*) have a similar signal. However, by preserving information about the polarity of Mz, on the PSIR image pericardial fluid appears very dark (*white arrow*) as its T1 relaxation is longer than myocardium time while adjacent pericardial fat (*black arrowhead*) appears bright as its T1 relaxation time is shorter than myocardium.

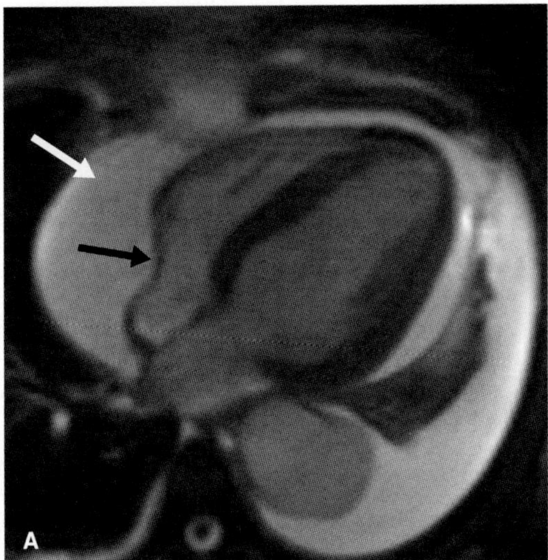

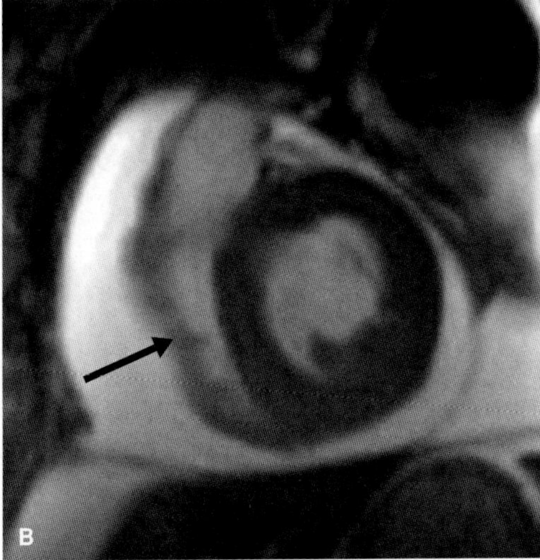

FIGURE 29.14. **A, B:** Cardiac tamponade due to large pericardial effusion in a 37-year-old woman with renal failure. **A:** Four-chamber SSFP cine sequence from a cardiac MRI shows a large pericardial effusion (*white arrow*) with diastolic flattening of the right atrium (*black arrow*). **B:** Short axis SSFP cines sequence shows early diastolic collapse of the right ventricle (*black arrow*). These findings are suggestive of cardiac tamponade which was confirmed on echocardiography.

Pericardial Tamponade

Pericardial tamponade occurs when the pressure in the pericardial space exceeds that of the right ventricle. Due to decreased right ventricular filling, tamponade can lead to hemodynamic compromise and rapid death. The development of tamponade depends on the distensibility of the pericardium and rapidity in the accumulation of the pericardial fluid. If the pericardium is distensible and the accumulation of an effusion is slow, a large pericardial effusion can be present without the development of tamponade. However, patients who rapidly develop an effusion are more susceptible to developing tamponade, especially if the pericardium is less compliant due to inflammation or scarring. In this instance, as little as 100 to 200 mL of fluid can lead to tamponade.

It is important to remember that tamponade is a clinical and physiologic diagnosis and cross-sectional imaging with CT or MRI should not be the first imaging choice in cases of suspected tamponade. The diagnosis is usually made based on clinical criteria in combination with characteristic cardiac findings on echocardiography, notably diastolic collapse of the right ventricular free wall, RA collapse, paradoxical motion of the interventricular septum, and a swinging motion of the heart in the pericardial sac. Although not normally performed in cases of tamponade, cardiac MRI can show similar imaging findings (Fig. 29.14).

While cross-sectional imaging should not play a primary role in the diagnosis of tamponade, CT still may be the first study performed in the emergency setting, especially in cases of trauma or if there is concern for vascular pathology such as an aortic dissection or pulmonary embolism. Typical findings of tamponade include a moderate to large pericardial collection with compression or flattening of the right atrium and/or right ventricular free wall (Fig. 29.15). Other nonspecific findings

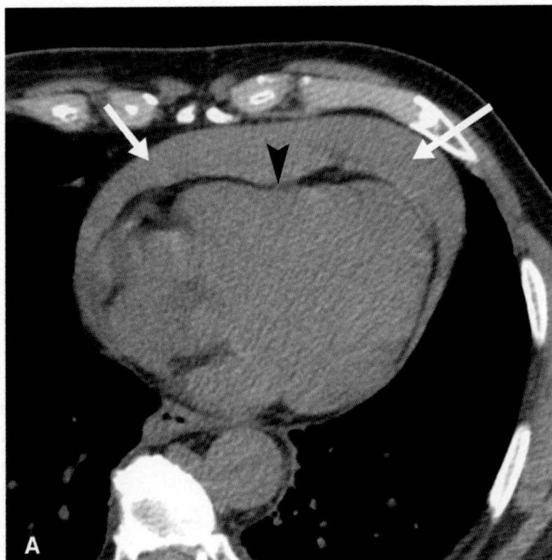

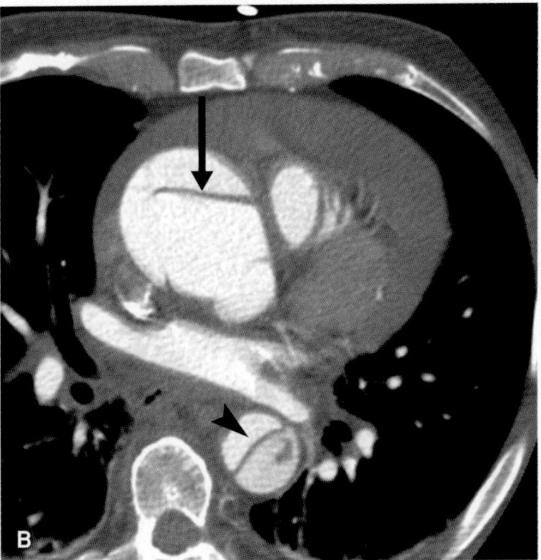

FIGURE 29.15. **A, B:** Cardiac tamponade in a 71-year-old woman with a Type A dissection. **A:** Axial CT from the noncontrast portion of a CT angiography shows a moderate size, high attenuation pericardial effusion due to hemopericardium. Mild compression of the free wall of the right ventricle (*black arrowhead*) raised the concern for pericardial tamponade which was confirmed on echocardiogram. **B:** Enhanced portion during arterial phase shows an intimal flap in the ascending aorta (*arrow*) and descending aorta (*arrowhead*).

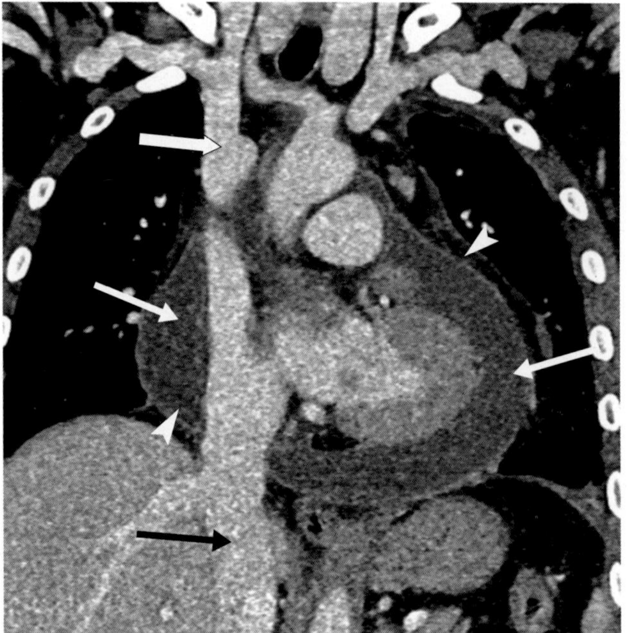

FIGURE 29.16. Cardiac tamponade on CT. Coronal oblique reconstruction in a 21-year-old man presenting to the emergency department with severe chest pain and shortness of breath shows a large pericardial effusion (*white arrows*) with enhancement of the pericardium (*white arrowheads*) due to acute pericarditis. The superior vena cava (*fat white arrow*) and inferior vena cava (*black arrow*) are both dilated due to increased right atrial pressures. Echocardiography confirmed cardiac tamponade. The pericarditis was thought to be viral in etiology as the patient had a recent history of upper respiratory tract infection and was otherwise in good health.

of increased right atrial pressure can be seen including dilation of the SVC, IVC, and azygos vein, as well as reflux of contrast into the hepatic veins (Fig. 29.16). In normal instances, the interventricular septum is bowed rightward toward the right ventricle. In cases of tamponade, leftward bowing or flattening of the interventricular septum can occur. However, this is a nonspecific finding as it can occur with numerous conditions causing either pressure or volume overload of the right ventricle. Although effusions are the most common cause of tamponade, it is important to remember that large volumes of air within the pericardial sac, which can occur with trauma or surgery, can cause tamponade as well (Fig. 29.17).

INFLAMMATION OF THE PERICARDIUM

Acute Pericarditis

There are many causes of pericardial inflammation. While many cases are labeled as idiopathic, it is assumed that a large percentage of these are viral in etiology (Fig. 29.16). However, pericarditis can be secondary to various pathogens including bacteria (Fig. 29.10F), fungi, parasites, and myobacterium (Fig. 29.10C). Acute pericarditis can also occur after postcardiac injury syndromes such as those that occur after myocardial infarction (Fig. 29.18), connective tissue diseases (systemic lupus erythematosus [SLE; Fig. 29.13B], rheumatoid arthritis [RA], scleroderma), hypersensitivity reaction, radiation therapy, chronic renal failure, pericardial trauma, surgical manipulation, and malignancy.

In acute pericarditis, the pericardium reacts by releasing excess fluid, fibrin, or cells in isolation or in combination depending on the cause and severity of the insult. The healing response can dramatically vary depending on the underlying cause. Patients with acute pericarditis due to tuberculosis, radiation, chronic renal failure, or collagen vascular disease are more likely to develop chronic pericardial fibrosis and adhesions than patients who develop acute pericarditis secondary to viral infection, sarcoidosis, or hypersensitivity reactions. However, the severity of injury and patient specific factors play a role. For instance, while many with idiopathic or viral pericarditis undergo complete resolution (Fig. 29.19),

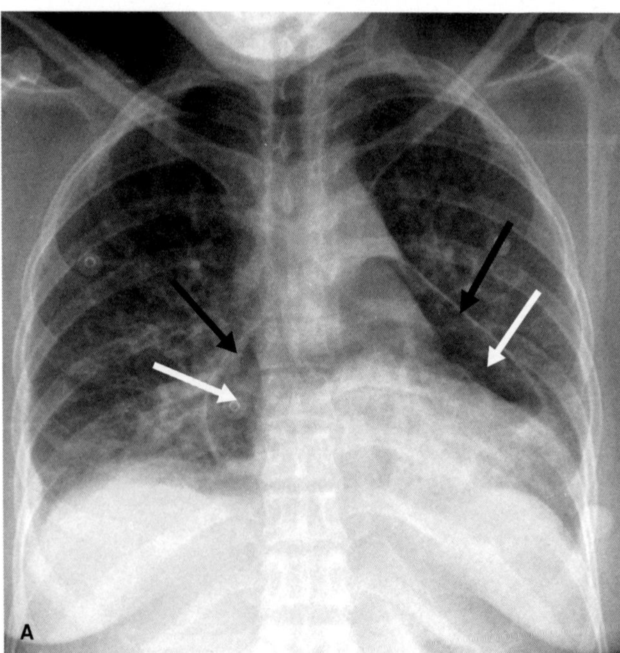

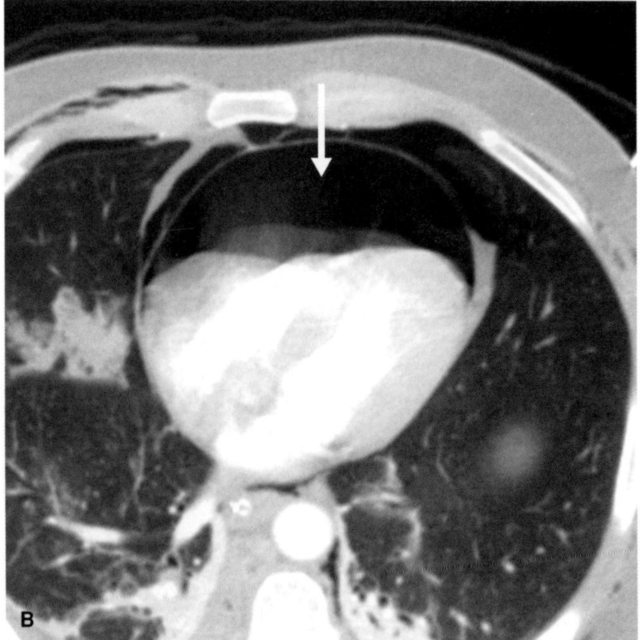

FIGURE 29.17. Cardiac tamponade due to pneumopericardium in a 33-year-old woman involved in a motor vehicle collision. **A:** Portable radiograph shows a large volume of intrapericardial air (*white arrows*) outlining the pericardium (*black arrows*). The heart is displaced inferiorly. **B:** Axial CT confirms large volume of intrapericardial air leading to cardiac compression and tamponade physiology.

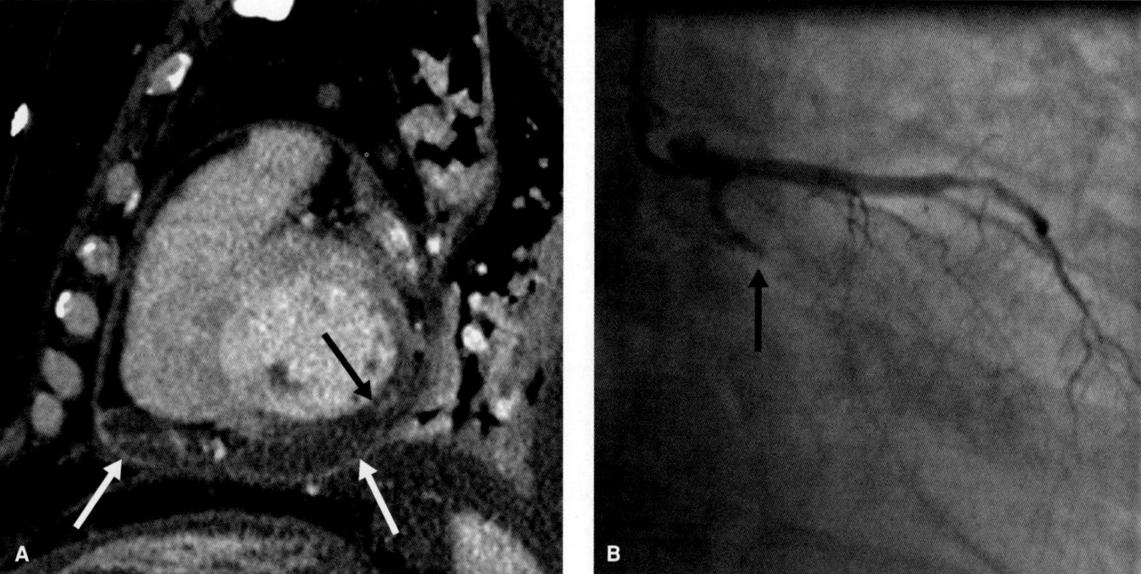

FIGURE 29.18. **A, B:** Dressler syndrome in a 55-year-old woman who had a left circumflex (LCx) myocardial infarction 3 weeks prior. **A:** Sagittal image of the heart shows pericardial thickening, fluid, and enhancement that is most pronounced inferiorly and along the lateral aspect of the left ventricle (*black arrow*). There is associated transmural hypoattenuation of the inferolateral and inferior segments of the left ventricle consistent with recent infarction (*white arrows*). **B:** Coronary angiogram obtained at time of acute myocardial infarction shows complete occlusion of the LCx (*arrow*).

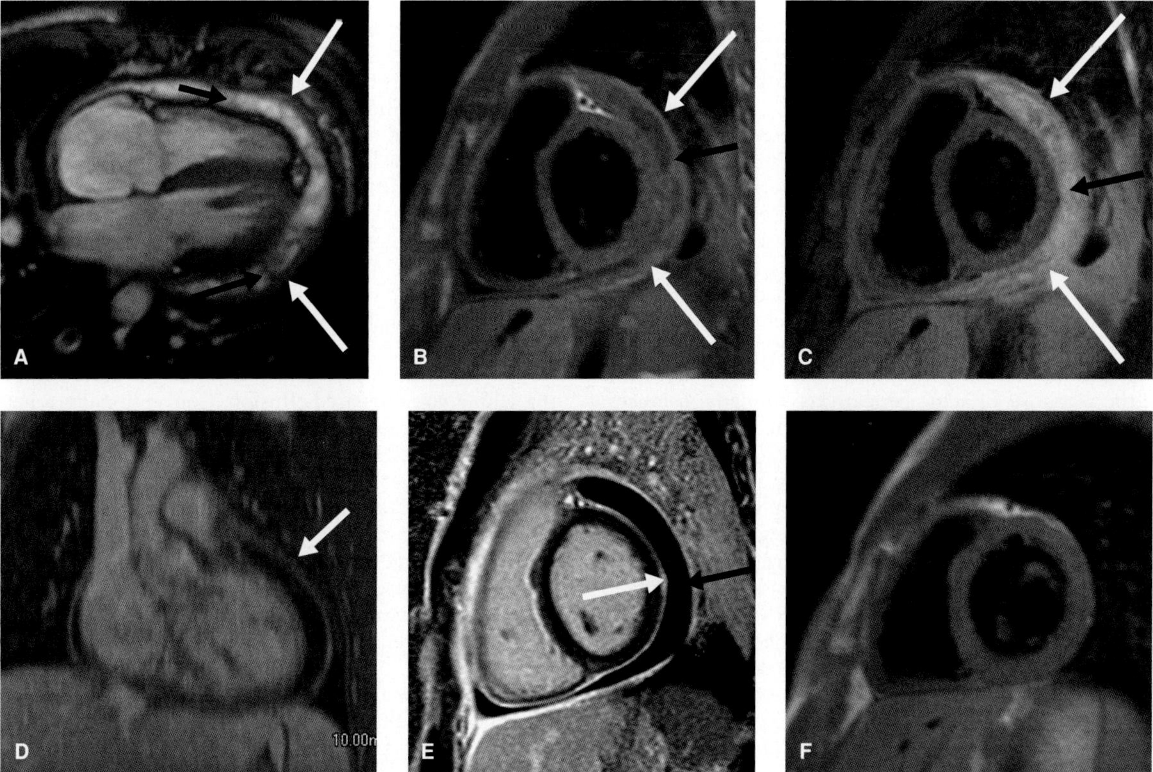

FIGURE 29.19. **A to F:** Idiopathic fibrinous pericarditis in a 21-year-old man with chest pain. **A:** Four-chamber SSFP image from a cardiac MRI shows a large, complex pericardial effusion with septations (*black arrows*) with associated pericardial thickening (*white arrows*). **B:** Short-axis T1-weighted and (**C**) spectral adiabatic inversion recovery (SPAIR) T2-weighted images shows severe pericardial thickening (*white arrows*). The signal of the thickening pericardium is isointense to slightly hyperintense to the underlying myocardium on the T1-weighted and SSFP sequences but is high in signal on the SPAIR sequence due to edema. In addition to thickening, the pericardial effusion shows fibrinous bands (*black arrows*). **D:** Coronal T1-weighted postcontrast VIBE imaging shows enhancement of the thickened pericardium (*white arrow*). The pericardial fluid does not demonstrate any significant enhancement. **E:** Phase sensitive inversion recovery (PSIR) delayed gadolinium enhancement imaging set at an inversion time of 300 ms shows enhancement of both the parietal (*black arrow*) and visceral (*white arrow*) pericardium. The pericardial fluid appears very low in signal on PSIR sequences. **F:** Short-axis T1-weighted image 2 months after pericardial window and anti-inflammatory therapy shows complete resolution. While some patients with fibrinous pericarditis may develop permanent pericardial thickening and fibrosis, others may have complete resolution.

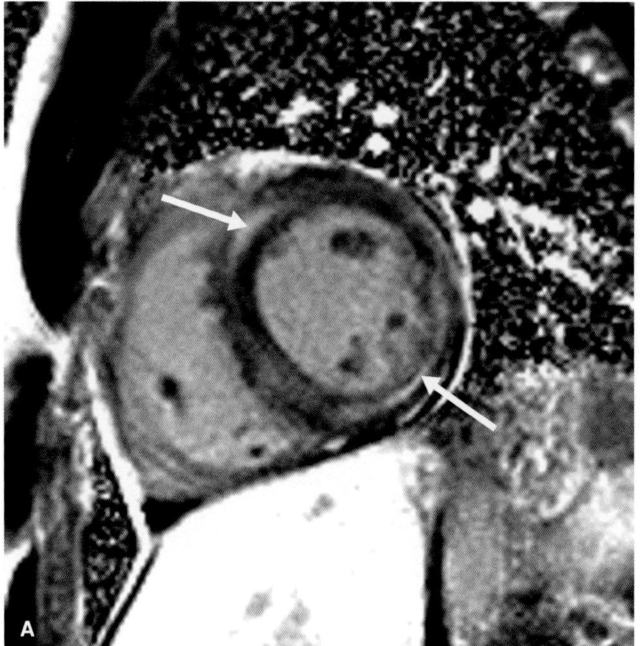

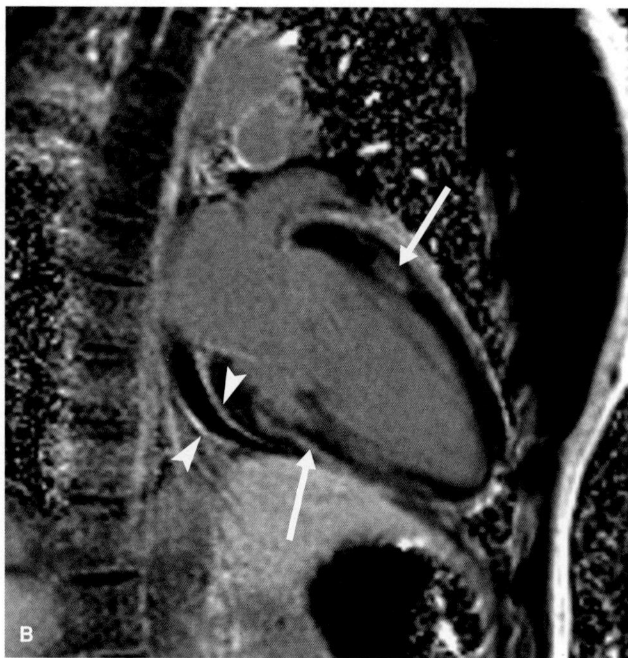

FIGURE 29.20. Myopericarditis in a 17-year-old man with elevated troponin levels but normal coronary arteries on cardiac catheterization. Short-axis (**A**) and two-chamber (**B**) phase sensitive inversion recovery (PSIR) delayed gadolinium enhancement imaging set at an inversion time of 300 ms shows extensive mid-myocardial and subepicardial enhancement consistent with myocarditis (*white arrows*). In addition, there is pericardial enhancement and a small pericardial effusion consistent with pericardial inflammation (*white arrowheads,* **B**) making the diagnosis of myopericarditis.

others may develop permanent pericardial adhesions, thickening, or calcification.

In the acute setting, many patients with acute pericarditis experience sharp chest pain which is usually worse on inspiration and when the patient is supine. A pericardial friction rub, due to fibrinous deposits, may be present on examination. ECG changes are often present and a small elevation of troponins is common.

On CT, the pericardium is usually thickened to greater than 4 mm in diameter and demonstrates either smooth or nodular enhancement (Figs. 29.10C, D, F; 29.16; 29.18; and 29.19). However, the lack of enhancement or thickening does not exclude the diagnosis of acute pericarditis. In many instances, there will be an associated pericardial effusion which may help one visualize the pericardial inflammation (Fig. 29.10B).

On MRI, the signal of the inflamed pericardium can vary depending on the severity of disease and pulse sequence utilized (Fig. 29.19). On T1-weighted, T2-weighted, and SSFP sequences, the pericardium will appear intermediate (grayish) in signal and will be thickened. Edema sensitive T2-weighted sequences such as a short-tau inversion recovery (STIR) may show pericardial edema and inflammation of the surrounding fat. In some cases, fibrinous bands can be seen in the pericardium. Postcontrast, the pericardium will often enhance. In cases of myopericarditis, delayed enhancement imaging can also show injury to the underlying myocardium (Fig. 29.20).

Fibrous Pericarditis

While the pericardium may return to normal after an episode of pericarditis, in some instances the pericardium becomes permanently injured due to the deposition of fibrous tissue with subsequent pericardial thickening and development of adhesions. If the adhesions are extensive, it can lead to obliteration of the pericardial space.

Certain etiologies of pericarditis are more likely to lead to chronic fibrous thickening. These include conditions that lead to relapsing episodes of pericarditis such as renal disease (Fig. 29.21) and certain collagen vascular diseases such as RA, SLE (Fig. 29.22), and scleroderma. Other etiologies of fibrous pericardial disease include radiation, infections (most notably tuberculosis), and pericardial injury due to cardiac surgery or trauma.

Calcium deposition in the pericardium represents an end-stage reaction to pericardial injury. While deposits may be focal (Fig. 29.21D), extensive calcification can occur that can lead to encasement of the entire heart (Fig. 29.23). The etiology of calcific pericarditis is the same as those that lead to fibrous pericarditis.

On CT, fibrous pericarditis manifests as pericardial thickening with a variable-sized effusion. Conventionally, a pericardial thickness of greater than 4 mm has been used to define pericardial thickening. However, it can often be difficult to accurately distinguish pericardial thickening from fluid, especially if both are coexistent. Pericardial enhancement may be present. Calcifications are best visualized on CT although extensive pericardial calcifications can be seen on chest radiography (Fig. 29.23).

On MRI, the pericardium will appear thickening and irregular with variable early enhancement (Fig. 29.24). However, delayed enhancement obtained 10 minutes after the administration of gadolinium can show enhancement from the deposition of fibrous tissue (Fig. 29.22). An MRI tagging sequence, which involves placing a grid of saturation lines over the heart and pericardium, can demonstrate adhesion between the visceral and parietal pericardium. In normal cases, the grid lines between the pericardial layers slip past each other during the cardiac cycle and the grid lines break. When the visceral and parietal pericardium are adherent to one another, the grid lines in the area of adhesions will remain intact (Fig. 29.24). Calcifications may be difficult to see but the pericardium but will appear low signal on all sequences and enhancement within the areas of calcification will be absent. While patients with pericardial fibrosis, adhesions, and calcification can remain asymptomatic, patients are at an increased risk of developing constrictive pericarditis (CP).

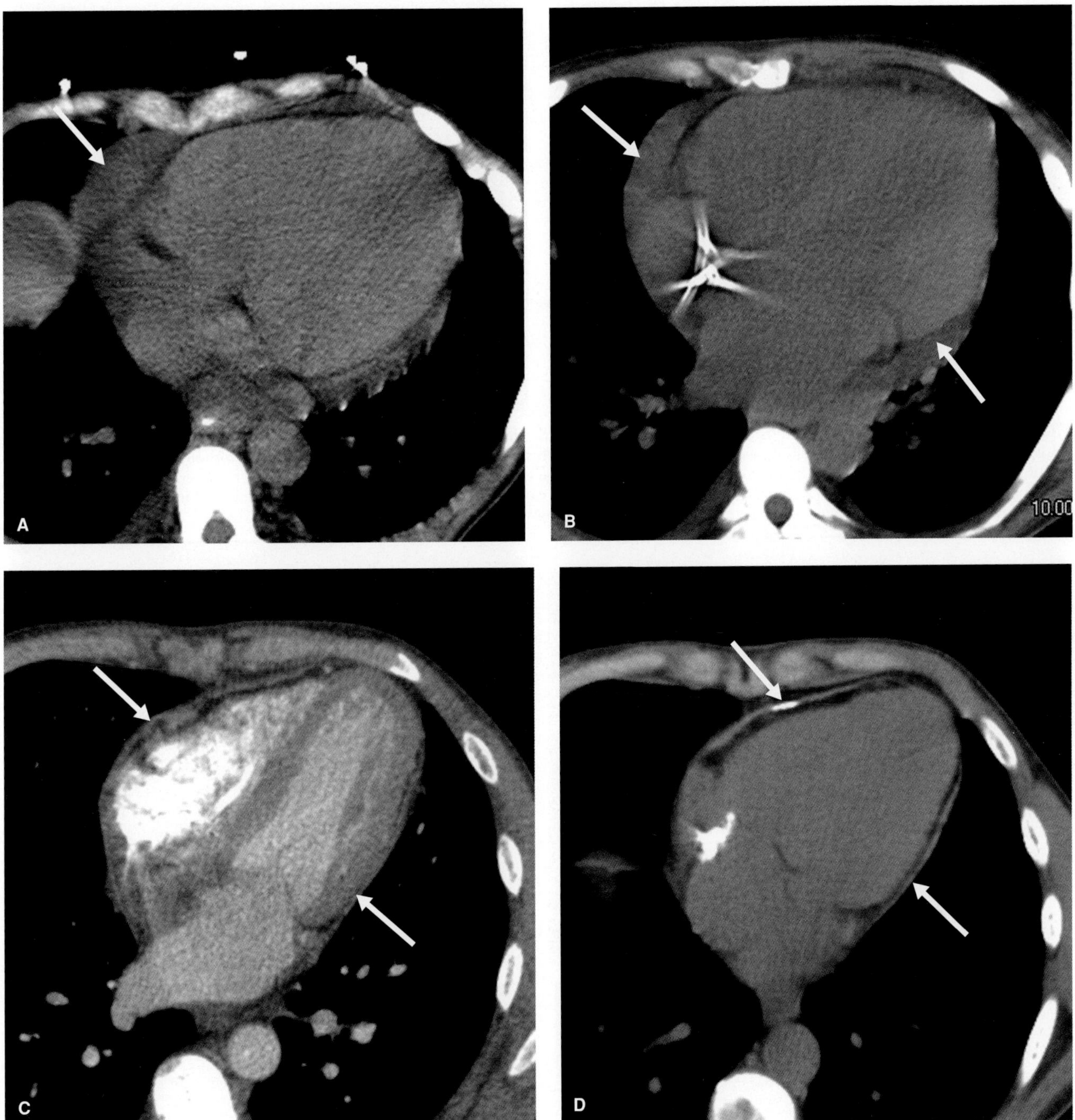

FIGURE 29.21. A to D: Progression of uremic pericarditis over 6 years from fibrinous pericarditis to fibrous pericarditis. **A, B:** Axial CT images from noncontrast CT scans in a patient with chronic renal failure obtained in 2005 (**A**) and 2006 (**B**) shows recurrent pericardial effusions (*white arrows*). Pericardial thickening and fibrinous strands in the pericardium were visible on echocardiogram during both episodes. Axial images from CT scans with contrast obtained in 2008 show diffuse pericardial thickening without a pericardial effusion (*white arrows*). Notice the more elongated shape of the ventricles compared to the prior studies which can be seen with pericardial constriction. **D:** Noncontrast study performed in 2011 shows increased thickening and calcification of the pericardium (*white arrows*). Pericardial stripping was performed on the patient in 2012 due to worsening symptoms of constrictive pericarditis. Pathology showed fibrous adherence of the visceral and parietal pericardium leading to obliteration of the pericardial space.

Constrictive Pericarditis

CP is a condition in which reduced compliance of the pericardium leads to elevated ventricular diastolic pressures. While CP is occasionally secondary to acute or subacute pericarditis, it occurs in cases of pericardial fibrosis, adhesions, and/or calcification.

The pathophysiology of CP is secondary to equalization of pressures in all cardiac chambers because the total cardiac volume is determined by the scarred and inelastic pericardium. Similar to tamponade, the heart is forced to operate in a noncompliant space leading to elevated systemic and pulmonary venous pressures which are required to maintain cardiac filling. The noncompliant space also leads to ventricular

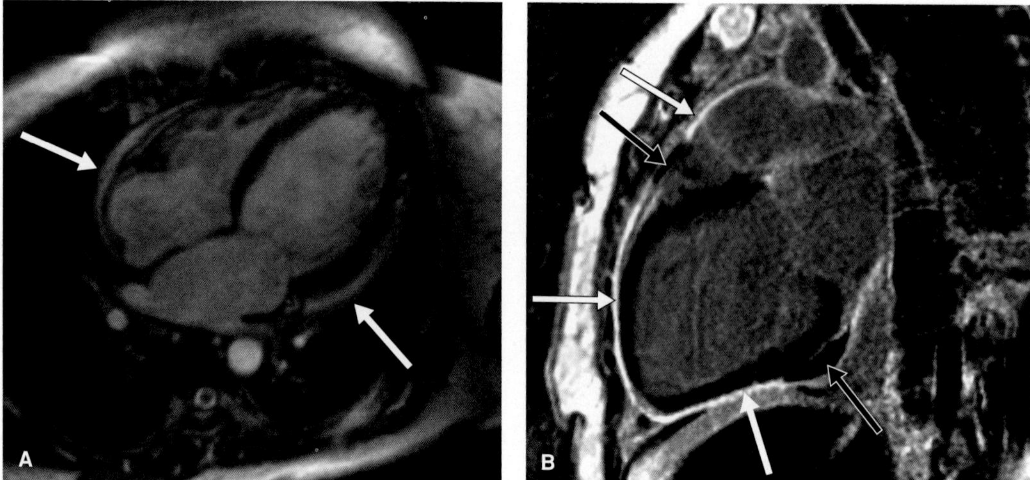

FIGURE 29.22. A, B: Fibrous pericarditis and nonischemic dilated cardiomyopathy in a 29-year-old woman with systemic lupus erythematosus (SLE). A: Four-chamber SSFP image shows a dilated left ventricle and diffuse pericardial thickening (*white arrows*) without effusion. The calculated ejection fraction was 28%. B: Two-chamber delayed–enhancement image shows extensive delayed enhancement of the pericardium (*white arrows*) due to the deposition of fibrous tissue which obliterates the pericardial cavity. Only a trace amount of pericardial fluid is present (*black arrows*). Lack of delayed myocardial enhancement suggests a nonischemic cardiomyopathy which is also common in SLE.

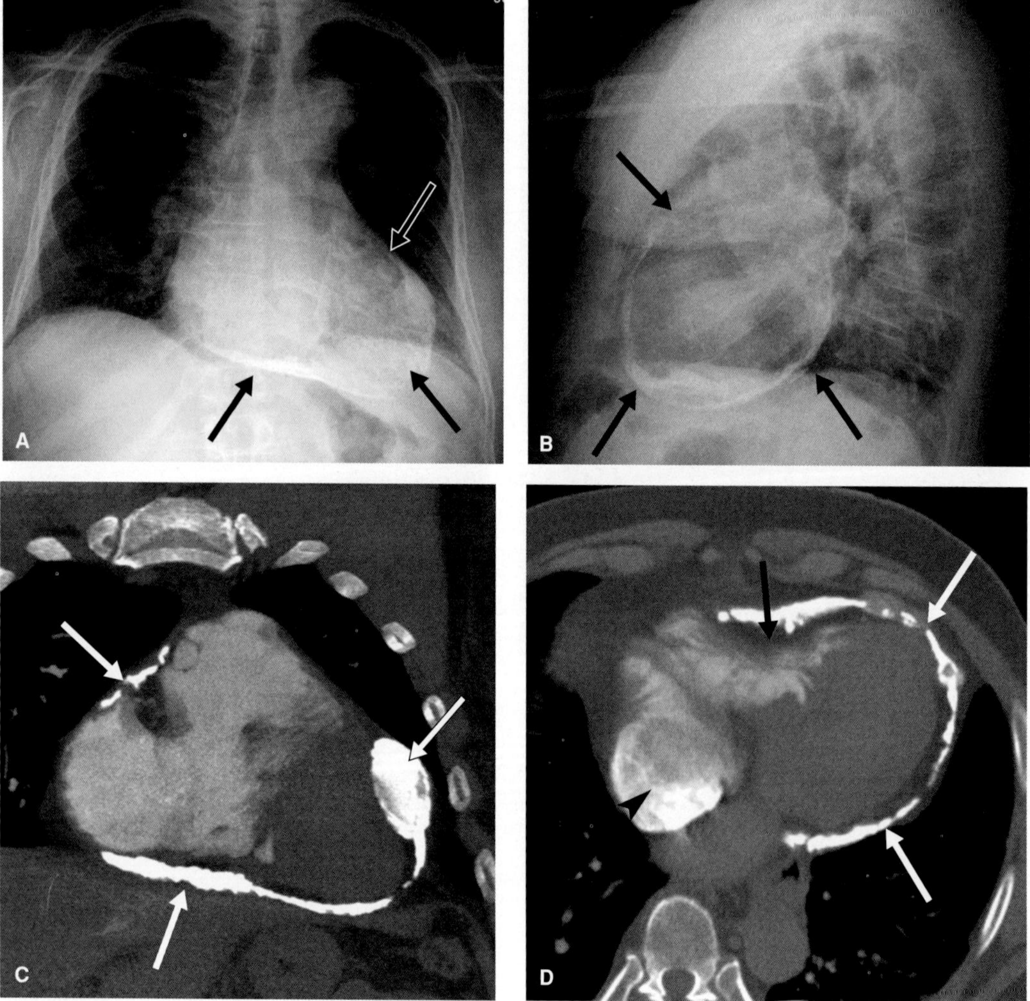

FIGURE 29.23. A to D: Diffuse pericardial calcification in a 70-year-old man with a history of tuberculous pericarditis and signs of constrictive pericarditis. A, B: PA (A) and lateral (B) radiographs demonstrate extensive circumferential pericardial calcification (*black arrows*). C: Coronal image from a contrast-enhanced CT shows the diffuse calcification (*white arrows*). D: Axial image through the inferior aspect of the heart again shows diffuse calcification (*white arrows*) with compression of the anterior wall of the right ventricle (*black arrow*) and dilation of the inferior vena cava (IVC, *black arrowhead*). The patient underwent pericardial stripping to alleviate his constrictive physiology.

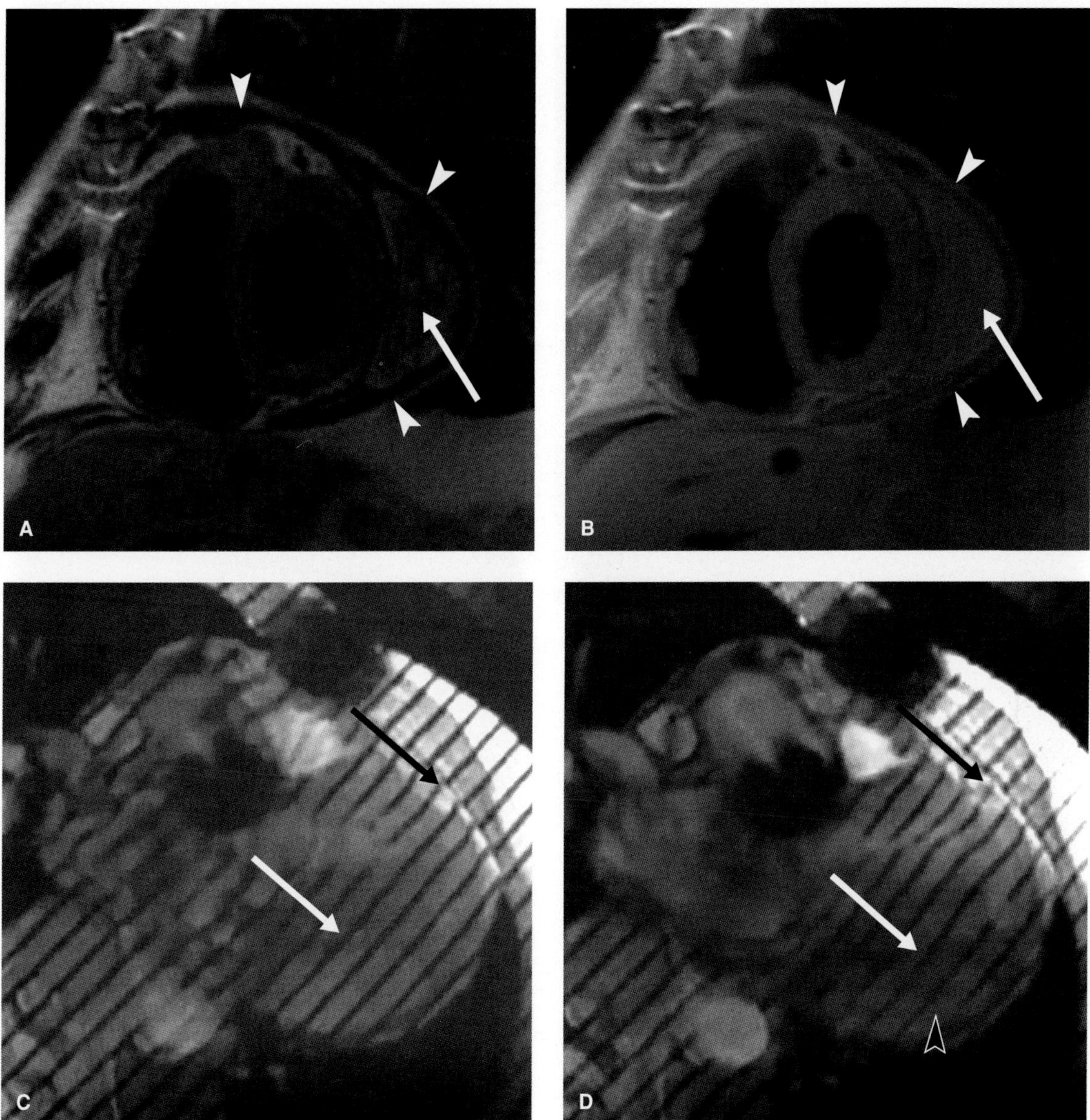

FIGURE 29.24. **A** to **D:** Fibrous pericarditis with pericardial adhesions in a 73-year-old woman who developed hemopericardium after coronary artery bypass and aortic valve replacement. **A, B:** Short-axis T2-weighted (**A**) and T1-weighted images (**B**) through the mid-cavity level shows pronounced pericardial thickening along the anterior, anterolateral, inferolateral, and inferior aspects of the pericardium which measures up to 9 mm in thickness (*white arrowheads*). The dark signal of the pericardium on T2 weighting is due to calcification. Sequela of chronic hematoma are present between the thickened parietal and visceral pericardium (*white arrows*). **C, D:** Axial gradient echo tagging sequence shows multiple grid lines. At the start of the sequence, during diastole (**C**), the anterior (*black arrow*) and posterior (*white arrow*) grid lines are intact. During systole (**D**) the grid lines between the endocardial and epicardial surfaces of the right ventricle and more anterior portions of the left ventricle break as the pericardium slides freely along the surface of the heart (*black arrow*). However, posteriorly, in the region of the chronic hematoma (*black arrowhead*), the grid lines between the endocardial and epicardial surfaces remain intact (*white arrow*) which signifies that the pericardium is scarred down and adherent to the underlying epicardium.

interdependence as the increased volume in one ventricle leads to decreased volume in the other ventricle.

CP typically manifests with symptoms of low cardiac output, which particularly affects the right side of the heart. Echocardiography is often obtained initially and can show findings of CP such as equalization of pressures during diastole and the decrease or reversal of blood flow in the hepatic veins during expiration. However, in some instances, the echocardiogram is of limited diagnostic yield or the results are equivocal and additional imaging may aid in the diagnosis.

CT and MRI are helpful techniques in making the diagnosis of CP. Thickening of the pericardium is well visualized with both techniques (Figs. 29.21 and 29.25). On CT, pericardial calcification is evident in up to 27% of patients with CP. Delayed gadolinium enhancement of the pericardium secondary to scarring is present in approximately one-half of patients with CP.

However, although pericardial thickening is a common imaging feature, the absence of pericardial thickening does not exclude the diagnosis as up to 28% of patients with CP demonstrate normal pericardial thickness on CT and 18% had normal thickness on histology. Moreover, patients with end-stage CP are more likely than those with reversible CP to have a normal diameter of the pericardium.

Other morphologic features may be visible on CT or MRI. Poor compliance of the pericardium can change the shape of the cardiac chambers as the ventricles may show a conical appearance (Figs. 29.21 and 29.25) and there may be atrial enlargement. Dilation of the IVC (Fig. 29.23D) and azygos

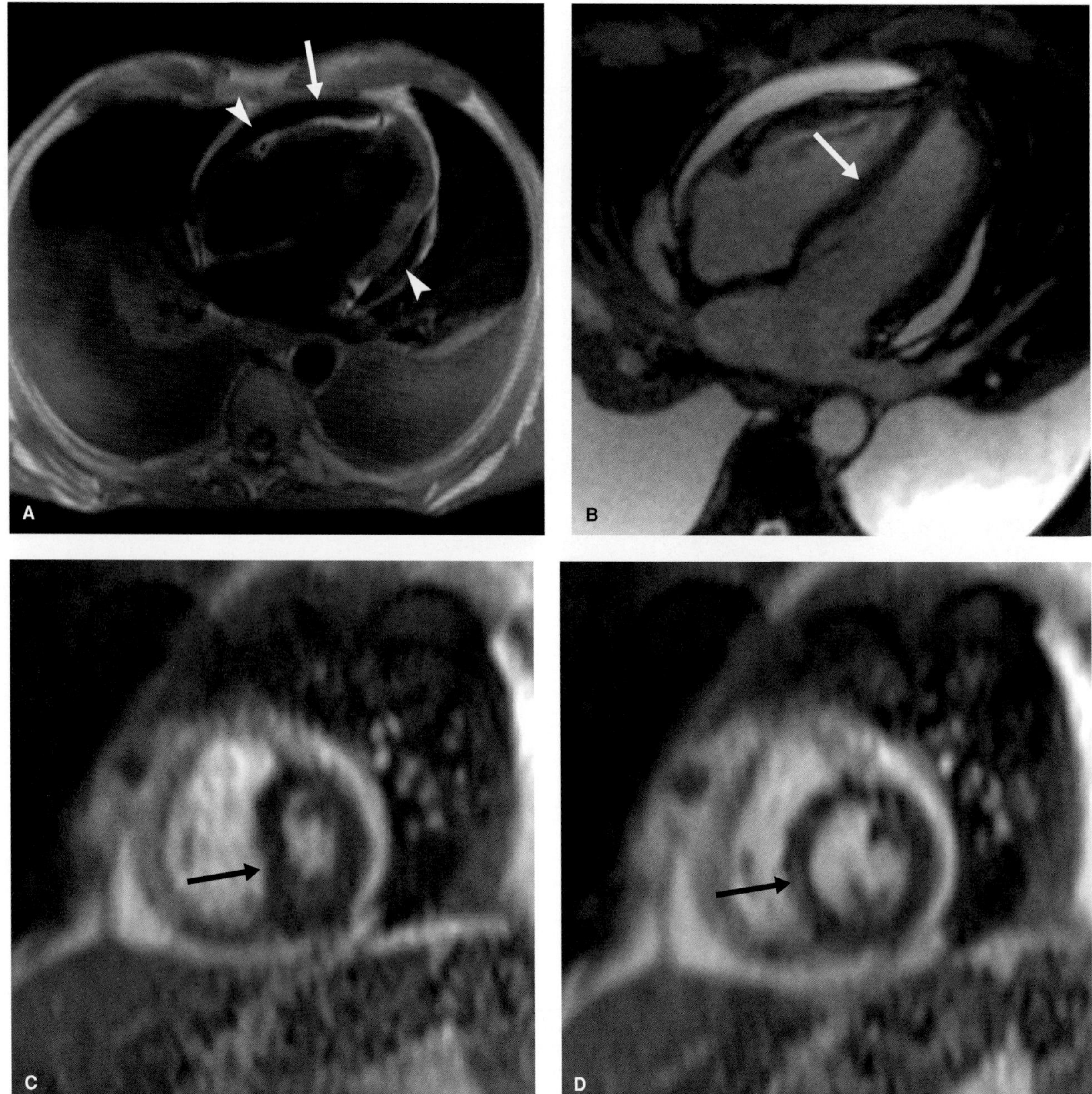

FIGURE 29.25. **A** to **D:** MRI findings in constrictive pericarditis in a 45-year-old man. **A:** Four-chamber axis T1-weighted image shows diffuse pericardial thickening best seen anteriorly (*white arrow*). A small to moderate pericardial effusion is present (*white arrowheads*). **B:** Four-chamber SSFP sequence show a septal bounce which is characteristic of constrictive pericarditis. During early diastole, increased right ventricular (RV) pressures from early RV filling causes bowing of the septum to the left (*arrow*). During mid diastole, increased left ventricular (LV) pressures due to later LV filling causes the septum to bounce back to the right. **C, D:** Free-breathing, nongated short-axis cine images obtained during deep respiration (**C**) and expiration (**D**) show the respiratory variation in septal morphology in constrictive pericarditis. On early inspiration (**C**), rapid increase of RV pressures due to increased right-sided venous return leads to dramatic flattening of the septum (*black arrow*). During expiration (**B**), LV pressures exceed RV pressures and the septum has a normal appearance (*black arrow*). This findings confirms ventricular interdependence and the diagnosis of constrictive pericarditis.

vein, ascites, pleural effusions, and peripheral edema are often present due to elevated right heart pressures.

On retrospectively gated cine MRI or cardiac CTA, ventricular interdependence leads to a classic septal bounce. In CP, rapid ventricular filling in early diastole is followed by abrupt termination of diastolic flow across the atrioventricular valves due to the noncompliant pericardium. Since right ventricular filling occurs slightly before left ventricular filling, the early increase in right ventricular pressures leads to paradoxical leftward motion of the septum in early diastolic filing. The septum will then rebound back toward the right during left ventricular filling and increased left ventricular pressures creating a septal bounce (Fig. 29.25). Although this early diastolic septal bounce can be seen in other conditions, it is often more pronounced in CP. While tagging sequences can demonstrate pericardial adhesions, patients without adhesions can have a constrictive physiology and patients with adhesions may not.

One of the best methods to make the diagnosis of CP on MRI is to demonstrate respiratory variation of the diastolic bounce using free-breathing, nongated cine MRI sequences

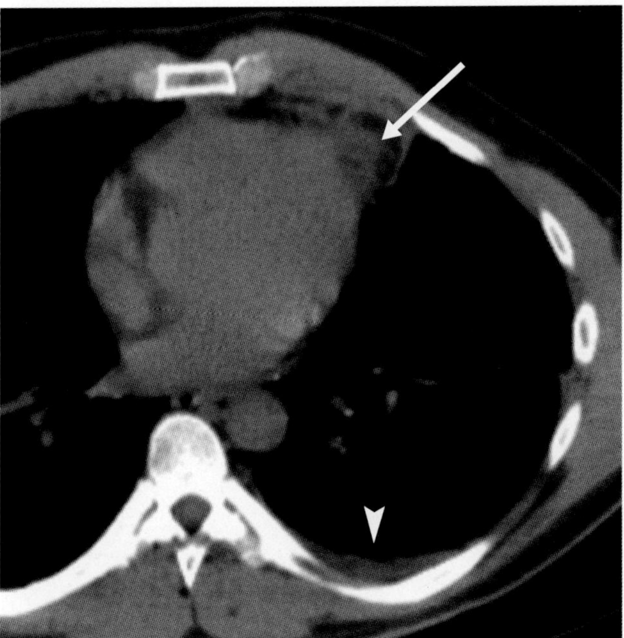

FIGURE 29.26. Epipericardial fat pad necrosis in a 45-year-old man with intense left-sided chest pain. Axial image shows an encapsulated fatty lesion adjacent and contiguous with the pericardium with associated pronounced inflammatory changes (*white arrow*). There is an associated small pleural effusion (*white arrowhead*) ipsilateral to the inflammatory changes. Although uncommon, this benign and self-limited entity should be recognized to prevent unnecessary intervention.

(Fig. 29.25). In patients with CP, during inspiration the negative intrathoracic pressure increases venous return to the right heart. However, since the right ventricular motion is limited by the noncompliant pericardium, the increased right ventricular pressures lead to pronounced flattening of the interventricular septum. On expiration, the opposite occurs as positive intrathoracic pressure increases pulmonary return resulting in a normal configuration of the septum of septal bowing to the right. This finding should be absent in restrictive cardiomyopathy and can help differentiate between the two.

Although pericardial thickening is a common finding in CP, pericardial effusions are usually not large. In rare instances, a patient may present with both a large pericardial effusion and a stiff, noncompliant pericardium, leading to both tamponade and constrictive physiologies, respectively. This syndrome is referred to as effusive CP and is a rare entity occurring in less than 7% of patients presenting with pericardial tamponade.

Epipericardial Fat Pad Necrosis

Epipericardial fat necrosis, also called pericardial fat necrosis, is an uncommon cause of acute chest pain that can mimic other conditions. The etiology is unknown but pathologic findings can resemble that seen with epiploic appendagitis adjacent to the colon and fat necrosis in the breast. It most commonly appears as an encapsulated fatty lesion with focal inflammation centered in the juxtapericardial fat (Fig. 29.26). Associated pleural and pericardial effusions as well as pericardial thickening are common. Recognition of this entity can prevent surgical intervention for a usually self-limiting process.

PERICARDIAL TUMORS

Primary pericardial tumors are quite rare and are often malignant. Primary pericardial mesothelioma, which arises from the mesothelial cells that line the pericardium, accounts for 50% of primary pericardial neoplasms. However, it is still extremely rare and in a necropsy series of 500,000 cases, the incidence was <0.0022%. Unlike pleural mesothelioma, the association between asbestos exposure and pericardial mesothelioma is unclear. However, in approximately one-third of

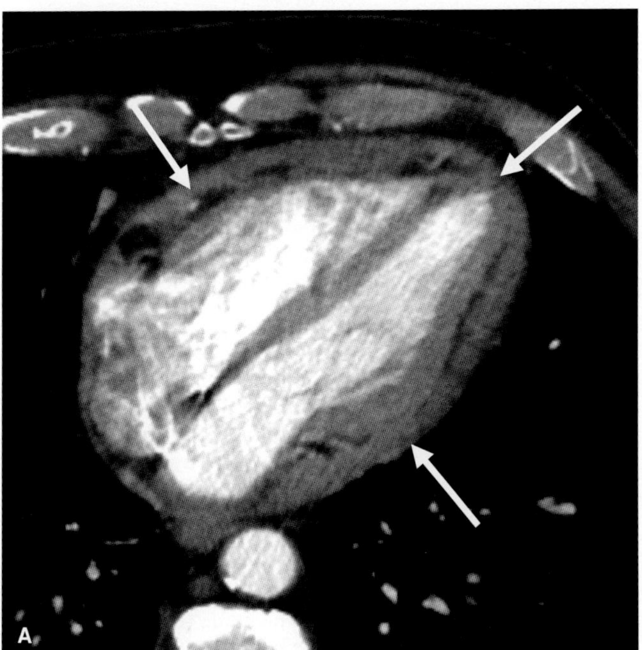

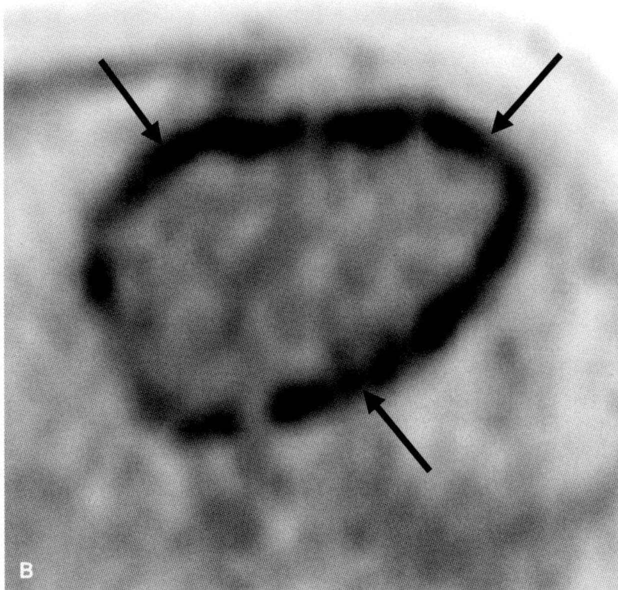

FIGURE 29.27. **A, B:** Pericardial mesothelioma in a 55-year-old man with shortness of breath. **A:** Axial CT image shows rind-like thickening of the pericardium. The entire heart is compressed, including the left ventricle. **B:** PET image at the same level shows diffuse FDG uptake in the pericardial thickening. Biopsy confirmed pericardial mesothelioma, which, although rare, is the most common primary pericardial tumor.

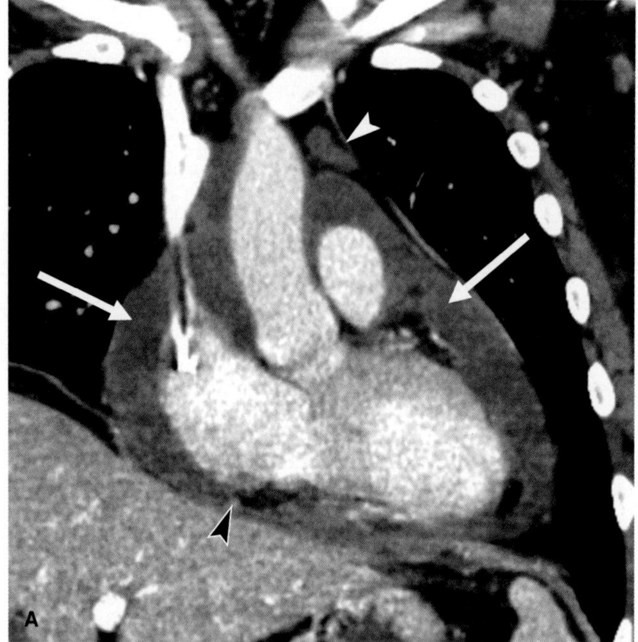

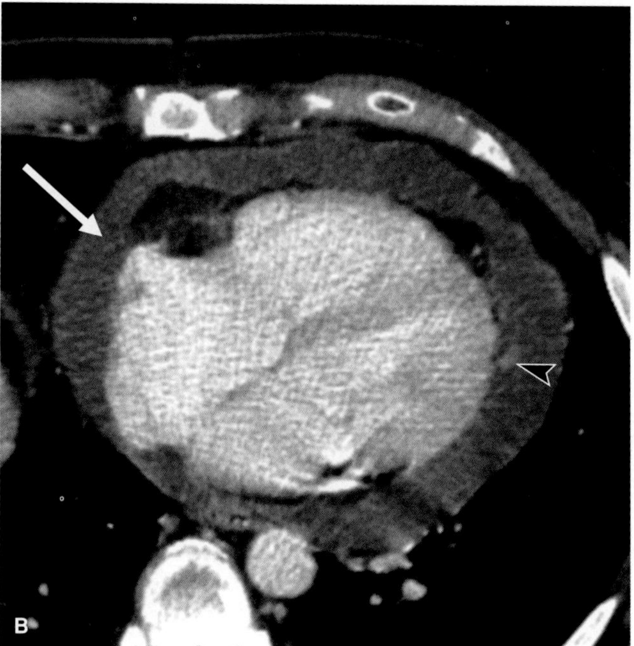

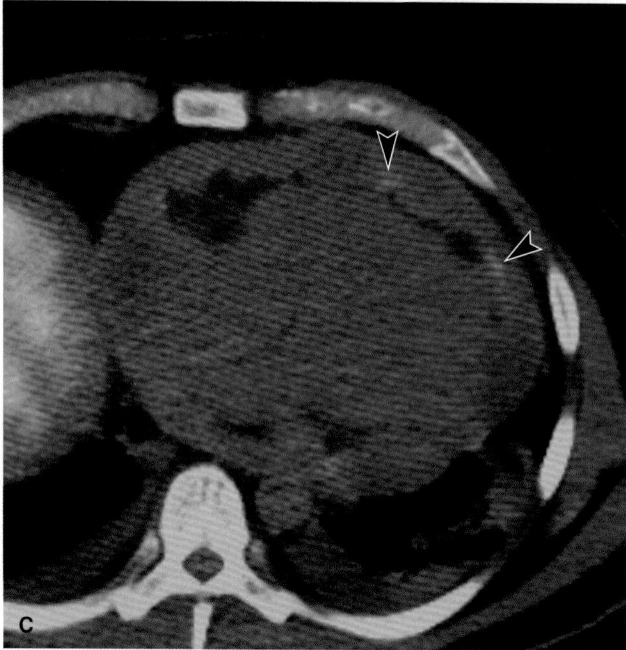

FIGURE 29.28. **A** to **C**: Pericardial angiosarcoma in a 50-year-old man. **A, B**: Coronal (**A**) and axial (**B**) CT images show a lobulated circumferential pericardial effusion with areas of pericardial enhancement and a few enhancing nodules (*black arrowheads*). There were enlarged adjacent lymph nodes (*white arrowhead*). **C**: Fused image from a PET-CT shows FDG uptake in the pericardium (*black arrowheads*) while much of the pericardial fluid shows minimal to no uptake. The patient did not demonstrate clinical findings suggestive of acute pericarditis. Subsequent pericardial biopsy showed angiosarcoma. There was no associated cardiac mass.

cases, patients have had a known exposure to asbestos. Similar to pleural mesothelioma, pericardial mesothelioma can be epitheliod, sarcomatoid, or biphasic on pathology. Early in the disease, CT and MRI demonstrate heterogeneous pericardial effusions and pericardial thickening that early in the disease it may be mistaken for acute or chronic pericarditis. As the disease progresses, masses fill the pericardium, often invading surrounding structures including the heart and vasculature (Fig. 29.27). Prognosis is poor and few patients survive longer than 12 months after diagnosis.

In addition to mesothelioma, primary pericardial sarcomas can occur and have numerous histologic subtypes (Fig. 29.28). While most lymphomas that involve the pericardium occur in those with system disease, primary pericardial lymphoma can occur. Its appearance is widely variable as it can appear as a solitary mass which can mimic other tumors. Additionally, a primary effusion lymphoma can occur in patients with HIV infection and appear as a large pericardial effusion (Fig. 29.29). Most intrapericardial germ cell tumors occur in children and are benign teratomas. However, malignant germ cell tumors do occur and should be considered in any pediatric patient with a heterogeneous intrapericardial mass, especially if it is located between the aortic root and left atrium (Fig. 29.30).

There are a wide variety of benign intrapericardial tumors. If fat is present in an intrapericardial tumor, teratomas or lipoblastomas should be considered in the pediatric population. In nonpediatric patients, if the lesion is composed entirely of fat, the diagnosis of a lipoma can be made (Fig. 29.31). Other benign pericardial tumors include lymphangiomas and hemangiomas. Lymphangiomas appear as localized or serpiginous masses primarily of fluid attenuation on CT. They may infiltrate around structures but are not invasive. Septations, which are usually absent with pericardial cysts may be present and

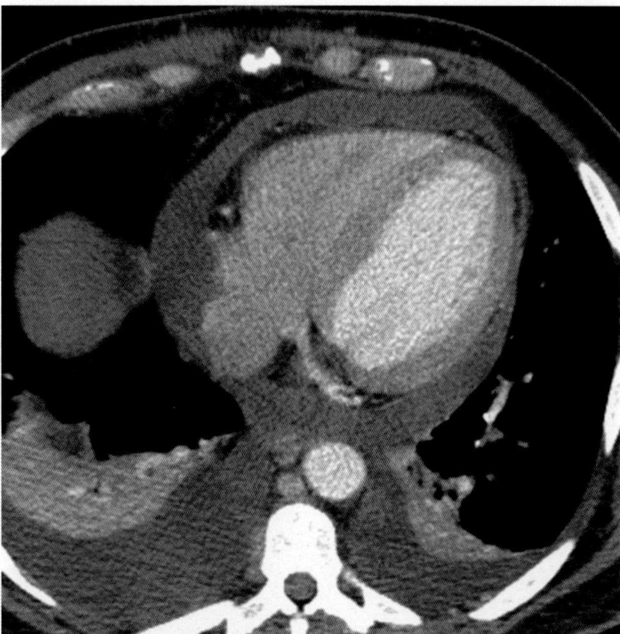

FIGURE 29.29. Primary pericardial effusion lymphoma in a 53-year-old man with HIV infection A. Axial image from a CT scan shows a moderate size pericardial effusion (*arrows*) and bilateral pleural effusions which did not resolve over many months. Pericardiocentesis and thoracentesis showed hemorrhagic fluid with numerous atypical lymphocytes consistent with a B-cell lymphoma. Lymphoma was not present anywhere else in the body.

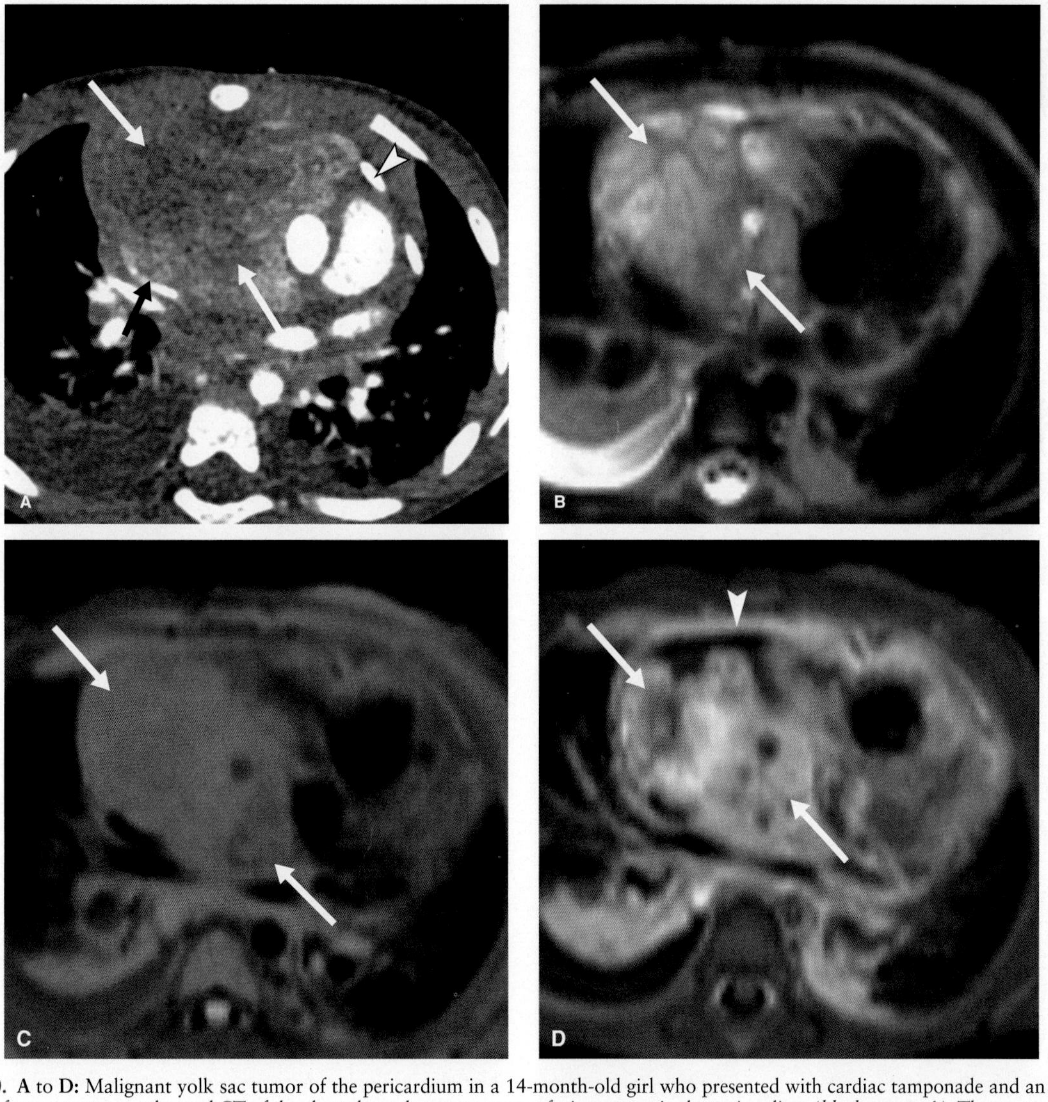

FIGURE 29.30. **A** to **D**: Malignant yolk sac tumor of the pericardium in a 14-month-old girl who presented with cardiac tamponade and an elevated AFP. **A**: Axial image from a contrast-enhanced CT of the chest shows heterogeneous soft tissue mass in the pericardium (*black arrow*, **A**). The mass compresses the superior vena cava (SVC, *black arrow*). A pericardial drain was placed to relieve the tamponade (*white arrowhead*). **B**: Axial SSFP T2-weighted imaging at the same level of the CT shows the very high-signal mass with cystic areas. **C**: T1-weighted images without contrast shows the mass is slightly hyperintense to myocardium. Areas of low signal represent cystic components. **D**: T1-weighted post contrast images show intense enhancement of the mass (*white arrows*) and adjacent pericardium (*white arrowhead*).

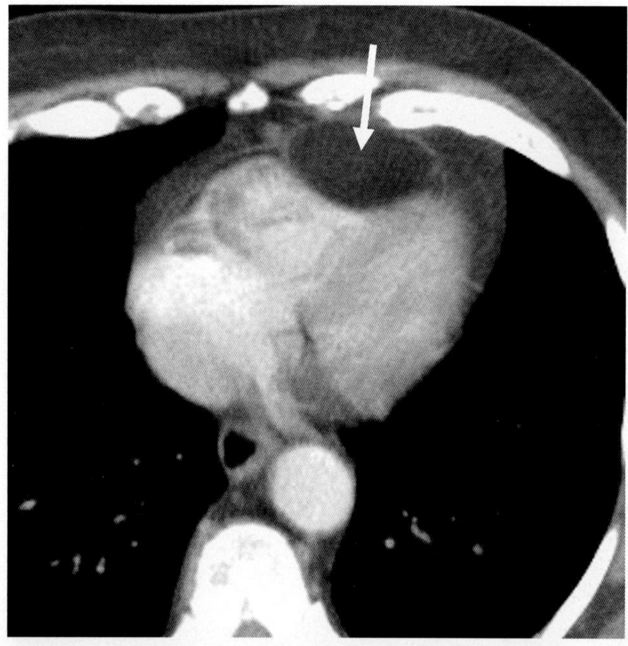

FIGURE 29.31. Incidental finding of an intrapericardial lipoma in a 77-year-old woman. Axial CT shows a fatty mass (*arrow*) located within the pericardium. Lipomas are benign lesions and can be located in the pericardium, heart, or mediastinum.

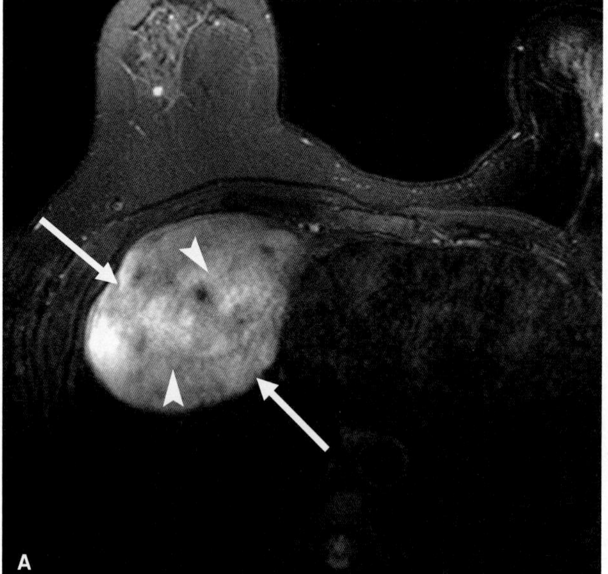

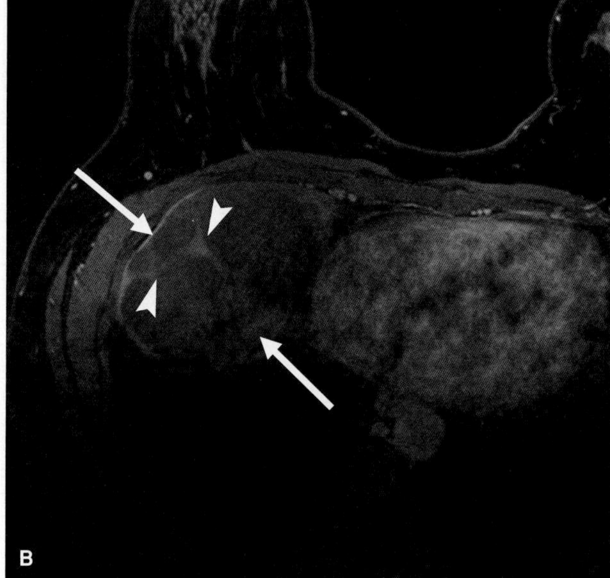

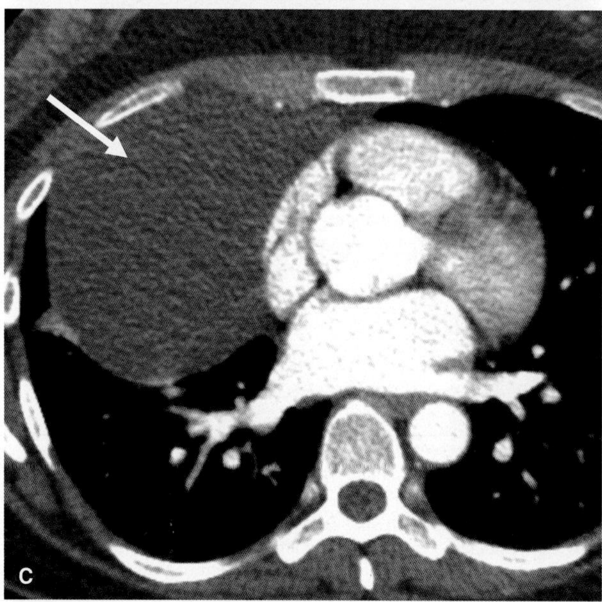

FIGURE 29.32. **A** to **C:** Incidental discovery of a pericardial lymphangioma in a 42-year-old woman with newly diagnosed breast cancer. **A:** Axial T2-weighted images from a breast MRI shows predominantly hyperintense but somewhat heterogeneous mass in the right cardiophrenic recess (*white arrows*) with internal septations (*white arrowheads*). **B:** Axial T1-weighted postcontrast image from the breast MRI shows enhancement of the septations and rim of the mass but no enhancement elsewhere. **C:** Axial image from a contrast-enhanced CT shows a smoothly marginated, fluid attenuation mass in the right cardiophrenic recess (*white arrow*). No enhancement was seen. Although the differential diagnosis on CT includes a pericardial cyst, the presence of enhancing septations and heterogeneous internal signal on MRI makes this unlikely. A pericardial lymphangioma was confirmed on resection.

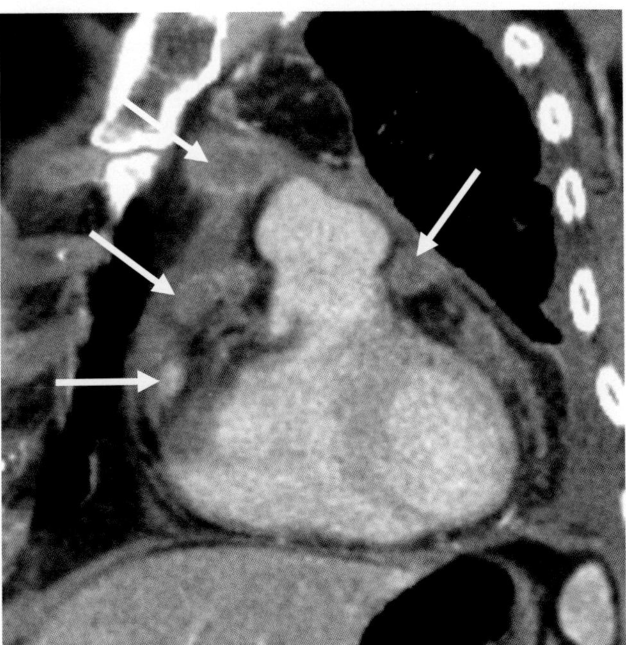

FIGURE 29.33. Pericardial metastases from lung cancer in a 58-year-old woman. Coronal oblique multiplanar reformat shows multiple enhancing pericardial masses (*white arrows*). Pleural metastases were also present. Pericardial metastases are much more common than primary pericardial tumors.

can show enhancement (Fig. 29.32). On MRI, they are high signal on T2-weighted images but can vary from low signal to high signal on T1-weighted images. The administration of contrast can help distinguish pericardial lymphangiomas from hemangiomas which can appear similar on precontrast imaging. Except for septations, lymphangiomas show no internal enhancement, while hemangiomas show nodular enhancement with progressive filling over time owing to their vascular nature. Other benign pericardial tumors include paragangliomas, fibromas, and teratomas.

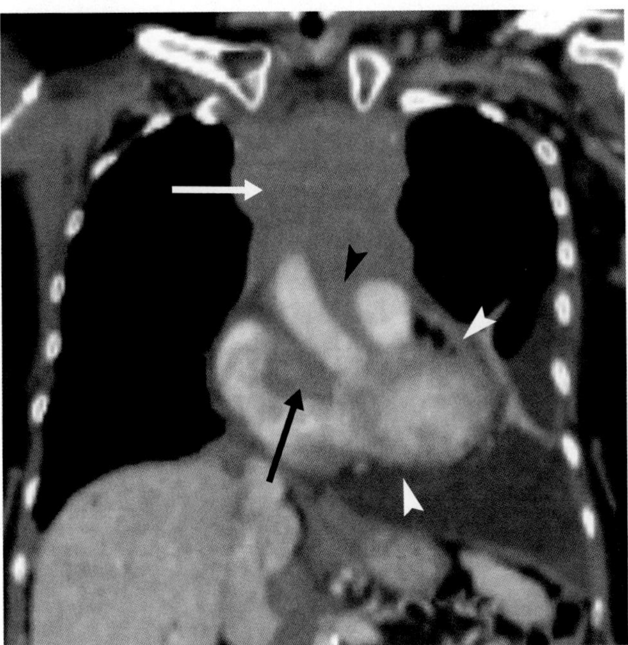

FIGURE 29.34. Pericardial metastases from lymphoma in a 67-year-old woman. Coronal oblique multiplanar reformat shows a very large confluent mediastinal mass (*white arrow*) invading into the pericardium (*black arrowhead*) and heart (*black arrow*). There is pericardial thickening and an effusion due to pericardial metastases (*white arrowheads*). A left pleural effusion is also present.

Secondary involvement of the pericardium by malignancy is much more common than primary pericardial neoplasms. Lung cancer (Fig. 29.33), breast cancer, and lymphoma (Fig. 29.34) are the most common malignancies to involve to the pericardium and can occur through direct invasion or metastatic spread. Other tumors that have a propensity to involve the pericardium include melanoma and renal cell carcinoma.

Symptoms of pericardial involvement by tumor are related to the extent of disease. Nonspecific symptoms of chest pain and shortness of breath are frequent. Effusions are often hemorrhagic and can be quite large leading to tamponade in 16% of patients. Diffuse involvement can encase the heart leading to pericardial constriction. CT and MRI may show the primary site of disease as well as the extent of pericardial involvement. Typically, pericardial thickening is present with a variable amount of pericardial nodularity. However, thickening may be absent, and the only finding is a pericardial effusion which may represent a mixture or fluid, hemorrhage, and malignant cells (Fig. 29.30). Enhancement of portions of the pericardium may be present after contrast administration using either CT or MRI.

Suggested Readings

Abbas AE, Appleton CP, Liu PT, Sweeney JP. Congenital absence of the pericardium: case presentation and review of literature. *Int J Cardiol* 2005;98:21–25.

Akiba T, Marushima H, Masubuchi M, Kobayashi S, Morikawa T. Small symptomatic pericardial diverticula treated by video-assisted thoracic surgical resection. *Ann Thorac Cardiovasc Surg* 2009;15:123–125.

Alter P, Figiel JH, Rupp TP, Bachmann GF, Maisch B, Rominger MB. MR, CT, and PET imaging in pericardial disease. *Heart Fail Rev* 2013;18:289–306.

Bogaert J, Francone M. Cardiovascular magnetic resonance in pericardial diseases. *J Cardiovasc Magn Reson* 2009;11:14.

Bogaert J, Francone M. Pericardial disease: value of CT and MR imaging. *Radiology* 2013;267:340–356.

Broderick LS, Brooks GN, Kuhlman JE. Anatomic pitfalls of the heart and pericardium. *Radiographics* 2005;25:441–453.

Bull RK, Edwards PD, Dixon AK. CT dimensions of the normal pericardium. *Br J Radiol* 1998;71:923–925.

Burazor I, Aviel-Ronen S, Imazio M, et al. Primary malignancies of the heart and pericardium. *Clin Cardiol* 2014;37:582–588.

Carretta A, Negri G, Pansera M, Melloni G, Zannini P. Thoracoscopic treatment of a pericardial diverticulum. *Surg Endosc* 2003;17:158.

Carsky EW, Mauceri RA, Azimi F. The epicardial fat pad sign: analysis of frontal and lateral chest radiographs in patients with pericardial effusion. *Radiology* 1980;137:303–308.

Chiles C, Woodard PK, Gutierrez FR, Link KM. Metastatic involvement of the heart and pericardium: CT and MR imaging. *Radiographics* 2001;21:439–449.

Choe YH, Im JG, Park JH, Han MC, Kim CW. The anatomy of the pericardial space: a study in cadavers and patients. *AJR Am J Roentgenol* 1987;149:693–697.

Choi YW, McAdams HP, Jeon SC, Seo HS, Hahm CK. The "High-Riding" superior pericardial recess: CT findings. *AJR Am J Roentgenol* 2000;175:1025–1028.

Cohen R, Mirrer B, Loarte P, Navarro V. Intrapericardial mature cystic teratoma in an adult: case presentation. *Clin Cardiol* 2013;36:6–9.

Cracknell BR, Ail D. The unmasking of a pyopericardium. *BMJ Case Rep* 2015;2015:pii: bcr2014207441.

Eisenberg MJ, Dunn MM, Kanth N, Gamsu G, Schiller NB. Diagnostic value of chest radiography for pericardial effusion. *J Am Coll Cardiol* 1993;22:588–593.

Feigin DS, Fenoglio JJ, McAllister HA, Madewell JE. Pericardial cysts. A radiologic-pathologic correlation and review. *Radiology* 1977;125:15–20.

Feng D, Glockner J, Kim K, et al. Cardiac magnetic resonance imaging pericardial late gadolinium enhancement and elevated inflammatory markers can predict the reversibility of constrictive pericarditis after anti-inflammatory medical therapy: a pilot study. *Circulation* 2011;124:1830–1837.

Francone M, Dymarkowski S, Kalantzi M, Bogaert J. Real-time cine MRI of ventricular septal motion: a novel approach to assess ventricular coupling. *J Magn Reson Imaging* 2005;21:305–309.

Francone M, Dymarkowski S, Kalantzi M, Rademakers FE, Bogaert J. Assessment of ventricular coupling with real-time cine MRI and its value to differentiate constrictive pericarditis from restrictive cardiomyopathy. *Eur Radiol* 2006;16:944–951.

Frank H, Globits S. Magnetic resonance imaging evaluation of myocardial and pericardial disease. *J Magn Reson Imaging* 1999;10:617–626.

Fred HL. Pericardial fat necrosis: a review and update. *Tex Heart Inst J* 2010; 37:82–84.

Giassi KS, Costa AN, Bachion GH, Kairalla RA, Filho JR. Epipericardial fat necrosis: who should be a candidate? *AJR Am J Roentgenol* 2016:1–5.

Groell R, Schaffler GJ, Rienmueller R. Pericardial sinuses and recesses: findings at electrocardiographically triggered electron-beam CT. *Radiology* 1999; 212:69–73.

Hammer MM, Raptis CA, Javidan-Nejad C, Bhalla S. Accuracy of computed tomography findings in acute pericarditis. *Acta Radiol* 2014;55:1197–1202.

Hiratzka LF, Bakris GL, Beckman JA, et al. 2010 ACCF/AHA/AATS/ACR/ASA/SCA/SCAI/SIR/STS/SVM guidelines for the diagnosis and management of patients with Thoracic Aortic Disease: a report of the American College of Cardiology Foundation/American Heart Association Task Force on Practice Guidelines, American Association for Thoracic Surgery, American College of Radiology, American Stroke Association, Society of Cardiovascular Anesthesiologists, Society for Cardiovascular Angiography and Interventions, Society of Interventional Radiology, Society of Thoracic Surgeons, and Society for Vascular Medicine. *Circulation* 2010;121:e266–e369.

Hynes JK, Tajik AJ, Osborn MJ, Orszulak TA, Seward JB. Two-dimensional echocardiographic diagnosis of pericardial cyst. *Mayo Clin Proc* 1983;58: 60–63.

Ishihara T, Ferrans VJ, Jones M, Boyce SW, Kawanami O, Roberts WC. Histologic and ultrastructural features of normal human parietal pericardium. *Am J Cardiol* 1980;46:744–753.

Jeudy J, Kirsch J, Tavora F, et al. From the radiologic pathology archives: cardiac lymphoma: radiologic-pathologic correlation. *Radiographics* 2012; 32:1369–1380.

Kar SK, Ganguly T. Current concepts of diagnosis and management of pericardial cysts. *Indian Heart J* 2017;69:364–370.

Kellman P, Arai AE, McVeigh ER, Aletras AH. Phase-sensitive inversion recovery for detecting myocardial infarction using gadolinium-delayed hyperenhancement. *Magn Reson Med* 2002;47:372–383.

Klein AL, Abbara S, Agler DA, et al. American Society of Echocardiography clinical recommendations for multimodality cardiovascular imaging of patients with pericardial disease: endorsed by the Society for Cardiovascular Magnetic Resonance and Society of Cardiovascular Computed Tomography. *J Am Soc Echocardiogr* 2013;26:965–1012. e15.

Kodama F, Fultz PJ, Wandtke JC. Comparing thin-section and thick-section CT of pericardial sinuses and recesses. *AJR Am J Roentgenol* 2003;181:1101–1108.

Kojima S, Yamada N, Goto Y. Diagnosis of constrictive pericarditis by tagged cine magnetic resonance imaging. *N Engl J Med* 1999;341:373–374.

LeWinter MM. Clinical practice. Acute pericarditis. *N Engl J Med* 2014; 371:2410–2416.

Little WC, Freeman GL. Pericardial disease. *Circulation* 2006;113:1622–1632.

Maisch B, Seferovic PM, Ristic AD, et al. Guidelines on the diagnosis and management of pericardial diseases executive summary; the task force on the diagnosis and management of pericardial diseases of the European Society of Cardiology. *Eur Heart J* 2004;25:587–610.

Myers RB, Spodick DH. Constrictive pericarditis: clinical and pathophysiologic characteristics. *Am Heart J* 1999;138:219–232.

Nasser WK. Congenital diseases of the pericardium. *Cardiovasc Clin* 1976;7: 271–286.

Natanzon A, Kronzon I. Pericardial and pleural effusions in congestive heart failure-anatomical, pathophysiologic, and clinical considerations. *Am J Med Sci* 2009;338:211–216.

National Clinical Guideline Centre. *Major Trauma: Assessment and Initial Management.* London: 2016:85–110.

Oh KY, Shimizu M, Edwards WD, Tazelaar HD, Danielson GK. Surgical pathology of the parietal pericardium: a study of 344 cases (1993–1999). *Cardiovasc Pathol* 2001;10:157–168.

O'Leary SM, Williams PL, Williams MP, et al. Imaging the pericardium: appearances on ECG-gated 64-detector row cardiac computed tomography. *Br J Radiol* 2010;83:194–205.

Peebles CR, Shambrook JS, Harden SP. Pericardial disease—anatomy and function. *Br J Radiol* 2011;84 Spec No 3:S324–S337.

Pineda V, Caceres J, Andreu J, Vilar J, Domingo ML. Epipericardial fat necrosis: radiologic diagnosis and follow-up. *AJR Am J Roentgenol* 2005;185: 1234–1236.

Pugatch RD, Braver JH, Robbins AH, Faling LJ. CT diagnosis of pericardial cysts. *AJR Am J Roentgenol* 1978;131:515–516.

Rajiah P. Cardiac MRI: Part 2, pericardial diseases. *AJR Am J Roentgenol* 2011; 197:W621–W634.

Restrepo CS, Lemos DF, Lemos JA, et al. Imaging findings in cardiac tamponade with emphasis on CT. *Radiographics* 2007;27:1595–1610.

Restrepo CS, Vargas D, Ocazionez D, Martinez-Jimenez S, Betancourt Cuellar SL, Gutierrez FR. Primary pericardial tumors. *Radiographics* 2013;33: 1613–1630.

Rienmuller R, Groll R, Lipton MJ. CT and MR imaging of pericardial disease. *Radiol Clin North Am* 2004;42:587–601, vi.

Riquet M, Le Pimpec-Barthes F, Hidden G. Lymphatic drainage of the pericardium to the mediastinal lymph nodes. *Surg Radiol Anat* 2001;23: 317–319.

Roberts WC. Pericardial heart disease: its morphologic features and its causes. *Proc (Bayl Univ Med Cent)* 2005;18:38–55.

Sagrista-Sauleda J, Angel J, Sanchez A, Permanyer-Miralda G, Soler-Soler J. Effusive-constrictive pericarditis. *N Engl J Med* 2004;350:469–475.

Shabetai R, Meaney E. Proceedings: haemodynamics of cardiac restriction and tamponade. *Br Heart J* 1975;37:780.

Shaffer K, Rosado-de-Christenson ML, Patz EF, Jr., Young S, Farver CF. Thoracic lymphangioma in adults: CT and MR imaging features. *AJR Am J Roentgenol* 1994;162:283–289.

Shah AB, Kronzon I. Congenital defects of the pericardium: a review. *Eur Heart J Cardiovasc Imaging* 2015;16(8):821–827.

Sharma R, Harden S, Peebles C, Dawkins KD. Percutaneous aspiration of a pericardial cyst: an acceptable treatment for a rare disorder. *Heart* 2007;93:22.

Spodick DH. Macrophysiology, microphysiology, and anatomy of the pericardium: a synopsis. *Am Heart J* 1992;124:1046–1051.

Suman S, Schofield P, Large S. Primary pericardial mesothelioma presenting as pericardial constriction: a case report. *Heart* 2004;90:e4.

Talreja DR, Edwards WD, Danielson GK, et al. Constrictive pericarditis in 26 patients with histologically normal pericardial thickness. *Circulation* 2003;108:1852–1857.

Thomason R, Schlegel W, Lucca M, Cummings S, Lee S. Primary malignant mesothelioma of the pericardium. Case report and literature review. *Tex Heart Inst J* 1994;21:170–174.

Thurber DL, Edwards JE, Achor RW. Secondary malignant tumors of the pericardium. *Circulation* 1962;26:228–241.

Truong MT, Erasmus JJ, Gladish GW, et al. Anatomy of pericardial recesses on multidetector CT: implications for oncologic imaging. *AJR Am J Roentgenol* 2003;181:1109–1113.

Verhaert D, Gabriel RS, Johnston D, Lytle BW, Desai MY, Klein AL. The role of multimodality imaging in the management of pericardial disease. *Circ Cardiovasc Imaging* 2010;3:333–343.

Vesely TM, Cahill DR. Cross-sectional anatomy of the pericardial sinuses, recesses, and adjacent structures. *Surg Radiol Anat* 1986;8:221–227.

Vogiatzidis K, Zarogiannis SG, Aidonidis I, et al. Physiology of pericardial fluid production and drainage. *Front Physiol* 2015;6:62.

Waller BF, Taliercio CP, Howard J, Green F, Orr CM, Slack JD. Morphologic aspects of pericardial heart disease: Part I. *Clin Cardiol* 1992;15: 203–209.

Wang ZJ, Reddy GP, Gotway MB, Yeh BM, Hetts SW, Higgins CB. CT and MR imaging of pericardial disease. *Radiographics* 2003;23 Spec No: S167–S180.

Welch TD, Ling LH, Espinosa RE, et al. Echocardiographic diagnosis of constrictive pericarditis: Mayo Clinic criteria. *Circ Cardiovasc Imaging* 2014;7:526–534.

Yared K, Baggish AL, Picard MH, Hoffmann U, Hung J. Multimodality imaging of pericardial diseases. *JACC Cardiovasc Imaging* 2010;3:650–660.

Zurick AO, Bolen MA, Kwon DH, et al. Pericardial delayed hyperenhancement with CMR imaging in patients with constrictive pericarditis undergoing surgical pericardiectomy: a case series with histopathological correlation. *JACC Cardiovasc Imaging* 2011;4:1180–1191.

CHAPTER 30 ■ THORACIC AORTA

KATHLEEN JACOBS, MICHAEL J. HOROWITZ, AND SETH KLIGERMAN

The thoracic aorta is a tubular, candy-cane–shaped structure that connects the left ventricle to the systemic circulation. It extends from the level of the aortic valve to the diaphragmatic hiatus where it transitions to the abdominal aorta, approximately at the level of T12. The thoracic aorta is anatomically divided into the aortic root, ascending aorta, transverse arch, and descending thoracic aorta (Fig. 30.1).

AORTIC ROOT ANATOMY AND VARIANTS

The aortic root extends from the aortic annular ring to the sinotubular junction. The aortic valve annulus is a fibrous oval ring where the leaflets of the aortic valve attach and extend superiorly toward the sinuses of Valsalva. The aortic annulus is coupled to the mitral annulus via aortomitral fibrous tissue, which is a defining feature of the left ventricle. This is in contradistinction to the pulmonary valve, which is supported by the muscular right ventricular outflow tract.

Superior to the annulus are the sinuses of Valsalva which are three anatomic bulges of the aorta (Fig. 30.2). The three leaflets of the aortic valve form the valve plane at the level of the sinuses. The coronary artery ostia arise from the sinuses of Valsalva above the valve plane but below the sinotubular junction. The sinuses are named based on their respective coronary artery. The right coronary artery (RCA) arises from the right sinus of Valsalva which is directed anteriorly, and the left main coronary artery arises from the leftward facing left sinus of Valsalva. The noncoronary sinus is usually directed posteriorly between the right and left atria. Above the sinuses of Valsalva is the sinotubular junction, which is an anatomic waist between the sinuses of Valsalva and tubular ascending aorta.

Dimensions of the aorta vary with age, gender, and body size in adults. The aorta is generally largest in diameter at the sinuses of Valsalva and progressively tapers distally. Reported normal diameter of the aortic root is 3.5 to 3.72 cm in females and 3.63 to 3.91 cm in males on CT, measured orthogonal to the aorta.

Aortic Valve

The aortic valve serves as both a physical and hemodynamic boundary between the left ventricle and aorta. The normal aortic valve is composed of three leaflets/cusps which insert into the annular ring and coapt and form a trileaflet valve plane just inferior to the sinuses of Valsalva (Fig. 30.2). The contact points between valve leaflets are termed the valve commissures, which are best visualized during end diastole when the aortic valve is closed.

Congenital anomalies of the aortic valve are not uncommon and include unicuspid, bicuspid, or quadricuspid valve morphologies. Bicuspid aortic valve is the most common congenital cardiovascular anomaly with a prevalence of 0.5% to 2%. There are two major morphologic types of bicuspid aortic valve. A true bicuspid valve with completely separate and symmetric valves without a fused raphe is less frequent, comprising approximately 7% of bicuspid aortic valves (Fig. 30.3).

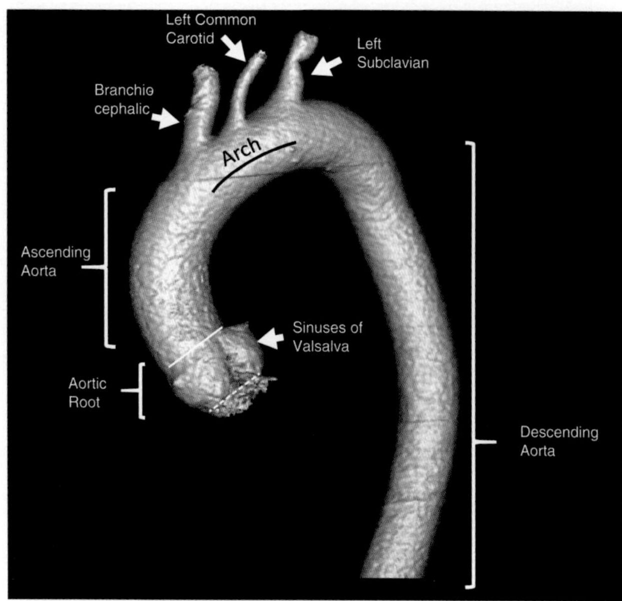

FIGURE 30.1. 3D Volume-Rendered Reformat of the Thoracic Aorta. Aortic root extends from the aortic valve annulus (*dashed line*) to the sinotubular junction (*solid line*) to the origin of the brachiocephalic artery. Normal three-vessel branching pattern of the aortic arch.

In 93% of cases, there is visible fusion between two leaflets or cusps. The fusion point between them is termed a raphe and appears as a dysmorphic, partially formed commissure below the valve plane. Of bicuspid valves with a raphe, fusion between the right and left coronary cusps is most common (70%) (Fig. 30.3), followed by fusion of the right and noncoronary cusps (28%), and fusion of the left and noncoronary cusps (1.4%).

Early development of aortic stenosis is a common complication in patients with a bicuspid aortic valve secondary to myxoid degeneration. This occurs in patients from 30 to 50 years, in contrast to senile aortic valve degeneration which occurs in patients 80 to 90 years old. Aortopathy and aneurysm formation are also associated with a bicuspid aortic valve. Due to the increased risk of rupture compared to the general population, guidelines recommend the repair of these aneurysms when they measure between 4.5 and 5 cm diameter versus 5.5 cm in the general population. Another common association with a bicuspid aortic valve is aortic coarctation, which is discussed below.

Unicuspid aortic valve has a reported incidence of 0.02%. Unicuspid aortic valve is defined by a single opening/commissure (i.e., unicommissural) usually in the left posterior position and has similar associations as bicuspid aortic valve (Fig. 30.4). Quadricuspid aortic valve has a clover-leaf morphology, is extremely rare, and more typically associated with early-onset regurgitation as opposed to stenosis (Fig. 30.5).

ASCENDING AORTA

The ascending aorta extends from the sinotubular junction to the origin of the right brachiocephalic artery (Fig. 30.1). The normal ascending aorta arises posterior and to the right of the main pulmonary artery (Fig. 30.6).

CT or MR evaluation of the aortic root and ascending aorta should use ECG gating to minimize cardiac motion artifact. It is important to reduce cardiac motion for multiple reasons including improved visualization of the valve/root anatomy, accurate measurement of the aorta in assessment for aneurysm, and to prevent false-positive diagnosis of aortic dissection. Gating technique (prospective vs. retrospective) will also vary depending on the indication of the study. For instance, evaluation of valvular function or dysfunction requires retrospective gating, while basic anatomic evaluation can be performed with prospective gating.

AORTIC ARCH ANATOMY AND VARIANTS

The aortic arch is a transverse segment from which the great vessels arise. The normal aortic arch is left sided and courses

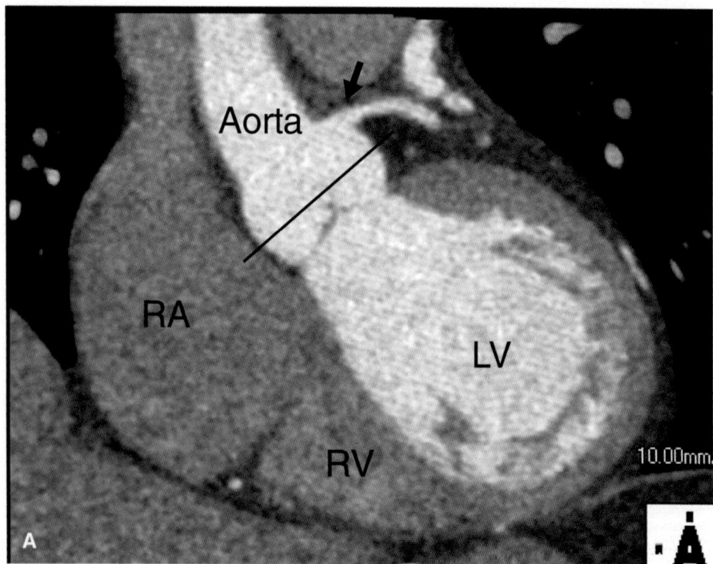

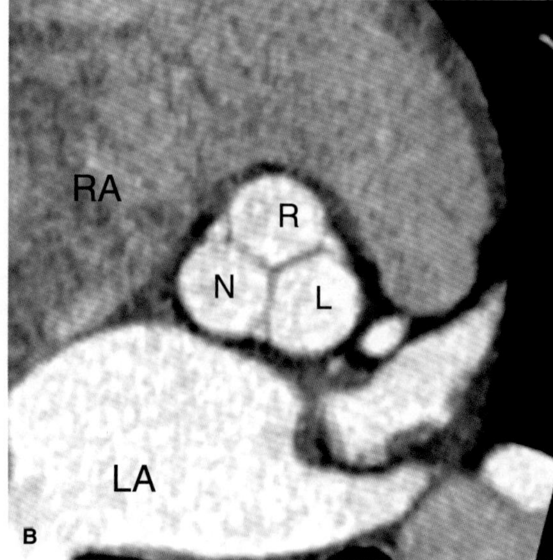

FIGURE 30.2. Coronal view through the aortic root (**A**), left coronary artery ostium indicated by *black arrow*. Orthogonal cross section through the **sinuses of Valsalva** (*black line*) produces a transverse view of the right (*R*), left (*L*), and noncoronary (*N*) cusps (**B**). Note that the normal noncoronary cusp is directed toward the interatrial septum between the left atrium (*LA*) and right atrium (*RA*). RV, right ventricle; LV, left ventricle.

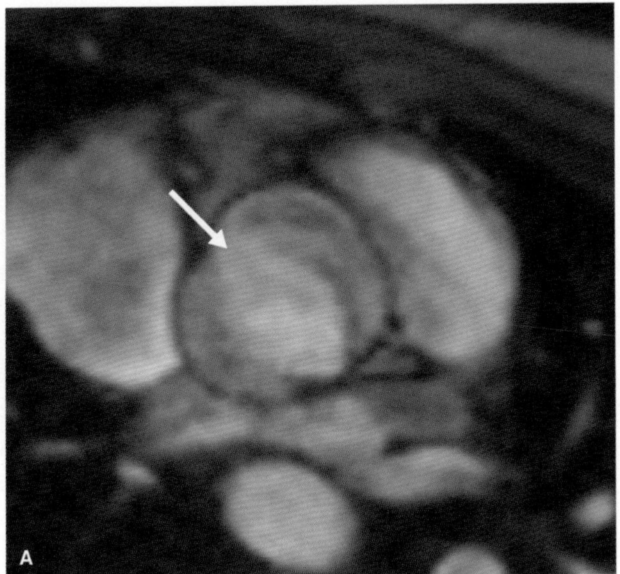

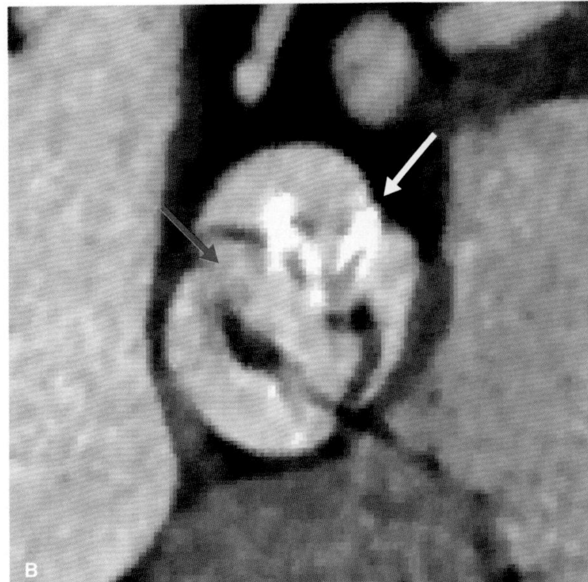

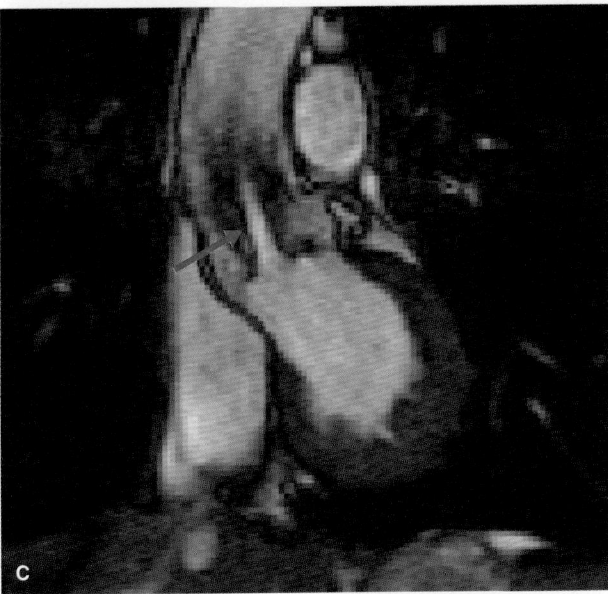

FIGURE 30.3. MR GRE image through the aortic valve during systole in a 23 year-old woman with Turners syndrome shows a true bicuspid aortic valve with two separate leaflets and a central fish mouth (*arrow*, **A**). There is no fused raphe. CT image through the aortic valve in a 51-year-old man with shortness of breath shows a thickened and partially calcified bicuspid aortic valve (*red arrow*) with fusion of the right and left coronary cusps. Calcified and thickened soft tissue is present inferior to the valve plane (*white arrow*) indicating the fused raphe (**B**). Oblique coronal MR GRE in this patient demonstrates flow acceleration across bicuspid aortic valve (*red arrow*, **C**).

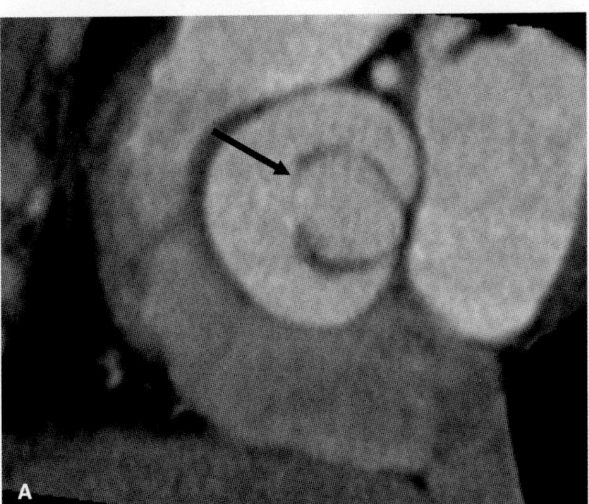

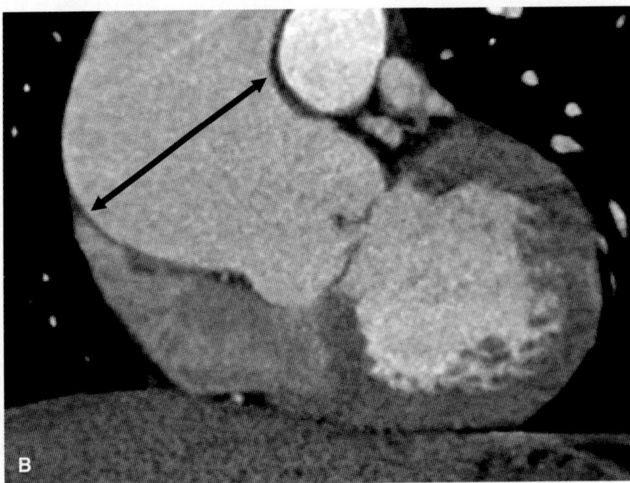

FIGURE 30.4. Unicuspid Aortic Valve. CT image transverse to the aortic valve demonstrates a single, eccentric opening/commissure (*arrow*, **A**), indicating an unicuspid valve. There is an associated aneurysmal dilation of the ascending aorta measuring up to 5.4 cm on coronal-oblique reformat (*double-headed arrow,* **B**).

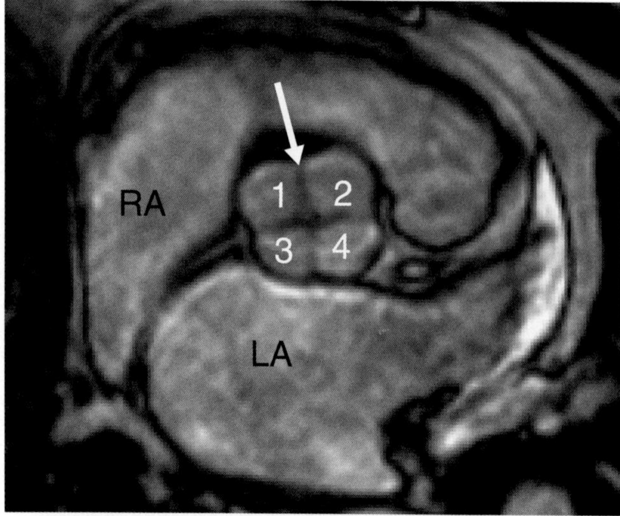

FIGURE 30.5. **Quadricuspid Aortic Valve.** Gradient echo MR image, transverse view of the aortic valve demonstrates the clover-leaf morphology of a quadricuspid valve (*arrow*) with four valve leaflets (1–4). LA, left atrium; RA, right atrium.

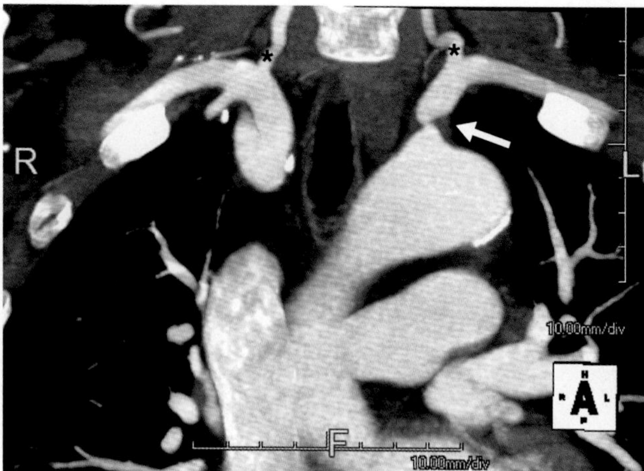

FIGURE 30.7. **Subclavian Steal.** Coronal MIP CT demonstrates narrowing of the proximal left subclavian artery secondary to large noncalcified atherosclerotic plaque (*arrow*). Normal origins of the vertebral arteries (*) from the ipsilateral subclavian arteries. Patient presented with diminished left upper extremity pulses.

above the pulmonary arteries toward the left (Fig. 30.6). Usually the aortic arch gives rise to three great vessels, occurring in 74% to 80% of the population (Fig. 30.1). The first vessel to branch from the aorta is the right brachiocephalic or innominate artery which bifurcates into the right common carotid artery and subclavian artery a few centimeters from its origin. The left common carotid artery and left subclavian artery are the second and third vessels to branch from the aortic arch, respectively.

The vertebral arteries normally arise from the proximal aspect of the subclavian arteries. Narrowing of the subclavian arteries proximal to the origin of the vertebral arteries, whether degenerative, inflammatory, or iatrogenic, can result in subclavian steal syndrome if there is hemodynamically significant obstruction. Findings on cross-sectional imaging of proximal subclavian narrowing with suggestive clinical history including symptoms of limb ischemia, differential arm pressures, or vertebrobasilar insufficiency should prompt concern for subclavian steal syndrome (Fig. 30.7).

The aortic isthmus is a physiologic narrowing of the aortic arch between the left subclavian artery origin and ligamentum arteriosum, the embryologic remnant of the ductus arteriosus (Fig. 30.8). Focal prominence of the aorta at the ligamentum arteriosum is a normal variant, termed a "ductus diverticulum" or "ductus bump" and should not be confused for an aneurysm or pseudoaneurysm. Distal to the ligamentum arteriosum, the aorta continues as the descending thoracic aorta

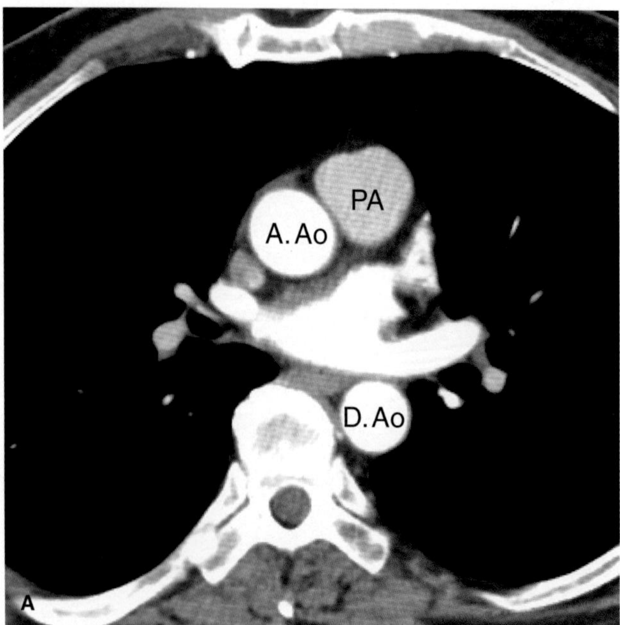

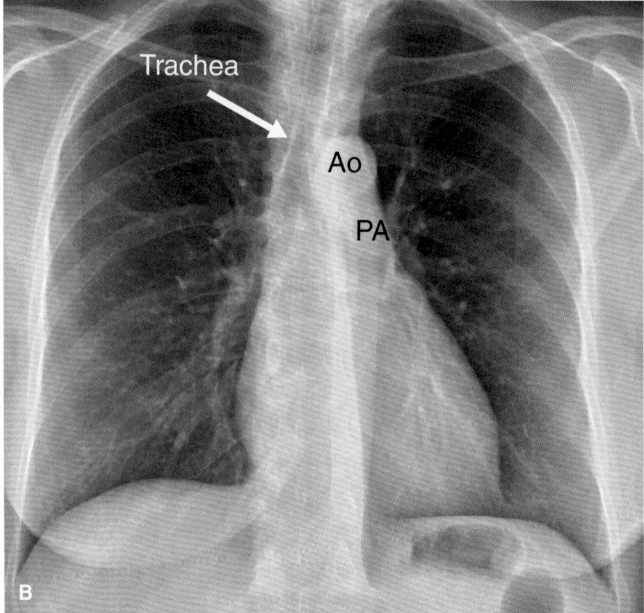

FIGURE 30.6. **Normal Ascending Aorta and Left Arch.** Axial CT image demonstrates ascending aorta (*A. Ao*) is located slightly posterior and to the right of the main pulmonary artery (*PA*) (**A**). Descending thoracic aorta (*D. Ao*) is to the left of the spine. PA chest radiograph demonstrates a normal left-sided aortic arch to the left of the trachea (*arrow*) and spine, positioned above the main pulmonary artery contour (**B**).

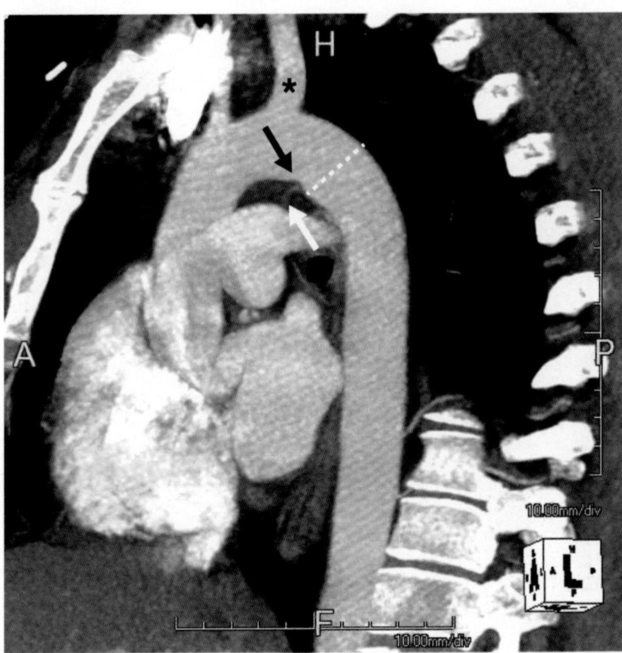

FIGURE 30.8. Sagittal MIP CT demonstrates focal narrowing of the distal aortic arch corresponding to the aortic isthmus (*black arrow*), just distal to the left subclavian artery takeoff (*). Note the focal prominence of the aorta (*dashed line*) at the origin of the ligamentum arteriosum (*white arrow*) which extends toward the left pulmonary artery. This is often referred to as a "ductus bump" or "ductus diverticulum."

abutting the left aspect of the thoracic spine and becoming the abdominal aorta at the diaphragmatic hiatus.

Left Arch Variants

Left aortic arch variants are common incidental findings usually of little clinical significance. Two-vessel aortic arch is characterized by common origin of the right brachiocephalic and left common carotid arteries and occurs in 13% to 20% of the population (Fig. 30.9). Although this is often termed a "bovine arch," this is a misnomer as a true bovine arch has only a single vessel from the aortic arch. A four-vessel arch in which the left vertebral artery has an independent origin from the aortic arch occurs in 5% to 6% of the population. In this case, the left vertebral artery originates between the left common carotid and subclavian arteries (Fig. 30.10).

Left aortic arch with aberrant right subclavian artery has a prevalence of 0.5% to 2%. Instead of the normal origin from the right brachiocephalic artery, the right subclavian artery arises distal to the left subclavian artery from the distal aortic arch and travels through the mediastinum behind the esophagus to supply the right upper extremity. On esophagram, the aberrant subclavian artery indents the posterior aspect of the esophagus (Fig. 30.11). In approximately 15% of cases, the aberrant right subclavian artery is associated with an aneurysm at its origin, termed a diverticulum of Kommerell. The diverticulum of Kommerell is an embryologic remnant of the dorsal aortic arch and can cause compressive symptoms on the esophagus if large. However, in most instances of an aberrant right subclavian artery, this diverticulum is absent or small. Additionally, this configuration does not form a vascular ring in the vast majority of instances. Only in the setting of a very rare right ligamentum arteriosum, which is a fibrous remnant of the ductus arteriosum, does a vascular ring occur with an aberrant right subclavian artery. In the absence of a diverticulum of Kommerell and vascular ring, an aberrant right subclavian artery is typically asymptomatic, but about 10% of patients can have dysphagia (aka "dysphagia lusoria") secondary to extrinsic compression of the esophagus.

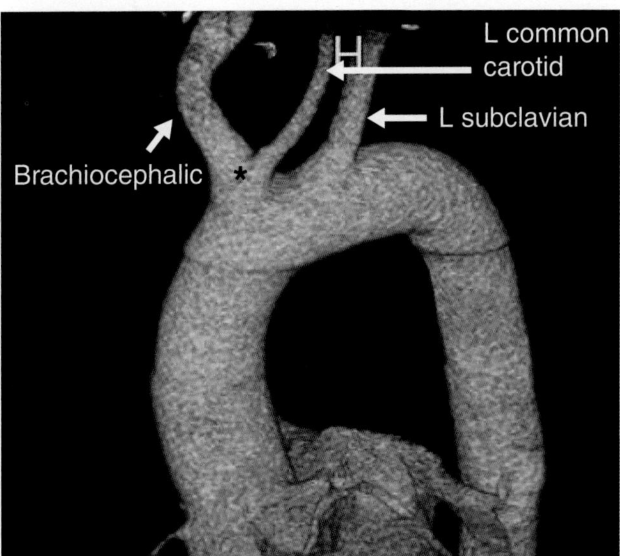

FIGURE 30.9. **Two-Vessel Arch.** 3D volume-rendered image of the aortic arch shows common origin (*) of the brachiocephalic artery and left common carotid artery.

Right Arch Variants

Right aortic arch has a prevalence of 0.05%. On frontal projection chest radiograph, the normal indentation of the left aortic arch on the left aspect of the trachea is absent, replaced

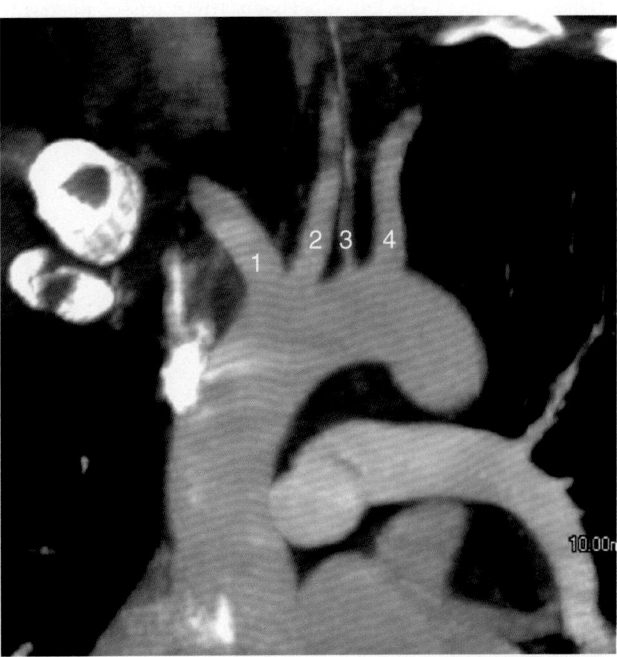

FIGURE 30.10. **Four-Vessel Arch.** Oblique sagittal MIP CT demonstrates separate origin of the left vertebral artery (*3*) between the left common carotid artery (*2*) and left subclavian artery (*4*). The brachiocephalic artery (*1*) is the first branch off the arch.

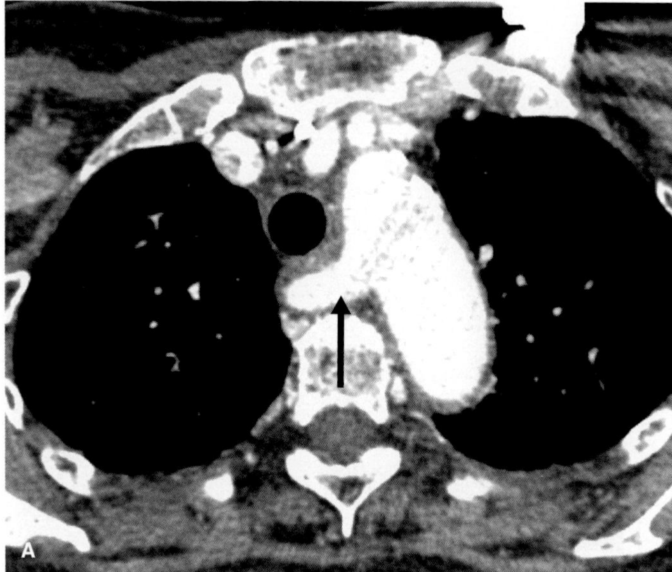

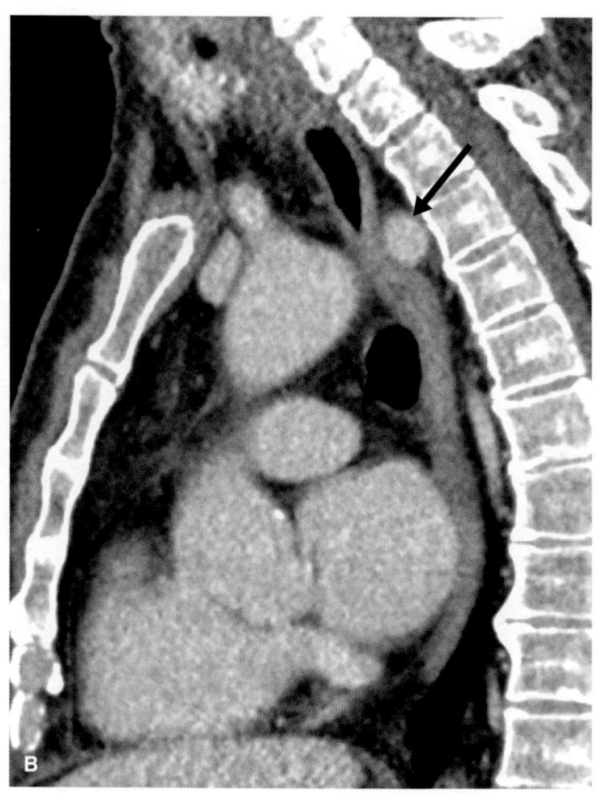

FIGURE 30.11. Left Arch and Aberrant Right Subclavian Artery. Axial (**A**) and sagittal CT (**B**) demonstrate the right subclavian artery arising from the distal arch (*arrow*) which indents the posterior esophagus corresponding to the aberrant right subclavian artery. This is a common anatomic variant that leads to no symptoms in the vast majority of patients.

by a rounded soft tissue structure abutting and indenting the inferior aspect of the right trachea (Fig. 30.12).

Right aortic arch can have variable arch branching patterns, but the most common are aberrant left subclavian artery and mirror-image branching. In right arch with aberrant left subclavian artery, the first branch from the aortic arch is the left common carotid artery, followed by the right carotid artery, right subclavian artery, and the aberrant left subclavian artery. The left subclavian artery passes posterior

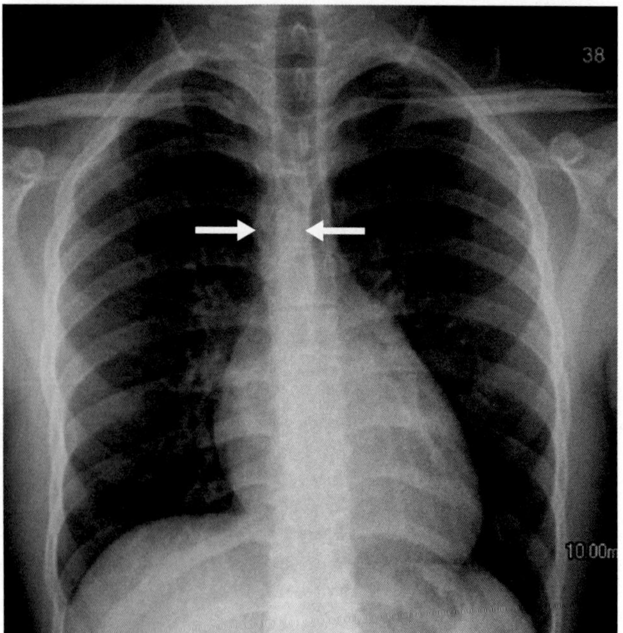

FIGURE 30.12. Right Arch. PA chest radiograph with a right aortic arch (*arrows*) indenting the right lateral aspect of the distal trachea.

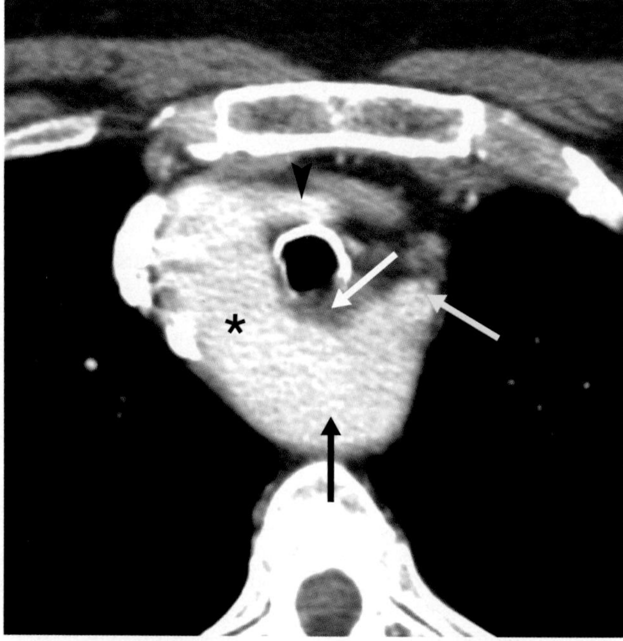

FIGURE 30.13. Right Arch and Aberrant Left Subclavian Artery. Axial CT scan in a patient with dysphagia shows a right aortic arch (*). The first vessel off the arch is the left common carotid artery (*black arrowhead*). The right common carotid and right subclavian arteries, which are the second and third vessels off the arch, respectively, are not seen on this image. The last vessel off the arch is the aberrant left subclavian artery (*yellow arrow*). This vessel courses posterior to the esophagus (*white arrow*) and trachea via a large 3.5-cm diverticulum of Kommerell (*black arrow*) which compresses the esophagus and slightly narrows the trachea. A left ligamentum arteriosum, which is not usually visualized, forms a vascular ring that can cause symptoms.

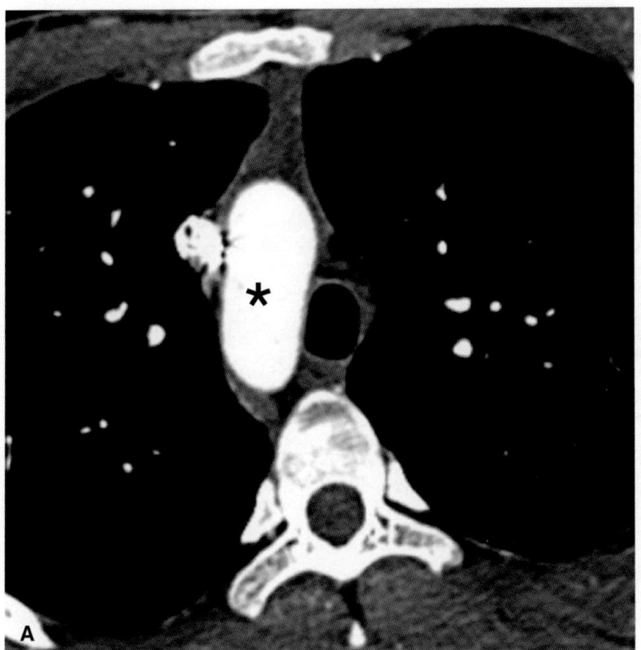

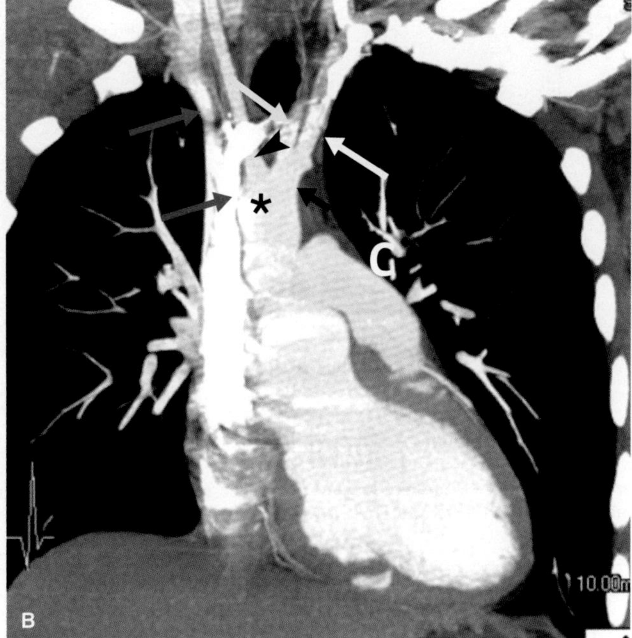

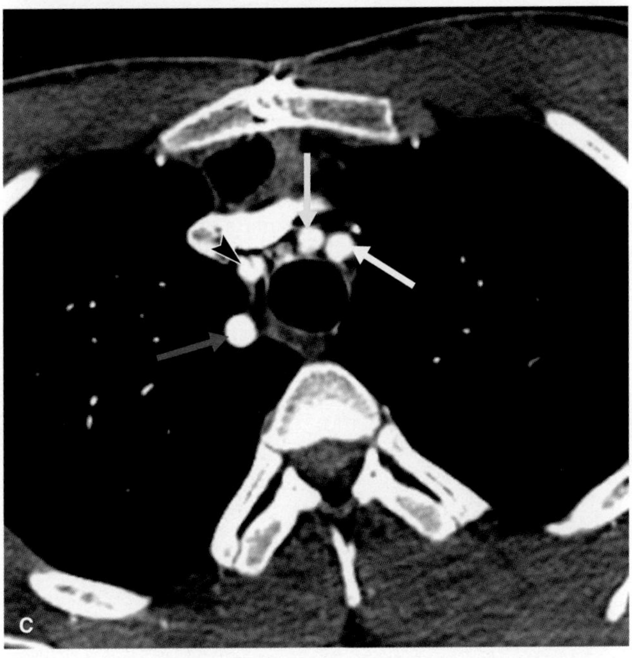

FIGURE 30.14. **Right Arch and Mirror-Image Branching. A:** Axial CTA images in a patient with repaired tetralogy of Fallot demonstrate a right aortic arch (*). **B:** A 20-mm coronal MIP image shows the right arch (*). The first branch off the right arch is the left brachiocephalic artery (*black arrow*), which divides into the left subclavian (*white arrow*) and left common carotid (*yellow arrow*) arteries. The next branch off the arch is the right common carotid artery (*black arrowhead*) and the last branch is the right subclavian artery (*red arrows*). **C:** Axial image above the arch shows the left subclavian (*white arrow*), left common carotid (*yellow arrow*), right common carotid (*black arrowhead*), and right subclavian (*red arrow*) arteries. There is no retroaortic subclavian artery.

to the esophagus, often with an associated diverticulum of Kommerell (Fig. 30.13). This is most commonly associated with left-sided ligamentum arteriosum which forms a vascular ring that can cause symptoms due to compression. However, the ligamentum itself is usually not visualized on imaging.

In right aortic arch with mirror-image branching, the first branch is the left brachiocephalic artery which divides into the left common carotid and subclavian arteries, followed by the right common carotid artery and right subclavian artery (Fig. 30.14). If an aberrant subclavian artery is present, there cannot be mirror-image branching. Congenital heart disease, especially tetralogy of Fallot, is commonly seen with right arch and mirror-image branching. Right aortic arch with isolated arch vessels is extremely rare and associated with congenital heart disease. Isolation indicates that the vessel arises from the pulmonary artery rather than the aorta.

Double Aortic Arch

Right aortic arch with aberrant left subclavian artery and double aortic arch represent the two most common vascular rings. Double aortic arch results from persistence of both right and left embryologic aortic arches. The common carotid and subclavian arteries arise from their ipsilateral arch, resulting in a four-vessel branching pattern. On frontal projection radiography, double aortic arch will present as bilateral indentations on the lower trachea (Fig. 30.15). Posterior indentation of the esophagus may be seen on esophagram, similar to that seen in cases of aberrant subclavian arteries (Fig. 30.16). On axial CT or MR images, there is symmetric, four-vessel branching at the thoracic inlet in contrast to right or left arch variants, which results in asymmetric vessel branching.

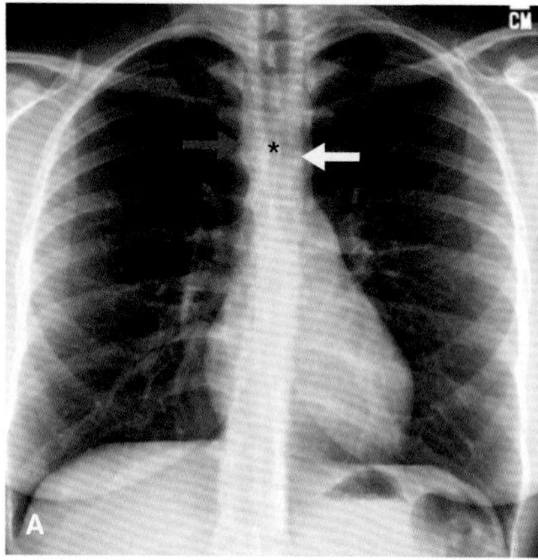
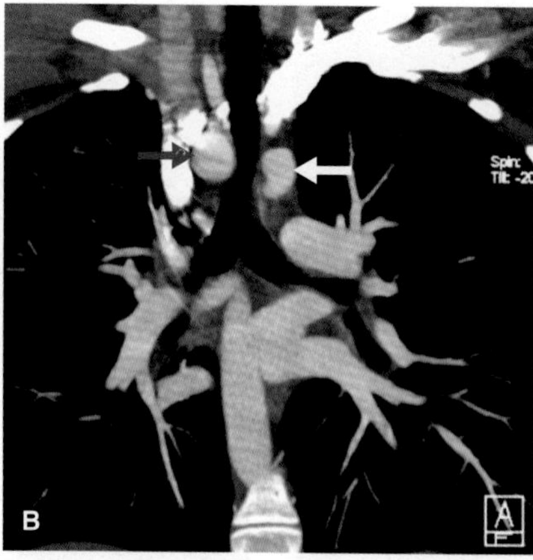
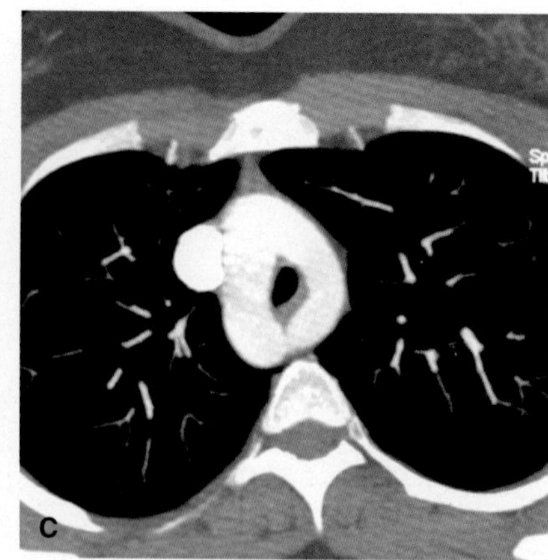

FIGURE 30.15. **Double Aortic Arch.** PA chest radiograph in an adult (**A**) with mild dysphagia demonstrates two bilateral indentations on the lower trachea (*), a slightly larger and more superior right indentation (*red arrow*) and slightly smaller and more inferior left indentation (*white arrow*). Coronal CT image (**B**) shows that the indentations represent a larger and more superior right aortic arch (*red arrow*) and smaller and more inferior left aortic arch (*white arrow*). Axial MIP image (**C**) shows the double aortic arch. The right arch is larger than the left arch, which is common.

The left arch is typically hypoplastic and located inferior to the dominant right arch (Fig. 30.15), with a left-sided descending thoracic aorta and ductus arteriosus. Since the right and left arches encircle the trachea and esophagus, patients present in childhood with findings of airway compromise, including wheezing and stridor (Fig. 30.16). Double aortic arch is uncommonly associated with congenital heart disease.

Cervical Aortic Arch

Cervical aortic arch is extremely rare, with case reports describing a high location of the aortic arch above the level of the clavicle (Fig. 30.17). It is most often associated with a right arch, although a left cervical arch can occur. While often presenting as an asymptomatic pulsatile mass in the neck or supraclavicular region, it can be associated with other aortic abnormalities, aneurysm formation, and congenital heart disease.

Interrupted Aortic Arch

Interrupted aortic arch occurs in 2 of every 100,000 births, characterized by discontinuity of the aortic arch in which there is complete absence or a fibrous remnant of the interrupted segment. There are three main types of interrupted aortic arch (A, B, and C) depending on location of interruption. Type A interruption occurs distal to the left subclavian takeoff at the isthmus, type B between the left common carotid and subclavian origins, and type C between the right

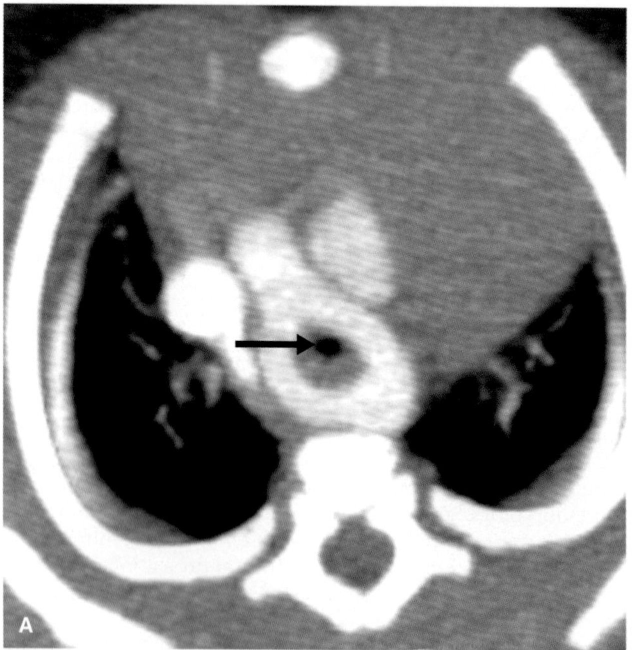
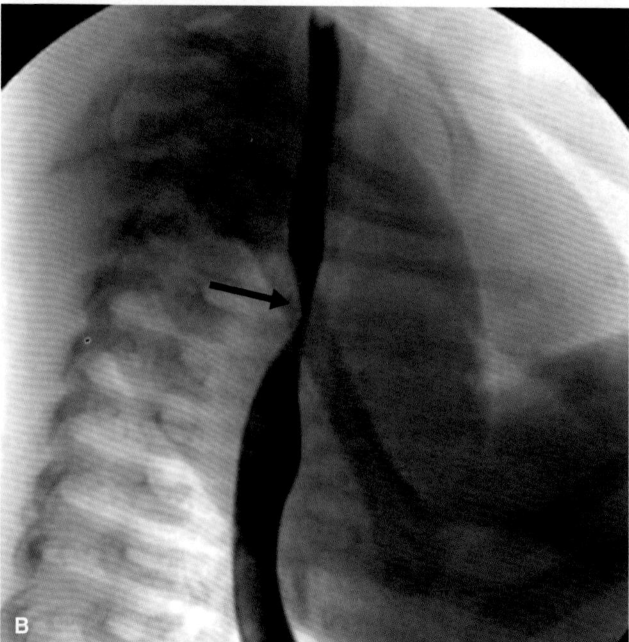

FIGURE 30.16. **Double Aortic Arch.** Axial MIP image in a 1-month-old baby with severe stridor and vomiting (**A**) shows a double aortic arch creating a vascular ring and causing compression of the trachea (*black arrow*). Additionally, lateral view from an esophagram (**B**) shows marked compression of the posterior wall of the esophagus (*black arrow*).

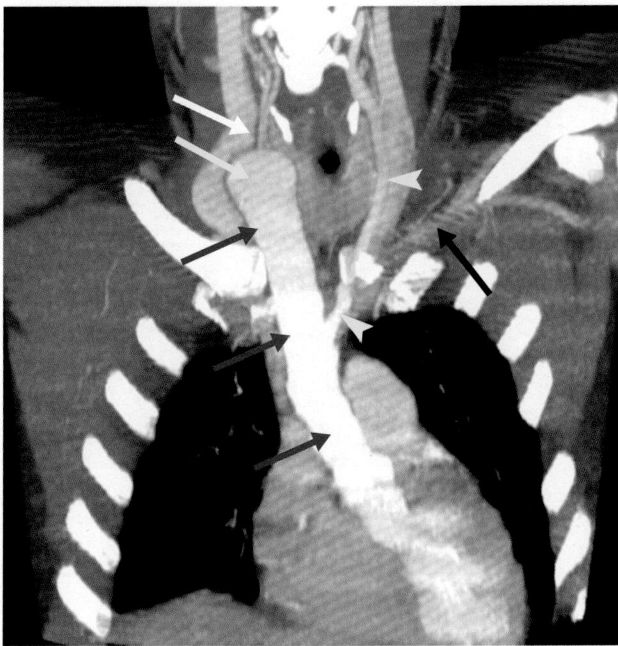

FIGURE 30.17. **Cervical Arch With Aberrant Left Subclavian Artery.** Coronal oblique MIP CT image shows the ascending aorta extending high into the right supraclavicular region (*red arrows*) with a right-sided cervical arch (*yellow arrow*). Similar to other right arches with an aberrant subclavian artery, the first vessel of the aorta is the left common carotid artery (*yellow arrowheads*) followed by the right common carotid artery (*white arrow*) and right subclavian artery (not visualized). The last branch off the aorta is the aberrant left subclavian artery (*black arrow*), the origin of which is not visualized in this view. (Courtesy of David Godwin, MD.)

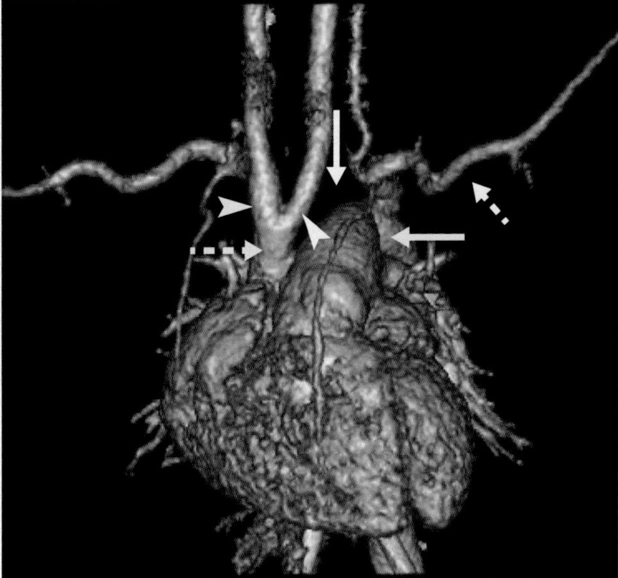

FIGURE 30.18. **Type B Interrupted Aortic Arch.** 3D VR shows a type B interrupted aorta arch with the ascending aorta (*dashed yellow arrow*) giving rise to the right brachiocephalic artery (*yellow arrowhead*) and left common carotid artery (LCCA, *white arrowhead*). The aortic arch is absent, or interrupted, after the origin of the LCCA (*white arrow*). The left subclavian artery (*dashed white arrow*) arises from the descending thoracic aorta which received flow through a large patent ductus arteriosus (*yellow arrow*).

brachiocephalic and left common carotid origins. Type B is most common (50% to 60%) and is associated with VSD, bicuspid aortic valve, and left ventricular outflow tract anomalies (Fig. 30.18). All types require a patent ductus arteriosus for survival. Methods of surgical repair are similar to those of aortic coarctation, described below. Please see "Postoperative Aorta" section for further discussion.

Circumflex Aorta

Circumflex aorta is an extremely rare anomaly which can occur with either a left- or right-sided aortic arch. The aortic arch travels posteriorly as usual but crosses the midline behind the esophagus, above the tracheal carina at the level of the distal arch/descending thoracic aorta, and continues distally contralateral to the aortic arch side (Fig. 30.19). A vascular ring can be present depending on the location of the ductus arteriosus.

Descending Thoracic Aorta

The descending thoracic aorta begins after the ligamentum arteriosum and transitions to the abdominal aorta after passing through the diaphragmatic hiatus. The descending thoracic aorta gives rise to multiple systemic vessels, including the intercostal and bronchial arteries.

AORTIC COARCTATION

Aortic coarctation is defined as focal narrowing of the aorta adjacent to the ductus arteriosus (i.e., juxtaductal) and often occurs with varying degrees of aortic arch hypoplasia. In very rare instances, it can involve the abdominal aorta. Aortic coarctation is a relatively common anomaly, representing

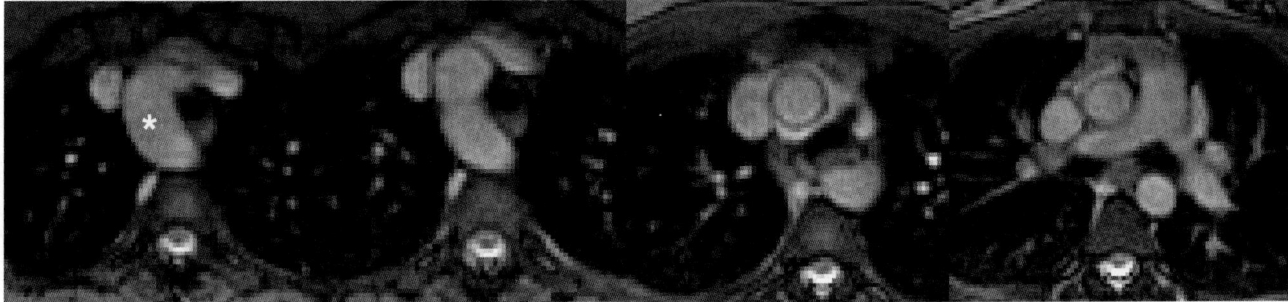

FIGURE 30.19. **Circumflex Aortic Arch.** Sequential axial MR GRE images demonstrate a right-sided arch (*) which passes behind the esophagus before continuing as a left-sided descending thoracic aorta.

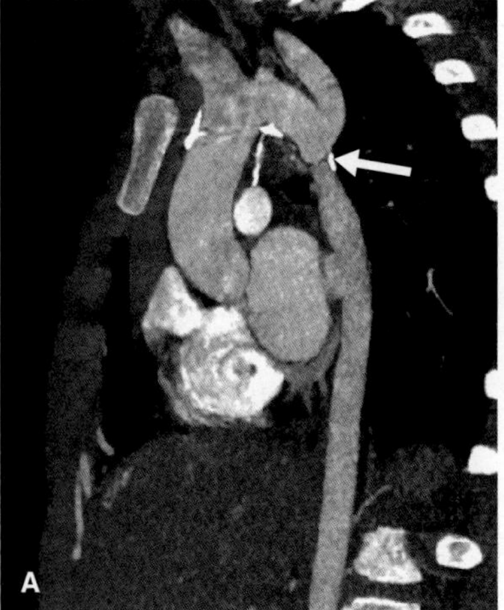

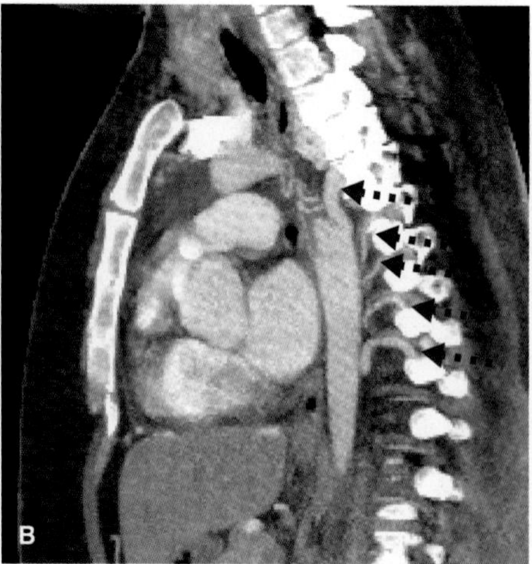

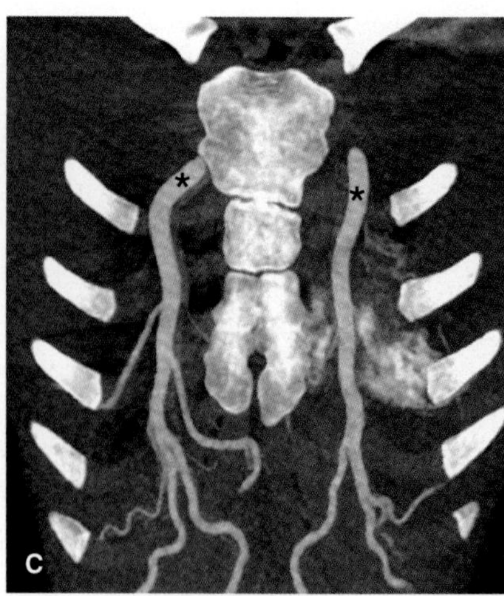

FIGURE 30.20. **Aortic Coarctation.** Sagittal CT (**A**), sagittal CT MIP (**B**), and coronal MIP (**C**). Focal narrowing of the proximal descending thoracic aorta corresponds to a postductal aortic coarctation (*white arrow*). Large collateral intercostal (**B**, *dashed black arrows*) and internal mammary arteries (**C**, *) are present.

approximately 6% to 8% of all congenital heart disease. There is a strong association with bicuspid aortic valve, which occurs in up to 75% of coarctation cases, and Turner syndrome. The etiology remains unclear but a common pathogenesis with bicuspid aortic valve has been proposed, including abnormalities of neural crest tissue migration, decreased in utero blood flow, and aortopathy with cystic medial necrosis.

There are two main types of aortic coarctation: preductal and postductal. Preductal coarctation tends to be more severe, involving a longer segment. It commonly presents in infancy, with systemic hypoperfusion following closure of the ductus arteriosus. Postductal coarctation usually presents in adulthood with hypertension and signs of left heart failure. To bypass the area of aortic narrowing, collateral systemic blood flow occurs via adjacent internal mammary and intercostal arteries which become enlarged (Fig. 30.20). Although classically there is differential blood pressure and asymmetric pulses between the right and left upper extremities (in the context of preductal coarctation) or between the upper and lower extremities (postductal coarctation), blood pressure between upper and lower extremities can potentially equalize in the setting of very extensive collateral formation.

Radiographic findings of aortic coarctation may only be apparent in severe cases. Indentation of the distal aortic arch with pre- and poststenotic dilation results in a "figure-of-3" sign on chest radiograph. Hypertrophied intercostal arteries result in bilateral central rib notching, involving the posterior fourth through eighth ribs (Fig. 30.21). Although CT best

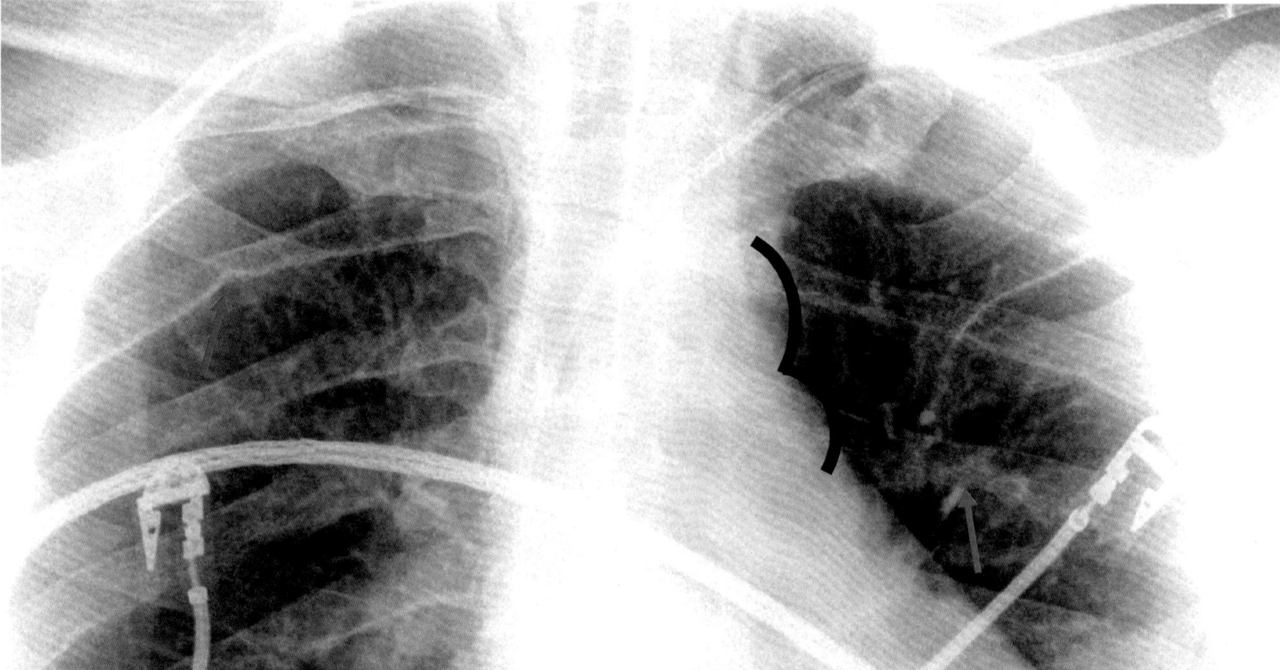

FIGURE 30.21. **Aortic Coarctation.** Coned down frontal chest radiograph in a patient with aortic coarctation demonstrates the "*figure-of-3*" sign with indentation of the 3 corresponding to the area of aortic narrowing. Inferior rib notching is also present due to hypertrophied intercostal collateral arteries (*arrows*).

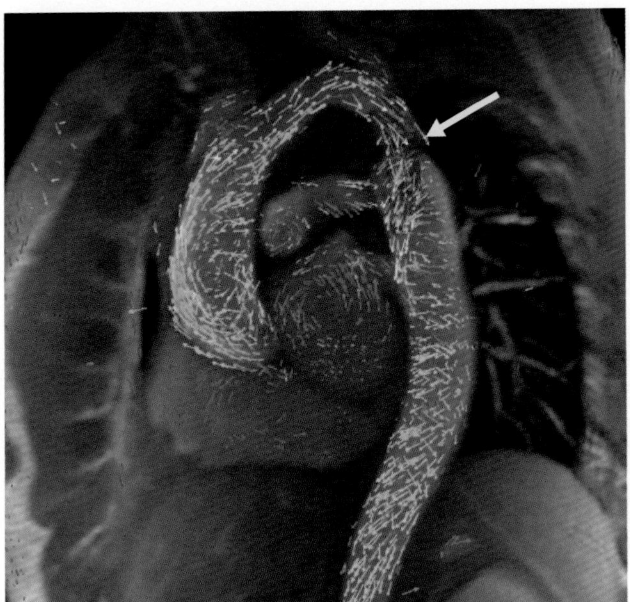

FIGURE 30.22. **Aortic Coarctation.** Four-dimensional phase-contrast, sagittal MPR demonstrates flow acceleration, indicated by red color flow (*yellow arrow*) across the coarctation in the proximal thoracic aortic; pressure gradient quantified as 31 mm Hg.

demonstrates anatomy, MRI and echocardiography allow quantitative evaluation of severity, including pressure gradient and flow acceleration across the coarctation (Fig. 30.22).

Aortic coarctation is treated with surgical repair, which typically involves resection of the narrowed segment and primary anastomosis or interposition graft. Additional repair techniques include subclavian flap or prosthetic patch aortoplasty to augment the coarcted segment, extra-anatomic bypass grafting, and endovascular balloon dilation. Intervention is recommended when the coarctation pressure gradient exceeds 20 mm Hg. Following surgical repair, there is a 72% to 74% reported 30-year survival. Postoperative complications include aneurysm formation, rupture with pseudoaneurysm formation, accelerated atherosclerotic disease, and increased cardiovascular morbidity. Restenosis can occur in up to 30% of patients. Treatment options in these patients include endovascular stenting, surgical resection, aortoplasty, and bypass grafting.

Pseudocoarctation

Congenital elongation with prominent kinking of the aorta at the aortic isthmus can mimic the appearance of coarctation and is termed pseudocoarctation (Fig. 30.23). Pseudocoarctation lacks the hemodynamic changes of true coarctation, such as a significant pressure gradient and arterial collateral formation. Although usually asymptomatic, pseudocoarctation can be associated with hypertension and aortic aneurysm. Like coarctations, it is associated with a bicuspid aortic valve. On chest radiograph, the superior mediastinum may appear widened with a superiorly positioned aortic arch (Fig. 30.23A).

ATHEROMA

The pathogenesis and consequences of atherosclerotic disease are more thoroughly discussed in the section of this text dedicated to coronary artery disease; however, it warrants mentioning here as it is so highly prevalent in the aorta. Risk factors for the development of aortic atherosclerotic disease include advanced age, heredity, hypertension, diabetes, smoking, hyperlipidemia, sedentary lifestyle, and endothelial dysfunction. Atheroma formation is a cyclical process that starts with lipoprotein phagocytosis by macrophages, which are then incorporated into the subintima of the aortic wall. Intracellular processes within the macrophage lead to the formation of "foam cells." Eventually, the macrophages die, with a resultant influx of additional white blood cells and fibroblasts. The result of this cycle is an intramural mass consisting of the inner extracellular lipid core with an outer layer of inflammatory cells and connective tissue that can narrow the arterial lumen. Similar to coronary artery plaques, noncalcified or mixed plaques with a thin fibrous cap and a large necrotic core are more likely to rupture and are termed vulnerable plaques. As plaques age and calcify, they generally become less prone to rupture.

Atherosclerotic disease involving the thoracic aorta is a common finding on chest radiograph and should follow the

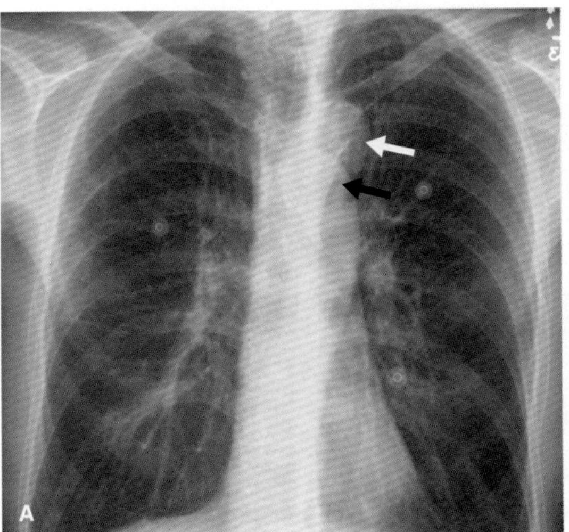

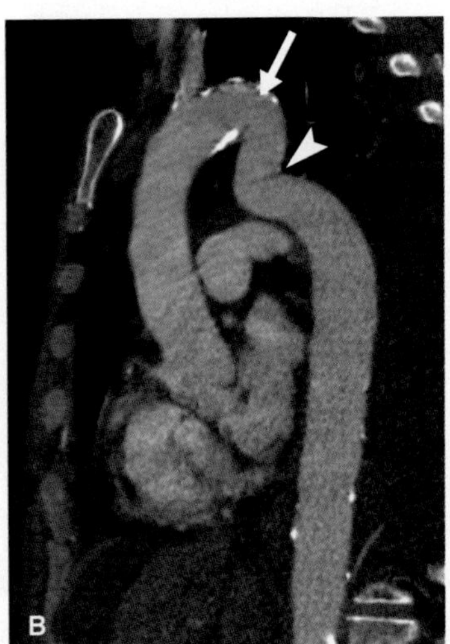

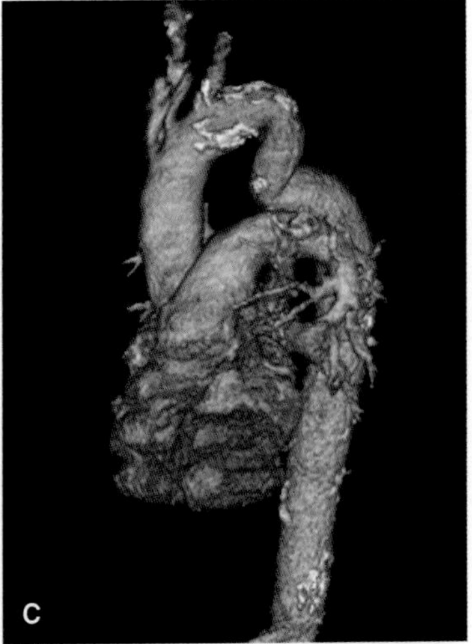

FIGURE 30.23. **Pseudocoarctation.** PA chest radiograph (**A**) demonstrates a rounded density (*white arrow*) superior to the aortic arch (*black arrow*). On sagittal CT (B), the aortic arch and proximal descending thoracic aorta are elongated and folded on themselves (*white arrow*), producing focal kinking (*white arrow*) but without significant narrowing. 3D VR of same patient (**C**).

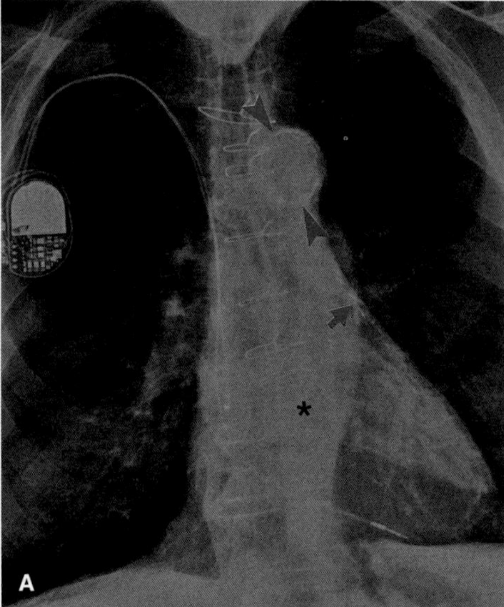

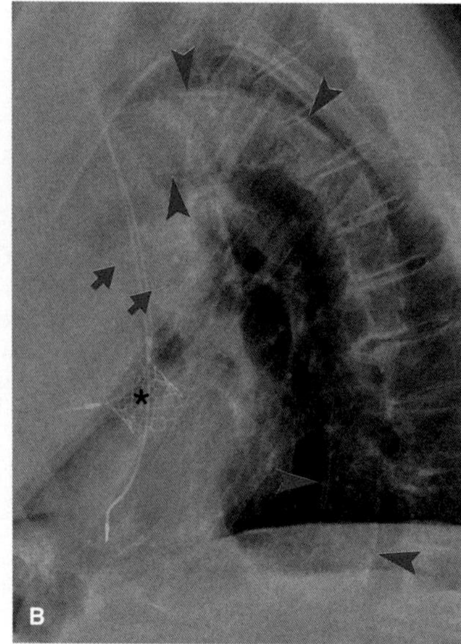

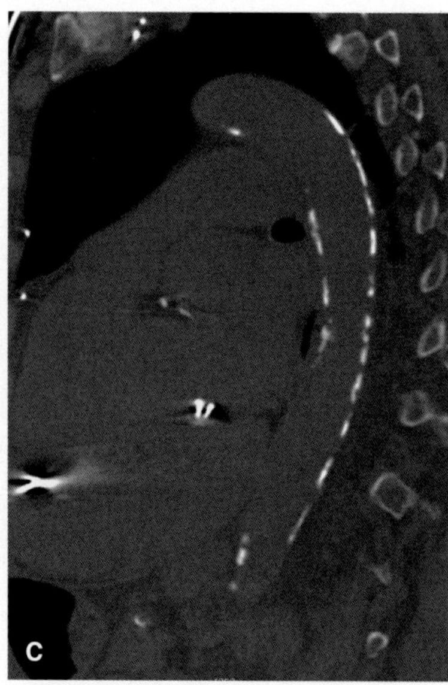

FIGURE 30.24. **Diffuse Thoracic Aortic Atherosclerotic Disease.** Frontal (**A**) and lateral (**B**) chest radiographs in a 95-year-old man demonstrate multifocal calcified plaques (*arrowheads*) along the thoracic aorta. The patient has had prior coronary artery bypass grafting indicated by the surgical clips (*arrows*) and transcatheter aortic valve intervention (TAVI, *). Sagittal nonenhanced chest CT in a different patient (**C**), a 79-year-old man, demonstrates multifocal calcifications along the descending aorta.

course of the aorta (Fig. 30.24). On chest CT, aortic atherosclerotic disease is a common finding and does not usually lead to direct hemodynamic compromise, given the large caliber of the aorta. However, given that atherosclerotic disease is a multifocal process, in the thorax there may be concomitant disease involving the subclavian or carotid arteries which can lead to hemodynamic compromise.

In some patients with severe atherosclerotic disease, thick layers of diffuse, predominantly noncalcified atherosclerotic plaques can layer much of the thoracic and abdominal aorta, which has been termed as "complex atheroma" by some authors (Fig. 30.25). These complex atheromas, which are an indirect sign of previous plaque rupture, are independent risk factors for the development of future ischemic events and should be mentioned as they may change medical or surgical management.

In certain areas, contrast can be seen extending between areas of complex plaque, toward the wall of the aorta, which some authors refer to as "plaque ulceration." This appearance can mimic a penetrating atherosclerotic ulcer (PAU), which is discussed in more detail below, but the distinction between the two is imperative. While plaque ulceration is an indirect sign of previous plaque rupture and can lead to thromboembolic events, a PAU is a sign of intimal disruption and lies in the "acute aortic syndrome" spectrum, which is also discussed below. In general, ulcerated plaque will not extend beyond the lumen of the aorta into the intima which is demarcated in areas by linear calcification due to atherosclerosis (Fig. 30.26). However, distinction between the two is not always easy, even among expert radiologists.

ANEURYSM

Sinus of Valsalva Aneurysm

Sinus of Valsalva aneurysms are abnormal dilations of the sinuses which can be congenital or acquired. Congenital aneurysm secondary to weakness in the fibroelastic elements is seen in connective tissue disorders such as Marfan, Ehlers–Danlos,

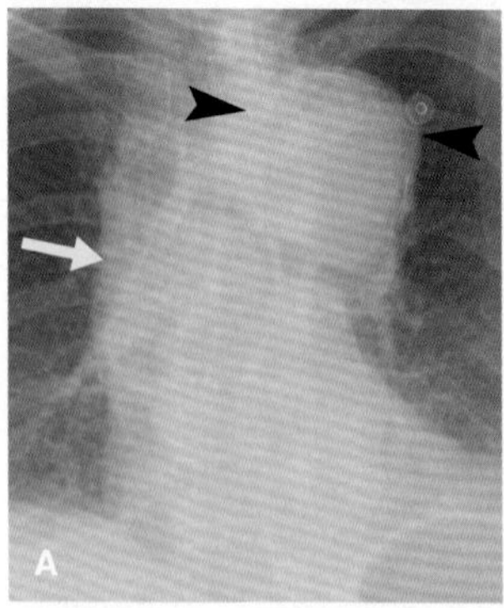

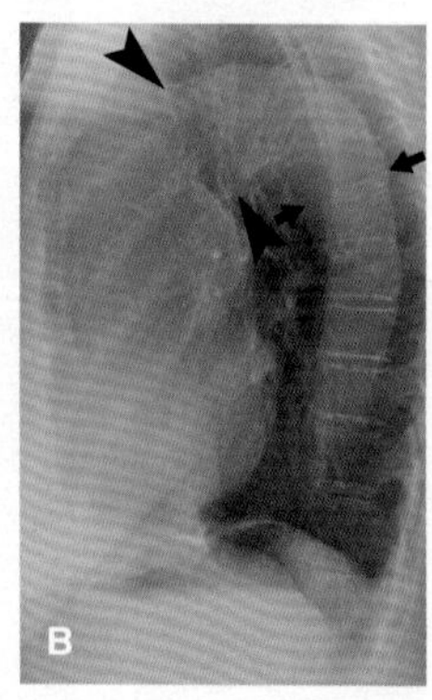

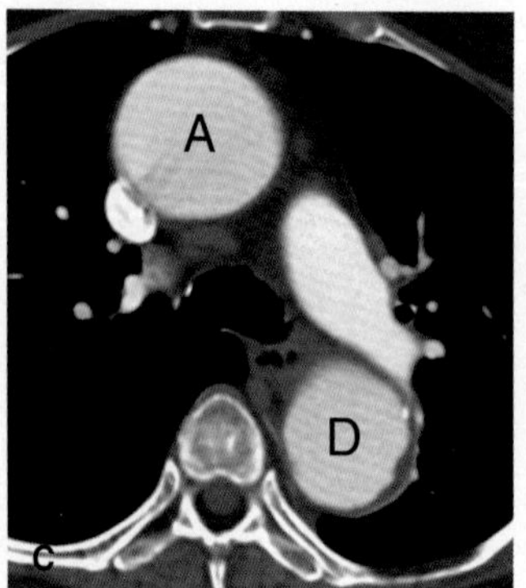

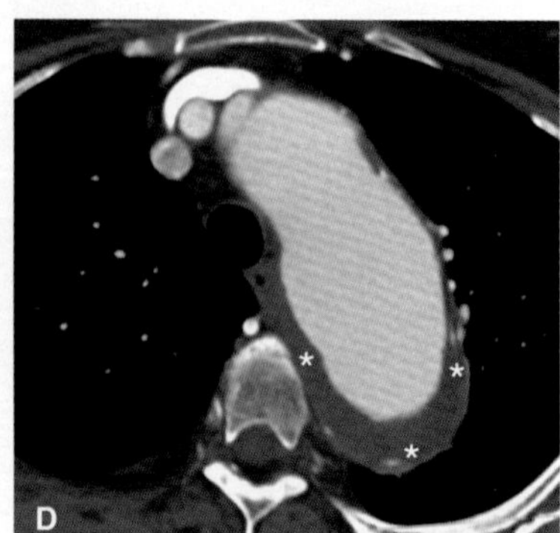

FIGURE 30.25. **Complex Atherosclerotic Plaque in a Patient With Aneurysmal Dilation of the Aorta.** Frontal (**A**) and lateral (**B**) chest radiographs in a 75-year-old woman demonstrate aneurysmal dilation of the ascending aorta (*yellow arrow*), aortic arch (*black arrowheads*), and descending thoracic aorta (*black arrows*). CT angiography at the level of the left pulmonary artery (**C**) shows aneurysmal dilation of the ascending (**A**) and descending (**D**) thoracic aorta. At the level of the aortic arch (**D**), the aortic aneurysm measures up to 5.8 cm. Layering mural thrombus (*) is present along the arch and descending thoracic aorta and should not be confused with intramural hematoma.

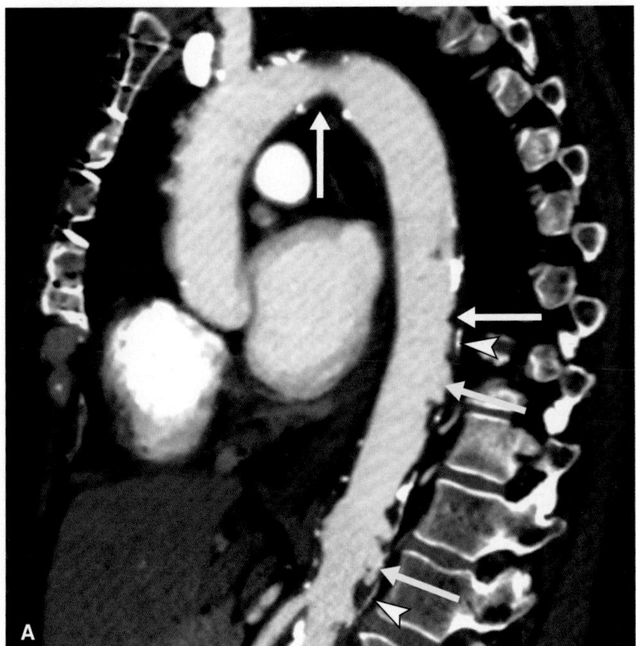

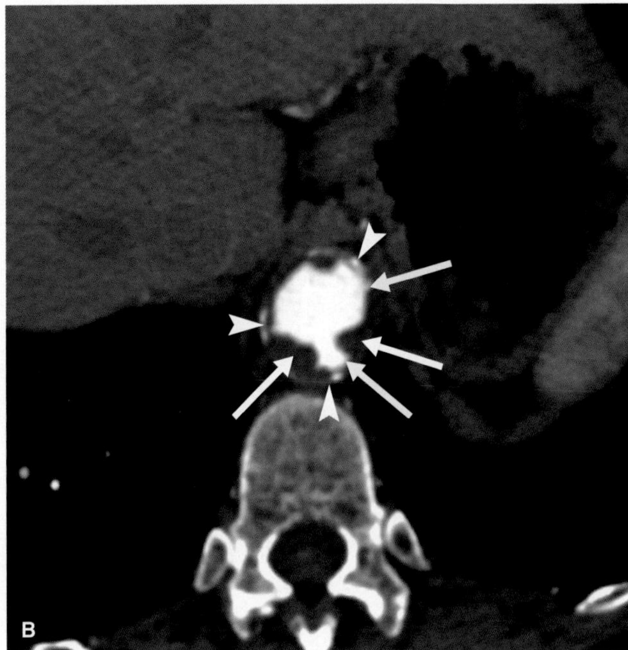

FIGURE 30.26. **Areas of Ulcerated Plaque in a 65-Year-Old Man.** Parasagittal (**A**) and axial (**B**) CT images of the aorta show extensive layering, mixed but predominantly noncalcified plaque throughout the thoracic aorta (*white arrows*). In certain areas, contrast can be seen extending into the plaque (*yellow arrows*) but does not extend beyond the intima, which is demarcated by a thin calcification along the aortic wall (*white arrowheads*). It is important to differentiate this ulcerated plaque from penetrating atherosclerotic ulcers, as they have different treatments.

and Loeys–Dietz syndromes (Fig. 30.27). Congenital aneurysms are also associated with bicuspid aortic valve and VSD. Acquired sinus of Valsalva aneurysms often represent pseudoaneurysms and result from bacterial aortic valve endocarditis or aortic surgery. Dilation of the sinuses may be diffuse and circumferential or eccentric, focally involving one of the coronary sinuses. The right sinus of Valsalva is involved in 70% of cases.

Symptoms are nonspecific but are usually secondary to complication such as rupture, aortic regurgitation, or compression of adjacent cardiovascular structures. Rupture often occurs into a cardiac structure, most commonly the right ventricle and right atrium. This results in a left-to-right shunt with development of heart failure. Early surgical or endovascular repair is essential, as mean survival after rupture is 1 to 2 years.

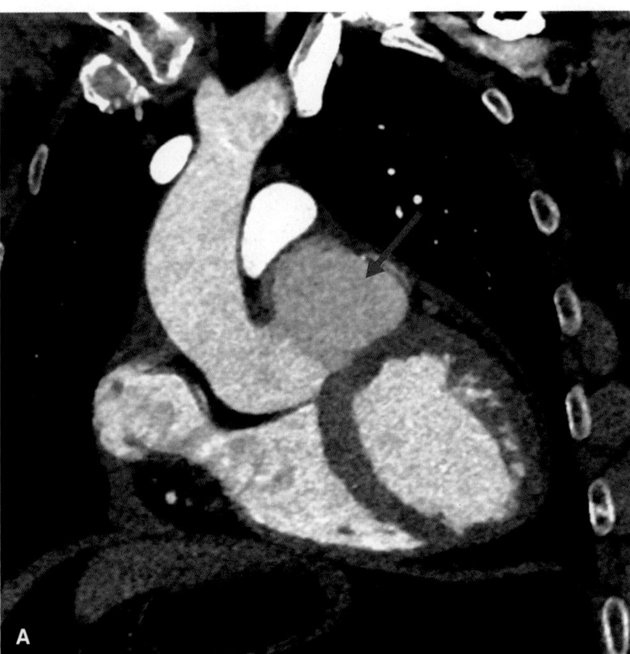

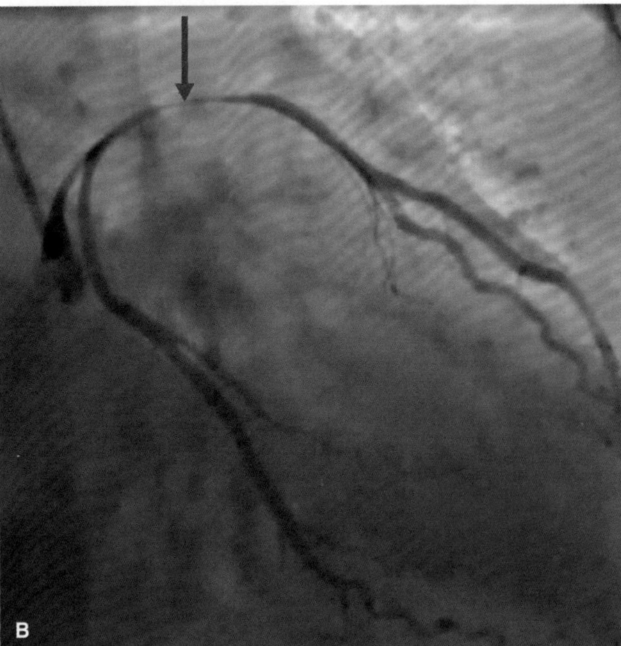

FIGURE 30.27. **Sinus of Valsalva Aneurysm.** Coronal oblique CTA in a patient with chest pain and no significant past medical history shows a large aneurysm arising from the left sinus of Valsalva (**A**, *arrow*). Still image from a coronary angiography shows that the large sinus of Valsalva aneurysm stretches and narrows the left anterior descending coronary artery (**B**, *arrow*). The patient's symptoms resolved after surgical repair.

Ascending Thoracic Aorta and Aortic Arch Aneurysms

Thoracic aortic aneurysms (TAAs), defined as aortic enlargement to greater than 4 cm with preservation of vessel wall integrity—that is, without intimal disruption—may occur anywhere along the vessel; 50% occur in the ascending aorta (proximal to the right brachiocephalic artery), 10% in the aortic arch, and 40% in the descending aorta (distal to the left subclavian artery). There are a multitude of risk factors for the development of TAA, but by far the highest association is with atherosclerosis, which is seen in 70% of cases. Aneurysms secondary to atherosclerotic disease are more commonly seen in the descending thoracic aorta but may occur anywhere along the thoracic and abdominal aorta (Fig. 30.28). Thus, imaging of the abdominal aorta is also indicated in these patients. Homocystinuria, Marfan syndrome, and other connective tissue disorders may result in dilation of the aortic annulus and proximal ascending aorta, termed annuloaortic ectasia. Ascending aortic aneurysm can also result from noninfective or infective aortitis. Giant cell arteritis (GCA), rheumatic fever, and relapsing polychondritis may result in ascending aortic aneurysms, while Takayasu arteritis may affect the ascending aorta, aortic arch, arch vessels, abdominal aorta, and/or pulmonary arteries. Infective aortitis may arise in the setting of bacterial endocarditis, with resultant aneurysm formation most often in the proximal ascending aorta. Historically, syphilis was a more common cause of ascending aortitis and aneurysm; incidence of syphilitic aortitis has decreased, but a number of other organisms (including *Streptococcus* and *Staphylococcus* spp.) can be implicated in infective aortitis ("mycosis") which may lead to formation of a "mycotic" aneurysm. Bicuspid valve is an independent risk factor for ascending TAA, unrelated to the presence of associated aortic stenosis.

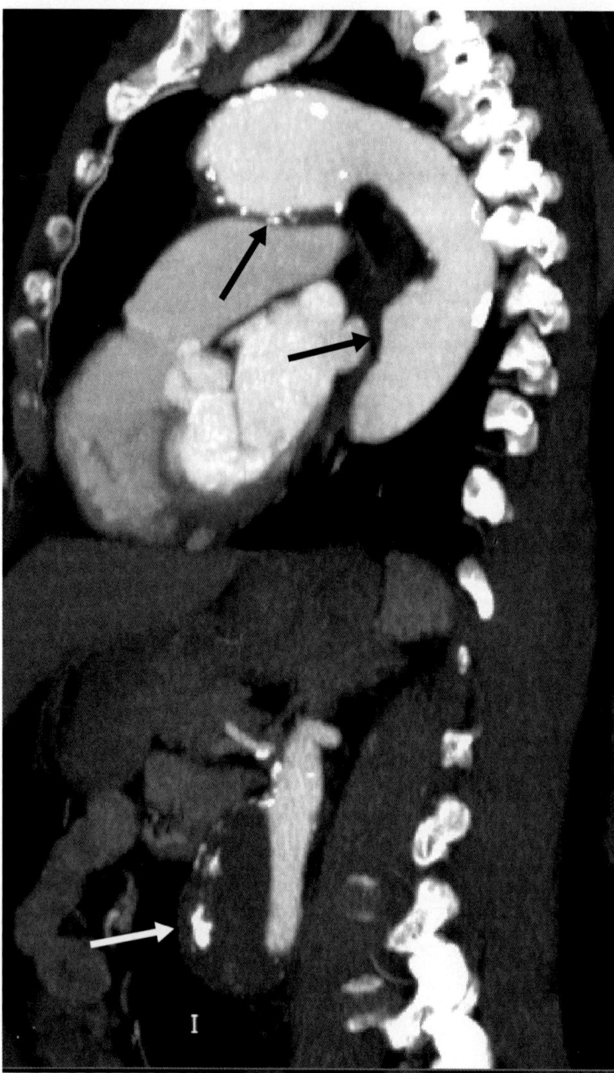

FIGURE 30.28. Multifocal Thoracoabdominal Aortic Aneurysm. Sagittal CT image in a 69-year old woman demonstrates multifocal aneurysms in the thoracic (*black arrows*) and infrarenal abdominal aorta (*white arrow*). Note layering mural thrombus in the abdominal aortic aneurysm.

Chest radiography may demonstrate dilation of the ascending aorta or arch (Fig. 30.25), with or without associated calcifications. Technique is also an important consideration; the ascending aortic contour may be exaggerated if the patient is rotated to the right and this should not be confused for an aneurysm. There may be tracheal deviation and/or left upper lobe atelectasis in the setting of an aortic arch aneurysm. CT angiography (CTA) has replaced traditional catheter angiography as the mainstay of imaging and has the benefit of extraluminal evaluation, though treatment cannot be concurrently performed as with catheter angiography. CTA will demonstrate typically fusiform and concentric focal dilation of the ascending aorta or arch (Fig. 30.29) to greater than 4 cm. Patients with Marfan syndrome may demonstrate dilation of the main pulmonary artery in addition to annuloaortic ectasia (Fig. 30.30). Aneurysms cause turbulent flow patterns with nonlaminar flow, often eventually resulting in discontinuous or circumferential mural thrombus formation (Fig. 30.25). Noncontrast imaging is not always routinely performed in follow-up imaging of known aneurysms, but some studies have suggested that focal crescentic hyperattenuation in mural thrombus may be a sign of impending rupture. Multiplanar (MPR) and three-dimensional reformats can be easily rendered, allowing for accurate orthogonal measurements and aiding with pre- and/or periprocedural planning and

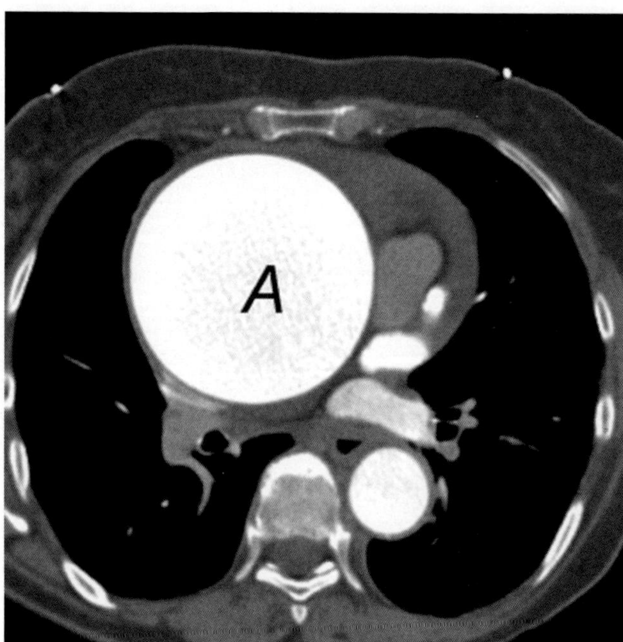

FIGURE 30.29. Ascending Thoracic Aortic Aneurysm. Axial CT in a 77-year-old woman demonstrates marked dilation of the ascending aorta measuring 7.7 cm consistent with aneurysm (*A*).

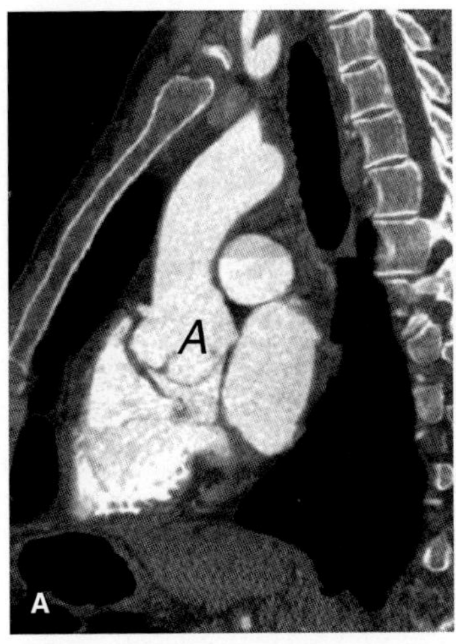

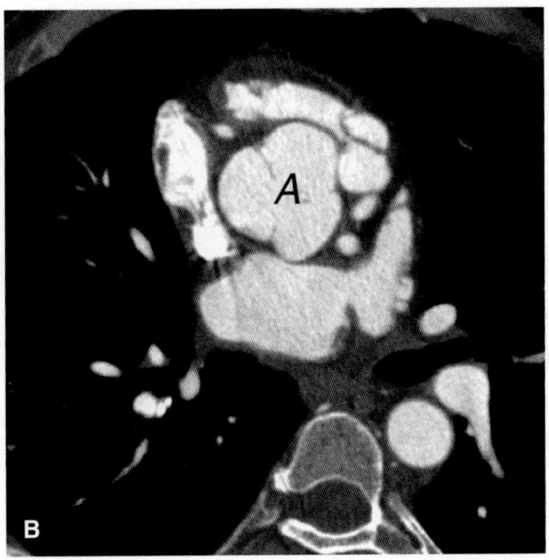

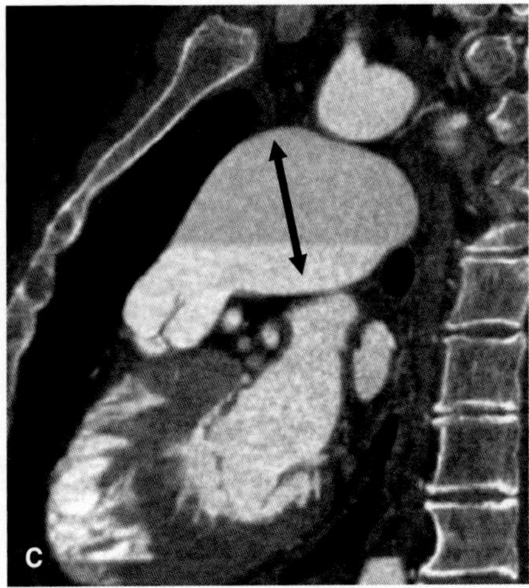

FIGURE 30.30. Marfan Syndrome With Aortic and Pulmonary Artery Involvement. Sagittal CT image (**A**) in a 59-year-old man demonstrates aortic annulus/root aneurysm (*A*), with characteristic "tulip" appearance of the dilated root. Axial oblique reformat through the sinuses of Valsalva (**B**) demonstrates aneurysmal dilation measuring 4.8 cm (*A*). Sagittal CT image (**C**) demonstrates aneurysmal dilation of the main pulmonary artery (*double-headed arrow*), which is one of the established criteria for the diagnosis of the syndrome.

navigation for interventionalists. These can be particularly helpful over time for risk stratification.

MR and MR angiography (MRA), like CT, are also highly sensitive and specific for aneurysm, along with mural thrombus and other associated complications. Cine sequences allow visualization of flow patterns, though further study is needed to determine the clinical usefulness of this information. MR may be the most appropriate modality in younger patients and/or those requiring more extensive follow-up imaging, given the lack of ionizing radiation; and non–contrast-enhanced imaging is likely adequate in patients with allergies or poor renal function.

Ascending aortic aneurysms may be complicated by dissection or rupture, and rupture is the leading cause of death in these patients. The risk of rupture increases with size, and ascending aortic aneurysms greater than 6 cm carry a risk of rupture of approximately 14%. Rupture carries a 97% to 100% mortality rate, if not emergently treated; the perioperative mortality associated with repair is not insignificant but is considerably lower in elective compared to emergent repair (9% vs. 22%). For this reason, early diagnosis is crucial, and patients with known aneurysms are monitored with regular, serial imaging to evaluate for size and interval growth. Ascending thoracic aneurysm diameter greater than 5.5 cm and/or interval growth (greater than 0.5 cm in 6 months or 1 cm in 1 year) are/is indication(s) for intervention, either surgical or endovascular. In the setting of connective tissue disease such as Marfan syndrome, there is a lower threshold for repair, usually greater than 5 cm.

Descending Thoracic Aortic Aneurysms

Aneurysms in the descending aorta are most commonly associated with atherosclerosis, though aneurysms secondary to other diseases including collagen vascular disease, infective aortitis, and autoimmune/inflammatory disease may occur in the descending aorta as well.

Chest radiography may demonstrate dilation of the descending aortic contour (Fig. 30.25); any associated calcifications will be displaced outward in a true aneurysm. CTA is highly sensitive and specific for aneurysm, with or without associated mural thrombus. MRA is also highly sensitive and specific for detection of aneurysms and their complications. Though hemodynamically unstable patients are unsuitable for MR imaging, it may be more appropriate in the setting of routine surveillance imaging, particularly given the lack of ionizing radiation.

Descending thoracic aortic aneurysms may be complicated by dissection, rupture, or fistula formation to the esophagus and/or airways; rupture is the leading cause of death. Risk factors for rupture include age, size greater than 5 cm, hypertension, smoking, and COPD. The rate of growth increases with aneurysm size and is estimated at 0.12 cm/yr for aneurysm diameter greater than 5.2 cm. Thus, aneurysms are monitored with serial imaging; size greater than 6.5 cm and/or interval growth (greater than 0.5 cm in 6 months or 1 cm in 1 year) are/is indication(s) for open surgical or endovascular treatment. Operative mortality is 5% to 12% with renal failure (5% to 13%) and spinal cord ischemia (4% to 30%, depending on the extent of disease/repair), among the major postoperative complications. As in the ascending aorta, aneurysms associated with connective tissue disease are managed more aggressively with earlier intervention.

ACUTE AORTIC SYNDROME

Acute aortic syndrome (AAS) includes aortic dissection, acute intramural hematoma (IMH), and PAU, which share the common classical clinical presentation of excruciating chest pain that may radiate to the back. While these have traditionally been classified as distinct entities, mounting evidence suggests that they may rather represent variants or a spectrum of disease, as described in more detail below. The three cannot be distinguished by clinical history or physical examination, and thus, imaging plays an integral role in diagnosis. Transesophageal echocardiography (TEE), multidetector CT (MDCT)/CTA, and MRA are all useful, highly sensitive, and specific. Owing to its ubiquity, rapid acquisition, and high accuracy, CTA is the most commonly employed modality in this setting, with a sensitivity and specificity of 100% and 98%, respectively, for thoracic aortic dissection. Careful consideration of imaging parameters and the manner of intravenous administration of contrast material for CTA is paramount. Noncontrast phase imaging is important to identify IMH, and timing of imaging relative to administration of the contrast material bolus is critical for optimal imaging. Two commonly used methods for ensuring arterial phase imaging are the timing/test bolus and

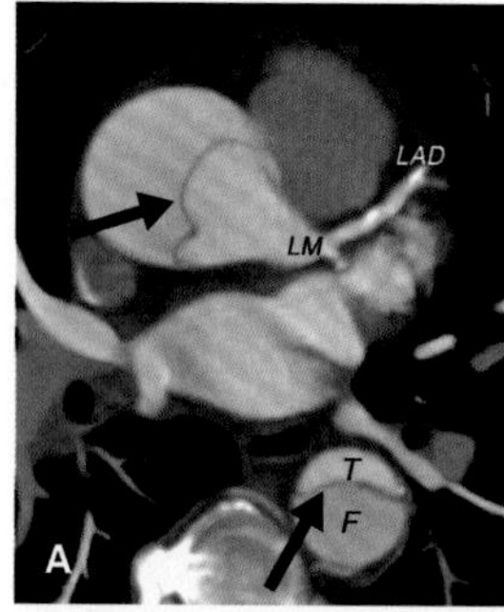

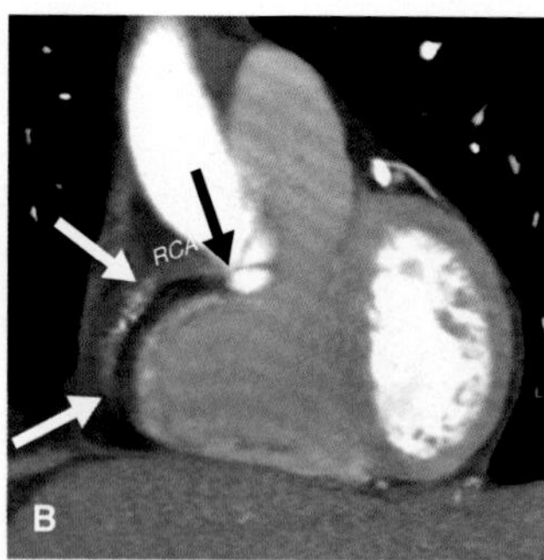

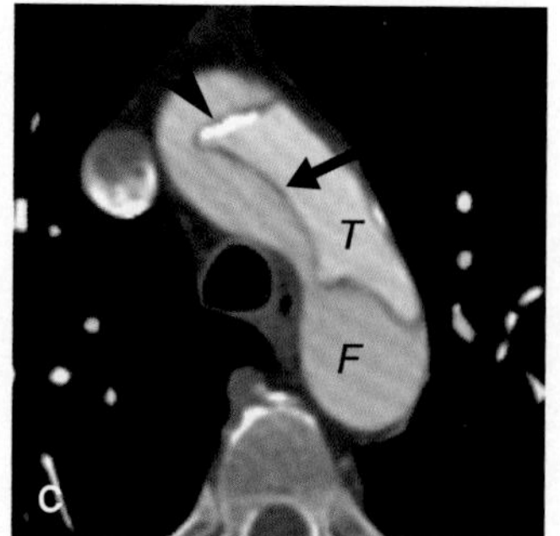

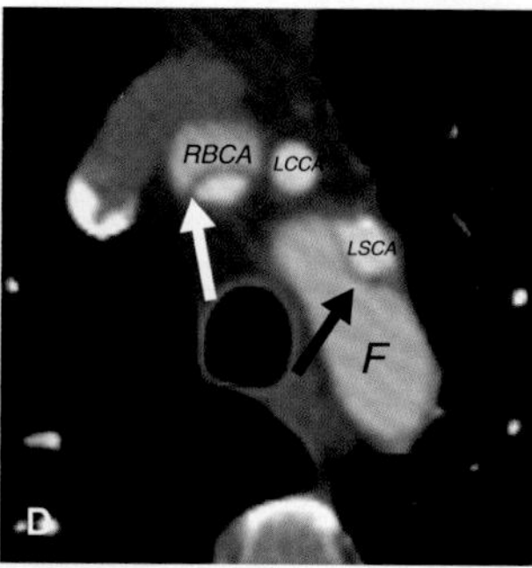

FIGURE 30.31. Type A Aortic Dissection, RCA Occlusion, and Propagation Into the Right Brachiocephalic Artery. Axial maximum intensity projection (MIP) CT image at the level of the left main coronary artery (**A**) demonstrates the proximal margin of the dissection flap (*arrow*) extending to the aortic root. The left main (*LM*) and left anterior descending (*LAD*) coronary arteries are patent. The dissection extends into the descending thoracic aorta with delineation of the flap (*arrow*), true (*T*), and false (*L*) lumens. Oblique coronal MIP image at the level of the right coronary artery (**B**) demonstrates the dissection flap (*black arrow*) extending into the ostium of the right coronary artery (*RCA*) leading to its occlusion (*white arrows*). Axial image at the level of the aortic arch (**C**) demonstrates the dissection flap (*arrow*), true (*T*), and false (*F*) lumens. Note inward displacement of intimal calcifications (*arrowhead*). Axial image at the level of the arch vessels (**D**) demonstrates propagation of the dissection flap into the right brachiocephalic artery (*RBCA, white arrow*). The left common carotid (*LCCA*) and subclavian (*LSCA*) arteries are supplied by the true lumen.

bolus tracking. With a test bolus, a small amount of contrast is administered and repeat axial images are obtained at a single level to assess the time to maximum opacification. Once this is determined, the full contrast bolus is administered, and imaging occurs with a scan delay as indicated by the timing bolus. With bolus tracking, a region of interest (ROI) is prescribed in the ascending aorta, the contrast bolus is administered, and when the Hounsfield Units in the ROI exceed a preset threshold, the scan is triggered. If there is concern for an ascending aortic dissection, prospective ECG gating should be employed to avoid false-positive diagnoses from motion or other artifacts at the aortic root. With gating and careful angiographic timing, the coronary arteries may also be evaluated for dissection propagation in this setting.

Aortic Dissection

Thoracic dissections are classified according to the Stanford system by their most proximal extent: type A dissections involve the ascending aorta (proximal to the innominate artery) and require immediate surgical management with stent–graft placement (Figs. 30.31 and 30.32). Type B dissections involve only the descending aorta (distal to the left subclavian artery) and are often managed medically unless there is evidence of end-organ ischemia or impending rupture, in which case surgical or endovascular stent grafting is indicated (Figs. 30.33 and 30.34). Dissections that involve the aortic arch but do not extend proximal to the innominate artery (Figs. 30.35 and 30.36) are rare,

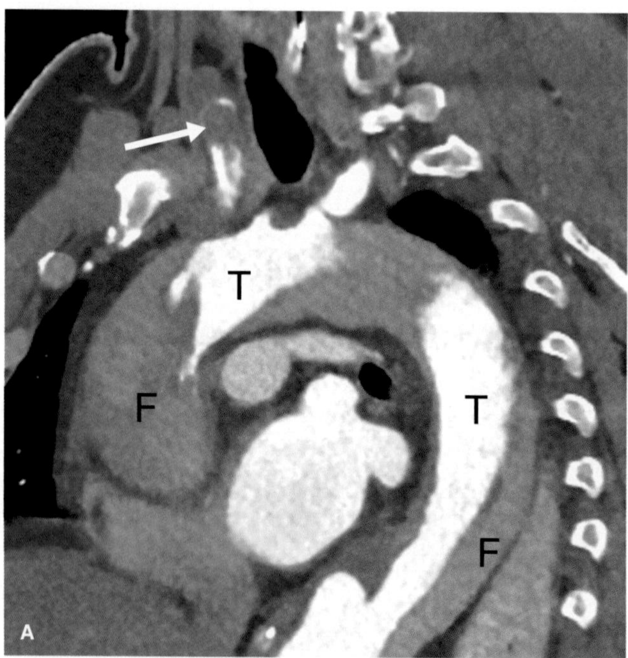

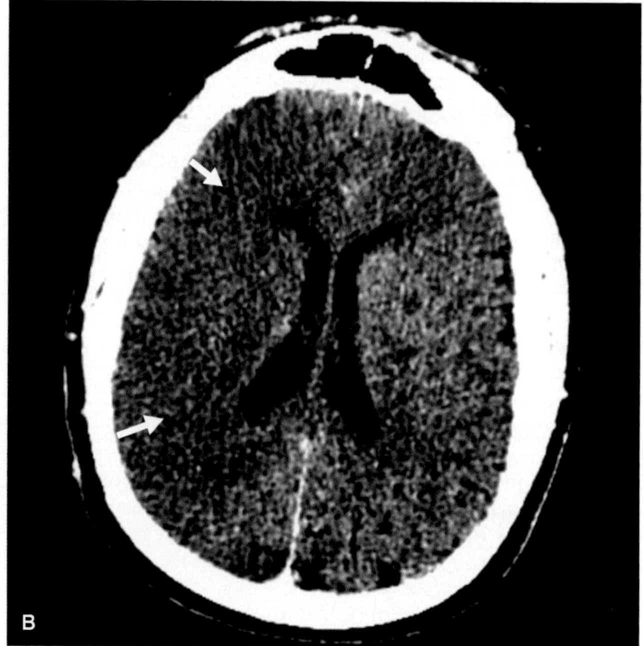

FIGURE 30.32. Type A Aortic Dissection With Occlusion of the Right Common Carotid Artery. Parasagittal CT reformat (**A**) demonstrates a type A dissection with very slow flow in the false lumen (*F*) compared to the true lumen (*T*). The dissection flap extends into and occludes the right common carotid artery (*white arrow*). Axial image from a head CT (**B**) shows relative hypoattenuation of nearly the entire right cerebral hemisphere (*white arrows*) due to right common carotid artery occlusion.

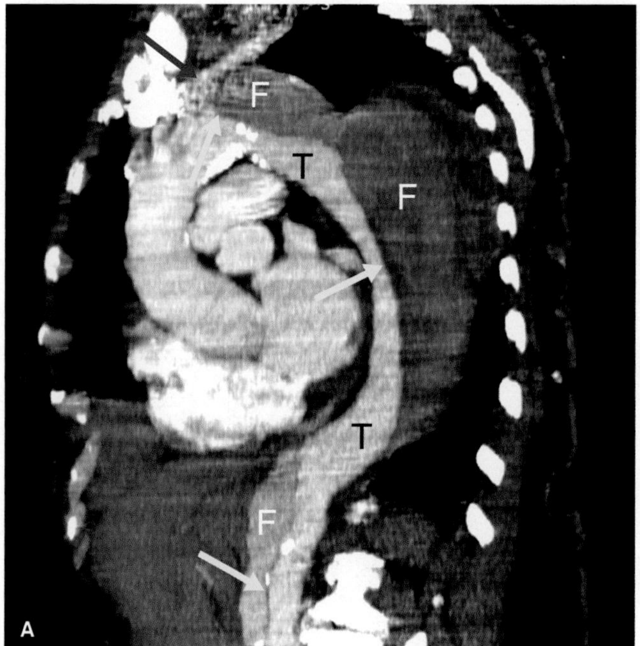

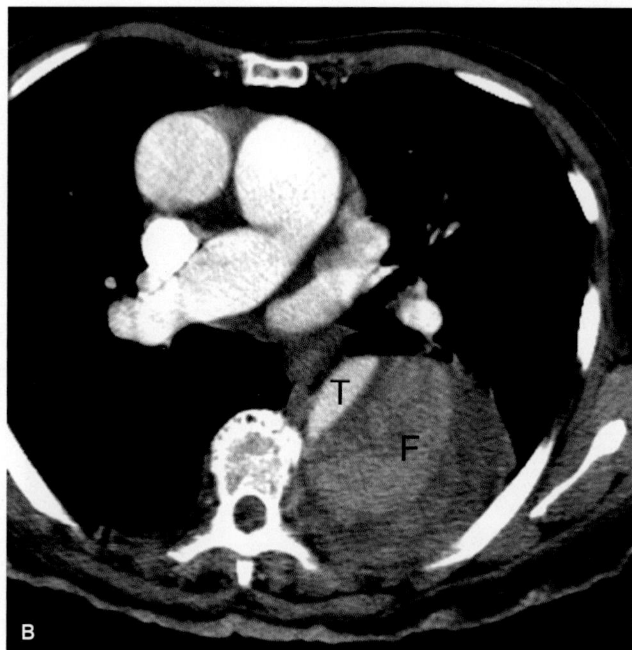

FIGURE 30.33. **Type B Aortic Dissection With Impending Rupture.** Parasagittal image from a CTA (**A**) shows the intimomedial flap (*yellow arrows*) extending to the level of the left subclavian artery (*red arrow*) but not involving the vessel or extending proximally into the aortic arch, consistent with a type B dissection. The true lumen (*T*) is smaller in size and shows increased contrast opacification compared to the false lumen due to the increased pressures within the false lumen. Axial image (**B**) shows the large size of the false lumen (*F*) compared to the true lumen (*T*). The maximum diameter of the aorta was 7.1 cm. Although most type B dissections are treated medically, this patient was treated surgically due to the large size of the aorta and the risk of subsequent aortic rupture.

comprising approximately 7% of all dissections. They are not specifically classified by the traditional surgical systems and have not been entirely characterized in the medical or surgical literature. For the purposes of reporting and to facilitate understanding among providers, they may be described as type B dissections with aortic arch involvement. Postoperative surveillance imaging in patients who undergo endovascular treatment is important to assess for the presence of endoleaks, discussed in more detail later in the chapter.

The pathogenesis of aortic dissection is a complex process involving degeneration of the aortic media, a dynamic structure that plays a vital role in regulating aortic compliance among other functions. This degeneration may be congenital, secondary to aberrant or defective protein production (e.g., in Marfan and Ehler–Danlos syndromes), or acquired, most commonly secondary to chronic hypertension which causes medial degeneration. Other risk factors include Turner syndrome and bicuspid aortic valve, cocaine and methamphetamine use, pregnancy, and aortitis. The altered microenvironment and function of the media predispose to the acute phase of dissection when the intima is disrupted, with resultant blood flow from the true aortic lumen into the media and formation of a second, false lumen. The intimomedial tear most commonly occurs along the right lateral wall of the ascending aorta, 1 to 2 cm from the sinotubular junction, or in the proximal descending aorta near the insertion of the ligamentum arteriosum, the sites of maximum shear stress. Once blood has entered the false lumen, it propagates longitudinally along the aortic wall, typically in retrograde fashion; a second, reentrance tear allows blood to circulate through the false lumen. This process also induces a robust inflammatory response—the aortic wall is friable and fragile in the acute phase, with a higher risk of rapid expansion and/or rupture compared to the chronic setting (Figs. 30.33 and 30.34). Dissections involving the ascending

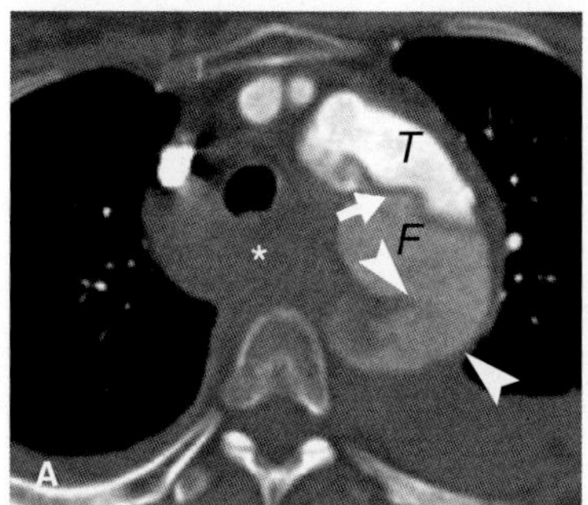

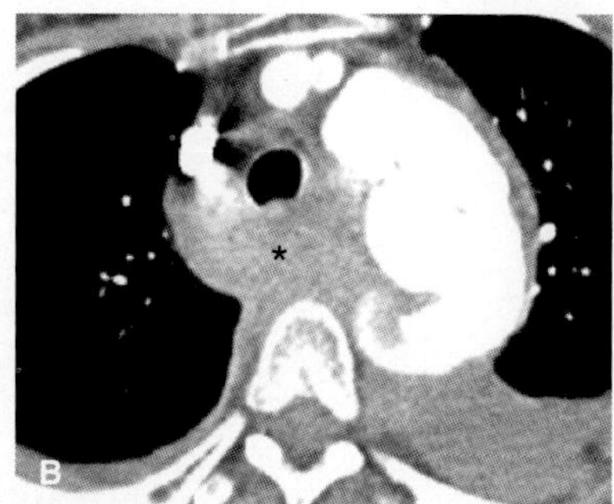

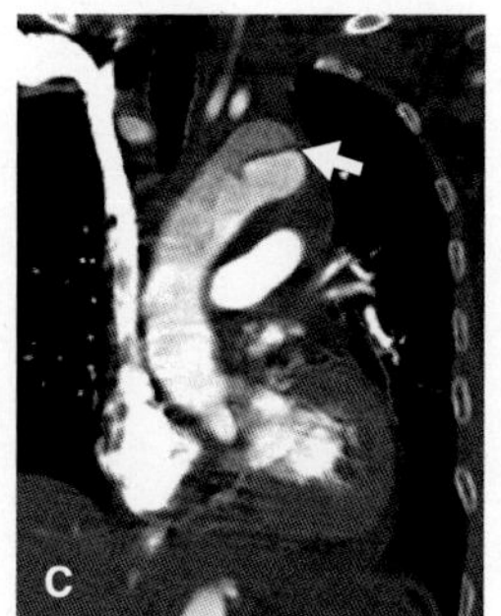

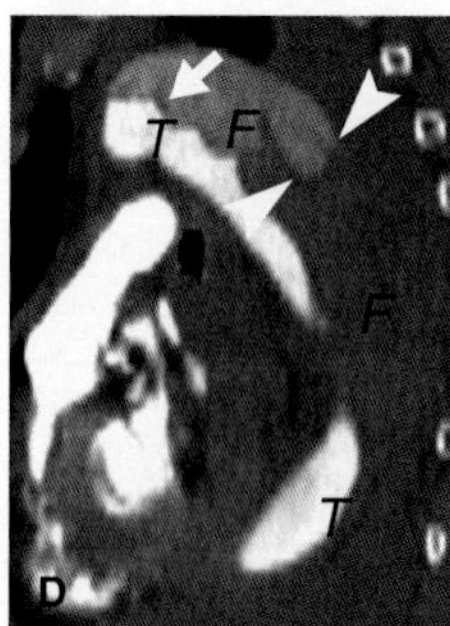

FIGURE 30.34. **Type B Aortic Dissection With Rupture.** Axial CT in the angiographic (**A**) window/level demonstrates the intimomedial flap (*arrow*), with delineation of the true (*T*) and false (*F*) lumens. The large area of contrast extravasation extending posteromedially from the posterior aspect of the pseudoaneurysm (*arrowheads*) represents rupture. The soft tissue window/level (**B**) shows the mediastinal hematoma (*) to better advantage; the esophagus is obscured. Coronal (**C**) and sagittal (**D**) reformats can be easily rendered from the original dataset at the workstation; the sagittal view demonstrates partial thrombosis of the false lumen (*F*) in the mid-distal descending thoracic aorta.

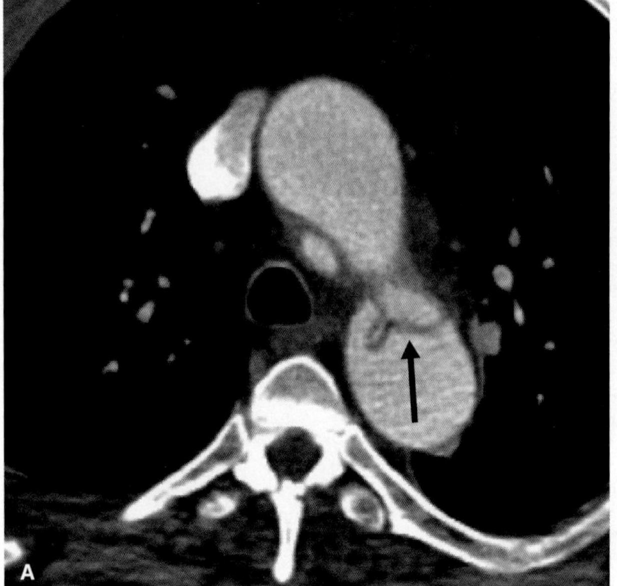

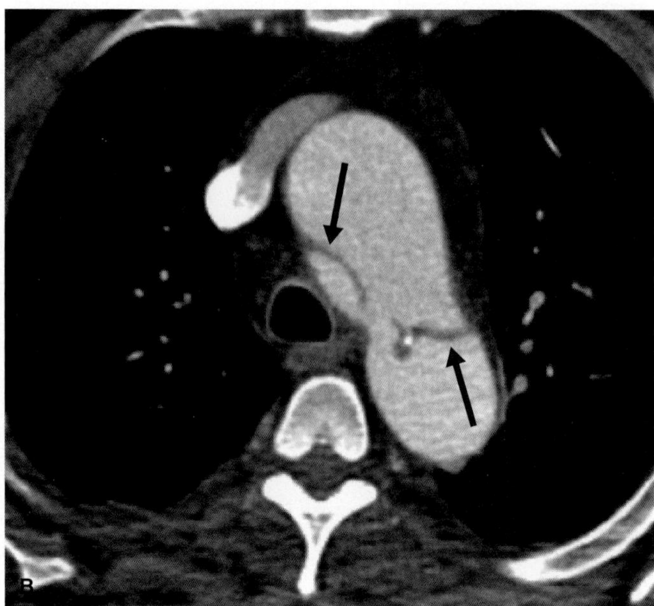

FIGURE 30.35. **Type B Dissection With Aortic Arch Involvement.** Axial CT images at the level of the lower (**A**) and mid-aortic arch (**B**) demonstrate a dissection flap (*arrows*) that extends to the proximal aspect of the arch but does not propagate beyond the origin of the right brachiocephalic artery and thus does not meet the definition of a type A dissection; dissections involving the arch have been incompletely characterized in the medical and surgical literature.

aorta may be complicated by severe aortic regurgitation, cardiac tamponade due to hemopericardium, and/or coronary artery occlusion depending on propagation (Fig. 30.31). Rupture into the right ventricle, left atrium, venae cavae, and pulmonary arteries is also possible, leading to large left-to-right shunts. Elsewhere, end-organ hypoperfusion/ischemia may result from propagation of the dissection flap into the arch or abdominal vessels (Fig. 30.32).

Chest radiographs (Fig. 30.37) are often the initial study but may be normal in up to 40% of cases. The frontal view may demonstrate tracheal deviation, mediastinal widening, loss of the aortic knob contour, enlargement of the ascending and/or descending aorta, pericardial effusion, or inward displacement of intimal calcifications which may be apparent if prior radiographs are available for comparison.

CTA should be performed in the setting of positive findings on chest radiographs or high clinical suspicion and is critical for diagnosis and treatment planning. On noncontrast imaging, there may be inward displacement of intimal calcifications. On angiographic phase imaging, the classic intimomedial flap is seen in the vast majority of cases. The true and false lumens can usually be distinguished by the relatively increased contrast enhancement and smaller size of the true lumen in relation to the false lumen, due to the increased pressures in the false lumen (Figs. 30.31 to 30.34). This increased pressure also causes the corners of the true lumen to demonstrate an acute angle with the intimal flap, which can help differentiate between the two. However, a later timing of the angiogram and/or fenestrations in the flap may confound these findings. In extremely rare cases, there may be circumferential intimal disruption ("shearing") with concentric true/false lumens. CTA is also useful to evaluate propagation of the dissection flap into branch vessels (Fig. 30.32).

MRI and MRA can be performed using abbreviated protocols with rapid, single breath-hold sequences with similar

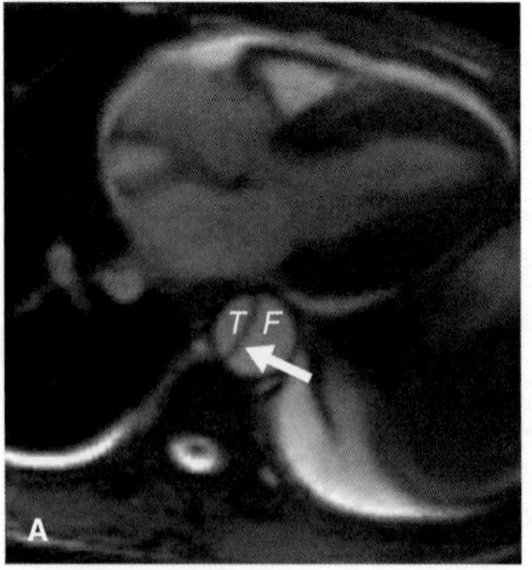

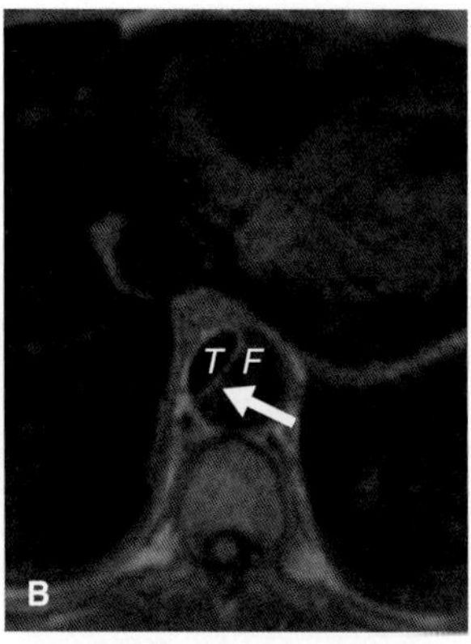

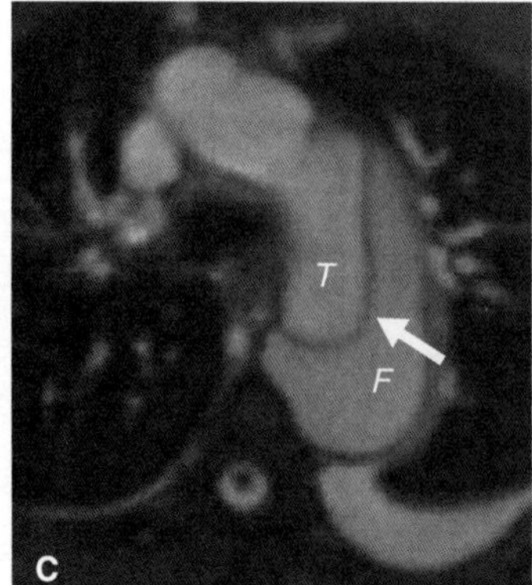

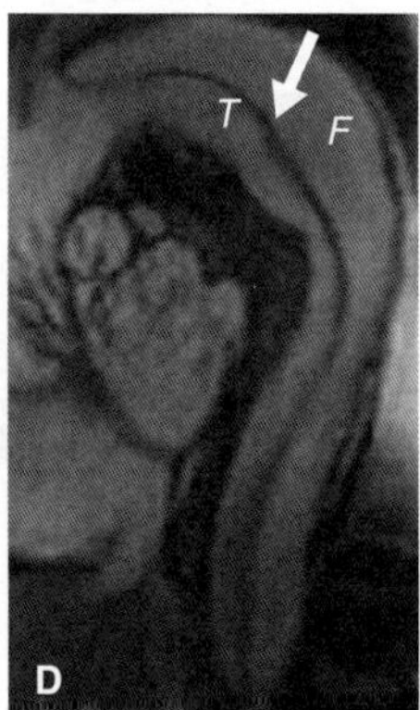

FIGURE 30.36. **Type B Dissection With Aortic Arch Involvement.** Axial balanced steady state free precession (bSSFP) gradient echo (**A, C**) and double inversion recovery (DIR) T2-weighted (**B**) MR images demonstrate the intimomedial dissection flap (*arrows*) with delineation of the true (*T*) and false (*L*) lumens. The true lumen (*T*) is smaller and demonstrates acute angles with the dissection flap, while the larger false lumen (*F*) demonstrates obtuse angles at interface with the flap. Note also the small pericardial and left pleural effusions, most evident in **A.** Sagittal reformat (**C**) shows the dissection extending into the arch but not involving the ascending aorta.

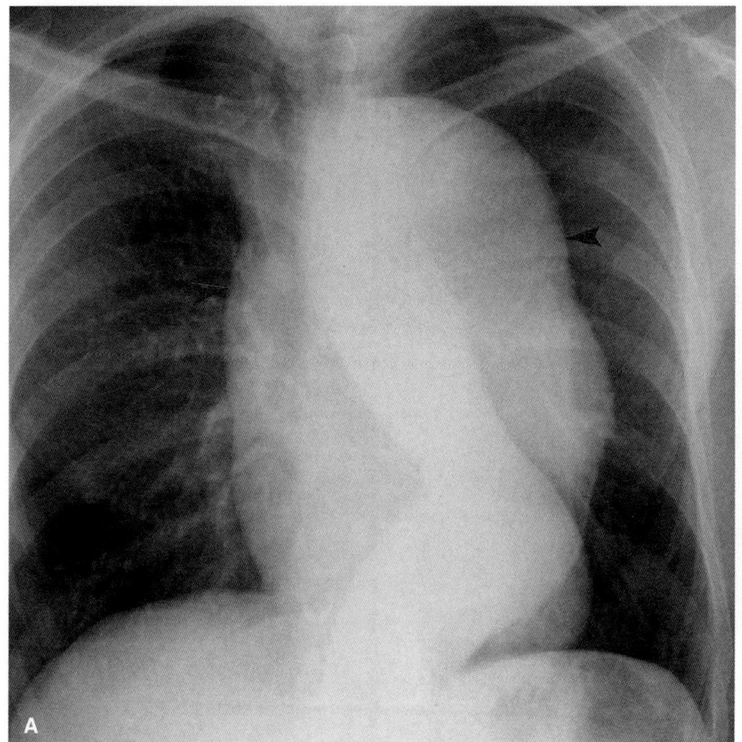

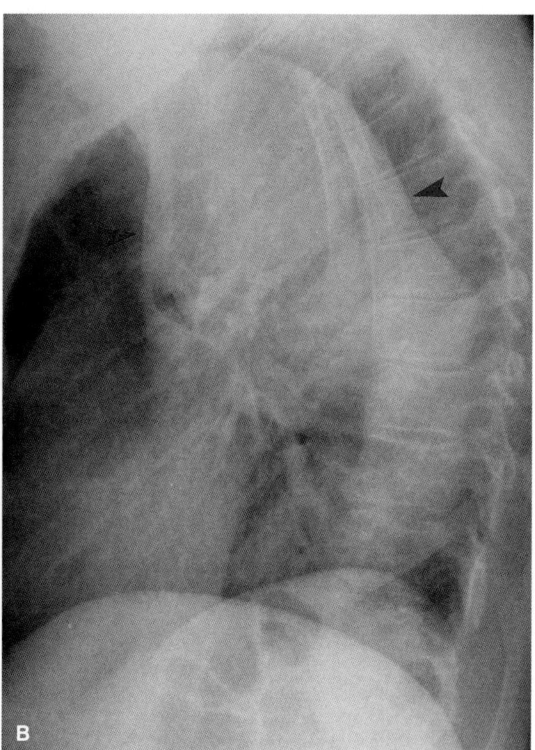

FIGURE 30.37. **Type A Thoracic Aortic Dissection.** Frontal (**A**) and lateral (**B**) chest radiographs in a 36-year-old man demonstrate a widened, lobulated mediastinal contour (between *arrowheads*).

sensitivity/specificity to CTA, with similar visualization of the intimomedial flap, true, and false lumens (Fig. 30.36). MR is also particularly useful in root dissections, where retrograde flow dephasing across the aortic valve on steady state free precession (SSFP) sequences is diagnostic of aortic regurgitation. As mentioned above, proximal aortic dissections may rupture into the pericardium, resulting in hemopericardium; in patients with possible tamponade, functional cinematic cardiac MR imaging with SSFP allows evaluation for gross visual inspection of wall motion through the cardiac cycle. Further, end-systolic and end-diastolic volumes can be quantified using postprocessing software to calculate stroke volumes and cardiac output. However, in most instances, patients with ascending dissections are unstable and require immediate surgical intervention.

Intramural Hematoma

IMH describes acute hemorrhage within the aortic wall and represents 5% to 15% of cases of AAS. IMH was traditionally thought to represent a distinct disease process that resulted from rupture of the vasa vasorum within the media, forming a hematoma without communication to the aortic lumen. TEE, however, provides the best images of the intima, and the common finding of intimal irregularity in cases of IMH suggests that an intimal "microtear" may be the inciting event, a theory corroborated by the fact that such tears are often found at the time of surgery and/or in pathologic analysis of IMH specimens.

On CT, IMH is characterized by continuous, often crescentic, hyperdense thickening of the aortic wall seen on noncontrast imaging (Fig. 30.38); there may also be inward

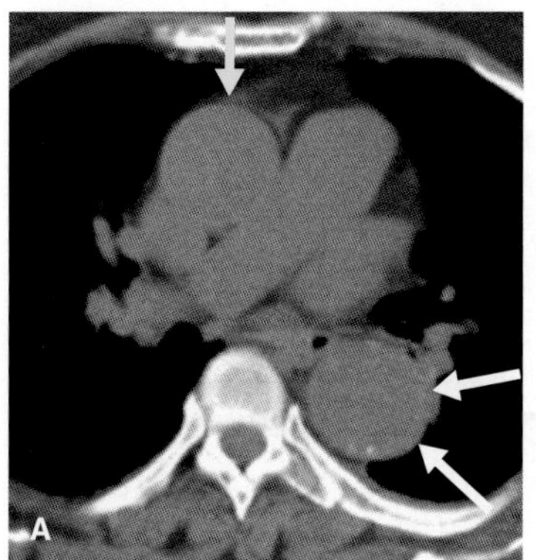

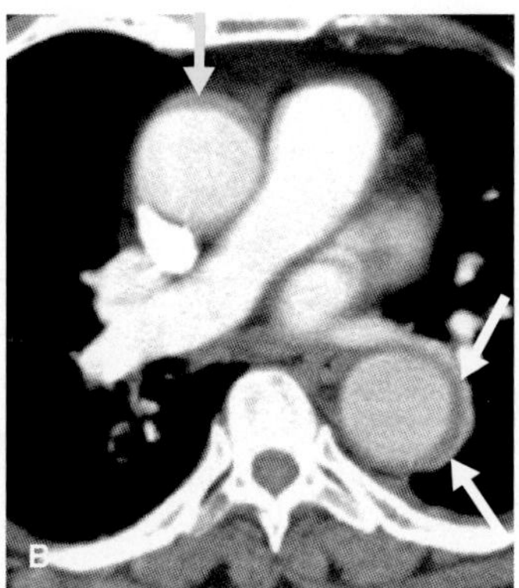

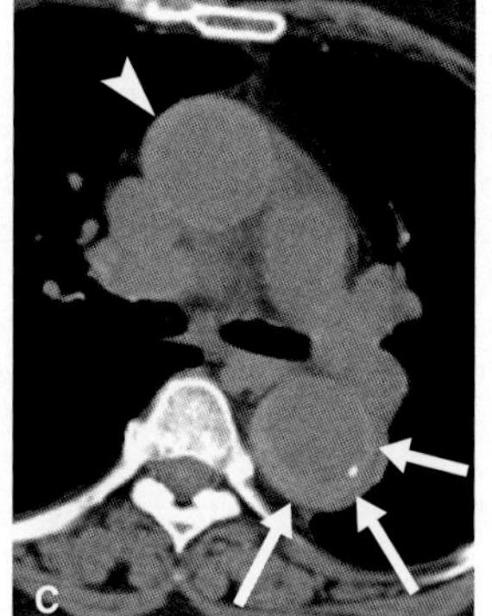

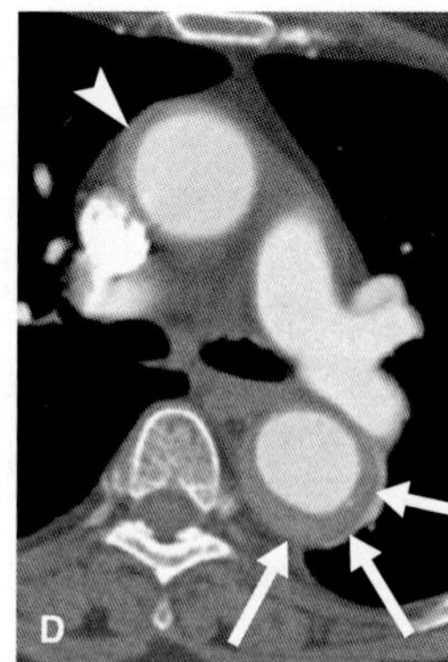

FIGURE 30.38. **Type B Progressing to Type A Intramural Hematoma (IMH).** Axial nonenhanced (**A**) and contrast-enhanced (**B**) CT images at the level of the right pulmonary artery in a 73-year-old woman demonstrate crescentic high attenuation intramural hematoma involving the descending thoracic aorta (*white arrows*), best seen on the non-contrast portion of the examination. The IMH extended to the level of the left subclavian artery but did not extend into the arch or ascending aorta. Motion artifact in the ascending aorta on the contrast portion of this non-gated study (*yellow arrow*, **B**), which is absent on the non-contrast portion (*yellow arrow*, **A**) should not be confused with an intimal flap or IMH. Axial nonenhanced (**C**) and contrast-enhanced (**D**) images at the level of the left pulmonary artery taken 4 days later demonstrate interval increase in IMH along the descending aorta (*arrows*), with new hyperattenuating crescentic thickening along the ascending aorta (*arrowheads*), consistent with progression to type A IMH.

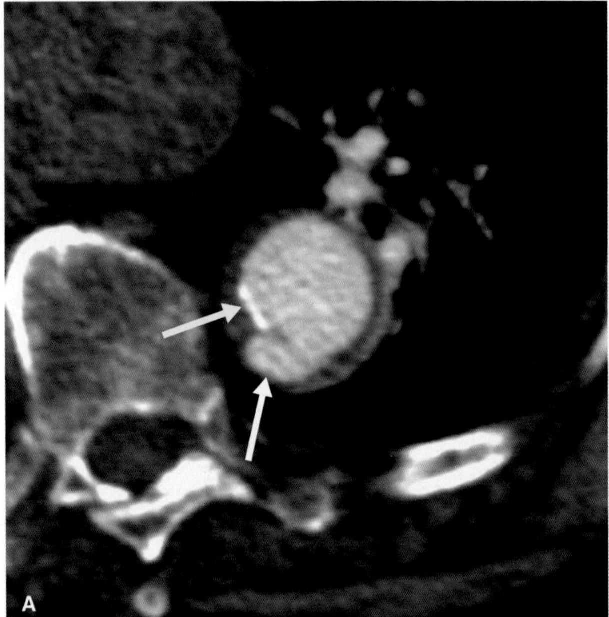

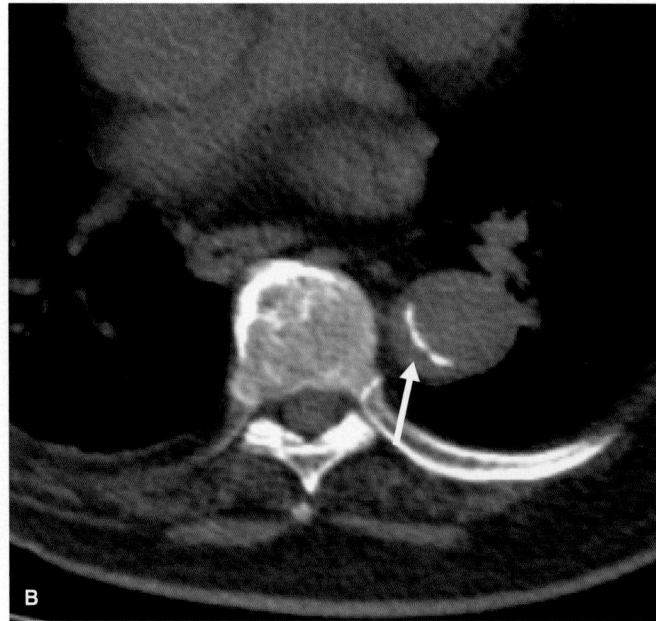

FIGURE 30.39. **Penetrating Atherosclerotic Ulcer (PAU).** Axial image from a CTA (**A**) in an 82-year-old man shows a contrast outpouching in the mid-descending thoracic aorta (*white arrow*) which extends beyond the calcified intima (*yellow arrow*), consistent with a PAU. Noncontrast CT image (**B**) just inferior to this level shows subtle high attenuation in the aortic wall (*white arrow*) due to adjacent hematoma. It is important to differentiate PAU from an ulcerated plaque, as the two have different treatments and outcomes.

displacement of atherosclerotic calcifications. On postcontrast imaging, the hyperdensity is often less apparent and can be overlooked or misdiagnosed. MR likewise demonstrates the crescentic wall thickening, which may demonstrate T1 and T2 signal abnormality depending on the age of the hemorrhage. Like dissection, IMH is classified by the Stanford system and is divided into type A and type B. Type B IMH is treated medically in most instances. Like those with type A aortic dissection, unstable patients with type A IMH usually undergo emergent surgery. However, there is debate regarding the treatment of patients with type A IMH who are clinically stable. This is secondary to the variable clinical course of IMH in which the hematoma may regress (10%), rupture (20% to 45%), or evolve into a frank aortic dissection (28% to 47%). Unfortunately, the course of a type A IMH is difficult to predict although if an IMH and PAU are seen concomitantly, this generally harbors a higher risk of progression. Given that some cases of type A IMH regress, some studies suggest initial medical therapy with surgery for those that progress to a frank dissection or expansion of the IMH. However, other studies show an increased mortality with this method. For this reason, serial imaging with CT or MR may be of critical importance in patient care, particularly in those with acute type A IMH who are treated medically. Like type A dissections, extension of the hematoma into the mediastinum or pericardium can occur with type A IMH.

Penetrating Atherosclerotic Ulcer

PAU describes internal erosion into the aortic media and typically manifests on the background of severe atherosclerotic disease. This most commonly occurs in the descending aorta, though ulceration may be seen anywhere along the thoracic aorta, with worse prognosis at the aortic root or along the proximal ascending aorta. PAU is thought to represent up to 7.5% of cases of AAS. On contrast-enhanced CT and on MRA with or without contrast, PAU manifests as a focal erosion into the aortic wall in the setting of typically severe atherosclerosis (Fig. 30.39) and may be distinguished from other causes of AAS by the focal vessel ectasia, absence of a flap, and lack of compression of the lumen from which the PAU arises. In some cases, it may be difficult to distinguish PAU from a background of complex atherosclerotic disease; however, PAU typically has a crater-like shape which extends beyond the calcified intima of the aorta, while complex ulcerated plaques are often more jagged appearing and do not extend beyond the intima. Progression of PAU is unpredictable but early identification is critical, as the ulcer can erode into the media with associated IMH (Fig. 30.40). When seen together, these findings herald poor prognosis, with further complications in up to 70% of patients, including formation of saccular aneurysms, aortic rupture, and dissection. Rupture appears to be more common than dissection in the setting of PAU. Treatment typically involves stent grafting, particularly in acute or symptomatic cases, with medical management and imaging surveillance reserved for asymptomatic patients or those with chronic, stable disease.

AORTIC PSEUDOANEURYSM

Aortic pseudoaneurysm is a focal irregular outpouching of the aorta secondary to intimomedial disruption, with extravasation contained by a variable amount of adventitia and by the surrounding mediastinal tissues. Pseudoaneurysms are most typically seen in the setting of traumatic aortic injury (TAI) or in the postoperative setting after cardiac or aortic vascular surgery, but they may also be seen in the setting of particularly aggressive/destructive infections and rare cases of ruptured dissection. Traumatic thoracic pseudoaneurysms are described in more detail later in the chapter, but most typically occur due to rapid deceleration/shearing forces at the sites of maximum traction; the most common such site is along the aortic isthmus, the narrowing between the distal arch and

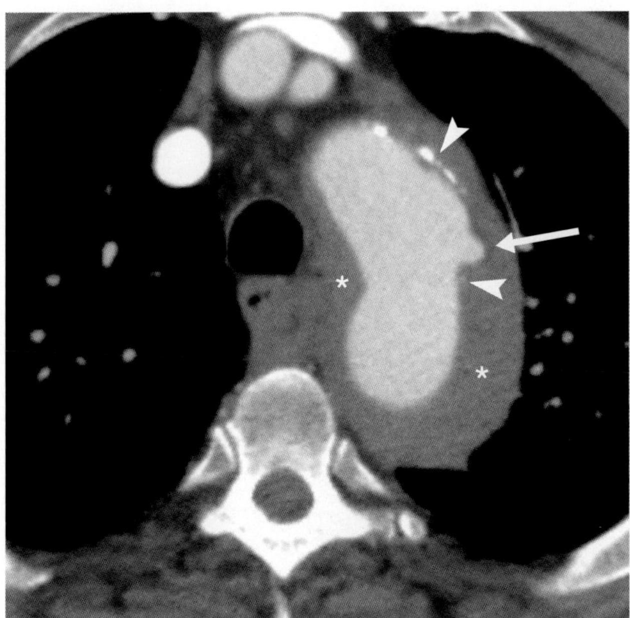

FIGURE 30.40. **Penetrating Atherosclerotic Ulcer (PAU) With Intramural Hematoma (IMH).** Axial CT image at the level of the aortic arch demonstrates the focal outpouching of contrast (*arrow*) extending beyond the surrounding intimal calcifications (*arrowheads*) consistent with a PAU. The PAU has eroded into the aortic media with surrounding intramural hematoma (*).

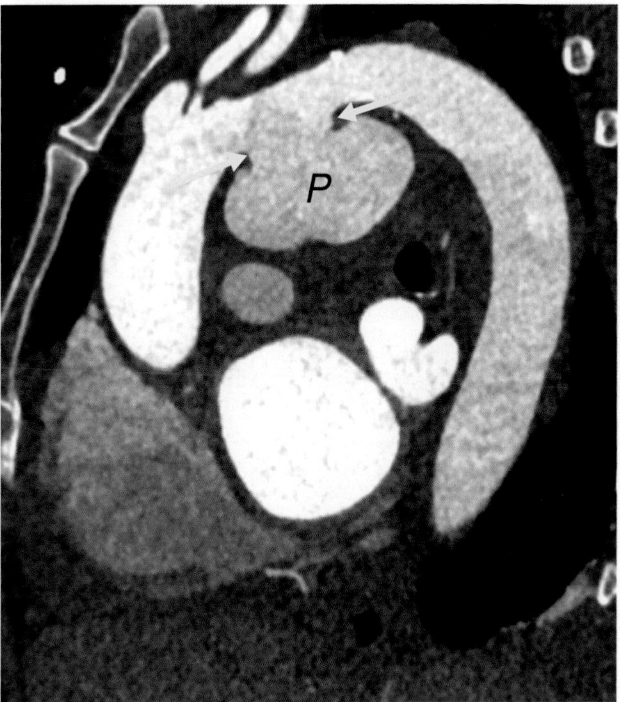

FIGURE 30.41. **Proximal Descending Aorta Pseudoaneurysm.** Sagittal CT image in a 68-year-old woman demonstrates a large saccular pseudoaneurysm (*P*) along the inferior aspect of the aortic arch and descending thoracic aorta. A relatively narrow neck (*yellow arrows*) connects the aorta to the pseudoaneurysm. This represents a contained aortic rupture.

ligamentum arteriosum. Postoperative pseudoaneurysms are typically seen along the ascending aorta at the sites of aortic puncture, cannulation, and/or cross-clamping. Thoracic aortic pseudoaneurysms may be complicated by aortoenteric and/or aortobronchial fistulas, mediastinal hemorrhage, hemothorax, and pulmonary hemorrhage.

Chest radiographs are of limited sensitivity and specificity for diagnosing pseudoaneurysms. Findings are similar to those in thoracic aortic aneurysm and may include widening of the mediastinal/aortic contour. Pseudoaneurysms of the aortic arch or proximal descending aorta may lead to tracheal deviation and/or left upper lobe atelectasis. Thoracic CTA is the primary imaging modality, with essentially 100% sensitivity and specificity for detecting pseudoaneurysms. The characteristic focal irregular outpouching/extravasation of contrast beyond the aortic lumen with a narrow neck (Figs. 30.41 and 30.42) is usually easily distinguishable from the concentric enlargement of a true aneurysm. CT is also particularly useful in assessing extent of mediastinal hematoma and associated complications. As discussed below, traumatic pseudoaneurysms are most common at the aortic isthmus.

As pseudoaneurysms represent contained aortic rupture, they must be treated emergently via either open surgical repair or endovascular covered stent placement. Untreated pseudoaneurysms progress (Fig. 30.43) eventually to aortic exsanguination and death.

AORTIC FISTULAS

Aortic rupture can occur in a multitude of settings including trauma, aortopathy, degenerative atherosclerosis, inflammation, and infection. The aorta can rupture and hemorrhage freely into the mediastinum or, rarely, communicate with a distinct anatomic space via a fistula. Aortic fistulas can form with the adjacent esophagus (i.e., aortoesophageal fistula) (Fig. 30.44), pleura (i.e., aortopleural fistula) (Fig. 30.45), bronchi (i.e., aortobronchial fistula) (Fig. 30.42), or other cardiovascular structures.

Aortoesophageal fistulas can occur with aneurysm rupture, PAU, foreign body ingestion with esophageal perforation, intrathoracic malignancies such as esophageal cancer, and postaortic endovascular stenting. Aortobronchial fistulas have been reported in cases of prior bronchial intervention such as stenting and thoracic surgery such as lobectomy. Patients with aortoesophageal and aortobronchial fistulas present most commonly with hematemesis and/or hemoptysis.

On imaging, extravasation of aortic contrast into an adjacent structure is pathognomonic but is not always seen. Secondary signs of aortic fistulas include a periaortic gas-containing collection mimicking an abscess, pseudoaneurysm, and effacement of the normal periaortic fat plane. Aortic fistulas are typically lethal if not surgically treated, although endovascular aortic repair may serve as a bridge to open repair in the emergent setting.

ACUTE TRAUMATIC AORTIC INJURY

Acute traumatic aortic injury (ATAI) represents a spectrum of disease from mild, focal injuries to the endothelium ("minimal intimal injury") to contusion/IMH to mural disruption with pseudoaneurysm or rupture. ATAI most often occurs secondary to high-energy blunt trauma—the classic scenario

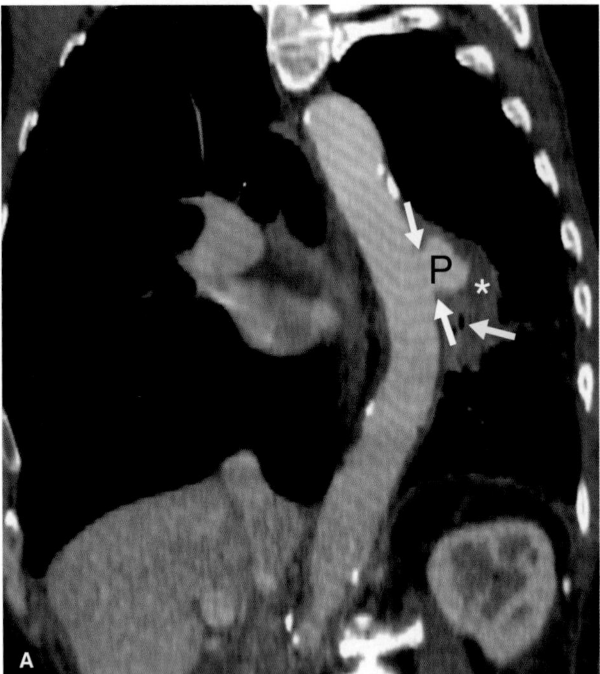

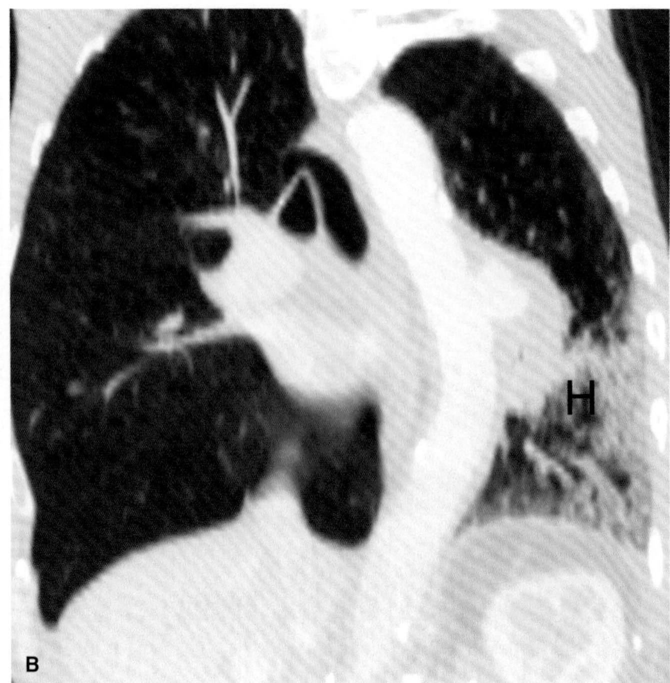

FIGURE 30.42. Descending Aortic Pseudoaneurysm Complicated by Aortobronchial Fistula and Pulmonary Hemorrhage. Coronal CT image (**A**) demonstrates the irregular margins of the pseudoaneurysm (*P, white arrows*) with adjacent hematoma (*). The neck of the pseudoaneurysm is narrower than the pseudoaneurysm itself. Air (*yellow arrow*) adjacent to the hematoma represents sequela of an aortobronchial fistula. Coronal CT image at the same level using lung algorithm (**B**) demonstrates the adjacent consolidative, reticular and ground-glass opacities representing pulmonary hemorrhage (*H*).

is a rapid deceleration injury in the setting of motor vehicle accident. The exact mechanism of injury is not known but may result from shearing forces and/or an "osseous pinch" between the manubrium and thoracic spine; the most common sites of injury are those of maximum traction: the aortic root, the aortic isthmus, and much less commonly the aorta at the level of the diaphragmatic aortic hiatus. While survival rates for those with isthmus injuries have improved over the past few decades, those with injuries located at the aortic root rarely survive.

Aortic injury with pseudoaneurysm is often asymptomatic; imaging is therefore key in rapid diagnosis. Chest radiography is almost invariably performed as part of the workup for trauma patients; while it is limited in sensitivity and specificity and often performed using portable technique, it may demonstrate superior mediastinal widening, apical cap, and/or loss of the normal aortic knob or descending aortic contour (Fig. 30.46). Positive findings on radiography and/or high clinical suspicion should prompt further imaging. Prior to the advent of modern CT scanners, direct catheter angiography was the preferred method at many trauma centers, with the ability to diagnose and treat with endovascular techniques in the same setting. However, CT has mostly supplanted angiography as a primary imaging modality, except in certain limited circumstances—

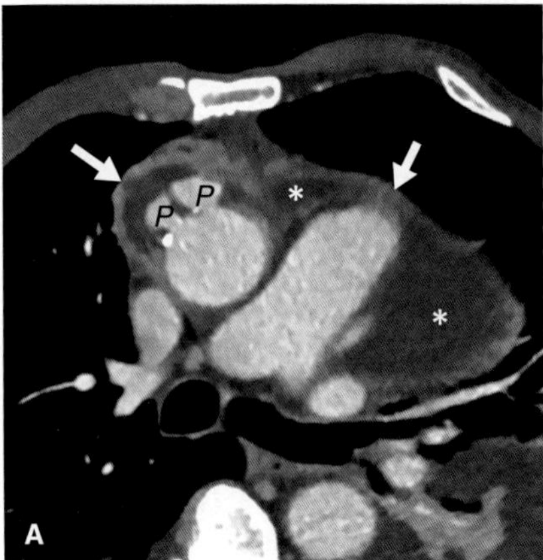

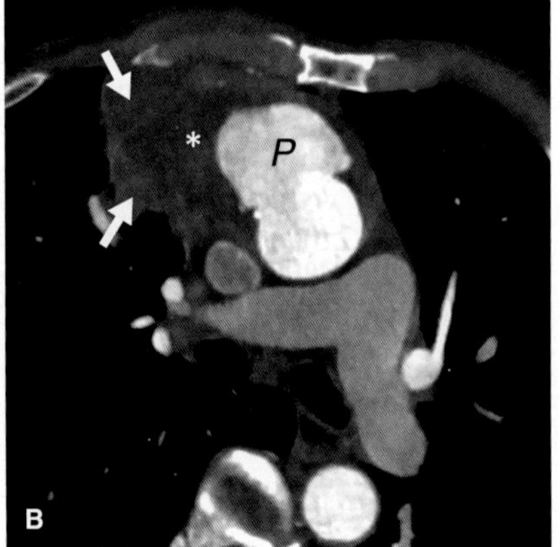

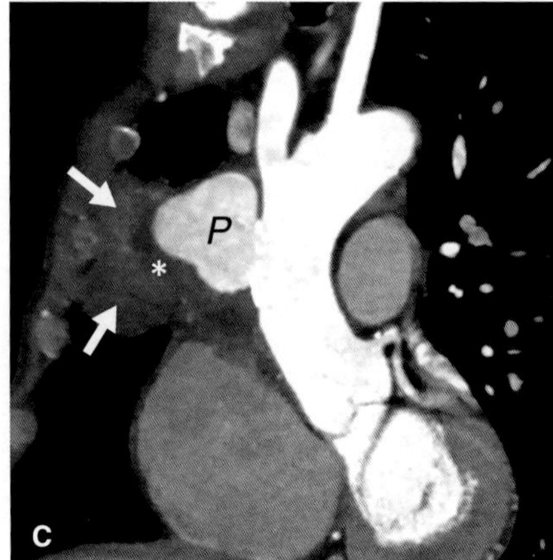

FIGURE 30.43. Ascending Aorta Pseudoaneurysm. Axial-oblique CT image at the time of presentation (**A**) demonstrates two narrow-necked pseudoaneurysms (*P*) along the ascending aorta. There is associated hemopericardium (*) causing pericardial inflammation (*white arrows*). The patient adamantly refused treatment and returned 3 months later with severe chest pain. Axial-oblique (**B**) and coronal-oblique (**C**) CT images demonstrate marked interval increase in size of the pseudoaneurysm (*P*). In addition to hemopericardium (*), there is now blood in the mediastinum (*white arrows*).

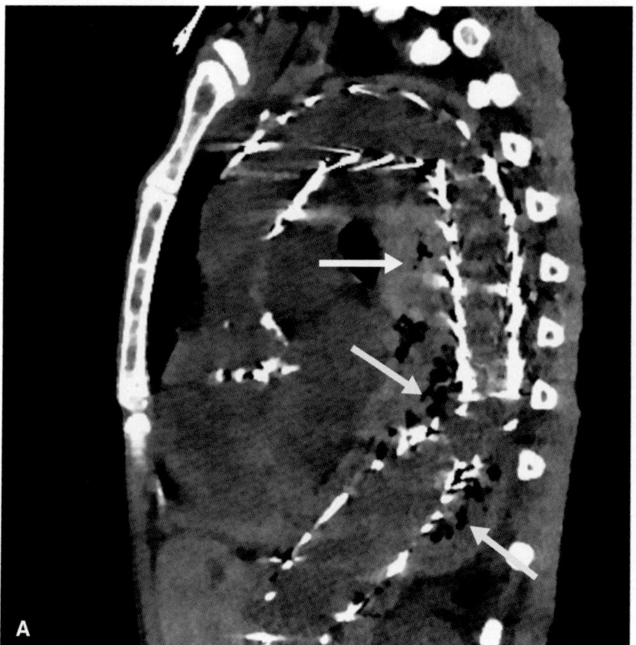

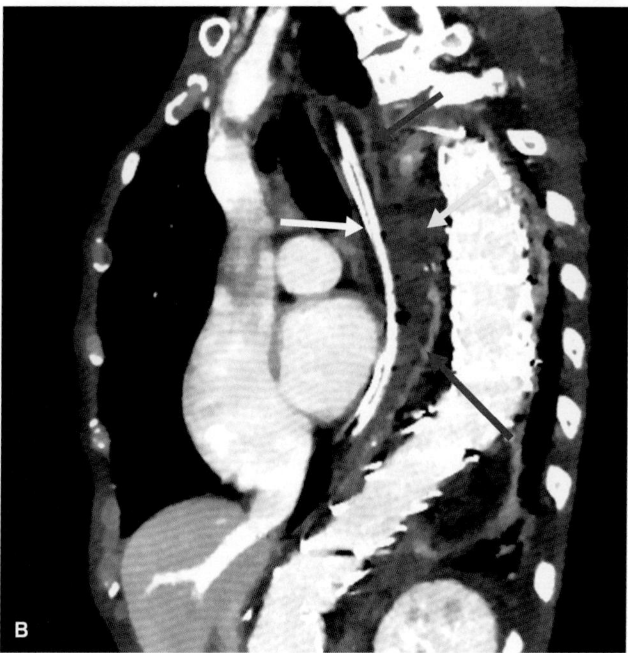

FIGURE 30.44. Aortoesophageal Fistula in a Woman Presenting With Hematemesis 3 Months After Endovascular Stent Placement. Noncontrast parasagittal CT image (**A**) shows a high-density mediastinal collection (*white arrow*) due to hematoma between the esophagus and descending thoracic aorta. Complex air and fluid collections are present, surrounding the thoracic endovascular stent (TEVAR, *yellow arrows*). Parasagittal contrast-enhanced image from the same study (**B**) shows absence of a large portion of the posterior wall of the esophagus (*yellows arrow*) with adjacent hemorrhage, air, and phlegmon. An esophagogastric tube is present (*white arrow*). The intact esophageal wall is seen both superior and inferior to the defect (*red arrows*).

for example, an unstable pelvic injury with high suspicion for vascular injury. TEE, intravascular ultrasound (IVUS), and MRA are typically secondary modalities due to higher invasiveness, longer imaging times, and limited availability. Transthoracic echocardiography (TTE) is an easier and more rapid modality but is useful only in the setting of ascending aortic injury.

As mentioned above, CT findings in ATAI may vary. On the mildest end of the spectrum is minimal intimal injury, which describes a focal hematoma/minimal filling defect at the luminal margin. ATAI may also manifest as IMH, which is described in greater detail above ("Acute Aortic Syndrome"). More severe injuries include traumatic pseudoaneurysm or even complete transmural disruption of all mural layers

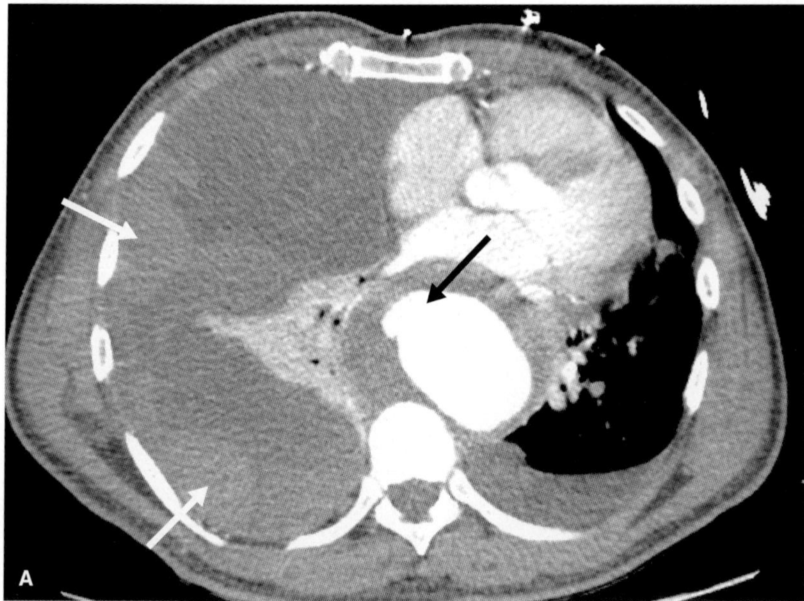

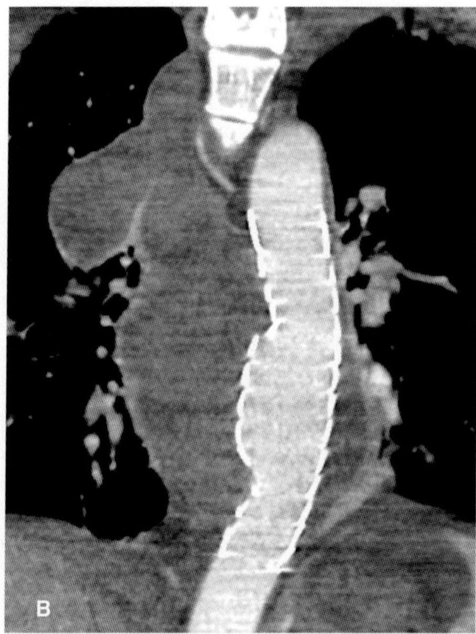

FIGURE 30.45. Aortopleural Fistula. Axial CT image (**A**) shows a distal descending thoracic aortic dilation with contour irregularity and periaortic hematoma compatible with a ruptured mycotic aneurysm (*black arrow*). Note the large right pleural effusion with heterogeneous high attenuation consistent with hemothorax (*white arrows*). Patient was emergently stented (**B**).

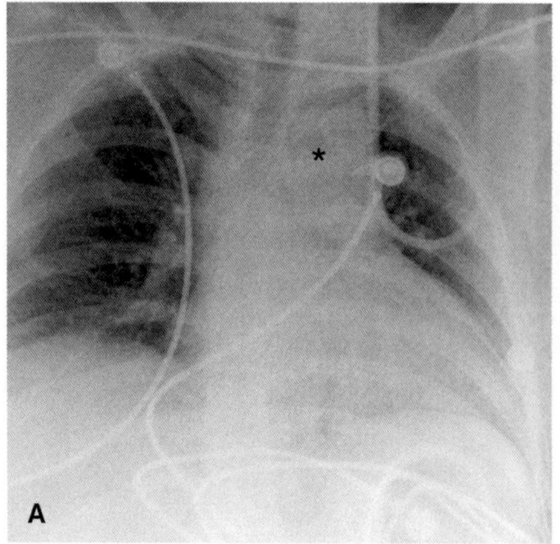

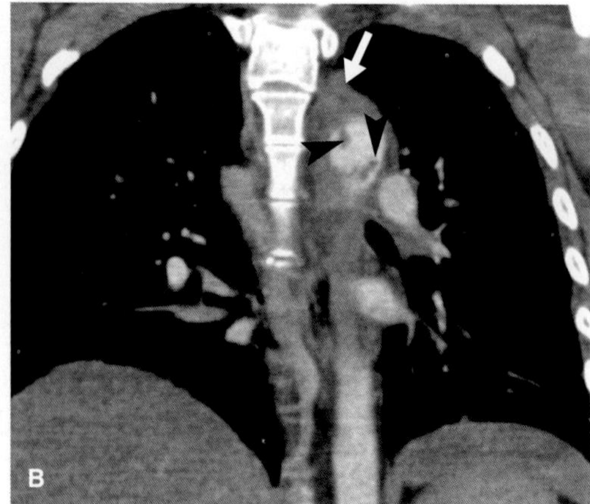

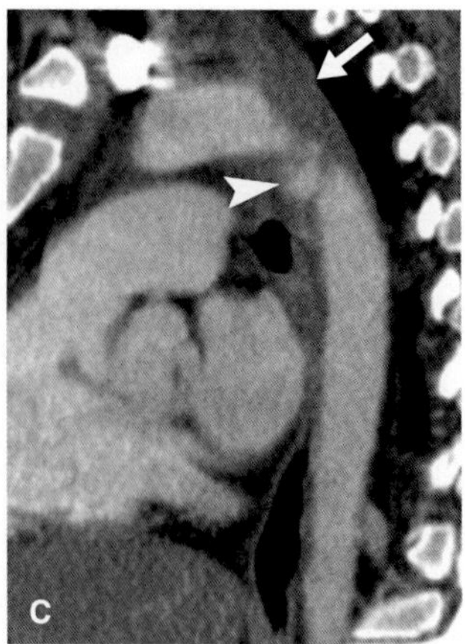

FIGURE 30.46. **Acute Traumatic Aortic Injury (ATAI).** Frontal chest radiograph (**A**) in a 42-year-old woman demonstrates mild superior mediastinal widening, most notably affecting the aortic contour(*). Coronal CT image (**B**) demonstrates disruption of the aorta (*arrowheads*) along the aortic isthmus with adjacent periaortic hematoma (*arrow*). Sagittal reformat (**C**) demonstrates aortic isthmic irregularity with a focal anterior bulge near the expected attachment of the ligamentum arteriosum (*arrowhead*) with surrounding periaortic hematoma (*arrow*) consistent with ATAI. This must not be confused for the physiologic ductus bump that can also be seen at this location.

with extravasation only contained by adjacent soft tissues (Figs. 30.46 and 30.47). These higher-grade injuries carry extremely high morbidity and mortality and are treated with open surgical repair or, increasingly, with endovascular stent grafting. Of particular note, a slight, smooth convex bulge in the aortic contour at the attachment of the ligamentum arteriosum called the "ductus bump" (Fig. 30.48) is physiologic and should not be confused for a traumatic pseudoaneurysm. The distinction is often easy, with a sharp, shouldered appearance, visible intimomedial fragment or mural irregularity in severe trauma; in less obvious cases, the presence of other findings, for instance adjacent mediastinal hematoma or fractures to the sternum and/or anterior ribs should raise concern for possible vascular injury.

Improved spatial resolution in CTA has allowed detection of milder aortic injuries, and management of these injuries varies by institution and physician preference. Though no large-scale studies are available, limited-case series suggest that these milder injuries are unlikely to progress to clinical significance and, in most cases, can likely be managed nonoperatively.

POSTOPERATIVE AORTA

It is important to be familiar with the normal postoperative imaging appearance of the aorta to understand appropriate imaging evaluation and avoid misdiagnosis. Evaluation of the postoperative aorta is typically performed with helical CTA, although MRI/MRA can also be used. MR may be limited by accessibility, long image acquisition time, and metallic artifacts from surgical material. For patients post aortic root or ascending aortic repair, ECG gating should be used to minimize motion artifact.

Aortic root and ascending aortic pathologies such as type A dissection and ascending aortic aneurysm are usually repaired by resecting the native aorta and placing an interposition synthetic or tissue graft, with or without concurrent aortic valve replacement. Graft containing an attached prosthetic valve is termed a composite graft (Fig. 30.49). Synthetic grafts are composed of polyethylene and appear slightly hyperattenuating to the aorta on noncontrast CT but hypoattenuating to the aorta on CTA. Tissue grafts will have the same attenuation as

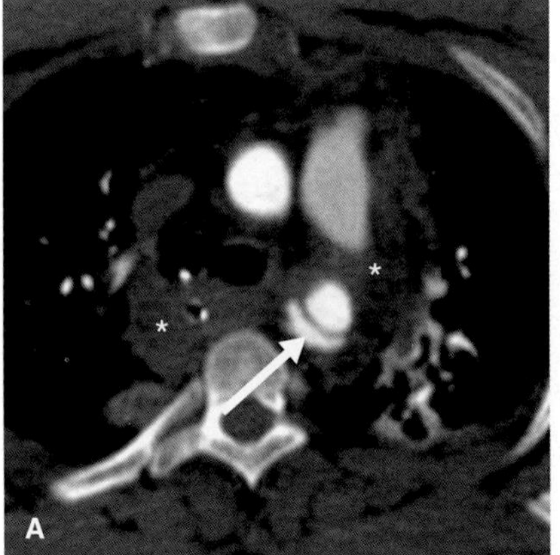

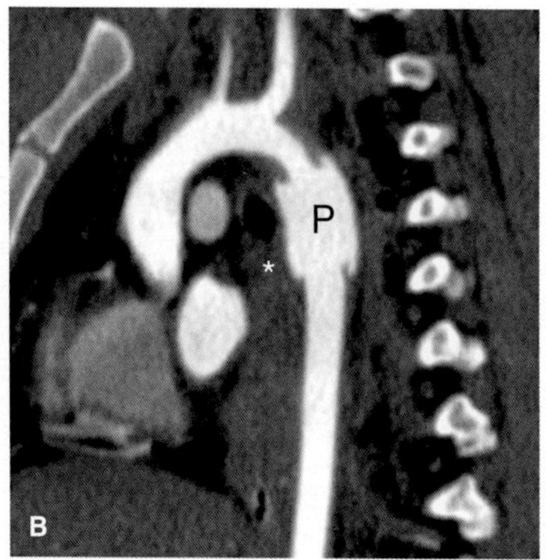

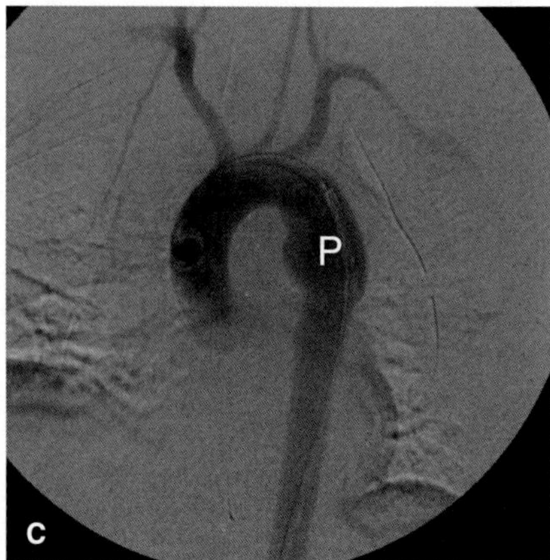

FIGURE 30.47. **Acute Traumatic Aortic Injury/Traumatic Pseudoaneurysm.** Axial CTA image at the level of the aortic isthmus (**A**) and parasagittal reformat (**B**) demonstrates a complete transection of the aorta (*white arrow*, **A**) contained by a large pseudoaneurysm (*P*, **B**) and surrounding mediastinal hematoma (*, **A**, **B**). Emergent catheter angiography mirrors the findings of the CTA with a pseudoaneurysm (*P*) at the aortic isthmus.

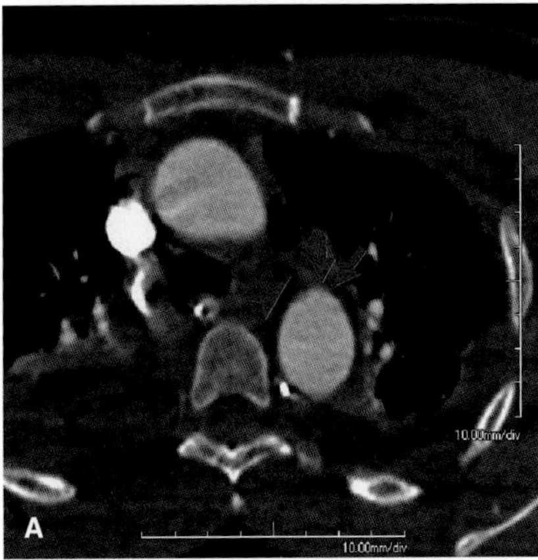

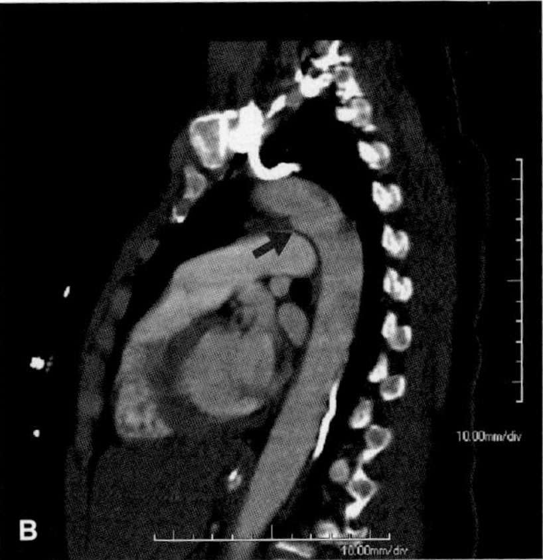

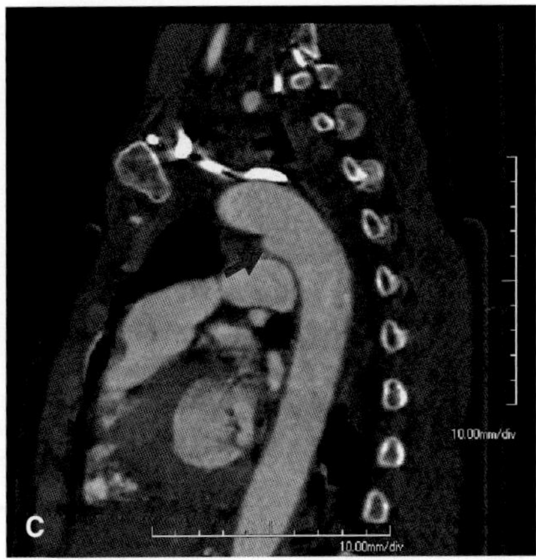

FIGURE 30.48. Physiologic Ductus Bump. Axial and sagittal CT images (**A, B**) in a trauma patient demonstrate a focal outpouching in the aortic contour (*arrows*) at the ligamentum arteriosum (*arrowhead*). Fortunately, this patient had a prior study for comparison; sagittal image from that study (**C**) demonstrates similar morphology representing the ductus bump. It is important to distinguish this finding from aortic injury in the setting of high-velocity injury. Note the absence of mediastinal hematoma or other evidence of blunt trauma in **A** and **B**.

normal aortic wall, but anastomotic margins of aortic repair are indicated by an abrupt caliber change in the aorta and foci of high attenuation surgical material. Graft repair of the aortic arch and descending thoracic aorta will have a similar imaging appearance, although aortic arch repair sometimes requires debranching of the aortic arch with reanastomosis or bypass grafting of great vessels.

Grafts may also be placed in the native aorta without resection, termed the inclusion technique, resulting in a soft tissue density surrounding the graft representing fluid and thrombosis within the native aorta. Atherosclerotic calcification of the native diseased aorta will remain and suggests this type of repair. "Elephant trunk" technique, in which the distal aspect of the graft is left floating in the native aorta, can mimic a dissection (Fig. 30.50).

Complications

In the immediate postoperative period, perigraft air can be normal and should eventually resolve by 6 weeks postsurgery. Perigraft fluid and soft tissue can also be normal, representing organizing hematoma/fibrosis or edema, and last for months to years following repair. Concern for graft infection should be raised when there is new or increasing perigraft air and fluid collection and contrast enhancement (Fig. 30.51). Rarely,

FIGURE 30.49. Composite Valve-Graft Repair. Coronal oblique CT shows repair of the aortic and ascending aorta with a mechanical aortic valve (*black arrow*) attached to a tubular synthetic graft (*solid white arrow*). Note high attenuation surgical material at the distal anastomosis (*dashed white arrow*) and normal widening of the coronary ostia at the site of coronary reimplantation (*).

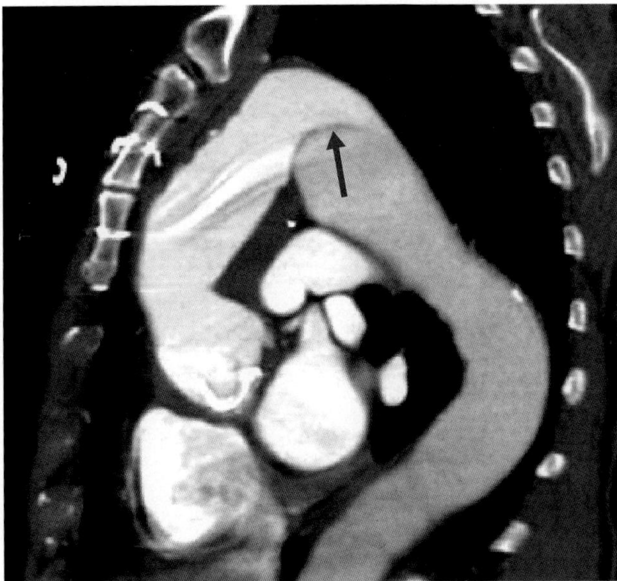

FIGURE 30.50. Elephant Trunk Repair. Sagittal oblique CT. Linear filling defect (*arrow*) in the proximal descending thoracic aorta corresponds to the distal aspect of an aortic graft which is left floating in the aorta. This should not be mistaken for a dissection flap.

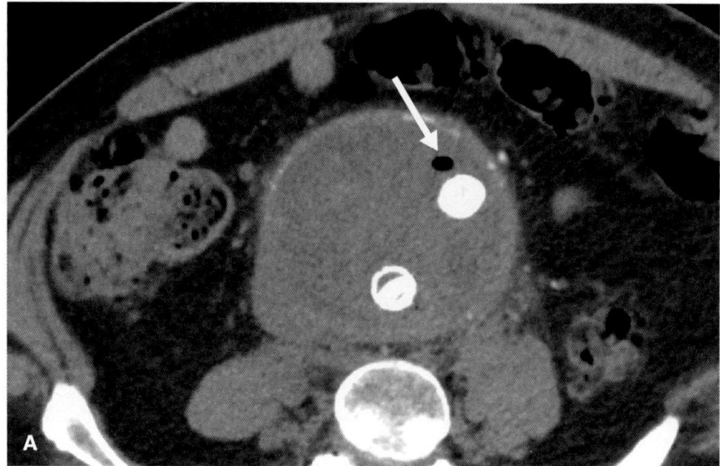

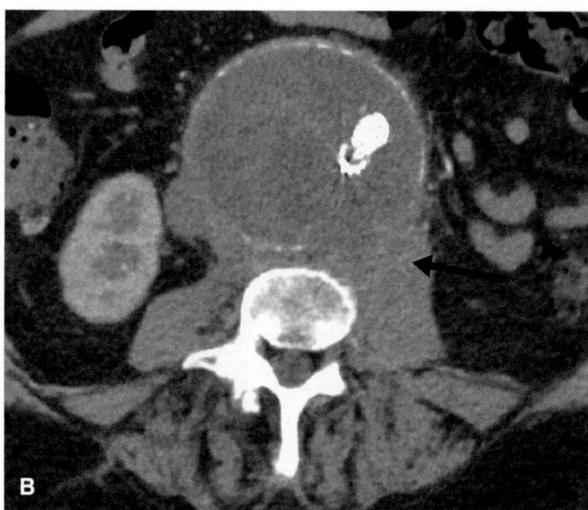

FIGURE 30.51. **Graft Infection With Perigraft Abscess.** Axial images through the lower abdomen in a patient 3 months status postendovascular stent repair of an abdominal aneurysm. Small focus of gas (*white arrow*, **A**) near the left common iliac artery is abnormal this late post repair. Contour irregularity of the left posterolateral abdominal aorta, which is contiguous with a left psoas abscess (*black arrow*, **B**).

increasing perigraft air can be caused by fistulization to an adjacent bronchus or esophagus (Fig. 30.44). Other signs of fistula include tethering to and contrast leak into the adjacent structure (Fig. 30.52).

Postoperative pseudoaneurysm is a contained rupture that manifests as a contrast-containing collection contiguous with the aortic lumen, usually occurring at the anastomotic margins (Fig. 30.52). Graft reinforcements such as felt and pledgets are hyperattenuating and can be mistaken for contrast leak, mimicking a pseudoaneurysm. In these instances, noncontrast comparison imaging is essential to distinguish contrast from surgical material.

Thoracic Endovascular Aortic Repair

Thoracic endovascular aortic repair (TEVAR) entails placement of a metallic stent–graft into the aorta via an endovascular approach. Indications for TEVAR include aortic dissection, PAU, pseudoaneurysm, and enlarging aneurysm. TEVAR may be preferred to open surgical repair depending on location of aortic pathology and whether the patient is a poor surgical candidate. Since stents are rigid compared to grafts, stent grafts are more easily placed within the straight descending thoracic aorta, as opposed to the curved ascending aorta and aortic arch. Stent–grafts are designed to expand within the aortic lumen and closely appose with the aortic wall, thereby occluding intimal tears or covering atherosclerotic ulcers or pseudoaneurysms. Stent grafts are usually covered with a synthetic membrane which is not visible on imaging. In some instances, the proximal end of a stent graft is placed in the aortic arch and occludes the left subclavian artery. In this instance, the subclavian artery will fill via retrograde flow from the left vertebral artery. Before this is done, the surgeons need to ensure that the basilar system is complete, allowing for collateralization and that the left vertebral artery does not arise directly from the aortic arch.

Endoleak complications of stent grafts in the thoracic aorta are the same as those in the abdominal aorta and occur in 29% of patients post TEVAR of TAAs. Endoleak is characterized by contrast external to the stent graft and represents continued blood flow within the excluded aortic lumen, which can result

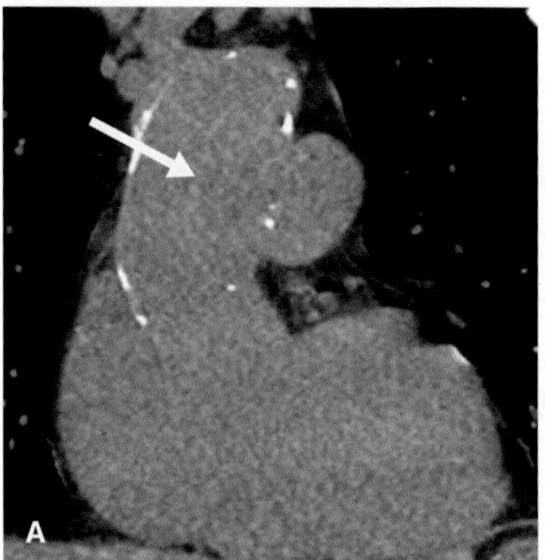

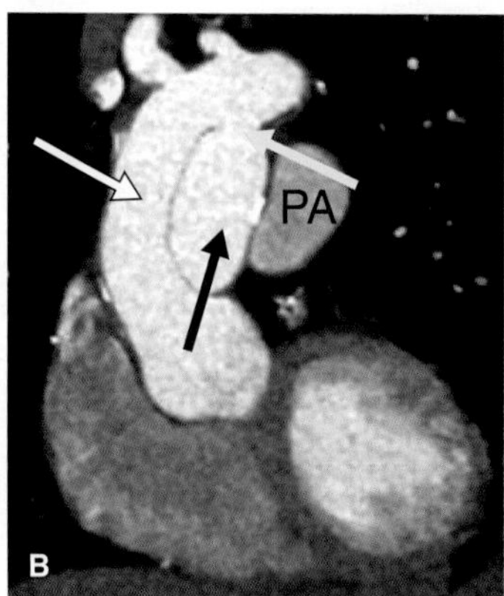

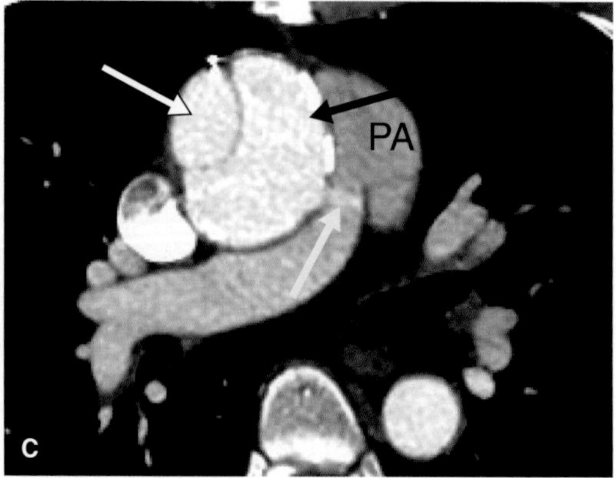

FIGURE 30.52. **Graft Pseudoaneurysm and Fistula.** Noncontrast coronal (**A**), arterial phase coronal (**B**), and arterial phase axial (**C**) images. On noncontrast CT (**A**), there is calcification of the synthetic graft material (*white arrow*). Postcontrast (**B, C**), there is a contrast-filled collection (*black arrows*) located between the graft (white arrows) and the pulmonary artery (*PA*). A defect is present at the distal anastomotic site of the graft (*yellow arrow*, **B**), with a large pseudoaneurysm extending inferiorly (*black arrow*, **B**). Axial image (**C**) shows that the pseudoaneurysm (*black arrow*, **C**) partially wraps around the repaired ascending aorta (*white arrow*, **C**). Interestingly, the pseudoaneurysm has fistulized with the right pulmonary artery (*yellow arrow*, **C**).

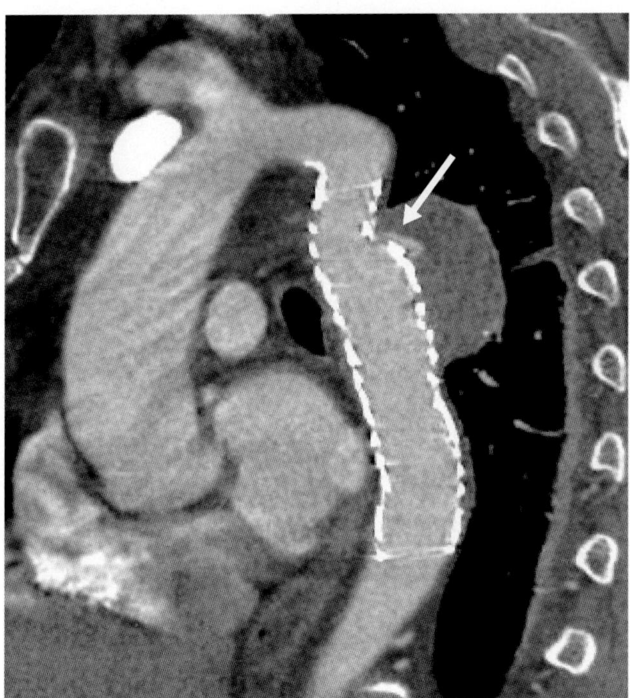

FIGURE 30.53. **Endoleak, Type I.** Patient status post remote repair of aortic coarctation with two overlapping stents. Small extravasation of contrast (*arrow*) at the junction of these two stents is compatible with a type I endoleak.

in expansion of an aortic aneurysm, pseudoaneurysm, or dissection false lumen with increased risk for rupture.

There are five types of endoleaks. Type I endoleak is most common and occurs at the proximal (type IA) or distal (type IB) margins of the stent graft. Contrast will be seen in the excluded aortic lumen, directly communicating with the proximal or distal end of the stented aorta (Fig. 30.53). Type II endoleak is retrograde opacification of the excluded aortic lumen through an aortic branch vessel such as an intercostal or bronchial artery within the thorax and inferior mesenteric or lumbar arteries in the abdomen. Type III endoleak results from device failure, with contrast leaking through a fracture or defect in the stent graft (Fig. 30.54). Type IV endoleak is caused by graft wall porosity and does not require repair. This is usually seen in anticoagulated patients as a blush of contrast around the stent graft on catheter angiography around the time of stent placement. Type V endoleak, also referred to as endotension leak, is a diagnosis of exclusion in which there is expansion of the excluded aortic lumen without a visible contrast leak. This presumably represents an occult type I to III endoleak. A small endoleak may only be detected on delayed images, so it is important to acquire delayed images in addition to angiographic phase images in post EVAR patients.

Additional complications of TEVAR include stent collapse, migration, and ischemia. Ischemic complications occur secondary to occlusion of branch vessels and occur in 30% to 50% of patients with type B aortic dissection.

AORTITIS

The term aortitis refers to inflammation of the aortic wall (specifically the media and/or adventitia), which may be focal/segmental or multifocal, may also affect large and small branch vessels, and is broadly classified into noninfectious and infectious causes.

The noninfectious causes are myriad and include numerous primary vasculitides, both large- (e.g., giant cell or Takayasu arteritis) and variable-vessel predominant varieties. Aortitis is also commonly seen in the setting of other rheumatic diseases including chronic ankylosing spondylitis, rheumatoid arthritis, and relapsing polychondritis; and aortic valve/vessel disease is an uncommon but known manifestation of IgG4-associated autoimmune disease, systemic lupus erythematosus (SLE), Behçet disease, and the seronegative arthritides—for example, reactive arthritis. Radiation-induced aortitis may manifest as thrombosis, pseudoaneurysm/rupture, stenosis, and accelerated calcification confined to the treated field. Finally, an idiopathic form of aortitis may result in acute and/or chronic periaortic inflammation, associated with the formation of "inflammatory" aortic aneurysms and chronic secondary retroperitoneal inflammation/fibrosis. It is likely that many cases previously thought to represent idiopathic disease were undiagnosed IgG4-associated disease, a multisystem disorder that has been better understood in the last decade.

The native aorta is resistant to infection, but vessel abnormality related to atherosclerosis, pre-existing aneurysm, cystic medial necrosis, or other disease renders the vessel more vulnerable. Classically, infectious aortitis was seen commonly in the setting of tertiary syphilis (also called "luetic" aortitis) and tuberculosis infection, in addition to other bacterial and viral

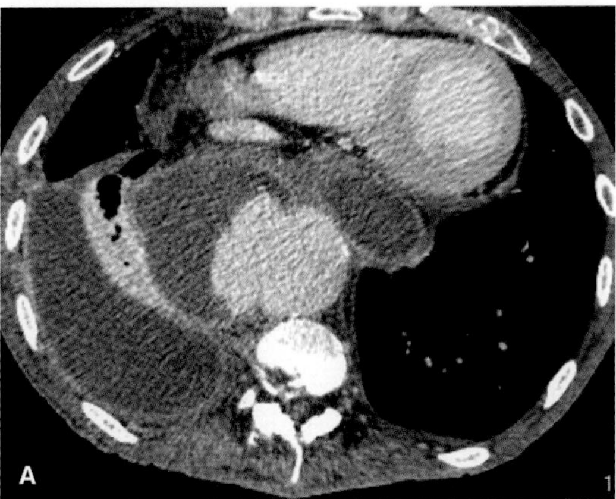

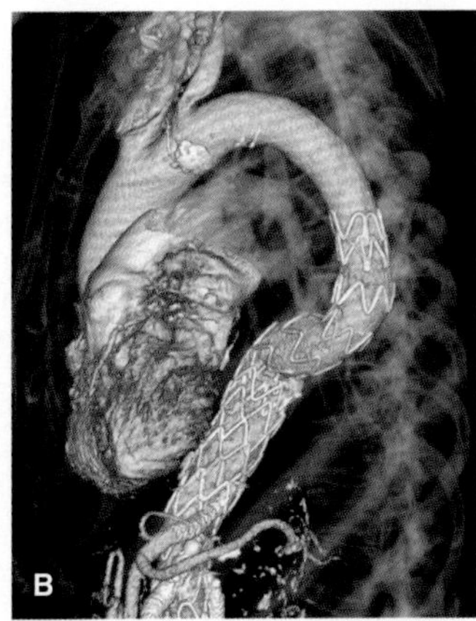

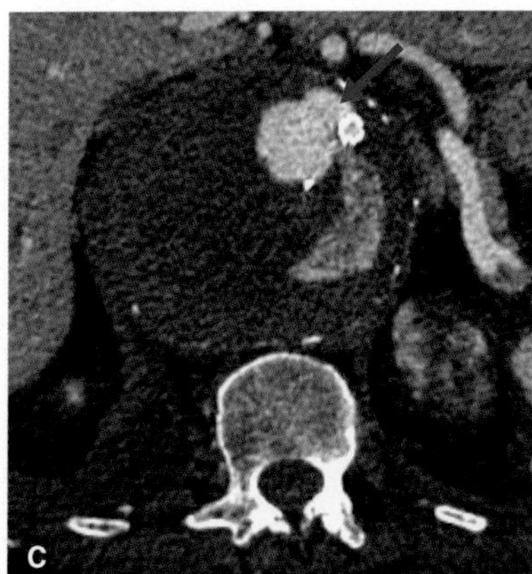

FIGURE 30.54. **Endoleak, Type III.** Patient presented with descending thoracic aortic aneurysm rupture into the mediastinum and pleura (axial CT, **A**). Postendovascular repair (3D VR, **B**) with extravasation of contrast through the graft near the ostium of a stented renal artery (*arrow*, axial CT, **C**).

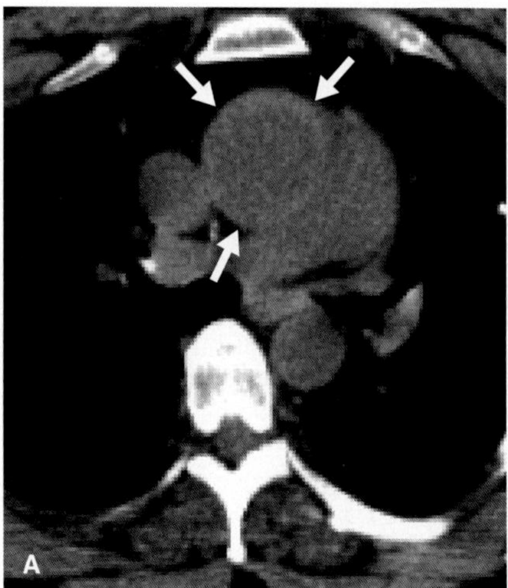

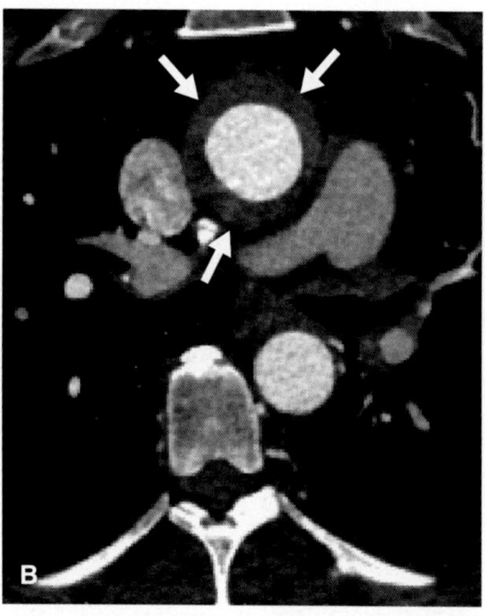

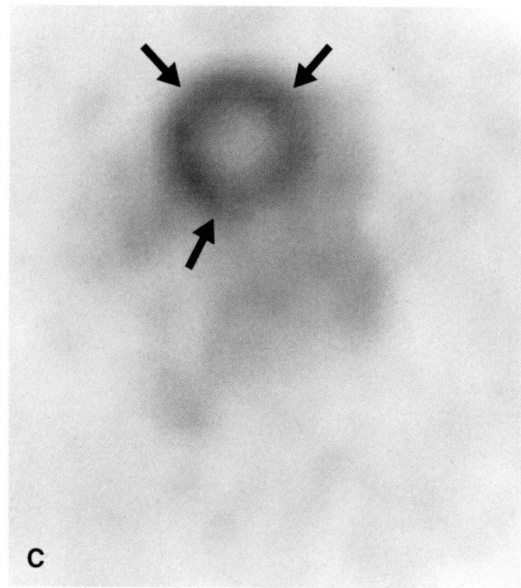

FIGURE 30.55. **Takayasu Arteritis.** Axial nonenhanced (**A**) and contrast-enhanced (**B**) CT images at the level of the right pulmonary artery in a 54-year-old man demonstrate hyperattenuating circumferential wall thickening along the ascending aorta (*arrows*). Attenuation-corrected PET image (**C**) at the same level demonstrates corresponding increased uptake that has been shown to correlate with active disease.

agents. With the advent and widespread availability of penicillin and effective tuberculosis treatment, however, infectious aortitis is now most commonly caused by *Staphylococcus aureus* and *Salmonella* but can also be seen in *Listeria, Clostridium septicum,* and *Campylobacter* infections. Involvement of the aorta most commonly occurs due to hematogenous seeding in the setting of high-grade bacteremia, but infection may also arise directly from adjacent structures—for example, the aortic root/aortic valve or para-aortic mediastinal lymph nodes—and may be caused by traumatic or iatrogenic inoculation.

Early diagnosis of aortitis (and vasculitis in general) may be difficult owing to the vague signs and symptoms, particularly in the acute phase. Given the common diagnostic uncertainty, imaging plays a vital role, both to confirm the presence of inflammatory sequela and to narrow the differential diagnosis, given patterns of findings. However, it is crucial to interpret these findings in the presenting clinical context, as different entities show considerable overlap at imaging and certain etiologies can demonstrate more suggestive signs or symptoms. For instance, GCA and Takayasu arteritis predominantly affect the ascending aorta, aortic arch, and branch vessels and may be indistinguishable on imaging alone. However, the populations most typically affected (patients over 50 for GCA and under 30 for Takayasu) are distinct and presentation may differ (e.g., temporal headache and symptoms of polymyalgia rheumatica in GCA).

Acute complications associated with aortitis include intraluminal thrombus and aneurysm formation. Infected aortic aneurysms are rare, encompassing 0.06% to 2.6% of all aneurysms, and may lead to severe hemorrhage/sepsis and death if untreated. Aortitis may also be complicated by dissection and rupture, which are more likely in the acute phase of inflammation. Luminal stenosis may occur in the acute inflammatory or the chronic fibrotic phase. Complete vascular occlusion may also occur, more often in branch vessels but even possibly in the aorta (most commonly in the distal abdominal aorta) and/or iliac vessels in severe cases. Aortoenteric fistula may develop between the aorta and adjacent structures—for example, esophagus, stomach, small or large bowel—a rare complication seen most often in the setting of infectious or inflammatory aneurysm.

CTA is one of the primary modalities used to assess for vasculitis. The inflammatory wall thickening (defined as greater than 3 mm) in aortitis may be circumferential or crescentic and may involve arch and other smaller branch vessels, depending on the etiology. Crescentic thickening may be difficult to distinguish from IMH, particularly on non–contrast-enhanced (NECT) imaging (Fig. 30.55). Classically, the wall thickening in IMH is confluent over the site of involvement and is often hyperattenuating. In aortitis, the thickening may be discontinuous or more variable along diseased segments. Intramural enhancement is a more specific sign of mural inflammation and may be reduced or absent after initiation of treatment—for example, corticosteroids in rheumatic disease. Patients with Takayasu arteritis often demonstrate multifocal areas of wall thickening/luminal narrowing along the aorta and arch vessels, as well as other vascular structures such as the coronary arteries and/or pulmonary arteries.

MR imaging has slightly worse spatial resolution than CTA but provides additional information owing to its superior soft tissue characterization (Fig. 30.56). Wall thickening is well seen and intramural T1 hypointensity and T2 hyperintensity due to mural edema suggests active disease. Periaortitis in idiopathic disease will demonstrate T1 hypointensity and T2 hyperintensity, while chronic periaortic fibrosis will typically be both T1 and T2 hypointense. Contrast-enhanced imaging with gadolinium-based agents can demonstrate similar intramural enhancement characteristics to contrast enhanced CT, which again may be less or not evident after appropriate treatment. Chronic periaortic fibrosis will demonstrate avid enhancement.

Nuclear medicine imaging, specifically PET-CT with ^{18}F-FDG, is a valuable tool for the assessment of aortitis. Mural thickening can be seen on the CT portion of the exam and FDG uptake in the aortic wall can be used to assess disease activity and treatment response (Figs. 30.55 and 30.56).

AORTIC TUMORS

Primary aortic tumors are exceedingly rare, with only about 150 cases reported, and typically carry a dismal prognosis due to advanced local and/or metastatic disease at the time of diagnosis as well as complications typically secondary to tumor embolization with distal vascular occlusion and end-organ ischemia/infarction. By histopathologic classification,

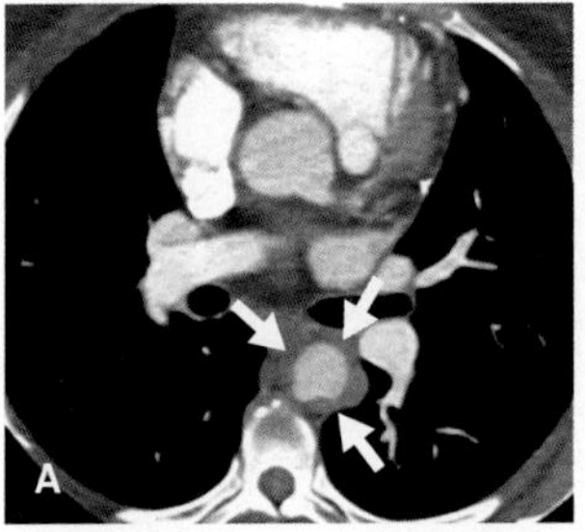
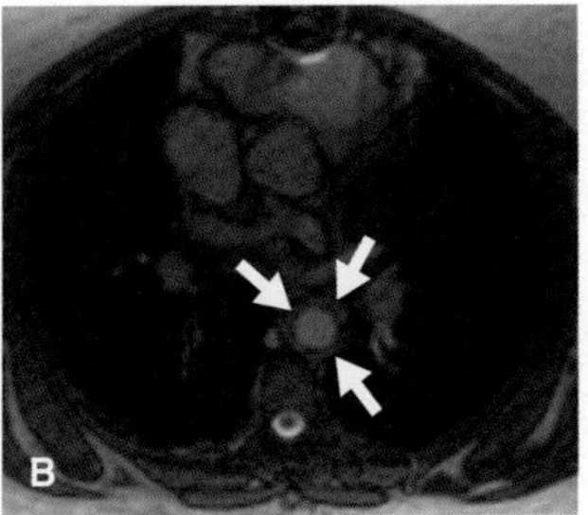
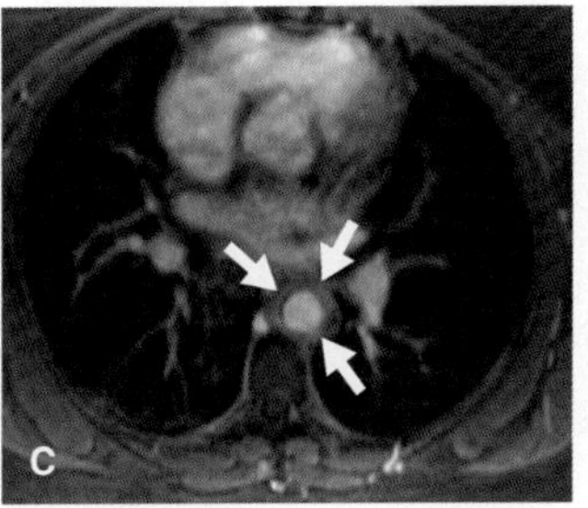
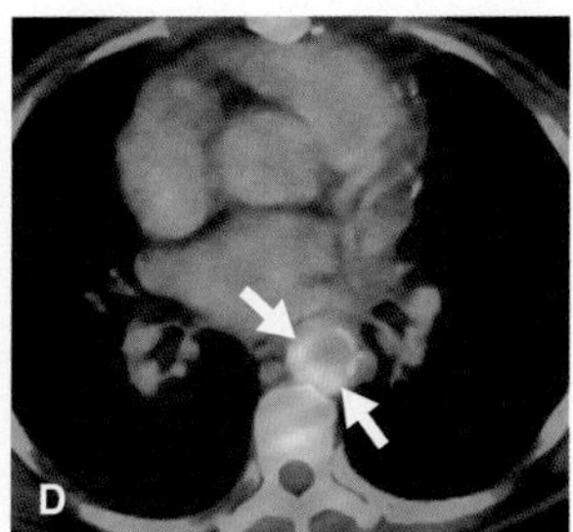

FIGURE 30.56. **Takayasu Arteritis.** Axial CT image at the level of the left coronary cusp (**A**) in a 39-year-old woman demonstrates irregular wall thickening along the descending aorta (*arrows*). Axial balanced steady state free precession (bSSFP) (**B**) and contrast-enhanced T1-weighted (**C**) MR images at the same level demonstrate irregular, hyperintense wall thickening with enhancement (*arrows*, noncontrast T1 image not shown). Axial fused PET-CT image at the same level (**D**) demonstrates corresponding increased uptake that has been shown to correlate with active disease.

tumors include leiomyosarcomas, hemangioendotheliomas, fibrosarcomas, myxoid sarcomas, and angiosarcomas. Tumors can also be characterized by their location—that is, intra- or extraluminal/periaortic.

Mural plaques in atherosclerosis and intramural thrombus associated with aneurysm are easily diagnosed when seen in the classic setting and with classic features—for example, a circumferential, smooth appearance. Focal, eccentric mural thrombus is less common but may be more difficult to differentiate from tumor, especially in the absence of associated atherosclerotic disease.

Most aortic tumors are sarcomas and will typically manifest on both CT and MR as an eccentric, pedunculated, and/or lobulated intramural filling defect (Fig. 30.57). Postcontrast enhancement may be absent or difficult to detect adjacent to bright intraluminal contrast. Subtraction images, more commonly performed with MR, can be invaluable in this setting to make subtle enhancement more apparent. An extraluminal tumor often appears on CECT and MR as an enhancing periaortic soft tissue rind that may be confused for a contained aortic rupture; lymphoproliferative disorder, for example, lymphoma; or inflammatory process, for example, retroperitoneal fibrosis.

In addition to primary cardiac tumors, tumors can embolize into the aorta. This can occur with a primary cardiac tumor, such as an atrial myxoma (Fig. 30.58). In addition, lung cancers and pulmonary metastases can invade into the left atrium through the pulmonary veins and embolize into the aorta or its branches.

CONCLUSION

Imaging plays a vital role in evaluation of the thoracic aorta, in delineating anatomy and anatomic variants, as well as in diagnosing the full spectrum of thoracic aortic disease including

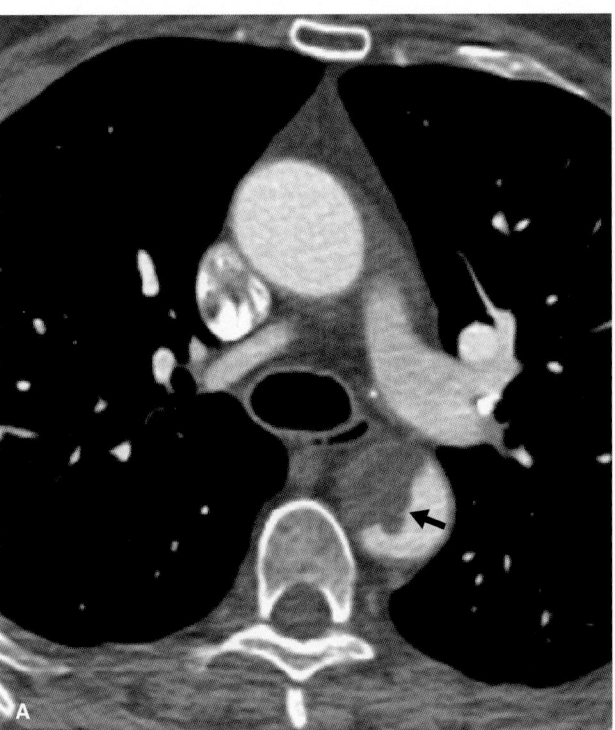
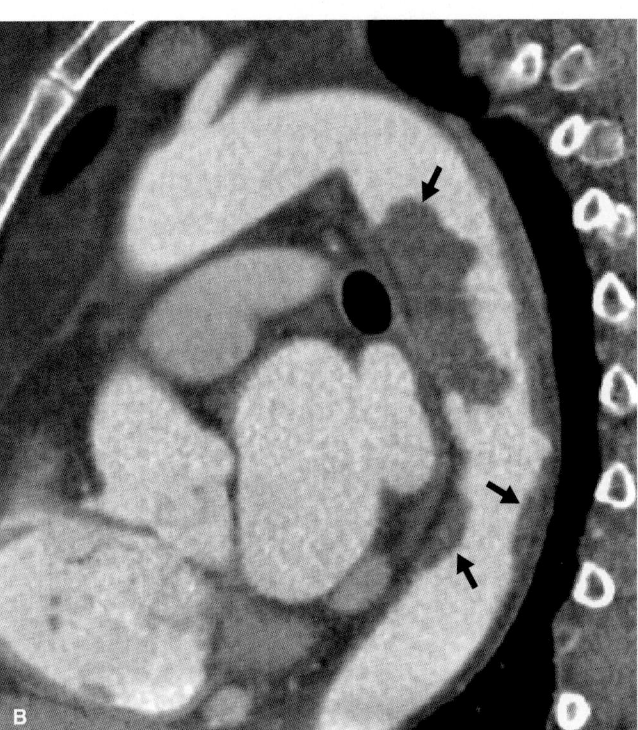

FIGURE 30.57. **Aortic Sarcoma.** Axial CT image at the level of the left pulmonary artery (**A**) and oblique sagittal reformat (**B**) in a 61-year-old woman demonstrate irregular mass-like thickening along the descending aorta (*arrows*) representing primary aortic sarcoma.

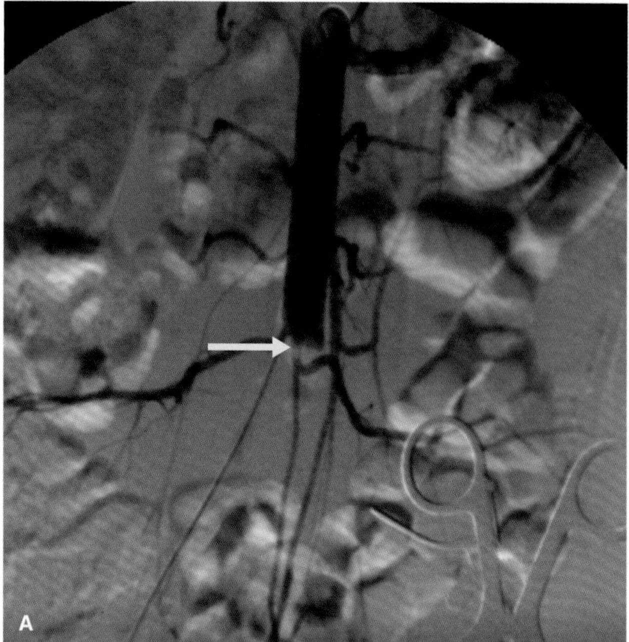

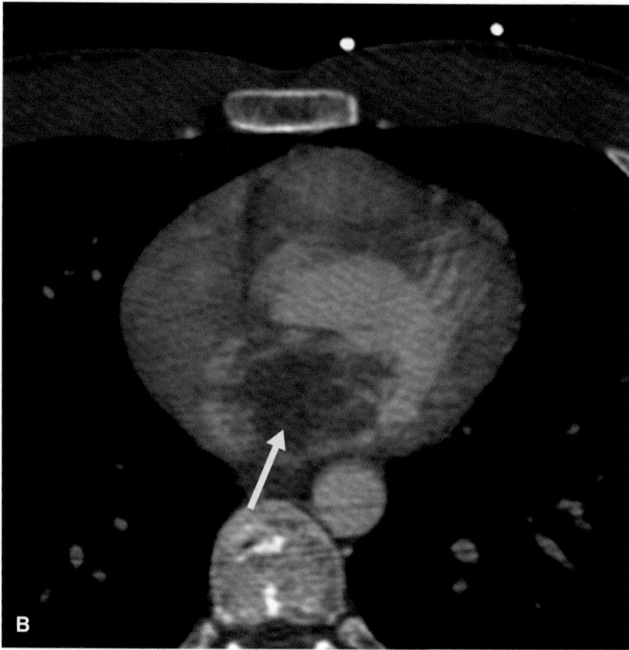

FIGURE 30.58. **Aortic Occlusion due to Tumor Embolization in a 34-Year-Old Man.** Image from a direct catheter angiography shows abrupt occlusion of the infrarenal abdominal aorta (*yellow arrow*, **A**). A tumor embolus was removed. Axial CT image from a contrast-enhanced CT of the chest shows a large left atrial myxoma (*yellow arrow*, **B**).

congenital, infectious, autoimmune/inflammatory, neoplastic, and iatrogenic etiologies. CTA and MRI have become the primary diagnostic modalities to assess the aorta, although knowledge of radiographic findings is important, as they are often the first imaging performed and can appropriately triage patients. It is imperative that the radiologist understands the imaging appearances of these numerous aortic variants and pathology to ensure appropriate patient care.

Suggested Readings

Agarwal PP, Chughtai A, Matzinger FR, Kazerooni EA. Multidetector CT of thoracic aortic aneurysms. *Radiographics* 2009;29(2):537–552.

Akashi H, Kawamoto S, Saiki Y, et al. Therapeutic strategy for treating aortoesophageal fistulas. *Gen Thorac Cardiovasc Surg* 2014;62(10):573–580.

Amarenco P, Cohen A, Tzourio C, et al. Atherosclerotic disease of the aortic arch and the risk of ischemic stroke. *N Engl J Med* 1994;331(22):1474–1479.

Backer CL, Ilbawi MN, Idriss FS, DeLeon SY. Vascular anomalies causing tracheoesophageal compression. Review of experience in children. *J Thorac Cardiovasc Surg* 1989;97(5):725–731.

Bennett CJ, Maleszewski JJ, Araoz PA. CT and MR imaging of the aortic valve: radiologic-pathologic correlation. *Radiographics* 2012;32(5):1399–1420.

Bortone AS, De Cillis E, D'Agostino D, Schinosa Lde L. Stent graft treatment of thoracic aortic disease. *Surg Technol Int* 2004;12:189–193.

Bricker AO, Avutu B, Mohammed TL, et al. Valsalva sinus aneurysms: findings at CT and MR imaging. *Radiographics* 2010;30(1):99–110.

Brown ML, Burkhart HM, Connolly HM, et al. Coarctation of the aorta: lifelong surveillance is mandatory following surgical repair. *J Am Coll Cardiol* 2013;62(11):1020–1025.

Bryant R 3rd, Wallen W, Rizwan R, Morales DL. Modified aortic uncrossing procedure: a novel approach for Norwood palliation of complex univentricular congenital heart disease with a circumflex aorta. *World J Pediatr Congenit Heart Surg* 2017;8(4):507–510.

de BALSAC R. Left aortic arch (posterior or circumflex type) with right descending aorta. *Am J Cardiol* 1960;5:546–550.

de Lutio di Castelguidone E, Merola S, Pinto A, Raissaki M, Gagliardi N, Romano L. Esophageal injuries: spectrum of multidetector row CT findings. *Eur J Radiol* 2006;59(3):344–348.

Eggebrecht H, Mehta RH, Dechene A, et al. Aortoesophageal fistula after thoracic aortic stent-graft placement: a rare but catastrophic complication of a novel emerging technique. *JACC Cardiovasc Interv* 2009;2(6):570–576.

Falk E. Why do plaques rupture? *Circulation* 1992;86(6 Suppl):III30–III42.

Fatima J, Duncan AA, Maleszewski JJ, et al. Primary angiosarcoma of the aorta, great vessels, and the heart. *J Vasc Surg* 2013;57(3):756–764.

Fernandes SM, Sanders SP, Khairy P, et al. Morphology of bicuspid aortic valve in children and adolescents. *J Am Coll Cardiol* 2004;44(8):1648–1651.

Freeman LA, Young PM, Foley TA, Williamson EE, Bruce CJ, Greason KL. CT and MRI assessment of the aortic root and ascending aorta. *AJR Am J Roentgenol* 2013;200(6):W581–W592.

Gomibuchi T, Seto T, Yamamoto T, et al. Surgical repair of cervical aortic arch with brain circulation anomaly through clamshell incision. *Ann Thorac Surg* 2017;104(3):e235–e237.

Goodman PC, Jeffrey RB, Minagi H, Federle MP, Thomas AN. Angiographic evaluation of the ductus diverticulum. *Cardiovasc Intervent Radiol* 1982;5(1):1–4.

Ha HI, Seo JB, Lee SH, et al. Imaging of Marfan syndrome: multisystemic manifestations. *Radiographics* 2007;27(4):989–1004.

Hanneman K, Newman B, Chan F. Congenital variants and anomalies of the aortic arch. *Radiographics* 2017;37(1):32–51.

Hartlage GR, Palios J, Barron BJ, et al. Multimodality imaging of aortitis. *JACC Cardiovasc Imaging* 2014;7(6):605–619.

Hata M, Hata H, Sezai A, Yoshitake I, Wakui S, Shiono M. Optimal treatment strategy for type A acute aortic dissection with intramural hematoma. *J Thorac Cardiovasc Surg* 2014;147(1):307–311.

Heinemann MK, Buehner B, Jurmann MJ, Borst HG. Use of the "elephant trunk technique" in aortic surgery. *Ann Thorac Surg* 1995;60(1):2–6; discussion 7.

Hermann DM, Lehmann N, Gronewold J, et al; Heinz Nixdorf Recall Study Investigative Group. Thoracic aortic calcification is associated with incident stroke in the general population in addition to established risk factors. *Eur Heart J Cardiovasc Imaging* 2015;16(6):684–690.

Hiratzka LF, Bakris GL, Beckman JA, et al; American College of Cardiology Foundation/American Heart Association Task Force on Practice Guidelines. 2010 ACCF/AHA/AATS/ACR/ASA/SCA/SCAI/SIR/STS/SVM guidelines for the diagnosis and management of patients with thoracic aortic disease: a report of the American College of Cardiology Foundation/American Heart Association Task Force on Practice Guidelines, American Association for Thoracic Surgery, American College of Radiology, American Stroke Association, Society of Cardiovascular Anesthesiologists, Society for Cardiovascular Angiography and Interventions, Society of Interventional Radiology, Society of Thoracic Surgeons, and Society for Vascular Medicine. *Circulation* 2010;121(13):e266–e369.

Hoang JK, Martinez S, Hurwitz LM. MDCT angiography after open thoracic aortic surgery: pearls and pitfalls. *AJR Am J Roentgenol* 2009;192(1):W20–W27.

Holloway BJ, Rosewarne D, Jones RG. Imaging of thoracic aortic disease. *Br J Radiol* 2011;84 Spec No 3:S338–S354.

Isner JM, Donaldson RF, Fulton D, Bhan I, Payne DD, Cleveland RJ. Cystic medial necrosis in coarctation of the aorta: a potential factor contributing to adverse consequences observed after percutaneous balloon angioplasty of coarctation sites. *Circulation* 1987;75(4):689–695.

Isselbacher EM. Thoracic and abdominal aortic aneurysms. *Circulation* 2005; 111(6):816–828.

Jakanani GC, Adair W. Frequency of variations in aortic arch anatomy depicted on multidetector CT. *Clin Radiol* 2010;65(6):481–487.

Johansson G, Markström U, Swedenborg J. Ruptured thoracic aortic aneurysms: a study of incidence and mortality rates. *J Vasc Surg* 1995;21(6):985–988.

Kaji S, Akasaka T, Horibata Y, et al. Long-term prognosis of patients with type a aortic intramural hematoma. *Circulation* 2002;106(12 Suppl 1):I248–I252.

Kappetein AP, Gittenberger-de Groot AC, Zwinderman AH, Rohmer J, Poelmann RE, Huysmans HA. The neural crest as a possible pathogenetic factor in coarctation of the aorta and bicuspid aortic valve. *J Thorac Cardiovasc Surg* 1991;102(6):830–836.

Karacan A, Türkvatan A, Karacan K. Anatomical variations of aortic arch branching: evaluation with computed tomographic angiography. *Cardiol Young* 2014;24(3):485–493.

Karaosmanoglu AD, Khawaja RD, Onur MR, Kalra MK. CT and MRI of aortic coarctation: pre- and postsurgical findings. *AJR Am J Roentgenol* 2015;204(3):W224–W233.

Kessler RM, Miller KB, Pett S, Wernly JA. Pseudocoarctation of the aorta presenting as a mediastinal mass with dysphagia. *Ann Thorac Surg* 1993;55(4):1003–1005.

Knight L, Edwards JE. Right aortic arch. Types and associated cardiac anomalies. *Circulation* 1974;50(5):1047–1051.

Ko SM, Song MG, Hwang HK. Bicuspid aortic valve: spectrum of imaging findings at cardiac MDCT and cardiovascular MRI. *AJR Am J Roentgenol* 2012;198(1):89–97.

Kovanen PT. Atheroma formation: defective control in the intimal round-trip of cholesterol. *Eur Heart J* 1990;11(Suppl E):238–246.

Layton KF, Kallmes DF, Cloft HJ, Lindell EP, Cox VS. Bovine aortic arch variant in humans: clarification of a common misnomer. *AJNR Am J Neuroradiol* 2006;27(7):1541–1542.

Lempel JK, Frazier AA, Jeudy J, et al. Aortic arch dissection: a controversy of classification. *Radiology* 2014;271(3):848–855.

Li PS, Tsai CL, Lin TC, Hung SW, Hu SY. Endovascular treatment for traumatic thoracic aortic pseudoaneurysm: a case report. *J Cardiothorac Surg* 2013;8:36.

Lowe GM, Donaldson JS, Backer CL. Vascular rings: 10-year review of imaging. *Radiographics* 1991;11(4):637–646.

Macura KJ, Corl FM, Fishman EK, Bluemke DA. Pathogenesis in acute aortic syndromes: aortic aneurysm leak and rupture and traumatic aortic transection. *AJR Am J Roentgenol* 2003;181(2):303–307.

Maddu KK, Shuaib W, Telleria J, Johnson JO, Khosa F. Nontraumatic acute aortic emergencies: part 1, acute aortic syndrome. *AJR Am J Roentgenol* 2014;202(3):656–665.

McMahon MA, Squirrell CA. Multidetector CT of aortic dissection: a pictorial review. *Radiographics* 2010;30(2):445–460.

Mohsen NA, Haber M, Urrutia VC, Nunes LW. Intimal sarcoma of the aorta. *AJR Am J Roentgenol* 2000;175(5):1289–1290.

Moreno PR, Purushothaman KR, Fuster V, et al. Plaque neovascularization is increased in ruptured atherosclerotic lesions of human aorta: implications for plaque vulnerability. *Circulation* 2004;110(14):2032–2038.

Moresco KP, Shapiro RS. Abdominal aortic coarctation: CT, MRI, and angiographic correlation. *Comput Med Imaging Graph* 1995;19(5):427–430.

Mosquera VX, Marini M, Pombo-Felipe F, et al. Predictors of outcome and different management of aortobronchial and aortoesophageal fistulas. *J Thorac Cardiovasc Surg* 2014;148(6):3020–3026, e1–e2.

Moustafa S, Mookadam F, Cooper L, et al. Sinus of Valsalva aneurysms—47 years of a single center experience and systematic overview of published reports. *Am J Cardiol* 2007;99(8):1159–1164.

Mullins CE, Gillette PC, McNamara DG. The complex of cervical aortic arch. *Pediatrics* 1973;51(2):210–215.

Nishimura RA, Otto CM, Bonow RO, et al. 2017 AHA/ACC focused update of the 2014 AHA/ACC guideline for the management of patients with valvular heart disease: a report of the American College of Cardiology/American Heart Association Task Force on Clinical Practice Guidelines. *Circulation* 2017;135(25):e1159–e1195.

Noor N, Sadat U, Hayes PD, Thompson MM, Boyle JR. Management of the left subclavian artery during endovascular repair of the thoracic aorta. *J Endovasc Ther* 2008;15(2):168–176.

Novaro GM, Mishra M, Griffin BP. Incidence and echocardiographic features of congenital unicuspid aortic valve in an adult population. *J Heart Valve Dis* 2003;12(6):674–678.

Ochoa VM, Yeghiazarians Y. Subclavian artery stenosis: a review for the vascular medicine practitioner. *Vasc Med* 2011;16(1):29–34.

Osgood MJ, Heck JM, Rellinger EJ, et al. Natural history of grade I-II blunt traumatic aortic injury. *J Vasc Surg* 2014;59(2):334–341.

Park KH, Lim C, Choi JH, et al. Prevalence of aortic intimal defect in surgically treated acute type A intramural hematoma. *Ann Thorac Surg* 2008;86(5):1494–1500.

Parmer SS, Carpenter JP, Stavropoulos SW, et al. Endoleaks after endovascular repair of thoracic aortic aneurysms. *J Vasc Surg* 2006;44(3):447–452.

Piciche M, De Paulis R, Fabbri A, Chiariello L. Postoperative aortic fistulas into the airways: etiology, pathogenesis, presentation, diagnosis, and management. *Ann Thorac Surg* 2003;75(6):1998–2006.

Polguj M, Chrzanowski L, Kasprzak JD, Stefańczyk Ł, Topol M, Majos A. The aberrant right subclavian artery (arteria lusoria): the morphological and clinical aspects of one of the most important variations—a systematic study of 141 reports. *Scientific World Journal* 2014;2014:292734.

Prescott-Focht JA, Martinez-Jimenez S, Hurwitz LM, et al. Ascending thoracic aorta: postoperative imaging evaluation. *Radiographics* 2013;33(1):73–85.

Restrepo CS, Ocazionez D, Suri R, Vargas D. Aortitis: imaging spectrum of the infectious and inflammatory conditions of the aorta. *Radiographics* 2011;31(2):435–451.

Riley P, Rooney S, Bonser R, Guest P. Imaging the post-operative thoracic aorta: normal anatomy and pitfalls. *Br J Radiol* 2001;74(888):1150–1158.

Rosenthal E. Coarctation of the aorta from fetus to adult: curable condition or life long disease process? *Heart* 2005;91(11):1495–1502.

Rozenblit AM, Patlas M, Rosenbaum AT, et al. Detection of endoleaks after endovascular repair of abdominal aortic aneurysm: value of unenhanced and delayed helical CT acquisitions. *Radiology* 2003;227(2):426–433.

Shih MC, Tholpady A, Kramer CM, Sydnor MK, Hagspiel KD. Surgical and endovascular repair of aortic coarctation: normal findings and appearance of complications on CT angiography and MR angiography. *AJR Am J Roentgenol* 2006;187(3):W302–W312.

Sievers HH, Schmidtke C. A classification system for the bicuspid aortic valve from 304 surgical specimens. *J Thorac Cardiovasc Surg* 2007;133(5):1226–1233.

Singh S, Hakim FA, Sharma A, et al. Hypoplasia, pseudocoarctation and coarctation of the aorta—a systematic review. *Heart Lung Circ* 2015;24(2):110–118.

Song JK. Diagnosis of aortic intramural haematoma. *Heart* 2004;90(4):368–371.

Stavropoulos SW, Charagundla SR. Imaging techniques for detection and management of endoleaks after endovascular aortic aneurysm repair. *Radiology* 2007;243(3):641–655.

Steenburg SD, Ravenel JG, Ikonomidis JS, Schönholz C, Reeves S. Acute traumatic aortic injury: imaging evaluation and management. *Radiology* 2008;248(3):748–762.

Stern A, Tunick PA, Culliford AT, et al. Protruding aortic arch atheromas: risk of stroke during heart surgery with and without aortic arch endarterectomy. *Am Heart J* 1999;138(4 Pt 1):746–752.

Sundaram B, Quint LE, Patel HJ, Deeb GM. CT findings following thoracic aortic surgery. *Radiographics* 2007;27(6):1583–1594.

Sundt TM. Intramural hematoma and penetrating atherosclerotic ulcer of the aorta. *Ann Thorac Surg* 2007;83(2):S835–S841; discussion S846–S850.

Svensson LG, Kouchoukos NT, Miller DC, et al; Society of Thoracic Surgeons Endovascular Surgery Task Force. Expert consensus document on the treatment of descending thoracic aortic disease using endovascular stent-grafts. *Ann Thorac Surg* 2008;85(1 Suppl):S1–S41.

Türkvatan A, Büyükbayraktar FG, Olçer T, Cumhur T. Congenital anomalies of the aortic arch: evaluation with the use of multidetector computed tomography. *Korean J Radiol* 2009;10(2):176–184.

Vilacosta I, San Roman JA. Acute aortic syndrome. *Heart* 2001;85(4):365–368.

Warnes CA. Bicuspid aortic valve and coarctation: two villains part of a diffuse problem. *Heart* 2003;89(9):965–966.

Warnes CA, Williams RG, Bashore TM, et al. ACC/AHA 2008 Guidelines for the Management of Adults with Congenital Heart Disease: a report of the American College of Cardiology/American Heart Association Task Force on Practice Guidelines (writing committee to develop guidelines on the management of adults with congenital heart disease). *Circulation* 2008;118(23):e714–e833.

Wu D, Shen YH, Russell L, Coselli JS, LeMaire SA. Molecular mechanisms of thoracic aortic dissection. *J Surg Res* 2013;184(2):907–924.

Ye C, Chang G, Li S, et al. Endovascular stent-graft treatment for Stanford type A aortic dissection. *Eur J Vasc Endovasc Surg* 2011;42(6):787–794.

Yuan J, Usman A, Das T, Patterson AJ, Gillard JH, Graves MJ. Imaging carotid atherosclerosis plaque ulceration: comparison of advanced imaging modalities and recent developments. *AJNR Am J Neuroradiol* 2017;38(4):664–671.

SECTION VI

VASCULAR AND INTERVENTIONAL RADIOLOGY

SECTION EDITORS: Juan C. Camacho and Akhilesh K. Sista

CHAPTER 31 ■ MEDICATIONS IN INTERVENTIONAL RADIOLOGY

RICARDO TADAYOSHI BARBOSA YAMADA, JONATHAN DAVID PERRY, HEATHER HARTUNG, AND MARCELO GUIMARAES

INTRODUCTION

Vascular and interventional radiology (VIR) is a dynamic specialty with continued advancement in the scope and complexity of procedures. In this context, medications play a major role, assisting patients before, during, and after the procedure. Different classes of medications are regularly used in VIR including but not limited to anticoagulants, opioids, benzodiazepines, antibiotics, and thrombolytics.

In addition, given the continuous development of newer agents (e.g., new oral anticoagulants), it is critical to maintain current knowledge of these frequently prescribed drugs. The underlying mechanisms of action, common dosages, contraindications, side effects, and possible interactions with other medications should be well understood.

Finally, the scenario in which those medications are used can also vary, ranging from outpatient clinical encounters to the critical care setting. Familiarity with drug utilization in these different scenarios is very important, and this chapter will outline the common medications utilized in VIR in light of current society guidelines.

MODERATE SEDATION (TABLE 31.1)

Moderate sedation is utilized for most VIR procedures, usually provided by a certified nurse under direct supervision of a physician. By definition, it is the administration of pharmacologic agents causing a minimally depressed level of consciousness in which the patient retains independent ability to maintain a patent airway, be aroused by physical and/or verbal stimulation, and maintain protective reflexes. A trained independent observer should be present during the entire procedure and recovery period.

The interventional radiologist should perform a thorough chart review to confirm patient eligibility to undergo moderate sedation. History and physical examination should be obtained including the patient's current medications and prior adverse or allergic reactions. History of substance abuse also needs to be investigated, since this may interfere with the patient's response to sedation.

Risk stratification is assessed by the American Society of Anesthesiology (ASA) classification system (Table 31.2). This system incorporates the patient's underlying diagnosis and overall severity of the disease. It is measured on a I to VI scale. For patients at level IV, anesthesia consultation is recommended, given the increased risk of patient decompensation during sedation.

Workup also includes evaluation of patient's airway according to Mallampati score. This ranges from 1 to 4 depending on visualization of the hard pallet, soft pallet, tonsils, and uvula as above (Table 31.3). This directly correlates with the level of difficulty of intubation should this be required. Anesthesia consultation is also recommended for patients with Mallampati score 4.

Moderate conscious sedation is composed of two major components: anxiolysis and analgesia. Benzodiazepines

TABLE 31.1

QUICK REFERENCE VIR MODERATE SEDATION MEDICATIONS AND REVERSAL AGENTS

Midazolam (Versed®)	Starting dose 0.5–1 mg IV; maintenance dose 0.5–1 mg
Fentanyl (Sublimaze®)	Starting dose 25–100 mcg IV; maintenance dose 25–75 mcg IV
Flumazenil (Romazicon®) Reversal agent for Midazolam	Starting dose 200 mcg IV; repeat as necessary up to 1 mg
Naloxone (Narcan®) Reversal agent for fentanyl	Starting dose 0.2–2 mg IV; repeat as necessary up to 2 mg. Option of continuous infusion 2 mcg/mg per hour

are used for anxiolysis, whereas opioids are utilized for analgesia.

Benzodiazepines

Midazolam (Versed®) is the most common benzodiazepine used for moderate sedation. The mechanism of action is through enhancement of the neurotransmitter GABA on $GABA_a$ receptors, leading to the anxiolytic effects as well as anterograde amnesia. Most concerning side effects are respiratory depression and hypotension, which are dose dependent. This is the reason for risk stratification before the procedure and the need for an independent provider. Those side effects can be resolved by reversal agents, which are listed later in this chapter.

The usual starting dose is 0.5 to 1 mg intravenously (IV) for medically naïve patients. Additional maintenance doses may be necessary based on the patient's response and duration of the procedure. Alternative routes of administration can be considered in the appropriate setting, including oral route for the pediatric population. Half-life is approximately 2 hours and onset of action is 3 to 5 minutes when given IV. Midazolam is a class D pregnancy medication and the main route of metabolism is via the liver. Other benzodiazepines include diazepam and lorazepam with much longer half-life and duration of action; therefore, these drugs are not frequently used for moderate sedation.

TABLE 31.2

AMERICAN SOCIETY OF ANESTHESIOLOGY (ASA) CLASSIFICATIONS

I	Healthy patient without systemic disease
II	Mild to moderate systemic disease or elderly
III	Severe systemic disease that is not incapacitating or chronic systemic disease
IV	Systemic disease that is a constant threat to life
V	Moribund patient not expected to survive 24 hours
VI	Brain dead patient undergoing anesthesia care for the purposes of organ donation
E	Modifier signifying emergent nature of procedure and suboptimal risk modification

TABLE 31.3

MALLAMPATI CLASSIFICATION

I	Visualization of soft palate, fauces, tonsillar pillars, and uvula
II	Visualization of soft palate, fauces, and portion of the uvula
III	Visualization of soft palate and base of the uvula
IV	Visualization of hard palate only

Opioids

Fentanyl (Sublimaze®) is the most common opioid used for analgesia during moderate sedation. Mechanisms of action involve binding of the medication to opioid receptors within the central nervous system causing hyperpolarization of nerves and blockage of pain sensation. This class of medications can also cause dose-dependent respiratory depression and hypotension, as well as histamine release leading to pruritus. Nausea and vomiting can also occur in certain patients.

The usual starting dosage is 25 to 100 mcg IV with additional maintenance doses of 25 to 75 mcg based on the duration of the procedure and the patient's opioid tolerance. Its half-life is approximately 4 hours and onset of action occurs a few minutes after intravenous administration. The duration of action is up to 60 minutes depending on the patient's tolerance.

Fentanyl is a class C pregnancy medication. There are many medications within this family of opioids that can also be considered during moderate sedation, but in general these have much longer durations of action and can be difficult to titrate in a procedural setting. These medications include morphine and hydromorphone and are commonly used in the management of postprocedure pain.

Given the risk of respiratory depression and hypotension with both midazolam and fentanyl, moderate conscious sedation should be performed by an independent provider, who must constantly monitor the patient's vital signs. If signs of oversedation to the level of airway endangerment are present, including decreased oxygen saturation, increased CO_2, bradycardia, hypotension, or complete loss of consciousness, reversal medications should be administered. The reversal agent of choice for midazolam is flumazenil (Romazicon®) and for fentanyl is naloxone (Narcan®). The duration of action of these medications is shorter than the half-life of most benzodiazepines and opioids; therefore, patients who have received the reversal agents should be monitored closely for recurrent symptoms, and repeat dosing may be required.

ANTIBIOTICS (TABLE 31.4)

Antibiotic coverage is a broad topic that is consistently debated across medical specialties and VIR is no exception. While specific practice recommendations vary based on institution, there are general guidelines that should be followed.

In order to determine whether antibiotics should be considered prior to intervention, the procedure should be classified as clean, clean-contaminated, contaminated, or dirty, similar to the surgical concept. A clean VIR procedure is defined as one in which the gastrointestinal (GI) tract, genitourinary (GU) tract, or respiratory tract are not entered. A clean-contaminated procedure is considered when the GI tract, GU tract, or biliary tree is entered and there are no signs of inflammation or infection. A contaminated procedure is one in which the GI or GU

TABLE 31.4

QUICK REFERENCE VIR PROPHYLACTIC ANTIBIOTICS

Cefazolin (Ancef®)	1 g IV, consider repeating in 2 hours if necessary
Ciprofloxacin (Cipro®)	400-mg IV prophylactic dose, 250–500 mg PO BID for 5–7 days in the setting of added coverage
Gentamicin (Garamycin®)	80-mg IV/IM prophylactic dose for transrectal biopsy or drainage
Ampicillin–sulbactam (Unasyn®)	1.5–3 g IV
Ceftriaxone (Rocephin®)	1 g IV

TABLE 31.5

QUICK REFERENCE VIR ANTIBIOTIC PROPHYLACTIC PROCEDURAL SUGGESTIONS

Cefazolin (Ancef®)	Arterial stent placement, uterine artery transcatheter arterial embolization, percutaneous gastrostomy and nephrostomy tube placement, percutaneous tumor ablation, subcutaneous venous access ports
Ciprofloxacin (Cipro®)	Percutaneous nephrostomy tube placement, transrectal percutaneous biopsy
Gentamicin (Garamycin®)	Percutaneous nephrostomy tube placement and transhepatic cholangiogram
Ampicillin–sulbactam (Unasyn®)	TIPS, percutaneous transhepatic cholangiogram, transcatheter arterial embolization
Ceftriaxone (Rocephin®)	Percutaneous nephrostomy tube placement, TIPS, percutaneous transhepatic cholangiogram

tracts are entered and there is evidence of inflammation or bacterial colonization. This is also a procedure where a break in sterile technique may have occurred. A dirty procedure is one in which there is entry to an infected site with frank purulent material or entry into a clinically infected GI or GU site.

It is generally accepted that clean procedures do not require antibiotic coverage (e.g., angiography). On the other hand, for contaminated or dirty procedures, where a catheter or needle causes communication between an infected space and the bloodstream, antibiotic coverage should be strongly considered. Clean-contaminated cases should be reviewed on an individual basis with attention to patient risk factors.

Prophylactic antibiotics should be administered within 1 hour prior to the beginning of the procedure. For inpatients concurrently receiving antibiotics—for example, patients with an abscess in need of percutaneous drainage—timing of the most recent antibiotic administration and organism coverage should be inspected. Additional preprocedural dosages may be required in certain cases.

According to the Society of Interventional Radiology (SIR) guidelines, there is consensus in only a few procedures regarding specific antibiotic type, but antibiotics are broadly recommended for many procedures in which, for example, a new device is placed or embolization is performed (Table 31.5). It is generally acceptable to use the above-listed antibiotics, although coverage is based on the individual case and local bacterial resistance profiles. If there has been significant embolization or ablation of tissue and postprocedural infection from tissue necrosis is also a concern, extended coverage over 5 to 7 days can also be provided.

It should be noted that antibiotic usage during subcutaneous venous access port placement remains controversial given recent meta-analysis suggesting no significant difference in infection rates in immunocompetent patients who received prophylactic antibiotics compared to control group.

VASODILATORS AND VASOCONSTRICTORS (TABLE 31.6)

Vasodilators

Vasodilators are primarily utilized to prevent and treat vasospasm induced by manipulation of endovascular devices (e.g., catheters, wires, sheaths). A common current usage is during radial artery access to prevent arterial spasm/occlusion caused by the access sheath.

These drugs can also be used to improve diagnostic accuracy of conventional angiogram. For example, they can improve pressure gradient measurement in the setting of significant arterial stenosis and differentiation between severe spasm and vasculitis. Vasodilators can also be used when performing "provocative" angiogram by inducing gastrointestinal bleeding when conventional arteriogram fails to identify the source of bleeding.

The most common vasodilators used for these purposes are nitroglycerin (NTG) and verapamil. The mechanism of action of NTG involves peripheral conversion to nitric oxide and subsequent accumulation of cyclic GMP leading to intracellular calcium ion extrusion and smooth muscle relaxation. NTG is administered in an IV bolus of 50 to 300 mcg/min according to patient blood pressure. The onset of action is immediate and the half-life is approximately 1 to 4 minutes.

Verapamil is a calcium channel blocker leading to decreased levels of intracellular calcium and subsequent smooth muscle relaxation. It is commonly administered at a dosage of 1 to 10 mg in a mixture of 10 mL saline solution IV. The typical onset of action is approximately 5 minutes, with a longer duration of action lasting approximately 10 to 20 minutes. Both of the above medications are pregnancy class C with metabolism via the liver and excretion via the kidneys. Care should be taken in patients with elevated intracranial pressures, pericardial effusion, pericardial tamponade, and those with severe systemic hypotension.

TABLE 31.6

QUICK REFERENCE VIR VASODILATORS AND VASOCONSTRICTORS

Nitroglycerin	50–300 mcg IV bolus
Verapamil	1–10 mg IV intra-arterial bolus in 10 mL saline
Vasopressin (ADH)	0.2–0.4 U/min intra-arterial infusion

Finally, vasodilators can be used as therapeutic agents for acute, nonocclusive mesenteric ischemia and cerebral arterial vasospasm caused by subarachnoid hemorrhage. The medication of choice for these scenarios can be papaverine. Mechanism of action is not well understood, but it is believed to involve accumulation of cyclic AMP and cyclic GMP causing nonselective smooth muscle relaxation. The typical dosage in the setting of nonocclusive mesenteric ischemia is 25 mg given intra-arterial with possible continuous infusion if necessary. Higher dosages diluted in saline are typically used for cerebral vasospasm. This is a pregnancy class C medication and the typical effective half-life is approximately 1 to 2 hours. As above, care should be taken in patients with symptomatic systemic hypotension.

Vasoconstrictors

Vasopressin is the most common vasoconstrictor used in VIR. It can be used as a therapeutic agent in the setting of diffuse GI bleeding or when the bleeding cannot be corrected via selective embolization. Also, vasopressin has been shown to decrease bleeding complication in uremic patients and may be used prior to percutaneous kidney biopsy in patients with renal dysfunction.

Vasopressin is an analog of antidiuretic hormone (ADH) and the mechanism of action involves smooth muscle contraction, most notably at the capillary and small arteriole level through cAMP pathway. When used for GI bleeding, vasopressin is given intra-arterially into the vascular distribution of the bleeding source at an initial dose rate of 0.2 U/min. Typically, infusion is continued for up to 24 hours with gradual tapering. Prior to percutaneous kidney biopsy, the usual dose is 0.3 g/kg IV 30 minutes before the procedure. The half-life of this medication is approximately 10 to 20 minutes, and it is metabolized by liver and excreted by the kidneys. Complications of administration include symptoms of severe hypertension from ADH-like effects and ischemia/infarction of distal tissue. Care should be taken in patients with coronary artery disease and severe peripheral arterial disease.

ANTICOAGULANTS (TABLE 31.7)

Managing anticoagulants in the setting of VIR procedures can be challenging and involves different scenarios. Patients may need to be prescribed anticoagulant drugs right after a procedure (e.g., post lower extremity venous thrombectomy) or it often occurs that these drugs need to be discontinued before the procedure to decrease bleeding risk. Knowledge of the mechanism of action and pharmacodynamics of those agents is recommended (Fig. 31.1). Also, bleeding risk stratification according to type of procedure should be well understood for appropriate periprocedural management.

According to the SIR guidelines, procedures are classified into three different categories according to bleeding risk. Category 1 includes low-risk procedures (nontunneled venous catheter placement, superficial biopsies, IVC filter placement, etc.). Category 2 includes moderate-risk procedures (arterial

TABLE 31.7

QUICK REFERENCE FOR VIR ANTICOAGULANTS AND REVERSAL AGENTS

Agent	Dose
Heparin	5,000 U IV loading, then 20–40,000 U/24-h IV infusion based on aPTT goal
LMWH (enoxaparin, Lovenox®)	1 mg/kg twice-daily SC therapeutic dose, 40-mg daily SC prophylactic dose
Fondaparinux (Arixtra®)	7.5 mg SC daily
Warfarin (Coumadin®)	2–5 mg daily, titrate based on INR goal
Dabigatran (Pradaxa®)	150 mg daily
Apixaban (Eliquis®)	5 mg twice daily
Edoxaban (Savaysa®)	60 mg daily
Rivaroxaban (Xarelto®)	20 mg daily prophylactic, 15 mg twice daily therapeutic
Protamine Reversal agent for heparin	2 mg/kg bolus or 1 mg/100 U UFH administered
Vitamin K Reversal agent for warfarin	5 mg daily oral or in 50 mL IV
Idarucizumab (Praxbind®) Reversal agent for dabigatran	5 g/100 mL IV

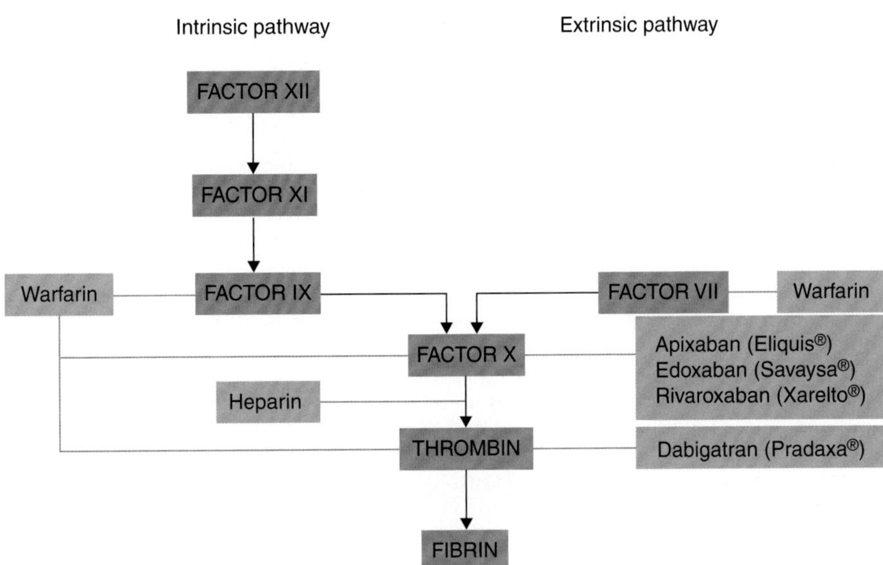

FIGURE 31.1. Simplified Coagulation Cascade Including Intrinsic and Extrinsic Pathways. Note the level of action of each anticoagulation drug.

angiography, intraperitoneal and lung biopsies, tunneled catheter placement, abscess drainage, chemoembolization, etc.). Category 3 includes high-risk procedures (TIPS, renal biopsy, radiofrequency ablation, biliary intervention in which a new tract is formed, etc.).

For category 2 and 3 procedures, an international normalized ratio (INR) of less than or equal to 1.5 and platelet count greater than 50,000 are recommended. While there are no consensus recommendations for category 1 procedures, it is generally recommended to maintain the above laboratory values whenever possible.

Heparin

Heparin is the most widely used anticoagulant with prophylactic or therapeutic intent. This medication is available in two forms: unfractionated heparin (UFH) and low–molecular-weight heparin (LMWH). The mechanism of action is the inhibition of thrombin and factor Xa through binding to antithrombin III. UFH is administered via continuous IV infusion and is titrated via aPTT (activated partial thromboplastin time), which should be 2 to 3 times normal value. Initial therapeutic dose of heparin is weight based (50 to 100 units/kg) and is typically 5,000 to 7,500 units IV loading dose for an average individual. This is followed by continuous IV infusion of up to 40,000 units/24 h based on aPTT. Dosages sometimes vary based on clinical indication. This a pregnancy class C medication with an onset of action of approximately 3 minutes and a half-life of approximately 30 minutes to 2.5 hours based on multiple complex metabolic factors.

LMWH (enoxaparin, Lovenox®) is a synthetic, shorter segment version of UFH and offers increased specific anti-Xa activity. Half-life is 4.5 hours, and route of administration is via subcutaneous injection (SC). Initial therapeutic dosages are also weight based and typically 1 mg/kg every 12 hours. Prophylactic dosages are typically 30 to 40 mg daily. Because of its increased binding specificity, it is not adequately monitored with aPTT or other currently available laboratory testing.

Fondaparinux (Arixtra®) is another synthetic form of LMWH with higher specific anti-factor Xa activity. Dosing for fondaparinux is weight based and typically 7.5 mg daily for standard 70-kg individuals. It is most commonly used for at least 5 days as a bridge to oral anticoagulation with warfarin and is also considered an alternative for patients with heparin-induced thrombocytopenia (HIT). This reaction occurs in approximately 1% of patients receiving heparin, most commonly UFH, and leads to antibody formation to heparin complexes and subsequent platelet consumption. Treatment is generally discontinuation of all heparin-containing products.

Infusion of UFH should be discontinued 2 hours before any procedure. For LMWH given for therapeutic purpose, the dose prior to categories 1 and 2 procedures should be held. For category 3 procedure, the last two doses should be held. Per manufacturer recommendations, fondaparinux should be held for up to 4 days due to its longer half-life of approximately 17 hours.

Protamine is the reversal agent for UFH. Its use has also been described for LMWH reversal; however, there is low efficacy and unpredictable effect in this setting and it is not routinely used.

Other direct thrombin inhibitors are also available in intravenous form, including bivalirudin and argatroban. Bivalirudin (Angiomax®) exhibits a similar route of renal excretion but has a much shorter half-life of approximately 1 hour and is primarily used in the setting of percutaneous coronary intervention. Argatroban (Acova®) is primarily metabolized by the liver. Both can be used in the setting of suspected heparin-induced thrombocytopenia.

Warfarin (Coumadin®)

Warfarin is the traditional oral anticoagulant used for long-term anticoagulation in patients with deep vein thrombosis, pulmonary embolism, atrial fibrillation, and other high-risk thromboembolic situations.

The mechanism of action is via inhibition of vitamin K epoxide reductase leading to inactivation of multiple coagulation factors and subsequent disruption of thrombin formation. Typical initial dose is 2 to 5 mg daily, with adjustments made based on INR. Goal INR for these patients is typically 2 to 3 but can vary based on indication for anticoagulation. The effective half-life is approximately 36 hours with clinical effects lasting up to 5 days. Metabolism occurs primarily by the liver, and there are many possible interactions with food and other medications that can decrease or increase drug bioavailability and therefore efficacy. This makes drug titration challenging, requiring constant patient monitoring with PT (prothrombin time) and INR.

Initial anticoagulation with warfarin should be "bridged" with heparin until therapeutic INR level is achieved. This is necessary given the delayed onset of action (usually 5 days) and the initial decreased levels of proteins C and S, leading to a prothrombotic effect.

Warfarin is not recommended during pregnancy except in very rare clinical circumstances. It is recommended to withhold warfarin for 5 days before any procedure and ensure that INR has fallen below 1.5, especially for category 2 and 3 procedures. Vitamin K is the reversal agent for warfarin and can be administered via oral or IV route. If more emergent correction of coagulopathy from warfarin is indicated, fresh frozen plasma should be given.

New Direct Oral Anticoagulants (NOACs)

The NOACs act by direct inhibition of either thrombin or factor Xa, with similar indications for atrial fibrillation and acute venous thromboembolism. Given its early onset of action, there is no need for initial heparin "bridging." Another advantage over warfarin is the more predictable response which eliminates the need for constant laboratory monitoring.

Dabigatran (Pradaxa®) is the direct thrombin inhibitor that blocks the conversion of fibrinogen to fibrin. Initial dose is 150 mg daily, with dose reduction based on baseline renal function. Peak plasma level is reached within 1 to 3 hours depending on coadministration with food. Half-life is approximately 14 to 17 hours and is primarily excreted by the kidneys. It is a pregnancy class C medication and contraindicated in patients with creatinine clearance of less than 30 mL/min and in those with severe hepatic dysfunction.

Apixaban (Eliquis®), edoxaban (Savaysa®), and rivaroxaban (Xarelto®) are direct factor Xa inhibitors blocking the formation of thrombin. Typical initial dosing is 5 mg twice daily for apixaban and 60 mg daily for edoxaban. Rivaroxaban can vary based on indication; however, the most common prophylactic dosage is 20 mg daily. Half-lives range from approximately 5 to 15 hours. These are pregnancy class B/C agents, primarily metabolized by the liver and with approximately 30% renal excretion. It is for this reason that care should also be taken in patients who have decreased hepatic and renal functions since the effective half-life can be prolonged.

PT/INR is not affected by NOACs and should not be used to monitor anticoagulation status. Dabigatran should be discontinued 24 to 48 hours before invasive procedures. In patients older than 75 years or with renal impairment, the drug should be held for 36 to 72 hours. For the factor Xa inhibitors,

TABLE 31.8

QUICK REFERENCE VIR ANTIPLATELET AND REVERSAL AGENTS

Aspirin	81–325 mg daily
Clopidogrel (Plavix®)	300-mg loading dose followed by 75 mg daily
Desmopressin (DDAVP, Minrin®) Reversal agent for aspirin and desmopressin	0.3–0.4 mcg/kg infusion

the drug should be discontinued 12 to 36 hours before the procedure and up to 48 hours in patients older than 75 years or with renal impairment. While there is no established recommendation for restarting NOACs, resuming therapy 12 to 24 hours post VIR intervention is generally appropriate.

While there are many NOAC reversal agents in clinical trials, the only currently FDA-approved agent is idarucizumab (Praxbind®) for dabigatran. In certain cases, dialysis can also be considered for partial reversal of dabigatran because of its primary excretion by the kidneys. Currently, there is no available reversal agent for apixaban, rivaroxaban, or other factor Xa inhibitors.

ANTIPLATELETS (TABLE 31.8)

Antiplatelet drugs are commonly used to decrease overall cardiovascular risk, including prevention of acute myocardial infarction and stroke. In addition, these medications are often utilized after intravascular stent placement to improve long-term patency. They act by blocking platelet activation or aggregation and thereby rendering circulating platelets nonfunctional (Fig. 31.2). Given their frequent utilization, it is important to have familiarity with the most common agents and discontinuation guidelines prior to VIR intervention.

Cyclooxygenase Inhibitors (NSAIDs)

Aspirin, or acetylsalicylic acid (ASA), is the most commonly used antiplatelet medication. Dose ranges from 81 to 325 mg daily depending on patient risk profile. The mechanism of action is binding of platelet cyclooxygenase leading to the inhibition of thromboxane A2 production and prevention of platelet aggregation. Occasionally, the phosphodiesterase inhibitor dipyridamole (Persantine®) is also used in conjunction with ASA in the setting of stroke prophylaxis and this can add to patient bleeding risk. For category 1 (low-risk) and 2 (moderate-risk) procedures, withholding ASA is not recommended. For category 3 (high-risk) procedures such as renal biopsy or areas where adequate vascular compression cannot be obtained, it is suggested to withhold ASA for 5 days. Because platelet life span is approximately 10 days, withholding aspirin will generally result in an increase in functional platelet counts to acceptable levels in patients with normal marrow function within that period of time.

Thienopyridines

Thienopyridines, also known as the adenosine diphosphate (ADP) receptor inhibitors, block ADP binding to platelet surface receptors, preventing platelet activation. The most widely used is clopidogrel (Plavix®) with a loading dose of 300 mg given once, followed by 75 mg daily. It is metabolized by the liver and has duration of action of up to 5 to 7 days following cessation.

Clopidogrel is commonly given in conjunction with ASA (dual antiaggregation) for high-risk patients or post intravascular stent placement. SIR guidelines currently recommend to withhold this medication for at least 5 days prior to any procedure, including category 1 procedures. However, recent retrospective review including 63 deep biopsies showed only one major bleeding episode in patients in whom clopidogrel/ASA were discontinued for less than 5 days (median = 3 days). This topic remains an area of continued debate within the medical literature. Other medications such as prasugrel (Effient®) and ticlopidine (Ticlid®) have a similar mechanism of action, with some differences in their side-effect profiles and length of platelet deactivation.

Glycoprotein IIb/IIIa Inhibitors

The glycoprotein IIb/IIIa inhibitors are represented by eptifibatide (Integrilin®), tirofiban (Aggrastat®), and abciximab (ReoPro®). They are administered IV and primarily used for acute coronary syndrome in patients undergoing coronary intervention. They act by blocking glycoprotein complexes which interact with fibrinogen and von Willebrand factor on the platelet surface. Loss of glycoprotein function prevents platelet aggregation.

It is unusual to prescribe these medications in the setting of VIR procedure, but it is still possible to encounter

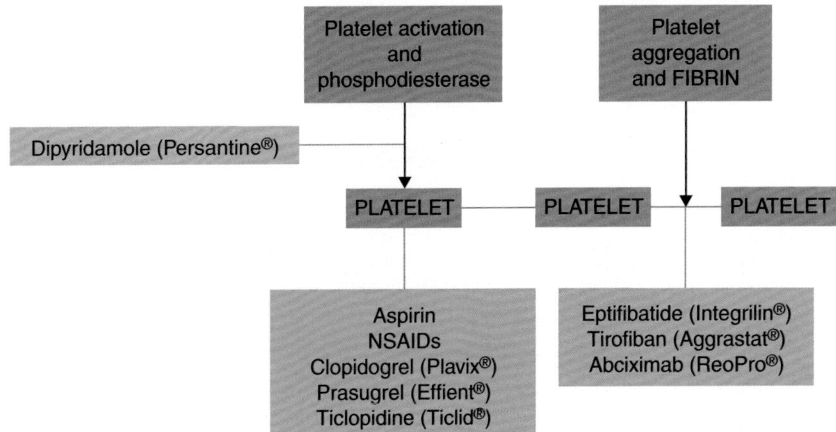

FIGURE 31.2. **Simplified Platelet Aggregation Diagram.** Note the level of action of each antiplatelet drug.

patients under the influence of these drugs after recent coronary intervention. Abciximab has the longest length of action of approximately 48 hours and should be held for at least 24 to 48 hours prior to a VIR procedure. Eptifibatide and tirofiban can be held for approximately 4 hours prior to procedure.

Desmopressin and platelet transfusion have been used with success in attempts to reverse the actions of cyclooxygenase inhibitors, glycoprotein IIb/IIIa inhibitors, and thienopyridines. PTT should be monitored after discontinuation of glycoprotein IIb/IIIa inhibitors with a goal of less than 50 seconds prior to any major VIR intervention.

While there are no definitive recommendations for resuming antiplatelet therapy following VIR procedures, it is generally accepted to restart medications within 24 hours after intervention. As usual, special consideration should be paid to the type of procedure performed and individual risk factors.

THROMBOLYTICS (TABLE 31.9)

Catheter-directed thrombolysis is a common VIR technique used to treat arterial, venous, and pulmonary thromboembolic disease. This technique involves local drug delivery within the thrombosed vessel instead of systemic infusion. This results in lower overall dose administration and lower risk of bleeding.

Streptokinase was the first medication administered for intravascular thrombus degradation. The mechanism of action involved activation of plasmin by both fibrin-dependent and fibrin-independent pathways leading to thrombolysis. Given the associated bacterial antigenic properties, it was later replaced by urokinase. This medication was isolated from human urine and therefore lacked the risks associated with bacterial antigens. Unfortunately, given manufacturing issues, the drug was discontinued by the Food and Drug Administration (FDA).

Currently, the plasminogen activator (TPA) is the class of drug available for thrombolysis. The mechanism of action is via fibrin-dependent interaction leading to intrathrombus plasminogen conversion into plasmin.

Alteplase (Activase®)

Alteplase was the first of these fibrin-selective agents. This medication was originally isolated from vascular endothelial cells, with the commercial recombinant form exhibiting small structural differences that allow for higher fibrin affinity. The usual initial dose is 0.25 to 1.0 mg/h, not exceeding 1.5 mg/h due to the significantly increased risk of bleeding. Half-life is approximately 5 minutes and the primary route of metabolism is hepatic. If this medication is used in conjunction with heparin, it is recommended to limit heparin to a subtherapeutic dosage.

TABLE 31.9

QUICK REFERENCE FOR VIR THROMBOLYTICS

Alteplase (r-tPA) (Activase®)	0.25–1.0 mg/h intravascular infusion, up to 40 mg maximum over 24 hours
Reteplase (r-PA) (Retavase®)	0.25–1.0 units/h intravascular infusion, up to 20 U maximum over 24 hours
Tenecteplase (TNKase®)	0.125–0.25 mg/h intravascular infusion

TABLE 31.10

QUICK REFERENCE VIR PROTHROMBOTIC

Thrombin	0.3–3 mL of 1,000 U/mL concentration

Reteplase (Retavase®)

Reteplase is a recombinant plasminogen activator created by a commercially derived deletion mutation of tPA leading to slightly decreased fibrin affinity. This decrease in surface affinity for fibrin is thought to allow for deeper thrombus penetration. Typical dose ranges from 0.25 to 0.5 units/h for intra-arterial intervention and up to 1 unit/h for venous system. No more than 20 units/24 h are recommended. Half-life is up to 16 to 20 minutes and primary metabolism is also hepatic.

Tenecteplase (TNKase®)

Tenecteplase is another modified t-PA agent, with the main differences lying in the medication half-life and area of fibrin affinity. Typical dosage is 0.125 to 0.25 mg/h continuous infusion with option for initial bolus of 1 to 5 mg. Half-life is biphasic with a terminal half-life of 90 to 130 minutes, significantly longer than other t-PA medications.

PROTHROMBOTICS (TABLE 31.10)

Thrombin is a prothrombotic agent that is used primarily to treat arterial pseudoaneurysms post catheterization. This drug promotes thrombus formation by converting fibrinogen into fibrin. It is available in human and bovine forms, with bovine being the cheapest and most widely used. The typical initial concentration is 1,000 units/mL and injection volume typically ranges from 0.3 to 3 mL. Injection is usually performed percutaneously by direct puncture of the pseudoaneurysmal sac under ultrasound guidance. There is a risk of thromboembolic event in case of drug extravasation into the systemic circulation. Thrombin injection should not be performed in the setting of local infection, and careful consideration should be taken in patients with distal ischemia such as that caused by peripheral arterial disease.

ADJUNCT MEDICATIONS (TABLE 31.11)

Nonsteroidal Anti-Inflammatory Drugs (NSAIDs)

NSAIDs are commonly used drugs given their analgesic and anti-inflammatory properties. As mentioned before, this class of medication inhibits cyclooxygenase activity, leading to decreased thromboxane and prostaglandin production.

They are frequently used for pain control after a procedure and prescribed for outpatient utilization upon discharge. Common drugs for this purpose are paracetamol, ibuprofen, and naproxen. In addition, they can also be given preemptively to minimize intra- and postprocedural pain and therefore lowering total dose of opioid. A common medication for this purpose is ketorolac (Toradol®). It can be given as a single dose (60 mg intramuscular) or scheduled IV doses of 15 to 30 mg every 6 hours, up to a total maximum dose of 60 to

TABLE 31.11

QUICK REFERENCE VIR ADJUNCT MEDICATIONS

Ketorolac (Toradol®)	15–30 mg every 6 hours, up to 60–120 mg/24 h based on weight and renal function
Ondansetron (Zofran®)	4 mg IV, up to 16 mg per dose
Diphenhydramine (Benadryl®, Dramin®)	25–50 mg IV, up to a maximum of 400 mg daily
Glucagon	0.25–1 mg IV given slowly over 1 minute
Meperidine (Demerol®)	25 mg IV every 15 minutes as needed up to 100 mg
Lidocaine	Up to 50 mL subcutaneous infiltration of 1% solution

120 mg based on the patient's weight. It can also be administrated orally. The main route of metabolism is via the liver and excretion is via the kidneys. The typical onset of action is approximately 10 minutes.

Care should be taken in patients who have a history of renal failure, hepatic failure, peptic ulcer disease, or GI bleeding. This medication is contraindicated in pregnancy.

Ondansetron (Zofran®)

Ondansetron is an antiemetic commonly used to treat nausea and vomiting related to the intervention (e.g., chemoembolization). These symptoms are also common side effects of opioids utilized during moderate sedation. The mechanism of action of ondansetron is antagonism of the $5HT_3$ histamine receptors. Usual initial dose is 4 mg IV given at the induction of moderate sedation or immediately when symptoms occur. This dose can be repeated up to 16 mg IV. It is a pregnancy class B medication metabolized by the liver, and those with liver dysfunction should not receive more than 8 mg. Occasionally, patients may experience ondansetron-related headache at higher dosages. Other antiemetics such as promethazine and scopolamine may also be considered, but these medications are generally avoided due to the larger side-effect profile as compared to ondansetron.

Diphenhydramine (Benadryl®, Dramin®)

Diphenhydramine is a versatile medication used in VIR given its multiple properties including sedative, antipruritic, and antiemetic. It is often used during moderate sedation to manage opioid-related side effects and assists with sedation at the same time. The mechanism of action is direct blockage of histamine-1 receptors. The initial dose is 25 to 50 mg IV up to a maximum of 400 mg daily. The geriatric population is at higher risk of side effects given the longer biologic half-life and increased risk of deep sedation and psychosis. Also, this medication has strong anticholinergic properties and should be avoided in patients with asthma, acute angle glaucoma, and urinary retention.

Glucagon

Glucagon is a peptide hormone secreted by the pancreas and plays a major role in maintaining serum glucose levels. Secondary effects are decreased bowel peristalsis, relaxation of the esophagus, and decreased pyloric opening. Some VIR procedures in the region of the abdomen and pelvis may require this medication to decrease motion artifact from bowel peristalsis during acquisition of digital subtracted images. This can be critical to define arterial and venous structures as well as localization of GI bleeding.

Other procedures that may benefit from this drug are percutaneous placement of feeding tubes. The full mechanism of action of glucagon remains unknown, but the peptide is similar in structure and function to that naturally produced within the pancreatic α-cells. The usual dose is 0.25 to 1 mg IV given slowly over 1 minute to decrease nausea and vomiting. The onset of action is within 1 minute and duration of action can last for up to 30 minutes. Higher dosages may be required when working in the colon, as this area is more resistant to glucagon effects. The peptide is a pregnancy class B medication and degraded primarily by the hepatic and renal systems. Care should be taken in patients with history of cardiac disease or pheochromocytoma as it is known to cause the release of catecholamines.

Meperidine (Demerol®)

Meperidine is an opioid with reduced sedative and analgesic properties compared with other members of the family. On the other hand, it has been shown to be very effective in the treatment of procedure-related rigors due to transient/worsening bacteremia.

The initial dose is 25 mg IV, with repeat dosing every 15 minutes as needed up to a total of 100 mg. This medication is metabolized by the liver and excreted via the kidneys. There is a significant risk of serotonin syndrome if the patient also uses serotonin reuptake–inhibiting medications.

Lidocaine

Local anesthesia is routinely provided during VIR procedures and lidocaine is the most commonly utilized drug. This medication is either injected intradermally or applied topically along the projected path of intervention. The mechanism of action is reversible binding to sodium channels causing stabilization of nerve membranes in the region of trauma, preventing propagation of painful stimulus. Most common presentation is 1% to 2% solution. Dosing of lidocaine can be repeated as necessary to achieve adequate local anesthesia, up to a total dose of approximately 50 mL of 1% solution. Onset of action is within 1 to 2 minutes of application and the duration of action is approximately 30 to 60 minutes. This medication can also be injected with 8.4% sodium bicarbonate to increase patient comfort, if available. Care should be taken to avoid intravenous injection, since local anesthetic systemic toxicity (LAST) that includes seizures and cardiovascular collapse can be elicited by inadvertent infusion.

Suggested Readings

American Society of Anesthesiologists Task Force on Sedation and Analgesia by Non-Anesthesiologists. Practice guidelines for sedation and analgesia by non-anesthesiologists. *Anesthesiology* 2002;96(4):1004–1017.

Geschwind J, Dake M. *Abrams' Angiography: Interventional Radiology*. 3rd ed. Philadelphia, PA: Lippincott Williams & Wilkins; 2014.

Jaffe TA, Raiff D, Ho LM, Kim CY. Management of anticoagulant and antiplatelet medications in adults undergoing percutaneous interventions. *AJR Am J Roentgenol* 2015;205(2):421–428.

Johnson E, Babb J, Sridhar D. Routine antibiotic prophylaxis for totally implantable venous access device placement: meta-analysis of 2,154 patients. *J Vasc Interv Radiol* 2016;27(3):339–343; quiz 344.

Kamath SD, McMahon BJ. Update on anticoagulation: what the interventional radiologist needs to know. *Semin Intervent Radiol* 2016;33(2):122–131.

Knuttinen MG, Emmanuel N, Isa F, et al. Review of pharmacology and physiology in thrombolysis interventions. *Semin Intervent Radiol* 2010;27(4):374–383.

Kumar P, Ravi R, Sundar G, Shiach C. Direct oral anticoagulants: an overview for the interventional radiologist. *Cardiovasc Intervent Radiol* 2017; 40(3):321–330.

Martin ML, Lennox PH. Sedation and analgesia in the interventional radiology department. *J Vasc Interv Radiol* 2003;14(9 Pt 1):1119–1128.

Mathis JM, Jensen ME, Dion JE. Technical considerations on intra-arterial papaverine hydrochloride for cerebral vasospasm. *Neuroradiology* 1997; 39(2):90–98.

Moran TC, Kaye AD, Mai AH, Bok LR. Sedation, analgesia, and local anesthesia: a review for general and interventional radiologists. *Radiographics* 2013;33(2):E47–E60.

Morrison HL. Catheter-directed thrombolysis for acute limb ischemia. *Semin Intervent Radiol* 2006;23(3):258–269.

O'Connor P, Kavian R, Lakshmi K, Ahmad I. Bleeding complications following CT-guided percutaneous native kidney biopsy with DDAVP (1-deamino-8-D-arginine vasopressin) pre-treatment. *J Vasc Interv Radiol* 2016;27(3):S132.

Olsen JW, Barger RL Jr., Doshi SK. Moderate sedation: what radiologists need to know. *AJR Am J Roentgenol* 2013;201(5):941–946.

Oppenheimer J, Ray CE Jr., Kondo KL. Miscellaneous pharmaceutical agents in interventional radiology. *Semin Intervent Radiol* 2010;27(4):422–430.

Patel IJ, Davidson JC, Nikolic B, et al. Consensus guidelines for periprocedural management of coagulation status and hemostasis risk in percutaneous image-guided interventions. *J Vasc Interv Radiol* 2012;23(6):727–736.

Patel IJ, Davidson JC, Nikolic B, et al. Addendum of newer anticoagulants to the SIR consensus guideline. *J Vasc Interv Radiol* 2013;24(5):641–645.

Pieper M, Schmitz J, McBane R, et al. Bleeding complications following image-guided percutaneous biopsies in patients taking clopidogrel—a retrospective review. *J Vasc Interv Radiol* 2017;28(1):88–93.

Stoeckelhuber BM, Suttmann I, Stoeckelhuber M, Kueffer G. Comparison of the vasodilating effect of nitroglycerin, verapamil, and tolazoline in hand angiography. *J Vasc Interv Radiol* 2003;14(6):749–754.

Stone JR, Wilkins LR. Acute mesenteric ischemia. *Tech Vasc Interv Radiol* 2015;18(1):24–30.

Sutcliffe JA, Briggs JH, Little MW, et al. Antibiotics in interventional radiology. *Clin Radiol* 2015;70(3):223–234.

Swischuk JL, Smouse HB. Differentiating pharmacologic agents used in catheter-directed thrombolysis. *Semin Intervent Radiol* 2005;22(2):121–129.

van Veen JJ, Maclean RM, Hampton KK, et al. Protamine reversal of low molecular weight heparin: clinically effective? *Blood Coagul Fibrinolysis* 2011;22(7):565–570.

Venkatesan AM, Kundu S, Sacks D, et al. Practice guidelines for adult antibiotic prophylaxis during vascular and interventional radiology procedures. Written by the Standards of Practice Committee for the Society of Interventional Radiology and Endorsed by the Cardiovascular Interventional Radiological Society of Europe and Canadian Interventional Radiology Association [corrected]. *J Vasc Interv Radiol* 2010;21(11):1611–1630; quiz 1631.

Weber AA, Braun M, Hohlfeld T, Schwippert B, Tschöpe D, Schrör K. Recovery of platelet function after discontinuation of clopidogrel treatment in healthy volunteers. *Br J Clin Pharmacol* 2001;52(3):333–336.

Zarrinpar A, Kerlan RK. A guide to antibiotics for the interventional radiologist. *Semin Intervent Radiol* 2005;22(2):69–79.

CHAPTER 32A ■ BASICS OF ANGIOGRAPHY AND ARTERIAL DISEASE – (ANGIOGRAPHY)

LOUIS G. MARTIN

Catheter-based angiography has been a favorite topic of mine since I first saw a cerebral arteriogram performed in 1964. It seemed unbelievable that a clinical diagnosis, in that case a subdural hematoma, could be diagnosed in a living patient by injecting a contrast agent into the carotid artery and recording it on x-ray film. The technical problems related to angiographic image quality became apparent when I performed my first arteriogram as a Neuroradiology fellow in 1969. "Performing" the perfect arteriogram involved much more than percutaneously placing a needle or catheter tip in the artery of interest, injecting contrast, and taking an x-ray. One by one I learned the importance of the focal spot of the x-ray tube, its distance from the patient, focused and nonfocused grids, film changers, the fluorescence of iodide crystals imbedded into the x-ray film, the contrast agent, needle and catheter properties, contrast media injectors, and many other factors that I won't list at this time. At that time, the quality of the recorded x-ray image was a goal in of itself. My contribution to the patient's care was determined, in a large part, by the quality "perfection" of the image that I was able to achieve. Being able to identify the most distal branches of the anterior choroidal artery or malposition of the lateral mesencephalic vein was of critical importance in the days before CT and MR.

We often take an entirely different approach in the present digital age. Do we really need a "perfect" arteriogram? How does patient risk modify our quest for perfection? Is expense a factor that should be considered? Can we choose an imaging modality based on the reported sensitivity and specificity? Do you really believe that a computerized angiography (CTA) or magnetic resonance angiography (MRA) could be 100% sensitive and over 85% specific? How do patient factors such as allergy, obesity, age, claustrophobia, tremors, tics, clotting disorders, renal insufficiency, other systemic diseases, and treatment goal modify what the "perfect angiogram" is for an individual patient? Of course, all these factors and many more need to be considered and each may at some time take precedence, but for the sake of discussion let's assume that there are no limitations imposed by the patient or a disease process on the quest for the "perfect angiogram." Let us search for it in the chronologic order that it has presented itself.

HISTORY OF ANGIOGRAPHY

The basics of cardiovascular physiology and anatomy have been known for thousands of years, but the first angiogram in a live patient was performed only 99 years ago. Why such a delay? It wasn't for lack of interest but lack of a means to visualize and record vascular flow and the lack of a nontoxic agent that could be injected into a living person and would opacify the bloodstream. Through the experience of hunting and warfare, a rudimentary knowledge of the cardiovascular system was most likely known to the caveman. The earliest known writings on the circulatory system are found in a 16th-century BC Egyptian medical document, the Ebers Papyrus, which contained over 700 prescriptions and remedies, both physical and spiritual. This knowledge was expanded by the Greeks, Romans, Arabs, Chinese and the 16th- to 19th-century scientists, such as Harvey and Hunter, whose work most of us have studied. Beginning in 1884 and continuing for almost 40 years, French physiologist Claude Bernard developed techniques for passing a catheter from a peripheral artery or vein into the cardiac chambers of live laboratory animals. He is credited with being the first to introduce a catheter into the femoral vein and advance it through the inferior vena cava into the right cardiac chambers. He lacked the means to visualize the course of the catheterization and record the event. This changed dramatically on December 1, 1895, the day the x-ray was discovered by Wilhelm Conrad Röntgen. In a matter of a few days, Röntgen discovered the x-ray and recorded the famous radiograph of his wife's hand (Fig. 32A.1).

The first mention of trying to opacify the circulatory system occurred shortly after Roentgen's discovery on November 8, 1895 of the x-ray; physicist Edward Haschek and physician T.O. Lindenthal performed the first angiogram in January 1896 by injecting Teichmann mixture—which consists of lime, cinnabar (mercury sulfide), and petroleum—into the a cadaveric hand and exposing it for nearly an hour under an early x-ray tube (Fig. 32A.2). In 1903, German surgeon O. Riethus conducted the first angiogram in a live animal by introducing buckshot into dogs' jugular veins and tracing them to the right heart and pulmonary circulation. Modern cardiovascular science was out of the starting block. The means to visualize

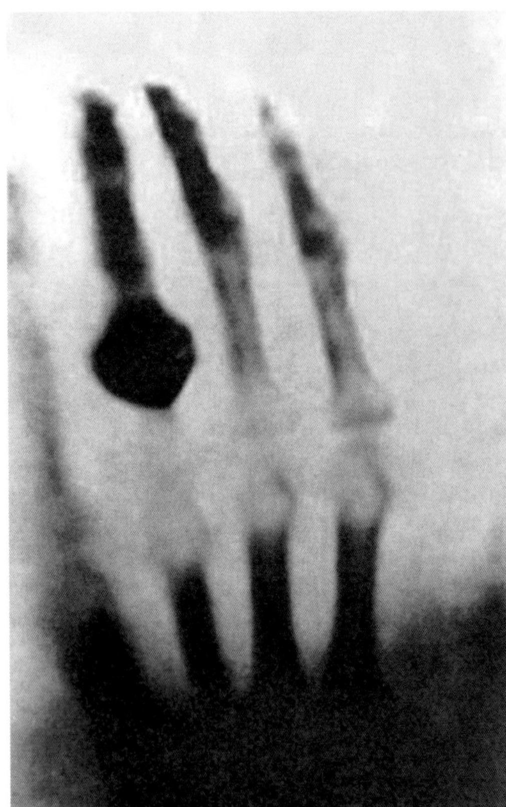

FIGURE 32A.1. Image of Mrs. Röntgen's hand.

the course of the catheter as it was being introduced into a blood vessel and to make a record of its location were now available, what was lacking was a contrast agent that could be safely injected into a living human blood vessel. During this time period, iodine compounds were being used to treat the osseous and aortic lesions associated with tertiary syphilis. E.D. Osborne, who was treating patients with syphilis at the Mayo Clinic, was the first to note that the renal collecting system and bladder were opacified on abdominal radiographs taken to evaluate osseous syphilitic involvement in patients

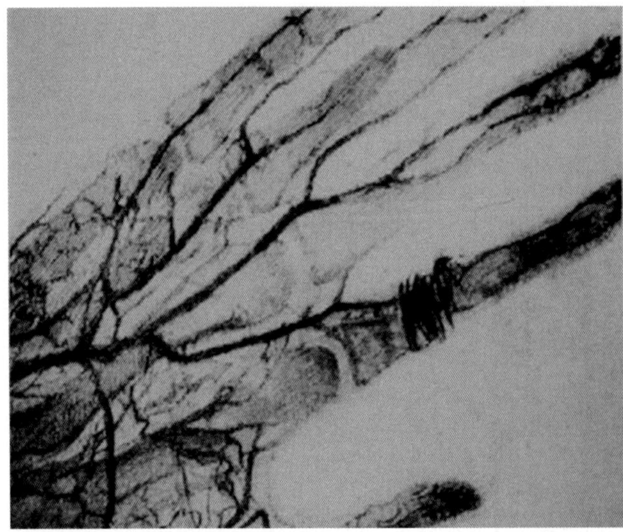

FIGURE 32A.2. The first angiogram.

treated with potassium iodide. "The major breakthrough was achieved three years later in 1925 and 1926, when Professor of Chemistry Arthur Binz and his assistant Curt Räth synthesized organic iodine preparations of pyridine at the Agricultural College in Berlin. Moses Swick, an American graduate of Columbia University Medical College, who was working in the Berlin laboratory of Professor von Lichtenberg used 5-iodo-2-pyridone *N*-ascetic acid, the sodium salt of a compound Arthur Binz had produced, later called Uroselectan. Using Uroselectan, Swick was able to produce the first reliably successful intravenous urograms.

The medical implementation of clinical diagnostic angiography was delayed because of the lack of a suitable nontoxic contrast agent. Two Parisian investigators, Jean-Athanase Sicard and Jacques Forestier performed the first arteriography in a human in 1923 by injecting Lipiodol, a contrast using poppy seed oil, into the femoral artery of an amputation patient. The same year, German physicians Joseph Berberich and Samson R. Hirsch performed the first angiogram in a patient using a water-soluble contrast agent, strontium bromide; however, they found it too painful for the patient and discontinued its use. At the same time, an American surgeon Barney Brooks was experimenting in animals with sodium iodide, the water-soluble contrast agent that would be used by Egas Moniz, who was the first to use a 22% sodium iodide solution to image the cerebral circulation in 1927. Moniz developed a carotid angiography technique, which involved making a surgical incision into the neck, cannulating the carotid artery and injecting contrast into it. His early images were rushed to Paris for presentation at a Neurologic conference. Instead of the praise he expected, the value of the angiogram was not appreciated and Moniz was chastised for endangering the patient. Development of angiography was continued by Moniz and his colleagues at the University in Lisbon. In 1929, Moniz's colleagues dos Santos, Lamas, and Pereira-Caldas published the first abdominal aortogram and reported a method for visualizing the abdominal aorta using a translumbar injection of contrast agent via a long needle (the dos Santos needle) inserted into the abdominal aorta through the patient's back. The contrast and detail of dos Santos' angiograms are comparable to those produced today, almost a hundred years later (Fig. 32A.3).

Moniz's concepts were rapidly expanded by dos Santos et al., who applied these techniques to the peripheral circulation, thus developing arteriography and aortography. dos Santos' group was the first to clearly delineate atherosclerotic lesions, arterial aneurysms, and patterns of arterial collateralization. Rapid developments in the basics of imaging blood vessels, contrast agents, catheters and catheterization techniques were developing simultaneously. Fritz Bleichröder found a way to put catheters into the arteries and veins of dogs and even put a catheter in his own vein without imaging in 1905. His work indicated that a catheter could stay in an artery for several hours without complications, so in 1912, he used the technique in four seriously ill women. The dramatic foundation of cardiac arteriography also occurred during this time period with the work of Werner Forssmann, who was then a surgical intern in Berlin. Defying his superiors, who refused to allow him to conduct cardiac catheterization experiments, he catheterized himself in 1929, advancing a urethral catheter from his basilic vein into his right ventricle under fluoroscopic guidance. It was not until 1941, when André Cournand performed his important studies on cardiopulmonary physiology, that the true potential of cardiac catheterization became apparent. Cournand, Forssmann, and D.W. Richards shared the Nobel Prize in Physiology and Medicine in 1956, for these important accomplishments.

Improvements in diagnostic arteriography evolved rapidly in the 1950s with the better access techniques of Seldinger.

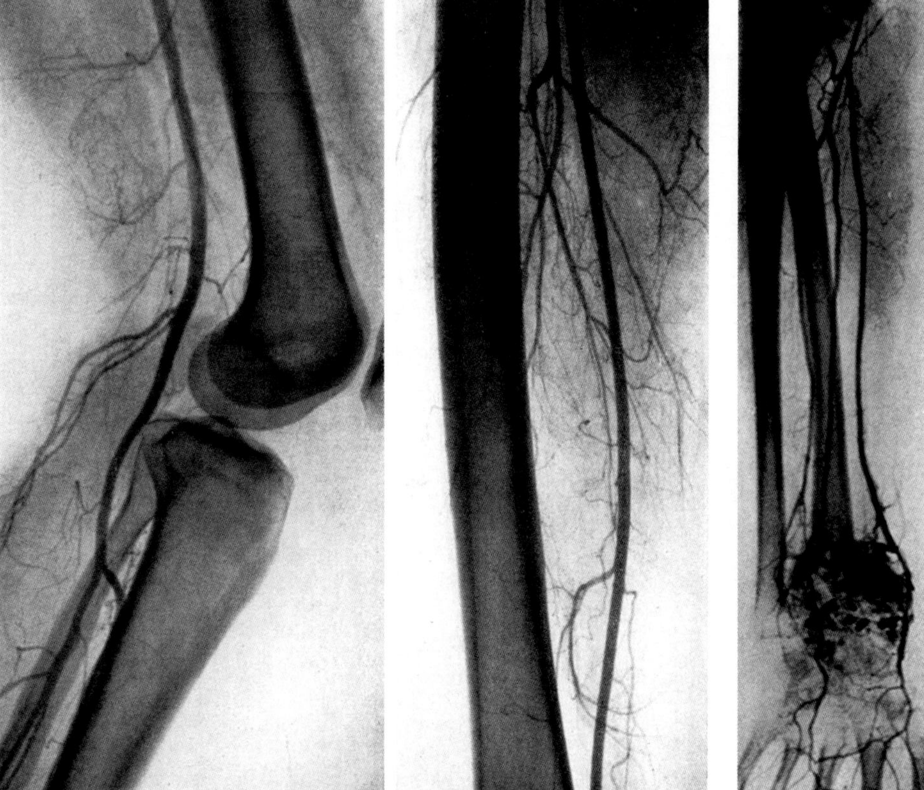

FIGURE 32A.3. **A–C:** Dos Santos' ability to achieve excellent contrast detail and special resolution almost 100 years ago is evident on these three peripheral arterial angiograms in which he used primitive x-ray equipment and thorotrast as the contrast agent.

Sven-Ivar Seldinger came upon the ingenious idea of his new technique in 1952 as a young resident at the Karolinska Institute. Seldinger has related the story about his discovery. The following is a quotation from "A Leaf out of the History of Angiography." Seldinger writes after giving a brief account on the state of the art in the early 1950s: "Thus, there was obviously a need for an improved percutaneous method for aortography, and one of the requirements to the solution was an increased bore of the catheter. Such an increase would be substantially beneficial. According to the law of Poiseuille, the rate of flow through a long narrow tube, all other factors constant, is approximately proportional to the fourth power of the diameter. When doubled, the time of injection could be divided by 16! There existed a puncture instrument, named after Cournand, consisting of an inner sharp needle in an outer blunt cannula, the leading edge of the needle protruding from the cannula by 1 or 2 mm. One alternative was to use a flexible catheter instead of the metal cannula, but it would certainly be tricky to handle an inner needle half a meter long. I avoided this trouble by cutting a side hole on a polyethylene catheter at such a level that a cutting needle of convenient length, when inserted through it, exceeded the tip of the catheter by 1 or 2 mm. After some moulding of the catheter and a minute incision in the skin, this instrument could be inserted into the artery by percutaneous puncture. Some obvious disadvantages were inherent in this technique. For instance, the thin-walled catheters were so flexible that it was sometimes impossible to advance them further into the vessel. This difficulty could be overcome: When intravascular position was obtained, the needle could be withdrawn from the side hole and replaced by a semi-flexible metal wire which was introduced through the entire length of the catheter to support it. Now! After an unsuccessful attempt to use this technique I found myself disappointed and sad, with three objects in my hand—a needle, a wire and a catheter—and... in a split second I realized in what sequence I should use them: Needle in, wire in—needle off—catheter on wire—catheter in—catheter advance—wire off. I have been asked how this idea turned up and I quote Phokion, the Greek: "I had a severe attack of common sense." With "beginner's luck," the first angiography performed with this technique was successful. A subclavian arteriography, with one single exposure, the catheter introduced through the brachial artery after puncture at the cubital level revealed a mediastinal parathyroid adenoma, unsuccessfully searched for by the surgeon at a former operative exploration."

THE X-RAY PHOTON

Although the contributions of these early investigators are invaluable to the 21st-century interventionalist, they just initiate our quest for the perfect angiogram. Let's follow the x-ray photons in their journey toward the angiographic image. Following their generation from a tungsten filament in the x-ray tube, the photons are directed toward the patient by a tungsten target which is imbedded in a copper anode (Fig. 32A.4). The photon is partially or completely absorbed by the patient's body as it passes through. The less it is absorbed the more it will activate photosensitive cesium iodide crystals that are imbedded on a film or plate. If the photons are completely

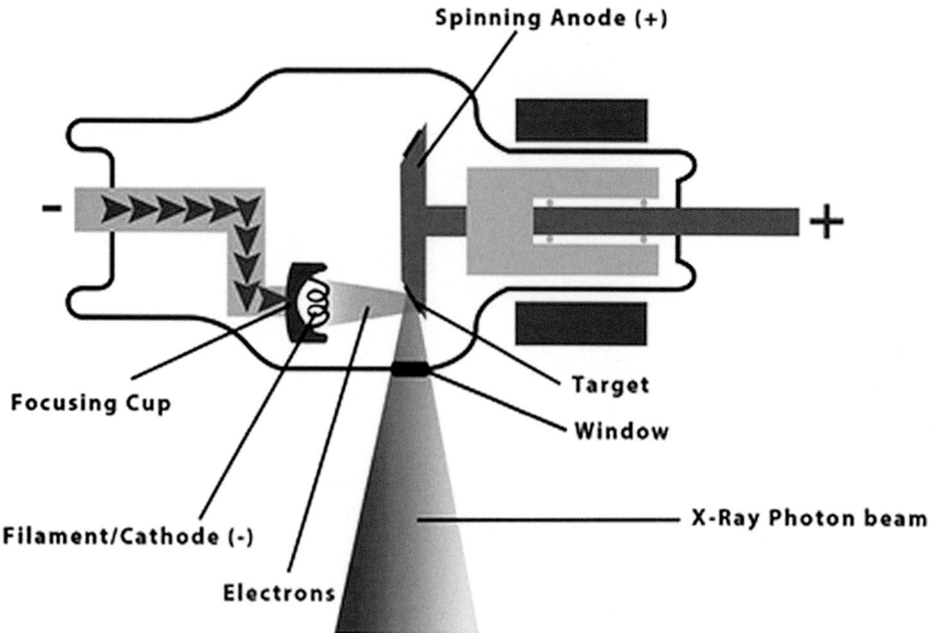

FIGURE 32A.4. The x-ray tube.

absorbed, as they may be by thick metal, there will be no fluorescence of the crystals.

The penumbra on an x-ray image is a zone of distortion surrounding the target, which is primarily caused by a double image of the subject which is directly related to the size of the tungsten target in the tube that generates the x-ray, called the source focal spot. Assuming that the distance between the subject and the x-ray film or fluoroscopic screen is constant, the distortion of the subject will be increased if the distance between subject and the source focal spot is decreased or the size of the source focal spot is increased. Theoretically, the clearest image will be obtained by using the smallest focal spot and the greatest distance between the focal spot and the subject. These factors are limited by overheating of the x-ray tube and the machinery that is available. Light photons produced by the sun are parallel when they strike the earth. Therefore, the shadow of an airplane will be the same size whether the plane is on the ground or 10,000 ft above it. This is not true for the photons generated by the x-ray tube, they diverge from one another. This causes blurring of the information recorded on the image intensifier or x-ray film. This blurring, which is most evident at the margins of the image but also affects its entirety, is called "the penumbra effect" (Fig. 32A.5). Additional blurring or image distortion can be caused by scatter of the photons passing through the body and physiologic or random patient motion. Photons which are scattered can be eliminated by filtering them with a grid before they contact the image intensifier or film. Basically, the grid is composed of strips of a metal which prevent photons from passing whose path are not parallel after they have passed through the body. Historically, the angiographic image was recorded on an x-ray film, at first a single film, then numerous films rapidly cycled by a film changer which were timed to record the opacified blood as it coursed through the tissue under investigation. Today, of course, all images are recorded digitally. Digital subtraction angiography was first described by Kruger et al. It has the obvious advantages of picture archiving, instant retrieval, electronic distribution or undistorted images, higher patient throughput, increased radiation dose efficiency, and reduction of irradiation of the patient. "The physical principles of digital radiography do not differ much from those of screen-film radiography. The digital detector is exposed to x-rays generated by a standard tube. Ultimately, the energy absorbed by the detector must be transformed into electrical charges, which are then recorded, digitized, and quantified into a gray scale that represents the amount of x-ray energy deposited at each digitization locus in the resultant digital image. After final image generation, images are sent to a digitized storage archive. A digital header file containing patient demographic information is linked to each image. The advantages of digital radiography are not realized completely unless images are viewed digitally on a computer workstation. Digital images can be manipulated during viewing with functions like

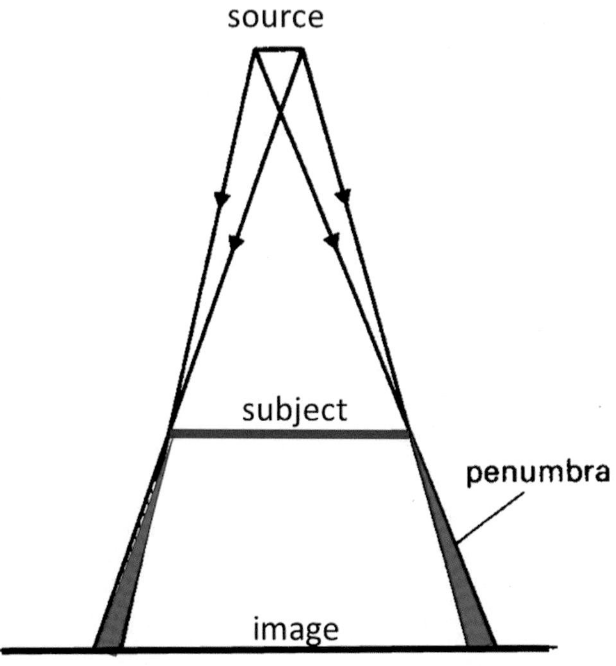

FIGURE 32A.5. Factors affecting the penumbra.

panning, zooming, inverting the gray scale, measuring distance and angle, and windowing." Technologic elements such as the power of the x-ray tube, its heat capacity, target size, parallel course of the photons, the thickness and orientation of the grid elements, the size and number of the fluorescent crystals, and others have a dramatic effect on the image quality as do physiologic elements such as motion and pharmacologic factors such as the contrast agent.

ANGIOGRAPHIC CONTRAST AGENTS

Most angiographic contrast agents are iodine based, the more iodine the more "dense" the x-ray effect. The iodine may be bound either in an organic (nonionic) compound or an ionic compound. Ionic agents were developed first, are cheaper, and are still in widespread use despite causing more side effects. Organic compounds have fewer side effects as they do not dissociate into component molecules. Many of the side effects are due to the hyperosmolar solution being injected, that is, they deliver more iodine atoms per molecule. There are many different molecules. Some examples of organic iodine molecules are iohexol, iodixanol, ioversol. Iodine-based contrast media are water soluble and harmless to the body. These contrast agents are sold as clear colorless water solutions, the concentration is usually expressed as mg I/mL. Modern iodinated contrast agents can be used almost anywhere in the body. Most often they are used intravenously or intra-arterially, but for various purposes they can also be in just about any body cavity or potential space. Modern iodinated contrast agents are safe drugs; adverse reactions exist but they are uncommon. The major side effects of radiocontrast are anaphylactoid reactions and contrast-induced nephropathy. The osmolality of the contrast agent is believed to be of great importance in contrast-induced nephropathy. Ideally, the contrast agent should be iso-osmolar to blood. Modern iodinated contrast agents are nonionic; the older ionic types caused more adverse effects and are not used much anymore. Iso-osmolar, nonionic contrast media may be the best according to a randomized controlled trial (Table 32A.1). Opacification during angiography requires the injection of adequate flow rates of contrast media. The injection pressure required to achieve a given flow rate of contrast is related to its viscosity. In order to reduce injection pressure to a level similar to low viscosity contrast media (ioxilan), high-viscosity contrast media (iodixanol) required a 1-Fr-size larger catheter.

Although these water-based angiographic contrast agents are by far the most commonly used, other non–water-based agents are also available. These include carbon dioxide (CO_2), gadolinium, ethiodol, and tantalum. "CO_2 gas is used as an alternative contrast to iodinated contrast material. The gas produces negative contrast because of its low atomic number and its low density compared with the surrounding tissues. When injected into a blood vessel, carbon dioxide bubbles displace blood, allowing vascular imaging. Because of the low density of the gas, a digital subtraction angiographic technique is necessary for optimal imaging. The gas bubble can be visible on a standard radiograph and fluoroscopic image. Because of the lack of nephrotoxicity and allergic reactions, CO_2 is increasingly used as a contrast agent for diagnostic angiography and vascular interventions in both the arterial and venous circulation. The gas is also used as a contrast agent for imaging of the nonvascular structures such as the bile duct, upper urinary tract, gastrointestinal tract, and peritoneal cavity. CO_2 is particularly useful in patients with renal insufficiency or a history of hypersensitivity to iodinated contrast medium. CO_2 should not be used as a contrast agent in the coronary and cerebral circulations because of the possibility of adverse effects secondary to a gas embolism."

Gadolinium is an FDA-approved contrast agent for MRI. Gadolinium, or gadodiamide, provides greater contrast between normal tissue and abnormal tissue in the brain and body. Gadolinium looks clear like water and is nonradioactive and hypoallergenic. After it is injected into a vein, gadolinium accumulates in the abnormal tissue that may be affecting the body or head. Gadolinium causes these abnormal areas to become very bright (enhanced) on the MRI. This makes it very easy to see. Gadolinium is then rapidly cleared from the body by the kidneys. Although it is not as radiodense, gadolinium has been substituted for iodinated contrast agents in patients with renal insufficiency having a catheter-based angiogram for many years. Recently, gadolinium has been identified as a cause of nephrogenic systemic fibrosis (NSF) in patients with a glomerular filtration rate less than 30 mL/min/1.73 m^2. The FDA has issued the following warning: "FDA ALERT [6/2006, updated 12/2006 and 5/23/2007: This updated Alert highlights FDA's request for addition of a boxed warning and new warnings about risk of nephrogenic systemic fibrosis (NSF) to the full prescribing information for all gadolinium-based

TABLE 32A.1

PROPERTIES OF COMMON IODINATED CONTRAST AGENTS

COMPOUND	NAME	TYPE	IODINE CONTENT	OSMOLALITY	OSMOLARITY	VISCOSITY (cP) AT 37°C
Diatrizoate	Hypaque 50	Ionic monomer	300	1,550	High	
Metrizoate	Isopaque Coronar 370	Ionic	370	2,100	High	
Ixoaglate	Hexabrix	Ionic dimer	320	580	Low	
Iopamidol	Isovue 370	Nonionic monomer	370	796	Low	4.7
Iohexol	Omnipaque 350	Nonionic	350	884	Low	6.3
Ioxilan	Oxilan 350	Nonionic	350	695	Low	
Iopromide	Ultravist 370	Nonionic	370	744	Low	4.6
Iodixanol	Visapaque 320	Nonionic dimer	320	290	Iso	11.4

contrast agents (GBCAs) (Magnevist, MultiHance, Omniscan, OptiMARK, ProHance). This new labeling highlights and describes the risk for NSF following exposure to a GBCA in patients with acute or chronic severe renal insufficiency (a glomerular filtration rate <30 mL/min/1.73 m^2) and patients with acute renal insufficiency of any severity due to the hepatorenal syndrome or in the perioperative liver transplantation period. In these patients, avoid the use of a GBCA unless the diagnostic information is essential and not available with non–contrast-enhanced magnetic resonance imaging. NSF may result in fatal or debilitating systemic fibrosis."

At present, gadolinium is rarely used for catheter-based angiography except in patients, with normal renal function, who have a severe allergy to iodinated contrast agents in whom CO_2 is not a good alternative. Ethiodol is used to opacify and alter the polymerization rate of n-butyl cyanoacrylate (n-BCA) and as a hepatic embolic agent. Tantalum is used rarely to opacify n-BCA instead of ethiodol.

THE CONTRAST INJECTOR

Features that the operator is able to select on the contrast injector are the volume to be injected, the injection rate, the maximum injection pressure, the time from the start of the injection to the maximum injector pressure (linear rise), a time delay in filming or contrast injection. If you select "NO" (zero) linear rise, the injector will exert the maximum pressure that you have selected immediately. This may have the effect of whipping the tip of the catheter, possibly dislodging it from the orifice of a selected vessel. A long linear rise may compromise the amount of contrast agent opacifying the vessel or organ of interest. It is necessary to begin imaging the area of interest before the arrival of contrast so that a subtracted image can be obtained. The imaging delay can be prolonged if the site of injection is very far distant from the area of interest; this limits the number of blank exposures and reduces the heat stress on the x-ray tube.

You may not get everything that you ask for. The injector will delay the injection or imaging, prolong the time to maximum injector pressure, and deliver the volume of contrast as prescribed; however, the flow rate and maximum pressure reached are interdependent and self-limiting. Assume that the injector flow rate has been set for 25 mL/s and the maximum pressure for 1,000 psi. In a high-resistance system, that is, injecting a relatively viscous contrast agent through a 100-cm 5-Fr catheter, the prescribed flow rate will not be reached at 1,000 psi. In this circumstance, the contrast injection through the catheter will be delivered at a lesser flow rate for a longer period of time until the selected volume is reached, for example, 17 mL/s until the prescribed volume is delivered. This may result in poor opacification of the vascular bed under study.

GUIDEWIRE USE AND CONSTRUCTION

Guidewires are used to reduce trauma to the endothelium of the aorta, vena cava, or their branches while the catheter is being introduced. In general, there are two types of guidewires: straight and curved each made of stainless steel or nitinol. The stainless steel guidewire has a metal core which is wrapped with a stainless steel outer wire (Fig. 32A.6). It is usually coated with Teflon and frequently heparinized. The core is tapered to make the tip less rigid than the shaft and may be solid or segmented from the tip so that it is "movable" within its outer wrapping. The shaft of the "movable guidewire" becomes softer as the core is withdrawn. The J-tipped guidewire (Fig. 32A.7) is named for its radius, that is, the leading end of a 3-mm J-tipped wire has a 6-mm diameter and the 5-mm curved wire has a 10-mm diameter, etc. The core of the nitinol wire is solid. The wire may be straight, curved, or angled and has a hydrophilic coating which makes it almost frictionless as it passes through the lumen of the blood vessel. It is important to visualize the tip of any guidewire as you advance it into the aorta, vena cava, or their branches. Hesitation in the forward movement of the guidewire tip may indicate that it has entered a nontarget vessel or gone beneath a subintimal plaque. It is especially important to keep the tip of the guidewire in the field of view when you are advancing a hydrophilic nitinol wire because its stiff shaft and finely tapered tip significantly increase the chance that you will enter and perforate a small side branch vessel. It is important to rotate the tip of the hydrophilic nitinol guidewire as you advance it to make sure that the tip is in the lumen of the desired vessel. If the tip does not rotate, it is an indication that it has entered a small branch vessel or undermined a plaque. The nitinol–hydrophilic wire can be your best friend or your worst enemy; I recommend exchanging it for a safer guidewire after it has helped you complete a selective catheterization. The J-tipped guidewires are generally considered safer than straight wires because their contact with the vessel wall is softened by their blunt leading margin. The endothelium can be damaged if the J-tip is advanced in a confined space. In this case, a Rosen guidewire which is a comparatively stiff

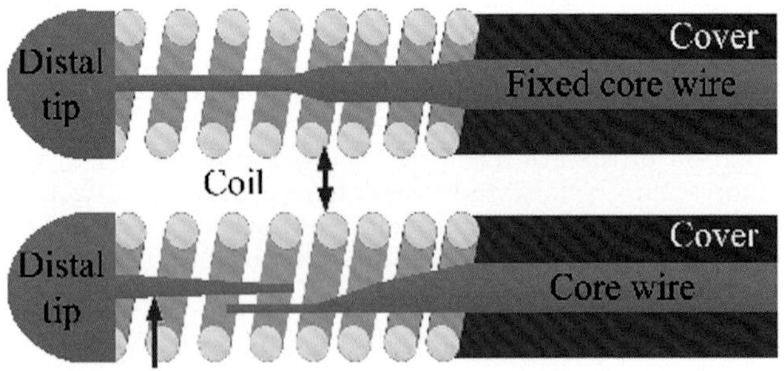

FIGURE 32A.6. Fixed and movable core stainless steel guidewire construction.

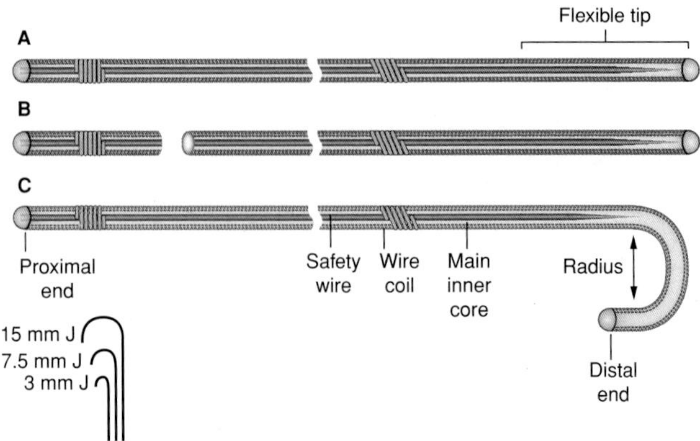

FIGURE 32A.7. J-tipped guidewires. (From https://www.dicardiology.com/article/understanding-design-and-function-guidewire-technology.)

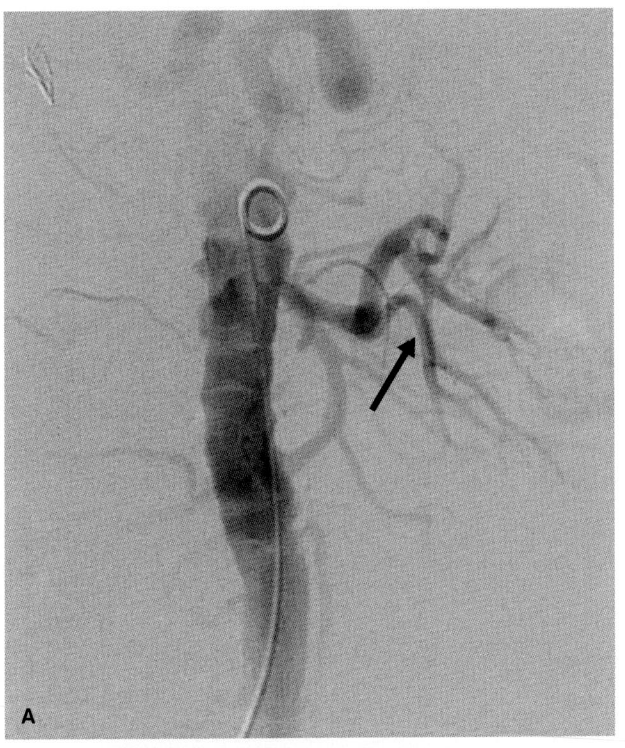

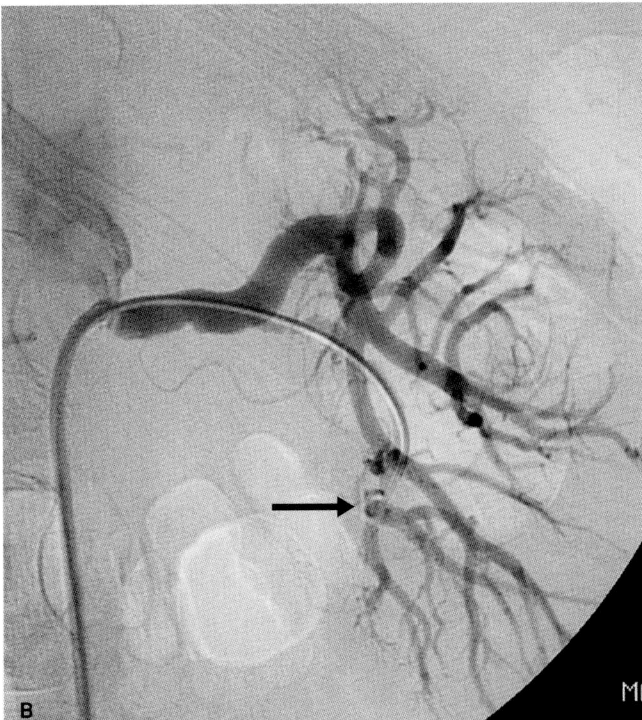

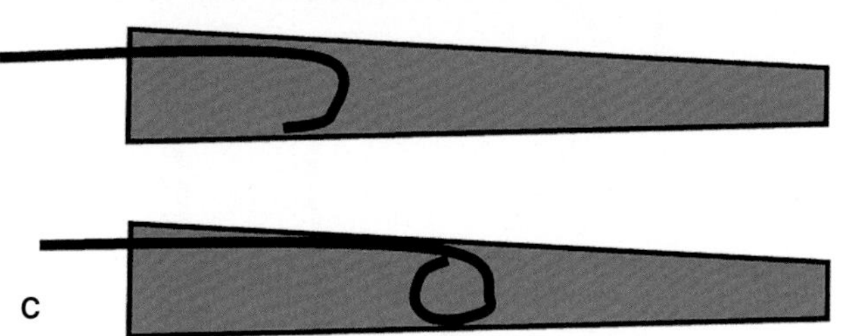

FIGURE 32A.8. **A:** Digital subtraction angiogram (DSA) abdominal aorta. Occlusion of the right renal artery, ostial stenosis of the left renal artery with normal filling of the dorsal and ventral (*arrow*) left renal artery branches. **B:** DSA of the left demonstrates that a 1.5-mm Rosen guidewire has been advanced into the ventral branch causing it to be occluded. Note that the J-tip of the guidewire (*arrow*) now forms an "O" and that the branch that the guidewire is in no longer is opacified. **C:** As the J-wire is advanced further into the vessel, the "J"-shaped tip becomes an "O."

J-tipped wire which has a 1.5-mm distal curve, that is, a 3-mm diameter, was advanced into a renal artery branch with a progressively diminishing diameter and occluded the vessel. The warning sign that this was occurring was that the "C"-shaped tip was transformed into an "O" configuration. This is called the "O" sign and should serve as a warning that if the guidewire is advanced any further, significant endothelial damage is likely (Fig. 32A.8C).

SELECTING THE "RIGHT" CATHETER

Catheters are designed for nonselective and selective use. The nonselective catheters are designed for rapid injection of a large volume of contrast over a short time to opacify large vessels such as the aorta, vena cava, and pulmonary artery. They usually have 6 to 12 side holes and frequently terminate in a "pig tail" which prevents the tip from entering a smaller branch vessel or dissecting underneath the intima during injection (Fig. 32A.9). Selective catheters usually have only a solitary end hole but may have one or two side holes. There are hundreds of catheters designed for use in selective cerebral, coronary, visceral angiography, etc. (Fig. 32A.10). How do you choose among them? Where do you start? Why are there so many? If one catheter worked in every situation there would only be one catheter. Most of the catheters are designed for a selective placement into a specific artery or vein. If the vascular system had a straight trunk and branches that originated at right angles (think of a pine tree), a catheter with a right-angled tip could be used to make all the necessary selective branch catheterizations. Reality is not quite that simple; the lumen of the parent vessel may be aneurysmal or stenotic and its course may have multiple angulations that affect the

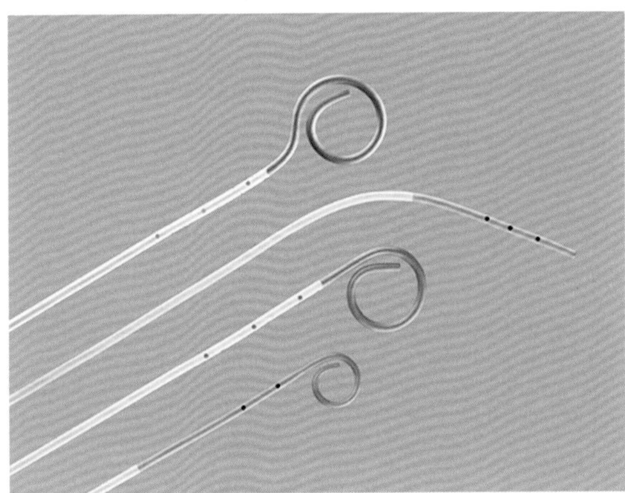

FIGURE 32A.9. Aortic flush catheters.

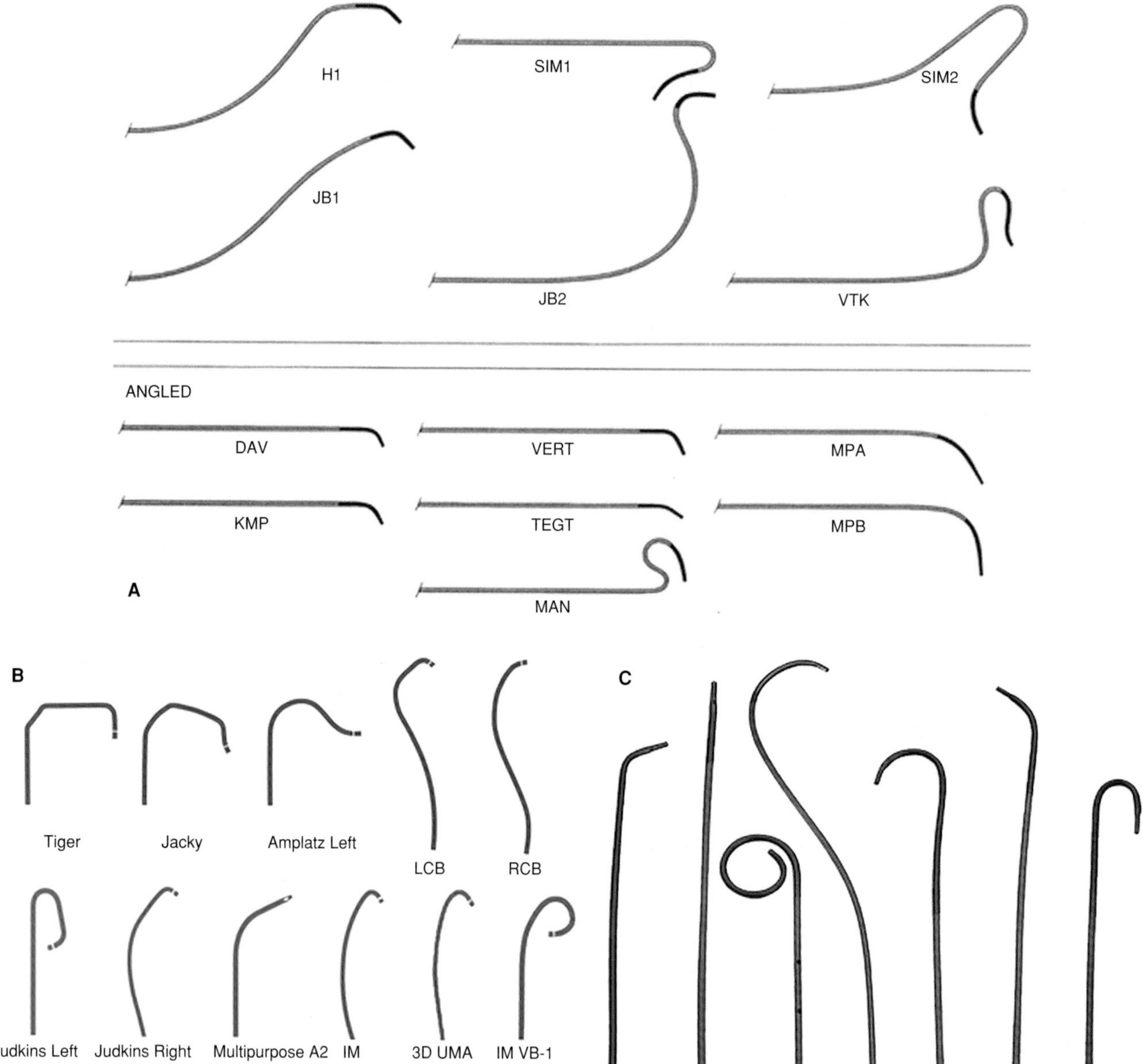

FIGURE 32A.10. **A:** Cerebral catheters. **B:** Coronary catheters. **C:** Visceral catheters.

course of the catheter. Let's take a look at Figures 32A.11 and 32A.12. Both patients are adults, but the patient in Figure 32A.11 has almost no atherosclerotic disease and very little angulation or ectasia, other than a fusiform aneurysm of the proximal splenic artery. There will be very little stress on the catheter used for selective catheterization of any of its pelvic or abdominal arterial branches. On the other hand, the patient in Figure 32A.12 has an infrarenal abdominal aortic aneurysm (AAA), extensive aortic ectasia, and exaggerated angulation of major arteries in the pelvis, abdomen, and thorax. While attempting to catheterize the superior mesenteric artery of this patient, the angiographer must advance his/her catheter through severe angles of the external and internal iliac arteries, through an AAA, then through a sharply angulated aorta between the AAA and the superior mesenteric artery (SMA) which could make selective catheterization of the SMA very difficult and the catheter position unstable. The difficulty could be greatly lessened by introducing a CHG 3 or 4 (Fig. 32A.10C) through a sheath that had been placed in the lower abdominal aorta, forming the catheter in the suprarenal aorta and retracting it until its tip makes contact with the SMA orifice.

Fifty to 60 years ago, most catheters were custom-made by the angiographer who chose catheter material of a desired French size, cut the catheter to the desired length from a role of tubing, flared one end, attached an injection hub to it, and tapered the distal end of the catheter over a flame or steam to conform to the size of the guidewire being used. The distal end of the catheter was then modified by the same heating and cooling manner to optimize its ability to selectively catheterize the desired vascular branch. If further modifications were necessary, they were made on the table during the angiography. Certain catheter designs became popular through personal communication among angiographers and published methods. Soon, medical supply companies began making catheters to the angiographer's specifications and still later a series of

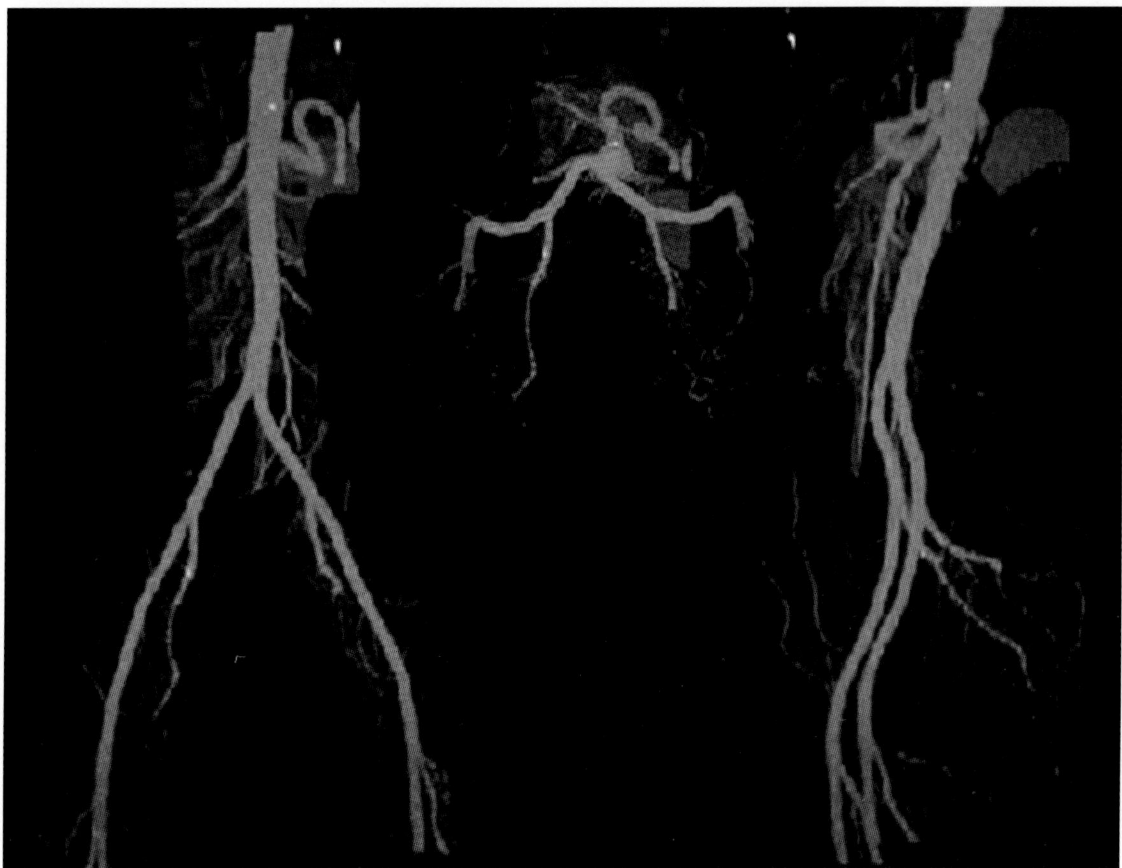

FIGURE 32A.11. Anterior-posterior, axial, and lateral views of a CT abdominal angiogram.

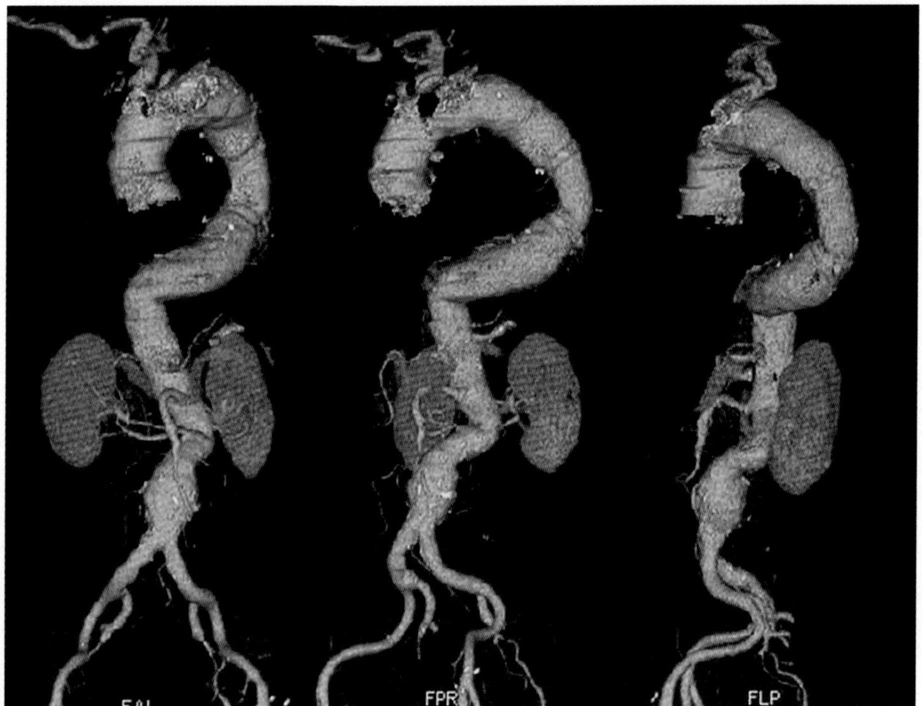

FIGURE 32A.12. CT angiogram of a patient with aortic ectasia, angulation, elongation, and an infrarenal abdominal aortic aneurysm.

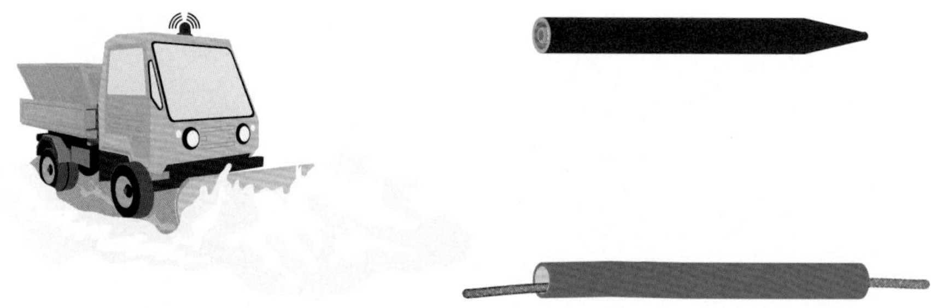

FIGURE 32A.13. The tip of a nontapered catheter scores, "Snow Plows," the vascular endothelium.

catheters to the design specifications of respected angiographers such as Chuang, Rösch, Judkins, and Amplatz were marketed by the supply companies. Let's look at the Chuang catheter set as an example (Fig. 32A.10). This set consists of a single catheter which is straight, five catheters with a simple curve, and eight with a double-angled reverse curve. These readily available catheters meet the needs of most angiographers, significantly reducing the necessity of reshaping catheters during the abdominal catheterization procedures.

Initially, vascular catheters were made of polyethylene, polyurethane, or Teflon. The Teflon material was too stiff to reshape but the polyethylene and polyurethane catheters could be reshaped after softening them with steam or a flame after which they were placed in cold saline to harden so they would maintain their shape. As you can imagine, it could be hard to control the tip of a long soft catheter, so the next evolution of the selective vascular catheter was placement of braided stainless steel wire in the body of the catheter to increase its response to torque. More recently, most of the selective catheters are made with a firmer synthetic tip that is bonded or glued onto the shaft which is strengthened by braided stainless steel wire. These latter catheters are designed to maintain their tip shape in normal body temperatures but sometimes kink if the tips are straightened or reshaped. The size of a vascular catheter is listed as the outer diameter in the French (Fr) catheter scale or "French units." The French catheter scale is commonly used to measure the outside diameter (OD) of needles as well as catheters. 1 "French" or "Fr" is equivalent to 0.33 mm = 0.013 in = 1/77 in of diameter. The size in French units is roughly equal to the circumference of the catheter in millimeters. Depending on the type of catheter material and its wall construction, its inner diameter (ID) may vary significantly. Most, but not all, catheters are tapered at the distal end so that the tip closely approximates the diameter of the guidewire that is used to introduce it. It is designed this way to protect the endothelium of the blood vessel that is being catheterized. Without the tapering, the endothelial surface cells would be scored or scraped by the edge of the catheter while it is being introduced (Fig. 32A.13).

Vascular catheters can be divided into two main groups, those used for nonselective and selective contrast injections. The larger the catheter ID and the "number" of side holes, the greater the volume of contrast that can be injected at a given time using a specific pressure. A multiside hole catheter may have up to 12 side holes. The end of this catheter is frequently curved or looped to confine the contrast injection to a limited portion of the vessel. The longer the catheter, the more resistance there is to flow through its lumen. A large lumen, multiside hole catheter may deliver 35 mL of contrast/s at 1,000 psi whereas a longer catheter or one with less side holes may deliver only 15 mL at the same pressure That explains the luminal diameter, length and number of side holes, but why so many different catheter configurations? Each has been designed to solve a potential vascular access problem. The catheter you choose to use should follow your initial evaluation of the patient's body habitus and conform to the patient's vascular anatomy as you have determined it to be after reviewing all available data, that is, CTAs, MRAs, and previous angiograms, etc.

CATHETER-BASED ARTERIOGRAPHY

The impact of switching from a film to digital format has had a monumental impact on catheter-based angiography; however, although contrast resolution has been vastly improved, spatial resolution hasn't. This is true of both digitally subtracted and nonsubtracted images (Fig. 32A.14). The resolution of the digital subtracted angiogram (DSA) is degraded by any subject movement that occurs between the image chosen for the mask and the subsequent images. These include vascular pulsations and patient movement which may be voluntary or nonvoluntary such as respiration, swallowing, and peristalsis. Iodinated contrast and CO_2 are both excellent digital contrast agents, but they each have angiographic limitations. Although iodinated contrast is water soluble and mixes with blood, the mixture is not homogeneous. The contrast tends to layer because it is denser and has a higher specific gravity than blood. This is most obvious when blood flow is slow as when it flows from a normal suprarenal aorta into a large infrarenal AAA or opacifies a vessel distal to an occlusion by collateral circulation. Likewise, because of their hyperdensity, iodinated contrast tends to opacify vascular branches that originate from the dependent or lower part of the parent vessel rather than those above. Since the patient is usually supine on the angiographic table, this means that the posterior vascular branches are usually denser and better defined than those which are anterior. Examples of this may include failure to opacify a patent inferior mesenteric artery originating from a large aneurysm or a patent femoropopliteal bypass graft distal to an occlusion of the external iliac artery. Conversely, vessels originating from the anterior margin of the parent vessel will be very well opacified by CO_2 which floats on the blood within the vessel. The greatest vascular definition will be attained when the contrast agent displaces or replaces all of the blood flowing into the vessel of interest. Reflux of contrast proximal to the tip of the catheter or needle through which it is injected is an indication that this has occurred. Vascular stenoses are best evaluated by orthogonal views, one of which maximizes the area of stenosis. This is not often practical for branches of the abdominal aorta and pelvic arteries where oblique views may be the best obtainable. A decrease in contrast density may be the only indication of an en face stenosis in the vessel of interest. The flow characteristics of the contrast agent can

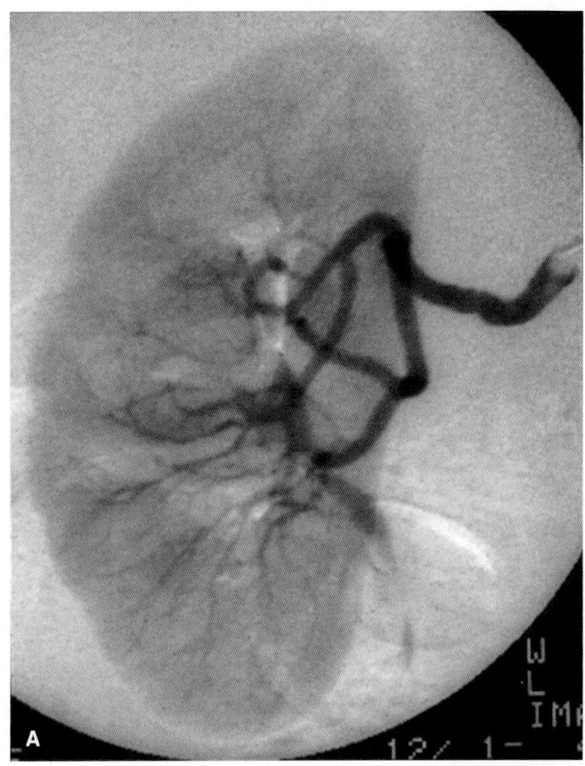

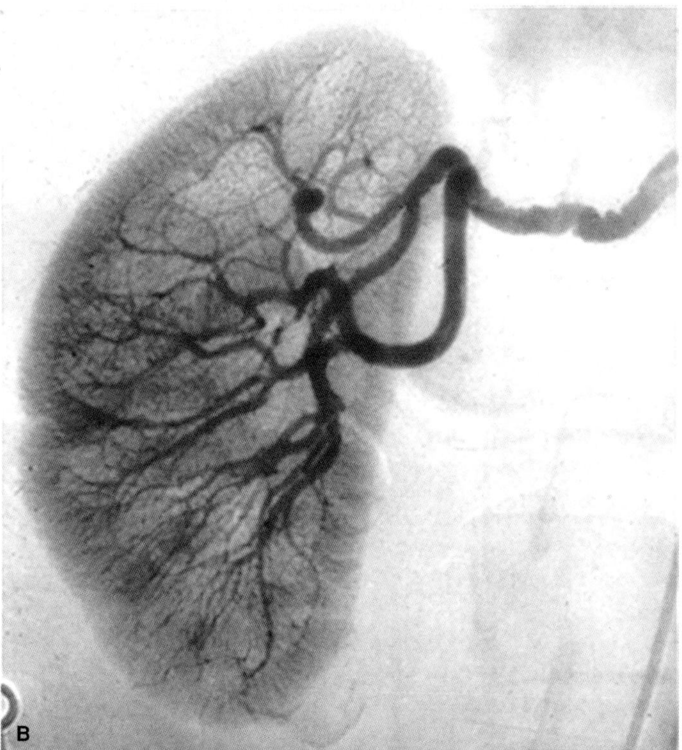

FIGURE 32A.14. **A:** Digital subtraction renal angiogram. **B:** Film screen angiogram of the same kidney; note the superior spatial resolution of the main renal artery and the small vessel detail compared to Figure 32A.6.

be evaluated by catheter-based angiography and may be very significant in evaluating an area of stenosis. This is not true of CTA or MRA.

The secrets for performing the perfect angiogram are not really secret at all. They are well known and widely practiced albeit occasionally compromised or ignored. Here are a few:

1. Make sure the patient is comfortable, cooperative, and pain free.
2. The patient must remain motionless during the angiogram. Nonionic, iso-osmolar contrast agents are practically painless; unfortunately, brand X which is less expensive isn't. Warn them that they may feel burning if you are using brand X.
3. Make sure the patient holds his/her breath while you are filming.
4. Make sure the YOU tell the patient that it is OK to breathe after the angiogram is recorded!

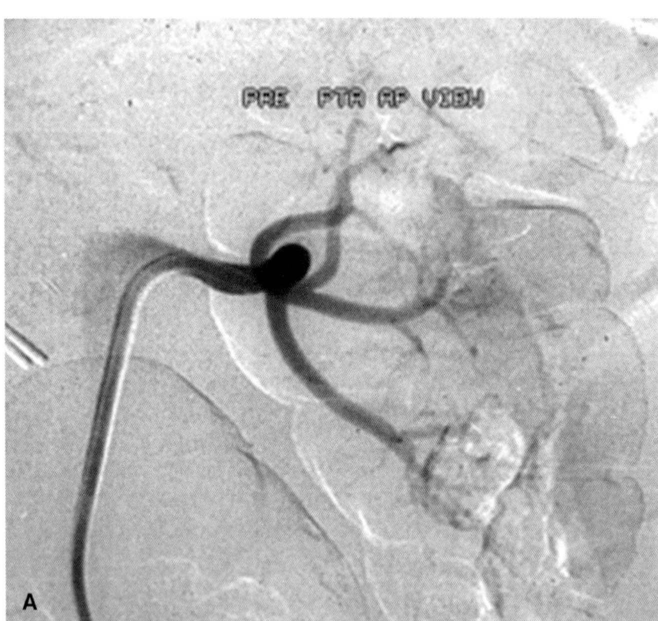

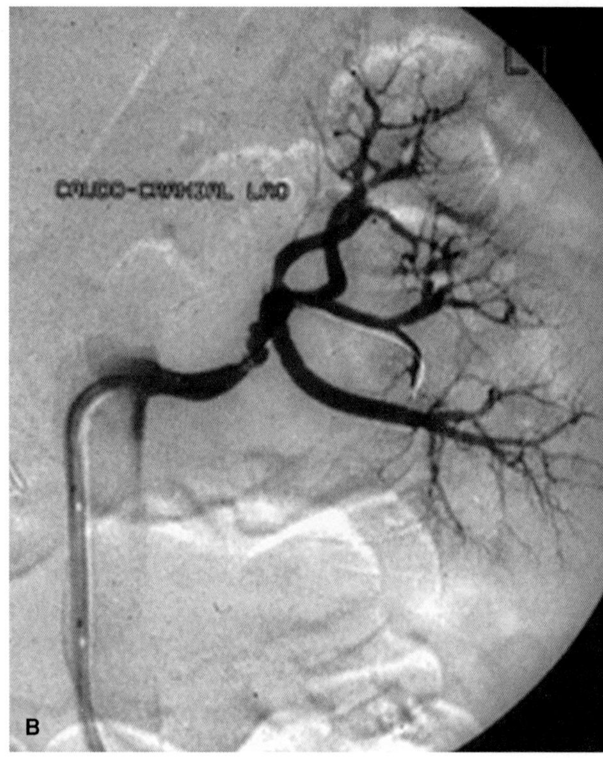

FIGURE 32A.15. **A:** Patient treated for FMD by PTA of the right renal artery returns with poorly controlled hypertension. The right renal artery was normal but how about the left? **B:** Steep left anterior oblique and craniocaudal angulation demonstrates the hidden stenosis.

5. Nonvoluntary motion such as peristalsis can be controlled with glucagon, if necessary.
6. Inject selectively into the vessel of interest, or at the very least, directly adjacent to its origin.
7. Don't occlude the vessel ostium with the catheter tip.
8. Inject enough contrast media to completely fill the vessel under examination.
9. The rate of imaging should mirror the rate of blood flow. Flow rate will depend on distal resistance. You have to film fast to characterize an arteriovenous fistula or malformation.
10. Ideally, imaging should begin before the contrast arrives in the vessel and not end before it passes.
11. Obtain orthogonal views when needed. Angle the x-ray tube and image intensifier to a position perpendicular to the origin of the vessel being evaluated, if possible. Complex angulations may be necessary to evaluate the origins of the renal, hypogastric, and superficial femoral arteries (Fig. 32A.15).
12. Frequently, a pressure measurement across a stenosis will tell more than multiple oblique views.
13. NEVER lose sight of the tip of a Glidewire. Thousands of "preventable" vascular perforations and intimal dissections have occurred because the angiographer broke this rule.
14. Slowly rotate the tip of the Glidewire as it is moved forward. Tactile resistance to forward motion, loss of the ability to rotate the wire, or failure of the wire to advance are signs to stop and reevaluate the situation.
15. The most valuable asset of a catheter-based contrast angiogram is that it is directly under the control of the angiographer. He or she knows exactly what information is needed and can adjust the examination to fit the clinical scenario and frequently treat the problem during the same procedure. Questions that arise during the examination can be immediately answered.
16. CTA, MRA, and Doppler US are wonderful screening procedures and may supply all the necessary information, but if they don't, take the patient to the angiography suite (Figs. 32A.16 and 32A.17).

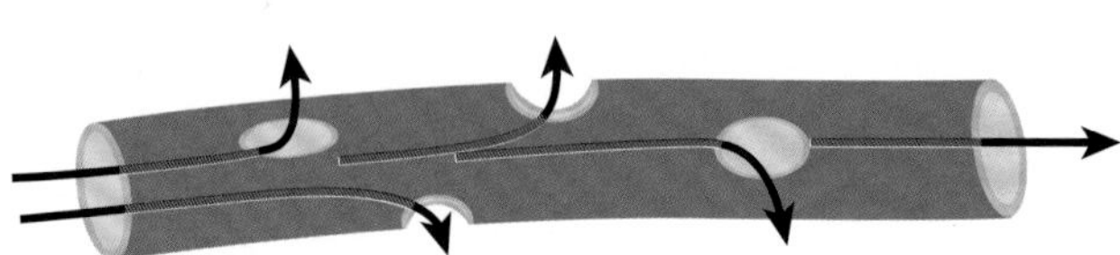

FIGURE 32A.16. When irrigating a multiside hole catheter, the injection must be forceful enough to clear all the side holes and the end hole.

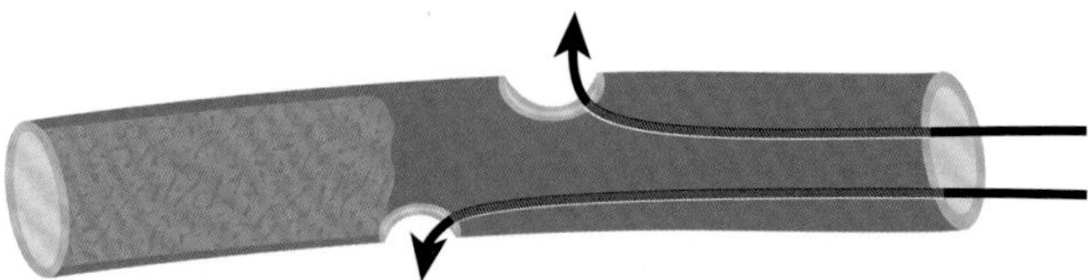

FIGURE 32A.17. Multiside hole catheters must be irrigated frequently because blood that quickly reenters the tip may potentially become an embolic thrombus. Multiside hole catheters should NOT be used for cerebral angiography!

Suggested Readings

Aspelin P, Aubry P, Fransson SG, Strasser R, Willenbrock R, Berg KJ; Nephrotoxicity in High-Risk Patients Study of Iso-Osmolar and Low-Osmolar Non-Ionic Contrast Media Study Investigators. Nephrotoxic effects in high-risk patients undergoing angiography. *N Engl J Med* 2003;348(6):491–499.

Bernard C. *Introduction à l' étude de la médecine expérimentale*. Paris: JB Baillière; 1865.

Cho KJ, Hawkins IF Jr. Carbon dioxide angiography. 2005. Available from http://www.emedicine.com/RADIO/topic870.htm.

Cho KJ, Hawkins IF Jr. Carbon dioxide angiography. 2016. Available from https://emedicine.medscape.com/article/423121-overview.

Cournand A. Cardiac catheterization; development of the technique, its contributions to experimental medicine, and its initial applications in man. *Acta Med Scand Suppl* 1975;579:3–32.

dos Santos R, Lamas A, Caldas J. Arteriografia des membros. *Medicina Contemanea* 1929;47:1.

dos Santos R, Lamas A, Pereira-Caldas J. Arteriografia da aorta e dos vasa abdominalis. *Medicina Contemanea* 1929;47:93–97.

FDA. Gadolinium-based contrast agents for magnetic resonance imaging. 2007. Available from https://www.fda.gov/Safety/MedWatch/SafetyInformation/.../ucm559709.htm.

Grainger RG. Intravascular contrast media—the past, the present and the future. Mackenzie Davidson Memorial Lecture, April 1981. *Br J Radiol* 1982;55(649):1–18.

Greene J, Linton O. *The History of Dotter Interventional Institute*. Portland, Oregon: Oregon Health and Science University; 2005.

Greitz T. Sven-Ivar Seldinger. *AJNR Am J Neuroradiol* 1999;20(6):1180–1181.

Korner M, Weber CH, Wirth S, Pfeifer KJ, Reiser MF, Treitl M. Advances in digital radiography: physical principles and system overview. *Radiographics* 2007;27(3):675–686.

Kruger RA, Mistretta CA, Crummy AB, et al. Digital K-edge subtraction radiography. *Radiology* 1977;125(1):243–245.

Linton OW. Medical applications of x rays. 1995. Available from http://www.slac.stanford.edu/pubs/beamline/25/2/25-2-linton.pdf.

McDaniel MC, Nelson MA, Voeltz MD, et al. High-viscosity contrast media require higher injection pressures in diagnostic coronary catheters. *Cardiovasc Revasc Med* 2007;8(2):140.

Moniz E. L'encéphalographie artérielle, son importance dans la localisation des tumeurs cérébrales. *Rev Neurol (Paris)* 1927;2:72–90.

Osborne ED, Sutherland CG, Scholl AJ Jr, Roundtree LG. Roentgenography of urinary tract during excretion of sodium iodid. *JAMA* 1923;80(6):368–373.

Seldinger SI. Catheter replacement of the needle in percutaneous arteriography; a new technique. *Acta Radiol* 1953;39(5):368–376.

Swick M. Darstellung der Niere und Harnwege in Roentgenbild durch intravenose Einbringung eines neuen Kontraststoffes: des Uroselectans. *Kliniche Wochenschrift* 1929;8(45):2087–2089.

CHAPTER 32B ■ PERIPHERAL ARTERIAL DISEASE

STEPHEN BRACEWELL, CARL GUNNAR FORSBERG, RICARDO TADAYOSHI BARBOSA YAMADA, CLAUDIO SCHONHOLZ, AND MARCELO GUIMARAES

INTRODUCTION

Peripheral arterial disease (PAD) describes atherosclerosis in noncardiac vessels, and is a common and often disabling disease that affects up to 12 million Americans. A diagnosis of PAD is associated with significantly higher costs of care. This chapter discusses the causes, diagnosis, imaging findings, and treatment of PAD, particularly in the lower extremities.

RISK FACTORS

Risk factors for PAD include age, hyperlipidemia, tobacco use, diabetes, and hypertension. Atherosclerosis can also be enhanced by systemic diseases such as homocystinuria, systemic lupus erythematosus, and rheumatoid arthritis. High levels of inflammatory markers, such as C-reactive protein, fibrinogen, and interleukin 6 have also been observed in PAD patients. African heritage and poor socioeconomic status have been postulated as additional risk factors. Men and women are equally affected in the United States; however, women appear to be at higher risk in lower-income countries. Of those presenting with advanced PAD—also known as critical limb ischemia—women appear to suffer worse outcomes, possibly due to underutilization of preventative care compared to men. Patients with other comorbid vascular disease, such as coronary artery disease, cerebrovascular disease, and chronic kidney disease, are also at increased risk.

PATHOGENESIS

The principal physiologic alteration of PAD is plaque formation due to atherosclerosis. Plaque formation is a multifaceted event, and there are several theories as to the exact pathophysiology. The most commonly accepted theory is the "response to injury." First, fat-laden macrophages known as "foam cells" deposit in the muscle well. Secretions from foam cells incite smooth muscle proliferation. This, in turn, leads to intimal disruption. At this stage, collagen is exposed in the lumen, leading to fibrous plaque and thrombus formation. Plaque formation is generally increased at arterial branch points and curvatures, possibly from disrupted laminar flow and increased lipid deposition. The most common area of disease is in the superficial femoral artery (SFA) within the adductor canal. Resultant luminal narrowing will ensue. As narrowing progresses, collateral vessels will be recruited.

CLINICAL PRESENTATION

History

Patients with symptomatic lower extremity PAD will generally present with a history of claudication or pain with ambulation over a set distance. Symptoms generally correlate with a narrowing at one level above the area of pain and discomfort. For example, buttock claudication will originate from aortoiliac disease, and thigh claudication from stenosis at the external iliac artery (EIA). Knee or calf pain is due to plaque in the common femoral arteries (CFAs) or SFAs. Patients may complain of foot pain at nighttime, worse with certain positions—which is classified as rest pain. A positive history of erectile dysfunction may serve as a clue for occult PAD. Occlusion at aortoiliac bifurcation can result in the Leriche syndrome, which can present clinically as impotence, buttock claudication, and absent femoral pulses. Some patients may have plaque detected incidentally on imaging, but may endorse no symptoms; this is classified as asymptomatic PAD, which outnumbers symptomatic PAD on an order of 3:1.

Common mimics of PAD and claudication include lumbar spinal stenosis and radiculopathy, which classically produces a back pain that can be magnified or alleviated by position (neurogenic claudication). Hip, knee, and foot arthritis can cause similar symptoms. Diabetic neuropathy also produces lower extremity pain which may manifest clinically like claudication. Nocturnal cramps are unlikely to originate from an arterial stenosis, and may originate from venous or musculoskeletal disease. In the absence of abnormal pulses, ankle–brachial indices (ABI) or imaging, these above entities are more likely to be the cause of a patient's presentation.

Physical Examination

In general, the initial assessment of PAD begins with the pulse examination. A typical pulse examination consists of palpation of the CFA just below the inguinal ligament. A strong pulse is described as 2+, a faint pulse as 1+, and absent as 0. The dorsalis pedis (DP) and posterior tibial (PT) arteries are also examined by palpation. A small portion of the population may lack a DP pulse due to anatomic variants, but a PT pulse should be present always. The popliteal artery can usually be palpated, but is dependent on patient position, habitus, and knee flexion. Typically it is easier to examine the popliteal pulse with the patient's knee slightly flexed by the examiner while the patient keeps the leg muscles relaxed. If pulses are unable to be palpated, a handheld Doppler probe is utilized. A normal triphasic signal can be heard in a vessel with no negligible stenosis. Moderate narrowing in the affected vessel results in an audible biphasic signal, and severe disease results in a monophasic signal. Other PAD examination signs in the lower extremities include pallor, hair loss, slow capillary refill, and nail changes. The Buerger test, which evaluates for gravity-dependent rubor, can be positive in PAD. One should closely scrutinize the lower extremities for ulcers or eschar, especially in between the digits. Dependent edema should also be evaluated.

IMAGING WORKUP

In the imaging workup of peripheral vascular disease, there are several imaging modalities that can be utilized both for diagnostic use and preoperative planning.

Vascular Doppler Ultrasound

Vascular Doppler ultrasound is often the initial screening test in the evaluation of PAD. Duplex Doppler sonography is generally performed on the DP, PT, popliteal, and superficial femoral arteries, as well as the aortoiliac vessels. The anatomic location of a lesion can be deduced by the change from a normal triphasic waveform on spectral Doppler imaging to a biphasic (moderate stenosis) or a monophasic waveform (severe stenosis/occlusion). Evaluation of triphasicity and waveform magnitude is essential in the evaluation for flow-limiting stenosis (Fig. 32B.1). In the acute setting, a dedicated lower extremity Doppler examination can allow for evaluation of acute occlusion, or acute limb ischemia (ALI). Advantages of vascular ultrasound include low cost, no need for contrast agents, and dynamic evaluation of vessels. Sonography can aid in determining the length of a stenosis, or an appropriate target for revascularization. It can also evaluate the patency of vascular grafts or stents. Limitations include limited evaluation of collateral vessel and degree of stenosis, especially in calcified plaque. Doppler signal intensity can also be influenced by external factors, such as vasospasm, body temperature, and medications. Finally, vascular ultrasound is time-consuming for the sonographer and operator dependent.

Ankle–Brachial Index and Pulse Volume Recording

A modification of vascular sonography includes addition of the ABI and pulse volume recording (PVR). The ABI is a critical element of the objective evaluation of PAD that can be performed in the absence of dedicated duplex sonography. Utilizing a handheld Doppler probe and blood pressure cuff, the ABI is calculated by comparing the highest occlusion pressure on either side at the ankle (DP or PT arteries) as the numerator, and the highest pressure in the arm (brachial artery) as the denominator. More precise values can be estimated with formal duplex sonography. The resting ABI can also be modified with stress, with changes in the ABI monitored before and after walking a set distance on a treadmill. Limitations of the ABI include false elevations in diabetics with heavily calcified vessel walls, which can be partially avoided with performing a toe–brachial index. Brachial artery occlusion values can be falsely deranged with subclavian or brachiocephalic artery stenosis. Common values for ABI in PAD are listed in Table 32B.1.

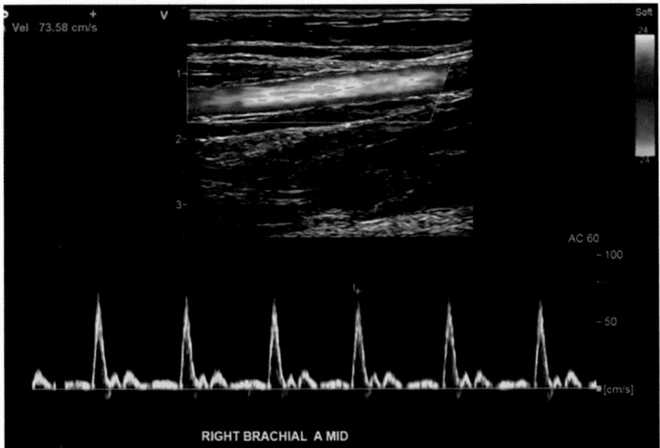

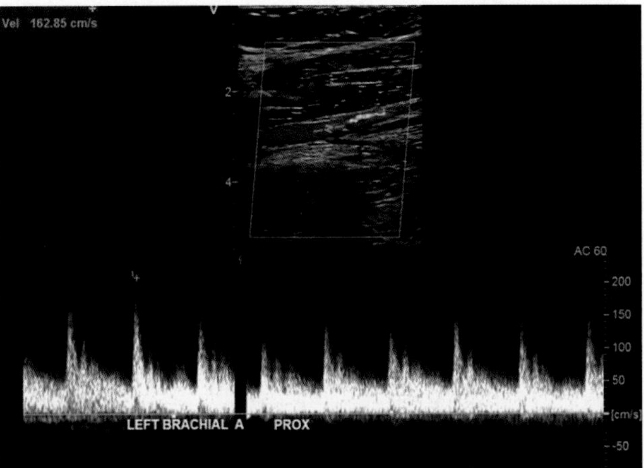

FIGURE 32B.1. Vascular Ultrasound. Young female smoker with upper extremity ischemia. Gray scale and duplex Doppler in a normal patient (**left**) and a symptomatic patient with Buerger disease (**right**) demonstrate turbulent flow and increased velocities in the brachial artery.

TABLE 32B.1

COMMON VALUES FOR ABI IN PAD

■ ANKLE–BRACHIAL INDEX	■ DEGREE OF CLAUDICATION
Greater than 1.1	No PAD
0.9–1.09	Asymptomatic PAD
0.7–0.89	Mild Claudication
0.5–0.69	Moderate to severe claudication
0.2–0.49	Rest pain, tissue loss

PVRs are performed by placing custom pneumatic cuffs at serial levels in the lower extremity, and measuring changes in the vascular waveform with applied pressure. The resultant image is a pulse waveform, and allows for evaluation of triphasicity and amplitude. This examination can also be modified with stress PVR. An example of a typical report from an ABI/PVR is demonstrated in Figure 32B.2.

Computed Tomography Angiography

CT angiography (CTA) of the lower extremities has emerged as an increasingly utilized, noninvasive alternative to digital subtraction angiography (DSA) for anatomic characterization

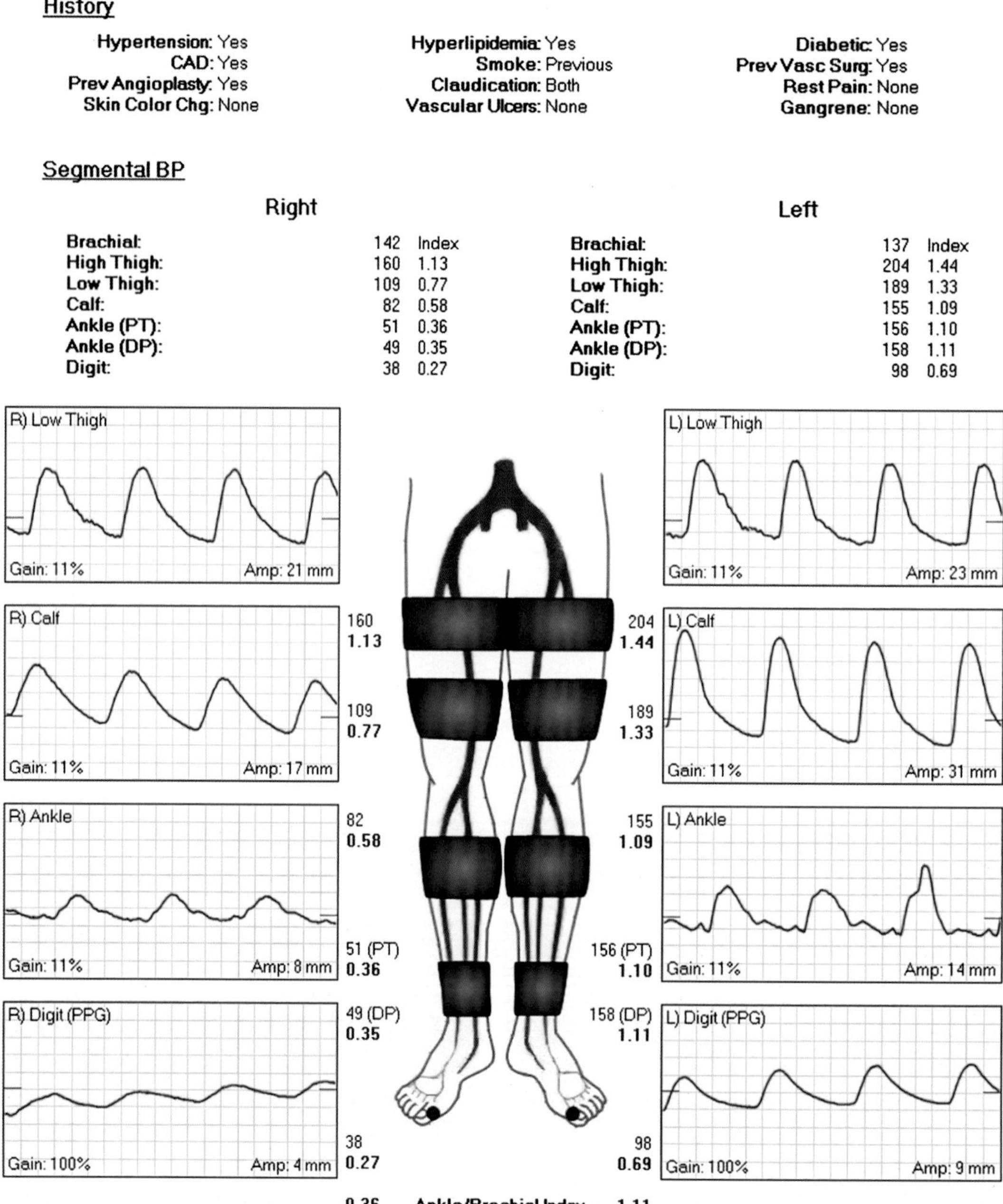

FIGURE 32B.2. **Ankle–Brachial Indices and Pulse Volume Recordings.** Elderly patient with moderate to severe claudication on the right due to a TASC A right SFA lesion, with ABIs and PVRs obtained. Note the asymmetry in ABIs and dampened, monophasic waveforms on the right compared to the left.

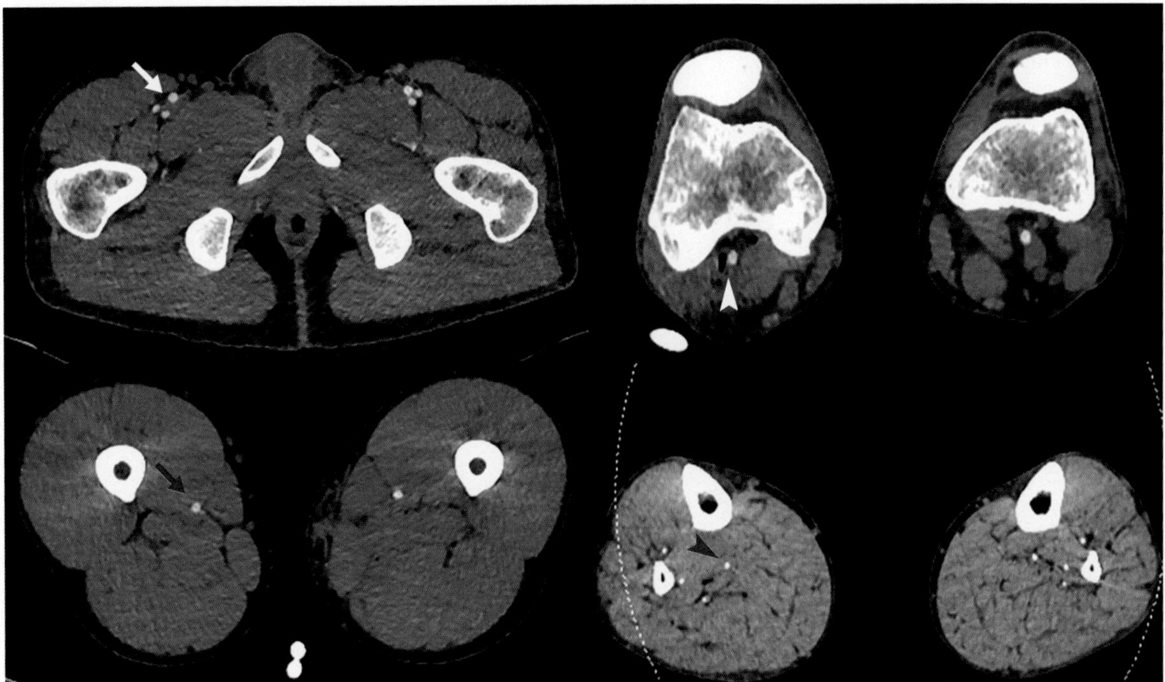

FIGURE 32B.3. Normal CTA With Runoff. CTA demonstrates normal appearance of the common femoral trifurcation (*white arrow*), SFA (*red arrow*), popliteal artery (*white arrowhead*), and three-vessel runoff (*red arrowhead*).

of PAD. Multidetector CT evaluation is generally performed from the abdominal aorta throughout both lower extremities in the arterial phase. A medium-sized bore peripheral intravenous cannula (ideally a 20 gauge) is generally required to achieve flow rate of 4 to 5 cc/s using a power injector. Slice thickness generally ranges between 2 and 3 mm, and arterial phase acquisition is followed by a delayed venous series at many centers. A three-dimensional (3D) reconstruction is typically performed at a separate workstation. This technique is particularly useful in the setting of acute trauma to evaluate for vascular injury (Fig. 32B.3). With appropriate parameters, CTA can allow for excellent evaluation of patency within surgical devices, such as grafts and metallic stents. CT allows for limited evaluation of the vessel wall, which is useful in conditions such as cystic adventitial disease or aneurysm. Other advantages of CTA include short examination time, excellent spatial resolution, and evaluation of other surrounding structures in the pelvis and lower extremity. Compared to MR, there are increased voxels per image. Disadvantages include radiation, contrast dose and cost (in comparison to a duplex ultrasound). Calcified lesions can cause blooming artifact, which often overestimates the degree of stenosis. CTA may also have low diagnostic accuracy (due to low resolution) in heavily calcified arteries below the knee.

Magnetic Resonance Angiography

Magnetic resonance angiography (MRA) provides a 3D alternative to CTA for evaluation of PAD (Fig. 32B.4). MRA allows for unlimited planes of acquisition, and can better evaluate runoff vessels due to the ability to detect vessels at lower velocities than other modalities. MRA is the study of choice in states where there is concern for inflammatory or degenerative changes of the vessel wall, as well as cystic adventitial disease. MRA is also an excellent noninvasive option for patients with allergies to iodinated contrast media, with the added benefit of no radiation dose. Typical sequences include a True FISP

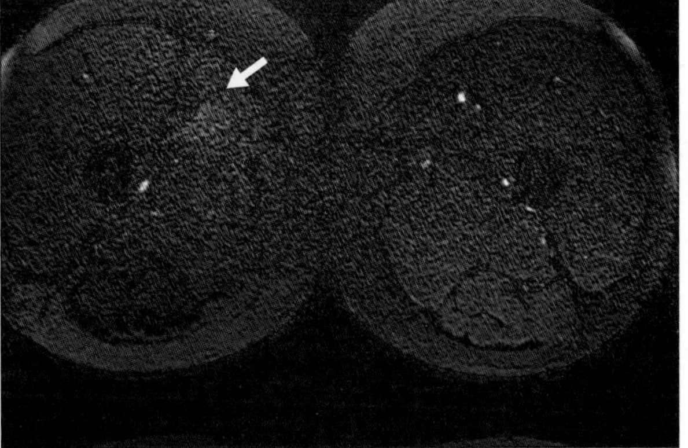

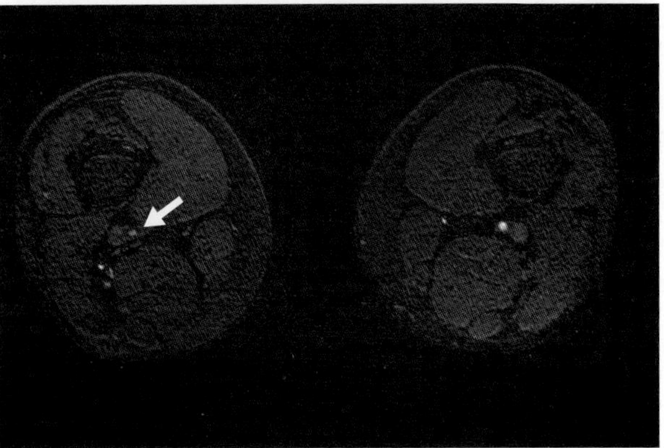

FIGURE 32B.4. Magnetic Resonance Angiography in SFA Occlusion. Patient with severe claudication underwent MRA of the lower extremities. Axial images at the mid-thigh demonstrate complete occlusion of the right SFA (*superior arrow*), with distal reconstitution at the level of the popliteal artery (*lower arrow*). An advantage of MRA is ability to detect slow flow in collaterals.

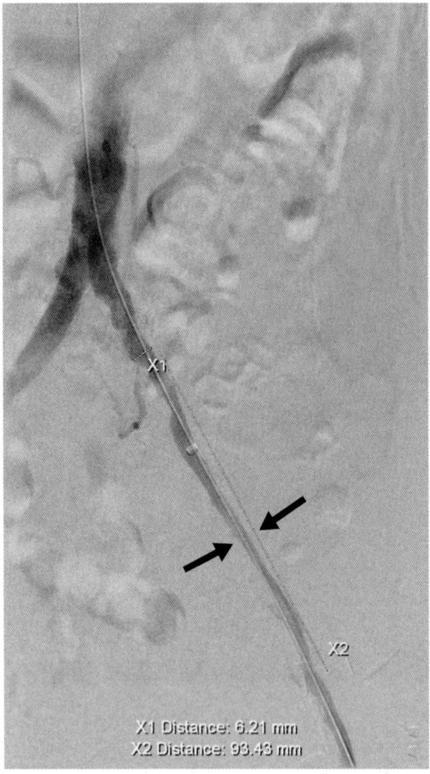

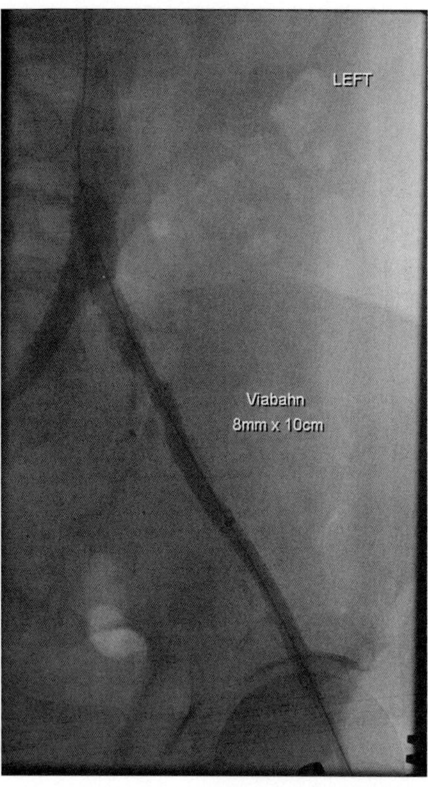

FIGURE 32B.5. **Angiographic Intervention of the Iliac Arteries.** Patient with claudication undergoes diagnostic and therapeutic angiography. DSA pre- and postintervention for TASC B. External Iliac stenosis (**left**, *arrows*). An excellent result is noted after angioplasty and VIABAHN stent placement.

localizer (Fast Imaging with Steady State Precession), followed by a contrast-enhanced T1 acquisition, followed by 3D MRA reconstructions. Disadvantages include risk of nephrogenic systemic fibrosis (in patients with glomerular filtration rate <30 mL/min), incompatibility due to implanted ferromagnetic devices, time of acquisition, and cost. Also, there may be significant artifact associated with vascular implants such as stents.

Digital Subtraction Angiography

DSA is the gold standard for imaging lower extremity PAD (Fig. 32B.5). Patients are brought to the angiography suite, administered conscious sedation, and typically the groin is prepped in a sterile fashion. Ipsilateral access is typically utilized for single-limb angiography. Alternatives include contralateral femoral access for an "up and over" technique around the aortic bifurcation or antegrade approach utilizing a "radial to peripheral approach." Current imaging systems offer up to a 2,022 × 2,022 pixel imaging matrix via a 31 × 31 cm detector. A typical angiographic run is timed at 4 fps for an initial 5 seconds, and then a reduced frame rate for additional time added to the series. The CFA is accessed via the Seldinger technique. A vascular access sheath is placed, via which a variety of diagnostic and interventional wires, catheters, and patency devices can be introduced. At the conclusion of the procedure, the sheath is removed, and hemostasis is achieved via closure devices or manual compression. Advantages include high spatial resolution and ability to immediately intervene on occlusions, stenosis, and vascular trauma. Additional dynamic factors, such as pressure gradients, can be measured intraoperatively. Additional diagnostic studies such as intravascular ultrasound (IVUS) can be performed. In cases of severe contrast allergy or acute kidney dysfunction, carbon dioxide (CO_2) angiography (only below the diaphragm in the arterial system) can be employed in selected patients (Figs. 32B.6 and 32B.7). DSA disadvantages include perioperative complications, contrast load (potential contrast-induced

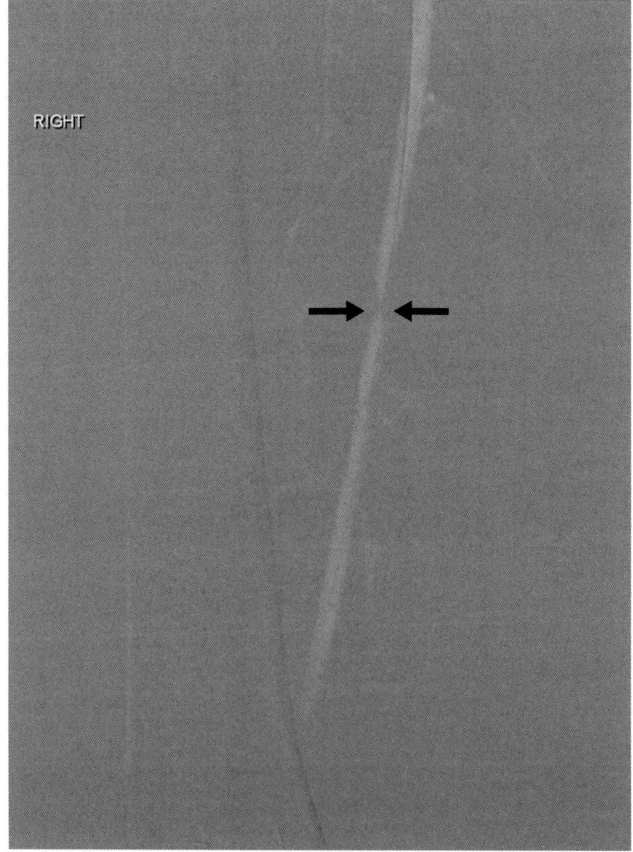

FIGURE 32B.6. **CO_2 Angiogram.** Patient with claudication and borderline end-stage renal disease who could not receive intravenous iodine contrast. CO_2 angiogram demonstrates multifocal short segment SFA lesions. Subsequent DEB angioplasty of the dominant lesions demonstrates improved luminal narrowing.

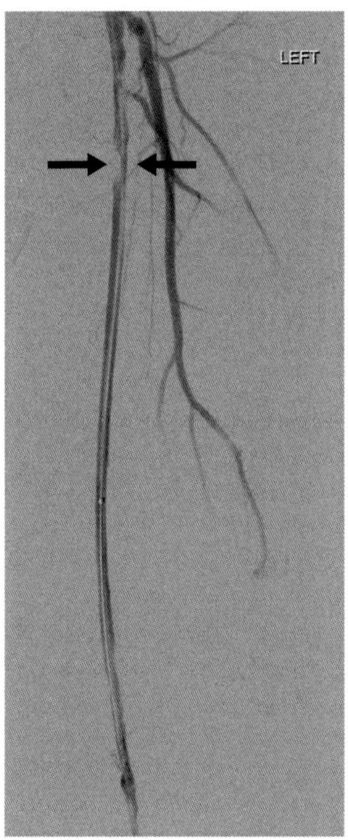

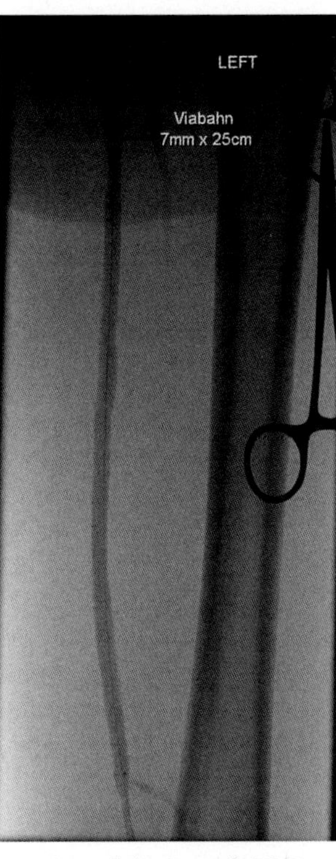

FIGURE 32B.7. **Angiographic Intervention of the Superficial Femoral Artery.** Symptomatic patient with claudication with TASC A proximal SFA lesion on DSA. There is near-complete resolution after angioplasty and VIABAHN stent placement.

nephropathy in patients with dehydration, diabetes mellitus, and creatinine >1.5) and radiation dose.

Imaging allows for preoperative planning, evaluation of collaterals, and evaluation of extent of disease. Once lesions are identified, they can be classified according to the TASC-II guidelines (Table 32B.2).

CLASSIFICATION OF PAD AND MEDICAL DECISION MAKING

After appropriate history, physical, and imaging evaluation, a patient's overall PAD status can be ascertained. The single most important factor to be determined is the presence of critical limb ischemia (CLI). This defines a chronic syndrome, which manifests as symptoms of near occlusion, rest pain, or end-stage tissue stages. CLI is not always preceded by a classic history of claudication, and tissue loss may be only manifestation. Less severe forms of PAD are most commonly stratified by the Rutherford classification. A simplified explanation of the Rutherford classification is demonstrated in Table 32B.3.

INTERVENTIONS

Once a patient is stratified in the spectrum of PAD, an appropriate treatment strategy can be determined. Regardless of the degree of symptoms, all patients should undergo risk modification. This entails tobacco cessation, blood pressure control, and increased physical activity. Medical therapy is also pursued with antiplatelet and statin therapy for high cholesterol. If a patient is symptomatic, there is evidence to support supervised exercise programs. FDA-approved medications for claudication, such as cilostazol and pentoxifylline, can be offered as part of maximizing medical therapy. Fortunately,

TABLE 32B.2

TASC-II GUIDELINES

■ LESION	■ AORTOILIAC	■ FEMORAL–POPLITEAL
TASC A	▪ Unilateral or bilateral short segment stenosis of CIA or EIA	▪ Single lesion up to 10 cm ▪ Single occlusion up to 5 cm
TASC B	▪ Up to 3 cm of the stenosis of infrarenal aorta ▪ Unilateral CIA or EIA occlusion, which does not extend into the origin of the internal iliac or CFA ▪ Single or multiple stenosis totaling 3–10 cm involving the EIA, but not extending into the CFA	▪ Multiple lesions up to 5 cm ▪ Single stenosis or occlusion up to 15 cm not involving the infrageniculate popliteal artery ▪ Single heavily calcified lesion up to 5 cm ▪ Single popliteal stenosis
TASC C	▪ Bilateral CIA occlusions ▪ Bilateral EIA up to 10 cm long, not including the CFA ▪ Unilateral EIA stenosis extending into the CFA ▪ Unilateral EIA occlusion that involves the origins of internal iliac and/or CFA ▪ Heavily calcified unilateral EIA occlusion	▪ Multiple stenoses or occlusions totaling 15 cm with or without heavy calcification ▪ Recurrent stenoses or occlusions after failing treatment
TASC D	▪ Infrarenal aortoiliac occlusion ▪ Diffuse disease involving the aorta and both iliac arteries requiring treatment ▪ Diffuse multiple stenoses involving the unilateral CIA, EIA, and CFA ▪ Unilateral occlusions of both CIA and EIA ▪ Bilateral occlusions of EIA ▪ Iliac stenoses in patients with AAA requiring treatment open surgery due to incompatibility with endograft	▪ Chronic total occlusions of CFA or SFA up to 20 cm, which involve the popliteal artery ▪ Chronic total occlusion of popliteal artery and proximal trifurcation vessels

CIA, common iliac artery; EIA, external iliac artery; CFA, common femoral artery; SFA, superficial femoral artery; AAA, abdominal aorta aneurysm.

TABLE 32B.3

RUTHERFORD CLASSIFICATION, SIMPLIFIED

0	Asymptomatic
1	Mild claudication
2	Moderate claudication
3	Severe claudication
4	Ischemic rest pain
5	Minor tissue loss
6	Major tissue loss

up to 80% of patients with PAD will not experience progression to CLI. If compliant with maximal medical therapy, these numbers improve to 95%.

Despite maximal medical therapy, or in cases of decompensated CLI, some patients will become candidates for revascularization. The most compelling indications for revascularization include rest pain, ischemic tissue changes, and claudication that limit the quality of life. Ischemic tissue changes can be objectively qualified by the Society of Vascular Surgery's Wifi Classification system, which takes into account the wound, ischemia, and foot infection. Other factors, such as the patient's functional status and comorbidities, factor into whether to intervene. If a patient is deemed a suitable candidate for revascularization, diagnostic testing as to the extent and location of the disease will dictate the course of intervention. Ideal candidates will proceed to endovascular therapy. More complex lesions may require a hybrid surgical and endovascular approach, or even surgical bypass. Recent data suggest that higher volumes of tissue recovered at endovascular revascularization are associated with improved outcomes pertaining to mortality and amputation.

The traditional intervention for isolated iliac, femoral, and popliteal disease is percutaneous transluminal angioplasty (PTA). In this method, a lesion is traversed percutaneously via fluoroscopic guidance with a guidewire. Once the lesion has been crossed, a PTA can be performed. PTA may involve single or combined use of a balloon (regular or drug eluting), stent placement, and atherectomy device (it is used to shave calcified plaques with the goal to increase the arterial wall diameter). Balloon PTA for PAD demonstrates acceptable results with a low complication profile. However, restenosis due to neointimal hyperplasia at 12-month follow-up may be as high as 50% depending on the vascular territory. The proximal and larger arteries (e.g., CIA) have better patency rates than distal arteries (infragenicular) following PTA. Newer angioplasty devices, such as the drug-eluting balloon (DEB) demonstrate promising results in preventing neointimal hyperplasia. Advantages of the DEB include the ability to intervene on vessels too small for stenting and it does not leave any metal or foreign body in place. Potential adverse effect of the DEB includes downstream migration of the drug microparticles.

Due to the aforementioned rate of restenosis and to the potential recoiling of the stenotic area with primary balloon PTA alone, there is increased utilization of vascular stents to maintain vessel patency after revascularization. Stents range in variety from regular, noncovered bare metal to bare drug eluting, some are covered, and the delivery system may be self-expanding or balloon expandable. Considerations in stent placement include vessel tortuosity, lesion length, lesion complexity, and patient ability to tolerate or be compliant with antiplatelet therapy. Limitations of stents include restenosis, thrombosis, potential stent fracture, and migration (Figs. 32B.5 to 32B.7).

OTHER PERIPHERAL VASCULAR DISORDERS

Acute Limb Ischemia

Contrary to CLI, ALI is a medical emergency, requiring prompt diagnosis and intervention for limb salvage. ALI typically occurs within 2 weeks of symptom onset and the incidence is estimated at 1.5 cases per 10,000 people per year. The classic "6 P's" (pulselessness, pallor, pain, paresthesia, poikilothermia, and paralysis) illustrate the presentation of a limb threatened by acute arterial occlusion. The two most common causes are arterial embolism and thrombosis. The most common presentation is lower extremity pain out of proportion to examination. Focused physical examination should be accompanied with a handheld Doppler, and there should be careful evaluation of compartment syndrome. Systolic perfusion pressure can also be measured by placing a Doppler probe on the dorsum of the foot, underneath a blood pressure cuff; with values of less than 50 mm Hg suggestive of ischemia.

The etiology of ALI can be divided into embolic and thrombotic, each of which has consequences in treatment and long-term management. The majority of emboli originate in the heart as the result of arrhythmia, valvular disease, and postmyocardial infarction motion abnormalities. Noncardiogenic embolism may originate from an aneurysm, or can be iatrogenic, namely after vascular access and arterial catheterization. Primary causes of arterial thrombosis include atherosclerosis, hypercoagulability, low flow states, and intravascular devices. Arterial occlusion can be confirmed on CTA or DSA. Imaging can allow for intervention planning, and can delineate whether there is an acute or subacute process, with well-developed collateral suggesting an acute or chronic process. Due to the many nonatherosclerotic causes of ALI, there may be negligible atherosclerotic disease. In either thrombosis or embolism, imaging can demonstrate acute cutoff of the occluded vessel or the meniscus sign.

Initial treatment of ALI begins with immediate patient systemic intravenous heparinization. Revascularization is the primary goal and this can be achieved via endovascular intervention or open surgery. Recent meta-analyses suggest equal rates of limb salvage and 1-year mortality between surgery and thrombolysis, although there is an increasing trend toward endovascular therapy. Adequate revascularization does not ensure a positive outcome for this patient population as 10% to 15% will undergo amputation of the affected limb and the 1-year mortality after ALI can be as high as 15% to 20%. Treated patients are also at risk of reperfusion injury, as free radicals formed during ischemia induce cellular damage. Resultant increased vascular permeability, microthrombi formation, and edema will ensue. Close inpatient assessment of the limb after revascularization is critical, and if compartment syndrome develops, an emergent fasciotomy is indicated. Follow-up angiography after revascularization is generally pursued to evaluate for continued patency or other critical lesions (Fig. 32B.8). Long-term management of ALI patients requires addressing the underlying cause of the thrombus formation (cardia arrhythmia) associated with systemic anticoagulation or use of antiplatelet agents, depending on the etiology of the initial event.

Vasospasm

The Raynaud phenomenon is the most common vasospastic disorder and is primarily a clinical diagnosis that relies upon patient history. The primary and secondary forms consist of a biphasic change of digits from white to blue in a cold environment, representing cyanosis followed by

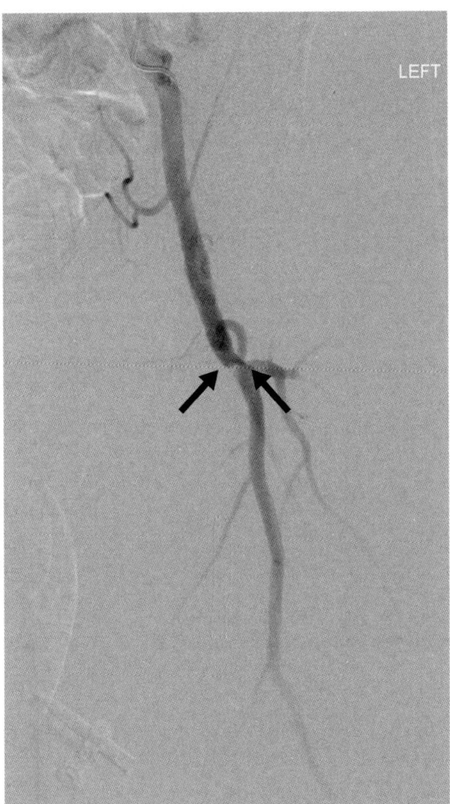

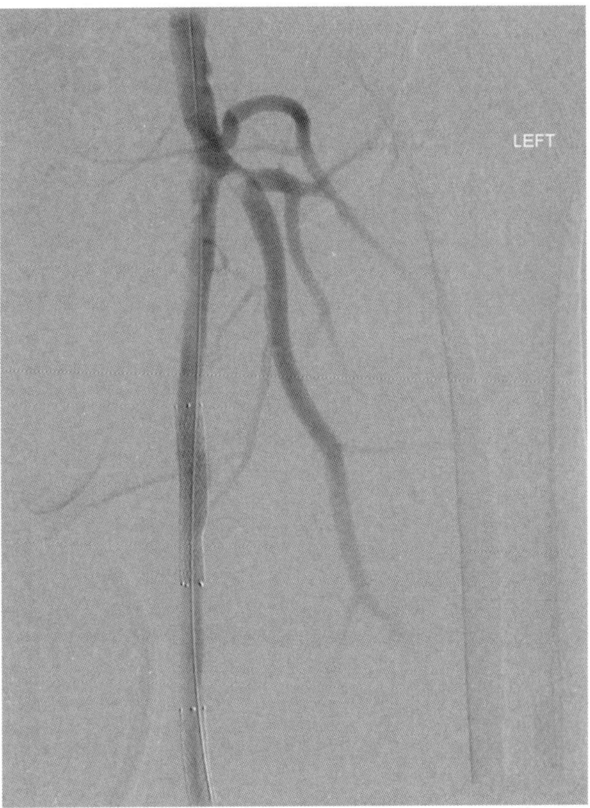

FIGURE 32B.8. **Thrombectomy for Acute Limb Ischemia.** Patient with prior SFA intervention presents with acute limb ischemia. CFA angiogram in a patient preintervention demonstrates abrupt cutoff of the left SFA (notice nonopacified SFA stent). Images after recanalization demonstrate restored patency. Lack of collateral vessels is more often seen in an acute rather than chronic occlusion.

revascularization. These events are usually limited to 15 to 20 minutes and range from mild to severe. Primary Raynaud phenomenon has no underlying cause, presents in a younger population (15 to 30 years of age), and up to half have a first-degree relative with the disorder. Secondary Raynaud phenomenon is characterized by a later onset with an underlying secondary cause that includes scleroderma, systemic lupus erythematosus, mixed connective tissue disease, Sjögren syndrome, and polymyositis. First line of treatment for both involves avoidance of cold in addition to decreasing stress and anxiety related to the condition. Calcium channel blockers are often the first form of pharmacotherapy for patients refractory to cold avoidance, but a recent Cochrane Review of CCBs in primary Raynaud phenomenon demonstrated moderate-quality evidence that these were minimally effective in decreasing the frequency of attacks and high-quality evidence that they did not affect attack severity. Imaging has a limited, if any, role in the diagnosis of this disorder, but acute exacerbations have been documented with angiography and display tapering of distal vessels with no intraluminal filling defects (Fig. 32B.9).

Ergotism is a rare vasospastic disorder caused by ingestion of ergot alkaloids. This class of drugs is currently used to treat migraines and postpartum hemorrhage. Lysergic acid diethylamide (LSD), a recreational drug, may trigger ergotism. The incidence is low, with only 0.01% of patients on these medications experiencing clinically relevant vasospasm. Certain medications, such as strong inhibitors of CYP3A4, taken in combination with ergot alkaloids, magnify these effects. Examples of common CYP3A4 inhibitors include protease inhibitors (Ritonavir), azole antifungals (Ketoconazole), and some macrolide antibiotics (Erythromycin). The vasospasm typically occurs in medium-sized arteries and can lead to claudication and even gangrene of the extremities. This spasm manifests as long smooth stenosis and can be demonstrated with angiography or duplex ultrasound. Treatment involves early withdrawal of the offending agent and supportive care but there are case reports of PTA intervention.

Trauma and vascular interventions can induce vasospasm as well. This is important to consider when directing devices in smaller arteries, namely in the radial and mesenteric arteries. The vasospasm can be resolved pharmaceutically with nitroglycerine or often with a "cocktail" of drugs that includes nitroglycerine, verapamil, and heparin.

Cystic Adventitial Disease

Cystic adventitial disease is a rare vascular disorder characterized by compression of a vessel, much more commonly an artery than a vein. The popliteal artery is involved in roughly 80% of these cases and presents as claudication of sudden onset. A notable physical examination finding is loss of distal pulses with sharp flexion of the knee. Typical patients are of young to middle age, with no cardiovascular risk factors, affecting males compared to females at a ratio of 4:1. Pathogenesis is unclear, but the most recent comprehensive review of this condition proposed an "articular theory" in which a capsular defect leads to tracking of synovial fluid along a vascular articular branch and this has been demonstrated on imaging of several cases of adventitial disease. Acceptable imaging modalities include catheter angiography,

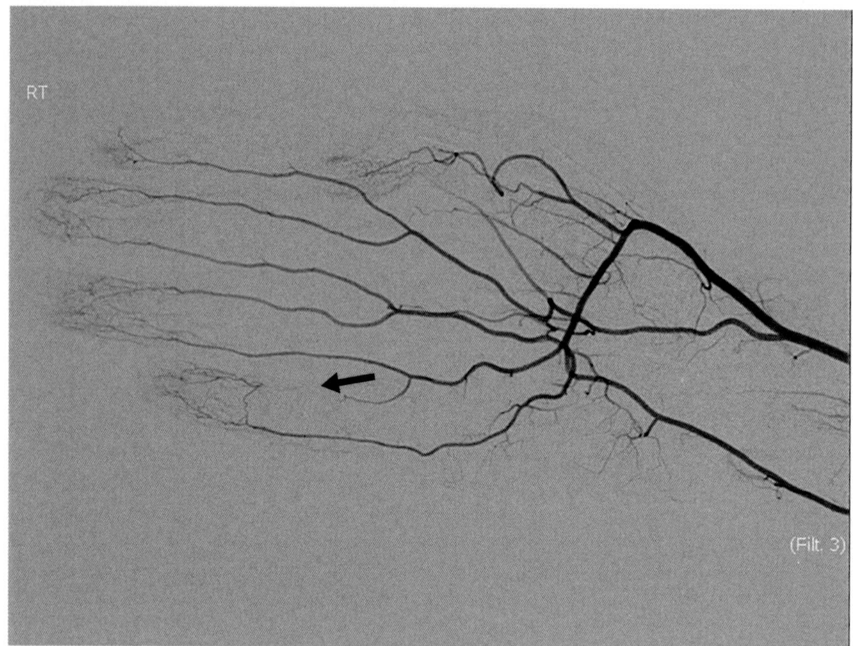

FIGURE 32B.9. **Raynaud Phenomenon.** Right upper extremity angiogram in a patient with intermittent pallor of the fifth digit. DSA demonstrates typical findings of Raynaud phenomenon, with nonopacification of the radial fifth proper digital artery (*arrow*).

US, CT, and MR. MRA is considered the gold standard. A "scimitar sign" can be demonstrated on MRA in which the T2 hyperintense cyst displaces the vessel and narrows the lumen. The preferred treatment is surgery, with percutaneous and endovascular interventions found to be a risk factor for cyst recurrence.

Mönckeberg Medial Sclerosis (MMS)

MMS is a common acquired disease, which involves the media in smaller muscular arteries in a local distribution. The prevalence of MMS is increased in patients with end-stage renal disease and type 2 diabetes, and can be diagnosed objectively with ABIs >1.3. MMS increases vessel stiffness and causes a loss of elasticity. Consequently, muscle perfusion may be decreased leading to arterial stasis and potential thrombosis. MMS can be observed on conventional radiography and CT due to concentric calcifications, but US can also demonstrate hyperechoic vessel walls.

Buerger Disease

Thromboangiitis obliterans (Buerger disease) is an inflammatory disorder of medium and small vessels of the extremities. Buerger disease is directly linked to tobacco use, and is more common in males. The prevalence in North America is estimated at 12.6/100,000 and the Eastern Asian, India, and the Middle East have a much higher prevalence due to increased tobacco consumption. Segmental inflammatory thrombi disrupt perfusion of distal arteries and veins leading to claudication, ischemic rest pain, ulcers, and eventually gangrenous lesions necessitating amputation (Fig. 32B.10).

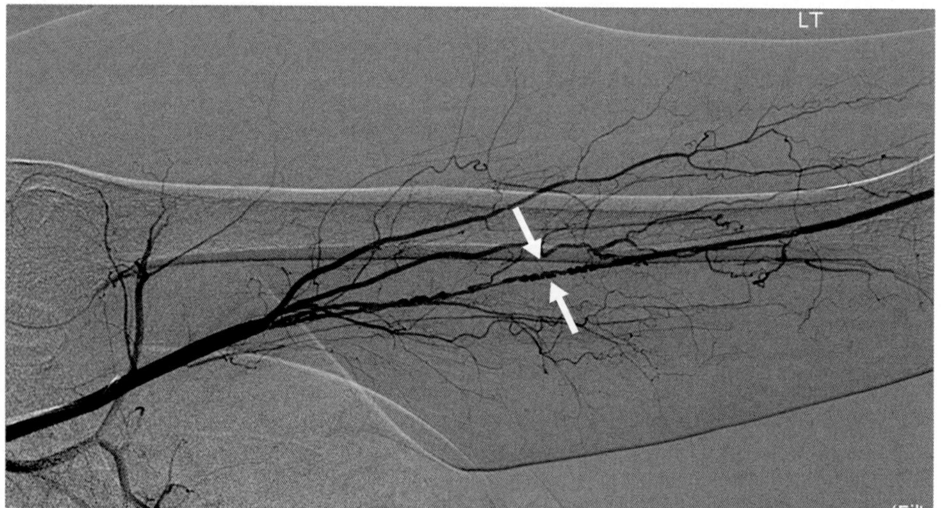

FIGURE 32B.10. **Buerger Disease.** Upper extremity angiogram in a young female smoker with digital ischemia. DSA demonstrates typical findings of Buerger disease, with corkscrew appearance of left brachial artery (*arrow*).

Smoking cessation is the only definitive treatment of the disease. Patients typically have multiple extremities affected even if they are only symptomatic in one. DSA can effectively display the vascular changes, such as segmental occlusive lesions, more severe distally, with "corkscrew collaterals" around these segments.

Impingement Syndromes

Thoracic outlet syndrome (TOS) encompasses symptomatic compression of the subclavian neurovascular bundle by overlying osseous structures. Compression can be due to abnormalities of the first rib, a cervical rib, hypertrophy of the anterior and middle scalene muscles, clavicular trauma, or an elongated transverse process of C7. Incidence is estimated to be 1 in 10,000, with roughly equal distribution in men and women. Younger patients are primarily affected with symptoms produced in certain positions, due to repetitive movement, or trauma. Untreated disease can result in disability at a young age.

TOS can be stratified into arterial, venous and neurogenic disease. There is higher incidence of neurogenic TOS, however, only the vascular manifestations will be discussed in this section. Venous TOS often presents as axillary and subclavian vein thrombosis (Paget–Schroetter syndrome) with discoloration, edema, and pain and occasionally pulmonary embolism. This presentation may be preceded by intense physical activity, resulting in the moniker "effort thrombosis." Treatment involves endovascular thrombolysis or thrombectomy and anticoagulation. Arterial TOS is the least common form of TOS (<3%) but generally carries the worst consequences if left untreated. Bony abnormalities in conjunction with arterial stenosis, occlusion, or poststenotic dilatation characterize this form of TOS. Patients present with upper extremity ischemia and or embolism. Treatment involves thrombectomy with possible thrombolysis and surgical decompression of the thoracic outlet with removal of the first cervical rib, scalenectomy, and possible arterial reconstruction. Diagnosis of TOS requires and adequate history and physical and supplemental imaging. A chest radiograph or CT can evaluate for bony abnormalities and exclude upper lobe neoplasia that can cause similar presentation. CTA and MRA are both helpful in the examination of TOS, and multiple sequences can be acquired with the patient in different positions (Fig. 32B.11). DSA can provide definitive imaging confirmation, especially if an intervention is already planned. It is important to note that stenosis alone is not adequate to diagnose TOS alone, as this can occur in certain positions in a large portion of the population.

Popliteal entrapment syndrome describes compression of the popliteal artery by the medial head of the gastrocnemius muscle. This rare syndrome manifests as intermittent claudication in young adults without atherosclerotic risk factors. Prompt diagnosis is paramount, as progressive arterial damage can lead to loss of limb. Occasionally, unaffected individuals may demonstrate dynamic occlusion of the vessel, so correlation with history of claudication is necessary. MRA is the preferred imaging modality due to excellent evaluation of the soft tissue surrounding the popliteal artery. To halt the progression of arterial damage, treatment requires surgical division of the musculotendinous structures compressing the artery with occasional vessel reconstruction.

May–Thurner syndrome is characterized by compression of the **left** common iliac vein between the **right** common iliac artery and a lumbar vertebral body. This syndrome is most common in young to middle-aged women (72% of cases). Extrinsic compression is often asymptomatic, but can cause left lower extremity DVT, postthrombotic syndrome, pain, edema, venous insufficiency, lipodermatosclerosis, and rarely pulmonary embolism. Symptomatic patients often present with left lower extremity DVT, which may be aggravated by immobility, pregnancy, dehydration, and infection. Affected patients may complain of a feeling of fullness in the affected extremity with activity. While venography is the gold standard for imaging, vascular ultrasound is a quick, safe, and cost-effective examination to assess DVT and evaluate for venous compression. MRV can provide more detailed anatomic definition, such as evaluation of vessel diameter and visualization of thrombi. IVUS provides the highest degree of sensitivity, given the risks associated with angiography. Endovascular treatment of the DVT can be pursued in appropriate candidates with possible thrombectomy and thrombolysis. An underlying cause of venous thromboembolism should be excluded, and anticoagulation is generally pursued, despite suboptimal results due to the anatomic obstruction. Once DVT resolution has been achieved, early stenting of the narrowed vessel is recommended followed by antiplatelet therapy in order to decrease the burden of rethrombosis and postthrombotic syndrome.

Inherited Disorders of the Vessel Wall

Marfan syndrome is an autosomal-dominant genetic disorder caused by a mutation in the fibrillin-1 gene (FBN1) with a prevalence of 1/5,000. This protein is a component of the extracellular matrix and patients present with skeletal (tall stature/arachnodactyly, pectus deformity), ocular (ectopia

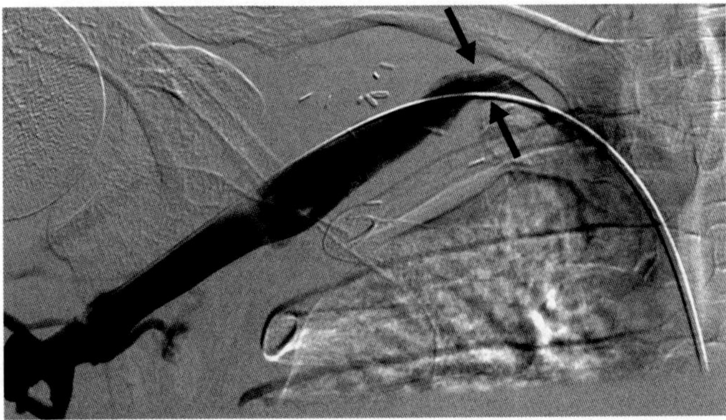

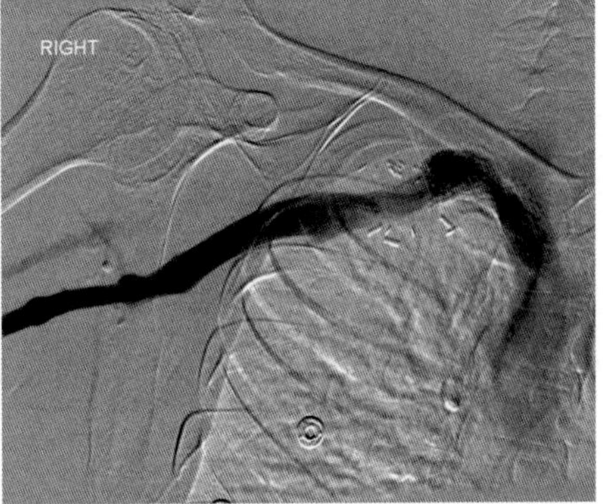

FIGURE 32B.11. **Venous Thoracic Outlet Syndrome.** Young male with severe upper extremity swelling which worsens with certain arm positions. Venogram pre and post intervention demonstrates narrowing of the right brachiocephalic vein at the first rib (*arrows*) with subsequent resolution after thrombectomy and stenting.

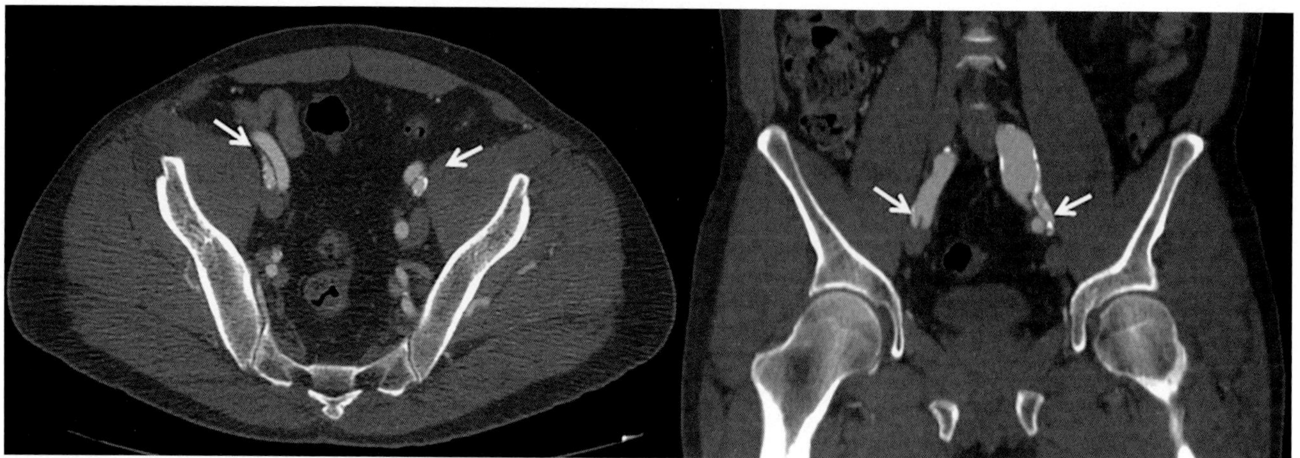

FIGURE 32B.12. **External Iliac Artery Dissection Secondary to Ehlers–Danlos Syndrome.** Middle-aged male with known Ehlers–Danlos syndrome and several other foci of intimal irregularity. CTA demonstrates bilateral external iliac artery dissection.

lentis), and cardiovascular deformities. Cardiovascular manifestations typically affect the cardiac valves and the thoracic aorta, with peripheral arteries less often involved. Patients with Marfan syndrome are recommended CTA or MRA of the entire aorta to assess for dilatation for screening, and annually if an abnormality is detected.

Ehlers–Danlos syndrome (EDS) is a collection of disorders characterized by specific mutations in the subtypes of collagen. Type IV or vascular EDS occurs due to an autosomal-dominant mutation of COL3A1 affecting the alpha chain of type III collagen with an estimated prevalence of 1/90,000. A clinical diagnosis is achieved with at least two of the four criteria: easy bruising, thin skin with visible veins, characteristic facial features, and rupture of arteries, uterus, or intestines. Vascular complications are common with 75% of patients experiencing at least one major event by the age of 40 years. Common complications of the disease include arterial dissection, spontaneous rupture, and aneurysm formation, with dissection and rupture accounting for the majority of deaths (Fig. 32B.12). Angiography is associated with a high complication rate due to the friable nature of these vessels, therefore noninvasive modalities such as MRA and CTA are preferred.

Loeys–Dietz syndrome (LDS) is a rare autosomal-dominant connective tissue disorder caused by mutations in several subtypes of the TGFBR gene. The syndrome is characterized by hypertelorism, bifid uvula/cleft palate, arterial tortuosity, and aortic aneurysm. LDS has systemic skeletal, skin, cardiovascular, and nervous system manifestations with arterial involvement being widespread and risk of dissection and aneurysm throughout. Prevalence is estimated at 1/1,000,000 and the mean age of death is approximately 26 years with the leading causes of mortality being aortic dissection and cerebral hemorrhage. Imaging should begin at an early age with annual echocardiograms and MRA of the head/neck/abdomen/pelvis with 3D reconstruction to assess aneurysm burden biannually if there is no apparent pathology. If abnormalities are noted, imaging should be scheduled more frequently and patients with severe craniofacial manifestations are at an increased risk of vascular pathology. Treatment involves aggressive blood pressure control and favors surgical intervention over an endovascular approach.

Fibromuscular dysplasia is a nonatherosclerotic, noninflammatory vascular disease of medium-sized vessels classified by the location of the lesion in the vessel wall. The most common locations include the renal, carotid, and vertebral arteries. Common presenting symptoms include refractory hypertension, headache, dizziness, and pulsatile tinnitus. Medial hyperplasia is the most common subtype of FMD and displays the characteristic "string of pearls" on imaging that consists of focal narrowing interspersed with small aneurysms (Fig. 32B.13). PTA has proven to be an effective treatment for FMD with surgical revascularization as a second-line treatment due to its increased rate of morbidity.

Acquired Disorders of the Arterial Wall

Just as in the thoracic and abdominal aorta, peripheral arterial aneurysms (PAAs) can form in the lower extremity arteries.

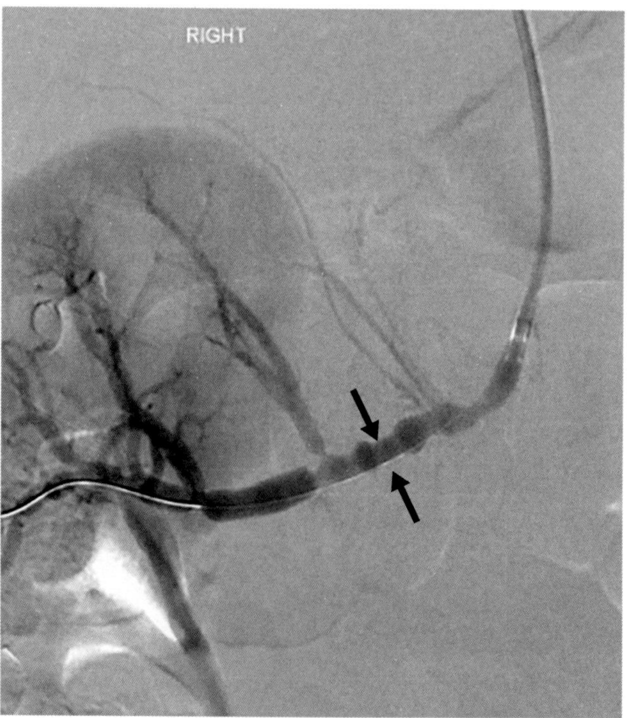

FIGURE 32B.13. **Fibromuscular Dysplasia.** Young female with unexplained renal dysfunction. Right renal angiogram demonstrates the typical beaded appearance of medial fibromuscular dysplasia (*arrows*).

Similar to aortic aneurysm, risk factors include age, sex, atherosclerosis, and hypertension. The most common site of PAA is the popliteal artery. A popliteal artery is considered aneurysmal if the diameter exceeds 2 cm, or there are symptoms such as knee pain or ALI. Aneurysms of the common iliac artery are often bilateral, and are associated with concomitant abdominal aneurysm. In general, the iliac and femoral arteries are considered aneurysmal if the vessel diameter exceeds 2 to 2.5 cm. Recent literature suggests that asymptomatic CFA and SFA aneurysms can be observed up to 3.5 cm in size. Serial imaging is best achieved with CTA. Treatment of PAA is varied, and there is increasing utilization of endovascular techniques such as exclusion by a covered stent or embolization. Complex cases may require open surgical or hybrid approach.

PAA may present in a rare congenital variant known as **persistent sciatic artery**. The sciatic artery is an important vessel in development, but naturally regresses as the CFA develops. In some patients, however, there is altered development of the CFA and the sciatic artery persists as the dominant blood supply to the lower extremity. This may be an incidental finding in some patients, whereas other affected patients can present with claudication or even ALI. CTA and DSA can reliably diagnose persistent sciatic artery, and treatment depends on whether the patient is symptomatic, or aneurysm size, if present (Figs. 32B.14 to 32B.16).

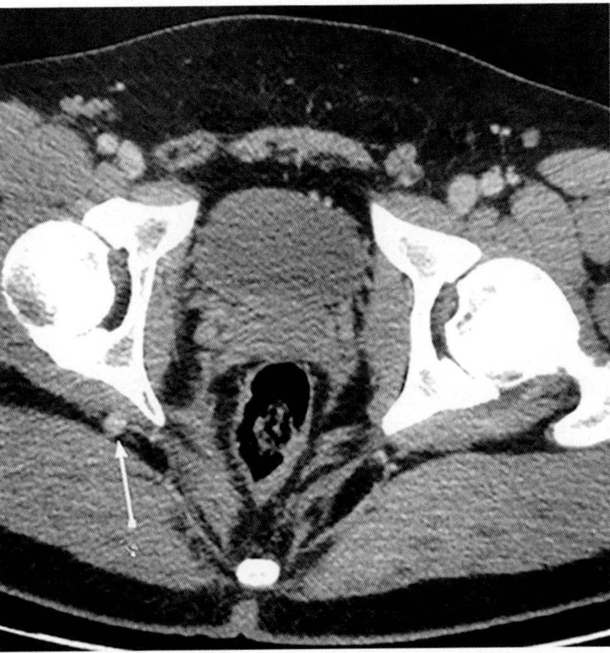

FIGURE 32B.14. Persistent Sciatic Artery. *White arrow* demonstrates incidental finding of persistent sciatic artery opacified by contrast on axial contrast enhanced CT.

Exercise-related endofibrosis is a rare condition most associated with competitive cycling. Repetitive motions at the hip associated with high-velocity, long-distance cycling can cause chronic impaction of the EIA bilaterally against a hypertrophied psoas muscle. Luminal endofibrosis can ensue from chronic trauma. Typical patients are young to middle-aged males with a long history of cycling. Symptoms can manifest as lower extremity cramping and numbness with activity. Imaging demonstrates narrowing and tortuosity of the EIA, more often on the left, but sometimes bilaterally. ABIs and vascular waveforms may decrease with activity. Treatment entails lifestyle modification and possible open surgical repair.

AVF/Pseudoaneurysm

Acquired vascular injuries, such as **pseudoaneurysm (PSA)** and **arteriovenous fistula (AVF)** can be encountered in the extremities after trauma, with vascular access–related trauma being one of the most common. AVF entails an abnormal connection from the artery to the adjacent vein, while PSA describes a defect in the arterial media and intima. In PSA, the sac contains only blood and the adventitia, compared to a true aneurysm, containing all three layers of the vessel wall. Symptoms vary, but there may be pain, limb ischemia, or obvious pulsatile lesions presenting at a variable period of time from the inciting event. Well-known risk factors include low femoral puncture, penetrating trauma, and severe fractures (Fig. 32B.17). If left untreated, AVF and PSA may serve as a source of thrombosis, embolism, infection, or high output failure. Due to only being contained by the adventitia, a PSA can rupture causing hemorrhage. Duplex Doppler ultrasound is the initial study of choice. In PSA, the neck, or defect in the vessel well, can be

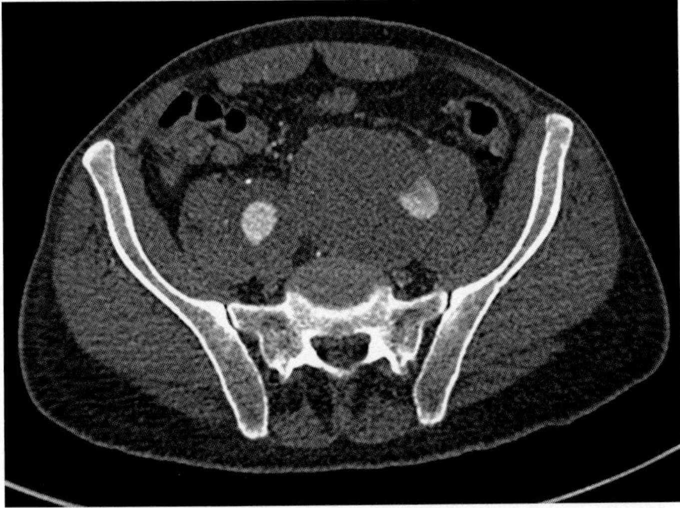

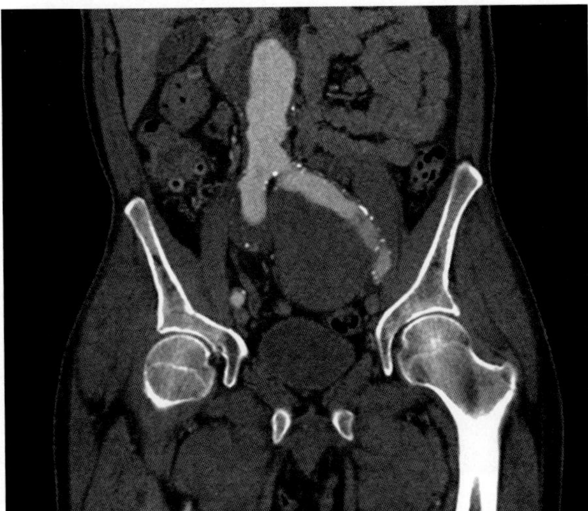

FIGURE 32B.15. Common Iliac Artery Aneurysm. Axial and Coronal MDCT CTA of bilateral external iliac artery aneurysms. Note the majority of the lumen is filled with mural thrombus.

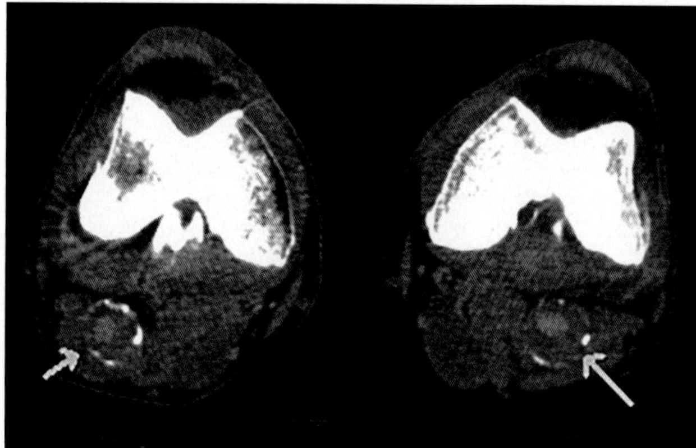

FIGURE 32B.16. **Popliteal Artery Aneurysm.** Elderly male with incidental aneurysm discovered on knee radiograph. CTA demonstrating bilateral popliteal artery aneurysms (*arrow*).

identified, as well as the "yin–yang" sign, describing the swirling of high-velocity blood on color flow. Ultrasound of AVF may demonstrate a connection from the artery to the vein, and possibly arterial waveforms in the adjacent vein on spectral Doppler. Other ultrasound findings in AVF include dampened arterial waveforms and decreased diastolic flow. Treatment of PSA can be obtained with image-guided thrombin injection of the neck, or excluding the defect with a covered stent. AVF can also be managed with endovascular exclusion in some scenarios, with some complex anomalies requiring surgery.

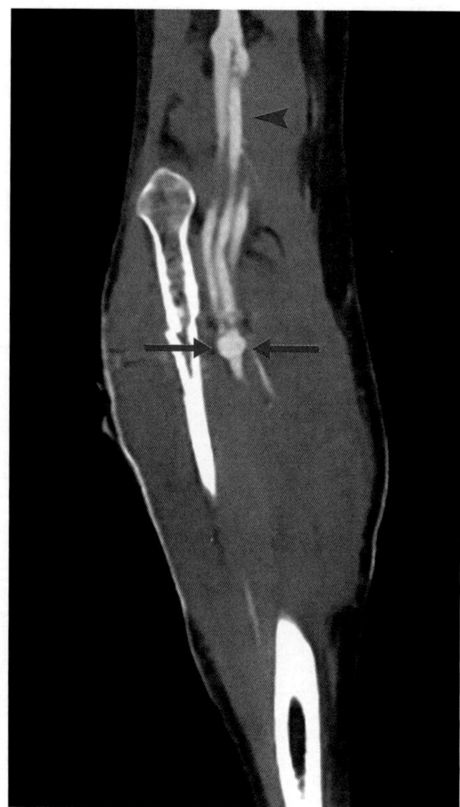

FIGURE 32B.17. **Traumatic Arteriovenous Fistula.** Young male who suffered penetrating ballistic wound of the lower extremity. CTA demonstrates arterial wall outpouching (*red arrows*) with venous contamination (*red arrowhead*), compatible with AVF of the TP trunk.

SUMMARY

PAD is a common illness with a significant disease burden. Risk factors include lifestyle choices, concomitant cardiovascular disease, autoimmune disease, and genetic syndromes. Imaging plays a wide role in the diagnosis and staging of PAD. Treatment ranges from medical management to surgical and endovascular techniques.

Suggested Readings

Ahn S, Min SK, Min SI, et al. Treatment strategy for persistent sciatic artery and novel classification reflecting anatomic status. *Eur J Vasc Endovasc Surg* 2016;52:360–369.

Altin RS, Flicker S, Naidech HJ. Pseudoaneurysm and arteriovenous fistula after femoral artery catheterization: association with low femoral punctures. *AJR Am J Roentgenol* 1989;152:629–631.

Barkat M, Torella F, Antoniou GA. Drug-eluting balloon catheters for lower limb peripheral arterial disease: the evidence to date. *Vasc Health Risk Manag* 2016;12:199–208.

Beridze N, Frishman WH. Vascular Ehlers-Danlos syndrome: pathophysiology, diagnosis, and prevention and treatment of its complications. *Cardiol Rev* 2012;20:4–7.

Berridge DC, Kessel DO, Robertson I. Surgery versus thrombolysis for initial management of acute limb ischaemia. *Cochrane Database Syst Rev* 2013;6:CD002784.

Bonow RO, Smaha LA, Smith SC, Mensah GA, Lenfant C. World Heart Day 2002: the international burden of cardiovascular disease: responding to the emerging global epidemic. *Circulation* 2002;106:1602–1605.

Buller LT, Jose J, Baraga M, Lesniak B. Thoracic outlet syndrome: Current concepts, imaging features, and therapeutic strategies. *Am J Orthop (Belle Mead NJ)* 2015;44:376–382.

Chu LC, Johnson PT, Dietz HC, Fishman EK. CT angiographic evaluation of genetic vascular disease: role in detection, staging, and management of complex vascular pathologic conditions. *AJR Am J Roentgenol* 2014;202:1120–1129.

Conte MS, Pomposelli FB, Clair DG, et al. Society for Vascular Surgery practice guidelines for atherosclerotic occlusive disease of the lower extremities: management of asymptomatic disease and claudication. *J Vasc Surg* 2015;61:2S–41S.

Craig P, Zuchowski A, Young S, Lunos S, Golzarian J, Rosenberg M. Results of endovascular management of May-Thurner syndrome in the acute, subacute, and chronic setting. *J Vasc Interv Radiol* 2017;28:S113.

Creager MA, Kaufman JA, Conte MS. Clinical practice. Acute limb ischemia. *N Engl J Med* 2012;366:2198–2206.

Dargon PT, Landry GJ. Buerger's disease. *Ann Vasc Surg* 2012;26:871–880.

Dawson J, Fitridge R. Update on aneurysm disease: current insights and controversies: peripheral aneurysms: when to intervene—is rupture really a danger? *Prog Cardiovasc Dis* 2013;56:26–35.

Deak Z, Treitl M, Reiser MF, Degenhart C. [Angiographic diagnosis of acral circulatory disorders of the upper extremities]. *Radiologe* 2010;50:879–886.

Desy NM, Spinner RJ. The etiology and management of cystic adventitial disease. *J Vasc Surg* 2014;60:235–245, 245.e1–245.e11.

Egorova NN, Guillerme S, Gelijns A, et al. An analysis of the outcomes of a decade of experience with lower extremity revascularization including limb salvage, lengths of stay, and safety. *J Vasc Surg* 2010;51:878–885, 885.e1.

Enezate TH, Omran J, Mahmud E, et al. Endovascular versus surgical treatment for acute limb ischemia: a systematic review and meta-analysis of clinical trials. *Cardiovasc Diagn Ther* 2017;7:264–271.

Ennis H, Hughes M, Anderson ME, Wilkinson J, Herrick AL. Calcium channel blockers for primary Raynaud's phenomenon. *Cochrane Database Syst Rev* 2016;2:CD002069.

Farsad K, Keller FS, Kandarpa K. Vascular access and catheter directed angiography. In: Kandarpa K, Machan L, Durham JD, eds. *Handbook of Interventional Radiologic Procedures*. 5th ed. Philadelphia, PA: Wolters Kluwer; 2016:14.

Fleischmann D, Hallett RL, Rubin GD. CT angiography of peripheral arterial disease. *J Vasc Interv Radiol* 2006;17:3–26.

Fong JK, Poh AC, Tan AG, Taneja R. Imaging findings and clinical features of abdominal vascular compression syndromes. *AJR Am J Roentgenol* 2014;203:29–36.

Gates J, Hartnell GG. Optimized diagnostic angiography in high-risk patients with severe peripheral vascular disease. *Radiographics* 2000;20:121–133.

Geraghty PJ, Mewissen MW, Jaff MR, Ansel GM; VIBRANT Investigators. Three-year results of the VIBRANT trial of VIABAHN endoprosthesis versus bare nitinol stent implantation for complex superficial femoral artery occlusive disease. *J Vasc Surg* 2013;58:386–395.e4.

Goksu E, Yuruktumen A, Kaya H. Traumatic pseudoaneurysm and arteriovenous fistula detected by bedside ultrasound. *J Emerg Med* 2014;46:667–669.

Insall RL, Davies RJ, Prout WG. Significance of Buerger's test in the assessment of lower limb ischaemia. *J R Soc Med* 1989;82:729–731.

Jaff MR, White CJ, Hiatt WR, et al. An update on methods for revascularization and expansion of the TASC lesion classification to include below-the-knee arteries: A supplement to the inter-society consensus for the management of peripheral arterial disease (TASC II). *Ann Vasc Dis* 2015;20:465–478.

Khawaja FJ, Kullo IJ. Novel markers of peripheral arterial disease. *Vasc Med* 2009;14:381–392.

Kock MC, Dijkshoorn ML, Pattynama PM, Myriam Hunink MG. Multi-detector row computed tomography angiography of peripheral arterial disease. *Eur Radiol* 2007;17:3208–3222.

Lanzer P, Boehm M, Sorribas V, et al. Medial vascular calcification revisited: review and perspectives. *Eur Heart J* 2014;35:1515–1525.

Lawrence PF, Harlander-Locke MP, Oderich GS, et al. The current management of isolated degenerative femoral artery aneurysms is too aggressive for their natural history. *J Vasc Surg* 2014;59:343–349.

Liegl CA, McGrath MA. Ergotism: Case report and review of the literature. *Int J Angiol* 2016;25:e8–e11.

Lo RC, Bensley RP, Dahlberg SE, et al. Presentation, treatment, and outcome differences between men and women undergoing revascularization or amputation for lower extremity peripheral arterial disease. *J Vasc Surg* 2014;59:409–418.e3.

MacCarrick G, Black JH 3rd, Bowdin S, et al. Loeys-Dietz syndrome: a primer for diagnosis and management. *Genet Med* 2014;16:576–587.

Medhekar AN, Mix DS, Aquina CT, et al. Outcomes for critical limb ischemia are driven by lower extremity revascularization volume, not distance to hospital. *J Vasc Surg* 2017;66:476–487.e1.

Mills JL, Conte MS, Armstrong DG, et al. The society for vascular surgery lower extremity threatened limb classification system: risk stratification based on wound, ischemia, and foot infection (WIfI). *J Vasc Surg* 2014;59:220–234. e1–2.

Mousa AY, AbuRahma AF. May-Thurner syndrome: update and review. *Ann Vasc Surg* 2013;27:984–995.

Murphy TP, Cutlip DE, Regensteiner JG, et al. Supervised exercise versus primary stenting for claudication resulting from aortoiliac peripheral artery disease: six-month outcomes from the claudication: exercise versus endoluminal revascularization (CLEVER) study. *Circulation* 2012;125:130–139.

Norgren L, Hiatt WR, Dormandy JA, et al. Inter-society consensus for the management of peripheral arterial disease. *Int Angiol* 2007;26:81–157.

O'Connell JB, Quiñones-Baldrich WJ. Proper evaluation and management of acute embolic versus thrombotic limb ischemia. *Semin Vasc Surg* 2009; 22:10–16.

O'Connor SC, Gornik HL. Recent developments in the understanding and management of fibromuscular dysplasia. *J Am Heart Assoc* 2014;3:e001259.

Olin JW. Thromboangiitis obliterans (Buerger's disease). *N Engl J Med* 2000;343:864–869.

Olin JW, Sealove BA. Peripheral artery disease: current insight into the disease and its diagnosis and management. *Mayo Clin Proc* 2010;85:678–692.

Owens C. *Rutherford's Vascular Surgery*. 8th ed. Philadelphia, PA: Saunders/ Elsevier; 2014.

Paravastu SC, Regi JM, Turner DR, Gaines PA. A contemporary review of cystic adventitial disease. *Vasc Endovascular Surg* 2012;46:5–14.

Patel NH, Krishnamurthy VN, Kim S, et al. Quality improvement guidelines for percutaneous management of acute lower-extremity ischemia. *J Vasc Interv Radiol* 2013;24:3–15.

Peach G, Schep G, Palfreeman R, Beard JD, Thompson MM, Hinchliffe RJ. Endofibrosis and kinking of the iliac arteries in athletes: a systematic review. *Eur J Vasc Endovasc Surg* 2012;43:208–217.

Pepin M, Schwarze U, Superti-Furga A, Byers PH. Clinical and genetic features of Ehlers-Danlos syndrome type IV, the vascular type. *N Engl J Med* 2000;342:673–680.

Pollak AW, Kramer CM. MRI in lower extremity peripheral arterial disease: recent advancements. *Curr Cardiovasc Imaging Rep* 2013;6:55–60.

Radke RM, Baumgartner H. Diagnosis and treatment of Marfan syndrome: an update. *Heart* 2014;100:1382–1391.

Ramachandra CJ, Mehta A, Guo KW, Wong P, Tan JL, Shim W. Molecular pathogenesis of Marfan syndrome. *Int J Cardiol* 2015;187:585–591.

Raptis CA, Sridhar S, Thompson RW, Fowler KJ, Bhalla S. Imaging of the patient with thoracic outlet syndrome. *Radiographics* 2016;36:984–1000.

Raval MV, Gaba RC, Brown K, Sato KT, Eskandari MK. Percutaneous transluminal angioplasty in the treatment of extensive LSD-induced lower extremity vasospasm refractory to pharmacologic therapy. *J Vasc Interv Radiol* 2008; 19:1227–1230.

Ring DH Jr., Haines GA, Miller DL. Popliteal artery entrapment syndrome: arteriographic findings and thrombolytic therapy. *J Vasc Interv Radiol* 10:713–721.

Rutherford RB, Baker JD, Ernst C, et al. Recommended standards for reports dealing with lower extremity ischemia: revised version. *J Vasc Surg* 1997;26:517–538.

Scully RE, Arnaoutakis DJ, DeBord Smith A, Semel M, Nguyen LL. Estimated annual health care expenditures in individuals with peripheral arterial disease. *J Vasc Surg* 2018;67:558–567.

Sinha S, Houghton J, Holt PJ, Thompson MM, Loftus IM, Hinchliffe RJ. Popliteal entrapment syndrome. *J Vasc Surg* 2012;55:252–262.e30.

Slovut DP, Olin JW. Fibromuscular dysplasia. *N Engl J Med* 2004;350:1862–1871.

Vemuri C, McLaughlin LN, Abuirqeba AA, Thompson RW. Clinical presentation and management of arterial thoracic outlet syndrome. *J Vasc Surg* 2017;65:1429–1439.

Watson JD, Gifford SM, Clouse WD. Biochemical markers of acute limb ischemia, rhabdomyolysis, and impact on limb salvage. *Semin Vasc Surg* 2014; 27:176–181.

Wigley FM, Flavahan NA. Raynaud's phenomenon. *N Engl J Med* 2016;375: 556–565.

Wooltorton E. Risk of stroke, gangrene from ergot drug interactions. *CMAJ* 2003;168:1015.

Yamada T, Ohta T, Ishibashi H, et al. Clinical reliability and utility of skin perfusion pressure measurement in ischemic limbs—comparison with other noninvasive diagnostic methods. *J Vasc Surg* 2008;47:318–323.

Zhong H, Gan J, Zhao Y, et al. Role of CT angiography in the diagnosis and treatment of popliteal vascular entrapment syndrome. *AJR Am J Roentgenol* 2011;197:W1147–W1154.

CHAPTER 33 ■ CENTRAL VENOUS CATHETERS

CLAYTON LI AND DIVYA SRIDHAR

BACKGROUND

Central venous catheters (CVCs) play an integral role in contemporary clinical practice. The first reported central venous catheterization was performed less than a century ago, in 1929 by Werner Forssmann, who boldly cannulated his own right atrium via a cephalic vein access. CVC technology took a leap forward in 1953, when Sven Ivar Seldinger introduced the technique of inserting the catheter over a guidewire to facilitate placement. Today, over 5 million CVCs are inserted annually in the United States alone.

CVCs by definition are a subset of vascular access devices; their unifying characteristic is that the catheter tip terminates in the central superior vena cava, at the cavoatrial junction, or in the central inferior vena cava. This distinguishes them from other vascular access devices, such as peripheral intravenous lines and midline catheters, which terminate in other veins. Most CVCs are 15 to 25 cm in length and are inserted through a central vein such as the internal jugular, subclavian, or femoral vein. Peripherally inserted central catheters (PICCs) are unique CVCs that are inserted through a peripheral access site, such as the basilic or brachial vein, and terminate near the cavoatrial junction.

CVCs' position in the central venous system permits a myriad of uses, many of which cannot be achieved with peripheral venous access. A major indication for central venous catheterization is establishing access for the administration of drugs that cannot safely be administered into the peripheral venous system due to pH, osmolarity, or vesicant or irritant properties. For example, most total parenteral nutrition (TPN) solutions are high osmolarity and therefore must be delivered directly to the central venous system where the high flow rate minimizes potentially damaging effects on local tissues. CVCs are also appropriate in situations when the need to change peripheral access sites every 3 to 4 days is pragmatically disadvantageous, such as when the patient has limited or fragile accessible peripheral veins or requires long-term intravenous therapy. Large-bore CVCs are also used to establish the high-flow access required for extracorporeal blood circuits for dialysis or plasmapheresis. Other indications for central venous access include monitoring oxygen saturation, central venous pressure, and pulmonary artery pressure. CVCs also allow for targeted temperature management and repeated blood sampling.

ELUCIDATING THE TYPES OF CENTRAL VENOUS CATHETERS

CVCs can be divided into four groups: nontunneled, tunneled, totally implantable, and peripherally inserted central catheters, each with a different profile of advantages and limitations. Nontunneled, tunneled, and totally implantable CVCs are also referred to as centrally inserted central catheters (CICCs).

■ CENTRAL VENOUS CATHETERS (CVCs)

Centrally inserted central catheter (CICC)			Peripherally inserted central catheter (PICC)
Nontunneled CVC	Tunneled CVC	Totally implantable CVC	

Nontunneled Central Venous Catheter

The nontunneled CVC can be thought of as the prototypic device that the other CVCs are based upon. These CVCs are designated as nontunneled because they exit the skin at the venous cannulation site. The nontunneled CVC is placed by directly accessing and cannulating one of the central veins, typically the internal jugular, subclavian, or femoral veins. The catheter is then advanced such that the tip rests in the superior vena cava or near the cavoatrial junction for jugular and subclavian access, and in the inferior vena cava for femoral access. Nontunneled CVCs are mainly used for temporary access to the central circulation.

One significant and unique advantage of nontunneled CVCs is that they can be placed emergently in nearly any clinical setting. Thus, they are ideal for quickly establishing venous access to infuse drugs or perform hemodynamic monitoring. Large-bore nontunneled CVCs can provide rapid temporary access for dialysis and plasmapheresis.

Nontunneled CVCs also have several disadvantages. Placement of the catheter is an invasive procedure which traditionally requires a physician; however, more recently, CVCs are beginning to be placed by specially trained nurses in some settings. Nontunneled CVCs also carry a risk of infection due to the proximity of the skin opening to the central venous entry point, more so than the less invasive peripheral intravenous catheters and the more protected tunneled central venous access. All CVCs also confer a risk of deep vein thrombosis (DVT), although this risk is less with CICCs versus PICCs.

Tunneled Central Venous Catheter

Tunneled CVCs are characterized by a physical separation between the site of insertion into the skin and the site of insertion into the accessed vein. They are otherwise similar to nontunneled CVCs. Like other CVCs, the tunneled CVC is inserted into a central vessel like the subclavian or internal jugular vein with its tip positioned at the cavoatrial junction (Fig. 33.1). The external end of the catheter travels through a shallow subcutaneous tunnel to exit at a site several centimeters away from the venipuncture site, typically in the infraclavicular area. A Dacron cuff attached to the catheter is positioned within the subcutaneous tunnel and helps to promote scarring and closure of the tunnel; once healed, the sealed tunnel aids in preventing infection and securing the catheter.

The physical separation of the skin insertion and venipuncture sites affords several advantages to the tunneled CVC. Tunneled CVCs are associated with a lower rate of infection compared with nontunneled CVCs, theoretically because the sealed subcutaneous tunnel limits transit of bacteria from the skin surface along the catheter. Tunneled CVCs are usually placed such that the catheter exits the skin in the infraclavicular area, which is an easier site to clean and maintain compared with the neck area. The configuration of the tunneled catheter is also preferable for many patients because it is more comfortable and aesthetically acceptable compared with catheters which exit from the neck, such as nontunneled CVCs inserted into the internal jugular vein. Finally, tunneled CVCs can provide an appropriate form of long-term venous access in patients with impending or chronic renal failure to aid in preserving the peripheral veins for potential arteriovenous fistula creation; nontunneled CVCs are not indicated for long-term access, and PICCs are contraindicated in these patients due to potential damage to upper extremity veins which may be required for dialysis access. Large-bore tunneled CVCs can be used for long-term dialysis access, although they may be more prone to infection than arteriovenous fistulas and grafts.

Totally Implantable Central Venous Catheters (Ports)

Totally implantable CVCs, also known as ports, are conceptually similar to tunneled CVCs, except that rather than exiting through the skin, the tunneled portion of the catheter attaches to an infusion port underneath the skin. Like the previously discussed tunneled CVCs, the catheter enters the venous system via a central vein with its tip at the cavoatrial junction (Fig. 33.2). A small subcutaneous pocket is created in the chest wall to accommodate the port reservoir, typically in the infraclavicular region. The catheter travels through a subcutaneous tunnel to connect the port site to the venipuncture site. Afterward, the skin over the port pocket is sutured closed. Once the incisions heal, the port system is entirely covered by skin, which protects the CVC from accidental dislodgement

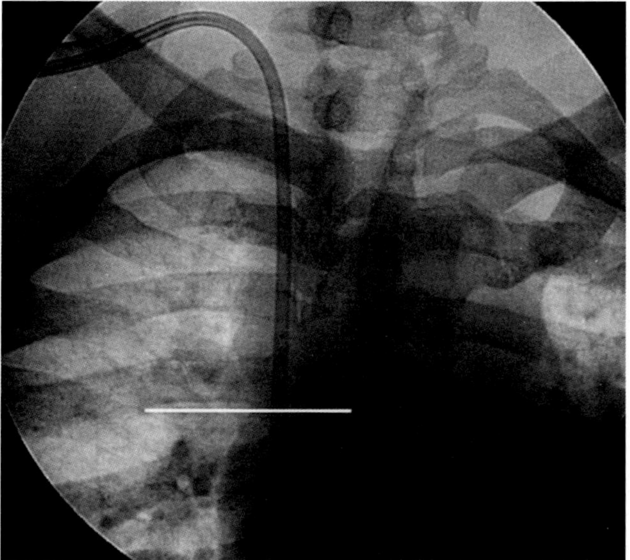

FIGURE 33.1. Fluoroscopic image of right internal jugular tunneled dialysis catheter with proximal tip at cavoatrial junction (*white line*) and distal tip in right atrium. Note the smooth curvature of the catheter at the venous insertion site, which helps avoid kinking and malfunction. (From Heberlein W. Principles of tunneled cuffed catheter placement. *Tech Vasc Interv Radiol* 2011;14[4]:192–197. Figure 33.1, p. 184.)

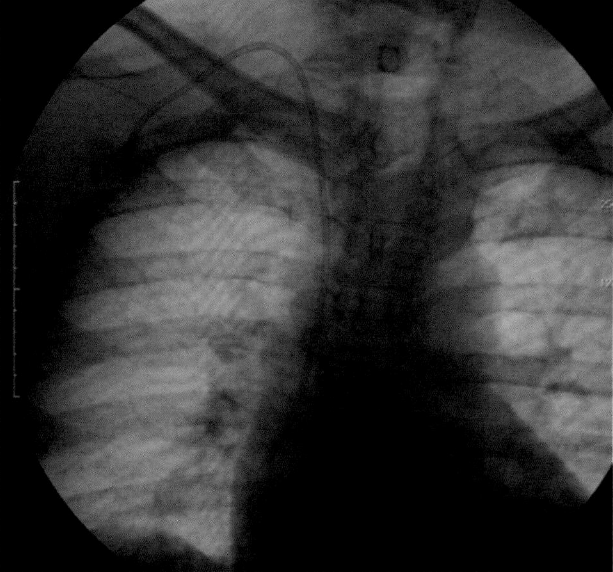

FIGURE 33.2. Fluoroscopic image of right internal jugular port reservoir and catheter, with the tip at the superior cavoatrial junction. Catheter tip position, as well as continuity of the catheter and port reservoir, should be noted in the reports for subsequent imaging. (From Gonda SJ, Li R. Principles of subcutaneous port placement. *Tech Vasc Interv Radiol* 2011;14[4]:198–203. Figure 9, p. 201.)

and infection, and permits safe immersion in water for swimming and bathing.

The port is used by advancing a specialized access needle through the skin into the reservoir using a sterile technique. The port reservoir is typically made of a firm material such as metal or plastic, but has a soft self-sealing septum anteriorly made of silicone or plastic; the septum is palpable beneath the skin. The specialized Huber access needle has a shallow bevel and slight angulation which combine to create a "noncoring" design; that is, the channel it creates through the septum has a tendency to seal itself rather than remove a core of material. Ports are ideal for therapies which require long-term intermittent access, such as chemotherapy. However, the need to access the port before each infusion makes them less ideal for treatments which require frequent access or infusion of large volumes, as with TPN. The low rates of extravasation and infection of ports also make them ideal for the administration of chemotherapeutic agents. Another advantage of ports is that they are more cosmetically appealing since they are concealed beneath the skin.

Peripherally Inserted Central Catheter

PICCs, unlike the previously described catheters, are inserted through a peripheral vein, most commonly the basilic, brachial, or cephalic vein in the medial upper arm. Then, like the other CVCs, the catheter is advanced such that the tip is within the central aspect of the superior vena cava or at the cavoatrial junction (Fig. 33.3).

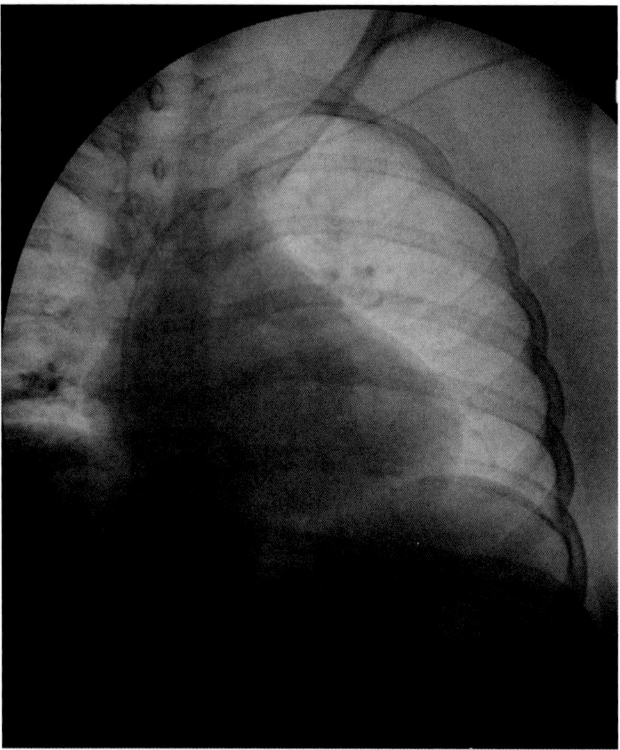

FIGURE 33.3. Fluoroscopic image of left upper extremity PICC with the tip just below the superior cavoatrial junction. PICC tip position will vary slightly with breathing and arm position; expiration and abduction of the arm will cause the PICC tip to appear more central, while inspiration and adduction of the arm will do the opposite. (From Chung HY, Beheshti MV. Principles of non-tunneled central venous access. *Tech Vasc Interv Radiol* 2011;14[4]:186–191. Figure 14, p. 101.)

Compared with other CVCs, PICCs have several advantages. Inserting a catheter into a vein in the arm is safer than accessing central vessels such as the subclavian or internal jugular vein with a lower risk of major bleeding, and without the risks of hemothorax and pneumothorax. In addition, many PICCs can be placed by teams of nurses trained in vascular access, without the direct supervision of a physician, increasing their availability and cost-effectiveness. The arm access site is more cosmetically appealing, easier to maintain and keep clean, and more manageable for patients to self-administer medications and fluids outside of the hospital setting.

However, PICCs are not without their disadvantages. Placement of multiple PICCs at the same site is associated with increased difficulty of placement, likely due to vessel scarring and stenosis. As a result, it is prudent to consider placing other types of CVCs in patients who have already had multiple PICCs placed in both arms. Placement is often difficult in pediatric patients due to narrow vasculature and may be associated with more complications due to the relatively large catheter size within these smaller vessels. PICCs are relatively contraindicated in patients with significant renal dysfunction due to associated risks of venous thrombosis and stenosis which could limit future options for peripheral access creation for hemodialysis.

VENIPUNCTURE TECHNIQUE AND RELEVANT ANATOMY

Internal Jugular Vein Approach

Cannulation of the right or left internal jugular vein is a common approach for CVC insertion due to both ease of access and low associated complication rates. Each internal jugular vein is formed by the ipsilateral sphenoid sinus as it exits the jugular foramen. From there, the internal jugular vein courses inferiorly lateral to the vagus nerve and internal carotid artery, then common carotid artery more inferiorly, within the carotid sheath. In the thorax, the internal jugular vein joins the subclavian vein to form the brachiocephalic trunk. The right internal jugular vein is typically preferred over the left because it offers a straighter course to the superior vena cava, and is often larger in caliber. Moreover, the right pulmonary apex is lower than the left, so the right pleural membranes are more distant from the right internal jugular vein, theoretically lessening the risk of pneumothorax.

Cannulation of the vein can be achieved using anatomic landmarks or ultrasound guidance; however, in contemporary practice, ultrasound guidance is used almost universally, given the ready availability and low cost of ultrasound, as well as the greater safety and better success rates associated with direct visualization during access. Using ultrasound, the internal jugular vein and needle can both be visualized continuously while attempting cannulation. Due to the relatively superficial location of the internal jugular vein, a high-frequency ultrasound probe should be used, generating a higher-resolution image. The probe is placed near the apex of the triangle formed by the heads of the sternocleidomastoid muscle. Practitioner preferences regarding probe orientation vary. The short-axis view is ideal when first inserting the needle into the skin because it shows the internal jugular vein and carotid artery simultaneously, allowing the practitioner to confirm the needle trajectory and avoid arterial puncture (Fig. 33.4). Once the needle entry into the jugular vein is confirmed, some operators prefer to change to the long-axis view to confirm wire advancement into the lumen of the internal jugular vein.

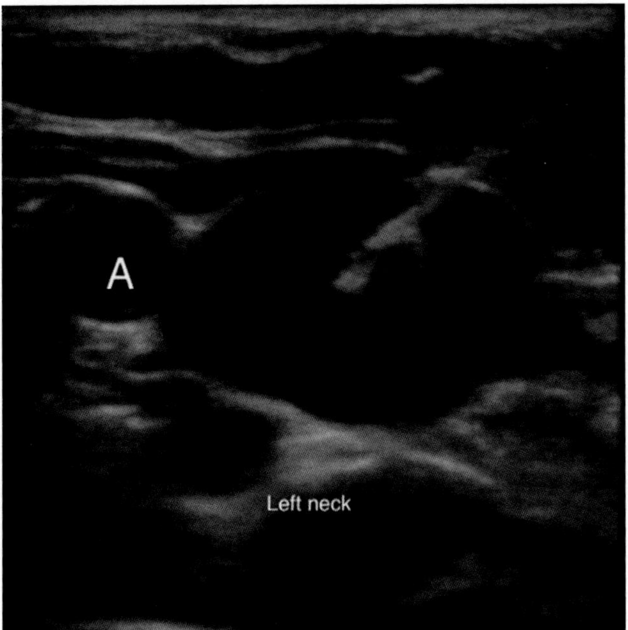

FIGURE 33.4. Echogenic needle tip within left internal jugular vein on short-axis ultrasound image; note proximity of the carotid artery (*A*). The short-axis view permits simultaneous visualization of the artery and vein, which may help avert inadvertent arterial puncture. (From Chung HY, Beheshti MV. Principles of non-tunneled central venous access. *Tech Vasc Interv Radiol* 2011;14[4]:186–191. Figure 3, p. 187.)

Subclavian Vein Approach

Cannulation of the subclavian vein is not as easily performed under ultrasound guidance, but can be a desirable approach to establishing central venous access because it is more comfortable for patients. Compared with internal jugular access, subclavian access has an overall similar rate of complications. Subclavian access is associated with a higher rate of insertion failure but a lower rate of catheter colonization by infectious organisms. Notably, the two approaches have shown no difference in the risk of bloodstream infection. The subclavian vein is the central continuation of the axillary vein from the lateral border of the first rib and delivers venous drainage from the arm to the central venous system. The subclavian vein courses anteroinferiorly alongside the subclavian artery, and the two are separated by the anterior scalene muscle. It is also located posterior to the clavicle and the subclavius muscle. In the superior thorax at the level of the sternoclavicular joint, the subclavian veins join the internal jugular veins on either side to form the brachiocephalic trunks. These then join to form the superior vena cava.

There exist both supra- and infraclavicular approaches to cannulating the subclavian vein. Ultrasound visualization can be challenging due to shadowing by the clavicle; often access into the subclavian vein near its confluence with the jugular vein can be achieved under ultrasound guidance via a supraclavicular approach. Infraclavicular access into the subclavian vein is more typically achieved using anatomic landmarks due to the difficulty of ultrasound visualization from this approach. The lung apex is in close proximity to the subclavian vein, and thus great care should be taken to ensure needle visualization throughout access and avoid advancement of the needle beyond the vein.

Femoral Vein Approach

Femoral venous access has historically been associated with a higher rate of infection due to difficulties in maintaining sterility at the groin. However, advances in skin sterilization and catheter maintenance have now brought it in line with other approaches. The femoral vein conducts the majority of the venous drainage from the lower extremity. It is a continuation of the popliteal vein proximal to the adductor hiatus, and ascends the thigh to the groin. Near the groin, it takes a superficial course through the femoral triangle, bordered by the inguinal ligament, sartorius muscle, and adductor longus. The femoral vein is most commonly accessed here, in the femoral triangle, as it courses medial to the femoral artery. From there, the femoral vein dives deep to the inguinal ligament to enter the pelvis as the external iliac vein.

Prior to femoral venous access, the patient is placed in the supine position; abduction and external rotation of the thigh will provide the best access to the femoral triangle. The femoral vein may be localized by palpating for the pulse of the femoral artery as it courses through the femoral triangle, just inferior to the inguinal ligament; the femoral vein will lie just medial to the artery, so the access needle should be directed medial to the femoral arterial pulse.

Although the femoral vein can be localized and accessed by palpation, the use of real-time ultrasound guidance is associated with a significantly higher rate of success. The short-axis sonographic view allows visualization of both the femoral artery and vein, which can help avert inadvertent arterial puncture. Once the needle trajectory is confirmed on short-axis view, the long-axis view may be used to visualize the needle and wire passage into the lumen of the vein.

POTENTIAL COMPLICATIONS

Mechanical Complications

Various mechanical complications can occur during the placement of CVCs. Increased complication rates are associated with very low or high BMI, prior surgery, prior radiation therapy, number of previous venipunctures or prior catheter placement, advanced age, and greater time needed to place the catheter. The most common mechanical complication is failure to place the catheter, followed by accidental arterial puncture. Pneumothorax is the most common major complication of subclavian venous catheterization and occurs in 1.5% to 2.3% of cases. The most frequent major complication of femoral venous catheterization is femoral and retroperitoneal hematoma, occurring in up to 1.3% of cases. Rarely, the thoracic duct can be inadvertently injured during placement of a CVC into the internal jugular or subclavian veins. Ultrasound guidance allows for visualization of the needle and vascular anatomy, including any variant findings, during placement and has been shown to decrease the mechanical complication rate and failure rate.

Even when the target vein is successfully cannulated, errors in catheter positioning can lead to complications. For example, CVCs which are erroneously advanced into the right atrium can cause arrhythmias and, in rare extreme cases, asystolic cardiac arrest. Mechanical complications can also occur delayed from the time of placement. For example, catheters that are not sufficiently secured can migrate due to accidental manipulation. If catheters are advanced too far, they can perforate the myocardium. Sometimes, catheters can fracture, with free pieces of the catheter potentially embolizing to other areas of the body.

Infection

As with any procedure, central line insertion carries a risk of infection. The Center for Disease Control and Prevention defines two terms referring to infection as a complication of central venous catheterization: catheter-related bloodstream infection and central line–associated bloodstream infection (CLABSI). Of the two, CLABSI is the broader and more commonly used term and only requires (1) laboratory evidence of bloodstream infection, that is positive blood culture, not related to infection at another site, (2) insertion of the central line at least 48 hours prior to blood culture, and (3) presence of the catheter at the time of blood culture or removal not more than 1 day before blood culture. By contrast, catheter-related blood infection is more difficult to establish, requiring proof that the infection originated from the catheter.

As with any other type of infection, CLABSI may be occult or may present with fever or leukocytosis. Inflammation and presence of purulent fluid at the insertion site are more specific but less sensitive signs. The suspicion for CLABSI is higher when blood cultures show organisms such as *Staphylococcus aureus* and coagulase-negative staphylococci which tend to be associated with CVC infection.

Infection related to CVCs can be caused by colonization of either the intra- or extraluminal surface of the catheter. The extraluminal surface can become colonized during insertion of the catheter, particularly if the skin surface is improperly sterilized prior to the procedure. In this scenario, microorganisms from the skin surface are brought into the body on the extraluminal surface of the catheter. The extraluminal surface can also become colonized after insertion due to migration of microorganisms along the catheter tract. Hematogenous spread from another location in the body can also cause colonization of the extraluminal surface. In contrast, intraluminal colonization can occur due to improper cleaning leading to contamination of the catheter hubs during use. Although infusion of contaminated fluids into the catheter can theoretically also cause intraluminal colonization, this occurs less frequently due to quality control.

Meta-analysis has shown that despite their peripheral site of insertion, PICCs are associated with a similar rate of CLABSI as centrally inserted CVCs.

To minimize intraluminal colonization and CLABSI, the catheter hub or access port should be decontaminated before and after each use. Patients' catheters should be regularly reviewed and promptly removed once they are no longer medically indicated. On a systems level, regular hand washing, full barrier precautions during insertion, cleaning the skin with chlorhexidine, avoidance of the femoral site for insertion, and removal of unnecessary catheters have been shown to significantly decrease the rate of CLABSI in the ICU setting.

The use of catheters coated with antiseptic agents like chlorhexidine–silver sulfadiazine and minocycline–rifampicin reduces the risk of CLABSI but has no effect on the rate of sepsis and mortality. Thus, antiseptic-impregnated catheters are only indicated for patients who require longer durations of treatment and are located in an environment where the risk of CLABSI is high. In addition, although the topic is controversial, some studies have shown multilumen catheters to be associated with increased incidence of CLABSI. Thus, catheters with the minimal number of lumens that is appropriate for patient care should be selected. Notably, antibiotic prophylaxis has been shown to have no effect on the risk of CLABSI and is therefore not recommended.

Occlusion

CVC lumen occlusion is a common problem, affecting up to 25% of CVCs that are placed. Occlusion is defined as the decreased ability to infuse solutions into or withdraw solutions from the CVC. Partial occlusion presents with reduced flow rate, increased resistance during manual administration of infusate, or sustained increase in pressure and activation of alarms when using infusion devices. Total occlusion is defined as complete inability to infuse fluid to or withdraw fluid from a CVC lumen.

Etiologies for CVC occlusion include (1) mechanical causes, (2) thrombosis, (3) chemical precipitates, and (4) lipid residues. Occlusion of CVCs has negative implications for patient care and creates additional costs for the health system. Patients are exposed to additional risk of morbidity and mortality, not only from potential interruptions in drug regimens or nutritional support, but also from potential complications of interventions required to restore CVC patency or replacement of the CVC.

Mechanical Causes of Occlusion. Mechanical problems related to the various components of the catheter can cause occlusion. Flow through the CVC may be impeded because it is kinked or damaged. The catheter hub may be damaged. Stopcocks and clamps can also contribute to occlusion. Many CVCs have a filter which may become clogged due to a drug incompatibility. If this is the case, caretakers should replace the filter and resolve the incompatibility.

Thrombosis. Occlusion, both partial and complete, commonly occurs due to fibrin deposition and eventually formation of thrombus. Fibrin can deposit within the catheter resulting in an intraluminal thrombus, at the distal tip of the CVC forming a fibrin tail, around the wall of the blood vessel forming a mural thrombus, and as a layer around the CVC forming a fibrin sheath. This accumulation of fibrin does not result from a single instance of stationary blood within the catheter but rather repeated reflux of blood into the CVC lumen resulting in a mature fibronectin and fibrin biofilm. Thrombosis has been reported to occur in 6.6% to 25% of femoral catheterizations and 10% to 50% of subclavian catheterizations.

When symptomatic, thrombosis can present with swelling, discomfort, erythema, and dilation of collateral vessels in the affected limb. Patients may also have a low-grade fever. The diagnosis is made using duplex ultrasonography or contrast venography. Notably, thrombosis may be asymptomatic and be found incidentally or during screening. Thrombosis can lead to further complications such as catheter and venous occlusion. Thromboembolism can also occur, particularly when the thrombosed catheter is removed. This can lead to subsequent pulmonary embolism or more rarely paradoxical embolus through a patent foramen ovale. Initiation of anticoagulation should be considered prior to removal of a catheter with an associated thrombosis. Thrombosis of a CVC is also associated with increased incidence of CLABSI.

There is not sufficient evidence to warrant anticoagulant prophylaxis as a means of preventing complications of catheter-associated thrombosis. A meta-analysis including noncancer patients on TPN and cancer patients showed that anticoagulant prophylaxis decreased the risk of catheter-related thrombosis but had no effect on the rate of pulmonary embolus or overall mortality. Therefore, anticoagulant prophylaxis is not recommended.

Once thrombosis has occurred, however, anticoagulant is warranted as it reduces the risk of embolism, recurrent thrombosis, and postthrombotic syndrome. The evidence supporting the use of thrombolytic therapy is less robust. A Cochrane review revealed only weak evidence supporting the beneficial effects of urokinase and alteplase in the treatment of CVC occlusion. Moreover, it found no evidence to support the safety of their use. In practice, however, low-dose intracatheter thrombolytic therapy is often used as an initial treatment for catheter occlusion, although not catheter-associated thrombosis, prior to attempting more invasive maneuvers or catheter replacement.

The previously mentioned findings apply to all types of CVCs. Studies looking specifically at PICCs have shown that they are associated with a 2.5-fold increased risk of DVT when compared with centrally inserted CVCs. Therefore, PICC placement should ideally be avoided in patients with a baseline hypercoagulable state.

Chemical Precipitate. Precipitation is also a cause of CVC occlusion, whether it is infusion of preformed precipitant or intraluminal precipitation from infusate. Precipitation is known to occur with TPN and various drugs.

TPN carries the risk of formation of crystalline precipitates, most commonly calcium phosphate. Visual inspection is one obvious strategy to prevent infusion of precipitates. However, this is complicated by the fact that certain types of TPN solutions, such as all-in-one and total-nutrient admixtures, are opaque thus making precipitates harder to visualize. Various pharmacologic strategies can be employed while making TPN solution to minimize the risk of calcium phosphate precipitation.

Once it has occurred, calcium phosphate precipitation can be treated by infusion of 0.1-N hydrochloric acid solution into the CVC. Hydrochloric acid solubilizes calcium and phosphate by converting the relatively dibasic calcium phosphate to the more soluble monobasic calcium phosphate and calcium chloride. These more soluble compounds will dissolve into a solution, resolving the occlusion. It should be noted that hydrochloric acid is a strong acid and should be handled carefully.

The drugs which have been associated with precipitation include diazepam, phenytoin, heparin, calcium gluconate, bicarbonate, mannitol, pentobarbital, and phenobarbital. Failure to flush with sodium chloride solution between administration of drug doses and heparin is one of the most common causes of precipitation since many drugs are incompatible with heparin. Precipitation is determined by the chemical principle that salts derived from weak acids are more soluble in acidic solution and salts derived from weak bases are more solid in basic solution. Precipitation occurs when the aforementioned drugs are mixed with flushing solutions or other drugs with an opposing pH. It follows then that the precipitant can theoretically be dissolved with a solution that has a similar pH. For example, acidic medications like calcium gluconate can be dissolved with hydrochloric acid whereas basic medications like phenytoin can be dissolved with sodium bicarbonate. However, this approach has not been completely evaluated and is not currently supported by research.

Lipid Residue. CVC lumen occlusion can also occur due to deposition of lipid residue from infusion of parenteral nutrition, which is administered to patients who cannot achieve adequate nutrition orally. All-in-one mixtures and total nutrient admixture leave behind lipid residue which accumulates over time and obstruct the lumen of the CVC. Factors which affect the likelihood of lipid residue deposition include the type of liquid emulsion used, the age of the lipid and parenteral nutrition, the material used in the catheter, and any concomitant therapy being infused into the catheter.

DEVICE SELECTION

Due to increasing usage of PICCs in hospital settings, the Michigan Appropriateness Guide for Intravenous Catheters was developed to better outline which CVC is most appropriate for any given clinical scenario.

Since peripheral forms of venous access are contraindicated for the infusion of peripherally incompatible infusate (caustic medications), PICCs are appropriate for this purpose regardless of duration of infusion. Nontunneled CVCs are appropriate for this purpose in patients who need infusion for less than 2 weeks.

For the administration of peripherally compatible infusate, nontunneled CVCs are only appropriate in critically ill patients or patients who require hemodynamic monitoring for treatment regimens less than 14 days. All other patients who require short durations of therapy should receive peripheral forms of venous access. PICCs are appropriate for peripherally compatible intravenous therapy lasting longer than 5 days.

Tunneled CVCs are appropriate if central venous access is needed for more than 14 days, and ports are appropriate if needed for more than 30 days. For shorter durations of use, the risks and discomforts of tunneled or implanted device placement are not warranted. If longer treatment duration is planned, however, tunneled devices and ports are preferred due to their lower rate of infection when compared with nontunneled catheters.

Patients with difficult venous access or who require frequent phlebotomy may receive a nontunneled CVC for infusion durations less than 14 days if they are critically ill, and PICCs for infusion durations longer than 5 days if a CICC is not warranted. For patients with difficult venous access who require infusions for longer than 30 days, both tunneled CVCs and ports are also appropriate.

CVCs are not the optimal catheter for fluid resuscitation. Rather, the ideal configuration is two large-bore peripheral IVs located within the antecubital fossae; the large caliber and short length maximize flow rates. However, it may be difficult to cannulate peripheral veins in patients who are severely dehydrated. For these patients, nontunneled CVCs are preferred over PICCs due to their larger caliber and shorter length.

Suggested Readings

Al Raiy B, Fakih MG, Bryan-Nomides N, et al. Peripherally inserted central venous catheters in the acute care setting: A safe alternative to high-risk short-term central venous catheters. *Am J Infect Control* 2010;38(2):149–153.

Arvaniti K, Lathyris D, Blot S, Apostolidou-Kiouti F, Koulenti D, Haidich AB. Cumulative evidence of randomized controlled and observational studies on catheter-related infection risk of central venous catheter insertion site in ICU patients: A pairwise and network meta-analysis. *Crit Care Med* 2017; 45(4):e437–e448.

Bouza E, Guembe M, Munoz P. Selection of the vascular catheter: can it minimise the risk of infection? *Int J Antimicrob Agents* 2010;36 Suppl 2:S22–S25.

Brass P, Hellmich M, Kolodziej L, Schick G, Smith AF. Ultrasound guidance versus anatomical landmarks for subclavian or femoral vein catheterization. *Cochrane Database Syst Rev* 2015;1:Cd011447.

Center for Disease Control and Prevention. Bloodstream infection event (central line-associated bloodstream infection and non-central line-associated bloodstream infection). 2017. Available from https://www.cdc.gov/nhsn/pdfs/pscmanual/4psc_clabscurrent.pdf.

Chong HY, Lai NM, Apisarnthanarak A, Chaiyakunapruk N. Comparative efficacy of antimicrobial central venous catheters in reducing catheter-related bloodstream infections in adults: Abridged Cochrane systematic review and network meta-analysis. *Clin Infect Dis* 2017;64(Suppl 2):S131–S140.

Chopra V, Anand S, Hickner A, et al. Risk of venous thromboembolism associated with peripherally inserted central catheters: a systematic review and meta-analysis. *Lancet North Am Ed* 2013;382(9889):311–325.

Chopra V, O'Horo JC, Rogers MA, Maki DG, Safdar N. The risk of bloodstream infection associated with peripherally inserted central catheters compared with central venous catheters in adults: a systematic review and meta-analysis. *Infect Control Hosp Epidemiol* 2013;34(9):908–918.

Chopra V, Ratz D, Kuhn L, Lopus T, Chenoweth C, Krein S. PICC-associated bloodstream infections: prevalence, patterns, and predictors. *Am J Med* 2014;127(4):319–328.

Chopra V, Ratz D, Kuhn L, Lopus T, Lee A, Krein S. Peripherally inserted central catheter-related deep vein thrombosis: contemporary patterns and predictors. *J Thrombosis Haemost* 2014;12(6):847–854.

Climo M, Diekema D, Warren DK, et al. Prevalence of the use of central venous access devices within and outside of the intensive care unit: results of a survey among hospitals in the prevention epicenter program of the Centers for Disease Control and Prevention. *Infect Control Hosp Epidemiol* 2003;24(12):942–945.

Eisen LA, Narasimhan M, Berger JS, Mayo PH, Rosen MJ, Schneider RF. Mechanical complications of central venous catheters. *J Intensive Care Med* 2006;21(1):40–46.

Hardy G, Ball P. Clogbusting: time for a concerted approach to catheter occlusions? *Curr Opin Clin Nutr Metab Care* 2005;8(3):277–283.

Hoffman T, Du Plessis M, Prekupec MP, et al. Ultrasound-guided central venous catheterization: A review of the relevant anatomy, technique, complications, and anatomical variations. *Clin Anat* 2017;30(2):237–250.

Li C, Babb J, Sridhar D. Assessing the effect of multiple peripherally inserted central catheter insertions in a pediatric population: a single-center retrospective review. *J Vasc Interv Radiol* 2016;28(2):S7–S8.

Marik PE, Flemmer M, Harrison W. The risk of catheter-related bloodstream infection with femoral venous catheters as compared to subclavian and internal jugular venous catheters: a systematic review of the literature and meta-analysis. *Crit Care Med* 2012;40(8):2479–2485.

Mermel LA, Allon M, Bouza E, et al. Clinical practice guidelines for the diagnosis and management of intravascular catheter-related infection: 2009 Update by the Infectious Diseases Society of America. *Clin Infect Dis* 2009; 49(1):1–45.

Merrer J, De Jonghe B, Golliot F, et al. Complications of femoral and subclavian venous catheterization in critically ill patients: a randomized controlled trial. *JAMA* 2001;286(6):700–707.

Meyer BM. Developing an alternative workflow model for peripherally inserted central catheter placement. *J Infus Nurs* 2012;35(1):34–42.

Miller DL, O'Grady NP; Society of Interventional Radiology. Guidelines for the prevention of intravascular catheter-related infections: recommendations relevant to interventional radiology for venous catheter placement and maintenance. *J Vasc Interv Radiol* 2012;23(8):997–1007.

O'Grady NP, Alexander M, Burns LA, et al; Healthcare Infection Control Practices Advisory Committee (HICPAC). Guidelines for the prevention of intravascular catheter-related infections. *Clin Infect Dis* 2011;52(9): e162–e193.

Parienti JJ, Mongardon N, Megarbane B, et al. Intravascular complications of central venous catheterization by insertion site. *N Engl J Med* 2015; 373(13):1220–1229.

Pegues D, Axelrod P, McClarren C, et al. Comparison of infections in Hickman and implanted port catheters in adult solid tumor patients. *J Surg Oncol* 1992;49(3):156–162.

Pittiruti M, Hamilton H, Biffi R, MacFie J, Pertkiewicz M; ESPEN. ESPEN guidelines on parenteral nutrition: Central venous catheters (access, care, diagnosis and therapy of complications). *Clin Nutr* 2009;28(4):365–377.

Ruesch S, Walder B, Tramer MR. Complications of central venous catheters: internal jugular versus subclavian access—a systematic review. *Crit Care Med* 2002;30(2):454–460.

Smith RN, Nolan JP. Central venous catheters. *BMJ* 2013;347:f6570.

Stephens LC, Haire WD, Kotulak GD. Are clinical signs accurate indicators of the cause of central venous catheter occlusion? *JPEN J Parenter Enteral Nutr* 1995;19(1):75–79.

Timsit JF, Bouadma L, Mimoz O, et al. Jugular versus femoral short-term catheterization and risk of infection in intensive care unit patients. Causal analysis of two randomized trials. *Am J Respir Crit Care Med* 2013;188(10):1232–1239.

van Miert C, Hill R, Jones L. Interventions for restoring patency of occluded central venous catheter lumens. *Cochrane Database Syst Rev* 2012;(4): CD007119.

Williams JF, Seneff MG, Friedman BC, et al. Use of femoral venous catheters in critically ill adults: prospective study. *Crit Care Med* 1991;19(4):550–553.

Yang RY, Moineddin R, Filipescu D, et al. Increased complexity and complications associated with multiple peripherally inserted central catheter insertions in children: The tip of the iceberg. *J Vasc Interv Radiol* 2012;23(3): 351–357.

Yokoe DS, Anderson DJ, Berenholtz SM, et al. A compendium of strategies to prevent healthcare-associated infections in acute care hospitals: 2014 updates. *Infect Control Hosp Epidemiol* 2014;35(8):967–977.

CHAPTER 34 ■ CHRONIC VENOUS DISEASE AND DEEP VEIN THROMBOSIS

AMISH PATEL, BEDROS TASLAKIAN, AND AKHILESH K. SISTA

LOWER EXTREMITY VENOUS DISEASE

Introduction

Venous disease of the lower extremities most commonly manifests as chronic venous insufficiency (CVI) or venous thromboembolism (VTE). CVI is divided into two types, superficial and deep, based on which venous system is involved. Likewise, VTE involves two related but separate conditions, deep venous thrombosis (DVT) and pulmonary embolism (PE). In recent decades, procedural techniques have evolved to become an important piece in the management of patients with CVI and VTE.

Anatomy

In the lower extremities, the venous system is divided into the superficial and deep veins based on their relationship to the muscular fascia. Veins that traverse the muscular fascia are known as perforating veins, connecting the deep and superficial veins (Fig. 34.1). Veins that connect deep veins to other deep veins, or superficial veins to other superficial veins, are known as communicating veins. The two main superficial veins of the lower extremity (Fig. 34.2) are the small saphenous vein (SSV) and the great saphenous vein (GSV). The small and great saphenous veins travel in their own respective saphenous compartments bound by fascial layers. In cross section, these veins with the surrounding fascial layers have an "Egyptian eye" appearance (Fig. 34.3). The SSV drains into the deep venous system at the popliteal vein, known as the saphenopopliteal junction (SPJ). The GSV drains into the deep system at the common femoral vein, known as the saphenofemoral junction (SFJ).

The majority of the deep veins of the lower extremity are named the same as their corresponding artery (Fig. 34.4). These include the paired anterior tibial, posterior tibial, and peroneal veins. However, there are two additional veins, the soleal and gastrocnemius veins, which do not have corresponding arteries. These veins form the popliteal vein, which becomes the femoral vein in the thigh. This vein merges with the deep femoral vein to form the common femoral vein. The common femoral vein passes under the inguinal ligament to become the external iliac vein. This merges with the internal iliac vein to become the common iliac vein. The bilateral common iliac veins converge on the right side of the body to become the inferior vena cava (IVC). The IVC receives each of the renal veins and the confluence of the hepatic veins, ultimately draining into the right atrium.

Unlike arteries, veins of the lower extremity contain valves that function to create unidirectional flow toward the heart. These valves are more concentrated in the calf and become more infrequent up to the groin. The central veins of the pelvis do not contain valves.

Like the lower extremity, the venous system of the upper extremity also contains superficial and deep veins. These are demonstrated in Figure 34.5.

SUPERFICIAL VENOUS DISEASE

Pathophysiology

When the valves of the veins of the lower extremity become dysfunctional, blood flow becomes bidirectional, resulting in prolonged periods of reflux. This results in venous hypertension, which is responsible for leg swelling and varicose transformation of saphenous vein branches.

Clinical Evaluation and Patient Selection

When evaluating any patient, a thorough history and physical is mandatory. Doing so will prevent misdiagnosis and

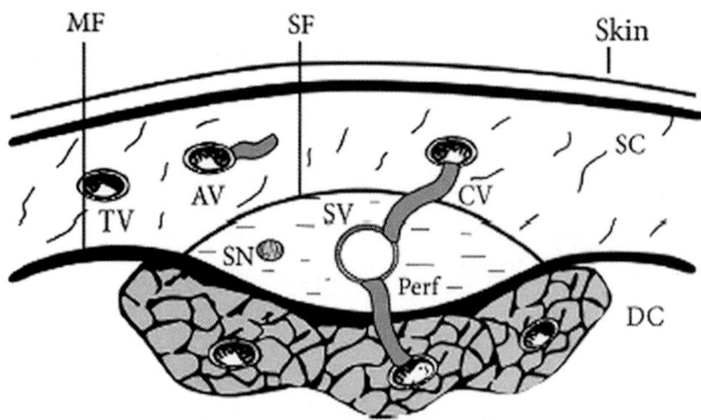

FIGURE 34.1. **Deep and Superficial Venous Compartments.** Muscular fascia (MF) separates the superficial compartment (SC) from the deep compartment (DC). The SC contains saphenous veins (SV), tributary veins (TV), and accessory veins (AV). Saphenous veins and accompanying nerves are contained within a saphenous compartment that is bound superficially by saphenous fascia (SF) and deeply by muscular fascia. The deep compartment is bound by muscular fascia and contains the deep veins. Perforator veins (Perf) traverse the superficial and the deep compartments. Communicating veins (CV) connect veins within the same venous compartment, either deep to deep or superficial to superficial. (Reprinted from Black CM. Anatomy and physiology of the lower-extremity deep and superficial veins. *Tech Vasc Interv Radiol* 2014;17(2):68–73, with permission from Elsevier.)

unnecessary procedures. When superficial venous disease is suspected, important history items are prior treatment, pregnancy history, family history of venous disease, and prior deep or superficial vein thrombosis. Symptoms of superficial venous insufficiency include leg heaviness, pain, fatigue, or swelling with standing. These symptoms are often relieved with leg elevation or exercise. On physical examination, patients will commonly have unsightly reticular or varicose veins, edema, or skin discoloration (Fig. 34.6). In the most severe cases, ulceration may develop. There are several scoring systems that function to standardize the reporting of clinical findings for patients with venous disease, both superficial and deep. Two commonly used systems are the Clinical, Etiologic, Anatomic, Pathophysiologic (CEAP, Table 34.1) classification and the revised venous clinical severity score (VCSS).

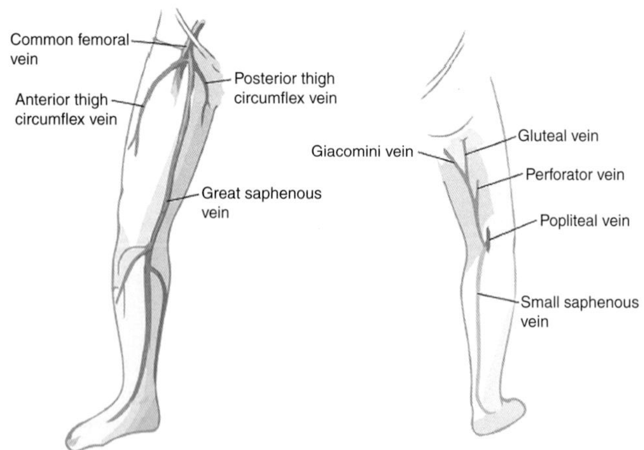

FIGURE 34.2. **Superficial Veins of the Lower Extremity.** (Reprinted from Winokur RS, Khilnani NM. Superficial veins: treatment options and techniques for saphenous veins, perforators, and tributary veins. *Tech Vasc Interv Radiol* 2014;17[2]:82–89, with permission from Elsevier.)

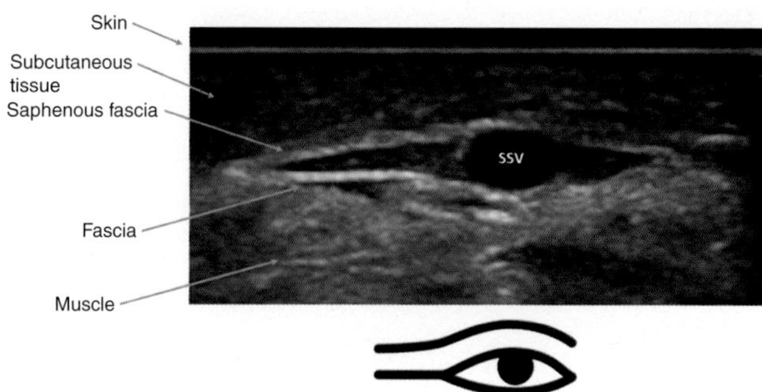

FIGURE 34.3. **The "Egyptian Eye" Appearance of the Small Saphenous Vein (SSV) With the Surrounding Fascial Layers.**

Imaging Evaluation

A Doppler ultrasound (US) will be the test of choice for patients with suspected superficial venous insufficiency. The study should be performed with a high-frequency linear transducer and with the patient in the standing position. The primary focus of the test is to evaluate the size and direction of flow within the veins. Although short periods of reflux are normal, retrograde flow exceeding 0.5 seconds in superficial veins is considered abnormal (Fig. 34.7). An SSV larger than 3 mm and a GSV larger than 5 mm are considered abnormal.

Treatment

Conservative treatment with graduated compression stockings (GCSs) and exercise should be first-line therapy for patients

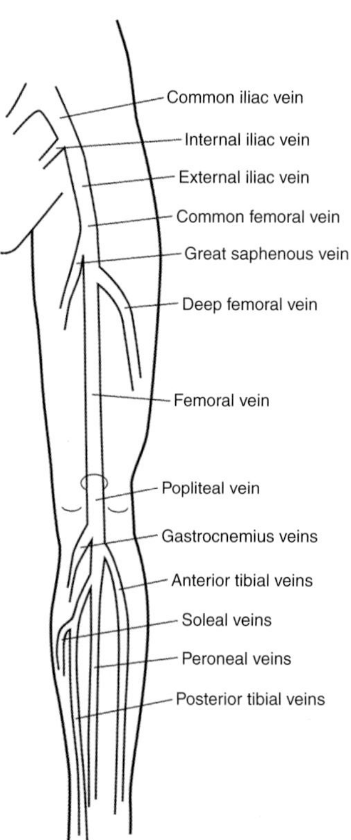

FIGURE 34.4. **Deep Veins of the Lower Extremity.** (Reprinted from Black CM. Anatomy and physiology of the lower-extremity deep and superficial veins. *Tech Vasc Interv Radiol* 2014;17[2]:68–73, with permission from Elsevier).

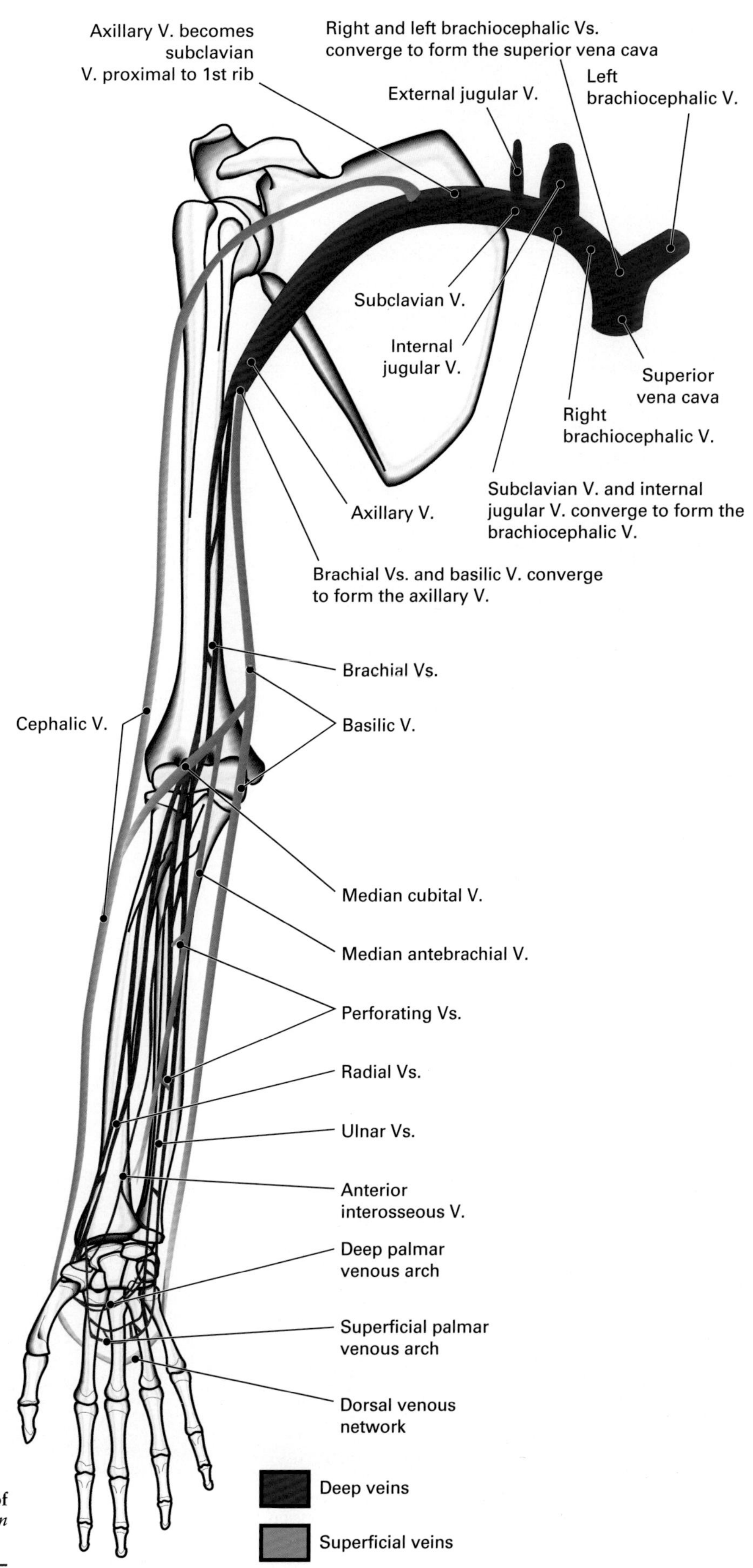

FIGURE 34.5. **Deep and Superficial Veins of the Upper Extremity.** (Olinger AB. *Human Gross Anatomy.* Wolters Kluwer; 2016.)

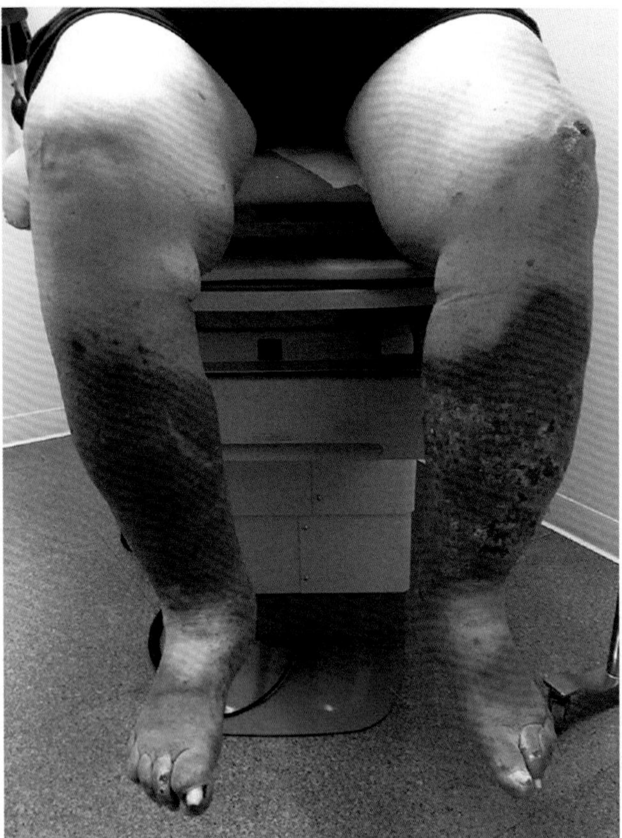

FIGURE 34.6. **Changes of Chronic Venous Insufficiency: Bilateral Lower Extremity Edema, Hyperpigmentation, and Ulcerations.**

presenting with mild or moderate symptoms. However, if the patient does not respond to or tolerate GCSs, or if ulcers are present, intervention may be necessary.

The goal of treatment is to eradicate the incompetent superficial vein, forcing blood to flow through the competent deep venous system. This was originally achieved by surgically removing the great or SSV. However, this is now more commonly achieved using venous ablation. This lesser invasive procedure comes in two forms, radiofrequency ablation (RFA) and endovenous laser ablation (ELVA). These catheter-based devices function by depositing energy into the wall of the vein thus resulting in venous occlusion (Fig. 34.8).

TABLE 34.1

CLINICAL PORTION OF CEAP CLASSIFICATION OF CHRONIC VENOUS DISEASE

C0	No visible signs of venous disease
C1	Telangiectasias or reticular veins
C2	Varicose veins
C3	Edema
C4a	Hyperpigmentation or venous eczema
C4b	Lipodermatosclerosis
C5	Healed venous ulceration
C6	Active venous ulceration

Often performed in an outpatient office setting using US guidance alone, the procedure can be done with or without intravenous sedation. With the patient in reverse Trendelenburg, the vein to be treated is accessed caudally with a needle and a wire. The device is then advanced cranially to 2 cm within the junction of the superficial vein with the deep vein (Fig. 34.7). Tumescent anesthesia using dilute lidocaine is then administered around the entire length of vein to be treated. This serves to collapse the vein around the device catheter and bring the vein into direct contact with the device, as well as create separation of the vein from adjacent nerves and skin. This is particularly important when treating the SSV because of its close proximity to the sural nerve and skin of the calf. The device is then activated and withdrawn through the vein, ablating it as it is removed. Newer devices use glue or foam sclerosant to seal the vein, doing so without the need of tumescent anesthesia. It is common for patients to experience bruising, soreness, or induration after ablation, but true complication of saphenous vein ablation is rare. However, deep vein thrombosis, skin burns, and nerve damage are not uncommon.

DEEP VENOUS THROMBOSIS

Pathophysiology

As the third most common cardiovascular disease, DVT carries significant societal cost and individual morbidity. The three factors involved in venous thrombosis, known as Virchow triad, are hypercoagulability, venous stasis, and venous endothelium

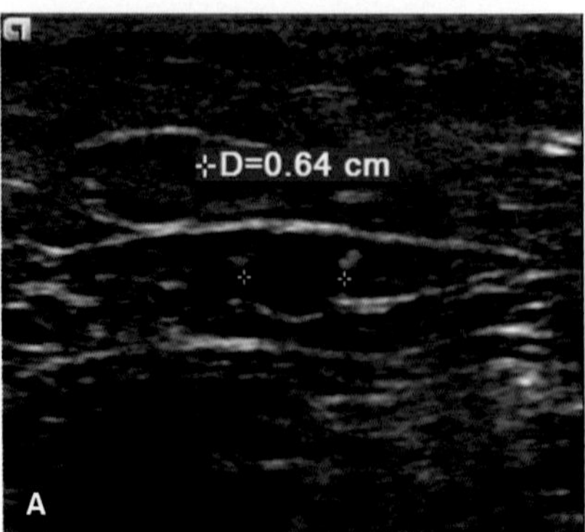

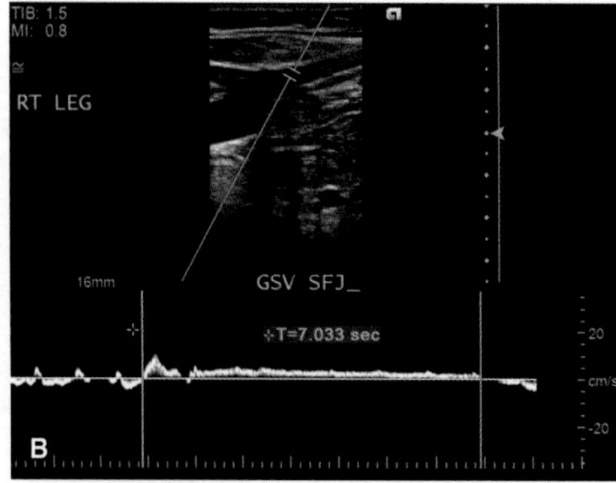

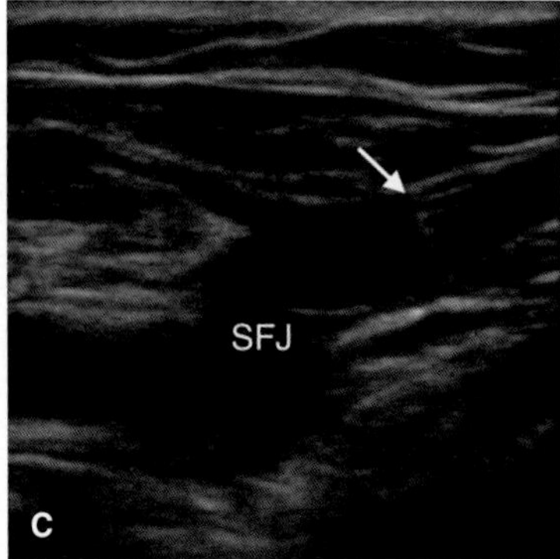

FIGURE 34.7. Transverse (**A**) and longitudinal (**B**) grayscale ultrasound at the level of the right saphenofemoral junction demonstrates an enlarged greater saphenous vein (0.64 cm) with 7.0 seconds of reflux, compatible with superficial venous insufficiency. In a different patient, intraprocedural ultrasound (**C**) demonstrates the laser filament (*arrow*) positioned 2–3 cm away from the saphenofemoral junction (SFJ).

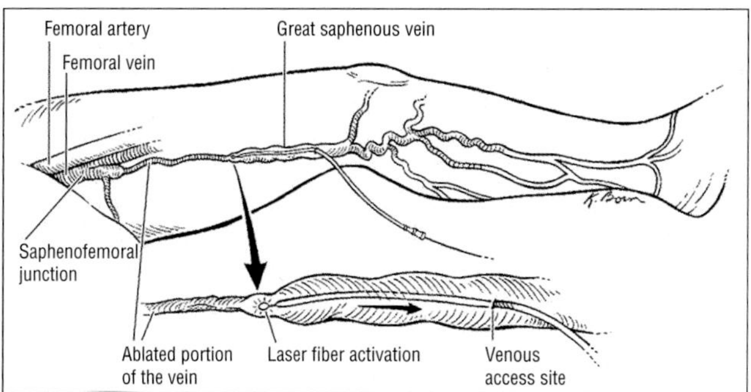

FIGURE 34.8. Endovenous Laser Ablation (EVLA) Treatment of the Great Saphenous Vein.

abnormality. There is a subset of patients with DVT whose cause is unknown and are said to have "unprovoked DVT." However, it is hypothesized that these patients have an underlying pathology which is not yet evident. Table 34.2 shows common causes of DVT.

The most worrisome consequence of DVT is PE because of its significant mortality. As such, treatment of DVT has traditionally been focused on PE prevention with anticoagulant medications. However, despite adequate anticoagulation, there can be incomplete clearance of thrombus that leads to chronic obstruction. In addition, the inflammatory response to thrombosis results in endothelial injury that renders valves of the deep veins nonfunctional. These consequences put the patient at risk for DVT again in the future. In fact, 30% of patients with "unprovoked DVT" will have recurrence within 8 years. The venous hypertension that results from chronic obstruction and reflux is known as postthrombotic syndrome (PTS). This condition shares many of the symptoms of venous hypertension from superficial venous insufficiency: leg swelling, heaviness, pain with standing, varicose veins, and in severe cases, ulceration. PTS develops in approximately 40% of patients, months to years after their first episode of symptomatic DVT. After recurrent ipsilateral DVT, the risk of PTS increases by two- to sixfold. The location of the DVT is also an important predictor of a patient's risk for developing PTS. Patients with proximal or "iliofemoral" DVT (thrombosis affecting the common femoral and/or iliac vein) are more likely to experience the severe symptoms of PTS such as venous ulcers. In order to bypass diseased veins, blood is shunted through uninvolved distal deep veins and superficial collaterals, which themselves become dilated and incompetent. This leads to worse venous hypertension and therefore edema, tissue injury, and skin ulceration.

TABLE 34.2

COMMON CAUSES OF DVT

Hypercoagulability
Factor V Leiden deficiency
Antithrombin III deficiency
Protein C or S deficiency
Oral contraceptive use
Pregnancy or postpartum state
Malignancy
Venous stasis
Prolonged immobilization
Recent surgery
Long travel
Foreign body
Central venous catheter
IVC filter
External compression
Pelvic lymphadenopathy or tumors
May–Thurner lesion
Endothelial abnormality
Trauma from venous catheter
Damage from IV medications

Clinical Evaluation and Patient Selection

When evaluating a patient with DVT, it is important to gather historical information that may uncover the underlying cause of thrombosis. This includes history of malignancy, family history of DVT or coagulopathy, recent surgery or long flight, presence of IVC filter, and medication usage. History of prior DVT, method of treatment, and outcome of that event are also important. The onset of symptoms is important because it allows the age of the clot to be determined, which may change the treatment approach.

Symptoms can include leg swelling, pain with forced dorsiflexion of the foot (Homans sign), and redness. A few patients will present with severe leg pain and discoloration that is the hallmark of phlegmasia (Fig. 34.9). This acute limb-threatening condition is the result of severe venous hypertension caused by the DVT. The initial stage of the disease is known as phlegmasia alba dolens and is characterized by a swollen, painful, and pale extremity. As thrombosis progresses and causes occlusion of collaterals, a blue discoloration develops in the extremity and the disease becomes known as phlegmasia cerulea dolens. If not recognized and treated promptly, the condition can progress to arterial compromise and limb loss. Thus, aggressive treatment of these patients is usually warranted. Since a usual component of endovascular treatment is thrombolytic medication, it is important to include a careful evaluation for potential risk factors that may increase the risk of major bleeding (Table 34.3). When considering a DVT intervention, patients can be grouped into three categories. Group 1 includes patients for whom urgent thrombolysis is required to prevent the life- or limb-threatening complications of acute DVT, such as phlegmasia cerulea dolens or progressive IVC thrombosis. Group 2 includes patients for whom thrombolysis is reasonable because of failure of medical management. This includes patients with progression of DVT or severe symptoms (pain and swelling) despite anticoagulation. Group 3 includes patients for whom thrombolysis is being considered to prevent PTS. Patients in group 1 will require the most aggressive approach in spite of significant risk factors, whereas the

TABLE 34.3

CONTRAINDICATIONS TO CATHETER-DIRECTED THROMBOLYSIS

Absolute
Active bleeding
Recent GI bleed (<3 months)
Recent stroke
Relative
Major recent trauma or surgery
Recent eye trauma or surgery
Uncontrolled hypertension
Pregnancy
Recent cardiopulmonary resuscitation
Thrombocytopenia or bleeding diathesis
Intracranial malignancy or vascular lesion

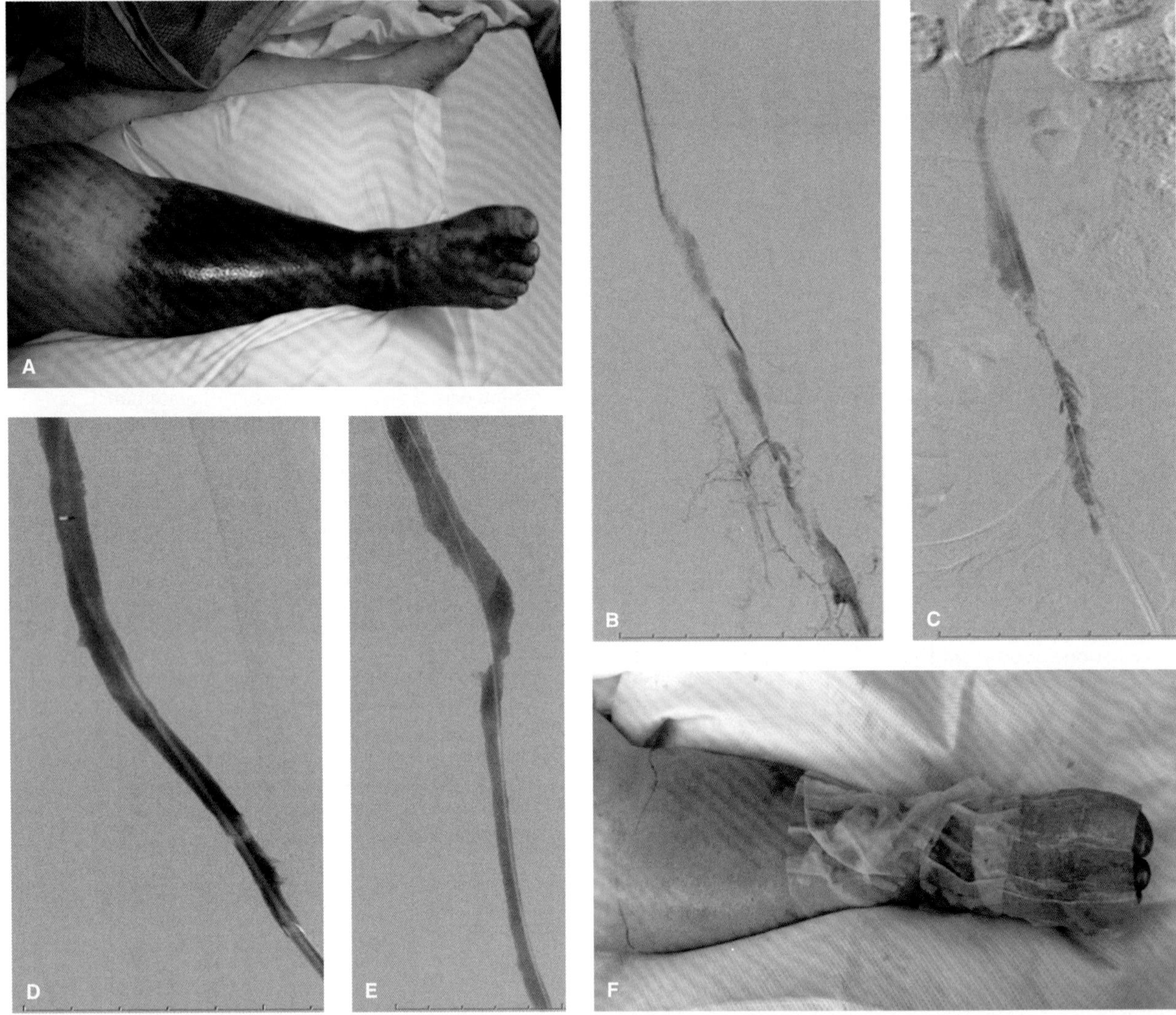

FIGURE 34.9. **Catheter-Directed Treatment of Phlegmasia. A:** Acutely swollen, mottled, cyanotic leg in the setting of an extensive occlusive DVT. **B, C:** Preintervention venograms demonstrate extensive thrombus along the length of the femoral (**B**) and iliofemoral (**C**) deep veins. **D, E:** After thrombolysis, angioplasty, and stent deployment, the flow through these segments is markedly improved. **F:** Appearance of the leg 10 days after treatment. (Courtesy of Brooke Spencer, MD.)

threshold for exclusion will be much higher for patients in groups 2 and 3.

Imaging Evaluation

Like superficial venous disease, the primary means of imaging evaluation for patients with DVT is ultrasonography. This test is readily accessible, easily performed, and has excellent sensitivity and specificity for the detection of infrainguinal DVT. For patients in whom ultrasonography is limited, because of intolerance to compression or obesity, computed tomographic (CT) or magnetic resonance (MR) venography can be performed. If there is suspicion for more central involvement of thrombus in the iliac veins or IVC, CTV or MRV can be considered.

Treatment

Medical Management. In general, anticoagulation alone will be the first-line therapy for treating patients with DVT. For the majority of patients, treatment starts with parenteral anticoagulant drug (unfractionated heparin, low–molecular-weight heparin [LMWH], or fondaparinux) given its ability to achieve therapeutic blood levels rapidly. Patients will then be transitioned to an oral or subcutaneous anticoagulant prior to discharge. Warfarin is an inexpensive oral anticoagulant, but its interaction with several medications and foods causes its efficacy to vary. As a result, it requires regular blood tests to allow appropriate titration. LMWH medications such as enoxaparin do not require blood test for dosing, but must be administered subcutaneously, making it a poor option for many patients. However, LWMH is the preferred anticoagulant in a patient with active cancer. Direct oral anticoagulants (DOACs) are a newer class of anticoagulation composed primarily of direct factor-Xa inhibitors and direct thrombin inhibitors. These medications do not require a blood test for dosing. However, unlike the other medications, there is currently no means for reversing the anticoagulant effect of DOACs, should a patient start bleeding or require emergent surgery. Regardless of the agent chosen, the length of treatment will be 3 months at minimum. If the patient has other risk factors or a history of prior DVT, the length of treatment may be longer or even lifelong.

Prevention of PTS is difficult, even with adequate anticoagulation. The use of elastic compression stockings, while low risk and somewhat helpful for symptom control, rarely prevents the development of PTS. It has been hypothesized that early elimination of thrombus from the vein with restoration of unobstructed flow prevents venous obstruction and valvular reflux, and subsequent PTS. Small randomized trials have shown that surgical venous thrombectomy and pharmacologic thrombolysis are associated with decreased rates of PTS compared to anticoagulation alone. However, the procedures are associated with higher rates of complications. A large randomized clinical trial (Acute Venous Thrombosis: Thrombus Removal With Adjunctive Catheter-Directed Thrombolysis [ATTRACT]) was performed to determine whether pharmacomechanical thrombolysis prevents PTS. The results show that pharmacomechanical thrombolysis does not prevent PTS and recurrent VTE, with increased risk of major bleeding (1.7% vs. 0.3%). However, it was evident that pharmacomechanical thrombolysis reduces the severity of PTS.

Pharmacologic thrombolysis can be achieved in many different ways. The thrombolytic medications can be injected systemically (i.e., into a peripheral vein), into veins near the clot in the effected extremity, or through infusion catheters embedded within the clot itself (Fig. 34.10). Studies have shown systemic infusion to be less effective when the thrombus is completely occlusive compared to when a channel exists

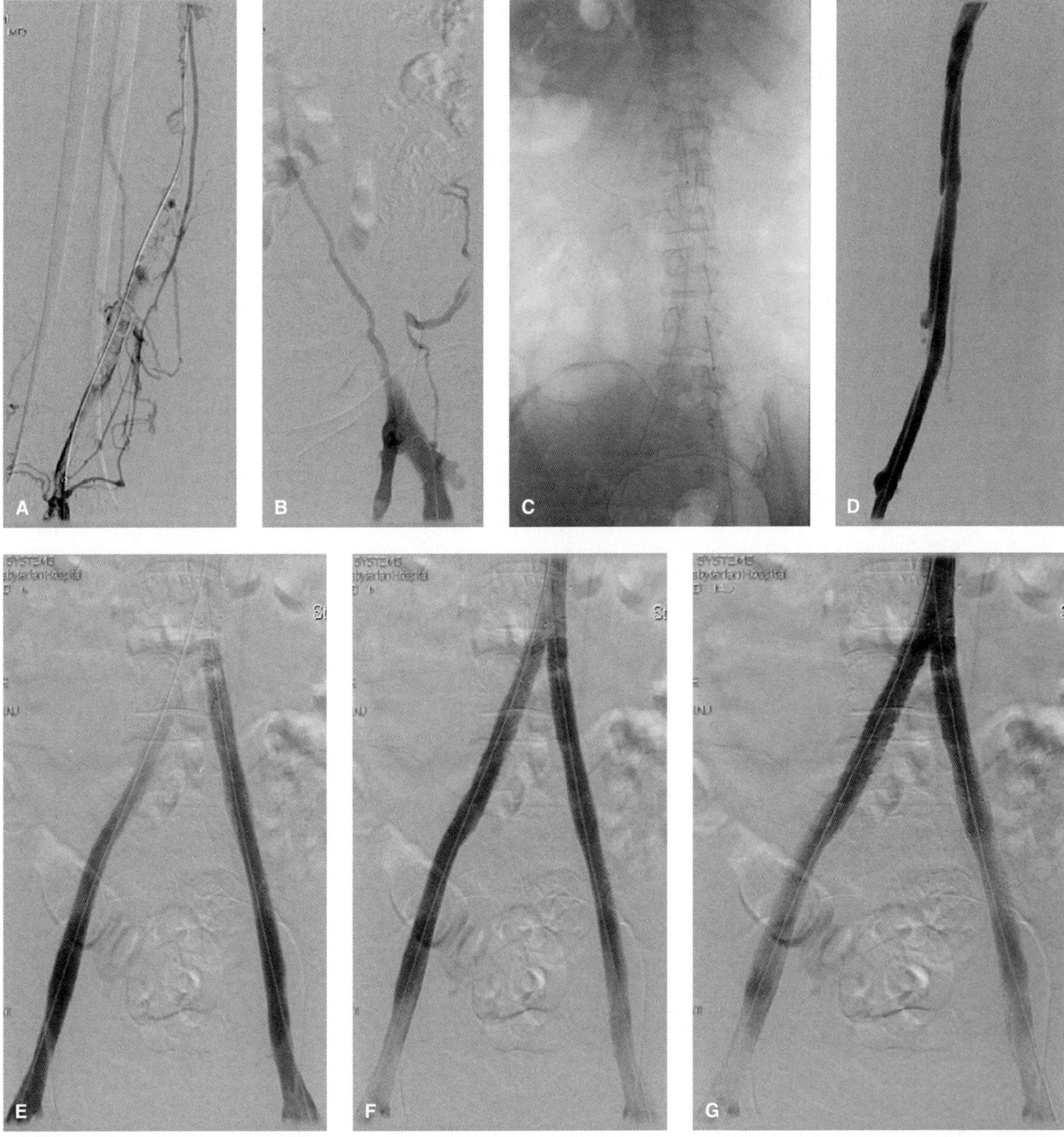

FIGURE 34.10. CDT and Stent Placement in a Patient With Progressive Bilateral DVTs in Spite of Anticoagulation. A: Left femoral venogram (patient prone) demonstrates extensive acute thrombus along the length of the vein. **B:** Right iliac venogram demonstrates no filling of the iliac vein. **C:** Fluoroscopic image depicts infusion catheters along the length of the left and right iliac thrombi. **D:** Postinfusion left femoral venogram demonstrates excellent patency. After stent placement, venogram of both iliacs demonstrates rapid inflow and outflow as evidenced by flow into the stents (E), through the stents (F), and washout of contrast from the stents (G). (Reprinted from Sista AK, Vedantham S, Kaufman JA, Madoff DC. Endovascular interventions for acute and chronic lower extremity deep venous disease: state of the art. *Radiology* 2015;276(1):31–53, with permission from RSNA.)

around the clot. Performing multiple injections of thrombolytic medication into the patent veins adjacent to a thrombosed segment has been studied, but has been shown to be ineffective. However, infusion of thrombolytic medication directly into the thrombus has been shown to be more safe and effective. This technique serves as the foundation for catheter-directed therapy (CDT) for DVT.

Interventional Therapies. CDT aims to introduce fibrinolytic medication at higher intrathrombus drug concentrations (increased efficacy) and decreased systemic exposure (increased safety). The procedure is commonly performed with moderate sedation. US guidance is used to access a deep vein in the affected limb. When possible, it is best to access a patent vein below the thrombosed venous segment. For isolated iliofemoral DVT, popliteal access is preferred since it is large, making access easier, and compressible, allowing for reliable hemostasis at the end of the procedure. If the popliteal vein is thrombosed, accessing one of the paired posterior tibial veins is preferred. This is done either in the calf or at the ankle. Internal jugular vein access is also an option, but traversing the valves of the femoropopliteal veins in a retrograde approach can be challenging. Venography is performed to delineate the extent of thrombosis. Based on the length of the thrombus, an appropriate length multiside hole infusion catheter is selected. Dilute thrombolytic drug is then infused into the thrombus for 6 to 24 hours. Commonly, recombinant tissue plasminogen activator (tPA) is used as the thrombolytic drug (rate of 0.5 mg to 1.0 mg an hour), but no lytic drug is currently approved by the U.S. Food and Drug Administration. During infusion, complete blood count, partial thromboplastin time, and fibrinogen levels are commonly drawn every 6 hours and used to determine the systemic effect of the thrombolytic drug and risk of bleeding. In conjunction with laboratory values, clinical signs of bleeding such as epistaxis or access site oozing may necessitate decreasing or terminating the thrombolytic infusion. Because of the bleeding risk, patients undergoing thrombolysis must be monitored in an elevated care setting, such as a step-down unit or an intensive care unit. However, some institutions have developed protocols which allow single setting or single-day thrombolysis, making use of elevated monitoring in the procedural recovery unit.

After thrombus removal, venography is performed to evaluate for residual thrombus or obstructive lesions. Residual thrombus can be treated with balloon maceration or mechanical thrombectomy. Obstructive lesions are treated with balloon angioplasty and/or stent placement. Stents are usually reserved for iliac lesions, but can be extended into the common femoral veins, using the level of the lesser trochanter of the femur as a landmark. Currently, no stent has U.S. Food and Drug Administration approval for treating venous disease. Usually, self-expanding bare-metal stents are preferred for their strength and ability to allow inflow from tributary veins.

Limitations to CDT include the cost of ICU observation during lysis (usually 1 to 3 days) and the risk of the procedure, namely bleeding and PE. Major bleeding is rare and can be reduced by routine use of US-guided venous access, which avoids inadvertent arterial puncture. Likewise, PE during CDT is so rare that the routine use of IVC filters is generally not necessary. An alternative to CDT is percutaneous mechanical thrombectomy (PMT), which does not rely on thrombolytic medications to remove thrombus. PMT devices aim to fragment thrombus or remove the thrombus entirely (Fig. 34.11). However, this carries the disadvantage of increased procedure time, increased venous valve trauma, and potential for thrombus embolization from mechanical manipulation. A hybrid of CDT and PMT, pharmacomechanical CDT (PCDT) aims to combine elements of both procedures to achieve better results. Many different combinations of medications and devices have been described, each with the aim of increasing the surface area of the thrombus, accelerating pharmacologic thrombolysis, and reducing bleeding complications. Regardless of the technique selected, all patients should receive usual medical management for DVT after successful thrombolysis, including anticoagulation, as described previously.

CHRONIC VENOUS DISEASE

Pathophysiology

Most commonly affecting the lower extremities, chronic venous disease is highly prevalent and often debilitating. This condition can result from superficial venous disease, prior DVT, and/or nonthrombotic obstruction, with some patients presenting with all three causes. The mechanisms of superficial venous disease and PTS have been discussed previously. Nonthrombotic causes include extrinsic compression, trauma, and congenital abnormalities. Extrinsic compression can be due to abdominopelvic neoplasms, lymphadenopathy, or lymphoceles that compress and subsequently obstruct the pelvic veins. Alternatively, extrinsic compression can be secondary to non-neoplastic causes such as May–Thurner syndrome and its variants. Congenital abnormalities like IVC atresia may also present in adolescence or adulthood as chronic venous disease.

Clinical Evaluation and Patient Selection

A complete and thorough history should be elicited from any patients with chronic venous disease. This includes a history of VTE, trauma, malignancy, central venous catheter placement, and IVC filter placement. It is important to enquire about the duration and severity of symptoms to exclude a superimposed acute thrombotic event. Chronic venous disease symptoms include long-standing pain, heaviness, and fatigue that worsen throughout the day. Physical examination findings include swelling, skin pigmentation, and dermatitis, and presence of active or healed ulceration. Baseline calf and thigh circumferences, as well as limb photography, are useful for tracking patient progression, as are the use of standardized classification systems like the Clinical Portion of CEAP (Table 34.1) or Villalta scale for PTS (Table 34.4). Patients

TABLE 34.4

VILLALTA SCALE FOR PTS

TYPE	FINDING
Symptoms	Cramps Itching Pins and needles Leg heaviness Pain
Signs	Pretibial edema Skin induration Hyperpigmentation Venous ectasia Redness Pain during calf compression Ulcer present?

Each symptom or sign is assigned a grade of none/minimal, mild, moderate, or severe, with 0–3 points assigned for each. The presence of an ulcer automatically confers severe PTS. A score greater than 5 is considered diagnostic for PTS.

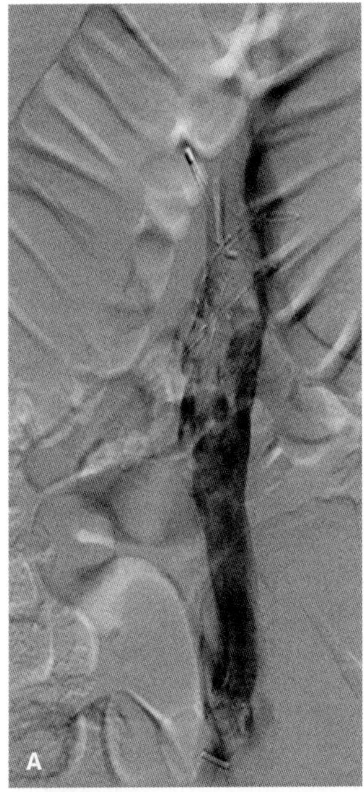
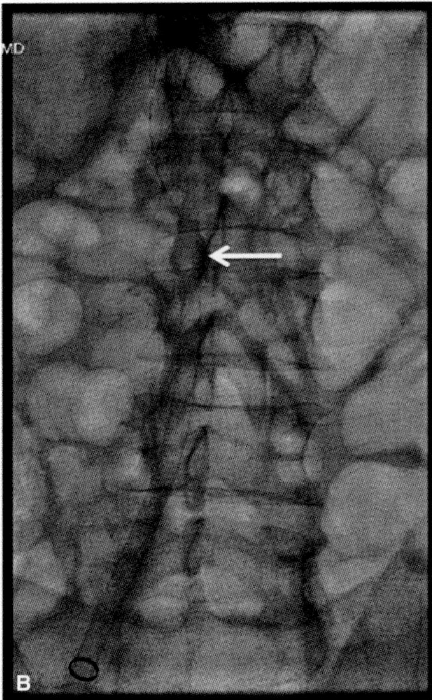
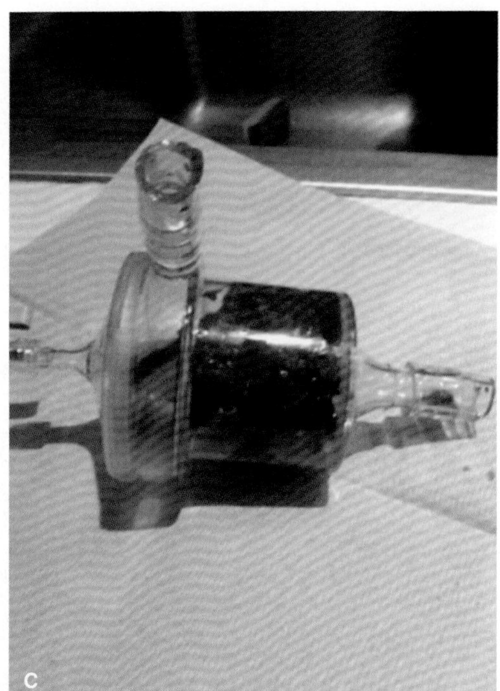
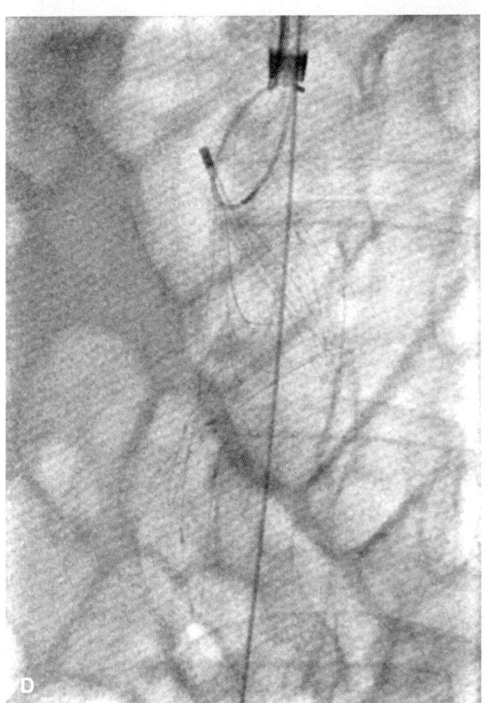
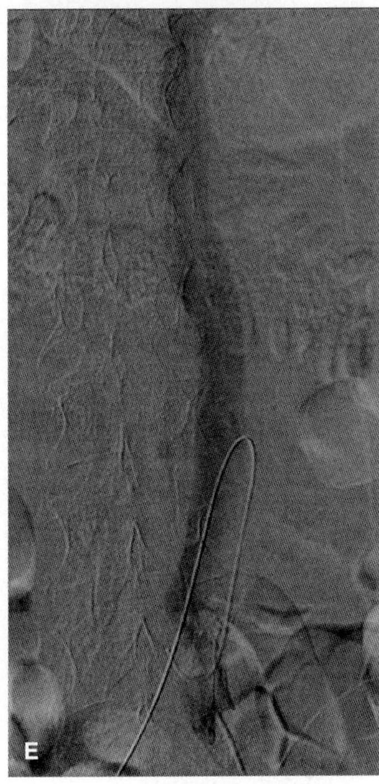

FIGURE 34.11. **Caval Thrombus Treated With a Large-Bore Aspiration Device, a Type of PMT. A:** IVC venogram demonstrates extensive caval thrombus and a malpositioned suprarenal IVC filter. **B:** Fluoroscopic image depicts the suction/aspiration device in the IVC. The *arrow* points to the balloon at the tip, which when inflated flares the tip. **C:** Photograph of the recirculation filter shows bulky extracted thrombus. **D:** Fluoroscopic image during filter retrieval shows a tip-deflecting wire grasping the malpositioned filter. The tip of the wire has been snared, and the filter is subsequently pulled through the sheath. **E:** IVC venogram obtained the next day after IVC filter removal demonstrates marked reduction in thrombus burden and free flow through the inferior vena cava. No lytic drug was used during this procedure owing to a hemorrhagic stroke in this patient 3 weeks earlier. (Reprinted from Sista AK, Vedantham S, Kaufman JA, Madoff DC. Endovascular interventions for acute and chronic lower extremity deep venous disease: state of the art. *Radiology* 2015;276(1):31–53, with permission from RSNA.)

with isolated calf swelling typically have femoropopliteal disease, with thigh swelling indicating more proximal iliofemoral involvement. Bilateral lower extremity involvement should raise suspicion of caval involvement, particularly if there is a history of IVC filter insertion.

Imaging Evaluation

Imaging is useful for determining the etiology of chronic venous disease as well as for planning treatment. Duplex US of the lower extremities can be used to evaluate for the presence of deep and superficial venous insufficiency as well as for superimposed acute DVT. CT or MR venography will evaluate for central thrombus and nonthrombotic causes of obstruction in the pelvis, where US evaluation is limited due to overlying gas-filled bowel. The diameter of the deep pelvic veins and IVC can be measured on MR and CT venography, with any abrupt change in caliber being suggestive of an underlying stenosis. However, these measurements can be affected by respiratory variation, position, and hydration, which may be falsely interpreted as stenotic lesions. Depending on the duration and severity of venous obstruction, the vein may appear diminished in size or entirely absent. Nevertheless, on conventional venography, there is frequently an infundibulum that leads into an atretic venous lumen.

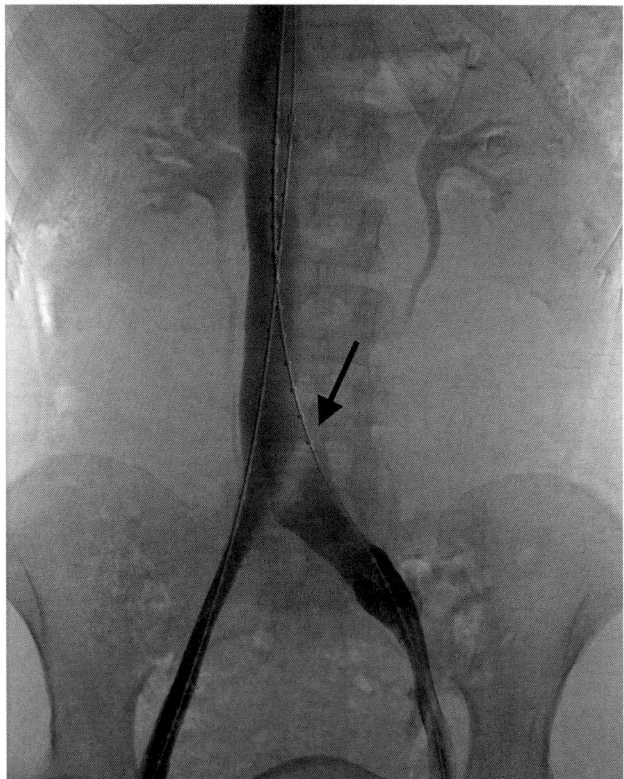

FIGURE 34.12. **May–Thurner Syndrome.** Inferior vena cavagram and pelvic venogram demonstrate flattening/effacement of the left common iliac vein with a tubular filling defect (*arrow*) indicative of external compression by the crossing right common iliac artery.

Treatment

Medical Management. Many patients with PTS have a persistent risk of thrombosis, either from underlying obstruction or thrombophilia, and require prolonged anticoagulation. Evaluation for adequate anticoagulation is essential since rethrombosis is a major risk factor for PTS. Compression stockings can be helpful in treating the symptoms of chronic venous disease but play an uncertain role in the prevention of PTS. Lifestyle modifications, including smoking cessation, exercise, and weight loss should be encouraged. If ulcers are present, aggressive treatment should be pursued, including referral to an infectious disease and wound care specialist, if necessary.

Interventional Therapies. In preparation for venous recanalization, usual patient workup will include complete blood count, basic metabolic panel, and coagulation parameters. Many interventionalists will perform this procedure with the patient fully anticoagulated given the risk of intraprocedural thrombosis. The procedure can be lengthy and if angioplasty is performed, painful. Thus, general anesthesia may be required. If popliteal access is needed, the patient will either be prone or in a frog-legged position.

May–Thurner compression is a controversial topic because the majority of patients with this anatomic variant are asymptomatic. May–Thurner syndrome is classically described as compression of the left common iliac vein between the vertebral body posteriorly and the crossing right common iliac artery anteriorly. Over time, this chronic compression is believed to lead to endothelial damage and stenosis. Although this obstruction can be visualized on conventional venography as a filling defect within the left common iliac vein (Fig. 34.12), intravascular ultrasound (IVUS) is more sensitive and specific

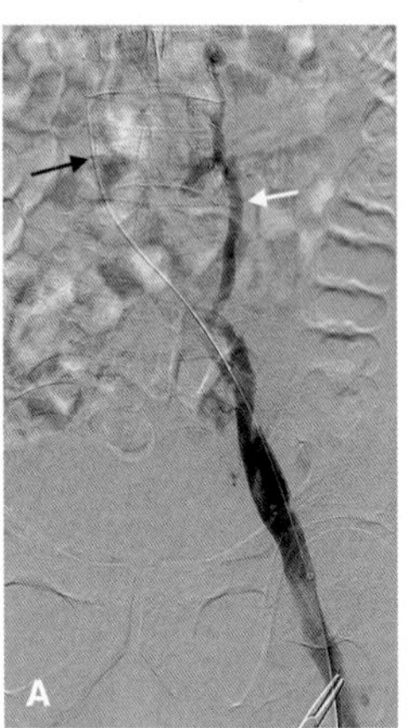

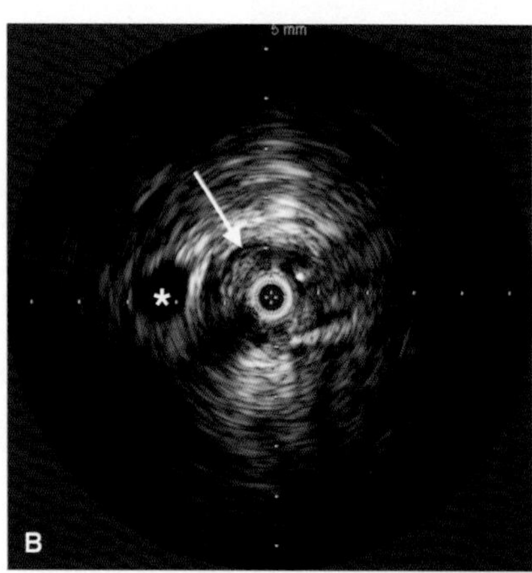

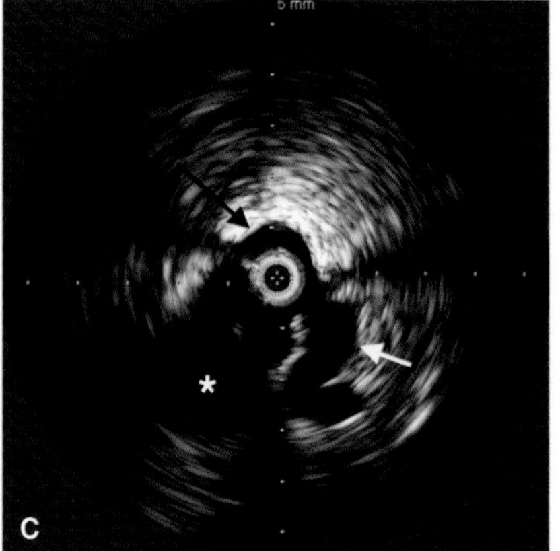

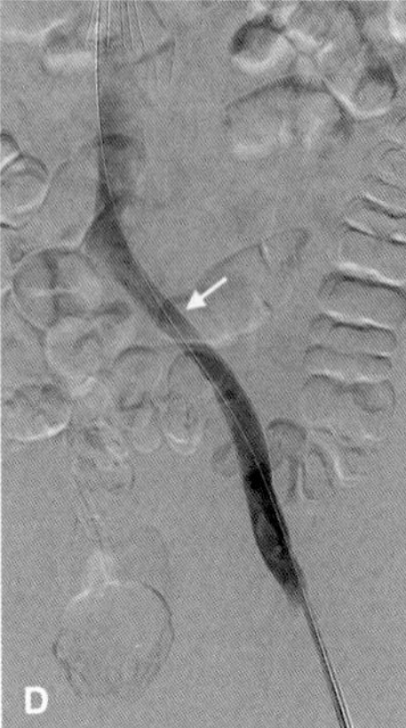

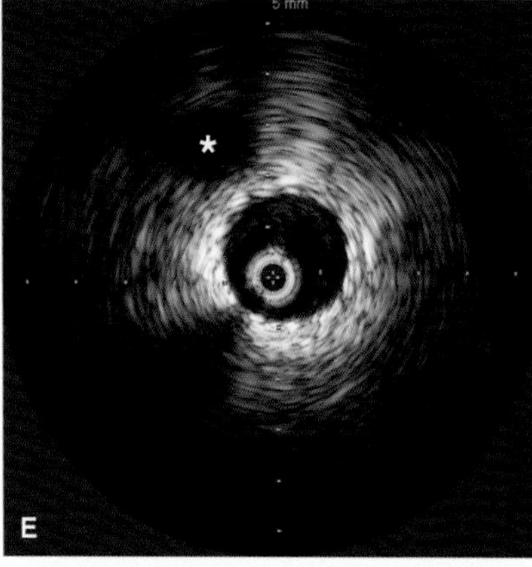

FIGURE 34.13. **Chronic Venous Occlusion.** Venogram from a left common femoral vein access (**A**) demonstrates a wire (*black arrow*) traversing a chronic occlusion of the left common iliac vein, with well-formed lumbar collateral (*white arrow*). IVUS at the level of the occlusion (**B**) demonstrates irregular echogenicity within the chronically occluded left common femoral vein (*white arrow*). IVUS above the occlusion (**C**) demonstrates a narrowed, but patent vein (*black arrow*) with supply from the tortuous lumbar collateral (*white arrow*). Venography (**D**) and IVUS (**E**) after stenting demonstrates markedly improved caliber and flow through the left common iliac vein (*white arrow*). The left common iliac artery (*asterisk*) is seen adjacent to the vein on IVUS images.

at identifying these lesions. This is also true for other causes of pelvic vein narrowing. When identified and found to correlate with the location of the patient's symptoms, the lesion is treated with angioplasty and stent placement (Fig. 34.13).

When not associated with venous thrombosis, treatment of iliac vein stenosis like May–Thurner is relatively straightforward. However, in the presence of thrombosis, recanalization becomes more challenging. Using a hydrophilic wire and a catheter, the occluded and stenotic segments are traversed, connecting normal vein peripherally to normal vein centrally. If acute thrombus is encountered, thrombolysis may be necessary, either with CDT or PCDT. In the absence of acute thrombus, serial balloon angioplasty of the diseased veins will be performed. As was mentioned previously, stenting is reserved for iliac vein segments and the common femoral veins. Stents can be extended caudally through the common femoral vein, if necessary. Angioplasty alone is the treatment of choice for chronically occluded femoropopliteal veins given the poor performance of stents in this area.

When IVC recanalization is planned in the presence of an IVC filter, the need for caval filtration should be determined (persistent risk of PE or contraindication to anticoagulation). If no longer needed, retrieval during recanalization should be considered. While planning for the intervention, the type of filter should be determined since different filters have a different propensity for fracture after long indwelling periods. Assessment for additional features such as filter position, wall penetration, and caval patency will help with retrieval planning. Retrieval will be more difficult for filters that have significant IVC wall contact or tilt resulting in embedding of the retrieval hook. The use of rigid bronchoscopy forceps may be necessary in these scenarios. However, IVC stenosis or occlusion associated with irretrievable filters can be treated with stent placement across the filter so as to displace the filter from the central lumen of the IVC. Stents with higher radial force should be selected in this scenario. This technique has been shown to have a similar patency rate compared to filter removal and stenting.

Chronic venous recanalization is generally safe, with most complications being access site bleeding. This is usually controlled with manual compression alone and does not necessitate stopping anticoagulation. Stenting of chronic occlusion is often painful, with patients complaining of back and flank pain for several days after the procedure. There is no consensus regarding the optimal use of anticoagulation after chronic venous recanalization. A typical regimen for patients will include a short period of enoxaparin followed by transition to an oral agent. Patients will likely require more prolonged anticoagulation after stent placement if their May–Thurner lesion is associated with thrombosis. Likewise, the use of antiplatelet agents after stent placement is also variable.

Suggested Readings

Amin VB, Lookstein RA. Catheter-directed interventions for acute iliocaval deep vein thrombosis. *Tech Vasc Interv Radiol* 2014;17(2):96–102.

Beckman MG, Hooper WC, Critchley SE, Ortel TL. Venous thromboembolism: a public health concern. *Am J Prev Med* 2010;38(4 Suppl):S495–S501.

Bergan JJ, Schmid-Schonbein GW, Smith PD, Nicolaides AN, Boisseau MR, Eklof B. Chronic venous disease. *N Engl J Med* 2006;355(5):488–498.

Bergqvist D, Jendteg S, Johansen L, Persson U, Odegaard K. Cost of long-term complications of deep venous thrombosis of the lower extremities: an analysis of a defined patient population in Sweden. *Ann Intern Med* 1997;126(6):454–457.

Black CM. Anatomy and physiology of the lower-extremity deep and superficial veins. *Tech Vasc Interv Radiol* 2014;17(2):68–73.

Brandjes DP, Büller HR, Heijboer H, et al. Randomised trial of effect of compression stockings in patients with symptomatic proximal-vein thrombosis. *Lancet* 1997;349(9054):759–762.

Caggiati A, Bergan JJ, Gloviczki P, et al. Nomenclature of the veins of the lower limbs: an international interdisciplinary consensus statement. *J Vasc Surg* 2002;36(2):416–422.

Chick JFB, Jo A, Meadows JM, et al. Endovascular iliocaval stent reconstruction for inferior vena cava filter-associated iliocaval thrombosis: approach, technical success, safety, and two-year outcomes in 120 patients. *J Vasc Interv Radiol* 2017;28(7):933–939.

Chitsike RS, Rodger MA, Kovacs MJ, et al. Risk of post-thrombotic syndrome after subtherapeutic warfarin anticoagulation for a first unprovoked deep vein thrombosis: results from the REVERSE study. *J Thromb Haemost* 2012;10(10):2039–2044.

Comerota AJ, Throm RC, Mathias SD, Haughton S, Mewissen M. Catheter-directed thrombolysis for iliofemoral deep venous thrombosis improves health-related quality of life. *J Vasc Surg* 2000;32(1):130–137.

Deroo S, Deatrick KB, Henke PK. The vessel wall: a forgotten player in post thrombotic syndrome. *Thromb Haemost* 2010;104(4):681–692.

Eklöf B, Rutherford RB, Bergan JJ, et al. Revision of the CEAP classification for chronic venous disorders: consensus statement. *J Vasc Surg* 2004; 40(6):1248–1252.

Garcia MJ, Lookstein R, Malhotra R, et al. Endovascular management of deep vein thrombosis with rheolytic thrombectomy: final report of the prospective multicenter PEARL (peripheral use of angiojet rheolytic thrombectomy with a variety of catheter lengths) registry. *J Vasc Interv Radiol* 26(6): 777–785.

Goldhaber SZ. Venous thromboembolism: epidemiology and magnitude of the problem. *Best Pract Res Clin Haematol* 2012;25(3):235–242.

Goldhaber SZ, Meyerovitz MF, Green D, et al. Randomized controlled trial of tissue plasminogen activator in proximal deep venous thrombosis. *Am J Med* 1990;88(3):235–240.

Johnson BF, Manzo RA, Bergelin RO, Strandness DE Jr. Relationship between changes in the deep venous system and the development of the postthrombotic syndrome after an acute episode of lower limb deep vein thrombosis: a one- to six-year follow-up. *J Vasc Surg* 1995;21(2):307–312; discussion 313.

Kahn SR. Measurement properties of the Villalta scale to define and classify the severity of the post-thrombotic syndrome. *J Thromb Haemost* 2009;7(5): 884–888.

Kearon C, Akl EA, Ornelas J, et al. Antithrombotic therapy for VTE disease: CHEST guideline and expert panel report. *Chest* 2016;149(2):315–352.

Kibbe MR, Ujiki M, Goodwin AL, Eskandari M, Yao J, Matsumura J. Iliac vein compression in an asymptomatic patient population. *J Vasc Surg* 2004; 39(5):937–943.

Lee AY, Levine MN, Baker RI, et al. Low-molecular-weight heparin versus a coumarin for the prevention of recurrent venous thromboembolism in patients with cancer. *N Engl J Med.* 2003;349(2):146–153.

Markel A, Manzo RA, Bergelin RO, Strandness DE Jr. Valvular reflux after deep vein thrombosis: incidence and time of occurrence. *J Vasc Surg* 1992;15(2): 377–382; discussion 383–384.

Meissner MH, Manzo RA, Bergelin RO, Markel A, Strandness DE Jr. Deep venous insufficiency: the relationship between lysis and subsequent reflux. *J Vasc Surg* 1993;18(4):596–605; discussion 606–608.

Mewissen MW, Seabrook GR, Meissner MH, Cynamon J, Labropoulos N, Haughton SH. Catheter-directed thrombolysis for lower extremity deep venous thrombosis: report of a national multicenter registry. *Radiology* 1999;211(1):39–49.

Neglén P, Hollis KC, Olivier J, Raju S. Stenting of the venous outflow in chronic venous disease: long-term stent-related outcome, clinical, and hemodynamic result. *J Vasc Surg* 2007;46(5):979–990.

Niedzwiecki G. Endovenous thermal ablation of the saphenous vein. *Semin Intervent Radiol* 2005;22(3):204–208.

Nunnelee JD. Review of an article: oral rivaroxaban for symptomatic venous thromboembolism. The EINSTEIN Investigators et al. *N Engl J Med* 2010; 363(26):2499–2510. *J Vasc Nurs* 2011;29(2):89.

Prandoni P, Frulla M, Sartor D, Concolato A, Girolami A. Vein abnormalities and the post-thrombotic syndrome. *J Thromb Haemost* 2005;3(2):401–402.

Prandoni P, Lensing AW, Prins MH, et al. Below-knee elastic compression stockings to prevent the post-thrombotic syndrome: a randomized, controlled trial. *Ann Intern Med* 2004;141(4):249–256.

Raju S. Long-term outcomes of stent placement for symptomatic nonthrombotic iliac vein compression lesions in chronic venous disease. *J Vasc Interv Radiol* 2012;23(4):502–503.

Raju S, Martin A, Davis M. The importance of IVUS assessment in venous thrombolytic regimens. *J Vasc Surg Venous Lymphat Disord* 2013;1(1):108.

Raju S, Neglén P. Percutaneous recanalization of total occlusions of the iliac vein. *J Vasc Surg* 2009;50(2):360–368.

Sista AK, Vedantham S, Kaufman JA, Madoff DC. Endovascular interventions for acute and chronic lower extremity deep venous disease: state of the art. *Radiology* 2015;276(1):31–53.

Sugimoto K, Hofmann LV, Razavi MK, et al. The safety, efficacy, and pharmacoeconomics of low-dose alteplase compared with urokinase for catheter-directed thrombolysis of arterial and venous occlusions. *J Vasc Surg* 2003; 37(3):512–517.

Turpie AG, Levine MN, Hirsh J, et al. Tissue plasminogen activator (rt-PA) vs heparin in deep vein thrombosis. Results of a randomized trial. *Chest* 1990; 97(4 Suppl):172S–175S.

Vasquez MA, Munschauer CE. Venous clinical severity score and quality-of-life assessment tools: application to vein practice. *Phlebology* 2008;23(6): 259–275.

Vedantham S. Interventional approaches to deep vein thrombosis. *Am J Hematol* 2012;87(Suppl 1):S113–S118.

Vedantham S. Treating infrainguinal deep venous thrombosis. *Tech Vasc Interv Radiol* 2014;17(2):103–108.

Vedantham S, Goldhaber SZ, Julian JA, et al. Pharmacomechanical catheter-directed thrombolysis for deep-vein thrombosis. *N Engl J Med* 2017;377(23): 2240–2252.

Vedantham S, Millward SF, Cardella JF, et al. Society of Interventional Radiology position statement: treatment of acute iliofemoral deep vein thrombosis with use of adjunctive catheter-directed intrathrombus thrombolysis. *J Vasc Interv Radiol* 2006;17(4):613–616.

Vedantham S, Thorpe PE, Cardella JF, et al. Quality improvement guidelines for the treatment of lower extremity deep vein thrombosis with use of endovascular thrombus removal. *J Vasc Interv Radiol* 2006;17(3):435–447; quiz 448.

Winokur RS, Khilnani NM. Superficial veins: treatment options and techniques for saphenous veins, perforators, and tributary veins. *Tech Vasc Interv Radiol* 2014;17(2):82–89.

Ye K, Lu X, Li W, et al. Long-term outcomes of stent placement for symptomatic nonthrombotic iliac vein compression lesions in chronic venous disease. *J Vasc Interv Radiol* 2012;23(4):497–502.

CHAPTER 35 ■ PULMONARY EMBOLISM

BEDROS TASLAKIAN, AMISH PATEL, AND AKHILESH K. SISTA

INTRODUCTION

Acute pulmonary embolism (PE) is the third leading cause of death among hospitalized patients . It has a reported annual mortality of approximately 100,000 to 180,000 patients. In patients who survive the initial insult, residual thrombus in the pulmonary vascular bed may lead to post-PE syndrome, which ultimately results in decreased exercise tolerance and impaired quality of life . Therefore, successful management of acute PE is essential and requires immediate recognition, accurate risk stratification, and early treatment. Societal guidelines classify PE into three major categories. Patients with "high-risk" or "massive" PE present with systemic hypotension and/or hemodynamic collapse, whereas patients with "intermediate" or "submassive" PE are hemodynamically stable but show signs of right heart strain. Low-risk PE, characterized by hemodynamic stability and no right-heart dysfunction, has excellent prognosis and low mortality rate of <1%, and is often adequately treated with therapeutic doses of anticoagulation alone. In contrast, patients with massive or submassive PEs have much higher mortality rates of 20% to 50% and 3% to 9%, respectively . The poor outcome associated with massive and submassive PE despite anticoagulation prompted physicians to explore different therapy escalation options such as surgical embolectomy, systemic thrombolysis, and catheter-directed therapy. Although treatment escalation with systemic thrombolysis may reduce mortality, it is also associated with a higher risk of hemorrhagic complications. Catheter-directed intervention is an alternative to systemic thrombolysis to rapidly debulk the central clot in patients with shock and can be achieved by catheter-directed mechanical or pharmacomechanical thrombectomy. Emerging evidence suggests catheter-directed thrombolysis (CDT), which uses a low-dose intraclot thrombolytic infusion, as an adjunct therapy in patients presenting with acute submassive PE. However, its safety, as well as short and long-term clinical outcomes compared to anticoagulation alone have yet to be evaluated in randomized controlled trials. In the absence of strong evidence, treatment approaches vary among institutions based on local expertise; however, the employment of these interventional techniques is of great interest.

This book chapter reviews clinical evaluation, risk stratification, and treatment strategies in patients who present with acute PE, in particular the use of catheter-directed therapies for massive and submassive PE. We also review the indications of inferior vena cava (IVC) filter placement in patients with venous thromboembolic disease (VTE) and describe the technique.

PATIENT EVALUATION AND RISK STRATIFICATION

The clinical diagnosis of PE can be challenging. Different strategies designed to predict the likelihood of PE are beyond the scope of this chapter. Several imaging modalities have been used for the diagnosis of PE; computed tomographic pulmonary angiography (CTPA) has become the method of choice for imaging the pulmonary vasculature in patients with suspected PE. Once PE is diagnosed, immediate prognostic assessment and risk stratification is imperative for rapid triaging to determine the need for treatment escalation beyond anticoagulation. Several institutions implemented multidisciplinary team approach via emerging PE response teams (PERT) given the complexity of management and various treatment options involving different areas of expertise. Timely evaluation of patient's clinical status, comorbidities, imaging and biomarker results, bleeding risk, and presence of concerning signs may help in selecting patients for treatment escalation (Fig. 35.1 and Table 35.1).

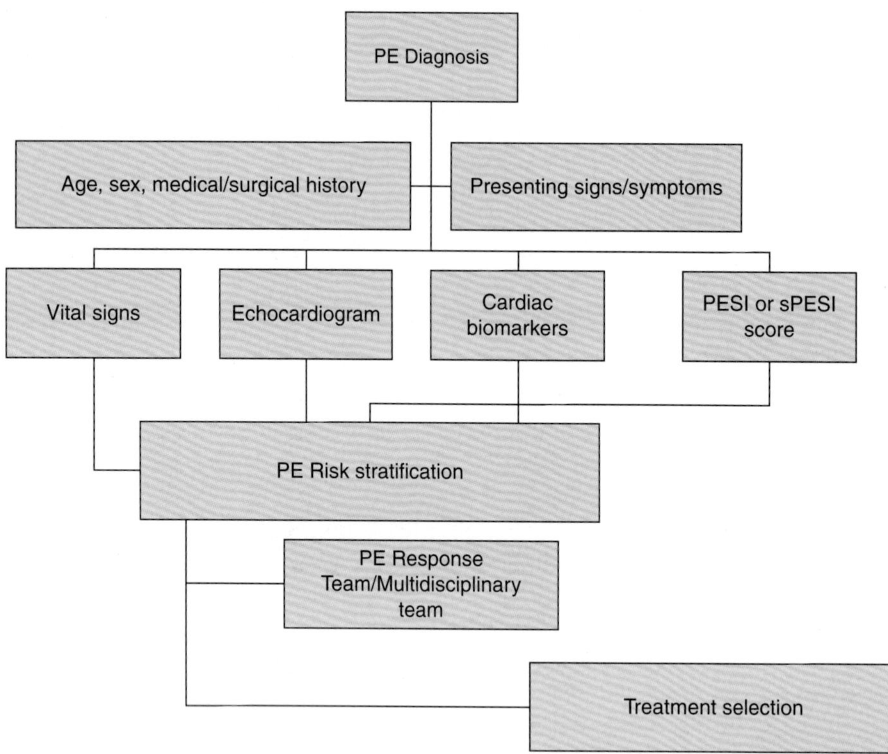

FIGURE 35.1. **Suggested Algorithm for Management of Acute PE.**

Clinical status and signs of right ventricular (RV) dysfunction and myocardial injury are the main predictors of short-term mortality in patients with acute PE. Persistent arterial hypotension and shock indicate acute RV failure and carry high risk of early death. Most of the deaths in hemodynamically unstable patients occur within the first hour of presentation. In hemodynamically stable patients, several predictors of death have been identified and different strategies have been proposed to optimize risk stratification and health resource utilization. Imaging and cardiac biomarkers are currently used for the assessment of RV overload. Echocardiography is routinely used for evaluation of RV function and size, in addition to the possibility of identifying RV thrombi and right-to-left shunt through a patent foramen ovale, both of which have shown an association with increased mortality in patients with acute PE. RV dysfunction and dilatation assessed by right-to-left ventricular diameter ratio of >0.9 are associated with increased risk for short-term death (Fig. 35.2). Elevated troponin, a marker of myocardial injury, is also associated with increased in-hospital mortality in patients with acute PE, even in hemodynamically stable patients. B-type natriuretic peptide (BNP) or N-terminal (NT)-proBNP reflect the severity of hemodynamic compromise and RV dysfunction. In addition, unfavorable outcome has been associated with syncope, tachycardia, and other routinely available clinical parameters related to pre-existing comorbidities and conditions. Therefore, clinical models based on simple and rapidly available information on patients' medical history and clinical status have been developed to determine mortality risk; the Pulmonary Embolism Severity Index (PESI) and its simplified version (sPESI) are the most extensively validated scoring systems (Table 35.2). Studies showed that patients in PESI classes III–V have up to 24.5% 30-day mortality and those with a sPESI ≥1 have a 30-day mortality rate approaching 11%.

Likewise, the American College of Chest Physicians (ACCP), the American Heart Association (AHA), and the European Society of Cardiology (ESC) have all adopted a risk-based prognostic stratification strategy to guide the management of acute PE (Table 35.3). The AHA classified acute PE into three major categories: massive, submassive, and low risk. In the 2014 guidelines of the ESC, a new model for PE risk stratification was proposed. The ESC's PE categories include high-risk, intermediate-risk, and low-risk PE. The ESC acknowledges the complexity of risk stratification and management of intermediate-risk (submassive) PE that encompasses a broad range of presentations, and further stratifies this group into "high-risk" and "low-risk" intermediate PE. The ESC also recognizes the role of different clinical parameters in PE risk stratification and includes the PESI and sPESI scores as valuable tools to assess mortality risk.

MANAGEMENT OF ACUTE PULMONARY EMBOLISM

Unless contraindicated, anticoagulation is the first-line therapy in patients with acute PE regardless of its severity. It allows the natural thrombolytic system to function unopposed, ultimately reducing the thromboembolic burden.

Management of Acute Low-Risk PE

Low-risk PE (normotensive with normal biomarker levels and no RV dysfunction on imaging) can be adequately treated with anticoagulation alone and have an excellent prognosis and short-term mortality rates of approximately 1%.

Management of Acute Massive (High-Risk) PE

In patients with acute PE and sustained hypotension or hemodynamic collapse, the goal is to achieve rapid central clot removal to relieve life-threatening RV strain and immediately improve pulmonary perfusion. Guidelines suggest treatment escalation with primary reperfusion particularly with

TABLE 35.1

CLINICAL PARAMETERS DURING ASSESSMENT OF ACUTE PE

CLINICAL PARAMETERS	COMMENTS
Presenting Symptoms	
Dyspnea, chest pain	Common presenting symptoms
Syncope, presyncope, cardiopulmonary arrest	Concerning symptoms. Although not included in risk stratification strategies, they may help in the decision to escalate therapy
Presenting Signs	
Vital Signs: blood pressure, heart rate, oxygen saturation, temperature	Used for risk stratification and calculation of shock index (heart rate/systolic blood pressure)
Persistent hypoxia, tachypnea, marked tachycardia, and an inability to ambulate short distances	Concerning signs. Although some of these signs are not included in risk stratification strategies, they may help in the decision to escalate therapy
Severe hypertension	Increased risk of bleeding with thrombolytic therapy
Past Medical and Surgical History	
History of hypertension	May represent an increased risk of bleeding with thrombolytic therapy History of hypertension in a patient who presented with a systolic blood pressure of 100 mm Hg might be concerning for severe hypotension (massive PE)
Recent surgery/intervention (type, date), active bleeding, intracranial pathology, stroke	To assess the risk of bleeding with thrombolytic therapy
Imaging Studies	
CT pulmonary angiography	Helps in selecting the best treatment strategy and assists interventionalist for preprocedural preparation Assess vascular anatomy, location/extent of PE, right ventricular/left ventricular ratio (risk stratification), contrast reflux into the inferior vena cava/hepatic veins (radiographic sign of elevated right heart pressures), flattening of the interventricular septum (radiographic sign of right ventricular strain)
Echocardiography	Risk stratification and treatment strategy selection (right ventricular/left ventricular ratio, right ventricular hypokinesis, moving right ventricular emboli
Lower extremity ultrasound	Assess presence and location/extent of venous thrombosis. Help in access site selection if catheter-based therapy is selected
Electrocardiogram	To rule out acute myocardial infarction, assess arrhythmias, and evaluate for right ventricular strain (P-pulmonale, right-axis deviation, RBBB, or S1Q3T3)
Laboratory Tests	
Troponin, B-natriuretic peptide	Risk stratification
Elevated lactate	Concerning results; may suggest organ hypoperfusion
Elevated liver enzymes	Concerning results; may suggest liver dysfunction secondary to acute right heart failure

systemic thrombolysis (100 mg of intravenous tPA [alteplase; Genentech, South San Francisco, CA] infusion over 2 hours). In patients with contraindications for thrombolysis, severe hemodynamic collapse that is likely to cause death before full dose IV tPA infusion can take effect, and when systemic thrombolysis fails to improve hemodynamic status, guidelines suggest treatment escalation with surgical embolectomy or percutaneous catheter-directed therapy (catheter embolectomy or pharmacomechanical thrombectomy) if appropriate expertise and resources are available.

Management of Acute Submassive (Intermediate-Risk) PE

Unlike with massive and low-risk PE, the optimal management for submassive PE is still largely uncertain. Submassive PE is associated with a higher rate of clinical deterioration and mortality than low-risk PE despite anticoagulation. Although anticoagulation alone remains standard of care in the treatment of submassive PE, the question remains whether treatment should be routinely escalated. Systemic thrombolysis in particular has been extensively studied in acute submassive PE, demonstrating a small mortality benefit and a lower rate of clinical deterioration at the expense of increased bleeding risk.

CDT has garnered significant interest in the treatment of submassive PE based on its potential to confer higher efficacy compared to anticoagulation due to its local infusion of medication into the clot. In addition, there is a lower risk of bleeding compared to systemic thrombolysis due to significantly lower overall dose. However, its use is based on a mediocre level of evidence on the clinical effectiveness and safety compared to anticoagulation and systemic thrombolysis. Only three prospective clinical trials examining CDT in the setting of submassive and massive

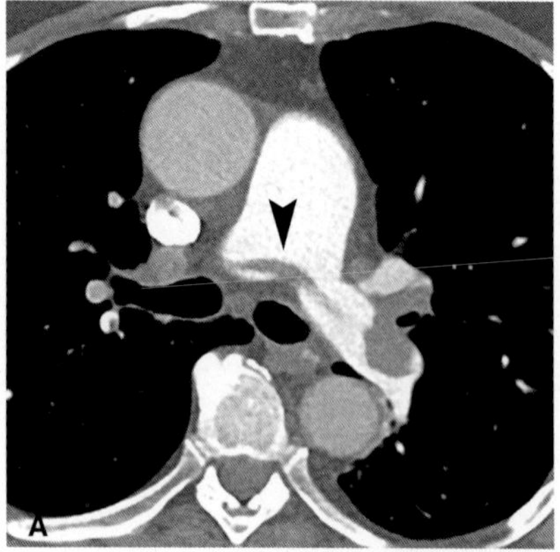

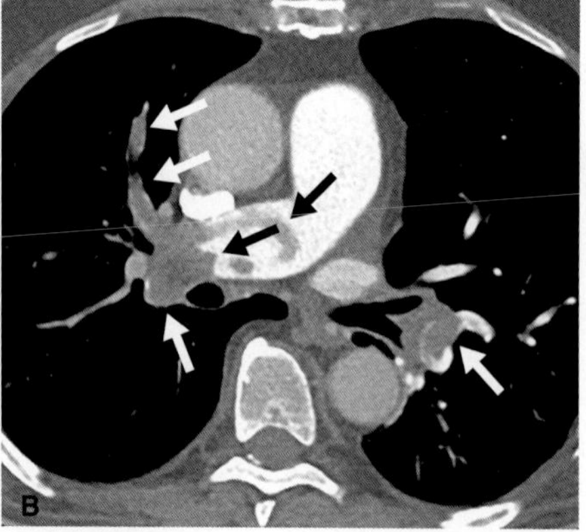

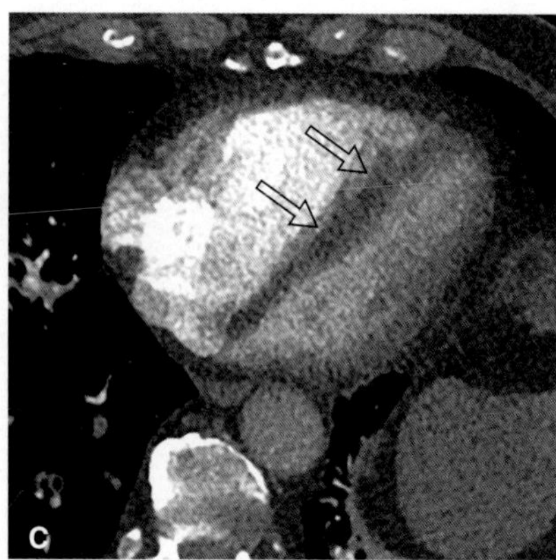

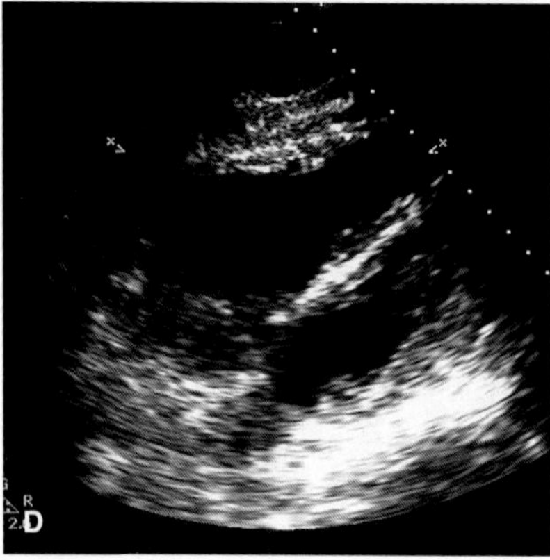

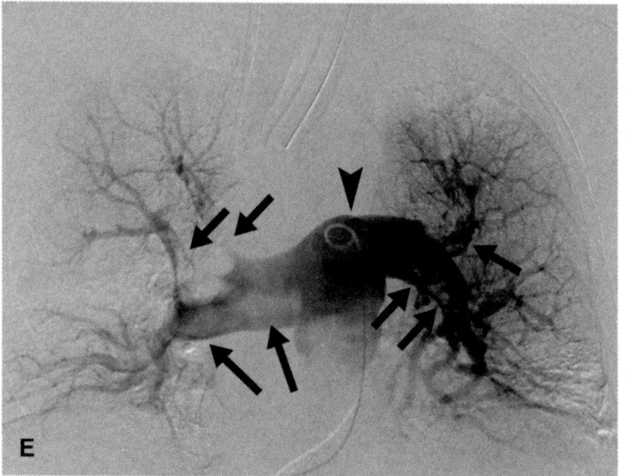

FIGURE 35.2. **A 78-Year-Old Man Presenting With Acute Dyspnea.** Initial evaluation revealed a dyspneic patient with a heart rate of 90 beats/min, a blood pressure of 140/87 mm Hg, and oxygen saturation of 85% to 90% on room air. **A, B:** Axial computed tomography pulmonary angiography (CTPA) showing acute saddle embolus (*arrowhead*) extending into the left and right main pulmonary arteries and their lobar branches (*arrows*). **C:** Axial CT image at the level of the ventricles shows a severely dilated right ventricle and flattening of the interventricular septum (*open arrows*); the right ventricle/left ventricle ratio on 4-chamber reformatted imaging was 2:1. **D:** Echocardiography performed at the emergency department shows a severely dilated and hypokinetic right ventricle. The cardiac biomarker levels were increased. The patient was transferred to the interventional radiology suite and pulmonary angiography (**E**) showed large filling defects in the main (*arrowhead*), left, and right pulmonary arteries and several lobar and segmental branches (*arrows*). (Reprinted with permission from Taslakian B, Sista AK. Catheter-directed therapy for pulmonary embolism: patient selection and technical considerations. *Interv Cardiol Clin* 2018;7(1):81–90.)

PE exist: Ultrasound Accelerated Thrombolysis of Pulmonary Embolism (ULTIMA), SEATTLE II, and Pulmonary Embolism Response to Fragmentation, Embolectomy, and Catheter Thrombolysis (PERFECT). Significant reductions in pulmonary artery (PA) pressures, and improved RV function and short-term pulmonary blood flow with CDT have been demonstrated. However, these studies are preliminary, and their data do not justify routine use of CDT for submassive PE. In addition, one of the largest knowledge gaps is whether CDT for submassive PE will prevent long-term morbidity and mortality.

CATHETER-DIRECTED THERAPY FOR ACUTE PE

Contraindications

Several relative and absolute contraindications for pulmonary angiography and catheter-directed intervention in the pulmonary circulation exist. However, in cases of severe PE requiring treatment escalation, a careful risk–benefit assessment, as well as knowledge of cardiopulmonary physiology and procedural pitfalls are essential to decrease the risk of procedure-related complications.

The risk of contrast reaction in patients with prior history can be adjusted by emergent prophylactic premedication; however, this risk should not delay treatment in cases of life-threatening massive PE and the procedure can potentially be performed without contrast injection.

Pulmonary hypertension is a relative contraindication to pulmonary angiography. Patients referred for interventional treatment of severe (massive and submassive) PE have at least some degree of pulmonary hypertension and RV strain. Therefore, careful assessment of the cardiopulmonary reserve and degree of pulmonary hypertension are important considerations prior to performing pulmonary angiography. Measurement of RV end diastolic pressure (RVEDP) and systolic PA pressure (PAP) is essential to determine the risk of angiography and obtain baseline preintervention pressure readings. The mortality associated with pulmonary angiography is increased (approximately 2% to 3%) in patients when the systolic PAP exceeds 55 mm Hg or RVEDP is greater than 20 mm Hg. Lower injection parameters, subselective injection, use of nonionic contrast media, and even avoiding angiography should be considered. In such cases, selective contrast injection into the main left or right PAs should be limited to a 20 to 30 mL volume at a rate of 10 to 15 mL/s. When preprocedural CTPA is available to demonstrate the location/extent of PA thrombus, injection of a large volume of contrast medium is usually unnecessary and angiography can be avoided altogether.

TABLE 35.2

PESI AND sPESI SCORING SYSTEMS FOR ACUTE PE

PULMONARY EMBOLISM SEVERITY INDEX (PESI)

CLINICAL FEATURES	NO. OF POINTS
Age	Score in years
Male gender	10
History of cancer	30
Heart failure	10
Chronic pulmonary disease	10
Pulse ≥110/min	20
Systolic blood pressure <100 mm Hg	30
Respiratory rate ≥30/min	20
Temperature <36°C	20
Arterial oxygen saturation <90% on room air	20
Altered mental status	60

PESI Classes

PESI Class I, <66 points (very low 30-day mortality; 0–1.6%)
PESI Class II, 66–85 points (low 30-day mortality risk; 1.7–3.5%)
PESI Class III, 86–105 points (moderate 30-day mortality risk; 3.2–7.1%)
PESI Class IV, 106–125 points (high 30-day mortality risk; 4.0–11.4%)
PESI Class V, >125 points (very high 30-day mortality risk; 10.0–24.5%)

SIMPLIFIED PULMONARY EMBOLISM SEVERITY INDEX (sPESI)

CLINICAL FEATURES	POINTS
Age >80	1
History of cancer	1
Chronic cardiopulmonary disease	1
Pulse ≥110/min	1
Systolic blood pressure <100 mm Hg	1
Arterial oxygen saturation <90%	1

sPESI Classes:

0 points, low risk (30-day mortality ~1.0%)
≥1 points, high risk (30-day mortality risk ~10.9%)

Jiménez D, Aujesky D, Moores L, et al. Simplification of the pulmonary embolism severity index for prognostication in patients with acute symptomatic pulmonary embolism. *Arch Intern Med* 2010;170(15):1383–1389. Carrier M, Righini M, Djurabi RK, et al. VIDAS D-dimer in combination with clinical pre-test probability to rule out pulmonary embolism. A systematic review of management outcome studies. *Thromb Haemost* 2009;101(5):886–892.

Because pulmonary intervention may precipitate right bundle branch block (RBBB), a pre-existing left bundle branch block (LBBB) is considered a relative contraindication. External pacing pads should be available, and the operator may elect to insert a transvenous pacing catheter prior to the procedure to treat complete heart block in the event that this complication occurs.

Because of the risk of major hemorrhage, catheter-directed infusion of thrombolytic agents may be contraindicated in patients with increased risk of bleeding (Table 35.4). In cases of high anticipated procedural risk, individualized risk assessment is essential preferably by reaching a multidisciplinary consensus on the best option for an individual patient, taking into account thrombus burden and location, imaging and biomarker results, bleeding risk, and clinical presentation (Table 35.5). In patients with recent surgeries, direct communication with the surgeon to conjunctly estimate the bleeding risk is recommended; surgeries might carry a lower than anticipated bleeding risk depending on the complexity of the surgery performed and surgical approach.

Procedure Preparation

Once a catheter-based intervention is selected, the procedure should be performed emergently or urgently based on the severity of the PE and patient's clinical status. Advance planning is the key for procedural success and avoiding complications. Review of available diagnostic imaging studies is essential to determine approach and choice of access vessel based on assessment of the relevant vascular anatomy, location/extent of pulmonary emboli, and presence/extent of deep venous thrombosis. If preprocedural lower extremity duplex is not available, a limited lower extremity ultrasound is strongly

TABLE 35.3

ACUTE PE RISK STRATIFICATION

■ AMERICAN HEART ASSOCIATION (AHA) RISK STRATIFICATION	
■ ACUTE PE CATEGORY	**■ DEFINITION**
Massive	Sustained hypotension (systolic blood pressure <90 mm Hg for >15 minutes or requiring inotropic support)[a] or Hemodynamic collapse (e.g., pulselessness or persistent profound bradycardia—heart rate <40 bpm, symptoms of shock)[a]
Submassive	Normotensive (systolic blood pressure >90 mm Hg) with either RV dysfunction[b,c] or myocardial injury[d]
Low risk	Normotensive with normal biomarker levels and no RV dysfunction on imaging
■ EUROPEAN SOCIETY OF CARDIOLOGY (ESC) RISK STRATIFICATION	
■ ACUTE PE CATEGORY	**■ DEFINITION**
High risk	Acute PE with sustained hypotension (SBP <90 mm Hg) or SBP drop >40 mm Hg for >15 minutes[a]
Intermediate risk	Normotensive with a PESI class III–V or sPESI ≥1
Intermediate–high risk	Evidence of both RV dysfunction[b] and elevated cardiac biomarker levels[c,d]
Intermediate–low risk	Absence of both or evidence of either RV dysfunction or elevated cardiac biomarker levels
Low risk	Normotensive, with PESI Class I–II or sPESI of 0, and absence of signs of RV dysfunction and myocardial injury[e]

[a]In the absence of other causes such as new-onset arrhythmias, hypovolemia, or sepsis.
[b]Imaging criteria of RV dysfunction: RV dilation (increased end-diastolic RV–LV diameter ratio >0.9); hypokinetic RV free wall; pulmonary hypertension as identified by increased velocity of the tricuspid regurgitation jet on echocardiography greater than 2.6 m/s; interventricular septal flattening; paradoxical motion toward the left ventricle; abnormal transmitral Doppler flow profile; tricuspid regurgitation; and loss of inspiratory collapse of the inferior vena cava; or combinations of the above.
[c]Markers of heart failure due to RV dysfunction: elevation of B-type natriuretic peptide (BNP >90 pg/mL) or elevation of N-terminal pro-BNP (>500 pg/mL).
[d]Markers of myocardial injury: elevated cardiac troponin I (>0.4 ng/mL) or troponin T (>0.1 ng/mL).
[e]Patients with PESI Class I–II, or with sPESI of 0, and elevated cardiac biomarkers or signs of RV dysfunction on imaging tests are classified into the intermediate–low-risk group.

TABLE 35.4

CONTRAINDICATIONS TO CATHETER DIRECTED THROMBOLYSIS

■ ABSOLUTE CONTRAINDICATIONS
Active bleeding
Recent GI bleed (<3 months)
Recent intracranial or intraspinal surgery (<3 months)
Recent cerebrovascular accident (<2 months)
Presence of active intracranial processes (e.g., aneurysm, vascular malformation, or neoplasm)
■ RELATIVE CONTRAINDICATIONS
Recent (<10 days) major general surgery, deep organ biopsy or puncture, or obstetrical delivery
Major internal bleeding within the past 6 months
Recent major trauma
Recent eye trauma or surgery
Uncontrolled severe hypertension (systolic blood pressure >200 mm Hg; diastolic blood pressure >110 mm Hg)
Pregnancy
Recent cardiopulmonary resuscitation
Thrombocytopenia or bleeding diathesis
Intracranial malignancy or vascular lesion
Hemorrhagic retinopathy

advised to evaluate the vascular access. The risk of arrhythmias and heart block should be evaluated by the operator after review of ECG findings.

Before starting the procedure, the operator should ensure the preparedness of the team, availability of all required equipment (Table 35.6), and the presence of an appropriate support team. It is essential to discuss the procedure plan and the anticipated course of the procedure and complications with the assistants, technologists, nurses, and anesthesia staff. If anesthesia is required, a specialized cardiac anesthesiologist is recommended. Medications that diminish ventricular preload and depress myocardial contractility, such as Propofol, should be avoided.

Percutaneous Catheter-Directed Therapy for Massive PE

In patients with hemodynamic collapse, the goal is rapid debulking of central clots to immediately restore blood flow to the pulmonary circulation, improve oxygenation, and relieve life-threatening RV dysfunction. Percutaneous catheter-directed PE intervention is a possible alternative to surgical embolectomy in high-risk patients. Several endovascular techniques exist to remove, macerate, and/or dissolve acute PEs with low-dose thrombolytic drugs. The choice of procedure and tools will differ based on the severity of the PE, operator preference, and estimated bleeding risk.

Percutaneous mechanical thrombectomy in patients with high risk of bleeding achieves central thrombus removal without fibrinolytic drug infusion. Mechanical thrombectomy techniques

TABLE 35.5

DIRECTIONS FOR INTERMEDIATE-RISK PE MANAGEMENT

■ INTERMEDIATE-RISK PE TYPE/PRESENTATION	■ NEED FOR TREATMENT ESCALATION WITH CDT
Intermediate–high-risk PE bordering on high risk: very sick patients with signs of organ hypoperfusion (e.g., elevated lactate and liver enzymes) or severe RV dysfunction	Frequently If there is a saddle embolus, consult cardiothoracic surgery, as embolectomy might be a viable option; systemic lysis may also be an option
Intermediate–high-risk PE (sPESI ≥1, with evidence of both RV dysfunction and elevated cardiac biomarker levels)	Possibly; particularly if there are concerning signs such as a severely hypokinetic RV and occlusive central clot, particularly if there is a lack of improvement in symptoms and hemodynamics with anticoagulation alone, and low bleeding risk
Intermediate–low-risk PE (sPESI ≥1, with absence of both or evidence of either RV dysfunction or elevated cardiac biomarker levels)	Infrequently May choose to undergo CDT in young or active patients with central thrombus and low risk of bleeding

Reprinted with permission from Taslakian B, Sista AK. Catheter-Directed Therapy for Pulmonary Embolism: Patient Selection and Technical Considerations. *Interv Cardiol Clin* 2018;7(1):81–90.

include: (1) pressurized saline injection through a catheter's tip (rheolytic embolectomy); (2) fragmentation of thrombus by a rotating device at the catheter tip (rotational embolectomy); (3) aspiration of the thrombus through a large-lumen end-hole catheter using a syringe and a hemostatic valve or aspiration devices (suction embolectomy) (Fig. 35.3); (4) rotation of a standard pigtail; or (5) balloon angioplasty and maceration of the thrombus. Macerated fragments can be continuously aspirated through a catheter port to decrease clot burden.

In patients with low risk of bleeding, a pharmacomechanical thrombectomy can be performed by mechanical clot fragmentation and in conjunction with catheter-directed intraclot injection of a low-dose thrombolytic drug. For further technical details on catheter-directed thrombolytic drug infusion or CDT, see the submassive PE section below (***Percutaneous Catheter-Directed Therapy for Submassive PE***). An advantage of pharmacomechanical thrombectomy with an extended thrombolytic infusion after mechanically debulking the central thrombus is the potential for reducing the risk of chronic PE formation. This is particularly true if there is residual elevation of PAPs with RV strain and the PE has been "downstaged" from massive to submassive PE. Data on thrombolytic therapy have suggested it may reduce the likelihood of developing chronic thromboembolic pulmonary hypertension (CTEPH).

The venous system may be accessed with direct ultrasound guidance from the internal jugular vein or common femoral vein with differing advantages and disadvantages depending on the individual device used. Several catheters can be used to catheterize the PAs (Table 35.6). As described earlier, pressure measurements should be obtained to establish a baseline and to determine the injection rate for angiography. Selective left and right pulmonary angiography is commonly performed at a left (20 degrees) and anteroposterior or slight right anterior oblique projection, respectively at an imaging rate of 4 to 6 frames per second. When a single projection is used, a repeat angiogram in a different angle may be required in select cases to help separate the distal branches. The contralateral oblique projection is valuable for separating out branches of the lower lobes. Detailed angiography is often unnecessary when preprocedural CTPA is available to evaluate the anatomy and location/extent of thrombus to shorten the procedure time and achieve rapid central clot removal in these hemodynamically unstable patients. A catheter/wire combination is then used to traverse the central thrombus.

Several devices have been described to effectively debulk the central thrombus in patients with massive PE. The most common technique is rotating pigtail catheter fragmentation using a standard 5-Fr catheter inserted over a wire exiting from a side hole at the outer curvature of the pigtail loop, leaving the loop free to rotate around the wire to provide stability. The clot is fragmented by placing the catheter distal to the clot and rotating the pigtail while retracting proximally. Additional clot maceration may be achieved with inflation of an angioplasty balloon slightly smaller than the largest PA diameter (usually <16-mm balloons). Adjunctive aspiration thrombectomy may be required to remove the clot with a large (>8 Fr) end-hole catheter or sheath or by using specialized catheters. Different new thrombus removal devices offer the potential for robust thrombus removal. Further details on these devices are beyond the score of this chapter; review articles are available for detailed description of these devices.

Percutaneous Catheter-Directed Therapy for Submassive PE

In submassive (intermediate-risk) PE, central clot fragmentation may lead to distal embolization resulting in acute elevation of PAP and RV afterload and therefore it is advised to avoid mechanical techniques in this group of patients. Infusion of fibrinolytic drug through an embedded catheter into the clot potentially exposes a larger surface area of the embolus, theoretically accelerating clot lysis. Schmitz-Rode et al. emphasized this mechanism by demonstrating proximal vortex formation by obstructing emboli which may divert systematically administered thrombolytic drugs away from the thrombus, thus minimizing efficacy and delivering a substantial dose to the systemic circulation. CDT instead delivers a substantially lower dose of fibrinolytic drug directly into the thrombus over an extended period of time (12 to 24 hours). Therefore, the rationale for CDT is to improve thrombolytic efficacy and safety compared to systemic thrombolysis, which is yet to be proven by randomized controlled trials.

Intraclot delivery of the thrombolytic drug can be achieved through a standard multisidehole catheter (Fig. 35.4). An alternative is the use of ultrasound-assisted CDT drug delivery catheter systems that use microsonic (high-frequency, low-intensity ultrasound) energy delivered through the catheter core which theoretically alters the local architecture of the clot and drives the thrombolytic agent deep into the blood clot to enhance thrombolysis. Ultrasound-assisted CDT was used in ULTIMA and SEATTLE II trials; however, investigators did not compare its efficacy with standard CDT. In the PERFECT registry there was no difference in technical or clinical success

TABLE 35.6

INTERVENTIONAL PE TREATMENT TRAY: EQUIPMENT NEEDED FOR CATHETER-BASED THERAPY

■ EQUIPMENT	■ PURPOSE
Vascular Access	
Vascular sheath (5–6 Fr, short)	To secure initial vascular access Will require two sheaths if plan for bilateral CDT
Micropuncture needle kit (Boston Scientific, Natick, MA or Cook Medical Inc., Bloomington, IN)	To reduce the risk of access site–related complications
Ultrasound for guidance and sterile ultrasound probe cover	To reduce the risk of access site–related complications
Pulmonary Catheterization and Angiography	
Cobra, angled pigtail (Grollman), or straight pigtail catheters (100 cm)	To catheterize the pulmonary artery
Balloon-tipped pulmonary artery catheter	Can be helpful in cases of severe tricuspid regurgitation or a severely dilated right ventricle To avoid entrapment behind a papillary muscle while crossing the tricuspid valve (less likely than nonballoon catheters to become entrapped underneath a tricuspid valve papillary muscle or chordae, thus avoiding damage to the tricuspid apparatus)
Pigtail catheter	To perform pulmonary angiography
Rosen wire (0.035 inch, 260 cm) Wholey wire (0.035 inch, 260 cm)	Start with an exchange length medium stiffness wire, to provide stability
Amplatz wire (0.035 inch, 260 cm)	Stiff wire to provide increased stability for catheter exchange or escalation to mechanical thrombectomy
Long Flexor sheath (5–6 Fr, 55 cm)	To provide a stable access for catheter-directed thrombolysis
Medications	
Intravenous unfractionated heparin (300–500 units/hour through the sheath)	To maintain subtherapeutic anticoagulation and prevent perisheath clot formation
tPA (alteplase; Genentech, South San Francisco, CA)	To perform thrombolysis; recommended total infusion dose is 1–2 mg/h for a total dose of 24 mg (half the dose through each catheter for bilateral catheters)
Contrast agent (nonionic, low-osmolality contrast)	To perform angiography
Infusion Catheters	
Cragg-McNamara® Valved Infusion Catheter (Covidien, Plymouth, MN)	Multisidehole catheter for intraclot infusion of thrombolytic agent
UniFuse™ Infusion Catheter (Angiodynamics, Latham, NY)	Multisidehole catheter for intraclot infusion of thrombolytic agent
Ultrasound-assisted EkoSonic® Endovascular System (EKOS, Bothell, WA)	Multisidehole catheter with an ultrasound emitting wire to perform ultrasound-assisted catheter-directed thrombolysis
Other Devices	
External pacemaker, internal venous pacemaker	To treat complete heart block if this complication occurs

Reprinted with permission from Taslakian B, Sista AK. Catheter-directed therapy for pulmonary embolism: patient selection and technical considerations. *Interv Cardiol Clin* 2018;7(1):81–90.

between ultrasound-assisted and standard CDT. It is unclear whether ultrasound-assisted CDT offers improved fibrinolysis and safety over standard multipurpose catheters, as there were no randomized trials comparing these two techniques.

A common femoral or internal jugular vein access is obtained preferably using ultrasound-guided, single-wall puncture to minimize the risk of access site complications. If bilateral PA infusion is required, a second venous access is obtained. The right internal jugular approach may be preferred in the presence of a large thrombus in the IVC, iliac vein, and/or femoral vein. The venous access can be initially secured with a 5-Fr or 6-Fr vascular sheath. After pressure measurement and pulmonary angiography, the access wire can be exchanged for a stiff wire (e.g., 0.035-in Rosen or Amplatz) to provide stability for subsequent long vascular sheath placement to traverse the pulmonary valve and allow for stability of infusion catheters for the duration of thrombolysis. Multisidehole catheters (infusion lengths of 10 to 20 cm) are passed over the wires via the sheaths and embedded within the thrombus. The tip of the catheter is commonly placed in a location that allows maximum thrombolytic delivery into the clot burden through the sideholes. The recommended total tPA infusion rate is 1 to 2 mg/h, for a total dose of 24 mg. Some operators advocate boluses of tPA of 1 to 4 mg during initial

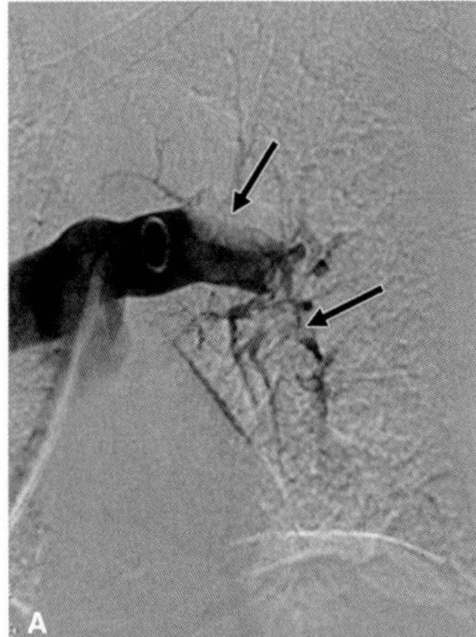

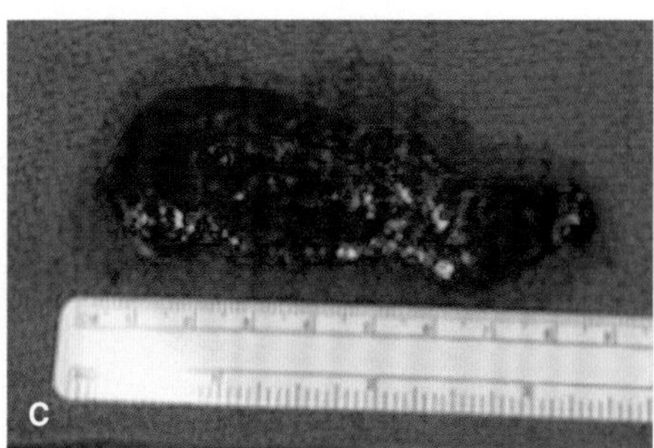

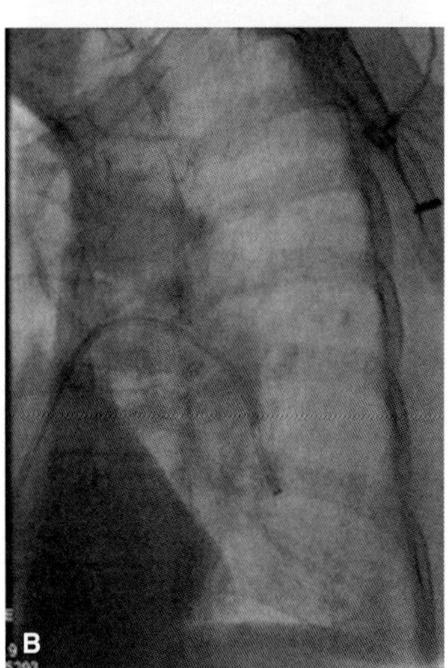

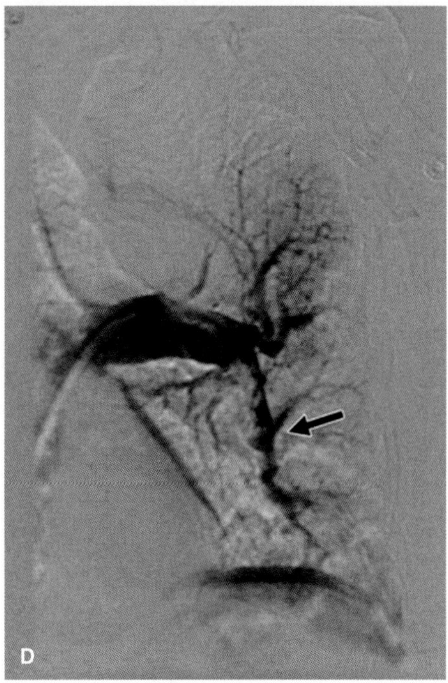

FIGURE 35.3. **Demonstration of Aspiration Thrombectomy With the CT 8 Device (Penumbra, Alameda, California) in a 73-Year-Old Woman With an Acute Submassive PE. A:** Bulky thrombus (*arrows*) in the left upper and lower lobe pulmonary arteries. **B:** Aspiration catheter embedded in the left lower lobe clot. **C:** The aspirated thrombus in various stages of organization. **D:** The immediate postextraction angiogram demonstrates improved perfusion to the left lower lobe (*arrow*). (Reprinted with permission from Sista AK, Kuo WT, Schiebler M, Madoff DC. Stratification, imaging, and management of acute massive and submassive pulmonary embolism. *Radiology* 2017;284(1):5–24.)

catheter placement. A common protocol infuses alteplase at a rate of 0.5 to 1 mg/h through each PA catheter if bilateral catheters are used. The recommended concentration for t-PA is 0.01 to 0.05 mg/mL of normal saline solution and the pump can be set accordingly to deliver the prescribed dose of tPA (e.g., infusion rate starting at 0.5 to 2 mg/h).

Postprocedural Management and Follow-Up Care

A structured approach to postprocedural care, including early identification and management of complications, specific instructions during monitoring period, effective inpatient rounds, and routine outpatient follow-up facilitates efficient and thorough management with an emphasis on quality and patient safety.

Following the procedure, the vascular sheaths and infusion catheters should be secured in place with sutures and dressing. A transfer to a monitored bed is required during the infusion period for close monitoring of vital signs and screening for potential complications. A detailed postprocedural order set that includes instructions for the observation period and specific criteria for nursing staff to alert the physicians is essential (Table 35.7). PAP measurements can be obtained through the long sheath, if used, during the monitoring period. Fibrinogen levels can be monitored, particularly if the infusion will be continued beyond 24 hours and in those patients at greater risk of bleeding. However, fibrinogen levels do not clearly correlate with bleeding. When fibrinogen levels drop below 100 mg/dL, most operators prefer to reduce (to half), or discontinue thrombolysis, or alternatively continue with transfusions of fresh frozen plasma if further thrombolysis is desired. Some operators may switch tPA infusion to normal saline if fibrinogen levels drop below 50 mg/dL. The duration of infusion varies between operators, but is usually limited to 12 to 24 hours. Posttreatment angiography and/or echocardiography can be performed to assess the clot burden and RV function.

During the procedure, full heparin anticoagulation may be continued (target anti-Xa goal of 0.3 to 0.5 units/mL). However, once thrombolytic infusion has been started, some operators prefer to discontinue full heparin anticoagulation and use subtherapeutic heparin infusions to minimize the risk of bleeding complications. During concomitant low-dose tPA infusion, a subtherapeutic heparin dose (e.g., 300 to 500 units/h through a peripheral IV site or the vascular sheath; partial thromboplastin time [PTT] <60 s) is desirable by some operators to minimize risk of perisheath clot formation. Once CDT is completed, full therapeutic anticoagulation should be resumed immediately and maintained for 7 to 10 days as a bridge to subsequent oral anticoagulation.

Interventionalists should participate in longitudinal follow-up for massive and submassive PE patients. Outpatient follow-up ensures adequate anticoagulation and recognition of signs and symptoms of long-term complications such as unresolved dyspnea and exercise intolerance. If an IVC filter was inserted during the procedure, the patient should be scheduled for filter retrieval once filtration is no longer indicated to spare

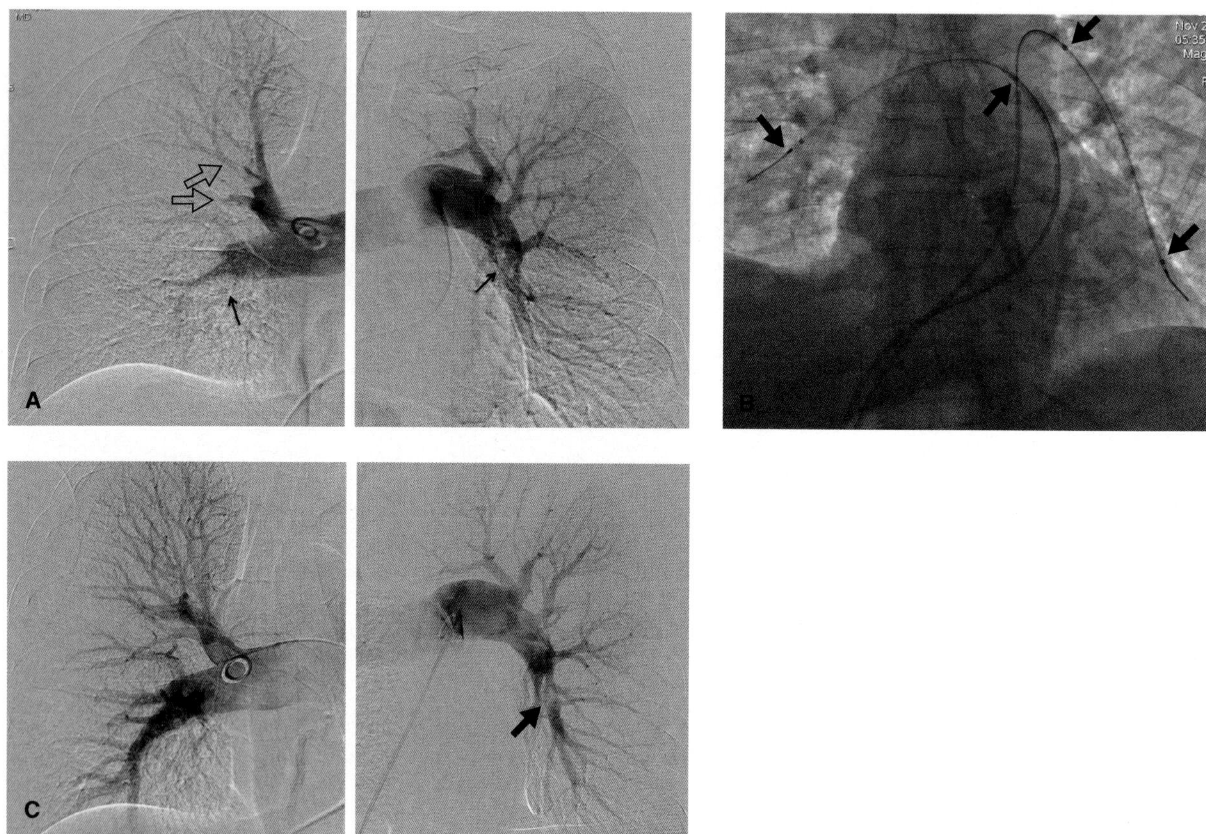

FIGURE 35.4. **Catheter-Directed Thrombolysis in Submassive PE. A:** Initial pulmonary angiograms in a 55-year-old man with submassive PE demonstrate poor perfusion and proximal thrombus (*black arrows*). Also note the vascular "cut-off" of the right upper lobe lateral segmental and middle lobar pulmonary arteries (*open arrows*). **B:** Bilateral 5-Fr, 10-cm infusion catheters embedded within the thrombus. The 10-cm infusion lengths are demarcated by the radiopaque markers (*arrows*). Multiple sideholes are present between the markers that infuse the thrombolytic agent. Recombinant tPA (0.5 mg per hour per catheter) was infused for a total of 22 hours. **C:** Post-CDT angiograms demonstrate improved perfusion with mild residual thrombus in the left lower lobe pulmonary artery (*arrow*). Pulmonary artery systolic pressure improved from 61 to 41 mm Hg after infusion. (Reprinted with permission from Sista AK, Kuo WT, Schiebler M, Madoff DC. Stratification, imaging, and management of acute massive and submassive pulmonary embolism. *Radiology* 2017;284(1):5–24.)

TABLE 35.7

POSTPROCEDURAL INFUSION INSTRUCTIONS

■ INSTRUCTIONS	■ RATIONALE
Keep patient on complete bed rest with legs extended (femoral access)	Minimize the risk of access site complications and dislodging the catheter
Keep patient fasting (or on clear liquid diet)	Depending on clinical status, other comorbidities, risk of aspiration, expected risk of bleeding and need to an emergency surgery, intubation, or reintervention to prevent or decrease the risk of aspiration
Check vascular access sites for signs of bleeding and hematoma formation	Early detection of access site complications
Perform serial neurologic examinations (every 2–4 hours)	Early detection of intracranial bleeding complications
Monitor complete blood count (CBC), fibrinogen, partial thrombin time (PTT) (e.g., every 4 hours)	Early detection of complications (bleeding, acute anemia, supratherapeutic levels of anticoagulation, hypofibrinogenemia)
Remove sheaths and perform manual compression for hemostasis (30–45 minutes) after thrombolytic infusion is stopped	This is the correct/recommended period to allow for rapidly obtaining hemostasis while minimizing the total amount of time that the patient is not therapeutically anticoagulated

Reprinted with permission from Taslakian B, Sista AK. Catheter-directed therapy for pulmonary embolism: patient selection and technical considerations. *Interv Cardiol Clin* 2018;7(1):81–90.

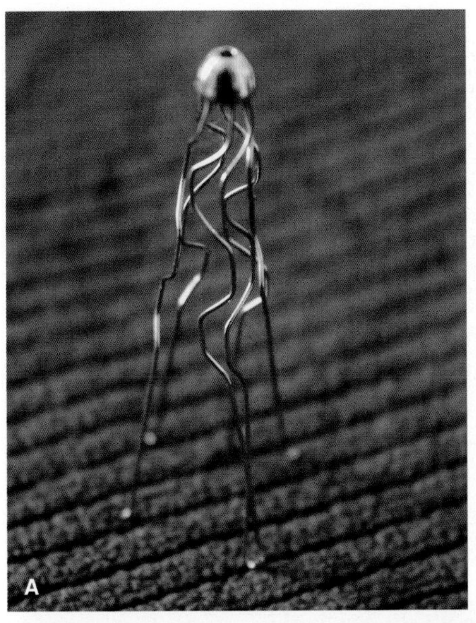

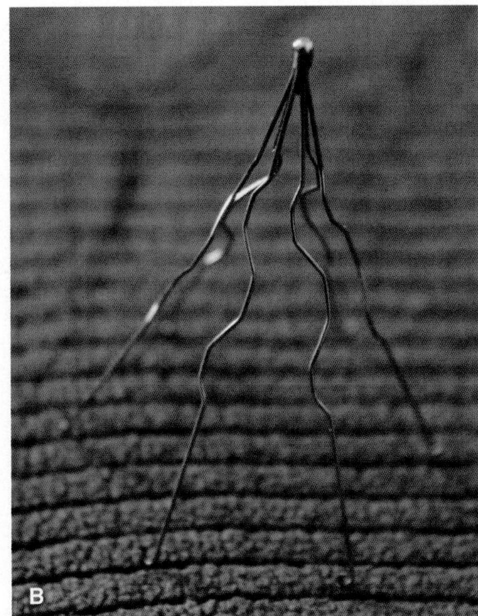

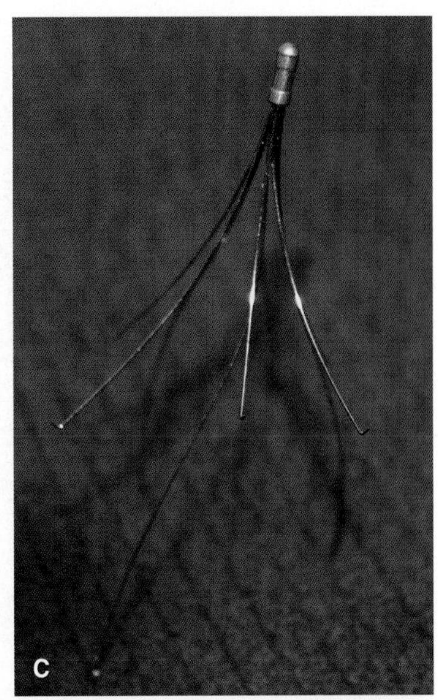

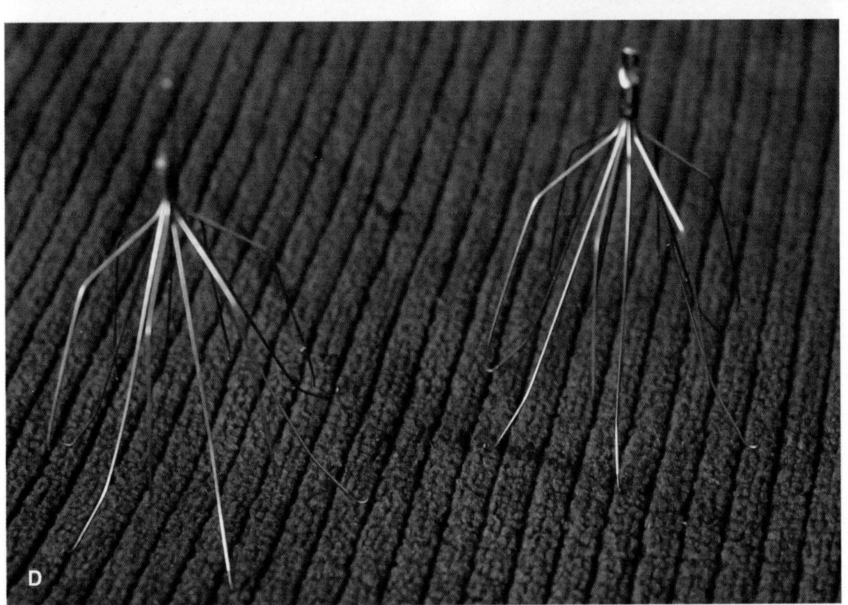

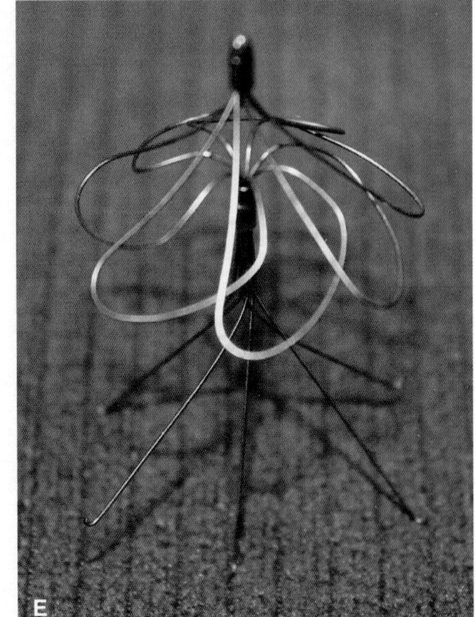

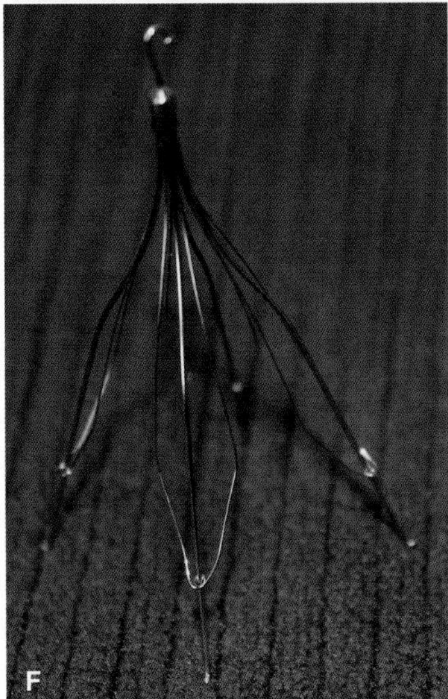

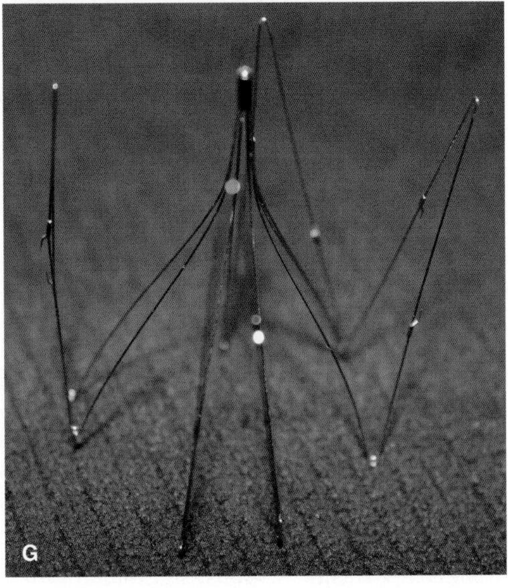

FIGURE 35.5. **Different IVC Filters.** **A:** Greenfield filter (stainless steel) (Boston Scientific, Natick, MA). **B:** Greenfield filter (Titanium) (Boston Scientific, Natick, MA). **C:** ALN filter (ALN International, Miami, FL). **D:** G2 (left) and Eclipse (right) filters (Bard Peripheral, Tempe, AZ). **E:** Simon Nitinol filter (Bard Peripheral, Tempe, AZ). **F:** Gunther Tulip filter (Cook Medical, Bloomington, IN). **G:** VenaTech LP filter (B. Braun, Sheffield, UK). *(continued)*

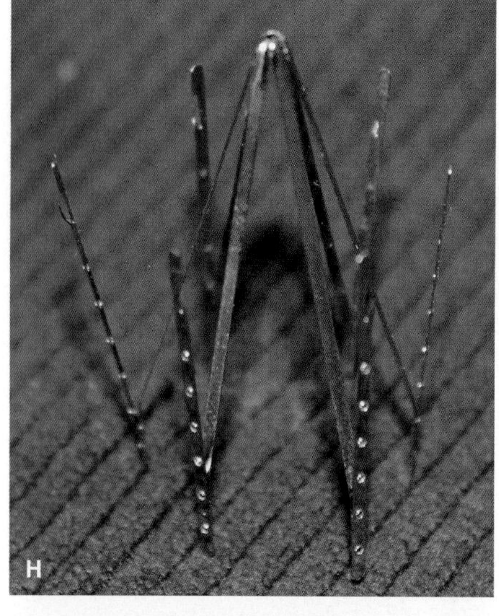

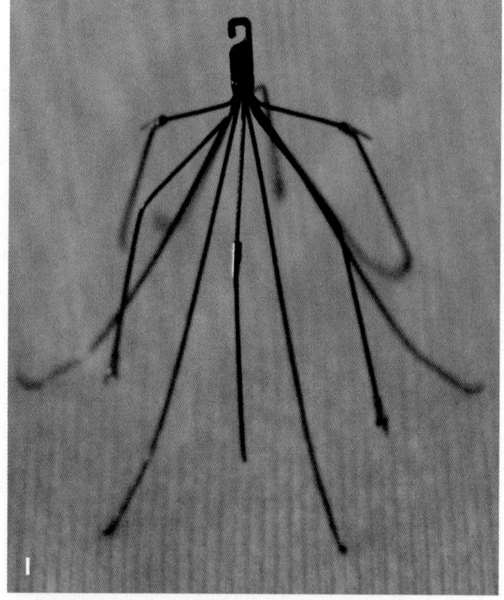

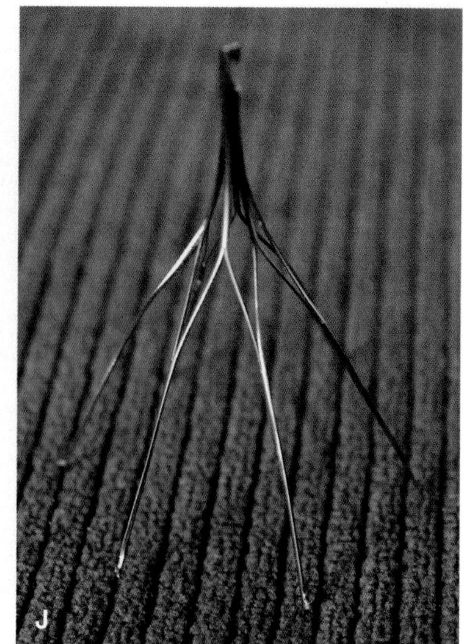

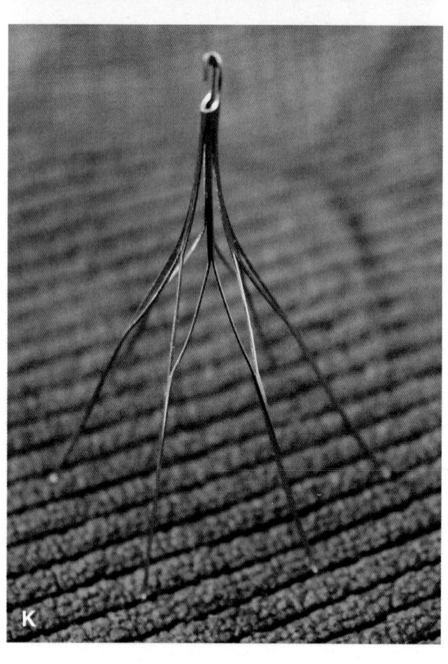

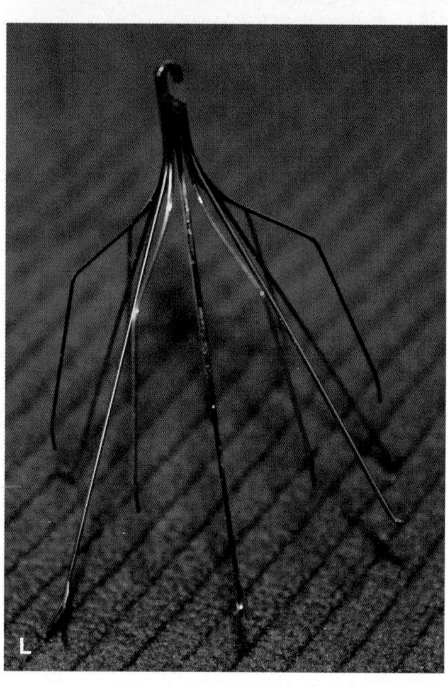

FIGURE 35.5. (*Continued*) **H:** VenaTech LGM filter (B. Braun, Sheffield, UK). **I:** Meridian filter (Bard Peripheral, Tempe, AZ). **J:** Option filter (Rex Medical, Conshohocken, PA). **K:** Option ELITE filter (Rex Medical, Conshohocken, PA). **L:** Denali filter (Bard Peripheral, Tempe, AZ).

patients the potential risks associated with long-term filter implantation.

IVC FILTERS

The goal of vena caval interruption, currently accomplished by percutaneous image-guided insertion of an IVC filter, is to prevent a symptomatic PE by capturing the clot. It is an important option in the management of selected patients with VTE. Several different IVC filter models have been used (Figs. 35.5 and 35.6). The current generation of IVC filter devices derives from the design and performance characteristics obtained from the Greenfield IVC filter. Most IVC filters have a conal shape to capture emboli within the center of the vein, allowing for dissolution of the trapped clot over time and para-axial venous blood flow. There are two general types of IVC filters currently available in the United States; permanent and optional. Permanent filters have been used since the 1970s and are placed in patients with a long-term need for mechanical prophylaxis against PE and absolute contraindications to anticoagulation. In recent years, there has been a trend toward the use of optional filters; these are permanent filters with the option to be removed if no longer clinically needed and can be entirely removed (retrievable filters) or converted to a caval stent (convertible filters), depending on the design. Most optional filters are designed to be removed and have a hook typically at the cranial tip of the filter that can be grasped with a snare.

Indications for IVC Filter Placement

The indication for caval filtration remains the main controversy for IVC filters. Anticoagulation remains the preferred treatment for VTE. Depending on the risk of PE and/or downsides of anticoagulation, the indications for IVC filters can be categorized into three main groups: absolute indications, relative indications, or prophylactic indications (Table 35.8). Although there is little controversy about the absolute indications, substantial differences about the relative and prophylactic indications exist. These are mostly based on "expert opinion," and case series, and not supported by prospective,

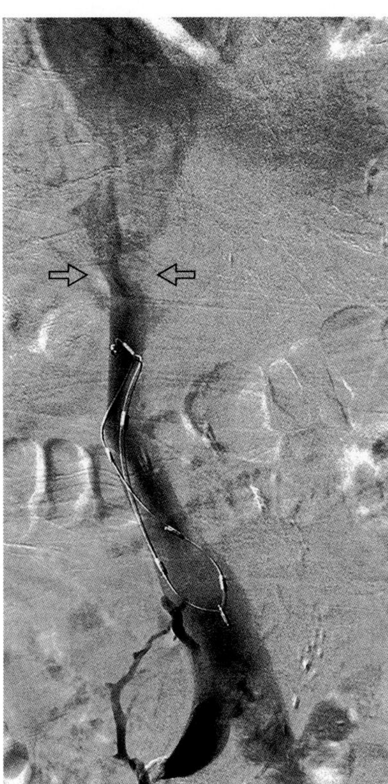

FIGURE 35.6. **Venogram Postplacement of a Crux Filter (Volcano Corporation, Rancho Cordova, CA).** The level of the renal veins is annotated with open arrows. Retrieval hooks on both the cranial and caudal ends of the filter allow filter removal from either a jugular or femoral access.

TABLE 35.8

INDICATIONS FOR INFERIOR VENA CAVA FILTERS

Absolute (Classic) Indications
Documented VTE with one of the following: ▪ Recurrent PE despite adequate anticoagulation ▪ Failure of anticoagulation (propagation/progression of DVT during therapeutic anticoagulation) ▪ Contraindication to anticoagulation ▪ Complication of anticoagulation ▪ Inability to achieve/maintain therapeutic anticoagulation ▪ Massive PE with residual DVT in a patient at risk for further PE
Relative (Extended) Indications
Documented VTE with one of the following: ▪ Iliocaval DVT ▪ Large, free-floating proximal thrombus ▪ Thrombolysis for iliocaval DVT ▪ VTE with limited cardiopulmonary reserve ▪ Poor compliance with anticoagulation ▪ High risk of complication of anticoagulation (e.g., frequent falls)
Prophylactic Indications
No documented VTE, but at risk of developing VTE and cannot receive anticoagulation or be monitored for the development of VTE ▪ Severe trauma ▪ Closed head injury ▪ Spinal injury ▪ Multiple long bone or pelvic fractures ▪ Surgical procedure in patient at high risk of VTE ▪ Medical condition with high risk of VTE

Kaufman JA, Kinney TB, Streiff MB, et al. Guidelines for the use of retrievable and convertible vena cava filters: report from the Society of Interventional Radiology multidisciplinary consensus conference. *J Vasc Interv Radiol* 2006;17:449–459.
Caplin DM, Nikolic B, Kalva SP, et al. Quality improvement guidelines for the performance of inferior vena cava filter placement for the prevention of pulmonary embolism. *J Vasc Interv Radiol* 2011;22(11):1499–1506.

randomized controlled trials. Based on the current available data, guidelines for IVC filter placement from the American College of Radiology (ACR) in conjunction with the Society of Interventional Radiology (SIR), AHA, ACCP, and ESC support IVC filter placement in patients with VTE and a contraindication to anticoagulation. In patients with submassive PE, there are no data to support the routine placement of IVC filters. Patients with massive PE and proximal DVT should receive IVC filters regardless of anticoagulation status, based on lower mortality associations with IVC filters in the International Cooperative Pulmonary Embolism Registry (ICOPER) and a national inpatient database survey.

Contraindications

There are very few contraindications for caval filtration. The main contraindication for an IVC filter is absence of a location to place the filter, such as occlusion or absence of the IVC. In these conditions, blood returns to the heart through multiple tortuous and small collateral venous networks preventing large blood clots from traveling to the pulmonary circulation. However, if a large collateral venous pathway develops over time, placement of a filter into the azygos or hemiazygos vein can be considered. Another contraindication to percutaneous IVC filter placement is lack of access to the IVC in cases when all possible venous access sites are occluded.

Coagulopathy is generally a contraindication for percutaneous procedures. However, due to availability of jugular delivery systems, relatively small size of filter placement sheaths, and the use of ultrasound guidance for access, IVC filters can be safely placed in almost every patient with coagulopathy. Other contraindications such as renal insufficiency and severe allergy to contrast media can be mitigated by the use of alternative contrast agents for venography such as gadolinium or CO_2.

Technique

Knowledge of venous drainage pathways, including congenital anomalies is essential. There are numerous, but rare variations in the venous anatomy of the abdomen and pelvis which may impact IVC filter placement (Table 35.9).

IVC filters are available in a jugular or femoral delivery system. For symmetric filters, one delivery system can be used for either approach. For nonsymmetric cone-shaped filters, selecting the appropriate delivery system (jugular or femoral) is important to avoid an upside-down placed filter. The most commonly used access sites are the right common femoral and right internal jugular veins because of straight alignment of the delivery system with the IVC to avoid filter tilting. However, new generations of filters can be placed from any vein including peripheral veins due to the low profile of the delivery systems combined with the high deformability of the mostly nitinol-based filters. If a peripheral vein is selected for access, a longer delivery sheath might be needed.

TABLE 35.9

VARIATIONS OF VENOUS ANATOMY OF THE ABDOMEN AND PELVIS

■ VENOUS ANATOMY VARIANT	■ COMMENTS
Absent IVC (0.15% of patients)	The blood is drained through the azygos system (azygos continuation). No IVC filter can be placed
Left-sided IVC (2% of patients)	Typically drain into the left renal vein, which crosses anterior to the aorta to join the right IVC
Duplicated IVC	Typically left accessory IVC with a left common iliac vein is present. Either a suprarenal IVC filter or two IVC filters, one in each IVC, have to be placed for appropriate caval filtration. Alternatively, a filter can be placed in each common iliac vein or a filter can be placed in the right-sided IVC and the left-sided IVC can be embolized
Circumaortic (5.5%) left renal vein	One left renal vein crosses anterior to the aorta and another crosses posterior to the aorta. IVC filters should be placed below the circumaortic renal vein because if the IVC filter is placed between the main left renal vein and the circumaortic renal vein, a possible conduit exists for clot from the lower extremity to bypass the filter
Retroaortic left renal vein (4.7%)	Do not impact IVC filter placement because no venous conduit exists for bypassing an infrarenal IVC filter

Preprocedural assessment of clinical data, indications, and contraindications is essential. Evaluation of available imaging studies, such as cross-sectional imaging, can provide detailed assessment of the venous anatomy and anomalies can be depicted to avoid incomplete filtration. In general, IVC filters are placed in an infrarenal position, to minimize the space between the filter tip and the inflow of the renal veins. The rationale is to limit the area of stagnant blood in case of filter thrombosis and avoid renal vein thrombosis. Placement at the level of the renal veins should be avoided because of the possibility that parts of the filter might engage with a renal vein, causing severe filter tilting. Therefore, placement of the filter tip about 1 cm below the renal veins has become more popular recently with optional filters. Some operators advocate positioning the filter with the hook at the level of the renal inflow to avoid thrombus formation on the hook and therefore rendering the retrieval easier (Fig. 35.7).

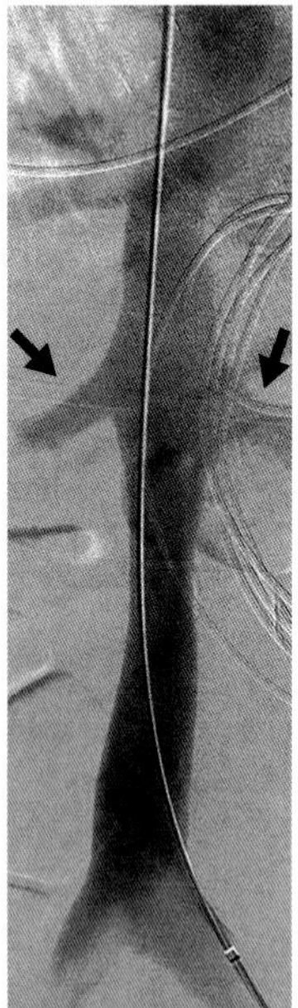

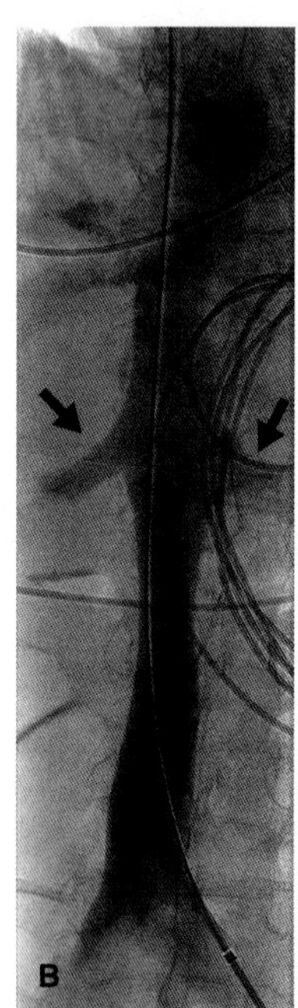

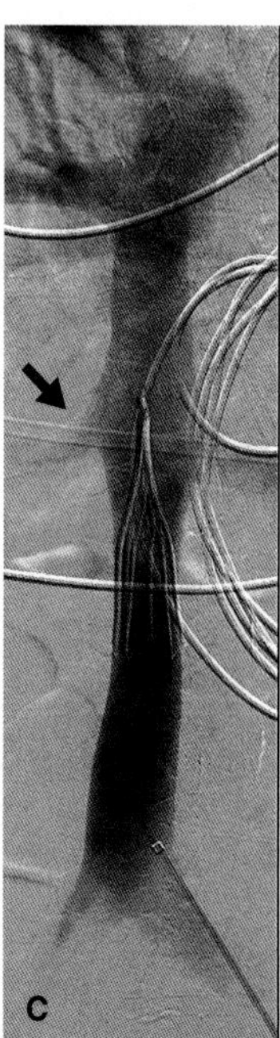

FIGURE 35.7. Filter Placement. A: Digital subtraction venography and **(B)** nonsubtracted IVC venogram prior to filter placement show contrast reflux within the renal veins (*arrows*). **C:** Digital subtraction venography post Option filter placement shows appropriate positioning of the filter with the hook at the level of the renal vein inflow (*arrow*) and without significant tilting.

After obtaining a venous access, venography should be performed to evaluate the venous anatomy and identify the location of the renal veins for accurate infrarenal placement of the IVC filter. When a cross-sectional imaging is not available, a jugular approach with venography performed from the left common iliac vein is advised to identify duplicate IVCs. Alternatively, a left common femoral approach can be selected in these cases. To avoid filter migration, the diameter of the IVC must be measured before placement. There is no minimally required IVC diameter for any device, but there is an upper diameter for each filter. Typically, for an IVC larger than 28 mm, only certain devices are approved. If the cava has a diameter >30 mm (megacava), two filters can be placed in the common iliac veins.

If an IVC thrombus is detected, the filter should be placed above the most cranial extension of the clot for maximal protection. When the clot is extending beyond the renal veins, a suprarenal filter placement is required (Fig. 35.8). Avoiding placement of the filter within the thrombus is also essential to avoid incomplete deployment and therefore filter migration.

During deployment, it is essential to unsheathe the filter while keeping the pusher and the filter in a stable position to avoid filter migration. A post deployment venography can be performed through the sheath for completion.

Complications

There are two different types of complications: procedure-related complications during filter placement or retrieval and device-related complications that occur during the dwell time of the filter (Table 35.10).

Follow-Up Care

In the case of optional filters, reevaluation within the time window of retrievability of a given device is essential. If the indication for caval filtration no longer exists, discontinuation of caval filtration should be considered to minimize device-related complications. Interventional radiologists should be

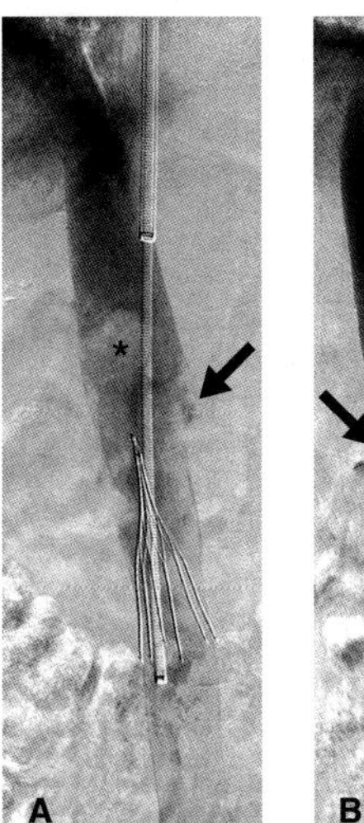

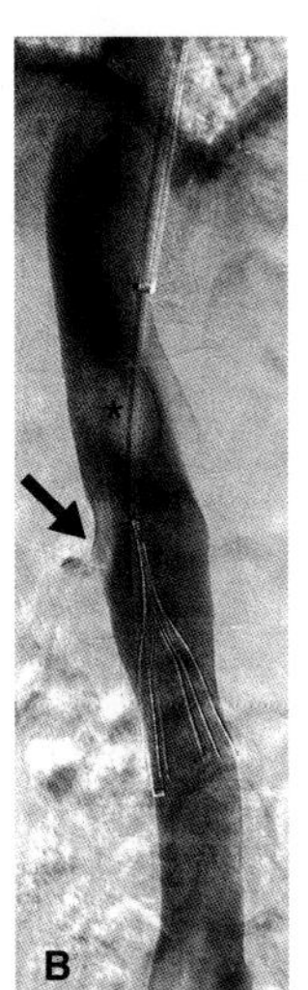

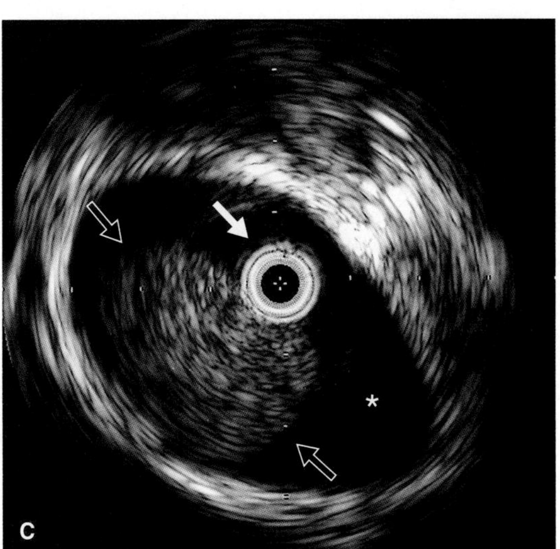

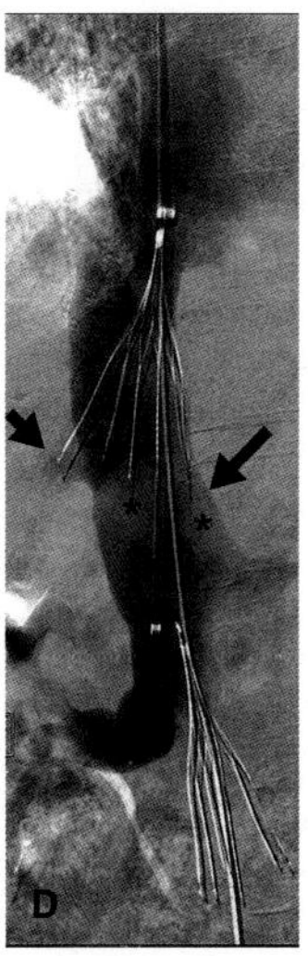

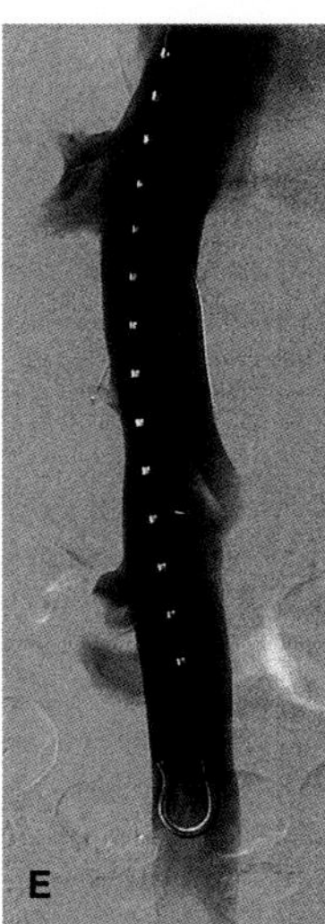

FIGURE 35.8. **Suprarenal Filter. A, B:** Digital subtraction IVC venography prior to Option filter retrieval show a thrombus (*asterisk*) extending cranial to the indwelling filter above the level of the renal veins (*arrows*). **C:** Intravascular ultrasound (IVUS) was performed to confirm the findings showing a large IVC thrombus (between *open arrows*). Note the IVUS probe (*arrow*) within the IVC lumen (*asterisk*). The filter cannot be retrieved in this setting. **D:** A second suprarenal Option filter was deployed above the most cranial extension of the thrombus (*asterisks*). The renal veins are identified (*arrows*). **E:** Digital subtraction venography after retrieval of the most caudal filter shows absence of thrombus within the IVC. The suprarenal filter was then retrieved.

actively involved in the follow-up care to increase the retrieval rate for optional filters.

Filter Retrieval

Retrievable filters have been shown to be safe, prevent fatal PE, and effectively provide a bridge to anticoagulation. Retrievable devices are designed to be removed when protection from PE is no longer needed, which mitigates the risk of filter-related DVT. The majority of retrievable filters are left in place permanently, with retrieval rates as low as 8.5%. Discontinuation of caval filtration is recommended when the indication for an IVC filter is no longer present and is not anticipated to recur. Depending on the design of the optional filter, either the hook at the tip or at the bottom is snared for retrieval. Complex filter retrieval techniques have been described to remove long-term indwelling filters and tilted filters adherent to the IVC wall. These are beyond the scope of this chapter and several review articles are available.

TABLE 35.10

COMPLICATIONS OF IVC FILTER PLACEMENT

■ COMPLICATION	■ COMMENTS
Procedure-Related Complications	
Contrast-induced nephropathy	Can be avoided by adequate hydration prior to and after the procedure, as well as the use of alternative contrast agents in high-risk patients
Contrast allergy	Can be avoided by premedication and the use of alternative contrast agents in patients with history of allergy to contrast media
Access site complications	Bleeding and thrombosis. The main bleeding risk comes from inadvertent arterial puncture. This can be minimized with ultrasound guidance, which is increasingly used, especially for the jugular approach
Caval injury	Particularly during filter retrieval
Device-Related Complications	
Filter migration	Observed in about 6% of cases, is mostly asymptomatic. Severe complications can occur, such as cardiac shock from intracardiac migration
Filter fracture	Rare (1%) and different based on filter design. Usually asymptomatic but can cause severe problems such as cardiac tamponade
Penetration of filter parts through the IVC	Usually asymptomatic. Aortic pseudoaneurysm and duodenal perforation have been reported from penetrating filters
Filter thrombosis or occlusion	
Filter-related deep venous thrombosis	

SUMMARY

Acute PE has various forms of presentation, each having a different rate of mortality and morbidity. Risk stratification and multidisciplinary team approach is essential in optimizing the treatment of patients presenting with acute PE. Catheter-directed intervention is gaining interest in the medical community as a treatment option for patients with massive and submassive PE. Further prospective randomized trials are needed to assess the clinical utility of CDT in patients with submassive PE, it's short- and long-term outcome and associated risk of bleeding.

Suggested Readings

Aujesky D, Obrosky DS, Stone RA, et al. Derivation and validation of a prognostic model for pulmonary embolism. *Am J Respir Crit Care Med* 2005;172(8):1041–1046.

Becattini C, Agnelli G, Germini F, Vedovati MC. Computed tomography to assess risk of death in acute pulmonary embolism: a meta-analysis. *Eur Respir J* 2014;43(6):1678–1690.

Becattini C, Vedovati MC, Agnelli G. Prognostic value of troponins in acute pulmonary embolism: a meta-analysis. *Circulation* 2007;116(4):427–433.

British Thoracic Society Standards of Care Committee Pulmonary Embolism Guideline Development Group. British Thoracic Society guidelines for the management of suspected acute pulmonary embolism. *Thorax* 2003; 58(6):470–483.

Caplin DM, Nikolic B, Kalva SP, et al. Quality improvement guidelines for the performance of inferior vena cava filter placement for the prevention of pulmonary embolism. *J Vasc Interv Radiol* 2011;22(11):1499–1506.

Carrier M, Righini M, Djurabi RK, et al. VIDAS D-dimer in combination with clinical pre-test probability to rule out pulmonary embolism. A systematic review of management outcome studies. *Thromb Haemost* 2009;101(5):886–892.

Casazza F, Becattini C, Bongarzoni A, et al. Clinical features and short term outcomes of patients with acute pulmonary embolism. The Italian Pulmonary Embolism Registry (IPER). *Thromb Res* 2012;130(6):847–852.

Chamsuddin A, Nazzal L, Kang B, et al. Catheter-directed thrombolysis with the Endowave system in the treatment of acute massive pulmonary embolism: a retrospective multicenter case series. *J Vasc Interv Radiol* 2008;19(3): 372–376.

Chatterjee S, Chakraborty A, Weinberg I, et al. Thrombolysis for pulmonary embolism and risk of all-cause mortality, major bleeding, and intracranial hemorrhage: a meta-analysis. *JAMA* 2014;311(23):2414–2421.

Coutance G, Cauderlier E, Ehtisham J, Hamon M, Hamon M. The prognostic value of markers of right ventricular dysfunction in pulmonary embolism: a meta-analysis. *Crit Care* 2011;15(2):R103.

Decousus H, Leizorovicz A, Parent F, et al. A clinical trial of vena caval filters in the prevention of pulmonary embolism in patients with proximal deep-vein thrombosis. Prevention du Risque d'Embolie Pulmonaire par Interruption Cave Study Group. *N Engl J Med* 1998;338(7):409–415.

Dinglasan LA, Oh JC, Schmitt JE, et al. Complicated inferior vena cava filter retrievals: associated factors identified at preretrieval CT. *Radiology* 2013; 266(1):347–354.

Elias A, Mallett S, Daoud-Elias M, Poggi JN, Clarke M. Prognostic models in acute pulmonary embolism: a systematic review and meta-analysis. *BMJ Open* 2016;6(4):e010324.

Engelberger RP, Spirk D, Willenberg T, et al. Ultrasound-assisted versus conventional catheter-directed thrombolysis for acute iliofemoral deep vein thrombosis. *Circ Cardiovasc Interv* 2015;8(1):e002027.

Fanikos J, Piazza G, Zayaruzny M, Goldhaber SZ. Long-term complications of medical patients with hospital-acquired venous thromboembolism. *Thromb Haemost* 2009;102(4):688–693.

Farquharson S. *Pulmonary Artery Thrombectomy and Thrombolysis. Procedural Dictations in Image-Guided Intervention*: Springer; 2016: 545–551.

Fava M, Loyola S, Bertoni H, Dougnac A. Massive pulmonary embolism: percutaneous mechanical thrombectomy during cardiopulmonary resuscitation. *J Vasc Interv Radiol* 2005;16(1):119–123.

Font C, Carmona-Bayonas A, Beato C, et al. Clinical features and short-term outcomes of cancer patients with suspected and unsuspected pulmonary embolism: the EPIPHANY study. *Eur Respir J* 2016:1600282.

Gibson NS, Sohne M, Kruip MJ, et al. Further validation and simplification of the Wells clinical decision rule in pulmonary embolism. *Thromb Haemost* 2008;99(1):229–234.

Greenfield LJ. Evolution of venous interruption for pulmonary thromboembolism. *Arch Surg* 1992;127(5):622–626.

Greenfield LJ, Proctor MC. Twenty-year clinical experience with the Greenfield filter. *Cardiovasc Surg* 1995;3(2):199–205.

Heit JA, Cohen AT, Anderson FA. Estimated annual number of incident and recurrent, non-fatal and fatal venous thromboembolism (VTE) events in the US. *Blood* 2005;106(11):267A.

Henzler T, Roeger S, Meyer M, et al. Pulmonary embolism: CT signs and cardiac biomarkers for predicting right ventricular dysfunction. *Eur Respir J* 2012;39(4):919–926.

Horlander KT, Mannino DM, Leeper KV. Pulmonary embolism mortality in the United States, 1979–1998: an analysis using multiple-cause mortality data. *Arch Intern Med* 2003;163(14):1711–1717.

Jaber WA, McDaniel MC. Catheter-based embolectomy for acute pulmonary embolism: devices, technical considerations, risks, and benefits. *Interv Cardiol Clin* 2018;7(1):91–101.

Jaff MR, McMurtry MS, Archer SL, et al. Management of massive and submassive pulmonary embolism, iliofemoral deep vein thrombosis, and chronic thromboembolic pulmonary hypertension: a scientific statement from the American Heart Association. *Circulation* 2011;123(16):1788–1830.

Jiménez D, Aujesky D, Moores L, et al. Simplification of the pulmonary embolism severity index for prognostication in patients with acute symptomatic pulmonary embolism. *Arch Intern Med* 2010;170(15):1383–1389.

Kabrhel C, Jaff MR, Channick RN, Baker JN, Rosenfield K. A multidisciplinary pulmonary embolism response team. *Chest* 2013;144(5):1738–1739.

Kaufman JA, Kinney TB, Streiff MB, et al. Guidelines for the use of retrievable and convertible vena cava filters: report from the Society of Interventional Radiology multidisciplinary consensus conference. *Surg Obes Relat Dis* 2006;2(2):200–212.

Kearon C, Akl EA, Comerota AJ, et al. Antithrombotic therapy for VTE disease: antithrombotic therapy and prevention of thrombosis, 9th ed: American College of Chest Physicians evidence-based clinical practice guidelines. *Chest* 2012;141(2 Suppl):e419S–e496S.

Kearon C, Akl EA, Ornelas J, et al. Antithrombotic therapy for VTE disease: CHEST guideline and expert panel report. *Chest* 2016;149(2):315–352.

Kline JA, Steuerwald MT, Marchick MR, Hernandez-Nino J, Rose GA. Prospective evaluation of right ventricular function and functional status 6 months after acute submassive pulmonary embolism: frequency of persistent or subsequent elevation in estimated pulmonary artery pressure. *Chest* 2009;136(5):1202–1210.

Klok FA, van Kralingen KW, van Dijk AP, et al. Quality of life in long-term survivors of acute pulmonary embolism. *Chest* 2010;138(6):1432–1440.

Konstantinides S, Geibel A, Kasper W, Olschewski M, Blümel L, Just H. Patent foramen ovale is an important predictor of adverse outcome in patients with major pulmonary embolism. *Circulation* 1998;97(19):1946–1951.

Konstantinides S, Torbicki A, Agnelli G, et al. 2014 ESC guidelines on the diagnosis and management of acute pulmonary embolism. *Eur Heart J* 2014;35(43):3033–3069.

Kucher N, Boekstegers P, Muller OJ, et al. Randomized, controlled trial of ultrasound-assisted catheter-directed thrombolysis for acute intermediate-risk pulmonary embolism. *Circulation* 2014;129(4):479–486.

Kucher N, Rossi E, De Rosa M, Goldhaber SZ. Massive pulmonary embolism. *Circulation* 2006;113(4):577–582.

Kuo WT. Endovascular therapy for acute pulmonary embolism. *J Vasc Interv Radiol* 2012;23(2):167–179. e4.

Kuo WT, Banerjee A, Kim PS, et al. Pulmonary Embolism Response to Fragmentation, Embolectomy, and Catheter Thrombolysis (PERFECT): Initial Results From a Prospective Multicenter Registry. *Chest* 2015;148(3): 667–673.

Kuo WT, Gould MK, Louie JD, Rosenberg JK, Sze DY, Hofmann LV. Catheter-directed therapy for the treatment of massive pulmonary embolism: systematic review and meta-analysis of modern techniques. *J Vasc Interv Radiol* 2009; 20(11):1431–1440.

Kuo WT, Robertson SW, Odegaard JI, Hofmann LV. Complex retrieval of fractured, embedded, and penetrating inferior vena cava filters: a prospective study with histologic and electron microscopic analysis. *J Vasc Interv Radiol* 2013;24(5):622–630.e1; quiz 631.

Le Gal G, Righini M, Sanchez O, et al. A positive compression ultrasonography of the lower limb veins is highly predictive of pulmonary embolism on computed tomography in suspected patients. *Thromb Haemost* 2006;95(6):963–966.

Marti C, John G, Konstantinides S, et al. Systemic thrombolytic therapy for acute pulmonary embolism: a systematic review and meta-analysis. *Eur Heart J* 2015;36(10):605–614.

Mauro MA, Murphy KP, Thomson KR, Venbrux AC, Morgan RA. *Image-Guided Interventions: Expert Radiology Series*. Philadelphia, PA: Elsevier Health Sciences; 2013.

Meyer G, Vicaut E, Danays T, et al. Fibrinolysis for patients with intermediate-risk pulmonary embolism. *N Engl J Med* 2014;370(15):1402–1411.

Mismetti P, Laporte S, Pellerin O, et al. Effect of a retrievable inferior vena cava filter plus anticoagulation vs anticoagulation alone on risk of recurrent pulmonary embolism: a randomized clinical trial. *JAMA* 2015;313(16): 1627–1635.

Nakazawa K, Tajima H, Murata S, Kumita SI, Yamamoto T, Tanaka K. Catheter fragmentation of acute massive pulmonary thromboembolism: distal embolisation and pulmonary arterial pressure elevation. *Br J Radiol* 2008;81(971):848–854.

Park B, Messina L, Dargon P, Huang W, Ciocca R, Anderson FA. Recent trends in clinical outcomes and resource utilization for pulmonary embolism in the United States: findings from the nationwide inpatient sample. *Chest* 2009;136(4):983–990.

Piazza G, Goldhaber SZ. Chronic thromboembolic pulmonary hypertension. *N Eng J Med* 2011;364(4):351–360.

Piazza G, Hohlfelder B, Jaff MR, et al. A Prospective, Single-Arm, Multicenter Trial of Ultrasound-Facilitated, Catheter-Directed, Low-Dose Fibrinolysis for Acute Massive and Submassive Pulmonary Embolism: The SEATTLE II Study. *JACC Cardiovasc Interv* 2015;8(10):1382–1392.

Poorthuis MH, Brand EC, Hazenberg CEVB, et al. Plasma fibrinogen level as a potential predictor of hemorrhagic complications after catheter-directed thrombolysis for peripheral arterial occlusions. *J Vasc Surg* 2017;65(5):1519–1527.e26.

PREPIC Study Group. Eight-year follow-up of patients with permanent vena cava filters in the prevention of pulmonary embolism: the PREPIC (Prevention du Risque d'Embolie Pulmonaire par Interruption Cave) randomized study. *Circulation* 2005;112(3):416–422.

Pulido T, Aranda A, Zevallos MA, et al. Pulmonary embolism as a cause of death in patients with heart disease: an autopsy study. *Chest* 2006;129(5):1282–1287.

Ray CE, Jr, Mitchell E, Zipser S, Kao EY, Brown CF, Moneta GL. Outcomes with retrievable inferior vena cava filters: a multicenter study. *J Vasc Interv Radiol* 2006;17(10):1595–1604.

Remy-Jardin M, Pistolesi M, Goodman LR, et al. Management of suspected acute pulmonary embolism in the era of CT angiography: a statement from the Fleischner Society 1. *Radiology* 2007;245(2):315–329.

Righini M, Roy PM, Meyer G, Verschuren F, Aujesky D, Le Gal G. The simplified Pulmonary Embolism Severity Index (PESI): validation of a clinical prognostic model for pulmonary embolism. *J Thromb Haemost* 2011; 9(10):2115–2117.

Rosenthal D, Wellons ED, Lai KM, Bikk A, Henderson VJ. Retrievable inferior vena cava filters: initial clinical results. *Ann Vasc Surg* 2006;20(1):157–165.

Schmitz-Rode T, Kilbinger M, Günther RW. Simulated flow pattern in massive pulmonary embolism: significance for selective intrapulmonary thrombolysis. *Cardiovasc Interv Radiol* 1998;21(3):199–204.

Segal JB, Streiff MB, Hofmann LV, Thornton K, Bass EB. Management of venous thromboembolism: a systematic review for a practice guideline. *Ann Intern Med* 2007;146(3):211–222.

Sharafuddin MJ, Hicks ME. Current status of percutaneous mechanical thrombectomy. Part II. Devices and mechanisms of action. *J Vasc Interv Radiol* 1998;9(1):15–31.

Sista AK, Friedman OA, Horowitz JM, Salemi A. Building a pulmonary embolism lysis practice. *Endovasc Today* 2013;12:61–64.

Sista AK, Horowitz JM, Goldhaber SZ. Four key questions surrounding thrombolytic therapy for submassive pulmonary embolism. *Vasc Med* 2016;21(1):47–52.

Sista AK, Kuo WT, Schiebler M, Madoff DC. Stratification, Imaging, and Management of Acute Massive and Submassive Pulmonary Embolism. *Radiology* 2017;284(1):5–24.

Sista AK, Miller LE, Kahn SR, Kline JA. Persistent right ventricular dysfunction, functional capacity limitation, exercise intolerance, and quality of life impairment following pulmonary embolism: Systematic review with meta-analysis. *Vasc Med* 2017;22(1):37–43.

Stein PD, Matta F, Keyes DC, Willyerd GL. Impact of vena cava filters on in-hospital case fatality rate from pulmonary embolism. *Am J Med* 2012; 125(5):478–484.

Tapson VF. Acute pulmonary embolism. *N Engl J Med* 2008;358(10): 1037–1052.

Taslakian B, Chawala D, Sista AK. A survey of submassive pulmonary embolism treatment preferences among medical and endovascular physicians. *J Vasc Interv Radiol* 2017;28(12):1693–1699.e2.

Taslakian B, Georges Sebaaly M, Al-Kutoubi A. Patient evaluation and preparation in vascular and interventional radiology: what every interventional radiologist should know (part 1: patient assessment and laboratory tests). *Cardiovasc Intervent Radiol* 2016;39(3):325–333.

Taslakian B, Georges Sebaaly M, Al-Kutoubi A. Patient evaluation and preparation in vascular and interventional radiology: what every interventional radiologist should know (part 2: patient preparation and medications). *Cardiovasc Intervent Radiol* 2016;39(4):489–499.

Taslakian B, Latson LA, Truong MT, et al. CT pulmonary angiography of adult pulmonary vascular diseases: technical considerations and interpretive pitfalls. *Eur J Radiol* 2016;85(11):2049–2063.

Taslakian B, Sridhar D. Post-procedural care in interventional radiology: what every interventional radiologist should know—part I: standard post-procedural instructions and follow-up care. *Cardiovasc Intervent Radiol* 2017;40(4): 481–495.

Torbicki A, Galié N, Covezzoli A. Right heart thrombi in pulmonary embolism: results from the International Cooperative Pulmonary Embolism Registry. *J Am Coll Cardiol* 2003;41(12):2245–2251.

Uflacker R. Interventional therapy for pulmonary embolism. *J Vasc Interv Radiol* 2001;12(2):147–164.

Vanni S, Nazerian P, Pepe G, et al. Comparison of two prognostic models for acute pulmonary embolism: clinical vs. right ventricular dysfunction guided approach. *J Thromb Haemost* 2011;9(10):1916–1923.

Verstraete M, Miller GA, Bounameaux H, et al. Intravenous and intrapulmonary recombinant tissue-type plasminogen activator in the treatment of acute massive pulmonary embolism. *Circulation* 1988;77(2):353–360.

Wood KE. Major pulmonary embolism: review of a pathophysiologic approach to the golden hour of hemodynamically significant pulmonary embolism. *Chest* 2002;121(3):877–905.

CHAPTER 36A ■ GASTROINTESTINAL INTERVENTIONS

MEREDITH McDERMOTT

MESENTERIC ANGIOGRAPHY AND INTERVENTION

Anatomy

The main arterial supply to the gastrointestinal tract comes from three main arteries: the celiac artery, the superior mesenteric artery (SMA), and the inferior mesenteric artery (IMA).

The celiac artery arises from the ventral surface of the aorta at the T12–L1 level. It immediately divides giving rise to the common hepatic, splenic, and left gastric arteries (Fig. 36A.1). The common hepatic artery runs to the right and divides into the proper hepatic artery and the gastroduodenal artery. The gastroduodenal artery runs inferiorly and branches into the right gastroepiploic artery and superior pancreaticoduodenal arteries. The right gastric artery is a small branch with variable origin; however, it typically arises from the proper or left hepatic artery. The splenic artery is usually the largest branch of the celiac trunk and has a tortuous course to the left, running along the superior aspect of the pancreas. It gives off several pancreatic branches supplying the neck, body, and tail of the pancreas. The left gastroepiploic artery and short gastric arteries are distal branches of the splenic artery. The short gastric arteries supply additional flow to the fundus of the stomach, and the left gastroepiploic runs along the greater curvature of the stomach to anastomose with the right gastroepiploic artery. The left gastric artery is the smallest branch of the celiac trunk and supplies the gastroesophageal junction, the fundus, and part of the body of the stomach along the lesser curvature with anastomoses to the right gastric and esophageal branches of the thoracic aorta.

The SMA originates just below the celiac trunk (usually within 2 cm) on the ventral surface of the aorta near the level of L1 (Fig. 36A.2). The SMA runs anteriorly over the left renal vein and third portion of the duodenum. It gives supply to the pancreas, duodenum, the entire small bowel, and proximal two-thirds of the colon. The first branch of the SMA is the inferior pancreaticoduodenal artery which further divides into anterior and posterior branches which anastomose with the superior pancreaticoduodenal arteries arising from the gastroduodenal artery. These branches form an arcade which supplies the head/uncinate process of the pancreas and the duodenum. The jejunal and ileal arteries arise from the left side of the SMA and supply the jejunum and most of the ileum, respectively. The middle colic, right colic, and ileocolic arteries all arise from the right side of the SMA. The middle colic is typically the second branch on the right after the inferior pancreaticoduodenal artery and divides into right and left branches which supply the transverse colon. The right and left branches anastomose with the right colic and left colic, with the latter originating in the IMA. The right colic arises next to supply the ascending colon; it divides into ascending and descending branches with anastomoses to the right colic and ileocolic arteries. The ileocolic artery also arises from the right side of the SMA and supplies the terminal ileum, cecum/appendix, and ascending colon. Its superior branch anastomoses with the right colic arterial branches.

The IMA originates at the L3–L4 level above the aortic bifurcation and gives supply to the distal transverse colon, descending colon, sigmoid colon, and rectum (Fig. 36A.3). The first branch of the IMA is the left colic artery which divides into ascending and descending branches. The ascending branch forms an anastomosis with the middle colic and supplies the distal transverse and descending colon. The descending branch forms an anastomosis with the sigmoid artery and supplies the remainder of the descending colon. The sigmoid arteries arise next and supply the lowest part of the descending colon and the sigmoid colon. The terminal branch of the IMA is the superior rectal artery which divides to run along both sides of the rectum and anastomoses with the middle and inferior rectal arteries of the internal iliac system.

There are several important collateral communications between the mesenteric vessels. The marginal artery of Drummond runs along the mesenteric border of the colon and supplies the vasa recta. It provides the anastomoses between SMA and IMA via connections between the right colic, middle colic, and left colic arteries. The arc of Riolan is a variable communication, also between the SMA and IMA, via anastomoses of the left colic and middle colic arteries which run more centrally within the mesentery. The arc of Buhler is a persistent fetal communication which sometimes exists between the celiac artery and the SMA. The various anastomotic connections between the mesenteric arteries are summarized in Table 36A.1.

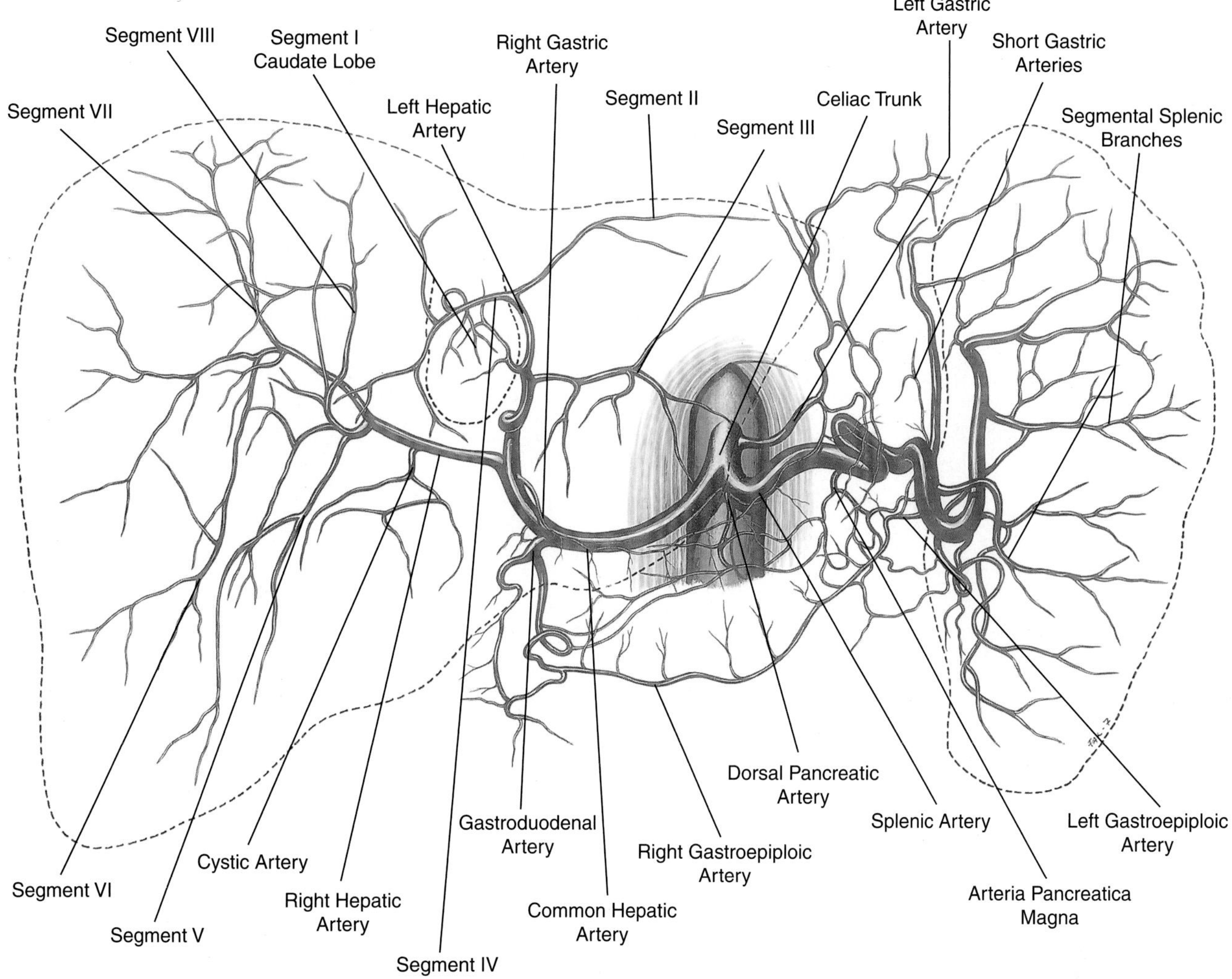

FIGURE 36A.1. Celiac Axis Anatomy. (From Uflacker R. *Atlas of Vascular Anatomy: An Angiographic Approach*. Philadelphia, PA: Lippincott Williams & Wilkins; 2007.)

Variations in the arterial anatomy of the gastrointestinal tract are common and important to be aware of when performing interventions. Variations are most common in the celiac axis and SMA. For common arterial variants, please refer to Table 36A.2.

GI Hemorrhage

GI bleeding is a common reason to perform angiography of the mesenteric vessels. The workup and management of GI bleeding includes nasogastric tube aspirate, upper endoscopy,

TABLE 36A.1

ANASTOMOTIC CONNECTIONS OF THE MESENTERIC VASCULATURE

Within vessel collaterals	Celiac artery	Right and left gastric arteries Right and left gastroepiploic arteries Left gastric and short gastric arteries
	SMA	Right, middle, and ileocolic arteries via marginal artery of Drummond
	IMA	Left colic, sigmoid, and superior rectal arteries via marginal artery of Drummond
Between vessel collaterals	Celiac and SMA	Superior and inferior pancreaticoduodenal arteries Arc of Bühler
	SMA and IMA	Middle colic and left colic via marginal artery of Drummond Middle colic and left colic via arc of Riolan

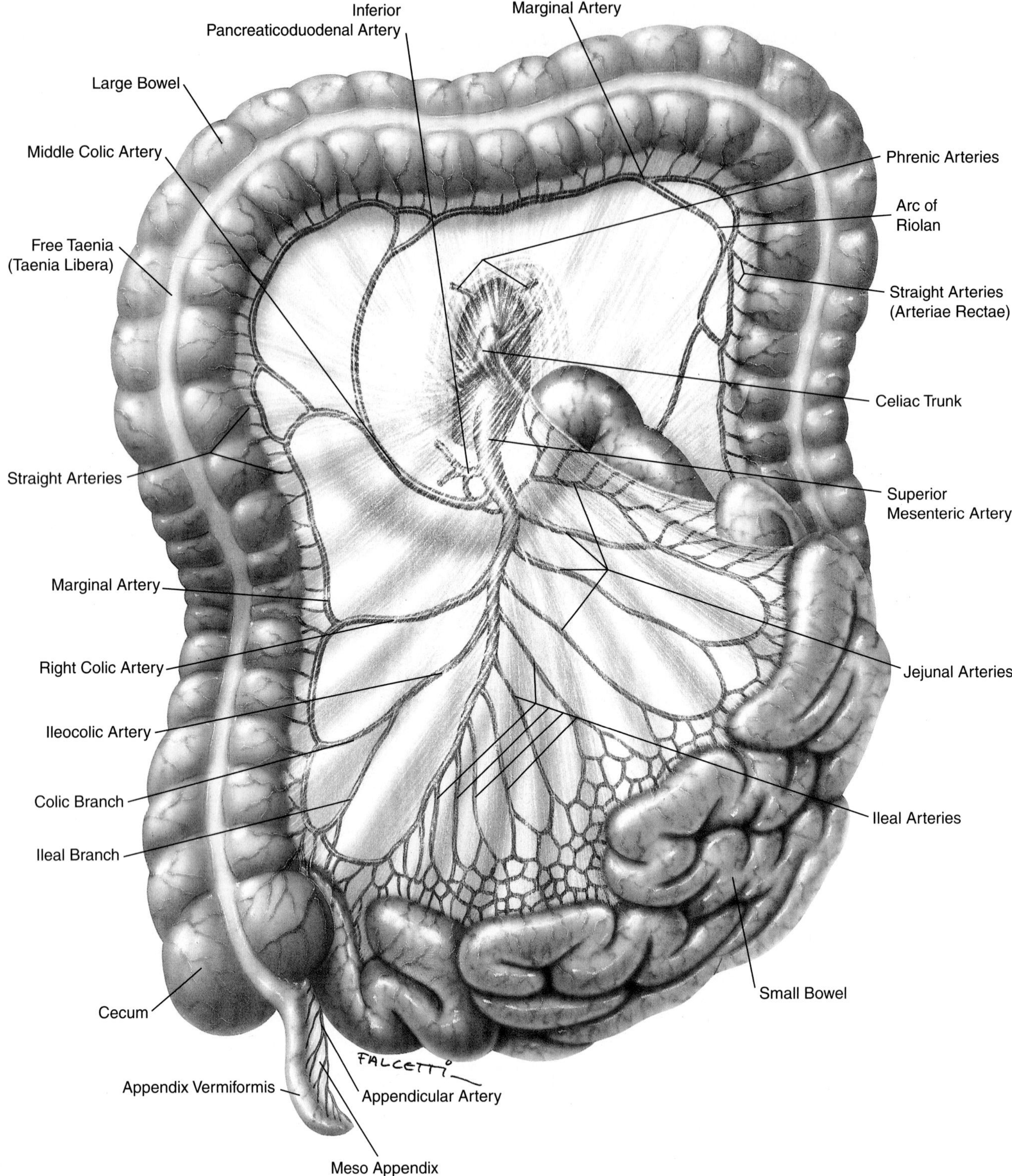

FIGURE 36A.2. **SMA Anatomy.** (From Uflacker R. *Atlas of Vascular Anatomy: An Angiographic Approach*. Philadelphia, PA: Lippincott Williams & Wilkins; 2007.)

colonoscopy, radionuclide imaging, CT angiography, conventional angiography, and surgery. The application of these different modalities often depends on the source/location of the bleed and the acuity and clinical status of the patient. The distinction between upper and lower GI bleeding is made based on the location of the bleed in relation to the ligament of Treitz, with upper GI bleeds occurring proximal to this location. Both upper and lower GI bleeding episodes are intermittent in nature, which can make diagnosis and treatment challenging. Diagnostic catheter angiography has a reported threshold sensitivity for bleeding of 0.5 mL/min in animal studies, which can limit its use if the patient is not actively bleeding. Noninvasive methods such as sulfur colloid scintigraphy (0.1 mL/min), red blood cell scintigraphy (0.2 to 0.4 mL/min), and MDCTA

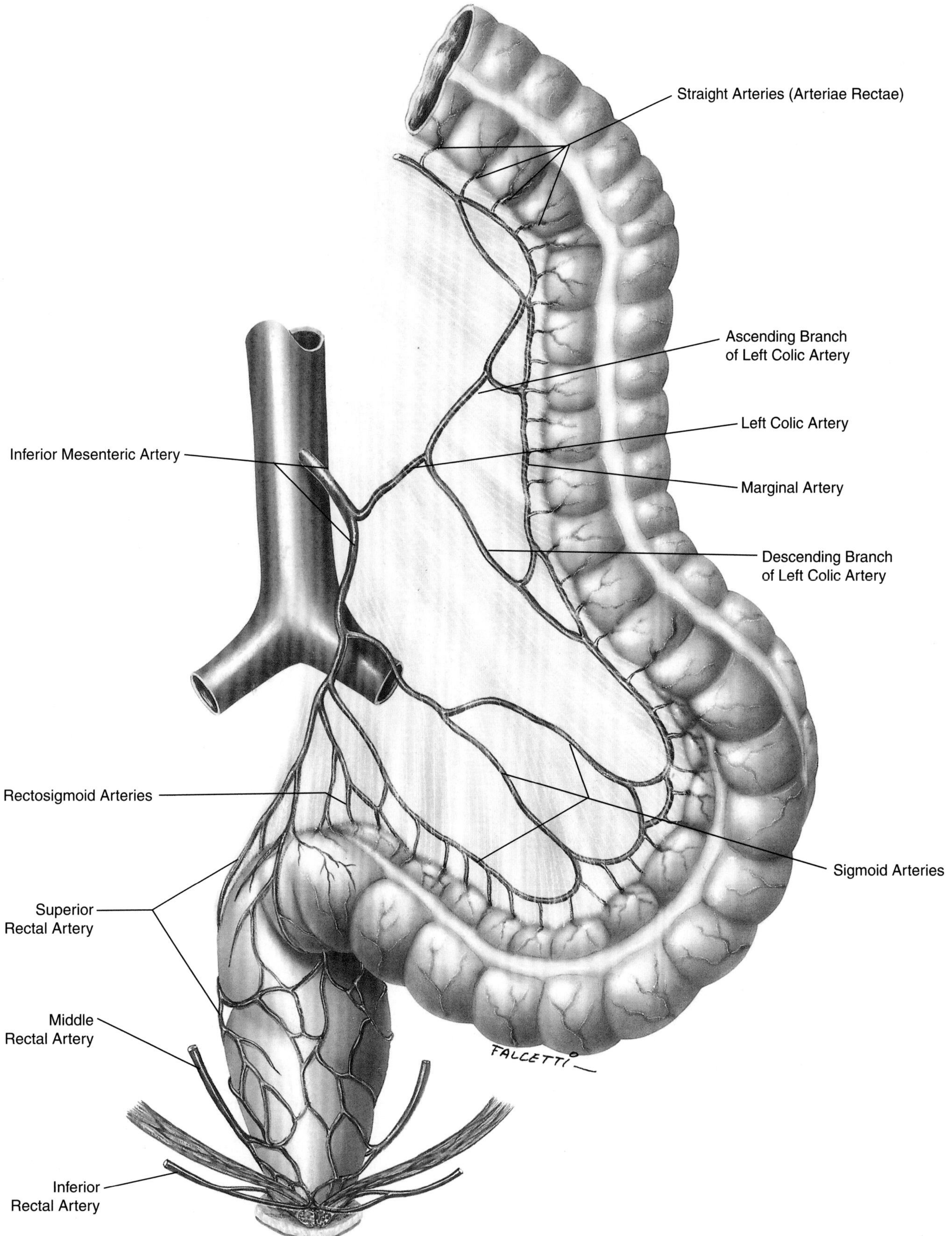

FIGURE 36A.3. **IMA Anatomy Image.** (From Uflacker R. *Atlas of Vascular Anatomy: An Angiographic Approach*. Philadelphia, PA: Lippincott Williams & Wilkins; 2007.)

TABLE 36A.2

COMMON VARIATIONS SEEN IN MESENTERIC ARTERIAL ANATOMY

Celiac artery variations	Left gastric arises directly from aorta Splenic artery arises directly from aorta Common hepatic arises directly from aorta
Hepatic artery variations	Accessory or replaced right hepatic artery arising from the SMA Proper hepatic artery arising from SMA Common hepatic artery arising from SMA Accessory or replaced left hepatic artery arising from left gastric
SMA variations	SMA arises from celiac artery (celiac–mesenteric trunk) Middle colic and right colic arise from common trunk Right colic and ileocolic arise from common trunk

(0.35 mL/min) are more sensitive and frequently used when no source of bleeding is identified on endoscopy. CT also has the advantage of demonstrating intra- and extraluminal pathology and signs of a recent bleed such as blood clot, pseudoaneurysm, or other vascular abnormalities which can direct subsequent angiography.

Upper GI Hemorrhage

Upper GI bleeding is common with an incidence of 100 per 100,000 adults per year and a mortality of 3% to 14%. Causes of upper GI bleeding are listed in Table 36A.3. The most common cause is peptic ulcer disease which is responsible for about 50% of cases. Patients with acute upper GI hemorrhage may present with hematemesis, blood from nasogastric tube lavage, melena, or in severe cases of upper GI bleed, hematochezia (bright red blood per rectum). Patients with more chronic bleeding may simply present with iron-deficiency anemia.

Endoscopy is the first-line therapy for upper GI bleeding because it allows for rapid identification and often treatment of the site of bleeding. For patients who fail endoscopy, angiography and embolization is typically the preferred second-line treatment. If the bleeding is well localized on endoscopy, then additional cross-sectional imaging may be deferred, especially in an unstable patient. Bleeding from the duodenum can usually be attributed to the gastroduodenal artery and the pancreaticoduodenal arcade, while gastric bleeding is typically related to the left gastric artery and, much less often, the right gastric artery. Metallic clips are also frequently placed during endoscopy which can aid in localizing the bleeding source. Extravasation of contrast material during angiography is a direct sign of bleeding. Indirect signs include pseudoaneurysm, truncated vessels, vessel irregularity, neovascularity, and arteriovenous shunting (Fig. 36A.4). In the upper GI tract, there is a rich collateral blood supply which allows for the prophylactic embolization of vessels even without direct or indirect signs of bleeding if a source is identified on endoscopy (Fig. 36A.5). This rich collateral supply can sometimes make embolization difficult, and care must be taken when embolizing the gastroduodenal artery to evaluate for retrograde filling from the SMA via the inferior pancreaticoduodenal arcade, which can become a continued source of bleeding even if the gastroduodenal artery appears to be under control (Fig. 36A.6). The choice of embolic agent depends on the abnormality, territory being treated, anatomy, and operator preference. Most commonly metallic coils and Gelfoam (a temporary occlusive agent) are used. Other liquid agents such as n-butyl cyanoacrylate or liquid polyvinyl alcohol copolymer can be used with success but often require more training to safely use. In certain lesions, such as tumors, particulate agents may be also of use. The technical success rate for upper GI bleeding embolization is greater than 90% with clinical success rate ranging between 75% and 90%.

TABLE 36A.3

COMMON CAUSES OF UPPER GASTROINTESTINAL HEMORRHAGE

Peptic ulcer disease (gastric and duodenal)
Esophageal and gastric varices (due to portal hypertension)
Gastritis/esophagitis
Mallory–Weiss tear
Dieulafoy lesion
Marginal ulcer (postanastomotic)
Aortoenteric fistula
Hemobilia (trauma, iatrogenic causes: biopsy, biliary drain, surgery)
Transpancreatic duct hemorrhage (pseudoaneurysms after pancreatitis)
Tumors

Transpapillary hemorrhage refers to bleeding into the biliary tree (hemobilia) or bleeding into the pancreatic duct; etiologies are detailed in Table 36A.3. Patients present with symptoms similar to that of upper GI bleeding. In the setting of hemobilia, catheter embolization is the primary treatment, and the abnormality is usually intrahepatic. Postpancreatitis abnormalities can include true aneurysms, pseudoaneurysms, or pseudocyst hemorrhages. The most commonly involved vessel is the splenic artery; however, any upper abdominal vessel can be a source of hemorrhage. Angiography and embolization is the preferred treatment in these patients as surgical mortality rates have been reported to be up to 56%.

Aortoenteric fistula is the term for a direct communication between the aorta and small bowel (usually duodenum), which is most frequently a complication of recent surgery for an abdominal aortic aneurysm. Angiography is performed with an aortic injection; however, rarely, contrast extravasation into the bowel is seen. Treatment is urgent surgery.

Lower GI Hemorrhage

Lower GI bleeding is far less common than upper GI bleeding with an incidence of around 20 cases per 100,000 and a mortality rate of about 10%. Causes of lower GI bleeding are listed in Table 36A.4. The most common cause of lower GI

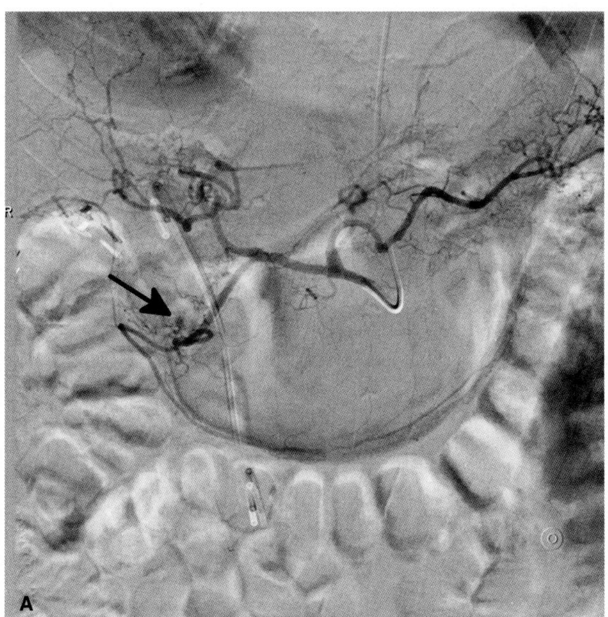

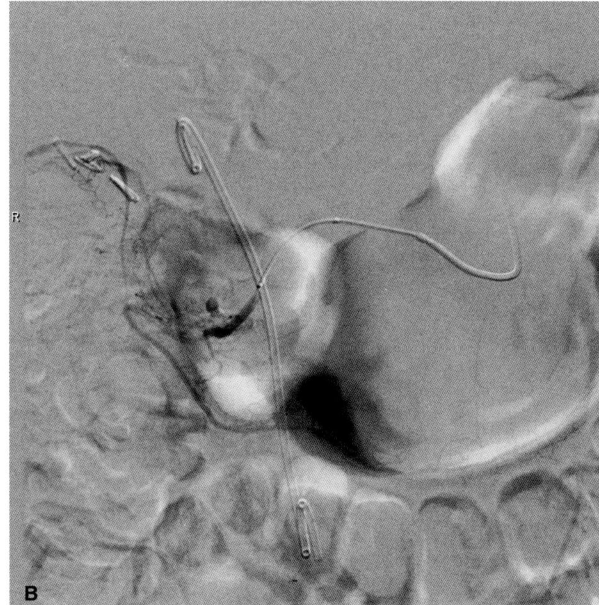

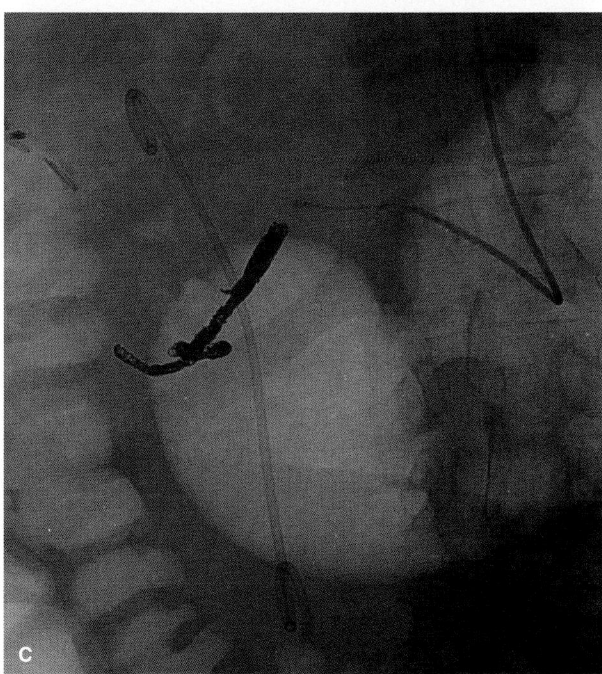

FIGURE 36A.4. **A:** Selective celiac angiogram demonstrates pseudoaneurysm, marked by the *arrow*, arising from the gastroduodenal artery. **B:** Subselective angiogram of the gastroduodenal artery again demonstrates appearance of pseudoaneurysm. **C:** Postembolization images demonstrate coils placed across the area of abnormality.

TABLE 36A.4

CAUSES OF LOWER GI BLEEDING

Diverticulosis	30%
Hemorrhoids	14%
Ischemia	12%
Inflammatory bowel disease	9%
Postpolypectomy	8%
Colon cancer/polyps	6%
Vascular ectasia	3%
Other causes	

bleeding is diverticulosis which accounts for about 30% of cases. The most common presentation of lower GI bleeding is hematochezia, followed by maroon stool and melena.

Lower GI bleeding is frequently self-limited, and the initial steps in treatment are resuscitation and careful observation as to whether the patient is bleeding briskly enough to warrant intervention. The actual volume of bleeding is not the best criterion for intervention. An analysis of 88 patients showed the following clinical factors are associated with positive angiography: systolic blood pressure <90 mm Hg, transfusion requirements of 5 or more units of blood, and hemoglobin drop of more than 5 g/dL from prior values. In such acutely bleeding patients, colonoscopy is often deferred due to the time required to adequately prep the patient for visualization. Furthermore, with heavy bleeding, the ability to clear blood during colonoscopy to visualize and treat a source is far more challenging. In more

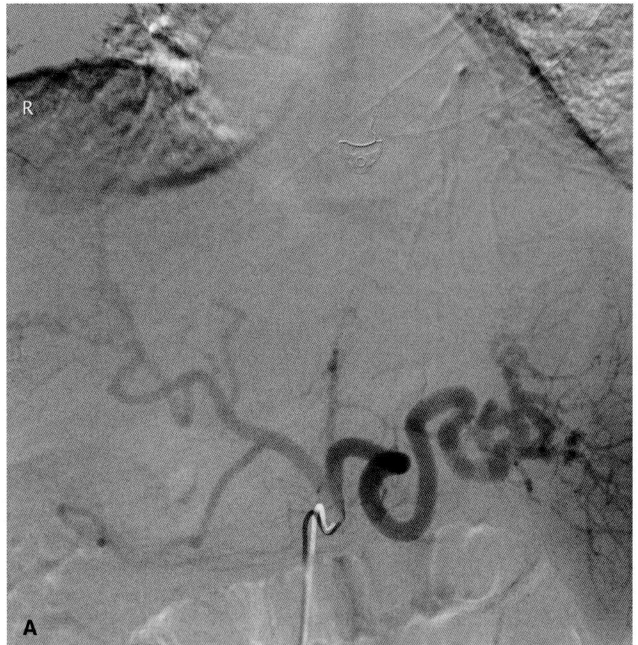

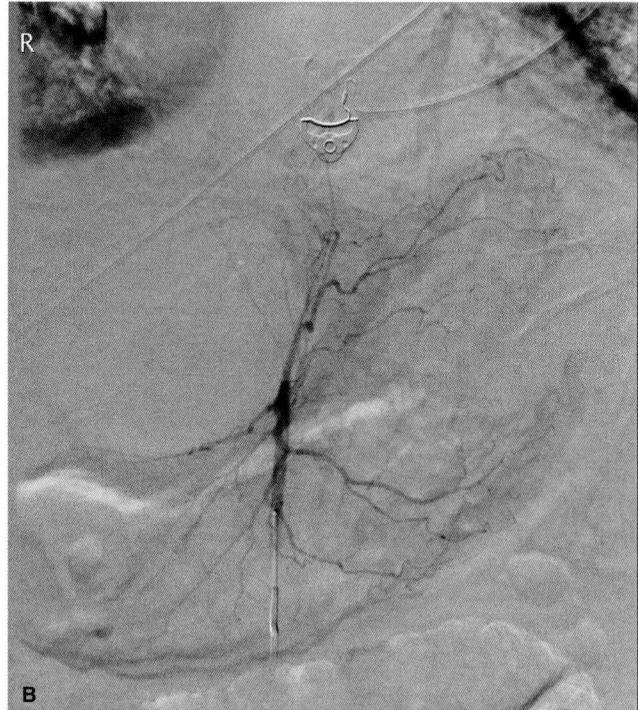

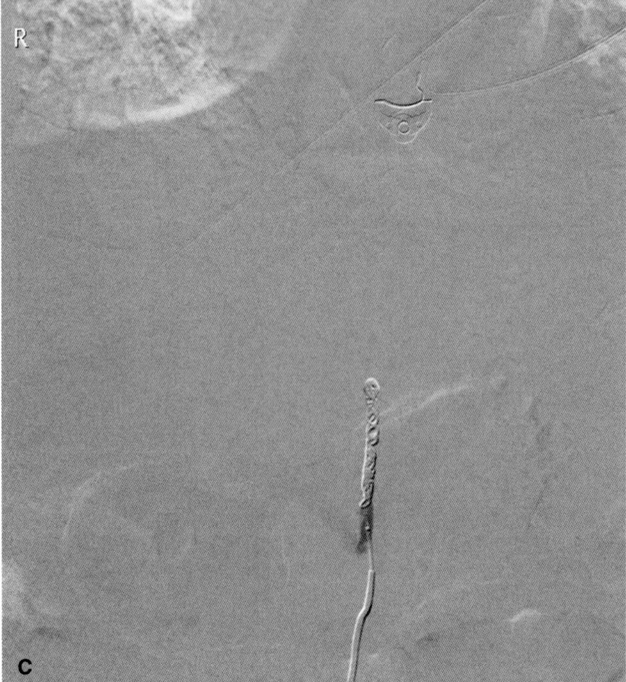

FIGURE 36A.5. **A:** Celiac angiogram in a patient with bleeding at the gastric fundus identified on endoscopy. **B:** Selective angiogram of the left gastric artery does not demonstrate any focal arterial abnormalities. **C:** Prophylactic coil embolization of the left gastric artery performed, based on endoscopic findings.

recent years, CT angiography has been proposed as a way to localize bleeding in the lower GI tract. Although slightly less sensitive than radionuclide scans, CTA can be performed quickly with better anatomic localization of bleeding. Depending on the location of the hemorrhage, the SMA (ascending and transverse colon) and IMA (descending/sigmoid colon and rectum) are the two main vessels which are interrogated. More selective angiography with a microcatheter may be required to identify the source of the bleed. Although there is some debate over the ideal level to treat lower GI bleeds, the general consensus is to embolize as close to the point of extravasation or abnormality as possible to limit the risk of bowel ischemia. Unlike in upper GI bleeding, the blood supply to the lower GI tract is less robust with less collateral flow. Findings on angiography will be similar to upper GI bleeding, with contrast extravasation being the only direct sign of bleeding (Fig. 36A.7). Other vascular abnormalities may indicate the site of bleeding, for example, angiodysplasia has a classic angiographic appearance with early opacification of an enlarged draining vein with persistent opacification of the vein and vascular tufts along the antimesenteric border of the colon (Fig. 36A.8). The technical success rate for lower GI bleeding embolization is around 90%, with a clinical success rate ranging between 60% and 100%.

Bleeding from the small bowel (ileum and jejunum) is far less common and accounts for only about 5% to 10% of all GI bleeding. The causes are more likely to be inflammatory bowel disease or Meckel diverticulum, and in patients over 40, the

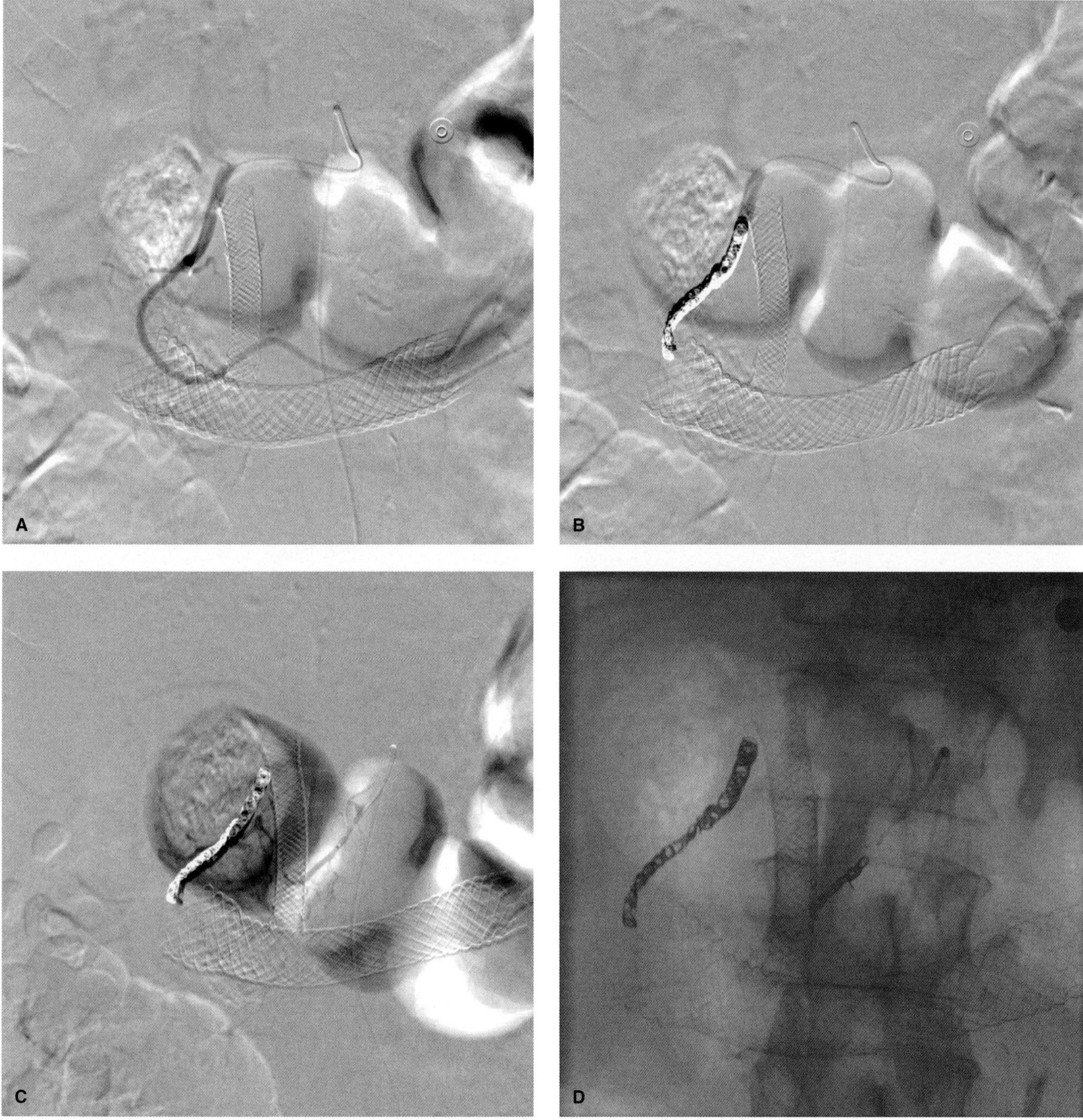

FIGURE 36A.6. **A:** Gastroduodenal artery angiogram performed in a patient with bleeding seen in the duodenum after stent placement in endoscopy. **B:** Coil embolization of the gastroduodenal artery performed. **C:** Evaluation of the inferior pancreaticoduodenal arcade demonstrates supply to the region of the duodenum. **D:** Coil embolization performed to prevent retrograde filling of the GDA territory.

causes are more likely angiodysplasia or other vascular lesions. Small bowel neoplasms and Dieulafoy lesions occur in both cohorts. Conventional angiography has largely been replaced in the workup of small bowel lesions by CT and MRI; however, it may still be a preferred treatment in acute hemorrhage.

Mesenteric Ischemia

Mesenteric ischemia can be caused by a variety of disorders resulting in bowel necrosis with a mortality rate as high as 70%. It can be divided into acute and chronic presentations.

In acute mesenteric ischemia (AMI), arterial embolism and thrombosis account for up to 80% of cases. The classic presentation is severe abdominal pain that is out of proportion to the physical examination. Associated symptoms can include nausea, diarrhea, and bloody stools. AMI is most often due to pathology of the SMA. The IMA tends to have a better collateral circulation, and the SMA is more susceptible to emboli (90% of emboli occur in the SMA) in comparison to the other mesenteric vessels. Arterial embolism accounts for 40% to 50% of cases of AMI and is typically cardiac in origin. The angiographic appearance of an embolus is an abrupt cutoff of the SMA with a sharp, round, filling defect about 4 to 6 cm

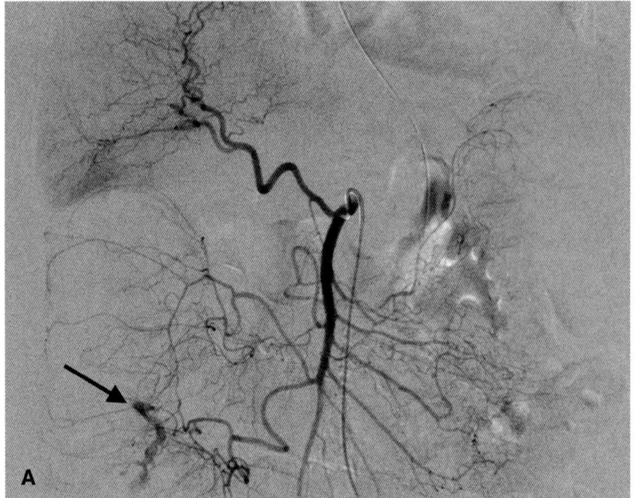

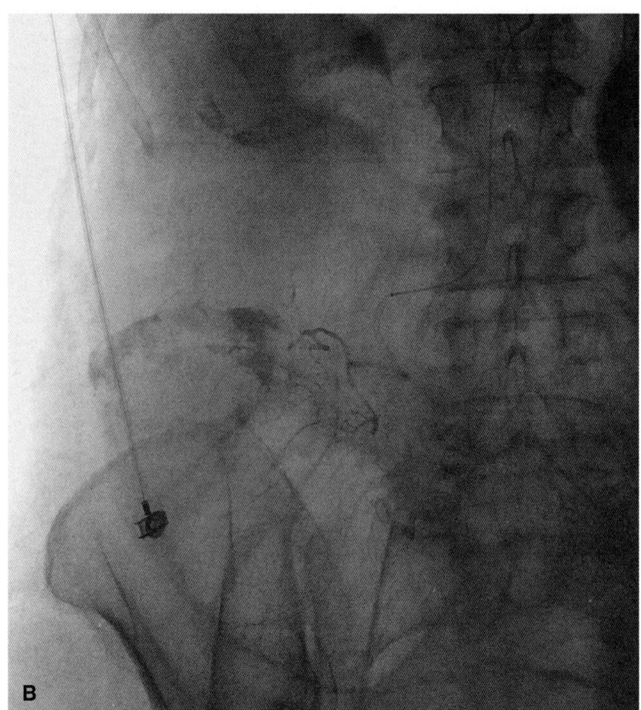

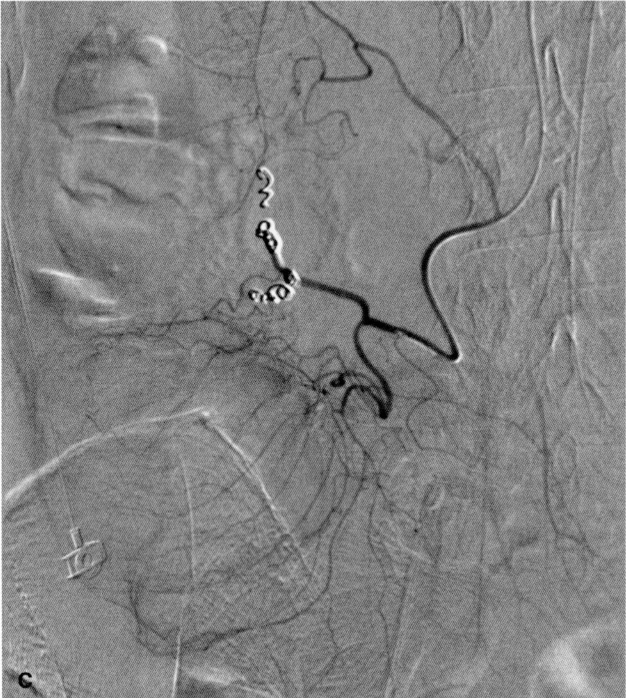

FIGURE 36A.7. **A:** Patient presenting with massive lower GI bleeding. SMA angiogram demonstrates active extravasation, marked by the *arrow*, from the ileocolic artery. **B:** Subselective angiogram of the ileocolic artery with a microcatheter confirms the previous finding. **C:** Selective coil embolization of two branches of the ileocolic artery performed with cessation of extravasation.

from the origin at a natural narrowing of the SMA near the takeoff of the middle colic artery. In comparison, thrombosis, which accounts for 25% to 30% of cases, is seen in patients with underlying atherosclerotic lesions and has a more insidious onset. The angiographic appearance is of a more tapered occlusion closer to the origin of the SMA, sometimes with collateral vessel formation. Historically, treatment of AMI included surgical exploration and revascularization. More recently, endovascular treatment options have shown favorable outcomes and include intra-arterial infusion of tissue plasminogen activator (tPA) to dissolve the clot, mechanical embolectomy, angioplasty, and stenting.

Nonocclusive mesenteric ischemia (NOMI) accounts for 20% to 30% of cases of AMI and is caused by conditions which result in low-flow states such as prolonged hypotension, dehydration, or use of vasopressors. Imaging with CTA, MRI, or conventional angiography will demonstrate diffuse arterial vasospasm, or sausage-like segmental narrowing. Secondary findings include delayed filling of distal branches and asymmetric bowel perfusion. Treatment should begin with correcting the underlying cause of hypotension or low-flow state. The other primary therapy is intra-arterial infusion of a vasodilator such as papaverine directly into the SMA. Treatment should continue until symptoms resolve.

Chronic mesenteric ischemia is relatively rare due to the rich collateral circulation of the bowel and will occur with high-grade stenosis of at least two of the three mesenteric arteries. Patients will typically present with postprandial pain and weight loss. Etiologies include atherosclerosis and vasculitis such as fibromuscular dysplasia. Diagnosis is typically made on cross-sectional imaging with CTA or MRA; however, conventional angiography remains the gold standard. The goal of treatment is to relieve the arterial obstruction and provide adequate flow into the affected mesenteric arterial bed. Surgical endarterectomy or bypass was the traditional treatment; however, endovascular management has taken on an increasing role, and occlusions or stenoses can be treated with angioplasty and stenting (Fig. 36A.9).

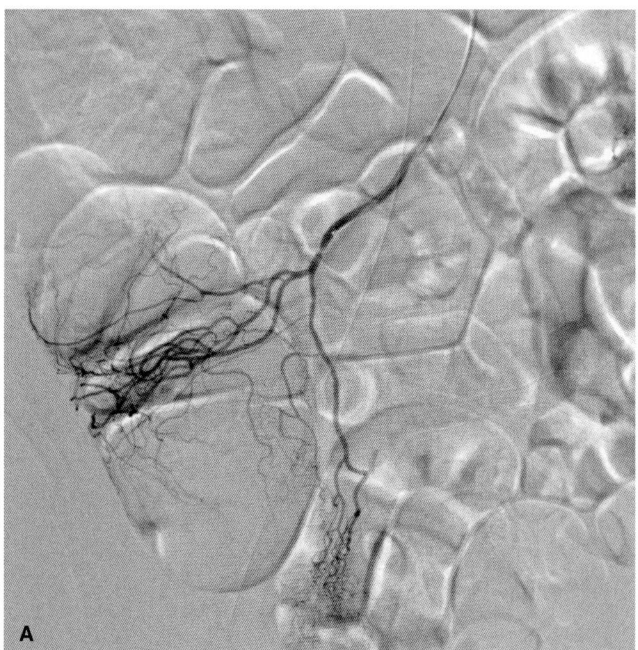

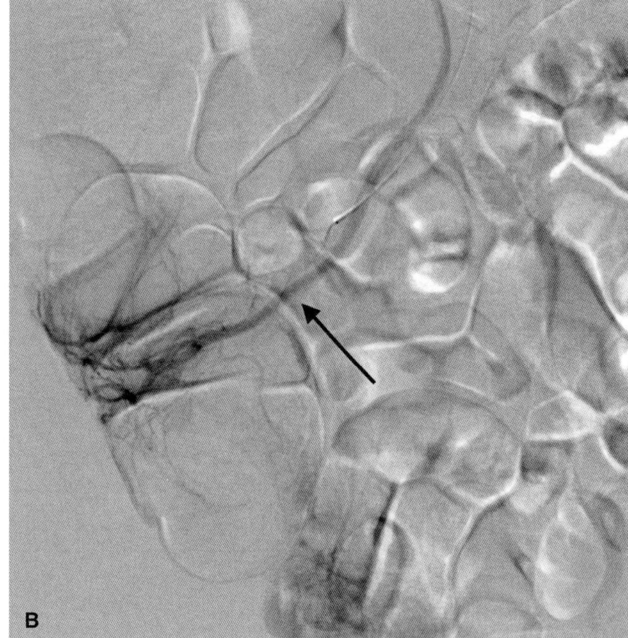

FIGURE 36A.8. A: Subselective angiogram of the ileocolic artery demonstrating a tangle of vessels in the right colon. **B:** Early-draining vein marked by the *arrow* consistent with angiodysplasia.

Mesenteric Aneurysms

True aneurysms of the mesenteric vessels are rare and account for only 0.1% to 0.2% of all arterial aneurysms. Different vascular territories may be involved, and the splenic artery is the most commonly affected, accounting for 60% of cases. Please refer to Table 36A.5 for the distribution of visceral aneurysms.

Given the low incidence, most mesenteric aneurysms are found incidentally on cross-sectional imaging. The absolute risk of rupture is unknown, and indications for treatment are not clear-cut due to lack of prospective data. Typically, aneurysms under 2 cm in size can be managed conservatively with observation alone. General guidelines for indications for intervention include aneurysms greater than 2 to 2.5 cm, symptomatic aneurysms, aneurysms in women of childbearing age or in patients who may require liver transplant, multiple hepatic aneurysms, or interval growth of more than 0.5 cm/yr. Treatment method is dependent on the location and individual anatomy and may include coil embolization, exclusion with a covered stent, thrombin injection, or other liquid embolic agents.

TABLE 36A.5

DISTRIBUTION OF VISCERAL ARTERIAL ANEURYSMS

Splenic	60%
Hepatic	20%
Superior mesenteric	5%
Celiac	4%
Gastric/gastroepiploic	4%
Jejunal/ileal/ileocolic	3%

Mesenteric Trauma

Trauma is another common indication for angiography of the mesenteric viscera. Typical angiographic findings include active extravasation, pseudoaneurysm, arteriovenous fistula, or more subtle findings such as truncated vessels or vessel irregularities. Injury to the liver and spleen may result from blunt or penetrating trauma; iatrogenic causes are not uncommon in the liver related to biopsy or biliary procedures. Indications for embolization are usually related to CT findings compatible with active bleeding or laceration to the viscera as well as the patient's clinical status. Splenic artery embolization may be performed proximally or distally depending on the type of injury (Fig. 36A.10). Hepatic artery embolization should be as selective as possible. In the setting of trauma, coils or temporary agents such as Gelfoam are typically the embolic agent of choice.

BILIARY INTERVENTIONS

Percutaneous Biliary Drainage

Percutaneous transhepatic biliary drainage (PTBD) is performed in the setting of biliary obstruction from both malignant and benign causes, and less commonly for biliary leaks. Biliary obstruction can result from extrinsic compression of the biliary ducts or from an internal obstructing mass. Please refer to Table 36A.6 for a list of common causes of malignant and benign biliary obstruction. The diagnosis can be made with a variety of imaging modalities; however, cross-sectional imaging with CT or MRI is most helpful to determine the exact nature and level of the obstruction, which is important for treatment planning.

Patients with biliary obstruction will typically present with classic signs and symptoms which are related to the absence of bile in the intestinal tract and the abnormal buildup of bilirubin and bile salts in the bloodstream which are summarized

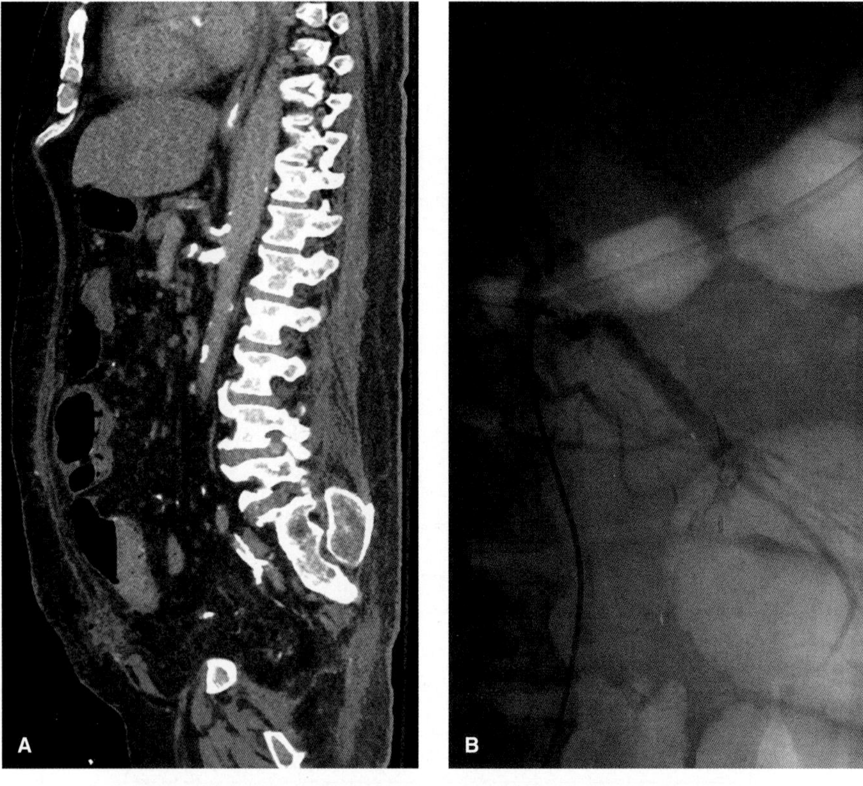

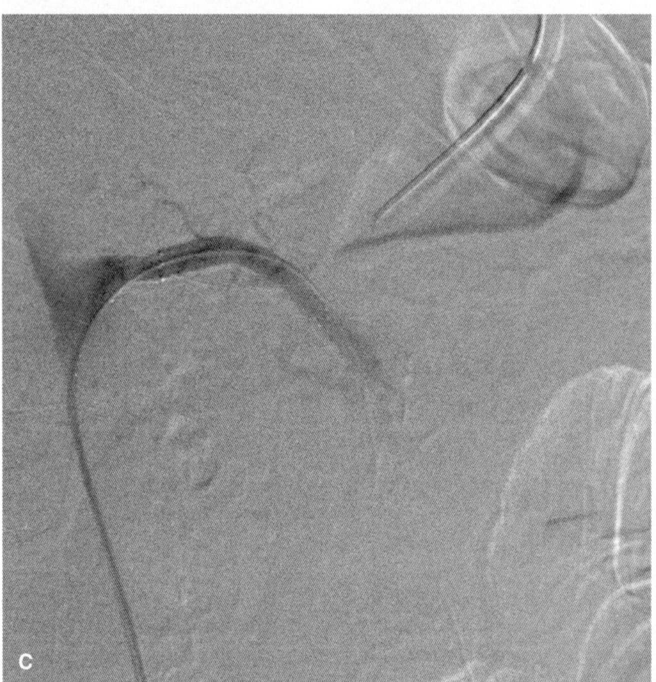

FIGURE 36A.9. **A:** CT demonstrating calcific atherosclerosis in both the celiac and SMA distributions. There are also bowel changes concerning for ischemic colitis. **B:** SMA angiogram demonstrating tight stenosis. **C:** Post-stent angiogram.

in Table 36A.7. Patients may also present more acutely with infection of the biliary system, termed cholangitis, with severity ranging from low-grade fevers to septic shock; however, this is an infrequent presentation in malignant biliary obstruction without a prior endoscopic or percutaneous intervention.

First-line treatment for biliary obstruction is typically with endoscopic retrograde cholangiopancreatography (ERCP) and stent placement by a gastroenterologist. If ERCP fails, or in the setting of altered gastrointestinal anatomy from prior surgery, then percutaneous biliary drainage is indicated. There are no absolute contraindications to PTBD; relative contraindications include coagulopathy and large volume ascites. An additional relative contraindication is a central or intrahepatic mass causing obstruction and isolation of several ducts, as

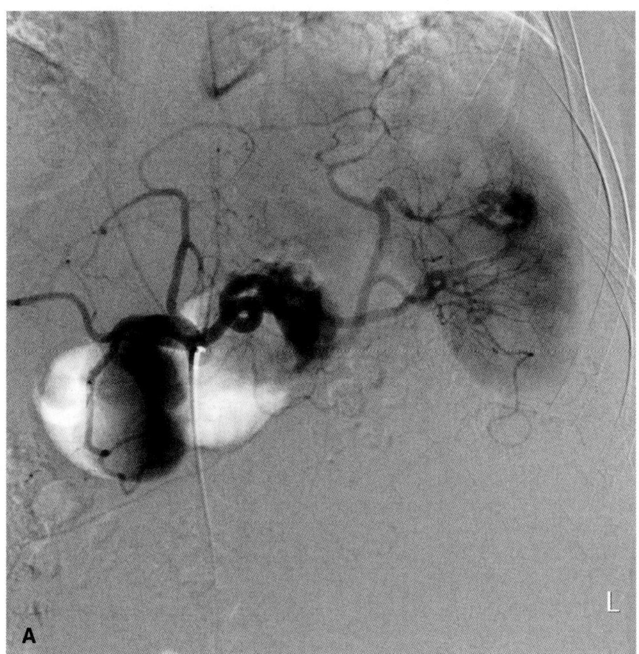

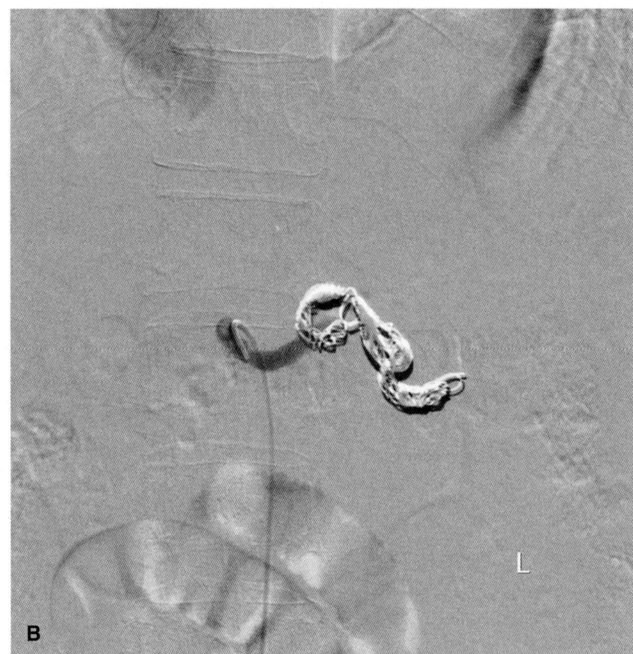

FIGURE 36A.10. **A:** Angiogram showing pseudoaneurysm secondary to trauma in the spleen. **B:** Mid-splenic artery embolization with coils performed.

any drainage is unlikely to improve the patient's symptoms. PTBD carries a high risk of bacteremia due to bacterial colonization of the biliary tree and subsequent manipulation during the procedure. Patients should be given broad-spectrum antibiotics with both gram-positive and gram-negative coverage prophylactically.

Biliary drainage may be performed via the right or left hepatic lobe and is performed with US and fluoroscopic guidance (Fig. 36A.11). Some obstructing masses necessitate bilateral drainage. For a right-sided biliary drain, needle entry should be near the midaxillary line, with a low intercostal approach at the 11th intercostal space. This level is chosen as it usually prevents transgression of the pleural space. A 21- or 22-gauge styleted needle is advanced into the liver under fluoroscopic guidance. The needle is then slowly withdrawn while contrast is gently injected until a biliary radical is identified. A bile duct is recognized by slow, nonpulsatile opacification of a tubular structure which does not wash out (unlike the hepatic vasculature). For a left-sided biliary drain placement, a subxiphoid approach is taken, usually under sonographic guidance, as dilated bile ducts will be easily visualized. Whether from the right or left, a more peripheral access to the biliary tree is preferred to avoid potential injury to the central vasculature. Once fine-needle access in a suitable duct is obtained, a guidewire is advanced and the tract is dilated. Attempts should be made to pass the point of obstruction with a guidewire and catheter. If the obstruction cannot be traversed, a locking loop catheter can be placed above the level of obstruction in the biliary tree which is considered an external biliary drain. If the obstruction can be traversed, then an internal–external biliary drainage catheter can be placed, which refers to a catheter with a locking loop and multiple side holes with the distal loop located in the duodenum. Internal–external biliary drains are often preferred because of catheter stability and simulation of normal physiologic flow of bile. External drainage may be preferable in a septic patient in whom minimal manipulation in the biliary tree is desired. Potential complications of PTBD are listed in Table 36A.8.

For patients with malignant biliary obstructions, self-expanding metallic stents can be placed in the biliary system to allow for internal drainage (Fig. 36A.12). The timing of stent placement often depends on the clinical situation and can be performed at the time of initial biliary drainage or at a later time via the previously obtained access. The stent is placed across the obstruction and may need to extend into the duodenum if the lesion involves the ampulla. Balloon dilation of the stricture is typically performed at the time of stent placement. Once adequate drainage is confirmed, external drains can be fully removed. Metallic stents are reserved for patients with a short life expectancy as they will eventually occlude over time, resulting in recurrence of symptoms.

TABLE 36A.6

EXAMPLES OF CAUSES OF BILIARY OBSTRUCTION

■ BENIGN	■ MALIGNANT
Calculi	Pancreatic cancer
Sclerosing cholangitis	Cholangiocarcinoma
Postsurgical stricture	Gallbladder cancer
Postinfection/inflammation	Lymphoma
	Metastases

TABLE 36A.7

SYMPTOMS OF BILIARY OBSTRUCTION

Jaundice and scleral icterus
Pruritus
Acholic stool (clay-colored stool)
Bilirubinuria (dark-colored urine)
Anorexia
Nausea
Fatigue

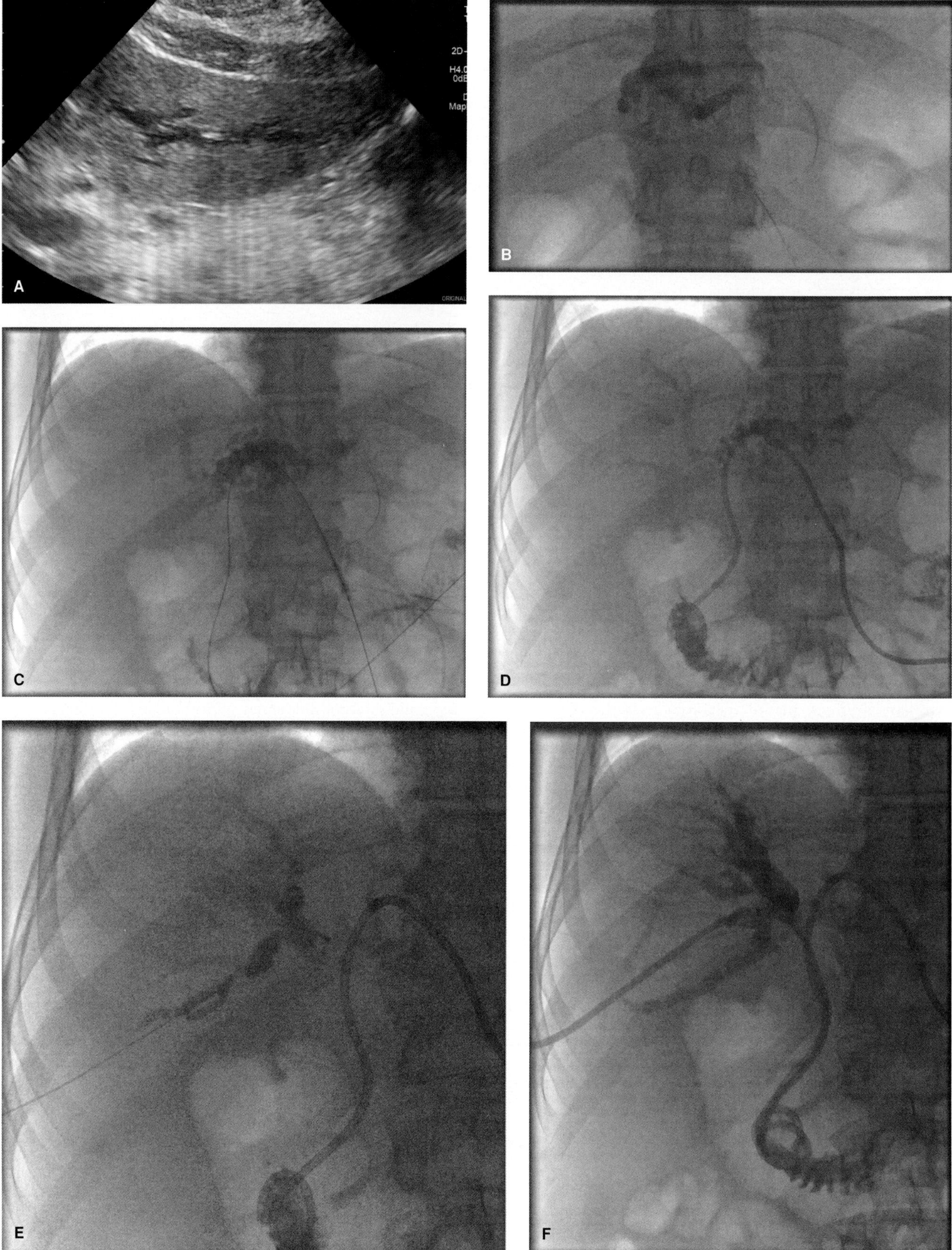

FIGURE 36A.11. **A:** US images demonstrate dilated left biliary ducts which have been accessed with a 22-gauge needle. **B:** Contrast injection confirms access to the biliary tree. **C, D:** A wire is passed through the obstruction and into the duodenum for eventual placement of an internal–external biliary drain. **E, F:** Access to a right hepatic duct is performed under fluoroscopic guidance with eventual placement of a right-sided internal–external drain in a patient with a hilar cholangiocarcinoma.

TABLE 36A.8

COMPLICATIONS OF BILIARY DRAINAGE

Sepsis
Hemorrhage
Pleural transgression (pneumothorax, empyema)
Bile leak
Catheter dislodgement
Catheter occlusion

Benign biliary strictures are not typically treated with permanent stenting, and there is a greater variation in how these lesions are managed. In general, treatment is with a combination of balloon dilation and long-term placement of internal–external biliary drains across the stricture.

Bile leak, or biliary injury, frequently related to surgery is another indication for percutaneous biliary drainage. Small leaks can often be treated conservatively with antibiotics and maintenance of operatively placed drains; however, large leaks can result in bilomas, fistulas, or bile peritonitis and require treatment. Drain placement is used to divert bile away from the site of the injury to allow for healing. ERCP with stent placement is the first-line treatment; however, PTBD is necessary when endoscopic means fail or in patients with altered anatomy such as hepaticojejunostomy. Technically, the procedure is performed in the same way as for obstruction; however, the biliary tree is often minimally or nondilated in this setting, which can make cannulation of a bile duct extremely challenging (Fig. 36A.13). Once biliary diversion is achieved, the catheter will likely have to stay in place for several weeks. If the site of injury does not heal despite diversion, surgical repair is required.

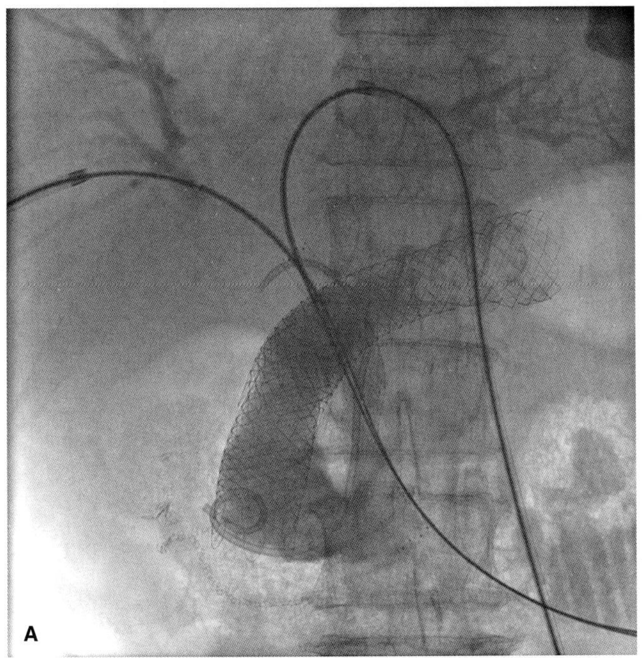

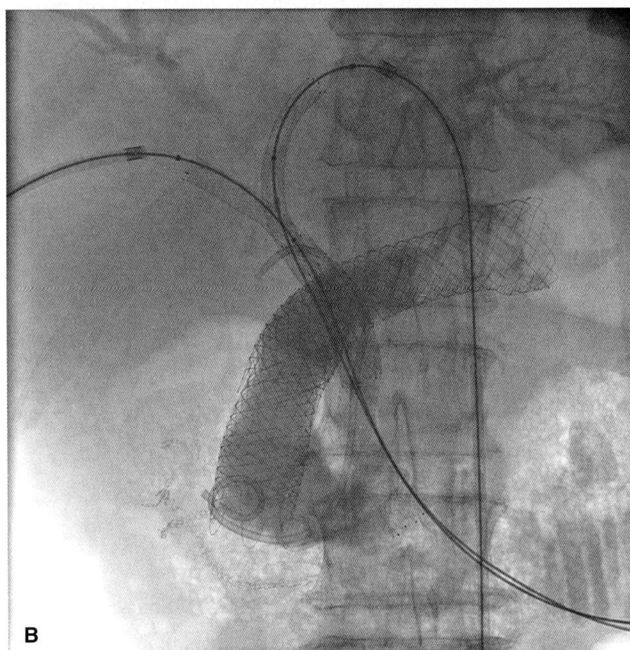

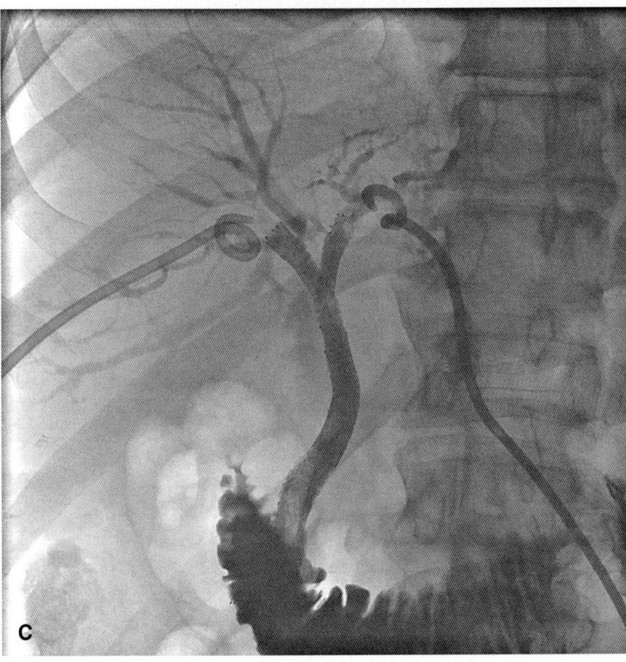

FIGURE 36A.12. **A:** A 10-mm self-expanding uncovered metallic stent placed in the common bile duct to allow for internal drainage. **B:** Six-millimeter stents used to extend into the right and left main hepatic duct due to hilar obstruction. **C:** Sometimes external drains are left in place as a safety measure to ensure internal drains are working adequately.

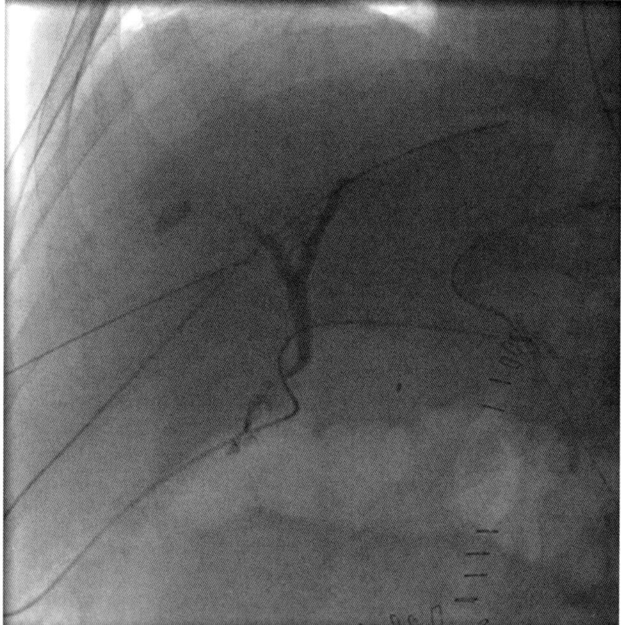

FIGURE 36A.13. **Percutaneous Biliary Drain Requested in a Patient With Recent Liver Transplant and Concern for Biliary Leak.** Image demonstrates decompressed biliary tree with no appreciable leak and rapid transit of contrast into the duodenum.

Percutaneous Cholecystostomy

Percutaneous cholecystostomy tube placement is a treatment option for both calculous and acalculous acute cholecystitis. It is usually reserved for acutely ill patients as a temporizing measurement before definitive surgery, in patients who have comorbidities which make them poor surgical candidates, or when patients have a delayed presentation. Symptoms of acute cholecystitis include fever, elevated white blood cell count, right upper quadrant pain, and the sonographic Murphy sign (pain in the right upper quadrant with pressure from the ultrasound probe). Diagnosis in a patient suspected of acute cholecystitis is confirmed with ultrasound or cross-sectional imaging with findings of gallbladder wall thickening, distention, and pericholecystic fluid/stranding. Similar to other biliary procedures, broad-spectrum antibiotics should be initiated, and any coagulopathy should be corrected prior to the procedure. The only absolute contraindication would be lack of safe access to the gallbladder.

TABLE 36A.9

COMPLICATIONS OF PERCUTANEOUS CHOLECYSTOSTOMY

Sepsis
Bile leak
Peritonitis
Hemorrhage
Abscess formation
Transgression of pleura
Bowel perforation

Percutaneous access to the gallbladder can be achieved under direct visualization with ultrasound complemented with fluoroscopy or less commonly under CT guidance (Fig. 36A.14). In critically ill patients, this procedure can be performed at the bedside with sonography alone. The approach can be transhepatic or transperitoneal. The transhepatic approach is preferred, and proposed advantages include decreased risk of intraperitoneal bile leakage, quicker tract maturation, and greater catheter stability. However, there are advantages for the transperitoneal route that include decreased risk of bleeding and liver contamination. With either approach, it is important to be aware of and exclude any interposed bowel. If possible, a subcostal approach is also preferred to avoid the pleural space. Potential complications are listed in Table 36A.9. Catheter placement can be performed by two techniques, the Seldinger technique or the trocar technique. The Seldinger technique involves fine-needle access with an 18- to 22-gauge needle and subsequent upsizing after bile aspiration and potentially contrast injection to confirm intraluminal positioning under fluoroscopy. In the trocar technique, the needle tip is placed within the drain and the entire system is advanced into the gallbladder. For either technique, an 8- or 10-Fr locking pigtail catheter is placed with contrast injection to confirm final position within the gallbladder.

Once the catheter is placed, it must remain in place for 3 to 6 weeks to allow for tract maturation unless the patient goes on to have surgery before that time. For acalculous cholecystitis, cholecystostomy can be the definitive treatment. Before

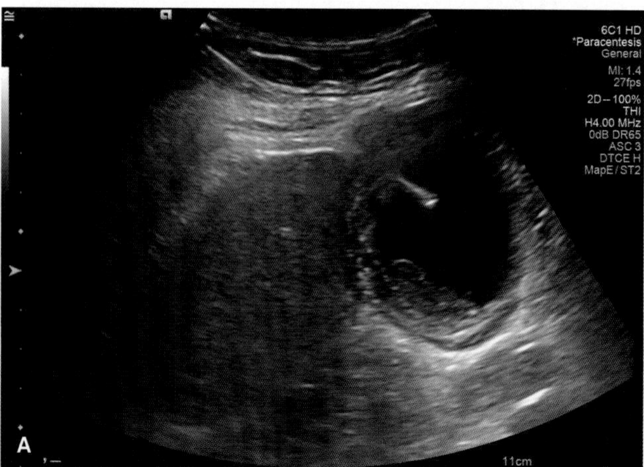

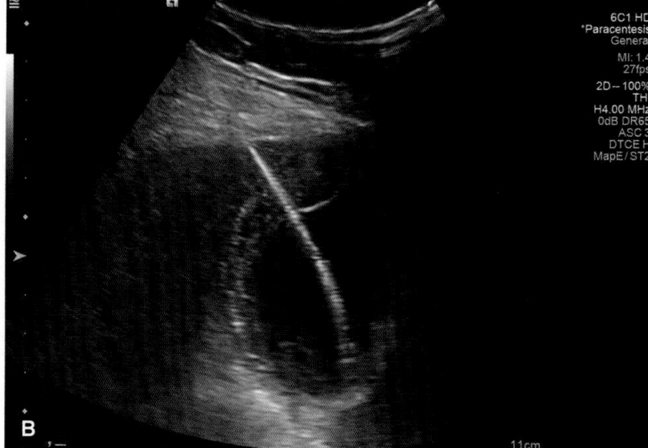

FIGURE 36A.14. **A:** US demonstrates dilated, thick-walled gallbladder with needle access via a short transhepatic route. **B:** US demonstrates wire coiling within the gallbladder lumen.

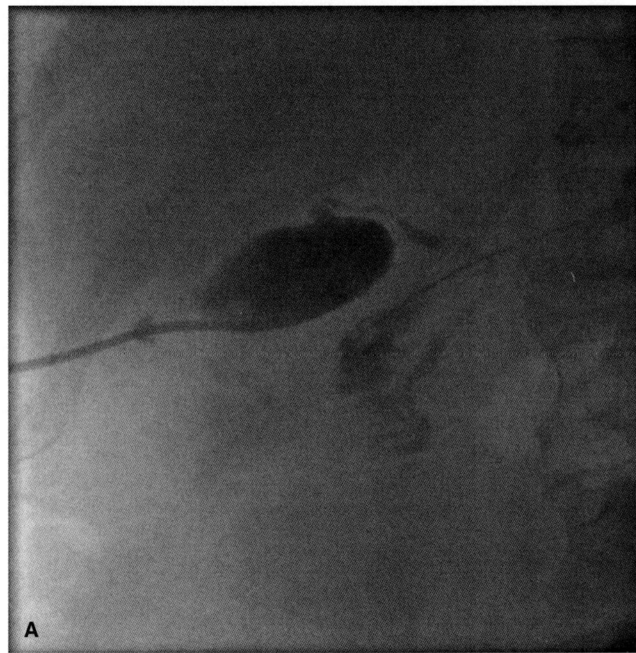

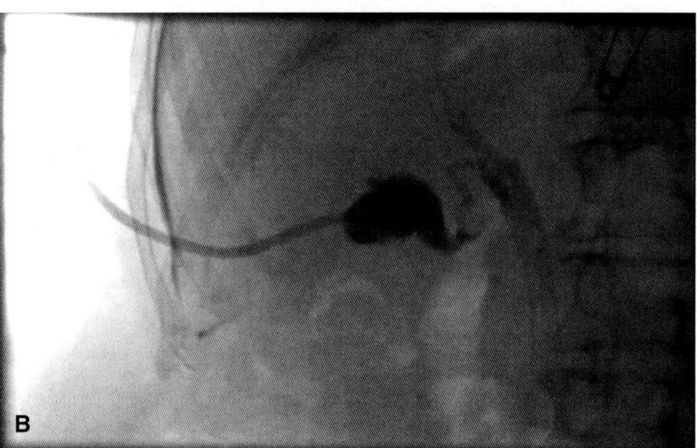

FIGURE 36A.15. **A:** Cholangiogram demonstrates drain well positioned within the gallbladder and no obstruction in the cystic or common bile duct. If this drain has been in place for 4 to 6 weeks, it may be safely removed. **B:** In contrast, this cholangiogram shows a stone lodged in the cystic duct; although contrast does pass around the stone, the drain should remain in place until definitive surgery can happen.

the catheter can be removed, a cholangiogram should be performed to evaluate the cystic and common bile ducts to confirm patency (Fig. 36A.15). Extraction of gallstones with or without lithotripsy through the mature percutaneous tract can be performed in patients with calculous cholecystitis, which could obviate the need for surgery.

PERCUTANEOUS ABSCESS DRAINAGE

Abdominal or pelvic abscess formation can occur spontaneously in association with a visceral infection or in the postoperative setting. Since first being introduced in the 1980s, percutaneous drainage of abscesses has become the primary treatment and can be safely performed in effectively every organ or space in the abdomen and pelvis, including intraperitoneal, retroperitoneal, liver, renal, pancreatic, splenic, subcutaneous, and deep pelvic abscesses. Symptoms of abscess formation include pain, nausea, fever, and elevated white blood cell count. Diagnosis is best made with contrast-enhanced cross-sectional imaging. A CT or MRI is also vital for intra-abdominal or pelvic collections to evaluate the surrounding anatomy, determine approach for drainage, and whether or not a percutaneous approach is feasible and safe.

The only absolute contraindication to drainage is lack of a safe percutaneous approach to the abscess. This can sometimes be mitigated by patient positioning or angulation of the CT gantry during drainage. Relative contraindications include coagulopathy, lack of patient cooperation, or severe cardiopulmonary compromise; most of these situations can, however, be corrected to allow for percutaneous drainage.

The choice of route and modality is dependent on the location of the collection to be drained. In general, the shortest and most direct route that is free of any intervening solid organs, bowel, or other vital structures is chosen. Access to the collection is performed under US or CT guidance, each of which has its advantages and disadvantages summarized in Table 36A.10. In general, US is quicker with real-time visualization of the access needle during placement; however, deeper

TABLE 36A.10

US VERSUS CT FOR PERCUTANEOUS ABSCESS DRAINAGE

■ ULTRASOUND		■ CT	
■ ADVANTAGES	■ DISADVANTAGES	■ ADVANTAGES	■ DISADVANTAGES
Real-time imaging	Requires significant operator experience	Less operator dependent	Not real-time
Faster	Cannot penetrate to deeper collections	Deeper collections easily visualized	Increased procedure time
Portable	Difficult to visualize abscesses with air	Intervening air, bone, fat less significant	Radiation exposure
Less expensive	Intervening bowel less visible	Bowel well visualized	
No radiation		Final catheter position better visualized	

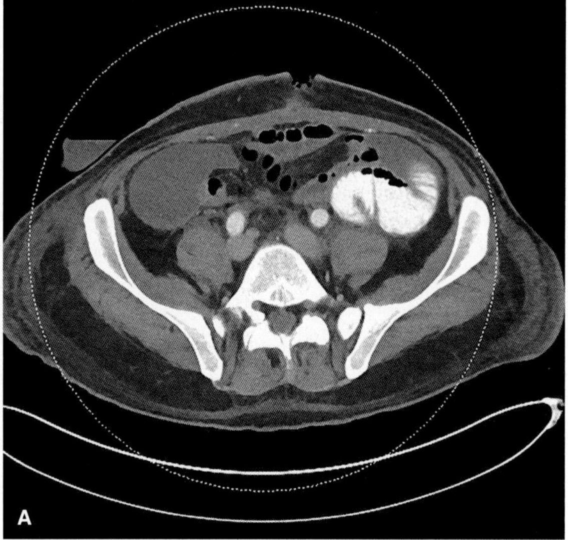

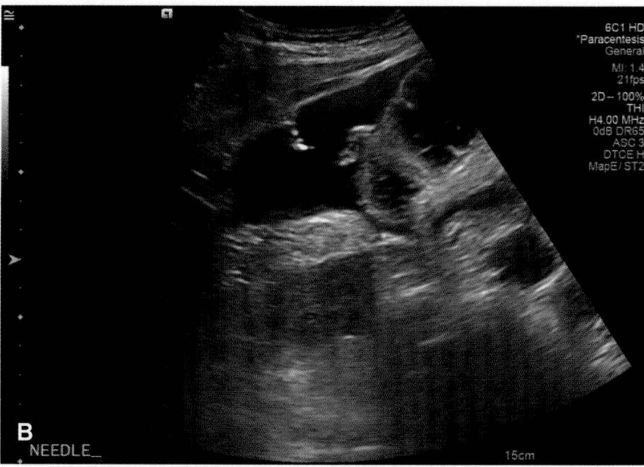

FIGURE 36A.16. **A:** CT demonstrates large right lower quadrant abscess which is superficial to the abdominal wall. **B:** US clearly demonstrates this abscess and nearby structures with real-time visualization of the access needle in the collection.

abdominal structures and bowel can be difficult to visualize (Fig. 36A.16). CT is not real-time and therefore slower; however, there is excellent visualization of the deeper intra-abdominal and pelvic structures. Fluoroscopy can also be used in conjunction with ultrasound to confirm appropriate positioning or to aid in catheter repositioning (Fig. 36A.17).

The catheter placement can be performed by either the Seldinger or trocar technique. In the Seldinger technique,

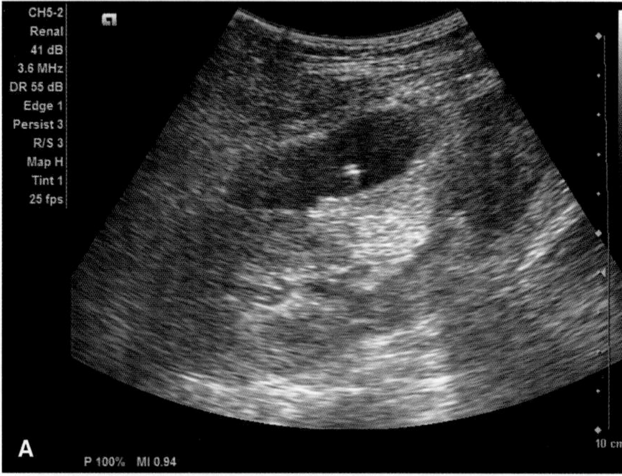

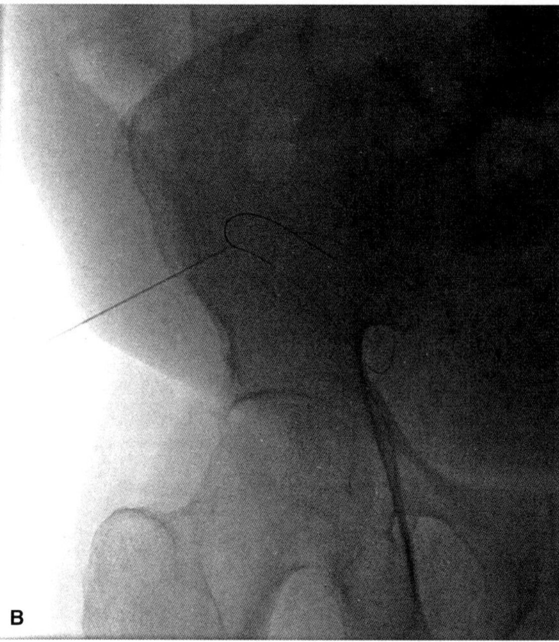

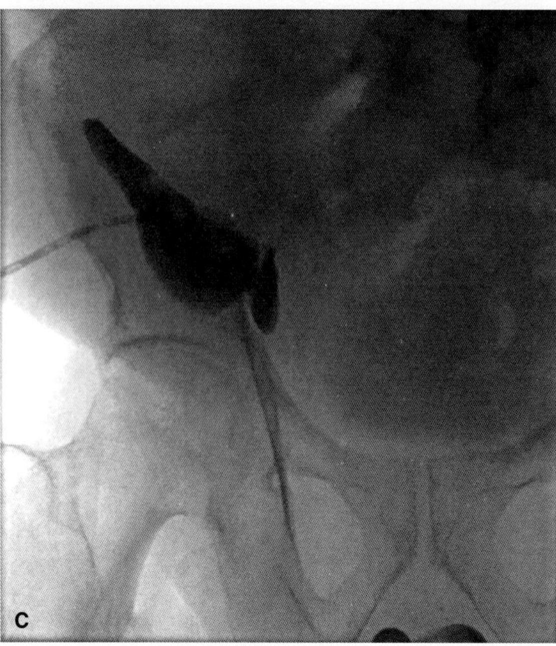

FIGURE 36A.17. **A:** Perirenal collection in a patient with a right lower quadrant renal transplant; US shows access needle in the collection. **B:** Fluoroscopic images show wire coiling in the collection. **C:** Injection confirms drain is well located in the collection.

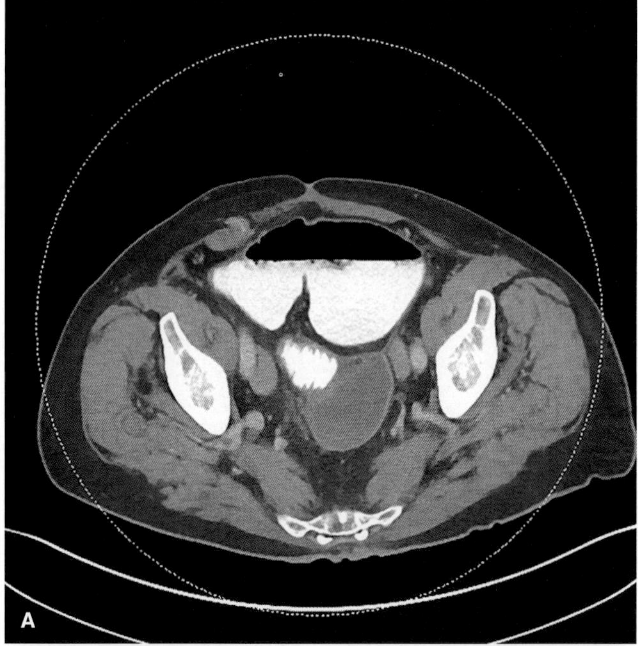

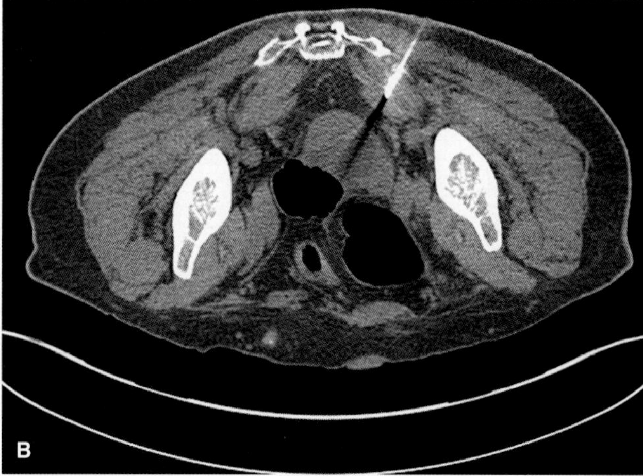

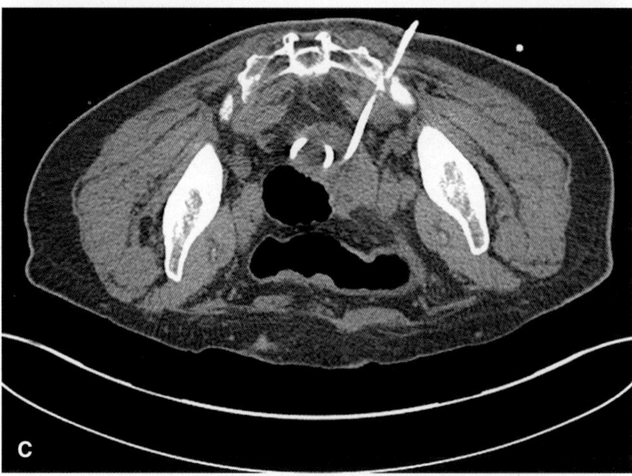

FIGURE 36A.18. **A:** CT demonstrates abscess in the deep pelvis with no safe approach anteriorly due to the intervening bowel. **B:** Transgluteal approach taken through the greater sciatic foramen; needle path should be as close to the sacrum as possible. **C:** Pigtail drainage catheter coiled within the abscess.

fine-needle access is obtained first with an 18- to 22-gauge needle followed by serial dilation over a guidewire to the desired drain size. The drain is mounted on a metallic stiffener to aid in passage through the intervening tissues. In the trocar technique, the catheter itself is placed directly into the collection using the metallic stiffener with an inner sharp trocar needle. The choice of method is often based on the size and location of the collection as well as operator preference. No randomized trial comparing the two methods has been performed. The size of catheter placed may depend on the type of fluid encountered; usually a locking pigtail catheter is placed ranging from 8 to 16 Fr.

Although most abdominal and pelvic collections can be drained by a straightforward approach, there are several locations which warrant special consideration. Deep pelvic collections are often inaccessible from an anterior or lateral approach due to the urinary bladder, uterus in women, and interposed bowel. In such cases, a transgluteal approach may be necessary during which a catheter is placed through the greater sciatic foramen (Fig. 36A.18). When using this approach, care must be taken to avoid the sciatic nerve and gluteal arteries, usually by choosing a path as close to the sacrum as possible. If no safe access point can be identified, some deep pelvic collections can be drained under sonographic guidance via a transvaginal or transrectal approach using a needle guide secured to the appropriate ultrasound probe (Fig. 36A.19). Subphrenic collections can be challenging because care must be taken in this location to avoid transgressing the pleural space. This can be accomplished by a subcostal approach, or if an intercostal approach is necessary, accessing as caudal as possible to minimize the risk of pleural effusion or empyema.

Major complications following percutaneous abscess drainage are rare and include bacteremia/sepsis, hemorrhage, bowel perforation, and pleural complication (pneumothorax, effusion, empyema, etc.). Minor complications are often related to issues with the drain itself, such as dislodgement, malposition, or obstruction.

Follow-up care after drainage catheter placement includes daily flushing and monitoring of fluid output. Removal of the catheter depends on clinical improvement in the patient, decreased output from the catheter, and resolution of the collection. Persistent high-volume output could indicate fistula formation, which can be confirmed with a contrast injection under fluoroscopic guidance. The catheter should remain in place until the fistula has resolved. Low output with a persistent collection on imaging may reflect obstruction of

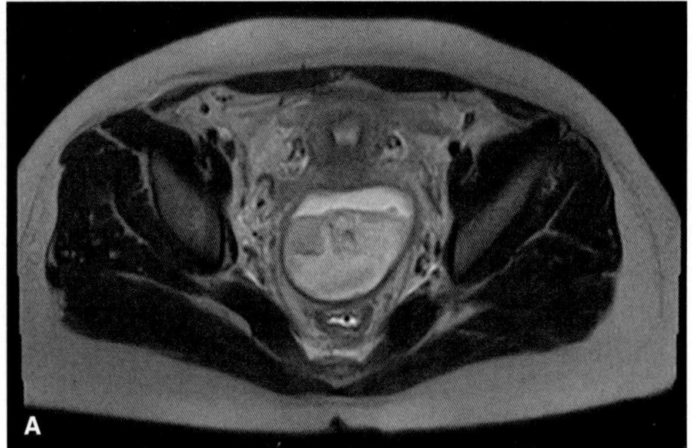

FIGURE 36A.19. **A:** MRI demonstrating deep pelvic abscess in a pregnant patient who wished to avoid any radiation exposure. **B:** Transrectal US demonstrates needle and wire within the abscess cavity.

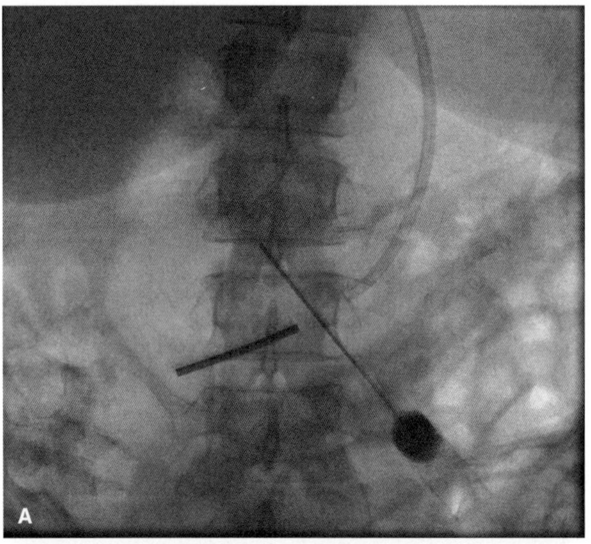

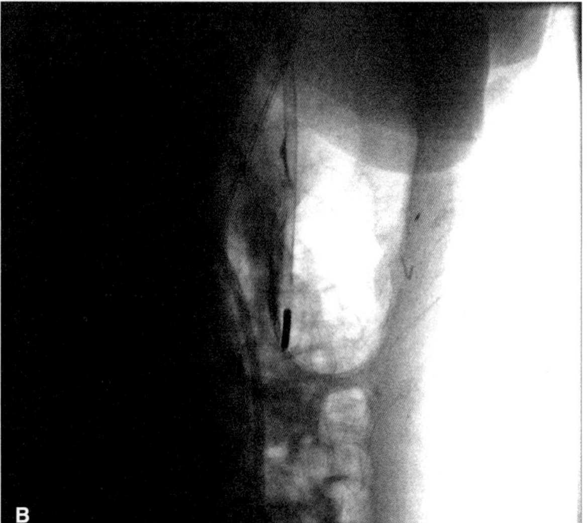

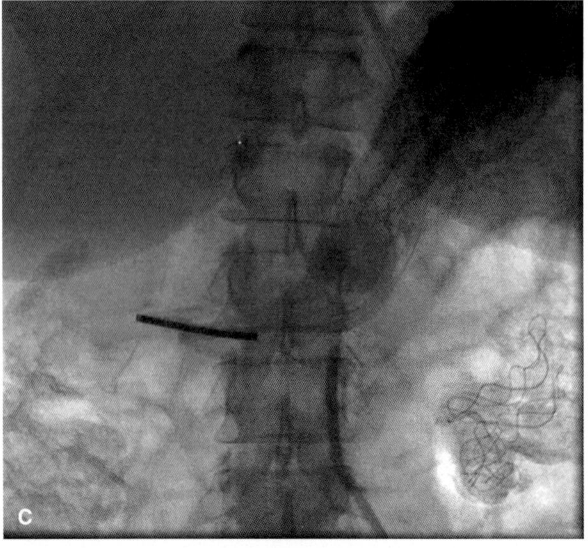

FIGURE 36A.20. **A:** T-fasteners are placed under fluoroscopic guidance to secure the stomach to the anterior abdominal wall. **B:** Position of T-fasteners confirmed with a lateral view; no other intervening structures identified. **C:** Balloon-retention gastrostomy tube is placed at the center of the T-fasteners. Final contrast injection demonstrates good position within the stomach with opacification of rugal folds.

the catheter, very complex/viscous material, or catheter malposition. Injection of tPA can be attempted to break up the complex material and facilitate drainage, or the drain can be adjusted under fluoroscopic guidance, as needed.

ENTERIC ACCESS

Gastrostomy Tube Placement

Enteral feeding tubes were traditionally placed by surgery or endoscopy; however, fluoroscopically guided placement has been a well-accepted method for many years with low morbidity and mortality. Percutaneous radiologic gastrostomy (PRG) placement is indicated in patients who cannot maintain adequate nutrition orally. These patients often have neurologic impairments, causing inability to swallow, or suffer from head and neck cancer. A less common indication for PRG placement is for gastrointestinal obstruction, which can be found in patients with abdominopelvic malignancies or diabetes-related gastroparesis. In this case, the tube is used to decompress the stomach. Contraindications to PRG are listed in Table 36A.11. The only absolute contraindications are gastric varices, which could result in severe hemorrhage, or lack of

TABLE 36A.11

CONTRAINDICATIONS TO PERCUTANEOUS GASTROSTOMY TUBE PLACEMENT

■ RELATIVE	■ ABSOLUTE
Coagulopathy	Gastric varices
Interposition of liver or colon—may be overcome through use of US or CT	No safe percutaneous window
Prior surgery affecting the stomach	
Ascites	

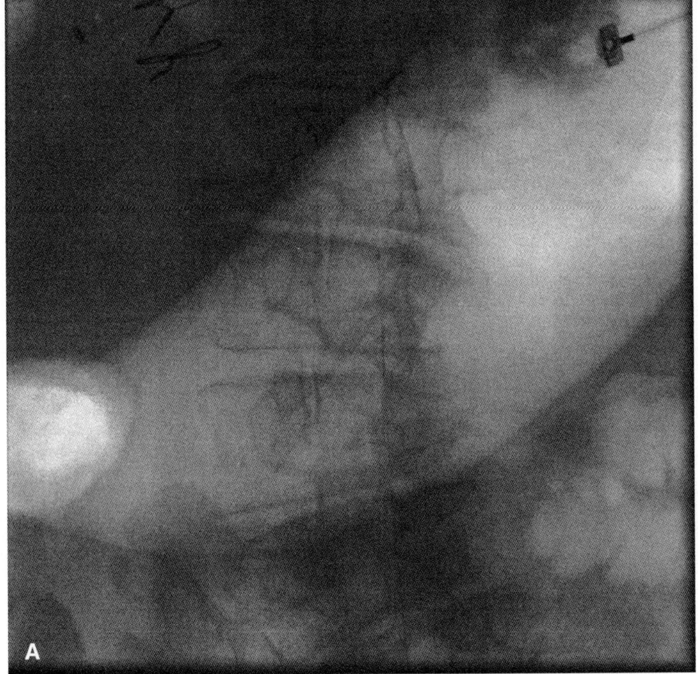

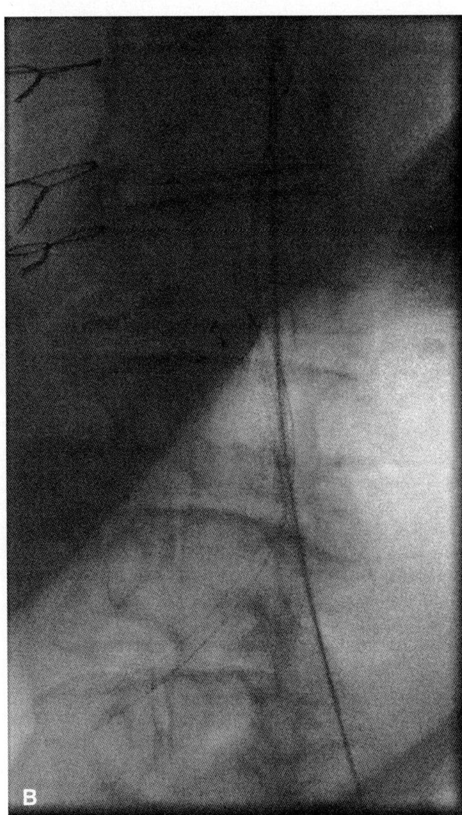

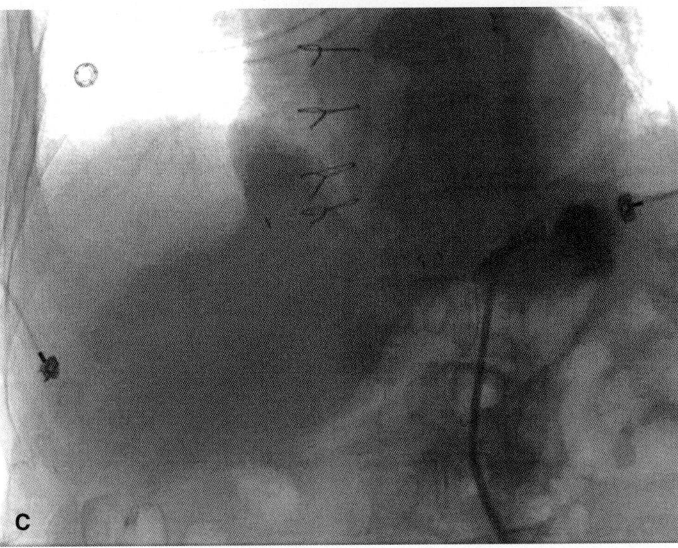

FIGURE 36A.21. **A:** Single 21-gauge needle access to the stomach is achieved under fluoroscopic guidance. **B:** Catheter and guidewire are directed through the gastroesophageal junction. **C:** Final images demonstrate good positioning of a mushroom-retention gastrostomy tube.

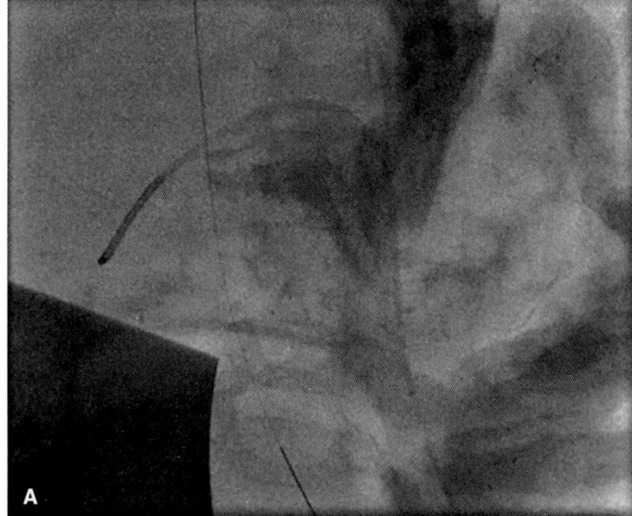

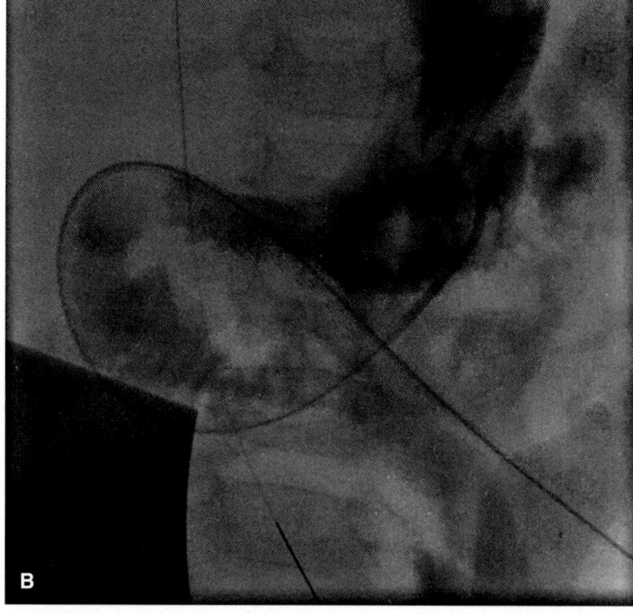

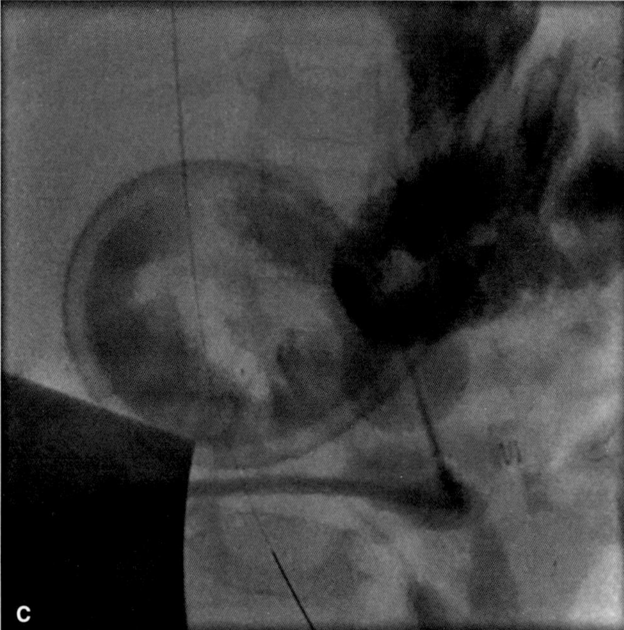

FIGURE 36A.22. **A:** Conversion of gastrostomy to gastrojejunostomy performed in a pediatric patient. Through the existing access, a wire and catheter are manipulated through the pylorus and into the duodenum. **B:** The access should be advanced into the jejunum. **C:** Exchange is then made for a gastrojejunostomy tube.

safe percutaneous access. Anatomic factors such as interposition of the colon sometimes preclude placement but may also be overcome with techniques such as CT guidance.

There are two general methods for the placement of PRG: the push method and the pull method. Both methods are performed primarily under fluoroscopic guidance. CT is sometimes used as an adjunct in difficult cases. For both methods, a nasogastric tube should be placed, or a 5-Fr catheter can be manipulated under fluoroscopic guidance into the stomach immediately prior to the procedure. The stomach is then insufflated with air via the nasogastric tube. The access site is chosen using fluoroscopy. In general, this should be to the left of midline over the antrum or mid-distal body of the stomach; however, the location may vary slightly based on other anatomic considerations. In the push method, gastropexy is first performed with T-fasteners to approximate the stomach to the anterior abdominal wall. Each T-fastener is placed under fluoroscopic guidance. The access for the tube itself is at the center of the T-fasteners and is usually performed with an 18-gauge needle. Aspiration of air can confirm positioning within the stomach. Tract dilation is performed over a stiff 0.035-in wire with subsequent placement of a balloon-retention gastrostomy tube; sizes generally range from 14 to 18 Fr on initial placement. Position is confirmed with contrast injection (Fig. 36A.20). In comparison, the pull method is performed with a single gastric puncture under fluoroscopic guidance (Fig. 36A.21). Then, a hydrophilic guidewire and catheter are manipulated through the gastroesophageal junction and up through the oral cavity. The hydrophilic guidewire is exchanged for a stiff guidewire, and the gastrostomy tube is passed through the oral cavity and pulled out through the percutaneous abdominal access.

Potential complications of gastrostomy tube placement include infection (both deep and superficial), peritonitis, GI hemorrhage, unintended GI perforation, and complications related to the tube itself, such as leaking, dislodgement, and obstruction.

Gastrojejunostomy

Gastrojejunostomy tube placement can be performed as a primary access for feeding or from conversion of an existing gastrostomy tube. Indications for placement include gastroesophageal reflux, aspiration, or large gastric residuals for which feeding beyond the ligament of Treitz may be helpful. In primary placement, the basic steps are the same as for the push method of PRG placement. Ideally, the access needle should be directed toward the pylorus to facilitate passage into the duodenum. The pylorus is typically passed with a combination of an angled 5-Fr catheter and hydrophilic guidewire, both of which are advanced into the jejunum. Exchange is made for a stiff wire, and the gastrojejunostomy tube is placed after tract dilation. Conversion of an existing gastrostomy tube can be technically challenging depending on the angulation of the tube at initial placement. The same process is performed, with cannulation of the pylorus and jejunum, using a 5-Fr catheter and guidewire (Fig. 36A.22).

Suggested Readings

Abbas SM, Bissett IP, Holden A, Woodfield JC, Parry BR, Duncan D. Clinical variables associated with positive angiographic localization of lower gastrointestinal bleeding. *ANZ J Surg* 2005;75(11):953–957.

Alexander AA, Eschelman DJ, Nazarian LN, Bonn J. Transrectal sonographically guided drainage of deep pelvic abscesses. *AJR Am J Roentgenol* 1994; 162(5):1227–1230.

Baron TH, Grimm IS, Swanstrom LL. Interventional approaches to gallbladder disease. *N Engl J Med* 2015;373(4):357–365.

Boley SJ, Brandt LJ, Veith FJ. Ischemic disorders of the intestines. *Curr Probl Surg* 1978;15(4):1–85.

Browning PD, McGahan JP, Gerscovich EO. Percutaneous cholecystostomy for suspected acute cholecystitis in the hospitalized patient. *J Vasc Interv Radiol* 1993;4(4):531–537.

Bulakba i N, Kurtaran K, Ustünsöz B, Somuncu I. Massive lower gastrointestinal hemorrhage from the surgical anastomosis in patients with multiorgan trauma: treatment by subselective embolization with polyvinyl alcohol particles. *Cardiovasc Intervent Radiol* 1999;22(6):461–467.

Chang YR, Ahn YJ, Jang JY, et al. Percutaneous cholecystostomy for acute cholecystitis in patients with high comorbidity and re-evaluation of treatment efficacy. *Surgery* 2014;155:615–622.

Covey AM, Brown KT. Palliative percutaneous drainage in malignant biliary obstruction. Part 1: indications and preprocedure evaluation. *J Support Oncol* 2006;4:269–273.

de Baere T, Chapot R, Kuoch V, et al. Percutaneous gastrostomy with fluoroscopic guidance: single-center experience in 500 consecutive cancer patients. *Radiology* 1999;210:651–654.

De Martino RR. Normal and variant mesenteric anatomy. In: Oderich GS, ed. *Mesenteric Vascular Disease*. New York: Springer Science+Business Media; 2015:9–23.

Defreyne L, De Schrijver I, Decruyenaere J, et al. Therapeutic decision-making in endoscopically unmanageable nonvariceal upper gastrointestinal hemorrhage. *Cardiovasc Intervent Radiol* 2008;31:897–905.

Dixon S, Chan V, Shrivastava V, Anthony S, Uberoi R, Bratby M. "Is there a role for empiric gastroduodenal artery embolization in the management of patients with active upper GI hemorrhage?" *Cardiovasc Intervent Radiol* 2013;36(4):970–977.

El Hamel A, Parc R, Adda G, Bouteloup PY, Huguet C, Malafosse M. Bleeding pseudocysts and pseudoaneurysms in chronic pancreatitis. *Br J Surg* 1991;78:1059–1063.

Ell C, May A. Mid-gastrointestinal bleeding: capsule endoscopy and push-and-pull enteroscopy give rise to a new medical term. *Endoscopy* 2006;38(1):73–75.

Eriksson LG, Sundbom M, Gustavsson S, Nyman R. Endoscopic marking with a metallic clip facilitates transcatheter arterial embolization in upper peptic ulcer bleeding. *J Vasc Interv Radiol* 2006;17:959–964.

Ernst O, Sergent G, Mizrahi D, Delemazure O, L'Herminé C. Biliary leaks: treatment by means of percutaneous transhepatic biliary drainage. *Radiology* 1999;211(2):345–348.

Fidelman N. Benign biliary strictures: diagnostic evaluation and approaches to percutaneous treatment. *Tech Vasc Interv Radiol* 2015;18(4):210–217.

Fidler J, Paulson EK, Layfield L. CT evaluation of acute cholecystitis: findings and usefulness in diagnosis. *AJR Am J Roentgenol* 1996;166(5):1085–1088.

Gayer C, Chino A, Lucas C, et al. Acute lower gastrointestinal bleeding in 1,112 patients admitted to an urban emergency medical center. *Surgery* 2009; 146(4):600–606; discussion 606–607.

Ghassemi KA, Jensen DM. Lower GI bleeding: epidemiology and management. *Curr Gastroenterol Rep* 2013;15(7):333.

Gillespie CJ, Sutherland AD, Mossop PJ, Woods RJ, Keck JO, Heriot AG. Mesenteric embolization for lower gastrointestinal bleeding. *Dis Colon Rectum* 2010;53(9):1258–1264.

Ginat D, Saad WE. Cholecystostomy and transcholecystic biliary access. *Tech Vasc Interv Radiol* 2008;11(1):2–13.

Hemp JH, Sabri SS. Endovascular management of visceral arterial aneurysms. *Tech Vasc Interv Radiol* 2015;18(1):14–23.

Huang CS, Lichtenstein DR. Nonvariceal upper gastrointestinal bleeding. *Gastroenterol Clin North Am* 2003;32:1053–1078.

Kennedy DW, Laing CJ, Tseng LH, Rosenblum DI, Tamarkin SW. Detection of active gastrointestinal hemorrhage with CT angiography: a 4(1/2)-year retrospective review. *J Vasc Interv Radiol* 2010;21(6):848–855.

Lawson AJ, Beningfield SJ, Krige JE, Rischbieter P, Burmeister S. Percutaneous transhepatic self-expanding metal stents for palliation of malignant biliary obstruction. *S Afr J Surg* 2012;50:54, 56, 58 passim.

Lee MJ, Dawson SL, Mueller PR, Krebs TL, Saini S, Hahn PF. Palliation of malignant bile duct obstruction with metallic biliary endoprostheses: technique, results, and complications. *J Vasc Interv Radiol* 1992;3:665–671.

Liao Z, Gao R, Xu C, Li ZS. Indications and detection, completion, and retention rates of small-bowel capsule endoscopy: a systematic review. *Gastrointest Endosc* 2010;71(2):280–286.

Lock G. Acute intestinal ischaemia. *Best Pract Res Clin Gastroenterol* 2001;15:83–98.

Loffroy R, Rao P, Ota S, De Lin M, Kwak BK, Geschwind JF. Embolization of acute nonvariceal upper gastrointestinal hemorrhage resistant to endoscopic treatment: results and predictors of recurrent bleeding. *Cardiovasc Intervent Radiol* 2010;33(6):1088–1100.

Malgor RD, Oderich GS, McKusick MA, et al. Results of single- and two-vessel mesenteric artery stents for chronic mesenteric ischemia. *Ann Vasc Surg* 2010; 24(8):1094–1101.

Neff CC, Mueller PR, Ferrucci JT Jr, et al. Serious complications following transgression of the pleural space in drainage procedures. *Radiology* 1984;152:335–341.

Nusbaum M, Baum S. Radiographic demonstration of unknown sites of gastrointestinal bleeding. *Surg Forum* 1963;14:374–375.

Ozbülbül NI. CT angiography of the celiac trunk: anatomy, variants and pathologic findings. *Diagn Interv Radiol* 2011;17(2):150–157.

Ozden I, Tekant Y, Bilge O, et al. Endoscopic and radiologic interventions as the leading causes of severe cholangitis in a tertiary referral center. *Am J Surg* 2005;189:702–706.

Papanicolaou N, Mueller PR, Ferrucci JT Jr, et al. Abscess-fistula association: radiologic recognition and percutaneous management. *AJR Am J Roentgenol* 1984;143:811–815.

Picus D, Hicks ME, Darcy MD, et al. Percutaneous cholecystolithotomy: analysis of results and complications in 58 consecutive patients. *Radiology* 1992;183(3):779–784.

Robert B, Chivot C, Rebibo L, Sabbagh C, Regimbeau JM, Yzet T. Percutaneous transgluteal drainage of pelvic abscesses in interventional radiology: a safe alternative to surgery. *J Visc Surg* 2016;153(1):3–7.

Roy-Choudhury SH, Gallacher DJ, Pilmer J, et al. Relative threshold of detection of active arterial bleeding: in vitro comparison of MDCT and digital subtraction angiography. *AJR Am J Roentgenol* 2007;189(5):W238–W246.

Ryan J, Hahn P, Boland G, McDowell RK, Saini S, Mueller PR Percutaneous gastrostomy with T-fastener gastropexy: results of 316 consecutive procedures. *Radiology* 1997;203(2):496–500.

Shin JH, Park AW. Updates on percutaneous radiologic gastrostomy/gastrojejunostomy and jejunostomy. *Gut Liver* 2010;4(Suppl 1):S25–S31.

Spira RM, Nissan A, Zamir O, Cohen T, Fields SI, Freund HR. Percutaneous transhepatic cholecystostomy and delayed laparoscopic cholecystectomy in critically ill patients with acute calculus cholecystitis. *Am J Surg* 2002;183:62–66.

Sreenarasimhaiah J. Diagnosis and management of intestinal ischaemic disorders. *BMJ* 2003;326:1372–1376.

Stampfl U, Hackert T, Radeleff B, et al. Percutaneous management of postoperative bile leaks after upper gastrointestinal surgery. *Cardiovasc Intervent Radiol* 2011;34(4):808–815.

Sutter CM, Ryu RK. Percutaneous management of malignant biliary obstruction. *Tech Vasc Interv Radiol* 2015;18(4):218–226.

van Leerdam ME. Epidemiology of acute upper gastrointestinal bleeding. *Best Pract Res Clin Gastroenterol* 2008;22(2):209–224.

van Overhagen H, Meyers H, Tilanus HW, Jeekel J, Lameris JS. Percutaneous cholecystostomy for patients with acute cholecystitis and an increased surgical risk. *Cardiovasc Intervent Radiol* 1996;19:72–76.

vanSonnenberg E, Ferrucci JT Jr, Mueller PR, Wittenberg J, Simone JF, Malt RA. Percutaneous radiographically guided catheter drainage of abdominal abscesses. *JAMA* 1982;247:190–192.

vanSonnenberg E, Mueller PR, Ferrucci JT Jr. Percutaneous drainage of 250 abdominal abscesses and fluid collections. Part I: results, failures, and complications. *Radiology* 1984;151:337–341.

Venkatesan AM, Kundu S, Sacks D, et al; Society of Interventional Radiology Standards of Practice Committee. Practice guidelines for adult antibiotic prophylaxis during vascular and interventional radiology procedures. Written by the Standards of Practice Committee for the Society of Interventional Radiology and endorsed by the Cardiovascular Interventional Radiological Society of Europe and Canadian Interventional Radiology Association [corrected]. *J Vasc Interv Radiol* 2010;21:1611–1630.

Wollman B, D'Agostino H, Walus-Wigle JR, Easter DW, Beale A. Radiologic, endoscopic, and surgical gastrostomy: an institutional evaluation and meta-analysis of the literature. *Radiology* 1995;197:699–704.

Yata S, Ihaya T, Kaminou T, et al. Transcatheter arterial embolization of acute arterial bleeding in the upper and lower gastrointestinal tract with N-butyl-2-cyanoacrylate. *J Vasc Interv Radiol* 2013;24(3):422–431.

Zuckier LS. Acute gastrointestinal bleeding. *Semin Nucl Med* 2003;33(4):297–311.

CHAPTER 36B ■ GENITOURINARY INTERVENTIONS

CASH JEREMY HORN

UTERINE ARTERY EMBOLIZATION

Uterine artery embolization (UAE) is a well-established treatment option for the management of symptomatic uterine fibroids. Compared to myomectomy and hysterectomy, UAE allows a minimally invasive approach with a short recovery time and a high technical and clinical success rate. The safety and efficacy of the procedure has been demonstrated in several randomized trials, with clinical outcomes similar to those of myomectomy. Of note, UAE can also be performed in the setting of postpartum hemorrhage to control bleeding, though this section will focus on its use in the treatment of symptomatic fibroids.

Knowledge of the pelvic arterial anatomy and its variations is critical when performing UAE. The internal iliac artery arises from the bifurcation of the common iliac artery in the region of the lumbosacral junction, and provides the majority of the blood supply to the pelvis. Although the anatomy of the internal iliac artery varies tremendously among individuals, it most commonly bifurcates into an anterior and posterior trunk. The posterior trunk gives off the superior gluteal artery, iliolumbar artery, and the lateral sacral artery. The anterior trunk gives off vesicular arteries, the middle hemorrhoidal artery, obturator artery, internal pudendal artery, inferior gluteal artery, and the uterine and vaginal arteries in females. There is variable origin of the uterine artery, which most commonly arises as the first or second branch of the inferior gluteal artery (Fig. 36B.1). Other variations include an origin directly from a trifurcation of the anterior division, or even directly from the internal iliac artery. There is a characteristic appearance of the uterine artery, which demonstrates a "U" shape on its descending segment then ascends in a tortuous manner.

Uterine fibroids are benign, smooth muscle vascular neoplasms that grow in size and increase in prevalence throughout a woman's reproductive life. They are common tumors, with a prevalence of approximately 40% to 60% in women aged 35, increasing to 70% to 80% in women aged 50. However, only approximately 25% of women with fibroids have symptoms severe enough to pursue treatment. Patients may present with heavy menstrual bleeding (menorrhagia), irregular periods (metorrhagia), bulk-related symptoms (urinary frequency, constipation, pelvic pressure), or pain. Fibroids may also lead to decreased fertility as well as complications during pregnancy. They may be single or multiple and are described by their location within the uterus (Table 36B.1).

Medical therapy has a limited role in the management of symptomatic fibroids. Hormonal manipulation (oral contraceptives, gonadotropin-releasing hormone agonists, antiprogestins, intrauterine devices) may reduce fibroid size and control symptoms; however, the efficacy of these medications is inconsistent and compliance is poor due to significant side effects.

Traditional surgical management includes hysterectomy and myomectomy. While hysterectomy offers definitive management, the in-hospital recovery time can take days to weeks and the complication rate is reported to be upward of 9%. Myomectomy (the surgical removal of individual fibroids with preservation of the uterus) has a shorter recovery time and lower overall complication rate than hysterectomy; however, the procedure is limited when there are multiple or large fibroids. In addition, the symptoms due to uterine fibroids often recur following myomectomy due to continued growth of unresected fibroids, with up to 25% of women requiring repeat intervention.

UAE is an alternative therapy for women with symptomatic uterine fibroids. Although there is no established guideline for UAE patient selection, many factors come into play when deciding the appropriate therapy including fibroid size and extent, as well as patient preference. Absolute contraindications to performing UAE include active pregnancy, active pelvic infection, or suspicion for gynecologic malignancy (unless the procedure is being planned for palliation prior to resection).

The location of the fibroids may also play a role in the decision of whether or not to pursue UAE: fibroids along the broad ligament as well as cervical fibroids may not respond well to UAE, likely related to vascular supply arising from arteries other than the uterine arteries. Early literature cautioned against performing UAE in the setting of pedunculated subserosal fibroids, with the concern of stalk necrosis and detachment of the pedunculated fibroid following the procedure. However, a large number of more recent studies have demonstrated that UAE can be safe and effective in the treatment of these fibroids.

The desire to maintain fertility should not preclude UAE. Earlier guidelines recommended that uterine embolization should not be the first choice for women with symptomatic fibroids who wished to become pregnant; however, there has been little evidence to support that advice. A single randomized controlled trial comparing UAE to myomectomy demonstrated superior reproductive outcomes after myomectomy in the first 2 years of follow-up. However, a number of limitations of the study led the Cochrane Review to conclude in 2012 that "there is very low-level evidence suggesting that myomectomy may be associated with better fertility outcomes than UAE, but more research is needed." Ever since the procedure was first described, it has been clear that uncomplicated pregnancies and deliveries could occur after UAE. The decision for the correct therapy in women

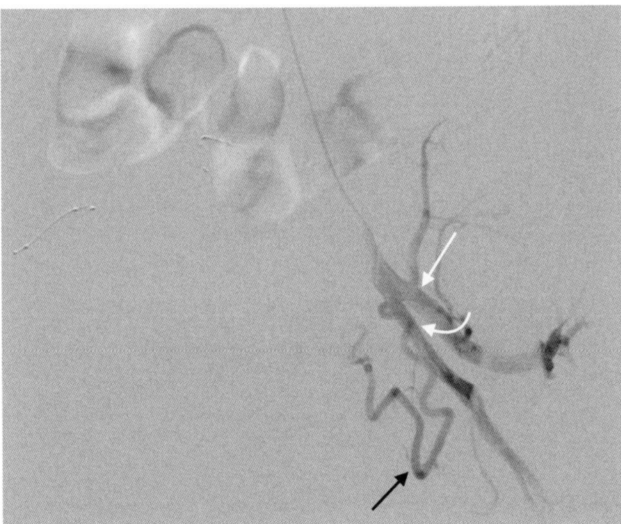

FIGURE 36B.1. Digital subtraction angiogram (DSA) of the left internal iliac artery in a left anterior oblique projection demonstrating bifurcation into the posterior division (*white arrow*) and anterior division (*curved white arrow*). The uterine artery (*black arrow*) arises as the first branch of the anterior division and demonstrates its characteristic U-shaped course and tortuous appearance.

TABLE 36B.1

FIBROID CLASSIFICATION

Submucosal	Located in the muscle beneath the endometrium and may distort the uterine cavity
Intramural	Located within the myometrium
Subserosal	Located on the surface of the uterus; may be pedunculated
Cervical	Located within the wall of the cervix

desiring future pregnancy therefore should be made on an individual basis based on the collaboration between the interventional radiologist, the gynecologist, and the patient, with UAE remaining a suitable choice for patients that are poor surgical candidates and those that refuse surgical management.

Preprocedural workup should include a consultation with the patient where a complete medical and gynecologic history can be obtained. At this time, the interventionalist can explain the procedure in greater detail, and decide whether additional testing or imaging needs to be obtained. If the patient is self-referred, it is recommended that she also be evaluated by a gynecologist to allow for a more complete discussion of treatment options other than UAE. During the consultation, it is important to review the patient's symptoms, pregnancy history, prior surgeries, history of pelvic infections, and her preferences regarding future pregnancy.

At most institutions, it has become routine to obtain a pelvic MRI prior to UAE. This allows identification of the location and extent of fibroid burden, while excluding other etiologies of abnormal uterine bleeding and/or pelvic pain, including adenomyosis. It also aids in the assessment of vascular supply and collateral vasculature, which may be beneficial in pretreatment planning. Preprocedural MRI should include contrast-enhanced imaging, which is essential in determining the vascularity and viability of the uterine fibroids (Fig. 36B.2). A lack of fibroid enhancement on pretreatment MRI may suggest poor response to UAE due to fibroid degeneration and lack of blood supply.

The UAE procedure can be performed in a standard IR fluoroscopy suite. An awareness of radiation exposure is crucial during this procedure, as most patients are young and otherwise healthy and would benefit from conscientious fluoroscopy. Techniques that can aid in reducing radiation dose can include using a low fluoroscopy pulse rate, utilization of collimation, and minimizing the use of magnification and digital subtraction angiography. The fluoroscopy time and dose should be recorded in the procedural report.

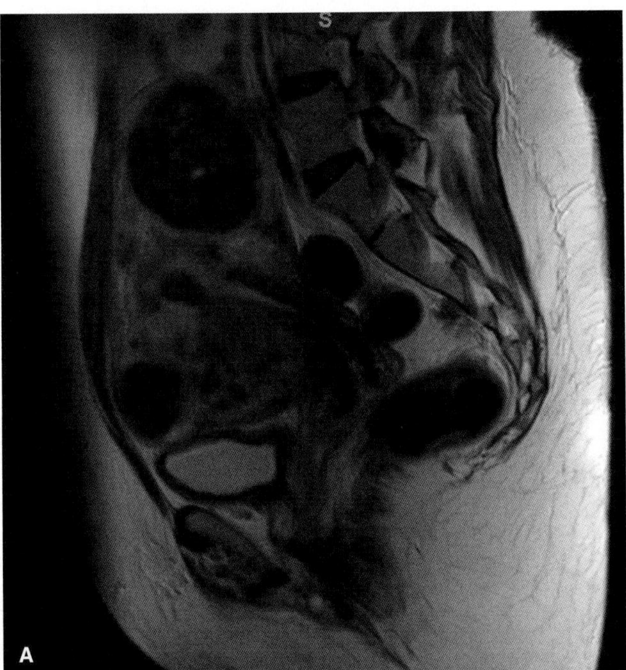

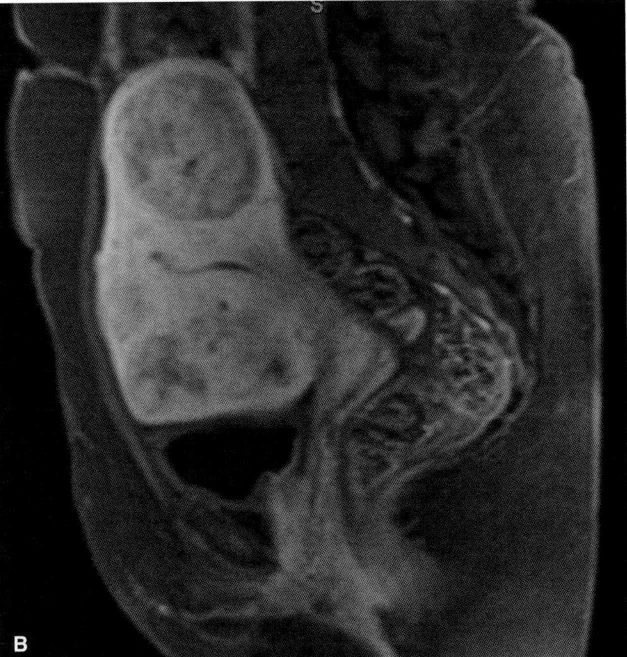

FIGURE 36B.2. A sagittal T2-weighted MRI (**A**) demonstrating multiple large uterine fibroids, resulting in a massively enlarged uterus. A sagittal T1-weighted postcontrast image (**B**) demonstrates heterogeneous enhancement of the fibroids.

UAE can be performed using conscious sedation, usually with a combination of midazolam and fentanyl. Prior to the embolization, it is recommended that the patient receives a single dose of prophylactic antibiotic, most frequently a broad-spectrum cephalosporin. Intravenous analgesics and nonsteroidal anti-inflammatory drugs (NSAIDs) should also be administered prior to or during the embolization.

Although there are variations in technique, the end goal never varies: a catheter is advanced into the bilateral uterine arteries, and embolic material is injected through the catheter until the desired endpoint of embolization is met. Arterial access can be obtained via the common femoral artery or the radial artery, depending on the operator's preference. Initial literature recommended flush abdominal aortography with the catheter positioned at the level of the renal arteries to identify collateral ovarian artery supply to the fibroid uterus. However, this is no longer routinely performed at our institution unless there is evidence of hypertrophic ovarian arteries on preprocedural imaging, or if the uterine arteries do not appear to be hypertrophied relative to the extent of fibroid burden (Fig. 36B.3).

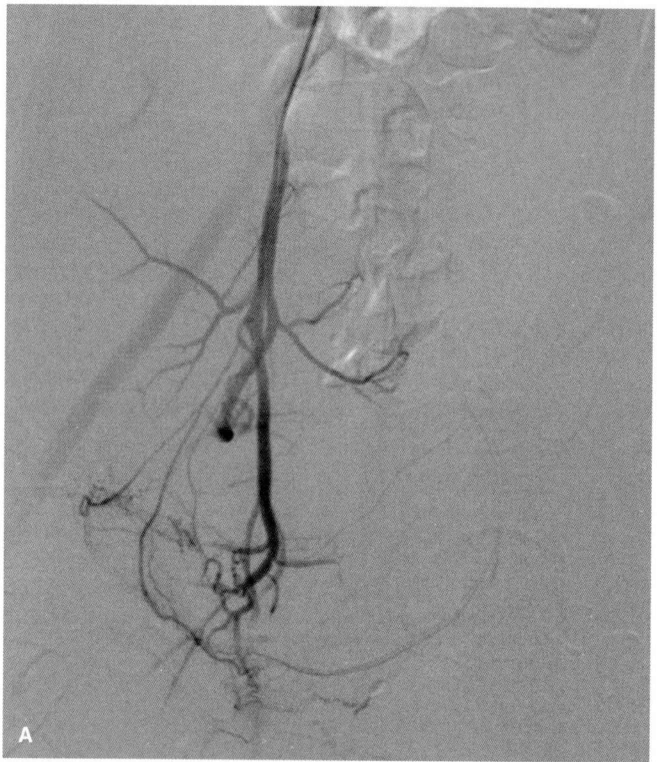

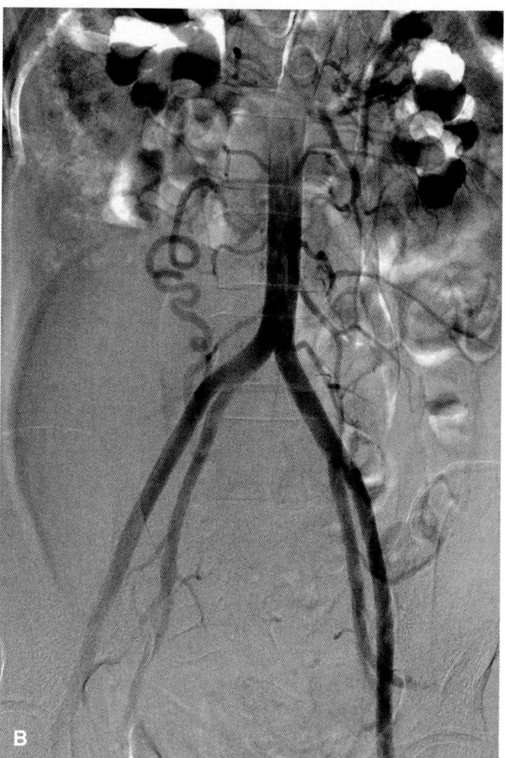

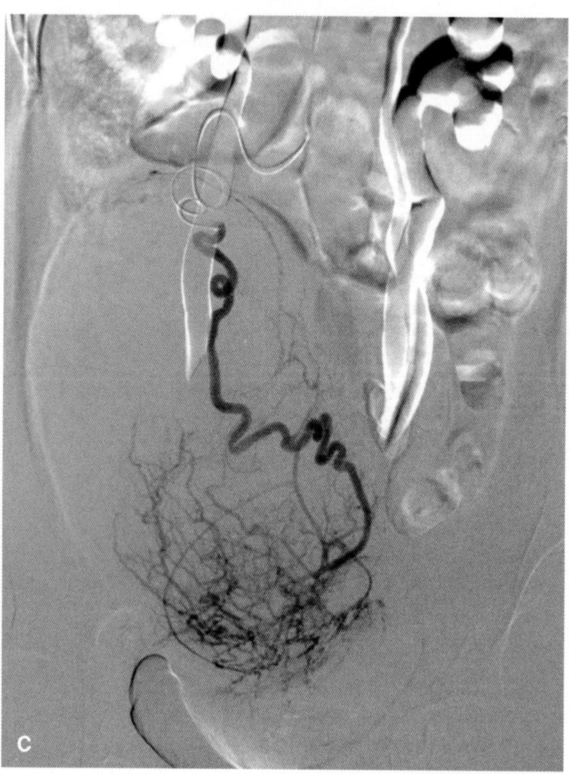

FIGURE 36B.3. **Ovarian Artery Fibroid Supply.** Right internal iliac angiogram (**A**) without evidence of right uterine artery hypertrophy. Subsequent flush aortogram (**B**) demonstrates a hypertrophic right ovarian artery arising directly from the aorta. Selective angiogram after catheterization with a microcatheter demonstrating fibroid supply arising from the hypertrophic right ovarian artery (**C**).

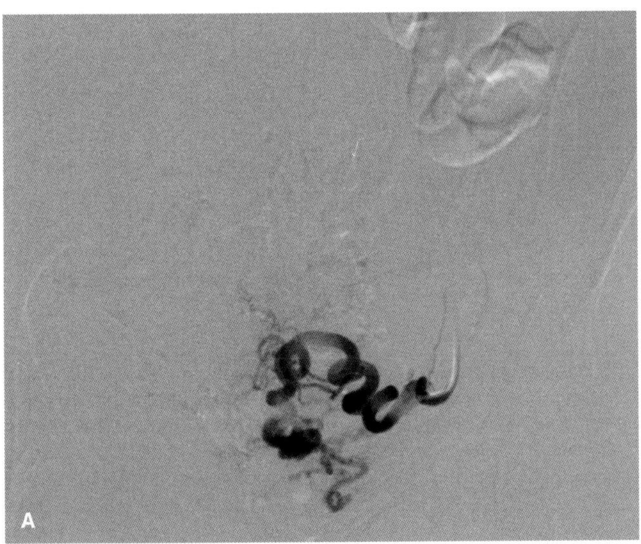

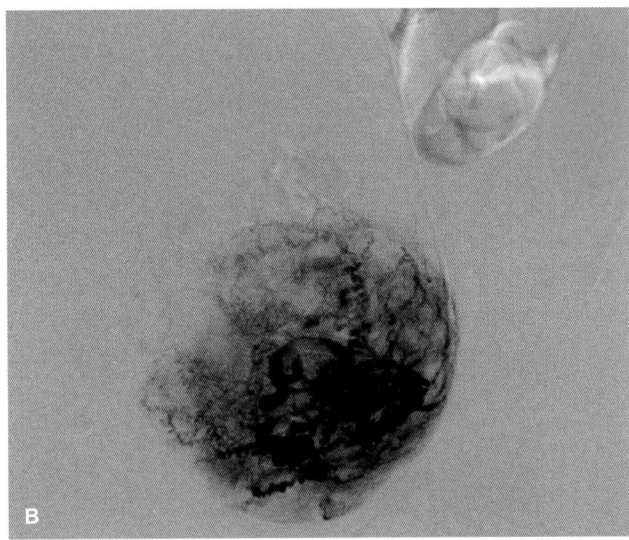

FIGURE 36B.4. Early image (**A**) from a left uterine artery angiogram showing the tip of the catheter in the transverse segment of the uterine artery. Late-phase image (**B**) from the same run showing filling of a large fibroid.

A diagnostic catheter is first advanced into the right or left internal iliac artery. Digital subtraction angiography or a roadmap image is performed in the 30-degree contralateral oblique position to identify the origin of the uterine artery. In cases where the uterine artery arises from a trifurcation of the internal iliac artery, the origin is best imaged by the ipsilateral anterior oblique projection. Once an adequate view of the origin of the uterine artery has been obtained, a wire is used to aid in advancing the diagnostic catheter into the artery. It is ideal to advance the catheter to the transverse segment of the uterine artery distal to the origin of any visible side branches. If the diagnostic catheter cannot be advanced due to arterial spasm or vessel tortuosity, a microcatheter can be used coaxially. Once the catheter tip is seated in the appropriate position, repeat contrast injection is performed to confirm catheter position and demonstrate fibroid blood supply. At this point, embolization may begin (Fig. 36B.4). In the past, the endpoint of embolization was stasis or near-stasis; however, newer research suggests that devascularization of the fibroid branch arteries with maintenance of slow antegrade flow in the main uterine artery is equally effective. This technique is then repeated on the contralateral side.

The choice of embolic agent is a matter of operator preference and training. Proximal occlusion of larger arteries with coils would allow distal filling via collaterals and would result in clinical failure, and is therefore not recommended. Nonspherical polyvinyl alcohol (PVA) was the first embolic agent used for UAE with good clinical success. A number of newer embolic agents have been described, including gelatin microspheres and spherical PVA, all with good clinical results. When using gelatin microspheres, the typical recommendation is to start with 500- to 700-μ–sized particles. The size of particles can be increased to 700 to 900 μ if there is still flow in the same uterine artery after two vials.

Following the procedure, the patient is monitored for several hours in the IR recovery suite. Pelvic pain and cramping is expected following UAE, and the symptoms can be severe. Appropriate management of patient expectations and adequate pain control are essential components of the UAE procedure. Every patient should be counseled beforehand on the symptoms to be expected following the procedure. The pelvic pain and cramping often starts intraprocedurally, and worsens during the first couple hours following the procedure. Depending on the institution, the patient may be given a PCA pump for pain management. Alternatively, the pain regimen may involve scheduled anti-inflammatory and opioid analgesics, with PRN narcotics available for breakthrough pain. Regardless of the medication regimen chosen, close patient observation is crucial. The majority of patients are discharged the same day as the procedure; if necessary, patients can be admitted overnight for pain management. The pain is most severe in the first 12 to 24 hours following the procedure, with the severity decreasing over the next 7 days. Patients are sent home with NSAIDs and oral narcotics on a PRN basis.

Postembolization syndrome is common following UAE, manifest by mild flu-like symptoms in the first few days following embolization. The overall complication rate following UAE is low, with serious adverse event rates of 0.66% in the initial hospital visit and 4.8% within 30 days in the largest registry assessing UAE complications and outcomes. The most commonly reported complications of UAE other than pain and postembolic syndrome are permanent amenorrhea and prolonged vaginal discharge. The reported rate of complications and suggested thresholds as described by the Society of Interventional Radiology (SIR) Quality Improvement Guidelines for Uterine Artery Embolization are shown in Table 36B.2.

TABLE 36B.2

COMPLICATIONS FOLLOWING UAE

■ COMPLICATIONS	■ REPORTED RATE (%)	■ SUGGESTED THRESHOLD (%)
Permanent amenorrhea		
Age <45 years	0–3	3
Age >45 years	20–40	45
Prolonged vaginal discharge	2–17	20
Fibroid expulsion	3–15	15
Septicemia	1–3	3
DVT/PE	<1	2
Nontarget embolization	<1	<1

Following the procedure, embolized fibroids decrease approximately 50% in size over the following 6 months. Patients begin to notice symptomatic improvement within one to two menstrual cycles, with the maximum benefit noted by the first 6 months to 1 year. Symptomatic improvement is slightly better with bleeding symptoms than with bulk symptoms, although both are successfully treated by UAE.

The largest current registry assessing the outcomes following UAE is the FIBROID registry sponsored by the SIR foundation, which enrolled a total of 72 practices performing UAE. Outcomes were assessed utilizing the Uterine Fibroid Symptom and Quality of Life (UFS-QOL) questionnaire, a uterine-specific survey developed to evaluate the symptoms of uterine fibroids and their impact on the quality of life (QOL). A higher score indicates more severe symptoms. At 1 year of follow-up, the UFS-QOL score had decreased from a baseline mean of 59.83 to a mean of 19.87 in 2,666 fibroid patients. This further decreased to 16.5 at 3 years. This is the largest of many studies that confirms high rates of symptomatic improvement following UAE.

Adenomyosis

Adenomyosis is a benign uterine disorder where endometrial tissue is found within the myometrium; it can present with menorrhagia and dysmenorrhea. On imaging, adenomyosis can be diffuse—affecting most of the uterus—or focal. It is best diagnosed on MRI, which demonstrates thickening of the junctional zone greater than 12 mm, either diffusely or focally (Fig. 36B.5). Hysterectomy is considered the definitive therapy for adenomyosis; medical management with hormonal manipulation has demonstrated poor and inconsistent efficacy. Although adenomyosis was once considered a contraindication to UAE, studies have recognized improvement in symptoms following the procedure. However, the clinical success for treating adenomyosis with UAE remains much lower than the success for treatment of fibroids, with approximately 50% of patients demonstrating either partial or complete resolution of their symptoms following UAE. The rate of recurrence is also higher, particularly with long-term follow-up. However, given the lack of good treatment options for adenomyosis other than hysterectomy, UAE is considered a reasonable technique in the management of adenomyosis.

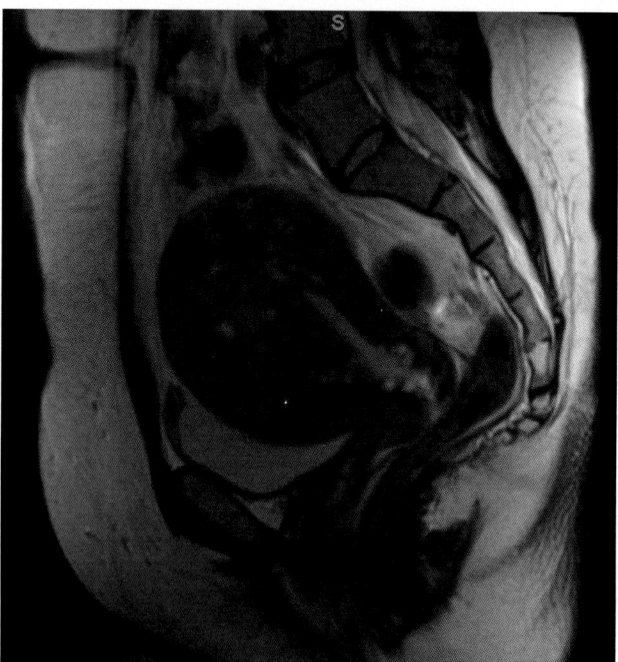

FIGURE 36B.5. Sagittal T2-Weighted MRI Demonstrating Diffuse Thickening of the Ill-Defined Junctional Zone, Particularly Within the Anterior Body, Compatible With Adenomyosis. Focal high-signal T2 regions within the junctional zone represent small foci of cystic change.

RENAL INTERVENTIONS—PERCUTANEOUS

Percutaneous nephrostomy (PCN) is one of the most common procedures performed by an interventional radiologist. It was originally described in 1955 as a means to decompress an obstructed kidney, and since that time it has been described in the management of various genitourinary pathologies. Hydronephrosis in the setting of urinary obstruction remains a common indication for PCN placement; however, access to the renal collecting system also plays a role in the management of renal stones and urinary leaks (Table 36B.3). While the reason for placement may vary, the basic technique for PCN placement remains the same regardless of the indication.

As with all interventional procedures, a fundamental knowledge of the genitourinary anatomy is essential when performing percutaneous renal interventions. This knowledge will contribute to the technical success of the procedure as well as minimize bleeding-related complications during access.

The kidneys are located in the retroperitoneum, usually between the lower thoracic and upper lumbar vertebral bodies. The right kidney usually is slightly lower than the left kidney, displaced inferiorly by the liver. The renal artery and vein enter each kidney at the renal hilum, where the renal vein is situated anteriorly. The renal pelvis is situated posterior to both the renal artery and vein at the renal hilum. At the level of the hilum, the renal artery divides into a larger anterior and smaller posterior division, which distribute throughout the collecting system. Because of this division, an avascular zone is created in the posterolateral region of each kidney (Fig. 36B.6), which in theory allows for an ideal entry point for access into the collecting system. In practice, however, this line is not able to be routinely identified and placement into any posterior calyx is usually adequate. Generally, posterior calyces in the mid to lower pole of the kidney are targeted for PCN access. Upper pole calyceal access caries an associated risk of pneumothorax, as the parietal pleural can come as low as the 12th rib posteriorly. Access directly into the renal pelvis is not recommended as there is increased risk of main renal artery injury.

The most common indications for PCN placement are described in Table 36B.3. Symptoms of urinary tract obstruction can include flank pain, nausea, and vomiting. If there is superimposed urinary tract infection, fever will also be present. When both kidneys are involved—or if there is a single functioning kidney—symptoms of acute renal failure may be present with laboratory values reflecting this. Imaging with ultrasound (US) or CT is nearly always performed prior to intervention to assess for the degree of dilatation of the collection system, to assess the anatomy of the target kidney, and to confirm the indication for placement.

The only true contraindication to PCN placement is an uncorrectable coagulopathy. According to the SIR consensus guidelines, the international normalized ratio (INR) should be less than 1.5 and platelet count >50,000 prior to PCN placement. PCN should also not be attempted if there is no safe percutaneous approach to the kidney due to interposed colon, spleen, or organ; however, this is rarely encountered in practice.

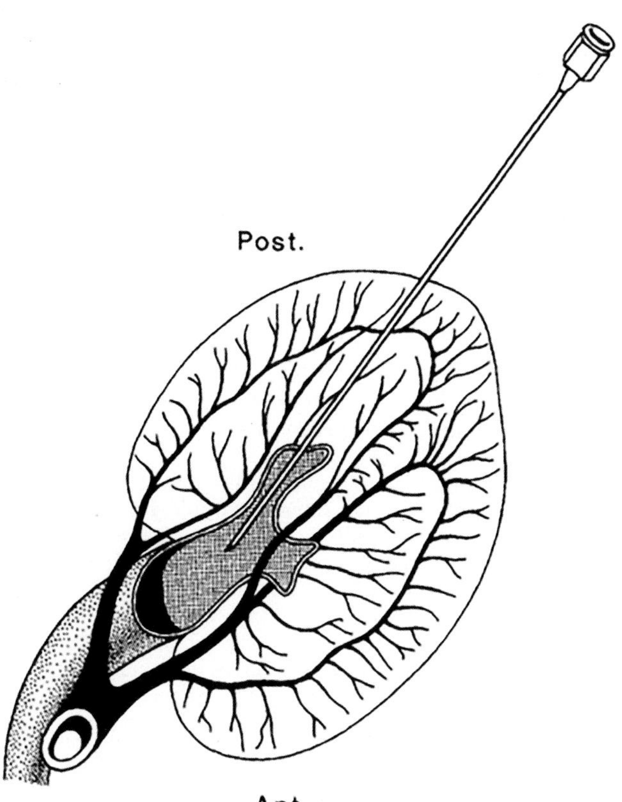

FIGURE 36B.6. **Cross-Section Diagram of a Kidney Showing the Needle Path for Percutaneous Nephrostomy Placement Through Brodel's Avascular Line.** (Redrawn from Castaneda-Zuniga WR, Tadavarthy SM, eds. *Interventional Radiology*. 2nd ed. Baltimore, MD: Williams & Wilkins; 1992:787, with permission.)

PCN placement can be performed in a standard interventional suite with conscious sedation. If there is a risk of patient instability, particularly in the setting of an infection, it is recommended that the procedure be performed in the presence of anesthesia. Broad-spectrum periprocedural antibiotics are administered with coverage for gram-negative organisms. The patient is most frequently placed prone on the angiographic table. If the patient is unable to lay prone due to abdominal surgery or discomfort, an oblique position may be necessary.

TABLE 36B.3

INDICATIONS FOR PERCUTANEOUS NEPHROSTOMY PLACEMENT

Renal obstruction (stones, malignant obstruction, extrinsic ureteral compression) Urosepsis or suspected infection Acute renal failure Pain
Urinary diversion Ureteral injury or leak Vesicular fistula Hemorrhagic cystitis
Access for urologic procedure Lithotripsy Antegrade ureteral stenting Urothelial biopsy Stone or foreign body retrieval

Access into the renal collecting system can be performed with US, fluoroscopy, or CT imaging. CT is rarely used but can be helpful in complex cases or in patients with anatomic anomalies that need to be taken into consideration. US guidance is the most commonly used technique to obtain access, allowing for real-time visualization of needle entry into the collecting system (Fig. 36B.7). Fluoroscopic access can be used to puncture directly into a radiopaque calyceal calculus, or if the collecting system is opacified by the intravenous administration of contrast material (intravenous pyelogram). This technique is particularly useful when attempting access into a nondilated system.

Several different access sets are available for access into the kidney, all of which include a 20- to 22-gauge needle with an inner stylet. Ideal skin entry site when targeting a posterior lower pole calyx is approximately 10 to 12 cm lateral to midline but medial to the posterior midaxillary line; further lateral than this increases the risk of colonic perforation. Once access into the collecting system is achieved, the inner stylet of the needle is removed and urine is aspirated to confirm location within the system and to send for culture. Contrast can then be injected through the needle to confirm the access site within a posterior calyx (Fig. 36B.7B). Care should be taken when injecting contrast to avoid overdistention, particularly in cases of infection, due to increased risk of sepsis. If the initial access site is deemed unfavorable, the first needle can be used to opacify the collecting system so that a second needle can be used to obtain more suitable access under fluoroscopic guidance.

Once appropriate needle access is obtained, a series of exchanges is performed until a drainage catheter is ultimately

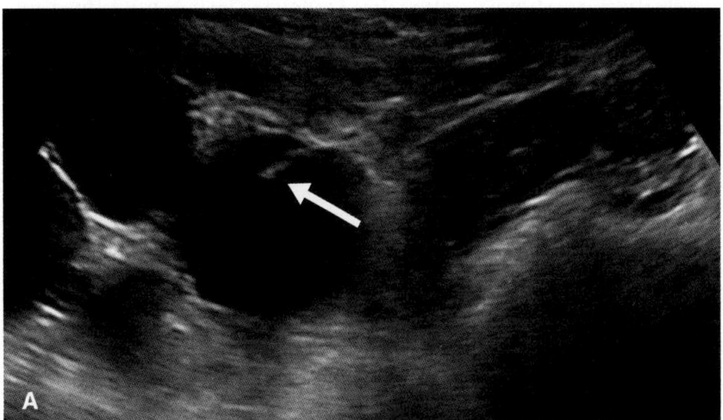

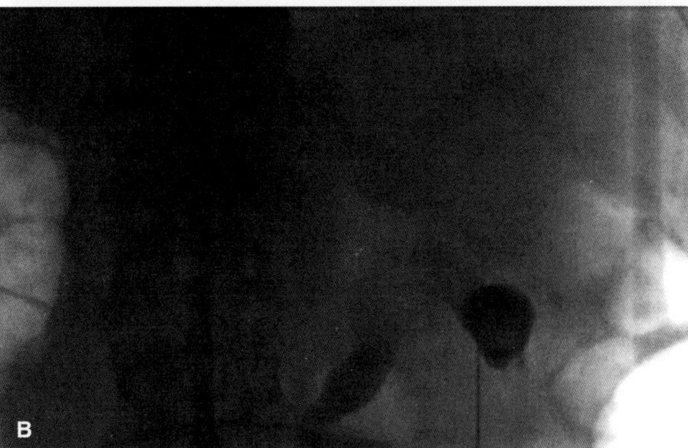

FIGURE 36B.7. **A:** Real-time grayscale ultrasound during percutaneous needle access into the lower pole calyx of a severely dilated right kidney. The echogenic tip of the needle can be visualized (*white arrow*). **B:** Injection of contrast through the needle under fluoroscopy demonstrates contrast filling of the lower pole calyx and proximal markedly dilated right ureter.

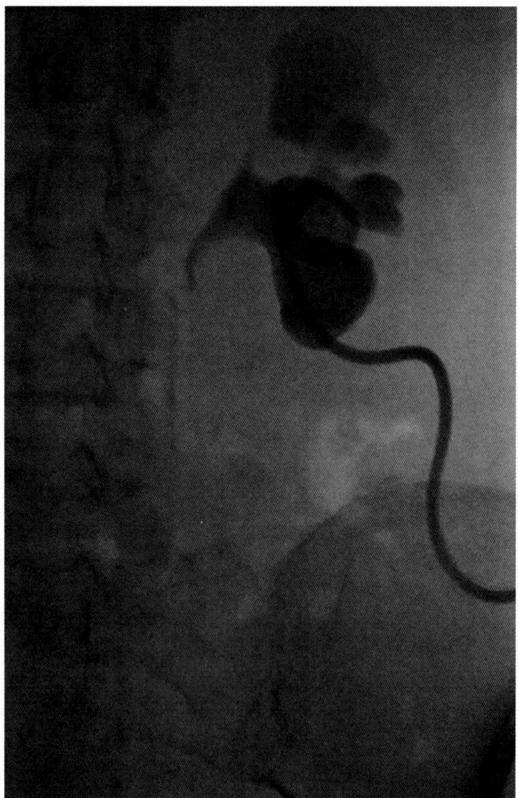

FIGURE 36B.8. Contrast Injection Through a Newly Placed Nephrostomy Catheter Shows the Pigtail Formed Within the Right Renal Pelvis (Patient Is Prone). There is moderate hydronephrosis with no contrast passing beyond the proximal right ureter.

placed through the calyx with the pigtail formed in the renal pelvis. Most commonly, an 8- to 12-Fr multipurpose pigtail catheter is placed; larger tubes can be useful in patients with pyonephrosis. Contrast can then be injected through the drain to confirm appropriate positioning (Fig. 36B.8). The catheter can then be attached to a gravity drainage bag, allowing decompression of the renal collecting system.

Major complications are rare following PCN placement. According to the SIR Standards of Practice Committee, minor and major complications occur in approximately 10% of patients (Table 36B.4). The most commonly reported complications are bleeding and sepsis. A small amount of hematuria can be normal in the first 48 hours after placement, with slow clearing of blood over this period. If the level of hematuria worsens or causes hemodynamic instability, imaging should be obtained to assess for arterial injury, including renal artery pseudoaneurysm or AV fistula.

Following placement, PCN catheters should be connected to a drainage bag. Routine flushing of the catheter is only necessary if output decreases or if output is purulent. Patients who require long-term external drainage should undergo routine scheduled catheter exchanges every 6 to 12 weeks.

TABLE 36B.4

COMPLICATIONS FOLLOWING PCN PLACEMENT

■ COMPLICATION	■ REPORTED RATE (%)
Septic shock requiring major increase in care	1–10
Septic shock in the setting of pyonephrosis	7–9
Hemorrhage requiring transfusion	1–4
Vascular injury requiring embolization or nephrectomy	0.1–1
Bowel transgression	0.2–0.5
Pleural complications	0.1–0.6

Nephroureterostomy and Ureteral Stent

If there is any concern for infection when placing a PCN, no further manipulation should be performed and the system should be allowed to decompress for several days until the patient is stabilized. If there is no sign of infection, an attempt can be made at time of PCN placement to access distal to the level of obstruction and place either an internal–external nephroureteral stent or an internal double-J ureteral stent. Both of these catheters allow drainage to the urinary bladder rather than to an external bag and are suitable options for patients that require long-term drainage, often allowing greater comfort for the patient.

A nephroureteral stent extends from the percutaneous access site in the skin similar to a PCN but extends through the renal pelvis and terminates in the urinary bladder. It has sideholes both in the urinary bladder and in the renal pelvis, and urine can drain externally to a bag or internally to the bladder (Fig. 36B.9A). Similarly, a primary double-J stent can be placed in the ureter at the time of access. Double-J stents can be placed retrograde (via cystoscopy) or antegrade (via existing PCN access). If placing a double-J stent during initial access, it is recommended to leave a PCN in place for 24 to 48 hours after placement of the stent to confirm that the patient tolerates internal drainage (Fig. 36B.9B).

RENAL INTERVENTIONS—VASCULAR

Renal Artery Stenosis

Renal artery stenosis (RAS) involves narrowing of one or both renal arteries. RAS can be asymptomatic but may also lead to impaired renal function due to ischemic nephropathy, cardiac decompensation, and renovascular hypertension (RVH). Although the majority of patients with hypertension (HTN) have primary (or essential) HTN, RVH is thought to be responsible for approximately 3% to 5% of cases of elevated blood pressure in the United States.

The pathophysiology for RVH involves decreased intrarenal arterial pressure due to the stenosis, which causes activation of the juxtaglomerular apparatus of the afferent arterioles, triggering the renin–angiotensin–aldosterone system (Fig. 36B.10). Increased renin production then leads to vasoconstriction of systemic arteries as well as sodium and water retention, both of which cause systemic HTN.

Although there can be a number of etiologies for RAS, the two most common causes are atherosclerosis and fibromuscular dysplasia (FMD):

- **Atherosclerosis:** Accounts for approximately 70% to 90% of the cases of RAS, most frequently seen in men over the age of 65. Obstruction or stenosis usually results from plaque within the aorta encroaching on the renal artery ostium, within 1 cm from the origin of the artery, leading to "ostial stenosis" (Fig. 36B.11). Less frequently, atherosclerotic stenoses can be seen more distally (>1 cm from the ostium) in the renal artery; these are described as "truncal"

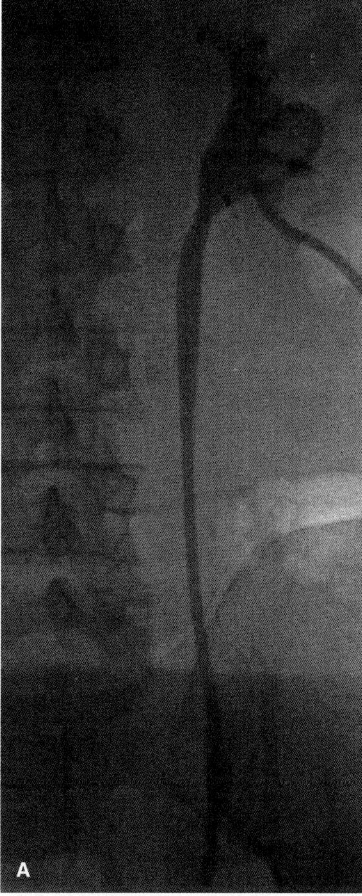

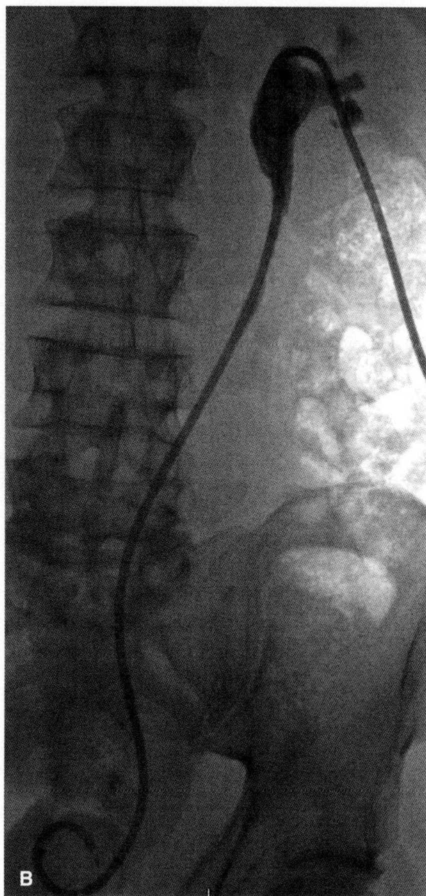

FIGURE 36B.9. **A:** Contrast injection through a right-sided percutaneous nephroureterostomy catheter. The proximal pigtail is formed within the right renal pelvis; the catheter then continues through the right ureter and terminates in the urinary bladder (not pictured). **B:** Simultaneous placement of a right percutaneous nephrostomy and internal double-J stent. The percutaneous nephrostomy was left in place for 24 hours prior to removal.

stenoses. Bilateral disease is common in atherosclerotic RAS. Risk factors for atherosclerosis include dyslipidemia, cigarette smoking, and age.

- **Fibromuscular Dysplasia:** As opposed to atherosclerotic RAS, FMD most frequently affects a younger population and is more common in females. It should be suspected in patients with difficult-to-control HTN at a young age; it rarely causes ischemic nephropathy. FMD is subdivided into an assortment of histologic patterns depending on the morphologic appearance of the layers of the arterial wall involved. Medial fibroplasia accounts for the majority of cases and causes web-like stenoses and aneurysms. The middle and distal main renal artery is most frequently involved, and often demonstrates a classic "string of beads" appearance on angiography (Fig. 36B.12). FMD affects both renal arteries about two-thirds of the time.
- **Other Causes:** RAS can also be seen in multiple vasculitides (Takayasu, Buerger, polyarteritis nodosa), thromboembolic disease, neurofibromatosis type 1, retroperitoneal fibrosis, and arterial dissection.

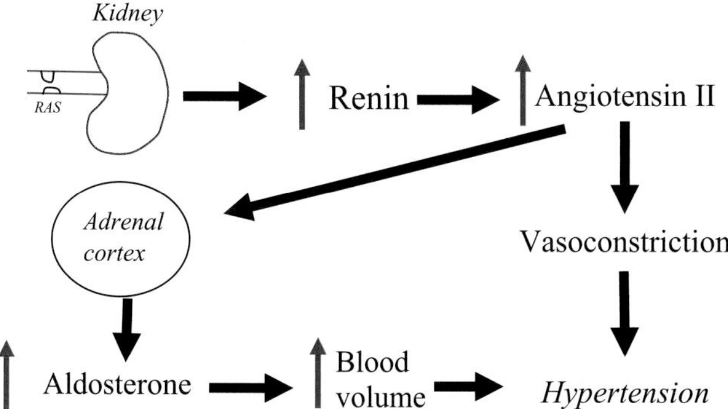

FIGURE 36B.10. **Renin–Angiotensin System Activation During Renal Artery Stenosis.** The juxtaglomerular apparatus in the kidney releases renin into the bloodstream in response to decreased renal perfusion in the setting of renal artery stenosis (RAS). Renin subsequently converts angiotensinogen (produced in the liver) into angiotensin I, which is further metabolized in the lungs to angiotensin II. Angiotensin II has a number of effects on the body, including increasing sympathetic activity, directly causing vasoconstriction, and causing the release of aldosterone by the adrenal gland. Aldosterone further causes hypertension by increasing the resorption of water in the renal tubules.

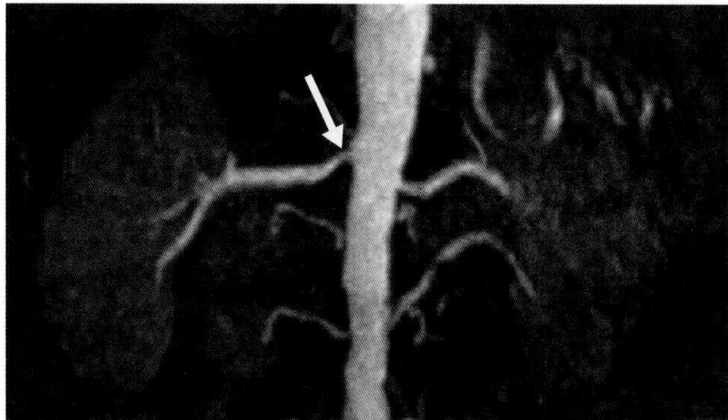

FIGURE 36B.11. Reconstructed images from an MRA of the abdomen demonstrating ostial stenosis of the right renal artery (*white arrow*), classic for atherosclerotic renal artery stenosis.

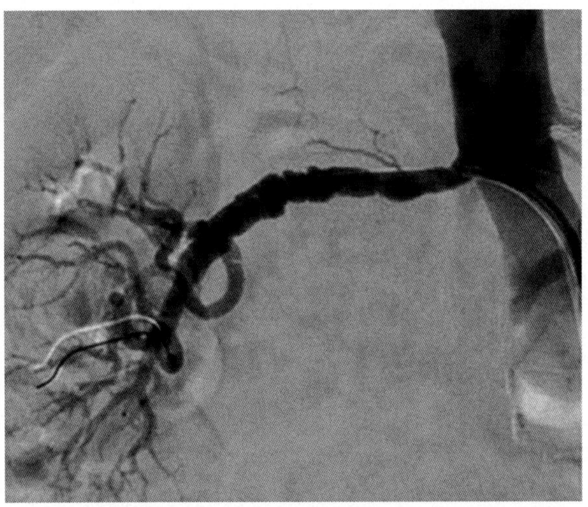

FIGURE 36B.12. Classic "string of beads" appearance of FMD on renal angiography. Postangioplasty angiogram (not pictured) demonstrated marked improvement of the irregularity and luminal narrowing. Translesional pressure gradient decreased to 6 mm Hg and hypertension improved following treatment, with patient able to discontinue antihypertensive medications.

Clinical signs that suggest the likelihood of renovascular disease as a cause of HTN are described in Table 36B.5, which are reflective of screening guidelines created by both SIR and the American Heart Association (Table 36B.5). Once clinical findings suggest RAS as a potential cause of HTN rather than primary HTN, a variety of tests can be employed for further evaluation. US, computed tomographic angiography (CTA), magnetic resonance angiography (MRA), and nuclear scintigraphy can all play a role in the screening assessment for RAS; however, angiography remains the gold standard once screening suggests an abnormality.

Color Doppler US is one of the most commonly used tools for screening for RAS. If the main renal artery is able to be visualized, signs of RAS include peak systolic velocity (PSV) greater than 180 cm/s and PSV renal/aortic ratio greater than 3.5. Turbulent flow in the poststenotic site may also be indicative of significant stenosis. A lack of detectable Doppler signal in the visualized renal artery is suggestive of complete renal artery occlusion. In addition, a "parvus et tardus" waveform (slowing of the time to peak systole) within the parenchymal arteries is suggestive of a more proximal stenosis.

TABLE 36B.5

INDICATIONS FOR SCREENING FOR RENAL ARTERY STENOSIS

Onset of HTN before the age of 30
Abdominal bruit
Resistant HTN
Recurrent pulmonary edema
Renal failure of unknown etiology
Coexisting diffuse atherosclerotic vascular disease
Acute renal failure precipitated by antihypertensive therapy
Malignant HTN causing end-organ damage
HTN with a unilateral small kidney
Unstable angina in the setting of suspected RAS

CTA and MRA can also detect RAS, both with high sensitivity and specificity. However, only angiography allows assessment of the hemodynamic significance of a stenosis by measuring the translesional pressure gradient. A pressure gradient of >20 mm Hg is considered hemodynamically significant and is correlated with significant renal hypoperfusion. In addition, angiography allows better assessment of accessory or branch renal arteries, which are not as well visualized on other diagnostic studies.

Again, knowledge of the vascular anatomy is essential prior to performing renal angiography. Each kidney is usually supplied by a single renal artery that arises from the aorta in the L1–L2 region. Frequently, there are either multiple renal arteries or early bifurcation of the renal artery. The right renal artery crosses posterior to the IVC and runs posterior to the right renal vein in the retroperitoneum. The left renal artery also courses posterior to the left renal vein. Both renal arteries give off a proximal branch that supplies the adrenal gland. After dividing into anterior and posterior divisions, the arteries further bifurcate into segmental, lobar, then interlobar arteries. The interlobar arteries divide into the arcuate arteries at the corticomedullary junction, which subsequently give off terminal interlobular arteries.

The management of patients with atherosclerotic RAS has been a topic of debate and research for many years. A number of trials have failed to consistently show improvement in blood pressure control, preservation of renal function, or decreased cardiovascular events following renal artery revascularization versus medical therapy alone. The presence of a significant atherosclerotic RAS does not on its own warrant treatment. However, there is still consensus that in the appropriately selected individuals, renal artery revascularization is the most appropriate strategy for management. In general, the patients most likely to benefit from renal artery intervention are those with uncontrolled RVH despite maximal medical therapy who have hemodynamically significant RAS as determined by translesional pressure gradient. A systolic translesional pressure gradient of greater than 20 mm Hg between the aorta and the renal artery distal to the lesion can be used to confirm severity of RAS.

Angioplasty and stent placement are the most common techniques employed to treat RAS. In the setting of atherosclerotic RAS requiring intervention, angioplasty alone is rarely employed due to clinical studies demonstrating markedly improved patency with renal artery stenting. Balloon-expandable stents are most frequently used, which allows for more precise deployment at the ostium of the artery.

As opposed to atherosclerotic RAS, FMD classically responds well to angioplasty alone (Fig. 36B.12); stenting is rarely required unless there is a dissection resulting from angioplasty. In either case, it is crucial to obtain pressure measurements in the aorta and across the lesion before and after treatment. The apparent luminal narrowing on angiography may over- or underestimate the actual resistance to flow. Angioplasty is considered successful when the systolic pressure gradient is less than 10 mm Hg. Technical success approaches 100% in the treatment of FMD-related RAS; high clinical success rates have also been reproduced in a number of studies.

Complications following angioplasty and stenting are usually minor, with overall reported complications rates of up to 35% (Table 36B.6). The most commonly reported complications include puncture-site–related complications and worsening renal function which is more likely in patients with already existing renal insufficiency. Renal artery rupture after angioplasty occurs in less than 1% of cases but can cause

TABLE 36B.6

COMPLICATIONS FOLLOWING RENAL ARTERY ANGIOPLASTY +/– STENTING

Access site complications (hematoma, pseudoaneurysm)	3–5%
Worsening renal insufficiency	5–10%
Renal artery dissection	5%
Cholesterol embolization (systemic)	1%
Renal artery rupture	<1%
Death	0–0.5%

complete renal infarction or death if not recognized immediately. This can be treated by temporary balloon occlusion across the site of rupture until more definitive therapy with a stent graft is performed.

Renal Angiomyolipoma

Angiomyolipoma (AML) is the most common benign tumor of the kidney. They are hypervascular tumors that can be solitary or multiple, and can be sporadic or associated with tuberous sclerosis complex. Most cases of AML are incidentally found on imaging; they are rarely symptomatic. When symptomatic, the AML can present as a palpable flank mass, hematuria, and flank pain. The vascular tissues within the tumor are prone to aneurysm formation and rupture. On imaging, there is characteristic macroscopic fat within the AML that can be detected on both CT and MRI. Angiography can demonstrate a hypervascular mass with tortuous vessels as well as intralesional aneurysms (Fig. 36B.13).

Renal AMLs greater than 4 cm in diameter have a significant risk of spontaneous hemorrhage. Therefore, the current guideline is to prophylactically embolize those AMLs that are greater than 4 cm to prevent the risk of bleeding. The goal of prophylactic renal AML embolization is selective devascularization of the AML to prevent growth of the mass or spontaneous aneurysmal rupture, while preserving normal renal parenchyma. Renal AML embolization is also performed in an emergent manner when spontaneous AML rupture has already occurred. Different embolic materials have been reported for AML embolization, most commonly either absolute ethanol or particles.

PROSTATE ARTERY EMBOLIZATION

Benign prostatic hyperplasia (BPH) is a common condition related to aging that can lead to a cluster of chronic symptoms collectively known as lower urinary tract symptoms (LUTS), including urinary frequency, urinary urgency, nocturia, hematuria, and decreased urinary stream. Treatment options for BPH traditionally include medical therapy, minimally invasive therapies (including transurethral ablations), or surgical therapies including open prostatectomy or transurethral resection of the prostate (TURP).

Medical therapy is often considered the first-line option for symptomatic patients; however, a large subset of patients does not respond to or cannot tolerate pharmacotherapy, in part owing to a number of side effects including sexual dysfunction. TURP has remained the "gold standard" surgical treatment for BPH for over half a century, owing to its high success rate in reducing LUTS. Over the past two decades, the TURP procedure has undergone significant technical improvements, with morbidity rates reported to be <1%. However, with a general shift toward minimally invasive treatment options, the number of TURPs performed has fallen in more recent years.

Embolization of the prostatic arteries was first described as a technique to control severe bladder and prostate hemorrhage as well as hematuria following TURP. In the early 2000s, a case report by DeMeritt et al. described a patient with BPH and refractory hematuria treated by prostatic artery embolization, who subsequently had alleviation in his LUTS and reduction in the volume of his prostate. This first introduced the idea that BPH could intentionally be treated by selective prostate artery embolization (PAE).

Over the past decade, a number of studies have demonstrated promising results in the treatment of BPH using PAE. A growing body of literature suggests that PAE enables reduction in prostate volume with improvements in urine flow parameters, QOL, and sexual function. With increasing experience by operators across the nation, technical success rates have been reported as high as

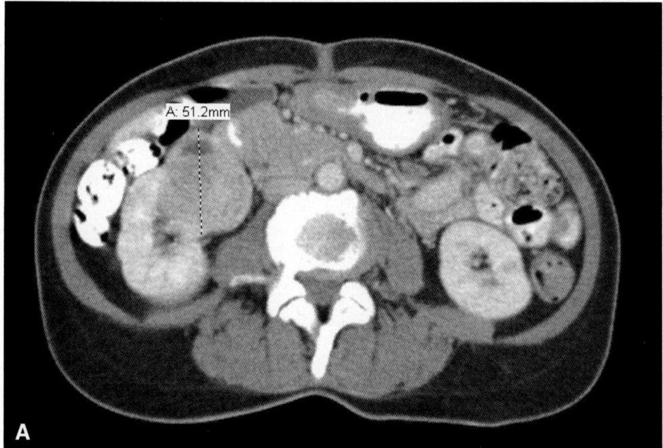

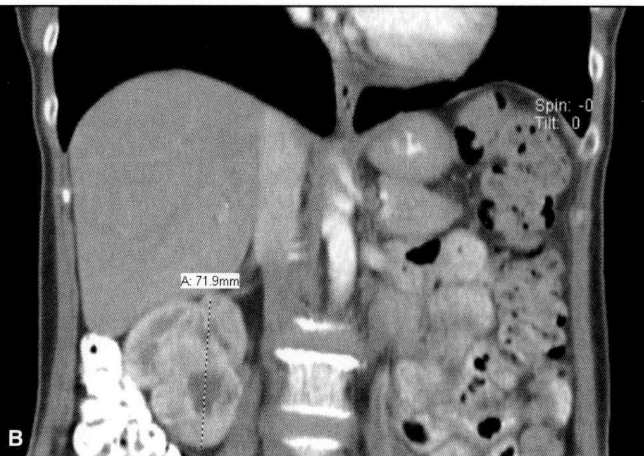

FIGURE 36B.13. Classic Appearance of Renal Angiomyolipoma. Axial (**A**) and coronal (**B**) contrast-enhanced CT images demonstrate a large hypervascular mass arising from lower pole of the right kidney. The mass contains large areas of macroscopic fat (demonstrated by areas measuring less than –20 HU), and measures up to 7.2 cm in craniocaudal dimension. (*continued*)

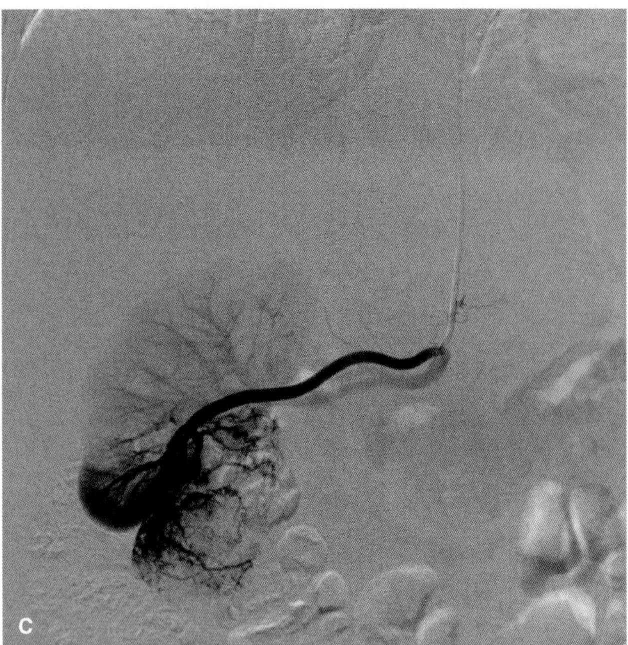

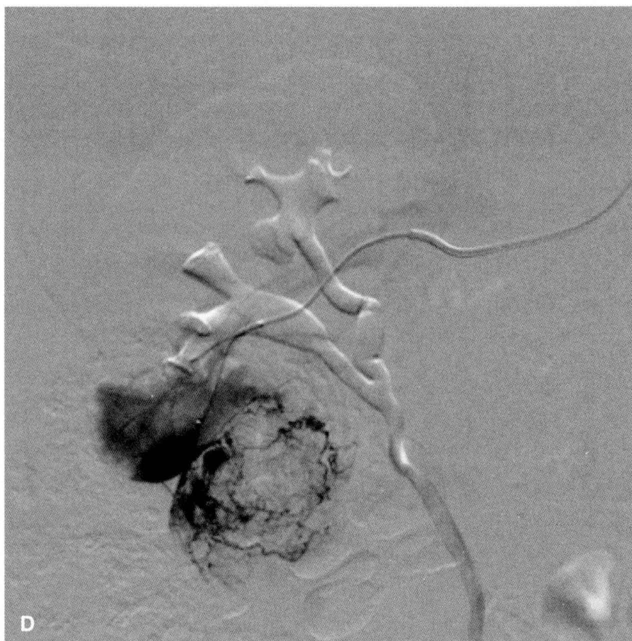

FIGURE 36B.13. (*Continued*) Angiography (**C, D**) demonstrates an accessory renal artery supplying the lower pole of the right kidney and the AML. Tortuous vessels are seen within the AML, with small aneurysmal components seen on more selective angiography (**D**). The mass was subsequently embolized with 500- to 700-μ gelatin particles.

98%, with clinical success rates reaching upward of 80% in the first month. In the only RCT to date comparing PAE to TURP, the authors found that all parameters—including improvement of the International Prostate Symptom Score (IPSS), QOL, peak urinary flow, and postvoid residual (PVR) urine volume—were improved by both treatment modalities.

The technique for PAE involves gaining arterial access with subsequent catheterization of the anterior division of the internal iliac artery. A thorough knowledge of the male pelvic arterial anatomy and its common variants is necessary in order to identify the prostatic artery (Fig. 36B.14). A Foley balloon catheter within the urinary bladder can help identify the region of the prostate during angiography. The prostate artery arises most commonly as a branch from the internal pudendal artery, superior vesical artery, obturator artery, or directly off the anterior division; however, a number of additional variants are possible. Digital subtraction angiography is used to confirm arterial anatomy and allow for superselective catheterization of the prostatic artery. Cone beam CT can be utilized to confirm targeting of the prostate gland. Most literature has described the use of various particles as the embolic material, with total stasis as the desired endpoint. Embolization is then performed on the contralateral side using the same technique.

Compared with traditional surgical therapies for BPH, PAE offers the advantage of being minimally invasive and does not result in the same incidence of erectile and/or ejaculatory dysfunction. It can be performed on an outpatient basis and requires only conscious sedation, and has a high success rate and a low rate of complications. The most common complications have included perineal pain, nausea, and vomiting. Hematuria, urinary tract infections, and hematospermia have been described as self-limiting adverse events within the first month after the procedure. Nontarget embolization is a more serious complication that could result in bladder ischemia and necrosis.

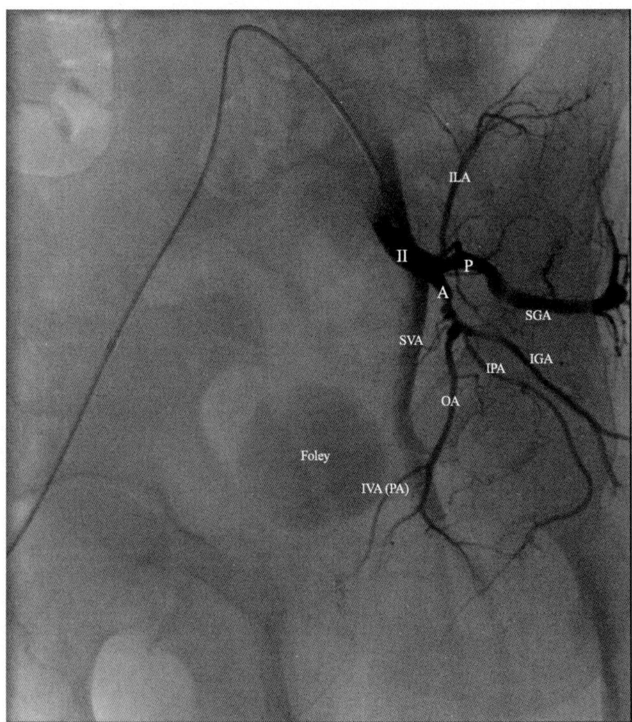

FIGURE 36B.14. **Left Internal Iliac Angiogram Performed During Prostate Artery Embolization (PAE) in the Left Anterior Oblique (LAO) Projection.** Labeled arteries are as follows: II, internal iliac; P, posterior division; A, anterior division; ILA, iliolumbar artery; SGA, superior gluteal artery; SVA, superior vesicular artery; IGA, inferior gluteal artery; IPA, internal pudendal artery; OA, obturator artery; IVA (PA), inferior vesicular artery (continuing as the prostatic artery distally).

Suggested Readings

Baird DD, Dunson DB, Hill MC, Cousins D, Schectman JM. High cumulative incidence of uterine leiomyoma in black and white women: ultrasound evidence. *Am J Obstet Gynecol* 2003;188(1):100–107.

Clarke-Pearson DL, Geller EJ. Complications of hysterectomy. *Obstet Gynecol* 2013;121(3):654–673.

Dariushnia SR, Nikolic B, Stokes LS, Spies JB; Society of Interventional Radiology Standards of Practice Committee. Quality improvement guidelines for uterine artery embolization for symptomatic leiomyomata. *J Vasc Interv Radiol* 2014;25(11):1737–1747.

DeMeritt JS, Elmasri FF, Esposito MP, Rosenberg GS. Relief of benign prostatic hyperplasia-related bladder outlet obstruction after transarterial polyvinyl alcohol prostate embolization. *J Vasc Interv Radiol* 2000;11(6):767–770.

Gao YA, Huang Y, Zhang R, et al. Benign prostatic hyperplasia: prostatic arterial embolization versus transurethral resection of the prostate—a prospective, randomized, and controlled clinical trial. *Radiology* 2014;270(3):920–928.

Goodwin SC, Spies JB, Worthington-Kirsch R, et al. Uterine artery embolization for treatment of leiomyomata: long-term outcomes from the FIBROID Registry. *Obstet Gynecol* 2008;111(1):22–33.

Gupta JK, Sinha A, Lumsden MA, Hickey M. Uterine artery embolization for symptomatic uterine fibroids. *Cochrane Database Syst Rev* 2012(5): CD005073.

Jones P, Rai BP, Nair R, Somani BK. Current status of prostate artery embolization for lower urinary tract symptoms: review of world literature. *Urology* 2015;86(4):676–681.

Mara M, Maskova J, Fucikova Z, Kuzel D, Belsan T, Sosna O. Midterm clinical and first reproductive results of a randomized controlled trial comparing uterine fibroid embolization and myomectomy. *Cardiovasc Intervent Radiol* 2008;31(1):73–85.

Martin LG, Rundback JH, Wallace MJ, et al. Quality improvement guidelines for angiography, angioplasty, and stent placement for the diagnosis and treatment of renal artery stenosis in adults. *J Vasc Interv Radiol* 2010; 21(4):421–430; quiz 230.

Pabon-Ramos WM, Dariushnia SR, Walker TG, et al. Quality improvement guidelines for percutaneous nephrostomy. *J Vasc Interv Radiol* 2016;27(3): 410–414.

Patel IJ, Davidson JC, Nikolic B, et al. Consensus guidelines for periprocedural management of coagulation status and hemostasis risk in percutaneous image-guided interventions. *J Vasc Interv Radiol* 2012;23(6):727–736.

Pelage JP, Cazejust J, Pluot E, et al. Uterine fibroid vascularization and clinical relevance to uterine fibroid embolization. *Radiographics* 2005;25(Suppl 1): S99–S117.

Spies JB, Myers ER, Worthington-Kirsch R, Mulgund J, Goodwin S, Mauro M; FIBROID Registry Investigators. The FIBROID Registry: symptom and quality-of-life status 1 year after therapy. *Obstet Gynecol* 2005;106(6): 1309–1318.

Tafur JD, White CJ. Renal artery stenosis: when to revascularize in 2017. *Curr Probl Cardiol* 2017;42(4):110–135.

Yu X, Elliott SP, Wilt TJ, McBean AM. Practice patterns in benign prostatic hyperplasia surgical therapy: the dramatic increase in minimally invasive technologies. *J Urol* 2008;180(1):241–245; discussion 245.

CHAPTER 37A ■ PORTAL HYPERTENSION

ERIC T. AALTONEN

PORTAL HYPERTENSION BACKGROUND

Definition of Portal Hypertension

Normal portal pressure is usually 5 to 10 mm Hg. Portal hypertension is defined as an absolute portal pressure greater than 11 mm Hg or more commonly a hepatic venous pressure gradient (HVPG) greater than or equal to 6 mm Hg. HVPG represents the difference in pressure between the portal veins and the systemic hepatic veins. Direct measurement of portal venous pressure is invasive and has been replaced with far less invasive indirect measurement using wedged hepatic venous pressure (WHVP). WHVP closely estimates portal venous pressures except in cases of prehepatic and presinusoidal causes of portal hypertension. WHVP is measured by placing a balloon occlusion catheter in a distal hepatic vein. When the balloon is inflated and fully occlusive, the WHVP is obtained; when the balloon is deflated, a free hepatic venous pressure (FHVP) is obtained. The difference between these two pressures is the HVPG. A normal HVPG is 1 to 5 mm Hg; however, portal hypertension is usually not clinically significant until HVPG is greater than 10 to 12 mm Hg.

Etiology of Portal Hypertension and Cirrhosis

There are several causes of portal hypertension and these can be categorized as prehepatic, hepatic, and posthepatic. Hepatic causes of portal hypertension can be further categorized as presinusoidal, sinusoidal, and postsinusoidal as shown in Table 37A.1. Cirrhosis accounts for 90% of portal hypertension in developed countries. Schistosomiasis is a leading cause of portal hypertension in the rest of the world. It is important to note that not all causes of portal hypertension are associated with increased HVPG. For example, pulmonary hypertension can result in elevated WHVP and FHVP which results in a normal HVPG. However, sinusoidal processes such as cirrhosis, by far the most common cause of portal hypertension in the United States, are associated with increased WHVP and normal FHVP with subsequent elevated HVPG. Cirrhosis is caused by chronic injury and is characterized by the development of intraparenchymal scar tissue. The liver responds to injury by creating regenerative nodules. The liver, therefore, can fully recover from an acute injury. However, if an insult is chronic, these nodules are eventually replaced over time with scar tissue leading to irreversible hepatic dysfunction. The most common causes of cirrhosis in the United States are hepatitis C, alcoholic liver disease, and nonalcoholic fatty liver disease (NAFLD). Worldwide, chronic hepatitis B infection is another significant cause of cirrhosis. With the advent of curative hepatitis C treatment, the incidence of cirrhosis secondary to hepatitis C is expected to decrease. However, there is a concurrent increase in the incidence of NAFLD and NAFLD cirrhosis due to rising obesity rates. The development of portal hypertension secondary to cirrhosis is multifactorial and caused by structural and dynamic changes which cause increased hepatic resistance.

Complications of Portal Hypertension

As stated previously, the complications of portal hypertension often do not manifest until the HVPG is greater than 10 mm Hg. These complications are listed in Table 37A.2 and all can result in significant patient morbidity and potential mortality as liver disease worsens. When the HVPG is greater than 10 mm Hg, this pressure recanalizes pre-existing vessels such as the umbilical vein and initiates angiogenesis to develop new venous varices. These varices are enlarged, tortuous vessels that bypass the diseased liver and drain blood from the portal circulation

TABLE 37A.1

CAUSES OF PORTAL HYPERTENSION

Prehepatic	Portal/splenic vein thrombosis Congenital portal vein stenosis Arteriovenous fistula
Hepatic	
Presinusoidal	Primary biliary cirrhosis Schistosomiasis
Sinusoidal	Cirrhosis Hepatic fibrosis Idiopathic (nodular regenerative hyperplasia) Polycystic liver disease
Postsinusoidal	Veno-occlusive disease
Posthepatic	Budd–Chiari syndrome Inferior vena cava web Hepatic vein thrombosis Heart failure Constrictive pericarditis Pulmonary hypertension

to the systemic circulation and the right side of the heart. Varices are extremely common in cirrhotic patients, as new esophageal varices develop and small varices become large at a rate of 8% annually. In advanced stages of portal hypertension, increased blood flow through these portosystemic collaterals leads to the release of vasodilators and systemic hypotension with consequent plasma volume expansion and increased cardiac output. This increased cardiac output then exacerbates portal hypertension in a cyclic fashion and can lead to the development of ascites and hepatorenal syndrome. Ascites, hepatorenal syndrome, and other sequelae of portal hypertension cause significant patient morbidity, but the highest mortality rates are associated with variceal bleeding. Varices are friable and at risk of hemorrhage when the HVPG is greater than 12 mm Hg. Risk of hemorrhage is further increased when varices are large, have thin overlying mucosa, and project into enteric lumen such as at the gastroesophageal junction. This hemorrhage is the most concerning complication of portal hypertension for an interventional radiologist as it can be acutely fatal if not properly treated. Proper treatment requires an understanding of portal venous and portosystemic collateral anatomy.

TABLE 37A.2

COMPLICATIONS OF PORTAL HYPERTENSION

Variceal hemorrhage
Ascites/hepatic hydrothorax
Spontaneous bacterial peritonitis
Splenomegaly
Thrombocytopenia
Hepatorenal syndrome
Hepatic encephalopathy
Portal hypertensive gastropathy
Cirrhotic cardiomyopathy

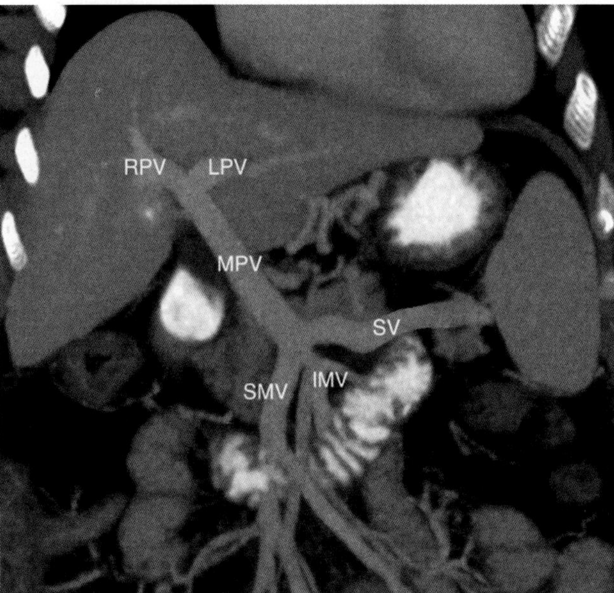

FIGURE 37A.1. **Portal Venous Anatomy.** Coronal maximum intensity projection (MIP) CT of the upper abdomen demonstrating the confluence of the splenic vein (SV), inferior mesenteric vein (IMV), and superior mesenteric vein (SMV) to form the main portal vein (MPV). The IMV typically flows into the splenic vein prior to confluence with the SMV but anatomy is variable. The main portal vein then branches into the right (RPV) and left (LPV) portal veins within the hepatic parenchyma.

PORTAL VENOUS AND PORTOSYSTEMIC COLLATERAL ANATOMY

Portal Venous Anatomy

The portal system drains the colon, small bowel, pancreas, stomach, and spleen. Branches from the right and transverse colon and small bowel converge to form the superior mesenteric vein (SMV). Branches from the sigmoid and left colon converge to form the inferior mesenteric vein (IMV). Typically, the IMV then drains into the splenic vein prior to its convergence with the SMV to form the main portal vein (Fig. 37A.1). The main portal vein then enters the liver and splits into left and right portal veins as it supplies approximately 70% of blood flow to the liver. In portal hypertension, collaterals to the systemic circulation reconstitute or form in several areas of the body (Fig. 37A.2) and blood flow reverses from hepatopetal to hepatofugal. The most common and clinically relevant varices are esophageal/gastroesophageal and gastric varices which occur at the distal esophagus/gastroesophageal junction and stomach, respectively.

Gastroesophageal Varices

Gastroesophageal varices form via hepatofugal blood flow, typically from the left gastric vein, toward the systemic azygos system. By definition, these varices cross the gastroesophageal junction (Fig. 37A.3). Gastroesophageal varices are common, occurring in approximately 50% of cirrhotic patients overall. The modified Child–Pugh score classifies liver disease and ranges from mild, class A, to severe, class C,

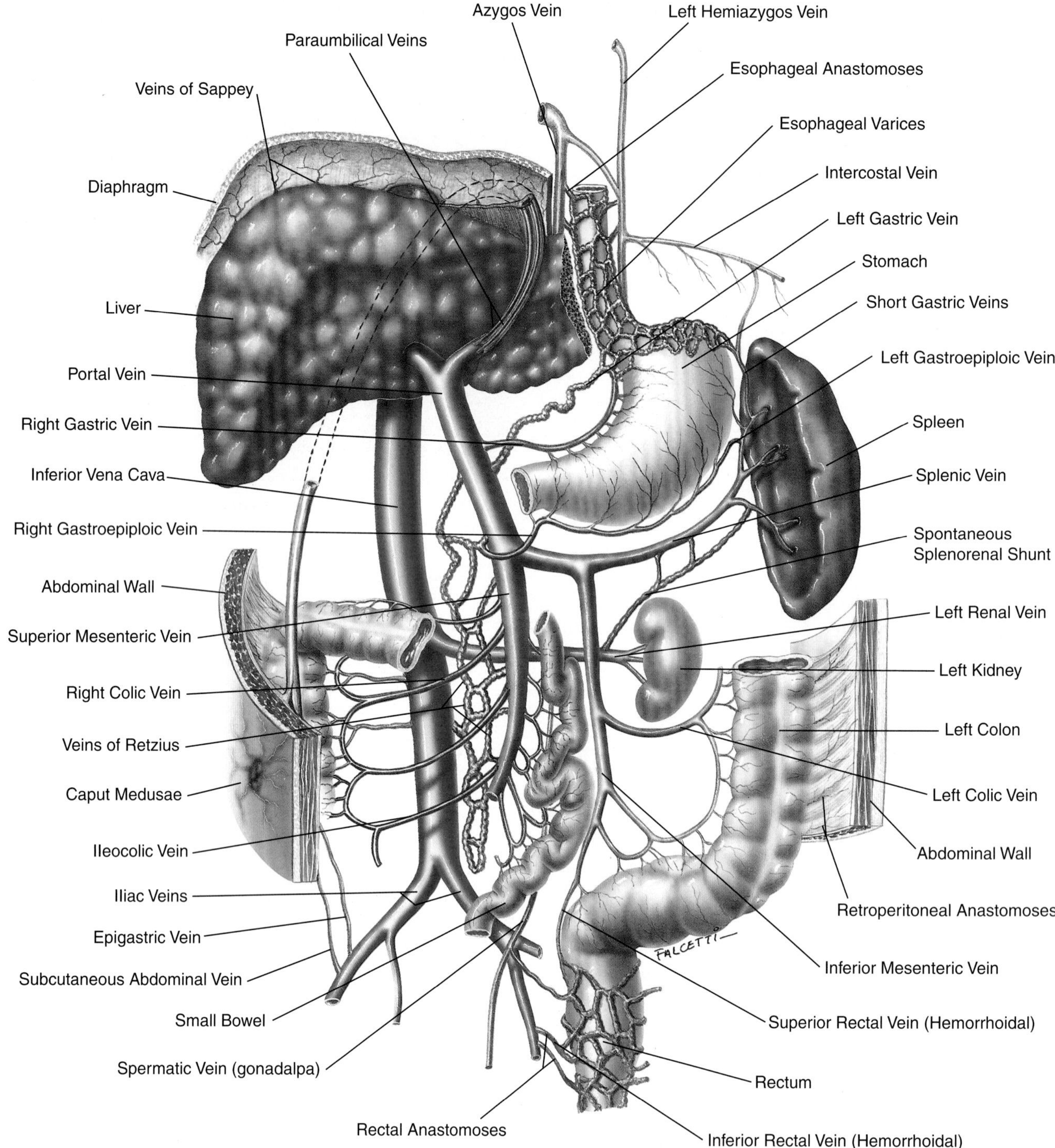

FIGURE 37A.2. Portosystemic Collaterals. Portosystemic collaterals can form in various locations throughout the body in the setting of portal hypertension. The most common locations are gastroesophageal varices formed from hepatofugal flow of the left gastric vein into the systemic azygos venous system and gastric varices formed from hepatofugal flow of short gastric and splenic veins into the systemic left renal vein via a gastrorenal or splenorenal (shown here) shunt. (From Uflacker, R. *Atlas of Vascular Anatomy: An Angiographic Approach*. 2nd ed. Philadelphia, PA: Lippincott Williams & Wilkins, 2007.)

disease. Approximately 40% of Child–Pugh class A patients have gastroesophageal varices, but the prevalence increases to 85% in Child–Pugh class C patients. Majority of variceal bleeding, 70% to 90%, is due to these varices. Gastroesophageal varices have an annual hemorrhage rate of 5% to 15% and associated mortality rate of 20%. First-line treatment for gastroesophageal varices is endoscopic management with ligation or banding in combination with supportive measures. When these interventions are unsuccessful, a transjugular intrahepatic portosystemic shunt (TIPS) may be required to control hemorrhage. TIPS has also been shown to prevent additional bleeding events and reduce mortality following gastroesophageal hemorrhage even when initial endoscopic management is successful.

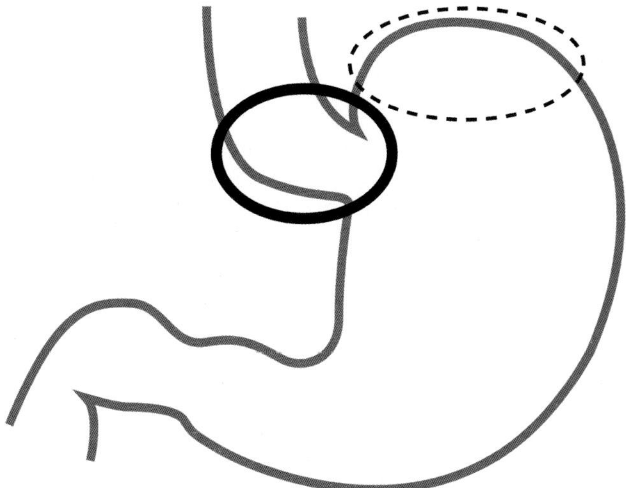

FIGURE 37A.3. **Location of Most Common Varices.** Gastroesophageal varices (*solid black oval*) arise from hepatofugal blood flow to the systemic azygos system. Gastric varices (*dashed black oval*) arise from hepatofugal blood flow in short gastric veins. Gastroesophageal varices are more common than gastric varices.

Gastric Varices

Gastric varices form via hepatofugal blood flow in the short gastric veins which often drain into a gastrorenal or splenorenal shunt to the left renal vein. Gastric varices have been classified as isolated at the fundus (IGV1) or isolated elsewhere in the gastric body or antrum (IGV2) according to the Sarin classification (Fig. 37A.3). Gastric varices have a similar hemorrhage rate but are less common than gastroesophageal varices, occurring in 5% to 30% of cirrhotic patients and accounting for 10% to 30% of overall variceal bleeding. However, gastric variceal bleeding, especially at the gastric fundus, is difficult to control endoscopically and is associated with a significantly higher mortality rate of 45% versus 20% for gastroesophageal varices. It is important to recognize that these varices can be treated with balloon-occluded retrograde transvenous obliteration (BRTO) when a shunt is present. The shunt consists of variceal drainage into the left inferior phrenic vein which then drains into the left renal vein, a gastrorenal shunt, or directly into the inferior vena cava, a gastrocaval shunt. A gastrorenal shunt is much more common, occurring 85% to 90% of the time. In addition to a gastrorenal or gastrocaval shunt, gastric varices often have additional systemic drainage via peridiaphragmatic veins such as the cardiophrenic vein.

MANAGEMENT OF PORTAL HYPERTENSION AND COMPLICATIONS

Portosystemic Shunt Creation

Initial treatment of symptomatic portal hypertension is medical therapy and endoscopic management of varices when present. If these methods prove ineffective, such as in the case of variceal bleeding or refractory ascites, portal decompression may be required. Historically, this decompression was achieved with a surgical portocaval shunt. Patients would undergo open surgery to create a direct communication between a component of the portal venous system, often the main portal vein, and the systemic system, often the inferior vena cava. Surgical shunts are effective but to minimize morbidity and mortality, appropriate candidates must have well-compensated liver disease. Unfortunately, the majority of patients with portal hypertension, especially cirrhotics, do not meet these criteria and another means of portal decompression is needed. TIPS creation is a minimally invasive endovascular procedure that mimics a side-to-side portocaval shunt and can be successfully performed in a much larger population of patients with liver disease. Indications and contraindications for TIPS creation are presented in Table 37A.3. The two most common indications are variceal bleeding and refractory ascites. The listed contraindications must take into account the setting in which a TIPS procedure is being performed. Emergent TIPS creation for acute variceal bleeding that cannot be controlled with endoscopy is a much different situation than elective TIPS creation for refractory ascites. If TIPS is the best or only life-saving option for a critically ill patient, the threshold for proceeding is much higher than for a stable patient. The model for end-stage liver disease (MELD) score is an objective measure of hepatic function using bilirubin, international normalized ratio (INR), creatinine, and more recently sodium. The MELD score is useful in determining the expected mortality of a TIPS procedure, and a score of 18 is often considered the threshold over which an elective TIPS may be deferred. For example, MELD score greater than 24 is associated with 60% 30-day mortality. Regardless of the MELD score, close collaboration with relevant specialists in hepatology, transplant surgery, and cardiology should be routine prior to any TIPS creation.

TABLE 37A.3

TIPS INDICATIONS AND CONTRAINDICATIONS

Indications	Acute gastroesophageal variceal bleeding refractory to medical/endoscopic treatment
	Recurrent gastroesophageal variceal bleeding
	Refractory ascites
	Hepatic hydrothorax
	Budd–Chiari syndrome
Contraindications	
Absolute	Severe hepatic failure
	Severe right heart failure
Relative	Portal vein thrombosis
	Polycystic liver disease
	Biliary obstruction
	Hepatic neoplasm
	Hepatic encephalopathy
	Sepsis
	Uncorrectable coagulopathy

TIPS Technique and Surveillance

Right internal jugular venous access is obtained and a combination of equipment is used to complete the procedure. Typically, the shunt is created between the right hepatic vein and the right portal vein (Fig. 37A.4). Much of this equipment, including the appropriate-angled catheters, portal access needle, and sheaths are available in packaged TIPS sets. An angled catheter is used to catheterize a hepatic vein, typically the right hepatic vein, and a sheath is advanced. A portal venogram is obtained in a number of ways (Fig. 37A.5) to visualize the intrahepatic portal venous structures. Venogram is extremely helpful in planning access to the portal system. Next, a curved needle is then advanced through the sheath

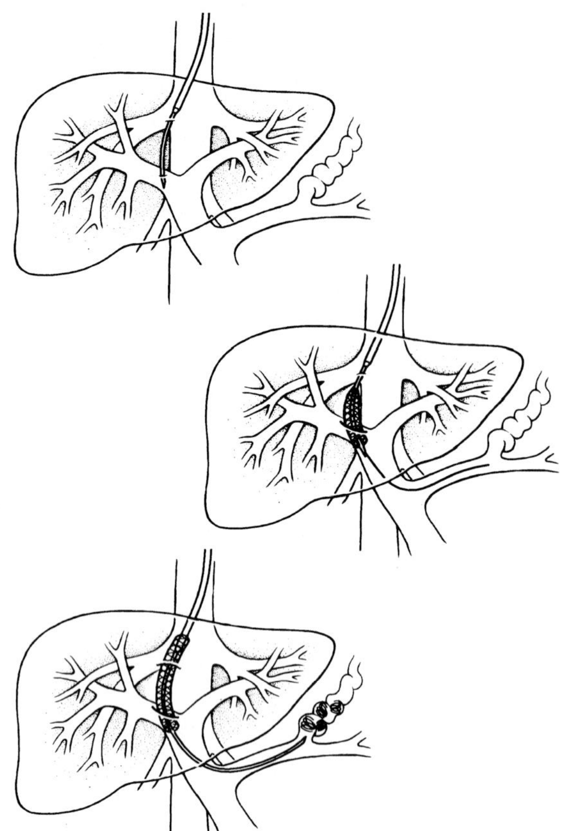

FIGURE 37A.4. Schematic of TIPS Creation. The needle is advanced through a sheath in the central right hepatic vein into the proximal right portal vein. Tortuous left gastric vein varices are present and represent hepatofugal flow away from the liver. The TIPS stent is deployed with the covered portion spanning the parenchymal tract, and the left gastric vein varices are embolized with coils.

and passes are made into the liver parenchyma toward the portal venous system. The direction and angle of needle entry is based on hepatic vein access and the portal venous target. The right portal vein is typically anterior of the right hepatic vein and requires the angled needle to be turned anteriorly, whereas the right portal vein is posterior of the middle hepatic vein and would require the needle to be turned in the opposite direction if advanced from middle hepatic vein access. Excessive needle passes, capsular punctures, and access to an extrahepatic portion of the portal vein should be avoided. Several modifications to the typical TIPS technique exist to mitigate these concerns and include the use of external or intravascular ultrasound to visualize needle passes. For example, a modified technique where the shunt is created directly between the portal vein and the inferior vena cava requires intravascular ultrasound to successfully pass the needle through the caudate lobe of the liver. Once access is gained into the portal venous system, pressure measurements are obtained to determine the HVPG. Portal venogram is performed to assess anatomy and presence of varices. The intraparenchymal tract is then dilated as needed to advance the sheath from the hepatic vein into the portal vein. A covered stent is then deployed across this tract and dilated (Fig. 37A.6). The size of the stent and extent of balloon dilation is often determined by the HVPG. Typically, a 10-mm stent will be placed and balloon dilation to 8 or 10 mm will be performed. Literature varies on the target HVPG to reach for adequate treatment of variceal bleeding. Many believe the gradient must be reduced to less than 12 mm Hg, as prior studies have shown that varices present with an HVPG below this level do not typically bleed. Other studies support a goal of 25% to 50% reduction in HVPG to prevent rebleeding. Adequate HVPG reduction for refractory ascites is also controversial. Similar to variceal bleeding, ascites does not usually develop until HVPG exceeds 12 mm Hg, and this is often referenced as a target threshold. For either indication, it is important to not reduce the HVPG below 5 mm Hg as this has been shown to increase the risk of hepatic encephalopathy. Following dilation of the stent, varices will often no longer be visible; hence, providers may prefer to embolize varices in advance of dilation if the indication was bleeding (Fig. 37A.7). Variceal embolization also promotes hepatopetal blood flow in the main portal vein and then through the stent. Hepatofugal steal from continued variceal filling can shorten stent patency, especially if there is an element of portal vein thrombosis. The advent of covered stents has led to increased primary patency rates. In-stent restenosis secondary to liver parenchymal neoendothelialization, bile inflammation, and fibroblast proliferation is reduced with a lining, usually of polytetrafluoroethylene (PTFE). TIPS surveillance is required as covered stents still develop in-stent restenosis, albeit at a slower rate, and also suffer from end stent intimal hyperplasia similar to that seen with covered dialysis grafts and coronary stents, especially at the hepatic venous end. Extension of the hepatic venous end of the stent to within 2 cm of the hepatocaval junction has been shown to improve patency. TIPS surveillance currently involves Doppler ultrasound to assess in-stent velocities. Ultrasound is usually performed at 1, 3, and 6 months postprocedure and then every 6 months. Abnormal velocities should be evaluated with venography and pressure measurements. Return of symptoms also warrants further evaluation; some advocate that routine TIPS surveillance is unnecessary when indication was refractory ascites and return of symptoms is clinically obvious. Primary patency rates vary in the literature but are significantly improved with surveillance and subsequent revision to maintain flow. One study demonstrated a primary patency rate of 64% and a primary assisted patency rate of 92% at 6 months.

TIPS Outcomes

Technical success rate with TIPS creation is over 95% with procedural mortality of less than 1%. Control of bleeding has a clinical success rate of approximately 90%. Improved control of ascites has a clinical success rate of 60% to 85%. Worsening hepatic encephalopathy is the most common complication, occurring in 15% to 30% of cases and is often treatable with conservative measures, though stent reduction may be required in certain refractory cases. Minor complications should occur in less than 4% of cases and include worsening encephalopathy, transient contrast-induced renal failure, transient pulmonary edema, and fever. Major complications should occur in less than 3% of cases and include hemobilia, hepatic artery injury, gallbladder puncture and hemoperitoneum related to needle passes, and renal failure requiring chronic dialysis. Survival is largely dependent on patient characteristic and indication, but one study with 10-year follow-up demonstrated survival rates of 55%, 46%, and 27% at 1 year, 2 years, and 5 years, respectively, with majority of patients having alcohol-related cirrhosis and suffering from gastroesophageal variceal bleeding.

Venous Recanalization

Inflow (portal) and outflow (hepatic) venous obstruction can be treated with recanalization. Anticoagulation is first-line treatment for portal vein thrombosis; however, depending

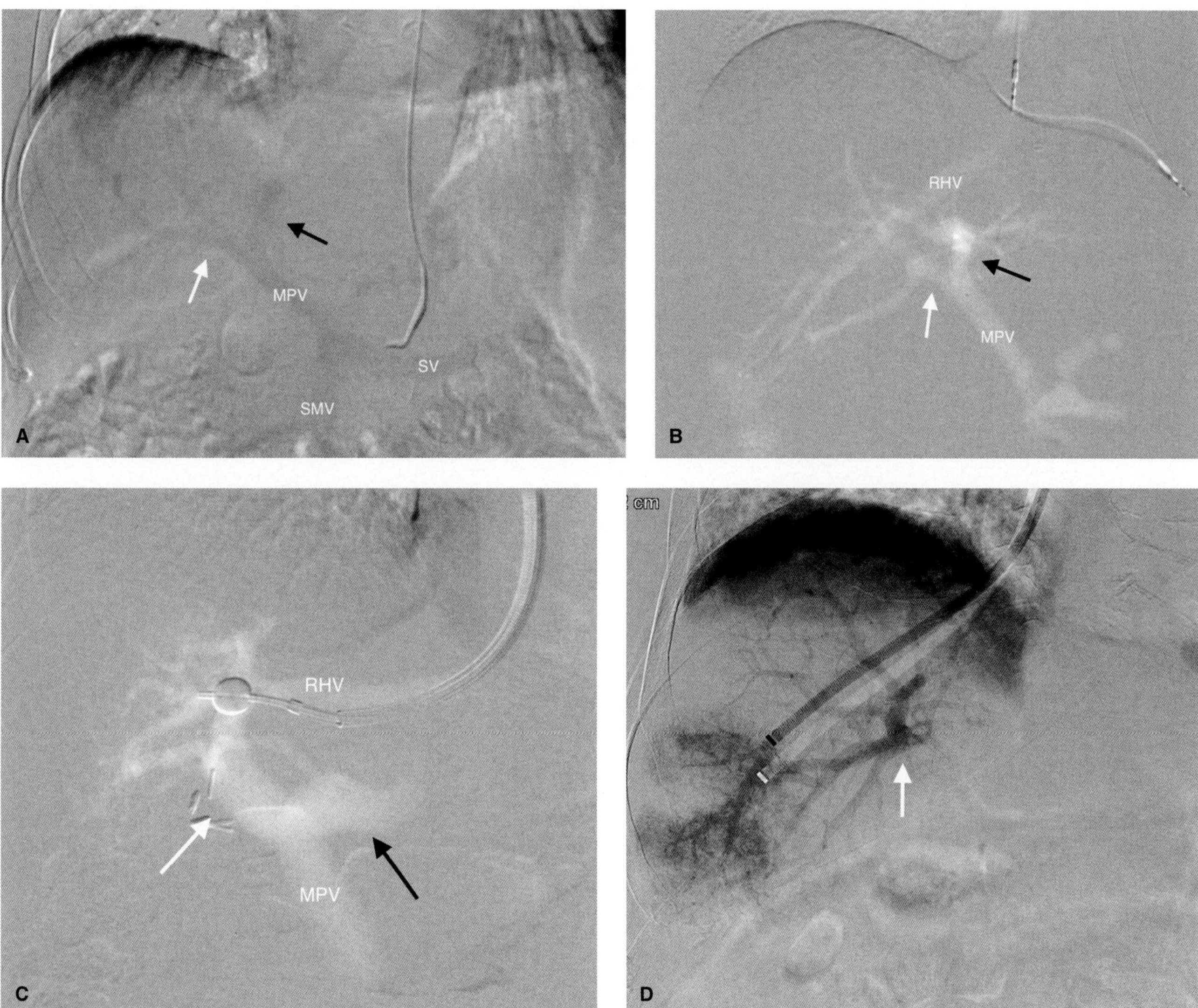

FIGURE 37A.5. Portal Venography for TIPS Planning. A: Indirect portal venogram obtained by contrast injection in the superior mesenteric artery. Main portal vein (MPV), splenic vein (SV), superior mesenteric vein (SMV), intrahepatic right (*white arrow*) and left (*black arrow*) portal veins are opacified. **B:** Wedged CO_2 venogram obtained by carbon dioxide injection with right hepatic vein catheter wedged in the distal hepatic parenchyma. Main portal vein (MPV), right hepatic vein (RHV), and intrahepatic right (*white arrow*) and left (*black arrow*) portal veins are opacified. **C:** Balloon-occluded CO_2 venogram obtained by carbon dioxide injection with right hepatic vein balloon occlusion. Main portal vein (MPV), right hepatic vein (RHV), and intrahepatic right (*white arrow*) and left (*black arrow*) portal veins are opacified. **D:** Wedged contrast venogram obtained by contrast injection with right hepatic vein sheath wedged in the distal hepatic parenchyma. Intrahepatic right (*white arrow*) portal vein and its branches are opacified. The main and left portal veins were not visualized due to known thrombosis.

on acuity and extent of thrombosis, percutaneous treatment options exist if anticoagulation fails. Acute portal vein thrombosis can be treated with pharmacomechanical thrombectomy and thrombolysis, but this is associated with a high morbidity rate and should be reserved for extensive disease. It is important to recognize that restoration of inflow will be short-lived if there is underlying liver disease and impaired outflow from the portal system. In these cases, TIPS creation is often required to provide adequate outflow and prevent rethrombosis of the portal vein. Chronic occlusion of the portal vein with cavernous transformation can be treated with recanalization of the portal vein remnant, often via a transhepatic or transsplenic vein approach; again TIPS is required to provide adequate outflow once the remnant portal vein is reopened (Fig. 37A.8). Budd–Chiari syndrome and associated portal hypertension result from the obstruction of hepatic vein outflow. Presentation can be acute, chronic, or asymptomatic, and etiology includes hepatic vein thrombosis, usually secondary to an underlying coagulopathy such as polycythemia vera, extrinsic venous compression, and hepatic vein or inferior vena cava membranous webs. Treatment depends on the nature of obstruction and as with all causes of portal hypertension, liver transplant is the definitive treatment and often the only option if acute thrombosis is accompanied by fulminant liver failure. Membranous webs can be treated with angioplasty and stent placement to maintain patency of the affected hepatic vein and/or inferior vena cava. Chronic thrombosis often demonstrates a spiderweb pattern of small hepatic vein collaterals during venography and can be treated with TIPS creation to bypass the thrombosed outflow (Fig. 37A.9).

Variceal Occlusion

As previously discussed, gastric varices are less common than gastroesophageal varices; however, bleeding from gastric

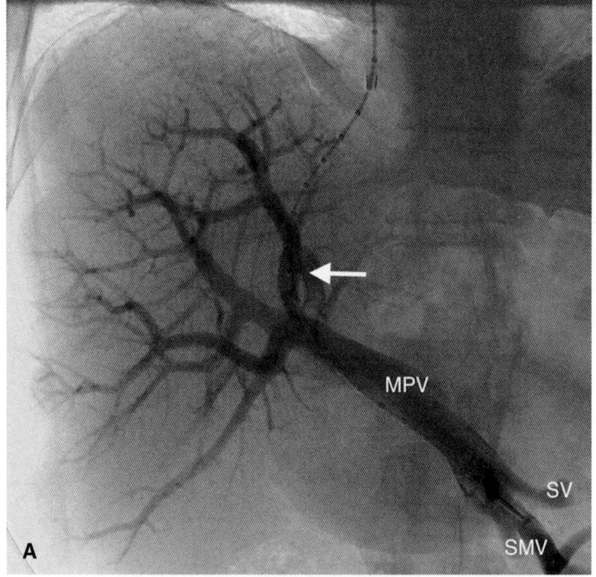

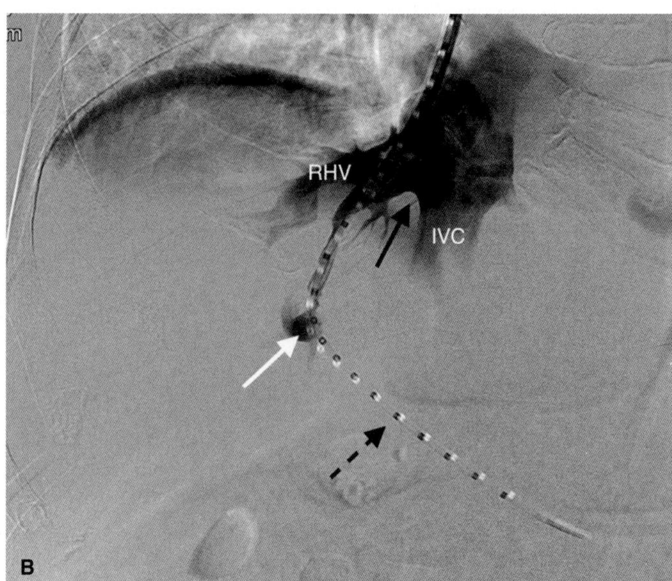

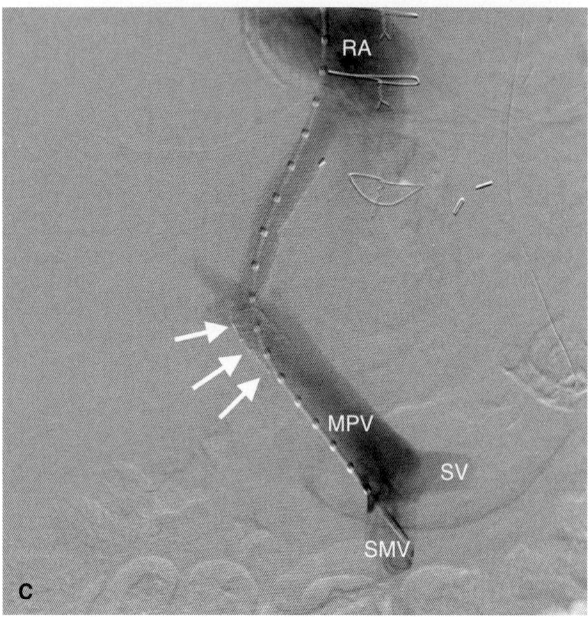

FIGURE 37A.6. TIPS Creation. A: Pre-TIPS portal venogram obtained by contrast injection in the superior mesenteric vein (SMV) just proximal of confluence with the splenic vein (SV). Confluence forms the main portal vein (MPV). Portal access via a branch of the right portal vein is indicated by the *white arrow*. **B:** Right hepatic venogram obtained by contrast injection in the central right hepatic vein (RHV). Small amount of contrast also seen in a right portal vein branch at portal access site (*white arrow*). Confluence with the inferior vena cava (IVC) is opacified (*solid black arrow*). The marking catheter (*dashed black arrow*) allows for accurate determination of TIPS length with systemic end ideally placed less than 2 cm from the IVC. **C:** Post-TIPS portal venogram (different patient from **A**) obtained by contrast injection in the superior mesenteric vein (SMV). Note the absence of intrahepatic portal vein branch opacification and filling of the right atrium (RA). *White arrows* denote the portion of the TIPS stent that is within the portal vein and is uncovered.

varices is usually more severe and more difficult to control due to the large size of these varices. Since endoscopic treatment is usually ineffective, endovascular occlusion of these varices is often considered first-line therapy for patients who have bled or are at risk of bleeding. Newly developed or rapidly growing varices and varices with red spots visible on endoscopy are considered high risk. Variceal occlusion is achieved by performing BRTO. Indication and contraindications for BRTO are presented in Table 37A.4. In addition to isolated gastric varices, an additional indication for BRTO is hepatic encephalopathy; however, there is not enough data currently available to confirm long-term efficacy. The reason why BRTO has shown improvement of hepatic encephalopathy and is contraindicated as listed in Table 37A.4 is because of the portal hemodynamic change created by the procedure. Isolated gastric varices drain to the systemic circulation through a shunt, typically to the left renal vein (Fig. 37A.10). This gastrorenal shunt may drain a large portion of blood from the portal circulation. When the shunt is closed, along with the varices, this diverted portal venous blood must either flow in a hepatopetal direction and perfuse the liver or travel through another collateral pathway to the systemic circulation. Increased blood flow to the liver may improve hepatic encephalopathy and potentially liver function. Whereas TIPS creation decompresses the portal venous system and leads to a decrease in HVPG, BRTO increases HVPG as the primary extrahepatic shunt to drain portal blood is closed. This increased portal hypertension can worsen gastroesophageal varices and ascites, especially in the setting of main portal vein thrombosis. For these reasons, appropriate patient selection is critical prior to BRTO. In certain scenarios, a combination of BRTO and endoscopic management of gastroesophageal varices or concurrent TIPS creation may be necessary.

BRTO Technique

Access for the retrograde approach to the gastrorenal shunt can be from the femoral vein or the internal jugular vein. From either approach, an angled catheter is used to catheterize the left renal vein and then the gastrorenal shunt. A long sheath or guiding catheter is often required to provide stability when

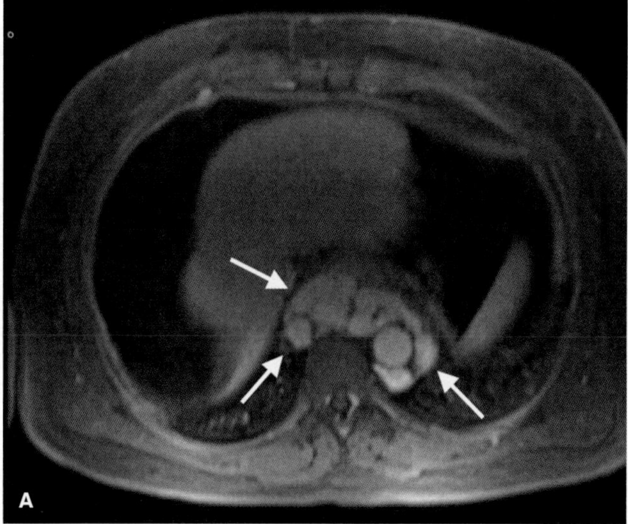

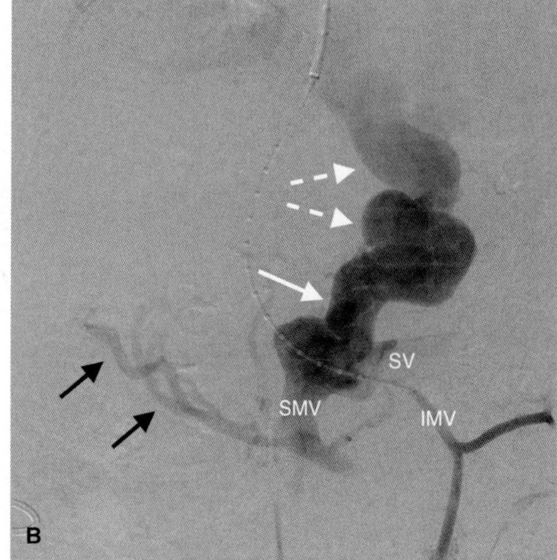

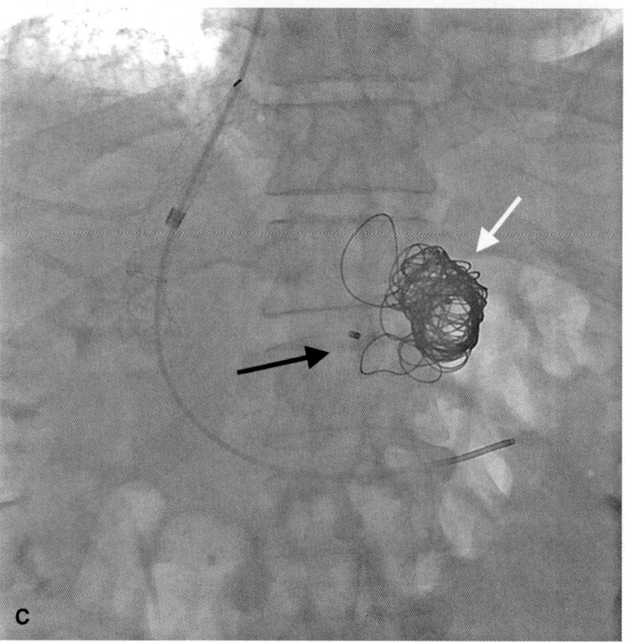

FIGURE 37A.7. **Large Gastroesophageal Varices. A:** Large gastroesophageal varices (*white arrows*) present on an MRI of the abdomen in a patient with a history of bleeding. **B:** Pre-TIPS portal venogram obtained by contrast injection in the inferior mesenteric vein (IMV) just proximal of confluence with the splenic vein (SV). The main portal vein is thrombosed. Superior mesenteric vein (SMV) and collaterals (*black arrows*) are present, as is a markedly enlarged left gastric vein (*solid white arrow*) and gastroesophageal varices (*dashed white arrows*). **C:** Post-TIPS image demonstrating embolization of left gastric vein with large coils (*white arrow*) and a vascular plug (*black arrow*). Additional embolization with hemostatic collagen powder was required given large volume of hepatofugal flow through the left gastric vein.

accessing the gastrorenal shunt. An angled catheter with a 10- to 20-mm balloon at the tip can be used if available or an exchange for a straight balloon catheter can be made once the gastrorenal shunt is accessed. Venography is then performed with the occlusion balloon inflated to assess for additional systemic drainage of the gastric varices via peridiaphragmatic veins (Fig. 37A.11). Systemic collaterals must be embolized with coils or liquid embolic agents to prevent nontarget embolization during gastric variceal obliteration with a sclerosing agent. Volume of sclerosant is determined by the volume of contrast necessary to opacify the varices during venography. Several sclerosing agents are available and have been shown to be effective. A common agent used in Japan is a 1:1 mixture of 10% ethanolamine oleate and contrast. The ethanolamine oleate causes hemolysis and release of free hemoglobin which can cause acute renal failure. To prevent renal damage, haptoglobin is often given systemically to bind free hemoglobin. A different agent is more commonly used in the United States, a 1:2:3 mixture of ethiodol, 3% sodium tetradecyl sulfate, and air to create a foam solution. Regardless of the agent used, the sclerosant must remain within the gastric varices for a period of time with the balloon inflated to prevent systemic migration of sclerosant or thrombosed blood. The duration of balloon occlusion ranges from 30 minutes to 24 hours. Many providers assess for residual flow after 30 to 60 minutes and inject additional sclerosant as needed. Depending on patient anatomy, occlusion of gastric variceal inflow, commonly from the left gastric vein, may be indicated. Access to the left gastric vein may be achieved through a percutaneous route or via a transhepatic route through a TIPS. When inflow is occluded for treatment, this procedure is known as balloon-occluded antegrade transvenous obliteration (BATO). Combination BRTO/BATO procedures and the use of plugs or coils to occlude variceal inflow and outflow are all variations of the basic BRTO technique. Contrast-enhanced CT 1 to 2 weeks following the procedure should be obtained to evaluate degree of variceal obliteration and to assess for nontarget thrombosis of the portal or systemic venous systems (Fig. 37A.12). If variceal filling persists, repeat BRTO may be needed. Serial endoscopy is another important aspect of patient follow-up. Endoscopy is used to evaluate the treatment response of gastric varices and screen for potential exacerbation of gastroesophageal varices. If gastroesophageal varices have increased in size, endoscopic treatment is warranted.

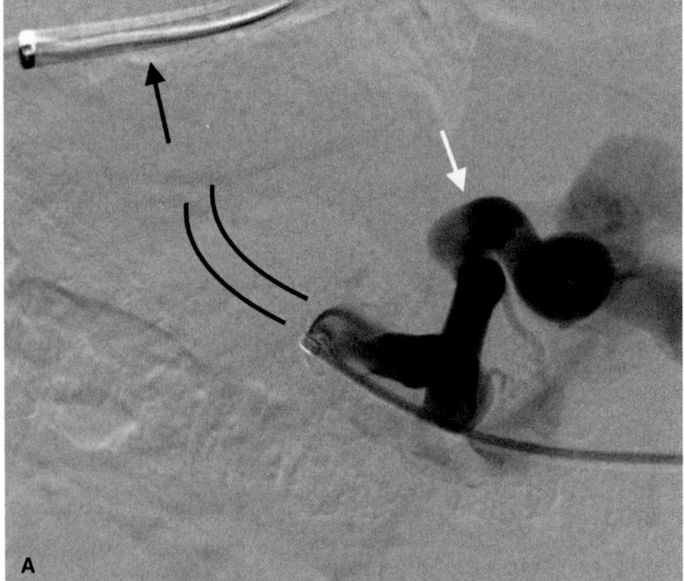

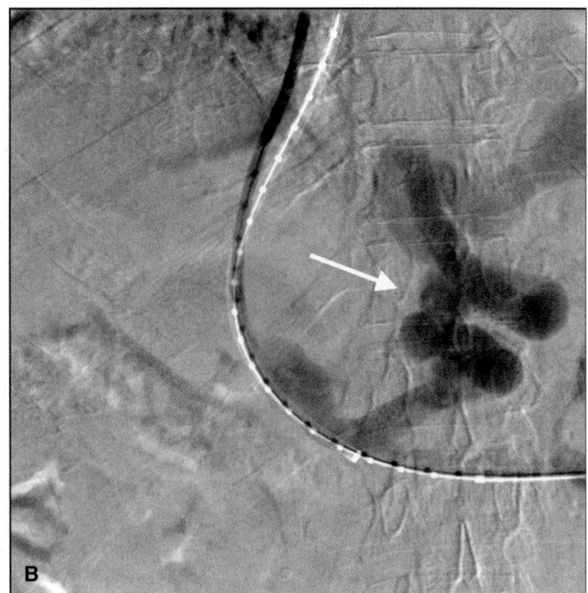

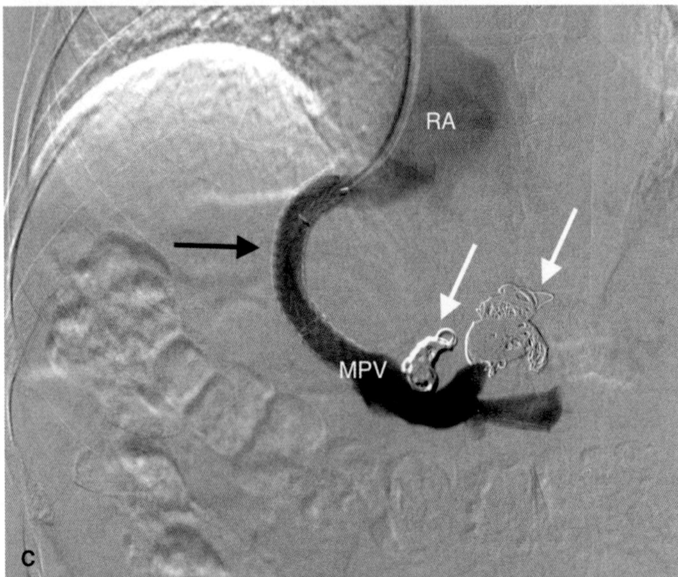

FIGURE 37A.8. **Portal Vein Recanalization and TIPS Creation.** **A:** Pre-TIPS portal venogram via a transsplenic percutaneous approach. Splenic vein and large gastroesophageal varices (*white arrow*) are opacified, but there is no opacification of the main portal vein (*black lines* outline expected region). A sheath is seen within the right hepatic vein at the top of the image (*black arrow*). **B:** Pre-TIPS portal venogram via a sheath advanced from the right hepatic vein. Gastroesophageal varices again seen (*white arrow*). **C:** Post-TIPS portal venogram. Varices have been embolized (*white arrows*) and the main portal vein (MPV) has been restored with contrast flowing through the TIPS stent (*black arrow*) into the right atrium (RA).

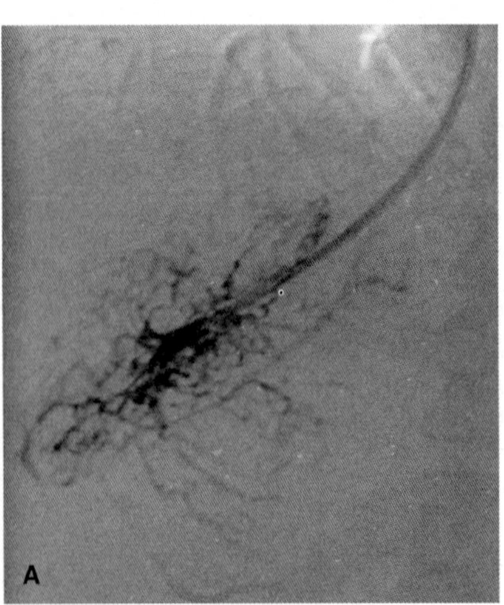

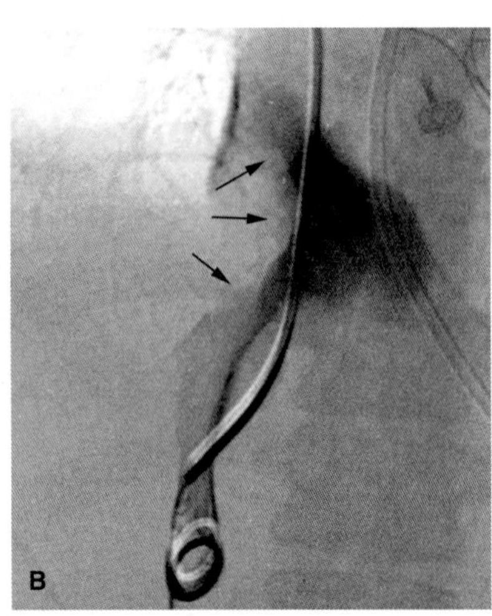

FIGURE 37A.9. **Budd–Chiari Syndrome.** **A:** Hepatic venogram demonstrates classic spiderweb appearance of Budd–Chiari syndrome. **B:** Venogram of the intrahepatic inferior vena cava (IVC) demonstrates mass effect (*black arrows*) on the IVC from the congested liver and thrombus extending from the hepatic veins.

TABLE 37A.4

BRTO INDICATION AND CONTRAINDICATIONS

Indication	Isolated gastric varices with active bleed, history of bleed, or high risk of bleed
Contraindications	High-risk esophageal varices Portal vein occlusion/thrombosis Refractory ascites Refractory hepatic hydrothorax

BRTO Outcomes

Technical success rate with BRTO ranges from 90% to 100%. Decreased size or complete resolution of gastric varices on endoscopy has a clinical success rate of 80% to 100% and control of bleeding has an even higher clinical success rate of 95% to 100%. BRTO is less invasive than TIPS creation as there is no hepatic needle puncture and as such has a very low procedural complication rate. Cardiogenic shock, atrial fibrillation, pulmonary embolism, and variceal rupture have been reported. The most common long-term complication is exacerbation of gastroesophageal varices, occurring in up to 58% of patients 3 years post procedure. However, these varices are often successfully managed with endoscopic treatment.

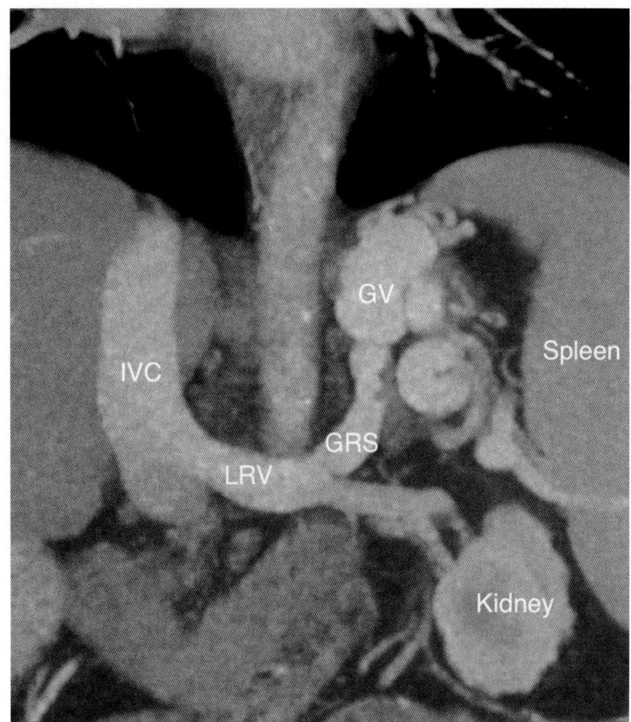

FIGURE 37A.10. Anatomy of Gastric Varices. Coronal maximum intensity projection (MIP) CT demonstrating gastric varices (GV), gastrorenal shunt (GRS), left renal vein (LRV), and inferior vena cava (IVC).

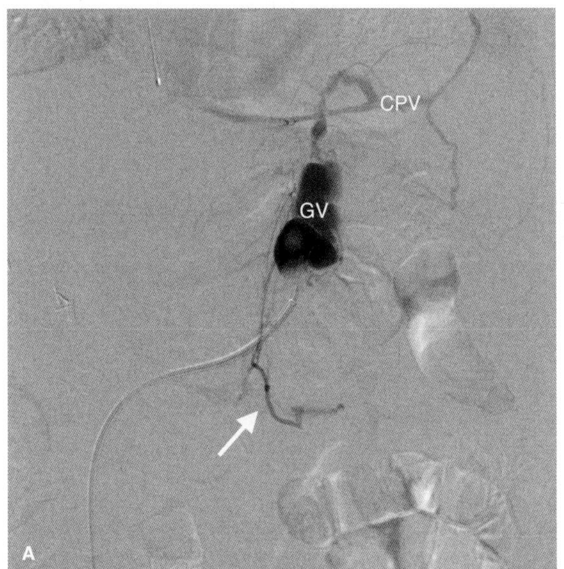

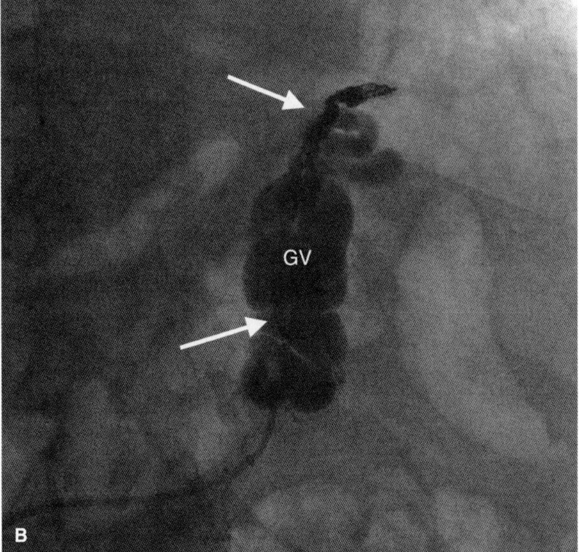

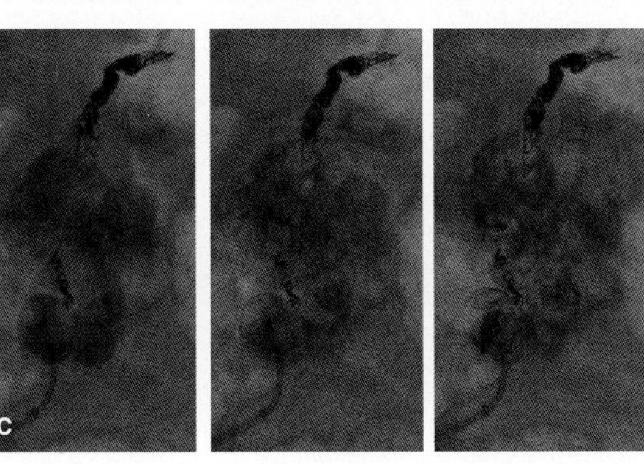

FIGURE 37A.11 BRTO Technique. A: Access to gastrorenal shunt is obtained from the right common femoral vein. A sheath is advanced into the left renal vein to the shunt to provide stability. The balloon is inflated and occlusive within the shunt, allowing opacification of the gastric varices (GV). Systemic drainage of the varices is noted via communication with the cardiophrenic vein (CPV) and smaller vessel extending inferiorly (*white arrow*). **B:** Following coil embolization of the systemic collaterals (*white arrows*), the gastric varices (GV) are again filled with contrast with the balloon inflated to estimate the volume of sclerosant required. Note that additional variceal filling is seen once the collaterals are embolized. **C:** Normal change in appearance of sclerosant (1:2:3 mixture of ethiodol, 3% sodium tetradecyl sulfate, and air) over 60-minute duration of balloon occlusion.

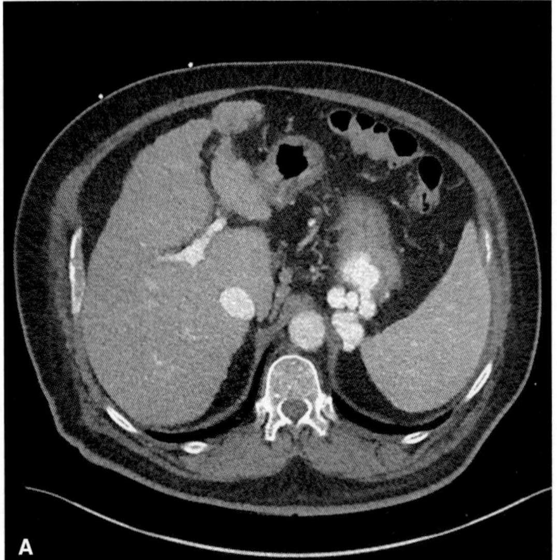

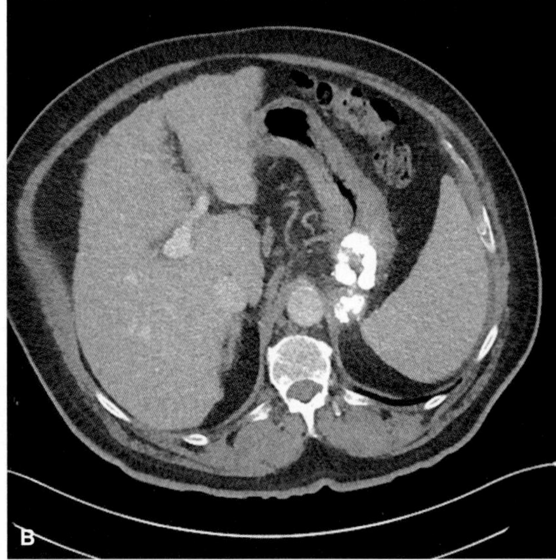

FIGURE 37A.12. **Pre- and Post-BRTO CT of Gastric Varices. A:** Venous phase CT of the abdomen demonstrates filling of large varices at the gastric fundus. Large gastrorenal shunt and no evidence of gastroesophageal varices make this patient an excellent candidate for BRTO. **B:** Post-BRTO venous phase CT of the abdomen demonstrates hyperdense sclerosant material within treated gastric varices and no residual venous filling.

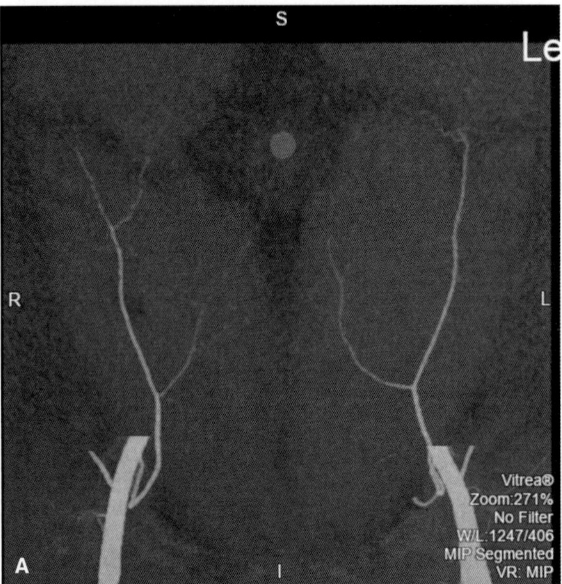

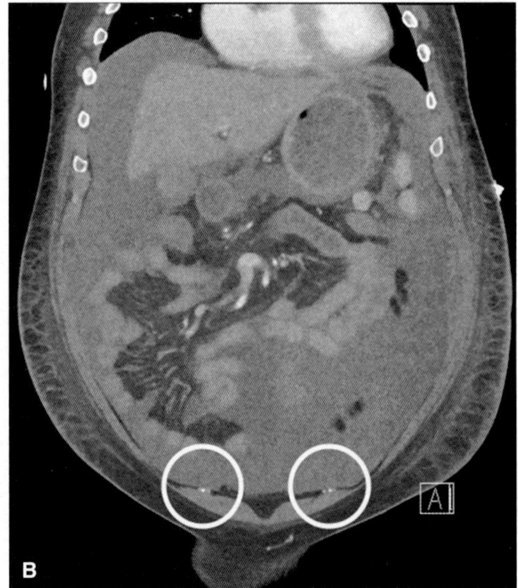

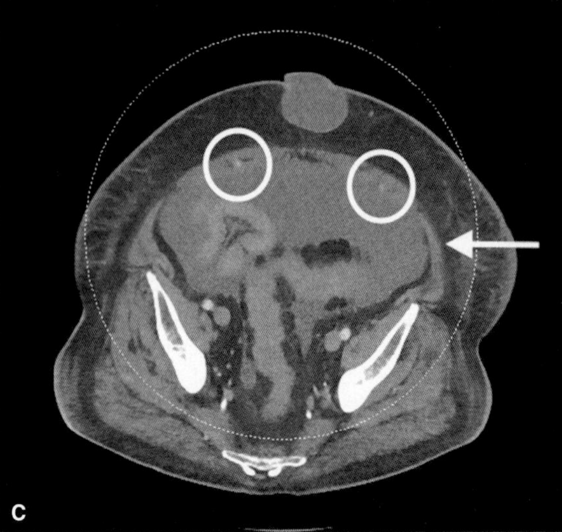

FIGURE 37A.13. **Inferior Epigastric Artery in Relation to Ascites. A:** Coronal maximum intensity projection (MIP) CT of the bilateral inferior epigastric arteries arising from the common femoral arteries (remainder of arterial system subtracted) and extending superiorly. **B:** Coronal CT with bilateral inferior epigastric neurovascular bundles (*white circles*) running superiorly along anterior abdominal wall musculature. **C:** Axial CT with bilateral inferior epigastric neurovascular bundles (*white circles*) running superiorly along anterior abdominal wall musculature. Approach to drain ascites should be lateral of these vessels to avoid the inferior epigastric artery (*white arrow*).

Ascites Drainage

Ascites refractory to medical management with diuretics and sodium restriction is an indication for TIPS creation; however, serial paracentesis and peritoneovenous shunt creation are far less invasive options. Serial paracentesis is performed by placing a small catheter percutaneously into the peritoneal cavity to drain ascites. The preferred location for paracentesis is the lateral right or left lower abdomen. Care should be taken to avoid the inferior epigastric artery as it courses superiorly along the anterolateral aspect of the abdomen from the ipsilateral common femoral artery (Fig. 37A.13). Other anatomic considerations include hepatomegaly, splenomegaly, abdominal wall edema, and bowel distention. Ultrasound guidance should be considered in these cases. Large-volume paracentesis, greater than 4 to 5 L of fluid removed, should be accompanied with intravenous albumin infusion of 6 to 8 g/L of ascites. Intravenous albumin is a plasma volume expander which reduces the incidence of circulatory dysfunction following large volume drainage. A meta-analysis demonstrated reduced mortality in cirrhotic patients receiving albumin for large-volume serial paracentesis. Unlike TIPS creation, serial paracentesis does not treat the underlying portal hypertension and instead provides temporary symptomatic relief. Peritoneovenous shunts also do not treat portal hypertension and remain controversial as some physicians consider them a third-line option for treatment of refractory ascites, behind paracentesis and TIPS creation, or second line if a patient is not a TIPS candidate. However, many believe the risk of placement outweighs any benefit. The shunt can be placed percutaneously and diverts ascites from the peritoneal cavity to the systemic venous circulation, usually via internal jugular vein access. Pleurovenous shunts can also be placed for refractory hepatic hydrothorax. These shunts follow a subcutaneous course similar to a ventriculoperitoneal shunt. A pump valve is required to prime the tubing and initiate flow of ascites from the peritoneum to the venous system. A one-way valve is also present to prevent reflux of venous blood into the shunt (Fig. 37A.14). Potential benefits of peritoneovenous shunt placement versus serial paracentesis (or pleurovenous shunts for serial thoracentesis) include improved quality of life and improved maintenance of blood volume and nutrient retention. These shunts remain controversial, however, because of high complication rates which include shunt occlusion, shunt leak, peritoneal infection, post-shunt coagulopathy, and pneumothorax. Infection is a particularly worrisome complication as bacterial peritonitis can jeopardize a patient's eligibility for liver transplantation. Despite shunt dysfunction occurring in up to 25% of patients, meticulous patient education and shunt care along with shunt revision to maintain patency have been effective. As a result, in the correct setting and in collaboration with hepatology and transplant surgery, peritoneovenous and pleurovenous shunts can play a role in the treatment of symptomatic ascites and hepatic hydrothorax.

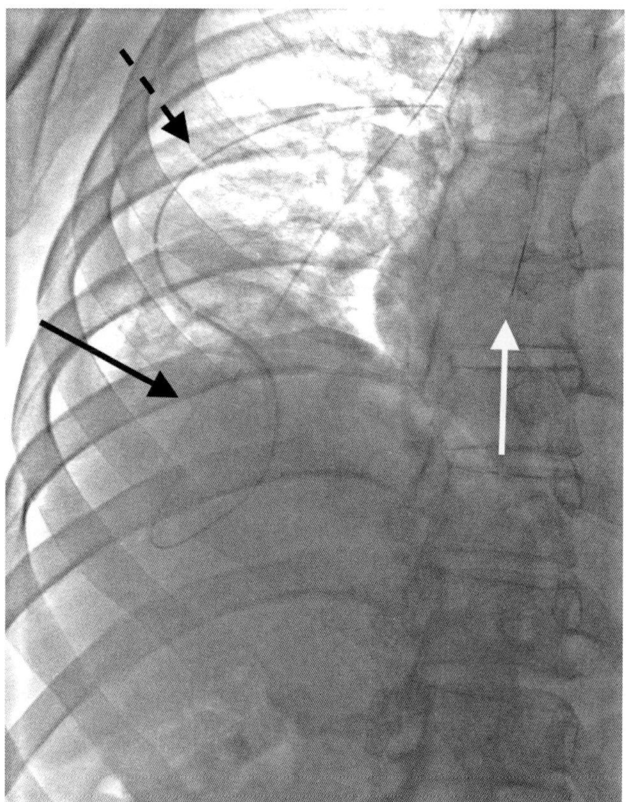

FIGURE 37A.14. **Pleurovenous Shunt.** Multi–side-hole portion of the shunt is within the left pleural effusion secondary to hepatic hydrothorax (*dashed black arrow*) and exits the pleural space to connect with a subcutaneous one-way valve and pump (*solid black arrow*). The shunt continues the subcutaneous course to the right internal jugular access site (not pictured). The intravenous distal tip of the shunt is seen overlying the cavoatrial junction (*white arrow*).

Partial Splenic Embolization

Splenomegaly with subsequent platelet sequestration and thrombocytopenia is associated with portal hypertension. Increased portal venous pressure creates impaired outflow from the splenic vein and leads to hypersplenism. While mechanisms are not fully understood, the congested spleen may then release cytokines that travel to the liver and worsen hepatic fibrosis which in turn worsens portal hypertension and leads to worsening splenomegaly. The purpose of partial splenic embolization (PSE) is to decrease the inflow and, therefore, the outflow from the spleen in an effort to reduce portal venous congestion and pressure. Reduced inflow also decreases the degree of platelet sequestration and can improve thrombocytopenia. PSE may be effective in reducing portal hypertension in select patients; one study demonstrated a greater than 20% decrease in portal venous pressure only when the spleen was at least half the volume of the liver. Patients with a spleen to liver ratio of less than 0.5 had no significant reduction in portal venous pressure. PSE is often performed in conjunction with other treatments such as TIPS, BRTO, or endoscopic variceal management. Hepatofugal portal flow is a contraindication to PSE due to increased risk of portal vein thrombosis. Particle embolization is typically performed with a goal of 50% to 70% reduction in splenic volume. Less aggressive embolization is ineffective and more aggressive embolization increases the risk of splenic abscess formation.

Suggested Readings

Bernardi M, Caraceni P, Navickis RJ, Wilkes MM. Albumin infusion in patients undergoing large-volume paracentesis: a meta-analysis of randomized trials. *Hepatology* 2012;55(4):1172–1181.

Berne RM, Koeppen BM, Stanton BA. *Berne & Levy Physiology*. 6th ed. Philadelphia, PA: Mosby/Elsevier; 2010.

Berzigotti A, Seijo S, Reverter E, Bosch J. Assessing portal hypertension in liver diseases. *Expert Rev Gastroenterol Hepatol* 2013;7(2):141–155.

Bratby MJ, Hussain FF, Lopez AJ. Radiological insertion and management of peritoneovenous shunt. *Cardiovasc Intervent Radiol* 2007;30(3):415–418.

Bureau C, Garcia-Pagan JC, Otal P, et al. Improved clinical outcome using polytetrafluoroethylene-coated stents for TIPS: results of a randomized study. *Gastroenterology* 2004;126:469–475.

Charon JP, Alaeddin FH, Pimpalwar SA, et al. Results of a retrospective multicenter trial of the Viatorr expanded polytetrafluoroethylene-covered stent-graft for transjugular intrahepatic portosystemic shunt creation. *J Vasc Interv Radiol* 2004;15(11):1219–1230.

Clark TW, Agarwal R, Haskal ZJ, Stavropoulos SW. The effect of initial shunt outflow position on patency of transjugular intrahepatic portosystemic shunts. *J Vasc Interv Radiol* 2004;15(2 Pt 1):147–152.

Colley DG, Bustinduy AL, Secor WE, King CH. Human schistosomiasis. *Lancet* 2014;383(9936):2253-2264.

Dariushnia SR, Haskal ZJ, Midia M, et al. Quality improvement guidelines for transjugular intrahepatic portosystemic shunts. *J Vasc Interv Radiol* 2016; 27(1):1–7.

Fukuda T, Hirota S, Sugimura K. Long-term results of balloon-occluded retrograde transvenous obliteration for the treatment of gastric varices and hepatic encephalopathy. *J Vasc Interv Radiol* 2001;12(3):327–336.

García-Pagán JC, Caca K, Bureau C, et al; Early TIPS (Transjugular Intrahepatic Portosystemic Shunt) Cooperative Study Group. Early Use of TIPS in patients with cirrhosis and variceal bleeding. *N Engl J Med* 2010;362: 2370–2379.

Garcia-Tsao G. Transjugular intrahepatic portosystemic shunt in the management of refractory ascites. *Semin Intervent Radiol* 2005;22:278–286.

Garcia-Tsao G, Bosch J. Varices and variceal hemorrhage in cirrhosis: a new view of an old problem. *Clin Gastroenterol Hepatol* 2015;13(12): 2109–2117.

Garcia-Tsao G, Sanyal AJ, Grace ND, Carey W; Practice Guidelines Committee of the American Association for the Study of Liver Diseases; Practice Parameters Committee of the American College of Gastroenterology. Prevention and management of gastroesophageal varices and variceal hemorrhage in cirrhosis. *Hepatology* 2007;46(3):922–938.

Groszmann RJ, Wongcharatrawee S. The hepatic venous pressure gradient: anything worth doing should be done right. *Hepatology* 2004;39(2): 280–282.

Hollingshead M, Burke CT, Mauro MA, Weeks SM, Dixon RG, Jaques PF. Transcatheter thrombolytic therapy for acute mesenteric and portal vein thrombosis. *J Vasc Interv Radiol* 2005;16(5):651–661.

Iwakiri Y, Groszmann RJ. Vascular endothelial dysfunction in cirrhosis. *J Hepatol* 2007;46(5):927–934.

Jung HS, Kalva SP, Greenfield AJ, et al. TIPS: comparison of shunt patency and clinical outcomes between bare stents and expanded polytetrafluoroethylene stent-grafts. *J Vasc Interv Radiol* 2009;20(2):180–185.

Kim T, Yang H, Lee CK, Kim GB. Vascular plug assisted retrograde transvenous obliteration (PARTO) for gastric varix bleeding patients in the emergent clinical setting. *Yonsei Med J* 2016;57(4):973–979.

LaBerge JM, Ferrell LD, Ring EJ, Gordon RL. Histopathologic study of stenotic and occluded transjugular intrahepatic portosystemic shunts. *J Vasc Interv Radiol* 1993;4(6):779–786.

Lee BB, Villavicencio L, Kim YW, et al. Primary Budd-Chiari syndrome: outcome of endovascular management for suprahepatic venous obstruction. *J Vasc Surg* 2006;43(1):101–108.

Li L, Duan M, Chen W, et al. The spleen in liver cirrhosis: revisiting an old enemy with novel targets. *J Transl Med* 2017;15(1):111.

Luca A, Miraglia R, Caruso S, Milazzo M, Gidelli B, Bosch J. Effects of splenic artery occlusion on portal pressure in patients with cirrhosis and portal hypertension. *Liver Transpl* 2006;12(8):1237–1243.

Malinchoc M, Kamath PS, Gordon FD, Peine CJ, Rank J, ter Borg PC. A model to predict poor survival in patients undergoing transjugular intrahepatic portosystemic shunts. *Hepatology* 2000;31(4):864–871.

Mancuso A, Fung K, Mela M, et al. TIPS for acute and chronic Budd-Chiari syndrome: a single-centre experience. *J Hepatol* 2003;38(6):751–754.

Martin LG. Percutaneous placement and management of peritoneovenous shunts. *Semin Intervent Radiol* 2012;29(2):129–134.

Merli M, Nicolini G, Angeloni S, et al. Incidence and natural history of small esophageal varices in cirrhotic patients. *J Hepatol* 2003;38(3):266–272.

Miyoshi H, Ohshiba S, Matsumoto A, Takada K, Umegaki E, Hirata I. Haptoglobin prevents renal dysfunction associated with intravariceal infusion of ethanolamine oleate. *Am J Gastroenterol* 1991;86(11):1638–1641.

Montgomery A, Ferral H, Vasan R, Postoak DW. MELD score as a predictor of early death in patients undergoing elective transjugular intrahepatic portosystemic shunt (TIPS) procedures. *Cardiovasc Intervent Radiol* 2005;28(3): 307–312.

Ninoi T, Nishida N, Kaminou T, et al. Balloon-occluded retrograde transvenous obliteration of gastric varices with gastrorenal shunt: long-term follow-up in 78 patients. *AJR Am J Roentgenol* 2005;184(4):1340–1346.

N'Kontchou G, Seror O, Bourcier V, et al. Partial splenic embolization in patients with cirrhosis: efficacy, tolerance and long-term outcome in 32 patients. *Eur J Gastroenterol Hepatol* 2005;17(2):179–184.

Orloff MJ, Isenberg JI, Wheeler HO, et al. Portal-systemic encephalopathy in a randomized controlled trial of endoscopic sclerotherapy versus emergency portacaval shunt treatment of acutely bleeding esophageal varices in cirrhosis. *Ann Surg* 2009;250(4):598–610.

Petersen BD, Clark TW. Direct intrahepatic portocaval shunt. *Tech Vasc Interv Radiol* 2008;11(4):230–234.

Riggio O, Masini A, Efrati C, et al. Pharmacological prophylaxis of hepatic encephalopathy after transjugular intrahepatic portosystemic shunt: a randomized controlled study. *J Hepatol* 2005;42(5):674–679.

Rossle M, Siegerstetter V, Olschewski M, Ochs A, Berger E, Haag K. How much reduction in portal pressure is necessary to prevent variceal rebleeding? A longitudinal study in 225 patients with transjugular intrahepatic portosystemic shunts. *Am J Gastroenterol* 2001;96(12):3379–3383.

Runyon BA. Management of adult patients with ascites due to cirrhosis: an update. *Hepatology* 2009;49(6):2087–2107.

Russo MW, Sood A, Jacobson IM, Brown RS Jr. Transjugular intrahepatic portosystemic shunt for refractory ascites: an analysis of the literature on efficacy, morbidity, and mortality. *Am J Gastroenterol* 2003;98(11):2521–2527.

Saad WE. Balloon-occluded retrograde transvenous obliteration of gastric varices: concept, basic techniques, and outcomes. *Semin Intervent Radiol* 2012;29(2):118–128.

Saad WE, Darcy MD. Transjugular intrahepatic portosystemic shunt (TIPS) versus balloon-occluded retrograde transvenous obliteration (BRTO) for the management of gastric varices. *Semin Intervent Radiol* 2011;28(3):339–349.

Saad WE, Kitanosono T, Koizumi J. Balloon-occluded antegrade transvenous obliteration with or without balloon-occluded retrograde transvenous obliteration for the management of gastric varices: concept and technical applications. *Tech Vasc Interv Radiol* 2012;15(3):203–225.

Sabri SS, Swee W, Turba UC, et al. Bleeding gastric varices obliteration with balloon-occluded retrograde transvenous obliteration using sodium tetradecyl sulfate foam. *J Vasc Interv Radiol* 2011;22(3):309–316.

Sanyal AJ, Freedman AM, Shiffman ML, Purdum PP 3rd, Luketic VA, Cheatham AK. Portosystemic encephalopathy after transjugular intrahepatic portosystemic shunt: results of a prospective controlled study. *Hepatology* 1994;20: 46–55.

Sarin SK, Lahoti D, Saxena SP, Murthy NS, Makwana UK. Prevalence, classification and natural history of gastric varices: a long-term follow-up study in 568 portal hypertension patients. *Hepatology* 1992;16:1343–1349.

Thornburg B, Desai K, Hickey R, et al. Portal vein recanalization and transjugular intrahepatic portosystemic shunt creation for chronic portal vein thrombosis: technical considerations. *Tech Vasc Interv Radiol* 2016;19(1):52–60.

Tripathi D, Helmy A, Macbeth K, et al. Ten years' follow-up of 472 patients following transjugular intrahepatic portosystemic stent-shunt insertion at a single centre. *Eur J Gastroenterol Hepatol* 2004;16(1):9–18.

Wong RJ, Aguilar M, Cheung R, et al. Nonalcoholic steatohepatitis is the second leading etiology of liver disease among adults awaiting liver transplantation in the United States. *Gastroenterology* 2015;148(3):547–555.

Zhu K, Meng X, Qian J, et al. Partial splenic embolization for hypersplenism in cirrhosis: a long-term outcome in 62 patients. *Dig Liver Dis* 2009; 41(6):411–416.

CHAPTER 37B ■ INTERVENTIONAL RADIOLOGY IN THE DIAGNOSIS AND MANAGEMENT OF POST LIVER AND KIDNEY TRANSPLANT COMPLICATIONS

PETER A. HARRI, PARDEEP K. MITTAL, AND JUAN C. CAMACHO

INTRODUCTION

Orthotopic liver transplantation (OLT) is the definitive treatment for patients with end-stage acute and chronic liver disease. Imaging in the postoperative period is fundamental to monitor complications. Often, these complications involve close collaboration of a multidisciplinary team, which includes diagnostic radiology, interventional radiology, transplant hepatology–nephrology, and transplant surgery. Clinical signs and symptoms of rejection are often nonspecific and only definitively diagnosed via a graft biopsy. However, radiology examinations can often identify other complications that can clinically mimic acute rejection, and interventional radiology plays a key role in their treatment when possible.

Like OLT, renal transplantation is the definitive treatment for chronic renal failure, and also close surveillance is needed to ensure proper graft function. This includes close serum creatinine monitoring in the immediate postoperative months, followed by decreasing frequency over time. If these levels are elevated, diagnostic imaging, like ultrasound of the allograft is immediately obtained.

For educational purposes, posttransplant complications may be divided into vascular, biliary/urinary, pathology extrinsic to the graft, and pathology intrinsic to the graft. Furthermore, vascular complications can be subdivided into those of inflow (involving the portal vein [PV] and hepatic artery [HA] for the liver, and renal artery [RA] for the kidney) and those of outflow (involving the inferior vena cava [IVC] and hepatic veins [HVs] for the liver, and the renal vein [RV] for the kidney). Biliary and urinary complications may be subdivided into leakage or obstruction. Extrinsic complications include fluid collections, such as bilomas, urinomas, lymphoceles, hematomas, or abscesses. Intrinsic complications (primary pathology affecting the transplanted organ) include graft dysfunction due to acute/chronic rejection, posttransplant lymphoproliferative disorder (PTLD), hepatocellular or renal cell carcinoma (RCC), recurrent primary sclerosing cholangitis, and/or cirrhosis (Tables 37B.1 and 37B.2; Fig. 37B.1).

In this chapter, the clinically relevant imaging findings are described as they are initially seen on screening ultrasonography (US) and subsequently on computed tomography (CT), magnetic resonance imaging (MRI), and scintigraphy and vascular-interventional imaging (i.e., cholangiography, nephrostogram, angiography). A brief overview of the available percutaneous interventional procedures is also provided.

OVERVIEW OF LIVER AND KIDNEY TRANSPLANT SURGICAL TECHNIQUES

To understand liver transplantation complications, a brief understanding of the surgery itself is necessary. In the case of liver transplantation, there are four anastomoses that are required: inflow—HA and PV, outflow—IVC, and biliary—bile duct. For kidney transplants in general, three anastomoses are required: inflow—RA, outflow—RV, and urinary—ureteral implantation into the urinary bladder. For both liver and kidney transplants, multiple surgical techniques have been described in detail.

However, the pertinent details for the practice of diagnostic and interventional radiology are the following:

TABLE 37B.1

POST KIDNEY TRANSPLANT COMPLICATIONS

■ VASCULAR	■ URINARY	■ EXTRINSIC PATHOLOGY	■ INTRINSIC PATHOLOGY
Arterial stenosis or thrombosis (inflow)	Urine leak	Hematoma	Delayed graft dysfunction
Renal vein thrombosis	Urinary obstruction	Abscess	Graft rejection (hyperacute, acute, and chronic)
Pseudoaneurysm (anastomosis or postbiopsy)		Urinoma	Posttransplant lymphoproliferative disorder
Arteriovenous fistula (postbiopsy)			

Liver Transplantation

1. The HA is commonly an end-to-end anastomosis; however, if the caliber of the recipient HA is too small, a jump graft from the recipient aorta (above the celiac trunk or below the renal arteries) using donor iliac artery is made (Fig. 37B.2). If there is replaced or accessory hepatic arterial vasculature in the recipient, anastomosis to the largest branch or two anastomoses may be necessary.
2. The PV anastomosis is also end-to-end between the donor and recipient PVs.
3. The IVC anastomosis has in general, two techniques. Historically, the recipient native liver and retrohepatic IVC was removed, and the donor IVC was implanted using two (proximal and distal) anastomoses. A newer, "piggyback," technique keeps the recipient native retrohepatic IVC in situ. This allows the donor suprahepatic IVC to be anastomosed to the recipient HV confluence.
4. The biliary anastomosis is normally an end-to-end choledochostomy; however, in diseased recipient biliary systems, a Roux-en-Y choledochojejunostomy may be required.
5. Livers can be transplanted whole from deceased nonrelated donors, also known as OLT. Newer living donor and split-liver transplantations can also be performed. The first split-liver transplant involves removing segments II and III (left lateral sector) and giving it to a smaller pediatric recipient. The larger segment stays with the living donor or is given to an adult recipient, in the case of a deceased donor. Newer techniques, which are more complex, allow for the right and left hepatic lobes to be split, and each given to an adult recipient (deceased donor) or the right lobe to one recipient (living donor).

Kidney Transplantation

1. The RA is normally anastomosed to the external iliac artery with an end-to-side anastomosis or the internal iliac artery with an end-to-end anastomosis (Fig. 37B.3). If the donor kidney has multiple renal arteries, the smaller arteries may be anastomosed to a larger donor artery that is then anastomosed to the recipient external or internal iliac artery, or multiple anastomoses from the donor renal arteries to the recipient iliac vessel can be made.
2. The RV is most commonly anastomosed to the recipient external iliac vein using an end-to-side anastomosis.
3. A myotomy to the urinary bladder is made for ureteral implantation. If the donor allograft has a duplicated collecting system, both ureters may be implanted, or the ureters may be joined together and implanted as a single unit.
4. Renal transplants can be performed extraperitoneally or intraperitoneally. Extraperitoneal transplantation is performed more commonly and is easier for biopsy and examination of the allograft. Intraperitoneal transplantation is quicker and easier to perform; however, it increases the difficulty of biopsy due to bowel interposition. In addition, while not common, torsion of the renal hilum is more common in the intraperitoneal approach.

VASCULAR COMPLICATIONS

Hepatic Inflow

Like the native liver, post-OLT hepatic inflow consists of the HA and the PV. However, in the post-OLT liver, the HA

TABLE 37B.2

POST LIVER TRANSPLANT COMPLICATIONS

■ VASCULAR	■ BILIARY	■ EXTRINSIC PATHOLOGY	■ INTRINSIC PATHOLOGY
Arterial stenosis or thrombosis (inflow)	Bile leak	Hematoma	Graft dysfunction
Portal stenosis or thrombosis (inflow)	Bile stenosis	Abscess	Graft rejection
Hypoperfusion/steal (inflow)	Biliary duct obstruction	Biloma	Posttransplant lymphoproliferative disorder
IVC or hepatic vein stenosis or thrombosis (outflow)			Hepatocellular carcinoma
Pseudoaneurysm (anastomosis or postbiopsy)			Primary sclerosing cholangitis

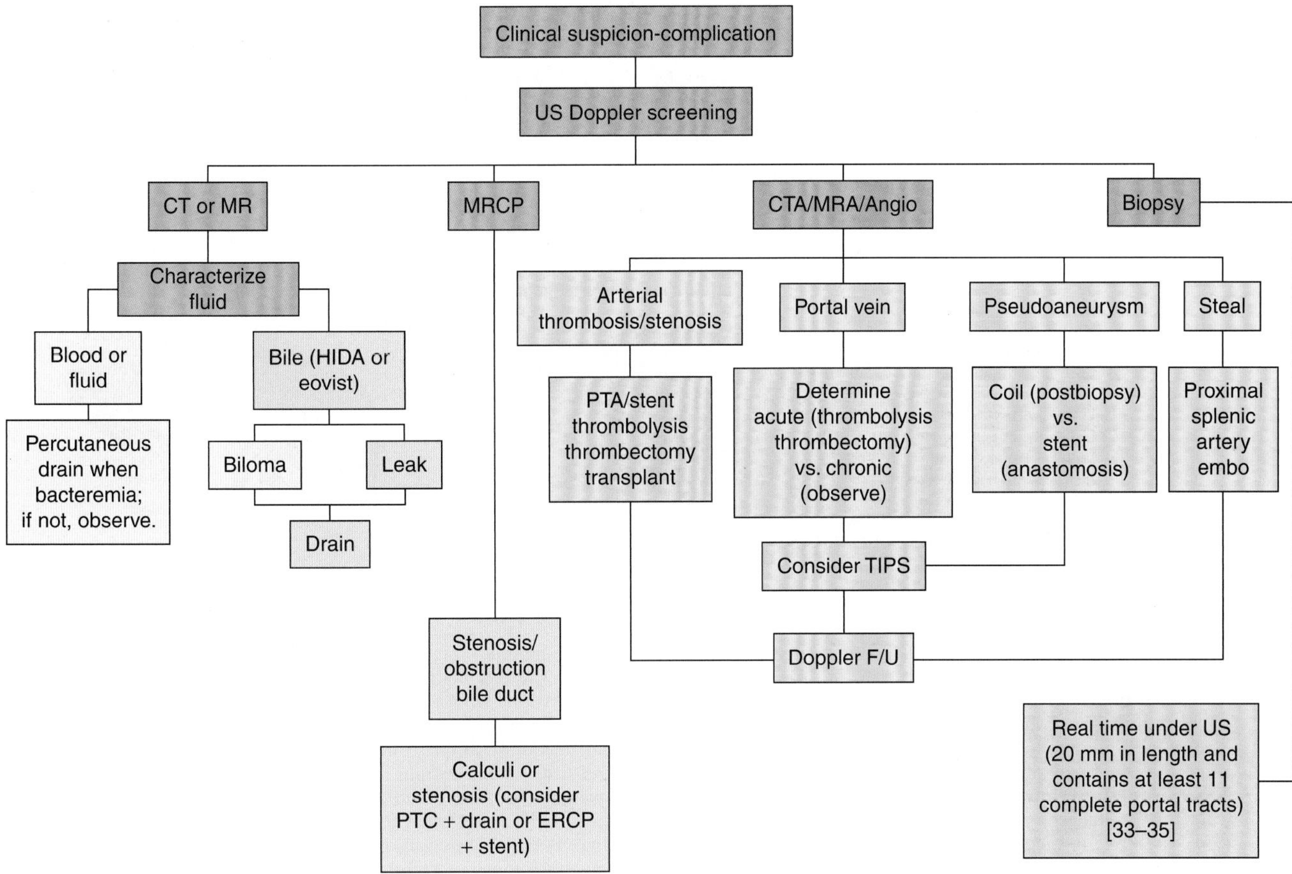

FIGURE 37B.1. General approach to screening and management of liver transplant complications.

has a critical role since the biliary tree entirely depends on the patency of the vessel. HA complications include stenosis, thrombosis, and pseudoaneurysms, while PV complications include stenosis and thrombosis. Splenic steal is also a common cause of arterial dysfunction and it is a poorly recognized/characterized entity.

Hepatic Artery Stenosis. HA stenosis is the second most common vascular complication of OLT and occurs in 2% to 11% of transplantations. HA stenosis usually occurs at the anastomotic site within the first few months following transplantation. Clinically, HA stenosis presents as worsening liver function tests. Risk factors for development of HA stenosis include allograft rejection, poor surgical technique, and clamp injury. If left untreated, HA stenosis may progress to HA thrombosis.

The initial examination of choice in the evaluation of HA stenosis is Doppler ultrasonography. Findings that suggest HA stenosis on Doppler ultrasonography include poststenotic resistive index (RI) of <0.5, tardus parvus waveform distal to the stenosis, and elevated peak systolic velocity (PSV) of >200 cm/s at the stenosis. Of note, in the first 3 days following OLT, increased RI (>0.8) is commonly seen and usually returns to normal within 72 hours. If HA stenosis is suggested by Doppler ultrasonography, further evaluation with CT angiography (CTA) or MR angiography (MRA) may be performed. CTA or MRA can confirm stenosis, occlusion, redundancy, kinking, or other HA abnormality. Once HA stenosis is confirmed, balloon angioplasty with or without stenting may be performed as the definitive treatment (Fig. 37B.2). Angioplasty in the first line of management and has a technical success rate of up to 90% with physiologic improvement in up to 60% of the cases. Stents are reserved for those unsuccessful dilatations, and some series report 93% patency up to 24 months if used as primary therapy (Fig. 37B.4).

Hepatic Artery Thrombosis. HA thrombosis is the most common vascular complication of OLT occurring in 2% to 12% of transplant recipients and usually occurs within the first 6 months following transplant. The initial imaging modality of choice is Doppler ultrasonography, which may demonstrate lack of arterial flow within the HA (Fig. 37B.3). Although Doppler ultrasonography may correctly diagnose 92% of cases, CTA or MRA is usually employed to confirm the diagnosis; furthermore, these imaging modalities may also demonstrate an area of hepatic infarction. Treatment usually consists of emergent thrombectomy/thrombolysis or retransplantation in severe cases.

Imaging of the HA is exceedingly important in the post-OLT patient. In the native liver, the biliary ducts are perfused via the HA and peribiliary collaterals; however, in the transplanted liver the biliary tree is perfused solely via the HA. Thus, the post-OLT biliary system is extremely sensitive to HA flow and any disruption in the HA may have profound effects upon the biliary system. Arterial ischemia commonly presents as biliary ductal dilatation but may also lead to biliary necrosis (Fig. 37B.5).

Hepatic Artery Pseudoaneurysm. Although a relatively uncommon post-OLT complication, pseudoaneurysm can be a potential source for major arterial hemorrhage if ruptured. Two types of HA pseudoaneurysm may be seen post-OLT—intrahepatic and extrahepatic. Intrahepatic pseudoaneurysms are usually iatrogenic secondary to injury from graft biopsy

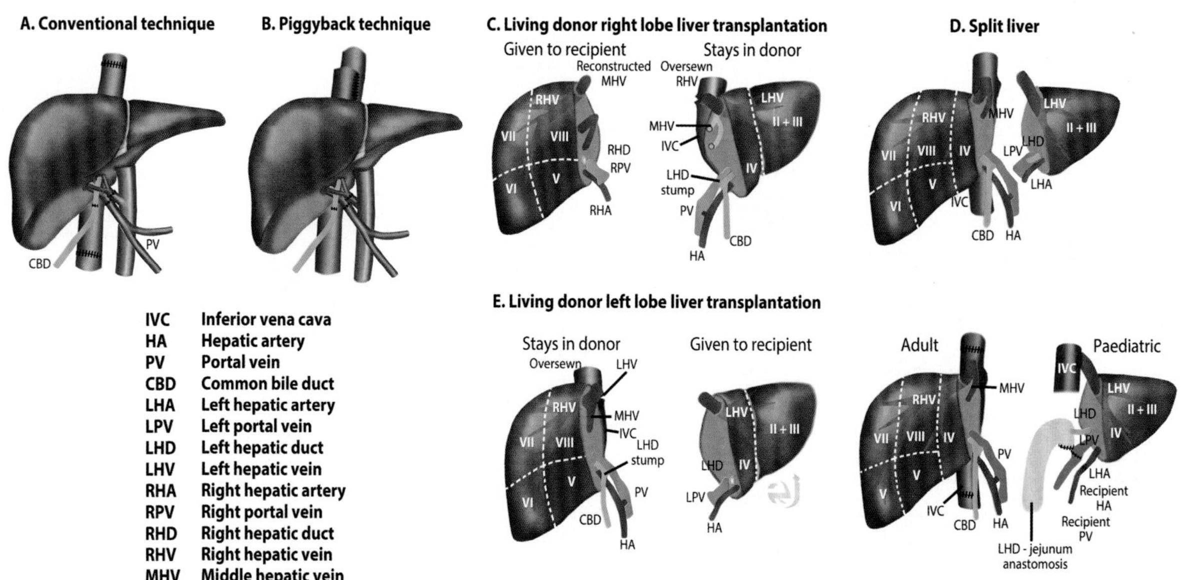

FIGURE 37B.2. **Different Available Surgical Techniques for Liver Transplantation. A:** In the conventional technique, five standard anastomoses are performed including the hepatic artery, the portal vein, two IVC anastomoses (suprahepatic and infrahepatic), and a choledochocholedochostomy. **B:** Modification of the conventional technique ("piggyback") in which the IVC anastomoses are replaced by a single anastomosis of the donor suprahepatic IVC to the recipient RHV and MHV confluence, with the recipient's native retrohepatic IVC remaining in situ. **C:** Living donor right lobe transplantation includes performing a conventional right hepatectomy followed by anastomoses of donor RHA and recipient HA (end-to-end), donor RPV and recipient PV (end-to-end), donor RHV and MHV to recipient retrohepatic IVC (end-to-side) or recipient hepatic vein confluence (end-to-end), and donor right hepatic duct to recipient jejunal limb with Roux-en-Y reconstruction. **D:** Split liver transplant involves dividing the donor liver into segments II and III which are given to a pediatric recipient performing the following anastomoses: donor LHA to recipient HA (end-to-end), donor LPV to recipient PV (end-to-end), donor LHV to recipient retrohepatic IVC (end-to-side), and a Roux-en-Y biliary reconstruction to the donor LHD. The remaining liver is transplanted in an adult with the same anastomoses as the "living donor right lobe transplantation" except that the biliary anastomosis is a choledochocholedochostomy. **E:** Living donor left lobe transplantation is performed with same anastomoses as the previously described "pediatric split liver," although sometimes segment IV is included in the donor liver. (Camacho JC, Coursey-Moreno C, Telleria JC, Aguirre DA, Torres WE, Mittal PK. Nonvascular post-liver transplantation complications: from US screening to cross-sectional and interventional imaging. *Radiographics* 2015;35[1]:87–104.)

or biliary procedure, but may also be secondary to an intrahepatic focus of infection. Intrahepatic pseudoaneurysms may resolve spontaneously or in some cases, require embolic therapy. Extrahepatic pseudoaneurysms usually occur at the anastomotic site and are frequently iatrogenic secondary to the surgical technique, although they can also be due to infection. These are treated with covered stenting or surgical revision.

FIGURE 37B.3. **Simplified Scheme of the Surgical Technique for Vascular Anastomoses in Renal Transplantation.** IVC, inferior vena cava; Ao, aorta; K, kidney graft; RV, renal vein; RA, renal artery; EIV, external iliac vein; EIA, external iliac artery.

Pseudoaneurysm can be detected with Doppler US, which will appear as a cystic mass usually along the course of the HA with internal turbulent flow. CTA, MRA, or conventional angiography can confirm the diagnosis with postcontrast imaging demonstrating internal enhancement (Fig. 37B.6).

Splenic Steal Syndrome (Hepatic Artery Hypoperfusion Syndrome). Splenic steal syndrome is a controversial diagnosis of HA hypoperfusion and may represent an underrecognized cause of graft ischemia. Splenic steal syndrome presents nonspecifically as graft dysfunction, and if overlooked, may lead to graft failure. Its incidence in the literature ranges widely from 0.6% to 10.1% in liver transplant recipients. Angiography is the gold standard diagnostic modality in the evaluation of splenic steal syndrome. The diagnosis is defined by sluggish or even reversed flow in the HA relative to the flow in the splenic artery in the absence of hepatic arterial stenosis, thrombosis, and/or kinking. The most objective angiographic definition includes visualization of the HA during the portal venous phase of the angiogram. Doppler ultrasound findings are nonspecific and include high arterial RI (>0.80). Management of HA hypoperfusion syndrome requires identification of the underlying predisposing factor. If there is preferential flow to the splenic artery, and if

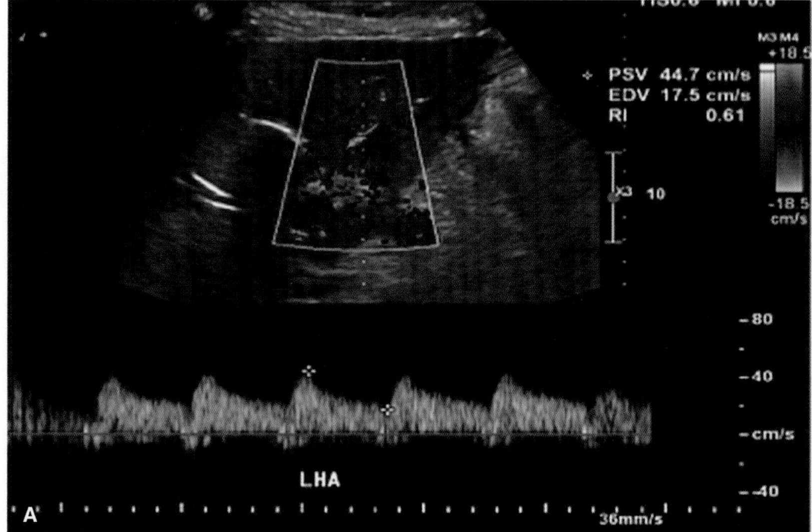

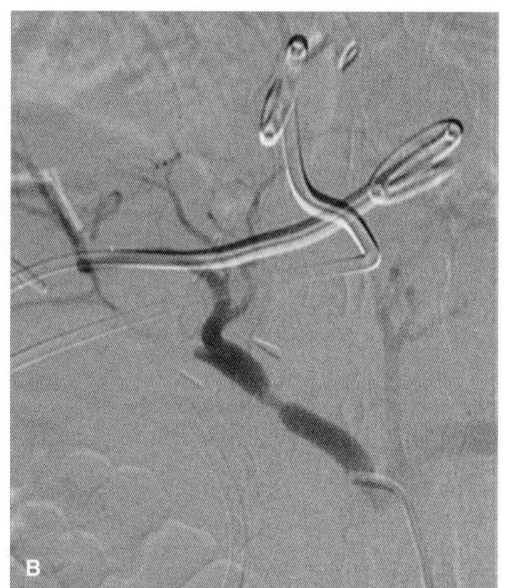

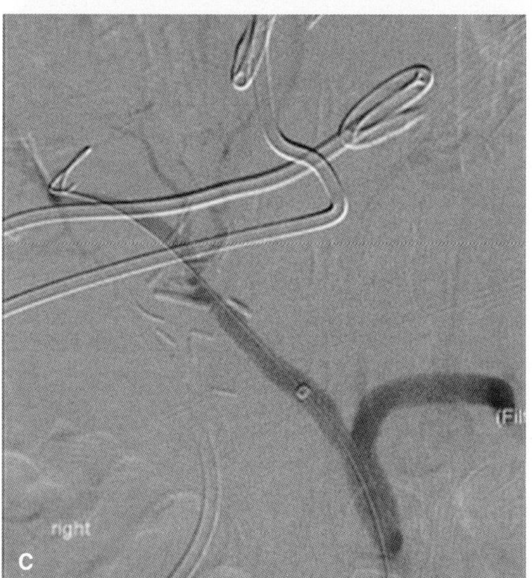

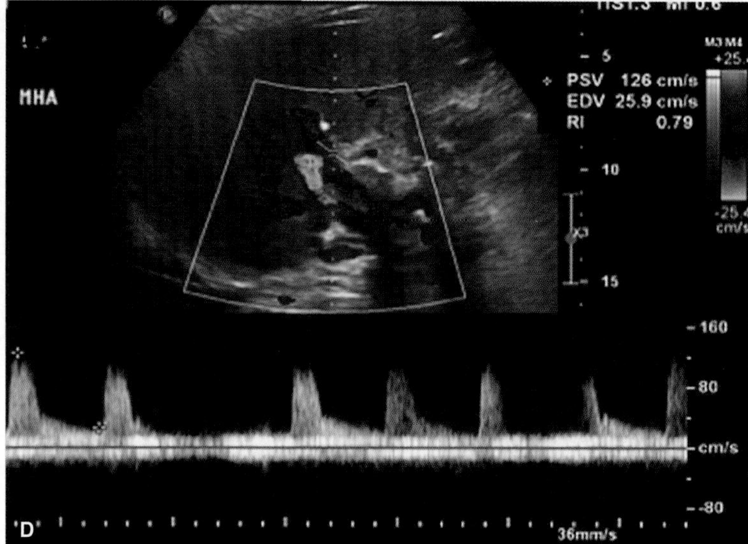

FIGURE 37B.4. **Hepatic Artery Stenosis. A:** Ultrasound Doppler intrahepatic tardus parvus waveform morphology. **B:** Angiogram demonstrates a focal stenosis of the common hepatic artery involving the anastomosis. **C:** Percutaneous stent placement was performed with resolution of the stenosis. **D:** End-result Doppler demonstrates a normalized waveform following intervention.

surgically feasible, an aortohepatic conduit can be created. A more common alternative is to restrict flow to the spleen with splenic artery banding, ligation, hourglass stents, and proximal embolization, which ultimately redirect flow, decreasing the hyperdynamic portal flow. These techniques have excellent results with low risk of splenic infarction (Fig. 37B.7).

Portal Vein Stenosis. PV stenosis has been reported in approximately 1% of post-OLT patients and usually occurs at the portal venous anastomosis. It is important to note that a mild reduction in PV caliber is to be expected at the anastomotic site and may be due to size discrepancy between donor and recipient PVs. Doppler ultrasonography is the initial imaging modality of choice and may demonstrate turbulent flow at the site of the anastomosis. In addition, spectral Doppler imaging will show high transanastomotic velocities (>125 cm/s) or a preanastomotic to postanastomotic velocity ratio of ≥3:1. Loss of the normal portal venous respiratory phasicity may also be observed.

Once PV stenosis is suggested by US, further evaluation with CTA/MRA may be pursued to better depict the area of focal narrowing. Ultimately, PV stenosis may be confirmed by transhepatic portography with a greater than 5 mm Hg pressure gradient across the region of stenosis as the diagnostic threshold (Fig. 37B.8). Definitive treatment is by angioplasty or stenting.

Portal Vein Thrombosis. PV thrombosis occurs in up to 1% to 2% of OLT patients. Initial evaluation with Doppler US may demonstrate no flow within the PV and may also show echogenic thrombus within the vessel lumen. PV thrombosis may be confirmed noninvasively by contrast-enhanced CT or MR, which will demonstrate a filling defect within the PV.

Postcontrast CT or MRI may also demonstrate transient hepatic attenuation or intensity difference (THAD/THID) (Fig. 37B.9). THAD/THID may occur in the setting of PV thrombosis due to the compensatory relationship between the dual hepatic blood supply. Namely, arterial flow to a region increases when portal flow is decreased or is interrupted. The relative increase in hepatic arterial supply causes a higher attenuation/intensity to the affected region. Multiple treatment

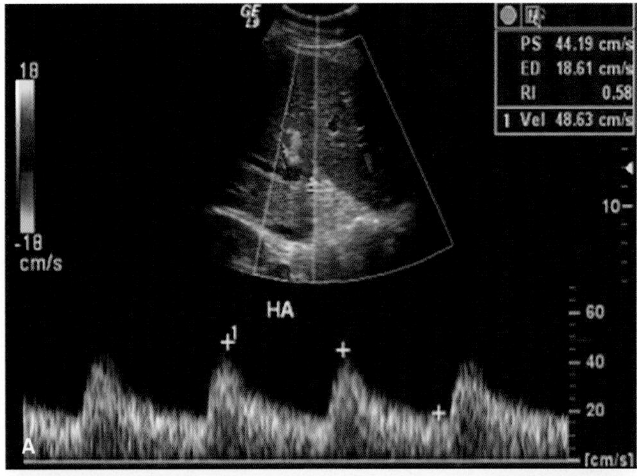

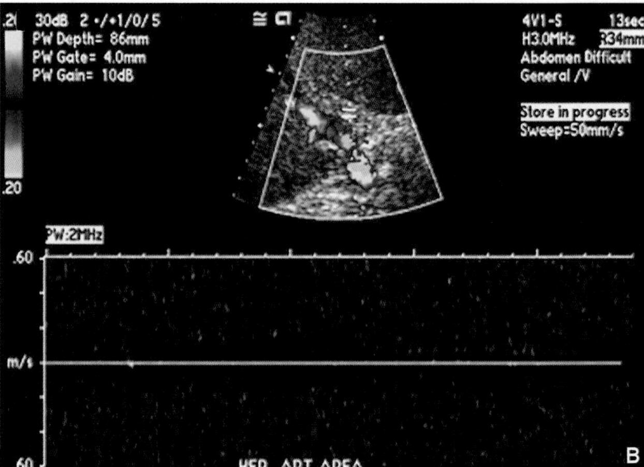

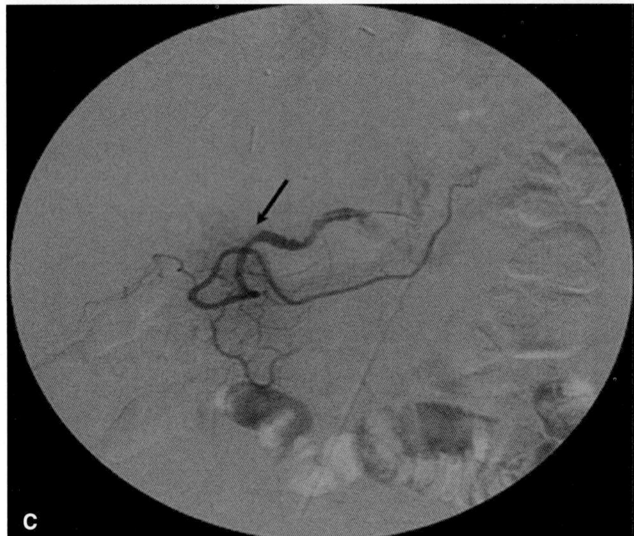

FIGURE 37B.5. **Acute Hepatic Artery Thrombosis. A:** Immediate postoperative ultrasound demonstrates normal low-resistance (RI 0.58) pulsatile flow in the main hepatic artery. **B:** Ultrasound performed after sudden increase in liver function tests demonstrates no flow in the hepatic artery. **C:** Emergent angiography reveals complete occlusion of the proper hepatic artery (*arrow*). The vessel extending inferiorly at the level of the arrow is the gastroduodenal artery.

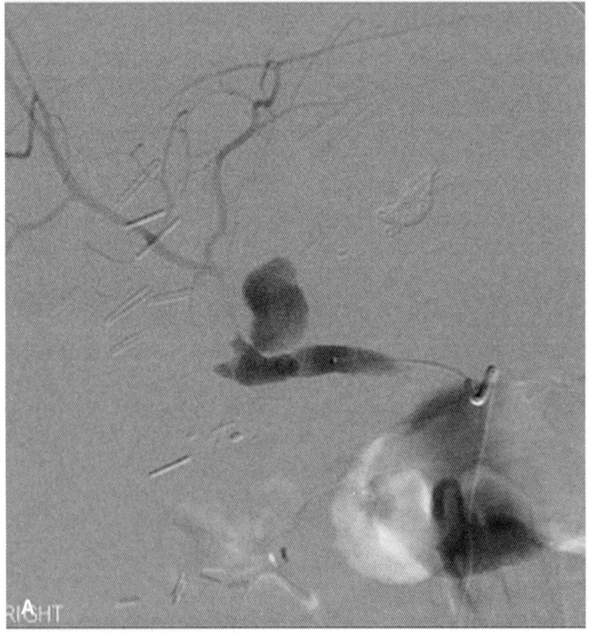

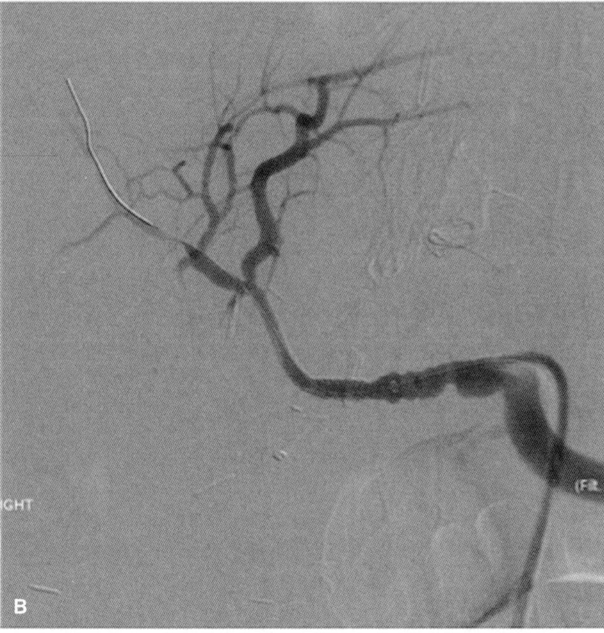

FIGURE 37B.6. **Hepatic Artery Pseudoaneurysm. A:** Celiac angiogram demonstrates active extravasation of contrast at the anastomosis with distal vasoconstriction. **B:** A covered stent was deployed and postprocedural angiogram shows pseudoaneurysm resolution with patency of the hepatic vessels.

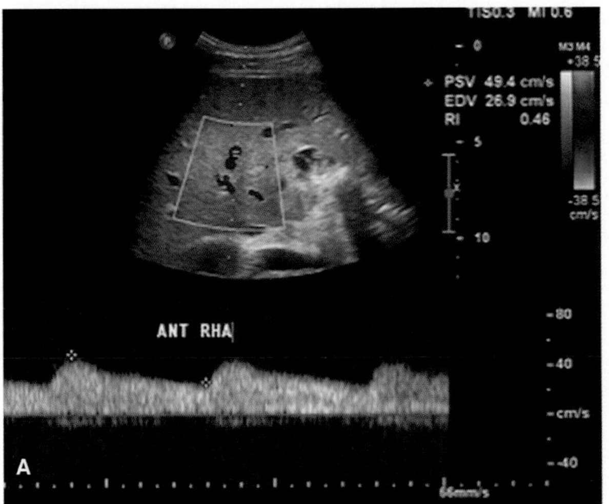

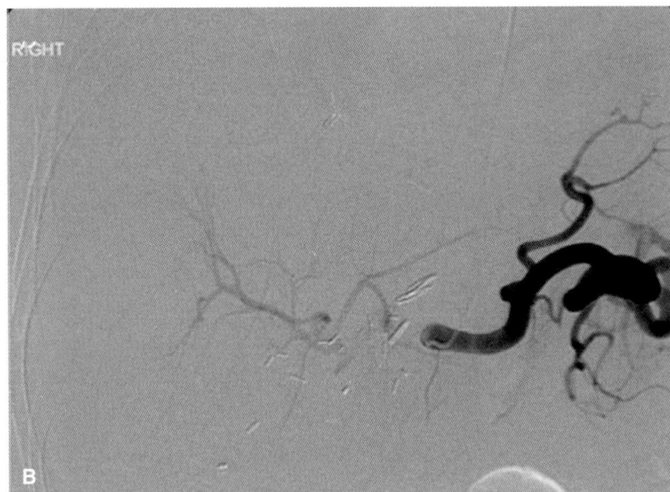

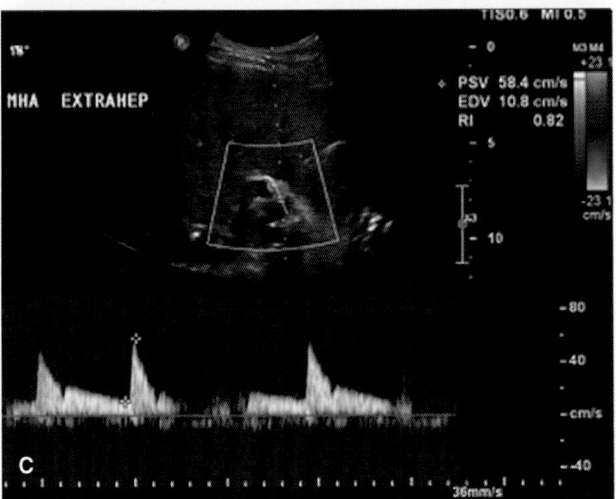

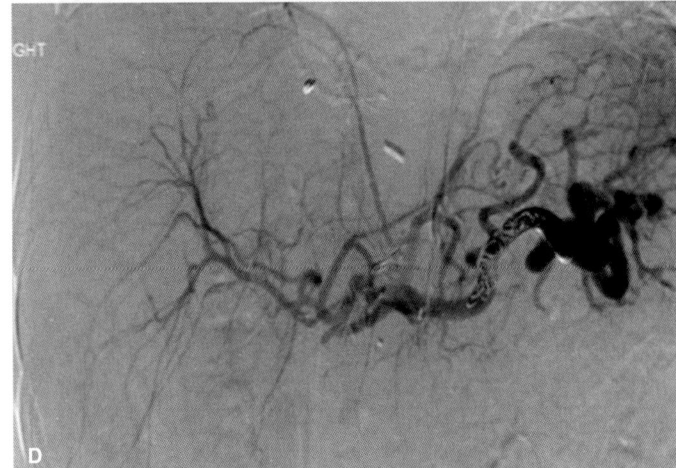

FIGURE 37B.7. **Splenic Steal Syndrome. A:** Ultrasound Doppler intrahepatic tardus parvus waveform morphology. **B:** Celiac angiogram demonstrates decreased intrahepatic vessels and predominant flow into an enlarged splenic artery. **C:** Following splenic artery embolization, Doppler ultrasound demonstrates normalization of the hepatic artery waveform. **D:** End-result celiac angiogram demonstrates opacification of intraparenchymal branches of the hepatic artery with significant flow redistribution.

options for PV thrombosis are available including anticoagulation, angioplasty, stenting, thrombectomy, or thrombolysis.

Hepatic Infarct. Hepatic infarcts are also important to discuss regarding the transplanted liver vascular supply. Hepatic infarcts are rare in the native liver as blood flow is maintained via the HA, PV, and collateral vessels. However, since collateral vessels are ligated in transplanted patients, the graft liver is more susceptible to ischemic injury. Eighty-five percent of infarcts in post-OLT recipients are associated with HA complications, but infarct secondary to PV occlusion can also be seen. Furthermore, infarcts can be complicated by abscess formation. At this point, percutaneous drainage is indicated to obtain cultures to direct proper antibiotic therapy and as definitive management.

Renal Inflow

Like a native kidney, a renal allograft is an end organ with only one blood supply, the RA. Complications affecting the RA after transplant are stenosis, thrombosis, pseudoaneurysm, and AV fistula.

Renal Artery Stenosis (RAS). RAS occurs after transplantation in 0.9% to 8% of patients. The clinical presentation of RAS after transplant includes a bruit heard over the graft, new-onset hypertension, and allograft dysfunction. Typical presentation occurs at 3 months to 2 years after transplantation, with stenosis most commonly found at the anastomosis. End-to-end anastomoses with the internal iliac arteries more commonly develop RAS than end-to-side anastomoses with the external iliac arteries. Common causes of RAS are atherosclerotic disease of the donor or recipient, arterial damage during organ harvest, surgical technique, and cytomegalovirus infection.

Doppler US is the most sensitive and specific diagnostic examination for transplant RAS. Diagnosis is made with PSV of greater than 200 to 300 cm/s at the anastomotic site; higher values have an increased specificity and positive predictive value. Tardus parvus waveforms can be seen distal to the stenosis in the main RA on spectral Doppler US. The ratio of main RA to external iliac artery can also be used with a ratio greater than 1.8 suggestive of RAS.

If the sonographic window is compromised or vessel tortuosity/kinking are suspected, CTA or MRA can be obtained for confirmation. A luminal narrowing of 50% or greater is considered hemodynamically significant. Angioplasty is

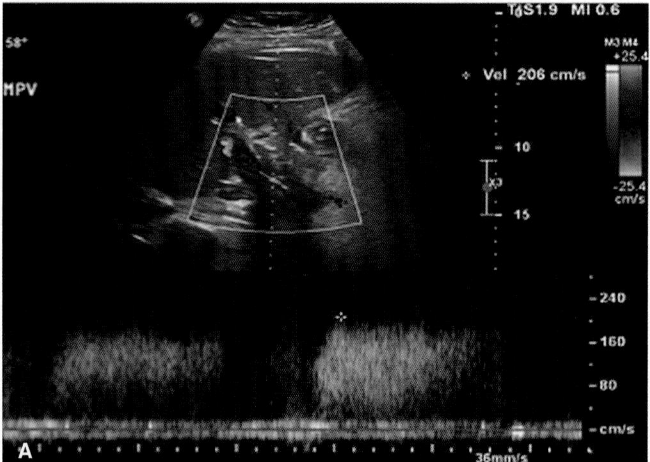

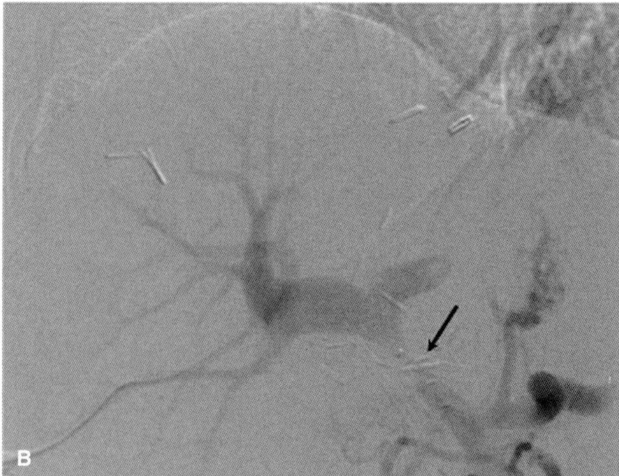

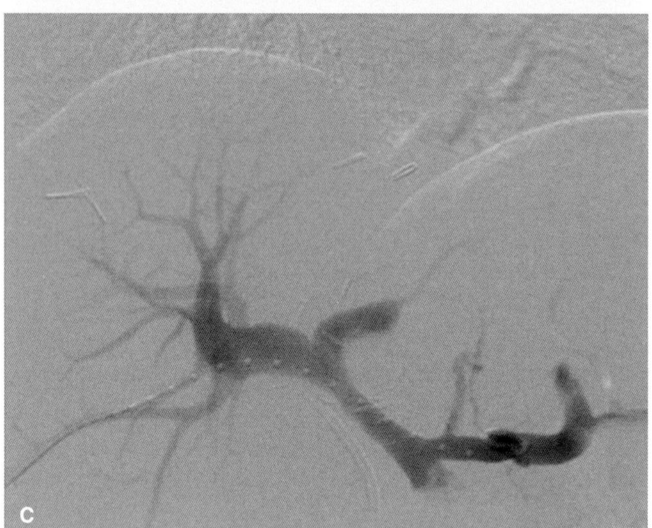

FIGURE 37B.8. **Portal Vein Stenosis. A:** Ultrasound performed to evaluate abnormal liver function tests demonstrates an elevated velocity (206 cm/s) at the portal vein anastomosis. **B:** Image from portal venogram performed via percutaneous approach demonstrates marked anastomotic narrowing (*arrow*). **C:** Portal venogram following angioplasty and stent placement was performed demonstrating resolution of the stricture.

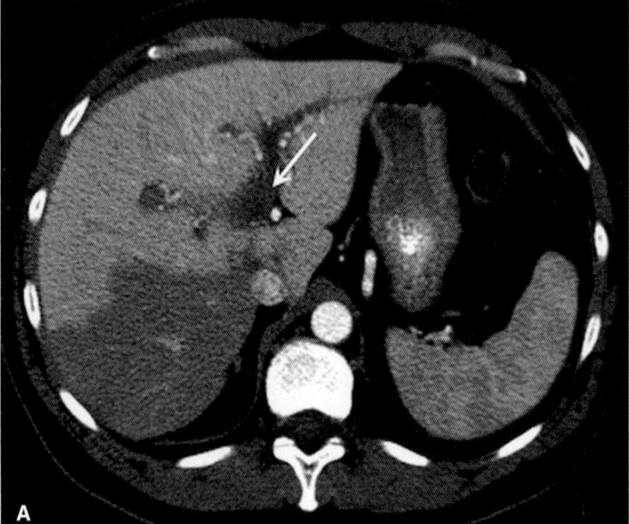

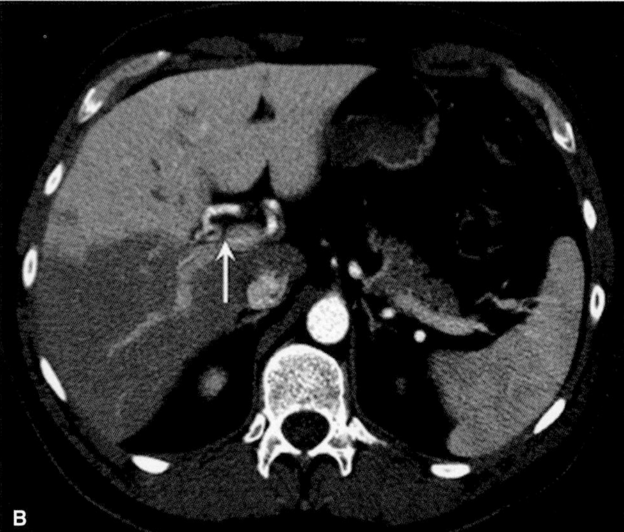

FIGURE 37B.9. **Transient Hepatic Attenuation Difference (THAD)—Portal Vein Thrombosis. A:** CTA of the abdomen in a delayed arterial phase demonstrates a thrombosed left portal vein (*arrow*) (**B**), while the right portal vein remains patent (*arrow*). The "normal" liver appears hypodense as it relies upon the normal liver circulation deriving most of its blood supply from the PV. The hyperdense "abnormal" liver, having lost its portal vein supply due to thrombosis, now relies solely upon the HA and demonstrates increased early enhancement.

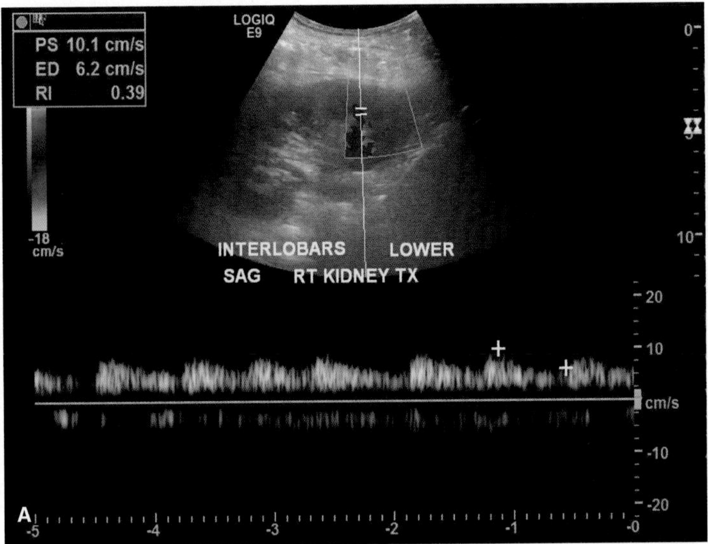

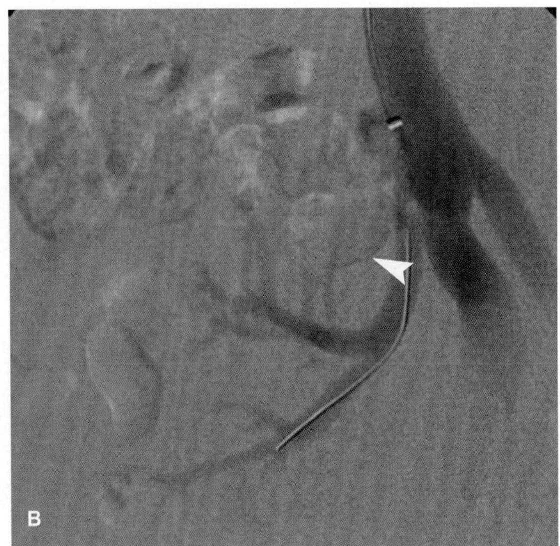

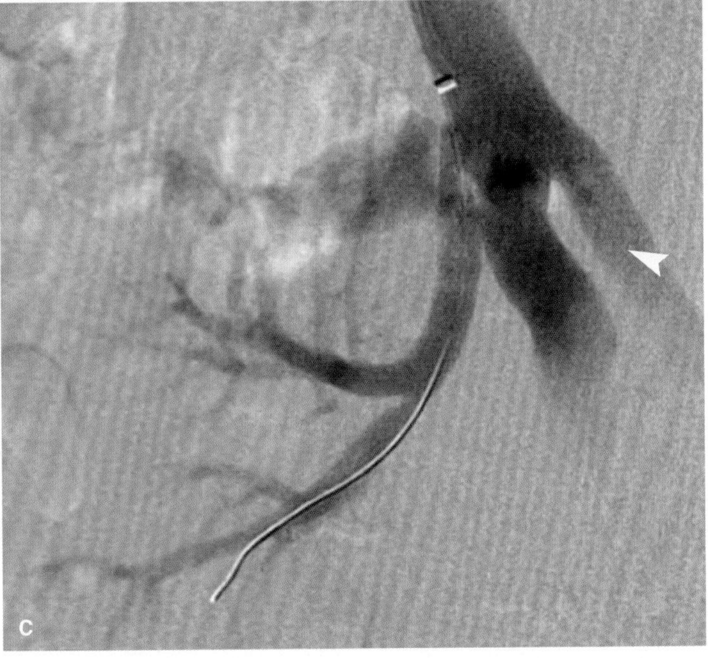

FIGURE 37B.10. **Renal Artery Stenosis. A:** Duplex renal sonography shows tardus parvus (slow and diminished upstroke during systole) with decreased resistive indices and decreased velocity. **B:** Renal artery angiogram confirms the proximal arterial stenosis (*arrow*). **C:** Following stent placement, renal artery angiogram demonstrates resolution of the anastomotic stricture (*arrow*).

appropriate treatment with stents used as second treatment after angioplasty (Fig. 37B.10).

Renal Artery Thrombosis. RA thrombosis typically occurs in the immediate postoperative period and presents with acute urine reduction and elevated creatinine. This occurs in 0.4% to 3.5% of recipients. Etiologies of RA thrombosis include vessel kinking, arterial dissection, hypercoagulable states, rejection, and immunosuppressive drug toxicity. No vascular flow is identified on Doppler or power Doppler US in RA thrombosis. Confirmatory contrast-enhanced CT or MRI will demonstrate lack of opacification of the RA and its branch vessels.

Quick treatment is required to prevent graft loss. Surgical thrombectomy can be attempted. Catheter-directed thrombolysis is contraindicated in the first 14 days after transplantation because of associated bleeding complications; however, it can be attempted if RA thrombosis occurs after the immediate postoperative period.

Renal Artery Pseudoaneurysm. Similar to the HA, pseudoaneurysms of the RA can occur at the site of anastomoses but are more common in the renal allograft after biopsy or from infection. On grayscale US, pseudoaneurysms appear as anechoic or hypoechoic cysts with turbulent, or “yin–yang,” flow on Doppler US. Spectral waveforms show “to-and-fro” flow that traverses above and below the baseline. Confirmatory CTA or MRA can be obtained but is not usually necessary. Treatment includes graded extrinsic pressure, direct percutaneous thrombin injection, or transcatheter embolization (Fig. 37B.11).

Arteriovenous Fistula. Arteriovenous fistulas (AVFs) are commonly complications due to laceration of adjacent arterial and venous structures during allograft biopsy that results in the creation of an abnormal communication between the two vessels. AVFs cannot usually be identified on grayscale US, so spectral waveform analysis is key. The arterial component of the fistula will have a high-velocity, low-impedance waveform; whereas, the venous component will be arterialized. If the AVF is large enough, the turbulent flow will propagate vibrations into the surrounding tissues causing a “soft tissue bruit,” or color flow artifact in the adjacent renal parenchyma

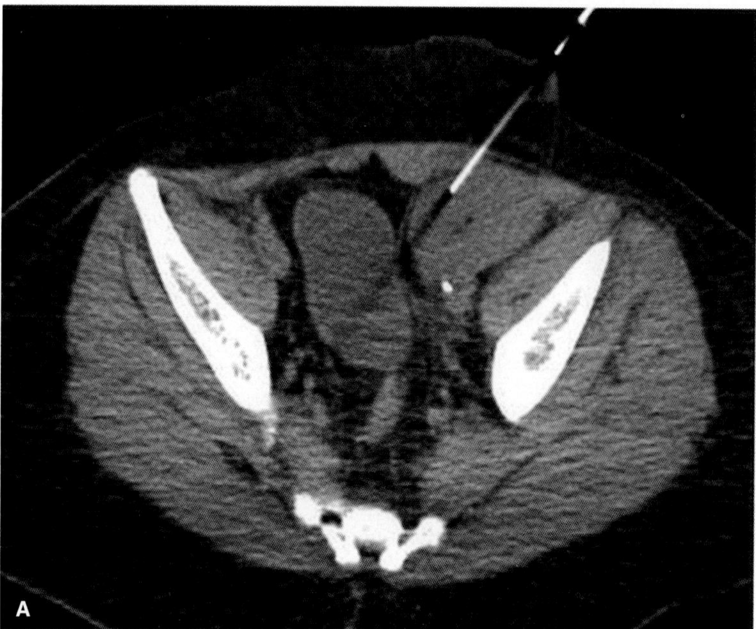

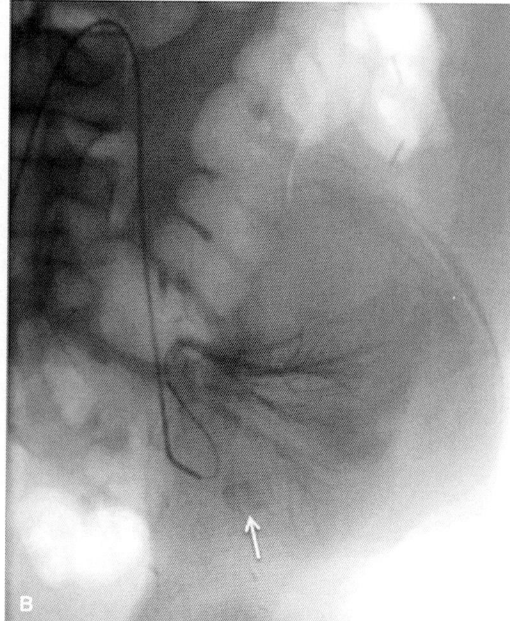

FIGURE 37B.11. Renal Artery Pseudoaneurysm. A: Axial noncontrast CT during percutaneous biopsy shows biopsy needle in the lower pole of the transplanted kidney. **B:** Renal artery angiogram after the patient presented with hematuria and flank pain confirms the presence of multiple small pseudoaneurysms following biopsy (*arrow*).

on color Doppler. Most AVFs are small and do not require intervention; however, treatment of large or symptomatic AVFs is controversial. Transcatheter embolization may be performed (Fig. 37B.12).

Hepatic Outflow

IVC Stenosis. IVC stenosis occurs in less than 1% of OLT patients and may be due to either anastomotic narrowing

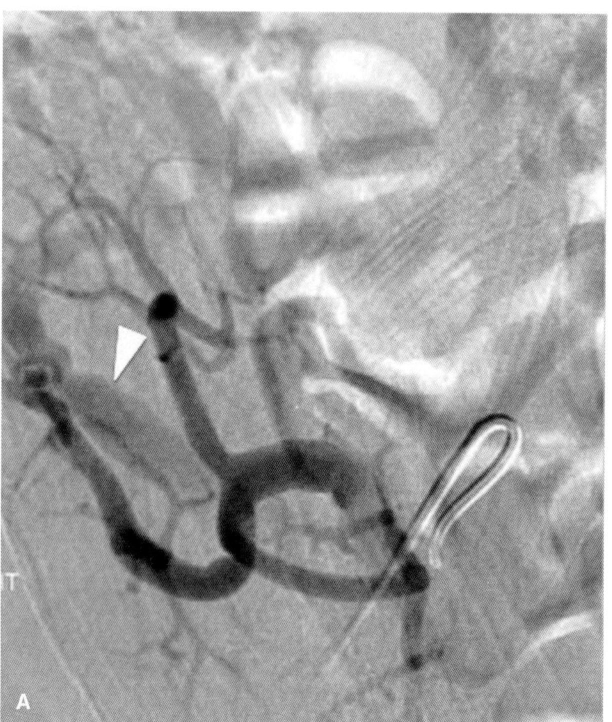

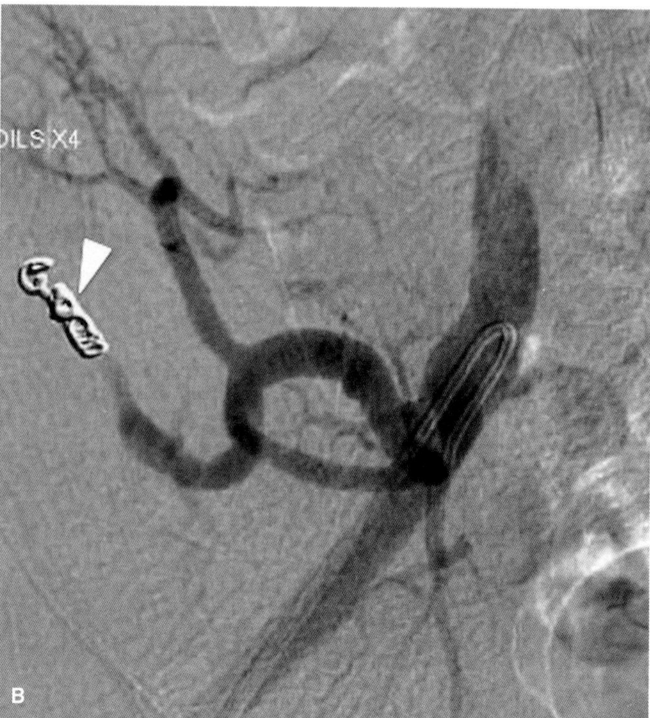

FIGURE 37B.12. Renal Artery Arteriovenous Fistula. A: Right renal artery angiogram demonstrates contrast enhancement of the renal vein (*arrowhead*). **B:** Renal artery angiogram following superselective coil embolization demonstrates complete closure of the fistulous tract (*arrowhead*).

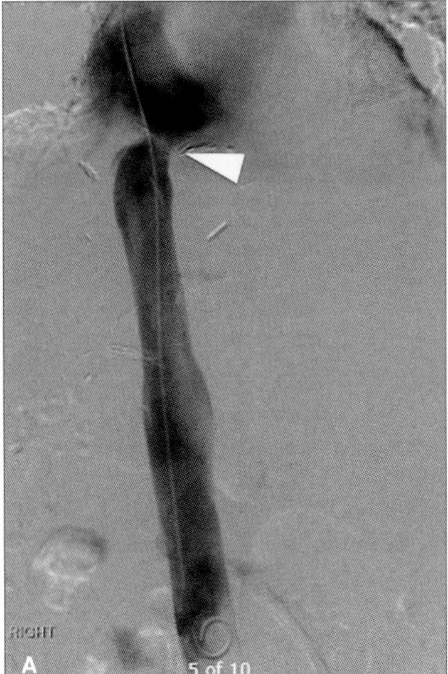

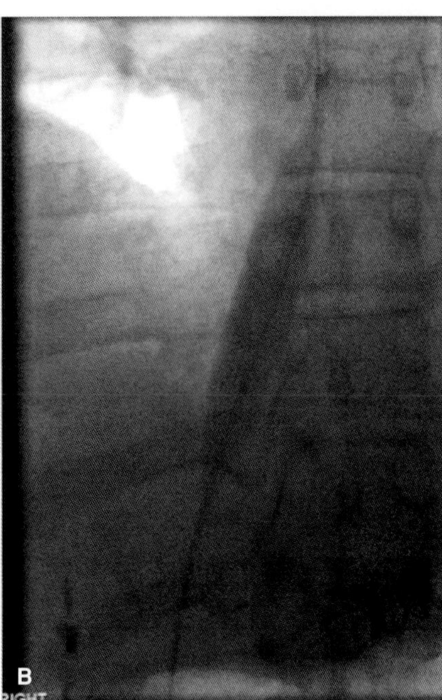

FIGURE 37B.13. **IVC Stenosis. A:** Inferior vena cavogram demonstrates stenosis and the cavoatrial junction (*arrowhead*). **B:** The stenosis is no longer seen after balloon dilation of the area with an Atlas balloon.

or extrinsic compression secondary to graft edema, adjacent fluid collections, or hematoma. In IVC stenosis, Doppler US demonstrates a three-to fourfold increase in velocity at the site of stenosis as compared to the nonaffected IVC. CT and MR venography may be used for confirmation of Doppler US findings and may show an area of focal narrowing (Fig. 37B.10) or imaging features of the Budd–Chiari syndrome (postsinusoidal hypertension), such as distention of the HVs, loss of respiratory phasicity within the HVs, hepatomegaly, ascites, and pleural effusions. Definitive treatment is usually with angioplasty or stenting (Fig. 37B.13).

IVC Thrombosis. IVC thrombosis is usually secondary to surgical factors or underlying hypercoagulable states. Doppler US will demonstrate echogenic intraluminal thrombus within the IVC. CT or MR venogram will confirm the diagnosis and will demonstrate low-density/intensity intraluminal thrombus.

Hepatic Vein Stenosis. HV stenosis usually occurs in living-donor OLT. Doppler US will demonstrate a pulsatility index of ≤0.5 as well as monophasic waveforms. This diagnosis is usually confirmed by the use of venography and treated with angioplasty of the stenosis (Fig. 37B.14).

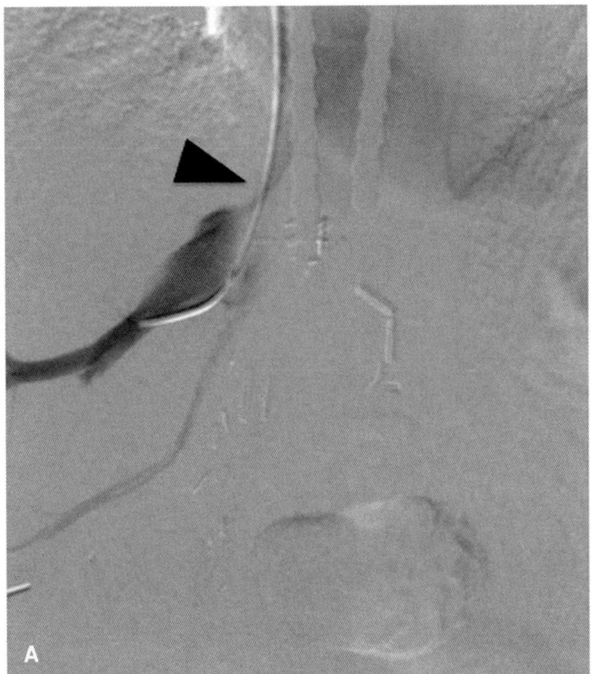

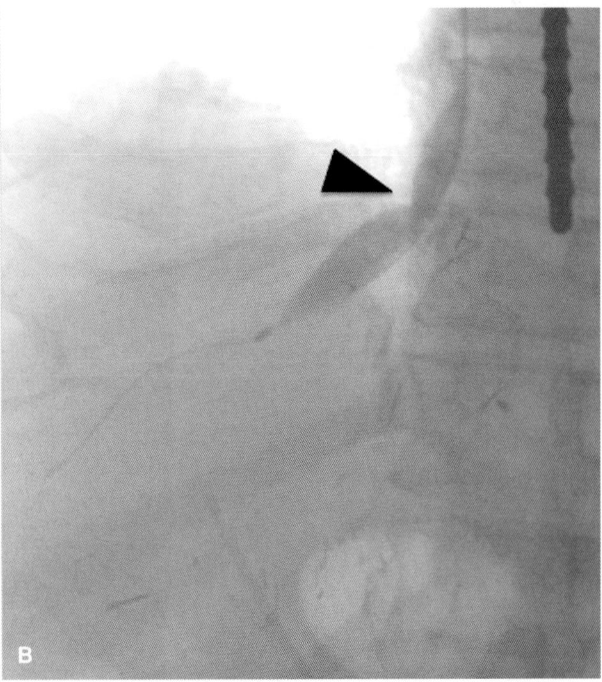

FIGURE 37B.14. **Hepatic Vein Stenosis. A:** Middle hepatic venogram demonstrates stenosis and the piggyback anastomosis (*arrowhead*). **B:** The stenosis causes a significant waist during balloon dilation of the area with an Atlas balloon (*arrowhead*).

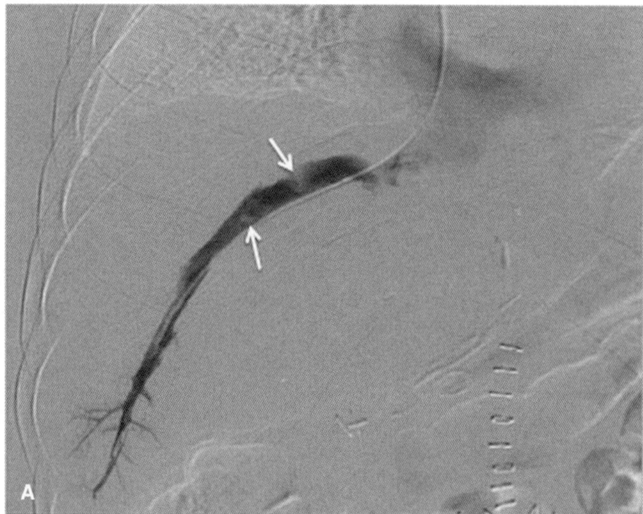

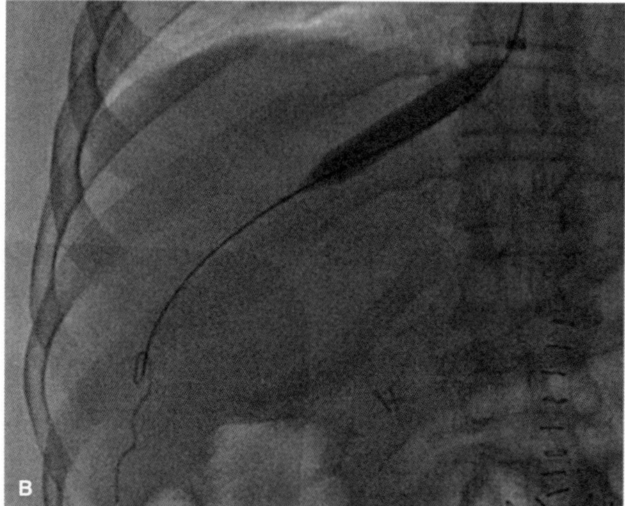

FIGURE 37B.15. **Hepatic Vein Thrombosis. A:** Right hepatic venogram demonstrates multiple filling defects inside the vein (*arrows*). **B:** Balloon maceration of the clot burden was performed with a Conquest balloon.

Hepatic Vein Thrombosis. Doppler US in HV thrombosis will show absent hepatic venous flow. CT or MR with contrast will confirm lack of venous flow within the HVs and may demonstrate intraluminal-filling defect suggestive of thrombus. In addition, CT and MR imaging may demonstrate a mosaic perfusion pattern characteristic of the Budd–Chiari syndrome (Fig. 37B.13). Treatment options include balloon angioplasty (Fig. 37B.15).

Renal Outflow

Renal Vein Thrombosis. Transplant RV thrombosis presents clinically with pain, fever, and swelling in the area of the graft with or without ipsilateral lower extremity edema. It occurs in 0.55% to 4% of patients, usually in the early postoperative period. Factors causing early RV thrombosis include prolonged ischemia, extrinsic vein compression, vein torsion, or hypercoagulable states. RV thrombosis occurring later than the postoperative period can be due to acute rejection or immunosuppressive drugs.

Doppler US is the best initial diagnostic examination to diagnose RV thrombosis. The RV will have an absence of flow, and the main RA typically demonstrates an extremely high-resistance waveform with reversal of diastolic flow. However, reversal of diastolic flow in the RA alone is not pathognomonic for RV thrombosis, as hydronephrosis, rejection, and extrinsic compression of the allograft can cause this as well. Clinical presentation and US are usually adequate for diagnosis, and contrast-enhanced CT or MR are not usually necessary; however, they will demonstrate a lack of opacification of the RV with internal thrombus present (Fig. 37B.16).

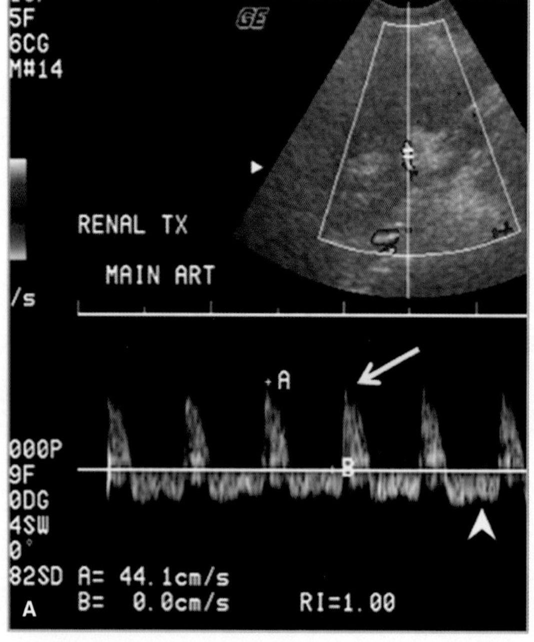

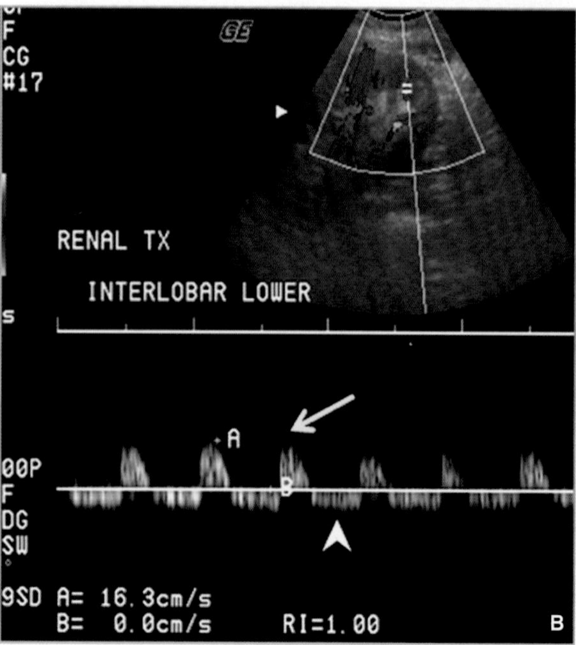

FIGURE 37B.16. **Renal Vein Thrombosis.** Duplex renal sonography (**A**) and (**B**) shows abnormal arterial waveform with broad systolic peak (*arrows*) and pandiastolic reversal (*arrowheads*).

Previously, the treatment was allograft removal due to concerns of transplant rupture or death. Surgical thrombectomy in the postoperative period is now attempted, and catheter-directed thrombolysis is used for later RV thrombosis. However, allografts are still often lost despite these efforts.

BILIARY COMPLICATIONS

As a whole, post-OLT biliary complications occur in up to 25% of patients, usually within the first few months following transplant and are second in incidence only to rejection. Complications of the biliary system may be divided into leakage and obstruction.

Biliary Leak

Biliary leaks occur in approximately 5% of liver transplant recipients and usually within the first few months following the transplant. Biliary leaks may first be identified via US or CT and appear as rounded fluid collections. Biliary leaks most commonly occur at the T-tube site if one was left behind, and can often be diagnosed via cholangiography (direct or MR), biliary scintigraphy, or aspiration of a fluid collection (biloma), which was previously identified on US or CT. Biliary leaks are confirmed by endoscopic retrograde cholangiopancreatography (ERCP), MRI with hepatobiliary contrast agents or HIDA scans; and treated by placement of a biliary stent. If ERCP is not possible, percutaneous transhepatic cholangiography with drain placement may be employed (Fig. 37B.17).

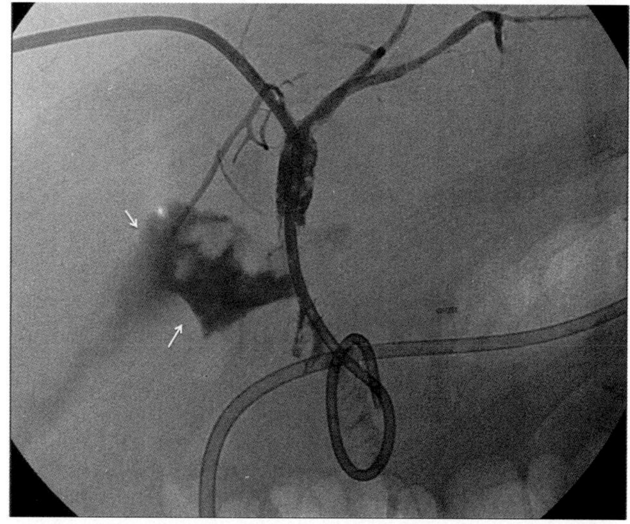

FIGURE 37B.17. **Biliary Leak.** Cholangiogram demonstrates active extravasation of contrasts at the anastomosis (*arrows*); finding consistent with a leak. An internal–external biliary drain was left in place to help controlling the leak.

Biliary Obstruction

Post-OLT biliary obstructions may be subdivided into strictures and stones/debris. Biliary strictures may be extrahepatic at the site of anastomosis, usually secondary to scar formation. Alternatively, biliary strictures may be intrahepatic secondary to ischemia, infection, or primary sclerosing cholangitis recurrence in selected cases. Imaging via direct cholangiography or magnetic resonance cholangiopancreatography (MRCP) usually demonstrates postobstructive dilatation of the donor common bile duct. Incomplete obstruction can be treated with balloon dilatation or stenting; whereas, complete obstruction requires surgical intervention (Fig. 37B.18).

Biliary obstruction secondary to stones/debris occurs in approximately 6% of OLT patients. Obstruction secondary

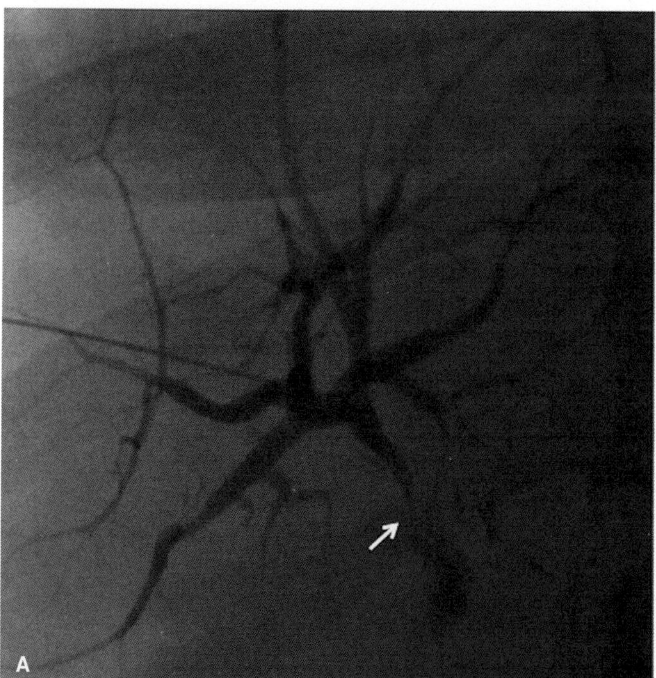

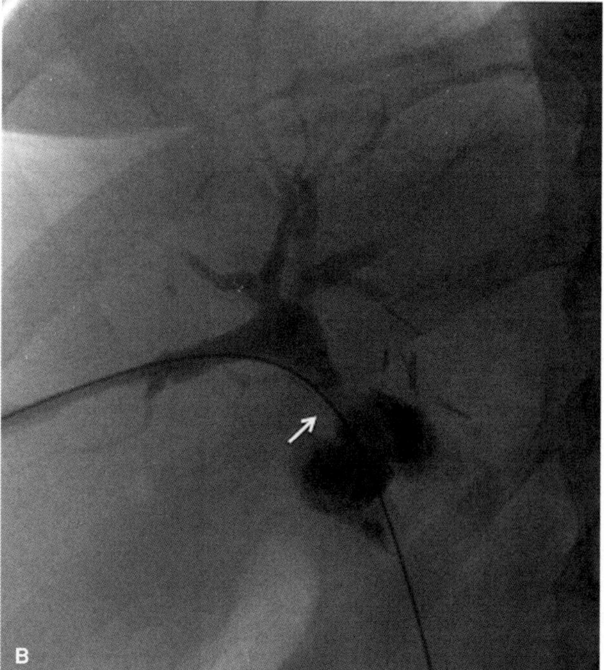

FIGURE 37B.18. **Enterobiliary Anastomotic Stricture. A:** Cholangiogram shows moderately dilated intrahepatic biliary radicals with a high-grade stricture at the hepaticojejunostomy (*arrow*). **B:** Following percutaneous management of the stricture, which included a large-bore percutaneous biliary drain as well as cholangioplasties, the cholangiogram now demonstrates a widely patent anastomosis (*arrow*).

to stones is usually a late complication seen years after OLT; whereas, obstruction secondary to debris is seen earlier and usually secondary to cholangitis, infection, rejection, or ischemia. MRCP may help to distinguish stones from debris. Treatment is via ERCP with endoscopic sphincterotomy and debris/stone removal with or without temporary stent placement (Fig. 37B.15). If ERCP is not possible, a percutaneous access can be obtained.

URINARY COMPLICATIONS

Urine Leak

Urine leak is often an early complication in the postoperative period, occurring 4 to 29 days after transplantation and in 1.1% to 6.5% of patients. Causes include direct injury during organ harvest or implantation and ischemic necrosis from vascular compromise. The most common site of leak is the distal ureter, followed by the urinary bladder, and then the proximal ureter/renal collecting system.

Urine leaks appear as fluid collections on imaging. On US, the fluid is anechoic to hypoechoic with or without internal debris. CT will demonstrate a low attenuating collection (<10 HU). MRI signal is T1 hypointense and T2 hyperintense; however, there may be heterogeneity due to internal debris. If renal function allows for iodinated contrast administration, delayed images (5 to 20 minutes) after injection can demonstrate the leak or at least accumulation of the concentrated contrast in the collection. Alternatively, technetium-99m scintigraphy or gadolinium-based contrast agents with MRI can be used (Fig. 37B.19).

Large urine leaks are percutaneously drained under image guidance. However, it is important to determine the location and size of the leak. Defects in the collecting system or ureter can be treated with a retrograde stent if small, but larger leaks require urethral reimplantation, ureteroureterostomy, and/or nephrostomy tube placement. Larger urinary bladder leaks require surgical repair, but smaller ones can be treated with catheter drainage. These interventions are almost always successful.

Urinary Obstruction

Urinary obstruction can be defined as primary, related to a primary collecting system stricture, or secondary, due to extrinsic compression from a crossing vessel or fluid collection. Primary urinary obstruction can occur early when related to technical or anatomic factors. Ureteral strictures also cause urinary obstruction and occur in 2.6% to 6.5% of patients. These occur later in a median time of 6 months, and are related to ischemia.

Renal US will demonstrate a dilated renal collecting system. Color Doppler should be used to confirm the anechoic tubular areas are dilated calyces, and not large vessels; vessels will demonstrate flow; whereas, hydronephrosis will remain anechoic (Fig. 37B.20). The entire ureter should be traced to determine the level of obstruction; in addition, the urethral jet should be monitored to determine if the obstruction is incomplete. High-resistance waveforms with possible reversal of diastolic flow can be seen in the RA.

Treatment for the obstruction is typically percutaneous nephroureteral stenting. However, there is often still the necessity for surgical repair or ureteral reimplantation.

EXTRINSIC COMPLICATIONS

Abdominal Fluid Collections

Following transplantation, postoperative hematomas, lymphoceles, and urinomas may be routinely identified in the

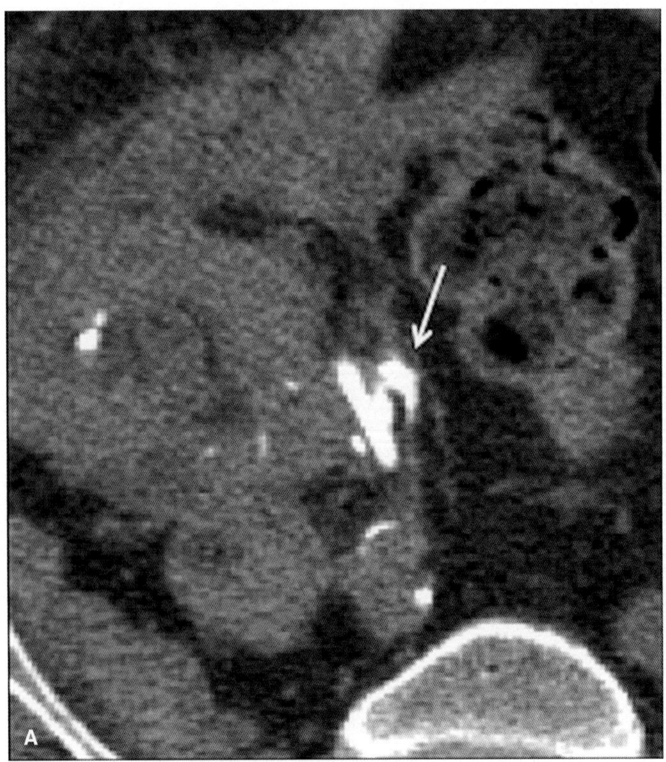

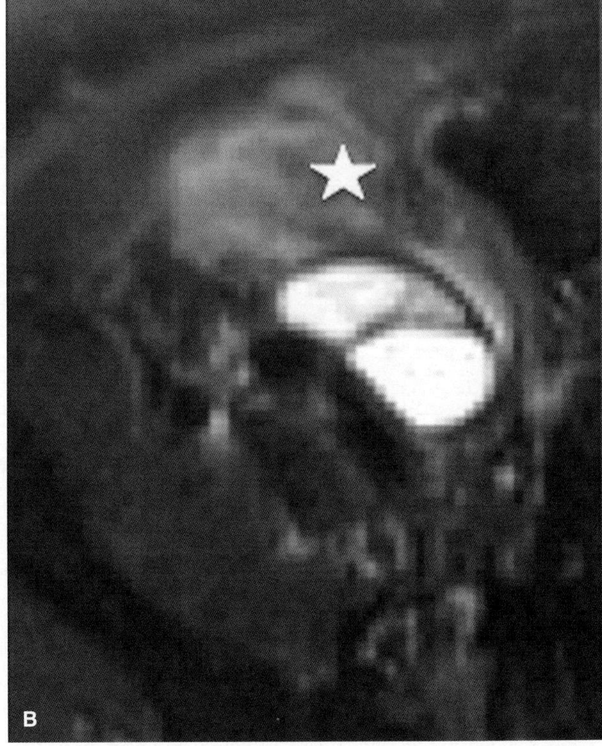

FIGURE 37B.19. Urine Leak and Urinoma. A: CT cystogram illustrates contrast leak from the ureter (*arrow*). **B:** Follow-up MRI axial T2WI reveals a small urinoma (*) at the site of ureteroureteric anastomosis.

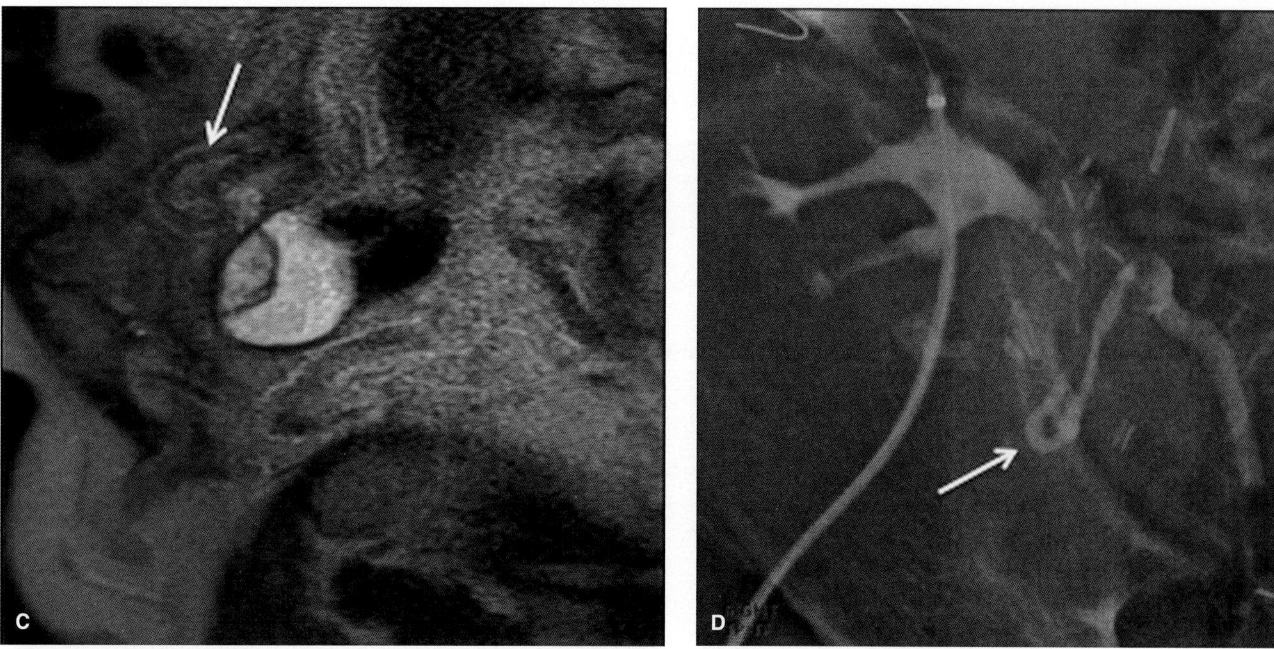

FIGURE 37B.19. (*Continued*) **C:** Sagittal T2WI reveals periureteric edema (*arrow*). **D:** Percutaneous nephrostogram shows no contrast leak, suggesting interval closure of the urine leak. Note tortuous course of ureter (*arrow*).

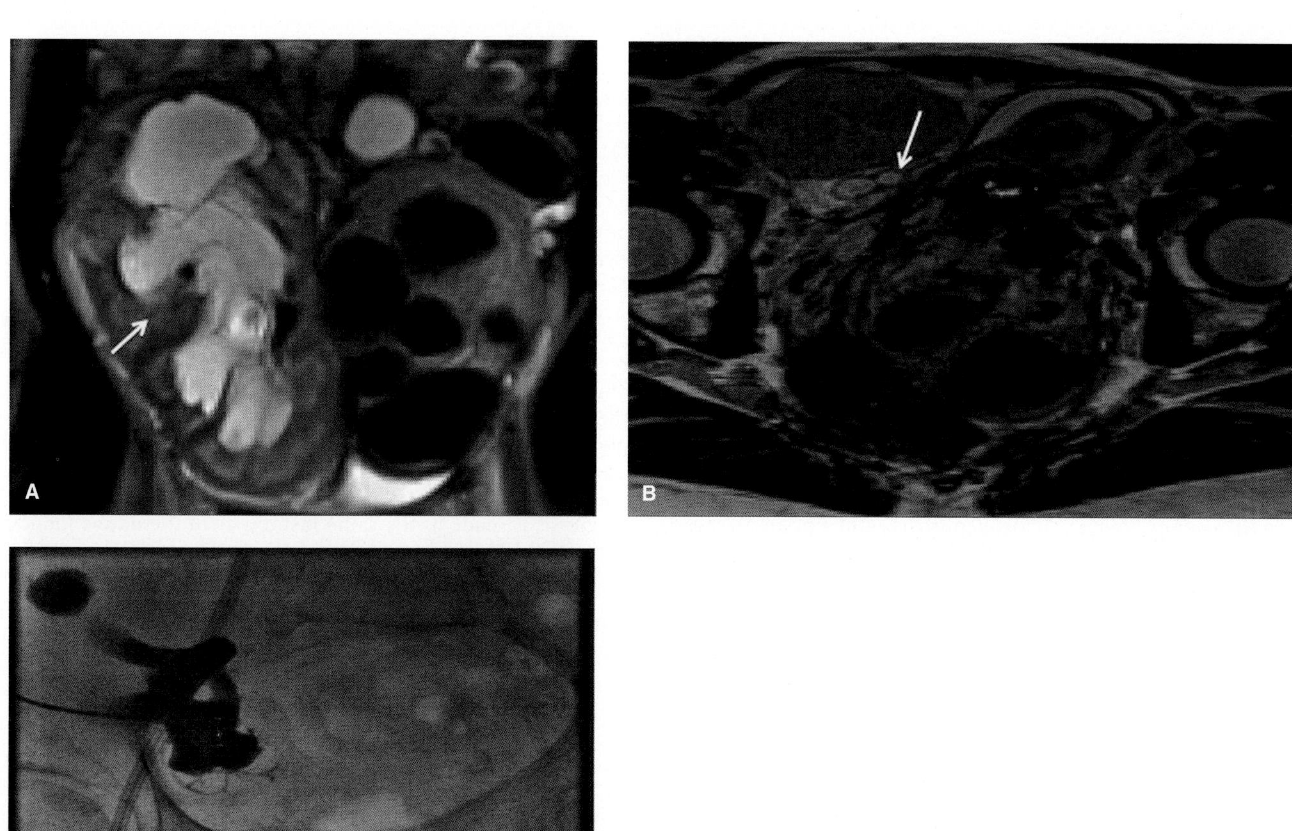

FIGURE 37B.20. **Ureteral Stricture Causing Urinary Obstruction. A:** Coronal T2WI demonstrates severe hydronephrosis (*arrow*). **B:** T2 SPACE sequence thin slices depict distal ureteral stricture (*arrow*). **C:** Percutaneous nephrostogram confirms obstruction without passage of contrast into the bladder.

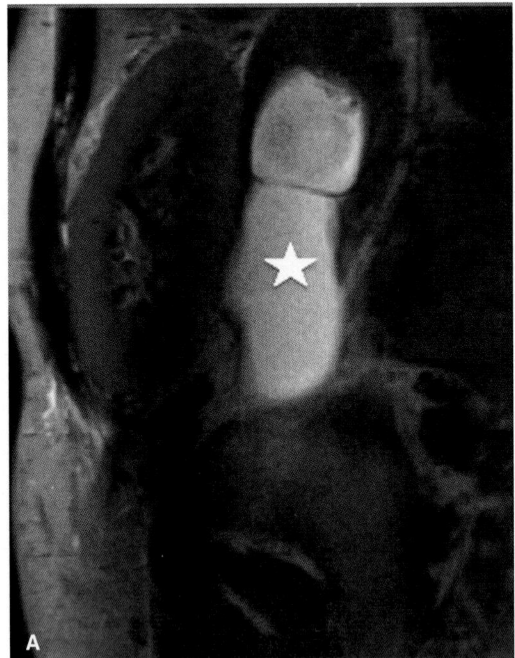

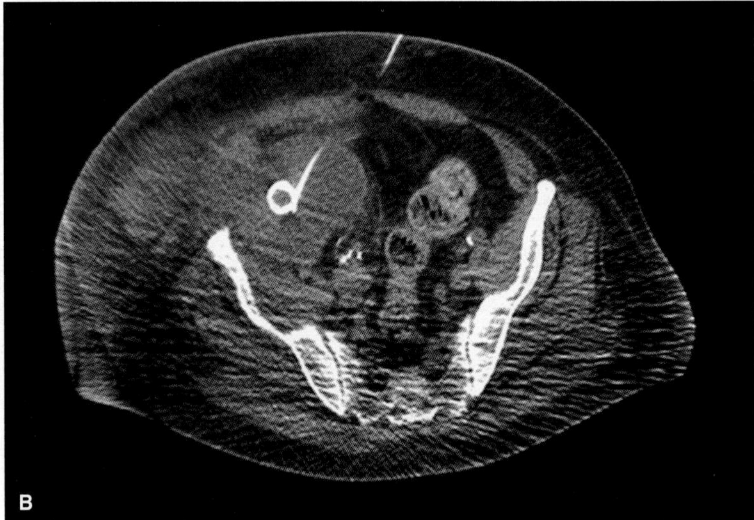

FIGURE 37B.21. **Lymphocele. A:** Sagittal T2WI shows posterior hyperintense peritransplant fluid collection (*) adjacent to the vessels. **B:** Percutaneous drainage confirmed the presence of a lymphocele.

perianastomotic regions (vascular, biliary, and urinary) but usually resolve within weeks. Intra- and perigraft fluid collections may first be identified by US but are more easily characterized by CT/MR (Fig. 37B.16). Differential considerations when evaluating intra-abdominal, perigraft fluid collections include loculated ascites, abscess, biloma/urinoma, lymphocele, or hematoma. These collections are usually amenable to image-guided aspiration and drainage, which can be both diagnostic and therapeutic (Fig. 37B.21).

Hematomas will have a heterogeneous appearance on US. On CT, the collection of blood will be greater than 40 HU, and on MRI, there will be areas of low-to-high T1- and T2-intensity depending on the age. Drainage of hematomas is not generally advised because the solid clot will not adequately drain through a catheter, and hematoma, which was previously sterile, may become infected. Lymphoceles are due to lymph leaking from recipient lymphatic channels. They can result in pain, edema, hydronephrosis, and impaired graft function. They develop in 3.3% of patients.

On US, lymphoceles are anechoic to hypoechoic and may contain septations. On CT and MRI, they are well circumscribed with low (less than 10 HU) attenuation and T1 hypointense/T2 hyperintense. Larger or symptomatic lymphoceles require treatment. Percutaneous drainage can be attempted but has a 30% recurrence rate and 17% infection rate. Surgical drainage with fenestration has a 7% recurrence rate. Urinomas and bilomas usually appear as well-circumscribed collections with similar imaging appearance and treatment.

INTRINSIC COMPLICATIONS

PTLD is caused by the Epstein–Barr viral infection in an immunocompromised host and usually arises 4 to 8 months posttransplantation. The clinical spectrum includes polyclonal proliferation of lymphocytes to high-grade monoclonal lymphoma (non-Hodgkin). Radiographically, PTLD may present as soft tissue masses within the allograft or bowel as well as hilar and retroperitoneal lymphadenopathy (Fig. 37B.22).

Hepatocellular carcinoma (HCC) is an uncommon post-OLT complication given the rigorous selection criteria for OLT recipients with early-stage HCC, according to the Milan or UCSF criteria. The diagnosis is made in the same fashion as in the native liver with MRI demonstrating a heterogeneous, hypervascular mass with contrast washout and presence of pseudocapsule that can have a tendency to invade venous structures (Fig. 37B.23).

RCC occurs twice as frequently in patients who have received a transplant. The overall incidence of malignancy after renal transplantation is three to five times higher than in the general population. Nonmelanoma skin cancer and lymphoma are the most common malignancies followed by RCC. The incidence of RCC is 0.5% to 1.5% among renal transplant patients occurring in the native kidneys or allograft. The diagnosis is made in the same fashion as in the native kidney with CT/MRI demonstrating a heterogeneous, hypervascular mass with contrast washout (Fig. 37B.24).

Primary sclerosing cholangitis tends to occur several years following OLT with imaging findings of hepatic atrophy, intrahepatic biliary ductal dilatation, and stenotic areas secondary to fibrosis. Cirrhosis recurrence is also uncommon and it has been reported in about 1.5% of liver transplants. In a significant number of adult patients who survived more than 12 months, a potentially treatable or preventable cause can be identified. The majority of cases are increasingly likely to be related to recurrent disease, particularly recurrent hepatitis C virus infection; however, in approximately 40% of cases, a treatable cause cannot be identified.

Allograft rejection/dysfunction is the most common post-OLT–related complication; however, it has no reliable imaging findings. Diagnosis is made via allograft biopsy usually under ultrasound guidance given that it is safe, inexpensive, and minimizes patient discomfort. However, on screening US, increasing resistive indices greater than 0.80 on Doppler US can be suggestive of such pathology.

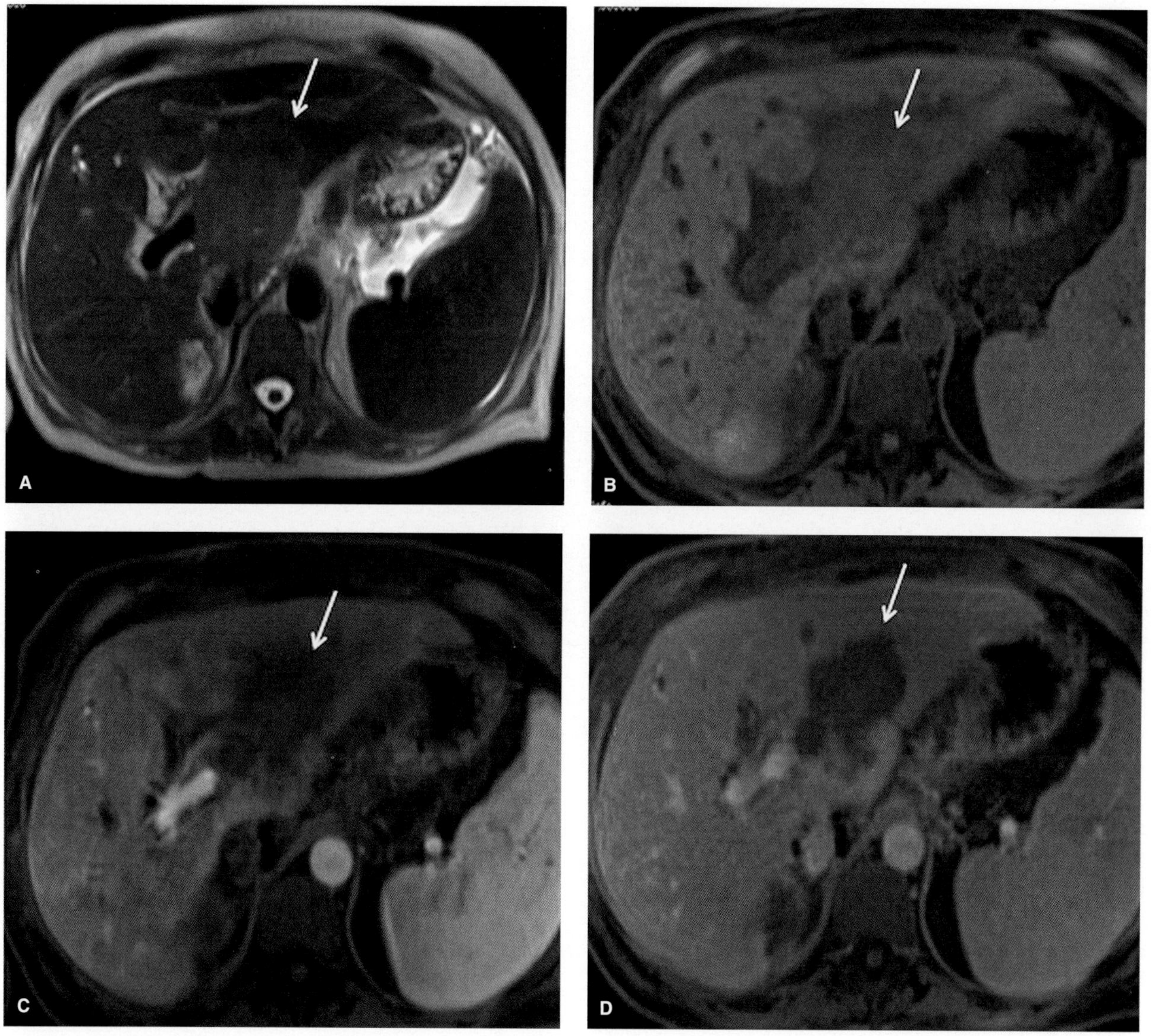

FIGURE 37B.22. **Posttransplant Lymphoproliferative Disease (PTLD). A:** Axial T2W image and axial T1W image (**B**) demonstrating intermediate high T2 signal soft tissue infiltrative periportal mass without significant arterial (**C**) or delayed enhancement (**D**) on axial contrast-enhanced T1W acquisitions (*arrows*). Biopsy confirmed PTLD in the graft.

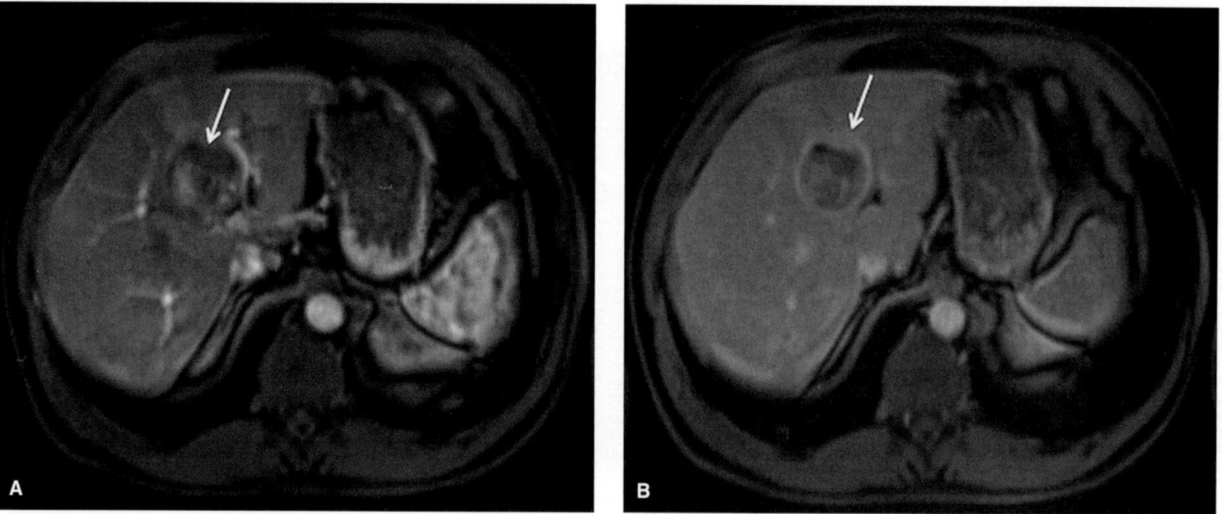

FIGURE 37B.23. **Hepatocellular Carcinoma. A:** Axial T1W arterial phase-contrast–enhanced MR demonstrates an arterially enhancing lesion (*arrow*) with washout (**B**) and delayed pseudo capsule on delayed acquisitions (*arrow*).

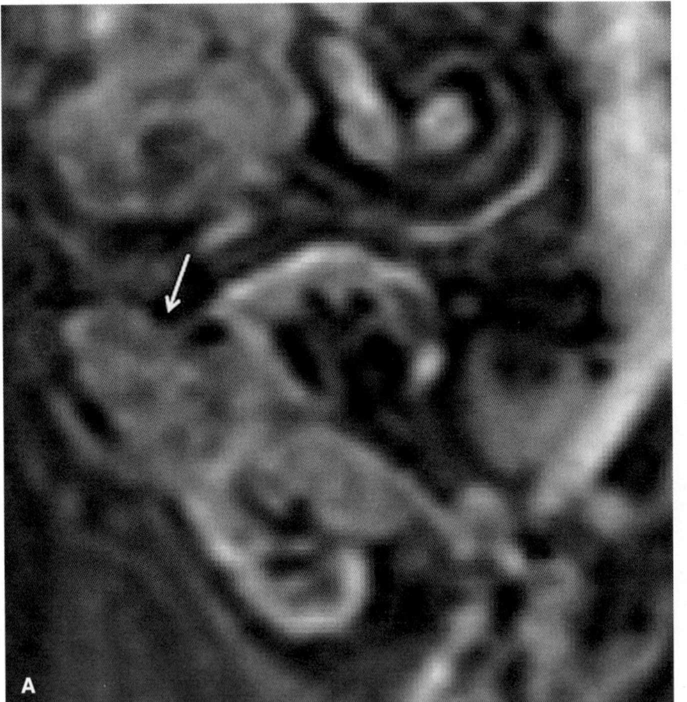

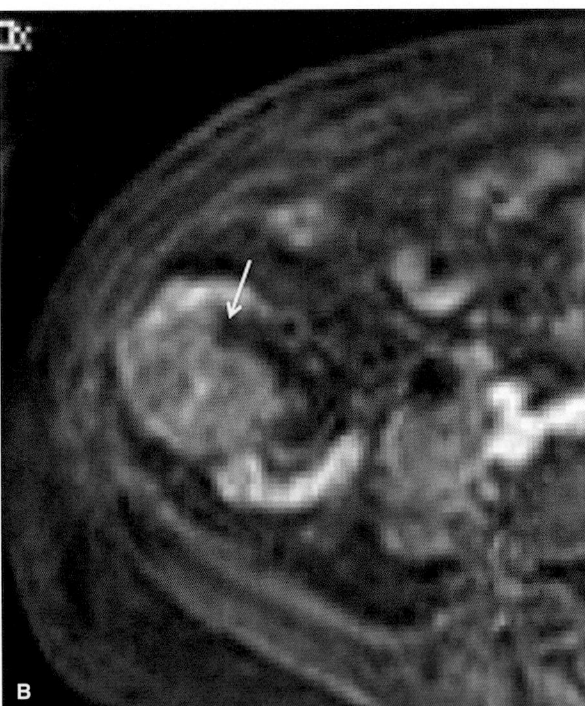

FIGURE 37B.24. **Renal Cell Carcinoma (RCC). A:** Coronal T1W image and axial T1W image (**B**) demonstrating intermediate signal intensity soft tissue renal mass (*arrows*). Biopsy confirmed RCC in the graft.

For kidney transplants, requiring dialysis within 1 week of renal transplantation is related to graft dysfunction. It can occur in up to 20% to 30% of patients and may be due to cold ischemia time or acute tubular necrosis (ATN). Biopsy, under US guidance, may be required to diagnose the underlying cause. Many patients who develop delayed graft function regain function but are at a 41% increased risk of graft loss. There are three types of renal graft rejection. Hyperacute rejection occurs immediately at the time of reperfusion in the operating room, with abrupt cessation of graft perfusion caused by cortical ischemia and small-vessel thrombosis. This causes complete loss of the allograft. Acute rejection can occur in the immediate postoperative period with deteriorating function; it occurs up to 33% of the time. Chronic rejection is seen as a slow deterioration of graft function over time. Acute and chronic rejections require biopsy, usually under US guidance, to diagnose; however, increasing resistive indices greater than 0.80 on Doppler US can be a clue (Fig. 37B.25).

CONCLUSION

Liver and kidney transplantation complications may demonstrate typical imaging manifestations and common patterns that guide diagnosis; however, findings may represent normal variants in the early posttransplantation period. Cross-sectional imaging modalities play a key role for patients with liver transplantation complications and their management decisions. Adequate knowledge of liver and kidney transplantation complications, including key imaging features and

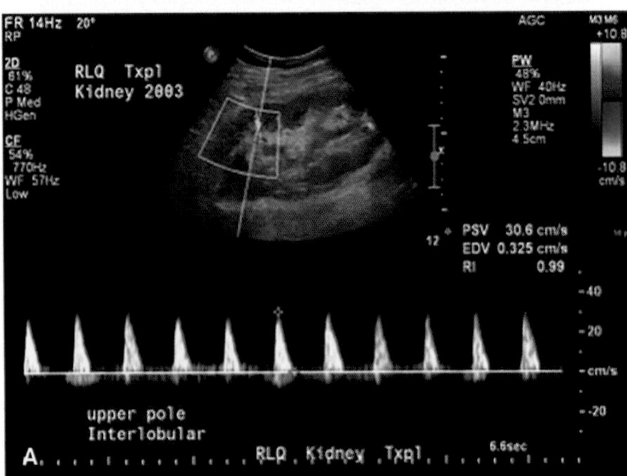

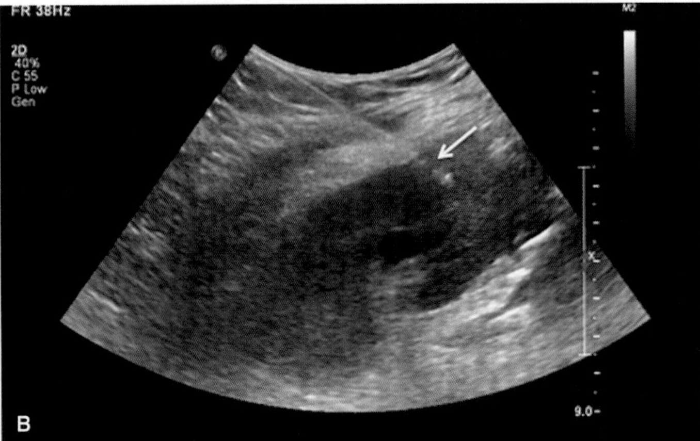

FIGURE 37B.25. **Acute Rejection. A:** Duplex renal sonography shows near-complete loss of diastolic flow and severely increased resistive indices. While this is sensitive for renal allograft dysfunction, it is not specific for rejection. **B:** US-guided percutaneous biopsy to evaluate for rejection should be performed. Note the needle tip in the lower pole of the graft (*arrow*).

potential interventional radiology procedures, is crucial. The spectrum of Doppler US findings and the confirmatory vascular-interventional imaging findings determine patient management (Fig. 37B.20).

Suggested Readings

Abbasoglu O, Levy MF, Vodapally MS, et al. Hepatic artery stenosis after liver transplantation—incidence, presentation, treatment, and long term outcome. *Transplantation* 1997:63(2):250–255.

Akbar SA, Jafri SZ, Amendola MA, Madrazo BL, Salem R, Bis KG. Complications of renal transplantation. *Radiographics* 2005;25(5):1335–1356.

Aydin C, Berber I, Altaca G, Yigit B, Titiz I. The outcome of kidney transplants with multiple renal arteries. *BMC Surg* 2004;4:4.

Bhargava P, Vaidya S, Dick AA, Dighe M. Imaging of orthotopic liver transplantation: review. *AJR Am J Roentgenol* 2011;196(3 Suppl):WS15–WS25; quiz S35–S38.

Biederman DM, Fischman AM, Titano JJ, et al. Tailoring the endovascular management of transplant renal artery stenosis. *Am J Transplant* 2015;15(4): 1039–1049.

Bischof G, Rockenschaub S, Berlakovich G, et al. Management of lymphoceles after kidney transplantation. *Transpl Int* 1998;11(4):277–280.

Broering DC, Schulte am Esch J, Fischer L, Rogiers X. Split liver transplantation. *HPB (Oxford)* 2004;6(2):76–82.

Caiado AH, Blasbalg R, Marcelino AS, et al. Complications of liver transplantation: multimodality imaging approach. *Radiographics* 2007;27(5):1401–1417.

Camacho JC, Moreno CC, Harri PA, Aguirre DA, Torres WE, Mittal PK. Posttransplantation lymphoproliferative disease: proposed imaging classification. *Radiographics* 2014;34(7):2025–2038.

Camacho JC, Moreno CC, Telleria JC, Aguirre DA, Torres WE, Mittal PK. Nonvascular post-liver transplantation complications: from US screening to cross-sectional and interventional imaging. *Radiographics* 2015;35(1): 87–104.

Cheng YF, Chen CL, Chen YS, et al. Interventional radiology in the treatment of post-liver transplant complications. *Transplant Proc* 2000;32(7):2196–2207.

Chong WK, Beland JC, Weeks SM. Sonographic evaluation of venous obstruction in liver transplants. *AJR Am J Roentgenol* 2007;188(6):W515–W521.

Crossin JD, Muradali D, Wilson SR. US of liver transplants: normal and abnormal. *Radiographics* 2003;23(5):1093–1114.

de'Angelis N, Landi F, Carra MC, Azoulay D. Managements of recurrent hepatocellular carcinoma after liver transplantation: a systematic review. *World J Gastroenterol* 2015;21(39):11185–11198.

de Morais RH, Muglia VF, Mamere AE, et al. Duplex Doppler sonography of transplant renal artery stenosis. *J Clin Ultrasound* 2003;31(3):135–141.

Dimitroulis D, Bokos J, Zavos G, et al. Vascular complications in renal transplantation: a single-center experience in 1367 renal transplantations and review of the literature. *Transplant Proc* 2009;41(5):1609–1614.

Dodd GD 3rd, Tublin ME, Shah A, Zajko AB, et al. Imaging of vascular complications associated with renal transplants. *AJR Am J Roentgenol* 1991;157(3):449–459.

Einecke G, Sis B, Reeve J, et al. Antibody-mediated microcirculation injury is the major cause of late kidney transplant failure. *Am J Transplant* 2009; 9(11):2520–2531.

Flint EW, Sumkin JH, Zajko AB, Bowen A. Duplex sonography of hepatic artery thrombosis after liver transplantation. *AJR Am J Roentgenol* 1988; 151(3):481–483.

Friedewald SM, Molmenti EP, DeJong MR, Hamper UM. Vascular and nonvascular complications of liver transplants: sonographic evaluation and correlation with other imaging modalities and findings at surgery and pathology. *Ultrasound Q* 2003;19(2):71–85; quiz 108–110.

Fulcher AS, Turner MA. Orthotopic liver transplantation: evaluation with MR cholangiography. *Radiology* 1999;211(3):715–722.

Fuller TF, Kang SM, Hirose R, Feng S, Stock PG, Freise CE. Management of lymphoceles after renal transplantation: laparoscopic versus open drainage. *J Urol* 2003;169(6):2022–2025.

Glockner JF, Forauer AR. Vascular or ischemic complications after liver transplantation. *AJR Am J Roentgenol* 1999;173(4):1055–1059.

Glockner JF, Forauer AR, Solomon H, Varma CR, Perman WH. Three-dimensional gadolinium-enhanced MR angiography of vascular complications after liver transplantation. *AJR Am J Roentgenol* 2000;174(5):1447–1453.

Golriz M, Klauss M, Zeier M, Mehrabi A. Prevention and management of lymphocele formation following kidney transplantation. *Transplant Rev (Orlando)* 2017;31(2):100–105.

Humar A, Ramcharan T, Kandaswamy R, Gillingham K, Payne WD, Matas AJ. Risk factors for slow graft function after kidney transplants: a multivariate analysis. *Clin Transplant* 2002;16(6):425–429.

Hurst FP, Abbott KC, Neff RT, et al. Incidence, predictors and outcomes of transplant renal artery stenosis after kidney transplantation: analysis of USRDS. *Am J Nephrol* 2009;30(5):459–467.

Ishigami K, Zhang Y, Rayhill S, Katz D, Stolpen A. Does variant hepatic artery anatomy in a liver transplant recipient increase the risk of hepatic artery complications after transplantation? *AJR Am J Roentgenol* 2004;183(6): 1577–1584.

Karami S, Yanik EL, Moore LE, et al. Risk of renal cell carcinoma among kidney transplant recipients in the United States. *Am J Transplant* 2016;16(12): 3479–3489.

Karlsen TH, Folseraas T, Thorburn D, Vesterhus M. Primary sclerosing cholangitis—a comprehensive review. *J Hepatol* 2017;67(6):1298–1323.

Kasiske BL, Vazquez MA, Harmon WE, et al. Recommendations for the outpatient surveillance of renal transplant recipients. American Society of Transplantation. *J Am Soc Nephrol* 2000;11(Suppl 15):S1–S86.

Keogan MT, McDermott VG, Price SK, Low VH, Baillie J. The role of imaging in the diagnosis and management of biliary complications after liver transplantation. *AJR Am J Roentgenol* 1999;173(1):215–219.

Klepanec A, Balazs T, Bazik R, Madaric J, Zilinska Z, Vulev I. Pharmacomechanical thrombectomy for treatment of acute transplant renal artery thrombosis. *Ann Vasc Surg* 2014;28(5):1314.e11–e14.

Ko GY, Sung KB, Lee S, et al. Stent placement for the treatment of portal vein stenosis or occlusion in pediatric liver transplant recipients. *J Vasc Interv Radiol* 2007;18(10):1215–1221.

Kornasiewicz O, Hołówko W, Grąt M, et al. Hepatic abscess: a rare complication after liver transplant. *Clin Transplant* 2016;30(10):1230–1235.

Laberge JM. Interventional management of renal transplant arteriovenous fistula. *Semin Intervent Radiol* 2004;21(4):239–246.

Le L, Terral W, Zea N, et al. Primary stent placement for hepatic artery stenosis after liver transplantation. *J Vasc Surg* 2015;62(3):704–709.

Li C, Kapoor B, Moon E, et al. Current understanding and management of splenic steal syndrome after liver transplant: a systematic review. *Transplant Rev (Orlando)* 2017;31(3):188–192.

Li C, Quintini C, Hashimoto K, et al. Role of Doppler sonography in early detection of splenic steal syndrome. *J Ultrasound Med* 2016;35(7):1393–1400.

Liu DY, Yi ZJ, Tang Y, Niu NN, Li JX. Three case reports of splenic artery steal syndrome after liver transplantation. *Transplant Proc* 2015;47(10): 2939–2943.

Llado L, Figueras J. Techniques of orthotopic liver transplantation. *HPB (Oxford)* 2004;6(2):69–75.

Mahmoud MZ, Al-Saadi M, Abuderman A, et al. "To-and-fro" waveform in the diagnosis of arterial pseudoaneurysms. *World J Radiol* 2015;7(5):89–99.

Mangus RS, Haag BW. Stented versus nonstented extravesical ureteroneocystostomy in renal transplantation: a metaanalysis. *Am J Transplant* 2004; 4(11):1889–1896.

Maraschio M, Giordano E. Extraperitoneal placement of the kidney prevents graft vascular kinking or rotation in simultaneous pancreas-kidney transplant (SPK). *Am J Transplant* 2016;16(Suppl 3). Available from http://atcmeetingabstracts.com/abstract/extraperitoneal-placement-of-the-kidney-prevents-graft-vascular-kinking-or-rotation-in-simultaneous-pancreas-kidney-transplant-spk. Accessed June 11, 2018.

Meersschaut V, Mortelé KJ, Troisi R, et al. Value of MR cholangiography in the evaluation of postoperative biliary complications following orthotopic liver transplantation. *Eur Radiol* 2000;10(10):1576–1581.

Mehrzad H, Mangat K. The role of interventional radiology in treating complications following liver transplantation. *ISRN Hepatol* 2012;2013:696794.

Moreno CC, Mittal PK, Ghonge NP, Bhargava P, Heller MT. Imaging complications of renal transplantation. *Radiol Clin North Am* 2016;54(2):235–249.

Moris D, Kakavia K, Argyrou C, et al. De novo renal cell carcinoma of native kidneys in renal transplant recipients: a single-center experience. *Anticancer Res* 2017;37(2):773–779.

Ng S, Tan KA, Anil G. The role of interventional radiology in complications associated with liver transplantation. *Clin Radiol* 2015;70(12):1323–1335.

Nghiem HV. Imaging of hepatic transplantation. *Radiol Clin North Am* 1998;36(2):429–443.

Nishida S, Nakamura N, Vaidya A, et al. Piggyback technique in adult orthotopic liver transplantation: an analysis of 1067 liver transplants at a single center. *HPB (Oxford)* 2006;8(3):182–188.

Ojo AO, Wolfe RA, Held PJ, Port FK, Schmouder RL. Delayed graft function: risk factors and implications for renal allograft survival. *Transplantation* 1997;63(7):968–974.

Olsen S, Burdick JF, Keown PA, Wallace AC, Racusen LC, Solez K. Primary acute renal failure ("acute tubular necrosis") in the transplanted kidney: morphology and pathogenesis. *Medicine (Baltimore)* 1989;68(3):173–187.

Orlic P, Vukas D, Drescik I, et al. Vascular complications after 725 kidney transplantations during 3 decades. *Transplant Proc* 2003;35(4):1381–1384.

Pallardó Mateu LM, Sancho Calabuig A, Capdevila Plaza L, Franco Esteve A. Acute rejection and late renal transplant failure: risk factors and prognosis. *Nephrol Dial Transplant* 2004;19(Suppl 3):iii38–iii42.

Pareja E, Cortes M, Navarro R, Sanjuan F, López R, Mir J. Vascular complications after orthotopic liver transplantation: hepatic artery thrombosis. *Transplant Proc* 2010;42(8):2970–2972.

Parera A, Salcedo M, Vaquero J, et al. Arterial complications after liver transplantation: early and late forms. *Gastroenterol Hepatol* 1999;22(8): 381–385.

Patel NH, Jindal RM, Wilkin T, et al. Renal arterial stenosis in renal allografts: retrospective study of predisposing factors and outcome after percutaneous transluminal angioplasty. *Radiology* 2001;219(3):663–667.

Peri L, Vilaseca A, Serapiao R, et al. Development of a pig model for laparoscopic kidney transplant. *Exp Clin Transplant* 2016;14(1):22–26.

Quiroga S, Sebastià MC, Margarit C, Castells L, Boyé R, Alvarez-Castells A. Complications of orthotopic liver transplantation: spectrum of findings with helical CT. *Radiographics* 2001;21(5):1085–1102.

Saad WE. Nonocclusive hepatic artery hypoperfusion syndrome (splenic steal syndrome) in liver transplant recipients. *Semin Intervent Radiol* 2012;29(2): 140–146.

Sanchez-Bueno F, Robles R, Ramírez P, et al. Hepatic artery complications after liver transplantation. *Clin Transplant* 1994;8(4):399–404.

Seyam M, Neuberger JM, Gunson BK, Hübscher SG. Cirrhosis after orthotopic liver transplantation in the absence of primary disease recurrence. *Liver Transpl* 2007;13(7):966–974.

Shah SA, Levy GA, Adcock LD, Gallagher G, Grant DR. Adult-to-adult living donor liver transplantation. *Can J Gastroenterol* 2006;20(5):339–343.

Sheng R, Orons PD, Ramos HC, Zajko AB. Dissecting pseudoaneurysm of the hepatic artery: a delayed complication of angioplasty in a liver transplant. *Cardiovasc Intervent Radiol* 1995;18(2):112–114.

Sheng R, Ramirez CB, Zajko AB, Campbell WL. Biliary stones and sludge in liver transplant patients: a 13-year experience. *Radiology* 1996;198(1):243–247.

Singh AK, Nachiappan AC, Verma HA, et al. Postoperative imaging in liver transplantation: what radiologists should know. *Radiographics* 2010;30(2): 339–351.

Soin AS, Friend PJ, Rasmussen A, et al. Donor arterial variations in liver transplantation: management and outcome of 527 consecutive grafts. *Br J Surg* 1996;83(5):637–641.

Stafford-Johnson DB, Hamilton BH, Dong Q, et al. Vascular complications of liver transplantation: evaluation with gadolinium-enhanced MR angiography. *Radiology* 1998;207(1):153–160.

Sterrett SP, Mercer D, Johanning J, Botha JF. Salvage of renal allograft using venous thrombectomy in the setting of iliofemoral venous thrombosis. *Nephrol Dial Transplant* 2004;19(6):1637–1639.

Streeter EH, Little DM, Cranston DW, Morris PJ. The urological complications of renal transplantation: a series of 1535 patients. *BJU Int* 2002;90(7):627–634.

Titton RL, Gervais DA, Hahn PF, et al. Urine leaks and urinomas: diagnosis and imaging-guided intervention. *Radiographics* 2003;23(5):1133–1147.

Troppmann C, Gillingham KJ, Benedetti E, et al. Delayed graft function, acute rejection, and outcome after cadaver renal transplantation. The multivariate analysis. *Transplantation* 1995;59(7):962–968.

Uflacker R, Selby JB, Chavin K, Rogers J, Baliga P. Transcatheter splenic artery occlusion for treatment of splenic artery steal syndrome after orthotopic liver transplantation. *Cardiovasc Intervent Radiol* 2002;25(4):300–306.

Uzochukwu LN, Bluth EI, Smetherman DH, et al. Early postoperative hepatic sonography as a predictor of vascular and biliary complications in adult orthotopic liver transplant patients. *AJR Am J Roentgenol* 2005;185(6): 1558–1570.

Watson CJ, Harper SJ. Anatomical variation and its management in transplantation. *Am J Transplant* 2015;15(6):1459–1471.

Williams GM, Hume DM, Hudson RP Jr, Morris PJ, Kano K, Milgrom F. "Hyperacute" renal-homograft rejection in man. *N Engl J Med* 1968; 279(12):611–618.

Wozney P, Zajko AB, Bron KM, Point S, Starzl TE. Vascular complications after liver transplantation: a 5-year experience. *AJR Am J Roentgenol* 1986; 147(4):657–663.

Yarlagadda SG, Coca SG, Formica RN Jr, Poggio ED, Parikh CR. Association between delayed graft function and allograft and patient survival: a systematic review and meta-analysis. *Nephrol Dial Transplant* 2009;24(3):1039–1047.

Yildirim S, Ayvazoglu Soy EH, Akdur A, et al. Treatment of biliary complications after liver transplant: results of a single center. *Exp Clin Transplant* 2015;13(Suppl 1):71–74.

Zhang L, Teng D, Chen G, et al. The risk factors of splenic arterial steal syndrome after orthotopic liver transplantation. *Zhonghua Wai Ke Za Zhi* 2015; 53(11):836–840.

CHAPTER 38 ■ IMAGE-GUIDED NEEDLE BIOPSIES AND PERSONALIZED MEDICINE

ANOBEL TAMRAZI, AISHWARYA GULATI, AND VIBHOR WADHWA

INTRODUCTION

Since time immemorial, physicians have attempted to tailor treatments to suit individual patients—from ancient Babylon to *Prakriti*-based Ayurveda to Hippocrates. Whereas previously, treatment was based on broader characteristics, we are now delving at the molecular and genomic level, ultimately aiming to treat the individual, not the group. Modern Personalized Medicine is the use of a combination of unique patient-specific characteristics (genomic, proteomic, metabolome, and microbiome) to predict disease susceptibility, disease prognosis, and ultimately, to provide the patient with the right treatment, at the right dose, and at the right time (Fig. 38.1) (1). This is an exciting opportunity for Radiologists, specifically those that perform image-guided procedures, to use their unique skills and gain minimally invasive access into different spaces or organs to acquire molecular analysis, which is essential in moving the field of medicine toward true Personalized Medicine.

In Personalized Medicine, biomarkers are often used to describe the biology of a patient's tumor. While the spectrum of definitions is vast, the National Institutes of Health Biomarkers Definitions Working Group defines a *biomarker* as "a characteristic that is objectively measured and evaluated as an indicator of normal biologic processes, pathogenic processes, or pharmacologic responses to a therapeutic intervention" (2). In light of the evolution of Oncology treatment options with Targeted and Immunotherapeutic Drugs, molecular and genetic analysis of tissue in addition to histologic diagnosis, is now necessary to guide therapy in a number of cancers such as lung, breast, melanoma, and colorectal. The biomarkers analyzed necessitate increased volume of samples and often repeat sampling from a patient's tumor during their treatment. Repeat tissue analysis is often necessary for prognostication and further guiding treatment in the event of drug resistance with imaging evidence of disease progression.

Radiologists are playing a direct and key role in changing the management of patients through their image-guided tissue sampling procedures. It has also been found in lung cancer trials that molecular and biomarker targeted therapies have a much higher chance of clinical success (3). Also, image-guided tissue biopsy may help reduce unnecessary surgery with thyroid and renal lesions as a substantial number of patients undergoing surgery are found to have benign pathology (4).

It is of note that delays in sample acquisition by Radiologists or inadequate samples have been shown to be a common cause of ineligibility in clinical trials for Oncology patients (5). The NCI-MATCH trial discovered in its interim survey that almost 15% biopsy samples were inadequate for molecular analysis and proved to be a major impediment in the treatment of patients for whom this trial was the last resort (6). Radiologists are in a unique position of identifying which site would be ideal for biopsy and ensuring adequate sample is obtained, while keeping in mind the risks of the procedure. Whether it is the study of imaging biomarkers or improvements and standardizations in the acquisition of tissue biopsy specimens in the near future, the Radiologist has a crucial role to play in the future of Personalized Medicine, especially in Oncology patients.

IMAGE-GUIDED NEEDLE BIOPSIES: MODALITIES AND EQUIPMENT

Percutaneous needle biopsy is a commonly used technique for obtaining tissue for both oncologic and nononcologic diagnoses. The critical element of the procedure is *image-guidance*—which allows the operator to visualize the target lesion and closely monitor the sampling needle, often in real time, and avoid vital structures, thus making the procedure safer and more accurate. Improved technologies within various imaging equipment used during interventions (Table 38.1) have made it possible to easily access tissues by augmenting the physician's understudying of spatial anatomy. For example, biopsy protocols on CT scanners allow for rapid visualization of target lesions and sampling needle in different planes allowing

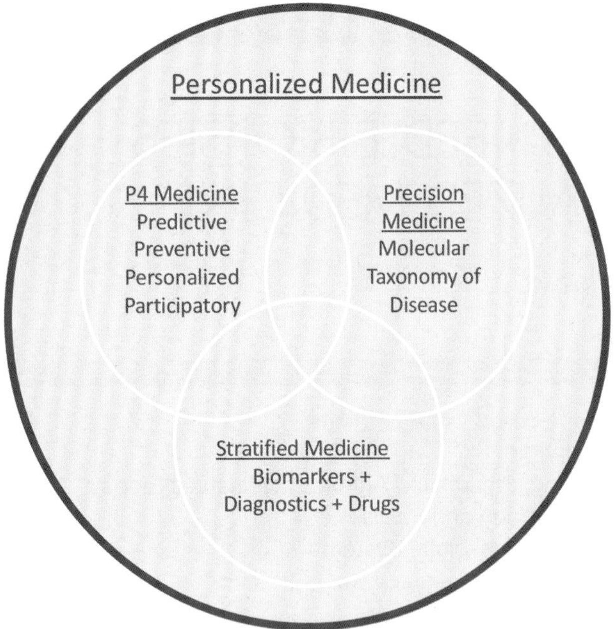

FIGURE 38.1. **The Spectrum of Personalized Medicine.** Personalized Medicine is a broad term encompassing a multifaceted approach to patient care. P4 Medicine is the systems-based approach to disease that aims to optimize wellness using patient data and provides strategies for patients toward their healthcare, encouraging their participation and responsibility. Precisions Medicine molecularly classifies a disease so as to guide diagnosis and treatment. Stratified Medicine classifies a patient population into subgroups on the basis of particular characteristics to best match a particular therapy to them. (Adapted with permission from the PHG Foundation. Many names for one concept or many concepts in one name? Available from http://www.phgfoundation.org/documents/311_1358522182.pdf.)

the Radiologist to make precise approach modifications to safely access the target lesion.

Advanced imaging technologies allow *fusion*, which is the overlay of different imaging datasets together, and *co-registration*—the spatial alignment of the two separate datasets. *Tracking* is another component of the navigation system which allows the visualization of the position of the needle in real time (7).

The choice of imaging modality, or use of combinations such as ultrasound and CT during a biopsy, is dependent upon a number of factors—lesion visualization, size, location, depth, surrounding tissue, patient body habitus, suitability of ionizing radiation, and physician preference.

The choice of the needle is also determined by a variety of factors such as nature of the target lesion, body tissues to be traversed, and amount of sample required. Broadly, there are two major needle sampling techniques—aspiration and core biopsy.

Aspiration techniques include fine needle aspiration (FNA), fine needle capillary sampling (FNCS), and large needle aspiration (LNA). Aspiration techniques are generally considered less traumatic and safer. In an FNA, a sample is acquired by applying gentle suction until tissue collected in the syringe. FNCS is essentially FNA without aspiration, wherein the needle is gently rotated within the target until sample ascends into the needle hub by capillary action. An LNA is similar to an FNA but performed with a larger bore needle and often useful to aspirate fluid for cytology. In Oncology patients, image-guided aspiration of fluid containing malignant cells, for example, pleural or peritoneal, may obviate the need of a tissue biopsy if enough malignant cells are obtained to establish a histopathologic diagnosis, and utilized for molecular and genetic analysis.

A core needle biopsy (CNB) procures a larger piece of tissue allowing for evaluation of architecture during histopathology analysis. It is usually done with a 16- to 21-gauge needle with an automated spring-loaded biopsy gun. CNB needles with a throw between 5 and 30 mm may be chosen depending on the target size and presence of vital/vascular organs beyond the margins of the target lesion. The needle length should be chosen as per the depth required based on the patient's imaging and the identified approach to the target lesion, keeping in mind that longer needles are more difficult to control. The CNB technique generally results in samples with more definitive diagnoses, but it also carries higher risk of complications.

However, the yield of both techniques may be sufficient for histologic as well as molecular diagnoses depending on the target tissue and amount of sample acquired during the biopsy.

For small, partially necrotic or incompletely visualized lesions, it may be helpful to have a cytopathologist or pathologist present during the biopsy procedure to evaluate aspiration or core tissue samples in real-time confirming the proper location of the needle within the most viable portion of the target lesion and also often giving feedback on how much more sample may be needed for definitive diagnosis and molecular diagnostic testing. Although, it's often not realistic, this has been shown to minimize false negatives and improve diagnostic accuracy (8).

PREPROCEDURE CLINICAL EVALUATION

It is important to know as the Radiologist performing the biopsy that you are a specialist and a consultant and thus consider independently the indication for the procedure and any possible alternatives to ensure that the patient does not undergo any unnecessary intervention and complication risks. A multidisciplinary evaluation, such as tumor boards, is helpful and may highlight the need for additional steps during the biopsy like fiducial marker placement for subsequent radiation therapy in nonsurgical patients. Always get to know the patient using a focused brief interaction prior to starting the case as that will help decision making during the procedure, especially for longer cases and cases resulting in various complications. For example, consider the patient's dependence on opioids for chronic pain, which may make them resistant to standard dosing of moderate sedation during biopsy procedures. This will ensure least number of complications during the case and also allows for establishing a connection with the patient, often leading to a higher patient satisfaction. The patient should be explained the procedure using simple layman's terms in order to mitigate patient anxiety. Informed consent must always be obtained after discussing the indication and alternatives to the procedure including possibilities of potential complications, nondiagnostic results and the sedation planned. Also, it is important to ensure that the patient is able to follow basic instructions and that vitals are within acceptable range. Prophylactic antibiotic use is generally not recommended for biopsy procedures performed by Radiologists.

It is very important to obtain a history of bleeding disorders and review all medications, especially anticoagulants, and decide upon their management. Temporary cessation versus bridging may be determined after a consultation with the treating specialist in patients with a history of prosthetic valves, stents, arrhythmias, recent pulmonary embolism, or CVA. This is especially important in the case of high bleeding

TABLE 38.1

COMMONLY USED IMAGING MODALITIES FOR PLANNING AND IMAGE-GUIDED TISSUE BIOPSY

■ MODALITY	■ REAL TIME	■ CURRENTLY PREFERRED FOR	■ LIMITATIONS	■ ADVANTAGES
Intervention				
Ultrasound	Yes	■ Superficial soft tissue lesions ■ Solid visceral organ lesions, most commonly liver, kidney, thyroid ■ Adenopathy in the neck, axilla, or groin ■ Omental and peritoneal lesions	■ Operator dependent ■ High susceptibility to artifacts ■ Unsuitable for lesions deep to bone or gas-filled organs like lung, bowel ■ Dense calcifications may obscure needle	■ Multiplanar ■ Cost effective ■ Nonionizing
CT	No	■ Thoracic ■ Pelvic ■ Musculoskeletal ■ Retroperitoneal ■ Deep abdominal viscera—liver, adrenal, pancreas	■ Ionizing radiation ■ Metal artifacts ■ Motion sensitive ■ Difficulty with angled approaches	■ Less operator dependent allowing visualization of the entire path to the lesion ■ Multiplanar ■ High geometric accuracy ■ C-arm CT available, but not widespread ■ CT Fluoroscopy may allow for more rapid maneuvering for small mobile lesions with the operator remaining within the suite
Fluoroscopy	Yes	■ Endoluminal biopsies, most often brush biopsies—bile ducts, ureters ■ Transjugular liver, renal biopsies ■ Bone lesions	■ Ionizing radiation ■ Not a cross-sectional modality, limiting visualization of adjacent structures	■ Widely available ■ Multiplanar
X-ray	Yes	Stereotactic—Breast	Ionizing radiation	Visualize and sample calcifications not seen on ultrasound
MRI	No	■ Breast ■ Prostate ■ Abdominal lesions	■ Higher cost ■ Requires open bore scanners and special needles ■ Slow	■ Nonionizing ■ Multiplanar ■ Different sequences allow better tissue visualization—fluid, fat, blood, restricted diffusion
Planning Only				
PET-CT	No	■ Suspected malignancies ■ Plan optimal biopsy site—based on maximal metabolic activity within the lesion	■ False positives such as infections, inflammation and even normal tissue like brown fat ■ Artifacts—Misregistration: superimposition of FDG activity on inappropriate anatomic structures on concurrent CT ■ Higher cost	■ Guides in the planning of the best location to sample, especially useful in areas of fibrosis and necrosis within a tumor ■ High sensitivity-may demonstrate malignant changes before structural changes on CT

TABLE 38.2

GUIDELINES FOR PERIPROCEDURE ANTICOAGULANT MANAGEMENT

		LAST DOSE–PROCEDURE INTERVAL (HOURS)		
DRUG	RENAL FUNCTION CrCl IN mL/min	LOW BLEEDING RISK	MODERATE–HIGH BLEEDING RISK	RESUME ANTICOAGULANT AFTER (hours)
Dabigatran	≥80 50–79 30–49 15–29 <15	≥24 ≥36 ≥48 ≥72 ≥96 and/or consider measuring dTT	≥48 ≥72 ≥96 ≥120 No data. Consider measuring dTT	Low bleeding risk: 24 High–moderate bleeding risk: 48–72
Rivaroxaban	≥30 15–29 <15	≥24 ≥36 [a]	≥48 [b] [b]	
Apixaban	≥30 15–29 <15	≥24 ≥36 [a]	≥48 [b] [b]	
Edoxaban	≥30 15–29 <15	≥24 ≥36 [a]	≥48 [b] [b]	
Warfarin	5 days			
ASA/Clopidogrel	5 days			
Dalteparin	24 hours			
LMWH	12 hours			
Heparin	1–2 hours			2–4

[a]Indicates no data. Consider measuring agent-specific anti Xa level and/or withholding ≥48 hours.
[b]Indicates no data. Consider measuring agent-specific anti Xa level and/or withholding ≥72 hours.
CrCl, creatinine clearance; dTT, diluted thrombin time.
Table courtesy of Stephanie Dizon, PharmD (10–14).

risk procedures such as CNB of kidney, or moderate bleeding risk like CNB of lung or liver (Table 38.2) (9–14). Low bleeding risk cases include aspirations and superficial biopsies, for example, thyroid and lymph nodes.

Lab work including platelets, PT/INR, and aPTT, should be obtained on a case-by-case basis considering patient history and factors that may affect bleeding complications. There is no consensus on the timeline or necessity of the lab work before the procedure. In the event of any clinical suspicion, or any change in medication, for example, the addition of drugs that may cause thrombocytopenia, or alter coagulation, labs should be repeated on the morning of the procedure.

It may also be reasonable to review renal function tests (BUN/creatinine) as most commonly used anticoagulants are renally excreted and their effects may not be directly monitored using standard INR testing.

TECHNIQUE

Most image-guided biopsies are performed on an outpatient basis under local anesthetic often with moderate sedation. The patient is placed in a comfortable position that allows access to the lesion. The target should be visualized using the imaging modality that will be used during the biopsy procedure and access approach identified on the patient's skin and marked. Strict sterile technique is to be followed at all times. Often the shortest and safest path to the lesion is preferred. Sometimes, it may be necessary to displace intervening structures such as bowel or lung tissue, which can often be accomplished by altering patient position and breathing instructions. Radiologists can achieve safe image-guided needle access in a tremendous number of anatomical locations for sampling procedures.

Ultrasound-Guided Needle Biopsy

Higher-frequency transducers are used for more superficial structures and lower frequencies for deeper. The head of the transducer probe must be covered with a sterile cover. The lesion is localized by scanning in multiple planes and the relationship between the lesion and major vessels/organs is mapped to avoid vascular injury and organ damage along the needle access path and also just beyond the target lesion if CNB is being utilized for sampling. The needle may be ideally inserted parallel to the transducer, which allows visualization of entire length of the needle, or perpendicular if needed to minimize risk of injury to major vessels along the access path, however only the tip of the needle is visualized. If the needle is not visualized, it is probably due to misalignment between the probe and the needle. If the inserted needle is no longer visualized, the needle depth should not be changed and only the US probe should be moved back and forth until the needle is clearly visualized to minimize risk of injury. Slight oscillation of the needle during insertion may allow visualization of the path of the needle, especially for smaller needles. Larger gauge and specific echogenic needles are better visualized on US.

Computed Tomography–Guided Needle Biopsy

A scan of the target area is first obtained with a localizing marker in place on the skin along the predicted access entry site (Fig. 38.2). The craniocaudal location of the safest access point to the target lesion is determined. The depth to the lesion is measured, and the optimum site of insertion in the mediolateral location and angle of insertion is planned. The needle is inserted parallel to the CT localizer light so that the entire needle is visualized in a single slice, minimizing total number of CT slices and radiation needed to visualize the target and needle tip. The needle is gradually advanced in stages, with serial scans being done to monitor its progression until the target lesion is reached. For lesions without a direct anteroposterior access pathway, one can angle the gantry of the CT scanner or approach the lesion from a craniocaudal access pathway as long as the needle is well visualized within intraprocedural images.

Sampling

Sampling is done when the needle is visualized to be in the correct position (Fig. 38.2).

For an FNA, when the target is reached, suction is applied and rotatory motions are made in the target area until material is seen filling the hub. Specimens are ideally obtained from different areas of the lesion for a more representative sampling of the target, especially if central necrosis or suspicious peripheral calcifications or thickening is noted within the target lesion. If an FNC technique is preferred, the needle is rapidly moved to and fro through the lesion to capture representative cells.

When performing a CNB, it is advisable to perform a test deployment of the device on the back table outside of the patient beforehand. In the coaxial systems, the introducer needle system with a trocar is first advanced adjacent to or just within the target lesion, allowing greater control and safety for the core biopsy needle and minimizing needle passes along

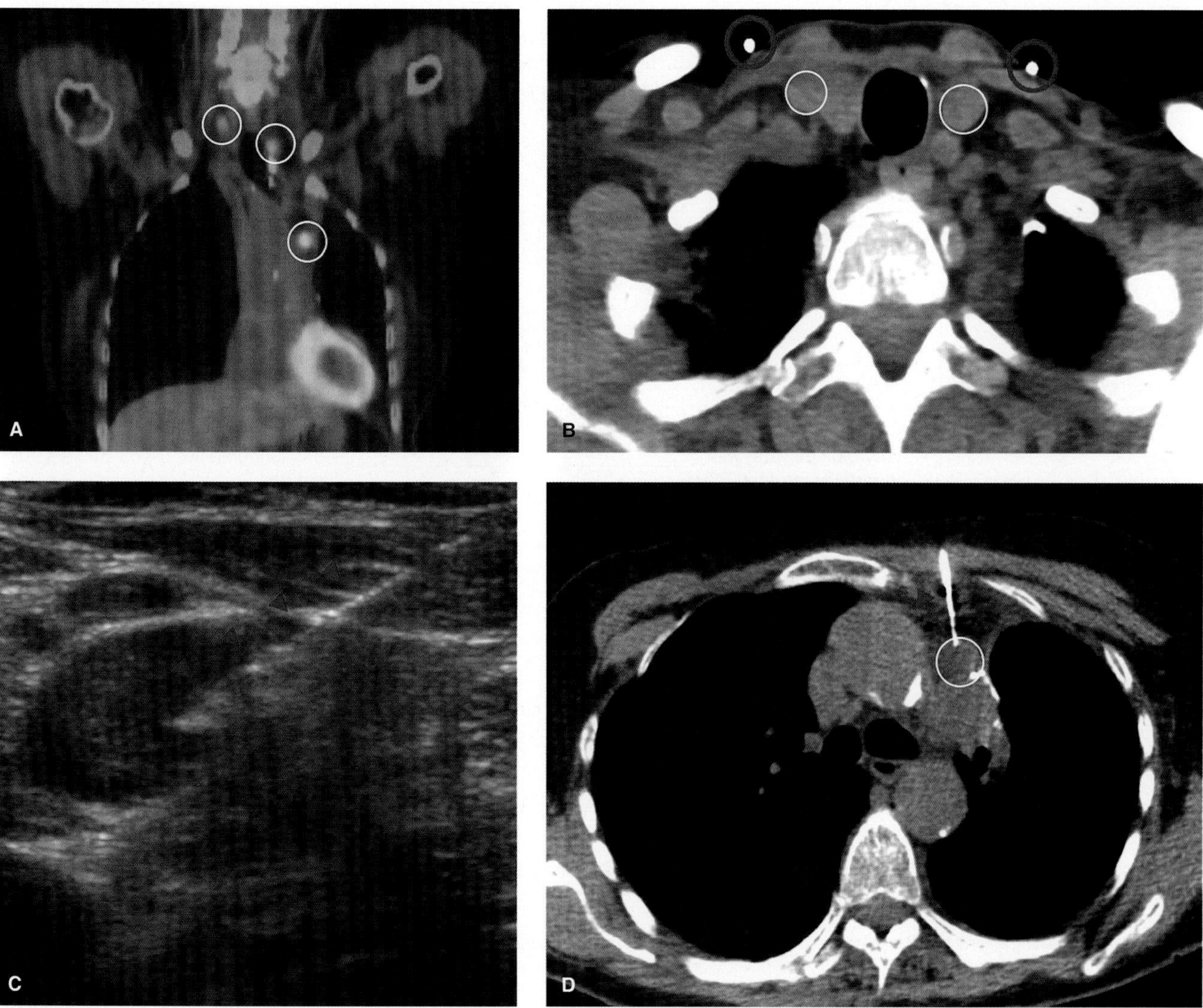

FIGURE 38.2. Combined US- and CT-Guided Biopsy. This 73-year-old female with a history of stage IIIA (pT1 pN2 cM0) adenocarcinoma of the upper left lung lobe underwent presumably curative lobectomy with mediastinal lymph node dissection. She also had a remote history of thyroid cancer treated by thyroidectomy. She presented 1 year later with FDG avid adenopathy in the mediastinum and bilateral supraclavicular nodal regions (*white circles* in **A**) concerning for recurrent lung cancer. Markers (*red circles* in **B**) were placed with CT to localize the FDG avid nodes (*white circles* in B). The left neck node was biopsied under US guidance (*arrowheads* indicate needle in **C**) and the mediastinal node was biopsied with CT guidance (*white circle* indicates lesion, *arrowhead* indicates needle in **D**). All the nodes were reactive in nature and no evidence of malignancy was detected.

the access path. It is important to keep in mind the initial position of the CNB tip and the excursion length (5 to 30 mm) of the needle to ensure that no surrounding soft tissues and vessels are damaged. It is helpful to obtain an intraprocedural image confirming ideal location of the needle relative to the target lesion as that will subsequently assure the clinical team that the proper lesion was sampled during the case, especially if a benign or unexpected diagnosis (e.g., radiation-induced changes, inflammatory changes but no malignancy) is finalized several days after the biopsy. As core samples are obtained, there is often obscuration of the target lesion to some extend due to focal hemorrhage or iatrogenic gas, and therefore it is essential that the biopsy needle is in the ideal location prior to initiation of obtaining core biopsy samples. Finally, it is important to remember that for larger lesions, attempts should be made to sample the tissue along its periphery, as the central part may be necrotic.

ORGAN-BASED CONSIDERATIONS

Thyroid

Thyroid nodules may be discovered by the patient, during a routine physical examination, or often during another imaging study. There is a high prevalence of thyroid nodules in the general population: 2% to 6% (palpation), 19% to 35% (ultrasound) and 8% to 65% (autopsy data) (15). The incidence of nodules increases with age and is more common in women (16).

A nodule with an elevated or normal TSH is first evaluated by a dedicated thyroid US study that includes an evaluation of cervical lymph nodes. While the risk of a nodule being malignant remains low (4.0% to 6.5%) (17), it is important to rule out treatable cancer in nodules that meet suspicious US imaging criteria for biopsy (Fig. 38.3) (18). FDG avid lesions, and hot nodules on sestamibi scans should undergo an FNA (19).

Aside from imaging stratified suspicious nodules, a biopsy may also be needed in case of rapid, diffuse enlargement of the gland, especially in those older than 50 years, to rule out malignancy.

Preprocedure planning remains the same as for any other biopsy, except that fasting is generally not required since these aspiration sampling cases are often done under local anesthetic only. The procedure is done with the patient in supine position with the neck slightly extended under real-time US-guidance to visualize the course and tip of the needle the entire time for each pass of the sampling procedure.

The American Thyroid Association recommends FNA as the procedure of choice in the evaluation of thyroid nodules,

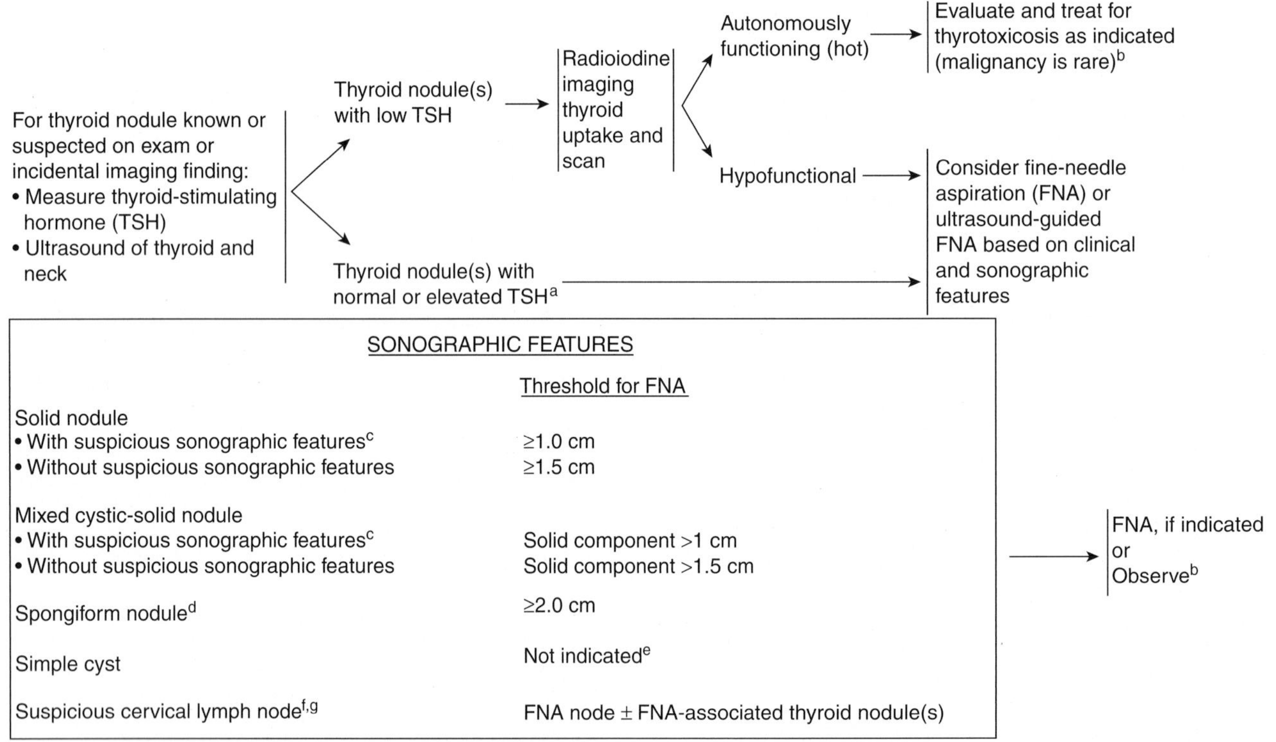

[a]Evaluate and treat for hypothyroidism as clinically indicated.
[b]For nodules not meeting criteria for FNA, or nodules that appear to be benign by ultrasound or FNA, surveillance should include repeat ultrasound after 6–12 months; if stable for 1–2 years, then subsequent ultrasound can be considered at 3- to 5-year intervals.
[c]Suspicious sonographic features include hypoechoic, microcalcifications, infiltrative margins, and taller than wide in the transverse plane. Sonographic features associated with a low risk of malignancy include spongiform nodules, isoechoic or hyperechoic solid nodules, and mixed solid-cystic nodules without any of the suspicious features listed above.
[d]Aggregation of multiple microcystic components in more than 50% of the volume of the nodule.
[e]Except as therapeutic modality.
[f]Tg washout may be helpful in diagnosis of lymph node metastases.
[g]Suspicious lymph node features may include hypoechoic, rounded, absence of fatty hilum, cystic or partially cystic, and/or microcalcifications.

FIGURE 38.3. **NCCN Guidelines for Thyroid Nodule Evaluation.** (From Bischoff L, Lamki Busaidy N, Byrd D, et al. NCCN Guidelines Version 2.2017 Thyroid Carcinoma 2017 with permission. Available from https://www.nccn.org/professionals/physician_gls/pdf/thyroid.pdf.)

when clinically indicated (20). Thyroid nodule FNA is generally done with 22- to 27-gauge needles (21).

There are four possible outcomes of an FNA—benign 50% to 90% (av. 70%), malignant 1% to 10% (av. 5%), indeterminate 10% to 30% (av. 20%), and nondiagnostic 2% to 20% (av. 10%) (22).

While there is no consensus among guidelines, a CNB, with an automated 18- to 21-gauge spring loaded needle with a short excursion distance (21) is usually recommended for previously repeatedly nondiagnostic FNA or for heavily calcified and degenerating low cellularity thyroid nodules (19,21,23).

Molecular analysis of an indeterminate lesion (Bethesda III–V) is now a possibility and would help avoid unnecessary thyroidectomy, which has been historically offered to these patients. Molecular biomarkers including BRAF, RET/PTC1, RET/PTC3, PAX8/PPARG, and RAS can be detected (23). Specific biomarker profiles are suggestive of a malignancy and would indicate thyroidectomy.

Postbiopsy Care and Complications. The area is bandaged and manual compression is applied as needed to achieve hemostasis. Pain at the site that may radiate up to the ear is the most common complication and is usually minor. An ice pack is often useful in decreasing patient discomfort. Hematoma is a complication that may rarely cause airway obstruction especially in coagulopathic patients. Discharge instructions are given to the patient with advice to contact the Radiologist performing the procedure and seek medical care at their closest emergency room in case of a neck swelling that continues to enlarge despite manual pressure.

Lung, Pleural and Anterior Mediastinal Biopsy

A lung biopsy may be required for the evaluation of suspicious pleuroparenchymal solid or ground glass focal or multifocal abnormalities in the proper clinical setting, including (24):

- New or enlarging solitary nodule or mass in a high-risk patient (smoking history, treated malignancy), which is not easily accessible for sampling by bronchoscopy (Fig. 38.4).
- Multiple nodules in a patient without a known malignancy or in prolonged remission with known malignancy.
- Persistent focal infiltrates of unknown etiology.
- Anterior mediastinal mass.
- Recurrent pleural effusions of unknown etiology or suspicious pleural masses or thickenings (25).

The preprocedure planning and evaluation remain the same as for other biopsies. Additionally, baseline oxygen requirement of the patient and severity of their COPD should be evaluated prior to the procedure as those patients are at higher risk of respiratory compromise during and immediately post-biopsy procedures, even with small pneumothorax or hemorrhage.

Exercise caution in young patients with an apparent lung nodule on a noncontrast CT chest that may reflect a pulmonary arteriovenous malformation (AVM), which should not be biopsied.

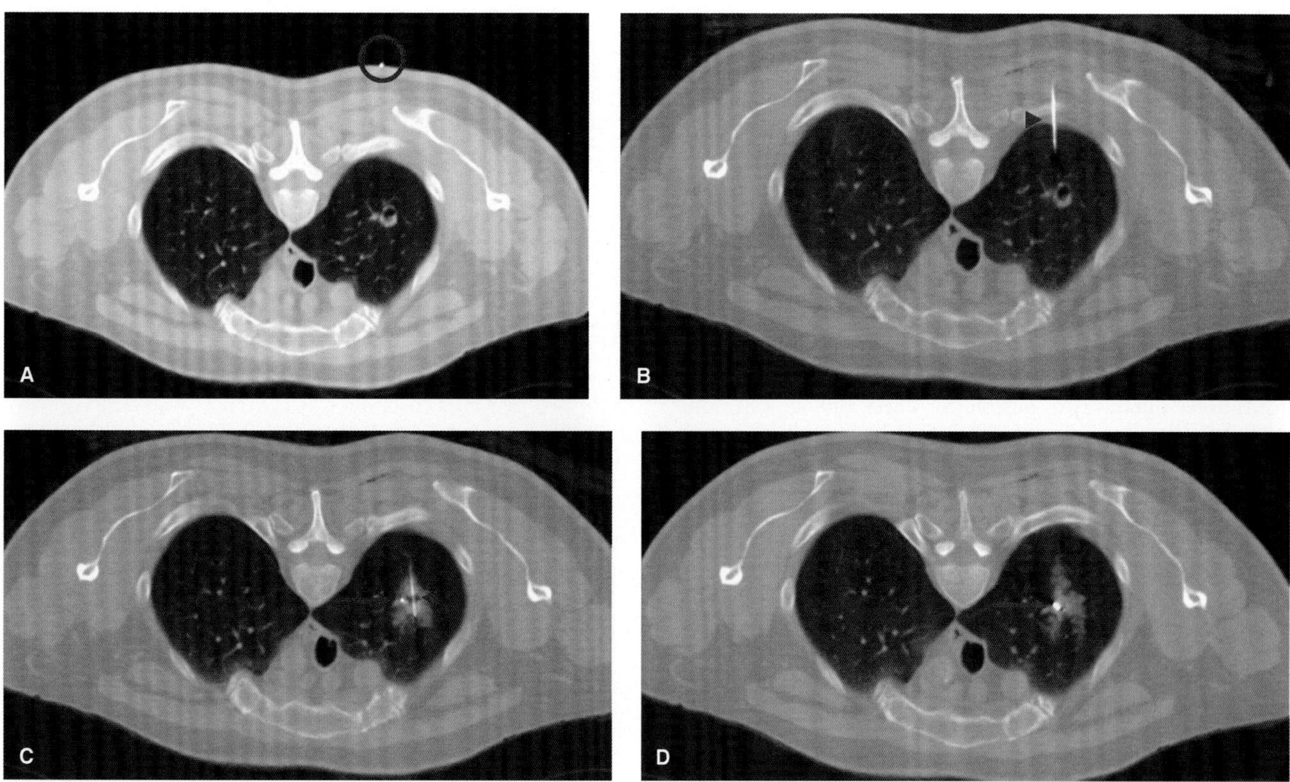

FIGURE 38.4. CT-Guided Lung Nodule Fiducial Marker Placement and Biopsy. This 70-year-old male with a history of smoking presented with a right upper lobe cavitary nodule with FDG avidity, suspicious for malignancy. A marker was placed to guide the cephalocaudal entry point (*circle* in **A**). The needle was advanced on the path planned taking care to not cross any fissures (*arrowhead* in **B**). The biopsy needle trough was visualized within the target: the nodular area within the cavitary lesion (*arrowhead* in **C**). A fiducial marker was placed (*arrow* in **C** and **D**). The lesion was completely obscured, as often is the case, postbiopsy due to the hematoma within the parenchyma. The final pathology report was squamous cell carcinoma.

TABLE 38.3

SOME COMMONLY USED FIXATIVE SOLUTIONS

■ SOLUTION	■ COMMON USES	■ MAIN COMPONENTS
Normal saline	Immunohistochemistry	0.9% NaCl
10% neutral-buffered formalin	Light microscopy Electron microscopy Most commonly used for molecular testing	40% formaldehyde Phosphate buffer
Roswell Park Memorial Institute medium (RPMI)	Flow cytometry for suspected lymphoma, e.g., lymphadenopathy or anterior mediastinal masses	Bicarbonate buffer Amino acids Vitamins D-glucose Glutathione
Methanol-water solution (e.g., CytoLyt)	Cytology samples to make cell blocks	Methanol
Alcohol	Cytology specimens, often thyroid	95% ethanol

The patient must be educated about the breathing technique that may be required during the procedure, especially for small targets (1-cm lung nodule). The patient is positioned depending on the access entry site identified. The needle access pathway should be via the superior aspect of the rib in order to avoid injury to the neurovascular bundle (intercostal artery), which runs along the inferior aspect of the rib. Crossing fissures should be avoided when possible to minimize risk of bronchopleural fistula requiring chest tube insertion. Pleural lesions/masses are often best visualized under CT-guidance, while pleural effusions can easily be visualized using US-guidance during sampling. For an anterior mediastinal mass, exercise caution to avoid the internal mammary vessels along the access pathway to the lesion. Additionally, since lymphoma is often within the differential diagnosis of an anterior mediastinal mass, samples must be placed in proper fixative solutions, not only formalin that would allow for flow cytometry (Table 38.3).

The sampling technique of choice is often CNB to allow histologic as well as molecular biomarker analysis in view of the rapidly evolving and advancing Personalized Medicine aspect of lung cancer.

Postbiopsy Care and Complications. After the procedure is done, the skin nick is cleaned and dressed, and a repeat scan is obtained to rule out the presence of a pneumothorax. Most institutions obtain two postbiopsy chest radiographs, one immediate baseline and a repeat 2- to 3-hour study, to ensure no enlarging pneumothorax. The patients are observed until the follow-up radiograph is obtained while fasting in case a chest tube insertion is needed (Fig. 38.5). The patient is discharged if the follow-up radiograph shows no evidence of developing pneumothorax (Fig. 38.6) (26), substantial hemorrhage and patient clinically not requiring additional supplemental oxygen to maintain proper ventilation. Discharge instructions are given to the patient with advice to contact the Radiologist performing the procedure and seek medical care at their closest emergency room in case of sudden or increased shortness of breath, fullness/heaviness in chest or excessive hemoptysis.

Pneumothorax. The most common complication of CT-guided lung biopsy is an iatrogenic pneumothorax, which has been reported to occur in as high as 54% of all lung biopsies with an average of 20% (27). Acute pneumothoraces may develop at the time of the procedure or often within 2 hours of the procedure, but delayed pneumothoraces have also been reported, post normal radiographs up to 24 hours after biopsy (24). While the influence of some factors remains debated, underlying smoking-related lung disease, smaller lesion size, shallow pleural puncture angle, depth and long needle path, number of pleural reflections along the access pathway, and patient age may increase the rate of pneumothorax development and the need and duration of a chest tube (27).

Although the rate of pneumothoraces can be substantial, only about 2% to 15% of all patients clinically require a

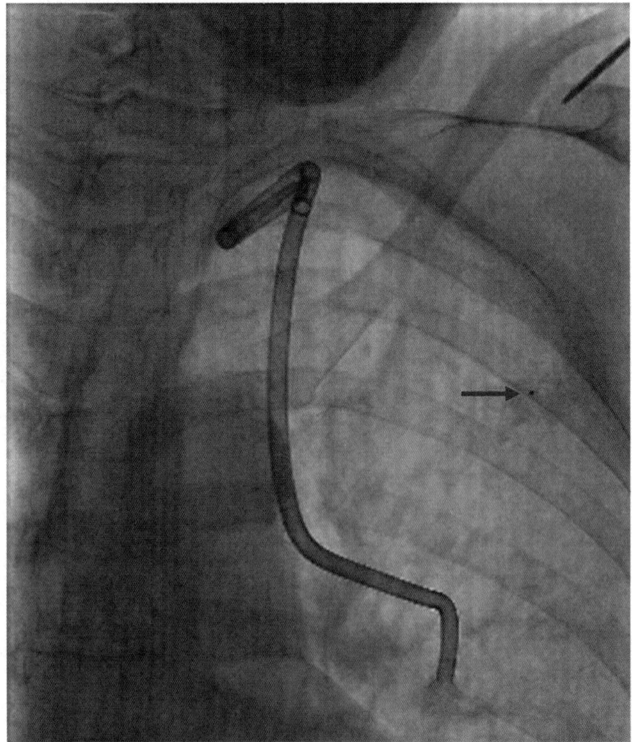

FIGURE 38.5. **Anterior Chest Wall Chest Tube Insertion for Pneumothorax.** This 62-year-old female presented with a single solid pleuroparenchymal FDG avid lesion in the setting of moderate emphysematous changes concerning for lung malignancy. Post-biopsy and fiducial marker placement (*arrow*), a pneumothorax developed for which a 10-Fr chest tube was inserted anteriorly with the pigtail along the apex.

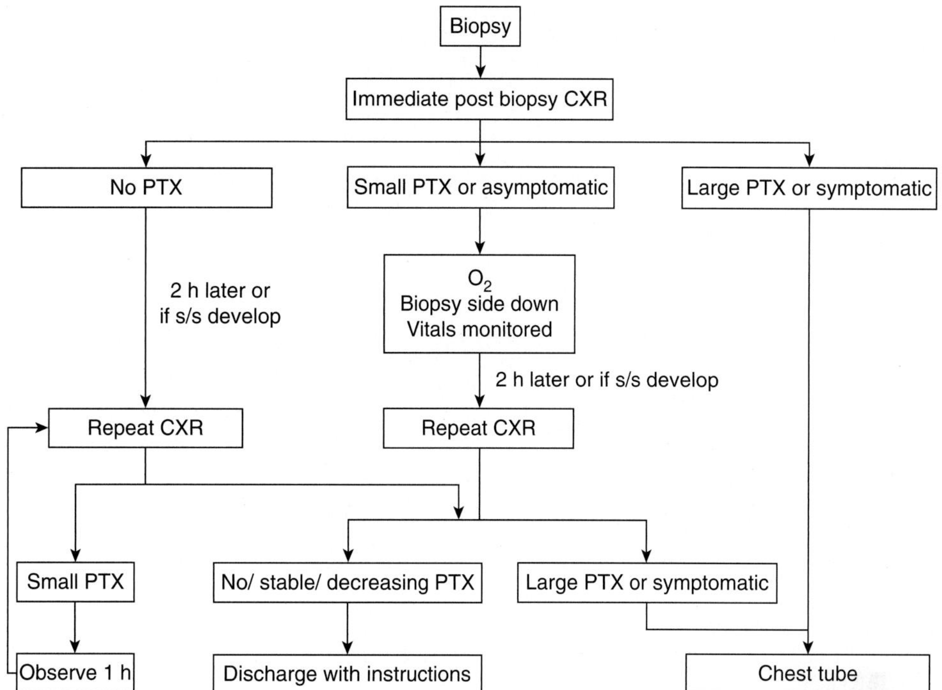

FIGURE 38.6. **Post Lung Biopsy Care and Pneumothorax Management.** Signs/symptoms (S/S) may include desaturation and shortness of breath. PTX, pneumothorax; CXR, expiratory chest x-ray. (Adapted from Brown KT, Brody LA, Getrajdman GI, et al. Outpatient treatment of iatrogenic pneumothorax after needle biopsy. *Radiology* 1997;205: 249–252.)

chest tube insertion to maintain proper ventilation (27). Hospitalization is often only necessary in cases of persistent bronchopleural fistulas. Most Interventionalists prefer an anteriorly placed 8- to 10-Fr chest tube with the pigtail strategically placed along the anterior apex of the pleural space under fluoroscopy- or CT-guidance to best decompress the pneumothorax and help resolve the persistent bronchopleural fistula (Fig. 38.5). Injection of an autologous blood patch may decrease likelihood of chest tube insertion (28–30).

Pulmonary Hemorrhage and Hemoptysis. Significant post-biopsy hemoptysis, defined as 30 to 50 mL, has been reported to occur only in <1% patients (27). Hemoptysis often simply requires reassurance and the patient lying in a decubitus position, with the biopsy side down. Mild hemoptysis is often transient (1 to 2 days) and focal parenchymal hemorrhage usually does not lead to substantial respiratory compromise, unless the patient has decreased respiratory reserve making them much more susceptible for rapid clinical decline post lung biopsy.

Air embolism, development of a hemothorax and tumor seeding of the pleura or chest wall are additional rare complications (31). To minimize air embolism during any central parenchymal lung tissue biopsy via the pulmonary veins, care must be taken to minimize introducing air through the introducer needle as the biopsy needle is placed and removed with each pass.

Abdomen and Pelvis

Liver Biopsy. A nontargeted liver biopsy may be indicated for diffuse parenchymal disease such as viral/autoimmune/alcoholic hepatitis, metabolic and storage diseases, unexplained hepatomegaly or abnormal LFTs, transplant rejection, and for drug-induced liver damage (32,33).

A targeted liver biopsy is performed for the evaluation of suspicious focal lesions. Benign focal lesions such as adenoma, hemangioma, and focal nodular hyperplasia (FNH) are often diagnosed on multiphase CT and MRI studies; however, biopsy may be required in the event of nonspecific imaging findings. Suspicious hypervascular lesions with venous phase washout in a cirrhotic liver are more likely to be hepatocellular carcinoma (HCC) often diagnosed based on their imaging features. Tissue biopsy can be considered in cases of suspicious lesions with atypical imaging features to exclude HCC. Suspected cholangiocarcinoma with delayed enhancement of desmoplastic tissue often require tissue biopsy for conclusive pathologist diagnosis and in some cases identification of treatment options. In case of multiple intrahepatic lesions, an accessible peripheral lesion may need to be biopsied in case metastasis is suspected from an occult primary.

Exercise caution in suspected hydatid cysts due to a possibility of anaphylaxis, ascites due to increased risk of bleeding, and functional neuroendocrine tumor metastasis due to possible hypertension.

Depending on the target lesion location, visualization and imaging features, either CT-, or US-, or MRI-guidance can be used to access and successfully sample the hepatic lesion (Table 38.1). US is generally preferred as it offers a real-time imaging modality allowing for accessing smaller lesions often mobile with patient breathing during the sampling procedure. In addition, some lesions may not be easily visualized using CT or US and in those cases where an interventional MRI unit may not be available, landmarks can be used from prior PET or MRI imaging to help access the target lesion under CT-guidance (Fig. 38.7).

General access pathway considerations during targeted or nontargeted liver biopsy include passage of the biopsy needle above the rib to avoid the intercostal artery, maintaining a fairly peripheral pathway of the biopsy needle toward the target and avoiding crossing the diaphragm or lung parenchyma to eliminate risks of pneumothorax. A medial subcostal or inferior access pathways with a peripheral preference within the liver parenchyma toward the target may decrease risk of bleeding. Also, a single passage through the hepatic capsule using a coaxial CNB technique is often utilized to minimize patient discomfort and risks of subcapsular hematoma. In case

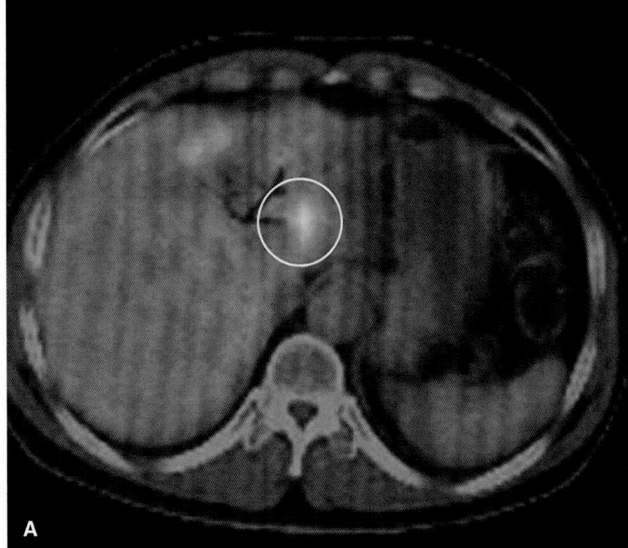

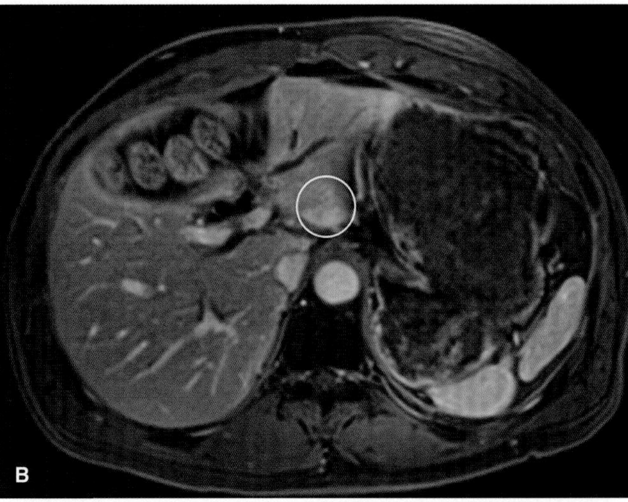

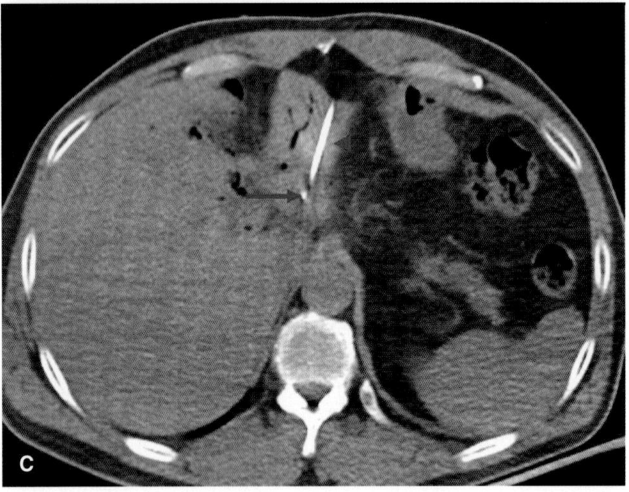

FIGURE 38.7. **Landmark-Based CT-Guided Biopsy.** This 52-year-old male with a history of pancreatic cancer postresection subsequently presented with caudate lobe metastasis and was treated with XRT. Currently, he presented with an FDG avid lesion within the posterior medial segment 3 with vague-associated MRI abnormality concerning for a new focus of metastatic disease (*white circles* in **A** and **B**). The lesion was not visible on CT or US. Anatomical landmarks with PET and MRI were used to perform the biopsy (*arrowhead* in **C**) and place fiducials (*arrow* in **C**). The final report revealed no evidence of malignancy and only nonspecific portal and lobular inflammation suggestive of postradiation changes.

of ascites, drainage of the fluid with paracentesis should be considered to best contain hepatic parenchymal hemorrhage through the capsule before the biopsy procedure.

In addition, if a nontargeted biopsy of the liver is needed clinically, a transjugular liver biopsy (TJLBX) approach with a lower bleeding risk profile can be considered, as the capsule of the liver is never crossed with the needle and small hepatic hemorrhage can decompress via the access pathway through the hepatic vein (Fig. 38.8). This fluoroscopic endovascular biopsy approach should be considered for patients with coagulopathy (graft vs. host disease (34), thrombocytopenia), those requiring hepatic venous pressure gradient measurement (prerenal transplant, suspected portal hypertension) and patients with substantial ascites requiring nontargeted liver biopsy.

Postbiopsy Care and Complications. Following an uncomplicated, outpatient liver biopsy, the patient is often observed for 4 to 6 hours post percutaneous and 1 to 2 hours post TJLBX. The majority of complications occur within 3 hours of the procedure (35). Discharge instructions are given to the patient with advice to contact the Radiologist performing the procedure and seek medical care at their closest emergency room in case of sudden or increased right upper quadrant pain, abdominal distention, or dizziness.

Pain. It is the most common complaint after a biopsy and is thought to be either due to bile leak or small hemorrhage, leading to capsular swelling and right upper quadrant discomfort, with possible referred right shoulder pain due to irritation of the diaphragm. A small amount of local anesthetic placed near the hepatic capsule during the biopsy prior to crossing the capsule with the coaxial needle may help limit postbiopsy pain associated with clinically insignificant bleeding.

Bleeding. Postbiopsy bleeding rarely can be clinically substantial and life threatening, manifesting as hemoperitoneum, intrahepatic hematoma, or hemobilia. The patient age, history of bleeding disorders, ascites, liver cirrhosis, amyloidosis, malignancy, renal failure, use of a larger bore needle, or an inexperienced operator all add to the risk of bleeding (35). The patient may manifest with worsening pain, hypotension, tachycardia, and a drop in hematocrit. Most patients with clinically significant postbiopsy bleeding will need to be admitted at least overnight for close monitoring and to ensure blood products and IV fluid are available, which often is sufficient for their care. If their hematocrit continues to drop or if they show signs of hemodynamic instability, they may require a CTA of the abdomen to look for active arterial extravasation and extent of the hemorrhage with potential arterial embolization of hepatic and or intercostal arteries that may be injured during the biopsy.

Needle Tract Seeding. This is a rare, but potentially devastating complication in which the extrahepatic tract of the

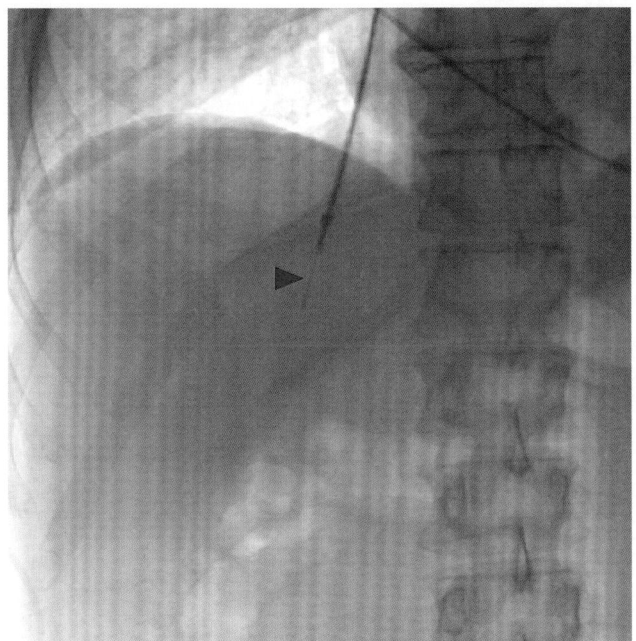

FIGURE 38.8. **Transjugular Liver Biopsy.** The internal jugular vein provided endovascular access into the hepatic vein. A biopsy needle is placed through the sheath in the hepatic vein to sample the parenchyma (*arrowhead*).

biopsy is seeded with malignant cells. It has been reported to occur following biopsy of liver metastasis or an HCC, with the reported incidence ranging from 0.6% to 5.1% (36–38). Needles of a smaller gauge, going through some normal liver parenchyma along the pathway access to the tumor and coaxial sampling technique may decrease the risk of needle tract seeding (39,40).

Percutaneous biopsy may also be complicated by pneumothorax, hemothorax, or an intercostal hemorrhage. Arrhythmias are rare complications possible after a TJLBX. Bile peritonitis, infection, pseudoaneurysm and intrahepatic AV fistulas and active arterial extravasation may occur after either of the approaches (35).

Renal Biopsy. A targeted renal biopsy may be indicated for the evaluation of a suspicious focal lesion. A nontargeted renal biopsy of the parenchyma may be needed to evaluate nephropathies, renal transplant rejection, or various systemic diseases that alter renal function including drug reactions (41).

Targeted renal biopsy referral should preferably come from Urology team after risk stratification of the lesion based on US or contrast-enhanced cross-sectional studies. Nontargeted renal biopsy referral should preferably come from Nephrology team after obvious clinical etiologies such as diabetes mellitus, chronic hypertension, and obstruction have been considered and ruled out.

Targeted renal biopsy remains underutilized prior to nephrectomies or lesion ablation due to the belief that no clear histopathologic distinction may be made between a benign and malignant disease, especially oncocytomas versus chromophobe renal cell carcinoma. However, improvements in immunohistochemistry and the advent of microRNA-based assays have made tissue diagnosis more definitive, potentially avoiding unnecessary surgery (42). Studies have shown that a substantial proportion of small solid renal lesions have a benign etiology (<1 cm/38.5%, 1 to 2 cm/19%, 2 to 3 cm/ 17%, and 3 to 4cm/13%) (4).

A percutaneous renal biopsy is usually performed under US-guidance. CT-guidance may be preferred in the case of a difficult to visualize focal lesion, marked obesity, or complicated renal anatomy (43). The major vessels and ureter must be visualized to avoid injury.

The prone position is usually preferred with ipsilateral side up decubitus as an alternative in those that cannot tolerate it (e.g., obesity, airway issues). The supine position is preferred for transplanted kidney biopsies as these are placed in the pelvis.

The nontargeted renal biopsy site for chronic kidney disease (CKD) patient is along the periphery of the kidney, which contains glomeruli, often with a 16-gauge coaxial CNB. Similar to the liver, a transjugular endovascular nontargeted renal biopsy technique is an option especially for morbidly obese patients that do not fit into the CT scanner gantry or are difficult to visualize their kidneys with US. However, unlike the TJLBX, this technique is not associated with decreased risk of bleeding and thus is a rarely utilized approach for renal biopsy in CKD (44).

Post-biopsy Care and Complications. After a renal biopsy, bed rest and close postprocedure monitoring for 24 hours is ideal as the majority of complications occur within this time (45). Post-biopsy imaging may be considered, but its utility is limited. However, the absence of a hematoma has been shown to have a negative predictive value for complications and may decrease the observation period required for a patient (46). Discharge instructions are given to the patient with advice to contact the Radiologist performing the procedure and seek medical care at their closest emergency room in case of sudden or increased ipsilateral biopsy side flank pain, increasing hematuria or dizziness.

Bleeding. Renal biopsy is considered to be a high bleeding risk procedure (9). In CKD patients, there is the possibility of an elevated bleeding time (BT) due to platelet dysfunction but the increased risk of bleeding remains controversial (47). Females, low baseline Hb <12 mg/dL, systolic blood pressure >130, elevated serum creatinine (>2 mg/dL), biopsies done for acute kidney injury, and the use of larger bore needles are all associated with a higher bleeding risk (48). It may present as a perinephric hematoma (10% to 90%) or transient gross hematuria (1% to 10%). Major bleeds may need transfusion (0.3% to 7.4%), superselective arterial embolization by Interventional Radiology or even rarely a nephrectomy (0.1% to 0.5%) (49), however most hematoma and hematuria in patients are usually self-resolving as Gerota's fascia helps tamponade the bleed. If a patient presents several days postprocedure with persistent hematuria but otherwise stable vitals, a CTA should be considered to rule out pseudoaneurysm or AV fistula.

Other rare complications include infection, urinary leak, adjacent organ injury, pneumothorax when the upper pole is sampled and possible tumor seeding, which has been reported to occur in less than 1:10,000 biopsies (50).

Other Abdominopelvic Biopsies. A **prostate biopsy** is usually performed as an outpatient procedure by a Urologist via Transrectal US in order to rule out malignancy. These procedures are not routinely performed by Radiologists and thus will not be addressed in detail in this chapter.

A **pancreatic** lesion is usually biopsied endoscopically by a Gastroenterologist due to more direct and shorter needle path, that precludes tumor seeding with decreased risk of adjacent organ injury and bleeding. However, a large pancreatic lesion may be easily accessible via a retroperitoneal percutaneous pathway for tissue biopsy. Postbiopsy complications can include pancreatitis, hemorrhage, and pancreatic duct fistulas (51).

A **splenic** mass biopsy is rarely performed but may be done in cases of a suspicious focal splenic lesion or diffuse splenomegaly with suspected malignancy. A suspicion of lymphoma is the most common indication. Hemorrhage is a serious potential complication as the spleen is a very hypervascular organ, but lesser number of passes and FNA with 20- to 23-gauge and CNB with 18-gauge needles have been shown to be relatively safer (52). A short biopsy path to the most peripheral location also minimizes bleeding risk (52).

A **gallbladder (GB) biopsy** is also rarely performed by Radiologists and carries the risk of rare serious complications like bile peritonitis and hemobilia, but some studies have shown it to be a safe procedure (53). A GB mass, or, less preferably, focally thickened GB wall suspicious for malignancy may be biopsied. An intrahepatic trajectory and perpendicular penetration into the GB are preferred to minimize leakage (53).

A CT-guided **adrenal biopsy** may be considered in the event of suspicious adrenal lesions with inconclusive imaging features. A reteroperitoneal posterior access approach is often utilized. At times an inferior to superior approach is used to avoid crossing the diaphragm and lung parenchyma. Exercise caution when a pheochromocytoma is suspected clinically, and approach only after pretreatment with alpha blockers (54). Hemorrhage, pneumothorax, and hypertensive crisis are rare complications (55).

Bowel lesions are nearly exclusively biopsied under endoscopic guidance by Gastroenterologists but may be accessed percutaneously if the lesion is large and along the outer surface of the bowel loop allowing for needle biopsy without causing a perforation and leak.

While the normal **omentum and peritoneum** are not visualized by US, any solid lesion or nodular thickening may be detected, especially in case of peritoneal carcinomatosis. A combination of CT- and US-guidance will likely be needed to safely access a peritoneal implant/lesion as these are quite mobile and patient position dependent during the procedure. Some institutions prefer to defer these cases to Surgeons for laparoscopic biopsy as image-guided percutaneous biopsy of these mobile lesions can be quite challenging with low yield of success.

Lymph node sampling by US or CT is effective for suspicious retroperitoneal, pelvic, neck, axillary, inguinal, submandibular, and parotid lymph nodes as small as 1 cm (Fig. 38.2). Smaller, superficial lesions near vital organs and vessels are often sampled via aspiration techniques using 21- to 25-gauge needles. Larger, fixed retroperitoneal lesions are sampled via CNB after carefully identifying critical structures like the ureter and adjacent vessels and ensuring the core biopsy needle does not penetrate beyond the target lesions toward vascular structures. As lymphoma often remains in the differential diagnosis of abnormal lymphadenopathy, samples need also to be placed in proper fixative solutions allowing for flow cytometry (Table 38.3).

Musculoskeletal System

A musculoskeletal biopsy may be indicated to establish diagnosis of a bone or soft tissue lesion with aggressive or indeterminate imaging features, to confirm metastasis in a patient with a known malignancy, determination of causal organism in case of infections to guide antibiotic therapy, and to determine the etiology of a pathologic fracture. Imaging studies can be very helpful before the procedure—an MRI may allow better delineation of myofascial compartments and neurovascular visualization, while CT may better depict bone destruction, erosion, or calcification.

Exercise caution for classic “do not touch” lesions including pseudotumor of the calcaneus, desmoid, and elastofibroma dorsi.

Bone Biopsy. Targeted bone lesion biopsy is sometimes needed to confirm the presence of a malignancy or to identify tumor biology by molecular biomarkers in metastatic patients with progression of disease. A suspicious solitary bone lesion in young patients without known primary malignancy is considered as Sarcoma unless proven otherwise, with the intent of treatment being limb salvage. A bone lesion biopsy is usually performed under CT-guidance which allows localization of the lesion and visualization of anatomic muscle compartments. Fluoroscopy may be used for larger lesions or transpedicular approach for vertebral body biopsy. Lesions close to the surface or with extra osseous soft tissue components may be biopsied via US.

Soft Tissue. Most suspected soft tissue lesions tend to be superficial and sampling can be performed using a high-frequency linear array probe. Color Doppler is used to visualize surrounding and intralesional vessels. The shortest path is preferred directed toward the target area. The risk of needle tract seeding, especially for soft tissue Sarcoma has been reported to be as high as 57.1% (56). A consultation with Surgeons prior to biopsy is suggested to determine a biopsy access pathway that would be eventually resected if Sarcoma is diagnosed due to a high rate of needle tract seeding.

SAMPLE ADEQUACY AND ANALYSIS

In this era of Personalized Medicine, especially in Oncology, it becomes of paramount importance that specimen yield (adequate sample acquired) is sufficient for both histopathologic and biomarker analysis, minimizing the need for repeat biopsies and delaying patient care including clinical trial enrollments. Inadequate sample amounts have been shown to be associated with higher rates of false negatives, delays in necessary biomarker analysis, and as demonstrated with NSCLC, can lead to inferior outcomes due to the initiation of inappropriate chemotherapy (57,58).

At least 50 viable cells per tissue section are required for fluorescent in situ hybridization (FISH) testing, and a minimum of ~200 ng of DNA or about 500 cells per histology section for DNA extraction for genotyping, although these numbers are decreasing due to improved sensitivity of molecular diagnostic platforms with newer genotyping techniques needing as low as 10 ng of DNA extracted from formalin-fixed and paraffin-embedded (FFPE) tissue and cytology specimens (7). Mutation analysis requires at least 10% malignant cell content (7). To put things into perspective, a good quality, nonhemorrhagic 21-gauge needle aspirate yields about 100 cells and CNB sample 500 cells (59). Unfortunately, for biomarker testing, there are no established guidelines on the amount of tissue needed due to the vast number of unknowns in this field: no objective criteria for biopsy site selection, type of sample acquisition device and technique used, evolving techniques of molecular analysis requiring differing amounts of tissue with none established as gold standard, different labs following their own protocols for the amount of tissue or proportion of tumor cells needed, and inherent tumor factors that can influence yield (7). Guidelines from the College of American Pathologists, International Association for the Study of Lung Cancer, and Association for Molecular Pathology state “ultimately, any specimen that meets the laboratory’s requirements for tumor content, fixation, and quality, as established during validation, may be chosen for analysis” (57). Keeping in mind these confounding factors, most Radiologists prefer to obtain 5 to 10 cores for both histologic and biomarker analysis.

TABLE 38.4

COMMON CANCER TYPES WITH ASSOCIATED PREDOMINANT BIOMARKERS WITH THEIR BIOMARKER BASED THERAPEUTIC AGENTS. THE FIELD OF ONCOLOGY IS NOW MOVING TOWARD DEFINING CANCER TYPES MOLECULARLY, NOT GEOGRAPHICALLY. THESE THERAPEUTIC AGENTS ACT BY VARIOUS MECHANISMS AND MAY BE KINASE INHIBITORS (KIs), MONOCLONAL ANTIBODIES (mABs) THAT MAY WORK AS IMMUNOMODULATORS AND UPREGULATE THE BODY'S OWN IMMUNE SYSTEM, OR MAY ACT ON VARIOUS TUMOR TARGETS DIRECTLY. THERE ARE ALSO OTHER AGENTS THAT ACT BY DIFFERENT MECHANISMS LIKE IMMUNOSUPPRESSION, AND HORMONE RECEPTOR ANTAGONISM AMONG OTHERS LISTED UNDER MISCELLANEOUS (MISC)

■ MALIGNANCY	■ MAJOR BIOMARKERS/MUTATIONS	■ THERAPEUTIC AGENT
Head and Neck	EGFR and KRAS -	mABs: Cetuximab
Melanoma	BRAFV600E	KIs: Vemurafenib
	BRAFV600E or V600K	KIs: Dabrafenib, Trametinib, Cobimetinib
	BRAF V600X	mABs: Nivolumab
	PD-L1	mABs: Pembrolizumab
Lung cancer (NSCLC)	EGFR	KIs: Afatinib, Erlotinib, Gefitinib
	EGFR T790M	KIs: Osimertinib
	EML4—ALK	KIs: Ceritinib, Crizotinib, Alectinib
	KRAS	KIs: Erlotinib, Gefitinib
	ROS1	KIs: Crizotinib
	PD-L1	mABs: Pembrolizumab
Breast	ESR1 and HER2-	Everolimus
	HER2	KIs: Lapatinib
		mABs: Pertuzumab, Trastuzumab, Trastuzumab-emtansine
	ESR1 and PGR	Misc: Tamoxifen, Anastrozole, Exemestane, Letrozole
Leukemia	t(15;17) PML-RARα	Tretinoin
	Ph	KIs: Imatinib, Dasatinib, Nilotinib, Bosutinib
	17p deletion	KIs: Ibrutinib
		Misc: Venetoclax
	Ph-	Blinatumomab
Lymphoma	17p deletion	KIs: Ibrutinib
	HIV- or HHV8-	mABs: Siltuximab
	BRAF V600X	mABs: Nivolumab
Gastric ACA	HER2	Trastuzumab
GIST	c-KIT	TKIs: Imatinib, Sunitinib
Pancreatic	EGFR and KRAS	TKIs like Erlotinib
Colorectal	EGFR and KRAS-	KIs: Cetuximab, Panitumumab
	ESR1 and PGR and HER2-	KIs: Palbociclib
		Misc: Fulvestrant
Renal	ESR1 and HER2-	Misc: Everolimus
	BRAF V600X	mABs: Nivolumab
Ovarian epithelial/ fallopian tube/ primary peritoneal	BRCA	KIs: Olaparib

ACA, adenocarcinoma; GIST, gastrointestinal stromal tumor; KIs, Kinase inhibitors; mABs, Monoclonal antibodies; Misc, Miscellaneous mechanisms including mTOR inhibitors and hormone receptor antagonists.
Twomey JD, Brahme NN, Zhang B. Drug-biomarker co-development in oncology—20 years and counting. *Drug Resist Updat* 2017;30:48–62.

Additionally, the biopsy samples need to be preserved in appropriate fixatives as per the analysis platform requirements and differential diagnosis of the suspicious lesion (Table 38.3).

CURRENT APPLICATIONS OF BIOMARKERS

Depending upon their utilization, biomarkers may be for diagnosis, predictive, prognostication, treatment monitoring, and to lesser extent screening. Predictive biomarkers inform of the potential response of a patient to a certain intervention including targeted or immunotherapeutic treatment options. The field of Oncology in particular is becoming increasingly reliant on biomarkers to guide therapy and is now moving towards defining cancer types molecularly, not geographically (Table 38.4) (60).

ETHICAL CONSIDERATIONS

As we unravel a patient's genetic information, there are many ethical issues that need to be considered. Currently in

Oncology, both tumor somatic mutations and patient's germline mutations can be analyzed in depth and are often included in a patient's medical record. The full impact and reachings of the genomic data obtained aren't completely known. This also raises the question of how much of the results obtained should be disclosed to the patient and to their relatives, for example, in patients with germline p53 mutations as noted in Li Fraumeni syndrome. Patients need to meet and discuss findings with Genetic Counselors. For many clinical trials, participation rests upon compulsory repeat biopsies with their inherent risks primarily for research purposes and not necessarily to determine next clinical treatment options. Samples are also often analyzed for research molecular markers beyond those for which there are current treatment agents (61,62).

The ethics and moral implications of biopsies for genetic analysis need to be looked into further keeping in mind both patient perspectives and scientific advancement. Consent for biopsies for genetic tissue analysis needs to be as explicit and as thorough as possible and currently often involves Institutional Review Board (IRB) panel–approved protocols to help with transparency and patient protection.

FUTURE TRENDS AND CONCEPTS

Radiologists are centrally positioned to play key roles in advancing the field of Personalized Medicine through improvements in both diagnostic imaging modalities and image-guided biopsy sample acquisition.

Advances in diagnostic imaging modalities include *Radiogenomics, or imaging genomics*, which is the study of the relationship between imaging phenotypes and the possible underlying genetic characteristics, which could potentially act as a guide to determine the ideal site to biopsy (7). *Quantitative radiology* is the measurement of the structural and biologic parameters from medical images, and obtaining objective data that practically provide a virtual biopsy and allow the measurement of disease status, severity, and treatment response and outcomes, for example, obtaining a virtual cortical biopsy in Alzheimer's patients that would help monitor disease progression (63). Theoretically, biomarkers may be mapped out to show the extent and severity of a disease and monitor it over time including emerging Molecular Imaging techniques via specific tracers that are being developed in the field of Nuclear Medicine. These developing fields will certainly improve and complement image-guided tissue sampling in the near future.

The main aim of the Radiologist performing image-guided biopsies is to sample the portion of the suspicious lesion that is most likely to provide highest histopathologic and molecular diagnostic yield. This can be done with advances in imaging modalities that allow intraprocedural identification of the ideal location to biopsy within the lesion or by devices that allow greater control and real-time feedback during sampling. *Optical molecular imaging* is an emerging modality that allows the characterization of tissue in real-time and thus may guide the Radiologist to the optimal biopsy site within the lesion during the procedure. The use of microbubble molecular tracers in sentinel lymph node biopsy in breast cancer patients, which enhances suspicious areas of the node, may be extrapolated and applied elsewhere as well (7). Other tracers, such as nanoparticles, are starting to emerge into clinical practice, especially in hollow organs specifically to aid with clear surgical margins during resection of colorectal cancers. The development of biopsy devices and smart needles that sense the molecular makeup of a lesion, for example, by a needle gamma detector, would allow for the detection of a molecular tracer during the biopsy, confirming the ideal site for sampling. Needles are also being developed with enhanced steering techniques, allowing greater control and maneuverability and thus making the path to a lesion safer (7). Shaft-based steering needles have precurved, telescoping, concentric tubes which can potentially be personalized for patients by measuring the required curvatures. There is also great interest in further development of robotically assisted MR-guided interventions in addition to the current Breast Radiologist MR-guided breast mass biopsy procedures (7).

It is important for Radiologists to be aware of a parallel universe to the tissue biopsy acquisition and analysis within the emerging field of *liquid biopsy*. Liquid biopsy platforms detect shed circulating tumor cells (CTCs), circulating tumor DNA (ct-DNA), and microvesicles containing RNA within a peripheral venous blood sample. As all shed markers are detected, it potentially provides a more comprehensive picture of tumor heterogeneity within the patient. It provides a much safer, noninvasive method of analyzing a patient's tumor burden and biology, allowing for safe repeated sampling as needed, potentially at lower costs. This is a rapidly evolving field with some early clinical applications mainly in metastatic stage IV patients with lung, colorectal, and melanoma malignancies.

The concept of personalized healthcare makes many promises that sound almost too good to be true and aims for eventually all medical decisions, investigations, treatments, dosages, or interventions to be singularly adapted to the patient. Biomedical imaging and image-guided interventions can enable the correlation of phenotype with molecular markers allowing precise care. For Personalized Medicine to realize its full potential, Radiologists must not only continue to evolve with it, but more importantly play a pivotal central role in helping shape the path.

References

1. PHG Foundation. Many names for one concept or many concepts in one name? Available from http://www.phgfoundation.org/documents/311_1358522182.pdf. Accessed September 29, 2017.
2. Atkinson AJ, Colburn WA, DeGruttola VG, et al. Biomarkers and surrogate endpoints: Preferred definitions and conceptual framework. *Clin Pharmacol Ther* 2001;69:89–95.
3. Falconi A, Lopes G, Parker JL. Biomarkers and receptor targeted therapies reduce clinical trial risk in non–small-cell lung cancer. *J Thorac Oncol* 2014;9:163–169.
4. Thompson RH, Kurta JM, Kaag M, et al. Tumor size is associated with malignant potential in renal cell carcinoma cases. *J Urol* 2009;181: 2033–2036.
5. Lim C, Sung M, Shepherd FA, et al. Patients with advanced non—small cell lung cancer: Are research biopsies a barrier to participation in clinical trials? *J Thorac Oncol* 2015;11:79–84.
6. Executive Summary. Interim analysis of the NCI-MATCH Trial. 2016. Available from https://dctd.cancer.gov/majorinitiatives/NCI-MATCH_Interim_Analysis_Executive_Summary.pdf. Accessed September 29, 2017.
7. Tam AL, Lim HJ, Wistuba II, et al. Image-guided biopsy in the era of personalized cancer care: Proceedings from the society of interventional radiology research consensus panel. *J Vasc Interv Radiol* 2016;27:8–19.
8. Hasanovic A, Rekhtman N, Sigel CS, Moreira AL. Advances in fine needle aspiration cytology for the diagnosis of pulmonary carcinoma. *Patholog Res Int* 2011;2011: Article ID 897292, 7 pages.
9. Patel IJ, Davidson JC, Nikolic B, et al. Consensus guidelines for periprocedural management of coagulation status and hemostasis risk in percutaneous image-guided interventions. *J Vasc Interv Radiol* 2012;23:727–736.
10. Ridout G, de la Motte S, Niemczyk S, et al. Effect of renal function on edoxaban pharmacokinetics and on population PK/PK-PD model. *J Clin Pharmacol* 2009;49:1091–130.
11. Baron TH, Kamath PS, McBane RD. Management of antithrombotic therapy in patients undergoing invasive procedures. *New Engl J Med* 2013;368: 2113–2124.
12. Nutescu EA. Oral anticoagulant therapies: Balancing the risks. *Am J Health Syst Pharm* 2013;70(10 Suppl 1):S3–S11.
13. Fleisher LA, Fleischmann KE, Auerbach AD, et al. 2014 ACC/AHA guideline on perioperative cardiovascular evaluation and management of patients undergoing noncardiac surgery. *Circulation* 2014;130:e278–e333.
14. Doherty JU, Gluckman TJ, Hucker WJ, et al. 2017 ACC expert consensus decision pathway for periprocedural management of anticoagulation

in patients with nonvalvular atrial fibrillation: A report of the American College of Cardiology Clinical Expert Consensus Document Task Force. *J Am Coll Cardiol* 2017;69:871–898.

15. Dean DS, Gharib H. Epidemiology of thyroid nodules. *Best Pract Res Clin Endocrinol Metab* 2008;22:901–911.
16. Kwong N, Medici M, Angell TE, et al. The influence of patient age on thyroid nodule formation, multinodularity, and thyroid cancer risk. *J Clin Endocrinol Metab* 2015;100:4434–4440.
17. Popoveniuc G, Jonklaas J. Thyroid Nodules. *Med Clin North Am* 2012; 96:329–349.
18. Bischoff ð L, Lamki Busaidy N, Byrd D, et al. NCCN Guidelines Version 2. 2017 Thyroid Carcinoma 2017. Available from https://www.nccn.org/professionals/physician_gls/pdf/thyroid.pdf. Accessed September 29, 2017.
19. Baloch ZW, Cibas ES, Clark DP, et al. The National Cancer Institute Thyroid fine needle aspiration state of the science conference: A summation. *Cytojournal* 2008;5:6.
20. Haugen BR, Alexander EK, Bible KC, et al. 2015 American Thyroid Association Management Guidelines for Adult Patients with Thyroid Nodules and Differentiated Thyroid Cancer. *Thyroid* 2015;26:1–133.
21. Na DG, Baek JH, Jung SL, et al. Core needle biopsy of the thyroid: 2016 consensus statement and recommendations from Korean society of thyroid radiology. *Korean J Radiol* 2017;18:217–237.
22. Dean DS, Gharib H. Fine-needle aspiration biopsy of the thyroid gland—thyroid disease manager. 2015. Available from http://www.thyroidmanager.org/chapter/fine-needle-aspiration-biopsy-of-the-thyroid-gland/. Accessed accessed September 29, 2017.
23. Gharib H, Papini E, Garber JR, et al. American Association of Clinical Endocrinologists, American College of Endocrinology, and Associazione Medici Endocrinologi Medical Guidelines for Clinical Practice for the Diagnosis and Management of Thyroid Nodules—2016 Update. *Endocr Pract* 2016;22:622–639.
24. Manhire A, Charig M, Clelland C, et al. Guidelines for radiologically guided lung biopsy. *Thorax* 2003;58(11):920–936.
25. Ghosh D, Howes TQ. How to do it: Ultrasound-guided pleural biopsy. *Breathe* 2007;4:151 LP–155.
26. Brown KT, Brody LA, Getrajdman GI, Napp TE. Outpatient treatment of iatrogenic pneumothorax after needle biopsy. *Radiology* 1997;205: 249–252.
27. Boskovic T, Stanic J, Pena-Karan S, et al. Pneumothorax after transthoracic needle biopsy of lung lesions under CT guidance. *J Thorac Dis* 2014;6(Suppl 1): S99–S107.
28. Wagner JM, Hinshaw JL, Lubner MG, et al. CT-guided lung biopsies: Pleural blood patching reduces the rate of chest tube placement for postbiopsy pneumothorax. *AJR Am J Roentgenol* 2011;197:783–788.
29. Malone LJ, Stanfill RM, Wang H, Fahey KM, Bertino RE.l. Effect of intraparenchymal blood patch on rates of pneumothorax and pneumothorax requiring chest tube placement after percutaneous lung biopsy. *Am J Roentgenol* 2013;200:1238–1243.
30. Graffy P, Loomis SB, Pickhardt PJ, et al. Pulmonary intraparenchymal blood patching decreases the rate of pneumothorax-related complications following percutaneous CT-guided needle biopsy. *J Vasc Interv Radiol* 2017; 28:608–613.e1.
31. Heerink WJ, de Bock GH, de Jonge GJ, Groen HJ, Vliegenthart R, Oudkerk M. Complication rates of CT-guided transthoracic lung biopsy: meta-analysis. *Eur Radiol* 2017;27:138–148.
32. Tannapfel A, Dienes HP, Lohse AW. The indications for liver biopsy. *Dtsch Ärztebl Int* 2012;109:477–483.
33. Marrero JA, Ahn J, Rajender Reddy K; Americal College of Gastroenterology. ACG clinical guideline: The diagnosis and management of focal liver lesions. *Am J Gastroenterol* 2014;109:1328–1347.
34. Kis B, Pamarthi V, Fan C-M, Rabkin D, Baum RA. Safety and utility of transjugular liver biopsy in hematopoietic stem cell transplant recipients. *J Vasc Interv Radiol* 2013;24:85–89.
35. Machado NO. Complications of liver biopsy—Risk factors, management and recommendations. In: Takahashi H, ed. Liver Biopsy. INTECH; 2011.
36. Takamori R, Wong LL, Dang C. Needle-tract implantation from hepatocellular cancer: Is needle biopsy of the liver always necessary? *Liver Transpl* 2000;6:67–72.
37. Liu YW, Chen CL, Chen Y Sen, Wang CC, Wang SH, Lin CC. Needle tract implantation of hepatocellular carcinoma after fine needle biopsy. *Dig Dis Sci* 2007;52:228–231.
38. Maturen KE, Nghiem HV, Marrero JA, et al. Lack of tumor seeding of hepatocellular carcinoma after percutaneous needle biopsy using coaxial cutting needle technique. *AJR Am J Roentgenol* 2006;187:1184–1187.
39. Shyamala K, Girish HC, Murgod S. Risk of tumor cell seeding through biopsy and aspiration cytology. *J Int Soc Prev Community Dent* 2014;4: 5–11.
40. Kim KR, Thomas S. Complications of image-guided thermal ablation of liver and kidney neoplasms. *Semin Intervent Radiol* 2014;31:138–148.
41. Uppot RN, Harisinghani MG, Gervais DA. Imaging-guided percutaneous renal biopsy: Rationale and approach. *AJRAm J Roentgenol* 2010; 194:1443–1449.
42. Fahy K, Augustine L, Sanden MO, Wassman ER. Clinicians' real world perceptions of pre-nephrectomy diagnostic biopsy performance as a driver of reduction in unnecessary surgeries in renal tumors. *J Kidney Cancer VHL* 2015;2:1–14.
43. Hogan JJ, Mocanu M, Berns JS. The native kidney biopsy: Update and evidence for best practice. *Clin J Am Soc Nephrol* 2016;11:354–356.
44. Misra S, Gyamlani G, Swaminathan S, et al. Safety and diagnostic yield of transjugular renal biopsy. *J Vasc Interv Radiol* 2008;19:546–551.
45. Whittier WL, Korbet SM. Timing of complications in percutaneous renal biopsy. *J Am Soc Nephrol* 2004;15:142–147.
46. Waldo B, Korbet SM, Freimanis MG, Lewis EJ. The value of post-biopsy ultrasound in predicting complications after percutaneous renal biopsy of native kidneys. *Nephrol Dial Transplant* 2009;24:2433–2439.
47. Stratta P, Canavese C, Marengo M, et al. Risk management of renal biopsy: 1387 Cases over 30 years in a single centre. *Eur J Clin Invest* 2007;37:954–963.
48. Corapi KM, Chen JLT, Balk EM, Gordon CE. Bleeding complications of native kidney biopsy: A systematic review and meta-analysis. *Am J Kidney Dis* 2012;60:62–73.
49. Chikamatsu Y, Matsuda K, Takeuchi Y, et al. Quantification of bleeding volume using computed tomography and clinical complications after percutaneous renal biopsy. *Clin Kidney J* 2017;10:9–15.
50. Andersen MF, Norus TP. Tumor seeding with renal cell carcinoma after renal biopsy. *Urol Case Rep* 2016;9:43–44.
51. Lewitowicz P, Matykiewicz J, Heciak J, Koziel D, Gluszek S. Percutaneous fine needle biopsy in pancreatic tumors: A study of 42 cases. *Gastroenterol Res Pract* 2012;2012:908963.
52. Sammon J, Twomey M, Crush L, Maher MM, O'Connor OJ. Image-guided percutaneous splenic biopsy and drainage. *Semin Intervent Radiol* 2012;29:301–310.
53. Venkataramu NK, Sood BP, Gupta S, Gulati M, Khandelwal N, Suri S. Ultrasound-guided fine needle aspiration biopsy of gall bladder malignancies. *Acta Radiol* 1999;40:436–439.
54. Sudheendra D, Wood BJ. Appropriate premedication risk reduction during adrenal ablation. *J Vasc Interv Radiol* 2006;17:1367–1368.
55. Sharma KV, Venkatesan AM, Swerdlow D, et al. Image-guided adrenal and renal biopsy. *Tech Vasc Interv Radiol* 2010;13:100–109.
56. Oliveira MP, Lima PM de A, da Silva HJ, de Mello RJ. Neoplasm seeding in biopsy tract of the musculoskeletal system. A systematic review. *Acta Ortop Bras* 2014;22:106–110.
57. Lindeman NI, Cagle PT, Beasley MB, et al. Molecular testing guideline for selection of lung cancer patients for EGFR and ALK tyrosine kinase inhibitors: Guideline from the College of American Pathologists, International Association for the study of lung cancer, and Association for Molecular Pathology. *Arch Pathol Lab Med* 2013;137:828–860.
58. Lim C, Tsao MS, Le LW, et al. Biomarker testing and time to treatment decision in patients with advanced nonsmall-cell lung cancer. *Ann Oncol* 2015;26:1415–1421.
59. Pirker R, Herth FJF, Kerr KM, et al. Consensus for EGFR mutation testing in non-small cell lung cancer: results from a European workshop. *J Thorac Oncol* 2010;5:1706–1713.
60. Twomey JD, Brahme NN, Zhang B. Drug-biomarker co-development in oncology—20 years and counting. *Drug Resist Updat* 2017;30:48–62.
61. Peppercorn J, Shapira I, Collyar D, et al. Ethics of mandatory research biopsy for correlative end points within clinical trials in oncology. *J Clin Oncol* 2010;28:2635–2640.
62. Lolkema MP, Gadellaa-van Hooijdonk CG, Bredenoord AL, et al. Ethical, legal, and counseling challenges surrounding the return of genetic results in oncology. *J Clin Oncol* 2013;31:1842–1848.
63. QIBA. Available from https://www.rsna.org/QIBA/. Accessed September 29, 2017.

CHAPTER 39 ■ INTERVENTIONAL MANAGEMENT OF HEPATIC MALIGNANCIES: GENERAL CONCEPTS FROM ANATOMY TO PRACTICE

SARAH H. ALLGEIER, NIMA KOKABI, AND JUAN C. CAMACHO

INTRODUCTION

Liver-directed therapies for hepatic malignancies are currently used as the primary treatment in some malignancies (i.e., hepatocellular carcinoma [HCC]), in combination with surgical or systemic therapies in the setting of other primary liver tumors (i.e., cholangiocarcinoma), or in the setting of liver-dominant metastatic disease. Interventional oncology as a subspecialty of interventional radiology has evolved tremendously and some of the current techniques, which initially were developed as palliative, now offer the possibility of curing disease that had limited treatment strategies in the past. Liver-directed therapies are accepted today as a fundamental part of robust transplantation programs that treat primary liver malignancies, and it has been demonstrated in the literature that such interventions improve patient outcomes. In the case of metastatic disease, ablative and intra-arterial therapies are often used as an adjunct to surgical resection, either to limit the extent of surgery or to treat bilobar disease. These minimally invasive therapies minimize systemic effects, preserve as much normal liver tissue as possible, and provide adequate tumor control. From the radiology residency perspective, it has therefore become imperative for trainees to understand and be able to apply these concepts into general radiology practice. The following chapter will review the principles behind the available intra-arterial and percutaneous therapies, the main applications in the liver, and the relevant mandatory anatomical concepts that a general radiology practitioner should know.

VASCULAR ANATOMY OF THE LIVER

Segmental Liver Anatomy

Since 1951 when Hjortsjö described the segmental pattern of bile duct branching, multiple hepatic segmentation systems have been proposed. Healey and Schroy described a five-segment system based on secondary bile duct and hepatic artery branching, Goldsmith and Woodburne described four segments based on second-order portal vein branching, and subsequently Couinaud described eight segments based on third-order portal vein branching. Bismuth then introduced a system which combined the Couinaud and Goldsmith and Woodburne systems into one. However, the Couinaud system, described by Claude Couinaud, a French surgeon and anatomist, is the most widely used. In this system, each segment has its own vascular inflow, outflow, and biliary drainage, allowing for surgical resection of individual segments without damage to adjacent segments. At the center of each segment, there is a branch of the portal vein, hepatic artery, and bile duct; and in the periphery of each segment are the hepatic veins.

According to Couinaud segmental liver anatomy, a plane created along the middle hepatic vein from the inferior vena cava to the gallbladder fossa divides the liver into the right and left lobes. The right hepatic vein divides the right lobe into anterior and posterior segments; and the falciform ligament divides the left lobe into medial and lateral segments. The main portal vein divides the liver into upper and lower segments (Fig. 39.1).

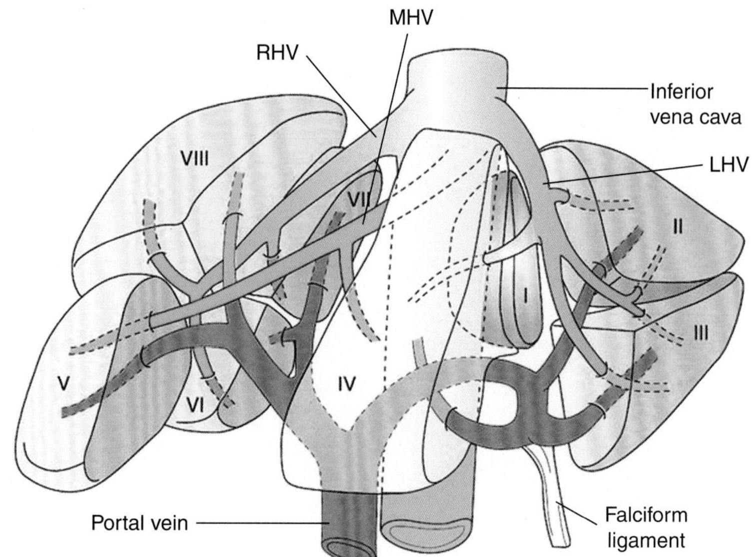

FIGURE 39.1. Couinaud segmental liver anatomy. LHV, left hepatic vein; MHV, middle hepatic vein; RHV, right hepatic vein. (From Greenfield LJ, Mulholland MW. (2017). *Greenfields surgery: scientific principles and practice*. Philadelphia, PA: Wolters Kluwer Health/Lippincott Williams & Wilkins, with permission.)

There are eight Couinaud liver segments. Segment I, the caudate lobe, is located posterior to the hepatic hilum and wraps around the inferior vena cava. The numbering of the segments then proceeds in a clockwise manner beginning with the upper lateral left lobe. The lateral left lobe is comprised of segments II (superior) and III (inferior). The medial left lobe is comprised of segment IV, often subdivided into segments IVA (superior) and IVB (inferior) according to Bismuth. The anterior right lobe is comprised of segments V (inferior) and VIII (superior). The posterior right lobe is comprised of segments VI (inferior) and VII (superior) (Fig. 39.2).

Hepatic Arterial Anatomy and Special Considerations for Intra-Arterial Therapy

Hepatic arteries typically provide more than 90% of hepatic tumor blood supply, whereas normal liver parenchyma is primarily supplied by the portal vein. For this reason, hepatic tumors can be effectively treated with various intra-arterial embolization therapies while surrounding normal liver is spared. Embolization is the process by which vascular flow is occluded using various materials and is utilized in the treatment of hemorrhage and, in the case of tumor therapy, to facilitate target tissue ischemia. Mastery of hepatic arterial anatomy is imperative to achieving optimal tumor therapy while avoiding complications related to nontarget embolization.

Classically, the celiac artery emerges from the aorta at approximately the level of T12 and the celiac trunk then branches into the common hepatic artery (CHA), left gastric artery (LGA), and splenic artery (SA). The CHA courses to the right along the superior edge of the pancreas and then branches into the gastroduodenal artery (GDA) and proper hepatic artery (PHA). The PHA courses right and upward and divides into the left (LHA) and right (RHA) hepatic arteries at the hepatic hilum. Conventional hepatic arterial anatomy, with the RHA and LHA arising from the PHA, is present in approximately 60% of patients (Fig. 39.3). Variations include replaced arteries, where the artery origin is from a different parent vessel, and accessory branches, which are present in addition to the primary vessel (Fig. 39.4).

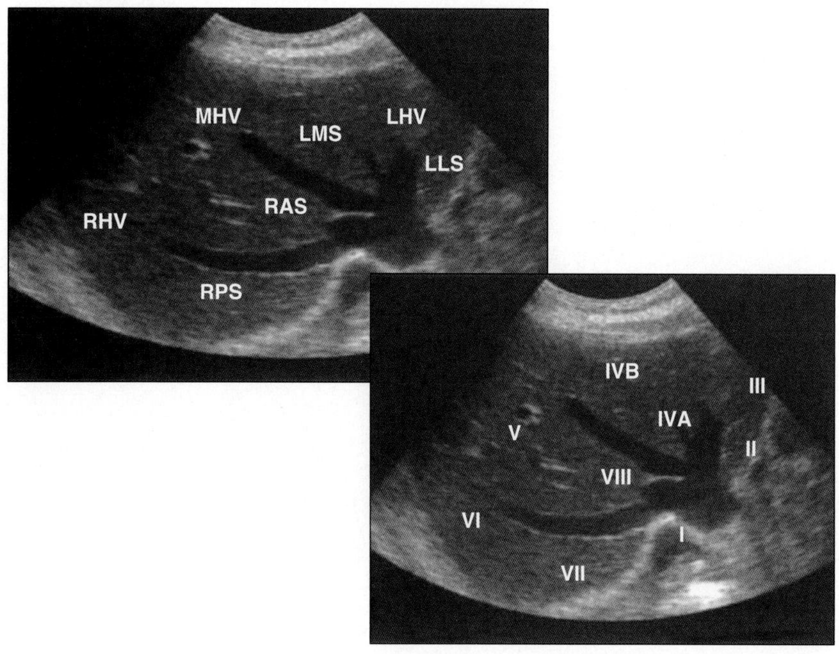

FIGURE 39.2. Couinaud segmental liver anatomy with ultrasound correlation. LHV, left hepatic vein; MHV, middle hepatic vein; RHV, right hepatic vein; LLS, left lateral segment; LMS, left medial segment; RAS, right anterior segment; RPS, right posterior segment.

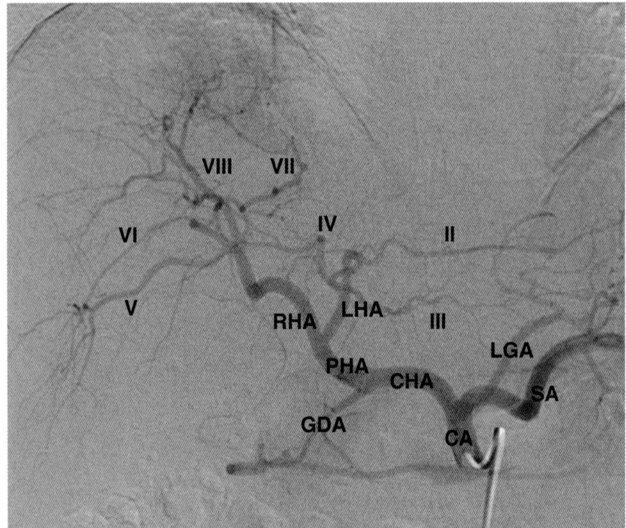

FIGURE 39.3. Celiac angiogram demonstrating conventional anatomy. CA, celiac artery; CHA, common hepatic artery; LGA, left gastric artery; SA, splenic artery; GDA, gastroduodenal artery; PHA, proper hepatic artery; LHA, left hepatic artery; RHA, right hepatic artery.

The LHA usually arises from the PHA, but when replaced it most commonly arises from the LGA (~5%), less commonly from the celiac trunk. Accessory LHAs may arise from the LGA, celiac trunk, RHA, or aorta. The LHA runs from the hepatic hilum to the umbilical portion of the left portal vein, then courses over the portal vein to form the arch of the LHA, after which it divides into the branches to segments II and III (Fig. 39.5).

The RHA usually arises from the PHA, but when replaced it most commonly arises from the superior mesenteric artery (SMA) (~12%) (Fig. 39.6), less commonly from the right phrenic artery or celiac trunk. Accessory RHAs may arise from the SMA, celiac trunk, GDA, right phrenic artery, or the aorta. The RHA divides into anterior and posterior branches, with the anterior branch taking a right upward course to supply segments V and VIII, and the posterior branch supplying segments VI and VII.

The segment IV branch has two main branching patterns. Classically it arises from the LHA, branching to the right

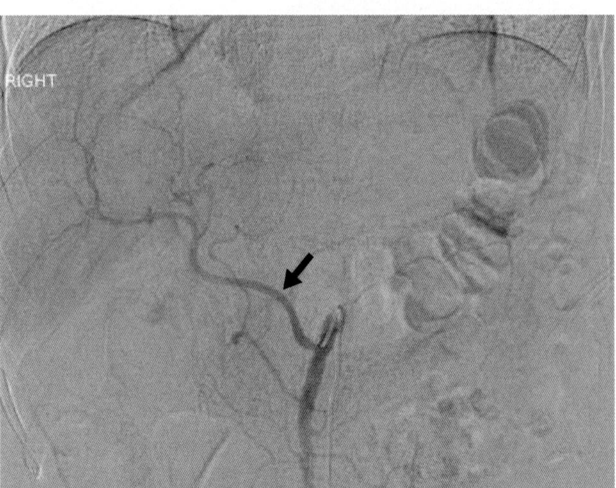

FIGURE 39.4. Superior mesenteric artery angiogram demonstrating a replaced common hepatic artery (*arrow*).

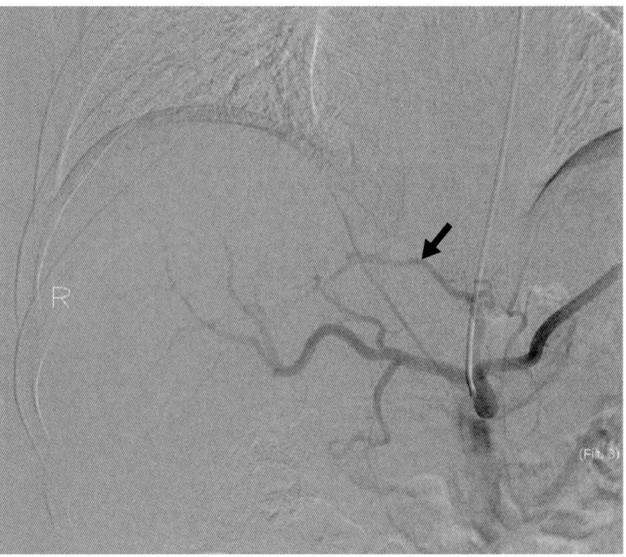

FIGURE 39.5. Celiac angiogram demonstrating a replaced left hepatic artery (*arrow*) from the left gastric artery.

from the proximal umbilical portion. However, it may also arise from the PHA, seen as a trifurcation of the PHA, and be termed the middle hepatic artery (MHA) (Fig. 39.7). The caudate lobe, segment I, is supplied by multiple small branches arising from the LHA and RHA.

When planning intra-arterial tumor therapy, it is important not only to determine which arteries are supplying the tumor but which arteries are in danger of nontarget therapy. The origins of these arteries may require prophylactic embolization to prevent nontarget therapy leading to complications including gastrointestinal ulceration, skin ulceration, and cholecystitis. Commonly encountered nontarget vessels include the GDA, RGA, accessory LGA, and the retroduodenal, supraduodenal, falciform, and cystic arteries, with the GDA and RGA being the most frequently prophylactically coil embolized in the setting of selective internal radiation therapy.

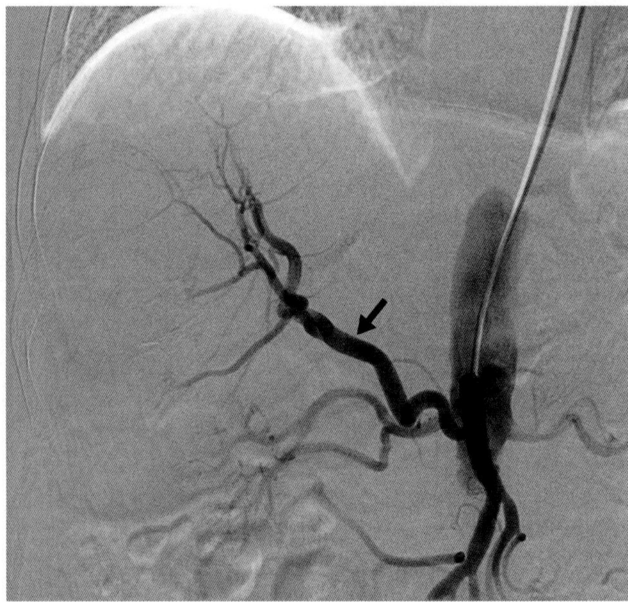

FIGURE 39.6. Superior mesenteric artery angiogram (SMA) demonstrating a replaced right hepatic artery (*arrow*).

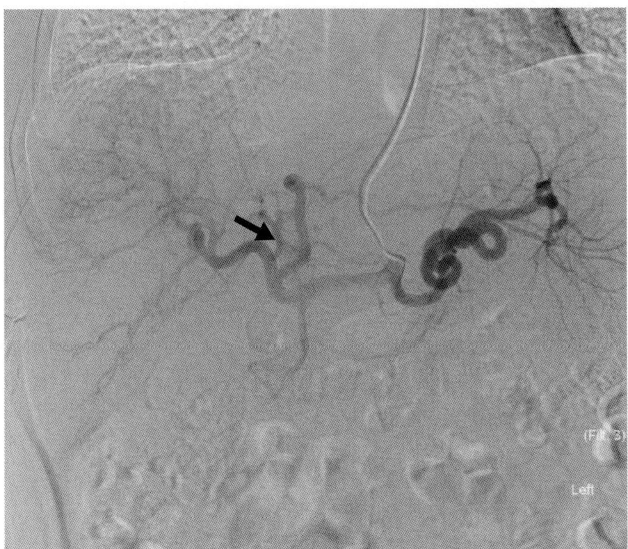

FIGURE 39.7. Celiac angiogram demonstrating a "middle hepatic artery" (*arrow*).

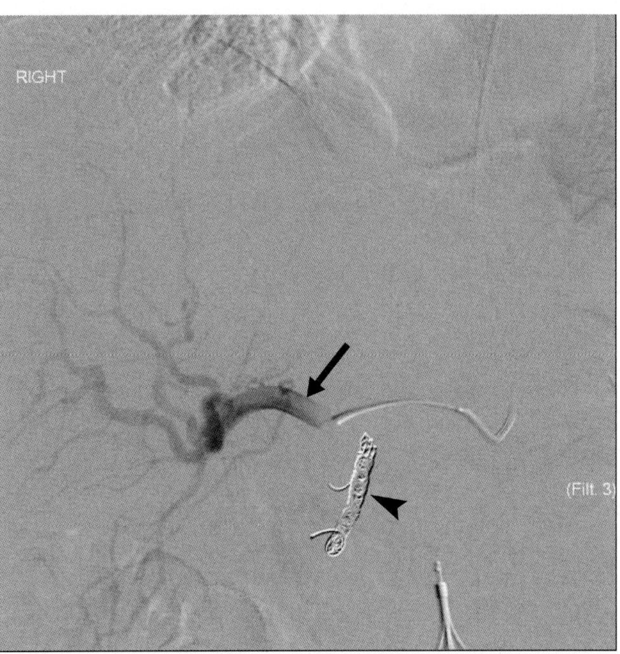

FIGURE 39.8. Selective right hepatic angiogram demonstrating antegrade flow in the right hepatic artery (*arrow*) with coil embolization of the gastroduodenal artery (*arrowhead*) during a selective internal radiation therapy work-up procedure.

The GDA typically arises at the terminus of the CHA and supplies the pylorus, proximal duodenum, and pancreatic head. It should be prophylactically coil embolized prior to intra-arterial therapy when the expected catheter position for delivery of therapeutics is not sufficiently distal to the GDA to prevent reflux and nontarget embolization (Fig. 39.8). However, in the instance of celiac trunk stenosis and resultant retrograde GDA flow to supply the celiac axis, prophylactic GDA embolization should not be performed. In some cases, retrograde GDA flow is seen but is due to decreased hepatic arterial resistance related to a large hepatic tumor burden. In this case, prophylactic GDA embolization should be performed as tumor embolization may lead to reversal of the retrograde GDA flow and subsequent nontarget embolization.

The RGA supplies the gastric antrum, pylorus, and proximal duodenal bulb and usually originates from the PHA, though it may originate from the LGA or CHA. It may require prophylactic coil embolization unless its origin is off the proximal CHA and nontarget embolization is unlikely (Fig. 39.9). The RGA often branches at an acute angle and can therefore be difficult to cannulate. In this case, retrograde access for prophylactic embolization via the LGA may be considered.

The supraduodenal artery supplies the proximal duodenum. The retroduodenal artery, also known as the posterosuperior pancreaticoduodenal artery, supplies the duodenal bulb and the pancreatic head and uncinate process. These vessels usually arise from the GDA but may arise from the CHA,

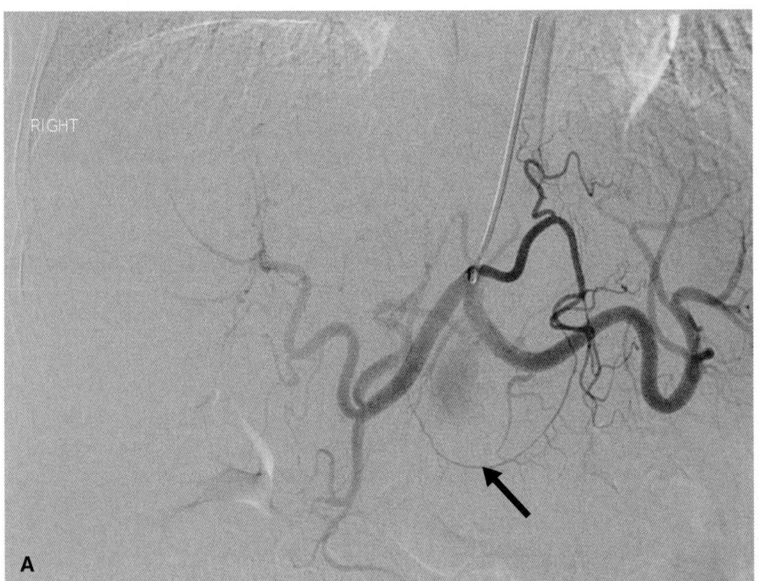

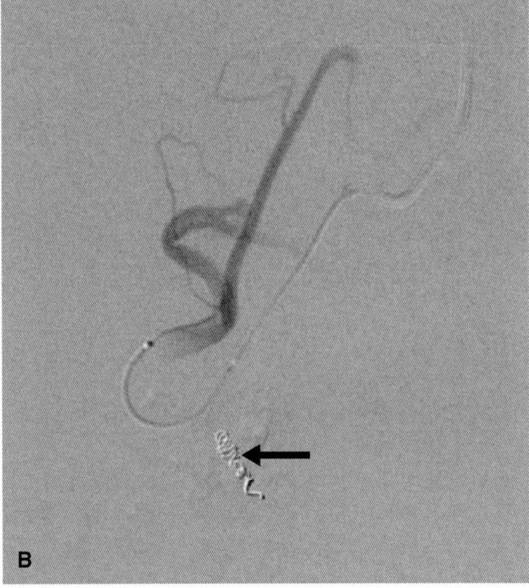

FIGURE 39.9. **A:** Celiac angiogram demonstrating a right gastric artery (*arrow*) originating off the proximal left hepatic artery. **B:** In order to protect the territory from nontarget embolization, coil embolization of the vessel was performed (*arrow*). Following embolization, left hepatic artery angiogram demonstrates antegrade flow with absence of flow through the right gastric artery.

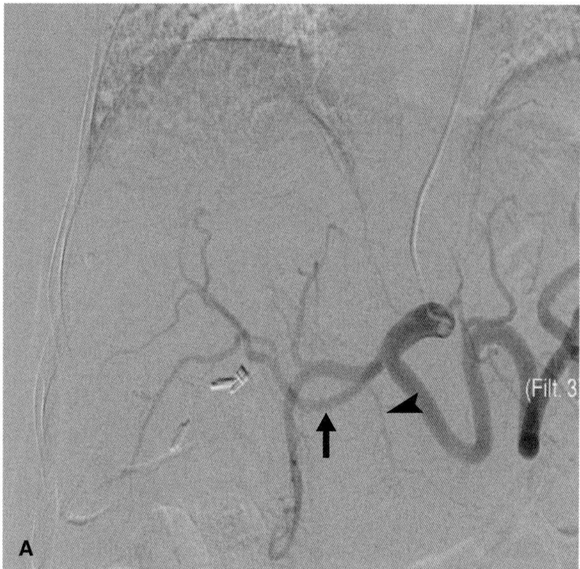

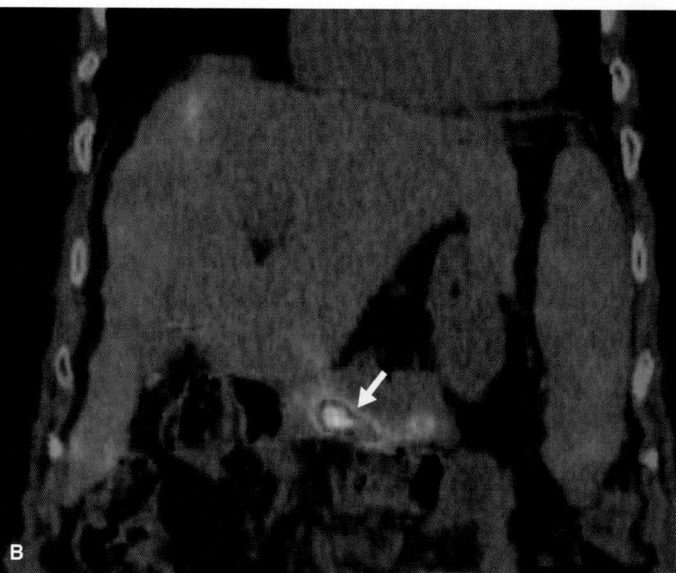

FIGURE 39.10. A: Celiac angiogram demonstrating the right hepatic artery originating directly from the celiac axis (*arrow*). A posterosuperior pancreaticoduodenal artery (PSPDA) is seen proximally from the right hepatic artery (*arrowhead*). B: Coronal ^{99m}Tc-MAA SPECT-CT demonstrating radiotracer activity in the duodenum and pancreas, indicating that the PSPDA must be prophylactically embolized prior to selective internal radiation therapy to prevent nontarget embolization.

PHA, or RHA, and should be prophylactically coil embolized if they originate from the hepatic circulation (Fig. 39.10).

An accessory LGA, when present, arises from the LHA and supplies the gastric cardia and fundus. If possible, it should be prophylactically coil embolized prior to LHA territory tumor embolization (Fig. 39.11).

The falciform artery is uncommon but, when present, it supplies the umbilical region of the anterior abdominal wall and most commonly originates from the MHA or LHA. When at risk it should be prophylactically coil embolized as nontarget embolization during tumor therapy can result in painful abdominal wall injury or skin ulceration (Fig. 39.12).

The cystic artery supplies the gallbladder and is typically the first branch of the RHA, subsequently bifurcating into deep and superficial branches that outline the gallbladder. While prophylactic coil embolization may rarely lead to ischemic cholecystitis, it is generally well tolerated and should be

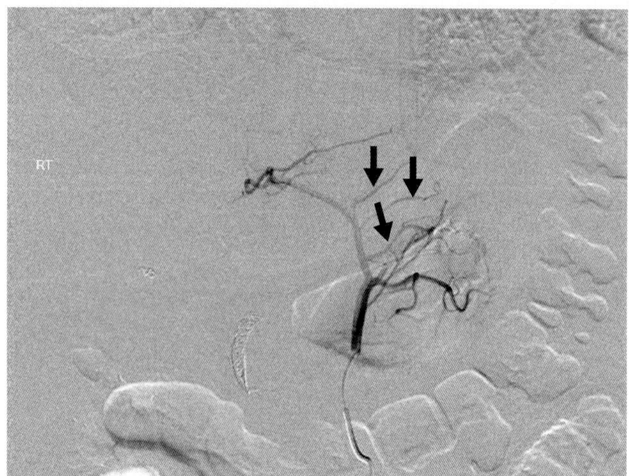

FIGURE 39.11. Selective left hepatic angiogram demonstrating multiple accessory left gastric arteries off the proximal left hepatic artery (*arrows*).

performed if there is sufficient risk of nontarget embolization. Permanent particle embolization of the cystic artery is generally not advised due to the high risk of ischemic cholecystitis. However, gelatin-sponge particles have been used in the past with variable success rates (Fig. 39.13).

In addition to determining the hepatic arterial branches supplying the tumor to be treated and identifying arteries that require prophylactic embolization to prevent nontarget tumor therapy, one must also evaluate for parasitized collateral vessels supplying the target tumor. Serosal liver tumors, especially large tumors, are more likely to have parasitized arterial supply. The likelihood of parasitization also increases with repeated embolizations. Commonly encountered parasitized collateral vessels include the phrenic, adrenal, internal mammary, omental, renal, renal capsular, adrenal, intercostal, lumbar, gastric, gastroduodenal, and cystic arteries, depending on the location of the tumor (Fig. 39.14).

The right inferior phrenic artery (RIPA) is the most commonly encountered extrahepatic collateral vessel to supply hepatic tumors (Fig. 39.15). It arises most commonly from the aorta or celiac trunk, supplies the right hemidiaphragm, and should be investigated when the targeted hepatic tumor involves the bare area of the liver (especially segments VII and VIII). While embolization of the RIPA is generally well tolerated, complications including shoulder pain, pleural effusion, and diaphragmatic weakness may occur.

Omental arteries are also commonly parasitized. They supply the greater omentum and typically arise from the right or left gastroepiploic artery. They can supply tumors anywhere in the liver and their embolization is well tolerated.

The cystic artery should be investigated when the target tumor lies near the gallbladder fossa. Due to the aforementioned risk of ischemic cholecystitis with cystic artery embolization, super-selective embolization of tumor-feeding branches is recommended when possible.

INTRA-ARTERIAL THERAPIES

Intra-arterial therapies exploit the fact that, while normal hepatic parenchyma receives two-thirds of its blood supply

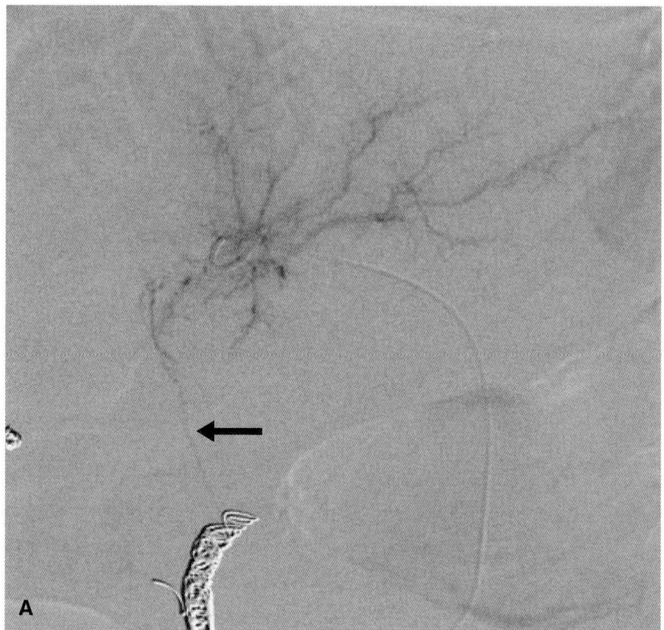

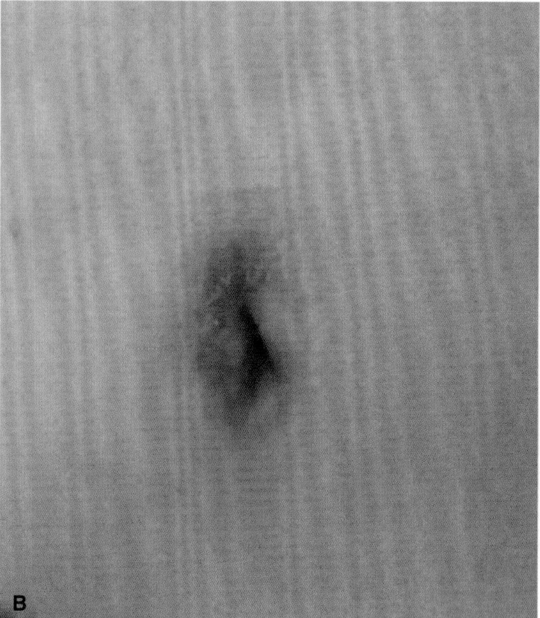

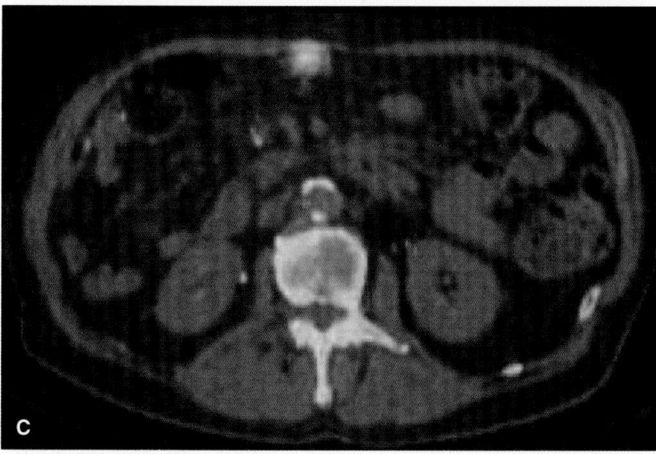

FIGURE 39.12. **A:** Selective left hepatic angiogram in a patient with metastatic colon cancer that underwent selective internal radiation therapy. The falciform artery was identified (*arrow*), but due to small size it could not be selected for embolization. An ice pack was placed in the umbilical region prior to treatment to facilitate vasoconstriction and limit nontarget embolization. **B:** Despite protection, the patient developed a grade 1 cutaneous radiation injury, which was treated conservatively and later granulated and resolved. **C:** ^{90}Y bremsstrahlung axial SPECT-CT demonstrates intense uptake extending to the umbilicus.

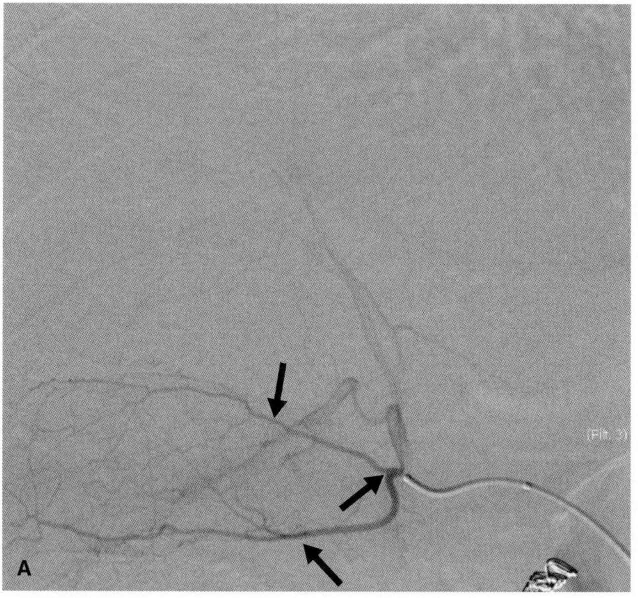

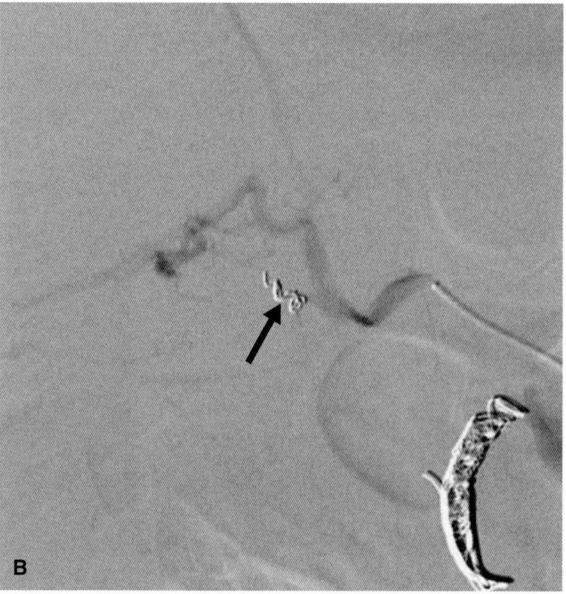

FIGURE 39.13. **A:** Right hepatic angiogram demonstrating the cystic artery (*arrow*) originating off the proximal right hepatic artery. **B:** In order to protect the territory from nontarget embolization, prophylactic coil embolization of the vessel was performed (*arrow*). Following coil embolization (*arrow*), right hepatic angiogram demonstrating antegrade flow with decreased flow through the cystic artery.

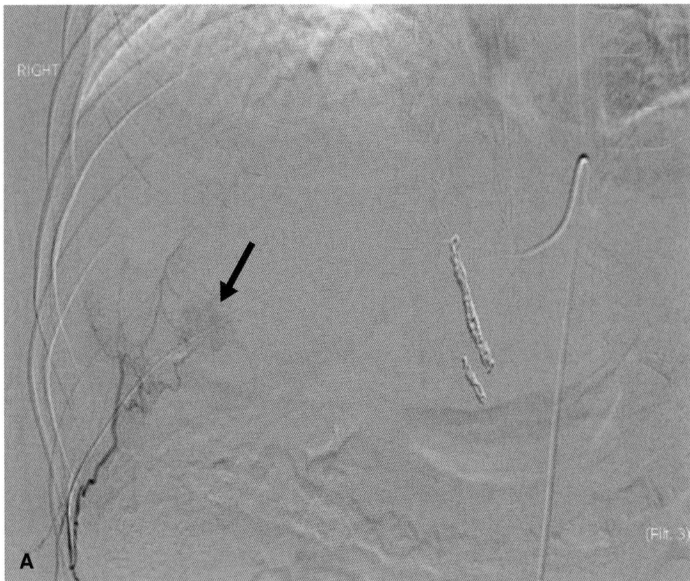

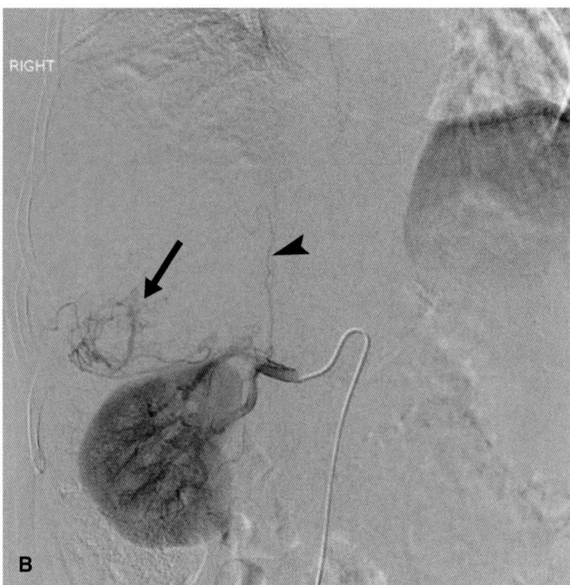

FIGURE 39.14. **A:** Right intercostal artery angiogram demonstrating tumor blush in segment VII (*arrow*) of the liver following multiple DEB-TACE therapies. **B:** Right renal angiogram demonstrating tumor blush in segment VI from parasitized flow from the right renal (*arrow*) and right adrenal (*arrowhead*) arteries.

from the portal vein and only one-third from the hepatic artery, most hepatic malignancies receive the majority of their blood supply from the hepatic artery and may parasitize flow from extrahepatic arteries (Fig. 39.16). In addition, tumors in general have a high vessel density secondary to angiogenesis. Therefore, the arterial system provides the perfect delivery vehicle for tumor-selective therapy in the liver.

Transarterial Chemoembolization

Transarterial chemoembolization (TACE) is used for palliation of unresectable hypervascular hepatic tumors, as an adjunctive therapy to resection or ablation, and as a bridge to transplantation. High-dose chemotherapy is delivered intra-arterially to the tumor bed while sparing surrounding hepatic parenchyma supplied mainly by the portal vein. However, tumors may also receive blood via the portal venules and surrounding hepatic sinusoids. This occurs as a result of portal flow reversal following hepatic artery embolization and may contribute to tumor survival posttreatment. TACE causes tumor ischemia, and the hypoxic stress stimulates vascular endothelial growth factor production by the residual tumor cells in an effort to recruit a new blood supply. Once this occurs, future treatments become increasingly challenging. Therefore, the best TACE outcomes are achieved when the peritumoral portal venules are embolized at the initial treatment session in addition to complete embolization of the hepatic arterial and parasitized extrahepatic arterial inflow. For larger tumors, for multifocal disease, or if complete response is not achieved after the first therapy,

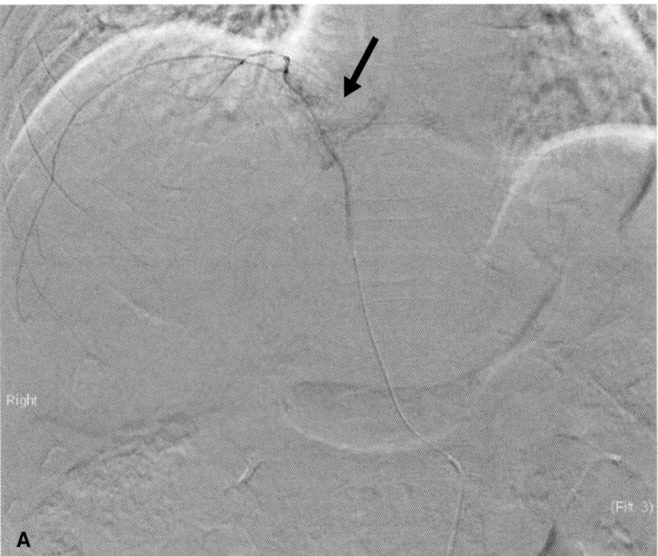

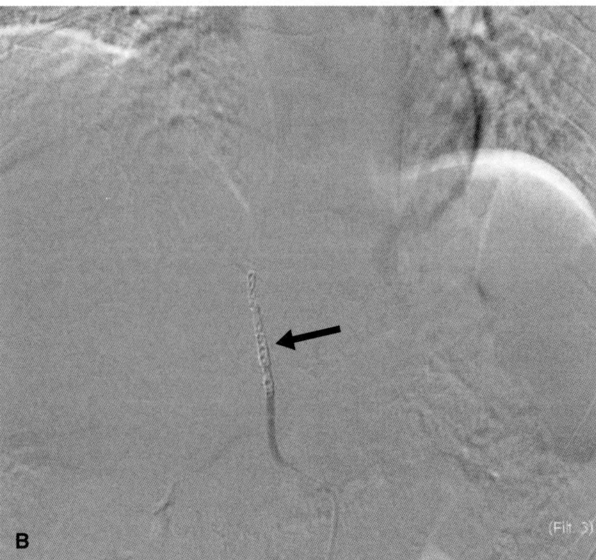

FIGURE 39.15. **A:** Right inferior phrenic artery (RIPA) angiogram demonstrating tumor blush in segment VIII from parasitized flow (*arrow*). **B:** Particle embolization of the RIPA was performed as therapeutic intervention as well as coil embolization to avoid recanalization (*arrow*).

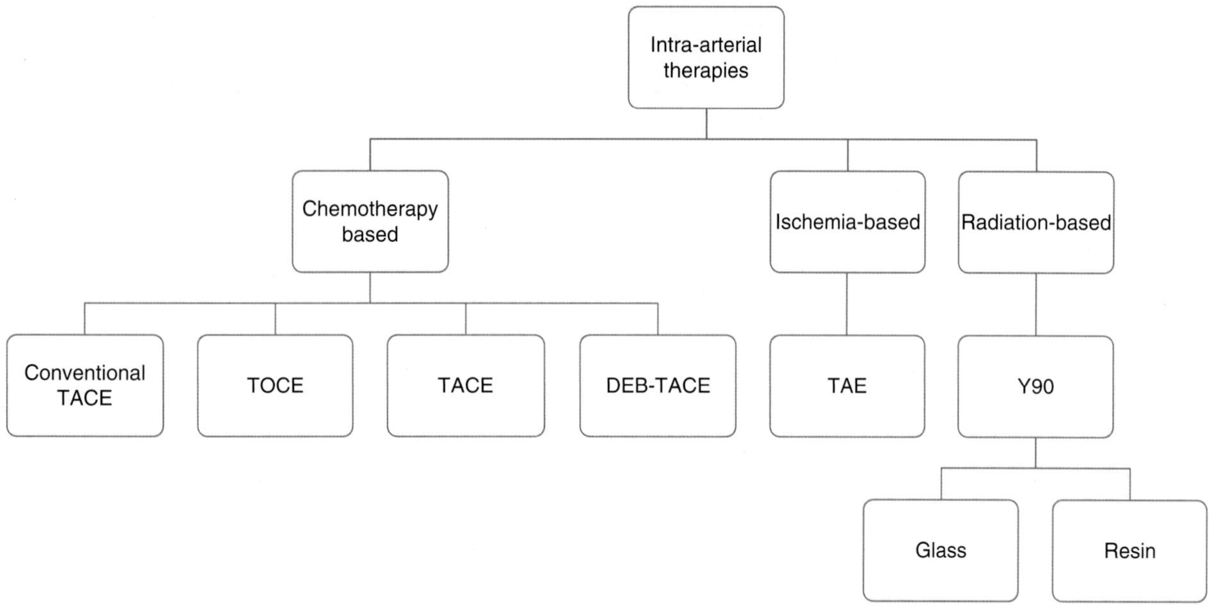

FIGURE 39.16. Scheme demonstrating the available intra-arterial therapies.

the best results are obtained when long-term arterial patency is maintained to allow repeated treatment. Appropriate choice of embolic agents is crucial in achieving these goals, and permanent embolic agents are not recommended.

Conventional TACE involves infusion of a mixture of chemotherapeutic agents with or without iodized oil, followed by embolization with particles to prevent rapid washout of the delivered chemotherapeutic agent (Fig. 39.17). The technique was originally described in the 1980s by Yamada, who delivered gelatin-sponge pieces impregnated with mitomycin C or doxorubicin intra-arterially, building on the work of Doyon, who first described transcatheter hepatic artery embolization to treat hepatic tumors. It was then determined that ethiodized oil added to the infused chemotherapy mixture engaged the chemotherapeutic agents and would be taken up and retained by many hepatic tumors, facilitating embolization and tumor necrosis. Ethiodized oil is a mixture of di-iodinated ethyl esters of fatty acids from poppy seed with an iodine content of 37% by weight. It is therefore opaque to x-rays, an excellent lipophilic vehicle for drug delivery, tumor-seeking due to a siphoning effect related to tumor hypervascularity and the lack of Kupffer cells in tumors, and induces transient embolization of tumor microvessels as it will eventually be cleared from the tissue. Because of its lipophilic nature, ethiodized oil distributes in both the tumor artery branches and the peritumoral portal venules, thus allowing dual embolization. As such, the degree of tumor staining with ethiodized oil is an independent prognostic factor.

The most widely used single chemotherapeutic agent is doxorubicin, and the most widely used combination of agents is cisplatin, doxorubicin, and mitomycin C. Embolic agents that have been employed in conjunction with ethiodized oil to perform TACE include gelfoam, polyvinyl alcohol (PVA) particles, and glass, starch, or trisacryl gelatin microspheres. However, the use of PVA particles is highly discouraged.

Biodegradable embolic agents such as gelfoam and starch microspheres that allow for initial complete embolization but long-term arterial patency, thus facilitating repeated transcatheter therapy, are known to be beneficial. Small embolic agents (less than 100 μm) are generally preferred as they can embolize end branches of the hepatic artery and prevent the development of collateral arterial flow to the treated tumor. However, if the embolic agents are too small, they can damage extratumoral liver tissue including the biliary system; and if they are too big, they can cause clogging of the delivery catheter or proximal artery embolization with failure of the embolic agent to reach the small vessels of the tumor vascular bed.

Variations on conventional TACE include transcatheter oily chemoembolization (TOCE), where the chemotherapeutic agent is mixed with ethiodized oil but no other embolic agent is used, transarterial embolization (TAE), where embolization is performed but no chemotherapeutic agent is delivered, and transarterial chemotherapy (TAC), where chemotherapy is infused without ethiodized oil or embolization particles. Regarding TOCE, Takayasu et al. demonstrated that the injection of cytotoxic drugs mixed with lipiodol but not followed by embolization does not show any substantial antitumor effect. Further, TAE, also called bland embolization, which simulates arterial ligation, has demonstrated similar overall survival benefit when compared to TACE. These findings suggest that ischemia plays a key role in tumor necrosis.

Drug-eluting bead TACE (DEB-TACE) is a newer iteration of TACE performed with biocompatible, nonresorbable polymers such as polyvinyl alcohol hydrogel that have been sulphonated to enable the reversible ionic binding of polar chemotherapeutic agents (Fig. 39.18). The beads then serve the dual purpose of embolic agent and chemotherapy reservoir, allowing the chemotherapy to slowly diffuse locally. The beads are available in multiple sizes and can be loaded with doxorubicin, epirubicin, or irinotecan, depending on the type of malignancy. These beads allow for fixed dosing and the ability to release the chemotherapeutic agents in a sustained and controlled manner. Significant reduction of peak plasma concentrations with DEB-TACE have been observed when compared with conventional TACE as mixed hydrophilic chemotherapeutics are lost from ethiodized oil within 4 hours, in contrast to days for drug-eluting beads.

Not all patients with unresectable primary or metastatic liver tumors will benefit from TACE. Gadolinium-enhanced magnetic resonance imaging (MRI) of the liver and multiphase computed tomography (CT) are useful in the biologic characterization of tumors and predictive efficacy of TACE. Overall survival has been shown to be significantly longer for patients with completely encapsulated HCC versus patients with incompletely or nonencapsulated tumors or infiltrative

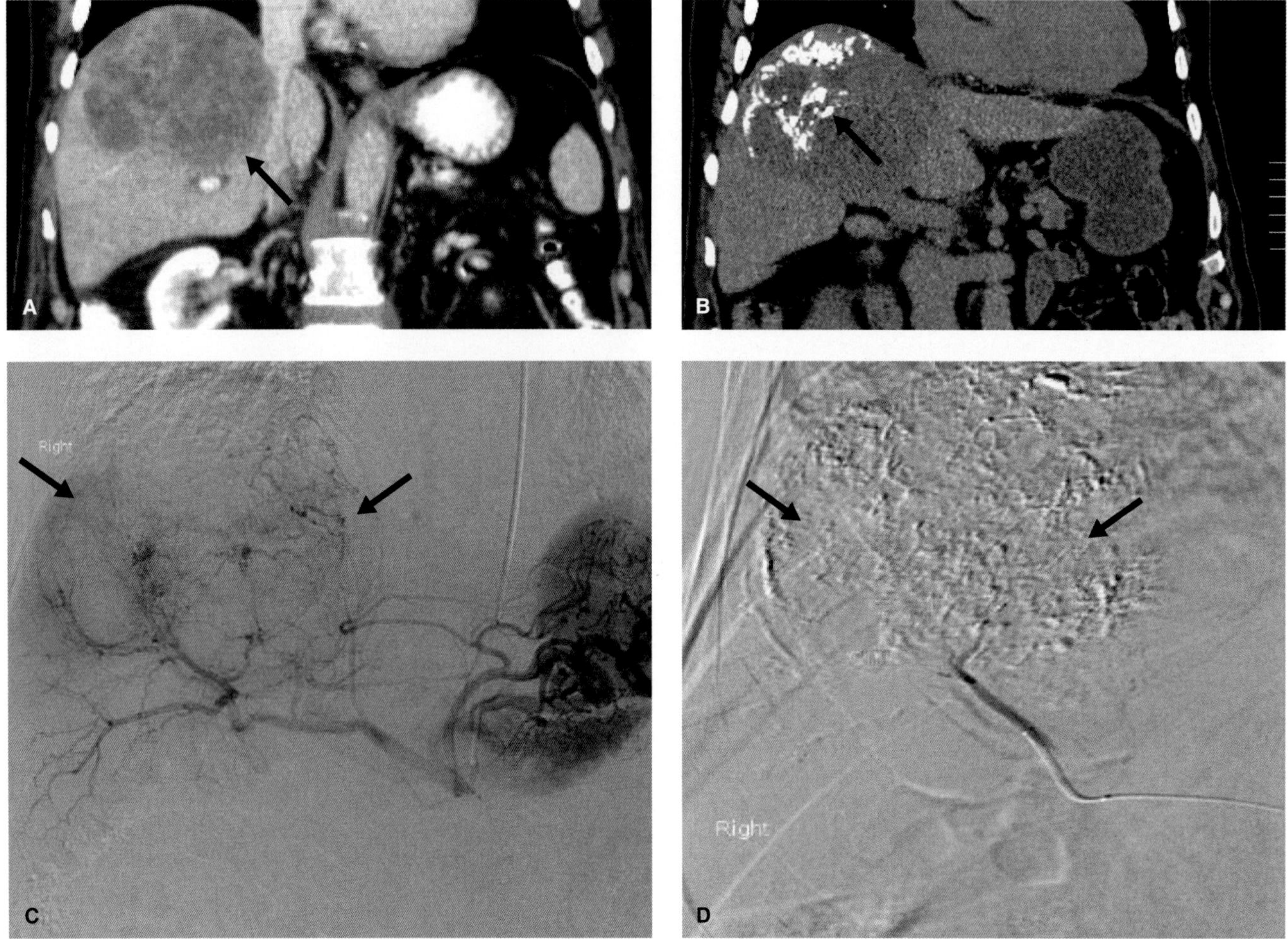

FIGURE 39.17. **Conventional TACE Case. A:** Coronal contrast-enhanced CT demonstrating a right lobe mass (*arrow*), known to be a hepatocellular carcinoma. **B:** Postprocedural noncontrast CT shows ethiodized oil deposition within the mass (*arrow*). **C:** Correlative celiac angiogram demonstrates a large right lobe mass and associated tumor blush (*arrows*). **D:** The territory was subsequently embolized with ethiodized oil containing chemotherapy to stasis (*arrows*).

presentations (Fig. 39.19). Gross vascular invasion, bile duct invasion, irregular tumor margin, peripheral ragged enhancement, and satellite nodules are associated with less favorable response to TACE after adjustment for tumor size, tumor number, and alpha-fetoprotein level (Table 39.1).

In patients with advanced liver disease, treatment-induced liver failure may offset any survival benefit related to tumor killing. Tumor burden, underlying liver function, and overall performance status should therefore be considered in patient selection, with the best candidates being those with preserved liver function and asymptomatic tumors without vascular invasion or extrahepatic metastases.

Absolute contraindications to TACE include tumor resectability, intractable systemic infection, or the combination of poor liver synthetic function and compromised hepatopedal portal vein flow. Relative contraindications include, but are not limited to, tumor burden involving greater than 50% of the liver, bilirubin greater than 2 mg/dL, lactate dehydrogenase greater than 425 U/L, aspartate aminotransferase greater than 100 U/L, the presence of extrahepatic metastases, poor performance status, cardiac or renal insufficiency, significant tumoral arteriovenous shunting, recent variceal bleeding, significant thrombocytopenia, portal vein thrombosis, and tumor invasion into the IVC and right atrium.

To perform the procedure, arterial access is achieved via the common femoral or radial artery. Digital subtraction angiograms of the superior mesenteric and celiac arteries are performed, one of which should have continuation into the portal venous phase. The angiograms are used to evaluate for variant vascular anatomy such as a replaced right hepatic artery, retrograde flow through the GDA, and patency and direction of flow of the portal vein. The base catheter or coaxially introduced microcatheter is then advanced into the desired hepatic artery branch and digital subtraction angiogram performed to demonstrate the tumor blush, to identify any arteriovenous shunting, and to determine whether pretherapy prophylactic coil embolization of branch arteries to adjacent organs (aka flow redistribution) is needed to avoid nontarget chemoembolization. Three-dimensional angiogram and cone-beam CT should be used in all cases, especially those with difficult vascular anatomy, to identify tumor feeders and avoid complications. The arterial branch or branches to the tumor bed are then selected and the chemotherapeutic and embolic agents delivered.

Frequent complications of TACE include pain, fever, nausea, fatigue, and elevated transaminases. This combination of symptoms is commonly referred to as postembolization syndrome and is usually self-limiting. However, care must be taken to rule out more serious complications such as septicemia, liver abscess, and nontarget chemoembolization leading to infarction and necrosis of the gallbladder, bowel, diaphragm, or skin (Fig. 39.20). All patients are treated prophylactically

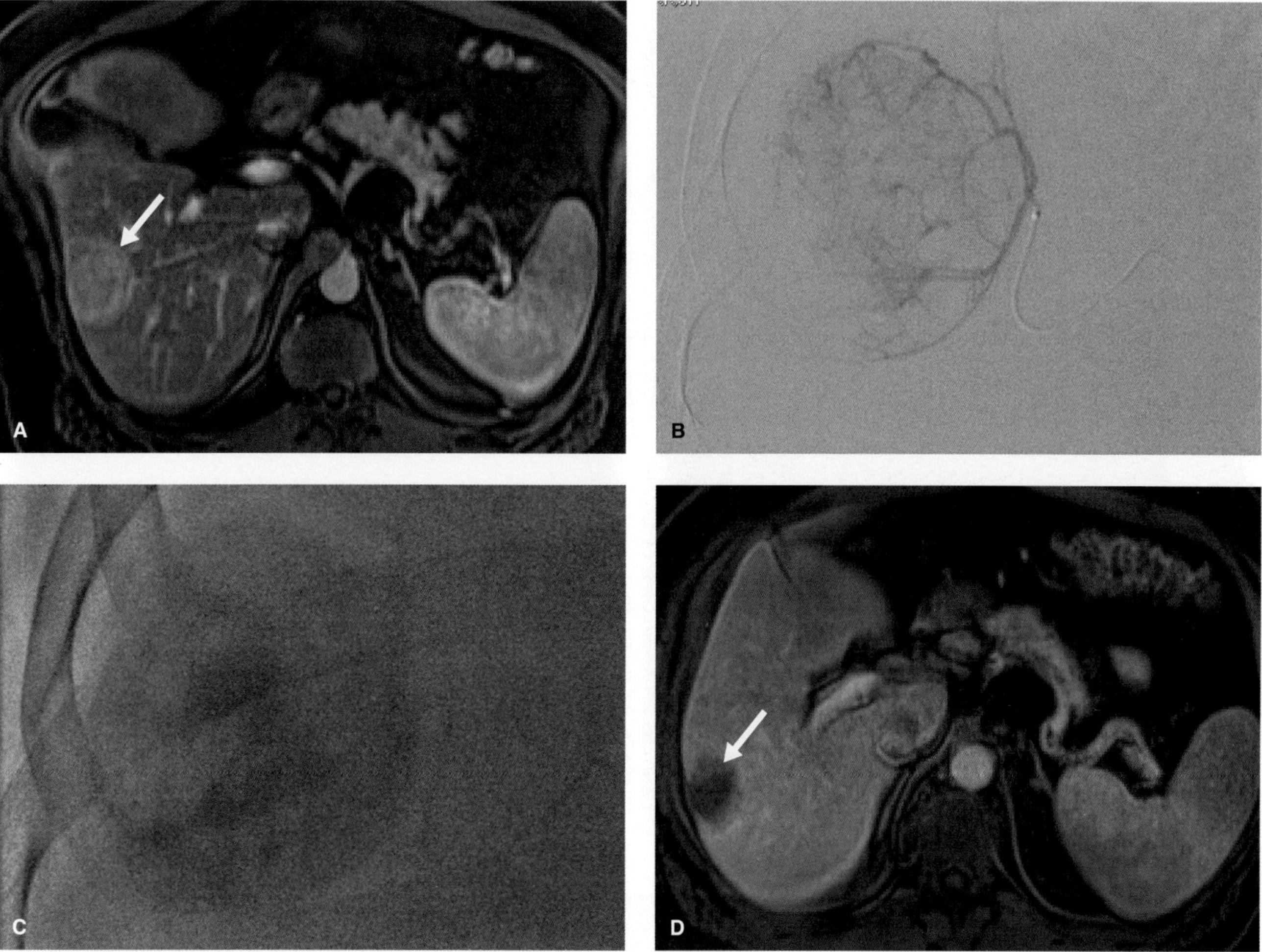

FIGURE 39.18. **DEB-TACE Case. A:** Axial T1W contrast-enhanced MRI image demonstrating a right lobe mass (*arrow*), known to be a hepatocellular carcinoma. **B:** Selective right hepatic angiogram demonstrating tumor blush. **C:** Correlative fluoroscopic spot image demonstrating tumor staining following embolization with drug-eluting beads. **D:** Postprocedural axial T1W contrast-enhanced MRI image demonstrating absence of enhancement within the threated tumor along with significant decrease in size of the lesion.

TABLE 39.1

PROGNOSTIC FACTORS FOR FAVORABLE TACE OUTCOME

Small tumor size/tumor burden
Preserved hepatic synthetic function
Child–Pugh A
Low MELD score
Complete HCC encapsulation
Absence of gross vascular invasion
Absence of bile duct invasion
Absence of irregular tumor margin
Absence of peripheral ragged enhancement
Absence of satellite nodules
Age <60 years
Serum albumin >3.5 g/dL
Alpha fetoprotein <400 ng/mL

with antibiotics to decrease the risk of hepatic abscess following TACE, with those patients having sphincter of Oddi dysfunction related to prior surgery or stent being at especially high risk (Table 39.2).

Transarterial Radioembolization (TARE) or Selective Internal Radiation Therapy (SIRT)

External beam irradiation has historically played a limited role in the treatment of hepatic tumors due to the radiosensitivity of normal hepatic parenchyma. Exposures above 70 Gy in noncirrhotic liver and 50 Gy in cirrhotic liver may result in a syndrome characterized by ascites, anicteric hepatomegaly, and elevated liver enzymes weeks to months later. SIRT, a form of brachytherapy in which intra-arterial injection of embolic particles loaded with a radioisotope is performed, has evolved to circumvent this issue. The technical aspects of performing the procedure are identical to TACE, with the exception that radioembolics are delivered in place of chemoembolics. However, while occlusion of medium and large size arteries in TACE results in tumor killing via ischemia, with delivered chemotherapeutic agents potentiating the effect, the antitumoral effect of SIRT is predominantly related to radiation delivery and the source of radiation must reach the

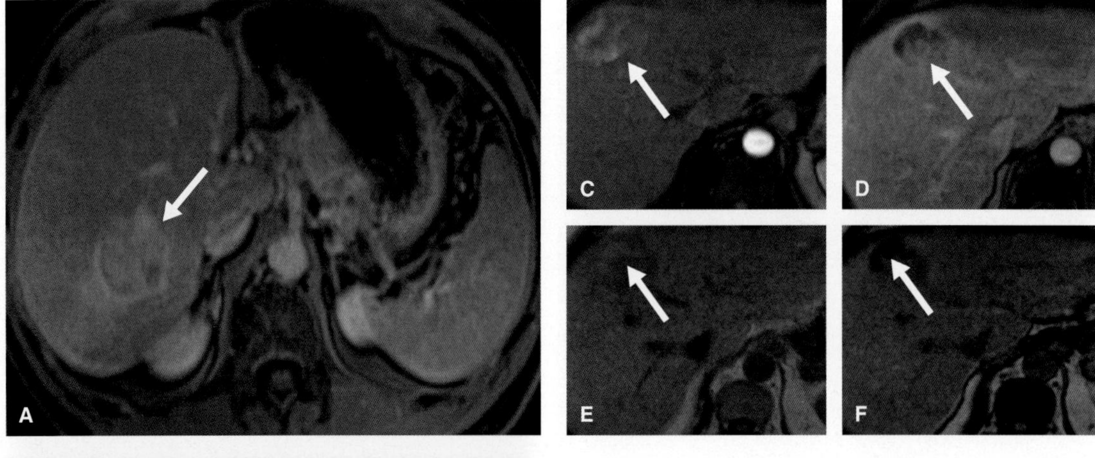

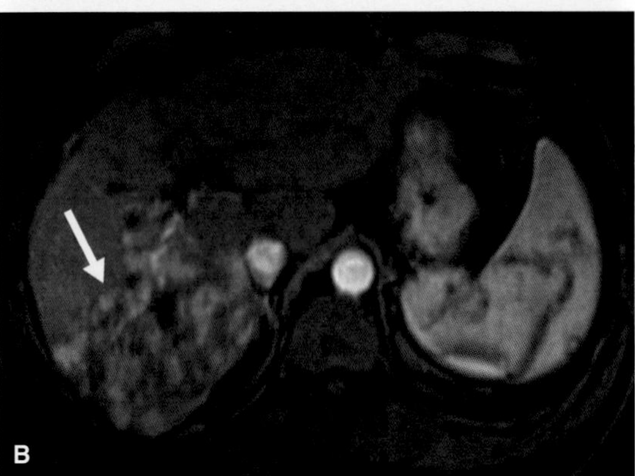

FIGURE 39.19. Examples of Different HCC Appearances. **A:** Axial T1W contrast-enhanced MRI image demonstrating an encapsulated right lobe mass (*arrow*), known to be a hepatocellular carcinoma. **B:** Axial T1W contrast-enhanced MRI image demonstrating a geographic area of arterial enhancement (*arrow*), known to be an infiltrative hepatocellular carcinoma. **C:** Axial T1W contrast-enhanced MRI image demonstrating an encapsulated arterially enhancing right lobe mass (*arrow*) with (**D**) washout (*arrow*), (**E**) increased T1 signal on the T1W in-phase gradient echo sequence, and (**F**) loss of signal intensity on the T1W out-of-phase gradient echo sequence, compatible with a well-differentiated hepatocellular carcinoma with areas of intracellular fat components.

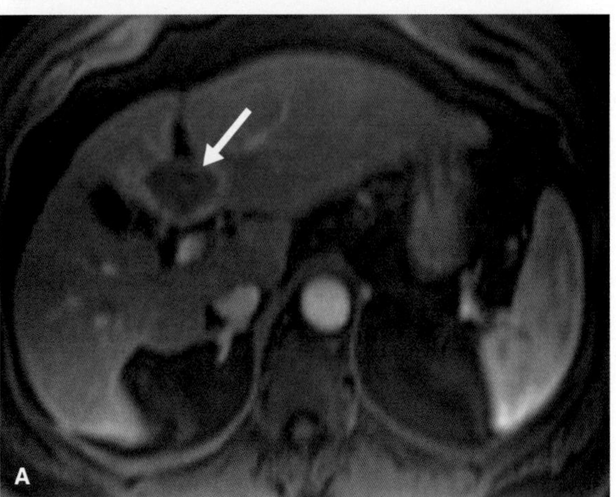

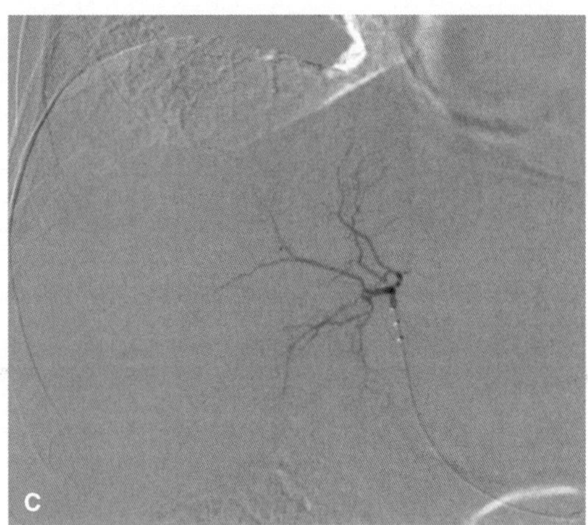

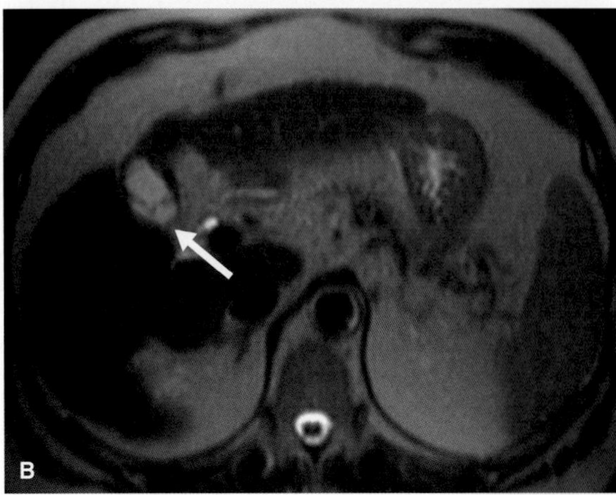

FIGURE 39.20. Chronic Cholecystitis Following DEB-TACE. **A:** Axial T1W contrast-enhanced MRI image demonstrating a left lobe mass (*arrow*), known to be a hepatocellular carcinoma. **B:** Selective left hepatic angiogram (segment IV branch) demonstrating tumor blush. **C:** Correlative T2W axial image 1 month following therapy demonstrating ischemic changes of the gallbladder wall (*arrow*) due to nontarget embolization.

TABLE 39.2

ADVANTAGES AND DISADVANTAGES OF EACH TRANSARTERIAL EMBOLIZATION METHOD

■ METHOD	■ ADVANTAGES	■ DISADVANTAGES
cTACE	■ Choice of chemotherapy ■ Choice of embolic agent ■ Tumor labeling on CT	■ Chemotherapy lost from ethiodized oil within 4 hours ■ Higher chemotherapy systemic peak plasma concentration resulting in increased side effects ■ Postembolization syndrome is severe ■ Variable dosing ■ Caution in portal vein thrombosis
DEB-TACE	■ Reduced chemotherapy systemic peak plasma concentration resulting in reduced side effects ■ Controlled release of chemotherapy over 7–10 days ■ Fixed dosing ■ Beads available in multiple sizes ■ Postembolization syndrome is tolerable	■ Can induce biliary duct necrosis
TOCE	■ Reduced postembolization syndrome ■ Tumor labeling on CT	■ Chemotherapy lost from ethiodized oil within 4 hours ■ Higher chemotherapy systemic peak plasma concentration resulting in increased side effects ■ Studies reporting lack of substantial antitumor effect ■ Variable dosing
TAE	■ Studies reporting similar overall survival benefit to TACE without adverse effects of chemotherapy ■ Choice of embolic agent	■ Severe postembolization syndrome
TAC	■ No postembolization syndrome ■ Choice of chemotherapy	■ Studies reporting lack of substantial antitumor effect ■ Higher chemotherapy systemic peak plasma concentration resulting in increased side effects ■ Variable dosing

tumor microvasculature to maximize beneficial effects. Therefore, in contrast with the particles used in TACE to embolize tumor-feeding vessels (typically 100 μm and larger), much smaller particles (25 to 35 μm) are used in SIRT to reach the tumor microvasculature.

Most patients treated by SIRT are poor candidates for TACE because of presence of vascular invasion, high tumor burden, or poor response to previous TACE. However, SIRT is also useful when options such as ablation and resection cannot be pursued due to factors including lesion location, patient comorbidities, and insufficient hepatic reserve. For example, the term *SIRT segmentectomy* refers to administration of a concentrated dose of radiation beads to two or fewer tumor-bearing hepatic segments, resulting in an ablative dose and segment resorption over time (Fig. 39.21). SIRT lobectomy, on the other hand, is used in patients with right lobe disease amenable to curative resection but where such resection cannot be performed due to an insufficient future liver remnant. While embolization of the portal vein to the lobe to be resected was traditionally used to induce hypertrophy of the future liver remnant, this method is suboptimal in cirrhotic livers and does not treat the tumors. In such cases, SIRT of right lobe disease not only treats the tumors but induces a more controlled diversion of portal venous flow to the left lobe as the right lobe atrophies, resulting in desired left lobar hypertrophy (Fig. 39.22).

Yttrium-90 (^{90}Y), a pure beta emitter that decays to stable zirconium with a physical half-life of 64.2 hours, is the radioisotope most commonly employed. Its emissions have a mean tissue penetration of 2.5 mm and maximum penetration of 11 mm, thus allowing for local high-dose radiation with less risk of radiation-induced hepatic necrosis than external beam therapy. One GBq (27 mCi) of ^{90}Y per kilogram of tissue provides a dose of 50 Gy. It has been reported in the literature that the lowest tumor dose necessary to generate a detectable response was 40 Gy and that doses up to 100 Gy to the uninvolved liver were tolerated without the development of venous occlusion or liver failure.

The two types of microspheres currently commercially available are SIR-Spheres® (Sirtex Medical Limited, Australia) and TheraSphere® (Biocompatibles, UK), which have several important differences. SIR-Spheres® was initially Food and Drug Administration (FDA) approved for the treatment of colorectal metastases in conjunction with intrahepatic floxuridine, an analog of 5-FU, while TheraSphere® was FDA approved for the treatment of unresectable HCC. SIR-Spheres® consists of biodegradable resin-based microspheres containing ^{90}Y and has an average diameter of 35 μm (range 20 to 60 μm). SIR-Spheres® has lower specific activity (50 Bq per microsphere at time of calibration), and a greater number of spheres per dose (approximately 40 to 80 million spheres/3 GBq vial). TheraSphere® is composed of nonbiodegradable glass microspheres ranging from 20 to 30 μm in diameter, with ^{90}Y as an integral constituent of the glass. TheraSphere® has higher specific activity (2,500 Bq per microsphere at time of calibration) and lower number of spheres per dose (1.2 million microspheres/3 GBq vial) (Table 39.3).

The biologic effects of SIRT depend on the absorbed dose, defined as the energy absorbed per unit mass of tissue, which depends on the amount of ^{90}Y injected, the tumoral vessel density, and hepatic artery hemodynamics. While the amount of ^{90}Y injected can be accurately determined, hemodynamics and vessel density are variable, thus making accurate dosimetry prediction impossible. However, in spite of this variability, most injected microspheres are preferentially absorbed into the tumor microvasculature in a 3:1 to 20:1 ratio compared with the normal liver, especially at the periphery of nodules.

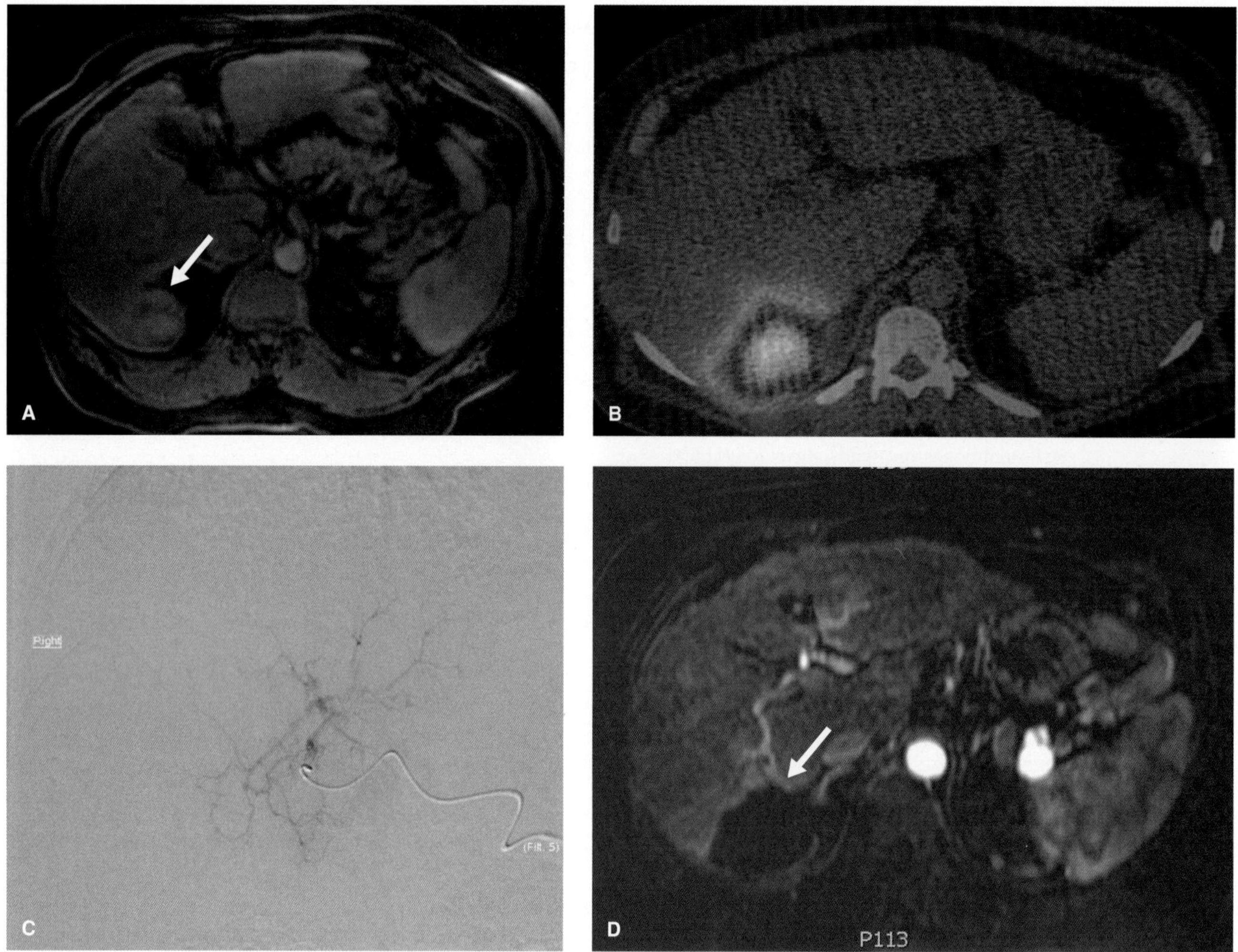

FIGURE 39.21. Radiation Segmentectomy. A: Axial T1W postcontrast image (arterial phase) demonstrates an exophytic arterially enhancing lesion within segment VII of the liver parenchyma (*arrow*) corresponding to a hepatocellular carcinoma. **B:** SPECT-CT ^{90}Y bremsstrahlung axial image confirming complete tumoral distribution by the therapy. **C:** Selective angiogram of the posterior segment VII branch of the right hepatic artery confirming adequate catheter position for ^{90}Y delivery. **D:** Axial T1W postcontrast image (arterial phase) demonstrating an absence of enhancement within the segment VII lesion (*arrow*).

SIRT is also technically challenging because of the risk of nontarget embolization. The two absolute contraindications to ^{90}Y microsphere treatment are significant hepatopulmonary shunting (usually >20%) that would result in >30 Gy being delivered to the lungs with a single infusion or 50 Gy for multiple infusions, and the inability to prevent deposition of microspheres to the gastrointestinal tract. For these reasons, a mandatory treatment simulation where the intra-arterial catheter is positioned as it would be during SIRT followed by injection of ^{99m}Tc macroaggregated albumin (MAA) is performed at a separate session prior to SIRT. Gamma camera imaging is then performed to determine the degree of hepatopulmonary shunting and estimate the dose of radiation that may be delivered to the target tumor areas. While the resulting estimates reflect the average rather than the actual dose to a given area, and there is variability in correlating between ^{99m}Tc-MAA and actual ^{90}Y microsphere deposition, activity measured with intraoperative probes has correlated with the actual dose of radiation delivered and with ^{99m}Tc-MAA planar scintigraphy.

Side effects are uncommon following SIRT. When they do occur, they often are the result of nontarget microsphere delivery. The postembolization syndrome that occurs following TACE is not observed, though patients may experience similar symptoms including fatigue, abdominal pain, nausea and vomiting, and low-grade fever transiently over the first several hours following SIRT. The transience of symptoms with SIRT as compared to TACE likely relates to the lack of significant ischemia with SIRT. Mild-to-moderate lymphopenia is commonly seen after radioembolization but is not associated with increased susceptibility to infections. However, a form of sinusoidal obstruction syndrome appearing 4 to 8 weeks after SIRT may occur in noncirrhotic patients, termed radioembolization-induced liver disease (REILD), and is characterized by jaundice, mild ascites, and moderate increases in gamma-glutamyl transpeptidase and alkaline phosphatase.

PERCUTANEOUS THERAPIES (TABLE 39.4)

Chemical Ablation

Ethanol Ablation. One of the first methods devised to ablate liver tumors involved percutaneous ethanol injection, termed ethanol ablation, which has been shown to safely achieve complete necrosis of small HCCs and has the advantage of

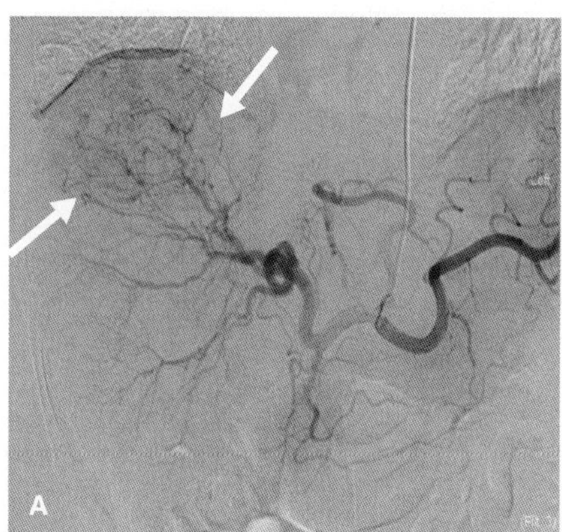
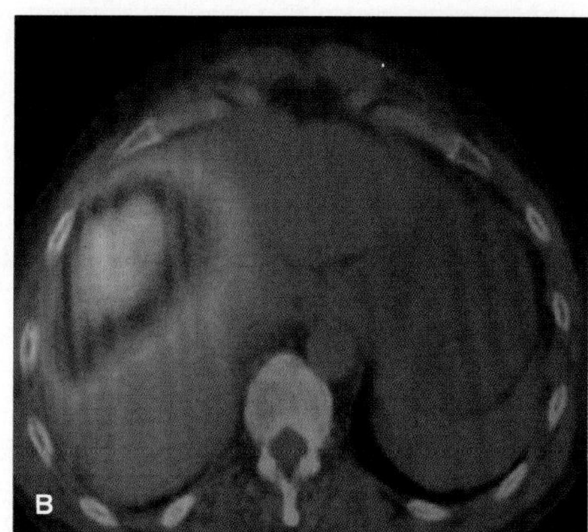
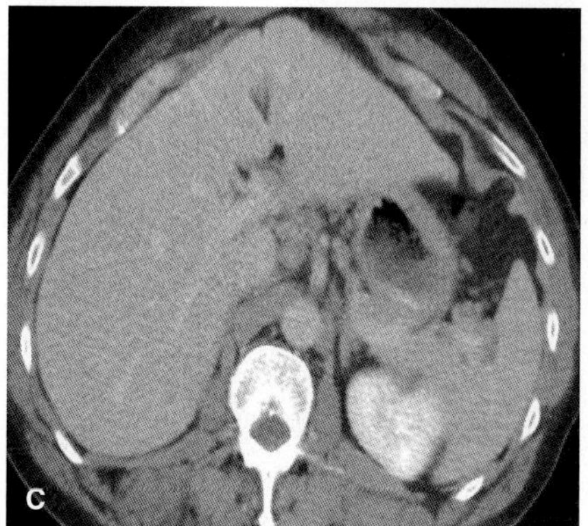
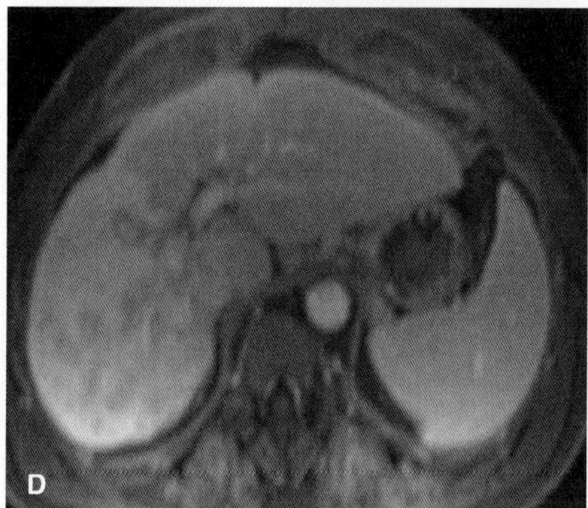
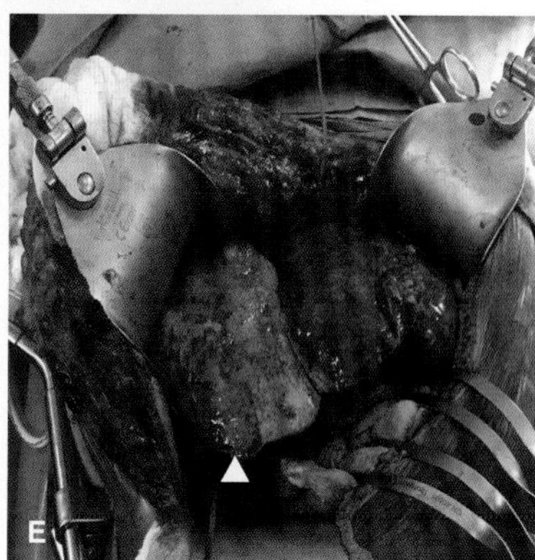

FIGURE 39.22. Radiation Lobectomy. A: Celiac angiogram demonstrating a large mass within segment VII and VIII of the liver with corresponding tumor blush (*arrows*). **B:** SPECT-CT ^{90}Y bremsstrahlung axial image confirming complete tumoral distribution by the therapy as well as counts within the normal liver. **C:** Preprocedural contrast-enhanced CT at the level of the portal vein demonstrating a small left lateral segment which will become the future liver remnant. **D:** Axial T1W postcontrast image demonstrating delayed enhancement of the right lobe corresponding to postprocedural fibrosis along with significant hypertrophy of the left lateral segment. **E:** Intraoperative view of the liver corroborating significant hypertrophy of the left lateral segment and fibrosis of the treated right lobe (*arrow*).

allowing treatment of tumors near sensitive organs and blood vessels. However, it typically requires multiple treatment sessions, one cannot be certain of the ablation zone, and there are high local progression and recurrence rates (Fig. 39.23).

Acetic Acid Ablation. Percutaneous acetic acid injection for ablation of tumors was first described in 1994. Acetic acid is a noxious chemical with better tissue diffusion than ethanol as well as better infiltration into tumor septae and capsules, proposed to decrease the number of repeat ablation sessions. It is generally considered safe, with rare side effects including transient hemoglobinuria, fever, and right upper quadrant abdominal pain. Segmental infarction and metabolic acidosis can occur at high doses.

TABLE 39.3

COMPARISON OF AVAILABLE SIRT PARTICLES

PARAMETER	SIR-SPHERES®	THERASPHERE®
Manufacturer	Sirtex Medical, Lane Cove, Australia	Biocompatibles UK Ltd, Farnham, Surrey, UK
Sphere composition	Resin	Glass
^{90}Y incorporation	Bound to resin on sphere surface	Embedded in glass matrix
Sphere size (µm)	32.5 ± 2.5 (range 20–60)	25 ± 5 (range 20–30)
Specific gravity (g/mL)	1.6	3.6
Specific activity/Sphere at calibration (Bq)	50 (range 40–80)	2500
Spheres/3 GBq dose (million)	40–80	1.2
Doses available (GBq)	3	3, 5, 7, 10, 15, 20
FDA approval	Unresectable metastatic colorectal cancer	Unresectable HCC

TABLE 39.4

ADVANTAGES AND DISADVANTAGES OF EACH ABLATION METHOD

■ ABLATION METHOD	■ ADVANTAGES	■ DISADVANTAGES
Ethanol ablation	■ Safe near sensitive organs ■ Not susceptible to heat-sink effect ■ Low complication rate ■ Well tolerated ■ No specialized equipment	■ Often requires multiple treatments ■ Cannot be sure of ablation zone ■ High local progression and recurrence rates
Acetic acid ablation	■ Safe near sensitive organs ■ Not susceptible to heat-sink effect ■ Better tissue diffusion and infiltration into tumor septae and capsules than ethanol ■ Low complication rate ■ Well tolerated ■ No specialized equipment	■ Often requires multiple treatments (though fewer than ethanol ablation) ■ High local progression and recurrence rates
Radiofrequency ablation	■ Single treatment often effective ■ Low local progression and recurrence rates for small lesions	■ Susceptible to heat-sink effect ■ Risk of damage to adjacent sensitive structures ■ Dependent on tissue conductivity ■ Efficacy decreases with increasing lesion size ■ Time consuming ■ Requires grounding pads ■ Requires multiple probes which can increase complications
Microwave ablation	■ Single treatment often effective ■ Less susceptible to heat-sink effect ■ Less time consuming ■ Low local progression and recurrence rates for small lesions ■ Less dependent on tissue characteristics ■ Often requires single probe	■ Risk of damage to adjacent sensitive structures
Cryoablation	■ Single treatment often effective	■ Higher complication rate including cryoshock ■ Higher local recurrence rate ■ Risk of damage to adjacent sensitive structures ■ Susceptible to heat-sink effect ■ Time consuming ■ Requires multiple probes which can increase complications
Irreversible electroporation	■ Safe near sensitive organs ■ Not susceptible to heat-sink effect ■ Low complication rate ■ Well tolerated	■ Dependent on tissue conductivity ■ High local progression and recurrence rates ■ Requires general anesthesia ■ Long procedural time ■ Caution in patients with arrhythmia
Laser ablation	■ Single treatment often effective ■ Can be used with MRI guidance	■ Susceptible to heat-sink effect ■ Risk of damage to adjacent sensitive structures ■ Efficacy decreases with increasing lesion size

Energy-Based Ablation

Radiofrequency Ablation. Radiofrequency ablation (RFA) utilizes a probe generating electromagnetic radiation within the radiofrequency spectrum, part of the electromagnetic spectrum bound by a low oscillation of 3 Hz and a high of 300 GHz, with most RFA probes generating electromagnetic radiation in the 300 to 500 kHz range. The probe is inserted within the target lesion, typically using CT or ultrasound guidance, and the circuit is closed by placing grounding pads on the patient's body, usually the thighs. A generator modulates the radiofrequency amplitude, and the resultant energy is locally deposited in the form of heat as a result of molecular frictional loss, resulting in coagulative tissue necrosis. Effective ablation requires good tissue conductivity, which allows heat transfer farther away from the probe and a larger ablation zone. Counterintuitively, a fast power increase will result in desiccation of the tissue around the probe, limiting heat conduction and decreasing the size of the ablation zone. The eventual ablation zone geometry depends on multiple factors including the type and shape of the probe, maximum temperature reached, duration of ablation, and proximity to blood vessels.

Lesion size is the most important determinant of RFA success, with reported complete ablation rates of about 90% for lesions up to 3 cm. For lesions >3 cm, the efficacy of RFA decreases with increasing lesion size. Complete ablation is possible for lesions of 3 to 5 cm but unlikely with lesions >5 cm. The rate of recurrence is nearly 0% for smaller lesions and >50% for lesions >5 cm. Lesion location is also a determinant

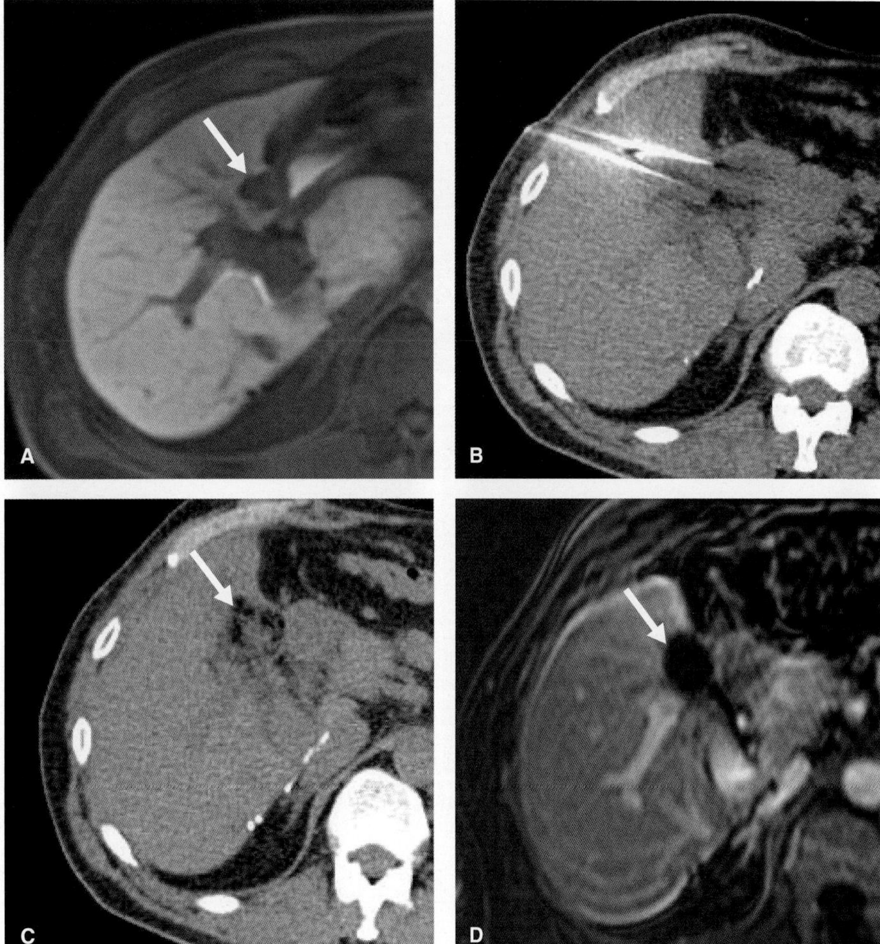

FIGURE 39.23. Percutaneous Ethanol Ablation. A: Axial T1W postcontrast image in the hepatobiliary phase demonstrating a lesion within the posterior aspect of segment III (*arrow*), in close proximity to the stomach, the portal vein and adjacent bile ducts, in a patient that underwent right hepatectomy due to metastatic colorectal cancer. **B:** CT image demonstrating needle placement within the lesion. **C:** Subsequent ethanol injection was performed, which was confirmed by noncontract CT (*arrow*). **D:** Axial T1W postprocedural image demonstrating absence of enhancement of the ablation cavity, compatible with lesion necrosis (*arrow*).

of RFA success. RFA of lesions near the hilum is generally avoided due to the risk of injury to the central biliary tree or hepatic vasculature. Additionally, lesions adjacent to blood vessels may show variable ablation response secondary to the heat-sink effect, whereby generated heat is dissipated by the adjacent flowing flood.

RFA may offer the same benefit as resection in selected patients. Child–Pugh class A or B patients with lesions up to 3 cm treated with RFA demonstrate similar overall survival rates to those treated with surgical resection. Although Child–Pugh class C patients may be safely treated with RFA, their life expectancy is determined by the progression of cirrhosis and a survival benefit is therefore unlikely. Liver transplantation for HCC offers the longest survival for the approximately 10% of patients who are candidates, and treatment with RFA while awaiting liver transplantation has been shown to be an independent prognostic factor for longer survival.

Deaths after RFA are uncommon and typically attributed to liver failure, and risk increases with larger ablation volumes and diminished hepatic reserve. Most patients treated with RFA for HCC may be discharged home on the day of the procedure after several hours of observation.

Microwave Ablation. Microwave ablation (MWA) refers to all electromagnetic methods of inducing tumor destruction via coagulative tissue necrosis by using devices with frequencies greater than or equal to 900 MHz. MWA uses an oscillating electromagnetic field that realigns polarized molecules such as water, generating kinetic energy, heat, and subsequent tumor necrosis through dielectric hysteresis. This creates an ablation zone around the needle in a column or rounded shape, depending on the type of needle used and the generating power. Compared to RFA, MWA shows more uniform tissue penetration, does not require grounding pads, is less prone to heat-sink effect, is not affected by tissue carbonization, and has a more predictable ablation zone (Fig. 39.24).

Cryoablation. Most cryoablation systems rely on the Joule–Thomson effect, whereby expansion of a cryogen (i.e., argon) at the cryoprobe tip causes the temperature to decrease. Cell death induced by cryoablation is caused by direct intracellular ice crystal formation resulting in damage to plasma membranes and organelles. The ice crystals continue to grow during thawing, maximizing cell killing. Tumor response depends on the rate of cooling, depth of hypothermia, rate of thawing, the number of freeze–thaw cycles, and delayed effects of postthaw ischemia. Repeated freeze–thaw cycles can improve the efficacy. The large diameter of currently available probes, the requirement of using multiple probes, the location of many tumors, and the risk of cryoshock syndrome, a clinical syndrome caused by circulating inflammatory cytokines and characterized by renal failure, disseminated intravascular coagulation, and adult respiratory distress syndrome, significantly limit its application in the liver.

Irreversible Electroporation. Irreversible electroporation (IRE) uses pulsed electric fields to induce cell death. At a specific electric potential threshold, the cell membrane lipid bilayer becomes inundated with pores, a change that is reversible at low current but which becomes permanent and results in cell death as the electric field strength is increased. Ablation of liver lesions using IRE was first described in 2005 by

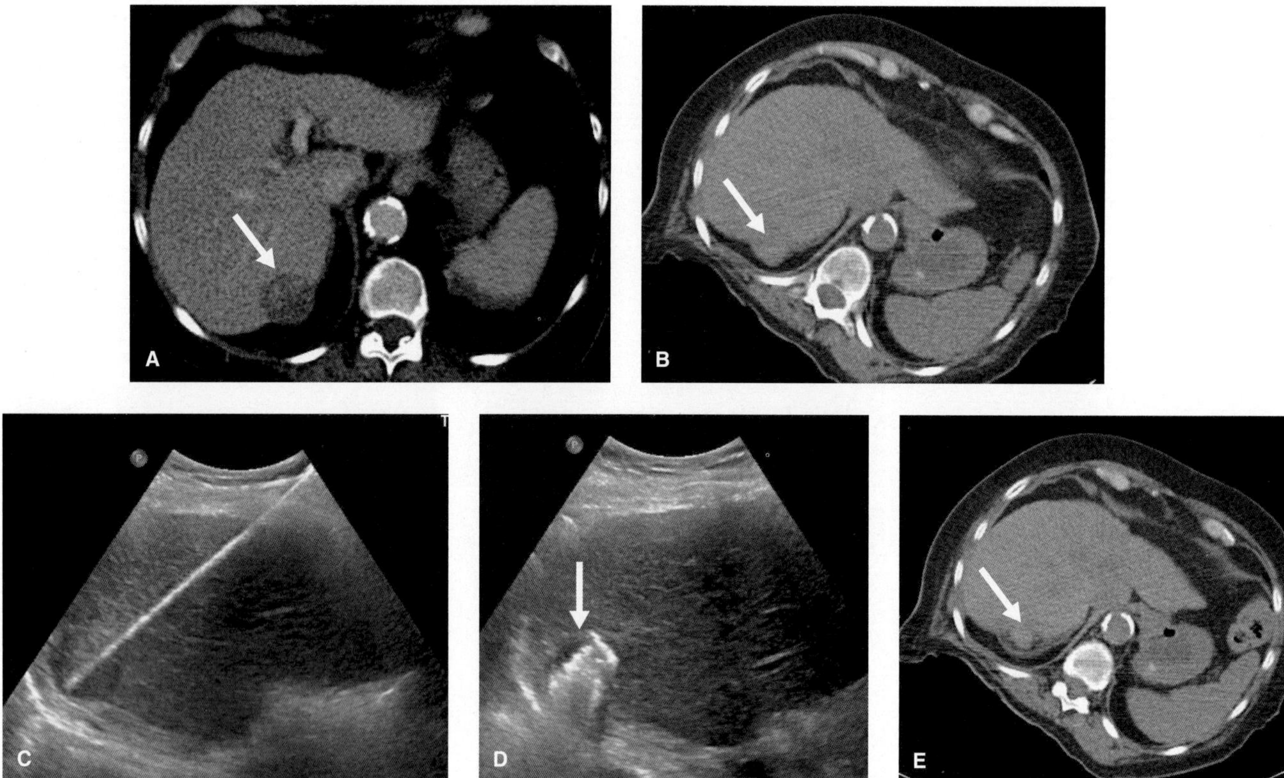

FIGURE 39.24. **Percutaneous Microwave Ablation. A:** Contrast-enhanced CT image demonstrating a lesion within the posterior right lobe (*arrow*). **B:** Noncontrast CT image demonstrating the exophytic lesion during the actual procedure (*arrow*). **C:** Subsequently, a microwave antennae was advanced into the lesion under direct ultrasound guidance. **D:** Immediate postprocedural ultrasound demonstrating expected post-procedural changes (*arrow*) with (**E**) the expected perilesional halo on noncontrast CT (*arrow*), indicating technical success and tissue retraction.

Davalos et al. IRE devices can deliver up to 3,000 V and 50 A through either unipolar or bipolar needle electrodes. Ablation zone size can be influenced by length of the electrode tip, distance between electrodes, pulse number, duration of pulses, and voltage applied. Electric fields are strongly influenced by the conductivity of the local environment, which depends on tissue heterogeneity and the presence of metal such as biliary stents. Since IRE does not depend on heating or cooling of target tissues, the technique is not limited by the heat-sink effect when performing ablation of tumors close to major blood vessels and does not appear to have deleterious effects on adjacent normal tissues including nerves and bile ducts. However, despite these advantages over thermal ablative techniques, multiple groups have suggested poor local control and high recurrence rates with IRE. Therefore, IRE should only be considered when thermal ablative techniques are contraindicated.

Laser Ablation. Laser ablation uses a laser to generate monochromatic light and a small flexible optical fiber to transport the light inside tissue where it is then converted to heat. Tumor cell exposure to temperatures ranging from 45° to 55°C for prolonged periods or temperatures higher than 60°C for short periods causes irreversible cell damage. Heat generation in the target tissue is influenced by multiple factors including laser light wavelength, laser power, laser energy, treatment time, the emission characteristics of the optical fiber, and characteristics of the tissue. Various invasive and noninvasive methods are available for real-time temperature monitoring with good spatial resolution, facilitating tumor

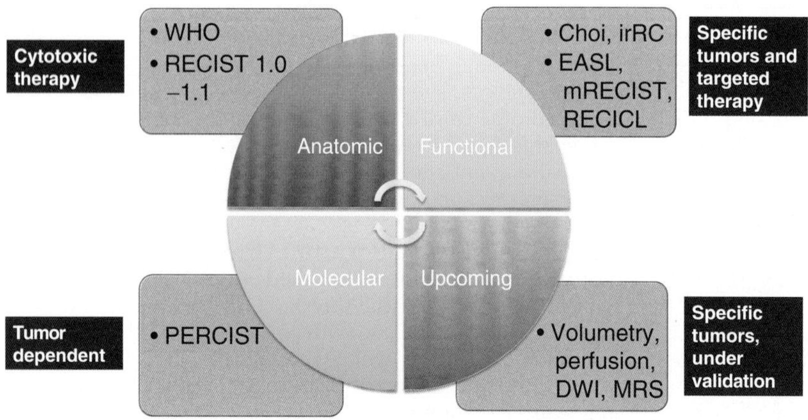

FIGURE 39.25. Scheme demonstrating the available follow-up criteria and their specific therapeutic targets.

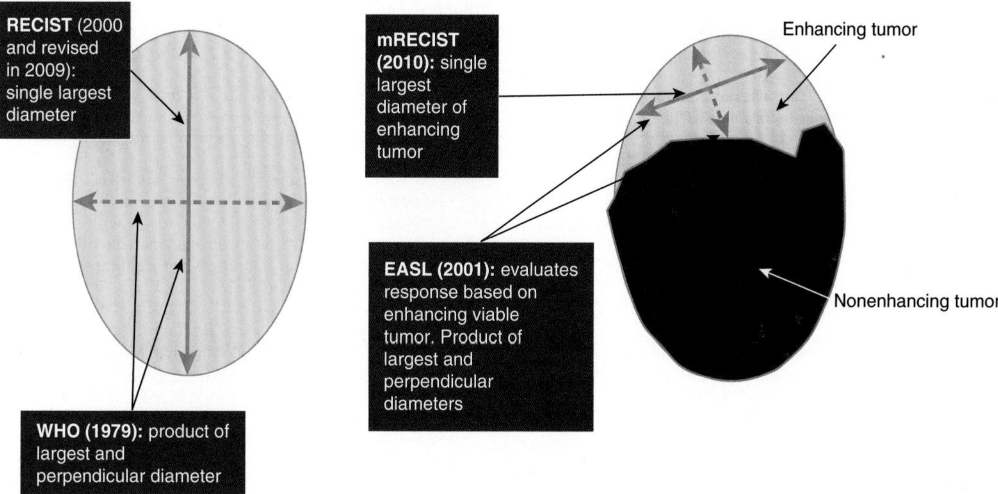

FIGURE 39.26. Scheme demonstrating the available anatomic criteria and their basic measuring strategies.

killing with sparing of as much normal tissue as possible. Additionally, nanoparticles are being developed for use in photothermal tumor ablation that highly absorb light and can be designed and delivered specifically to tumor cells.

PRINCIPLES OF ASSESSING TREATMENT RESPONSE

Assessment of tumor response is crucial in patients undergoing locoregional liver cancer therapies. Conventional methods, such as classical Response Evaluation Criteria in Solid Tumors (RECIST) criteria, have no predictive value in HCC patients treated with TACE or SIRT as they rely solely on tumor shrinkage as a measure of antitumor activity, an assumption that is only valid with cytotoxic drugs. TACE and SIRT induce direct tumor necrosis and their anticancer activity is predictive to a reduction in viable tumor, as identified by contrast-enhanced CT or MRI. The Clinical Practice Guidelines jointly issued by the European Association for the Study of Liver Disease (EASL) and the European Organization for Research and Treatment of Cancer (EORTC) therefore state that assessment of response in HCC should be based on modified RECIST (mRECIST) criteria by performing contrast-enhanced CT or MRI 4 weeks after treatment to assess residual viable tumor burden as well as for vascular invasion, lymph nodes, ascites, pleural effusion, and new lesions. Tumor response measured by mRECIST after TACE has been shown to correlate with survival outcomes (Figs. 39.25 and 39.26).

If complete tumor necrosis is not achieved after the first TACE, a second TACE may be performed as some feeding arteries may have been missed. However, patients that do not respond to two consecutive sessions of TACE should be considered for alternative therapies, and those that show no tumor response following TACE have a worse prognosis.

All response criteria that measure the tumor dimensionally (RECIST and mRECIST), presume that lesion diameter directly correlates with lesion volume. This assumption is based on the belief that tumors grow and shrink in a spherical manner, which is not entirely accurate. Therefore, quantification by volumetry can be a more accurate reflection of the actual tumor size and additional methods have been developed in order to quantify such a change.

Also, quantitative imaging techniques allow robust evaluation of hepatic tumor response. In addition to size changes, various biologic and functional parameters such as diffusion and perfusion can be quantified. Measurement of these parameters is especially important for the evaluation of tumor response to novel targeted therapies including SIRT, in which a change in functional status sometimes precedes anatomic modification.

Other biomarkers have been explored including AFP. Preprocedural AFP has not been demonstrated to be a prognostic marker of clinical response following intervention. AFP elevation may be seen in the immediate postprocedure period secondary to cellular lysis rather than disease progression, and while decrease in AFP following treatment is indicative of response, it is unreliable and AFP monitoring should not be substituted in place of dynamic imaging studies.

CONCLUSION

Management of hepatic malignancies requires a multidisciplinary approach and the ability to translate basic anatomical and radiologic concepts into daily clinical practice. Decisions are often based on the tumor burden, liver function, imaging findings, and patient presentation, including a judicious evaluation of patient performance status. Locoregional therapies offer multiple options with different treatment objectives. Currently, ablation therapies including SIRT segmentectomy can be used in a potentially curative manner. The remaining therapies are typically used in a palliative or downstaging setting. Each of the available locoregional treatments offers specific advantages and must be individualized to each patient in order to achieve the desired optimal outcome.

Suggested Readings

Arch-Ferrer JE, Smith JK, Bynon S, et al. Radio-frequency ablation in cirrhotic patients with hepatocellular carcinoma. *Am Surg* 2003;69(12):1067–1071.

Basile A, Tsetis D, Montineri A, et al. MDCT anatomic assessment of right inferior phrenic artery origin related to potential supply to hepatocellular carcinoma and its embolization. *Cardiovasc Intervent Radiol* 2008;31(2):349–358.

Bismuth H. Surgical anatomy and anatomical surgery of the liver. *World J Surg* 1982;6(1):3–9.

Brown KT, Do RK, Gonen M, et al. Randomized trial of hepatic artery embolization for hepatocellular carcinoma using doxorubicin-eluting microspheres compared with embolization with microspheres alone. *J Clin Oncol* 2016; 34(17):2046–2053.

Brown KT, Nevins AB, Getrajdman GI, et al. Particle embolization for hepatocellular carcinoma. *J Vasc Interv Radiol* 1998;9(5):822–828.

Camma C, Di Marco V, Orlando A, et al; Unità Interdipartimentale Neoplasie Epatiche (U.I.N.E) Group. Treatment of hepatocellular carcinoma in compensated cirrhosis with radio-frequency thermal ablation (RFTA): a prospective study. *J Hepatol* 2005;42(4):535–540.

Camma C, Schepis F, Orlando A, et al. Transarterial chemoembolization for unresectable hepatocellular carcinoma: meta-analysis of randomized controlled trials. *Radiology* 2002;224(1):47–54.

Cannon R, Ellis F, Hayes D, Narayanan G, Martin RC 2nd. Safety and early efficacy of irreversible electroporation for hepatic tumors in proximity to vital structures. *J Surg Oncol* 2013;107(5):544–549.

Carr BI. Hepatic arterial 90Yttrium glass microspheres (Therasphere) for unresectable hepatocellular carcinoma: interim safety and survival data on 65 patients. *Liver Transpl* 2004;10(2 Suppl 1):S107–S110.

Charpentier KP, Wolf F, Noble L, Winn B, Resnick M, Dupuy DE. Irreversible electroporation of the liver and liver hilum in swine. *HPB (Oxford)* 2011;13(3):168–173.

Chung JW, Kim HC, Yoon JH, et al. Transcatheter arterial chemoembolization of hepatocellular carcinoma: prevalence and causative factors of extrahepatic collateral arteries in 479 patients. *Korean J Radiol* 2006;7(4):257–266.

Clark TW. Complications of hepatic chemoembolization. *Semin Intervent Radiol* 2006;23(2):119–125.

Coster HG. A quantitative analysis of the voltage-current relationships of fixed charge membranes and the associated property of "punch-through". *Biophys J* 1965;5(5):669–686.

Couinaud C. *Le foie: études anatomiques et chirurgicales*. Masson & Cie; 1957.

Covey AM, Brody LA, Maluccio MA, Getrajdman GI, Brown KT. Variant hepatic arterial anatomy revisited: digital subtraction angiogram performed in 600 patients. *Radiology* 2002;224(2):542–547.

Crucitti A, Danza FM, Antinori A, et al. Radiofrequency thermal ablation (RFA) of liver tumors: percutaneous and open surgical approaches. *J Exp Clin Cancer Res* 2003;22(4 Suppl):191–195.

Davalos RV, Mir IL, Rubinsky B. Tissue ablation with irreversible electroporation. *Ann Biomed Eng* 2005;33(2):223–231.

Doyon D, Mouzon A, Jourde AM, Regensberg C, Frileux C. [Hepatic, arterial embolization in patients with malignant liver tumours (author's transl)]. *Ann Radiol (Paris)* 1974;17(6):593–603.

Dumortier J, Chapuis F, Borson O, et al. Unresectable hepatocellular carcinoma: survival and prognostic factors after lipiodol chemoembolisation in 89 patients. *Dig Liver Dis* 2006;38(2):125–133.

Forner A, Ayuso C, Varela M, et al. Evaluation of tumor response after locoregional therapies in hepatocellular carcinoma: are response evaluation criteria in solid tumors reliable? *Cancer* 2009;115(3):616–623.

Furuta T, Maeda E, Akai H, et al. Hepatic segments and vasculature: projecting CT anatomy onto angiograms. *Radiographics* 2009;29(7):e37.

Georgiades CS, Hong K, Geschwind JF. Radiofrequency ablation and chemoembolization for hepatocellular carcinoma. *Cancer J* 2008;14(2):117–122.

Gillmore R, Stuart S, Kirkwood A, et al. EASL and mRECIST responses are independent prognostic factors for survival in hepatocellular cancer patients treated with transarterial embolization. *J Hepatol* 2011;55(6): 1309–1316.

Goldsmith NA, Woodburne RT. The surgical anatomy pertaining to liver resection. *Surg Gynecol Obstet* 1957;105(3):310–318.

Goseki N, Nosaka T, Endo M, Koike M. Nourishment of hepatocellular carcinoma cells through the portal blood flow with and without transcatheter arterial embolization. *Cancer* 1995;76(5):736–742.

Gruttadauria S, Foglieni CS, Doria C, Luca A, Lauro A, Marino IR. The hepatic artery in liver transplantation and surgery: vascular anomalies in 701 cases. *Clin Transplant* 2001;15(5):359–363.

Guglielmi A, Ruzzenente A, Sandri M, et al. Radio frequency ablation for hepatocellular carcinoma in cirrhotic patients: prognostic factors for survival. *J Gastrointest Surg* 2007;11(2):143–149.

Gulec SA, Mesoloras G, Dezarn WA, McNeillie P, Kennedy AS. Safety and efficacy of Y-90 microsphere treatment in patients with primary and metastatic liver cancer: the tumor selectivity of the treatment as a function of tumor to liver flow ratio. *J Transl Med* 2007;5:15.

Hasegawa S, Yamasaki N, Hiwaki T, et al. Factors that predict intrahepatic recurrence of hepatocellular carcinoma in 81 patients initially treated by percutaneous ethanol injection. *Cancer* 1999;86(9):1682–1690.

Healey JE Jr, Schroy PC. Anatomy of the biliary ducts within the human liver; analysis of the prevailing pattern of branchings and the major variations of the biliary ducts. *AMA Arch Surg* 1953;66(5):599–616.

Hiatt JR, Gabbay J, Busuttil RW. Surgical anatomy of the hepatic arteries in 1000 cases. *Ann Surg* 1994;220(1):50–52.

Hjortsjo CH. The topography of the intrahepatic duct systems. *Acta Anat (Basel)* 1951;11(4):599–615.

Huo TI, Huang YH, Wu JC, et al. Sequential transarterial chemoembolization and percutaneous acetic acid injection therapy versus repeated percutaneous acetic acid injection for unresectable hepatocellular carcinoma: a prospective study. *Ann Oncol* 2003;14(11):1648–1653.

Idee JM, Guiu B. Use of Lipiodol as a drug-delivery system for transcatheter arterial chemoembolization of hepatocellular carcinoma: a review. *Crit Rev Oncol Hematol* 2013;88(3):530–549.

Izzo F. Other thermal ablation techniques: microwave and interstitial laser ablation of liver tumors. *Ann Surg Oncol* 2003;10(5):491–497.

Kadir S, Brothers MF. *Atlas of Normal and Variant Angiographic Anatomy*. 1st ed. 1991, Philadelphia, PA: Saunders. xi, 529 pp.

Kennedy AS, Nutting C, Coldwell D, Gaiser J, Drachenberg C. Pathologic response and microdosimetry of (90)Y microspheres in man: review of four explanted whole livers. *Int J Radiat Oncol Biol Phys* 2004;60(5):1552–1563.

Kim HC, Chung JW, Lee W, Jae HJ, Park JH. Recognizing extrahepatic collateral vessels that supply hepatocellular carcinoma to avoid complications of transcatheter arterial chemoembolization. *Radiographics* 2005;25 Suppl 1: S25–S39.

Kim W, Clark TW, Baum RA, Soulen MC. Risk factors for liver abscess formation after hepatic chemoembolization. *J Vasc Interv Radiol* 2001;12(8): 965–968.

Kim BK, Kim KA, An C, et al. Prognostic role of magnetic resonance imaging vs. computed tomography for hepatocellular carcinoma undergoing chemoembolization. *Liver Int* 2015;35(6):1722–1730.

Kim HC, Kim TK, Sung KB, et al. CT during hepatic arteriography and portography: an illustrative review. *Radiographics* 2002;22(5):1041–1051.

Kingham TP, Karkar AM, D'Angelica MI, et al. Ablation of perivascular hepatic malignant tumors with irreversible electroporation. *J Am Coll Surg* 2012;215(3):379–387.

Knesaurek K, Machac J, Muzinic M, DaCosta M, Zhang Z, Heiba S. Quantitative comparison of yttrium-90 (^{90}Y)-microspheres and technetium-99m (^{99m}Tc)-macroaggregated albumin SPECT images for planning 90Y therapy of liver cancer. *Technol Cancer Res Treat* 2010;9(3): 253–262.

Koda M, Murawaki Y, Mitsuda A, et al. Predictive factors for intrahepatic recurrence after percutaneous ethanol injection therapy for small hepatocellular carcinoma. *Cancer* 2000;88(3):529–537.

Konno T, Maeda H, Iwai K, et al. Effect of arterial administration of high-molecular-weight anticancer agent SMANCS with lipid lymphographic agent on hepatoma: a preliminary report. *Eur J Cancer Clin Oncol* 1983;19(8): 1053–1065.

Kusano S, Matsubayashi T, Ishii K. [The evaluation of the angiographic "umbilical point" of the left hepatic artery (author's transl)]. *Nihon Igaku Hoshasen Gakkai Zasshi* 1976;36(1):7–12.

Lau WY, Leung TW, Ho S, et al. Diagnostic pharmaco-scintigraphy with hepatic intra-arterial technetium-99m macroaggregated albumin in the determination of tumour to non-tumour uptake ratio in hepatocellular carcinoma. *Br J Radiol* 1994;67(794):136–139.

Lee AJ, Gomes AS, Liu DM, Kee ST, Loh CT, McWilliams JP. The road less traveled: importance of the lesser branches of the celiac axis in liver embolotherapy. *Radiographics* 2012;32(4):1121–1132.

Lencioni R, Bartolozzi C, Caramella D, et al. Treatment of small hepatocellular carcinoma with percutaneous ethanol injection. Analysis of prognostic factors in 105 Western patients. *Cancer* 1995;76(10):1737–1746.

Lencioni R, Llovet JM. Modified RECIST (mRECIST) assessment for hepatocellular carcinoma. *Semin Liver Dis* 2010;30(1):52–60.

Lewis AL, Gonzalez MV, Lloyd AW, et al. DC bead: in vitro characterization of a drug-delivery device for transarterial chemoembolization. *J Vasc Interv Radiol* 2006;17(2 Pt 1):335–342.

Lewis AL, Taylor RR, Hall B, Gonzalez MV, Willis SL, Stratford PW. Pharmacokinetic and safety study of doxorubicin-eluting beads in a porcine model of hepatic arterial embolization. *J Vasc Interv Radiol* 2006;17(8): 1335–1343.

Liapi E, Geschwind JF, Transcatheter arterial chemoembolization for liver cancer: is it time to distinguish conventional from drug-eluting chemoembolization? *Cardiovasc Intervent Radiol* 2011;34(1):37–49.

Liu DM, Salem R, Bui JT, et al., Angiographic considerations in patients undergoing liver-directed therapy. *J Vasc Interv Radiol* 2005;16(7):911–935.

Livraghi T, Giorgio A, Marin G, et al. Hepatocellular carcinoma and cirrhosis in 746 patients: long-term results of percutaneous ethanol injection. *Radiology* 1995;197(1):101–108.

Livraghi T, Goldberg SN, Lazzaroni S, et al. Hepatocellular carcinoma: radio-frequency ablation of medium and large lesions. *Radiology* 2000; 214(3):761–768.

Llovet JM. Updated treatment approach to hepatocellular carcinoma. *J Gastroenterol* 2005;40(3):225–235.

Loffroy R, Estivalet L, Favelier S, et al. Interventional radiology therapies for liver cancer. *Hepatoma Research* 2016;2(1):1–9.

Lu MD, Chen JW, Xie XY, et al. Hepatocellular carcinoma: US-guided percutaneous microwave coagulation therapy. *Radiology* 2001;221(1): 167–172.

Lu DS, Siripongsakun S, Kyong Lee J, et al., Complete tumor encapsulation on magnetic resonance imaging: a potentially useful imaging biomarker for better survival in solitary large hepatocellular carcinoma. *Liver Transpl* 2013;19(3):283–291.

Ludwig JM, Camacho JC, Kokabi N, Xing M, Kim HS. The role of diffusion-weighted imaging (DWI) in locoregional therapy outcome prediction and response assessment for hepatocellular carcinoma (HCC): the new era of functional imaging biomarkers. *Diagnostics (Basel)* 2015;5(4): 546–563.

Lunderquist A. Arterial segmental supply of the liver. An angiographic study. *Acta Radiol Diagn (Stockh)* 1967:Suppl 272:1+.

Mantatzis M, Kakolyris S, Amarantidis K, Karayiannakis A, Prassopoulos P. Treatment response classification of liver metastatic disease evaluated on imaging. Are RECIST unidimensional measurements accurate? *Eur Radiol* 2009;19(7):1809–1816.

Matsui O, Kadoya M, Kameyama T, et al. Benign and malignant nodules in cirrhotic livers: distinction based on blood supply. *Radiology* 1991;178(2):493-497.

McWilliams JP, Kee ST, Loh CT, Lee EW, Liu DM. Prophylactic embolization of the cystic artery before radioembolization: feasibility, safety, and outcomes. *Cardiovasc Intervent Radiol* 2011;34(4):786–792.

Michels NA. Variational anatomy of the hepatic, cystic, and retroduodenal arteries; a statistical analysis of their origin, distribution, and relations to the biliary ducts in two hundred bodies. *AMA Arch Surg* 1953;66(1):20–34.

Miyayama S, Matsui O. Superselective conventional transarterial chemoembolization for hepatocellular carcinoma: rationale, technique, and outcome. *J Vasc Interv Radiol* 2016;27(9):1269–1278.

Miyayama S, Matsui O, Kameyama T, et al. [Angiographic anatomy of arterial branches to the caudate lobe of the liver with special reference to its effect on transarterial embolization of hepatocellular carcinoma]. *Rinsho Hoshasen* 1990;35(3):353–359.

Mondazzi L, Bottelli R, Brambilla G, et al. Transarterial oily chemoembolization for the treatment of hepatocellular carcinoma: a multivariate analysis of prognostic factors. *Hepatology* 1994;19(5):1115–1123.

Murphy KP, Maher MM, O'Connor OJ. Abdominal ablation techniques. *AJR Am J Roentgenol* 2015;204(5):W495–W502.

Ohnishi K. Comparison of percutaneous acetic acid injection and percutaneous ethanol injection for small hepatocellular carcinoma. *Hepatogastroenterology* 1998;45 Suppl 3:1254–1258.

Ohnishi K, Ohyama N, Ito S, Fujiwara K. Small hepatocellular carcinoma: treatment with US-guided intratumoral injection of acetic acid. *Radiology* 1994;193(3):747–752.

Riaz A, Gates VL, Atassi B, et al. Radiation segmentectomy: a novel approach to increase safety and efficacy of radioembolization. *Int J Radiat Oncol Biol Phys* 2011;79(1):163–171.

Ruzicka FF Jr, Rossi P. Normal vascular anatomy of the abdominal viscera. *Radiol Clin North Am* 1970;8(1):3–29.

Salem R, Mazzaferro V, Sangro B. Yttrium 90 radioembolization for the treatment of hepatocellular carcinoma: biological lessons, current challenges, and clinical perspectives. *Hepatology* 2013;58(6):2188-2197.

Sancho L, Rodriguez-Fraile M, Bilbao JI, et al. Is a technetium-99m macroaggregated albumin scan essential in the workup for selective internal radiation therapy with yttrium-90? An analysis of 532 patients. *J Vasc Interv Radiol* 2017;28(11):1536–1542.

Sangro B. Chemoembolization and radioembolization. *Best Pract Res Clin Gastroenterol* 2014;28(5):909-919.

Sangro B, Carpanese L, Cianni R, et al; European Network on Radioembolization with Yttrium-90 Resin Microspheres (ENRY). Survival after yttrium-90 resin microsphere radioembolization of hepatocellular carcinoma across Barcelona clinic liver cancer stages: a European evaluation. *Hepatology* 2011;54(3):868–878.

Sangro B, D'Avola D, Iñarrairaegui M, Prieto J. Transarterial therapies for hepatocellular carcinoma. *Expert Opin Pharmacother* 2011;12(7):1057–1073.

Sangro B, Gil-Alzugaray B, Rodriguez J, et al. Liver disease induced by radioembolization of liver tumors: description and possible risk factors. *Cancer* 2008;112(7):1538–1546.

Sangro B, Inarrairaegui M, Bilbao JI. Radioembolization for hepatocellular carcinoma. *J Hepatol* 2012;56(2):464-473.

Schena E, Saccomandi P, Fong Y. Laser ablation for cancer: past, present and future. *J Funct Biomater* 2017;8(2):E19.

Schoellnast H, Monette S, Ezell PC, et al. Acute and subacute effects of irreversible electroporation on nerves: experimental study in a pig model. *Radiology* 2011;260(2):421–427.

Seidenfeld J, Korn A, Aronson N. Radiofrequency ablation of unresectable primary liver cancer. *J Am Coll Surg* 2002;194(6):813–828; discussion 828.

Shiina S, Tagawa K, Niwa Y, et al. Percutaneous ethanol injection therapy for hepatocellular carcinoma: results in 146 patients. *AJR Am J Roentgenol* 1993;160(5):1023–1028.

Shim JH, Lee HC, Kim SO, et al. Which response criteria best help predict survival of patients with hepatocellular carcinoma following chemoembolization? A validation study of old and new models. *Radiology* 2012;262(2):708–718.

Silk M, Tahour D, Srimathveeravalli G, Solomon SB, Thornton RH. The state of irreversible electroporation in interventional oncology. *Semin Intervent Radiol* 2014;31(2):111–117.

Silk MT, Wimmer T, Lee KS, et al. Percutaneous ablation of peribiliary tumors with irreversible electroporation. *J Vasc Interv Radiol* 2014;25(1):112–118.

Song SY, Chung JW, Kwon JW, et al. Collateral pathways in patients with celiac axis stenosis: angiographic-spiral CT correlation. *Radiographics* 2002;22(4):881–893.

Stafford RJ, Fuentes D, Elliott AA, Weinberg JS, Ahrar K. Laser-induced thermal therapy for tumor ablation. *Crit Rev Biomed Eng* 2010;38(1):79–100.

Stroehl YW, Letzen BS, van Breugel JM, Geschwind JF, Chapiro J. Intra-arterial therapies for liver cancer: assessing tumor response. *Expert Rev Anticancer Ther* 2017;17(2):119–127.

Stulberg JH, Bierman HR. Selective hepatic arteriography. Normal anatomy, anatomic variations, and pathological conditions. *Radiology* 1965;85: 46–55.

Tacher V, Radaelli A, Lin M, Geschwind JF. How I do it: cone-beam CT during transarterial chemoembolization for liver cancer. *Radiology* 2015; 274(2):320–334.

Takayasu K, Arii S, Ikai I, et al; Liver Cancer Study Group of Japan. Overall survival after transarterial lipiodol infusion chemotherapy with or without embolization for unresectable hepatocellular carcinoma: propensity score analysis. *AJR Am J Roentgenol* 2010;194(3):830–837.

Tancredi T, McCuskey PA, Kan Z, Wallace S. Changes in rat liver microcirculation after experimental hepatic arterial embolization: comparison of different embolic agents. *Radiology* 1999;211(1):177–181.

Tang Y, Taylor RR, Gonzalez MV, Lewis AL, Stratford PW. Evaluation of irinotecan drug-eluting beads: a new drug-device combination product for the chemoembolization of hepatic metastases. *J Control Release* 2006;116(2):e55–e56.

Thomson KR, Cheung W, Ellis SJ, et al. Investigation of the safety of irreversible electroporation in humans. *J Vasc Interv Radiol* 2011;22(5):611–621.

Varela M, Real MI, Burrel M, et al. Chemoembolization of hepatocellular carcinoma with drug eluting beads: efficacy and doxorubicin pharmacokinetics. *J Hepatol* 2007;46(3):474–481.

Vouche M, Lewandowski RJ, Atassi R, et al. Radiation lobectomy: time-dependent analysis of future liver remnant volume in unresectable liver cancer as a bridge to resection. *J Hepatol* 2013;59(5):1029-1036.

Wang YX, De Baere T, Idée JM, Ballet S. Transcatheter embolization therapy in liver cancer: an update of clinical evidences. *Chin J Cancer Res* 2015;27(2):96–121.

Wang B, Xu H, Gao ZQ, Ning HF, Sun YQ, Cao GW. Increased expression of vascular endothelial growth factor in hepatocellular carcinoma after transcatheter arterial chemoembolization. *Acta Radiol* 2008;49(5):523–529.

Yamada R, Nakatsuka H, Nakamura K, et al. Hepatic artery embolization in 32 patients with unresectable hepatoma. *Osaka City Med J* 1980;26(2):81–96.

Yamada R, Sato M, Kawabata M, Nakatsuka H, Nakamura K, Takashima S. Hepatic artery embolization in 120 patients with unresectable hepatoma. *Radiology* 1983;148(2):397–401.

Yamagami T, Nakamura T, Iida S, Kato T, Nishimura T. Embolization of the right gastric artery before hepatic arterial infusion chemotherapy to prevent gastric mucosal lesions: approach through the hepatic artery versus the left gastric artery. *AJR Am J Roentgenol* 2002;179(6):1605–1610.

Yokoyama T, Egami K, Miyamoto M, et al. Percutaneous and laparoscopic approaches of radiofrequency ablation treatment for liver cancer. *J Hepatobiliary Pancreat Surg* 2003;10(6):425–427.

Yoon CJ, Chung JW, Cho BH, et al., Hepatocellular carcinoma in the caudate lobe of the liver: angiographic analysis of tumor-feeding arteries according to subsegmental location. *J Vasc Interv Radiol* 2008;19(11):1543–1550; quiz 1550.

Yu H, Burke CT. Comparison of percutaneous ablation technologies in the treatment of malignant liver tumors. *Semin Intervent Radiol* 2014;31(2): 129–137.

SECTION VII

GASTROINTESTINAL TRACT

SECTION EDITOR: William E. Brant

CHAPTER 40 ■ ABDOMEN AND PELVIS

WILLIAM E. BRANT AND JENNIFER POHL

IMAGING METHODS

Conventional radiographs of the abdomen remain a mainstay for the assessment of the acute abdomen. CT, US, and MR provide comprehensive evaluation of the abdomen including the peritoneal cavity, retroperitoneal compartments, abdominal and pelvic organs, blood vessels, and lymph nodes.

COMPARTMENTAL ANATOMY OF THE ABDOMEN AND PELVIS

Knowledge of the complex compartmental anatomy of the abdomen and pelvis is fundamental to understanding the effects of pathologic processes and to correctly interpret imaging studies. Understanding the shape and extent of anatomic compartments and their normal variations may clarify imaging findings that would otherwise be incomprehensible or lead to misdiagnosis. Fundamental considerations include constant anatomic landmarks, ligaments and fascia that define compartments, and normal variations in size and appearance of the various compartments and recesses. Identifying the precise compartment that an abnormality is in determines to a great extent the origin of the abnormality.

The peritoneal cavity is divided into the greater peritoneal cavity and the lesser peritoneal cavity (the lesser sac) (Figs. 40.1 and 40.2). Within both portions of the peritoneal cavity are numerous recesses in which pathologic processes tend to loculate. The *right subphrenic space* communicates around the liver with the anterior subhepatic and posterior subhepatic space (*Morison pouch*). Morison pouch (the right hepatorenal fossa) is the most dependent portion of the abdominal cavity in a supine patient and it preferentially collects ascites, hemoperitoneum, metastases, and abscesses. The right subphrenic and subhepatic spaces communicate freely with the pelvic peritoneal cavity via the right paracolic gutter.

The *left subphrenic space* communicates freely with the left subhepatic space, but is separated from the right subphrenic space by the falciform ligament and from the left paracolic gutter by the phrenicocolic ligament. The left subphrenic (perisplenic) space distends with fluid from ascites and with blood from splenic trauma. It is a common location for abscesses and for disease processes of the tail of the pancreas. The left subhepatic space (gastrohepatic recess) is affected by diseases of the duodenal bulb, lesser curve of the stomach, gallbladder, and left lobe of the liver.

The *falciform ligament* consists of two closely applied layers of peritoneum extending from the umbilicus to the diaphragm in a parasagittal plane. The caudal free end of the falciform ligament contains the ligamentum teres, which is the remnant of the obliterated umbilical vein. Paraumbilical veins (portosystemic collateral vessels) that enlarge within the falciform ligament are a specific sign of portal hypertension. The reflections of the falciform ligament separate over the posterior dome of the liver to form the coronary ligaments, which define the "*bare area*" of the liver not covered by peritoneum. The coronary ligaments reflect between the liver and diaphragm and prevent access of ascites and other intraperitoneal processes from covering the bare area of the liver.

The *lesser omentum*, composed of the gastrohepatic and hepatoduodenal ligaments, suspends the stomach and duodenal bulb from the inferior surface of the liver. The lesser omentum separates the gastrohepatic recess of the left subphrenic space from the lesser sac. The lesser omentum transmits the coronary veins (which dilate as varices) and contains lymph nodes (which enlarge with involvement by gastric carcinoma and lymphoma). The *lesser sac* is the isolated peritoneal compartment between the stomach and the pancreas. It communicates with the rest of the peritoneal cavity (the greater sac) only through the small foramen of Winslow. Pathologic processes in the lesser sac usually occur because of disease in adjacent organs (pancreas, stomach) rather than spread from elsewhere in the abdominal cavity. The lesser sac is normally collapsed but can become huge when filled with fluid.

The *greater omentum* is a double layer of peritoneum that hangs from the greater curvature of the stomach and descends in front of the abdominal viscera separating bowel from the anterior abdominal wall. The greater omentum encloses fat and a few blood vessels. It serves as fertile ground for implantation of peritoneal metastases, and assists in loculation of inflammatory processes of the peritoneal cavity such as abscesses and tuberculosis.

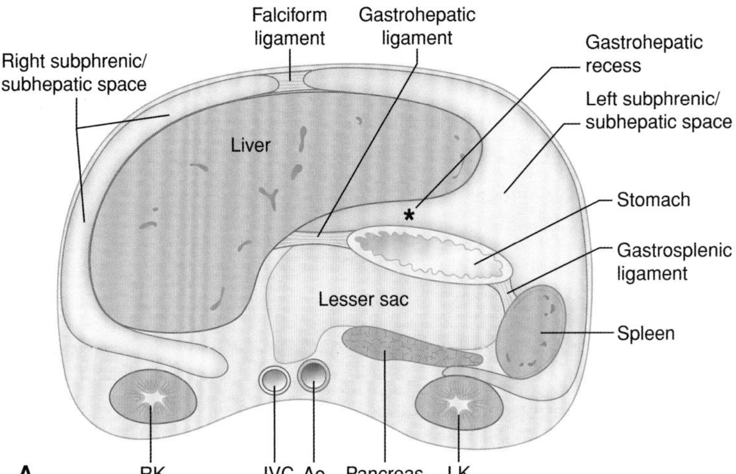

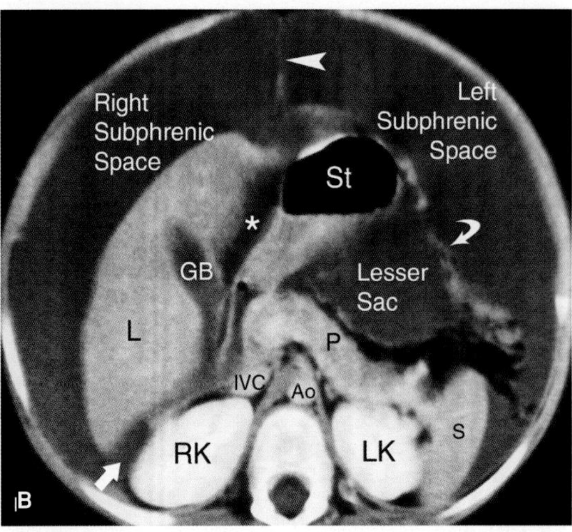

FIGURE 40.1. **Anatomy of the Peritoneal Cavity. A:** Diagram of an axial cross-section of the abdomen illustrates the recesses of the greater peritoneal cavity and the lesser sac. **B:** CT scan of a patient with a large amount of ascites nicely demonstrates the recesses of the greater peritoneal cavity and the lesser sac. The lesser sac is bounded by the stomach (*St*) anteriorly, the pancreas (*P*) posteriorly, and the gastrosplenic ligament (*curved arrow*) laterally. The falciform ligament (*arrowhead*) separates the right and left subphrenic spaces. Fluid from the greater peritoneal cavity extends into Morison pouch (*arrow*) between the liver and the right kidney. Fluid in the gastrohepatic recess (*) separates the stomach from the liver (*L*). *S,* spleen; *GB,* gallbladder; *RK,* right kidney; *IVC,* inferior vena cava; *Ao,* aorta; *LK,* left kidney.

The retroperitoneal space between the diaphragm and the pelvic brim is divided into anterior pararenal, perirenal, and posterior pararenal compartments by the anterior and posterior renal fascia (Fig. 40.3). The *anterior pararenal space* extends between the posterior parietal peritoneum and the anterior renal fascia. It is bounded laterally by the lateroconal fascia. The pancreas, duodenal loop, and ascending and descending portions of the colon are within the anterior pararenal space. Disease in the anterior pararenal space usually originates from these organs (pancreatitis, perforating/penetrating ulcer, diverticulitis).

The anterior and posterior renal fascias encompass the kidney, adrenal gland, and perirenal fat within the *perirenal space.* The anterior renal fascia is thin and consists of one layer of connective tissue. The posterior renal fascia is thicker, consisting of two layers of connective tissue. The anterior layer of the posterior renal fascia is continuous with the anterior renal fascia. The posterior layer of the renal fascia is continuous

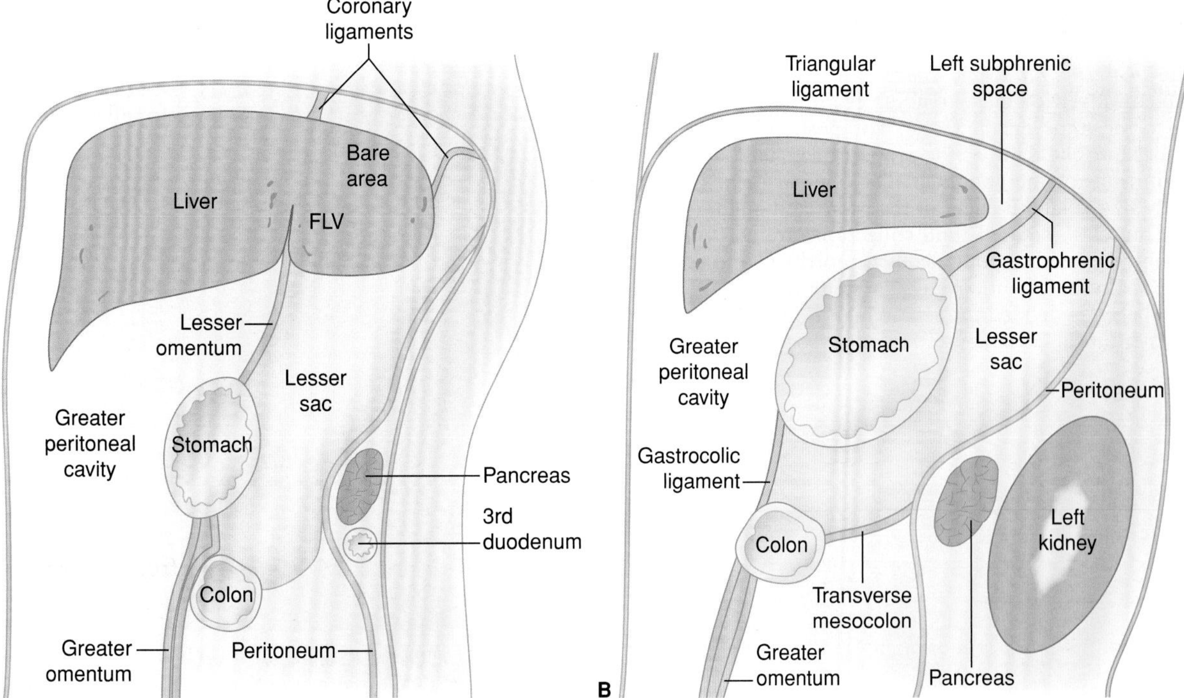

FIGURE 40.2. **The Lesser Sac.** Sagittal plane diagrams of the medial (**A**) and lateral (**B**) aspects of the lesser sac illustrate its position posterior to the stomach and anterior to the posterior parietal peritoneum covering the pancreas. Note that projections of the lesser sac extend to the diaphragm, resulting in the potential for disease processes in the lesser sac to cause pleural effusions. The coronary ligaments reflect between the liver and the diaphragm producing a bare area of liver not covered by peritoneum.

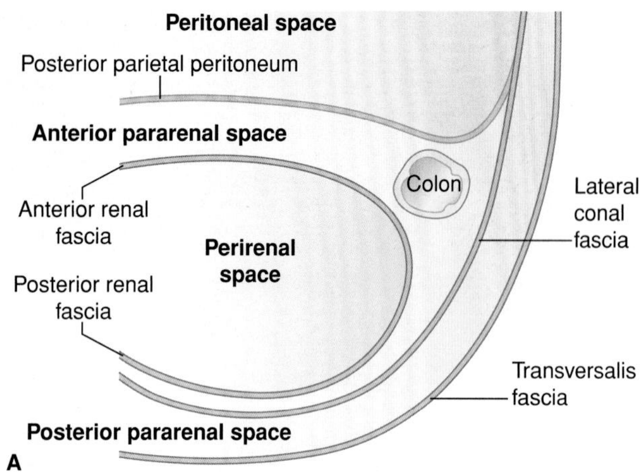

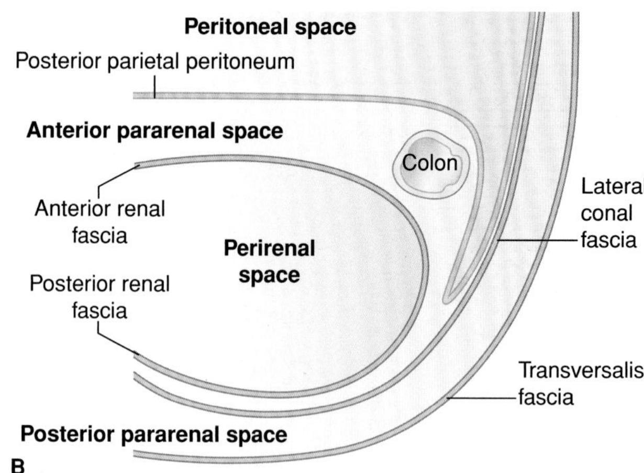

FIGURE 40.3. **Retroperitoneal Compartmental Anatomy.** Diagrams illustrate two normal variations of the reflections of the posterior parietal peritoneum around the descending colon. In (**A**) the colon is entirely retroperitoneal and in (**B**) the peritoneum forms a deep pocket lateral to the colon, allowing intraperitoneal fluid to extend far posteriorly. Fluid or disease processes in the anterior pararenal space from the pancreas or colon may also extend posteriorly to the kidney by separating the two layers of the posterior renal fascia.

with the lateroconal fascia, forming the lateral boundary of the anterior pararenal space. The anterior and posterior layers of the posterior renal fascia may be separated by inflammatory processes, such as pancreatitis, extending from the anterior pararenal space. The renal fascia is bound to the fascia surrounding the aorta and vena cava usually preventing spread of disease to the contralateral perirenal space. However, disease processes arising in the perivascular space, such as hemorrhage from aortic aneurysm rupture, may extend into the perirenal space. Fluid collections in the perirenal space are usually renal in origin (infection, urinoma, hemorrhage). Bridging septa extend between the renal fascia and the renal capsule tends to cause loculations of fluid processes in the perirenal space. The right perirenal space is open superiorly to the bare area of the liver allowing spread of disease processes (infection, tumor) between the kidney and liver.

The *posterior pararenal space* is a potential space, usually filled only with fat, extending from the posterior renal fascia to the transversalis fascia. The posterior pararenal fat continues into the flank as the properitoneal fat "stripe" seen on plain films of the abdomen. The compartment is limited medially by the lateral edges of the psoas and quadratus lumborum muscles. Isolated fluid collections are rare and most commonly caused by spontaneous hemorrhage into the psoas muscle as a result of anticoagulation therapy.

The pelvis is divided into three major anatomic compartments: peritoneal cavity, extraperitoneal space, and perineum (Fig. 40.4). The *peritoneal cavity* extends to the level of the vagina, forming the pouch of Douglas (*cul-de-sac*) in females, or to the level of the seminal vesicles, forming the rectovesical pouch in males. The broad ligaments reflect over the uterus, fallopian tubes, and parametrial uterine vessels and serve as the anterior boundary of the rectouterine pouch of Douglas. The cul-de-sac is the most dependent portion of the peritoneal cavity and collects fluid, blood, abscesses, and intraperitoneal drop metastases. The *extraperitoneal space of the pelvis* is continuous with the retroperitoneal space of the abdomen, extends to the pelvic diaphragm, and includes the retropubic space (of Retzius). Pathologic processes from the pelvis spread preferentially into the retroperitoneal compartments of the abdomen. The *perineum* lies below the pelvic diaphragm. The ischiorectal fossa serves as its anatomic landmark (Fig. 40.5).

Peritoneum
Iliopsoas
Rectum
Iliac vessels
Peritoneal cavity
Extraperitoneal space
Ureter
Obturator internus
Levator ani
Ischiorectal fossa (perineum)
Rectum

FIGURE 40.4. **Compartmental Anatomy of the Pelvis.** Diagram in the coronal plane illustrates the major anatomic compartments of the pelvis.

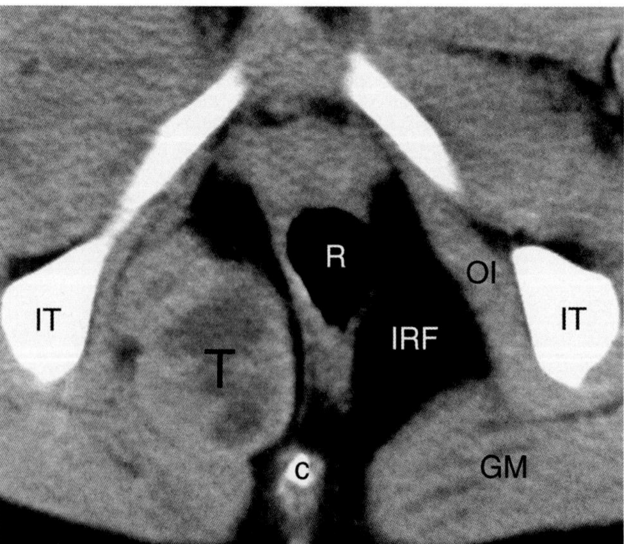

FIGURE 40.5. **Perineal Tumor.** A CT scan of a 12-year-old girl with a history of a rhabdomyosarcoma of the right leg demonstrates a tumor metastasis (*T*) in the right ischiorectal fossa. The left ischiorectal fossa (*IRF*) shows its normal appearance as a triangle of fat bordered by the rectum (*R*), obturator internus muscle (*OI*), and the gluteus muscles (*GM*). The ischiorectal fossa is entirely below the levator ani and is part of the perineum. *c*, tip of the coccyx; *IT*, ischial tuberosities.

FLUID IN THE PERITONEAL CAVITY

Fluid in the peritoneal cavity originates from many different sources and varies greatly in composition. Ascites is serous fluid in the peritoneal cavity most commonly caused by cirrhosis, hypoproteinemia, or congestive heart failure. Exudative ascites results from inflammatory processes such as abscess, pancreatitis, peritonitis, or bowel perforation. Hemoperitoneum results from trauma, surgery, or spontaneous hemorrhage. Neoplastic ascites is associated with intraperitoneal tumors. Urine, bile, and chyle may also spread freely within the peritoneal cavity.

Conventional radiographic diagnosis of ascites requires that at least 500 cc of fluid be present. Findings are (a) diffuse increase in density of the abdomen (gray abdomen), (b) indistinct margins of the liver, spleen, and psoas muscles, (c) medial displacement of gas-filled colon, liver, and spleen away from the properitoneal flank stripe, (d) bulging of the flanks, (e) increased separation of gas-filled small bowel loops, and (f) "dog's ears" appearance of symmetric densities in the pelvis due to fluid spilling out of the cul-de-sac on either side of the bladder. CT demonstrates fluid density in the recesses of the peritoneal cavity. The CT density of the fluid gives a clue as to its composition. Serous ascites has attenuation values near water (–10 to +10 H). Exudative ascites is usually above +15 H and acute bleeding into the peritoneal cavity averages +45 H. US is sensitive to small amounts of fluid in the peritoneal recesses. Care must be taken with US to examine the most gravity-dependent portions of the peritoneal cavity (Morison pouch and the pelvis). Simple ascites is anechoic, while exudative, hemorrhagic, or neoplastic ascites often contains floating debris. Septations in ascites are associated with an inflammatory or malignant process. MR shows limited specificity for defining the type of fluid present. Serous fluid is low signal intensity on T1WI and markedly increased in signal intensity on T2WI. Hemorrhagic fluid shows high signal intensity on both T1WI and T2WI. Serous ascites is commonly bright on gradient-echo images due to fluid motion.

Pseudomyxoma peritonei ("jelly belly") refers to gelatinous ascites that occurs as a result of intraperitoneal spread of mucin-producing cells resulting from rupture of appendiceal mucocele, or intraperitoneal spread of benign or malignant mucinous cysts of the ovary or mucinous adenocarcinoma of the colon or rectum. Conventional radiographs may demonstrate punctate or ring-like calcifications scattered through the peritoneal cavity. CT demonstrates mottled densities, septations, and calcifications within the fluid. The mucinous fluid is typically loculated and causes mass effect on the liver and bowel (Fig. 40.6). US demonstrates intraperitoneal nodules that range from hypoechoic to strongly echogenic.

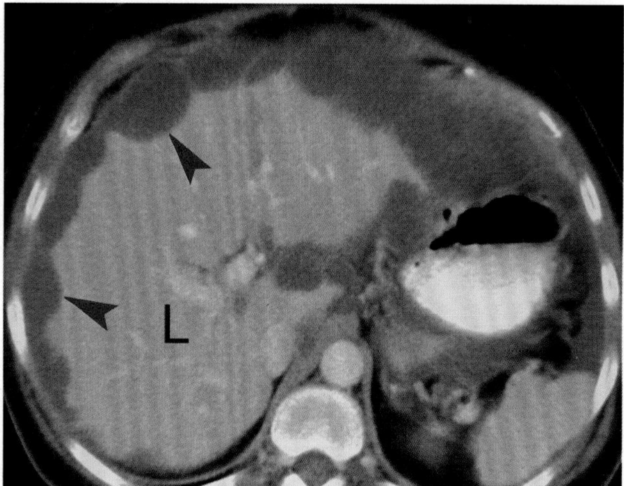

FIGURE 40.6. **Pseudomyxoma Peritonei.** A CT scan of a 60-year-old man with intraperitoneal spread of mucinous adenocarcinoma of the colon shows loculations (*arrowheads*) of fluid indenting the surface of the liver (*L*) giving evidence of mass effect. The attenuation of the fluid measured 32 H indicating exudative ascites.

PNEUMOPERITONEUM

Free air within the peritoneal cavity is a valuable sign of bowel perforation, most commonly caused by duodenal or gastric ulcer perforation. However, additional causes of pneumoperitoneum include trauma, recent surgery or laparoscopy, and infection of the peritoneal cavity with gas-producing organisms. Postoperative pneumoperitoneum usually resolves in 3 to 4 days. Serial images demonstrate a progressive decrease in the amount of air present. Failure of progressive resolution, or an increase in the amount of air present, suggests a leak of bowel anastomosis or sepsis. Pneumoperitoneum in the absence of a ruptured viscus may occur with air introduced through the female genital tract by orogenital insufflation, or associated with pulmonary emphysema, alveolar rupture, and dissection of air into the peritoneal cavity.

Conventional radiographs show pneumoperitoneum best on images obtained with the patient in the standing or sitting position. Upright chest radiographs are the most sensitive for free air. Small amounts of air are clearly demonstrated beneath the domes of the diaphragm. Left lateral decubitus and cross-table lateral views may be used with very ill patients to demonstrate air outlining the liver. Signs of pneumoperitoneum on supine radiographs (Fig. 40.7) include the following: (a) gas on both sides of the bowel wall (Rigler sign), (b) gas outlining the falciform ligament, (c) gas outlining the peritoneal cavity (the "football sign"), and (d) triangular or linear localized extraluminal gas in the right upper quadrant. On CT, small amounts of extraluminal gas may be confused with gas within the bowel and can be surprisingly difficult to recognize. Images should be examined at lung windows to detect free intraperitoneal air. The peritoneal recess between the liver and diaphragm (Fig. 40.8) is a good place to look for pneumoperitoneum on CT.

ABDOMINAL CALCIFICATIONS

Intra-abdominal calcifications may be an important sign of intra-abdominal disease and should be searched for on every imaging study of the abdomen. CT and US are more sensitive to detection of calcifications than are conventional radiographs. However, the high spatial resolution of conventional radiography commonly provides characteristic findings that allow a specific diagnosis of the nature of the calcification.

Vascular calcifications are common in the aorta and iliac vessels (see Fig. 40.12) of older individuals. Plaque-like vascular calcifications overlie the lumbar spine and sacrum and commonly require detailed inspection to detect. Aneurysms of the aorta are manifest by luminal diameter exceeding 3 cm as measured between calcifications in the aortic wall (Fig. 40.9). Ring-like calcified aneurysms most commonly involve the splenic or renal arteries. *Phleboliths* are calcified thrombi in veins most commonly visualized in the lateral aspects of the pelvis. They are round or oval calcifications up to 5 mm size that commonly contain a central lucency. They may be mistaken for urinary tract calculi.

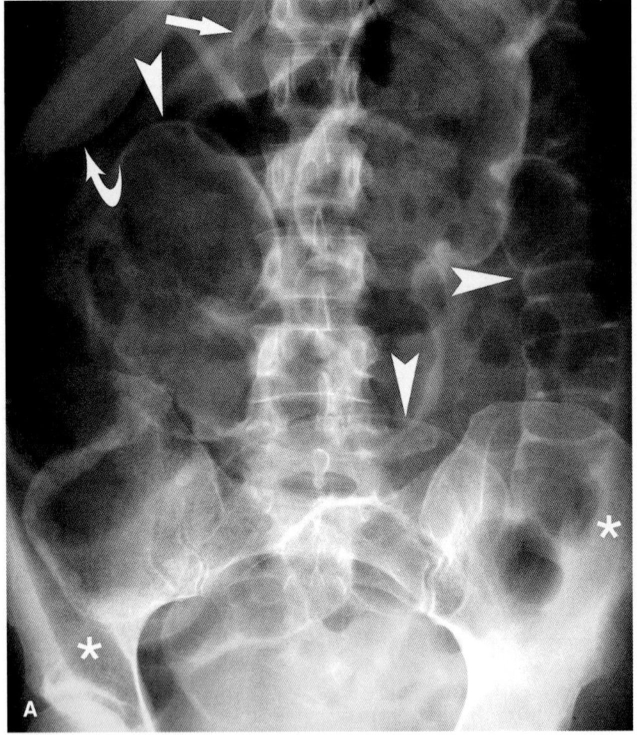

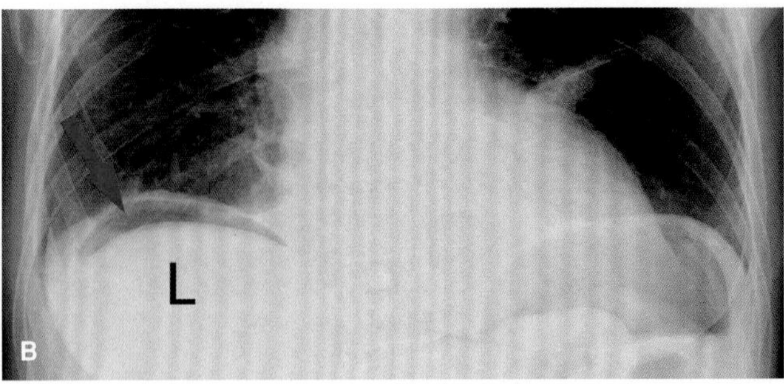

FIGURE 40.7. **Pneumoperitoneum: Conventional Radiograph.** **A:** Supine abdominal radiograph in a patient with a perforated gastric ulcer demonstrates visualization of both sides of the bowel wall (Rigler sign) (*arrowheads*), free air outlining the falciform ligament (*arrow*), free air outlining the edge of the liver (*curved arrow*), and free air outlining the pericolic gutters (*). **B:** Erect chest radiograph in a different patient shows a crescent-shaped band of gas (*arrow*) between the liver (*L*) and the diaphragm. Pneumoperitoneum was caused by a perforated sigmoid colon diverticulitis.

Calcified lymph nodes result most commonly from granulomatous diseases such as tuberculosis or histoplasmosis. The calcification is usually mottled and 10 to 15 mm in size. Mesenteric nodes are the most commonly calcified.

Gallstones and Gallbladder. Only about 15% of gallstones contain sufficient calcium to be identified on conventional radiography. Most calcified gallstones contain calcium bilirubinate and have a laminated appearance with a dense outer rim and more radiolucent center. When multiple gallstones are present, they are commonly faceted. Calcifications in the gallbladder wall (*porcelain gallbladder*) (Fig. 40.10) are plaque like and oval in configuration conforming to the size and shape of the gallbladder. Milk of calcium bile is a suspension of radiopaque crystals within gallbladder bile. Layering of the suspension can be demonstrated on erect radiographs.

Urinary Calculi. About 85% of urinary calculi are visible on conventional radiographs. They range in size from punctate up to several centimeters. Most characteristic are the staghorn calculi, which assume the shape of the renal collecting system (Fig. 40.11). Renal calculi are differentiated from gallstones on radiographs by oblique projections that confirm their posterior position, as opposed to the more anterior positions of gallstones. Ureteral calculi may be seen anywhere along the course of the ureter, but are most common at the areas of

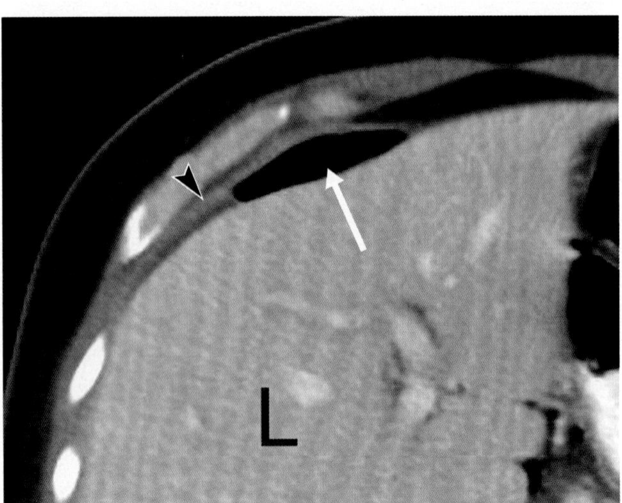

FIGURE 40.8. **Pneumoperitoneum: CT.** A collection of air (*arrow*) is seen within the peritoneal space between the liver (*L*) and the diaphragm (*arrowhead*). This is a prime area to search to detect small amounts of free intraperitoneal air on CT. This patient had a torn jejunum as a result of trauma from a motor vehicle collision.

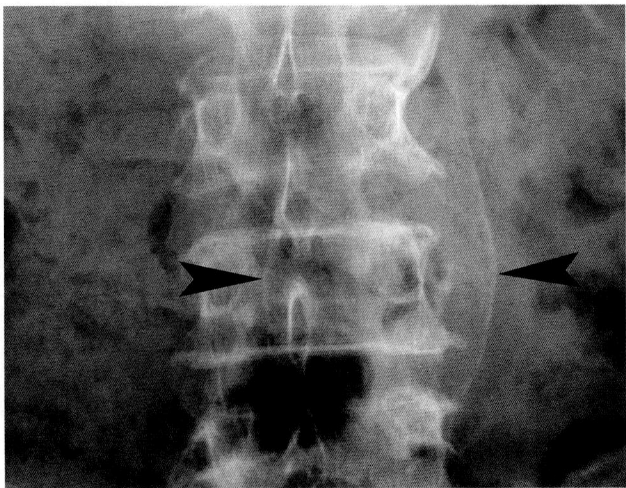

FIGURE 40.9. **Abdominal Aortic Aneurysm.** Conventional radiograph demonstrates an aneurysm of the abdominal aorta evidenced by wide separation of calcifications in the aortic wall (*arrowheads*). Calcification in the wall overlying the spine may be difficult to visualize. A radiograph taken with the patient in left posterior oblique position will project the aorta away from the spine and make visualization of aortic wall calcifications easier.

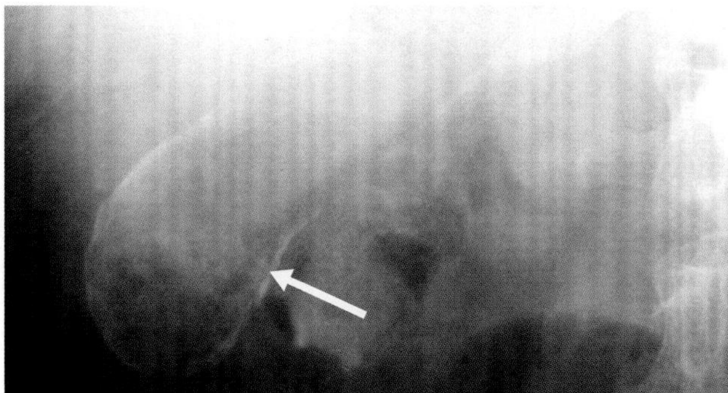

FIGURE 40.10. **Porcelain Gallbladder.** Cone-down radiograph of the right upper quadrant of the abdomen demonstrates calcification in the wall of the gallbladder (*arrow*). This finding is indicative of chronic obstruction of the cystic duct, chronic gallbladder inflammation, and an increased risk of gallbladder carcinoma.

narrowing: the ureteropelvic junction, the pelvic brim, and the vesicoureteral junction. Bladder calculi (Fig. 40.12) are single or multiple, commonly laminated, may be any size, and usually lie near the midline of the pelvis. Calculi within bladder diverticula may be eccentric to the bladder. CT has become the imaging method of choice to document urinary tract stones.

Liver and spleen granulomas are usually multiple, small, and dense. They are healed foci of tuberculosis, histoplasmosis, or other granulomatous disease.

Appendicoliths and enteroliths are concretions within the lumen of the bowel. Most are round or oval and have concentric laminations. Appendicoliths are strongly indicative of acute appendicitis in patients presenting with acute abdominal pain. Enteroliths are most common in the colon and often due to calcium deposition on an undigestible material such as a fruit pit.

Epiploic appendagitis results from inflammation believed to be due to torsion of the colonic appendages, resulting in vascular occlusion and ischemia. The resultant fat necrosis often calcifies resulting in a mobile oval-shaped calcification.

Calcified adrenal glands are associated with adrenal hemorrhage in the newborn, tuberculosis, and Addison disease.

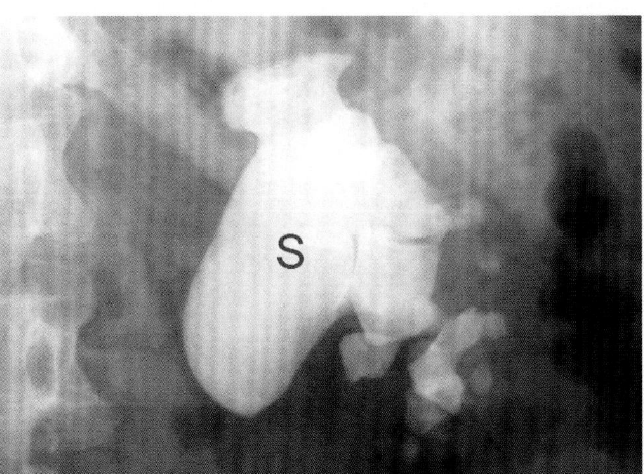

FIGURE 40.11. **Staghorn Calculus.** Conventional radiograph reveals a large calculus occupying the collecting system of the left kidney and assuming its shape. Staghorn calculi (*S*) are usually composed of struvite and form in the presence of chronic urinary infection.

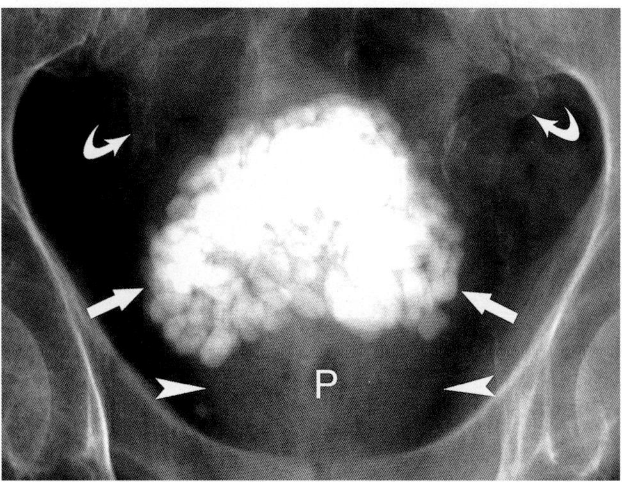

FIGURE 40.12. **Bladder Calculi.** Numerous calculi (*arrows*) in the bladder are evident on this conventional radiograph of the pelvis. The large prostate (*P*, between *arrowheads*), responsible for urinary stasis leading to stone formation, makes a mass impression on the layering stones. Also evident are atherosclerotic calcifications in the iliac arteries (*curved arrows*).

The calcification is mottled and in the location of the adrenal glands on either side of the first lumbar vertebra (Fig. 40.13).

Pancreatic calcification is associated with chronic alcohol-induced pancreatitis and hereditary pancreatitis. The calcifications are due to pancreatic calculi and are usually coarse and of varying size (Fig. 40.14).

Calcified cysts may be found in the kidneys, spleen, liver, appendix, and the peritoneal cavity. Calcification in the wall of a cyst is curvilinear or ring shaped (Fig. 40.15). *Echinococcus* cysts commonly calcify and may be found in any intra-abdominal organ as well as within the peritoneal cavity.

Tumor Calcification. A wide variety of different tumors of abdominal organs may contain calcifications. The coarse "popcorn" calcifications of uterine leiomyomas are most characteristic. Benign cystic teratomas may form teeth or bone. Calcified peritoneal metastases of ovarian or colon mucinous cystadenocarcinoma may outline the peritoneal cavity (Fig. 40.16). Renal cell carcinoma calcifies in up to 25% of cases.

Soft tissue calcifications may be seen with hypercalcemic states, idiopathic calcinosis, and old hematomas. Calcified injection granuloma from quinine, bismuth, and calcium salts of penicillin are commonly evident in the buttocks. Cysticercosis causes characteristic "rice-grain" calcifications in muscles.

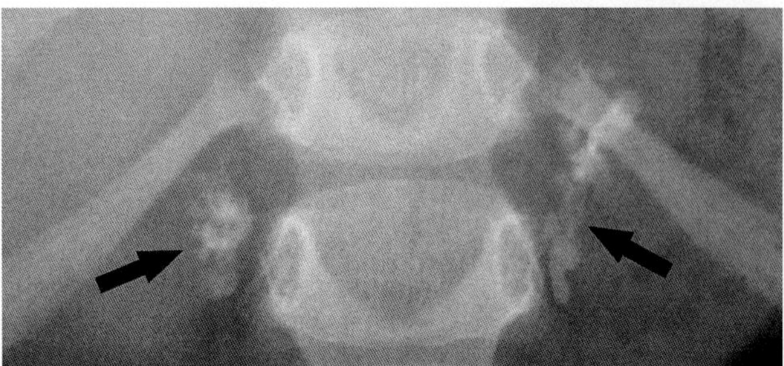

FIGURE 40.13. **Adrenal Calcifications.** Conventional radiograph of the abdomen in a 4 year old demonstrates calcification of both adrenal glands (*arrows*) resulting from bilateral adrenal hemorrhage as an infant.

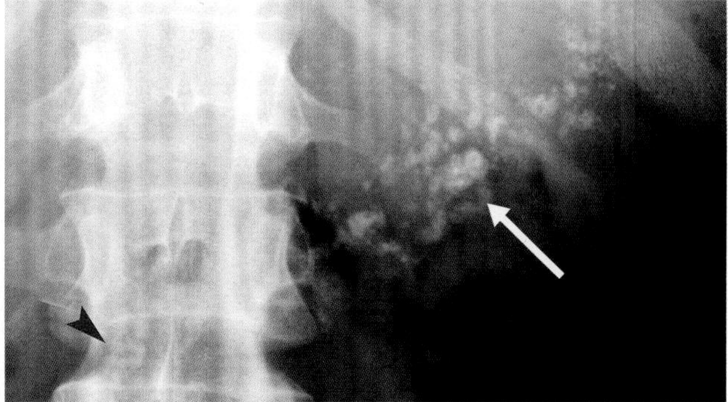

FIGURE 40.14. **Pancreatic Calcifications.** Coarse and punctate calcifications (*arrow*) extend upward across the left upper quadrant in this patient with chronic alcoholic pancreatitis. Calcifications in the pancreatic head (*arrowhead*) are obscured by the spine.

Bowel contents may include bone, pits, seeds, birdshot, or medications containing iron or other heavy metals that result in abdominal opacities.

Peritoneal calcifications may be nodular or sheet like and result most commonly from peritoneal dialysis, previous peritonitis, or peritoneal carcinomatosis (Fig. 40.16).

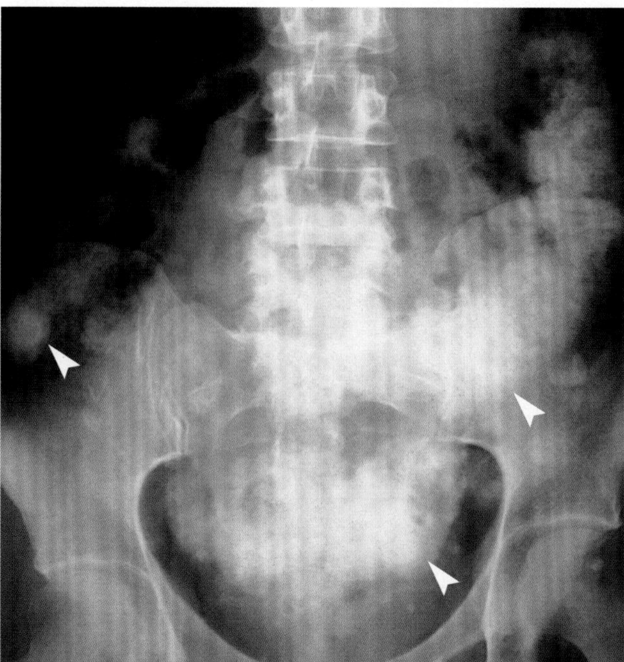

FIGURE 40.16. **Tumoral Calcifications.** Radiograph of the abdomen demonstrates cloud-like calcifications (*arrowheads*) in the distribution of peritoneal recesses. These calcifications were caused by intraperitoneal spread of a papillary serous cystadenocarcinomas of the ovary.

ACUTE ABDOMEN

The differential diagnosis of patients presenting with acute abdominal pain is extremely broad (Table 40.1). Accurate and efficient diagnosis requires cooperation between the referring physician and the radiologist to select the imaging method most likely to provide the correct diagnosis. Routine assessment of the acute abdomen commonly includes the "acute abdomen series," which consists of an erect posterior–anterior chest radiograph, and supine and erect or decubitus radiographs of the abdomen. The chest radiograph provides optimal detection of pneumoperitoneum and intrathoracic diseases that may present with abdominal complaints. The supine abdominal film permits diagnosis of many acute abdominal conditions, and the horizontal-beam abdominal film adds confidence to the diagnosis. CT or US is routinely obtained to provide a definitive diagnosis.

Normal Abdominal Gas Pattern. Interpretation of conventional abdominal radiographs routinely includes assessment of gas, fluid, soft tissue, fat, and calcium densities. Normal gas in the abdomen is predominantly swallowed air (Fig. 40.17). Air–fluid levels are seen in normal patients commonly in the stomach, often in the small bowel, but never in the colon distal to the hepatic flexure. Normal air–fluid levels in the small bowel should not exceed 2.5 cm in width. Small bowel gas usually appears as multiple small, random gas collections scattered throughout the abdomen. Small bowel gas is increased in patients who chronically swallow air or drink carbonated beverages. A normal intestinal gas pattern varies from no intestinal gas to gas within three to four variably shaped small intestinal loops measuring less than 2.5 to 3 cm in diameter. The normal colon contains some gas and fecal material and varies in diameter from 3 to 8 cm, with the cecum having the largest diameter. Complete absence of gas in the small bowel may be seen in patients with bowel obstruction with fluid rather than air filling the dilated bowel loops. The term "nonspecific abdominal gas pattern" has no precise meaning and should not be used.

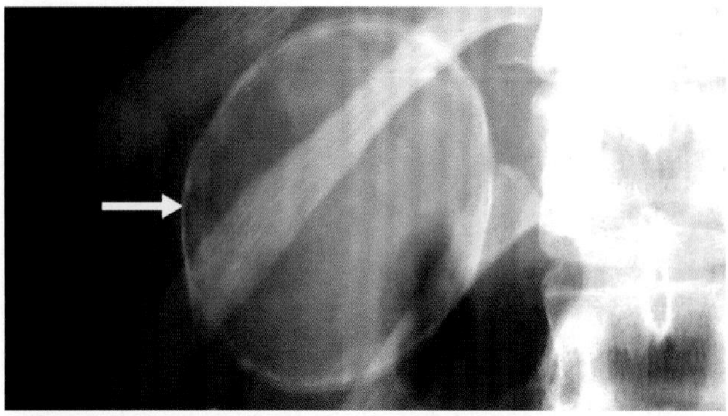

FIGURE 40.15. **Calcified Renal Cyst.** Conventional radiograph shows the rim calcification (*arrow*) characteristic of wall calcification in a renal cyst.

Dilated Bowel. Small bowel is dilated when it exceeds 2.5 to 3.0 cm in diameter. The colon is dilated when it exceeds 5 cm in diameter, and the cecum is dilated when it exceeds 8 cm diameter. In adults, dilated small bowel can usually be differentiated from dilated large bowel by assessment of location and anatomic

TABLE 40.1

COMMON CAUSES OF ACUTE ABDOMEN

Appendicitis	Peritonitis
Acute cholecystitis	Intraperitoneal abscess
Acute pancreatitis	Retroperitoneal abscess
Acute diverticulitis	Bowel obstruction
Acute ulcerative colitis	Urinary tract infection
Pseudomembranous colitis	Urinary tract obstruction
Amebiasis	Pelvic inflammatory diseases
Acute intestinal ischemia	Tubo-ovarian abscess

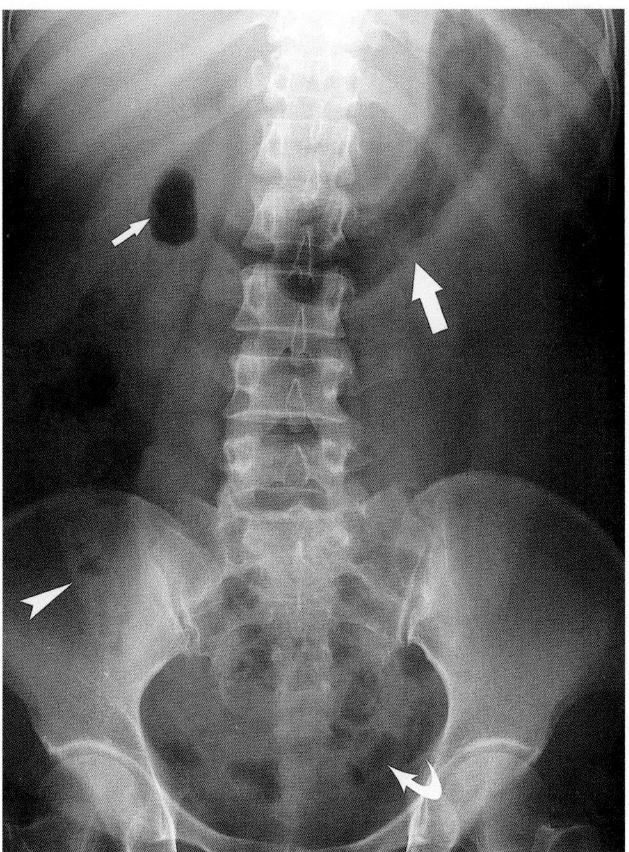

FIGURE 40.17. Normal Bowel Gas Pattern. Supine radiograph shows the normal distribution of gas in the stomach (*large arrow*) and duodenum (*small arrow*). The normal mottled pattern of stool is seen in the distribution of the right colon (*arrowhead*). A few gas collections within small bowel (*curved arrow*) are seen in the pelvis.

features. Small bowel is more central in the abdomen and is characterized by valvulae conniventes, which cross the entire diameter of the lumen. Dilated small bowel rarely exceeds 5 cm in diameter although large bowel is not considered dilated until it exceeds 5 cm diameter. Large bowel is more peripheral in the abdomen and is characterized by haustra that extend only partway across the lumen. Large bowel contains fecal material that has a characteristic mottled appearance. The cecum, which has the largest normal diameter of the large bowel, always dilates to the greatest extent irrespective of the site of obstruction.

TABLE 40.2

COMMON CAUSES OF ADYNAMIC ILEUS

Drugs Atropine, glucagon, morphine, barbiturates, phenothiazines
Metabolic causes Diabetes mellitus, hypothyroidism, hypokalemia, hypercalcemia
Inflammation Intraluminal: gastroenteritis Extraluminal: peritonitis, pancreatitis, appendicitis, cholecystitis, abscess
Postoperative: resolves in 4–7 days
Posttrauma
Postspinal injury

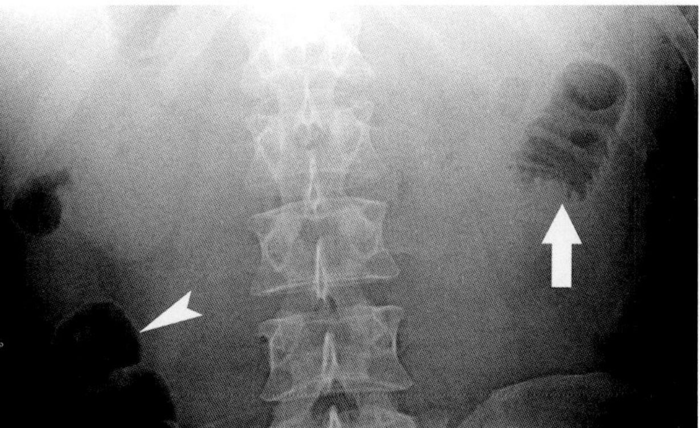

FIGURE 40.18. Sentinel Loop. Daily serial radiographs on this patient demonstrated a persistent loop of dilated small bowel (*arrow*) in the same location. This sentinel loop was caused by acute pancreatitis. Normal gas pattern is present in the right colon (*arrowhead*). The abdomen was otherwise devoid of intestinal gas.

Adynamic Ileus. The word "ileus" means stasis and does not differentiate mechanical obstruction from nonmechanical stasis. The terms "adynamic ileus," "paralytic ileus," and "nonobstructive ileus" are used interchangeably and refer to stasis of bowel contents because of decreased or absent peristalsis. Common causes of adynamic ileus are listed in Table 40.2. Adynamic ileus typically demonstrates diffuse symmetric, predominantly gaseous, distention of bowel. The small bowel, stomach, and colon are proportionally dilated without an abrupt transition. More bowel loops are dilated than with obstruction. Occasionally adynamic ileus may result in a gasless abdomen with dilated loops of bowel that are filled only with fluid. US is useful in confirming decreased or absent peristalsis, although examination may be difficult if large amounts of gas are present.

Sentinel loop refers to a segment of intestine that becomes paralyzed and dilated as it lies next to an inflamed intra-abdominal organ. In essence, it is a short segment of adynamic ileus that appears as an isolated loop of distended intestine that remains in the same general position on serial images (Fig. 40.18). A sentinel loop alerts one to the presence of an adjacent inflammatory process. A sentinel loop in the right upper quadrant suggests acute cholecystitis, hepatitis, or pyelonephritis. In the left upper quadrant, pancreatitis, pyelonephritis, or splenic injury may be suspected. In the lower quadrants, diverticulitis, appendicitis, salpingitis, cystitis, or Crohn disease is the cause of a sentinel loop.

Toxic megacolon is a manifestation of fulminant colitis characterized by extreme dilation of all or a portion of the colon. In this state, peristalsis is absent and the large bowel loses all tone and contractility. The patient has progressive abdominal distention and is toxic, febrile, and obtunded. Bowel sounds and bowel movements are absent. The bowel wall becomes like "wet blotting paper," and the risk of perforation is extreme. Mortality approaches 20% in toxic megacolon. Acute ulcerative colitis is the most common cause of toxic megacolon (Table 40.3). Conventional radiographs demonstrate distention of the colon with

TABLE 40.3

CAUSES OF TOXIC MEGACOLON

Ulcerative colitis: 75% of cases	Amebic colitis
Pseudomembranous colitis	Ischemic colitis
Crohn colitis	Bacterial colitis: cholera, typhoid

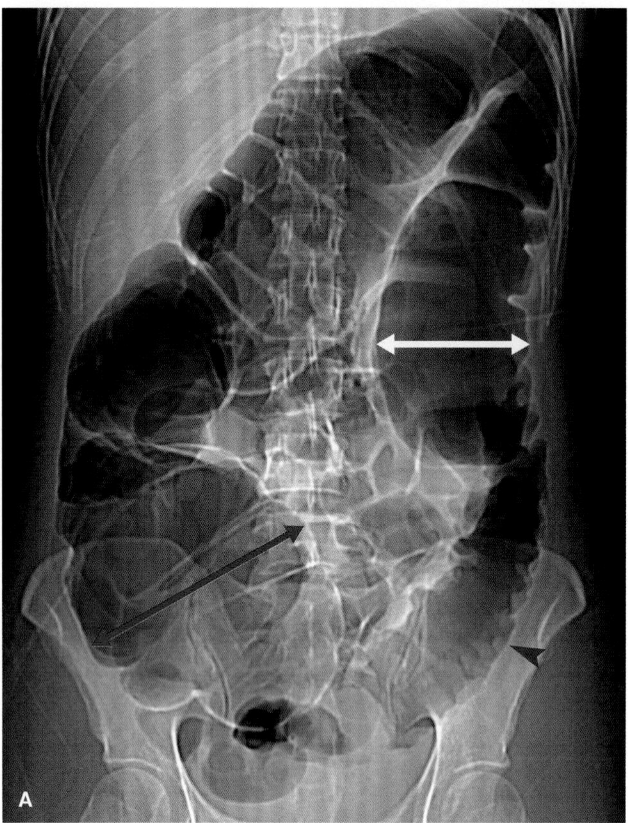

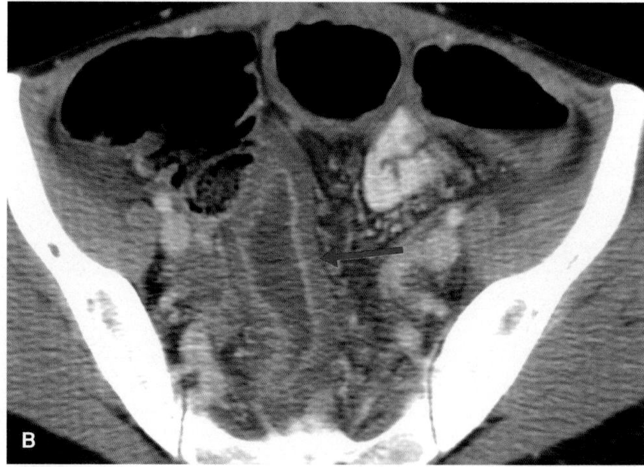

FIGURE 40.19. **Toxic Megacolon. A:** Supine radiograph of the abdomen demonstrates marked dilation of the colon with the cecum measuring 14 cm (*red line*) and the descending colon measuring 7 cm (*white line*) in diameter. The mucosal pattern of the lower descending colon is strikingly nodular (*arrowhead*). **B:** Corresponding CT showed marked thickening of the wall of the colon (*arrow*). Toxic megacolon was related to ulcerative colitis. The colon perforated just prior to surgery.

absent haustra. Dilation of the transverse colon up to 15 cm diameter is often the most striking finding. The diagnosis is suggested when the diameter of the colon exceeds 5 cm and the mucosa appears abnormal (Fig. 40.19). Pseudopolyps due to islands of edematous mucosa surrounded by extensive ulceration appear as soft tissue nodules within the air-distended colon. CT demonstrates a distended colon filled with air and fluid. The wall of the colon is thin but has an irregular nodular contour; air may be seen within the colon wall. Barium enema is absolutely contraindicated because of risk of perforation.

Mechanical bowel obstruction means stasis of bowel contents above a focal lesion. The obstruction may be due to obturation (occlusion by a mass in the lumen), stenosis due to intrinsic bowel disease, or compression of the lumen by extrinsic disease. The goal of imaging is to confirm the presence of obstruction, identify its level, and demonstrate its cause. Radiographs can confirm the presence of bowel obstruction 6 to 12 hours before the diagnosis can usually be made clinically (Fig. 40.19). When bowel obstruction occurs, the lumen of the bowel proximal to the obstruction progressively dilates because of continued secretions, swallowed fluid, air, and food, and eventual cessation of absorption. Stasis results in the overgrowth of bacteria and production of toxins that may injure the mucosa. Compromise of blood supply may occur because of distention of the bowel wall and increased intraluminal pressure. A variety of terms used clinically must be understood. *Complete obstruction* means the lumen is totally occluded and *partial obstruction* means some bowel contents pass through. *Simple obstruction* refers to blockage of the luminal contents without interference of blood supply. *Strangulation obstruction* means that the blood supply to the bowel wall is impaired. Most strangulation obstructions are *closed-loop obstructions*, which mean blockage of a bowel loop segment at both ends. This occurs with incarcerated hernias and volvulus.

Emphysematous infections of abdominal and pelvic organs with gas-forming organisms are detectable on conventional radiographs and may be confirmed by CT or US (see Figs. 41.49, 47.41, and 48.21). Gas within the parenchyma of solid organs or within the wall of hollow viscera may represent infection, fistula, infarction, or recent surgery or instrumentation. Prompt and accurate diagnosis is essential because infected patients are often septic, immunocompromised, or diabetic. Emphysematous infections result in bubbles and streaks of air that must be differentiated from normal gas collections. Emphysematous cholecystitis, emphysematous pyelonephritis and pyelitis, and emphysematous cystitis are described and illustrated in appropriate chapters. Other organs affected include gas gangrene of the uterus and emphysematous pancreatitis.

Fournier gangrene is the term applied to necrotizing fasciitis of the perineum, perianal and genital regions. Polymicrobial organisms cause rapid tissue destruction. Radiographs and CT show bubbles and streaks of gas in affected soft tissues (Fig. 40.20).

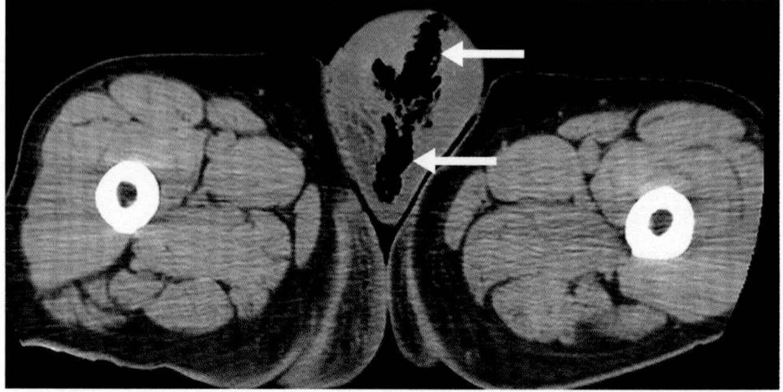

FIGURE 40.20. **Fournier Gangrene.** CT shows prominent pockets of gas (*arrows*) in the subcutaneous tissues of the perineum and scrotum characteristic of this condition.

SMALL BOWEL OBSTRUCTION

Small bowel obstruction accounts for 20% of surgical admissions for acute abdominal pain and 80% of all intestinal tract obstruction. The causes of small bowel obstruction are listed in Table 40.4. In the Western world, postsurgical adhesions account for 75% of small bowel obstruction, whereas in developing nations, 80% of small bowel obstructions are caused by incarcerated hernia, but only 10% are caused by adhesions. Patients present clinically with crampy abdominal pain, abdominal distention, and vomiting. Conventional radiographs are diagnostic in only 50% to 60% of cases. Findings of small bowel obstruction on conventional radiography are (a) dilated loops of small bowel (>3 cm) disproportionate to more distal small bowel or colon, (b) small bowel air–fluid levels that exceed 2.5 cm in width, (c) air–fluid levels at differing heights (>5 mm) within the same loop ("dynamic air–fluid levels") (strong evidence of obstruction) (Fig. 40.21), (d) two or more air–fluid levels, and (e) small bubbles of gas trapped between folds in dilated, fluid-filled loops producing the "string of pearls" sign, a row of small gas bubbles oriented horizontally or obliquely across the abdomen. The level of obstruction is determined by dilated loops above the obstruction and normal or empty loops below the obstruction. Stepladder or hairpin loops of small bowel are most characteristic. Inguinal hernias, easily overlooked clinically in the obese, may be evident on radiographs. CT has become the imaging method of choice to confirm small bowel obstruction and to identify its cause. CT reveals the cause of obstruction in 70% to 90% of cases. CT diagnosis is based upon demonstration of a transition site between small bowel loops dilated with fluid or air and collapsed bowel loops distal to the obstruction (Fig. 40.22). Sagittal and coronal reformations are invaluable in clearly demonstrating transition zones. A potential pitfall is the common finding of a collapsed descending colon even in patients with adynamic ileus. Bowel obstruction should not be diagnosed in this setting unless an obstructing lesion is visualized at the splenic flexure. The "small bowel feces" sign is a strong CT evidence of bowel obstruction. Particulate feculent matter mixed with gas bubbles is seen within dilated small bowel. Abrupt beak-like narrowing, without other lesion evident, is indicative of adhesions as the cause of obstruction. Other causes, including tumor, abscess, inflammation, hernia, and intussusception have characteristic findings.

TABLE 40.4

CAUSES OF SMALL BOWEL OBSTRUCTION

Adhesions Postsurgical Postinflammatory
Incarcerated hernia
Malignancy: usually metastatic
Intussusception
Volvulus
Gallstone ileus
Parasites: ascaris
Foreign body
Tumors of the small bowel
Crohn disease
Radiation enteritis

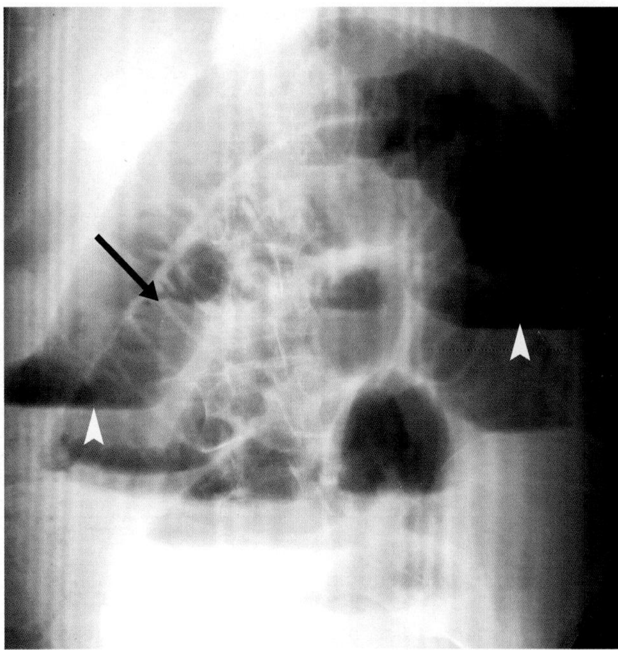

FIGURE 40.21. **Small Bowel Obstruction—Conventional Radiograph.** Erect radiograph of the abdomen reveals dilated air-filled loops of small bowel containing air–fluid levels at different heights within the same loop (*arrowheads*). Note the valvulae conniventes (*arrow*) that extend across the entire diameter of the bowel lumen. The small bowel obstruction was due to adhesions.

Strangulation obstruction is associated with changes in the bowel wall and mesentery due to impairment of blood supply. CT findings are (a) circumferential wall thickening (>3 mm), (b) edema of the bowel wall (target or halo appearance of lucency in the bowel wall), (c) lack of enhancement of the bowel wall (most specific sign), (d) haziness or obliteration of the mesenteric vessels, and (e) infiltration of the mesentery with fluid or hemorrhage. Because most cases are due to closed-loop obstruction, findings of that condition are commonly present as well.

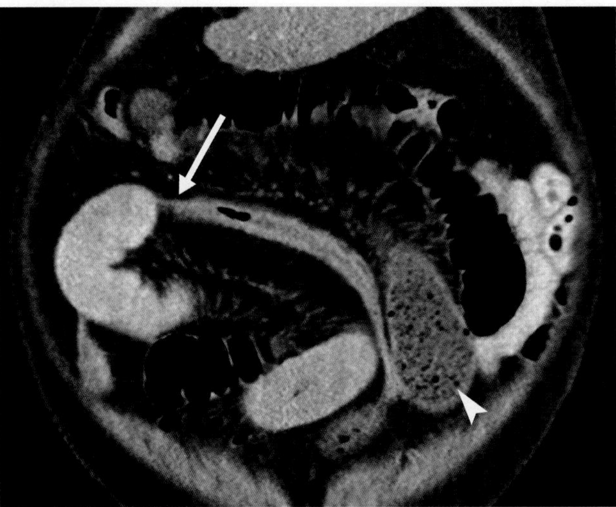

FIGURE 40.22. **Small Bowel Obstruction—CT.** Coronal plane reconstructed CT demonstrates abrupt transition (*arrow*) between dilated and nondilated small bowel in this patient with radiation enteritis causing small bowel obstruction. The small bowel feces sign (*arrowhead*) is also evident.

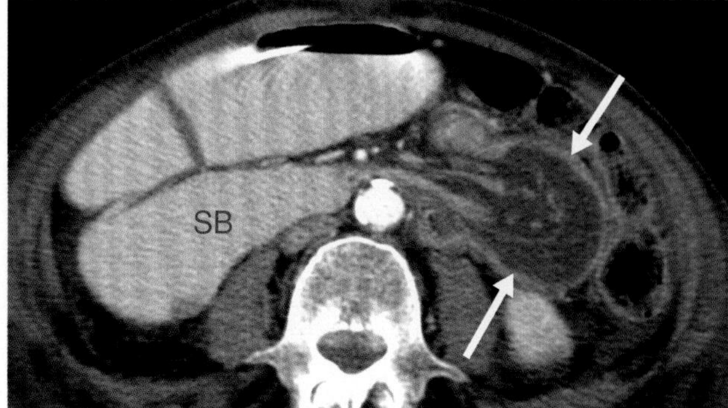

FIGURE 40.23. Enteroenteric Intussusception. CT shows small bowel obstruction with dilated proximal small bowel (*SB*) extending to an area of jejuno-jejunal intussusception (*arrows*). The lead point proved to a metastatic lesion from malignant melanoma to small bowel.

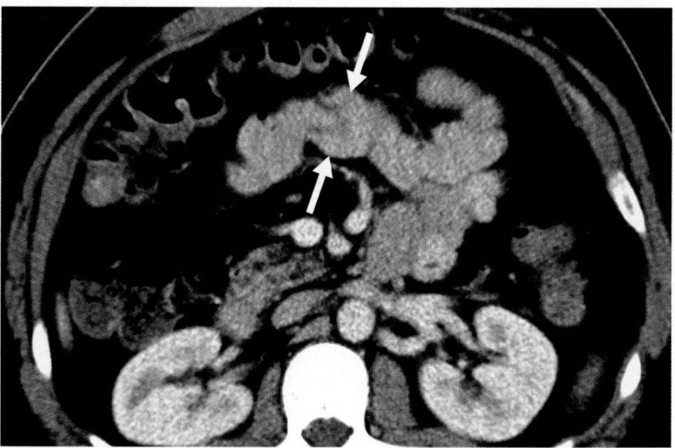

FIGURE 40.24. Transient Intussusception. CT in an asymptomatic patient studied for other reasons shows a short segment enteroenteric intussusception (*arrows*) without proximal small bowel dilatation.

Small bowel volvulus and closed-loop obstruction are indicated by these signs on CT: (a) radial distribution of dilated small bowel with mesenteric vessels converging toward a focus of torsion, (b) U- or C-shaped dilated small bowel loop, (c) "beak" sign at the site of torsion seen as fusiform tapering of a dilated bowel loop, (d) "whirl" sign of tightly twisted mesentery seen with volvulus. The presence of a whirl sign in a patient with small bowel obstruction correlates strongly with the need for surgery.

Intussusception is a major cause of small bowel obstruction in children, but is less common in adults. In adults, intussusception is often chronic, intermittent, or subacute, and is usually caused by a polypoid tumor, such as lipoma. Additional causes are malignant tumor, Meckel diverticulum, lymphoma, mesenteric nodes, and foreign bodies. Enteroenteric intussusception occurs with small bowel tumors and sprue. Ileocolic intussusception is usually idiopathic in children, but is caused by a mass in adults. Colocolic intussusception is common in adults but rare in children. Conventional radiographs demonstrate small bowel obstruction and a soft tissue mass. Barium studies demonstrate barium trapped between the intussusceptum and the receiving bowel forming a coiled spring appearance. CT is usually diagnostic, demonstrating a characteristic target-like intestinal mass (Fig. 40.23). On transverse section, the inner central density is the invaginating loop surrounded by fat-density mesentery that is enveloped by the receiving loop. US exhibits a similar "donut" configuration of alternating hyperechoic and hypoechoic rings representing alternating mucosa, muscular wall, and mesenteric fat tissues in cross-section. Asymptomatic, incidental, short segment (<3.5 cm), jejunal or ileal, *transient intussusception* without associated small bowel obstruction is a common and incidental finding on CT (Fig. 40.24).

Gallstone ileus is a cause of mechanical small bowel obstruction that should be suspected in any elderly female with small bowel obstruction. It is the cause of 24% of small bowel obstruction in patients over age 70. Because it is a disease of the elderly, insidious in onset, and difficult to diagnose, mortality is increased fivefold over mortality for small bowel obstruction due to adhesions. Bowel obstruction is caused by a large gallstone that erodes through the gallbladder wall and passes into the intestine, creating a cholecystoduodenal fistula. The gallstone most commonly lodges in the distal ileum. Causative gallstones are typically single, faceted, and 2 to 5 cm in size. Specific radiographic signs are present in only about half the patients. Rigler triad consists of (a) dilated small bowel loops (80% of cases), (b) air in the biliary tree or gallbladder (67%), and (c) calcified gallstone in an ectopic location (50%).

LARGE BOWEL OBSTRUCTION

Large bowel obstruction is predominantly a condition of older adults, accounting for about 20% of all bowel obstruction. The cecum dilates to the greatest extent, irrespective of the site of large bowel obstruction. When the cecum exceeds 10 cm in diameter, it is at high risk for perforation with attendant risks of peritonitis and septic shock. The common causes of large bowel dilatation and obstruction are listed in Table 40.5. Most colonic obstructions occur in the sigmoid colon where the bowel lumen is narrower and stool is more formed. Conventional radiographs are commonly diagnostic in large bowel obstruction, demonstrating dilation of the colon from the cecum to the point of obstruction. The colon distal to the obstruction is devoid of gas. When the ileocecal valve is competent, the small bowel usually contains little gas; the colon is unable to decompress into the small bowel and gaseous distention of the cecum is progressive. When the ileocecal valve is incompetent, gaseous distention of the small bowel is present; the colon can decompress into the ileum and jejunum, and risk of perforation of the cecum is reduced. Air–fluid levels distal to the hepatic flexure are strong evidence of obstruction unless the patient has had an enema.

Sigmoid volvulus is most common in the elderly and in individuals on high-residue diets. Sigmoid volvulus causes 3% to 8% of large bowel obstruction in adults and has a reported mortality of 20% to 25%. The sigmoid colon twists around its mesentery, resulting in a closed-loop obstruction. The proximal

TABLE 40.5

CAUSES OF LARGE BOWEL DILATATION

Obstruction:
Colon carcinoma (50–60%)
Metastatic disease, especially pelvic malignancies
Diverticulitis
Volvulus—cecal, sigmoid, transverse
Fecal impaction
Amebiasis
Ischemia
Adhesions
Pseudo-obstruction
Ogilvie syndrome
Adynamic ileus
Toxic megacolon

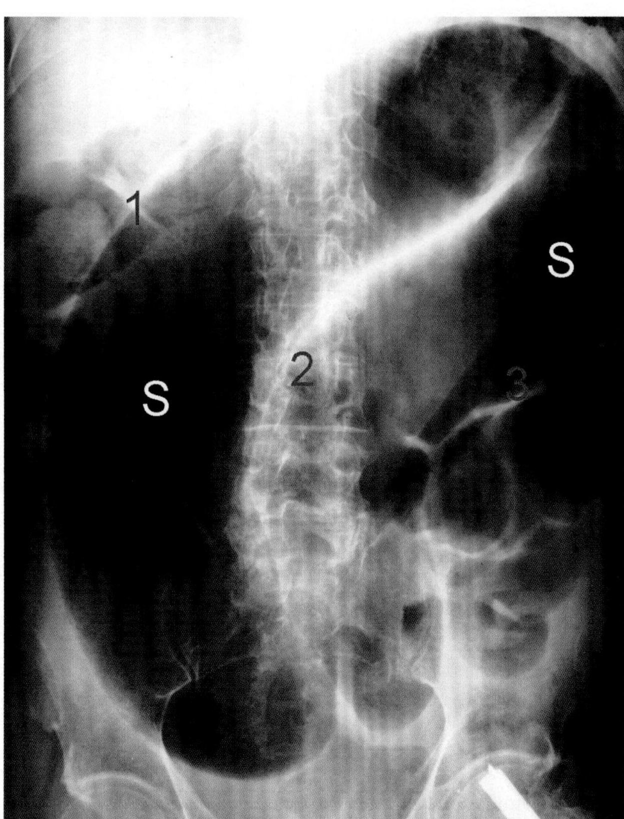

FIGURE 40.25. **Sigmoid Volvulus.** Radiograph of the abdomen demonstrates the characteristic massive dilation of the sigmoid colon (*S*) arising from the pelvis and extending to the left diaphragm. The three lines representing the walls of the twisted loop converging to the left lower quadrant are evident (*1, 2, 3*).

colon dilates while the rectum empties. Conventional radiographs are usually diagnostic. The sigmoid colon appears as a large gas-filled loop without haustral markings, arising from the pelvis and extending high into the abdomen and often to the diaphragm. The three lines formed by the lateral walls of the loop and the summation of the two opposed medial walls of the loop converge inferiorly into the left iliac fossa (Fig. 40.25). The apex of the distended sigmoid colon may extend cephalad to the transverse colon ("northern exposure sign"). Proximal colonic dilatation is present in half of the cases. Water-soluble enema demonstrates obstruction that tapers to a beak at the point of the twist, usually approximately 15 cm above the anal verge. Mucosal folds spiral into the beak at the point of obstruction. CT shows (a) an inverted, dilated, U-shaped sigmoid colon; (b) absence of gas in the rectum; (c) transition zones between dilated and collapsed bowel occur at the point of twisting; (d) oblique lines created by the orientation of the transition zones create the "x-marks the spot sign" appreciated on sequential images; and (e) a single beak-shaped transition point corresponding to the beak sign seen on enema. As a closed-loop obstruction the bowel is prone to ischemia and perforation, signs of which must be carefully sought.

Cecal volvulus causes 1% to 3% of large bowel obstruction in adults and occurs most frequently in the 30 to 60 age group. Cecal volvulus is a closed-loop obstruction that may result in ischemia, necrosis, and perforation. Three types of cecal volvulus are described. The most common type is the twist and invert with the cecum displaced to the left upper quadrant. An axial twist of the cecum about the long axis of the ascending colon results in the cecum remaining in the right lower quadrant. *Cecal bascule* refers to a folding of the cecum to a position anteromedial to the ascending colon, rather like folding the toe of a sock back on itself. Bascule accounts for about one-third of cases. Classic radiographic findings are (a) coffee bean–shaped loop of gas-distended bowel having haustral markings directed toward the left upper quadrant, (b) apex of the cecum in the left upper quadrant, (c) cecal distention greater than 10 cm in diameter (Fig. 40.26), and (d) collapse of the distal colon. Proximal small bowel dilatation may or may not be present. CT is increasingly used to confirm the diagnosis. Findings include the following: (a) cecum in the upper mid and left abdomen; (b) volvulus in the right lower quadrant seen as an area of swirling of the bowel and mesenteric fat ("whirl sign"); (c) appendix is displaced to the left upper quadrant; (d) two transition points are present, one for the entering loop and one for the exiting loop; (e) when the loops are completely wound around each other an "x-marks the spot" sign is present formed by the crossing configuration of the transition zones; (f) cecum is distended >10 cm; and (g) distal large bowel is decompressed. Images should be examined carefully for evidence of ischemia. A contrast enema demonstrates a beak- or fold-like termination at the point of obstruction in the ascending colon. Mortality rates of 20% to 40% are reported because of delays in diagnosis.

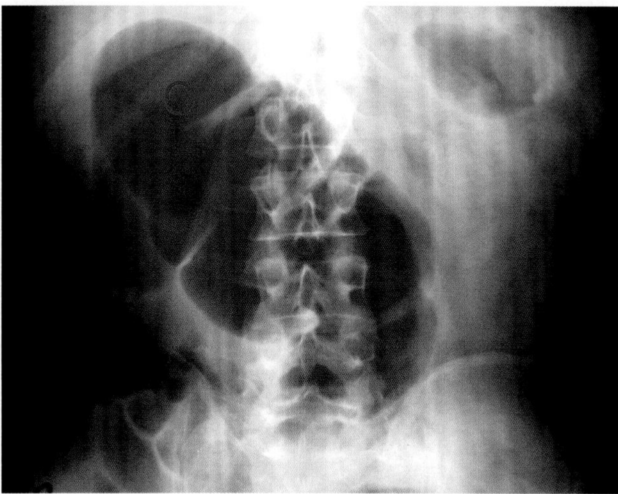

FIGURE 40.26. **Cecal Volvulus.** Supine abdominal radiograph demonstrates displacement of the dilated cecum (C) to the epigastrium. The more distal colon is collapsed. The diagnosis was confirmed at surgery.

Fecal impaction is the most common cause of large bowel obstruction in elderly and bedridden patients. Stercoral colitis is a rare inflammation of the wall of the colon caused by fecal impaction. Pressure on the colon wall may lead to ischemic necrosis and colon perforation. Radiographs demonstrate a large mass of stool having a characteristic mottled appearance in the distal colon. Following disimpaction, colonoscopy, or barium enema should be performed to search for an obstructing carcinoma that may have caused the fecal impaction.

Colonic pseudo-obstruction (Ogilvie syndrome) is a clinical disorder of acute colonic distention with abdominal pain and distention but without the presence of mechanical obstruction. Despite the absence of obstruction colonic distention may be progressive leading to ischemia, necrosis, and perforation. Pathophysiology is uncertain. Most current theories favor an imbalance in autonomic innervation of the colon. Conventional radiographs demonstrate dilatation of the colon most commonly from cecum to splenic flexure, occasionally to the rectum. CT demonstrates the same findings with additional evaluation for wall thickening associated with colitis or findings of colonic ischemia. The cecum dilates the most. Cecal dilatation >10 cm warrants colonic decompression by colonoscopy or tube cecostomy. Recurrent and chronic forms of the condition have been described.

BOWEL ISCHEMIA AND INFARCTION

Bowel ischemia, potentially leading to infarction, is a true emergency with high associated morbidity and mortality. Insufficient blood supply to small or large bowel may be transient and reversible or lethal. Causes include arterial occlusion of the mesenteric arteries by thrombus, embolus, volvulus, vasculitis, or external compression; hypotension related to congestive heart failure, sepsis, or blood loss; vasoconstrictive medications such as ergotamine, digitalis, or norepinephrine; and impaired venous drainage caused by venous thrombosis, tumor, adhesions, or volvulus. Ischemic injury starts at the mucosa and extends progressively through the bowel wall to the serosa. Contrast-enhanced MDCT is the imaging method of choice. Findings of bowel ischemia include (a) circumferential or nodular thickening (>5 mm) of the bowel wall with infiltration of low-density edema or high-density blood resulting from mucosal injury; (b) "thumbprinting" resulting from this nodular infiltration of the bowel wall; (c) dilatation of the bowel lumen (>3 cm for small bowel; >5 cm for colon; >8 cm for cecum); (d) pneumatosis intestinalis (see following paragraph); (e) edema or hemorrhage into the mesentery; (f) engorged mesenteric vessels; (g) thrombosis of mesenteric arteries or veins; (h) poor enhancement of the bowel wall along its mesenteric border which is evidence of ischemia; (i) poor or absent mucosal enhancement with thinning of the bowel wall, an evidence of bowel infarction; and (j) ascites which is commonly present.

Pneumatosis intestinalis refers to the presence of gas within the bowel wall. It may occur as a benign entity without clinical significance or may be an important finding of bowel ischemia. It is a radiographic sign, not a specific disease. Causes of pneumatosis intestinalis may be lumped into four categories: (1) bowel necrosis, usually associated with other radiographic and clinical signs of bowel ischemia; (2) mucosal disruption caused by ulcers, mucosal biopsies, trauma, enteric tubes, inflammatory bowel disease; (3) increased mucosal permeability related to immunosuppression in acquired immune deficiency syndrome (AIDS), organ transplantation, or chemotherapy; and (4) pulmonary disease resulting in alveolar disruption and dissection of air along interstitial pathways to the bowel wall. Causes of the latter include chronic obstructive pulmonary disease, asthma, cystic fibrosis, mechanical ventilation, and chest trauma. Interpretation of the imaging finding of pneumatosis must be correlated with the clinical condition of the patient. Pneumatosis in asymptomatic patients is very likely benign and incidental. Pneumatosis in seriously ill patients with abdominal pain or distention is more likely to be a sign of bowel ischemia. Pneumatosis appears on radiographs or CT as cystic air bubbles (few millimeters to several centimeters) or linear streaks of air within the bowel wall, especially in its most gravity-dependent aspect (Fig. 40.27). On CT air bubbles within the lumen may mimic pneumatosis but should always be seen adjacent to the nondependent bowel wall. Turning the patient and rescanning may clarify the diagnosis. Air may also be evident within mesenteric vessels or within portal veins in the liver.

ABDOMINAL TRAUMA

CT of the abdomen and pelvis is an integral part of the emergency evaluation of victims of blunt abdominal trauma. CT characterizes the precise nature of traumatic injury and is used to direct therapy, especially in patients with coexisting injuries, head trauma, or who have impaired consciousness due to injury, drugs, or alcohol. Candidates for CT are patients with a history of significant blunt trauma who are hemodynamically stable. Focused abdominal sonograms for trauma ("FAST" scans) may be used to detect the presence of intraperitoneal fluid to triage trauma patients for CT. CT findings of traumatic injury include the following: (a) hemoperitoneum—acute blood within the peritoneal cavity measuring 30 to 45 H (Fig. 40.28); (b) sentinel clot—a focal collection of clotted blood (>60 H) that may be seen in the peritoneal cavity adjacent to an injured organ (Fig. 40.28); (c) active bleeding evidenced by extravasated contrast (85 to 370 H) (Fig. 40.29)

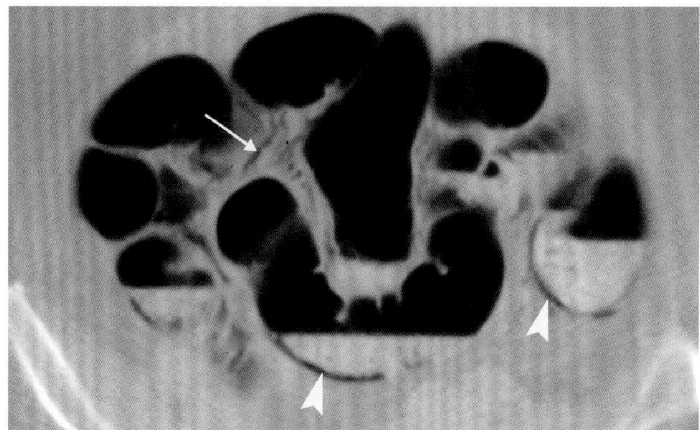

FIGURE 40.27. **Pneumatosis Intestinalis—Colon Infarction.** CT viewed with lung windows reveals air in the dependent wall (*arrowheads*) of the colon and air within mesenteric veins (*arrow*). This patient had a total infarction of the colon.

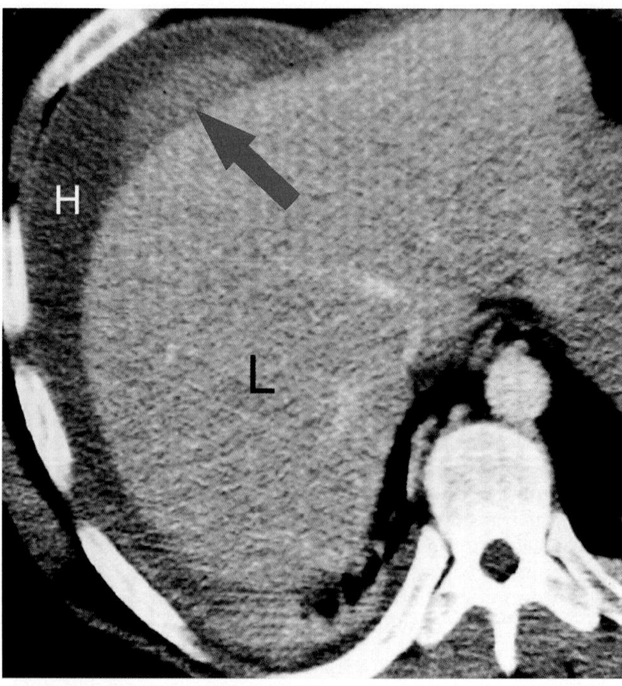

FIGURE 40.28. **Hemoperitoneum and Sentinel Clot.** CT scan shows high attenuation fluid in the peritoneal recesses indicating hemoperitoneum (*H*). A sentinel clot (*arrow*) stands out as a high attenuation collection within the lower attenuation liquid blood. The location of the clot suggests injury to the liver (*L*). A laceration of the left lobe of the liver, not evident on the CT, was found at surgery.

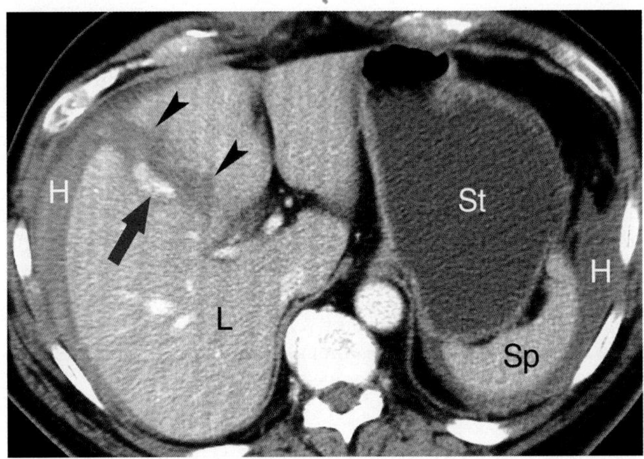

FIGURE 40.29. **Active Hemorrhage—Liver Laceration.** CT shows a jagged laceration (*arrowheads*) of the liver (*L*) filled with blood. A focus of continuing active hemorrhage (*arrow*) is seen as an ill-defined collection of high attenuation contrast agent. Hemoperitoneum (*H*) is evident in the peritoneal recesses. *Sp*, spleen; *St*, stomach.

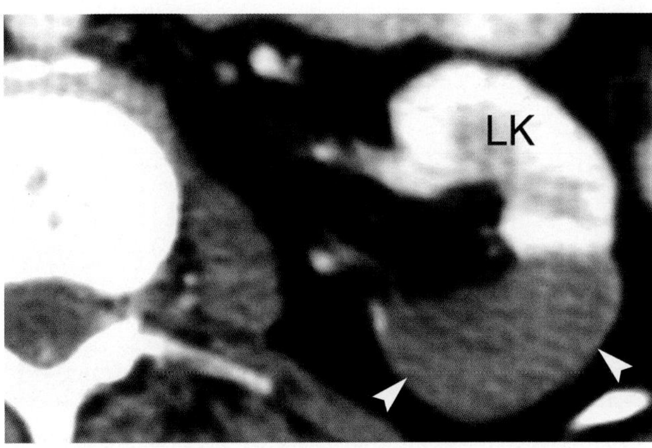

FIGURE 40.30. **Renal Infarction.** Postcontrast CT reveals a lack of enhancement (*arrowheads*) of the posterior portion of the left kidney (*LK*), which occurred as a result of an intimal tear and thrombosis of a branch renal artery occurring during a motor vehicle collision. Note the defect in enhancement extends to the capsule of the kidney indicating acute renal vascular injury.

seen during arterial phase of scanning with MDCT; (d) free air; (e) free contrast within the peritoneal cavity which may result from oral contrast leaking from injured bowel or intravenous contrast leaking from a ruptured bladder; (f) subcapsular hematomas appearing as crescent-shaped collections confined by the capsule of the injured organ; (g) intraparenchymal hematomas appearing as irregularly shaped low-density areas within a contrast-enhanced solid organ; (h) lacerations appearing as jagged linear defects (Fig. 40.29) defined by lower-density blood within a contrast-enhanced injured organ; (i) absence of organ enhancement reflecting damage to the organ's arterial supply; and (j) infarctions seen as zones of decreased contrast enhancement that extend to the capsule of a solid organ (Fig. 40.30).

LYMPHADENOPATHY

The abdomen and pelvis contain more than 230 lymph nodes that may be involved in a wide variety of neoplastic and inflammatory diseases. CT, US, and MR are effective at evaluation of the entire abdominopelvic lymphatic system. PET CT is increasingly utilized to demonstrate tumor involvement of a lymph node. Criteria for pathologic involvement are based primarily on alterations in node size (Table 40.6). Short-axis measurements of lymph node size are preferred to determine abnormal enlargement. Morphologic patterns of pathologic lymphadenopathy include single enlarged nodes, multiple separate lobulated enlarged nodes, or bulky conglomerate masses of lymph nodes (Fig. 40.31). Calcification in enlarged nodes may be seen with inflammatory adenopathy, mucinous carcinomas, sarcomas, and treated lymphoma. CT optimized to detect adenopathy includes contrast opacification of blood vessels and the gastrointestinal (GI) tract. Normal nodes are oblong in shape, homogeneous in configuration, and have short-axis diameters below the limits listed in Table 40.6. Most pathologically enlarged nodes have CT densities slightly less than skeletal muscle. Low-density nodal metastases are commonly seen with nonseminomatous testicular carcinoma, tuberculosis, and occasionally lymphoma. US is almost equal to CT in accuracy for detection of lymphadenopathy, however, a skillful dedicated examination is required. Lymphoma typically produces hypoechoic or even anechoic lymphadenopathy. Masses of retroperitoneal nodes may silhouette segments of the normally echogenic wall of the aorta (the "sonographic silhouette sign"). The "sandwich sign" refers to entrapment of

TABLE 40.6

ABDOMINAL AND PELVIS LYMPHADENOPATHY: UPPER LIMITS OF NORMAL NODE SIZE BY LOCATION

NODE LOCATION	MAXIMUM DIMENSION (mm)	COMMENTS
Retrocrural	6	May enlarge from disease above or below the diaphragm
Retroperitoneal	10	Multiple nodes 8–10 mm in size are usually abnormal
Gastrohepatic ligament	8	Must differentiate lymphadenopathy from coronary varices
Porta hepatis	6	May cause biliary obstruction
Celiac and superior mesenteric artery	10	Also called preaortic nodes
Pancreaticoduodenal	10	Commonly involved by lymphoma and GI carcinoma
Perisplenic	10	Involved by lymphoma and GI carcinoma
Mesenteric	10	In the small bowel mesentery
Pelvic	15	Most commonly involved by pelvic tumors

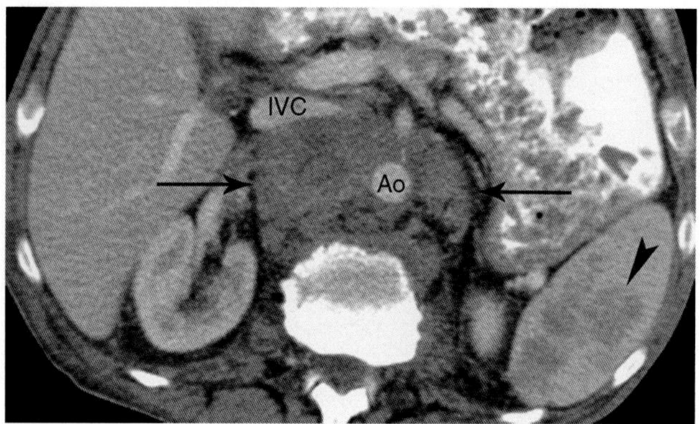

FIGURE 40.31. **Hodgkin Lymphoma.** CT shows bulky confluent adenopathy (*arrows*) in the retroperitoneum surrounding the aorta (*Ao*) and displacing the inferior vena cava (*IVC*) anteriorly. Masses of lymphoma (*arrowhead*) are also present in the spleen.

mesenteric vessels by masses of enlarged lymph nodes in the mesentery. MR usually provides excellent differentiation of lymph nodes from blood vessels because of flow void within vessels. On T1WI, lymph nodes show low signal intensity compared to surrounding fat. On T2WI, lymph nodes show high signal intensity compared to muscle. Fat-saturation technique highlights pathologic adenopathy on T2WI. PET CT has assumed a primary role in the imaging and staging of lymphomas sometimes identifying sites of extranodal disease even when CT shows no lesion.

Hodgkin lymphoma is responsible for 20% to 40% of all lymphoma and is characterized histologically by the presence of the Reed–Sternberg cell. Hodgkin lymphoma has a bimodal age distribution most commonly affecting patients aged 25 to 30 and over 50 years. At presentation, abdominal adenopathy is present in about 25% of cases. The spleen is involved in about 40% of cases and the liver in about 8%. Involvement of the GI tract and urinary tract is much less common with Hodgkin than with non-Hodgkin lymphoma.

Non-Hodgkin lymphoma is responsible for 60% to 80% of lymphoma. Non-Hodgkin lymphoma is a heterogeneous group of disorders with a confusing array of changing names and classifications. Disease severity ranges from indolent to very aggressive. Non-Hodgkin lymphomas are particularly common in immunocompromised patients. The non-Hodgkin lymphomas commonly involve extranodal sites. Solid organ involvement affects primarily the spleen, liver, pancreas, kidneys, adrenal glands, and testes. Manifestations include (a) solitary or multiple homogeneous well-defined nodules; (b) confluent masses; (c) mild uniform contrast enhancement of nodules and masses; (d) diffuse involvement producing only organomegaly; and (e) organ invasion from adjacent tissue. GI involvement includes (a) wall involvement deep to the mucosa that may be missed at endoscopy; (b) circumferential wall thickening; (c) luminal dilatation, narrowing, or cavitation; (d) nodules, polyps, and ulcers; and (e) impaired peristalsis. At presentation, abdominal adenopathy is present in about 50% of cases. The spleen is involved in about 40% of cases and the liver in about 14%.

Posttransplantation lymphoproliferative disorder ("PTLD") is a spectrum of lymphoid hyperplasias and neoplasias in patients who have received solid organ transplants and immunosuppressive therapy. Up to 20% of transplant recipients may be affected. The disorder results from an Epstein–Barr virus-induced proliferation of B lymphocytes that is usually opposed by functioning T cells. However, T-cell function is limited by the immunosuppressive therapy of transplantation. The proliferation ranges from polyclonal, benign, and reversible to aggressive and difficult-to-treat monoclonal lymphoma. Extranodal involvement in solid organs with discrete solitary, multiple, or infiltrative masses is most common. GI involvement is similar to that seen with non-Hodgkin lymphoma and includes wall thickening, luminal narrowing, eccentric extraluminal mass, luminal ulceration, and stranding in the mesentery. Lymph node enlargement occurs near the transplanted organ but may also occur at remote sites, that is, in the abdomen but associated with a heart or lung transplant. CT may reveal lymphadenopathy before the patient becomes symptomatic. Treatment is reduction of immunosuppressive therapy.

ABDOMINOPELVIC TUMORS AND MASSES

Peritoneal mesothelioma is an uncommon primary tumor of the peritoneal membrane. One-third of all mesotheliomas arise from the peritoneum with most of the remainder arising from the pleura. All are closely associated with asbestos exposure. CT demonstrates nodular, irregular peritoneal and omental thickening and masses, which merge to large plaques and cake-like thickening of the omentum, "omental cake." Adjacent bowel may be invaded and become fixed. US demonstrates the sheet-like superficial masses. Rare multilocular cystic forms of the tumor also occur. Prognosis is poor although has improved with cytoreductive surgery and hyperthermic intraperitoneal chemotherapy (HIPEC).

Peritoneal metastases are most commonly associated with ovarian, colon, stomach, or pancreas carcinoma. The preferential sites for tumor implantation are the pelvic cul-de-sac, right paracolic gutter, and the greater omentum. CT demonstrates tumor nodules on peritoneal surfaces; "omental cake" (Fig. 40.32), which displaces bowel away from the anterior abdominal wall; tumor nodules in the mesentery; thickening and nodularity of the bowel wall due to serosal implants; and ascites that is commonly loculated. US may directly visualize the peritoneal tumors, and demonstrates secondary signs of malignant ascites including echogenic debris in the fluid, septation, and matted bowel loops.

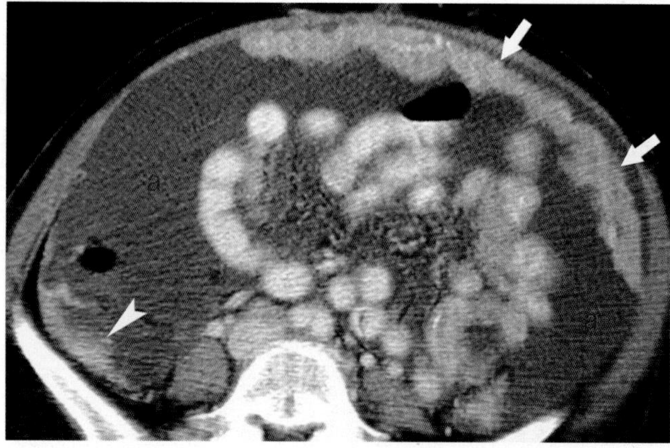

FIGURE 40.32. **Peritoneal Metastases.** A CT scan demonstrates intraperitoneal spread of ovarian carcinoma. The tumor is implanted on the omentum (*arrows*), causing the appearance of "omental cake" as the thickened omentum floats in ascites (*a*) between bowel loops and the abdominal wall. Nodules of tumor (*arrowhead*) are implanted on the peritoneal surface.

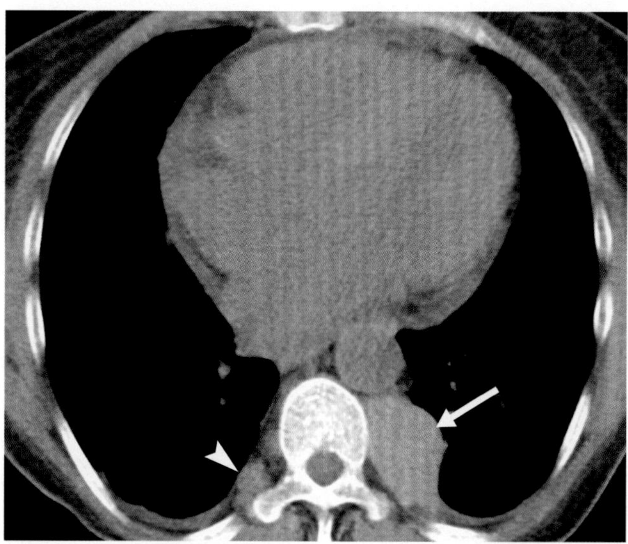

FIGURE 40.33. **Extramedullary Hematopoiesis.** CT without contrast shows a slightly high attenuation left paraspinal mass (*arrow*) and a smaller right paraspinal mass (*arrowhead*). Cardiomegaly is evident. The patient also had massive hepatosplenomegaly. Extramedullary hematopoiesis was induced by sickle cell disease.

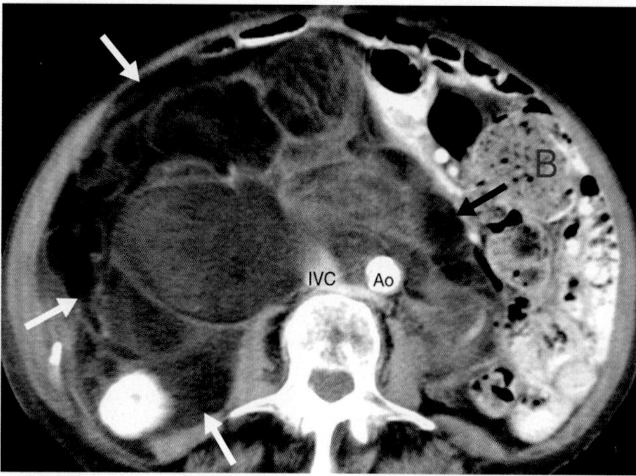

FIGURE 40.34. **Liposarcoma.** CT shows a large liposarcoma (*arrows*) that arose in the retroperitoneum as a mottled fat-density mass that distorts the inferior vena cava (*IVC*), surrounds the aorta (*Ao*), and displaces small and large bowel (*B*) laterally.

Extramedullary hematopoiesis occurs when the primary sites of hematopoiesis in the bone marrow fail as a result of myelofibrosis or when hemolytic anemias overwhelm blood cell production (sickle cell disease and thalassemia). The most obvious manifestations are homogeneous, well-marginated paraspinal masses that favor the thoracic spine (Fig. 40.33). They are bilateral, relatively symmetric and enhance mildly, and homogeneously postcontrast. Diffuse involvement of the liver and spleen may cause massive hepatosplenomegaly without affecting organ function. It rarely causes a presacral mass mimicking a chordoma.

Lymphangiomas are benign cystic lesions that arise from lymphatic vascular channels. The cystic mass contains septations and multiple loculations containing chylous, serous, hemorrhagic, or mixed fluid. Lesions occur in the omentum, mesentery, mesocolon, and retroperitoneum. CT shows a fluid-density mass with enhancing wall and septa. US shows better the multilocular nature of the mass. Fluid contains echogenic debris. MR shows low signal on T1WI and high signal on T2WI for serous lymphangiomas. Those complicated by infection or hemorrhage are high signal on T1WI.

Primary retroperitoneal neoplasms arise in the retroperitoneal tissues outside of the retroperitoneal organs. Many tumors grow to large size before discovery. Tumors displace and compress abdominal and pelvic organs. Benign lipomas rarely arise in the retroperitoneum. Other tumors that contain distinct fat density may be liposarcomas (Fig. 40.34), the most common sarcoma of the retroperitoneum, or teratomas. Other fat-containing mass lesions include adrenal myelolipoma, angiomyolipoma, omental infarction, and mesenteric panniculitis. Cystic tumors that enhance minimally are likely lymphangiomas. Other considerations include neurogenic tumors such as schwannomas, neurofibromas, and ganglioneuromas; lymphoma; desmoid tumors; and malignant mesenchymomas.

Retroperitoneal fibrosis is a rare condition manifest by formation of a fibrous plaque in the lower retroperitoneum that encases and compresses the aorta, inferior vena cava, and ureters. Two-thirds of cases are idiopathic. Methysergide, an ergot prescribed for migraine headache, is a cause of 12% of cases. Small foci of metastatic malignancy that elicit a fibrotic reaction in the retroperitoneum account for another 8% to 10%. Inflammatory aneurysms, which induce a rind of perianeurysmal fibrosis, are responsible for 5% to 10% of cases. Other possible causes include tuberculosis, syphilis, actinomycosis, and fungi. About 15% of patients have additional fibrosing processes including mediastinal fibrosis, Riedel fibrosing thyroiditis, sclerosing cholangitis, and fibrotic orbital pseudotumors. The fibrotic plaque is usually located over the anterior surfaces of the L4 and L5 vertebrae. In the early stages the plaque is highly cellular and edematous; when mature, it consists of dense hyalinized collagen with few cells. Cases induced by malignancy have a few malignant cells scattered within the collagen. The hallmark of retroperitoneal fibrosis is smooth extrinsic narrowing of one or both ureters in the region of L4–5. Proximal hydronephrosis results from impairment of ureteral peristalsis. The process may extend into the pelvis and cause a teardrop configuration to the bladder and narrowing of the sigmoid colon. CT demonstrates a fibrous plaque (Fig. 40.35)

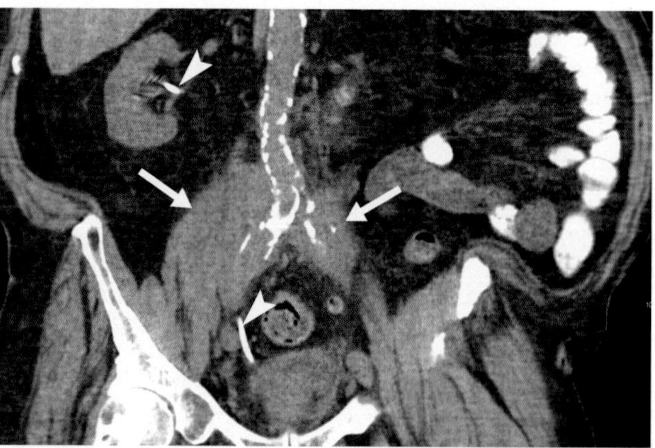

FIGURE 40.35. **Retroperitoneal Fibrosis.** Coronal plane reconstructed CT performed without intravenous contrast shows poorly marginated soft tissue (*arrows*) encasing the distal aorta and common iliac vessels. The right ureter was enveloped and obstructed by the fibrosing process. A ureteral stent (*arrowheads*) is in place. The left kidney is absent.

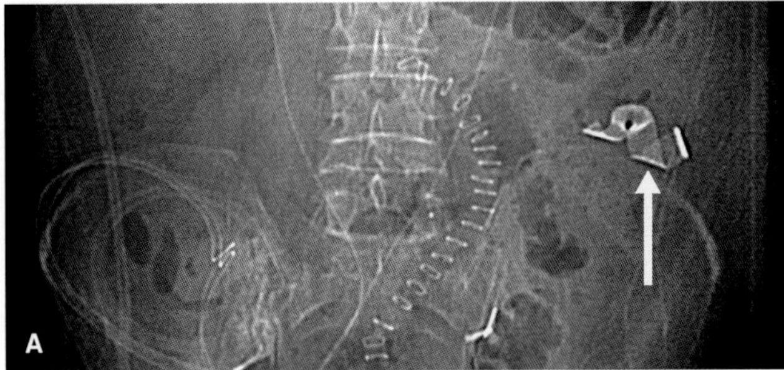

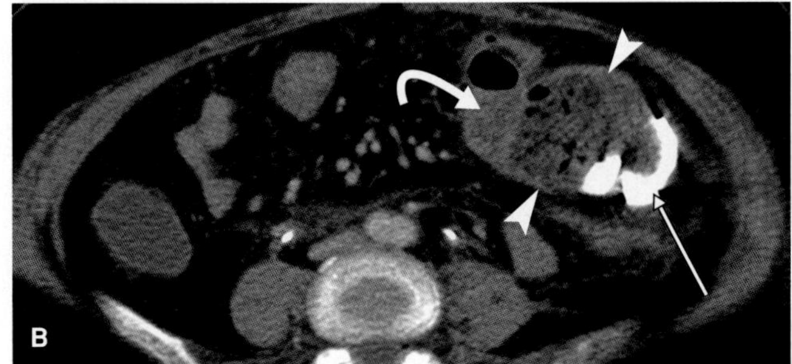

FIGURE 40.36. **Retained Surgical Sponge.** **A:** Digital radiograph of the abdomen taken at bedside reveals the characteristic radiopaque tape (*arrow*) that marks a surgical sponge inadvertently left within the abdominal cavity. Metallic cutaneous staples identify the patient as having had recent surgery. **B:** CT reveals the difficulty of identifying the surgical sponge if the radiopaque marker (*straight arrow*) was not present. The sponge (between *arrowheads*) contains fluid, blood, and air bubbles producing a pattern very similar to stool in the colon. The descending colon (*curved arrow*) is displaced medially.

that envelops the vena cava, aorta, and often the ureters. The plaque may be midline or asymmetric, well or poorly defined, localized or expansive. On MR the plaque is typically of low signal intensity on both T1WI and T2WI. Plaque that shows high signal intensity on T2WI should be considered suspicious for malignancy as a cause, although early edematous plaques may have the same appearance. On US, retroperitoneal fibrosis is easily confused with lymphoma. Both appear as confluent hypoechoic masses encasing the cava and aorta. Typically, lymphoma extends behind the vessels and displaces them anteriorly, but retroperitoneal fibrosis does not.

Foreign bodies may be ingested or inserted, enter the abdomen or pelvis as a result of penetrating trauma, or be left behind at surgery. Recognition is important to avoid complications, which include hemorrhage, abscess formation, septicemia, bowel perforation or obstruction, or embolization. Many orally ingested foreign bodies are radiopaque, such as coins, pins, and parts of toys. Most will pass through the intestinal tract causing only minimal mucosal damage. Large or elongated pointed objects may impinge at flexures or narrowed areas of the GI tract such as the pylorus, duodenojejunal junction, ileocecal valve, or appendix. Button batteries such as those used in watches and hearing aids contain highly toxic substances that can erode or perforate the bowel, or cause heavy metal poisoning if the battery ruptures. These should be followed to ensure they pass entirely through the bowel. Endoscopic or surgical removal should be considered if they fail to progress. Objects inserted into the vagina, rectum, or urethra can be removed manually or endoscopically. Retained bullets and shotgun pellets may lead to abscess formation or lead intoxication. CT is utilized to determine their exact position, complications, and the difficulty of removal. Wooden foreign bodies are usually not visualized on conventional radiographs. CT shows high attenuation of the wooden object. US demonstrates high echogenicity with acoustic shadowing. MR shows wood to have variable intensity usually less than that of skeletal muscle on T1WI and T2WI. Retained surgical sponges (*gossypiboma*) are a rare but dreaded complication of surgery. Retained sponges may be asymptomatic, cause an abscess, or generate a granulomatous response inducing fibrosis and calcification. Sponges are usually detectable because of an incorporated tape- or string-like radiopaque marker (Fig. 40.36). CT shows a soft tissue density mass, frequently containing air bubbles.

Radiologists should be familiar with an ever-expanding number of medical devices that appear in images of the abdomen and pelvis including intestinal tubes, postoperative apparatus, genitourinary devices, and monitoring instruments and attachments.

Abscesses occur within the peritoneal cavity because of spillage of contaminated material from perforated bowel or as a complication of surgery, trauma, pancreatitis, sepsis, or AIDS. Development of an abscess is commonly insidious, and the clinical presentation is often nonspecific and confusing. The pelvis is the most common site for abscess formation. Radiographic findings include soft tissue mass, collection of extraluminal gas, displacement of bowel, localized or generalized ileus, elevation of the diaphragm, pleural effusion, and atelectasis or consolidation at the lung bases. A focal collection of extraluminal gas is the most specific sign of abscess but is uncommon. CT shows a loculated fluid collection often with internal debris and fluid–fluid levels. The walls of the fluid collection are often thick and irregular. Gas within the fluid collection is strong evidence of abscess (Fig. 40.37). Fascia adjacent to the abscess is thickened, and fat surrounding the abscess may be increased in density and contain soft tissue strands due to inflammation. US demonstrates a focal fluid collection often containing echogenic fluid, floating debris, and septations. However, completely anechoic fluid collections may also be infected. A thickened wall is usually evident. Gas within the fluid collection is evidenced by echogenic foci producing comet-tail or reverberation artifacts. CT- or US-guided needle aspiration confirms the diagnosis, provides material for culture, and offers the opportunity for percutaneous catheter drainage.

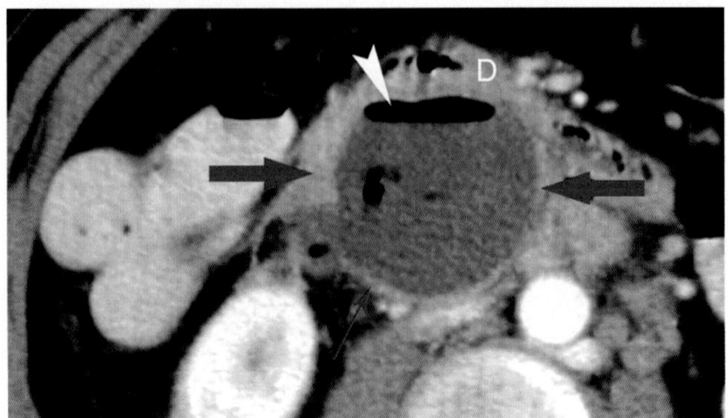

FIGURE 40.37. **Abscess.** CT reveals an abscess (between *fat arrows*) in the retroperitoneum. The abscess contains fluid and gas (*arrowhead*). Note the discrete enhancing wall (*skinny arrow*) of the abscess. Duodenum (*D*) containing intraluminal gas is displaced anteriorly and is draped over the collection.

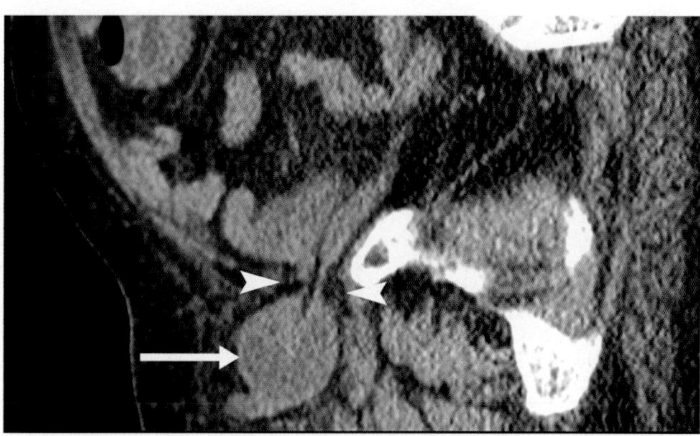

FIGURE 40.38. **Incarcerated Inguinal Hernia.** In a patient with acute right pelvic pain, a sagittal plane reconstructed CT shows a loop of small bowel (*arrow*) extending into the inguinal canal (between *arrowheads*). The bowel contained within the hernia is swollen and edematous with thickened bowel walls, signs of incarceration that were confirmed at surgery.

HERNIAS OF THE ABDOMINAL WALL

A hernia of the abdominal wall is a protrusion of bowel, omentum, or mesentery through a defect in the wall of the abdomen or pelvis. While many are diagnosed clinically by physical examination, imaging is used to identify hernias when they are not palpable or clinically suspected. *Incarceration* refers to hernias that are not reducible. *Strangulation* refers to hernias associated with bowel obstruction and bowel ischemia. *Richter hernias* entrap only a portion of the bowel wall without compromising viability. *Inguinal hernias* are most common in children and adults. Indirect inguinal hernias extend through the internal inguinal ring into the inguinal canal lateral to the inferior epigastric vessels. Direct inguinal hernias occur medial to the inferior epigastric vessels directly into the inguinal canal through a weakness in its floor (Fig. 40.38). *Incisional hernias* are complications of surgery with herniation through the surgical incision. *Parastomal hernias* occur in association with surgically created stomas. *Lumbar hernias* occur through defects in the lumbar musculature posterolaterally below the 12th rib and above the iliac crest. *Spigelian hernias* occur in the lower abdominal wall lateral to the rectus abdominis and inferior to the umbilicus through a defect in the aponeurosis of the transversus abdominia and internal oblique muscles.

HIV AND AIDS IN THE ABDOMEN

AIDS is caused by infection with human immunodeficiency virus (HIV), a member of the Lentivirus subgroup of retroviruses. Rapid and accurate testing for HIV now identifies most patients with HIV infection prior to their developing the clinical manifestations of AIDS. Antiretroviral treatment (ART) delays progression to AIDS and death from infection. HIV binds to CD4 lymphocytes and monocytes, enters the cells, replicates to produce viral DNA, and incorporates into host DNA to allow further replication and involvement of more host cells. HIV transmission is primarily through sexual contact. Worldwide more heterosexual men and women are now infected than homosexual men. Transmission of infection by blood products now occurs almost exclusively in intravenous drug users. Children may be infected perinatally. Progression from HIV infection to AIDS generally requires 8 to 10 years in nontreated patients. Death occurs 1 to 2 years after diagnosis of AIDS. AIDS remains a worldwide epidemic with 35 million dead and 70 million infected. Although HIV infection is not curable, patients on ART have now lived for decades with the disease and without progression to AIDS. UNAIDS/WHO estimates indicate that more than 18 million people were receiving ART in mid-2016.

Primary infection with HIV causes only minor symptoms which may resemble infectious mononucleosis, or other viral syndrome, with fevers, myalgias, transient adenopathy, and skin rash. This is the stage of active viral replication and dissemination. With development of the immune response, usually within 3 months, virus levels dramatically decrease and the patient enters a clinically "silent" period. However, the CD4 receptor–coated T lymphocytes, which are primarily responsible for cell-mediated immunity, gradually but progressively, decrease in number in the peripheral blood. Immune system activation is impaired. A CD4+ T-cell count below 200 cells/mm^3 (normal = 800 to 1,000 cells/mm^3) is diagnostic of AIDS.

AIDS is characterized by multiple opportunistic infections and aggressive malignancies, most commonly Kaposi sarcoma (KS) and AIDS-related lymphoma. Infection by multiple organisms at multiple sites is the rule. AIDS in the abdomen is characterized by multiple coexisting diseases with multicentric involvement. Up to 90% of patients with AIDS develop complaints related to the GI or hepatobiliary systems. Genitourinary tract disease affects 38% to 68% of AIDS patients. Manifestations of infectious and neoplastic processes in AIDS patients are effectively demonstrated by abdominal imaging techniques. Patients with abdominal disease and AIDS may present with dysphagia, abdominal pain, diarrhea, fever, or progressive weight loss with muscle wasting. CT and US are the most useful modalities for evaluating the solid visceral organs, adenopathy, and the peritoneal cavity.

Opportunistic infections are caused by organisms that are usually effectively controlled by normal cellular immunity. *Pneumocystis jiroveci pneumonia* (PJP), formerly known as *Pneumocystis carinii pneumonia* (PCP), is the most common opportunistic infection in persons with HIV infection. Extrapulmonary *Pneumocystis* infection affects the liver, spleen, kidney, pancreas, and lymph nodes. *Mycobacterium avium-intracellulare* and *M. tuberculosis* are also frequent infections. Atypical mycobacterium is a cause of bulky abdominal adenopathy, hepatosplenomegaly, and focal lesions in the liver and spleen. *Candida albicans* and cytomegalovirus are common causes of esophagitis as well as gastric antritis and duodenitis. *Cryptosporidium* and *Isospora belli* are protozoans, previously found only in animals that infect the GI tract and cause severe diarrhea. *Cryptosporidium* and cytomegalovirus are causes of AIDS-related cholangitis. Herpes virus, *Toxoplasma gondii, Entamoeba histolytica, Giardia lamblia,* and *Cryptococcus neoformans* are additional pathogens in AIDS patients.

Kaposi sarcoma occurs as the most common malignancy associated with AIDS and may also occur in organ transplant patients. Classic KS and endemic African KS are primarily diseases of the skin diagnosed and treated on a clinical nonimaging basis. AIDS and organ transplant–related KS frequently disseminate, have internal manifestations, and are staged by imaging. The typical lesion is a vascular nodule on the skin or mucous membranes, in the GI tract, or in any solid visceral organ. The tumor is always multicentric and arises from lymphatic epithelium found in all organs and tissues. Most common organs involved are lymph nodes, lung, GI tract, liver, and spleen. Most patients with internal involvement have multiple lesions on the skin. Lymphadenopathy is a common feature. In the GI tract KS causes nodules, plaques, polypoid lesions, and thickened folds. Multiple nodules are seen in the liver and spleen. The skeletal system may be involved usually by direct extension of tumor from the skin.

AIDS-related lymphomas are extremely aggressive neoplasms that respond poorly to therapy and commonly involve extranodal sites. Median survival is only 5 to 6 months. Extranodal involvement is found at presentation in most patients, with the most common locations being the central nervous system (27%), bone marrow (22%), GI tract (17% to 54%), liver (12% to 29%), kidney (11%), and spleen (7%). Focal hepatic lesions are hypodense on postcontrast CT and vary from innumerable small lesions (<1 cm in size) to large solitary masses up to 15 cm in diameter. Hepatosplenomegaly is minimal or absent unless focal lesions are present. Spleen and renal lesions appear as hypodense nodules 1 to 3 cm in diameter. Evidence of GI tract involvement includes focal or diffuse wall thickening, which is often striking, and eccentric homogeneous masses. Rectal and perianal involvement is particularly common. Retroperitoneal or mesenteric lymph node enlargement is seen in only 64% of patients. Lymphoma may be the initial AIDS-defining illness.

Suggested Readings

Brant WE. Abdominal trauma. In: Webb WR, Brant WE, Major NM, eds. *Fundamentals of Body CT*. 4th ed. Philadelphia, PA: Saunders Elsevier; 2015:175–187.

Caiafa RO, Vinuesa AS, Izquierdo RS, Brufau BP, Ayuso Colella JR, Molina CN. Retroperitoneal fibrosis: role of imaging in diagnosis and follow-up. *Radiographics* 2013;33:535–552.

Chen MY, Bechtold RE, Bohrer SP, Dyer RB. Abdominal calcification on plain radiographs of the abdomen. *Radiologist* 1999;7:65–83.

Childers BC, Cater SW, Horton KM, Fishman EK, Johnson PT. CT evaluation of acute enteritis and colitis: is it infectious, inflammatory, or ischemic? *Radiographics* 2015;35:1940–1941.

Craig WD, Fanburg-Smith JC, Henry LR, Guerrero R, Barton JH. Fat-containing lesions of the retroperitoneum: radiologic-pathologic correlation. *Radiographics* 2009;29:261–290.

Fernandes T, Oliveira MI, Castro R, Araújo B, Viamonte B, Cunha R. Bowel wall thickening at CT: simplifying the diagnosis. *Insights Imaging* 2014;5:195–208. (Pictorial review).

Jaffe T, Thompson WM. Large-bowel obstruction in the adults: classic radiographic and CT findings, etiology, and mimics. *Radiology* 2015;275: 651–663.

Keraliya AR, Tirumani SH, Shinagare AB, Ramaiya NH. Beyond PET/CT in Hodgkin lymphoma: a comprehensive review of the role of imaging at initial presentation, during follow-up and for assessment of treatment-related complications. *Insights Imaging* 2015;6:381–392.

Meyers MA, Charnsangavj C, Oliphant M. *Meyers' Dynamic Radiology of the Abdomen: Normal and Pathologic Anatomy*. 6th ed. Secaucus, NJ: Springer; 2011.

Paulson EK, Thompson WM. Review of small-bowel obstruction: the diagnosis and when to worry. *Radiology* 2015;275:332–342.

Peterson CM, Anderson JS, Hara AK, Carenza JW, Menias CO. Volvulus of the gastrointestinal tract: appearances at multimodality imaging. *Radiographics* 2009;29:1281–1293.

Stavros AT, Rapp C. Dynamic ultrasound of hernias of the groin and anterior abdominal wall. *Ultrasound Quarterly* 2010;26:135–169.

Vilaça AF, Reis AM, Vidal IM. The anatomic compartments and their connections as demonstrated by ectopic air. *Insight Imaging* 2013;4: 759–772.

CHAPTER 41 ■ LIVER, BILIARY TREE, AND GALLBLADDER

WILLIAM E. BRANT AND JENNIFER POHL

LIVER

Imaging Methods. CT, MR, and US produce high-quality diagnostic images of the liver parenchyma. Dynamic bolus contrast-enhanced multidetector computed tomography (MDCT) is the current method of choice for most hepatic imaging. Fast imaging techniques that control motion have increased the role of MR as a problem solver and often as the primary hepatic imaging modality. US is used as a screening method for patients with abdominal symptoms and suspected diffuse or focal liver disease. Color flow and spectral Doppler are used to assess hepatic vessels and tumor vascularity. Radionuclide imaging is used in the characterization of cavernous hemangiomas and focal nodular hyperplasia (FNH).

MDCT of the liver is performed using a three- or four-phase protocol of multiple scans of the entire liver. Initial noncontrast images are followed by rapid bolus intravenous contrast injection by a mechanical injector. Immediate images are optimally obtained during peak hepatic arterial enhancement phase to detect hypervascular tumors and other lesions supplied primarily by the hepatic artery. Arterial phase enhancing lesions, like hepatocellular carcinoma (HCC), are high attenuation on a background of lower attenuation, minimally enhanced, parenchyma. Maximum enhancement of the liver parenchyma is attained during portal venous phase to demonstrate hypovascular lesions as low attenuation masses on a background of brightly enhanced parenchyma. Because about two-thirds of the hepatic blood supply comes from the portal vein, maximum enhancement of the liver parenchyma occurs at 60 to 120 seconds following hepatic arterial enhancement allowing time for contrast to past through the spleen and gastrointestinal tract into the portal veins. Further delayed images are obtained several minutes after contrast injection to document "washout" of HCC, late contrast fill-in of hemangioma and delayed enhancement of cholangiocarcinoma.

Hepatic MR imaging is performed with a broad array of fast spin-echo, breath-hold gradient recall, short-time inversion-recovery, fat-suppressed, in-phase/out-of-phase, and diffusion-weighted pulse sequences. The goal is to maximize lesion detection by using the striking contrast resolution of MR while minimizing motion artifact by rapid scan breath-hold sequences. Dynamic contrast enhancement is achieved with MR by repeating full liver scans multiple times in the first minutes following gadolinium injection. Two major classes of gadolinium-based contrast agents are in use. Extracellular agents, such as gadopentetate dimeglumine (Magnevist®), are akin to iodine-based contrast agents used in CT. Liver-specific contrast agents such as gadoxetate disodium (Eovist®) have conventional properties of the extracellular agents as well as being taken up by hepatocytes, which improves detection and characterization of small lesions. Diffusion-weighted MR has emerged as a method of hepatic lesion detection and characterization in patients who cannot receive intravenous contrast. MR spectroscopy is used for quantitation of liver fatty infiltration and other diffuse hepatic diseases. MR and US elastography are used to assess for liver fibrosis.

US is used as a rapid screening modality to detect diseases of the liver, biliary tree, and gallbladder. Contrast-enhanced US is used to characterize liver lesions. Hepatic US imaging is reviewed in Chapter 50.

Radionuclide imaging of the liver is inferior to CT, MR, or US for lesion detection but offers functional information in characterizing lesions such as FNH. Radionuclide blood pool imaging is very useful for definitive diagnosis of cavernous hemangioma. Hepatic radionuclide imaging is reviewed in Chapter 72A.

Fine-needle aspiration for cytology or core needle biopsy for histology, guided by US or CT, is the popular and safe method to obtain tissue diagnoses.

Anatomy

Surgical Liver Segments. The vascular anatomy that defines the surgical approach to lesion resection is the anatomy most relevant to liver imaging. A numbering system developed by Couinaud (pronounced "kwee-NO") is commonly used internationally and provides standardized identification of hepatic segments (Fig. 41.1; Table 41.1). The International Hepato-Pancreato-Biliary Association (IHPBA) (Brisbane 2000

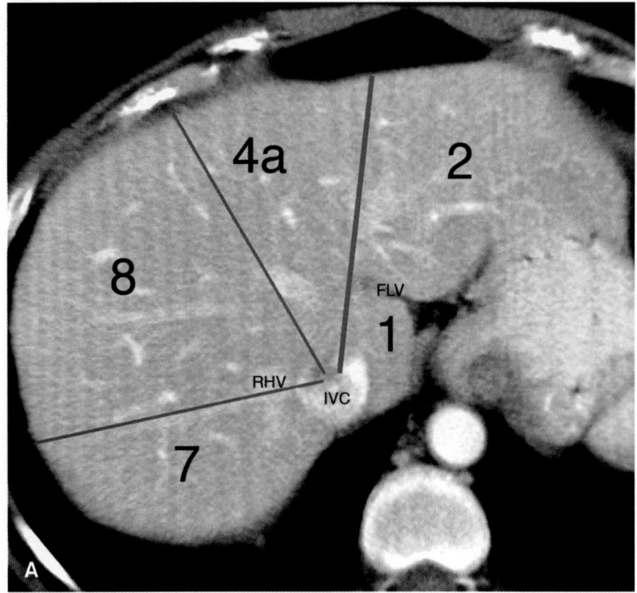

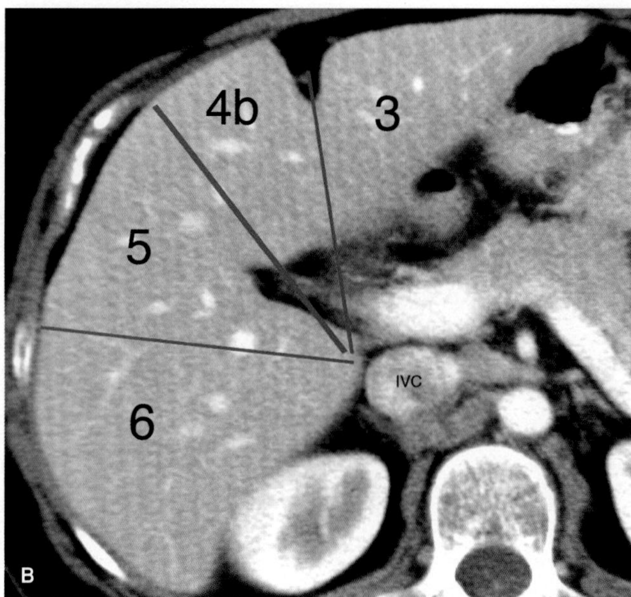

FIGURE 41.1. **Couinaud Liver Segments. A:** Superior portion of the liver. **B:** Inferior portion of the liver. CT scans illustrate the Couinaud classification of numbering of liver segments. The longitudinal plane of the right hepatic vein (*RHV*) divides *8* from *7* in the superior portion of the liver and *5* from *6* in the inferior portion of the liver. The longitudinal plane of the middle hepatic vein through the gallbladder fossa separates *4a* from *8* in the superior liver and *4b* from *5* in the inferior liver. The longitudinal plane of the left hepatic vein and fissure of the ligamentum teres separate *4a* from *2* in the superior liver and *4b* from *3* in the inferior liver. The axial plane of the left portal vein separates *4a* superiorly from *4b* inferiorly and *2* superiorly from *3* inferiorly in the left lobe. The axial plane of the right portal vein separates *8* and *7* superiorly from *5* and *6* inferiorly in the right lobe. The caudate lobe (*segment 1*) extends between the fissure of the ligamentum venosum (*FLV*) anteriorly and the inferior vena cava (*IVC*) posteriorly.

conference) adopted this segment terminology for liver resections. The 8 segments have separate vascular inflow, outflow, and biliary drainage and can each be resected without damaging the remaining segments. Division of the liver into 8 segments is based on a concept of 3 longitudinal planes and 2 transverse planes. A longitudinal plane through the middle hepatic vein, inferior vena cava (IVC), and gallbladder fossa divides the liver into right and left lobes. A longitudinal plane through the right hepatic vein divides the right lobe into anterior (**8** and **5**) and posterior (**7** and **6**) segments. A longitudinal plane through the left hepatic vein divides the left lobe into medial (**4a** and **4b**) and lateral (**2** and **3**) segments. A transverse plane through the left portal vein divides the left lobe into superior (**4a** and **2**) and inferior (**4b** and **3**) segments. An oblique transverse plane through the right portal vein divides the right lobe into superior (**8** and **7**) and inferior (**5** and **6**) segments. Segment **1** is the caudate lobe which extends between the fissure of the ligamentum venosum and the IVC. Hepatic venous drainage from the caudate lobe is directly into the IVC via small veins.

Blood supply to the liver is approximately two-thirds via the portal vein and one-third via the hepatic artery. When intravenous contrast is administered as a bolus during rapid CT scanning, the maximum liver parenchymal enhancement will be delayed 1 to 2 minutes following initiation of injection. This delay reflects the transit time of contrast agent through the gastrointestinal tract and spleen before accessing the liver through the portal vein. Tumors, which are supplied primarily by the hepatic artery, will enhance maximally during the early hepatic arterial phase, while the liver parenchyma enhances maximally during the portal venous phase.

TABLE 41.1

INTERNATIONAL NOMENCLATURE FOR ANATOMIC SEGMENTS OF THE LIVER

■ INTERNATIONAL NOMENCLATURE LIVER SEGMENTS	■ NUMBER
Caudate lobe	1
Left lateral superior segment	2
Left lateral inferior segment	3
Left medial superior segment	4a
Left medial inferior segment	4b
Right anterior inferior segment	5
Right anterior superior segment	8
Right posterior inferior segment	6
Right posterior superior segment	7

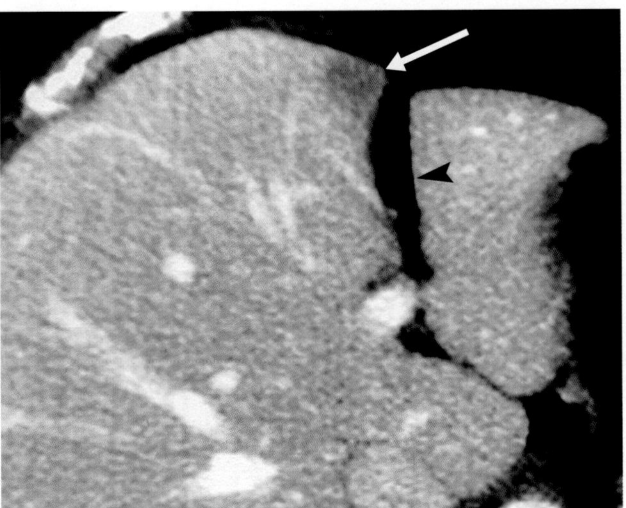

FIGURE 41.2. **Perfusion Defect.** A common perfusion defect (*arrow*) is seen in segment 4b adjacent to the fissure of the ligamentum teres (*arrowhead*). This perfusion defect is related to "third inflow" from paraumbilical systemic veins. Focal fatty infiltration is commonly seen in this location as well. Importantly, this normal variant must not be mistaken for a neoplasm.

Perfusion abnormalities are seen on postintravenous contrast CT and MR because of variations in hepatic arterial and portal venous blood supply to various areas of the liver. This dual blood supply has a compensatory relationship: arterial flow increases when portal venous flow decreases and increased portal venous flow compensates for decreased hepatic arterial flow. Transient enhancement differences are seen during either arterial phase imaging or portal venous phase imaging on MDCT and dynamic MR. These abnormalities have been termed "THADs" (transient hepatic attenuation differences) or "THIDs" (transient hepatic intensity differences) and "THEDs" (transient hepatic enhancement differences). Typically these perfusion alterations show the following findings relative to liver parenchyma: (a) hyperenhancement in the arterial phase, (b) isoenhancement in portal venous and delayed phase, (c) isoattenuation on unenhanced CT, and (d) isointensity on MR unenhanced T1WI, T2WI, and diffusion-weighted images. They may be rounded, wedge-shaped, diffuse, lobar, segmental, peritumoral, subcapsular, or patchy. There is no associated mass effect, vessels traverse them without distortion, and underlying liver parenchyma is preserved.

Portal venous flow may be altered by (a) portal venous blockade by tumor or thrombus; (b) extrinsic compression caused by ribs, diaphragmatic slips, or tumors on the liver capsule; or (c) "*third inflow*" from systemic veins in the pericholecystic, parabiliary, and epigastric–paraumbilical venous systems (Fig. 41.2). Systemic venous blood drains into hepatic sinusoids altering normal intrahepatic blood flow. This results in focal areas of increased or decreased enhancement during the various phases of parenchymal enhancement. Hepatic arterial flow may also be increased by (a) hypervascular tumors; (b) arterioportal shunting caused by cirrhosis, benign or malignant tumor, or arterioportal fistula; (c) inflammation of adjacent organs (cholecystitis, pancreatitis); or (d) aberrant hepatic arterial supply. Regional differences in blood supply related to these factors explain patterns of enhancement abnormalities as well as altered patterns of diffuse liver disease such as focal fatty deposition and focal fatty sparing in diffuse fatty infiltration.

On unenhanced CT, the attenuation of normal liver parenchyma is equal to or greater than the attenuation of normal spleen parenchyma. Following bolus intravenous contrast administration, the normal parenchymal enhancement is less than that of the spleen during arterial phase and equal to or greater than that of the spleen during portal venous phase.

On MR T1WI, the normal liver is of slightly higher signal intensity than the spleen, and most focal lesions appear as lower intensity defects. With T2WI, the normal liver is less than or equal to the spleen in signal strength, and most lesions appear as high intensity foci.

Diffuse Liver Disease

Hepatomegaly. Enlargement of the liver is usually judged subjectively on imaging studies. Rounding of the inferior border of the liver and extension of the right lobe of the liver inferior to the lower pole of the right kidney are evidence of hepatomegaly. A liver length of greater than 15.5 cm, measured in the midclavicular line, is considered enlarged. *Reidel lobe* is a normal variant of hepatic shape found most often in women. It refers to an elongated inferior tip of the right lobe of the liver. When a Reidel lobe is present the left lobe of the liver is correspondingly smaller in size. The liver is overall not enlarged. The left lobe of the liver may, as a normal variant, be elongated and surround a portion of the spleen. Causes of hepatomegaly are listed in Table 41.2.

Fatty liver (hepatic steatosis) is the most common abnormality demonstrated by hepatic imaging. It is prevalent in 15% of the general population, in 50% of patients with hyperlipidemia or high alcohol consumption, and in up to 75% of patients with severe obesity. Causes are many but two of the most common are alcoholic liver disease and nonalcoholic fatty liver disease related to the "metabolic syndrome" of insulin resistance, obesity, diabetes, hyperlipidemia, and hypertension. Other causes include viral

TABLE 41.2

CAUSES OF HEPATOMEGALY

Vascular congestion
Congestive heart failure
Hepatic vein thrombosis
Metabolic/diffuse infiltration
Fatty infiltration
Alcohol
Drugs/chemotherapy
Hepatic toxins
Gaucher disease and lipidoses
Carbohydrate
Glycogen storage diseases
Diabetes mellitus
Iron
Hemochromatosis
Amyloid
Amyloidosis
Tumor/cellular infiltrate
Diffuse metastases
Diffuse hepatocellular carcinoma
Lymphoma
Extramedullary hematopoiesis
Systemic mastocytosis
Cysts
Polycystic disease
Inflammation/infection
Hepatitis
Sarcoidosis
Tuberculosis
Malaria

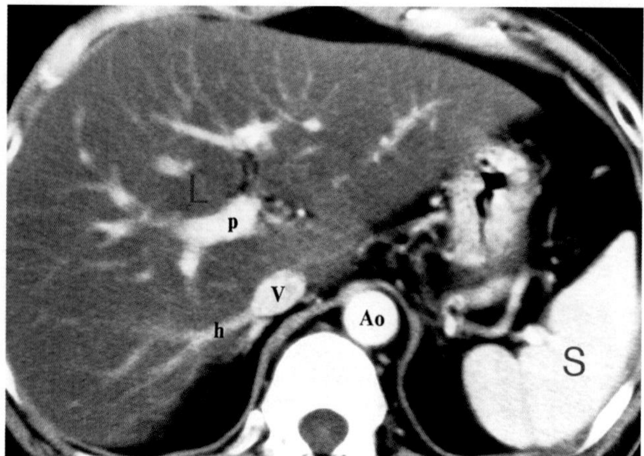

FIGURE 41.3. **Diffuse Fatty Liver—CT.** Portal venous phase CT reveals the density of the enhanced liver parenchyma (*L*) to be significantly less than the density of the enhanced splenic parenchyma (*S*). Portal (*p*) and hepatic (*h*) veins run their normal courses without displacement or distortion. *V*, inferior vena cava; *Ao*, aorta.

hepatitis, drugs (especially steroids and chemotherapy agents), nutritional abnormalities, radiation injury, cystic fibrosis, and storage disorders. All conditions injure hepatocytes by altering hepatocellular lipid metabolism with defects in free fatty acid metabolism resulting in accumulation of triglycerides within hepatocytes. Fatty liver is initially reversible but may progress to steatohepatitis (cell injury, inflammation, fibrosis) with further progression to cirrhosis.

Nonalcoholic fatty liver disease includes a continuum of liver disease that extends from simple fatty liver through nonalcoholic steatohepatitis (NASH) to cirrhosis. NASH is diagnosed by MR or US elastography showing liver fibrosis or by liver biopsy showing inflammation and fibrosis in addition to hepatic steatosis. Patients at risk for this increasingly common condition include those with type II diabetes and the "metabolic syndrome" described previously.

On US the normal liver parenchyma is equal to, or slightly more echogenic, than the renal cortex and spleen parenchyma. Intrahepatic blood vessels and small portal triads in the liver periphery are well defined. Reliable US findings of fatty liver include liver echogenicity distinctly greater than that of the renal cortex, loss of visualization of normal echogenic portal triads in the periphery of the liver, and poor sound penetration with loss of definition of the diaphragm (see Fig. 50.5B). All three findings must be present to make an unequivocal US diagnosis.

On CT, fat infiltration lowers the attenuation of the hepatic parenchyma and makes the liver appear less dense than the spleen on unenhanced images. The liver normally has a slightly higher attenuation than the spleen or blood vessels. On unenhanced CT, fatty liver is diagnosed when the liver attenuation is 10 H less than the spleen attenuation, or when the liver attenuation is less than 40 H. When fatty liver is severe blood vessels may appear brighter than the dark liver on unenhanced CT. On postcontrast images (Fig. 41.3), the normal spleen enhances maximally 1 to 2 minutes before maximal liver enhancement and is thus transiently brighter than the normal liver on arterial phase. Care must be taken to assess the phase of contrast enhancement of the liver. Fatty livers enhance less than normal livers. Comparison of CT and US findings may yield the diagnostic "flip-flop" sign with fatty liver being dark on unenhanced CT and bright on US.

MR T1- and T2-weighted images show no significant abnormalities with fat infiltration. Gradient echo (GRE) imaging with fat and water molecules in-phase and out-of-phase is the MR method most sensitive to diagnosis of fatty liver. On in-phase images, the signal from water and fat molecules are additive. On out-of-phase images, the signals from water and fat cancel out each other. A loss of signal intensity between in-phase and out-of-phase images is indicative of fatty liver (Fig. 41.4). This is the same technique used to characterize benign adrenal adenomas (see Chapter 47). This opposed-phase chemical shift GRE technique is more sensitive to detection of the microscopic intracellular fat characteristic of fatty liver than fat-saturation MR techniques, which have greater sensitivity for macroscopic fat. Iron deposition in the liver will also cause a loss of signal on out-of-phase MR imaging and is a potential pitfall in MR diagnosis of fatty liver in patients with cirrhosis. MR spectroscopy is used to quantify liver fat.

Characteristic features of fatty deposition on all modalities include lack of mass effect (no bulging of the liver contour or displacement of intrahepatic blood vessels) and angulated geometric boundaries between involved and uninvolved parenchyma. Areas of fat deposition may be multifocal with interdigitating fingers of normal and abnormal parenchyma. Fatty changes can develop within 3 weeks of hepatocyte insult and may resolve within 6 days of removing the insult. Patterns of fatty infiltration are strongly related to hepatic blood flow.

Diffuse fatty liver involving the entire liver is the most common pattern (Figs. 41.3 and 41.4). Most cases show homogeneous fat deposition, though slight heterogeneity is common and adds to the confidence of diagnosis.

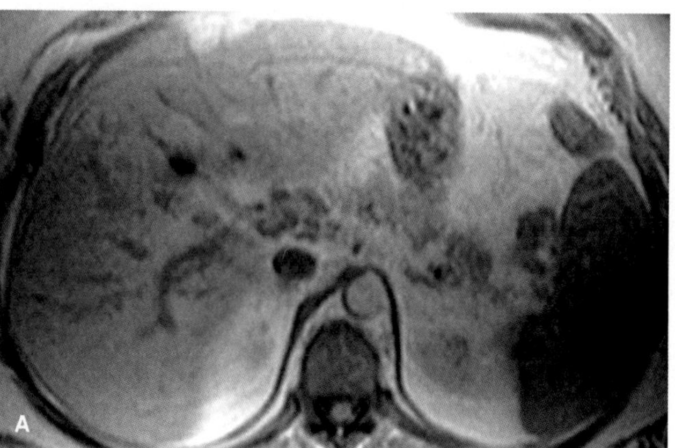

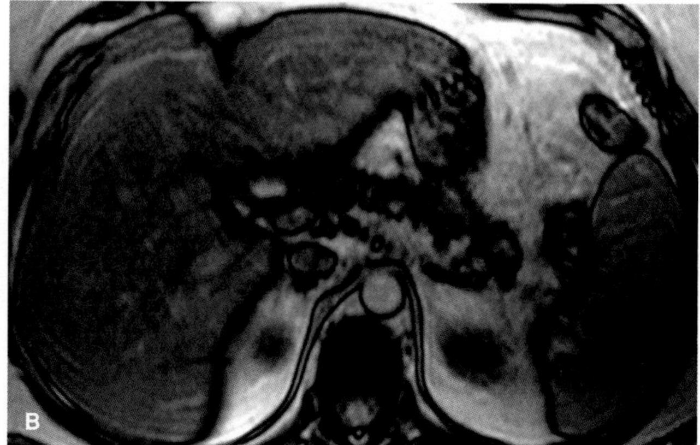

FIGURE 41.4. **Diffuse Fatty Liver—MR. A:** In-phase gradient recall MR. **B:** Out-of-phase gradient recall MR. The out-of-phase image shows distinct loss of signal (darkening) of the entire liver parenchyma compared to the in-phase image. The out-of-phase MR image is easily recognized by the *black line* surrounding soft tissue structures at the interface with abdominal fat.

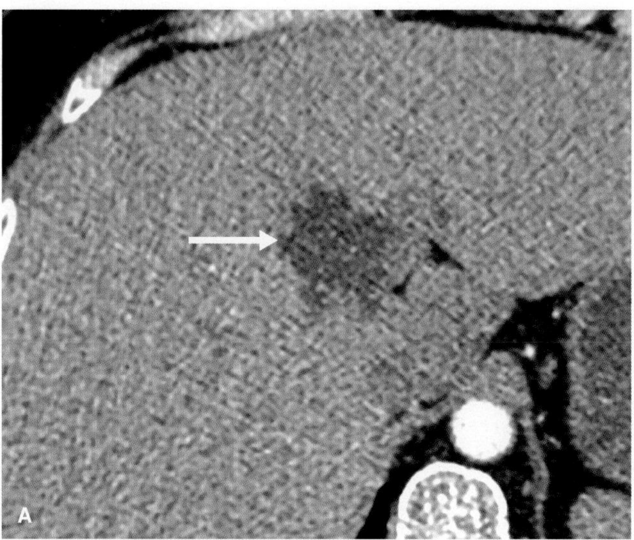

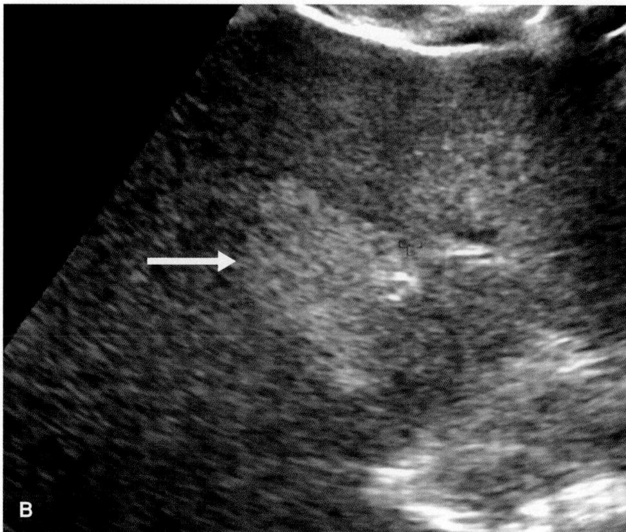

FIGURE 41.5. **Focal Fatty Liver. A:** CT following intravenous contrast administration shows a low attenuation focal mass (*arrow*) with irregular margins near the porta hepatis. **B:** US in the same patient shows the mass (*arrow*) to be highly echogenic confirming its identity as focal fatty infiltration. This is an example of the "flip-flop" sign of fatty tissue on CT and US.

Focal fatty liver involves a usually small, subsegmental, geographic, or fan-shaped portion of the liver with the same imaging features as diffuse fat deposition. Vessels run their normal course through the area of involvement. Focal fat may simulate a liver tumor, however, the area of involvement has imaging features characteristic of fat (Fig. 41.5). Focal fat is most common adjacent to the falciform ligament, the gallbladder fossa, and the porta hepatis. These are areas prone to altered hepatic blood flow with systemic inflow, and focal fat deposition may be related to higher concentrations of insulin in these areas.

Focal sparing in a diffusely fatty infiltrated liver may be the most confusing pattern because spared areas of normal parenchyma may convincingly simulate a liver tumor (Fig. 41.6). The fat-spared area is most commonly in segment 4. The fat-spared area is hypoechoic relative to the rest of the liver on US and is of higher attenuation than the rest of the liver on CT ("flip-flop" sign). The remainder of the liver demonstrates features characteristic of diffuse fatty infiltration (CT attenuation ≤40 H). MR shows diffuse signal loss on out-of phase images compared to in-phase images with fat-spared areas showing less signal loss than the rest of the liver.

Multifocal fatty liver is an uncommon pattern of fat deposition throughout the liver in atypical locations (Fig. 41.7). Fat foci may be round or oval and mimic metastatic disease or other liver nodules. Confluence of the fatty nodules to form larger masses is common. Chemical shift MR is the most reliable method to make the diagnosis and is particularly useful when CT and US are equivocal.

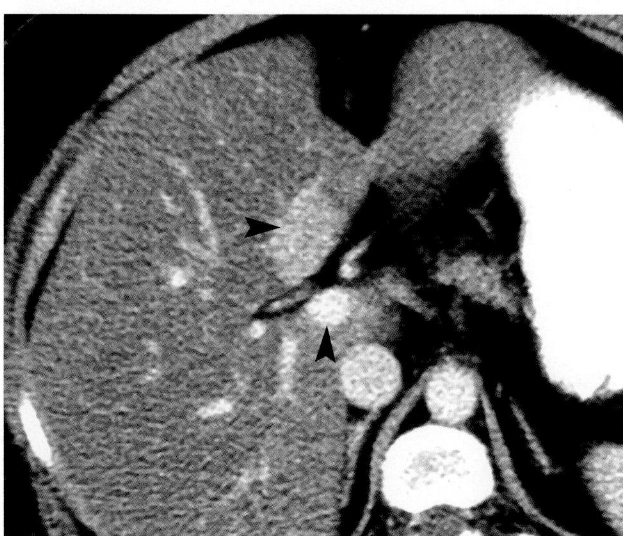

FIGURE 41.6. **Fatty Infiltration With Focal Sparing.** Postcontrast CT shows diffuse low attenuation of the liver with two areas (*arrowheads*) of normal liver attenuation near the porta hepatis. In-phase/out-of-phase MR confirmed diffuse fatty liver with focal sparing.

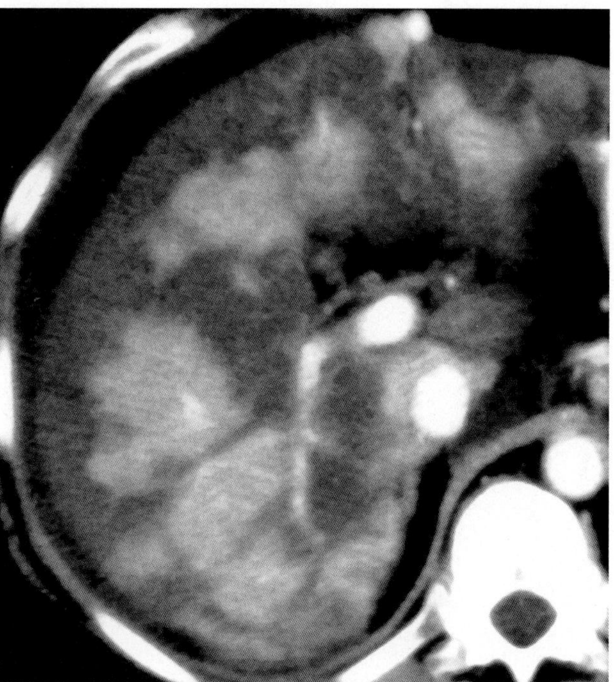

FIGURE 41.7. **Multifocal Fatty Liver.** Postcontrast CT demonstrates multiple geographic areas of decreased attenuation extending to liver capsule representing multifocal fat deposition.

Perivascular fatty liver is seen as halos of fat surrounding the portal veins, hepatic veins, or both. The cause of this unusual pattern is unknown.

Subcapsular fatty liver is seen only in patients with renal failure on peritoneal dialysis and only when insulin is added to the dialysate. High concentrations of insulin in the subcapsular liver lead to fat deposition.

Acute viral hepatitis most commonly causes no abnormalities on hepatic imaging. In some patients, diffuse edema lowers the parenchyma echogenicity and causes the portal venules to appear unusually bright on US. In acute fulminant hepatitis, areas of necrosis show as ill-defined areas of low density on CT. MR T2WI may show increased signal around the portal triads caused by periportal edema.

Chronic hepatitis is characterized pathologically by portal and perilobular inflammation and fibrosis. Causes include chronic viral infection and hepatitis B and C. Imaging studies are insensitive to early pathologic changes. Fatty changes are minimal and the liver is usually not enlarged. Perihepatic lymph nodes are commonly visualized. US may show a subtle coarse increase in hepatic echogenicity. The primary role of imaging patients with chronic hepatitis is to detect HCC. Core biopsy of the liver parenchyma, often guided by US, is used to stage the disease. MR and US elastography quantitate fibrosis.

Cirrhosis is characterized pathologically by diffuse parenchymal destruction, fibrosis with alteration of hepatic architecture, and innumerable regenerative nodules (RN) that replace normal liver parenchyma. Causes of cirrhosis include hepatic toxins (alcohol, drugs, aflatoxin from a grain fungus), infection (viral hepatitis, especially types B and C), biliary obstruction, and heredity (Wilson disease). In the United States, 75% of patients with cirrhosis are chronic alcoholics. In Asia and Africa, most cases of cirrhosis are due to chronic active hepatitis. A variety of morphologic alterations are seen on imaging studies. These include (Fig. 41.8) (a) hepatomegaly (early); (b) atrophy or hypertrophy of hepatic segments; (c) coarsening of hepatic parenchymal texture; (d) nodularity of the parenchyma, often most noticeable on the liver surface; (e) hypertrophy of the caudate lobe and left lobe with shrinkage of the right lobe; (f) regenerating nodules (Fig. 41.9); and (g) enlargement of the hilar periportal space (>10 mm) reflecting parenchymal atrophy. Extrahepatic signs of cirrhosis include the presence of portosystemic collaterals as evidence of portal hypertension, splenomegaly, and ascites. The pathologic changes of cirrhosis are irreversible, but disease progression can be limited or stopped by eliminating the causative agent (stop drinking alcohol). Transjugular intrahepatic portosystemic shunts (TIPS) are effective treatment for portal hypertension and long-term control of esophageal variceal bleeding. Liver transplantation is well established as effective treatment for end-stage liver disease.

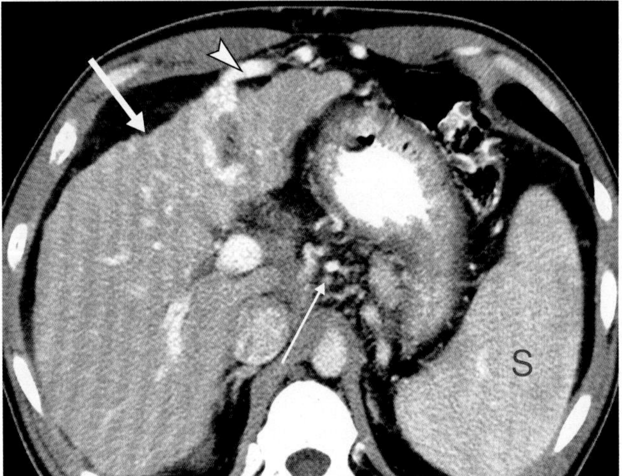

FIGURE 41.8. **Cirrhosis and Portal Hypertension.** A CT scan reveals atrophy of the liver with diffuse nodularity of its surface (*fat arrow*) and splenomegaly (*S*). Numerous enhancing portosystemic collateral vessels are evident including gastrohepatic (*skinny arrow*), and gastric varices. A dilated periumbilical vein (*arrowhead*) is seen coursing out of the fissure of the ligamentum teres into the falciform ligament.

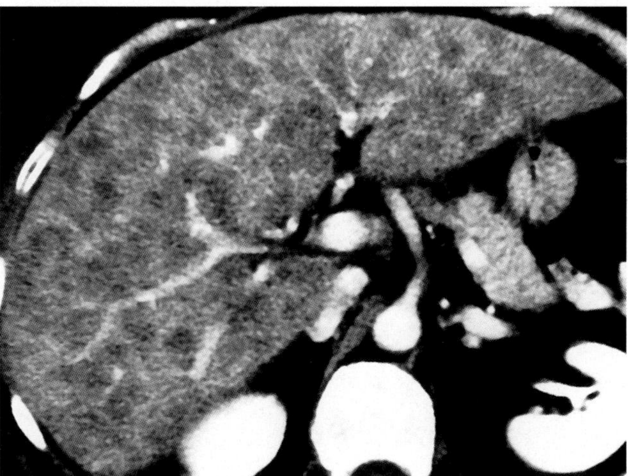

FIGURE 41.9. **Regenerative Nodules in Cirrhosis.** CT image filmed at a narrow window shows innumerable low-density small nodules evident throughout the liver in this patient with cirrhosis. Needle biopsy confirmed benign regenerative nodules.

US demonstrates heterogeneous parenchyma with coarsening of the echotexture and decreased visualization of small portal triad structures. High-frequency detailed scanning of the liver surface reveals fine nodules (82% to 95% specific for cirrhosis). Echogenicity of the liver parenchyma is not significantly increased unless fatty deposition is also present. US elastography is used to quantitate liver fibrosis.

CT may be normal in the early stages, or reveal parenchymal inhomogeneity with patchy areas of increased and decreased attenuation. Fine or coarse nodularity of the liver surface is characteristic.

MR shows heterogeneous parenchymal signal on T1WI and T2WI. High signal fibrosis on T2WI is the predominant cause of the heterogeneous appearance. MR elastography may be more reliable than US elastography to grade liver fibrosis.

Mimics of cirrhosis are conditions that cause diffuse hepatic nodularity or portal hypertension including pseudocirrhosis of treated breast cancer metastases, miliary metastases, sarcoidosis, schistosomiasis, Budd–Chiari syndrome, nodular regenerative hyperplasia, idiopathic portal hypertension, portal vein obstruction, and biliary obstruction.

Nodules in Cirrhosis. Nodules are a constant feature of cirrhosis (Table 41.3), and the challenge is to differentiate ubiquitous

TABLE 41.3

CAUSES OF NODULES IN A CIRRHOTIC LIVER

Regenerative nodules
Dysplastic nodules
Hepatocellular carcinoma
Confluent fibrosis
Focal fat infiltration
Focal fat sparing
Metastases (rare in cirrhosis)

benign nodules from HCC. HCC may arise de novo or as a stepwise process from an RN to low-grade dysplastic nodule to high-grade dysplastic nodule to small HCC to large HCC.

RN (Fig. 41.9) are the most common nodules and are a regular pathologic feature of cirrhosis due to attempted repair of hepatocyte injury. RN are composed primarily of hepatocytes that are surrounded by coarse fibrous septations. Small RN (<3 mm) produce the micronodular pattern of cirrhosis. Larger RN (>3 mm) produce the macronodular pattern of cirrhosis. Very large RN (up to 5 cm) mimic a mass. RN are supplied by the portal vein and thus show no enhancement on arterial phase postcontrast imaging. RN, because they consist of proliferating hepatocytes, are typically indistinct on US, CT, and MR imaging. MR typically shows heterogeneity without distinct nodules on T1WI and T2WI. Uncommonly, RN are hyperintense to liver on T2WI reflecting the accumulation of fat, protein, or copper. RN that accumulate iron (*siderotic nodules*) are low signal intensity on T1WI and T2WI. Infarction of RN results in a high signal on T2WI. A useful diagnostic feature is that in any given cirrhotic liver the RN tend to be uniform in size and other imaging features. Nodules that are different from background nodules in imaging appearance are more likely to be dysplastic nodules (DN) or HCCs.

DN show foci of low- or high-grade dysplasia. Low-grade DN show minimal atypia, have no mitosis, and are not premalignant. Low-grade DN are supplied by the portal vein and show no arterial phase enhancement postcontrast. Low-grade dysplasia typically progresses to high-grade dysplasia. High-grade DN show moderate atypia, have occasional mitosis, and may secrete alpha-fetoprotein (AFP), but are not frankly malignant. They are, however, considered premalignant. High-grade DN receive increasing blood supply by the hepatic artery and show arterial phase enhancement overlapping the appearance of small HCC. Low-grade DN have similar imaging characteristics as RN. They are indistinct and isointense to liver on US, CT, and T1- and T2-weighted MR. DN are almost never hyperintense on T2WI, differentiating them from HCC. Only very rare infarction of DN results in high signal on T2WI. DN may disappear on imaging follow-up.

Siderotic nodules describe cirrhotic nodules that are high in iron content and appear as low signal nodules on both T1WI and T2WI. CT is insensitive to iron content in cirrhosis nodules. The nodules may be regenerative or dysplastic but are seldom malignant. Siderotic nodules may be considered benign when they are <20 mm in diameter, homogeneous on all image sequences, and isoenhance compared to background cirrhotic nodules in all phases. Iron-rich nodules that are ≥20-mm diameter, heterogeneous on one or more MR sequences, or enhance differently from liver parenchyma on one or more phases may be HCC.

Small HCC, defined as <2-cm diameter, overlaps the appearance of high-grade DN. Detection leading to treatment of small HCC is a major goal of hepatic imaging in cirrhosis (Fig. 41.10).

The Liver Imaging Reporting and Data System (LI-RADS) was created by the American College of Radiology in 2011 and updated several times as a system for standardized interpretation, reporting, and data collection of CT, MR, and contrast-enhanced ultrasound imaging to be applied only for patients with cirrhosis or high risk for HCC. The system utilizes a defined lexicon and a scoring algorithm to characterize individual lesions (Table 41.4). The LI-RADS score for a liver lesion is an indication of its relative risk for HCC. Major criteria for diagnosis of HCC utilized by LI-RADS include (a) hyperenhancement in arterial phase definitely greater than background liver; (b) "washout" defined as visual hypointensity of the lesion compared with background liver on portal

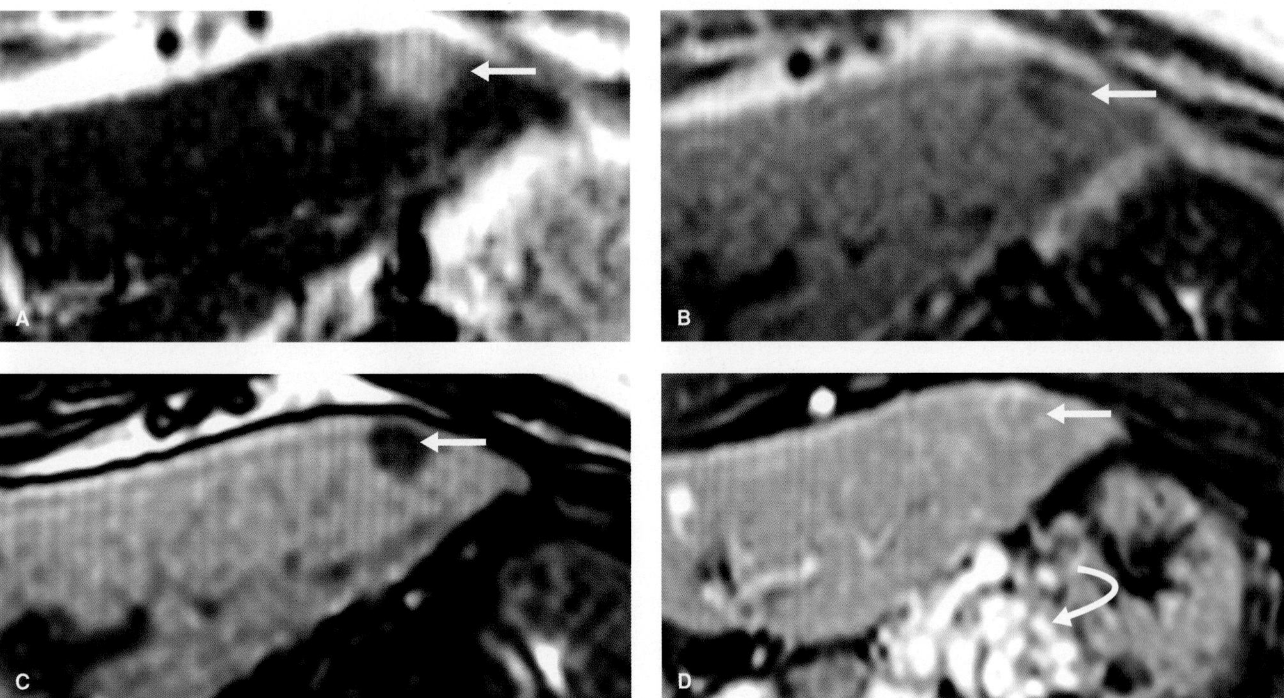

FIGURE 41.10. **Small Hepatocellular Carcinoma.** MR images show findings characteristic of a small hepatocellular carcinoma (*arrows*). **A:** Axial T2WI shows a hyperintense, poorly marginated, 1.8-cm nodule in the left hepatic lobe. Hyperintensity on T2WI is rare for dysplastic or regenerative nodules but is highly characteristic of HCC. **B:** T1-weighted in-phase image shows the low signal ill-defined nodule. **C:** T1-weighted out-of-phase image shows distinct loss of signal indicating the presence of intracellular fat, a finding seen in HCC and hepatic adenomas. **D:** Post-contrast arterial phase image shows ring-like peripheral enhancement of the lesion. Arterial phase enhancement is a key finding in the imaging diagnosis of HCC. Prominent early enhancement of a tangle of portosystemic collateral vessels (*curved arrow*) is also present in this patient with advanced cirrhosis and intrahepatic arterioportal shunting. (*continued*)

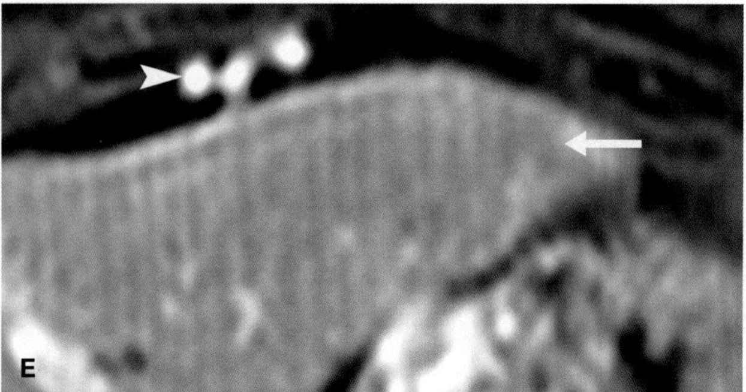

FIGURE 41.10. (*Continued*) E: Portal venous phase postcontrast image shows early washout of contrast from the nodule, which has become slightly hypointense to the enhanced hepatic parenchyma. This is another key finding of HCC on postcontrast images. Also noted is enhancement of paraumbilical collateral vessels (*arrowhead*), a specific sign of advanced portal hypertension.

venous and delayed phases; (c) peripheral rim of hyperenhancement of the capsule or pseudocapsule of the lesion on portal venous or delayed-phase images; and (d) threshold growth defined as diameter increase of the mass by 5 mm or more, 50% increase in diameter compared to prior examination ≤6 months, 100% increase in diameter compared to prior examination at >6 months, or a new 10-mm lesion regardless of time interval. Threshold is optimally assessed on similar studies or MR sequences.

Ancillary signs of HCC by LI-RADS criteria include (a) mild to moderate hyperintensity on T2WI; (b) restricted diffusion on MR; (c) rim of perilesional enhancement termed corona enhancement; (d) mosaic architecture; (e) "nodule within a nodule" appearance of HCC developing within a dysplastic nodule seen as a high signal focus within a low intensity nodule. The high signal focus enhances avidly on arterial phase; (f) intralesional fat; (g) intralesional iron sparing; (h) intralesional fat sparing; and (i) diameter increase less than that defined as threshold growth.

LI-RADS criteria favoring a benign nodule include (a) homogeneous marked hyperintensity on T2WI; (b) homogeneous marked hypointensity on T2- or T2*-weighted images; (c) intralesional vessels without distortion; (d) nodule enhancement parallels blood pool; (e) decrease in diameter, and (f) stable diameter for >2 years.

US is commonly used as an inexpensive and widely available method to survey the liver of patients with cirrhosis and chronic viral hepatitis for evidence of HCC. On US small HCC appears as well-circumscribed hypoechoic nodules in the cirrhotic liver. Contrast-enhanced US may show arterial phase enhancement with portal venous phase washout.

Hypertrophic pseudomass describes a bulging hypertrophied expanse of the liver surrounded by atrophic fibrotic liver parenchyma. The lesion may mimic a tumor. Imaging features that favor pseudomass over tumor include preservation of hepatic architectures and presence of undistorted vessels traversing the lesion. On MR hypertrophic pseudomasses are mildly hyperintense on T1WI, mildly hypointense on T2WI, and hypoenhancement on delayed-phase images.

Confluent fibrosis describes mass-like areas of fibrosis found in livers with advanced cirrhosis. Extensive fibrosis produces a wedge-shaped mass radiating from the porta hepatis associated with parenchymal atrophy and flattening or retraction of the liver capsule. Volume loss of the affected portion of the liver is a key feature. The central portion of the right hepatic lobe is most often involved. The lesion is low attenuation on noncontrast CT. On arterial phase postcontrast CT most lesions (60%) show little to no enhancement while the remainder isoenhance with liver parenchyma. On portal venous phase most lesions are hypodense or isodense to liver parenchyma, while 17% showed hyperenhancement

TABLE 41.4

LI-RADS CATEGORIES AND MANAGEMENT

LI-RADS CATEGORY	EXAMPLES	MANAGEMENT
LR-1 Definitely benign	Hemangioma, cyst, cystic biliary hamartoma, focal fat deposition or sparing, perfusion alteration, vascular anomalies, definite confluent fibrosis, hypertrophic pseudomass	Continued routine surveillance, as appropriate
LR-2 Probably benign	Findings are less certain than for LR-1: Persistent perfusion alteration, probable confluent fibrosis, pseudomass, cirrhosis-associated nodule, focal scars	Continued routine surveillance, as appropriate
LR-3 Intermediate probability for HCC		Variable follow-up (depends on clinical considerations)
LR-4 Probably HCC		Additional imaging, biopsy, treatment, or close follow-up
LR-5 Definitely HCC		Treat without biopsy Radiologic TNM staging
LR-TIV Definitely tumor invading vein		Treat without biopsy Radiologic TNM staging
LR-5 Treated Posttreatment observation		Close follow-up to assess treatment response. Retreat if needed
OM Other malignancy	Cholangiocarcinoma, lymphoma, metastases	Biopsy, additional imaging, treatment, or close follow-up

LI-RADS, Liver Imaging Reporting and Data System; *HCC*, hepatocellular carcinoma; *TNM*, American Joint Committee on Cancer tumor/node/metastases staging.
Adapted from American College of Radiology LI-RADS v2017.

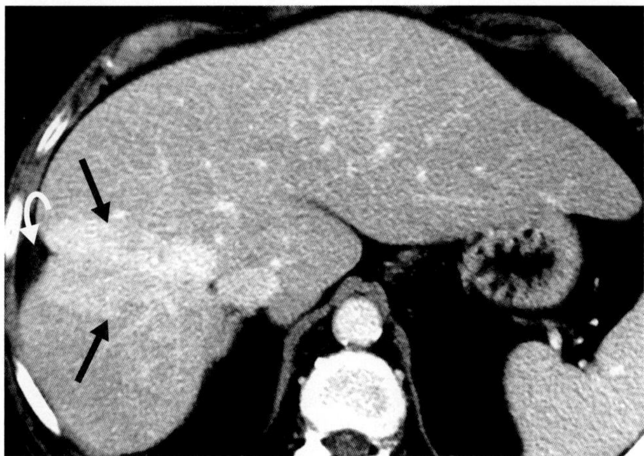

FIGURE 41.11. **Confluent Fibrosis.** Portal venous phase postcontrast CT image shows a mass-like enhancing lesion (*straight arrows*) extending from the portal hepatis to a prominent area of parenchymal atrophy with overlying retraction (*curved arrow*) of the liver capsule. This is an example of the minority of cases of confluent fibrosis that show contrast enhancement. Most cases (80%) of confluent fibrosis are hypoattenuating on noncontrast images and show no enhancement.

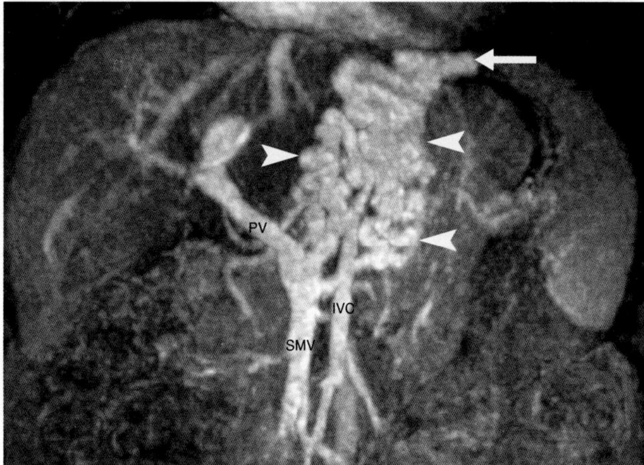

FIGURE 41.12. **Portosystemic Collaterals.** Coronal MR in a patient with advanced portal hypertension shows prominent perigastric (*arrowheads*) collaterals extending to distal periesophageal varices (*arrow*). These large collaterals may become a source of brisk gastric hemorrhage. *PV*, portal vein; *SMV*, superior mesenteric vein; *IVC*, inferior vena cava.

(Fig. 41.11). On MR the areas of fibrosis are hypointense to liver parenchyma on T1WI. On T2WI signal intensity depends on the chronicity of the fibrosis. Acute fibrosis has high fluid content and appears bright on T2WI. Chronic fibrosis is low in fluid content and appears dark on T2WI. Postcontrast MR shows negligible enhancement on arterial phase and late enhancement on delayed venous phase.

Portal hypertension is a pathologic increase in portal venous pressure that results in the formation of portosystemic collateral vessels that divert blood flow away from the liver and into the systemic circulation. Causes of portal hypertension include progressive vascular fibrosis associated with chronic liver disease, especially cirrhosis, portal vein thrombosis or compression, and parasitic infections (schistosomiasis). Portal hypertension carries the risk of hemorrhage from varices and hepatic encephalopathy. The signs of portal hypertension include (Figs. 41.8 and 41.10) (a) visualization of portosystemic collaterals (coronary, gastroesophageal, splenorenal, paraumbilical, hemorrhoidal, and retroperitoneal) (Fig. 41.12); (b) increased portal vein diameter (>13 mm); (c) increased superior mesenteric and splenic vein diameters (>10 mm); (d) portal vein thrombosis; (e) calcifications in the portal and mesenteric veins; (f) edema in the mesentery, omentum, and retroperitoneum; (g) splenomegaly due to vascular congestion; (h) ascites; and (i) reversal of flow in any portion of the portal venous system (hepatofugal flow).

Portal vein thrombosis may occur as a complication of cirrhosis, or be caused by portal vein invasion or compression by tumor (Fig. 41.13), hypercoagulable states, or inflammation (pancreatitis). The cause is unknown in 8% to 15% of patients. On CT the thrombus is seen as a hypodense plug within the portal vein. On US the thrombus may be of variable echogenicity depending upon chronicity. Malignant thrombus in the portal vein is contiguous with and extends from the primary tumor. The portal vein is expanded, filled with tumor in vein of the same imaging characteristics, including enhancement, as the primary tumor. Color Doppler may show blood vessels extending from the primary tumor into the tumor in vein. Bland thrombus fills a portal vein of near-normal size. On MR bland thrombus is of low signal because of its hemosiderin content. Bland thrombus does not enhance. The thrombus is hyperintense on T1WI when acute and isointense when chronic. Signal in the thrombus is increased on T2WI. Portal hypertension is exacerbated, or may be caused, by portal vein thrombosis. *Cavernous transformation of the portal vein* develops when small collateral veins adjacent to the portal vein expand and replace the obliterated portal vein. These collateral veins appear as a tangle of small vessels surrounding the thrombosed portal vein.

Budd–Chiari syndrome refers to a group of disorders characterized by obstruction to hepatic venous outflow involving one or more hepatic veins. Hepatic venous obstruction causes

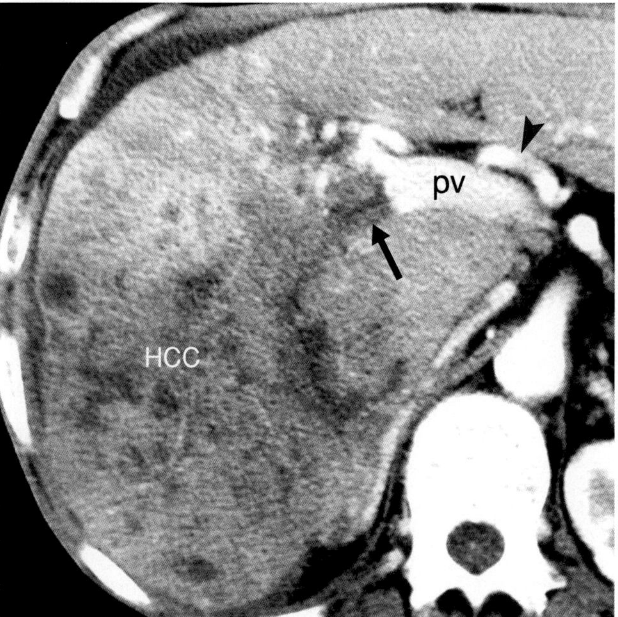

FIGURE 41.13. **Portal Vein Thrombosis—Hepatocellular Carcinoma.** Contrast-enhanced CT demonstrates multiple hypodense nodules typical of the multinodular appearance of hepatocellular carcinoma (*HCC*) replacing the right hepatic lobe. The portal vein (*pv*) is invaded by tumor (*arrow*), seen as a filling defect with the vein. The hepatic artery (*arrowhead*) is enlarged because of cirrhosis and portal hypertension.

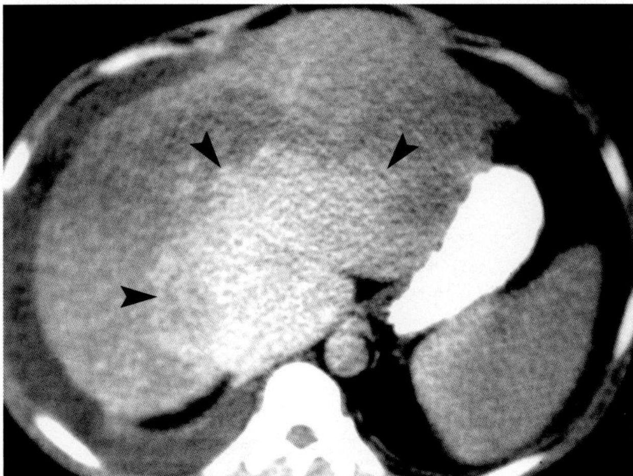

FIGURE 41.14. **Budd–Chiari Syndrome.** Early-phase CT images show the markedly heterogeneous liver with prominent central (*arrowheads*) and weak peripheral enhancement that is characteristic of Budd–Chiari syndrome. Both the right and left lobe are affected indicating occlusion of the right, middle, and left hepatic veins.

increased pressure in the hepatic sinusoids resulting in liver congestion, portal hypertension, and decreased hepatic perfusion. Diagnosis is urgent because of rapid progression to liver dysfunction, hepatocyte necrosis, and cirrhosis. Causes include coagulation disorders (the most common cause in Western countries), membranous webs obstructing the hepatic veins or IVC (most common in Asian countries), and malignant tumor invasion of the hepatic veins. In the acute stage the liver is enlarged and edematous. Blood flow to the right and left hepatic lobes is severely impaired resulting in a characteristic "flip-flop" pattern on contrast-enhanced CT. On early images, the central liver enhances prominently while the peripheral liver enhances weakly (Fig. 41.14). On delayed images, the periphery of the liver is enhanced, while contrast has washed out of the central liver. The caudate lobe is spared because of its separate venous drainage to the IVC. The caudate lobe is characteristically enlarged and enhances normally. Thrombus may be seen in the hepatic veins, or they may be reduced in caliber and difficult to visualize. Comma-shaped intrahepatic collateral vessels may be seen on CT or MR (the "comma sign"). Multiple benign hepatic nodules up to 3 cm size commonly develop. Most are detected by prominent contrast enhancement during arterial phase or mild contrast enhancement during portal venous phase.

In the acute stage of Budd–Chiari syndrome, MR shows in the periphery of the liver moderately low signal on T1WI, moderately high signal on T2WI, and decreased in enhancement on both early and late postcontrast images. In subacute and chronic stages, MR shows increasing heterogeneity of the liver periphery on both T1WI and T2WI with the comma-shaped venous collaterals.

Passive hepatic congestion is a common complication of congestive heart failure and constrictive pericarditis. Hepatic venous drainage is impaired and the liver becomes engorged and swollen. Chronic congestion leads to liver fibrosis and cirrhosis. Findings include distention of the hepatic veins and IVC, reflux of intravenous contrast into the hepatic veins and IVC, increased pulsatility of the portal vein, and inhomogeneous contrast enhancement of the liver. Secondary findings commonly present include hepatomegaly, cardiomegaly, pleural effusions, and ascites.

Hemochromatosis may be primary resulting from a hereditary disorder that increases dietary iron absorption, or secondary due to excessive iron intake usually from multiple blood transfusions or chronic diseases including cirrhosis, myelodysplastic syndrome, and certain anemias. MR is the imaging method of choice for this condition because of its high sensitivity and specificity. The susceptibility effect of iron, best appreciated on T2* images, causes loss of signal in tissues with excessive iron accumulation.

The *parenchymal pattern* of iron deposition is seen with increased iron absorption of primary hemochromatosis and with secondary hemochromatosis caused by chronic anemias (thalessemia, congenital dyserythropoietic anemias, sideroblastic anemia). This pattern shows decreased MR signal in the liver, pancreas, and heart. The spleen and bone marrow are spared.

The *reticuloendothelial pattern* of iron deposition is seen in secondary hemochromatosis with iron overload caused by blood transfusions. The excess iron accumulation occurs in reticuloendothelial cells in the liver, spleen, and bone marrow. MR shows diffuse decreased signal in all three areas (Fig. 41.15).

The *renal pattern* of iron deposition is rare but dramatic, occurring only in patients with intravascular hemolysis caused by mechanical heart valves. Excess iron deposition occurs in the proximal convoluted tubules of the renal cortex causing loss of cortical signal on T1WI and T2WI, reversing the normal corticomedullary differentiation pattern.

CT is sensitive to only severe cases of hemochromatosis. Excess iron increases hepatic parenchymal attenuation above 72 H on noncontrast images. Wilson disease (copper deposition), and treatment with amiodarone (iodine deposition) or colloidal gold also increase hepatic parenchymal attenuation on CT. Coexisting fatty infiltration will lower hepatic parenchymal attenuation and the sensitivity of CT for hemochromatosis.

Long-standing hemochromatosis places the patient at risk for cirrhosis, HCC, and colorectal carcinoma.

Gas in the portal venous system may be an ominous imaging sign associated with bowel ischemia in adults (Fig. 41.16) and necrotizing enterocolitis in infants. Additional, less ominous, causes include recent colonoscopy, enema administration, gastrostomy tube placement, abdominal trauma, inflammatory bowel disease, perforated gastric ulcer, necrotizing pancreatitis, diverticulitis, and abdominal abscess. CT reveals air in branching tubular structures extending to the liver capsule. Air is commonly evident within the mesenteric and central portal veins. Conventional radiographs show streaks of low density in the periphery of the liver. In distinction, air in the

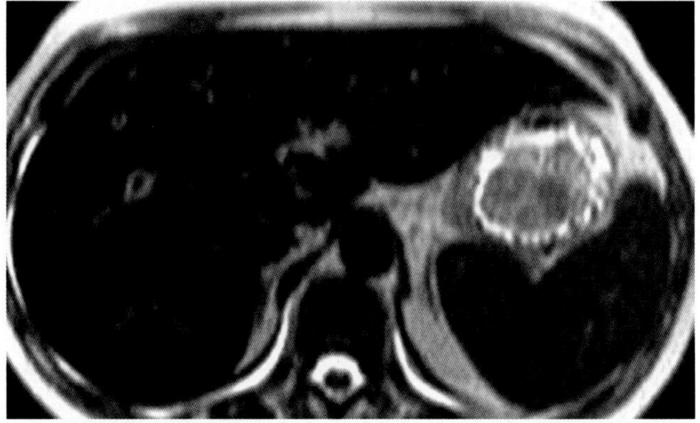

FIGURE 41.15. **Hemochromatosis—Reticuloendothelial Pattern.** T2-weighted MR images demonstrate markedly low signal intensity in the liver, spleen, and bone marrow of the vertebral body. The low signal is caused by iron deposition in the reticuloendothelial system in this case of secondary hemochromatosis caused by multiple blood transfusions.

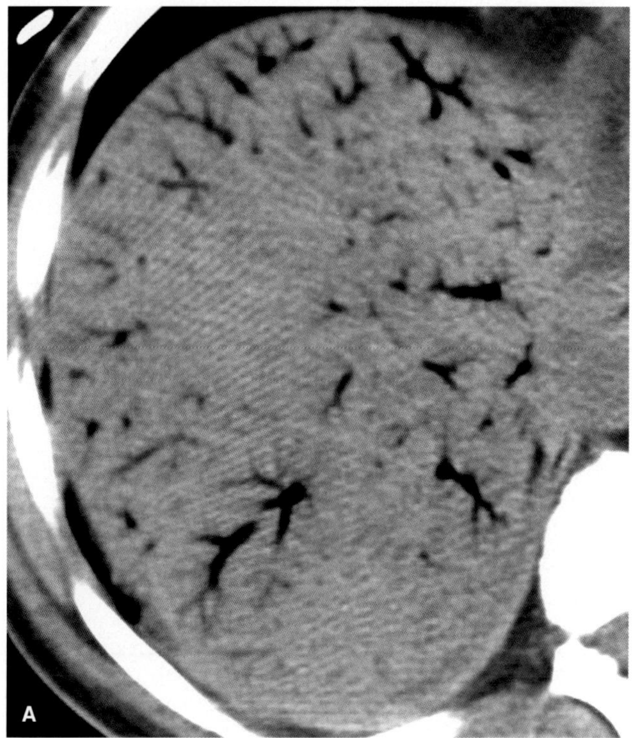

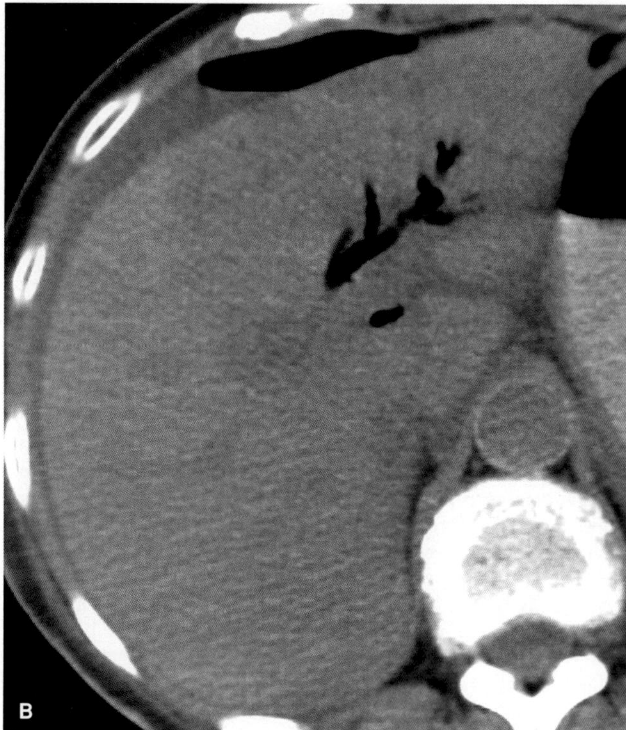

FIGURE 41.16. **Portal Venous Gas versus Pneumobilia. A:** Noncontrast CT reveals gas in the portal vein as air-density tubular structures extending to the periphery of the liver. In this case portal venous gas was associated with infarction of the small bowel. **B:** Gas in the biliary tree is central and does not extend into the peripheral 2 cm of the liver. Because gas rises to the highest accessible location, pneumobilia is usually seen on CT in the anterior portions of the liver.

biliary tree is more central, not extending to within 2 cm of the liver capsule.

Liver Masses

A major challenge of liver imaging is to differentiate common and benign liver masses, such as cavernous hemangioma and simple hepatic cysts, from malignant masses such as metastases and HCC. US can definitively characterize hepatic cysts; however, benign and malignant solid masses overlap in sonographic appearance. CT can characterize most cysts and cavernous hemangiomas but only with optimal technique and multiphase contrast administration. On MR, simple cysts and hemangiomas are hypointense on T1WI and extremely hyperintense on T2WI. These benign masses are typically homogeneous and have sharp outer margins. Malignant lesions on MR tend to be inhomogeneous with unsharp outer margins, peritumoral edema, and central necrosis. Most focal lesions are hypointense on T1WI and hyperintense on T2WI. Hyperintensity of focal lesions on T1WI may be due to the presence of fat, blood, proteinaceous material, or melanin in melanoma metastases (Table 41.5). Diffuse hypointensity of liver, due to diffuse edema or iron overload, may make any lesion appear relatively hyperintense. Hypointensity on T2WI is commonly due to acute fibrosis (Table 41.6). Dynamic postcontrast CT and MR are utilized to provide the most definitive characterization of hepatic masses by assessing tumor blood flow during arterial, portal venous, delayed, and equilibrium phases of contrast enhancement.

In normal liver parenchyma the most common hypervascular lesions are hemangiomas, FNH, hepatic adenoma, and hypervascular metastases. In fibrotic liver and cirrhosis the most common hypervascular lesions are HCC and DN. THADs must be differentiated from true hypervascular masses.

TABLE 41.5

CAUSES OF HYPERINTENSITY IN FOCAL LIVER LESIONS ON MR T1WI

Fat deposits
Focal fat infiltration
Fat deposition in tumor
Hepatoma
Lipoma
Angiomyolipoma
Hepatic adenoma
Blood
Hematoma
Hemorrhage into tumor
Proteinaceous material
Proteinaceous fluid in cysts
Necrosis/hemorrhage in tumor
Abscess
Hematoma
Copper
Intratumoral copper in hepatoma
Melanin
Melanoma metastasis
Contrast enhancement
Gadolinium administration
Lipiodol administration
Ghosting artifact
Due to blood flow in adjacent vessels
Hypointensity of liver parenchyma
Edema due to passive hepatic congestion
Iron deposition in hepatocytes

TABLE 41.6

CAUSES OF HYPOINTENSITY IN FOCAL LIVER LESIONS ON MR T2WI

Fibrous capsule
Hepatoma (24–42% of HCC)
Hepatic adenoma
Focal nodular hyperplasia (rare)

Fibrous central scar
Fibrolamellar hepatocellular carcinoma
Focal nodular hyperplasia

Metastases are the most common malignant masses in the liver. Metastases are 20 times more common than primary liver malignancies. Of all patients who die of malignancy, 24% to 36% have liver involvement. Hepatic metastases most commonly originate from the gastrointestinal tract, breast, and lung. A wide spectrum of appearance of metastatic disease is seen on all imaging studies (Fig. 41.17). Metastases may be uniformly solid, cystic, necrotic, hemorrhagic, or calcified; they may be avascular, hypovascular, or hypervascular; they are commonly irregular and poorly marginated but may be sharp and well defined. Most characteristic is band-like peripheral enhancement creating a "target lesion" on postcontrast CT and MR images. Metastatic disease must be considered in the differential of virtually all hepatic masses (Table 41.7). Multiplicity of lesions favors metastatic disease. Metastases are extremely rare in cirrhotic livers.

Hypovascular metastases are usually low signal on T1WI and isointense or hyperintense on T2WI. Postcontrast images show delayed enhancement. On CT hypovascular metastases are most apparent on portal venous phase images when the background liver is maximally enhanced and the metastatic lesions are of low attenuation (Fig. 41.17A). The most common hypovascular metastases are colorectal, lung, prostrate, gastric, and uroepithelial carcinomas.

Hypervascular metastases overlap the appearance of HCC. MR and CT show arterial phase enhancement (Fig. 41.17B) with rapid washout on portal venous and delayed images. These metastases may be overlooked if arterial phase postcontrast images are not obtained. Hypervascular metastases are associated with primary neuroendocrine tumors (pancreatic islet cell tumors, carcinoid tumor, pheochromocytoma), renal cell carcinoma, thyroid carcinoma, melanoma, some sarcomas, and choriocarcinoma.

TABLE 41.7

CAUSES OF MULTIPLE SMALL (10 mm) LESIONS IN THE LIVER

Regenerative nodules in cirrhosis
Microabcesses (immunocompromised patient)
Multiple bacterial abscesses
Histoplasmosis
Lymphoma
Kaposi sarcoma (AIDS patient)
Hepatocellular carcinoma (multinodular form)
Sarcoidosis
Gamna–Gandy bodies (portal hypertension)
Metastases
Breast carcinoma
Lung carcinoma
Ovarian carcinoma
Gastric carcinoma
Malignant melanoma
Prostate carcinoma

Cavernous hemangioma is second only to metastases as a common cause of a liver mass. It is the most common benign liver neoplasm, found in 7% to 20% of the population and more commonly in women. Up to 10% of patients have multiple lesions easily mistaken for metastases. Many hemangiomas are discovered incidentally on hepatic imaging performed for other reasons. The tumor consists of large, thin-walled, blood-filled vascular spaces separated by fibrous septa. Blood flow through the maze of vascular spaces is extremely slow, resulting in characteristic imaging findings. Thrombosis within the vascular channels may result in central fibrosis and calcification. Most lesions are less than 5 cm in size, cause no symptoms, and are considered benign incidental findings. Larger lesions, "giant hemangiomas" (>5 cm), occasionally

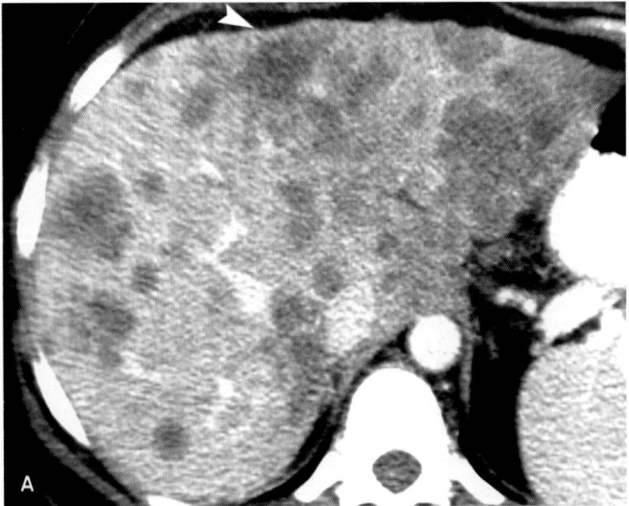

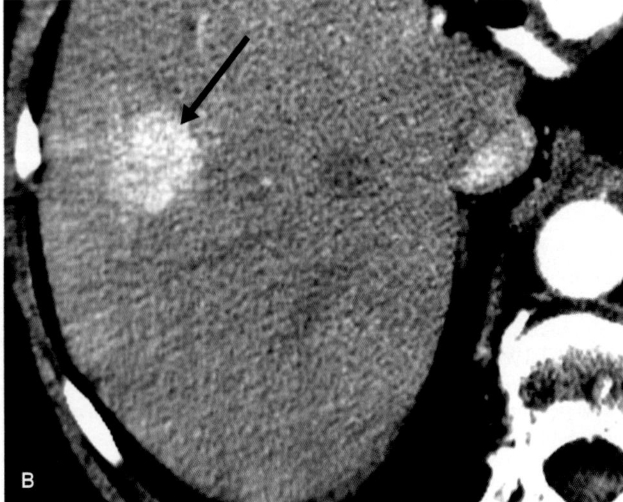

FIGURE 41.17. Metastases. A: Hypovascular metastases from adenocarcinoma of the colon appear as numerous low attenuation nodules of varying size on this portal venous phase postcontrast CT. Note how the metastatic disease causes nodularity of the liver contour (*arrowhead*) and the resemblance to regenerative nodules in cirrhosis seen in Figure 41.9. **B**: Hypervascular metastasis (*arrow*) from renal cell carcinoma shows bright enhancement on this arterial phase postcontrast CT image. While metastases are usually multiple, solitary metastases also occur.

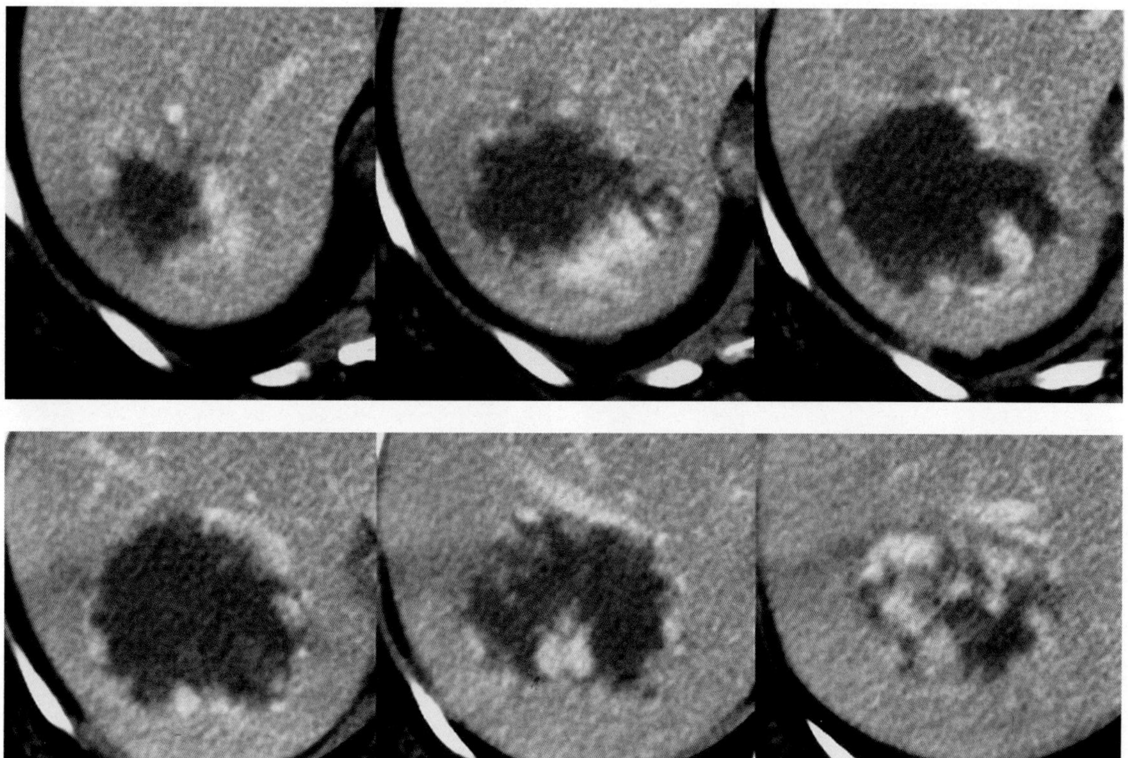

FIGURE 41.18. Cavernous Hemangioma. Images from a contrast-enhanced MDCT demonstrate the discontinuous nodular pattern of enhancement from the periphery of the lesion characteristic of cavernous hemangioma.

cause symptoms by mass effect, hemorrhage, or arteriovenous shunting. The size of most cavernous hemangiomas is stable over time. Enlargement of a lesion is cause for reassessment. In livers with progressive cirrhosis hemangiomas become more fibrotic and smaller.

US demonstrates a well-defined, uniformly hyperechoic mass in 80% of patients. In a patient with no history of malignant disease and normal liver chemistries, only follow-up is generally recommended. No Doppler signal is obtained from most cavernous hemangiomas because the flow is too slow.

CT generally shows a well-defined, round, oval, or lobulated hypodense mass on unenhanced scans. Because the lesion consists mostly of blood, attenuation of the hemangioma is similar to that of blood vessels within the liver. The characteristic pattern of enhancement with bolus intravenous contrast is discontinuous nodular enhancement from the periphery of the lesion (Fig. 41.18) that gradually becomes isodense or hyperdense compared to the liver parenchyma. The degree of contrast enhancement parallels that of hepatic blood vessels during all postcontrast phases. The contrast enhancement persists for 20 to 30 minutes following injection because of slow flow within the lesion.

MR demonstrates a well-defined homogeneous mass that is hypointense on T1WI and markedly hyperintense with increasing amounts of T2 weighting. Areas of fibrosis remain dark on all image sequences. However, on standard MR appearance of cavernous hemangiomas overlaps that of cysts, abscesses, and hypervascular metastases. A specific diagnosis is made by administering intravenous gadolinium. The most common pattern of enhancement (80%) demonstrates a well-marginated mass with discontinuous peripheral nodular enhancement leading to progressive fill-in of the lesion on delayed imaging (>5 minutes). Brightness of enhancement parallels the blood pool. Central areas of fibrosis, usually seen only in giant hemangiomas (>5 cm) do not enhance. Small capillary hemangiomas (<1.5 cm) fill-in more rapidly and the peripheral nodular enhancement may not be evident depending upon timing of the images. These "flash hemangiomas" retain contrast on delayed images while other small early-phase enhancing lesions, such as HCC and hypervascular metastases, show early and progressive contrast washout.

Radionuclide scanning using technetium-labeled red blood cells as a blood pool agent is extremely accurate in the diagnosis of cavernous hemangioma. Hemangiomas are characterized by prolonged intense activity within the lesion on delayed images.

Biopsy may be required in atypical cases. Percutaneous biopsy can be safely performed using small needles (20 gauge and smaller). The characteristic finding is blood with normal epithelial cells and no malignant cells. Biopsy with large bore needles has been associated with hemorrhage and death.

Hepatocellular carcinoma (hepatoma) is the most common primary malignancy of the liver. It ranks as the fifth most common tumor in the world and the third most common cause of cancer-related death (following lung and gastric cancer). The tumor is becoming increasingly common in the United States as well as worldwide.

Risk factors include cirrhosis, chronic hepatitis, and a variety of carcinogens (sex hormones, aflatoxin, thorotrast). In the United States, most HCCs (80%) are found in patients with cirrhosis (usually due to alcohol abuse). In Asia, most HCCs are found in patients with chronic active viral hepatitis. Elevation in serum AFP is found in 90% of patients and is strongly suggestive of hepatoma in patients with cirrhosis. Detection of HCC on a background of cirrhosis and RN is a major imaging challenge that has led to the development of LI-RADS.

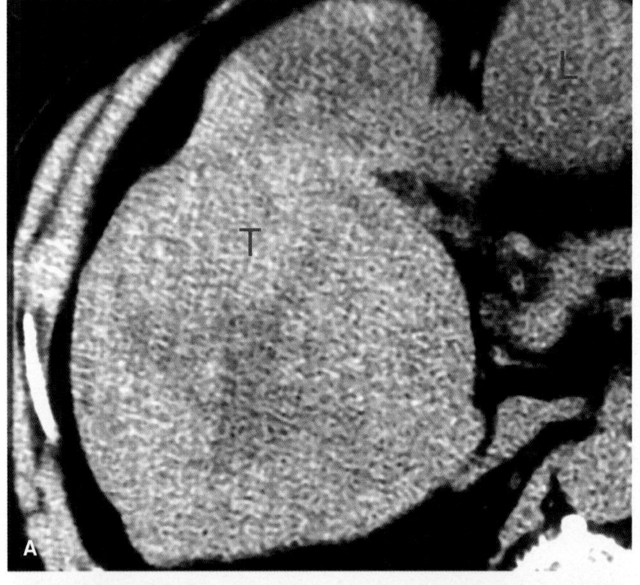

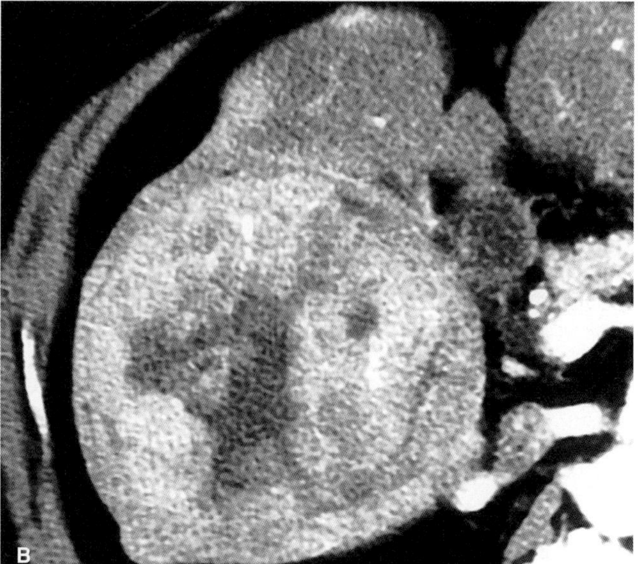

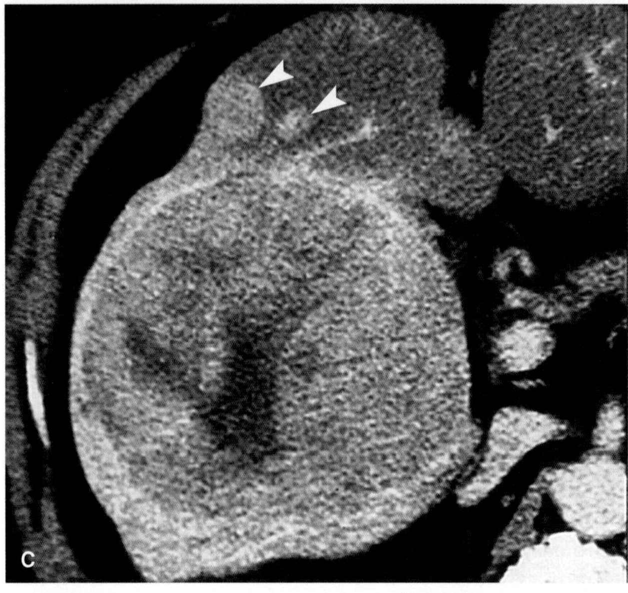

FIGURE 41.19. Hepatocellular Carcinoma—Solitary Massive Appearance—CT. Three-phase MDCT demonstrates the enhancement pattern of a large solitary hepatocellular carcinoma in the right lobe. The tumor (*T*) is slightly hyperdense to cirrhotic liver parenchyma (*L*) on the unenhanced scan (**A**) and shows intense enhancement on the early arterial phase (**B**) scan with contrast washout on delayed portal venous phase (**C**) scan. The central low density is due to necrosis. Note the satellite lesions (*arrowheads*).

Large hepatomas (>2 cm) demonstrate three major growth patterns that affect their imaging appearance: solitary massive (Figs. 41.19 and 41.20), multinodular (Fig. 41.13), and diffuse infiltrative. Solitary massive HCC is a single large mass with or without satellite nodules. Multinodular HCC appears as multiple discrete nodules involving a large area of the liver. Diffuse HCC manifests as innumerable tiny indistinct nodules throughout the liver distorting the parenchyma but not causing a discrete mass. It is difficult to differentiate from the distorted parenchyma of cirrhosis.

HCC has variable intensity on T1WI and T2WI. High intensity on T1WI reflects the accumulation of fat, glycogen, or copper within the tumor. Fat shows signal loss on opposed-phase or fat-saturation images. Moderate high signal on T2WI is quite specific for HCC as DN are not high signal unless infarcted. Arterial phase enhancement reflects neoangiogenesis with supply from the hepatic artery. This is considered an essential characteristic for diagnosis. Arterial phase enhancement is homogeneous for small lesions and heterogeneous for large lesions. The American Association for the Study of Liver Diseases (AASLD), the United Network for Organ Sharing, and LI-RADS consider arterial phase enhancement as an essential imaging finding for radiologic diagnosis of HCC.

Large HCCs have the following characteristic features: (a) the hallmark finding of HCC consisting of heterogeneous enhancement during arterial phase with rapid washout of contrast during portal venous and delayed phase; (b) peritumoral arterial phase enhancement related to portal vein compression or occlusion by the tumor with compensatory increase in hepatic arterial supply appearing wedge shaped and confined to the segment of the liver with compromised portal venous supply; (c) a mosaic pattern (80% to 90% of HCC) of confluent small nodules separated by thin septations and necrotic areas, best seen on T2-weighted MR; (d) distinct tumor capsule (60% to 80%) seen on CT, T1WI, and T2WI as a hypointense rind up to 4 mm thick consisting of an inner fibrous layer and an outer tissue layer of compressed bile ducts and blood vessels; (e) extracapsular extension (40% to 80%) of tumor with satellite lesions (Fig. 41.19) or tumor projection through the capsule; (f) vascular invasion (25%) of tumor into the portal veins or, less commonly hepatic veins, seen as enhancing tumor and lack of flow within the blood vessels;

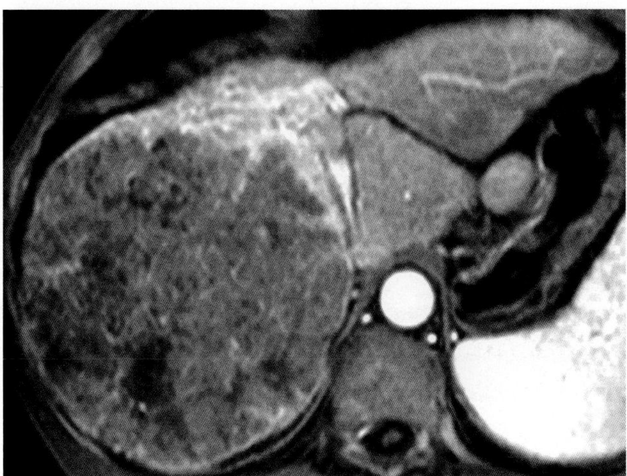

FIGURE 41.20. Hepatocellular Carcinoma—Solitary Massive Appearance—MR. Postcontrast T1-weighted MR image shows the typical mosaic pattern of large hepatocellular carcinomas. Note the heterogeneous enhancement most pronounced in the periphery of the tumor.

(g) occluded veins have expanded lumens, ill-defined walls, and show restricted diffusion on diffusion-weighted MR; (h) calcifications (punctate, stippled, or rim-like) in approximately 10% of cases; (i) fatty metamorphosis within the tumor (Table 41.8) best seen on chemical shift MR; (j) arterioportal shunting seen as early or prolonged enhancement of the portal vein, or as a wedge-shaped area of parenchymal enhancement adjacent to the tumor; and (k) excessive copper accumulation within the tumor causing the tumor to appear hyperdense on CT and T1WI on MR.

Focal nodular hyperplasia is a benign solid mass consisting of abnormally arranged hepatocytes, bile ducts, and Kupffer cells. FNH is second to hemangioma as the most common benign liver tumor. Most lesions are solitary, less than 5 cm in diameter, and are hypervascular with a central fibrous scar containing thick-walled blood vessels. Lesions are lobulated and well circumscribed but lack a capsule. These are benign lesions without risk of malignant transformation. They do not require treatment but must be differentiated from hepatic adenoma and fibrolamellar carcinoma.

Unlike hepatic adenoma, hemorrhage, necrosis, and infarction are extremely rare. Similar to hepatic adenoma, FNH is found most commonly in women, but is twice as common as hepatic adenoma and is not related to oral contraceptive use. Most tumors (80% to 95%) are solitary. Because of the presence of Kupffer cells, most (50% to 70%) FNH will show normal or increased radionuclide activity on technetium-99m sulfur colloid liver–spleen scans. This finding is highly indicative of FNH.

TABLE 41.8

FAT-CONTAINING LESIONS IN THE LIVER

Hepatic adenoma
Hepatocellular carcinoma
Focal fatty deposition
Lipoma
Teratoma
Liposarcoma (primary or metastatic)
Postoperative packing material (omentum)
Focal intrahepatic extramedullary hematopoiesis

US images show the mass to very subtle, blending with surrounding parenchyma because the lesion consists of the same elements. A slight bulge in the liver contour or subtle alteration of parenchymal echogenicity may be the only clues to the presence of a lesion. Color Doppler may show the central vascularity.

CT also shows a subtle, slightly hypoattenuating lesion on unenhanced images. Postcontrast shows characteristic intense homogeneous enhancement in arterial phase sometimes with visualization of large feeding vessels. Contrast washes out early on portal venous phase. The lesion is isointense and commonly near-invisible on delayed-phase equilibrium images.

On MR (Fig. 41.21), FNH appears homogeneous and isointense to slightly hypointense to normal parenchyma on T1WI and isointense to slightly hyperintense on T2WI. A key to diagnosis is to recognize that the lesion is near isointense to liver parenchyma on all precontrast MR sequences. The central scar, if present, is hypointense on T1WI and hyperintense on T2WI. FNH shows characteristic very intense homogeneous enhancement on arterial phase postcontrast images. The lesion becomes isointense on portal venous phase images. The central scar and radiating septa enhance on delayed postcontrast images. Hepatocyte-specific MR contrast agents show uptake within FNH appearing iso- to hyperintense to parenchyma on MR imaging obtained 1 to 3 hours after contrast administration.

Hepatic adenomas are rare, benign tumors that carry a risk of life-threatening hemorrhage and potential for malignant degeneration. Surgical removal of the tumor is advocated. They are found most commonly in women on long-term oral contraceptives. Additional risk factors include androgenic steroid intake and glycogen storage disease. The tumor consists of sheets and cords of benign hepatocytes without a distinct acinar architecture. The hepatocytes occasionally contain abundant fat, detectable by imaging studies. Kupffer cells are present in some tumors but are nonfunctional, thus hepatic adenomas appear as cold defects on technetium sulfur colloid radionuclide scans, allowing differentiation from FNA. The characteristic poor connective tissue support makes the tumors susceptible to hemorrhage. Most tumors are solitary (21% are multiple), smooth, and encapsulated. They do not have central scars. Tumor size is commonly 8 to 15 cm but may be up to 30 cm size. Areas of necrosis, hemorrhage, and fibrosis are common.

US shows a well-circumscribed tumor that is usually heterogeneous depending on presence of fat, necrosis, hemorrhage, or rarely calcification. High fat content or acute intratumoral hemorrhage makes the lesions appear hyperechoic. Contrast-enhanced US shows prominent arterial phase enhancement.

CT shows well-circumscribed tumors that are often low in attenuation because of internal fat, necrosis, or old hemorrhage. Calcifications in areas of old hemorrhage or necrosis are present in 15% of tumors. Postcontrast scans show intense homogeneous enhancement during arterial phase that becomes isodense with liver on portal venous and delayed-phase scans.

MR appearance (Fig. 41.22) varies with fat content and internal hemorrhage, both of which produce bright foci on T1WI. Fat suppression sequences or opposed-phase chemical shift imaging darken fat within the lesion and provide differentiation from FNH, which does not contain fat. On T2WI most are hyperdense to liver and are commonly heterogeneous because of hemorrhage or necrosis. Postcontrast arterial phase images show heterogeneous enhancement, usually not as avid as FNH. Delayed contrast washout is typical. With hepatocyte-specific contrast administration adenomas are hypointense to liver parenchyma on delayed images obtained at 1 to 3 hours.

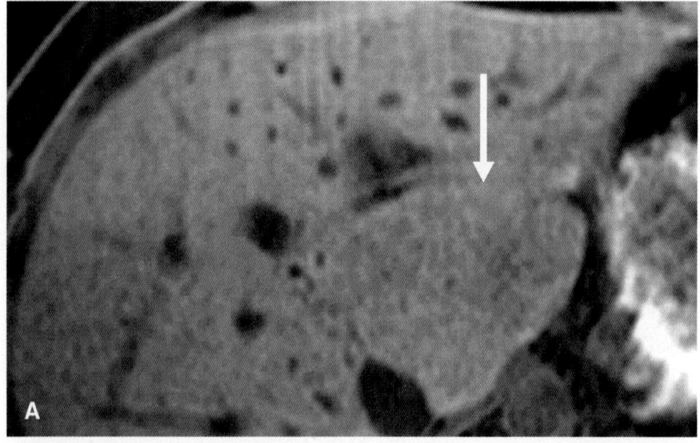

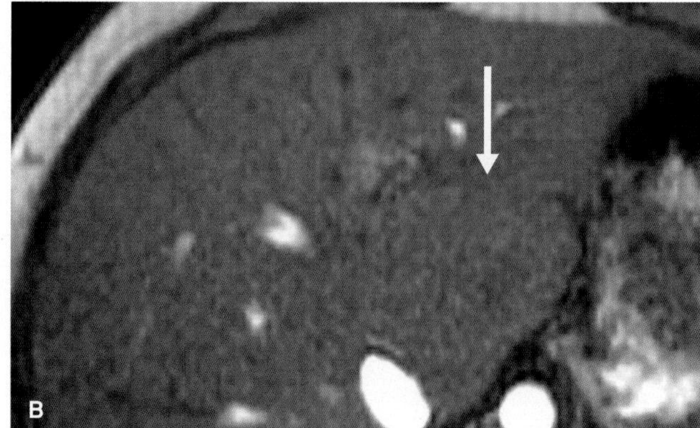

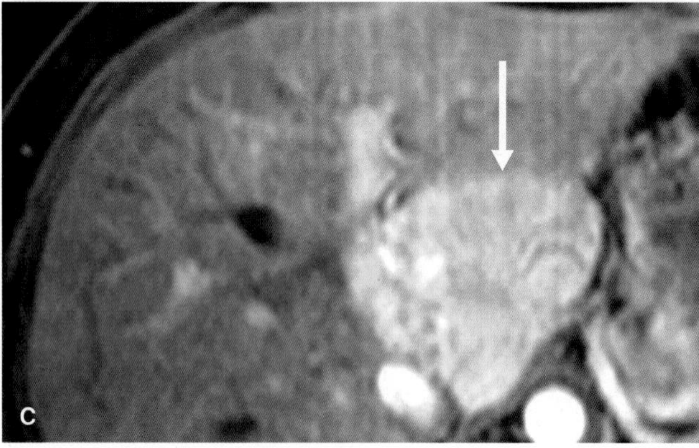

FIGURE 41.21. **Focal Nodular Hyperplasia—MR.** The lesion (*arrows*), consisting of liver elements, is isointense with the hepatic parenchyma on T1WI (**A**) and gradient recall 2D time-of-flight image (**B**). The lesion is clearly depicted by intense enhancement during arterial phase (**C**) postgadolinium administration. The findings are typical of focal nodular hyperplasia. This lesion lacks a central scar.

Liver adenomatosis is considered a separate clinical entity characterized by the presence of multiple adenomas (>10) in an otherwise normal liver in patients, usually young women without risk factors for hepatic adenomas.

Fibrolamellar carcinoma is a hepatocellular malignancy with clinical and pathologic features that are distinct from HCC. Tumors typically present as a large liver mass in an adolescent or young adult (mean age, 23 years) with none of the risk factors for HCC, and without elevation of AFP levels. Cords of tumor are surrounded by prominent fibrous bands that emanate from a central fibrotic scar. The surrounding liver is usually normal without features of cirrhosis or chronic liver disease. The characteristic appearance is a large, lobulated hepatic mass with central scar and calcifications. The central scar with radiating septa mimics the appearance of FNH. Satellite tumor nodules are occasionally present (10% to 15%). Hemorrhage and necrosis are uncommon (10%), but are occasionally massive resulting in a multicystic appearance of the tumor. Although the tumor is less aggressive than HCC, stage at presentation tends to be advanced with malignant adenopathy present. Aggressive surgical management is indicated.

US shows a large lobulated well-defined mass with mixed echogenicity. The central scar is echogenic, if visible.

On CT (Fig. 41.23), the tumor is low attenuation precontrast. The central scar is variably evident (20% to 71%). Calcification may be evident within the fibrous scar. The tumor

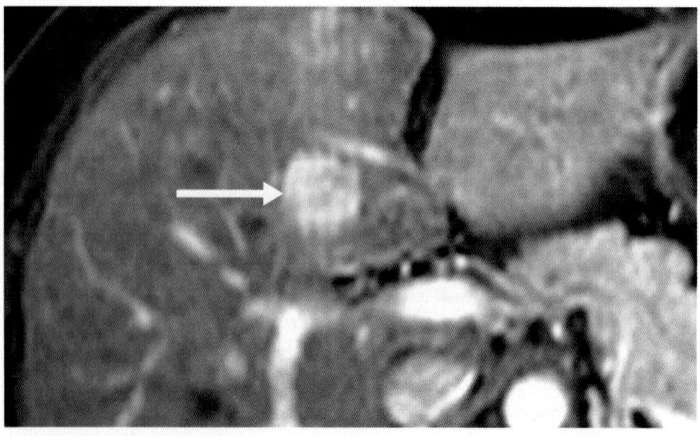

FIGURE 41.22. **Hepatic Adenoma—MR.** Postgadolinium, T1-weighted, fat-suppressed MR image shows intense homogeneous enhancement during arterial phase of a biopsy-proven hepatic adenoma (*arrow*). The MR appearance closely resembles a small hepatocellular carcinoma but the lesion is most often found in a normal liver.

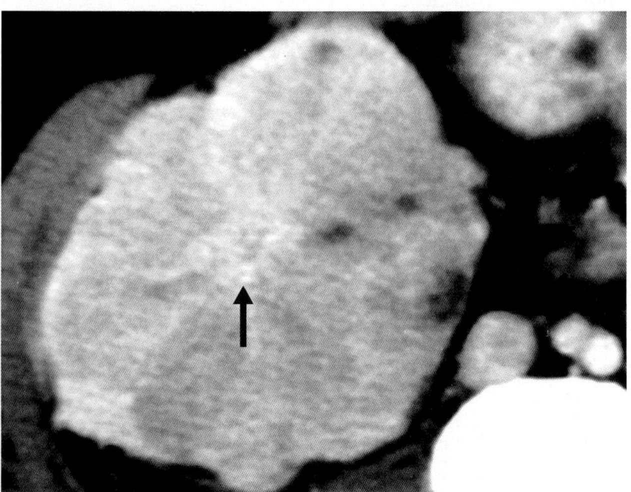

FIGURE 41.23. **Fibrolamellar Hepatocellular Carcinoma—CT.** Delayed postcontrast image demonstrates a large enhancing tumor extending caudally from the right lobe of the liver. A characteristic enhancing stellate central scar (*arrow*) is present.

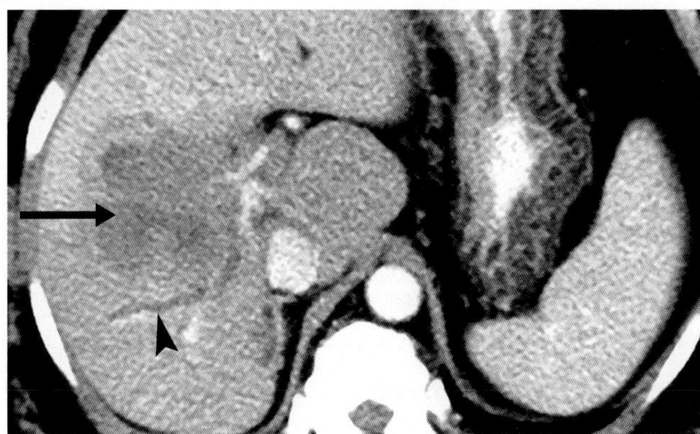

FIGURE 41.24. **Primary Hepatic Lymphoma—CT.** A poorly marginated hypodense, minimally enhancing mass (*arrow*) extends from the porta hepatis occluding blood vessels and causing biliary dilatation (*arrowhead*). Initial diagnosis was cholangiocarcinoma, but biopsy showed B-cell lymphoma.

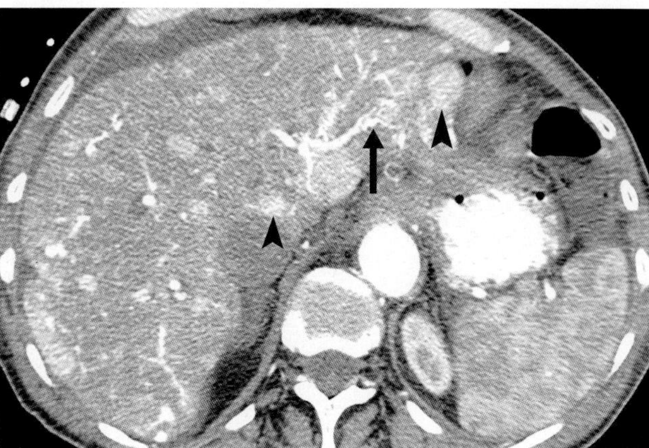

FIGURE 41.25. **Hereditary Hemorrhagic Telangiectasia—CT.** Arterial phase image reveals a nodular contour to the liver (pseudocirrhosis), multiple enhancing confluent vascular masses (*arrowheads*), and tortuous enlarged hepatic arteries (*arrow*).

enhances prominently and heterogeneously on both arterial and portal venous phases. Enhancement of the scar is most evident on delayed scans.

MR shows a usually homogeneous hypointense mass (86%) or an isointense mass (14%) on T1WI. On T2WI the mass is usually hyperintense and much more heterogeneous. The fibrous scar (seen in 80%) is hypointense on all image sequences. Gadolinium enhancement shows the same pattern as CT.

Lymphoma involving the liver is usually diffusely infiltrative and undetectable by imaging methods. The multiple nodule pattern found in 10% of cases resembles metastatic disease. Some cases present as a large poorly defined hypodense mass (Fig. 41.24) with or without satellite nodules. On MR, lymphoma lesions are hypodense on T1WI and of variable intensity on T2WI. Lesions enhance poorly or not at all.

Hematomas show the evolution and breakdown of blood products. Subacute hematomas are bright on T1WI (effect of methemoglobin). Chronic hematomas are dark on T2WI (effect of hemosiderin). Postcontrast images may show rim enhancement.

Hereditary hemorrhagic telangiectasia (Osler–Weber–Rendu syndrome) is an autosomal dominant disorder of fibrovascular dysplasia resulting in multiple telangiectasias and arteriovenous malformations. Telangiectasias are thin-walled dilated vascular channels that appear on the skin and mucous membranes as well as throughout the body in multiple organs. Patients present with epistaxis and intestinal bleeding. About 30% of patients have diffuse telangiectasias and multiple arteriovenous fistulas in the liver. These can result in pain, jaundice, portal hypertension, and high-output cardiac failure. Nodular transformation of the liver parenchyma without fibrosis occurs and is called pseudocirrhosis (Fig. 41.25). Telangiectases appear as hypervascular rounded masses resembling an asterisk, usually a few millimeters in size. They may become confluent to form large vascular masses. Dilated and tortuous intra- and extrahepatic arteries are usually evident.

Peliosis hepatis is a rare disorder associated with chronic wasting from cancer or tuberculosis, or associated with use of oral contraceptives or anabolic steroids. Cystic dilatation of the hepatic sinusoids and multiple small (1 to 3 mm) blood-filled spaces characterize the lesions. MR shows variable hypointense or hyperintense signal due to hemorrhage on T1WI. On T2WI lesions are hyperintense. Postcontrast images show no significant arterial phase enhancement with progressive delayed enhancement on portal venous and delayed-phase images.

Benign hepatic cyst is a common hepatic mass, found in 5% of the population. Cysts range in size from microscopic to 20 cm. Hepatic cysts do not communicate with the biliary tree. Tiny cysts are responsible for many of the "hypoattenuating lesions too small to characterize" seen on MDCT. Larger cysts tend to occur in clusters with cysts of varying size resulting in sharply defined, but lobulated, margins and septations.

US accurately characterizes hepatic cysts. Typical cysts are anechoic with thin walls and may have fine thin septa. Posterior acoustic enhancement confirms their fluid nature. Occasionally, hepatic cysts have internal debris, especially if they have internal hemorrhage or previous infection.

CT shows low internal attenuation near water, thin walls, and thin septa without enhancing solid components (Fig. 41.26).

MR shows homogeneous low internal signal on T1WI and homogeneous intense high internal signal on T2WI. Cysts do not enhance following contrast administration.

Polycystic liver disease is in the spectrum of autosomal dominant polycystic disease and occasionally occurs in the absence of polycystic kidneys. The number and size of cysts increase over time and may eventually result in massive hepatomegaly

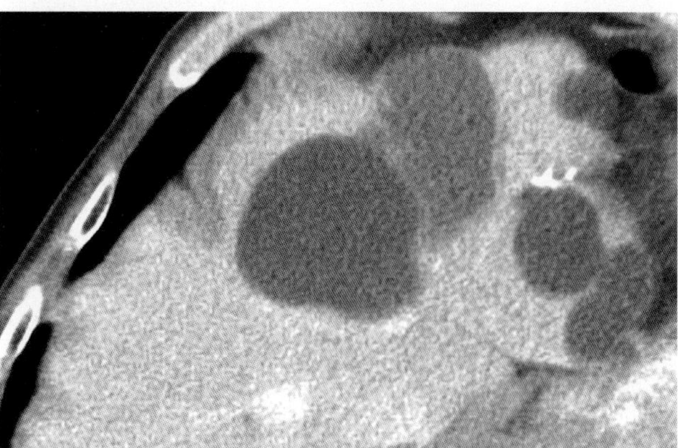

FIGURE 41.26. **Hepatic Cysts—CT.** Multiple hepatic cysts are an incidental finding on this postcontrast CT in a 78-year-old patient. The cysts are unilocular, well-defined, homogeneously low in attenuation, and without solid or enhancing components.

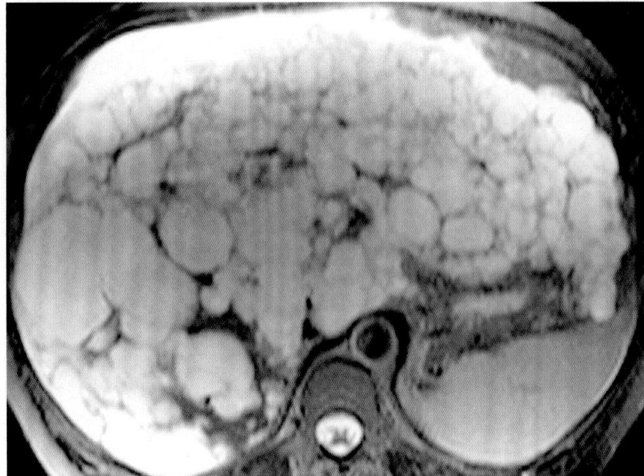

FIGURE 41.27. **Polycystic Liver Disease—MR.** Axial T2WI shows near-complete replacement of the liver parenchyma by innumerable cysts of varying size. This patient has a variant of autosomal dominant polycystic disease.

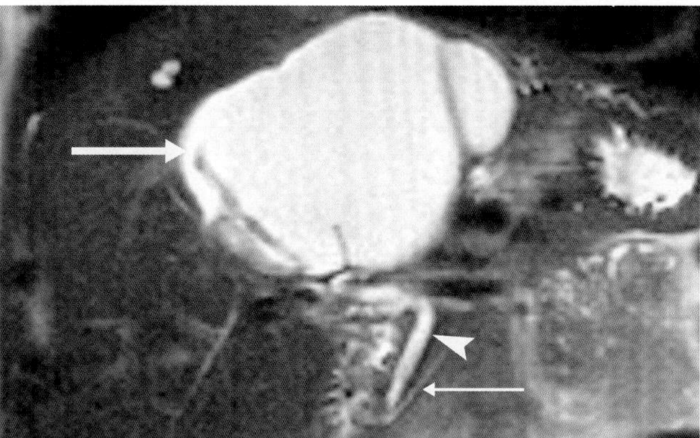

FIGURE 41.29. **Biliary Cystadenoma—MR.** Coronal T2WI shows a large cystic mass (*large arrow*) with prominent septations. No mural nodules or papillary projections were identified. Surgical removal confirmed a benign biliary cystadenoma. Because of the potential of malignant transformation and the difficulty in differentiating benign from malignant lesions by imaging, surgical removal is routinely recommended. Coronal T2WI nicely demonstrates the distal common bile duct (*arrowhead*) and pancreatic duct (*skinny arrow*) near the ampulla.

and affect hepatic function (Fig. 41.27). Cysts are prone to hemorrhage and infection.

Bile duct hamartomas (von Meyenburg complexes) are small benign neoplasms consisting of dilated cystic branching bile ducts embedded within fibrous tissue. They appear as multiple tiny (<1 cm) cystic lesions throughout the liver, best recognized on MR. They are low signal on T1WI, high signal on T2WI (Fig. 41.28), and show peripheral enhancement postcontrast. CT shows widespread tiny cystic lesions. The cysts are usually too small to be seen with US.

Biliary cystadenoma/cystadenocarcinoma is a rare cystic neoplasm of the biliary epithelium. Cystadenomas are premalignant and on a continuum of disease with cystadenocarcinomas. Tumors typically contain mucin and appear as large (up to 35 cm) multiloculated cystic mass. Fine septations are seen in cystadenomas. Cystadenocarcinomas may have mural nodules and papillary projections. The presence of thick, coarse calcification suggests malignancy. Differentiation of benign from malignant lesions by imaging may not be possible. Treatment is surgical in any case.

US shows the large multicystic mass, septations, and mural nodules and papillary projections, if present. CT shows enhancement of the wall and any solid components. Calcifications are well shown by CT and favor cystadenocarcinoma. MR depicts the mass as multiseptated cystic with low signal on T1WI and high signal on T2WI (Fig. 41.29). Complications such as hemorrhage or infection change the signal characteristics of the fluid. Calcifications are easily overlooked with MR. Postcontrast images demonstrate enhancement of the rim and internal solid components.

Pyogenic abscess is usually caused by *Escherichia coli, Staphylococcus aureus, Streptococcus,* or anaerobic bacteria. Patients present with fever and pain. Destruction of liver parenchyma results in a solitary cavity or a tight group of individual loculated abscesses (Fig. 41.30). Lesions may be echogenic and appear solid on US. A peripheral rim enhances with contrast. Gas is present within the lesion in 20% of cases. Diagnosis is confirmed by percutaneous aspiration. Catheter or surgical drainage is often indicated.

Amebic abscess, caused by *Entamoeba histolytica* infection, is usually solitary with thick nodular walls. The lesion may be indistinguishable from pyogenic abscess (Fig. 41.31),

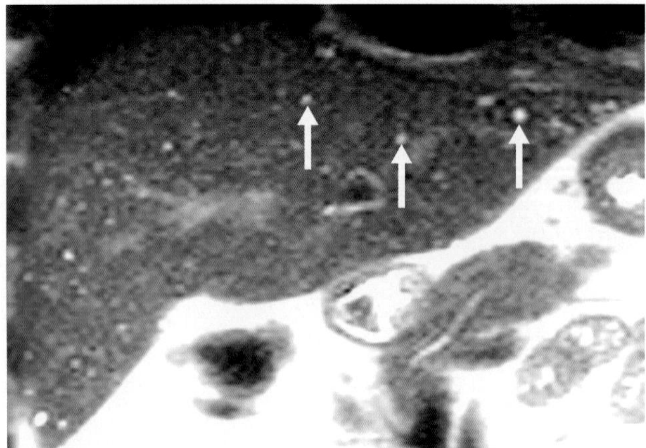

FIGURE 41.28. **Biliary Hamartomas—MR.** Coronal plane T2WI shows innumerable tiny cysts (*arrows*) scattered throughout the liver parenchyma. These von Meyenburg complexes are small benign neoplasms without clinical significance or malignant potential.

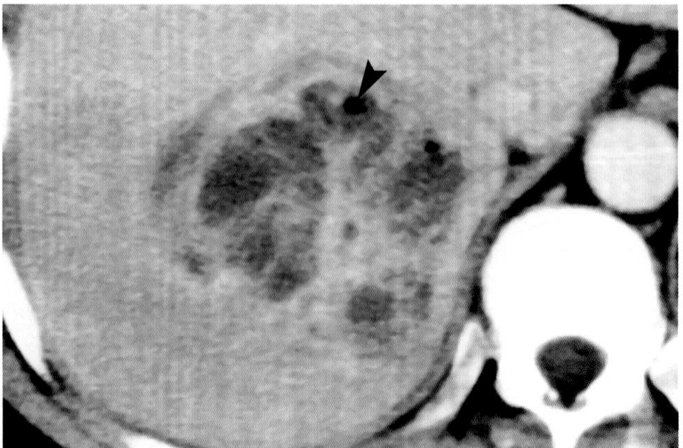

FIGURE 41.30. **Pyogenic Abscess—CT.** Postcontrast scan shows multiple low-density areas separated by enhancing septa and representing abscess locules. Air bubbles (*arrowhead*) are evident within the lesion.

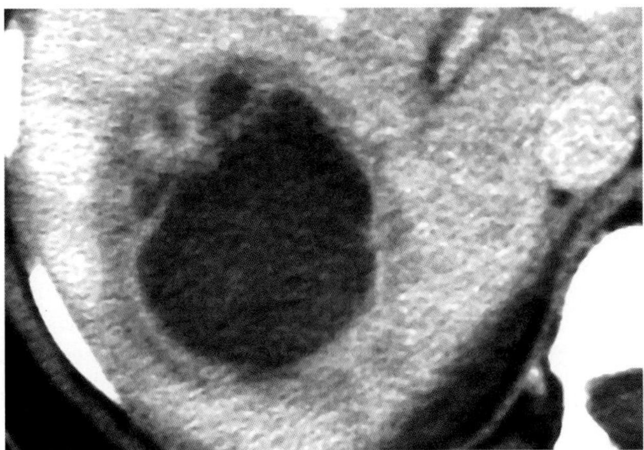

FIGURE 41.31. **Amebic Abscess—CT.** Postcontrast CT image reveals a thick-walled fluid collection in the right hepatic lobe. Differentiation of amebic from pyogenic liver abscess is made by history, serology, or image-guided aspiration.

however, the patient often resides or has travelled to endemic areas (India, Africa, the Far East, Central and South America). Intestinal amebic infection usually causes no symptoms but liver abscesses present with abdominal pain, fever, and weight loss. Amebic abscesses commonly occur in the right lobe of the liver causing elevation of the right hemidiaphragm, and may rupture through the diaphragm into the pleural space. In the United States, the diagnosis is typically confirmed by serology and the patient is treated with metronidazole or tinidazole. In endemic areas, the diagnosis is confirmed by aspiration of "anchovy paste" material and the patient is treated by repeated aspiration or catheter drainage.

Hydatid cyst is due to infestation with *Echinococcus granulosus* or *E. multilocularis* tapeworm. The parasite is endemic in central and northern Europe, the Mediterranean, northern Asia, China, Japan, Turkey, and parts of North America. The liver is the most common organ affected (95%). Single or multiple cystic masses usually have well-defined walls that commonly calcify (50%). The cyst wall and septations usually enhance. Daughter cysts may be visualized within the parent cyst (75%) (Fig. 41.32). Diagnostic aspiration carries a risk of anaphylactic reaction. Treatment is mebendazole or surgical excision.

Cystic/necrotic tumor must always be considered for atypical cystic masses. Metastases may be necrotic or predominantly cystic. HCC is occasionally cystic. Undifferentiated embryonal sarcomas are multicystic and seen in older children, adolescents, and young adults.

Tiny hypoattenuating lesions on MDCT are detected with increased frequency related to thinner collimation, improved resolution, and rapid, multiphase, postcontrast scanning (Fig. 41.33). Lesions smaller than 1 cm are difficult to characterize and often too small to biopsy. Differential diagnoses include cysts, hemangiomas, and metastases. Statistically most of these tiny lesions are benign. In a patient with known malignancy follow-up scans are needed to exclude metastatic disease.

BILIARY TREE

Imaging Methods. Imaging of the biliary tree uses assorted techniques that differ in degrees of invasiveness. US is the preferred screening method for biliary obstruction because of its low cost, high accuracy in detecting biliary dilatation,

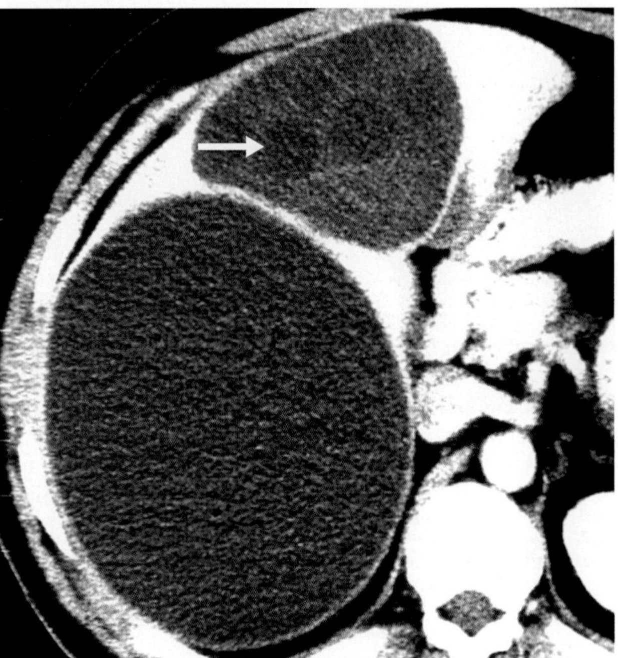

FIGURE 41.32. **Hydatid Cyst—CT.** Two large well-defined cystic masses in the liver are caused by infestation with *Echinococcus granulosus*. Daughter cysts (*arrow*) are faintly visible in the smaller lesion.

and convenience. However, US is limited by inconsistent visualization of the distal common bile duct and low sensitivity for determining the cause of obstruction. CT with or without contrast demonstrates biliary dilatation. Unenhanced MDCT has a reported sensitivity of 88% in detection of stones in the common bile duct. Standard MR can also demonstrate biliary

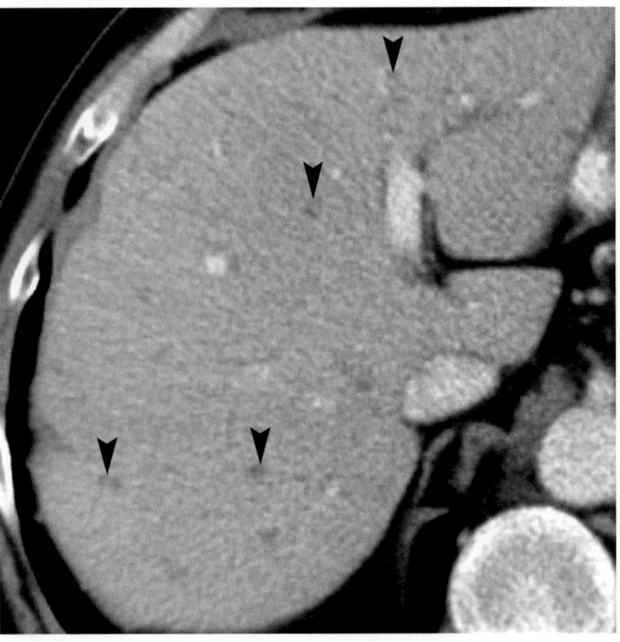

FIGURE 41.33. **Too Small to Characterize.** MDCT shows multiple tiny low attenuation lesions (*arrowheads*) that are too small to definitively characterize. Even in patients with known malignancy these lesions are usually benign. However, on follow-up in some patients, they will prove to be early metastatic lesions. They are usually identified on high-quality postcontrast CT only. Image-guided biopsy can usually not be performed because the lesions cannot be identified on US or noncontrast CT.

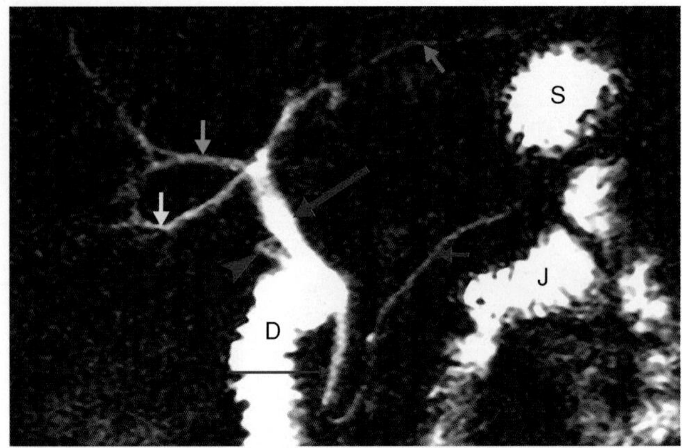

FIGURE 41.34. Normal MRCP. Image from an MRCP in a patient who has had a cholecystectomy shows the cystic duct remnant (*red arrowhead*), common bile duct (*skinny red arrow*), common hepatic duct (*fat red arrow*), pancreatic duct (*small red arrow*), left hepatic duct (*small blue arrow*), anterior branch of the right hepatic duct (*small yellow arrow*), and posterior branch of the right hepatic (*small green arrow*). Relatively static fluid in the stomach (*S*), duodenum (*D*), and jejunum (*J*) is high signal on this maximum intensity projection (MIP) T2WI with prolonged acquisition time.

dilation, and appears more effective than CT or US in demonstrating associated tumors.

MR cholangiopancreatography (MRCP) provides excellent visualization of the biliary tree by taking advantage of the high water content of bile and its relative stasis compared to flowing blood. MRCP is performed using heavily T2-weighted sequences with acquisition times slower than for moving blood, producing high signal in the biliary tree and signal voids in nearby blood vessels. Extreme T2 weighting demonstrates bright bile ducts with dark surrounding soft tissues (Fig. 41.34). However, any static fluid will also be bright on MRCP images, so ascites, hepatic and renal cysts, and fluid in the bowel may obscure the biliary tree. "Thick slab" MRCP uses slice thickness of 40 to 60 mm with fat saturation to improve visualization of the biliary tree. High resolution three-dimensional acquisitions and maximum intensity projection (MIP) images produce impressive displays of the entire biliary tree. MRCP is combined with standard MR of the liver to produce a comprehensive examination for detection and staging of tumors. Similar to contrast cholangiography, stones are seen as hypodense filling defects (Table 41.9).

Endoscopic retrograde cholangiography (ERCP) is now used primarily to guide therapy such as stent placement for biliary strictures, stone extraction, or sphincterotomy. Direct contrast injection of the biliary tree during ERCP produces higher resolution images than MRCP, but duct visualization is limited to the ducts that can be filled retrograde. Ducts proximal to a high-grade obstruction are not visualized. Morbidity for ERCP-guided therapy approaches 8% including hemorrhage, duodenal perforation, acute pancreatitis, infections, and stent-related complications.

Percutaneous transhepatic cholangiography (PTC) is mainly used to guide therapy when the biliary tree cannot be accessed endoscopically. Operative cholangiography is used to visualize nonpalpable bile duct stones at surgery, and T-tube cholangiography is used to visualize common duct stones following surgery.

Radionuclide imaging, utilizing technetium-99m iminodiacetic acid, is useful for showing the patency of biliary-enteric anastomoses and for demonstrating bile leaks and fistulae. Scintigraphy has the greatest sensitivity for early obstruction.

CT cholangiography is performed using agents such as iopanoic acid formerly used for oral cholecystography. Hepatobiliary agents for MRCP such as gadoxetate disodium (Eovist®) are utilized for contrast-enhanced cholangiogram, bile leak, suspected gallbladder obstruction, and hepaticojejunostomy evaluations.

TABLE 41.9

CAUSES OF FILLING DEFECTS IN THE BILE DUCTS

Biliary stones
Air bubbles
Blood clots
Neoplasms Cholangiocarcinoma Ampullary carcinoma Granular cell myoblastoma Mesenchymal tumor
Parasites Ascaris lumbricoides Liver fluke

Anatomy of the Biliary Tract. The bile ducts arise as bile capillaries between hepatocytes and join progressively larger branches until two main trunks are formed draining the right and left lobes of the liver. The ducts of the left hepatic lobe are more anterior than those of the right hepatic lobe. This relationship must be kept in mind when contrast cholangiography is performed. Contrast agents flow to the most dependent portions of the biliary tree and may not opacify nondependent ducts. Failure to fill ducts before gravitational repositioning must not be interpreted as evidence of obstruction.

The right and left hepatic ducts combine to form the *common hepatic duct* (CHD) that courses with the portal vein and hepatic artery in the porta hepatis. The *cystic duct* courses posteriorly and inferiorly from the gallbladder to join the CHD and form the *common bile duct* (CBD). The location of the junction of the cystic duct and CHD is variable and often not apparent on routine cross-section imaging resulting in the less-specific term "*common duct.*" The CBD runs ventral to the portal vein and to the right of the hepatic artery, descending from the porta hepatis along the free right margin of the hepatoduodenal ligament to the duodenal bulb. The distal third of the CBD turns caudally and descends in the groove between the descending duodenum and the head of the pancreas just anterior to the IVC. The CBD tapers distally as it ends in the *sphincter of Oddi*, which protrudes into the duodenum as the *ampulla of Vater*. The CBD and the pancreatic duct share a common orifice in 60% of individuals and have separate orifices in the remainder. However, because of their close proximity, tumors of the ampulla region generally obstruct both ducts. The CHD and CBD are considered to be extrahepatic bile ducts (EHBD).

Normal intrahepatic bile ducts (IHBD) are occasionally seen on US and on postcontrast MDCT with thin (≤3 mm) collimation. Normal IHBD do not exceed 40% of the diameter of the adjacent portal vein, or 2 mm in diameter in the central liver, or 1.8 mm in diameter in the peripheral liver. The normal extrahepatic CBD is routinely visualized and does not exceed 6 to 7 mm in internal diameter. Normal ducts appear larger on contrast cholangiography studies because of distention by forceful contrast injection and magnification of conventional radiography. Increased CBD diameter has been attributed to aging and previous cholecystectomy. These relationships are, however, controversial. Care must be taken to differentiate an enlarged common duct from an enlarged hepatic artery. Color Doppler is useful to make this differentiation on US. Contrast enhancement of blood vessels makes differentiation easy on CT.

MRCP and cholangiographic studies demonstrate IHBD branches that parallel the portal veins and correspond to the Couinaud segments of the liver. The right hepatic duct drains segments 5 to 8 and is formed by the junction of the more horizontal coursing right posterior duct draining 6 and 7 and the more vertically coursing right anterior duct draining 5 and 8. The left hepatic duct is formed by segmental ducts draining segments 2, 3, and 4. The duct of the caudate lobe (segment 1) joins either the right or left hepatic duct. Normal anatomy of the biliary tree is present in only 58% of the population. Variations include drainage of the right posterior duct into the left hepatic duct (13% to 19%), triple confluence with the right posterior, right anterior, and left hepatic ducts uniting at a single position (11%), and anomalies of the cystic duct including low insertion on the CBD, long parallel course with the CHD, and insertion on the medial rather than lateral side of the CBD. These anomalies have significant importance to the biliary surgeon.

Biliary Dilatation

CT, US, and MR are highly effective at demonstrating the anatomic finding of biliary dilatation, which is usually equated with biliary obstruction. However, biliary obstruction may be present intermittently or in the early stage without biliary dilation being present. Alternatively, biliary dilatation may be present without obstruction, such as after surgical decompression or bypass. Patients with clinical evidence of biliary obstruction (i.e., elevated alkaline phosphatase and direct hyperbilirubinemia) may not have biliary dilation. Hepatitis causes swelling of hepatocytes, which blocks biliary capillaries and causes intrahepatic cholestasis without surgical obstruction.

Imaging signs of biliary dilation include (a) multiple branching tubular, round, or oval structures that course toward the porta hepatis, (b) diameter of IHBD larger than 40% of the diameter of the adjacent portal vein (Fig. 41.35), (c) dilation of the common duct greater than 6 mm, and (d) gallbladder diameter greater than 5 cm, when obstruction is distal to the cystic duct. The "double duct" sign refers to dilatation of both the common bile duct and the pancreatic duct in the head of the pancreas. Dilatation of both ducts is usually caused by a tumor at the ampulla. Benign disease is responsible for approximately 75% of cases of obstructive jaundice in the adult, while malignant disease causes the remainder. Gradual tapering of a dilated common duct suggests benign stricture. Gallstones may be identified in the bile duct surrounded by a crescent of bile. Abrupt termination of a dilated common duct is characteristic of a malignant process.

Infected bile is present in up to 10% of cases of complete biliary obstruction and 60% of cases of partial or intermittent biliary obstruction. Intravenous antibiotic therapy is warranted prior to biliary interventional procedures in the obstructed patient.

Causes of biliary dilation and obstruction (Table 41.10) include the following.

Choledocholithiasis is responsible for approximately 20% of cases of obstructive jaundice in the adult (Fig. 41.36). Gallstones are present in the gallbladder in 10% of the population, but the presence of stones in the gallbladder does not necessarily mean that stones are the cause of ductal obstruction. In addition, 1% to 3% of patients with choledocholithiasis will have no stones in the gallbladder.

The sensitivity of US for stones in the bile ducts ranges from 20% to 80%. Stone detection by US is much improved when the CBD is dilated and the pancreatic head is well visualized. CT sensitivity is 70% to 80% with stones appearing as intraluminal masses of varying attenuation (Fig. 41.33). Contrast studies and MRCP have the highest sensitivity for stone detection (95% to 99%) and demonstrate stones as dark filling defects within bright bile (Fig. 41.37). MRCP may miss stones smaller than 3 mm because they are lost within high signal fluid.

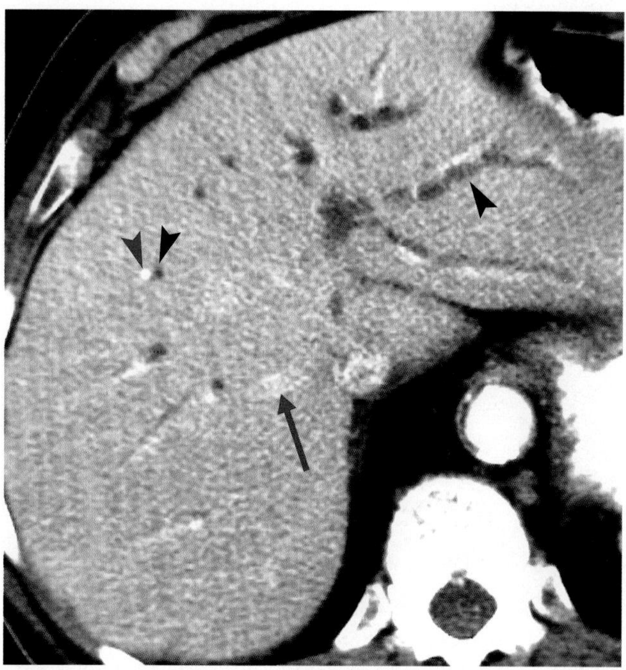

FIGURE 41.35. **Biliary Dilation—CT.** Scan demonstrates dilated intrahepatic ducts (*black arrowheads*) easily differentiated from portal veins (*red arrowhead*) and hepatic veins (*arrow*) by contrast enhancement of the blood vessels. Note that the diameter of the bile ducts clearly exceeds 40% of the diameter of the adjacent portal vein. Biliary dilatation in this patient was caused by adenocarcinoma of the head of the pancreas.

Imaging signs of stones within the bile ducts include (a) stones layer dependently within allowing a crescent of bile to outline the anterior portion of the stone (the "crescent sign"); (b) stones are usually geometric or angulated in shape and lamellated in appearance; and (c) periductal edema and thickening and enhancement of the wall of the bile duct occur with

TABLE 41.10

CAUSES OF BILIARY TRACT OBSTRUCTION

BENIGN—75%
Benign stricture
Surgery/instrumentation
Trauma
Stone passage
Pancreatitis
Cholangitis
Choledochal cyst
Stone impacted in duct
Parasite (ascariasis)
Liver cyst
MALIGNANT—25%
Pancreatic carcinoma
Ampullary/duodenal carcinoma
Cholangiocarcinoma
Metastasis

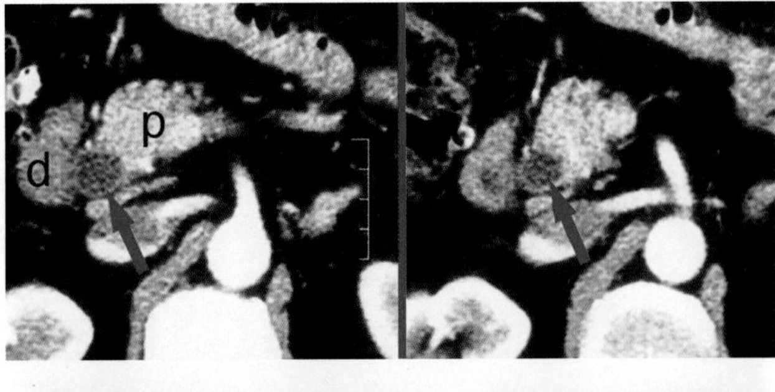

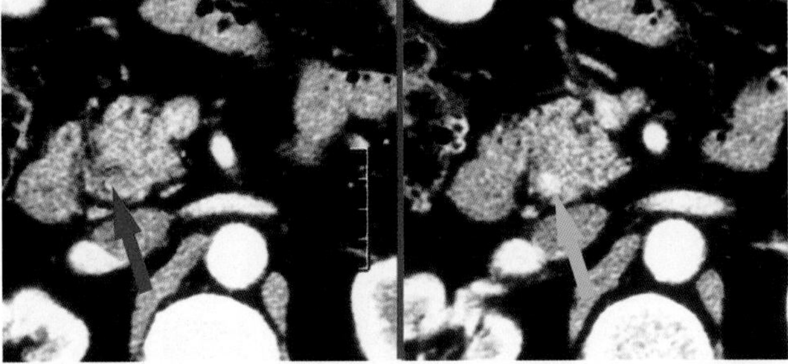

FIGURE 41.36. **Obstructing Stone in Common Bile Duct—CT.** Serial CT images obtained from a jaundiced patient demonstrate dilatation of the common bile duct (*red arrows*) due to an obstructing high-density gallstone (*green arrow*) impacted in the distal common bile duct. This stone is high attenuation indicating calcium content. On CT, stones vary from fat density to calcium density. The bile duct above the calcific stone is low attenuation due to its bile content. Note the course of the common bile duct in relationship to the head of the pancreas (*p*) and descending duodenum (*d*).

impacted stones or infection. Wall thickening and enhancement are also seen with tumors.

Benign stricture is the cause of 40% to 45% of obstructive jaundice in the adult. Causes of benign stricture include trauma, surgery, prior biliary interventional procedures, recurrent cholangitis, chronic pancreatitis, previous passage of stones through the bile ducts, radiation therapy, and perforated duodenal ulcer. The wall of the involved CBD enhances minimally with benign strictures, while hyperenhancement of the CBD during portal venous phase is evidence of malignant stricture.

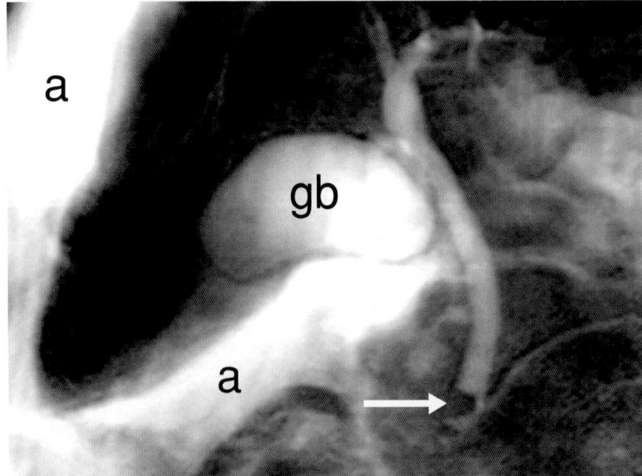

FIGURE 41.37. **Choledocholithiasis—MR.** MRCP image demonstrates two stones (*arrow*) seen as filling defects in the distal common bile duct. Ascites (*a*) outlines the liver. A normal gallbladder (*gb*) is evident.

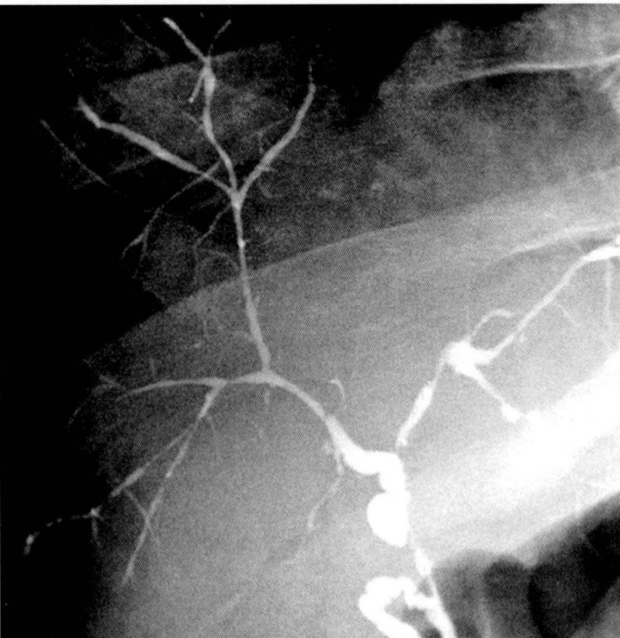

FIGURE 41.38. **Primary Sclerosing Cholangitis—ERCP.** Radiograph from an ERCP demonstrates the focal irregular strictures and focal mild dilatation of intrahepatic bile ducts typical of early-stage primary sclerosing cholangitis.

Pancreatitis is responsible for approximately 8% of cases of biliary obstruction. Inflammation, fibrosis, and inflammatory masses narrow the bile ducts.

Primary sclerosing cholangitis (PSC) is associated with a history of ulcerative colitis (50% to 70% of cases). PSC is an idiopathic, fibrosing, chronic inflammatory disease characterized by insidious onset of jaundice with progressive disease affecting both IHBD and EHBD. Imaging findings include (a) IHBD dilatation, (b) IHBD strictures, and (c) EHBD wall thickening, wall enhancement, and stenosis. Alternating dilation and stenosis (Fig. 41.38) produce a characteristic beaded pattern of intrahepatic ducts that serves as a key diagnostic finding. Small saccular outpouchings (duct diverticula), demonstrated on cholangiography, are also considered to be pathognomonic. Complications include biliary cirrhosis (50%) and cholangiocarcinoma.

HIV-associated cholangitis is characterized by thickening of the walls of the bile ducts and the gallbladder due to inflammation and edema. Infection by opportunistic organisms, most commonly Cytomegalovirus and *Cryptosporidium*, as well as reaction to the human immunodeficiency virus itself, are implicated as the cause of observed disease. Bile ducts are commonly dilated in association with stenosis at the ampulla. Ulcers in the common duct, inflammatory changes in the duodenum, and additional evidence of infection with opportunistic organisms are commonly associated. The incidence of this disease has decreased with use of antiretroviral agents to treat HIV infection.

Acute bacterial cholangitis occurs in the setting of biliary obstruction and is life-threatening with mortality as high as 65%. Patients present with fever, pain, and jaundice (the Charcot triad). Infection is usually polymicrobial with gram-negative rods predominating. Findings include biliary dilatation, usually caused by a stone in the duct, associated with peribiliary contrast enhancement and periductal edema reflecting spread of the inflammatory process to adjacent parenchyma

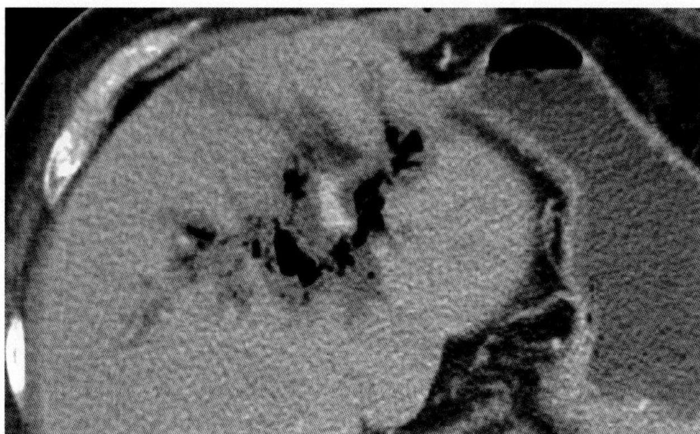

FIGURE 41.39. **Acute Bacterial Cholangitis—CT.** Postcontrast image demonstrates irregular collections of air expanding bile ducts surrounded by low attenuation edema. Pyogenic cholangitis resulted in necrosis of the bile ducts.

(Fig. 41.39). Treatment is urgent and based upon relieving the obstruction and antibiotics.

Recurrent pyogenic cholangitis has previously been called Oriental cholangiohepatitis because it is an endemic disease in Southeast Asia. It is characterized by recurrent attacks of jaundice, abdominal pain, fever, and chills. IHBD and EHBD are dilated and filled with soft pigmented stones and pus. The disease is associated with parasitic infestation (*Clonorchis sinensis*, *Ascaris lumbricoides*) and nutritional deficiency. Findings include intraductal stones, severe extrahepatic biliary dilation, focal strictures, pneumobilia, and straightening and rigidity of intrahepatic ducts. Complications include liver abscess, biloma, pancreatitis, cholangiocarcinoma, and atrophy of the liver parenchyma.

Caroli disease is an uncommon congenital anomaly of the biliary tract characterized by saccular ectasia of the IHBD without biliary obstruction. Only one hepatic lobe or segment, or the entire liver may be affected. The EHBD are spared in 50% of cases. Findings include (a) saccular dilatation of IHBD giving the appearance on cross-sectional imaging of scattered intrahepatic cysts that communicate with the biliary tree (Fig. 41.40); (b) enhancing fibrovascular bundles are seen centrally within many of the dilated ducts producing the

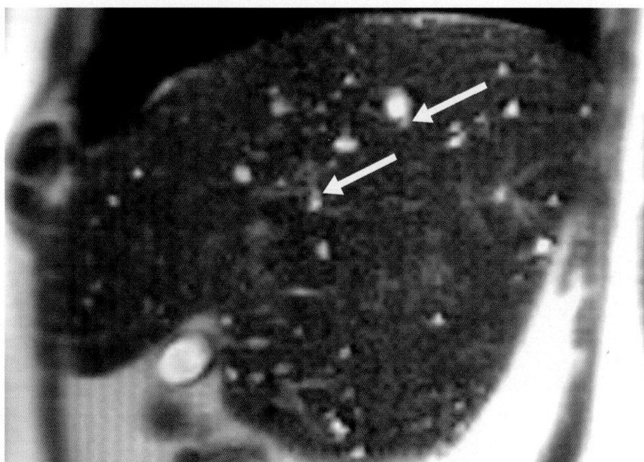

FIGURE 41.40. **Caroli Disease—MR.** Sagittal T2WI shows numerous small high signal cystic lesions scattered throughout the liver. Careful inspection on this and other images shows connection (*arrows*) between the cystic lesions and the biliary tree.

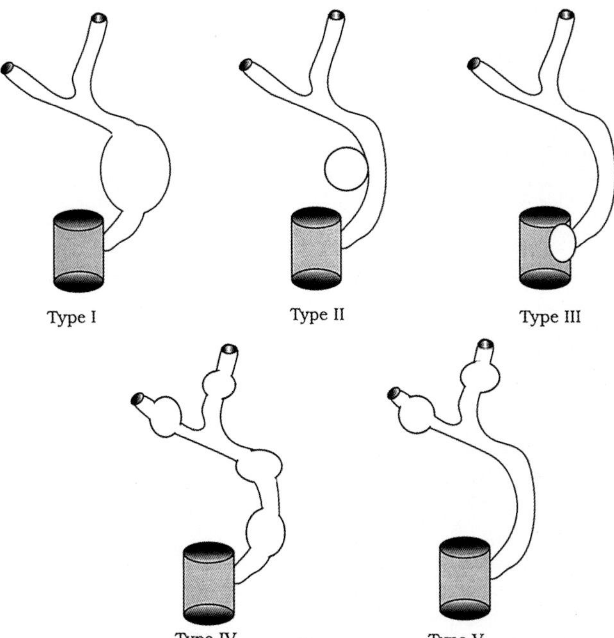

FIGURE 41.41. **Classification of Congenital Biliary Cysts.** Type I choledochal cysts (80% to 90% of cases) are focal, saccular or fusiform, dilatations of the common bile duct. Type II cysts (2%) are true diverticuli of the common bile duct. Type III cysts (1.4% to 5%) are termed choledochoceles and are dilatations of the terminal intraduodenal portion of the common bile duct. Type IV cysts (19%) refer to multiple intra- and extrahepatic bile duct cysts. Caroli disease is classified Type V.

characteristic "central dot sign"; (c) segmental distribution of the bile duct abnormality with normal appearance of unaffected liver segments; (d) cholangiography shows a characteristic pattern of focal biliary narrowing and saccular dilatation; and (e) dilatation of the CBD (10 to 30 mm) in half the cases. The disease is associated with medullary sponge kidney and autosomal recessive polycystic kidney disease. Complications include pyogenic cholangitis, liver abscess, and biliary stones. Cholangiocarcinoma develops in 7% of cases. Most cases present in childhood. Autosomal recessive inheritance is evident in many cases.

Choledochal cysts are uncommon congenital anomalies of the biliary tree characterized by cystic dilation of the bile ducts. Many (60%) present in infancy or childhood, while the remaining are not discovered until adulthood. Some are discovered during fetal US. The condition is much more common in females (70% to 84% of cases). Patients present with abdominal pain, mass, and jaundice. The Todani classification (1977) is typically used to describe choledochal cysts (Fig. 41.41). Type I lesions are most common (80% to 90%), are confined to the EHBD, and appear as fusiform or saccular dilatations (Fig. 41.42) of the CHD, CBD, or segments of each. Type II lesions are diverticula of the CBD attached by a narrow stalk. Type III lesions are termed choledochoceles and are focal dilatations of the intraduodenal portion of the CBD, closely resembling ureteroceles. Type IV lesions are defined as multiple focal dilatations of the IHBD and EHBD usually with a focal large cystic dilatation of the CBD. Type V lesions referred to Caroli disease, which is more appropriately classified as a disease separate from choledochal cyst.

Pancreatic and ampullary carcinomas are the cause of 20% to 25% of cases of biliary obstruction in the adult. Metastatic disease, from lung, breast, gastrointestinal tumors, and lymphoma, accounts for 2% of cases.

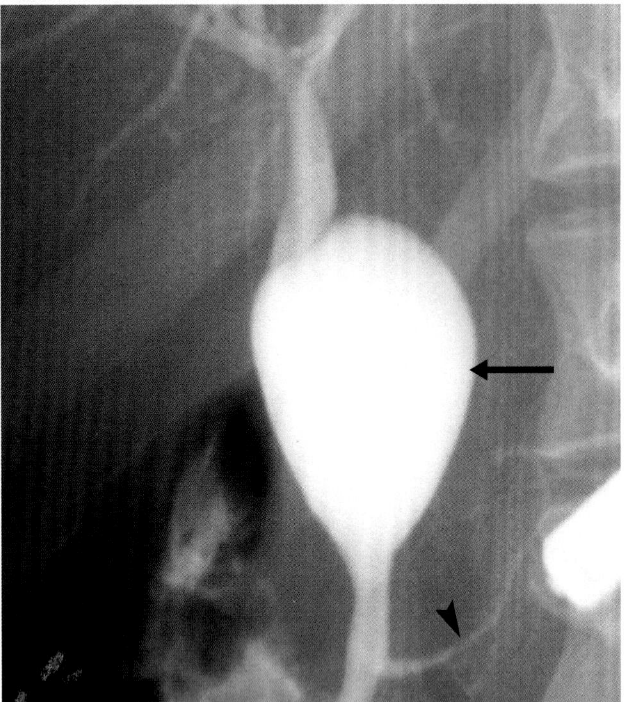

FIGURE 41.42. Choledochal Cyst—Type I—ERCP. Radiograph from endoscopic retrograde cholangiography demonstrates saccular dilation (*arrow*) of the common bile duct typical of the most common form of choledochal cyst, type I. Additionally noted is the accessory pancreatic duct (of Santorini) (*arrowhead*).

Metastases may present as intraductal filling defects. Colorectal cancers are the most common primary tumors associated with intraluminal biliary metastases. Findings that favor metastases over cholangiocarcinoma are the presence of a contiguous parenchymal mass and expansion of the duct at the site of the intraluminal mass in a patient with known colorectal cancer.

Cholangiocarcinoma is the second most common malignant primary hepatic tumor. Tumors arise from the epithelium of bile ducts and are usually adenocarcinomas (90%). Growth patterns include mass-forming, periductal infiltrating, and intraductal polypoid. Cross-sectional imaging is used to detect adenopathy and hepatic metastases. Prognosis is poor, with less than 20% of tumors being resectable.

Peripheral cholangiocarcinoma (10%) presents as an intrahepatic hypodense mass sometimes (25%) causing peripheral biliary dilatation (Fig. 41.43). MDCT demonstrates a homogeneous low attenuation mass with delayed, mild, thin, incomplete, rim-like enhancement. Additional findings may include capsular retraction and satellite nodules. Findings which favor peripheral cholangiocarcinoma over HCC include (a) arterial phase target enhancement, (b) portal venous and delayed-phase central enhancement, (c) retraction of the liver surface, (d) biliary obstruction disproportionate to the size of the mass, and (e) elevated cancer antigen 19-9 (CA 19-9) and carcinoembryonic antigen (CEA).

Hilar cholangiocarcinoma (Klatskin tumor) (25%) occurs near the junction of the right and left bile ducts (Fig. 41.44). The tumor is usually small, poorly differentiated, aggressive, and causes obstruction of both ductal systems. Surgical resection is the only hope for cure. Imaging plays a vital role in determining surgical candidates.

Extrahepatic cholangiocarcinoma (65%) causes stenosis or obstruction of the common bile duct in most cases (95%) and presents as an intraductal polypoid mass in 5%.

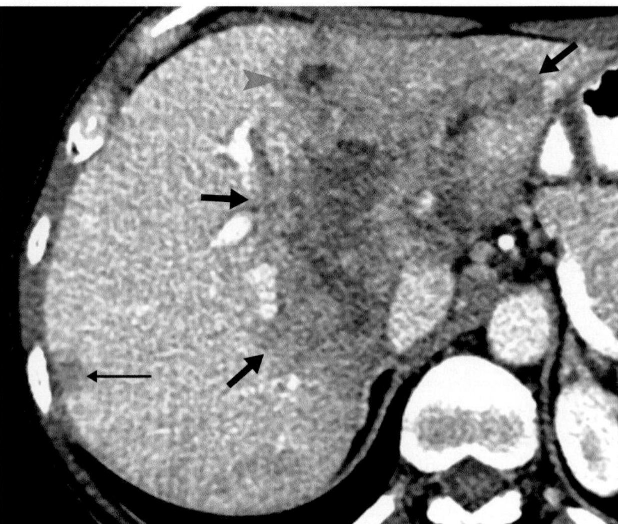

FIGURE 41.43. Cholangiocarcinoma—Peripheral—CT. Postcontrast CT shows a low attenuation tumor (*fat arrows*) with ill-defined margins infiltrating the central liver and obstructing portal and hepatic veins. Satellite lesions (*blue arrowhead*) and metastases (*skinny arrow*) are evident.

Infiltrating cholangiocarcinoma shows thickening of the wall of the involved bile duct with hyperenhancement during arterial phase. Predisposing conditions include choledochal cyst, ulcerative colitis, Caroli disease, *Clonorchis sinensis* infection, and PSC. The tumor may be infiltrative, desmoplastic, and

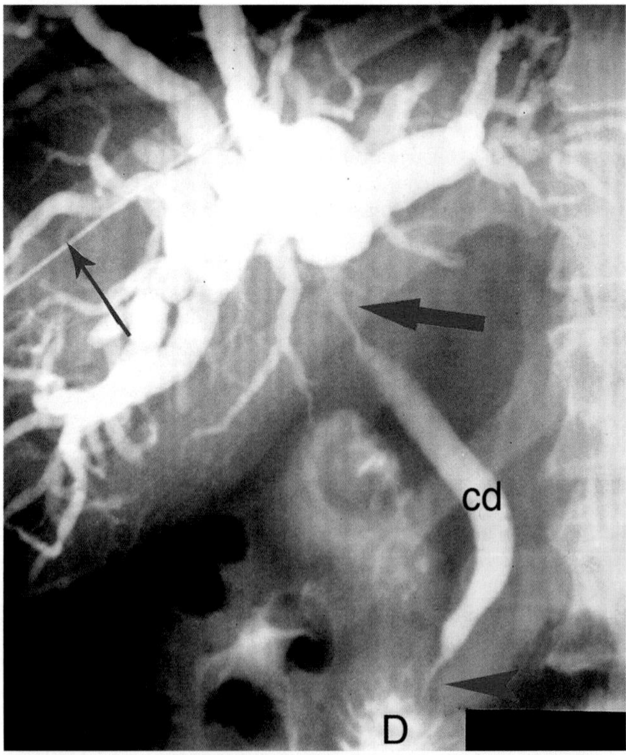

FIGURE 41.44. Cholangiocarcinoma—Hilar—PTC. Percutaneous transhepatic cholangiogram demonstrates abrupt focal narrowing (*fat arrow*) of the proximal common bile duct (*cd*) near the bifurcation. The intrahepatic bile ducts are diffusely and markedly dilated. The common bile duct shows normal narrowing at the ampulla of Vater (*arrowhead*). The PTC needle (*long arrow*) is evident. *D*, duodenum.

TABLE 41.11

CAUSES OF GAS IN THE BILIARY TRACT

Postsurgical
Sphincterotomy
Choledochoduodenostomy
Choledochojejunostomy
Biliary-enteric fistula
Cholecystoduodenal fistula (gallstone erodes into CBD)
Choledochoduodenal fistula (ulcer penetrates CBD)
Surgery/trauma
Tumor erosion with fistula
Infection
Emphysematous cholecystitis
Pyogenic cholangitis

small, making imaging detection as well as needle biopsy difficult. Abrupt stricture with thickening of duct wall may be the only findings.

Intraductal papillary mucinous tumor of the bile ducts may produce a large amount of mucin that markedly dilates the biliary tree and impairs the flow of bile. The tumors are intraductal, polypoid, and characterized by innumerable tiny frond-like papillary projections. The entire biliary tree is distended by mucin. Pathologically the tumors are classified as adenomas, dysplastic, or adenocarcinomas.

Gas in the Biliary Tract

Gas in the biliary tract (pneumobilia) is most commonly encountered in the patient with a surgically created biliary-enteric anastomosis, or who has had a sphincterotomy to facilitate stone passage (Table 41.11). Other causes are:

Cholecystoduodenal fistula is most commonly due to erosion of a gallstone through the gallbladder and into the duodenum. When the gallstone is large, it may cause small bowel obstruction, that is, "*gallstone ileus.*" The gallstone may also erode into the colon and pass spontaneously in the feces. Cholecystoduodenal fistula is most common in women because of the higher incidence of gallstones.

Choledochoduodenal fistula is caused by a penetrating peptic ulcer eroding into the common bile duct (Fig. 41.45).

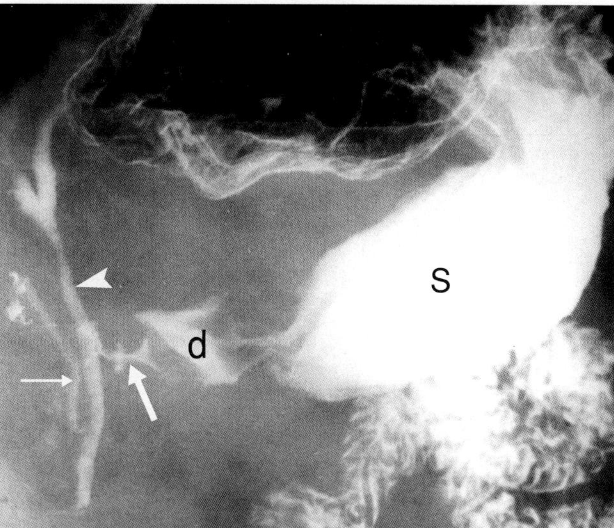

FIGURE 41.45. Choledochoduodenal Fistula—UGI. An upper gastrointestinal series demonstrates filling of the bile ducts due to a penetrating duodenal ulcer that created a fistula (*large arrow*) between the duodenum (*d*) and the common hepatic duct (*arrowhead*). The cystic duct (*small arrow*) is evident. *S*, stomach.

GALLBLADDER

Imaging Methods. US is the imaging method of choice for the gallbladder. It offers high anatomic detail, accuracy, convenience, and cost efficiency. Gallbladder US is reviewed in detail in Chapter 50. Cholescintigraphy utilizing a biliary-specific radionuclide has sensitivity and specificity comparable to US for the diagnosis of acute cholecystitis. Oral cholecystograms (OCG) have been abandoned in favor of other imaging methods. However, oral biliary contrast agents, previously used for OCG, are currently utilized for CT cholangiography. Conventional radiographs demonstrate calcified gallstones, porcelain gallbladder, and emphysematous cholecystitis. CT, as the imaging method of choice for the acute abdomen, frequently provides imaging diagnosis of gallbladder disease. MR and MRCP provide high-quality images to complement indeterminate findings on CT or US.

Anatomy. The gallbladder lies on the underside of the liver in the fossa formed by the junction of the left and right lobes. While the position of the fundus is inconsistent, the neck of the gallbladder is invariably positioned in the porta hepatis and major interlobar fissure. The gallbladder fundus frequently causes a mass impression on the top of the duodenal bulb. Kinking and folding of the gallbladder are common and generally easily recognized by careful image analysis. The so-called *phrygian cap*, which is descriptive of folding of the gallbladder fundus, is a common normal variant. Septa within the gallbladder may be partial or complete. The spiral valves of Heister are small folds in the cystic duct.

The normal gallbladder is well distended with bile following a 4-hour fast and is easily visualized by all imaging modalities. A gallbladder greater than 5 cm in diameter is considered enlarged (hydropic) while a gallbladder less than 2 cm in diameter is considered contracted. The length of the gallbladder is highly variable. The normal gallbladder wall does not exceed 3 mm in thickness, measured from gallbladder lumen to liver parenchyma, when the gallbladder is distended. The normal gallbladder lumen filled with bile is free of particulate debris and is fluid density on imaging studies.

Gallstones are present in 8% of the general population and 15% of the population aged 40 to 60. Approximately 85% of gallstones are predominantly cholesterol, while 15% are predominantly bilirubin (pigment stones) related to hemolytic anemia. Approximately 10% of stones are sufficiently radiopaque to be detected by conventional radiographs as laminated or faceted calcifications. Fissures within gallstones may contain nitrogen gas that appears on radiographs as branching linear lucencies resembling a "crow's foot." Gallstones are most common in women (female:male = 4:1), and in patients with hemolytic anemia, diseases of the ileum, cirrhosis, and diabetes mellitus.

US detects 95% of all gallstones (see Fig. 50.23) whereas CT detects only 80% to 85% (Fig. 41.46A). Gallstones vary in CT attenuation from fat density to calcium density. Up to 20% of gallstones are isodense with bile and not detected by CT, while some gallstones are missed because of their small size or volume averaging with adjacent bowel. Care must

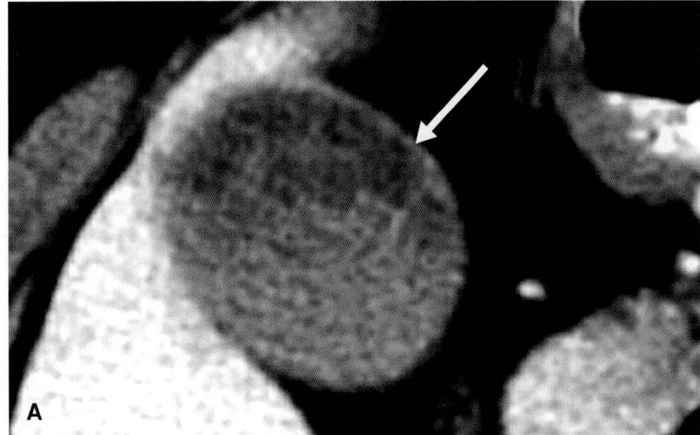

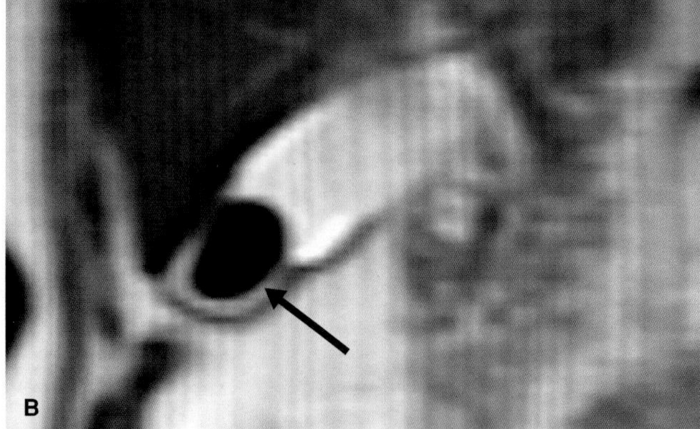

FIGURE 41.46. **Cholelithiasis. A:** CT reveals numerous subtle low attenuation floating gallstones (*arrow*) within the gallbladder. The stones are close to isodense with bile. Stones may be overlooked on CT because they are isodense with bile or because of small size. **B:** Coronal plane T2-weighted MR shows a large gallstone (*arrow*) as a filling defect within high signal bile.

be taken to avoid interpreting contrast in adjacent bowel as cholelithiasis. Contrast studies, MRCP, and T2-weighted MR demonstrate gallstones as "filling defects," rounded or faceted dark objects within high-density bile (Fig. 41.46B).

Differential considerations for lesions in the gallbladder that may be mistaken for gallstones include the following.

Sludge balls or tumefactive biliary sludge result from biliary stasis. The bile thickens and forms layers of bile and mobile toothpaste-like masses that move with changes in patient position. The presence of sludge indicates lack of bile turnover, which may occur because of obstruction, or simply lack of oral food intake.

Cholesterol polyps are common (4% to 7% of the population) benign, polypoid masses that result from accumulation of triglycerides and cholesterol in macrophages in the gallbladder wall. They are of no clinical significance. Polyps 5 mm and smaller are routinely dismissed as benign cholesterol polyps.

Adenomatous polyps are potentially premalignant. Virtually all polypoid gallbladder cancers found on large series of cholecystectomy specimens are larger than 10 mm. This has led to the common recommendation to follow at 6- to 12-month intervals gallbladder polyps in the range of 5 to 10 mm. This is based on the theory of adenoma-to-carcinoma development found in the gastrointestinal tract.

Gallbladder carcinoma may present as a polypoid mass. Gallbladder polyps larger than 10 mm should be considered for surgical removal because of risk of cancer. Gallstones are usually present.

Adenomyomatosis may be focal and presents as a polypoid mass fixed to the gallbladder wall.

Acute Cholecystitis. Acute inflammation of the gallbladder is caused by gallstones obstructing the cystic duct in 90% of cases. *Acalculous cholecystitis* occurs nearly always in patients with predisposing conditions listed subsequently.

US findings combined with clinical assessment are usually diagnostic (see Fig. 50.26). Confident US diagnosis of acute cholecystitis requires the presence of three findings: cholelithiasis, edema of the gallbladder wall seen as a band of echolucency in the wall, and a positive sonographic Murphy sign.

Scintigraphic diagnosis of acute cholecystitis is based on obstruction of the cystic duct with nonvisualization of the gallbladder. See Chapter 71A.

CT demonstrates (Fig. 41.47): gallstones, distended gallbladder, thickened gallbladder wall, subserosal edema, high-density bile, intraluminal sloughed membranes, inflammatory stranding in pericholecystic fat, pericholecystic fluid, blurring of the interface between gallbladder and liver, and prominent arterial phase enhancement of the liver adjacent to the gallbladder.

MR findings are similar: (a) gallstones, often impacted in the neck, (b) wall thickening (>3 mm) with edema, (c) distended gallbladder, and (d) pericholecystic fluid.

Acalculous cholecystitis causes special problems in diagnosis because the cystic duct is often not obstructed. Inflammation may be due to gallbladder wall ischemia or direct bacterial infection. Patients at risk for acalculous cholecystitis include those with biliary stasis due to lack of oral intake, posttrauma, postburn, postsurgery, or on total parenteral nutrition. Scintigraphy usually demonstrates lack of gallbladder visualization. Although this finding is 90% to 95% sensitive for acalculous cholecystitis, it is only 38% specific. False-positive conditions for nonvisualization include hyperalimentation and prolonged severe illness, which are predisposing conditions for acalculous cholecystitis. US demonstrates a distended tender gallbladder with thickened wall but without stones. Many patients are too ill to elicit a reliable sonographic Murphy sign.

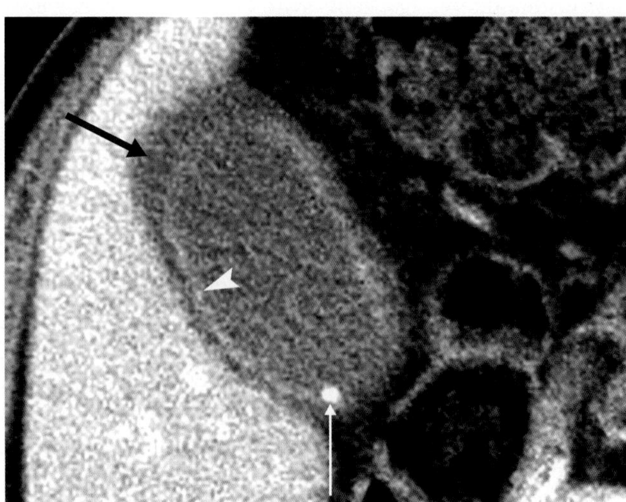

FIGURE 41.47. **Acute Cholecystitis—CT.** Postcontrast image demonstrates fluid (*fat arrow*) around the enhancing mucosa (*arrowhead*) of the gallbladder and a small high attenuation gallstone (*skinny arrow*) within the gallbladder lumen in a patient with acute, severe right upper quadrant pain. Surgery confirmed acute cholecystitis.

Sludge is the term used to describe the presence of thick particulate matter in highly concentrated bile (see Fig. 50.22). Calcium bilirubinate and cholesterol crystals precipitate in the bile when biliary stasis is prolonged because of a lack of oral intake or biliary obstruction. Sludge appears as echodense bile on US, as high attenuation bile on CT, and as layering bile of different signal on MR. Since sludge may be found in a fasting, but otherwise normal patient, its presence is not definitive evidence of gallbladder disease. Pus, blood, and milk of calcium are additional causes of thick bile.

Complications of acute cholecystitis include the following.

Gallbladder empyema describes the gallbladder distended with pus in a patient, often diabetic, with rapid progression of symptoms suggesting an abdominal abscess.

Gangrenous cholecystitis indicates the presence of necrosis of the gallbladder wall. The patient is at risk for gallbladder perforation. Findings include mucosal irregularity and asymmetric thickening of the gallbladder wall with multiple lucent layers, indicating mucosal ulceration and reactive edema.

Perforation of the gallbladder is a life-threatening complication seen in 5% to 10% of cases. Perforation may occur adjacent to the liver resulting in pericholecystic abscess, into the peritoneal cavity resulting in generalized peritonitis, or into adjacent bowel resulting in biliary-enteric fistula. Overall mortality is as high as 24%. A focal pericholecystic fluid collection suggests pericholecystic abscess. Gas is often present within the gallbladder lumen if the perforation extends into bowel.

Emphysematous cholecystitis results from infection of the gallbladder with gas-forming organisms, usually *E. coli* or *Clostridium perfringens*. Approximately 40% of patients are diabetic. Gallstones may or may not be present. Gas is demonstrated within the wall or within the lumen of the gallbladder by conventional radiography or CT (Fig. 41.48). On US, intramural gas has an arc-like configuration difficult to differentiate from calcification and porcelain gallbladder.

Mirizzi syndrome refers to the condition of biliary obstruction resulting from a gallstone in the cystic duct eroding into the adjacent common duct and causing an inflammatory mass that obstructs the common duct. Visualization of a stone at the junction of the cystic duct and the CHD in a patient with biliary obstruction and gallbladder inflammation suggest the diagnosis.

Chronic cholecystitis includes a spectrum of pathology that shares the presence of gallstones and chronic gallbladder inflammation. Patients with chronic cholecystitis complain of recurrent attacks of right upper quadrant abdominal pain and

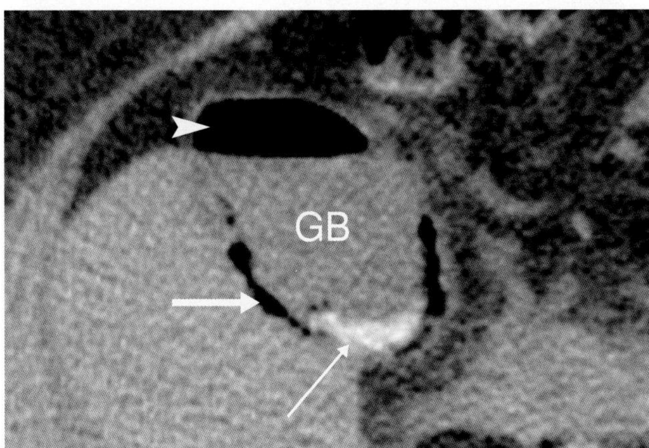

FIGURE 41.48. **Emphysematous Cholecystitis—CT.** Scan of a patient with diabetes, fever, and sepsis reveals air in the lumen (*arrowhead*) and wall (*fat arrow*) of the gallbladder (*GB*) indicative of emphysematous cholecystitis. Numerous tiny layering gallstones (*skinny arrow*) are present within the gallbladder.

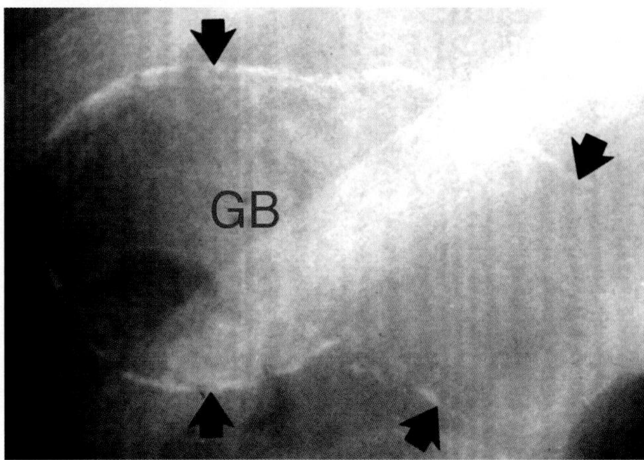

FIGURE 41.49. **Porcelain Gallbladder.** Conventional radiograph of the right upper quadrant of the abdomen shows calcification (*arrows*) in the wall of the gallbladder (*GB*). This finding is indicative of chronic obstruction of the cystic duct with chronic cholecystitis. The risk of gallbladder carcinoma is increased.

biliary colic. Imaging findings include gallstones, thickening of the gallbladder wall, contraction of the gallbladder lumen, delayed visualization of the gallbladder on cholescintigraphy, and poor contractility. Variants of chronic cholecystitis include the following.

Porcelain gallbladder describes the presence of dystrophic calcification in the wall of an obstructed and chronically inflamed gallbladder (Fig. 41.49). The condition is associated with gallstones in 90% of cases. Porcelain gallbladder carries a 10% to 20% risk of gallbladder carcinoma. Cholecystectomy is usually indicated.

Milk of calcium bile, also called limy bile, is associated with an obstructed cystic duct, chronic cholecystitis, and gallstones. Particulate matter with a high concentration of calcium compounds is precipitated in the bile, making the bile radiopaque on radiographs or CT. Dependent layering of bile can be demonstrated on conventional radiographs. The bile is extremely echogenic on US and gallstones may be visualized within it.

Xanthogranulomatous cholecystitis is an uncommon variant of chronic cholecystitis characterized by nodular deposits of lipid-laden macrophages in the gallbladder wall and proliferative fibrosis. Imaging findings include marked wall thickening (2 cm), fat-density nodules in the wall, and narrowing of the lumen. Cholelithiasis is frequently present. The condition is difficult to differentiate from gallbladder carcinoma. Preservation of linear enhancement of the mucosa on postcontrast MR favors xanthogranulomatous cholecystitis over carcinoma.

Thickening of the gallbladder wall is present when the wall thickness measured on the hepatic aspect of the gallbladder exceeds 3 mm in patients who have fasted at least 8 hours. Conditions associated with wall thickening include the following.

Acute and chronic cholecystitis. Wall thickening is a usual feature of acute cholecystitis and is present in 50% of cases of chronic cholecystitis.

Hepatitis causes reduction in bile flow, which results in reduced gallbladder volume and thickening of the gallbladder wall in approximately half of the patients.

Portal venous hypertension and congestive heart failure may cause wall thickening by passive venous congestion.

AIDS is associated with thickening of the gallbladder wall and the walls of the bile ducts. Opportunistic organisms are sometimes present.

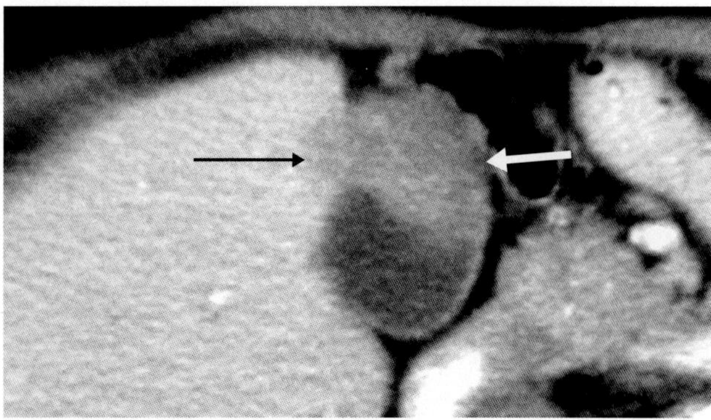

FIGURE 41.50. Gallbladder Carcinoma. Postcontrast CT shows an enhancing soft tissue mass (*fat arrow*) within the lumen of the gallbladder. Direct invasion of tumor into the adjacent liver parenchyma is evident (*skinny arrow*).

Hypoalbuminemia is associated with thickened gallbladder wall in 60% of patients.

Gallbladder carcinoma usually presents as a focal mass but may cause only focal wall thickening.

Adenomyomatosis is a benign condition of the gallbladder characterized by wall thickening caused by hyperplasia of the mucosa and smooth muscle. It may localize usually in the fundus, segmental, or diffuse involving the entire gallbladder. Outpouchings of mucosa into or through the muscularis form characteristic Rokitansky–Aschoff sinuses (see Fig. 50.28), which are diagnostic of adenomyomatosis. US shows "comet-tail" reverberation artifacts emanating from inspissated bile within these sinuses in the thickened gallbladder wall. MRCP shows a "pearl necklace" appearance of the gallbladder wall caused by bright fluid within the sinuses. CT shows wall thickening with tiny cystic spaces. The condition has no malignant potential. Coexisting gallstones are commonly present.

Gallbladder Carcinoma. Adenocarcinoma of the gallbladder may be overlooked or misdiagnosed preoperatively. The presence of gallstones in 70% to 80% of cases masks the findings of cancer, especially with US examination. Gallbladder carcinoma is a tumor of elderly women (>60 years, female:male = 4:1). Patients present with pain, anorexia, weight loss, and jaundice. Calcification of the gallbladder wall (porcelain gallbladder) is a risk factor. Imaging findings include (a) intraluminal soft tissue mass (Fig. 41.50); (b) focal or diffuse thickening of the gallbladder wall; (c) soft tissue mass replacing the gallbladder; (d) gallstones; (e) extension of tumor into the liver, bile ducts, and adjacent bowel; (f) dilated bile ducts; and (g) metastases to periportal and peripancreatic lymph nodes and liver. Most tumors are unresectable at discovery.

Suggested Readings

Liver

American College of Radiology. CT/MRI LI-RADS—Liver imaging reporting and data system. https://www.acr.org/Quality-Safety/Resources/LIRADS/LIRADS-v2017

Bächler P, Baladron MJ, Menias C, et al. Multimodality imaging of liver infections: differential diagnosis and potential pitfalls. *Radiographics* 2016;36(4):1001–1023.

Bandali MF, Mirakhur A, Lee EW, et al. Portal hypertension: imaging of portosystemic collateral pathways and associated image-guided therapy. *World J Gastroenterol* 2017;23(10):1735–1746.

Choi BI, Lee JM, Kim TK, Dioguardi Burgio M, Vilgrain V. Diagnosing borderline hepatic nodules in hepatocarcinogenesis: imaging performance. *AJR Am J Roentgenol* 2015;205(1):10–21.

Expert Panel on Gastrointestinal Imaging; Horowitz JM, Kamel IR, Arif-Tiwari H, et al. ACR appropriateness criteria chronic liver disease. *J Am Coll Radiol* 2017;14(11S):S391–S405.

Ferral H, Behrens G, Lopera J. Budd-Chiari syndrome. *AJR Am J Roentgenol* 2012;199(4):737–745.

Huber A, Ebner L, Heverhagen JT, Christe A. State-of-the-art imaging of liver fibrosis and cirrhosis: A comprehensive review of current applications and future perspectives. *Eur J Radiol Open* 2015;2:90–100.

Jha P, Poder L, Wang ZJ, Westphalen AC, Yeh BM, Coakley FV. Radiologic mimics of cirrhosis. *AJR Am J Roentgenol* 2010;194(4):993–999.

Jo PC, Jang HJ, Burns PN, Burak KW, Kim TK, Wilson SR. Integration of contrast-enhanced US into a multimodality approach to imaging of nodules in a cirrhotic liver: How I do it. *Radiology* 2017;282(2):317–331.

Kim HJ, Kim AY, Kim TK, et al. Transient hepatic attenuation differences in focal hepatic lesions: dynamic CT features. *AJR Am J Roentgenol* 2005;184(1):83–90.

Kouri BE, Abrams RA, Al-Refaie WB, et al. ACR appropriateness criteria radiologic management of hepatic malignancy. *J Am Coll Radiol* 2016; 13(3):265–273.

Lee SS, Park SH. Radiologic evaluation of nonalcoholic fatty liver disease. *World J Gastroenterol* 2014;20(23):7392–7402.

Strasberg SM, Phillips C. Use and dissemination of the Brisbane 2000 nomenclature of liver anatomy and resections. *Ann Surg* 2013;257(3):377–382.

Vilgrain V, Lagadec M, Ronot M. Pitfalls in liver imaging. *Radiology* 2016; 278(1):34–51.

Wells ML, Fenstad ER, Poterucha JT, et al. Imaging findings of congestive hepatopathy. *Radiographics* 2016;36(4):1024–1037.

Biliary Tree and Gallbladder

Akisik MF, Jennings SG, Aisen AM, et al. MRCP in patient care: a prospective survey of gastroenterologists. *AJR Am J Roentgenol* 2013;201(3): 573–577.

Bonatti M, Vezzali N, Lombardo F, et al. Gallbladder adenomyomatosis: imaging findings, tricks and pitfalls. *Insights Imaging* 2017;8(2):243–253. (Pictorial review).

Castaing D. Surgical anatomy of the biliary tract. *HPB (Oxford)* 2008;10(2):72–76. (Review article).

Charalel RA, Jeffrey RB, Shin LK. Complicated cholecystitis—the complementary roles of sonography and computed tomography. *Ultrasound Q* 2011;27(3):161–170. (Pictorial essay).

Costi R, Gnocchi A, Di Mario F, Sarli L. Diagnosis and management of choledocholithiasis in the golden age of imaging, endoscopy, and laparoscopy. *World J Gastroenterol* 2014;20(37):13382–13401.

Katabathina VS, Flaherty EM, Dasyam AK, et al. "Biliary diseases with pancreatic counterparts": cross-sectional imaging findings. *Radiographics* 2016;36(2):374–392.

Mellnick VM, Menias CO, Sandrasegaran K, et al. Polypoid lesions of the gallbladder: disease spectrum with pathologic correlation. *Radiographics* 2015;35(2):387–399. (Review article).

Nikolaidis P, Hammond NA, Day K, et al. Imaging features of benign and malignant ampullary and periampullary lesions. *Radiographics* 2014;34(3): 624–641. (Review article).

Patel NB, Oto A, Thomas S. Multidetector CT of emergent biliary pathologic conditions. *Radiographics* 2013;33(7):1867–1888.

Santiago I, Loureiro R, Curvo-Semedo L, et al. Congenital cystic lesions of the biliary tree. *AJR Am J Roentgenol* 2012;198(4):825–835. (Pictorial essay).

Shanbhogue AK, Tirumani SH, Prasad SR, Fasih N, McInnes M. Benign biliary strictures: a current comprehensive clinical and imaging review. *AJR Am J Roentgenol* 2011;197(2):W295–W306.

Tonolini M, Pagani A, Blanco R. Cross-sectional imaging of common and unusual complications after endoscopic retrograde cholangiopancreatography. *Insights Imaging* 2015;6(3):323–338. (Pictorial review).

Woldenberg N, Masamed R, Petersen J, Jude CM, Kadell BM, Patel MK. Murphy's law: what can go wrong in the gallbladder. *Radiographics* 2015;35(4):1031–1032. (Online digital presentation).

CHAPTER 42 ■ PANCREAS AND SPLEEN

WILLIAM E. BRANT AND JENNIFER POHL

PANCREAS

Imaging Techniques

CT, US, and MR provide high-quality images of the pancreatic parenchyma and are used as the primary imaging modalities for the pancreas (Fig. 42.1). MDCT optimizes contrast enhancement for detection of small tumors and provides the capability of CT angiography (CTA) to detect vascular involvement by pancreatic tumor. Improved MR techniques and the use of gadolinium enhancement have increased its capability to detect and characterize pancreatic lesions and to serve as the primary imaging modality in many practices. MR cholangiopancreatography (MRCP) offers an excellent noninvasive method of imaging the pancreatic duct as well as the biliary system. Secretin administration during MRCP increases pancreatic secretions and improves visualization of the pancreatic duct. Endoscopic retrograde cholangiopancreatography (ERCP) provides excellent visualization of the lumen of the pancreatic duct (Fig. 42.2), which is usually affected by any mass lesion of the pancreas. This procedure is performed by endoscopic cannulation of the bile and pancreatic ducts, followed by injection of a contrast agent and fluoroscopy. Because of the increasing excellence of MRCP, ERCP is now performed primary to guide interventional procedures such as stent placement. Arteriography is now routinely performed using CTA and MR angiographic (MRA) techniques. US- and CT-guided biopsy and drainage procedures play a major role in the diagnosis and treatment of pancreatic diseases. Endoscopic US is an important adjunct to characterize pancreatic tumors by imaging and endoscopic US-guided fine needle aspiration.

Anatomy

The pancreas is a tongue-shaped organ, approximately 12 to 15 cm in length, that lies within the anterior pararenal compartment of the retroperitoneum (Fig. 42.1). The pancreas is posterior to the left lobe of the liver, the stomach, and the lesser sac. It is anterior to the spine, the inferior vena cava, and the aorta. Pancreatic tissue is best recognized by identification of the vessels around it. The neck, body, and tail of the pancreas lie ventral to the splenic vein, with the tail extending into the hilum of the spleen. The splenic vein and pancreas are anterior to the superior mesenteric artery (SMA). Just to the right of the SMA, the head of the pancreas wraps around the junction of the superior mesenteric vein (SMV) and the splenic vein, with the uncinate process of the pancreatic head extending under the SMV just anterior to the inferior vena cava. The splenic artery courses through the pancreatic bed in an often tortuous course. Atherosclerotic splenic artery calcifications are easily mistaken for pancreatic calcifications. The lumen of the splenic artery may be mistaken for pancreatic cysts or a dilated pancreatic duct on CT without contrast or on US.

Maximum dimensions for pancreatic size are a 3.0-cm diameter for the head, 2.5-cm diameter for the body, and 2.0-cm diameter for the tail. The gland is somewhat larger in young patients and progressively decreases in size with age. Because the gland is not encapsulated, fatty infiltration between the lobules in older patients gives the pancreas a delicate, feathery appearance on CT. The pancreatic duct is visualized with thin-slice CT and with US. It normally measures 3 to 4 mm in diameter in the head and tapers smoothly to the tail. Images from ERCP show the normal duct to be a bit larger owing to magnification effect and distention resulting from contrast injection (Fig. 42.2). The duodenum cradles the pancreatic head in the C-loop. Many pancreatic abnormalities show secondary effects on the duodenum, and occasionally on the stomach and colon.

On MR, the pancreas is well seen on fat-suppressed T1WI. High protein content in the exocrine pancreas results in high signal of the pancreatic parenchyma, which is difficult to differentiate from fat on non–fat-suppressed T1WI. Tumors are typically of lower signal than pancreatic parenchyma on T1WI. On T2WI, pancreatic tissue is variable in signal intensity from as low as the liver is to as high as fat. Cystic lesions are bright and easily seen on T2WI. Gadolinium will enhance the parenchyma, whereas adenocarcinoma enhances poorly and remains low signal on postcontrast T1WI.

Pancreatitis

Acute pancreatitis is generally diagnosed clinically. The role of imaging is to clarify the diagnosis when the clinical picture is confusing, to assess its severity, to determine prognosis, and to detect complications. Per-case mortality is 6%. Inflammation of the pancreatic tissue leads to disruption of small pancreatic ducts, resulting in leakage of pancreatic secretions.

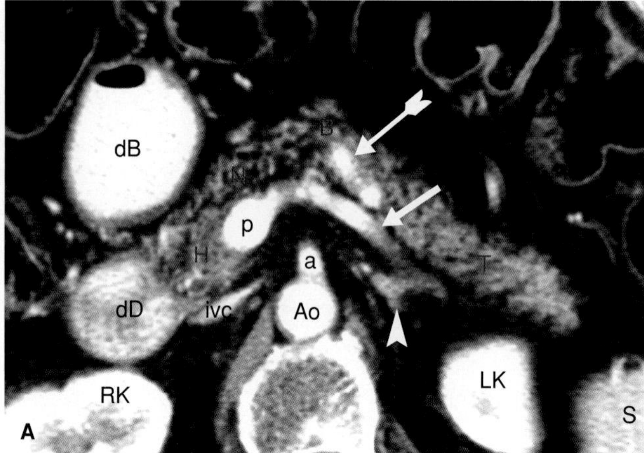

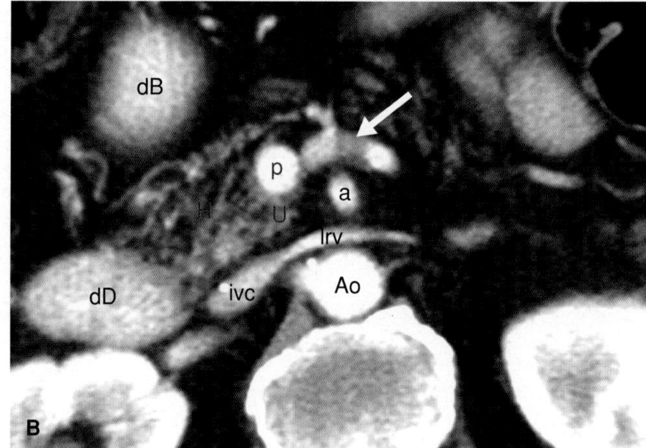

FIGURE 42.1. **Normal Pancreas—CT.** Postcontrast images from a 75-year-old man show the normal lacy appearance of the pancreas in older patients. Because the pancreas lacks capsule normal retroperitoneal fat infiltrates between the lobules of the pancreas. **A:** Image through the head (*H*), neck (*N*), body (*B*), and tail (*T*) of the pancreas. **B:** Image just inferior to (**A**) through head (*H*) and uncinate process (*U*) of the pancreas. The vascular landmarks that assist in identification of the pancreas are evident. The majority of the pancreas lies anterior to the splenic vein (*arrow without tail*) while the splenic artery (*arrow with tail*) courses through the pancreatic parenchyma. The junction of the splenic vein and superior mesenteric vein forms the portal confluence (*p*), which marks the location of the neck of the pancreas just anterior. The superior mesenteric artery (*a*) arises from the aorta (*Ao*) posterior to the splenic vein and courses caudally just to the left of the superior mesenteric vein. The superior mesenteric artery is normally surrounded by a collar of clear fat. Other landmarks are the inferior vena cava (*ivc*), left renal vein (*lrv*), duodenal bulb (*dB*), descending duodenum (*dD*), spleen (*S*), right kidney (*RK*), left kidney (*LK*), and left adrenal gland (*arrowhead*).

Because the pancreas lacks a capsule, the pancreatic juices have ready access to surrounding tissues. Pancreatic enzymes digest fascial layers, spreading the inflammatory process to multiple anatomic compartments. Causes of acute pancreatitis are listed in Table 42.1.

Imaging studies of acute pancreatitis may be normal in mild cases. Contrast-enhanced MDCT provides the most comprehensive initial assessment and is recommended as the initial imaging study. US is useful for follow-up of specific abnormalities, such as fluid collections. MR is used especially in patients in whom intravenous iodinated or gadolinium contrast agents are contraindicated.

The Atlanta classification for acute pancreatitis was developed by a multispecialty expert panel in 1992 and updated in 2012 to provide uniform definitions of terminology and to simplify clinical and morphologic classification of the disease. Two morphologic types are defined: *interstitial edematous pancreatitis* and *acute necrotizing pancreatitis.* A number of imprecisely used terms are discouraged including phlegmon, organized necrosis, pancreatic abscess, and intrapancreatic pseudocyst.

Interstitial edematous pancreatitis appears on contrast-enhanced CT as localized or diffuse enlargement of the pancreas with normal homogeneous parenchymal enhancement or slightly heterogeneous enhancement due to edema. Mild fat stranding

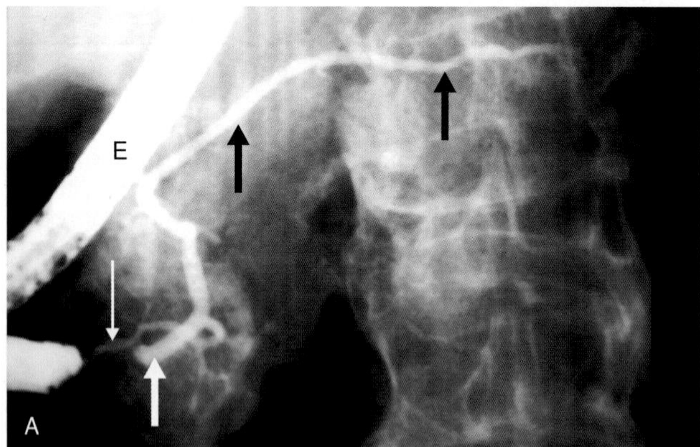

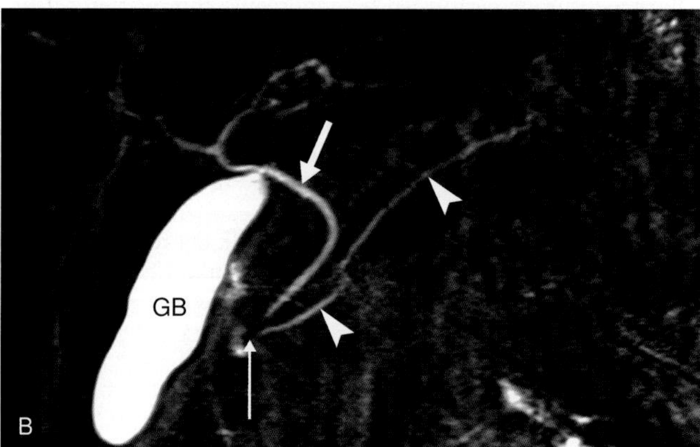

FIGURE 42.2. **Normal Pancreatic Ducts. A:** Radiograph from an ERCP demonstrates the main duct of Wirsung (*fat arrows*) and the accessory duct of Santorini (*skinny arrow*). In this patient, the main duct drained separately into the major papilla (of Vater) with a different orifice for the common bile duct. The accessory duct drained into the minor papilla. Both ampullae were cannulated endoscopically and injected before this radiograph. A number of different variants of pancreatic duct anatomy exist. This variant is found in about 35% of individuals. Embryologically, the main duct is formed by the entire duct of the ventral pancreatic bud and the distal portion of the duct of the dorsal pancreatic bud. The main duct may join the common bile duct or have a separate orifice in the major papilla. The proximal portion of the duct of the dorsal pancreatic bud may be obliterated or persist as the accessory duct. *E,* endoscope. **B:** Image from an MRCP in a different patient. MRCP offers the obvious advantage of being noninvasive. The pancreatic duct (*arrowheads*) and the common bile duct (*fat arrow*) have adjoining orifices into the ampulla (*skinny arrow*). The normal gallbladder (*GB*) is well shown.

TABLE 42.1

CAUSES OF ACUTE PANCREATITIS

Alcohol abuse—most common cause of chronic pancreatitis
Gallstone passage/impaction—most common cause of acute pancreatitis

Metabolic disorders
- Hereditary pancreatitis—autosomal dominant
- Hypercalcemia
- Hyperlipidemia—types I and V
- Malnutrition

Trauma
- Blunt abdominal trauma
- Surgery
- ERCP

Penetrating ulcer

Malignancy
- Pancreatic adenocarcinoma
- Lymphoma

Drugs—steroids, tetracycline, furosemide, many others

Infection
- Viral—mumps, hepatitis, infectious mononucleosis, AIDS
- Parasites—ascariasis, clonorchis
- Tuberculosis

Structural
- Choledochocele
- Pancreas divisum

Idiopathic—20% of cases of acute pancreatitis

and peripancreatic inflammatory changes may be present with varying volumes of peripancreatic fluid (Fig. 42.3).

Acute necrotizing pancreatitis is divided into three forms by CT appearance. *Pancreatic parenchymal necrosis with peripancreatic necrosis* (Fig. 42.4) is most common (75% to 80%) appearing as a lack of parenchymal enhancement associated with nonliquefied heterogeneous areas of nonenhancement in peripancreatic tissues, most commonly in the lesser sac and retroperitoneum. *Peripancreatic necrosis alone* occurs in 20% of patients. *Pancreatic parenchymal necrosis alone* occurs in 5% of patients. Necrosis is best determined by CT at 72 hours following onset of symptoms.

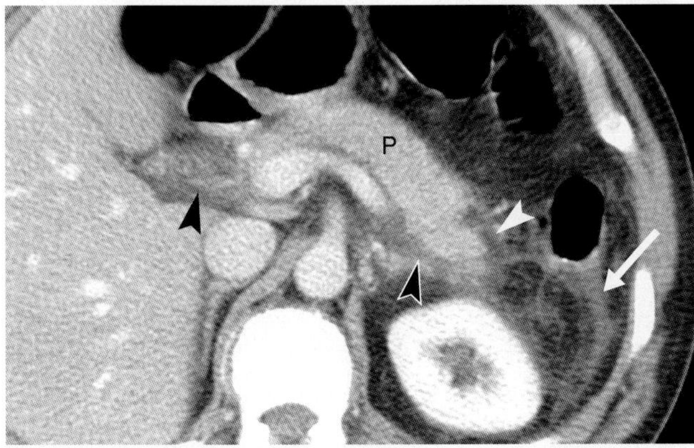

FIGURE 42.3. **Interstitial Edematous Pancreatitis.** Postcontrast CT shows a mildly edematous pancreas (*P*) with inflammatory stranding into the peripancreatic fat (*arrowheads*) with fluid (*arrow*) extending around Gerota fascia.

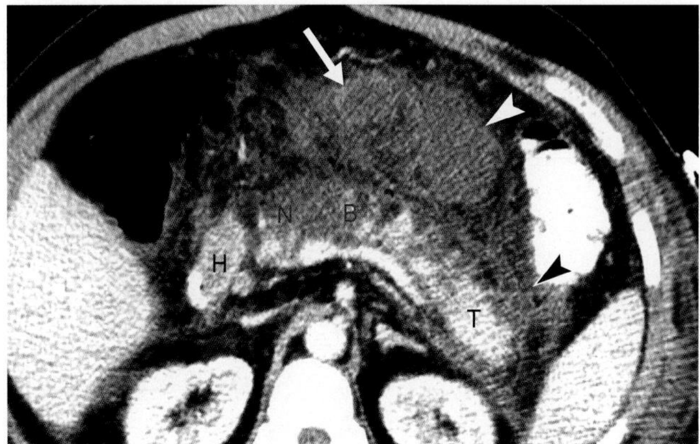

FIGURE 42.4. **Acute Necrotizing Pancreatitis.** CT scan performed with rapid bolus administration of intravenous contrast demonstrates enhancement of only the head (*H*) and tail (*T*) of the pancreas. The neck (*N*) and body (*B*) of the pancreas show no enhancement, a finding indicative of necrosis. Inflammatory fluid (*arrowheads*) extends into the lesser sac and peripancreatic tissues. Foci of nonliquefied areas of nonenhancement are present (*arrow*). These findings are indicative of *pancreatic parenchyma necrosis with peripancreatic necrosis.*

Collections associated with interstitial pancreatitis are classified as "*acute peripancreatic fluid collections*" when shown on CT in the initial 4 weeks as nonencapsulated, nonenhancing, low attenuation, liquefied collections without solid components. Walls are imperceptible. "*Pseudocysts*" are defined as simple collections with perceptible walls seen after 4 weeks (Fig. 42.5). These collections usually do not require drainage. Infection is uncommon but may be suspected if gas is seen within the collection on CT. Drainage is often required for infected fluid collections.

Collections associated with necrotizing pancreatitis are classified as "*acute necrotic collections*" (ANC) if seen on CT in the first 4 weeks. These appear as heterogeneous collections containing hemorrhage, fat, or necrotic fat within or surrounding necrotic pancreatic parenchyma. The collection may be peripancreatic or intraparenchymal or both. An enhancing wall may develop around an ANC and if seen after 4 weeks the collection is termed "*walled-off necrosis*" (WON). WONs appear heterogeneous in attenuation and complex because of variable necrotic tissues and debris (Fig. 42.6).

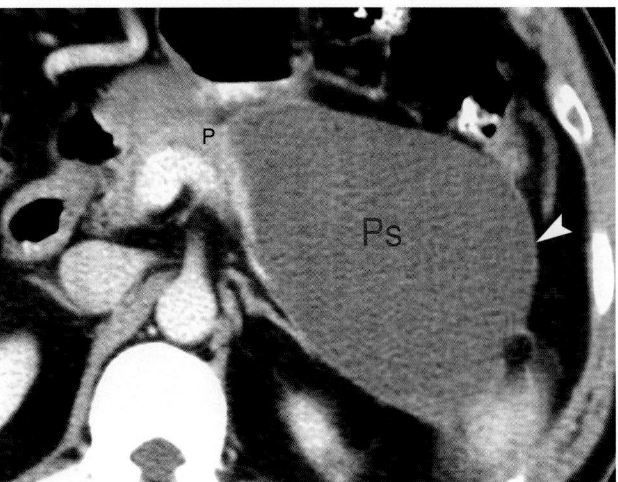

FIGURE 42.5. **Pseudocyst.** Postcontrast CT performed 6 weeks following onset of acute pancreatitis shows a large well-defined fluid collection (*Ps*) with discrete thin wall (*arrowhead*) occupying the body and tail region of the pancreas (*P*).

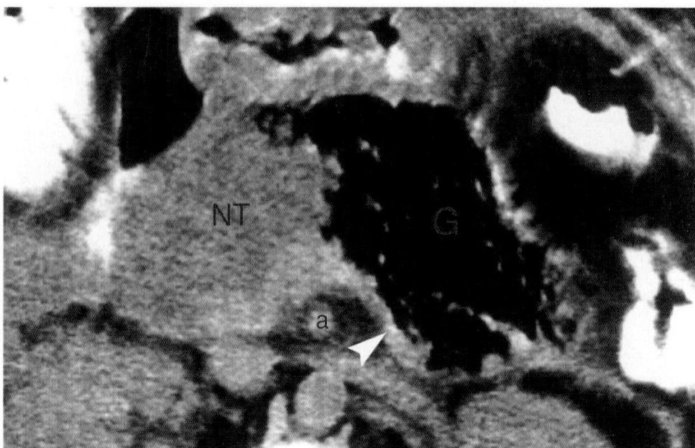

FIGURE 42.6. **Infected Walled-Off Necrosis (WON).** CT performed without contrast because of renal failure shows a large collection of gas (*G*) occupying the bed of necrotic body and tail of the pancreas. A large mass of necrotic tissue (*NT*) occupies the head and neck region of the pancreatic bed. Anatomic landmarks include the superior mesenteric artery (*a*) and splenic vein (*arrowhead*). Gas within necrotic tissue is highly indicative of infection but fistulous communication with bowel is another consideration. With renal failure lasting more than 48 hours, this case would be classified as *severe pancreatitis*.

TABLE 42.2

COMPLICATIONS OF ACUTE PANCREATITIS

- **Pancreatic fluid collections**—collections of enzyme-rich pancreatic juice.
  - ***Acute peripancreatic fluid collection*** (observed within 4 weeks of onset of acute pancreatitis without necrosis): 50% resolve spontaneously. May be intrapancreatic, anterior pararenal space, lesser sac, or extend anywhere in the abdomen, into solid organs, or even into the chest.
    - *Acute necrotic collections* (ANC) (observed within 4 weeks with necrosis): may be sterile or infected.
  - ***Pseudocyst*** (thin-walled collection persisting after 4 weeks without necrosis): round or oval, encapsulated pancreatic fluid collection encased by a distinct fibrous capsule; about 50% will spontaneously resolve; the remainder will require catheter or surgical drainage.
    - *Walled-off necrosis* (WON) (persisting after 4 weeks with necrosis): may be sterile or infected.
- **Secondary infection**—most common 2–3 weeks after onset of disease and associated with increased mortality (32% of cases).
- **Hemorrhage**—resulting from erosion of blood vessels and tissue necrosis. CT shows high attenuation blood in the retroperitoneum.
- **Pseudoaneurysm**—autodigestion of arterial walls by pancreatic enzymes results in pulsatile mass that is lined by fibrous tissue and maintains communication with parent artery.
- **Disconnection of the pancreatic duct**—caused by pancreatic necrosis resulting in a viable segment of the pancreas (most common in the neck) being disconnected from the intestinal tract and a persistent fistula with continuing leakage of fluid into peripancreatic spaces.
- **Pancreatic ascites**—leakage of pancreatic secretions into peritoneal cavity.

Infection is more common in necrotic tissue and is highly likely if gas is present within the collection. Image-guided needle aspiration is used to confirm the diagnosis and direct drainage catheter placement.

The severity of acute pancreatitis is termed mild, moderate, or severe based on the presence of organ failure and complications. If no organ dysfunction or acute complications are present cases are classified as *mild*. Most will cases will appear on imaging as acute interstitial pancreatitis without other findings. Cases are classified as *moderate* severity if organ failure develops but lasts less than 48 hours. Complications (Table 42.2) may or may not be present. *Severe* cases have single or multi-organ failure for 48 hours or longer.

Pancreas divisum is a common congenital variant of pancreatic anatomy that serves as a predisposition to pancreatitis (Fig. 42.7). The ventral and dorsal ductal systems of the pancreas fail to fuse. As a result the major portion of the pancreatic secretions from the body and tail drain via the dorsal pancreatic duct (Santorini) into the minor papilla while the minor portion of pancreatic secretions from the head and uncinate process (ventral duct of Wirsung) drain into the duodenum through the major papilla in association with the common bile duct. Relative obstruction at the minor papilla results

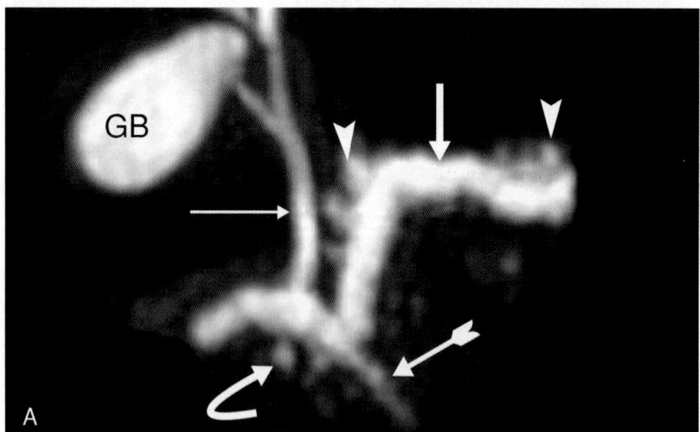

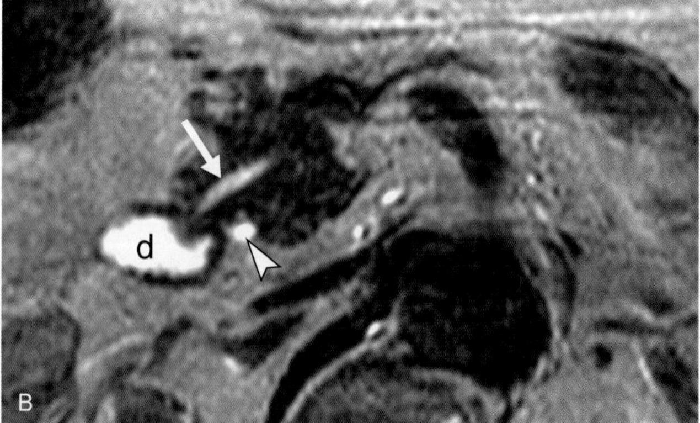

FIGURE 42.7. **Pancreas Divisum. A:** Image from a thick slab MRCP reveals marked enlargement and tortuosity of the main pancreatic duct (*fat arrow*) with dilation of side branches (*arrowheads*) highly indicative of chronic pancreatitis. The dilated main duct is seen to bypass the descending common bile duct (*skinny arrow*) to enter the duodenum at the narrow minor papilla. The common bile duct continues caudad to enter the major papilla (*curved arrow*). In this patient the ventral duct (*arrow with a tail*) from the pancreatic head and uncinate process join the dorsal duct to drain into the minor papilla. This duct is also dilated indicating chronic pancreatitis. *GB*, gallbladder. **B:** Axial T2-weighted MR image from a different patient shows the main pancreatic duct (*arrow*) bypassing the descending common bile duct (*arrowhead*) to enter the duodenum (*d*) at the minor papilla. This patient has pancreas divisum but without evidence of pancreatitis.

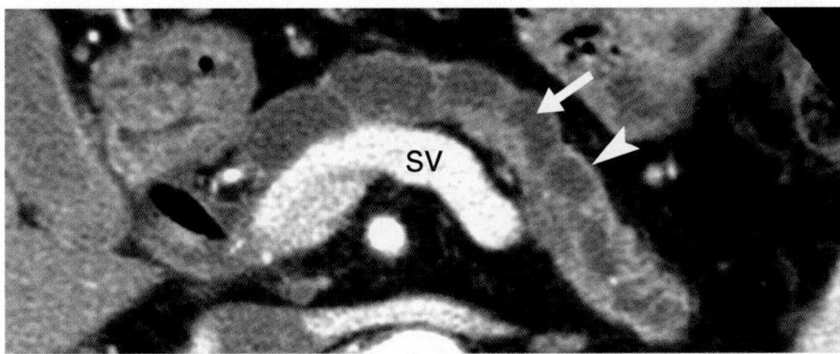

FIGURE 42.8. **Chronic Pancreatitis.** Postcontrast CT demonstrates marked beaded dilation of the pancreatic duct (*arrow*) associated with atrophy (*arrowhead*) of the pancreatic parenchyma. These are characteristic findings of chronic pancreatitis. The splenic vein (*SV*) confirms the location of the pancreas.

in pancreatitis in 5% to 15% of patients with pancreas divisum. The anomaly is found in 6% of the general population and 10% to 20% of patients with a history of acute recurrent pancreatitis. MRCP and ERCP are most reliably used to make the diagnosis.

Chronic pancreatitis is caused by recurrent and prolonged bouts of acute pancreatitis that cause parenchymal atrophy and progressive fibrosis. Both the exocrine and endocrine function of the pancreas may be impaired. The most common causes are alcohol abuse (70%) and biliary stone disease (20%). Many of the remaining patients may have autoimmune pancreatitis that responds to steroid therapy. The clinical diagnosis is often vague, so imaging is used both to confirm the diagnosis and to detect complications. The morphologic changes of chronic pancreatitis include (a) dilation of the pancreatic duct (70% to 90% of cases), usually in a beaded pattern of alternating areas of dilation and constriction (Fig. 42.8); (b) decrease in visible pancreatic tissue because of atrophy; (c) calcifications (40% to 50% of cases) in the pancreatic parenchyma that vary from finely stippled to coarse, usually associated with alcoholic pancreatitis (Fig. 42.9); (d) fluid collections that are both intra- and extrapancreatic; (e) focal mass-like enlargement of the pancreas owing to benign inflammation and fibrosis; (f) stricture of the bile duct because of fibrosis or mass in the pancreatic head resulting in proximal bile duct dilation; and (g) fascial thickening and chronic inflammatory changes in surrounding tissues. Differentiation between an inflammatory mass resulting from chronic pancreatitis and that of pancreatic carcinoma frequently requires image-directed biopsy. MR reveals the fibrosis and parenchymal atrophy as a loss of the bright signal of pancreas parenchyma normally seen on T1-weighted fat-suppressed images. Parenchymal enhancement on MR is heterogeneous and early and increases on delayed images. MRCP and ERCP demonstrate the characteristic changes in the pancreatic duct. Calcifications are demonstrated by CT, US, and conventional radiographs but are easily overlooked on MR.

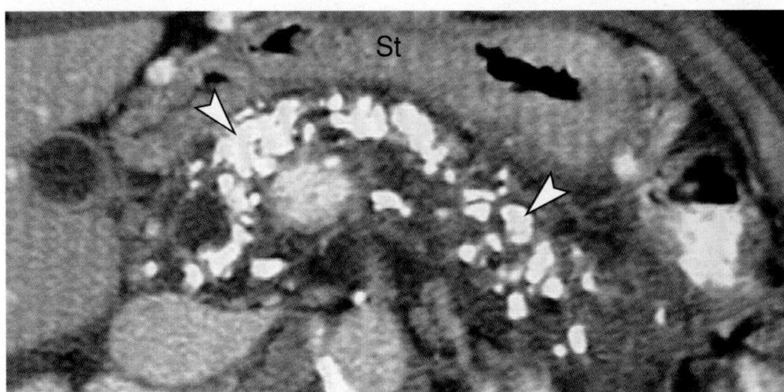

FIGURE 42.9. **Chronic Pancreatitis.** CT in a patient with a history of chronic alcohol abuse reveals innumerable coarse calcifications (*arrowheads*) throughout the pancreas. This finding is most common in chronic pancreatitis caused by alcoholism. *St*, stomach.

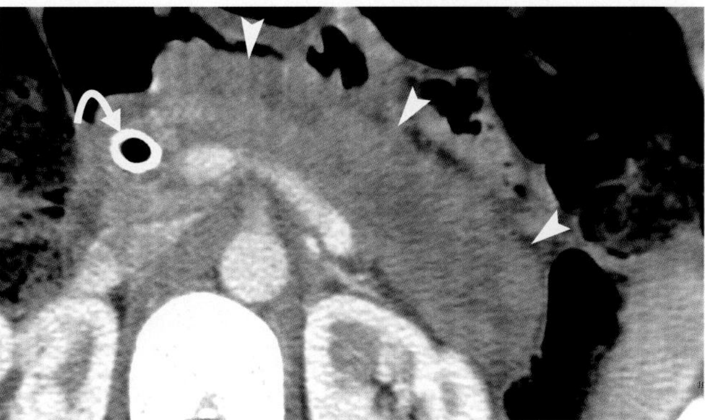

FIGURE 42.10. **Autoimmune Pancreatitis.** Contrast-enhanced CT shows the pancreas (*arrowheads*) to be enlarged with decrease in attenuation and loss of its normal lobulated borders. The common bile duct was narrowed sufficiently to result in jaundice and to warrant treatment with a wallstent (*curved arrow*).

Autoimmune pancreatitis (lymphoplasmacytic sclerosing pancreatitis) is a unique form of pancreatitis caused by autoimmune disease associated with elevation of IgG4. The disease is most common in men aged 40 to 65. Presentation is often obstructive jaundice with history of recurrent mild abdominal pains. Extrapancreatic manifestations occur in 30% of patients and may include inflammatory bowel disease, especially ulcerative colitis, long-segment bile duct strictures, lung nodules, lymphadenopathy, lymphocytic infiltrates in the liver and kidneys, retroperitoneal fibrosis, and Sjögren syndrome.

Periductal infiltration by lymphocytes and plasma cells with accompanying dense fibrosis results in diffuse enlargement of the pancreas and masses closely simulating adenocarcinoma. Differentiation is important because autoimmune pancreatitis is effectively treated with oral steroids. Findings which favor a diagnosis of autoimmune pancreatitis include (Fig. 42.10) (a) diffuse or focal swelling of the pancreas with characteristic tight halo of edema; (b) extensive peripancreatic stranding and edema are absent; (c) diffuse or segmental narrowing of the pancreatic duct and/or the common bile duct; (d) absence of dilation of the pancreatic duct and absence of parenchymal atrophy proximal to the pancreatic mass (these findings are typically present with adenocarcinoma); (e) fluid collections and parenchymal calcifications are typically absent; (f) peripancreatic blood vessels are usually not involved; and (g) the kidneys are involved in one-third of cases showing round, wedge-like, or diffuse peripheral patchy areas of decreased contrast enhancement. Imaging findings normalize following steroid treatment.

Groove pancreatitis is an uncommon form of pancreatitis that may also mimic adenocarcinoma. Fibrosis in the groove between the head of the pancreas, the descending duodenum, and the common bile duct produces an inflammatory mass that obstructs the common bile duct. The disease is most common in middle-aged men with a long history of alcohol abuse. The cause is unknown. Characteristic findings include (a) sheet-like mass in the pancreaticoduodenal groove, (b) atrophy and fibrotic changes in the pancreatic head, (c) small cysts along the wall of the duodenum, (d) duodenal wall thickening and luminal narrowing, (e) tapering stenosis of the common bile and pancreatic ducts, (f) widening of the space between the distal ducts and the wall of the duodenum (rarely seen with adenocarcinoma), and (g) enhancement is delayed but progressive.

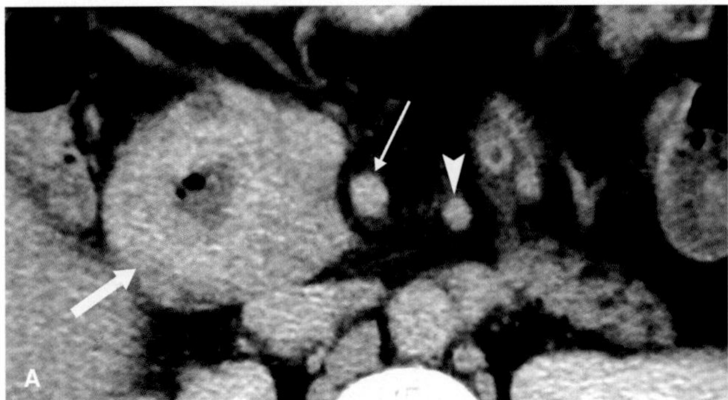

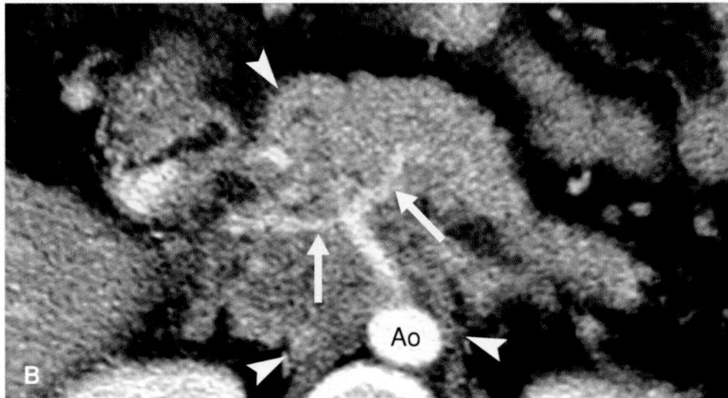

FIGURE 42.11. **Pancreatic Carcinoma. A: Resectable.** This adenocarcinoma (*fat arrow*) of the pancreatic head proved to be surgically resectable. Central necrosis produced low density and air bubbles in the middle of the lesion. The superior mesenteric artery (*arrowhead*) and vein (*skinny arrow*) are spared of involvement. **B: Nonresectable.** Adenocarcinoma of the pancreas (*arrowheads*) envelopes the aorta (*Ao*) and celiac axis and its branches (*arrows*) encasing and narrowing the arteries. This cancer is not resectable by CT criteria.

Solid Lesions of the Pancreas

Pancreatic adenocarcinoma (ductal carcinoma) is a highly lethal tumor that is usually unresectable at presentation. The average survival time of a patient with this disease is only 6 to 12 months. It accounts for 3% of all cancers and is second only to colorectal cancer as the most common digestive tract malignancy. Radiographic assessment of resectability is critical because surgical resection offers the only hope of cure, yet the surgery itself carries a high morbidity. Less than 20% of patients are candidates for surgery. MR and CT have comparable overall performance for determination of potential resectability. Scanning by CT or MR should include rapid bolus contrast injection, thin slices, and angiography to provide accurate tumor staging. Adenocarcinoma appears as a hypodense mass distorting the contour of the gland. Associated findings include obstruction of the common bile duct and pancreatic duct and atrophy of pancreatic tissue proximal to the tumor. Metastases commonly go to regional nodes, liver, and the peritoneal cavity. Signs of *resectability* (Fig. 42.11A) include (a) isolated pancreatic mass with or without dilation of the bile or pancreatic ducts; (b) no extrapancreatic disease; and (c) no encasement of celiac axis or SMA. Signs of *potential resectability* include (a) absence of involvement of the celiac axis or SMA; (b) regional nodes may be involved; and (c) limited peripancreatic extension of tumor may be present. Signs of *unresectability* include (a) encasement of the celiac axis or SMA (Fig. 42.11B); (b) occlusion of the superior mesenteric or portal vein without a technical option for reconstruction; and (c) liver, peritoneal, lung, or any other distant metastases. Evidence of arterial encasement that indicates unresectability include (a) tumor abutting >180 degrees of the circumference of the artery; (b) tumor abutment focally narrowing the artery; and (c) occlusion of the artery by tumor. As noted previously, consideration should be given to alternative diagnoses of chronic, autoimmune, or groove pancreatitis. Image-guided biopsy can confirm the diagnosis in patients whose tumors are deemed to be unresectable. Tumor recurrence following the Whipple procedure is best detected with MDCT. MR shows low signal infiltrative tumor surrounded by high signal–enhanced parenchyma on postcontrast T1WI. MRCP defines ductal anatomy with dilation proximal to the stricturing tumor. MRA and MRV are excellent in identifying vascular involvement by tumor.

Chronic pancreatitis may produce a mass that mimics pancreas carcinoma. Beaded dilation of the pancreatic duct is characteristic of chronic pancreatitis while smooth ductal dilation is most frequent with carcinoma. Calcifications within the mass are common with chronic pancreatitis and are very rare with adenocarcinoma. Neuroendocrine tumors more commonly contain calcifications. As many as 14% of patients with pancreatic adenocarcinoma also have chronic pancreatitis. Image-guided biopsy is usually needed to provide a definitive diagnosis, but a negative biopsy is not always definitive because of sampling errors.

Neuroendocrine (islet cell) tumors may be functioning producing hormones resulting in distinct clinical syndromes, or may be nonfunctional and grow to large size before presenting clinically. Insulinomas present with episodic hypoglycemia. Gastrinomas present with peptic ulcers, diarrhea caused by gastric hypersecretion, or Zollinger–Ellison syndrome. Other neuroendocrine tumors include glucagonoma (diabetes mellitus and painful glossitis), somatostatinoma (diabetes and steatorrhea), and VIPoma (massive watery diarrhea). Functioning tumors vary in malignant potential from 10% for insulinoma to 60% for gastrinoma and to 80% for glucagonoma. Functioning neuroendocrine tumors are usually less than 3 cm size and require strict attention to technique for accurate preoperative identification. Most small neuroendocrine tumors cannot be identified on precontrast CT. Because the lesions tend to be hypervascular, bolus contrast administration during rapid, thin-slice, MDCT scanning through the pancreatic bed offers the best chance of lesion visualization. The tumor stands out as an enhancing nodule within the pancreas (Fig. 42.12). MR shows functional tumors as low signal on T1WI, high signal on T2WI, and homogeneously hyperintense on postcontrast images. Intraoperative sonography has proved extremely

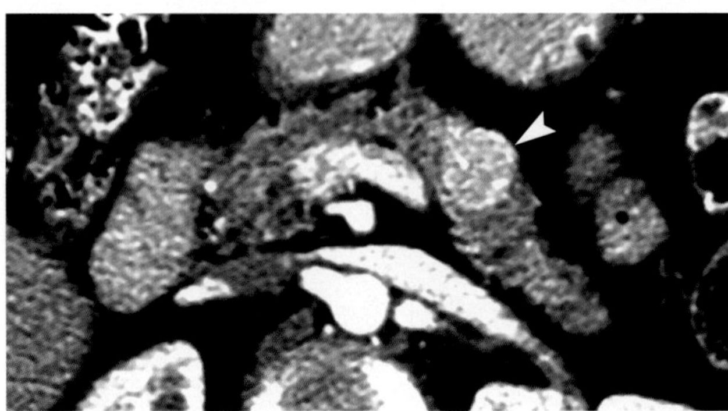

FIGURE 42.12. **Neuroendocrine Tumor—Insulinoma.** A small insulin-secreting tumor (*arrowhead*) in the distal body of the pancreas is identified by bright enhancement during arterial phase of contrast injection by MDCT.

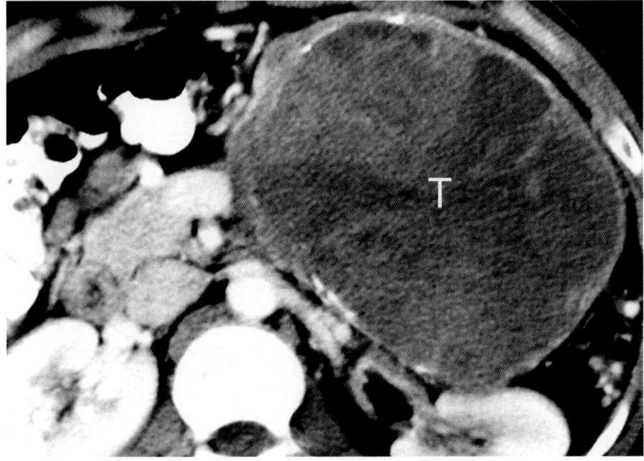

FIGURE 42.13. **Nonfunctioning Malignant Neuroendocrine Tumor.** A huge tumor mass (*T*) arises from the tail of the pancreas. This tumor grew to large size before producing symptoms. Note the heterogeneous attenuation characteristic of large neuroendocrine malignancies.

valuable for tumor localization during surgery. The lesions appear as hypoechoic masses within the pancreas.

Up to 80% of nonfunctioning tumors are malignant. Nonfunctioning neuroendocrine tumors tend to be much larger (6- to 20-cm diameter) (Fig. 42.13) than functioning tumors. Imaging findings include coarse calcifications, cystic degeneration, necrosis, local and vascular invasion, and metastases. MR shows heterogeneous masses generally low signal on T1WI, heterogeneous high signal in cystic and necrotic areas on T2WI, and heterogeneously hyperenhancing on dynamic postcontrast images (Fig. 42.14).

Metastases to the pancreas are most frequent with renal cell carcinoma and bronchogenic carcinoma. Lesions may appear as a solitary, well-defined, heterogeneously enhancing mass (Fig. 42.15), as diffuse heterogeneous enlargement of the pancreas, or as multiple nodules. Tumors have no predilection for any particular portion of the pancreas. On MR most lesions are low signal on T1WI and high signal on T2WI. Melanoma metastases are characteristically hyperintense on T1WI because of the paramagnetic properties of melanin.

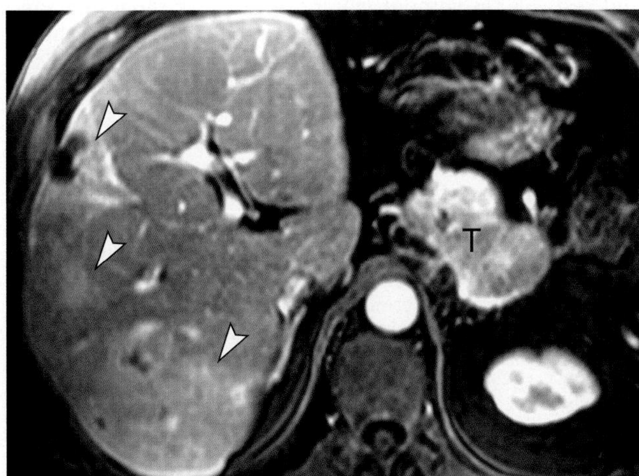

FIGURE 42.14. **Malignant Islet Cell Tumor.** Fat-suppressed T1-weighted early phase postcontrast MR demonstrates bright enhancement of the primary tumor (*T*) as well as its metastases (*arrowheads*) in the liver.

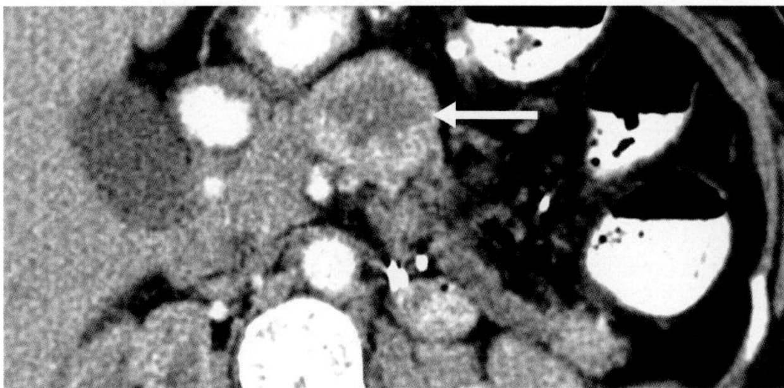

FIGURE 42.15. **Metastasis to the Pancreas.** Postcontrast CT reveals an avidly enhancing mass (*arrow*) with low attenuation necrotic center in the neck of the pancreas. This proved to be metastatic disease from renal cell carcinoma.

Lymphoma may involve the pancreas as a primary site (rare) or by direct extension from disease in the retroperitoneum. On CT most lesions are homogeneous, of lower attenuation than muscle, and show limited enhancement. Lesions be a localized, well-defined mass or be infiltrating diffusely enlarging or replacing the gland. Attenuation may be so low as to appear cystic. Peripancreatic lymph nodes are often enlarged.

Fatty lesions of the pancreas include diffuse fatty infiltration, focal fatty infiltration, focal fatty sparing, and lipoma. Diffuse infiltration is associated with aging and obesity and is seen with pancreatic atrophy. Fat infiltrates between the lobules of pancreatic parenchyma (Fig. 42.16). Focal fatty sparing in diffuse infiltration may simulate a pancreatic mass, especially when it involves the head or uncinate process. Focal fatty infiltration may involve any portion of the pancreas. Lipomas are rare, usually solitary, fat-density masses that are usually incidental findings but may occasionally obstruct the pancreatic or bile ducts.

Cystic fibrosis is now commonly seen in adults as treatment has continued to improve. The pancreas in teenage and adult patients is commonly entirely replaced by fat in association with exocrine insufficiency. *Pancreatic cystosis* refers to the unusual occurrence of macrocysts of varying size distributed throughout the pancreas in patients with cystic fibrosis. The cysts are true cysts developing from functional remnants of pancreatic ducts. Additional findings include acute pancreatitis and calcifications in the pancreas.

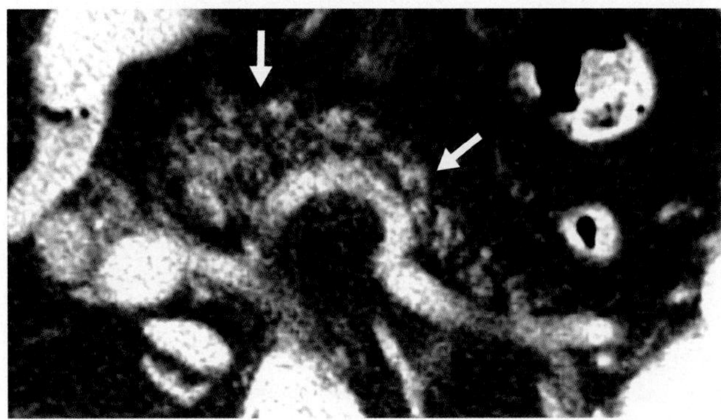

FIGURE 42.16. **Diffuse Fatty Infiltration Pancreas.** CT shows diffuse fatty infiltration between the lobules of the pancreas (*arrows*) in a 70-year-old obese patient.

Cystic Lesions of the Pancreas

A current challenge of pancreatic imaging is to differentiate potentially aggressive cystic neoplasms from benign pseudocysts and other nonaggressive cystic lesions. As the use of imaging expands cystic lesions of the pancreas are commonly revealed as incidental findings on US, CT, and MR performed for other reasons. Cystic neoplasms include primary cystic tumors (5% to 10% of cystic lesions) and cystic degeneration of solid tumors.

Pancreatitis-associated fluid collections are the most common pancreatic cystic lesions representing up to 85% to 90% of cystic lesions. Most are unilocular fluid collections confined by a fibrous wall that does not contain epithelium (Fig. 42.5). They arise after episodes of acute pancreatitis or are insidiously associated with chronic pancreatitis. Some occur with no history or findings of pancreatitis. Most are symptomatic causing abdominal pain. Findings include (a) fluid-density unilocular cyst associated with findings of acute or chronic pancreatitis; (b) complex cystic mass with internal hemorrhage, infection, or gas; (c) most are round or oval with a thin or thick wall that may enhance, however, cyst contents do not enhance; (d) septations and lobulated contours are unusual and more often associated with serous cystadenoma; (e) some lesions may be infected showing the presence of gas and debris within the lesion (Fig. 42.6); and (f) serial imaging usually shows involution of noninfected collections. Cyst fluid aspiration commonly reveals elevated amylase levels.

Serous cystadenomas are benign tumors not requiring treatment. Tumors occur most commonly in women (especially >60 years of age) and are distributed uniformly throughout the head, body, and tail of the pancreas. Patients with von Hippel–Lindau syndrome may develop multiple tumors and at a younger age. Tumors show three major imaging appearances: (a) most common is honeycomb microcysts (microcystic adenoma) with innumerable small cysts 1 mm to 2 cm size (Fig. 42.17); (b) a macrocystic form with larger cysts is seen in 10% overlapping the appearance of mucinous cystadenoma (see Fig. 42.21); (c) innumerable tiny cysts may make the lesion appear solid (Fig. 42.18). A central stellate scar that may calcify is a highly diagnostic feature. The lesions do not communicate with the pancreatic duct. Diagnosis is confirmed by aspiration of clear fluid without mucin and without tumor markers seen with cystic mucinous neoplasms of the pancreas such as carcinoembryonic antigen (CEA) or carbohydrate antigen (CA 19-9, CA 72-4, CEACAM6).

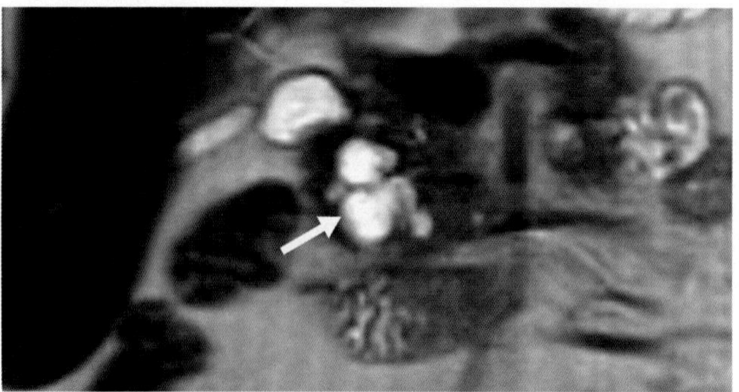

FIGURE 42.17. Serous Cystadenoma—Microcystic Appearance. Coronal plane T2-weighted MR image shows a mass (*arrow*) in the pancreatic head composed of numerous small cysts of varying size. Careful inspection of multiplane images showed no communication with the pancreatic duct. Endoscopic US-guided aspiration confirmed serous fluid within the small cysts.

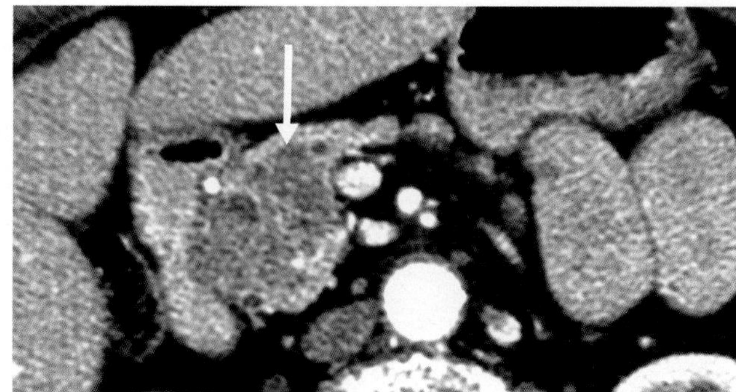

FIGURE 42.18. Serous Cystadenoma—Solid Appearance. Enhanced CT shows a mass (*arrow*) in the pancreatic head consisting of innumerable cysts that are so small the low attenuation mass appears almost solid.

Cystic mucinous neoplasms of the pancreas are classified as intraductal papillary mucinous neoplasm (IPMN) and mucinous cystic neoplasm (MCN). Both tumor types are characterized pathologically by mucin-producing epithelial tumor cells that tend to form papillae and grow as cystic lesions. Both tumor types show pathologic progression from low-grade dysplasia (adenoma) to high-grade dysplasia (carcinoma in situ) to invasive carcinoma. Thus, even benign lesions are considered premalignant.

International consensus guidelines for management of mucinous tumors of the pancreas were established in 2006 and revised in 2012 (Fukuoka guidelines). Morphologic classification of tumors is based on radiographic features. Contrast-enhanced MDCT or MR with MRCP is recommended for cysts ≥10 mm and cysts producing symptoms to check for “high-risk stigmata” or “worrisome features.” Invasive cancer is rare in asymptomatic cysts <10 mm size. “Worrisome features” on imaging include cysts ≥3-cm diameter; enhancing thickened cyst walls; main pancreatic duct diameter 5 to 9 mm; mural nodules without enhancement; abrupt narrowing of the main pancreatic duct with proximal atrophy of pancreatic parenchyma; and regional lymphadenopathy. “High-risk stigmata” on imaging include common bile duct obstruction with jaundice associated with cystic tumor in the pancreatic head; enhancement of solid components; and main pancreatic duct diameter ≥10 mm. The Fukuoka guidelines recommend resection without further testing for cystic lesions with high-risk stigmata. Cystic lesions with worrisome features and cysts >3 cm without worrisome features should undergo endoscopic US for further characterization. Cysts ≤3 cm should undergo routine surveillance with MCDT or MR with MRCP.

Intraductal papillary mucinous neoplasms are intraductal neoplasms that arise in the main pancreatic duct or its branches. Mucin secretion causes dilation of affected ducts. Dysplastic changes range from low grade to invasive carcinoma sometimes within a single cystic lesion. IPMNs are classified into three morphologic types: branch duct (BD-IPMN), main duct (MD-IPMN), and mixed type. BD-IPMN is most common in the uncinate process arising in branches of the main pancreatic duct to form grape-like collections of small cysts (5- to 20-mm diameter) that communicate with the ductal system (Fig. 42.19). Some lesions consist of a single unilocular cyst. The cysts have thin walls with flat or papillary lining that produces tenacious mucin. Invasive carcinoma is found in 17%. MD-IPMN is characterized by diffuse or segmental dilation of the main pancreatic duct >5-mm diameter without evidence of other causes of obstruction. The diffusely or partially dilated, tortuous and irregular, main pancreatic duct is filled with mucin produced by tumor cells (Fig. 42.20). Mucin may be extruded from the ampulla. Most tumors arise in the head of the pancreas and progress along the duct often involving the entire pancreas. Segmental

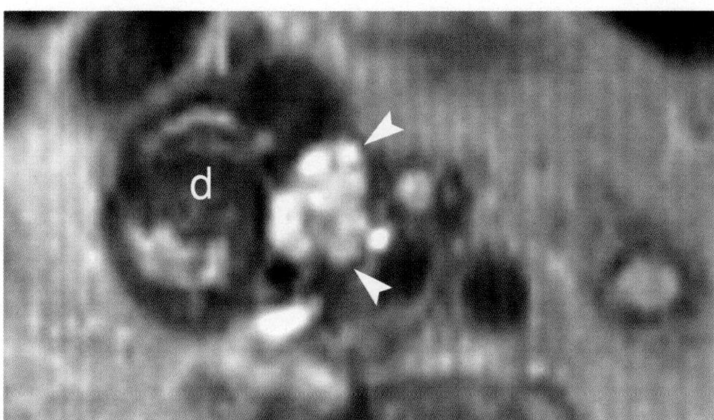

FIGURE 42.19. Intraductal Papillary Mucinous Neoplasm—Branch Duct Type. T2-weighted axial plane MR image shows a multilobulated cystic mass (*arrowheads*) with "bunch of grapes" appearance occupying the head of the pancreas. Multiple images confirmed communication of the cystic mass with the pancreatic ductal system. Pathology after surgical removal confirmed IPMN. *d*, duodenum.

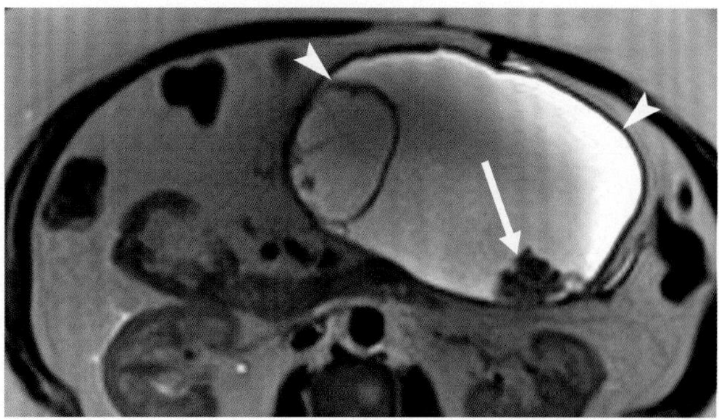

FIGURE 42.21. Mucinous Cystic Neoplasm (Cystadenocarcinoma). Precontrast T1-weighted MR shows a very large cystic mass (*arrowheads*) arising from the tail of the pancreas. A frond-like papillary projection (*arrow*) showed enhancement on subsequent postcontrast images. This focus proved to be adenocarcinoma in a mucinous cystic neoplasm.

dilation is most common in the body and tail of the pancreas. Uninvolved pancreas may become atrophic proximal to tumor involvement developing findings of chronic obstructive pancreatitis. Invasive carcinoma is found in 44% of MD-IPMN. Mixed-type IPMN meets criteria for both MD-IPMN and BD-IPMN. Invasive carcinoma is found in 45% of mixed-type IPMN. Patients who develop IPMN average 60 to 70 years of age with about equal male to female incidence. Ovarian stroma is not found in IPMN.

Mucinous cystic neoplasm occurs nearly always in women (F:M = 19:1) with mean age of 45 years. The presence of ovarian stroma in addition to mucin-producing epithelial tumor cells is specific to this tumor. MCNs do not arise from or communicate with the pancreatic duct. The prevalence of invasive carcinoma is less than 15% with no malignancy found in MCNs of <4 cm without mural nodules. The risk of malignancy increases with the patient's age. Imaging shows a cystic lesion larger than 2 cm nearly always in the pancreatic tail. Tumors are multilocular with a few compartments or uncommonly unilocular. Papillary projections of solid tumor are common (Fig. 42.21). Peripheral eggshell calcification is an uncommon but highly specific finding. MRCP reveals no communication with pancreatic ducts. Endoscopic US-guided fluid aspiration revealing mucin confirms the diagnosis of mucinous neoplasm. Metastases to the liver tend to be cystic.

It is currently generally accepted, and recommended by Fukuoka guidelines, that MD-IPMNs, mixed-type IPMNs, and MCNs, and should be resected if the patient is "surgically fit" because of their high malignant potential. BD-IPMN >3-cm diameter and without high-risk stigmata can be observed with MDCT or MR/MRCP follow-up initially at 3 to 6 months and then annually.

Solid pseudopapillary tumor of the pancreas is a rare (1% to 2% of pancreatic neoplasms) low-grade malignancy that presents as a large (mean 9 cm) encapsulated mass with a mixture of fluid, hemorrhagic, necrotic, and solid components (Fig. 42.22). It is not truly papillary or cystic. Pseudopapillae are formed by layers of epithelial cells that cover a fibrovascular core. Cells degenerate and fall off the pseudopapillae contributing to debris within the tumor. It occurs most frequently in young women (F:M = 9:1) (mean age 30 to 35 years). Approximately 15% demonstrate low-grade malignant elements.

Patients are often asymptomatic even though the lesions may exceed 20 cm in size. These lesions most closely resemble neuroendocrine tumors. CT shows a heterogeneous well-encapsulated tumor with variable cystic and solid components. Solid areas, usually in the periphery, enhance. Peripheral calcifications may be present. MR shows heterogeneous low signal on T1WI, heterogeneous high signal on T1WI, and enhancement of solid tissue.

Cystic change in solid tumors is far less common than pancreatic pseudocysts or primary pancreatic cystic neoplasms. Cystic change that rarely occurs in neuroendocrine tumors is the result of tumor degeneration. Cystic neuroendocrine neoplasms tend to be larger, more symptomatic, and more likely to be nonfunctional

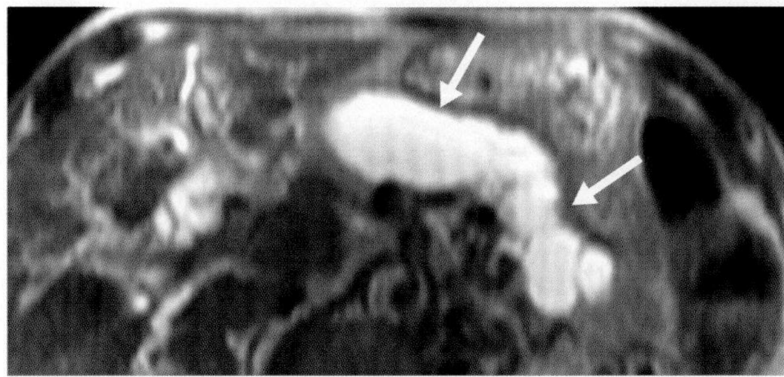

FIGURE 42.20. Intraductal Papillary Mucinous Neoplasm—Main Duct Type. T2-weighted axial plane MR shows massive irregular tortuous dilation of the main pancreatic duct (*arrows*). No discernible pancreatic parenchyma is evident. Endoscopy revealed mucin extruding from the major papilla. Chronic obstruction caused by the tumor results in diffuse pancreatic atrophy.

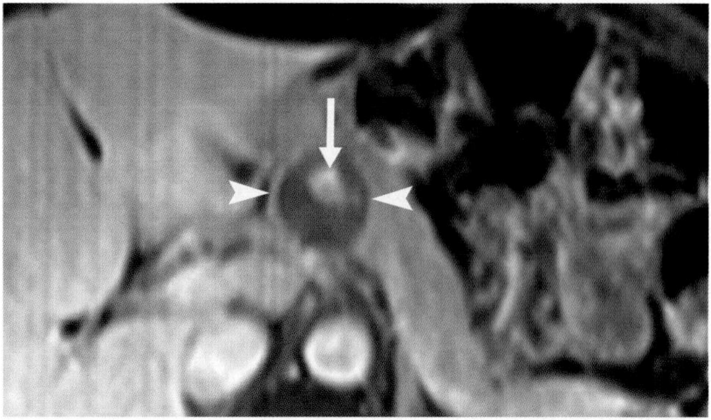

FIGURE 42.22. Solid Pseudopapillary Tumor. Axial T1-weighted postcontrast MR image shows a well-encapsulated low signal tumor (*arrowheads*) in the neck of the pancreas. A solid component (*arrow*) enhances.

than solid neuroendocrine tumors. Cystic change in adenocarcinoma is usually the result of necrosis, hemorrhage, or formation of pseudocysts adjacent to the neoplasm. Cystic change in solid tumors is suggested by the presence of vascularized enhancing soft tissue elements within the tumors.

Cystic teratomas arise rarely in the pancreas and usually have characteristic hair, fat, calcifications, and cystic and solid components. MR is the optimal modality for imaging characterizations of cystic lesions. Endoscopic US-guided aspiration of cyst fluid confirms mucinous, serous, hemorrhagic, or infected cyst contents.

Duodenal diverticula filled with fluid may mimic a cystic pancreatic tumor or an abscess.

Tiny simple cysts are common incidental findings in the pancreas demonstrated with high sensitivity by MR. Unilocular cysts smaller than 10 mm are virtually always benign pseudocysts or retention cysts.

SPLEEN

Imaging Techniques

CT and US remain the major techniques used to image the splenic parenchyma although MR plays an increasing role. Gadolinium enhancement improves the specificity of spleen MR. Technetium-99m sulfur colloid radionuclide scanning images both the liver and the spleen and can be used to confirm the presence of functioning splenic tissue, important in the diagnosis of splenosis.

Anatomy

The spleen is the body's largest lymphoid organ. Although it serves as a site of blood formation in the fetus, there is no hematopoietic activity in the normal adult spleen. The spleen sequesters abnormal and aged red and white blood cells and platelets and serves as a reservoir for red blood cells. The spleen occupies the left upper quadrant of the abdomen just below the diaphragm, posterior and lateral to the stomach. Its diaphragmatic surface is smooth and convex, conforming to the shape of the diaphragm, whereas its visceral surface has concavities for the stomach, kidney, colon, and pancreas. Spleen size varies with age, nutrition, and hydration. The spleen is relatively large in children, reaching adult size by age 15. The average spleen dimensions in adults are 12 cm in length, 7 cm in width, and 3 to 4 cm in thickness. In older adults, the spleen progressively decreases in size with age. The splenic artery and vein course through the pancreas to the splenic hilum, where they divide into multiple branches. Splenic arteries are end arteries without anastomoses or collateral supply. Occlusion of the splenic artery or its branches produces infarction. US demonstrates a midlevel homogeneous echo pattern for the splenic parenchyma. On noncontrast CT, the normal spleen density is less than or equal to the density of normal liver. On MR the spleen signal intensity is lower than hepatic parenchyma on T1WI images and higher than liver parenchyma on T2WI.

Following intravenous contrast injection the enhancement pattern of the spleen reflects the normal low-resistance fast-flow circulation, as well as the high-resistance slow-flow filtering circulation, which functions to clear aging and damaged blood cells. During arterial phase contrast enhancement appears as alternating bands of high and low density, the arciform enhancement pattern. Delayed postcontrast images show homogeneous enhancement of the splenic parenchyma.

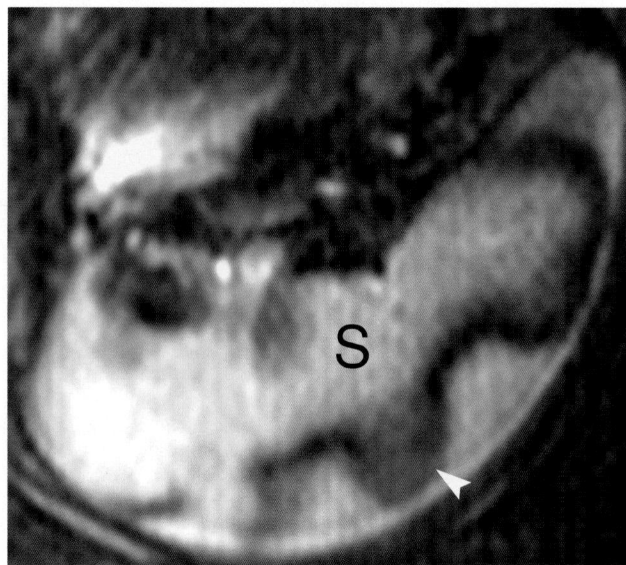

FIGURE 42.23. **Transient Pseudomasses in Spleen.** Early T1-weighted image from a contrast-enhanced dynamic MR shows the normal arciform pattern of splenic enhancement with pseudomass formation (*arrowhead*). On delayed images the spleen (*S*) showed normal uniform enhancement. This appearance results from the uneven diffusion of contrast agent through the pulp of the spleen.

Transient pseudomasses may be formed during the arciform enhancement phase on postcontrast CT and MR (Fig. 42.23). Irregular defects in parenchymal enhancement may closely simulate splenic lesions. One or 2 minutes later, the entire spleen becomes homogeneously enhanced. Diffuse liver disease is associated with more prominent splenic pseudomasses during early enhancement.

Lobulations and clefts in the splenic contour are common and must not be mistaken for masses or splenic fractures.

Accessory spleens are found in 10% to 16% of normal individuals. These appear as round masses, 1 to 3 cm in size, and of the same imaging features as normal splenic parenchyma (Fig. 42.24). They may be single or multiple and are usually located near the splenic hilum. Technetium sulfur colloid

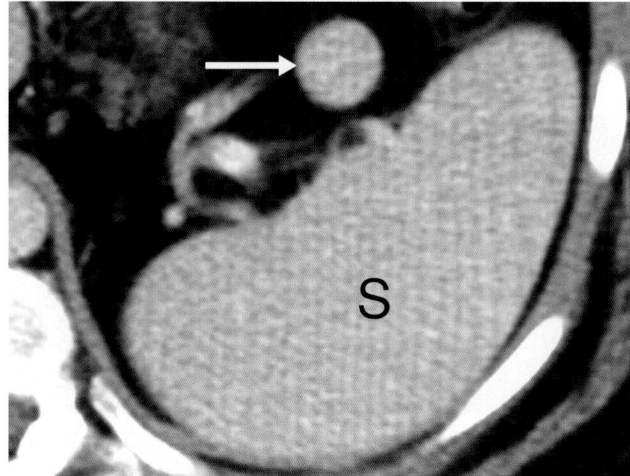

FIGURE 42.24. **Accessory Spleen.** An accessory spleen (*arrow*) is seen in the splenic hilum. Accessory spleens have the same imaging and enhancement characteristics as the parent spleen (*S*).

radionuclide scans can be used to confirm suspected accessory spleens as functioning splenic tissue.

Wandering spleen is the term applied to a normal spleen positioned outside of its normal location in the left upper quadrant. Laxity of the splenic ligaments, commonly found in association with abnormalities of intestinal rotation, allows the spleen to be positioned anywhere in the abdominal cavity. A wandering spleen may present as a palpable abdominal mass, although most cause no symptoms. Because of lax ligaments the spleen may rotate and torse causing acute or recurrent abdominal pain. The diagnosis is made by recognizing the normal shape and tissue texture of the spleen, noting the absence of normal spleen in the left upper abdomen, and by identifying the blood supply from splenic vessels. Radionuclide scans confirm functioning splenic tissue.

Splenosis refers to multiple implants of ectopic splenic tissue that may occur after traumatic splenic rupture. Splenic tissue can implant anywhere in the abdominal cavity, or even in the thorax if the diaphragm has been ruptured. Splenosis complicates 40% to 60% of traumatic splenic injuries. The splenic implants are usually multiple and vary in size and shape. The tissue fragments enlarge over time and may simulate peritoneal metastases. Functioning splenic tissue is confirmed by radionuclide scanning.

Splenic Regeneration. After splenectomy, remaining accessory spleens, or splenules resulting from traumatic peritoneal seeding of splenic tissue may enlarge and resume the function of the resected spleen. When the spleen is removed, bits of nuclear material, called Howell–Jolly bodies, are routinely seen in red cells on peripheral blood smears. Absence or disappearance of these Howell–Jolly bodies from peripheral blood is a clinical sign of splenic regeneration. Imaging studies demonstrate single or multiple rounded well-defined spleen-like masses (Fig. 42.25) in the abdominal cavity in patients with a history of splenectomy.

Polysplenia is a rare congenital anomaly that features multiple small spleens, usually located in the right abdomen and associated with situs ambiguous. Both lungs are two-lobed. Most patients also have cardiovascular anomalies.

Asplenia (Ivemark syndrome) is the congenital absence of the spleen, found in association with bilateral right-sidedness, midline liver, and bilateral three-lobed lungs. Major cardiac anomalies are present in 50% of cases. Most patients die before 1 year of age.

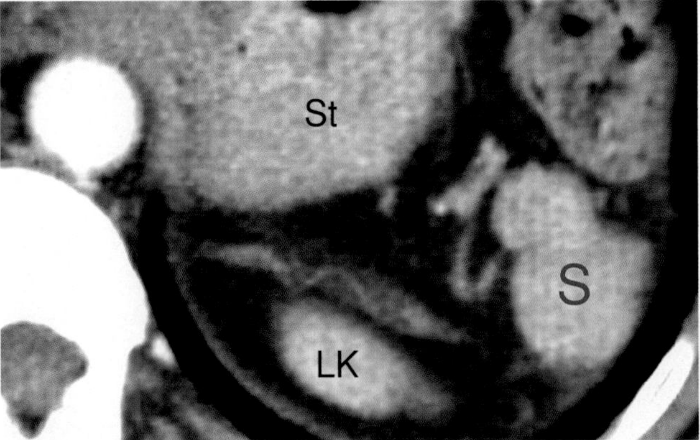

FIGURE 42.25. **Splenic Regeneration.** Hypertrophy of remnants of splenic tissue deposited on the diaphragm after traumatic splenic rupture has created a homogeneously enhancing mass of functioning splenic tissue (*S*). This patient has a history of splenectomy. *LK*, left kidney; *St*, stomach.

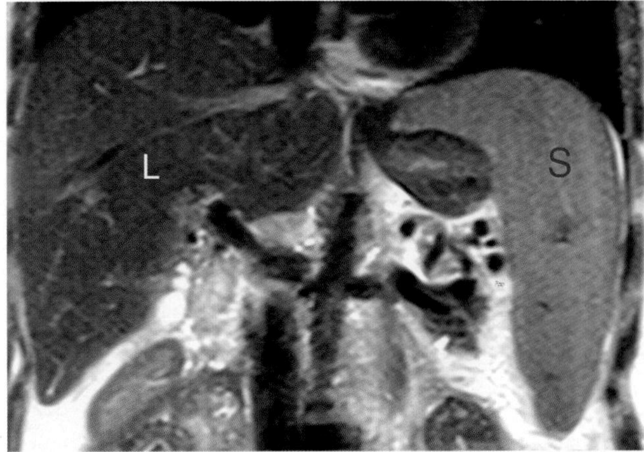

FIGURE 42.26. **Splenomegaly.** Coronal T2-weighted image of a patient with cirrhosis shows the spleen (*S*) to be enlarged measuring 20 cm in length. The spleen is larger than the liver (*L*) and extends into the central abdomen.

Splenomegaly. The diagnosis of splenic enlargement on imaging studies is usually made subjectively. Although quantitative methods have been attempted, none have proved popular. Findings that suggest splenomegaly are any spleen dimension greater than 14 cm, projection of the spleen ventral to the anterior axillary line, inferior spleen tip extending more caudally than the inferior liver tip, or inferior spleen tip extending below the lower pole of the left kidney. Enlarged spleens frequently compress and displace adjacent organs, especially the left kidney (Fig. 42.26). The causes of splenomegaly are exhaustive (Table 42.3). Most do not produce a change in spleen imaging features, so differentiation is based upon other

TABLE 42.3

CAUSES OF SPLENOMEGALY

Congestive
Portal hypertension (50% of cases)
Portal vein thrombosis
Myeloproliferative disorders
Leukemia
Lymphoma (30% of cases)
Polycythemia vera
Idiopathic thrombocytopenia purpura
Sickle cell disease (in infants)
Thalassemia major
Hereditary spherocytosis
Myelofibrosis
Infection
Malaria (universal in endemic areas)
Schistosomiasis (in endemic areas)
Infectious mononucleosis
Subacute bacterial endocarditis
AIDS
Intravenous drug abuse
Infiltrative
Systemic lupus erythematosus
Amyloidosis
Gaucher disease

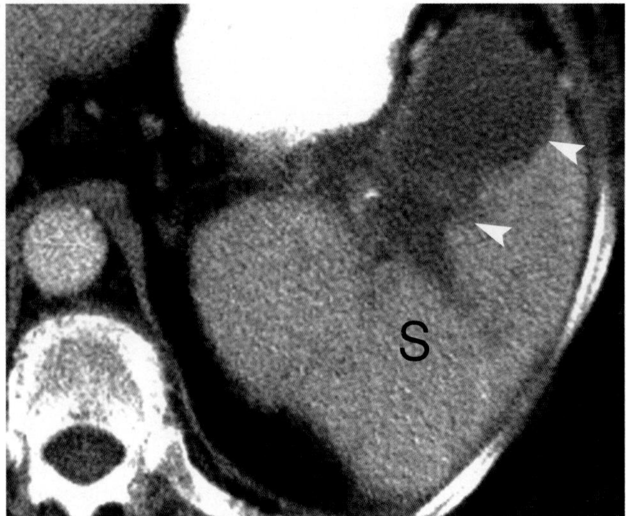

FIGURE 42.27. **Lymphoma.** Contrast-enhanced CT demonstrates a lobulated low attenuation mass (*arrowheads*) within the parenchyma of the spleen (*S*). The lesion resembles splenic infarction because it extends all the way to the splenic capsule.

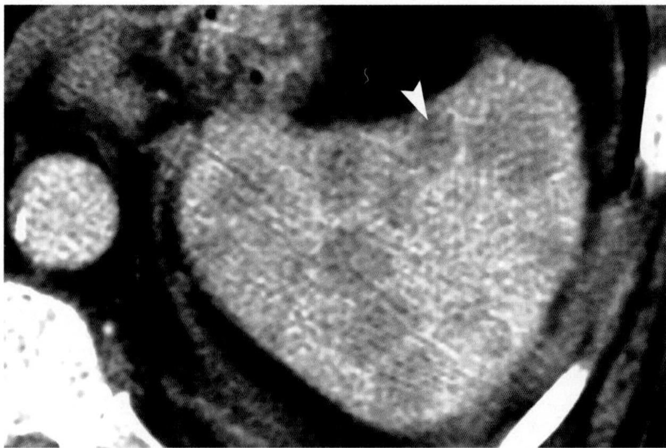

FIGURE 42.28. **Metastases.** Numerous metastases (*arrowhead*) from malignant melanoma are seen as low attenuation nodules on this post-contrast CT.

imaging findings or on clinical evaluation. MR offers no significant benefit to the differential diagnosis of splenomegaly. Mild to moderate splenomegaly is seen with portal hypertension, AIDS, storage diseases, collagen vascular disorders, and infection. More marked splenomegaly is usually associated with lymphoma, leukemia, infectious mononucleosis, hemolytic anemia, and myelofibrosis.

Solid Lesions of the Spleen

Lymphoma is the most common malignant tumor involving the spleen either as primary splenic lymphoma or as part of systemic disease. Patterns of involvement visible on imaging studies include diffuse splenomegaly, multiple masses of varying size, miliary nodules resembling microabscesses, large solitary mass (Fig. 42.27), and direct invasion from adjacent lymphomatous nodes. Adenopathy is frequently evident elsewhere in the abdomen. On CT splenic lymphoma is low attenuation. On MR it is low to intermediate signal intensity on T1WI and mild to moderate high signal intensity on T2WI. Lesions are hypoenhancing on both modalities. Diffuse infiltrative lymphoma may appear normal on all imaging studies. Lymphoma is a common predisposing condition for splenic infarction.

Metastases are found in the spleen on autopsy series in up to 7% of patients who die of cancer. Most splenic metastases are microscopic and are not detected by imaging studies. The most common tumors to metastasize to the spleen are malignant melanoma and lung, breast, ovary, prostate, and stomach carcinoma. Most are spread by hematogenous dissemination and reflect widespread disease. On CT metastases appear as single or multiple low-density masses (Fig. 42.28). On MR, metastases are low intensity on T1WI and high intensity on T2WI. The increased signal intensity of the lesions parallels the increased signal intensity of the normal splenic parenchyma on T2WI, and the lesions may not be evident. Contrast enhancement is recommended for both CT and MR demonstration of metastases. Calcification is rare. Melanoma metastases commonly appear cystic.

Infarction is produced by occlusion of the main or branch splenic arteries. Causes of infarction include emboli (arising from endocarditis, atherosclerotic plaques, or cardiac valve thrombi), sickle cell disease, pancreatitis, pancreatic tumors, and arteritis. Additional predisposing conditions include myeloproliferative disorders, hemolytic anemias, and sepsis. Infarcts classically appear as wedge-shaped defects in the splenic parenchyma. Multiple infarcts may fuse, however, and the wedge shape may be lost. The key finding is extension of the abnormal parenchymal zone to an intact splenic capsule (Fig. 42.29). Splenomegaly, especially due to lymphoma, is a predisposing condition. Complications of splenic infarctions include subcapsular hematomas, infection, and splenic rupture with hemoperitoneum.

Gamna–Gandy bodies (also called siderotic nodules) are small foci of hemosiderin resulting from focal hemorrhages

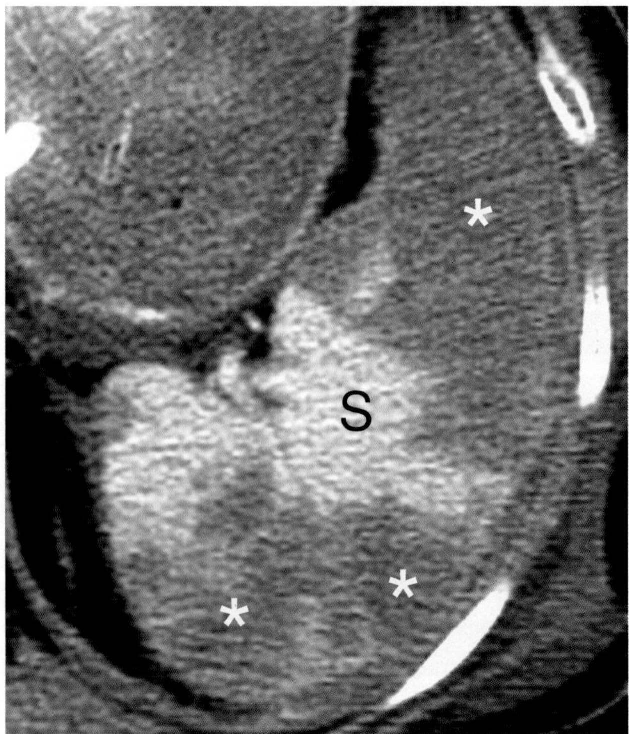

FIGURE 42.29. **Splenic Infarction.** Postcontrast CT in a patient with chronic lymphocytic leukemia shows multiple infarctions (*) within the spleen (*S*). Note how each lesion extends to the splenic capsule.

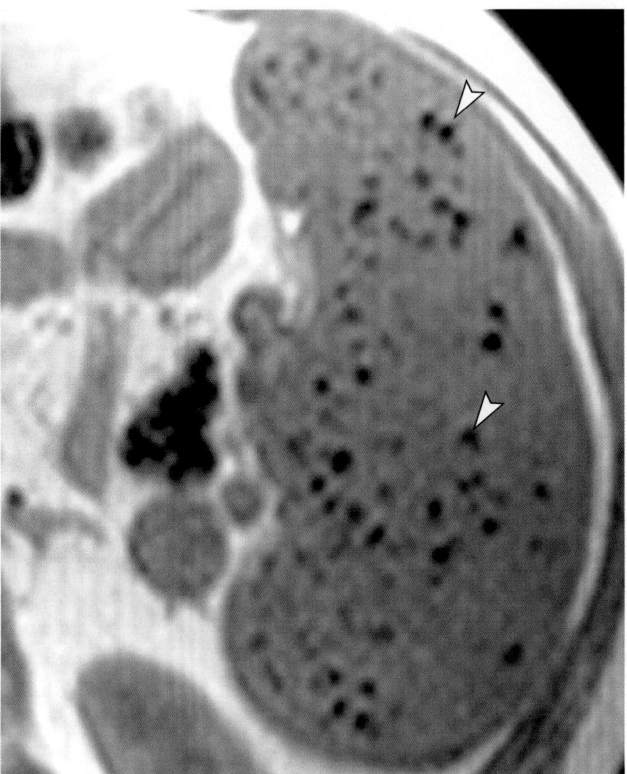

FIGURE 42.30. **Gamna–Gandy Bodies.** Axial plane T1-weighted MR image shows numerous low signal nodules (*arrowheads*) throughout the splenic parenchyma in a patient with splenomegaly and portal hypertension. These represent hemosiderin deposits from previous tiny intraparenchymal hemorrhages.

in the spleen caused by portal hypertension. They are seen best on MR as multiple small low-intensity nodules on T1WI- (Fig. 42.30) and T2*-weighted images. Signal intensity is low because of hemosiderin content. They do not enhance.

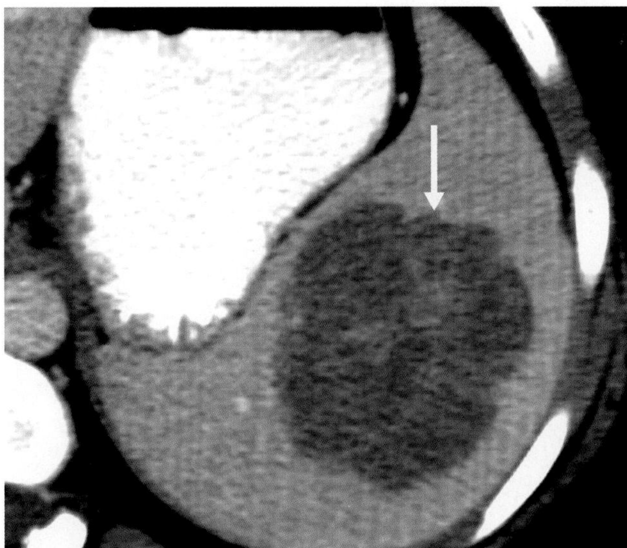

FIGURE 42.31. **Hemangioma Spleen.** Postcontrast CT shows this splenic hemangioma (*arrow*) to be an inhomogeneous, minimally enhancing, lobulated, low attenuation mass. This lesion is likely largely fibrotic.

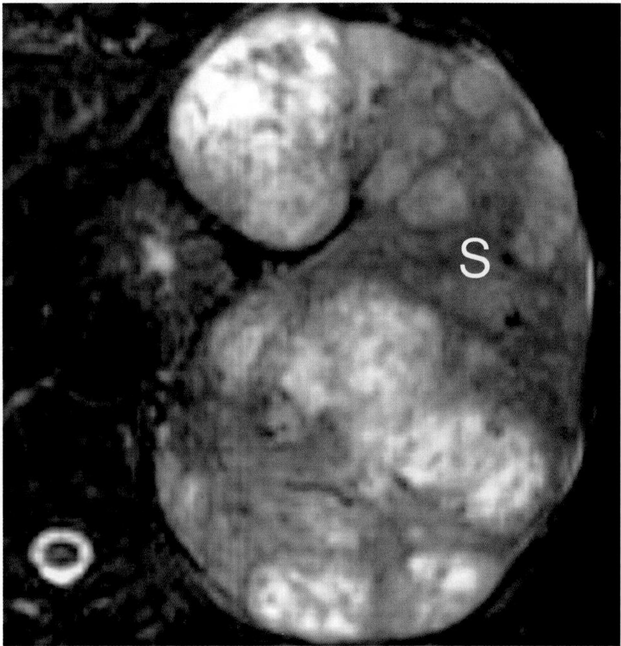

FIGURE 42.32. **Angiosarcoma Spleen.** Axial plane MR T2WI shows near-complete replacement of the parenchyma of the spleen (*S*) with numerous heterogeneous high signal nodules of various sizes. Pathology confirmed near-complete involvement of the spleen with angiosarcoma.

Hemangioma is the most common primary neoplasm of the spleen, found in 14% of patients on autopsy series. Like in the liver the tumor consists of vascular channels of varying size lined by a single layer of endothelium and demonstrates similar findings on noncontrast imaging studies. US shows a well-defined hyperechoic mass. On CT the lesion may appear solid and may have central punctate or peripheral curvilinear calcification. On MR the lesion is low in signal intensity on T1WI and high in signal intensity on T2WI. The contrast enhancement pattern is variable (Fig. 42.31). The nodular enhancement from the periphery described for liver hemangiomas is infrequently seen with splenic hemangiomas. More commonly peripheral rim-like enhancement progressively fills in. Hemangiomas may undergo thrombosis leading to fibrosis, hemorrhage, or infarction.

Angiosarcoma is very rare but is still the most common malignancy arising in the spleen. The tumor is aggressive, usually presenting with widespread metastases, especially to the liver. One-quarter of the cases present with spontaneous splenic rupture. CT shows multiple heterogeneous hypervascular masses of varying size. Internal hemorrhage and necrosis is common. MR shows heterogeneous high and low signal on T1WI and T2WI (Fig. 42.32) with heterogeneous hyperenhancement in solid areas. Patients with thorotrast exposure are at increased risk.

Cystic Lesions of the Spleen

Posttraumatic cysts are false cysts with fibrous walls that lack an epithelial lining. The walls are thick and commonly (30% to 40%) become calcified (Fig. 42.33). The internal fluid may be complex with blood products, cholesterol crystals, or cellular debris. Posttraumatic cysts result from previous hemorrhage, infarction, or infection. They account for 80% of all splenic cysts.

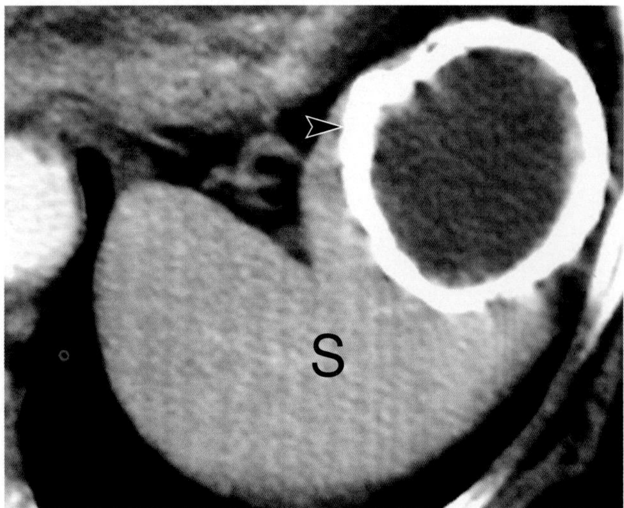

FIGURE 42.33. **Posttraumatic Splenic Cyst.** The well-defined cyst (*arrowhead*) with thick, densely calcified walls seen in the spleen (*S*) on this CT scan is the result of an old intrasplenic hemorrhage.

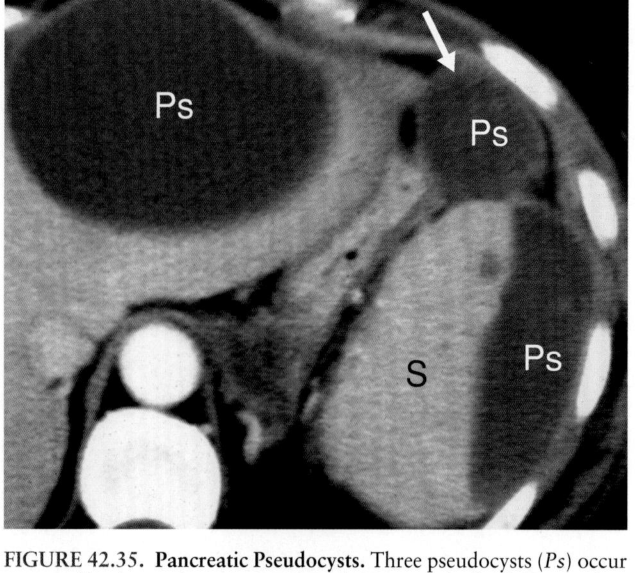

FIGURE 42.35. **Pancreatic Pseudocysts.** Three pseudocysts (*Ps*) occur as complications of acute pancreatitis. Pancreatic fluid dissected to subcapsular locations in the spleen and liver with one collection developing in the peritoneal cavity (*arrow*).

Epidermoid cysts are true epithelial-lined cysts that are probably developmental in origin. They have the same appearance as posttraumatic cysts but less frequently have calcification in their walls (5%) (Fig. 42.34). Most are found incidentally in asymptomatic individuals.

Pancreatic fluid collections and pseudocysts extend beneath the splenic capsule by tracking along the pancreatic tail to the splenic hilum. Splenic subcapsular pancreatic fluid collections develop in 1% to 5% of patients with pancreatitis (Fig. 42.35). Internal debris and hemorrhage are commonly present. Imaging studies demonstrate associated findings of pancreatitis.

Bacterial abscesses occur most commonly in spleens that are already diseased. They present with vague symptoms but have a high mortality when left untreated. They result from hematogenous spread of infection (75%), trauma (15%), or infarction (10%). Abscesses (Fig. 42.36) appear as single or multiple low-density masses with ill-defined, often thick, walls. US commonly demonstrates internal echoes resulting from inflammatory debris. Abscesses are low intensity on T1WI and high intensity on T2WI. They may contain gas or demonstrate air–fluid levels. Perisplenic fluid collections and left pleural effusions are common. Image-guided aspiration confirms the diagnosis. Treatment is by catheter drainage or splenectomy.

Microabscesses are found in patients with compromised immune systems attributable to AIDS, organ transplantation, lymphoma, or leukemia. The causes of microabscesses include fungi, tuberculosis, *Pneumocystis jiroveci,* histoplasmosis, and cytomegalovirus. Imaging studies demonstrate multiple small

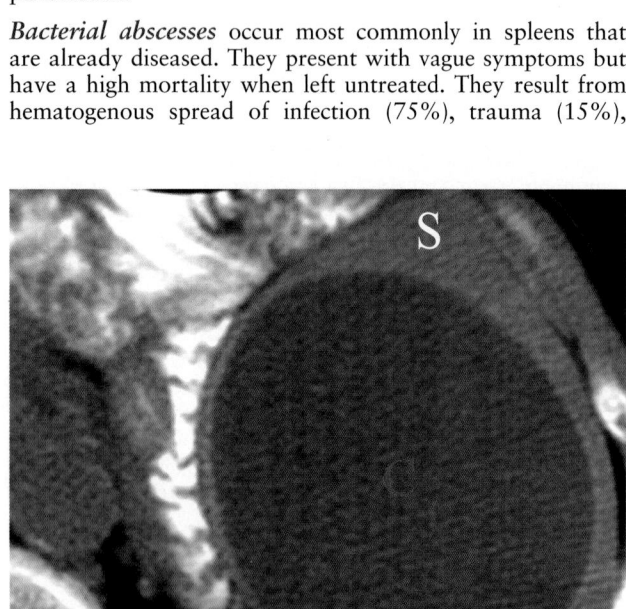

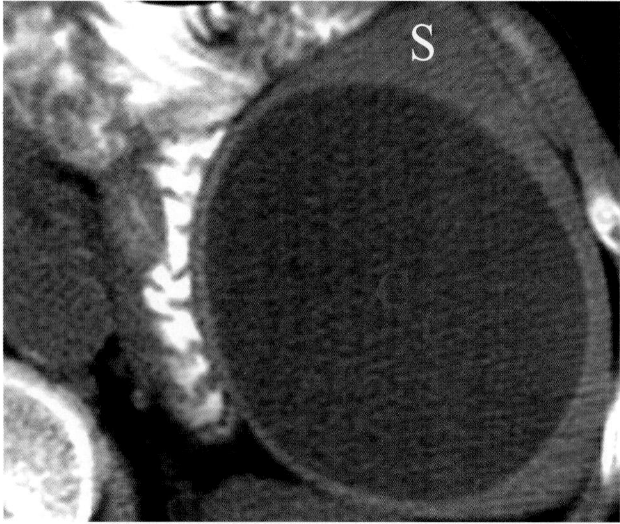

FIGURE 42.34. **Epidermoid Cyst Spleen.** CT without intravenous contrast shows a large well-defined homogenous benign appearing cyst (C) within the spleen (*S*).

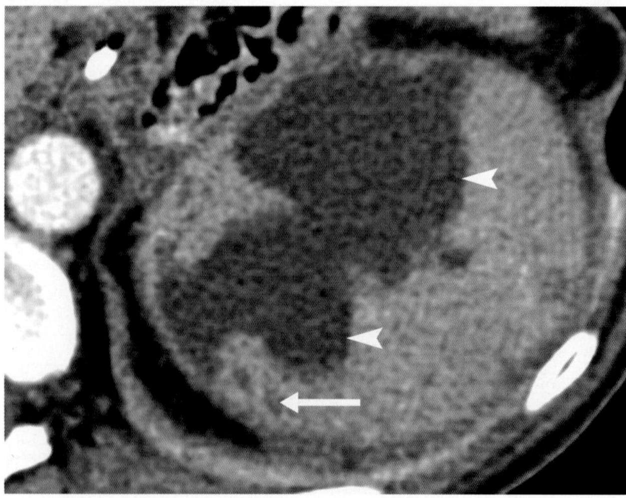

FIGURE 42.36. **Splenic Abscess.** Postcontrast CT shows confluent low attenuation collections (*arrowheads*) in the spleen proven by US-guided percutaneous aspiration to be a bacterial abscess. Small satellite collections (*arrow*) are also present.

TABLE 42.4

CAUSES OF MULTIPLE SMALL (10-mm) LESIONS IN THE SPLEEN

Microabcesses (immunocompromised patient)
Multiple bacterial abscesses
Histoplasmosis
Lymphoma
Kaposi sarcoma (AIDS patient)
Sarcoidosis
Gamna–Gandy bodies (portal hypertension)
Metastases Breast carcinoma Lung carcinoma Ovarian carcinoma Gastric carcinoma Malignant melanoma Prostate carcinoma

defects in the spleen, usually 5 to 10 mm, up to 20 mm, in size. The differential diagnosis of multiple small low-density splenic defects is listed in Table 42.4.

Hydatid cysts in the spleen are found in only 2% of patients with hydatid disease. Hydatid cysts are usually also present in the liver or lung. The lesions consist of spherical mother cysts that contain smaller daughter cysts and have internal septations and debris representing hydatid sand. Ring-like calcifications in the wall are usually prominent in the chronic stage.

Suggested Readings

Pancreas

Baker ME, Nelson RC, Rosen MP, et al. ACR appropriateness criteria—acute pancreatitis. *Ultrasound Q* 2014;30(4):267–273.

Chen FM, Ni JM, Zhang ZY, Zhang L, Li B, Jiang CJ. Presurgical evaluation of pancreatic cancer: a comprehensive imaging comparison of CT versus MRI. *AJR Am J Roentgenol* 2016;206(3):526–535.

Expert Panel on Gastrointestinal Imaging; Qayyum A, Tamm EP, Kamel IR, et al. ACR appropriateness criteria—staging of pancreatic ductal adenocarcinoma. *J Am Coll Radiol* 2017;14(11S):S560–S569.

Foster BR, Jensen KK, Bakis G, Shaaban AM, Coakley FV. Revised Atlanta classification for acute pancreatitis: a pictorial essay. *Radiographics* 2016;36(3):675–687. (Atlanta classification 2012).

Freeny PC, Saunders MD. Moving beyond morphology: new insights into the characterization and management of cystic pancreatic lesions. *Radiology* 2014;272(2):345–363.

Horger M, Lamprecht HG, Bares R, et al. Systemic IgG4-related sclerosing disease: spectrum of imaging findings and differential diagnosis. *AJR Am J Roentgenol* 2012;199(3):W276–W282. (Pictorial essay).

Kim KW, Krajewski KM, Nishino M, et al. Update on the management of gastroenteropancreatic neuroendocrine tumors with emphasis on the role of imaging. *AJR Am J Roentgenol* 2013;201(4):811–824. (Review).

Madhani K, Farrell JJ. Autoimmune pancreatitis: an update on diagnosis and management. *Gastroenterol Clin North Am* 2016;45(1):29–43.

Manning MA, Srivastava A, Paal EE, Gould CF, Mortele KJ. Nonepithelial neoplasms of the pancreas: radiologic-pathologic correlation, part 1—benign tumors: From the radiologic pathology archives. *Radiographics* 2016;36(1):123–141.

Murphy KP, O'Connor OJ, Maher MM. Updated imaging nomenclature for acute pancreatitis. *AJR Am J Roentgenol* 2014;203(5):W484–W469. (Atlanta classification 2012).

Raman SP, Salaria SN, Hruban RH, Fishman EK. Groove pancreatitis: spectrum of imaging findings and radiology-pathology correlation. *AJR Am J Roentgenol* 2013;201(1):W29–W39.

Seo N, Byun JH, Kim JH, et al. Validation of the 2012 international consensus guidelines using computed tomography and magnetic resonance imaging: branch duct and main duct intraductal papillary mucinous neoplasms of the pancreas. *Ann Surg* 2016;263(3):557–564.

Tanaka M, Fernandez-del Castillo C, Adsay V, et al. International consensus guidelines 2012 for the management of IPMN and MCN of the pancreas. *Pancreatology* 2012;12(3):183–197.

Spleen

Ahmed S, Horton KM, Fishman EK. Splenic incidentalomas. *Radiol Clin North Am* 2011;49(2):323–347.

Chapman J, Bhimji S. *Splenomegaly. National Center for Biotechnology Information (NCBI) Bookshelf.* Treasure Island, FL: Stat Pearls Publishing; 2017.

Dhyani M, Anupindi SA, Ayyala R, Hahn PF, Gee MS. Defining an imaging algorithm for noncystic splenic lesions identified in young patients. *AJR Am J Roentgenol* 2013;201(6):W893–W899.

Kaza RK, Azar S, Al-Hawary MM, Francis IR. Primary and secondary neoplasms of the spleen. *Cancer Imaging* 2010;10:173–182.

Lake ST, Johnson PT, Kawamoto S, Hruban RH, Fishman EK. CT of splenosis: patterns and pitfalls. *AJR Am J Roentgenol* 2012;199(6):W686–W693. (Pictorial essay).

Mortele KJ, Mortele B, Silverman SG. CT features of the accessory spleen. *AJR Am J Roentgenol* 2004;183(6):1653–1657.

Saboo SS, Krajewski KM, O'Regan KN, et al. Spleen in haematological malignancies: spectrum of imaging findings. *Br J Radiol* 2012;85(1009):81–92.

Singh AK, Shankar S, Gervais DA, Hahn PF, Mueller PR. Image-guided percutaneous splenic interventions. *Radiographics* 2012;32(2):523–534.

Thipphavong S, Duigenan S, Schindera ST, Gee MS, Philips S. Nonneoplastic, benign, and malignant splenic diseases: cross-sectional imaging findings and rare disease entities. *AJR Am J Roentgenol* 2014;203(2):315–322.

Urritia M, Mergo PJ, Ros LH, Torres GM, Ros PR. Cystic lesions of the spleen: radiologic-pathologic correlation. *Radiographics* 1996;16(1):107–129.

CHAPTER 43 ■ PHARYNX AND ESOPHAGUS

WILLIAM E. BRANT

IMAGING METHODS

Barium pharyngography, barium swallow, and barium esophagography are studies dedicated to evaluation of swallowing disorders and suspected lesions of the pharynx and esophagus. The upper gastrointestinal (UGI) series, also called a barium meal, is an extended barium examination of the alimentary tract from the pharynx and esophagus to the ligament of Treitz.

Air-contrast techniques provide optimal imaging for structural lesions of the pharynx. The standing patient takes one swallow of barium suspension while being observed fluoroscopically for obstruction, stricture, aspiration, leak, or delayed emptying. Additional swallows are evaluated in upright lateral and anteroposterior (AP) projections. Video images are recorded digitally for later review. A single swallow of thick high-density barium is used to coat the pharynx. Lateral and AP views of the pharynx are recorded with the patient phonating "eee" and "aaahh" to distend and collapse the pharynx and optimize visualization of mucosal detail. Speech-language pathologists commonly collaborate with the radiologist in performing these studies and reviewing the video images.

The esophagus is studied in similar fashion, observing a single solid column swallow of barium suspension for peristalsis, obstruction, stricture, and delayed emptying in the upright position and then again in prone right anterior oblique position. A single swallow of thick high-density barium coats the esophagus. Distention of the esophagus is attained by having the patient ingest gas-producing crystals to assess mucosal detail. Video fluoroscopic images are recorded digitally to review swallowing dynamics and motility.

CT and MR are used to stage malignancies of the pharynx and esophagus and to clarify findings seen with other imaging methods. The cross-sectional techniques complement barium studies and endoscopy of the pharynx and esophagus by demonstrating the wall, blood vessels, and adjacent structures to determine extent of disease. CT and MR are limited in evaluation of the mucosa and generally cannot differentiate inflammatory and neoplastic conditions. Endoscopic sonography is useful for demonstration of tumor penetration of the esophageal wall.

This chapter reviews the pharynx as studied by barium examination and for assessment of swallowing disorders. Cross-sectional imaging of the pharynx and neck is reviewed in Chapter 8, Head and Neck Imaging.

ANATOMY

The pharynx extends from the nasal cavity to the larynx and is arbitrarily divided into three compartments (Fig. 43.1). The *nasopharynx* extends from the skull base to the soft palate. Its function is entirely respiratory. The nasopharynx is not considered further in this chapter. The *oropharynx* is posterior to the oral cavity and extends from the soft palate to the hyoid bone. The *hypopharynx* (laryngopharynx) extends from the hyoid bone to the cricopharyngeus muscle. The base of the tongue forms the anterior boundary of the oropharynx. The outline of the surface of the tongue is nodular because of the presence of lymphoid tissue forming the lingual tonsils and the circumvallate papillae, which contain taste buds. The lingual tonsils may hypertrophy and mimic a neoplasm. The epiglottis and aryepiglottic folds separate the larynx from the oropharynx and hypopharynx. The *valleculae* are two symmetrical pouches formed in the recess between the base of the tongue and the epiglottis. They are divided medially by the median glossoepiglottic fold and bounded laterally by the lateral glossoepiglottic folds. The *piriform sinuses* are deep, symmetrical, lateral recesses formed by the protrusion of the larynx into the hypopharynx.

The esophagus extends from the cricopharyngeus muscle at the level of C5–6 to the gastroesophageal junction (GEJ). The esophagus is a muscular tube formed by an outer longitudinal muscle layer and an inner circular muscle layer lined by stratified squamous epithelium. The esophagus lacks a serosal layer, which allows for rapid spread of tumor into adjacent tissues. The proximal one-third of the esophagus is predominantly striated muscle, whereas the distal two-thirds, below the level of the aortic arch, is predominantly smooth muscle. Normal extrinsic impressions on the esophagus are made by the aortic arch, the left mainstem bronchus, and the left atrium. The normal esophageal mucosa is smooth and featureless when fully distended on air-contrast barium studies. With partial collapse, multiple longitudinal folds, 1 to 2 mm in thickness, become evident. Multiple regular, transverse folds, 1 mm thick, result from contraction of the longitudinal fibers in the muscularis mucosa. This pattern is called *feline esophagus* because it is typical of a normal esophagus in cats. In humans, it may be an early sign of dysmotility or esophagitis (see Fig. 43.22).

On cross-sectional imaging, the esophagus appears as an oval of soft tissue density usually surrounded by fat. In most cases (>60%), the esophagus is collapsed and contains no air. Normal air or contrast within the esophagus is located

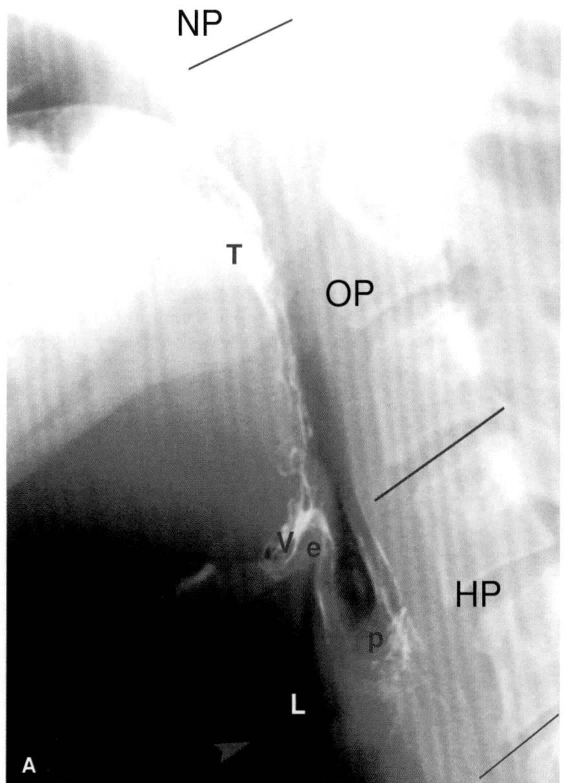

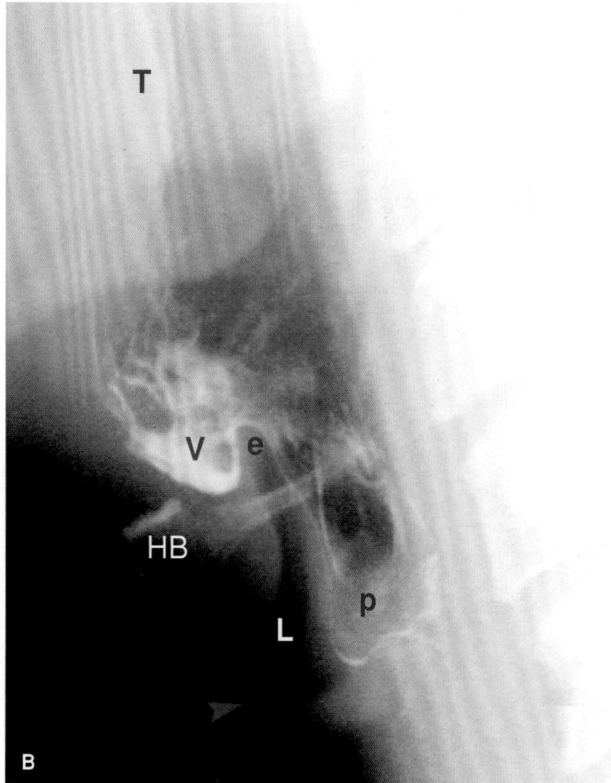

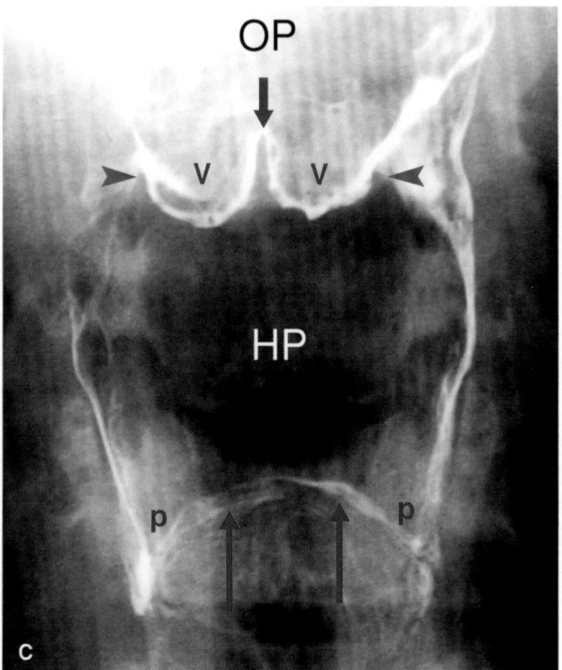

FIGURE 43.1. Double-Contrast Pharyngogram. Three radiographs of the pharynx coated with barium demonstrate normal anatomic structures: (**A**) nondistended lateral view; (**B**) distended lateral view, obtained by having the patient phonate "eee…"; and (**C**) frontal (anteroposterior) view. The nasopharynx (*NP*) extends from the skull base to the soft palate. The oropharynx (*OP*) spans from the soft palate to the hyoid bone (*HB*). The hypopharynx (*HP*) extends from the hyoid bone to the cricopharyngeus muscle (C5–6), which demarcates the pharynx and esophagus. The epiglottis (*e*) closes during swallowing to protect the larynx (*L*) from aspiration. The cricoid cartilage makes a prominent impression on the hypopharynx (*skinny arrows*). The base of the tongue (*T*) has a normal lobulated appearance due to nodular lymphoid tissue. The valleculae (*V*) are recesses between the tongue and epiglottis, bordered by the median glossoepiglottic fold (*fat arrow*) and the lateral glossoepiglottic folds (*blue arrowheads*). The piriform recesses (*p*) extend laterally and posterior to the larynx. The piriform recesses are commonly slightly asymmetric in size. The laryngeal ventricle (*red arrowheads*) is faintly visualized outlined by air between the false vocal cords above and the true vocal cords below.

centrally within its lumen. Eccentric contrast or air should be considered abnormal. Distention of the upper esophagus more than 10 mm or the lower esophagus more than 20 mm is abnormal. Air–fluid levels in the esophagus are always abnormal. The lower esophageal sphincter (LES) is normally closed. Normal thickness of the wall of the esophagus as seen on CT and MR is 2 to 4 mm.

Anatomy of the esophagogastric region is complex (Fig. 43.2). The length of the esophagus is tubular, and its termination is saccular. The saccular termination is called the *esophageal vestibule*. The tubulovestibular junction is formed by a symmetrical muscular ring called the *A ring*. The *B ring* is an asymmetrical mucosal ring or notch that occurs at the junction of esophageal squamous epithelium with gastric columnar epithelium. This squamocolumnar junction is also marked by the *Z line,* a thin ragged line of demarcation seen on double-contrast views of the lower esophagus. The B ring and the Z line are considered to be radiographic markers of the GEJ. The *LES* is a physiologic rather than an anatomic structure. It is a 2- to 4-cm long high-pressure zone located in the esophageal vestibule. It is defined manometrically but is without a distinct anatomic correlate. At rest the LES is tightly

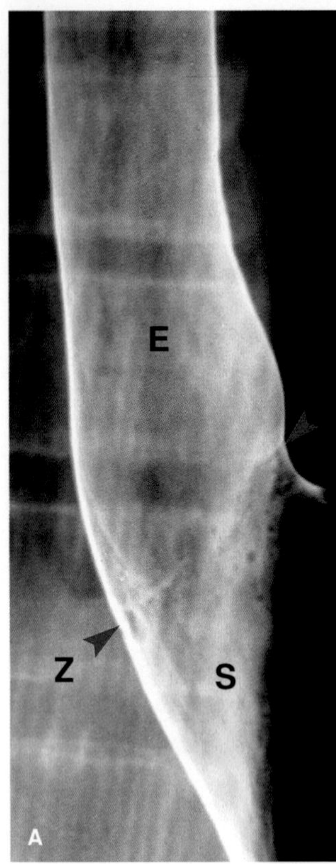

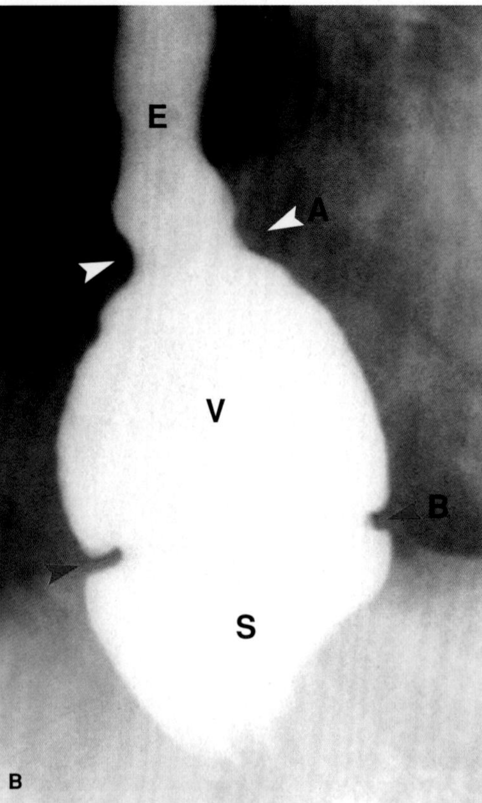

FIGURE 43.2. **Anatomy of the Gastroesophageal Junction.** Radiographs from an air-contrast barium study (**A**) and a single-contrast barium study (**B**) demonstrate the physiologic and anatomic landmarks of the gastroesophageal junction. The Z line (*Z, red arrowheads*), seen best on the double-contrast study, marks the junction of the squamous epithelium of the esophagus (*E*) and the columnar epithelium of the stomach (*S*). The single-contrast study demonstrates the esophageal vestibule (*V*) demarcated by the muscular A ring (*A, white arrowheads*) and the mucosal fold of the B ring (*B, red arrowheads*). The vestibule marks the location of the lower esophageal sphincter. The Z line and the B ring are markers of the gastroesophageal junction. Their location relative to the esophageal hiatus in the diaphragm varies with swallowing and other physiologic motions. The air-contrast study shows the featureless mucosal pattern of the well-distended normal esophagus.

closed with a pressure higher than gastric pressure to prevent reflux of gastric contents into the esophagus. Malfunction of the LES results in gastroesophageal reflux disease (GERD). The act of swallowing generates peristalsis in the esophagus, which results in relaxation of the LES allowing passage of swallowed liquids and solids into the stomach.

The esophageal hiatus is an angled opening in the diaphragm, formed by the edges of the diaphragmatic crura. On CT and MR, the crura appear as often prominent, teardrop-shaped structures of muscle density. With normal breathing, the proximal vestibule and A ring lie in the thorax. The mid-vestibule is in the esophageal hiatus, and the distal vestibule and B ring are in the abdomen. With swallowing, the vestibule opens and moves upward and the B ring may be seen 1 cm above the diaphragm.

NORMAL SWALLOWING AND MOTILITY

The normal process of swallowing can be divided into oral, pharyngeal, and esophageal phases. The oral stage involves mastication, formation of a bolus, and voluntary transport of the bolus from the oral cavity into the pharynx. The soft palate elevates and the tongue depresses to accommodate the bolus and channel it into the oropharynx. The oropharynx and hypopharynx receive the bolus and conduct it to the esophagus. Breathing is halted while the larynx elevates, the laryngeal vestibule closes, and the epiglottis and aryepiglottic folds close over the opening into the larynx and deflect the bolus through the lateral piriform recesses.

The functional upper esophageal sphincter (UES), formed by the cricopharyngeus and other pharyngeal muscles, opens to receive the bolus. Peristalsis conveys ingested material through the tubular esophagus to the stomach. *Primary peristalsis* is composed of a rapid wave of inhibition that opens the sphincters, followed by a slow wave of contraction that moves the bolus. Normal peristalsis will clear the esophagus completely with each swallow. Primary peristalsis appears as a stripping wave that traverses the entire esophagus from top to bottom. *Secondary peristalsis* is initiated by distention of the esophageal lumen. The peristaltic wave starts in the mid-esophagus and spreads simultaneously up and down the esophagus to clear reflux or any part of a bolus left behind. Secondary waves have the same appearance as primary waves except that they start at the point of the retained barium bolus. *Tertiary waves* are nonproductive contractions associated with motility disorders. Irregular contractions follow one another at close intervals from the top to the bottom of the esophagus. These nonperistaltic contractions cause a corkscrew or beaded appearance of the esophageal barium column. These waves are not effective in clearing material from the esophagus. The functional LES at the level of the esophageal vestibule relaxes and opens in response to swallowing, primary peristalsis, and proximal esophageal dilation.

MOTILITY DISORDERS

Difficulty with swallowing occurs in all age groups but has an increasingly high prevalence with age, especially age over 65. Swallowing disorders may lead to aspiration pneumonia, airway obstruction, dehydration, weight loss, and reduced quality of life. Symptoms of abnormal oral or pharyngeal swallowing include difficulty initiating swallowing, globus sensation (lump in throat), cervical dysphagia, nasal regurgitation, hoarseness, coughing, or choking. Coughing after a swallow may indicate aspiration of material into the airway. However, aspiration is silent in half of the patients. Symptoms suggesting esophageal dysfunction include heartburn, dysphagia, "indigestion," and chest pain. Dysphagia is defined as the awareness of swallowing difficulty during the passage

TABLE 43.1

CAUSES OF PHARYNGEAL SWALLOWING DYSFUNCTION

Cause
Aging (primary presbyphagia)
Neurologic disease
Cerebrovascular accident
Multiple sclerosis
Movement disorders
Neurodegenerative diseases
Central nervous system infections
Muscle disease
Muscular dystrophies
Myasthenia gravis
Structural abnormalities
Pharyngeal webs
Zenker diverticulum
Tumors
Medications
Radiation
Gastroesophageal reflux
Trauma
Postsurgical changes
Malignancy
Oral cavity
Pharynx
Larynx

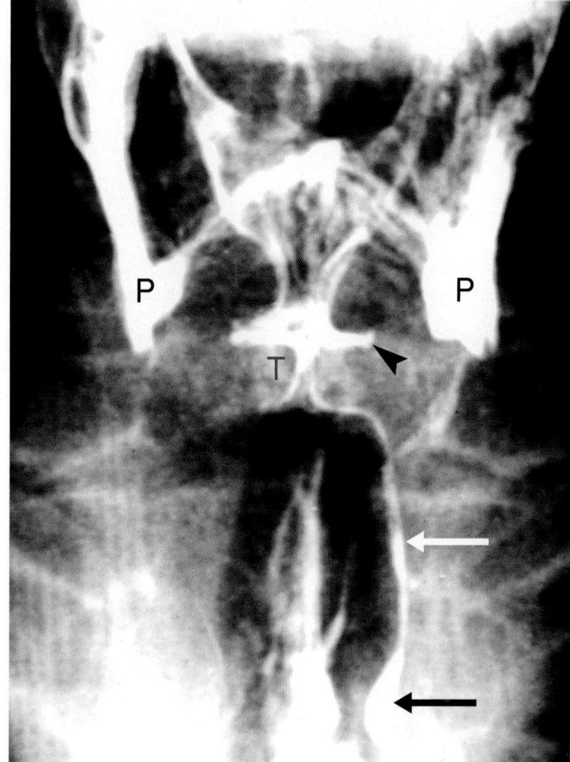

FIGURE 43.3. **Aspiration.** Frontal radiograph taken during barium pharyngography demonstrates the appearance of aspiration. Barium coats the surface of the false cords (*F*), the intervening laryngeal ventricle (*arrowhead*), and the true vocal cords (*T*). Barium coating to this level would be diagnostic of *laryngeal penetration*. However, barium coating is seen in the proximal trachea (*arrows*) indicating that *aspiration* has occurred. Barium is also seen pooling in the piriform recesses (*P*). This is a normal finding.

of solids or liquids from mouth to stomach. Patients complain of food "sticking in the throat" and of painful swallowing (odynophagia). These symptoms may be caused by anatomic abnormalities, tumors, or motility disorders. The patient's subjective assessment of the location of the abnormality is not reliable. Detailed dynamic barium studies of the entire oropharyngeal–esophageal pathway with videofluoroscopy are needed for complete evaluation. Radiographic findings of functional abnormalities of the pharynx and esophagus increase in prevalence with age, may not correlate with specific symptoms, and must be interpreted with caution. Causes of pharyngeal swallowing dysfunction are listed in Table 43.1.

Aspiration, resulting in pneumonia, is a major problem with the elderly, especially those in nursing homes. Aspiration is evident when the ingested bolus passes through the vocal cords into the proximal trachea (Fig. 43.3). *Laryngeal penetration* is defined as entry of barium into the laryngeal vestibule without passage below the vocal cords. Either finding may precipitate a cough. Mortality from aspiration pneumonia is reported as high as 65% in patients over age 65. Up to 20% of stroke patients with aspiration die within 1 year of having a stroke.

Cricopharyngeal achalasia is attributable to failure of complete relaxation of the UES, commonly resulting in dysphagia and aspiration. Barium studies demonstrate a shelf-like impression (*cricopharyngeal bar*) on the barium column at the pharyngoesophageal junction at the level of C5–6. The cricopharyngeus muscle is normally closed between swallows and relaxes to open completely for the passage of the bolus with swallowing. The cricopharyngeal bar seen during swallowing indicates dysfunction and incomplete opening. The pharynx is distended, and barium may overflow into the larynx and trachea. Because some normal individuals have a prominent cricopharyngeal impression, controversy exists as to how prominent the impression must be to be considered significant. Narrowing of the lumen greater than 50% is generally accepted as a definite cause of dysphagia. Cricopharyngeal dysfunction is commonly associated with GERD, Zenker diverticulum, and neuromuscular disorders of the pharynx.

Achalasia of the esophagus is a disease of unknown etiology characterized by (1) absence of peristalsis in the body of the esophagus, (2) marked increase in resting pressure of the LES, and (3) failure of the LES to relax with swallowing. The abnormal peristalsis and LES spasm result in a failure of the esophagus to empty. Pathologically, cases show a deficiency of ganglion cells in the myenteric plexus (Auerbach plexus) throughout the esophagus. The clinical presentation is insidious, usually at age 30 to 50 years, with dysphagia, regurgitation, foul breath, and aspiration. Imaging findings include (a) uniform dilation of the esophagus, usually with an air–fluid level present; (b) absence of peristalsis, with tertiary waves common in the early stages of the disease; (c) tapered "beak" deformity at the LES because of failure of relaxation (Fig. 43.4); (d) findings of esophagitis including ulceration; and (e) increased incidence of epiphrenic diverticula and esophageal carcinoma. Treatment of achalasia is balloon dilation or Heller myotomy. Diseases that may mimic esophageal achalasia include the following.

Chagas disease is caused by the destruction of ganglion cells of the esophagus due to a neurotoxin released by the protozoa, *Trypanosoma cruzi,* endemic to South America, especially eastern Brazil. The radiographic appearance of the esophagus is identical to achalasia. Associated abnormalities include cardiomyopathy, megaduodenum, megaureter, and megacolon.

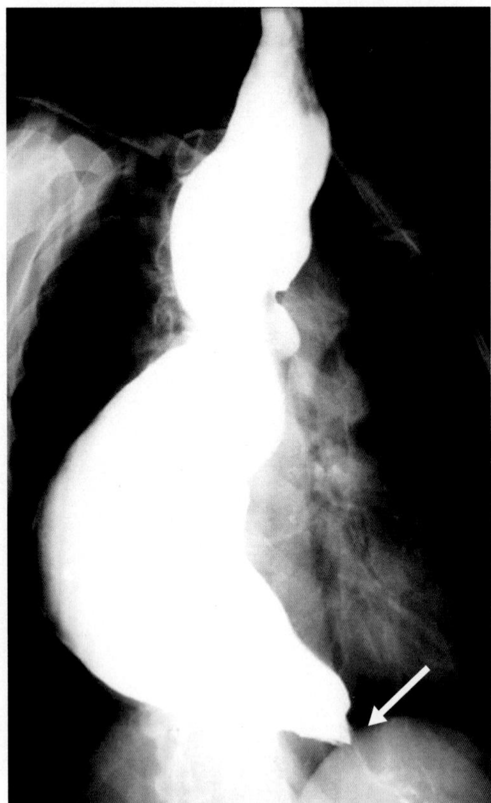

FIGURE 43.4. **Achalasia.** Upright radiograph from air-contrast barium esophagography shows 1-cm long smooth, tapered narrowing (*arrow*) of distal esophagus with proximal dilation of the esophagus. Note standing column of barium on this upright view. Short length of narrowed segment is characteristic of primary achalasia.

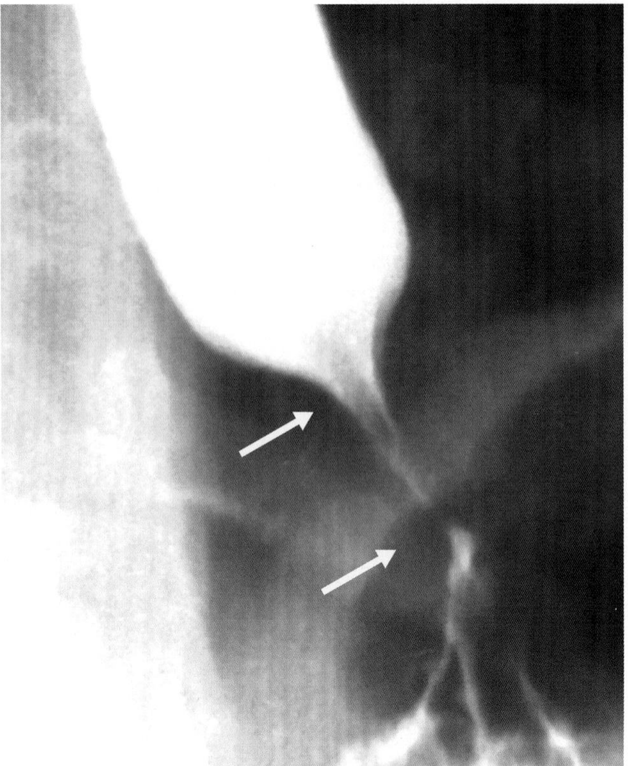

FIGURE 43.5. **Pseudoachalasia—Carcinoma of Esophagus.** Spot radiograph from barium esophagram shows 4-cm long tapered narrowing (*arrows*) of distal esophagus with esophageal diameter proximally of 4 cm. Endoscopy and biopsy confirmed carcinoma of the esophagus.

Carcinoma of the GEJ may mimic achalasia, but tends to involve a longer (>3.5 cm) segment of the distal esophagus, is rigid, and tends to show more irregular tapering of the distal esophagus and mass effect (Fig. 43.5). When findings of achalasia are present on barium studies, it is important to evaluate the gastric cardia and fundus to rule out an underlying malignant tumor at the GEJ as the cause of these findings. The cardia and fundus are however not adequately evaluated in all patients because of delayed emptying of barium from the esophagus. Therefore, it is important to be aware of the limitations of barium studies in evaluating the cardia and fundus in patients with suspected achalasia.

Peptic strictures are usually associated with normal primary peristalsis. A hiatal hernia is usually present.

Diffuse esophageal spasm is a syndrome of unknown cause characterized by multiple tertiary esophageal contractions (Fig. 43.6), thickened esophageal wall, and intermittent dysphagia and chest pain. Primary peristalsis is usually present, but the contractions are infrequent. Most patients are middle aged. The LES is frequently dysfunctional and the condition commonly improves with injection of *Clostridium botulinum* toxin at the GEJ or with endoscopic balloon dilation of the LES. Diffuse esophageal spasm is characterized on barium studies by intermittently absent or weakened primary esophageal peristalsis with simultaneous, nonperistaltic contractions that compartmentalize the esophagus, producing a classic corkscrew appearance. CT reveals circumferential thickening (5 to 15 mm) of the wall of the distal 5 cm of the esophagus in 20% of patients.

Neuromuscular disorders are a common cause of abnormalities of the oral, pharyngeal, or esophageal phases of swallowing. The most common cause of neurologic dysfunction is cerebrovascular disease and stroke. Additional causes include parkinsonism, Alzheimer disease, multiple sclerosis, neoplasms of the central nervous system, and posttraumatic central nervous system injury. Diseases of striated muscle, such as muscular dystrophy, myasthenia gravis, and dermatomyositis, predominantly affect the pharynx and proximal third (striated muscle portion) of the esophagus.

Scleroderma is a systemic disease of unknown cause characterized by progressive atrophy of smooth muscle and progressive fibrosis of affected tissues. Women are most commonly affected, usually aged 20 to 40 years at the onset of disease. The esophagus is affected in 75% to 80% of patients. Imaging findings (Fig. 43.7) include (a) weak to absent peristalsis in the distal two-thirds (smooth muscle portion) of the esophagus; (b) delayed esophageal emptying; (c) a stiff dilated esophagus that does not collapse with emptying; and (d) wide-gaping LES with free gastroesophageal reflux. Despite free reflux, tight strictures of the distal esophagus are uncommon.

Postoperative states, including surgery for malignancy of the tongue, larynx, and pharynx, commonly impair swallowing function as well as alter the morphology. Surgical resection is aimed at providing at least a 1-cm margin free of tumor and often results in removing large blocks of tissue and functionally altering the structures that remain.

Esophagitis frequently results in abnormal esophageal motility and visualization of tertiary esophageal contractions.

Gastroesophageal reflux disease (GERD) is a major health problem in the United States and Western countries with a prevalence of 10% to 20% of the adult population. GERD occurs as a result of incompetence of the LES. The resting pressure of the LES is abnormally decreased and fails to increase with

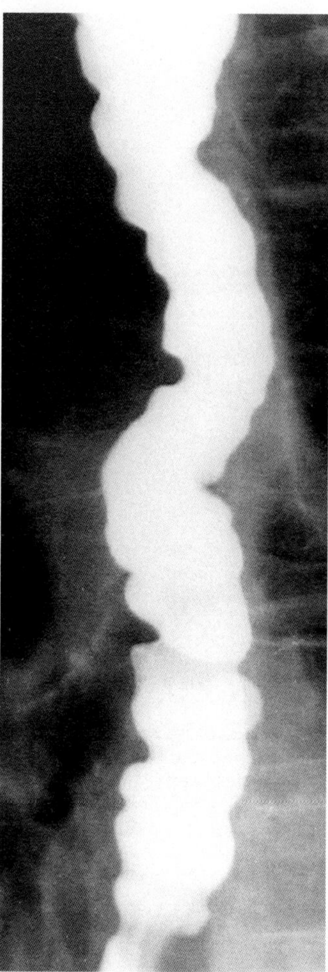

FIGURE 43.6. **Diffuse Esophageal Spasm.** Image from a barium esophagram demonstrates numerous ineffective tertiary contractions throughout the esophagus. The lower esophageal sphincter was dysfunctional, not opening appropriately on fluoroscopic examination.

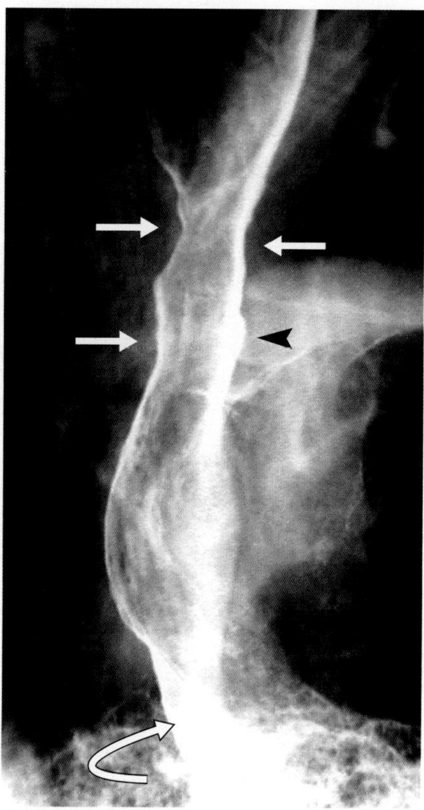

FIGURE 43.7. **Scleroderma.** Air-contrast esophagram in a patient with scleroderma demonstrates a stiff distal esophagus without peristalsis. The gastroesophageal junction (*curved arrow*) is gaping and free gastroesophageal reflux was observed. Reflux esophagitis has resulted in mild stricturing (*white arrows*) of the esophagus and focal ulcers (*arrowhead*).

raised intra-abdominal pressure. As a result, increases in intra-abdominal pressure exceed LES pressure, and gastric contents are allowed to reflux into the esophagus. Symptoms of GERD include substernal burning pain ("heartburn"), postural regurgitation (especially in supine position), dysphagia, and odynophagia. Complications of GERD include reflux esophagitis (RE), stricture, development of Barrett esophagus, and esophageal dysmotility. The radiographic diagnosis of GERD may be difficult because 20% of normal individuals show spontaneous reflux on UGI examination, and patients with pathologic GERD may not demonstrate reflux without provocative tests. Findings associated with GERD on barium esophagrams include (a) hiatal hernia, associated with presence of RE; (b) shortening of the esophagus, a finding of importance to treating GERD surgically; (c) impaired esophageal motility; (d) gastroesophageal reflux, often demonstrated only by provocative maneuvers such as Valsalva, leg raising, and cough; and (e) prolonged clearance time of refluxed gastric contents. Low-volume reflux that clears rapidly is not considered a significant finding. Monitoring of esophageal pH for 24 hours in an ambulatory patient is the most sensitive means of diagnosing GERD. GERD is managed medically with agents that inhibit gastric acid production or surgically with fundoplication.

Hiatus hernia is often considered synonymous with GERD. However, most patients with hiatus hernia do not have gastroesophageal reflux or evidence of esophagitis. Hiatus hernia is therefore not likely as a primary cause of reflux. On the other hand, up to 90% of patients with GERD have a hiatus hernia. The presence of hiatus hernia delays the clearance of reflux and promotes development of RE. An area of controversy is the definition of hiatus hernia and the criteria used for diagnosis. The simplest definition is protrusion of any portion of the stomach into the thorax. Using that definition hiatus hernia is highly prevalent affecting 40% to 60% of adults. Three types of hiatal hernia are described. The most common (95%) is the *sliding hiatus hernia,* with the GEJ, marked by the B ring and Z line displaced more than 1 cm above the hiatus. The esophageal hiatus is often abnormally widened to 3 to 4 cm (Fig. 43.8). The upper limit of normal hiatal width is 15 mm, most easily measured by CT. The gastric fundus may be displaced above the diaphragm and present as a retrocardiac mass on chest radiographs. The presence of an air–fluid level in the retrocardiac mass suggests the diagnosis. Small, sliding hiatus hernias commonly reduce in the upright position. The mere presence of a sliding hiatus hernia is of limited clinical significance in most cases. The function of the LES and the presence of pathologic gastroesophageal reflux are the crucial factors in producing symptoms and causing complications. Much less common is the *paraesophageal hiatus hernia,* in which the GEJ remains in normal location, while a portion of the stomach herniates above the diaphragm (Fig. 43.9). The *mixed or compound hiatal hernia* is the most common type of paraesophageal hernia (Fig. 43.10). The GEJ is displaced into the thorax with a large portion of the stomach, which is usually abnormally rotated. Paraesophageal hernias, especially

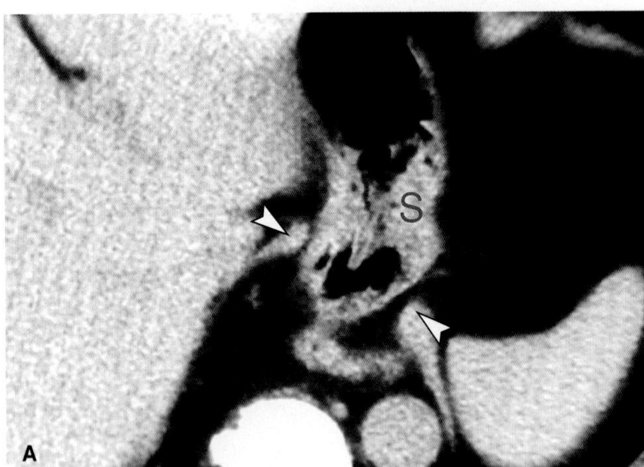

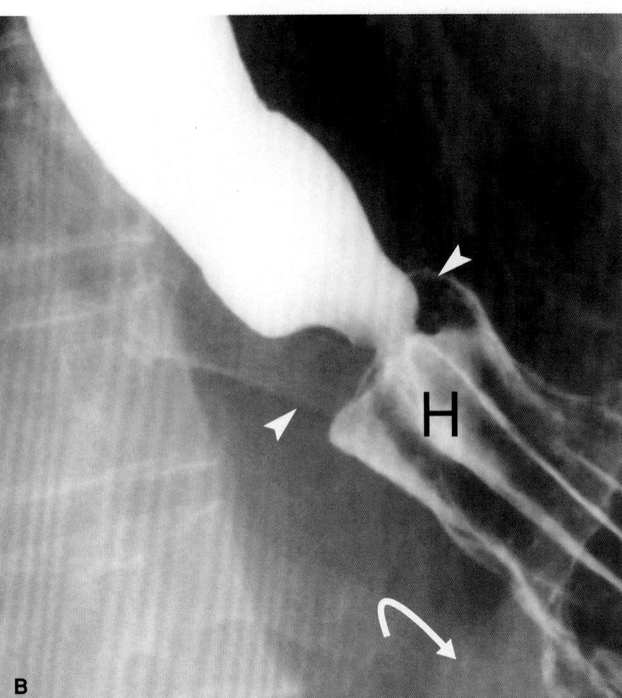

FIGURE 43.8. **Sliding Hiatus Hernia. A:** CT demonstrates a 26-mm gap between the crura (*arrowheads*) of the diaphragm. The normal esophageal hiatus should not exceed 15 mm. The stomach (*S*) extends through the hiatus and is positioned both above and below the diaphragm. The GEJ was seen at a higher level in the thorax. **B:** Radiograph from a barium esophagram shows a small sliding hiatus hernia (*H*) with gastric folds extending to the level of the B ring marking the gastroesophageal junction (*arrowheads*). The GEJ is well above the level of the left hemidiaphragm (*curved arrow*).

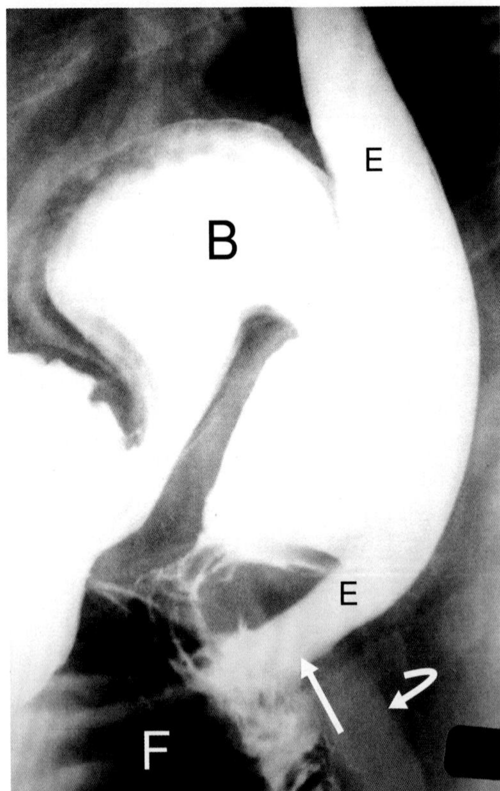

FIGURE 43.9. **Paraesophageal Hiatal Hernia.** Radiograph from an upper GI series shows the characteristic findings of paraesophageal hiatal hernia. The gastroesophageal junction (*straight arrow*) and fundus (*F*) of the stomach are below the diaphragm (*curved arrow*) while a portion of the body (*B*) of the stomach herniates through the esophageal hiatus into the chest and then doubles back into the abdomen. *E*, esophagus.

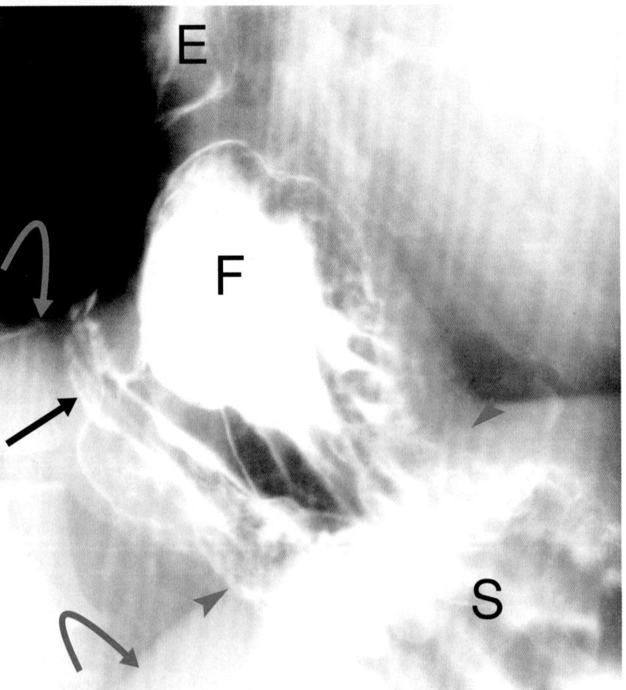

FIGURE 43.10. **Compound Hiatus Hernia.** Left posterior oblique view from an upper GI series demonstrates a large hiatus hernia. The fundus (*F*) of the stomach (*S*) extends well above the level of the left hemidiaphragm (*red curved arrow*). The widened (6 cm) esophageal hiatus makes an impression (*arrowheads*) on the body of the stomach. The gastroesophageal junction (*black arrow*) is 5 cm above the left hemidiaphragm. The distal esophagus is bowed around the herniated stomach. The right hemidiaphragm (*blue curved arrow*) projects well above the left hemidiaphragm on this view. *E*, esophagus.

when large with most of the stomach in the thorax, are at risk for volvulus, obstruction, and ischemia.

OUTPOUCHINGS

Lateral pharyngeal diverticula are protrusions of pharyngeal mucosa through areas of weakness of the lateral pharyngeal wall, most common in the region of the tonsillar fossa and thyrohyoid membrane. They reflect increased intrapharyngeal pressure and are seen most commonly in wind instrument players. Pouches of sufficient size to retain food and liquid may be associated with laryngeal penetration and aspiration.

Zenker diverticulum arises in the hypopharynx just proximal to the UES. It is located in the posterior midline at the cleavage plane, known as Killian dehiscence, between the circular and oblique fibers of the cricopharyngeus muscle. The diverticulum has a small neck that is higher than the sac, resulting in food and liquid being trapped within the sac (Fig. 43.11). The distended sac may compress the cervical esophagus. Symptoms include dysphagia, halitosis, and regurgitation of food. They are rarely found in patients under age 40.

Killian–Jamieson diverticula originate on the anterolateral wall of the proximal cervical esophagus in a gap just below the cricopharyngeus and lateral to the longitudinal tendon of the esophagus (i.e., the Killian–Jamieson space). Killian–Jamieson diverticula are less common and considerably smaller than Zenker diverticulum and appear on pharyngoesophagography as persistent left-sided or, less frequently, bilateral (25%) outpouchings from the proximal cervical esophagus below the cricopharyngeus (Fig. 43.12). Killian–Jamieson diverticula also are less likely to cause symptoms and are less likely to be associated with overflow aspiration or gastroesophageal reflux than is Zenker diverticulum.

Mid-esophageal diverticula may be pulsion or traction diverticula. Pulsion diverticula occur as a result of disordered esophageal peristalsis (Fig. 43.13). Traction diverticula occur because of fibrous inflammatory reactions of adjacent lymph nodes and contain all esophageal layers (Fig. 43.14). Most mid-esophageal diverticula have large mouths, empty well, and are usually asymptomatic.

Epiphrenic diverticula occur just above the LES, usually on the right side. They are rare and usually found in patients with

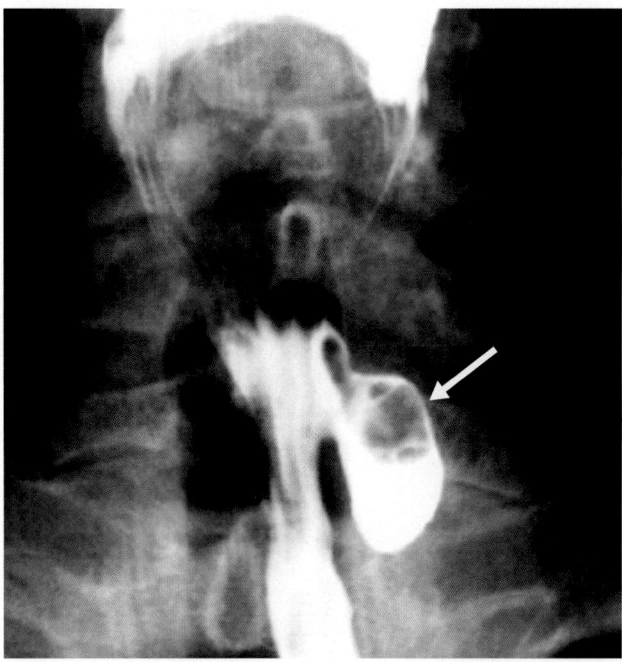

FIGURE 43.12. **Killian–Jamieson Diverticulum.** Spot radiograph obtained with patient in frontal position shows a left-sided Killian–Jamieson diverticulum (*arrow*) with wide neck.

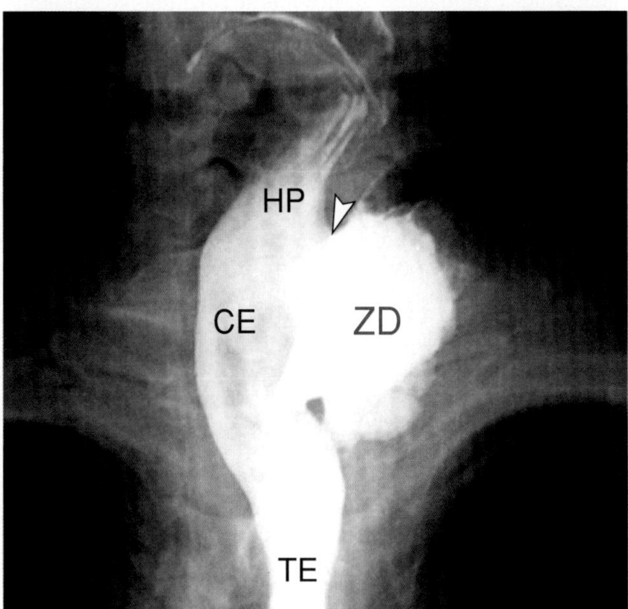

FIGURE 43.11. **Zenker Diverticulum.** Barium esophagram demonstrates the characteristic barium-filled outpouching indicating a Zenker diverticulum (*ZD*) at the junction of the hypopharynx (*HP*) and cervical esophagus (*CE*). Note that the neck of the diverticulum (*arrowhead*) is at a more cephalad location than its base, encouraging the trapping of food and liquid. *TE*, thoracic esophagus.

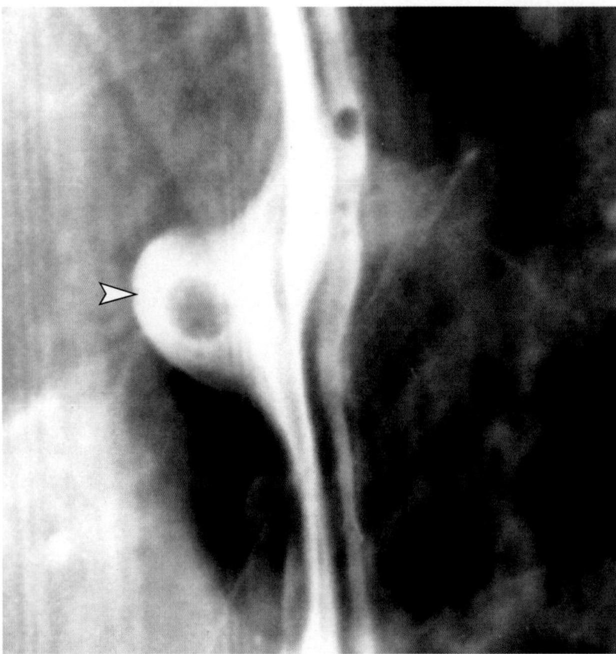

FIGURE 43.13. **Pulsion Diverticulum.** A barium esophagram demonstrates a persistent mucosal outpouching (*arrowhead*) in the mid-esophagus. The patient was asymptomatic. Pulsion diverticula are formed when the mucosa and submucosa herniate through the muscularis as a result of disordered esophagus peristalsis.

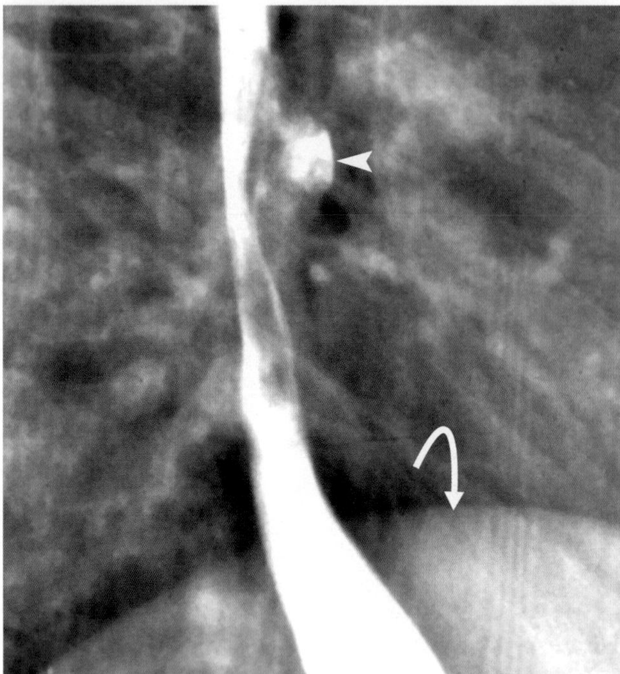

FIGURE 43.14. **Traction Diverticulum.** Double-contrast esophagram shows a small traction diverticulum (*arrowhead*) extending from the mid-esophagus caused by fibrosis induced by a mediastinal mass. The *curved arrow* indicates the diaphragm.

esophageal motility disorders (Fig. 43.15). Because of a small neck, higher than the sac, they may trap food and liquids and cause symptoms.

Sacculations are small outpouchings of the esophagus that usually occur as a sequela of severe esophagitis (Fig. 43.16). They are thought to result from the healing and scarring of ulcerations. Sacculations tend to change in size and shape during fluoroscopic observation. Smooth contours help to differentiate sacculations from ulcerations.

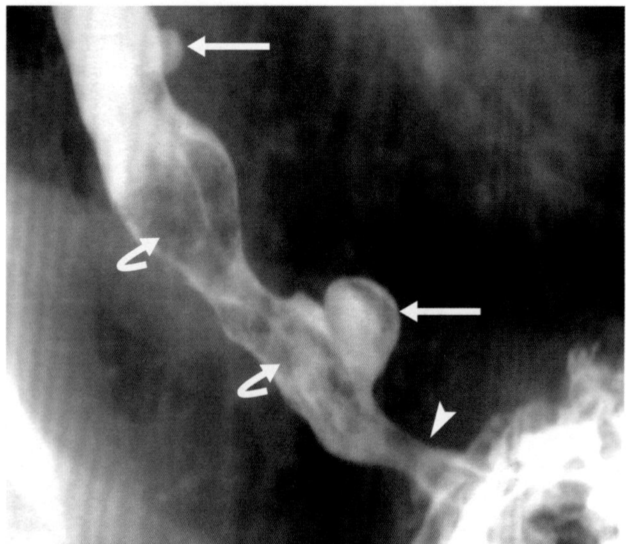

FIGURE 43.15. **Epiphrenic Diverticula.** A stricture (*arrowhead*) of the distal esophagus has resulted in the formation of two pulsion diverticula (*arrows*). The filling defects (*curved arrows*) in the barium column are caused by retained boluses of meat proximal to the stricture.

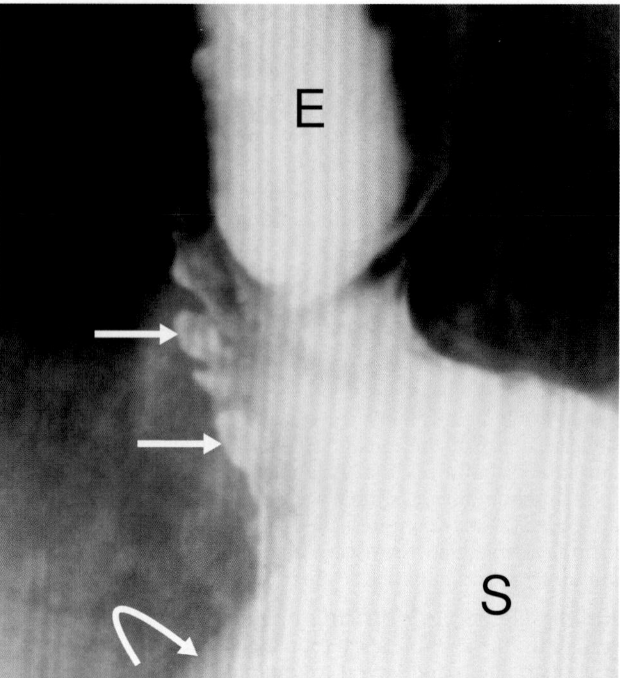

FIGURE 43.16. **Reflux Esophagitis—Sacculations.** A barium esophagram demonstrates stiffness and narrowing of the distal esophagus just above the level of the diaphragm (*curved arrow*). Several prominent sacculations (*arrows*) are present, indicating long-standing and severe esophagitis. *E*, distal esophagus; *S*, stomach.

Intramural pseudodiverticula are the dilated excretory ducts of deep mucous glands of the esophagus. They appear as flask-shaped barium collections that extend from the lumen or as lines and flecks of barium outside the esophageal wall. They tend to occur in clusters and in association with strictures. Liner tracks of barium ("intramural tracking") commonly bridge adjacent pseudodiverticula.

ESOPHAGITIS

Esophagitis is a common disease with many causes. Radiologic evaluation will detect most cases of moderate to severe esophagitis but will demonstrate less than half the cases of mild esophagitis. Attention to excellent technique and use of double-contrast studies are essential. Radiographic signs of esophagitis include (a) thickened esophageal folds (>3 mm), (b) limited esophageal distensibility (asymmetric flattening), (c) abnormal motility, (d) mucosal plaques and nodules, (e) erosions and ulcerations, (f) localized stricture, and (g) intramural pseudodiverticulosis (barium filling of dilated 1 to 3 mm submucosal glands). Ulcers are a hallmark finding of esophagitis. Small ulcers (<1 cm) are found with RE, herpes, acute radiation, drug-induced esophagitis, and benign mucous membrane pemphigoid. Larger ulcers (>1 cm) are characteristic of cytomegalovirus, human immunodeficiency virus (HIV), Barrett esophagus, and carcinoma. CT usually reveals nonspecific findings of thickening of the wall (>5 mm) and target sign with hypoattenuating thickened wall and high attenuation enhancing mucosa.

Reflux esophagitis is the result of esophageal mucosal injury caused by exposure to gastroduodenal secretions. The severity depends on the concentration of caustic agents including acid, pepsin, bile salts, caffeine, alcohol, and aspirin, as well as the duration of contact with the esophageal mucosa. The findings

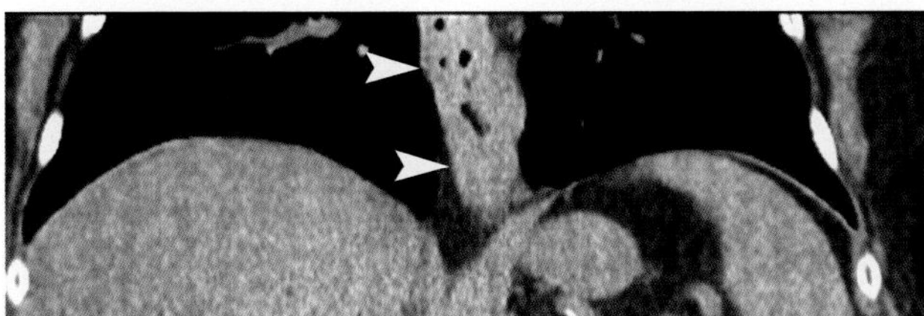

FIGURE 43.17. **Reflux Esophagitis—CT.** A CT performed without intravenous contrast unexpectedly showed marked irregular wall thickening (*arrowheads*) of the distal esophagus as seen on this coronal image. Subsequent endoscopy confirmed severe reflux esophagitis.

of RE are always most prominent in the distal esophagus and GEJ (Fig. 43.16). Early changes of RE include mucosal edema, which is manifest as a granular or nodular pattern of the distal esophagus. In contrast to the distinct borders of *Candida* plaques and nodules, RE nodules have poorly defined borders. Inflammatory exudates and pseudomembrane formation may mimic fulminant *Candida* esophagitis; however, the patient has symptoms of reflux rather than severe odynophagia. RE is the most common cause of esophageal ulcerations. The ulcers appear as discrete linear, punctate, or irregular collections of barium, usually surrounded by a radiolucent mound of edema. Prominence of the ulcerations in the distal rather than proximal or mid-esophagus is the key to differentiating RE ulcers from those of herpes or drug-induced esophagitis. Complications of RE include ulceration, bleeding, stricture, and Barrett esophagus. Wall thickening and irregular narrowing of thc lumen may be evident on CT (Fig. 43.17, Table 43.2).

Barrett esophagus is an acquired condition of progressive columnar metaplasia of the distal esophagus caused by chronic gastroesophageal reflux. Columnar rather than squamous epithelium lines the distal esophagus. The prevalence of Barrett esophagus in patients with RE is about 10%, but increases to 37% in patients with scleroderma and 40% in patients with RE strictures. It is premalignant, with a 30 to 40 times increased risk of developing adenocarcinoma, resulting in a 15% prevalence of adenocarcinoma in patients with Barrett

TABLE 43.2

CAUSES OF ESOPHAGEAL WALL THICKENING (≥5 mm)

- **Esophagitis** (circumferential)
  - Reflux esophagitis
  - Barrett esophagus
  - Infectious esophagitis
  - Crohn disease
  - Prolonged esophageal intubation
  - Postirradiation scarring
  - Epidermolysis bullosa
  - Eosinophilic esophagitis
- **Benign tumors** (asymmetric, focal)
  - Leiomyoma
  - Granular cell tumors
  - Hemangiomas (phleboliths characteristic)
  - Fibroepithelial polyps
- **Malignant tumors** (asymmetric, focal)
  - Adenocarcinoma
  - Squamous cell carcinoma
  - Lymphoma
  - Metastatic disease
- **Esophageal varices**
- **Intramural hematoma**
- **Diffuse esophageal spasm**

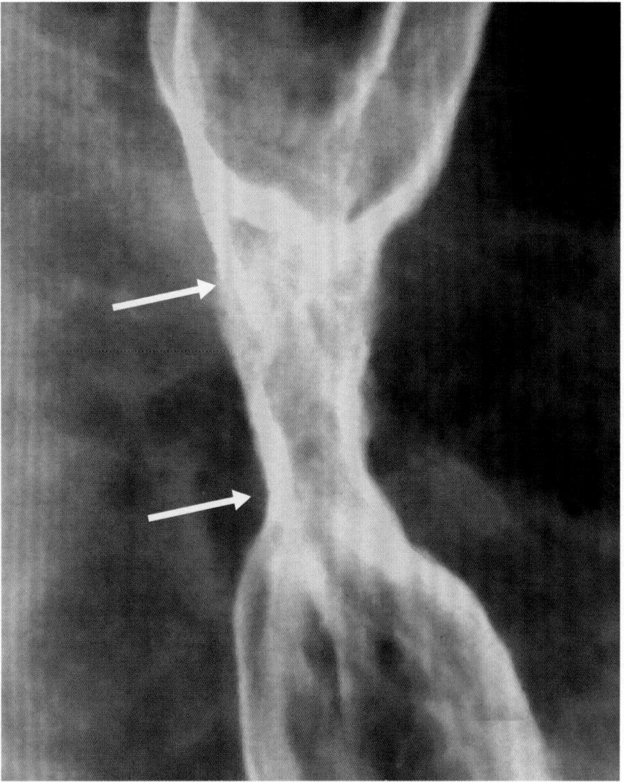

FIGURE 43.18. **Barrett Esophagus.** Air-contrast esophagram shows a focal area of moderate narrowing (*arrows*) in the mid-esophagus with distinctive reticular pattern which results from intestinal metaplasia in Barrett mucosa.

esophagus. Clinical presentation is usually indistinguishable from RE. Adenocarcinoma may develop at any age. The characteristic radiographic appearance of Barrett esophagus is a high (mid-esophageal) stricture or deep ulcer in a patient with GERD (Fig. 43.18). A reticular mucosal pattern of the esophageal mucosa, resembling areae gastricae of the stomach, is also suggestive. The diagnosis is confirmed by endoscopy and biopsy.

Infectious esophagitis is found most commonly in patients with compromised immune systems. It is increasingly common because of the use of steroids, cytotoxic drugs, and prevalence of AIDS.

*Candida albicans*is by far the most common cause of infectious esophagitis and is highly prevalent in immunocompromised patients. Additional risk factors include diabetes, malignancy, radiation, chemotherapy, and steroid treatment. *Candida* of the oropharynx (thrush) is commonly present and is usually evident on physical examination. Odynophagia is a prominent symptom. Discrete plaque-like lesions demonstrated by air-contrast esophagrams are most characteristic (Fig. 43.19). The plaques appear as longitudinally oriented linear or irregular discrete filling defects etched in white with intervening normal-appearing mucosa. The lesions may be tiny and nodular, or giant and coalescent with pseudomembranes. Ulcers tend to be small (<1 cm) and may be punctate, round, oval, or linear. Fulminant disease produces the "foamy esophagus" with a pattern of tiny bubbles at the top of the barium column.

Herpes simplex esophagitis begins as discrete vesicles that rupture to form discrete mucosal ulcers. The ulcers may be linear, punctate, or ring-like and have a characteristic radiolucent halo. Discrete ulcers on a background of normal mucosa

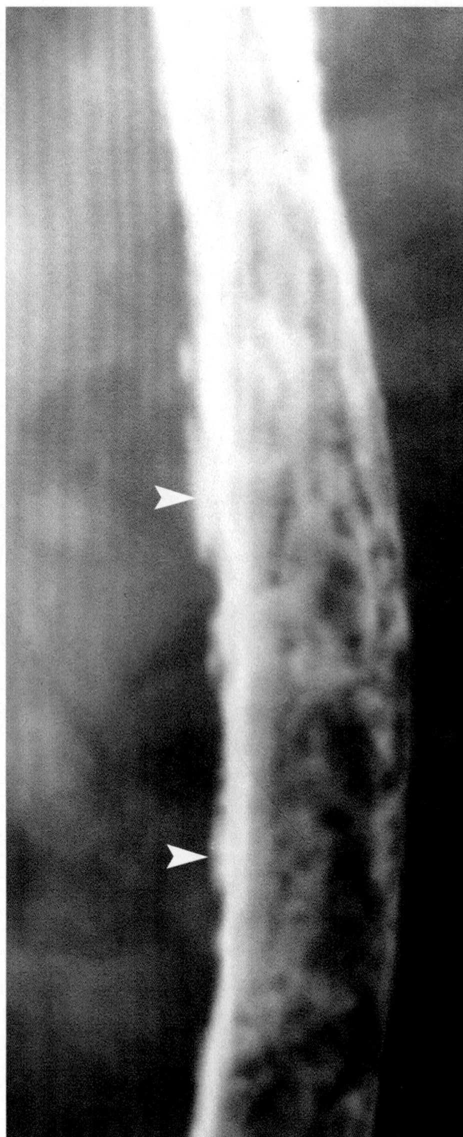

FIGURE 43.19. **Candida Esophagitis.** Barium esophagram in an immunocompromised patient on chemotherapy demonstrates "shaggy" esophageal mucosa caused by multiple confluent plaques and shallow ulcers (*arrowheads*) produced by *Candida albicans* esophagitis.

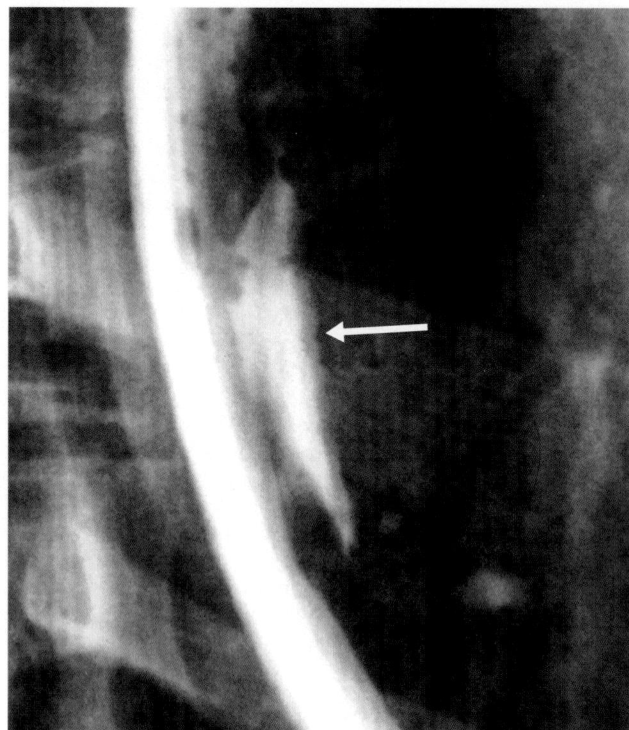

FIGURE 43.20. **Cytomegalovirus Esophagitis.** A large flat mucosal ulcer (*arrow*) in the distal esophagus is characteristic of cytomegalovirus esophagitis in a patient with AIDS.

involving the mid-esophagus are most characteristic of herpes. Nodules and plaques are usually absent.

Cytomegalovirus is a cause of fulminant esophagitis in patients with AIDS. Cytomegalovirus esophagitis is characteristically manifest as one or more large, flat mucosal ulcers (Fig. 43.20). Endoscopic biopsy or culture confirms the diagnosis.

HIV esophagitis causes giant ulcers and severe odynophagia. Electron microscopy reveals HIV particles in the ulcers. The ulcers are large, flat, and usually in the mid-esophagus similar to those with cytomegalovirus esophagitis.

Tuberculosis. The esophagus is the least common portion of the gastrointestinal (GI) tract to be involved by tuberculosis. Manifestations include ulceration, stricture, sinus tract, and abscess formation (Fig. 43.21).

Drug-induced esophagitis is the result of intake of oral medications that produce a focal inflammation in areas of contact with the mucosa. Drugs that cause this condition include tetracycline, doxycycline, quinidine, aspirin, indomethacin, ascorbic acid, potassium chloride, and theophylline. The radiographic appearance may be identical to herpes esophagitis, with discrete ulcers separated by normal mucosa in the

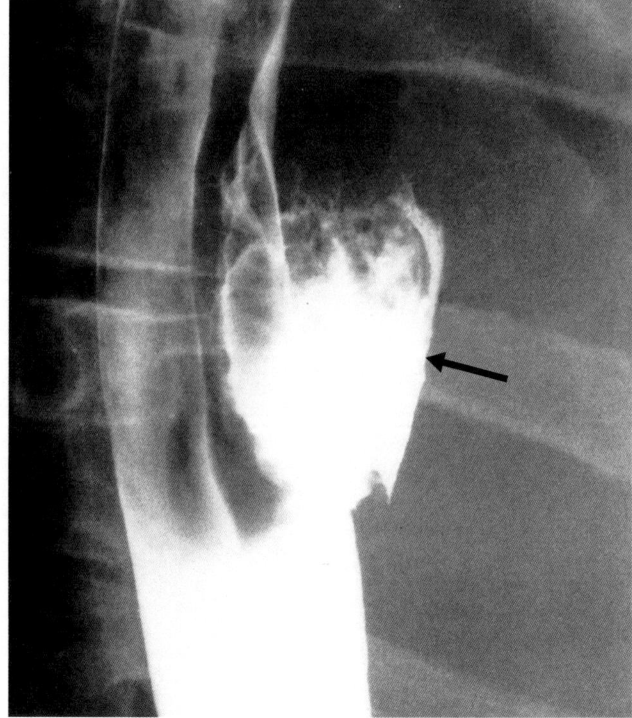

FIGURE 43.21. **Tuberculous Esophagitis.** Tuberculosis in an immunocompromised patient has ulcerated the esophagus and causes a periesophageal abscess (*arrow*).

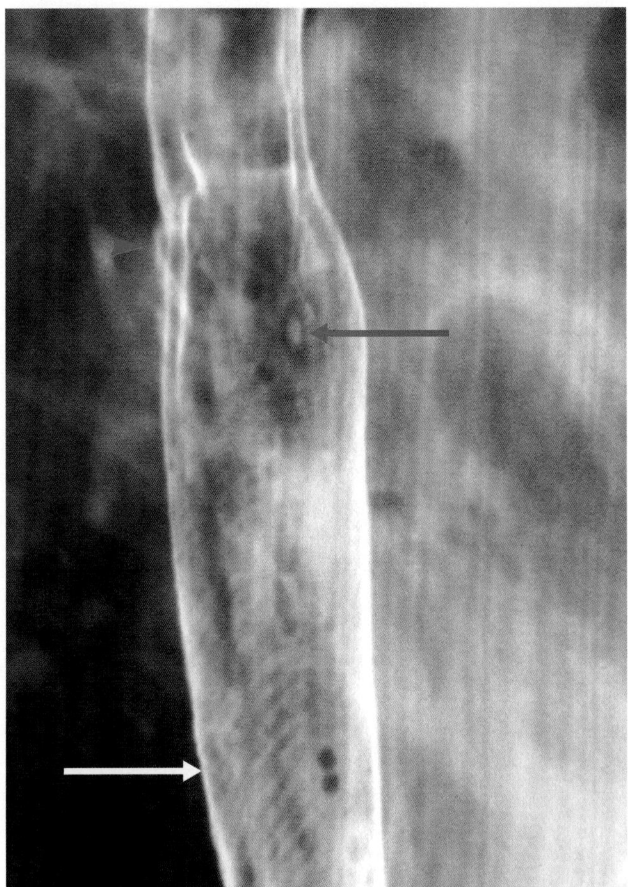

FIGURE 43.22. **Drug-induced Esophagitis—Feline Esophagus.** Air-contrast esophagram demonstrates discrete shallow aphthous ulcers en face (*red arrow*) and in profile (*arrowhead*). The ulcers were caused by stasis of tetracycline capsules in the esophagus. Multiple regular, thin, transverse folds (*white arrow*) in the distal esophagus are typical of *feline esophagus*, a finding suggestive of esophagitis.

mid-esophagus (Fig. 43.22). The diagnosis is suggested by a history of recent drug ingestion. Healing usually occurs within 7 to 10 days of discontinuing the offending medication.

Corrosive ingestion usually occurs as an accident in children or a suicide attempt in adults. Alkaline agents (liquid lye) produce deep (full-thickness) coagulation necrosis. Acid agents tend to produce more superficial injury. Ulceration, esophageal perforation, and mediastinitis may complicate the acute injury. Late complications are fibrosis and long or multiple strictures.

Crohn disease may rarely manifest as discrete aphthous ulcers (Fig. 43.22) in the esophagus. Involvement of the small or large bowel by Crohn disease is virtually always present. Crohn disease of the esophagus should not be considered unless Crohn disease of the bowel is already evident.

Radiation esophagitis occurs in patients with a history of thoracic radiation therapy for malignant disease. Acute radiation may cause shallow or deep ulcers in the area of involvement. With the development of fibrosis, the peristaltic wave is interrupted and a long smooth stricture may develop within the radiotherapy field. Risk depends on total dose, treatment time, and radiotherapy technique. Simultaneous radiotherapy and doxorubicin hydrochloride (Adriamycin) chemotherapy greatly accentuate esophageal inflammation. UGI shows a variable length segment of esophageal narrowing multiple discrete ulcers or a granular mucosal pattern within the radiation field.

ESOPHAGEAL STRICTURE

Strictures are defined as any persistent intrinsic narrowing of the esophagus. The most common causes are fibrosis induced by inflammation and neoplasm. Because radiographic findings are not reliable in differentiating benign from malignant strictures, all should be evaluated endoscopically. Distal esophageal strictures are caused by GERD, scleroderma, and prolonged nasogastric intubation. Upper and middle esophageal strictures most commonly results from Barrett esophagus, mediastinal radiation, caustic ingestion, and skin diseases associated with mucosal ulceration such as pemphigoid, erythema multiforme, and epidermolysis bullosa dystrophica. Benign strictures typically show smoothly tapering concentric narrowing (Fig. 43.18). Malignant strictures are characteristically abrupt, asymmetric, eccentric narrowings with irregular, nodular mucosa. Tapered margins may occur with malignant lesions because of the ease of submucosal spread of tumor.

Esophagitis. Chronic inflammation induces progressive fibrosis that eventually narrows the esophageal lumen. Acute and chronic findings of esophagitis commonly overlap.

Reflux esophagitis (GERD) is the most common cause of esophageal stricture. Reflux strictures are usually confined to the distal esophagus and may be tapered, smooth, and circumferential (the classic appearance) (Fig. 43.23) or asymmetric and irregular. Small smooth sacculations and fixed transverse

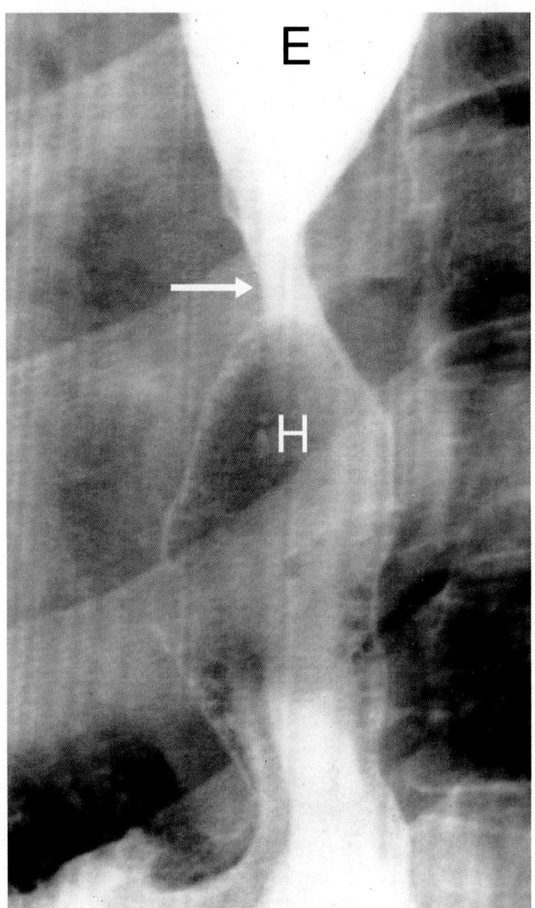

FIGURE 43.23. **Benign Stricture Resulting from Reflux Esophagitis.** A short, narrowed area (*arrow*) of the distal esophagus (*E*) extends to the top of a hiatus hernia (*H*) in this patient with chronic gastroesophageal reflux. Note the tapered margins and concentric shape of the stricture typical for a benign stricture.

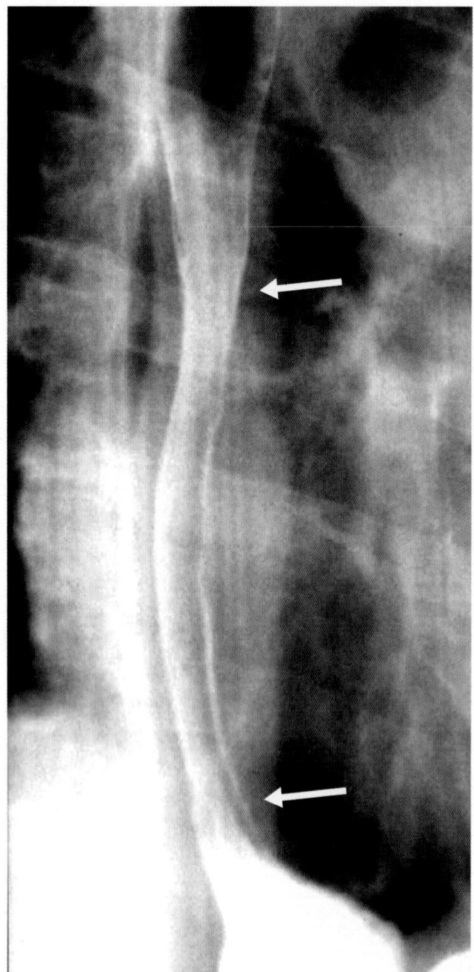

FIGURE 43.24. **Nasogastric Intubation Stricture.** Double-contrast esophagram shows a long segment of narrowing (*arrows*) in the distal esophagus. This stricture developed 4 months after prolonged nasogastric intubation.

folds are characteristic and caused by scarring. Most RE strictures are 1 to 3 cm in length. A *Schatzki ring* is a pathologic fixed ring-like stricture at the level of the B ring, caused by RE. Typical Schatzki rings are 2 to 4 mm in length. Long-segment stricture may be induced by long-term nasogastric intubation (Fig. 43.24). Nasogastric tubes prevent closure of the LES, resulting in continuous bathing of the distal esophagus with acid reflux from the stomach. Zollinger–Ellison syndrome can lead to severe RE because of the high acid content of refluxed gastric contents.

Barrett esophagus strictures tend to be high in the mid-esophagus and may be smooth and tapered or ring-like narrowings. The high position is because of a tendency for strictures to occur at the squamocolumnar junction, which has been displaced to a position well above the GEJ.

Corrosive strictures are long and symmetrical. They commonly develop years after the initial injury.

Alkaline reflux esophagitis may occur in patients who have undergone partial or total gastrectomy. Reflux of bile or pancreatic secretions into the esophagus results in the development of severe alkaline reflux esophagitis and distal esophageal strictures whose length and severity increase rapidly over a short period of time. Performing a Roux-en-Y reconstruction at the time of the surgery helps prevent reflux of bile and pancreatic secretion into the esophagus. An alkaline reflux stricture should be suspected when barium examination performed in patients who have undergone partial or total gastrectomy or gastrojejunostomy reveals a long stricture in the distal esophagus.

Eosinophilic esophagitis is an increasingly common diagnosis made most often in young men with a history of allergies. Some have a peripheral eosinophilia. Patients present with a long-standing history of dysphagia and food impaction. Barium studies demonstrate smooth long-segment narrowing of the esophagus or a series of ring-like strictures, called the "ringed esophagus." CT reveals circumferential wall thickening and submucosal edema. Biopsy reveals eosinophilic infiltration of the wall of the esophagus. The cause may be related to ingested food allergens. Treatment is steroids.

Radiation strictures are confined to the radiotherapy field usually following doses of 50 to 60 Gy. Strictures appear 3 to 6 months after radiation treatment. They are smooth and tapered and usually in the upper or mid-esophagus.

Neoplasm. An irregular, ulcerated, circumferential narrowing with nodular shoulders is most typical of malignant stricture (Fig. 43.25). Infiltrative tumors may cause smooth, rigid narrowing of the esophagus without a clear zone of transition. The mucosa may not be altered until tumor spread is substantial. Because longitudinal spread of tumor along the length

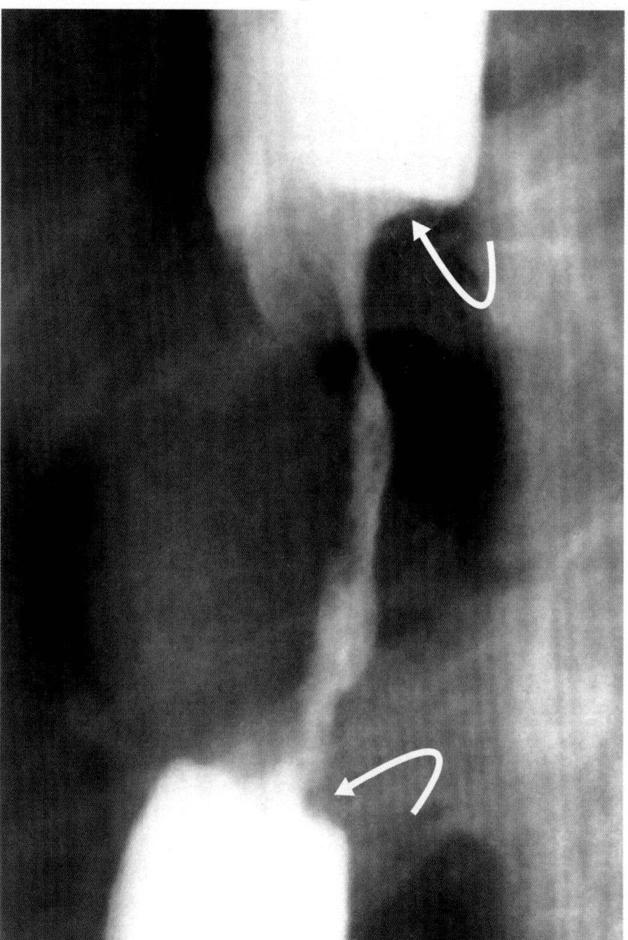

FIGURE 43.25. **Malignant Stricture.** A squamous cell carcinoma of the mid-esophagus causes an abrupt narrowing with irregular mucosa. The prominent shoulders (*curved arrows*) are characteristic of tumor. Differential diagnosis of strictures of the upper and mid-esophagus includes Barrett esophagus, mediastinal irradiation, caustic ingestion, and drug-induced esophagitis.

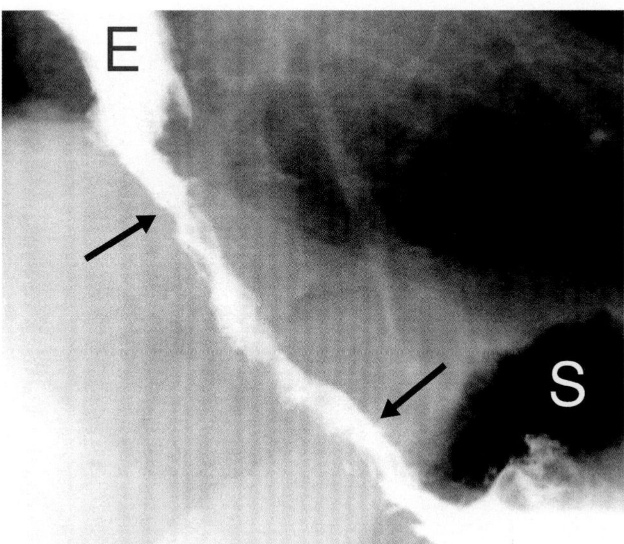

FIGURE 43.26. **Long Stricture Resulting From Esophageal Carcinoma.** A long-segment stricture (*arrows*) of the distal esophagus (*E*) is apparent on this barium esophagram. The column of barium is abruptly narrowed to a thin markedly irregular channel. Differential diagnosis of long-segment strictures of the esophagus includes reflux esophagitis, caustic ingestion, complicated scleroderma, and radiation esophagitis. *S*, stomach.

of the esophagus is typical, long-segment strictures caused by carcinoma are common (Fig. 43.26).

Webs are thin (1 to 2 mm), delicate membranes that sweep partially across the lumen (Fig. 43.27). They occur in both the pharynx and esophagus and are commonly multiple. Pharyngeal webs arise most commonly from the anterior wall of the hypopharynx. Esophageal webs may occur anywhere, but they are most common in the cervical esophagus just distal to the cricopharyngeus impression. Most are incidental findings; however, they occasionally cause sufficient obstruction to result in dysphasia.

Extrinsic Compression. Malignancy or inflammation in the mediastinum may encase the esophagus and narrow its lumen. Causes include lung carcinoma, lymphoma, metastasis to mediastinal nodes, tuberculosis, and histoplasmosis.

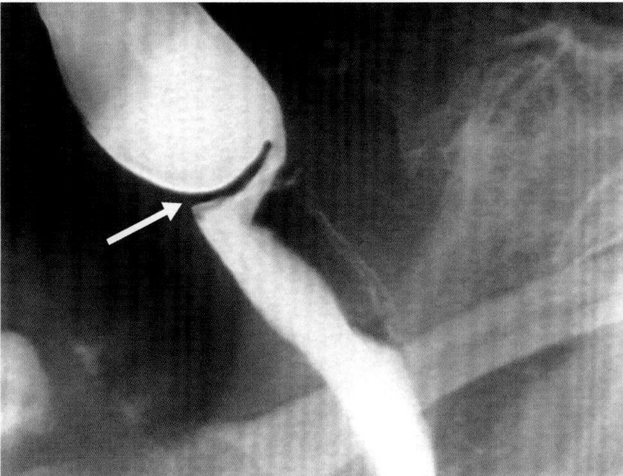

FIGURE 43.27. **Esophageal Web.** Lateral oblique view from a barium esophagram reveals a thin membrane (*arrow*) that extends partially across the lumen of the proximal esophagus, leaving only a narrow passage for food. The esophagus is dilated proximal to the web.

ENLARGED ESOPHAGEAL FOLDS

Esophagitis. Thick folds occur most commonly with RE. Additional findings associated with esophagitis, such as ulcerations and nodules, are commonly present.

Varices appear as serpiginous filling defects (Fig. 43.28A) that change in size with changes in intrathoracic pressure and that collapse with esophageal peristalsis and distention. They are best demonstrated on UGI with mucosal relief views. CT with bolus contrast enhancement demonstrates varices as enhancing vascular structures within and adjacent to esophageal wall near the GEJ. MR is also effective in demonstrating varices as vascular spaces, with signal void because of flowing blood (Fig. 43.28B).

Uphill varices refer to the portosystemic collateral veins that enlarge because of portal hypertension. Coronary vein collaterals connect with gastroesophageal varices that drain into the inferior vena cava via the azygos system. Uphill varices are usually only present in the distal esophagus.

Downhill varices are formed as a result of obstruction of the superior vena cava with drainage from the azygos system through esophageal varices to the portal vein. Downhill varices usually predominate in the proximal esophagus.

Lymphoma may infiltrate the submucosa and thicken the folds. Lymphoma rarely involves the esophagus directly and is virtually never primary in the esophagus.

Varicoid carcinoma causes thick, tortuous, longitudinal folds that resemble varices but are rigid and persistent.

MASS LESIONS/FILLING DEFECTS

Pharyngeal carcinomas are well demonstrated by air-contrast pharyngography. Barium studies may detect tumors difficult to visualize endoscopically. Radiographic signs include (a) intraluminal mass seen as a filling defect, abnormal luminal contour, or focal increased density; (b) mucosal irregularity owing to ulceration or mucosal elevations; and (c) asymmetrical distensibility due to infiltrating tumor or extrinsic nodal mass. Most pharyngeal tumors are squamous cell carcinomas (SCCs) that may arise on the base of the tongue, palatine tonsil, posterior pharyngeal wall, or the piriform sinus (Fig. 43.29). Laryngeal tumors may impress on the pharynx or extend into it. Staging is best performed by CT or MR.

Pharyngeal retention cysts are benign lesions that typically involve the valleculae and should not be mistaken for pharyngeal neoplasms. They appear as small, smooth, well-defined, round, or oval filling defects best appreciated on frontal views. They arise from dilation of mucus glands caused by chronic inflammation. They are never malignant.

Lymphoma of the pharynx is usually manifest as a large, bulky tumor of the lingual or palatine tonsils. Lymphoma constitutes 15% of oropharyngeal tumors.

Esophageal Carcinoma. Most (80%) of esophageal neoplasms are malignant, primarily adenocarcinoma or SCC. In the United States, adenocarcinoma is now the most common cell type of esophageal cancer, related to the increasing incidence of GERD. SCC risk factors are smoking and alcohol consumption. Presenting signs and symptoms include dysphagia, weight loss, bleeding leading to anemia, chest or epigastric pain, cough, and recurrent pneumonia. Adenocarcinoma arises from malignant transformation of columnar epithelium

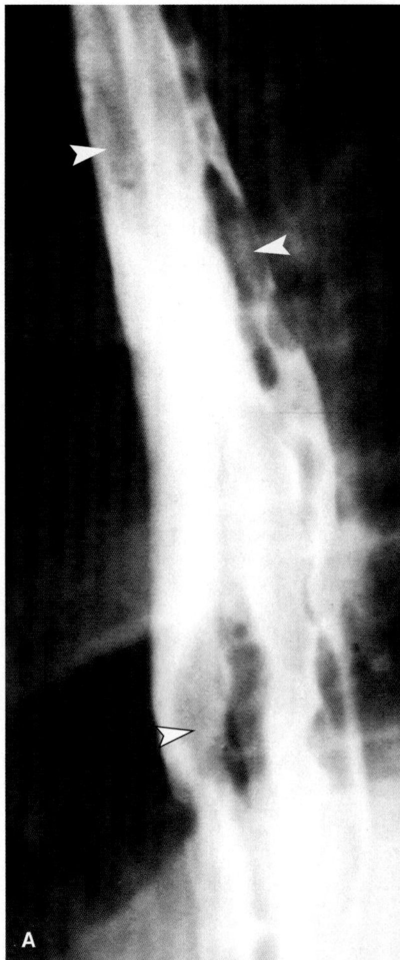

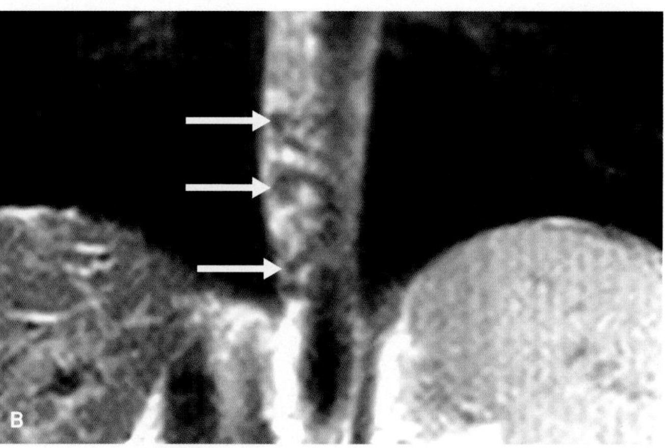

FIGURE 43.28. **Varices. A:** A single-contrast barium esophagram demonstrates sinuous tubular and nodular filling defects (*arrowheads*) in the esophagus. This patient has cirrhosis, portal hypertension, and a history of upper gastrointestinal bleeding. **B:** Coronal MR shows esophageal varices as tortuous tubular vessels (*arrows*).

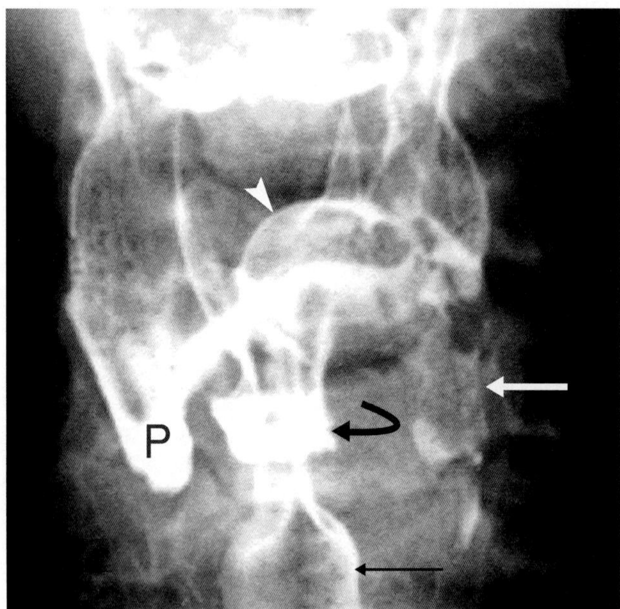

FIGURE 43.29. **Carcinoma in the Piriform Recess.** Frontal view from a barium pharyngogram demonstrates a mass mostly filling and obliterating the left piriform recess (*fat arrow*) and bulging into the hypopharynx (*arrowhead*). The right piriform recess (*P*) has a normal appearance. The presence of the mass has caused aspiration. Barium is seen filling the larynx (*curved arrow*) and extending into the trachea (*skinny arrow*).

of Barrett esophagus in the lower third of the esophagus. SCC arises from the stratified squamous epithelium that lines the entire esophagus. Imaging features of the two cell types are indistinguishable, except that adenocarcinoma is almost always distal, usually invades the GEJ, and is much more likely to invade the stomach. Tumors assume four basic imaging patterns. An annular constricting lesion, appearing as an irregular ulcerated stricture, is most common (Figs. 43.25 and 43.26). The polypoid pattern causes an intraluminal filling defect (Fig. 43.30). The infiltrative variety grows predominantly in the submucosa and may simulate a benign stricture. The least common pattern is that of an ulcerated mass. The tumor spreads quickly by direct invasion into adjacent tissues because of the lack of a serosal covering on the esophagus. Lymphatic spread may go to nodes in the neck, mediastinum, or below the diaphragm, depending on the location of the primary tumor in the esophagus. Hematogenous spread is to lung, liver, and adrenal gland.

The diagnosis is usually made by endoscopy and biopsy. CT and endoscopic US are used primarily to define the extent of disease and determine surgical resectability (Fig. 43.31). Findings include irregular thickening of the esophageal wall (>5 mm), eccentric narrowing of the lumen, dilation of the esophagus above the area of narrowing, invasion of periesophageal tissues, and metastases to mediastinal lymph nodes and the liver. Obliteration of the fat space between the aorta, esophagus, and vertebral body is highly indicative of tumor spread. PET-CT is used primarily for demonstration of distant metastases, although fludeoxyglucose (FDG) uptake is avid for primary tumors of both cell types.

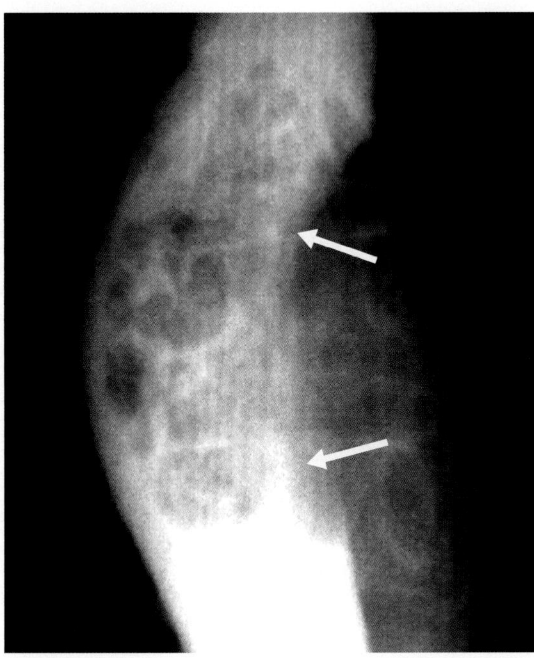

FIGURE 43.30. **Polypoid Squamous Cell Carcinoma.** This esophageal carcinoma appears as a polypoid mass (*arrows*) in the mid-esophagus on barium esophagram. Barium outlines the lobulations in the tumor.

Gastric adenocarcinoma may spread from the fundus and GEJ into the distal esophagus. Adenocarcinoma of the distal esophagus may be either primary esophageal or primary gastric (Fig. 43.32).

Leiomyoma, while rare, is still the most common benign neoplasm of the esophagus, accounting for 50% of all benign esophageal neoplasms. Gastrointestinal stromal tumors (GISTs), common in the rest of the GI tract, are rare in the esophagus. The tumor is firm, well encapsulated, and arises in the wall. Ulceration is rare. Most cause no symptoms and are discovered incidentally. Men aged 25 to 35 years are affected most commonly (male-to-female ratio = 2:1). On barium esophagram, most are small and appear as smooth, well-defined wall lesions, although rarely they may be pedunculated or polypoid. Coarse calcifications are occasionally present and strongly indicative of leiomyoma (Fig. 43.33). CT demonstrates a smooth, well-defined mass of uniform soft tissue density. The esophageal wall is eccentrically thickened. Leiomyosarcoma of the esophagus is exceedingly rare, accounting for less than 1% of esophageal malignancy. Malignant lesions are typically heterogeneous with a large exophytic component.

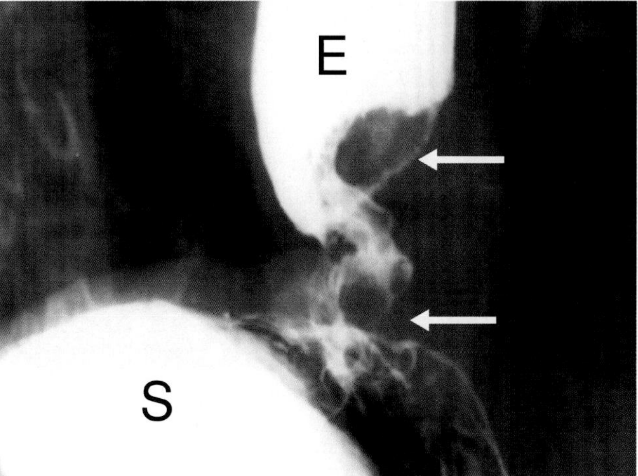

FIGURE 43.32. **Adenocarcinoma in Barrett Esophagus.** A tumor in the distal esophagus (*E*) forms nodular (*arrows*) narrowing of the barium column. Endoscopy confirmed adenocarcinoma arising in Barrett esophagus. *S*, stomach.

Fibrovascular polyps are a rare cause of esophageal filling defect. They are benign and composed of fatty and fibrous tissue with accompanying blood vessels. Long polyps may be regurgitated into the pharynx or mouth obstructing the airway. They appear as large elongated intraluminal masses in the upper esophagus.

Esophageal duplication cysts are congenital abnormalities that are usually incidental findings presenting without symptoms. Most (60%) occur in the lower esophagus. CT shows a well-defined cystic mass (Fig. 43.34). Barium examination will show extrinsic or intramural compression due to close contact with the esophagus. Differential diagnosis include bronchogenic and neurenteric cyst.

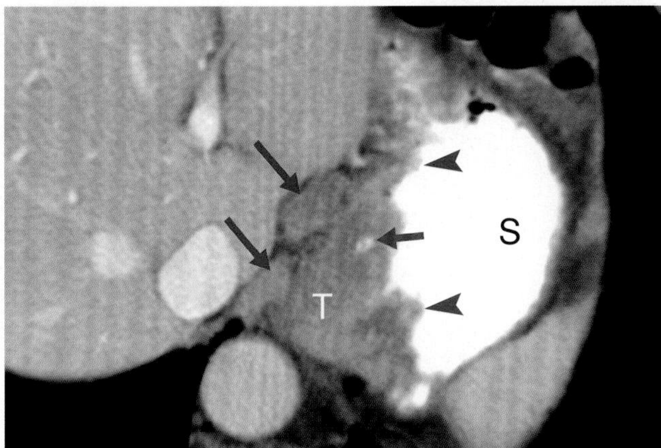

FIGURE 43.31. **Esophageal Adenocarcinoma—CT.** Postintravenous contrast CT image shows a large tumor (*T*) of the distal esophagus invading the fundus (*arrowheads*) of the stomach (*S*). Two metastatic lymph nodes (*red arrows*) are evident. The lumen (*blue arrow*) of the distal esophagus is markedly narrowed.

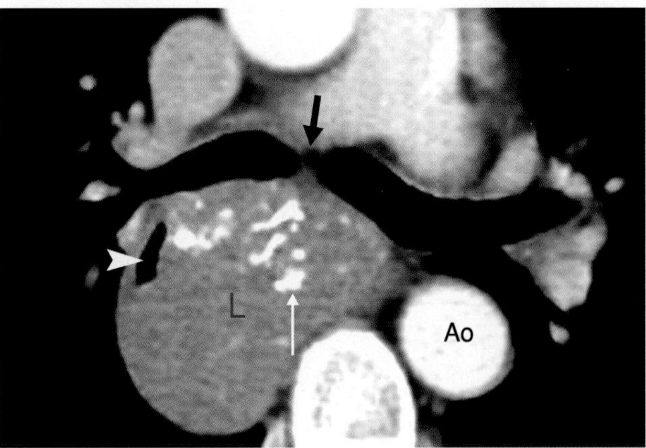

FIGURE 43.33. **Leiomyoma Esophagus.** Postcontrast CT at the level of the carina (*fat arrow*) shows a large eccentric tumor (*L*) arising from the esophagus. The lumen (*arrowhead*) of the esophagus is narrowed and displaced. The tumor contains coarse calcifications (*skinny arrow*) characteristic of leiomyoma. *Ao*, descending thoracic aorta.

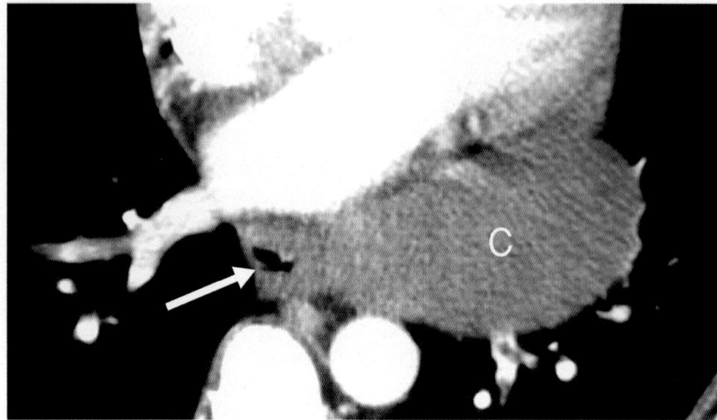

FIGURE 43.34. **Esophageal Duplication Cyst.** CT reveals a periesophageal well-defined oval cystic mass (*C*). Appearance is typical of an esophageal duplication cyst. Though large and displacing the esophagus (*arrow*) the patient was asymptomatic.

Extrinsic lesions may invade the esophagus or simulate an esophageal mass or filling defect. Causes include mediastinal adenopathy, lung carcinoma, and vascular structures.

Aberrant right subclavian artery arises from the aorta distal to the left subclavian artery. To reach its destination, it must cross the mediastinum behind the esophagus. It causes a characteristic upward-slanting linear filling defect on the posterior aspect of the esophagus (Fig. 43.35).

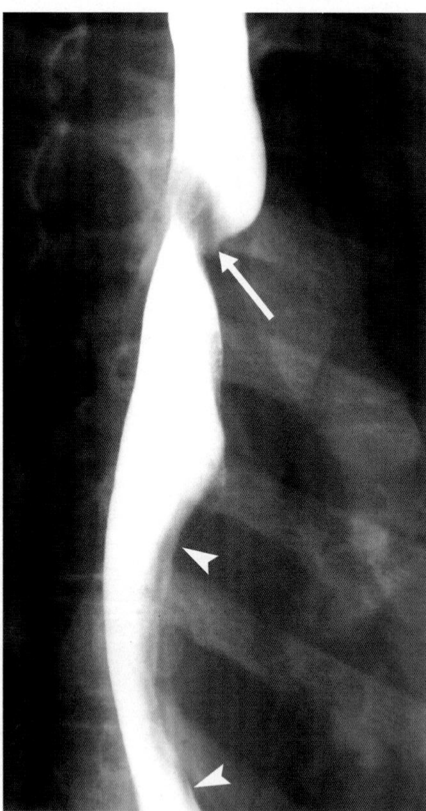

FIGURE 43.35. **Aberrant Right Subclavian Artery.** Frontal view from a barium esophagram reveals an aberrant right subclavian artery that arises from the aortic arch distal to the left subclavian artery and crosses behind the esophagus, causing a tubular extrinsic impression (*arrow*) on the esophagus slanting upward and to the patient's right. The normal smooth impression of the left atrium (*arrowheads*) on the esophagus is also evident.

ESOPHAGEAL PERFORATION AND TRAUMA

Esophageal perforation is a life-threatening event requiring prompt diagnosis and treatment. More than half the cases are related to esophageal instrumentation. Bleeding can be profuse, and infection is a great risk. Conventional radiographs demonstrate subcutaneous, cervical, or mediastinal emphysema within 1 hour of perforation. Chest radiographs may show a widened mediastinum and pleural effusion or hydropneumothorax. Contrast studies should be performed initially with low-osmolar water-soluble agents and, if negative, followed by repeating the study with barium. The key finding is focal or diffuse extravasation of contrast outside the esophagus. CT demonstrates fluid collections, extraluminal contrast, and air in the mediastinum (Fig. 43.36).

Trauma. Endoscopy, esophageal dilation procedures, or any type of instrumentation may perforate the esophageal wall. Knife and bullet wounds may perforate the esophagus. Blunt trauma may tear the esophagus by an explosive increase in intraesophageal pressure.

Boerhaave syndrome refers to rupture of the esophageal wall as a result of forceful vomiting. The tear is virtually always in the left posterior wall near the left crus of the diaphragm. Esophageal contents usually escape into the left pleural space or into the potential space between the parietal pleura and left crus. Tears may result in intramural dissections and hematomas in the wall of the esophagus.

Mallory–Weiss tear involves only the mucosa and not the full thickness of the esophagus. The tears are usually caused by violent retching. Endoscopy usually identifies the lesion. The lesion is commonly missed on UGI. When seen, the tear appears as a longitudinally oriented barium collection, 1 to 4 cm in length, in the distal esophagus. It may be a cause of copious hematemesis.

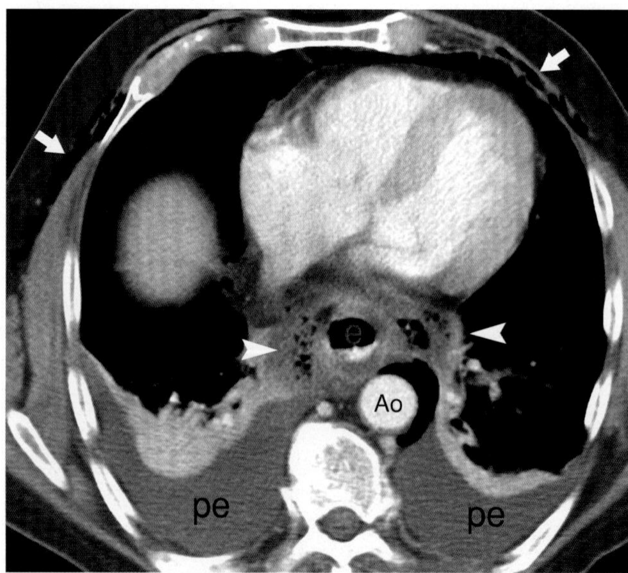

FIGURE 43.36. **Esophageal Perforation.** CT scan through the lower thorax shows bubbles of air and fluid in the mediastinum (*arrowheads*) and around the thoracic aorta (*Ao*). Air and contrast distend the esophagus (*e*). Air has dissected into the subcutaneous tissues (*fat arrows*). Bilateral pleural effusions (*pe*) are also evident. Esophageal perforation occurred during endoscopic esophageal stenting.

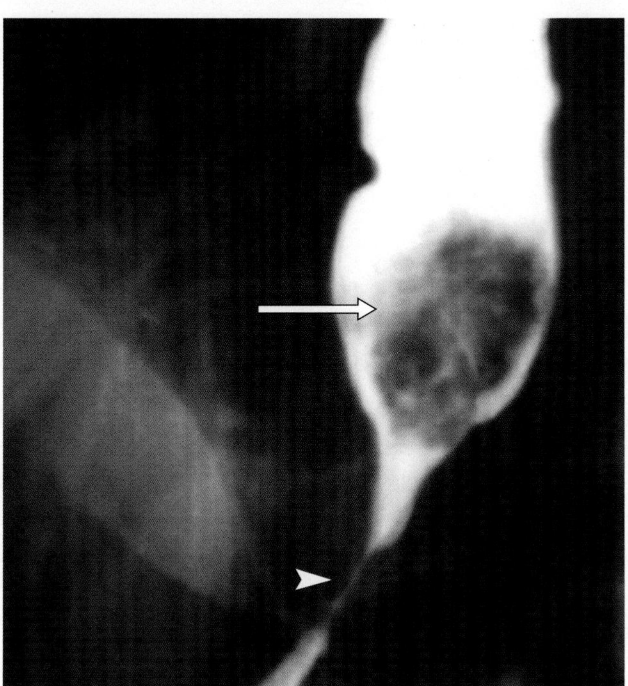

FIGURE 43.37. **Food Impaction.** Single-contrast esophagram shows a polypoid filling defect (*arrow*) representing a bolus of food just proximal to a stricture (*arrowhead*) in the distal esophagus.

Foreign-body impaction in adults is usually attributable to bones or boluses of meat. Children may ingest any foreign object including toys, coins, and jewelry. Bones usually lodge in the pharynx, most often near the cricopharyngeus muscle. Meat impacts in the distal or mid-esophagus. Perforation occurs in only 1% of cases, but the risk increases if impaction persists more than 24 hours. Bones in the pharynx are difficult to differentiate from calcification of the thyroid and cricoid cartilages. Contrast studies show nonopaque foreign bodies as filling defects (Fig. 43.37). Impacted foreign bodies may be removed by use of a Foley balloon catheter or wire basket or by gaseous distention of the esophagus with gas-producing crystals. CT demonstrates the nature of the foreign body and frequently any associated pathology that predisposed to impaction.

Suggested Readings

Carucci LR, Turner MA. Dysphagia revisited: common and unusual causes. *Radiographics* 2015;35:105–122.

Edmonds CE, Levine MS. A clinical/pattern approach for barium esophagography. *Appl Radiol* 2015;1:12–22. (Pictorial review).

Hong SJ, Kim TJ, Nam KB, et al. New TNM staging system for esophageal cancer: what chest radiologists need to know. *Radiographics* 2014;34:1722–1740.

Jaffer NM, Ng E, Au FW, Steele CM. Fluoroscopic evaluation of oropharyngeal dysphagia: anatomic, technical, and common etiologic factors. *AJR Am J Roentgenol* 2015;204:49–58. (Pictorial review).

Levine MS, Carucci LR, DiSantis DJ, et al. Consensus statement of Society of Abdominal Radiology disease-focused panel on barium esophagography in gastroesophageal reflux disease. *AJR Am J Roentgenol* 2016;207:1009–1015.

Lewis RB, Mehrotra AK, Rodriquez P, Levine MS. Esophageal neoplasms: radiologic-pathologic correlation. *Radiographics* 2013;33:1083–1108.

Madan R, Bair RJ, Chick JF. Complex iatrogenic esophageal injuries: an imaging spectrum. *AJR Am J Roentgenol* 2015;204:W116–W125. (Structured review).

Marini T, Desal A, Kaproth-Joslin K, Wandtke J, Hobbs SK. Imaging of the oesophagus: beyond cancer. *Insights Imaging* 2017;8:365–376. (Pictorial review).

Tao TY, Menias CO, Herman TE, McAlister WH, Balfe DM. Easier to swallow: pictorial review of structural findings of the pharynx at barium pharyngography. *Radiographics* 2013;33:E189–E208. (Pictorial review).

CHAPTER 44 ■ STOMACH AND DUODENUM

WILLIAM E. BRANT

IMAGING METHODS

Commonplace use of endoscopy has diminished utilization of fluoroscopy to study the upper gastrointestinal (GI) tract. CT, MR, and US are used to evaluate the extraluminal component of disease. Nonetheless a high-quality upper gastrointestinal (UGI) series provides excellent evaluation of the stomach and duodenum and remains part of the radiologic armamentarium. To attain a high sensitivity for the examination and to avoid missing significant pathology, multiple techniques must be used for the UGI. Single-contrast technique involves filling and distending the stomach and duodenum with barium suspension followed by compression procedures to demonstrate abnormalities of the distal stomach and duodenum. Mucosal relief technique entails using small amounts of barium to coat the mucosa without distending the bowel to demonstrate abnormalities such as varices. Double-contrast technique, using high-density barium suspensions to coat the mucosa and ingestible effervescent granules to distend the stomach and duodenum, is optimal for demonstration of subtle features of the mucosal surface. As with any radiographic examination, attention to detail and tailoring the examination to address the clinical problem are essential in producing optimal results.

CT, with use of air-contrast distention techniques, is a valuable adjunct to endoscopy and barium studies to document abnormalities of the wall of the stomach and duodenum and to determine the extent of extraluminal disease. Optimal distention of the stomach and duodenum is mandatory for accurate CT interpretation. Gastric and duodenal distention may be attained by filling the organs with water, positive contrast agents, or by ingesting effervescent granules to cause gaseous distention. The patient is positioned to optimize distention of the GI tract portion of greatest interest.

ANATOMY

The GI tract is essentially a hollow tube consisting of four concentric layers of tissue. The innermost layer exposed to the lumen is the *mucosa*. The mucosa consists of epithelium supported by loose connective tissue of the lamina propria and a thin band of smooth muscle called the muscularis mucosae. The *submucosa* provides connective tissue support for the mucosa. The submucosa contains the primary vascular and lymphatic channels, lymphoid follicles, and autonomic nerve plexuses. The major muscular structure of the bowel wall is the *muscularis propria*, comprised of inner circular and outer longitudinal layers. The *serosa* or adventitia is the outer covering of the bowel. Lymphoid tissue in the GI tract is located in the mucosa (epithelium and lamina propria), the submucosa, and the mesenteric lymph nodes. As the major component of the mucosa-associated lymphoid tissue (MALT), lymphoid tissue plays a major role in host immune defenses and is a site of significant disease.

The appearance and position of the stomach and duodenum vary considerably from one individual to another. The terms used to describe the anatomic divisions of the stomach and duodenum are illustrated in Figure 44.1. *Cardia* refers to the region of the gastroesophageal junction (GEJ). The *fundus* is that portion of the stomach above the level of the GEJ. The *body* of the stomach is the central two-thirds portion from the cardia to the *incisura angularis*. The incisura angularis is the acute angle formed on the lesser curvature that marks the boundary between the body and the antrum. The parietal cells, which produce hydrochloric acid, and the chief cells, which produce pepsin precursors, are located in the fundus and body. The *antrum* is the distal one-third of the stomach, and contains gastrin-producing cells but no acid-secreting cells.

The *pylorus* is the junction of the stomach with the duodenum, and the pyloric canal is the channel through the pylorus. The *duodenal bulb*, or cap, is the pyramidal first portion of the duodenum. The gallbladder frequently makes a prominent impression on the top of the bulb. The duodenum bulb, like the stomach, is covered on all surfaces by visceral peritoneum. The remainder of the duodenum is retroperitoneal and within the anterior pararenal compartment. The second or descending portion of the duodenum is lateral to the head of the pancreas. The common bile duct and pancreatic duct pierce the medial aspect of the descending duodenum at the ampulla of Vater. The third or horizontal portion of the duodenum passes to the left between the superior mesenteric vessels and the inferior vena cava and aorta. The fourth or ascending portion of the duodenum ascends on the left side of the aorta to the level of L2 and the ligament of Treitz, where it turns abruptly ventrally to form the duodenal–jejunal flexure.

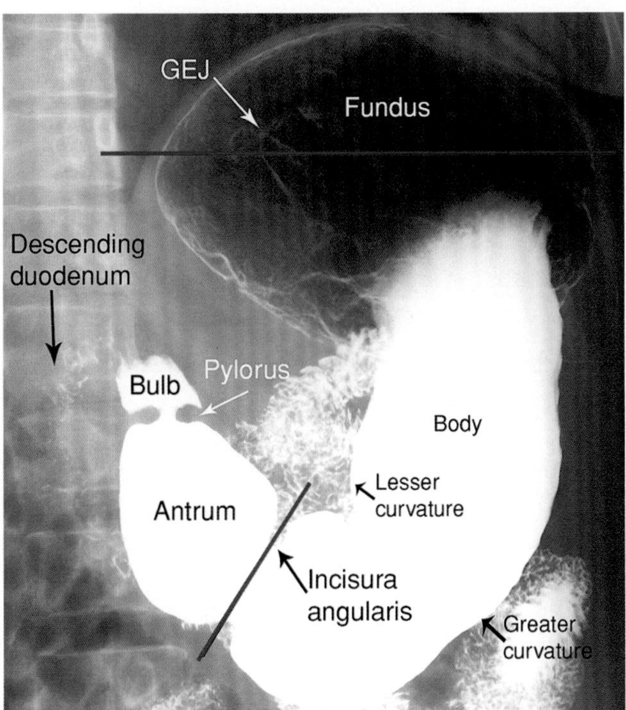

FIGURE 44.1. Anatomy of the UGI Tract. A prone right anterior oblique radiograph of the stomach taken during a UGI series demonstrates normal radiographic anatomy. The *fundus* is that portion of the stomach above the level of the gastroesophageal junction (*GEJ*). The *incisura angularis* is the angular notch on the *lesser curvature* that serves as a landmark dividing the *body* and *antrum* of the stomach. The *greater curvature* serves as the attachment for the greater omentum. The partially contracted *pylorus* is the valve between the stomach and duodenum. The *bulb* is the pyramidal-shaped first portion of the duodenum. The *descending duodenum* is faintly outlined by barium on *this* image.

The term *areae gastricae* refers to the detailed pattern of the gastric mucosa as demonstrated by double-contrast technique (Fig. 44.2). Normal areae gastricae varies from a fine reticular pattern to a coarse nodular pattern. The hallmark of normal is the regularity of the pattern in all areas in which it is visualized. The term *rugae* refers to the gastric mucosal folds that produce distinct radiolucent ridges when the stomach is partially distended. Rugae are composed of mucosa, the lamina propria, the muscularis mucosae, and portions of the submucosa. Disease in any of these structures may cause thickening of the gastric folds. Rugal folds are most prominent in the fundus and proximal gastric body and are usually absent in the antrum. The *lesser curvature* of the stomach is attached to the liver by the lesser omentum. The greater omentum attaches to the *greater curvature* of the stomach. The lesser sac is the intraperitoneal space posterior to the stomach and anterior to the pancreas.

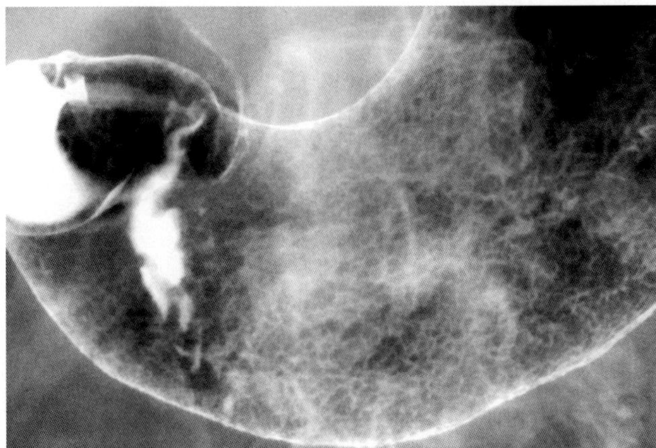

FIGURE 44.2. Normal Areae Gastricae. Double-contrast technique provides distention of the stomach with coating of its mucosa to demonstrate the normal pattern of areae gastricae produced by small polygonal mounds of normal gastric mucosa.

On CT the normal gastric wall when well distended in the antrum is 5 to 7 mm thick and in the body 2 to 3 mm thick. The wall of the normal duodenal is less than 3 mm thick. Both organs must be fully distended to accurately assess wall thickness. A prominent pseudotumor, caused by inadequate distention, is often seen on CT near the GEJ.

STOMACH

Helicobacter pylori Infection

Helicobacter pylori infection is the major cause of chronic gastritis, duodenitis, benign gastric and duodenal ulcers, gastric adenocarcinoma, and MALT lymphoma. *H. pylori* is a gram-negative spiral bacillus that colonizes the stomachs in as many as 80% of individuals in some populations. It will infect only gastric-like epithelium and is usually localized to the gastric antrum, living on surface epithelial cells beneath the mucous coat. It survives in gastric acid by using a powerful urease enzyme to break down urea into ammonia and bicarbonate, creating a more alkaline environment for itself. The prevalence of infection increases with age (>50% of Americans older than age 60) and is high in lower socioeconomic populations and in developing countries. Infection is chronic and causes a superficial gastritis, which is most commonly asymptomatic. Approximately 70% of peptic gastric ulcers, 95% of duodenal ulcers, and 50% of gastric adenocarcinoma are caused by this infection. Double-contrast technique demonstrates enlarged areae gastricae in 50% of patients with *H. pylori* infection. Diagnosis of *H. pylori* infection is made by serology, urease breath tests, and endoscopic biopsy. Treatment is usually a combination of two to four drugs including one or more antibiotics, H2 blockers to decrease acid secretion, and occasionally a bismuth compound. Cure rates of 90% are reported although antibiotic resistance is emerging. Although spontaneous elimination of infection is rare, treatment of asymptomatic infected individuals is not currently recommended.

Gastric Mass Lesions/Filling Defects

Gastric carcinoma is the third most common GI malignancy, following colon and pancreatic carcinoma. Most (95%) are adenocarcinomas; the remainder is diffuse anaplastic (signet ring) carcinoma, squamous cell carcinoma, or rare cell types. Predisposing factors include smoking, pernicious anemia, atrophic gastritis, and gastrojejunostomy. *H. pylori* infection increases the risk of gastric carcinoma sixfold and is the cause of approximately half of gastric adenocarcinoma cases. Peak age is from 50 to 70 years with males predominating 2:1. The incidence of gastric carcinoma is as much as five times higher in Japan, Finland, Chile, and Iceland than in the United States. Mortality is high with a 5-year survival rate of 10% to 20%.

The tumor has four common morphologic growth patterns. One-third is polypoid masses that present as filling defects within the gastric lumen (Fig. 44.3). Many of these are

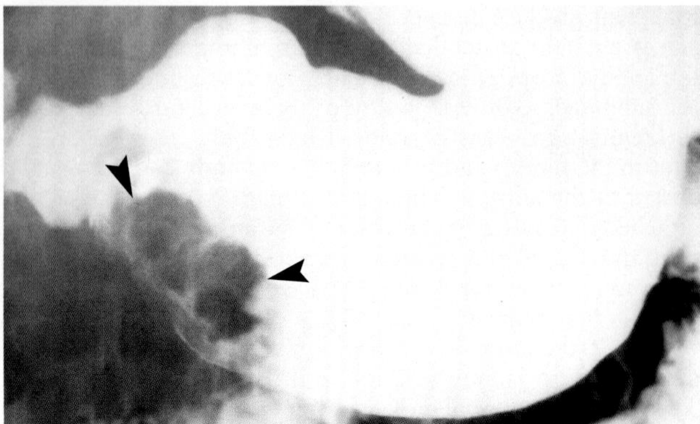

FIGURE 44.3. **Polypoid Gastric Carcinoma.** Single-contrast technique UGI series reveals a lobulated filling defect (*arrowheads*) in the antrum of the stomach.

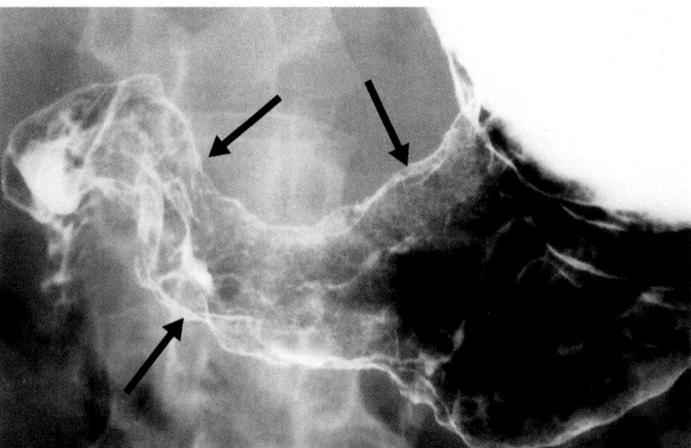

FIGURE 44.5. **Scirrhous Carcinoma—Double-Contrast UGI.** Double-contrast technique in a different patient shows the nodular and irregular mucosa (*arrows*) in the fixed and narrowed distal stomach. Scirrhous carcinoma may also be termed linitis plastica.

broad-based and papillary in configuration. Another third are ulcerative masses presenting as malignant gastric ulcers. The remainder are infiltrating tumors, focal plaque-like lesions with central ulcer, or diffusely infiltrating (15%) with poorly differentiated carcinomatous cells producing bizarre thickened folds and thickened rigid stomach wall, so-called scirrhous carcinomas (Figs. 44.4 and 44.5). The terms "linitis plastica" and "water bottle stomach" may be applied to describe the resulting stiff narrowed stomach. Additional causes of narrowed stomach are listed in Table 44.1.

The tumor spreads by direct invasion through the gastric wall to involve perigastric fat and adjacent organs, or it may seed the peritoneal cavity. Lymphatic spread is to regional lymph nodes including perigastric nodes along the lesser curvature, celiac axis, and hepatoduodenal, retropancreatic, mesenteric, and para-aortic nodes. Hematogenous metastases involve the liver, adrenal glands, ovaries, and, rarely, bone and lung. Intraperitoneal seeding presents as carcinomatosis or Krukenberg ovarian tumors. PET-CT is most effective in demonstration of metastatic lymph nodes and distant spread of tumor.

Early gastric cancers appear on barium studies as (a) gastric polyps with risk of malignancy increased for lesions larger than 1 cm, (b) superficial plaque-like lesions or nodular mucosa, or (c) shallow, irregular ulcers with nodular adjacent mucosa. These lesions are most sensitively detected on double-contrast studies.

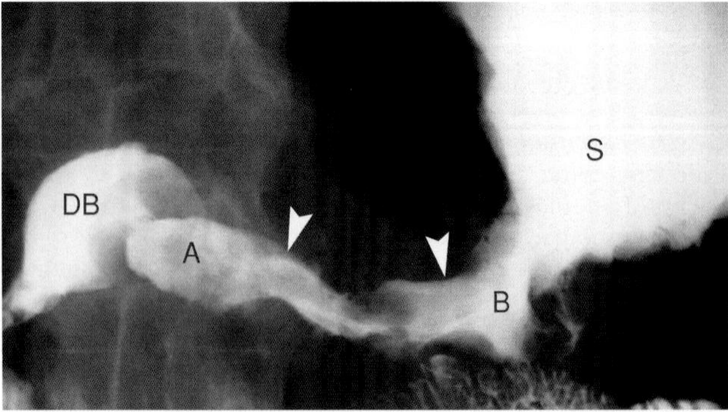

FIGURE 44.4. **Scirrhous Carcinoma—Single-Contrast UGI.** Radiograph from UGI shows fixed nodular narrowing (*arrowheads*) of the body (*B*) and antrum (*A*) of the stomach (*S*). No peristalsis through this portion of the stomach was observed at fluoroscopy. Biopsy yielded undifferentiated adenocarcinoma. *DB*, duodenal bulb.

CT and MR are used to determine the extent of tumor to facilitate preoperative planning (Fig. 44.6). Findings include (a) focal, often irregular, wall thickening (>1 cm); (b) diffuse wall thickening due to tumor infiltration (linitis plastica) (contrast enhancement is common); (c) intraluminal soft tissue mass; (d) bulky mass with ulceration; (e) rare, large, exophytic tumor resembling leiomyosarcoma; (f) extension of tumor into perigastric fat; (g) regional lymphadenopathy; and (h) metastases in the liver, adrenal, and peritoneal cavity. Mucinous adenocarcinomas frequently contain stippled calcifications. Early cancers appear on CT and MR as polypoid lesions or focal mucosal thickening that enhances with contrast. Advanced cancers (Fig. 44.7) show thicker walls, ulceration, and extension into perigastric fat. Findings used to differentiate malignant gastric neoplasms are listed in Table 44.2. Transmural extension, intraperitoneal spread, or distant metastases limit treatment to palliative surgery or chemotherapy.

Lymphoma accounts for 2% of gastric neoplasms. The stomach is the most common site of involvement of primary GI lymphoma, accounting for approximately 50% of cases. Risk

TABLE 44.1

NARROWED STOMACH

Neoplastic
Gastric adenocarcinoma (linitis plastica)
Lymphoma (antral narrowing + extension into duodenum)
Metastases (linitis plastica due to breast carcinoma)
Kaposi sarcoma (AIDS)
Inflammatory
H. pylori gastritis (usually antral narrowing)
Corrosive ingestion (usually acid)
Radiotherapy (>4,500 rads)
AIDS (*Cryptosporidium* infection) (narrowed antrum + small bowel involvement)
Eosinophilic gastroenteritis (narrowing + wall thickening)
Infection (tuberculosis or syphilis; both are rare)
Crohn disease (rare)
Sarcoidosis (usually asymptomatic)
Extrinsic compression
Pancreatitis
Pancreatic carcinoma
Omental cake

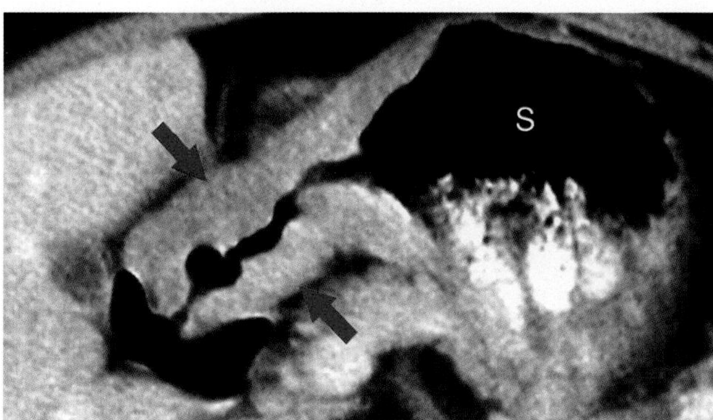

FIGURE 44.6. **Scirrhous Carcinoma—CT.** Axial CT image demonstrates nodular thickening (*arrows*) of the antrum of the stomach (*S*) caused by poorly differentiated gastric adenocarcinoma. The outer margin of the stomach is well defined, giving evidence against extension of tumor through the wall. Note the fixed irregular narrowing of the gastric lumen.

factors for gastric lymphoma include chronic infection with *H. pylori*, Epstein–Barr virus, hepatitis B virus, or *Campylobacter jejuni*, as well as celiac disease, atrophic gastritis, and inflammatory bowel disease. Most (80%) gastric lymphomas are B-cell type especially MALT type, which are more indolent and have a better prognosis than B-cell lymphomas. Because lymphoma remains confined to the bowel wall for prolonged periods of time, it has a better prognosis than carcinoma with 5-year survival in the 62% to 90% range.

Lymphoma demonstrates four morphologic patterns: polypoid solitary mass, ulcerative mass, multiple submucosal nodules (Fig. 44.8), and diffuse infiltration (Fig. 44.9).

UGI findings include the following: (a) polypoid lesions, (b) irregular ulcers with nodular thickened folds, (c) bulky tumors with large cavities, (d) multiple submucosal nodules that commonly ulcerate and create a target or "bull's-eye" appearance, (e) diffuse but pliable wall and fold thickening, and (f) rarely, linitis plastica appearance of diffuse, stiff narrowing

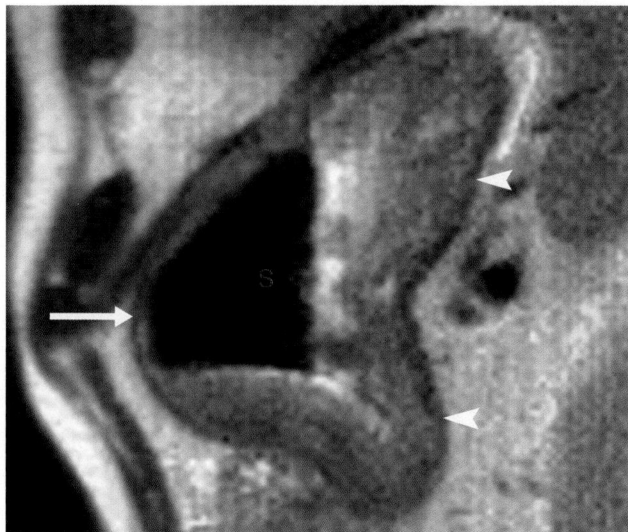

FIGURE 44.7. **Gastric Carcinoma—MR.** Sagittal T2-weighted MR reveals diffuse asymmetric irregular thickening (*arrowheads*) of the gastric wall proven by endoscopic biopsy to be adenocarcinoma. Compare the posterior wall (*arrow*) of the stomach (*S*) to the normal anterior wall (*arrowheads*).

TABLE 44.2

GASTRIC MALIGNANCIES

■ TUMOR	■ IMAGING FEATURES
Gastric adenocarcinoma	Focal wall thickening (>1 cm suggests malignancy) Diffuse wall thickening (linitis plastica) Large mass Ulcerated mass that is predominantly intraluminal Soft tissue stranding from mass into perigastric fat Adenopathy, peritoneal implants, distant metastases
Gastric lymphoma	Marked wall thickening (4–5 cm) Circumferential wall thickening without luminal narrowing Homogeneous attenuation of tumor Multiple polyps with ulceration Extensive adenopathy, especially if below the renal hila Transpyloric tumor spreads to the duodenum
Malignant GIST	Large, heterogeneous exophytic mass (>5 cm) Extensive ulceration of the mass Prominent necrosis, hemorrhage, liquefaction Calcification within the tumor
Metastases to stomach	Wall thickening similar to primary carcinoma Focal intramural mass Ulcerated mural nodule Direct invasion of the stomach from adjacent tumor

(Fig. 44.9). Multiplicity of lesions favors MALT lymphoma as the diagnosis.

CT is the primary imaging modality used to stage lymphoma. CT findings that are helpful in differentiating gastric lymphoma from carcinoma include (a) more marked thickening of the wall (may exceed 3 cm) (Fig. 44.10), (b) involvement of additional areas of the GI tract (transpyloric spread of lymphoma to the duodenum in 30%), (c) absence of invasion

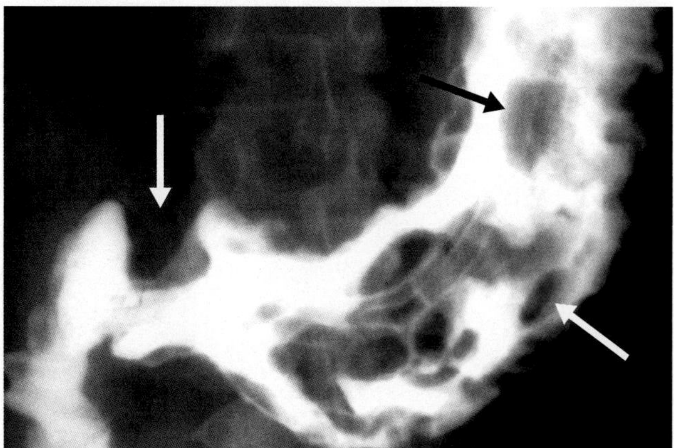

FIGURE 44.8. **Gastric Lymphoma—Multinodular.** UGI series shows multiple smoothly marginated polypoid nodules (*arrows*) of varying size and shape in the stomach. Multiple polypoid nodules may also be seen with gastric carcinoma.

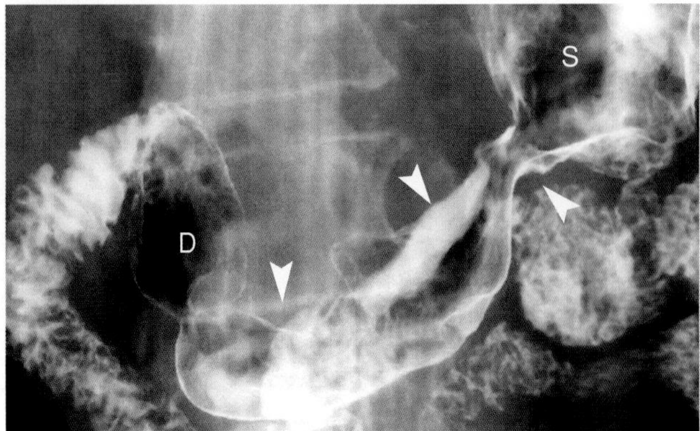

FIGURE 44.9. Gastric Lymphoma—Infiltrating. UGI series reveals striking nodular narrowing of the body and antrum (*arrowheads*) of the stomach (*S*). This linitis plastica appearance is much less common with lymphoma than with adenocarcinoma. *D*, duodenal bulb.

of the perigastric fat, (d) absence of luminal narrowing and obstruction despite extensive involvement, and (e) more widespread and bulkier adenopathy.

Gastrointestinal stromal tumors (GISTs) are the most common mesenchymal tumor to arise from the GI tract. Most, but not all, tumors previously classified as leiomyomas, leiomyosarcomas, and leiomyoblastomas are now classified as GISTs. Approximately 60% to 70% of GISTs arise in the stomach and 10% to 30% of these are malignant. True leiomyomas and leiomyosarcomas are very rare in the stomach.

Long-term silent growth to a large size is characteristic. The overlying mucosa is commonly ulcerated. Dystrophic calcification is relatively common in both benign and malignant tumors and helps differentiate these lesions from other gastric tumors. Histologic differentiation of benign from malignant tumors is difficult; the differentiation is based upon size, gross appearance, and behavior of the tumor. On UGI, GISTs appear as submucosal nodules and masses (Fig. 44.11). Ulceration causes a bull's-eye appearance and may be responsible for significant bleeding (Fig. 44.12).

CT is useful in characterizing the tumors because they are predominantly extraluminal. Benign tumors are smaller (4 to 5 cm, average size), are homogeneous in density, and

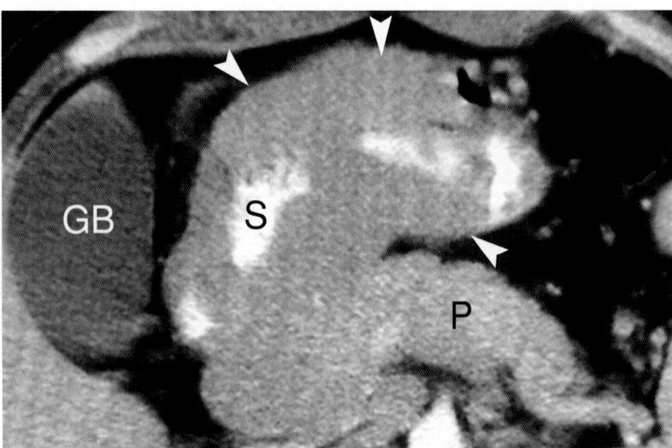

FIGURE 44.10. Gastric Lymphoma—Marked Wall Thickening. CT demonstrates marked thickening (*arrowheads*) of the gastric wall with homogeneous minimally enhancing tumor. The gastric tumor blends into and involves the pancreas (*P*). The lumen of the stomach (*S*) is irregularly narrowed. *GB*, gallbladder.

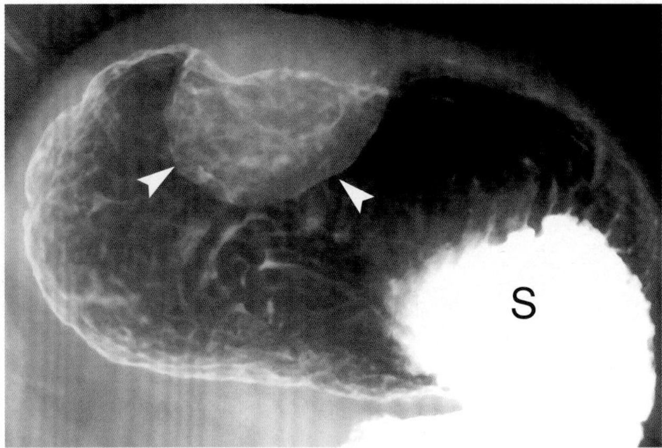

FIGURE 44.11. GI Stromal Tumor. A benign GIST (*arrowheads*) demonstrates the characteristic findings of a submucosal mass on a UGI series. The mass protrudes into the lumen of the stomach (*S*). The surface of the mass is coated with barium and outlined by air in the fundus. The margin of the lesion is very well defined. A significant portion of the tumor extends outside the lumen, better appreciated with CT, MR, or US.

show uniform diffuse enhancement. Malignant tumors tend to be larger (>10 cm) with central zones of low density caused by hemorrhage and necrosis and show irregular patterns of enhancement (Fig. 44.12).

Metastasis may present as submucosal nodules or ulcerated masses (Fig. 44.13). Most are hematogenous metastases. Rich blood supply results in common involvement of the stomach and small bowel. Common primary tumors are melanoma and breast and lung carcinoma. Breast cancer metastases may cause linitis plastica.

Kaposi sarcoma, when disseminated in patients with AIDS, involves the GI tract in 50% of patients. Double-contrast studies demonstrate flat masses with or without ulceration, polypoid masses, irregularly thickened folds, multiple submucosal masses, and linitis plastica. CT demonstrates enhancing adenopathy in the porta hepatis, mesentery, and retroperitoneum. Bleeding is a common symptom and may require embolization.

Villous tumors are adenomatous polypoid masses that produce multiple frond-like projections. Most are solitary and 3 to 9 cm in size although giant tumors may be as large as 15 cm. Malignant potential is high and varies with size of the lesion (50% for 2- to 4-cm lesions, 80% for lesions >4 cm). Barium trapped in the clefts between fronds produces a characteristic soap bubble appearance. The tumors are mobile and deform with compression. All should be treated as malignant lesions.

Polyps are lesions that protrude into the lumen as sessile or pedunculated masses. Their appearance on double-contrast UGI series depends on whether they are on the dependent or nondependent surface. A polyp on the dependent surface appears as a radiolucent filling defect in the barium pool; a polyp on the nondependent surface is covered with a thin coat of barium. The x-ray beam catches its margin in tangent, resulting in a lesion whose margins are etched in white. The *bowler hat sign* is produced by the acute angle of attachment of the polyp to the mucosa. The *Mexican hat sign* consists of two concentric rings and is produced by visualizing a pedunculated polyp end on. Polyps are commonly multiple (Table 44.3).

Hyperplastic polyps account for 80% of gastric polyps. Most are less than 15 mm in diameter. They are not neoplasms, but rather hyperplastic responses to mucosal injury, especially gastritis. They may be located anywhere in the

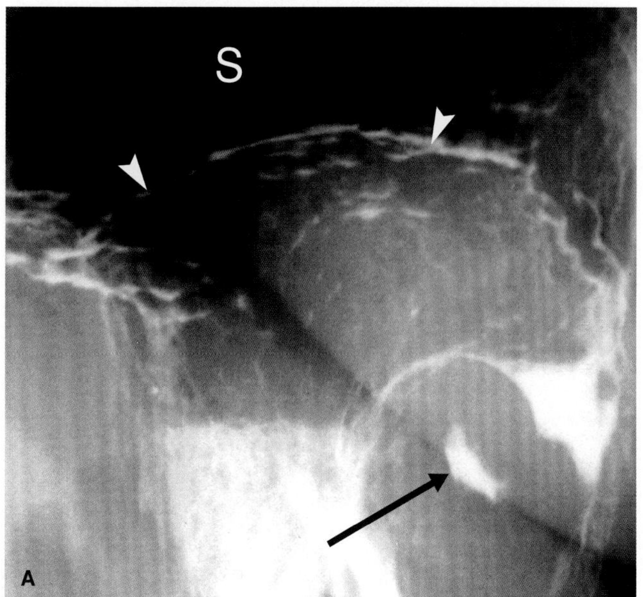

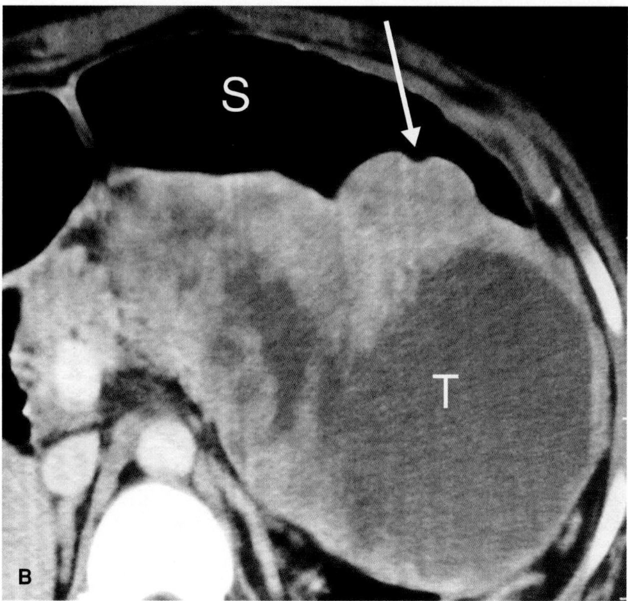

FIGURE 44.12. **Malignant GI Stromal Tumor. A:** Radiograph in lateral upright position from a UGI series demonstrates a huge mass (*arrowheads*) impressing into the lumen of the stomach (*S*). A mound of tumor contains an irregular ulcer (*arrow*) that collects barium within its crater. **B:** CT of the same patient reveals the tumor (*T*) to be heterogeneous with large low attenuation areas representing necrosis. The ulcer (*arrow*) and tumor mound protruding into the lumen of the stomach (*S*) are evident.

stomach, are frequently multiple, have no malignant potential, but are indicative of chronic gastritis.

Adenomatous polyps account for 15% of gastric polyps and are true neoplasms with malignant potential. Most are solitary, located in the antrum, and are larger than 2 cm in diameter. Polyps that are larger than 1 cm, lobulated, or pedunculated should have biopsies taken of them because of the risk of malignancy.

Hamartomatous polyps occur in Peutz–Jeghers syndrome. They have no malignant potential.

Lipomas are submucosal neoplasms composed of mature benign fatty tissue. UGI reveals a smooth well-defined submuscosal lesion that occasionally ulcerates. CT provides a definitive diagnosis by demonstration of a sharply circumscribed wall mass with uniform fat attenuation.

Ectopic pancreas is a common intramural lesion, usually found in the antrum. Lobules of heterotopic pancreatic tissue, up to 5 cm in size, are covered by gastric mucosa. Most are nipple- or cone-shaped with small central orifices.

Bezoar/Foreign Body. The term "bezoar" refers to an intraluminal gastric mass consisting of accumulated undigested material. Bezoars may be composed of a wide variety of substances: trichobezoars are composed of hair (Fig. 44.14); phytobezoars are composed of fruit or vegetable products; pharmacobezoars consist of tablets and semi-solid masses of drugs. Stones may be ingested or form with the bezoar. Any ingested foreign body may produce an intraluminal filling defect.

TABLE 44.3

MULTIPLE GASTRIC FILLING DEFECTS

Hyperplastic polyps
Adenomatous polyps (especially with polyposis syndromes)
Metastases
Lymphoma
Varices

Thickened Gastric Folds/Thickened Wall

Normal gastric folds are thicker and more undulated in the proximal stomach and along the greater curvature. They have a smooth contour and taper distally. Gastric distention causes the folds to become thinner, straighter, and less prominent. Normal rugal folds consist of both mucosa and submucosa and may become thickened by disease processes that infiltrate these layers. Key points:

- Irregular, focal (<5 cm length), asymmetric bowel wall thickening suggests malignancy.

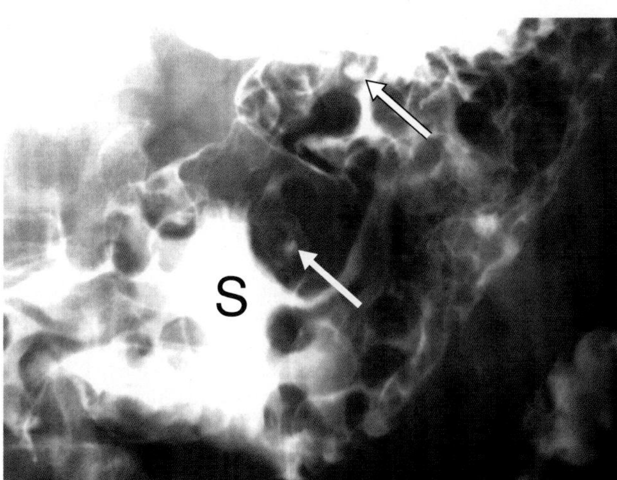

FIGURE 44.13. **Metastases to the Stomach.** Metastases from malignant melanoma produce innumerable polypoid nodules protruding into the stomach (*S*). Some are ulcerated (*arrows*) producing a target appearance.

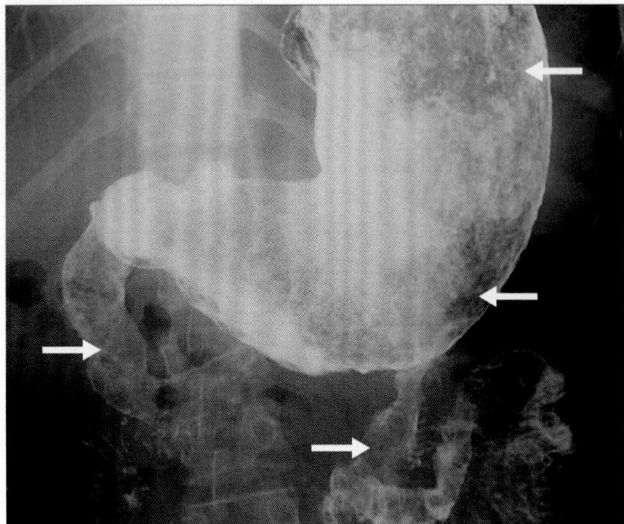

FIGURE 44.14. **Trichobezoar.** Radiograph from an upper GI series performed in an 11-year-old girl with abdominal pain shows a large mottled streaky filling defect (*arrows*) in the stomach extending through the entire duodenum. Surgery confirmed a hairball (trichobezoar) forming a cast of the stomach and duodenum. This young girl had compulsive trichotillomania (hair pulling) and trichophagia (hair swallowing).

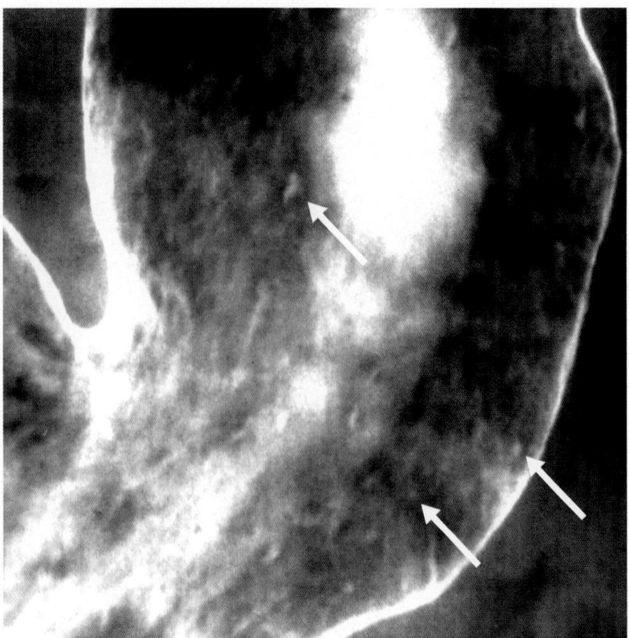

FIGURE 44.15. **Erosive Gastritis—Aphthous Ulcers.** Double-contrast UGI series demonstrates numerous aphthous ulcers (*arrows*) throughout the gastric mucosa. The characteristic appearance of aphthous ulcers is a persistent small collection of barium surrounded by a tiny lucent mound of edema. This patient had a recent heavy intake of alcohol.

- Regular, homogeneous, symmetric bowel wall thickening suggests a benign process.
- Diffuse bowel wall thickening (>6 cm in length) is usually caused by benign inflammatory, ischemic, or infectious diseases.
- Following intravenous contrast administration, bowel wall thickening that shows alternating densities of high and low attenuation (target appearance) is nearly always benign and secondary to inflammation or ischemia. The low-density layer is indicative of bowel wall edema.
- Perigastric fat stranding disproportionally more severe than the degree of wall thickening suggests an inflammatory process.

Gastritis is a convenient label used to describe a wide variety of diseases affecting the gastric mucosa. Most of these diseases are inflammatory. Gastritis is much more common than gastric ulcers. The hallmarks of gastritis are thickened folds and superficial mucosal ulcerations (erosions). The thickened folds are usually caused by mucosal edema and superficial inflammatory infiltrate. *Erosions* are defined as defects in the mucosa that do not penetrate beyond the muscularis mucosae. *Aphthous ulcers* (also called varioliform erosions) are complete erosions that appear as tiny central flecks of barium surrounded by a radiolucent halo of edema (Fig. 44.15). Incomplete erosions appear as linear streaks and dots of barium. Erosions heal without scarring. Barium precipitates may mimic erosions, appearing as distinct punctate barium spots but without the distinctive radiolucent halo of a true erosion. Gastritis is commonly accompanied by duodenitis. CT findings include (a) wall thickening of the distal stomach and duodenum, often with target appearance indicating wall edema, (b) involved mucosa may enhance avidly, and (c) edematous stranding in the perigastric and periduodenal fat.

Helicobacter pylori gastritis is the most common form of gastritis and is the most common cause of thickened gastric folds. Although most people who are infected with *H. pylori* are asymptomatic, most have gastritis endoscopically and pathologically. Almost all patients with benign gastric and duodenal ulcers have *H. pylori* gastritis. UGI findings of *H. pylori* gastritis include (a) thickening (<5 mm) of gastric folds, (b) nodular folds, (c) erosions, (d) antral narrowing, (e) inflammatory polyps, (f) antral narrowing, and (g) enlarged areae gastricae.

Erosive gastritis is most often caused by alcohol, aspirin, and other nonsteroidal anti-inflammatory agents, or steroids. Double-contrast UGI findings include (a) erosions (aphthous ulcers) (Fig. 44.15), (b) thickened, nodular folds in the antrum, (c) limited distensibility of the antrum, and (d) wall stiffness and limited peristalsis.

Crohn gastritis characteristically involves the gastric antrum and proximal duodenum. Early-stage disease manifests as aphthous ulcers identical to those seen with erosive gastritis. More advanced disease shows antral narrowing, wall thickening, and fistulas.

Atrophic gastritis is a chronic autoimmune disease that destroys the fundic mucosa but spares the antral mucosa. Destruction of parietal cells results in decreased acid and intrinsic factor production that lead to vitamin B_{12} deficiency and pernicious anemia. Antibodies to parietal cells and intrinsic factors are found in peripheral blood samples. Characteristic UGI findings are (a) decreased or absent folds in the fundus and body ("bald fundus"), (b) narrowed, tube-shaped stomach (fundal diameter <8 cm), and (c) small (1 to 2 mm) or absent areae gastricae.

Phlegmonous gastritis is an acute, often fatal, bacterial infection of the stomach. α-Hemolytic streptococci are the most common cause, but a variety of other bacteria have also been identified. It may arise as a complication of septicemia, gastric surgery, or gastric ulcers. Multiple abscesses are formed in the gastric wall, which is markedly thickened. The rugae are swollen. Barium may penetrate into abscess crypts in the gastric wall. Peritonitis develops in 70% of cases. Healing usually results in a severely contracted stomach.

Emphysematous gastritis is a form of phlegmonous gastritis caused by gas-producing organisms, usually *Escherichia coli*,

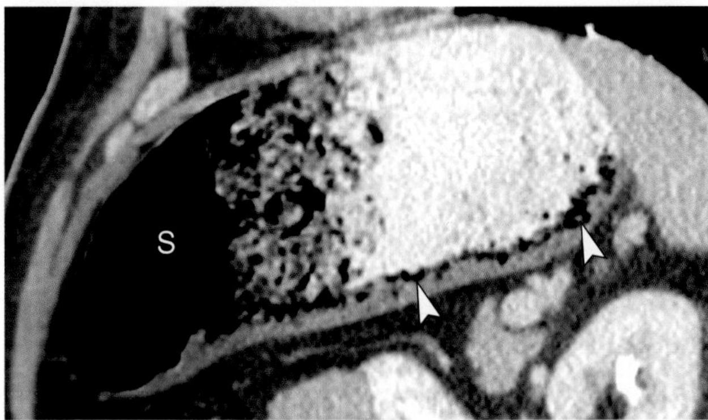

FIGURE 44.16. **Emphysematous Gastritis.** Sagittal CT scan shows numerous air bubbles (*arrowheads*) in the submucosal layer of the wall of the stomach (*S*), which is distended by air and oral contrast media.

Clostridium welchii, or mixed infections with *Staphylococcus aureus.* Most cases are caused by caustic ingestion, alcohol abuse, surgery, trauma, or ischemia. Multiple gas bubbles are apparent within the wall of the stomach (Fig. 44.16). Gastric folds are thickened and edematous.

Eosinophilic gastroenteritis is a rare disease characterized by diffuse infiltration of the wall of the stomach and small bowel by eosinophils. Any or all layers of the wall may be involved. The condition is associated with a peripheral eosinophilia as high as 60%. Initially, the folds are markedly thickened and nodular, especially in the antrum. When chronic, the antrum is narrowed with a nodular "cobblestone" mucosal pattern. Ascites and pleural effusions may be present.

Ménétrier disease, also called giant hypertrophic gastritis, is a rare condition characterized by excessive mucus production, giant rugal hypertrophy, hypoproteinemia, and hypochlorhydria. Pathologically patients have mucosa thickened by hyperplasia of epithelial cells. UGI findings include (a) markedly enlarged (>10 mm in the fundus) and tortuous but pliable folds in the fundus and body, especially along the greater curvature, with sparing of the antrum, and (b) hypersecretion that has diluted the barium and impaired mucosal coating. CT demonstrates nodular markedly thickened folds (Fig. 44.17) with smooth serosal surface and normal gastric wall thickness between folds.

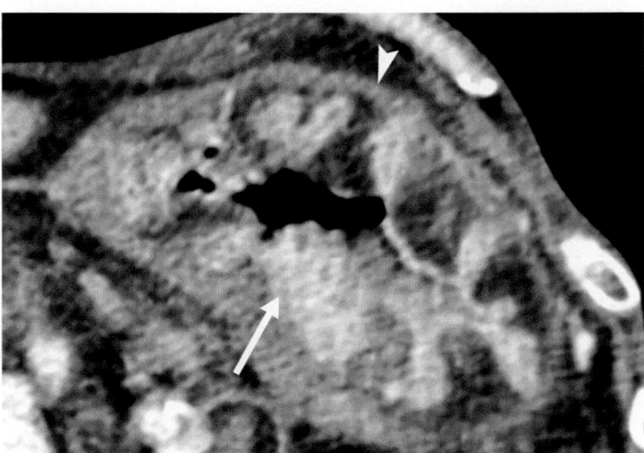

FIGURE 44.17. **Ménétrier Disease.** Axial plane postcontrast CT reveals marked thickening of the mucosal folds (*arrow*) in the stomach. The thickened folds are heterogeneous with enhancing areas and fat density. The thickness of the muscular portions (*arrowhead*) of the stomach wall is normal in some areas.

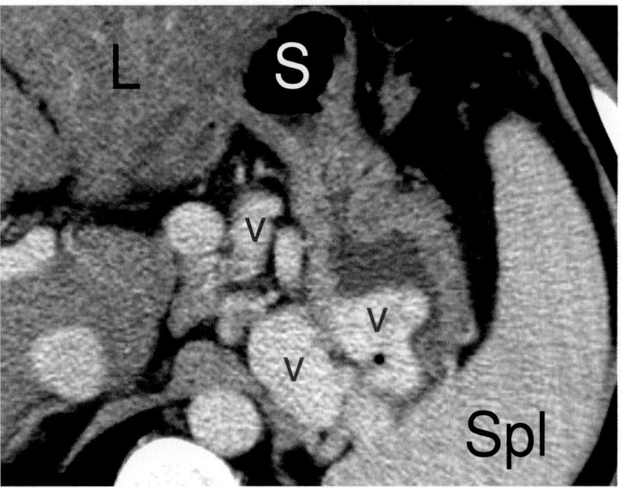

FIGURE 44.18. **Gastric Varices.** Helical CT with bolus intravenous contrast reveals enhancing varices (*v*) outside the stomach (*S*) in the gastrohepatic ligament and protruding into the gastric lumen. The liver (*L*) is nodular in contour indicating the presence of cirrhosis. The spleen (*Spl*) is enlarged providing further evidence of portal hypertension.

Varices appear as smooth, lobulated filling defects resembling thickened folds. They are most common in the fundus and usually accompany esophageal varices. Isolated gastric varices occur with splenic vein occlusion. MDCT with bolus contrast enhancement is an excellent method for confirming the presence of gastric varices as well as demonstrating their cause (Fig. 44.18). CT shows well-defined clusters of rounded and tubular enhancing vessels. Additional findings of portal hypertension may be evident.

Neoplasm. Lymphoma and superficial spreading gastric carcinoma may produce distorted rigid gastric folds that are commonly ulcerated and appear nodular. The distal stomach is the most common location for neoplasms.

Gastric Ulcers

An ulcer is defined as a full-thickness defect in the mucosa. It frequently extends to the deeper layers of the stomach, including the submucosa and muscularis propria. About 95% of ulcerating gastric lesions are benign. Gastroduodenal endoscopy is the diagnostic method of choice. However, it is invasive, not available everywhere, and often cannot be performed in urgent situations.

Signs of an ulcer as demonstrated by a double-contrast UGI series include (a) a barium-filled crater on the dependent wall (Fig. 44.19), (b) a ring shadow caused by barium coating the edge of the crater on the nondependent wall, (c) a double ring shadow if the base of the ulcer is broader than the neck, and (d) a crescentic or semilunar line when the ulcer is seen on tangent oblique view. Some ulcers may be linear or rod-shaped. Ulcers are multiple in about 20% of patients. Careful assessment of radiographic findings allows differentiation of benign from malignant ulcers on double-contrast barium studies.

Peptic Ulcer Disease. Benign gastric ulcers are caused by *H. pylori* infection and by chronic use of nonsteroidal anti-inflammatory medications. The effects of the two conditions are additive for development of peptic disease. Alcohol and smoking are other exacerbating factors. Duodenal ulcers are usually associated with increased production of acid. Gastric ulcers occur with normal or even decreased acid levels. However, hydrochloric

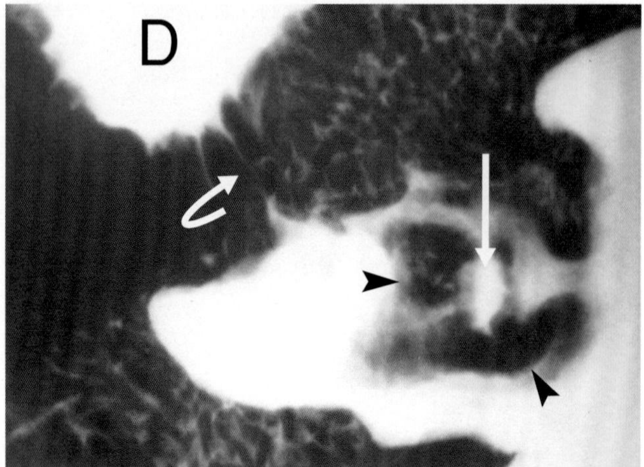

FIGURE 44.19. **Benign Gastric Ulcer.** Spot radiograph from a UGI demonstrates a benign gastric ulcer (*arrow*) in the antrum. Prominent, nodular folds (*arrowheads*) surround the ulcer crater. The normal contracted pyloric channel (*curved arrow*) is seen as a thin line of barium. *D*, normal distended duodenal bulb.

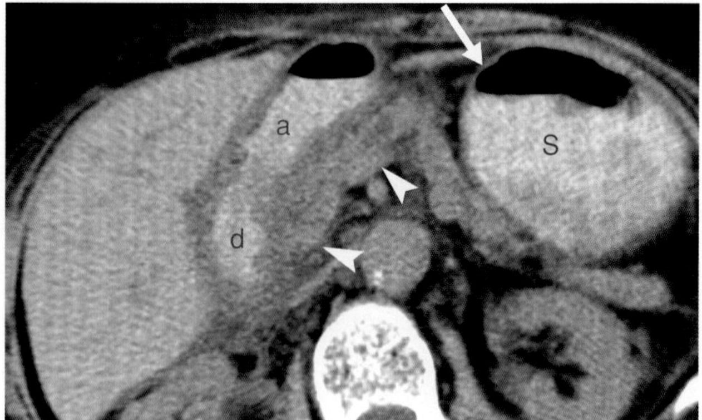

FIGURE 44.20. **Erosive Gastroduodenitis.** CT performed without intravenous contrast marked thickening (*arrowheads*) of the wall of the gastric antrum (*a*) and duodenum (*d*). Edema extends into periduodenal and periantral fat and adjacent tissue. The remainder of the stomach (*S*) is normal in appearance with a thin wall (*arrow*). Endoscopy showed numerous mucosal erosions in the antrum and duodenum.

acid must be present for peptic ulceration to occur. Patients usually present with aching or burning pain within several hours after eating. Some patients with ulcers may be asymptomatic. The major complications of peptic ulcer disease are bleeding, obstruction, and perforation. Bleeding occurs in 15% to 20% of patients and is manifest by melena, hematemesis, or hematochezia. Gastric outlet obstruction complicates approximately 5% of cases. Ulcers may perforate into the free abdominal cavity or penetrate into adjacent organs. Free perforations usually present with an acute abdomen. Ulcer penetration into an adjacent organ is usually heralded by a marked increase in abdominal pain.

Benign Ulcers. Most (95%) gastric ulcers currently diagnosed in the United States are benign. The hallmark of benign ulcers and the basis for most radiographic signs of benignancy is mucosa that is intact to the very edge of an undermining ulcer crater. About two-thirds of all gastric ulcers evaluated on double-contrast barium studies can be unequivocally diagnosed as benign. Demonstration of complete and sustained healing is reliable radiographic evidence of benign ulcer. Signs of benignancy include (a) a smooth ulcer mound with tapering edges, (b) an edematous ulcer collar with overhanging mucosal edge (Fig. 44.19), (c) an ulcer projecting beyond the expected lumen, (d) radiating folds extending into the crater, (e) depth of ulcer greater than width, (f) sharply marginated contour, and (g) Hampton line (a thin, sharp, lucent line that traverses the orifice of the ulcer). Hampton line, best demonstrated on spot films obtained with compression, is caused by an overhanging gastric mucosa in an undermined ulcer. CT shows (a) wall thickening usually involving both the antrum and duodenum, (b) edema and edematous stranding extending into periantral and periduodenal fat or involving adjacent organs (Fig. 44.20), and (c) deep ulcers that may show focal discontinuity of mucosal enhancement and/or outpouching of the lumen.

The size, depth, and location of the ulcer, and the contour of the ulcer base are of no diagnostic value in differentiating benign from malignant ulcers. The differential diagnosis of benign ulcer includes *H. pylori* peptic disease, gastritis, hyperparathyroidism, radiotherapy, and Zollinger–Ellison syndrome.

Malignant ulcers demonstrate signs that are the antithesis of benign ulcers. About 5% of gastric ulcers can be diagnosed as unequivocally malignant on UGI. Evidence of irregular tumor mass or infiltration of the surrounding mucosa is evidence of malignancy. Signs of malignancy include (a) an ulcer within the lumen of the stomach, (b) an ulcer eccentrically located within the tumor mound, (c) a shallow ulcer with a width greater than its depth, (d) nodular, rolled, irregular, or shouldered edges, and (e) Carmen meniscus sign (describes a large flat-based ulcer with heaped-up edges that fold inward to trap a lens-shaped barium collection that is convex toward the lumen) (Fig. 44.21). The differential diagnosis of malignant ulcer includes gastric adenocarcinoma, lymphoma, leiomyoma, and leiomyosarcoma.

Equivocal ulcers have indeterminate radiographic findings. While most are benign, endoscopy and biopsy are required. Equivocal ulcers may show the following findings: (a) coarse areae gastricae abutting the ulcer; (b) nodular ulcer collar; and (c) mildly irregular folds extending to the ulcer edge. CT is useful in demonstrating the extent of the tumor mass and the degree of involvement of the gastric wall.

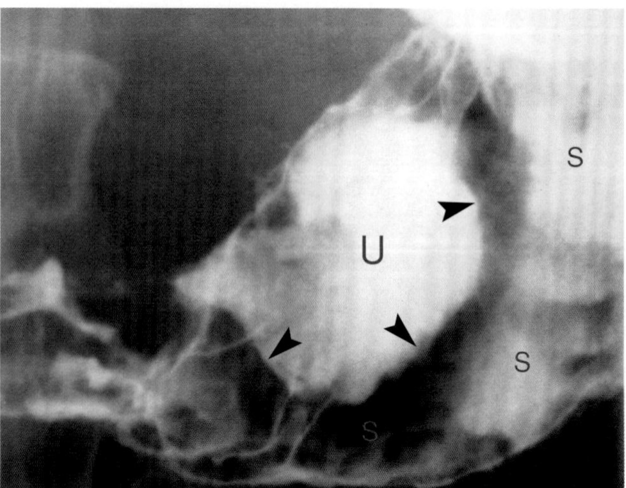

FIGURE 44.21. **Malignant Gastric Ulcer—Carmen Meniscus Sign.** A large, flat malignant ulcer (*U*) traps barium within its rounded edges, seen as a band of lucency (*arrowheads*) surrounding the barium collection. The barium collection is convex toward the lumen (*S*) of the stomach.

DUODENUM

Duodenal Mass Lesions/Filling Defects

In the duodenal bulb, 90% of tumors are benign. In the second and third portions of the duodenum, tumors are 50% benign and 50% malignant. In the fourth portion of the duodenum, most tumors are malignant. Small, benign tumors of the duodenum usually present as smooth, polypoid filling defects. CT is helpful, but not specific, in predicting malignancy. Biopsy is required. Signs of malignancy include the following: (a) central necrosis, (b) ulceration or excavation, (c) exophytic or intramural mass, and (d) evidence of tumor beyond the duodenum.

Duodenal adenocarcinoma, although being the most frequent malignant tumor of the duodenum, is a rare lesion (1.5% of GI neoplasms). Malignant tumors are most common in the periampullary region and are rare in the bulb. Morphologic patterns include polypoid mass, ulcerative mass, and annular constricting lesion. Metastases to regional lymph nodes are present in two-thirds of patients at presentation. CT and MR demonstrate an enhancing intramural or exophytic soft tissue mass with frequently a bilobed "dumbbell" shape. Central necrosis and ulceration occur. Regional adenopathy, hepatic metastases, and local extent of tumor are demonstrated for surgical planning (Fig. 44.22).

Metastases to the duodenum may occur in the wall or subserosa of the duodenum presenting with wall thickening (Fig. 44.23). As the tumor grows, it may extend into the lumen and present as an intraluminal mass that may ulcerate. The most common primaries are breast, lung, and other GI malignancies. The duodenum may be invaded by tumors of adjacent organs including the pancreas and kidney.

Lymphoma in the duodenum usually presents as nodules with thickened folds. The nodules associated with lymphoma are distinctly larger than those seen with benign lymphoid hyperplasia.

Duodenal adenoma presents as a polypoid lesion that may be pedunculated or sessile. Adenomas account for about half of the neoplasms of the duodenum. Multiple adenomatous polyps are associated with polyposis syndromes. Villous adenomas have a high incidence of malignant degeneration and a characteristic "cauliflower" appearance on double-contrast UGI series.

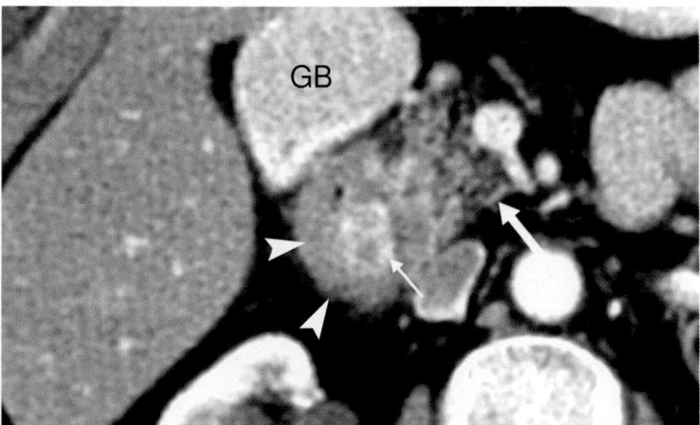

FIGURE 44.22. **Adenocarcinoma Duodenum.** CT following administration of oral and intravenous contrast shows a circumferential tumor (*arrowheads*) arising in the second portion of the duodenum constricting the lumen (*skinny arrow*). Subtle stranding extending from the tumor into the periduodenal fat suggests tumor extension, confirmed at surgery. The tumor also invades the pancreas (*fat arrow*). *GB*, gallbladder.

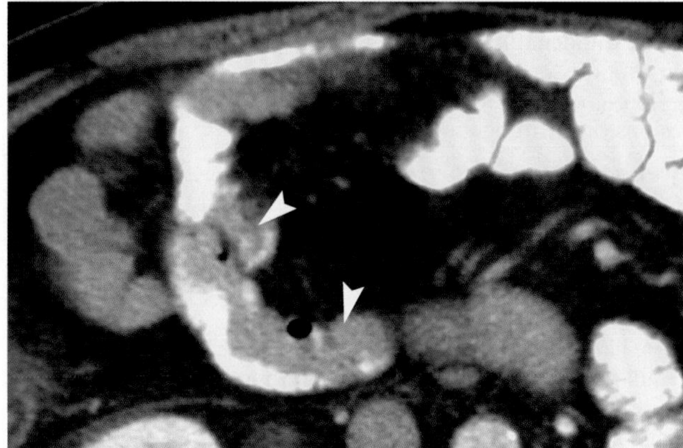

FIGURE 44.23. **Metastasis to Duodenum.** Axial image from MDCT shows asymmetric wall thickening (*arrowheads*) of the second and third portions of the duodenum. Endoscopy confirms metastatic renal cell carcinoma.

GISTs of the duodenum present as an intramural, endoluminal, or exophytic mass, most commonly in the second or third portion of the duodenum (Fig. 44.24). Ulceration is common. Malignant tumors range up to 20 cm size and are most common in the more distal duodenum. Malignant GISTs are the second most common primary malignant tumor of the duodenum.

Lipoma of the duodenum is a soft tumor that may grow to a large size. A definitive diagnosis can be made by CT or MR demonstration of a uniform fat density mass.

Lymphoid hyperplasia presents as small (1 to 3 mm) polypoid nodules diffusely throughout the duodenum. The condition is usually benign, especially in children. It is associated with immunodeficiency states in some adults. No evidence supports the concept that lymphoid hyperplasia is a precursor to lymphoma.

Gastric mucosal prolapse/heterotopic gastric mucosa. Gastric mucosa may prolapse through the pylorus during peristalsis and cause a lobulated mass at the base of the duodenal bulb. The diagnosis is suggested by characteristic location and change in configuration with peristalsis, which may be observed on UGI. Heterotopic gastric mucosa in the duodenal bulb is common on endoscopy (12%) but seen infrequently

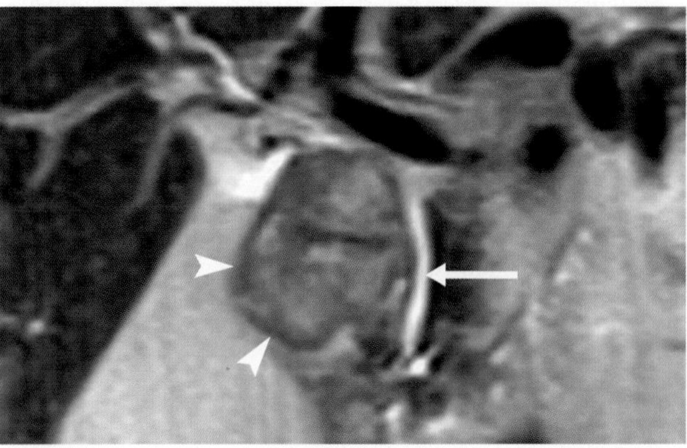

FIGURE 44.24. **Gastrointestinal Stromal Tumor—Duodenum.** Coronal T2-weighted MR shows a large rounded mass (*arrowheads*) arising in the descending duodenum displacing and bowing the common bile duct (*arrow*). Most tumors of the duodenum are not discovered until they are large enough to produce symptoms.

on imaging. The lesion has the appearance of areae gastricae in the duodenal bulb, or as clusters of 1- to 3-mm plaques on the smooth duodenal bulb mucosa. It may also appear as a solitary polyp that is indistinguishable from other polypoid lesions of the duodenum.

Brunner gland hyperplasia/hamartoma. Brunner glands are located in the submucosa of the proximal two-thirds of the duodenum and secrete an alkaline substance that buffers gastric acid. Nomenclature is confusing in the literature. Lesions, usually multiple and smaller than 5 mm, are termed hyperplasia. Lesions larger than 5 mm are termed hamartomas. Larger lesions are more likely to be symptomatic. All lesions are benign and without cellular atypia. Diffuse nodular gland hyperplasia is a common cause of multiple nodules, often with a cobblestone appearance. Brunner gland hamartoma usually presents as a solitary nodule and is identical in appearance to other benign duodenal nodules. CT shows well-defined enhancing nodules. Because Brunner glands are located deep in the wall of the duodenum they may be overlooked on endoscopy.

Ectopic pancreas may also occur in the duodenum, most commonly in the proximal descending portion. A solitary mass with a central dimple is most characteristic.

Extrinsic mass impressions on the duodenum may be made by the gallbladder; masses in the liver, pancreas, adrenal gland, kidney, or colon; pancreatic fluid collections; adenopathy; or aneurysms.

Thickened Duodenal Folds

The valvulae conniventes, or Kerckring folds, of the small bowel begin in the second portion of the duodenum and continue throughout the remainder of the small bowel. The valvulae conniventes are permanent circular folds of mucosa supported by a core of fibrovascular submucosa. They are normally several millimeters wide and remain visible even with full distention of the duodenum. Folds greater than 2 to 3 mm wide are usually considered thickened.

Normal Variant. Thickened folds are a nonspecific radiographic finding that may be found in normal individuals. The radiographic diagnosis of a pathologic condition is more confident when there are additional findings.

Duodenitis refers to inflammation of the duodenum without discrete ulcer formation. The major cause of duodenitis is *H. pylori* infection. Alcohol and anti-inflammatory medications are additional causes. UGI findings include (a) thickening (>4 mm) of the proximal duodenal folds, (b) nodules or nodular folds (enlarged Brunner glands), (c) deformity of the duodenal bulb, and (d) erosions. CT shows nonspecific wall thickening and inflammatory changes (Fig. 44.25).

Pancreatitis and cholecystitis thicken the duodenal folds by paraduodenal inflammation. Both may also cause mass impressions on the duodenal lumen. CT or US demonstrates the extent and nature of the paraduodenal process.

Crohn disease of the duodenum usually involves the first and second portions and is almost always associated with contiguous involvement of the stomach. Duodenal involvement is manifest by thickened folds, aphthous ulcers, erosions, and single or multiple strictures.

Parasites. Giardiasis is caused by an overgrowth of the parasite *Giardia lamblia* in the duodenum and jejunum. Many patients are asymptomatic carriers, but patients with invasion of the gut wall have abdominal pain, diarrhea, and malabsorption. Giardiasis is a frequent cause of traveler's diarrhea. Imaging findings include (a) distorted thickened folds in the duodenum and jejunum, (b) hypermotility and spasm, and (c) increased secretions. Strongyloidiasis is caused by infection with the nematode,

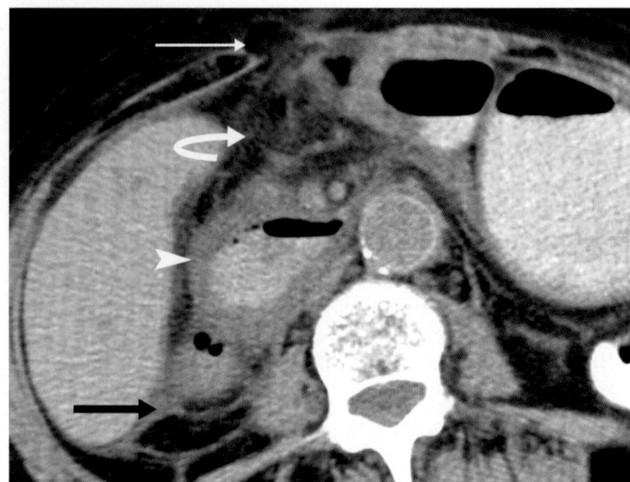

FIGURE 44.25. Erosive Duodenitis. Axial CT shows marked diffuse circumferential thickening of the wall of the duodenum (*arrowhead*). The inflammatory process extends posteriorly into the retroperitoneum (*fat arrow*) and anteriorly (*curved arrow*) into the periduodenal and perigastric fat, even extending into a fat-containing incisional hernia (*skinny arrow*). Endoscopy revealed erosive gastroduodenitis.

Strongyloides stercoralis, found in all areas of the world but most common in the warm, moist regions of the tropics. As with giardiasis, many patients are asymptomatic carriers. Invasion of the intestinal wall causes vomiting and malabsorption. The UGI findings include edematous folds, spasm, dilation of the proximal duodenum, and diffuse mucosal ulceration.

Lymphoma presents with nodular thickened folds.

Intramural hemorrhage is caused by trauma, anticoagulation, and bleeding disorders. The regular pattern of thickened folds resembles a stack of coins. Partial or complete duodenal obstruction is usually present. Mural hematomas may result in a large mass (Fig. 44.26). The fixed retroperitoneal position of the third portion of the duodenum makes it susceptible to blunt abdominal trauma and compression against the lumbar spine.

Duodenal Ulcers and Diverticuli

Duodenal ulcers are caused by *H. pylori* infection in 95% of cases. Additional causes include anti-inflammatory

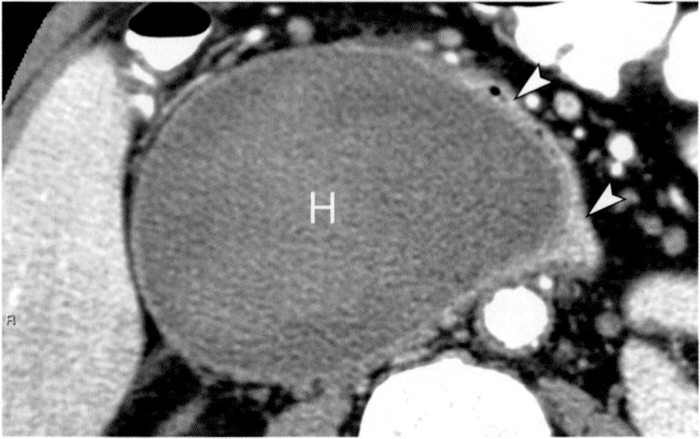

FIGURE 44.26. Duodenal Hematoma. Postintravenous contrast CT following blunt trauma to the abdomen reveals a large hematoma (*H*) in the wall of the duodenum displacing the duodenum (*arrowheads*) and compressing the lumen. Blunt trauma to the abdomen compresses the duodenum against the spine often resulting in hemorrhage.

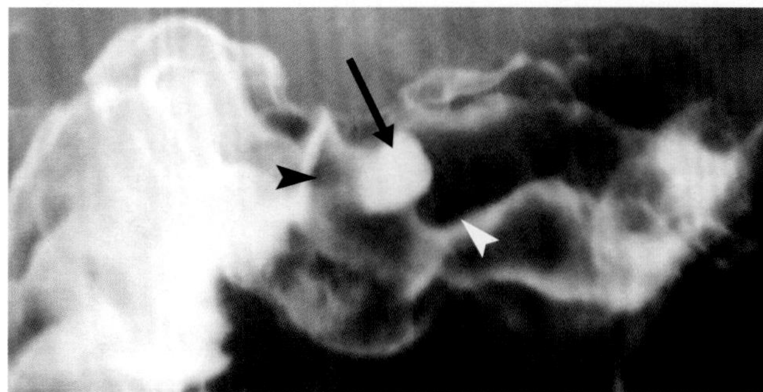

FIGURE 44.27. **Peptic Ulcer—Duodenum.** An upper GI series demonstrates a persistent barium collection (*arrow*) in the duodenal bulb. A well-defined ulcer collar (*arrowheads*) formed by mounds of edema is present.

medications, Crohn disease, Zollinger–Ellison syndrome, viral infections, or penetrating pancreatic cancer. Duodenal ulcers are associated with acid hypersecretion. Most (95%) are in the duodenal bulb with the anterior wall being most often involved. Imaging diagnosis of a duodenal ulcer depends upon demonstration of the ulcer crater or niche (Fig. 44.27). En face, the crater appears as a persistent collection of barium or air. In profile, ulcers project beyond the normal lumen. Thickened folds often radiate toward the ulcer crater, which may be surrounded by a mound of edema. Although the shape is usually round or oval, linear ulcers also occur. Most duodenal ulcers are smaller than 1-cm diameter. Giant ulcers larger than 2 cm resemble diverticuli or a deformed bulb. Ulcer craters have no mucosal lining and therefore no mucosal relief pattern, and do not contract with peristalsis. Ulcer scarring may cause a pattern of radiating folds with a central barium collection that is indistinguishable from an acute ulcer. Endoscopy may be required to make the differentiation. Postbulbar ulcers represent about 5% of the total, but are more commonly associated with serious upper GI hemorrhage. Most involve the second and third portions of the duodenum, which are frequently narrowed. Complications of duodenal ulcer disease include obstruction, bleeding, and perforation. Bleeding from a duodenal ulcer is most efficiently diagnosed endoscopically. Perforation may be manifest by pneumoperitoneum or a localized retroperitoneal gas collection. Peptic duodenal ulcer is not a premalignant condition.

Zollinger–Ellison syndrome is caused by a gastrin-secreting neuroendocrine tumor (gastrinoma). Gastrinomas are found

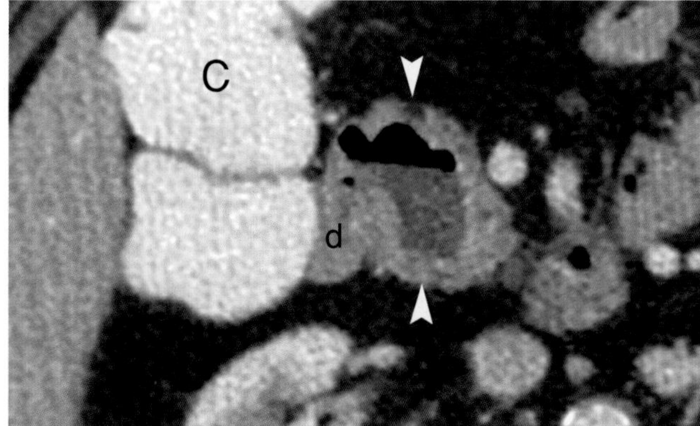

FIGURE 44.28. **Duodenal Diverticulum.** Axial CT shows fluid and gas filling a duodenal diverticulum (*arrowheads*) extending from the second portion of the duodenum (*d*). The hepatic flexure of the colon (C) is filled with orally administered contrast media.

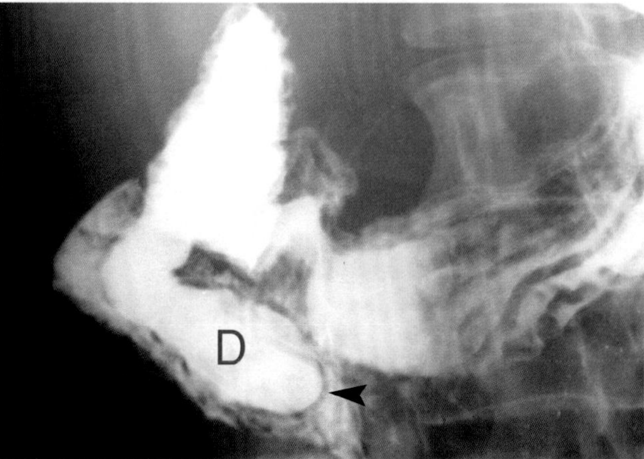

FIGURE 44.29. **Intraluminal Duodenal Diverticulum.** A UGI series demonstrates a barium-filled "sock" (*D*) within the lumen of the descending duodenum. The radiolucent wall of the diverticulum (*arrowhead*) is outlined by barium, both within the diverticulum and within the lumen of the duodenum.

in the pancreas (75%), duodenum (15%), and in 10% in extraintestinal sites (liver, lymph nodes, and ovary). The tumor is malignant in 60% of cases. Gastrinomas also occur as part of the hereditary syndrome of multiple endocrine neoplasia, type I (MEN-I). Continuous gastrin secretion results in marked hyperacidity and multiple peptic ulcers in the duodenum, stomach, and jejunum. UGI studies show pathognomonic findings of (a) multiple peptic ulcers in the stomach, duodenal bulb, and, most characteristically, in the postbulbar duodenum; (b) hypersecretion with high-volume gastric fluid diluting the barium and impairing mucosal coating; and (c) thick edematous folds in the stomach, duodenum, and proximal jejunum.

Duodenal diverticula are common and usually incidental findings. They may be multiple and may form in any portion of the duodenum, but are most common along the inner aspect of the descending duodenum (Fig. 44.28). Diverticula are differentiated from ulcers on a UGI series by demonstration of mucosal folds entering the neck of the diverticulum and change in appearance with peristalsis. On conventional abdominal radiographs, duodenal diverticuli may be seen as abnormal air collections. On CT they may be filled with fluid and mimic a pancreatic pseudocyst, or they may contain air and fluid and mimic a pancreatic abscess. Rare complications include perforation and hemorrhage. Diverticuli adjacent to the ampulla of Vater may rarely obstruct the common bile duct or pancreatic duct.

Intraluminal diverticula are caused by a thin, incomplete, congenital diaphragm that is stretched by moving intraluminal contents to form a "windsock" configuration within the duodenum (Fig. 44.29). The diverticulum is partially obstructing eventually resulting in postprandial epigastric pain and fullness. Some patients present with vomiting or GI bleeding.

Duodenal Narrowing

Annular pancreas is the most common congenital anomaly of the pancreas. Pancreatic tissue encircles the descending duodenum and narrows its lumen (Fig. 44.30). The abnormality occurs when the bilobed ventral component of the pancreas fuses with the dorsal pancreas on both sides of the duodenum. Although it often presents in childhood, especially in children with Down syndrome, about half of the cases do not present until adulthood. Symptomatic adults present with

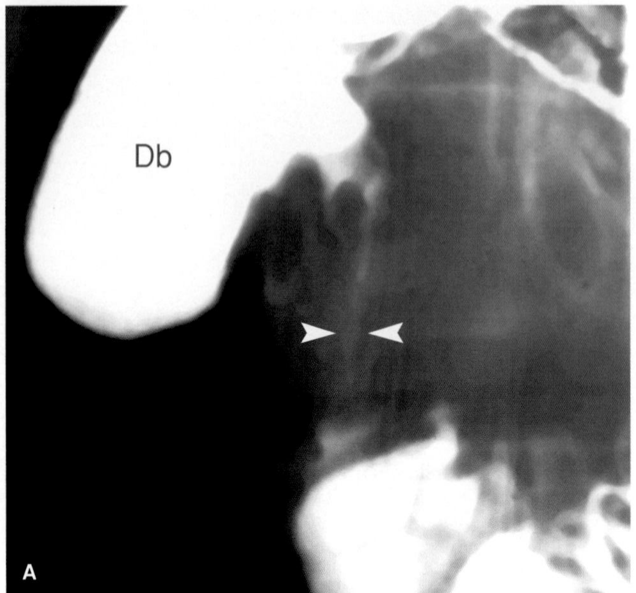

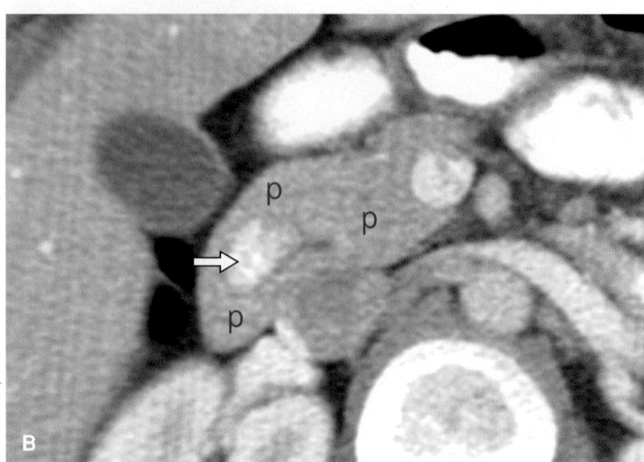

FIGURE 44.30. **Annular Pancreas. A:** Radiograph from an upper GI series demonstrates a 3-cm long circumferentially narrowed segment (*arrowheads*) of the descending duodenum. No ulceration was evident. *Db*, duodenal bulb. **B:** CT of a different patient shows pancreatic tissue (*p*) encircling the descending duodenum and constricting its lumen (*arrow*).

nausea, vomiting, abdominal pain, and occasionally jaundice. The UGI series typically demonstrates eccentric or concentric narrowing of the descending duodenum. Annular pancreas is associated with a high incidence of postbulbar peptic ulceration in adults. CT confirms the diagnosis by demonstration of pancreatic tissue encircling the duodenum. Endoscopic retrograde cholangiopancreatography demonstrates an annular pancreatic duct encircling the duodenum.

Duodenal adenocarcinoma can present as a circumferential constricting lesion with tumor shoulders giving evidence of mass effect. Ulceration is common. CT demonstrates the extent of the lesion.

Pancreatic carcinoma may also encircle and obstruct the pancreas. Jaundice with dilation of the bile and pancreatic ducts are usually present.

Lymphoma causes marked wall thickening and bulky paraduodenal lymphadenopathy that may narrow the lumen.

Postbulbar ulcer is commonly associated with narrowing of the lumen of the second and third portions of the duodenum.

Extrinsic compression, because of inflammation or tumor in adjacent organs, especially the pancreas, may constrict the duodenal lumen.

Upper Gastrointestinal Hemorrhage

UGI hemorrhage refers to bleeding with the site of origin proximal to the ligament of Treitz. This hemorrhage has an average mortality of 8% to 10%. Causes in an approximate order of frequency are (a) duodenal ulcer, (b) esophageal varices, (c) gastric ulcer, (d) acute hemorrhagic gastritis, (e) esophagitis, (f) Mallory–Weiss tear, (g) neoplasm, (h) vascular malformation, and (i) vascular enteric fistula.

Barium studies should be avoided in patients in the acute stages of UGI hemorrhage. Endoscopy is much more accurate than a UGI series in demonstrating the bleeding site (95% vs. 45%). The UGI series may identify a lesion but does not indicate whether that lesion is responsible for the bleeding. Also, retained barium in the GI tract following a UGI series will usually make performing angiography impossible. MDCT angiography may show the bleeding site as a focus of contrast extravasation. MDCT performed in the setting of UGI bleeding should be performed with intravenous contrast only. Oral contrast may obscure the bleeding site. Conventional angiography is used to localize active bleeding sites and provide therapy by infusion of vasoconstrictors or performance of transcatheter embolization.

Suggested Readings

Cai PQ, Lv XF, Tian L, et al. CT characterization of duodenal gastrointestinal stromal tumors. *AJR Am J Roentgenol* 2015;204:988–993.

Carbo AI, Sangster GP, Caraway J, Heldmann MG, Thomas J, Takalkar A. Acquired constricting and restricting lesions of the descending duodenum. *Radiographics* 2014;34:1196–1217.

Cloyd JM, George E, Visser BC. Duodenal adenocarcinoma: advances in diagnosis and surgical management. *World J Gastrointest Surg* 2016;8:212–221.

Fernandes T, Oliviera MI, Castro R, Araújo B, Viamonte B, Cunha R. Bowel wall thickening at CT: simplifying the diagnosis. *Insights Imaging* 2014;5:195–208. (Pictorial review).

Guniganti P, Bradenham CH, Raptis C, Menias CO, Mellnick VM. CT of gastric emergencies. *Radiographics* 2015;35:1909–1921.

Kim JH, Eun HW, Goo DE, Shim CS, Auh YH. Imaging of various gastric lesions with 2D MPR and CT gastrography performed with multidetector CT. *Radiographics* 2006;26:1101–1118.

McNeeley MF, Lalwani N, Dhakshina MG, et al. Multimodality imaging of diseases of the duodenum. *Abdom Imaging* 2014;39:1330–1349.

Rakita D, Hines JJ, Davidoff S, Sideridis K, Yacobozzi M, Friedman B. CT imaging of endoscopy-confirmed gastric pathology. *Appl Radiol* 2014: 18–28.

Re GL, Federica V, Midiri F, et al. Radiological features of gastrointestinal lymphoma. *Gastroenterol Res Pract* 2016;2016:1–9. (Review article) http://dx.doi.org/10.1155/2016/2498143

Sheybani A, Menias CO, Luna A, et al. MRI of the stomach: a pictorial review with focus on oncologic applications and gastric motility. *Abdom Imaging* 2015;40:907–930.

Tonolini M, Ierardi AM, Bracchi E, Magistrelli P, Vella A, Carrafiello G. Non-perforated peptic ulcer disease: multidetector CT findings, complications, and differential diagnosis. *Insights Imaging* 2017;8:455–469. (Pictorial review).

CHAPTER 45 ■ MESENTERIC SMALL BOWEL

WILLIAM E. BRANT

IMAGING METHODS

Disease of the mesenteric small intestine is relatively rare. Detailed radiographic study of the small bowel is justified only when clinical suspicion of small bowel disease is high. Small bowel disease is usually manifest by four major symptoms: colic, diarrhea, malabsorption, and bleeding. Colic is defined as recurrent and spasmodic abdominal pain with periods of relief every 2 to 3 minutes. Diarrhea caused by small bowel disease is less urgent than that caused by colon disease. Malabsorption is manifest by steatorrhea, foul-smelling stools, and weight loss. Bleeding from small bowel disease is usually occult and manifest by anemia. The majority of the mesenteric small intestine is out of traditional reach of the endoscopist, giving diagnostic radiology a primary role in its evaluation. The development of capsule endoscopy provides a limited but safe and well-accepted method for small bowel endoscopy. Traditional fluoroscopic methods of small bowel evaluation are being supplemented and replaced by CT and MR enteroclysis and enterography. Fluoroscopic methods are limited to evaluation of the lumen of the small bowel while the cross-sectional methods of CT and MR provide added information about the wall of the small bowel, its mesentery, and adjacent structures and tissues.

Small bowel follow-through (SBFT) is the traditional method (Fig. 45.1) for radiographic examination of the small bowel tacked onto a standard upper GI series. The patient is asked to continue drinking barium while a series of supine abdominal films are obtained until the terminal ileum and cecum are filled with barium. Fluoroscopic examination of the small bowel is then performed. This study is notoriously insensitive. It is limited by overlap of bowel loops, poor distention, flocculation of barium, intermittent barium filling, and unpredictable transit time. Visualization of the distal ileum may be improved with a double-contrast technique by insufflating the colon with air (SBFT with peroral pneumocolon).

Fluoroscopic enteroclysis, or the small bowel enema, is a more sensitive fluoroscopic method for detailed small bowel examination (Fig. 45.2). This study provides more uniform distention of the bowel, even distribution of barium, superior anatomic detail, and shorter overall examination time. The study is performed by passing a specially designed 12- to 14-Fr enteroclysis catheter through the mouth or nose and into the distal duodenum or proximal jejunum. A guidewire is used for directional control of the catheter during manipulation under fluoroscopy. The study may be performed single contrast using approximately 600 mL of barium or double contrast using 200 mL of barium followed by 1,000 mL of methylcellulose to advance the barium and distend the bowel. The small bowel lumen and mucosal surface are best demonstrated by barium studies.

CT enteroclysis improves upon barium enteroclysis by demonstrating the extraluminal component of bowel disease, the mesentery, adjacent solid organs, the peritoneal cavity, and the retroperitoneum. Patients prepare with a low-residue diet on the day before the examination followed by an overnight fast. Similar to fluoroscopic enteroclysis an 8- to 13-Fr nasojejunal catheter is advanced beyond the ligament of Treitz under fluoroscopic guidance. A choice is made between using high attenuation enteric contrast agents without intravenous contrast agents or low attenuation enteric contrast agents with intravenous contrast enhancement. High attenuation contrast agents include 4% to 15% water-soluble iodinated contrast agents and dilute barium solution. Low attenuation enteric agents include water and methylcellulose. Two liters of enteric agent is infused at 100 to 150 cc/min under fluoroscopic observation. Glucagon or other antispasmodic agent is administered intravenously. The patient is moved to the CT table and additional 500 to 1,000 cc of enteric contrast is infused at the same rate during CT scanning. Thin-slice MDCT allows for high-resolution reconstructions in axial, coronal, and sagittal planes.

CT enterography is performed in a manner similar to CT enteroclysis except the 1.5 to 2.0 L of enteric contrast is given orally instead of by enteric tube injection (Fig. 45.3). Either high or low attenuation enteric contrast agents may be used. Low attenuation enteric agents allow for use of intravenous contrast to assess bowel wall and lesion enhancement. CT enterography tends to have less reliable and less complete distention of the small bowel but is easier to perform and has higher patient acceptance.

MR enteroclysis and MR enterography are performed in a similar manner to CT enteroclysis and CT enterography (Fig. 45.3). While more expensive and somewhat less available MR small bowel studies offer the significant advantage of lack of ionizing radiation. This is particularly important in the study of patients with Crohn disease who are young and undergo many imaging examinations. Tissue contrast is also superior with MR. MR enterography is most commonly used with MR enteroclysis reserved for patients with low-grade small bowel obstruction or who are unable to ingest large volumes of enteric agents orally. A wide variety of enteric agents are available but the most popular are biphasic agents that are low signal intensity on T1WI and high signal intensity on T2WI. Biphasic agents include water, methylcellulose, low-density barium, and polyethylene glycol.

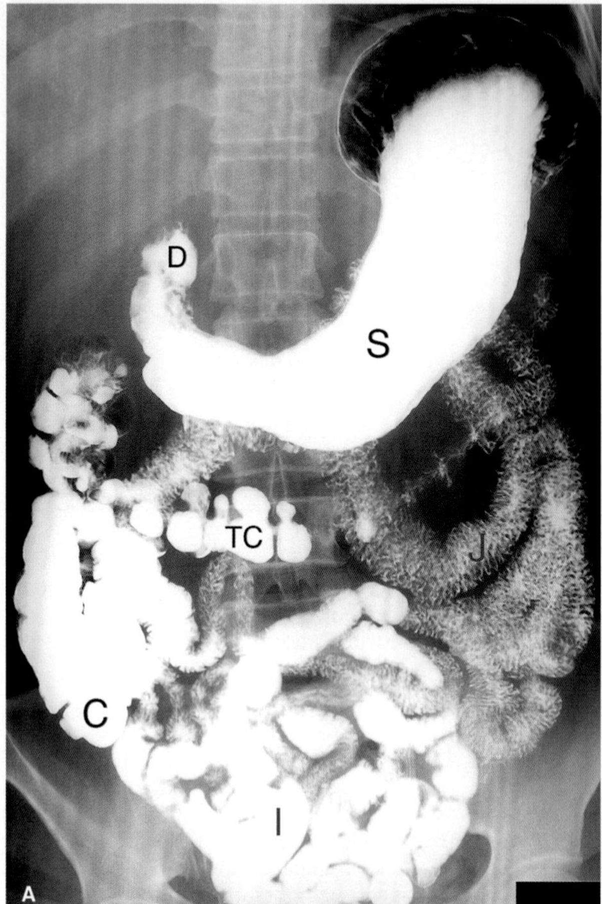

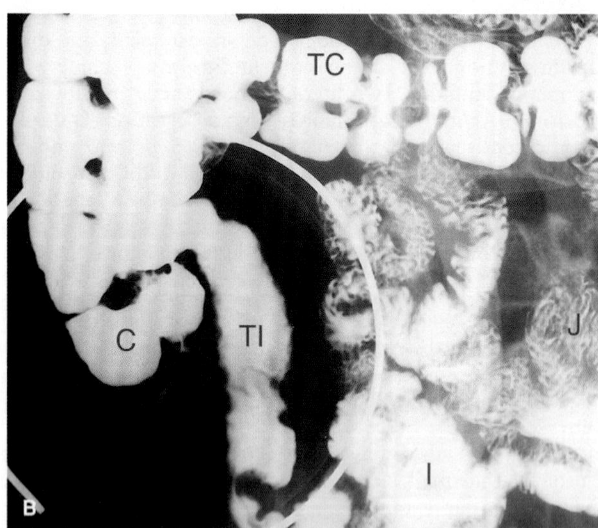

FIGURE 45.1. Normal Small Bowel Follow-Through. A: Prone abdominal radiograph. **B:** Spot-compression view of the terminal ileum. The small bowel is demonstrated on an upper GI series by having the patient ingest additional barium and by taking additional radiographs to document passage of barium through the small bowel into the colon. The loops of jejunum (*J*) have a delicate feathery appearance in the left upper abdomen, whereas the loops of ileum (*I*) are coarse and featureless in the right lower abdomen. Barium has filled portions of the cecum (*C*), ascending and transverse colon (*TC*), identified by its haustral folds. Colonic haustral folds extend only partway across the bowel lumen, and small bowel folds extend completely across the bowel lumen. Spot compression provides separation of bowel loops in the right lower quadrant to optimally demonstrate the terminal ileum (*TI*). *S*, stomach; *D*, duodenum.

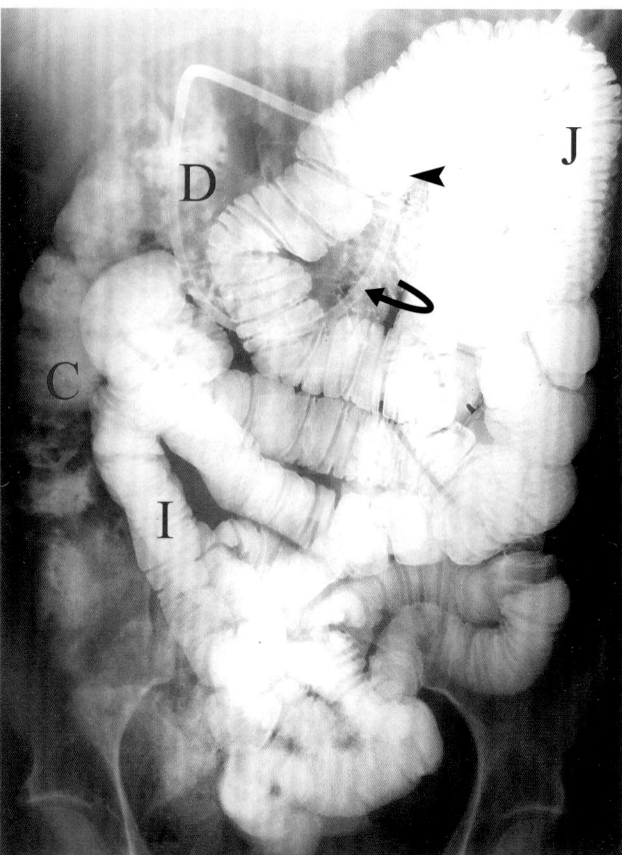

FIGURE 45.2. Normal Small Bowel Enteroclysis. The enteroclysis catheter (*curved arrow*) has been passed through the C-loop of the duodenum to the location of the ligament of Treitz (*arrowhead*), using fluoroscopy to guide catheter manipulation. The enteroclysis technique provides uniform distention of the jejunum (*J*) and ileum (*I*). Barium fills portions of the ascending colon (*C*). Note the small bowel folds crossing the entire diameter of the small bowel lumen. *D*, duodenum.

Patients are asked to ingest 1,200 to 2,000 cc of enteric agent in the hour before MR scanning. Spasmolytic agents reduce peristalsis and motion artifacts. Breath-hold fast gradient echo sequences are obtained in axial, sagittal, and coronal planes. Intravenous contrast may be utilized to assess for inflammatory hyperenhancement and tumor vascularity. Preliminary studies using state-of-the-art techniques indicate equivalent sensitivities for CT and MR enterography. Diagnostic findings of small bowel disease on MR and CT are listed in Table 45.1.

Capsule endoscopy involves the use of a swallowable video capsule 26 mm long by 11-mm diameter and weighing 4 g. The capsule contains a video camera, four light-emitting diodes as light source, a radio transmitter, and batteries. Patients fast for 10 hours prior to ingesting the capsule. A sensor array is placed on the patient's abdomen and attached to a portable battery powered recorder that can be worn around the waist. The capsule is swallowed and color video images are recorded at a rate of 2 per second up to approximately 50,000 images over an 8-hour battery life span. The patient resumes normal activities including eating while the capsule transits the intestinal tract. The capsule is excreted naturally and discarded. Capsules cost approximately $1,500. Images are reviewed on a work station. Capsule endoscopy is able to visualize the entire small bowel mucosa and may detect mucosal lesions, ulcers, and tumors missed by imaging examinations. Significant limitations include limited ability to localize, biopsy, or treat lesions and limited use in patients with small bowel obstruction or strictures.

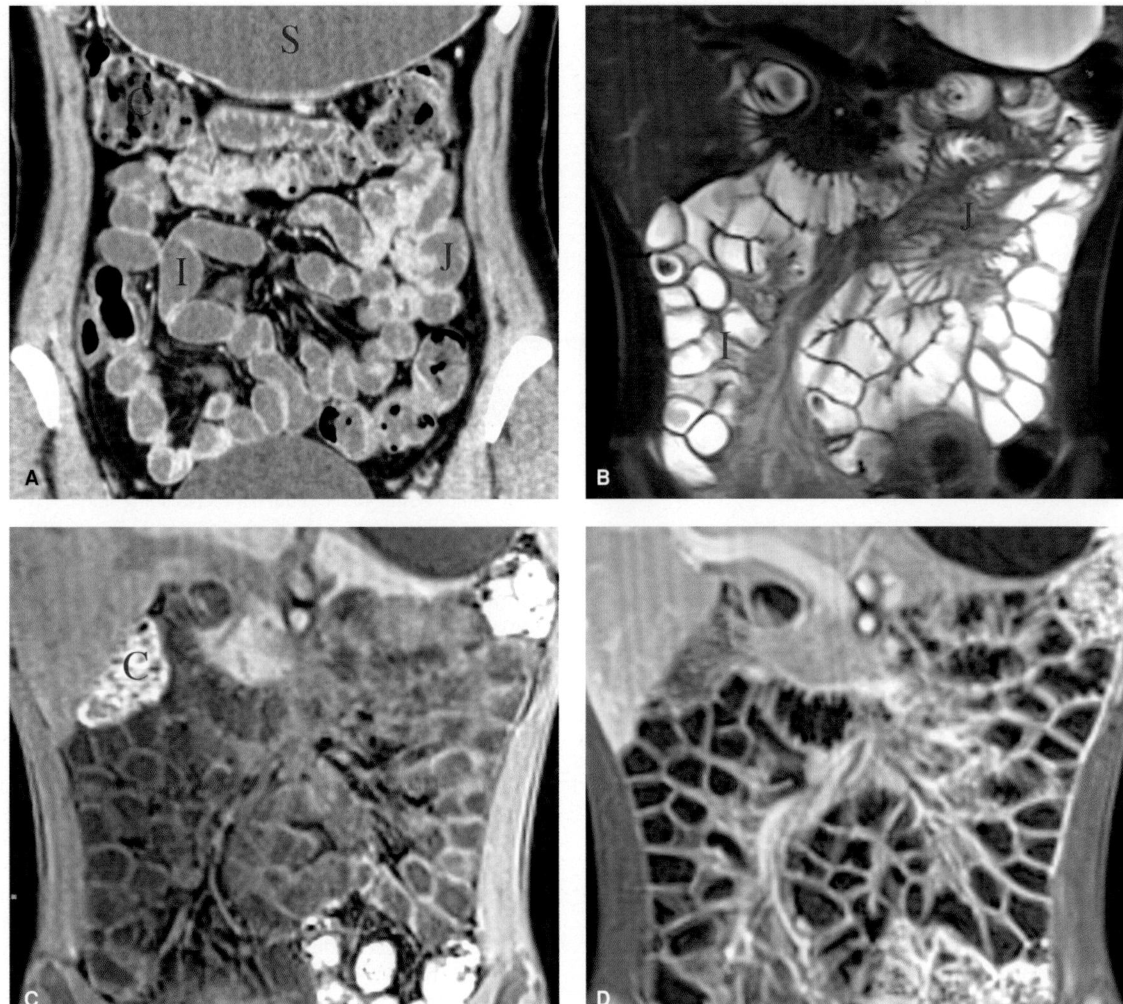

FIGURE 45.3. **CT and MR Enterography. A: CT Enterography.** Representative coronal image of the jejunum (*J*), ileum (*I*), and portion of the stomach (*S*) from a normal examination performed to assess for inflammatory bowel disease is shown. The bowel is distended with low attenuation methylcellulose given orally. Glucagon was administered intravenously to inhibit bowel peristalsis. Intravenous iodinated contrast material enhances the bowel wall. The colon (*C*) contains stool and gas. **MR Enterography.** Representative T2-weighted (**B**), T1-weighted precontrast (**C**), and T1-weighted postintravenous contrast (**D**) coronal images from an MR enterography examination show the normal MR appearance of the jejunum (*J*) and ileum (*I*). Stool-filled colon (*C*) is also evident. The bowel is distended with orally ingested low-density barium, which acts as a biphasic intraluminal contrast agent with high signal intensity on T2-weighted images and low signal intensity on T1-weighted images.

TABLE 45.1

DIAGNOSTIC FINDINGS ON CT AND MR OF THE GASTROINTESTINAL TRACT

■ BENIGN LESION	■ NEOPLASTIC LESION
Circumferential thickening	Eccentric thickening
Symmetrical thickening	Asymmetric thickening
Thickening <1 cm	Thickening >2 cm
Segmental or diffuse involvement	Focal soft tissue mass
Thickened mesenteric fat	Abrupt transition
Wall is homogeneous soft tissue density	Lobulated contour
"Double halo sign": dark inner ring/bright outer ring	Spiculated outer contour
"Target sign": bright inner-dark, middle-bright outer	Luminal narrowing Regional adenopathy Liver metastases

ANATOMY

The mesenteric small intestine is a tube approximately 7 m long that lies totally within the greater peritoneal cavity. The *jejunum* is arbitrarily defined as the proximal two-fifths of the mesenteric intestine, while the *ileum* is the distal three-fifths. The jejunum and ileum are suspended from the posterior abdominal wall by the small bowel mesentery. The small bowel mesentery is composed of connective tissue, blood vessels, and lymphatic vessels, and is covered by peritoneum, which reflects from the posterior parietal peritoneum. The root of the small bowel mesentery extends obliquely from the ligament of Treitz, just left of the L2 vertebra, to the cecum, near the right sacroiliac joint. On CT the mesentery is defined by its normal vascular structures outlined by fat between loops of bowel. Normal mesenteric lymph nodes may be seen as soft tissue density nodules 5 mm or less in size. The concave border of the small bowel loops is the mesenteric border where the mesentery attaches. The convex border, facing away from the mesentery, is called the antimesenteric border. Identification of the border involved by disease can be of diagnostic value.

TABLE 45.2

NORMAL SMALL BOWEL MEASUREMENTS

	NORMAL VALUES	
FEATURE	JEJUNUM	ILEUM
Diameter of lumen	<3.0 cm	<2.0 cm
Normal fold thickness	2–3 mm	1–2 mm
Diameter of lumen on enteroclysis	<4.0 cm	<3.0 cm
Normal fold thickness on enteroclysis	1–2 mm	1–1.5 mm
Number of folds	4–7 per inch	2–4 per inch
Depth of folds	8 mm	8 mm
Thickness of bowel wall	3 mm	3 mm

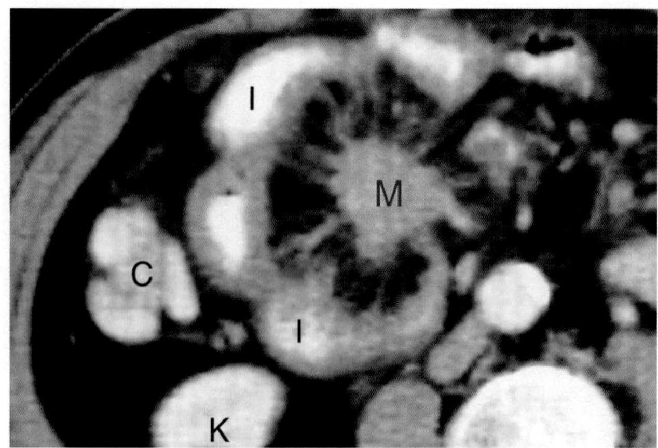

FIGURE 45.4. **Carcinoid Tumor.** CT scan shows classic "sunburst" appearance of a mesenteric (*M*) fibrosis with radiating strands due to carcinoid tumor arising in the ileum (*I*). *C*, ascending colon; *K*, right kidney.

On imaging studies (Figs. 45.1 to 45.3), the jejunum has a feathery mucosal pattern, more prominent valvulae conniventes, a wider lumen, and a thicker wall. The ileum has a less featured mucosal pattern, thinner, less frequent folds, narrower lumen, and a thinner wall. The transition between jejunum and ileum is gradual, and all loops are freely mobile. The ileum has larger and more numerous lymphoid follicles in the submucosa. Villi are finger-like projections that extend from the entire mucosal surface of the small bowel. They are composed of loose connective tissue of the lamina propria. Tiny capillaries and lymphatic vessels (lacteals) extend to the submucosal vessels. The combination of valvulae conniventes and villi greatly expands the absorptive surface area of the small intestine. The caliber of the normal small bowel lumen is less than 3 cm in the jejunum tapering to less than 2 cm in ileum (Table 45.2). Normal jejunal folds measure 2 to 3 mm thick while normal ileum folds measure 1 to 2 mm thick. Enteroclysis typically distends the normal jejunum to 4 cm and the normal ileum to 3 cm with the folds appearing 1 mm thinner in each portion of the mesenteric small bowel. Normal lymph nodes seen in the mesentery are less than 4 mm in diameter.

SMALL BOWEL FILLING DEFECTS/MASS LESIONS

Neoplasms of the small intestine are rare accounting for only 2% to 3% of GI tumors. Benign neoplasms are about equal to malignant neoplasms in overall frequency. However, when the patient presents with symptoms, malignancy is three times more common. Presenting afflictions include obstruction, pain, weight loss, bleeding, and palpable mass. CT and MR enterography findings that suggest malignant small bowel lesions include (a) solitary lesions; (b) nonpedunculated lesions; (c) long-segment lesions; (d) presence of mesenteric fat infiltration; and (e) presence of enlarged mesenteric lymph nodes (>1-cm short-axis diameter).

Carcinoid tumors are the most common neoplasm of the small intestine, accounting for about one-third of all small bowel tumors. They are considered a low-grade malignancy that may recur locally or metastasize to the lymph nodes, liver, or lung. They arise from endocrine cells (enterochromaffin or Kulchitsky cells) deep in the mucosa. These cells produce vasoactive substances including serotonin and bradykinins. About 20% of all carcinoid tumors arise in the small bowel, most commonly in the ileum where 30% are multiple. Only 7%, those with liver metastases, present with carcinoid syndrome (cutaneous flushing, abdominal cramps, and diarrhea) because the liver inactivates the vasoactive substances. The tumors grow slowly but cause a marked fibrotic response of the bowel wall and mesentery because the serotonin produced by the tumor induces an intense local desmoplastic reaction. Complications include stricture, obstruction, and bowel infarction induced by fibrosis of the mesenteric vessels. The tumors may be pedunculated and cause intussusception. Imaging signs of fibrosis and metastases resemble the findings of Crohn disease and overshadow demonstration of the primary tumor. Barium studies show (a) luminal narrowing, (b) thickened and spiculated folds, (c) separation of bowel loops by mesenteric mass or (d) bowel loops drawn together by fibrosis, and (e) primary lesion appearing as small (<1.5 cm) mural nodule or intraluminal polyp. CT and MR findings that are highly indicative of carcinoid tumor are (Fig. 45.4) (a) sunburst pattern of radiating soft tissue density in the mesenteric fat due to mesenteric fibrosis, (b) bowel wall thickening, (c) primary lesion appearing as a small, lobulated soft tissue mass, occasionally with central calcification, usually in the distal ileum, (d) marked contrast enhancement of the primary tumor mass, and (e) enlarged mesenteric nodes and liver masses due to metastatic disease.

Adenocarcinoma of the small bowel is about half as common as carcinoid tumor. It is most frequent in the duodenum (50%) and proximal jejunum, and is uncommon in the distal ileum, where carcinoid is most common. Most patients are symptomatic at presentation, and 30% have a palpable mass. Patients with adult celiac disease, Crohn disease, and Peutz–Jeghers syndrome are at increased risk for small bowel carcinoma. Complications include bleeding, obstruction, and intussusception. Prognosis is poor, with a 5-year survival of 20%. Metastatic spread is by intraperitoneal seeding, lymphatic channels to regional nodes, and portal veins to the liver. Morphologically the tumor may be infiltrating producing strictures (most common in the jejunum); polypoid producing filling defects (most common in the duodenum); or ulcerating. Barium studies typically show a characteristic "apple core" stricture of the small bowel (Fig. 45.5). CT and MR (Fig. 45.6) demonstrate (a) solitary mass in the duodenum or jejunum (up to 8-cm diameter), (b) an ulcerated lesion, or (c) abrupt irregular circumferential narrowing of the bowel lumen with abrupt edges to the wall thickening. Differential diagnosis of annular constricting lesions of the small bowel is listed in Table 45.3.

Lymphoma is responsible for about 20% of all small bowel malignant tumors. The GI tract, being the largest immunologic organ in the body, is the most common site for extranodal origin of lymphoma, and the small bowel is commonly involved. The

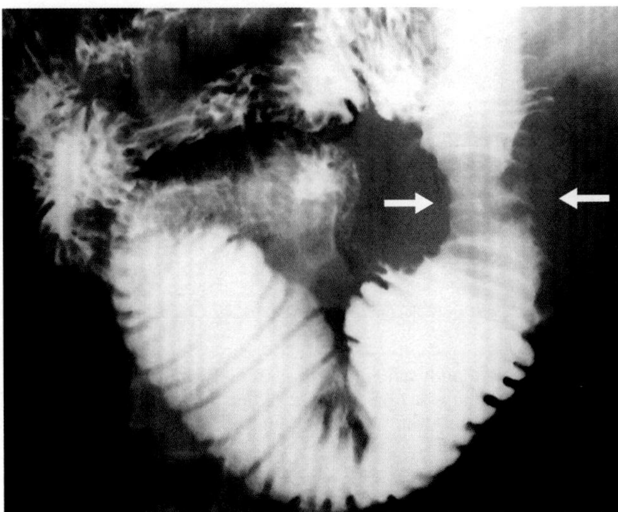

FIGURE 45.5. **Adenocarcinoma of the Jejunum—SBFT.** Small bowel follow-through study demonstrates a fixed constricting lesion (*arrows*) of the jejunum. The folds in the involved area are thickened and effaced. This is an "apple core" lesion similar to those seen with colorectal adenocarcinoma.

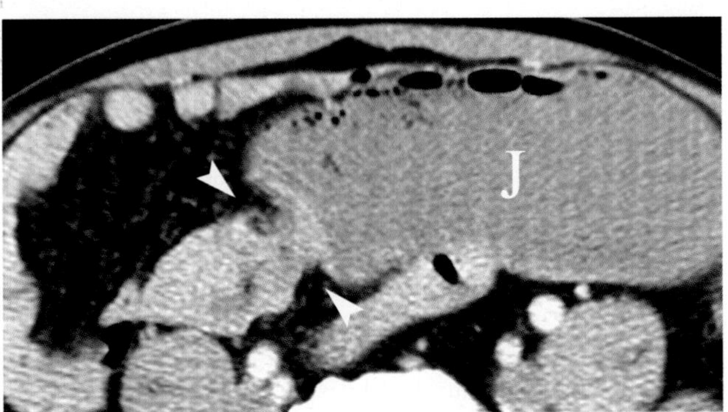

FIGURE 45.6. **Adenocarcinoma of the Jejunum—CT.** CT image from another patient demonstrates similar tumor narrowing (*arrowheads*) of the wall of the jejunum (*J*) resulting in constriction of the lumen. The proximal jejunum is greatly dilated indicating small bowel obstruction caused by the tumor.

TABLE 45.3

ANNULAR CONSTRICTING LESIONS OF THE SMALL BOWEL

Small bowel adenocarcinoma
Annular metastases
Intraperitoneal adhesions
Malignant gastrointestinal stromal tumors
Lymphoma (rare)

World Health Organization periodically changes the classification of lymphoma. The latest classification (2016) includes mature B-cell neoplasms (which include mantle cell and Burkitt lymphoma), mature T-cell/natural killer cell neoplasms, Hodgkin lymphoma, posttransplant lymphoproliferative disorder, and histiocytic and dendritic cell neoplasms. GI lymphomas are a heterogeneous group of entities with different cell lineage and biologic behavior. Most are lymphomas of B-cell type with 8% to 10% of T-cell origin. GI lymphoma involves the ileum with its high concentration of lymphoid cells in 60% to 65% of cases and the jejunum in 20% to 25%. Infections due to *Helicobacter pylori*, HIV, *Epstein–Barr virus*, hepatitis B virus, and others are risk factors for GI lymphoma. Presenting symptoms include abdominal pain, weight loss, anorexia, GI bleeding, and bowel perforation.

Morphologic patterns of involvement show wide variation including diffuse infiltration, exophytic mass, polypoid/nodular mass, and multiple nodules. Multiple sites of involvement are seen in 10% to 25% of cases. Aneurysmal dilation of the lumen is a feature of lymphoma due to replacement of the muscularis and destruction of the autonomic plexus by tumor without inducing fibrosis. As a result, obstruction is uncommon. Barium studies most commonly reveal (a) wall thickening with irregular, distorted folds due to submucosal infiltration of cells (Fig. 45.7); (b) fold thickening may be smooth and regular in early stages due to lymphatic blockage in the mesentery; (c) folds become effaced in later stages with greater cell infiltration into the bowel wall; (d) narrowed, widened, or normal lumen; (e) cavitary lesions containing fluid and debris; (f) polypoid masses that may cause intussusception; and (g) rare multiple filling defects that are larger than 4 mm, variable in size, and nonuniform in distribution. Shallow ulceration is common. CT and MR demonstrate (a) circumferential wall thickening involving a long segment of small bowel, (b) effacement of folds, (c) solid nodule, often polypoid (Fig. 45.8), (d) eccentric wall thickening (Fig. 45.9),

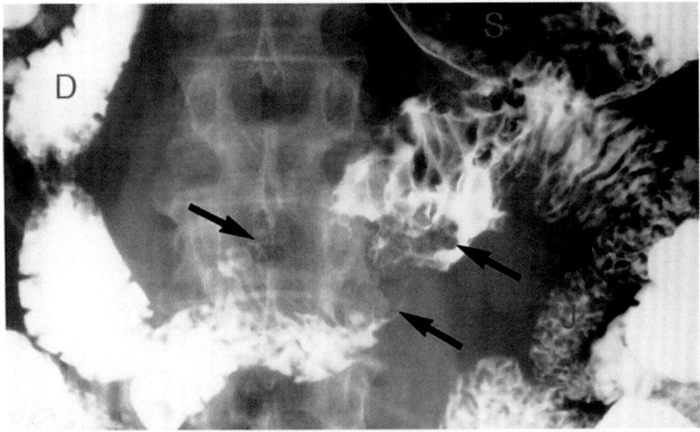

FIGURE 45.7. **B-Cell Lymphoma—UGI.** A UGI series demonstrates polypoid filling defects (*arrows*) in the third portion of the duodenum (*D*) caused by masses of lymphoma in the bowel wall. The duodenal C-loop is widened and the jejunum (*J*) is displaced laterally. *S*, stomach.

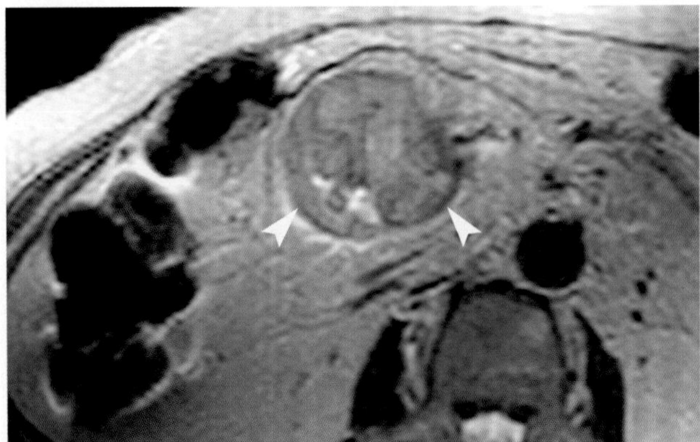

FIGURE 45.8. **B-Cell Lymphoma—MR.** T2-weighted MR reveals the solid nodule (*arrowheads*) pattern of lymphoma. This nodule arose in the jejunum.

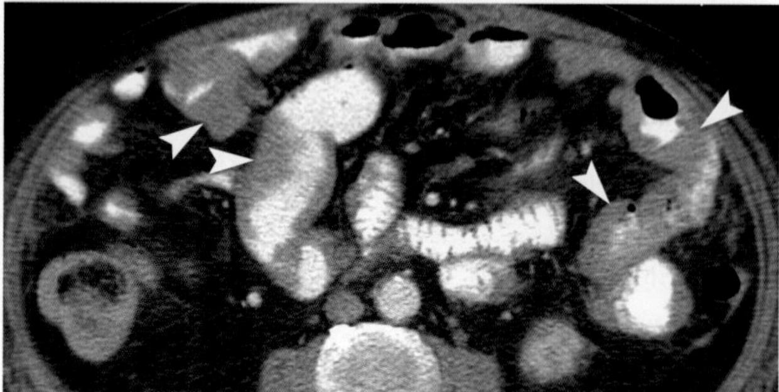

FIGURE 45.9. **B-Cell Lymphoma—CT.** CT image shows eccentric wall thickening (*arrowheads*) of multiple loops of small bowel.

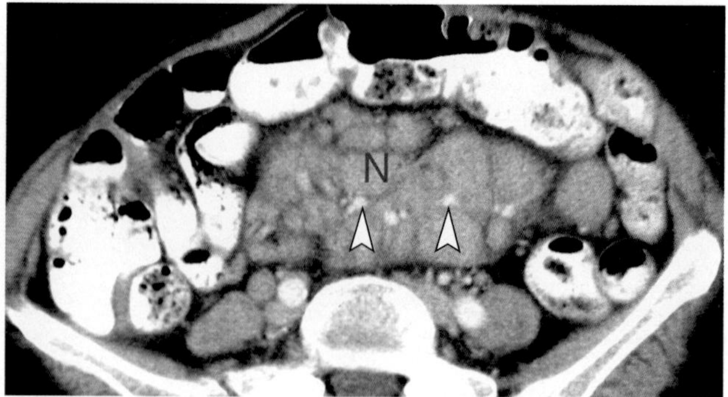

FIGURE 45.10. **Sandwich Sign—Mesenteric Lymphoma.** CT demonstrates confluent masses of enlarged lymph nodes (*N*) in the small mesentery producing the "sandwich sign" by engulfing mesenteric blood vessels (*arrowheads*).

(e) aneurismal dilation (lumen >4 cm), and (f) stenosis of the lumen (rare). Exophytic lymphoma is generally of uniform soft tissue density and enhances little, if any, with intravenous contrast administration. This is a differentiating finding in comparison with GISTs and adenocarcinoma, which usually enhance prominently. CT and MR readily demonstrate associated findings of lymphoma including mesenteric and retroperitoneal adenopathy and hepatosplenomegaly. The mesentery may show a large confluent mass encasing multiple bowel loops or enlarged individual nodes (Fig. 45.10). The "sandwich sign" refers to the sparing of rind of fat surrounding mesenteric vessels that are encased by lymphomatous nodes.

Burkitt lymphoma in North America usually presents with intestinal involvement, especially of the ileocecal area in children and young adults. The malignancy is aggressive, with rapid doubling time and poor prognosis. Imaging studies show bulky ileocecal mass.

AIDS-related lymphoma is an aggressive high-grade non-Hodgkin lymphoma with poor prognosis. Extranodal involvement, including small bowel lymphoma, is common. Adenopathy may be caused by lymphoma, Kaposi sarcoma, or *Mycobacterium avium-intracellulare* infection. The radiographic findings are identical to those seen in immunocompetent patients.

Nodular lymphoid hyperplasia may involve the entire small bowel. The condition is differentiated from lymphoma by the uniform small size of the nodules (2 to 4 mm) and even distribution through the area of involvement. Lymphoid hyperplasia confined to the terminal ileum and proximal colon is usually considered incidental and may be related to recent viral infection. Diffuse lymphoid hyperplasia is associated with hypogammaglobulinemia, especially low IgA.

Metastases to the small bowel are more common than primary neoplasms. The two most frequent routes of spread are by peritoneal seeding, usually involving the mesenteric border, and by hematogenous spread, which usually implants on the antimesenteric border. Intraperitoneal implantation on the small bowel serosa is most commonly due to ovarian carcinoma in women, and colon, gastric, and pancreatic carcinoma in men. The mesenteric border of the small bowel is favored by the flow of fluid along the small bowel mesentery from the left upper to the right lower abdomen. Implantation is most common along the terminal ileum, cecum, and ascending colon. Peritoneal implants on the parietal peritoneum, and omentum (omental cake), as well as in the pouch of Douglas, are demonstrated by CT. Barium studies demonstrate nodules and tethering of folds due to mesenteric fibrosis. Hematogenous metastases are deposited along the antimesenteric border where the submucosal blood vessels arborize. Common primary malignancies are melanoma, lung, breast, and colon carcinoma, and embryonal cell carcinoma of the testes. Imaging studies demonstrate mural nodules of uniform or varying size anywhere in the small bowel (Fig. 45.11). They may appear as target lesions, or ulcerate or cavitate. Direct extension to involve the small bowel is seen with malignancies of the pancreas and colon.

Kaposi sarcoma in AIDS patients commonly involves the small intestine. About half of the patients with skin lesions have intestinal lesions as well. Barium studies demonstrate multiple mural nodules, often centrally umbilicated. CT demonstrates mesenteric, retroperitoneal, and pelvic adenopathy.

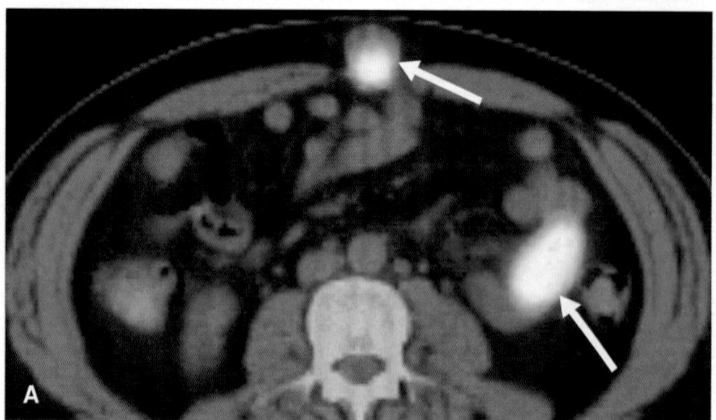

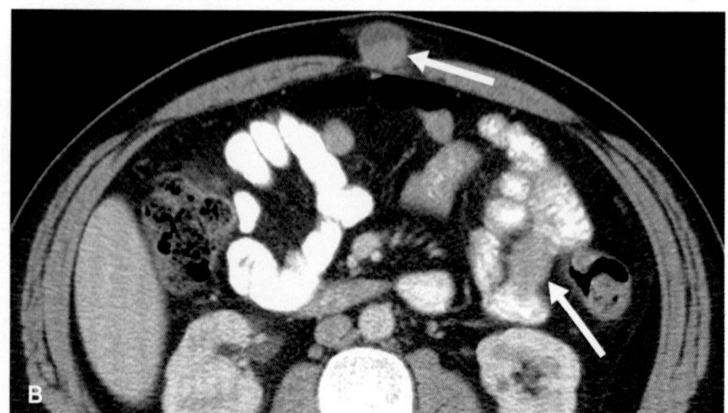

FIGURE 45.11. **Metastasis to Jejunum. A:** Fused axial image from a restaging PET-CT demonstrates intense FDR activity (*arrows*) in the mid-jejunum and the anterior abdominal wall. **B:** Diagnostic CT with intravenous and oral contrast demonstrates the corresponding lesions (*arrows*). The primary tumor was melanoma.

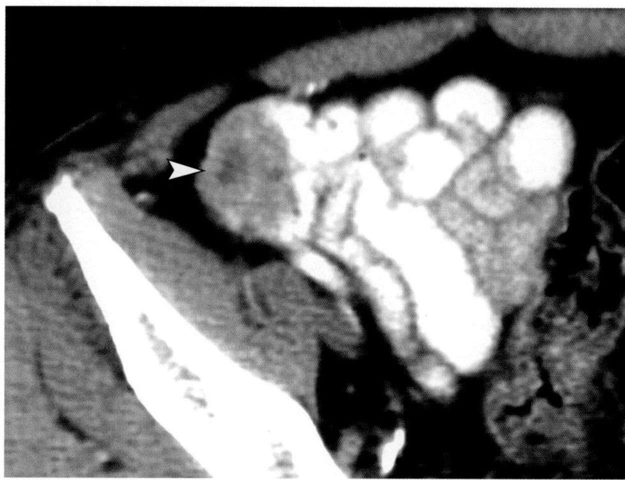

FIGURE 45.12. **Malignant GI Stromal Tumor of the Ileum.** Contrast-enhanced CT reveals a heterogeneous solid tumor (*arrowhead*) in the distal ileum. The tumor is exophytic and does not obstruct the small bowel.

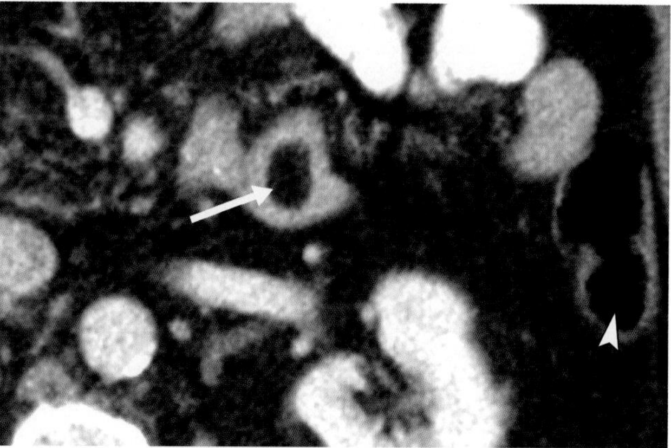

FIGURE 45.13. **Small Bowel Lipoma.** A fat density mass (*arrow*) within a loop of proximal ileum is the cause of partial small bowel obstruction. Note that the lesion is isoattenuating with adjacent mesenteric fat and is not as low in density as the gas within the colon (*arrowhead*). CT demonstration of a mass of pure fat density is diagnostic of lipoma.

Gastrointestinal stromal tumors (GISTs). As in the stomach, most tumors previously classified as leiomyomas and leiomyosarcomas are now classified as GISTs. Approximately 30% of GISTs arise in the jejunum and ileum and tend to be more aggressive than gastric tumors of the same size. GISTs account for 10% of primary small bowel neoplasms. Tumors present with obstruction or intestinal bleeding. Barium studies show a well-defined submucosal mass with smooth mucosa. Tumors that exceed 2 cm in size tend to ulcerate whether they are benign or malignant. On CT, benign GISTs are homogeneous with attenuation similar to muscle. Malignant GISTs tend to be larger (>5 cm) and heterogeneous with prominent areas of low attenuation necrosis and hemorrhage (Fig. 45.12). Nodal metastases are uncommon. Calcification is infrequent. MR shows the solid portions of the lesions to be low signal on T1WI and high signal on T2WI. Small solid tumors are round and show distinct arterial contrast enhancement. Larger tumors are lobulated and show mild gradual enhancement in solid areas. Hemorrhage shows characteristic MR signal dependent on its age.

Adenoma accounts for about 20% of benign small bowel neoplasms. It is more common in the duodenum than in the mesenteric small intestine. The tumor is a benign proliferation of glandular epithelium, and has the potential for malignant degeneration. Barium studies demonstrate an intraluminal polyp with a finely lobulated surface.

Lipoma is most common in the ileum. The tumor arises from the fat of the submucosa. Lipomas account for about 17% of benign small bowel tumors. Most are asymptomatic incidental findings, although some cause bleeding or intussusception. CT and MR demonstrate characteristic fat density (–50 to –100 H) tumor is diagnostic (Fig. 45.13).

Hemangioma is usually solitary and submucosal, projecting into the lumen as a polyp. These tumors are located predominantly in the jejunum. About two-thirds present with occult bleeding and anemia. Barium studies demonstrate a small polyp. The occasional presence of a calcified phlebolith suggests the diagnosis. They account for less than 10% of benign small bowel tumors.

Polyposis syndromes cause multiple polypoid lesions of the small bowel. The differential diagnosis includes metastases, lymphoma, nodular lymphoid hyperplasia, Kaposi sarcoma, and carcinoid tumors.

Peutz–Jeghers syndrome is an autosomal dominant inherited condition consisting of multiple hamartomatous polyps in the small intestine (most common), colon, and stomach associated with melanin freckles on the facial skin, palmar aspects of the fingers and toes, and mucous membranes. Hamartomatous polyps are a nonneoplastic, abnormal proliferation of all three layers of the mucosa, epithelium, lamina propria, and muscularis mucosae. The polyps are most common in the jejunum, are usually pedunculated, and are variable in size up to 4 cm. Patients are at increased risk for intussusception, GI tract adenocarcinoma, and extraintestinal malignancy (breast, pancreas, ovary). Barium studies demonstrate myriad polyps in involved areas of small intestine, separated by normal bowel segments.

Cronkhite–Canada syndrome involves the small bowel in about half the cases with multiple inflammatory polyps. The colon and stomach are always involved.

Gardner syndrome of inherited adenomatous polyposis coli usually includes a few adenomatous polyps in the small bowel.

Juvenile GI polyposis is most common in the colon but occasionally involves the small bowel. Inflammatory polyps containing cysts filled with mucin develop secondary to chronic irritation. Most are round, smooth, and pedunculated.

Ascariasis is caused by infestation with the roundworm *Ascaris lumbricoides*. Ascariasis is found worldwide, but is most common in Asia and Africa. Endemic areas in the United States include rural southern Appalachia and the Gulf Coast states. Infestation is acquired by ingesting food or water contaminated with *Ascaris* eggs. The eggs hatch in the small bowel. Larvae penetrate the wall and migrate through the vascular system to the lungs, where they molt and grow before migrating up the bronchi and trachea to the larynx where they are again swallowed. Worms mature in the small bowel, especially in the jejunum, and may reach 15 to 35 cm in size. New generations of infective ova are excreted in feces. A large bolus of worms may obstruct the small bowel, especially in children, or cause intussusception. Worms can be identified on conventional abdominal radiographs in 70% of cases. Barium studies demonstrate worms as long linear filling defects (Fig. 45.14). Barium ingested by the worms may be seen in their intestinal tract as a long, string-like white line.

MESENTERIC MASSES

Masses arising in the small bowel mesentery frequently present as a palpable abdominal mass. The mesenteric fat may be

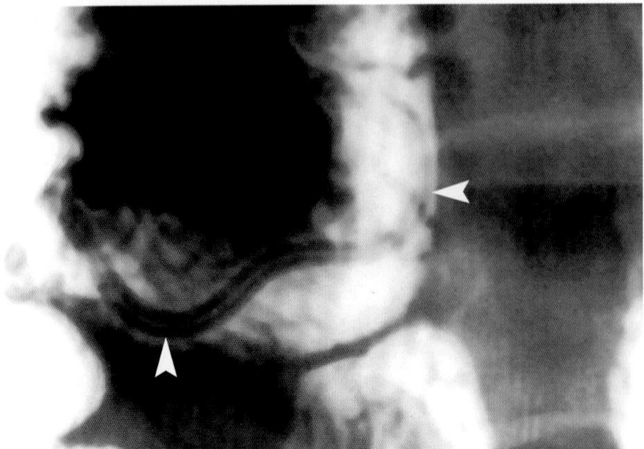

FIGURE 45.14. **Ascaris Infestation.** Cone-down radiograph from an SBFT examination reveals an adult ascaris worm (*arrowheads*) in the distal ileum. The worm has ingested barium, which outlines the worm's intestinal tract. Tangles of a mass of these large worms in distal ileum are a common cause of small bowel obstruction in endemic areas.

infiltrated by edema, hemorrhage, or inflammatory cells. The disorders may be diseases of the small intestine or be primary to the mesentery itself. CT, US, and MR provide the most diagnostic information.

Lymph nodes in the mesentery are common findings on CT or MR imaging of the abdomen. Normal mesenteric lymph nodes are less than 5 mm in short-axis diameter. Enlarged lymph nodes are associated with neoplastic, inflammatory, and infectious disease and may be the only imaging manifestation. Number and distribution of lymph nodes are as important as size. Enlarged lymph nodes may represent lymphoma or metastatic disease from the breast, lung, pancreas, or GI tract. Inflammatory lymph nodes are associated with appendicitis, diverticulitis, pancreatitis, or cholecystitis. Infectious lymphadenopathy is associated with *Yersinia enterocolitica* infections of the terminal ileum, tuberculosis, HIV, and Whipple disease.

Lymphoma causing bulky adenopathy is the most common solid mesenteric mass. Confluent adenopathy surrounds mesenteric vessels and fat producing the "sandwich sign" (Fig. 45.10). Adenopathy is commonly present in the retroperitoneum and elsewhere. The sandwich sign is specific to mesenteric lymphomas.

Metastases may implant in the mesentery and produce a large mesenteric mass without impingement of the bowel lumen or may implant adjacent to bowel narrowing the bowel lumen. Carcinoid and small bowel adenocarcinoma metastases produce a prominent desmoplastic reaction in the mesentery while melanoma produces no mesenteric retraction.

Mesenteric desmoid tumors (mesenteric fibromatosis) are benign but locally aggressive, solid, fibrous, mesenteric tumors. They may be solitary (28%) or multiple (72%) and associated with Gardner syndrome. Tumors commonly recur after surgical resection. US and CT demonstrate a homogeneous solid mass with well-defined (68%) or infiltrative borders (Fig. 45.15). Attenuation is similar to muscle. On MR tumors demonstrate low signal on T1WI and variable high signal on T2WI related to fibrous content of the tumors. Calcifications generally do not occur. Tumors commonly also occur within the muscles of the anterior abdominal wall or in the psoas muscles.

GISTs may arise primarily in the mesentery or omentum or may be found as metastases from tumors arising elsewhere. On CT tumors appear as large, well-defined masses with prominent areas of low density representing hemorrhage and necrosis.

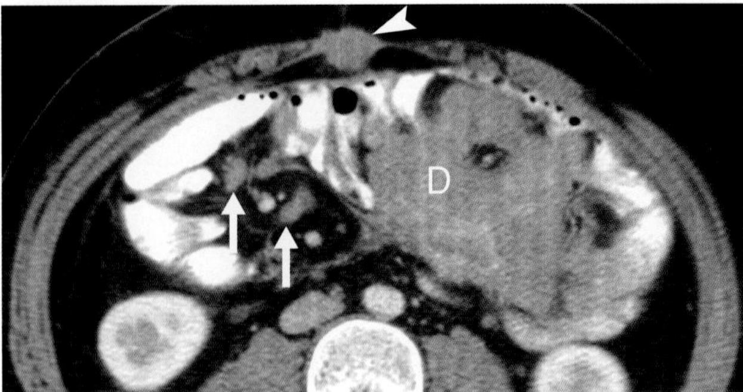

FIGURE 45.15. **Mesenteric Desmoid.** Multiple desmoid tumors are evident on this CT image. A large desmoid (*D*) infiltrates the mesentery displacing bowel loops. Two smaller desmoid tumors (*arrows*) appear as soft tissue nodules within the mesentery. Another desmoid tumor (*arrowhead*) expands the linea alba in the midline of the anterior abdominal wall.

Mesenteric cysts are lymphangiomas that arise in the root of the small bowel mesentery. Most are thin walled and multiloculated with internal fluid that may be chylous, serous, or bloody. US demonstrates a well-defined cyst with internal debris, and fluid-debris or fluid-fat levels. CT shows a cystic mass, displacing loops of small bowel anteriorly and laterally. On MR, cyst contents are hyperintense on T2WI and hypointense on T1WI when serous, or hyperintense on T1WI when chylous or hemorrhagic (Fig. 45.16).

GI duplication cyst is a congenital, partial, or complete replica of the small bowel. Most arise from the distal small bowel and may communicate with the normal intestinal lumen at one or both ends, or not at all. They are lined by intestinal epithelium. US, CT, and MR reveal a thick-walled cyst with usually serous contents. Malignancies, primarily adenocarcinoma, may arise within duplication cysts.

Mesenteric teratoma is heterogeneous with cystic and solid components. Demonstration of calcium or fat is a clue to radiographic diagnosis.

Mesenteric panniculitis (sclerosing mesenteritis) is an uncommon inflammatory condition affecting the root of the mesentery with variable inflammation, fat necrosis, and fibrosis. Lesions may be solitary or multifocal within the mesentery. Cause is unknown but the disease is associated with other idiopathic inflammatory disorders including retroperitoneal fibrosis and sclerosing cholangitis. Patients commonly present

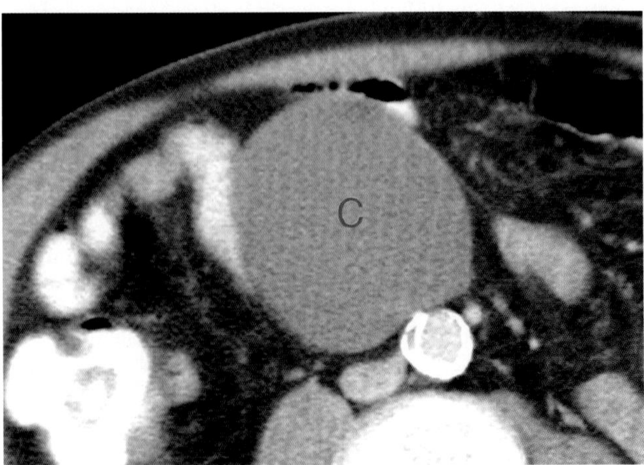

FIGURE 45.16. **Mesenteric Cyst.** Postcontrast CT reveals a thin-walled simple cyst (C) arising the small bowel mesentery.

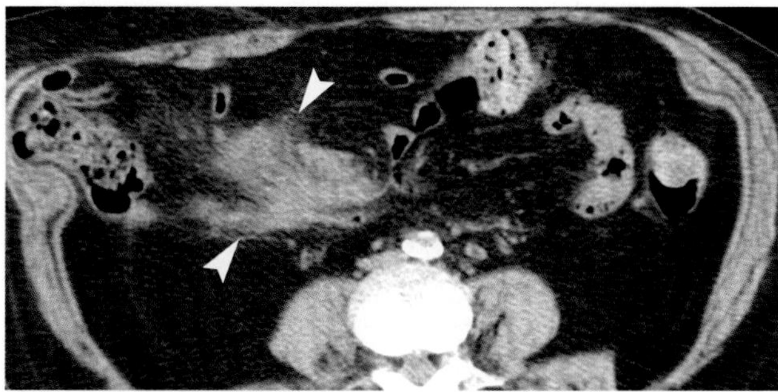

FIGURE 45.17. **Mesenteric Panniculitis.** CT without contrast shows a fibrosing lesion (*arrowheads*) in the mesentery. Borders are ill defined as the mass infiltrates and surrounds the mesenteric blood vessels.

with abdominal pain. CT shows localized increase in fat density in the mesentery (Fig. 45.17).

This finding has been termed "*misty mesentery*" and may be caused by mesenteric infiltration by edema, inflammatory cells, neoplastic cells, or fibrosis. Mesenteric panniculitis can be diagnosed as the cause of misty mesentery if other causes are excluded. Mesenteric edema may occur with portal hypertension, cardiac or renal failure, or hypoproteinemia. Inflammation of the mesentery may be associated with pancreatitis, inflammatory bowel disease, or other GI inflammatory disorders. Hemorrhage into the mesentery occurs with trauma, ischemia, and anticoagulation therapy. Lymphoma in early stages may increase the density of the mesenteric fat.

TABLE 45.4

CAUSES OF DILATED SMALL BOWEL

Obstruction (has transition zone between dilated and nondilated bowel)
Adhesions (75% of small bowel obstruction)
Postsurgical
Postperitonitis
Incarcerated hernia
Volvulus
Extrinsic tumor
Congenital stenosis
Intraluminal lesion
Tumor: usually malignant
Intussusception
Foreign body
Gallstone ileus
Bezoar
Ascaris (bolus of worms)
Meconium
Muscle dysfunction (no transition zone)
Adynamic ileus
Surgery
Trauma
Peritoneal inflammation
Ischemia
Drugs
Opiates
Barbiturates
Anticholinergics
Vagotomy
Diabetic neuropathy
Metabolic disorders
Electrolyte imbalance
Collagen diseases
Scleroderma
Dermatomyositis
Malabsorption syndromes
Celiac disease
Chronic idiopathic pseudo-obstruction

DIFFUSE SMALL BOWEL DISEASE

Students of radiology dread learning about diseases of the small bowel because they are numerous, obscure, confusing, and lead to long lists of differential diagnosis (see Tables 45.4 to 45.7). A few common diseases cause the majority of small bowel abnormalities that most radiologists will encounter in routine practice. The rest of the list must be known to pass *The Boards*. Five rules, learned well, simplify the problem.

Rule #1. Dilation of the small bowel lumen means small bowel obstruction or dysfunction of small bowel muscle.

Rule #2. Thickening of small bowel folds means infiltration of the submucosa.

Rule #3. Uniform, regular, straight thickening means infiltration by fluid (edema or blood).

Rule #4. Irregular, distorted, nodular thickening means infiltration by cells or nonfluid material.

Rule #5. The specific diagnosis requires matching the small bowel pattern with the clinical data.

The normal values for small bowel luminal diameter and fold anatomy are given in Table 45.2.

TABLE 45.5

THICKENED SMALL BOWEL FOLDS: STRAIGHT AND REGULAR

Intestinal edema (diffuse)
Hypoproteinemia
Congestive heart failure
Portal hypertension
Lymphatic obstruction
Tumor infiltration (lymphoma)
Radiation
Fibrosis of the mesentery
Lymphangiectasis
Zollinger–Ellison syndrome
Lactase deficiency
Intestinal edema (short segment)
Crohn disease
Eosinophilic gastroenteritis
Hemorrhage into bowel wall (long segment)
Trauma
Ischemia
Anticoagulant therapy
Bleeding disorders
Vasculitis
Henoch–Schonlein syndrome
Connective tissue disease
Radiation
Thromboangiitis obliterans
Stomach and small bowel involved
Ménétrier disease
Zollinger–Ellison syndrome
Crohn disease
Lymphoma
Eosinophilic gastroenteritis

TABLE 45.6

THICKENED SMALL BOWEL FOLDS: IRREGULAR AND DISTORTED

Proximal (predominantly duodenum + jejunum)
Giardiasis
Strongyloides
Whipple disease
Eosinophilic gastroenteritis
Zollinger–Ellison syndrome
Distal (predominantly ileum)
Lymphoma
Crohn disease
Yersinia/Campylobacter infection
Salmonella infection
Tuberculosis
Behçet disease
Cystic fibrosis
AIDS-related infections
Diffuse
Lymphoma
Polyposis syndromes
Amyloidosis
Histoplasmosis
Systemic mastocytosis
Waldenström macroglobulinemia
Lymphoma
Stomach and small bowel involved
Lymphoma
Crohn disease
Eosinophilic gastroenteritis
Whipple disease
Tuberculosis
Mastocytosis

Dilated small bowel lumen (Table 45.4). The hallmark of mechanical bowel obstruction is a point of transition between dilated bowel and nondilated bowel at the site of obstruction. With muscle dysfunction, the small bowel dilation is diffuse with no transition point. If no coexisting mucosal disease is present, the small bowel folds are straight and regular (Fig. 45.18). See Chapter 40 for an expanded discussion of this topic.

Thickened folds: straight and regular (Table 45.5). Infiltration of edema fluid or hemorrhage into the submucosa results in uniform straight thickening of the folds (Fig. 45.19). Hemorrhage usually causes thicker folds than edema and may result in scalloping or "thumbprinting" of some folds.

Thickened folds: irregular and distorted (Table 45.6). This is the most difficult category of abnormality because many conditions are unusual. The distribution of fold abnormality helps to limit the differential diagnosis (Fig. 45.20).

Some conditions are included in several categories. Early Crohn disease is characterized by edema and regular folds. More advanced Crohn disease has inflammatory cell infiltrate and irregular folds. Lymphoma in the mesentery obstructs lymphatics and causes edema, and lymphoma in the bowel wall causes nodular, irregular folds. Lymphoma and Crohn disease are the two most commonly encountered small bowel diseases.

Scleroderma affects the small bowel in 60% of patients producing atrophy of the muscularis by the process of progressive collagen deposition resulting in flaccid, atonic, often greatly dilated small bowel. The valvulae conniventes are normal or thinned (Fig. 45.21). A "hide-bound" appearance of thinned folds tethered together is produced by contraction of the

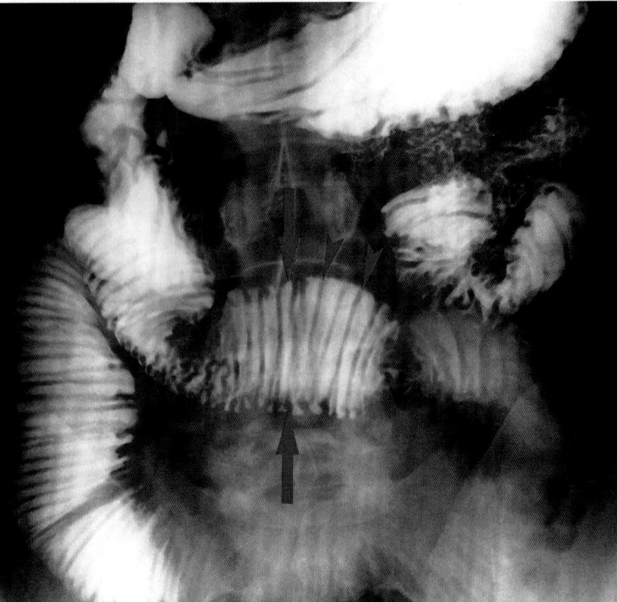

FIGURE 45.18. Dilated Small Bowel, Normal Folds. SBFT examination reveals dilation of the small bowel lumen (>5 cm between *arrows*) with normal thickness of well-defined folds (*arrowheads*). The cause was small bowel obstruction caused by adhesions.

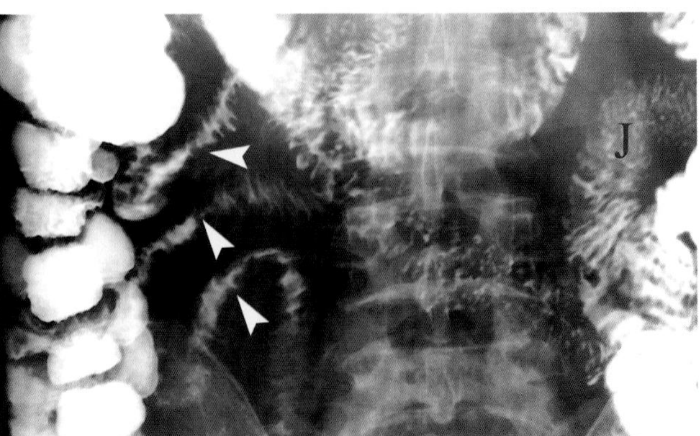

FIGURE 45.19. Thickened Folds—Regular and Straight. Barium examination demonstrates a striking separation of multiple loops of ileum (*arrowheads*), indicating thickening of the bowel walls. The folds in involved loops are thickened and nodular due to edema and hemorrhage resulting from ischemia. A repeat study 1 month later documented complete resolution of all findings. *J*, jejunum.

TABLE 45.7

TINY SMALL BOWEL NODULES

Nodular lymphoid hyperplasia (2–4 mm)
Lymphoma (>4 mm)
Amyloidosis
Whipple disease (1–2 mm)
Mycobacterium avium-intracellulare infection
Lymphangiectasia
Systemic mastocytosis (<5 mm)

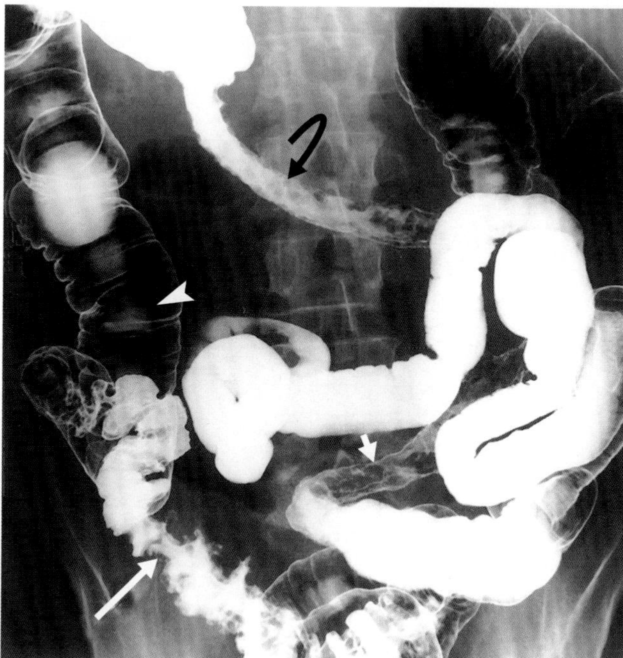

FIGURE 45.20. **Thickened Folds—Irregular.** Crohn disease of the ileum causes thickened folds (*large arrow*) that are irregular and distorted. A more proximal segment of jejunum (*small arrow*) is effaced and narrowed. The transverse colon (*curved arrow*) is narrowed, stiffened, and has multiple inflammatory polyps producing filling defects. This is an excellent example of "skip lesions" characteristic of Crohn disease.

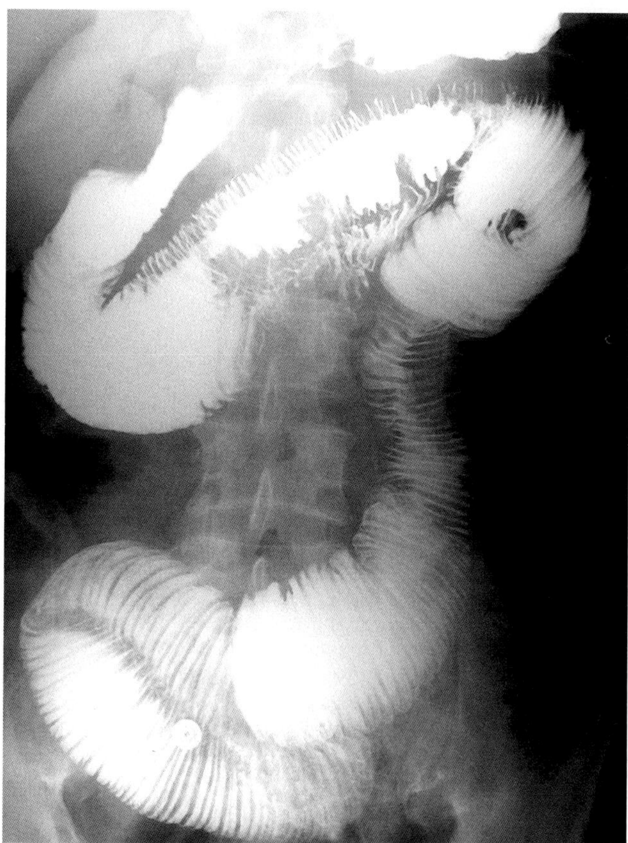

FIGURE 45.21. **Scleroderma.** Radiograph from an SBFT examination demonstrates dilation of the jejunum with thin normal folds, an appearance commonly seen with scleroderma. Luminal dilation is caused by smooth muscle dysfunction in the bowel wall.

longitudinal muscle layer to a greater extent than the circular muscle layer. Excessive contraction of the mesenteric border of the small bowel results in formation of mucosal sacculations along the antimesenteric border. The jejunum and duodenum are more severely involved than the ileum. The diagnosis is confirmed by skin changes and characteristic involvement of the esophagus. Malabsorption eventually occurs. High-resolution chest CT is required to document pulmonary involvement.

Adult celiac disease (nontropical sprue) presents with malabsorption, steatorrhea, and weight loss. Gluten, an insoluble protein found in wheat, rye, oats, and barley, acts as a toxic agent to the small bowel mucosa. The mucosa becomes flattened and absorptive cells decrease in number; villi disappear. The submucosa, muscularis, and serosa remain normal. Findings and symptoms resolve with a strict gluten-free diet. Complications of celiac disease include small bowel intussusception, lymphoma, ulcerative jejunoileitis, cavitating lymphadenopathy syndrome, and pneumatosis intestinalis. The classic radiographic findings (Fig. 45.22) are as follows: (a) dilated small bowel, (b) normal or thinned folds, (c) a decreased number of folds per inch in the jejunum, and (d) an increased number of folds per inch in the ileum (≥5). Findings are best demonstrated by standard or CT enteroclysis. Five or more folds per inch in the jejunum make the diagnosis unlikely. Fluid excess is often evident in the ileum. Distention of small bowel loops with increased volume of intraintestinal fluid is seen on conventional MDCT. CT enterography findings include (a) reversed jejunoileal fold pattern with loss of folds in the jejunum and increased number of folds in the ileum; (b) small bowel dilation; (c) increased separation of small bowel folds; (d) mesenteric lymphadenopathy; and (e) engorgement of mesenteric vessels. Transient nonobstructing intussusceptions may be observed.

Tropical sprue has similar clinical and radiographic findings as nontropical sprue but is confined to India, the Far East,

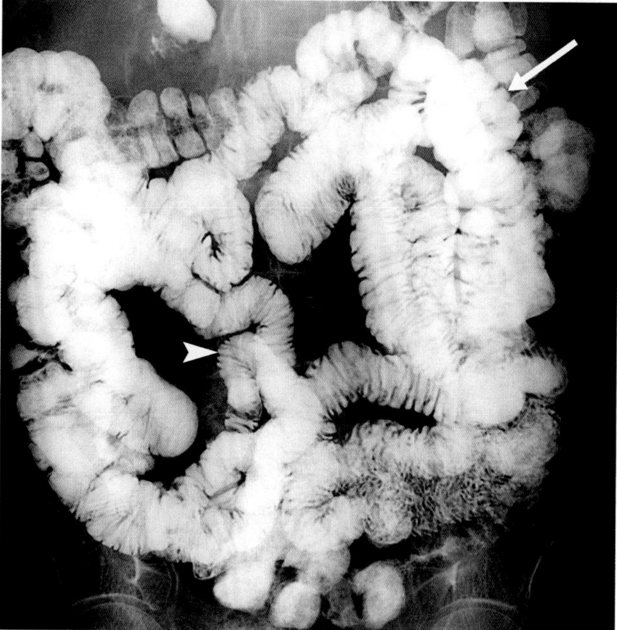

FIGURE 45.22. **Adult Celiac Disease.** Small bowel enteroclysis examination demonstrates mild dilation of the lumen of the small bowel. The number of folds in the jejunum (*arrow*) in the left upper quadrant is decreased, while the number of folds in the ileum (*arrowhead*) in the right lower quadrant is increased. The folds are of normal thickness, less than 3 mm. This patient with malabsorption became asymptomatic on a gluten-free diet.

and Puerto Rico. Illness starts with acute diarrhea, fever, and malaise and transitions to chronic steatorrhea, weight loss, malaise, and nutrient and vitamin deficiencies. The cause is unknown but the disease responds to administration of folate and antibiotics.

Lactase Deficiency. Lactase is required within the absorptive cells of the jejunum to properly digest disaccharides. Several population groups, including Chinese, Arabs, Bantu, and Eskimos, may become totally deficient in lactase during adult life. Secondary lactase deficiency may develop with alcoholism, Crohn disease, and drugs such as neomycin. The nondigested lactose in the small bowel causes increased intraluminal fluid and dilated small bowel with normal folds.

Intestinal ischemia may result from embolism or thrombosis of the superior mesenteric artery or vein. Patients may present with an acute abdomen or vague symptoms. Arterial occlusion may be due to embolus, vasculitis, trauma, or adhesions. Venous thrombosis results from hypercoagulability states (neoplasms, oral contraceptives), inflammation (pancreatitis, peritonitis, abscess), or stasis (portal hypertension, congestive heart failure). Conventional radiographs demonstrate gaseous distention, thickened mucosal folds (thumbprinting) (Fig. 45.19), and, in some cases, intramural or portal venous gas. MDCT with intravenous contrast is the diagnostic imaging method of choice. CT findings (Fig. 45.23) of acute intestinal ischemia include (a) diffuse thickening of the bowel wall, usually to 8 to 9 mm, rarely exceeding 15 mm; (b) thinning of the bowel wall may occur in acute arterial occlusion caused by loss of intestinal muscle tone and tissue volume loss with vessel constriction; (c) low attenuation of the bowel wall is caused by edema; (d) high attenuation of the bowel wall is caused by intramural hemorrhage; (e) lack of or decreased bowel wall enhancement is highly specific for acute ischemia; (f) pneumatosis of the thickened bowel wall may indicate transmural infarction; (g) dilation of the bowel wall occurs with adynamic ileus; (h) mesenteric vessels with emboli or thrombi fail to enhance following intravenous contrast administration; and (i) mesenteric fat stranding and ascites are commonly present.

Radiation enteritis occurs when large doses of radiation are given to adjacent organs. The small bowel is the most radiosensitive organ in the abdomen. Long segments of bowel may be involved, with thickening of folds and bowel wall. Peristalsis is impaired. Progressive fibrosis leads to tapered strictures commonly involving long segments. The bowel may be kinked and obstructed by adhesions. Fistulas to the vagina or other organs may also result. CT demonstrates wall thickening and increased density of the mesentery, and fixation of bowel loops

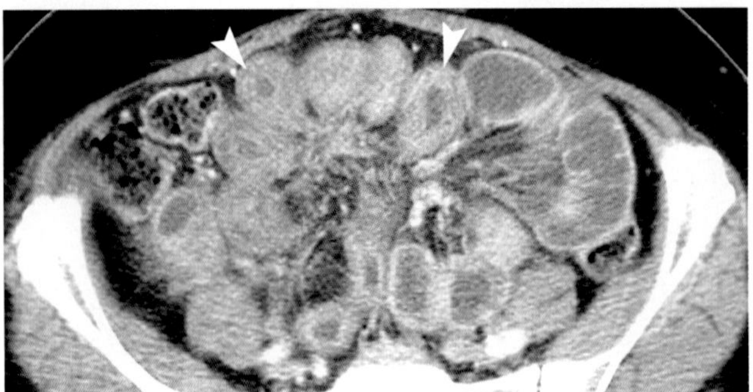

FIGURE 45.23. Intestinal Ischemia. CT demonstrates circumferential thickening (*arrowheads*) of numerous small bowel loops caused by intestinal ischemia as a result of occlusion of mesenteric vessels by metastatic carcinoid tumor. The characteristic, benign, "target" appearance of bowel wall thickening is evident. The mesentery is edematous and congested.

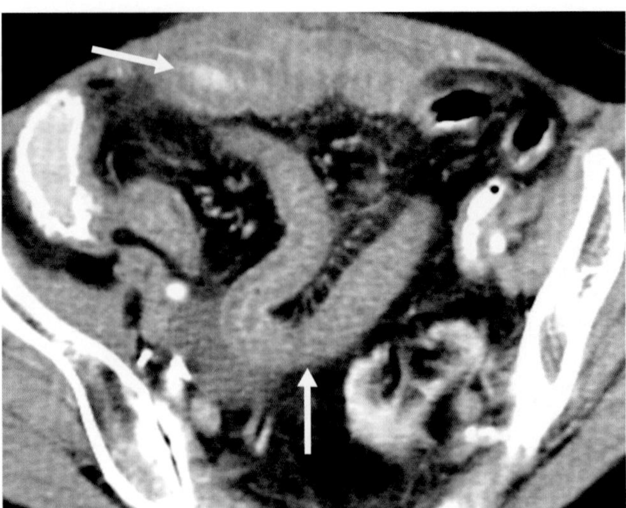

FIGURE 45.24. Radiation Enteritis. CT image through the pelvis in a patient with cervical carcinoma treated with high-dose external beam radiation reveals long segments of small bowel (*arrows*) with wall thickening and infiltrated mesentery.

(Fig. 45.24). Diagnosis is confirmed by researching the radiation field and dose.

Lymphangiectasia refers to gross dilation of the lymphatic vessels in the small bowel mucosa and submucosa. The primary form is a congenital lymphatic blockage, often associated with asymmetric edema of the extremities. Despite being congenital, symptoms often do not occur until young adulthood. Patients present with protein-losing enteropathy, diarrhea, steatorrhea, and recurrent infection. Secondary lymphangiectasia refers to lymphatic obstruction due to radiation, congestive heart failure, or mesenteric node involvement by malignancy or inflammation. The diagnosis is confirmed by jejunal biopsy. Barium study findings include diffuse fold thickening that is most pronounced in the jejunum, increased intraluminal fluid, and groups of tiny (1 mm) nodules due to distended villi. The pattern closely resembles Whipple disease (Table 45.7). CT helps the differentiation by revealing thickening of the bowel wall and mesenteric adenopathy in secondary lymphangiectasia.

Eosinophilic gastroenteritis virtually always affects the gastric antrum, as well as all or part of the small bowel. Intense infiltration of eosinophils in the lamina propria causes thickening of the bowel wall and mucosal folds, often with luminal narrowing. Barium studies show thickened and straightened folds. Thickening of the bowel wall is evidenced by wide separation between bowel loops. CT shows thickened distorted folds in the distal stomach and proximal small bowel. Most patients have a history of allergic disorders. The disease is self-limited but recurrences are frequent.

Amyloidosis is a disease complex associated with extracellular infiltration of an amorphous protein material in body tissues. The disease may be primary or associated with multiple myeloma (10% to 15%), rheumatoid arthritis (20% to 25%), or tuberculosis (50%). Most cases are systemic, but 10% to 20% are localized. The small bowel is the most common site of GI involvement. Amyloid deposits are seen throughout the wall of the small bowel, especially within the walls of small blood vessels resulting in ischemia and infarction. Deposits in the muscularis impair motility. Diffuse, irregular thickened folds may be seen throughout the small bowel. Nodules are sometimes present. CT demonstrates symmetric wall thickening of affected bowel without luminal dilation or hypersecretion. Small mesenteric lymph nodes may be evident. Diagnosis is confirmed by biopsy.

Systemic mastocytosis is a myeloproliferative neoplasm characterized by infiltration of mast cells in the skin, bones, lymph nodes, liver, spleen, and GI tract. Urticaria pigmentosa is the characteristic skin manifestation. Osteoblastic bone changes are found in 70% of cases. Lymphadenopathy and hepatosplenomegaly are often present. The bowel wall and mucosal folds are thickened, and mucosal nodules up to 5 mm size are often evident (Table 45.6).

Whipple disease is an uncommon systemic disorder affecting the GI tract, joints, central nervous system, and lymph nodes. The disease is caused by Whipple bacilli, gram-positive, rod-shaped bacteria that are found within macrophages in many organs and tissues. Patients may present with arthritis, neurologic symptoms, or steatorrhea. Generalized lymphadenopathy is usually present. Enteroclysis demonstrates irregularly thickened folds most prominent in the jejunum. Demonstration of tiny (1 mm) sand-like nodules spread diffusely over the mucosa or in small groups is strong evidence of the disease. Increased luminal fluid is usual. CT reveals thick folds especially in the jejunum without significant dilation. Low-density or fat density nodes in the mesentery are characteristic.

AIDS Enteritis. In addition to lymphoma and Kaposi sarcoma, AIDS patients are predisposed to multiple opportunistic infections of the GI tract. Infective agents usually occur in combination and in multiple GI sites.

Cryptosporidium and *Isospora belli* are protozoans that may infest the proximal intestine and cause a cholera-like diarrhea with life-threatening fluid loss. Barium studies show thickened folds and marked increased fluid.

Cytomegalovirus causes disease in the small bowel and colon as well as the lungs, liver, and spleen. Mucosal ulceration with bleeding and perforation are the major intestinal manifestations. Barium studies show thickened folds, loop separation, ulcers, and fistulae.

Mycobacterium avium-intracellulare is a common systemic infection in AIDS, involving lung, liver, spleen, bone marrow, lymph nodes, and intestinal tract. Barium studies show thickened, nodular folds with a sand-like mucosal pattern. CT demonstrates retroperitoneal and mesenteric adenopathy and focal lesions in the liver and spleen.

Candida, Amoeba histolytica, Giardia, Strongyloides, herpes simplex, and *Campylobacter* may also occur in AIDS patients.

SMALL BOWEL EROSIONS AND ULCERATIONS

Crohn disease is a common inflammatory disease of uncertain etiology that may involve the GI tract from the esophagus to the anus. The disease is characterized by erosions, ulcerations, full-thickness bowel wall inflammation, and formation of noncaseating granulomas. Patients present, usually in their teens, 20s, and 30s, with diarrhea, abdominal pain, weight loss, and often fever. The typical course is one of remissions, relapse, and progression of disease. Patterns of GI involvement include colon and terminal ileum (55%), small bowel alone (30%), colon alone (15%), and proximal small bowel without terminal ileum (3%). Imaging hallmarks of Crohn disease are (a) aphthous erosions (see Fig. 44.15), (b) confluent deep ulcerations, (c) thickened and distorted folds (Fig. 45.20), (d) fibrosis with thickened walls, contractures, and stenosis, (e) involvement of the mesentery, (f) asymmetric involvement both longitudinally and around the lumen, (g) skip areas of normal intervening bowel between disease segments (Fig. 45.20), and (h) fistula and sinus tract formation. Aphthous ulcers are shallow, 1- to 2-mm depressions usually surrounded by a well-defined halo.

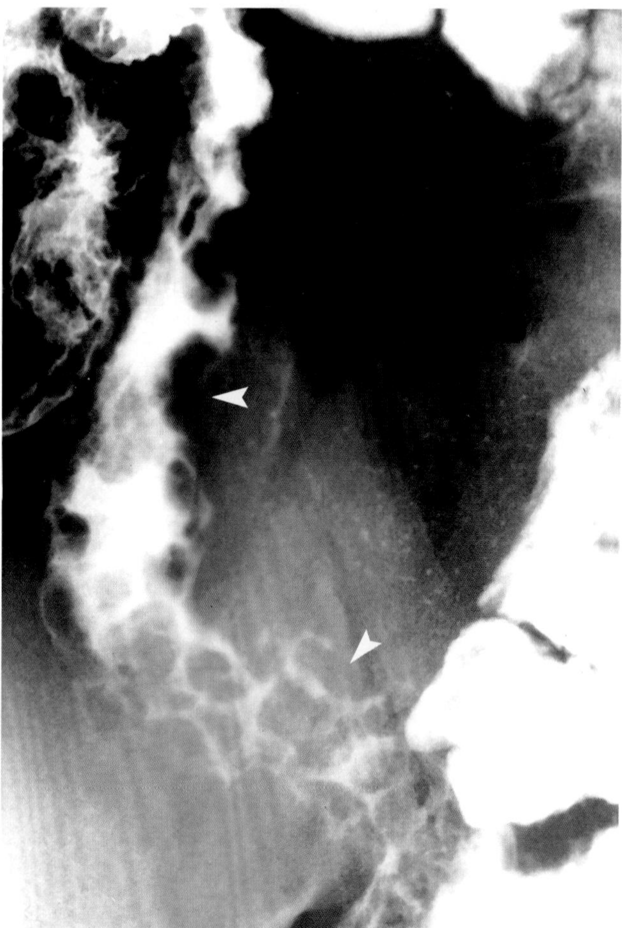

FIGURE 45.25. **Crohn Disease: Cobblestone Pattern.** Coned-down view of the terminal ileum from an SBFT reveals cobblestone pattern (*arrowheads*) of ulcerations and fissures between mounds of unaffected mucosa.

Deep ulcerations are larger and often linear, forming fissures between nodules of elevated edematous mucosa ("cobblestone pattern") (Fig. 45.25). Fibrosis and progressive thickening of the bowel wall narrow the lumen, particularly of the terminal ileum, producing the "string sign" (Figs. 45.26 to 45.28). Mesenteric involvement is best demonstrated by CT or MR. Ulceration along the mesenteric border may extend between the leaves of the mesentery. The mesenteric fat is infiltrated; the mesentery is thickened and retracted. CT and MR enterography (Fig. 45.28) are used to determine disease activity. Findings indicative of active inflammation include (a) wall thickening (>3 mm); (b) a layered pattern of wall enhancement; (c) the "comb sign" of fibrofatty proliferation around inflamed bowel segments with engorged mesenteric vessels forming the comb (Figs. 45.27 and 45.28); and (d) on MR high signal intensity of the thickened bowel wall on T2WI with fat saturation. Diffusion-weighted MR enterography shows restricted diffusion in acutely inflamed small bowel.

Complications of Crohn disease are common and well shown by CT and MR. Obstruction is usually partial and due to strictures or areas of severe ulceration and spasm. Fistulae are formed in 19% of patients with small bowel disease. Fistulae are abnormal communications between two epithelial-lined organs. Most frequent are ileocolonic and ileocecal, but enterocutaneous, enterovesical, and colovesical fistulae are also common. Sinus tracts extend into inflammatory extraluminal masses from the bowel lumen (Fig. 45.26).

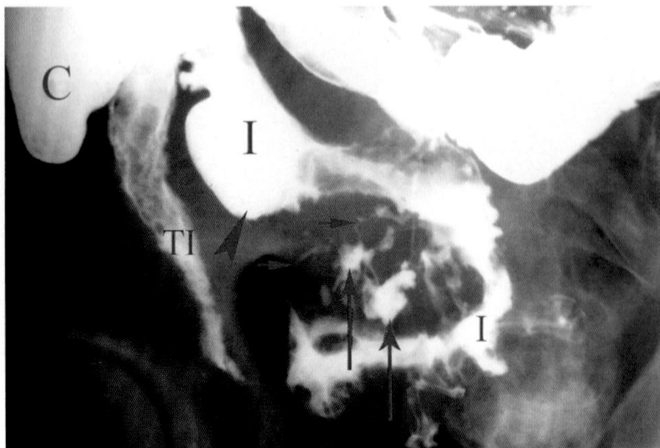

FIGURE 45.26. **Crohn Disease.** A small bowel study in a patient with long-standing Crohn disease demonstrates numerous sinus tracts and fistulas (*short arrows*) with extraluminal abscesses (*long arrows*). Fistulous connections extended between loops of small bowel as well as between ileum and the right ureter (not shown). The distal ileum (*I*) demonstrates irregular narrowing and separation from adjacent loops. Asymmetric involvement of a portion of the ileum has resulted in the formation of a sacculation (*arrowhead*). The terminal ileum (*TI*) is narrowed and stiffened with a thick wall evidenced by separation from adjacent loops. C, cecum.

Abscess and phlegmon formation in the mesentery, peritoneal cavity, retroperitoneum, and abdominal wall are common. Free perforation occurs in 3% of cases. Most perforations are confined and form sinus tracts or fistulae. Carcinomas of the small and large bowel are increased in frequency with a prevalence of about 0.5% in Crohn disease patients. Derangements of intestinal absorption cause megaloblastic anemia (vitamin B_{12} deficiency) and an increased incidence of gallstones and renal stones. Up to 20% of patients have arthritis or spondylitis that mimics ankylosing spondylitis.

Yersinia enterocolitis is caused by infection with the gram-positive bacilli, *Y. enterocolitica*,or *Y. pseudotuberculosis*. Infection causes acute enteritis with abdominal pain, fever, and often bloody diarrhea that mimics acute appendicitis or acute Crohn disease. Children and young adults are most often affected. The infection runs a self-limited course of 8 to 12 weeks. Diagnosis is confirmed by stool culture. Imaging

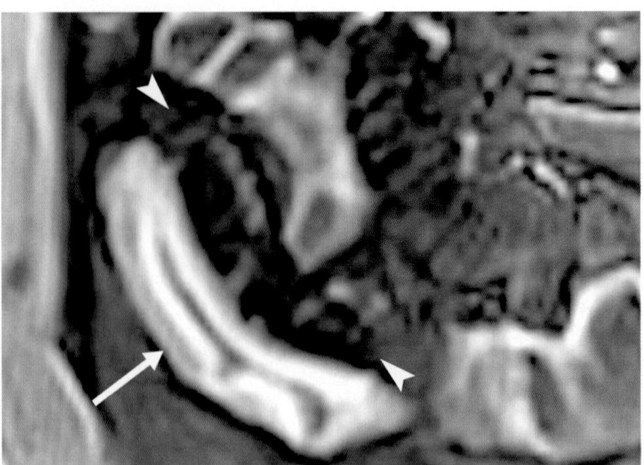

FIGURE 45.28. **Crohn Disease—Terminal Ileitis—MR.** Coronal plane postintravenous contrast T1WI from MR enterography examination shows the thickened and enhancing wall (*arrow*) of the terminal ileum narrowing the lumen. Again evident is the adjacent fibrofatty proliferation (*arrowheads*).

findings are most pronounced in the distal 20 cm of the ileum. They include aphthous ulcers, nodules up to 1 cm in size, wall thickening, and thickened folds that become effaced with increasing edema. Nodular lymphoid hyperplasia may appear during the resolution stage.

Campylobacter fetus jejuni infection is clinically and radiographically similar to *Yersinia* enterocolitis. The disease usually lasts 1 to 2 weeks, but relapses are common. Diagnosis is by stool culture.

Behçet disease is a multisystem disease due to a small vessel vasculitis that affects eyes, joints, skin, central nervous system, and the intestinal tract. Prominent clinical features include relapsing iridocyclitis, mucocutaneous ulcerations, vesicles, pustules, and mild arthritis. Intestinal disease most commonly involves the ileocecal region, where Crohn disease is closely mimicked with aphthous erosions, deep ulceration, stenosis, and fistula formation. Complications include bowel perforation and peritonitis. The cause is unknown and there is no cure. The disease is most common in the Middle East, especially Turkey, and Asia.

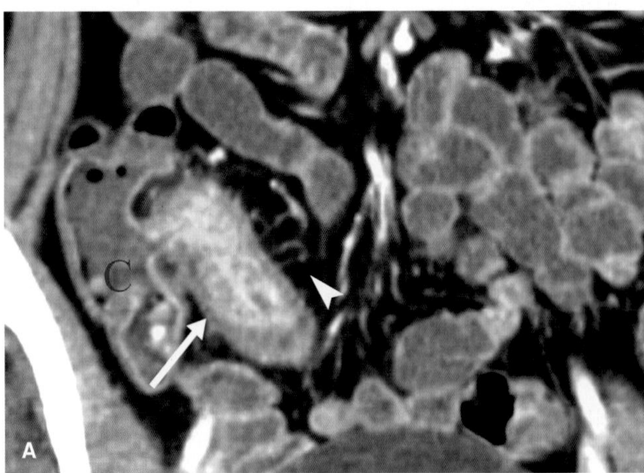

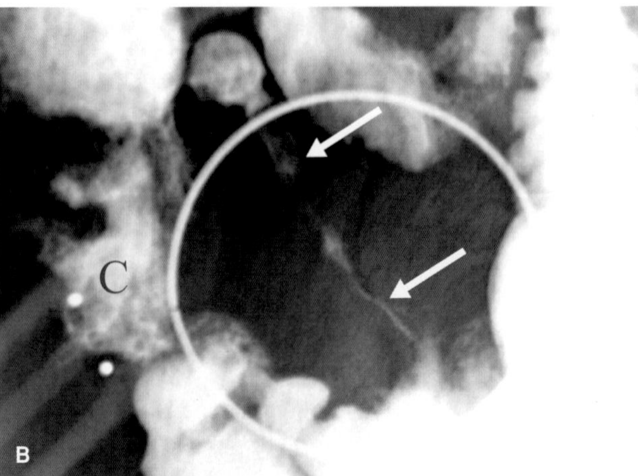

FIGURE 45.27. **Crohn Disease—Terminal Ileitis. A:** Image of the right lower quadrant from CT enterography shows the marked circumferential wall thickening of the terminal ileum (*arrow*) that narrows the lumen producing the "string sign" seen on barium studies. Note the characteristic fibrofatty proliferation (*arrowhead*) adjacent to the diseased ileum. Stretching of the mesenteric vessels through the fibrofatty proliferation produces the "comb sign." **B:** Spot-compression view of the terminal ileum from enteroclysis examination of the same patient shows the string sign (*arrows*). C, cecum.

Tuberculosis presents as peritonitis or focal infection of the gut, most commonly involving the ileocecal area, closely mimicking Crohn disease. Less than half of the patients have concurrent evidence of pulmonary tuberculosis. Barium studies demonstrate inflamed mucosa with transverse and stellate ulcers. The affected bowel becomes rigid and narrowed with nodular mucosa. The ileocecal valve is stiff and gaping with narrowed terminal ileum and cecum. CT shows characteristic findings of mesenteric adenopathy, high-density ascites, and peritoneal thickening and enhancement accompanying the bowel wall thickening.

SMALL BOWEL DIVERTICULA

Small bowel diverticula are most common in the jejunum along the mesenteric border. They are outpouchings of mucosa through the bowel wall and between the leaves of the mesentery. They are commonly multiple and often asymptomatic. However, because of stasis of bowel contents within them, bacterial overgrowth may occur, resulting in deconjugation of bile salts and malabsorption. Vitamin B_{12} absorption may also be impaired, resulting in megaloblastic anemia. Additional complications include obstruction, acute diverticulitis, hemorrhage, and volvulus. Conventional radiographs may reveal featureless ovoid collections of air. Barium studies show the outpouchings, most with a neck smaller in diameter than the outpouching itself (Fig. 45.29). The diverticulum lacks mucosal folds and does not contract because of the lack of muscle within its wall. On CT diverticula appear as discrete, round or ovoid, structures outside the expected lumen of the small bowel. They may be filled with air, fluid, or contrast and have a thin smooth wall.

Meckel diverticulum is the most common congenital anomaly of the GI tract, present in 2% to 3% of the population. The diverticulum varies from 2 to 8 cm in length, and is located on the antimesenteric border of the ileum up to 2 m from the ileocecal valve. The tip of the diverticulum may be attached to the umbilicus by a remnant of the vitelline duct. Ectopic gastric mucosa is present in up to 62% of cases. Peptic secretions may cause ulceration and bleeding. Other complications are intussusception, volvulus, and perforation. Radionuclide (Tc-99m pertechnetate) scanning for ectopic gastric mucosa is the test of choice but is less reliable in adults than in children, and is negative when the diverticulum does not contain gastric mucosa. Enteroclysis is then the best method to demonstrate the diverticulum, which appears as a blind sac attached to the antimesenteric border of the ileum. On CT, Meckel diverticulitis appears as a blind-ending pouch of variable size and wall thickness with inflammatory changes in adjacent mesentery (Fig. 45.30).

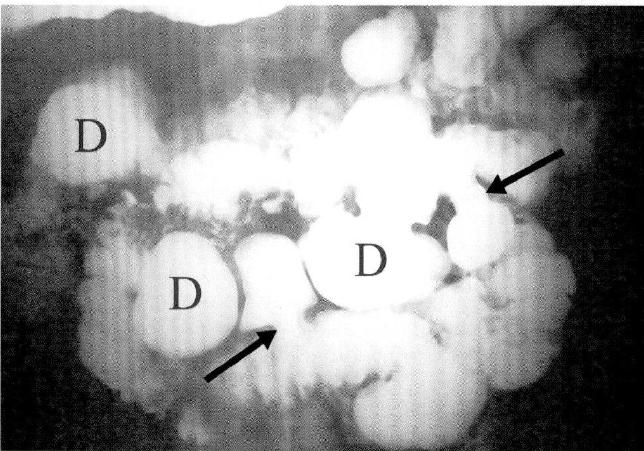

FIGURE 45.29. Small Bowel Diverticula. A small bowel series demonstrates numerous diverticula (*D*) extending from the duodenum and jejunum. The narrow necks (*arrows*) of two diverticula are shown particularly well.

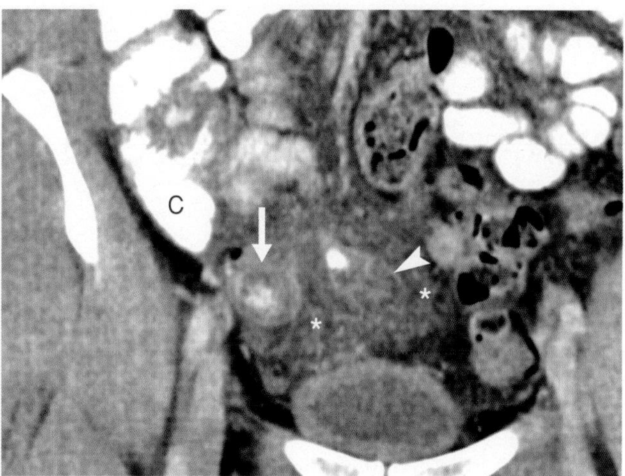

FIGURE 45.30. Meckel Diverticulitis. Coronal CT shows a fecalith (*skinny arrow*) obstructing a Meckel diverticulum (*arrowhead*) causing diverticulitis with marked inflammation in adjacent fat (*) including involvement of nearby bowel (*fat arrow*) in the inflammatory process. *C*, cecum.

Pseudodiverticula or sacculations are outpouchings along the antimesenteric border of the small bowel that result from disease of the small bowel. They occur most commonly in association with Crohn disease or scleroderma. With fibrosis and contraction of the mesenteric border of the bowel, the unsupported antimesenteric border becomes pleated and forms sacculations.

Suggested Readings

Childers BC, Cater SW, Horton KM, Fishman EK, Johnson PT. CT evaluation of acute enteritis and colitis: Is it infectious, inflammatory, or ischemic? *Radiographics* 2015;35:1940–1941. (Online digital presentation).

Fernandes T, Oliveira MI, Castro R, Araújo B, Viamonte B, Cunha R. Bowel wall thickening at CT: simplifying the diagnosis. *Insights Imaging* 2014;5:195–208. (Pictorial review).

Ganeshan D, Bhosale P, Yang T, Kundra V. Imaging features of carcinoid tumors of the gastrointestinal tract. *AJR Am J Roentgenol* 2013;201:773–786.

Kaushal P, Somwaru AS, Charabaty A, Levy AD. MR enterography of inflammatory bowel disease with endoscopic correlation. *Radiographics* 2017;37:116–131.

Kawamoto S, Raman SP, Blackford A, Hruban RH, Fishman EK. CT detection of symptomatic and asymptomatic Meckel diverticulum. *AJR Am J Roentgenol* 2015;205:281–291.

Lo Re G, Vernuccio F, Midiri F, et al. Radiologic features of gastrointestinal lymphoma. *Gastroenterol Res Pract* 2016;2016:1–9. (Review article) http://dx.doi.org/10.1155/2016/2498143

Lou L, Teng J, Qi H, Ban Y. Sonographic appearances of desmoid tumors. *J Ultrasound Med* 2014;33:1519–1525.

McLaughlin PD, Filippone A, Maher MM. The "misty mesentery": mesenteric panniculitis and its mimics. *AJR Am J Roentgenol* 2013;200:W116–W123. (Structured resident review).

McLaughlin PD, Maher MM. Nonneoplastic diseases of the small intestine: differential diagnosis and Crohn disease. *AJR Am J Roentgenol* 2013;201:W174–W182. (Structured resident review).

McLaughlin PD, Maher MM. Primary malignant disease of the small intestine. *AJR Am J Roentgenol* 2013;201:W9–W14. (Structured resident review).

Nougaret S, Lakhman Y, Reinhold C, et al. The wheel of the mesentery: imaging spectrum of primary and secondary mesenteric neoplasms—how can radiologists help plan treatment? *Radiographics* 2016;36:412–413. (Online digital presentation).

Swerdlow SH, Campo E, Pileri SA, et al. The 2016 revision of the World Health Organization classification of lymphoid neoplasms. *Blood* 2016;127:2375–2390.

Yi MH, Lee JM, Baek JH, Han JK, Choi BI. MRI features of gastrointestinal stromal tumors. *AJR Am J Roentgenol* 2014;203:980–991.

CHAPTER 46 ■ COLON AND APPENDIX

WILLIAM E. BRANT

COLON

Imaging Methods

The primary imaging methods for detection and characterization of colon abnormalities have continued to evolve over time. The persistently expanding availability of colonoscopy has reduced the role of barium enema in imaging the colon. On the other hand, the use of CT to image the abdomen and pelvis continues to increase, making CT often the method of initial detection of colon disease. CT and MR colonography challenge the role of traditional colonoscopy for polyp and cancer detection. Once a possible neoplastic lesion is discovered, however, colonoscopy or proctoscopy is needed for biopsy. The single-contrast barium enema is still occasionally used for the evaluation of colonic obstruction, fistulas, and in old, seriously ill or debilitated patients. The double-contrast (air-contrast) barium enema (Fig. 46.1) is favored for detection of small lesions (<1 cm), for documentation of inflammatory bowel disease, and for detailed imaging evaluation of the rectum. Colonoscopy is limited by occasional failure to reach the right colon. Then barium enema or CT or MR colonoscopy is utilized to complete the examination. As elsewhere in the GI tract, CT complements colonoscopy and barium examinations by demonstrating intramural and extracolonic components of disease. It is excellent for demonstrating extrinsic inflammatory and neoplastic processes that affect the colon: abscesses, sinuses, and fistulas.

CT and MR imaging are utilized for initial staging of colorectal carcinoma. Both methods have limitations especially in determining involvement of regional lymph nodes. Significant improvements have been made in preoperative CT and MR staging with use of thin-slice MDCT, and high-resolution and diffusion-weighted MR techniques. PET-CT aids in the detection of metastatic disease to lymph nodes and distant metastases but is limited in assessment of local disease by physiologic and iatrogenic uptake of FDG by the colon. Transrectal US is more accurate than CT or MR in determining local tumor extent of rectal carcinomas, and is used in the evaluation of other rectal and perirectal disease.

CT colonography (Fig. 46.2) has become a viable alternative to invasive colonoscopy to screen for colorectal cancer. The procedure begins with diligent bowel preparation identical to that used for invasive colonoscopy. A rectal tube is inserted and the colon is insufflated with carbon dioxide or room air. MDCT of the entire extent of the colon with the patient in supine position is obtained in a single breath-hold utilizing 1.25- to 2.5-mm collimation and a reconstruction interval of 1 mm. The scan is repeated with the patient in prone position. Commercially available software programs that provide endoluminal display and "fly-through" capabilities provide three-dimensional volume rendering image processing. Image viewing and interpretation are usually performed using both standard two-dimensional axial CT reconstructions and the three-dimensional volume rendered images on a computer workstation.

MR colonography offers the advantage of screening for colorectal carcinoma without the use of ionizing radiation. Dark lumen MR colonography with filling and distention of the lumen with air, water, or other low signal intensity agents, fecal tagging agents, 3-Tesla magnets, and optimal pulse sequences shows great promise. The same bowel preparation is needed as for colonoscopy or CT colonography. The bowel must be well distended with either bright lumen or dark lumen agents. Dark lumen agents are generally preferred because intravenous contrast agents can be effectively utilized. Limitations are expense and artifact such as from hip prostheses.

Anatomy

The large intestine consists of the cecum and appendix, colon, rectum, and anal canal. It is approximately 1.5 m in length from the ileum to the anus. The large intestine is characterized by the *taenia coli,* three longitudinal bands of muscle that traverse the colon shortening it to form haustra, the sacculations created by puckering of the bowel wall. The major functions of the large intestine are the formation, transport, and evacuation of feces. These functions require mobility, absorption of water, and secretion of mucus. Infrequent peristalsis transports feces from the ascending and transverse colon to the sigmoid colon where fecal material is stored until defecation. The cecum and ascending colon absorb water from the highly liquid material received from the ileum. Mucus secreted by mucosal goblet cells protects the mucosa from injury, and is secreted in profuse amounts when the mucosa is irritated or injured. The cecum is the large blind pouch that extends below the level of the ileocecal valve. The cecum generally lies in the right iliac fossa but may be quite mobile. It is usually

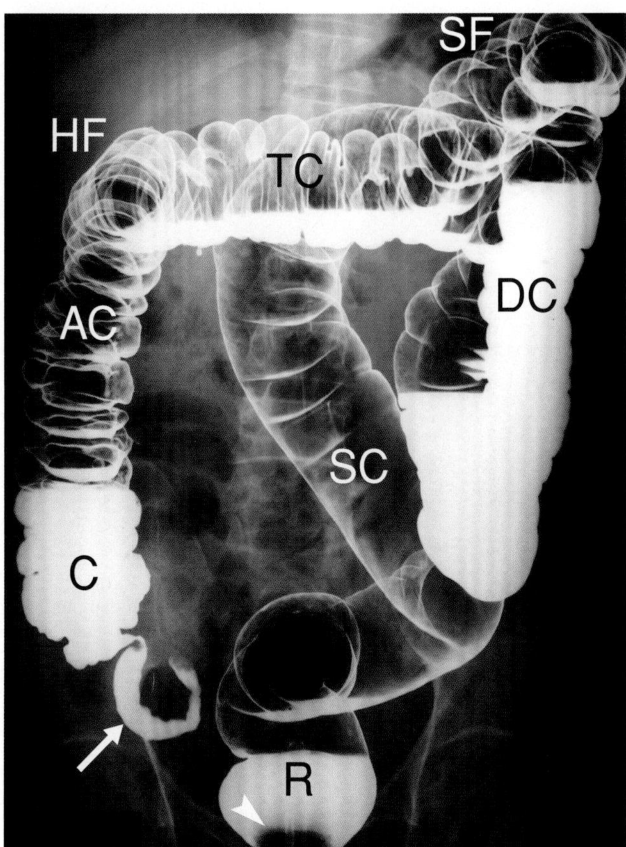

FIGURE 46.1. **Double-Contrast Barium Enema.** An upright radiograph from a double-contrast barium enema demonstrates normal colon anatomy. The appendix (*fat arrow*) extends from the cecum (*C*). The ascending colon (*AC*) extends to the hepatic flexure (*HF*), the coils of which must be examined by multiple oblique views. The transverse colon (*TC*) extends to the splenic flexure (*SF*), which continues as the descending colon (*DC*). This patient has a long sigmoid colon (*SC*) that extends high into the abdomen. The transverse colon is relatively short. Patients with a short sigmoid colon usually have a long redundant transverse colon. The distended balloon at the tip of the enema catheter causes a lucent filling defect (*arrowhead*) in the rectum (*R*). A tiny intramural diverticulum (*skinny arrow*) is seen in the proximal transverse colon.

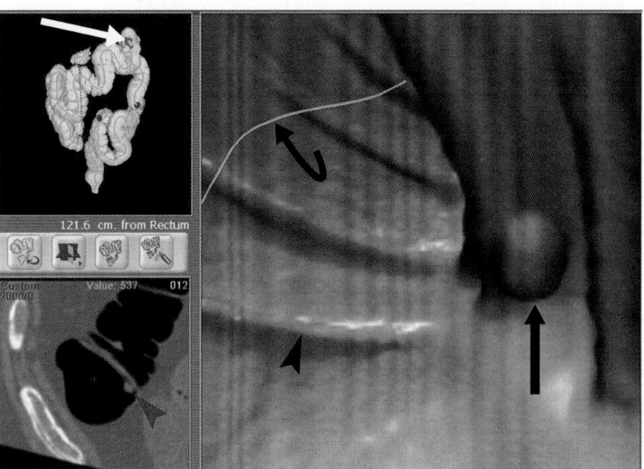

FIGURE 46.2. **Polyp on CT Colonography.** Three-dimensional reconstructed image on the right shows a 7-mm polyp (*black straight arrow*) extending into the lumen of the colon. Multiple normal appearing folds (*black arrowhead*) are evident. The *green line* (*black curved arrow*) shows the colon "fly-through" path. Image at the top left shows a three-dimensional reconstruction of the entire colon with the matching *green line* showing the fly-through path. The location of this polyp is shown as the *blue thumbtack* (*white arrow*) in the splenic flexure, 121.6 cm from the rectum. The *red dots* show additional polyps discovered on this examination. Thin-section source CT image on the lower left shows the polyp (*red arrowhead*).

covered on all sides by peritoneum (intraperitoneal), but may be fixed extraperitoneally, covered only on its ventral surface by peritoneum. The appendix is a long worm-like tube that hangs from near the apex of the cecum. The ileocecal valve consists of two lips that project into the cecum forming a sometimes prominent mass. The ascending colon is extraperitoneal, lying in the anterior pararenal space, covered only on its ventral surface by peritoneum. The hepatic flexure forms two curves. The proximal, more posterior curve is closely related to the descending duodenum and right kidney. The more distal anterior curve is closely related to the gallbladder. The transverse colon is intraperitoneal and suspended from the transverse mesocolon that arises from the peritoneum covering the pancreas and sweeps transversely across the upper abdomen. The transverse mesocolon limits the superior extent of the small bowel loops. The splenic flexure is closely related to the tail of the pancreas and the caudal aspect of the spleen. The splenic flexure is anchored to the diaphragm by the phrenicocolic ligament, which serves as a boundary between disease processes of the left subphrenic space and the left paracolic gutter. The descending colon, like the ascending colon, is extraperitoneal within the anterior pararenal space and is covered by peritoneum only on its ventral surface. The sigmoid colon forms a redundant loop of variable length from the distal descending colon in the left iliac fossa to the rectum. The sigmoid colon is completely intraperitoneal and is suspended by the sigmoid mesocolon that allows considerable mobility. The sigmoid colon penetrates the peritoneum at the level of vertebrae S2 to S4 to continue as the extraperitoneal rectum. The rectum extends for approximately 12 cm in close relationship with the sacrum. Peritoneum forming the pouch of Douglas covers the ventral and lateral aspects of the rectum. The anal canal is 3 to 4 cm long and is invested by the sphincter ani and levator ani muscles. A series of vertical folds form the rectal columns of Morgagni, beneath which are the veins that when dilated, are hemorrhoids. The colon is recognized on imaging studies by its course, haustral markings, and fecal content. The thickness of the wall of the normal colon does not exceed 5 mm.

Colon Polyps and Mass Lesions

Polyps. The term "polyp" is generic for a lesion that protrudes from the mucosal surface of the GI tract (Fig. 46.2). The term does not imply a histologic diagnosis. *Filling defect* refers to radiolucency in a contrast media pool caused by a protruding mass lesion. On CT and barium enema examinations, filling defects maybe polyps, tumors, plaques, air bubbles, feces, mucus, or foreign objects. Protrusions from the mucosa that produce filling defects in pools of contrast media or are etched in white when coated by barium and outlined by air on double-contrast studies. Polyps may be pedunculated and on a stalk, or sessile (Fig. 46.3). They may appear as "bowler hats" (Fig. 46.4) when viewed obliquely. Air bubbles rise to the highest point of a contrast column, but fecal material usually remains dependent. Plaques are flat lesions that barely rise above the mucosal surface.

Colorectal adenocarcinoma is the most common malignancy of the GI tract, the fourth most common malignant tumor, and

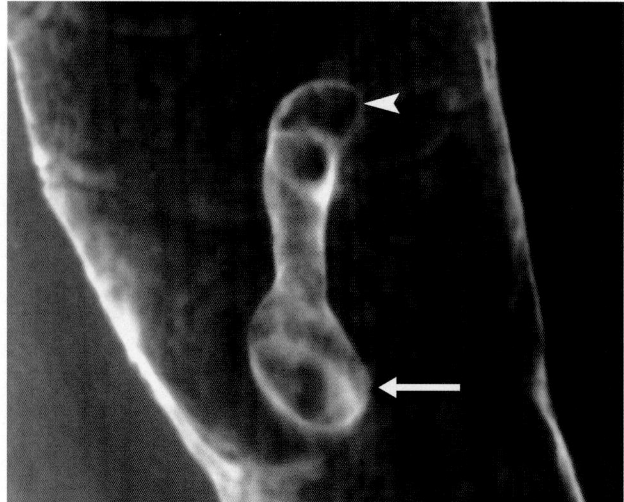

FIGURE 46.3. **Pedunculated Polyp.** Double-contrast barium enema demonstrates a long-stalked pedunculated polyp with a bulbous tip (*arrow*) arising (*arrowhead*) from the mucosa of the descending colon.

the second most frequent cause of cancer death in the United States. Approximately 50% arise in the rectum and rectosigmoid area. Another 25% occur in the sigmoid colon, and the remaining 25% are evenly distributed throughout the remainder of the colon. Nearly all cancers of the colon are adenocarcinomas arising from pre-existing adenomas. Most tumors are annular constricting lesions, 2 to 6 cm in diameter, with raised everted edges and ulcerated mucosa (Fig. 46.5). Polypoid tumors are less common, some having the frond-like appearance of villous carcinoma (Fig. 46.6). Infiltrating scirrhous tumors, so common in gastric carcinoma, are rare in the large intestine, unless the patient has ulcerative colitis. The tumor spreads by direct invasion through the bowel wall into pericolonic fat (Fig. 46.7) and adjacent organs, lymphatic channels to regional nodes, and hematogenously through the portal veins to the liver and systemic circulation. Intraperitoneal seeding from a tumor that penetrates the colon wall may also occur. Obstruction is the most frequent complication. Other complications are uncommon but include perforation (Fig. 46.8), intussusception, abscess, and fistula formation. Up to 20% of patients have a second tumor of the large bowel at diagnosis, usually an adenoma or another carcinoma. Approximately 5% of patients will have a second colorectal carcinoma either simultaneously or subsequently diagnosed. Patients with ulcerative colitis, Crohn disease, familial adenomatous polyposis

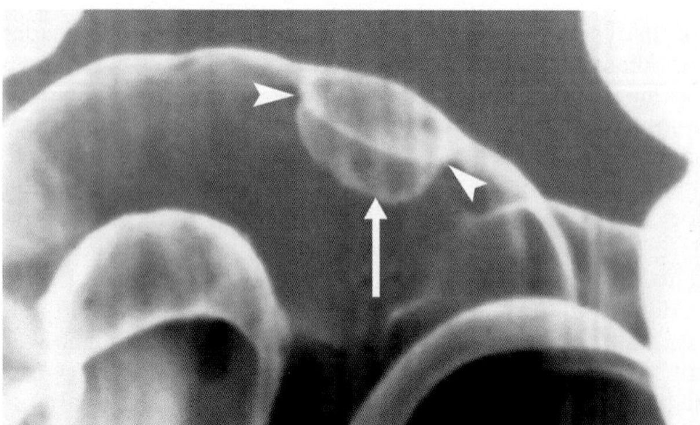

FIGURE 46.4. **Bowler Hat Sign** is produced by barium coating both the body of the polyp (*arrow*) and the recesses (*arrowheads*) between the base of the lesion and the normal colonic mucosa.

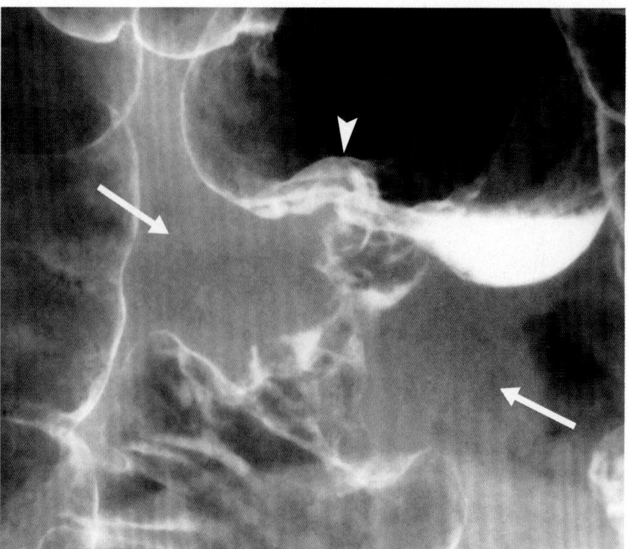

FIGURE 46.5. **Colon Carcinoma—Barium Enema.** Radiograph of the sigmoid colon from a double-contrast barium enema demonstrates a characteristic "apple core" constricting lesion of colon carcinoma. The lumen is markedly narrowed and shoulders of the tumor cause a mass impression on the adjacent distended lumen (*arrowhead*). The size of the tumor (between *arrows*) can be surmised from the marked narrowing of the lumen.

syndrome, and Peutz–Jeghers syndrome are at increased risk of colon carcinoma.

Local disease staging is best evaluated with transrectal or colonoscopic US. CT and MR are used for more advanced disease and to detect recurrence. Microscopic invasion through the bowel wall and tumor involvement of normal sized lymph nodes is not well detected by CT or MR. Diffusion-weighted MR shows improved detection of lymph node metastases. Cross-sectional imaging findings include (a) polypoid primary tumor (usually >1 cm) (Fig. 46.6); (b) "apple core" lesions with bulky, irregular thickening of the colon wall and irregular narrowing of the lumen (Fig. 46.9); (c) cystic, necrotic, and hemorrhagic areas within the tumor mass, especially when the tumor is large; (d) linear soft tissue stranding into the pericolonic fat often indicative of tumor extension through the bowel wall; (e) enlarged regional lymph nodes (>1 cm)

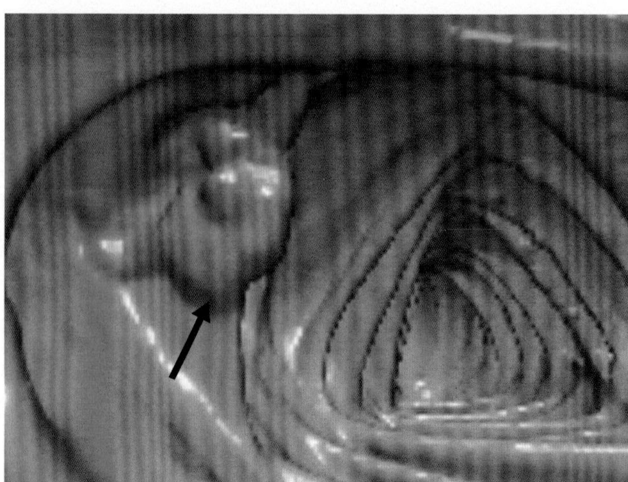

FIGURE 46.6. **Colon Carcinoma—CT Colonography.** A colon carcinoma (*arrow*) has the CT colonography appearance of a multinodular villous polyp.

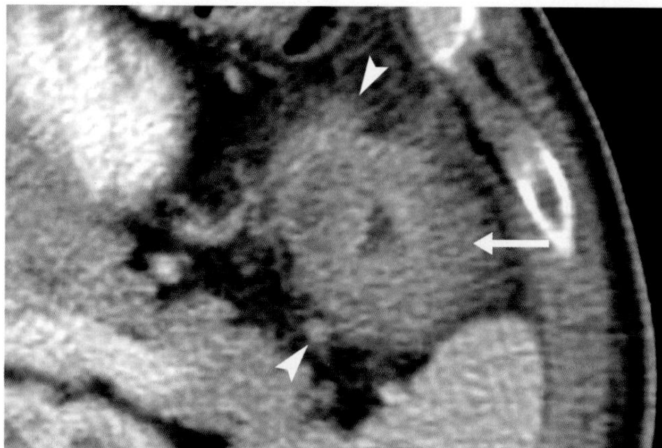

FIGURE 46.7. **Colon Carcinoma—CT.** Axial plane MDCT image shows circumferential thickening (*arrow*) of the wall of the colon near the splenic flexure. Nodules of tumor (*arrowheads*) in the pericolonic fat are signs of tumor invasion through the colon wall, a finding confirmed at surgery.

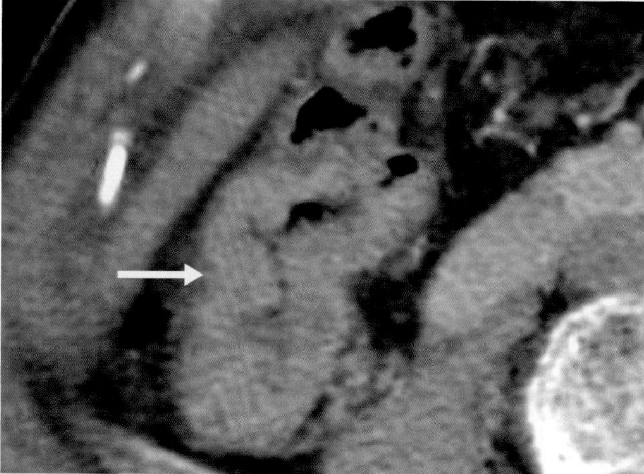

FIGURE 46.9. **Colon Carcinoma Wall Thickening.** Axial image from MDCT shows marked circumferential nodular wall thickening (*fat arrow*) of the ascending colon. The lumen (*skinny arrow*) is dramatically and irregularly narrowed.

representing lymphatic spread of tumor; and (f) distant metastases, especially in the liver. When tumors cause colonic obstruction edema and/or ischemia may thicken the wall of the uninvolved colon proximal to the tumor.

A variety of improved therapies in the past decade have increased survival of advanced (stage IV) and metastatic colon cancer from 6 months to 2 years increasing the importance of CT and MR imaging in these patients. Tumor recurrences are most common (a) at the operative site, near the bowel anastomosis, (b) in lymph nodes that drain the operative site, (c) in the peritoneal cavity, and (d) in the liver and distant organs. The entire abdominal cavity must be surveyed to detect tumor recurrence. CT, MR, and PET-CT are utilized to demonstrate response to therapy and tumor recurrence.

Polyps and Colon Cancer. Because the majority of colorectal cancers are believed to arise from pre-existing adenomatous polyps, the detection of colon polyps is a major indication for

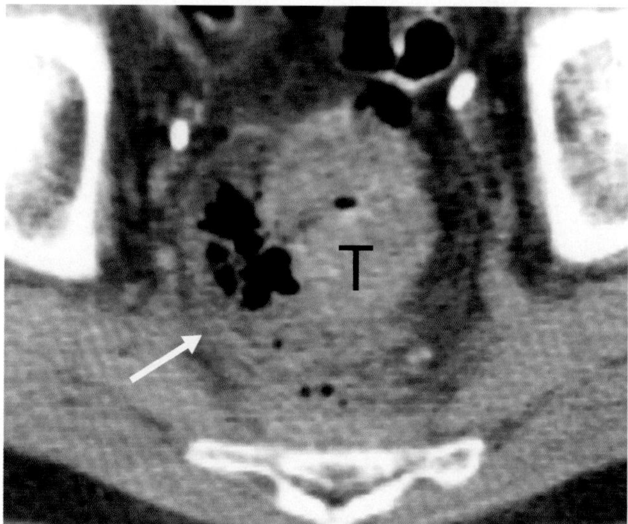

FIGURE 46.8. **Rectal Carcinoma With Perforation.** An aggressive rectal carcinoma (*T*) markedly thickens the wall of the rectum and narrows its lumen to a tiny channel (*skinny arrow*). The tumor has perforated the wall of the rectum resulting in a perirectal abscess (*fat arrow*) shown on CT as soft tissue and fluid density with air bubbles replacing the perirectal fat.

colonoscopy and imaging studies of the colon. The following "rules of thumb" can be applied. Polyps less than 5 mm are almost all hyperplastic, with a risk of malignancy less than 0.5%. Polyps 5 to 10 mm size are 90% adenomas, with a risk of malignancy of 1%. Polyps 10 to 20 mm in size are usually adenomas, with a risk of malignancy of 10%. Polyps larger than 20 mm are 50% malignant.

Hyperplastic polyps are nonneoplastic mucosal proliferations. They are round and sessile. Nearly all are less than 5 mm in size.

Adenomatous polyps are distinctly premalignant and a major risk for development of colorectal carcinoma. Adenomatous polyps are neoplasms with a core of connective tissue. Approximately 5% to 10% of the population older than 40 years have adenomatous polyps.

Hamartomatous polyps (juvenile polyps) represent 1% of colon polyps. They are a common cause of rectal bleeding in children. The Peutz–Jeghers polyp is type of hamartomatous polyp.

Inflammatory polyps are usually multiple and associated with inflammatory bowel disease (Fig. 46.10). They account for less than 0.5% of colorectal polyps.

Familial adenomatous polyposis syndrome is approximately two-thirds inherited and one-third spontaneous. The inheritance pattern is autosomal dominant with high

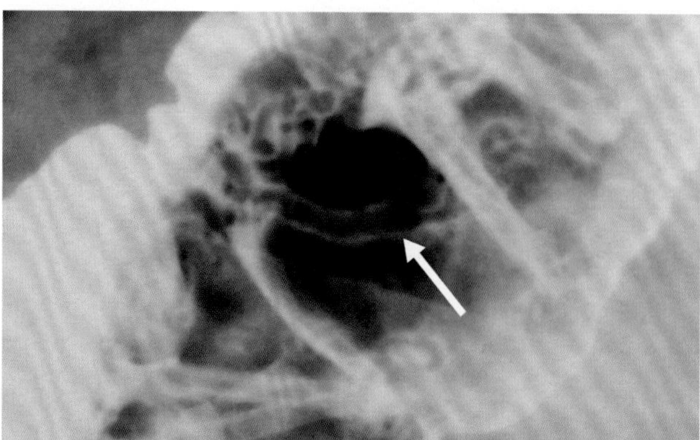

FIGURE 46.10. **Postinflammatory Filiform Polyps.** Detail view from an air-contrast barium enema in a patient with ulcerative colitis shows the characteristic worm-like appearance of postinflammatory filiform polyps (*arrow*). Numerous polyps are present.

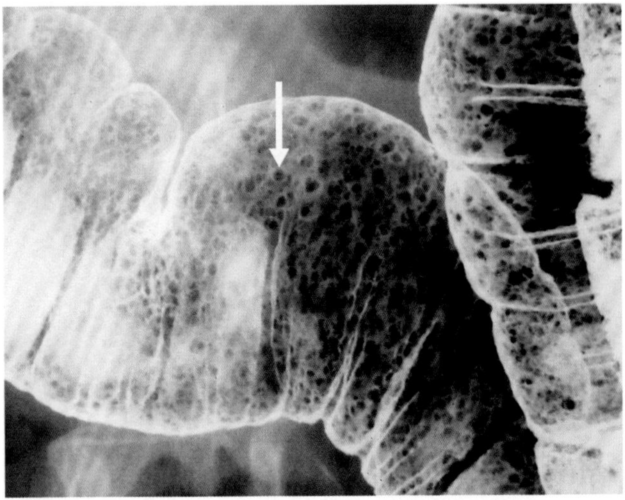

FIGURE 46.11. Familial Adenomatous Polyposis Syndrome. Cone-down image from a double-contrast barium enema reveals the colonic mucosa to be carpeted with innumerable small polyps seen as tiny filling defects (*arrow*).

penetrance. The polyps are tubulovillous adenomas which usually are evident by age 20. Colorectal cancer will eventually develop in nearly all patients, so total colectomy with rectal mucosectomy and ileoanal pouch construction is the current recommended therapy. Polyps typically carpet the entire colon (Fig. 46.11). Patients are at risk for numerous extracolonic manifestations including carcinomas of the small bowel, thyroid carcinoma, and mesenteric fibromatosis. Patients with associated bone and skin abnormalities including cortical thickening of the ribs and long bones, osteomas of the skull, supernumerary teeth, exostoses of the mandible, and dermal fibromas, desmoids, and epidermal inclusion cysts have been diagnosed as *Gardner syndrome*. Those with associated tumors of the central nervous system have been grouped as *Turcot syndrome*. These are variations of the same disease.

Hamartomatous Polyposis Syndromes. Hamartomatous polyps are nonneoplastic growths with a smooth muscle core covered by mature glandular epithelium. The hamartomatous polyps associated with the various syndromes have minor histologic differences. These lesions carry no risk of malignant transformation. However, patients with the hamartomatous polyposis syndromes may also develop adenomatous polyps, which do carry a risk of malignancy.

Peutz–Jeghers syndrome predominantly involves the small bowel, but most cases have gastric and colon polyps as well. The condition is autosomal dominant with incomplete penetrance. Dark pigmented spots on the skin and mucous membranes are characteristic. Risk of carcinoma arising from coexisting adenomatous polyps is 2% to 20%. Patients are also at risk for breast cancer, uterine and ovarian cancer, and early age cancer of the pancreas.

Cowden disease is a syndrome of multiple hamartomas including hamartomatous polyposis of the GI tract, with goiter and thyroid adenomas and increased risk of breast cancer and transitional cell carcinoma of the urinary tract. The syndrome is autosomal dominant and affects mainly Caucasians. All patients have mucocutaneous lesions with facial papules, oral papillomas, and palmoplantar keratoses.

Cronkhite–Canada syndrome is a disease of older patients with a mean age of onset of 60 years. Polyps are distributed throughout the stomach, small bowel, and colon. Associated skin findings include nail atrophy, brownish skin pigmentation, and alopecia. Patients present with watery diarrhea and protein-losing enteropathy.

Lymphoid hyperplasia may involve the colon. The normal lymphoid follicular pattern of diffuse tiny nodules 1 to 3 mm in diameter with characteristic umbilication is most common in the terminal ileum and cecum but may involve any portion of the colon. The nodular lymphoid hyperplasia pattern of diffuse nodules larger than 4 mm is associated with allergic, infectious, and inflammatory disorders.

Lymphoma. The colon is less commonly involved with lymphoma than the stomach or small bowel. Most are non-Hodgkin B-cell lymphoma. Involvement of the cecum or rectum is most common with anal and rectal lymphoma frequent in AIDS patients. Morphologic patterns include small to large nodules that may ulcerate, excavitate and perforate, and diffuse infiltration of the bowel wall resulting in bulbous folds and thickened bowel wall (Fig. 46.12). As in the small intestine, marked narrowing of the lumen is uncommon and aneurysmal dilation occurs when transmural disease destroys innervation. The diffuse multinodular form may be difficult to differentiate from nodular lymphoid hyperplasia. Lymphoma nodules vary in size although lymphoid hyperplasia nodules are uniform in size.

Gastrointestinal stromal tumors (GISTs) account for nearly all mesenchymal tumors of the colon. True colonic leiomyomas and leiomyosarcomas are very rare. GISTs are much less common in the colon than in the stomach and small bowel accounting for only 7% of the total. As in the remainder of the GI tract, they may appear as exophytic, mural, or intraluminal masses. Ulceration is relatively frequent. Hemorrhage, cystic change, necrosis, and calcification are more common in larger tumors (Fig. 46.13).

Lipoma is the most common submucosal tumor of the colon. It is most frequent in the cecum and ascending colon. Nearly 40% present with intussusception. Barium studies demonstrate a smooth, well-defined elliptical filling defect, usually 1 to 3 cm in diameter. The tumors are soft and change shape with compression. CT or MR demonstration of a fat density tumor is definitive (Fig. 46.14).

Extrinsic lesions commonly cause mass effect on the colon that may simulate intrinsic disease (Fig. 46.15).

Endometriosis commonly implants on the sigmoid colon and rectum. Defects are frequently multiple and of variable

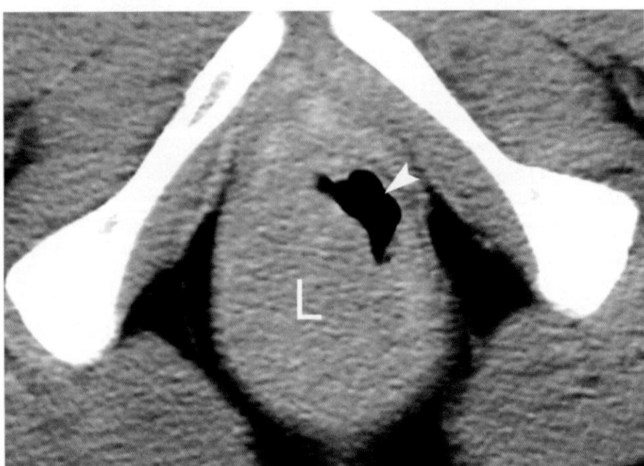

FIGURE 46.12. Rectal Lymphoma. CT demonstrates a prominent mass of lymphoma (*L*) that causes irregular narrowing of the lumen (*arrowhead*) of the rectum. Note the homogeneous attenuation of the lymphomatous mass. This CT appearance is indistinguishable from adenocarcinoma of the rectum.

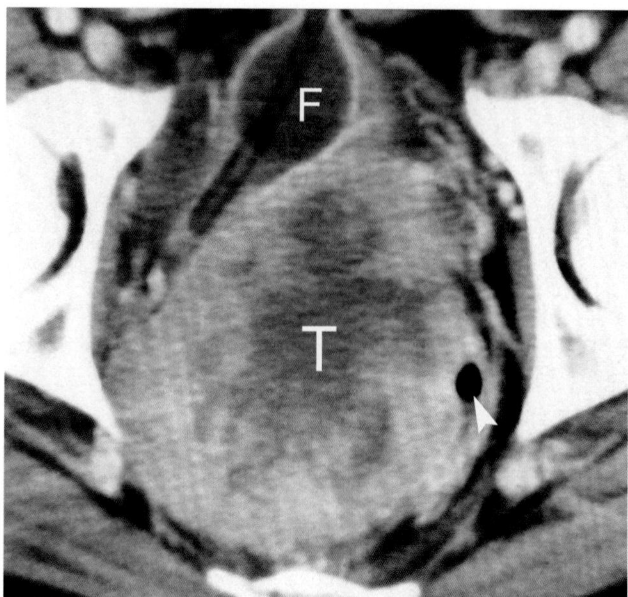

FIGURE 46.13. **Malignant GIST of the Rectum.** A CT scan shows a large tumor (*T*) with an irregular low-density area of central necrosis arising exophytically in the wall of the rectum narrowing the lumen (*arrowhead*), which is displaced laterally and anteriorly. The tumor obstructed the bladder outlet, necessitating placement of a suprapubic Foley catheter (*F*).

size. Lesions are commonly within the cul-de-sac. Barium studies demonstrate sharply defined defects that compress but do not usually encircle the lumen. CT demonstrates complex cystic pelvic masses with high-density fluid components. Multiple pelvic organs may be incorporated into the mass. MR demonstrates masses with signal characteristics of hemorrhage.

Benign pelvis masses such as ovarian cysts, cystadenomas, teratomas, and uterine fibroids produce smooth extrinsic mass impressions on the colonic wall. The colon is displaced but not invaded.

Malignant pelvic tumors and metastases may involve the colon by contiguous spread, spread along mesenteric fascial planes, by intraperitoneal seeding, through lymphatic channels, or by embolus through blood vessels. The involved colon demonstrates thickening of the wall, separation of folds, spiculation, angulations, narrowing, and serosal plaques. Metastases often cannot be differentiated from primary tumors by imaging methods. Crohn disease and metastatic disease may

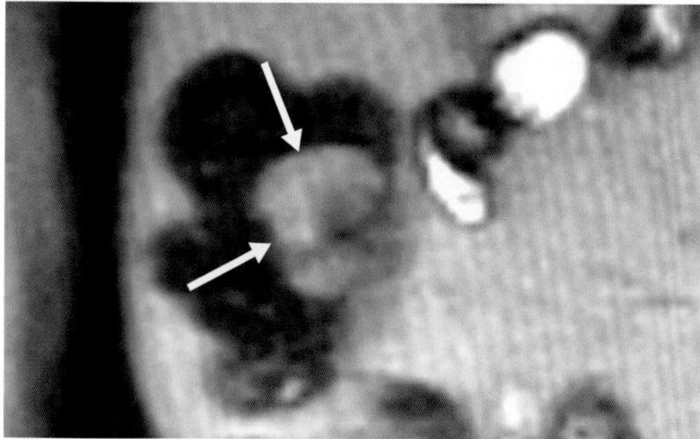

FIGURE 46.14. **Lipoma of the Colon.** Coronal T2-weighted MR shows the smooth rounded surface and fat density of a lipoma (*arrows*) arising from the wall of the ascending colon.

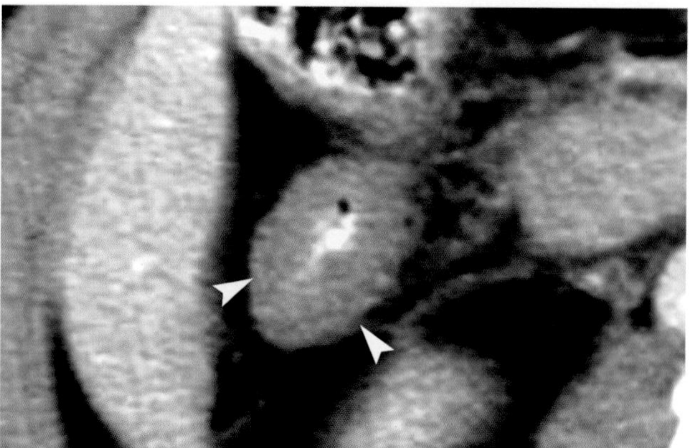

FIGURE 46.15. **Metastases to Colon.** Metastases (*arrowheads*) from breast carcinoma to the ascending colon mimic colon carcinoma.

also look exactly alike radiographically. CT or MR demonstrates contiguous involvement of the colon and rectum by pelvic tumors.

Extrinsic inflammatory processes, such as appendicitis, pelvic abscess, diverticular abscess, and pelvic inflammatory disease, cause mass effect, asymmetric tethering, and spiculation.

Colon Inflammatory Disease

Ulcerative colitis is an uncommon idiopathic inflammatory disease involving primarily the mucosa and submucosa of the colon. The peak age for its appearance is 20 to 40 years, but onset of disease after age 50 is common. The disease consists of superficial ulcerations, edema, and hyperemia. The radiographic hallmarks of ulcerative colitis are granular mucosa, confluent shallow ulcerations, symmetry of disease around the lumen, and continuous confluent diffuse involvement (Table 46.1). An early fine, granular pattern is produced by mucosal hyperemia and edema that precedes ulceration. Superficial ulcers spread to cover the entire mucosal surface. The mucosa is stippled with barium adhering to the superficial ulcers. *Collar button ulcers* (Fig. 46.16) are deeper ulcerations of thickened edematous mucosa with crypt abscesses extending in the submucosa. A coarse granular pattern is produced later by the replacement of diffusely ulcerated mucosa with granulation tissue. Late changes include a variety of polypoid lesions. *Pseudopolyps* are mucosal remnants in areas of extensive ulceration.

Inflammatory polyps are small islands of inflamed mucosa. *Postinflammatory polyps* are mucosal tags that are seen in quiescent phases of the disease. *Filiform polyps* are postinflammatory polyps with a characteristic worm-like appearance. They are typically seen in an otherwise normal appearing colon. *Hyperplastic polyps* may occur during healing after mucosal injury. Involvement typically extends from the rectum proximally in a symmetric and continuous pattern. The terminal ileum is nearly always normal. Rare *backwash ileitis* may produce an ulcerated but patulous terminal ileum. CT findings include (a) wall thickening, often with "halo sign" of low-density submucosal edema (Figs. 46.17 and 46.18), (b) narrowing of the lumen of the colon, and (c) pseudopolyps, and pneumatosis coli with megacolon. Complications of ulcerative colitis include (a) strictures, usually 2 to 3 cm or more in length and commonly involving the transverse colon and rectum, (b) colorectal adenocarcinoma, with an approximate risk of 1% per year of disease, (c) toxic megacolon (2% to 5% of cases) may be the initial manifestation, and (d) massive hemorrhage. Associated extraintestinal diseases include sacroiliitis

TABLE 46.1

ULCERATIVE COLITIS VERSUS CROHN COLITIS

■ ULCERATIVE COLITIS	■ CROHN COLITIS
Circumferential disease	Eccentric disease
Regional (continuous disease)	Skip lesions (discontinuous disease)
Symmetric disease	Asymmetric disease
Predominantly left-sided	Predominantly right-sided
Rectum nearly always present (95%)	Rectum normal in 50%
Confluent shallow ulcers	Confluent deep ulcers
No aphthous ulcers	Aphthous ulcers early
Collar button ulcers	Transverse and longitudinal ulcers
Small bowel not involved except for terminal ileum	Involves any small bowel segment
Terminal ileum usually normal	Terminal ileum usually diseased
Terminal ileum patulous	Terminal ileum narrowed
Ileocecal valve open	Ileocecal valve stenosed
No pseudodiverticula	Pseudodiverticula
No fistulae	Fistulae common
High risk of cancer	Low risk of cancer
Risk of toxic megacolon	Low risk of toxic megacolon

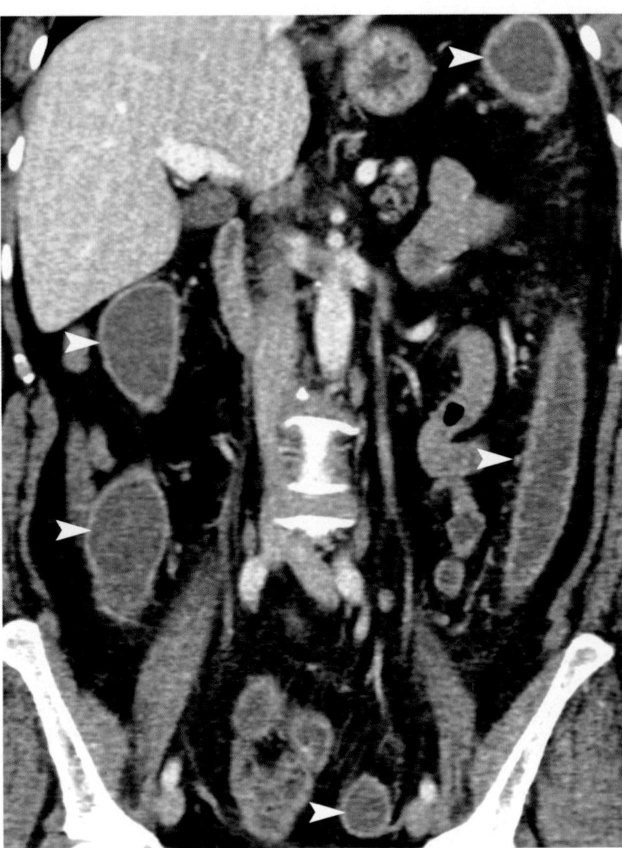

FIGURE 46.17. **Ulcerative Colitis—CT.** Coronal CT enterography reveals involvement of the entire colon (*arrowheads*) by ulcerative colitis. Note the circumferential and uniform wall thickening. The rectum was involved. The terminal ileum was normal.

mimicking ankylosing spondylitis (20% of cases), eye lesions including uveitis and iritis (10% of cases), cholangitis, and an increased incidence of thromboembolic disease.

Crohn disease involves the colon in two-thirds of all cases and is isolated to the colon in approximately one-third of all cases. Hallmarks of Crohn colitis include early aphthous ulcers, later confluent deep ulcerations, predominant right colon disease, discontinuous involvement with intervening regions of normal bowel, asymmetric involvement of the bowel

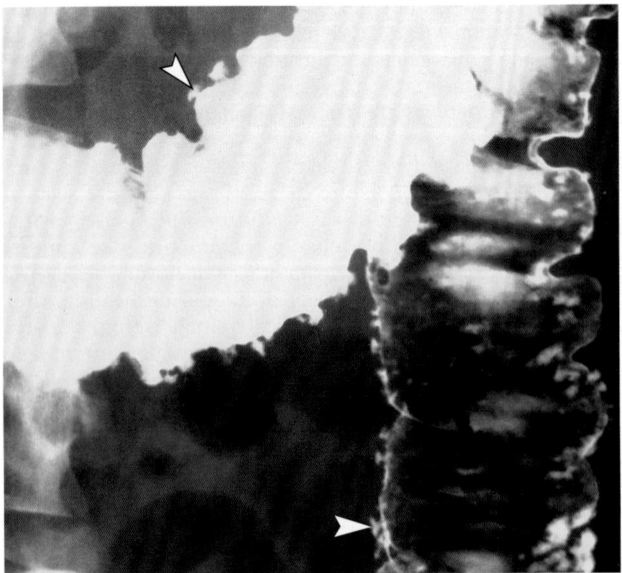

FIGURE 46.16. **Ulcerative Colitis—Collar Button Ulcers.** Double-contrast barium enema shows a pattern of continuous involvement of the colon with innumerable submucosal collar button ulcers (*arrowheads*).

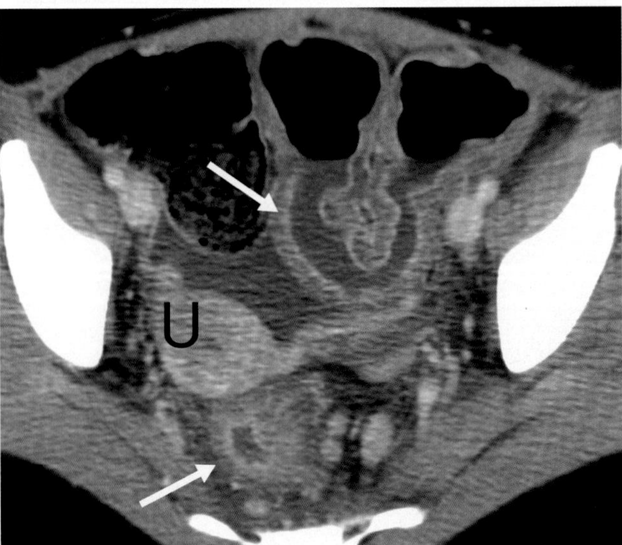

FIGURE 46.18. **Ulcerative Colitis—CT.** Image through the pelvis shows marked circumferential thickening (*arrows*) of the wall of the sigmoid colon and rectum. Inflammatory reaction extends into the pericolic tissues. Free intraperitoneal fluid is seen anterior to the uterus (*U*).

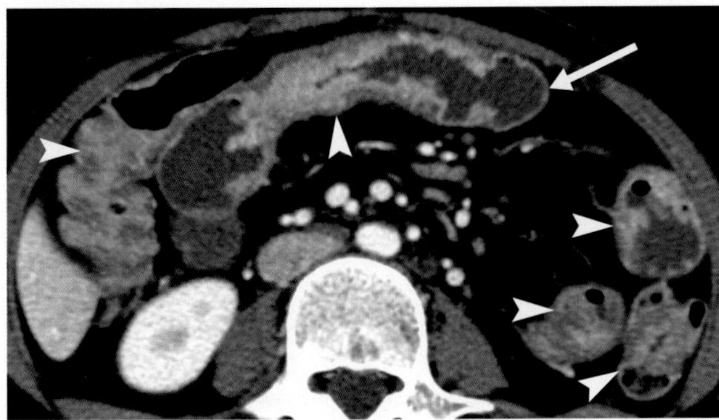

FIGURE 46.19. **Crohn Colitis—CT.** Scan through the upper abdomen demonstrates multiple loops of colon (*arrowheads*) with asymmetric and nodular wall thickening characteristic of Crohn colitis. Note that some sections of bowel (*arrow*) have normal wall thickness indicating skip lesions.

wall, strictures, fistulas, and sinus formation (Figs. 46.19 and 46.20; Table 46.1). Pseudodiverticula of the colon are formed by asymmetric fibrosis on one side of the lumen, causing saccular outpouches on the other side. Involvement of the rectum is characterized by deep rectal ulcers and multiple fistulous tracts to the skin. Both MR and CT show intense mucosal enhancement reflecting hyperemia of active inflammation.

Infectious colitis may be caused by a variety of bacteria (*Salmonella, Shigella, Escherichia coli*), parasites, viruses (cytomegalovirus, herpes), and fungi (histoplasmosis, mucormycosis). Most cause a pancolitis with edema and inflammatory wall thickening with infiltration of pericolonic fat. Pericolonic fluid and intraperitoneal fluid may be present (Fig. 46.21).

Toxic megacolon is a potentially fatal condition characterized by marked colonic distention and risk of perforation. It occurs as a complication of fulminant colitis often caused by ulcerative colitis, Crohn disease, pseudomembranous colitis, use of antidiarrheal drugs, and hypokalemia. Transmural inflammation causes deep ulcers that may extend to the serosa surface, large areas of denuded mucosa, and loss of muscle tone. Radiographic findings include (a) marked dilation of the colon (transverse colon >6 cm) with absence of haustral markings (Fig. 46.22), (b) edema and thickening of the colon wall, (c) pneumatosis coli, and (d) evidence of perforation. Barium studies should be avoided because of risk of perforation.

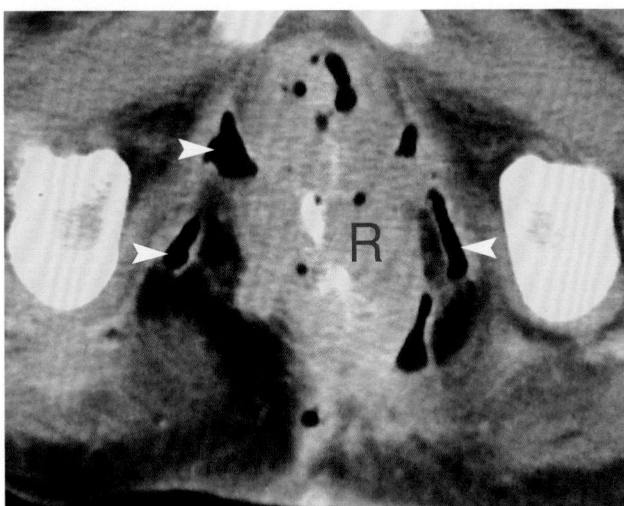

FIGURE 46.20. **Crohn Colitis—Perianal Fistulas.** Scan through the rectum shows multiple perirectal tracts of air (*arrowheads*) indicating fistulas extending into the ischiorectal fossae marking the perineum. The rectum (*R*) is extensively involved with nodular wall thickening and inflammation.

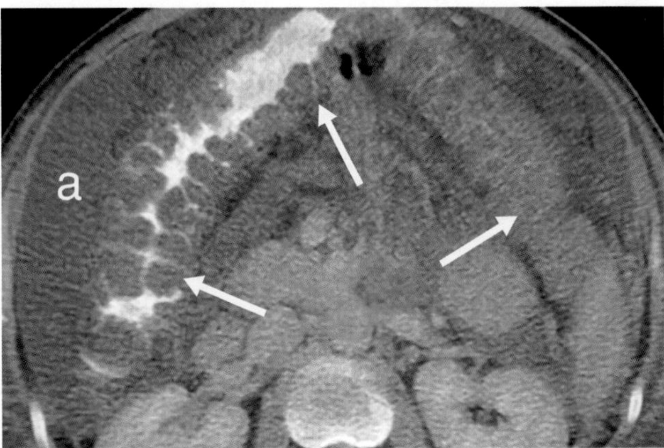

FIGURE 46.21. **Infectious Colitis.** CT demonstrates marked thickening of the wall (*arrows*) of the colon. Pericolonic fat is diffusely infiltrated and ascites (*a*) is present. This patient was proven to have colitis caused by cytomegalovirus (CMV).

Pseudomembranous colitis is an inflammatory disease of the colon, and occasionally involving the small bowel, characterized

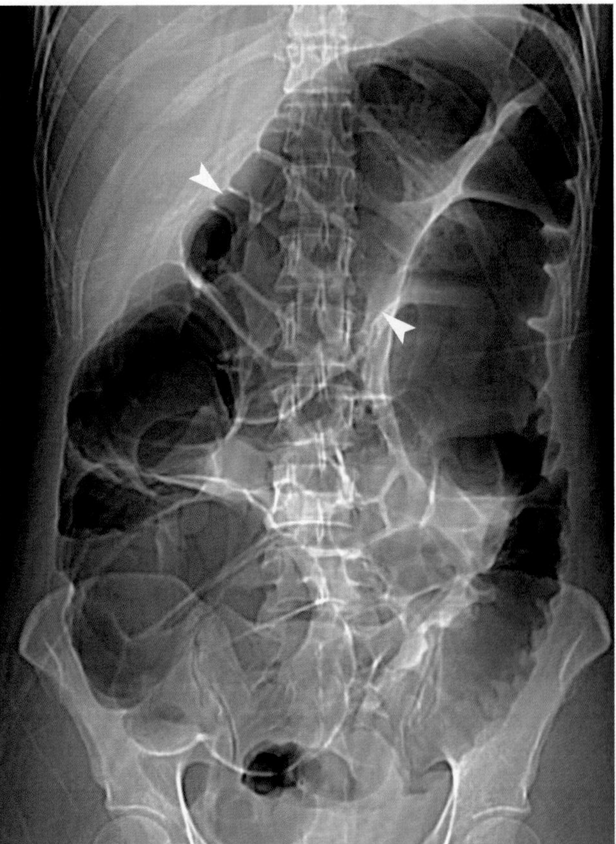

FIGURE 46.22. **Toxic Megacolon.** CT scanogram in a patient with history of ulcerative colitis presenting with fever, abdominal pain, and distention shows diffuse marked dilation of the colon. The transverse colon measures (between *arrowheads*) more than 10 cm in diameter. The bowel perforated and the patient died.

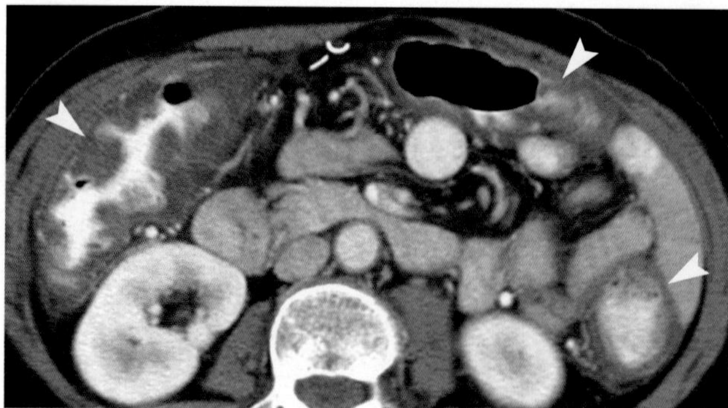

FIGURE 46.23. **Pseudomembranous Colitis.** The wall of the colon (*arrowheads*) is markedly and diffusely thickened trapping intraluminal contrast between the folds producing the "accordion sign" at the hepatic flexure. This patient developed *Clostridium difficile* colitis following broad spectrum antibiotic therapy.

by the presence of a pseudomembrane of necrotic debris and overgrowth of *Clostridium difficile*. There are many contributing causes including antibiotics (any that change bowel flora), intestinal ischemia (especially following surgery), irradiation, long-term steroids, shock, and colonic obstruction. The disease presents as fulminant inflammatory bowel disease with diarrhea and foul stools. Conventional radiographs may reveal (a) dilated colon, (b) nodular thickening of the haustra, and (c) ascites. The colon may be greatly dilated, and toxic megacolon has been reported. Barium enema demonstrates an irregular lumen with thumbprint indentations similar to ischemic colitis. Superficial ulcers are common. Plaque-like defects on the mucosal surface are due to the pseudomembranes. The colitis is frequently patchy in distribution with sparing of the rectum. The condition is commonly first detected on CT which shows (a) marked wall thickening up to 30 mm (average 15 mm) with halo or target appearance, (b) characteristic stripes of intraluminal contrast media trapped between nodular areas of wall thickening (the "accordion sign") (Fig. 46.23), (c) mild pericolonic fat inflammation disproportionate with the marked colonic wall inflammation, and (d) ascites (35%).

Amebiasis is an infection by the protozoan parasite *Entamoeba histolytica*. The disease is worldwide but particularly common in South Africa, Central and South America, and Asia. At least 5% of the population of the United States harbor amebae. Encysted amebae are ingested with contaminated food and water. The cyst capsule is dissolved in the small bowel, releasing trophozoites that migrate to the colon and burrow into the mucosa, forming small abscesses. The infection can spread throughout the body by hematogenous embolization or direct invasion. Amebic colitis produces dysentery with frequent bloody mucoid stools. Barium studies demonstrate a disease that closely mimics Crohn colitis with aphthous ulcers, deep ulcers, asymmetric disease, and skip areas. The cecum and rectum are the primary sites of colonic disease. The terminal ileum is characteristically not involved. Complications include strictures, amebomas consisting of a hard fixed mass of granulation tissue that may simulate carcinoma, toxic megacolon, and fistulas, particularly following surgical intervention. Amebic liver abscess results from the spread of infection through the portal system and may be complicated by diaphragm perforation, pleural effusion, and thoracic disease.

Typhlitis (neutropenic colitis) is a potentially fatal infection of the cecum and ascending colon usually seen in patients who are neutropenic and immunocompromised by chemotherapy. Concentric, often marked, thickening of the wall of the cecum

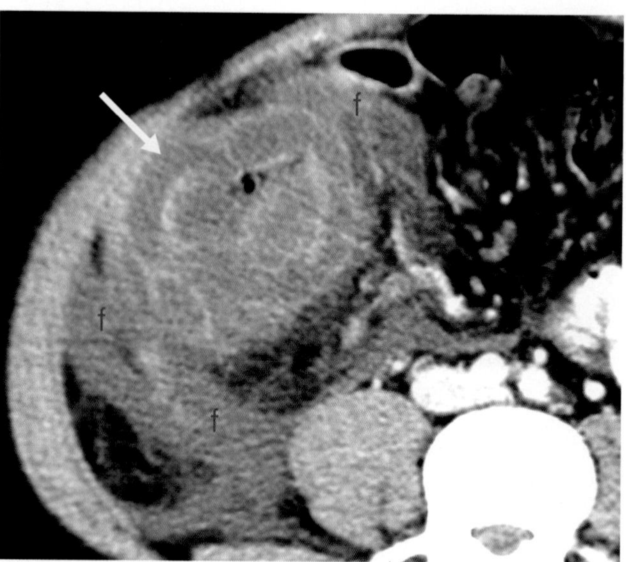

FIGURE 46.24. **Typhlitis.** The wall of the cecum (*arrow*) is markedly thickened and edematous demonstrating the target sign. The pericecal fat is infiltrated with fluid (*f*). The mucosa enhances weakly indicating ischemia. This patient was neutropenic because of chemotherapy.

and ascending colon with prominent pericolonic inflammatory changes are characteristic (Fig. 46.24). Patients are at risk for colon ischemia.

Ischemic colitis mimics ulcerative colitis and Crohn colitis both clinically and radiographically. The causes of ischemic colitis include arterial occlusion caused by arteriosclerosis, vasculitis, or arterial emboli; venous thrombosis due to neoplasm, oral contraceptives, and other hypercoagulation conditions; and low flow states such as hypotension, congestive heart failure, and cardiac arrhythmias. The pattern of involvement generally follows the distribution of a major artery and is the clue to diagnosis. The superior mesenteric artery supplies the right colon from the cecum to the splenic flexure. The inferior mesenteric artery supplies the left colon from the splenic flexure to the rectum. The splenic flexure region and descending colon are watershed areas most susceptible to ischemic colitis. Early changes include thickening of the colon wall, spasm, and spiculation. As blood and edema accumulate within the bowel wall, multiple nodular defects are produced in a pattern called "thumbprinting" (Fig. 46.25). Progression of the disease results in ulcerations, perforation, scarring, and stricture. CT demonstrates symmetrical or lobulated thickening of the bowel wall with an irregularly narrowed lumen. Submucosal edema may produce a low-density ring bordering on the lumen (target sign). Air in the abnormal bowel wall (pneumatosis) is highly suggestive of ischemia. Thrombus may occasionally be demonstrated within the superior mesenteric artery or vein.

AIDS-associated colitis occurs most commonly in AIDS patients with CD4 lymphocyte counts below 200. Causative organisms are most commonly cytomegalovirus or cryptosporidiosis, although the human immunodeficiency virus itself may cause ulceration and colitis. Right colon disease is most common with wall thickening and ulceration.

Radiation colitis may be indistinguishable radiographically from early ulcerative colitis (Fig. 46.26). The diagnosis is made by confirmation of the involved colon being within an irradiation field. The rectosigmoid region is most commonly involved due to radiation of pelvic malignancy. Colitis is produced by a slowly progressive endarteritis that causes ischemia and fibrosis.

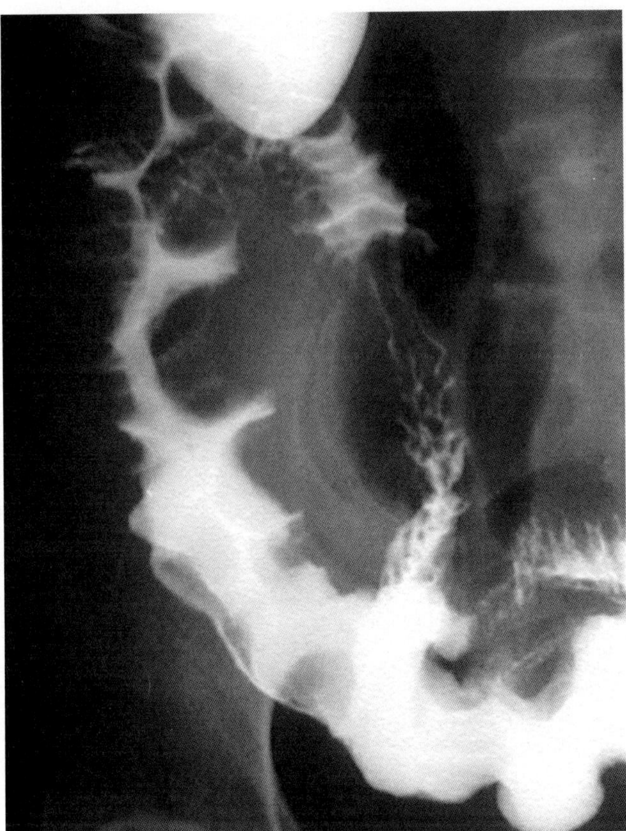

FIGURE 46.25. **Ischemic Colitis.** Barium enema shows thumbprinting pattern involving the proximal portion of a redundant transverse colon.

Radiographic findings include thickened folds, spiculation, ulceration, stricture, and occasionally fistula formation. Fibrosis results in a rigid, featureless bowel. Healing may include formation of pseudopolyps and postinflammatory polyps.

Cathartic colon is due to chronic irritation of the mucosa by laxatives including castor oil, bisacodyl, and senna. The involved colon may be dilated and without haustra, or narrowed. The right colon is most commonly affected. Bizarre contractions are often observed. The diagnosis is made by clinical history.

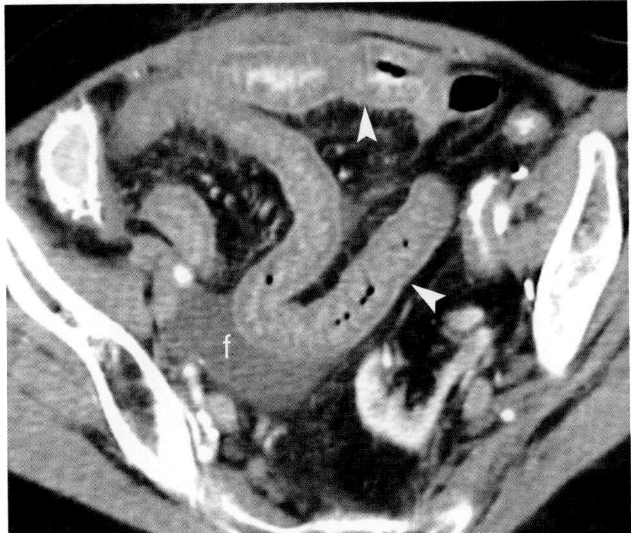

FIGURE 46.26. **Radiation Colitis.** The wall of the sigmoid colon (*arrowheads*) is thickened and stiffened by radiation colitis. The patient is 3 years post radiation therapy for cervical carcinoma. Free intraperitoneal fluid (*f*) is present.

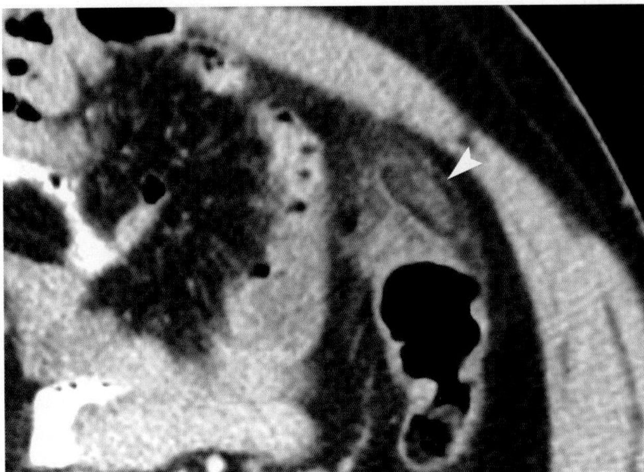

FIGURE 46.27. **Epiploic Appendagitis.** CT shows pericolonic inflammation adjacent to the descending colon with a "ring sign" (*arrowhead*) of inflammation surrounding central fat, a finding characteristic of epiploic appendagitis.

Tuberculous colitis is increasingly common especially in immunocompromised patients. Imaging findings mimic Crohn disease: (a) marked thickening of the wall of the colon and terminal ileum; (b) markedly enlarged lymph nodes, often with low central attenuation or calcification; (c) common fistulae and sinus tracts; (d) colitis may be segmental or diffuse; (e) short strictures may mimic colon cancer; and (f) thickening of the peritoneum and extensive abdominal adenopathy suggest the disease.

Epiploic appendagitis is a cause of abdominal pain that may mimic appendicitis, diverticulitis, and colitis. The epiploic appendages are pedunculated fatty structures that occur in rows on the external aspect of the colon adjacent to the anterior and posterior taenia coli. They occur in greatest concentration in the cecum and sigmoid colon sparing the rectum. Epiploic appendagitis is caused by ischemic infarction of these structures, often resulting from torsion. Patients present with focal abdominal pain, tenderness, and low-grade fever. Diagnosis is usually made by CT showing (a) 1- to 4-cm ovoid mass with central fat density and surrounding inflammation abutting the wall of the colon; (b) a hyperdense enhancing rim surrounds the mass ("ring sign") (Fig. 46.27); (c) inflammatory changes may extend into the adjacent peritoneum; (d) a central high attenuation dot is often present representing the central thrombosed vessels; and (e) infracted tissue may eventually calcify.

Diverticular Disease

Colon diverticulosis is an acquired condition in which the mucosa and muscularis mucosae herniate through the muscularis propria of the colon wall, producing a saccular outpouching. Colon diverticula are classified as false diverticula because the sacs lack all of the elements of the normal colon wall. The condition is rare under age 25, but increases with age thereafter to affect 50% of the population over age 75. The major risk factor for diverticulosis is a low-residue diet, typical of Western countries. The condition is very uncommon in cultures where a high-residue diet is the norm, such as African native

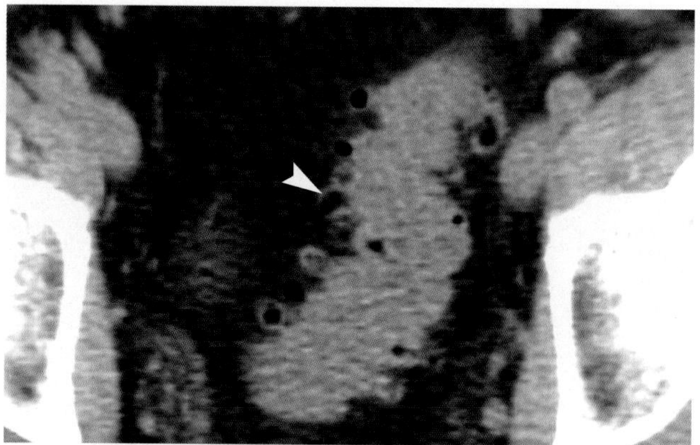

FIGURE 46.28. **Diverticulosis.** A noncontrast CT scan demonstrates air-filled outpouchings (*arrowhead*) representing diverticuli in the sigmoid colon. Note the absence of soft tissue stranding or fluid in the adjacent fat indicating that no inflammation is present.

populations. The formation of diverticular sacs is usually associated with thickening of the muscularis propria, including both the circular muscle and the taenia coli. Severely affected portions of bowel are usually shortened in length, resulting in crowding of the thickened circular muscle bundles. Muscle dysfunction associated with diverticulosis may result in pain and tenderness without evidence of inflammation. Diverticulosis without diverticulitis is a cause of painless colonic bleeding that may be brisk and life threatening. Conventional abdominal radiographs demonstrate diverticula as gas-filled sacs parallel to the lumen of the colon. Barium studies show diverticula as barium- or gas-filled sacs outside the colon lumen. Sacs vary in size from tiny spikes to 2 cm in diameter. Most are 5 to 10 mm in diameter. They may occur anywhere in the colon but are most common and usually most numerous in the sigmoid colon. Some sacs are reducible and may disappear with complete filling of the lumen. Others may contain fecal residue. The associated muscle abnormality is seen as thickening and crowding of the circular muscle bands with spasm and spiked irregular outline of the lumen. CT demonstrates the muscle hypertrophy as a thickened colon wall and distorted luminal contour. The diverticula are shown as well-defined gas-, fluid-, or contrast-filled sacs outside the lumen (Fig. 46.28).

Acute diverticulitis is inflammation of diverticula, usually with perforation and intramural or localized pericolic abscess. Diverticulitis eventually complicates approximately 20% of the cases of diverticulosis. Clinical signs include painful mass, localized peritoneal inflammation, fever, and leukocytosis. Complications of diverticulitis include bowel obstruction, bleeding, peritonitis, and sinus tract and fistula formation. Diverticulitis is a less common cause of colon obstruction than is colon carcinoma. Obstruction due to diverticulitis is often temporarily relieved by smooth muscle relaxants such as glucagon. Colon bleeding is more often associated with diverticulosis than diverticulitis. Most diverticular abscesses are quickly walled off and confined, but free perforation with pus and air in the peritoneal cavity and diffuse peritonitis may occur. Sinus tracts may lead to larger abscess cavities in the peritoneal or retroperitoneal compartments. Fistulas are most common to the bladder (Fig. 46.29), vagina, or skin, but may develop to any lower abdominal organ including fallopian tubes, small bowel, and other parts of the colon. Diverticulitis of the right colon may be mistaken clinically for acute appendicitis. Diverticulitis is efficiently diagnosed radiographically by barium enema or CT. Barium enema examination is considered safe except when signs of free intraperitoneal perforation or sepsis are present. Hallmarks of diverticulitis on barium enema

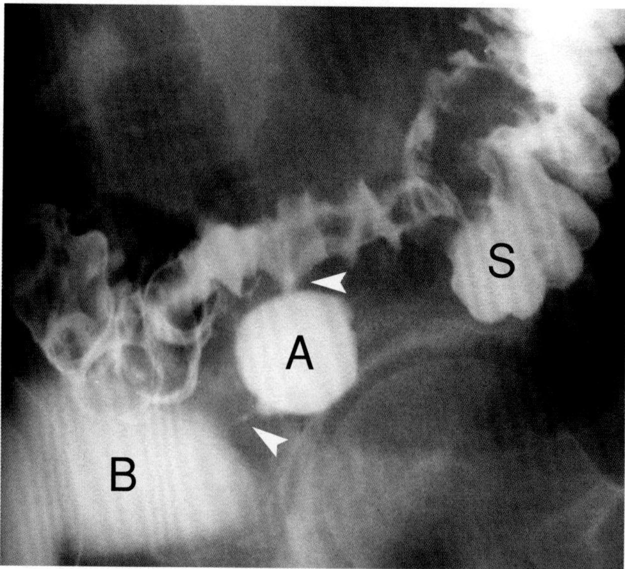

FIGURE 46.29. **Diverticular Abscess and Colovesical Fistula.** Single-contrast barium enema demonstrates barium filling a diverticular abscess (*A*) and opacifying the bladder (*B*). Thin columns of barium (*arrowheads*) outline fistulous tracts extending from the bowel lumen to abscess and from abscess to the bladder. The lumen of the sigmoid colon (*S*) is irregularly narrowed by the inflammatory process.

include deformed diverticular sacs, demonstration of abscess, and extravasation of barium outside the colon lumen. The smooth outline of the involved sacs is deformed by inflammation and perforation. The resulting abscess causes extrinsic mass effect on the adjacent colon. The colon lumen is narrowed but tapers at the margins of narrowing in distinction with the abrupt narrowing of carcinoma. Barium leaks into the abscess cavities, or forms tracks paralleling the colon lumen and often connecting multiple perforated sacs (the "double track sign"). CT excels at demonstrating the paracolic inflammation and abscess associated with diverticulitis, as well as complications such as colovesical fistula. CT findings are (a) localized wall thickening (Fig. 46.30); (b) inflammation of pericolonic fat;

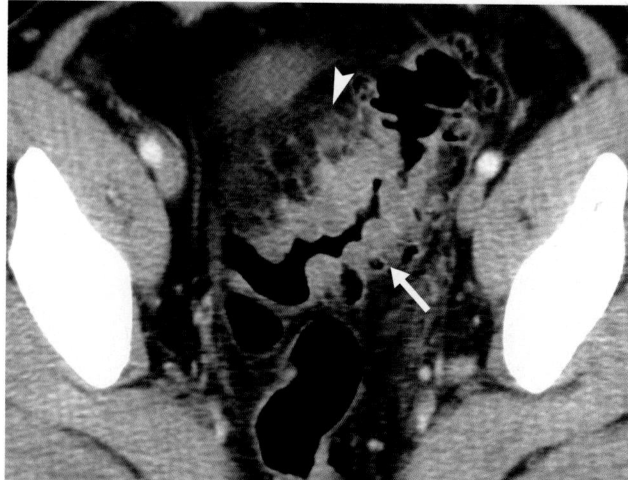

FIGURE 46.30. **Diverticulitis.** A CT scan demonstrates focal marked thickening of the wall (*arrow*) of the sigmoid colon. Stranding into the adjacent fat (*arrowhead*) is indicative of inflammation. Because of the close resemblance of diverticulitis to colon carcinoma on CT this patient must be followed to confirm complete resolution.

TABLE 46.2

CAUSES OF LOWER GASTROINTESTINAL HEMORRHAGE

■ CAUSE	■ PERCENTAGE OF CASES
Colon diverticula	40%
Angiodysplasia	17–30%
Colon carcinoma	7–16%
Polyps	8%
Rectal trauma/fissure/ hemorrhoids	7%
Duodenal ulcer	Rare
Meckel diverticulum	Rare
Bowel ischemia	Rare

(c) pericolonic abscess; (d) diverticula at or near the site of inflammation; and (e) common involvement of the adnexa with fluid collections and fistulae.

Lower Gastrointestinal Hemorrhage

Although upper GI hemorrhage is usually readily diagnosed by gastric aspirate and endoscopy, lower GI hemorrhage is difficult to localize, even during surgery. The common causes of lower GI hemorrhage are listed in Table 46.2. Radionuclide imaging studies are often selected as the screening examination of choice for confirming the presence of, and often localizing, lower GI bleeding. Technetium-99m sulfur colloid or Tc-99m-red blood cell studies are capable of detecting bleeding at rates below 0.1 mL/min. A negative scintigraphic study usually precludes the need for urgent angiography. Angiography requires bleeding rates of 0.5 mL/min or greater. However, angiography is more specific than scintigraphy in demonstrating the anatomic cause of bleeding and offers the possibility of nonoperative treatment by embolization. Colonoscopy is usually unrewarding because of the large quantities of sticky, melanotic stool. Barium enema is not used to evaluate acute hemorrhage because it usually cannot locate the source of bleeding and it will interfere with any subsequently needed angiographic procedure. CT angiography performed with intravenous contrast and without intraluminal contrast shows promise in the detection of hemorrhage by documenting intraluminal extravasation of intravenously administered contrast. CT angiography frequently also provides etiologic and anatomic detail. This information is useful to the interventional radiologist or surgeon as they may be able to identify the culprit mesenteric vessel or assess the condition of the femoral arteries prior to attempted therapy.

Angiodysplasia refers to ectasia and kinking of mucosal and submucosal veins of the colon wall. The condition results from a chronic intermittent obstruction of the veins where they penetrate the circular muscle layer. A maze of distorted, dilated vascular channels replaces the normal mucosal structures and is separated from the bowel lumen only by a layer of epithelium. Angiodysplasia is acquired, and probably related to aging. The average age of affected patients is 65 years. Bleeding is usually chronic, resulting in anemia, but may be acute and massive. Angiography demonstrates a tangle of ectatic vessels without an associated mass.

APPENDIX

Imaging Methods

MDCT, US, and MR have assumed primary roles in the diagnosis of acute appendicitis. US and MR are favored in children to avoid exposure to radiation.

Anatomy

The appendix arises from the posteromedial aspect of the cecum at the junction of the taenia coli, approximately 1 to 2 cm below the ileocecal valve. The appendix is a blind-ended tube that is 4 to 5 mm in diameter and approximately 8 cm in length, although it may be up to 30 cm long. Its mucosa is heavily infiltrated with lymphoid tissue, which when enlarged may mimic acute appendicitis. The appendix is quite variable in position: it may be pelvic, retrocecal, or retrocolic, and intra- or extraperitoneal in location. The appendix always arises from the cecum on the same side as the ileocecal valve. A posterior position of the ileocecal valve indicates a posterior position of the appendix. On CT, US, and MR the normal appendix appears as a thin-walled tube usually less than 6 mm in diameter (Fig. 46.30).

Acute Appendicitis

Acute appendicitis is the most common cause of acute abdomen. Often the clinical diagnosis is straightforward with abdominal pain (most patients), nausea (61% to 92%), anorexia (75%), and vomiting. However, atypical presentations in up to one-third of patients cause diagnostic problems. The most difficult patients are women of childbearing age, in whom ruptured ovarian cysts and pelvic inflammatory disease may mimic acute appendicitis. Acute appendicitis results from obstruction of the appendiceal lumen. Continued mucosal secretions cause dilation and increased intraluminal pressure that impairs venous drainage and results in mucosal ulceration. Bacterial infection causes gangrene and perforation with abscess. Most periappendiceal abscesses are walled off, but free perforation and pneumoperitoneum occasionally occur.

Conventional radiographs demonstrate an appendiceal calculus (appendicolith or fecalith) in approximately 14% of patients with acute appendicitis. An appendicolith is formed by calcium deposition around a nidus of inspissated feces. The resultant calcification is usually laminated with a radiolucent center. Appendiceal abscess or periappendiceal inflammation may result in a visible soft tissue mass in the right lower quadrant. The lumen of the cecum, as outlined by gas, will be deformed; localized ileus may be evident. Barium enema examination is frequently nonspecific and is now seldom used in favor of US, MR, and CT. Complete filling of the appendix to its bulbous tip is strong evidence against appendicitis. However, nonfilling of the appendix, as would be expected with luminal obstruction, has no diagnostic value of its own. Mass impression on the cecum has many causes besides appendicitis.

US, using the graded compression technique, is quite accurate in providing a definitive diagnosis and is commonly the imaging technique of choice in women of childbearing age and in children. Slow-graded compression is applied with a near-focus transducer to the area of maximum tenderness. The normal appendix has a diameter of less than 6 mm when compressed (Fig. 46.31). US signs of acute appendicitis are (a) a noncompressible appendix larger than 6 mm in diameter, measured outer wall to outer wall (Fig. 46.32); (b) visualization of a shadowing appendicolith; (c) inflamed periappendiceal fat

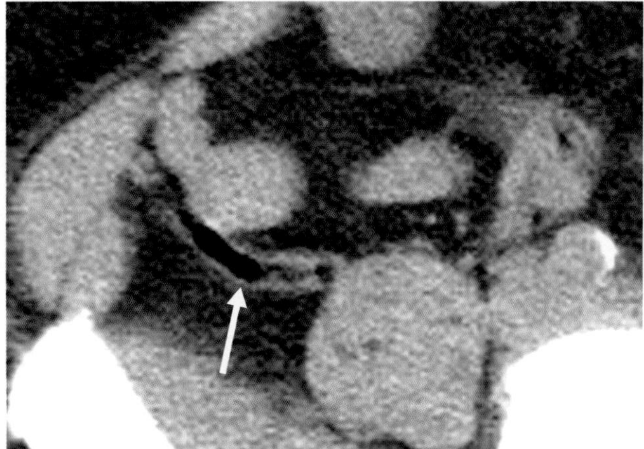

FIGURE 46.31. **Normal Appendix.** A noncontrast CT image shows a normal appendix (*arrow*) as a small gas-filled tubular structure with a blind end.

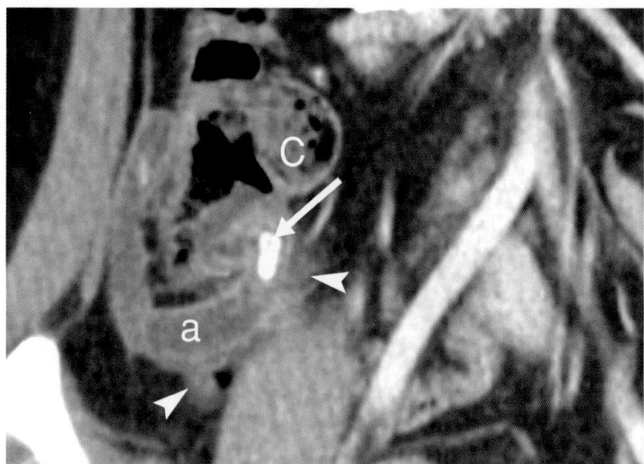

FIGURE 46.33. **Acute Appendicitis—CT.** Coronal CT image shows a dilated appendix (*a*) measuring 8 mm in diameter with irregularly thickened and indistinct wall. Fluid and stranding (*arrowheads*) in the periappendiceal fat is indicative of inflammation. An appendicolith (*arrow*) is seen in the lumen of the appendix. C, cecum.

becomes more echogenic and fixed moving with the appendix during compression; and (d) color Doppler shows increased vascularity in the wall of the appendix. With perforation, sonography demonstrates a loculated pericecal fluid collection, a discontinuous wall of the appendix, and prominent pericecal fat. When the US examination is negative for appendicitis, an alternate diagnosis, such as hemorrhagic ovarian cyst, can frequently be suggested based on visualized abnormalities.

CT is the usual imaging method of choice in men, in older patients, and when periappendiceal abscess is suspected. Definitive CT diagnosis of acute appendicitis is based on finding: (a) an abnormally dilated (>6 mm) appendix (Fig. 46.33), (b) enhancing appendix surrounded by inflammatory stranding or abscess, or (c) pericecal abscess or inflammatory mass with a calcified appendicolith. An inflammatory mass is seen as indurated soft tissue with a CT density greater than 20 H. A liquefied mass less than 20 H in CT density is evidence of abscess (Fig. 46.34). Abscesses larger than 3 cm generally require surgical or catheter drainage. Smaller abscesses commonly resolve on antibiotic treatment alone.

MR competes with US as the diagnostic method of choice for appendicitis in pregnant women and in children. Findings are similar to CT (Fig. 46.35): (a) dilated appendix larger than 6 to 7 mm diameter; (b) periappendiceal inflammation seen as high signal intensity on fat-suppressed T2WI; (c) thickened wall of the appendix; (d) appendicolith seen as focal area of low signal intensity in the lumen of the appendix; and (e) periappendiceal phlegmon or fluid collection high in signal intensity on T2WI.

Mucocele of the Appendix

Mucocele refers to distention of all or a portion of the appendix with sterile mucus. The lumen is obstructed by appendicolith, foreign body, adhesions, or tumor. Some cases are due to mucinous cystadenomas or cystadenocarcinomas of the appendix. Continued secretion of mucus produces a large (up to 15 cm), well-defined cystic mass in the right lower quadrant (Fig. 46.36). Appendiceal dilation greater than 13 mm suggests possible mucocele. Peripheral calcification may be present. Rupture of the mucocele may result in pseudomyxoma

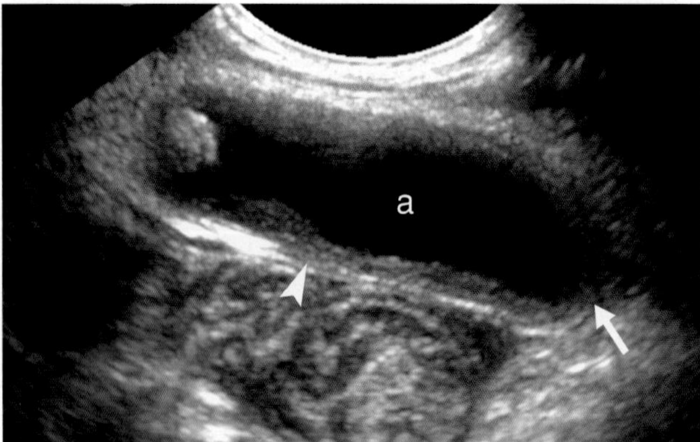

FIGURE 46.32. **Acute Appendicitis—US.** Graded compression US demonstrates a distended appendix with a diameter (*a*) of 10 mm. The wall of the appendix (*arrowhead*) is irregularly thickened by inflammation and edema. An obstructing appendicolith (*thin arrow*) is present. US may reveal noncalcified appendicoliths. The blunt tip (*fat arrow*) confirms identification of this tubular structure as the appendix. Surgery confirmed an acutely inflamed appendix.

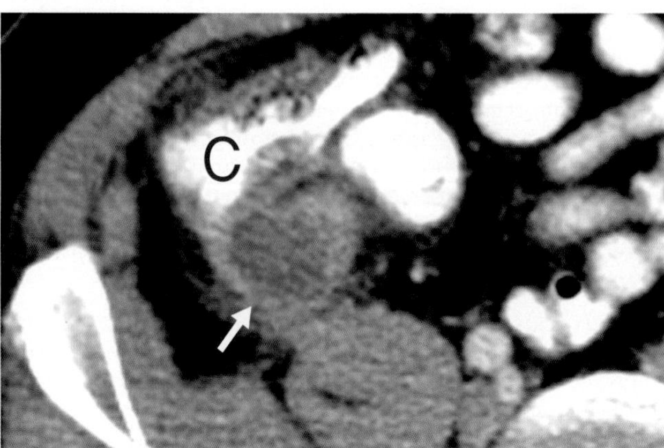

FIGURE 46.34. **Appendiceal Abscess.** CT demonstrates a thick-walled fluid collection (*arrow*) adjacent to the cecum (C). Inflammatory stranding is seen in the nearby fat. The appendix was not visualized. Surgery revealed a ruptured appendix with a focal abscess.

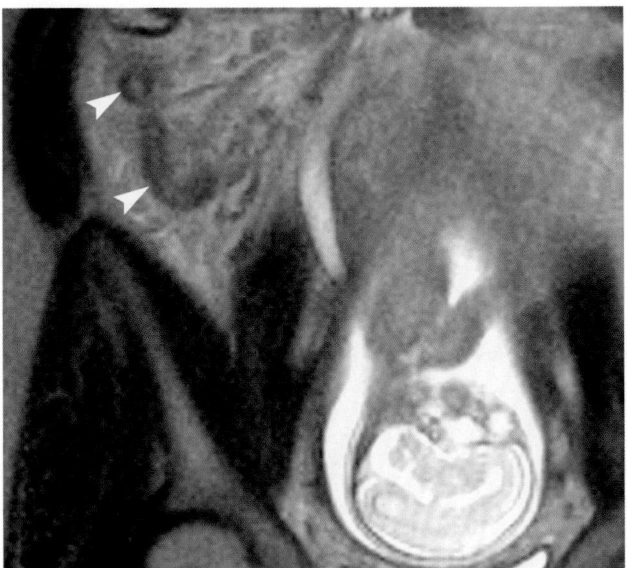

FIGURE 46.35. **Acute Appendicitis—MR.** Coronal plane T2-weighted MR in a 19-year-old woman with pregnancy at 22-week gestational age shows a dilated thick-walled appendix (*arrowheads*) with surrounding inflammation. Surgery revealed gangrenous appendicitis. MR offers excellent diagnostic images without use of radiation, an especially important consideration in pregnant patients.

peritonei. Gelatinous implants spread throughout the peritoneal cavity, causing adhesions and mucinous ascites.

Appendiceal Tumors

Carcinoid is the most common tumor of the appendix, accounting for 85% of all tumors. The appendix is the most common location for carcinoid tumor, accounting for 60% of all carcinoids. Most occur near the tip and are round, nodular tumors up to 2.5 cm size. Most are solitary and have less tendency to metastasize than carcinoids elsewhere in the GI tract. Carcinoid syndrome is rare and the mesenteric reaction seen with small bowel carcinoid is usually absent.

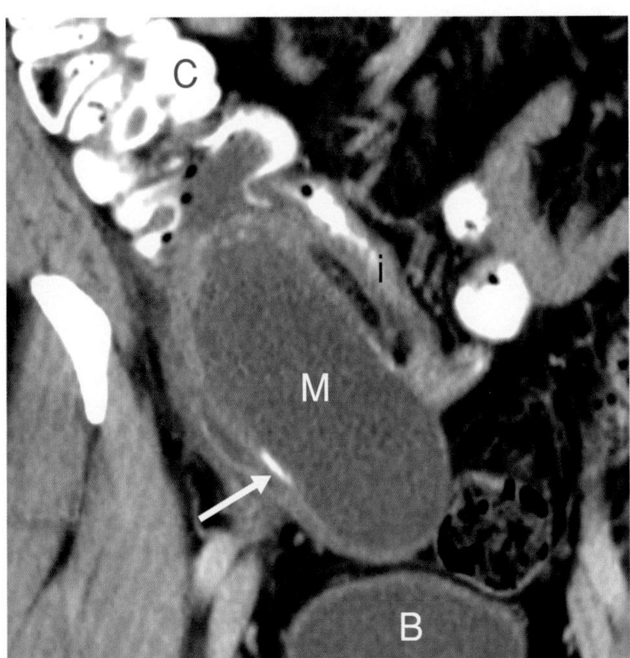

FIGURE 46.36. **Appendiceal Mucocele.** Coronal plane CT reveals a tubular cystic mass (*M*) with calcification in its wall (*arrow*) in the right lower quadrant of the abdomen. Landmarks include the cecum (*C*) and terminal ileum (*i*). *B*, bladder.

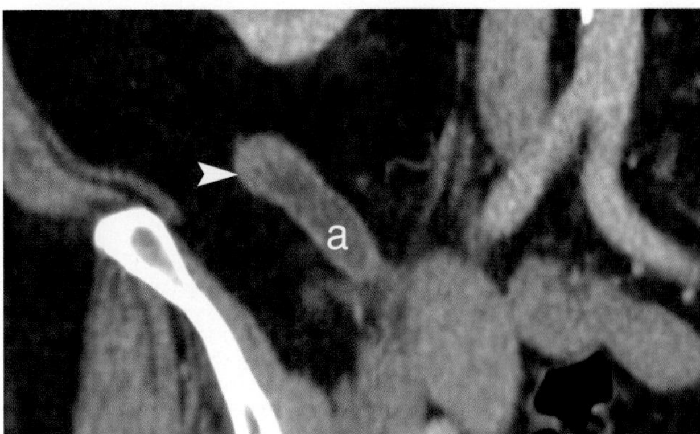

FIGURE 46.37. **Carcinoma of the Appendix.** Coronal CT in a 67-year-old patient with right lower quadrant pain shows a dilated appendix (*a*) with a subtle soft tissue mass (*arrowhead*) in its bulbous tip. Surgical removal confirmed a carcinoma of the appendix.

Adenomas occur in the appendix usually in association with familial multiple polyposis. Isolated adenomas are usually mucinous cystadenomas associated with mucocele of the appendix.

Adenocarcinoma of the appendix is rare and is usually discovered in the clinical setting of suspected appendicitis in an older adult (Fig. 46.37). Imaging demonstrates a soft tissue mass within or replacing the appendix.

Suggested Readings

Colon

Almeida AT, Melao L, Viamonte B, Cunha R, Pereira JM. Epiploic appendagitis: an entity frequently unknown to clinicians—diagnostic imaging, pitfalls, and look-alikes. *AJR Am J Roentgenol* 2009;193:1243–1251.

Childers BC, Cater SW, Horton KM, Fishman EK, Johnson PT. CT evaluation of acute enteritis and colitis: Is it infectious, inflammatory, or ischemic? *Radiographics* 2015;35:1940–1941. (Online digital presentation).

Feuerstein JD, Ketwaroo G, Tewani SK, et al. Localizing acute lower gastrointestinal hemorrhage: CT angiography versus tagged RBC scintigraphy. *AJR Am J Roentgenol* 2016;207:578–584.

Flor N, Maconi G, Cornalba G, Pickhardt PJ. The role of radiologic and endoscopic imaging in the diagnosis and follow-up of colonic diverticular disease. *AJR Am J Roentgenol* 2016;207:15–24.

Lewis RB, Mehrotra AK, Rodriguez P, Manning MA, Levine MS. Gastrointestinal lymphoma: radiologic and pathologic findings. *Radiographics* 2014;34:1934–1953.

Nerad E, Lahaye MJ, Maas M, et al. Diagnostic accuracy of CT for local staging of colon cancer: a systematic review and meta-analysis. *AJR Am J Roentgenol* 2016;207:984–995.

Onur MR, Akpinar E, Karaosmanoglu AD, Isayev C, Karcaaltincaba M. Diverticulitis: a comprehensive review with usual and unusual complications. *Insights Imaging* 2017;8:19–27. (Pictorial review).

Sinaei M, Swallow C, Milot L, Moghaddam PA, Smith A, Atri M. Patterns and signal intensity characteristics of pelvic recurrence of rectal cancer at MR imaging. *Radiographics* 2013;33:E171–E187.

Sinha R, Verma R, Verma S, Rajesh A. MR enterography of Crohn disease: Part 1, rationale, technique, pitfalls. *AJR Am J Roentgenol* 2011;197:76–79.

Sinha R, Verma R, Verma S, Rajesh A. MR enterography of Crohn disease: Part 2, imaging and pathologic findings. *AJR Am J Roentgenol* 2011;197: 80–85.

Spada C, Stoker J, Alarcon O, et al. Clinical indications for computed tomographic colonography: European Society of Gastrointestinal Endoscopy (ESGE) and European Society of Gastrointestinal and Abdominal Radiology (ESGAR) guideline. *Eur Radiol* 2015;25:331–345.

Tirumani SH, Kim KW, Nishino M, et al. Update on the role of imaging in the management of metastatic colorectal cancer. *Radiographics* 2014;34:1908–1928.

Yee J, Kim DH, Rosen MP, et al. ACR appropriateness criteria colorectal cancer screening. *J Am Coll Radiol* 2014;11:543–551.

Yu MH, Lee JM, Baek JH, Han JK, Choi BI. MRI features of gastrointestinal stromal tumors. *AJR Am J Roentgenol* 2014;203:980–991.

Appendix

Chin CM, Lim KL. Appendicitis: atypical and challenging CT appearances. *Radiographics* 2015;35:123–124. (Online digital presentation).

Duke E, Kalb B, Arif-Tiwari H, et al. A systematic review and meta-analysis of diagnostic performance of MRI for evaluation of acute appendicitis. *AJR Am J Roentgenol* 2016;206:508–517.

Purysko AS, Remer EM, Leão Filho HM, Bittencourt LK, Lima RV, Racy DJ. Beyond appendicitis: common and uncommon gastrointestinal causes of right lower quadrant pain at multidetector CT. *Radiographics* 2011;31: 927–947.

Smith MP, Katz DS, Lalani T, et al. ACR appropriateness criteria—right lower quadrant pain—suspected appendicitis. *Ultrasound Q* 2015;31:85–91.

Ung C, Chang ST, Jeffrey RB, Patel BN, Olcott EW. Sonography of the normal appendix—its varied appearance and techniques to improve its visualization. *Ultrasound Q* 2013;29:333–341.

SECTION VIII

GENITOURINARY TRACT

SECTION EDITOR: William E. Brant

CHAPTER 47 ■ ADRENAL GLANDS AND KIDNEYS

WILLIAM E. BRANT

ADRENAL GLANDS

Imaging Methods

The current major challenge of adrenal imaging is to provide noninvasive characterization of the many adrenal nodules found incidentally on CT or MR performed for other purposes. Up to 5% of patients who undergo MDCT of the abdomen will have an incidental adrenal lesion, an "incidentaloma." The predominant consideration is to determine if the lesion is a benign nonfunctioning adrenal adenoma or is it a metastasis. Within the differential diagnosis are subclinical pheochromocytomas, or functioning cortical adenomas causing unrecognized hyperaldosteronism or Cushing syndrome. Additional considerations include myelolipoma, adrenal carcinoma, hemorrhage, cyst, neuroblastoma, and ganglioneuroma. The adrenal glands are routinely imaged in patients with known malignancy, especially lung cancer, in order to detect metastatic disease. Many adrenal lesions in patients with known malignancy are benign. In patients with adrenal endocrine syndromes diagnosed clinically, imaging is used to find and characterize the causative lesion. MDCT remains the imaging modality of choice while MR, PET, PET-CT, US, scintigraphy, adrenal vein sampling, and image-guided adrenal biopsy all have significant roles.

Anatomy

The adrenal glands are composed of an outer cortex and an inner medulla that are functionally independent and anatomically distinct. The cortex secretes steroid hormones including cortisol, aldosterone, androgens, and estrogens. The medulla produces catecholamines.

The adrenal glands lie within the perirenal space surrounded by fat. The right adrenal gland is located posterior to the inferior vena cava (IVC) at the level where the IVC enters the liver. The right adrenal gland is between the right lobe of the liver and the right crus of the diaphragm just above the upper pole of the right kidney. The left adrenal gland lies just medial and anterior to the upper pole of the left kidney, posterior to the pancreas and splenic vessels, and lateral to the left crus of the diaphragm. On cross-sectional imaging, the adrenal glands appear triangular, linear, or inverted V- or Y-shaped (Fig. 47.1). Each limb is smooth in outline and uniform in thickness with straight or concave borders. The limbs are 4 to 5 cm in length and 5 to 7 mm in thickness. The adrenal glands are of uniform soft tissue density on CT and US. On MR, the normal adrenal is hypointense, about equal to striated muscle, on T1WI. On T1WI and T2WI, the adrenals are isointense or slightly hypointense compared with the liver (Fig. 47.1B). Chemical shift MR imaging is used to demonstrate intracellular fat in benign adrenal adenomas by utilizing in-phase (IP) and out-of-phase (OP) gradient-recalled sequences. Intracellular fat demonstrates a loss of signal on OP images compared to IP images because of signal cancellation effect resulting from fat and water occupying the same voxel. Fat saturation MR technique is used to demonstrate macroscopic fat seen in adrenal myelolipomas. Macroscopic fat shows a loss of signal intensity on fat saturation images compared to pulse sequences of the same technique without fat saturation.

Adjacent structures may cause problems in adrenal imaging by mimicking adrenal masses. Tortuous splenic vessels, splenic lobulations, pancreatic projections, exophytic upper pole renal masses, portosystemic venous collaterals, retroperitoneal adenopathy, gastric diverticuli, and portions of the stomach may all cause adrenal pseudotumors. Judicious use of oral and intravenous contrast on CT, or supplemental US or MR studies, will reveal the true nature of these conditions.

The Incidental Adrenal Mass

In patients without a known malignancy most small (<4 cm) adrenal nodules are benign nonhyperfunctioning adrenal cortical adenomas (Fig. 47.2). Less than 3% of lesions are malignant. In patients with a known malignancy the incidence of metastasis to the adrenal rises to 50%. These lesions are just as important to characterize in order to provide accurate tumor staging. Steady technical advances allow noninvasive imaging characterization of the majority of these nodules. Table 47.1 provides a summary of currently accepted criteria for characterization of adrenal lesions on CT, MR, and PET-CT.

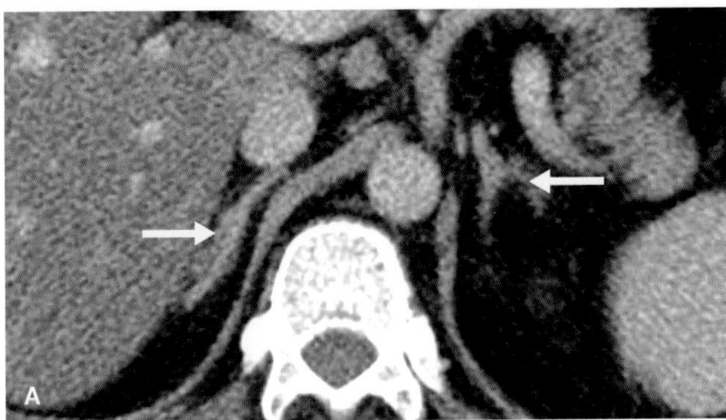

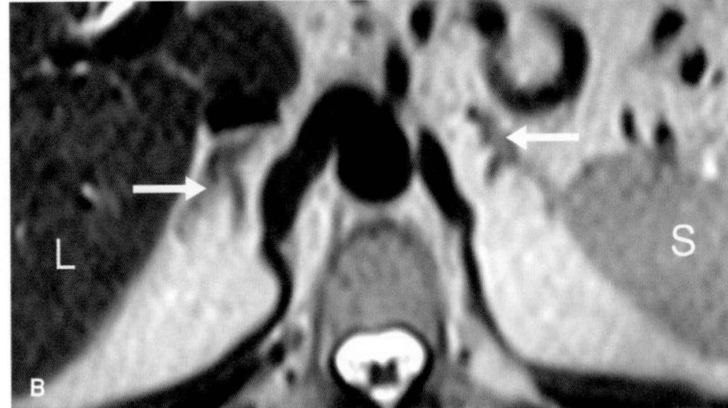

FIGURE 47.1. Normal Adrenal Glands. Contrast-enhanced axial CT (**A**) and axial T2-weighted MR image (**B**) show the normal appearance of the adrenal glands (*arrows*). *L*, liver; *S*, spleen.

Adrenal cortical adenomas are the most common adrenal mass found in 4% to 6% of the population and increasing in incidence with age. Most (94%) are nonhyperfunctioning, truly incidental, findings. Approximately 6% of adenomas secrete excess hormone and cause clinical or subclinical manifestations of one of the adrenal endocrine syndromes. Function of an adenoma cannot be determined by its imaging appearance but is assessed clinically. Cortical adenomas accumulate cholesterol, fatty acids, and other fatty substances, which serve as precursors of cortical hormones. Fat accumulation in 70% of adenomas is sufficient for them to be classified by imaging as *lipid-rich adenomas*. The remaining 30% are termed *lipid-poor adenomas*. Attenuation of adenomas on unenhanced CT has a range of −20 to +30 HU. Attenuation of less than +10 H on unenhanced CT is highly specific for lipid-rich adenomas. Enhancement on postcontrast CT and MR is unpredictable and often heterogeneous. However, benign adenomas are characterized on adrenal protocol MDCT by rapid washout of the contrast agent.

Adrenal metastases are exceedingly common, found in 27% of patients with malignant disease on autopsy series. The most common primary tumors are lung, breast, melanoma, gastrointestinal, thyroid, and renal. Small lesions (<4 cm) tend to be homogeneous, well defined, and difficult to distinguish from benign, nonfunctioning adenomas. To complicate the issue, even in patients with known primary malignancy, about 50% of small adrenal masses are benign adenomas and not metastases. On CT and MR, larger lesions (>4 cm) generally show features characteristic of malignancy, including inhomogeneous density, irregular shape, thick irregular margination, internal hemorrhage or necrosis, and invasion of adjacent structures (Fig. 47.3). Small lesions show the malignant features listed in Table 47.1.

Characterization. *Stability over time* is a well-recognized feature of benign adenoma. Detection of a small adrenal nodule should instigate a search for previous imaging studies. Absence of change in size and appearance of a small adrenal lesion for 6 months are generally accepted as evidence of benignancy. Stability for 1 to 2 years increases the confidence of a benign diagnosis. An increase in size of the lesion over 6 months is strong evidence of malignancy, though hemorrhage into a benign lesion causes an abrupt increase in size.

Clinical evaluation is recommended with increasing frequency as subclinical adrenal endocrine syndromes are recognized. Patients with hypertension should be evaluated for Cushing and Conn syndromes. Cushing syndrome is excluded in the absence of hypertension and obesity.

MDCT is the imaging modality of choice. CT without contrast successfully and accurately characterizes as benign in the 70% of patients with lipid-rich adenomas by demonstrating a CT attenuation of less than +10 H. Careful adherence to proper technique is essential when measuring CT attenuation (Fig. 47.2). Measurement is made on a thin section through the center of the lesion. The range-of-interest (ROI) cursor

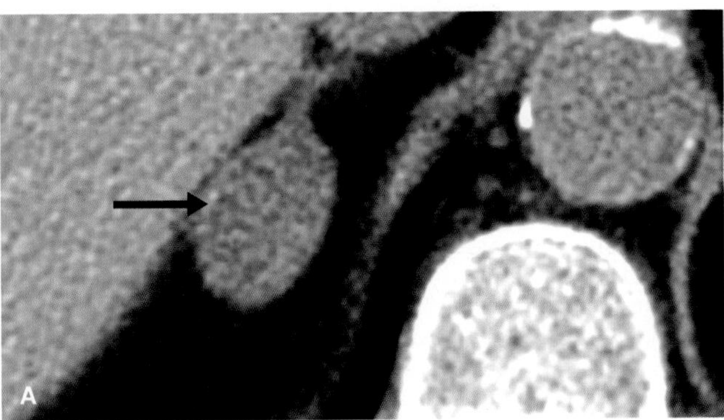

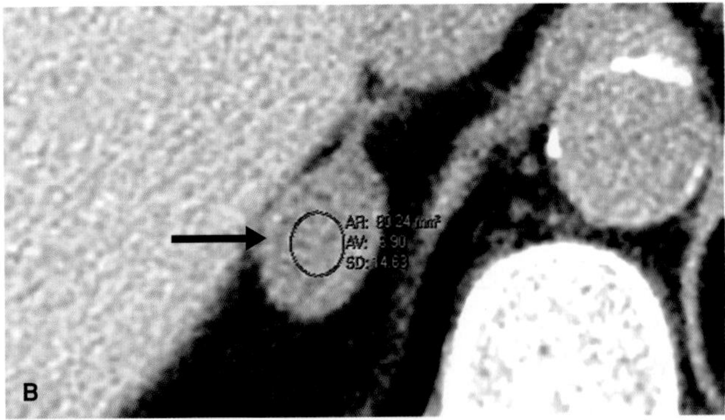

FIGURE 47.2. Incidentaloma. A: Image from MDCT performed without contrast to assess for ureteral stones shows a 30- × 17-mm nodule (*arrows*) arising from the right adrenal gland. The nodule is sharply marginated, oval, and homogeneous in attenuation. **B:** Range-of-interest (ROI) measurement on the same image shows an average (*AV*) attenuation of 6.90 HU with a standard deviation (*SD*) of 14.63 and area (*AR*) of 80.24 mm^2. This attenuation measurement combined with the imaging features of the lesion is diagnostic of benign lipid-rich cortical adenoma. Note that this 5 mm thick slice was selected because it was at the center of the lesion. The ROI cursor is centered within the cross-sectional area of the lesion and the ROI measures greater than 50% of the cross-sectional area. ROI measurements must be made according to the standards established for adrenal lesion characterization on CT.

TABLE 47.1

IMAGING FINDINGS OF MALIGNANT AND BENIGN ADRENAL LESIONS

■ FINDINGS OF MALIGNANCY	■ FINDINGS OF BENIGN LESION	■ SENSITIVITY (%)	■ SPECIFICITY (%)	■ REFERENCE
Irregular border and shape, heterogeneous nodule, size >4 cm	Smooth, round, homogeneous nodule size <4 cm			Garrett
	Macroscopic fat (attenuation <–30 HU): myelolipoma			Craig
Noncontrast CT Unenhanced attenuation >10 HU Indeterminate lesion—do contrast enhanced CT	**Noncontrast CT** Unenhanced attenuation <10 HU Benign lipid-rich adenoma	85	100	Garrett
Contrast-enhanced CT Slow-contrast washout APW <52% at 10 minute RPW <38% at 10 minute APW <60% at 15 minute RPW <40% at 15 minute Probably malignant	**Contrast-enhanced CT** Rapid contrast washout APW >52% at 10 minute RPW >38% at 10 minute APW >60% at 15 minute RPW >40% at 15 minute Benign lipid-poor adenoma	98 98	100 100	Garrett
Chemical shift MR No signal loss on opposed phase Indeterminate lesion—do contrast-enhanced CT Postcontrast washout MR has low sensitivity for lipid-poor benign adenoma	**Chemical shift MR** Decreased signal on opposed phase Benign lipid-rich adenoma	81–100	94–100	Elsayes Seo
PET-CT[a] CT attenuation >10 HU SUV_{max} >3.1 SUV ratio >1.0 FDG uptake visually brighter in the lesion than in the liver Metastatic lesion	**PET-CT**[a] CT attenuation <10 HU SUV_{max} <3.1 SUV ratio <1.0 FDG uptake not as bright as the liver Benign lesion	97 97 97	86 74 100	Boland

[a]PET is not recommended for adrenal lesion <1 cm size.

APW, absolute percentage washout; RPW, relative percentage washout; SUV, standardized uptake value; SUV_{max}, maximum SUV; SUV_{avg}, average SUV; SUV ratio, nodule SUV_{max}/liver SUV_{avg}.

Adapted and expanded from Miller JC, Blake MA, Boland GW, Copeland PM, Thrall JH, Lee SI. Adrenal masses. *J Am Coll Radiol* 2009;6(3):206–211.

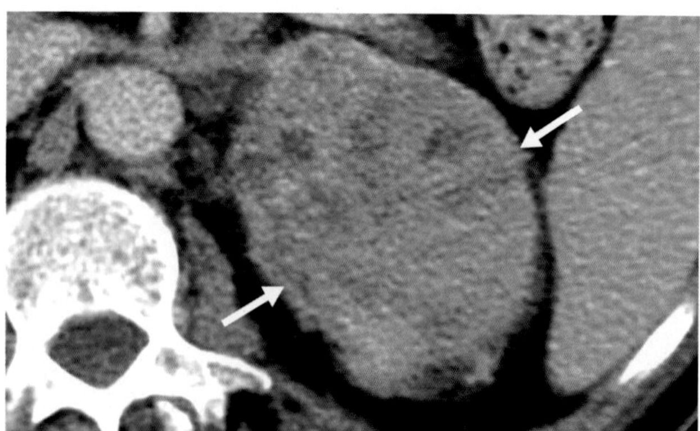

FIGURE 47.3. Adrenal Metastasis. Image from MDCT in a patient with lung cancer reveals a large (6 × 5 cm) solid mass (*arrows*) replacing the left adrenal gland. The mass is irregular in shape, poorly marginated with tissue strands extending into the adjacent fat, and has heterogeneous attenuation. These features are highly indicative of malignancy, and in this patient, metastatic lung cancer in the adrenal gland.

should cover at least half of the lesion surface area, avoiding areas of necrosis or hemorrhage. Measurements of attenuation below +10 H effectively exclude malignancy. Attenuation measurements above +10 H indicate indeterminate lesions that may be lipid-poor adenomas or malignancies. Unfortunately many CT examinations, on which incidental adrenal nodules are detected, are performed only after intravenous contrast administration. Perfusion differences between benign adenomas and metastasis provide a second reliable set of criteria for diagnosis. Adenomas are characterized by rapid washout of contrast agent while metastasis shows slow-contrast washout (Figs. 47.4 and 47.5). Percentage washout measurements are made on images taken at 60 to 75 seconds following the onset of intravenous contrast injection (enhanced attenuation). Delayed attenuation measurements are made on images obtained at 10 or 15 minutes following contrast injection. Absolute and relative percentage washout calculations are made (Table 47.2). Benign lesions show >60% absolute percentage washout and >40% relative percentage washout at 15 minutes. A number of studies have looked at calculating washout values from 10- and from

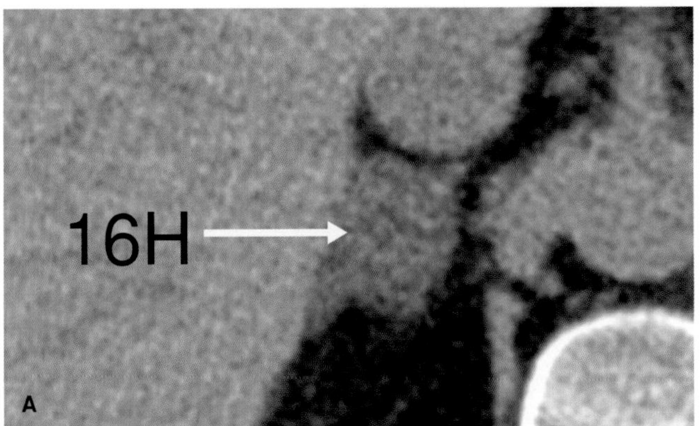

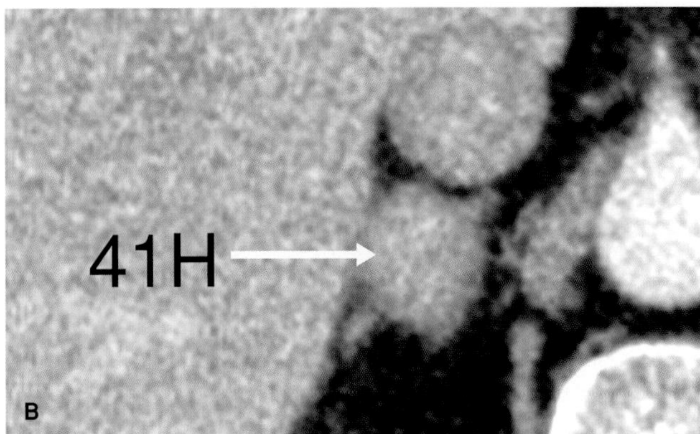

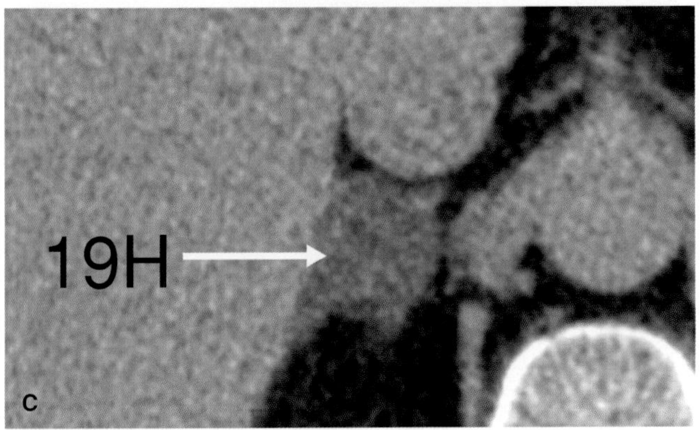

FIGURE 47.4. **Benign Lipid-Poor Adrenal Adenoma—CT.** **A:** Precontrast scan shows a small right adrenal mass (*arrows*) with attenuation of 16 H, too high to characterize the lesion as a lipid-rich adrenal adenoma. **B:** Image at 1-minute postintravenous contrast administration shows enhancement attenuation of the lesion at 41 H. **C:** Delayed image obtained at 15-minute postcontrast administration delayed attenuation of 19 H. Absolute percentage washout (APW) calculates to 88% (see Table 47.2). Relative percentage washout calculates to 53%. These findings characterize this lesion as a lipid-poor adrenal adenoma (see Table 47.1).

15-minute delay images. It seems to make little practical difference. The 60% APW and 40% RPW criteria are easier to remember and seem to work effectively using either 10- or 15-minute delayed images.

MR characterization depends on chemical shift techniques that detect intracellular lipid. Chemical shift MR relies on the different precession frequencies of fat protons versus water protons. When fat and water molecules occupy the same voxel, the MR signal from fat and water tend to cancel out each other reducing signal intensity. Chemical shift MR consists of IP sequences when fat and water signals are additive and opposed-phase sequences when fat and water signals are subtractive. A reduction in signal intensity on opposed-phase images as compared to IP images is indicative of intracellular fat. When evaluating adrenal nodules the chemical shift MR finding of signal drop indicates a benign lipid-rich adenoma (Fig. 47.6). Though some studies indicate a slight increase in the sensitivity of MR as compared to noncontrast CT, both modalities characterize essentially the same subset of lipid-rich adenomas.

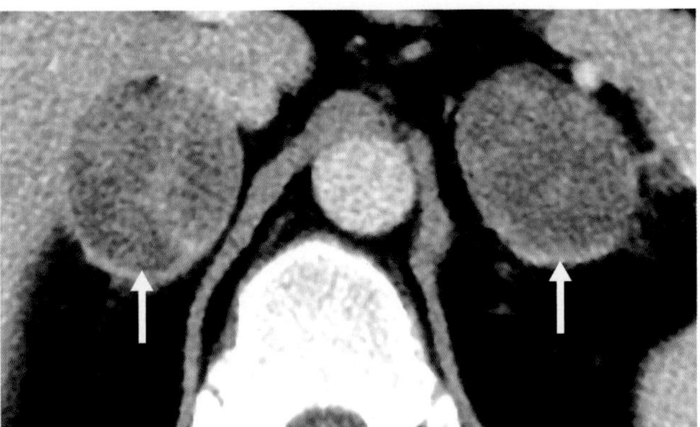

FIGURE 47.5. **Adrenal Metastases.** Contrast-enhanced CT demonstrates bilateral inhomogeneous adrenal masses (*arrows*). Adrenal protocol CT with delayed images showed minimal contrast washout at 15 minutes indicating a high likelihood of malignancy. The lesions are metastases from lung carcinoma.

MR offers limited capability to characterize lipid-poor adenomas, which are categorized along with metastases as indeterminate lesions when they fail to show signal loss on opposed-phase images. Contrast washout techniques following gadolinium enhancement on MR have so far not been successful in definitively characterizing incidentalomas. Patients with lesions not characterized by chemical shift MR should be considered for repeat study with contrast-enhanced CT or PET-CT.

PET-CT shows high sensitivity in detection of malignant lesions, which because of high metabolic activity accumulate FDG. Hemorrhage or necrosis within a metastasis may cause falsely negative FDG uptake. Some metastases are false negative on PET including those from neuroendocrine tumors and bronchoalveolar lung carcinoma. Some benign lesions including occasional adenomas, infectious, and inflammatory lesions may show slightly increased activity. Of PET positive adrenal lesions about 5% are false positive. Lesions smaller than 1 cm are not accurately evaluated by PET. Lesions that are brighter, that is, show more FDG uptake than the liver are considered to be malignant (Fig. 47.7). SUV_{max} greater than 3.1 correlates with malignancy.

Lesions not categorized by CT, MR, or PET-CT are considered for follow-up imaging in 4 to 6 months or for image-guided biopsy. Biopsy should be performed only if the result of the biopsy will affect further therapy. CT-guided adrenal biopsy is safe with hemorrhage and pneumothorax as unusual complications. Biopsy may be performed using a transhepatic approach or with decubitus positioning with the adrenal lesion side down to diminish the risk of pneumothorax. Caution should be used and biopsy generally avoided if the lesion is likely to be a pheochromocytoma. Percutaneous biopsy of a pheochromocytoma may precipitate a hypertensive crisis.

TABLE 47.2

ADRENAL NODULE PERCENTAGE WASHOUT FORMULAS

PERCENTAGE WASHOUT	FORMULAS
Absolute percentage washout	$\frac{\text{Enhanced attenuation} - \text{Delayed attenuation}}{\text{Enhanced attenuation} - \text{Unenhanced attenuation}} \times 100$
Relative percentage washout	$\frac{\text{Enhanced attenuation} - \text{Delayed attenuation}}{\text{Enhanced attenuation}} \times 100$

Note: Enhanced attenuation is measured at 60–75 seconds following onset of intravenous contrast injection. Delayed attenuation is measured at 10 or at 15 minutes following onset of intravenous contrast administration.
Adapted from Caoili EM, Korobkin M, Francis IR, et al. Adrenal masses: characterization with combined unenhanced and delayed enhanced CT. *Radiology* 2002;222(3):629–633; Blake MA, Kalra MK, Sweeney AT, et al. Distinguishing benign from malignant adrenal masses: multi-detector row CT protocol with 10-minute delay. *Radiology* 2006;238(2):578–585.

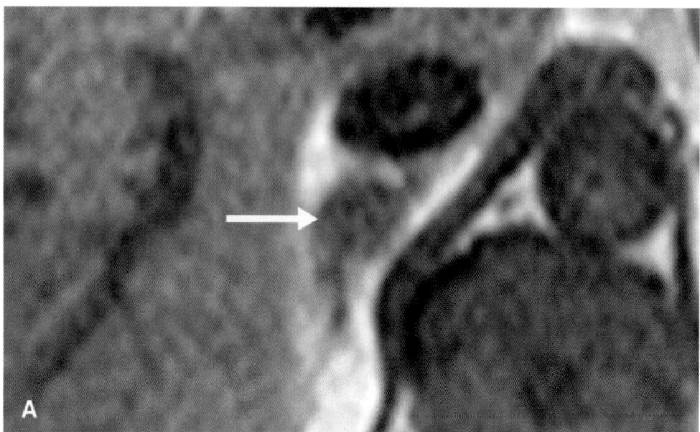

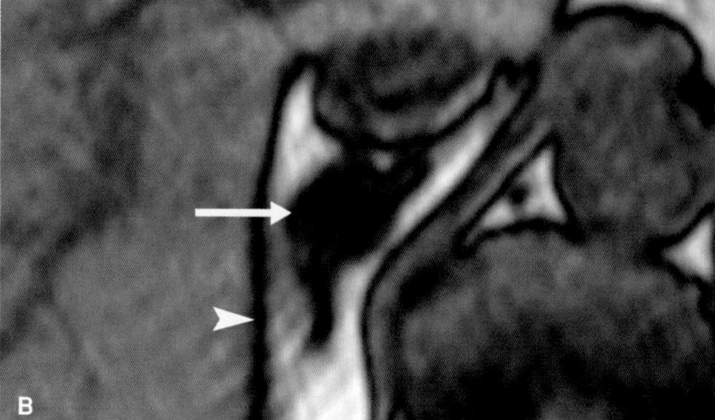

FIGURE 47.6. **Benign Lipid-Rich Adrenal Adenoma—MR.** Chemical shift MR imaging is used to characterize a lipid-rich adenoma in a patient with a history of renal cell carcinoma. **A:** In-phase MR image shows a small right adrenal mass (*arrows*) with signal intensity slightly less than that of the liver. **B:** Opposed-phase MR image shows the distinct loss of signal intensity caused by intracellular fat that characterizes lipid-rich adrenal adenomas. Note the black band (*arrowhead*) at interfaces between soft tissue and fat produced by chemical shift artifact. This finding allows immediate recognition of the opposed-phase MR image.

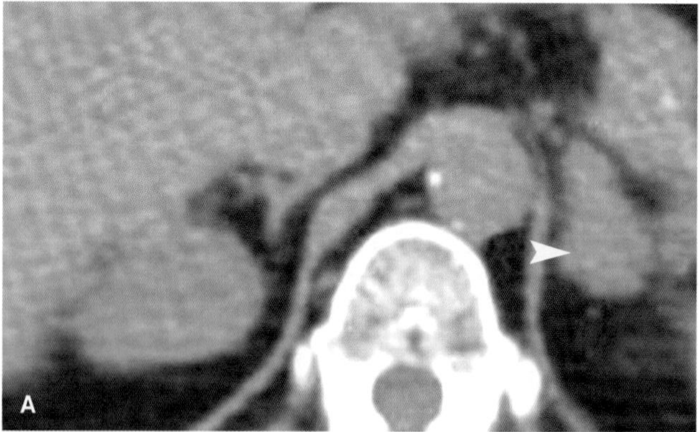

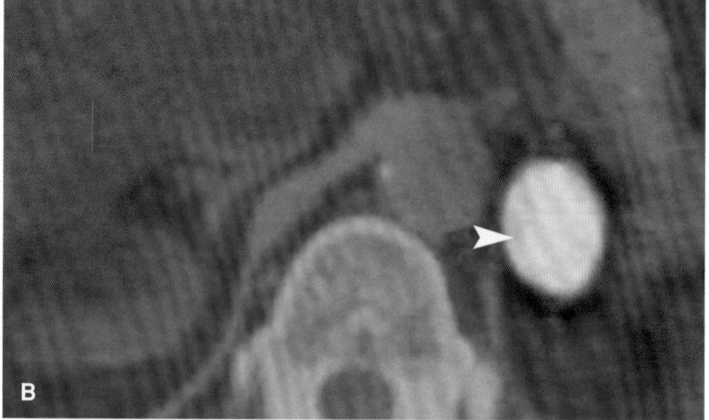

FIGURE 47.7. **Adrenal Metastasis—PET-CT.** **A:** Unenhanced CT image from PET-CT shows a small nodule (*arrowhead*) arising from the left adrenal gland. CT attenuation was 23 H. **B:** The corresponding PET image from PET-CT shows marked FDG uptake within the lesion (*arrowhead*) indicating metastatic disease in this patient with lung cancer. Note that the radionuclide activity within the adrenal lesion is substantially higher than the radionuclide activity in the liver (*L*).

Adrenal Endocrine Syndromes

Cushing syndrome is caused by excessive amounts of hydrocortisone and corticosterone released by the adrenal cortex. Clinical signs include hypertension, truncal obesity, easy bruisability, generalized weakness, diabetes mellitus, and oligomenorrhea. Adrenal hyperplasia causes 70% of cases of noniatrogenic Cushing syndrome. The hyperplasia is stimulated in 90% of cases by a pituitary microadenoma that produces adrenocorticotropic hormone (ACTH). MR of the sella turcica is recommended for suspected pituitary adenomas. In 10% of cases, the source of ACTH is ectopic, usually from lung malignancies. Benign adrenal adenomas cause 20% of cases of Cushing syndrome, and adrenal carcinoma causes the remaining 10%. A subclinical form of Cushing syndrome has been associated with the presence of small adrenal adenomas found incidentally. It may be more common than classic Cushing syndrome. Clinical evaluation for hypertension, type 2 diabetes, and obesity is often recommended. Atrophy of the contralateral adrenal gland may be present due to inhibition of ACTH.

Conn syndrome, produced by elevated levels of aldosterone, causes 1% to 2% of systemic hypertension. The clinical diagnosis is made by findings of persistent hypokalemia, increased serum and urine aldosterone, and decreased renin activity in the plasma. A solitary, benign, hyperfunctioning adrenal cortical adenoma is the cause of 80% of cases, and adrenal hyperplasia is the cause of the remaining 20%. Adenomas are treated with surgical resection, whereas hyperplasia is treated medically. Adenomas that produce Conn syndrome tend to be small (<2 cm); therefore, strict attention to excellent MDCT technique using thin slices is necessary for accurate localization. Adrenal venous sampling is used to confirm the site of excess aldosterone secretion and to differentiate adenoma from hyperplasia in problem cases.

Adrenogenital syndrome usually occurs in newborns and infants who have an enzyme deficiency (11β- or 22-hydroxylase) leading to deficient production of cortisol and aldosterone, and an excess of precursors, especially androgens. These infants have adrenal hyperplasia, which is usually well demonstrated by US. Both adrenal adenomas and carcinomas may be a cause of masculinizing or feminizing syndromes in older patients.

Addison disease refers to primary adrenal insufficiency, which occurs only after 90% of the adrenal cortex is destroyed. The most common cause (60% to 70%) in the United States is idiopathic atrophy, which is probably an autoimmune disorder. The adrenal glands shrink and may not be detectable with imaging methods. Additional causes involve destruction of the glands by tuberculosis, histoplasmosis, infarction, disseminated fungal infection, lymphoma, or metastatic tumor. Adrenal calcification suggests prior tuberculosis or histoplasmosis. Bilateral enlargement is seen with active infection. Lymphoma and metastases replace the glands with tumor.

Pheochromocytoma is a rare catecholamine-secreting tumor that causes hypertension, headaches, and tremors. Paroxysmal attacks are characteristic but not always present. Pheochromocytoma is said to follow the "rule of tens": 10% are bilateral, 10% are extra-adrenal, 10% are malignant, 10% are familial, and 10% are detected as "incidental" findings (Fig. 47.8). Pheochromocytoma is associated with multiple endocrine neoplasia (MEN II), von Hippel–Lindau syndrome, and neurofibromatosis. Pheochromocytoma is the most common adrenal tumor to spontaneously hemorrhage (Fig. 47.9). CT is the usual imaging method of choice for detecting the tumor when clinical manifestations are present. The literature has traditionally advised against the use of intravenous contrast media in patients with pheochromocytoma because of a presumed risk of precipitating adrenergic crisis. More recent experience indicates no significant risk with nonionic contrast media. Most tumors are larger than 2 cm in diameter. Tumors vary from purely solid to complex to predominantly cystic. Calcification is rare, but usually "eggshell" in configuration when present. Most tumors enhance avidly and washout slowly similar to malignant lesions. Findings are variable, however, as some lesions show poor contrast enhancement or rapid washout seen with benign lesions. On MR high signal (a "light bulb" lesion) on T2WI is characteristic but seen in only 70%. Chemical shift MR shows no change in signal intensity between IP and opposed-phase images. If no lesion is found in the adrenal, scanning is extended to include the chest and remainder of the abdomen and pelvis. Extra-adrenal sites for pheochromocytoma include the organ of Zuckerkandl near the bifurcation of the aorta, the bladder (Fig. 47.10), and the para-aortic sympathetic chain. Radionuclide scans using ^{131}I- or ^{123}I-metaiodobenzylguanidine (MIBG) are also effective in localizing pheochromocytoma. PET-CT shows increased FDG uptake in most tumors including some that are MIBG negative. Atypical appearance of the tumor is relatively common on all imaging modalities.

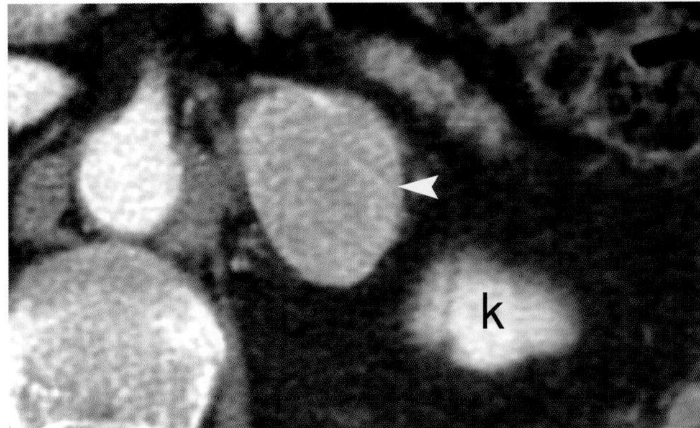

FIGURE 47.8. "Incidental" Pheochromocytoma. Postcontrast MDCT image in a patient with blunt abdominal trauma from a motor vehicle collision revealed a left adrenal mass (*arrowhead*). Subsequent clinical evaluation indicated evidence of pheochromocytoma. Adrenalectomy confirmed the diagnosis. Pheochromocytoma is quite variable in imaging appearance. This lesion closely resembles an adrenal cortical adenoma. *k*, top of left kidney.

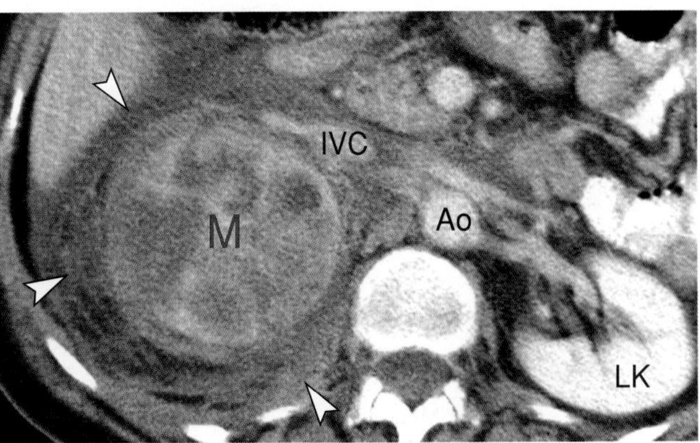

FIGURE 47.9. Pheochromocytoma With Spontaneous Hemorrhage. Postcontrast CT shows a heterogeneous adrenal mass (*M*) with hemorrhage (*arrowheads*) into the perinephric space. The inferior vena cava (*IVC*) is displaced anteriorly by the mass and hemorrhage. *Ao*, aorta; *LK*, left kidney.

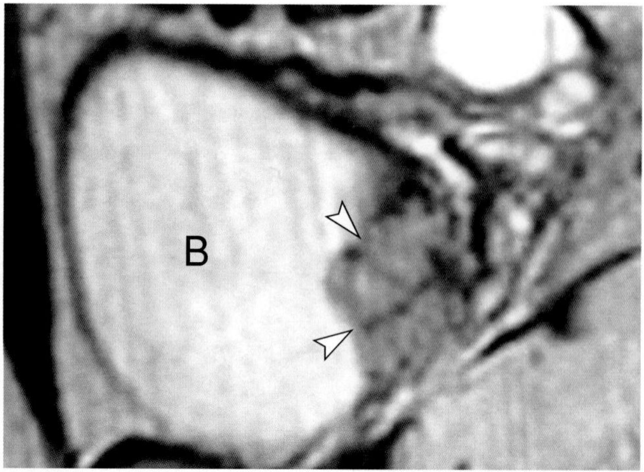

FIGURE 47.10. **Pheochromocytoma in Bladder Wall.** T2-weighted sagittal plane MR image demonstrates a lobulated mass (*arrowheads*) in the posterior wall of the bladder (*B*). Surgical excision confirmed a pheochromocytoma.

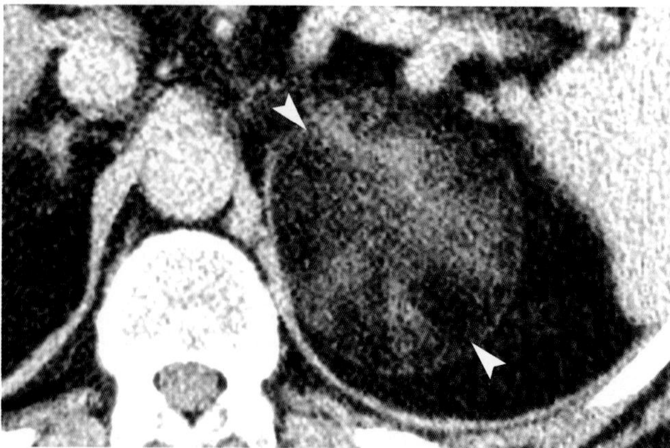

FIGURE 47.12. **Adrenal Myelolipoma.** The lesion (between *arrowheads*) of the left adrenal gland has large internal areas of fat density identical to surrounding retroperitoneal fat. Inhomogeneous attenuation is common and results from bone marrow hemopoietic tissue mixed with macroscopic fat.

Benign Adrenal Lesions

Adrenal hyperplasia is the cause of 70% of the cases of Cushing syndrome and 20% of the cases of Conn syndrome. Adrenal hyperplasia is important to differentiate from adrenal adenoma as a cause of endocrine syndromes. The syndrome is usually treated medically when hyperplasia is causative, whereas surgical removal of hyperfunctioning adrenal adenomas is usually curative. Half of the cases of biochemically hyperplastic glands will appear anatomically normal on CT and MR. In the remainder of cases, both glands will be diffusely enlarged but maintain their normal adrenal shape (Fig. 47.11). Uncommonly, hyperplasia may appear nodular and mimic solitary or multiple adenomas. In diffuse hyperplasia, the limbs of the adrenal glands are longer than 5 cm and exceed 10 mm thickness. Chemical shift MR occasionally shows a loss of signal on opposed-phase images. Metastatic disease, tuberculosis, and histoplasmosis may also cause diffuse adrenal enlargement and mimic the appearance of adrenal hyperplasia.

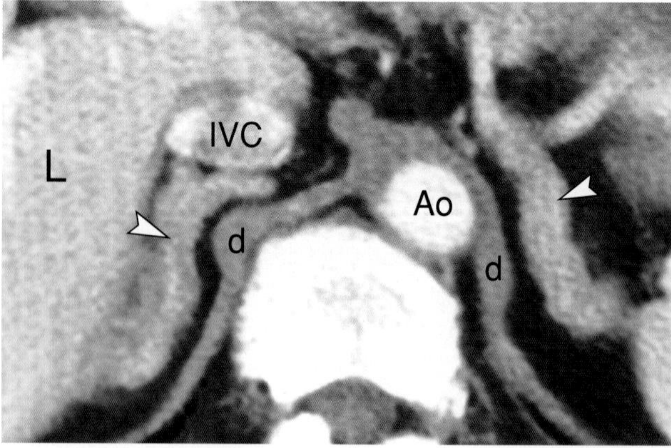

FIGURE 47.11. **Adrenal Hyperplasia.** The limbs of both adrenal glands (*arrowheads*) are thickened and somewhat nodular. Differential considerations include hyperplasia, metastases, and granulomatous disease. Note the anatomic landmarks for the adrenal glands: *d*, crura of the diaphragm; *L*, right lobe of the liver; *IVC*, inferior vena cava; *Ao*, aorta.

Adrenal myelolipomas are rare, nonfunctioning benign tumors arising from bone marrow elements in the adrenal gland. The tumors have no malignant potential. They range in size up to 30 cm and are frequently inhomogeneous because of their mixed components of marrow fat and hemopoietic tissue. Large lesions (>5 cm) have a tendency to hemorrhage. Calcifications are present in 20%. Identification of regions of macroscopic fat (−30 to −100 H) within the tumor by CT or by fat saturation MR is definitive in making the diagnosis (Fig. 47.12). CT attenuation <−30 H is definitive. MR shows high signal fat on T1WI and T2WI. Fat saturation pulse sequences showing decreased signal confirm the diagnosis. Chemical shift MR is usually not useful as the macroscopic fat cells have little intracellular water. PET typically shows no avid FDG uptake. On US they may be extremely echogenic and blend in with retroperitoneal fat.

Adrenal hemorrhage is most common in newborn infants, usually induced by episodes of hypoxia, birth trauma, or septicemia. Most cases are bilateral. In children, adrenal hemorrhage may be associated with child abuse. In adults, blunt trauma (80%) and infection are the most common causes of adrenal hemorrhage. Unilateral hemorrhage is most common in adults, with the right adrenal most frequently affected. Bilateral hemorrhage may cause adrenal insufficiency. On unenhanced CT hemorrhage shows high attenuation (50 to 90 H). Hemorrhage on CT is hypodense compared with the liver and spleen on contrast-enhanced studies (Fig. 47.13). Stranding in the periadrenal fat and thickening of the adjacent fascia are additional findings. MR is highly sensitive and specific for adrenal hemorrhage with imaging features dependent on the age of the hemorrhage. Acute hemorrhage is isointense on T1WI and low intensity on T2WI. Subacute hemorrhage is bright on T1WI and either dark or bright on T2WI. Old hemorrhage with hemosiderin content is low signal on both T1WI and T2WI. US demonstrates a hypoechoic mass that shrinks and becomes less echogenic over time.

Adrenal calcifications, in both children and adults, most commonly result from adrenal hemorrhage (Fig. 47.14). Tuberculosis and histoplasmosis may cause diffuse adrenal calcification associated with Addison disease. Adrenal tumors that calcify include neuroblastoma and ganglioneuroma in children and adrenal carcinoma, pheochromocytoma, and ganglioneuroma in adults. Adrenal pseudocysts attributable to previous hemorrhage are the most common calcified adrenal

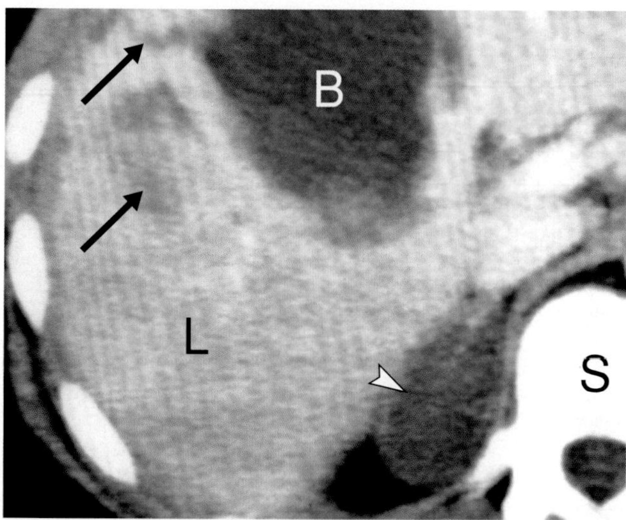

FIGURE 47.13. **Adrenal Hemorrhage.** Postcontrast CT shows post-traumatic hemorrhage (*arrowhead*) into the right adrenal gland. Blunt trauma to the abdomen compresses the right adrenal gland between the liver (*L*) and the spine (*S*) resulting in adrenal hemorrhage. This patient also has areas of fracture and hemorrhage (*arrows*) within the liver as well as a biloma (*B*).

masses in adults. Wolman disease is a rare, autosomal recessive lipid disorder associated with enlarged calcified adrenal glands, hepatomegaly, and splenomegaly.

Adrenal cysts are rare lesions that usually produce no symptoms and are discovered incidentally. True cysts are lined with endothelium or epithelium. Pseudocysts have a fibrous wall without lining cells and usually result from adrenal hemorrhage or infarction. Echinococcus may produce parasitic cysts. Adrenal cysts are more common in women and may be found at any age. Cysts can be classified as uncomplicated and benign when they have thin walls (<3 mm) with or without calcification, internal water density, size less than 5 to 6 cm, and show no internal enhancement on CT. Calcification in cyst walls and septa is a common finding in all types of cysts (Fig. 47.15). Endothelial cysts tend to be multilocular with septal calcification. Hemorrhagic pseudocysts are usually unilocular with calcification in the wall. US demonstrates thin-walled anechoic cysts that may be septated. Uncomplicated cysts have uniform low signal intensity contents on T1WI,

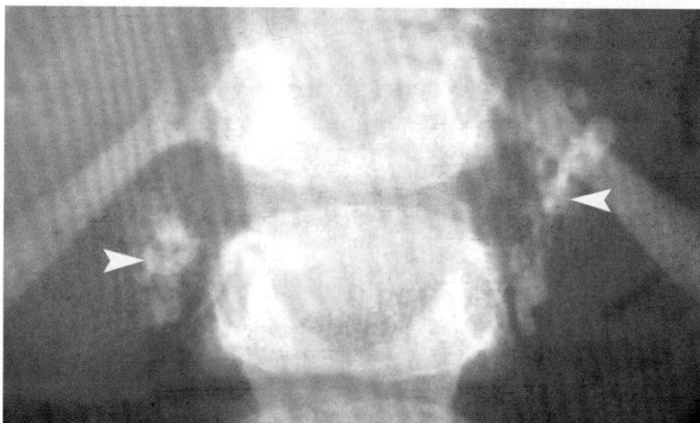

FIGURE 47.14. **Adrenal Calcification.** Conventional radiograph of the abdomen in a 4-year-old child demonstrates calcification of both adrenal glands (*arrowheads*) resulting from bilateral adrenal hemorrhage as an infant.

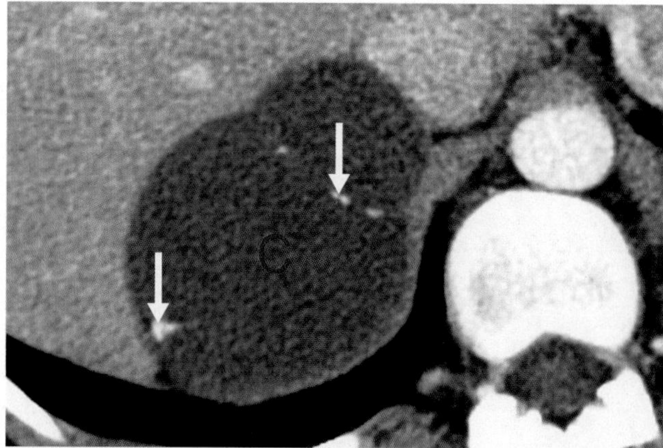

FIGURE 47.15. **Posthemorrhagic Adrenal Cyst.** CT shows a well-defined fluid density cyst (C) of the right adrenal gland. Calcification (*arrows*) is evident in the wall and in the septation.

uniform high signal intensity contents on T2WI, and show no internal enhancement with gadolinium. Cysts that are larger than 6 cm, have thick walls or solid components, show internal contrast enhancement on CT or MR, are inhomogeneous on MR, have echogenic fluid or internal debris on US, or produce symptoms should be considered for surgical removal. These lesions may be cysts complicated by hemorrhage or may be tumors with cystic degeneration, such as metastases and pheochromocytoma. Percutaneous biopsy of the cyst wall is difficult, and percutaneous aspiration of cyst fluid may not be reliable to exclude malignancy.

Ganglioneuroma is a rare benign tumor of the adrenal medulla or paravertebral sympathetic chain. Most, even when large, are asymptomatic. Imaging shows a usually homogeneous, often very large (>20 cm) mass with mild heterogeneous enhancement.

Malignant Adrenal Lesions

Adrenal carcinoma is an uncommon but lethal tumor, occurring with a frequency of one to two cases per million people. Most are large (>6 cm) and invasive at presentation. About half of the carcinomas are hyperfunctioning and cause endocrine syndromes, most commonly Cushing syndrome, and rarely Conn syndrome, virilization, or feminization. The typical CT appearance is a large mass (4 to 20 cm), with areas of central necrosis and hemorrhage, showing irregular contrast enhancement. On delayed postcontrast CT scans, enhancement washout is significantly less than benign adrenal adenomas and is similar to the poor washout of adrenal metastases. Adrenal tumors larger than 4 to 5 cm in size should be removed because of the significant risk of carcinoma. Calcification is present in 30% of the tumors. Hepatic and lymph node metastases are common. Tumor thrombus in the renal vein or IVC may be evident. Large tumors may be difficult to differentiate from hepatic masses. On MR, T1WI demonstrates an inhomogeneous large mass, predominantly hypointense compared with liver. Signal intensity is increased on T2WI especially in areas of necrosis (Fig. 47.16). Gadolinium enhancement or gradient echo imaging is useful to detect tumor thrombus. US with Doppler is also excellent for the evaluation of tumor thrombosis. PET-CT shows markedly FDG avidity not only in the tumor but also in metastatic lesions, some of which may be overlooked on MR and CT.

Lymphoma is rare as a primary adrenal lesion but systemic non-Hodgkin lymphoma involves the adrenal in 4% of cases.

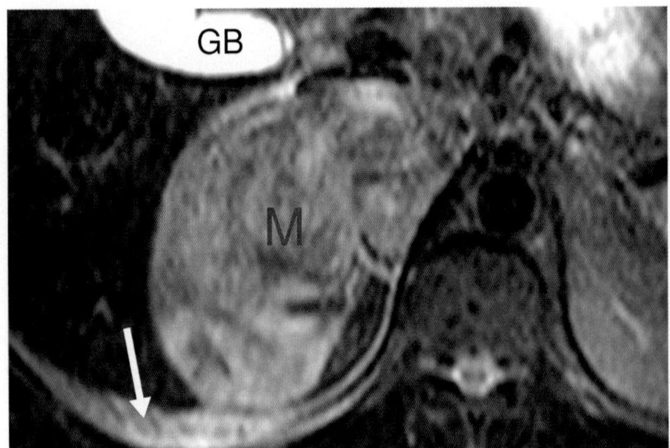

FIGURE 47.16. **Adrenal Carcinoma.** T2-weighted MR image with fat suppression shows a large inhomogeneous mass (*M*) replacing the right adrenal gland. Areas of high and low signal intensity represent necrosis and hemorrhage. The patient has a malignant right pleural effusion (*arrow*). *GB*, gallbladder.

Retroperitoneal lymphoma may totally encase the gland. On CT lymphoma shows washout characteristics similar to other malignancies. MR shows heterogeneously bright signal on T2WI. PET-CT shows increased FDG uptake.

Collision tumor refers to the coexistence of histologically distinct neoplasms that exist separately in the same region. Metastatic disease may deposit onto a previously characterized adrenal adenoma. Increase in size of the lesion or significant change in its imaging characteristic suggests this rare lesion.

KIDNEYS

Imaging Methods

The CT urogram ("CT-IVP") performed with MDCT has supplanted the traditional intravenous pyelogram (IVP) as the imaging method of choice in the evaluation of hematuria. With the ability to perform rapid thin-slice high-resolution scans and to reformat the images in multiple anatomic planes, the CT-IVP offers optimal evaluation of the renal parenchyma with satisfactory assessment of the collecting systems, ureters, and bladder. The traditional IVP based on conventional radiography offers higher spatial resolution to demonstrate the contrast-filled pelvicalyceal systems and ureters, however assessment of the renal parenchyma and any portion of the collecting system that is not filled with contrast is very limited (Fig. 47.17). As a result in most institutions it has been many years since a traditional IVP was performed. The CT urogram is usually performed as a multistage study using thin slices (0.5 to 1.5 mm). Precontrast scans are obtained from the kidneys through the bladder to detect urinary stones and calcifications and to provide a baseline to assess for enhancement of lesions. Following intravenous contrast administration, arterial phase scans through the kidneys show early enhancement of renal tumors. The renal cortex enhances before the renal medulla resulting in the characteristic *corticomedullary phase* appearance. Because the medulla is unenhanced small medullary lesions may be missed during this phase. Some protocols skip the corticomedullary phase. At approximately 120 seconds following onset of contrast injection the renal parenchyma is normally uniformly enhanced (the *nephrogram phase* scan). A *pyelogram-phase* scan at 3 to 5 minutes shows contrast filling of the collecting system and ureters. Thin-slice acquisition allows reformatting into three-dimensional images of the collecting systems and ureters mimicking the traditional IVP but with the improved parenchymal contrast resolution of CT. For evaluation of a known renal mass the MDCT examination may be limited to the kidneys omitting scans of the pelvis.

The MR urogram is a high-quality substitute for the CT urogram, especially useful when CT is equivocal or when intravenous contrast should not be administered because of impaired renal function. MR urography provides effective evaluation of the uroepithelium even without intravenous contrast by utilizing heavily T2WI showing the collecting system and ureters as static collections of fluid. This technique provides the best images when the ureters and collecting system are dilated. The collecting systems may be difficult to visualize unless filled with urine or contrast agent. Hydration and administration of diuretics are helpful in increasing urine output when the system is not dilated. The excretory MR urogram is performed pre- and postcontrast in a similar fashion to the CT urogram. Precontrast T1WI demonstrates a high signal cortex and a lower signal medulla. Urine in the collecting system is low signal. With T2WI, both the cortex and medulla brighten, but corticomedullary differentiation is often lost. Urine in the collecting system is high signal. After gadolinium administration dynamic postcontrast sequences are obtained through the kidneys during arterial, nephrogram, and pyelogram phases to evaluate the renal parenchyma. Subtraction images are essential for recognition of low-grade enhancement. Excretory phase T1WI images are obtained of the collecting system, ureters, and bladder as gadolinium is excreted into the urine. Gadolinium shortens the T1 relaxation time of urine making it bright as gadolinium initially mixes in the urine. However, as the gadolinium concentration increases T2* effects reduce signal intensity and the urine darkens impairing the quality of the study. Oral hydration, diuretics, and use of low-dose gadolinium agents minimize this effect. Three-dimensional reconstructions and maximum intensity projections (MIP) create the urographic images (Fig. 47.18). Diffusion-weighted MR, especially using 3 Tesla magnets, shows promise in improving MR characterization of renal lesions.

US is used to screen for hydronephrosis, assess kidney size, and characterize lesions thought to be cysts. Color Doppler US is valuable in the assessment of tumor vascularity and extension of renal tumors into the venous system.

Anatomy

The kidneys are located within the cone of renal fascia (Gerota fascia), surrounded by the fat of the perirenal space. The kidney is made up of lobes that consist of a pyramid-shaped medulla surrounded by cortex except at the apex of the pyramid. The cortex consists of all the glomeruli, proximal and distal convoluted tubules, and accompanying blood vessels. The *peripheral cortex* is immediately beneath the renal capsule, and the *septal cortex* extends down between the pyramids as the columns of Bertin. Prominent intrarenal septal cortex may simulate a renal mass. The medullary pyramids consist of the collecting tubules and the long, straight portions of the loops of Henle, as well as accompanying blood vessels. The apex of each pyramid is directed at the renal sinus and projects into a calyx. The term *papilla* refers to the innermost zone of the medulla, closest to the draining calyx. The kidneys gradually increase in size from birth to age 20. Renal length is relatively stable at 9 to 13 cm from ages 20 to 50 and gradually decreases thereafter.

Simple calyces are cup-shaped structures that drain one renal lobe. *Compound calyces* drain several renal lobes and are more complex in shape. Compound calyces are more common at the poles of the kidney and are more prone to intrarenal reflux. The shape of each calyx is determined by the shape

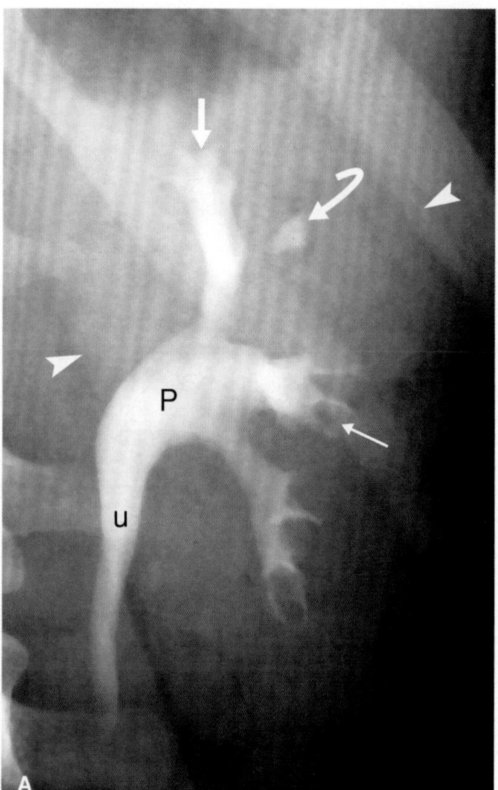

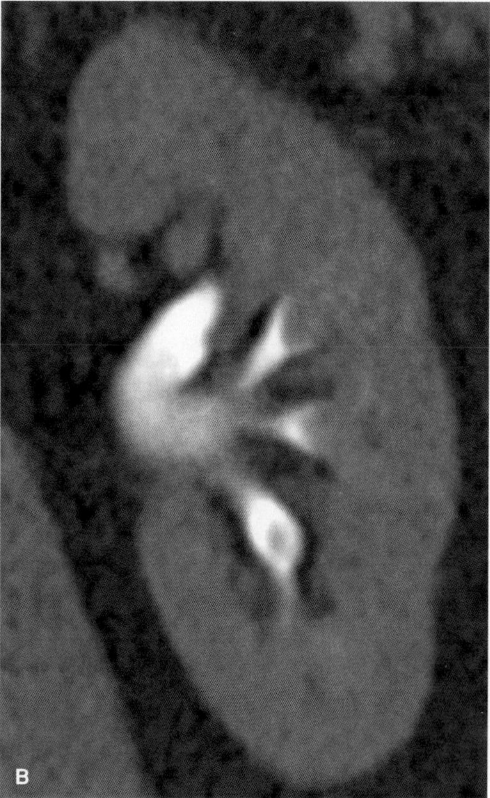

FIGURE 47.17. **Conventional Excretory Urogram Versus CT Urogram. A:** A radiograph of the left kidney taken 5 minutes after intravenous contrast injection during a conventional IVP demonstrates the enhanced renal parenchyma (between *arrowheads*) and the filled pelvis (*P*), ureter (*u*), and calyces (*skinny arrow*). The calyces are sharp and show the normal cup shape that accepts the apex of the medullary pyramids. Upper pole calyces (*thick arrow*) are usually compound because of drainage of multiple pyramids. Oblique views may be needed to confirm the normal appearance of calyces oriented anteriorly or posteriorly (*curved arrow*). The normal kidney is equal in length to between three and four vertebral bodies. **B:** Coronal plane reconstructed tomographic pyelogram-phase image from a CT-IVP shows similar anatomy. The detail of the calyces seen with the conventional IVP is clearly sharper than that shown with the CT-IVP. The spatial resolution of conventional radiography is significantly higher than that of CT. However CT offers the major advantage of markedly increased contrast resolution compared to conventional radiography allowing much higher sensitivity for detection of parenchymal renal lesions.

of the papilla. Disease of the papilla is reflected in the appearance of the calyx. The minor calyces join to form major calyces (infundibula), which drain into the renal pelvis and then into the ureter. The appearance of the calyces and pelvis varies widely from patient to patient, and often from one kidney to another, even in the same patient. About 1% of the renal collecting systems and ureters are bifid or completely duplicated.

The main renal arteries originate laterally from the aorta, just below the origin of the superior mesenteric artery. The right renal artery courses posterior to the IVC, whereas the left renal artery courses posterior to the left renal vein. The main renal artery divides into ventral and dorsal branches as it enters the renal hilum. These branches divide into segmental arteries that supply separate portions of the kidney. Each is an end artery without anastomoses. Supplied segments of the kidney are therefore highly subject to infarction caused by emboli or occlusion. Interlobar arteries arise from segmental arteries and course in the columns of Bertin. Arcuate arteries are continuations of the interlobar arteries and course parallel to the renal capsule at the corticomedullary junction. Arcuate arteries give rise to intralobular arteries. Arterial divisions down to the level of the arcuate artery are demonstrable by color Doppler US.

The tight fibrous capsule that covers the kidney produces a sharp renal margin on CT and MR. Perirenal fat continues into the renal sinus, outlining blood vessels and the collecting system. The renal fascia is commonly visualized on CT, especially when the fascia is thickened. Connective tissue septa extending between the renal capsule and the renal fascia subdivide the perirenal space into compartments and may be seen as linear strands in the perirenal fat.

Congenital Renal Anomalies

Renal agenesis is associated with uterine anomalies in females and ipsilateral seminal vesicle cysts in males. Ipsilateral adrenal agenesis is found in 10% of cases. In the remainder, the adrenal gland may appear enlarged. Compensatory hypertrophy and congenital anomalies of the remaining kidney are often evident. Vesicoureteral reflux is present in 24% of cases.

Horseshoe kidney is the most common renal fusion anomaly. The lower poles of the kidneys are joined across the midline by a fibrous or parenchymal band. As a result of fusion, the kidneys are malrotated, with the renal pelvises directed more anteriorly and the lower pole calyces directed medially. The fused kidney is low in position in the abdomen because normal ascent is prevented by renal tissue encountering the inferior mesenteric artery in the midline (Fig. 47.19). Renal

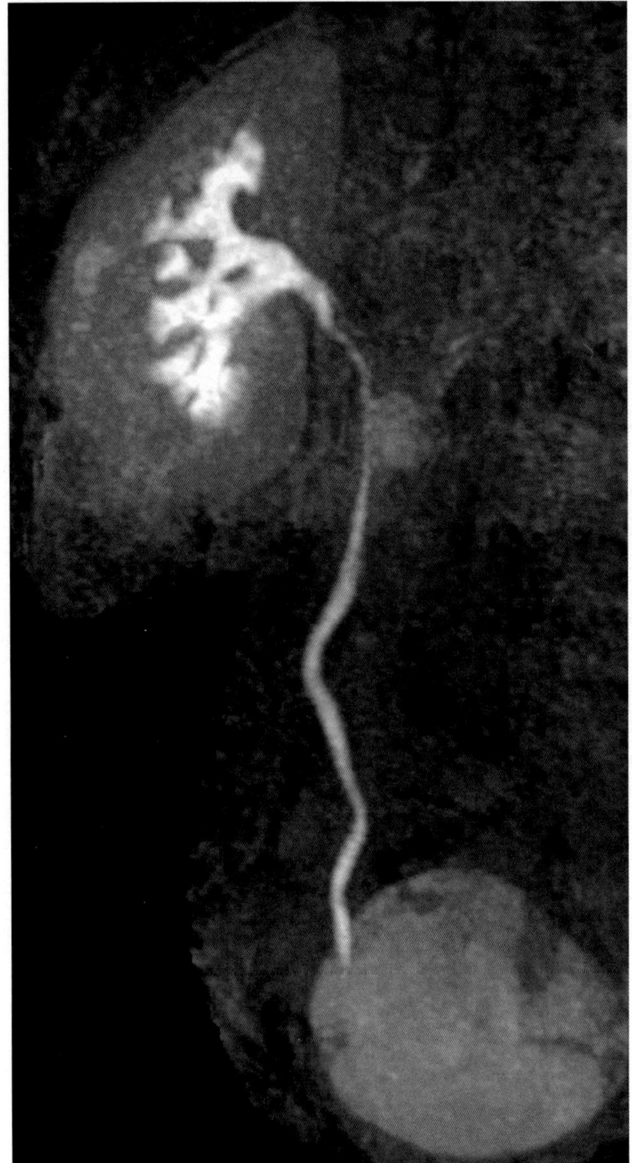

FIGURE 47.18. **MR Urogram.** A maximum intensity projection (MIP) image shows a normal right kidney, collecting system, ureter, and bladder.

arteries are frequently multiple and ectopic in origin. Complications include increased susceptibility to trauma because of low position in the abdomen and urinary stasis leading to stones and infection. The midline isthmus of the kidney is identified by cross-sectional imaging.

Crossed-fused renal ectopia may present as an abdominal mass because the two kidneys are fused (upper pole of the ectopic kidney to lower pole of the opposite kidney) on the one side of the abdomen. Renal arteries are invariably aberrant. Demonstration that one kidney is absent from its normal location and that the ureters insert in their normal locations in the bladder trigone confirms the diagnosis.

Solid Renal Masses

Renal cell carcinoma (RCC) accounts for 85% of all renal neoplasms. It is most common in men (3–5:1) and usually presents at age 50 to 70 years. RCC is now known to represent a family of related tumors with differing pathologic properties, prognoses, and imaging characteristics. Pathologies include conventional clear cell adenocarcinoma (80%), multilocular clear cell carcinoma (5%), papillary RCC (15%), chromophobe RCC (5%), renal medullary carcinoma (<1%), and others. Chromophobe tumors have the best prognosis. Predisposing conditions for RCC include von Hippel–Lindau disease, hereditary papillary RCC, acquired renal cystic disease associated with long-term dialysis, cigarette smoking, renal transplantation, and HIV infection. Most tumors are solitary but some (6%) are multifocal, and a few (4%) are bilateral. Any solid renal mass should be considered suspect for RCC (Fig. 47.20). Hemorrhage and necrosis are common. Cystic and multicystic forms (5% to 10%) (Figs. 47.21 and 47.22) are also seen.

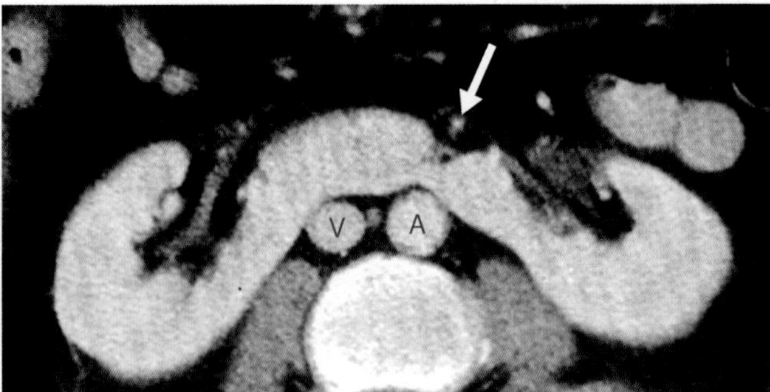

FIGURE 47.19. **Horseshoe Kidney.** Image from a post contrast CT demonstrates the two kidneys extending across the spine anterior to the IVC (*V*) and aorta (*A*) and joined at their lower poles. The kidneys are low in position in the abdomen stopped in their ascent by the inferior mesenteric artery (*arrow*).

Staging (see Renal cell carcinoma TMN staging online reference in Suggested Readings) is critical to the selection of expanding options for treatment. Small RCC (<3 cm) have been treated with laparoscopic partial nephrectomy or percutaneous radiofrequency ablation with good results. Prognosis is related to stage and tumor type but varies unpredictably in individual cases. Radiologic evaluation involves tumor detection and characterization as well as staging. Important findings include

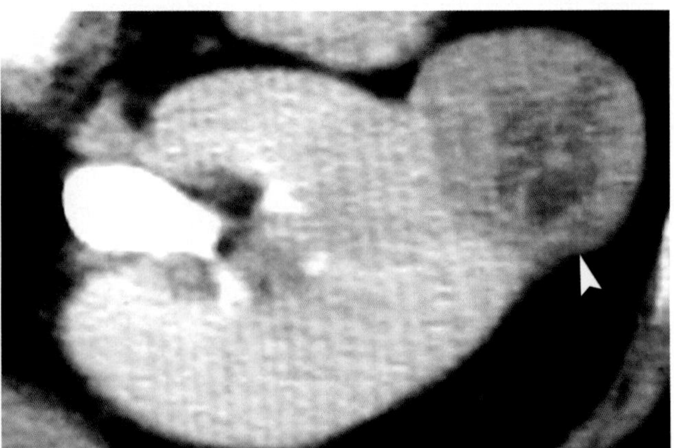

FIGURE 47.20. **Renal Cell Carcinoma.** Pyelogram-phase image from a CT urogram shows an exophytic solid mass (*arrowhead*) projecting from the lateral aspect of the kidney. The mass shows heterogeneous enhancement less than that of the renal parenchyma during this phase. Pathology revealed a conventional clear cell carcinoma. Low attenuation areas within the tumor proved to be foci of necrosis and hemorrhage.

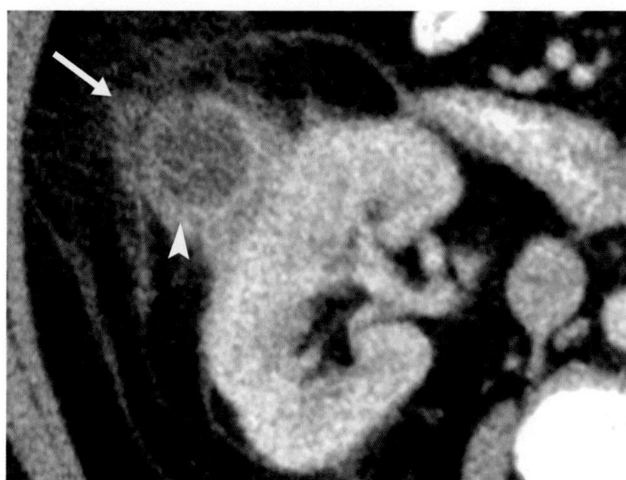

FIGURE 47.21. **Cystic Renal Cell Carcinoma.** Axial postcontrast image from MDCT reveals a cystic tumor (*arrowhead*) projecting from the lateral aspect of the right kidney. The lesion has shaggy thick walls with indistinct stranding extending into the perirenal fat. A distinct nodule (*arrow*) of enhancing soft tissue extends from the tumor into the perirenal fat. While soft tissue stranding is nonspecific, a distinct tumor nodule in the perirenal fat is highly indicative of tumor extension outside of the renal capsule.

extension beyond Gerota capsule, tumor invasion of the renal vein (20% to 30%) and IVC (4% to 10%), and distant metastases. Chest CT, brain MR, and radionuclide bone scans are important in demonstrating distant metastases in patients with aggressive tumors or symptoms to suggest disease at those sites.

MDCT without and with intravenous contrast administration is the tumor evaluation and staging method of choice. Diagnosis depends on demonstration of tumor enhancement. Avid heterogeneous tumor enhancement is seen with clear cell carcinoma. Papillary and chromophobe tumors show a lesser degree and a more peripheral pattern of enhancement. Tumors are slightly hypointense to renal parenchyma on noncontrast CT and are easily overlooked if they are entirely intrarenal. Even with enhancement most tumors are heterogeneously lower in attenuation than enhanced renal parenchyma. Low-density areas within the tumor reflect hemorrhage and necrosis (Fig. 47.20). CT is not accurate in the differentiation of stage I and stage II tumors, but this is of limited treatment significance. Stranding densities in the perirenal fat are usually attributable to edema or fibrosis from previous inflammation and are not a reliable sign of tumor spread. Discrete soft tissue nodules in the perirenal fat are highly predictive of tumor spread into the fat (Fig. 47.21). Bland thrombus appears as a filling defect within and often expanding the contrast-opacified renal vein or IVC. Tumor thrombus is detected as an enhancing mass within the vein. Cystic and multilocular cystic forms of RCC (Figs. 47.21 and 47.22) are Bosniak III and IV lesions characterized by nodular thickening of the wall and septa that enhance with contrast.

On MR, clear cell RCC is isointense or slightly hypointense compared with renal parenchyma on T1WI. Hyperintensity on T1WI usually reflects tumoral hemorrhage, but fat-suppression sequences should be used to ensure the high signal is not because of fat. Most RCCs are heterogeneous on T2WI, reflecting areas of tumor necrosis, hemorrhage, and hemosiderin. Because the MR imaging characteristics of RCC is so variable, diagnosis depends on showing enhancement of the mass regardless of its signal intensity. Clear cell carcinoma is hypervascular and enhances avidly. Papillary RCC tends to be hypointense on both T1WI and T2WI and shows low-level homogeneous enhancement postcontrast. MR angiography effectively shows venous invasion (Fig. 47.23).

The staging accuracy of MR and CT is about equal. US demonstrates solid RCCs as a heterogeneous hypoechoic or mildly hyperechoic mass. Areas of hemorrhage and necrosis appear cystic. Doppler US of the renal vein and IVC shows tumor thrombus by demonstration of echogenic material in the vein associated with partial or complete absence of blood flow.

Angiomyolipoma (AML) is an uncommon (1% to 3% of renal neoplasms) benign mesenchymal tumor composed of varying amounts of fat, smooth muscle, and abnormal blood vessels lacking elastic tissue. Most (80%) are solitary unilateral tumors discovered most commonly in middle-aged women. Most of the remaining 20% are found in patients with tuberous sclerosis. AML in patients with tuberous sclerosis are commonly multicentric and bilateral. Because of the abnormal thin-walled vessels, AMLs are prone to hemorrhage, which may be massive. Large solitary lesions are usually recommended for surgical removal. Follow-up of small lesions reveals slow growth. Imaging studies reflect the tissue composition of the tumor and can range from almost purely fat density to nearly homogeneously solid muscle density. Tumors may be as large as 20 cm and may be predominantly exophytic, mimicking nonrenal tumors.

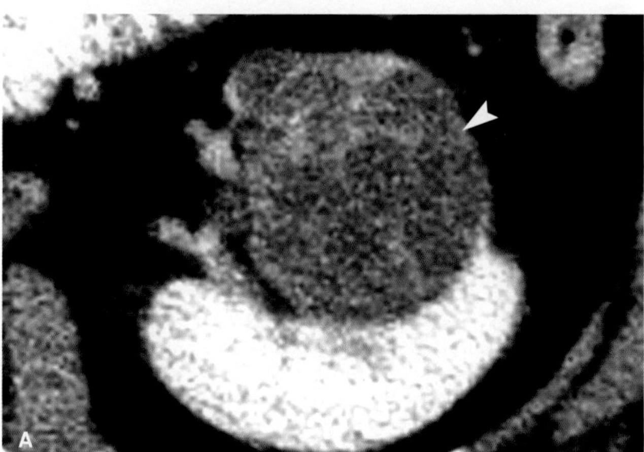

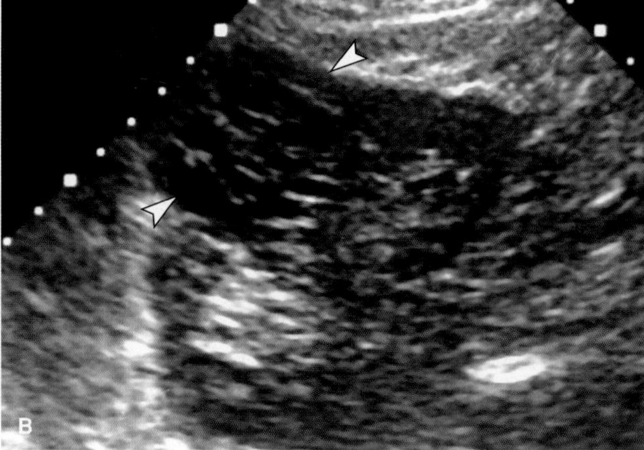

FIGURE 47.22. **Multicystic Renal Cell Carcinoma. A:** Contrast-enhanced CT scan reveals a low attenuation, well-defined mass (*arrowhead*) in the left kidney. Subtle enhancement of internal septations is present. **B:** A US image in a different patient shows a multicystic mass (between *arrowheads*) arising from the lateral aspect of the left kidney. In both patients the thin septations were lined by clear cells typical of renal carcinoma.

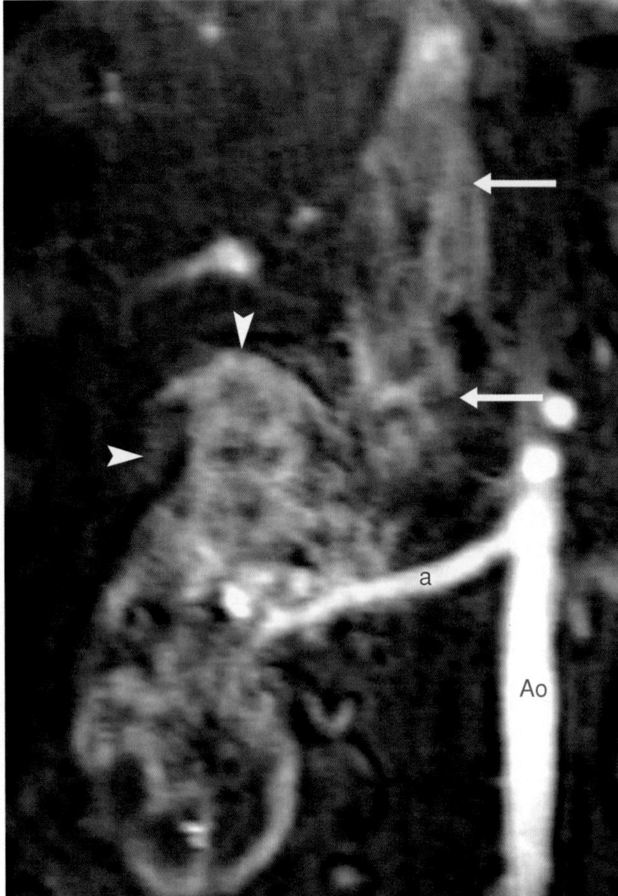

FIGURE 47.23. Tumor Thrombus in Renal Vein and Inferior Vena Cava. Coronal plane image from an MR angiogram shows an irregularly enhancing mass (*arrowheads*) replacing the upper pole of the right kidney. Enhancing tumor thrombus (*arrows*) extends continuously from the renal mass through the renal vein and into the lumen of the inferior vena cava. Enhancement differentiates tumor thrombus from bland thrombus. The right renal artery (*a*) and aorta (*Ao*) are well shown.

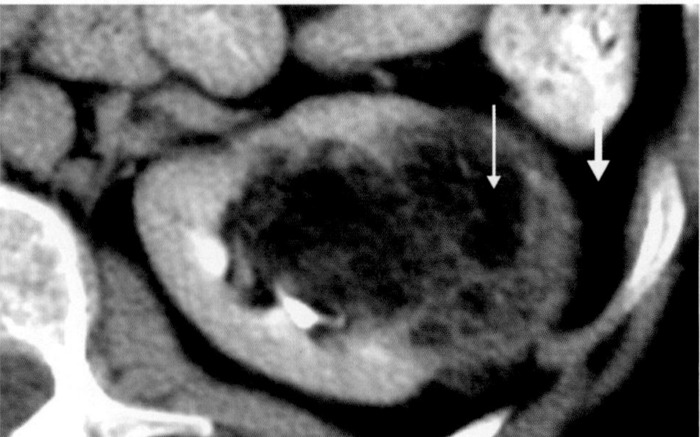

FIGURE 47.24. Angiomyolipoma—CT. Postcontrast CT demonstrates a tumor infiltrating and extending outside of the left kidney. Areas of fat density (*thin arrow*) are mixed with strands and foci of soft tissue density. The appearance is characteristic of angiomyolipoma. Compare the fat density regions within the tumor (*thin arrow*) with retroperitoneal fat (*thick arrow*).

MDCT is the usual diagnostic method of choice. CT demonstration of even small quantities of fat density within the tumor is considered diagnostic of AML (Fig. 47.24). Compare low-density areas within the tumor to retroperitoneal fat. Thin-section MDCT may be needed to convincingly show fat. On the other hand tiny tumors may be conspicuous because of their fat content. Smooth muscle and vascular components of the tumor are seen as nodules and strands of soft tissue density. Vascular areas of the tumor may show striking contrast enhancement. Lipid-poor AMLs may be indistinguishable from RCC by imaging methods. In a few reported cases, fat has been detected in association with calcification in an RCC. In these cases, the calcification was shown histologically to be ossification with associated marrow fat. Fat density in a solid renal tumor without calcification is diagnostic of AML.

MR diagnosis is also based on the demonstration of fat within the tumor. Decrease in signal in fat-containing areas on fat-suppression images is the most reliable finding. Chemical shift MR may demonstrate the characteristic India ink artifact at the interface between fat within the tumor and renal parenchyma (Fig. 47.25). Typically lipid-rich AML shows no significant change in signal between IP and opposed-phase images. However, low signal on opposed-phase images is a clue to the presence of scant amount of fat in lipid-poor AML, reflecting coexistence of fat and water within the MR voxels. This finding may also be seen in clear cell RCC that contain fat. On standard T1WI and T2WI, the signal intensity depends on the amount of bulk fat present, with more fat producing brighter signal. Enhancement postcontrast varies with the amount of vascularized soft tissue present within the tumor. The presence of central necrosis is important in differentiation of RCC from lipid-poor AML as necrosis is common with RCC but is rare with AML. Also RCC may contain intracellular fat but macroscopic fat characteristic of AML has been reported in RCC only in the presence of calcification.

US characteristically demonstrates a strikingly hyperechoic solid mass (see Fig. 50.62). Echogenicity of the tumor often exceeds renal sinus fat. Small tumors are common incidental findings. Because small RCC (<3 cm) may appear as echogenic renal masses that overlap the US appearance of AML, these lesions must be definitively characterized by CT or MR.

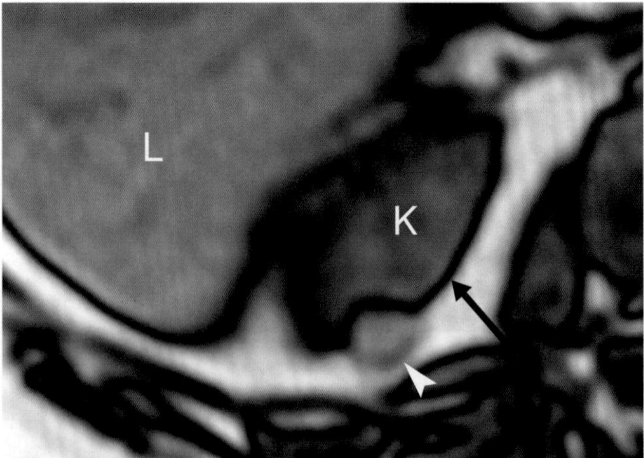

FIGURE 47.25. Angiomyolipoma—MR. An axial out-of-phase T1-weighted gradient echo MR image reveals a small predominantly fat density AML (*arrowhead*) extending from the right kidney (*K*). Note the black line "India ink" artifact (*arrow*) that marks the boundary of soft tissue of the kidney and liver (*L*) with adjacent fat. The artifact is caused by signal from water in soft tissue and signal from fat within the same voxel cancelling each other out. The artifact is present between the renal parenchyma and the mass but is absent between the mass and retroperitoneal fat indicating that the renal mass contains abundant fat.

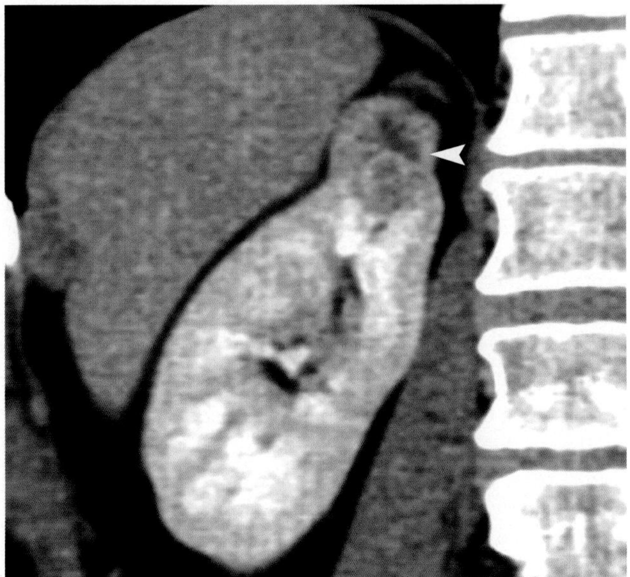

FIGURE 47.26. **Oncocytoma.** Coronal plane MDCT image shows a pathologically proven oncocytoma (*arrowhead*) that mimics a renal cell carcinoma.

Oncocytoma is a rare (3% to 5% of renal neoplasms), well-encapsulated, benign tumor composed of eosinophilic cells called oncocytes. Oncocytoma is the benign member of the family of renal cancer tumors. Tumors may be large (up to 25 cm), but they average 5 to 8 cm. Hemorrhage and necrosis are rare. Most are solitary, but 6% are multiple or bilateral. Large tumors demonstrate a stellate central scar that is suggestive of the diagnosis. MR shows low tumor signal on T1WI and higher tumor signal on T2WI overlapping the appearance of RCC. If a central scar is present, it appears as stellate low signal on both T1WI and T2WI. Oncocytomas are not reliably distinguished from RCC by all imaging methods and must be surgically removed to confirm the diagnosis (Fig. 47.26).

Lymphoma. Although primary renal lymphoma is rare, the kidney is commonly involved by direct invasion from retroperitoneal lymphoma or by metastatic lymphoma. Most cases are non-Hodgkin lymphoma (Fig. 47.27). Patterns of renal involvement include diffuse disease enlarging the kidney, multiple bilateral solid renal masses, solitary bulky tumor, perirenal tumor surrounding the kidney, and tumor invasion from the retroperitoneum into the renal sinus. CT shows lymphoma as homogenous and poorly enhancing. Extensive retroperitoneal adenopathy favors the diagnosis. On MR lymphoma is iso- or slightly hypointense to renal parenchyma on T1WI, hypointense on T2WI, and shows minimal heterogeneous enhancement postcontrast.

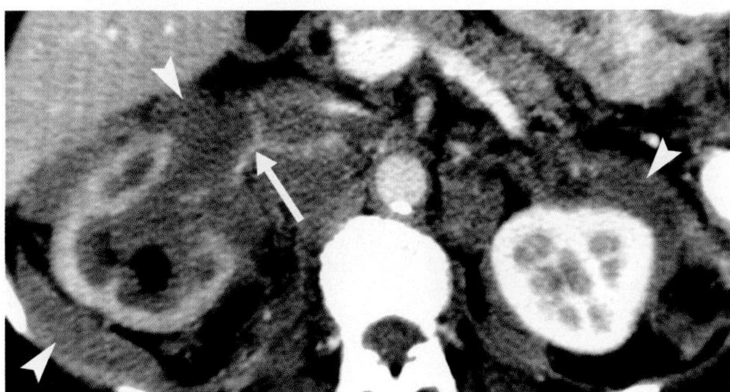

FIGURE 47.27. **Renal Lymphoma.** Non-Hodgkin lymphoma (*arrowheads*) infiltrates the perirenal space partially surrounding both kidneys. Note the impaired contrast enhancement of the right kidney caused by lymphomatous involvement of the right renal blood vessels (*arrow*). The tumor infiltrates the sinus and parenchyma of the right kidney.

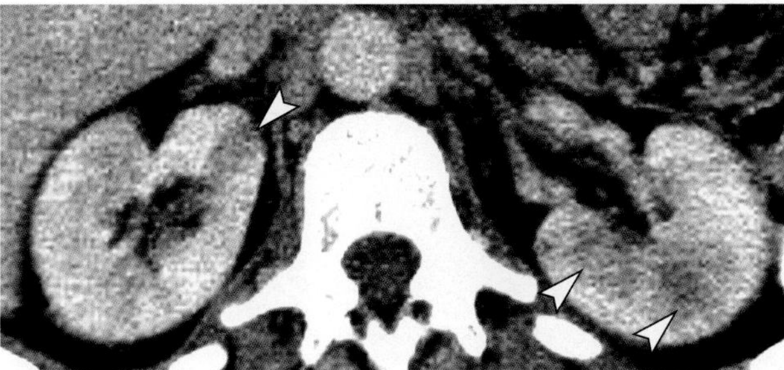

FIGURE 47.28. **Metastases to the Kidney.** In a patient with lung cancer the ill-defined low attenuation lesions (*arrowheads*) in the renal parenchyma of both kidneys represent metastatic disease. Metastases are typically infiltrative and poorly defined.

Metastases. The kidneys are a frequent site of hematogenous metastases; however, most are detected late in the course of malignancy. Most metastases appear as multiple, bilateral, small, irregular infiltrative renal masses (Fig. 47.28). Some are large, solitary, and not distinguishable from RCC. Common primary tumors include lung, breast, and colon carcinoma, and melanoma.

Cystic Renal Masses

Simple renal cyst is the most common renal mass. They are found in half the population older than age 55. Small cysts are asymptomatic. Large cysts (>4 cm) occasionally cause obstruction, pain, hematuria, or hypertension. Cysts are commonly multiple and bilateral. US, CT, and MR can each make a definitive diagnosis. US criteria for simple renal cyst are (a) round or oval anechoic mass, (b) increased through transmission, (c) sharply defined far wall, and (d) thin or imperceptible cyst wall. Definitive CT signs are (a) sharp margination with the renal parenchyma, (b) no perceptible wall, (c) homogeneous attenuation near water density (–10 to +10 H), and (d) absence of contrast enhancement (Fig. 47.29). MR criteria

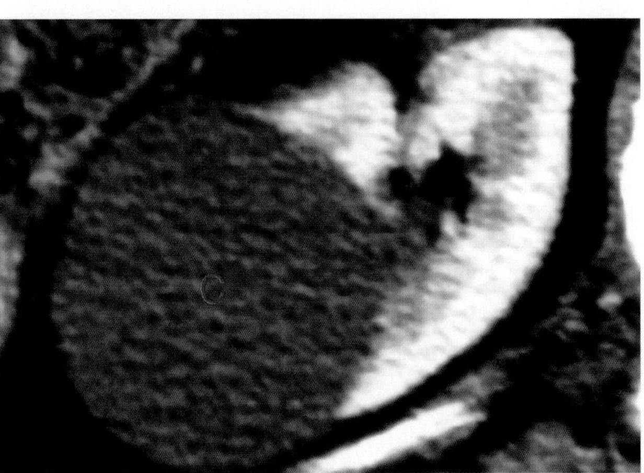

FIGURE 47.29. **Simple Renal Cyst.** A large cyst (C) arising from the right kidney shows characteristic CT features. The cyst is of uniform low density, has a sharp margin with the renal parenchyma, and its wall is imperceptible.

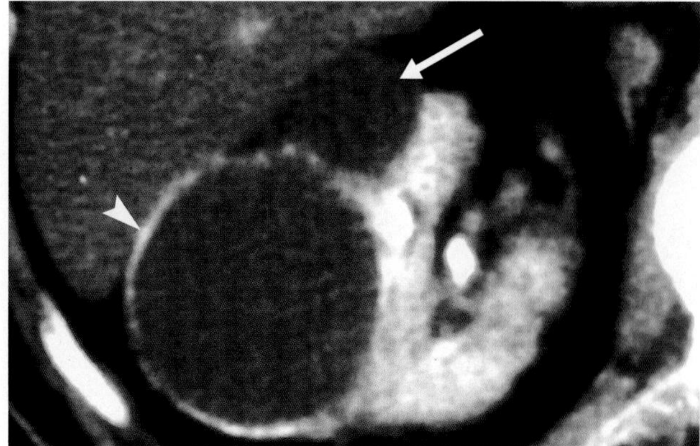

FIGURE 47.30. **Complicated Renal Cyst.** Postcontrast MDCT demonstrates a small simple renal cyst (*arrow*) and a larger renal cyst with a thin wall complicated by a thin rim of calcification (*arrowhead*). This larger cyst is classified as a benign renal cyst, Bosniak II.

are (a) homogeneous, sharply defined round or oval mass, (b) homogeneous low signal intensity similar to urine on T1WI, (c) homogeneous high signal intensity similar to urine on T2WI, and (d) no enhancement after gadolinium administration. Simple renal cysts are benign Bosniak category I lesions and once confidently characterized no further follow-up is needed.

Complicated Cyst. Simple renal cysts may become complicated by hemorrhage or infection. The resulting change in imaging characteristics may make differentiation from cystic renal tumors difficult. Bosniak developed in 1986 a classification system for cystic masses that with minor modification has been accepted and used worldwide. The Bosniak classification is used to determine the management of these lesions. The classification system was originally applied to CT but is currently utilized with MR as well.

Category I lesions are simple cysts with the imaging findings just listed. CT, MR, and US are definitive when all characteristic findings are present.

Category II lesions are benign, with no further imaging or follow-up needed. Three types of cysts are in this category: (a) cysts with delicate thin septations no more than 1 to 2 mm thick, (b) cysts with delicate thin calcification in the wall or septum (Fig. 47.30), and (c) "high-density" cysts that are hyperdense (60 to 100 H) on CT because of high concentration of protein or blood breakdown products and are of size of less than 3 cm. When cysts contain proteinaceous or hemorrhagic fluid MR shows high signal intensity on T1WI and lower signal on T2WI. MR may show more septations than CT but does not show calcifications as well as CT, especially if the calcification is hairline thin and in the wall of the cyst.

Category IIF lesions are those that are very likely benign but require additional follow-up imaging to confirm benignancy. These lesions may have many thin septa or minimal smooth thickening of the walls or septa but without measurable contrast enhancement. Cysts with thick or nodular calcification in the wall or septa are included in this category as are totally intrarenal nonenhancing high-density cysts <3 cm. Bosniak has recommended imaging follow-up of IIF lesions at 3, 6, and 12 months.

Category III lesions are indeterminate lesions that may be benign or malignant. Most should be treated surgically. Findings include thick irregular calcification, irregular margins, thick or enhancing septa, areas of nodularity, thick walls, and multilocular mass (Fig. 47.22). Lesions in this category include multilocular cystic nephroma, multilocular clear cell RCC, and complex benign hemorrhagic or chronically infected cysts.

Category IV lesions are clearly malignant necrotic cystic neoplasms or tumors that arise in the wall of a cyst. Findings include irregular solid nodules, irregular thick shaggy walls, and nodular septations (Fig. 47.21). CT or MR demonstration of enhancement of solid areas following contrast administration makes the diagnosis of malignancy.

Small renal lesions may be particularly difficult to classify. Thin-section MDCT with bolus contrast enhancement and great attention to detail will assist in correct classification of lesions. MR signal intensity depends on the amount of blood or proteinaceous material present within the cyst. Cyst fluid with signal characteristics similar to urine suggests a simple cyst. Higher signal intensity on T1WI suggests a complicated cyst, which may be indistinguishable from a solid mass. Because of its higher contrast resolution but lower spatial resolution, MR imaging may result in a higher Bosniak classification than MDCT of the same lesion.

Renal abscess usually results from pyelonephritis complicated by liquefactive necrosis of the renal parenchyma. A focal renal mass with a thick wall is the most common appearance. Associated inflammatory changes include stranding densities in the perirenal space and thickening of the renal fascia (Fig. 47.31). Renal abscesses may extend into the perirenal space and be associated with perirenal fluid collections.

Renal cell carcinoma may appear as a predominantly cystic or multiloculated cystic mass (Figs. 47.21 and 47.22). Malignant tumor cells line the walls and septa. Thick walls, thick septations, and contrast enhancement are usually evident. These are Bosniak III or IV lesions.

Multilocular cystic nephroma, also called adult cystic nephroma or mixed epithelial and stromal tumor ("MEST"), is an uncommon benign neoplasm consisting of a cluster of noncommunicating cysts of varying size separated by connective tissue septations of varying thickness. The tumor has a thick capsule with thin septations. Imaging features would be classified as a Bosniak III or IV lesion (Fig. 47.32). They are discovered most commonly in middle-aged women (40 to 60 years). Surgical excision is usually recommended because the lesion is indistinguishable from multicystic RCC. A similar, but now thought to be distinct tumor, is the pediatric cystic nephroma, usually found in boys aged 3 months to 4 years.

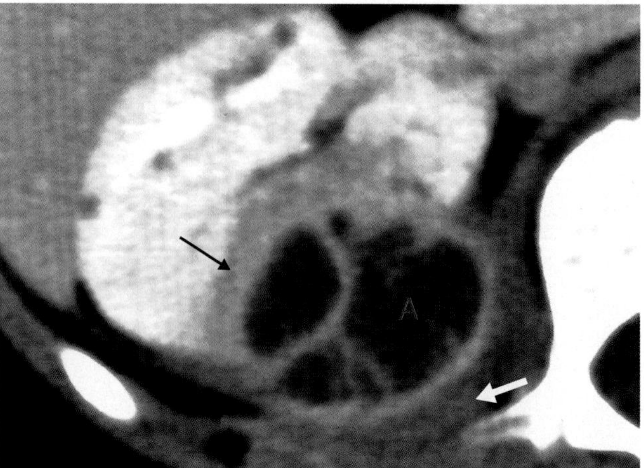

FIGURE 47.31. **Renal Abscess.** The right renal abscess (*A*) has characteristic thick walls and septations and internal fluid density. Edema reduces the CT density of the renal parenchyma adjacent to the mass (*thin arrow*) and infiltrates the perirenal space (*thick arrow*). This patient also has multiple small renal cysts associated with autosomal dominant polycystic disease.

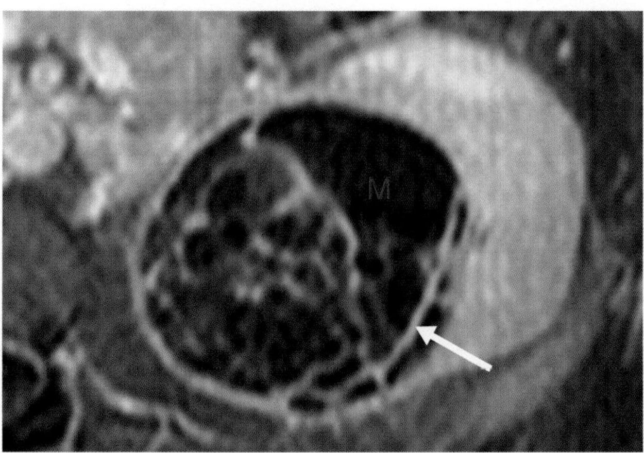

FIGURE 47.32. **Multilocular Cystic Nephroma.** Axial postgadolinium contrast-enhanced T1-weighted gradient echo fat saturation MR image shows a multiloculated cystic mass (*M*) with numerous enhancing septations (*arrow*) arising the left kidney in a middle-aged woman. Pathology revealed a benign multilocular cystic nephroma.

Renal Cystic Disease

Autosomal dominant polycystic disease is transmitted by autosomal dominant inheritance but usually manifests clinically later in life. Renal parenchyma is progressively replaced by multiple noncommunicating cysts of varying size (Fig. 47.33; see Fig 50.58). Renal volume increases with the number and size of the renal cysts. The cysts are commonly complicated by internal hemorrhage, often spontaneous, infection, and rupture. The condition can be detected in neonates and children, but most patients present clinically between ages 30 and 50 years with hypertension and renal failure. Imaging diagnosis is confirmed by demonstration of cysts in the liver (60% of patients), pancreas (10% of patients), and often in other organs. Extrarenal cysts seldom cause clinical problems. Associated cardiovascular abnormalities include intracranial aneurysms (20% of patients), mitral valve prolapse, bicuspid aortic valve, aortic aneurysms, and dissections. CT shows the innumerable cysts to have varying attenuation of internal fluid reflecting previous episodes of hemorrhage or infection. MR is even more sensitive to these changes showing increased signal on T1WI and usually decreased signal on T2WI.

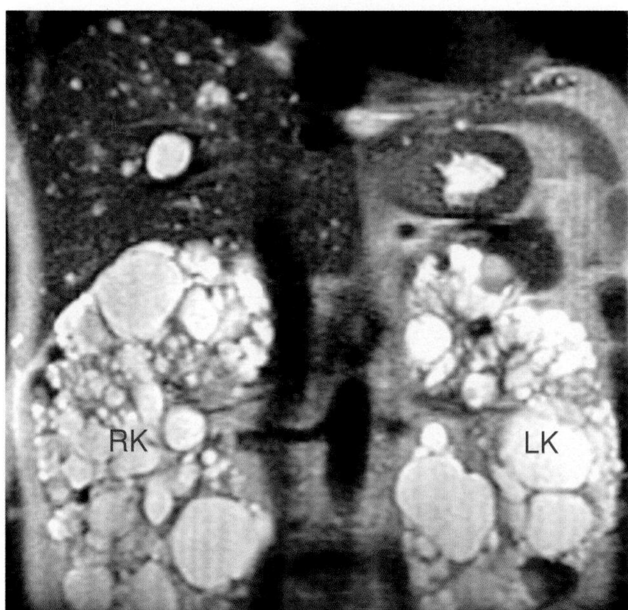

FIGURE 47.33. **Adult Dominant Polycystic Disease.** T2-weighted MR in coronal plane shows extensive replacement of the renal parenchyma with innumerable noncommunicating cysts of various sizes. Cysts are also seen in the liver (*L*). Both kidneys (*RK, LK*) are massively enlarged.

Multiple simple cysts must be differentiated from adult polycystic disease. Patients with multiple simple cysts are usually older, have fewer cysts, and typically have no renal failure and no family history of renal cystic disease. Cysts are not found in other organs.

von Hippel–Lindau disease is a rare, inherited, multisystem disease associated with development of multiple renal cysts (60% of patients), multiple and bilateral RCC (24% to 45%), adrenal pheochromocytomas (up to 60%), pancreatic cysts (serous cystadenomas) (50% to 90%), and pancreatic adenocarcinomas. Associated lesions include retinal angiomas and cerebellar hemangioblastomas. The RCC that develop may be cystic clear cell lesions. RCC develops at a young age (mean 30 to 36 years). The disease is inherited with an autosomal dominant pattern that is not expressed in every individual with the gene.

Tuberous sclerosis is a neurocutaneous syndrome that combines multiple simple renal cysts and multiple AML (55% to 75%). The AMLs are multiple and bilateral. Cutaneous, retinal, and cerebral hamartomas are associated. This condition also has an autosomal dominant inheritance pattern.

Acquired uremic cystic kidney disease is the term applied to the development of multiple cysts in the native kidneys of patients on long-term hemodialysis. The incidence exceeds 90% in patients after 5 to 10 years of hemodialysis. Affected kidneys are usually small, reflecting the chronic renal disease. Cysts are predominantly cortical and rarely exceed 2 cm size (Fig. 47.34). Cyst hemorrhage occurs in up to 50%. Solid renal adenomas and RCC (7%) also develop and are prone to spontaneous hemorrhage. Cysts usually regress after renal transplant but the increased risk of RCC persists.

Autosomal recessive polycystic kidney disease usually presents in the neonate and is detectable in the fetus. The condition is bilateral, relatively symmetrical, and is characterized by marked enlargement of the kidneys and occasionally the liver. Affected patients have a combination of cystic renal disease and hepatic fibrosis. The disease runs a spectrum from severe renal disease at birth (infantile polycystic disease) to relatively mild renal disease with development of hepatic fibrosis and liver failure in childhood (juvenile polycystic disease). The primary defect in the kidneys is fusiform dilatation and lengthening of the collecting tubules (Fig. 47.35; see Fig. 50.59). The

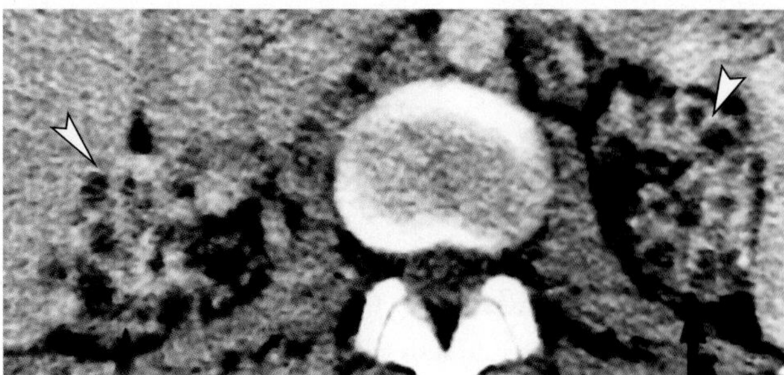

FIGURE 47.34. **Acquired Uremic Cystic Kidney Disease.** Noncontrast CT reveals both kidneys (*arrowheads*) are small and contain numerous small cysts. The patient has been on hemodialysis for 8 years.

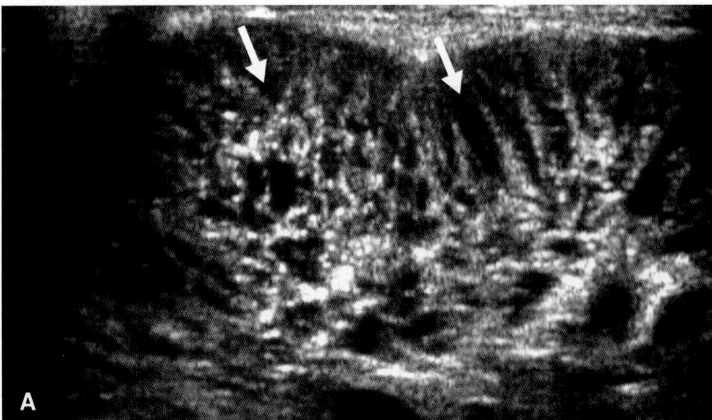

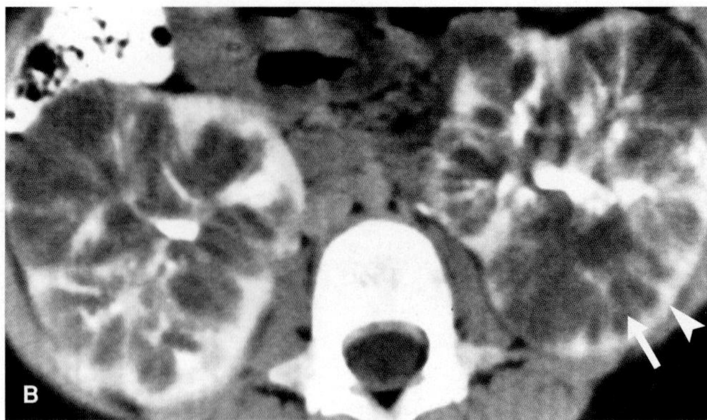

FIGURE 47.35. **Autosomal Recessive Polycystic Disease.** **A:** High-resolution US image of the massively enlarged right kidney in a newborn infant shows the innumerable dilated and elongated collecting tubules (*arrows*) that characterize this condition. **B:** Contrast-enhanced CT in a 5-year-old child shows massive kidneys. The enhanced cortex (*arrowhead*) is thinned and nonenhanced collecting tubules (*arrow*) in the medulla are enlarged. No discrete cysts are evident.

early prognosis depends on the number of abnormal nephrons. Most newborn infants who present in renal failure die in the neonatal period. Infants with a larger number of normal nephrons have mild renal impairment and present at age 3 to 5 years with progressive liver failure and portal hypertension. The hepatic defects consist of an excessive number of dilated, irregular bile ducts associated with fibrosis of the portal tracts. US is used to make the diagnosis in most cases by showing both kidneys to be large and echogenic centrally with a sonolucent rim of compressed cortex. Visualized cysts are generally small (<5 mm). Children with less severe renal disease develop larger cysts. In the older children, who develop liver disease, US shows an enlarged echogenic liver, cystic dilatation of intrahepatic bile ducts, splenomegaly, dilated portal vein, and enlarged portosystemic collateral vessels.

Medullary sponge kidney refers to dysplastic dilatation of the collecting tubules in the papilla (Fig. 47.36; see Fig. 50.55). The dilatation is cylindrical or saccular in configuration. The condition causes urinary stasis in the papilla, which results in stone formation and occasionally infection. Most patients are asymptomatic. There is no genetic predisposition and no risk of renal failure. The kidneys remain normal in size. The condition is usually bilateral and symmetrical but may be focal, unilateral, or asymmetrical. Striations or saccular contrast collections in the papilla on CT or MR urography are most characteristic. Stones in the papilla cause increased echogenicity in the medulla on US.

Uremic medullary cystic disease presents with renal failure, anemia, and salt wasting. The basic defect is progressive tubular atrophy with glomerular sclerosis and medullary cyst formation. The medullary cysts are generally too small to be visualized by current imaging methods. Kidney size is normal or small. Renal parenchymal echogenicity is usually increased.

Multicystic dysplastic kidney is usually diagnosed in utero or at birth. The classic multicystic dysplastic kidney appears as a mass of noncommunicating cysts of varying size. With time, the kidney progressively atrophies, so in the adult a nubbin of tissue, which is often calcified, is all that remains (Fig. 47.37). The ureter is usually atretic.

Renal Vascular Diseases

Renal arteriovenous malformations (AVM) and arteriovenous fistulas (AVF) may be congenital (25%) or acquired

FIGURE 47.36. **Nephrocalcinosis in Medullary Sponge Kidney.** Conventional radiograph demonstrates innumerable calcifications in the medullary regions of both kidneys. The stones form in dilated collecting tubules in the medullary pyramids producing this characteristic pattern in this patient with medullary sponge kidney.

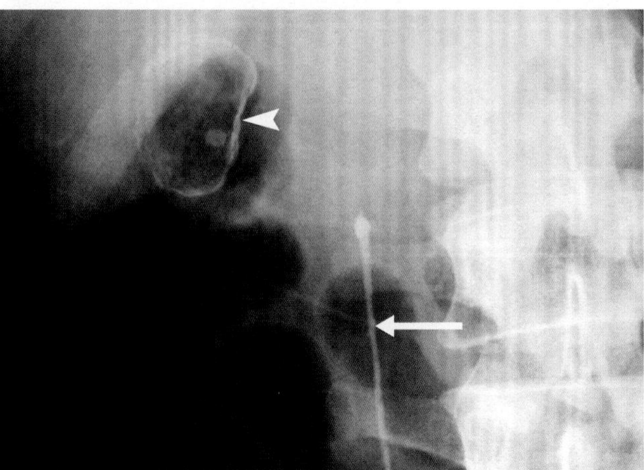

FIGURE 47.37. **Multicystic Dysplastic Kidney.** Conventional radiograph shows evidence of multicystic dysplastic kidney in a 27-year-old male with normal renal function. The residual right kidney (*arrowhead*) is atrophic and entirely calcified. The atretic right ureter (*arrow*) is also calcified. At US, the left kidney was hypertrophied but normal in appearance.

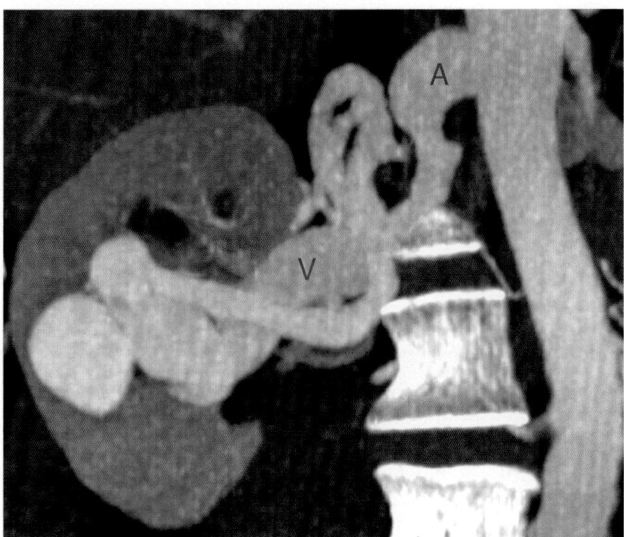

FIGURE 47.38. **Renal Arteriovenous Malformation.** Coronal plane image from a CT angiogram dramatically demonstrates the tangle of large vessels within the right kidney with enlarged supplying arteries (*A*) and draining veins (*V*).

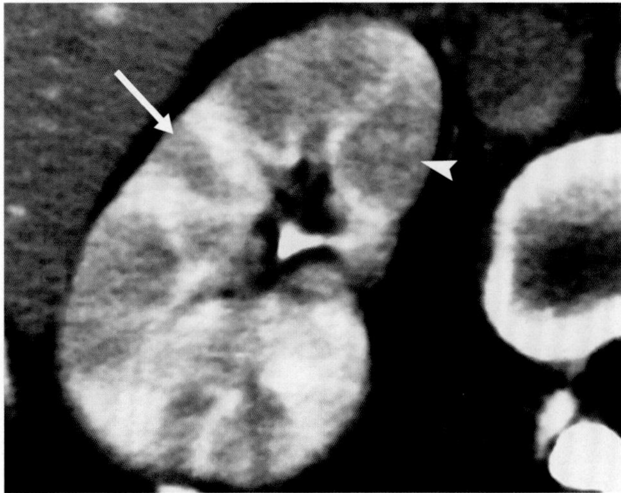

FIGURE 47.39. **Acute Pyelonephritis.** Edema and swelling associated with acute renal infection cause wedge-shaped (*arrow*) and mass-like (*arrowhead*) low attenuation defects in the enhanced parenchyma of the right kidney.

(75%). Congenital AVM are classified as cirsoid supplied by multiple arteries or cavernous supplied by one artery. They consist of a nest of torturous vessels that lie just beneath the uroepithelium and frequently cause hematuria. Acquired lesions are predominantly fistulous connections between the intrarenal arteries and veins caused by renal biopsy, penetrating trauma, nephron-sparing surgery, or malignant tumors. CT without contrast may show blood in the collecting system and a focus of cortical atrophy. Postcontrast CT shows filling of a network of vascular structures (Fig. 47.38). Renal veins are dilated if the shunt is large. Doppler US shows the nest of vessels with mixed color, turbulence, and tissue vibration artifact. MR angiography is less sensitive for slow-flow lesions but effectively demonstrates feeding and draining vessels of high-flow lesions.

Renal Infections

Acute pyelonephritis is usually the result of ascending urinary tract infection caused by gram-negative organisms, especially *Escherichia coli.* Uncomplicated infection requires no imaging and often shows no imaging abnormalities. Imaging evaluation is indicated in patients who fail to respond to treatment or are severely ill. CT is more sensitive than US in demonstrating the subtle changes in the renal parenchyma associated with uncomplicated pyelonephritis. Complications are well demonstrated by CT or US. Predisposing factors include diabetes, obstruction, immune system compromise, drug abuse, chronic debilitating disease, and incomplete antibiotic treatment. CT is normal in some patients with mild uncomplicated pyelonephritis. In most patients, edema causes diffuse or focal swelling. Areas of high attenuation on precontrast scans suggest hemorrhagic inflammation. Contrast enhancement reveals streaks and wedges of low attenuation extending to the renal capsule (the "*striated nephrogram*") (Fig. 47.39), often associated with thickened septa in perinephric fat and thickening of Gerota fascia. Inflammatory low-density masses may form in the renal parenchyma. A variety of confusing terms, including lobar nephronia and focal bacterial nephritis, have been applied to these masses. The Society of Uroradiology recommends abandoning these terms and using only the terms "acute pyelonephritis" with or without "focal, multifocal, or diffuse swelling." Complications of acute pyelonephritis include intrarenal (Fig. 47.31) and perirenal abscess (Fig. 47.40). MR findings are similar to those of CT with renal enlargement due to edema and hemorrhage, and perinephric fluid collections. Obstructing calculi and gas are well demonstrated by CT but are more easily overlooked on MR.

Emphysematous pyelonephritis is a form of acute pyelonephritis with gas in the renal parenchyma. Most cases occur in patients with diabetes, obstruction often caused by calculi, or immune compromise. The condition is rapidly progressive, destroys renal parenchyma, and is often life threatening. Mixed flora infection with gram-negative organisms is most common. Conventional radiographs and CT demonstrate streaks and

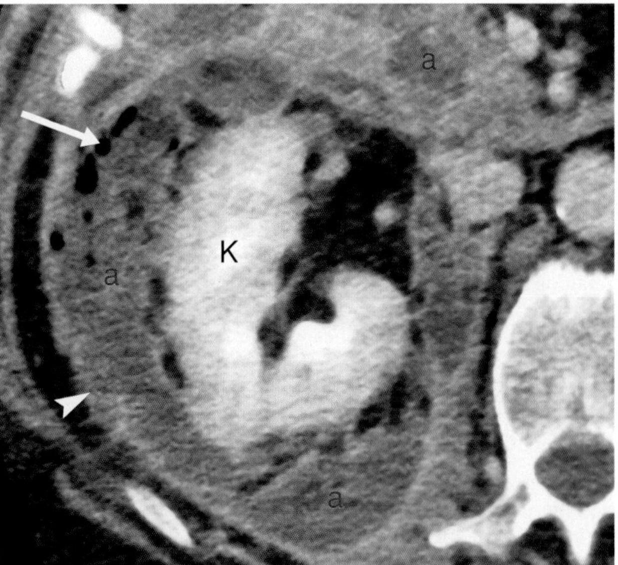

FIGURE 47.40. **Perirenal Abscess.** Contrast-enhanced CT scan reveals low-density fluid collection (*a*) in the perirenal space between the right kidney (*K*) and the thickened renal fascia (*arrowhead*). Gas bubbles (*arrow*) are seen within the perirenal abscess.

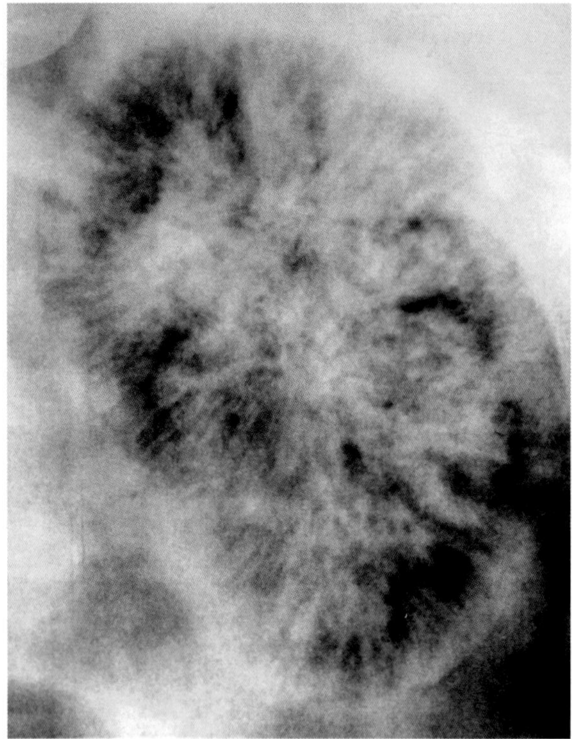

FIGURE 47.41. **Emphysematous Pyelonephritis.** Conventional radiograph of the left kidney shows striations in the renal parenchyma caused by interstitial gas. This finding is indicative of life-threatening infection.

collections of gas within the renal parenchyma (Fig. 47.41). *Emphysematous pyelitis* refers to infection with gas confined to the renal collecting system, sparing the parenchyma. The infection is less aggressive and morbidity is not as high.

Chronic Pyelonephritis and Reflux Nephropathy. Chronic pyelonephritis refers to chronic interstitial nephritis caused by infection. In children, vesicoureteral reflux of infected urine is the most common cause of chronic pyelonephritis. Intrarenal reflux, usually most prominent at the upper pole within compound calyces, damages the papilla, resulting in calyceal blunting with overlying cortical scarring. This process of progressive renal injury associated with reflux is referred to as *reflux nephropathy*. Adults may show stable residual findings of this childhood disease. Chronic pyelonephritis in adults is usually associated with calculi and chronic obstruction. Neurogenic bladder, ileal conduits, and other causes of urinary stasis are predisposing conditions. Both reflux nephropathy of childhood and chronic pyelonephritis in adults show similar imaging findings. The hallmark is a focal cortical scar that overlies a blunted calyx (Fig. 47.42). The disease is classically lobar, with normal lobes with normal calyces interposed between diseased lobes. These findings were traditionally well demonstrated on conventional excretory urography but now require careful inspection of CT and MR urograms. More prominent findings are demonstrable on US.

Xanthogranulomatous pyelonephritis is a rare chronic destructive granulomatous process that may diffusely involve an obstructed kidney or present as a focal renal mass. An obstructing stone, often a staghorn calculus, is usually present (Fig. 47.43; see Fig. 50.67). The kidney is chronically infected, most commonly with *Proteus mirabilis*, *Pseudomonas*, *Klebsiella*, and *E. coli*. It does not function in the affected areas. Renal parenchyma is destroyed and replaced by xanthoma cells, which are lipid-laden macrophages. CT and

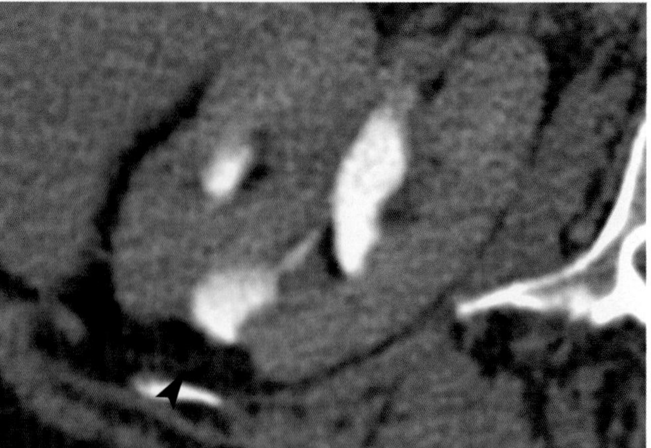

FIGURE 47.42. **Reflux Nephropathy.** Image of the right kidney from a CT urogram of an adult patient shows the characteristic findings of reflux nephropathy. A deep cortical scar overlies a blunted calyx (*arrowhead*). In adults these findings usually reflect renal injury that occurred during childhood.

US demonstrate focal or diffuse hydronephrosis and a complex mass with areas of high and low density. Inflammatory changes characteristically extend into perinephric fat. Since renal function is destroyed excretion of contrast is rarely evident. MR shows dilated calyces compressing and intrarenal abscesses replacing renal parenchyma. Fluid within the calyces and abscesses is intermediate high signal on both T1WI and T2WI. Calculi appear as areas of signal void but are more difficult to recognize on MR than on CT.

Renal tuberculosis may follow primary pulmonary tuberculosis by as much as 10 to 15 years. Active pulmonary tuberculosis is present in only 10% of cases of renal tuberculosis. Only 30% show any chest radiograph evidence of prior tuberculosis. The urinary tract is the most frequent site of extrapulmonary tuberculosis. Patients present with asymptomatic hematuria or sterile pyuria. Imaging studies often initially suggest the diagnosis

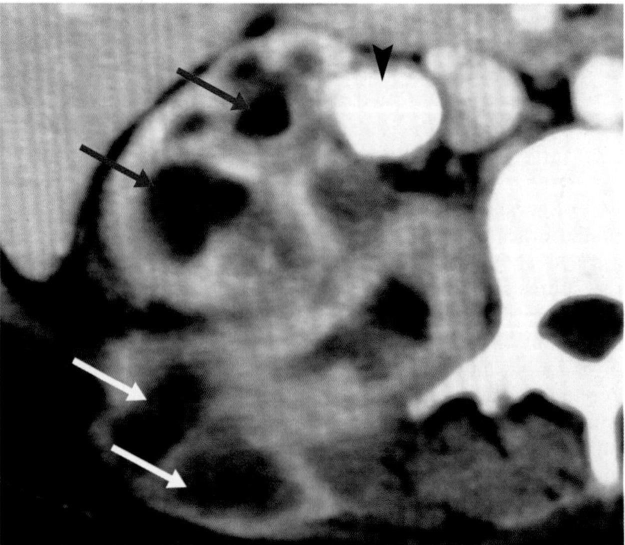

FIGURE 47.43. **Xanthogranulomatous Pyelonephritis.** Postcontrast CT shows a poorly functioning right kidney with a large obstructing stone (*arrowhead*) occupying the renal pelvis. Calyces (*red arrows*) are dilated and the parenchyma is atrophic and replaced by inflammatory tissue. Indolent abscess (*white arrows*) extends through the renal capsule and perirenal space into the subcutaneous tissues.

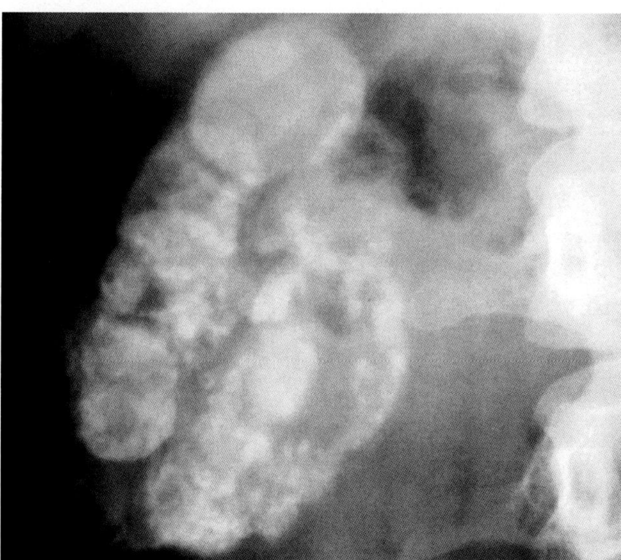

FIGURE 47.44. **End-Stage Renal Tuberculosis.** The right kidney is small, nonfunctioning, and completely calcified because of chronic tuberculous infection. This appearance has been called a "putty kidney" reflecting the physical texture of caseous necrosis mixed with calcification.

when it is unsuspected clinically. The hallmarks of renal tuberculosis are papillary necrosis, parenchymal destruction, and cavity formation leading to uneven caliectasis, fibrosis and scarring of the collecting system and the renal parenchyma, parenchymal masses owing to granuloma formation, strictures of the collecting system and ureters, and widely variant patterns of calcification (found in 40% to 70% of cases). The diagnosis is confirmed by positive urine culture or histology of a surgical specimen. End-stage nonfunctional tuberculous kidneys may be hydronephrotic sacs or appear as atrophic and calcified masses in the renal bed (Fig. 47.44).

Renal Parenchymal Disease

Renal Failure. In patients with renal failure, US is usually requested to assess renal size, exclude hydronephrosis, and to identify renal parenchymal disease. Bilateral hydronephrosis is a rare, but potentially reversible, cause of renal failure. Patients with acute renal failure and large or normal-sized kidneys often require biopsy for definitive diagnosis of renal parenchymal disease. Patients with small (<9 cm) kidneys usually have irreversible end-stage renal disease and generally do not benefit from biopsy. Measurements of renal cortical thickness are unreliable in assessing residual renal function. Sonographic signs of renal parenchymal disease include a diffuse increase in parenchymal echogenicity often associated with loss of corticomedullary differentiation.

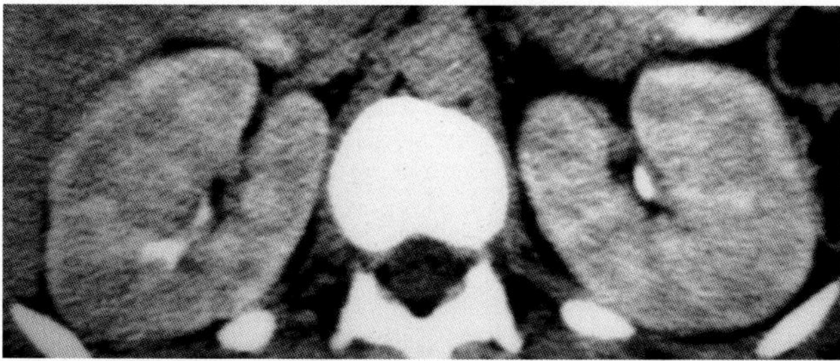

FIGURE 47.45. **HIV Nephropathy.** Postcontrast CT shows the mottled striated nephrogram seen with HIV nephropathy.

TABLE 47.3

CAUSES OF MEDULLARY NEPHROCALCINOSIS

Hyperparathyroidism
Medullary sponge kidney
Renal tubular acidosis (distal form)
Milk-alkali syndrome
Hypervitaminosis D
Hypercalcemic/hypercalciuric states

HIV-associated renal disease includes HIV nephropathy, opportunistic infections, lymphoma, Kaposi sarcoma, and renal disease secondary to antiretroviral therapy. HIV nephropathy is the primary cause of renal failure in HIV infected patients. Characteristic findings of HIV nephropathy on US are normal or enlarged, highly echogenic, kidneys in the setting of renal failure. Occasionally the presence of these characteristic findings may allow the radiologist to suggest the diagnosis of HIV infection before it is recognized clinically. CT shows enlarged kidney with high attenuation medullary regions on noncontrast scans and a striated nephrogram on postcontrast scans (Fig. 47.45). MR shows renal enlargement and loss of corticomedullary differentiation. Opportunistic infections are caused by *Pneumocystis carinii, P. jirovecii, Mycobacterium avium-intracellulare, M. tuberculosis, Candida albicans,* and *Aspergillus.* Imaging findings associated with infection include renal abscesses, multiple renal microabscesses, calcifications, and parenchymal areas of hypoperfusion. HIV-associated lymphoma is predominantly non-Hodgkin and shows the full spectrum of lymphoma findings in the kidney. Kaposi sarcoma causes renal enlargement associated with irregular cortical low attenuation areas on CT. Antiretroviral therapy, especially indinavir, is associated with development (in up to 20% of patients) of unusual calculi that cause obstruction, hydronephrosis, and pain. On CT the calculi are low in attenuation and may be overlooked as they are the only urinary calculi that are not high attenuation on noncontrast CT. Indinavir-induced crystals precipitate in the tubules and cause defects in enhancement in the renal parenchyma and parenchymal atrophy.

Nephrocalcinosis

Nephrocalcinosis is a broad term that refers to pathologic deposition of calcium in the renal parenchyma. Nephrocalcinosis is usually bilateral and the result of systemic disorders.

Cortical nephrocalcinosis is unusual, representing less than 5% of nephrocalcinosis. Causes include acute cortical necrosis precipitated by severe ischemia, chronic glomerulonephritis, and primary hyperoxaluria.

Medullary nephrocalcinosis is far more common and is usually related to hypercalcemic or hypercalciuric states (Table 47.3). Note that echogenic renal pyramids may result from medullary nephrocalcinosis, as well as other causes (Fig. 47.37).

Suggested Readings

Adrenal

Bassignani MJ. Adrenal and retroperitoneal MR imaging. In: Brant WE, de Lange EE. *Essentials of Body MRI.* New York: Oxford University Press; 2012:194–215.

Bessell-Browne R, O'Malley ME. CT of pheochromocytoma and paraganglioma: risk of adverse events with IV administration of nonionic contrast material. *AJR Am J Roentgenol* 2007;188(4):970–997.

Garrett RW, Nepute JC, Hayek ME, Albert SG. Adrenal incidentalomas: clinical controversies and modified recommendations. *AJR Am J Roentgenol* 2016;206(6):1170–1178.

Lattein GE Jr, Sturgill ED, Tujo CA, et al. Adrenal tumors and tumor-like conditions in the adult: radiologic-pathologic correlation. *Radiographics* 2014;34(3):805–829.

Poghosyan T. Urinary Tract MR Imaging. In: Brant WE, de Lange EE. *Essentials of Body MRI*. New York: Oxford University Press; 2012:162–193.

Shin YR, Kim KA. Imaging features of various adrenal neoplastic lesions on radiologic and nuclear medicine imaging. *AJR Am J Roentgenol* 2015; 205(3):554–563.

Taffel M, Haji-Momenian S, Nikolaidis P, Miller FH. Adrenal imaging: a comprehensive review. *Radiol Clin North Am* 2012;50(2):219–243.

Wagner-Bartak NA, Baiomy A, Habra MA, et al. Cushing syndrome: diagnostic workup and imaging features, with clinical and pathologic correlation. *AJR Am J Roentgenol* 2017;209(1):19–32.

Renal

Al-Katib S, Shetty M, Jafri SM, Jafri SZ. Radiologic assessment of native renal vasculature: a multimodality review. *Radiographics* 2017;37(1):136–156.

Bai X, Wu CL. Renal cell carcinoma and mimics: pathologic primer for radiologists. *AJR Am J Roentgenol* 2012;198(6):1289–1293.

Bosniak MA. The Bosniak renal cyst classification: 25 years later. *Radiology* 2012;262(3):781–785.

Chung AD, Schieda N, Shanbhogue AK, Dilauro M, Rosenkrantz AB, Siegelman ES. MRI evaluation of the urothelial tract: pitfalls and solutions. *AJR Am J Roentgenol* 2016;207(6):W108–W116.

Das CJ, Ahmad Z, Sharma S, Gupta AK. Multimodality imaging of renal inflammatory lesions. *World J Radiol* 2014;6(11):865–873.

Ng CS, Wood CG, Silverman PM, Tannir NM, Tamboli P, Sandler CM. Renal cell carcinoma: diagnosis, staging, surveillance. *AJR Am J Roentgenol* 2008; 191(4):1220–1232.

Renal cell carcinoma TMN staging. https://www.cancer.org/cancer/kidney-cancer/detection-diagnosis-staging/staging.html.

Schieda N, Hodgdon T, El-Khodary M, Flood TA, McInnes MD. Unenhanced CT for the diagnosis of minimal-fat renal angiomyolipoma. *AJR Am J Roentgenol* 2014;203(6):1236–1241.

Surabhi VR, Menias CO, George V, Matta E, Kaza RK, Hasapes J. MDCT and MR urogram spectrum of congenital anomalies of the kidney and urinary tract diagnosed in adulthood. *AJR Am J Roentgenol* 2015;205(3): W294–W304.

Wolin EA, Hartman DS, Olson JR. Nephrographic and pyelographic analysis of CT urography: differential diagnosis. *AJR Am J Roentgenol* 2013; 200(6):1197–1203.

Wood CG 3rd, Stromberg LJ 3rd, Harmath CB, et al. CT and MR imaging for evaluation of cystic renal lesions and diseases. *Radiographics* 2015; 35(1):125–141.

CHAPTER 48 ■ PELVICALYCEAL SYSTEM, URETERS, BLADDER, AND URETHRA

WILLIAM E. BRANT

PELVICALYCEAL SYSTEM AND URETER

Imaging Methods

As described in Chapter 47 the CT urogram ("CT-IVP") is now the imaging method of choice for evaluation of hematuria and as a screening examination of the pelvicalyceal system and ureters. Thin-slice MDCT acquisitions are reformatted in longitudinal planes to provide visualization of the collecting system comparable to the traditional intravenous pyelogram (IVP), also called the excretory urogram. The CT urogram is limited by lower spatial resolution than the IVP, which is based on traditional radiography (see Fig. 47.17). The CT urogram is also limited when contrast opacification of the collecting system and ureters is incomplete. However, the improved contrast resolution and demonstration of soft tissues make CT urogram a high-quality diagnostic study despite its limitations. The MR urogram may be substituted for the CT urogram (see Fig. 47.18). The MR urogram may be performed with gadolinium administration producing a full evaluation similar to the CT urogram. However, whenever contrast administration is contraindicated, an MR urogram can be performed without contrast by utilizing heavily T2WI. The high signal from urine in the collecting systems, ureters, and bladder closely resembles a contrast-enhanced study (see Fig. 48.8).

Retrograde pyelography, performed by cystoscopic catheterization of the ureteral orifice followed by injection of contrast, is independent of renal function, provides high-quality images of the ureter and the collecting system, and is another alternative commonly utilized by urologists. When a percutaneous nephrostomy catheter has been placed in the collecting system, antegrade pyelography is an additional choice. US is the imaging method of choice for screening for hydronephrosis but is limited in its ability to demonstrate small uroepithelial tumors. MDCT, utilizing thin slices and performed without intravenous or oral contrast agents, has replaced conventional radiographs and the traditional IVP for the diagnosis of renal stones in the kidneys and ureters.

Anatomy

The collecting tubules of a medullary pyramid coalesce into a variable number of papillary ducts that pierce the tip of the papilla and drain into the receptacle of the collecting system called a *minor calyx*. The projection of a papilla into the calyx produces a cup shape. The sharp-edged portion of the minor calyx projecting around the sides of a papilla is called the *fornix* of the calyx. Compound calyces, usually found at the poles of the kidney, are formed by the projection of two or more papilla into the calyx. *Infundibula* extend between minor calyces and the renal pelvis. The renal pelvis is triangular, with its base within the renal sinus. The apex of the pelvis extends outward and downward to join the ureter. A so-called *extrarenal pelvis* is predominantly outside the renal sinus and is larger and more distensible than the more common intrarenal pelvis, which is surrounded by renal sinus fat and other structures (Fig. 48.1). An extrarenal pelvis is a normal variant that should not be confused with hydronephrosis. There is endless variety in the size and arrangement of calyces and in the shape and appearance of the renal pelvis.

The ureters have an outer fibrous adventitia that is continuous with the renal capsule and with the adventitia of the bladder. The muscularis, responsible for ureteral peristalsis, consists of outer circular and inner longitudinal muscle bundles. The mucosa lining the entire pelvicalyceal system, ureters, and bladder is *transitional epithelium*, also termed *uroepithelium*. The ureters enter the bladder at an oblique angle. When the bladder wall contracts the ureteral orifices are closed. The ureters propel urine by active peristalsis, which

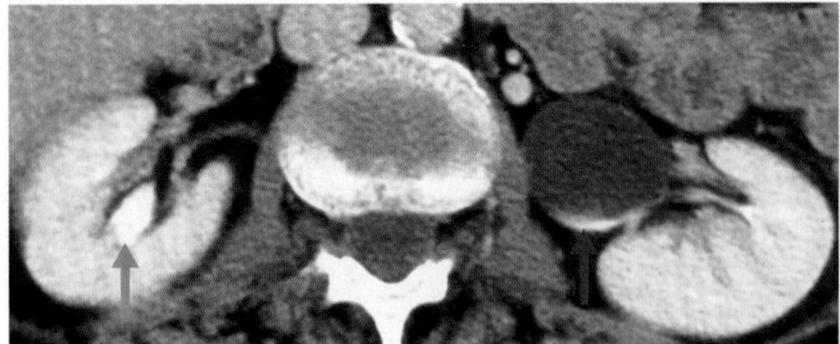

FIGURE 48.1. **Extrarenal Pelvis.** The position of the left renal pelvis (*red arrow*) outside of the renal sinus enables the pelvis to distend with urine and to be larger than the normal right renal pelvis (*blue arrow*). The extrarenal pelvis is a normal variant, not to be mistaken for hydronephrosis.

can be visualized fluoroscopically and by US. Jets of urine opacified by contrast are frequently seen within the bladder on CT. Because of peristalsis, the diameter of the ureter at any particular instant is highly variable. Three main points of ureteral narrowing, where calculi are likely to become impacted, are (a) the ureteropelvic junction (UPJ), (b) the site at which the ureter crosses the pelvic brim, and (c) the ureterovesical junction (UVJ).

Congenital Anomalies

Ureteral duplication occurs in 1% to 2% of the population (Fig. 48.2). Unilateral duplication is six times more common than bilateral duplication. The *Weigert–Meyer rule* states that with complete ureteral duplication, the ureter draining the upper pole passes through the bladder wall to insert inferior and medial to the normally placed ureter draining the lower pole. In females the ectopic ureter may insert into the lower bladder, upper vagina, or urethra. In males it may insert into the lower bladder, prostatic urethra, seminal vesicles, vas deferens, or ejaculatory duct. The upper pole ureter often ends as an ectopic ureterocele reflecting obstruction because of its ectopic insertion. The lower pole ureter inserts in, or near, the normal location in the bladder trigone and is subject to vesicoureteral reflux because of distortion of its passage through the bladder wall by the ectopic ureterocele. ("Upper pole obstructs; lower pole refluxes.") Complications of complete duplication include urinary tract infection, vesicoureteral reflux, and UPJ obstruction of the lower pole system. Reflux into the lower pole collecting system in childhood may produce scarring and deformity of the lower pole of the kidney.

CT or MR urography commonly demonstrates poor function or nonfunction of the obstructed upper pole system (Fig. 48.3). The lower pole system is displaced inferiorly and commonly shows a "drooping lily" appearance. Reflux nephropathy of the lower pole system may be evident. Cystic dilation of the upper pole system is usually associated with marked parenchymal thinning. The upper pole ureter is commonly tortuous and dilated. The ectopic ureterocele and its associated dilated ureter may simulate a multiseptated cystic mass in the pelvis.

Bifid renal pelvis occurs in 10% of the population. Separate pelvises draining the upper and lower poles join at the UPJ. This anomaly has no pathologic consequences.

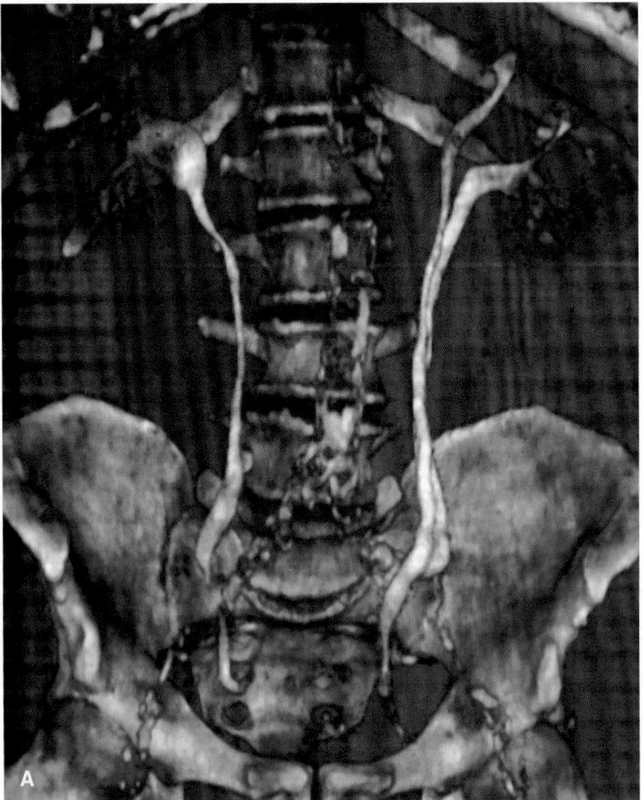

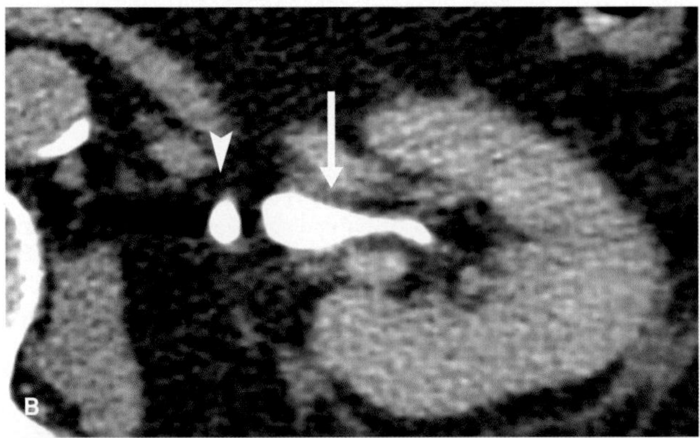

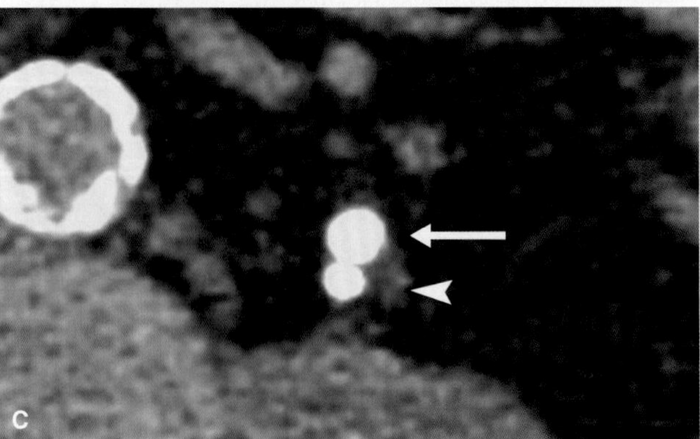

FIGURE 48.2. **Ureteral Duplication. A:** Reconstructed three-dimensional pyelogram-phase image from thin-slice MDCT urogram shows complete duplication of the left renal collecting system and ureter. **B:** Axial image from the same study shows the upper pole ureter (*arrowhead*) bypassing the origin of the lower pole ureter (*arrow*). Although this patient's upper pole ureter inserted ectopically in the lower bladder, no obstruction was present. **C:** Axial image at the level of the midureters shows the lower pole ureter (*arrow*) anterior to the upper pole ureter (*arrowhead*). The duplicated ureters tend to meander and twist about each other as they course to the bladder.

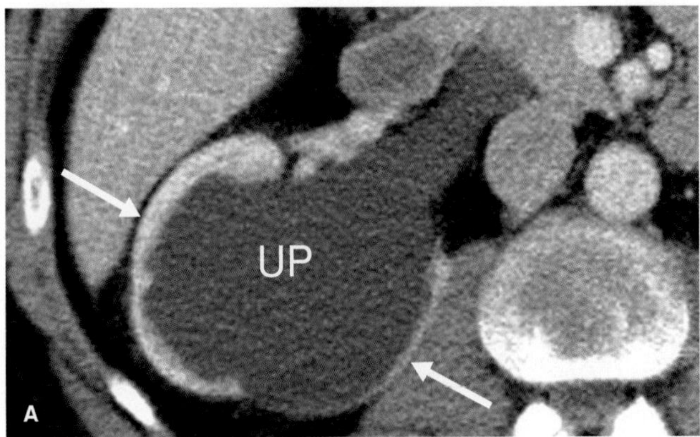

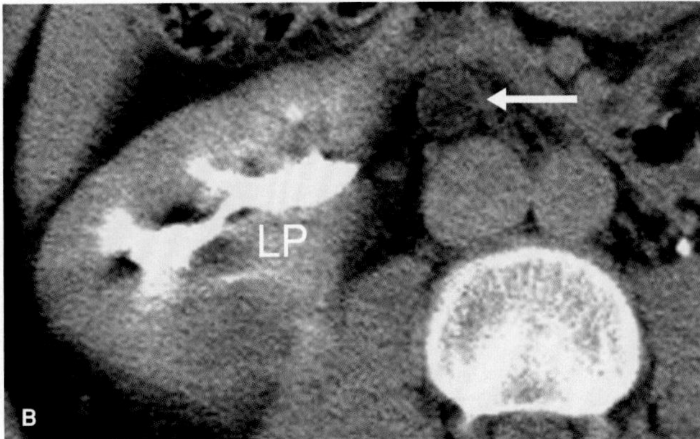

FIGURE 48.3. **Obstructed Duplication. A:** CT urogram pyelogram-phase image through the upper pole (*UP*) of the right kidney shows marked dilation of the calyces, pelvis, and ureter. The upper pole parenchyma (*arrows*) enhances but is markedly atrophic. **B:** Image through the lower pole (*LP*) shows contrast excretion into the nondilated lower pole collecting system. The markedly dilated upper pole ureter (*arrow*) courses past the origin of the lower pole ureter.

Ureteropelvic junction obstruction is a common congenital anomaly that may go undiagnosed until adulthood. The amount of hydronephrosis and parenchymal atrophy present depends on the severity of obstruction. The condition is bilateral in 30% of cases but is often not symmetrical. US demonstrates pelvicaliectasis with sharply defined narrowing at the UPJ. The ureter is not dilated. In 15% to 20% of cases, an aberrant renal vessel causes the obstruction. MDCT is effective in demonstrating the crossing vessel. In the majority of cases, the precise cause is unknown.

Retrocaval ureter is a developmental variant in which the right ureter passes behind the inferior vena cava at the level of L3 or L4 vertebra. The ureter exits anteriorly between the cava and the aorta to return to its normal position. The condition is associated with varying degrees of urinary stasis and proximal pyeloureterectasis. The anomaly is due to faulty embryogenesis of the inferior vena cava, with abnormal persistence of the right subcardinal vein anterior to the ureter instead of the right supracardinal vein posterior to the ureter.

Renal Stone Disease

Routine use of noncontrast CT has revolutionized the imaging evaluation of renal stone disease, near completely replacing radiographs and conventional excretory urography in diagnosis of acute ureteral obstruction by renal stones.

Nephrolithiasis refers to the presence of calculi in the renal collecting system. Nearly 10% of the population will form a renal stone in their lifetime. Sufficient calcium oxalate or calcium phosphate is present in 80% of renal calculi for them to be radiopaque on conventional radiographs. Brushite (2% to 4%) is a unique form of calcium phosphate stones that tends to recur quickly if patients are not treated aggressively. Brushite stones are resistant to treatment with shock wave lithotripsy. Struvite (magnesium ammonium phosphate) stones, formed in the presence of alkaline urine and infection, make up another 5% to 15% of renal calculi and are also radiopaque on radiographs. Struvite is the most common component of staghorn calculi (Fig. 48.4). Cystine stones comprise 1% to 2% of renal stones, are mildly radiopaque, and are found only in patients with congenital cystinuria. Uric acid and xanthine stones (5% to 10%) are radiolucent on conventional radiographs. A major advantage of noncontrast CT is that (nearly) all stones are opaque on CT (Table 48.1). The primary limitation of CT is small size of the stone rather than its attenuation. High CT attenuation makes calculi (>200 H) easy to differentiate from other collecting system lesions such as tumors, hematoma, fungus balls, or sloughed papilla, which are all usually <50 H. Dual-energy CT has been successfully used to determine the chemical composition of stones.

Complications of renal calculi include urinary obstruction, ureteral stricture, chronic renal infection, and loss of renal function. Acute flank pain is a common complaint of patients seeking emergency medical treatment. Renal colic, caused by a calculus obstructing the ureter, is the most common cause of acute flank pain and is the usual major consideration for

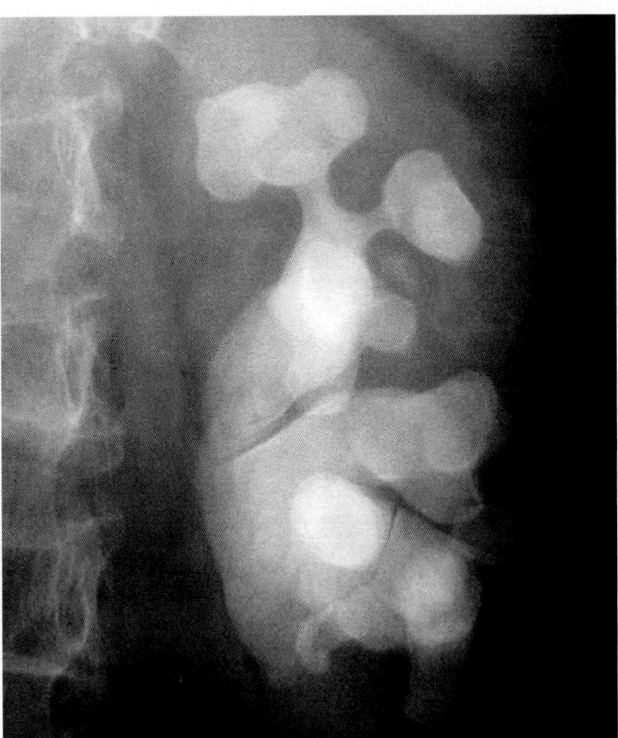

FIGURE 48.4. **Staghorn Calculus.** A conventional radiograph (without administration or any radiographic contrast agent) demonstrates a complex calculus creating a cast of the collecting system of the left kidney. This staghorn calculus, named (imprecisely) for its resemblance to the antlers of a male deer, is formed in the presence of obstruction with chronic infection and is composed of struvite.

TABLE 48.1

URINARY TRACT STONES

■ COMPOSITION	■ FREQUENCY	■ CONVENTIONAL RADIOGRAPH APPEARANCE	■ CT APPEARANCE (ATTENUATION)
Calcium oxalate	40–60%	Radiopaque	Opaque (1,700–2,800 H)
Calcium phosphate	20–60%	Radiopaque	Opaque (1,200–1,600 H)
Brushite	2–4%	Radiopaque	Opaque (1,700–2,800 H)
Uric acid	5–10%	Radiolucent	Opaque (200–450 H)
Struvite	5–15%	Radiopaque	Opaque (600–900 H)
Cystine	1–2.5%	Mildly radiopaque	Opaque (600–1,100 H)
Indinavir calculus	Only in HIV patients taking Indinavir	Radiolucent	Soft tissue attenuation (15–30 H)

Adapted from Kambadakone AR, Eisner BH, Catalano OA, Sahani DV. New and evolving concepts in the imaging and management of urolithiasis: urologists' perspective. *Radiographics* 2010;30:603–623.

diagnostic imaging. Although most calculi can be detected on conventional radiographs, difficulties in localizing the calcification to the ureter and differentiation from other calcifications limit the sensitivity of radiography for ureteral stones to as low as 45% with a specificity of only 77%. Noncontrast CT has a sensitivity of 97% and specificity of 96% for ureteral calculi. US has a sensitivity for stone detection of only 24% compared to unenhanced CT. An additional advantage of noncontrast CT in the diagnosis of acute flank pain is demonstration of pathology other than a ureteral stone. Among the numerous possibilities are acute appendicitis, incarcerated hernia, ovarian cyst, diverticulitis, and pyelonephritis.

Noncontrast renal stone CT is an MDCT scan of the urinary tract performed without oral or intravenous contrast in order to detect obstructing ureteral stones and to document stone burden (Fig. 48.5). The thin-slice (~1 mm) capability of MDCT is optimal for this indication. Nearly all stones are visible on unenhanced CT as high attenuation (>200 H), geometric or oval, opaque objects (Table 48.1). Stones appear as white dots on CT scans displayed with soft tissue window settings. The single exception is the soft tissue attenuation (15 to 30 H) crystalline calculus associated with treatment of HIV patients with the antiretroviral drug, indinavir. These calculi may cause ureteral obstruction but should be considered only in this very limited clinical circumstance.

The classic appearance of ureterolithiasis is a high attenuation stone within the ureter associated with proximal dilation and distal contraction of the ureter. A halo of soft tissue surrounding the calculus (the *tissue rim sign*) confirms the stone location within the ureter. Findings of ureteral obstruction include (a) mild dilation of the pelvicalyceal system and ureter (>3 mm) proximal to the stone; (b) slight decrease in attenuation of the affected kidney caused by edema; and (c) perinephric soft tissue stranding representing edema in the perinephric and periureteral fat. Sagittal and coronal reformatted images assist in confirming the diagnosis. Focal perinephric fluid collections represent forniceal rupture caused by high-grade obstruction coupled with high urine output. Pitfalls in diagnosis include (a) peripelvic cysts or extrarenal pelvis simulating hydronephrosis; (b) pre-existing stranding in the perinephric fat caused by previous inflammation, especially common in older patients; (c) atherosclerotic calcifications; (d) recent stone passage without a stone currently present; and (e) phleboliths. Phleboliths are calcifications within thrombosed veins, particularly common in the pelvis. Differentiation from stones is made by (a) location not along the course of the ureter; (b) absence of a tissue rim sign; (c) presence of a *tail sign,* a tubular tail extending from the calcification representing a thrombosed vein; and (d) relatively low attenuation of phleboliths with a mean value of 160 H. The probability that a calcification represents a phlebolith is less than 3% when the attenuation is >300 H. High attenuation in the renal pyramids is a sign of dehydration and must not be mistaken for stones. Stones less than 6 mm in size are likely to pass spontaneously through the ureter within 6 weeks. Stones larger than 6 mm are more likely to remain lodged in the ureter and require intervention for removal. Calculi are most likely to be found at the three points of ureteral narrowing previously described.

Hydronephrosis

Hydronephrosis is defined as dilation of the upper urinary tract. Hydronephrosis is not synonymous with obstruction but has a number of causes that are reviewed in this section. The terms *caliectasis, pyelectasis*, and *ureterectasis* are more precise in describing dilation of portions of the urinary tract. US is an excellent screening modality for determining the presence of urinary tract dilation.

Peripelvic cysts mimic hydronephrosis on noncontrast CT, MR, and on US. These are multiple or multilobulated cysts that occupy the renal sinus. They contain clear fluid and may be lymphatic or posttraumatic in origin. Because of the tight confines of the renal sinus as they enlarge they develop rounded projections that resemble pyelectasis and caliectasis. On CT they are low attenuation similar to urine. On MR the fluid is low signal on T1WI and high signal on T2WI. On US they are thin walled and anechoic (see Fig. 50.52). With contrast filling of the collecting structures the diagnosis becomes obvious. The enhanced collecting systems are stretched, narrowed, and displaced by the renal sinus cystic mass. Peripelvic cysts are asymptomatic and require no follow-up.

Obstruction. The causes of obstruction include stone, stricture, tumor, and extrinsic compression. The degree of dilation produced by obstruction is variable. In general, the more proximal and the more chronic the obstruction, the greater is the degree of dilation (Fig. 48.6). Acute obstruction produced by an impacted stone often produces minimal dilation. US demonstrates hydronephrosis as separation of normal sinus

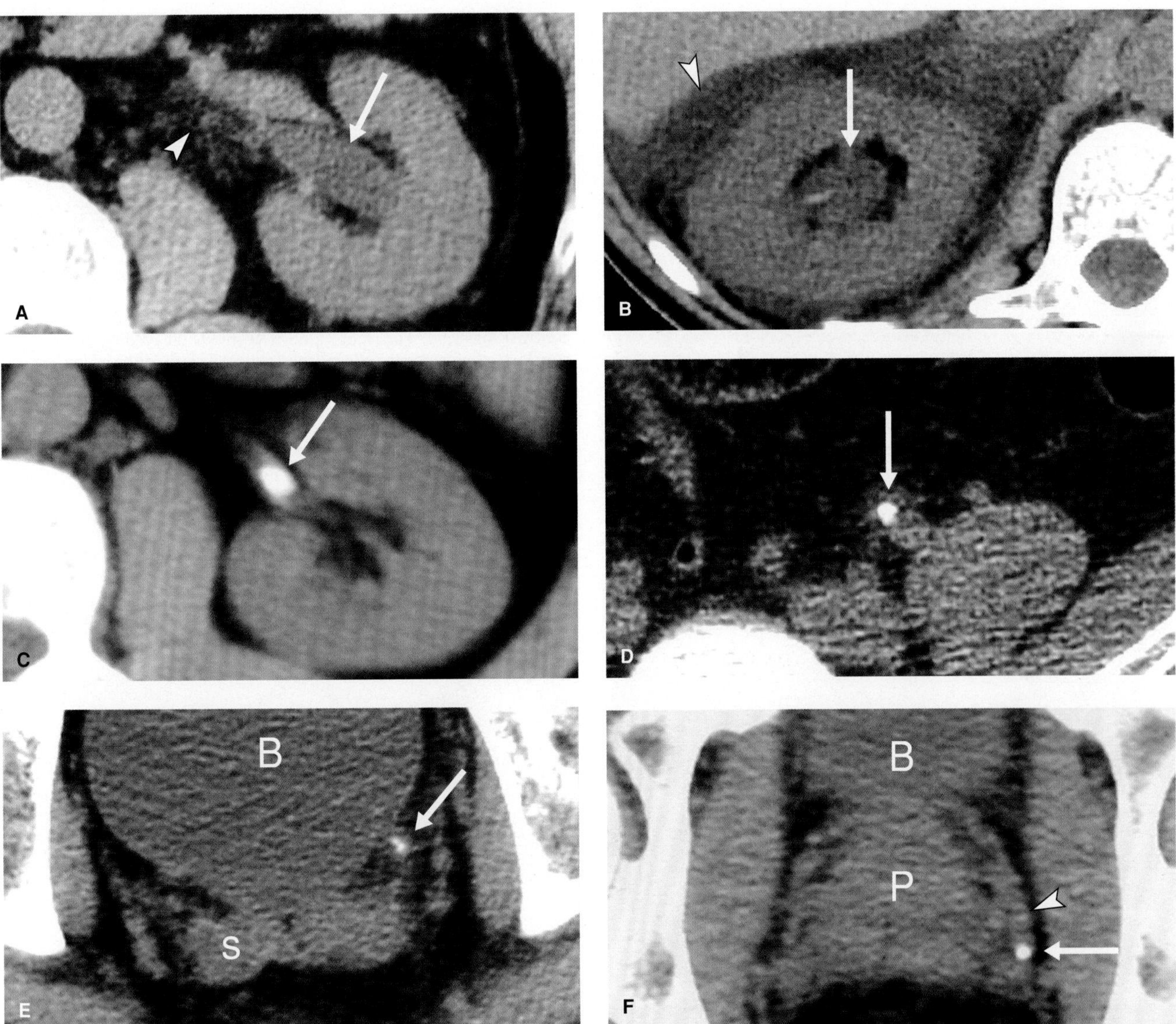

FIGURE 48.5. **Noncontrast Renal Stone CT. A:** CT image through the kidneys in a patient with left flank pain demonstrates mild enlargement of the left renal pelvis (*arrow*). Streaks and strands of edema (*arrowhead*) are seen in the fat adjacent to the renal pelvis. **B:** CT in a different patient with a stone in the distal ureter shows mild hydronephrosis (*arrow*) associated with fluid in the perinephric space (*arrowhead*). These findings indicate rupture of the collecting system at a fornix resulting from high-grade obstruction and high urine output. **C:** A stone (*arrow*) at the ureteropelvic junction is apparent in this patient. Absence of hydronephrosis or edema in the perinephric fat indicates that obstruction is very low grade. Note the rim of tissue around the stone is somewhat obscured by bloom artifact from the marked high attenuation of the stone. **D:** A stone in the left ureter (*arrow*) has impacted at the level of the pelvic brim. Note the irregular shape characteristic of renal stones. The rim of soft tissue density surrounding the stone represents the swollen wall of the ureter (tissue rim sign). **E:** CT at the level of the seminal vesicles (*s*) shows a high-density stone (*arrow*) in the distal left ureter. The "tissue rim sign" is evident. "All" urinary tract stones appear "white" on CT viewed at soft tissue windows. **F:** A more caudal image at the level of the base of the prostate (*P*) shows a phlebolith (*arrow*), not to be mistaken for a ureteral stone. The location is below the level of the distal ureter and the calcification lacks a tissue rim sign. The tubular structure (*arrowhead*) extending from the calcification represents the thrombosed vein (the tail sign). *B*, bladder.

echogenicity by anechoic urine in the collecting system. The calyces become enlarged and blunted and are seen to connect with the dilated renal pelvis. Medullary pyramids may be hypoechoic, especially in children, and must be differentiated from dilated calyces. Pyramids are more peripheral, surrounded by more echogenic cortex, and do not connect with the renal pelvis. Postcontrast MDCT signs of obstruction include (Fig. 48.7) (a) increasingly dense nephrogram with time, (b) delay in appearance of contrast in the collecting system, and (c) dilated pelvicalyceal system and ureter to the point of obstruction. *Pyelosinus reflux* may result from rupture of a fornix precipitated by contrast-induced diuresis superimposed on the increased hydrostatic pressure of an obstructed pelvicalyceal system. Urine and contrast extravasate into the renal sinus and perirenal space. Delay in opacification of the obstructed kidney and dependent layering of unopacified urine over heavier contrast media may also be evident. The location and cause of obstruction can usually be identified (Fig. 48.8).

Pyonephrosis refers to infection in an obstructed kidney. Pyonephrosis can result in rapid destruction of the renal parenchyma and must be treated promptly by relief of obstruction by ureteral stent or nephrostomy tube placement and antibiotics. US classically demonstrates a dilated collecting system filled with layering echogenic pus and debris. Shadowing

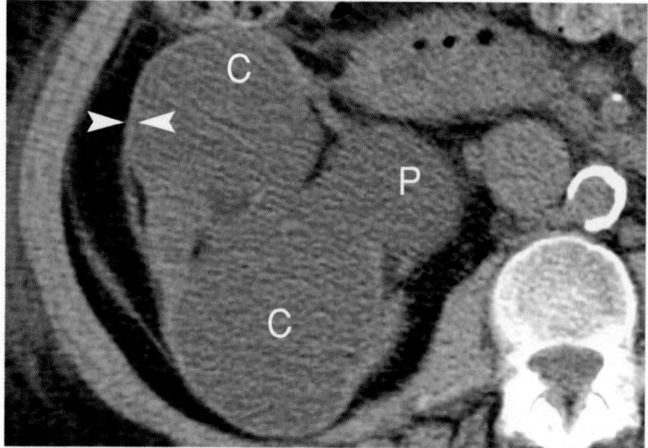

FIGURE 48.6. **Chronic Obstruction.** Image from a noncontrast renal stone CT shows marked dilation of the calyces (*C*) and renal pelvis (*P*). The renal parenchyma (between *arrowheads*) is markedly thin. A subsequent radionuclide renal scan showed no function in the right kidney. Findings are indicative of chronic proximal high-grade obstruction.

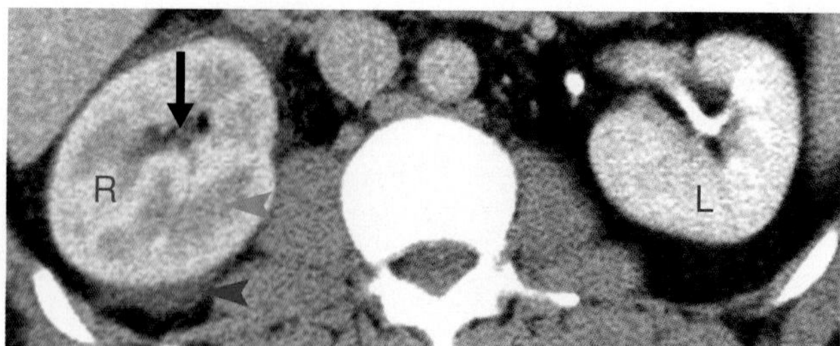

FIGURE 48.7. **Obstruction—Right Kidney.** Pyelogram-phase image from a CT urogram shows contrast filling the renal pelvis of the left kidney (*L*) on this scan performed at 4 minutes following intravenous contrast injection. The right kidney (*R*) shows delayed excretion with contrast enhancement only of the cortex. The medulla (*blue arrowhead*) is not enhanced and the collecting system (*arrow*) is not opacified with contrast. This patient had high-grade obstruction from a stone impacted at the ureterovesical junction. Note the presence of perirenal fluid (*red arrowhead*) indicating rupture at the fornix of an obstructed calyx caused by high renal output in the setting of high-grade obstruction.

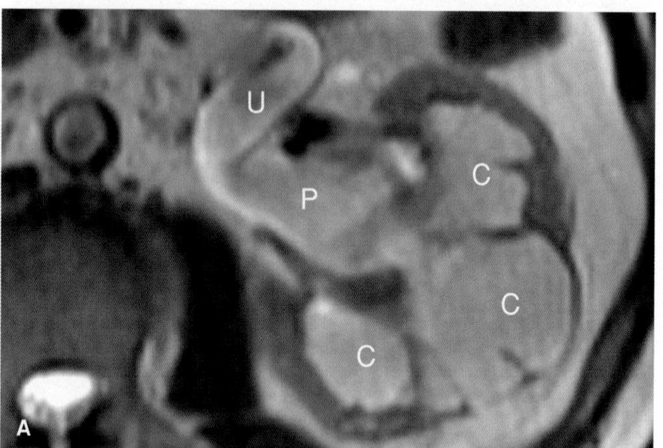

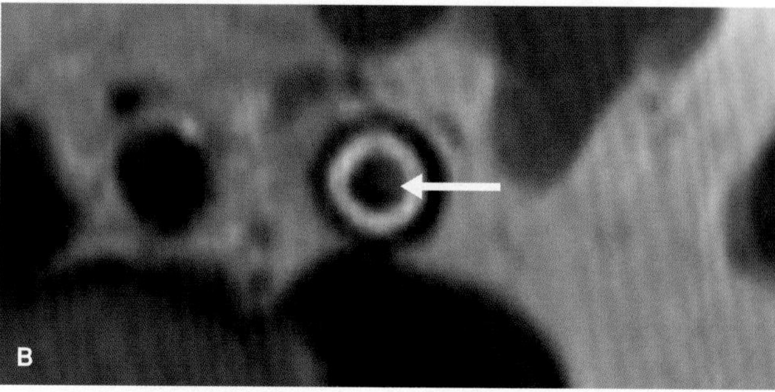

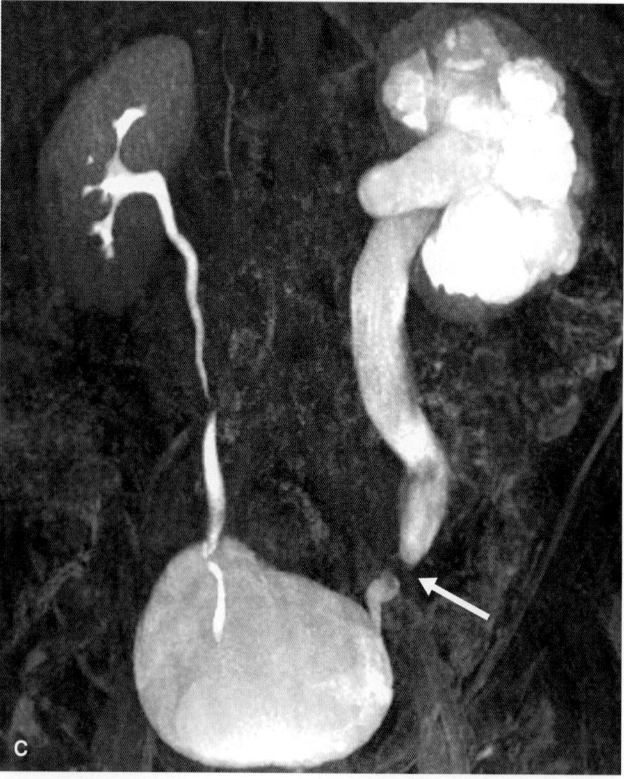

FIGURE 48.8. **Chronic Obstruction Due to Ureteral Stone.** **A:** T2-weighted axial plane MR image shows advanced hydronephrosis with dilation of the calyces (*C*), renal pelvis (*P*), and ureter (*U*). **B:** Axial plane T2WI of the distal ureter shows the stone (*arrow*) as a focus of black signal void surrounded by bright urine confined by the low signal wall of the ureter. **C:** T1-weighted coronal plane MR image obtained approximately 5 minutes following intravenous gadolinium administration shows the obstructed left kidney, the normal right kidney, the normal bladder, and the obstructing stone (*arrow*) in the distal left ureter. This figure illustrates use of the noncontrast as well as the postcontrast MR urogram.

calculi may also be evident. CT is better than US in demonstrating the site and cause of obstruction. CT demonstrates thickening (>2 mm) of the wall of the renal collecting system and urine of higher than normal attenuation reflecting the presence of pus.

Vesicoureteral reflux is a common cause of hydronephrosis in children. The basic defect is an abnormal ureteral tunnel at the UVJ and associated urinary tract infection allowing infected urine from the bladder to reflux up the ureter. In adults, vesicoureteral reflux is usually associated with neurogenic bladder or bladder outlet obstruction. Chronic vesicoureteral reflux of infected urine to the level of the kidney causes reflux nephropathy. Vesicoureteral reflux is confirmed by demonstrating retrograde filling of the ureters on voiding cystourography or radionuclide cystography.

Congenital megaureter is due to an aperistaltic segment of the lower ureter 5 to 40 mm in length causing a functional obstruction and resulting in dilation of the proximal ureter. Ureteral dilation exceeds 7 mm. The aperistaltic segment of the ureter demonstrates smoothly tapered narrowing without evidence of mechanical obstruction.

Prune belly syndrome, also called Eagle–Barrett syndrome, is a congenital disorder manifest by absence of the abdominal wall musculature, urinary tract anomalies, and cryptorchidism. Nearly all patients are males. The ureters are markedly dilated and tortuous, the bladder is large and distended, and the posterior urethra is dilated.

Polyuria, associated with acute diuresis and diabetes insipidus, may cause mild to severe hydronephrosis.

Mass or Filling Defect in Pelvicalyceal System or Ureter

Calculi are the most common cause of filling defects in the contrast-filled collecting system or ureter. Most calculi (>85%) are radiopaque on conventional radiographs. Noncontrast CT demonstrates nearly all calculi as high-density objects with a CT density of >200 H. The presence of contrast agent in the collecting system commonly obscures detection of calculi on CT. On MR, stones are seen as foci of absent signal within the collecting system (Fig. 48.8).

Blood clots cause nonradiopaque filling defects that can be differentiated from soft tissue tumors by their change in appearance over time. Attenuation values on CT are usually 40 to 80 H (Fig. 48.9).

Transitional cell carcinoma (TCC) accounts for 85% to 90% of all uroepithelial tumors and is the second most common primary renal malignancy (10% of renal malignancies). Most (85%) have a papillary growth pattern that is exophytic, polypoid, and attached to the mucosa by a stalk. These lesions cause a distinct filling defect in the collecting system (Fig. 48.10) or ureter. A stippled pattern of contrast material within the interstices of the papillary lesion is characteristic. Nonpapillary tumors are nodular or flat and tend to be infiltrating and aggressive. They cause strictures of the collecting system or ureter rather than a focal mass. Most TCC occur in men (4:1) aged 60 and older. A variety of chemical agents used in the textile and plastic industries, drugs including cyclophosphamide and phenacetin, chronic urinary stasis (horseshoe kidney), and smoking play a role in the etiology of these tumors. The tumor metastasizes most commonly to regional lymph nodes, liver, lung, and bone. TCC exhibits a strong tendency toward multiplicity. Patients with upper tract TCC have

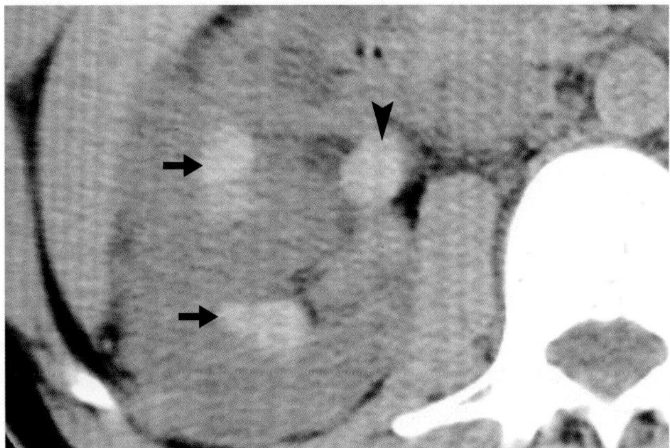

FIGURE 48.9. **Hemorrhage Into Collecting System.** Image from noncontrast renal stone CT in a patient with acute right flank pain shows the calyces (*short arrows*) and renal pelvis (*arrowhead*) filled with high attenuation material measuring 55 H. This patient on supratherapeutic doses of anticoagulants hemorrhaged into his right renal collecting system.

multicentric tumors in 20% to 44% of cases, and those with TCC of the ureter develop bladder TCC in 20% to 37% of cases. Careful evaluation of the entire urinary tract is essential both at initial diagnosis and for follow-up. Standard treatment of upper tract TCC is total nephroureterectomy and excision of a cuff of the bladder surrounding the ureteral orifice.

CT shows three typical appearances of TCC of the upper urinary tract: (a) focal intraluminal mass (Fig. 48.10), (b) thickening of the wall and narrowing of the lumen of the ureter or collecting system (Fig. 48.11), and (c) mass infiltrating the renal sinus and renal parenchyma (Fig. 48.12). Tumors in the ureter show similar findings (Fig. 48.13) but tend to be smaller at presentation because they cause early ureteral obstruction. On unenhanced CT, TCC attenuation is 8 to 30 H appearing slightly hyperdense to urine and slightly hyperdense to unenhanced renal parenchyma (Fig. 48.14). The much lower attenuation of TCC enables clear differentiation from calculi (>200 H) and usually from blood clots (40 to 80 H). Most focal masses are small (5 to 10 mm). Enhancement, usually low grade, following intravenous contrast administration confirms a neoplasm. Wall thickening and luminal narrowing are usually symmetric and show low-level enhancement postcontrast. These findings are not specific and may also be seen with stone passage, hemorrhage,

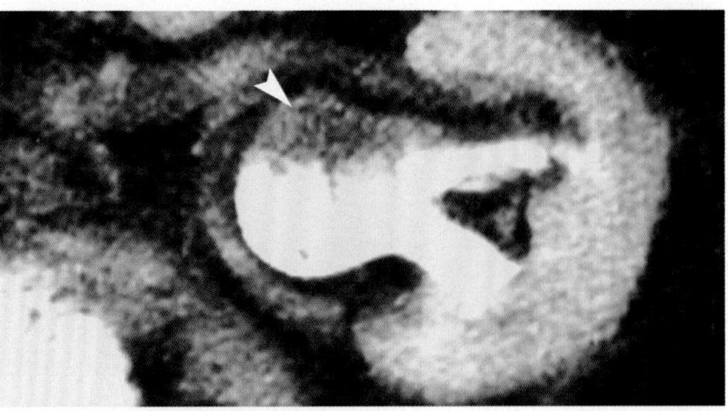

FIGURE 48.10. **Transitional Cell Carcinoma—Renal Pelvis—Intraluminal Mass.** Pyelogram-phase image from a CT urogram shows an intraluminal mass (*arrowhead*) in the left renal pelvis. This lesion proved to be a papillary transitional cell carcinoma.

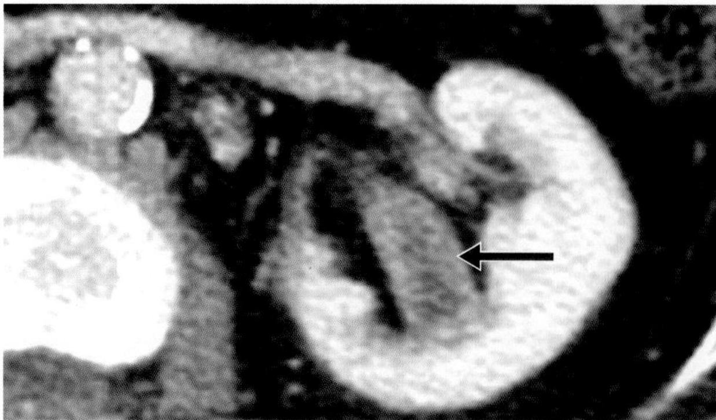

FIGURE 48.11. **Transitional Cell Carcinoma—Renal Pelvis—Wall Thickening.** Nephrogram-phase image from a CT urogram demonstrates circumferential wall thickening (*arrow*) of the renal pelvis caused by transitional cell carcinoma.

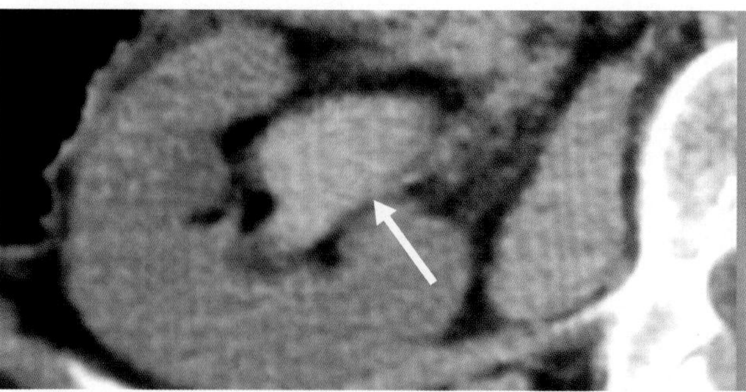

FIGURE 48.14. **Transitional Cell Carcinoma—Noncontrast CT.** Image from a noncontrast renal stone CT shows an intermediate attenuation mass (*arrow*) distending the right renal pelvis. Differential diagnosis would include blood clot versus tumor. Ureteroscopic-directed biopsy revealed transitional cell carcinoma.

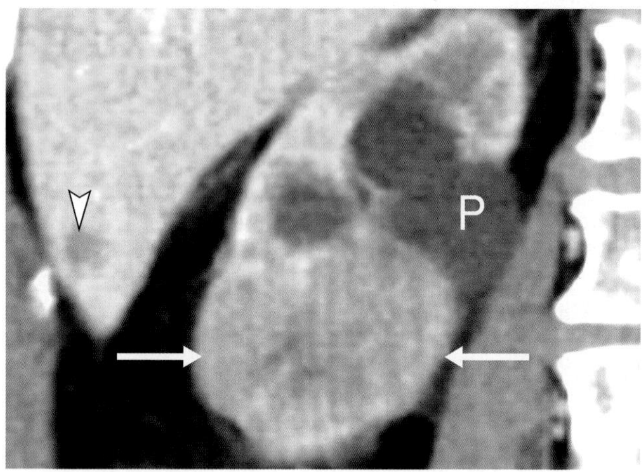

FIGURE 48.12. **Transitional Cell Carcinoma—Renal Pelvis—Infiltrative Tumor.** Coronal reformatted pyelogram-phase image from a CT urogram shows an enhancing tumor (between *arrows*) infiltrating the collecting system and renal parenchyma of the lower pole of the right kidney. Note that the tumor infiltration does not distort the shape of the kidney. The tumor obstructs upper pole collecting system and pelvis (*P*) causing hydronephrosis. A metastasis (*arrowhead*) in the liver is also evident. Biopsy confirmed stage IV transitional cell carcinoma.

or infection. Ureteroscopic-guided biopsy is usually required. The aggressive infiltrative form of TCC in the kidney extends from the renal pelvis infiltrating the renal sinus and the renal parenchyma while preserving the renal contour (Fig. 48.12). CT stages the tumor by demonstration of the extent of the tumor, including invasion of the kidney or surrounding structures, lymphadenopathy, and distant metastases.

On MR, TCC is usually isointense compared to the renal medulla on T1WI. Small tumors may not be detected. Large tumors obliterate fat within the renal sinus and infiltrate the parenchyma. On T2WI, TCC is outlined by high signal urine within the collecting system. Intermediate signal is seen within the tumor. Enhancement on postcontrast images is indicative of tumor and differentiates TCC from blood clots. Subtraction images may be needed to appreciate TCC enhancement. TCC in the renal pelvis or infundibulum commonly causes proximal caliectasis.

US demonstrates renal TCC as a discrete, slightly hypo- or hyperechoic mass within the renal sinus. Small lesions may be subtle and easily missed. Overall US is less sensitive for detection of TCC than CT or MR urography. The absence of acoustic shadowing from the lesion usually provides differentiation from calculi, although a few high-grade tumors may cast acoustic shadows.

Retrograde pyelography or excretory urography shows the tumor as an intraluminal filling defect within the contrast-filled collecting system or ureter. The defect may be irregular, stippled, or smooth. A missing or "amputated"

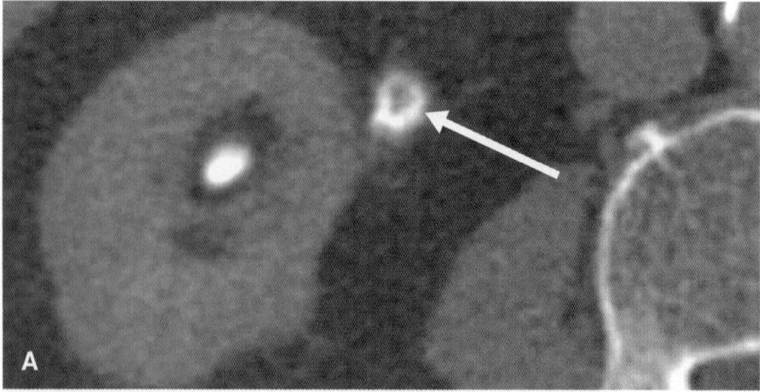

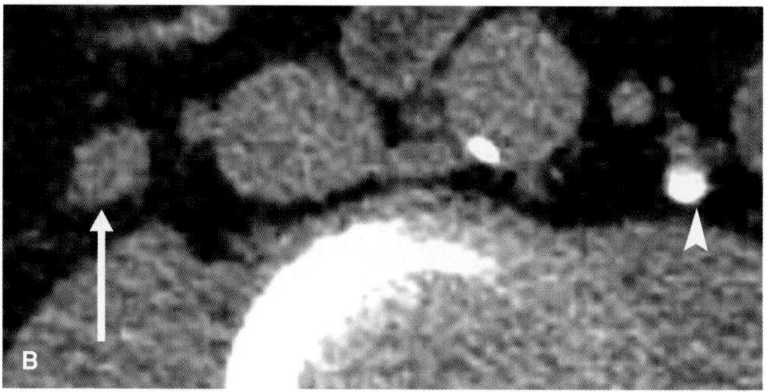

FIGURE 48.13. **Transitional Cell Carcinoma—Ureter. A:** Pyelogram-phase image from a CT urogram in a patient with hematuria reveals a polypoid mass seen as a filling defect (*arrow*) in the proximal right ureter. Biopsy confirmed transitional cell carcinoma. **B:** Postcontrast CT in a different patient demonstrates an enlarged right ureter (*arrow*) with ill-defined margins. This image was obtained at the level of a ureteral stricture. The ureter above this level was distended and filled with contrast. Surgery confirmed TCC. The left ureter (*arrowhead*) is filled with contrast and is normal in appearance.

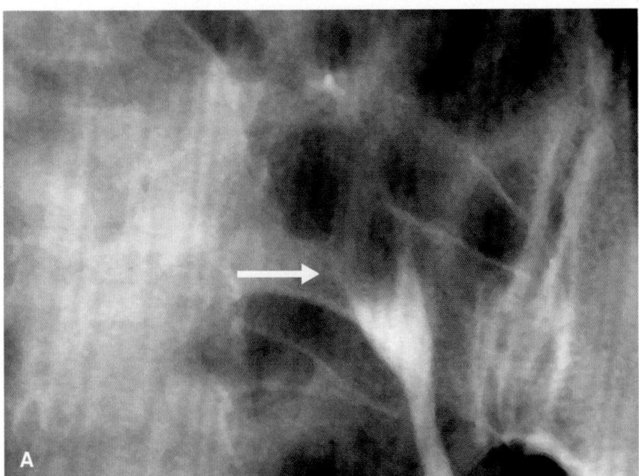

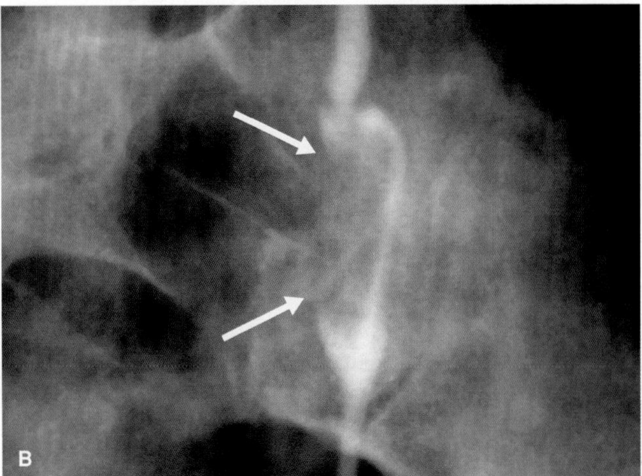

FIGURE 48.15. Transitional Cell Carcinoma—Ureter. A: A retrograde ureterogram demonstrates widening of the ureter (*arrow*) distal to an obstructing tumor. The distal ureter assumes a *champagne glass* configuration because of the slow growth of the tumor. **B:** Additional contrast administration demonstrates the full extent of the tumor (between *arrows*).

calyx that is completely obstructed by tumor will not fill with contrast administered retrograde. Tumors may also cause focal strictures and "apple core" lesions in the ureters. Tumors in the ureter may demonstrate a "champagne glass" sign (Fig. 48.15) of ureteral dilation distal to a filling defect. This sign distinguishes tumor from a calculus that impacts in the ureter and causes distal spasm and narrowing.

Squamous cell carcinoma accounts for 10% of uroepithelial tumors. Chronic infection, calculi, and phenacetin abuse are major predisposing factors. Most tumors are infiltrating and superficially spreading, producing stricture or subtle filling defects. Imaging appearance is indistinguishable from TCC.

Metastases are a rare cause of a collecting system mass. Common primary tumor sites are the breast, skin (melanoma), lung, stomach, and cervix.

Papillary necrosis is ischemic necrosis of the tips of the medullary pyramids. Causes include infection, tuberculosis, sickle cell trait and disease, diabetes, and analgesic nephropathy. Necrotic papilla may remain in situ, slough into the collecting system causing a mobile filling defect, or disappear, resulting in a contrast collection in the papilla or a blunted calyx (Fig. 48.16). Sloughed papilla may obstruct the ureter and cause renal colic.

Fibroepithelial polyp is a benign fibrous polyp covered by transitional epithelium. It is most common in young adult men. The polyp is mobile and hangs from the mucosa by a long, thin stalk.

Pyeloureteritis cystica is a benign process of submucosal cyst formation associated with chronic urinary tract infection. Multiple, small (2 to 3 mm), smooth, round filling defects in the ureter are characteristic. Cysts in renal pelvis tend to be larger, up to 2 cm.

Leukoplakia is a rare inflammatory condition of the uroepithelium related to chronic urinary tract infection and calculi. Squamous metaplasia with keratinization and desquamation results in irregular plaques in the renal pelvis, proximal ureter, and bladder. A key clinical feature is passage of flakes of desquamated epithelium in the urine. Leukoplakia is considered a premalignant condition in the bladder, but not in the ureter.

Malacoplakia is another rare inflammatory granulomatous condition of the uroepithelium associated with chronic infection, especially due to *Escherichia coli*. Smooth submucosal nodules composed of histiocytes produce multiple smooth nodules in the distal ureter and bladder. This condition is not premalignant but can be aggressive extending outside of the urinary system.

Stricture of Pelvicalyceal System or Ureter

A stricture is a fixed narrowing of the pelvicalyceal system or ureter. A diagnosis of ureteral stricture should never be made unless dilation of the ureter or pelvis above the point of narrowing is present. Active peristalsis and the numerous normal kinks and bends in the ureter mimic strictures but lack the combination of fixed narrowing with proximal dilation.

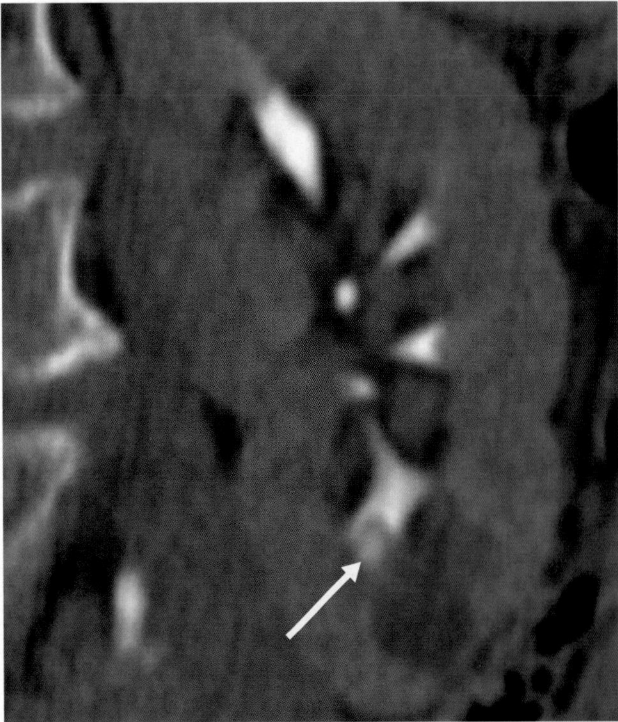

FIGURE 48.16. Papillary Necrosis. Coronal plane reformatted pyelogram-phase image from a CT urogram shows a focus of papillary necrosis (*arrow*) filling with contrast at the lower pole.

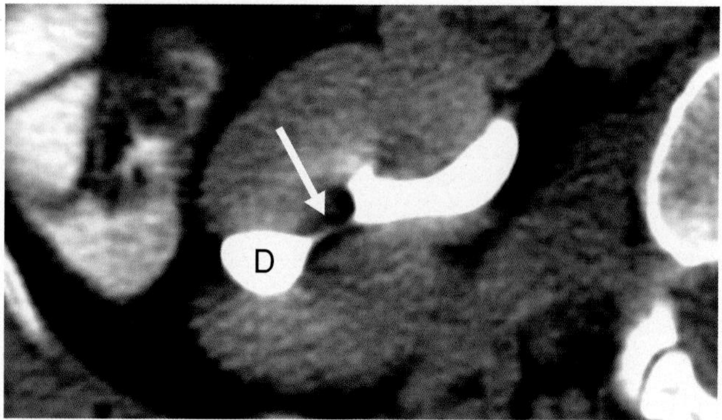

FIGURE 48.17. **Calyceal Diverticulum.** Pyelogram-phase image from a CT urogram demonstrates a cavity (*D*) that fills with contrast and is connected to the collecting system by a thin channel (*arrow*). This calyceal diverticulum is associated with a deep scar in the renal parenchyma.

Inflammation From Stone. An impacted calculus may cause inflammation, which results in scarring and fibrosis producing a stricture.

Posttraumatic strictures result from surgery and instrumentation.

Uroepithelial Tumor. The infiltrating growth pattern of TCC characteristically causes strictures of the collecting system or ureters. These account for 15% of TCC. Squamous cell carcinoma is usually manifest as a stricture of the pelvis or ureter.

Tuberculosis and schistosomiasis are two chronic inflammatory processes that are characterized by fibrosis and strictures. Differentiation from TCC may be difficult by imaging studies but may be suggested by history.

Extrinsic encasement by tumor or inflammatory processes is a common cause of stricture. Causes include lymphoma, cervical carcinoma, colon carcinoma, endometriosis, Crohn disease, diverticulitis, and pelvic inflammatory disease.

Papillary Cavities

Calyceal diverticuli are uroepithelium-lined cavities in the renal parenchyma that communicate via a narrow channel with the fornix of a nearby calyx (Fig. 48.17). They may be congenital, developing from a ureteral bud remnant, or acquired because of infection, reflux, or rupture of a cyst.

Papillary necrosis may result in cavities at the papillary tips that fill with contrast on both antegrade and retrograde studies (Fig. 48.16). Larger cavities cause blunting of the calyces.

BLADDER

Imaging Methods

The CT urogram is often the first imaging test obtained in the evaluation of hematuria. Images of the empty and partially contrast-filled bladder are obtained and demonstrate many bladder lesions. However, small lesions (<5 mm) and lesions at the bladder base near the prostate and urethra are easily overlooked. Direct cystoscopy is required in most instances to provide complete diagnostic evaluation of the bladder. Cystoscopic-guided biopsy provides definitive diagnosis of lesions seen on imaging studies or through the cystoscope. CT and MR are used to stage known bladder neoplasms.

The traditional cystogram, performed by instilling contrast agents directly into the bladder and taking a series of conventional radiographs, provides a more detailed examination. Fluoroscopic examination is performed during bladder filling to detect reflux from the bladder into the ureters. Radiographs are obtained in frontal, lateral, and oblique positions. Radiographs obtained during voiding demonstrate the bladder outlet and urethra. Postvoid radiographs document residual urine.

CT cystogram may be performed using similar technique. A minimum of 250 cc of contrast agent is instilled into the bladder via a catheter. CT is sensitive to small amounts of contrast that may leak into the perivesical tissues. Air instilled into the bladder has also been used to perform "CT cystoscopy." Patients are scanned in supine and prone positions to outline lesions that project into the lumen.

US examination of the pelvis is routinely preformed using the urine-filled bladder as a sonographic window to pelvic organs. Intraluminal masses, calculi, bladder wall thickness, and bladder emptying can be reliably assessed by US (see Chapter 51).

Anatomy and Anomalies

The normal filled urinary bladder is oval, with the floor parallel to, and 5 to 10 mm above, the superior aspect of the symphysis pubis. The size and shape of the bladder vary with the degree of bladder filling. The superior surface is covered by peritoneum, which extends to the side walls of the pelvis. The sigmoid colon and loops of small bowel, as well as the uterus in females, lie on top of the bladder and may cause mass impressions on the bladder dome. The inferior surface is extraperitoneal. Anteriorly, the bladder is separated from the symphysis pubis by fat in the extraperitoneal space of Retzius. Posteriorly, the bladder is separated from the uterus by the uterovesical peritoneal recess in females and from the rectum by the rectovesical peritoneal recess in males. The lining mucosa of the bladder is loosely attached to the muscular coat, so when the bladder is contracted, the mucosa appears wrinkled. The bladder wall has four layers: an outer connective tissue adventitia, smooth muscle consisting of circular muscle fibers sandwiched between inner and outer layers of longitudinal fibers, submucosal connective tissue (the lamina propria), and the mucosa of transitional epithelium. The *trigone* is a triangle at the bladder floor formed by the two ureteral orifices and the internal urethral orifice. With voiding, the trigone descends 1 to 2 cm and transforms from a flat surface into a cone with the urethra at the apex. On MR T1WI, the bladder wall is often indistinguishable from low-intensity urine. On T2WI, the low-intensity bladder wall is well outlined by high-intensity urine and perivesical fat. Chemical shift artifact at water–fat interfaces may interfere with assessment of tumor invasion of the bladder wall.

Bladder exstrophy results from a congenital deficiency in development of the lower anterior abdominal wall. The bladder is open, and its mucosa is continuous with the skin. Epispadias and wide diastasis of the symphysis pubis are associated. Ureteral obstruction, umbilical, and inguinal hernias are common. Management includes urinary diversion, bladder augmentation, and skin grafting.

Urachal remnant conditions may be discovered in asymptomatic adult patients on CT or US examinations performed for other reasons. The urachus is the vestigial remnant of the urogenital sinus and allantois. It is a tubular structure that extends from the bladder dome to the umbilicus along the anterior abdominal wall. The median umbilical ligament is its obliterated residual.

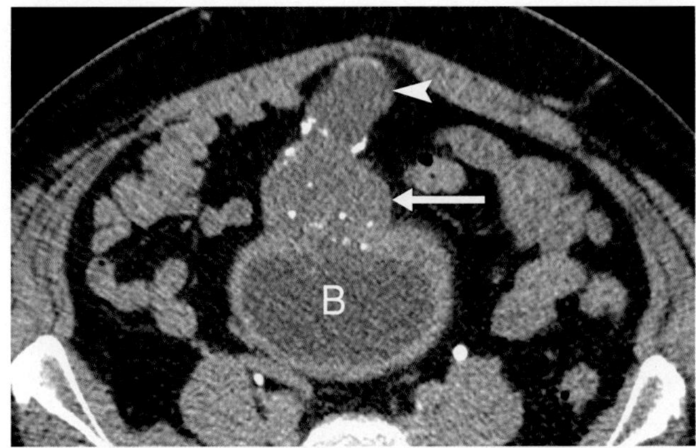

FIGURE 48.18. **Urachal Carcinoma.** Early postcontrast CT urogram image shows a urachal diverticulum (*arrowhead*) extending from the midline dome of the bladder (*B*) to the midline of the anterior abdominal wall. A solid mass (*arrow*) occupies the proximal aspect of the diverticulum. Several high attenuation stones and dystrophic calcifications are seen within the mass proven on biopsy to be adenocarcinoma. The wall of the bladder is thickened.

Patent urachus accounts for 50% of cases. The persistent communication between the bladder and umbilicus causes a urine leak usually resulting in discovery during the neonatal period. Some patients are asymptomatic until an obstructive lesion of the lower urinary tract opens the unobliterated urachus resulting in an umbilical-urinary fistula.

Umbilical-urachal sinus (15% of cases) is a blind-ended dilation of urachus at the umbilical end that may cause a persistent umbilical discharge. Imaging shows a tubular structure in the midline abdominal wall extending caudally from the umbilicus.

Vesical-urachal diverticulum (5%) is an outpouching of the bladder in the anterior midline location of the urachus. This is seen in adults with bladder outlet obstruction as a fluid-filled sac extending cranially from the bladder in midline abdominal wall. Stasis of urine in the diverticulum may result in infection, stone formation, and a risk of carcinoma developing within the diverticulum.

Urachal cyst (30%) develops if the urachus is closed at both ends but remains patent in the middle. Imaging shows a fluid-filled cyst in the midline abdominal wall usually in the lower third region of the urachus. Infection may complicate the usually simple nature of the fluid and may result in calcification of the cyst wall.

Urachal carcinoma is usually an adenocarcinoma (90%) and represents 0.5% of bladder carcinoma. Tumors are seen most commonly at ages 40 to 70. They are asymptomatic until they present with local invasion or metastatic disease (Fig. 48.18).

Thickened Bladder Wall/Small Bladder Capacity

The normal wall of a well-distended bladder should not exceed 5 to 6 mm in thickness. The following conditions are associated with abnormal thickening of the bladder wall and, often, reduced bladder capacity.

Benign prostatic hypertrophy affects 50% to 75% of men older than age 50. Prostate enlargement projects into the base of the bladder, uplifting the bladder trigone and causing "J-hooking" of the distal ureters (Fig. 48.19). Chronic bladder outlet obstruction results in thickening and trabeculation of the bladder wall. Prostate calcifications and bladder stones may be present. Prostate carcinoma must also be considered as a cause of prostate enlargement, although imaging methods cannot reliably differentiate benign enlargement from malignancy.

Urethral stricture and posterior urethral valves cause chronic obstruction to the outflow of urine from the bladder. The bladder wall thickens reflecting muscle hypertrophy in an attempt to overcome the obstruction. Voiding or retrograde urethrography demonstrates the urethral abnormality.

Neurogenic bladder may be spastic or atonic. Causes include meningomyelocele, spinal trauma, diabetes mellitus, poliomyelitis, central nervous system tumor, and multiple sclerosis. Neurogenic bladders are prone to urinary stasis, chronic infection, and stone formation. Most neurogenic bladders eventually become trabeculated, thick walled, and reduced in capacity.

Cystitis. Inflammation of the bladder has many causes, including infection (bacteria, adenovirus, tuberculosis, schistosomiasis), drugs (cyclophosphamide), radiation, and autoimmune reaction. CT shows bladder wall thickening and perivesical edema (Fig. 48.20). MR demonstrates mucosal edema and inflammation as high signal intensity on T2WI, easily differentiated from normal low signal bladder wall.

Cystitis cystica is characterized by multiple fluid-filled submucosal cysts. Most cases are associated with bladder infection.

Cystitis glandularis is a further progression of cystitis cystica with proliferation of mucous secreting glands in the lamina propria. The cysts vary in size and may obstruct the ureteral orifice. Cystitis glandularis may be a precursor of adenocarcinoma of the bladder.

Bullous edema of the bladder wall is usually associated with chronic irritation from indwelling catheters. Grape-like cysts elevate the mucosa.

Interstitial cystitis is a chronic, idiopathic inflammation of the bladder found most often in women. The bladder capacity is progressively diminished, and the bladder wall thickens and becomes trabeculated and fibrotic.

Hemorrhagic cystitis is characterized by hemorrhage into the mucosa and submucosa. It is caused by bacterial or adenovirus infection.

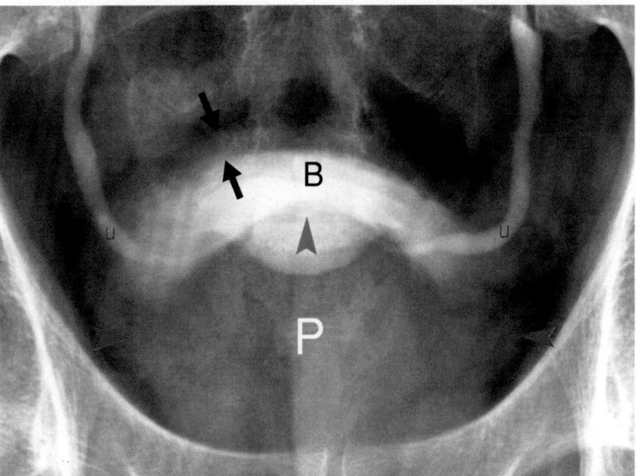

FIGURE 48.19. **Benign Prostatic Hypertrophy.** A radiograph from an excretory urogram shows marked uplifting of the bladder base because of massive enlargement of the prostate (*P*, between *red arrowheads*). The trigone (*blue arrowhead*) and ureteral orifices are markedly elevated, resulting in a J-shaped appearance to the distal ureters (*u*). The bladder wall is thickened (between *arrows*) and the bladder (*B*) mucosal pattern is prominent.

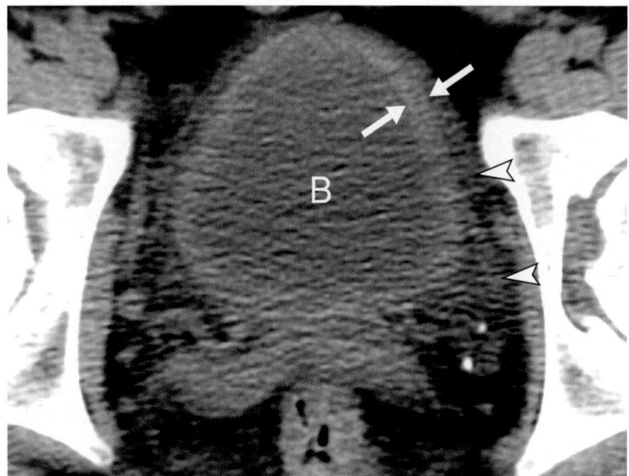

FIGURE 48.20. **Cystitis.** CT without contrast in a man with pyuria and hematuria shows thickening (between *arrows*) of the wall of the bladder (*B*) and edema (*arrowheads*) in the fatty tissues adjacent to the bladder. Urine culture confirmed cystitis caused by *E. coli.*

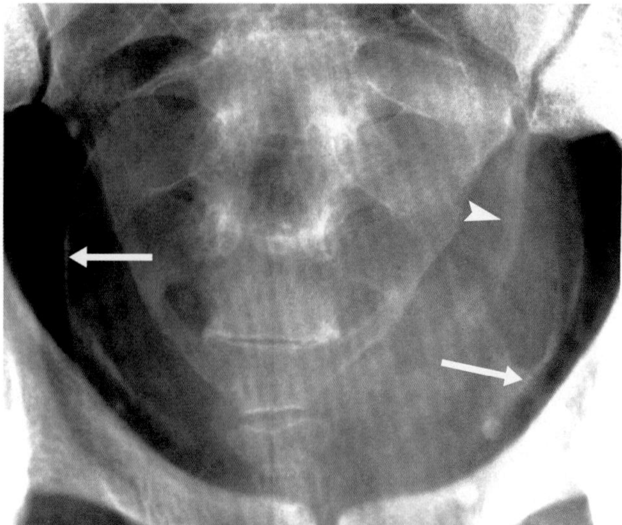

FIGURE 48.22. Schistosoma Haematobium. Conventional radiograph demonstrates calcification in the wall of the bladder (*arrows*) and in the wall of the left ureter (*arrowhead*). The bladder is filled with urine. The patient is a 25-year-old Egyptian male.

Eosinophilic cystitis is an infiltration of the bladder wall by eosinophils. The cause is uncertain. The bladder wall is greatly thickened and frequently nodular.

Emphysematous cystitis is a form of bladder inflammation with gas within the bladder wall (Fig. 48.21). It is associated with poorly controlled diabetes mellitus, bladder outlet obstruction, and infection with *E. coli,* which ferment sugar in the urine to release carbon dioxide and hydrogen gasses. Gas within the bladder lumen is seen with emphysematous cystitis, instrumentation, and vesicocolic fistula.

Calcified Bladder Wall

Schistosomiasis of the urinary tract is caused by infestation with *Schistosoma haematobium.* The disease is most prevalent in North Africa, the Nile Valley, and Egypt. The larval cercariae of the blood fluke penetrate the skin of humans in infected water, enter the lymphatic vessels, and circulate eventually to the portal venous system, where the organism matures into adulthood. Adult females migrate to the vesical venous plexus and lay their eggs in the wall of the urinary bladder and ureter. The eggs incite a fibrosing granulomatous reaction that results in beaded stenosis and irregular dilation of the ureters, and calcification of the walls of the distal ureters and bladder. The calcification is entirely the result of calcification of the eggs embedded within the wall (Fig. 48.22). The ureters become aperistaltic, resulting in vesicoureteral reflux. Eventually, the bladder may become shrunken, fibrotic, and contracted. Fistulas may develop in the perineum and scrotum. Renal disease develops slowly due to functional obstruction and reflux.

Tuberculosis affects the kidneys primarily and the ureters and bladder secondarily. Calcification affects the ureters proximally and may eventually extend into the distal ureters and bladder. Tuberculous infection of the bladder causes wall thickening and reduced capacity. Calcification of the bladder wall is uncommon and patchy.

Cystitis. Postirradiation cystitis, chronic infection, and cyclophosphamide-induced cystitis cause curvilinear or flocculent bladder wall calcification.

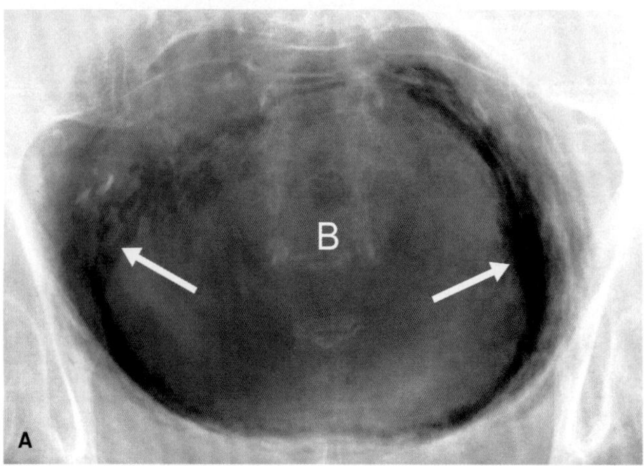

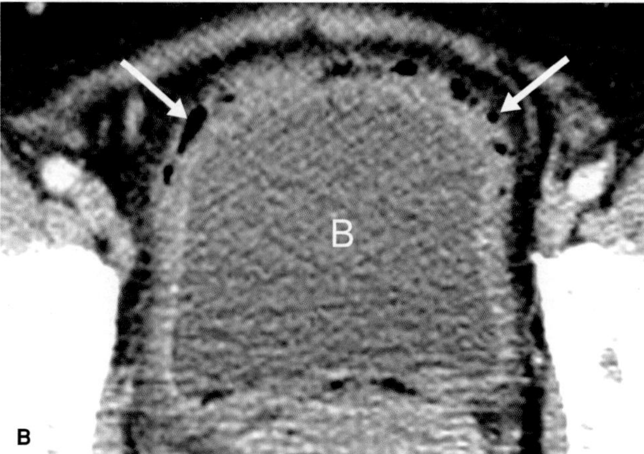

FIGURE 48.21. **Emphysematous Cystitis. A:** Air in the bladder wall is seen as a pattern of layering linear lucencies (*arrows*) outlining the bladder (*B*) on this conventional radiograph in a 67-year-old man with cystitis due to *Escherichia coli.* **B:** CT in a different patient with diabetes shows streaks and bubbles of air (*arrows*) in the wall of the bladder (*B*).

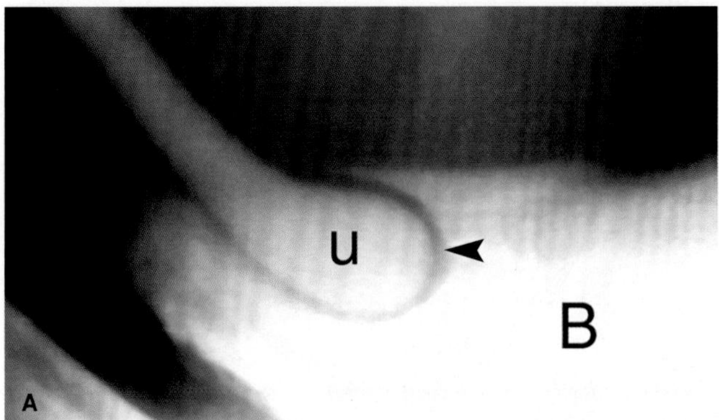

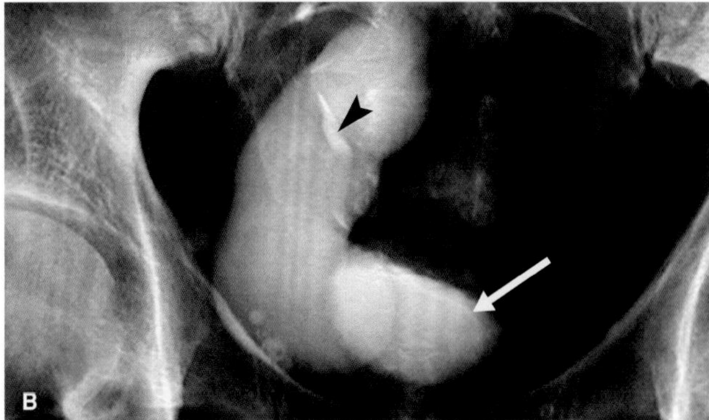

FIGURE 48.23. **Simple and Ectopic Ureteroceles. A:** Radiograph from a traditional excretory urogram demonstrates mild dilation of the right ureter associated with a simple ureterocele (*u*) that protrudes into the lumen of the bladder (*B*). The radiolucent wall of the ureterocele (*arrowhead*) is outlined by contrast within the ureterocele and contrast within the bladder lumen. The wall of the ureterocele is made up of the wall of the ureter and the bladder mucosa. **B:** Radiograph from another excretory urogram shows a normal ureter (*arrowhead*) from the normal lower pole of the kidney and a dilated ureter with ectopic ureterocele (*arrow*) from the obstructed upper pole of the kidney. The ectopic ureter inserts medial and caudad to the normal insertion of the upper pole ureter, following the Weigert–Meyer rule.

Neoplasm. Transitional cell and squamous cell carcinomas of the bladder may rarely calcify (1% to 7% incidence). Tumor calcification may be punctate or curvilinear and is best demonstrated by CT.

Bladder Wall Mass or Filling Defect

Simple ureterocele is a cystic dilation of the intravesicular segment of the ureter caused by a congenital prolapse of the distal ureter into the bladder lumen at the normal insertion site of the ureter into the trigone. It is usually an incidental finding in adults, although large, simple ureteroceles may be associated with ureter obstruction, infection, and stone formation. Contrast studies demonstrate a rounded filling defect in the bladder at the ureteral insertion (Fig. 48.23A). A "cobra head" or "spring onion" appearance is characteristic. A radiolucent halo is produced by the wall of the ureter outlined both inside and outside by contrast. US demonstrates a cystic mass at the ureteral orifice. Peristalsis of the ureter causing alternate filling and emptying of the ureterocele is seen on real-time US.

Ectopic ureterocele is usually associated with ureteral duplication. Females with ectopic ureters are prone to urinary incontinence because the ureter may insert distal to the external sphincter into the vestibule, uterus, or vagina. In males, the ectopic ureter usually inserts proximal to the external sphincter; no incontinence results. Large ectopic ureteroceles may obstruct the opposite ureter or cause bladder outlet obstruction because of their mass effect. The ectopic ureterocele appears as a cystic mass at the ectopic site of ureter insertion. The ureter is dilated and tortuous (Fig. 48.23B).

Transitional cell carcinoma of the bladder is the most common urinary tract neoplasm. TCC of the bladder is 50 times more common than TCC of the ureter. Although bladder tumors commonly develop in patients with primary TCC of the renal pelvis or ureter, only 2% to 4% of patients with bladder carcinoma have TCC of the ureter. Nonetheless, all patients with TCC deserve detailed screening of the entire uroepithelium. Risk factors for bladder urothelial tumors include tobacco use, arsenic ingestion, Balkan nephropathy, phenacetin abuse, cyclophosphamide treatment, exposure to aromatic amintes, schistosomiasis, and recurrent urinary tract infections and stones. Bladder cancers are classified as superficial (papillary tumors confined to the mucosa and associated with a high likelihood of multiplicity and recurrence following resection) or invasive (penetrating into and through the bladder wall resulting in local extension and metastases). Cross-sectional imaging and cystoscopy are used to stage known bladder carcinoma according to the TMN system. Bladder carcinoma spreads by direct invasion through the bladder wall, by lymphatic spread to regional lymph nodes, and by hematogenous spread most commonly to bones, liver, and lung. Approximately 5% of patients have distant metastases at initial diagnosis. The hallmark of TCC is multiplicity and recurrence. CT and MR are approximately equal in capability of staging bladder cancer.

CT demonstrates TCC as a soft tissue nodule or papillary mass projecting into the bladder lumen, or as a focal thickening of the bladder wall. The bladder should be well distended to avoid missing small or flat lesions. Calcification is present in 5% of tumors. Enhancing tumor is best seen against a background of low attenuation urine distending the bladder (Fig. 48.24). Tumor enhancement peaks during the first 60 seconds following contrast injection allowing the optimal identification of tumor invasion. When contrast has filled the bladder, tumor is seen as low attenuation polypoid or plaque-like mural nodule against a background of high attenuation contrast-opacified urine. Perivesical spread is seen as soft tissue density tumor in the perivesical fat. Previous biopsy, inflammation, and postradiation changes make image interpretation more difficult.

MR reveals TCC on T1WI as being of intermediate signal equal to muscle, higher signal than urine. T1WI are optimal for detection of tumor invasion through the bladder wall seen as intermediate signal tumor nodule extending into bright fat. On T2WI, the tumor is of lower signal than the bright urine but higher signal than normal bladder wall muscle. Intact low signal bladder wall deep to the tumor is evidence of the absence of muscle invasion. When the tumor is at or near the UVJ the presence of a dilated ureter is evidence of muscle invasion. With gadolinium administration the tumor enhances more than the normal bladder wall or postbiopsy inflammatory tissue. Involved lymph nodes are often normal in size but may be judged as suspicious by their location. Biopsy is often necessary to determine nodal metastases. Coronal and sagittal plane images improve the accuracy of staging on MR.

US demonstrates exophytic tumors as polypoid masses extending from the bladder wall (see Fig. 51.51). Infiltrating tumors may show as focal thickening of the bladder wall. Tumors may be difficult to recognize in the presence of diffuse bladder wall thickening and trabeculation.

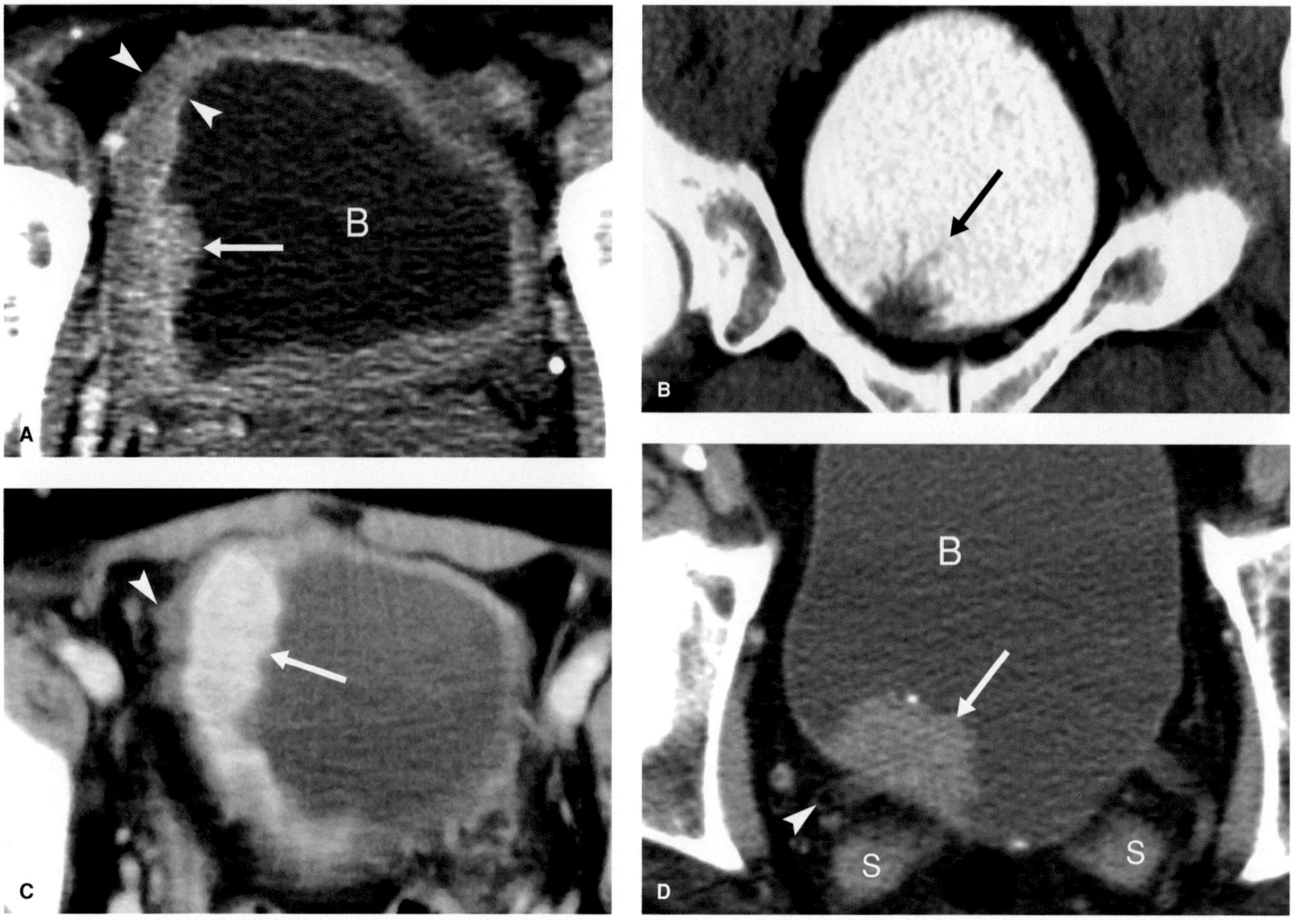

FIGURE 48.24. **Transitional Cell Carcinoma. A**: CT urogram image demonstrates a flat mucosal lesion (*arrow*) arising from the right lateral wall of the bladder (*B*). Contrast enhancement of the lesion is slightly greater than that of the bladder wall revealing the extent of the tumor. This is a T1 lesion, confined to the bladder wall. The bladder wall is thickened (between *arrowheads*) and irregular because of muscle hypertrophy induced by the chronic obstruction of an enlarged prostate. On this early phase CT image the bladder is distended with low attenuation urine. **B**: Coronal plane delayed image from CT urogram reveals the papillary growth pattern of a transitional cell carcinoma (*arrow*) well outlined by contrast-opacified urine. **C**: Early postcontrast image from a CT urogram shows enhancement of the tumor (*arrow*) and distinct enhancing nodules (*arrowhead*) of soft tissue extending into the perivesical fat. This is strong CT evidence of spread of tumor through the bladder wall, making this a pT3b stage lesion. **D**: Early-phase postcontrast CT urogram image shows an enhancing tumor (*arrow*) involving the right ureterovesical junction (*arrowhead*). This a stage T2 lesion. *S*, seminal vesicles; *B*, bladder.

Squamous cell carcinoma accounts for 4% of bladder malignancy. It tends to develop in bladders chronically irritated by stones and infection and is highly associated with bladder schistosomiasis. Tumors appear as an enhancing bladder mass or as focal or diffuse thickening of the bladder wall. Papillary tumor forms characteristic of TCC are not seen. Most tumors have invaded the bladder wall and many have metastasized to distant sites at the time of diagnosis.

Adenocarcinoma is rare, accounting for less than 1% of bladder malignancy. Most cases are associated with bladder exstrophy or urachal remnants. Adenocarcinoma metastases to the bladder are more common than primary bladder adenocarcinoma.

Benign bladder tumors include leiomyoma, hemangioma, pheochromocytoma, and neurofibroma. They produce well-defined bladder masses and smooth filling defects.

Blood clots in the bladder are usually irregular in shape, move with changes in patient position, and change in size and appearance over time.

Bladder stones may migrate from the kidney or form primarily within the bladder (Fig. 48.25) because of urinary stasis or a

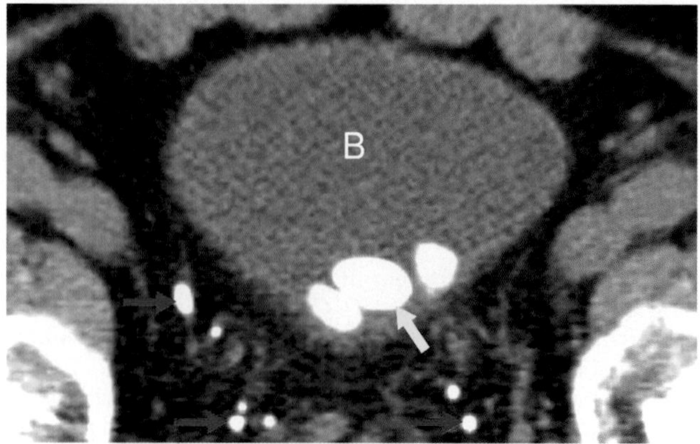

FIGURE 48.25. **Bladder Stones.** Multiple high attenuation stones (*yellow arrow*) are seen within the lumen of the bladder (*B*) on this noncontrast CT. Contrast opacification of the bladder may obscure the presence of bladder stones. This patient has a neurogenic bladder resulting in chronic urine stasis within the bladder. Numerous phleboliths (*red arrows*) are also evident.

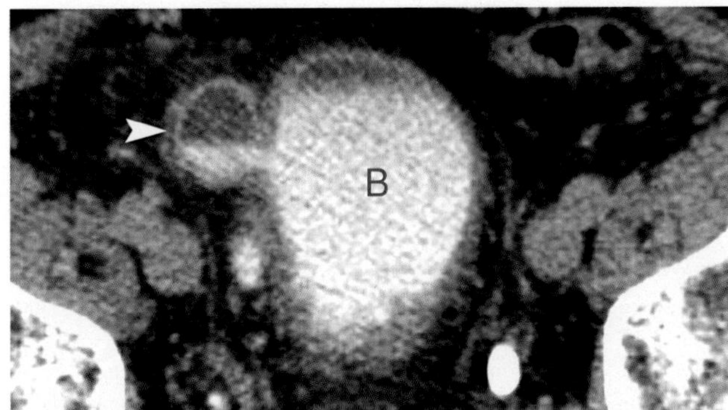

FIGURE 48.26. **Bladder Diverticulum.** Delayed-phase image from a CT urogram shows a bladder diverticulum (*arrowhead*) partially filled with contrast-opacified urine. The narrow neck of the diverticulum is apparent. *B*, bladder.

foreign body. Solitary stones are most common. Stones must be removed to cure chronic bladder infection. Chronic bladder stones increase the risk of developing bladder carcinoma.

Malacoplakia is most common in the bladder producing hematuria and signs of urinary tract infection. Lesions vary from nodules to papillary masses to ulcerated plaques. The inflammatory mass can extend through the bladder wall and even destroy bone.

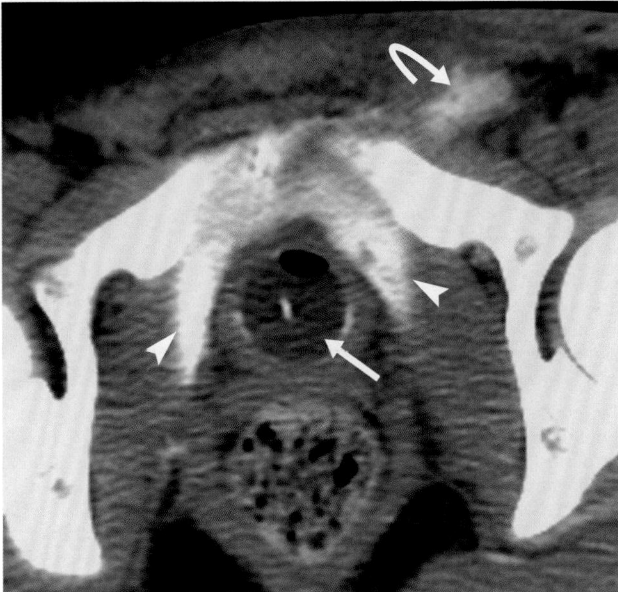

FIGURE 48.27. **Extraperitoneal Bladder Rupture.** Image from a CT cystogram performed in a patient with a pelvic fracture reveals contrast extravasation (*arrowheads*) from the bladder into the retropubic space of Retzius indicating bladder rupture into the extraperitoneal compartment. Contrast has also tracked into the subcutaneous tissues (*curved arrow*). Contrast was instilled into the bladder via a Foley catheter (*arrow*).

Bladder Outpouchings and Fistulas

Bladder diverticula are herniations of the bladder mucosa between interlacing muscle bundles. Most are located posterolaterally near the UVJ (Fig. 48.26). Diverticula may contain stones or tumor and occasionally do not fill on cystograms. Complications of bladder diverticula include urinary stasis, infection, stone formation, vesicoureteral reflux, and bladder outlet obstruction.

Vesicocolonic fistula most commonly occurs as a complication of diverticulitis. Additional causes include colon or bladder carcinoma, ulcerative colitis, and Crohn disease. The bladder is chronically infected, and the patient may complain of pneumaturia and fecaluria. The diagnosis is often made clinically. Barium enema and cystography detect only 35% of vesicocolonic fistulae. The fistulous tract is occasionally demonstrated by CT.

Vesicovaginal fistula is usually a complication of gynecologic surgery, especially for cervical carcinoma. Obstetric injury is an occasional cause.

Vesicoenteric fistula is almost always attributable to Crohn disease.

Bladder Trauma

Susceptibility of the bladder to traumatic injury depends largely on the degree of bladder filling at the time of injury. A distended bladder is more prone to injury than a collapsed bladder. Traditional or CT cystography defines the nature and extent of bladder injury.

Extraperitoneal bladder rupture (80% of bladder ruptures) results from puncture of the bladder by a spicule of bone from a pelvic fracture. Contrast extravasates into extraperitoneal compartments, most commonly the retropubic space of Retzius (Fig. 48.27). Contrast extravasation may extend into the anterior abdominal wall, thigh, and scrotum. Conventional or CT cystography with distention of the bladder to at least 250 mL is required to exclude bladder rupture.

Intraperitoneal bladder rupture (20% of bladder ruptures) results from blunt trauma applied to a distended bladder. The sudden rise in intravesical pressure results in rupture of the bladder dome and extravasation of urine into the peritoneal space. Contrast material flows into the paracolic gutters and outlines the loops of the bowel (Fig. 48.28). Intraperitoneal bladder rupture may clinically mimic acute renal failure. Urine output is decreased or absent, and serum creatinine is increased because of absorption of urine by the peritoneal surface.

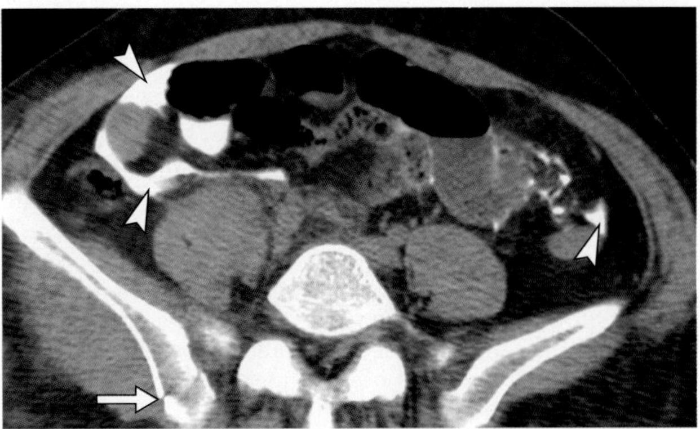

FIGURE 48.28. **Intraperitoneal Bladder Rupture.** Image from a CT cystogram demonstrates extravasation of contrast from the bladder into the intraperitoneal space. Contrast (*arrowheads*), enveloping loops of bowel, confirms its intraperitoneal location. This finding on a CT cystogram is diagnostic of intraperitoneal bladder rupture. A fracture (*arrow*) of the ilium is evident.

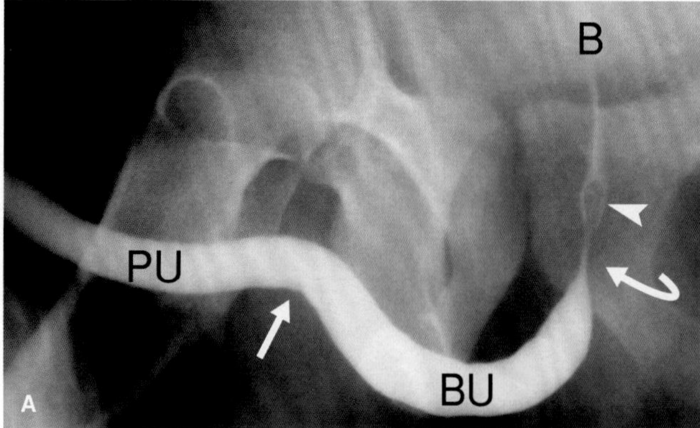

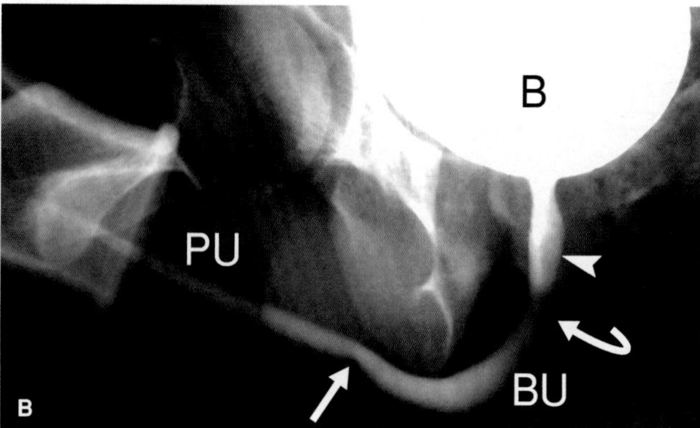

FIGURE 48.29. **Normal Male Urethra.** **A:** Retrograde urethrogram. **B:** Voiding cystourethrogram. The anterior urethra consists of the penile and bulbous urethra. The penile urethra (*PU*) extends from the urethral meatus to the suspensory ligament of the penis (*straight arrows*) at the penoscrotal junction. The bulbous urethra (*BU*) extends from the penoscrotal junction to the urogenital diaphragm (*curved arrows*) marked by the tip of the cone on the RUG and the slight narrowing of urethral caliber on the VCUG. The posterior urethra consists of the membranous urethra and the prostatic urethra. The membranous urethra (*curved arrows*) is only 1 cm in length and is entirely within the muscle of the urogenital diaphragm. On a retrograde urethrogram the membranous urethra extends between of the tip of cone and the verumontanum. The verumontanum (*arrowheads*) is a nodular structure that produces a filling defect on the urethrograms by bulging into the prostatic urethra. The prostatic urethra extends from the inferior aspect of the verumontanum to the base of the bladder (*B*).

URETHRA

Imaging Methods

The urethra is studied by retrograde and voiding urethrography (Fig. 48.29). The retrograde urethrogram is a simple study of the male anterior urethra. Contrast medium is injected into the anterior urethra by means of a syringe or catheter that occludes the meatal orifice. Radiographs are exposed in the right posterior oblique projection. The anterior urethra normally distends fully because of resistance of the external sphincter at the level of the urogenital diaphragm. Complete filling of the posterior urethra is not possible because contrast runs freely into the bladder. Voiding cystourethrography is performed by filling the bladder with contrast via a catheter. The catheter is removed, and radiographs are obtained while the patient urinates into a basin on the fluoroscopy table. The voiding urethrogram demonstrates distention of both the posterior and anterior urethra. Radiographic study of the female urethra may be conducted by voiding cystourethrogram or by retrograde urethrogram with a specially designed double-balloon catheter. The female urethra is also well studied by transrectal or perineal US and by CT and MR.

Anatomy

The male urethra is divided into posterior and anterior portions by the inferior aspect of the urogenital diaphragm (Fig. 48.29). The posterior urethra consists of the *prostatic urethra* within the prostate gland, from the bladder neck to urogenital diaphragm, and the short *membranous urethra,* which is totally contained within the 1 cm thick urogenital diaphragm. The anterior urethra extends from the urogenital diaphragm to the external urethral meatus. It consists of the *bulbous urethra* extending from the urogenital diaphragm to the penoscrotal junction, and the *penile urethra* extending to the urethral meatus. The anterior urethra is entirely contained within the corpus spongiosum penis except for the proximal 2 cm of the bulbous urethra, called the *pars nuda*. This unprotected portion of the urethra is particularly susceptible to straddle injury. The prostatic urethra runs vertically through the prostate over a length of 3 to 4 cm. An oval filling defect in the midportion of the posterior wall is the *verumontanum.* The ejaculatory ducts open into the urethra on either side of the verumontanum, and the prostatic glands empty into the urethra by multiple small openings that surround the verumontanum. The *utricle*, a mullerian remnant, is a small, saccular depression in the middle of the verumontanum. The distal end of the verumontanum marks the beginning of the membranous urethra, which extends to the apex of the cone of the bulbous urethra. The voluntary external urethral sphincter within the urogenital diaphragm entirely surrounds the membranous urethra. *Cowper glands* are pea-sized accessory sex glands within the urogenital diaphragm on either side of the membranous urethra. Their ducts empty into the bulbous urethra 2 cm distally (Fig. 48.30).

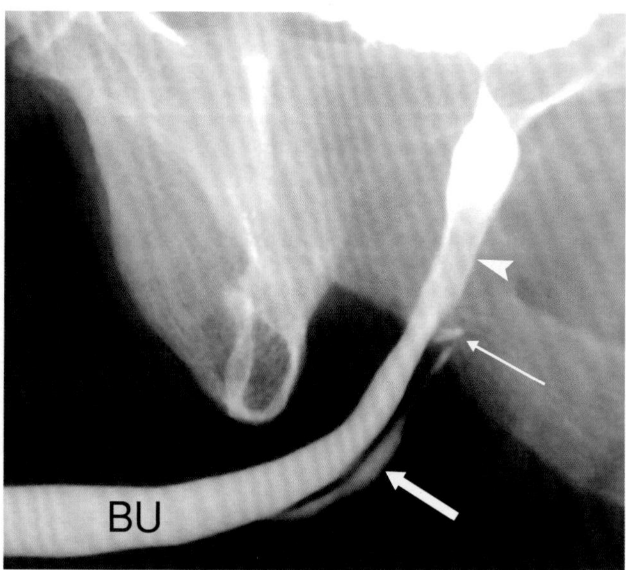

FIGURE 48.30. **Cowper Glands.** Radiograph from a voiding cystourethrogram shows filling of the ducts to Cowper glands. The glands (*skinny arrow*) are in the urogenital diaphragm and their ducts (*fat arrow*) drain into the bulbous urethra (*BU*). The verumontanum (*arrowhead*) produces its usual filling defect in the contrast column.

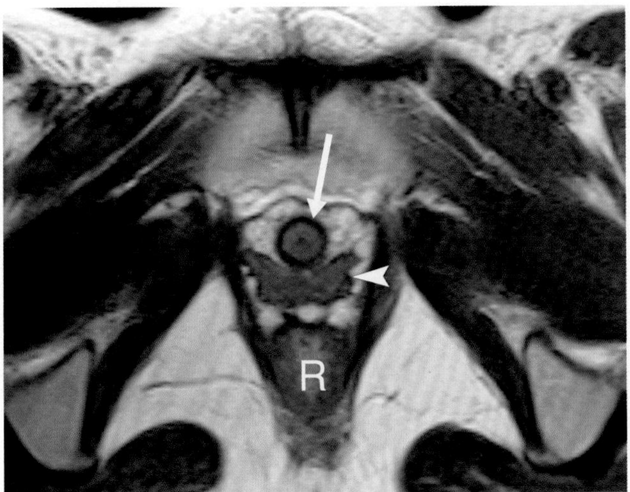

FIGURE 48.31. **Normal Female Urethra.** T2-weighted MR demonstrates the zonal anatomy of the female urethra (*arrow*) in the anterior wall of the vagina (*arrowhead*). The outer smooth layer is low signal (dark), the submucosal layer is moderately bright, and the central mucosa is dark. The rectum (*R*) is seen posteriorly.

On retrograde urethrography, the bulbous urethra tapers to a cone shape as the urethra enters the external sphincter. The apex of the cone marks the division between the membranous and bulbous urethra. The penoscrotal junction that divides the bulbous and penile urethra is marked by the suspensory ligament of the penis, which causes a normal bend in the urethra. The entire anterior urethra is lined by the *glands of Littre* (see Fig. 48.32), whose secretions lubricate the urethra. Cowper ducts and the utricle occasionally fill with contrast during urethrography in a normal patient. The filling of these structures with contrast occurs much more commonly in the presence of urethral strictures. Visualization of the glands of Littre is always abnormal and associated with chronic inflammation and urethral stricture. Reflux of contrast into the prostatic ducts is also abnormal and is associated with prostatitis and distal urethral stricture.

The female urethra varies in length from 2.5 to 4 cm. The urethra is embedded in the anterior wall of the vagina and is lined throughout by periurethral glands. On MR, the urethra is isointense with the vaginal muscle on T1WI. On T2WI, the normal urethra demonstrates a characteristic target appearance (Fig. 48.31) with dark inner and outer rings and a middle zone of high signal intensity. The middle zone corresponds to highly vascular submucosa and enhances markedly with gadopentetate administration. The dark inner zone is mucosa, and the dark outer zone is urethral smooth muscle.

Pathology

Urethral strictures are abnormal narrowings of the urethra resulting from fibrous scar tissue. They may involve the entire urethra or only a small portion. Abrupt, short-segment strictures are usually traumatic. Long-segment strictures may be either traumatic or inflammatory (Fig. 48.32). Causes of traumatic urethral strictures include instrumentation, indwelling catheters, prostatectomy procedures, chemical injury (podophyllin), saddle injuries (usually of the bulbous urethra), and pelvic fractures. Most inflammatory strictures are attributable to gonorrhea. Bacteria become sequestered in the glands of Littre and incite the formation of granulation tissue and fibrosis. Additional etiologies include chlamydia, mycoplasma, tuberculosis, and schistosomiasis. Complications of urethral strictures include the following:

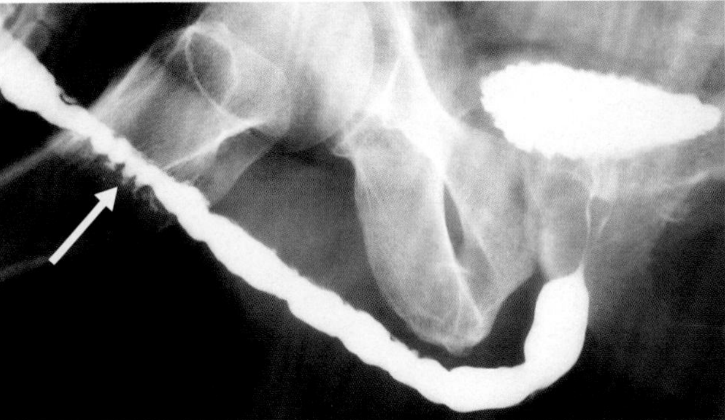

FIGURE 48.32. **Urethral Strictures, Glands of Littre.** Retrograde urethrogram demonstrates multiple strictures in the penile and bulbous urethra. Filling of the glands of Littre (*arrow*) is evidence of urethritis. This patient had a history of multiple episodes of gonorrhea.

- *Periurethral abscess* usually develops on the ventral surface and may drain into the lumen or onto the skin, creating a periurethral fistula.
- *False passage* is the most common complication of urethral stricture. It is usually iatrogenic because of attempted passage of catheters or instruments past the obstruction.
- *Stasis and infection* may cause disease of the more proximal urinary tracts including hydronephrosis, bladder hypertrophy, calculi, and chronic inflammation.
- *Carcinoma of the urethra* occurs as a complication of chronic urethritis and stricture. Carcinomas may appear as a filling defect in the urethra or as a change in appearance of the stricture. Most are squamous cell carcinomas and most involve the anterior urethra. MR is the imaging method of choice for showing extent of tumor (Fig. 48.33). Rare

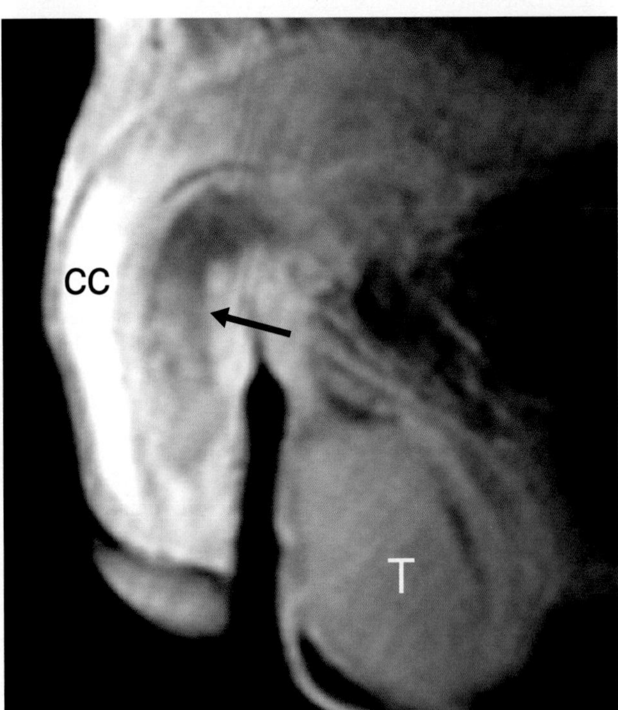

FIGURE 48.33. **Carcinoma of the Penile Urethra.** Sagittal plane MR image shows recurrent squamous cell carcinoma as abnormal low signal (*arrow*) filling and distending the penile urethra within the corpus spongiosum. This patient has already experienced partial resection of the tip of his penis for carcinoma. One of the corpora cavernosa (*CC*) is seen anteriorly. A normal testis (*T*) is also shown.

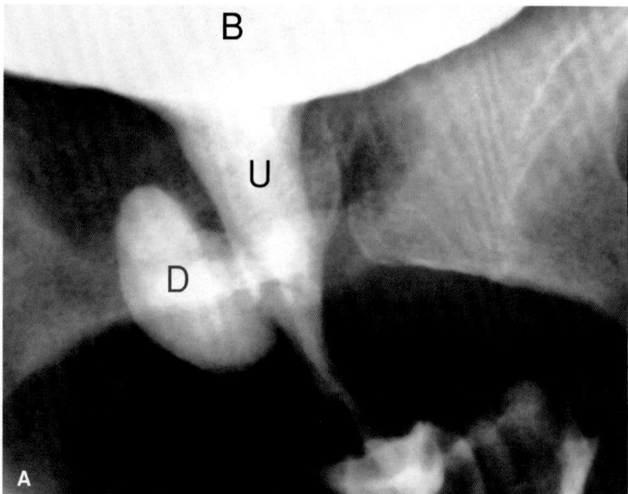

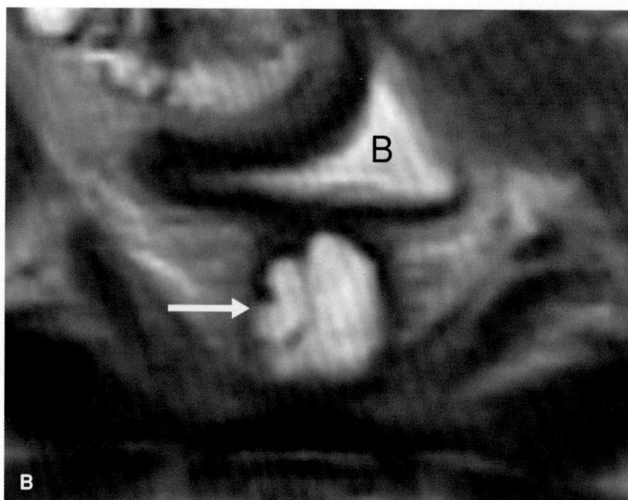

FIGURE 48.34. **Diverticulum of the Female Urethra. A:** Voiding cystourethrogram in a woman with recurrent urinary tract infections fills a urethral diverticulum (*D*). *B,* bladder; *U,* female urethra. **B:** Coronal T2-weighted MR image of a different woman shows a large diverticulum (*arrow*) of the urethra beneath the bladder (*B*) and posterior to the symphysis pubis.

tumors of the posterior urethra are usually TCC that occur as part of multiple uroepithelial neoplasia.

Posterior urethral valves are usually discovered on prenatal US. Mild cases may be not present until adulthood. A thick valve-like membrane extends obliquely across the urethral lumen from the verumontanum to the distal prostatic urethra obstructing the flow of urine. Findings of bladder outlet obstruction are present with bladder wall hypertrophy and usually bilateral hydronephrosis. Characteristically the membrane flattens to allow passage of a catheter into the bladder, but balloons and obstructs urine flow with voiding. Previous classification of posterior urethral valves into 3 types is no longer accepted. Variations in appearance are now believed secondary to trauma related to attempts at catheterization.

Urethral diverticuli are smooth, sac-like outpouchings of the urethra. They may be congenital or the result of infection or trauma. Because they serve as a site of urinary stasis, stone formation and recurrent infection are common complications.

Diverticulum of the female urethra is an uncommon cause of recurrent urinary tract infection. They are believed to arise from infection of the periurethral glands. Most extend from the posterolateral wall of the midportion of the short female urethra. Up to one-third of patients have multiple or complex diverticuli. On a voiding cystourethrogram the diverticulum is demonstrated on postvoid radiographs after voided urine and contrast fills the diverticulum (Fig. 48.34). Transrectal or transperineal US shows a cystic mass filled with complex fluid closely related to the urethra in the anterior vaginal wall. CT shows a low attenuation periurethral mass. T2-weighted MR shows the lesion best as a high signal mass.

Traumatic injury to the male posterior urethra occurs in about 10% of pelvic fractures. The junction between the prostatic and membranous urethra is the most common site of injury. Injury is suspected in patients with pelvic fractures or when blood is present at the urethral meatus. Retrograde urethrography should precede attempts at urethral catheterization. If a bladder catheter has already been inserted, the urethra can be studied by inserting a small (8F) pediatric feeding tube adjacent to the catheter and injecting contrast. The classification of posterior urethral injury is as follows: (a) *Type 1* is contusion without imaging findings; (b) *Type 2* is a stretch injury with elongation of the urethra without extravasation; (c) *Type 3* is partial disruption with extravasation of contrast agent from the urethra with opacification of the bladder; (d) *Type 4* is a complete disruption of the urethra without opacification of the bladder and with urethral separation of <2 cm; (e) *Type 5* is a complete disruption of the urethra without opacification of the bladder and with urethral separation of >2 cm (Fig. 48.35).

A "straddle injury," falling astride a fixed object commonly injures the bulbous urethra. Instrumentation, foreign body insertion, or direct trauma to the penis may injure the penile urethra. Long-term bladder catheterization may injure any portion of the urethra. Autodigestion of the urethra because of drainage of pancreatic exocrine enzymes has been reported as a complication of pancreatic transplantation with pancreatic drainage into the bladder. Complications of urethral injury are common and include stricture, incontinence, impotence, and pelvic and perineal sinus tracts and fistulas.

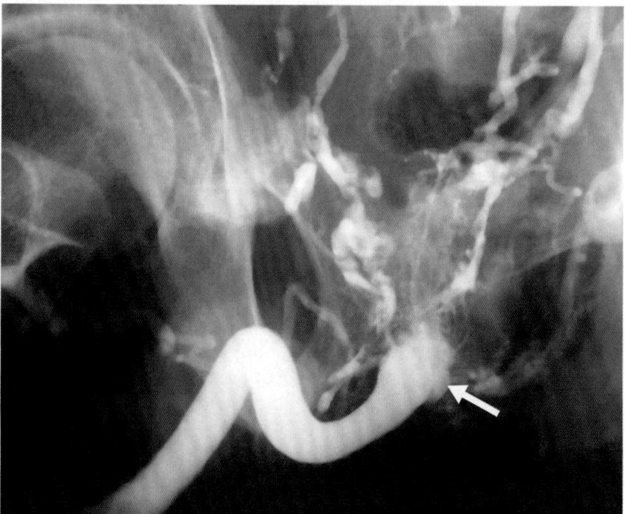

FIGURE 48.35. **Traumatic Urethral Transection.** Radiograph from a retrograde urethrogram shows transection of the urethra at the level of the urogenital diaphragm (*arrow*). Contrast extravasates into adjacent tissues and intravasates into pelvic veins.

Suggested Readings

Berrocal T, Lopez-Pereira P, Arjonilla A, Gutierrez J. Anomalies of the distal ureter, bladder, and urethra in children: embryologic, radiologic, and pathologic features. *Radiographics* 2002;22(5):1139–1164.

Chaudhari VV, Patel MK, Douek M, Raman SS. MR imaging and US of the female urethral and periurethral disease. *Radiographics* 2010;30(7):1857–1874.

Cheng PM, Moin P, Dunn MD, Boswell WD, Duddalwar VA. What the radiologist needs to know about urolithiasis: Part 1—pathogenesis, types, assessment, and variant anatomy. *AJR Am J Roentgenol* 2012;198(6):W540–W547.

Cheng PM, Moin P, Dunn MD, Boswell WD, Duddalwar VA. What the radiologist needs to know about urolithiasis: Part 2—CT findings, reporting, and treatment. *AJR Am J Roentgenol* 2012;198(6):W548–W554.

Chung AD, Schieda N, Shanbhogue AK, Dilauro M, Rosenkrantz AB, Siegelman ES. MRI evaluation of the urothelial tract: pitfalls and solutions. *AJR Am J Roentgenol* 2016;207(6):W108–W116.

de Haas RJ, Steyvers MJ, Fütterer JJ. Multiparametric MRI of the bladder: ready for clinical routine? *AJR Am J Roentgenol* 2014;202(6):1187–1195.

Jinzaki M, Kikuchi E, Akita H, Sugiura H, Shinmoto H, Oya M. Role of computed tomography urography in the clinical evaluation of upper tract urothelial carcinoma. *Int J Urol* 2016;23(4):284–298.

Kawashima A, Sandler CM, Wasserman NF, LeRoy AJ, King BF Jr, Goldman SM. Imaging of urethral disease: a pictorial review. *Radiographics* 2004;24 Suppl 1:S195–S216.

Raman SP, Fishman EK. Bladder malignancies of CT: the underrated role of CT in diagnosis. *AJR Am J Roentgenol* 2014;203(2):347–354.

Surablhi VR, Menias CO, George V, Matta E, Kaza RK, Hasapes J. MDCT and MR urogram spectrum of congenital anomalies of the kidney and urinary tract diagnosed in adulthood. *AJR Am J Roentgenol* 2015;205(3):W294–W304.

Verma S, Rajesh A, Prasad SR, et al. Urinary bladder cancer: role of MR imaging. *Radiographics* 2012;32(2):371–387.

Wolin EA, Hartman DS, Olson JR. Nephrographic and pyelographic analysis of CT urography: differential diagnosis. *AJR Am J Roentgenol* 2013;200(6):1197–1203.

CHAPTER 49 ■ GENITAL TRACT—CT, MR, AND RADIOGRAPHIC IMAGING

WILLIAM E. BRANT

FEMALE GENITAL TRACT

The primary modality for imaging of the female genital tract is US using transabdominal, transvaginal, and Doppler techniques. Sonography of the genital tract is reviewed in Chapter 51. MR and CT are used to stage and follow-up pelvic malignancies and to supplement US by providing additional characterization of lesions. MR, because of its excellent capacity to differentiate tissue types, is particularly useful in making an imaging diagnosis of pelvic disease. Diffusion-weighted MR has potential to aid in the discrimination between benign and malignant lesions and to provide improved detection of peritoneal metastases and tumor recurrence. MDCT with isotropic voxel acquisition allows for multiplanar reformatted images of high quality to improve recognition of anatomic variants and complex pathology. In addition, many uterine and adnexal lesions may be discovered incidentally by pelvic CT or MR performed for other reasons. Hysterosalpingography (HSG) is combined with US, CT, and MR to diagnose congenital anomalies of the female genital tract and mechanical causes of infertility. The HSG is performed by cannulating the cervix and injecting a contrast agent into the cavity of the uterus and fallopian tubes. Free communication of these lumina with the peritoneal cavity is evidenced by free spill of the contrast agent into the peritoneal cavity outlining loops of bowel. Sonohysterography is an alternative to HSG. Isotonic saline is injected into the uterine cavity while the uterus is examined sonographically. Virtual HSG is an emerging MDCT technique that offers the potential of high-resolution images depicting both the internal and external surfaces of the uterus and fallopian tubes.

Anatomy

The uterus is a pear-shaped muscular organ located between the bladder and rectum. The anterior and posterior surfaces of the uterus are covered by peritoneum, the folds of which extend laterally to the pelvic sidewalls forming the *broad ligament*. Peritoneum reflecting off the uterus and the bladder forms a shallow anterior vesicouterine pouch. A "bare area" of extraperitoneal space is present between the lower uterus and bladder. This is an important area for direct spread of tumor from one organ to the other. Posteriorly the peritoneum reflects onto the rectum and forms a deep recto-uterine pouch or cul-de-sac. The peritoneum completely covers the uterus and the posterior vaginal fornix. Only the thin wall of the vagina separates the vaginal cavity from the cul-de-sac, allowing transvaginal access to the intraperitoneal space for US-guided culdocentesis or biopsy. The uterus, cervix, and upper one-third of the vagina are derived from the Müllerian ducts, while the lower two-thirds of the vagina arise from the urogenital sinus. *Parametrium* refers to the connective tissue adjacent to the uterus between the folds of the broad ligament and adjacent to the vagina. Uterine vessels and lymphatics pass through the parametrium. The broad ligament covers the fallopian tubes hanging over them like a sheet folded on a clothesline enveloping the vessels of the parametrium. The broad ligament is well outlined when fluid is present in the pelvic peritoneal cavity. The fundus of the uterus is that portion that extends cephalad from the origin of the fallopian tubes. The body extends from the fallopian tubes to the isthmus, a slight constriction that marks the location of the internal cervical os. The cervix is cylindrical in shape and 3 to 4 cm in length. Its lower portion, including the external os, protrudes into the vagina and is surrounded by the vaginal fornices. The ureters pass 2 cm lateral to the supravaginal portion of the cervix. The ***vagina*** is a muscular tube that is a flattened oval shape on cross-sectional images. The urethra is a prominent tubular structure that courses in the anterior wall of the vagina.

Ovaries vary in size and appearance depending on the woman's age, hormonal status, and stage of the menstrual cycle. The adult ovary is oval with maximal dimensions of 5 × 3 × 2 cm. Abnormalities of size are best determined by calculating ovarian volume using the formula (length × width × thickness × 0.52). Maximum ovarian volume is 9 cc before menarche, 22 cc in menstruating women, and 6 cc in postmenopausal women. The location of the ovaries is variable in different patients and even in the same patient at different times depending on degree of bladder filling and the presence and size of other structures in the pelvis. The typical location is lateral, superior, or posterior to the uterine fundus, or in the cul-de-sac. When the uterus is retroverted the ovaries are anterior or lateral to the uterus. The pelvic ureters form an important anatomic landmark that assist in the recognition of the origin of pelvic masses. The ovaries are anterior to the ureters, so an ovarian mass will displace the ureter posteriorly or

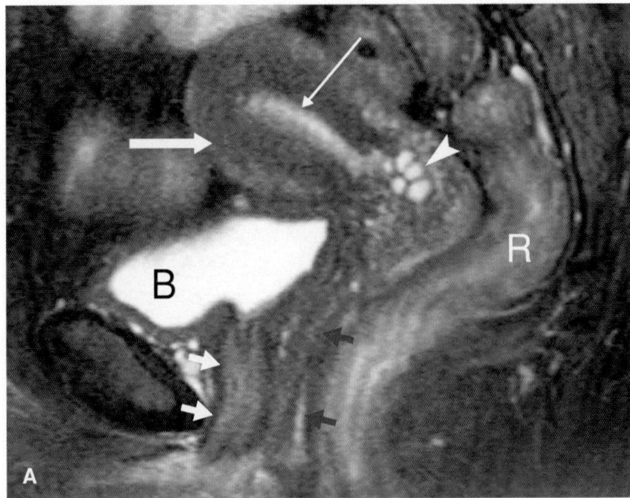

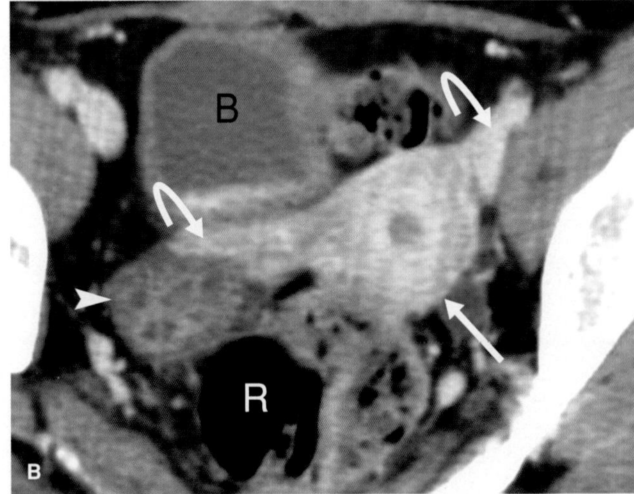

FIGURE 49.1. **Normal Uterus. A:** Sagittal T2-weighted MR image shows the uterus (*large arrow*), and the high signal intensity endometrium (*skinny arrow*) surrounded by the low signal intensity junctional zone myometrium. Multiple nabothian cysts (*arrowhead*) are present in the endocervical canal. The vagina (*short red arrows*) is shown as a low signal intensity muscular tube with the urethra (*short white arrows*) coursing in its anterior wall. High signal urine identifies the bladder (*B*) anteriorly. The rectum (*R*) is seen posteriorly. **B:** Axial postcontrast CT image shows the uterus (*arrow*) in transverse plane with enhancing endometrium surrounding a small volume of low attenuation fluid in the uterine cavity. The broad ligaments (*curved arrows*) enveloping the enhancing fallopian tubes and parametrial vessels extend laterally from the uterus to the right ovary (*arrowhead*). The bladder (*B*) containing low attenuation urine without contrast creates a fluid layer with high attenuation urine containing excreted contrast. The rectum (*R*) containing gas is seen posteriorly.

posterolaterally. Iliac lymph nodes are lateral to ureters, so adenopathy will displace the ureters medially or anteromedially.

Normal MR Anatomy. The internal anatomy of the uterus is depicted best on T2WI. On T2WI, the *endometrium* appears as a high signal intensity central stripe surrounded by the low signal intensity *junctional zone* myometrium (Fig. 49.1). The endometrium may normally be up to 14 mm in thickness in women of menstrual age. The bulk of the *myometrium* is intermediate signal intensity. The low signal intensity of inner junctional zone of the myometrium on T2WI is due to lower water content. On T1WI, the entire uterus is low in signal intensity and the internal anatomy of the uterus is poorly demonstrated. With gadolinium enhancement, uterine zonal anatomy becomes evident on T1WI. The cervix is largely composed of collagenous tissues that are low in signal intensity on both T1WI and T2WI, providing a dark background for visualization of hyperintense cervical carcinomas. The endocervical epithelium and mucus are homogeneous high signal on T2WI. High-resolution MR using surface or intravaginal coils shows two zones in the cervical fibromuscular stroma, a darker inner zone contiguous with the uterine junctional zone and an intermediate signal outer zone distinctly darker than the myometrium. Vaginal anatomy is also best seen on T2WI, which shows the muscular vaginal wall as low in signal with the epithelium and mucus as high in signal. Aqueous vaginal gel may be inserted for MR scanning to distend the vagina and optimize evaluation of the vagina and cervix. The normal ovaries of fertile women are easily identified by the bright signal of the follicles on T2WI (Fig. 49.2). The follicles are low or intermediate in signal on T1WI. The cortex of the ovary in the premenopausal woman is darker in the signal than the medulla on T2WI. The postmenopausal ovary is more difficult to identify because of the absence of follicles and the cortex and medulla being nearly equal in signal on both T1WI and T2WI.

MR is sensitive to physiologic changes that affect the uterus and ovary during the menstrual cycle. Signal intensity of the myometrium is highest during late proliferative and early secretory phases and is lowest during menstruation and early proliferative phase. Low-intensity myometrial lesions such as leiomyomas and adenomyomas are best demonstrated when the myometrium has the highest signal intensity in midmenstrual cycle. The ovaries vary in size and appearance during the menstrual cycle and are largest with a dominant follicle just prior to ovulation.

Normal CT Anatomy. Because the position of the uterus is so variable on axial plane CT the outline of the uterus often appears lobulated or bulbous solely because of position (Fig. 49.1). The uterus is uniform in soft tissue attenuation and its internal anatomy is not well demonstrated by unenhanced CT. Because the myometrium is highly vascular, the uterus enhances more than most other pelvic organs. Fluid in the uterine cavity is usually low density. The ovaries are easily mistaken for unopacified bowel loops in the pelvis. Ovarian follicles are recognized by their fluid attenuation (Fig. 49.2). The vagina is seen in cross-section as a flattened ellipse of soft tissue density between the bladder and rectum. Normal fallopian tubes are usually not evident on CT. Multiplanar reformatted MDCT images are of great value in interpretation of complex pelvic anatomy and pathology.

Hysterosalpingography is primarily used for the evaluation of infertility to demonstrate the morphology and patency of the uterine canal and fallopian tubes (Fig. 49.3). Contrast injected into the uterine cavity outlines the endocervical canal, uterine cavity, and lumen of the fallopian tubes with free spill of contrast into the peritoneal cavity in the normal patient. The uterine cavity is sharply defined and triangular in shape with normal mild concavity in the fundal region. The size of the cavity varies with parity. The endocervical canal is cylindrical in shape, 3 to 4 cm in length, and 1 to 3 cm in width. Folds in the endocervical mucosa form a normal serrated appearance. The normal fallopian tubes are 10 to 12 cm in length extending from the cornua of the uterus. The lumen is thread-like (1 to 2 mm) until it reaches the ampulla where it expands to 5 to 10 mm and rugal folds become visible. Patency of the tubes is confirmed by dispersal of contrast within the peritoneal cavity outlining loops of bowel.

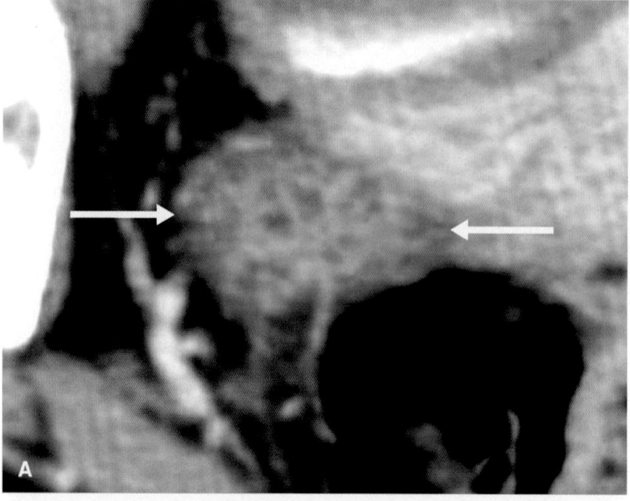

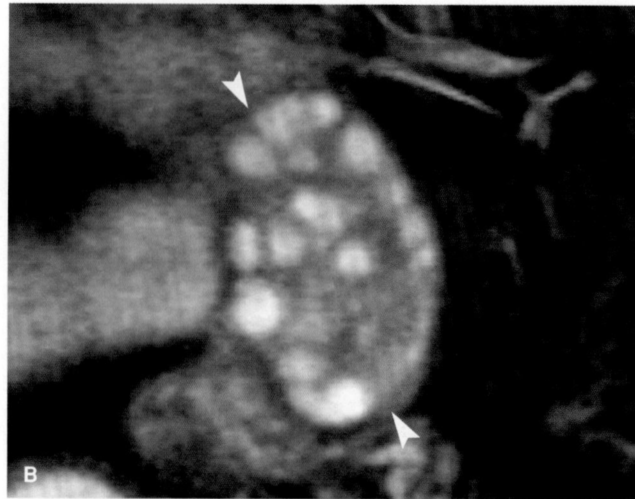

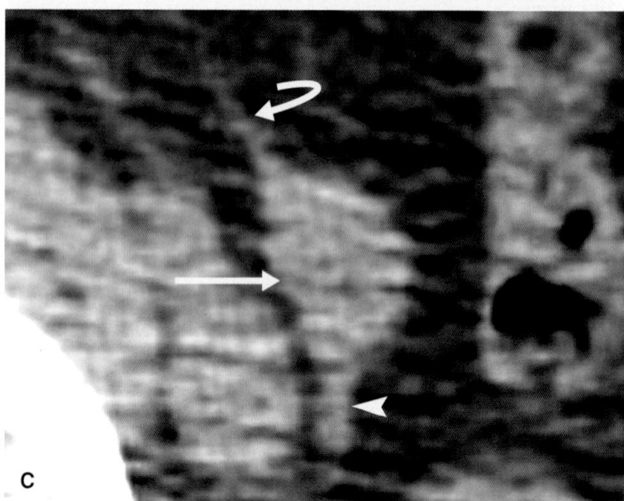

FIGURE 49.2. **Normal Ovaries. A**: Axial postcontrast CT image shows a normal ovary (between *arrows*) with follicles in a menstrual age woman. Follicles serve as an anatomic landmark to recognize the ovary. **B**: Coronal T2-weighted MR image of a 38-year-old woman shows the normal oval shape of the ovary (between *arrowheads*) marked by high signal intensity thin-walled follicles. **C**: Axial CT image of a postmenopausal woman shows the small oval soft tissue appearance of the normal postmenopausal ovary (*straight arrow*) without follicles. The identity of the ovary is confirmed by recognizing the suspensory ligament of the ovary (*curved arrow*) and the uteroovarian ligament (*arrowhead*).

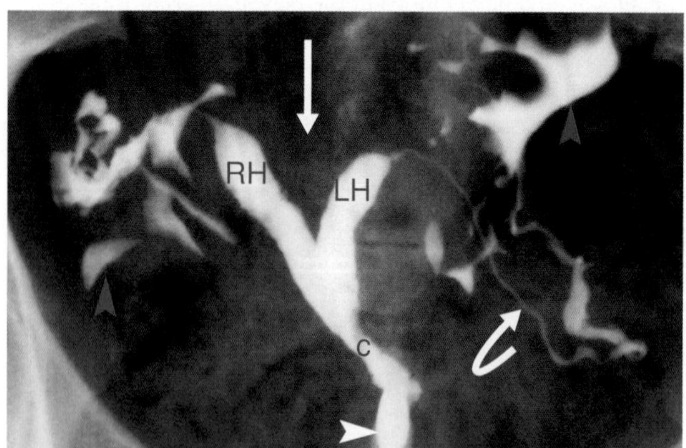

FIGURE 49.3. **Septate Uterus.** HSG demonstrates two horns of the uterine cavity (*RH, LH*) separated by a muscular septum (*arrow*). The delicate lumen of the left fallopian tube is well demonstrated (*curved arrow*), while the lumen of the right fallopian tube is obscured by the superimposed contrast. Free spill of contrast into the peritoneal cavity is evident (*red arrowheads*), confirming the patency of the fallopian tubes. Iodinated contrast agent was injected into the uterus after placing a cannula (*white arrowhead*) into the cervix (*c*).

Congenital Anomalies

Congenital anomalies of the female genital tract are a common cause of infertility, seen in up to 9% of women evaluated for infertility or repeated spontaneous abortion. In addition, unrecognized anomalies may be mistaken for other types of pathology, such as leiomyoma. Most anomalies result from arrested development or incomplete fusion of the paired Müllerian duct that forms the uterus, cervix, and fallopian tubes. Urinary tract abnormalities are found in 20% to 50% of patients with uterine anomalies. Arrested Müllerian duct development may result in uterine aplasia or unicornuate uterus with a single fallopian tube. Ipsilateral renal agenesis is found in 5% to 20% of patients with these anomalies. Failure of complete fusion of the Müllerian duct results in varying degrees of duplication, from *uterus didelphys*, with two uteri, two cervices, and two vaginas; to *bicornuate uterus* with two uterine horns, one (*unicollis*) or two (*bicollis*) cervices, and one vagina; to an *arcuate* (septate) uterus with a midline septum dividing the uterus into two cavities (Figs. 49.3 and 49.4). Uterine anomalies should be suspected when the uterus appears abnormal in size, contour, or position. The classification of the anomaly is made by a combination of physical examination and MR examination. HSG is used to demonstrate the uterine cavity and fallopian tubes.

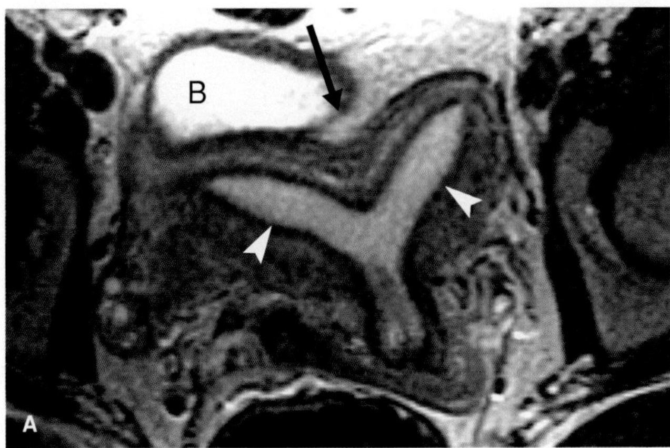

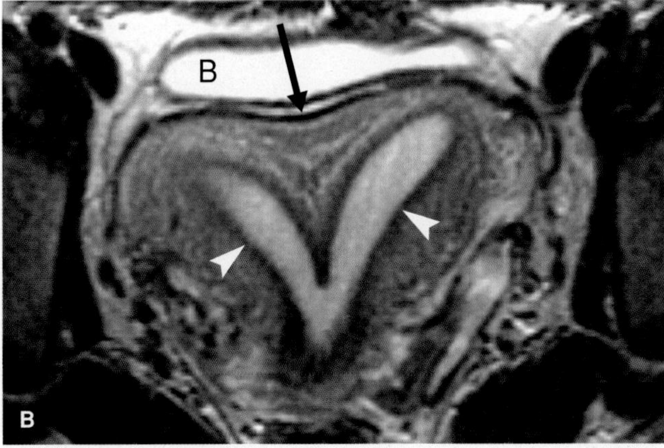

FIGURE 49.4. **Uterine Anomalies. A:** Bicornuate uterus. **B:** Septate uterus. T2-weighted axial images of the uterus in two patients demonstrate the characteristic difference between a bicornuate uterus, (**A**), with a surface indentation at the fundus (*arrow*) dividing the uterus into two separate horns (*arrowheads*) and a septate uterus, (**B**), showing a thick muscular septum and only a slight surface indentation at the fundus (*arrow*). Two uterine cavities (*arrowheads*) are present in both cases. Uterine anomalies represent a continuous spectrum of abnormality. *B*, bladder.

Benign Conditions

Leiomyomas are the most common uterine tumor affecting 50% of women of reproductive age. Most women are asymptomatic but the tumors may cause excessive bleeding, pelvic pain, mass symptoms, and infertility. Tumors are benign and made up of smooth muscle and a variable amount of fibrous tissue. Tumors with scant fibrous tissue enhance brightly while those with abundant fibrous tissue enhance poorly. Most tumors are intramural (within the myometrial wall), while others are submucosal (beneath the endometrium) or subserosal (beneath the serosa). Subserosal or submucosal tumors may be pedunculated and on long stalks. Submucosal tumors are prone to ulcerate resulting in severe menorrhagia. MR provides the best characterization of size, number, and location. Leiomyomas are usually low signal compared to myometrium on both T1WI and T2WI, although visualization is best on T2WI (Fig. 49.5). Areas of degeneration and cystic change cause inhomogeneous high internal signal. The tumors are well demarcated from adjacent myometrium by a discrete rim of low signal. Contrast enhancement does not improve leiomyoma detection or characterization. On CT, leiomyomas appear as homogeneous or heterogeneous masses that may be hypodense, isodense, or hyperdense relative to enhanced myometrium. Coarse calcifications within the mass are common and characteristic (Fig. 49.6). Cystic degeneration produces interior low density. Diffuse enlargement of the uterus and lobulation of its contour are common. Pedunculated leiomyomas may appear as adnexal rather than uterine masses. Lipoleiomyomas contain macroscopic fat detected on CT (Fig. 49.7), or by MR using fat-suppression sequences.

Adenomyosis is a benign disease of the uterus characterized by the presence of ectopic endometrial glands and stroma within the myometrium eliciting surrounding myometrial hypertrophy. Patients present with dysmenorrhea or menorrhagia. The disease may be focal or diffuse. MR provides the best detection of the disease. *Diffuse disease* is indicated by regular or irregular thickening of the junctional zone myometrium >12 mm. The low signal abnormality corresponds to myometrial hypertrophy. Half of the patients also demonstrate high signal foci within the myometrium corresponding to islands of endometrial glands with cystic change or hemorrhage (Fig. 49.8). *Focal disease* is evidenced by low signal masses within the myometrium on T2WI. These masses are isointense to myometrium on T1WI. High signal foci occasionally seen on T1WI represent hemorrhage. Differentiation from leiomyomas is difficult. Leiomyomas are characteristically well circumscribed while adenomyomas are poorly defined with vague margination. Adenomyosis is not routinely evident on CT. US findings are usually subtle and nonspecific.

Nabothian cysts are retention cysts of the mucous-secreting glands of the cervical epithelium. They are common, benign, and generally of no clinical significance. On MR they appear as bright, round, well-defined structures in the cervix on T2WI (Fig. 49.1A). On T1WI, they are isointense to urine or muscle. Small size and sharp margins differentiate nabothian cysts from *adenoma malignum*, a multicystic form of adenocarcinoma of the cervix. This malignancy appears as multicystic mass with numerous small cysts on a background of enhancing solid tissue.

Physiologic ovarian cysts and normal ovarian follicles contain simple fluid that is low signal on T1WI and high signal on T2WI. A uniform, thin, dark wall is evident on T2WI. Gadolinium enhancement of the cyst wall is common but not constant. On CT, they are well defined, thin walled, and have homogeneous internal density near water. Size less than 3 cm is indicative of physiologic ovarian follicle (Fig. 49.9). The corpus luteum is a normal physiologic ovarian structure that develops at the site of the dominant follicle following ovulation. A normal corpus luteum is smaller than 3 cm, and has a diffusely thick wall and prominent peripheral blood flow. A crenulated, collapsed cyst appearance is usual. Central hemorrhage is often present.

Hemorrhagic functional ovarian cysts appear high signal on T1WI if a large amount of methemoglobin is present. If predominantly intact red blood cells are present, the cyst appears low signal on T2WI. Thus hemorrhagic cysts may be low signal on both T1WI and T2WI, high signal on T1WI and low signal on T2WI, or low signal on T1WI and high signal on T2WI. Layering of blood products may be present. The absence of gadolinium enhancement differentiates internal blood clot adherent to the cyst wall from a solid nodule. On CT, hemorrhagic cysts appear as thin-walled cysts with internal density near water or higher in attenuation depending on the physical state of the blood products (Fig. 49.9). Atypical cysts can be followed with US to determine if they resolve after one or two menstrual cycles.

Endometriosis is the presence of endometrial tissue in locations outside of the uterus. The endometrial implants respond

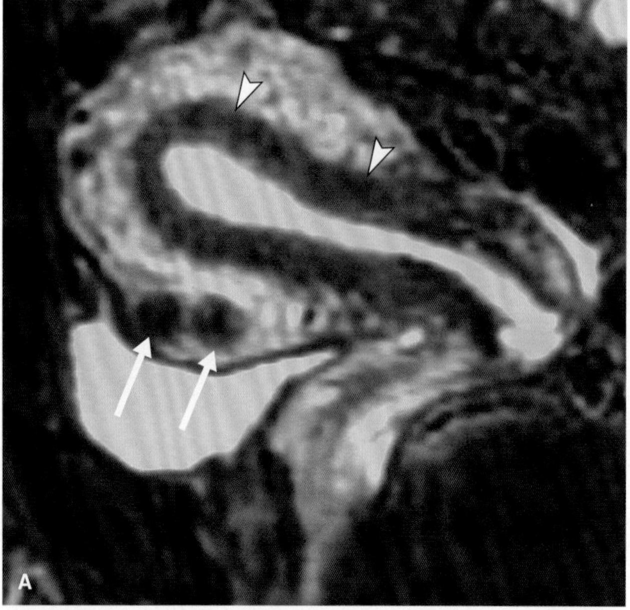

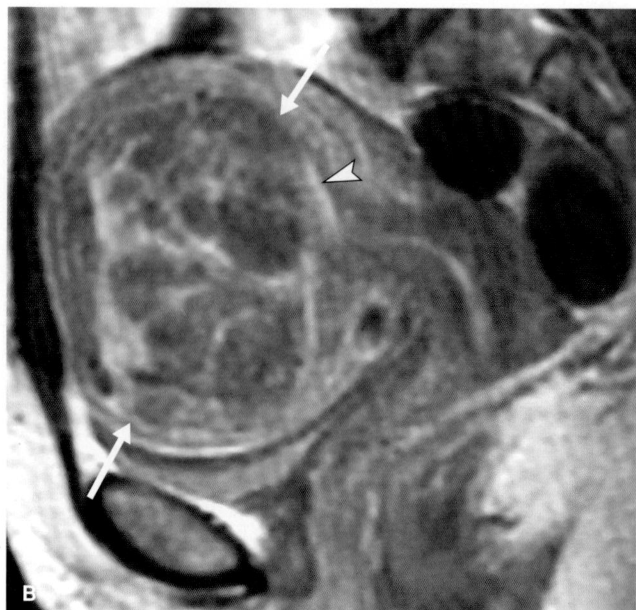

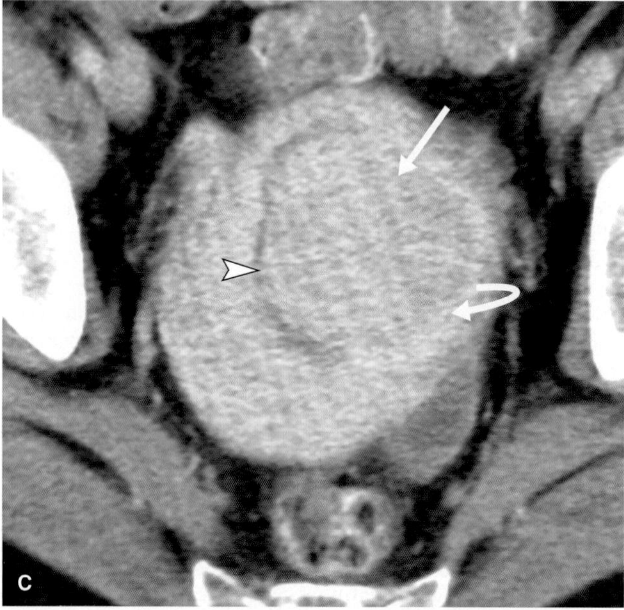

FIGURE 49.5. Leiomyomas. A: Sagittal T2-weighted MR image of the uterus shows two low signal intensity leiomyomas (*arrows*) in the anterior wall of the uterus. The junctional zone myometrium (*arrowheads*), having lower water content, is much lower in signal intensity than the adjacent myometrium. **B:** Sagittal T2-weighted MR image of the uterus of a different patient shows a very large leiomyoma (between *arrows*) with degenerative changes expanding the uterine fundus. The endometrial cavity (*arrowhead*) is greatly distorted and displaced by the leiomyoma. **C:** Axial postcontrast CT image shows a large submucous leiomyoma (*arrow*) abutting and displacing the uterine cavity (*arrowhead*) in this woman with menorrhagia. The leiomyoma shows enhancement equal to that of the normal myometrium. The tumor is pedunculated with attachment (*curved arrow*) to the left lateral posterior uterine wall.

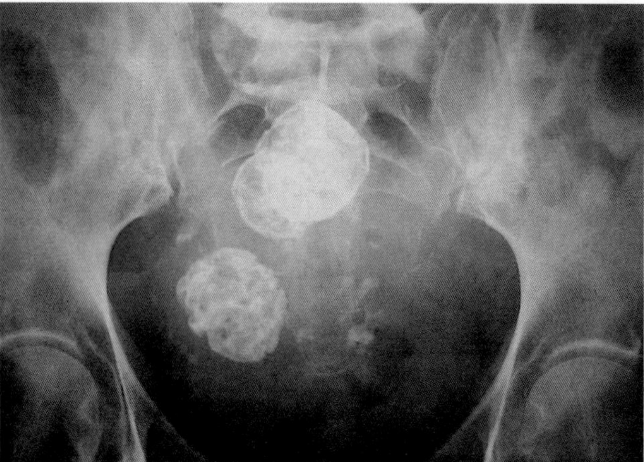

FIGURE 49.6. Leiomyoma Calcifications. Conventional radiograph of the pelvis reveals multiple leiomyomas with characteristic "popcorn" calcifications.

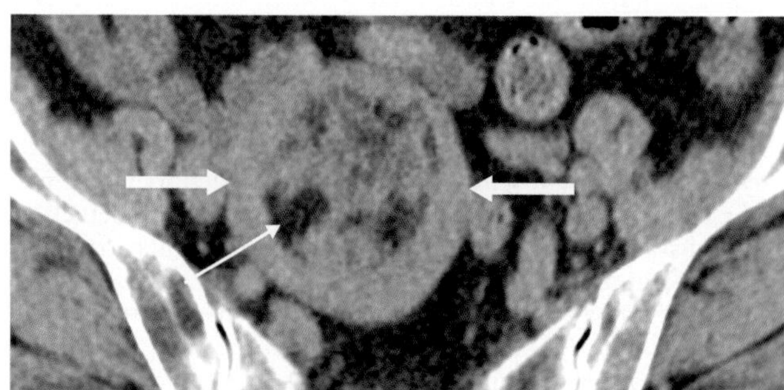

FIGURE 49.7. Lipoleiomyoma. Axial CT performed without contrast demonstrates a fat-containing myometrial tumor in the uterus (between *fat arrows*). Distinct fat attenuation (*skinny arrow*), equal to that of nearby pelvic fat, confirms the diagnosis of lipoleiomyoma.

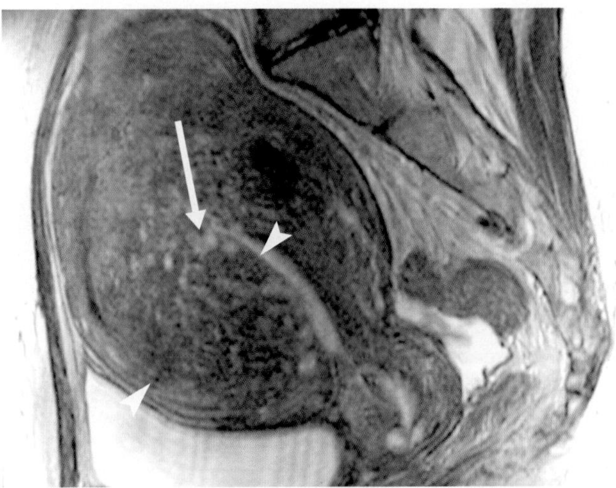

FIGURE 49.8. **Adenomyosis.** T2-weighted sagittal plane MR image shows marked widening of the junctional zone myometrium (between *arrowheads*), a key finding of adenomyosis. Tiny cystic deposits of endometrium seen as high signal intensity round foci (*arrow*) within the fibrotic lesion are also characteristic.

to cyclic hormonal stimulation resulting in recurrent bleeding, inflammation, and fibrosis. Hallmarks of disease include numerous tiny implantations of endometrial tissue on peritoneal surfaces, development of endometriomas (endometrial cysts filled with hemorrhage), and formation of adhesions between surrounding tissues. The most common sites of involvement are the ovaries, the cul-de-sac, and peritoneal reflections over the uterus, fallopian tubes, bladder, and rectosigmoid colon. All imaging modalities have high sensitivity for detection of endometriomas. Deep pelvic endometriosis is a cause of severe pelvic pain with tiny deposits of endometrium on peritoneal surfaces in recesses, pelvic organs, and other extraperitoneal sites. MR shows hypointense thickening and nodularity of ligaments and the walls of the vagina and rectum on T2WI. Endometriomas ("chocolate cysts") contain blood products of various ages reflecting recurrent episodes of bleeding corresponding to the menstrual cycle. They are characteristically multiple, bilateral, and located in the cul-de-sac. MR shows the cysts to be homogeneous high intensity on T1WI and characteristically low signal on T2WI, a finding termed "*T2 shading*" (Fig. 49.10). Loss of signal on T2WI is caused by the presence of methemoglobin within the cysts. Iron concentration and viscosity increase within the cysts as water is resorbed. The "shaded" fluid may layer dependently

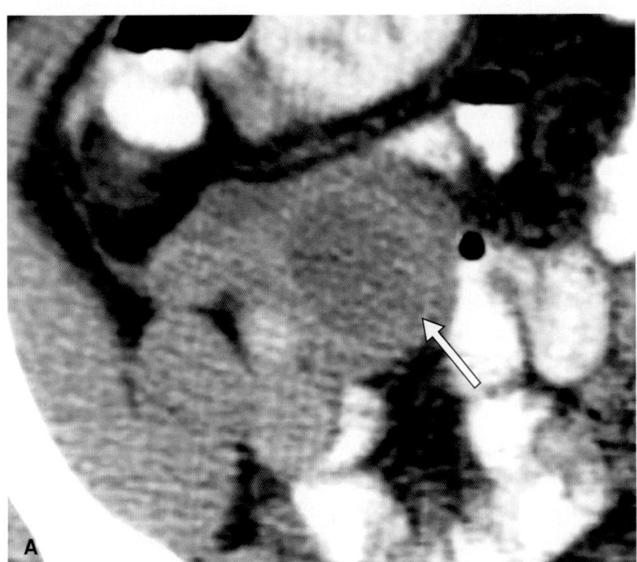

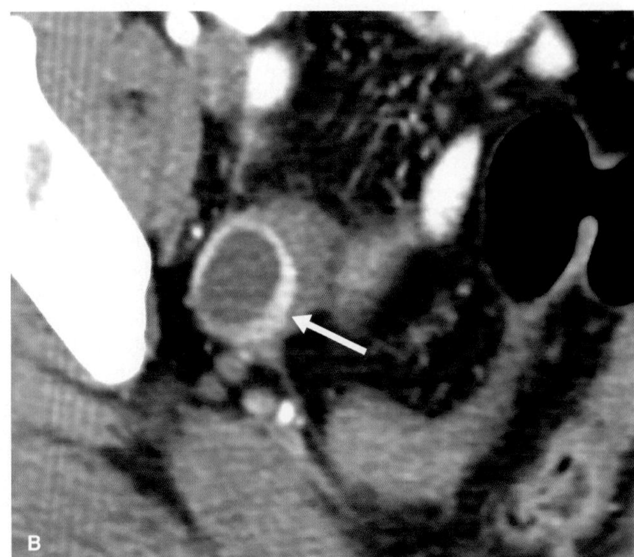

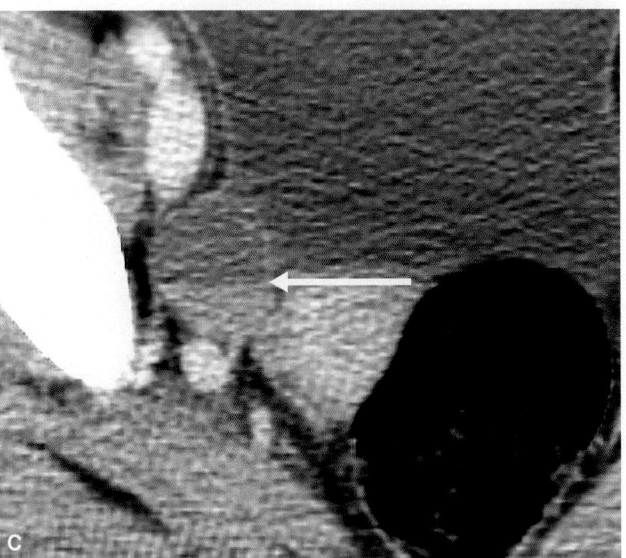

FIGURE 49.9. **Physiologic Ovarian Cysts. A:** Postcontrast CT reveals a thin-walled 2.6-cm cyst (*arrow*) arising from the right ovary in a 28-year-old woman. The appearance and size of this ovarian cyst are consistent with being a dominant follicle. This is a physiologic cyst and no follow-up is needed. **B:** Postcontrast CT in a 26-year-old woman shows an 18-mm right ovarian cyst (*arrow*) with intense rim enhancement. This appearance is consistent with a normal benign corpus luteum. A diagnosis of mittelschmerz was made after appendicitis was ruled out on this CT. **C:** Another CT performed for right lower quadrant pain in a 34 year old revealed a 3-cm right ovarian cyst with a fluid–fluid layer (*arrow*) yielding a diagnosis of hemorrhagic ovarian cyst as a cause for her pain. The dependent high attenuation fluid represents blood. Follow-up pelvic US in 10 weeks confirmed complete resolution.

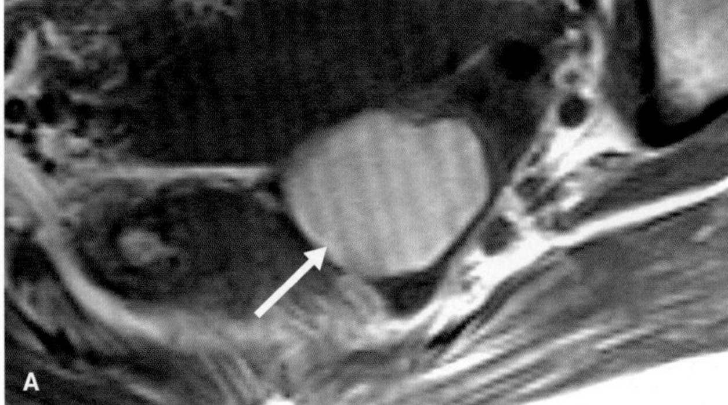

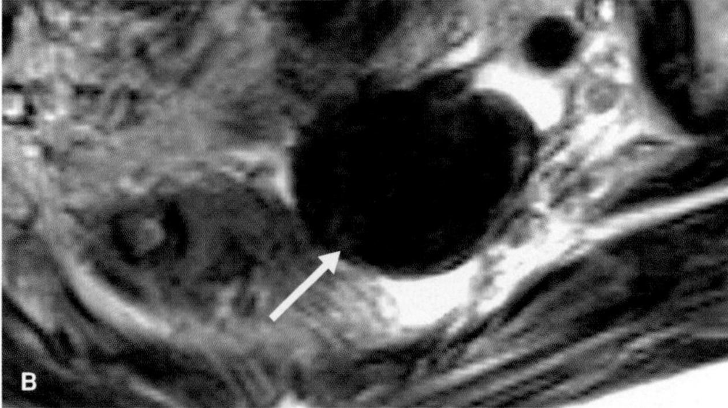

FIGURE 49.10. **Endometrioma—MR. A:** T1WI. **B:** T2WI. A cystic mass (*arrows*) in the cul-de-sac is high signal intensity on TIWI and shows characteristic loss of signal on T2WI (T2 shading). The loss of signal is caused by the presence of methemoglobin within the cyst resulting from multiple episodes of internal hemorrhage.

within the cyst. Cysts may appear heterogeneous because of the varying age of contained blood products. The cyst wall is usually low signal representing fibrous tissue or hemosiderin. Fat-saturation T1WI improves visualization of small implants on peritoneal surfaces. On CT, endometriomas appear as complex cystic pelvic masses, frequently with relatively high attenuation fluid components. Inflammation and fibrosis are prominent. Multiple pelvic organs may be incorporated into a mass. Hydrosalpinx is a common associated finding (30%). Endometriosis may involve bowel, the urinary tract, or occur outside the pelvis and in surgical scars. Malignant transformation of endometriosis is a rare occurrence.

Hydrosalpinx is a common adnexal mass that may occur as an isolated lesion or as a component of a complex adnexal mass. Occlusion of the fallopian tube, caused by infection, surgery, tumor, or endometriosis, results in fluid accumulation and dilatation of the tube. The most common cause is pelvic infection. Imaging of isolated hydrosalpinx demonstrates a sausage-, C-, or S-shaped adnexal structure distended with fluid of variable character that may be serous fluid, hemorrhage (hematosalpinx), or pus (pyosalpinx) (Fig. 49.11). Tortuosity, dilatation, and folding of the tube may resemble an ovarian tumor. Multiplanar images and identification of a normal ovary on the ipsilateral side assist in confirming the diagnosis. MR is sensitive to the nature of the fluid within the tube showing low signal on T1WI with high signal on T2WI for simple serous fluid. Proteinaceous fluid, hemorrhage, or pus causes high signal on T1WI. Pelvic inflammatory disease, endometriosis, or fallopian tumor may incorporate hydrosalpinx as a component of a complex cystic and solid adnexal mass. Hydrosalpinx is a common finding on HSG performed for infertility (Fig. 49.11A).

Pelvic inflammatory disease is a common affliction of women of reproductive age. The usual causative organisms are a mixture of anaerobic and aerobic bacteria from the vagina. Uncommon organisms include actinomycosis and tuberculosis. Endometritis and myometritis are treated medically. Imaging is performed to detect *tuboovarian abscess* and pyosalpinx, complications that may require surgical treatment. Early findings include pelvic and edema and stranding in the parametrium and paraovarian tissues. Pyosalpinx appears as a thick-walled edematous tube that contains complex fluid. Tuboovarian abscess appears as a thick-walled fluid-filled adnexal mass that incorporates the ovary and commonly a dilated fallopian tube (Fig. 49.12). Gas bubbles are occasionally present within the collection and are highly indicative of abscess. Adenopathy and ascites may be present.

Peritoneal inclusion cyst is an increasingly common and difficult to treat cause of chronic pelvic pain. Adhesions from previous surgery or inflammatory process entrap the ovary within a fluid collection that extends into peritoneal recesses. Continuing

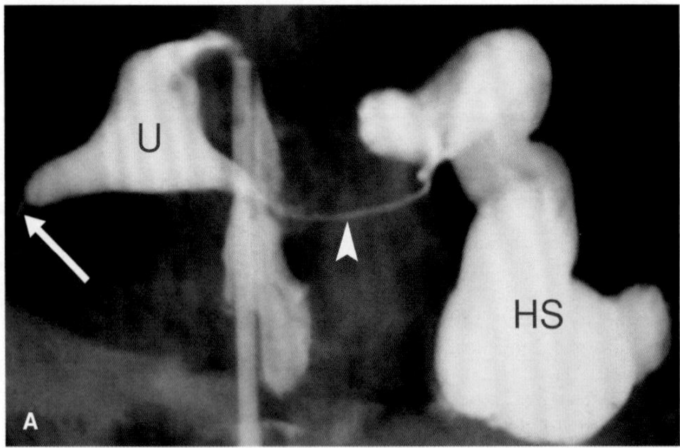

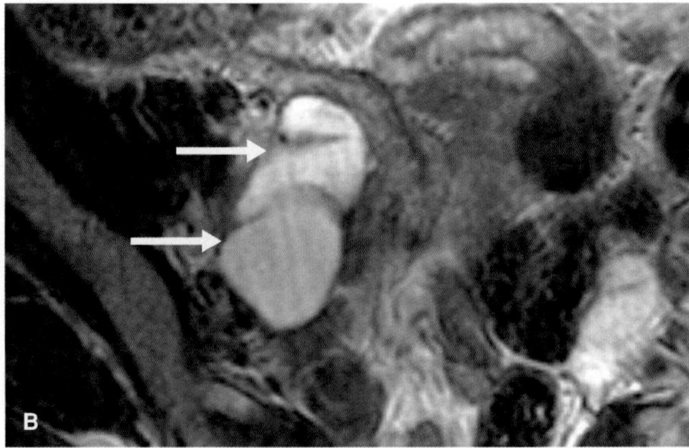

FIGURE 49.11. **Hydrosalpinx. A:** HSG demonstrates a retroflexed uterus (*U*) with the fundus directed posteriorly and inferiorly. The right fallopian tube is occluded at the isthmus (*arrow*). The left fallopian tube is massively dilated at its distal end, forming a hydrosalpinx (*HS*). The proximal portion (*arrowhead*) of the left fallopian tube is normal. No peritoneal spill of the injected contrast agent is present indicating bilateral total tubal occlusion. **B:** Axial T2-weighted MR in a different patient demonstrates a similar appearance of hydrosalpinx (*arrows*) as a dilated twisted convoluted tube on the right.

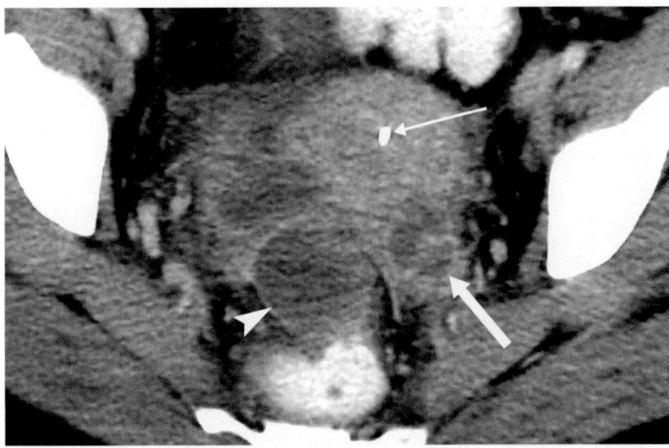

FIGURE 49.12. **Tuboovarian Abscess.** Postcontrast CT in a patient with fever, pelvic pain, and vaginal discharge shows a complex fluid collection enveloping the ovary (*fat arrow*), dilated fallopian tube (*arrowhead*), and uterus containing an IUD (intrauterine device) (*skinny arrow*). Note the extension of edema and inflammation into pelvic fat and the poor margination of involved organs. These are classic findings of tuboovarian abscess.

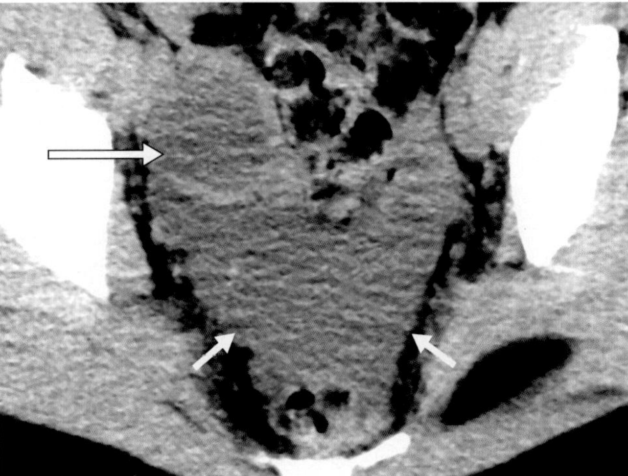

FIGURE 49.13. **Peritoneal Inclusion Cyst.** CT reveals a loculated fluid collection partially enveloping the right ovary (*large arrow*) and extending into the recesses of the peritoneal cavity (*small arrows*) in a patient with chronic pelvic pain. Attempts at needle and catheter drainage were unsuccessful. The patient became asymptomatic following oophorectomy.

secretion of fluid by the active ovary is not absorbed by the diseased peritoneal surfaces producing pain and pressure systems. Imaging shows a fluid collection that includes the ovary. The fluid is usually simple and characteristically extends into peritoneal recesses giving the collection an angled or pointed rather than spherical or oval shape (Fig. 49.13). Effective treatment generally requires removal of the ovary.

Benign cystic teratoma, ordermoid cyst, is the most common germ cell neoplasm of the ovary. Lesions contain mature elements derived from ectoderm, mesoderm, or endoderm resulting in a broad range of appearance. Mean patient age at discovery is 30 years. Most lesions are discovered incidentally while the patients are asymptomatic. The cysts are filled with liquid sebaceous material that is fat density on MR and CT. Internal contents include the Rokitansky nodule, which commonly includes hair, teeth, bone, or cartilage. US features are usually characteristic, but lesions may be discovered or further characterized by MR or CT. MR shows the sebaceous material as very high intensity on T1WI. Signal is usually decreased on T2WI approximating fat signal. Fat content is confirmed by in-phase and out-of-phase gradient recall images or frequency selective fat saturation images. CT demonstration of fat density within a cystic adnexal mass is definitive (Fig. 49.14). CT and conventional radiographs show bone and teeth formation within the mass. Atypical lesions mimic a wide variety of other adnexal pathology including ovarian malignancy.

Fibrotic ovarian tumors account for 4% of ovarian tumors. Because they are solid masses and are commonly associated with ascites (40% of cases), they may mimic ovarian cancers (Fig. 49.15). Tissue types include fibromas, thecomas, and fibrothecomas arising from ovarian stroma. Meigs syndrome is defined as the association of ascites and pleural effusion with an ovarian fibroma. The syndrome resolves following surgical removal of the tumor. US demonstrates a solid mass with poor sound transmission. CT shows a solid mass with minimal enhancement. MR shows a well-defined ovarian mass that is predominantly low signal on both T1WI and T2WI. Scattered high signal areas within the mass on T2WI represent focal edema or cystic change.

Adnexal torsion is a gynecologic emergency resulting from twisting of the ovary, fallopian tube, or most commonly both structures restricting blood supply. Failure to promptly relieve torsion and restore blood supply results in infarction. Patients

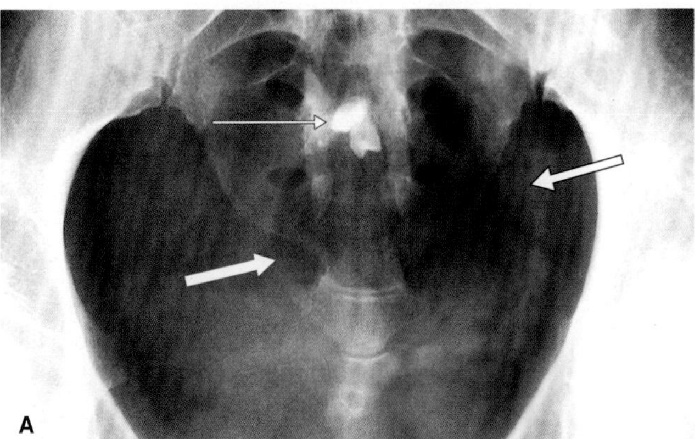

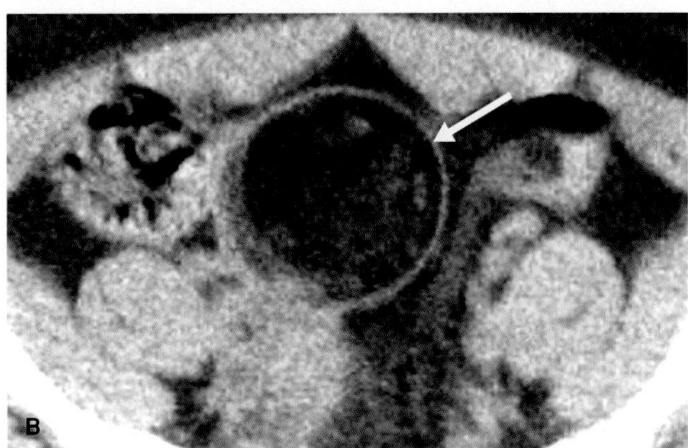

FIGURE 49.14. **Benign Cystic Teratoma. A:** Conventional radiograph of the pelvis in a young woman demonstrates several well-formed teeth (*skinny arrow*). A subtle, well-defined mass of fat density is also present (*fat arrows*). These findings are diagnostic of benign cystic teratoma. **B:** CT performed without contrast of a 28-year-old woman reveals a fat-density mass (*arrow*) diagnostic of a benign cystic teratoma.

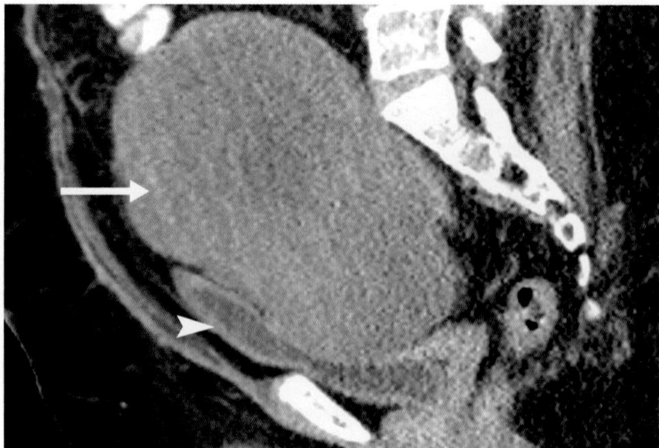

FIGURE 49.15. **Ovarian Fibroma.** Sagittal reformatted image from a CT scan demonstrates a very large lobulated homogeneous solid mass (*arrow*) arising from the pelvis and compressing the bladder (*arrowhead*). The patient had small pleural effusions and ascites that resolved after resection of the benign ovarian fibromas.

present with pain, nausea, vomiting, and leukocytosis. Diagnosis is most effectively made by US (see Figure 51.27). Key findings include a smooth-walled adnexal mass, which serves as a nidus for twisting (Fig. 49.16). The torsed mass demonstrates concentric wall thickening. The involved fallopian tube appears as an amorphous mass or as a tube with thickened walls. The uterus is deviated toward the torsed adnexa. Signs of hemorrhagic infarction of the torsed adnexa include marked thickening of the wall of the adnexal mass (>10 mm), hemorrhage within the mass and within the twisted tube, and hemoperitoneum.

Gynecologic Malignancy

Ovarian cancer represents 3% of all malignancy in women, but accounts for 15% of all cancer deaths. There are more than 20 histologic types of ovarian malignancy, however, epithelial (70%) and germ cell (15%) tumors account for the majority. Approximately 40% of ovarian tumors are malignant, two-thirds are cystic, and 25% are bilateral. The peak age of onset of ovarian cancer is 55 to 59. Ovarian malignancy has an insidious onset and a silent growth pattern that results in advanced disease at presentation in 70% of cases. CA 125 is a serologic marker for ovarian cancer found to be elevated in 80% of women with ovarian cancer. Unfortunately, it is more likely to be abnormal in advanced cancers and is elevated in only 25% to 50% of stage I ovarian cancers. Survival correlates directly with the stage of disease, which also determines treatment. MR and CT signs of ovarian malignancy are similar to those listed for US in Chapter 51. Wall thickness greater than 3 mm, nodularity, vegetations, solid components, evidence of invasion of adjacent structures, ascites, contrast enhancement of the peritoneum, and adenopathy are evidence of malignancy (Fig. 49.17). Ovarian carcinoma spreads primarily by peritoneal seeding with small tumor nodules implanting on the peritoneum, mesentery, and omentum, and malignant ascites (Fig. 49.18). Secondary patterns of spread include direct extension to adjacent structures, lymphatic metastases to pelvic and retroperitoneal nodes, and late hematogenous spread to lung, liver, and bones. CT is used primarily for follow-up of known ovarian cancer. Because ovarian cancer is usually staged with surgical laparotomy, initial radiographic tumor staging is indicated only in clearly advanced cases. Initial treatment is total abdominal hysterectomy, bilateral salpingo-oophorectomy, omentectomy, and tumor debulking. Both CT and MR are relatively poor in the detection of peritoneal metastases. The presence of ascites is highly predictive of the presence of peritoneal metastases. A careful search for focal peritoneal thickening and tiny nodules should be conducted. Thickening of the bowel wall and distortion of bowel loops suggest intestinal involvement. No imaging method can reliably differentiate benign from malignant ovarian masses. This is not surprising because many cases are borderline malignant, even histologically.

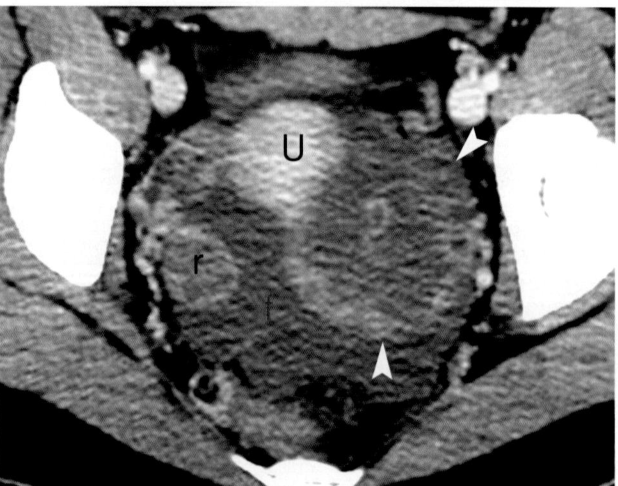

FIGURE 49.16. **Ovarian Torsion.** Axial postcontrast CT image shows a large cystic mass (*arrowheads*) arising from the left ovary with thickened poorly enhancing walls associated with a large volume of fluid (*f*) in the cul-de-sac. The patient was experiencing intermittent severe pelvic pain. Surgery reveals torsion of the left adnexa with a serous cystadenoma serving as the nidus for torsion. *U*, uterus; *r*, right ovary.

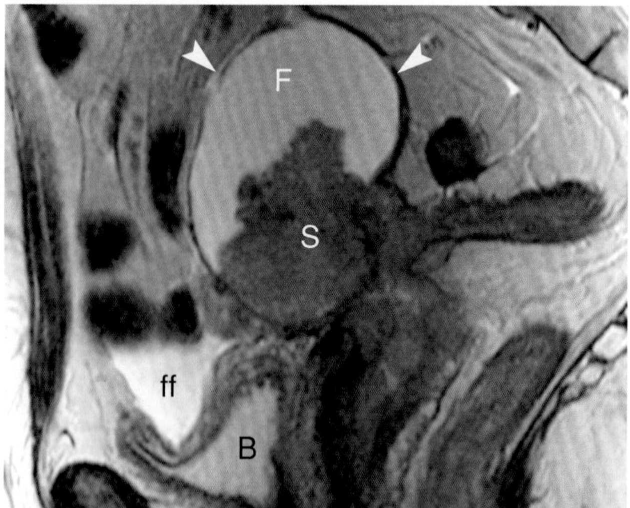

FIGURE 49.17. **Cystadenocarcinoma Ovary.** Sagittal plane MR T2WI in a 63-year-old woman demonstrates a cystic adnexa mass (*arrowheads*) with a prominent solid component (*S*) highly indicative of malignancy. The fluid content (*F*) of the mass was high signal on both T1WI and T2WI indicating internal hemorrhage or high protein content. Free intraperitoneal fluid (*ff*) is also present indicating high likelihood of intraperitoneal metastases. *B*, bladder.

Metastases to the ovary occur by peritoneal spread, direct extension, or hematogenous dissemination and account for 10% of ovarian malignancies. Most metastases to the ovaries originate as colon cancers (65%) with other common primary

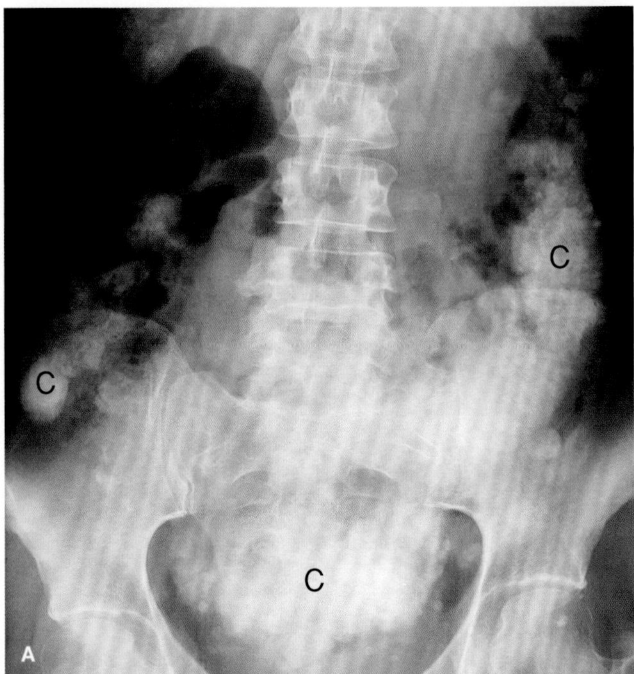

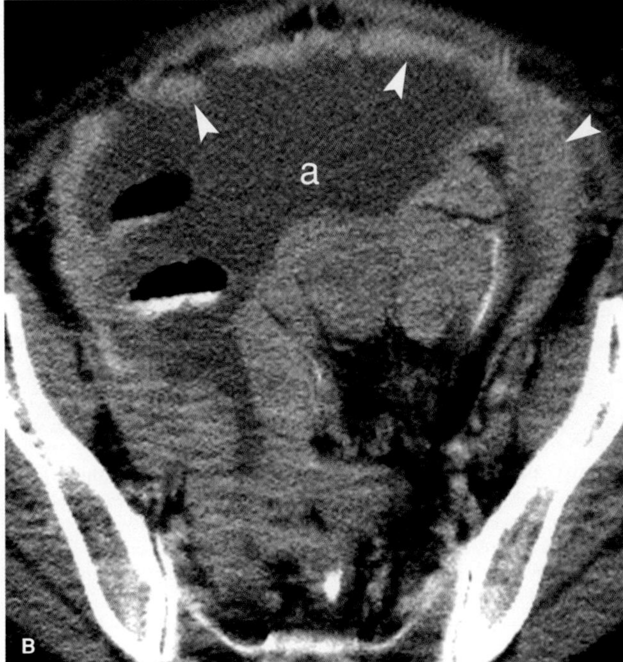

FIGURE 49.18. **Peritoneal Metastases From Ovarian Carcinoma. A:** Conventional radiograph of the abdomen demonstrates calcified implants of ovarian carcinoma (*C*) throughout the peritoneal cavity. The pathologic diagnosis was metastatic papillary serous cystadenocarcinoma of the ovary. **B:** CT image reveals nodular tumor implants (*arrowheads*) on the parietal peritoneum well outlined by ascites (*a*). The patient had metastatic ovarian carcinoma.

tumors being stomach, breast, lung, and pancreas. Most metastases are solid, bilateral, and enhance avidly. Cystic metastases are usually indistinguishable from ovarian primary tumors (Fig. 49.19). The term "Krukenberg tumor" is properly applied only to mucinous tumors metastatic to the ovary from a mucinous gastric carcinoma. Ovarian lymphoma produces large bilateral solid ovarian masses that show minimal enhancement.

Cervical cancer is the most common gynecologic malignancy. Squamous carcinoma accounts for 95% and adenocarcinoma for 5% of these cases. The peak age of onset is 45 to 55 years, but it is the second most common malignancy in women aged 15 to 34. Cervical cancer spreads predominantly by direct extension to involve the vagina, paracervical and parametrial tissues, and the bladder and rectum. Obstruction of the ureters is particularly common because of their proximity to the cervix. Lymphatic metastases to the pelvic, inguinal, and retroperitoneal nodes are common. Hematogenous metastases to the lung, bone, and brain occur only late in the course of the disease.

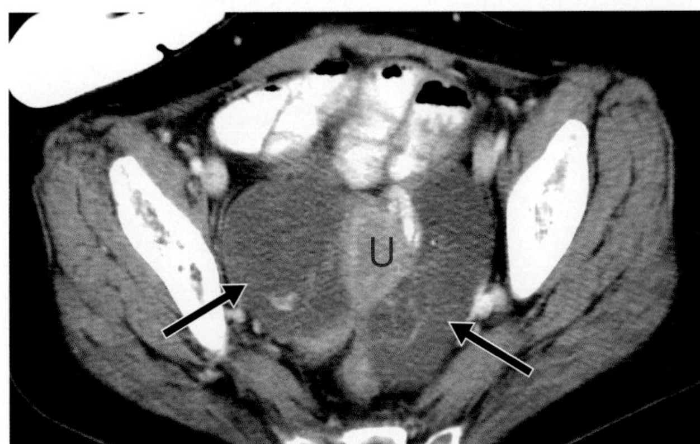

FIGURE 49.19. **Metastases to the Ovary.** Cystic metastases (*arrows*) replace and enlarge both ovaries compressing the uterus (*U*) in this patient with mucinous adenocarcinoma of the colon. The patient has had a colectomy and has an ileostomy bag.

MR is usually preferred to CT for staging of proven disease. On T1WI, cervical carcinoma is isointense with the myometrium. On T2WI, the tumor is higher in signal compared with the low signal of normal cervical tissue. A continuous rind of low signal cervical stroma surrounding the tumor is reliable evidence of the absence of parametrial invasion (Fig. 49.20). Signs of side wall invasion include tumor abutting or extending to within 3 mm of pelvic musculature. High-intensity signal in the parametrium on T2WI is evidence of parametrial invasion. Vaginal involvement is evidenced by loss of the normal thin rind of vaginal muscle on T2WI. Local staging by CT is limited by the fact that up to 50% of tumors are isodense to cervical tissue on both contrast and noncontrast scans (Fig. 49.21). Visible tumor is heterogeneously hypodense on postcontrast scans. Both MR and CT use node enlargement (>10 mm in short axis) as the primary criterion for involvement. This is inherently inaccurate because cervical cancer is known to involve nodes without enlarging them. Central necrosis within a lymph node is highly predictive of tumor involvement regardless of node size. Lymphatic spread involves internal and external iliac, presacral, and para-aortic nodes. Distant metastases most commonly involve liver, lung, and bone. Imaging studies should include the kidneys to assess for obstruction. PET-CT may prove to the optimal imaging modality to determine the extent of disease and to demonstrate residual or recurrent tumor. However, its use is impaired by pitfalls and artifacts, and its role in cervical cancer is not yet fully determined.

Endometrial carcinoma is now the most common invasive gynecologic malignancy. Histologically it is 95% adenocarcinoma and 5% sarcoma. The peak age at onset is 55 to 62 years, with postmenopausal vaginal bleeding as the key symptom. The tumor spreads initially by invasion into the

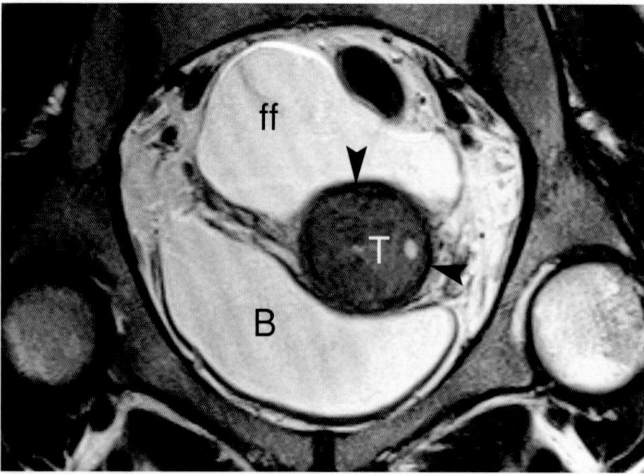

FIGURE 49.20. Cervical Carcinoma—MR. This T2-weighted MR image was obtained in an oblique coronal plane in order to image the cervix in transverse orientation. The tumor (*T*) appearing dark gray has nearly completely replaced the normal cervix seen only as a black rim (*arrowheads*). No parametrial invasion is evident. Free intraperitoneal fluid (*ff*) is seen in the cul-de-sac. *B*, bladder.

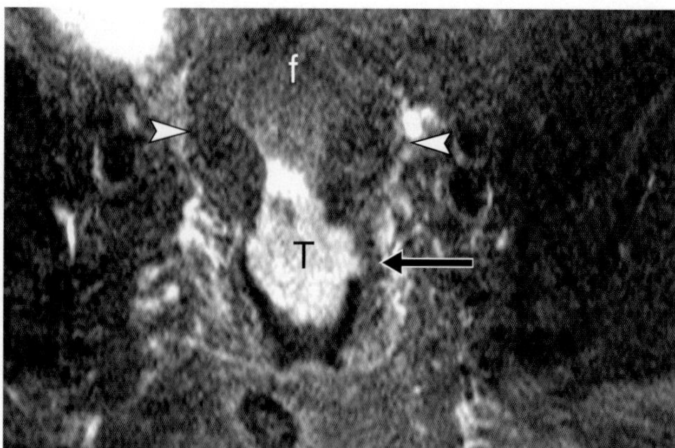

FIGURE 49.22. Endometrial Carcinoma—MR. Axial plane T2-weighted MR image through the uterus (between *arrowheads*) using fat saturation shows endometrial carcinoma (*T*) invading more than 50% of the thickness of the myometrium (*arrow*). This tumor is distinctly high signal compared to myometrium on this T2WI. *f*, fundus of the uterus.

myometrium and cervix, followed by lymphatic spread to the pelvic and retroperitoneal nodes, then continued direct spread into the broad ligaments, parametrium, and ovaries. Peritoneal seeding will occur with penetration of the uterine serosa. Hematogenous spread to the lung, bone, liver, and brain occurs late in the course of the disease. Prognosis and treatment depend on stage of the disease with the most critical factors being the depth of myometrial invasion and the involvement of lymph nodes. Lymph node metastases are unlikely if myometrial invasion is less than 50%. MR staging is more accurate than CT staging. On MR, the signal from tumor is similar to that of endometrium. Tumor is isointense to myometrium on T1WI and hyperintense to myometrium on T2WI (Fig. 49.22). Evidence of tumor includes thickening and poor definition of the endometrium. Large tumors appear as a polypoid mass that expands the uterine cavity. Tumor enhancement with gadolinium is variable and may be less than or greater than enhancement of myometrium and endometrium. Invasion of myometrium is determined on postcontrast T2WI. An intact junctional zone myometrium is evidence of the absence of myometrial invasion. Pitfalls for myometrial invasion include thinning of the myometrium by rapidly expanding tumors. Cervical invasion is determined on sagittal T2WI and postcontrast sequences with enhancing tumor seen within the dark tissue of the cervix. T1WI shows parametrial invasion into fat. Invasion of the bladder and rectum is evidenced by disrupted tissue planes and tumor signal with bladder or rectal wall on T2WI. On CT, the depth of myometrial invasion is determined on postcontrast images. The tumor enhances less than myometrium (Fig. 49.23). Obstruction of the cervix results in filling of the uterine cavity with fluid of variable density. Cervical involvement appears as heterogeneous enlargement of the cervix. Parametrial invasion appears as irregular margins of the uterus, parametrial soft tissue stranding, or parametrial mass. CT and MR evidence of nodal metastases are lymph nodes larger than 10 mm in short axis.

Uterine sarcomas are the most aggressive of the uterine tumors. Sarcomas may be suspected when uterine masses are large and heterogeneous. Malignant *mixed Müllerian tumors* are large solid tumors with prominent necrosis and hemorrhage that expand the uterine cavity and invade the myometrium. They appear as an intracavitary mass. Lymphatic and peritoneal spread are common. *Leiomyosarcomas* usually present as a rapidly growing pelvic mass. The uterus is

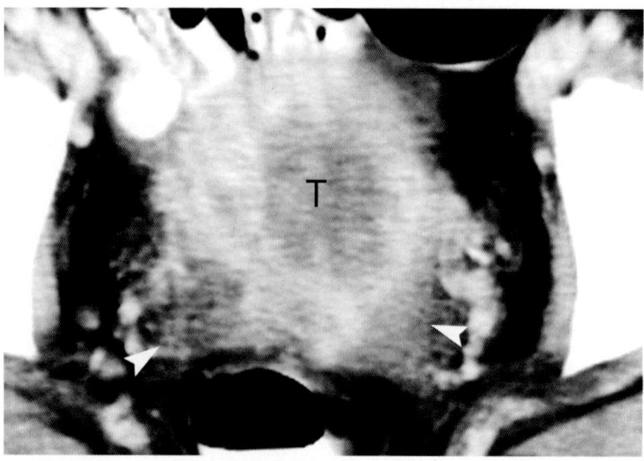

FIGURE 49.21. Cervical Carcinoma—CT. Heterogeneous tumor (*T*) has completely replaced the cervix on this CT scan. Stranding densities (*arrowheads*) into the paracervical fat indicate parametrial invasion by tumor.

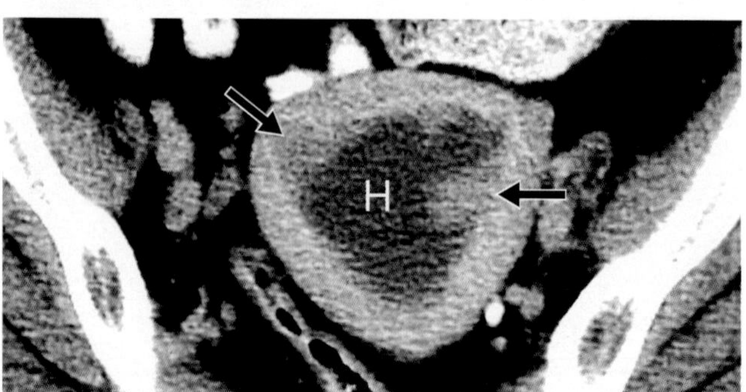

FIGURE 49.23. Endometrial Carcinoma—CT. Postcontrast CT image shows enhancing tumor nodules (*arrows*) invading the myometrium and extending into the uterine cavity being partially outlined by low attenuation hemorrhagic fluid (*H*). Tumor invasion is difficult to assess because the tumor is nearly isointense with enhanced myometrium.

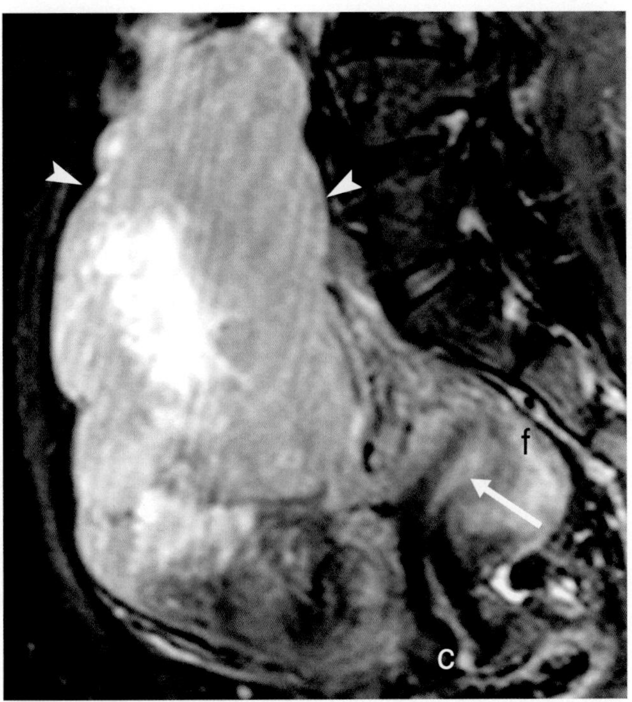

FIGURE 49.24. **Leiomyosarcoma.** T2WI shows a huge heterogeneous tumor mass (*arrowheads*) arising from the anterior wall of the retroflexed uterus. Note that the uterine cavity (*arrow*) is intact. The exophytic myometrial origin and heterogeneity of the mass are indicative of either a degenerated leiomyoma or a leiomyosarcoma. The latter diagnosis was confirmed at surgery. *f*, fundus of the uterus; *c*, cervix.

enlarged with a markedly heterogeneous mass with extensive necrosis, hemorrhage, and frequent calcifications (Fig. 49.24). Imaging differentiation from a degenerated benign leiomyoma is not possible unless signs of malignant spread of tumor are evident. *Endometrial stromal sarcomas* appear as polypoid endometrial masses that invade the myometrium.

Fallopian tube carcinoma is very rare accounting for only about 1% of gynecologic malignancy. Tumor types include serous adenocarcinoma, endometrioid carcinoma, and transitional cell carcinoma. Most tumors arise in the ampulla and occlude the tube causing hydrosalpinx (Fig. 49.25). Most

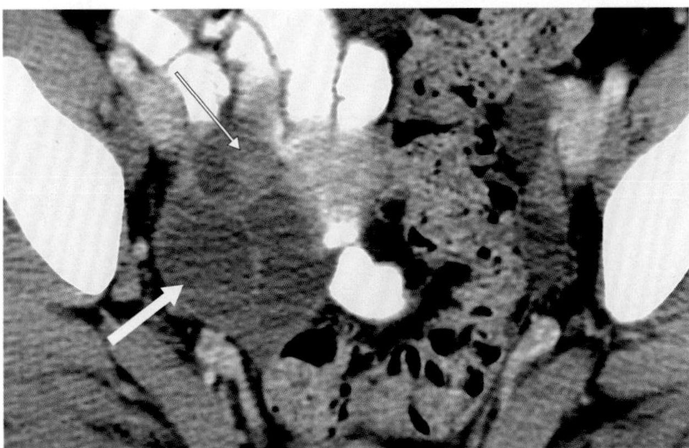

FIGURE 49.25. **Carcinoma of the Fallopian Tube.** Postcontrast CT shows a right sided hydrosalpinx (*fat arrow*). Close inspection reveals a papillary soft tissue attenuation nodule (*skinny arrow*) within the lumen of the dilated tube. Surgical resection confirmed adenocarcinoma of the fallopian tube.

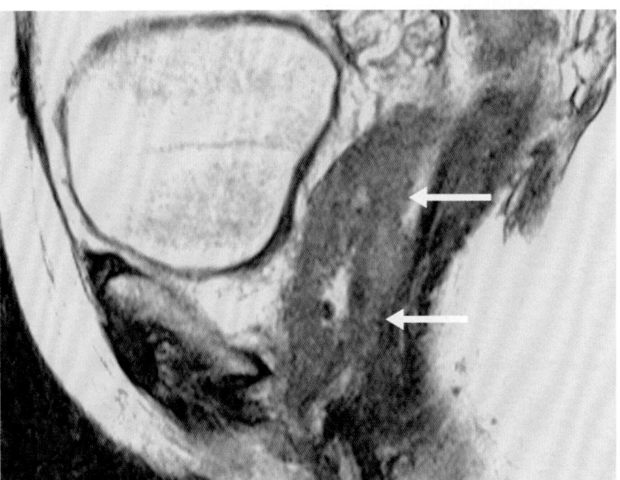

FIGURE 49.26. **Carcinoma of the Vagina.** Sagittal T2-weighted MR in a patient with previous hysterectomy shows marked nodular circumferential thickening (*arrows*) of the entire vagina. Biopsy revealed adenocarcinoma.

tumors are small. On MR, the small solid lesions are low signal on T1WI and high signal on T2WI. Most show enhancement with intravenous contrast administration. Fluid in the distended tube is usually complex reflected by high signal on T1WI.

Vaginal malignancies are also rare accounting for another 1% of gynecologic malignancies. Most are squamous cell carcinomas (85%) usually arising from the posterior wall of the upper third of the vagina. The remaining tumor types are adenocarcinoma, melanoma, and sarcoma. The vagina is much more commonly involved by direct spread of cervical, uterine, or rectal cancers. Primary vaginal malignancies produce a circumferential constricting lesion of the vagina (Fig. 49.26) or an ulcerated mass. MR shows low signal on T1WI and intermediate signal on T2WI. Use of vaginal gel during MR imaging greatly improves tumor visualization.

MALE GENITAL TRACT

Testes and Scrotum

US, supplemented by color Doppler, remains the initial imaging method of choice to evaluate the testes and scrotal contents. MR using surface coils offers excellent spatial resolution, greater tissue contrast, and wider field of view, but has the disadvantages of greater cost and lesser availability. MR is the choice for additional characterization of scrotal lesions when US findings are insufficient to determine for treatment. CT is the imaging method of choice for the staging of testicular neoplasms and in locating undescended testes that are not found by US. MR offers a staging alternative to CT. Radionuclide imaging provides useful information about perfusion, but with limited anatomic detail. This chapter reviews MR and CT imaging. Scrotal US is reviewed in Chapter 51.

Normal MR Anatomy. Because of high fluid content, the testes are of uniform low to intermediate signal on T1WI and uniform high signal on T2WI (Fig. 49.27). The tunica albuginea forms a well-defined 1 mm thick rim low in signal on T1WI and T2WI. Testicular masses are well depicted as lower in signal intensity than the bright testicular parenchyma on T2WI. Septations are often visualized radiating from the mediastinum to the tunica albuginea. A small amount of fluid is normally present in the

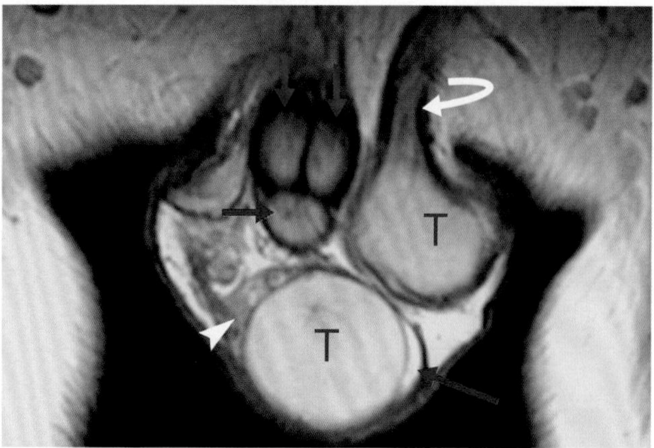

FIGURE 49.27. **Normal MR Anatomy: Male.** Coronal plane T2-weighted MR shows both testes (*T*) and the penis in cross-section. The testes are high in signal because of their high fluid content. The epididymis (*arrowhead*) is also high signal on T2WI but less than that of the testes. The left testis is suspended on the spermatic cord (*curved arrow*). The paired corpora cavernosa (*blue arrows*) are well demonstrated. The corpus spongiosum (*red arrow*) contains the urethra. A small amount of fluid (*long red arrow*) is present between the layers of the tunica vaginalis.

scrotum between the layers of the tunica vaginalis. The epididymis is isointense to the testes on T1WI and brightens on T2WI, though to a lesser extent than the testis. Postcontrast images depict homogeneous enhancement of the testis and avid hyperenhancement of the epididymis. The scrotum is intermediate signal reflecting the dartos muscle. The spermatic cord appears as numerous tubular structures representing the arteries and veins with MR signal determined by blood flow.

Undescended Testis. CT and MR are used to localize undescended testes not demonstrated by US to be within the inguinal canal. The testis, if present, will be seen between the lower pole of the kidney and the internal inguinal ring. In 3% to 5% of cases, the testis is congenitally absent. The undescended testis appears as an oval soft tissue mass up to 4 cm in size (Fig. 49.28). Because the undescended testis is usually atrophic, MR may show low or intermediate, instead of high signal, on T2WI. Undescended testis in the adult may be complicated by testicular tumor.

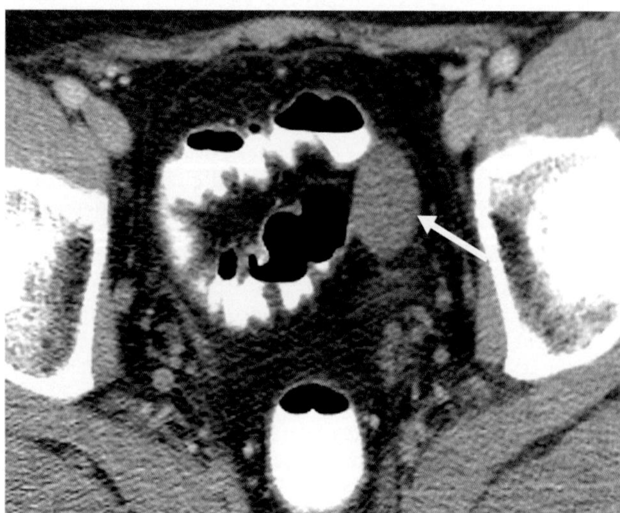

FIGURE 49.28. **Undescended Testis.** An undescended left testis (*arrow*) is found in the pelvis of a 40-year-old male. The testis is mildly atrophic.

Neoplasms. Diagnosis of testicular neoplasms is made by physical examination and US. The primary tumor in the testis may be clinically occult, yet is effectively demonstrated by US. Only in the rare case of an indeterminate lesion on US will MR of the testis be performed for further characterization. On MR, seminomas (60% of germ cell neoplasms) are homogeneous and hypointense to normal testis on T2WI. Nonseminomatous germ cell neoplasms (40%) are heterogeneous with areas of necrosis and hemorrhage but are still primarily low signal to normal testis on T2WI. Both tumor types enhance moderately showing prominent fibrovascular septa. Lymphoma, seen primarily in men >60 years, replaces testicular parenchyma with infiltrative tumor low in signal on T1WI and T2WI, and with low-level enhancement. Neither US nor MR can reliably differentiate benign from malignant testicular tumors.

With current treatment methods 95% of patients with germ cell testes neoplasms can be cured. Selection of proper treatment depends on staging, which relies primarily on CT, though MR offers an alternative accurate staging method. Lymphatic spread of tumor is most common, with a usual pattern of orderly ascending nodal involvement. Initial spread is along gonadal lymphatic vessels following the testicular veins to renal hilar nodes. Lymphatic metastases may also follow the external iliac chain to the para-aortic nodes. The internal iliac and inguinal nodes are rarely involved. Extensive metastatic involvement of the lymph nodes mimics lymphoma in young males. Hematogenous spread to the lungs usually follows lymphatic spread, except with choriocarcinoma, which spreads hematogenously early.

Scrotal Fluid Collections. Simple hydroceles show signal characteristics of water, low signal on T1WI and high signal on T2WI. Hematoceles and pyoceles show high signal on T1WI, reflecting complex fluid and high protein content. *Epididymal cysts* show the signal of simple fluid. *Spermatoceles* commonly contain fat and high protein causing high signal on T1WI, and layering debris may be evident. *Varicoceles* appear as serpiginous tubular structures in the spermatic cord. Signal intensity corresponds to slow blood flow. CT shows hydroceles as low attenuation fluid within the scrotum and varicoceles as enhancing tubular structures (Fig. 49.29).

Epididymitis/Orchitis. Orchitis causes inhomogeneous signal on both T1WI and T2WI, indistinguishable from tumor. With epididymitis, the epididymis is enlarged but signal intensity on T2WI is unpredictable and may be increased, decreased, or normal. Dilated vessels in the spermatic cord reflect hypervascularity. Hydrocele is usually present. Inflamed tissue shows avid enhancement.

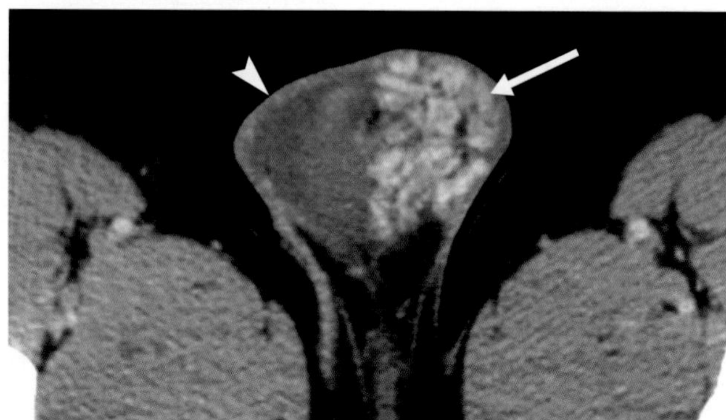

FIGURE 49.29. **Varicocele and Hydrocele.** Axial postcontrast CT through the scrotum reveals a large hydrocele (*arrowhead*) on the right and a very large enhancing varicocele (*arrow*) on the left.

Testicular torsion is best evaluated with Doppler US or scintigraphy. With acute torsion, MR may demonstrate a characteristic twisted pattern of torsion of the spermatic cord with impaired blood flow evident. The testis appears heterogeneous on all image sequences. Enhancement is diminished if blood flow is currently compromised but is intense if detorsion has occurred.

Prostate

Multiparametric MRI (mp-MRI) of the prostate has revolutionized imaging for detection and staging of prostate cancer. In 2012, the European Society of Urogenital Radiologists (ESUR) developed prostate MR imaging guidelines and suggested a PI-RADS (Prostate Imaging Reporting and Data System) structured reporting system. PI-RADS has been further refined by international consensus to version 2. Further refinement of this standardized reporting system is expected.

Current use of mp-MRI consists of a combination of high-resolution T2WI to assess anatomy with diffusion-weighted MRI (DWI) and MR spectroscopic imaging (MRSI) to improve specificity of lesion detection. Dynamic contrast-enhanced MRI (DCE-MRI) with gadolinium administration provides highly sensitive cancer detection. Each imaging method is assigned a PI-RADS score from 1 to 5 based on imaging findings and location. PI-RADS 1 indicates clinically significant cancer is highly unlikely. PI-RADS 2 indicates clinically significant cancer is unlikely. PI-RADS 3 indicates clinically significant cancer is equivocal. PI-RADS 4 indicates clinically significant cancer is likely. PI-RADS 5 indicates clinically significant cancer is highly likely. Recommendations for treatment are based on overall PI-RADS scoring. The details of PI-RADS scoring are complex and beyond the scope of this basic review. The reader is referred to Suggested Readings.

CT has no current role in the detection of prostate cancer as CT findings of benign and malignant disease overlap extensively. CT is also inferior to MRI for the staging of prostate cancer beyond the prostate. Transrectal US (TRUS) is used primarily to guide biopsy of areas of the prostate considered suspicious for cancer. However, TRUS underestimated the grade and the extent of prostate cancers. The role of PET-CT in prostate cancer is limited by the low metabolic activity of the tumor and high normal radionuclide activity in the bladder obscuring the prostate gland and surrounding tissues. Elevated serum prostate-specific antigen (PSA) (>3 to 4 ng/mL) has low specificity for prostate cancer, only 36%. A normal PSA does not exclude the presence of prostate cancer. These factors support the current enthusiasm for mp-MRI.

Normal MR Anatomy. The prostate is divided into three glandular zones surrounding the urethra (Fig. 49.30). The *peripheral zone* contains approximately 70% of prostate tissue and is draped around the remainder of the gland like a catcher's glove holding a baseball. Most prostate cancers (70%) arise in the peripheral zone. The *transitional zone* consists of two small areas of periurethral glandular tissue. Although it contains only 5% of prostatic tissue in the normal young man, it is the site of benign prostatic hypertrophy and may enlarge greatly in the older man. The *central zone* consists of the glandular tissue at the base of the prostate through which course the ducts of the vas deferens and seminal vesicles and the ejaculatory ducts. Although the central zone makes up 25% of glandular tissue, only 10% of cancers arise there. The anterior portion of the prostate is occupied by nonglandular tissue called the anterior *fibromuscular stroma.* The *base* of the prostate is that portion adjacent to the base of the bladder and the seminal vesicles (base to base). The *apex* of the prostate rests on the urogenital diaphragm. Prominent veins are frequently visualized in the periprostatic tissues. Lymphatic drainage of the prostate goes to regional pelvic lymph nodes with channels to para-aortic and inguinal nodes. Periprostatic venous connections to vertebral veins offer a route for the hematogenous spread of tumor to the axial skeleton. On T1WI, the prostate gland is uniform intermediate to low signal similar to skeletal muscle. The high signal periprostatic fat defines the margin of the prostate. Periprostatic veins and neurovascular bundles are low signal. On T2WI, the internal structure (zonal anatomy) of the prostate is demonstrated (Fig. 49.31). The peripheral zone is high in signal due to higher water content and looser acinar structure. The central zone is lower in signal due to more compact muscle fibers and acinar structure. The central and transitional zones become heterogeneous with age and the development of benign prostatic hyperplasia (BPH). The anterior fibromuscular stroma is low in signal and has poorly defined margins.

Normal CT Anatomy. The prostate gland is seen at the base of the bladder, just posterior to the symphysis pubis, as a homogeneous rounded soft tissue organ up to 4 cm in maximal diameter. Prostate zonal anatomy is not demonstrated by CT. A well-defined plane of fat separates the prostate from the obturator internus muscle.

Prostate carcinoma is the third leading cause of cancer death in men. Approximately one in six men will develop clinical prostate carcinoma in their lifetime. Despite the high prevalence and importance of prostate disease, treatment remains controversial. The primary issue is differentiating lethal from nonlethal disease. Nearly 50% of men older than 75 years of age will have prostate carcinoma on biopsy or autopsy. However, many of these cancers will not affect the patient's life span. The tumor is uncommon before age 50 and increases in incidence thereafter. The Gleason histologic grading system is used to assess the degree of differentiation of the tumor. A grade 1 is well differentiated and a grade 5 is anaplastic. The Gleason score varies from 2 to 10 and adds the Gleason grade for the predominant and the secondary portions of the tumors. Most tumors are adenocarcinoma (95%). Prostate cancer spreads

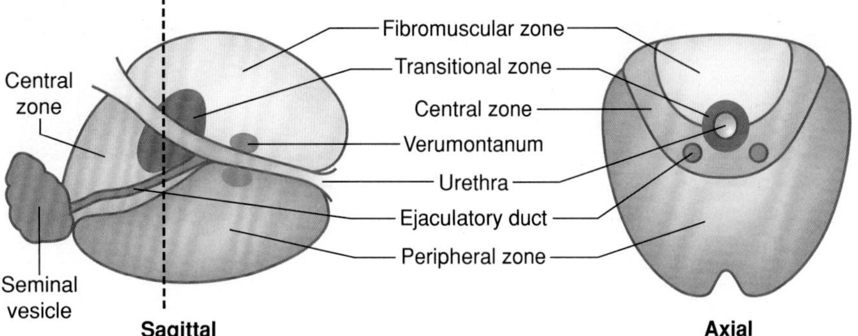

FIGURE 49.30. Zonal Anatomy of the Prostate. The anatomy is illustrated in midsagittal plane (*left*) and axial plane (*right*) at the level of the vertical *dashed line* on the left.

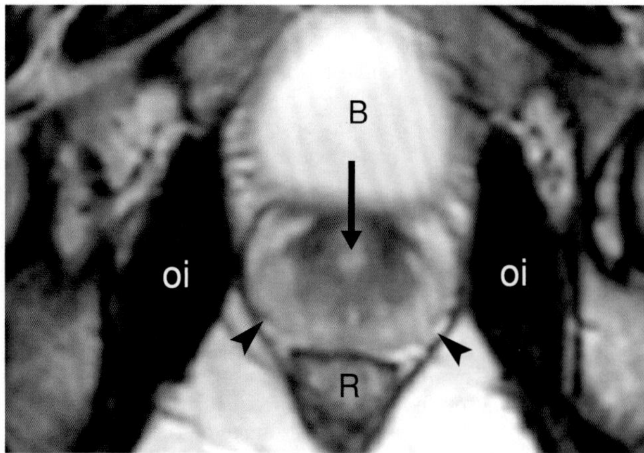

FIGURE 49.31. **Normal Prostate—MR.** Axial plane T2-weighted MR of a normal prostate in a 40-year-old man demonstrates the high-intensity peripheral zone (*arrowheads*), the urethra (*long arrow*), and the lower-intensity transitional zone surrounding the urethra. *B*, bladder; *r*, rectum; *oi*, obturator internus muscle.

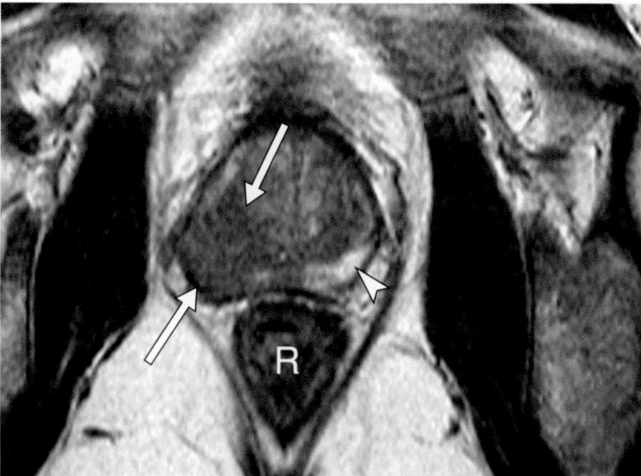

FIGURE 49.32. **Prostate Carcinoma.** Axial T2-weighted MR image of the prostate shows a low signal intensity adenocarcinoma (between *arrows*) replacing most of the peripheral zone and extending into the central gland of the prostate on the right. The peripheral zone on the left (*arrowhead*) remains normal high signal intensity. *R*, rectum.

by local extension, lymphatic vessels to regional nodes, and by hematogenous dissemination. Involvement of lymph nodes by metastatic disease is unreliably detected by conventional MR or CT because 70% of involved lymph nodes are small (<8 mm). Penetration of tumor through the capsule or into the seminal vesicles greatly worsens the prognosis. Involvement of the axial skeleton by hematogenous metastases is common. Metastases to the lungs, liver, and kidneys occur in the terminal phases of the disease.

On MR T2WI, cancers appear as areas of ill-defined low signal within the high signal peripheral zone (Fig. 49.32). Prostatitis, hemorrhage, scars, and posttreatment changes may have a similar appearance. In the transitional zone tumors are more difficult to detect overlapping the normal signal characteristics of transitional zone tissue. Cancer appears as an indistinct mass with homogeneous signal intensity, an appearance described as the "erased charcoal sign." Water-drop or lenticular shape is typical. Signal intensity is lower with high-grade cancers than with low-grade cancers. Criteria for extracapsular extension on T2WI include irregularity and thickening of the neurovascular bundle, loss of capsular enhancement, loss of visualization of the capsule, focal bulges of the capsule, and obliteration of the angle between the rectum and prostate. Prostate cancer shows intense early enhancement and variable early washout on DCE-MRI. On DWI, cancers show markedly hypointense focal abnormality on calculated apparent diffusion coefficient (ADC) maps and markedly hyperintense foci on high–*b*-value images. MRSI shows cancers have lower levels of citrate and higher levels of choline than benign prostate tissue. On T1WI, cancers are isointense with benign prostate tissue. T1WI is best used for assessing invasion of periprostatic fat and for detecting enlarged lymph nodes.

Benign prostatic hyperplasia begins at near age 40 and eventually occurs in all men. Hypertrophy and hyperplasia occur in glandular tissue in the transitional and periurethral zones accompanied by proliferation of supporting smooth muscle and stromal cells. The end result is focal or diffuse enlargement of the prostate (Fig. 49.33). Pressure on the

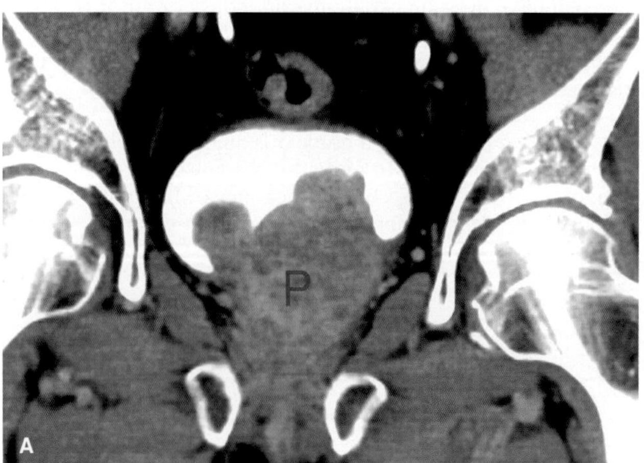

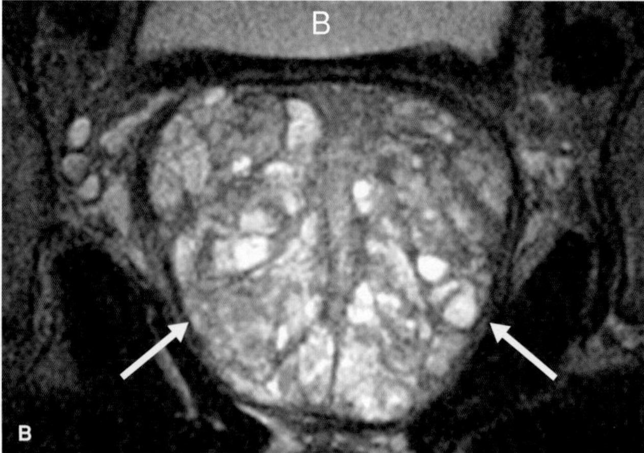

FIGURE 49.33. **Benign Prostatic Hypertrophy. A:** Postcontrast CT scan reformatted into coronal plane reveals marked nodular enlargement of the prostate gland (*P*) uplifting the bladder base. Despite marked hypertrophy of the prostate the bladder wall is only minimally thickened and the patient had only mild bladder outlet obstruction symptoms illustrating the clinical point that it is not the overall size of the prostate that matters but exactly where the hypertrophy occurs and how much narrowing of the urethra that it causes. **B:** T2-weighted MR image in axial plane shows marked diffuse enlargement of the prostate gland (*arrows*) with heterogeneous signal, nodules, and cystic change. The normal zonal anatomy of the prostate is not evident. *B*, bladder.

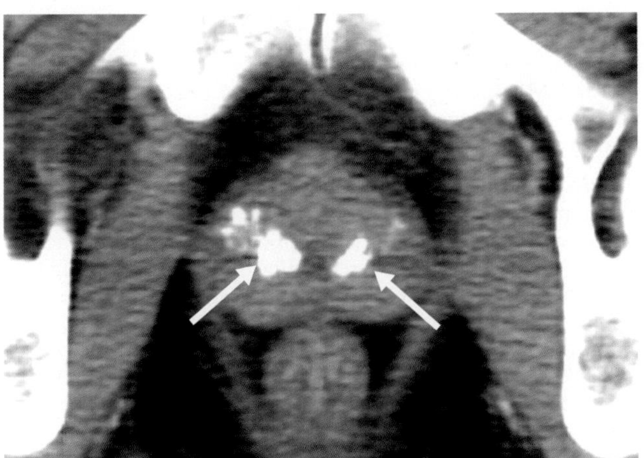

FIGURE 49.34. **Prostate Calcifications.** Axial postcontrast CT shows a mildly enlarged prostate with prominent coarse calcifications (*arrows*) typical of calcification associated with benign prostate hypertrophy.

urethra obstructs bladder outflow and results in symptoms of hesitancy, decreased force and caliber of the urine stream, dribbling, frequency, nocturia, and postvoid residual. This progressive process is combated by hypertrophy of the bladder wall musculature (see Fig. 48.19). Advanced symptoms require medical therapy, balloon dilatation, stents, or transurethral resection of the prostate (TURP). CT findings of BPH include (a) enlargement of the prostate, commonly with lobulated contour and visible high and low attenuation nodules; (b) coarse calcifications (Fig. 49.34); (c) cystic degeneration; and (d) bladder wall thickening and trabeculation.

MR shows prostate enlargement with heterogeneous central gland on T2WI (Fig. 49.31). Areas of cystic degeneration are low signal on T1WI and high signal on T2WI. The stromal component of BPH can have low signal on T2WI mimicking cancer in the transitional zone. On diffusion-weighted ADC images, BPH shows restricted diffusion because of its highly cellular nature. On contrast-enhanced MRI, BPH shows increased abnormal perfusion.

Prostate abscess occurs as a common complication of bacterial prostatitis. Patients present with fever, dysuria, pelvic pain, and tenderness on transrectal prostate examination. Sepsis or failure to improve on antibiotic treatment suggests development of an abscess. US, CT, and MR show a complex fluid collection with prominent peripheral vascularity and inflammatory changes (Fig. 49.35).

Cystic lesions of the prostate and periprostatic tissues are uncommon but often prominent findings on prostate imaging. Congenital lesions include *Müllerian duct* and *prostatic utricle cysts* (Fig. 49.36) that occur in the midline in the upper half of the prostate. While these are separate entities they are indistinguishable by imaging. Small cysts are incidental findings. Larger cysts may cause bladder outlet obstruction symptoms, pain, and hematuria. CT shows a well-defined midline cyst of variable size. These cysts are high signal on T2WI. Prostate *retention cysts* result from obstruction of the prostatic ductule. They may occur anywhere in the gland and are usually small and asymptomatic. *Cysts associated with BPH* are the most common cysts of the prostate. Cystic appearance of *prostatic carcinoma* is rare but may be suspected if a cystic lesion shows rapid growth. *Abscesses* may complicated bacterial prostatitis and may be drained using TRUS guidance.

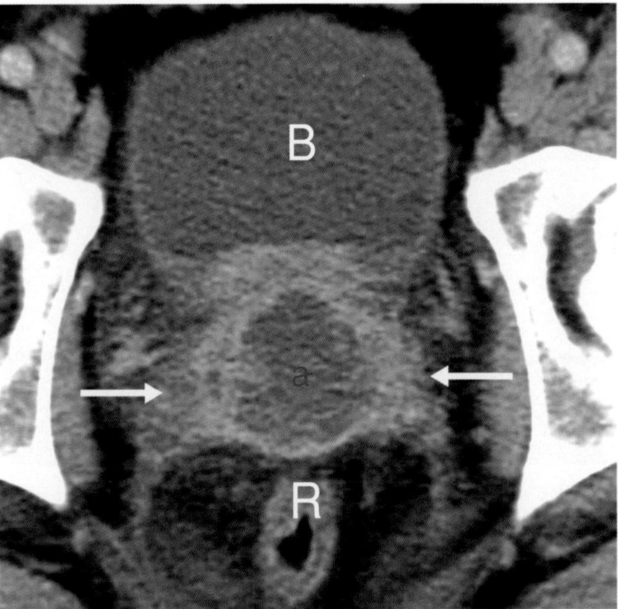

FIGURE 49.35. **Prostate Abscess.** Axial postcontrast CT shows a large irregular fluid collection (*a*) replacing and expanding most of the prostate gland representing an abscess. Periprostatic tissues (*arrows*) are infiltrated and edematous reflecting inflammation. *B*, bladder; *R*, rectum.

Seminal Vesicles

While primary tumors are rare, the seminal vesicles are commonly involved by tumors of the bladder, prostate, and rectum. Cysts and absence of the seminal vesicles are associated with ipsilateral renal dysgenesis or agenesis.

Anatomy. The seminal vesicles are paired elongated sac-like glands located in the posterior groove between the bladder base and the prostate. They produce 60% to 80% of the fluids passed during ejaculation. The dilated ampulla portion of the vas deferens courses just superior to the seminal vesicles. The vas deferens joins the ducts of the seminal vesicles to form the ejaculatory duct, which courses through the prostate gland

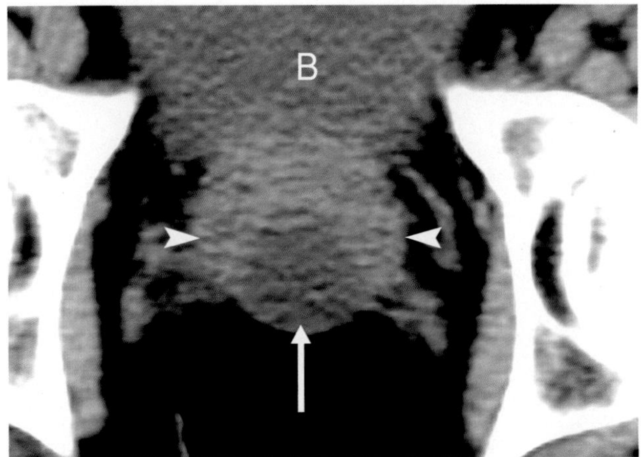

FIGURE 49.36. **Utricle/Müllerian Duct Cyst.** Axial CT without contrast shows a well-defined cyst (*arrow*) exactly in the midline of the prostate (between *arrowheads*). The patient was asymptomatic. This is an incidental finding of utricle cyst/Müllerian duct cyst. *B*, bladder.

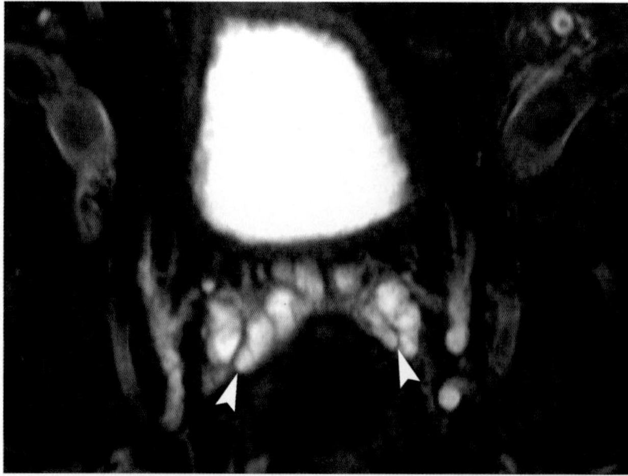

FIGURE 49.37. Normal Seminal Vesicles. T2-weighted axial plane MR with fat saturation shows the normal high signal intensity of the fluid-filled seminal vesicles (*arrowheads*).

to empty into the urethra at the level of the verumontanum. Normal seminal vesicles are 3 cm in length and 8 mm in diameter. Slight asymmetry is common. They contain fluid that is low to intermediate signal on T1WI and very high signal on T2WI (Fig. 49.37). The wall of the glands is 1 to 2 mm thick. The vas deferens is 3 to 5 mm in diameter. CT shows the fluid containing seminal vesicles as "bow-tie" in appearance on axial imaging. The seminal vesicles serve as a landmark for the lowest extent of the peritoneal cavity and for the location of the ureteral junctions with the bladder.

Pathology. Unilateral agenesis of the seminal vesicles is highly associated with ipsilateral renal agenesis (80% of cases). Bilateral seminal vesicle agenesis may be seen in some patients with cystic fibrosis. Hypoplasia occurs in association with cryptorchidism and hypogonadism. Cysts occur in patients with autosomal dominant polycystic disease and in association with developmental anomalies of the genitourinary tract. The extremely rare primary neoplasms include cystadenoma, cystadenocarcinoma, and sarcomas. Tumor involvement by prostate, bladder, or rectum carcinoma appears as contiguous solid tumor extending from the organ of origin to the seminal vesicles obliterating intervening fat planes. Bilateral calcification of the vas deferens is very highly associated with the presence of diabetes (Fig. 49.38).

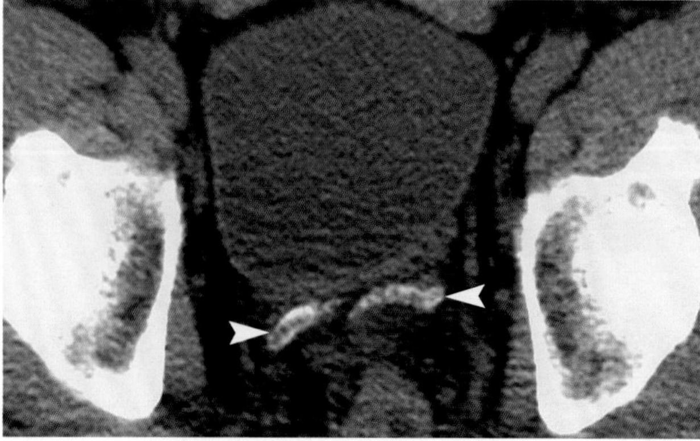

FIGURE 49.38. Calcification of the Vas Deferens. CT without contrast shows calcification of the bilateral vas deferens (*arrowheads*). This finding is almost universally associated with the presence of diabetes mellitus.

Penis

US and MR are the imaging modalities of choice for abnormalities of the penis. Indications include trauma, priapism, and tumors.

Anatomy. Both US and MR clearly delineate the anatomy of the penis (Fig. 49.27). The paired corpus cavernosa and the single corpus spongiosum containing the urethra are enveloped by the tough fibrous covering of the tunica albuginea. Buck fascia encases the corpora and deep vessels of the penis and fuses proximally with the deep urogenital fascia. A loose outer dartos facial layer is continuous with Colles fascia in the perineum. Hematomas or fluid collections within Buck fascia remain confined to the penis, while those external to Buck fascia may extend to the scrotum or anterior abdominal wall. Blood supply extends as branches of the internal pudendal artery, which arises from the internal iliac artery. Cavernosal arteries are imbedded within and supply the corpora cavernosa. Dorsal penile arteries and veins supply the glans penis, skin of the penis, and distal corpus spongiosum. The bulbar artery supplies the urethra and proximal corpus spongiosum.

Pathology. Penile fractures are uncommon and best evaluated initially by US, which demonstrates defects in the tunica albuginea and associated hematoma, usually confined within Buck fascia. On MR, the tunica albuginea is low signal and well demonstrated on both T1WI and T2WI. T1WI may detect subtle fractures obscured by high signal hematoma on T2WI. Diagnosis and surgical treatment are urgent as delay may result in erectile disorders and deformity. Painful penile induration, focal or generalized priapism, is most often caused by Peyronie disease, a connective tissue disorder, which produces plaques in the tunica albuginea resulting in penile curvature and deformity. Peyronie disease may present with acute pain or with chronic deformity. US and MR demonstrate focal fibrotic plaques causing thickening of the tunica albuginea. On MR, the plaques are low signal in concert with the tunica albuginea on both T1WI and T2WI. Contrast enhancement may be evident in the acute phase. Calcification may occur in the plaques in the chronic phase. Penile neoplasms are often accurately staged by clinical examination. MR is most accurate for imaging staging and for demonstrating adenopathy and tumor recurrence. Most tumors are squamous cell carcinomas or rare sarcomas. The cancers appear as an ill-defined infiltrating mass low in signal on both T1WI and T2WI. With intravenous contrast tumors enhance to a greater extent than the corpora.

Suggested Readings

Female Genital Tract

Agostinho L, Cruz R, Osírio F, Alves J, Setúbal A, Guerra A. MRI for adenomyosis: a pictorial review. *Insights Imaging* 2017;8:549–556.

Allen BC, Hosseinzadeh K, Qasem SA, Varner A, Leyendecker JR. Practical approach to MRI of female pelvic masses. *AJR Am J Roentgenol* 2014;202:1366–1375.

Arleo EK, Schwartz PE, Hui P, McCarthy S. Review of leiomyoma variants. *AJR Am J Roentgenol* 2015;205:912–921.

Bérangeer-Gilbert S, Sakly H, Ballester M, et al. Diagnostic value of MR imaging in the diagnosis of adnexal torsion. *Radiology* 2016;279:461–470.

Coutinho A Jr, Bittencourt LK, Pires CE, et al. MR imaging in deep pelvic endometriosis: a pictorial essay. *Radiographics* 2011;31:549–567.

Javadi S, Ganeshan DM, Qayyum A, Iyer RB, Bhosale P. Ovarian cancer, the revised FIGO staging system, and the role of imaging. *AJR Am J Roentgenol* 2016;206:1351–1360.

Lalwani N, Prasad SR, Vikram R, Shanbhogue AK, Huettner PC, Fasih N. Histologic, molecular, and cytogenetic features of ovarian cancers: implications for diagnosis and treatment. *Radiographics* 2011;31:625–646.

Micco M, Sala E, Lakhman Y, Hricak H, Vargas HA. Imaging features of uncommon gynecologic cancers. *AJR Am J Roentgenol* 2015;205:1346–1359.

Moyle PL, Kataoka MY, Nakai A, Takahata A, Reinhold C, Sala E. Nonovarian cystic lesions of the pelvis. *Radiographics* 2010;30:921–938.

Olpin JD, Moeni A, Willmore RJ, Heilbrun ME. MR imaging of Müllerian fusion anomalies. *Magn Reson Imaging Clin N Am* 2017;25:563–675.

Revzin MV, Mathur M, Dave HB, Macer ML, Spektor M. Pelvic inflammatory disease: multimodality imaging approach with clinical-pathologic correlation. *Radiographics* 2016;36:1579–1796.

Sahin H, Abdullazade S, Sanci M. Mature cystic teratoma of the ovary: a cutting edge overview on imaging features. *Insights Imaging* 2017;8:227–241.

Simpson WL Jr, Beitia LG, Mester J. Hysterosalpingography: a reemerging study. *Radiographics* 2006;26:419–431.

Takeuchi M, Matsuzaki K. Adenomyosis: usual and unusual imaging manifestations, pitfalls, and problem-solving MR imaging techniques. *Radiographics* 2011;31:99–115.

Takeuchi M, Matsuzaki K, Nishitani H. Manifestations of the female reproductive organs on MR images: changes induced by various physiologic states. *Radiographics* 2010;30:1147–1148.

Male Genital Tract

Barentsz JO, Richenberg J, Clements R, et al. ESUR prostate MR guidelines 2012. *Eur Radiol* 2012;22:746–757.

Barrett T, Haider MA. The emerging role of MRI in prostate cancer active surveillance and ongoing challenges. *AJR Am J Roentgenol* 2017;208:131–139.

Boonsirikamchai P, Choi S, Frank SJ, et al. MR imaging of prostate cancer in radiation oncology: what radiologists need to know. *Radiographics* 2013;33:741–761.

Li Y, Mongan J, Behr SC, et al. Beyond prostate adenocarcinoma: expanding the differential diagnosis in prostate pathologic conditions. *Radiographics* 2016;36:1055–1075.

Mohrs OK, Thoms H, Egner T, et al. MRI of patients with suspected scrotal or testicular lesions: diagnostic value in daily practice. *AJR Am J Roentgenol* 2012;199:609–615.

Moreno CC, Small WC, Camacho JC, et al. Testicular tumors: what radiologists need to know—differential diagnosis, staging, and management. *Radiographics* 2015;35:400–415.

Parker RA 3rd, Menias CO, Quazi R, et al. MR imaging of the penis and scrotum. *Radiographics* 2015;35:1033–1050.

Purysko AS, Rosenkrantz AB, Barentsz, Weinreb JC, Macura KJ. PI-RADS version 2: a pictorial update. *Radiographics* 2016;36:1354–1372.

Rosenkrantz AB, Tenaja SS. Radiologist, be aware: ten pitfalls that confound the interpretation of multiparametric prostate MRI. *AJR Am J Roentgenol* 2014;202:109–120.

Vargas HA, Akin O, Franiel T, et al. Normal central zone of the prostate and central zone involvement by prostate cancer: clinical and MR imaging implications. *Radiology* 2012;262:894–902.

SECTION IX

ULTRASONOGRAPHY

SECTION EDITOR: William E. Brant

CHAPTER 50 ■ ABDOMEN ULTRASOUND

WILLIAM E. BRANT

Ultrasound (US) is firmly established as a primary imaging modality for comprehensive evaluation of the abdomen including the abdominal organs, the peritoneal cavity, and the retroperitoneum. Its role includes screening for disease, evaluation and follow-up of known abnormalities, and guidance of biopsy, aspiration, and catheter drainage procedures. Comprehensive examination includes the use of Doppler and color flow imaging, as well as specialized techniques of transvaginal or transrectal US to demonstrate pelvic extension of disease. This chapter provides the basics for understanding effective use of US in examining the abdomen.

PERITONEAL CAVITY

Normal US Anatomy. The normal peritoneal cavity is a potential space best appreciated when fluid is present. The peritoneal membrane lines the abdominal cavity and covers, in whole or in part, the intra-abdominal organs. Numerous peritoneal ligaments, folds, and recesses are visualized when outlined by fluid within the peritoneal cavity. US examination for the presence of fluid includes inspection of the subdiaphragmatic and subhepatic regions, the pericolic gutters, and the pelvic cul-de-sac. Tiny volumes of intraperitoneal fluid are best detected by transvaginal US examination of the cul-de-sac. The focused assessment with sonography for trauma (FAST) scan has been defined to evaluate the peritoneal spaces for bleeding after trauma. This examination has been expanded to include the pleural and pericardial space to detect the presence of effusions. Firm transducer pressure and changes in patient position are needed to inspect between bowel loops for fluid collections. Solid organs and fluid serve as sonographic windows to the abdomen, and gas in the bowel, ribs, spine, and bony pelvis serve as obstacles.

Intraperitoneal Fluid. Fluid within the peritoneal cavity flows, under the effect of gravity, along peritoneal reflections to peritoneal recesses (Fig. 50.1). The hepatorenal recess (Morison pouch) and the pelvic cul-de-sac are the two most dependent recesses in the supine patient. They connect via the paracolic gutters. Fluid outlining intraperitoneal organs provides an opportunity to evaluate organ surface abnormalities, such as the fine nodularity of cirrhosis. Transudative ascites, urine, and bile are anechoic. Fluid with echogenic particles, layering debris, or septations may be exudative ascites, hemorrhage, pus, malignant ascites, or spilled gastrointestinal contents.

Free intraperitoneal fluid outlines recesses and compartments which retain their normal geometric shape. Loops of bowel float and sway freely within free fluid. Loculated fluid collections, abscesses, and cystic masses create their own space, displace bowel and adjacent organs, and are usually more round and tense.

Intraperitoneal Abscess. Although CT is commonly preferred for detection of small intraperitoneal abscesses, US readily demonstrates most abscesses and is effectively used to guide aspiration and catheter drainage (Fig. 50.2). Because abscesses most commonly form in the dependent recesses, the pelvis must be included in every examination. Abscesses appear as loculated collections of fluid that may be anechoic to densely echogenic. As loculated collections they displace bowel and abdominal organs. Fluid levels, internal debris, septations, thick walls, and gas within the abscess are common. Gas is brightly echogenic and associated with reverberation artifact and acoustic shadowing. An abscess containing extensive gas may be mistaken for gas-filled bowel and overlooked. Some abscesses appear solid. Changes in patient position show shifting of the particle pattern when liquid. Doppler and color flow US show the absence of internal blood vessels within echogenic fluid collections or the presence of blood flow within solid tissue.

Intraperitoneal Tumor. Metastases are the most common tumor of the peritoneal surface. Fluid and gravity distribute malignant cells throughout the peritoneal cavity where they implant upon visceral or parietal peritoneal surfaces. The greater omentum is fertile ground and thickens with tumor implantation to form "omental cake," a layer of solid tissue separating bowel from contact with the anterior abdominal wall (Fig. 50.3). Metastatic implants appear as hypoechoic solid masses of varying size on peritoneal surfaces. Ascites is usually present, commonly containing septations and echogenic debris. The most common tumors of origin are ovarian, colon, pancreas, and gastric carcinoma.

Primary peritoneal tumors include mesothelioma, desmoids, carcinoids, primary peritoneal serous papillary carcinoma, and lymphoma. These appear as predominantly hypoechoic solid masses. Acoustic shadows may arise from dense fibrous tissue or calcifications.

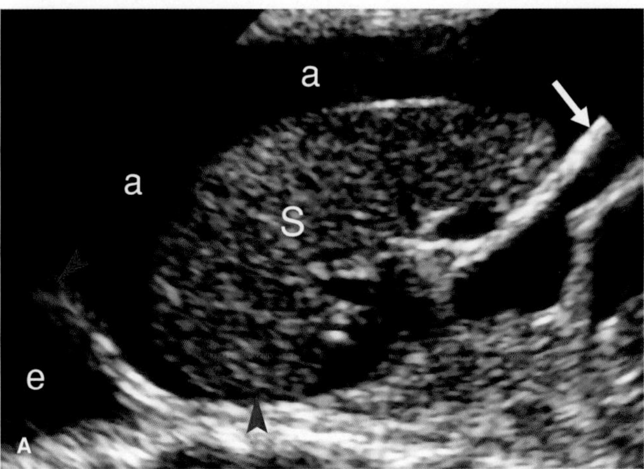

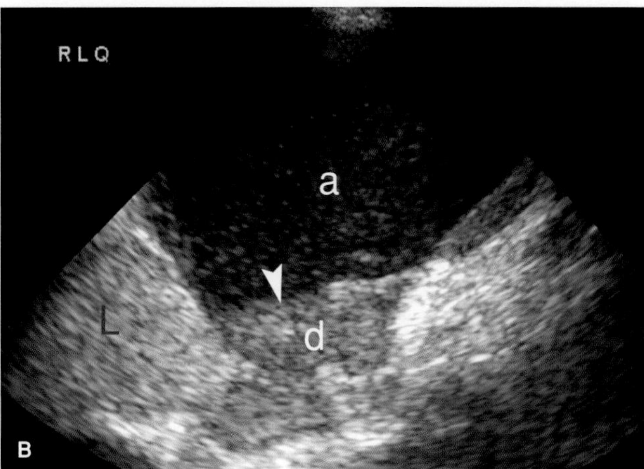

FIGURE 50.1. **Ascites. A:** Longitudinal US image shows anechoic ascites (*a*) surrounding the spleen (*S*). Fluid outlines the gastrosplenic ligament (*arrow*). Note the small bare area of the spleen (*blue arrowhead*) where reflections of the peritoneum from the spleen to the diaphragm prevent access of intraperitoneal fluid. A left pleural effusion (*e*) is seen above the diaphragm (*red arrowhead*). **B:** US image of the right lower quadrant (*RLQ*) of the abdomen reveals ascites (*a*) containing echogenic particulate matter. A fluid–fluid layer (*arrowhead*) is present between fluid ascites (*a*) and layering debris (*d*). This exudative ascites resulted from a bowel perforation. *L*, edge of the liver.

RETROPERITONEUM

Normal US Anatomy. The retroperitoneum is that portion of the abdomen behind the posterior parietal peritoneum. The anatomy of its three compartments is described in Chapter 40. US of the abdominal aorta and inferior vena cava (IVC) are discussed in Chapter 54. The crura of the diaphragm must not be mistaken for retroperitoneal adenopathy. Both are hypoechoic linear bands of muscle. The right crus is larger, more lobular, and inserts lower, extending to L3 vertebral body. The left crus is more uniform in thickness inserting on L1 and L2 vertebral bodies. The crura serve as landmarks for identification of the adrenal gland. The psoas and quadratus lumborum muscles show the typical hypoechoic pattern of muscle with longitudinally oriented echogenic fibrous strands dividing muscle bundles. Echogenic retroperitoneal fat surrounds and defines organs, vessels, and other structures.

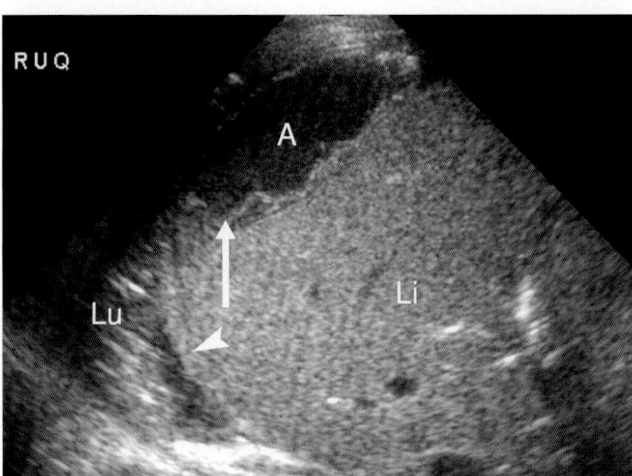

FIGURE 50.2. **Right Subphrenic Abscess.** Longitudinal US image of the right upper quadrant (*RUQ*) reveals a subphrenic abscess (*A*) displacing and indenting the liver (*Li*). The abscess contains echogenic fluid (pus) and is bounded by an inflammatory membrane (*arrow*). Atelectatic lung (*Lu*) and a tiny pleural effusion are present above the diaphragm (*arrowhead*).

Retroperitoneal Adenopathy. Enlarged individual lymph nodes are homogeneous, hypoechoic, and round or oval (Fig. 50.4). Accentuated sound transmission may be present, and some enlarged solid nodes are so hypoechoic they appear cystic. Solitary nodes larger than 1.5 cm in short-axis diameter, or multiple nodes larger than 1.0 cm, are considered to be pathologically enlarged. Lymphoma is characterized by confluence of enlarged nodes to form a solid mass which surrounds vessels and organs. Causes of retroperitoneal adenopathy are lymphoma (most common), tumor metastases (testicular, renal, pelvic, gastrointestinal malignancies and melanoma), and infection, especially in AIDS patients.

Retroperitoneal tumors are most commonly of mesenchymal origin and include liposarcoma, leiomyosarcoma, and malignant fibrous histiocytoma. These are aggressive tumors that invade organs and muscles and are difficult to remove surgically. Most are large, heterogeneous, and partially cystic. Germ cell tumors in the retroperitoneum may be primary or secondary, and benign or malignant. The sonographic features of the various tumors overlap and US examination does not yield a

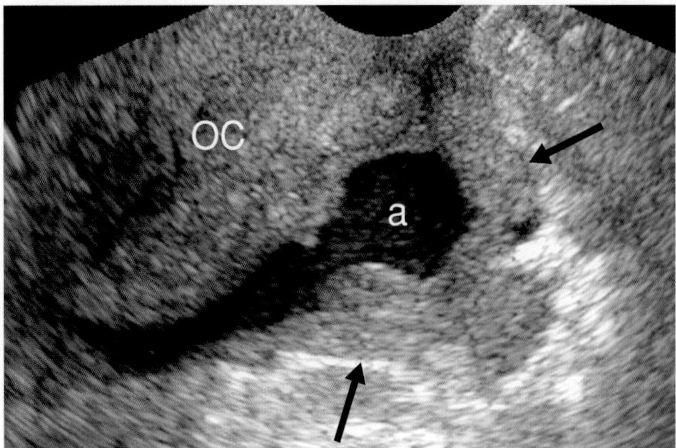

FIGURE 50.3. **Peritoneal Metastases.** US image shows solid tumor implanted on the omentum creating "omental cake" (*OC*). Solid tumor causes lumpy thickening of the peritoneal surfaces (*arrows*). Malignant ascites (*a*) contains floating echogenic debris. The primary tumor was ovarian carcinoma.

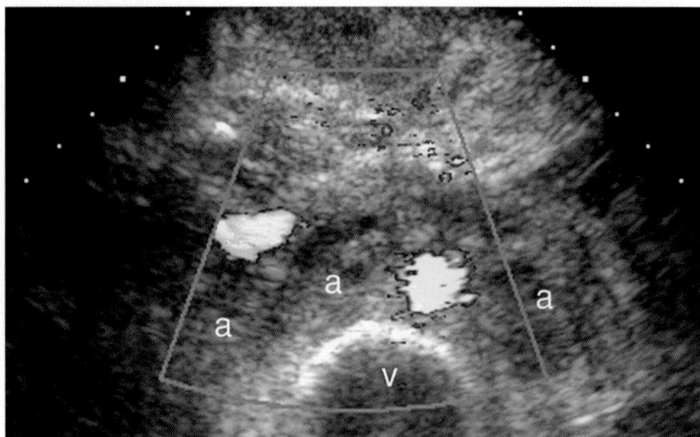

FIGURE 50.4. **Adenopathy—Lymphoma.** An axial plane US demonstrates confluent adenopathy (*a*) enveloping the inferior vena cava (*blue*) and the abdominal aorta (*yellow*). This appearance is typical of lymphoma. A vertebral body (*v*) casts an acoustic shadow posterior to the vessels.

specific diagnosis. Benign lipoma may be suggested when the tumor is isoechoic to retroperitoneal fat.

Retroperitoneal fluid collections include hemorrhage, infection, urinoma, pancreatic fluid collections, and cystic masses (lymphoceles, lymphangiomas, renal cysts, and teratomas). Portosystemic collaterals and other enlarged blood vessels are differentiated by Doppler US. As within the peritoneal cavity, retroperitoneal fluid may be anechoic or echogenic, with particulate cellular debris and layering fluid levels. Echogenic clotted blood may appear as a solid mass. Absence of internal vascularity on Doppler examination and change in appearance with time are distinguishing features.

LIVER

US is an efficient imaging method to screen patients for diffuse and focal hepatic disease. For focal liver metastases, its sensitivity approaches that of CT and MR; however its images are more difficult to reproduce for follow-up comparisons, and benign and malignant nodules cannot usually be distinguished. Contrast-enhanced US imaging shows promise in improving the ability of US to characterize benign and malignant hepatic lesions. Color Doppler US is valuable in the assessment of liver vasculature, the diagnosis of portal and hepatic vein thrombosis and portal hypertension, and in evaluating the vascularity of liver tumors.

Normal US Anatomy. The echogenicity of the liver parenchyma is homogeneous and equal to or slightly greater than that of the kidney (Fig. 50.5A). The surface of the normal liver is smooth and the inferior margin of the liver is sharp edged. The lobar and segmental anatomy of the liver are described and illustrated in Chapter 41. The hepatic veins are seen as echolucent tubes with thin walls that converge into the IVC. The portal veins, hepatic arteries, and bile ducts, encompassed by fibrofatty tissue, form the portal triads which are normally visualized as echogenic foci throughout the liver. Spectral and color flow Doppler US are essential to US examination of the liver to characterize mass lesions, demonstrate collateral vessels, and detect vascular abnormalities.

Fatty infiltration causes an increase in echogenicity of the liver making affected areas distinctly more echogenic than normal renal parenchyma. Fatty infiltration also increases the attenuation of the US beam diminishing visualization of the diaphragm and commonly requiring a lower-frequency transducer to examine deep portions of the liver (Fig. 50.5B). The hepatic echotexture appears coarsened and visualization of the portal triads is decreased. The various patterns of fatty infiltration are reviewed in Chapter 41. The "flip-flop" pattern of fatty infiltration as seen on US compared with CT is useful in confirming the diagnosis of focal fatty infiltration and focal fat sparing. Fat infiltrated areas are bright on US and dark on CT. Focally sparred areas within diffuse fatty infiltration are dark on US and bright on CT.

Acute hepatitis results in diffuse hepatic edema which reduces the echogenicity of the liver, resulting in a "*starry sky*" appearance. The portal triads appear unusually bright on the darkened background of edematous parenchyma. The starry sky appearance has also been described with diffuse leukemic or lymphomatous infiltrate, toxic shock syndrome, and diffuse decrease in glycogen stores in the liver.

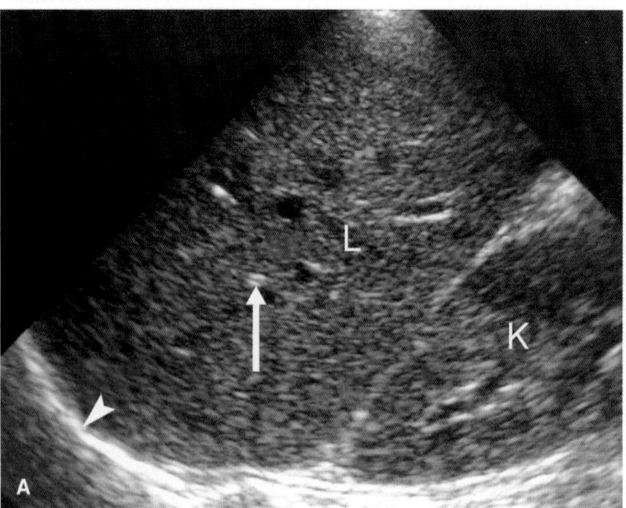

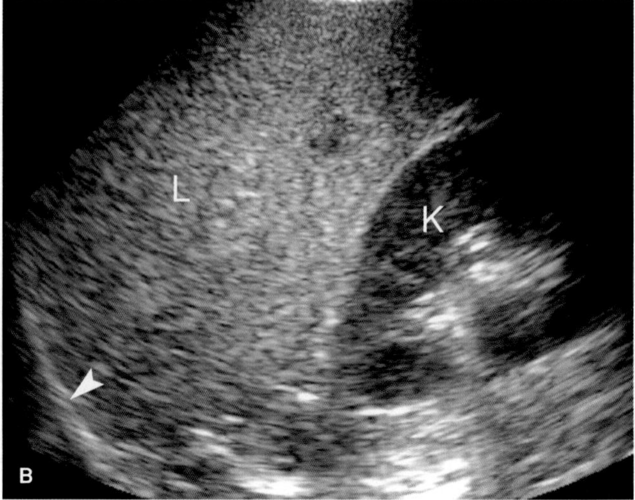

FIGURE 50.5. **Normal and Diffuse Fatty Liver. A:** Longitudinal US image demonstrates normal liver (*L*) and right kidney (*K*). The liver parenchyma is of uniform echogenicity, approximately equal to the parenchymal echogenicity of the kidney. The liver is well visualized to the level of the diaphragm (*arrowhead*). Small portal triad structures (*arrow*) are seen throughout the liver parenchyma. **B:** Diffuse fatty infiltration of the liver (*L*) markedly increases liver parenchymal echogenicity compared to that of the kidney (*K*). No portal triads are seen and the diaphragm (*arrowhead*) is less well visualized.

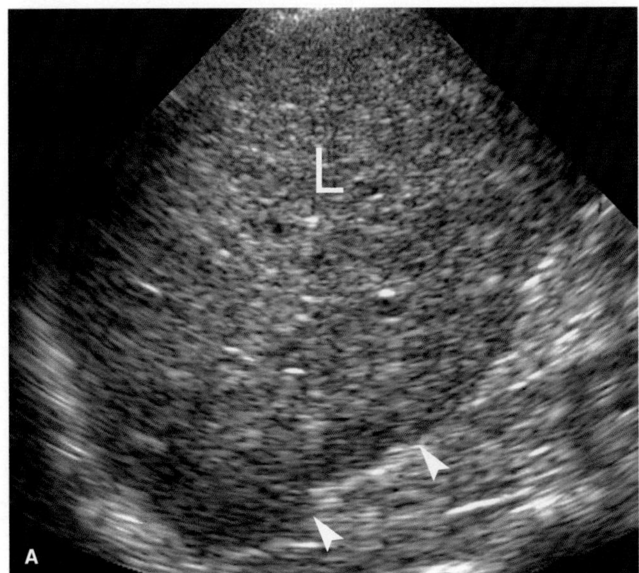

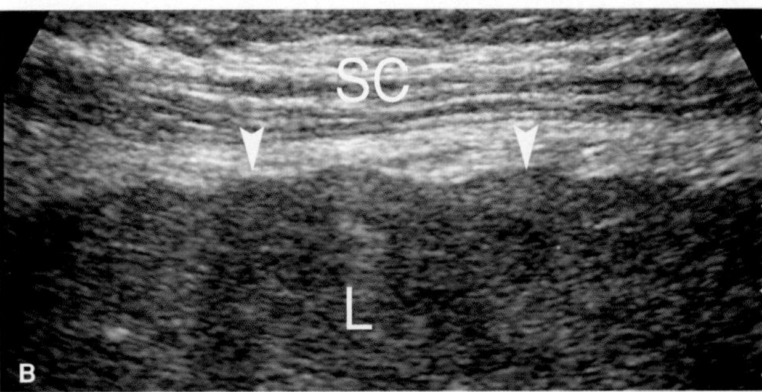

FIGURE 50.6. **Cirrhosis. A:** Longitudinal US image of the liver (*L*) shows coarsening of the echotexture, loss of visualization of portal triads, and nodularity characteristic of cirrhosis. The deep surface of the liver (*arrowheads*) shows the nodular contour typical of cirrhosis. Cirrhosis coarsens hepatic echotexture. Fatty infiltration increases hepatic echogenicity. **B:** A linear array transducer produces a detailed image of the liver (*L*) surface showing the nodular contour (*arrowheads*) of cirrhosis. *SC*, subcutaneous tissues. This technique is helpful in revealing the morphologic changes of cirrhosis.

Passive hepatic congestion refers to stasis of blood in the liver due to congestive heart failure. US findings include hepatomegaly, distention of the IVC and hepatic veins, and pulsatile portal vein flow seen on Doppler due to transmission of right atrial activity through congested sinusoids. Ascites, right pleural effusion, and pericardial effusion are often present.

Cirrhosis. US reflects the morphologic changes in the liver associated with cirrhosis. Hepatic echotexture is usually coarsened and heterogeneous with numerous vague nodules commonly evident (Fig. 50.6). The surface of the liver examined with high-frequency transducers shows abnormal fine or coarse nodularity. Echogenicity is increased in proportion to the degree of fatty infiltration. With alcoholic cirrhosis the right lobe is shrunken, and the left lobe and caudate lobe are enlarged. Advanced cirrhosis results in a small liver with a markedly nodular contour. The normal triphasic Doppler waveform of the hepatic veins is flattened in cirrhosis with loss of the reverse flow component caused by atrial systole. US is insensitive (<45%) to detection of malignancy in cirrhotic livers, however US demonstration of a discrete focal mass is highly predictive of malignancy.

US elastography techniques have emerged as an effective modality to stage the severity of fibrosis in chronic liver disease. It can be used to differentiate patients with little or no fibrosis from patients with severe fibrosis or cirrhosis. Biopsy can generally be avoided in these patients.

Portal Hypertension. US evidence of portal hypertension includes demonstration of portosystemic collateral vessels, dilation of the portal vein (>13 mm), dilation of the splenic and superior mesenteric veins (>10 mm), splenomegaly, and ascites. The hepatic artery is often enlarged and tortuous. Doppler demonstration of reversed (hepatofugal) flow in the portal vein is diagnostic of portal hypertension (Fig. 50.7). Flow in a dilated paraumbilical vein traversing the falciform ligament and anterior abdominal wall is also highly specific for portal hypertension. Color Doppler is very useful in the detection of splenorenal, retroperitoneal, and coronary vein collaterals.

Portal vein thrombosis is evidenced by the presence of echogenic clot within an enlarged portal vein (Fig. 50.8). Color Doppler confirms complete occlusion or demonstrates residual flow around the thrombus. The thrombus itself varies in appearance from anechoic to hyperechoic, depending upon the age of the thrombus. Tumor thrombus from invasion of the portal vein by hepatoma is confirmed by spectral Doppler demonstration of arterial waveforms within the thrombus in the portal vein. Cavernous transformation of the portal vein refers to formation of multiple tortuous collateral vessels that develop in the porta hepatis in response to chronic portal vein thrombosis.

Cysts are common and easily identified and characterized by US (Fig. 50.9). Benign hepatic cysts have US characteristics of simple cysts: anechoic fluid, thin walls, posterior acoustic enhancement. Thin septations are common. Size ranges from millimeters to 20 cm. Small cysts may mimic vessels on quick inspection. Doppler is useful to improve detection and confirm their avascular nature. *Biliary cystadenomas* are rare multilocular cystic lesions with malignant potential. US reveals a

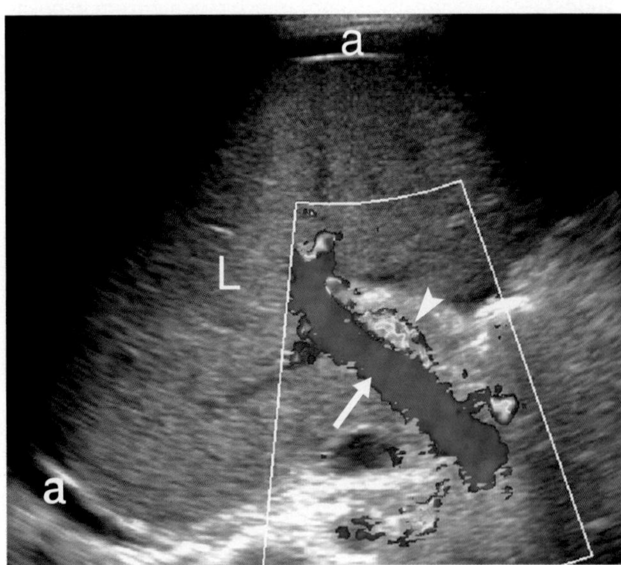

FIGURE 50.7. **Reversed Flow in the Portal Vein.** Color Doppler image through the porta hepatis shows reversed flow (out of the liver, *L*) in the portal vein (*arrow*, *blue*). The hepatic artery (*arrowhead*) is dilated and tortuous. Flow within the hepatic artery (*arrowhead*) is mixed in color due to aliasing. The predominant color is red indicating normal flow direction into the liver. Reversed flow in the portal vein is indicative of advanced portal hypertension. A small volume of ascites (*a*) surrounds the liver.

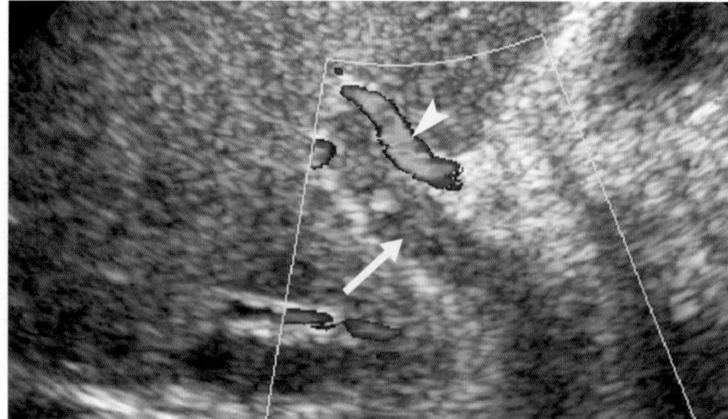

FIGURE 50.8. **Portal Vein Thrombosis.** Color Doppler US image through the porta hepatis shows echogenic thrombus (*arrow*) completely filling the portal vein. The hepatic artery (*arrowhead*) is mildly dilated and shows blood flow into the liver (*red*) and aliasing (*green*).

solitary cystic mass with thick walls, mural nodules, and multiple internal septations. *Biliary cystadenocarcinomas* have a similar appearance and cannot be differentiated from benign lesions by imaging alone. Both benign and malignant forms show slow growth.

Cavernous hemangiomas are commonly identified on hepatic sonograms. The classic US appearance is a sharply marginated homogeneous hyperechoic mass (Fig. 50.10). Doppler usually shows no internal blood flow although, on occasion, with high sensitivity settings very low–velocity flow is detected. Large lesions may contain hypoechoic thrombosis, fibrosis, and calcification. Most lesions remain stable in size over time, but about 2% show enlargement. Classic-appearing lesions in patients with normal liver function tests usually require no follow-up. Atypical lesions should have a 6-month follow-up US or be confirmed with other imaging modalities as discussed in Chapter 41.

Metastases vary greatly in appearance ranging from hypo- to hyperechoic and from homogeneous to heterogeneous to calcified (Fig. 50.11). Metastatic disease must be considered in the differential diagnosis of all solid and atypical cystic lesions in the liver. In 90% of cases metastatic disease is multifocal in the liver.

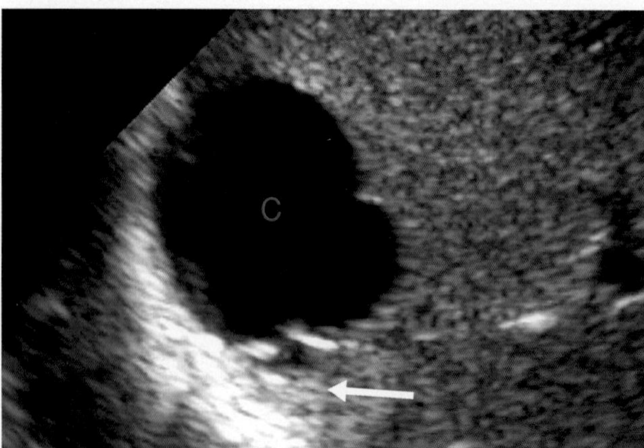

FIGURE 50.9. **Benign Hepatic Cyst.** A hepatic cyst (C) has sharply defined wall and anechoic contents. Benign hepatic cysts tend to occur in clusters, have thin septations, and lobulated contours. No solid nodular component is evident. Accentuated through-transmission (*arrow*) is evident.

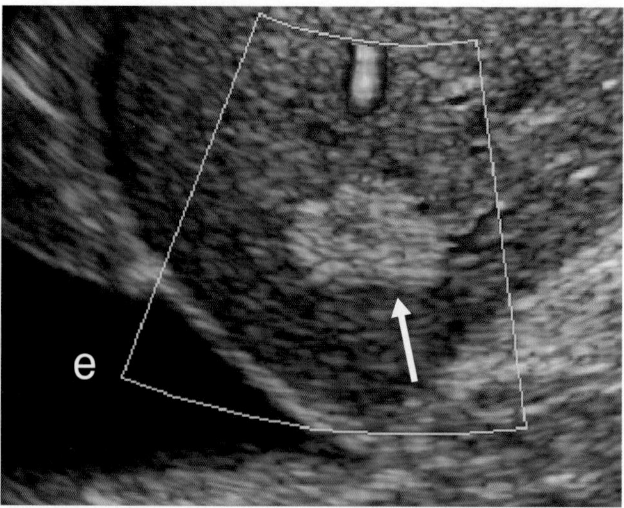

FIGURE 50.10. **Cavernous Hemangioma.** Power Doppler image shows the characteristic US appearance of a cavernous hemangioma (*arrow*). The mass is highly echogenic compared to surrounding liver, has sharply defined but lobulated borders, and shows no internal blood flow. Power Doppler is particularly sensitive to detection of slow flow. This patient also has a pleural effusion (*e*).

Lymphoma in the liver is suggested by the presence of multiple hypoechoic liver nodules in the presence of lymphadenopathy and splenomegaly.

Hepatocellular carcinoma (HCC) may be solitary, multifocal, or diffuse (Fig. 50.12). Detection in the diseased liver is commonly difficult with US. Most HCCs are hypervascular with prominent vascularity shown by color Doppler. Contrast-enhanced US shows arterial phase enhancement with washout during portal venous phase. Tumor invasion of the portal and hepatic veins is common. HCC may be hyperechoic with internal fat to hypoechoic and heterogeneous due to nonliquefactive necrosis. Any solid mass detected by US in a diseased liver, including echogenic lesions resembling hemangioma, is suspicious for HCC.

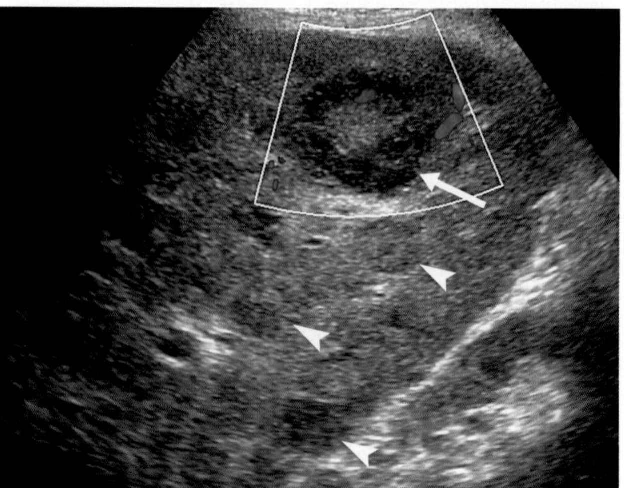

FIGURE 50.11. **Metastases.** Color Doppler shows limited vascularity to a liver mass lesion (*arrow*) with a target appearance commonly seen with metastatic disease. Numerous smaller nodules (*arrowheads*) seen throughout the liver show poor margination and variable echogenicity. Biopsy confirmed squamous cell carcinoma metastatic to the liver.

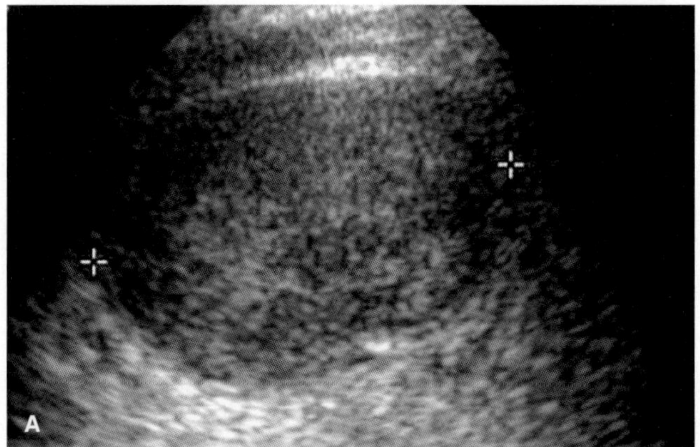

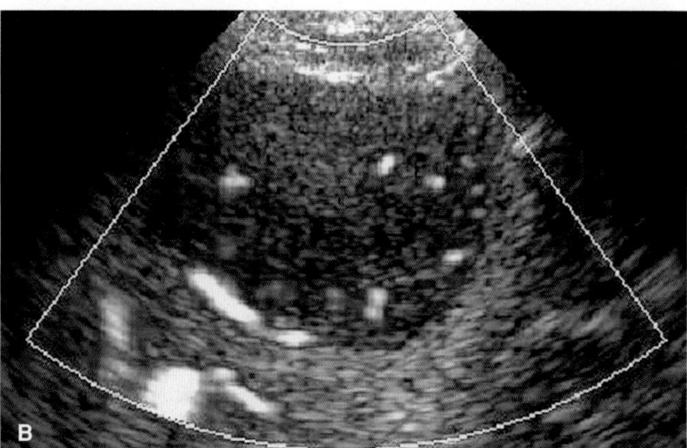

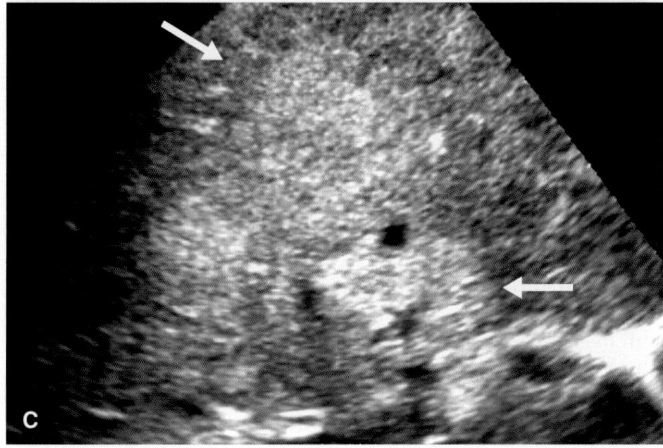

FIGURE 50.12. **Hepatocellular Carcinoma. A:** A well-differentiated hepatocellular carcinoma appears as a well-defined mass (between *cursors*, +) within an echogenic cirrhotic liver. **B:** Power Doppler interrogation of the same lesion as in **A** shows prominent internal blood flow commonly found with hepatocellular carcinoma. **C:** A poorly differentiated hepatocellular carcinoma appears as multiple poorly defined echogenic masses (*arrows*) within a cirrhotic liver.

Abscesses usually appear as complex fluid collections containing echogenic fluid, fluid–fluid layers, or gas (Fig. 50.13). Healed abscesses commonly calcify.

Microabscesses occur most commonly in immunocompromised patients with fungal or parasitic septicemia. Target lesions with central echogenic spot and peripheral hypoechoic halo are common. The differential diagnosis of multiple small (<10 mm) lesions in the liver is given in Table 40.6.

Other masses, including hepatic adenoma, focal nodular hyperplasia, sarcoma, and peripheral cholangiocarcinoma, have a varied and nonspecific sonographic appearance. They range from hypo- to hyperechoic and may contain areas of internal hemorrhage, necrosis, fibrosis, or calcification. Characterization of these nonspecific masses is often best performed with three-phase contrast-enhanced MDCT. The final diagnosis often depends on percutaneous biopsy.

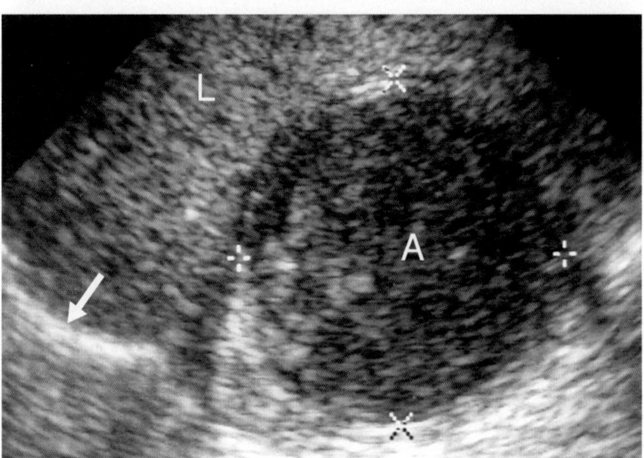

FIGURE 50.13. **Amebic Abscess.** A well-defined hypodense mass (*A*, between *calipers*) is seen in the right lobe of the liver (*L*). Note the proximity to the right hemidiaphragm (*arrow*). Amebic abscesses in the liver may rupture through the diaphragm into the right pleural space.

Transjugular intrahepatic portosystemic shunt (TIPS) has become a commonly performed procedure for the treatment of the complications of portal hypertension. However, shunt dysfunction is common (up to 80% in the first year) and US is the method of choice to evaluate for shunt patency and malfunction (Fig. 50.14). Both bare and covered expansile wire stents are used to create a shunt between the portal and hepatic venous systems. Bare stents have a high incidence of failure and are routinely evaluated with Doppler 24 hours after shunt placement. Covered stents have a lower TIPS malfunction rate. Covered stents transiently block sound transmission because of air bubbles in the graft for up to a week following placement. Routine US surveillance of covered TIPS is usually performed 7 to 14 days following placement. Doppler US is used to confirm patency and flow direction in the main portal vein and right and left portal branches, and to measure flow velocities in the portal venous end, midportion, and hepatic venous end of the TIPS. In a normally functioning TIPS flow direction in the portal vein is antegrade (hepatopetal—toward the TIPS) while in the right and left branches of the portal vein flow in most cases becomes retrograde (hepatofugal—toward the TIPS) after TIPS placement. Within the TIPS, spectral Doppler shows turbulent venous waveforms with normal flow velocities of 95 to 200 cm/s. Flow velocities of 50 to 95 cm/s are considered to be indicative of insignificant TIPS stenosis. Flow velocities below 50 cm/s, or a focal jet within the TIPS or at the hepatic vein outflow >200 cm/s, indicate significant TIPS stenosis. Conversion of hepatofugal to hepatopedal (away from the TIPS) flow in the

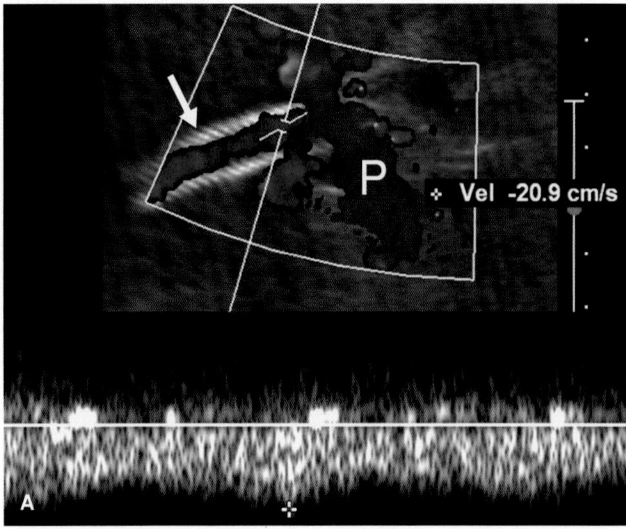

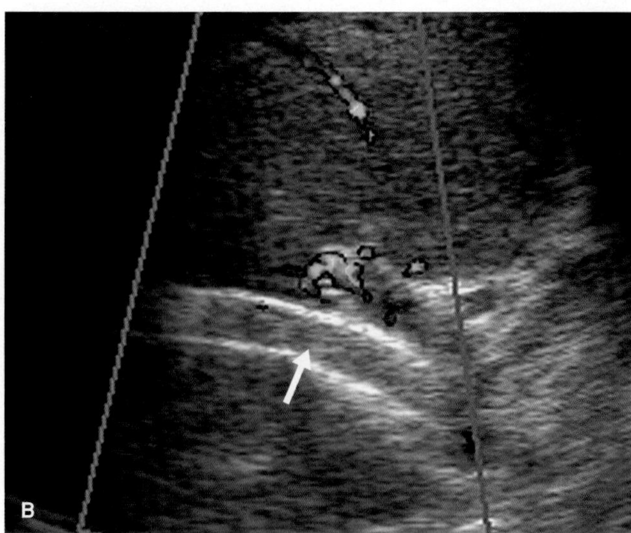

FIGURE 50.14. Transjugular Intrahepatic Portosystemic Shunt (TIPS) Malfunction. A: Color and spectral Doppler assessment of a TIPS (*arrow*) show abnormally low-velocity flow (20.9 cm/s) at the portal venous end (*P*). On further Doppler interrogation this finding was shown to be caused by high-grade stenosis at the hepatic venous end. **B:** TIPS in another patient is completely occluded, showing no blood flow on color Doppler imaging. The TIPS is filled with echogenic thrombus (*arrow*). Note the highly reflective walls of the stents in both patients.

right or left branches of the portal vein is an indirect sign of TIPS malfunction. With TIPS occlusion thrombus fills the lumen of the shunt. TIPS malfunction is addressed angiographically.

Liver Transplants. US with Doppler is the imaging method of choice for postoperative evaluation of liver transplants (Fig. 50.15). Liver transplantations are performed using living donors (either right lobe or left lobe transplants) or cadaveric full liver transplants in both adults and children. Peritransplant fluid collections are common in the immediate posttransplant period. Simple anechoic fluid collections include ascites, bile, and lymph. Fluid with particulate matter is usually pus or

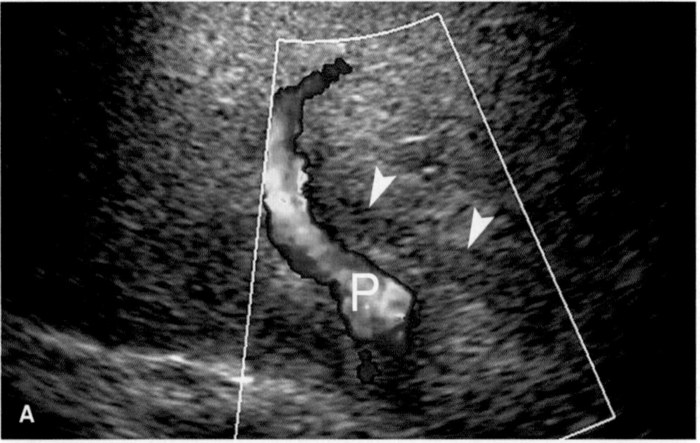

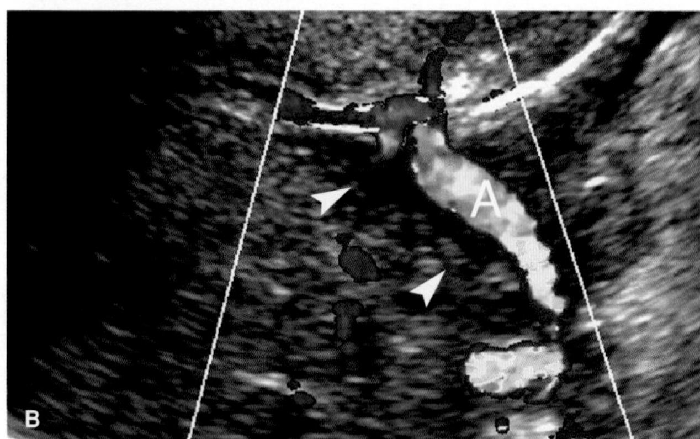

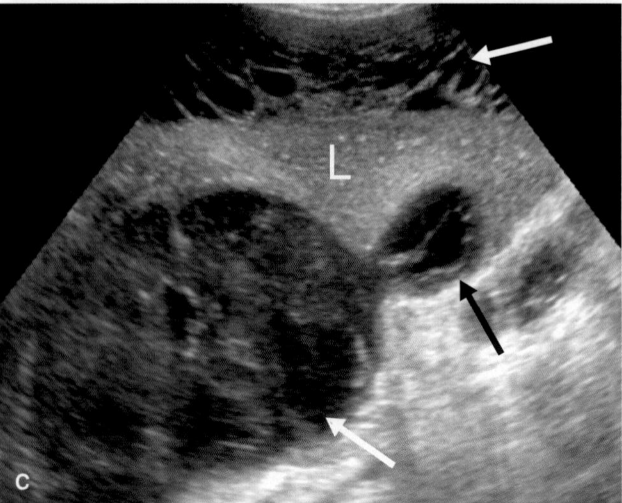

FIGURE 50.15. Liver Transplant. A: The hepatic artery (*arrowheads*) of the liver transplant is filled with thrombus and shows no flow on color Doppler imaging. This constitutes a surgical emergency requiring immediate revascularization to save the transplant. The portal vein (*P*) is widely patent. **B:** In this patient 2 days post liver transplant the portal vein (*arrowheads*) is completely occluded and filled with thrombus. The hepatic artery (*A*) is widely patent. This uncommon complication also requires correction with thrombolysis, angioplasty, or stent placement. **C:** Multiple complex septated fluid collections (*arrows*) surround and indent the transplant liver (*L*). The patient did not become infected and all fluid collections spontaneously resolved. Peritransplant hematomas and seromas are common following liver transplantation.

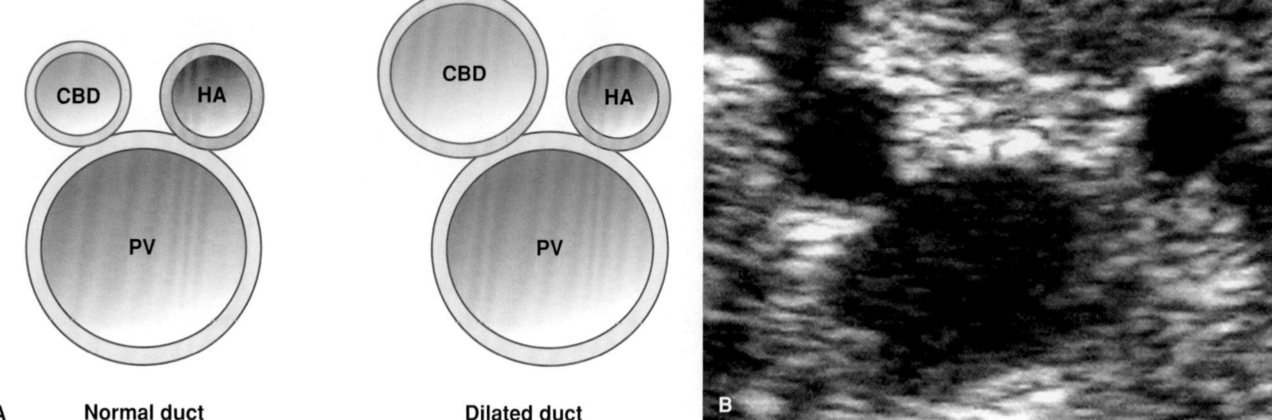

FIGURE 50.16. **"Mickey Mouse" Configuration of the Portal Triad. A:** A drawing demonstrates the anatomic relationships of the common bile duct (*CBD*), hepatic artery (*HA*), and portal vein (*PV*). Dilation of the common bile duct enlarges Mickey's right ear. **B:** US image of normal Mickey Mouse.

blood. Hepatic artery complications account for 60% of vascular complications and include thrombosis, stenosis, and pseudoaneurysms. Thrombosis and stenosis of the portal vein or IVC are uncommon. Bile leaks, bile duct anastomotic strictures, necrosis of bile ducts, and stones in the bile ducts account for 25% of complications. Posttransplantation lymphoproliferative disorder may occur 4 to 12 months following transplantation. Focal solid hypoechoic masses may be seen within or adjacent to the transplanted liver. HCC is a risk for the immunocompromised posttransplant patient.

BILE DUCTS

Normal US Anatomy. Intrahepatic bile ducts run in the portal triads in the company of the portal veins and hepatic arteries. Normal intrahepatic ducts are visualized with current high-resolution US. Intrahepatic ducts normally do not exceed 2 mm in diameter in the central liver or 40% of the diameter of the adjacent portal vein. The junction of the right lobe and left lobe bile ducts to form the common hepatic duct marks the division between the intra- and extrahepatic portions of the biliary tree. The junction of the cystic duct with the common hepatic duct marks the commencement of the common bile duct. Because this junction is seldom visualized with US, the generic term "common duct" is used to identify the duct in the porta hepatis. The common duct courses anterior to the main portal vein, the right portal vein, and the right hepatic artery in the portal region. The hepatic artery is commonly tortuous in the porta hepatis, but the common duct runs a straight course parallel to the portal vein. This straight portion of the common duct is routinely measured, although the normal limit of diameter for the adult population remains controversial. All agree that a common duct diameter ≤6 mm is normal for an adult. Some studies suggest that the normal duct dilates with age (1 mm per decade; an 8-mm duct would be normal for an 80-year-old patient) and that the duct dilates following cholecystectomy. Other studies refute these claims. It seems appropriate that an asymptomatic patient with a duct >7 mm could be followed for evidence of change. A symptomatic patient deserves further evaluation with magnetic resonance cholangiopancreatography (MRCP) or endoscopic retrograde cholangiopancreatography (ERCP).

As the portal triad structures course through the free edge of the hepatoduodenal ligament, a "Mickey Mouse" configuration is formed with the common duct forming Mickey's right ear (Fig. 50.16). The normal common bile duct can be traced descending adjacent to the pancreatic head to its insertion at the ampulla of Vater. Normal variants that may cause confusion include a "replaced" right hepatic artery arising from the superior mesenteric artery and coursing between the portal vein and IVC to the porta hepatis. An elongated gallbladder neck may be mistaken for a dilated common duct. Low insertion of the cystic duct causes the appearance of two common ducts. Doppler identification of vascular structures is helpful in confusing cases.

Dilation of the Biliary Tree. Dilated intrahepatic ducts are tortuous like the branches of an oak tree, exceed 40% of the diameter of the adjacent portal vein, and are visualized in the periphery of the liver. US shows "too many tubes" in the liver, and color Doppler US offers rapid differentiation of patent blood vessels and dilated bile ducts (Fig. 50.17). Dilated extrahepatic ducts exceed 6 to 7 mm in diameter, and appear as enlargement of Mickey's right ear in the hepatoduodenal ligament. The dilated duct should be followed to the level of obstruction, where careful evaluation will demonstrate the cause of obstruction in 80% of patients. Echogenic material within dilated bile ducts is seen with biliary stasis and hemobilia.

Choledocholithiasis. Stones in the bile ducts appear as echogenic objects within the lumen of the duct (Fig. 50.18).

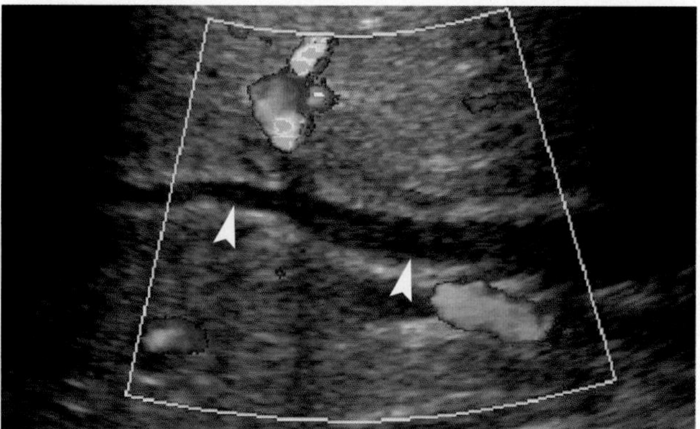

FIGURE 50.17. **Bile Duct Dilation.** Color Doppler US makes it easy to differentiate dilated bile ducts (*arrowheads*) from blood vessels showing blood flow in color.

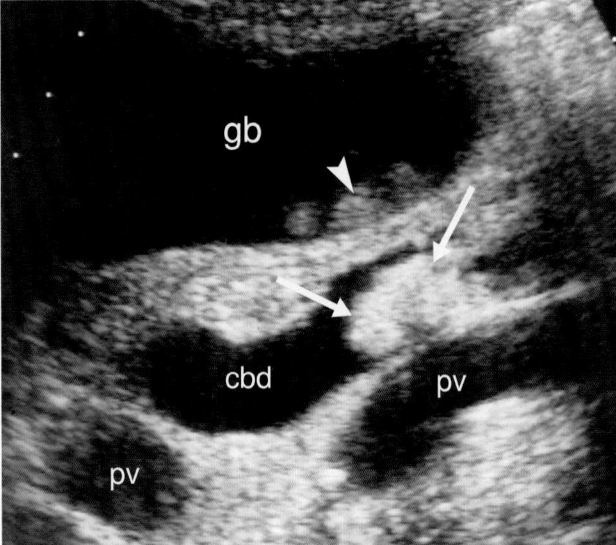

FIGURE 50.18. **Choledocholithiasis.** US image of the porta hepatis demonstrates a large stone (*arrows*) obstructing the common bile duct (*cbd*) and resulting in its dilation (13-mm diameter). The gallbladder (*gb*) is dilated and contains several nonshadowing sludge balls (*arrowhead*) formed as a result of biliary stasis. *pv*, portal vein.

Unfortunately, not all intraluminal stones will cast a distinct acoustic shadow. Technique must be optimized to demonstrate shadowing. Nonetheless, US detection of obstructing common duct stones is only about 75% sensitive. Abrupt termination of a dilated common duct is an indication for MR cholangiography. Calcification in the hepatic artery may mimic the appearance of stones or gas in the biliary tree.

Gas in the biliary tree is most commonly the result of surgical procedures, such as sphincterotomy or choledochoenterostomy (see Table 41.9). Additional causes include gas-producing infection, fistulous connection with the intestinal tract (gallstone ileus, perforating duodenal ulcer), and trauma. Air in bile ducts causes bright linear or globular reflections often with shadowing and ring-down artifacts (Fig. 50.19). Air will move in the biliary tree with changes in patient positioning. Ducts are usually dilated when air is present.

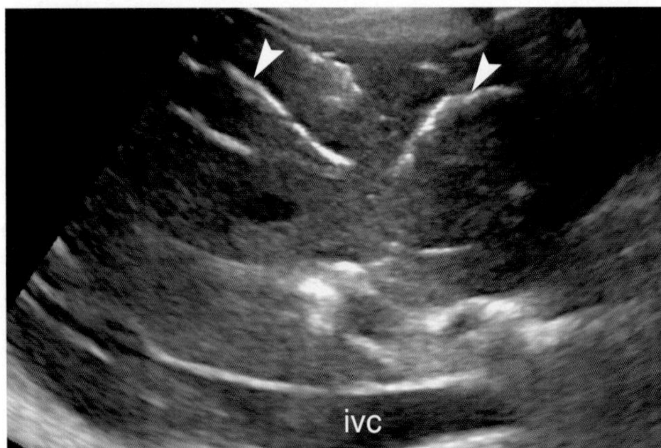

FIGURE 50.19. **Gas in the Biliary Tree.** Longitudinal image of the liver shows a series of bright linear echoes (*arrowheads*) corresponding to gas in the intrahepatic biliary tree. The linear echoes moved and changed in appearance with alterations in patient position. This patient had undergone a sphincterotomy because of gallstone disease. The inferior vena cava (*ivc*) is evident.

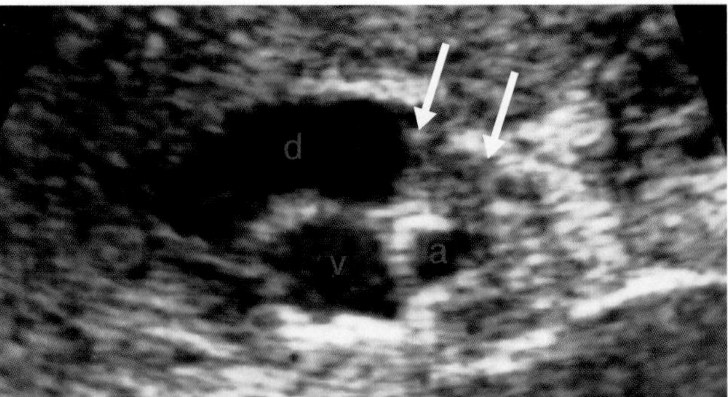

FIGURE 50.20. **Cholangiocarcinoma.** Tumor (*arrows*) obstructs and dilates the common bile duct (*d*) in the porta hepatis. *v*, portal vein; *a*, hepatic artery.

Cholangiocarcinoma. Hilar cholangiocarcinoma (Klatskin tumor) and extrahepatic cholangiocarcinoma tend to be small (<3 cm) when they present with biliary obstruction. US demonstrates the tumor as a focal mass at the point of obstruction (Fig. 50.20), nodular thickening of the bile duct wall, or polypoid intraluminal mass. The visualized mass is most commonly isoechoic with the liver parenchyma but may be hypo- or hyperechoic. Abrupt termination of a dilated duct without a mass being seen may be the only finding. Adjacent portal veins may be invaded and obstructed by tumor.

Recurrent pyogenic cholangiohepatitis, also referred to as "oriental" cholangiohepatitis is related to infestation of the biliary tree by parasites. Causative organisms include *Clonorchis sinensis*, *Opisthorchis viverrini* and *felineus*, and *Fasciola hepatica*. US reveals bile ducts that are focally dilated or stenotic. Flukes in the bile ducts appear as nonshadowing echogenic foci. Gallstones may or may not be present as well. Debris ("biliary mud") may fill and layer within dilated ducts. Most patients originate from Southeast Asian countries where the disease is endemic.

AIDS-related cholangitis features dilated intra- and extrahepatic bile ducts with thickening of the walls of the bile ducts and gallbladder. Sludge is commonly seen, but stones are usually not present. A unique finding is an echogenic nodule representing edema of the papilla of Vater at the termination of the dilated common bile duct.

Biliary Ascariasis. Worms that colonize the intestinal tract may find their way into the biliary tree and gallbladder. Living worms may obstruct the biliary tree and gallbladder and cause cholangitis, cholecystitis, and pancreatitis with a high associated mortality. Worms are seen by US as moving tubular echogenic structures with an echolucent core.

Congenital Biliary Cysts. The classification of congenital biliary cysts is illustrated in Chapter 41. US is excellent in demonstrating the morphology of cystic masses and their relationship to the biliary tree.

GALLBLADDER

Normal US Anatomy. The gallbladder is found on the undersurface of the liver with the gallbladder neck positioned in the interlobar fissure. Normal bile is anechoic. The normal wall does not exceed 3 mm in thickness (Fig. 50.21). The mucosa is echogenic and the smooth muscle layer of the wall is hypoechoic. The diameter of the gallbladder is less than 4 cm in 96% of normals. Length of the gallbladder is highly variable

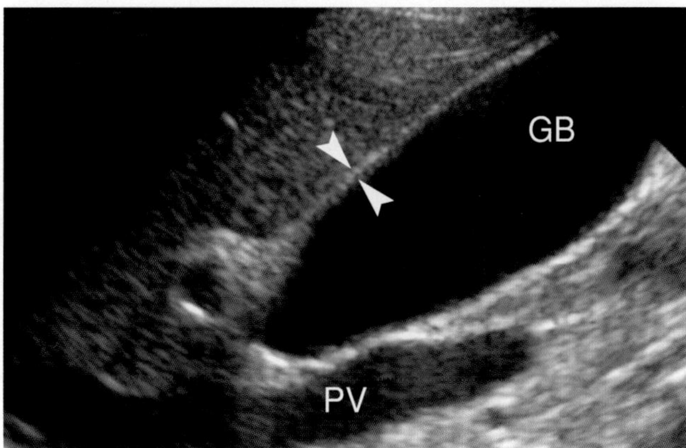

FIGURE 50.21. **Normal Gallbladder.** Sagittal image shows the normal appearance of the gallbladder (*GB*) distended with normal anechoic bile by a 4-hour fast. The gallbladder wall is routinely measured (*arrowheads*) between the lumen of the gallbladder and the parenchyma of the liver. This standardized measurement includes the wall of the gallbladder, the capsule of the liver, and any tissue, edema, or fluid between the two. The normal measurement does not exceed 3 mm. The portal vein (*PV*) is evident beneath the gallbladder.

and measurement is not diagnostically useful. Most patients are examined after an overnight fast although a 4-hour fast is usually sufficient to ensure gallbladder distention. Patients are examined in multiple positions to displace gallstones and demonstrate their mobility. The neck region should be carefully examined to avoid overlooking impacted stones. Normal folds in the gallbladder neck and cystic duct may cause acoustic shadows and mimic gallstones.

Echogenic Bile. Bile becomes echogenic when it is highly concentrated and cholesterol crystals and calcium bilirubinate granules precipitate as *sludge*. Sludge commonly layers in the gallbladder and may become quite viscous and form tumefactive sludge or "sludge balls" (Fig. 50.22). Sludge balls usually move within the gallbladder but do not cast acoustic shadows. Floating cholesterol crystals are seen as bright reflectors with short comet tail artifacts. Air in bile has a similar appearance. Sludge is not definitive evidence of gallbladder disease but is indicative of prolonged lack of bile turnover in the gallbladder. Prolonged fasting is the most common cause, but sludge is usually present with gallbladder and biliary obstruction. Sludge is not produced by the routine overnight fast advised in preparation for gallbladder examination. Additional causes of echogenic bile are blood, pus, and parasites.

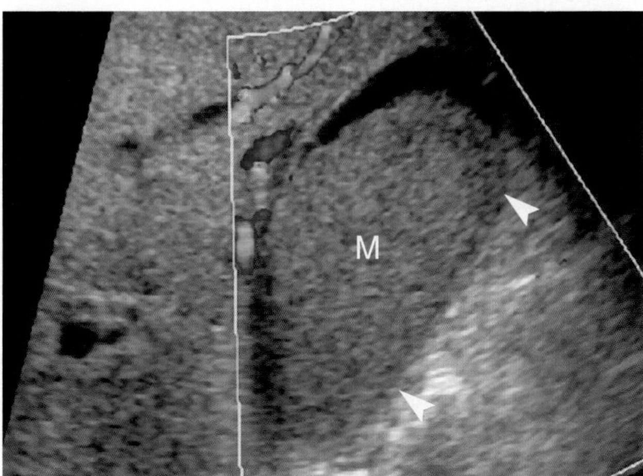

FIGURE 50.22. **Echogenic Bile—Large Sludge Ball.** Highly concentrated echogenic bile fills the gallbladder (*arrowheads*) producing an echogenic mass (*M*). Color Doppler US is essential to verify the lack of blood flow within the mass confirming echogenic bile and excluding gallbladder carcinoma.

TABLE 50.1

CAUSES OF GALLBLADDER WALL THICKENING

Contracted gallbladder after eating
Gallbladder disease
Acute cholecystitis
Chronic cholecystitis
Adenomyomatosis
Gallbladder carcinoma
AIDS cholangiopathy
Sclerosing cholangitis
Nonbiliary disease
Hypoproteinemia
Ascites
Edema due to congestive heart failure
Hepatitis
Portal hypertension
Portal lymph node obstruction
Cirrhosis

Thickened Gallbladder Wall. The gallbladder wall is considered thickened when it exceeds 3 mm as measured between the gallbladder lumen and the liver parenchyma. Causes of thickening include gallbladder disease and nonbiliary processes (Table 50.1). The most common causes are ascites, hypoproteinemia, and cholecystitis. Correlation of imaging findings and clinical presentation will usually determine the cause.

Gallstones. US is the imaging method of choice for detection of gallstones with a sensitivity of greater than 90%. Gallstones appear within the gallbladder lumen as echogenic objects which cast acoustic shadows and move with changes in patient position (Fig. 50.23). When these findings are present, specificity for gallstones is 100%. However, the demonstration of acoustic shadowing is strongly dependent on technique. When shadows are not evident with a suspected gallstone, a switch to a higher-frequency transducer with focal zone adjusted at the depth of the stone will commonly demonstrate the elusive shadow.

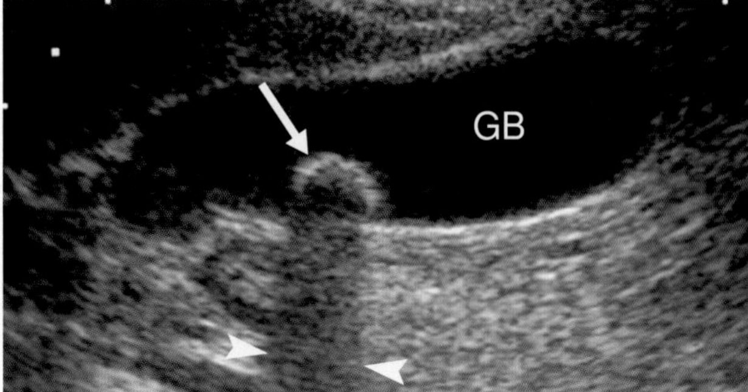

FIGURE 50.23. **Gallstone.** US demonstrates an echogenic mass (*arrow*) within the gallbladder (*GB*). The mass casts a prominent acoustic shadow (between *arrowheads*) caused by absorption of sound. Moving the patient into the upright position resulted in a change in position of the gallstone—the "rolling stone" sign.

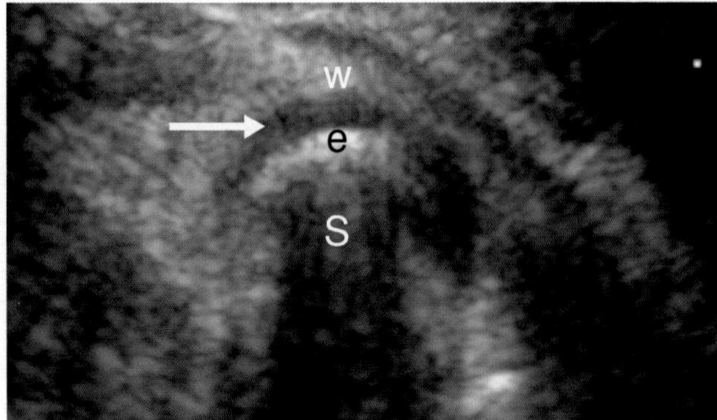

FIGURE 50.24. **Wall-Echo-Shadow Sign.** A thin layer of bile (*arrow*) separates the gallbladder wall (*w*) from the bright echo (*e*) of gallstones, which fill the gallbladder and cast a dense acoustic shadow (*S*). This appearance has also been called the "double-arc shadow sign."

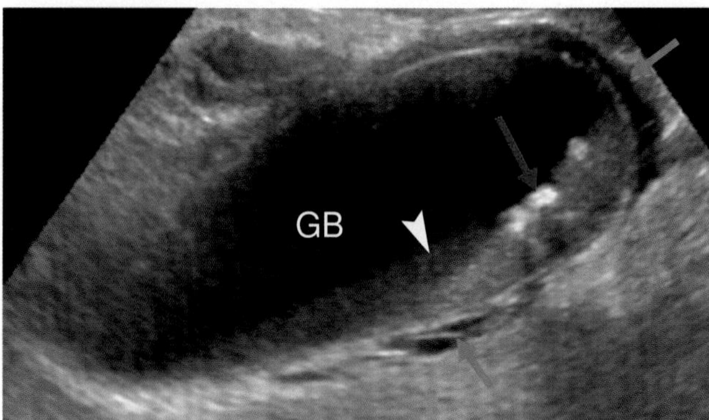

FIGURE 50.26. **Acute Cholecystitis.** US image through the long axis of the gallbladder (*GB*) demonstrates layering sludge (*arrowhead*) containing small shadowing gallstones (*red arrow*). The gallbladder wall (*blue arrows*) is thickened and edematous. The layering echogenic bile gives evidence of bile stasis. A sonographic Murphy sign was present. At surgery a gallstone was impacted in the gallbladder neck.

Gallstones may be nonmobile due to adhesion to the gallbladder wall, but acoustic shadowing should be demonstrable. Cholesterol polyps and adenomatous polyps are nonmobile, nonshadowing, soft tissue nodules attached to the gallbladder wall. Sludge balls appear as echogenic foci that move, or are adherent to the wall, but do not shadow.

Wall-Echo-Shadow (WES) Sign. When the gallbladder is completely filled with gallstones, a confident diagnosis becomes more difficult because the gallbladder resembles an air-filled loop of bowel. The WES sign is definitive evidence of a stone-filled gallbladder (Fig. 50.24). Gallstones produce a "clean" dark shadow, and air in bowel produces a "dirty" brighter shadow.

Polyps appear as echogenic nonshadowing nodules that extend from the gallbladder wall (Fig. 50.25). Most are cholesterol polyps, which are usually smaller than 1 cm and are commonly multiple. Adenomatous polyps are rare and indistinguishable by US from cholesterol polyps. Polyps larger than 1 cm may be malignant.

Acute Cholecystitis. US is commonly performed in patients who present with acute right upper quadrant pain. US evidence of acute cholecystitis includes (Fig. 50.26) (a) gallstones, (b) thickened gallbladder wall, (c) focal gallbladder tenderness elicited by transducer pressure directly over the gallbladder (positive sonographic Murphy sign), (d) pericholecystic fluid, (e) dilated gallbladder, and (f) Doppler evidence of wall hyperemia. A positive Murphy sign is highly predictive of acute cholecystitis (92%). A negative or equivocal Murphy sign is evidence against acute cholecystitis. A striated appearance of a thickened gallbladder wall is evidence of gangrenous cholecystitis. Pericholecystic fluid collections larger than 1 cm are evidence of gallbladder perforation. The absence of gallstones is not evidence against cholecystitis in patients who are at risk for *acalculous cholecystitis*. These patients usually have a prolonged illness associated with major surgery, trauma, burns, prolonged hospitalization, parenteral nutrition, and sepsis.

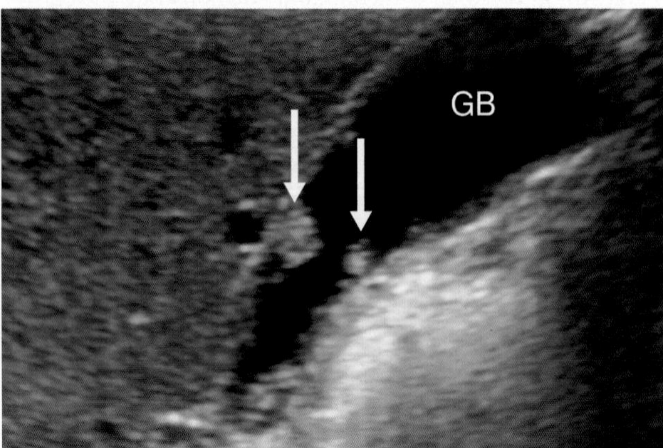

FIGURE 50.25. **Cholesterol Polyp.** Echogenic nodules (*arrows*) extend from the wall of the gallbladder (*GB*) projecting into the lumen. The nodules do not cast acoustic shadows and do not move with changes in patient position. The presence of multiple cholesterol polyps has been called *cholesterolosis* of the gallbladder.

Emphysematous cholecystitis is usually due to ischemia in elderly diabetics. Gas develops in the gallbladder wall and lumen in association with gas-producing bacterial infection of the gallbladder. Perforation occurs commonly and mortality is high. The diagnosis is suggested on US by bright reflections in the gallbladder wall associated with ring-down artifact. Gas bubbles in the lumen move and produce comet tail artifacts. Air may be present in the bile ducts. The diagnosis is confirmed by CT or radiographic confirmation of air in the gallbladder. Immediate surgery is indicated.

Gallbladder Carcinoma. Because gallstones are usually present, the signs of gallbladder carcinoma may be obscured during US examination. Three major patterns of disease have been described. A mass replacing the gallbladder is the most common appearance (40% to 65% of cases). A normal gallbladder is not evident. The mass is strikingly heterogeneous due to enveloped gallstones, tumor, and necrotic debris. Diffuse or focal thickening of the gallbladder wall is the second pattern seen in 20% to 30% of cases. The wall is thicker and more irregular than walls thickened by other causes. The least common pattern (5% to 10%) is a soft tissue mass within the gallbladder lumen. An intraluminal mass larger than 10 mm is suspicious for cancer (Fig. 50.27). Cholesterol polyps are usually less than 5 mm in size. Benign adenomatous polyps uncommonly exceed 10-mm diameter. Additional findings associated with gallbladder cancer include biliary obstruction, adenopathy, liver metastases, and invasion of adjacent structures.

Porcelain gallbladder refers to calcification of the gallbladder wall complicating chronic cholecystitis. US demonstrates a highly echogenic wall with acoustic shadowing. Porcelain gallbladder is a predisposing condition to gallbladder carcinoma.

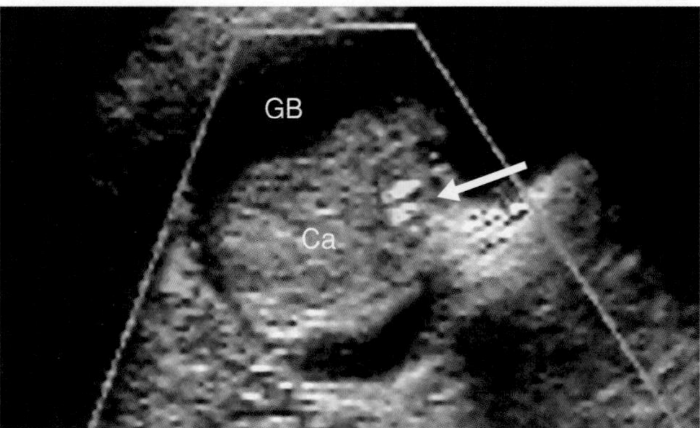

FIGURE 50.27. Gallbladder Carcinoma. Color Doppler image of the gallbladder (*GB*) reveals a large polypoid mass (*Ca*) with blood flow (*arrow*) extending through the stalk of its attachment to the gallbladder wall. These findings are characteristic of a polypoid gallbladder carcinoma.

Adenomyomatosis appears on US as focal or diffuse thickening of the gallbladder wall. The gallbladder fundus is nearly always involved. Rokitansky–Aschoff sinuses are a characteristic morphologic feature (Fig. 50.28). These are pockets of mucosa within the hypertrophied smooth muscle wall. These pockets commonly contain precipitated cholesterol crystals which are very echogenic and produce comet tail artifacts. This benign condition has no malignant potential, but may mimic gallbladder carcinoma on US studies.

SPLEEN

Normal US Anatomy. The spleen is best visualized with US with a posterolateral intercostal approach with the patient supine. With the patient in a right lateral decubitus position, the spleen may be difficult to visualize because of expansion of the left lung. When the spleen is large an anterior subcostal approach with the patient in deep inspiration is also useful. The splenic parenchyma is homogeneous and normally more echogenic than the liver (Fig. 50.29). In children the normal spleen may appear reticulonodular rather than entirely homogeneous. Its borders are smooth, sharply defined, and commonly lobulated. Doppler demonstrates the splenic artery and vein in the splenic hilum and their branches within the spleen.

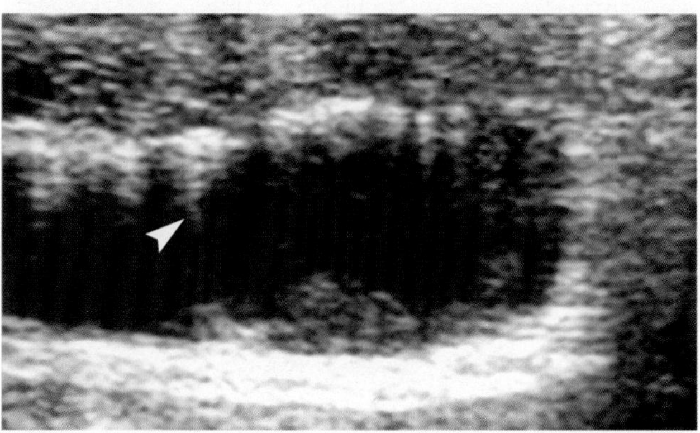

FIGURE 50.28. Adenomyomatosis. V-shaped comet tail artifacts (*arrowhead*) extend from the gallbladder wall thickened due to adenomyomatosis. The comet tail reverberation artifacts are caused by precipitation of cholesterol crystals within Rokitansky–Aschoff sinuses.

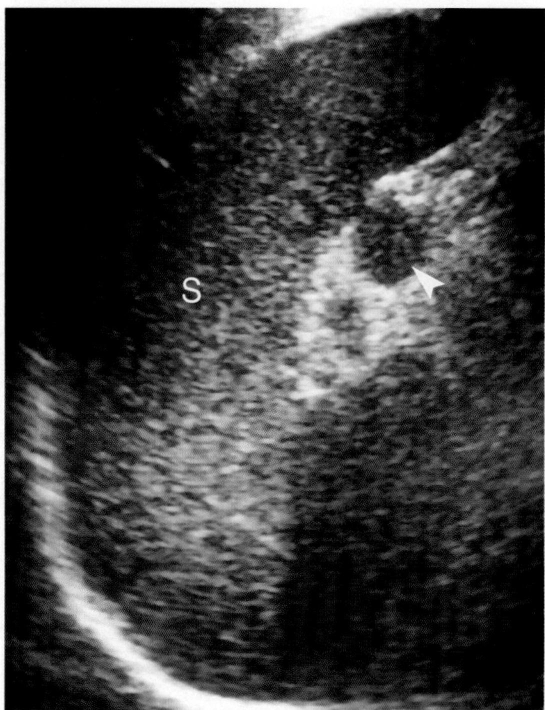

FIGURE 50.29. Normal Spleen With Splenule. A well-defined nodule (*arrowhead*) with the same echotexture as the splenic parenchyma is seen in the splenic hilum. The appearance and location are typical of splenules. The spleen (*S*) has a normal US appearance.

Accessory spleens (splenules) appear as rounded, well-defined masses, in or near the splenic hilum (Fig. 50.29). They are homogeneous and isoechoic with spleen parenchyma. Blood supply by branches of the splenic artery or vein is diagnostic.

Wandering spleen refers to an ectopic spleen that is predisposed to torsion because of laxity of the suspensory ligaments of the spleen. The wandering spleen may present as an abdominal mass or as a cause of severe abdominal pain. The diagnosis is made by confirming the normal echotexture of splenic tissue and the normal blood supply of the spleen.

Splenosis refers to splenic tissue that has been transplanted to an ectopic location as a result of trauma. If the spleen has been removed the ectopic splenic tissue may regenerate and be mistaken for an abdominal mass. US reveals multiple lobulated masses of variable size with sonographic appearance of splenic tissue (Fig. 50.30). The absence of Howell–Jolly bodies on a peripheral blood smear confirms the presence of functioning splenic tissue in a patient with a history of splenectomy. Radionuclide sulfur colloid imaging shows uptake in the splenic tissue.

Splenomegaly is evidenced by splenic length >14 cm or thickness >6 cm. The parenchyma usually remains homogeneous and normal in appearance no matter what the cause of splenic enlargement (see Table 42.3).

Posttraumatic cysts account for 80% of cystic lesions of the spleen. Most are well defined, anechoic, with accentuated through-transmission. Thick walls with ring-like calcification are common.

True epithelial cysts are indistinguishable from posttraumatic cysts although calcification in the wall is less common.

Pancreatic fluid collections are nearly always subcapsular in location (Fig. 50.31). Fluid tracks from the pancreas to the

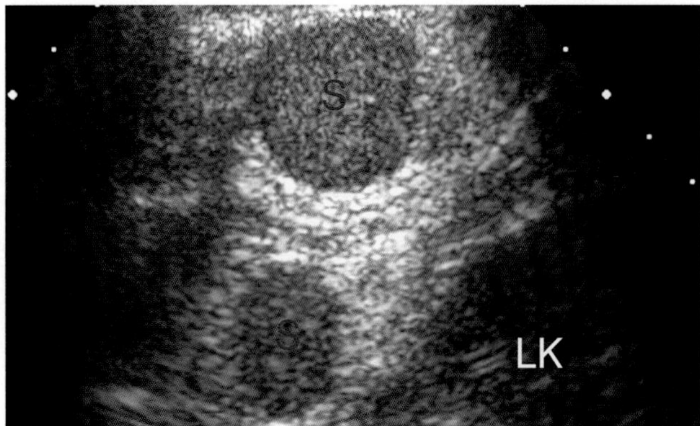

FIGURE 50.30. **Splenosis.** Longitudinal image of the left upper quadrant of the abdomen shows two well-defined left subphrenic masses (*S*) above the left kidney (*LK*) in a patient with a history of splenectomy following traumatic spleen rupture. These two masses and several smaller nodules all showed uptake on radionuclide sulfur colloid images confirming splenic tissue.

spleen along the course of the splenic artery and vein. Associated findings of pancreatitis confirm the diagnosis.

Aneurysms of the splenic artery are common and present as a hypoechoic mass in the region of the splenic hilum. Atherosclerotic calcification in the aneurysm wall is usually present. Doppler reveals arterial blood flow. Rupture causes a high mortality. Pseudoaneurysms of the splenic artery are usually caused by pancreatitis. Real-time scanning reveals a cystic-appearing mass with thin, noncalcified walls. Doppler demonstrates internal arterial flow and communication with the splenic artery.

Abscesses usually demonstrate echogenic fluid, layering debris, and air although some contain anechoic fluid (Fig. 50.32). US-guided percutaneous aspiration for diagnosis and catheter placement for treatment are safe procedures.

Microabscesses are most common in immunocompromised patients. High-frequency transducers reveal multiple tiny hypoechoic lesions. Common causes are *Mycobacterium tuberculosis*, *M. avium-intracellulare*, *Candida*, and *Pneumocystis carinii*. The differential diagnosis is listed in Table 41.4.

Lymphoma. Hypoechoic lesions in the spleen in patients with lymphoma are very likely to be foci of lymphoma (Fig. 50.33). Lesions range from numerous and small to solitary and large. However, the spleen may be enlarged without lymphoma involvement or appear normal and still be diffusely infiltrated.

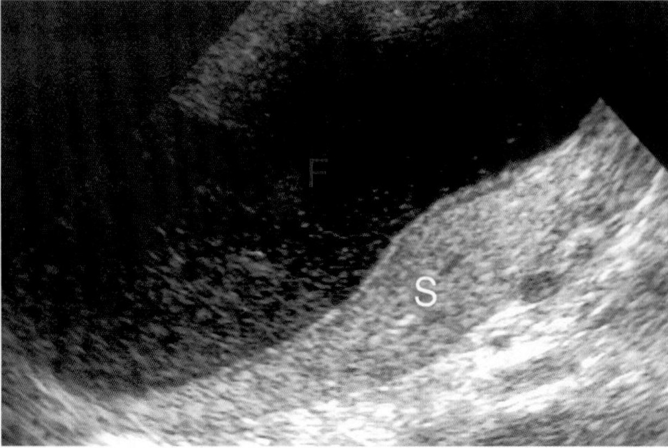

FIGURE 50.31. **Subcapsular Pancreatic Fluid Collection in the Spleen.** Pancreatic fluid (*F*) due to acute pancreatitis has tracked beneath the splenic capsule and compressed the splenic parenchyma (*S*).

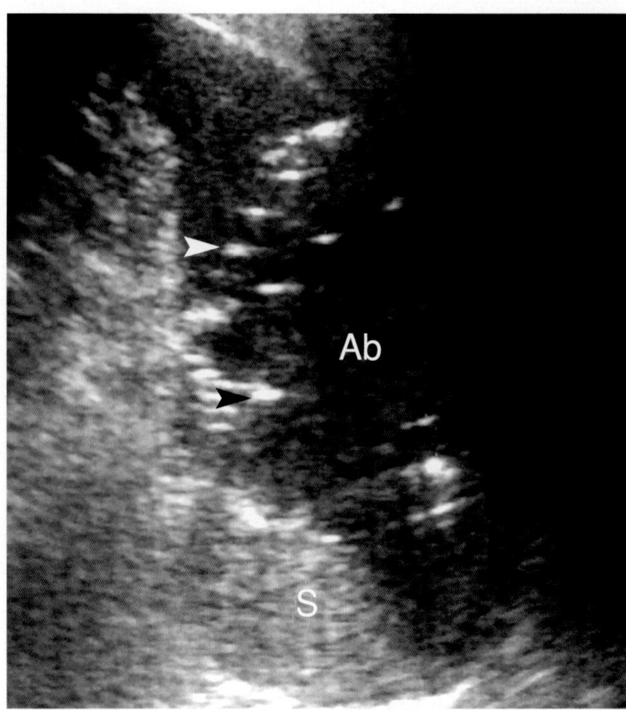

FIGURE 50.32. **Splenic Abscess.** Coronal plane US image demonstrates extensive destruction of the splenic parenchyma by a large abscess (*Ab*) containing air bubbles (*arrowheads*) seen as mobile echogenic foci distributed through the fluid of the abscess. Only a small remnant of normal splenic parenchyma (*S*) remains.

Infarctions appear hypoechoic or anechoic and are often wedge shaped and most characteristically extend to the splenic capsule (Fig. 50.34). Parenchymal borders may be sharply defined or irregular. Hemorrhage associated with infarction may dissect beneath the capsule or the capsule may rupture resulting in hemoperitoneum. Most patients with infarction

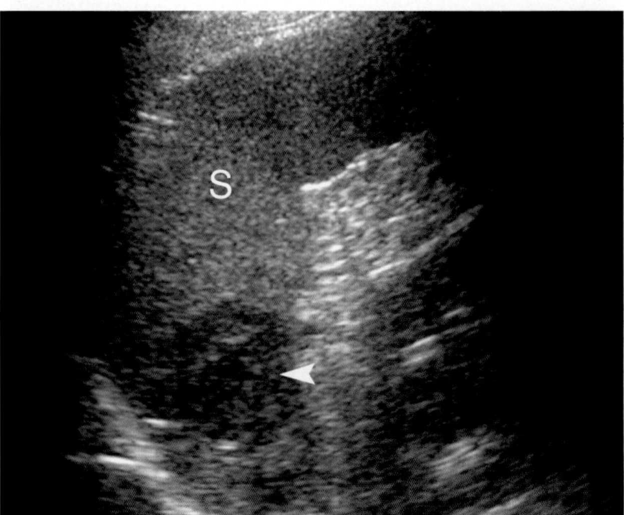

FIGURE 50.33. **Lymphoma in the Spleen.** Image of the spleen (*S*) reveals a heterogeneous hypoechoic mass (*arrowhead*) with irregular margins. This appearance is typical when lymphomatous involvement of the spleen is seen on US.

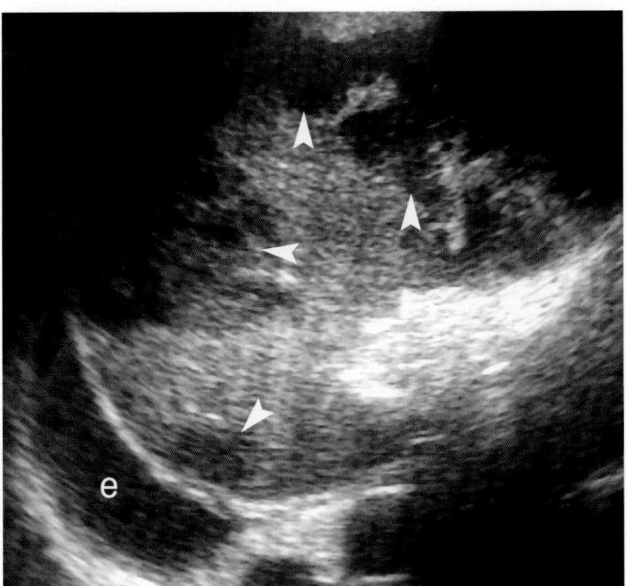

FIGURE 50.34. **Splenic Infarctions.** Acute splenic infarctions (*arrowheads*) appear as irregular or wedge-shaped, peripheral, hypoechoic regions in the spleen. An associated pleural effusion (*e*) is also evident.

have a predisposing cause such as splenomegaly or lymphoma involving the spleen.

Hemangiomas are usually homogeneous and hyperechoic, but have a much more variable appearance than they have in the liver. A complex mass appearance with multiple cystic areas has been described. Calcifications occur in areas of fibrosis.

Metastases are nonspecific in appearance, usually hypoechoic and multiple.

Angiosarcoma of the spleen appears as a heterogeneous mass with disorganized color flow enlarging the spleen.

Hematoma. Sonography is now commonly used to screen for free intraperitoneal blood in patients with blunt abdominal trauma. Splenic lacerations and subcapsular and intraparenchymal hematomas are commonly demonstrated. The US appearance of the hematoma varies with age and composition. Most are well defined and hypoechoic.

PANCREAS

Normal US Anatomy. The pancreas may be a difficult organ to image with US. Vascular landmarks are the key to its identification (Fig. 50.35). The body and tail of the pancreas are immediately anterior to the splenic vein as it courses from the splenic hilum toward the liver. The neck of the pancreas is anterior to the junction of the splenic vein with the superior mesenteric vein that marks the commencement of the portal vein. The head of the pancreas envelops this confluence and lies anterior to the IVC. It is important to remember that a portion of the pancreatic head, the uncinate process, lies caudal to level of the splenic vein, between the superior mesenteric vein and the IVC. This portion of the pancreas must not be overlooked because it includes the distal common bile duct, the termination of the pancreatic duct, and the ampulla of Vater. This is a common location for gallstone impaction and tumor.

The echogenicity of the pancreas depends upon the amount of fatty infiltration. In children and young adults, the pancreas is about equal in echogenicity to the liver. In older adults, the pancreas becomes more echogenic as fat progressively infiltrates between the lobules of pancreatic parenchyma. The pancreatic duct is commonly seen in normal individuals. The normal duct does not exceed 3 mm in diameter and tapers progressively toward the tail.

The left lobe of the liver serves as the best sonographic window to the pancreas. The distal stomach lies between the liver and the pancreas. The hypoechoic muscular wall of the stomach should not be mistaken for the pancreatic duct. Gas in the stomach, or more often in the transverse colon, commonly prevents visualization of the pancreas, especially if the left lobe of the liver is small. Progressive transducer pressure is most effective in displacing gas to visualize the pancreas. The tail of the pancreas can be visualized through the spleen by concentrating on the region of the splenic hilum.

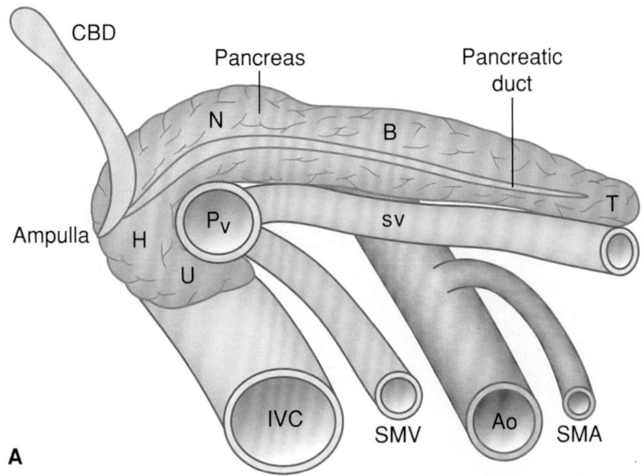

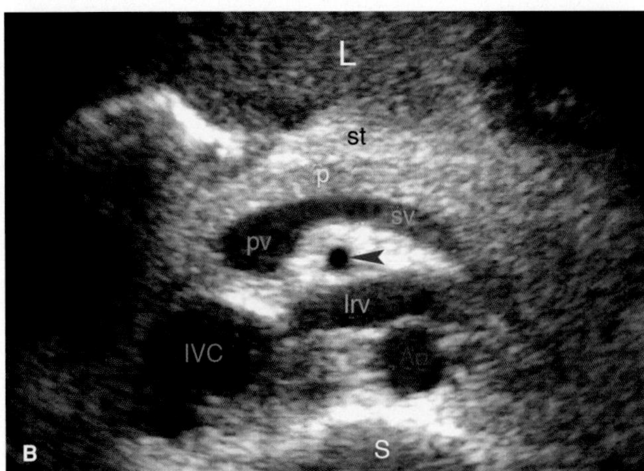

FIGURE 50.35. **Normal Pancreas Anatomy.** A diagram (**A**) and a US in transverse plane (**B**) demonstrate the normal anatomy of the pancreas. The majority of the pancreas lies anterior to the splenic vein (*sv*) and its junction with the superior mesenteric vein (*SMV*) forming the portal vein (*pv*). The head (*H*) and uncinate process (*U*) of the pancreas cradle the origin of the portal vein. The pancreatic neck (*N*) is anterior to the sv–SMV confluence, and the uncinate process and inferior vena cava (*IVC*) are posterior to the confluence. The superior mesenteric artery (*SMA, arrowhead*) arises from the aorta (*Ao*) dorsal to the splenic vein. The left renal vein (*lrv*) passes between the SMA and aorta to the inferior vena cava. The left lobe of the liver (*L*) offers a good sonographic window to the pancreas. The stomach (*st*) and lesser sac (collapsed) are anterior to the pancreas. *CBD*, common bile duct; *S*, spine; *B*, body of the pancreas; *T*, tail of the pancreas; *p*, pancreas.

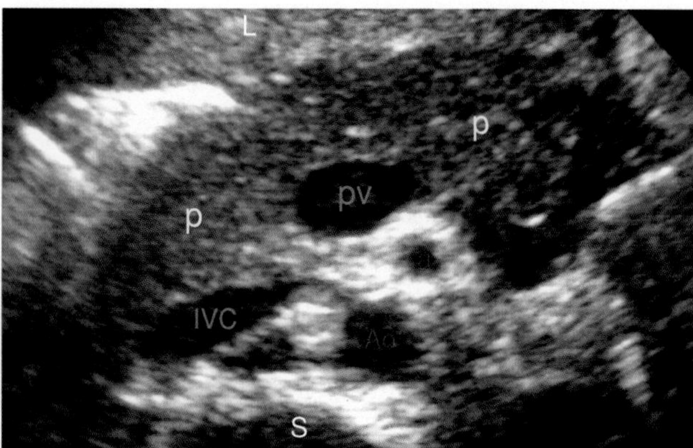

FIGURE 50.36. **Acute Pancreatitis.** Axial plane US image reveals a diffuse decrease in the echogenicity of the pancreatic parenchyma (*p*) compared to the liver (*L*) because of diffuse edema of acute inflammation. The normal pancreas is more echogenic than the normal liver (Fig. 50.35B). No discrete fluid collections were evident. *pv*, portal vein; *a*, superior mesenteric artery; *IVC*, inferior vena cava; *Ao*, aorta; *S*, spine.

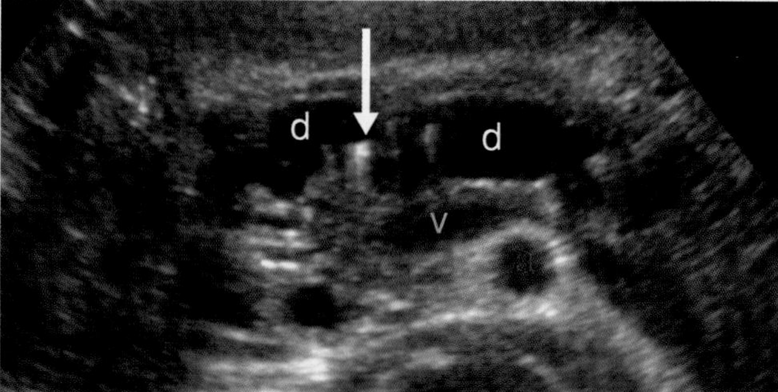

FIGURE 50.38. **Chronic Pancreatitis.** Axial plane image shows beaded dilation of the pancreatic duct (*d*) and pancreatic calcifications (*arrow*) with ring-down artifact. Anatomic landmarks of the pancreas are the splenic vein (*v*) and the superior mesenteric artery (*a*).

Acute Pancreatitis. US findings include diffuse glandular enlargement, decrease in echogenicity due to edema, and poorly defined gland margins (Fig. 50.36). In mild cases, the US examination may be normal. Focal pancreatitis most commonly involves the pancreatic head. US examination should include documentation of the presence of gallstones and dilation of the biliary tree. The ampullary region should be carefully examined for an impacted gallstone. US is excellent for detection and follow-up of fluid collections (Fig. 50.37). Fluid accumulates most commonly around the pancreas, in the lesser sac, and in the splenic hilum. Examination should be extended into the pelvis, especially if fluid is seen tracking caudal to the pancreas. Discrete cystic collections should be examined with Doppler to detect pseudoaneurysms. The splenic, portal, and superior mesenteric veins are examined for evidence of thrombosis.

Chronic Pancreatitis. Because of fibrosis and diffuse glandular atrophy, the pancreas is reduced in size and is increased in echogenicity making its identification with US more difficult. Calcifications produce focal echodensities and, often, acoustic shadowing. The pancreatic duct shows a pattern of alternating dilation and constriction. Calcifications are commonly seen within the duct (Fig. 50.38). Signs of acute pancreatitis are commonly superimposed on chronic pancreatitis. A mass of solid fibrinous tissue caused by chronic pancreatitis may be indistinguishable from adenocarcinoma. Ductal dilation may be present. A major use of US is to guide percutaneous biopsy to provide pathologic differentiation of this common clinical problem.

Adenocarcinoma appears as a hypoechoic mass or as a subtle alteration of acoustic texture in the pancreas (Fig. 50.39). Biliary and pancreatic ductal obstruction is easily identified. Sudden termination of dilated ducts in a hypoechoic mass is characteristic. Doppler is used to differentiate the pancreatic and biliary ducts from vessels, and to detect the vascular encasement or invasion that commonly makes the tumor nonresectable. The liver and retroperitoneum should be carefully examined for metastatic nodules and adenopathy.

Pancreatic neuroendocrine (islet cell) tumors are predominantly hypoechoic compared to pancreatic parenchyma. Cystic degeneration, hemorrhage, fibrosis, and calcification cause wide variation in appearance. Transabdominal US detects 20% to 75% of insulinomas and only 20% to 30% of gastrinomas. Endoscopic US improves detection to 77% to 94% range. Intraoperative US demonstrates 75% to 100% of small tumors and serves as a major aid to the surgeon having difficulty identifying small hormone secreting tumors.

Metastases, especially from colon carcinoma, may mimic pancreatic adenocarcinoma.

Lymphoma commonly involves the peripancreatic lymph nodes causing multiple or confluent hypoechoic masses.

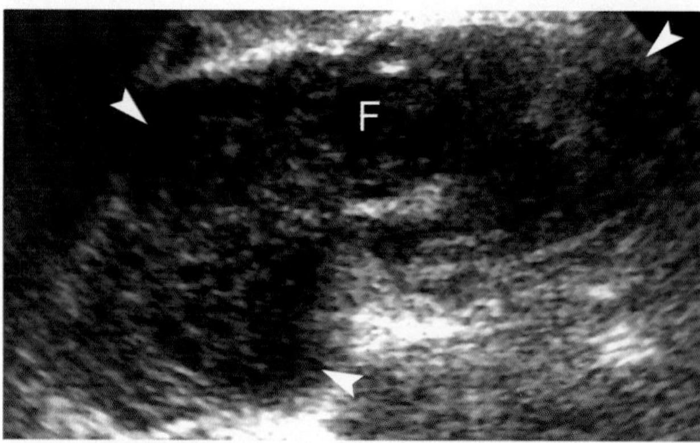

FIGURE 50.37. **Necrotizing Pancreatitis.** Transverse image through the bed of the pancreas (*arrowheads*) shows that the anatomic landmarks for the pancreas are obliterated and replaced by heterogeneous fluid (*F*) in this patient with acute severe necrotizing pancreatitis.

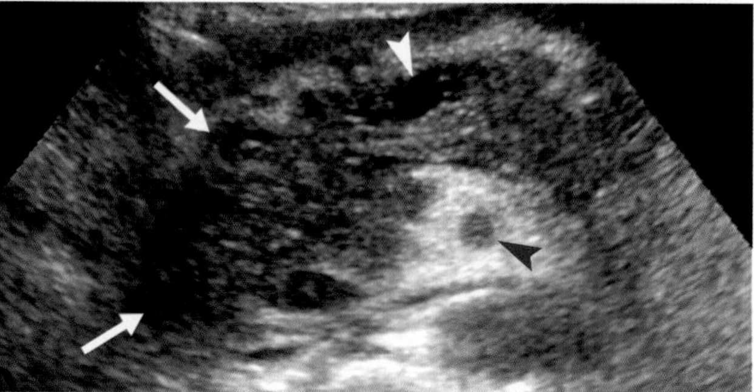

FIGURE 50.39. **Adenocarcinoma of the Pancreas.** The tumor is seen as a subtle hypoechoic mass (*arrows*) enlarging the head of the pancreas. The tumor margins are poorly defined. The pancreatic duct (*white arrowhead*) is dilated and terminates abruptly as it encounters the tumor. The superior mesenteric artery (*red arrowhead*) and its surrounding collar of echogenic fat are preserved.

Abscess. US demonstrates a fluid collection that is usually ill defined and contains echogenic fluid. Gas bubbles that move, shadow, and cause comet tail artifacts are strong evidence of infection. Any pancreatitis-associated fluid collection may become infected. US is used to guide aspiration and catheter drainage.

Multiple pancreatic cysts are seen in patients with autosomal dominant polycystic disease and those with von Hippel–Lindau syndrome. Solitary true epithelial-lined cysts are rare.

Pseudoaneurysms develop in the peripancreatic region most commonly as a complication of pancreatitis with enzyme erosion of arterial walls. US demonstrates a discrete cystic mass in close proximity to an artery. Doppler US confirms arterial flow extending into and out of the lumen of the pseudoaneurysm. A small neck of connection with the parent artery can be identified by flow jets.

Pseudocysts develop as complications of acute or chronic pancreatitis. Most appear as well-defined, smooth-walled, anechoic fluid collections. Multiple loculations and internal septations are common. Internal debris and fluid–fluid levels are indicative of hemorrhage or infection. Acute fluid collections often occupy the space available and are irregular or lobulated in shape. More chronic collections are usually oval or spherical and tend to have thicker, more distinct walls. US is an excellent, nonradiation, way to provide imaging follow-up of pseudocysts to confirm resolution or to provide guidance for drainage. Differentiation from cystic neoplasms may be difficult when a cystic lesion is discovered in a patient without a history or imaging findings of pancreatitis.

Cystic pancreatic neoplasms include serous cystadenoma (microcystic adenoma), mucinous cystic neoplasms, intraductal papillary mucinous tumor, and papillary epithelial neoplasm. See Chapter 42 for more complete description. Thin-slice MDCT and MR with MRCP are the imaging methods of choice to characterize these lesions. Endoscopic US has emerged as crucial to this evaluation by providing greater anatomic detail of the lesions as well as guidance for aspiration of fluid (for mucin content) and needle biopsy. *Serous cystadenoma* consists of a network of small cysts with a honeycomb or solid appearance on US (Fig. 50.40). *Mucinous cystic neoplasms* consist of larger cysts with internal septa, papillary projections, and discrete solid components well shown by endoscopic US. *Intraductal papillary mucinous tumors* produce focal multicystic masses (branch duct type) or marked diffuse dilation of the pancreatic duct (main duct type). Communication with the pancreatic ductal system is shown by MRCP or ERCP. *Papillary epithelial neoplasms* range from purely cystic to solid with a well-defined wall. Internal hemorrhage with necrosis of these tumors is common.

Pancreas transplants are performed with increasing frequency, often combined with renal transplants in patients with diabetes. US plays a key role in postoperative evaluation. Surgical techniques for pancreas transplantation evolve rapidly. In most cases the pancreas and a portion of the duodenum are transplanted as a unit either into the pelvis with exocrine drainage of the pancreas through a duodenovesical anastomosis or into the abdomen with a duodenoduodenal anastomosis. Complications of pancreas transplantation include vascular anastomotic leaks, stenosis, or thrombosis; pancreatitis; perigraft fluid collections, which may be hematomas, seromas, or pancreatitis-associated fluid; exocrine leaks, and allograft rejection.

GASTROINTESTINAL TRACT

US is highly effective but generally underutilized in evaluation of the gastrointestinal tract (GIT). Its well-defined utility in several specific conditions is reviewed in other chapters: appendicitis in Chapters 46 and 69, intussusception in children in Chapter 69, and pyloric stenosis in Chapter 69. The bowel should be included in every US examination of the abdomen especially in the setting of acute abdominal pain. Gas within the bowel is an obstacle to US examination, but the GIT is a common site of disease and bowel wall thickening and fluid-filled or solid mass lesions create their own windows for US evaluation.

Normal US Anatomy. Normal GIT has a recognizable gut signature on US examination that allows it to be differentiated from other structures within the abdomen. US reveals multiple layers with a target-like appearance (Fig. 50.41). The lumen has variable liquid, solid, and gas contents. The lining layer of the lumen is the thin mucosal membrane best recognized as the surface of the thicker and echogenic submucosa. The submucosa is bounded by the well-defined hypoechoic layer of muscle, the muscularis propria. The surface of the bowel is a thin layer of echogenic serosa. Doppler US of the normal bowel wall shows little to no blood flow. Tumors and inflammation involving the bowel wall may be highly vascular. Wall thickness is dependent upon luminal distention and muscle contraction. Peristalsis is a normal feature and its presence or absence aids in diagnosis. Graded compression with the US transducer is routinely beneficial to move gas out of the way, improve visualization and assess rigidity of suspected abnormalities, and to confirm the source of localized pain or tenderness.

Adenocarcinoma of the GIT is evident on US when the tumors are large or exophytic. Small mucosal tumors are not evident. US shows a lobulated hypoechoic solid mass often enveloping pockets of gas (Fig. 50.42).

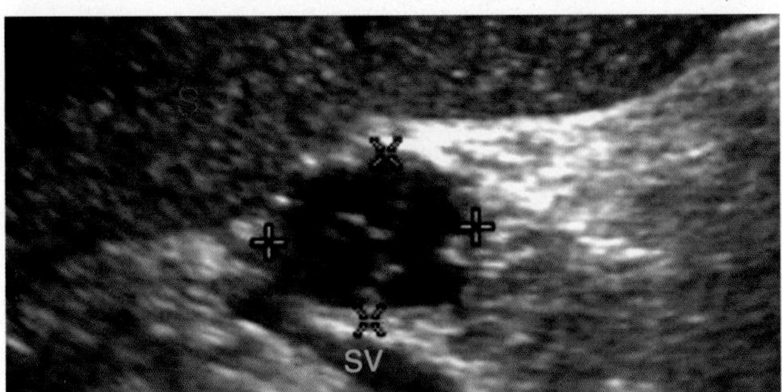

FIGURE 50.40. Serous Cystadenoma of the Pancreas. US image through the spleen (*S*) reveals a small tumor (between *cursors*, ×, +) of the pancreatic tail consisting of multiple small cysts. *sv*, splenic vein.

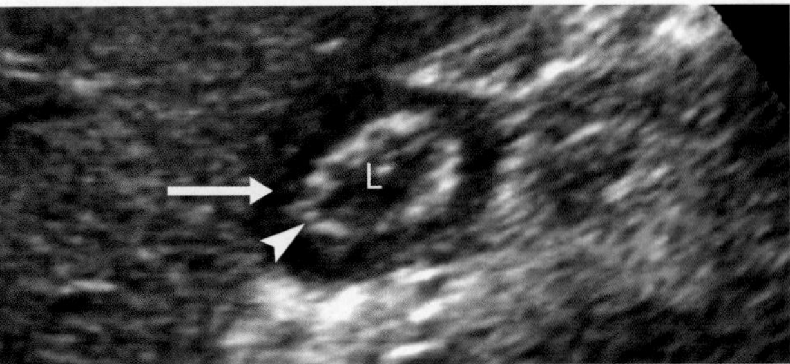

FIGURE 50.41. Normal Gut Signature. Transverse image of the antrum of the stomach shows the characteristic hypoechoic layer of muscularis propria (*arrow*) with underlying echogenic layer of submucosa (*arrowhead*). Liquid contents in the lumen (*L*) of the stomach complete the target appearance.

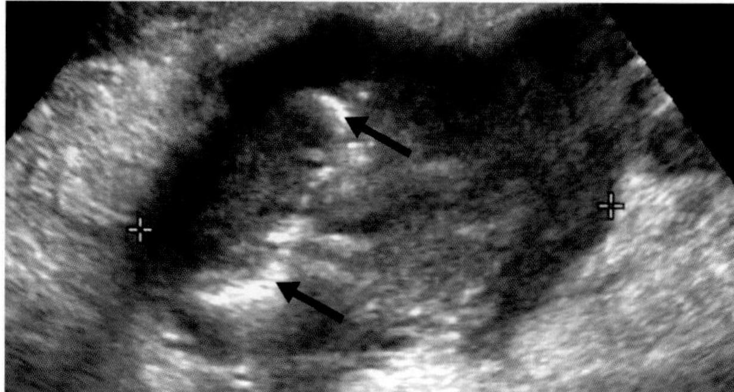

FIGURE 50.42. **Carcinoma of the Colon.** Transverse image shows a lobulated mass (between *cursors*, +) with irregular border in the location of the ascending colon. Bright echoes (*arrows*) emanate from gas trapped within the lumen, a useful US landmark for recognizing masses involving the bowel. Surgery confirmed a large lobulated partially obstructing carcinoma of the colon.

Gastrointestinal stromal tumors are frequently large, round, well-defined, extraluminal masses with central cystic areas of hemorrhage or necrosis. Larger size and increased intratumoral heterogeneity are associated with malignancy.

Lymphoma produces large, strikingly hypoechoic lobulated masses that may envelop the bowel without obstructing it. Regional adenopathy may be striking.

Metastases to the GIT are usually multiple, hypoechoic nodules often associated with exudative ascites with floating particulate matter and peritoneal implantation of tumor.

Inflammatory bowel disease produces circumferential thickening of the bowel wall with impaired peristalsis and frequent involvement of the mesentery. Doppler shows hyperemia in the thickened wall. Rigid narrowing produces strictures and obstruction. Extension of disease outside of the GIT includes inflammatory masses, fluid collections, and fistulas.

Diverticulitis produces an inflammatory mass that is often indistinguishable from a neoplasm. Wall thickening may be concentric or asymmetric. Pericolonic fat inflammation increases fat echogenicity and produces mass effect. Pericolonic abscesses of variable size and often containing gas are common (Fig. 50.43).

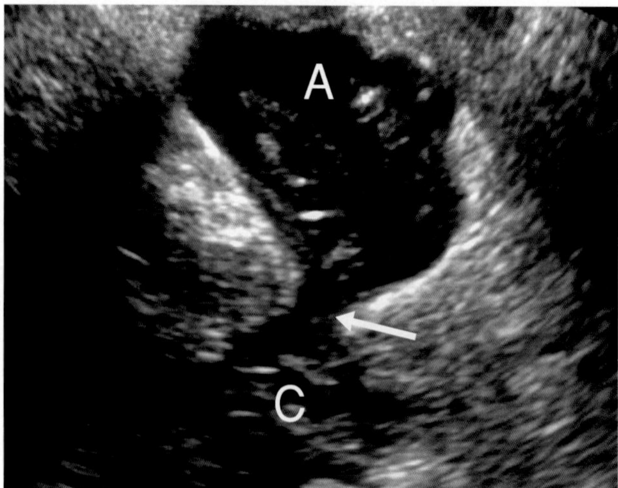

FIGURE 50.43. **Diverticulitis Abscess.** Transverse image in the lower left flank shows a fluid collection proven to be an abscess (*A*) connecting to the lumen of the descending colon (*C*) via a perforated diverticulum (*arrow*). US was used to guide aspiration confirming the presence of pus and subsequent catheter placement for drainage.

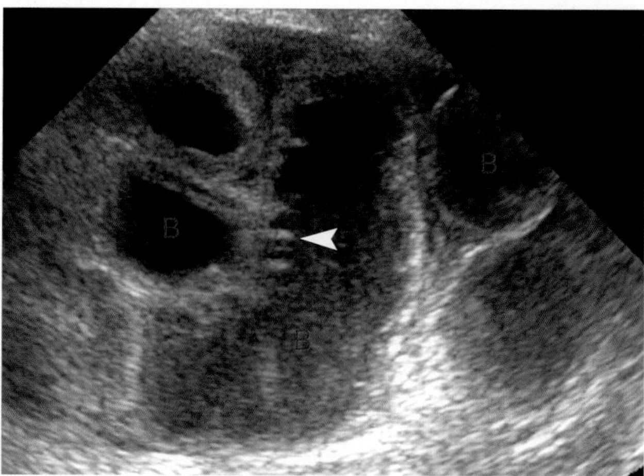

FIGURE 50.44. **Small Bowel Obstruction.** US clearly reveals multiple fluid-filled loops of small bowel (*B*). The characteristic keyboard appearance of the valvulae conniventes (*arrowhead*) serves as a sonographic landmark of small bowel. Vigorous peristalsis was observed on real-time US examination.

Bowel obstruction is diagnosed with US in coordination with conventional radiographs. Radiographs show dilated loops of bowel filled with gas, while US shows dilated loops of bowel filled with fluid. Valvulae conniventes produces prominent sonographic landmarks in fluid-filled bowel appearing like a row of piano keys (Fig. 50.44). US shows hyperperistalsis associated with mechanical obstruction or absence of peristalsis associated with adynamic ileus. However, high-grade complete obstruction of long duration may also result in aperistalsis.

Intussusception in adults is nearly always associated with a lead mass. US shows the characteristic concentric layers of bowel wall, bowel lumen, and echogenic mesenteric fat pulled into the lumen of the receiving bowel loop (Fig. 50.45). Color Doppler provides assessment for ischemia.

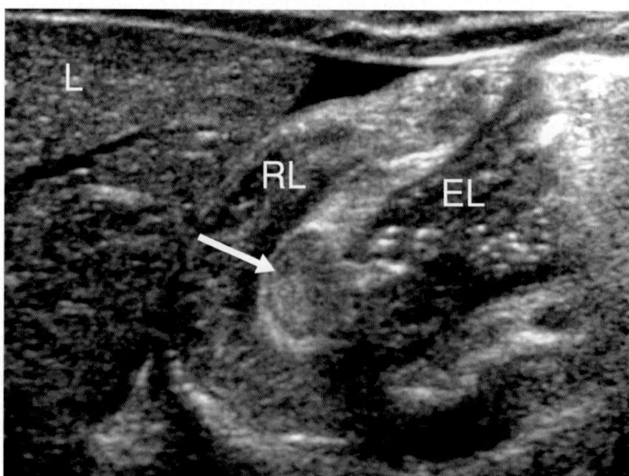

FIGURE 50.45. **Ileocolic Intussusception in an Adult.** US image of the right upper quadrant of a patient with abdominal pain reveals the characteristic multilayer appearance of intussusception. The receiving loop (*RL*) forms the outer portion of the mass while the entering loop (*EL*) forms the inner portion of the mass. The lead point, in this case an enlarged lymph node (*arrow*) is surrounded by echogenic fat-containing mesentery dragged inside of the receiving loop along with the entering loop. The patient's point of maximum tenderness and the location of the mass are near the liver (*L*).

Endoscopic ultrasonography is performed with high-frequency US transducers combined with fiberoptic endoscopes or colonoscopes. Intraluminal US provides high-resolution images of the bowel wall and nearby surrounding tissues. Guidance can be provided for biopsy or aspiration of wall lesions or extraluminal lesions not seen optically. Malignancies of the rectum and anal canal may be effectively staged.

ADRENAL GLANDS

Normal US Anatomy. The normal adrenal glands may be difficult to visualize sonographically in the adult, but are usually quite prominent in the newborn (Fig. 50.46). Scan planes to image the right adrenal gland include longitudinal in the long axis of the right kidney and transverse in a plane just superior to the upper pole of the right kidney. The Y- or V-shaped adrenal gland is seen just posterior to the IVC as the IVC enters the liver between the right lobe of the liver and the right crus of the diaphragm. The left adrenal is best seen between the upper pole of the left kidney and the aorta on an angled coronal plane. The adrenals are hypoechoic compared to retroperitoneal fat and isoechoic compared to the crura of the diaphragm. The medulla is seen as a thin echogenic line surrounded by the hypoechoic cortex. The limbs of the normal adult adrenal gland are 4 to 5 cm in length and 5 to 7 mm in width. In infants the adrenal glands normally appear large due to persistence of the "fetal" portion of the gland. The fetal cortex rapidly involutes in the first 3 weeks of life.

Although CT is more sensitive than US for detection of small adrenal masses, US is useful for characterizing adrenal masses as cystic, follow-up of presumed benign adrenal masses, and confirming the origin of large retroperitoneal masses. Most mass lesions in the adrenal gland discovered on US examination will require further characterization by adrenal protocol CT or MR.

Adrenal hyperplasia appears as bilateral diffuse enlargement, or as multiple bilateral small nodules. Hyperplastic glands are seen with the adrenal endocrine syndromes. The differential diagnosis of bilateral enlarged adrenal glands includes infection (especially tuberculosis, histoplasmosis, and cytomegalovirus), metastatic disease, and lymphoma. Patients with AIDS may have adrenal enlargement due to mycobacterial, fungal, or viral infection.

Adrenal adenomas appear as solid, homogeneous, adrenal masses with echogenicity similar to renal parenchyma (Fig. 50.47). US offers no specific findings that differentiate

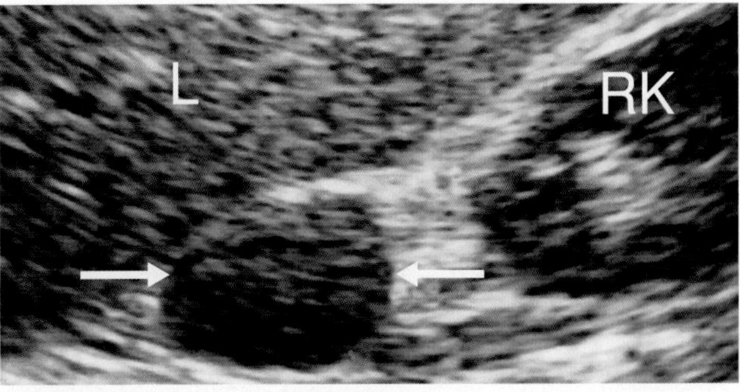

FIGURE 50.47. **Benign Adrenal Adenoma.** Longitudinal US demonstrates a homogeneous 3.5-cm mass (between *arrows*) arising from the right adrenal gland. The mass is outlined by echogenic fat. This is a nonhyperfunctioning adrenal adenoma that was discovered incidentally and was characterized by CT. *L*, liver; *RK*, right kidney.

benign from malignant masses. Masses larger than 4 cm should be considered suspicious for malignancy.

Adrenal carcinomas are indistinguishable from adenomas when the tumor is small (<4 cm). Larger carcinomas are inhomogeneous with areas of necrosis, hemorrhage, and calcification. Real-time imaging and Doppler are useful to detect tumor invasion of adrenal or renal veins and the IVC.

Pheochromocytoma arising in the adrenal gland can usually be demonstrated by US, because most are large (5 to 6 cm). Most are sharply marginated and predominantly solid, with cystic areas of necrosis and hemorrhage commonly present (Fig. 50.48). Predominantly cystic pheochromocytomas are less common.

Adrenal myelolipoma appears as a highly echogenic mass in the adrenal bed. They may be easily overlooked. Mixed hyper- and hypoechoic areas correspond to fatty and myeloid elements within the tumor. The diagnosis is confirmed by demonstration of internal fat density by CT or MR. Other echogenic masses in the adrenal region include renal angiomyolipoma (AML), teratoma, lipoma, and liposarcoma.

Adrenal Cysts. US may be utilized to differentiate benign cysts from cystic tumors. Benign adrenal cysts include pseudocysts resulting from previous adrenal hemorrhage; endothelial cysts being a form of lymphangioma; and rare epithelial cysts. Other cystic adrenal lesions include hydatid

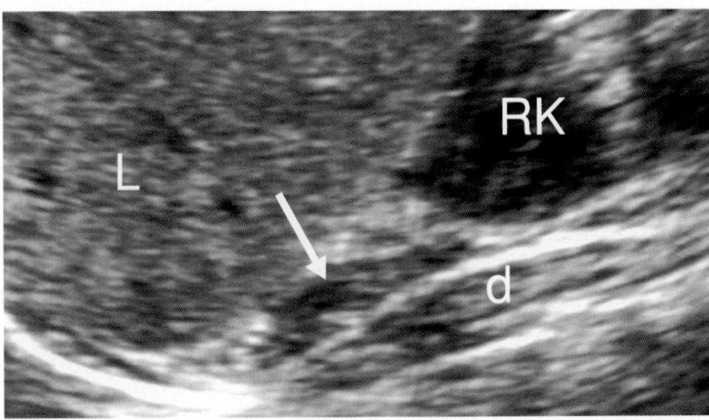

FIGURE 50.46. **Normal Adrenal Gland.** Longitudinal image reveals the normal right adrenal gland (*arrow*) in an adult. Sonographic landmarks for the right adrenal gland include the liver (*L*), the upper pole of the right kidney (*RK*), and the right crus of the diaphragm (*d*).

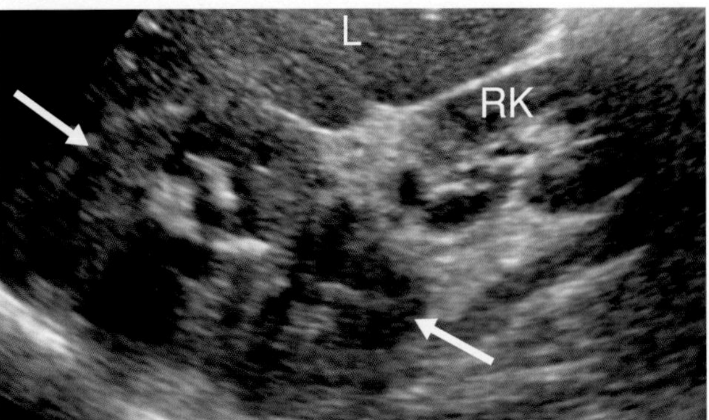

FIGURE 50.48. **Pheochromocytoma.** Longitudinal plane US in a patient with biochemically proven pheochromocytoma demonstrates the adrenal tumor (*arrows*) posterior to the liver (*L*) and superior to the right kidney (*RK*). The tumor is heterogeneous in echogenicity with highly echogenic shadowing foci of calcification.

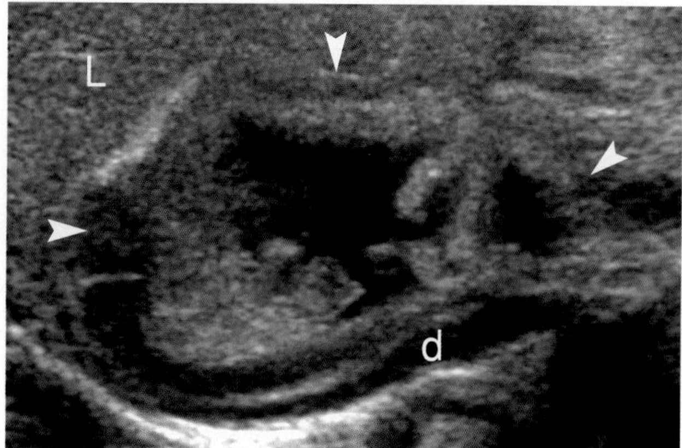

FIGURE 50.49. Adrenal Hemorrhage. The adrenal gland in an adult injured in a motor vehicle collision is markedly enlarged by a lobulated heterogeneous mass (*arrowheads*) representing adrenal hemorrhage with solid clot and liquid blood. *L*, liver; *d*, right crus of the diaphragm.

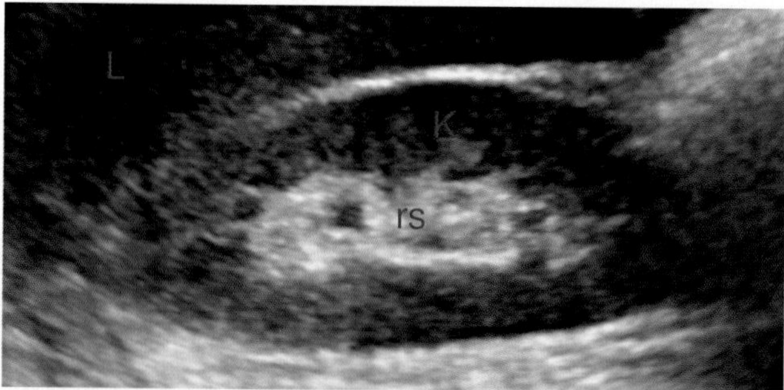

FIGURE 50.50. Normal Kidneys. A long-axis US view of the right kidney (*K*) in an adult obtained through the liver (*L*) demonstrates echogenicity of the normal renal parenchyma approximately equal to the echogenicity of the normal liver. The renal sinus (*rs*), containing vessels, the collecting system, and fat, is hyperechoic compared to the renal parenchyma. The margins of the kidney are outlined by echogenic perirenal fat.

cysts, and cystic degeneration of adrenal tumors including metastases, adrenal cortical carcinoma, and pheochromocytoma. Uncomplicated benign cysts have thin walls and septa (<3 mm), anechoic internal fluid, and demonstrate accentuated through-transmission. Calcification in walls and septa is common in all types of benign cysts. Echogenic internal fluid or debris, thick walls, solid components, and large size (>6 cm) suggest possible malignancy.

Adrenal Hemorrhage. US initially demonstrates hyperechoic, mass-like enlargement of the adrenal gland (Fig. 50.49). With time, the adrenal mass rapidly becomes hypoechoic and progressively decreases in size. The gland may return entirely to normal or evolve into a pseudocyst that commonly develops calcifications in its walls within 2 to 4 weeks of the hemorrhage. Eventual collapse of the pseudocyst results in coarsely calcified adrenal glands. In the neonate, adrenal hemorrhage is usually bilateral and due to hypoxic stress. In the adult, adrenal hemorrhage is usually unilateral and right sided (85%). Most adult cases of adrenal hemorrhage are associated with blunt abdominal trauma.

Adrenal calcifications commonly occur as a result of previous adrenal hemorrhage. Additional causes include tumor (neuroblastoma, adrenal carcinoma, pheochromocytoma), infection (tuberculosis, histoplasmosis), and Wolman disease.

KIDNEYS

Normal US Anatomy. On US examination the renal cortex is isoechoic or slightly hypoechoic compared to the liver and is distinctly hypoechoic compared to the spleen (Fig. 50.50). The medullary pyramids are visualized as hypoechoic cone-shaped structures surrounded by the more echogenic cortex. This corticomedullary differentiation is striking in the newborn and becomes less noticeable with age. Lucent pyramids should not be mistaken for hydronephrosis. The central renal sinus contains fat, blood vessels, the collecting system, and lymphatics. Central sinus echogenicity is usually the same as perirenal fat. Blood vessels appear as lucent tubular structures with flow demonstrated by Doppler. In well-hydrated normal patients, minimally dilated collecting structures may be visualized. The contour of the kidney is smooth and may be lobulated by the normal renal lobes. Adult kidneys range from 9 to 13 cm in length. The *junctional parenchymal defect* is a normal anatomic variant caused by incomplete fusion of the upper and lower poles of the kidney. Sonography demonstrates a wedge-shaped echogenic defect in the renal parenchyma at the junction of the upper and middle thirds of the kidney. Perirenal fat may be hypoechoic and mistaken for perirenal fluid collections or even enlarged kidneys. Normal but hypoechoic fat may be recognized by regular linear echoes representing fibrous septa, lack of acoustic enhancement that is characteristic of fluid, and bilateral symmetry. Hypoechoic fat in the renal sinus may suggest tumor or hydronephrosis.

Obstruction. US is commonly the imaging method of first choice for the diagnosis of urinary obstruction. Beware, there are numerous pitfalls in using US to make this diagnosis. The key US finding in obstruction is hydronephrosis. Hydronephrosis is recognized as fluid distention of the collecting system with communication between round fluid-filled calyces and the dilated renal pelvis (Fig. 50.51). A dilated ureter appears as a fluid-filled tube extending from the renal pelvis. However, in acute obstruction such as from a stone impacted in the ureter, the degree of collecting system dilation may be slight even though the obstruction is severe. Moreover, the presence of hydronephrosis does not always mean obstruction. Additional causes of pelvicaliectasis are listed in Table 50.2. An asymmetric elevation in the resistive index (RI >0.70 on the obstructed side) obtained from spectral Doppler of the arcuate artery favors obstruction over other causes of pelvicaliectasis. Structures that may mimic hydronephrosis include peripelvic cysts (Fig. 50.52), multiple simple cysts in the renal sinus, and an extrarenal pelvis. An *extrarenal pelvis* is one that extends

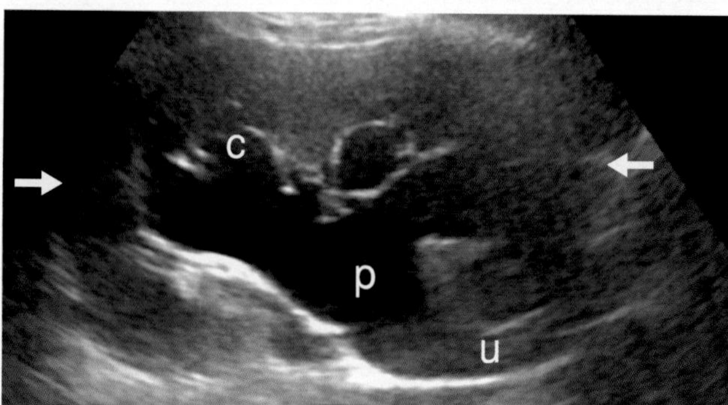

FIGURE 50.51. Hydronephrosis. Coronal plane US of the kidney (between *arrows*) reveals the characteristic appearance of hydronephrosis with interconnection of dilated calyces (*c*), pelvis (*p*), and proximal ureter (*u*).

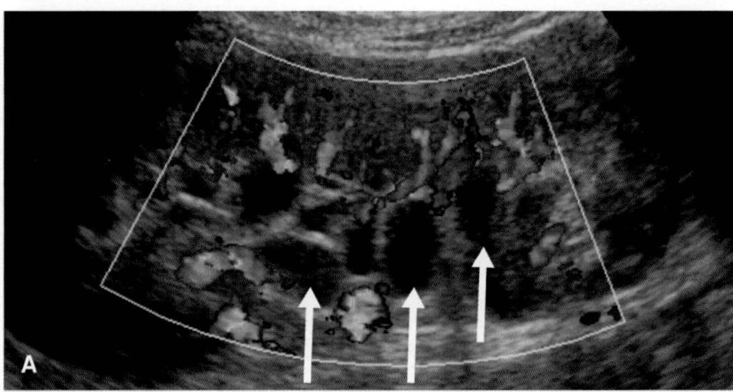

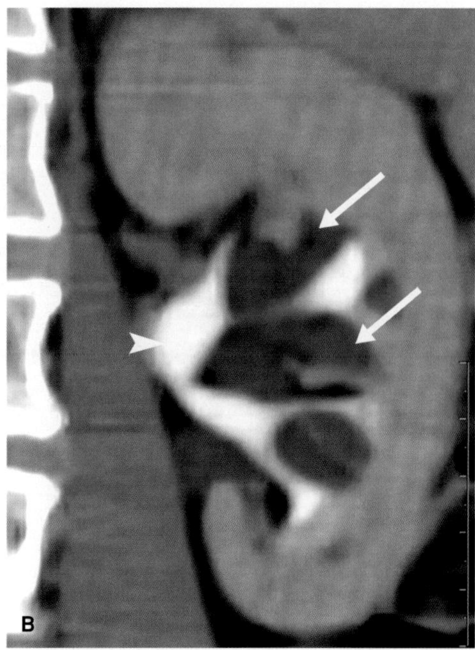

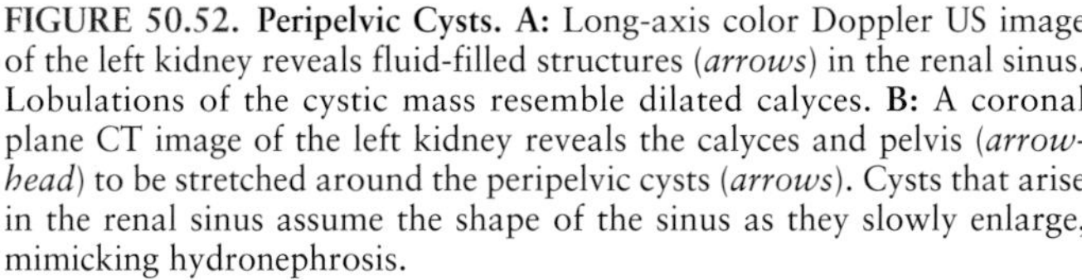

FIGURE 50.52. **Peripelvic Cysts. A:** Long-axis color Doppler US image of the left kidney reveals fluid-filled structures (*arrows*) in the renal sinus. Lobulations of the cystic mass resemble dilated calyces. **B:** A coronal plane CT image of the left kidney reveals the calyces and pelvis (*arrowhead*) to be stretched around the peripelvic cysts (*arrows*). Cysts that arise in the renal sinus assume the shape of the sinus as they slowly enlarge, mimicking hydronephrosis.

outside the renal sinus. This type of pelvis is commonly fluid filled but is a normal variant not associated with dilated calyces or ureter. Comparison with previous studies may help in making the correct diagnosis. The ureterovesical junction should be examined with color Doppler to detect the presence or absence of a ureteral jet.

Stones. All renal stones, regardless of composition, appear on US as bright echogenic foci (Fig. 50.53). Stones as small as 5 mm may be identified if they cast an acoustic shadow. However, when acoustic shadowing is not evident, often due to technical factors, small stones may be overlooked because they blend in with echogenic renal sinus fat. Technical factors that improve the capability to demonstrate shadowing include imaging the stone in the focal zone of the transducer, centering the stone within the US beam, and using high-frequency transducers. Color and power Doppler twinkling artifact is a feature of stones (Fig. 50.54) that may aid detection and should be recognized to avoid mistaking the artifact for a vascular abnormality. The *twinkling sign* appears as a rapidly changing mosaic of color displayed distal to a strong reflector, like a renal or bladder stone. Twinkling artifact results from internal machine noise and is seen more commonly in modern high-resolution US machines.

Nephrocalcinosis refers to calcification in the renal medullary pyramids causing the pyramids to appear echogenic rather than echolucent (Fig. 50.55). US is highly sensitive to even faint calcification that may not be visible on conventional radiographs. Acoustic shadowing is present only when calcification is dense. Common causes include furosemide therapy in the newborn, hypercalciuric states such as hyperparathyroidism, medullary sponge kidney, and renal tubular acidosis.

Diffuse Renal Parenchymal Disease. US is commonly used to evaluate patients with acute and chronic renal failure. Rarely, bilateral renal obstruction will be a cause of acute renal failure. Causes of bilateral obstruction include leaking abdominal aortic aneurysm, tumor (especially cervical carcinoma), and retroperitoneal fibrosis. These rare cases will benefit from relief of obstruction. In the remainder of patients, US reveals the size and morphology of the kidneys. End-stage renal disease is associated with small echogenic, often difficult to visualize, kidneys (Fig. 50.56; Table 50.3). When the kidneys are smaller than 9 cm in adults, reversible renal disease is unlikely and renal biopsy is seldom justified. Diffuse and focal renal parenchymal thinning and scarring provide rough estimates of renal parenchymal loss. Enlarged kidneys (>13 cm) suggest an infiltrative process such as acute glomerulonephritis, leukemia, lymphoma, or renal vein thrombosis (edema).

TABLE 50.2

CAUSES OF PELVICALIECTASIS

Obstruction
Vesicoureteral reflux
Distended bladder
Relieved obstruction with persistent dilation
Pregnancy
Diabetes insipidus
Active diuresis
Extrarenal pelvis (dilated pelvis without caliectasis)

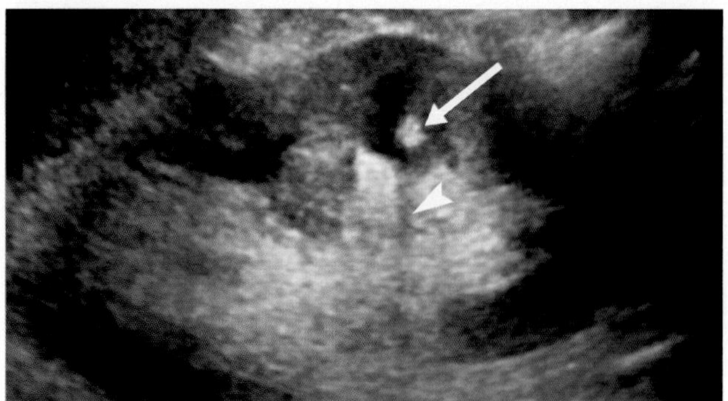

FIGURE 50.53. Renal Calculus. A 5-mm calculus is identified in the kidney appearing as an echogenic focus (*arrow*) with acoustic shadowing (*arrowhead*). Note that the echogenicity of the stone is very close to the echogenicity of the renal sinus. The stone would be difficult to identify without the presence of the acoustic shadow.

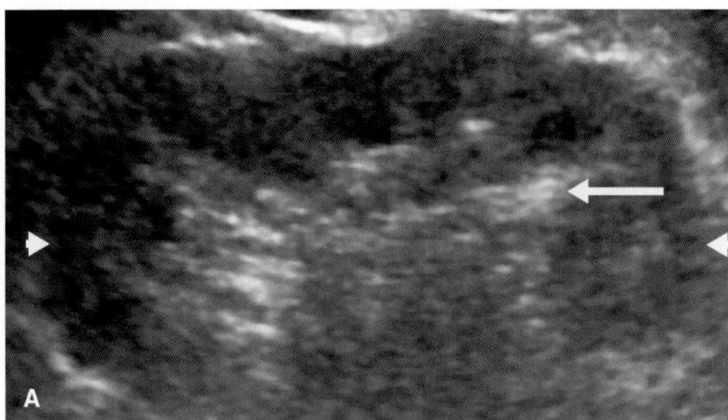

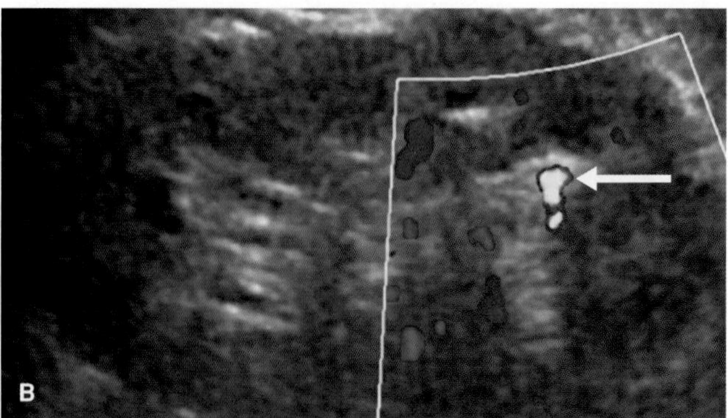

FIGURE 50.54. **Renal Calculus Identified by Twinkling Artifact. A:** A renal calculus (*long arrow*) is nearly impossible to appreciate on this longitudinal image of the kidney (between *short arrows*) in a difficult-to-image patient. The echogenic stone blends in with the echogenic renal sinus and no acoustic shadow is evident. **B:** Color Doppler image in the same plane shows the characteristic disorganized color of the twinkling artifact (*arrow*) identifying the highly reflective stone. The twinkling artifact can be effectively used to identify calculi and other highly reflective objects.

AIDS nephropathy is characterized by enlarged diffusely echogenic kidneys. Enlarged kidneys are an indication for Doppler examination of the renal veins to exclude thrombosis, and may warrant a renal biopsy to detect a treatable condition. US may demonstrate an unsuspected condition such as a form of renal cystic disease. Spectral Doppler waveforms of the renal arteries showing bilateral elevation of the resistive index (RI >0.7) are associated with an unfavorable outcome.

Renal Masses. Sonography plays a significant role in both the detection and characterization of renal masses. US is used to determine if a mass is a simple cyst, a complicated cyst, a complex mass, or an entirely solid mass. Doppler is used to demonstrate the internal vascularity to characterize a neoplasm. Contrast-enhanced US improves characterization.

Simple cysts are diagnosed accurately and easily by US (Fig. 50.57). Characteristic findings are (a) anechoic contents, (b) well-defined far wall, (c) acoustic enhancement deep to the lesion, and (d) imperceptibly thin walls. Small cysts may have artifactual internal echoes due to slice-thickness limitations. Acoustic enhancement may depend upon optimizing technique. All cysts should have a sharply defined back wall. Cysts with thin septations or thin peripheral curvilinear calcifications still qualify as benign cysts.

Complicated cysts have any of the following findings which disqualify their characterization as a simple cyst: internal debris, echogenic clot, fluid-debris levels, thick septations, thick walls, blood vessels in septations, thick or coarse calcification. Differential diagnosis of a complicated cystic mass includes hemorrhage or infection in simple cyst, cystic tumor, abscess, obstructed upper pole duplication, calyceal diverticulum, lymphoma, aneurysm, and pseudoaneurysm. Several studies indicate that US with contrast enhancement is equivalent to contrast-enhanced CT in characterizing complex renal cysts according to the Bosniak classification (see Chapter 47).

Peripelvic cysts form in the renal sinus, are multilobed, and may closely resemble hydronephrosis (Fig. 50.52). Peripelvic cysts are differentiated from hydronephrosis by demonstration of lack of communication with each other or dilated renal pelvis, echogenic fat between the tip of the medullary pyramid and the cyst, and lack of a dilated ureter. Problem cases require excretory urography or CT.

Renal cystic disease is discussed in detail in Chapter 47. US is a reliable, safe, and accurate method to demonstrate size, number, and characteristics of cysts in the kidney as well as other organs (Figs. 50.58 to 50.60).

Renal cell carcinoma (RCC) is, by far, the most common solid renal mass in adults (Fig. 50.61). On US, 50% are hyperechoic compared to renal parenchyma, 30% are isoechoic, 10% are hypoechoic, 5% to 10% are predominantly cystic, and 20% to 30% have coarse, punctate, central calcification.

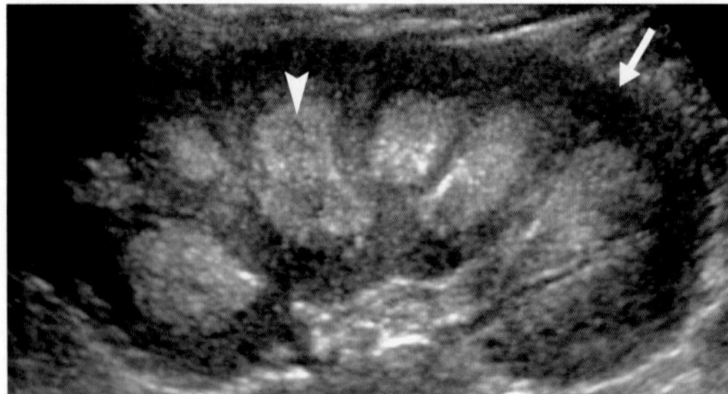

FIGURE 50.55. **Medullary Nephrocalcinosis.** Longitudinal US of the kidney demonstrates abnormally increased echogenicity of the medullary pyramids (*arrowhead*). Compare to the normal appearance of the kidneys in Figure 50.50. The echogenicity of the cortex (*arrow*) is normal. Medullary nephrocalcinosis usually does not cause acoustic shadowing.

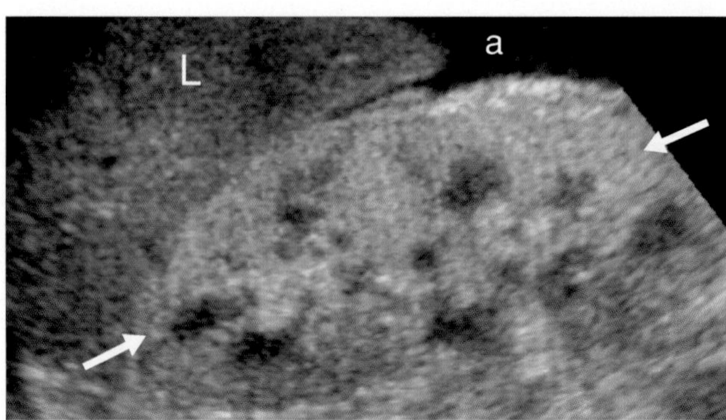

FIGURE 50.56. **End-Stage Kidney.** The echogenicity of the renal parenchyma of the kidney (between *arrows*) exceeds the echogenicity of the liver parenchyma (*L*). In this patient with advanced renal failure, both kidneys were small (<9 cm in length) and diffusely echogenic. This patient has ascites (*a*).

TABLE 50.3

MEDICAL RENAL DISEASES WITH ECHOGENIC RENAL PARENCHYMA IN ADULTS

Acute glomerulonephritis
Chronic glomerulonephritis
Hypertensive nephrosclerosis
Diabetic glomerulosclerosis
Lupus nephritis
Lymphoma
AIDS
Amyloidosis

Highly echogenic RCC may be confused with AML although RCC tends to be more heterogeneous and may have cystic components. CT or MR is indicated to demonstrate fat within echogenic tumors. Isoechoic tumors are detected when they distort the renal contour. Tumors become cystic because of necrosis and internal hemorrhage. Doppler demonstration of internal vascularity is strong evidence of RCC.

With detection of a solid renal mass the US examination should be extended to detect tumor invasion of the renal vein and IVC (Fig. 50.61B). Signs of tumor thrombus include echogenic mass in vein, enlarged vein, enlarged collateral vein, lack of or displacement of venous flow on color Doppler, and arterial Doppler signal within the vein due to tumor neovascularity.

Angiomyolipoma. The classic US appearance, seen in 80% of cases, is a uniformly hyperechoic renal mass with sharp borders (Fig. 50.62). The echogenicity of the mass is at least equal to that of renal sinus fat. Tumors which lack substantial fat are often indistinguishable from other renal tumors. Weak acoustic shadowing in the absence of calcification is seen with AML but not with RCC. AML is typically hypervascular but rarely has any cystic components. Definitive diagnosis is made by CT or MR demonstration of fat within the tumor. Calcification in the tumor is extremely rare.

Transitional cell carcinoma (TCC) is easy to overlook on US examination because fat within the renal sinus may be hypoechoic and simulate a renal pelvis tumor. Tumors may

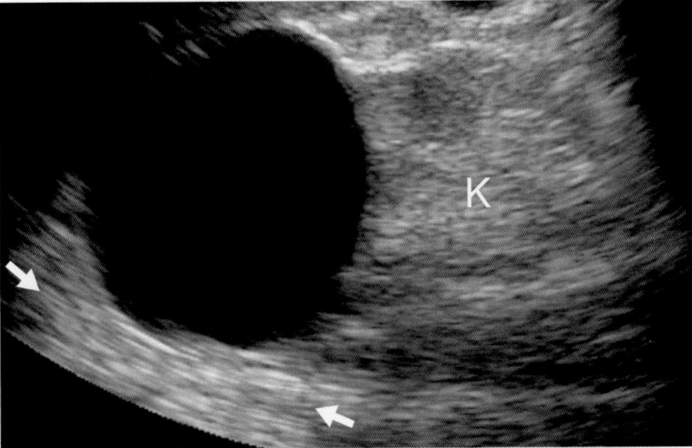

FIGURE 50.57. **Simple Renal Cyst.** Longitudinal image of the kidney (*K*) shows a simple renal cyst containing anechoic fluid and having imperceptibly thin walls, sharp interface with the renal parenchyma, and demonstrating accentuated sound transmission (between *arrows*).

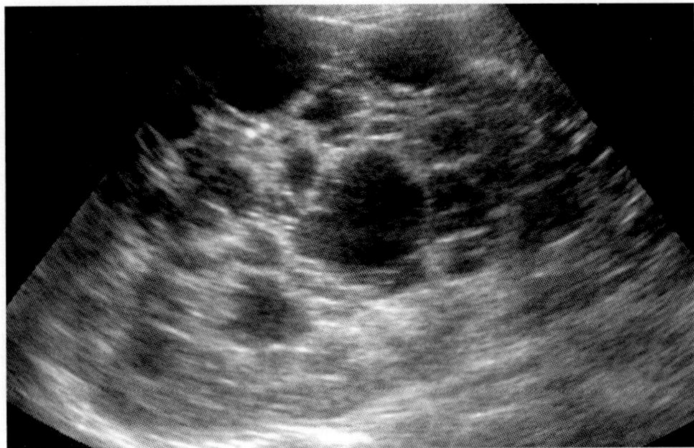

FIGURE 50.58. **Autosomal Dominant Polycystic Disease.** The kidney is greatly enlarged with its parenchyma near completely replaced by innumerable cysts of varying size. Both kidneys had the same appearance characteristic of advanced changes of autosomal dominant polycystic disease.

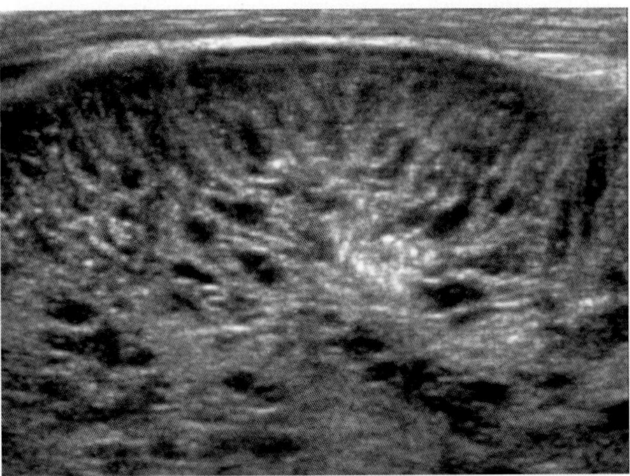

FIGURE 50.59. **Autosomal Recessive Polycystic Disease.** High-frequency (12 MHz) image of the parenchyma of the kidney in a newborn shows dilation of the collecting tubules that characterizes this condition.

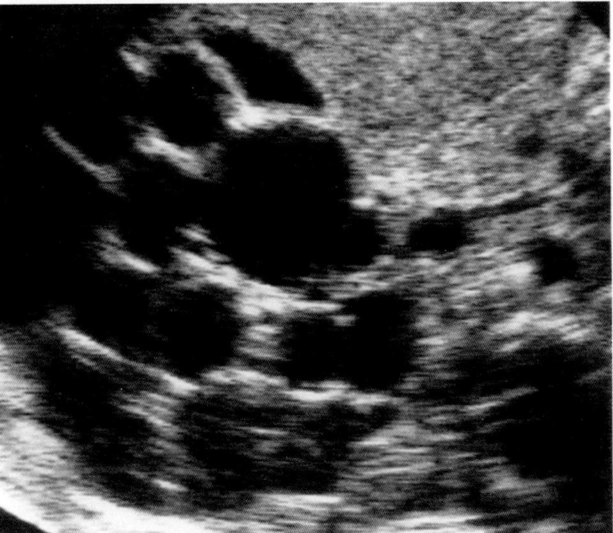

FIGURE 50.60. **Multicystic Dysplastic Kidney.** The right kidney is totally replaced by cysts of varying size, the classic appearance of multicystic dysplastic kidney. The left kidney appeared normal. A radionuclide scan demonstrated absent function on the right and normal function on the left.

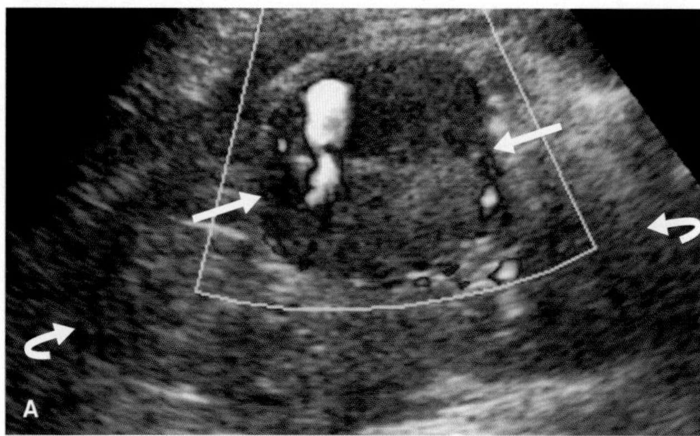

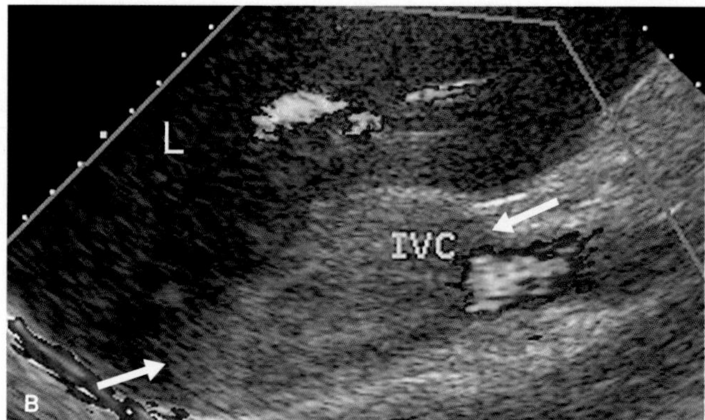

FIGURE 50.61. Renal Cell Carcinoma. A: A US image in the long axis of the kidney (between *curved arrows*) reveals a solid, hypervascular mass (between *straight arrows*). **B:** Longitudinal color Doppler image through the liver (*L*) shows tumor thrombus (between *arrows*) from a right renal cell carcinoma distending the inferior vena cava (*IVC*) and occluding blood flow.

be small, infiltrative, or stenosing. Hypoechoic renal sinus fat appears poorly marginated, central and bilaterally symmetric in location, shows posterior acoustic shadowing and poor definition of the posterior margin, and has sinus vessels coursing through it on color Doppler sonography. Renal sinus tumors (Fig. 50.63) tend to have relatively well-defined boundaries, are eccentric in location within the renal sinus, have well-seen posterior margin, show no acoustic shadowing, and displace renal sinus vessels on color Doppler US. Focal pelviectasis or caliectasis may be caused by a small TCC. TCC may also appear as soft tissue nodule within a dilated pelvis.

Lymphoma typically produces multiple hypoechoic masses, each of which has a uniform pattern of fine low-level echoes reflecting the homogeneous cellular structure. Doppler demonstration of internal vessels differentiates lymphoma from cysts containing echogenic fluid. Growth patterns include single dominant mass, multiple masses, diffuse infiltration causing renal enlargement, and invasion of the renal sinus from confluent retroperitoneal adenopathy.

Acute pyelonephritis frequently produces no US abnormalities. Severe cases alter the echogenicity of the renal parenchyma due to edema, local inflammation, and hemorrhage into renal tissue (Fig. 50.64). Mass-like areas of focal inflammation have been called lobar nephronia, focal nephritis, and a variety of other names that mostly cause confusion. These finding should be viewed as US evidence of severe pyelonephritis and probably nothing more. US is performed in patients with urinary tract infection to detect hydronephrosis, renal abscess, or perirenal abscess. Color flow Doppler increases the sensitivity of US examination by demonstrating edematous areas of pyelonephritis as foci of *decreased* parenchymal blood flow (Fig. 50.64B). This finding correlates with the foci of decreased enhancement characteristic of pyelonephritis on CT. Flow is decreased in inflamed areas by the pressure of edema confined by the strong renal capsule.

Pyonephrosis refers to infection within a dilated and obstructed renal collecting system. Echogenic debris, often with a shifting urine-debris level (Fig. 50.65), is seen within a dilated pelvicalyceal system in an infected patient. Gas in the collecting system produces shifting echogenic foci with shadowing and reverberation artifact. About 10% of cases of pyonephrosis are indistinguishable from uncomplicated hydronephrosis, so guided aspiration for diagnosis is indicated in clinically suspicious cases. Pyonephrosis is an indication for urgent percutaneous or surgical drainage.

Renal abscess appears as a poorly marginated intrarenal cystic mass containing echogenic fluid (Fig. 50.66). The appearance may change rapidly over a few days with extension of infection into and beyond the perirenal space. Small abscesses may be effectively treated with antibiotics, but larger abscesses

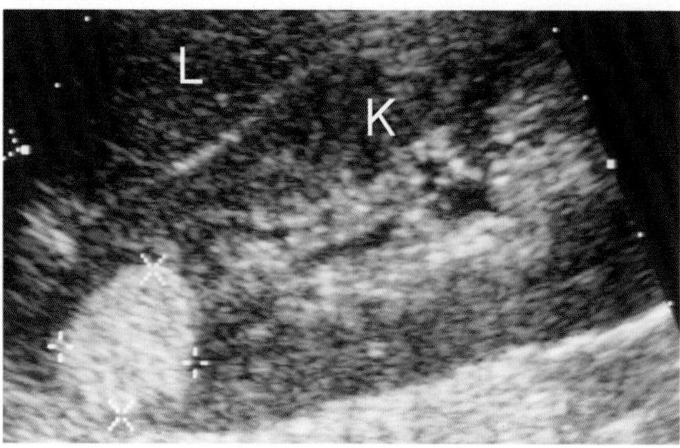

FIGURE 50.62. Angiomyolipoma. A US image through the long axis of the right kidney (*K*) demonstrates a well-defined, uniformly hyperechoic tumor (between *calipers*) in the upper pole. This appearance is strongly suggestive of angiomyolipoma. *L*, liver.

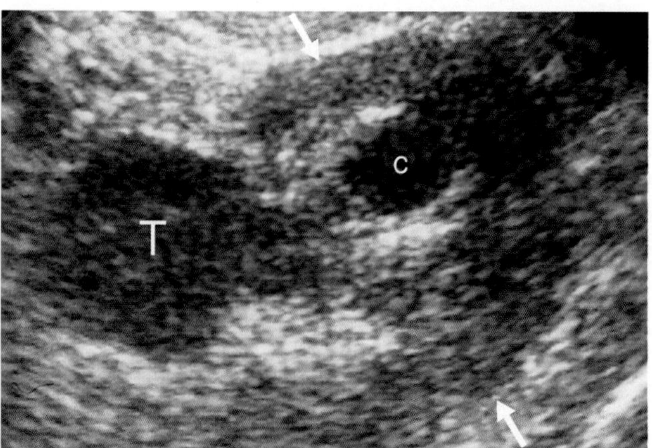

FIGURE 50.63. Transitional Cell Carcinoma. A US image of the left kidney (between *arrows*) in transverse plane shows the tumor (*T*) as a hypoechoic mass. The echogenicity of the mass is only slightly greater than that of a dilated calyx (*c*).

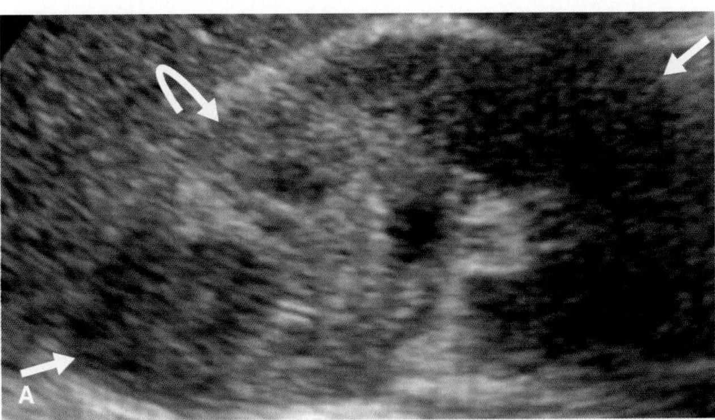

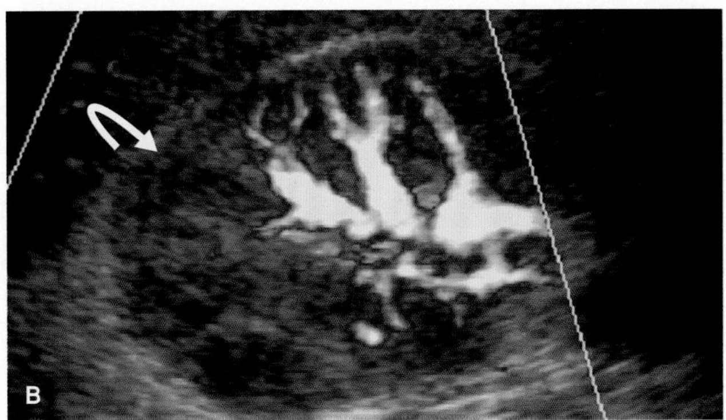

FIGURE 50.64. Acute Pyelonephritis. A: Longitudinal image of the kidney (between *arrows*) shows a focal area of increased echogenicity (*curved arrow*) that indicates inflammation and hemorrhage due to acute bacterial infection. **B:** Power Doppler image in the same plane shows focal *decreased* blood flow in the affected area (*curved arrow*). Blood flow is decreased because edema due to infection is confined within the renal capsule increasing pressure and inhibiting flow.

(>2 cm) may require percutaneous drainage. Extensive perirenal abscess usually requires surgical drainage.

Renal tuberculosis is characterized by the multiplicity of findings present including parenchymal scarring, calcification, intraparenchymal cavities with echogenic contents, and dilated calyces without accompanying dilation of the renal pelvis. US findings are seldom specific.

Xanthogranulomatous pyelonephritis is suggested by US demonstration of a shadowing stone in the renal pelvis, dilated collecting structures commonly filled with echogenic debris, mass-like distortion and enlargement of the kidney, and extension of disease into the perirenal space (Fig. 50.67). The renal parenchyma is frequently hypoechoic reflecting edema and inflammation.

Reflux nephropathy is suggested by US findings of focal renal parenchyma thinning with an underlying echogenic scar extending from the renal sinus toward the periphery, or a dilated calyx beneath the parenchymal thinning. The process is distinctly focal with the remainder of the kidney usually appearing normal.

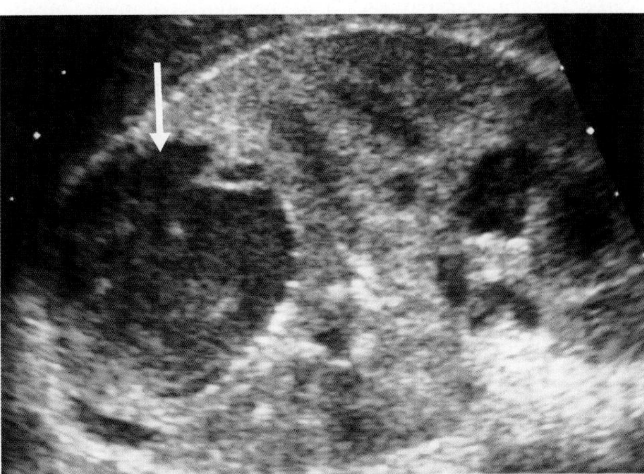

FIGURE 50.66. Renal Abscess. A cystic mass (*arrow*) in the upper pole of the kidney contains heterogeneous echogenic fluid. US-guided aspiration yielded coliform bacteria.

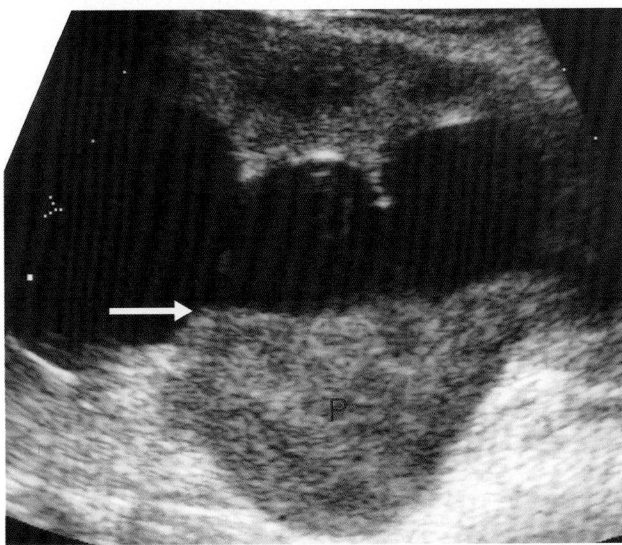

FIGURE 50.65. Pyonephrosis. US view of the left kidney with the patient in right lateral decubitus position reveals layering (*arrow*) of pus (*P*) in a dilated, obstructed collecting system.

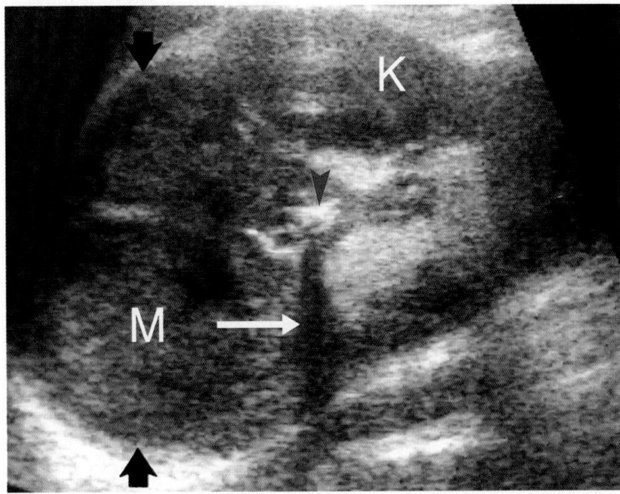

FIGURE 50.67. Xanthogranulomatous Pyelonephritis. Long-axis US of the right kidney (*K*) reveals a hypoechoic mass (*M*, between *black arrows*) enlarging the upper pole. An obstructing stone (*arrowhead*) casting an acoustic shadow (*red arrow*) is seen in the renal sinus. The kidney was chronically infected and was surgically removed, confirming xanthogranulomatous pyelonephritis.

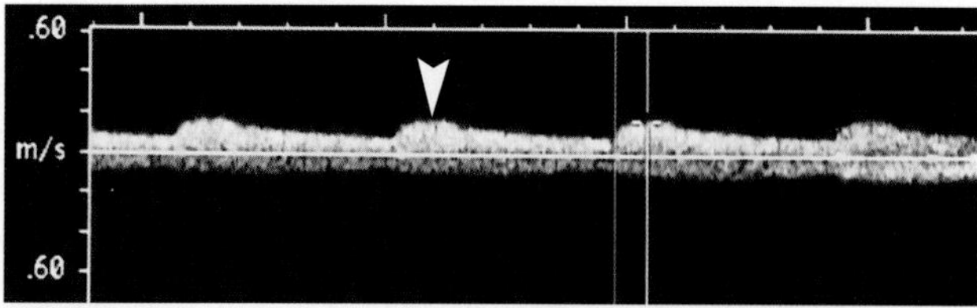

FIGURE 50.68. **Renal Artery Stenosis.** Doppler spectrum obtained from an intrarenal artery at the hilum reveals tardus–parvus waveform with delayed and stunted peak systolic velocities (*arrowhead*).

Arteriovenous fistula may be suspected following a renal biopsy but is rare in any other circumstance. Color Doppler shows a focal tangle of vessels with increased flow at the biopsy site. With large fistulas spectral Doppler of the hilar renal arteries shows a high-velocity low-resistance waveform while spectral Doppler of the renal vein shows arterial pulsations.

Renal artery stenosis (RAS) is the most common curable cause of hypertension accounting for 5% of hypertensive population. Atherosclerosis at the origin of the renal artery is the cause for 90% of the cases of renovascular hypertension while fibromuscular dysplasia in mid to distal renal artery accounts for 10%. US examination for RAS is challenging with visualization of the renal arteries limited by bowel gas and obesity. Accessory renal arteries are easily overlooked. However, with dedication and experience the US examination is successful in 80% to 90% of cases with specificity and sensitivity for RAS in 90% to 95% range. US is used primarily to screen for RAS and to follow-up on treatment for RAS. Examination is performed with real-time US of the kidneys and color flow and spectral Doppler of the renal arteries. A variety of criteria are used to diagnose significant RAS: (a) renal artery to abdominal aorta peak systolic velocity ratio >3.5; (b) main renal artery to interlobar renal artery peak systolic velocity ratio >5.0; (c) peak systolic velocity in the renal artery >180 to 200 cm/s (normal peak systolic velocity in the renal arteries is 60 to 100 cm/s); (d) tardus–parvus waveforms in the distal renal artery at the hilum (Fig. 50.68); (e) RI <0.45 in the intrarenal arteries; (f) RI > 0.7 in the intrarenal arteries. Additional findings include tissue vibration artifact at the site of stenosis and turbulent flow downstream from stenosis. A positive US for RAS is an indication for MRA or catheter angiography. Atherosclerotic disease is usually treated with an endovascular stent and fibromuscular dysplasia is routinely treated with angioplasty.

Renal vein thrombosis occurs in clinical settings of nephrotic syndrome, dehydration, trauma, coagulopathy, thrombosis of the IVC, or extension of RCC into the renal vein. It is more common in the pediatric than in the adult population. Patients are asymptomatic or present with flank pain and hematuria. Acute complete thrombosis causes an enlarged, hypoechoic, edematous kidney. US diagnosis is based on visualization of clot within the renal vein (Fig. 50.69). Color Doppler may confirm complete occlusion or document diversion of flow around the thrombus. Waveforms in the renal artery are diminished in velocity and show a high-resistance pattern with little to no forward flow in diastole. Incomplete venous thrombosis usually does not enlarge the kidney. Enlarged venous collateral vessels may be seen when renal vein thrombosis is chronic.

Renal transplantation is an increasingly common procedure associated with progressive decrease in surgical complications. US is essential to the immediate postoperative and long-term evaluation of renal transplants. US examination includes the morphology and size of the transplant kidney, detection of hydronephrosis, evaluation of the ureterovesical anastomosis, and Doppler assessment of the renal artery and vein and their anastomoses. US guidance is used to perform transplant biopsy and to aspirate and drain perirenal fluid. Increased size of the transplant kidney is seen with acute rejection, renal vein thrombosis, infection, and infiltration associated with posttransplant lymphoproliferative disorder. Decreased size of the kidney occurs with ischemia and chronic rejection. Dilation of the collecting system occurs with ureteral anastomosis stenosis, denervation of the collecting system and ureter, and bladder outlet obstruction. Peritransplant fluid collections are common and include hematoma, seroma, urinoma, abscess, and lymphocele. Vascular complications occur in up to 10% of patients and include renal artery or renal vein stenosis (usually at the anastomosis), kinking, compression, thrombosis, pseudoaneurysms, and rare intrarenal arteriovenous fistulae. Renal artery anastomotic stenosis is indicated by downstream tardus–parvus waveforms (Fig. 50.68), jets on color flow imaging and flow velocities >2 m/s near the anastomosis. Be aware of accessory artery anastomoses, which may be necessary in 20% of transplants. Vein stenosis shows a focal jet on color flow US. A fourfold increase in peak velocity indicates significant venous stenosis. Renal vein occlusion is rare but is an emergency associated with rapid failure of the transplant (Fig. 50.69). Thrombus is visualized within the renal vein on color flow imaging. Resistive indices are commonly calculated from the spectral waveform of the renal artery. RI is elevated (>0.70) with significantly impaired renal function. The finding is nonspecific and may occur with acute rejection, acute tubular necrosis, obstructive hydronephrosis, and compression of the kidney by adjacent mass or fluid collection.

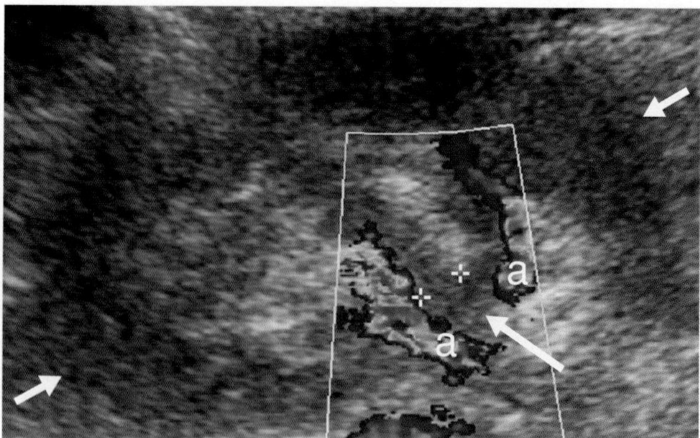

FIGURE 50.69. **Renal Vein Thrombosis in a Transplant Kidney.** Color Doppler US of a transplant kidney (between *small arrows*) on the second postoperative day shows blood flow in the renal arteries (*a*) but thrombus (*large arrow*) and no flow in the renal vein (between *cursors*, +). Acute thrombosis of the renal vein in a transplant kidney is a surgical emergency requiring immediate correction to save the kidney.

Suggested Readings

Ahn SE, Moon SK, Lee DH, et al. Sonography of gastrointestinal tract diseases: correlation with computed tomographic findings and endoscopy. *J Ultrasound Med* 2016;35:1543–1571.

American Institute of Ultrasound in Medicine. *AIUM Practice Parameter for the Performance of an Ultrasound Examination of the Abdomen and/or Retroperitoneum.* Laurel, MD: AIUM; 2017. Available from http://www.aium.org/resources/guidelines/abdominal.pdf.

American Institute of Ultrasound in Medicine. *AIUM Practice Parameter for the Performance of the Focused Assessment with Sonography for Trauma (FAST) Examination.* Laurel, MD: AIUM; 2014. Available from http://www.aium.org/resources/guidelines/fast.pdf.

Arslanoglu A, Seyal AR, Sodagari F, et al. Current guidelines for the diagnosis and management of hepatocellular carcinoma: a comprehensive review. *AJR Am J Roentgenol* 2016;207:W88–W98.

Barr RG, Ferraioli G, Palmeri ML, et al. Elastography assessment of liver fibrosis: society of radiologists in ultrasound consensus conference statement. *Ultrasound Q* 2016;32:94–107.

Benter T, Klühs L, Teichgräber U. Sonography of the spleen. *J Ultrasound Med* 2011;30:1281–1293.

Finstad TA, Tchelepi H, Ralls PW. Sonography of acute pancreatitis: prevalence of findings and pictorial essay. *Ultrasound Q* 2005;21:95–104; quiz 150, 153–154.

Foley WD, Quiroz FA. The role of sonography in imaging of the biliary tract. *Ultrasound Q* 2007;23:123–135.

Gerstenmaier JF, Gibson RN. Ultrasound in chronic liver disease. *Insights Imaging* 2014;5:441–455.

Go S, Kamaya A, Jeffrey B, Desser TS. Duplex Doppler ultrasound of the hepatic artery: a window to diagnosis of diffuse liver pathology. *Ultrasound Q* 2016;32:58–66.

Heller MT, Tublin ME. Detection and characterization of renal masses by ultrasound: a practical guide. *Ultrasound Q* 2007;23:269–278.

Manning MA, Srivastava A, Paal EE, Gould CF, Mortele KJ. Nonepithelial neoplasms of the pancreas: radiologic-pathologic correlation, Part 1—benign tumors: from the radiologic pathology archives. *Radiographics* 2016;36:123–141.

Mellnick VM, Menias CO, Sandrasegaran K, et al. Polypoid lesions of the gallbladder: disease spectrum with pathologic correlation. *Radiographics* 2015;35:387–399. Erratum: *Radiographics* 2015;35:1316.

Muradali D, Goldberg DR. US of gastrointestinal tract disease. *Radiographics* 2015;35:50–70.

Shapira-Rootman M, Mahamid A, Reindrop N, Nachtigal A, Zeina AR. Sonographic diagnosis of complicated cholecystitis. *J Ultrasound Med* 2015;34:2231–2236.

Sidhar K, McGahan JP, Early HM, Corwin M, Fananapazir G, Gerscovich EO. Renal cell carcinomas: sonographic appearance depending on size and histologic type. *J Ultrasound Med* 2016;35:311–320.

Stapa RZ, Jakubowski WS, Dobruch-Sobczak K, Kasperlik-Zatuska AA. Standards of ultrasound imaging of the adrenal glands. *J Ultrason* 2015;15:377–387.

Tamm EP, Kim EE, Ng CS. Imaging of neuroendocrine tumors. *Hemat Oncol Clin North Am* 2007;21:409–432; vii.

Thipphavong S, Duigenan S, Schindera ST, Gee MS, Philips S. Nonneoplastic, benign, and malignant splenic diseases: cross-sectional imaging findings and rare disease entities. *AJR Am J Roentgenol* 2014;203:315–322.

Tirkes T, Sandrasegaran K, Patel AA, et al. Peritoneal and retroperitoneal anatomy and its relevance for cross-sectional imaging. *Radiographics* 2012;32:437–451.

van Breda Vriesman AC, Engelbrecht M, Smithuis RH, Puylaert JB. Diffuse gallbladder wall thickening: differential diagnosis. *AJR Am J Roentgenol* 2007;188:495–501.

CHAPTER 51 ■ GENITAL TRACT AND BLADDER ULTRASOUND

WILLIAM E. BRANT

FEMALE GENITAL TRACT

Ultrasound (US) is the primary imaging modality for evaluation of the female genital tract and pelvis. Indications for pelvic US examination include infertility, pelvic pain, disorders of menstruation, abnormal or limited physical examination, suspicion of mass or infection, localization of intrauterine contraceptive device (IUD), and guidance for interventional procedures. US is used as an adjunct to physical examination to confirm the presence or absence of a pelvic mass, and to evaluate its size, contour, and character, determine the organ of origin, evaluate for involvement of other organs, and detect the presence of ascites, hydronephrosis, and metastases. The US examination is usually initiated with a transabdominal approach using the distended urinary bladder as a window to the pelvis. The transvaginal US is performed with the bladder empty and provides the most detailed evaluation. Color flow US is used to identify pelvic blood vessels, identify vascular lesions of the pelvis, and to demonstrate tumor vascularity. Saline infusion sonohysterography (SHG) utilizes real-time US imaging of the uterus during injection of the uterine cavity with sterile saline to detect and characterize abnormalities of the uterus and endometrium.

Uterus

Normal US Anatomy. The uterus in the postpubertal woman is smoothly contoured and pear shaped (Fig. 51.1). The myometrium is uniform midlevel echogenicity with the endometrium distinctly more echogenic. The thickness of the endometrial echo varies with menstrual state. The innermost myometrium, called the *junctional zone,* may appear as a thin hypoechoic layer adjacent to the echogenic endometrium. Maximum normal uterine dimensions in the adult woman are 9 cm in length, 6 cm in width, and 4 cm in anteroposterior diameter. Following menopause, the uterus atrophies to approximately 6 × 2 × 2 cm. The prepubertal, infantile, uterus is cigar shaped. The cervix makes up about one-third the length of the uterus in the adult woman and about two-thirds of the length of the uterus in the prepubertal girl. Normal uterine positions in the pelvis include tilted forward (anteverted—most common), tilted backward toward the sacrum (retroverted), or folded anteriorly (anteflexed) or posteriorly (retroflexed) (Fig. 51.1C). The normal uterus may also be tilted right or left toward the pelvic side walls. The position of the uterus is altered by the degree of bladder filling and the presence of pelvic masses. The retroverted or retroflexed uterus appears more globular on transabdominal scanning. The normal vagina appears as a flattened muscular tube with echogenic mucosa.

The US examination must always be correlated with the state of the menstrual cycle, which affects the normal brightness and thickness of the endometrium (Fig. 51.1). At the end of menstruation, the endometrium is discrete and thin (2 to 3 mm). During the *proliferative phase* the endometrium assumes a three-line appearance 4 to 8 mm thick. The basal endometrium, adjacent to the junctional zone myometrium, remains echogenic while the functional endometrium, which will thicken and eventually slough with menstruation, is relatively hypoechoic during the first half of the menstrual cycle. The three lines are formed by the anterior and posterior basal endometrium and the echogenic stripe that marks the uterine cavity. Measurement of endometrial thickness is defined by the added thickness of the anterior and posterior endometrium. Any fluid or blood within the uterine cavity is excluded. At midcycle the endometrium normally measures 8 to 10 mm in double-layer thickness. From ovulation to menstruation through the *secretory phase* the endometrium progressively thickens up to 14 mm and becomes more uniformly echogenic. The junction zone myometrium appears as a hypoechoic halo surrounding the bright endometrium. In the normal postmenopausal woman, the echogenic endometrium does not exceed 5 to 7 mm in thickness. During the normal fertile years, pregnancy must always be considered in evaluation of the female genital tract. Abnormalities of the first trimester of pregnancy are reviewed in Chapter 52.

Arcuate artery calcifications are seen as discrete echogenic foci in the outer third of the myometrium of postmenopausal women. They are seen more commonly in women who are diabetic or hypertensive.

Congenital anomalies of the uterus result from impaired development, fusion, or resorption of the paired Müllerian

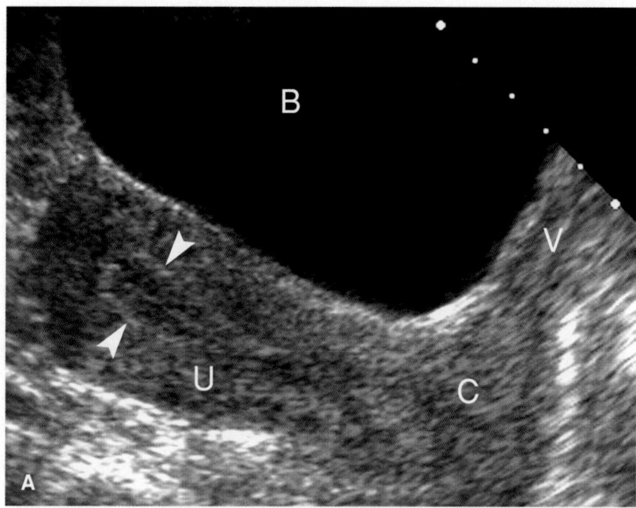

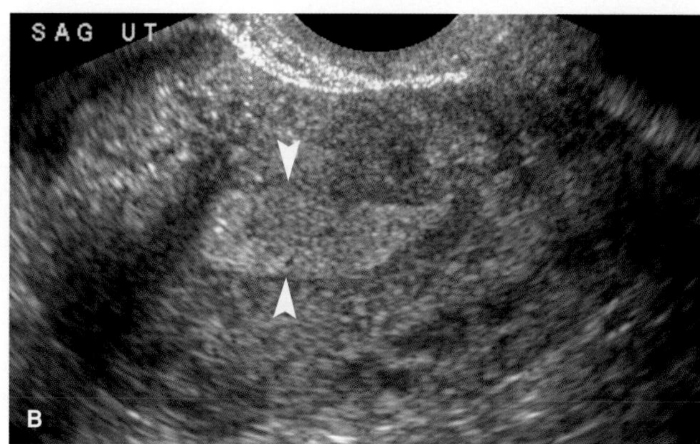

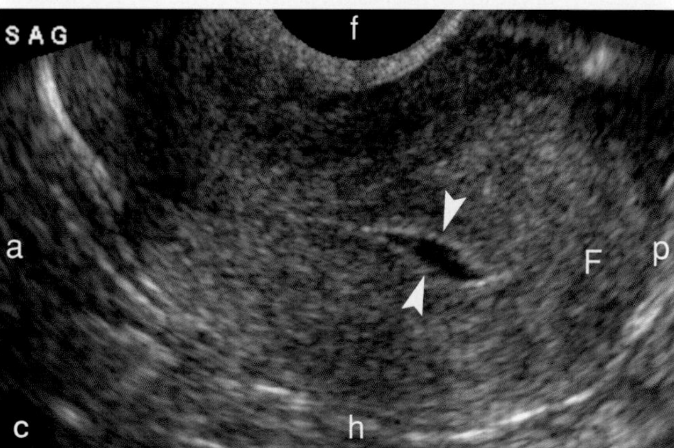

FIGURE 51.1. **Normal Uterus.** **A:** Transabdominal sagittal plane image through the urine-filled bladder (*B*) demonstrates the smooth contour and pear shape of the normal uterus (*U*). The endometrium (between *arrowheads*) is more echogenic than the surrounding myometrium. This image demonstrates the typical three-layer appearance of proliferative phase endometrium. The cervix (*C*) protrudes into the upper vagina (*V*) at the intersection between the long axis of the uterus and the axis of the vagina. **B:** Transvaginal sagittal plane image of the uterus demonstrates the improved resolution of this technique. The endometrium (between *arrowheads*) is more sharply defined and the myometrium is more clearly evaluated. This image demonstrates the typical uniformly echogenic appearance of secretory phase endometrium. **C:** Transvaginal sagittal plane image shows a retroflexed uterus. The uterine fundus (*F*) is directed posteriorly (*p*) toward the sacrum. Note the change in orientation when the transducer is placed endovaginally. The patient's head (*h*) is located toward the bottom of the image; her feet (*f*) are located toward the top of the image; her anterior abdominal wall (*a*) is located to the left of the image; and her sacrum is located posteriorly (*p*) toward the right of the image. This patient is at day 5 of her menstrual cycle having just completed menstruation. Her endometrium (between *arrowheads*) is at its thinnest. A small amount of residual menstrual fluid is in the uterine canal.

ducts that evolve into the structures of the female reproductive tract. Müllerian duct anomalies are frequently associated with infertility. MR provides the most comprehensive imaging characterization. Uterine anomalies are reviewed more extensively in Chapter 49. US may define two uterine horns, two distinct endometrial cavities, and an abnormal shape of the uterus. The kidneys should be examined for associated anomalies such as renal agenesis.

Leiomyomas (fibroids) are exceedingly common benign smooth muscle tumors of the myometrium that develop in women of all ages. They are suspected when the uterus is enlarged or altered in contour. Leiomyomas are virtually always multiple. They may be completely within the myometrium, subserosal, or submucosal in location. Leiomyomas may also be pedunculated and predominantly extrauterine, simulating an adnexal mass. Color flow US demonstration of vascular supply contiguous with the myometrium (the bridging sign) is definitive in confirming uterine origin of these exophytic leiomyomas. Uncomplicated leiomyomas may be isoechoic, hypoechoic, or hyperechoic compared to normal myometrium (Fig. 51.2). A characteristic finding is "Venetian blind" shadowing, a pattern of spaced dark linear echoes (shadows) emanating from the leiomyoma, caused by increased absorption of sound by fibrous tissue within the tumor. This finding may be particularly useful in the differentiation of submucous leiomyomas from endometrial polyps. Atypical appearance of leiomyomas may result from atrophy, internal hemorrhage, cystic degeneration, fibrosis, and calcification. A "popcorn" pattern of calcification is characteristic and definitive on plain film radiographs. Lipoleiomyomas contain fat in addition to smooth muscle and connective tissue resulting in highly echogenic uterine masses. Retroposition of the uterus and uterine anomalies, such as a bicornuate uterus, must be differentiated from leiomyoma. Leiomyomas may cause menorrhagia or vaginal bleeding unrelated to menstrual cycles. Exophytic tumors may torse and may be a cause of acute pelvic pain. The tumors are responsive to female hormones and commonly accelerate in growth during pregnancy. Correspondingly, they involute with menopause. Symptomatic leiomyomas are treated with gonadotropin-releasing hormone analogs, selective uterine artery embolization, or focused US

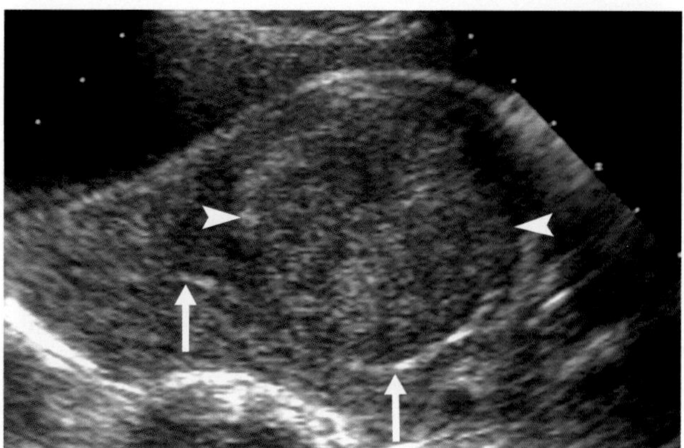

FIGURE 51.2. **Leiomyoma.** Transvaginal image of the uterus shows a hypoechoic leiomyoma (between *arrowheads*) displacing the endometrium (*arrows*) and impinging on the uterine cavity.

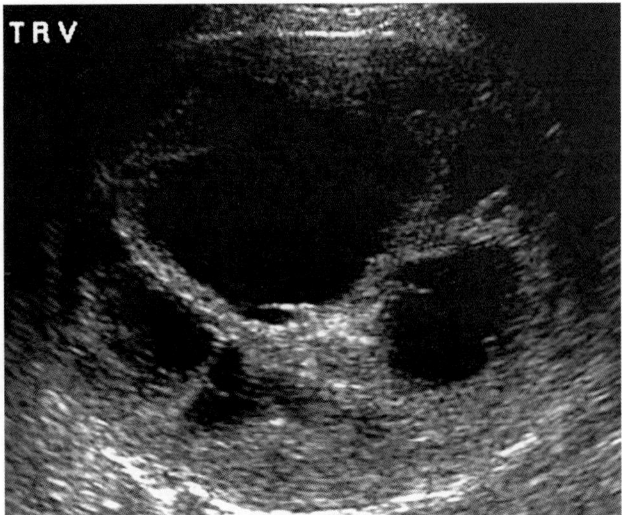

FIGURE 51.3. **Leiomyomasarcoma.** Transverse US image of the uterus in a 48-year-old woman with rapid uterine enlargement shows a heterogeneous mass with prominent cystic areas expanding the uterus. This proved to be a leiomyosarcoma. However, cystic degeneration in a benign leiomyoma may have an identical appearance.

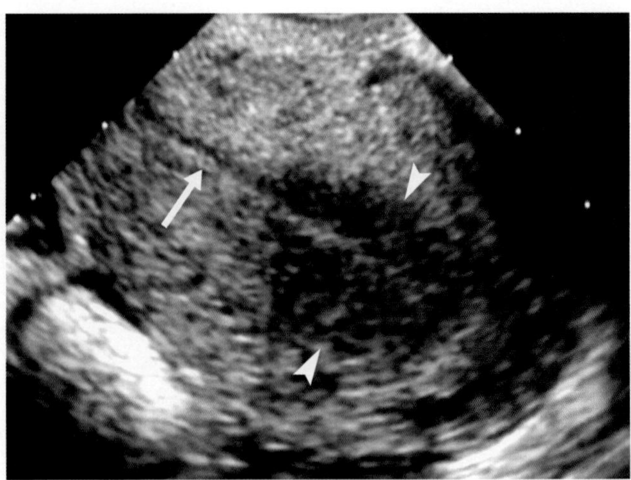

FIGURE 51.4. **Adenomyosis.** The junctional zone myometrium is irregularly thickened (*arrowheads*), poorly marginated, and markedly hypoechoic on this transvaginal US image in a woman with abnormal vaginal bleeding and pelvic pain. MR and pathology at hysterectomy confirmed adenomyosis. The endometrium (*arrow*) is thin and normal in appearance.

ablation, all of which may result in tumor necrosis, internal hemorrhage, and cystic changes. No imaging modality can reliably differentiate the very common benign leiomyoma from the quite rare leiomyosarcoma.

Leiomyosarcoma is a malignant tumor composed entirely of smooth muscle. It is a primary sarcoma of the uterus. It is a rare tumor difficult to diagnose clinically. Rapid increase in size of a uterine lesion or onset of vaginal bleeding in a postmenopausal women is the most diagnostic clinical feature. Imaging features overlap with benign leiomyomas (Fig. 51.3). Diagnosis is made histologically.

Adenomyosis is the condition of diffuse or focal invasion of the myometrium by benign endometrium ("internal endometriosis"). It is found commonly in multiparous women over age 30. The diffuse form is most common with islands of endometrium scattered throughout the myometrium. The localized form results in a mass, an adenomyoma, within the myometrium. A broad spectrum of sonographic appearance is related to the distribution of ectopic endometrium, the presence and number of cysts within the ectopic endometrium, and the amount of associated myometrial hypertrophy. The most common US findings are (1) diffuse abnormal hypoechoic or heterogeneous echotexture of the myometrium (Fig. 51.4), (2) poor definition or nodularity of the junction between endometrium and myometrium, (3) subendometrial echogenic nodules, (4) subendometrial myometrial cysts (1 to 5 mm), and (5) subendometrial hypoechoic linear striations. The uterus is usually enlarged. Leiomyomas are commonly present as well, frequently masking the coexistence of adenomyosis. MR provides the best detection and characterization of adenomyosis. See Chapter 49.

Thickened Endometrium. The thickness of the endometrium must always be correlated with age, menstrual history, and stage of the menstrual cycle. The full thickness of the echogenic endometrium, including both anterior and posterior endometrium, is measured perpendicular to the long axis of the uterus. In women having active menstrual cycles, the endometrium may measure up to 14 to 16 mm during the secretory phase. However, in postmenopausal women the endometrium normally does not exceed 5 mm in thickness.

Postmenopausal bleeding (PMB) occurs in 10% of postmenopausal women. The presence of endometrial cancer in 10% of women with PMB demands accurate evaluation. The most common cause of PMB is endometrial atrophy (70%) associated with a thin endometrium. Other common causes of PMB are associated with a thickened endometrium (Table 51.1). Transvaginal US is routinely used to assess the appearance and to measure the thickness of the endometrium. An endometrial thickness of 5 mm is generally accepted as a cutoff value. In the presence of PMB the endometrium should be biopsied if double-layer thickness exceeds 5 mm. The risk of cancer is minute if the endometrial thickness is <5 mm. SHG is used commonly to further characterize lesions shown on US and to assess whether they are amenable to hysteroscopic resection.

Endometrial atrophy is characterized by a uniformly thin endometrium with double-layer thickness less than 5 mm (Fig. 51.5). Thin endometrium is a normal and expected finding in postmenopausal women. However in some women the thin endometrium leads to superficial erosion and bleeding occurs.

The causes of thickening of the endometrium include:

1. *Endometrial carcinoma* may appear as diffuse thickening of the endometrium or as a focal endometrial mass.

TABLE 51.1

CAUSES OF POSTMENOPAUSAL BLEEDING

Common
Endometrial atrophy (70%)
Endometrial polyps (2–12%)
Endometrial hyperplasia (5–10%)
Endometrial carcinoma (10%)
Submucosal leiomyoma
Uncommon
Cervical carcinoma
Cervical polyps
Cervicitis
Tamoxifen therapy
Vaginal mucosal atrophy
"Rogue" ovulations

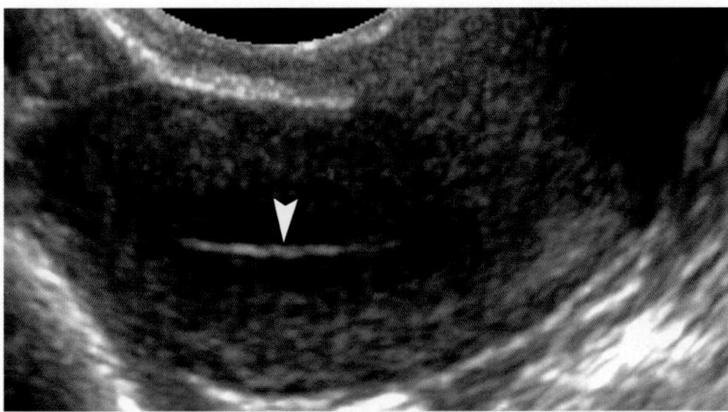

FIGURE 51.5. **Endometrial Atrophy.** Transvaginal sonogram in longitudinal plane reveals a very thin endometrium (*arrowhead*) measuring only 2 mm in a postmenopausal woman with vaginal bleeding. This is diagnostic of endometrial atrophy as the source of her bleeding. No biopsy is necessary.

Endometrial thickness >15 mm is strongly associated with carcinoma (Fig. 51.6). The endometrium is commonly heterogeneous, has uneven thickness, and an ill-defined interface with the adjacent myometrium. PMB is the most common presenting symptom.

2. *Endometrial hyperplasia* is caused by unopposed or prolonged estrogen stimulation and is most common in peri- and postmenopausal women. The endometrium is thickened and inhomogeneous with small cysts commonly present. Only biopsy can differentiate endometrial hyperplasia from endometrial cancer.

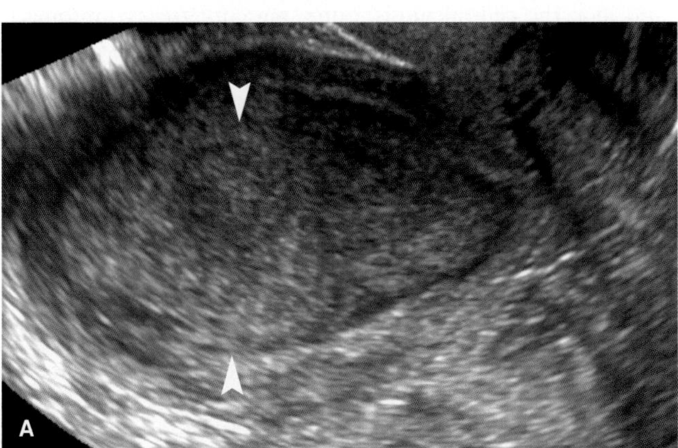

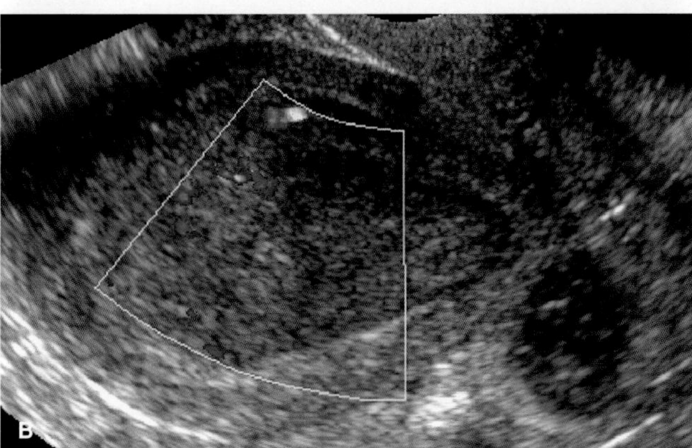

FIGURE 51.6. **Endometrial Carcinoma. A:** Transvaginal US in a 72-year-old woman with vaginal bleeding reveals a markedly thickened endometrium measured at 29 mm between *arrowheads*. **B:** Color Doppler image shows blood flow within the heterogeneous endometrial tissue. US findings are highly indicative of malignancy. Biopsy confirmed endometrial carcinoma.

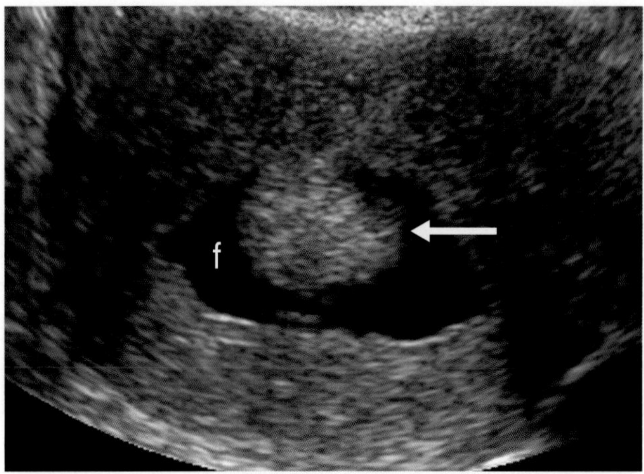

FIGURE 51.7. **Endometrial Polyp.** Transvaginal image in transverse plane taken during an SHG clearly reveals the polypoid nature of the endometrial mass (*arrow*). Sterile saline fluid (*f*) injected into the uterine cavity distends the uterine cavity.

3. *Endometrial polyps* result from focal hyperplasia or adenomatous neoplasia of the endometrium. They are most common between ages 30 and 60. Malignant transformation is reported in 1% to 4%. About 20% are multiple. US demonstrates a focal echogenic polypoid mass in the endometrium (Fig. 51.7) or diffuse endometrial thickening. Compared to submucosal leiomyomas endometrial polyps are homogeneously echogenic, smaller (<20 mm), and have a single feeding vessel.
4. *Tamoxifen*, used as an adjunct therapy for breast cancer, increases the risk of endometrial carcinoma two- to sevenfold. It is also associated with an increased incidence of endometrial polyps, endometrial hyperplasia, and sometimes striking cystic changes in the endometrium (Fig. 51.8).
5. *Submucosal leiomyomas* cause abnormal bleeding by erosion of the overlying endometrium. The most common symptom is bleeding throughout the menstrual cycle. Compared to endometrial polyps submucosal leiomyomas tend to be more hypoechoic, larger (>20 mm), and have multiple

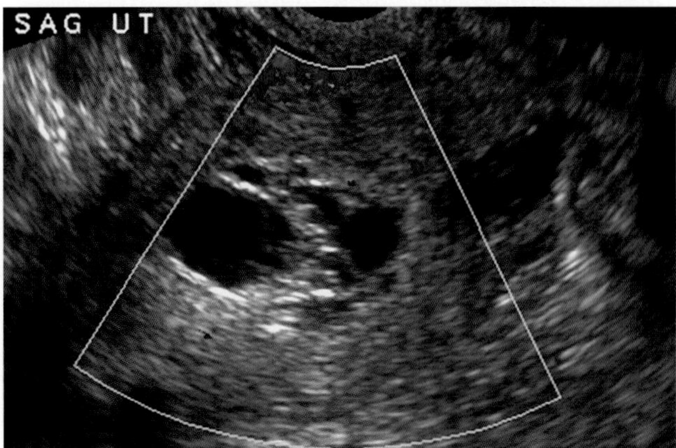

FIGURE 51.8. **Cystic Changes in the Endometrium.** Sagittal plane transvaginal color Doppler US image of the uterus shows advanced cystic changes in the endometrium in a patient taking tamoxifen therapy for breast cancer. Very little blood flow to the endometrium is evident. Biopsy showed benign endometrial hyperplasia.

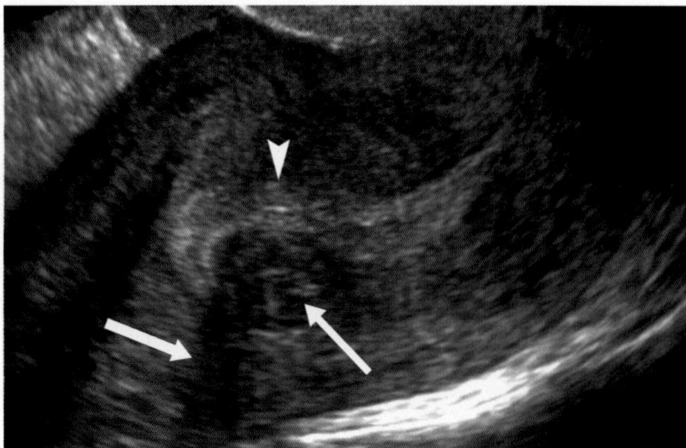

FIGURE 51.9. Submucosal Leiomyoma. Transvaginal image of the uterus in sagittal plane shows a hypoechoic mass (*long arrow*) abutting and distorting the endometrium (*arrowhead*). Acoustic shadowing (*fat arrow*) and low echogenicity compared to the endometrium are highly indicative of leiomyoma. The patient presented with brisk vaginal bleeding throughout the menstrual cycle.

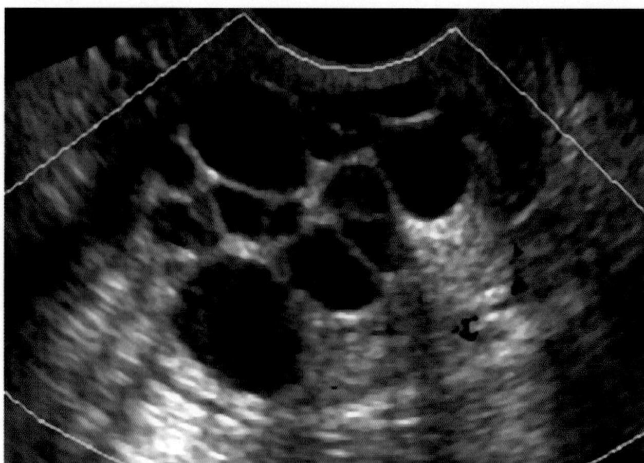

FIGURE 51.11. Nabothian Cysts. Transverse color Doppler image shows enlargement of the cervix caused by numerous Nabothian cysts. No blood flow within the cysts or within the cyst walls is demonstrated.

feeding vessels. Acoustic shadows emanating from the mass favor leiomyoma (Fig. 51.9). Lesions that protrude more than 50% of their diameter into the uterine cavity can generally be removed hysteroscopically.

The precise diagnosis is determined by endometrial biopsy. Pregnancy must never be forgotten as a possibility.

Fluid in the endometrial cavity may be blood, mucus, or purulent material. Hematometra refers to blood in the endometrial cavity and hematocolpos describes blood filling the vagina. In postmenopausal women causes of fluid in the uterine cavity include cervical stenosis (Fig. 51.10), cervical carcinoma, endometrial carcinoma, endometrial polyps, and pyometrium. In premenopausal women causes include congenital obstruction due to imperforate hymen; vaginal septum; vaginal or cervical atresia; acquired cervical obstruction due to instrumentation, radiation, or carcinoma; menorrhagia; and pregnancy.

Nabothian cysts result from obstruction of the ducts of mucous-secreting glands of the epithelial lining of cervix and are commonly visualized on transvaginal US. They are usually anechoic, frequently multiple (Fig. 51.11), and vary in size 2 to 3 mm up to 4 cm. They are nearly always asymptomatic.

Uterine arteriovenous malformations (AVMs) are composed of a tangle of vessels of various sizes consisting of both arteries and veins but without an intervening capillary network. Congenital AVMs have a central nidus with multiple feeding arteries, large branches external to the uterus, and draining veins. AVMs acquired as a result of trauma, surgical procedures, gestational trophoblastic disease, or endometrial or cervical cancer tend to have single or few intrauterine artery feeders and lack the central nidus. Some patients are asymptomatic while others have intermittent, sometimes torrential, bleeding. US shows a heterogeneous uterus with tubular anechoic spaces in the myometrium (Fig. 51.12). Color Doppler US shows a bright color mosaic of the vascular tangle. Spectral Doppler arterial waveforms are of high velocity and low resistance characteristic of arteriovenous shunting. Angiographic embolization is the treatment of choice.

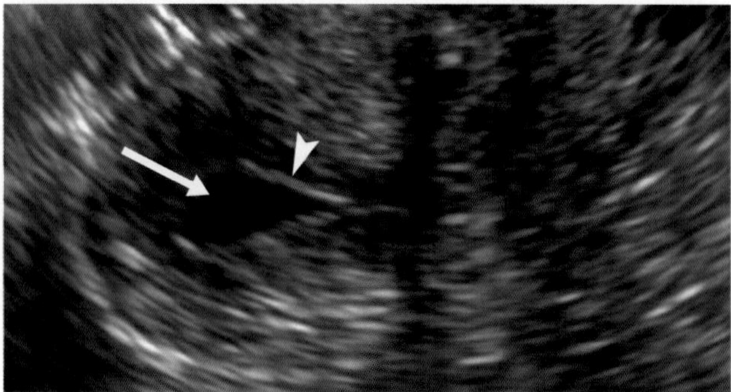

FIGURE 51.10. Fluid in the Endometrial Cavity. Anechoic fluid (*arrow*) is evident within the uterine cavity on this transvaginal US image of the uterus of a 75-year-old woman. The endometrium (*arrowhead*) is thin and normal. This patient has atrophic cervical stenosis.

Intrauterine contraceptive devices currently used in the United States include the T-shaped copper-wrapped ParaGard® IUD and the hormone impregnated T-shaped Mirena®, Kyleena®, Liletta®, and Skyla® IUDs. Complications include expulsion, malposition, uterine perforation, infection, and pregnancy. Copper-wrapped IUDs produce prominent acoustic shadowing and reverberation echoes that make identification and localization easy. The hormone impregnated IUDs are less echogenic and more difficult to identify requiring careful US examination especially if the uterus is distorted by the presence of leiomyomas. The normal position of the IUD is centered within the uterine canal with the T-shape portion abutting the fundus. If the IUD is low in position in the mid or lower uterus, it is ineffective as a contraceptive (Fig. 51.13). Malposition with penetration of the myometrium or even perforation of the uterus is associated with pelvic pain. Expulsion of the IUD may not be noticed by the patient, except for absence of the IUD string, and is confirmed with US. If a pregnancy occurs, it is more likely to be ectopic. Infection (pelvic inflammatory disease [PID]) may complicate the use of IUDs.

Ovaries and Adnexa

Normal US Anatomy. The term *adnexa* refers to the ovaries, fallopian tubes, broad ligament, and ovarian and uterine vessels, all of which may be involved in pathologic conditions. US demonstrates the ovaries as oval soft tissue structures with multiple small cystic follicles. The ovaries average 4 × 3 × 2 cm in size, with a maximum of 5 cm in any one dimension. The

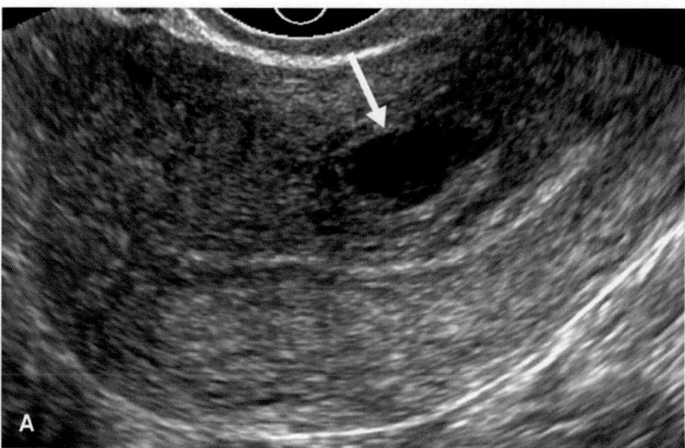

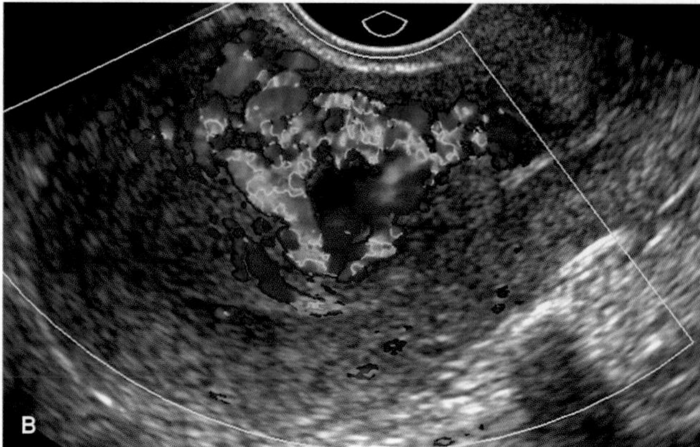

FIGURE 51.12. Uterine Arteriovenous Malformation. A: Gray scale US reveals a cystic appearing mass (*arrow*) in the anterior wall of the uterus. **B:** Color Doppler US image in the same longitudinal plane demonstrates the bright network of tangled blood vessels that make up an AVM.

maximum ovarian volume for an adult woman, calculated by the standard formula (length × width × height × 0.52), is 22 cc. The ovaries show characteristic morphologic changes with the menstrual cycle. Following menstruation, the ovaries are at their smallest with the follicles measuring less than 5 mm. During the estrogen phase, follicles enlarge to 10 to 15 mm size with one dominant follicle attaining 20 to 30 mm size by midcycle (Fig. 51.14). Rupture of the dominant follicle releases the ovum and the *corpus luteum* forms at the site of the dominant follicle. Ovulation releases fluid which pools in the cul-de-sac. All remaining follicles normally involute following ovulation. Hemorrhage into the corpus luteum or any follicle produces a *hemorrhagic functional cyst*. The ovaries vary widely in location, but usually lie in a shallow ovarian fossa in the angle between the external iliac vessels anteriorly and the ureter posteriorly with the fallopian tubes draped over and around them. The fallopian tubes are not visualized unless enlarged, however the broad ligament is clearly seen when it is outlined by fluid in the pelvis. *Postmenopausal ovaries* are atrophic, lack follicles, and are often difficult to visualize. Mean ovarian volume decreases from 8 cc at age 40 to 44 to less than 1 cc at age 70. Maximum ovarian volume in a postmenopausal woman is 6 cc. In infants up to 24 months of age the ovaries are small with mean volume of 1 cc and maximum volume of 3 cc. Focal *calcifications* in otherwise normal appearing ovaries are a common and benign finding.

Follicles are normal physiologic structures on the ovary. Follicles are thin walled, contain anechoic fluid, and are arranged around the periphery of the ovary (Fig. 51.14). Normal follicles range up to 15 mm size while the dominant follicle may be 30 mm in diameter just prior to ovulation. Follicles should be called follicles and should not be called cysts because "cyst" implies a pathologic finding.

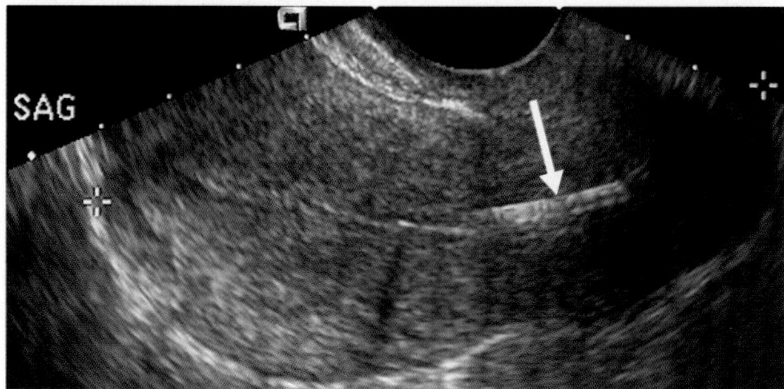

FIGURE 51.13. IUD Low in Position. Sagittal plane transvaginal image of the uterus shows the IUD (*arrow*) aberrantly positioned in the lower uterine segment. The IUD is seen as a bright linear echo with reverberation artifact. An IUD in this position is ineffective as a contraceptive.

Corpus lutea are formed by rupture and collapse of the dominant follicle during ovulation. The corpus luteum function is the secretion of progesterone and estrogen. It initially appears as solid, vascular portion of the ovary (collapsed cyst appearance) (Fig. 51.15). It forms a small cystic mass (<3 cm) often with internal echoes, fluid levels, or mesh-like internal structure (hemorrhagic cyst appearance). Its walls are typically thicker than the wall of normal follicles. Color Doppler shows an intensely vascular "ring of fire." If pregnancy does not occur, the normal corpus luteum involutes. If it fails to involute, or if hemorrhage occurs, it may enlarge to 4 to 5 cm to become a functional ovarian cyst or a hemorrhagic ovarian cyst. If pregnancy occurs the corpus luteum persists as a physiologic cystic structure through 16- to 18-week gestation.

Functional ovarian cyst is the most common ovarian mass (Table 51.2). Small cysts, up to 3 cm, should generally be considered to be normal follicles. Pathologic *follicular cysts* up to 20 cm result from excessive accumulation of fluid or internal hemorrhage. They basically represent follicles or corpus lutea that fail to regress. Functional cysts may rupture or undergo torsion. Diagnosis is made by the demonstration of a round, smooth, usually unilocular ovarian cyst (Fig. 51.16) that resolves on follow-up examination after one or two menstrual cycles. Anechoic thin-walled cysts (simple cysts) that fail to resolve after two menstrual cycles may be neoplasms (cystadenomas or benign cystic teratomas), however they are extremely unlikely to be malignant. The Society of Radiologists in Ultrasound recommends yearly follow-up of "simple" adnexal cysts >5 cm.

Hemorrhagic ovarian cysts result from hemorrhage into a follicle or the corpus luteum. Patients present with pelvic pain, often abrupt in onset, pelvic mass, or may be asymptomatic. Hemorrhagic ovarian cysts are common in premenopausal women and very rare in postmenopausal women unless they are taking hormone replacement therapy. US shows a broad spectrum of findings (Fig. 51.17): (1) the key finding is a cystic mass with internal echoes; (2) accentuated through-transmission reflects its cystic nature; (3) wall thickness is variable (2 to 20 mm); (4) blood flow in the wall is commonly prominent and does not differentiate hemorrhagic cyst from tumor; (5) internal echogenicity depends upon the physical state of

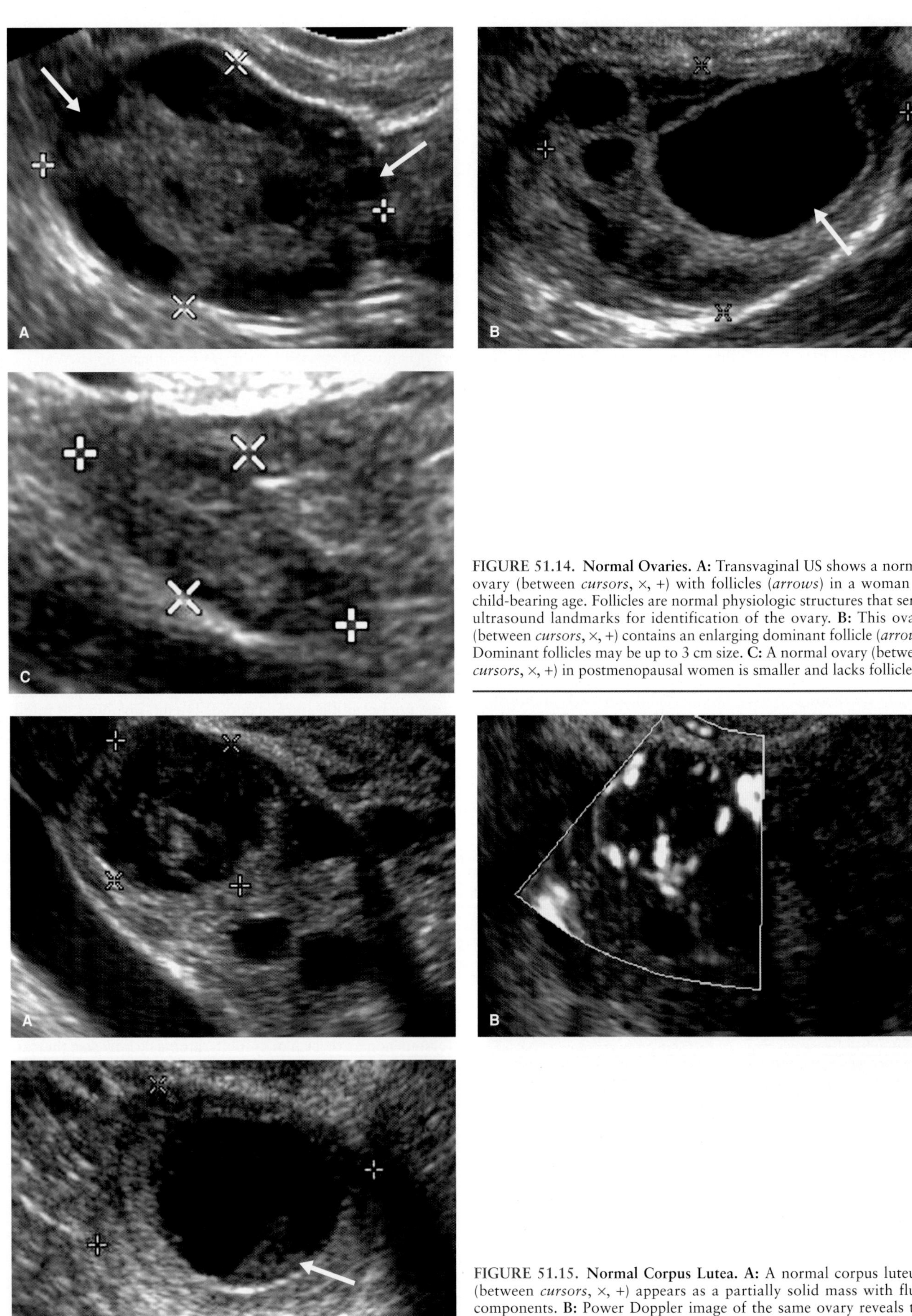

FIGURE 51.14. **Normal Ovaries. A:** Transvaginal US shows a normal ovary (between *cursors*, ×, +) with follicles (*arrows*) in a woman of child-bearing age. Follicles are normal physiologic structures that serve ultrasound landmarks for identification of the ovary. **B:** This ovary (between *cursors*, ×, +) contains an enlarging dominant follicle (*arrow*). Dominant follicles may be up to 3 cm size. **C:** A normal ovary (between *cursors*, ×, +) in postmenopausal women is smaller and lacks follicles.

FIGURE 51.15. **Normal Corpus Lutea. A:** A normal corpus luteum (between *cursors*, ×, +) appears as a partially solid mass with fluid components. **B:** Power Doppler image of the same ovary reveals the intense vascularity of the normal corpus luteum. **C:** In a different woman the corpus luteum (between *cursors*, ×, +) has reformed as a cyst. Echogenic material (*arrow*) within the cyst is a small blood clot.

TABLE 51.2

CAUSES OF AN OVARIAN MASS

■ CYSTIC OVARIAN MASS	■ SOLID OVARIAN MASS
Functional ovarian cyst	Fibroma (benign)
Hemorrhagic ovarian cyst	Brenner tumor (nearly always benign)
Endometrioma	Thecoma/Fibrothecoma (benign)
Cystic teratoma (97% benign)	Pedunculated leiomyoma
Serous cystadenoma/ cystadenocarcinoma (60% benign)	Dysgerminoma (Malignant germ cell tumor)
Mucinous cystadenoma/ cystadenocarcinoma (85% benign)	Granulosa cell tumor (85–90% benign)
Clear cell carcinoma	Sertoli–Leydig tumor (80–90% benign)
Endometrioid carcinoma	Metastasis
Necrotic metastasis	

the hemorrhage; (6) the cyst may appear solid but color flow US shows no internal blood vessels; (7) retracting clots adherent to the wall mimic neoplastic papillary projections but lack blood flow; and (8) a web-like pattern of lacy internal echoes representing fibrin strands is characteristic. Particulate matter within hemorrhagic cysts may demonstrate *acoustic streaming* described as the movement of particulate matter in fluid in the direction of the sound beam away from the transducer. Endometriomas, which may otherwise appear identical to hemorrhagic cysts, do not show acoustic streaming. Rupture of a hemorrhagic cyst causes acute pain and results in hemoperitoneum. Follow-up US usually shows complete resolution within two menstrual cycles.

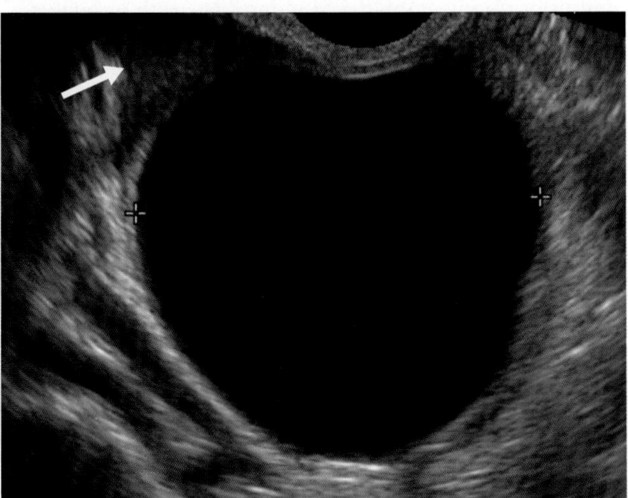

FIGURE 51.16. Functional Ovarian Cyst. Transvaginal US demonstrates a well-defined, thin-walled, anechoic ovarian cyst (between *calipers*, +) in a 36-year-old woman. A small portion of the ovary (*arrow*) is visible on this image. The appearance is typical of functional ovarian cyst. On follow-up US examination 10 weeks later the cyst had resolved.

Postmenopausal ovarian cysts are benign serous inclusion cysts found in 15% of asymptomatic postmenopausal women. US features are (1) small size <5 cm, (2) smooth thin walls of uniform thickness <3 mm, (3) anechoic fluid contents, and (4) absence of septations, nodules, or any soft tissue component. Over time these cysts commonly change size or disappear. Cysts with these characteristics in postmenopausal women are extremely unlikely to be malignant. The Society of Radiologists in Ultrasound recommends yearly follow-up of postmenopausal cysts >1 cm.

Pelvic inflammatory disease refers to acute or chronic inflammation of the fallopian tubes, ovaries, and pelvic peritoneum. Patients are usually in their teens and 20s and present with pain, fever, and vaginal discharge. Causes of PID include gonococcus, chlamydia, anaerobic bacteria, and tuberculosis. The disease runs a spectrum from endometritis to salpingitis to hydrosalpinx and tuboovarian abscess. In acute PID, US demonstrates a complex ill-defined adnexal mass that often includes a dilated, pus-filled fallopian tube, swollen ovary, and adhesions to adjacent structures (Fig. 51.18). Echogenic, purulent, fluid is usually present in the cul-de-sac. Chronic PID manifests as hydrosalpinx or peritoneal inclusion cyst.

Endometriosis is the occurrence of aberrant functioning endometrial tissue outside the uterus. Patients are commonly aged 25 to 35 and present with infertility and chronic pelvic pain. Many cases involve tiny (1 to 2 mm) implants of endometrial tissue on the peritoneum that are not visualized by US. These deposits are functionally active during the menstrual cycle resulting in inflammation and adhesions in the pelvis. Adhesions may produce a complex mass that mimics a tuboovarian abscess. Larger deposits form cystic masses filled with old, echogenic blood, a condition termed "chocolate cyst" or endometrioma. *Endometriomas* have a wide range of appearance as single, or characteristically multiple, adnexal masses with diffuse low-level internal echoes (Fig. 51.19). As mentioned, endometriomas may be identical in appearance to hemorrhagic functional ovarian cysts but do not demonstrate acoustic streaming. Doppler shows variable blood flow in the wall of the endometrioma but not within echogenic material within the cyst. Other appearances of endometrioma include solid mass without internal blood flow, a cystic mass with hyperechoic foci in the wall, a simple cyst mimicking a functional ovarian cyst, or a mass with calcific foci mimicking a teratoma. Deposits of endometrial tissue with surgical scars in the abdominal wall characteristically produce cyclic pain corresponding to menstruation.

Ovarian tumors whether benign or malignant, are most commonly predominantly cystic. The tumors most frequently encountered are the epithelial tumors: serous and mucinous cystadenoma and cystadenocarcinoma, and benign cystic teratoma. US is used to differentiate functional ovarian cysts from ovarian tumors, and to provide findings used to assess the risk of malignancy.

Benign cystic teratomas, also called dermoid cysts, are benign germ cell tumors usually discovered in patients aged 10 to 30. They are the most common ovarian neoplasm and are bilateral in 15% to 25% of cases. Although predominantly cystic, the presence of mature ectodermal elements results in formation of bone, teeth, and hair that give them a complex and varied appearance. Most tumors can be accurately diagnosed by US (Fig. 51.20). Three appearances are most common. The most characteristic appearance is a cystic mass with complex fluid and a mural nodule, the "dermoid plug." Fluid-fluid levels, representing fatty sebum floating on aqueous liquid are common. Another classic finding is the "tip of the iceberg" appearance of an amorphous echogenic mass that fades into acoustic reverberation and shadowing. The third common

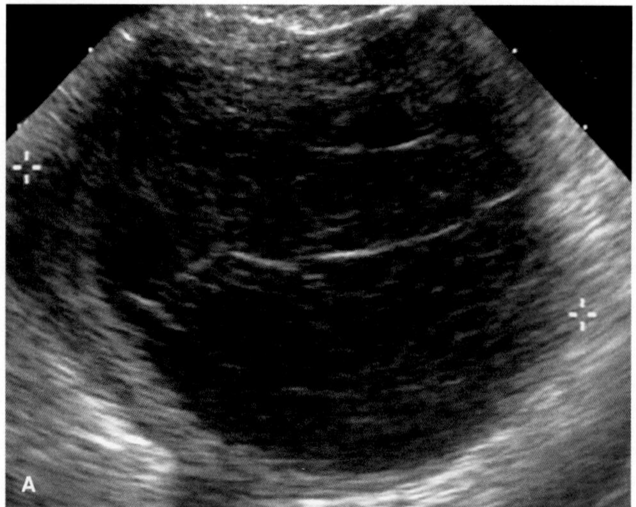

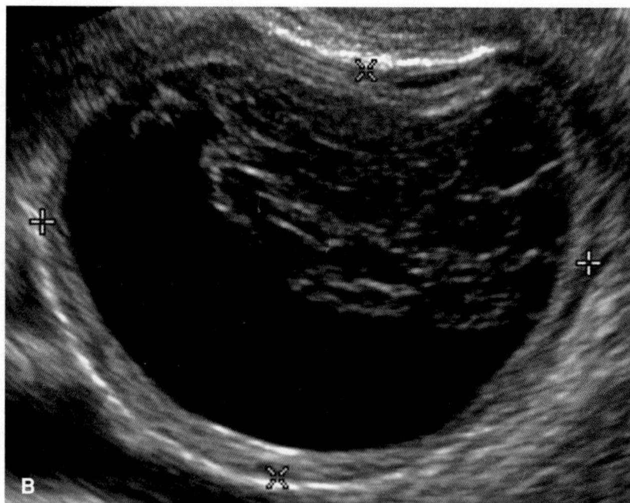

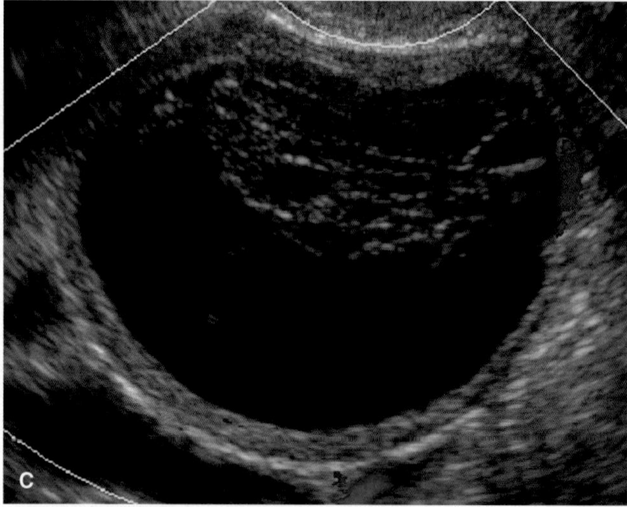

FIGURE 51.17. **Hemorrhagic Functional Cysts. A:** Transvaginal US shows the complex internal echogenicity of a hemorrhagic functional cyst (between *calipers*, +). The lacy internal appearance is characteristic of fibrin strands within evolving hemorrhage. **B:** Cystic ovarian mass in another woman shows nondependent echogenic material within the cyst (between *cursors*, ×, +). **C:** Color Doppler image of the same ovary as in **B** shows blood flow in the wall of the cyst but none in the solid appearing material within the cyst, confirming adherent blood clot in a hemorrhagic cyst. Follow-up US confirmed complete resolution in both cases.

pattern appears as multiple fine echogenic strands representing hair within the cyst cavity. Other appearances include the appearance of a simple cyst; a cystic mass containing multiple echogenic floating balls; or a solid mass with predominance of thyroid tissue (struma ovarii) that may cause thyrotoxicosis. The diagnosis of benign teratoma can often be confirmed by a conventional radiograph that demonstrates teeth or bone. CT or MR confirmation of fat content is also definitive.

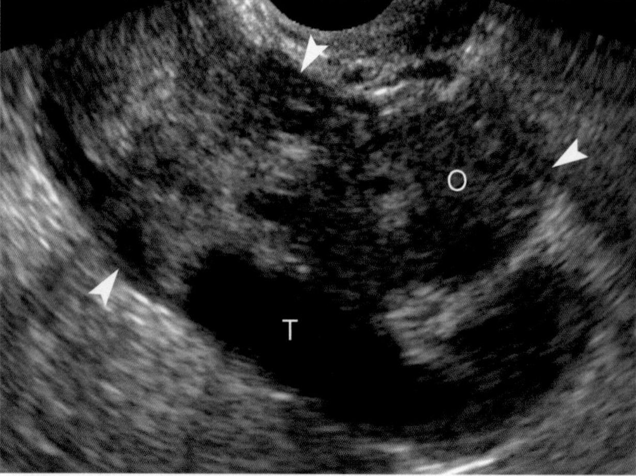

FIGURE 51.18. **Tuboovarian Abscess.** US of the adnexa reveals a complex mass (*arrowheads*) enveloping the ovary (*O*) and fallopian tube (*T*). Physical examination reveals marked pelvic tenderness with fixation of the pelvic organs.

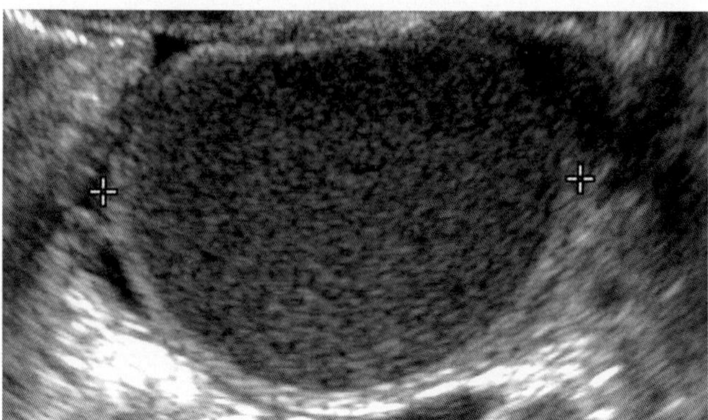

FIGURE 51.19. **Endometrioma.** Transvaginal sonogram shows an adnexal cyst (between *calipers*, +) with uniform thin wall and homogeneous fine internal echoes. This appearance may be seen with either a hemorrhagic ovarian cyst or an endometrioma. Endometrioma should be suspected if the cyst fails to resolve within 2 months.

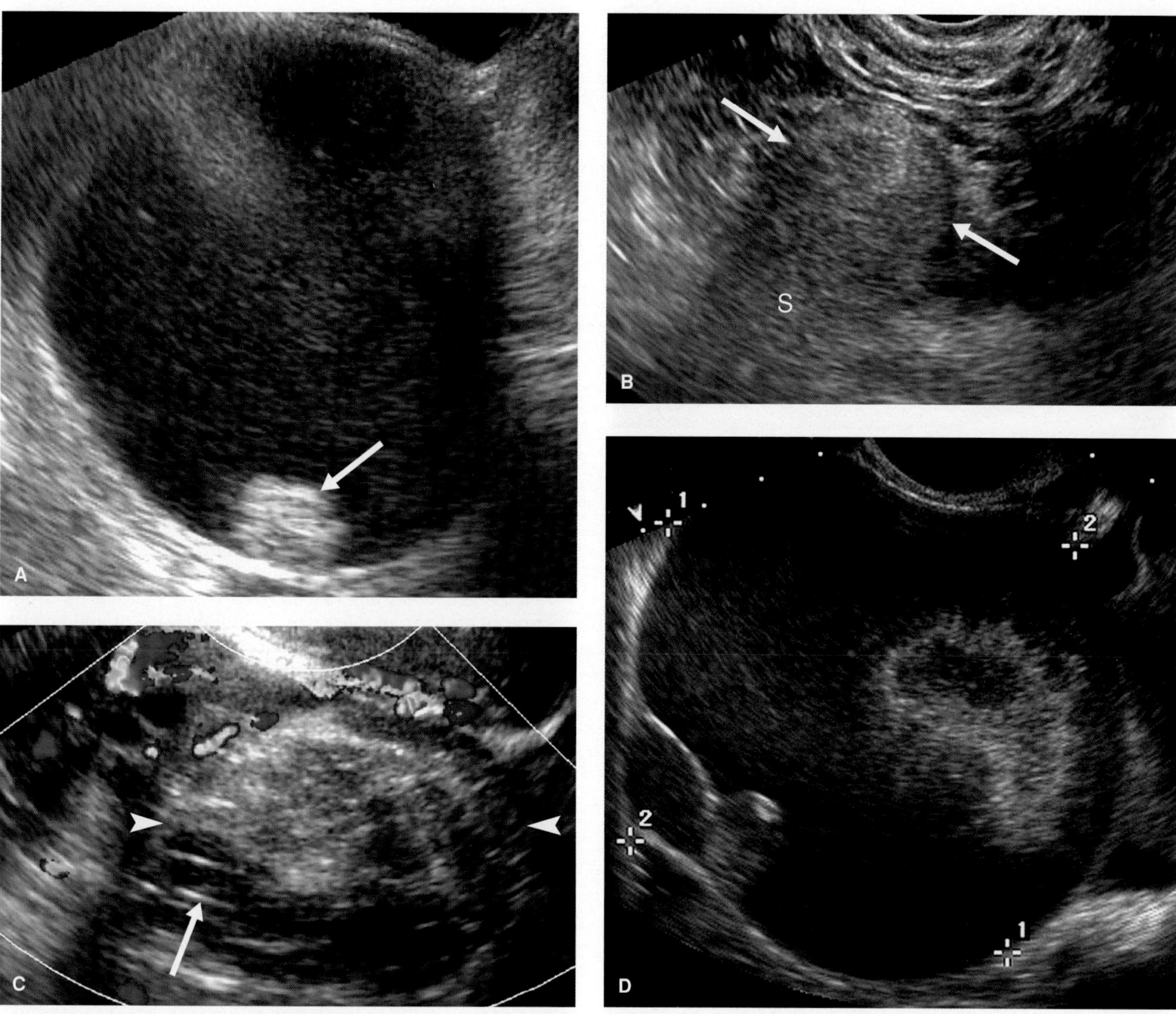

FIGURE 51.20. **Benign Cystic Teratomas. A:** An ovarian mass in a young woman is predominantly cystic with floating echoes within the fluid. An echogenic nodule (*arrow*) represents a dermoid plug. **B:** Transvaginal US in a patient with a palpable adnexal mass reveals an echogenic mass (between *arrows*) with indistinct margins that fade into acoustic shadowing (*S*) and reverberation. This is the typical "tip of the iceberg" appearance of a benign cystic teratoma. **C:** A complex ovarian mass (between *arrowheads*) with prominent echogenic components shows no internal blood flow. Avascular strands (*arrow*) represent hair characteristically found in benign cystic teratomas. **D:** Transvaginal image of an ovarian mass (between *calipers*, +) reveals a bizarre spiculated structure suspended within fluid containing floating particulate matter. A bizarre appearance of an ovarian mass should always bring to mind cystic teratoma as a possible diagnosis.

Epithelial tumors arise from the epithelial covering of the ovary. As a group they account for 65% to 75% of all ovarian neoplasms. Most present as predominantly cystic masses. Pathologic differentiation of benign and malignant forms is sometimes difficult resulting in some being classified as "borderline" malignant or tumor of "low malignant potential." Bilateral tumors are common and more frequent with malignant types.

Serous cystadenoma and cystadenocarcinoma comprise 30% of all ovarian neoplasms and 40% of all ovarian malignancies. Serous cystadenomas are thin-walled, usually unilocular, cysts with anechoic fluid mimicking in appearance a functional ovarian cyst. Serous cystadenocarcinomas are multiloculated with thick walls, thick septa, and papillary projections into fluid. Doppler usually documents blood flow within septa and papillary projections.

Mucinous cystadenoma and cystadenocarcinoma comprise 20% of ovarian neoplasms. About 85% are benign. Mucinous tumors may be huge, filling the pelvis and extending high into the abdomen. Most have multiple septations (Fig. 51.21) and contain fluid that is echogenic because of the presence of mucin. Rupture spreads mucin-secreting cells throughout the peritoneal cavity and may result in pseudomyxoma peritonei.

Endometrioid tumors are nearly always malignant. Most are cystic masses with papillary projections.

Other epithelial cell types include clear cell carcinoma (unilocular cyst with a mural nodule), Brenner tumor (solid, benign), and undifferentiated epithelial tumor (aggressive, ill defined, cystic, or solid).

Germ cell tumors include the benign cystic teratoma previously described, and malignant germ tumors (2.6% of ovarian malignancies) including dysgerminomas which consist of undifferentiated germ cells, yolk sac (endodermal sinus) tumor, and immature teratoma. Most present in adolescence with abdominal pain and pelvic mass. Malignant lesions appear as solid heterogeneous masses or mixed cystic and solid tumors.

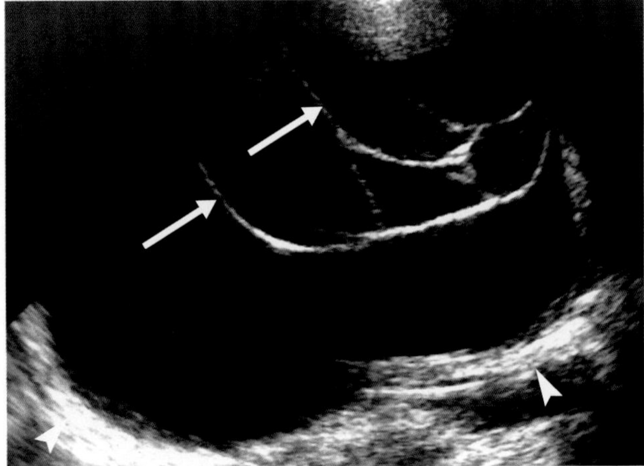

FIGURE 51.21. **Benign Mucinous Cystadenoma.** This ovarian tumor caused a huge mass, filling the pelvis and lower abdomen. US confirms a cystic mass (between *arrowheads*) with a network of fine septations (*arrows*). The absence of detectable solid components suggests a benign tumor.

Stromal tumors include Sertoli–Leydig cell tumors (which may cause masculinization and are malignant in 10% to 20% of cases), thecoma (which produces estrogen), and fibromas (which are associated with ascites and pleural effusions—Meigs syndrome). US reveals a solid hypoechoic mass that causes often striking sound attenuation. Pedunculated leiomyomas have a similar appearance. Physical connection to and vascular supply from the uterus differentiate leiomyomas from solid stromal tumors of the ovary.

Metastases to the ovary occur most commonly with gastrointestinal and breast carcinomas. A *Krukenberg tumor* is a metastasis to the ovary from a mucin-producing tumor of the gastrointestinal tract. Most metastases to the ovary are bilateral and solid. Cystic metastases may be indistinguishable from a primary ovarian tumor.

Signs of Malignancy. Since most pelvic masses are discovered, or initially evaluated, by US, every effort must be made to assess the risk of malignancy. Transvaginal US is essential in the evaluation. The following signs correlate with an increased risk of malignancy:

1. Solid tissue within a cystic mass—the more solid tissue presents the greater the risk of malignancy. Solid tissue includes thick walls (>3 mm), irregular wall thickness, thick septations (>3 mm), papillary projections, and solid nodules (Fig. 51.22). Malignancy is very unlikely in the absence of visible solid tissue. Unilocular cysts or cysts with thin septations are nearly always benign. Thick-walled, multilocular, masses with solid nodules are usually malignant. Heterogeneous solid vascularized tissue making up a portion of an ovarian mass is usually indicative of malignancy. Well-defined homogeneous entirely solid masses that transmit sound poorly are likely to be benign ovarian fibromas.
2. Size greater than 10 cm correlates with a 64% risk of malignancy in postmenopausal women. Masses less than 5 cm are more likely to be benign.

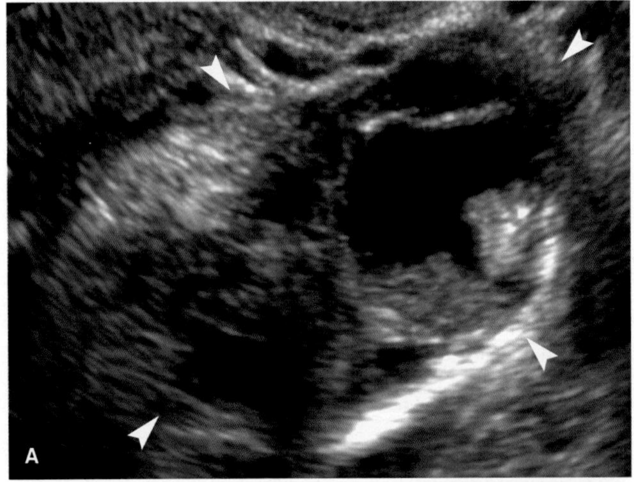

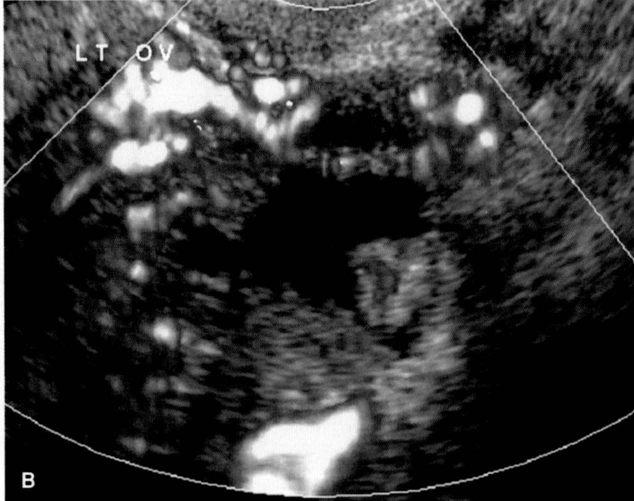

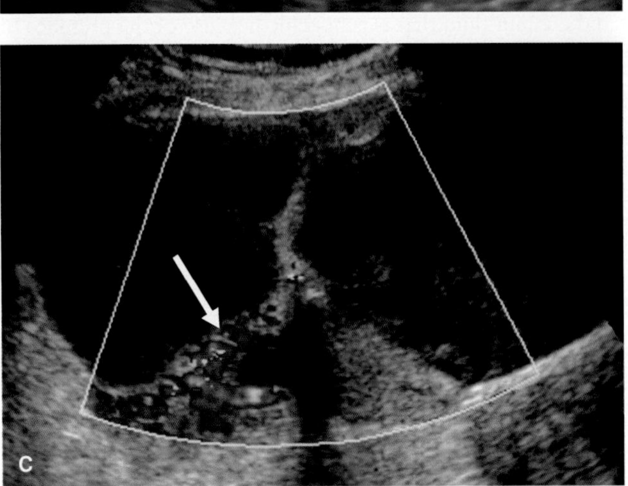

FIGURE 51.22. **Ovarian Carcinoma. A:** The ovary of a postmenopausal woman is replaced by a complex mass (between *arrowheads*) with prominent solid components. **B:** Power Doppler confirms prominent vascularity within the solid components of the same mass. This appearance is highly indicative of ovarian carcinoma. **C:** Color flow US image of a different tumor shows prominent blood flow with the septa (*arrow*) of a cystic mass. This finding is highly indicative of neoplasm, in this case ovarian carcinoma.

3. Color flow US demonstration of blood vessels within papillary projections is evidence of neoplasm and provides differentiation from avascular blood clots adherent to the cyst wall. Vascularized papillary projections are more common with malignant neoplasms.
4. Color flow US demonstration of blood vessels within septations is strong evidence of neoplasm. Hemorrhagic functional cysts may be complex in appearance but the septa are fibrin strands that lack vascularity. Blood flow in the wall of cystic masses is commonly seen in both benign and malignant lesions.
5. Age and clinical findings. The risk of malignancy of an ovarian mass increases with the patient's age from 24% at age 50 to 60 to 60% above at age 80. Germline mutations increase the risk of ovarian cancer, 39% to 46% for BRCA1 and 12% to 20% for BRCA2. The biochemical marker CA 125 is elevated in 50% of patients with stage 1 ovarian cancer and in 90% of patients with more advanced disease.
6. Extension of tumor outside the ovary to the uterus, broad ligament, or other pelvic organs is strong evidence of malignancy. However, inflammatory processes, such as tuboovarian abscess and endometriosis, may produce similar extension of disease.
7. Ascites, even in the absence of visualized tumor implants, is an ominous finding in the presence of an adnexal mass. Peritoneal implants from ovarian carcinoma are commonly minute and may not be detected by US or other imaging methods.
8. Evidence of metastatic spread including tumor implants on peritoneal surfaces, omental cake, and enlarged lymph nodes are clear signs of malignancy (Fig. 51.23).

Nonovarian cystic masses in the pelvis include abscess from appendicitis or diverticulitis, urachal cysts in the midline above the bladder, lymphocele in patients with prior pelvic node dissection, and neural origin cysts like meningoceles that extend anteriorly from the sacrum. Sonographic demonstration of a separate ovary on the same side as the adnexal mass suggests the diagnosis of nonovarian mass.

Paraovarian cysts account for 10% to 20% of all adnexal masses. They arise from remnants of the Wolffian duct and are covered by layers of the broad ligament. They have the appearance of a simple cyst separate from the ovary, thin walled, unilocular, well defined, containing anechoic fluid.

Peritoneal inclusion cysts are relatively common inflammatory pseudocysts of the peritoneal cavity that result from adhesions that envelop an ovary. Diseased peritoneum loses its ability to absorb fluid. Secretions from an active ovary confined by adhesions produce an expanding pelvic fluid collection. Patients present with pain or a pelvic mass. Most have a history of previous pelvic surgery, infection, trauma, or endometriosis. US demonstrates a complex collection of fluid occupying pelvic recesses and containing the ovary within the loculated fluid (Fig. 51.24). The presence of the ovary within or at the periphery of the mass is critical to the correct diagnosis. Septations, loculations, and particulate matter within contained fluid are common.

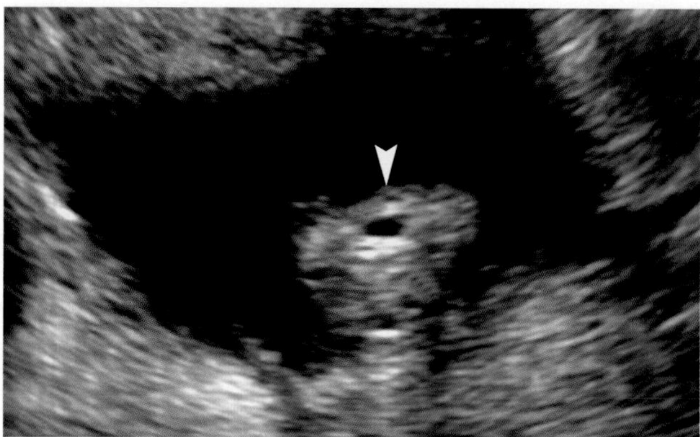

FIGURE 51.24. Peritoneal Inclusion Cyst. Sonogram reveals a fixed pelvic fluid collection with angulated boundaries and fluid occupying peritoneal recesses. The collection encloses the ovary (*arrowhead*) identified by the presence of follicles.

Polycystic ovary syndrome is a clinical and biochemical diagnosis based on findings of oligo- or anovulation, obesity, clinical and/or biochemical signs of hyperandrogenism (hirsutism), and polycystic ovaries. US only defines the morphology of the ovaries and does not by itself confirm or exclude the diagnosis. Polycystic ovaries are enlarged and contain multiple follicles (typically >12 follicles per ovary) (Fig. 51.25). The visualized follicles are 3 to 8 mm in size with no dominant follicle (>10 cc) present. Ovarian volume exceeds 10 cm^3. Patients with anovulatory menstrual cycles, especially young female athletes, may have ovaries with multiple follicles but lack the clinical features of polycystic ovary syndrome.

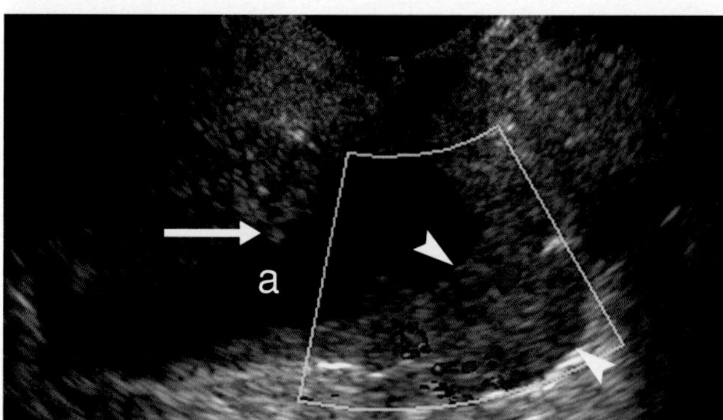

FIGURE 51.23. Metastatic Ovarian Carcinoma—Peritoneal Implants. An oblique US image of the right flank shows nodular soft tissue thickening (between *arrowheads*) of the parietal peritoneum indicative of tumor implant on the peritoneal surface. Prominent blood flow is shown by color Doppler. Ascites (*a*) outlines a peritoneal deposit (*arrow*) on the surface of the liver. This patient has ovarian carcinoma that has spread throughout the peritoneal cavity.

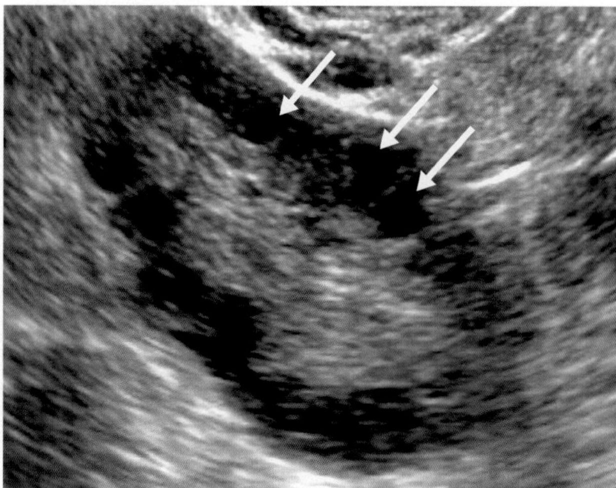

FIGURE 51.25. Polycystic Ovary Syndrome. The ovary of a woman with clinical features of polycystic ovary syndrome is enlarged with innumerable follicles (*arrows*) in the periphery.

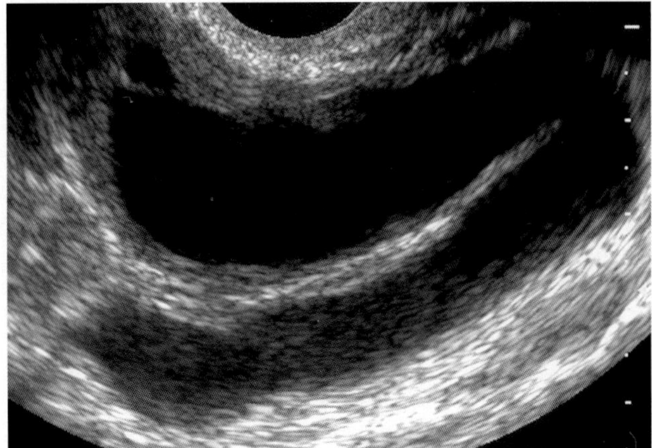

FIGURE 51.26. Hydrosalpinx. Transvaginal US demonstrates the tubular nature of an adnexal mass confirming hydrosalpinx.

Hydrosalpinx can produce a large complex cystic mass. US shows a thin- or thick-walled tubular mass that is commonly elongated and folded on itself (Fig. 51.26). The diagnosis is suggested when the mass appears elongated or tubular rather than spherical or oval. Folds in the dilated fallopian tube may simulate septa in an ovarian tumor but are characteristically incomplete in hydrosalpinx. The presence in a tubular collection of a "waist" described as diametrically opposed indentations in the wall has been reported as highly indicative of hydrosalpinx. Fluid within the dilated tube is commonly echogenic. Hydrosalpinx is often caused by PID or endometriosis. *Carcinoma of the fallopian tube* is rare. US shows a tubal mass with vascularized papillary projections or a large solid adnexal mass separate from the ovary.

Adnexal torsion is a result of axial rotation of the ovary and/or the fallopian tube about its vascular pedicle causing acute severe pelvic pain due to arterial occlusion and venous stasis. The torsed ovary becomes swollen, hemorrhagic, and often necrotic depending on the severity of torsion. The torsed tube becomes distended with fluid that is often echogenic. An ovarian cyst or mass usually serves as the lead point for torsion (Fig. 51.27). Torsion of the fallopian tube along with the ovary adds to the complexity of the adnexal mass. Clinically all patients have pain and 85% have nausea and vomiting. US reveals an enlarged ovary appearing as a swollen hemorrhagic edematous mass with peripheral follicles. Free fluid is frequently present in the cul-de-sac. Additional findings include echogenic debris within follicles, unusual position of the ovary, and twisted appearance of the ovarian pedicle. Doppler evaluation is not reliable due to normal variations in adnexal flow and the common occurrence of intermittent torsion. Typical findings show absence of venous flow (67%) with absence of arterial flow seen in less than half (46%). Even if flow is present torsion should be suspected if the ovary is enlarged and the patient has pain. Torsion is virtually excluded if the ovary is normal, regardless of the Doppler findings. Postmenopausal patients with torsion may have ovarian carcinoma (20%).

MALE GENITAL TRACT

Testes and Scrotum

US is the imaging method of first choice for examination of the testes and scrotum. Indications include suspicion of scrotal mass, scrotal pain, trauma, undescended testes, detection of varicocele in infertile men, and search for occult primary tumor or testicular involvement by lymphoma or leukemia. The scrotum is examined with a linear array transducer with frequency of 5 MHz or higher. The testes are documented and measured in long and transverse planes. The size and echogenicity of each epididymis and testes should be compared to the opposite side. Vascularity of scrotal structures is assessed with Doppler US.

Normal US Anatomy. The normal testis is ovoid and smooth, measuring approximately 3.5 cm in length and 2.0 to 3.0 cm in diameter (Fig. 51.28). It is covered by a dense fibrous capsule called the *tunica albuginea.* The testis consists of 250 lobules made up of seminiferous tubules that are the site of spermatozoa development. The seminiferous tubules unite to form the tubuli recti, the rete testes, and finally the efferent ductules, which exit the testis at the *mediastinum.* The mediastinum is an invagination of the tunica albuginea on the posterior surface of the testes that provides access for the testicular vessels and exit for efferent ductules. The efferent ductules carry seminal fluid to the epididymis. The epididymis is a highly convoluted tubule that is tightly applied to the posterior aspect of the testis. The *head of the epididymis* is the enlarged (7- to 8-mm diameter) superior portion of the epididymis adjacent to

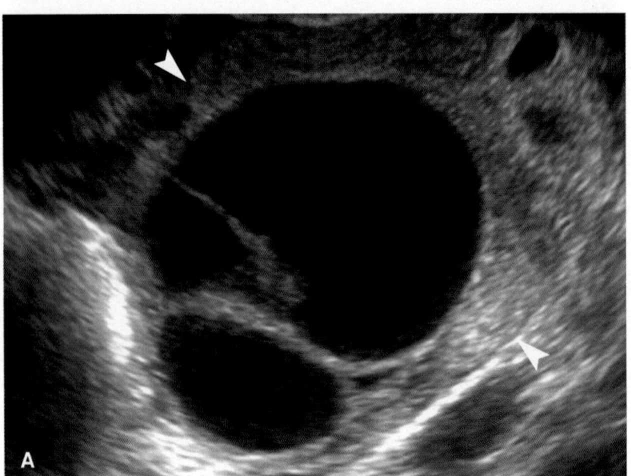

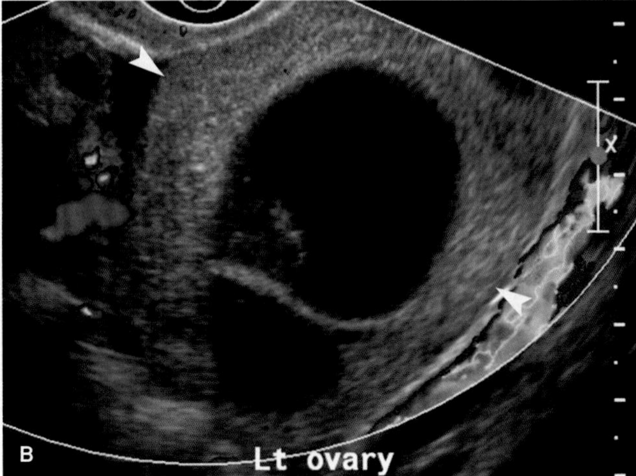

FIGURE 51.27. Adnexal Torsion. A: Gray scale US image shows an enlarged edematous ovary (between *arrowheads*) containing a cystic mass in a woman with acute onset of severe pelvic pain. **B:** Color Doppler US image shows no blood flow with the ovary (between *arrowheads*), but prominent blood flow in adjacent vessels. The ovarian mass which served as a nidus for torsion proved to be a hemorrhagic ovarian cyst.

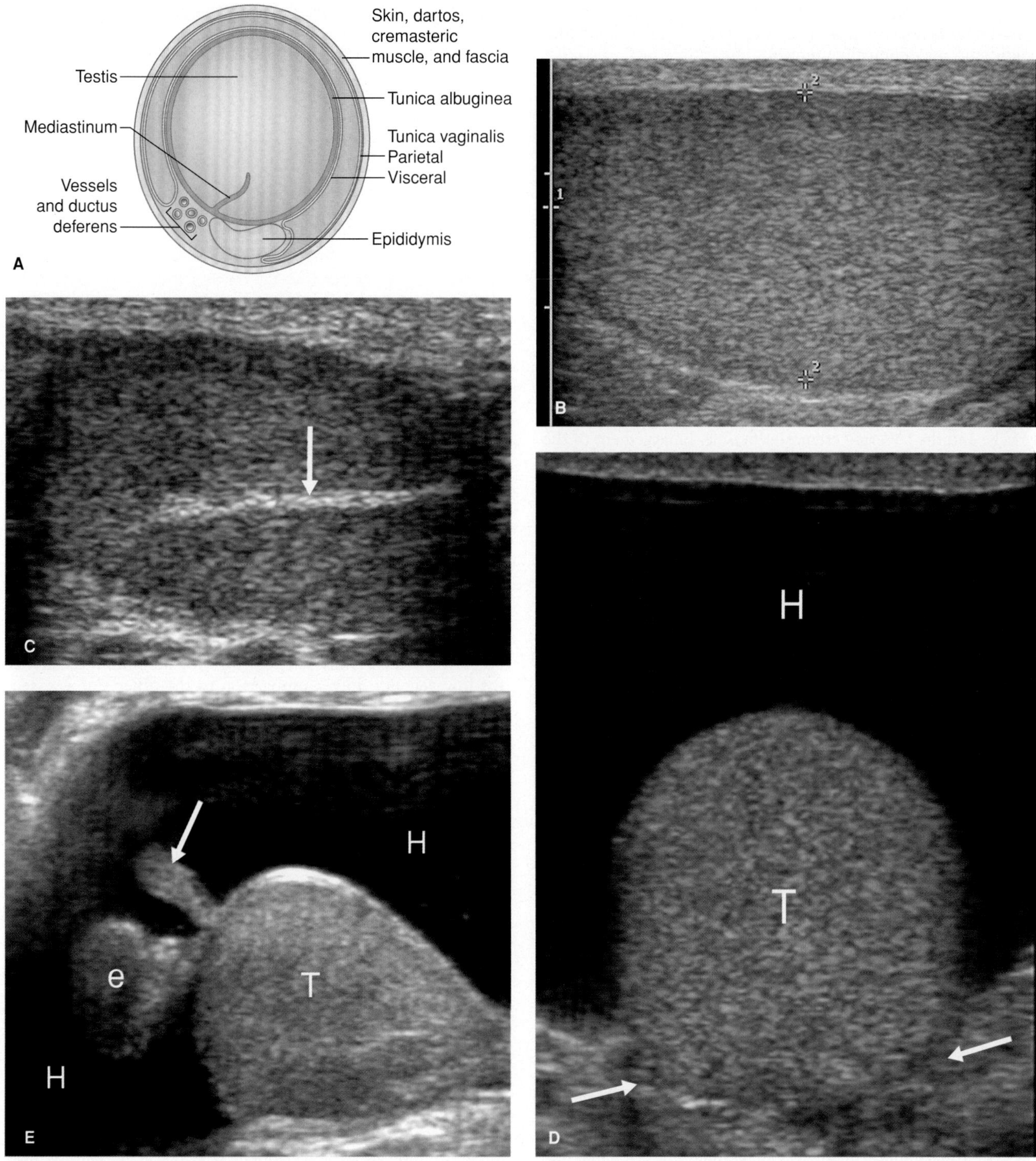

FIGURE 51.28. Normal Scrotal Anatomy. A: Drawing of a cross-section of the scrotum demonstrates the testis encapsulated by the tunica albuginea and largely surrounded by the potential space lined by the tunica vaginalis. The testis is attached to the scrotal wall posteriorly, where the testicular blood vessels, ductus deferens, and epididymis reside. **B:** The normal testis (between *calipers*) is of uniform midlevel echogenicity. **C:** The mediastinum of the testis appears as a brightly echogenic line (*arrow*) where the tunica albuginea infolds to allow entry and exit of blood vessels and the efferent ductules. **D:** The bare area (*arrows*) where the testis (*T*) attaches to the posterior wall of the scrotum is clearly shown in this patient with a large hydrocele (*H*). The epididymis courses in the bare area. **E:** The head of the epididymis (*e*) and appendix epididymis (*arrow*) are outlined by fluid of a hydrocele (*H*). Both structures are at the upper pole of the testis (*T*).

the superior pole of the testes. The *body of the epididymis* is a convoluted tube 1 to 2 mm in diameter that courses caudally along the posterior-lateral testis. The *tail of the epididymis* is the pointed lower extremity of the epididymis at the lower pole of the testis. The *ductus deferens* is the continuation of the epididymis that ascends as a straightened tube along the posterior-medial aspect of the testis to become a component of the spermatic cord and traverse the inguinal canal. The *appendix testis* is a Müllerian duct remnant seen as a small, oval structure just beneath the head of the epididymis. The *appendix epididymis* is a small, stalked appendage of the epididymal head. Torsion of the appendix testis or appendix epididymis may clinically mimic testicular torsion.

The scrotum consists of many layers of different tissue. The thickness of the scrotal skin is usually 3 to 6 mm, with a maximum of 8 mm. The *tunica vaginalis* is a peritoneal membrane that forms a closed serous sac that covers the medial, anterior, and lateral aspects of the testis and the lateral aspect of the epididymis. This space normally contains 1 to 2 mL of fluid. Excessive fluid in this space is termed a *hydrocele*. The tunica vaginalis leaves a bare area posteriorly that anchors the testis to the scrotal wall. Absence of this anchor of the testis to the scrotal wall is a congenital condition called a *bell clapper deformity* that predisposes to testicular torsion. A midline septum divides the scrotum into two separate compartments.

The spermatic cord is formed at the internal inguinal ring, courses through the inguinal canal and abdominal wall, and suspends the testes in the scrotum. The spermatic cord consists of the ductus deferens; the testicular, deferential, and external spermatic arteries; the pampiniform plexus of veins; lymphatic vessels; and the covering cremaster muscle. Enlargement of the pampiniform plexus of veins is termed a *varicocele*. Color flow and power Doppler US evaluate arterial flow in the spermatic cord and testes. After entering the testis, the testicular artery forms the capsular arteries, which course just beneath the tunica albuginea. The capsular arteries give rise to the centripetal branches, which flow toward the mediastinum through the testicular parenchyma. Because vascularity of the testes is quite variable, color flow images of one testis should always be compared to equivalent color flow images of the opposite testis.

US demonstrates the normal testes to be homogeneous in echogenicity with an echotexture similar to the thyroid. The mediastinum is seen as a prominent echogenic line along the posterior aspect of the testis. Fluid in the space formed by the tunica vaginalis provides the best visualization of the components of the epididymis. The epididymis has a coarser, more heterogeneous appearance than the testis.

Undescended Testis. About 3% of full-term newborns have an undescended testis. Most of these testes will spontaneously descend by 1 year of age, leaving 1% with cryptorchidism. Spontaneous descent after 1 year of age is unlikely. To preserve fertility, orchiopexy is recommended by 2 years of age. Long-term retention of an undescended testis is associated with a dramatically increased risk of testicular neoplasm, especially seminoma. The undescended testis may be located anywhere along the course of descent, from the lower pole of the kidney to the superficial inguinal ring. Most (70% to 80%) are within the inguinal canal and can be identified by US. The remainder, located in the abdomen, are best demonstrated by CT or MR. The inguinal canal runs an oblique, medially directed course through the flat muscles of the abdominal wall between the deep and superficial inguinal rings. The deep inguinal ring is located midway between the anterior superior iliac spine and the symphysis pubis. The superficial inguinal ring is located just above the pubic crest. Most undescended testes are atrophic, as small as 1 cm in size, and appear hypoechoic compared to normal testis. The bulbous termination of the *gubernaculum*, called the pars *infravaginalis gubernaculi*, must not be mistaken for the undescended testis. The gubernaculum is a cord-like structure that guides the testes into the scrotum during descent. The gubernaculum atrophies after normal testicular descent, but when descent is incomplete the pars infravaginalis gubernaculi persists as a fibrous or gelatinous mass. Correct identification of the testis is assured by demonstration of the testicular mediastinum.

Acute scrotal pain is a common indication for US examination (Table 51.3). Doppler US is the diagnostic imaging method of first choice.

TABLE 51.3

CAUSES OF ACUTE PAINFUL SCROTUM

Common
Acute epididymitis/orchitis
Acute testicular torsion
Uncommon
Torsion of appendix epididymis
Torsion of appendix testis
Incarcerated inguinal hernia
Hemorrhage into a testicular tumor

Testicular torsion is twisting of the testis on the spermatic cord resulting in impairment of blood supply. Venous and lymphatic flow are impaired before arterial flow is obstructed resulting in edema and swelling. Prolonged termination of arterial flow results in infarction. Torsion occurs only in patients who have the congenital "bell clapper deformity." The testis and epididymis lack their normal attachment to the posterior wall of the scrotum. Suspended by the spermatic cord they can rotate within the tunica vaginalis. Most patients are adolescents aged 12 to 20. Time is of the essence for surgical correction of torsion. If surgery is performed within 6 hours 90% of testes are salvaged. If surgery is delayed for 24 hours or more nearly all testes will be lost to infarction. Characteristic US findings are a swollen hypoechoic testis and epididymis lacking blood flow (Fig. 51.29). Doppler imaging must be performed carefully with settings for maximum sensitivity for low velocity flow. Comparison to the other side is essential because of the wide range of normal testicular vascularity. Classic findings are absent venous and arterial flow in the testis and increased resistive index on the affected side with low velocity or reversed flow in diastole. Flow to tissues surrounding the testis is increased in the presence of testicular infarction (Fig. 51.29B). Torsion may be transient or incomplete complicating the diagnosis. Presence of arterial flow on color or power Doppler does not exclude torsion. With partial torsion spectral Doppler may show asymmetry of the waveform of the testicular artery and reversed or absent flow during diastole.

Torsion of the appendix testis or appendix epididymis is a common cause of acute scrotal pain in children. Presentation mimics testicular torsion. US demonstrates an enlarged (>5 mm) hypoechoic, spherical mass medial or posterior to the epididymal head. Color Doppler shows no flow within the mass but increased flow around the mass. Hydrocele and thickening of the scrotal wall may be seen. The testes are normal in appearance. Treatment is symptomatic with spontaneous resolution expected.

Acute Epididymo-Orchitis. Although testicular torsion is most common in patients under 20 years, acute epididymitis is most common after age 20. The onset of pain and swelling is more gradual with epididymitis. Pyuria is commonly present. *Escherichia coli, Staphylococcus aureus*, gonococcus, and tuberculosis are the most common causative organisms. US demonstrates thickening and enlargement of the epididymis associated with decreased echogenicity indicating edema. Color Doppler demonstrates diffuse increased blood flow on the affected side as compared to the opposite side (Fig. 51.30). Hypervascularity may be confined to the epididymis or the testis, or involve both. Hydrocele is common. Inflammatory changes in the testis occur in 20% of cases. The inflamed testis is hypoechoic due to edema.

Scrotal Masses. US is 80% to 95% accurate in differentiating intra- from extratesticular masses. The majority of intratesticular

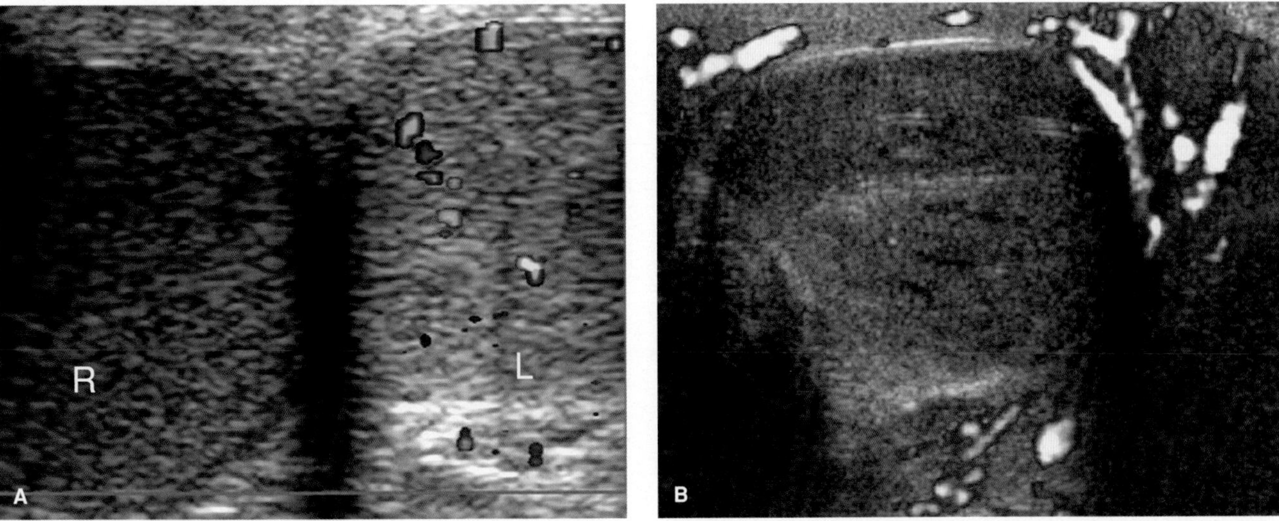

FIGURE 51.29. **Testicular Torsion. A:** Color Doppler image of both testes in a patient with right scrotal pain shows the right testis (*R*) to be edematous and swollen decreasing its echogenicity compared with the normal left testis (*L*). Color Doppler shows no blood flow on the right and normal blood flow on the left. **B:** Power Doppler image of the painful testis in another patient shows no flow in the affected testis and increased flow in the peritesticular tissues. Note the marked heterogenicity of the testis. At surgery this testis proved to be totally infarcted and could not be salvaged.

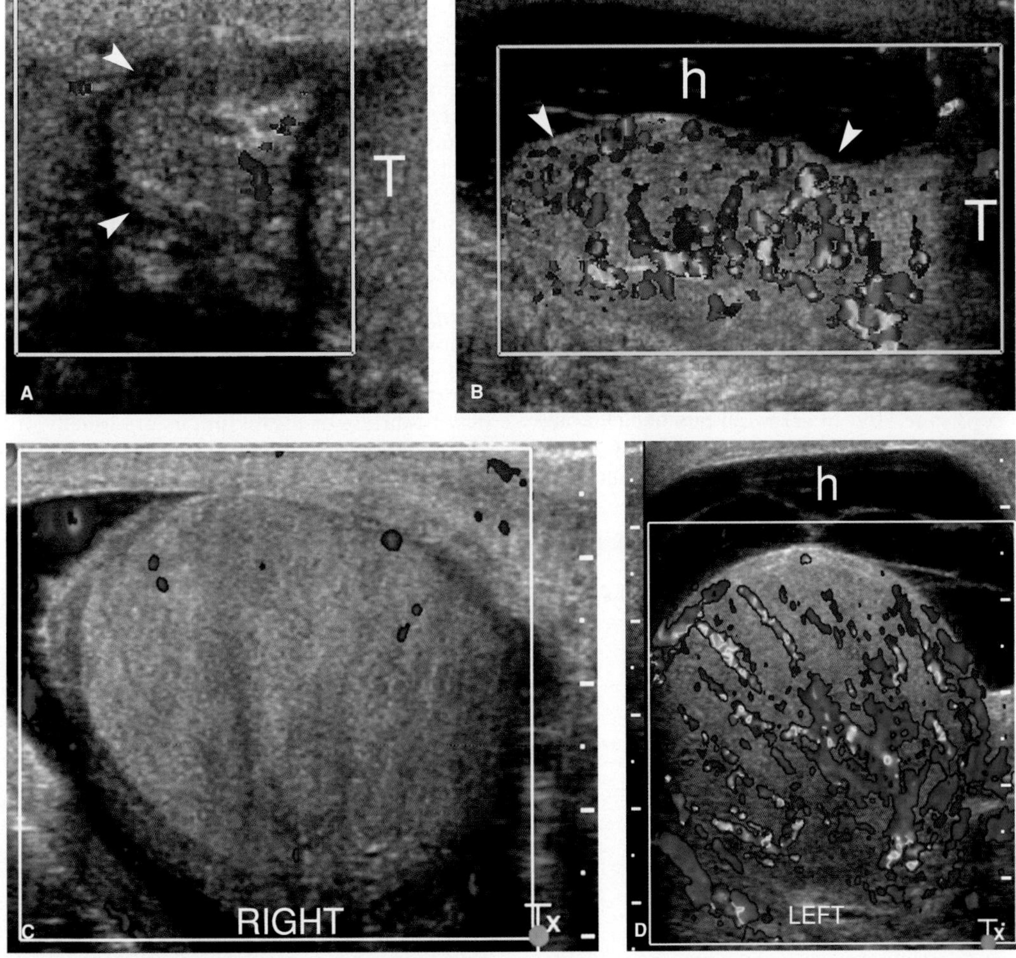

FIGURE 51.30. **Acute Epididymo-Orchitis. A:** Color Doppler image shows the normal size, appearance, and vascularity of the epididymis (between *arrowheads*) on the right in a patient with left scrotal pain. *T*, upper pole of the right testis. **B:** In the same patient the epididymis (between *arrowheads*) on the painful side is markedly enlarged and has dramatically increased blood flow indicative of acute epididymitis. A complex hydrocele (*h*) is present on the painful side. *T*, upper pole of the left testis. **C, D:** Dual color Doppler images in the same patient show normal vascularity in the asymptomatic right testis and marked increased vascularity in the painful left testis. The inflammatory hydrocele (*h*) with fibrin strands crossing the space of the tunica vaginalis is evident.

TABLE 51.4

DIFFERENTIAL DIAGNOSIS OF INTRATESTICULAR LESIONS

Malignant
Primary germ cell tumor
Seminoma
Nonseminoma
Embryonal cell carcinoma
Teratoma
Choriocarcinoma
Mixed cell tumor
Secondary malignancy
Leukemia and lymphoma
Metastasis
Benign
Inflammatory
Orchitis
Epididymo-orchitis
Mumps
Abscess
Torsion/infarction
Gonadal stromal tumor
Leydig cell tumor
Sertoli cell tumor
Cysts
Cyst of the tunica albuginea
Benign testicular cyst
Trauma/hemorrhage

masses are malignant (Table 51.4). Every intratesticular lesion should be considered to be potentially malignant until it is proven to be benign. Most extratesticular lesions are benign and are caused by inflammation or trauma (Table 51.5).

Primary testicular neoplasms constitute 4% to 6% of all male genitourinary tumors and 1% of all male malignancies. Most (95%) are germ cell tumors. These are the most common neoplasm in males aged 15 to 44. Most present as a painless mass, however 15% present with acute pain or pain following trauma.

Seminomas constitute 50% of germ cell tumors. They are less aggressive and are sensitive to radiation therapy. Seminomas are histologically monotonous, consisting of sheets of uniform cells intermixed with fibrous strands. Reflecting the histology, US demonstrates the tumor to be homogeneous and hypoechoic (Fig. 51.31).

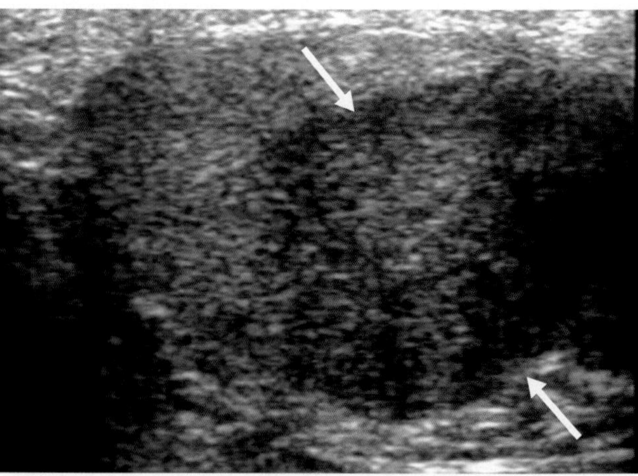

FIGURE 51.31. **Seminoma.** A homogeneous hypoechoic mass (between *arrows*) replaces a large portion of the testis. This appearance is typical of seminoma.

Nonseminomatous tumors include a variety of germ cell malignancies that are more aggressive and are resistant to radiation therapy. Cell types include embryonal cell carcinoma, teratoma, and choriocarcinoma. Most tumors are of mixed cell type. All appear as heterogeneous masses because of mixed cellularity as well as the presence of hemorrhage and necrosis. US shows irregular areas of high and low echogenicity, cystic areas, and calcification (Fig. 51.32). A hydrocele is present in 15% of patients with germ cell tumors. Both CT and MR are excellent methods for initial tumor staging and follow-up.

Lymphoma, leukemia, and metastases from other primary tumors are more common than germ cell tumors in patients over age 50. The testis serves as a sanctuary for disease because of ineffective access of chemotherapy. Involvement of the testis may be diffuse or focal. Tumors are usually of lower echogenicity than normal parenchyma (Fig. 51.33). Careful comparison with the opposite testis may be necessary for detection of

TABLE 51.5

DIFFERENTIAL DIAGNOSIS OF EXTRATESTICULAR LESIONS

Extrinsic to epididymis
Scrotal fluid collections
Hydrocele
Hematocele
Pyocele
Varicocele
Scrotal hernia
Epididymal lesions
Cystic
Spermatocele
Epididymal cyst
Abscess
Solid
Sperm granuloma
Epididymitis
Sarcoidosis
Adenomatoid tumor

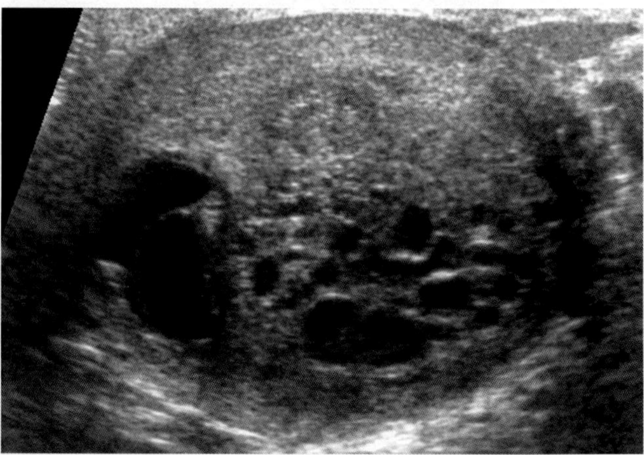

FIGURE 51.32. **Mixed Germ Cell Tumor.** The testis of this patient is largely replaced by a much more heterogeneous tumor with prominent cystic areas. Heterogeneous testicular neoplasms are usually nonseminomatous mixed germ cell tumors.

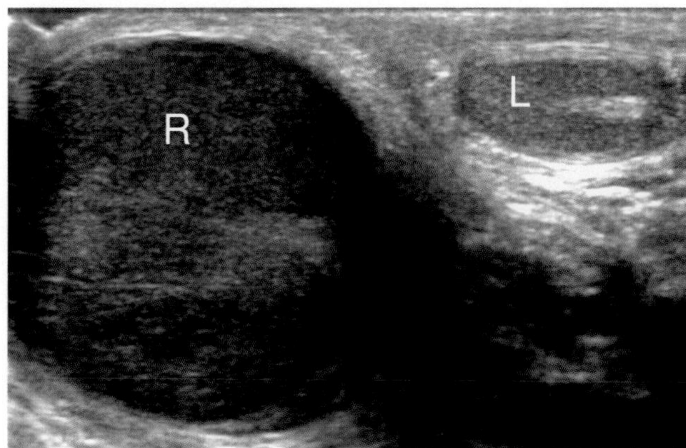

FIGURE 51.33. **Lymphoma Testis.** The right testis (*R*) is markedly enlarged and diffusely decreased in echogenicity compared to the normal left testis (*L*) in this 6-year-old boy with non-Hodgkin lymphoma.

lesions. Renal cell and prostate carcinoma are the most common tumors to metastasize to the testis.

Gonadal Stromal Tumors. Leydig and Sertoli cell tumors account for 3% to 6% of all testicular tumors; 3% are bilateral; up to 15% are malignant. They appear as small, solid masses.

Testicular microlithiasis appears on US as diffuse, punctate, nonshadowing, hyperechoic foci throughout the testicular parenchyma (Fig. 51.34). Most patients (67%) have bilateral microlithiasis. It is a benign condition of microcalcifications within the seminiferous tubules, but is associated with an incidence of testicular carcinoma as high as 40%. Nearly all tumors are bilateral. Additional associations include cryptorchidism and infertility.

Cysts. Benign testicular cysts are incidental findings in 8% to 10% of males. Cysts of the tunica albuginea are well defined, small (2 to 5 mm in diameter), and peripheral. Both types are filled with serous fluid (Fig. 51.35). The cyst wall is imperceptible.

Dilated rete testis may mimic a complex intratesticular mass. US demonstrates multiple small spherical or tubular cystic structures in the region of the mediastinum of the testis (Fig. 51.36). Nearly all cases are associated with abnormalities

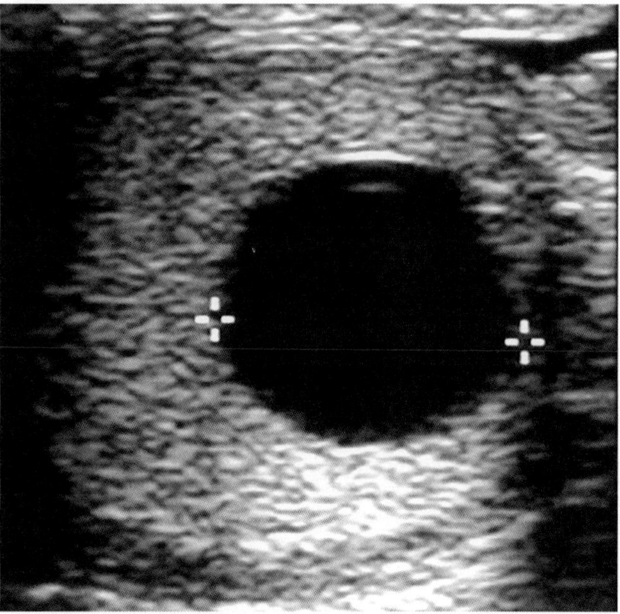

FIGURE 51.35. **Testicular Cyst.** A benign testicular cyst appears as a well-defined, spherical, uniformly anechoic mass (between *cursors,* +) within the testis. Care must be taken to differentiate simple testicular cysts from cystic necrosis within testicular tumors.

of the epididymis including spermatocele, epididymal cysts, or history of epididymitis or vasectomy.

Orchitis and Abscess. Most inflammations of the testis are associated with epididymitis. Mumps is an additional cause of orchitis. The testis with orchitis is enlarged with edematous areas that may be irregular in outline. A fluid-filled mass suggests abscess formation. Testicular abscess may rupture through the tunica albuginea and result in a pyocele.

Infarction. Testis infarction may result from torsion or trauma. The infarct appears as a focal low-density area or diffuse low density of the entire testis (Fig. 51-29B). With time, the testis shrinks and becomes fibrotic. Segmental infarctions appear as wedge-shaped avascular intratesticular lesions.

Trauma/Hemorrhage. In the setting of scrotal trauma, the role of imaging is to detect a ruptured testis. Most (90%)

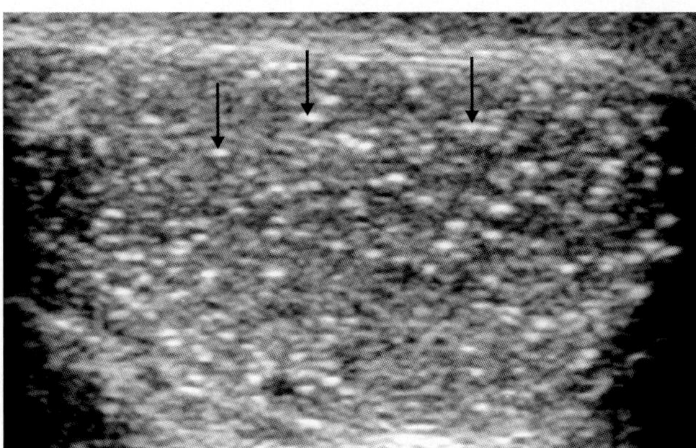

FIGURE 51.34. **Testicular Microlithiasis.** Innumerable tiny echogenic spots (*tiny arrows*) are evident throughout the testicular parenchyma. This benign condition is associated with a significant risk of testicular carcinoma.

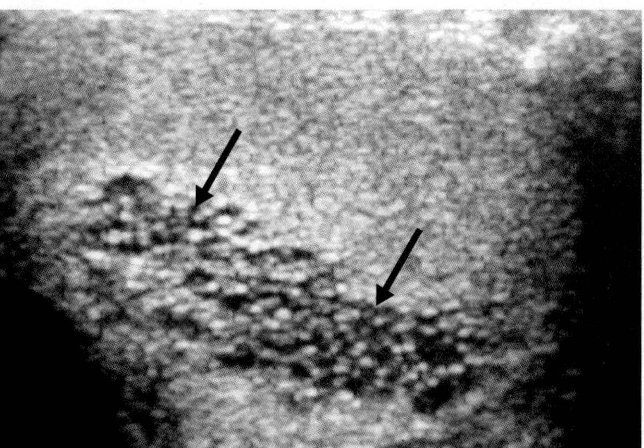

FIGURE 51.36. **Dilated Rete Testis.** A complex appearing mass (*arrows*) is made up of numerous tiny cystic tubular structures and is located in the mediastinum of the testis. Doppler showed no blood flow within the dilated tubules.

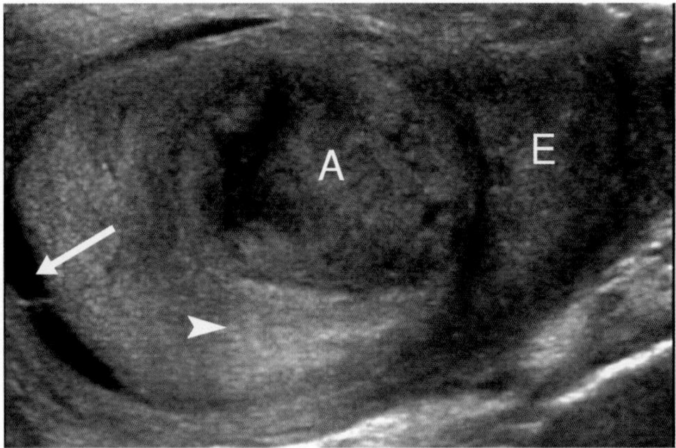

FIGURE 51.37. **Testicular Abscess.** A testicular abscess (*A*) developed as a result of untreated epididymo-orchitis. The epididymis (*E*) is enlarged. Note the accentuated through transmission (*arrowhead*) that indicates fluid in the abscess. A small complex hydrocele (*arrow*) is also present.

ruptured testes can be salvaged by surgery performed in the first 72 hours following trauma. The normal shape and clear definition of the testis are lost (Fig. 51.37). The testis appears heterogeneous, with contour abnormality and absence of normal vasculature. Hematocele is usually present. Normal vascular clefts should not be mistaken for a fracture. Intratesticular hematomas may be treated conservatively provided that testicular fracture has been excluded (Fig. 51.38). Hematomas appear as an avascular mass of variable echogenicity that decreases in size over time.

Scrotal Fluid Collections. A *hydrocele* is the accumulation of serous fluid between the visceral and parietal layers of the tunica vaginalis (Figs. 51.28 and 51.30). It is the most common cause of painless scrotal swellıng. Although many cases are idiopathic, hydrocele may accompany malignant tumors,

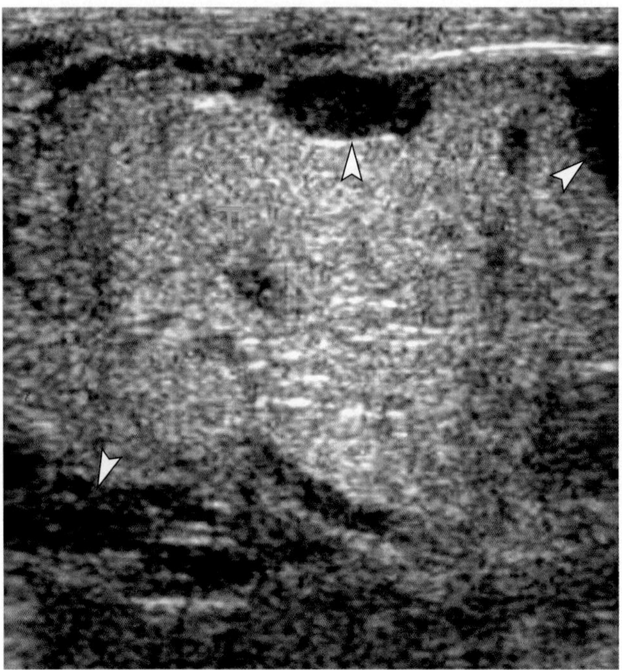

FIGURE 51.38. **Fractured Testis.** The testis (*T*) is heterogeneous and its normal shape is disrupted. Multiple areas of hemorrhage (*arrowheads*) are evident. This man was injured in a motorcycle accident.

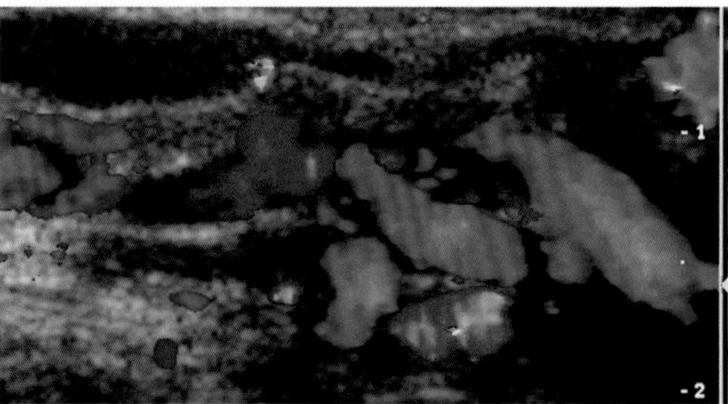

FIGURE 51.39. **Varicocele.** Sagittal color Doppler image of the spermatic cord demonstrates a network of curving tubular structures shown by spectral Doppler to be veins. These were shown to dilate even more by having the patient perform a Valsalva maneuver.

torsion, and inflammation. *Hematoceles* result from bleeding caused by trauma or surgery. *Pyoceles* usually result from rupture of an abscess into the space between the layers of the tunica vaginalis. Internal septations and loculations are common with hematoceles and pyoceles.

Scrotal calculi appear as mobile echogenic foci that move freely in the space between the layers of the tunica vaginalis. Most are small (2 to 10 mm). The larger ones have been called "scrotal pearls." Cause is uncertain, possibly related to prior episodes of epididymitis. They are considered incidental and of no clinical significance.

Varicoceles are dilated serpiginous veins of the pampiniform plexus (Fig. 51.39). They occur in 15% to 20% of males and are the most common correctable cause of male infertility. Acute onset of a varicocele in an adult male aged 40 or older may be a sign of neoplastic obstruction of the ipsilateral gonadal or renal vein. Varicoceles become more obvious with US examination performed during the Valsalva maneuver.

Scrotal hernias may contain omentum, small bowel, or colon. The herniated mass extends through the inguinal canal to the scrotum (Fig. 51.40). Omentum in the hernia is echogenic and contains blood vessels shown by color Doppler. Bowel in the hernia appears as a tubular mass containing fluid and air bubbles. Peristalsis is identified by movement of air bubbles.

Cystic Epididymal Lesions. Spermatoceles arise from obstructed efferent ductules at the epididymal head. They contain sperm and cellular debris. *Epididymal cysts* contain clear serous fluid and may occur anywhere along the course of the epididymis. Loculations and septations within the cysts are common (Fig. 51.41). Spermatoceles range in size up to several centimeters.

Solid Epididymal Lesions. Sperm granuloma form when sperm extravasates into the soft tissues surrounding the epididymis. *Chronic epididymitis,* resulting from incompletely resolved acute epididymitis, causes an irregular, hard, tender mass. *Sarcoidosis* may cause a painless, solid epididymal mass and involve the testis. *Adenomatoid tumors* are benign, slow-growing epididymal neoplasms.

Fournier gangrene is a rapidly progressive polymicrobial necrotizing fasciitis involving the scrotum and perineum. A high mortality rate (up to 75%) makes it a surgical emergency. It is primarily a disease of older men (aged 50 to 70) usually with predisposing factors such as diabetes, immunodeficiency syndromes, and poor hygiene. Infection spreads rapidly along fascial planes causing obliterative arteritis and rapid tissue necrosis. Gas in the scrotal wall and superficial tissues of the

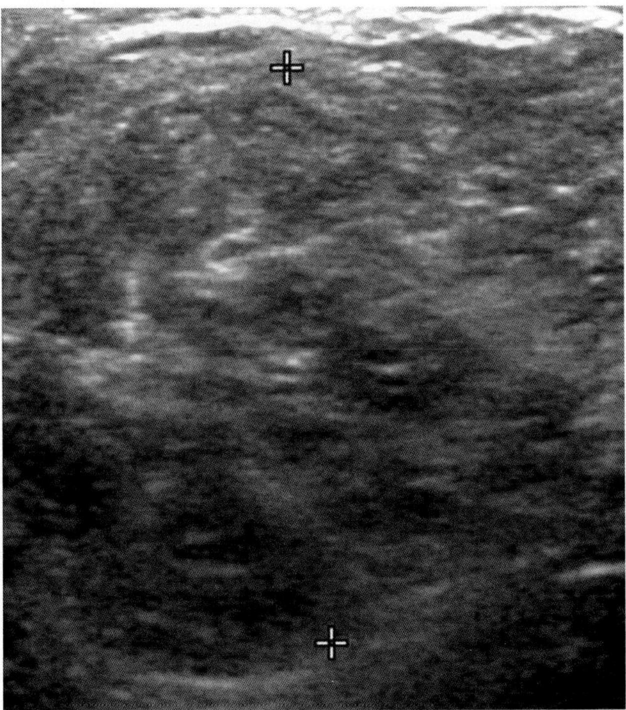

FIGURE 51.40. **Incarcerated Inguinal Hernia.** Longitudinal image through the inguinal canal reveals a mixed echogenicity solid mass (between *cursors*, +) that was not reducible. This appearance is typical of an inguinal hernia containing omentum. The clinical diagnosis was testicular torsion.

perineum is the US hallmark (Fig. 51.42, see Fig. 40.20). The scrotal wall is thickened but the testes and epididymis remain normal.

Prostate

The major indication for transrectal US of the prostate gland is to guide needle biopsy for diagnosis of prostate cancer. Early enthusiasm for use of transrectal US as a screening examination for prostate cancer has been dampened by well-documented sensitivity of only 60% for US examination alone. MR has proven to be increasingly useful in the detection and staging of prostate cancer. Additional indications for US include detection of abscess, infertility with suspicion of obstruction of the ejaculatory ducts or atresia of the seminal vesicles, and for examination of the posterior urethra.

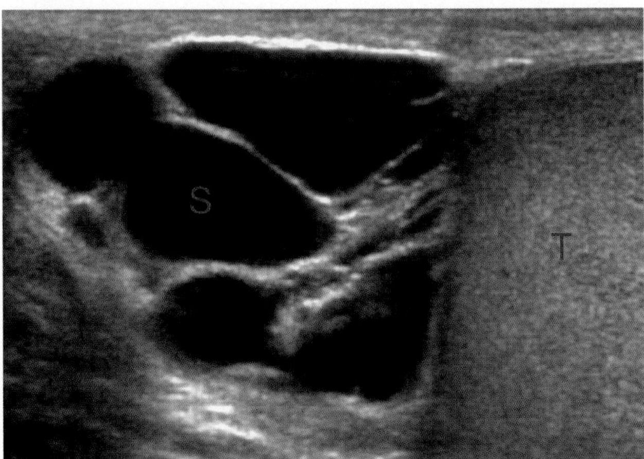

FIGURE 51.41. **Spermatocele.** US image displays a complex, septated extratesticular cyst mass (*S*) at the superior pole of the testicle (*T*) characteristic of a spermatocele.

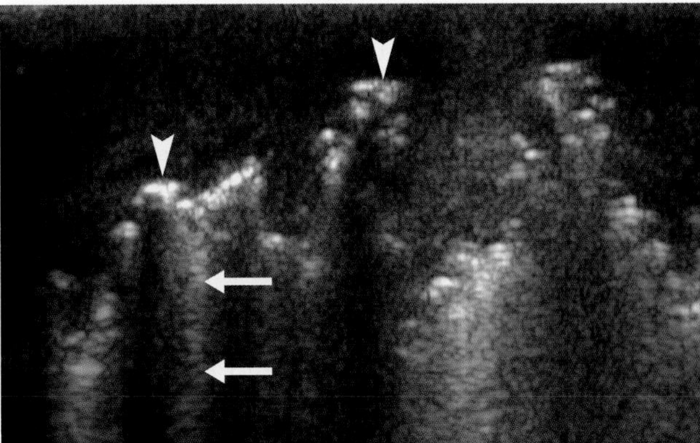

FIGURE 51.42. **Fournier Gangrene.** US image of the swollen scrotum of a 75-year-old man with diabetes reveals brightly echogenic foci (*arrowheads*) that produce bright reverberation artifacts (*arrows*). This should be recognized as air within the soft tissue.

Normal US Anatomy. On transabdominal US through the distended bladder the prostate is seen as a rounded organ at the base of the bladder (Fig. 51.43). Enlargement of the prostate elevates the base of the bladder. The urethral orifice can be identified as a V-shaped indentation in the prostate. The zonal anatomy of the prostate is described in Chapter 49. On transrectal US, the central and peripheral zones are nearly equal in echogenicity and are usually distinguished mainly by position. It is useful to describe the gland on US as having a *peripheral zone* and an *inner gland* comprised of the central and transitional zones and their pathologic alterations. The anterior fibromuscular stroma is seen as a hypoechoic area at the anterior superior aspect of the gland. US measurements are used to calculate the volume of the prostate gland using the formula width × height × length × 0.52. Larger than 30 cc

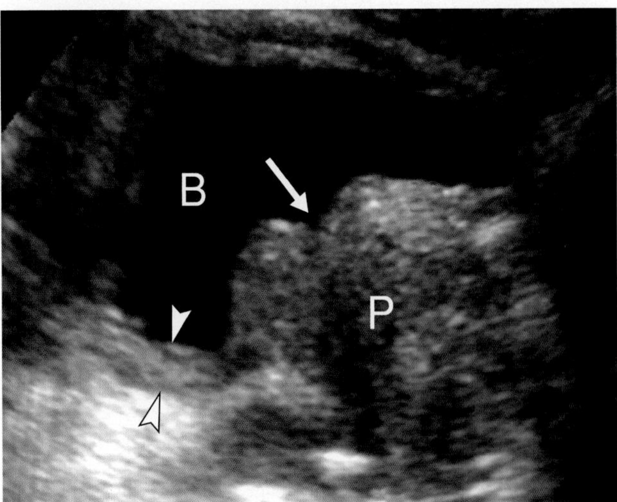

FIGURE 51.43. **Enlarged Prostate.** Midline sagittal US image shows an enlarged prostate (*P*) protruding into and elevating the base of the urine-filled bladder (*B*). The urethral orifice (*arrow*) forms a V-shaped depression in the prostate. The bladder wall is markedly thickened (between *arrowheads*).

(or 30 g) is considered enlarged. The seminal vesicles are seen as hypoechoic, lobulated, tubular structures in the groove between the base of the bladder and the base of the prostate.

Prostate Carcinoma. Unfortunately US has proven incapable of differentiating malignant from benign prostatic disease. US findings associated with prostate cancer include distinct hypoechoic nodule, poorly marginated hypoechoic area in the peripheral zone, mass effect on surrounding tissues, asymmetric enlargement of the prostate, deformation of prostatic contour, heterogeneous area in the homogeneous gland, and focal increased vascularity in the peripheral zone with color flow US. All findings are nonspecific. However, US-guided needle biopsy has proven effective in the diagnosis of prostate cancer. Core biopsies are usually obtained transrectally using US guidance to direct sampling from different areas of the gland, always including all four quadrants as well as being directed at suspicious areas.

Benign prostatic hyperplasia is a nodular hypertrophy of the glandular tissue of the transitional zone, usually beginning in the fifth decade of life. The transitional zone becomes enlarged and heterogeneous and compresses the urethra and the central zone (Fig. 51.44). Discrete nodules, some with cystic changes, may be visualized. The enlargement is often marginated circumferentially by a pseudocapsule. The size of the prostate exceeds 30 g (cc). The prostatic urethra becomes elongated, tortuous, and compressed, causing bladder outlet obstruction. Stasis of urine may lead to the formation of bladder stones. The bladder base is commonly elevated and the bladder wall is often thickened.

Prostatic calcifications occur with increasing frequency in older men. Corpora amylacea refers to echogenic proteinaceous debris within dilated prostatic ducts. Calcifications occur with prostatitis and benign hypertrophy and are of no clinical significance.

Acute prostatitis is usually caused by *E. coli* infection. The gland is swollen and edematous. Prostatic abscess is demonstrated by US as a focal collection of echogenic fluid within the gland (Fig. 51.45). Septations may be present. Transrectal US may be used to direct needle aspiration of a suspected abscess.

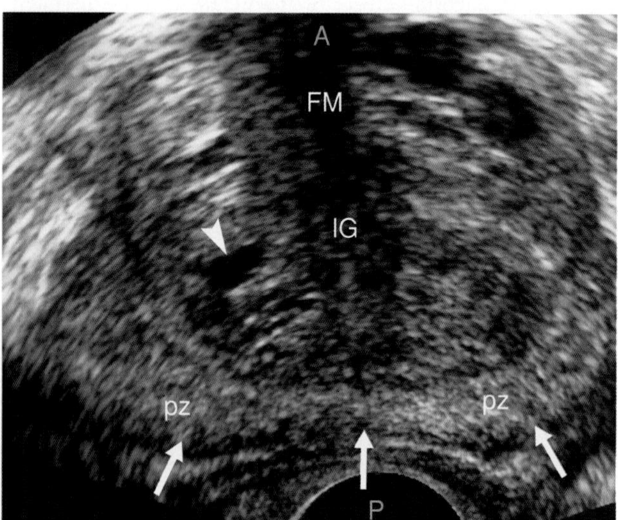

FIGURE 51.44. Benign Prostatic Hypertrophy. Transrectal US images of the prostate are routinely viewed inverted. The transducer is at the bottom, rather than the top of the image. Transrectal axial US view through the midprostate demonstrates excellent differentiation of a normal peripheral zone (*pz, arrows*). The inner gland (*IG*) demonstrates enlargement and heterogeneity that is characteristic of benign prostatic hypertrophy. A small prostatic cyst is evident (*arrowhead*). The hypoechoic fibromuscular zone (*FM*) is anterior. *A*, anterior; *P*, posterior.

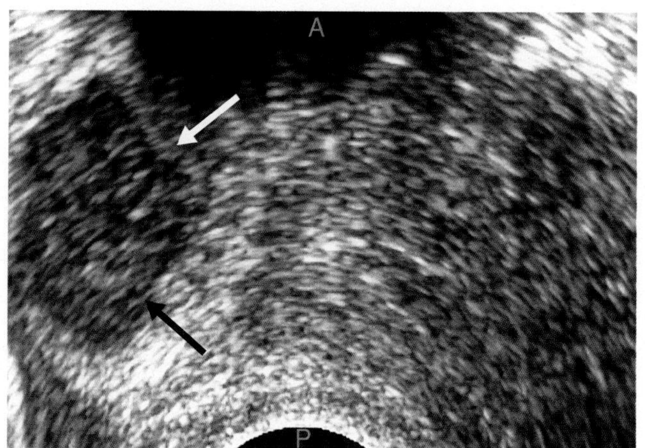

FIGURE 51.45. Prostate Abscess. Transverse transrectal US reveals an abscess (*arrows*) in the right side of the prostate gland in a patient with fever, pelvic pain, and pyuria. The abscess contained purulent debris seen on real-time US as floating particulate matter. *A*, anterior; *P*, posterior.

Prostatic cysts are relatively common findings on prostate imaging examinations (Table 51.6). Utricle cysts and Müllerian duct cysts arise in the midline verumontanum and are indistinguishable in their imaging appearance (Fig. 51.46). Both may be asymptomatic or associated with urinary urgency, obstructive symptoms, or hematuria. Cystic degeneration of benign prostatic hypertrophy (Fig. 51.44) and retention cysts occur away from the midline and rarely cause symptoms. Cysts of the seminal vesicle are associated with ipsilateral renal agenesis and autosomal dominant polycystic disease. Ejaculatory duct cysts occur with obstruction of the ejaculatory duct, which may be a cause of infertility.

TABLE 51.6

CYSTIC LESIONS OF THE PROSTATE

Müllerian duct cyst (midline)
Utricle cyst (midline)
Cystic degeneration of benign prostatic hypertrophy
Retention cysts
Seminal vesicle cyst
Ejaculatory duct cyst

BLADDER

The full bladder is used as an acoustic window to the pelvis for evaluation of the genital tract. Abnormalities of the bladder may be mistaken for abnormalities of other organs of the pelvis. Alternatively, large cystic masses may be mistaken for the bladder. US is valuable for evaluation of bladder wall, distal ureters, intravesical, and extravesical masses.

Normal US Anatomy. The urine-filled bladder is thin walled and contains anechoic urine. The normal bladder wall measures 3 mm when the bladder is distended and 5 mm when

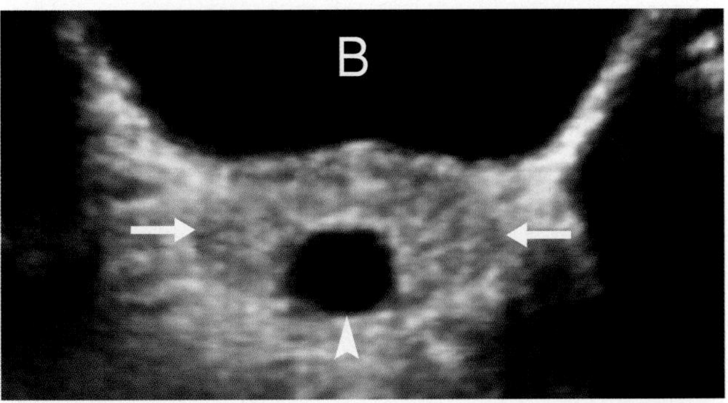

FIGURE 51.46. Utricle Cyst. Transverse view of the prostate (between *arrows*) through the urine-filled bladder (*B*) shows a midline cystic mass (*arrowhead*) within the prostate. This is the typical location and appearance of a utricle cyst.

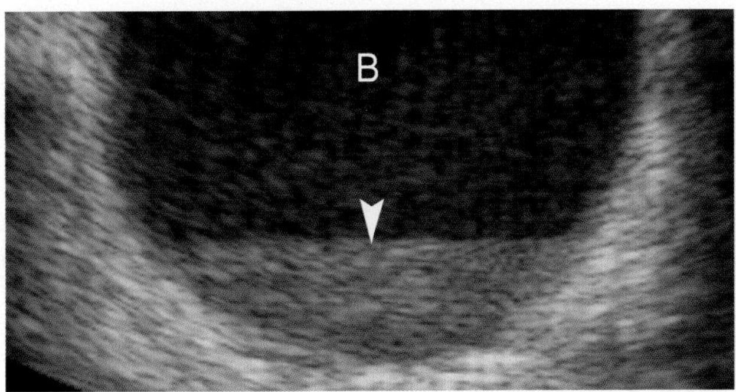

FIGURE 51.48. Cystitis—Echogenic Urine. Transverse image through the bladder (*B*) reveals echogenic particulate matter suspended in the urine and a fluid layer (*arrowhead*) of debris. Urinalysis showed numerous white blood cells in this patient with cystitis.

collapsed. The volume of bladder contents may be calculated by the standard formula for volume of a prolate ellipse (length × width × height × 0.52). US measurements are used to calculate postvoid urine residual and overdistended bladder volumes when the bladder is neurogenic or obstructed. Ureteral jets (Fig. 51.47) are spurts of urine into the bladder due to ureteral peristalsis. They are best visualized by color Doppler but are occasionally seen on gray scale US as swirling microbubbles. Visualization of ureteral jets confirms patency of the ureter.

Echogenic urine is caused by suspended particulate matter. Causes include concentrated urine with crystalline debris, hematuria, and pyuria (Fig. 51.48).

Bladder diverticula appear as fluid-filled sacs that project from the bladder wall. Bladder mucosa herniates through a defect in the bladder wall producing a fluid-filled mass that communicates with the main bladder lumen through a small orifice (Fig. 51.49). The wall of the diverticulum lacks a muscle layer and is thinner than the bladder wall. The orifice may be inconspicuous and requires a diligent search to detect. Color Doppler may be used to detect a jet of urine flow through the diverticular orifice when pressure is applied to the lower abdomen. Diverticula may not empty completely with voiding and serve as a site of urine stasis predisposing to infection and stone formation. US may demonstrate echogenic urine with layering debris due to stasis or infection and shadowing stones within the diverticulum or bladder. The presence of a soft tissue mass within the diverticulum suggests a complicating carcinoma.

Simple ureteroceles produce small oval fluid-filled masses projecting into the bladder lumen (Fig. 51.50). The size of the ureterocele changes as it fills and empties with ureteral peristalsis. The location at the ureterovesical junction is confirmed by observing ureteral jets that originate from the ureterocele.

Ectopic ureteroceles are found with ureteral duplication and appear as fluid-filled masses of variable size in the bladder lumen. The ectopic ureterocele commonly remains unchanged in size after voiding. The distal ureter is dilated and tortuous.

Bladder carcinoma appears as a polypoid mass or as focal, multifocal, or diffuse thickening of the bladder wall. An irregular papillary surface of the tumor may be evident. Tumors may be single or multiple, and occur with increased incidence within diverticula. Tumor can be differentiated from blood clot by Doppler demonstration of blood vessels within the mass (Fig. 51.51). Bladder carcinoma is difficult to differentiate from benign bladder wall thickening unless a polypoid mass is present. Early stage tumors are usually not demonstrated with US.

Bladder stones appear as brightly echogenic objects that cast acoustic shadows. Most stones will move with changes in patient position but some are adherent to the bladder wall. Stones may also be seen in the distal ureter, in ureteroceles, and in diverticula.

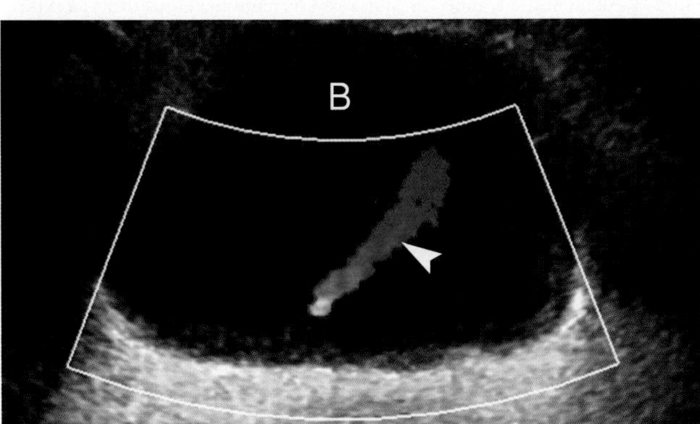

FIGURE 51.47. Ureteral Jet. Transverse image through the urine-filled bladder (*B*) shows a normal ureteral jet (*arrowhead*) emanating from the right ureteral orifice. This finding confirms patency of the right ureter.

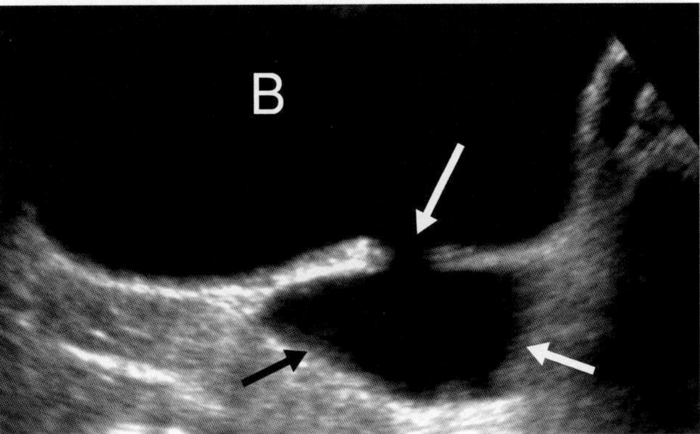

FIGURE 51.49. Bladder Diverticulum. Axial plane image through the bladder (*B*) shows a urine-filled diverticulum (*arrows*) with a narrow neck (*long arrow*) connecting it to the bladder.

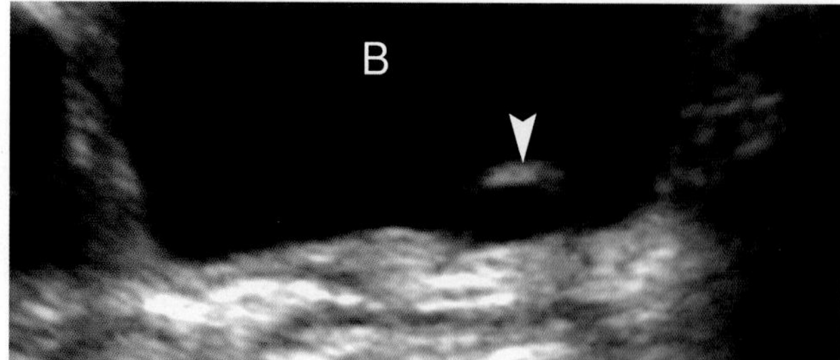

FIGURE 51.50. **Simple Ureterocele.** Transverse image through the bladder (*B*) displays a fluid-filled mass (*arrowhead*) protruding from the posterior bladder wall in the area of the trigone. Over time this mass was observed to increase and decrease in size. Ureteral jets confirmed its location at the ureterovesical junction. This is the classic US appearance of a simple ureterocele. Examination of the kidneys revealed no hydronephrosis.

Foreign bodies are usually echogenic and linear, angulated, or geographic in appearance, rather than round or oval like stones. Many will cast acoustic shadows and move within the bladder.

Blood clots produce layering fluid-debris levels when small or heterogeneous masses when large. Doppler shows no internal vascularity. Clots change in appearance and size with time.

Bladder outlet obstruction causes muscle hypertrophy and trabeculation of the bladder wall. US demonstrates thickening of the wall and marked irregularity of its luminal surface. Causes include prostate enlargement, neurogenic bladder, urethral stricture, ectopic ureterocele, tumors, and blood clots.

Cystitis due to any cause may produce focal or diffuse thickening of the bladder wall, often associated with layering or mass-like echogenic debris within the urine (Fig. 51.48). The mucosa may be raised and echolucent due to edema. Air within the bladder wall (emphysematous cystitis) or lumen produces bright echoes with acoustic shadowing or ring-down artifact.

Urethral diverticuli present with symptoms of urine dribbling, recurrent urinary infections, and dyspareunia. US reveals a cystic mass below the bladder containing echogenic urine (Fig. 51.52).

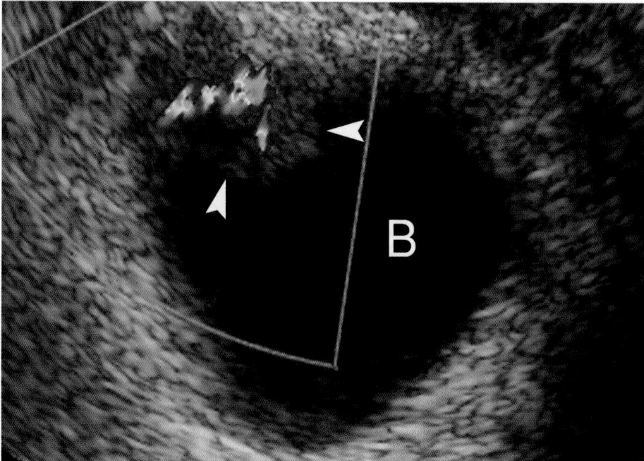

FIGURE 51.51. **Transitional Cell Carcinoma Bladder.** Transverse image through a partially filled bladder (*B*) demonstrates an echogenic polypoid mass (*arrowheads*) with blood flow extending from the bladder wall. Color Doppler demonstration of blood flow identifies this lesion as a neoplasm rather than a blood clot. Cystoscopic biopsy confirmed malignancy.

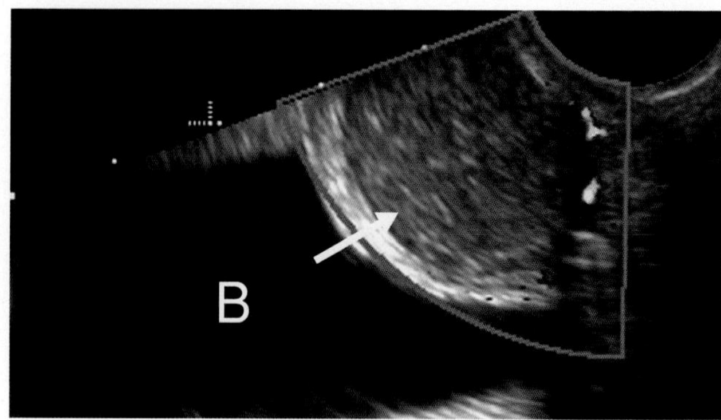

FIGURE 51.52. **Urethral Diverticulum.** Transvaginal US in a woman with a history of recurrent urinary tract infections shows a well-defined cystic mass (*arrow*) containing echogenic fluid inferior to the base of the bladder (*B*). Color Doppler confirms the cystic nature of the mass by demonstrating the lack of blood vessels within the echogenic material.

Suggested Readings

Female Genital Tract

American Institute of Ultrasound in Medicine. AIUM practice parameter for the performance of ultrasound of the female pelvis. Laurel, MD. 2014. Available from http://www.aium.org/resources/guidelines/femalepelvis.pdf.

Boortz HE, Margolis DJ, Ragavendra N, Patel MK, Kadell BM. Migration of intrauterine devices: radiologic findings and implications for patient care. *Radiographics* 2012;32:335–352.

Caserta MP, Bolan C, Clingan MJ. Through thick and thin: a pictorial review of the endometrium. *Abdom Radiol* 2016;41:2312–2329.

Early HM, McGahan JP, Scoutt LM, et al. Pitfalls of sonographic imaging of uterine leiomyoma. *Ultrasound Q* 2016;32:164–174.

Lahwani N, Prasad SR, Vikram R, Shanbhogue AK, Huettner PC, Fasih N. Histologic, molecular, and cytogenetic features of ovarian cancers: implications for diagnosis and treatment. *Radiographics* 2011;31:625–646.

Lee TT, Rausch ME. Polycystic ovarian syndrome: role of imaging in diagnosis. *Radiographics* 2012;32:1643–1657.

Levine D, Brown DL, Andreotti RF, et al. Management of asymptomatic ovarian and other adnexal cysts imaged at US Society of Radiologists in Ultrasound consensus conference statement. *Ultrasound Q* 2010;26:121–131.

Menakaya U, Reid S, Infante F, Condous G. Systematic evaluation of women with suspected endometriosis using a 5-domain sonographically based approach. *J Ultrasound Med* 2015;34:937–947.

Revzin MV, Mathur M, Dave HB, Macer ML, Spektor M. Pelvic inflammatory disease: multimodality imaging approach with clinical-pathologic correlation. *Radiographics* 2016;36:1579–1596.

Sahin H, Abdullazade S, Sanci M. Mature cystic teratoma of the ovary: a cutting edge overview on imaging features. *Insights Imaging* 2017;8:227–241.

Sakhel K, Abuhamad A. Sonography of adenomyosis. *J Ultrasound Med* 2012; 31:805–808.

Shaaban AM, Rezvani M, Elasyes KM, et al. Ovarian malignant germ cell tumors: cellular classification and clinical and imaging features. *Radiographics* 2014;34:777–801.

Male Genital Tract

American Institute of Ultrasound in Medicine. AIUM practice parameter for the performance of an ultrasound evaluation of the prostate (and surrounding structures). Laurel, MD. 2015. Available from http://www.aium.org/resources/guidelines/prostate.pdf.

American Institute of Ultrasound in Medicine. AIUM practice parameter for the performance of scrotal ultrasound examinations. Laurel, MD. 2015. Available from http://www.aium.org/resources/guidelines/scrotal.pdf.

Bertolotto M, Derchi LE, Secil M, et al. Grayscale and color Doppler features of testicular lymphoma. *J Ultrasound Med* 2015;34:1139–1145.

Coursey Moreno CC, Small WC, Camacho JC, et al. Testicular tumors: what radiologists need to know—differential diagnosis, staging, and management. *Radiographics* 2015;35:400–415.

Lee JC, Bhatt S, Dogra VS. Imaging of the epididymis. *Ultrasound Q* 2008;24:3–16.

Li Y, Mongan J, Behr SC, et al. Beyond prostate adenocarcinoma: extending the differential diagnosis in prostate pathologic conditions. *Radiographics* 2016;36:1055–1075.

Rafailidis V, Apostolou D, Charsoula A, Rafailidis D. Sonography of the scrotum—from appendages to scrotolithiasis. *J Ultrasound Med* 2015;34:507–518. (Pictorial essay).

Sadeghi-Nejad H, Simmons M, Dakwar G, Dogra V. Controversies in transrectal ultrasonography and prostate biopsy. *Ultrasound Q* 2006;22:169–175.

Sharmeen F, Rosenthal MH, Wood MJ, Tirumani SH, Sweeney C, Howard SA. Relationship between the pathologic subtype/initial stage and microliths in testicular germ cell tumors. *J Ultrasound Med* 2015;34:1977–1982.

Shebel HM, Farg HM, Kolokythas O, El-Diasty T. Cysts of the lower male genitourinary tract: embryologic and anatomic considerations and differential diagnosis. *Radiographics* 2013;33:1125–1143.

Wasnik AP, Maturen KE, Shah S, Pandya A, Rubin JM, Platt JF. Scrotal pearls and pitfalls—ultrasound findings of benign scrotal lesions. *Ultrasound Q* 2012;28:281–291. (Pictorial essay).

Bladder

Bala KG, Chou Y-H. Ultrasonography of the urinary bladder. *J Med Ultrasound* 2010;18:105–114.

Bharwani N, Stephens NJ, Heenan SD. Imaging of bladder cancer. *Cancer* 2008;20:97–111.

Wong-You-Cheong JJ, Woodward PJ, Manning MA, Sesterhenn IA. Neoplasms of the urinary bladder: radiologic-pathologic correlation. *Radiographics* 2006;26:553–580.

CHAPTER 52 ■ OBSTETRIC ULTRASOUND

WILLIAM E. BRANT

Imaging Methods. Ultrasound (US) remains the imaging method of choice for dating the pregnancy, monitoring fetal growth, assessing fetal well-being, and evaluating fetal anatomy and maternal pelvic organs. Transvaginal US is particularly useful in the assessment of first-trimester pregnancy and in the demonstration of fetal anatomic structures deep in the pelvis. Modern US offers superb anatomic detail in real time, keeping up with the frequently vigorous motion of the fetus. Three-dimensional (3D) volume US may shorten examination times and may provide additional diagnostic information for a variety of conditions including facial anomalies, neural tube defects, and cardiac and skeletal malformations. MR is used with increasing frequency as a supplement to US imaging when the US examination is equivocal, or when additional anatomic information is needed for appropriate treatment. MR offers excellent detail of maternal pelvic organs, unobscured by bone, gas, or fat. Demonstration of fetal anatomy is limited by fetal motion but may be overcome by fetal sedation and fast scan techniques.

Standards for the performance of obstetric ultrasound examinations have been published by the American Institute of Ultrasound in Medicine (AIUM) and endorsed by the American College of Radiology (ACR), Society of Radiologists in Ultrasound (SRU), and the American College of Obstetricians and Gynecologists (ACOG). Similar guidelines have been published by the International Society of Ultrasound in Obstetrics and Gynecology (ISUOG). In the first trimester, the location and appearance of the gestational sac are documented. The presence or absence of a yolk sac and embryo is confirmed. If an embryo is present, the crown-rump length (CRL) is measured and fetal cardiac activity is documented. Fetal number is determined and the uterus and adnexa are thoroughly examined. Whenever possible the fetal neck region should be examined and nuchal translucency (NT) measured. Increasingly, first-trimester US is also being used to detect fetal anomalies. The guidelines for the second and third trimester define a *standard* examination to include fetal presentation, amniotic fluid volume, cardiac activity, placental position, fetal measurements (biometry), fetal number, fetal anatomic survey, maternal cervix, and adnexa. A standard fetal anatomic survey includes the head, face, neck, upper lip, cerebellum, choroid plexus, cisterna magna, lateral cerebral ventricles, midline falx, cavum septum pellucidi, four-chamber heart, outflow tracts, stomach, kidneys, bladder, umbilical cord insertion site, umbilical cord vessel number, the entire spine, and presence or absence of the arms or legs. Fetal gender is determined when medically indicated. A *limited* examination is performed to answer a specific question such as to verify fetal position or to confirm fetal cardiac activity. Limited examinations are performed generally only when a prior complete examination is on record. When a fetal anomaly is suspected, a *specialized* examination is performed. Specialized examinations may include fetal echocardiography, biophysical profile, or fetal Doppler sonography.

Use of Doppler in Pregnancy. Evaluation of fetal and maternal circulation by color flow and spectral Doppler adds significantly to obstetric diagnosis. However, because all forms of Doppler involve the use of significantly higher levels of acoustic energy than conventional B-mode imaging, these modalities should be used with caution. Energy output from Doppler can be 10 to 15 times more intense than that of B-mode US. When modern US equipment is used at maximum power settings for Doppler examinations, acoustic outputs are sufficient to produce obvious biologic effects, including tissue heating, cavitation, and tissue disruption. Potential cavitation and tissue disruptive effects are most significant in the first trimester when embryologic tissues are tiny and loosely tethered. Thermal effects are more significant in the second and third trimesters when bone is present increasing sound absorption and heating. The International Perinatal Doppler Society and other organizations issue cautions and guidelines for use of Doppler in pregnancy. US exposures should be as low as reasonably achievable (ALARA), limiting output control and reducing the amount of time that the beam is focused on one site. Doppler US should be used only when the potential medical benefit outweighs any potential risk. Obstetric US should not be used for nonmedical reasons such as nonmedical photos or videos. When imaging the normal embryo in the first trimester, all forms of Doppler should be avoided. In particular, Doppler should not be used to document normal embryonic cardiac activity. M-mode US or recording of real-time US by cine loop provides the same documentation at much lower energies.

The presence of a pregnancy is confirmed by a positive serum human chorionic gonadotropin (hCG) test. Serum hCG is measured by use of the World Health Organization 3rd or 4th International Standard. A serum pregnancy test is defined as positive with values above 5 mIU/mL.

FIRST TRIMESTER

The first trimester covers the period from conception to the end of the 13th menstrual week. This includes the entire embryonic period (0 to 10 weeks) and is a time of dynamic growth and the differentiation and development of most organ systems. The embryo and fetus have the greatest risk of maldevelopment, injury, and death during this period because of chromosome abnormalities or external factors such as infection, drugs, or radiation. About 40% of implanted zygotes are menstrually aborted, and another 25% to 35% of surviving embryos will threaten to abort during the first trimester.

Normal Early Pregnancy

Normal Early Pregnancy (Table 52.1). The first US evidence of an intrauterine pregnancy is visualization of a *gestational sac*. Gestational sacs as small as 2 to 3 mm, corresponding to 4.5 to 5 weeks gestational, can be seen with current high-resolution US. Two signs have been described that are highly specific for and differentiate a normal gestational sac from *pseudogestational sac,* which is often associated with an ectopic pregnancy. The ***intradecidual sign*** describes a tiny well-defined cystic structure implanted within the echogenic decidua seen as early as 4.5 weeks (Fig. 52.1). The term *decidua* refers to the endometrium of the pregnant uterus. This sign has a sensitivity of 60% to 68% with specificity for gestational sac of 97% to 100%. The normal gestational sac appears on US as a smoothly contoured, round or oval, fluid-containing structure positioned within the endometrium near the fundus of the uterus. The normal sac has an echogenic border greater than 2 mm thick, which represents the choriodecidual reaction. The ***double decidua sign*** is produced by visualization of three layers of decidua early in pregnancy (Fig. 52.2). Hormones of pregnancy, progesterone and others, act on the endometrium to enlarge stromal cells and increase vascularity to promote implantation and development of the gestation. The *decidua vera (parietalis)* lines the endometrial cavity, and the *decidua capsularis* covers the gestational sac.

TABLE 52.1

NORMAL FIRST-TRIMESTER ULTRASOUND FINDINGS

- No visible findings up to 5 weeks GA
- 2–3 mm gestational sac appears at approximately 5 weeks GA
  - The intradecidual sign or double decidua sign may be present but is absent in at least 35% of cases. Their absence does not exclude an intrauterine pregnancy
- Yolk sac appears at approximately 5.5 weeks GA (>8-mm mean sac diameter) and provides definitive evidence of a gestational sac
- Embryo is visible at approximately 6 weeks GA with mean sac diameter 10 mm
  - The double bleb sign may be seen earlier
- Embryonic cardiac activity is visible at approximately 6 weeks GA. Transvaginal US may be needed to visualize
- Normal embryonic heart rate from 6.2–7 weeks GA is 100–120 beats per minute. After 7 weeks mean heart rate is 137–144 beats per minute
- Only M-mode US, not Doppler, should be used to document embryonic cardiac activity and heart rate

Adapted from Doubilet PM, Benson CB, Bourne T, et al. Diagnostic criteria for nonviable pregnancy early in the first trimester. *Ultrasound Q* 2014;30:3–9; Lane BF, Wong-You-Cheong JJ, Javitt MC, et al. ACR appropriateness criteria first trimester bleeding. *Ultrasound Q* 2013;29:91–96.

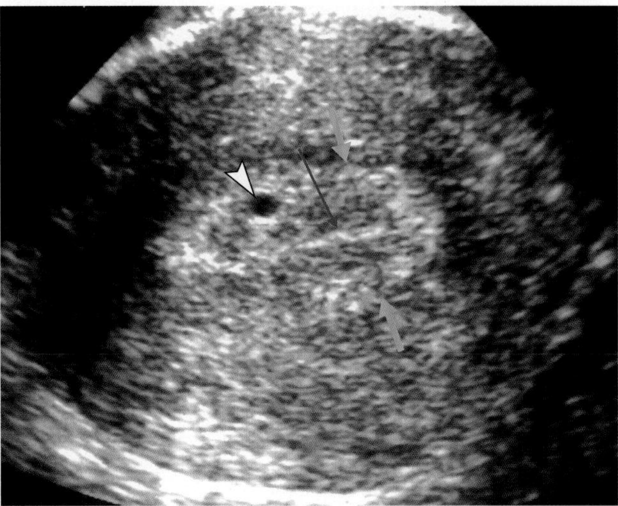

FIGURE 52.1. **Intradecidual Sign.** Transvaginal US image of the uterus in a transverse plane demonstrates a tiny gestational sac (*arrowhead*) implanted within the thickened decidual (between *blue arrows*). Note the eccentric position of the gestational sac entirely within the decidua and distinctly separate from the echogenic line (*thin red arrow*) that marks the collapsed uterine cavity. The size of the sac corresponds to a pregnancy of approximately 4.5 weeks menstrual age.

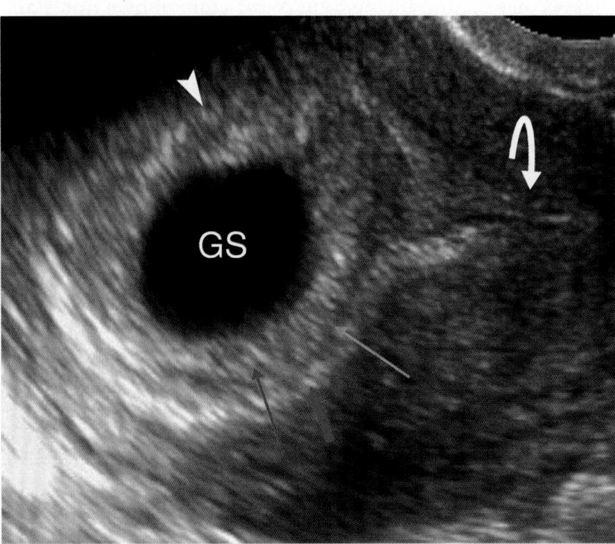

FIGURE 52.2. **Double Decidua Sign.** A magnified longitudinal endovaginal US image of the uterus demonstrates an intrauterine gestational sac (*GS*) and the normal layers of decidua that produce the double decidua sign. The decidua capsularis (*thin red arrow*) covers the gestational sac. The decidual vera (*short fat red arrow*) lines the uterine cavity. These two decidual surfaces are separated by a dark line (*thin blue arrow*) representing the uterine cavity. The uterine cavity continues into the lower uterine segment (*curved arrow*), which is lined by the thickened echogenic decidua vera. The site of implantation (*arrowhead*) on the anterior wall of the uterine cavity shows only one layer of decidua basilis, which is joining with the chorionic villi of the gestational sac to produce an anterior placenta.

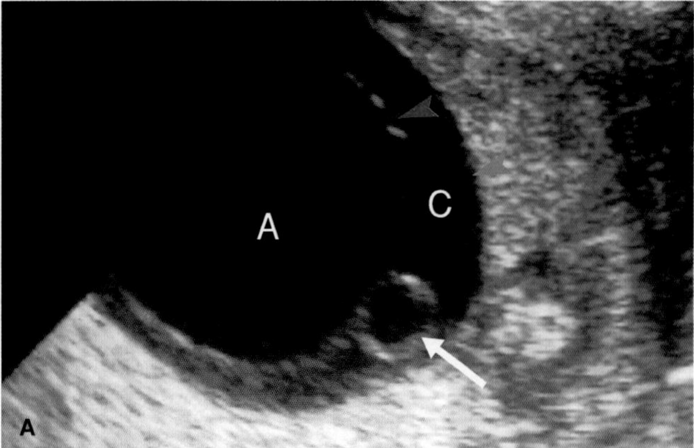

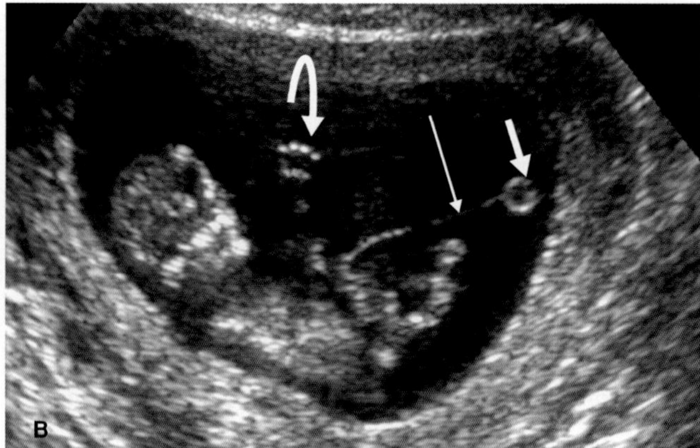

FIGURE 52.3. **Yolk Sac. A:** The yolk sac (*arrow*) is shown within the gestational sac by transvaginal US. The normal yolk sac is less than 6 mm in diameter, spherical, and fluid filled with a thin wall. The yolk sac is in the chorionic fluid space (*C*) between the thin membrane of the amnion (*red arrowhead*) and the chorion (*blue arrowhead*) that defines the limit of fluid within the gestational sac. The embryo develops within the amniotic space (*A*). **B:** Image of an 11-week embryo shows the vitelline duct (*long thin arrow*) extending from the umbilicus to the yolk sac (*short arrow*). The fingers (*curved arrow*) of the developing infant are also well shown.

The *decidua basalis* contributes to the formation of the placenta at the site of implantation. A small amount of fluid in the endometrial cavity separates the decidua vera from the decidua capsularis, enabling visualization of the "double decidua." The free margin of the gestational sac consists of chorion and decidua capsularis and is normally at least 2 mm thick. The double sac is not complete because of placental attachment to the uterine wall. The double decidua sign is 64% sensitive and nearly 100% specific for early intrauterine pregnancy. The ***yolk sac*** is the first structure seen with US within the gestational sac and is definitive in identifying a gestational sac. It is a 2- to 6-mm diameter, spherical, cystic structure (Fig. 52.3) that is connected to the mid-gut of the embryo by a thin stalk, the *vitelline duct*. A Meckel diverticulum is a remnant of the connection of the vitelline duct (also called the *omphalomesenteric duct*) to the distal ileum. The yolk sac is the earliest site of blood cell formation in the embryo. It floats freely in fluid between the amniotic and chorionic membranes. It is generally the earliest structure visualized within the gestational sac and serves as definitive evidence of early pregnancy. The yolk sac should always be visualized in normal pregnancy in gestational sacs of 8-mm mean sac diameter (MSD) by transvaginal US. The yolk sac is seen at 5.5 weeks and usually disappears by 12 weeks gestational age (GA). The ***embryo*** is first visible as a plate-like structure at the periphery of the yolk sac. The embryo develops within the amniotic cavity while the yolk sac resides in the chorionic cavity. The appearance of two adjacent cystic structures, the amnionic sac containing the embryo and the yolk sac, has been termed the *double bleb sign*. Embryos as small as 2 mm can be detected by transvaginal US (Fig. 52.4). The earliest embryonic cardiac activity can be detected by careful inspection of the embryonic disc by real-time US at approximately 6 weeks GA. The embryo, the amniotic cavity, and the chorionic cavity enlarge proportionally until about 10 weeks GA when fetal urine production begins. The amniotic cavity then enlarges faster than the chorionic cavity with fusion of the amnion and chorion at 14 to 16 weeks.

To estimate GA before an embryo is visible, *MSD* is measured. Once an embryo is visualized, *CRL* measurement is obtained. See Fetal Measurements and Growth.

The ***corpus luteum*** develops on the ovary at the site of the dominant follicle from which ovulation occurred. The corpus luteum secretes estrogens, progesterone, and other hormones that are essential for establishing and maintaining pregnancy. The wide range of normal appearance of the corpus luteum on US must be recognized for accurate diagnoses of abnormalities of the first trimester (Fig. 52.5). Immediately following ovulation the corpus luteum appears as an area of focal hemorrhage on the ovary. It soon develops into a cystic structure averaging 2 to 5 cm in size and containing clear fluid or fluid with floating internal echoes or clots of hemorrhage. Color Doppler shows an intense vascularized ring surrounding the corpus luteum and supplying blood flow to support its production of hormones. Acute hemorrhage into the corpus luteal cyst may be a cause of pelvic pain in the first trimester. While a corpus luteum may resemble an ectopic pregnancy, remember that most ectopic pregnancies occur in the tube while the corpus luteum is an ovarian structure. In up to one-third of cases the corpus luteum may be seen on the ovary opposite to the side of an ectopic pregnancy in the tube.

Normal developmental anatomy of the embryo in the first trimester includes cystic appearance of the rhombencephalon and herniation of the gut into the base of the umbilical cord. Between 6 and 8 weeks GA the hindbrain (rhombencephalon) forms a prominent cystic structure (Fig. 52.6) that becomes

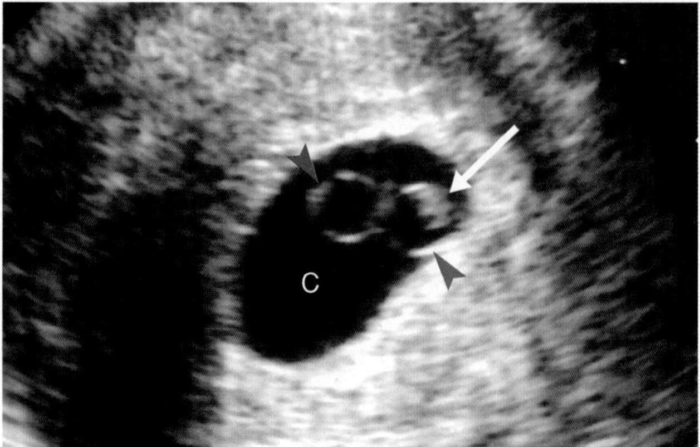

FIGURE 52.4. **Early Embryo—Double Bleb Sign.** The double bleb is formed by the yolk sac (*red arrowhead*) and the amniotic sac (*blue arrowhead*) suspended in the fluid of the early chorionic sac (*C*). The embryo is seen as a tiny disc-like structure (*arrow*) within the amniotic sac. Early cardiac activity can frequently be observed in the tiny embryo.

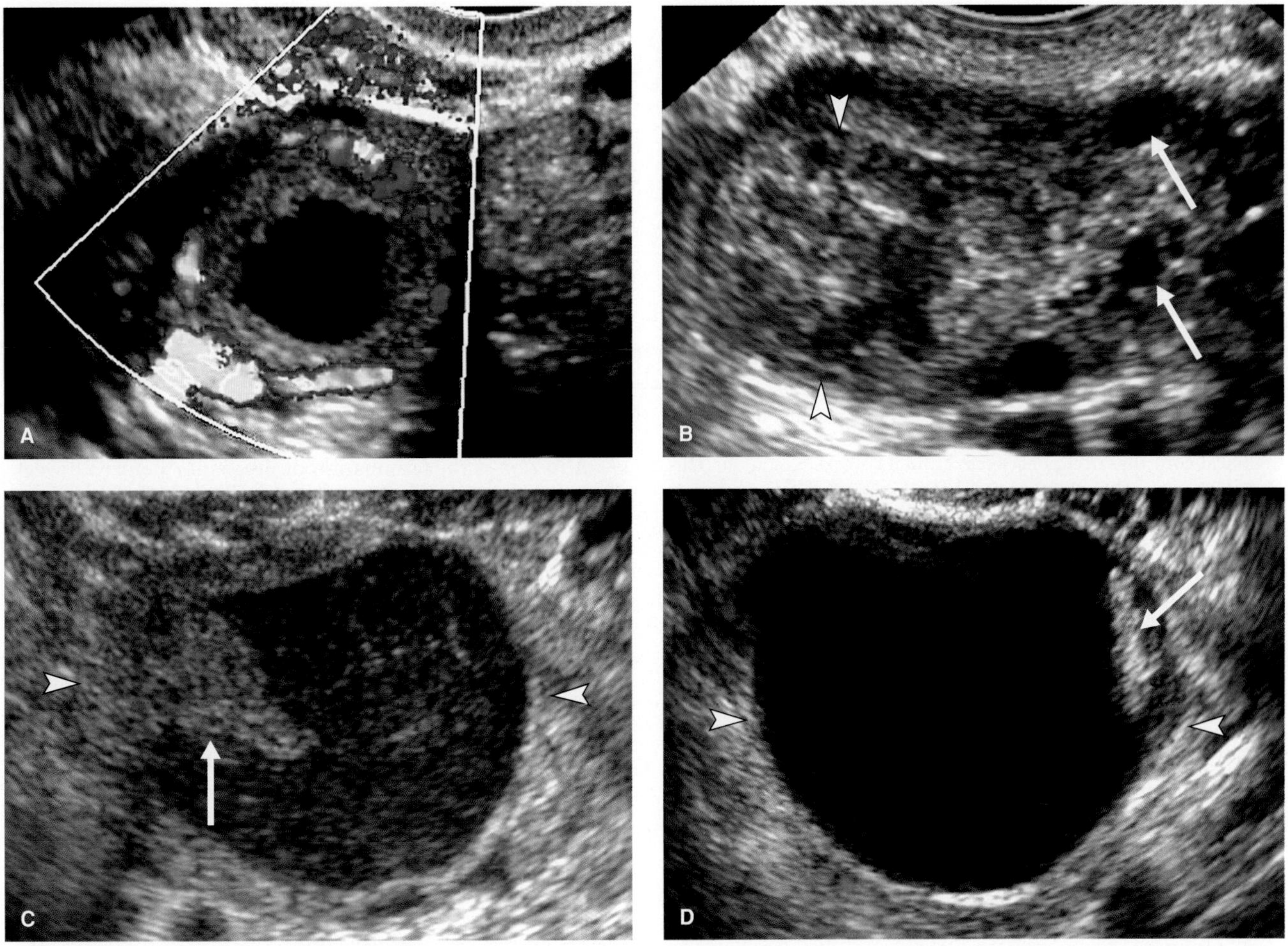

FIGURE 52.5. **Corpus Luteum. A:** Transvaginal color Doppler image of the ovary reveals a 3-cm cyst surrounded by an intense ring of vascularity ("ring of fire") characteristic of the corpus luteum. The corpus luteum secretes hormones essential for the development of the pregnancy. **B:** Transvaginal image of the ovary shows the collapsed cyst appearance of the corpus luteum (between *arrowheads*) that occurs just after ovulation. Note the follicles (*arrows*) that confirm the location of the structure on the ovary. **C:** Being highly vascular, the corpus luteum is prone to internal hemorrhage creating a hemorrhagic ovarian cyst (between *arrowheads*). Note the echogenic clot (*arrow*) and particulate fluid within the cyst. **D:** A hemorrhagic corpus luteal cyst (between *arrowheads*) may enlarge to become a prominent pelvic structure and be a source of adnexal pain in early pregnancy. This corpus luteal cyst measures 5 cm in diameter. Blood clots (*arrow*) within the cyst may simulate an ectopic pregnancy containing an embryo.

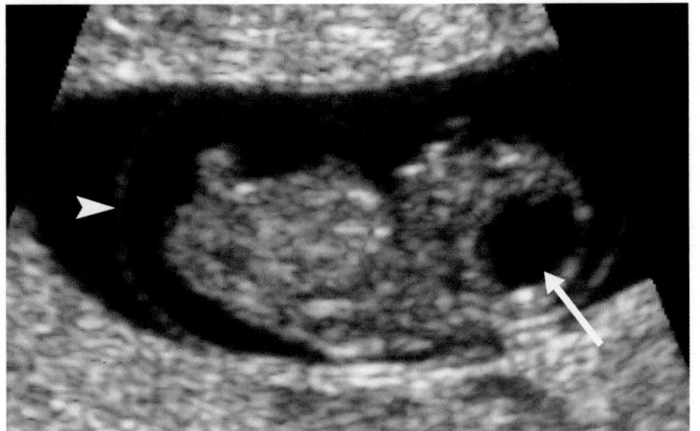

FIGURE 52.6. **Normal Cystic Rhombencephalon.** A 7-week embryo has a prominent cystic structure (*arrow*) within the cranium. This is the normal cystic phase of development of the rhombencephalon that is seen between 6 and 8 weeks gestational age. Development of the rhombencephalon results in normal structures in the posterior fossa. The amnion (*arrowhead*) is evident.

the normal fourth ventricle. Between 9 and 11 weeks GA the mid-gut herniates into the base of the umbilicus forming a physiologic omphalocele seen as a protruding midline anterior abdominal wall mass 6 to 9 mm in size (Fig. 52.7). These normal developmental landmarks must not be mistaken for anomalies.

Problematic Early Pregnancy

The most common clinical problem encountered in the first trimester is a pregnant woman presenting with vaginal bleeding or pelvic pain. Of confirmed pregnancies, approximately 25% fail and 1% to 2% are ectopic. US is used to evaluate the normal development of the pregnancy and to differentiate the various causes of vaginal bleeding. As a result of multiple studies that indicated that some early normal pregnancies were being diagnosed as nonviable using US criteria developed over the previous 30 years, the SRU organized a multispecialty conference in 2012 to create new consensus guidelines for early pregnancies of uncertain viability and unknown location (Tables 52.1 to 52.3). These new guidelines were published in

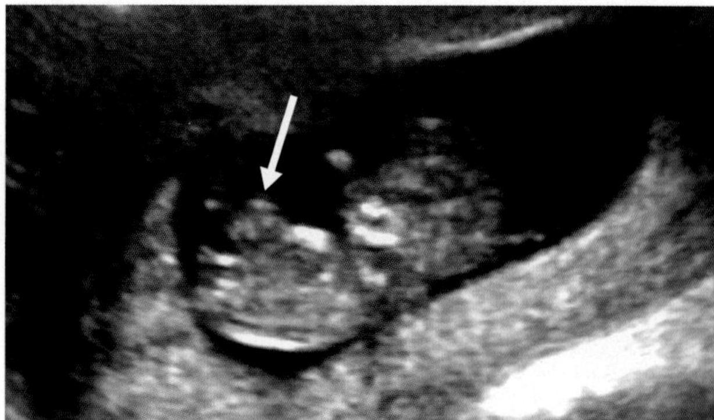

FIGURE 52.7. **Normal Mid-Gut Herniation.** A 10-week embryo shows a prominent bulge (*arrow*) at the level of the umbilicus. This is caused by the normal herniation of the mid-gut into the base of the umbilical cord that occurs between 9 and 11 weeks' gestation. This normal structure should not exceed 1 cm in size.

2013 and have been validated by subsequent studies. The new terminologies recommended for reporting early first-trimester pregnancies presenting with pelvic pain and vaginal bleeding are viable pregnancy, nonviable pregnancy, intrauterine pregnancy of uncertain viability, pregnancy of unknown location, and ectopic pregnancy.

Viable pregnancy can potentially result in the liveborn baby. At the time of US examination for vaginal bleeding, most viable pregnancies appear normal (Table 52.1).

Nonviable pregnancy cannot possibly result in a liveborn baby (Table 52.2). Nonviable pregnancies include failed intrauterine pregnancies and ectopic pregnancies.

TABLE 52.2

CRITERIA FOR NONVIABLE FIRST-TRIMESTER PREGNANCY

- **Diagnostic of pregnancy failure** (nonviable pregnancy)
  - No embryonic heartbeat with crown-rump length ≥7 mm
  - No embryo with mean sac diameter ≥25 mm
  - No embryo with heartbeat ≥2 weeks after US that showed a gestational sac without a yolk sac
  - No embryo with heartbeat ≥11 days after US that showed a gestational sac with a yolk sac
- **Suspicious but not diagnostic of pregnancy failure** (pregnancy of uncertain viability)
  - Crown-rump length <7 mm with no heartbeat
  - Mean sac diameter 16–24 mm with no embryo
  - No embryo with heartbeat 7–13 days after US that showed a gestational sac without a yolk sac
  - No embryo with heartbeat 7–10 days after US that showed a gestational sac with a yolk sac
  - Empty amnion
  - Yolk sac larger than 7 mm
  - Less than 5-mm difference between mean sac diameter and crown-rump length
  - If these findings are present a follow-up US examination in 7–10 days is appropriate

Adapted from Doubilet PM, Benson CB, Bourne T, et al. Diagnostic criteria for nonviable pregnancy early in the first trimester. *Ultrasound Q* 2014;30:3–9; Lane BF, Wong-You-Cheong JJ, Javitt MC, et al. ACR appropriateness criteria first trimester bleeding. *Ultrasound Q* 2013;29:91–96.

TABLE 52.3

CLINICAL RISK FACTORS FOR ECTOPIC PREGNANCY

- Tubal ligation
- Previous tubal surgery
- Pelvic inflammatory disease/salpingitis
- Previous ectopic pregnancy
- Presence of an intrauterine device
- Endometriosis
- In vitro fertilization
- History of smoking prior to conception
- Previous endometrial or myometrial surgery

Abortion is the termination of pregnancy before 20 weeks GA. *Spontaneous abortion* is the termination of pregnancy by natural causes. Approximately 10% to 15% of all known pregnancies end in spontaneous abortion. Up to 60% of spontaneous abortions have chromosomal abnormalities. A number of clinical terms are used to describe abortion. *Threatened abortion* refers to the occurrence of vaginal bleeding and uterine cramping with a closed cervical os in early pregnancy. Threatened abortion complicates roughly 25% of all pregnancies. *Inevitable abortion* presents with cervical dilation and fetal or placental tissues within the cervical os. With *complete abortion,* all uterine contents have been expelled. *Incomplete abortion* refers to the presence of residual products of conception within the uterus. In a *missed abortion,* the fetus has died but remains within the uterus. *Habitual abortion* is defined as three or more successive spontaneous abortions. *Anembryonic pregnancy* or *blighted ovum* is a pregnancy in which the embryo has died and is no longer visible, or never developed.

"Empty" Gestational Sac. A gestational sac without an embryo demonstrated by US may be a very early intrauterine pregnancy or a nonviable intrauterine pregnancy (anembryonic pregnancy) (Fig. 52.8). An empty gestational sac must be differentiated from a pseudogestational sac associated with ectopic pregnancy (see Fig. 52.13). A gestational sac is considered

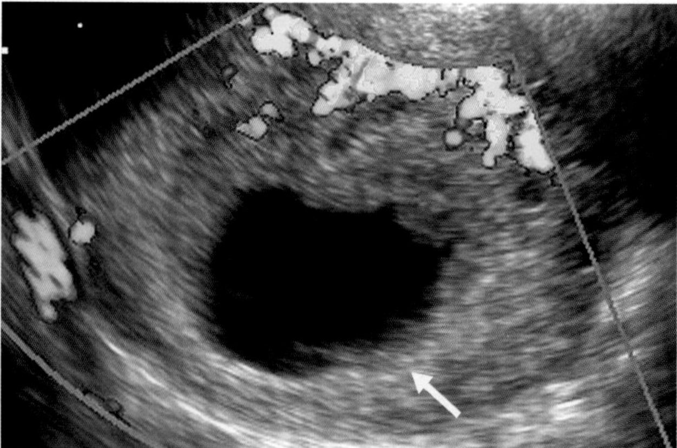

FIGURE 52.8. **Failed Pregnancy.** An empty gestational sac, measuring 27 mm in MSD, is demonstrated within the uterus by transvaginal US. The margin of the sac is irregular in contour and the decidual reaction (*arrow*) is poorly defined and only weakly echogenic. Color Doppler shows blood flow only in the myometrium. By the 2013 revised criteria an embryo should always be seen on transvaginal US when the MSD is ≥25 mm. Doppler US should be used with caution, especially in the first trimester, and only when the pregnancy is believed to be abnormal.

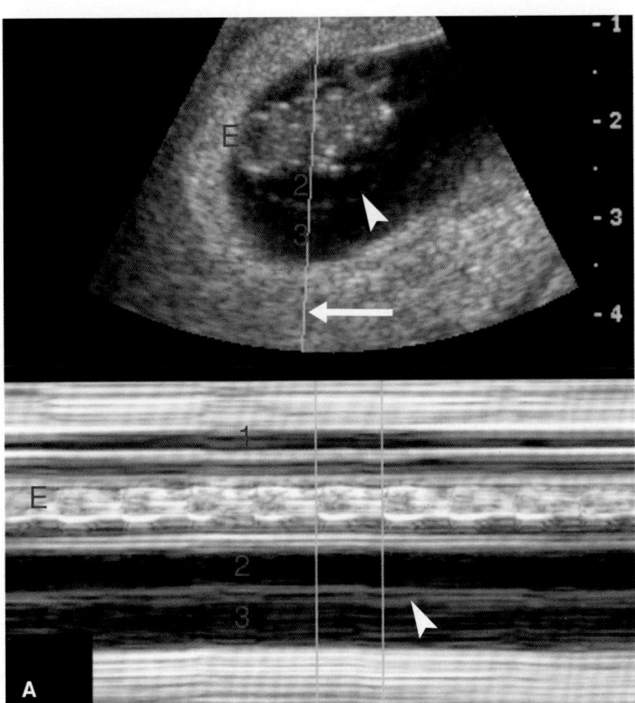

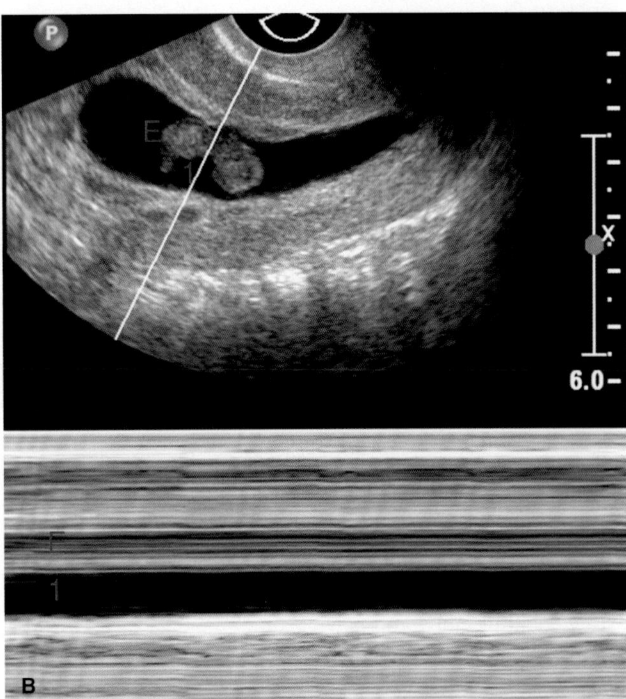

FIGURE 52.9. **Normal Embryonic Heartbeat and Embryonic Demise. A:** M-mode US is used to document the normal heartbeat of an 8-week embryo (CRL = 17 mm). The white line (*arrow*) shows the path of the pencil-beam M-mode sound wave passing through the embryo (*E*). The M-mode beam can be steered to the desired orientation. The M-mode trace is displayed in the lower half of the image. The heartbeat is evident as wavy lines at the level of the embryo (*E*). The number *1*, indicating fluid superficial to the embryo is displayed as the dark band (*1*) in the M-mode tracing. The number *2* indicates the amniotic fluid just deep to the embryo. The *arrowhead* indicates the amniotic membrane seen as a wavy echogenic line in the M-mode tracing. The number *3* indicates the chorionic fluid outside the amniotic membrane (*arrowheads*). **B:** M-mode US is used to document the absence of heartbeat in this deceased 8-week embryo (*E*) (CRL = 19 mm). No cardiac activity was visualized on real-time transvaginal US examination. The M-mode beam was steered through the proper location of the heart (*E*). No activity is present. The number *1* indicates the fluid deep to the embryo as the dark band on the M-mode tracing.

to be abnormal if it demonstrates the following features: large size (>25-mm MSD) without an embryo or yolk sac, distorted shape, irregular contour, thin or weak choriodecidual reaction, absence of a double decidual sac, or abnormal position. Large sac size without visualized yolk sac or embryo and a distorted sac contour have a reported 100% specificity and positive predictive value for identification of nonviable pregnancy. Most authors recommend allowing a 1- to 2-mm margin of error and repeating any equivocal scans in several days.

Embryonic or fetal demise is diagnosed by US confirmation of the absence of cardiac activity in an embryo ≥7-mm CRL on transvaginal US (Fig. 52.9). Transvaginal US may demonstrate cardiac activity even in embryos as small as 1.5-mm CRL. Transvaginal US may also visualize small, normal, living embryos (<7-mm CRL) without demonstrating cardiac activity. Embryos smaller than 7-mm CRL without cardiac activity should be rescanned in a few days to confirm viability. M-mode US is used to document visualized cardiac activity.

Intrauterine pregnancy of uncertain viability is the term used for the presence of an intrauterine gestational sac with no embryonic heartbeat and no findings of definite pregnancy failure (Table 52.2). The appearance of an early gestational sac on transvaginal US is highly variable. The intradecidual and double decidua signs are often absent. Prognosis for the pregnancy is unrelated to their absence. All round or oval intrauterine fluid collections in a pregnant patient should be treated as a gestational sac and potential viable pregnancy until proven otherwise (Fig. 52.10).

Pregnancy of unknown location describes the situation of a woman with a positive urine or serum pregnancy test and no intrauterine or ectopic pregnancy on transvaginal US examination. The major diagnostic considerations are early intrauterine pregnancy, occult ectopic pregnancy, and completed spontaneous abortion. A single quantitative hCG

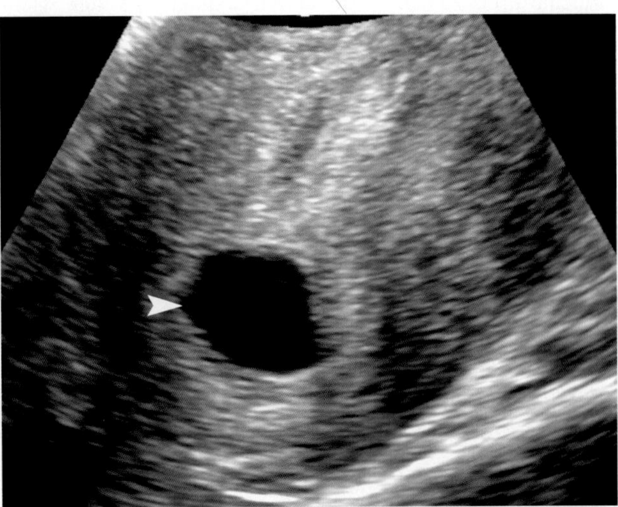

FIGURE 52.10. **Intrauterine Pregnancy of Uncertain Viability.** Transverse US of the uterus reveals a nonspecific intrauterine fluid collection (*arrowhead*) measuring 14-mm MSD. By the 2013 SRU criteria this should be considered a potentially viable intrauterine pregnancy until proven otherwise. Follow-up US in 7 to 10 days is advised.

determination does not differentiate between these conditions. About 8% of early pregnancies may fall into this category by US examination. US findings include the following:

- Empty uterus without an intrauterine fluid collection and no evidence of ectopic pregnancy. If a single hCG level is ≥3,000 IU/mL, a viable intrauterine pregnancy is unlikely; however these findings are not definitive.
- A nonspecific intrauterine fluid collection with smooth rounded or oval contours and with no yolk sac or embryo and normal adnexa. This is most likely an intrauterine pregnancy but ectopic pregnancy is not completely excluded. The intrauterine fluid collection may a pseudogestational sac.

For both findings, follow-up US and hCG determination in 7 to 10 weeks are recommended as long as the patient is hemodynamically stable.

Ectopic pregnancy occurs in only 2% of all pregnancies, but it is the major cause of pregnancy-related maternal deaths (9% to 14% of maternal mortality). Misdiagnosis of ectopic pregnancy remains one of the most common areas for medical malpractice litigation. About half of ectopic pregnancies are initially asymptomatic but subsequently rupture and present with vaginal bleeding and pelvic pain.

Patients at high risk for ectopic pregnancy include those with a history of pelvic inflammatory disease, tubal surgery, endometriosis, ovulation induction, previous ectopic pregnancy, or use of intrauterine device (IUD) for contraception (Table 52.3). Most ectopic pregnancies occur in the fallopian tube. Uncommon sites for ectopic implantation include the interstitial portion of the tube, abdominal cavity, ovary, and cervix. All patients with a positive pregnancy test (serum β-hCG), and vaginal bleeding, pelvic pain, or adnexal mass must be considered at risk for ectopic pregnancy.

A completely confident diagnosis of ectopic pregnancy can be made sonographically only when a living embryo or a gestational sac containing a yolk sac, is positively demonstrated to be in a position outside of the uterus. In any other circumstance, we are dealing with a situation of relative risk (Table 52.4). When an intrauterine pregnancy is documented by US, the risk of coexisting ectopic pregnancy is extremely low, estimated at 1 in 30,000. Concurrent intra- and extrauterine pregnancies (termed *heterotopic pregnancy*) do occur, however, especially in patients taking ovulation-inducing drugs. The risk of ectopic pregnancy is high when the uterus is empty (no gestational sac) and an adnexal mass, other than a corpus luteal cyst, is demonstrated. Similarly, an ectopic pregnancy is likely when the uterus is empty and a moderate or large amount of echogenic fluid or blood clots are seen in the cul-de-sac. Even when the US examination is entirely normal, but without definitive evidence of intrauterine pregnancy, a patient with a positive pregnancy test remains at risk for ectopic pregnancy. The role of US, then, is to demonstrate findings that determine relative risk. This assessment, in conjunction with clinical history and physical examination, determines the risk of ectopic pregnancy and the next step in the patient's evaluation.

US findings in ectopic pregnancy include demonstration of an extrauterine gestational sac appearing as a fluid-containing structure with an echogenic ring, the ***tubal ring sign*** (40% to 68% of ectopic pregnancies) (Fig. 52.11). A living or dead embryo might be evident. The ectopic gestational sac must be differentiated from a corpus luteum, which develops on the ovary at the site of ovulation. Clotted blood from hemorrhage

TABLE 52.4

FINDINGS OF ECTOPIC PREGNANCY

- **Most specific (100% specific, but low sensitivity, 18–26%)**
  - Live embryo with heartbeat outside of the uterus
- **Adnexal mass separate from the ovary (89–100% of cases)**
  - Tubal ring (echogenic ring surrounding gestational sac, 40–68% of cases)
    - Highly specific if embryo and yolk sac are present
    - Less specific if yolk sac and no embryo
  - Complex adnexal mass separate from ovary
  - Ring-of-fire sign (hypervascular ring on color Doppler)
    - Not specific
    - More likely to be a corpus luteum
- **Complex free fluid in the pelvis**
  - Strongly indicative of ectopic pregnancy rupture
- **Intrauterine findings in ectopic pregnancy**
  - Normal endometrium (86% of cases)
  - Pseudogestational sac (10–20% of cases)
    - Fluid collection within the uterine cavity
    - Central location surrounded by thick echogenic decidua
    - Angular or teardrop shape common
  - Decidual cyst—thin-walled cyst at junction of endometrium and myometrium

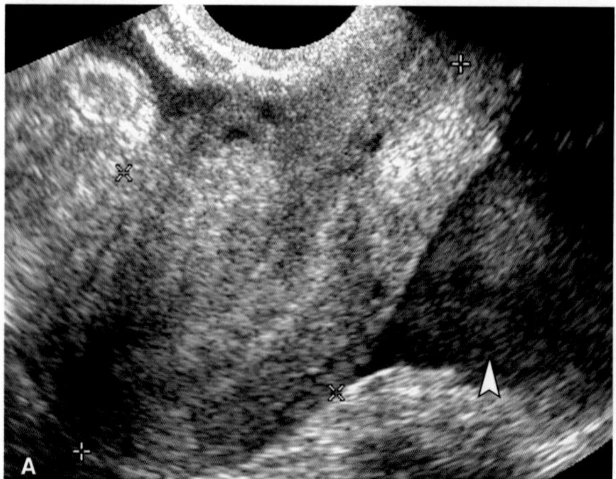

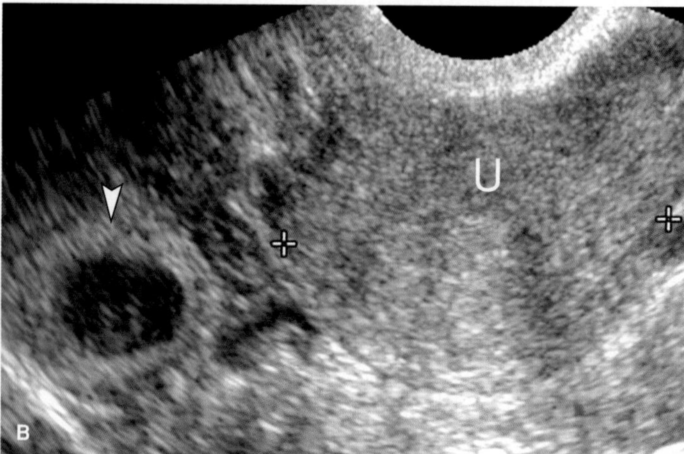

FIGURE 52.11. Ectopic Pregnancy. A: Transvaginal US in a longitudinal plane demonstrates an empty uterus (between *calipers*, +, ×) in a pregnant patient. Echogenic blood (*arrowhead*) distends the cul-de-sac. **B:** Transverse transvaginal image reveals a tubal ring sign (*arrowhead*) in the right adnexa highly indicative of ectopic pregnancy. *U*, uterus (between *calipers*, +).

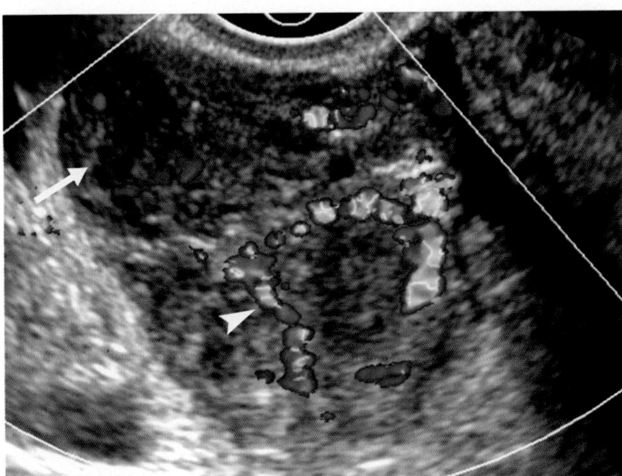

FIGURE 52.12. **Tubal Ectopic Pregnancy—"Ring of Fire."** Transvaginal US shows a circular ring (*arrowhead*) of intense vascularity surrounding a mass in the fallopian tube. This has been termed the "ring of fire" characteristic of ectopic pregnancy. The adjacent ovary (*arrow*) shows less intense vascularity surrounding the corpus luteum. Careful real-time US examination is required to confirm the ovary and the tubal mass are separate structures.

within a corpus luteal cyst may simulate an embryo. A key differentiating finding is whether the cystic mass arises from the ovary (Fig. 52.12). Most ectopic pregnancies occur within the fallopian tube and can be shown on real-time transvaginal US to be separate from the ovary. Implantation of ectopic pregnancy on the ovary is a rare event. Corpus luteal cysts always arise from the ovary. Hematosalpinx or ruptured ectopic pregnancy may appear as an amorphous solid or complex adnexal mass (a hematoma) lacking an embryo or sac. Blood in the cul-de-sac usually appears as echogenic fluid but may be entirely echolucent if liquid, or echogenic and solid-appearing if clotted. Moderate or large volumes of echogenic fluid or blood clots in the cul-de-sac are highly predictive of ectopic pregnancy. A small volume of anechoic fluid in the cul-de-sac is a common and normal finding.

In the presence of an ectopic pregnancy, the lining of the uterus will be thickened and echogenic reflecting the conversion of endometrium to decidua induced by the hormones of pregnancy. Blood in the uterine cavity produces cystic-appearing mass termed a ***pseudogestational sac*** in 10% to 20% of ectopic pregnancies (Fig. 52.13). A true gestational sac is

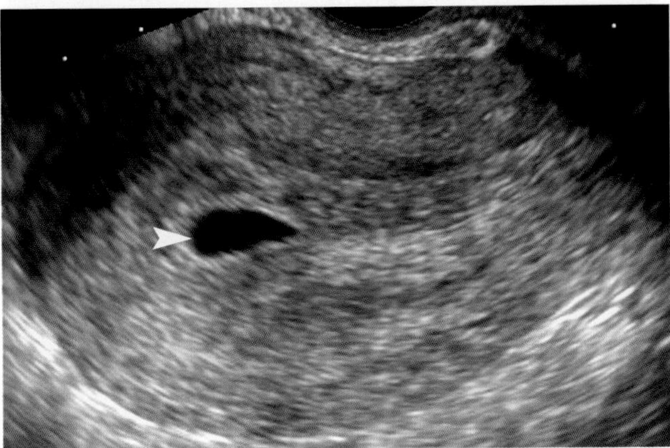

FIGURE 52.13. **Pseudogestational Sac.** Fluid within the endometrial cavity (*arrowhead*) in a patient with an ectopic pregnancy mimics an intrauterine gestational sac.

differentiated from "pseudosac" by the presence of a yolk sac or embryo. A double decidua sign suggests a true gestational sac, but is not totally reliable. Pseudosacs are located centrally within the uterine canal whereas a normal true gestational sac is eccentrically implanted within the decidua. Doppler studies demonstrate absent or minimal peritrophoblastic flow with pseudosacs and high-velocity, low-impedance flow with true gestational sacs. Serum hCG levels in most ectopic pregnancies are <3,000 IU/mL, often <1,000 IU/mL. However, hCG levels are variable and are not predictive of rupture of the ectopic pregnancy.

Ectopic pregnancies occur in the following locations:

Fallopian tube (95%), most commonly in the ampullary portion of the tube (70% of tubal pregnancies).

Interstitial (2% to 4%) are associated with a high incidence of severe maternal hemorrhage. Implantation is in the myometrial portion of the fallopian tube which allows development of the pregnancy up to 16 weeks with large supplying arteries. A fundal gestational sac is eccentric and the adjacent myometrium is thinned to less than 5 mm. It can be confused with a pregnancy in one horn of a bicornuate uterus.

Ovarian (<3%) are difficult to differentiate from a corpus luteum. Implantation is on the ovarian parenchyma. Occurs most commonly with IUD in place.

Abdominal (~1%) may occur as a result of secondary implantation of a ruptured ectopic pregnancy in the peritoneal cavity. Is associated with marked increase in maternal mortality because the growth of the pregnancy is unrestricted. The placenta is outside of the uterine cavity. The pregnancy is not surrounded by myometrium.

Cesarean scar (<1%) are prone to rupture because of thinness of the scar and surrounding myometrium. Implantation is in the thinned lower uterine segment. No adnexal mass is present. Hysterectomy may be necessary.

Cervical (<1%) are associated with previous dilation and curettage. The uterus is hourglass shaped with an enlarged cervix containing the gestational sac.

Heterotopic (<0.01) intrauterine and ectopic pregnancies are very rare natural occurrences but occur more commonly with in vitro fertilization.

Therapeutic options for ectopic pregnancy include medical management using methotrexate as a cell-growth inhibitor. This has become increasingly popular because tubal patency can be preserved. Other options include surgical resection, and local injection of the ectopic pregnancy with methotrexate or potassium chloride. Up to 15% of ectopic pregnancies resolve spontaneously.

Quantitative serum hCG levels have been correlated with US findings to assist in the identification of abnormal pregnancies. Previously defined discriminatory levels for hCG values have been determined to be not entirely valid. The SRU committee advises that single hCG level should not be used to exclude a potentially normal intrauterine pregnancy or to make a definitive diagnosis of failed or ectopic pregnancy. Serial hCG levels may be more helpful but have been shown to vary as well. In general, quantitative hCG levels are expected to double approximately every 2 days.

Subchorionic hemorrhage is a common finding, 18% to 22% of bleeding pregnant patients, before 20 weeks GA. All cases are believed to develop because of venous bleeding from separation of the margin of the placenta. The hematoma collects preferentially beneath the chorion because the chorion is more easily separated from the myometrium than the placenta. Patients may be asymptomatic if the hematoma remains confined, or may present with vaginal bleeding if the hematoma leaks through the cervix. In most patients, a subchorionic

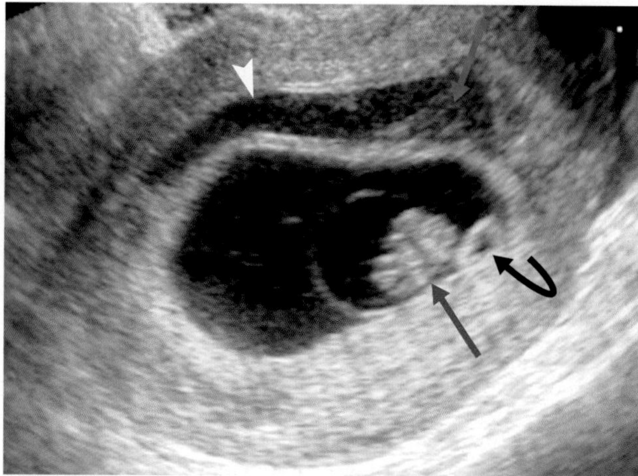

FIGURE 52.14. **Subchorionic Hemorrhage.** Hemorrhage (*arrowhead*) is seen in the uterine cavity between the decidua capsularis and the decidua vera. Some of the blood is clotted and appears more echogenic (*blue arrow*) than the liquid blood. A live embryo (*red arrow*) was present within its amnionic sac. The yolk sac (*curved arrow*) is partially visualized.

hematoma is an innocent finding; however, an increased rate of spontaneous abortion has been reported associated with large hematomas (encirclement of more than two-thirds of the circumference of the gestational sac), advanced maternal age (>35 years), and early GA (<8 weeks). The US appearance of the hemorrhage varies with age (Fig. 52.14). Acute bleeding is anechoic to hypoechoic. With clotting, it becomes hyperechoic and heterogeneous. With lysis, the hematoma reverts to being hypoechoic to anechoic. *Implantation bleeding* is a nonspecific term that refers to small collections of blood at the site of attachment of the chorion to the endometrium. These are in essence small areas of subchorionic hemorrhage that occur early in pregnancy. US follow-up is warranted to assess for progression.

Retained Products of Conception (RPOC). Following a spontaneous or induced abortion, or even a normal delivery, the patient may continue to have vaginal bleeding caused by incomplete expulsion of the pregnancy. The most common US appearance of RPOC is an echogenic mass within the uterine cavity representing retention of a portion of the placenta (Fig. 52.15). The mass, like the normal placenta, is more echogenic than the myometrium. A polypoid or pedunculated mass of retained placental tissues has been termed a *placental polyp*. Blood clots appear as hypoechoic masses without blood flow within the uterine cavity. Variants in appearance of RPOC include irregular thickening of the endometrium (>10 mm), highly reflective structures with shadowing representing fetal parts or calcified placental remnants, or mixed echogenicity masses representing necrotic tissue. Color Doppler findings are highly variable showing little or no vascularity within devascularized RPOC, or striking blood flow within the mass (Fig. 52.15B) and the myometrium resembling a uterine arteriovenous malformation. High-velocity blood flow (peak systolic velocity >60 cm/s) in retained trophoblastic tissue is associated with heavy bleeding during surgical removal.

Gestational Trophoblastic Disease

Gestational trophoblastic disease is a group of neoplasms that range from benign to highly malignant. All are derived from abnormal placental tissues and occur as sequelae to pregnancy. Both benign and malignant tumors produce hCG. Marked elevation of serum hCG levels is characteristic, and serial measurement is a sensitive and reliable indicator of tumor activity. Gestational trophoblastic disease complicates about 1 in 1,000 to 2,000 pregnancies in the United States but has a much higher incidence in the Far East and in Latin America. Women over age 40 and those with a prior history of molar pregnancy are also at increased risk.

Hydatidiform mole is the most common (80%) and most benign form of the disease but maintains a potential for malignant sequelae. The placenta demonstrates edema and proliferation of trophoblasts. The villi become swollen and vesicular, resembling a bunch of grapes. Patients present with hyperemesis, pregnancy-induced hypertension, and vaginal bleeding. The uterus may be enlarged (50%), normal (35%), or small

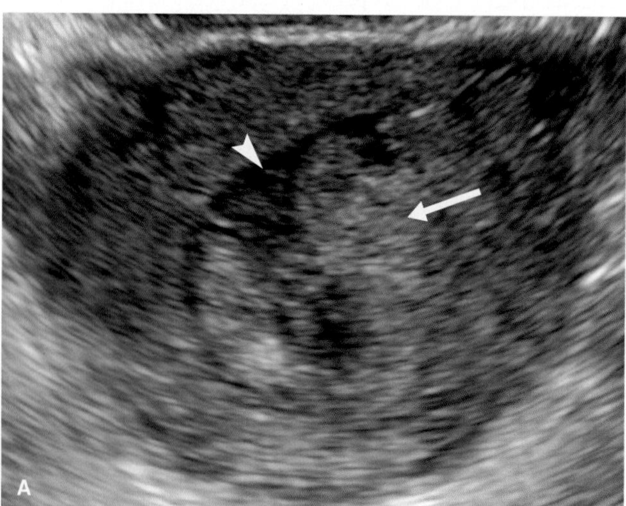

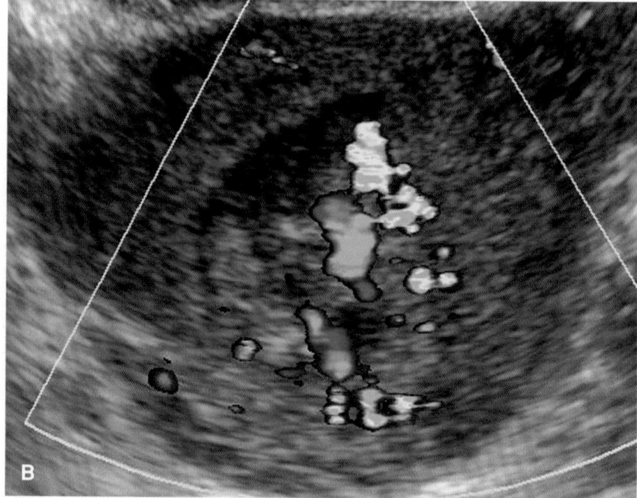

FIGURE 52.15. **Retained Products of Conception. A:** Transverse image of the uterus in a woman with continuing bleeding following a spontaneous abortion reveals echogenic material (*arrow*) representing retained placenta and echolucent material (*arrowhead*) representing blood and clots within the uterine cavity. **B:** Transverse color Doppler image of the uterus in the same patient documents continuing blood flow to the retained placenta.

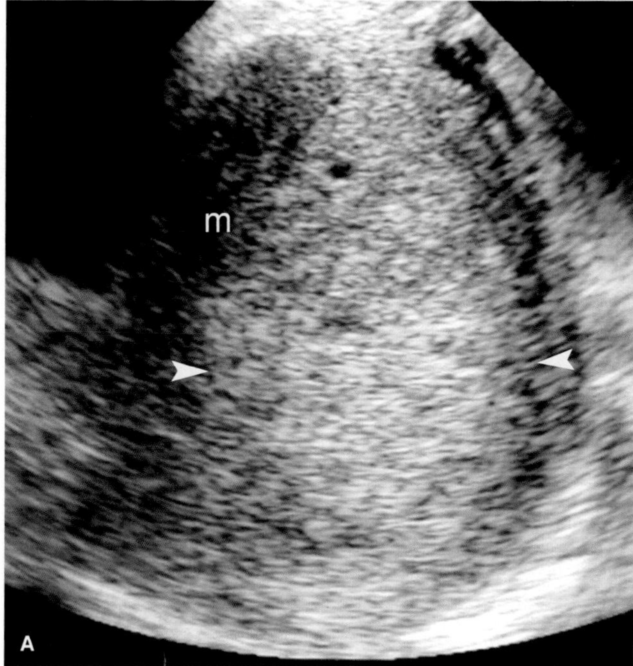

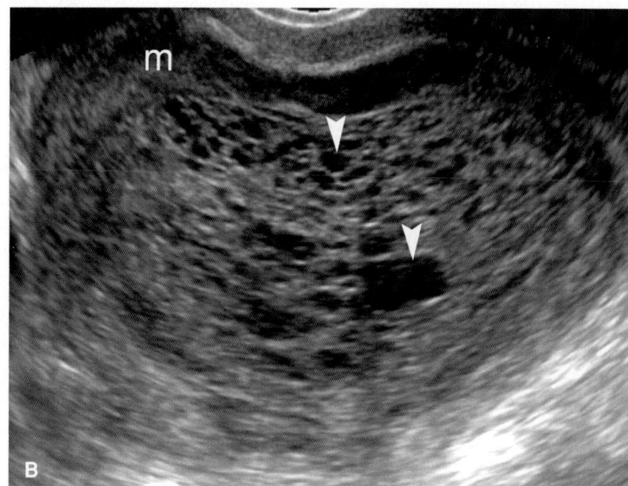

FIGURE 52.16. **Hydatidiform Mole. A:** Transvaginal US shows the "snowstorm" appearance of a molar pregnancy (between *arrowheads*) filling the uterine cavity in the first trimester. **B:** In another patient examined early in the second trimester, more discrete cysts are seen within the molar tissue (*arrowheads*). *m*, myometrium.

(15%) for dates. Two types of hydatidiform mole exist. *Complete mole* (classic mole) (70%) involves the entire placenta, lacks a fetus, and is diploid in karyotype. *Partial mole* (30%) involves only a portion of the placenta and is associated with an abnormal fetus that is triploid in karyotype (due to fertilization of an ovum by two sperm). This condition is lethal to the fetus. Rarely, a normal fetus may coexist with a complete mole in a twin pregnancy. Prognosis for the normal fetus in these cases is grim because of maternal complications of the mole.

US of complete mole in the first trimester classically shows the uterus to be filled with an echogenic, solid, highly vascular mass, often described as "snowstorm" in appearance. The tiny vesicles that make up the mole are too small to be resolved as discrete cysts but cause innumerable sound-reflective interfaces that produce the brightly echogenic appearance (Fig. 52.16). As the vesicles enlarge in the second trimester individual cysts 2 to 30 mm in size become apparent producing a "bunch-of-grapes" appearance. Partial mole demonstrates vesicular changes in only a portion of the placenta. The associated triploid fetus has multiple anomalies. The classic appearance of mole is not always evident. Molar pregnancy may occasionally appear as an anechoic fluid collection that mimics anembryonic pregnancy. *Theca lutein cysts* are seen as large, septated, bilateral cysts massively enlarging the ovaries in 25% to 65% cases of molar pregnancy (Fig. 52.17). Theca lutein cysts result from hyperstimulation of the ovaries by high circulating levels of hCG and are most commonly seen in molar pregnancy in the second trimester.

Invasive mole (chorioadenoma destruens) refers to invasion of molar tissue into, but usually not beyond, the myometrium. It is seen in about 10% of patients and usually becomes evident after treatment for hydatidiform mole. US shows penetration of the echogenic trophoblastic tissue into the myometrium. MR is more sensitive than US in demonstrating the muscle-invasive disease seen as focal myometrial masses, dilated vessels, and areas of hemorrhage and necrosis.

Choriocarcinoma is a highly aggressive malignancy that forms only trophoblasts without any villous structure. Choriocarcinoma is locally invasive, spreads into the myometrium and parametrium, and hematogenously metastasizes to any site in the body. Serum hCG levels that rise or plateau in the 8 to 10 weeks following evacuation of molar pregnancy suggest invasive or metastatic gestational trophoblastic disease. Choriocarcinoma at any site produces a highly echogenic solid mass.

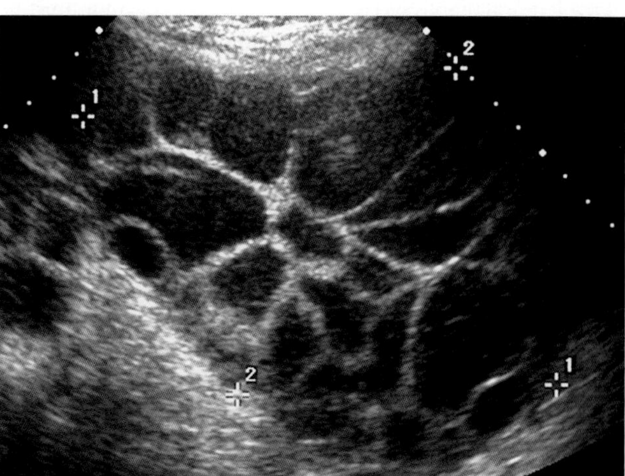

FIGURE 52.17. **Theca Lutein Cysts.** Transabdominal image demonstrates the ovary (between *calipers*, +) to be greatly enlarged by numerous cysts in this patient with a twin pregnancy following infertility therapy. The hCG level was greatly elevated. This ovary measured 16 × 12 × 8 cm in size.

FETAL MEASUREMENTS AND GROWTH

Dating the pregnancy and determining the appropriateness of fetal growth are essential to obstetric care. Clinical dating is based on history of the mother's last menstrual period (LMP) and physical examination assessment of uterine size. Sonographic dating is based on measurements of the gestational sac and the embryo or fetus. Serial measurements of fetal parameters are used to document growth. By convention, pregnancies are dated from the first day of the LMP. The terms *gestational age* (GA), which is the clinical standard, and *menstrual age* are usually considered to be synonymous terms and are based on the average 28-day menstrual cycle. Conception is assumed to occur 14 days following the LMP. Term is 40 weeks, with an acceptable range of 37 to 42 weeks.

Gestational sac size is used in the first trimester to estimate GA when no embryo is visualized. The gestational sac diameter is measured in three orthogonal planes, and the results are averaged. The MSD is accurate to within approximately 1 week menstrual age.

Crown-rump length is measured from the top of the head to the bottom of the torso of the visualized embryo or fetus (Fig. 52.18). The CRL is useful until about 12 weeks GA, when other fetal measurements become more accurate. Charts provide GA estimations accurate to approximately 0.5 week menstrual age.

Biparietal diameter (BPD) is measured on an axial image of the fetal head at the level of the third ventricle and thalamus (Fig. 52.19). By convention, the measurement is made from the outer table of the near cranium to the inner table of the far cranium. The measurement is affected by head shape and provides an inaccurate estimate of GA if significant *dolichocephaly* (elongated skull) or *brachycephaly* (round skull) is present.

Head circumference (HC) is the outer perimeter of the fetal cranium measured in the same plane as the BPD (Fig. 52.19). The HC measurement is relatively independent of head shape.

Abdominal circumference (AC) is the outer perimeter of the fetal abdomen measured on an axial plane image at the level of the intrahepatic portion of the umbilical vein (Fig. 52.20).

Femur length (FL) is the measurement of the ossified portion of the femoral diaphysis (Fig. 52.21). The entire femur must be imaged, and the femoral shaft must be centered in the beam so that it casts an acoustic shadow.

GA estimates are most accurate in early pregnancy and become progressively less accurate as the pregnancy advances.

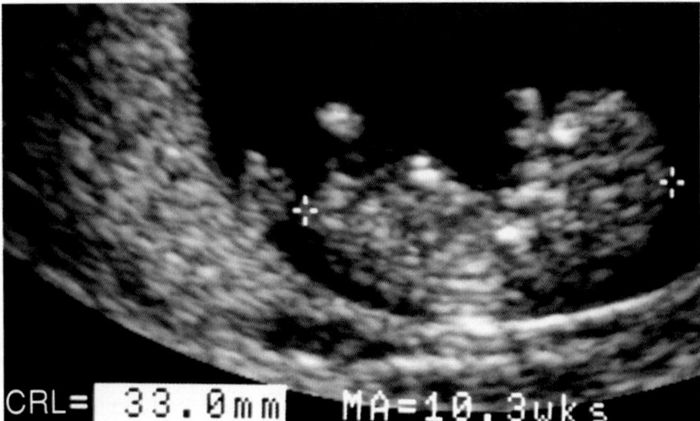

FIGURE 52.18. Crown-Rump Length. The CRL is measured from the top of the head to the bottom of the torso (between *cursors*, +).

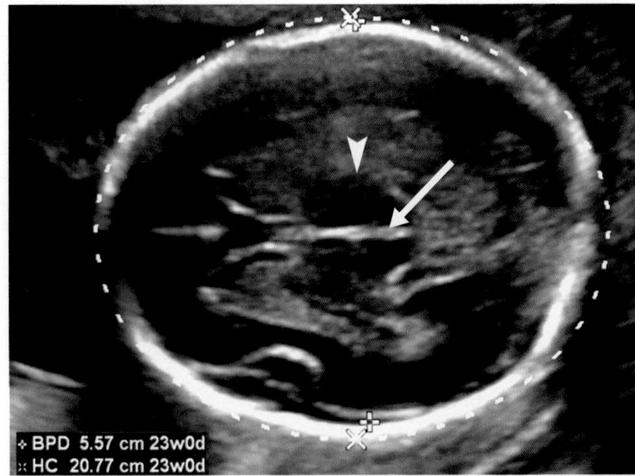

FIGURE 52.19. Transthalamic (BPD/HC) Plane. Axial image of the fetal cranium demonstrates the paired thalami (*arrowhead*) on either side of the midline third ventricle (*long arrow*). The BPD is measured in this plane from the outer surface of the near cranium to the inner surface of the far cranium (*cursors*, +). The head circumference is measured as an outer perimeter measurement of the cranium in the same plane (*elliptical dashed line, cursors*, ×).

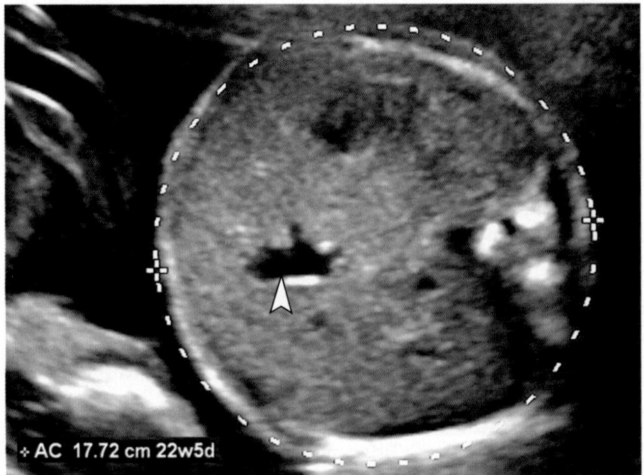

FIGURE 52.20. Abdominal Circumference. The correct plane of measurement of the abdominal circumference is an axial plane showing a round abdomen at the level of the umbilical vein (*arrowhead*) junction with the left portal vein. The elliptical dashed line and cursors (+) show measurement of the abdominal circumference at 17.72 cm corresponding to 22 weeks 5 days gestational age.

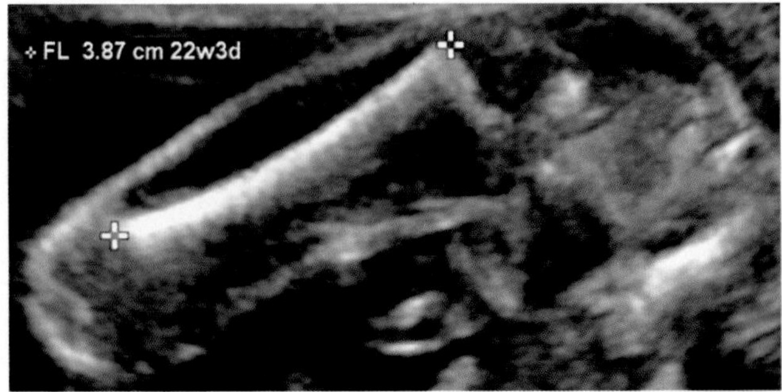

FIGURE 52.21. Femur Length. The FL is the measurement of the ossified portion of the femoral diaphysis (between *calipers*, +).

The composite age, calculated by averaging the GA estimates of multiple parameters, is more accurate than any single parameter. Fetal anomalies may make individual parameters inaccurate for estimation of GA. Body parts with structural anomalies should be excluded from the composite GA estimation. The composite of BPD, HC, AC, and FL measurements predicts GA accurate to about 1.1 weeks at 12 to 18 weeks, 1.8 weeks at 24 to 30 weeks but is accurate to only about 3.1 weeks at 36 to 42 weeks. GA is assigned at the time of the first US and is not changed thereafter. All subsequent US examinations are compared with the first examination to assess fetal growth.

Intrauterine Growth Retardation (IUGR). Fetuses with impaired intrauterine growth have an increased risk of intrauterine demise and a perinatal mortality four to eight times greater than normal growth fetuses. Half the survivors have significant morbidity, including intrapartum fetal distress, hypoglycemia, hypocalcemia, meconium aspiration pneumonia, impaired immune function, retarded neurologic development, and learning disabilities. A fetus or newborn is considered small for gestational age (SGA) if its weight is below the 10th percentile for GA. This definition will encompass normal infants who are constitutionally small as well as infants with IUGR who are pathologically small. The challenge is to separate the growth-restricted fetuses from those who are normal. Impaired growth may be caused by factors that are intrinsic to the fetus or related to a hostile fetal environment (Table 52.5). Fetuses with intrinsic insults have fixed defects and will not benefit from early delivery. The pattern of growth impairment occurs early in the second trimester and tends to be *symmetrical* in that the head, abdomen, and femur are all proportionally small. Fetuses exposed to an extrinsically impaired growth environment (uteroplacental insufficiency) will usually benefit from therapy that usually includes early delivery. Growth impairment occurs in the late second and third trimesters and tends to be *asymmetrical* in that the fetal abdomen is disproportionally small relative to the head and femur. The AC is small because of diminished glycogen stores in the fetal liver and decreased or absent subcutaneous fat.

Many US criteria have been proposed to diagnose IUGR, but none individually is highly accurate. A multiparameter approach using estimated fetal weight (EFW), amniotic fluid volume, and the presence or absence of maternal hypertension has the greatest accuracy for diagnosis. The first step in diagnosis is to establish an accurate GA. An early US provides assignment of GA, which should not be changed on subsequent examinations. When the initial US is not obtained until the third trimester, GA is assigned on the basis of BPD, HC, and FL measurements, recognizing the imprecision of GA estimations in the third trimester. EFW is determined from established charts with those based upon 3 or 4 biometric measurements being the most accurate. The error range of these weight predictions is large, as high as 18% depending upon the chart used. IUGR is diagnosed confidently when the EFW is below the 5th percentile for GA and is excluded when the EFW is above the 20th percentile for GA. When the EFW is between the 5th and 20th percentile, IUGR is diagnosed if oligohydramnios or maternal hypertension is present, and it is likely not present if the amniotic fluid volume is normal or elevated and the mother is normotensive. US follow-up of fetuses with IUGR should be performed weekly or biweekly and includes measurement of growth parameters, assessment of amniotic fluid volume, biophysical profile score, and umbilical cord Doppler. Normal fetal weight gain in the third trimester is 100 to 200 g/wk. An amniotic fluid index of 5 cm or less (oligohydramnios) is strongly predictive of poor outcome.

TABLE 52.5

CAUSES OF INTRAUTERINE GROWTH RETARDATION

- Uteroplacental insufficiency (80%) (prone to asymmetric IUGR)
  - Maternal causes
    - Demographics
      - Advanced maternal age
      - Young maternal age
      - Nulliparous
    - Chronic maternal diseases
      - Severe anemia
      - Renal failure
      - Diabetes
      - Preeclampsia
      - Vascular diseases
      - Chronic heart disease
    - Deficient nutrients
      - Maternal starvation
      - Smoking
      - Alcohol
      - Illicit drugs (cocaine, heroin)
      - High altitude
  - Placental causes
    - Extensive placental infarctions
    - Chronic partial abruption
      - Low-lying placenta, placenta previa
      - Placentitis (malaria)
- Fetal causes (20%) (prone to symmetric IUGR)
  - Chromosome abnormalities (trisomy, triploidy)
  - Congenital anomalies (heart, urinary, neurologic)
  - Viral infection (rubella, CMV, toxoplasmosis)

Biophysical profile is a test to identify compromised fetuses. Four parameters assess for acute hypoxia: reactive fetal heart rate (nonstress test), respiratory activity, gross motor movements, and fetal tone. One parameter, the amniotic fluid volume, evaluates for chronic hypoxia. A variety of different techniques are used for assessment and scoring. A score of 2 is given for a normal response, and 0 is given for an abnormal response. The fetus is at extreme risk for fetal demise within 1 week with a total score of 0 or 2, and it is at no immediate risk with a total score of 8 or 10.

Fetal arterial Doppler US provides another method of assessment of fetal well-being and prediction of perinatal morbidity and mortality related to IUGR. The umbilical artery (UA) circulation to the placenta is normally low impedance manifest by high blood flow velocities in late diastole on spectral Doppler waveforms. Destruction of blood vessels within the placenta by diseases that cause placental insufficiency increases the vascular resistance in the placental circulation and causes a decrease in flow velocities in late diastole on UA Doppler. A systolic-to-diastolic ratio (see Chapter 54) of 4 or greater, or the absence of forward flow in diastole, is strongly predictive of severe fetal compromise. Reversal of flow in diastole is a particularly ominous finding indicative of high risk for fetal demise within 1 to 7 days if the fetus is left in utero (Fig. 52.22). The middle cerebral artery (MCA) carries more than 80% of fetal cerebral blood flow and is accessible to Doppler interrogation. In the normal fetal brain, the MCA circulation shows a high vascular resistance pattern with little or no forward flow in late diastole. When the fetus is exposed to hypoxia brain-sparing redistribution of blood flow occurs increasing flow velocities in the MCA during both systole and diastole.

Fetal macrosomia is defined as EFW above the 90th percentile for GA or a fetal weight above 4,000 g. Risk factors include maternal diabetes, maternal obesity, previous history

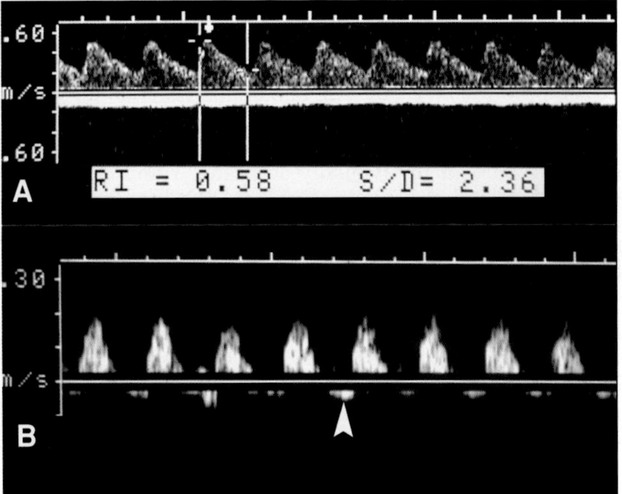

FIGURE 52.22. **Umbilical Artery Doppler. A: Normal.** Spectral Doppler tracing from an umbilical artery shows a normal pattern with forward flow maintained throughout diastole and a low vascular resistance with RI = 0.58. **B: Fetal Distress.** Spectral Doppler in a severely growth-retarded fetus shows a high vascular resistance pattern with flow toward the placenta during systole and reversal of blood flow direction in diastole (*arrowhead*). This finding is highly indicative of severe fetal distress. This fetus died 4 days after this examination.

of macrosomic infant, and excessive weight gain during pregnancy. Complications of macrosomia are manifest at delivery and include shoulder dystocia, traumatic delivery, fractures, brachial plexus injury, perinatal asphyxia, neonatal hypoglycemia, and meconium aspiration.

THE FETAL ENVIRONMENT

Uterus and Adnexa in Pregnancy

Uterine leiomyomas are the most common solid pelvic masses encountered during pregnancy. Fibroids commonly enlarge and undergo cystic degeneration induced by hormonal stimulation as the pregnancy advances. They are associated with bleeding, premature uterine contractions, malpresentation, and mechanical obstruction during labor. Spontaneous pregnancy loss is higher in patients with multiple fibroids than with a single fibroid. Leiomyomas must be differentiated from uterine contractions. Contractions are transient, although they may persist up to an hour. Contractions typically appear homogeneous and isoechoic with the myometrium. They bulge the inner, but generally not the outer, margin of the uterine wall. Leiomyomas are persistent, more heterogeneous, may have calcifications, and typically bulge the outer margin of the uterine wall. Doppler US demonstrates splaying of myometrial vessels around leiomyomas but no vessel displacement in areas of myometrial contraction.

Corpus luteal cysts are the most common cystic pelvic masses found in pregnancy. Internal hemorrhage causes enlargement up to 10 to 15 cm size, internal echoes, and septations (Fig. 52.5). Most of these cysts regress by 16 to 18 weeks GA. Differential diagnosis includes benign cystic teratoma, cystadenoma, hydrosalpinx, and paraovarian cyst.

Theca lutein cysts form due to an exaggerated corpus luteum response to high levels of hCG. They appear as bilateral multicystic enlargement of the ovaries (Fig. 52.17). They occur with gestational trophoblastic disease, pregnancy with more than one fetus, or associated with the use of ovulation-inducing drugs.

Cervical incompetence may be congenital or may result from cervical lacerations, excessive cervical dilation, or therapeutic abortion. The incompetent cervix is incapable of retaining a pregnancy to term. Preterm delivery is the single most common cause of a poor neonatal outcome. An obstetric history of recurrent spontaneous loss of pregnancy in the second trimester establishes the diagnosis. US is used to measure and follow cervical length and appearance. Scans are best performed transvaginally or translabially from the introitus with the bladder empty. A full urinary bladder compresses the lower uterus and falsely elongates the length of the cervix. The normal cervical length is 26 to 50 mm throughout gestation. Cervical length is measured in sagittal plane between the internal os marked by a V-shaped notch and the external os marked by a triangular echodensity (Fig. 52.23). The endocervical canal is seen as a thin hypo- or hyperechoic line. The relative risk of preterm delivery increases as cervical length decreases, with the greatest risk for cervical lengths of less than 2.5 cm. Cervical dilation is measured between the anterior and posterior surface of the cervical canal. Dilation of the cervical canal >8 mm is indicative of cervical incompetence. Membranes may be seen bulging into the cervical canal. Sutures associated with cervical cerclage used to treat cervical incompetence are seen on US as echogenic linear structures with acoustic shadowing.

Placenta and Membranes

Normal placenta is first apparent on US at about 8 weeks as a focal thickening at the periphery of the gestational sac. The disc-like shape of the placenta becomes evident by 12 weeks, and by 18 weeks the placenta is finely granular and homogeneous with a smooth covering chorionic membrane along its fetal surface. The *retroplacental complex* of decidual and myometrial veins forms a prominent sonographic landmark (Fig. 52.24). As the gestation advances, the placenta becomes more heterogeneous, with focal echolucencies owing to venous

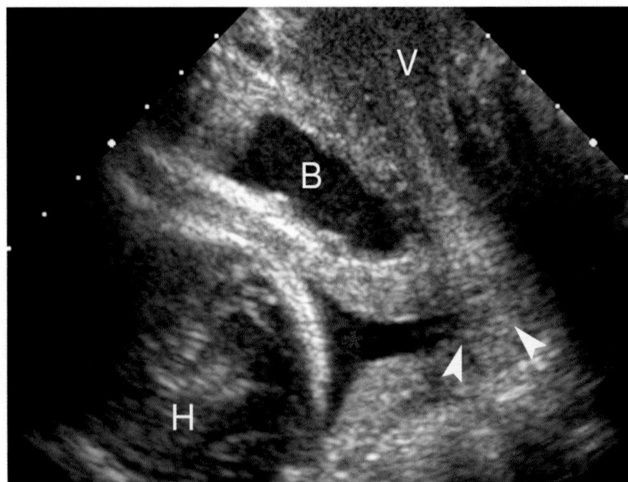

FIGURE 52.23. **Cervical Incompetence.** The cervix is best evaluated with a translabial view with the bladder (*B*) empty. The transducer, placed at the introitus, is aimed down the long axis of the vagina (*V*). The cervix, measured between the internal os and the external os (*arrowheads*), is shortened to 9 mm in this patient with a history of multiple spontaneous abortions in the second trimester. The cervix is also dilated allowing amniotic fluid (*) to enter the endocervical canal. The fetal head (*H*) is presenting at the internal cervical os.

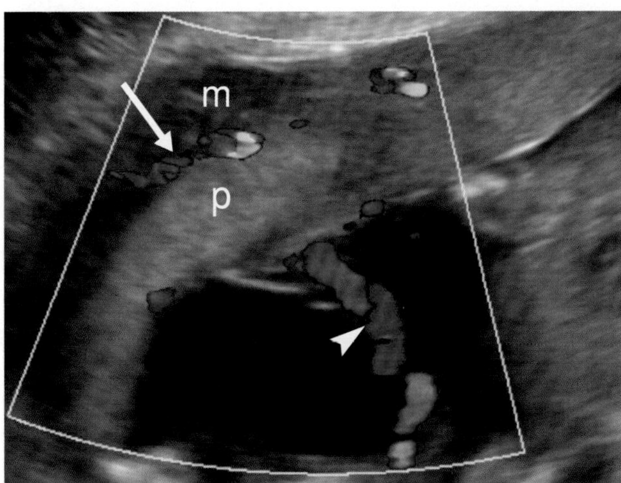

FIGURE 52.24. Normal Placenta and Umbilical Cord Insertion. A color Doppler transabdominal scan demonstrates a normal placenta (*p*) and the insertion site of the cord onto the placenta (*arrowhead*). The retroplacental complex of veins (*arrow*) appears as a network of vessels in the myometrium (*m*) beneath the placenta.

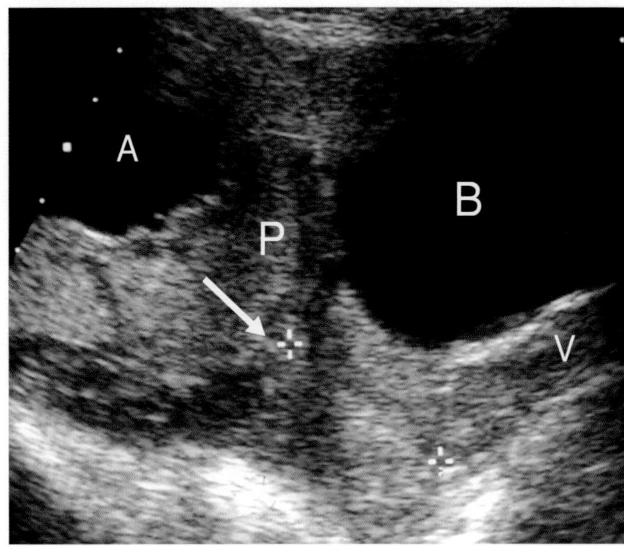

FIGURE 52.25. Placenta Previa. Transabdominal US shows a normal cervix (between *cursors*, +) measuring 34 mm. The placenta (*P*) covers the internal os (*arrow*). *A*, amniotic cavity; *B*, bladder; *V*, vagina.

lakes and areas of fibrin deposition. Septations become prominent US features throughout the placenta and cause undulations of the placental surface. Calcifications occur along the septations and are dispersed randomly throughout the placenta. These are normal changes of placental aging and should not be interpreted as indicators of disease. Grading of the placenta based on these normal changes in US appearance has not proven to be clinically useful. The normal placenta has a maximum thickness of 4 cm and a minimal thickness of 1 cm. Thick placentas are associated with maternal diabetes, maternal anemia, hydrops from immune and nonimmune causes, chronic uterine infections, and placental abruption. Thin placentas are associated with preeclampsia, placental insufficiency, IUGR, and trisomies 13 and 18.

Placenta previa is present when a part or all of the placenta covers the internal cervical os. Placenta previa is seen at term in 0.3% to 0.6% of live births. Placenta previa is suggested by US in as many as 45% of pregnancies examined in the first and second trimesters. These cases are the result of low implantation of the placenta and filling of the bladder, distorting the lower uterine segment and cervix. As the pregnancy progresses, the muscular portion of the cervix elongates and increases the distance from the margin of the placenta to the cervical os. Risk factors for placenta previa include scarring of the lower uterine segment associated with previous cesarean section, previous placenta previa, and multiple previous pregnancies. Patients usually present with painless vaginal bleeding in the third trimester. Bleeding is initiated by the effacement of the cervix and dilation of the cervical os, which disrupts the vascular bed of the placenta. US confirmation of placenta previa is performed transperineally, with the bladder empty to allow optimal identification of both the edge of the placenta and the internal os of the cervix. When the placenta covers the entire cervical os, placenta previa is complete (Fig. 52.25). When an edge of the placenta covers a portion of the cervical os, the previa is partial or marginal.

Vasa previa is present when placental blood vessels, or the umbilical cord, are adherent to the membranes that cover the cervix (Fig. 52.26). Risk factors include placenta previa, low-lying placenta, multiple gestation, *succenturiate lobe* (an accessory lobe separate from the main placenta), and *velamentous cord insertion* (the umbilical cord inserts into the chorioamniotic membranes at the margin of the placenta). The vessels tear as the cervix dilates resulting in fetal hemorrhage and death. Color Doppler is used to identify blood vessels fixed in place over the internal cervical os.

Placental abruption is defined as the premature separation of a normally positioned placenta from the myometrium. Separation is associated with hemorrhage from the maternal vessels at the base of the placenta. Abruption complicates 0.5% to 1.3% of pregnancies and is implicated in 15% to 25% of perinatal deaths. Risk factors include maternal hypertension, smoking, cocaine abuse, and previous history of abruption. *Subchorionic hemorrhage* (marginal abruption) occurs because of a separation at the edge of the placenta. Bleeding is usually venous and preferentially accumulates beneath the chorionic membrane adjacent to the placenta. *Retroplacental hemorrhage* occurs with more central abruption. Bleeding is usually arterial and accumulates beneath the placenta as an anechoic or mixed hypoechoic mass (Fig. 52.27). The hemorrhage may

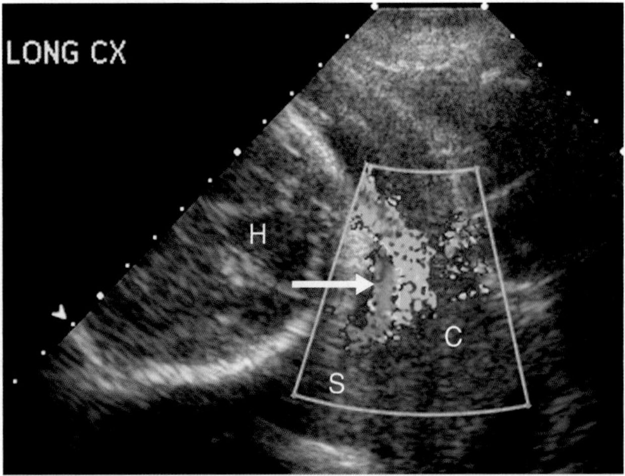

FIGURE 52.26. Vasa Previa. Transabdominal scan shows the vessels (*arrow*) associated with velamentous insertion of the umbilical cord into a succenturiate lobe of the placenta (*P*) covering the cervical os (*C*). The fetal head (*H*) is presenting.

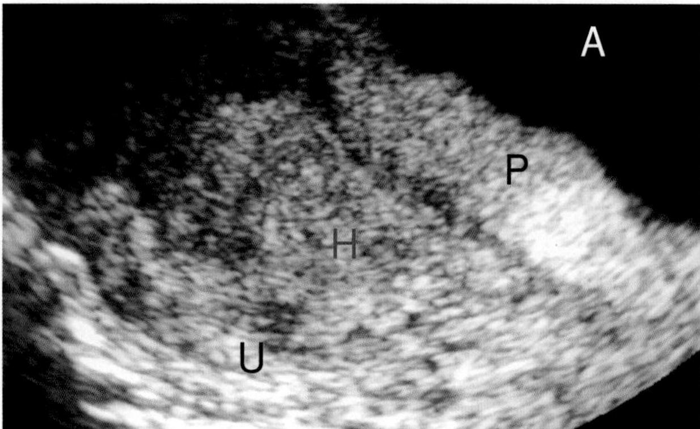

FIGURE 52.27. **Placental Abruption.** The placenta (*P*) is displaced away from the wall of the uterus (*U*) by an echogenic hematoma (*H*). Note the absence of visualization of the retroplacental complex of veins. *A*, amniotic cavity.

be isoechoic and difficult to differentiate from the placental tissue. The diagnosis is suggested by demonstrating disruption of the retroplacental complex of veins and thickening of the placenta (>4 cm).

Placenta accreta is an abnormal adherence of the placenta to the uterine wall. Invasion of the uterine wall by the placenta is referred to as *placenta increta* and penetration of the uterine wall is *placenta percreta.* Failure of the abnormally adherent placenta to separate completely from the myometrium after delivery results in copious hemorrhage. Scarring of the uterus results in the defective formation of decidua. Risk factors include prior cesarean section, prior placenta accreta, and prior placenta previa. The incidence of placenta accreta is rising with the increasing frequency of cesarean sections. US is 50% to 80% sensitive in making the diagnosis. Placenta previa is usually present (88%). The placenta itself appears full of holes, indistinct parallel vascular channels called *lacunae,* which show turbulent blood flow on color Doppler. These are distinct from normal placental vascular lakes, which are more rounded and have organized laminar flow. The myometrium appears thinned and the sharp hypoechoic line demarcating the placenta from the myometrium is lost. The normal retroplacental complex of vessels is focally or completely absent. Color Doppler shows gaps in the normal continuous blood flow pattern of the myometrium. Vascularity of the myometrium is increased and may extend to and produce nodularity of the bladder mucosal surface. MR is proving to be the imaging method of choice. MR is particularly useful when the placenta is posterior and difficult to see with US. MR shows focal thinning or absence of the myometrium at the site of placental attachment, mass effect of the placenta causing an outward bulge of the uterus, and nodularity of the interface between the placenta and the myometrium.

Chorioangioma is a benign vascular placental mass supplied by the fetal circulation. It is the most common tumor of the placenta. It appears on US as a solid hypoechoic, sometimes septated, mass within the placenta, usually close to the chorionic surface. Spectral Doppler demonstration of arterial waveforms at the fetal heart rate in vessels supplying the tumor is diagnostic. Color Doppler shows prominent internal vascularity and large feeding vessels. Most tumors are small and not clinically significant. Large lesions (>5 cm) with vascular shunting may cause fetal high-output cardiac failure and fetal hydrops.

Umbilical Cord. The normal umbilical cord consists of two arteries and one vein surrounded by Wharton jelly (Fig. 52.28). It has a normal diameter of 1 to 2 cm. A *single-artery umbilical cord* is found in about 1% of pregnancies and has a 10% to 20% association with congenital malformations. A detailed fetal survey and fetal echocardiography are indicated. Associated anomalies include cardiac, urinary tract, and central nervous system (CNS) malformations, omphalocele, trisomy 13, and trisomy 18. Masses in the umbilical cord include allantoic cysts, hematomas, hemangiomas, umbilical artery aneurysms, and teratomas. Encirclement of the fetal neck by the umbilical cord (nuchal cord) is usually a benign finding but may be associated with cord compression, bradycardia, and very rarely fetal death.

Placental membranes consist of an outer layer (*chorion*) and an inner layer (*amnion*) (Fig. 52.3A). These membranes commonly remain separated by a layer of fluid until 14 to 16 weeks GA when the two membranes fuse. The amnion is visualized on US as a thin membrane floating in fluid. The chorion is identified as the membrane confining fluid within the gestational sac. Occasional persistence of chorioamniotic separation into the third trimester is believed to be of no clinical significance.

Amniotic band syndrome is caused by the early (generally before 10 weeks GA) disruption of the amnion, enabling the fetus to enter the chorionic cavity (Fig. 52.29). The fetus

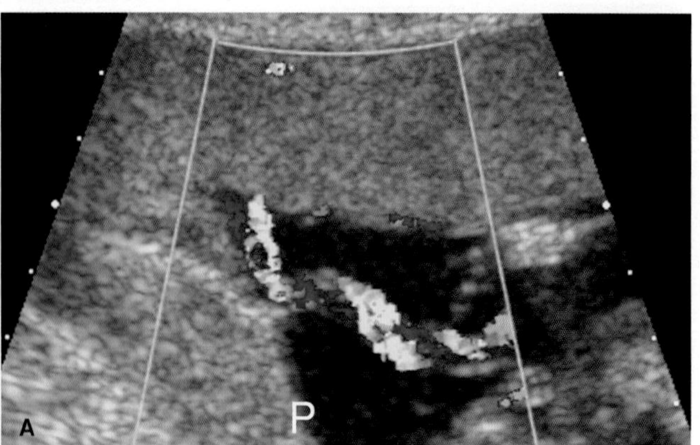

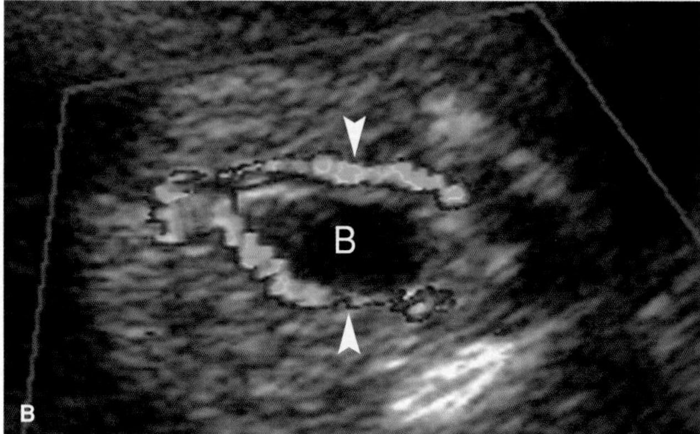

FIGURE 52.28. **Normal Umbilical Cord. A:** Color Doppler image shows the normal spiral ("barber pole") appearance of the three-vessel umbilical cord as it extends from the placenta (*P*). **B:** Transverse color Doppler image through the fetal pelvis shows the bladder (*B*) encompassed by the two umbilical arteries (*arrowheads*) as they course to join the fetal internal iliac arteries. This view provides a handy way to confirm the presence of a three-vessel cord with two umbilical arteries.

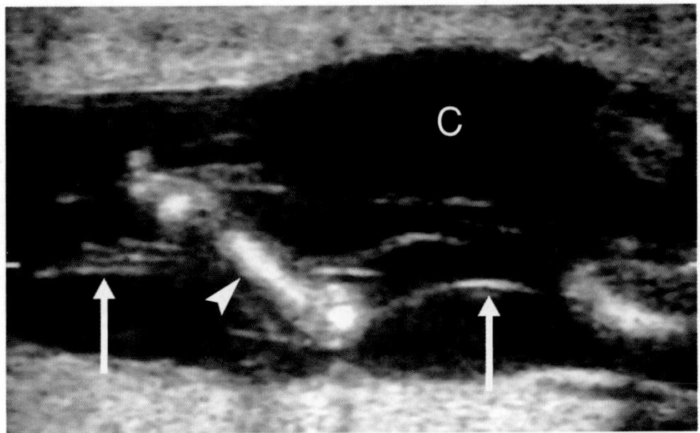

FIGURE 52.29. **Amniotic Band Syndrome.** The forearm (*arrowhead*) of a fetus at 15 weeks GA is entangled within fibrous bands (*arrows*) that extend across the chorionic cavity (C).

becomes entangled in fibrous bands that develop within the chorionic cavity. Entrapment of fetal parts results in amputation deformities that range from mild to incompatible with life. Typical abnormalities include asymmetrical absence of the cranium resembling anencephaly, encephaloceles, gastroschisis and truncal defects, spinal deformities, and extremity amputations. The amniotic bands trapping the fetus may be visualized.

Amniotic sheets (uterine synechia) are membranous structures that project into the uterine cavity. They demonstrate a characteristic appearance with a bulbous-free edge, thinner mid-portion, and a thickened base (Fig. 52.30). The fetus is able to move freely about the sheet of tissue. No fetal deformities are associated with this condition, which makes it distinct from the amniotic band syndrome. The amniotic sheets arise from folding of the chorioamniotic membranes over an intrauterine adhesion. Patients at risk for amniotic sheets include those with prior history of dilation and curettage, therapeutic abortion, or endometritis. An increased rate of adverse obstetric outcomes has been reported including increased rates of nuchal cords, breech presentation, low birth weight, and preterm delivery.

Amniotic Fluid

Normal amniotic fluid is essentially a dialysate of maternal serum in early pregnancy. As the pregnancy advances, fetal urine becomes the major source of amniotic fluid. The composition of amniotic fluid is dynamic, with turnover of the entire volume every 3 hours. The fetus swallows amniotic fluid at a rate up to 450 mL per 24 hours. Transudate from the fetal lungs contributes a small volume. Water crosses placental membranes in response to osmotic gradients. Amniotic fluid is essential in promoting normal development and maturation of the fetal lungs. Suspended particles in amniotic fluid visualized by US are attributable to normal vernix (desquamated fetal skin), blood, or meconium.

Amniotic fluid index is a rough US measurement of amniotic fluid volume obtained by measuring the vertical diameter of the deepest pockets of fluid in the four quadrants of the uterus and adding these values together. Pockets are selected that do not include fetal parts or umbilical cord. Normal values are 5 to 20 cm.

Polyhydramnios is an excessive amount of amniotic fluid, traditionally defined as greater than 2 L of fluid at delivery. US is used to confirm excessive fluid any time in pregnancy. Because amniotic fluid volume is difficult to measure accurately, the diagnosis is usually made subjectively by visual inspection. The visual proportion of fluid relative to the size of the fetus is greatest early in the second trimester and decreases progressively to term. Polyhydramnios is suggested by large pockets of fluid relative to the size of the fetus and the age of the pregnancy. An amniotic fluid index greater than 20 cm or a single fluid pocket greater than 8 cm deep is strongly suggestive of polyhydramnios. Another clue is failure of the fetal abdomen to be in contact with both anterior and posterior uterine wall after 24 weeks GA. Excessive fluid is associated with preterm labor, premature rupture of membranes, and substantial maternal discomfort. About 60% of cases are idiopathic, 15% to 20% are related to maternal disease (diabetes mellitus, preeclampsia, anemia, obesity), and 20% to 25% are associated with fetal anomalies. About half of all fetuses with anomalies will have polyhydramnios. Gross polyhydramnios has a higher association with fetal anomalies than mild polyhydramnios. Associated anomalies include anencephaly, encephalocele, gastrointestinal obstructions, abdominal wall defects, achondroplasia, and hydrops (isoimmunization).

Oligohydramnios refers to an abnormally low amniotic fluid volume. Fluid pockets are small or absent, fetal parts are crowded, fetal surface features such as the face are difficult to visualize, and the amniotic fluid index measures less than 5 cm. Measurement of the largest fluid pocket in the vertical direction of less than 1 cm is indicative of severe oligohydramnios. Causes of oligohydramnios include premature rupture of

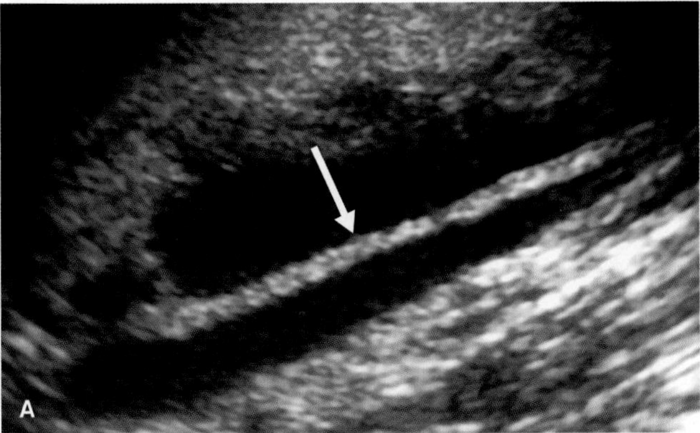

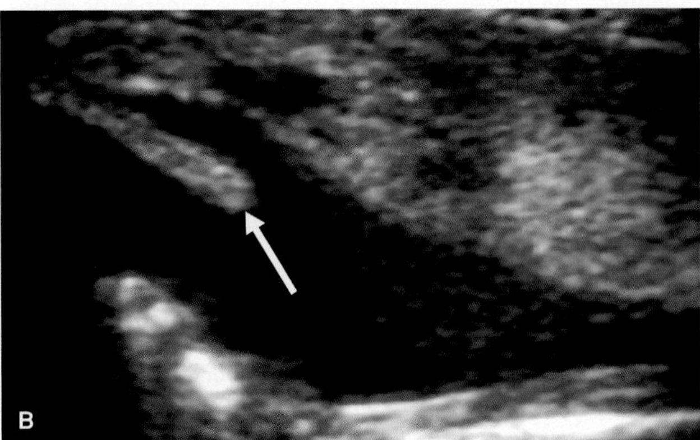

FIGURE 52.30. **Amniotic Sheet. A:** A fibrous band, covered by chorioamniotic membranes (*arrow*), extends across the amniotic cavity. The uterine synechia forms a shelf-like structure that partially compartmentalizes the uterine cavity. The fetus has free access to both compartments. **B:** The characteristic free edge (*arrow*) of the amniotic sheet is demonstrated.

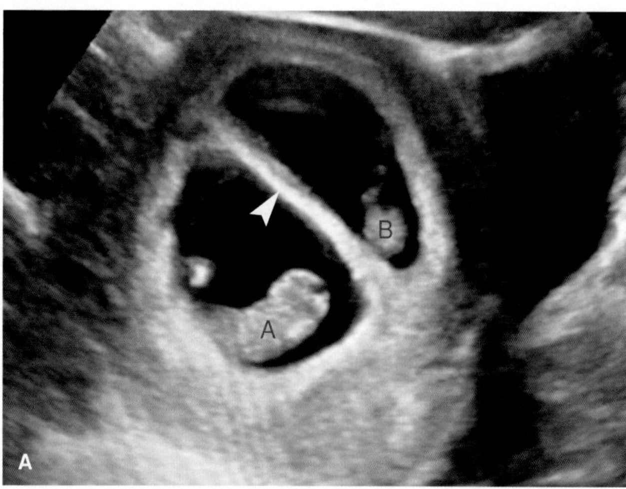

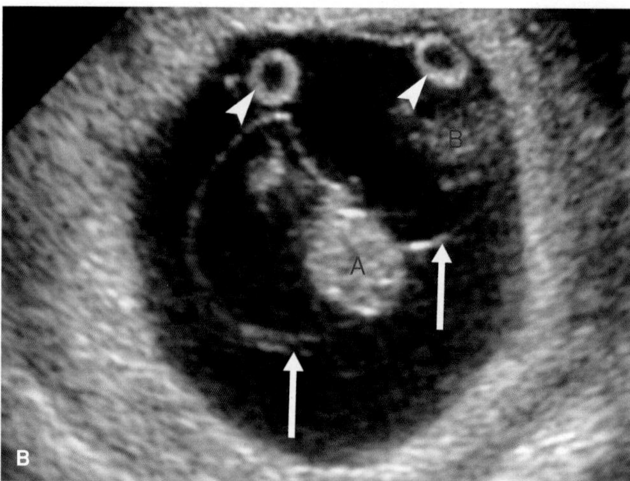

FIGURE 52.31. **Chorionicity in Twins. A:** Dichorionic diamniotic twins (*A, B*) are separated at 9 weeks gestational age by a thick layer (*arrowhead*) consisting of two fused chorionic membranes. **B:** Monochorionic diamniotic twins (*A, B*) are separated by two thin amniotic layers (*arrows*). Two yolk sacs (*arrowheads*) are evident.

membranes (with leakage of fluid out the vagina), IUGR, renal anomalies (lack of urine output), fetal death, eclampsia, and postdate pregnancies. A major complication of severe oligohydramnios is fetal lung immaturity.

Multiple Pregnancy

Twins occur in 32 of every 1,000 births. Morbidity and mortality are significantly increased in twin pregnancy compared with singleton pregnancy. Triplet and higher-order multiple births have even higher rates. Twins account for 12% to 13% of all neonatal deaths. Morbidity associated with multiple pregnancy includes prematurity (up to 60% of twins), polyhydramnios, increased incidence of congenital anomalies, growth restriction, and cord accidents. Relative risk is increased if the fetuses share a placenta (monochorionic twins, 20%) as opposed to each fetus having its own placenta (dichorionic twins, 80%) (Fig. 52.31). Twins that share a single amniotic cavity (monoamniotic twins) have the highest risk for morbidity, including conjoined twinning and intertwining of the umbilical cords. Chorionicity is best determined between 11 and 14 weeks GA. Visualization of two separate placentas, or determination that the twins are of different sex, is definitive proof of lower-risk dichorionic twinning. The presence of two yolk sacs is evidence of diamniotic twins. Unfortunately, about half of dichorionic twins will have a fused placenta. Visualization of a membrane separating the twins confirms diamniotic twins. Monochorionic twins usually have vascular anastomoses at the placental level, making them at risk for twin transfusion syndrome and twin embolization syndrome. One-third of twin pregnancies are monochorionic. The following complications occur only in monochorionic twin pregnancies:

Twin-to-twin transfusion syndrome (TTTS) results from shunting of blood from one twin to the other through vascular connections in the placenta. The abnormality ranges in severity from minor discordance in growth to severe IUGR in one twin, with hydropic fluid overload in the other twin. Severe disparity in amniotic fluid volume may be present, with one twin experiencing polyhydramnios while the other twin is virtually anhydramniotic ("a stuck twin" compressed against the uterine wall by the amnion). The mortality rate is as high as 70%.

Twin anemia–polycythemia sequence (TAPS) occurs in up to 5% of monochorionic diamniotic twins. Tiny arteriovenous anastomoses in the placenta allow slow transfusion of blood from the donor twin to the recipient twin resulting in anemia in the donor and polycythemia in the recipient. The placenta may show an echogenic thickened section supplying the donor and a thin hypoechoic section supplying the recipient. Severity ranges from mild with birth of two healthy babies to severe with intrauterine death of both twins. Cerebral injury may occur in both twins.

Twin reversed arterial perfusion (TRAP) sequence is rare occurring in 1% of monochorionic twins. A large arteriovenous anastomosis usually near a common cord insertion site results in a pump twin who perfuses a severely malformed acardiac twin. High-output cardiac failure develops in the pump twin who is driving blood through both fetuses. Arterial perfusion in the acardiac twin is reversed and in whom the heart is missing or deformed. Usually only a torso with deformed legs is present as the upper body does not develop. Doppler US shows blood flow entering the acardiac twin through the UA and exiting through the umbilical vein. Untreated, the pump twin dies in up to 75% of cases.

Twin embolization syndrome is an uncommon complication of the death of one twin in utero. Blood products from the dead twin are shunted through placental interconnections to the live twin, resulting in disseminated intravascular coagulopathy and multifocal tissue infarction.

FETAL ANOMALIES

General

All pregnancies carry a 2% to 3% risk of fetal anomalies regardless of risk factors. While chromosome abnormalities account for only 10% of birth defects, they are particularly important because of the severity of the associated anomalies. A detailed fetal anatomic US survey performed at the optimum time of 18 to 22 weeks GA will detect the majority of serious structural birth defects. Many fetal anomalies can be detected by skilled examiners in the first trimester by transvaginal US.

Aneuploidy screening tests are available for all trimesters of pregnancy. Aneuploidy is defined as having one or more

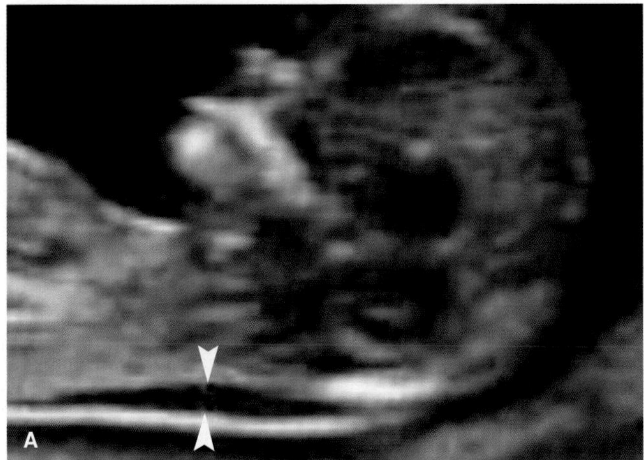

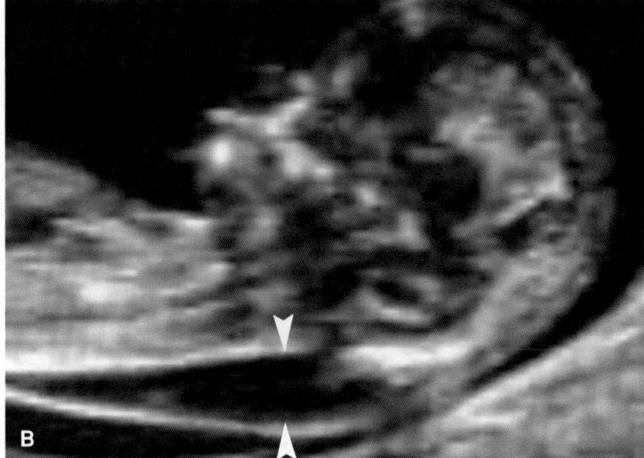

FIGURE 52.32. **Nuchal Translucency. A:** Normal nuchal translucency measurement of 2.6 mm. The measurement is precisely taken between the inner borders of the translucency (*arrowheads*). **B:** Abnormal nuchal translucency measurement of 3.9 mm (between *arrowheads*). Measurements greater than 3 mm are 85% predictive of the presence of Down syndrome.

extra, or missing, chromosomes in a cell. The presence of extra, or missing, genetic material often results in a nonviable pregnancy or a neonate that does not survive after birth. Risk factors for aneuploidy include advancing maternal age, history of prior aneuploid fetus, and presence of fetal anomalies. The most common aneuploidies are trisomy 21 (Down syndrome), trisomy 18, and trisomy 13.

First-trimester aneuploidy screening generally performed between 11 and 14 weeks GA includes NT measurement, serum free β-hCG or total hCG, and pregnancy-associated plasma protein A (PAPP-A) analyte levels. Using these results in correlation with maternal age, weight, race, number of fetuses, and prior history of aneuploidy, a specific risk estimate for aneuploidy can be calculated.

Nuchal translucency refers to the normal echolucent space between the spine and the overlying skin at the back of the fetal neck. US measurement is performed between 11 and 14 weeks GA (CRL 45 to 84 mm). On a carefully positioned midsagittal image cursors are precisely placed to measure the width between the inner borders of the NT (Fig. 52.32). Care must be taken to distinguish between the amnion and the fetal skin. A measurement of 3 mm or more is associated with fetal aneuploidy and structural malformations. The 3-mm measurement is 85% predictive of Down syndrome with a 5% false-positive rate. Risk of adverse pregnancy outcome increases with the degree of NT widening.

Quadruple marker screen is best performed between 16 and 18 weeks GA and includes screening for open neural tube defects as well as aneuploidy. The four maternal plasma substances measured in the quad screen are hCG, alpha fetoprotein (AFP), dimeric inhibin A, and unconjugated estriol. Results are correlated with maternal age, weight, race, presence of diabetes, and number of fetuses to calculate a risk estimate. Inaccurate GA dating decreases the accuracy of the quad screen. *Penta screen* testing adds hyperglycosylated hCG to the quad screen testing. Its efficacy is not fully determined at the present time.

Cell-free DNA screening evaluates short segments of fetal DNA derived from the placenta in maternal plasma. The amount of fetal DNA in maternal blood increases throughout pregnancy and is cleared within hours after delivery. Testing can be performed from 10 weeks GA throughout pregnancy and can be used to determine aneuploidy, fetal sex, as well as the presence of an Rh-positive fetus in an Rh-negative mother. The detection rate for Down syndrome is 98% with less than 0.5% false positives. Detection rates for trisomies 18 and 13 are lower.

US screening detects major fetal anatomic abnormalities, which may indicate the presence of a chromosome abnormality. "Genetic sonograms" may also be undertaken to detect soft sonographic markers for Down syndrome (Table 52.6). US findings are correlated with maternal serum screening (quad screen) results as integrated screening to determine risk of trisomies and other chromosome abnormalities. Fetuses with structural anomalies detected on US have an 11% to 35% risk of associated chromosome abnormality. Fetal conditions with significant high risk of associated chromosome abnormality include holoprosencephaly, Dandy–Walker syndrome, cystic hygroma, cardiac malformations, omphalocele, duodenal atresia, facial anomalies, and early symmetric IUGR.

Absent Nasal Bone. In the normal fetus the nasal bone is seen as a bright echogenic line projecting between the tip of

TABLE 52.6

SONOGRAPHIC MARKERS FOR TRISOMY 21

- Nuchal translucency ≥3.0 mm
  - Measured in first trimester 11–14 weeks GA
- Nuchal fold ≥5.0 mm
  - Measured in second trimester 18–22 weeks GA
- Absent nasal bone
  - Also associated with trisomies 13 and 18 and other abnormalities
- Echogenic intracardiac focus
  - Discrete focus in either ventricle as bright as bone
- Short femur
  - <0.9 multiples of the median length for GA
- Short humerus
  - <0.9 multiples of the median length for GA
- Pyelectasis
  - Anteroposterior diameter of renal pelvis ≥4 mm
- Hyperechoic bowel
  - Fetal bowel as bright as bone

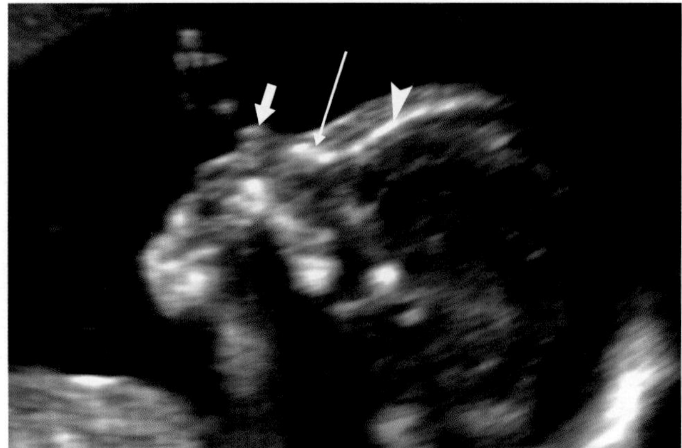

FIGURE 52.33. **Normal Nasal Bone.** Midline sagittal image shows the facial profile of the fetus. The normal nasal bone (*thin arrow*) is seen as a bright echogenic line between the frontal bone (*arrowhead*) and the nose (*fat arrow*).

the nose and the frontal bone (Fig. 52.33). Absence of the echogenic nasal bone at 11 to 14 weeks GA is found in 60% to 73% of fetuses with Down syndrome. Absence is also associated with trisomies 13 and 18, Turner syndrome, B-cell immunodeficiency, and other abnormalities. It may also be absent in normal euploid fetuses with a 5.8% prevalence in African Americans, a 2.8% prevalence in Caucasians, and a 2.1% prevalence in Asians.

Nuchal fold refers to the thickness of skin overlying the back of the neck and occipital bone seen in the second trimester when the NT is no longer present. The nuchal fold is measured on an axial US image at the level of the thalamus and cerebellar hemispheres. Measurement is made between the occipital bone and the skin surface (Fig. 52.34). Thickness ≥6 mm has a reported sensitivity of 33% for Down syndrome with a false-positive rate of 0.1%. The thickness measurement is considered reliable only between 15 and 20 weeks GA when normal skin thickness is relatively constant. Recent studies have concluded that the threshold value of 6 mm may be valid up to 24 weeks GA. Nuchal fold thickness continues to increase normally as the fetus grows.

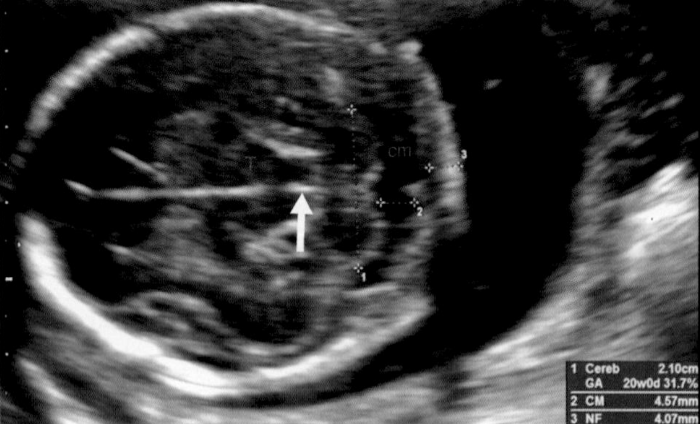

FIGURE 52.34. **Transcerebellar Plane—Nuchal Fold.** The landmarks of the transcerebellar plane are the thalamus (*T*), the inferior portion of the third ventricle (*arrow*) near where it joins the aqueduct, and the cisterna magna (*cm*). Measurements which are routinely made at this level include the transverse cerebellum (*1*), which in mm approximates the GA, the anteroposterior dimension of the cisterna magna (*2*), which is normal between 2 and 11 mm, and the thickness of the nuchal fold (*3*) in the second trimester, which is normal at <6 mm.

Prenatal Diagnostic Testing for Genetic Disorders. In contrast to prenatal genetic screening, prenatal diagnostic testing is used to determine if a specific genetic disorder is present. Fetal cells may be obtained by amniocentesis or chorionic villous sampling for traditional karyotype analysis to specifically identify trisomies and many chromosome abnormalities. Chorionic villous sampling is performed between 10 and 13 weeks GA by transcervical or transabdominal US-guided needle puncture of the placenta. Amniocentesis is generally performed between 15 and 20 weeks GA by US-guided puncture of the uterus to obtain an amniotic fluid sample. Both invasive procedures are associated with a low incidence of pregnancy loss. Fetal US, echocardiography, and MRI may also show fetal structural abnormalities that are highly indicative of a genetic disorder.

Trisomy 21, Down syndrome, is the most common chromosome abnormality, increasing in incidence and currently occurring in 1 of 800 births. Although women older than age 35 have a 1 in 250 risk of carrying a fetus with trisomy 21, 80% of fetuses with Down syndrome are born to younger women. In addition to biochemical screening of maternal serum, various sonographic markers indicate that trisomy 21 may be present (Table 52.6). Major structural defects found in Down fetuses include congenital heart disease (endocardial cushion defect, ventricular septal defect, tetralogy of Fallot), duodenal atresia, ventriculomegaly, and tracheoesophageal atresia.

Trisomy 18 is the second most common chromosome anomaly, occurring in 1 of 3,000 births. Prognosis is extremely poor enhancing the importance of early detection. A large number of structural abnormalities may occur, but the most common identified by US are IUGR (74%), complex congenital heart disease (52%), choroid plexus cysts (47%), congenital diaphragmatic hernia, omphalocele, neural tube defects, Dandy–Walker complex, clenched hands, and single UA.

Central Nervous System, Face, and Neck

Anomalies of the CNS occur in 1 of 1,000 live births. Survivors are often severely handicapped and require long-term care. Effective US screening for CNS anomalies can be performed by examination of three crucial axial planes through the fetal brain. The *transthalamic plane* is used to measure the BPD and HC (Fig. 52.19). Abnormalities of head shape, microcephaly, macrocephaly, and major structural abnormalities are evident in this plane. The third ventricle varies in appearance from a single echogenic line to a slit-like structure less than 3.5 mm in width. The *transventricular plane* is an axial plane at the level of the ventricular atria (Fig. 52.35). The dominant landmark is the echogenic choroid plexus, which normally fills the atrium nearly completely. Measurements of atrial diameter made perpendicular to the walls do not normally exceed 10 mm. The *transcerebellar plane* is an axial scan in approximately 10 to 15 degrees of inclination from the canthomeatal line. The anatomic landmarks include the inferior portion of the third ventricle and the cerebellar hemispheres outlined by fluid in the cisterna magna (Fig. 52.34). The normal cisterna magna measures 2 to 11 mm in width. A small cisterna magna (<2 mm) suggests a Chiari II malformation, but may also be seen with massive ventriculomegaly. A large cisterna magna (>11 mm) may be a normal variant (megacisterna magna) or indicate Dandy–Walker malformation, arachnoid cyst, or cerebellar hypoplasia. When these three planes are anatomically normal, the risk of CNS anomaly is minute (0.005%). An algorithm for sorting out fetal CNS anomalies is given in Table 52.7. MR plays an important supporting role in the characterization of fetal brain anomalies.

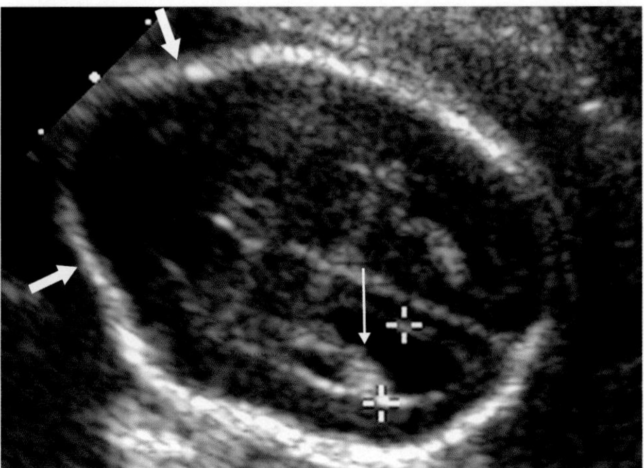

FIGURE 52.35. Transventricular Plane—Early Ventriculomegaly. The choroid plexus (*skinny arrow*) hangs dependently in the atrium of the downside lateral ventricle. The ventricular atrium is measured from its medial wall to its lateral wall (between *cursors*, +). The normal ventricular atrium does not exceed 10 mm in width at any time during pregnancy. The diameter of the atrium in this case measures 12 mm indicating mild ventriculomegaly. This fetus has a spina bifida defect with associated Arnold–Chiari II malformation as the cause of ventriculomegaly. Note the bossing of the frontal bones (*thick arrows*) giving the outline of the cranium an appearance similar in shape to a lemon (lemon head).

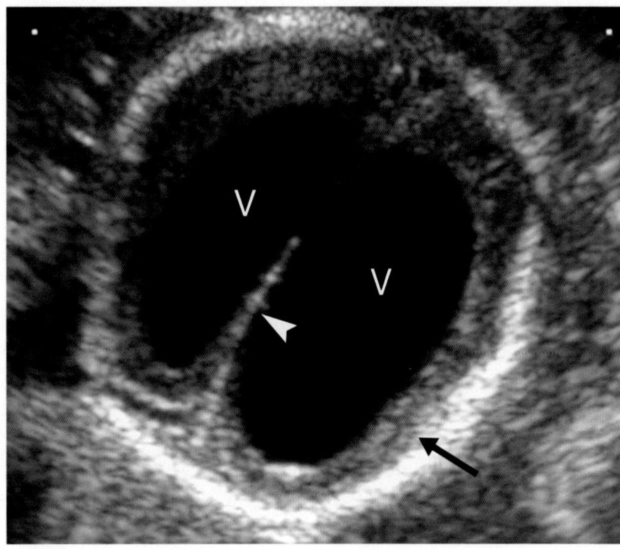

FIGURE 52.36. Ventriculomegaly. An axial image of the fetal brain of an infant with aqueduct stenosis demonstrates marked enlargement of the lateral ventricles (*V*). The falx (*arrowhead*) is seen as an echogenic stripe in the midline. A rind of cortex (*arrow*) is present. These latter two findings differentiate ventriculomegaly from hydranencephaly and holoprosencephaly.

Ventriculomegaly is an anatomic finding with many causes that can be grouped into the categories of obstructive hydrocephalus (obstruction to flow of cerebrospinal fluid), cerebral atrophy (ex vacuo), and maldevelopment (such as agenesis of the corpus callosum). Ventriculomegaly detected in utero carries a poor prognosis. Up to 80% of fetuses with ventriculomegaly have associated anomalies. The US signs of ventriculomegaly include diameter of the ventricular atrium >10 mm (Fig. 52.35), separation of choroid plexus from the ventricular wall by >3 mm, and a "dangling choroid." The choroid plexus hangs dependently in the ventricle and marks the position of the lateral ventricular wall. The most common causes of ventriculomegaly in the fetus are Chiari II malformation and aqueductal stenosis (Fig. 52.36).

Anencephaly is the most common fetal neural tube defect. US findings include absence of the cranial vault and cerebral hemispheres above the level of the orbits (Fig. 52.37). The cerebral

TABLE 52.7

ALGORITHM FOR DIAGNOSIS OF CONGENITAL BRAIN ABNORMALITIES

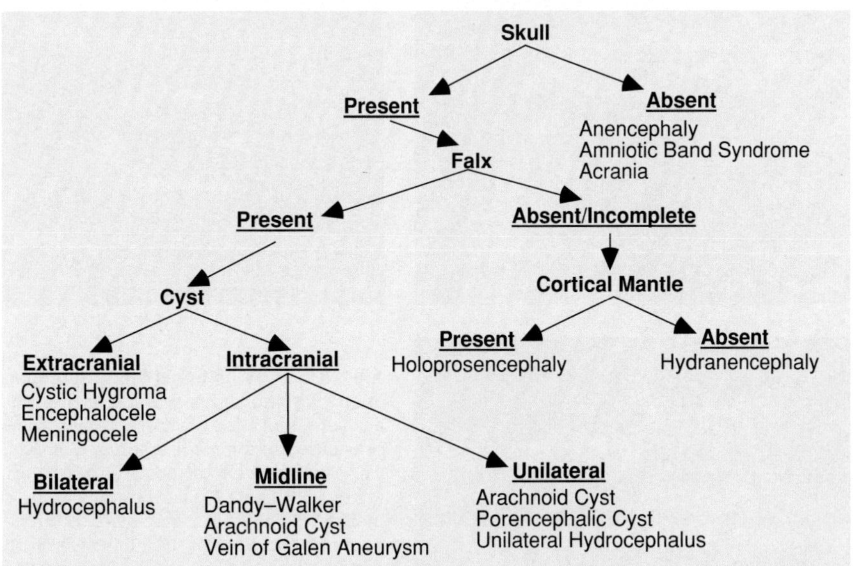

From Carrasco CR, Stierman ED, Hornsberger HR, Lee TG. An algorithm for prenatal ultrasound diagnosis of congenital CNS abnormalities. *J Ultrasound Med* 1985;4:163–168.

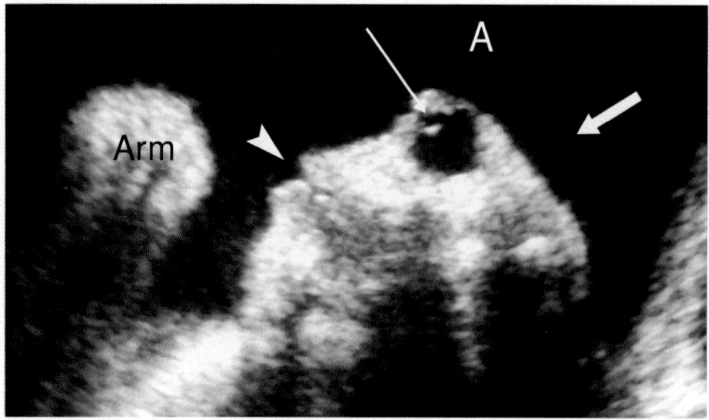

FIGURE 52.37. Anencephaly. A sagittal image through the head of a fetus demonstrates absence of the cranial vault (*thick arrow*) and brain above the level of the eye (*skinny arrow*). The mouth and lips are evident (*arrowhead*). The volume of amniotic fluid (*A*) is increased. Polyhydramnios is common in the presence of anencephaly. *Arm*, fetal arm.

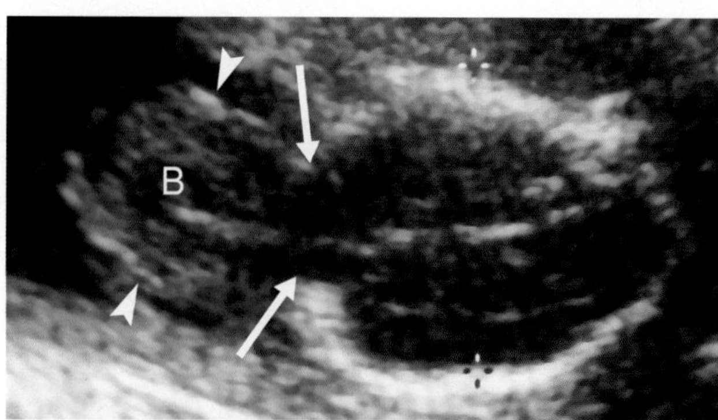

FIGURE 52.38. Encephalocele. Axial US image through the fetal skull demonstrates herniation of brain tissue (*B*) through a large defect (*arrows*) in the skull, forming an occipital encephalocele (between *arrowheads*). The intracranial contents are reduced and the BPD (between *cursors*, +) is less than expected for gestational age because of the encephalocele.

hemispheres may be replaced by an amorphous neurovascular mass (area cerebrovasculosa). The condition is inevitably fatal.

Cephaloceles are fluid- and/or brain tissue–filled sacs that protrude through a defect in the bony calvarium. They are found in the occipital (75%), frontoethmoid (13%), and parietal (12%) regions. Meningoceles contain only cerebrospinal fluid, whereas encephaloceles contain brain tissue (Fig. 52.38).

Spina bifida refers to a spectrum of spinal abnormalities resulting from failure of the complete closure of the neural tube. The condition ranges from simple nonfusion of the vertebral arches with intact skin (spina bifida occulta), to protruding sacs containing only cerebrospinal fluid (meningocele), to sacs with spinal cord or nerve roots (myelomeningocele), to a totally open spinal defect (myeloschisis). Spina bifida may occur anywhere in the spine but most often occurs in the lumbosacral region. Detection is a focus of biochemical and US prenatal screening. US findings (Fig. 52.39) include outward splaying, rather than inward convergence, of the laminae; defect in the soft tissues overlying the bony abnormality; and a protruding sac containing fluid and often neural tissues. The associated functional neuromuscular defect often results in club foot deformities and dislocated hips. Associated cranial abnormalities of the Chiari II malformation provide clues to the presence of the spinal defect. Ventriculomegaly is present in 75% of cases. The "lemon sign" refers to bossing of the frontal bones, causing a lemon-shaped appearance to the head in the axial plane (Fig. 52.35). The "banana sign" is produced by compression of the cerebellar hemispheres into a banana shape. The cisterna magna is small or obliterated.

Chiari II malformation is associated with 95% of myelomeningoceles. The cranial abnormality consists of caudal displacement of the cerebellar tonsils, pons, and medulla. The fourth ventricle is elongated, the posterior fossa is small, and the cisterna magna is obliterated.

Holoprosencephaly refers to a spectrum of disorders characterized by a failure of the prosencephalon to divide and form

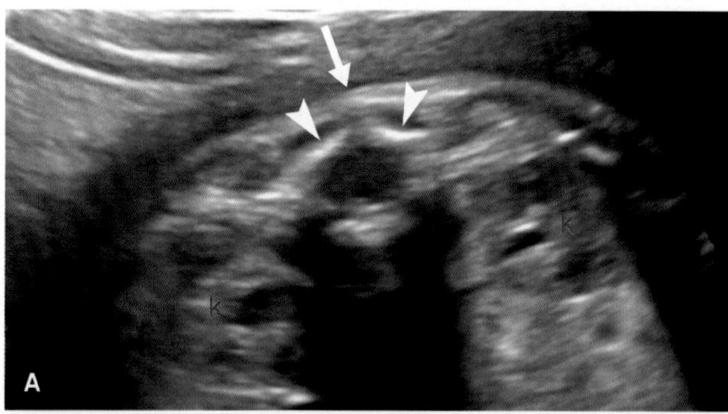

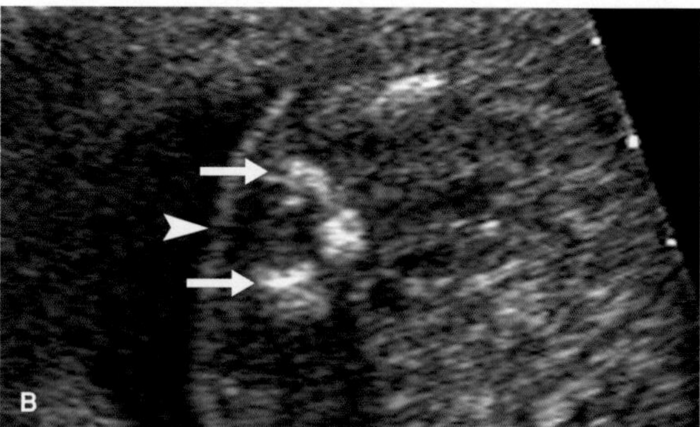

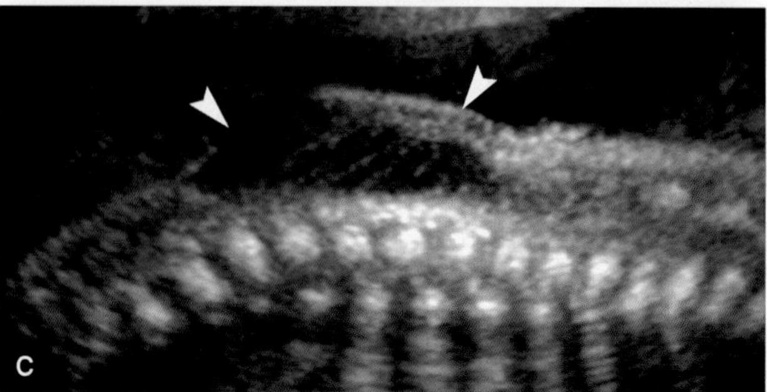

FIGURE 52.39. Normal Spine and Spina Bifida. A: Normal Spine. Posterior transverse image through a normal fetal spine at the level of the kidneys (*k*) demonstrates normal converging orientation of the ossified portions of the lamina (*arrowheads*). The skin overlying the posterior aspect of the vertebra is intact (*arrow*). **B: Spina Bifida.** Posterior transverse image through a lumbar spina bifida defect demonstrates abnormal divergence of ossified portions of the lamina (*arrows*) posteriorly. The skin surface (*arrowhead*) remains intact. **C: Meningomyelocele.** In a different patient with spina bifida, a mass (*arrowheads*) of dysmorphic spinal tissue bulges beneath intact skin.

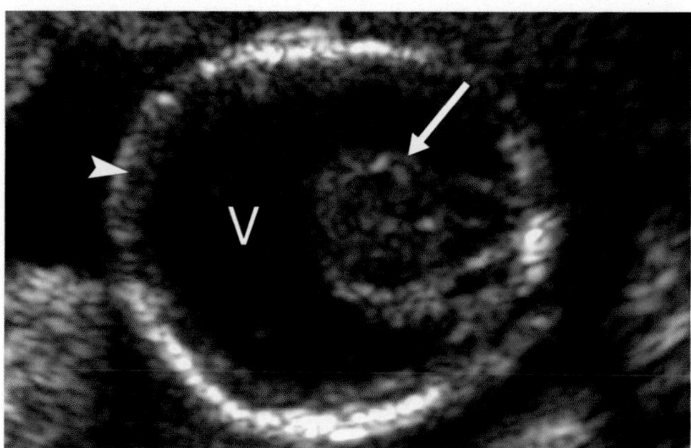

FIGURE 52.40. **Holoprosencephaly.** Image through the cranium of a fetus reveals a single large midline ventricle (*V*) and fused thalami (*arrow*). A thin rim of cortex (*arrowhead*) is present. These findings are characteristic of alobar holoprosencephaly. The fetal face should be examined for associated defects such as midline cleft and proboscis.

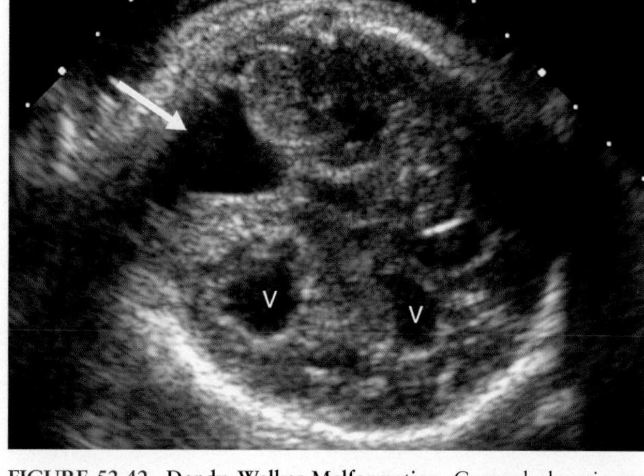

FIGURE 52.42. **Dandy–Walker Malformation.** Coronal plane image demonstrates cystic enlargement of the posterior fossa (*arrow*). The lateral ventricles (*V*) are enlarged indicating associated hydrocephalus.

the separate right and left hemispheres and thalami. Associated facial anomalies including hypotelorism, cyclopia, and proboscis are common. *Alobar* holoprosencephaly is the most severe form and demonstrates absence of the falx and interhemispheric fissure with a single midline ventricle (Fig. 52.40). The *semilobar* and *lobar* forms demonstrate greater degrees of midline separation.

Hydranencephaly refers to total destruction of the cerebral cortex, believed to be caused by the occlusion of the internal carotid arteries. The cranial vault contains fluid, but no cortical mantle of brain tissue is visible (Fig. 52.41). The falx may be present but is usually incomplete. The brainstem and structures supplied by the vertebral arteries appear normal.

Dandy–Walker malformation results from the maldevelopment of the roof of the fourth ventricle. The cisterna magna is enlarged and communicates directly with the fourth ventricle through its absent roof. The posterior fossa is enlarged, and the tentorium is elevated. The cerebellar hemispheres are usually hypoplastic (Fig. 52.42). Hydrocephalus is usually present. The condition varies in severity across a broad spectrum. Less severe abnormalities are called Dandy–Walker variants. Arachnoid cysts and large cisterna magna are differentiated by their lack of communication with the fourth ventricle.

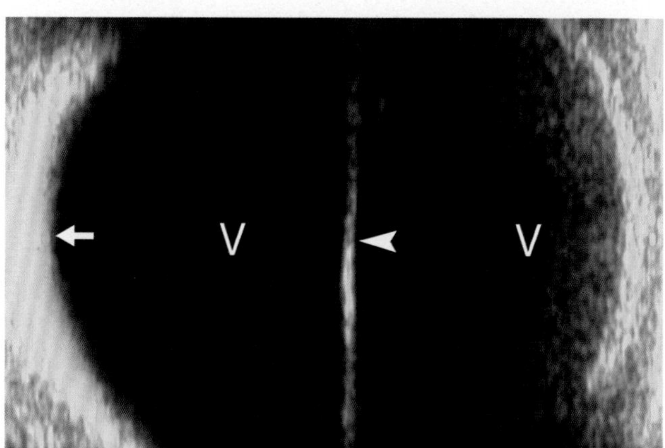

FIGURE 52.41. **Hydranencephaly.** Axial sonogram through the brain of a near-term fetus demonstrates two massive ventricles (*V*), a well-defined midline falx (*arrowhead*), and total absence of detectable cortical tissue (*arrow*). These findings are characteristic of hydranencephaly.

Choroid plexus cysts are found in 1% to 3% of normal fetuses during the second trimester. The cysts themselves cause no clinical problem and nearly always resolve. Because they are present in up to 30% to 50% of fetuses with trisomy 18, their discovery causes concern for the presence of chromosome abnormality. They are not associated with Down syndrome. In nearly all cases, detailed US examination, which should include echocardiography and examination of the fetal hands, will demonstrate additional structural abnormalities that justify amniocentesis for karyotyping. Trisomy 18 is unlikely and amniocentesis is not indicated if detailed US examination of the fetus is normal.

Cleft lip and cleft palate account for 13% of all congenital anomalies found in the United States. *Lateral cleft* is most common and involves both lip and palate in 50% of cases, the lip alone in 25%, and the palate alone in 25%. The condition is bilateral in 20% to 25% of cases. Up to 60% of affected fetuses have additional anomalies including polydactyly, congenital heart disease, and trisomy 21. US diagnosis is made on demonstration of a groove extending from one of the nostrils through the lip (Fig. 52.43). *Median cleft* is a completely different entity associated with holoprosencephaly and accounting for less than 0.7% of all cases of cleft lip. A coronal plane sonogram of the face demonstrates a wide central defect in the upper lip and palate. Diagnosis of facial anomalies is aided by use of 3D US.

Cystic hygroma is a fluid collection in the fetal neck caused by failure of the lymphatic system to develop normal connections with the venous system in the neck. US demonstrates a bilateral nuchal cystic mass with a prominent midline septum that represents the nuchal ligament (Fig. 52.44). Cystic hygroma is associated (70%) with karyotype abnormalities including Down syndrome (most), Turner syndrome, trisomy 18, and trisomy 13. Generalized lymphangiectasia and fetal hydrops may occur and are always fatal when they do.

Chest and Heart

Fetal hydrops refers to the pathologic accumulation of fluid in body cavities and tissues. US demonstrates ascites, pleural and

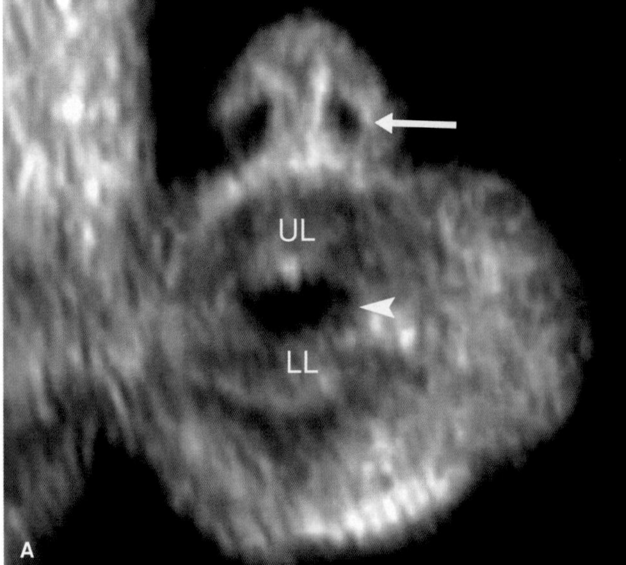

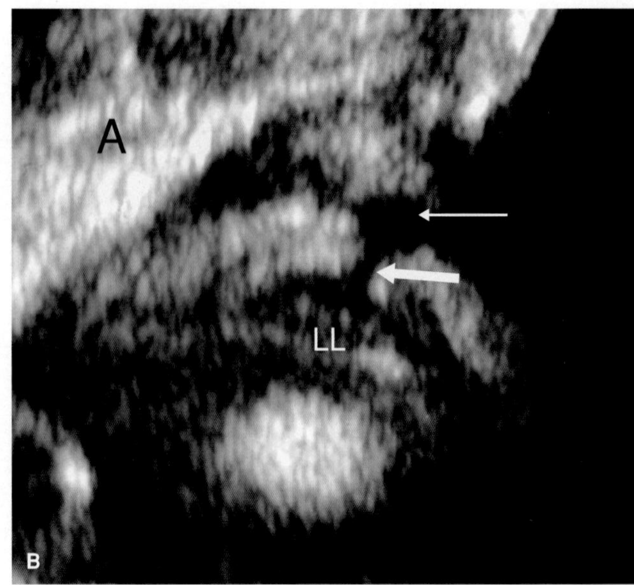

FIGURE 52.43. Normal Face View and Cleft Lip. A: Normal Face View. Coronal view of a normal fetal face ("up your nose" view) shows both nares (*arrow*), an open mouth (*arrowhead*), and the muscles of the upper (*UL*) and lower (*LL*) lips. **B: Lateral Cleft Lip.** Matching coronal view of another fetus reveals a cleft (*thick arrow*) in the left upper lip extending into the left nares (*skinny arrow*). The mouth is slightly open. The lower lip (*LL*) is apparent. An arm (*A*) extends across the face.

pericardial effusions, and subcutaneous edema (Fig. 52.45). *Immune hydrops* is caused by blood group incompatibility between mother and fetus. Current treatment, including fetal transfusion, is highly successful. *Nonimmune hydrops* is caused by a host of conditions including cardiac disorders, infections, chromosomal anomalies, twin pregnancy, urinary obstruction, and umbilical cord complications. The cause of many cases is not identified. The prognosis for nonimmune hydrops remains poor.

Congenital diaphragmatic hernia is a disorder in which abdominal contents protrude into the thorax through defects in the diaphragm. The majority (85%) occur on the left side (Fig. 52.46). Contents of the hernia usually include stomach, bowel, and portions of the liver. US findings include fluid-filled, solid, or multicystic mass in the chest; displacement of the heart and mediastinum; absence of the stomach in the abdomen; and polyhydramnios. Chromosome anomalies and associated defects, especially cardiac and CNS, are common. Mortality is high (70%) because of pulmonary hypoplasia.

Cystic adenomatoid malformation is a congenital hamartomatous lesion of the lung, usually affecting one lobe. The lesion consists of single or multiple cysts that vary in size from microscopic to larger than 2 cm size. Type I lesions appear on US as single or multiple cysts larger than 2 cm size. Type II lesions consist of multiple smaller cysts of uniform size less than 2 cm. Type III lesions appear as echogenic solid masses because the cysts are microscopic (Fig. 52.47). Mixed forms are common and classification does not determine prognosis.

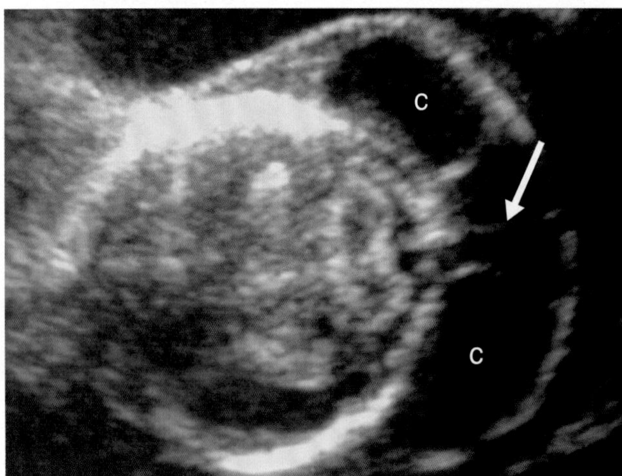

FIGURE 52.44. Cystic Hygroma. A multiseptated cystic mass (*c*) extends over the occipital region of the fetal skull. Cystic hygroma is differentiated from occipital cephalocele by demonstration of the midline septum (*arrow*) due to the nuchal ligament and by absence of a bony defect in the skull.

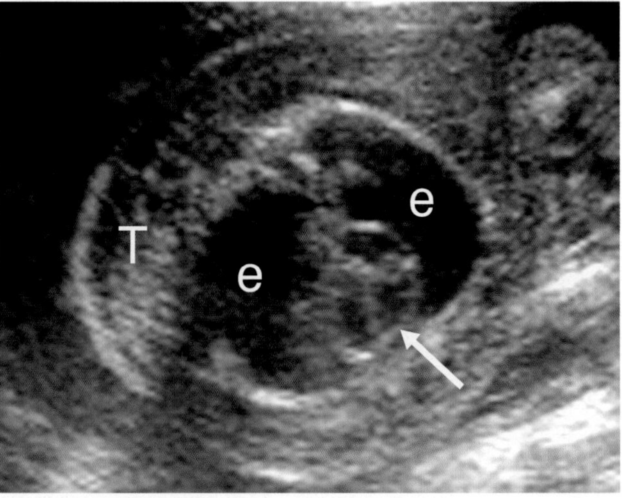

FIGURE 52.45. Fetal Hydrops. A: A transverse image through the fetal thorax at the level of a four-chamber view of the heart (*arrow*) demonstrates large bilateral pleural effusions (*e*). The skin surrounding the thorax is markedly thickened (*T*).

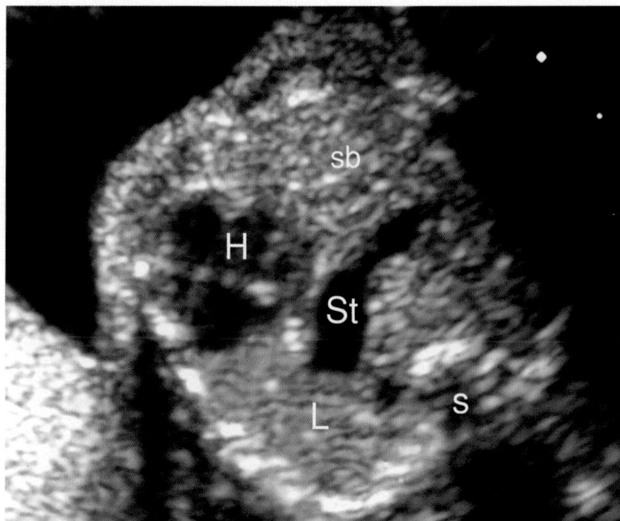

FIGURE 52.46. **Congenital Diaphragmatic Hernia.** Axial plane image of the fetal thorax shows stomach (*St*) and small bowel (*sb*) herniated into the left thorax. The heart (*H*) is shifted markedly into the right thorax and is abnormally rotated. Only a small volume of compressed right lung (*L*) is present. Severe pulmonary hypoplasia is likely and the prognosis for this fetus is grim. The spine (*s*) is seen posteriorly.

Polyhydramnios and fetal hydrops may occur. Some of these lesions resolve spontaneously in utero.

Pulmonary sequestration is a mass of lung tissue supplied by systemic arteries and separated from its normal bronchial and pulmonary vascular connections. *Intralobar sequestrations* (75%) are contained within the pleural covering of an otherwise normal lobe of the lung. Pulmonary venous drainage is maintained. US detection in the fetus is rare. *Extralobar sequestrations,* though less common (25%), are much more frequently evident on fetal US. These are accessory lobes, contained within their own pleura, and supplied by both systemic arteries and veins. US demonstrates a homogeneous echogenic solid lung mass that displaces the mediastinum. Color Doppler is used to demonstrate the systemic supplying artery arising from the thoracic aorta. Hydrops may occur.

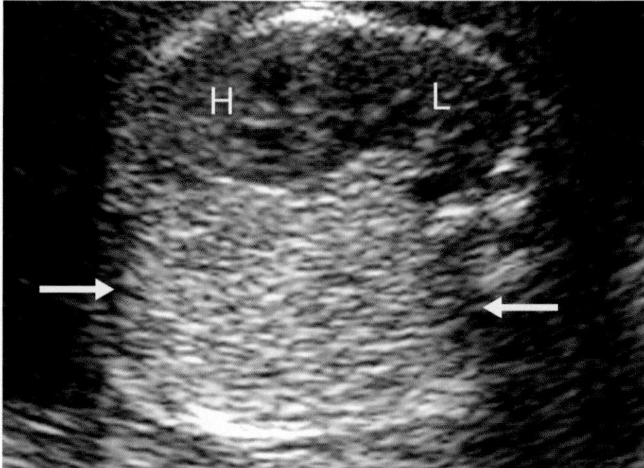

FIGURE 52.47. **Cystic Adenomatoid Malformation.** An echogenic solid-appearing mass (between *arrows*) is seen in the right thorax displacing and compressing the heart (*H*). A small portion of the compressed left lung (*L*) is evident. The appearance is characteristic of type III cystic adenomatoid malformation.

Fetal Cardiac Anomalies. Congenital heart disease is a major cause of neonatal morbidity and mortality and is the most common major anomaly in the neonate affecting 1 in 200 live births. Precise US diagnosis of fetal heart abnormalities usually requires a detailed examination with specialized US equipment and a high level of scanning expertise (fetal echocardiography). Routine screening views of the heart (Fig. 52.48) include the four-chamber heart view, right ventricular outflow tract (RVOT), and left ventricular outflow tract (LVOT). The four-chamber view is obtained on an axial scan through the fetal chest just above the diaphragm. The apex of the normal heart is directed at the left anterior chest wall at a 45-degree angle on the same side as the fetal stomach. Deviation from this position suggests a cardiac malformation or a thoracic mass. Pericardial effusions appear as an anechoic band surrounding the myocardium. The ventricles are approximately equal in size and slightly smaller than their corresponding atria. Motion of the atrioventricular valves is observed in this plane. Papillary muscles in the ventricles may be echogenic and prominent. Discrepancies in chamber size or valve motion suggest cardiac malformations. The LVOT view is obtained by angling the transducer from the position of the four-chamber view toward the right shoulder. The normal LVOT view shows the aortic valve and origin of the aorta from the left ventricle. The RVOT view is obtained by angling the transducer slightly from the LVOT view. The normal RVOT view shows the origin of the pulmonary artery to the bifurcation into right and left pulmonary arteries. Any abnormalities on these screening views are an indication for fetal echocardiography.

Abdomen

Normal Fetal Abdomen. The abdomen of the fetus is significantly different from the abdomen of the older child or adult. The abdomen of the fetus is large relative to its body length compared with the adult. The liver is large, and the left lobe is larger than the right lobe. The umbilical vein is an important US landmark. Half the blood it carries goes directly to the inferior vena cava via the ductus venosus. The remainder perfuses the liver via the left portal vein. The adrenal glands are up to 20 times larger in relative size because of the presence of the "fetal zone." The pelvis is relatively small, and pelvic organs extend into the lower abdomen. Swallowing begins at 11 to 12 weeks GA. The fetal stomach should be filled with swallowed fluid by 18 weeks GA. The small bowel is moderately echogenic, centrally located, and blends with the liver. By the third trimester, peristalsis in small bowel loops can be observed. The visualized small bowel loops are normally less than 6 mm in diameter and less than 15 mm in length. The colon is visualized after 20 weeks as a tubular structure around the periphery of the abdomen. The colon progressively fills with meconium but does not exceed 23 mm in diameter. Normal fetal kidneys are seen as paired, slightly hypoechoic structures adjacent to the spine (Fig. 52.39A). The renal sinus appears as an echogenic stripe. Fetal lobulation causes an undulating contour of the kidneys. The length of normal fetal kidneys in millimeters is approximately equal to GA in weeks. The bladder should be observed to fill and empty. Because amniotic fluid is predominantly urine, a normal amniotic fluid volume implies at least one functioning kidney.

Absent Stomach. By 18 weeks GA the fluid-filled stomach is normally seen in the left upper quadrant of the fetal abdomen. If not evident, the patient should be reexamined an hour or so later to see if it fills. If the stomach is still not seen a significant abnormality may be present. Causes include obstruction

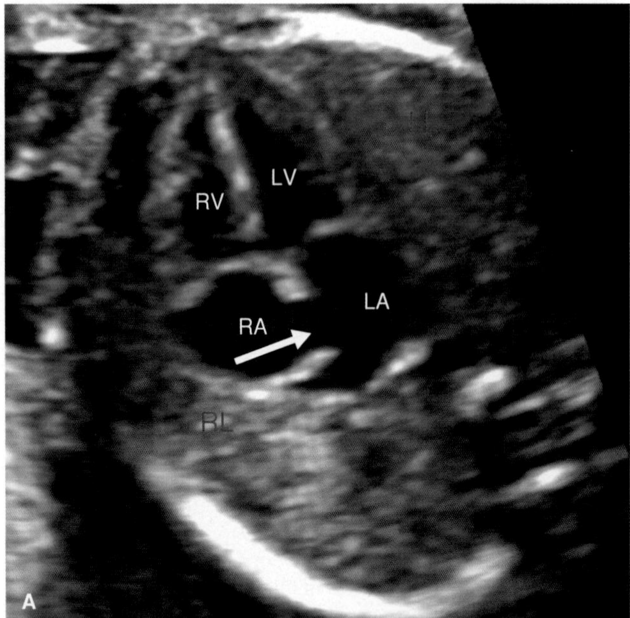

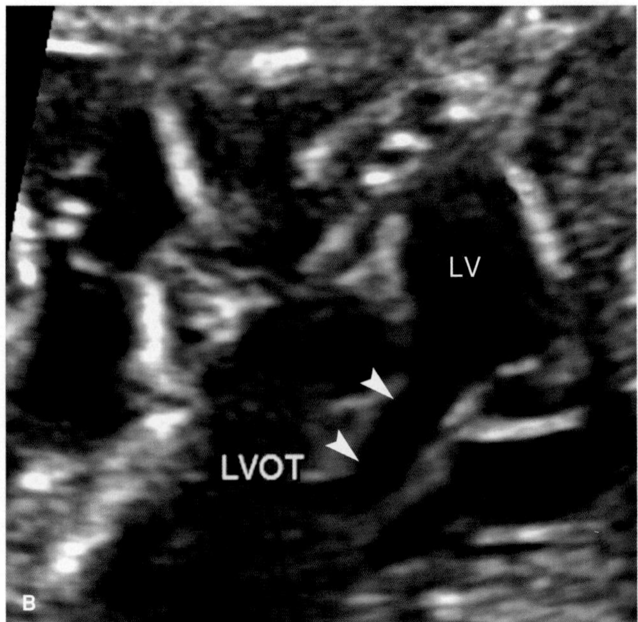

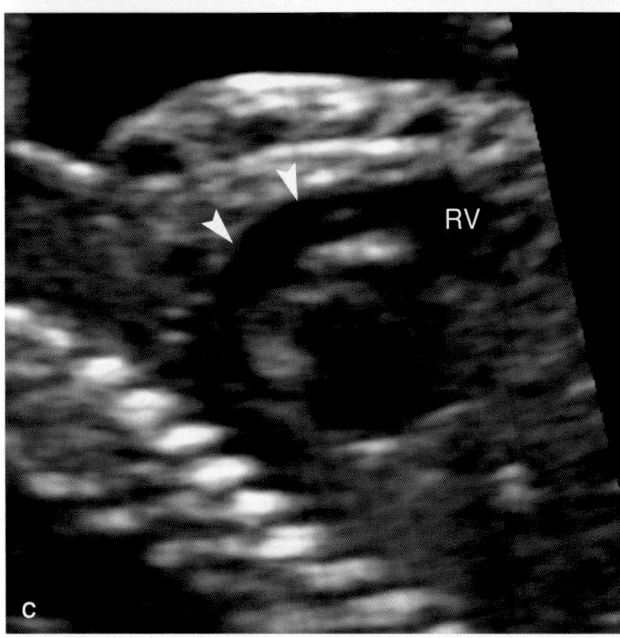

FIGURE 52.48. **Normal Screening Views of the Fetal Heart. A: Four-Chamber View.** Axial sonogram through the fetal chest demonstrates the normal heart and lungs (L) in an 18-week fetus. The right ventricle (*RV*) and left ventricle (*LV*) are approximately equal in size, as are the right atrium (*RA*) and left atrium (*LA*). The patent atrial septum (*arrow*) is apparent. The heart normally occupies about one-third of the cross-sectional area of the thorax. The developing lungs are fluid filled and moderately echogenic. *RL*, right lung; *LL*, left lung. **B: Left Ventricular Outflow Tract View.** This view shows the origin of the aorta (*arrowheads*) from the left ventricle (*LV*). The aortic valve can be visualized on real-time US. **C: Right Ventricular Outflow Tract View.** The pulmonary artery trunk (*arrowheads*) is shown from its origin from the right ventricle (*RV*).

(esophageal atresia, chest mass), impaired swallowing (facial clefts and neuromuscular disorders), low amniotic fluid volume, and stomach in an abnormal location (diaphragmatic hernia).

Double bubble is descriptive of fluid distention of the stomach and proximal duodenum (Fig. 52.49). Fluid distention of the duodenum is abnormal and indicative of duodenal atresia or stenosis, annular pancreas, or volvulus. Down syndrome is commonly present. Half the cases have additional anomalies.

Bowel obstruction is suggested by dilation of the small bowel of greater than 6 mm (Fig. 52.50). Causes include jejunal or ileal atresia or stenosis, volvulus, meconium ileus, and enteric duplication. A dilated and tortuous ureter should not be misinterpreted as dilated bowel.

Meconium ileus causes small bowel obstruction by impaction of abnormally thick meconium in the distal ileum. Meconium ileus is nearly always associated with cystic fibrosis. The presence of dilated bowel filled with echogenic meconium suggests cystic fibrosis.

Meconium peritonitis results from perforation of a bowel segment. Spillage of meconium into the peritoneal cavity causes a sterile peritonitis that results in calcifications on peritoneal surfaces, loculated fluid-filled masses within the peritoneal cavity (meconium pseudocysts), ascites, bowel dilation, and polyhydramnios. The cause is commonly not identified but may be due to vascular insult to small bowel. Identified causes include meconium ileus (cystic fibrosis), bowel atresia, and volvulus.

Echogenic Bowel. Meconium, consisting of desquamated cells, proteins, and bile pigments, fills the distal small bowel by 15 to 16 weeks. Its US appearance ranges from echolucent to moderately echogenic. Small bowel is considered abnormally echogenic when its echogenicity is equal to or greater than that of adjacent bone. High-frequency transducers (>5 MHz) are

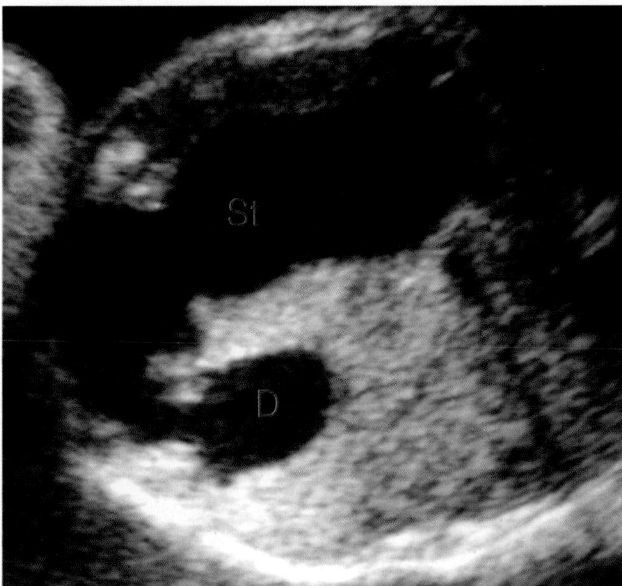

FIGURE 52.49. **"Double Bubble."** Fluid distention of the stomach (*St*) and the duodenal bulb (*D*) is caused by obstruction at the level of the descending duodenum.

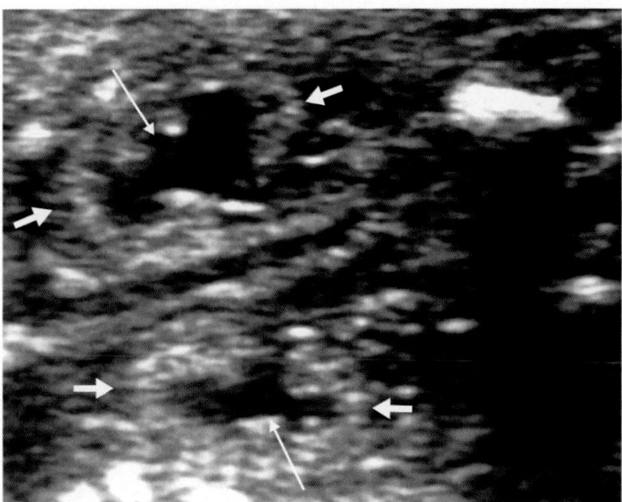

FIGURE 52.51. **Hydronephrosis.** Coronal plane image through the fetal abdomen reveals bilateral hydronephrosis (*skinny arrows*) resulting from posterior urethral valves. Calyces and the renal pelvis are dilated. Both kidneys (between *short arrows*) are normal in size, determined by comparing renal lengths in mm to gestational age in weeks (approximately equal).

more likely to make bowel appear abnormally echogenic than lower-frequency transducers (≤5 MHz). In any case this finding is often normal, but may serve as a marker of significant abnormality. Associations include cystic fibrosis, chromosome abnormalities (trisomy 21, trisomy 18), small bowel atresia, volvulus, and fetal viral infection (cytomegalovirus).

Urinary Obstruction. The most common causes of hydronephrosis in the fetus are ureteropelvic junction obstruction, ectopic ureterocele, and posterior urethral valves (Fig. 52.51). Dilation of the renal pelvis greater than 10-mm AP diameter or greater than 50% of the AP diameter of the kidney in axial section, or unequivocal caliectasis is definitive evidence of significant hydronephrosis. Assessment of bladder filling and amniotic fluid volume is necessary to determine the severity of obstruction.

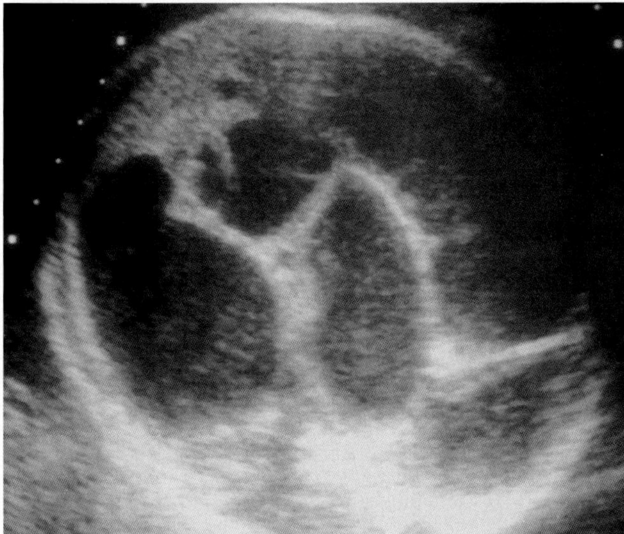

FIGURE 52.50. **Small Bowel Obstruction.** Ileal atresia was the cause of markedly dilated loops of small bowel seen throughout the abdomen.

Minimal dilation of the renal pelvis is most often due to physiologic vesicoureteral reflux that is normal during the second and third trimesters. A fluid-filled renal pelvis larger than 3 mm warrants attention because it may be a sonographic marker of aneuploidy (Down syndrome) or an early indicator of congenital urinary obstruction. A detailed fetal anatomic survey is indicated. Finding of additional abnormalities may warrant further tests for chromosome abnormality. Because some significant urinary tract obstructions may show only mild dilation in the second trimester, follow-up US in the third trimester is warranted to detect development of caliectasis or progression of pyelectasis. Elective postnatal US examinations of equivocal cases should be performed at 1 to 2 weeks of age to avoid underestimation of hydronephrosis because of the normal oliguria that occurs during the early postnatal period.

Renal cystic disease is commonly detected in utero. *Multicystic dysplastic kidney* appears as multiple noncommunicating cysts of varying size. Because affected kidneys do not function, bilateral multicystic dysplastic kidney is associated with severe oligohydramnios and is not compatible with life. Massive enlargement of both kidneys associated with oligohydramnios (Fig. 52.52) suggests *autosomal recessive polycystic disease*. The kidneys are predominantly echogenic with a sonolucent rim. Discrete cysts are usually not evident. *Autosomal dominant polycystic kidney disease* is occasionally detected in utero. The kidneys are enlarged but lack the sonolucent rim of autosomal polycystic kidney disease. Occasional discrete cysts are visualized. *Obstructive uropathy* such as posterior urethral valves may result in cystic renal dysplasia. Affected kidneys are hydronephrotic, with increased parenchymal echogenicity and parenchymal cysts of varying size. The kidneys may be dysplastic without cysts being visualized by US.

Gastroschisis results from a defect in the anterior abdominal wall nearly always on the right side of the umbilicus. The defect is usually 2 to 4 cm in size. Bowel herniates through the defect and floats freely in the amniotic fluid with no covering membrane (Fig. 52.53). Small defects may be associated with bowel ischemia, resulting in thickening of the wall of the herniated bowel. The cord insertion site is normal. Gastroschisis

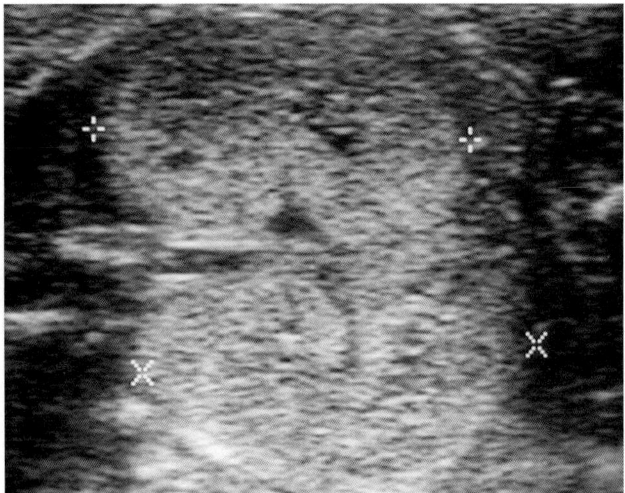

FIGURE 52.52. **Autosomal Recessive Polycystic Kidney Disease.** Coronal plane image in a 22-week fetus shows two markedly enlarged, highly echogenic kidneys (between *cursors*, +, ×) filling and distending the abdomen. Each kidney exceeded 5 cm in length. Severe oligohydramnios were present. This appearance is characteristic of the infantile form of autosomal recessive polycystic disease.

is most commonly an isolated defect without chromosomal anomaly or risk of recurrence. Postnatal repair is usually successful, so the prognosis is excellent when no other anomalies are present.

Omphalocele is a more serious abdominal wall defect that is about equal in frequency to gastroschisis. The defect is midline at the umbilicus with herniation of abdominal contents into the base of the umbilical cord (Fig. 52.53C). Both liver and bowel are commonly present in the herniation. A membrane consisting of peritoneum and amnion covers the omphalocele. The umbilical cord inserts through the membrane. Associated anomalies are common (67% to 88%), including cardiac, CNS, urinary tract, and gastrointestinal malformations. Chromosome anomalies are found in up to 40% of cases. The ventral wall defect may include the heart (ectopia cordis).

Sacrococcygeal Teratomas. While teratomas may occur anywhere in the fetus, the sacrococcygeal area is the most common site (70% to 80%). Females are more commonly affected (4:1). Mortality rates for the fetus are as high as 50%. US demonstrates a heterogeneous, mixed cystic or solid mass. In 15%, the lesion may be purely cystic mimicking a meningocele. Components of the mass may be entirely external to the pelvis, entirely internal within the pelvis and abdomen, or both internal and external to the pelvis. Solid tumors show prominent vascularity. Tumor growth is often rapid. Associated findings include hydrops, polyhydramnios, and additional anomalies. Obstetric complications include premature delivery, dystocia, and tumoral hemorrhage. Postnatal issues include malignant degeneration.

Skeleton

Skeletal dysplasias are a heterogeneous group of disorders of skeletal growth resulting in bones of abnormal size, density, and shape. US findings that are highly associated with the presence of a generalized skeletal dysplasia include shortening of extremity bones, fractures, bowing of long bones (Fig. 52.54), demineralization, and a small thorax. Finding of short FL

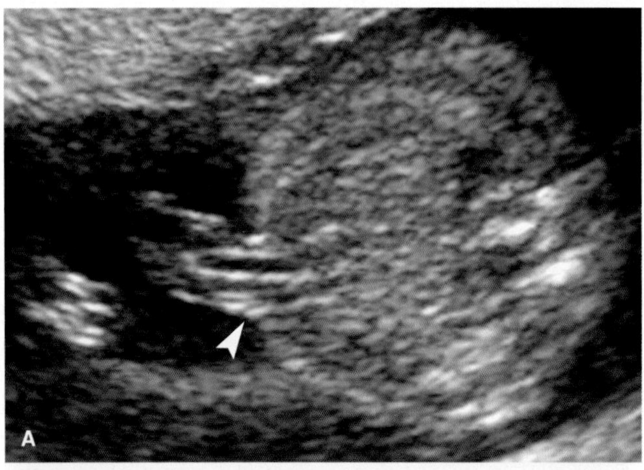

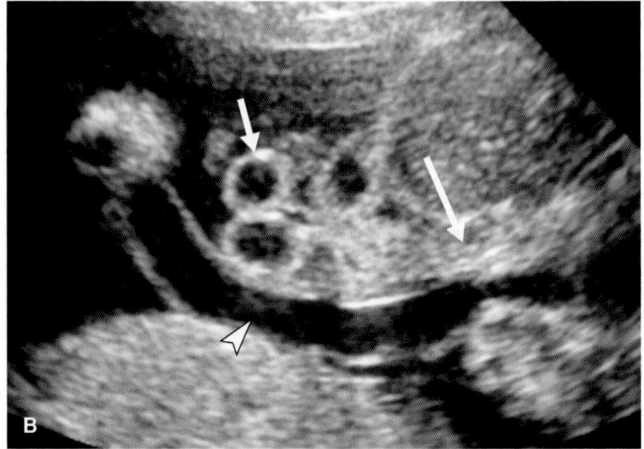

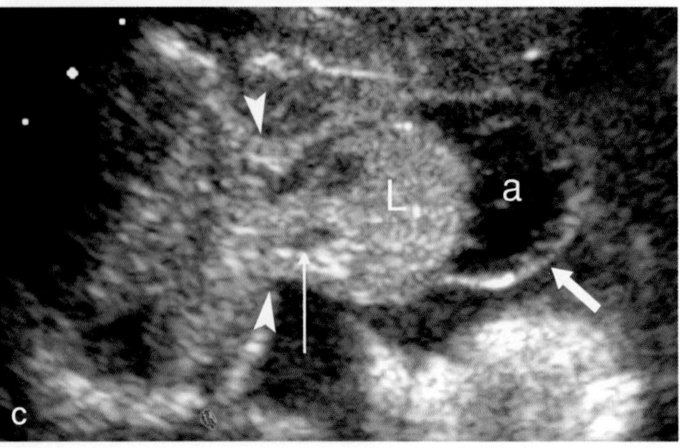

FIGURE 52.53. **Normal Umbilical Cord Insertion Site, Gastroschisis, Omphalocele. A: Normal.** Axial image through the fetal abdomen at the level of the umbilicus shows the normal cord insertion site (*arrowhead*). **B: Gastroschisis.** Axial image through the abdomen of another fetus shows loops of bowel (*short arrow*) extending through a defect in the anterior abdominal wall (*long arrow*) just to the right of the insertion site of the umbilical cord (*arrowhead*). **C: Omphalocele.** Axial image of another fetus at the level of the umbilicus shows liver (*L*) herniating through a defect (between *arrowheads*) in the anterior abdominal wall. The defect involves the umbilical cord (*skinny arrow*). A covering membrane (*short fat arrow*) is easily seen because it is outlined by ascites (*a*) within the omphalocele and amniotic fluid.

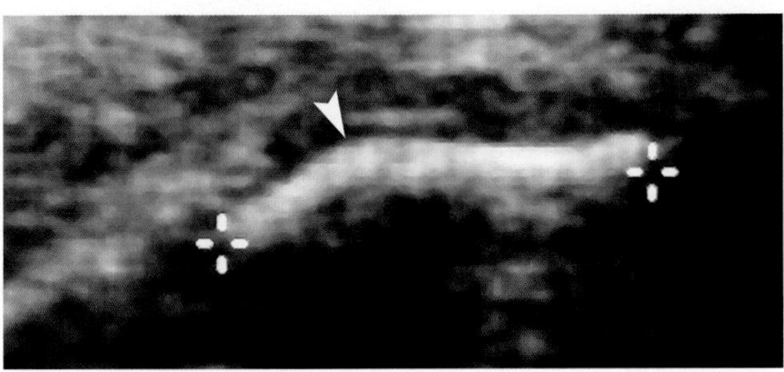

FIGURE 52.54. **Micromelic Dwarf.** A longitudinal image of the femur (between *cursors,* +) demonstrates poor mineralization, central bowing (*arrowhead*), and length that is markedly short for gestational age.

mandates detailed bone examination with measurement of all long bones. A ratio of FL to foot length of less than 1 suggests a skeletal dysplasia, whereas a ratio greater than 1 is usually associated with a constitutionally small or growth-retarded fetus. Additional findings that help categorize the skeletal dysplasia include polydactyly, abnormal head shape, spine anomalies, midface hypoplasia, abnormal bone configuration, ventriculomegaly, polyhydramnios, and hydrops. Precise diagnosis of a skeletal dysplasia may be difficult unless there is a family history. An algorithmic approach is recommended.

Thanatophoric dwarfism is the most common lethal skeletal dysplasia. Distinguishing features include small thorax, cloverleaf skull, large head, hydrocephalus, and polyhydramnios. *Achondroplastic dysplasia* is an autosomal dominant trait that is lethal in homozygous form and nonlethal in heterozygous form. Because at least one parent must have the condition, the US diagnosis is made on the basis of proximal limb shortening. *Osteogenesis imperfecta* is a heterogeneous group of disorders with both autosomal dominant and recessive inheritance patterns. The hallmark of the disease is osteoporosis that may manifest on US as diminished bone echogenicity. Additional features include bone thickening with fractures and callus formation, bone bowing, a small chest, and protuberant abdomen.

Examination of the fetal hands and feet may yield characteristic findings that suggest a variety of syndromes and chromosome abnormalities. Clenched hands with overlapping index fingers suggest trisomy 18. Polydactyly with polycystic kidneys suggests Meckel–Gruber syndrome. Hypoplasia of the middle phalanx of the fifth digit in association with femur and humerus shortening suggests Down syndrome.

Suggested Readings

First Trimester

American Institute of Ultrasound in Medicine. AIUM practice parameter for the performance of obstetric ultrasound examinations. Laurel, MD. 2013. Available from http://www.aium.org/resources/guidelines/obstetric.pdf.

Barnett SB, Maulik D, Society IPD. Guidelines and recommendations for safe use of Doppler ultrasound in perinatal applications. *J Matern Fetal Med* 2001; 10:75–84.

Chukas A, Tirada N, Restrepo R, Reddy NI. Uncommon implantation sites of ectopic pregnancy: thinking beyond the complex adnexal mass. *Radiographics* 2015;35:946–959.

Doubilet PM, Benson CB, Bourne T, et al. Diagnostic criteria for nonviable pregnancy early in the first trimester. *Ultrasound Q* 2014;30:3–9.

Histed SN, Deshmukh M, Masamed R, Jude CM, Mohammad S, Patel MK. Ectopic pregnancy: a trainee's guide to making the right call. *Radiographics* 2016;36:2236–2237. Available from http://media.rsna.org/media/journals/rg/presentations/2016/36.7.Histed/index.html.

International Society of Ultrasound in Obstetrics and Gynecology. ISUOG practice guidelines: performance of first-trimester fetal ultrasound scan. *Ultrasound Obstet Gynecol* 2013;41:102–113. Available from https://www.isuog.org/uploads/assets/uploaded/00bceab5-21e0-4ab5-85e6795e01d06d62.pdf

Lane BF, Wong-You-Cheong JJ, Javitt MC, et al. ACR appropriateness criteria first trimester bleeding. *Ultrasound Q* 2013;29:91–96.

Ranade M, Aquilera-Barrantes I, Quiroz FA. Gestational trophoblastic disease and choriocarcinoma. *Ultrasound Q* 2015;31:221–223.

Rodgers SK, Chung C, DeBardeleben JT, Horrow MM. Normal and abnormal US findings in early first-trimester pregnancy: review of the Society of Radiologists in Ultrasound 2012 consensus panel recommendations. *Radiographics* 2015;35:2135–2148.

Sellmyer MA, Desser TS, Maturen KE, Jeffrey RB Jr, Kamaya A. Physiologic, histologic, and imaging features of retained products of conception. *Radiographics* 2013;33:781–796.

Tan S, Pektas MK, Arslan H. Sonographic evaluation of the yolk sac. *J Ultrasound Med* 2012;31:87–95. (Pictorial essay).

Second and Third Trimester

American College of Obstetricians and Gynecologists. Practice Bulletin No. 163 Summary: screening for fetal aneuploidy. Summary published. *Obstet Gynecol* 2016;127:979–981.

American College of Obstetricians and Gynecologists. Practice Bulletin No. 162 Summary: prenatal diagnostic testing for genetic disorders. Summary published. *Obstet Gynecol* 2016;127:976–978.

Blask AN, Fagen K. Prenatal imaging of the gastrointestinal tract with postnatal imaging correlation. *Ultrasound Q* 2016;32:15–24. (Review article).

Dukhovny S, Wilkins-Haug L, Shipp TD, Benson CB, Kaimal AJ, Reiss R. Absent fetal nasal bone—what does it mean for the euploid fetus? *J Ultrasound Med* 2013;32:2131–2134.

Expert Panel on Women's Imaging: Glanc P, Nyberg DA, Khati NJ, et al. ACR appropriateness criteria—multiple gestations. *J Am Coll Radiol* 2017; 14:S476–S489.

Gün I, Muhçu M, Müngen E, Kiliç S, Atay V. Effect of an amniotic sheet on pregnancy outcomes. *J Ultrasound Med* 2013;32:807–813.

Hiersch L, Melamed N, Aviram A, Bardin R, Yogev Y, Ashwal E. Role of cervical length measurement for preterm delivery prediction in women with threatened preterm labor and cervical dilatation. *J Ultrasound Med* 2016;35:2631–2640.

Khalil A, Rodgers M, Baschat A, et al. ISUOG practice guidelines: role of ultrasound in twin pregnancy. *Ultrasound Obstet Gynecol* 2016;47:247–263.

Khurana A, Burt A, Beck G, et al. Fetal cardiac screening sonography: methodology. *Radiographics* 2017;37:360–361. (Online video presentation).

Kilcoyne A, Shenoy-Bhangle AS, Roberts DJ, Sisodia RC, Gervais DA, Lee SI. MRI of placenta accreta, placenta increta, and placenta percreta: pearls and pitfalls. *AJR Am J Roentgenol* 2017;208:214–221.

Magann EF, Sandlin AT, Ounpraseuth ST. Amniotic fluid and the clinical relevance of the sonographically estimated amniotic fluid volume—oligohydramnios. *J Ultrasound Med* 2011;30:1573–1585.

Mehta TS, Levine D. Ultrasound and MR imaging of fetal neural tube defects. *Ultrasound Clinics* 2007;2:187–201.

Moshiri M, Zaidi SF, Robinson TJ, et al. Comprehensive imaging review of abnormalities of the umbilical cord. *Radiographics* 2014;34:179–196.

Nelson DB, Dashe JS, McIntire DD, Twickler DM. Fetal skeletal dysplasias—sonographic indices associated with adverse outcomes. *J Ultrasound Med* 2014;33:1085–1090.

Sandlin AT, Chauhan SP, Magann EF. Amniotic fluid and the clinical relevance of the sonographically estimated amniotic fluid volume—ployhydramnios. *J Ultrasound Med* 2013;32:851–863.

Sheppard C, Platt L. Nuchal translucency and first trimester risk assessment. a systematic review. *Ultrasound Q* 2007;23:107–116.

Winter TC, Kennedy AM, Woodward PJ. Holoprosencephaly: a survey of the entity, with embryology and fetal imaging. *Radiographics* 2015;35:275–290.

Zaidi SF, Moshiri M, Osman S, et al. Comprehensive imaging review of abnormalities of the placenta. *Ultrasound Q* 2016;32:25–42.

Zelop CM, Javitt MC, Glanc P, et al. ACR appropriateness criteria growth disturbances—risk of intrauterine growth restriction. *Ultrasound Q* 2013; 29:147–151.

CHAPTER 53 ■ CHEST, THYROID, PARATHYROID, AND NEONATAL BRAIN ULTRASOUND

WILLIAM E. BRANT

CHEST

Ultrasound (US) is an excellent supplement to conventional film radiography and CT for the problem-solving evaluation of diseases of the chest. US can be effectively used to guide interventional procedures in the thorax, especially at the patient's bedside. US can image into and through pleural effusions and lung consolidation to evaluate the thorax opacified on radiographs. Its portability allows evaluation of critically ill patients who are impractical to be moved for a CT. US examination of the chest must always be correlated with available chest radiography or CT.

Pleural Space

Normal US Anatomy. Air in the lungs completely reflects the US beam and prohibits examination deeper into the chest. However, when pleural fluid displaces air-filled lungs away from the chest wall, disease in the pleural space can be optimally evaluated with US. The pleural space is examined by a direct intercostal approach, with the US transducer applied directly to the chest, or by an abdominal approach imaging through the diaphragm from the abdomen. The ribs are used as sonographic landmarks for direct chest imaging (Fig. 53.1). A linear array transducer applied to the chest wall shows the ribs as curving echoes that cast acoustic shadows. The visceral pleura–air-filled lung interface is seen within 1 cm of the rib echo as a bright echogenic surface that moves with respiration (the "*gliding sign*"). The moving lung surface is well visualized when the transducer is turned parallel to the intercostal space. The tiny normal amount of fluid in the pleural space is seen just superficial to the gliding pleura. From the abdomen, the diaphragm is seen as a bright, curving interface due to complete sound reflection from the air-filled lung above it (Fig. 53.2). Organs beneath the diaphragm (liver, spleen) are artifactually reproduced above the diaphragm due to multipath sound reflection (the "*mirror-image*" *artifact*).

Pleural fluid displaces the lung away from the chest wall allowing visualization of the pleural space (Figs. 53.1C and 53.2B). Most pleural fluid is anechoic or hypoechoic with floating particulate matter. The fluid separates the visceral and parietal pleural surfaces. From an abdominal approach, hypoechoic fluid is seen above the diaphragm, the inside of the thorax is visualized, and the mirror-image artifact is not present. Septations not evident on CT are commonly visualized by US. Collapsed or consolidated lung moves with respiration within the fluid in the pleural space. Fluid that appears echogenic, contains floating particles or layering debris, or is septated is an exudate (Fig. 53.3). Fluid that is anechoic may be a transudate, exudate, or even empyema. Loculations of pleural fluid and suspected empyemas can be localized and evaluated with US visualization used to guide needle aspiration and drainage catheter placement.

Pleural thickening complicates inflammatory and malignant disease of the thorax. US demonstrates uniform, undulating, or plaque-like thickening of the pleura (Fig. 53.4). The visceral pleura is easily evaluated. The parietal pleura is partially obscured by reverberation artifact in the near field.

Pleural Masses. Pleural metastases or tumors such as mesotheliomas are seen as nodular pleural thickening or hypoechoic soft tissue masses in the pleural space projecting from the pleural surface (Fig. 53.5).

Pneumothorax can be diagnosed by US. Pneumothorax produces a highly echogenic reflective line, very similar to that of air-filled lung but lacking the "gliding sign" associated with respiratory movement. Pneumothorax is also indicated by loss of visualization of a previously visualized lung lesion that occurs during an invasive procedure.

Lung Parenchyma

Normal US Anatomy. The normal air-filled lung with its covering visceral pleura completely blocks transmission of US into the thorax. The gliding visceral surface of the lung is easily seen, but reverberation artifact is displayed deep to that surface. However, consolidation, atelectasis, or tumor that extends to the visceral pleural surface produces a window for US examination. When scanning the thorax from the

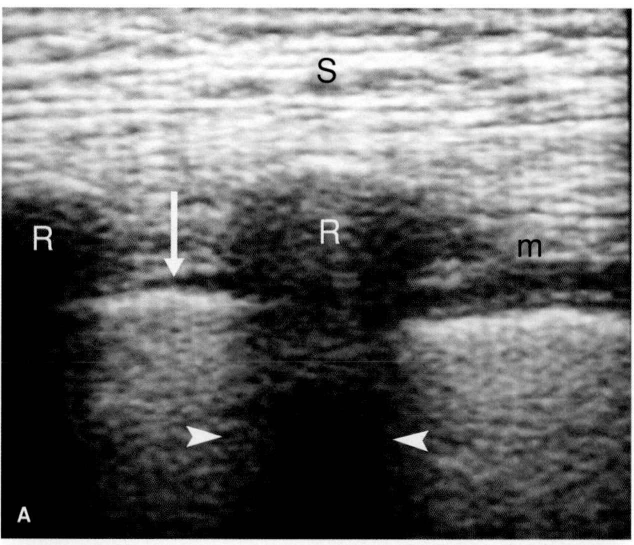

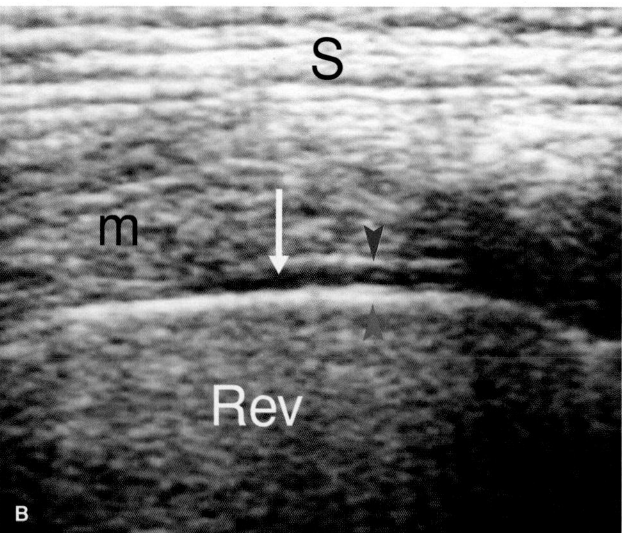

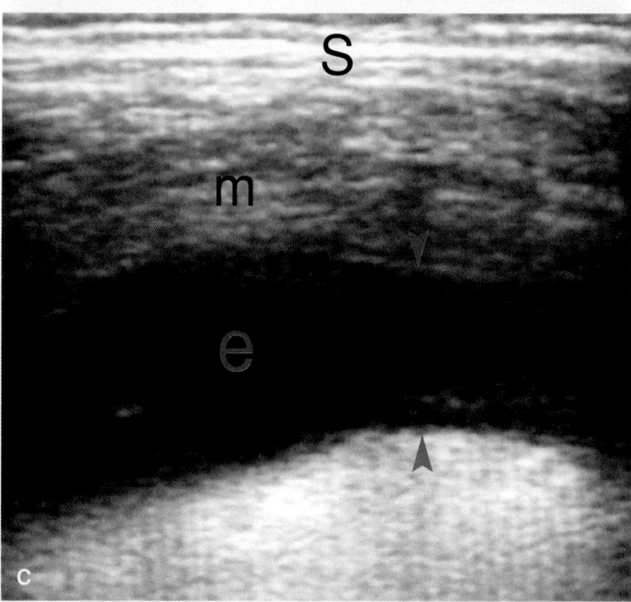

FIGURE 53.1. Pleural Space: Intercostal Scan. A: Longitudinal US image of the chest shows a rib (*R*) and its acoustic shadow (between *arrowheads*). The pleural space is approximately 1 cm deep to the surface of the rib (*arrow*). Intercostal muscle (*m*) is seen between the ribs. B: Aligning the transducer parallel to the ribs in the intercostal space enables improved visualization of the pleural space (*arrow*). The visceral pleura–air-filled lung interface (*blue arrowhead*) is identified by its movement with respiration—the "gliding sign." The visceral pleura is separated from the parietal pleura (*red arrowhead*) by a thin layer of pleural fluid in the pleural space (*arrow*). The air-filled lung is obscured by reverberation artifact (*Rev*). C: A pleural effusion (*e*) separates the visceral pleura (*blue arrowhead*) from the parietal pleura (*red arrowhead*). *m*, intercostal muscle; *S*, subcutaneous fatty tissue.

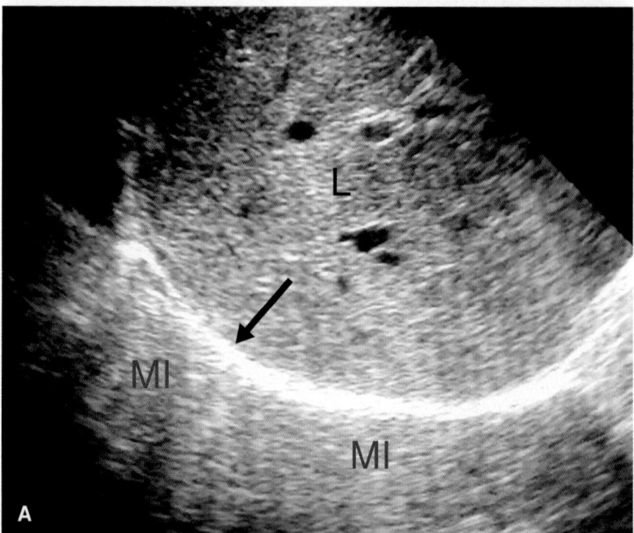

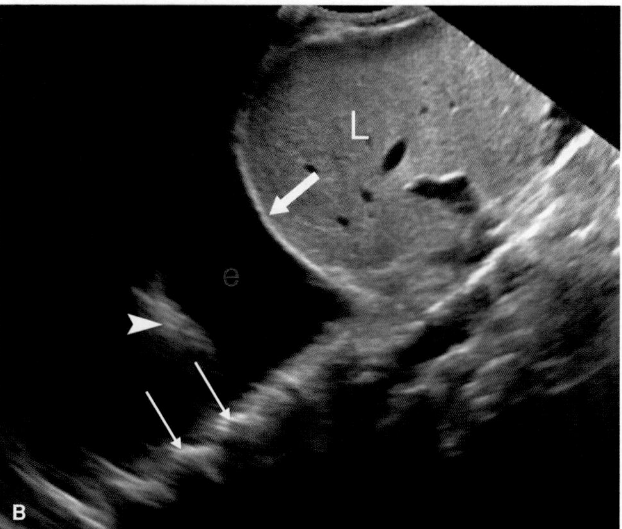

FIGURE 53.2. **Pleural Space: Abdominal Scan.** A: Examination of the chest is performed from an abdominal approach using the liver (*L*) or spleen as a sonographic window. The diaphragm is seen as a bright curving line (*arrow*). Normal air-filled lung causes the liver to be reproduced as a mirror-image artifact (*MI*) above the diaphragm. B: A large pleural effusion (*e*) eliminates the mirror-image artifact and allows visualization of the chest wall characterized by ribs and rib shadows (*skinny arrows*) through the diaphragm (*fat arrow*) and pleural space. Pleural effusions are always accompanied by atelectasis of the lung (*arrowhead*). *L*, liver.

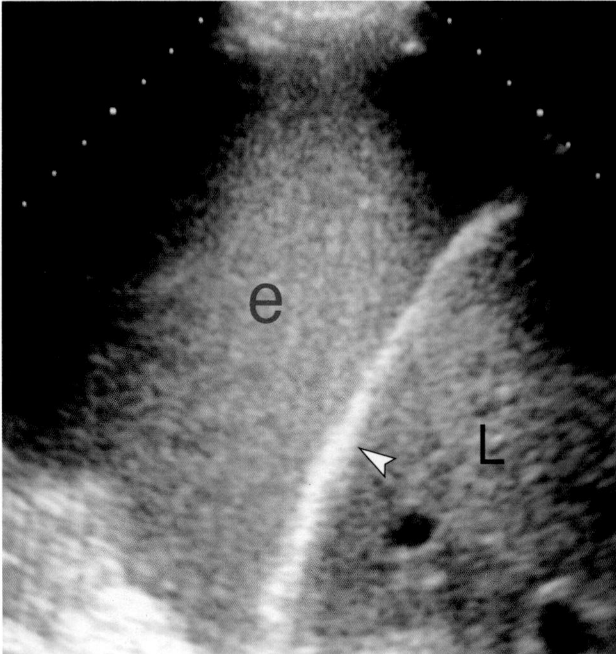

FIGURE 53.3. **Echogenic Pleural Effusion.** An empyema associated with right lower-lobe pneumonia appears on US as an echogenic effusion (*e*). Innumerable moving floating particles were observed within the fluid on real-time US examination confirming its liquid nature. The liver (*L*) is very similar in echogenicity. The diaphragm (*arrowhead*) is seen as a curving, brightly echogenic line.

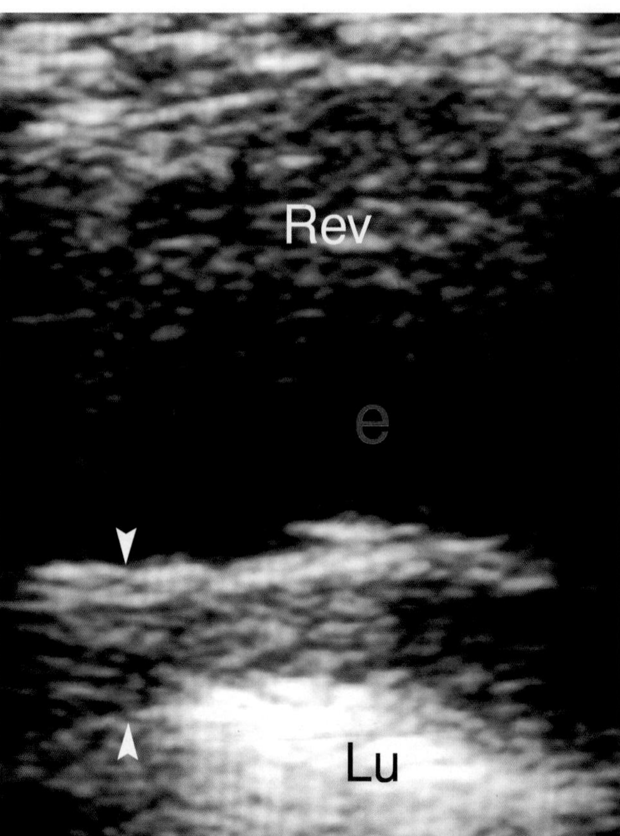

FIGURE 53.4. **Pleural Thickening.** Intercostal US image demonstrates a moderate-volume pleural effusion (*e*). The visceral pleura (between *arrowheads*) is thickened because of chronic inflammation. The parietal pleura is obscured in the near field by reverberation artifact (*Rev*). The air-filled lung (*Lu*) is brightly echogenic.

abdomen, the normal air-filled lung produces a mirror-image artifact.

Consolidation refers to filling of the air spaces of the lung with fluid and inflammatory cells. This process "solidifies" the lung and provides a medium for sound transmission (Fig. 53.6). The consolidated lung appears solid and hypoechoic, with echogenicity similar to liver. *Sonographic air bronchograms* and *sonographic air alveolograms* may be seen within the consolidated lung. Air-filled bronchi produce bright branching linear reflections. Air trapped in the alveoli surrounded by the consolidated lung produces globular bright echoes with comet tail artifacts. *Sonographic fluid bronchograms* appear as anechoic fluid-filled tubes extending from the hilum of the lung. Color flow US demonstrates pulmonary vessels extending through the consolidated lung.

Atelectasis. Collapse of the air spaces with absorption of air also results in solidification of the lung. With atelectasis, the lung volume is decreased and bronchi and pulmonary blood vessels are crowded together. Collapsed lung always accompanies large pleural effusions (Fig. 53.7). The atelectatic lung is wedge shaped and sharply defined by its covering pleura.

Lung masses and lung nodules completely surrounded by air-filled lung are not visualized by US, but those that extend to the visceral pleura or are accompanied by peripheral consolidation or atelectasis may be seen and evaluated (Fig. 53.8). US guidance may be effectively used to aspirate or biopsy lung masses in areas difficult to access with CT or fluoroscopy. Central tumor necrosis, hemorrhage within tumors, and lung abscesses are effectively evaluated.

Pulmonary sequestration is a congenital partition of lung tissue that does not communicate with the bronchial tree. Most occur at the lung base. *Intralobar sequestrations* are within the visceral pleura. *Extralobar sequestrations* are invested by their own separate pleura. US is used to confirm the diagnosis by demonstration of a feeding artery arising from the aorta. Extralobar sequestrations drain via a systemic vein, whereas intralobar sequestrations connect to the pulmonary veins.

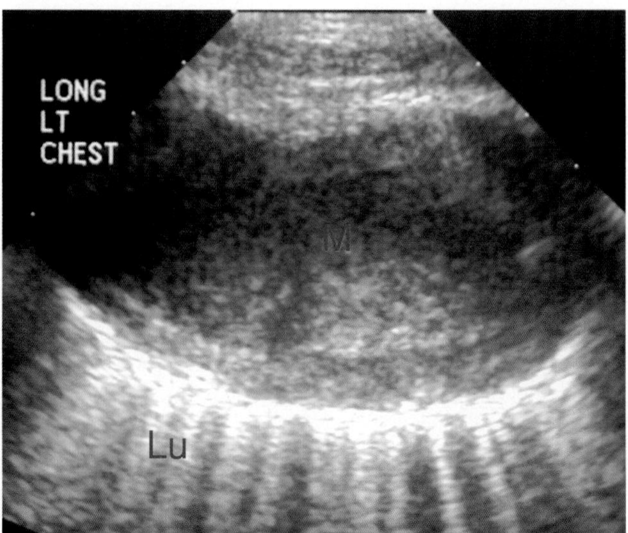

FIGURE 53.5. **Mesothelioma.** Intercostal US shows a solid mass (*M*) projecting from the parietal pleura and displacing air-filled lung (*Lu*) away from the chest wall. US-guided percutaneous biopsy confirmed mesothelioma.

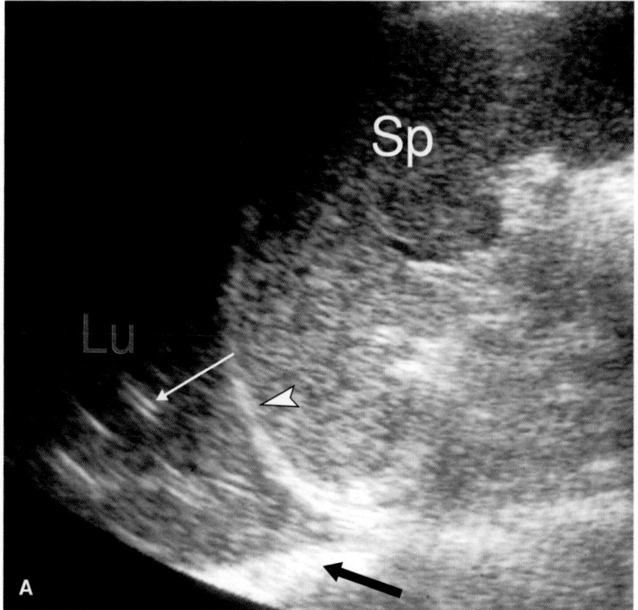

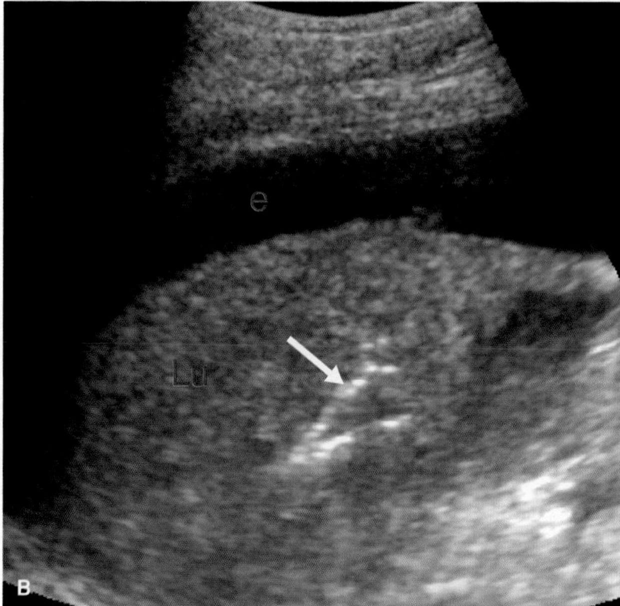

FIGURE 53.6. Lung Consolidation. **A:** US image obtained using the spleen (*Sp*) as a sonographic window in a patient with left upper quadrant pain reveals an unsuspected pneumonia in the left lower lobe of the lung (*Lu*). Inflammatory fluid and cells consolidate the lung replacing air and allowing visualization of the chest wall (*fat arrow*) through the airless lung. Sonographic fluid bronchograms (*skinny arrow*) are seen within the pneumonia. The diaphragm (*arrowhead*) produces a bright curving echo. **B:** Intercostal US image in a different patient shows the solid-appearing consolidated lung (*Lu*) through a parapneumonic pleural effusion (*e*). Sonographic air bronchograms (*arrow*) appear as linear, highly echogenic branching structures.

Mediastinum

Normal US Anatomy. The superior and anterior mediastinum are effectively evaluated with US using a parasternal or supramanubrial approach. The posterior mediastinum is less accessible because of the spine and lungs. Large lesions create sonographic windows to the mediastinum. Imaging downward into the superior mediastinum from just above the sternal manubrium demonstrates the innominate veins and the arteries arising from the aortic arch. Doppler US assists in the identification of vessels.

Vascular Lesions. Elongation and tortuosity of the brachiocephalic artery is a common cause of mediastinal widening in older adults. This diagnosis is easily confirmed by US, which

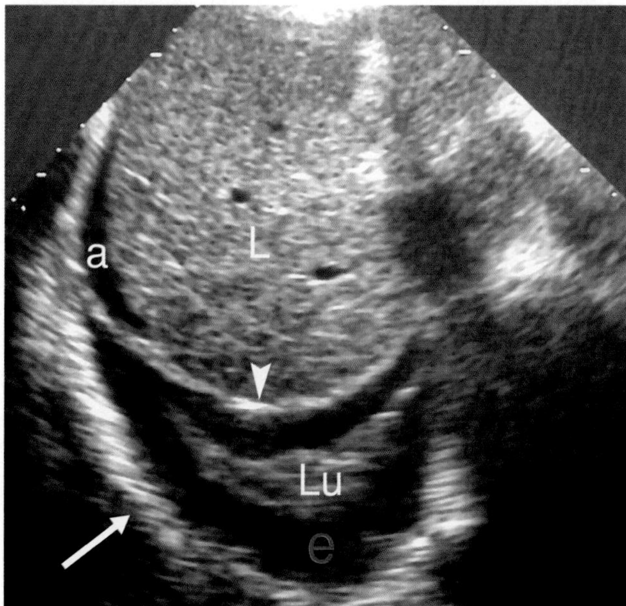

FIGURE 53.7. **Atelectasis.** A transverse image through the liver (*L*) reveals a pleural effusion (*e*) surrounding a tongue of collapsed lung (*Lu*). The patient also has ascites (*a*). The diaphragm (*arrowhead*) produces a thin, curving bright echo. The chest wall (*arrow*) produces a thick, curving bright echo.

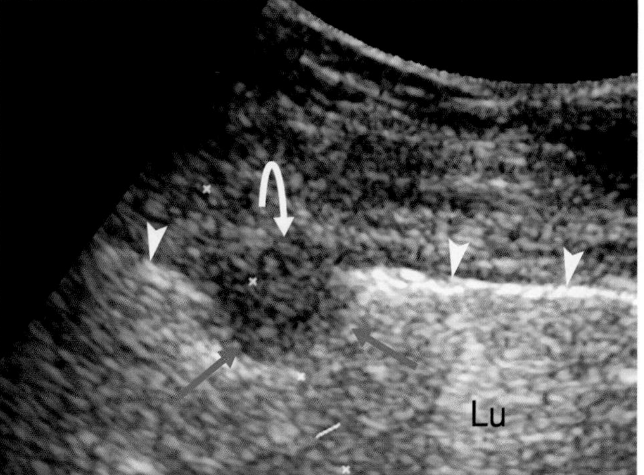

FIGURE 53.8. **Peripheral Lung Nodule.** Intercostal US scan shows a 1-cm peripheral lung nodule (*blue arrows*) abutting the pleural surface. Note how the bright echo from the visceral pleura–air-filled lung interface (*arrowheads*) is obliterated over the mass (*curved arrow*). The echogenic air-filled lung (*Lu*) provides a bright background on which to clearly visualize the nodule. Fine-needle biopsy precisely guided (*row of ×'s*) by US visualization revealed metastatic squamous cell carcinoma in this patient with a primary tumor in the neck.

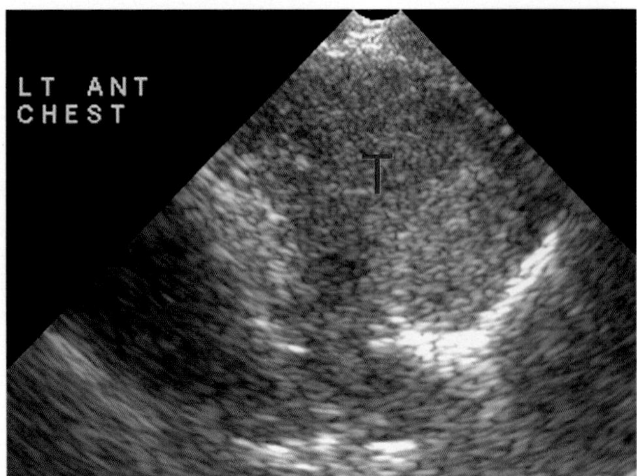

FIGURE 53.9. Mediastinal Mass. A left parasternal US image shows a large solid mediastinal mass (*T*). US-guided fine-needle and core biopsy were easily performed and confirmed a malignant thymoma.

can also exclude other masses of the superior mediastinum. The many blood vessels of the mediastinum are easily identified by color Doppler.

Mediastinal Masses. Thymic masses, substernal extension of thyroid enlargement, adenopathy, and other mediastinal masses are effectively demonstrated by US, which can confirm their cystic or solid nature and vascularity. Lesions that can be visualized by US can usually be biopsied using US guidance to avoid critical structures (Fig. 53.9). Continuation of thyroid tissue into the mediastinum is a straightforward diagnosis. Enlarged lymph nodes are usually homogeneous and hypoechoic. Confluent adenopathy due to lymphoma produces a solid, homogeneous, hypoechoic mass that encompasses and displaces blood vessels.

THYROID

Imaging of the thyroid gland remains a controversial topic. Thyroid nodules are exceedingly common, although thyroid cancer is uncommon and death from thyroid malignancy is rare. CT, MR, and US performed for other reasons commonly reveal thyroid nodules, which require further evaluation. High-resolution US is extremely sensitive in detecting thyroid nodules; however, imaging signs to differentiate benign from malignant lesions overlap and are of limited sensitivity and specificity. Since 2005, authors and several professional committees of radiologists, endocrinologists, and internists have attempted to define multiparameter algorithms that differentiate nodules that warrant biopsy or follow-up from incidental benign nodules that can be safely ignored. In 2012, an American College of Radiology committee was convened to address this problem. This committee developed Thyroid Imaging, Reporting, and Data System (TI-RADS). Guidance for use of this system was published in 2015 and 2017. TI-RADS is the most common decision algorithm in current use. Further modifications of TI-RADS are likely as its use is investigated.

US is used to precisely guide percutaneous fine-needle aspiration (FNA) and core biopsy of thyroid nodules, to screen patients at high risk for thyroid cancer, to identify recurrent disease in patients with known thyroid cancer, and to determine if palpable nodules arise from the thyroid gland. CT and MR supplement US by staging of invasive thyroid cancers, evaluating for postoperative recurrence of thyroid cancer, and demonstrating extension of goiter into the thorax. Radionuclide imaging, discussed in a subsequent chapter, evaluates the physiologic function of the gland. US-guided FNA of thyroid nodules is safe, accurate, and inexpensive. Complications, primarily hematoma and pain, are rare and minor.

Normal US Examination and Anatomy. The thyroid gland consists of paired lobes of near-equal size (5 × 2 × 2 cm) connected across the trachea by a thin thyroid isthmus (Fig. 53.10). The thyroid parenchyma is homogeneous with fine medium-level echogenicity greater than muscle. Anatomic landmarks include the midline air-filled trachea, which casts an air shadow; the common carotid artery and internal jugular vein, which parallel the lateral edge of the thyroid lobes; the longus colli muscles posteriorly; and the sternohyoid, sternothyroid, and sternocleidomastoid muscles anteriorly. Small pools of colloid (*colloid cysts*) are routinely visualized within the normal gland. The thyroid lobes are often mildly asymmetric in size. The esophagus commonly protrudes from behind the trachea, nearly always on the left side, and must not be mistaken for a thyroid or parathyroid mass or lymph node (Fig. 53.11). The superior thyroid artery and vein are imaged between the upper pole of the thyroid and the longus colli. The recurrent laryngeal nerve and inferior thyroid artery and vein are seen posterior to the lower poles. The thyroid is easily imaged with the patient in a supine position, with the neck extended by placement of a pillow beneath the shoulders.

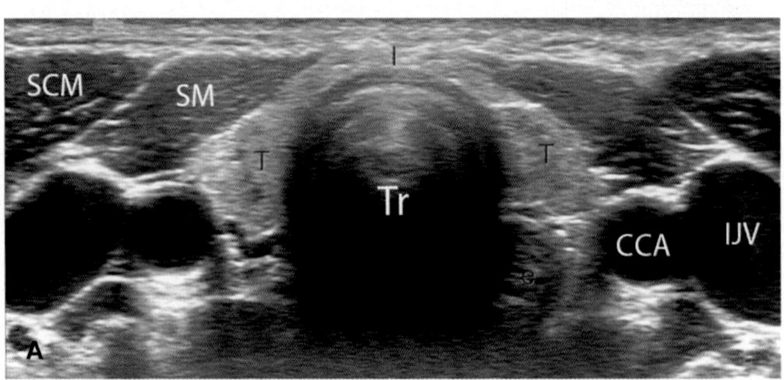

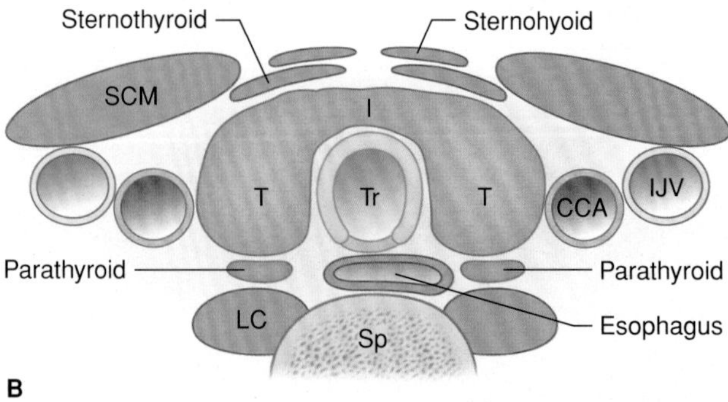

FIGURE 53.10. Normal Thyroid Ultrasound Anatomy. A: Transverse US image. **B:** Corresponding drawing. Symmetric lobes of homogeneous thyroid tissue (*T*) are seen on either side of the trachea (*Tr*). A thin isthmus (*I*) of thyroid tissue crosses anterior to the trachea. Anatomic landmarks include the common carotid arteries (*CCA*), internal jugular veins (*IJV*), sternocleidomastoid muscles (*SCM*), strap muscles (*SM, sternothyroid, sternohyoid*), longus colli muscle (*LC*), and the spine (*Sp*). The *esophagus* (*e*) is partially obscured by the acoustic shadow of the air-filled trachea but extends out to left beyond the acoustic shadow. The location of the *parathyroid* glands is shown on the drawing, deep to the thyroid lobes resting on the longus colli muscles.

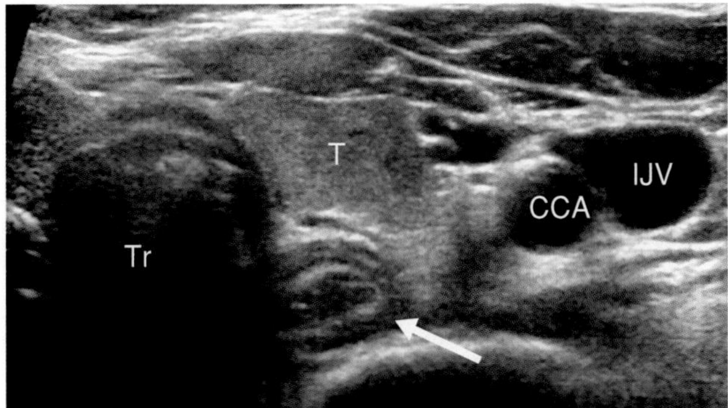

FIGURE 53.11. Normal Esophagus. Transverse US image of the thyroid gland (*T*) reveals an apparent nodule (*arrow*) deep to the thyroid and extending laterally from the acoustic shadow of the trachea (*Tr*). Having the patient swallow confirms this structure to be the normal esophagus. Note the multilayered echo pattern characteristic of the gastrointestinal tract. The esophagus should not be mistaken for a thyroid or parathyroid lesion. *CCA*, common carotid artery; *IJV*, internal jugular vein.

High-frequency (7 to 15 MHz) linear array transducers are recommended. The lobes of the thyroid gland are imaged and measured in longitudinal and transverse planes. The isthmus is imaged in transverse plane and its thickness is recorded. The number, location, size in three dimensions, and characteristics of nodules are documented. The neck is examined for adenopathy or other abnormalities.

Thyroid Nodules

The Problem. Thyroid nodules are extremely common: 4% to 8% of adults have palpable nodules, as many as 68% have nodules on high-resolution US examination, and 50% have nodules at autopsy. Thyroid nodules increase in frequency with age and are much more common in women. Thyroid cancer, on the other hand, affects only 0.1% of the population. Thyroid cancer is less than 1% of all cancer and is the cause of less than 0.5% of all cancer deaths. Most thyroid cancers are slow growing and have low morbidity and mortality. The ratio of benign thyroid nodules to thyroid cancer can be estimated at as high as 500:1. The challenge of imaging studies and clinical evaluation is to establish the likelihood of malignancy and to select out for surgery only those patients with thyroid malignancy.

TI-RADS assesses US features of thyroid nodules by composition, echogenicity, shape, margin, presence of echogenic foci, and size (Table 53.1). TI-RADS risk categories are benign, not suspicious, minimally suspicious, moderately suspicious, or highly suspicious for malignancy (Table 53.2). TI-RADS incorporates most of the US features included in recommendations previously published by other authors and societies. Like previous guidelines, TI-RADS does not recommend biopsy for any nodules under 1 cm in size. There is no TI-RADS category for a normal thyroid gland. Shear wave elastography, while showing some promise, is unproven and not included in TI-RADS.

Evaluation of Thyroid Nodules. A *thyroid nodule* is a discrete lesion sonographically distinct from the surrounding thyroid parenchyma. Nodules are characterized based upon their US appearance, independent of whether they are solitary nodules or are found within a multinodular gland. The decision to biopsy is based upon US characteristics and the patient's individual clinical risks. Physical examination finding of a firm, hard, rapidly growing, or fixed nodule is evidence in favor of biopsy. Age younger than 20 years or older than 70 years, male gender, history of neck irradiation, and family or personal history of thyroid cancer increase the risk of thyroid cancer. Published guidelines, such as TI-RADS, are meant to be flexible advice and are not rigid criteria. Features of thyroid nodules incorporated into TI-RADS include the following (Table 53.1):

- *Cystic* or almost completely cystic nodules are nearly always benign (Fig. 53.12).
- *Spongiform* lesions, defined as consisting of >50% tiny cysts, are almost always benign.
- *Mixed cystic and solid lesions*: The appearance of the solid component is most important. Solid tissue that is eccentric or has other suspicious characteristics such as decreased

TABLE 53.1

TI-RADS CATEGORIES FOR ULTRASOUND FINDINGS OF THYROID NODULES

■ COMPOSITION[a]	■ ECHOGENICITY[a]	■ SHAPE[a]	■ MARGIN[a]	■ ECHOGENIC FOCI[b]
Cystic, almost completely cystic 0 points	Anechoic 0 points	Wider than tall 0 points	Smooth 0 points	None or large (>1 mm) comet tail artifacts in cystic components 0 points
Spongiform Small cysts >50% 0 points	Hyperechoic or isoechoic 1 point	Taller than wide 3 points	Ill-defined 0 points	Macrocalcifications (cause acoustic shadowing) 1 point
Mixed cystic/solid 1 point	Hypoechoic 2 points		Lobulated or irregular 2 points	Peripheral (rim) calcifications (complete or incomplete) 2 points
Solid 2 points	Very hypoechoic (less echogenic than strap muscles) 3 points		Extrathyroidal extension 3 points	Punctate echogenic foci 3 points

[a]Choose one.
[b]Choose all that apply.
Adapted from Tessler FN, Middleton WD, Grant EG, et al. ACR thyroid imaging, reporting and data system (TI-RADS): white paper of the ACR TI-RADS Committee. *J Am Coll Radiol* 2017;14:587–595.

TABLE 53.2

TI-RADS SCORING, CLASSIFICATION, AND RECOMMENDATIONS

■ TI-RADS LEVEL SCORING	■ CLASSIFICATION	■ RECOMMENDATIONS
TR1: 0 points	Benign	No FNA recommended
TR2: 2 points	Not suspicious	No FNA recommended
TR3: 3 points	Mildly suspicious for malignancy	FNA if ≥2.5 cm US F/U if ≥1.5 cm at 1, 3, and 5 years
TR4: 4–6 points	Moderately suspicious for malignancy	FNA if ≥1.5 cm US F/U if ≥ 1 cm at 1, 2, 3, and 5 years
TR5: 7 or more points	Highly suspicious for malignancy	FNA if ≥1 cm US F/U if ≥0.5 cm yearly for 5 years

FNA, fine-needle aspiration; *F/U*, follow-up.
Follow-up can stop at 5 years if no significant change in the nodule.
Adapted from Tessler FN, Middleton WD, Grant EG, et al. ACR thyroid imaging, reporting and data system (TI-RADS): white paper of the ACR TI-RADS Committee. *J Am Coll Radiol* 2017;14:587–595.

echogenicity, lobulation, or punctate echogenic foci is more suspicious for malignancy (Fig. 53.13).

- *Color Doppler*: The prominence of blood flow within a nodule does not differentiate benign from malignant nodules. However, the presence of blood flow does allow differentiation of solid tissue from echogenic debris and hemorrhage (Fig. 53.14).
- *Echogenicity* of a nodule is determined by comparison to adjacent thyroid tissue. *Very hypoechoic* is determined by comparison to strap muscles. Uniform hyperechogenicity is highly predictive of benign nodules, especially in a patient with Hashimoto thyroiditis.
- *Shape:* Taller-than-wide shape is highly predictive of malignancy but is not frequently present.
- *Margins:* An echolucent halo surrounding a nodule does not discriminate benign from malignant, nor does poor definition of a nodule's margin. Lobulated or irregular margins with spiculated edges or protrusions into the surrounding thyroid tissue increase risk of malignancy (Fig. 53.14).
- *Extrathyroidal extension* may be minimal or extensive. Minimal extension is defined by bulging of the thyroid contour, abutment of the thyroid border, or loss of the echogenic border of the thyroid. Extensive extension refers to invasion of adjacent tissue or blood vessels and is highly predictive of malignancy with a poor prognosis.
- *Echogenic foci* may refer to dystrophic calcification, precipitated colloid, or psammomatous calcifications. *Large comet tail artifacts* refer to echogenic foci with V-shaped echoes longer than 1 mm extending deep from the focus (Fig. 53.12). These caused by inspissated colloid, usually occur in cystic nodules and are strong indicators of a benign nodule. *Macrocalcifications* are coarse dystrophic calcifications that cause acoustic shadowing. Their presence is a weak indicator of malignancy. *Peripheral calcification* extending completely or partially along the rim of a nodule is a stronger predictor of malignancy. *Punctate echogenic foci* (Fig. 53.15) are tiny and nonshadowing. They are closely associated with papillary carcinoma and occur both in the primary tumor and within lymph nodes containing metastatic disease.

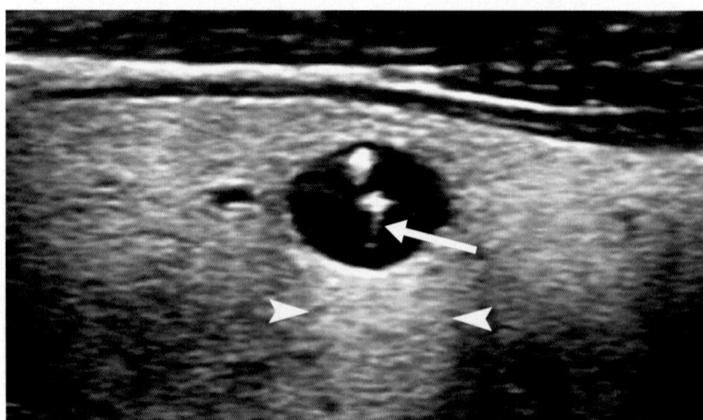

FIGURE 53.12. Colloid Cyst—Comet Tail Artifact. A cyst within the right thyroid lobe shows floating punctate echogenic foci with a tapering tail (*arrow*). This is an example of a *large comet tail artifact* and is characteristic of inspissated colloid and a benign lesion. Note the sharply defined walls and accentuated through-transmission (*arrowheads*) characteristic of a cyst and a benign thyroid lesion.

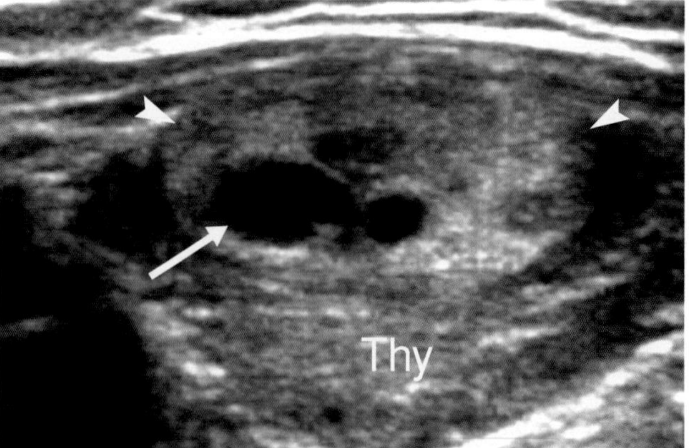

FIGURE 53.13. Mixed Cystic and Solid Nodule—Adenomatous Nodule. Longitudinal image of the thyroid gland reveals a mixed cystic (*arrow*) and solid nodule (between *arrowheads*) measuring 18 mm in greatest dimension. US-guided fine-needle aspiration biopsy yielded a cytologic diagnosis of "colloid nodule," indicating visualization of benign thyroid cells and thyroid colloid. Colloid nodules are the usual cytologic term for adenomatous nodules. Note the homogeneous pattern of the visualized normal thyroid parenchyma (*Thy*).

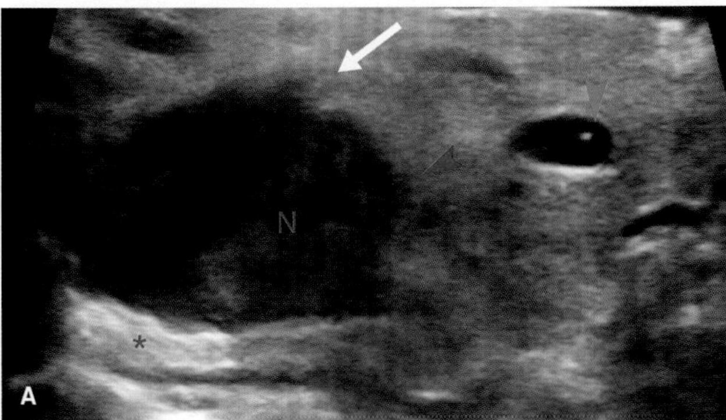

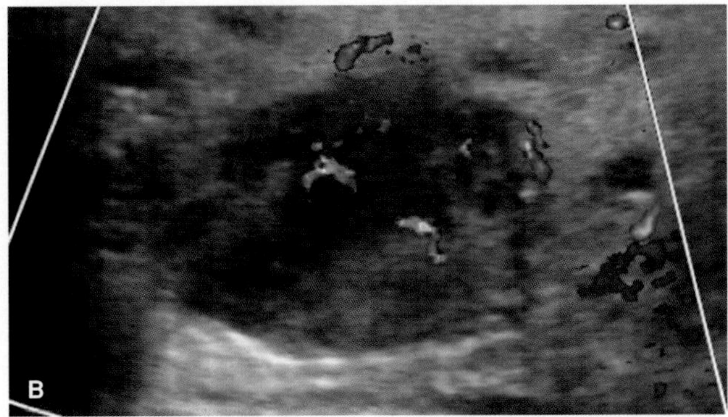

FIGURE 53.14. **Hypoechoic, Lobulated, and Spiculated Margins—Papillary Carcinoma.** **A:** Gray scale US image. **B:** Color Doppler US image. The nodule (*N*) is distinctly but heterogeneously hypoechoic to surrounding thyroid tissue. The margins are both spiculated (*red arrowhead*) and lobulated (*arrow*). Accentuated through-transmission (*) suggested a cystic component to the nodule. However, color Doppler confirms the presence of blood vessels in the solid tissue. A small colloid cyst (*blue arrowhead*) is also present. US-guided fine-needle aspiration confirmed papillary carcinoma.

- *Size* alone is not a predictor of malignancy. However, biopsy of small nodules less than 1 cm is not recommended by any Society because very small cancers are very likely to be slow growing and not clinically significant.
- *Growth:* TI-RADS defines significant growth on follow-up examinations as a 20% increase in at least two nodule dimensions with a minimal increase of 2 mm, or a 50% or larger increase in volume of the nodule. Comparison should be made to the earliest available scan showing the nodule.

Benign Thyroid Nodules

Adenomatous nodules, also called *colloid nodules*, are the most common thyroid nodules. They are not neoplasms but benign growths resulting from cycles of hyperplasia and involution of the thyroid tissue. They are usually multiple and associated with diffuse enlargement of the thyroid gland. Individual nodules are iso- or hypoechoic to the thyroid parenchyma and commonly show degenerative changes with prominent cystic components, necrosis, hemorrhage, and calcification (Fig. 53.13).

Follicular adenoma is the most common benign neoplasm. Autonomous hyperfunctioning adenomas are a cause of hyperthyroidism, but most adenomas cause no alteration of overall thyroid function. Most are solitary, solid, and well encapsulated. They may be hypo-, hyper-, or isoechoic to the thyroid parenchyma (Fig. 53.16). Hyperfunctioning adenomas are commonly strikingly hypervascular on color flow US. Degenerative changes include focal necrosis, hemorrhage, edema, infarction, fibrosis, and calcification. Differentiation from follicular carcinoma is difficult; therefore, an FNA cytologic diagnosis of follicular neoplasm is commonly considered an indication for surgical removal and histologic determination of the presence of cancer.

True thyroid cysts are extremely rare, epithelial-lined, simple cysts. Most cystic nodules found in the thyroid are actually cystic degeneration of an adenomatous nodule or a follicular adenoma.

Hemorrhage may occur into an adenomatous nodule or a follicular adenoma, or spontaneously into normal parenchyma. Patients present with sudden neck pain and subsequent swelling. US reveals a hypoechoic nodule with internal debris. Color Doppler shows no flow within the debris to differentiate hemorrhage from solid tissue.

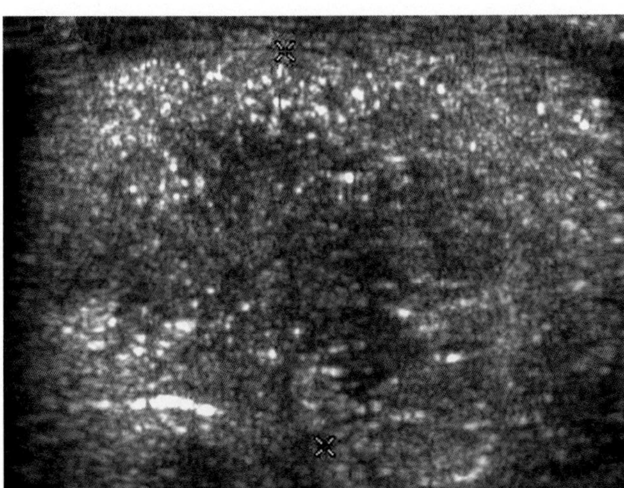

FIGURE 53.15. **Punctate Echogenic Foci—Papillary Carcinoma.** Longitudinal image reveals a solid nodule containing numerous punctate, nonshadowing echogenic foci characteristic of papillary carcinoma of the thyroid gland. The presence of punctate echogenic foci in a thyroid nodule is highly indicative of malignancy. Biopsy proved papillary carcinoma.

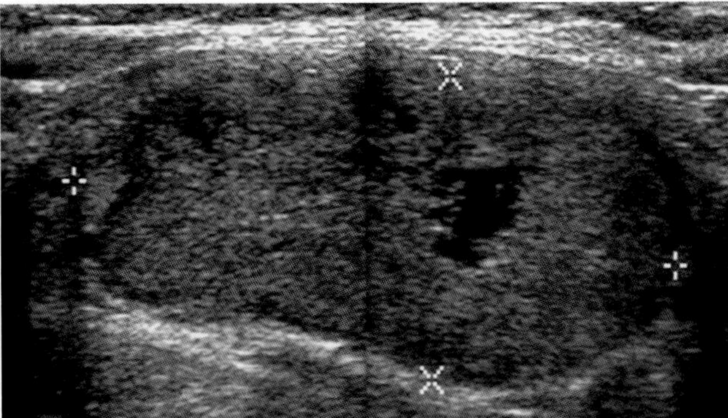

FIGURE 53.16. **Follicular Neoplasm.** US-guided fine-needle aspiration yielded abundant follicular cells from this large thyroid nodule (between *cursors*, ×, +). Because a diagnosis of follicular carcinoma could not be excluded, this lesion was surgically removed. No histologic evidence of malignancy was present. Follow-up showed no recurrence and no evidence of metastatic disease.

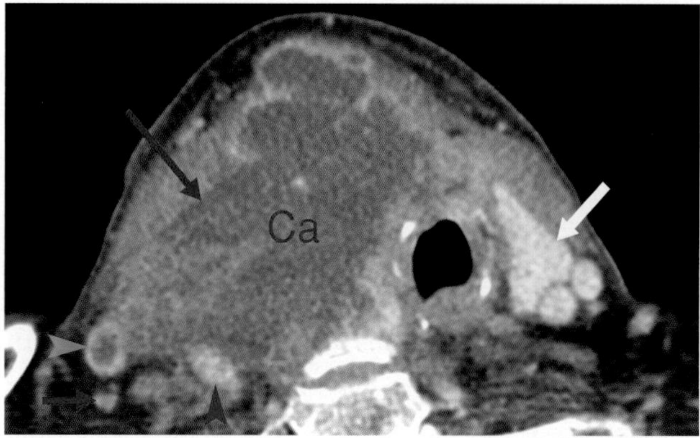

FIGURE 53.17. **Anaplastic Thyroid Carcinoma.** Postcontrast CT of a 90-year-old woman shows a huge right neck mass (*Ca*) displacing the trachea leftward, invading the sternocleidomastoid muscle (*long red arrow*), common carotid artery (*red arrowhead*), and internal jugular vein (*blue arrowhead*) resulting in its thrombosis. Multiple lymph nodes (*short red arrow*) involved with metastatic disease are evident. The left lobe of the thyroid (*thick arrow*) and its adjacent vessels are displaced leftward. Biopsy confirmed aggressive anaplastic carcinoma.

Malignant Thyroid Nodules

Papillary thyroid carcinoma (75% to 80% of thyroid cancer) is one of the least aggressive cancers in humans. Most patients are female (4:1). Nodules are hypoechoic (Fig. 53.14) and commonly multiple. Punctate echogenic foci (Fig. 53.15), representing psammoma bodies, are common (42%) and highly indicative of malignancy. Some tumors show the characteristic microcalcifications in the thyroid parenchyma without a discrete mass present. Involved cervical nodes may contain similar calcifications. The tumor spreads commonly to regional nodes, but rarely (2% to 3%) to the lungs or bones. Five-year survival is 95% to 99%.

Follicular thyroid carcinoma (10% to 20%) is also a slow-growing malignancy, but invasion of blood vessels is characteristic with common hematogenous spread to the lungs and bones. Lymphatic spread to cervical nodes is uncommon. The sonographic features of follicular carcinoma are very similar to those of follicular adenoma. Most tumors are solitary, isoechoic, and ill defined. Cystic areas, hemorrhage, and necrosis are common. Features that favor carcinoma over adenoma include larger size, hypoechoic appearance, and absence of cystic change. Clinical features that favor malignancy are male gender and older age. Five-year survival is about 65%.

Medullary thyroid carcinoma (3% to 5%) is a neuroendocrine malignancy that arises from parafollicular C cells that secrete calcitonin, which serves as a tumor marker. About 20% of cases are familial and associated with multiple endocrine neoplasia (MEN2). US appearance is similar to papillary carcinoma, with coarse internal calcifications common (80%). Five-year survival is 65%.

Anaplastic thyroid carcinoma (1% to 2%) is a lethal malignancy of the elderly. The tumor grows rapidly and metastasizes widely (Fig. 53.17). US shows an ill-defined, heterogeneous, hypoechoic, solid mass. Nodal metastases are commonly present. Five-year survival is less than 4%.

Thyroid Cancer Staging. When using US, CT, or MR for initial staging of thyroid malignancy or follow-up for recurrence, one must consider the common routes of spread of the specific type of malignancy to optimally plan the imaging study. The impressive contrast resolution of MR makes it excellent for determining involvement of muscles, larynx, esophagus, and other cervical structures by large invasive tumors. Recurrence of tumor may be demonstrated by T2WI, which shows a high signal intensity tumor, brighter than muscle. Fibrosis in the thyroid bed has low signal intensity, less than or equal to muscle. Lymph node involvement is determined primarily by size criteria. Normal lymph nodes in the neck are less than 7 mm in diameter.

Recurrence of Thyroid Cancer. Post total thyroidectomy, US is used to detect the recurrence of thyroid cancer. The US appearance of lesions in the thyroid bed is not specific and requires either imaging follow-up or US-guided FNA (Fig. 53.18). Besides, recurrence of cancer nodules in the thyroid bed may represent benign lymph nodes, fibrosis, suture granulomas, or fat necrosis.

Lymphoma accounts for 4% of thyroid malignancy and is most common in elderly women. Most cases are of the diffuse large B-cell variety. A solitary strikingly hypoechoic mass is most common, although some cases demonstrate multiple nodules. Associated enlarged cervical nodes are common. Nearly all patients with primary thyroid lymphoma also have Hashimoto thyroiditis.

Metastasis. Metastatic disease to the thyroid gland is rare. The most common primary tumors to metastasize to the thyroid are lung, breast, head and neck, kidney, and malignant melanoma. Metastases may present as discrete nodules or diffuse infiltration of the gland. Cervical adenopathy is commonly present (70%).

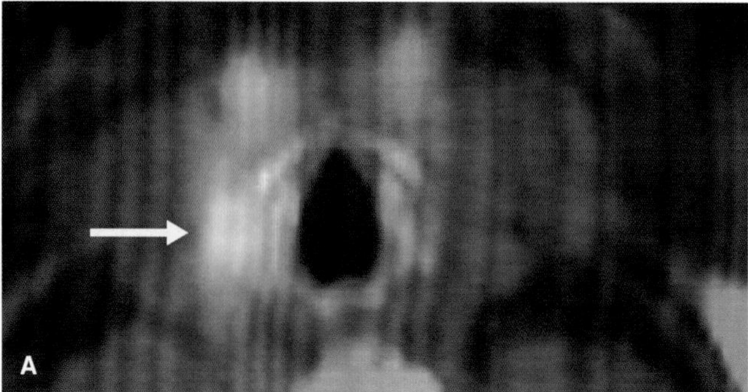

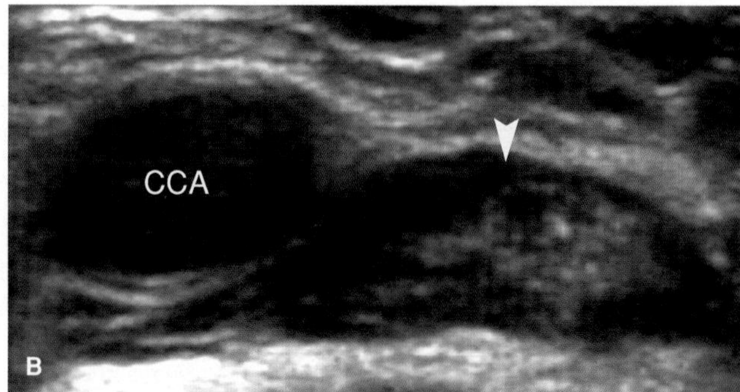

FIGURE 53.18. **Recurrent Thyroid Cancer. A:** PET-CT in a patient with a history of follicular carcinoma of the thyroid post total thyroidectomy shows several areas of increased radionuclide activity, with the area of greatest activity in the right thyroid bed (*arrow*). **B:** US of the right thyroid bed shows a mixed echogenicity solid nodule (*arrowhead*) in the area corresponding to the hot spot indicated by the *arrow* in (A). US-guided fine-needle aspiration confirmed recurrent follicular carcinoma. *CCA*, right common carotid artery.

Diffuse Thyroid Disease

The diagnosis of most diffuse diseases of the thyroid is made clinically and US is seldom indicated. US can be helpful when thyroid enlargement is asymmetric and a neoplasm is suspected.

Goiter is a general term that means diffuse thyroid enlargement. Goiter may be associated with increased, decreased, or normal thyroid function. The range of normal thyroid size is great. Thyroid enlargement is best judged subjectively. Helpful US signs of thyroid enlargement are thickening of the isthmus greater than 3 mm and outward bulge of the anterior surface of the gland. US measurement is useful in assessing and following thyroid gland size in determining response to therapy.

Nontoxic goiter is caused by iodine deficiency, goitrogens in the diet (soybeans and cruciferous vegetables), or deficiency of thyroid enzymes. US shows an enlarged gland with homogeneous parenchyma. Nontoxic goiter is not necessarily associated with thyroid dysfunction.

Adenomatous goiter, also called multinodular goiter, affects about 5% of the population of the United States. Adenomatous hyperplasia is the cause of 80% of thyroid nodules. Adenomatous goiter refers to the generalized enlargement of the thyroid that occurs when multiple hyperplastic nodules are present. US shows coarsening and heterogeneity of the thyroid parenchyma, with coarse calcifications commonly present. Each nodule must be individually evaluated for signs of malignancy.

Hashimoto thyroiditis (chronic lymphocytic thyroiditis) is an autoimmune disease that affects primarily women. About 10% to 15% of patients become clinically hypothyroid. It is the most common cause of hypothyroidism and goiter in adults in the United States. Circulating antithyroid antibody is associated with diffuse lymphocytic infiltration of the gland. US demonstrates diffuse thyroid enlargement with inhomogeneous, low echogenicity parenchyma. Characteristic linear echogenic lines represent fibrosis. No normal parenchyma is present. A pattern of multiple tiny nodules, 1 to 6 mm size, is highly indicative of the disease (Fig. 53.19). Patients are at risk for development of lymphoma. Focal lesions in patients with Hashimoto thyroiditis may represent hyperplastic nodules, papillary carcinoma, or lymphoma.

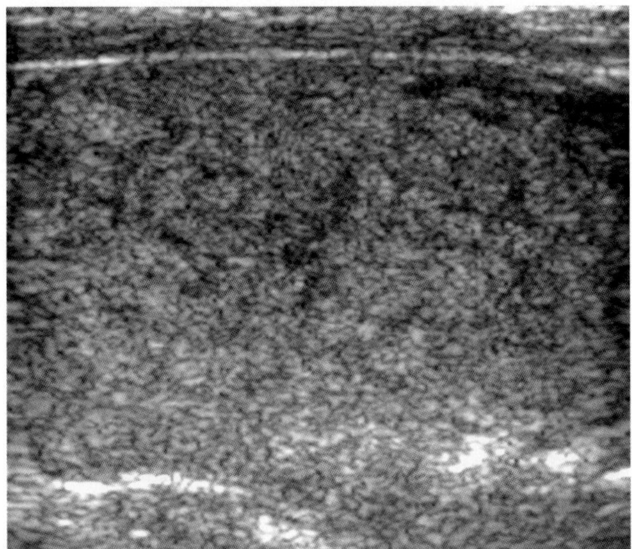

FIGURE 53.19. **Hashimoto Thyroiditis.** Longitudinal image through one lobe of the thyroid shows heterogeneous parenchyma with a myriad of indistinct tiny nodules. This is the characteristic US appearance of the disease.

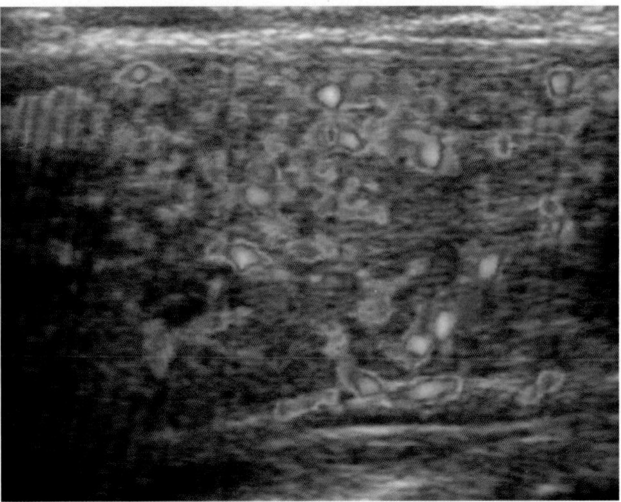

FIGURE 53.20. **Acute Graves Disease.** Color flow US image through one lobe of the thyroid gland in a patient with hyperthyroidism and exophthalmos shows the intense hypervascularity characteristic of Graves disease "thyroid inferno."

Graves disease is the most common cause of hyperthyroidism. The gland is usually enlarged two- to threefold, homogeneous, smooth or lobulated in contour, and usually without nodules. Echotexture is normal or diffusely hypoechoic. Color Doppler US demonstrates striking diffuse increased vascularity with multiple areas of intense intrathyroid flow, the "thyroid inferno" (Fig. 53.20). Extrathyroidal blood vessels may be prominent.

Subacute thyroiditis, also called de Quervain or granulomatous thyroiditis, presents with thyroid pain and hyperthyroidism following a viral upper respiratory infection. Radioiodine uptake is usually decreased or absent in the acute stages. The disease runs a subacute course of a few weeks to a few months. Affected focal or multifocal portions of the gland are swollen, edematous, poorly defined, and hypoechoic on US.

Acute suppurative thyroiditis is a rare bacterial infection of the thyroid gland. Often only a portion of the gland is involved. US is helpful in the detection and aspiration of abscesses.

Riedel thyroiditis is a rare inflammatory disease of progressive fibrosis that eventually destroys the thyroid gland and commonly extends into the neck. The gland is diffusely enlarged and inhomogeneous. US is used to show extension of fibrosis into the neck, with encasement of cervical blood vessels.

PARATHYROID

The primary indication for parathyroid imaging is preoperative localization of parathyroid adenomas or hyperplastic parathyroid glands in the setting of clinically diagnosed hyperparathyroidism. Preoperative localization has become essential as minimally invasive parathyroidectomy and sonographically guided ethanol ablation techniques have become treatments of choice. Preoperative imaging is particularly useful in patients with previous neck surgery. US, CT, MR, and

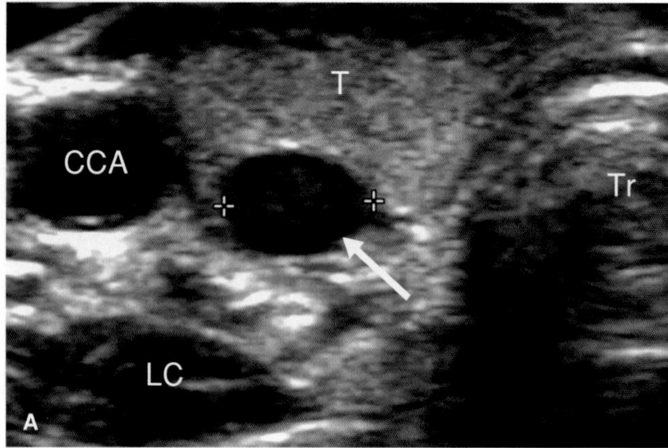

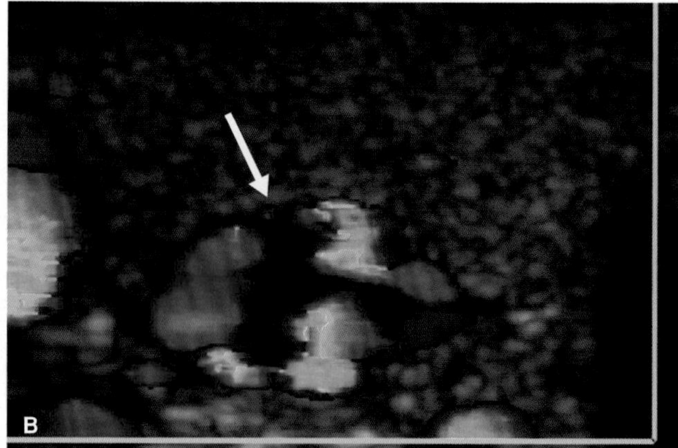

FIGURE 53.21. **Parathyroid Adenoma. A:** Transverse US image shows the characteristic markedly low echogenicity of a parathyroid adenoma (*arrow*, between calipers, +) in typical location, deep to the thyroid lobe (*T*), superficial to the longus colli muscle (*LC*), medial to the common carotid artery (*CCA*), and lateral to the acoustic shadow of the trachea (*Tr*). **B:** Color Doppler US shows the marked hypervascularity within the nodule (*arrow*) characteristic of parathyroid adenomas.

radionuclide imaging have all been used in this setting. Of these, radionuclide imaging is the most sensitive and accurate (see Chapter 72D Endocrine Gland Scintigraphy). However, because up to 90% of abnormal parathyroid glands are located in the neck, US is able to demonstrate the majority. Imaging has no role in hypoparathyroidism.

Normal US Anatomy. Normal parathyroid glands are flat disks measuring only 5 × 3 × 1 mm in size and are not usually demonstrated by any imaging method. Most enlarged glands are found beneath the thyroid lobes between the trachea and carotid sheath. The esophagus commonly protrudes out from behind the trachea, particularly on the left side. This normal structure should not be mistaken for a thyroid or parathyroid lesion (Fig. 53.11). Ectopic glands may be found in the neck or upper mediastinum between the upper pole of the thyroid and the thymus.

Hyperparathyroidism

Primary hyperparathyroidism is a common disease that affects women two to three times more often than men. More than half the patients are above the age of 50. A single benign hyperfunctioning adenoma is the cause in 85% of cases. Multiple-gland enlargement (two adenomas or hyperplasia) is responsible for 14% and parathyroid carcinoma is the cause of 1%. Most cases of hyperplasia involve all glands, although usually asymmetrically. The diagnosis is suspected on the basis of unexplained hypercalcemia and is confirmed by elevated serum parathyroid hormone level. Patients with hyperparathyroidism have a fourfold increase in the prevalence of renal stone disease. In secondary and tertiary hyperparathyroidism, elevated parathormone levels are caused by diffuse or nodular glandular hyperplasia. *Secondary hyperparathyroidism* occurs as a result of chronic hypocalcemia in patients with chronic renal failure. The parathyroid glands are overstimulated and become hyperplastic. When the chronically overstimulated glands become autonomous, the term *tertiary hyperparathyroidism* is used. Parathormone may also be produced by nonendocrine tumors such as renal cell and bronchogenic carcinoma.

Parathyroid adenomas appear on US as homogeneous, hypoechoic, solid, oval, and well-defined masses (Fig. 53.21), 8 to 15 mm in size. Color Doppler demonstrates hypervascularity. On MR T1WI, adenomas show low intensity similar to muscle. On T2WI, the adenomas show high intensity similar to or greater than fat. Because adenomas may be isointense with fat, T2WI alone provides an incomplete examination. CT is best performed with intravenous contrast to demonstrate the contrast-enhancing parathyroid nodules. Rarely, parathyroid adenomas may show cystic degeneration or calcification. Thyroid nodules may appear similar to parathyroid adenomas on US and degenerated parathyroid adenomas may mimic cystic thyroid masses. US may be used to guide needle biopsy. Cells of parathyroid origin can usually be readily differentiated from thyroid cells cytologically. An effective method of confirming parathyroid tissue on FNA is to request laboratory analysis of fluid aspirated from suspected parathyroid nodules. Parathyroid tissue will have extremely high levels of parathormone.

Parathyroid hyperplasia affects all the parathyroid glands, but the degree of enlargement is frequently asymmetric. Hyperplastic glands have the same imaging characteristics as parathyroid adenomas.

Parathyroid carcinoma is distinguished by larger size (>2 cm) than parathyroid adenomas. Tumors are usually more heterogeneous with cystic degeneration and occasional calcification (Fig. 53.22). The contour is lobulated or ill defined. Color

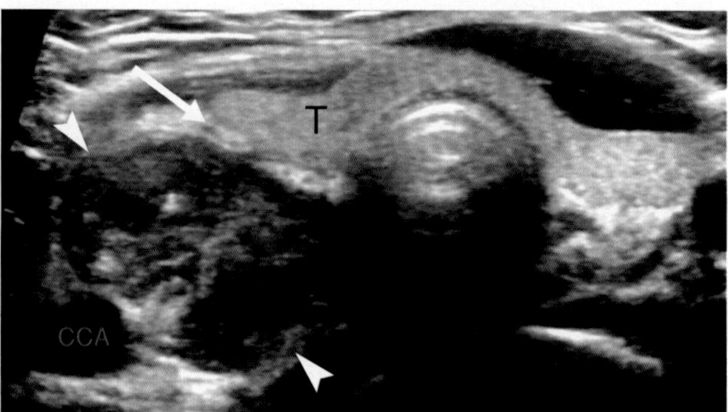

FIGURE 53.22. **Parathyroid Carcinoma.** Transverse US image of a patient with hyperparathyroidism reveals a heterogeneous lobulated solid mass (between *arrowheads*) in the area typical of parathyroid tissue. Punctate calcification is present. Note the uplifted right lobe of the thyroid gland (*T*) with a distinct plane of separation (*arrow*) from the nodule. Surgery confirmed a parathyroid carcinoma. *CCA*, common carotid artery.

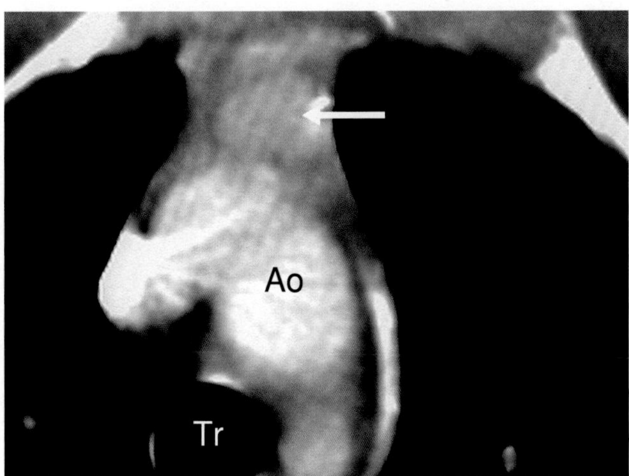

FIGURE 53.23. **Ectopic Parathyroid Adenoma.** Contrast-enhanced CT of the chest confirms the presence of an ectopic parathyroid adenoma (*arrow*) in the mediastinum just anterior to the top of the aortic arch (Ao). *Tr*, trachea.

flow US is useful to demonstrate invasion of adjacent vessels or muscle. The diagnosis is most commonly confirmed at surgical resection.

Ectopic parathyroids are best localized by radionuclide imaging. CT or MR is usually needed to show the anatomic relationships when they are located in the mediastinum (Fig. 53.23).

NEONATAL NEUROSONOGRAPHY

Sonography of the neonatal brain has become an integral part of the care of the neonate, allowing detailed evaluation of intracranial structures to be performed at the infant's bedside. The standard examination is relatively simple to perform, takes only a few minutes, and requires no sedation. The fact that the examination can be performed portably in the nursery where the infant can be kept warm and well monitored offers great advantage over CT and MR brain imaging. Indications for neonatal head US include evaluation for hemorrhage and brain injury due to hypoxia, especially in the premature infant; detection and follow-up of hydrocephalus and other sequelae of infection; and screening for congenital brain abnormalities. There are no contraindications to neurosonography.

Normal US Anatomy. Routine cranial sonograms are performed through the anterior fontanelle. The anterior fontanelle remains open until about 2 years of age, but examinations may be difficult after 12 to 14 months of age because of its smaller size. Standard views are taken in coronal and sagittal planes and are frequently supplemented by views in the axial plane through the thin squama of the temporal bone or through the posterior fontanelle, open sutures, or the foramen magnum. Examinations are performed at the bedside, keeping the infant warm, covered, and monitored in the isolette. The infant is positioned to optimize access to the anterior fontanelle. High-frequency, 5 to 10 MHz, sector transducers with a wide angle of view are preferred. The transducer is thoroughly cleansed with alcohol between each patient. In the coronal plane (Fig. 53.24), the brain is examined from anterior to the frontal horns to the occipital cortex. Standard views are recorded through the frontal horns, third ventricle, and trigone. Sagittal views (Fig. 53.25) include midline and parasagittal scans obtained 10 degrees laterally through the frontal horns and bodies of the lateral ventricles and 20 degrees laterally through the temporal horns. Axial views (Fig. 53.26) through the temporal bone provide excellent demonstration of the third ventricle, the cortex abutting the inside of the cranium, and the circle of Willis for Doppler studies. Key anatomic landmarks to be identified on every cranial US include the lateral, third, and fourth ventricles; cavum septum pellucidum/cavum vergae; corpus callosum; choroid plexus in the temporal horn, atrium, and body of the lateral ventricles and in the roof of the third ventricle; cerebellar vermis; and caudate nucleus, thalamus, and caudothalamic groove. The posterior fontanelle and foramen magnum can be effectively used as US windows to the posterior fossa.

Hypoxic–Ischemic Brain Injury

Premature infants, born at less than 32 weeks gestational age or with birth weight less than 1,500 g, are extremely susceptible to ischemic brain injury. Subependymal hemorrhage in the residual germinal matrix and periventricular leukomalacia are the two most common forms of hypoxic brain injury in premature infants. They are responsible for a 5% to 15% incidence of cerebral palsy (spastic motor deficits) (Fig. 53.27) and a 25% to 50% incidence of cognitive disabilities in surviving premature infants. Cranial sonograms are routinely performed on premature infants to detect these brain injuries and to monitor for treatable complications.

Germinal matrix is a fragile gelatinous mass of tissue found in the fetal brain between the ependyma lining the ventricles and the caudate nucleus. The germinal matrix is highly vascular and is a major source of hemorrhage when it becomes ischemic. The germinal matrix is the source of neuroblasts and spongioblasts, which migrate outward to the brain surface to form the glial cells of the cortex. The germinal matrix involutes so that by 32 weeks of gestational age, it is only present at the caudothalamic groove. By 35 to 36 weeks it has involuted completely, so only premature infants are susceptible to germinal matrix hemorrhage (GMH).

Germinal matrix hemorrhage (GMH), also called subependymal or periventricular–intraventricular hemorrhage, occurs in the residual germinal matrix overlying the frontal horn and body of the lateral ventricles. The incidence of GMH is reported at 67% in infants born at 28 to 32 weeks' gestation and at 80% of infants born between 23 and 24 weeks' gestation. Most hemorrhages originate in the region of the *caudothalamic groove* (Fig. 53.25B) where the germinal matrix is most prominent in the premature infant. The hemorrhage may remain confined but commonly ruptures into the ventricle resulting in intraventricular hemorrhage, ependymitis, and hydrocephalus. Most (97%) GMH occur in the first week after birth. Ventriculomegaly may develop in the first 2 weeks after hemorrhage and may persist for 3 to 6 months. Acute hemorrhage is anechoic. As fibrin is quickly deposited, the clot becomes homogeneously echogenic. A commonly used grading system for classifying the severity of hemorrhage is described in Table 53.3. US demonstrates confined subependymal hemorrhage as a focus of bright echogenicity anterior to the caudothalamic groove (grade I) (Fig. 53.28). On coronal views the echogenic clot is at the floor of the frontal horn, obscuring the caudate nucleus. Hemorrhage into the ventricle is seen as echogenic clots extending into the ventricles, without (grade II) (Fig. 53.29) or with (grade III) (Fig. 53.30) ventricular enlargement. Hemorrhage frequently has the same echogenicity as the choroid plexus. Hemorrhage is differentiated from choroid plexus by location and appearance. Because no choroid plexus is present in the frontal and occipital horns of the lateral ventricles, any echogenic foci in these locations

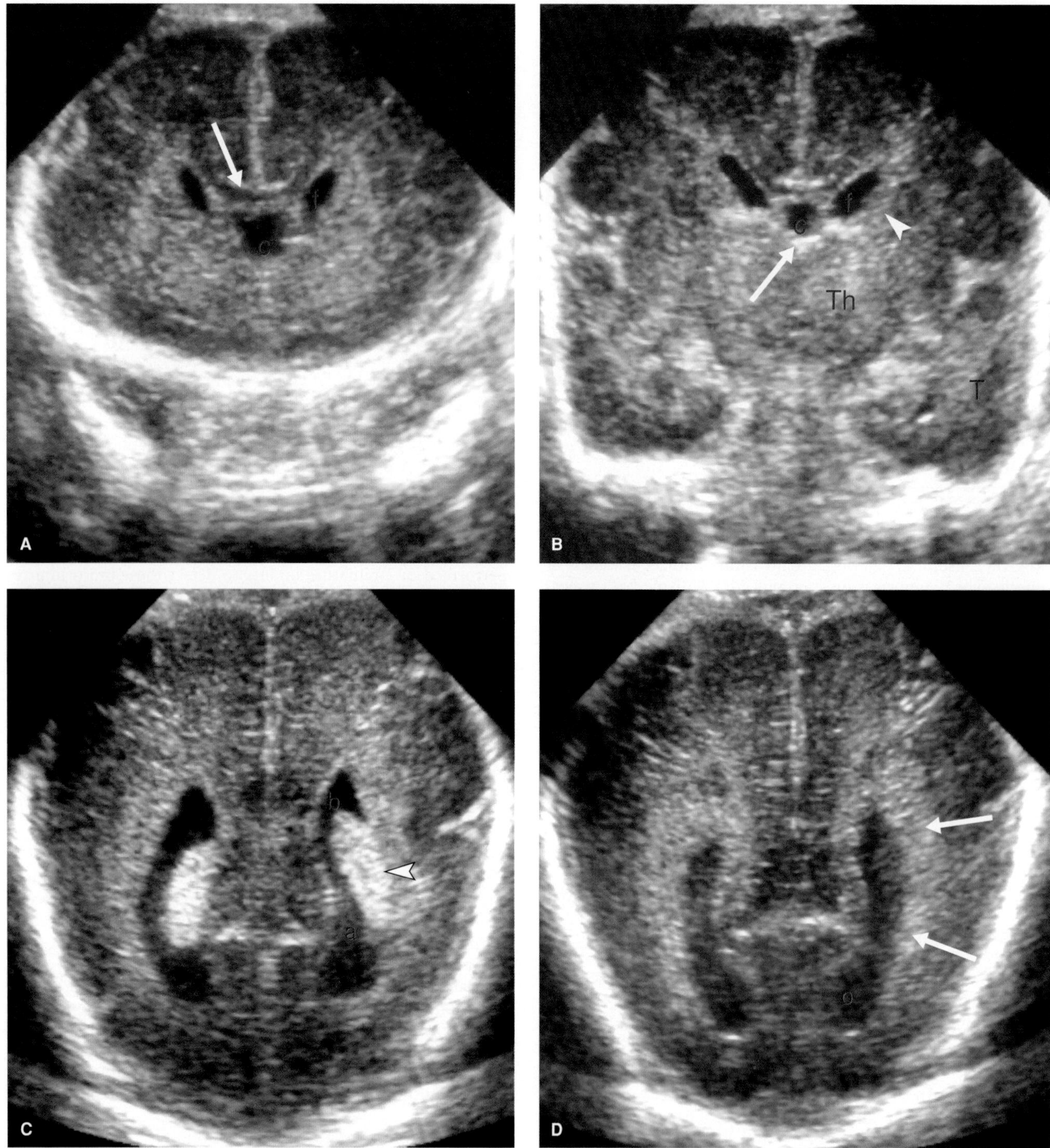

FIGURE 53.24. Normal Cranial US: Coronal Plane. The normal brain of a 29-week premature infant is imaged in coronal plane through the anterior fontanelle. **A:** Anterior image shows frontal horns of the lateral ventricles (*f*), cavum septum pellucidum (*c*), and corpus callosum (*arrow*). **B:** Midline image shows choroid plexus in the roof of the third ventricle (*arrow*), cavum septum pellucidum (*c*), frontal horns of the lateral ventricle (*f*), and caudate nucleus (*arrowhead*). The third ventricle is slit like between the lobes of the thalamus (*Th*) and inferior to its choroid plexus. The location of the third ventricle can be inferred but is not discretely visualized on this image. *T*, temporal lobe. **C:** Posterior image through the body (*b*) and atria (*a*) (trigone) of the lateral ventricles demonstrates the choroid plexus (*arrowhead*), which lies dependently against the down (left) side of the ventricles. The choroid plexus can shift with gravity. In this case, the infant was lying on his left side when this examination was performed. **D:** More posteriorly angled image shows the occipital horns (*o*) of the lateral ventricles and the moderately echogenic normal periventricular white matter (*arrows*). The periventricular white matter tracts are perpendicular to the ultrasound beam and thus appear more echogenic than the rest of the brain. Note the paucity of sulci and gyri on all images characteristic of the premature brain.

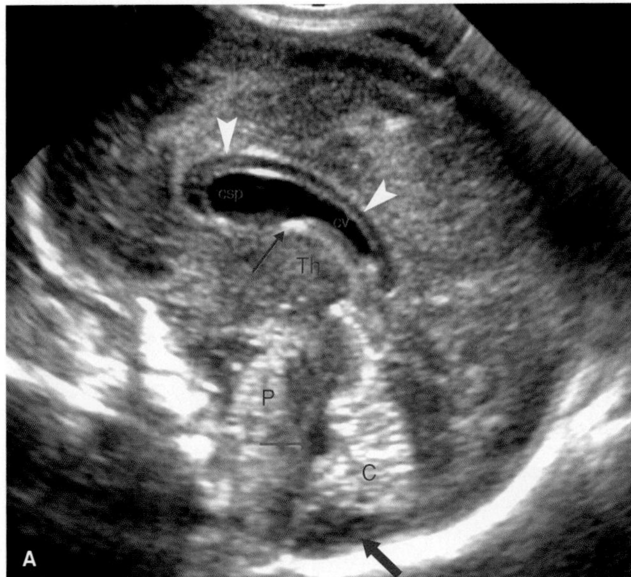

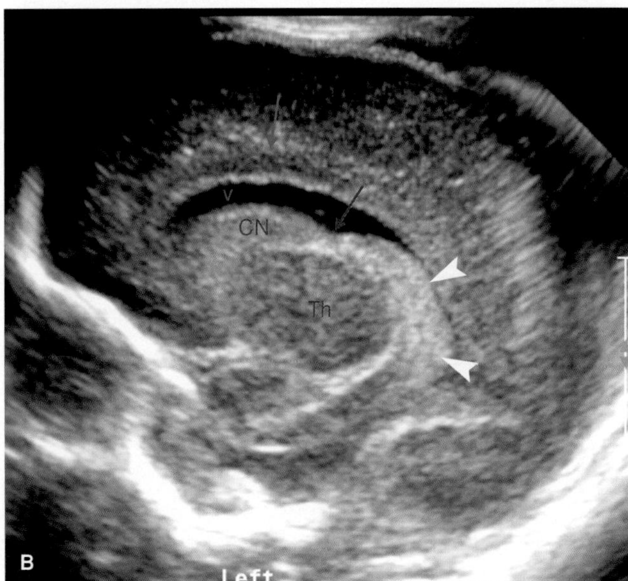

FIGURE 53.25. Normal Cranial US: Sagittal and Angled Sagittal Plane. **A:** Midline sagittal image shows the corpus callosum (*arrowheads*), cavum septum pellucidum (*csp*) anteriorly, cavum vergae (*cv*) posteriorly, echogenic choroid plexus in the roof of the third ventricle (*red skinny arrow*), echogenic cerebellar vermis (*C*), the triangular-shaped fourth ventricle (*blue skinny arrow*), and the cisterna magna (*red fat arrow*). The echogenic pons (*P*) is part of the brainstem. *Th*, thalamus. **B:** Laterally angled sagittal image shows the lateral ventricle (*v*), the echogenic caudate nucleus (*arrowheads*) which fills the atrium of the lateral ventricle, the caudate nucleus (*CN*), the thalamus (*Th*), and the caudothalamic groove (*red arrow*). The caudothalamic groove is a landmark for the location of the foramen of Monro. No choroid plexus is located anterior to the foramen of Monro. Echogenic foci overlying the caudate nucleus anterior to the caudothalamic groove are caused by germinal matrix hemorrhage in the premature infant. The linear tracts of the periventricular white matter (*blue arrow*) are parallel to the ultrasound beam in this image and are thus near isoechoic with the rest of the brain.

likely represent hemorrhage. Asymmetric enlargement of the choroid plexus is suspicious for hemorrhage. Parenchymal hematomas (Fig. 53.31) (grade IV) result from hemorrhagic infarction caused by obstruction of the medullary veins by the GMH. The sonographic appearance of hematomas follows a predictable evolution. The hematoma is initially densely echogenic, then becomes progressively echolucent centrally as it shrinks, maintaining an echogenic rim. Small cysts may form (Fig. 53.32). Eventually the clots resolve completely. Cellular debris from the hemorrhage is seen as echogenic material floating within the intraventricular cerebrospinal fluid. Hydrocephalus is a common sequelae of GMH. Hydrocephalus may result from obstruction of cerebrospinal fluid pathways by clot, organizing ependymitis, or arachnoid granulation obstruction. Spastic paralysis results from injury to the corticospinal tracts as they course in close proximity to the site of hemorrhage. Cognitive defects and learning disorders may also result from the brain injury.

Periventricular leukomalacia refers to lesions caused by hypoxic–ischemic injury in the periventricular white matter, primarily in premature infants. The periventricular white matter, at the angles of the lateral ventricles, is in a watershed zone between the arterial blood supply of the basal

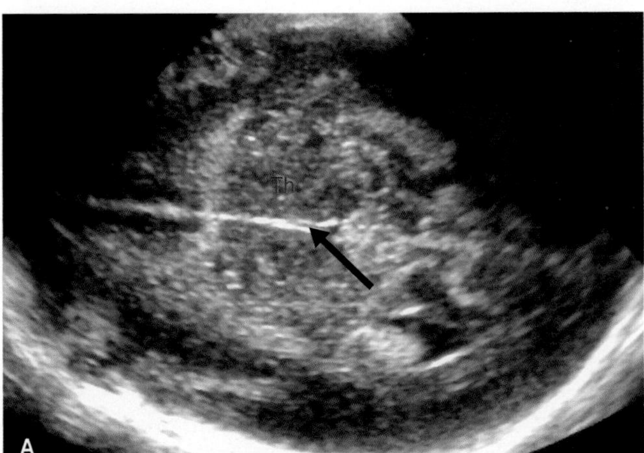

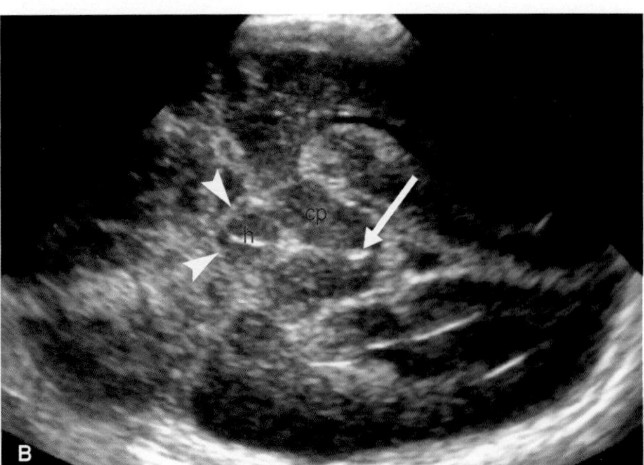

FIGURE 53.26. Normal Cranial US: Axial Plane. **A:** Axial plane image through the squama of the temporal bone shows both lobes of the walnut-shaped thalamus (*Th*). The slit-like third ventricle (*arrow*) lies between the halves of the thalamus. **B:** Image at a slightly lower level shows the hypothalamus (*h*) and heart-shaped cerebral peduncles (*cp*). The aqueduct of Sylvius is seen as an echogenic dot (*arrow*) posteriorly. The circle of Willis surrounds the hypothalamus in the suprasellar cistern (*arrowheads*).

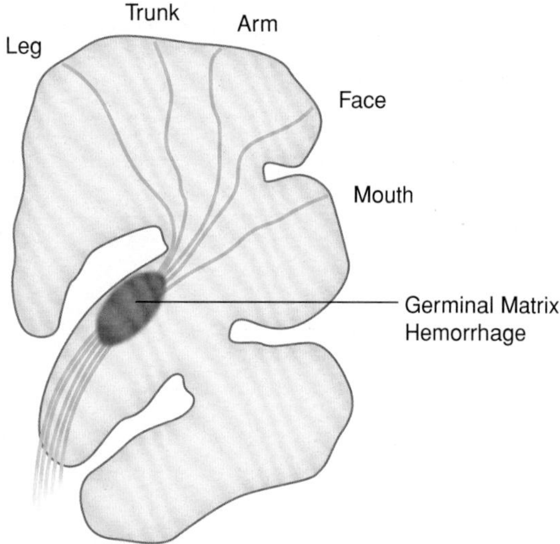

FIGURE 53.27. **Corticospinal Tracts.** Drawing of the left brain in coronal plane shows the corticospinal tracts (*yellow lines*) extending from the motor cortex of the parietal lobe coursing in close proximity to foci of hemorrhage arising from the germinal matrix. The risk of spastic motor defects resulting from germinal matrix hemorrhage is high.

TABLE 53.3

PAPILE CLASSIFICATION OF GERMINAL MATRIX HEMORRHAGE

GRADE	DESCRIPTION
I	Small hemorrhage confined to germinal matrix area (Fig. 53.28)
II	Small hemorrhage with extension into lateral ventricles with less than 50% ventricular dilatation, usually transient (Fig. 53.29)
III	Large hemorrhage that fills and dilates the ventricles with blood (Fig. 53.30)
IV	Intraparenchymal periventricular hemorrhagic venous infarction caused by obstruction of the medullary veins draining the periventricular white matter (Fig. 53.31)

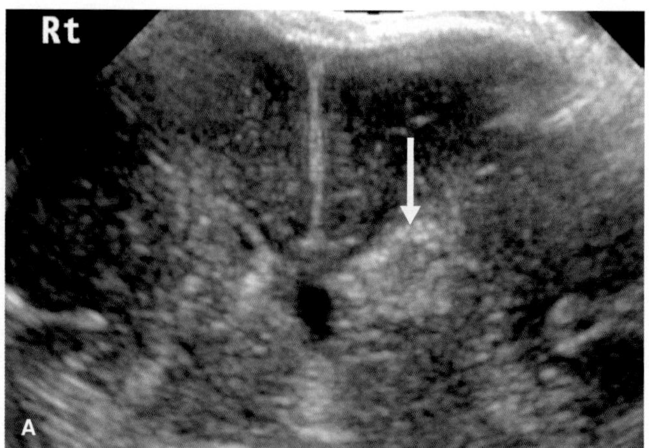

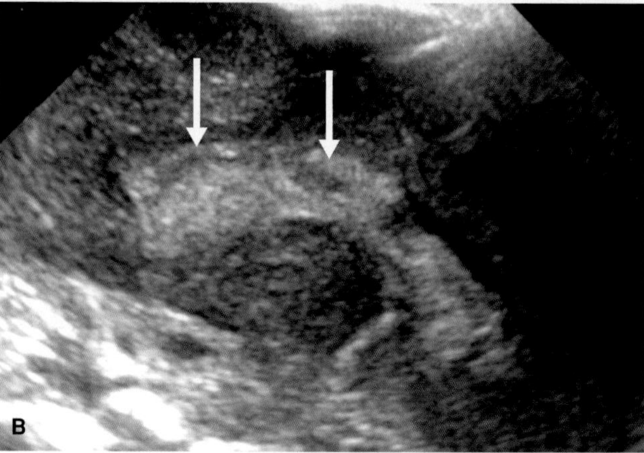

FIGURE 53.29. **Grade II Germinal Matrix Hemorrhage.** Coronal (**A**) and left-angled parasagittal (**B**) views show germinal matrix hemorrhage (*arrows*) extending from the subependymal region into the left lateral ventricle.

ganglia and the immature arterial supply to the cerebral cortex. After 34 weeks gestational age, maturation of cerebral arterial supply moves the watershed zones from the periventricular area to the cortex between the cerebral artery territories. Hypoxia in the premature infant may cause infarction of the periventricular white matter, followed by necrosis, cyst

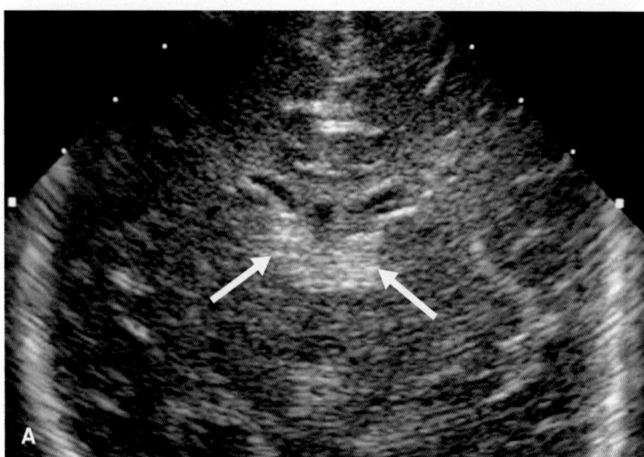

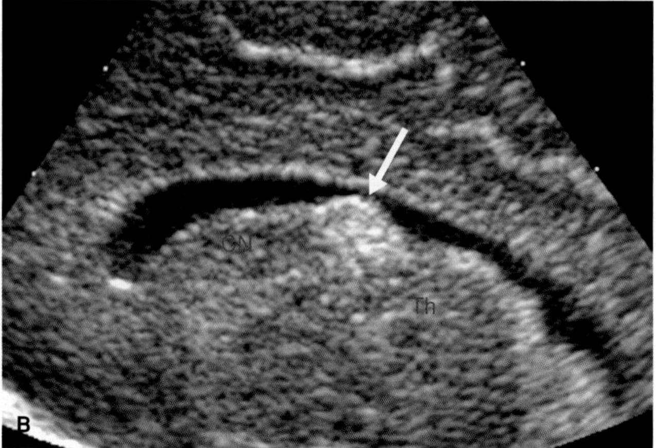

FIGURE 53.28. **Grade I Germinal Matrix Hemorrhage. A:** Coronal US through the anterior fontanelle of a premature twin shows bilateral grade I GMH as echogenic foci (*arrows*) underlying the frontal horns of the lateral ventricles. **B:** Left-angled parasagittal view shows the echogenic hemorrhage (*arrow*) just anterior to the caudothalamic groove. *CN*, caudate nucleus; *Th*, thalamus.

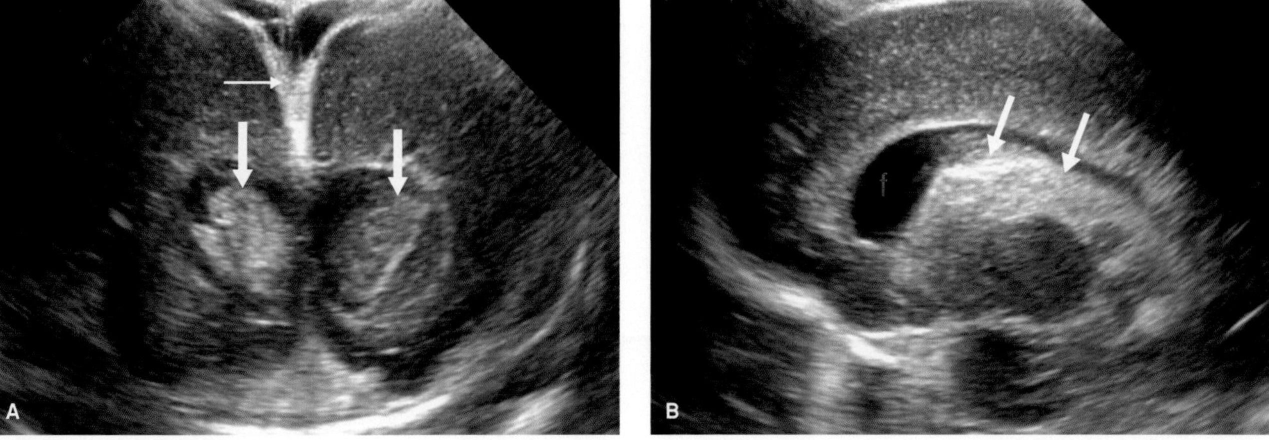

FIGURE 53.30. **Grade III Germinal Matrix Hemorrhage. A:** Coronal US shows bilateral hemorrhage (*fat arrows*) filling and dilating both frontal horns of the lateral ventricles. The hemorrhage has extended into the cerebrospinal fluid spaces and has caused meningeal inflammation seen as echogenic thickening (*skinny arrow*) in the midline sagittal fissure. **B:** A left parasagittal view shows hemorrhage (*arrows*) filling and dilating the left lateral ventricle and encompassing the choroid plexus. The echogenicity of clot and choroid plexus is nearly identical. The frontal horn (*f*) is dilated.

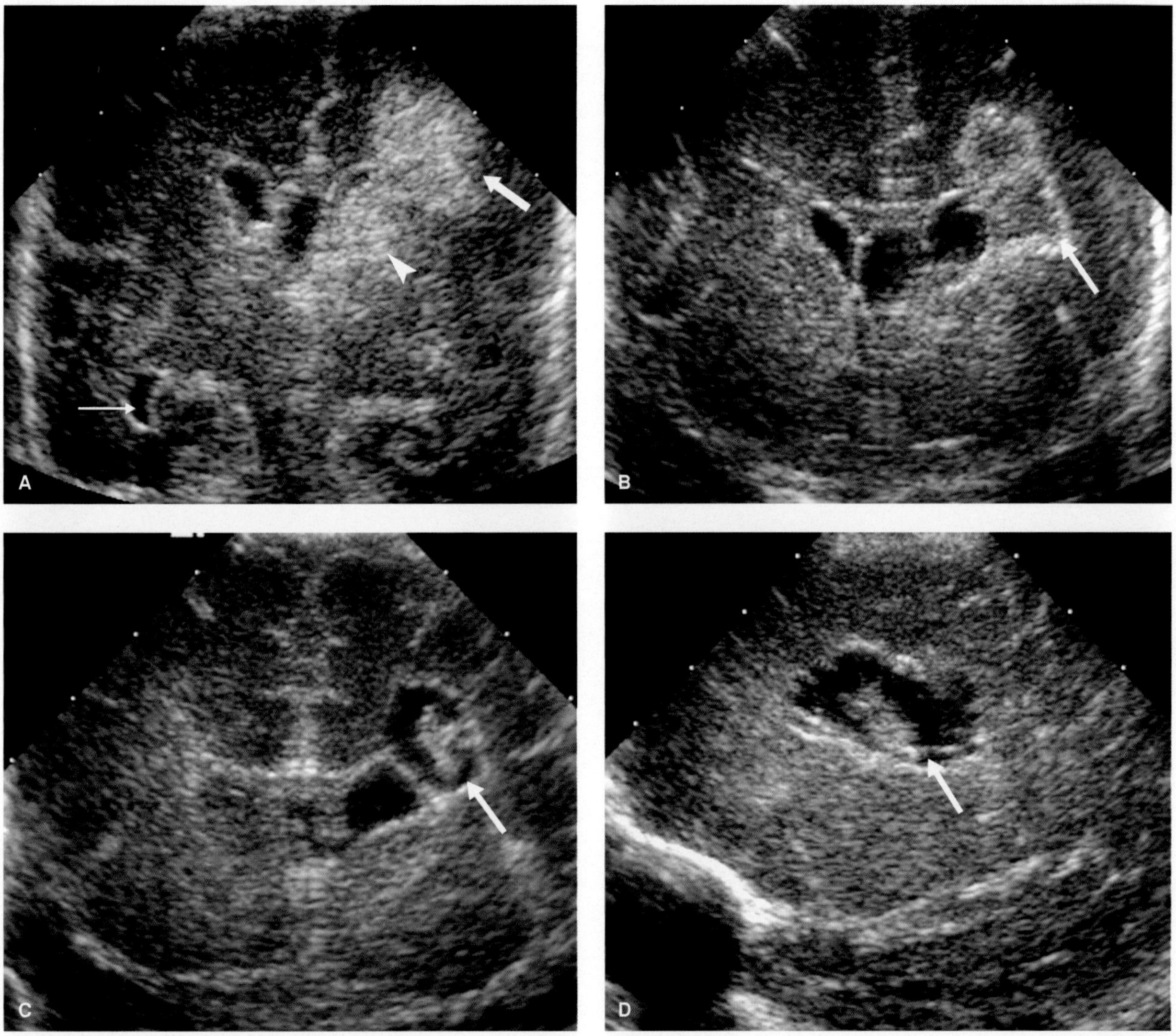

FIGURE 53.31. **Grade IV Germinal Matrix Hemorrhage Resulting in Porencephaly. A:** Coronal brain image on the third day of life for a premature infant shows germinal matrix hemorrhage in the caudate nucleus (*arrowhead*) extending into the periventricular brain parenchyma (*fat arrow*). The temporal horn (*skinny arrow*) of the right lateral ventricle is dilated. **B:** Two weeks later, the hemorrhage (*arrow*) has evolved and now shows a low echogenicity center with an echogenic rim. **C:** At 6 weeks after initial hemorrhage, the parenchymal infarction has evolved into an area of porencephaly (*arrow*) still containing some clot. **D:** Left-angled parasagittal image obtained during the same examination as image (C) shows the size of brain destruction (*arrow*) resulting in porencephaly.

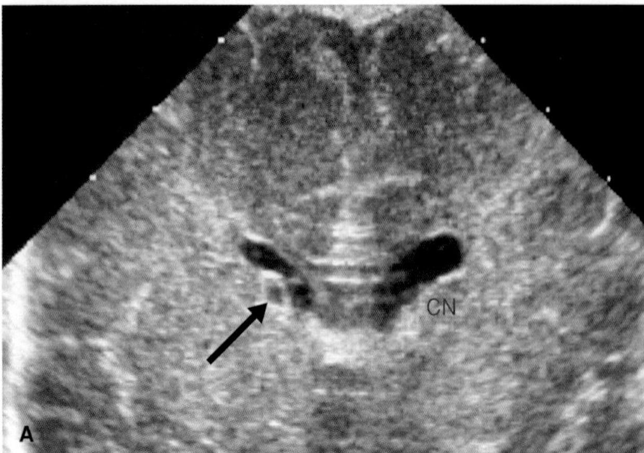

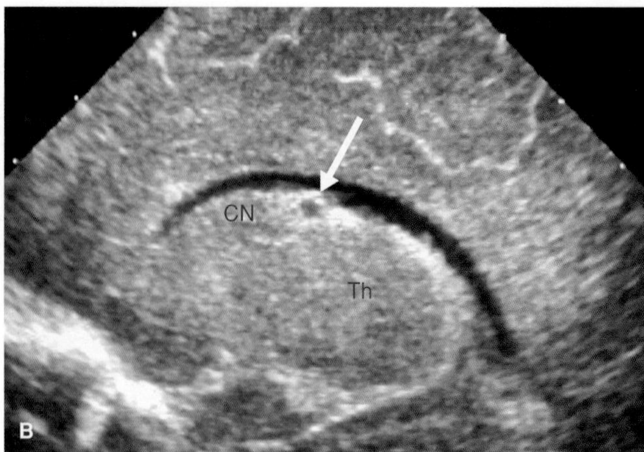

FIGURE 53.32. **Evolved Grade I Germinal Matrix Hemorrhage. A:** Coronal US at 3 weeks of age shows evolution of a grade I GMH into a subependymal cyst (*arrow*). Note its characteristic location overlying the caudate nucleus (*CN*) in the frontal horn of the lateral ventricle. **B:** Right-angled parasagittal view shows the cyst just anterior to the caudothalamic groove (*arrow*). *CN*, caudate nucleus; *Th*, thalamus.

formation, and gliosis. This injury results from arterial infarction, whereas the parenchymal injury from GMH results from venous infarction. The initial injury is usually not detected by US unless the damaged area of brain becomes echogenic due to hemorrhage (Fig. 53.33). In this case, US demonstrates foci of increased echogenicity in the periventricular white matter at the lateral angles of the lateral ventricles. This finding resolves in 2 to 4 weeks when periventricular cysts may be visualized (Fig. 53.33B). Within 2 to 4 months, these cysts may enlarge, coalesce and form porencephalic cysts, resolve completely, or result in ventriculomegaly due to brain atrophy.

Neonatal hypoxic–ischemic encephalopathy occurs primarily in the full-term newborn as a result of systemic hypoxia or reduced cerebral blood flow. Many cases are caused by asphyxia during birth, which is the cause of 23% of neonatal deaths worldwide. Mortality is 25% to 50% when severe. In addition to brain injury, multiorgan dysfunction occurs, including feeding difficulties, reduced myocardial contractility, pulmonary hypertension, and renal failure. MR is the imaging method of first choice. See Chapter 66, Pediatric Neuroradiology. Diffusion-weighted MR shows evidence of brain injury in the first 24 to 48 hours. US has low sensitivity (50%) for detecting findings of hypoxic brain injury. The primary US finding is diffuse cerebral edema seen as decreased visibility of the sulci and gyri, slit-like ventricles, obliteration of cerebrospinal fluid spaces, and diffuse increased parenchymal echogenicity. A slit-like lateral ventricle as an isolated finding is a common normal variant in premature infants. Severe hypoxia may cause cystic areas of brain destruction and diffuse brain atrophy resulting in microcephaly.

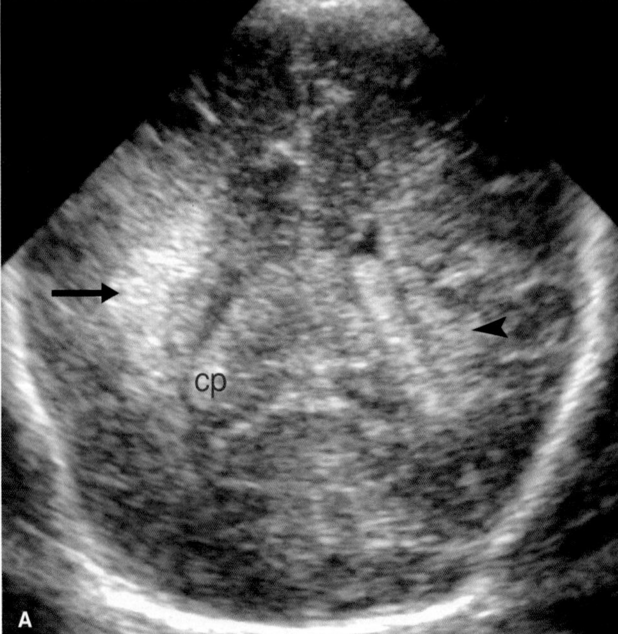

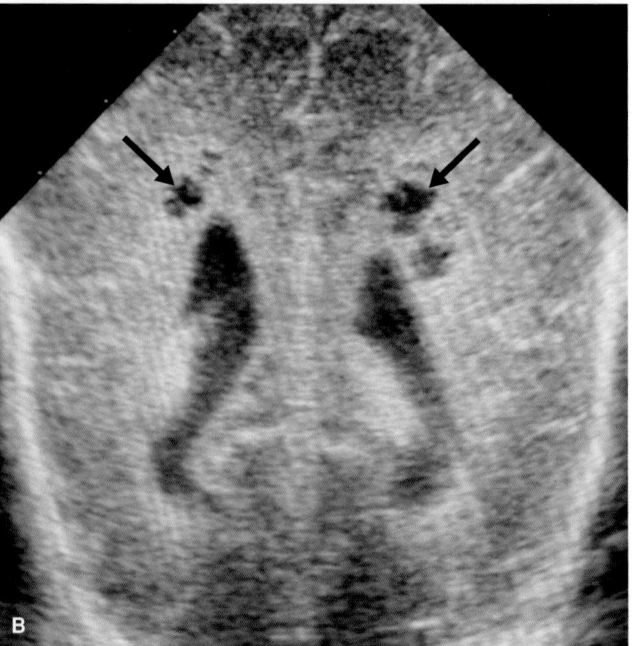

FIGURE 53.33. **Periventricular Leukomalacia. A:** Posteriorly angled coronal image shows asymmetric echogenicity in the periventricular white matter characteristic of the hemorrhage that causes periventricular leukomalacia. Compare the affected right side (*arrow*) with the unaffected left side (*arrowhead*). Compare as well to the normal echogenicity of the aligned periventricular white matter tracts in Figure 53.24D. *cp*, choroid plexus. **B:** Similarly angled posterior coronal image of a different patient several weeks post white matter ischemia shows the cysts (*arrows*) that develop in areas of white matter infarction.

Neurodevelopmental deficits are caused by the brain parenchymal injury due to GMH, PVL, or diffuse hypoxia. Spastic diplegia or quadriplegia is caused by injury to the corticospinal tracts. Developmental delay, learning disabilities, and mild mental retardation also occur. Severe mental retardation is uncommon. More severe long-term prognosis is associated with grade III and grade IV GMH, persistence of ventriculomegaly, large parenchymal cysts, and brain atrophy.

Infection

Meningitis occurs as a result of hematogenous spread of bacteria from respiratory infections or direct spread from ear or sinus infections. *Haemophilus influenzae, Escherichia coli,* and group B streptococcus are the most common causative organisms. Bacteria in the subarachnoid space cause inflammation of the pia and arachnoid. US findings (Fig. 53.34) in meningitis include (a) echogenic sulci, (b) echogenic debris in the ventricles, (c) enlarged ventricles, often due to obstruction by inflammatory exudate, (d) increased echogenicity and shaggy thickening of the ependyma, and (e) transient extra-axial fluid collections. US may be used to detect complications including persistent hydrocephalus, abnormal parenchymal echogenicity representing infarction or cerebritis, and brain abscess.

TORCH organisms cause congenital infections affecting the central nervous system. TORCH refers to *Toxoplasma gondii,* other conditions including syphilis, rubella, cytomegalovirus (CMV), and herpes simplex type 2. Congenital CMV infection is the most common and may cause severe brain destruction. Necrotizing periventricular infection causes periventricular calcification, subependymal cysts, and microcephaly. Toxoplasmosis causes scattered brain calcifications, especially in the basal ganglia, multicystic encephalopathy, and porencephaly. Herpes causes cystic periventricular encephalomalacia, hemorrhagic infarction, and scattered brain calcifications, as well as retinal dysplasia. Rubella uncommonly causes recognizable brain injury, but microcephaly, vasculopathy, and massive calcification have been reported.

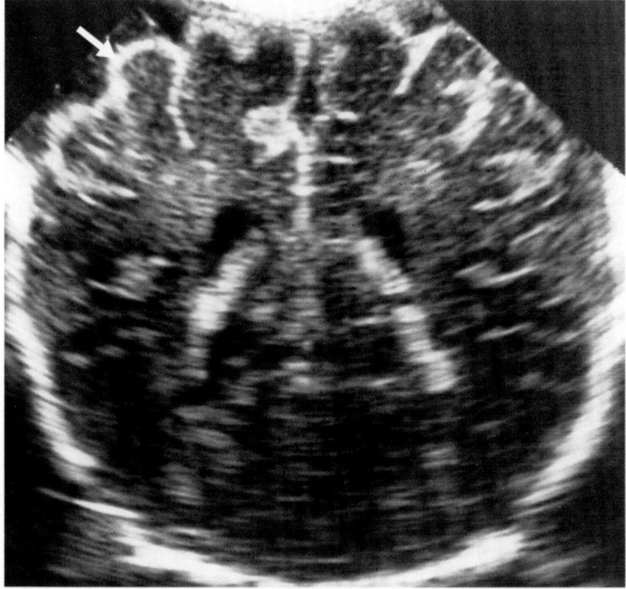

FIGURE 53.34. **Meningitis.** Posteriorly angled coronal US shows marked increased echogenicity of the gyri and sulci (*arrow*) associated with diffuse brain atrophy causing increased extra-axial fluid spaces (*).

Congenital Brain Abnormalities

Congenital brain abnormalities are among the most common human malformations. With obstetric US being routine, most brain abnormalities are detected or suspected in utero. Anomalies of the face, head, or other organ systems in the newborn suggest possible brain anomalies. Cranial US in the neonate can be used in these settings to screen for or confirm suspected abnormalities at the infant's bedside. Comprehensive and specific diagnoses are best performed by MR. Discussions of the classifications and findings of various brain malformations are provided in Pediatric Neuroradiology, Chapter 66.

Suggested Readings

Chest Ultrasound

Goh Y, Kapur J. Sonography of the pediatric chest. *J Ultrasound Med* 2016;35:1067–1080. (Pictorial essay).

Husain LF, Hagopian L, Wayman D, Baker WE, Carmody KA. Sonographic diagnosis of pneumothorax. *J Emerg Trauma Shock* 2012;5:76–81.

Jarmakani M, Duguay S, Rust K, Conner K, Wagner JM. Ultrasound versus computed tomographic guidance for percutaneous biopsy of chest lesions. *J Ultrasound Med* 2016;35:1865–1872.

Nations JA, Smith P, Parrish S, Browning R. Sonographic findings of hydropneumothorax. *Ultrasound Q* 2016;32:280–282. (Pictorial essay).

Wongwaisayawan S, Suwannanon R, Sawatmongkorngul S, Kaewlai R. Emergency thoracic US: the essentials. *Radiographics* 2016;36:640–659.

Thyroid Ultrasound

American Institute of Ultrasound in Medicine. AIUM practice parameter for the performance of a thyroid and parathyroid ultrasound examination. Laurel, MD. 2013. Available from http://www.aium.org/resources/guidelines/thyroid.pdf.

Debnam JM, Kwon M, Fornage BD, Krishnamurthy S, Clayman GL, Edeiken-Monroe BS. Sonographic evaluation of intrathyroid metastases. *J Ultrasound Med* 2017;36:69–76.

Klang K, Kamaya A, Tahvildari AM, Jeffrey RB, Desser TS. Atypical thyroid cancers on sonography. *Ultrasound Q* 2015;31:69–74.

Middleton WD, Teefey SA, Reading CC, et al. Multiinstitutional analysis of thyroid nodule risk stratification using the American College of Radiology Thyroid Imaging Reporting and Data System. *AJR Am J Roentgenol* 2017;208:1331–1341.

Oppenheimer DC, Giampoli E, Montoya S, Patel S, Dogra V. Sonographic features of nodular Hashimoto thyroiditis. *Ultrasound Q* 2016;32:271–276.

Tessler FN, Middleton WD, Grant EG, et al. ACR thyroid imaging, reporting and data system (TI-RADS): white paper of the ACR TI-RADS Committee. *J Am Coll Radiol* 2017;14:587–595.

Wang Z, Fu B, Xiao Y, Liao J, Xie P. Primary thyroid lymphoma has different sonographic and color Doppler features compared to nodular goiter. *J Ultrasound Med* 2015;34:317–323.

Xie C, Cox P, Taylor N, LaPorte S. Ultrasonography of thyroid nodules: a pictorial review. *Insights Imaging* 2016;7:77–86.

Parathyroid Ultrasound

Chandramohan A, Sathyakumar K, John RA, et al. Atypical ultrasound features of parathyroid tumours may bear a relationship to their clinical and biochemical presentation. *Insights Imaging* 2014;5:103–111.

Devcic Z, Jefffrey RB, Kamaya A, Desser TS. The elusive parathyroid adenoma: techniques for detection. *Ultrasound Q* 2013;29:179–187.

Kluijfhout WP, Pasternak JD, Beninato T, et al. Diagnostic performance of computed tomography for parathyroid adenoma localization; a systematic review and meta-analysis. *Eur J Radiol* 2017;88:117–128.

Sung JY. Parathyroid ultrasonography: the evolving role of the radiologist. *Ultrasonography* 2015;34:268–274.

Neonatal Brain Ultrasound

American Institute of Ultrasound in Medicine. AIUM practice parameter for the performance of neurosonography in neonates and infants. Laurel, MD. 2014. Available from http://www.aium.org/resources/guidelines/neurosonography.pdf.

Bhat V, Bhat V. Neonatal neurosonography: a pictorial essay. *Indian J Radiol Imaging* 2014;24:389–400.

Cassia GS, Faingold R, Bernard C, Sant'Anna GM. Neonatal hypoxic-ischemic injury: sonography and dynamic color Doppler sonography perfusion of the brain and abdomen with pathologic correlation. *AJR Am J Roentgenol* 2012;199:W743–W752.

Daneman A, Epelman M. Neurosonography: in pursuit of an optimized examination. *Pediatr Radiol* 2015;45:S406–S412.

Maller VV, Cohen HL. Neurosonography: assessing the premature infant. *Pediatr Radiol* 2017;47:1031–1045.

Riccabona M. Neonatal neurosonography. *Eur J Radiol* 2014;83:1495–1506.

CHAPTER 54 ■ VASCULAR ULTRASOUND

WILLIAM E. BRANT

Spectral Doppler (SD) US and color flow vascular imaging supplement gray scale US by identifying blood vessels, confirming the presence of blood flow, determining flow direction, detecting vessel stenosis and occlusion, assessing the perfusion of organs and tumors, and characterizing blood flow dynamics to detect physiologic abnormalities. This chapter reviews the basics of vascular US examination and Doppler interpretation.

DOPPLER BASICS

Doppler effect refers to the change in the frequency of sound waves that occurs due to motion of a sound source, a sound reflector, or a sound receiver. Johann Doppler of Salzburg, Austria, described this phenomenon in 1842. In medical diagnosis, the Doppler effect is used to confirm blood flow by detecting the change in frequency of US waves that occurs when sound is reflected from moving clumps of red blood cells (RBCs). The echoes reflected from RBCs are very weak, having signal intensities up to 10,000 times less than that of contiguous soft tissue; thus, Doppler US instruments require a high sensitivity to weak signals and instrument settings must be routinely optimized.

Doppler shift is the change in frequency between the US waves emitted by the transducer and the US waves returning to the transducer after reflection from moving RBCs (Fig. 54.1). This shift in sound frequency results from the Doppler effect. The reflected sound frequency increases when blood flow direction is toward the Doppler signal and decreases when the direction of blood flow is away from the Doppler signal. An increase in frequency is termed a positive Doppler shift; the sound waves are compressed by encountering RBCs moving toward the sound source. A decrease in frequency is termed a negative Doppler shift, as the reflected sound waves are stretched by RBCs moving away from the sound source. The presence of a Doppler shift within a blood vessel confirms the presence of blood flow. The direction of the Doppler shift toward higher or lower frequency indicates the direction of blood flow. Doppler shift frequencies are within the range of human hearing and produce distinctive audible sound patterns that characterize normal and abnormal arterial and venous blood flow.

Doppler Equation. The Doppler equation describes, in mathematical form, the relationship between the Doppler frequency shift (ΔF) and the velocity (V) of the moving RBCs that produce the shift.

$$\Delta F = (Fr - Ft) = \frac{2(V)(Ft)(\cos\theta)}{C}$$

$\Delta F = (Fr - Ft)$ = the Doppler frequency shift
Ft = frequency of the transmitted Doppler US beam (the transducer frequency)
Fr = frequency of the reflected US beam (shifted by RBC motion)
V = RBC velocity (blood flow velocity)
θ = the Doppler angle = the angle between the direction of blood flow and the direction of the Doppler US beam
C = speed of sound in tissue (assumed to be constant at 1,540 m/s)

The frequency shift (ΔF) is proportional to the following: (a) the velocity (V) of the moving RBCs, (b) the frequency of the transmitted Doppler US beam (Ft), and (c) the cosine of the angle between the incident Doppler US beam and the direction of blood flow. This angle is called the Doppler angle and is symbolized by the Greek letter theta (θ). The direction of blood flow is assumed to be parallel to the walls of the visualized blood vessel being interrogated (Fig. 54.2). The Doppler US beam can be steered by controls on the US unit. The direction of the Doppler beam is indicated on the US image by a dotted or dashed line.

The fact that the Doppler frequency shift is directly proportional to the *cosine* of the Doppler angle has important implications (Table 54.1). First, the largest frequency shift—that is, the largest Doppler signal—will be obtained when the Doppler US beam is directed straight down the barrel of the vessel ($\theta = 0°$, cosine $0° = 1$). Second, no Doppler shift will occur when the Doppler US beam is directly perpendicular to blood flow ($\theta = 90°$, cosine $90° = 0$). Small errors in Doppler angle estimation cause only small errors in velocity calculations at small Doppler angles, but small errors in Doppler angle estimation cause large errors in velocity calculations at angles close to 90°. **As a general rule, Doppler scanning should be performed to keep Doppler angles at 60° or less.**

By algebraic manipulation we can rewrite the Doppler equation as follows:

$$V = \frac{(\Delta F)(C)}{2(Ft)(\cos\theta)}$$

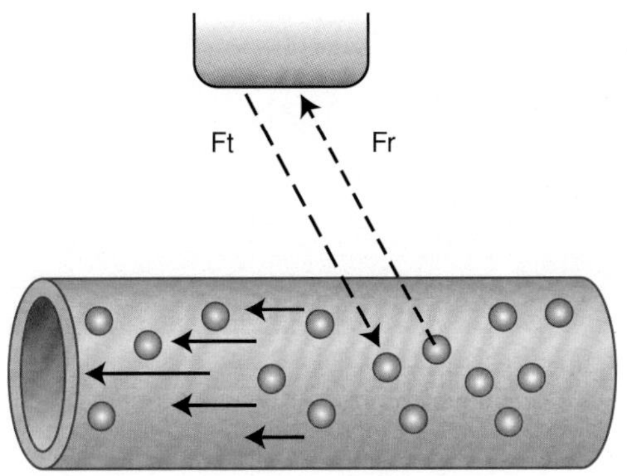

FIGURE 54.1. **Doppler Frequency Shift.** The transmitted Doppler US beam (*Ft*) encounters red blood cells moving toward it within a visualized blood vessel. The RBC motion causes an increase in frequency of the returning echo (*Fr*) due to the Doppler effect. The US instrument detects and measures the frequency of the returning Doppler signal, confirming the presence of blood flow and its direction by the presence and direction of the Doppler frequency shift.

TABLE 54.1

COSINE VALUES

■ ANGLE	■ COSINE
0°	1
10°	0.98
20°	0.93
30°	0.87
40°	0.77
50°	0.64
60°	0.50
70°	0.34
80°	0.17
90°	0

The US unit detects and measures the frequency of the Doppler beam reflected from moving RBCs (*Fr*) and calculates the Doppler frequency shift ($\Delta F = Ft - Fr$). The transmission frequency (*Ft*) is determined by the transducer chosen to perform the examination. The speed of sound in human tissue is assumed to be constant (C). The operator communicates the Doppler angle to the US unit by aligning the Doppler angle "wings" to be parallel with the walls of the vessels examined (Figs. 54.2 and 54.3).

Because depth of a structure in a US image is measured by the time delay between transmission of the US into tissue and the return of the echo from the structure, we can limit Doppler information to a selected Doppler "*sample volume*" by use of a "time window." The length of the time window determines the size of the sample volume, and the time delay of the time window determines its depth. Thus, we can restrict Doppler information to a small portion of a single visualized vessel. On most Doppler US units, the size and location of the Doppler sample volume is indicated by two short parallel lines along the Doppler beam indicator line (Figs. 54.2 and 54.3). Simultaneous gray scale imaging and Doppler scanning is called duplex US. Both SD and color Doppler (CD) imaging are examples of duplex imaging.

Doppler Spectral Display. Returning Doppler signals are processed using a fast Fourier transform spectrum analyzer that

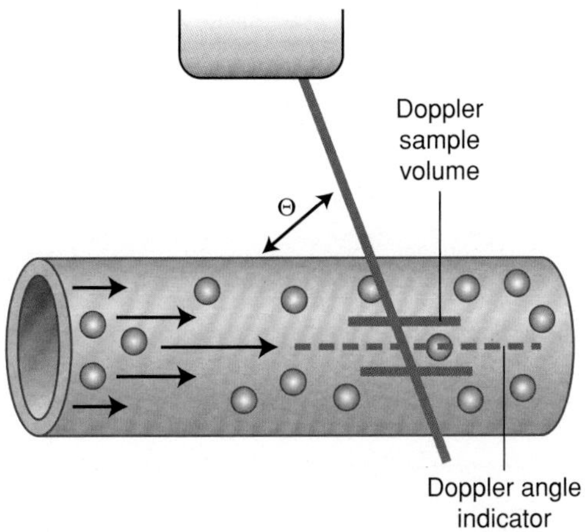

FIGURE 54.2. **Doppler Angle.** The Doppler angle, *q*, is defined as the angle between the Doppler US beam and the direction of blood flow, which is assumed to be parallel to the walls of the blood vessel. The Doppler sample volume is within the two parallel lines of the Doppler sample volume indicator. The Doppler angle indicator is displayed as a *dashed line* within the sample volume. The US unit has control knobs that are used to set the size of the Doppler sample volume and to align the Doppler angle indicator with the blood vessel walls.

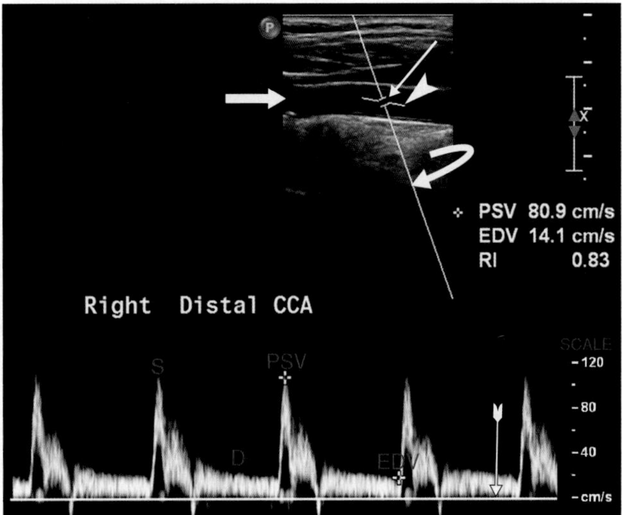

FIGURE 54.3. **Duplex Doppler US.** Duplex Doppler image shows a typical display of duplex Doppler US. The upper portion of the image displays the interrogated vessel; in this case the right distal common carotid artery (*fat arrow*), the orientation of the Doppler beam (*curved arrow*), the location and size of the Doppler sample volume (*skinny arrow*), and the setting of the Doppler angle indicator (*arrowhead*). The Doppler angle indicator is routinely aligned by the operator to be parallel to the walls of the blood vessel. The bottom portion of the image shows the Doppler velocity spectrum of the interrogated vessel. The spectrum is displayed above the zero baseline (*arrow with tail*) indicating blood flow toward the Doppler beam; in this case in the normal direction toward the brain. The Doppler spectrum displays the range of blood flow velocities obtained only from the Doppler sample volume. The Doppler angle corrected velocity *scale* in cm/s is displayed on the right. Systole (*S*) shows the highest velocity while lower velocities are displayed during diastole (*D*). Cursors (+) have been placed to measure peak systolic velocity (*PSV*) and end-diastolic velocity (*EDV*) used to calculate the resistance index (RI).

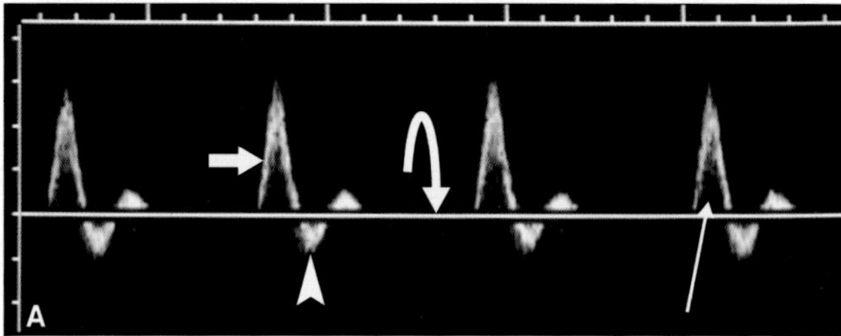

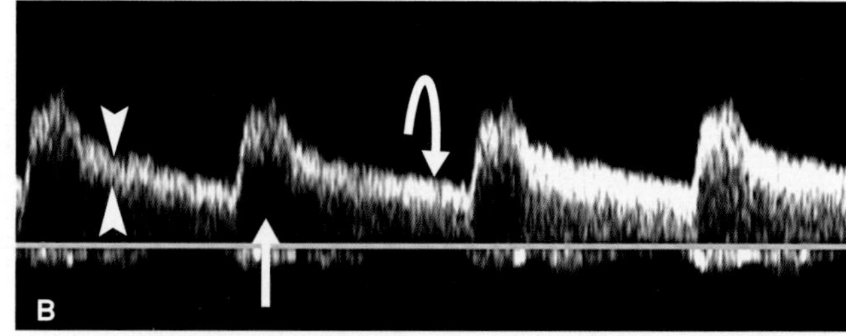

FIGURE 54.4. **High-Resistance and Low-Resistance Doppler Spectrum.** **A:** A high-resistance waveform is characterized by rapid systolic upstroke (*fat arrow*), low flow velocities or no flow during diastole (*curved arrow*), and, commonly, reversal of flow direction (*arrowhead*) in early diastole. This Doppler spectrum was obtained from the common femoral artery. Note the narrow Doppler spectrum and the "systolic window" (*skinny arrow*). **B:** A low-resistance waveform is characterized by relatively high flow velocities throughout all of diastole (*curved arrow*). The narrow spectrum (between *arrowheads*) and clean systolic window (*straight arrow*) is characteristic of laminar blood flow. This Doppler spectrum was obtained from the renal artery. Arteries that supply organs typically show low-resistance waveforms that represent continuous blood flow throughout the cardiac cycle.

sorts the range and mixture of Doppler frequency shifts into individual components and displays them as a function of time on a velocity (or frequency shift) scale (Fig. 54.3). Analysis is performed rapidly enough to be displayed in real time. The horizontal scale (x axis) of the Doppler spectrum represents time in seconds. The vertical scale (y axis) represents blood flow velocity in m/s or cm/s. Because velocity and Doppler frequency shift are directly related mathematically, Doppler frequency shift may alternatively be used on the vertical scale without changing the appearance of the Doppler spectrum. Since blood flow velocity provides the most diagnostically useful information, velocity is the usual choice for the vertical axis. Each pixel (dot) in the spectral display represents a group of RBCs moving at a specific velocity at a given moment in time. The more RBCs moving at that specific velocity and time, the brighter the pixel. Flow toward the Doppler beam (positive frequency shift) is displayed above the zero baseline, and flow away from the Doppler beam (negative frequency shift) is displayed below the zero baseline. Peaks of higher velocity occur during ventricular systole and periods of lower velocity represent ventricular diastole.

Spectral Waveforms. Different blood vessels have unique flow characteristics that can be recognized by the Doppler spectral waveform (Doppler "signature") they produce. Factors that affect the appearance of the spectral waveform include: cardiac contraction, vessel compliance, and downstream vascular resistance. Cardiac arrhythmias are reflected in the periodicity of the systolic peaks and the velocities reached during each cardiac contraction. A major determinant of the spectral waveform's appearance is the resistance to blood flow offered by the vascular bed supplied by the artery being studied. Arteries can be categorized as high resistance or low resistance based upon their Doppler spectral waveform. *High-resistance* spectral waveforms are characterized by velocities that increase sharply with systole, decrease rapidly with cessation of ventricular contraction, and show little or no forward flow during diastole (Fig. 54.4A). Blood flow direction may reverse briefly during early diastole producing a triphasic waveform. Blood flow in high-resistance arteries is always under considerable pressure and encounters constricted arterioles that impede forward blood flow. Pulse pressures traveling down the arterial tree are highly reflected, which results in minimal flow to the capillary bed during diastole. Diastolic flow velocity is low, absent, or reversed, and pulse pressure is high. The ratio of systolic velocity to diastolic velocity (pulsatility) is high. Arteries that normally show a high-resistance pattern Doppler waveform include arteries that supply primarily skeletal muscles at rest including the iliac, femoral, popliteal, subclavian, and brachial arteries. The external carotid artery (ECA) waveform is relatively high resistance in appearance. *Low-resistance* spectral waveforms are characterized by a slower increase in flow velocity with onset of systole and a gradual decrease in velocity during diastole, with continued forward flow throughout the cardiac cycle (Fig. 54.4B). Arteries that supply vital organs characteristically have a low-resistance waveform. Lower vascular resistance promotes blood flow. These arteries include the internal carotid, hepatic, and renal arteries. The superior mesenteric artery waveform has a high-resistance pattern during fasting and a low-resistance pattern after eating, thus reflecting opening of the intestinal tract arterioles and increased intestinal blood flow induced by food in the gut. The common carotid artery (CCA), with 70% of its blood flow going to the internal carotid artery (ICA), has a low-resistance spectral waveform.

Laminar Blood Flow. Most normal arteries and large veins have a laminar pattern of blood flow. Blood flow velocity is highest at the center of the vessel and progressively diminishes closer to the vessel wall (Fig. 54.5). The Doppler waveform of laminar flow is characterized by a "*narrow spectrum*"—a narrow band of blood flow velocities throughout the cardiac cycle with a "window" beneath the spectral trace in systole (Fig. 54.4B). Large arteries such as the aorta have "plug" flow characterized by uniform flow velocities extending from the center to near the vessel wall. At vessel bifurcations, the division of blood flow results in a small area of normal reversed blood flow near the vessel wall opposite the flow divider (Fig. 54.6). Tortuous blood vessels demonstrate normal slowing of blood

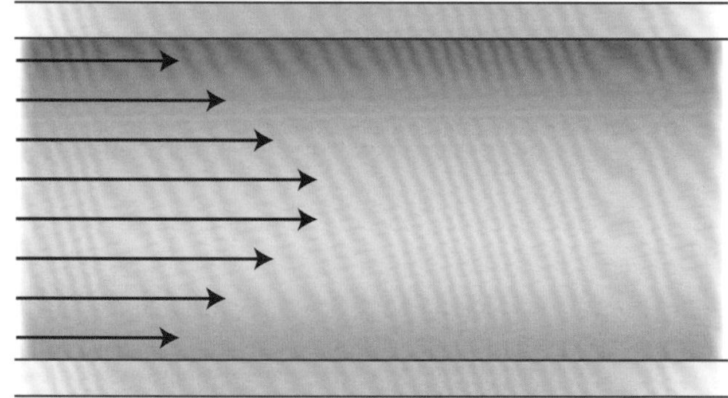

FIGURE 54.5. **Laminar Blood Flow.** Blood flow in most normal arteries is arranged in an orderly layering pattern with the highest velocity in the midstream and the lowest velocity near the vessel wall.

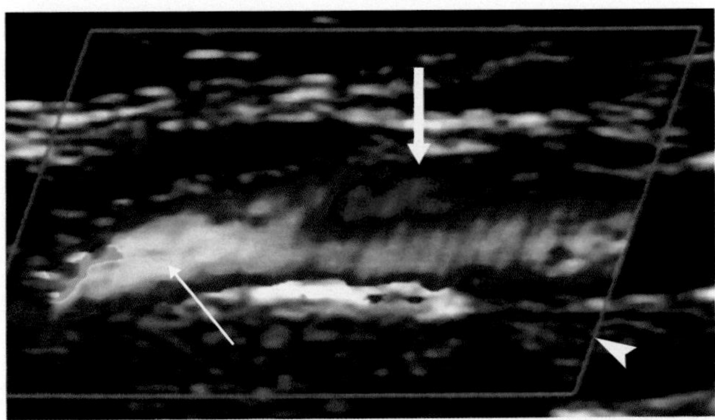

FIGURE 54.6. Normal Flow Reversal at Bifurcation. Flow in the internal carotid artery is shown in red with areas of higher flow velocity shown in yellow. A normal area of blood flow reversal (*fat arrow*) is seen in the carotid bulb. Note how the true color change, indicating reversal in the direction of flow, is outlined in black. The color Doppler interrogation area (sample volume) is shown on the image by the box outlined in white (*arrowhead*). The orientation of the Doppler beam is indicated by the angle of the sides of the box. Higher velocity centered in the middle of the vessel, shown in yellow (*thin arrow*), is indicative of laminar blood flow in the artery.

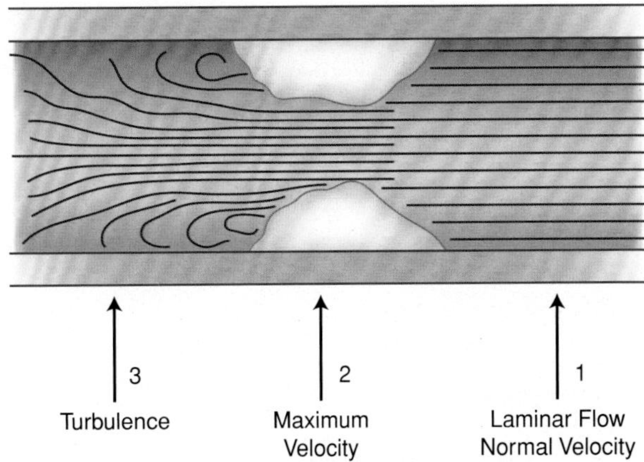

FIGURE 54.7. Assessing Arterial Stenosis. To assess a vessel plaque for stenosis, Doppler spectra are obtained: (1) proximal to the plaque where blood flow velocity is normal and flow is laminar, (2) in the area of the plaque where flow usually remains laminar but where flow velocity is at maximum, and (3) downstream from the plaque where turbulence and eddy currents are detected.

flow on the inner aspect of the curve, with acceleration of blood flow on the outer aspect of the curve. The highest velocities are seen at the outer aspect of the curving vessel, rather than at midlumen. Blood flow velocity returns to a laminar distribution a short distance downstream from the curve.

Disturbed Blood Flow. Turbulent and disturbed spectral waveforms are usually, but not always, indicative of pathologic changes in blood flow. Disturbed blood flow is a loss of the normal orderly laminar flow pattern. Characteristic SD signs of disturbed blood flow are: increased velocity, spectral broadening, simultaneous forward and reverse flow, and fluctuations of flow velocity with time. Peak systolic velocity (PSV) increases with severity of vessel stenosis. *Spectral broadening* is widening of the spectral waveform that reflects a broader range of flow velocities within the Doppler sample volume. Spectral broadening increases with the severity of flow disturbance. However, normal spectral broadening occurs when the size of the Doppler sample volume is large compared to the size of the vessel or when the sample volume is placed near the vessel wall instead of midlumen. Flow velocity fluctuation and simultaneous forward and reverse flow characterize turbulence. Turbulence is most pronounced just downstream from a severe vessel stenosis where eddy currents are produced as the high-velocity flow slows and occupies a larger vessel area.

Velocity Ratios. Blood flow velocity calculations are dependent upon accurate estimation of the Doppler angle. When the Doppler angle cannot be determined due to poor visualization of the interrogated blood vessel or the vessel's tortuosity (as with the umbilical artery in the cord), velocity cannot be accurately calculated. When the Doppler angle indicator is not displayed, the US instrument calculates Doppler velocities using Doppler equation by assuming the Doppler angle is 0° (cosine 0° = 1). Velocity ratios can be calculated from the spectral waveform and can be used to estimate vascular resistance and hemodynamics. The ratios are independent of absolute velocity measurements. The velocity ratios in common use are listed in Table 54.2.

Assessing Arterial Stenosis. Acute narrowing of the blood vessel lumen disturbs laminar flow. Doppler characterization of vessel stenosis is based upon changes in blood flow pattern and velocity. To assess the degree of stenosis, Doppler spectra are routinely obtained in three areas of the vessel lumen (Fig. 54.7): (1) proximal to stenosis, (2) at the point of maximal stenosis, and (3) 1 to 2 cm downstream from the stenosis. Laminar flow is generally present proximal to the stenosis. Within the stenotic zone, velocity is increased but usually remains laminar. The severity of stenosis correlates best with the highest blood flow velocity during peak systole (PSV). PSV may be in a very small region, and a careful search of the vessel is needed. In the poststenotic zone, flow spreads out, causing turbulence and eddy currents to occur and produce broadening of the Doppler spectrum. Downstream from

TABLE 54.2

DOPPLER VELOCITY RATIOS

$$\text{A/B ratio (systolic/diastolic ratio)} = \frac{\text{Peak systolic velocity}}{\text{End-diastolic velocity}}$$

$$\text{Resistance index (RI) (Pourcelot index [PoI])} = \frac{\text{Peak systolic velocity} - \text{end-diastolic velocity}}{\text{Peak systolic velocity}}$$

$$\text{Pulsatility index (PI)} = \frac{\text{Peak systolic velocity} - \text{end-diastolic velocity}}{\text{Temporal mean velocity}}$$

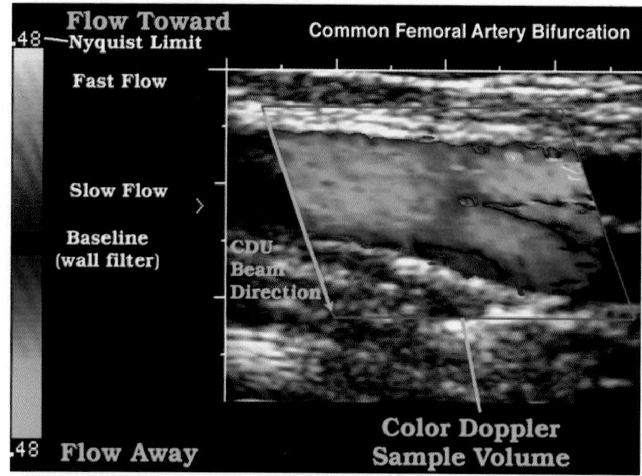

FIGURE 54.8. Color Doppler Image. This color Doppler image shows the bifurcation of the common femoral artery. The color map on the left side of the image shows red as the dominant color above the baseline, indicating flow relatively toward the CD beam direction. Blue is the dominant color, indicating flow relatively away from the CD beam direction. Higher flow velocities are displayed in brighter colors transitioning to yellow in the "toward" direction and to green in the "away" direction. The CD sample volume is indicated in the image by an angled box (parallelogram). The orientation of the CD ultrasound beam is shown by the angled sides of the box. Mean Doppler shift is determined only within the box and is displayed in the appropriate color if present. The background image is displayed in gray scale.

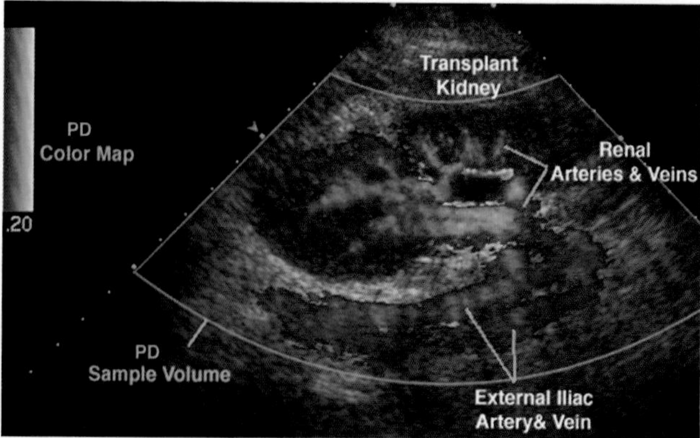

FIGURE 54.9. Power Doppler Image. This power Doppler (*PD*) image of a transplanted kidney nicely shows blood flow in the arteries and veins supplying the renal transplant as well as within the external iliac artery and vein. While power Doppler is highly sensitive to presence of blood flow, it does not show the direction of flow. The shape of the power Doppler sample volume is determined by the nature of the transducer used, in this case a sector transducer.

severe stenosis (>50%), the Doppler signals are dampened producing the *tardus–parvus* waveform. Flow velocities show a slow rise during systolic (tardus) and low PSV (parvus). The systolic waveform is rounded rather than pointed.

Color Flow US. Currently, two techniques are routinely used to produce color flow US images. *CD imaging* superimposes Doppler flow information on a standard gray scale B-mode real-time US image. The B-mode image is displayed in shades of gray, and the Doppler flow information is displayed on the same image in color (Fig. 54.8). Most of the same principles and limitations of SD apply to CD imaging. *Power Doppler* (PD) displays color flow information obtained from integration of the power of the Doppler signal, rather than the Doppler frequency shift itself. PD displays information more directly related to the number of moving RBCs than to their velocity (Fig. 54.9). PD is relatively angle independent and is more sensitive to slow flow than is CD.

On the CD image, flow directed toward the transducer is usually colored red whereas flow away from the transducer is usually colored blue. The operator may arbitrarily change the coloring of the Doppler information. The color map used is displayed as part of the color US image. Faster blood flow velocities are colored in lighter shades, while slower blood flow is colored in darker shades. Color shading is dependent on mean velocities, not peak velocities. Thus, peak velocities cannot be estimated from the color image alone and must be determined from SD. A normal laminar flow pattern will demonstrate lighter shades in the midstream and darker shades near the vessel walls, reflecting rapid flow in the middle of the vessel and slower flow near its walls. Disturbed flow, such as turbulence, is indicated by a wide range of colors in a scrambled pattern.

Changes in color within a blood vessel on a CD image may be caused by: (a) change in the Doppler angle, (b) change in blood flow velocity, (c) aliasing, or (d) artifact. A change in Doppler angle causes a change in Doppler frequency shift, which, on a CD image, produces a change in the color displayed. Variations in the Doppler angle may be caused by divergence of US beams emanating from sector or curved array transducers, a blood vessel curving through the color image, or a combination of both. CD images are used to detect changes in blood flow velocity for further analysis by SD. To interpret a CD image, inspect the color map for color display orientation, then analyze the image for variations in Doppler angle and blood flow velocity.

Doppler Artifacts. A variety of artifacts distort Doppler information and limit the information provided.

Aliasing is a limitation of pulsed Doppler US that occurs with both SD and CD. Aliasing happens with high-velocity blood flow and improper velocity scale and baseline settings. Aliasing on spectral displays is seen as a "wraparound" of peak velocities to the opposite end of the scale (Fig. 54.10). The highest velocities are cut off one side of the scale and artifactually displayed on the opposite side of the scale. Aliasing on CD "wraps around" high velocities onto the opposite color scale (Fig. 54.11). For example, velocities too high for the red scale setting are artifactually displayed as shades of blue. Color aliasing must be distinguished from true color changes caused by flow reversal or changes in the Doppler angle. True color

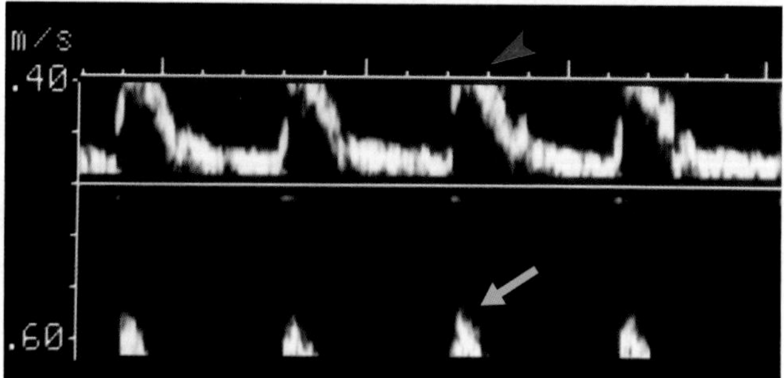

FIGURE 54.10. Aliasing on Spectral Doppler. The high-velocity peaks of the spectral Doppler display are cut off at the top (*red arrowhead*), "wrapped around," and displayed at the bottom (*green arrow*) of the spectral display. The spectral Doppler scale on the left is set with a Nyquist limit of 0.40 m/s, too low for the peak velocities encountered within the interrogated blood vessel. Aliasing in this case could be corrected by increasing the scale in the "toward" direction or by dropping the baseline.

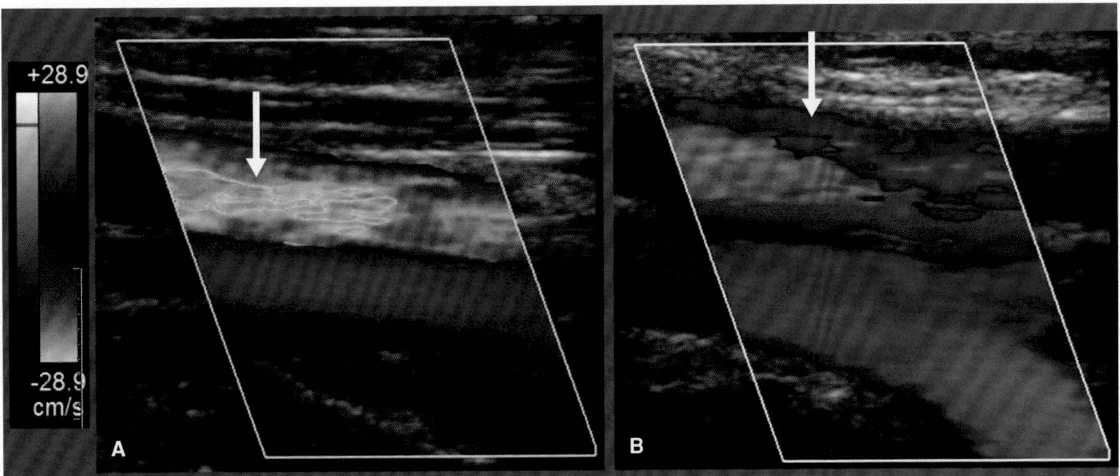

FIGURE 54.11. **Aliasing Versus Flow Reversal on Color Doppler Imaging.** The color map on the left shows that blue is the "toward" color and red is the "away" color. **A: Aliasing.** This image of the common femoral artery (in red) and vein (in blue) shows a patch of blue (*arrow*) in the femoral artery representing aliasing. Note that the blue in the artery is a light shade and that it is surrounded by a light shade of yellow. When the mean flow velocity exceeds the Nyquist limit, in this case 28.9 cm/s, aliasing occurs and the color display wraps around to the lightest colors on the opposite end of the scale, in this case from light yellow to light blue. The highest mean velocities in the femoral artery are aliased and displayed in light blue. **B: Flow reversal.** In this image of the femoral artery and vein in the same patient but taken later in the cardiac cycle, normal reversal of flow (*arrow*) in early diastole is displayed in dark blue etched in black. True flow reversal goes through the baseline (shown on the image as the black border) and involves the darker color shades.

changes are always surrounded by a black border, whereas color shifts related to aliasing lack this black border.

Aliasing occurs when the pulse Doppler sampling rate is too low for a given Doppler signal frequency, thus resulting in an inaccurate frequency measurement. The US instrument measures the frequency of returning Doppler signal piece by piece by a series of pulses. The rate at which pulses can be transmitted (the *pulse repetition frequency* or PRF) is limited by the depth of the vessel interrogated. Deeper vessels require more time for the US beam to travel to the vessel and for the echo to return. To avoid aliasing, the PRF must be at least twice the frequency of the signal to be detected. The maximum frequency that can be accurately detected without aliasing is called the *Nyquist limit* and is equal to one-half the PRF. The Nyquist limit is displayed at the top and bottom of the SD scale and the color map. On CD images, aliasing may be helpful and serve as a tag for high velocities associated with significant stenosis. Aliasing may be eliminated by proper adjustment of the Doppler scale and baseline settings, by using a lower Doppler transmission frequency, or by increasing the Doppler angle.

Incorrect Doppler Gain. When the Doppler gain is set too low, Doppler information may be lost and blood flow may not be demonstrated. The CD image with too high gain demonstrates color in nonflow areas and random color noise. Correct gain settings are attained by turning up the gain setting until noise appears on the image and then slightly lowering the setting.

Velocity Scale Errors. Velocity range settings that are too high may obscure low-velocity flow, which is lost in noise and the wall filter near the baseline. Vessels that are patent but with very slow flow may be considered thrombosed. When velocity scale settings are too low, aliasing occurs. Such aliasing is corrected by adjusting scale and baseline settings.

Color Flash. Any motion of a reflector relative to the transducer produces a Doppler shift (see Fig. 54.26). Rapid movement of the transducer itself may produce a Doppler shift and a flash of color projected over the gray scale image. Most Doppler US instruments incorporate motion discriminators that suppress color flash in hyperechoic but not in hypoechoic areas. Color flash is accentuated in cysts, the gallbladder, and other hypoechoic nonvascular structures. High color sensitivity settings accentuate color flash.

Tissue Vibration Artifact. Tissue vibration may produce color display in perivascular tissues indicating flow where none is present. Tissue vibration artifact is produced in nonflow areas by bruits, arteriovenous fistulas (AVFs), and shunts.

Fluid Motion. Color signal can be produced on CD images by motion of fluids other than blood. Motion of fluid within cysts and bowel may be misinterpreted as blood flow. Ureteral peristalsis produces a jet of color in the bladder that confirms patency of the ureter.

CAROTID ULTRASOUND

Stroke follows heart disease and cancer as a leading cause of death in the United States. Stroke is caused by emboli from the heart or from unstable plaques in carotid vessels or stenosis of the carotid arteries caused by extensive atherosclerotic plaque. For decades, carotid imaging has concentrated on demonstrating the severity of stenosis in the carotid arteries as a primary determinant of risk of stroke and indication for therapy. More recently, histologic and imaging studies have also concentrated on the morphology of plaques in the carotid arteries as being a major risk factor for thrombosis and emboli causing ischemic stroke. These studies have resulted in the concept of the "vulnerable plaque."

The North American Symptomatic Carotid Endarterectomy Trial (NASCET, 1991) demonstrated significant benefit of endarterectomy in appropriate symptomatic patients with 70% to 90% stenosis of the ICA. The Asymptomatic Carotid Atherosclerosis Study (1995) showed benefit of endarterectomy with reduced risk of stroke in asymptomatic patients with greater than 60% stenosis of the ICA. Carotid stenting and carotid angioplasty are additional treatments for carotid stenosis. Advances in medical therapy have also been proven effective in reducing the risk of stroke and preventing progression of the severity of carotid stenosis. Medical therapy includes moderate- to high-potency statin drugs, tight control of low-density lipoprotein (LDL) levels, control of systolic and diastolic hypertension, control of diabetes mellitus, and cessation of smoking.

Doppler US, MR angiography, and CT angiography are the primary imaging methods used for assessment of atherosclerotic disease in the carotid arteries. Doppler US has the advantages of wider availability, lower cost, absence of radiation, and lack of need for intravenous contrast media. Each modality can determine the severity of stenosis and demonstrate features of the vulnerable plaque. Contrast-enhanced MR may currently be the most sensitive modality for diagnosis of the vulnerable plaque. The United States Preventive Services Task Force (2015) recommends against any type of screening of asymptomatic adults for carotid artery stenosis. However, Doppler US is recommended for detection of carotid disease in symptomatic adults. Symptoms include transient ischemic attack, stroke, or other neurologic signs or symptoms. Screening of asymptomatic individuals for carotid atherosclerotic disease remains controversial.

Carotid Anatomy. The right CCA arises from the bifurcation of the inominate artery. The left CCA arises from the aortic arch. The CCAs ascend anterolaterally up the neck, medial to the jugular vein, and lateral to the thyroid. Each artery measures 6 to 8 mm in diameter. US of the CCA demonstrates the three layers of the normal vessel wall: the echogenic intima, hypoechoic media, and echogenic adventitia. The distance between these two echogenic lines (intima–media thickness) is normally less than 1 mm. The CCA dilates normally at the common carotid bulb and bifurcates into the ICA and ECA near the angle of the jaw. The ECA usually (70%) assumes an antero*medial* course off the carotid bulb. It overlaps the ICA in 20% of patients and is lateral to the ICA in 10%. The ECA has branch vessels that supply the head and face. It measures 3 to 4 mm in diameter. The ICA assumes a postero*lateral* course off the carotid bulb and measures 5 to 6 mm in diameter. The arterial wall between the ICA and ECA at their origin is the flow divider. The vertebral artery (VA) arises as the first branch of the subclavian artery, ascends in the transverse foramen of vertebrae C6 to C2, and crosses the posterior arch of C1 to enter the foramen magnum and form the basilar artery. Sonographic characteristics that aid in the differentiation of the ICA and ECA are listed in Table 54.3. Doppler waveforms of the normal carotid arteries are shown in Figure 54.12.

Technique. The American Institute of Ultrasound in Medicine provides guidelines for carotid US examination using gray scale imaging, Doppler spectral analysis, and CD imaging. The common, internal, external, and vertebral arteries are examined as completely as possible. Transducer frequencies >5 MHz should be used for imaging and >3 MHz for Doppler flow analysis. Atherosclerotic plaques are documented as to their extent, location, and characteristics, with attention devoted to identifying "vulnerable plaques." CD is used to detect areas of narrowing and to select locations for SD interrogation. Blood flow velocity measurements are documented at a minimum of one site in the CCA, ECA, and VA and two sites in the ICA. Maximum peak systolic and diastolic velocities are recorded for both ICAs. Direction of blood flow in each VA is recorded.

TABLE 54.3

ICA VERSUS ECA

■ INTERNAL CAROTID ARTERY	■ EXTERNAL CAROTID ARTERY
Larger (6 mm diameter)	Smaller (3–4 mm diameter)
No branches	Has branch vessels
Usually posterolateral	Usually anteromedial
Courses posteriorly to mastoid	Courses anteriorly to face
Low-resistance flow pattern	High-resistance flow pattern
Carotid bulb at origin	"Temporal tap" maneuver

Plaque Evaluation. Carotid plaques are most commonly found within 2 cm of the carotid bifurcation. Injury to the vascular endothelium results in the deposition of a fatty streak in the wall of the artery. Plaque growth results from progressive deposition of lipids, proliferation of smooth muscle cells, inflammation, neovascularity, and migration of fibrocytes.

Intima–media thickness is an index of the presence of atherosclerosis and a determinant of risk for stroke (Fig. 54.13). The thickness of the echogenic intima and hypoechoic media is measured in the wall of the CCA, carotid bulb, and ICA. Normal thickness is less than 1 mm. Thickening greater than 1 mm is associated with aging as well as increased risk of stroke and ischemic heart disease. Serial wall thickness measurements have been used to monitor the clinical response to specific treatments for atherosclerosis.

The "vulnerable plaque." Histologic studies show that rupture-prone atherosclerotic plaques have a distinct morphology. A lipid-rich necrotic core is covered by a thin, inflamed fibrous cap. The plaques show intimal neovascularity, fibrous cap fissures, and have a high macrophage count. They may have intraplaque hemorrhage. Plaques with this morphology in the carotid arteries are prone to rupture, thrombosis, and embolization leading to stroke. Similar plaques in the coronary arteries may lead to unstable angina, myocardial infarction, and sudden death. Rupture of the fibrous cap exposes the highly thrombogenic lipid matrix core to activated platelets and coagulation factors leading to thrombosis. High-resolution US shows an echolucent lipid core (Fig. 54.14). The fibrous cap may be evident as a thin, echogenic membrane. Progressive lipid necrosis results in the plaque appearing increasingly heterogeneous. The larger the plaque, the greater the risk of rupture and stroke. As the plaque increases in size, the shearing forces of blood flow cause repeated episodes of fissuring and intraplaque hemorrhage with interval healing.

Hemorrhage within the carotid plaque further increases the risk of plaque rupture and stroke. However, intraplaque hemorrhage on US does not significantly change the echolucent appearance of the vulnerable plaque.

Ulceration is a severe complication of vulnerable carotid plaques. Ulceration increases the risk of thrombosis, carotid occlusion, embolism, and stroke. Ulcerated plaques show an irregular plaque surface with focal depression (Fig. 54.15). Recesses 2 mm deep and 2 mm long are likely to be ulcerated. CD often shows reversed flow caused by eddy currents at the level of the recess. Three-dimensional US may improve detection of ulceration.

Calcification of carotid plaques is common but not directly to the risk of stroke. However, it may cause acoustic shadowing and block Doppler interrogation as well as angiographic visualization of carotid stenosis. The presence of calcified plaque is a well-established marker of significant cardiovascular disease.

Carotid Stenosis. Duplex Doppler US is well established in screening for carotid stenosis with sensitivity and specificity exceeding 90%. However, studies must be performed to the

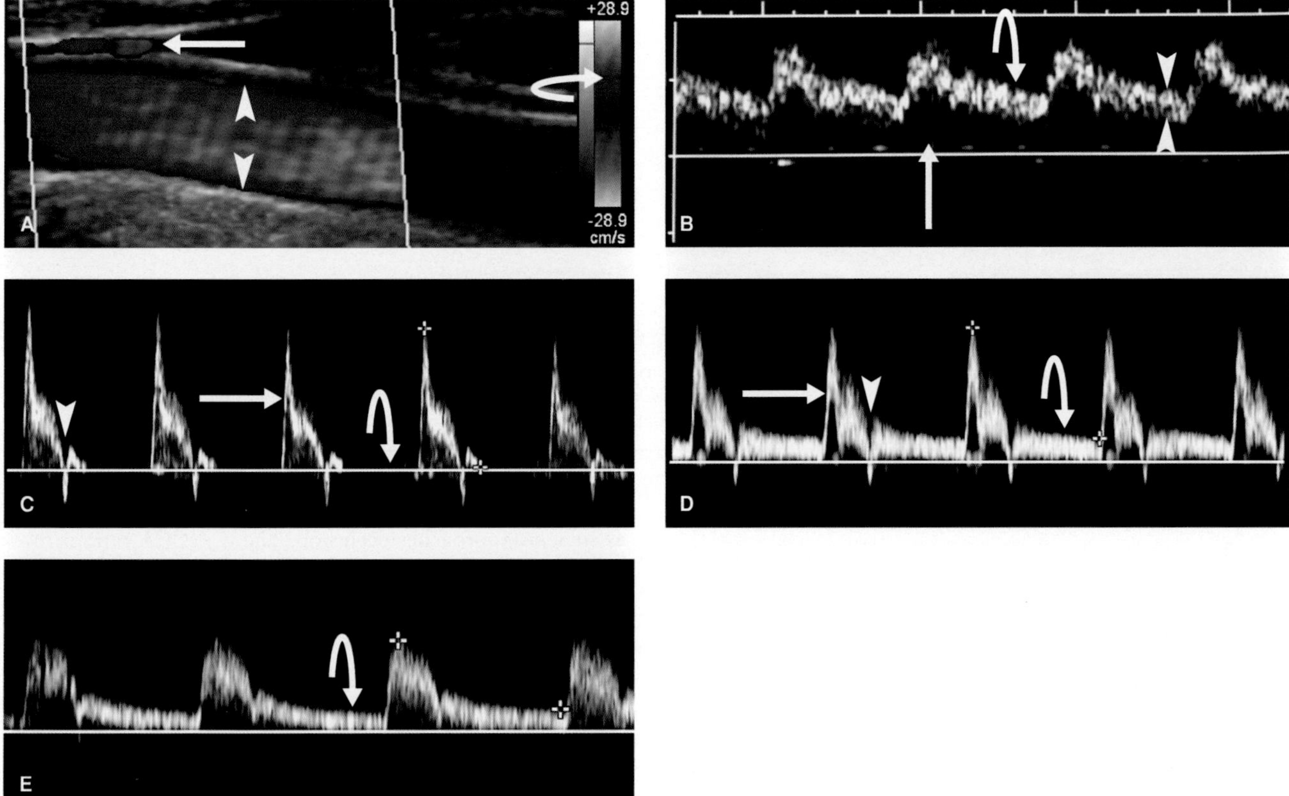

FIGURE 54.12. Normal Carotid Doppler Waveforms. A: Common carotid artery. Correlation with the color map on the right shows blood flow toward the transducer (*curved arrow*) is red merging to yellow in color, confirming blood flow toward the head. Color extending wall to wall (*arrowheads*) confirms blood flow throughout the vessel lumen. Brighter color merging to yellow toward the middle of the lumen confirms normal laminar flow. Motion of the vessel wall caused by normal vessel pulsation results in artifactual color outside the vessel lumen (*straight arrow*). This appearance is normal for the CCA, ICA, and ECA, with the exception of normal flow reversal in the bulb of the ICA as shown in Figure 54.6. **B: Internal carotid artery**. The normal waveform is low resistance shown by the high flow velocities maintained throughout diastole (*curved arrow*), providing the brain with constant blood flow throughout the cardiac cycle. The narrow spectrum (between *arrowheads*) and clean systolic window (*straight arrow*) is characteristic of laminar blood flow. **C: External carotid artery.** The normal waveform is high resistance with sharp upstroke at the onset of systole (*straight arrow*) and little to no blood flow during diastole (*curved arrow*). An early diastolic notch (*arrowhead*) is common and normal. **D: Common carotid artery**. The normal waveform shows features of both the ICA and ECA. Approximately 70% of the CCA blood flow goes to the ICA. The systolic upstroke (*straight arrow*) is sharp, similar to the ECA. Forward flow is maintained at relatively high velocity throughout diastole (*curved arrow*) similar to the ICA. An early diastolic notch (*arrowhead*) is present similar to the ECA. **E: Vertebral artery**. The normal Doppler waveform is low resistance similar to that of the ICA, with forward flow maintained throughout diastole (*curved arrow*).

highest standards with quality equipment to achieve reliable results.

ICA Stenosis. A variety of criteria exist for grading ICA stenosis including PSV, end-diastolic velocity (EDV), and PSV ICA to CCA ratio (Table 54.4; Fig. 54.16). Color flow mapping of the ICA aids in identifying areas of suspected high flow (aliasing) significantly shortening the examination time. PSV is the most accurate parameter for a stenosis greater than 50% and less than 90%. A stenosis less than 50% is more accurately graded with gray scale and color flow imaging in the transverse plane. At approximately 50% stenosis, spectral broadening of the ICA waveform and a mild increase in PSV are noted. Above 90% to 95% stenosis, the PSV falls

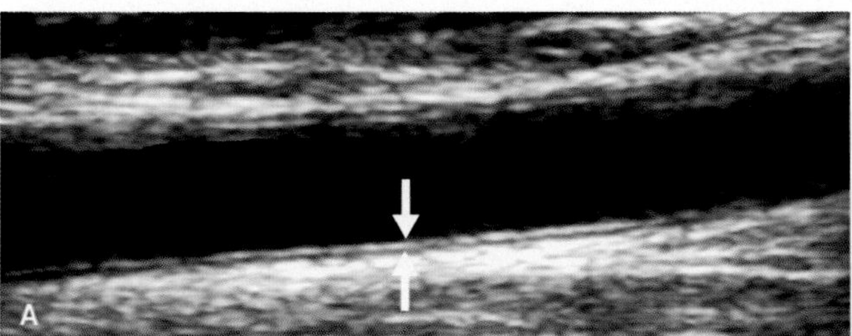

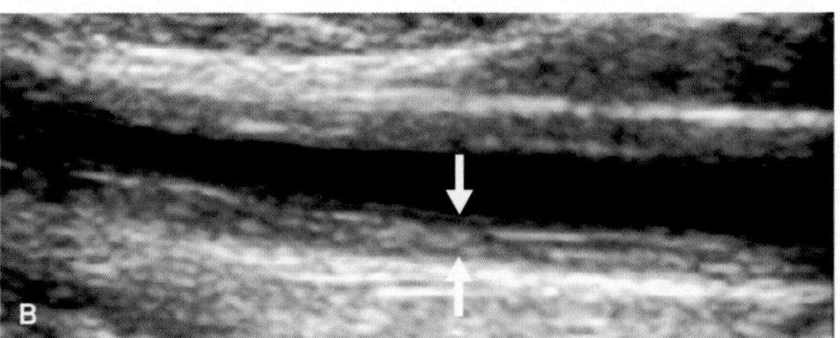

FIGURE 54.13. Intima–Media Thickness. A: Normal. The normal thickness of the intima–media complex (between *arrows*) is less than 1 mm. The normal intima has a smooth, well-defined luminal surface. **B: Thickened.** Thickening of the intima–media complex (between *arrows*) is indicative of atherosclerosis and is associated with increased risk of stroke and ischemic heart disease. In this case the intima–media complex measures 3 mm.

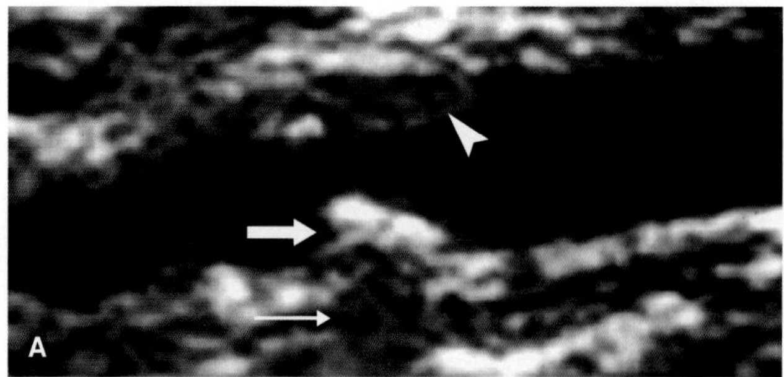

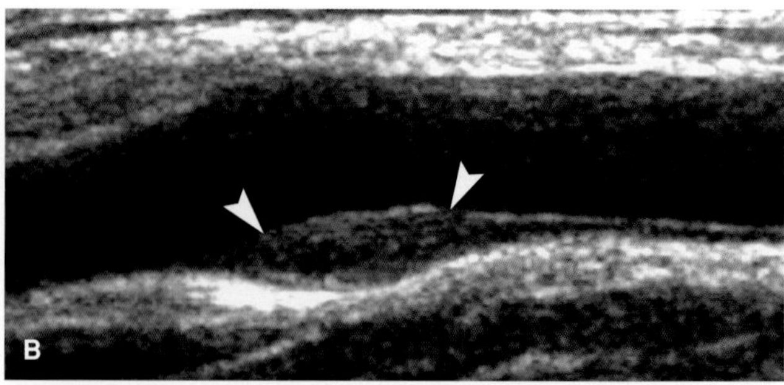

FIGURE 54.14. Vulnerable Plaque. A: The ICA is severely narrowed by two plaques. The upper plaque (*arrowhead*) may be considered a high-risk vulnerable plaque because its core is echolucent consistent with lipid or hemorrhage. The lower plaque (*thick arrow*) is heavily calcified and may be considered a stable plaque, although it contributes significantly to narrowing of the lumen. The calcified plaque casts an acoustic shadow (*thin arrow*). **B:** Image of the mid ICA shows the typical appearance of a vulnerable plaque (*arrowheads*) with hypoechoic core and a thin, echogenic covering membrane. The slight heterogeneity of the core is attributable to lipid necrosis.

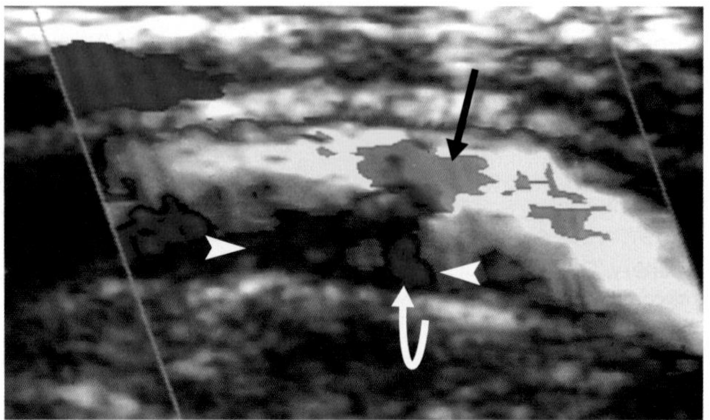

FIGURE 54.15. Ulcerated Plaque. Color flow image of the ICA demonstrates a heterogeneous plaque (between *arrowheads*) with a vortex of color flow reversal extending into the plaque (*curved arrow*). This represents an angiographically proven ulcer crater. Area of blue–green color shift (*black arrow*) represents aliasing due to increased flow velocity caused by stenosis.

as stenosis approaches occlusion. The ICA/CCA ratio is most helpful when the CCA velocities are abnormal (Table 54.5). The EDV (>100 cm/s) helps in distinguishing high grade from lesser degrees of stenosis (Fig. 54.17). Since the NASCET study, many investigators have published revised criteria for grading ICA stenosis. These studies demonstrate the wide variability between the vascular laboratories. Most vascular labs in North America have adopted the NASCET criteria (percent stenosis) for grading carotid disease. Since the lumen diameter of the distal ICA varies among normal individuals and is affected by perfusion pressure, many investigators believe residual lumen diameter is more accurate and a better predictor of stroke. A residual lumen diameter of <1.5 mm suggests a hemodynamically significant stenosis in most patients. For example, a 1.5-mm residual lumen diameter represents a 75% NASCET stenosis if the distal lumen measures 6 mm but only a 62% stenosis if it measures 4 mm. Each vascular US laboratory must develop its own criteria that correlate with conventional angiography, MR angiography, CT angiography, clinical outcomes data, and the desired sensitivity and specificity at their institution. Due to the lack of standardization of performance of carotid duplex examinations, the Society of Radiologists in Ultrasound in 2003 developed a consensus statement, which serves as a useful guide. Their conclusions are shown in Table 54.4.

TABLE 54.4

SOCIETY OF RADIOLOGISTS IN ULTRASOUND CONSENSUS PANEL FOR GRAY SCALE AND DOPPLER ULTRASOUND CRITERIA FOR CAROTID ARTERY STENOSIS

DEGREE OF STENOSIS (%)	ICA PSV (cm/s)	PLAQUE ESTIMATE (%)	ICA/CCA PSV RATIO	ICA EDV (cm/s)
Normal	<125	None	<2	<40
<50	<125	<50	<2	<40
50–69	125–230	≥50	2–4	40–100
≥70 but < near occlusion	>230	≥50	>4	>100
Near occlusion	High, low, or undetectable	Visible	Variable	Variable
Total occlusion	Undetectable	Visible, no detectable lumen	Not applicable	Not applicable

PSV, peak systolic velocity; ICA, internal carotid artery; EDV, end-diastolic velocity; CCA, common carotid artery.
From Grant EG, Benson CB, Moneta GL, et al. Carotid artery stenosis: grayscale and Doppler ultrasound diagnosis—Society of Radiologists in Ultrasound consensus conference. *Ultrasound Q* 2003;19:190–198.

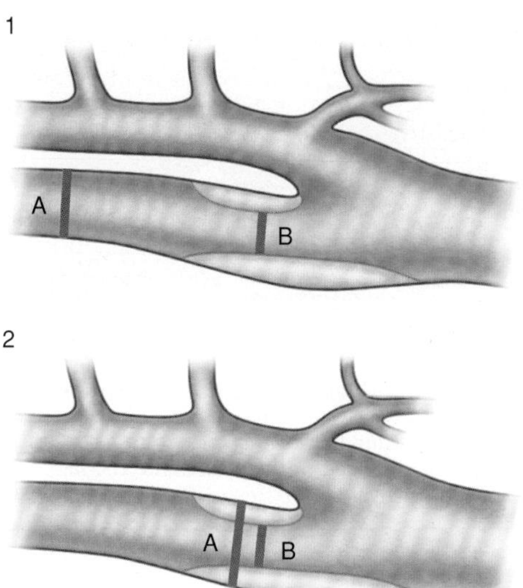

FIGURE 54.16. **Percent Carotid Stenosis** is determined by the ratio of carotid diameter *A* minus carotid diameter *B* divided by carotid diameter *A* (% carotid stenosis = [*A* – B]/A × 100%). **1**: The North American Symptomatic Carotid Endarterectomy Trial (NASCET) defined diameter *A* as being the normal diameter of the internal carotid artery downstream from the carotid bulb. **2**: The traditional definition of diameter *A*, used by the European Carotid Stenosis Trial (ECST), is the normal diameter of the carotid bulb. Most laboratories now use the NASCET method for defining carotid stenosis.

CCA Stenosis. The normal velocity in the CCA is 50 to 100 cm/s in the population over age 50. No specific velocity criteria exist for grading CCA stenosis. However, many vascular labs use ICA parameters (Table 54.4). Along with gray scale and color flow imaging, a *PSV ratio* can be used to estimate the percent stenosis. The velocity at the stenosis is divided by the velocity proximal to the stenosis (Table 54.6). If a significant stenosis exists in the extreme proximal portion of the CCA or at its origin, the CCA may have a tardus–parvus waveform (Fig. 54.18).

TABLE 54.5

CAUSES OF ABNORMAL COMMON CAROTID ARTERY (CCA) VELOCITIES

■ SYMMETRIC CCA VELOCITIES	
■ **BILATERAL LOW** **<50 cm/s**	■ **BILATERAL HIGH** **>100 cm/s**
Low cardiac output Congestive heart failure Cardiomyopathy Pericardial effusion	High cardiac output Hypertension Hyperthyroid Bradycardia
Wide diameter arteries	Narrow diameter arteries
■ **ASYMMETRIC CCA VELOCITIES**	
■ **UNILATERAL LOW** **<50 cm/s**	■ **UNILATERAL HIGH** **>100 cm/s**
Severe proximal stenosis	Technical (i.e., tortuous)
Severe distal stenosis or occlusion	CCA stenosis
Wide-diameter CCA	Narrow-diameter CCA
Long-segment stenosis	Contralateral severe stenosis

ECA Stenosis. Because the ECA predominantly supplies the face, the degree of stenosis (or occlusion) does not affect clinical management or stroke reduction. However, a significant ECA stenosis can alter the waveform of the CCA and cause elevated flow velocities in the ICA. A high-grade ECA stenosis may cause a neck bruit.

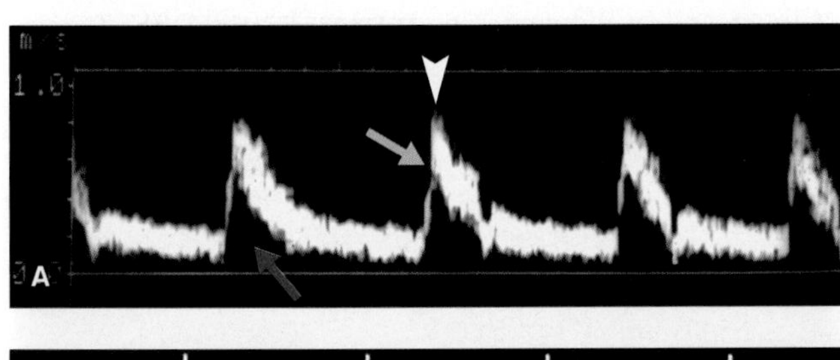

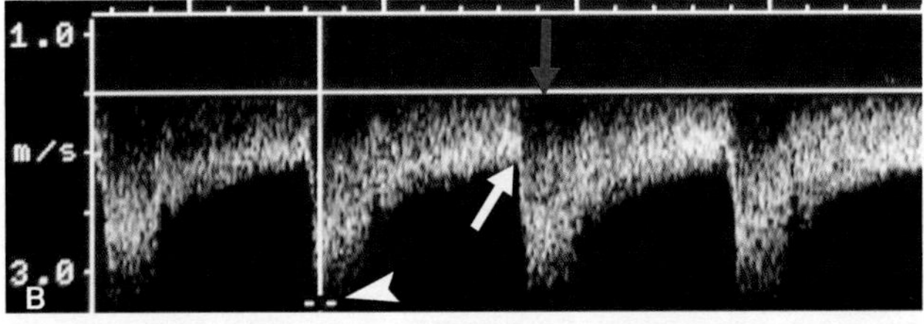

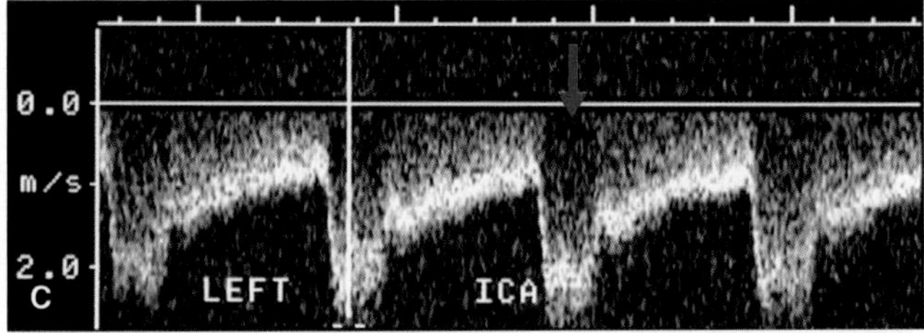

FIGURE 54.17. **Internal Carotid Artery Stenosis—Spectral Doppler Findings. A:** Normal spectral Doppler waveform from the common carotid artery just proximal to the bifurcation shows a normal PSV (*arrowhead*) of 0.86 cm/s. Note the nearly vertical rise (*green arrow*) to peak systole. The clear "systolic window" (*red arrow*) indicates normal laminar flow within the CCA. Compare to the tardus–parvus waveform in Figure 54.18. **B:** Waveform obtained from the narrowed lumen of the ICA adjacent to a prominent plaque shows a PSV (*arrowhead*) of 3.57 m/s with a calculated ICA/CCA ratio of 4.15. The end-diastolic velocity (EDV) (*white arrow*) is 1.25 m/s. These findings indicate severe stenosis (>70% diameter stenosis). Note the widening of the Doppler spectrum with partial filling in of the systolic window (*red arrow*) indicative of disturbed flow. **C:** Waveform obtained in the ICA downstream from the plaque shows further spectral broadening (*red arrow*) indicative of turbulence. PSV remains high at 2.70 m/s.

TABLE 54.6

PEAK SYSTOLIC VELOCITY RATIO TO ESTIMATE PERCENT ARTERIAL STENOSIS

■ VELOCITY RATIO	■ DIAMETER STENOSIS (%)
2:1	50
3.5:1	75
7:1	90

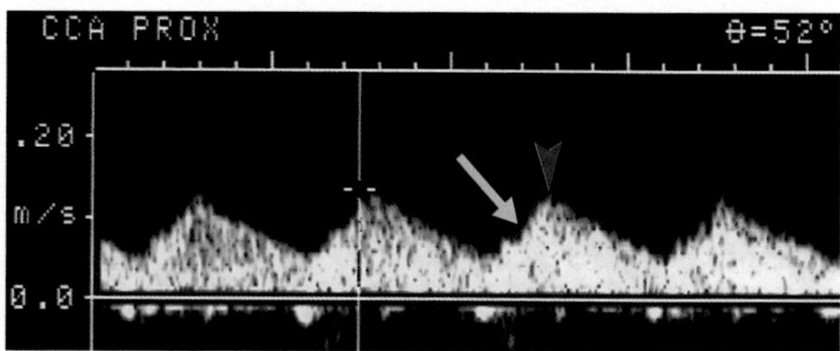

FIGURE 54.18. **Tardus–Parvus Waveform.** The tardus–parvus waveform is commonly demonstrated on spectral Doppler downstream from a significant arterial stenosis. Tardus refers to delayed or prolonged early systolic acceleration (*green arrow*). Parvus refers to diminished amplitude and rounding of the systolic peak (*red arrowhead*). This waveform was obtained in the proximal CCA in a patient with an angiographically proven severe stenosis at the origin of the CCA.

Vertebral Artery Stenosis. No well-established velocity parameters exist for determination of VA stenosis. Because treatment is limited and the VA origin and size is so variable, the detection of stenosis is not clinically useful. Analysis is usually limited to confirming the presence and normal direction of blood flow.

Carotid Occlusion. The clinical spectrum of complete thrombosis of the ICA ranges from being entirely asymptomatic to devastating stroke and death. Asymptomatic occlusion may have a relatively benign course, while symptomatic occlusions are associated with increased risk of future stroke.

CCA occlusion is easily identified on duplex scanning. No spectral waveform or color flow can be elicited within the CCA. Echogenic clot can often be seen filling the lumen. Antegrade flow is usually present in the ipsilateral ICA secondary to retrograde flow through the ECA to the carotid bifurcation and into the ICA. Spectral analysis in this situation demonstrates reversed flow in the ECA.

ICA occlusion is suggested when no flow is identified in the vessel with spectral analysis and color flow imaging (Fig. 54.19). On gray scale, the ICA diameter may be small and filled with echogenic thrombus. A brief systolic pulse (followed by a flow reversal) is usually present at the proximal end of the obstruction due to the "thumping" of blood against the occlusion (called "thud flow"). The CCA waveform has a high-resistance flow pattern with decreased diastolic flow velocity, more characteristic of the ECA. This pattern is often called "*externalization of the CCA*" (Fig. 54.19). If the patient has well-developed ipsilateral ECA to ICA collateral flow intracranially, the CCA may not be externalized. In this circumstance, the ECA waveform becomes more low resistance or ICA-like, often called "*internalization of the ECA*," because it then supplies brain parenchyma (Fig. 54.20). Differentiation of an internalized ECA from a patent ICA is made most confidently by identification of ECA branches.

ICA Near Occlusion. The distinction between total occlusion of the ICA and trickle flow is of critical importance. Patients with trickle flow are candidates for carotid endarterectomy and those with total occlusions are not. Despite advances in carotid US, 5% to 7% of trickle flow is not detected on gray scale, SD, CD, or PD imaging. Therefore, confirmatory imaging with catheter angiography, CT, or MR angiography is still recommended to exclude a "string sign" of trickle flow when the Doppler suggests occlusion.

VA occlusion limits collateral circulation through the circle of Willis and may make lesser degrees of ICA stenosis more clinically significant. VA occlusion may also produce symptoms of vertebrobasilar insufficiency, such as difficulties with balance, walking, and swallowing. No treatment is available.

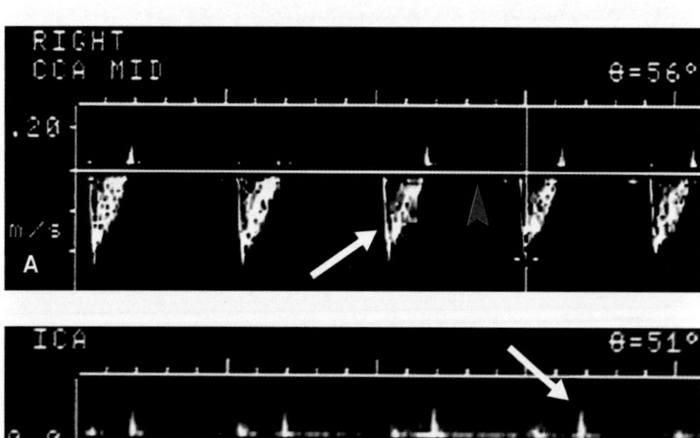

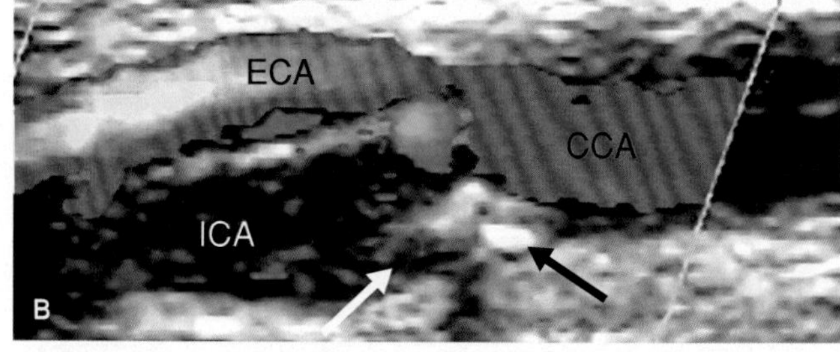

FIGURE 54.19. **Internal Carotid Artery Occlusion. A:** Spectral Doppler waveform (*white arrow*) in the mid CCA illustrates "externalization" of the CCA. The CCA waveform resembles the high-resistance ECA waveform. Note the absence of forward flow during diastole (*red arrowhead).* **B:** Longitudinal color Doppler image of the carotid bifurcation shows blood flow in the common carotid artery (*CCA*) and external carotid artery (*ECA*) but no flow in the internal carotid artery (*ICA*). The ICA is filled with echogenic thrombus. A prominent partially calcified plaque (*arrows*) is evident at the internal carotid bulb. **C:** Spectral Doppler waveform of the ICA at the proximal end of the occlusion shows the typical bidirectional flow. Antegrade flow (*red arrowhead*) slams into the occlusion resulting in flow reversal (*white arrow*). During scanning, an audible carotid "thump" could be heard.

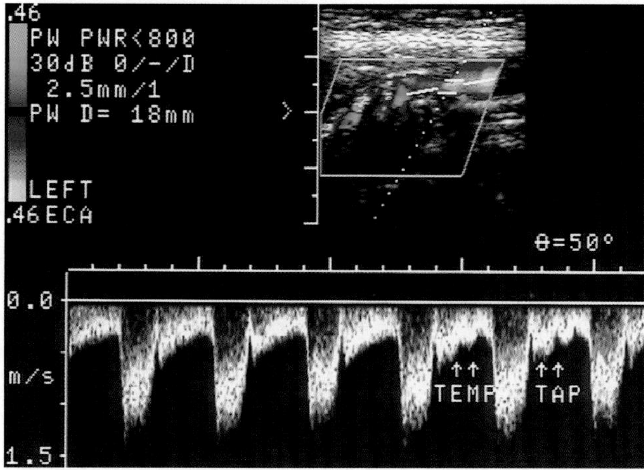

FIGURE 54.20. **"Internalization" of the External Carotid Artery.** Color and spectral Doppler demonstrate "internalization" of the ECA waveform due to ICA occlusion. The external carotid artery provides collateral flow to the internal carotid artery circulation intracranially bypassing the occluded ICA in the neck. The temporal tap (*arrows*) confirms that the artery visualized is the ECA. The superficial temporal artery (a branch of the ECA) is palpated over the temporal bone. A gentle tapping on the artery is transmitted to the ECA and displayed on its waveform as a series of small spikes.

Subclavian steal syndrome results from inominate or subclavian artery occlusion or severe stenosis proximal to the origin of the VA. In this circumstance, the ipsilateral upper extremity receives blood from the CCA through the circle of Willis and down the VA, partially or completely reversing its flow. With occult steal, SD shows predominantly antegrade flow in the VA with midsystolic deceleration and reversed flow only in late systole. Partial steal shows partially reversed flow on SD. Full steal shows reversed flow in VA throughout the cardiac cycle (Fig. 54.21). Doppler findings in steal are accentuated by having the patient exercise the affected arm. Patients may experience symptoms of vertebrobasilar insufficiency and pain in the arm with exercise. In addition to atherosclerosis, subclavian steal may result from trauma or malignancy.

Common Pitfalls. The following may lead to errors in the performance and interpretation of carotid Doppler US.

Angle of Insonation. Ensure that the angle of insonation is less than 60°. Spectral analysis with angles of interrogation >60° cause large errors in velocity calculation. Insonation angles of 45° to 60° can be obtained in most cases with transducer manipulation by the operator.

Tortuous and Narrow Vessels. The laminar flow pattern is disrupted as blood flows through a sharp bend. Reporting of the higher velocity at the outer bend in a tortuous vessel may overestimate the degree of stenosis or falsely suggest a stenosis when none is present. SD sample volumes should be placed away from the vessel wall and within the zone of maximal flow velocity as shown by CD.

Carotid Bulb. Normal flow reversal is usually noted in the carotid bulb opposite the flow divider (Fig. 54.6). This should not be mistaken for pathologic flow.

Calcified Plaque. Dense calcification can make it impossible to obtain velocities in portions of the ICA because of acoustic shadowing. As a result, a significant stenosis may not be detected. Color flow imaging is helpful in this situation. If the color flow into and out from behind the plaque is homogeneous, the presence of a significant stenosis is unlikely. However, if flow proximal to the plaque is homogeneous and flow distal to the plaque shows turbulence, a significant stenosis should be suspected.

Unilateral high-grade carotid stenosis may result in elevated flow velocities in the contralateral CCA and ICA. Flow is increased and velocities elevated to maintain cerebral perfusion.

Bilateral ICA stenosis causes physiologic flow alterations that complicate determining which side represents the more significant disease.

Tandem Lesions. The presence of more than one high-grade stenotic lesion can lead to interpretation errors. A significant intracranial ICA lesion causes a reduction in PSV with absence of diastolic flow in the cervical portion of the ICA. Alternatively, a significant proximal CCA lesion lowers the PSV and increases the diastolic flow. In either circumstance, a stenosis in the cervical ICA may be underestimated.

Mistaking ECA for ICA When ICA Is Occluded. Remember the ECA waveform may be internalized due to collateral flow. Use the temporal tap maneuver and look for branch vessels to identify the ECA (Fig. 54.20).

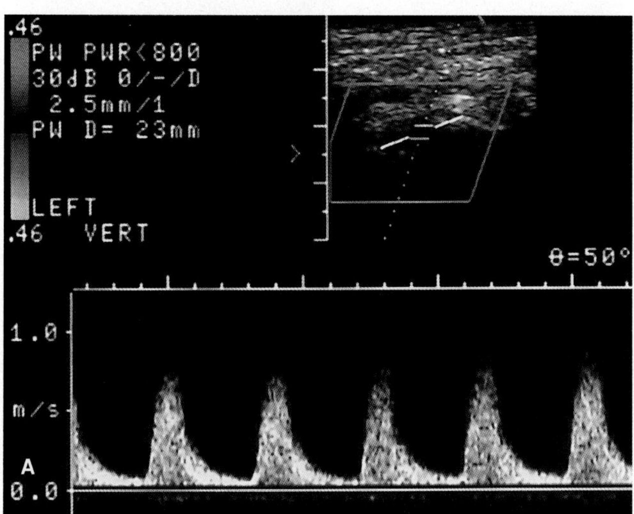

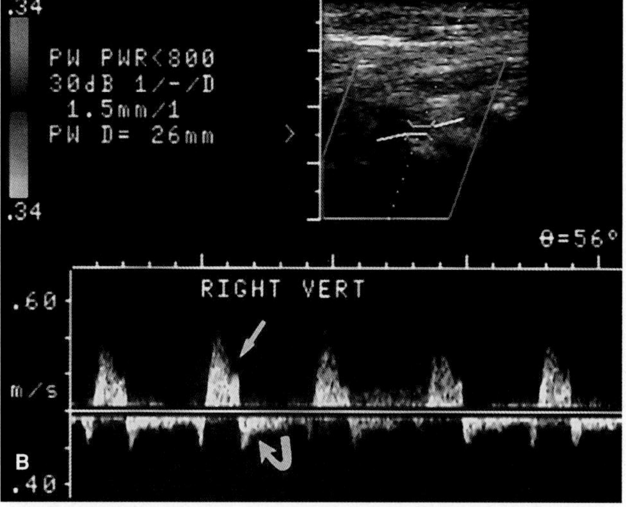

FIGURE 54.21. **Subclavian Steal. A:** Flow is reversed in the left vertebral artery (flow is away from the brain). **B:** Partial subclavian steal, in another patient, results in reversed flow during systole (*arrow*) and antegrade flow during diastole (*curved arrow*).

Near Occlusion of the ICA. As the ICA approaches occlusion, the PSV and EDV may approach normal. The severity of the stenosis can be grossly underestimated if gray scale and color flow imaging are not performed.

Tardus–parvus waveforms are typically seen distal to a severe arterial stenosis. Systolic acceleration is delayed and PSV is diminished (Fig. 54.18). The systolic upstroke is flattened and the peak at maximum systolic velocity is rounded. Findings are most pronounced as the waveform is obtained farther distal from the stenosis.

Low PSV in both common carotid arteries is associated with decreased cardiac output or an aneurysm of the thoracic aorta (Table 54.5). If PSV is extremely low and accompanied by absent or reversed flow during diastole, one should suspect a distal high-grade stenosis or occlusion. Additional considerations with this finding include carotid dissection, arteritis, bilateral intracranial arterial spasm, and elevated intracranial pressure.

Postendarterectomy. Following endarterectomy, the vein or graft patch sutures may remain visible along the arterial wall. A patulous carotid artery at the operative site is common. Complications include restenosis (~10% to 15% within the first year due to intimal hyperplasia), intimal flaps, and clamp strictures. Intraoperative US can be used to assess surgical result prior to closure. The postendarterectomy waveform often has a high-resistance flow pattern like the ECA. Turbulent flow is often noted due to the absence of the smooth endothelial lining.

Post–carotid stent placement alters SD unpredictably. Carotid US should be performed immediately after stent placement to establish a baseline. A change from baseline on serial CD and spectral analysis may indicate restenosis.

Takayasu arteritis (aortoarteritis) causes uniform thickening of the wall of all arteries involved. The lumen is smoothly narrowed by the wall thickening. Arterial calcification is rare and more typical of atherosclerotic disease if present. Vessel occlusion and aneurysmal dilatation can occur. The disease most commonly affects the subclavian arteries, aortic arch, and CCA.

Carotid dissection should be considered in any patient with smooth tapering ICA stenosis or ICA occlusion in the absence of atherosclerotic plaque. Dissection originates from a tear in the intima that allows blood to enter and dissect the arterial wall. The false lumen may end blindly, in which case the blood clots and becomes an intramural hematoma or the false channel may reconnect distally with the true lumen allowing blood to flow through two channels. In either case, blood in the vessel wall narrows the true lumen reducing flow and possibly leading to occlusion. US demonstrates a thin or thick flap separating the two lumens, smooth tapering narrowing of the true lumen, and possible thrombosis of the false lumen, true lumen, or both.

Radiation injury to the carotids occurs in portions of the arteries exposed to the radiation field. US shows diffuse and often severe wall thickening and narrowing of the lumen. Development of atherosclerotic plaques is accelerated. Significant stenosis and occlusion may occur.

Fibromuscular dysplasia may affect the carotid arteries, in addition to the renal arteries. The classic "string-of-beads" appearance is most common, though it may also cause long-segment stenosis of the ICA. Patients tend to be younger (25 to 50 years) than those with atherosclerotic disease. Women predominate 3 to 1.

Valvular Heart Disease. Significant aortic stenosis produces a tardus–parvus waveform in the aorta that is continued into the carotid arteries. Aortic insufficiency produces a *bisferious pulse* with two prominent systolic peaks and a midsystolic drop in velocity.

ABDOMINAL VESSELS

Anatomy

Abdominal Aorta. The abdominal aorta enters the abdomen through the aortic hiatus of the diaphragm and descends just to the left of midline and anterior to the spine. It bifurcates into the bilateral common iliac arteries at approximately the level of L4. The aorta has five main branches (Fig. 54.22). Three originate from the ventral aorta: the celiac axis, the superior mesenteric artery, and the inferior mesenteric artery. The left and right renal arteries originate from the aorta laterally. The proximal aorta measures 2.3 cm in diameter in men and 1.9 cm in women. It tapers progressively from its cranial to its caudal extent. Spectral analysis demonstrates a triphasic waveform. CD is useful to identify thrombus.

Inferior Vena Cava. The IVC courses toward the heart just to the right of midline and to the right of the aorta. As it reaches the liver, the IVC is contained in a deep groove on its posterior surface. It traverses the diaphragm and empties into the right atrium. The sonographically detectable branches include the hepatic and renal veins. The renal veins are anterior to their corresponding arteries and enter the IVC at right angles. The left renal vein is three times longer than the right. The hepatic veins enter the IVC from the posterior surface of the liver. Many embryologic variations of the IVC exist, including an interrupted IVC that does not extend above the renal arteries, a left-sided IVC, and a duplicated IVC. The left renal vein can be retroaortic or circumaortic. Spectral analysis of the IVC demonstrates the classic "sawtooth" pattern from cardiac and respiratory pulsations similar to the hepatic veins. Distally near the common iliac veins there is a more phasic pattern similar to the proximal extremities.

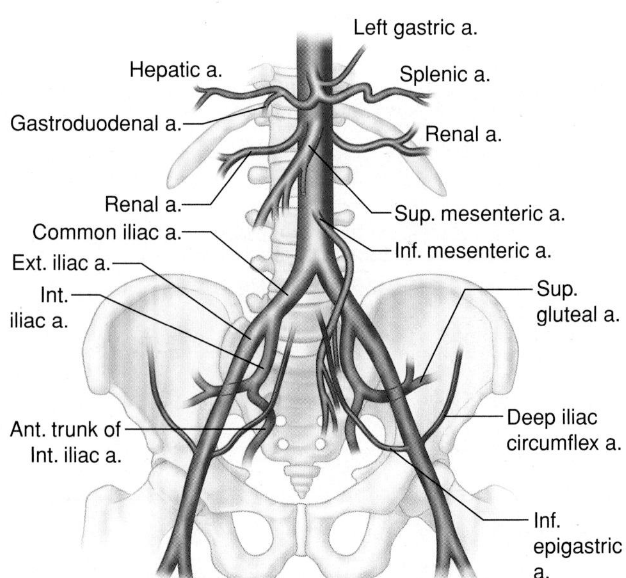

FIGURE 54.22. **Normal Abdominal Aorta and Major Arterial Branch Anatomy.**

TABLE 54.7

AORTIC ANEURYSM RUPTURE

SIZE (cm)	RUPTURE RATE (%)
<4	10
4–7	25
7–10	45
>10	60

Pathology

Abdominal Aorta Aneurysm (AAA). More than 95% of AAA involve the infrarenal aorta. AAAs which involve the renal arteries are much more difficult to repair. Most AAAs are fusiform and enlarge at the rate of 2 to 4 mm per year. Surgery is generally recommended for aneurysms >5 cm based on Darling's autopsy data of aneurysm rupture rates shown in Table 54.7. Additional complications include obstruction of the ureters, compression of the IVC, infection, thrombosis, dissection, and distal emboli. Aneurysm size, growth rate, clinical risk factors, and procedural morbidity and mortality rates are important factors in the decision for treatment. Endovascular aortic stent graft techniques compete with surgery as a treatment option.

Duplex US is the imaging modality of choice for diagnosis and follow-up of asymptomatic AAA because it is highly accurate and cost effective. The aorta is imaged from the diaphragm to the iliac bifurcation using a 3.5- to 5-MHz transducer in both the longitudinal and transverse planes. Limitations include patient obesity, bowel gas, and difficulty identifying the origins of the renal arteries. An AAA is defined as a focal enlargement of the aorta greater than 3 cm in the anteroposterior (AP) diameter (Fig. 54.23). The AP dimension of the aorta should be measured in both the transverse and longitudinal planes to assure accuracy. Many atherosclerotic aortas are tortuous, and if measured obliquely, measurement errors occur. The AP dimension can be overestimated in the transverse plane and underestimated in the longitudinal plane. The width and length of the aneurysm are also reported. The normal aorta normally tapers from proximal to distal. If it enlarges distally, it is technically considered aneurysmal regardless of the absolute measurement.

Intraluminal thrombus is usually present and ranges in appearance from hypoechoic to hyperechoic (Fig. 54.23B). CD demonstrates the size of the lumen and the abnormal, often swirling, slow flow associated with most AAAs. Inflammatory aneurysms have a hypoechoic ring surrounding the aorta corresponding to the perianeurysmal fibrosis.

Rupture of an AAA is a medical emergency, with 50% mortality requiring urgent diagnosis and treatment. US is often used in the emergency setting to make this diagnosis. Findings include (Fig. 54.24): (a) heterogeneous fluid or clotted periaortic and retroperitoneal hematoma, (b) deformity with irregular contour of the AAA, (c) inhomogeneity and focal discontinuity of the intraluminal thrombus, and (d) focal discontinuity of the outer wall of the AAA.

Infected (mycotic) AAA appears as an irregular AAA with indistinct wall, perianeurysmal edema, and perianeurysmal soft tissue mass, usually in a debilitated or drug-abusing patient with clinical signs of infection.

Inflammatory AAA is an atherosclerotic AAA with a thickened fibrotic wall and perianeurysmal adhesions and fibrosis that may obstruct ureters and involve adjacent structures. Repair of inflammatory AAA is associated with increased morbidity and mortality.

Dissection of the abdominal aorta can be diagnosed with US when an intimal flap is identified or CD shows flow in the false lumen (Fig. 54.25). Chronic dissection appears as a thickened aortic wall with thrombus in the false lumen.

Following AAA repair, the aortic graft demonstrates discrete echogenic walls. US is used to confirm patency of the graft, assess for perigraft fluid collections, and to evaluate for anastomotic stenosis or aneurysm. Perigraft fluid collections

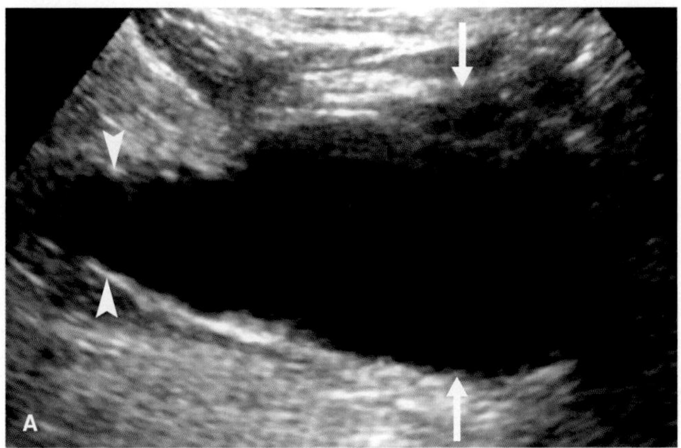

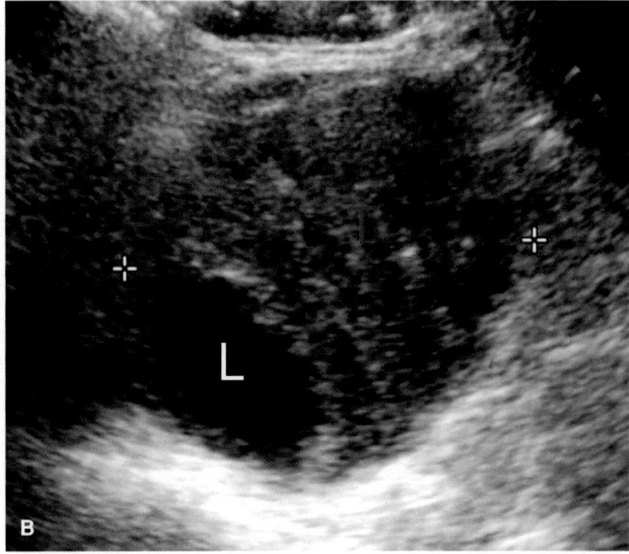

FIGURE 54.23. **Abdominal Aortic Aneurysm (AAA). A:** Longitudinal image of the distal aorta demonstrates dilatation of the lumen from 2.8 cm proximally (between *arrowheads*) to 4.9 cm distally (between *arrows*). The irregularity of the luminal surface is caused by atherosclerotic plaques. **B:** Transverse image of a distal AAA shows the large amount of thrombus (*T*) that commonly forms within large AAA (between cursors, +) as a result of slow flow within the aneurysm. The residual lumen (*L*) is echolucent representing flowing blood.

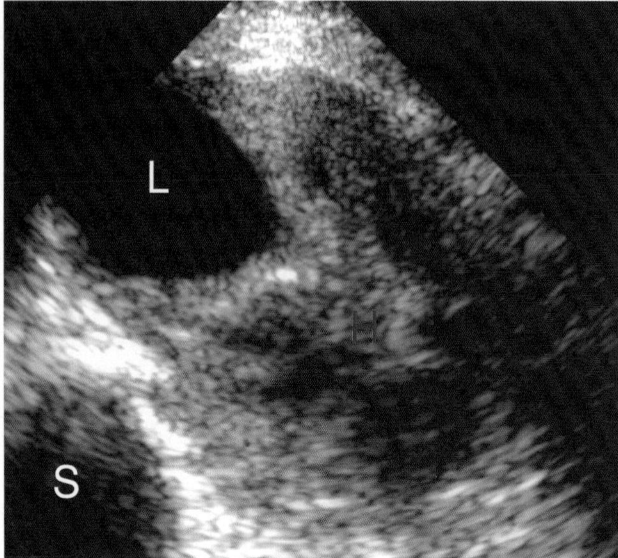

FIGURE 54.24. **Ruptured Abdominal Aortic Aneurysm.** Transverse image of the distal aorta shows the hypoechoic lumen (*L*) of the aneurysm with a large, mixed echogenicity hemorrhage (*H*) extending into the retroperitoneum. A vertebral body of the lower lumbar spine (*S*) is seen posteriorly.

seen more than 3 months after surgery may indicate hemorrhage or infection.

Iliac Artery Aneurysm. Approximately two-thirds of AAAs extend into the common iliac arteries; however, extension into the external iliac artery is uncommon. A common iliac artery aneurysm is diagnosed when the AP diameter exceeds 15 mm. Isolated iliac artery aneurysms are rare. Common iliac artery aneurysms can rupture or erode into the adjacent iliac vein, colon, or ureter.

IVC thrombosis usually extends from the peripheral veins. Bilateral lower extremity edema is present, and if acute, patients typically experience severe pain. Other clinical symptoms and signs are related to organ involvement such as renal

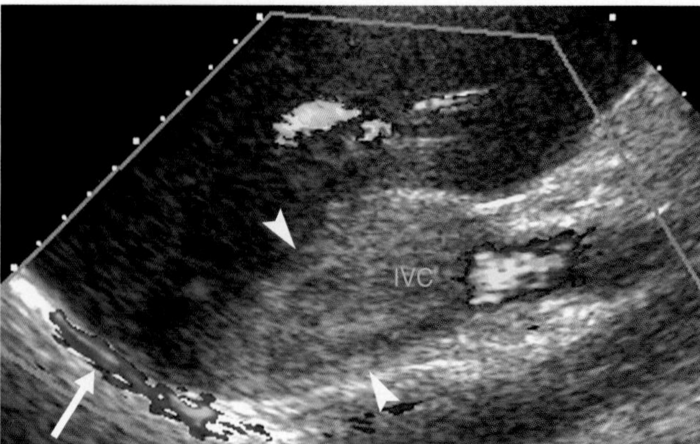

FIGURE 54.26. **Tumor Thrombus in Inferior Vena Cava.** Longitudinal color Doppler image of the inferior vena cava (*IVC*) shows echogenic thrombus (between *arrowheads*) distending the lumen. Spectral Doppler US of the thrombus (not shown) confirmed arterial blood flow within the clot indicating tumor extension into the IVC in this patient with renal cell carcinoma of the right kidney. The blue color along the diaphragm (*arrow*) is color flash artifact caused by motion of solid tissue.

failure or bowel ischemia. Gray scale US demonstrates intraluminal clot (Fig. 54.25) that acutely expands the diameter of the IVC. Remember that congestive heart failure also distends the hepatic veins and IVC and that slow-flowing blood can be mistaken for clot. Doppler demonstrates the absence of flow in complete occlusion or flow diverted around the thrombus with partial obstruction. In partial thrombosis, the spectral waveform is usually blunted with loss of the transmitted cardiac pulsation and respiratory phasicity. Extrinsic compression from any retroperitoneal process such as lymphadenopathy, hepatomegaly, retroperitoneal fibrosis, or hematoma can cause obstruction and thrombosis of the IVC.

Tumor extension into the IVC causes a tumor thrombosis (Fig. 54.26), which appears similar to bland thrombus. Demonstration of arterial flow in the mass within the lumen of the IVC confirms the presence of tumor thrombosis. The most common tumor to extend into the IVC is renal cell carcinoma. Other tumors which invade the IVC include hepatoma,

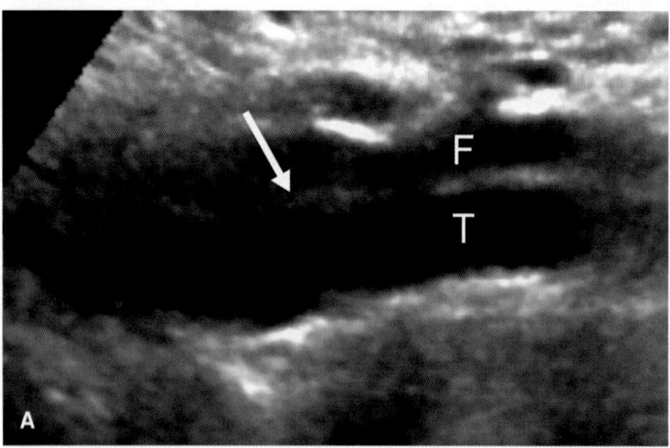

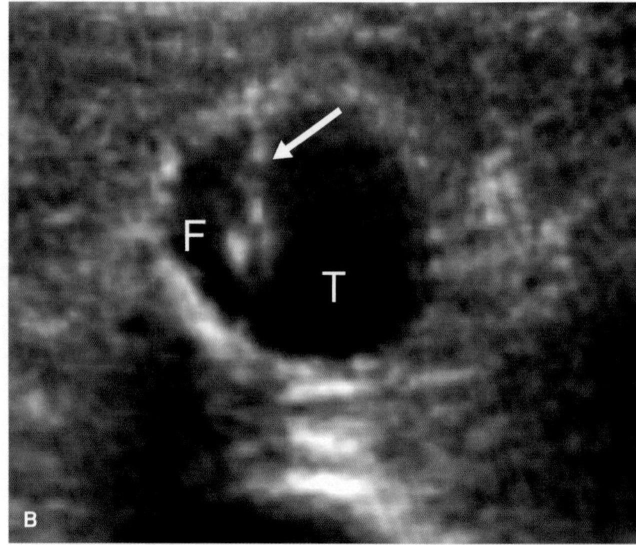

FIGURE 54.25. **Aortic Dissection.** Longitudinal (**A**) and transverse (**B**) images of the abdominal aorta demonstrate a prominent intimal flap (*arrow*) that separates the true lumen (*T*) from the false lumen (*F*). Echogenic clot is commonly present within the false lumen when the dissection is chronic.

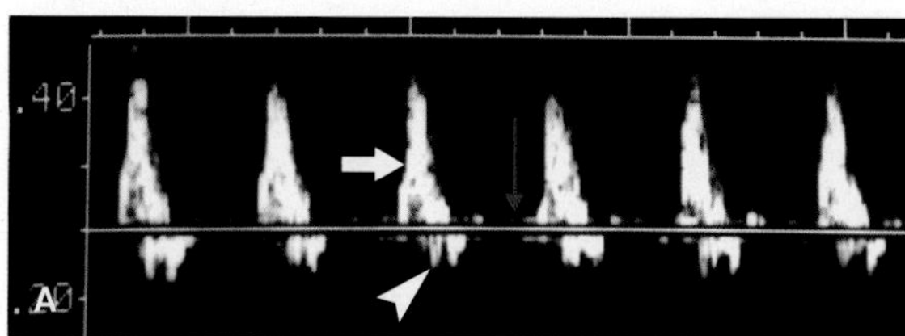

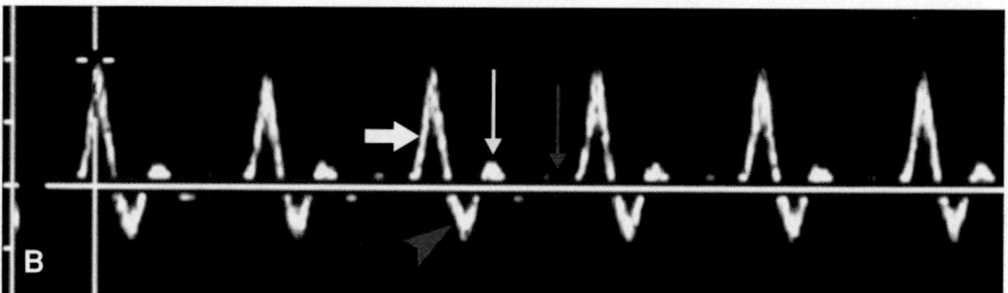

FIGURE 54.27. **Normal Extremity Artery Waveforms. A: Subclavian artery.** Ventricular systole causes a rapid rise in blood flow velocity followed by a sharp drop in velocity as the aortic valve closes. Blood flow direction reverses in early diastole because of high vascular resistance in the arm at rest. Typical of high-resistance waveforms, there is little to no forward blood flow in diastole. **B: Superficial femoral artery.** A triphasic high-resistance waveform is characteristic with the leg at rest. The first phase is a rapid rise to peak velocity in systole (*fat arrow*). The second phase is postsystole reversal of flow (*arrowhead*) reflecting high downstream vascular resistance. The third phase is low-velocity forward flow (*skinny yellow arrow*) in early diastole caused by elastic recoil of the vessel wall. No flow occurs in late diastole (*skinny red arrow*).

adrenal carcinoma, pheochromocytoma, lymphoma, angiomyolipoma, and atrial myxoma. Leiomyosarcoma is the most common primary tumor of the IVC.

PERIPHERAL ARTERIES

In the extremities, duplex US is the diagnostic modality of choice to screen for complications of arterial puncture, arterial bypass grafts, and dialysis grafts and is an adjunct in the evaluation of atherosclerotic peripheral vascular disease.

Anatomy. In the upper extremity, the right subclavian artery arises from the inominate artery and the left subclavian artery originates directly from the aortic arch. Their origins can usually be identified with US by using a supraclavicular approach. The subclavian arteries lie superficial to the subclavian veins. The distal subclavian artery is obscured by the clavicle but may be imaged by an infraclavicular approach. The subclavian artery continues as the axillary artery. The axillary artery becomes the brachial artery, which courses along the medial aspect of the arm. At the elbow, the brachial artery branches into the ulnar and radial arteries, which continue into the hand forming the palmar arches. The Doppler waveforms are high resistance at rest showing little to no blood flow in diastole (Fig. 54.27A). Blood flow direction is reversed in early diastole, reflecting high vascular resistance in the contracted arteries and arterioles. PSV is 110 cm/s in the proximal subclavian artery and decreases to 85 cm/s in the axillary artery.

In the lower extremity, the femoral and popliteal arteries (Fig. 54.28) travel with an accompanying vein. The patient is imaged supine using a 5- to 10-MHz linear transducer. The common femoral artery arises at the inguinal ligament and quickly bifurcates into the profunda femoris (deep femoral artery [DFA]) and superficial femoral artery (SFA). The SFA travels along the anteromedial thigh through the adductor (Hunter's) canal and becomes the popliteal artery. Below the knee, the popliteal artery branches into the anterior tibial artery and a short tibioperoneal trunk that quickly bifurcates into the peroneal and posterior tibial arteries. The anterior tibial artery descends anteriorly and terminates in the dorsalis pedis artery. The peroneal artery terminates above the ankle, while the posterior tibial artery continues behind the medial malleolus to supply the plantar surface of the foot. The normal Doppler waveform in each of these arteries is a high-resistance, triphasic pattern (Fig. 54.27B). The first phase is the high-velocity component of ventricular systole. PSV decreases from proximal to distal, averaging about 110 cm/s in the femoral artery and 70 cm/s in the popliteal artery. The second phase is postsystolic reversal of flow due to the high resistance of the arterioles with the muscles of the leg at rest. The third phase is a small amount of forward flow in early diastole due to elastic recoil of the vessel wall.

Pseudoaneurysm is a contained rupture of an artery wall with a persistent connection (neck) to the artery resulting in a pulsatile mass containing swirling blood flow. Most arise from the common femoral artery as a complication of arterial puncture, surgery, or trauma. The use of large-bore catheters, long indwelling catheter time, and routine postprocedure anticoagulation have increased the incidence of pseudoaneurysm from arterial puncture to as high as 6%.

US reliably differentiates pseudoaneurysms from other groin masses (Fig. 54.29). Gray scale US demonstrates a predominantly echolucent mass that may contain internal echoes or mural thrombus. The mass is located immediately adjacent to the artery. CD demonstrates the connection to the artery and documents flow within the mass in the typical "yin–yang" pattern. SD over the neck shows the characteristic "to and fro" spectral waveform (Fig. 54.30). US is commonly used to guide treatment using sustained direct compression or thrombin injection to thrombose the pseudoaneurysm.

Arteriovenous fistula (AVF) results from simultaneous puncture of the artery and vein. Less common than pseudoaneurysms,

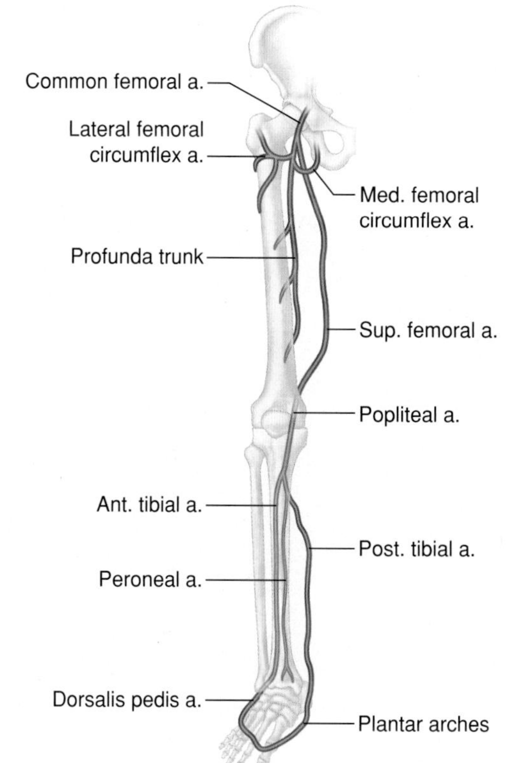

FIGURE 54.28. **Normal Lower Extremity Arterial Anatomy.**

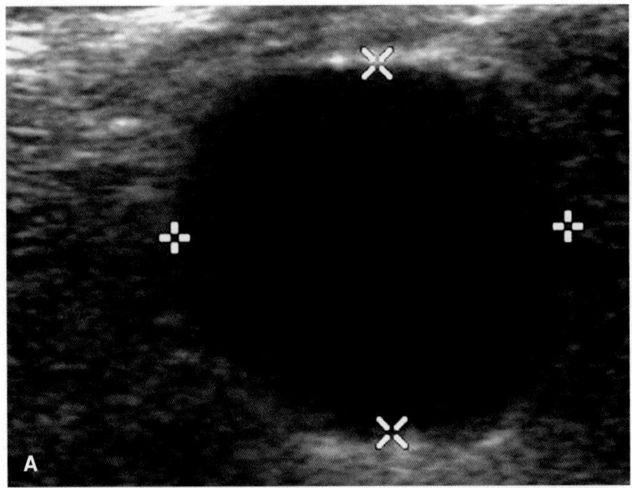

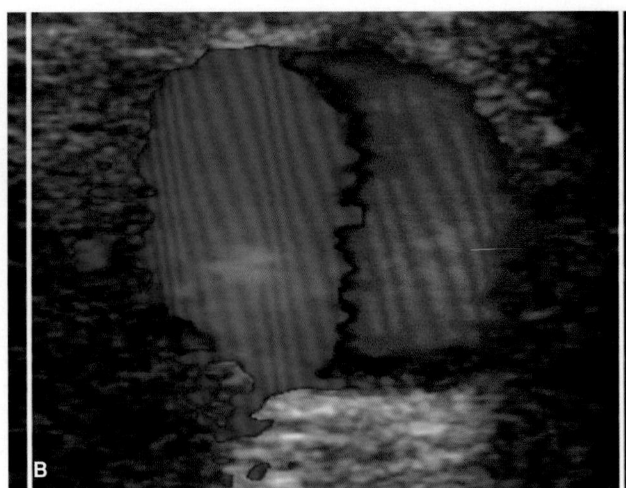

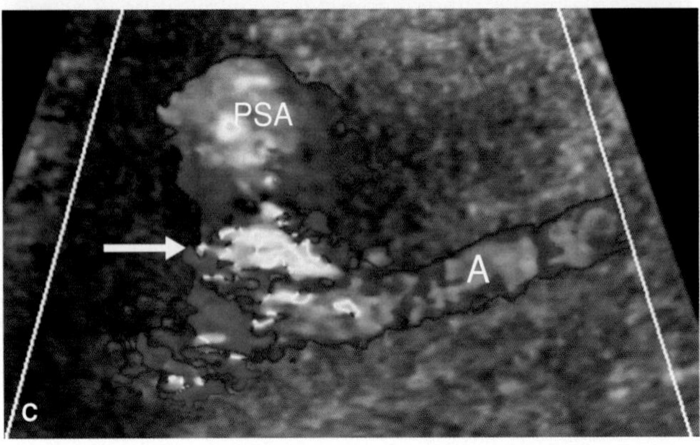

FIGURE 54.29. **Pseudoaneurysm.** **A:** An echolucent mass with thrombus (between *cursors*, +, ×) is seen in the groin at the site of arterial puncture for cardiac catheterization. **B:** Color Doppler image demonstrates complete filling of the mass with color, indicating active blood. The characteristic swirling or "yin–yang" flow represents flow in and out of the pseudoaneurysm. **C:** Longitudinal color Doppler image demonstrates the broad neck (*arrow*) of the pseudoaneurysm (*PSA*) with turbulent blood flow into the mass. The pseudoaneurysm arises from the common femoral artery (*A*).

AVFs are often small and resolve spontaneously. With a large AVF, SD shows a low-resistance waveform with increased diastolic flow in the feeding artery, distinctly abnormal for an extremity artery in a resting limb. The draining vein is distended and demonstrates high-velocity pulsatile flow. These characteristic findings are usually only present within several centimeters of the fistula (Fig. 54.31). SD waveforms are obtained in the artery and vein just above and just below the suspected site of the fistula. CD shows a heterogeneous disorganized color pattern overlying the fistula due to soft tissue vibration artifact, a CD bruit. When the AVF is small, Doppler US may be normal.

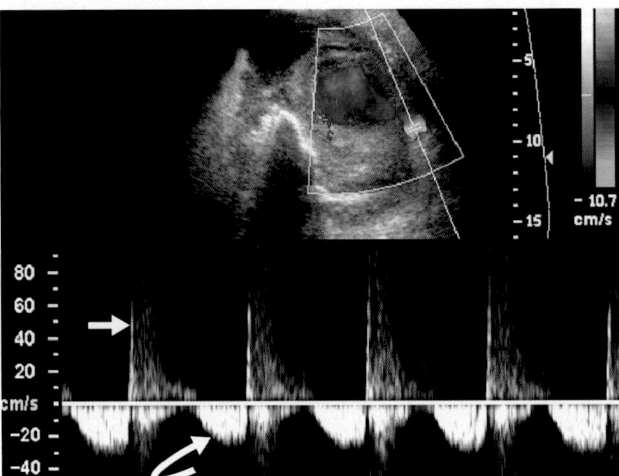

FIGURE 54.30. **Pseudoaneurysm.** Spectral Doppler tracing over the neck of a pseudoaneurysm showing the characteristic "to and fro" waveform. During systole, blood flows into the pseudoaneurysm (*straight arrow*) and during diastole (*curved arrow*) blood flows out of the pseudoaneurysm.

Hematoma. Perivascular masses occurring immediately following arterial puncture are most commonly hematomas. Sonographically, hematomas range from anechoic to hypoechoic with a complex echo pattern. No internal flow can be demonstrated on CD or SD. Hematomas cannot be distinguished from thrombosed pseudoaneurysms, seromas, or abscesses.

Aneurysms of the peripheral arteries are most common in the popliteal arteries (70% to 85%). AAA is also present in 20% to 40% of patients with popliteal aneurysms. Patients present with a popliteal fossa mass or lower extremity ischemia symptoms. US demonstrates a focal, usually fusiform, bulge of the arterial lumen. Treatment of peripheral artery aneurysms is usually recommended when the aneurysm exceeds 2 cm in diameter. Treatment may be surgical repair or an endovascular stent graft.

Stenosis and Occlusion. In most circumstances, the diagnosis of significant peripheral arterial occlusive disease is made on clinical grounds based on the symptom of claudication and physical examination findings. Doppler US may be used to screen for stenosis or occlusion prior to CT, MR, or catheter angiography. Peripheral arterial US is performed with a linear 5- to 10-MHz transducer. Gray scale imaging locates the vessels and evaluates plaque. CD identifies areas of narrowing and turbulent flow. Doppler spectra are obtained just proximal to the plaque, at the area of maximum stenosis, and just downstream from the plaque. PSV ratios are used to grade the severity of stenosis comparing PSV upstream from the plaque to PSV in the area of maximum stenosis. Minor stenosis (<50% diameter narrowing) has a PSV ratio <2 with a biphasic or

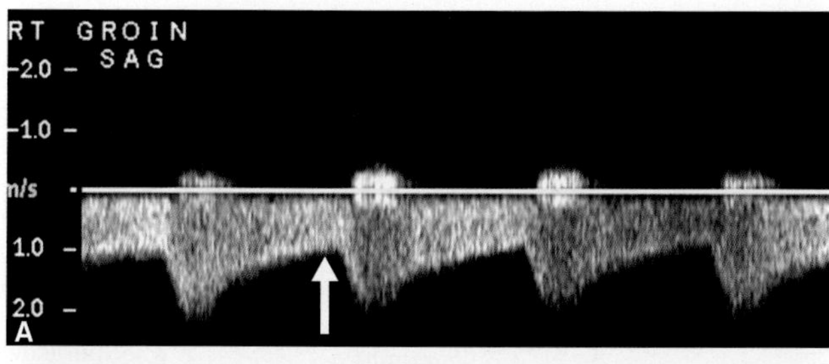

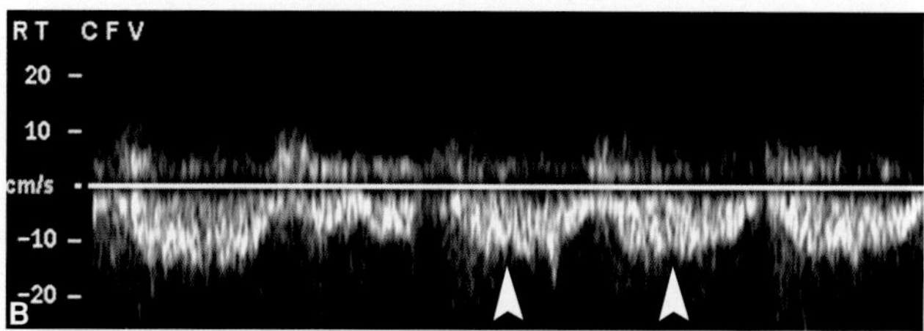

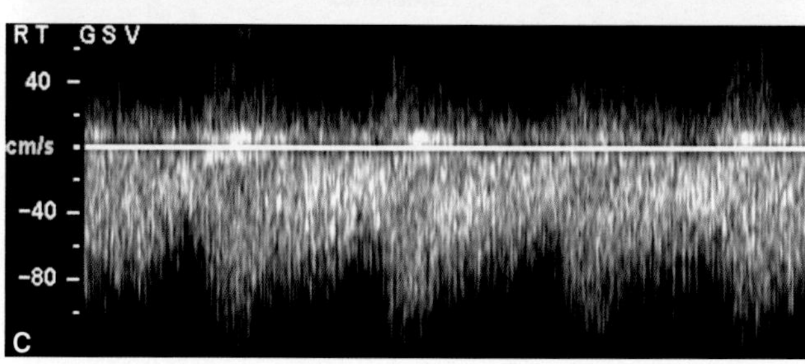

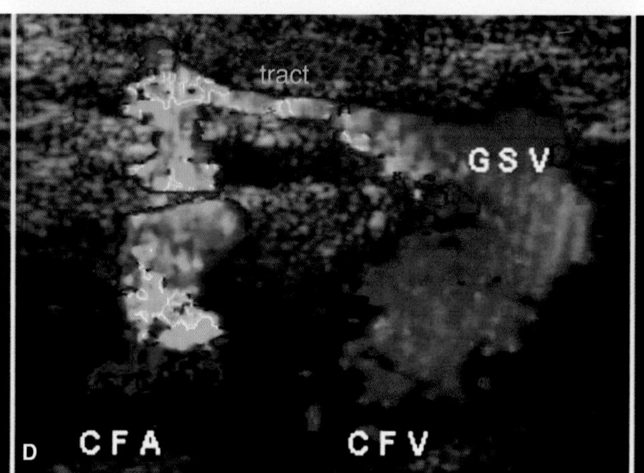

FIGURE 54.31. **Arteriovenous Fistula.** The ultrasound examination for an arteriovenous fistula complicating an arterial puncture should begin with obtaining Doppler spectra from the artery and vein just *above* the puncture site. These images were obtained from a patient with a persistent bruit heard at the puncture site for cardiac catheterization. **A:** Doppler spectrum from the common femoral artery just above the puncture site shows an abnormal low-resistance pattern manifest by high-velocity flow in diastole (*arrow*). The common femoral artery at rest should show a high-resistance Doppler spectrum (Fig. 54.27B). **B:** Doppler spectrum from the common femoral vein just above the puncture site shows abnormal pulsatility (*arrowheads*). **C:** Doppler spectrum from the greater saphenous vein shows marked turbulence as well as abnormal pulsatility. **D:** Color Doppler image reveals the fistulous *tract* between the common femoral artery (*CFA*) and the greater saphenous vein (*GSV*) near its junction with the common femoral vein (*CFV*).

triphasic waveform and little or no turbulence. Moderate stenosis (50% to 75%) shows a PSV ratio >2 with a monophasic waveform and moderate or marked poststenotic turbulence. Severe stenosis (>75%) shows a PSV ratio >2.5 with EDV in the stenotic zone higher than systolic velocity in the prestenotic zone. Poststenotic waveforms show the tardus–parvus appearance. As with the carotid arteries, complete occlusion may not be accurately differentiated from string flow. Occluded vessels show no flow on SD or CD, with intraluminal thrombus or termination of the vessel, with inability of US to demonstrate its course. Occluded arteries are often reconstituted by collateral vessels and should be searched for downstream.

Graft Surveillance. In contrast to native vessels, sonography has established itself as the noninvasive modality of choice in monitoring peripheral bypass grafts. About 30% of arterial grafts show signs of failure by the second year. US is used for early detection of impaired graft patency (Table 54.8). Graft failure is most common at the site of anastomosis to the native artery with development of a pseudoaneurysm or anastomotic stenosis (Fig. 54.32). The anastomosis is often patulous, with the graft being slightly larger than the native artery. This normal finding should not be mistaken for a pseudoaneurysm. Flow velocities within the graft vary depending upon the caliber of the graft and downstream runoff. Waveforms vary from monophasic to triphasic. New grafts show continuous diastolic flow caused by lack of autoregulation in downstream arterioles. Moderate graft stenosis (50% to 75% diameter stenosis) shows PSV ratio >2.5, with PSV in the area of maximum stenosis >150 cm/s. Severe graft stenosis (>75%) shows a PSV ratio >3.5, with PSV in the area of maximal stenosis >300 cm/s

TABLE 54.8

PRINCIPLES OF VEIN GRAFT SURVEILLANCE

Examine the entire graft with color Doppler to identify significant flow abnormalities
Interrogate suspicious areas with spectral Doppler
PSV >180 cm/s indicates ~50% stenosis
Velocity ratio >2 indicates ~50% stenosis
Flow rate <45 cm/s suggests impending graft failure
Marked velocity changes on serial examinations suggest stenosis
Waveform change from triphasic to monophasic is consistent with either proximal or distal stenosis

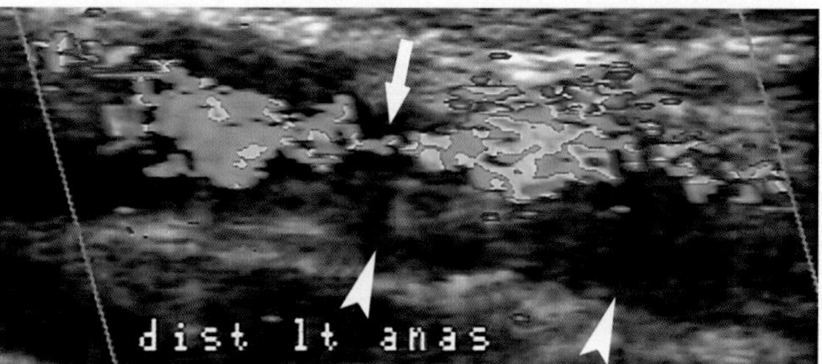

FIGURE 54.32. **Synthetic Graft Anastomotic Stenosis.** Longitudinal color Doppler image at the distal anastomosis of an aortofemoral graft. Prominent fibrointimal hyperplasia (*arrowheads*) markedly thickens the wall of the graft and causes a significant stenosis (*arrow*) at the anastomosis. The velocity proximal in the graft is 0.53 m/s and at the anastomosis 1.80 m/s. Using the values in Table 54.6, this represents about a 75% diameter stenosis, which was confirmed by catheter arteriogram.

and EDV >100 cm/s. Moderate stenosis is generally followed for evidence of progression. Severe stenosis usually mandates graft revision prior to occlusion.

VENOUS ULTRASOUND

Lower Extremity

Duplex US is clearly recognized as the diagnostic modality of choice for the evaluation of the lower extremity for deep venous thrombosis (DVT). Multiple studies demonstrate a sensitivity of 95% and a specificity of 98%. The D-dimer laboratory test is 99% sensitive for thrombosis but only 50% specific. Other imaging modalities such as MR venography and contrast venography are reserved for instances when duplex is nondiagnostic, pelvic or IVC clot is suspected, or if calf clot will be treated. CT venography is performed in conjunction with CT pulmonary angiography in some institutions.

Anatomy. The deep venous system of the lower extremity consists of veins that parallel the arteries both anatomically and in name (Fig. 54.33B). In the calf, the anterior tibial, posterior tibial, and peroneal veins converge just below the knee to form the popliteal vein. The popliteal vein continues into the thigh through the adductor canal as the superficial femoral vein. For clarity and to emphasize the fact that, despite its name, the superficial femoral vein is actually a deep vein, we call the superficial femoral vein simply the femoral vein (FV). Near the groin, the profunda femoris vein joins the FV to form the common femoral vein (CFV). The CFV ascends medial to the artery into the pelvis and becomes the external iliac vein. The internal iliac vein joins the external iliac vein to become the common iliac vein over the sacrum. The common iliac veins join to form the IVC. The popliteal and FV are partially or completely duplicated in about 25% of individuals. The calf veins have many normal variations. Thrombus within the deep venous system from the popliteal vein to the CFV and above places the patient at risk for pulmonary embolism. Thrombosis of the deep veins of the calf is not a risk factor for pulmonary embolism but does place the patient at risk for extension of thrombus into the deep veins of the thigh.

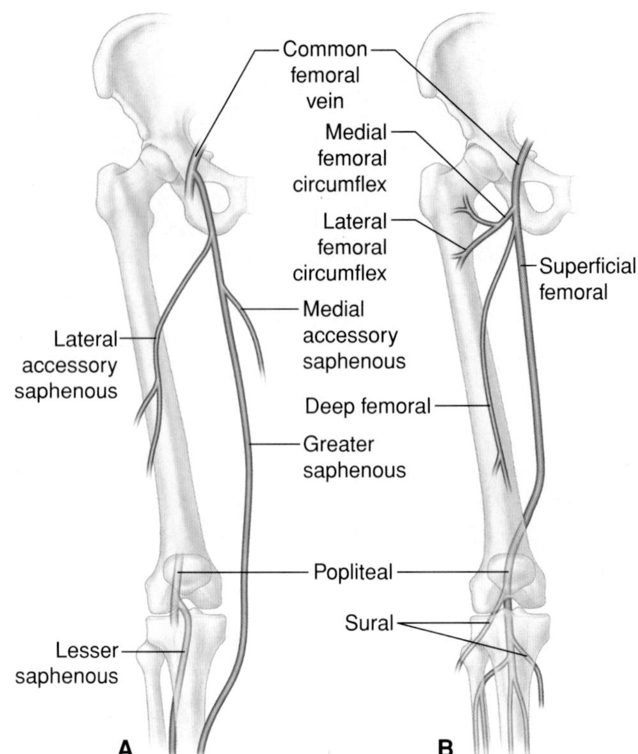

FIGURE 54.33. **Lower Extremity Venous Anatomy. A:** Superficial system. **B:** Deep system.

The greater and lesser saphenous veins comprise the superficial venous system of the lower extremity (Fig. 54.33A). The greater saphenous vein (GSV) originates on the medial side of the ankle, ascends anteromedially along the thigh, and empties into the CFV at the inguinal ligament. The lesser saphenous vein (LSV) originates laterally at the ankle and ascends

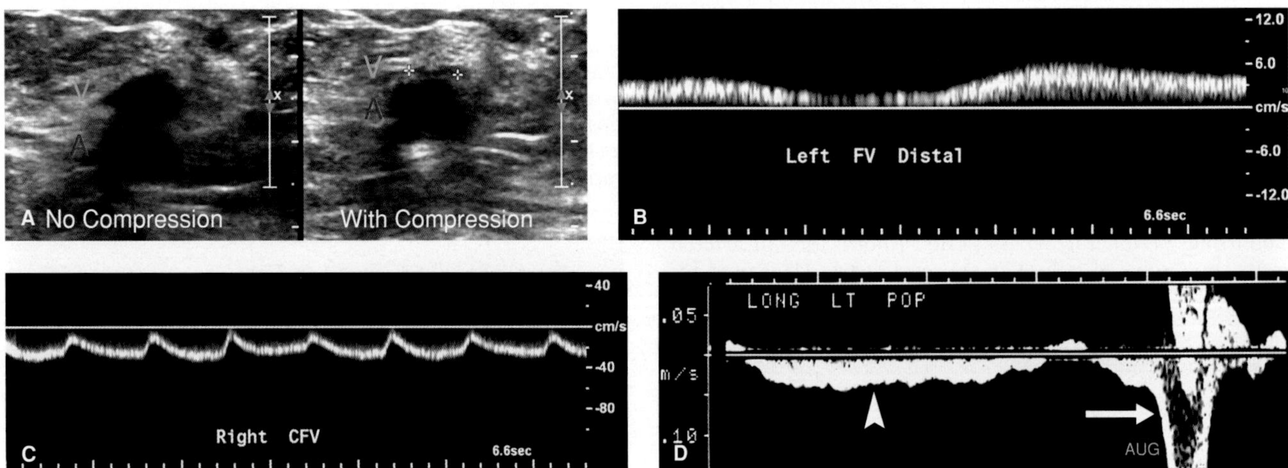

FIGURE 54.34. **Normal Venous US Examination. A:** Transverse gray scale images of a normal popliteal vein (*V*) and artery (*A*) without compression (*left*) and with compression (*right*) demonstrate normal complete wall-to-wall compression of the vein. Our sonographers routinely identify the normal compressed vein with cursors (+) placed horizontally. If the vein does not compress normally, they place the cursors vertically. **B:** Doppler waveform of a femoral vein shows the normal phasic change in velocity of venous flow with respiration. **C:** Doppler spectrum of a common femoral vein shows the normal phasic change in velocity of venous flow with cardiac pulsations. These respiratory and cardiac phasic changes in venous flow velocity in the lower extremity confirm patency of the venous system between the site of US examination and the thorax. **D:** Doppler spectrum of a popliteal vein shows normal respiratory phasicity (*arrowhead*) and normal augmented flow (*arrow*, *AUG*) induced by squeezing the patient's calf. Patency of the vein both above and below the site of US examination is confirmed.

posteriorly along the calf. It usually empties into the popliteal vein or rarely into the profunda femoris or GSV. Small perforating veins containing valves connect the superficial to the deep system in the calf and lower thigh. Flow is directed from the superficial to deep system.

Venous US Technique. The deep veins of the lower extremity are examined from the inguinal ligament (junction of the GSV with the CFV) through the popliteal fossa. Examination of the CFV/FV is performed in the supine position with a linear 5- to 7.5-MHz transducer in a slight reverse Trendelenburg position. In the transverse plane, compression and release of the veins are performed every 1 cm to the popliteal fossa (Fig. 54.34). Behind the knee, the popliteal vein is examined in a similar fashion with the patient prone and knee flexed at 15°. If a thrombus is present, longitudinal views are performed to determine its extent. SD interrogation demonstrates respiratory and cardiac phasicity (Fig. 54.34) confirming the absence of thrombi or venous obstruction in the abdomen and pelvis. Patency of the vein below the site of US examination can be confirmed by squeezing the calf or having the patient plantar flex the foot. This augmentation maneuver normally produces a brief burst of increased venous flow velocity. CD evaluation confirms vein patency and unidirectional flow and is particularly useful in areas or in patients difficult to examine (e.g., the adductor canal and obese patients). The increased sensitivity of PD to slow flow can be effectively used to augment the CD examination.

Because of the many anatomic variations and duplications of the calf veins, duplex US is time consuming and probably does not have the diagnostic accuracy needed to exclude a small thrombus. Most clinicians do not anticoagulate an isolated calf DVT since they are not a cause of pulmonary emboli and often spontaneously resolve. For these reasons, duplex US of the calf veins is not routinely performed. Up to 20% of calf vein DVT propagates to the popliteal or FV. Serial evaluation every 3 to 5 days is therefore important in patients who remain symptomatic with conservative therapy to diagnose clot propagation and prevent pulmonary embolus.

Deep Venous Thrombosis (DVT). Risk factors for developing DVT include prolonged immobilization, age, pregnancy, oral contraceptive use, surgery, trauma, myocardial infarction, congestive heart failure, malignancy, polycythemia, prior DVT, or any other hypercoagulable state. The clinical presentation and physical examination findings are unreliable in making the diagnosis. Differential diagnoses include Baker cyst, cellulitis, popliteal artery aneurysm, edema from multiple causes (congestive heart failure, lymphatic, renal failure, etc.), chronic venous insufficiency (CVI), extrinsic venous compression, superficial thrombophlebitis, and hematomas. The importance of making the diagnosis cannot be underestimated since 90% of pulmonary emboli arise in the lower extremities and untreated DVT results in pulmonary embolus in up to 50% of cases.

Acute DVT. The most accurate US criterion for the diagnosis of DVT is loss of compressibility of the vein (Fig. 54.35). Thrombus within the vein prevents its compression. The veins of the deep venous system are generally easily compressible with light pressure. The maximum pressure required to obliterate a

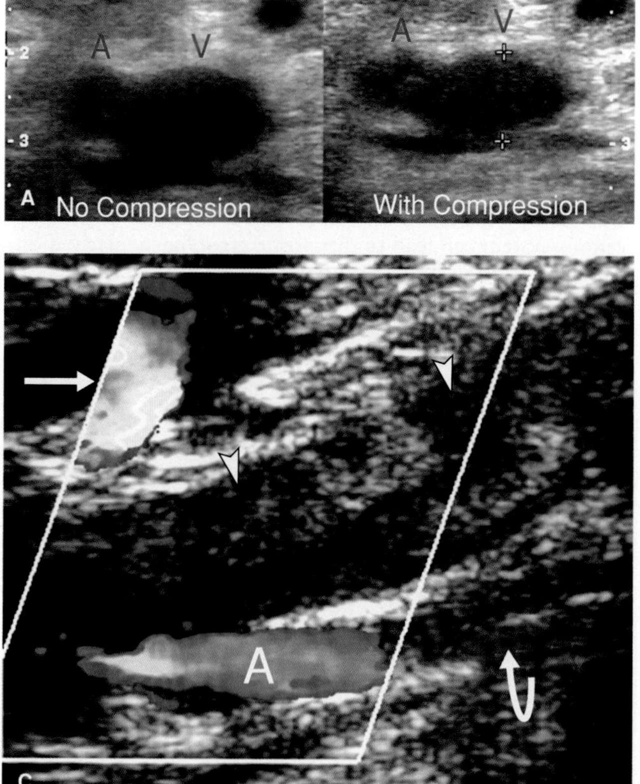

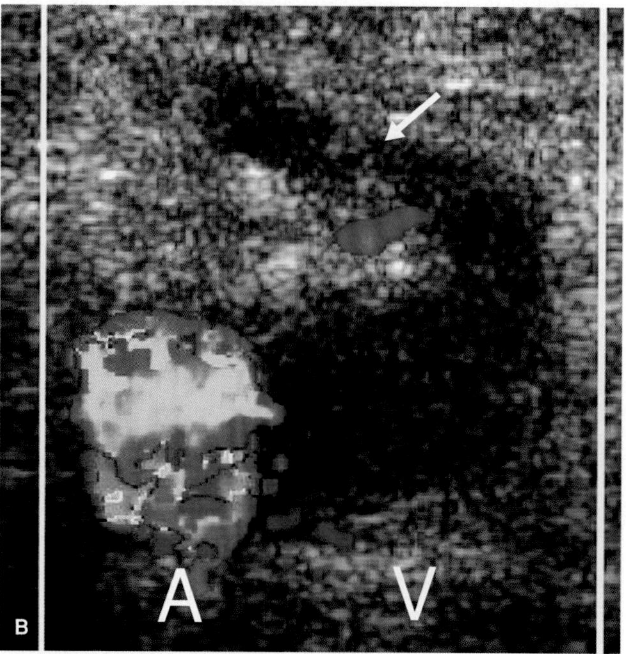

FIGURE 54.35. **Deep Venous Thrombosis—Lower Extremity. A:** Transverse gray scale US images of the common femoral vein (*V*) and artery (*A*) without compression (*left*) and with transducer compression (*right*) demonstrate hypoechoic acute thrombus (between *cursors*, +) within the vein. **B:** Transverse color Doppler image of the common femoral artery (*A*) and vein (*V*) shows flow within the artery and hypoechoic thrombus with no blood flow in the vein. The clot extends into the greater saphenous vein (*straight arrow*), part of the superficial venous system of the leg. **C:** Longitudinal color Doppler image shows extension of occlusive thrombus (*arrowheads*) into the deep femoral (*curved arrow*) vein. Flow in the deep femoral artery (*A*) and superficial femoral artery (*arrow*) is shown in blue.

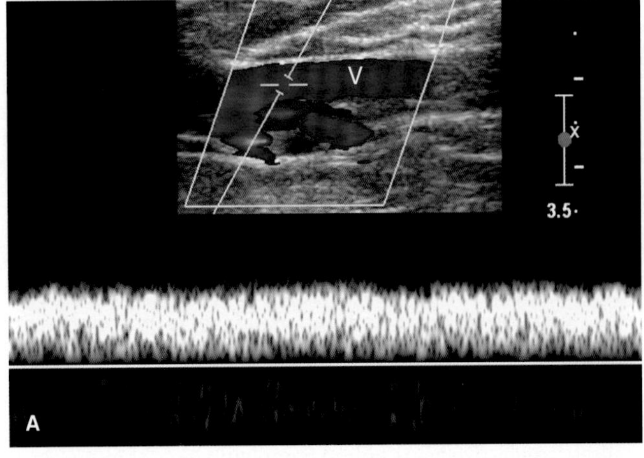

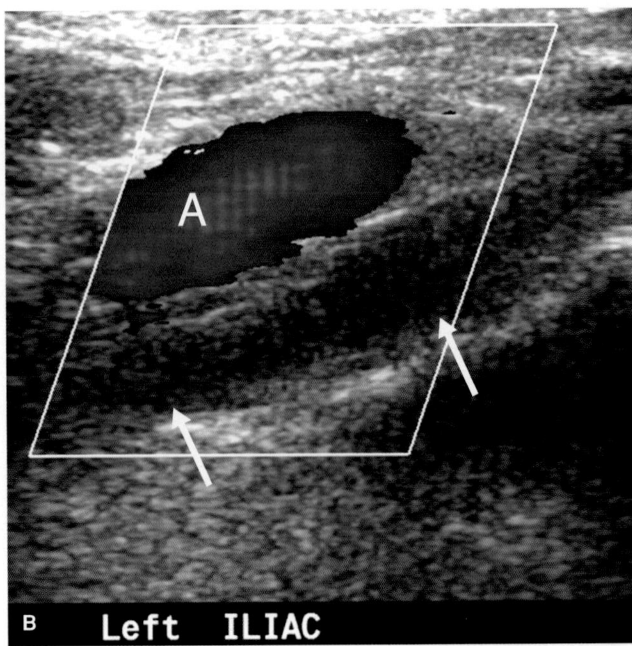

FIGURE 54.36. **Loss of Phasicity—Thrombosis of the Iliac Vein. A:** Spectral Doppler of the patent common femoral vein (*V*) shows venous flow at a constant velocity without the normal phasic velocity changes caused by respiration and cardiac motion. **B:** Color Doppler image of the ipsilateral external iliac artery (*A*) and adjacent vein shows occlusive thrombus (*arrows*) filling the vein. Commonly, deep venous thrombus in the pelvis cannot be directly visualized with US, and the diagnosis must be inferred from abnormal Doppler spectra obtained from the femoral veins.

normal vein in any patient is less than that required to deform the shape of the adjacent artery. Other findings of acute DVT include distention of the vein and direct visualization of intraluminal thrombus. A significant number of acute clots are isoechoic to flowing blood stressing the importance of the dynamic compression examination. CD demonstrates an intraluminal defect or color void. Several studies have shown that CD may be as accurate as compression US. SD exhibits a lack of augmentation of signal when the clot is between the point of Doppler interrogation and manual compression of the leg. SD may also show a loss of respiratory phasicity caudad to the clot. If the respiratory phasicity is lost in the CFV, an iliac vein or IVC thrombosis should be suspected (Fig. 54.36). Loss of augmentation of signal in the CFV with release of Valsalva is also suggestive of a more cephalad obstruction. A complete evaluation utilizes all the above techniques.

It is important to realize the limitations of US diagnosis. The iliac and pelvic veins are not adequately evaluated in most patients. Obesity and severe edema can cause technically inadequate examinations. The adductor canal can be difficult to visualize even in thin patients. The saphenous vein or collaterals can be mistaken for the SFV. Duplications of the deep venous system can lead to diagnostic error, particularly if one system is clotted and the other is patent. Extrinsic venous

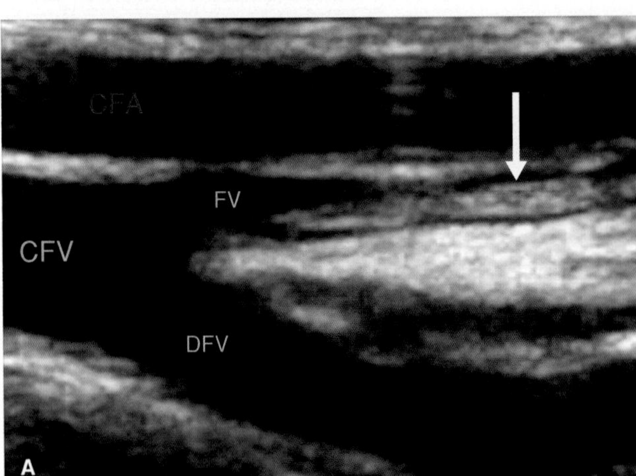

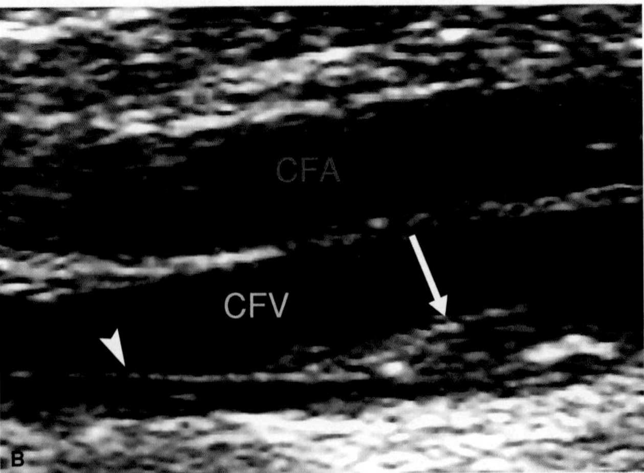

FIGURE 54.37. **Chronic Deep Venous Thrombosis. A:** Longitudinal image of the common femoral artery (*CFA*) and the common femoral vein (*CFV*). The CFV is formed by the junction of the deep femoral vein (*DFV*) (profunda femoris vein) and the (superficial) femoral vein (FV). Chronic thrombus (*arrow*) floats freely in the FV. Note the contracted echogenic appearance of the clot as well as the normal diameter of the affected vein. The chronic thrombus does not completely occlude the vein. Remember that the superficial femoral vein is considered a deep vein and that acute thrombus in the FV is a risk for pulmonary embolus. **B:** Longitudinal image of the common femoral artery (*CFA*) and common femoral vein (*CFV*) in a different patient shows chronic thrombus (*arrow*) appearing as an echogenic mass within the vein narrowing the lumen. An echogenic fibrin strand (*arrowhead*) extends from the thrombus floating freely within the vein.

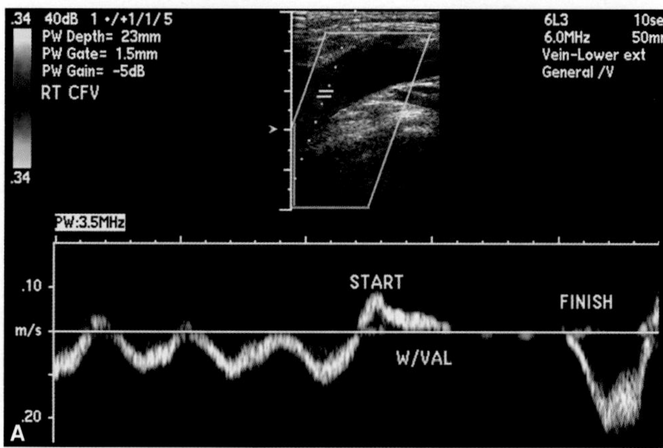

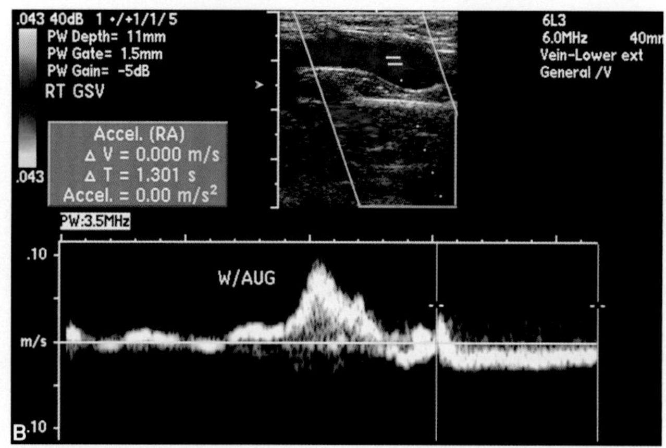

FIGURE 54.38. **Venous Insufficiency. A: Normal.** Duplex imaging in the CFV near its junction with GSV. The patient performs a Valsalva (start). No flow is noted during Valsalva. The patient breathes (finish) and "augmented" flow is noted toward the heart (normal). No reversed flow (reflux) is noted. **B: Reflux.** Duplex interrogation in the GSV just prior to joining the CFV. Calf augmentation is performed (W/AUG). Note the flow toward the feet (reversed) in the GSV for longer than 1 second following the augmentation (flow below baseline between cursors). Prolonged reversed flow is indicative of venous insufficiency.

compression by nodes or tumor can cause loss of respiratory phasicity and augmentation.

Chronic DVT. The distinction between acute and chronic DVT is difficult on all imaging modalities. Six months following a DVT, 50% of patients have persistent abnormalities on US. Typically, chronic clot is not associated with an expanded lumen as the clot shrinks with time. Chronic clot appears more echogenic than an acute clot (Fig. 54.37). Echogenic strands are often noted in the lumen. The walls of the vein also appear thickened, irregular, and echogenic, and the vein is incompletely compressible. CD often demonstrates collateral vessels. A baseline venous US obtained just prior to discontinuing anticoagulation therapy is helpful in distinguishing acute from chronic DVT on future examinations. Otherwise, with recurrent symptoms, a chronic DVT may be inadvertently diagnosed as an acute or recurrent DVT, subjecting the patient to long-term anticoagulation therapy. If a clot appears chronic and unchanged from baseline, an interval follow-up US in 2 to 3 days is performed to assess for change. Acute clot superimposed on chronic changes remains a difficult US diagnosis.

Chronic venous insufficiency (CVI) is extremely common, affecting up to 20% of American adults, especially women. Findings include varicose veins, dermatitis, skin discoloration, stasis ulcers, leg swelling, and symptoms of pain, muscle cramping, and itching. Previous DVT is the most important risk factor. A variety of effective minimally invasive percutaneous therapies are available. Duplex US is the key imaging modality for diagnosis, mapping of varicose veins, and locating the level and source of venous reflux. US is also used to guide most percutaneous therapies. Normal venous blood flow in the lower extremities is from the superficial to the deep venous system. Doppler US demonstrates reversal of flow from the deep to the superficial venous system in CVI. CVI US examination is often begun with a routine US to exclude DVT. Clinical inspection of the location of varicosities helps to focus the CVI examination. Examination is performed with the patient standing. CD or SD is used to detect retrograde flow. The CFV, FV, popliteal vein, GSV, and LSV are examined. Three techniques are used to elicit venous reflux. Augmentation technique involves manually squeezing the leg to increase venous return toward the heart (Fig. 54.38). With the release of pressure, blood drops back toward the feet. Transient (<0.5 second) reflux from deep to superficial system is normal. However, a prolonged reflux (>1 second) is indicative of CVI. The Valsalva maneuver increases intra-abdominal pressure and forces venous blood back toward the feet. Retrograde flow indicates CVI. The third technique, direct retrograde compression, involves squeezing the leg just above the site of Doppler examination which forces blood toward the feet if CVI is present.

Vein mapping using duplex US is a valuable adjunct to the vascular surgeon in preoperative evaluation for autologous vein grafts. The GSV is most commonly used for vein grafts but any vein can be used as long as the diameter is >3 mm and without varicosities. The course of the vein is marked with a permanent marker and all branch points are labeled. The exam is time consuming, and it is important to communicate with the vascular surgeon to make certain the desired veins are mapped and adequate for the procedure planned.

Upper Extremity

Although not as well studied, duplex US is a useful screening modality for the venous evaluation of the upper extremity, particularly for DVT and symptoms suggestive of thoracic outlet syndrome.

Anatomy. The superficial venous system is the primary drainage pathway for the upper extremity (Fig. 54.39). The basilic

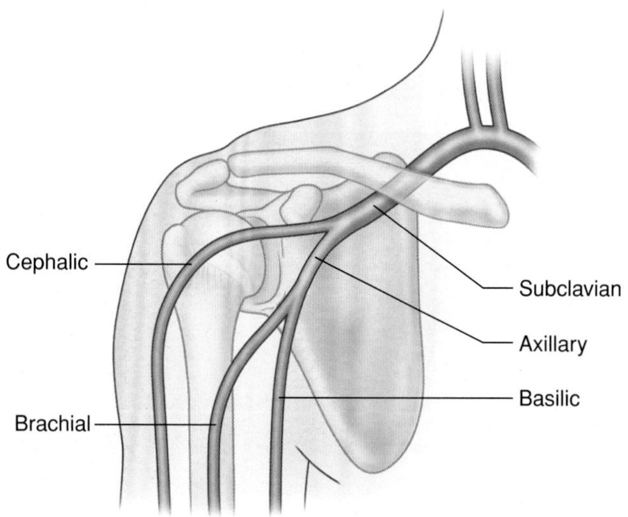

FIGURE 54.39. **Upper Extremity Venous Anatomy.**

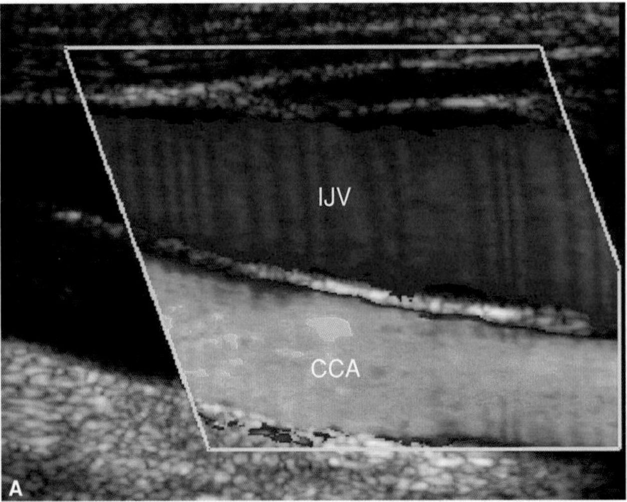

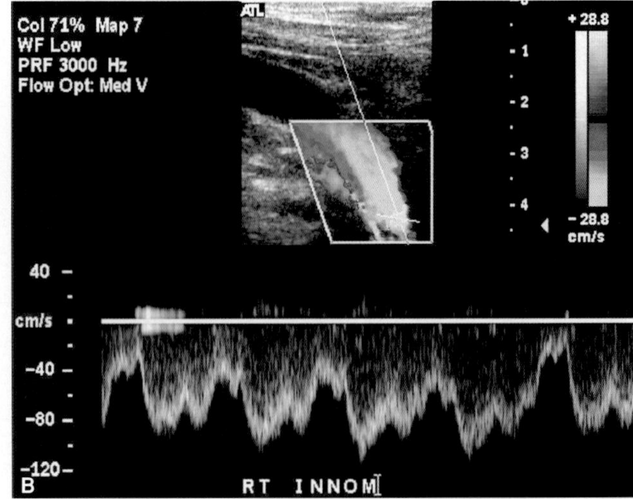

FIGURE 54.40. **Normal Upper Extremity Venous US. A:** Color Doppler image shows normal wall-to-wall color flow in the internal jugular vein (*IJV*) in blue and in the common carotid artery (*CCA*) in red. **B:** Normal venous waveform in the innominate vein demonstrates respiratory phasicity and transmitted cardiac pulsations.

vein courses along the ulnar side of the forearm and medial upper arm and continues as the axillary vein. The cephalic vein ascends on the radial aspect of the forearm and continues laterally to the shoulder. The cephalic vein joins the axillary vein just below the clavicle. The axillary vein continues as the subclavian vein at the lateral border of the first rib. After it receives the internal jugular vein, it continues as the brachiocephalic vein to the superior vena cava. The deep system consists of small, paired brachial veins that course with the artery and empty into the basilic vein.

Venous US Technique. A complete evaluation of the upper extremity includes the bilateral evaluation of the axillary, subclavian, inominate, and internal jugular veins (Fig. 54.40).

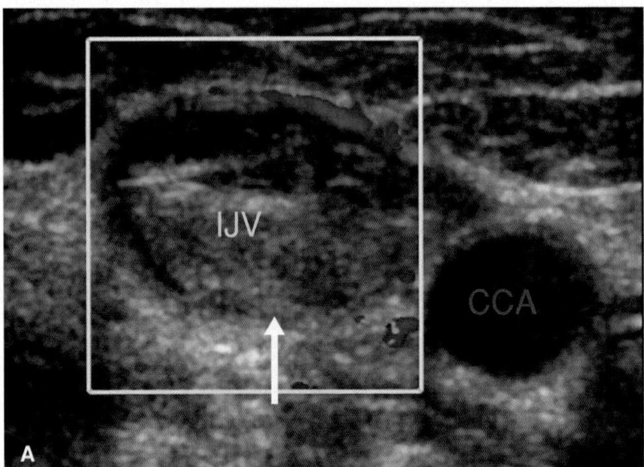

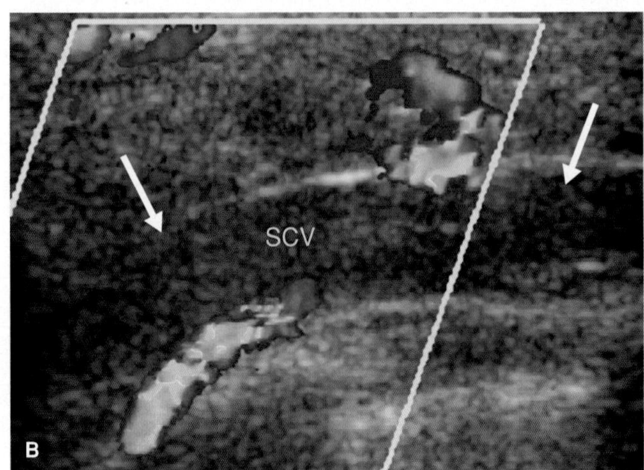

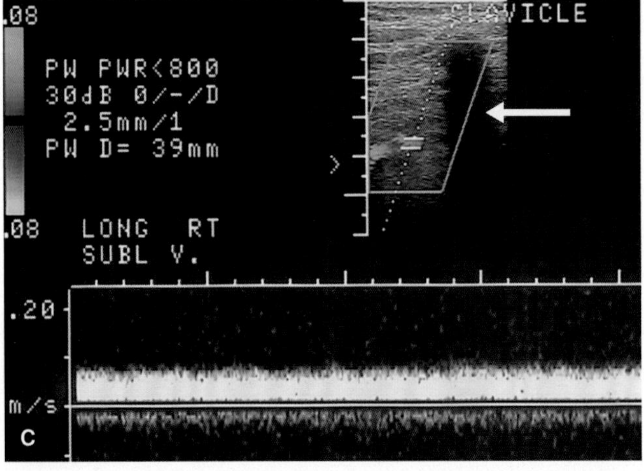

FIGURE 54.41. **Upper Extremity Venous Thrombosis. A:** Transverse image of the right internal jugular vein (*IJV*) and common carotid artery (*CCA*) reveals occlusive thrombus (*arrow*) filling and distending the vein. **B:** Longitudinal image of the subclavian vein (*SCV*) shows hypoechoic thrombus (*arrows*) occluding blood flow and filling the vein. **C:** The proximal right subclavian vein has a blunted, monophasic waveform suggesting a central obstruction. CT with intravenous contrast revealed a left brachiocephalic vein thrombosis. Note the acoustic shadow (*arrow*) from the clavicle obscuring a portion of the subclavian vein.

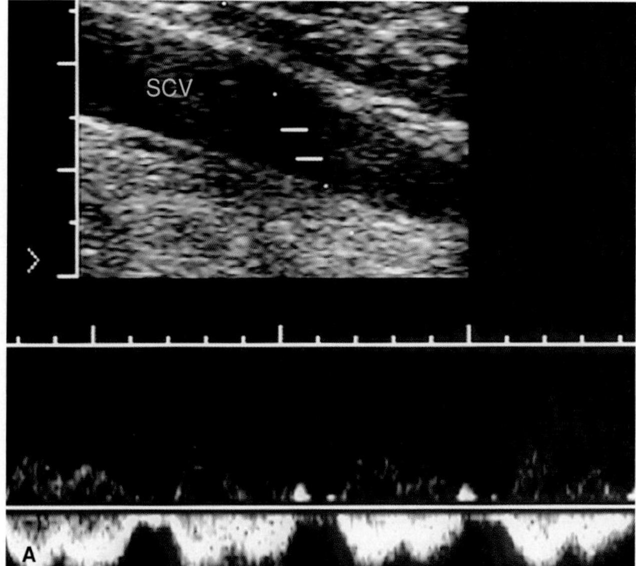

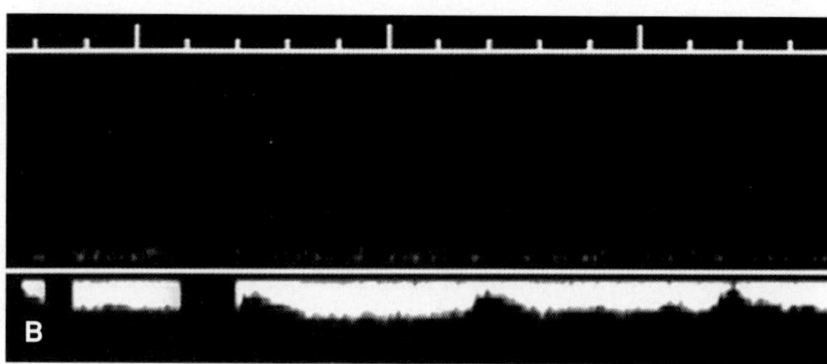

FIGURE 54.42. **Thoracic Outlet Syndrome: Venous. A:** The subclavian vein (*SCV*) waveform is normal with phasic flow while the arm is at the patient's side. **B:** With the arm abducted, the Doppler spectrum becomes blunted (more monophasic) due to compression of the vein. The contralateral side demonstrated no blunting of the waveform with abduction.

The basilic, cephalic, brachial, forearm veins and symptomatic areas are examined as clinically indicated. The same criteria used for the lower extremity can be applied in the upper extremity above the elbow (Fig. 54.41). Evaluation of the central veins, especially the subclavian, is restricted due to the overlying clavicle limiting visualization and compression. CD is the mainstay of evaluation of the central veins. In lieu of compression, the "sniff" test and the Valsalva maneuver are useful in the subclavian vein. With sniffing, the diameter of the subclavian vein will decrease and often completely collapse. With Valsalva, the vein will increase in diameter. These maneuvers are performed bilaterally and the response compared. Duplex evaluation of the venous waveforms reveals normal respiratory phasicity and transmitted cardiac pulsations in the central veins. The farther from the thoracic inlet, the more monophasic the waveform. Loss of the normal pulsatility (monophasic waveform) centrally when compared to the contralateral side suggests a proximal central obstruction (Fig. 54.41C).

Upper extremity DVT (Fig. 54.41) is usually the result of a current or previous indwelling catheter. A coexistent ipsilateral internal jugular vein clot is often present. Venous stasis in the upper extremity due to extrinsic compression or thoracic outlet syndrome is less common. In contrast to the lower extremity, upper extremity DVT is associated with pulmonary embolism in only 12% of cases. The diagnosis of DVT employs the same principles as that for the lower extremity, in addition to the techniques described in the previous paragraphs.

Thoracic Outlet Syndrome. The most common presentation for a patient with thoracic outlet syndrome is pain due to compression of the brachial plexus. Venous obstruction resulting in arm swelling is more common than arterial obstruction. Venous compression occurs on the subclavian vein as it passes

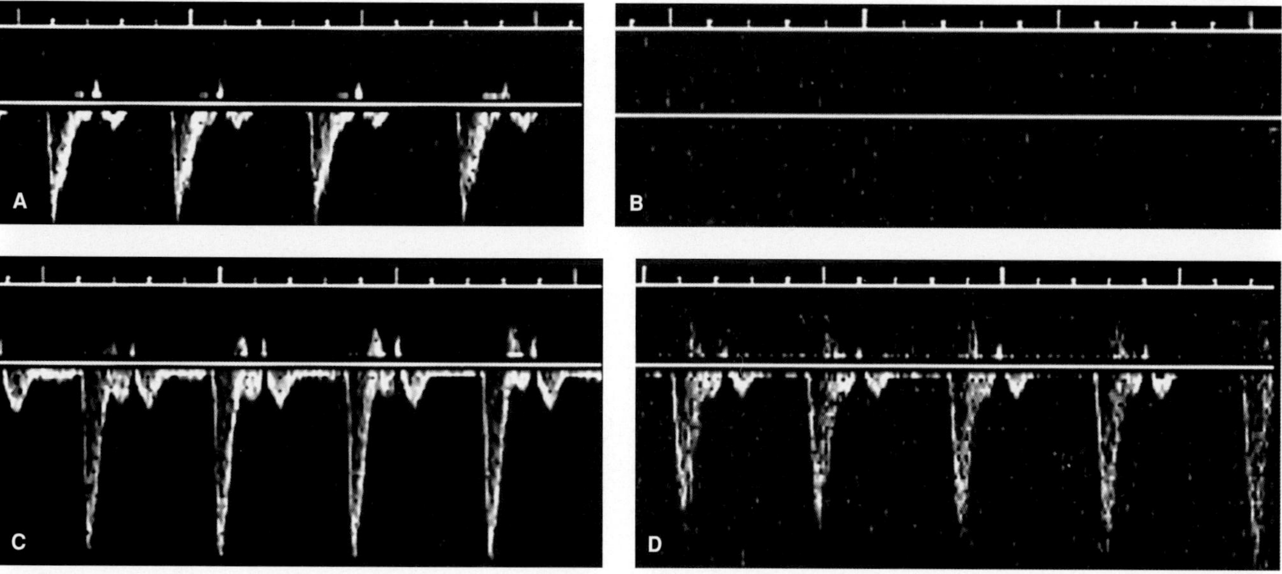

FIGURE 54.43. **Thoracic Outlet Syndrome: Arterial. A:** With the arm at the patient's side, the waveform in the left subclavian artery is a normal triphasic high-resistance pattern. **B:** Abduction of the left arm causes complete obliteration of the left radial pulse on physical examination. The Doppler tracing confirms the clinical finding demonstrating complete absence of flow in the subclavian artery. **C:** For comparison, the right subclavian artery has normal triphasic, high-resistance waveform with the arm at the patient's side. **D:** With abduction of the right arm, the spectral waveform does not change, indicating the absence of thoracic outlet syndrome.

between the first rib and scalene muscles at the thoracic inlet (Fig. 54.42). Intermittent arm swelling, effort thrombosis, and pain are the usual symptoms. If frank clot is not identified, the patient should be examined with the arm at the side and at various degrees of abduction. Using SD and CD, compression is likely if flow ceases or a dampening of the waveform occurs. No dampening is seen on the unaffected side. Arterial thoracic outlet syndrome (3% of cases) presents with ischemia resulting in claudication, pallor, paresthesias, decreased upper extremity pulses, and coolness of the arm. Causes include damage to the subclavian artery at the level of the first rib and emboli to the subclavian artery. A blunted arterial waveform or absent flow is seen if the subclavian artery is affected (Fig. 54.43).

Suggested Readings

Ali MU, Fitzpatrick-Lewis D, Miller J, et al. Screening for abdominal aortic aneurysm in asymptomatic adults. *J Vasc Surg* 2016;64:1855–1868.

American Institute of Ultrasound in Medicine. AIUM practice parameter for the performance of peripheral arterial ultrasound examinations using color and spectral Doppler imaging. Laurel, MD: American Institute of Ultrasound in Medicine; 2014. Available from http://www.aium.org/resources/guidelines/peripheralArterial.pdf.

American Institute of Ultrasound in Medicine. AIUM practice parameter for the performance of diagnostic and screening ultrasound examinations of the abdominal aorta in adults. Laurel, MD: American Institute of Ultrasound in Medicine; 2015. Available from http://www.aium.org/resources/guidelines/abdominalAorta.pdf.

American Institute of Ultrasound in Medicine. AIUM practice parameter for the performance of peripheral venous ultrasound examinations. Laurel, MD: American Institute of Ultrasound in Medicine; 2015. Available from http://www.aium.org/resources/guidelines/peripheralVenous.pdf.

American Institute of Ultrasound in Medicine. AIUM practice parameter for the performance of ultrasound examination of the extracranial cerebrovascular system. Laurel, MD: American Institute of Ultrasound in Medicine; 2016. Available from http://www.aium.org/resources/guidelines/extracranial.pdf.

American Institute of Ultrasound in Medicine. AIUM practice parameter for the performance of physiologic evaluation of extremity arteries. Laurel, MD: American Institute of Ultrasound in Medicine; 2017. Available from http://www.aium.org/resources/guidelines/extremityArteries.pdf.

Boote EJ. AAPM/RSNA physics tutorial for residents: topics in US: Doppler US techniques: concepts of blood flow detection and flow dynamics. *Radiographics* 2003;23:1315–1327.

Braun RM, Bertino RE, Milbrandt J, Bray M. Ultrasound imaging of carotid artery stenosis: application of the Society of Radiologists in Ultrasound consensus criteria to a single institution clinical practice. *Ultrasound Q* 2008;24:161–166.

Catalano O, Siani A. Ruptured abdominal aortic aneurysm: categorization of sonographic findings and report of 3 new signs. *J Ultrasound Med* 2005; 24:1077–1083.

Chin EE, Zimmerman PT, Grant EG. Sonographic evaluation of upper extremity deep venous thrombosis. *J Ultrasound Med* 2005;24:829–838.

DeMarco JK, Huston J 3rd. Imaging of high-risk carotid artery plaques: current status and future directions. *Neurosurg Focus* 2014;36:E1.

Deurdulian C, Emmanuel N, Tchelepi H, Grant EG, Malhi H. Beyond the bifurcation: there is more to cerebrovascular ultrasound than internal carotid artery stenosis! *Ultrasound Q* 2016;32:224–240. (Review article).

Gaitini D, Razi NB, Ghersin E, Ofer A, Soudack M. Sonographic evaluation of vascular injuries. *J Ultrasound Med* 2008;27:95–107.

Gaitini D, Soudack M. Diagnosing carotid stenosis by Doppler sonography: state of the art. *J Ultrasound Med* 2005; 24:1127–1136. (Review article).

Ginat DT, Bhatt S, Sidhu R, Dogra V. Carotid and vertebral artery Doppler ultrasound waveforms: a pictorial review. *Ultrasound Q* 2011;27:81–85.

Gonçalves I, den Ruijter H, Nahrendorf M, Pasterkamp G. Detecting the vulnerable plaque in patients. *J Intern Med* 2015;278:520–530.

Grant EG, Benson CB, Moneta GL, et al. Carotid artery stenosis: grayscale and Doppler ultrasound diagnosis—Society of Radiologists in Ultrasound consensus conference. *Ultrasound Q* 2003;19:190–198.

Khilnani NM. Duplex ultrasound evaluation of patients with chronic venous disease of the lower extremities. *AJR Am J Roentgenol* 2014;202: 633–642.

Kuhn JE, Lebus V GF, Bible JE. Thoracic outlet syndrome. *J Am Acad Orthop Surg* 2015;23:222–232.

Øygarden H. Carotid intima-media thickness and prediction of cardiovascular disease. *J Am Heart Assoc* 2017;6:e005313.

Rafailidis V, Chryssogonidis I, Tegos T, Kouskouras K, Charitanti-Kouridou A. Imaging of the ulcerated carotid atherosclerotic plaque: a review of the literature. *Insights Imaging* 2017;8:213–225.

Rubens DJ, Bhatt S, Nedelka S, Cullinan J. Doppler artifacts and pitfalls. *Radiol Clin North Am* 2006;44:805–835.

Shaf Z, Masoomi R, Thapa R, et al. Optimal medical management reduces risk of disease progression and ischemic events in asymptomatic carotid stenosis patients: a long-term follow-up study. *Cerebrovasc Dis* 2017;44:150–159.

Thorisson HM, Pollak JS, Scoutt L. The role of ultrasound in the diagnosis and treatment of chronic venous insufficiency. *Ultrasound Q* 2007;23:137–150.

U.S. Preventative Services Task Force. Screening for asymptomatic carotid artery stenosis: recommendation statement. *Am Fam Physician* 2015; 91:716I–716K.

Wood MM, Romine LE, Lee YK, et al. Spectral Doppler signature waveforms in ultrasonography: a review of normal and abnormal waveforms. *Ultrasound Q* 2010;26:83–99. (Review article).

SECTION X
MUSCULOSKELETAL RADIOLOGY

SECTION EDITORS: Clyde A. Helms and Emily N. Vinson

CHAPTER 55 ■ BENIGN LUCENT BONE LESIONS

CLYDE A. HELMS AND EMILY N. VINSON

A benign, bubbly, lucent lesion of the bone is one of the more common skeletal lesions a radiologist encounters. The differential diagnosis can be quite lengthy and is usually structured on how the lesion looks to the radiologist, using his or her experience as a guide. This method, called pattern identification, certainly has merits, but it can lead to a very long differential diagnosis and many erroneous conclusions if not tempered with some logic.

In general, if a differential diagnosis will yield the correct diagnosis 95% of the time, most would consider it a useful differential list; however, it would not be appropriate to accept a 1-in-20 miss rate for fractures and dislocations. In general, the shorter the differential diagnosis list, the more helpful it is to the clinicians and the easier it is to remember. A shorter differential list will usually have a lower accuracy rate than a long list; however, many times the longer lists contain such rare entities that the accuracy does not really increase substantially. For most of the entities in bone radiology, a 95% accurate differential is acceptable. If one wants to be more accurate than that, simply add more diagnoses to the list of differential possibilities.

When the differential diagnosis is long, as in the differential for bubbly, lucent lesions of bone, it can be difficult to recall all of the entities that should be mentioned. A mnemonic can be helpful in recalling long lists of information and is recommended.

FEGNOMASHIC

FEGNOMASHIC is a mnemonic that serves as a nice starting point for discussing possibilities that appear as benign, lucent lesions in bone. This mnemonic has been in general use for many years. By itself, it is merely a long list—15 entities—and needs to be coupled with other criteria to shorten the list into manageable form for each particular case. For instance, the age of the patient will help add or eliminate many of the possibilities. If multiple lesions are present, only-half a dozen entities need to be discussed. Methods of narrowing the differential are discussed later in this chapter.

The first step in approaching a benign, lucent bone lesion is to be certain it is really benign. The criteria for differentiating benign from malignant are covered in Chapter 56. Once it is established that the lesion is truly a benign, cystic lesion, FEGNOMASHIC will enable a differential diagnosis that is at least 95% accurate. Memorizing the 15 entities in this differential is easily done (Table 55.1).

The next step after learning the names of all of the lesions is getting some idea of each lesion's radiographic appearance. This is when experience becomes a factor. For the medical student or first-year resident, it is difficult to go beyond saying that they all look lucent, bubbly, and benign. The fourth-year resident should have no trouble differentiating between a unicameral bone cyst and a giant cell tumor because he or she has seen examples of each many times before and knows their appearance.

After getting a feel for what each lesion looks like radiographically and overcoming the frustration that builds when one realizes that many of them look alike, one should try to learn ways to differentiate each lesion from the others. I have developed a number of keys that I call discriminators, which will help to differentiate each lesion. These discriminators are 90% to 95% useful (I will mention when they are more or less accurate, in my experience) and are by no means intended to be absolutes or dogma. They are guidelines but have a high accuracy rate.

Textbooks rarely state that a finding "always" or "never" occurs. They temper descriptions with "virtually always," "invariably," "usually," or "characteristically." I have tried to pick out findings that come as close to "always" as I can, realizing that I will only be approximately 95% accurate. That is good enough for most radiologists.

The following is only a brief description of each entity, as more complete descriptions are readily available in any skeletal radiology text. What is emphasized here are the points that are unique for each entity, thereby enabling differentiation from the others. Table 55.1 is a synopsis of these discriminators.

FIBROUS DYSPLASIA

Fibrous dysplasia is a benign congenital process that can be seen in a patient of any age and can look like almost any

TABLE 55.1

DISCRIMINATORS FOR BENIGN LYTIC BONE LESIONS—MNEMONIC: FEGNOMASHIC

LETTER	REPRESENTS	CHARACTERISTICS
F	*Fibrous dysplasia*	No periosteal reaction
E	*Enchondroma*	1. Calcification present (except in phalanges) 2. Painless (no periostitis)
	Eosinophilic granuloma	Younger than age 30
G	*Giant cell tumor*	1. Physes closed 2. Abuts the articular surface (in long bones) 3. Well defined with a nonsclerotic margin (in long bones) 4. Eccentric
N	*Nonossifying fibroma*	1. Younger than age 30 2. Painless (no periostitis)
O	*Osteoblastoma*	Mentioned when ABC is mentioned (especially in the posterior elements of the spine)
M	*Metastatic diseases and myeloma*	Older than age 40
A	*Aneurysmal bone cyst*	1. Expansile 2. Younger than age 30
S	*Solitary bone cyst*	1. Central 2. Younger than age 30
H	*Hyperparathyroidism (brown tumor)*	Must have other evidence of HPT
	Hemangiomas	Rare. May be multiple
I	*Infection*	Always mention
C	*Chondroblastoma*	1. Younger than age 30 2. Epiphyseal
	Chondromyxoid fibroma	No calcified matrix

ABC, aneurysmal bone cyst; HPT, hyperparathyroidism.

pathologic process radiographically. It can be wild-looking, a discrete lucency, patchy, sclerotic, expansile, multiple, and many other descriptions. It is, therefore, difficult to look at a bubbly lytic lesion and unequivocally say it is or is not fibrous dysplasia. It would be better if the FEGNOMASHIC differential started on a positive note, say, with giant cell tumor or chondroblastoma, for which there are some definite criteria. Because fibrous dysplasia is first on the list, we might as well deal with it.

How do you know whether to include or exclude fibrous dysplasia if it can look like almost anything? Experience is the best guideline. In other words, look in a few texts and find as many different examples as possible; get a feeling for what fibrous dysplasia looks like.

Fibrous dysplasia will not have periostitis associated with it; therefore, if periostitis is present, one may safely exclude fibrous dysplasia. Fibrous dysplasia virtually never undergoes malignant degeneration and should not be a painful lesion unless there is a fracture. An occult fracture may occur in long bones with fibrous dysplasia; therefore, it is not unusual to have it present with pain and no obvious fracture seen in a long bone. Pain in a flat bone, such as the ribs or skull (non–weight-bearing bones), should not occur with fibrous dysplasia.

Fibrous dysplasia can be either monostotic (most commonly) or polyostotic and has a predilection for the pelvis, proximal femur, ribs, and skull. When it is present in the pelvis, it is invariably present in the ipsilateral proximal femur (Figs. 55.1 and 55.2). I have seen only one case in which the pelvis was involved with fibrous dysplasia and the proximal femur was spared. The proximal femur, however, may be affected alone, without involvement in the pelvis (Fig. 55.3).

Fibrous dysplasia often involves the ribs. It typically has an expansile, lytic appearance in the posterior ribs (Fig. 55.4) and a sclerotic appearance in the anterior ribs.

The classic description of fibrous dysplasia is that it has a ground-glass or smoky matrix. This description confuses people as often as it helps them, and I do not recommend using ground-glass appearance as a buzz word for fibrous dysplasia. Fibrous dysplasia is often purely lytic and becomes hazy or takes on a ground-glass look as the matrix calcifies (Fig. 55.5). It can go on to calcify significantly, and then it presents as a sclerotic lesion. Also, I often see lytic lesions with a pathologic diagnosis other than fibrous dysplasia that have a distinct ground-glass appearance; therefore, the ground-glass quality can be misleading.

Adamantinoma. When a lesion is encountered in the tibia that resembles fibrous dysplasia, an adamantinoma should also be mentioned. An adamantinoma is a malignant tumor that radiographically and histologically resembles fibrous dysplasia (Fig. 55.6). It occurs almost exclusively in the tibia and the jaw (for unknown reasons) and is rare. Because it is rare,

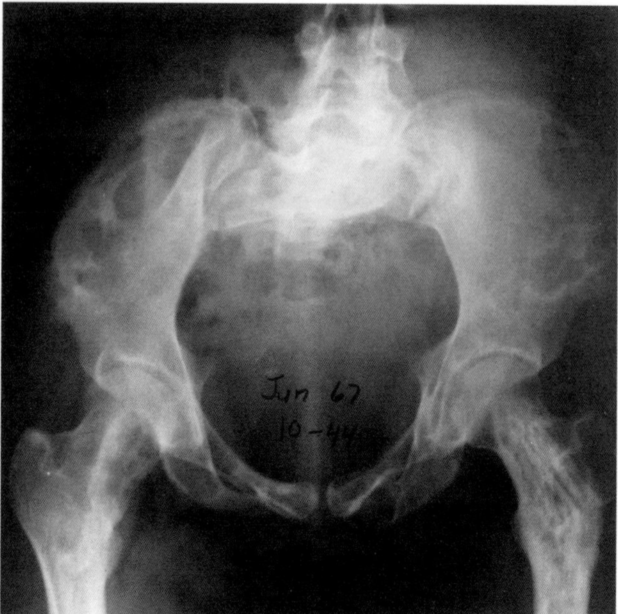

FIGURE 55.1. Fibrous Dysplasia. This patient has polyostotic fibrous dysplasia with diffuse involvement of the pelvis as well as the proximal femurs.

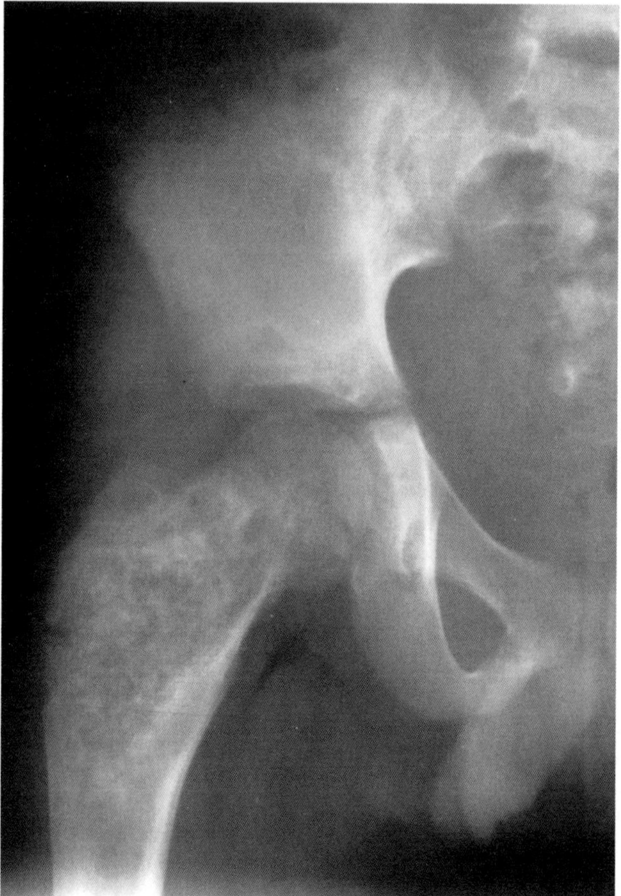

FIGURE 55.2. Fibrous Dysplasia. This patient has polyostotic fibrous dysplasia with the involvement of the right femur as well as the supraacetabular portion of the ilium. When the pelvis is involved with fibrous dysplasia, the ipsilateral femur on the affected side is invariably also involved.

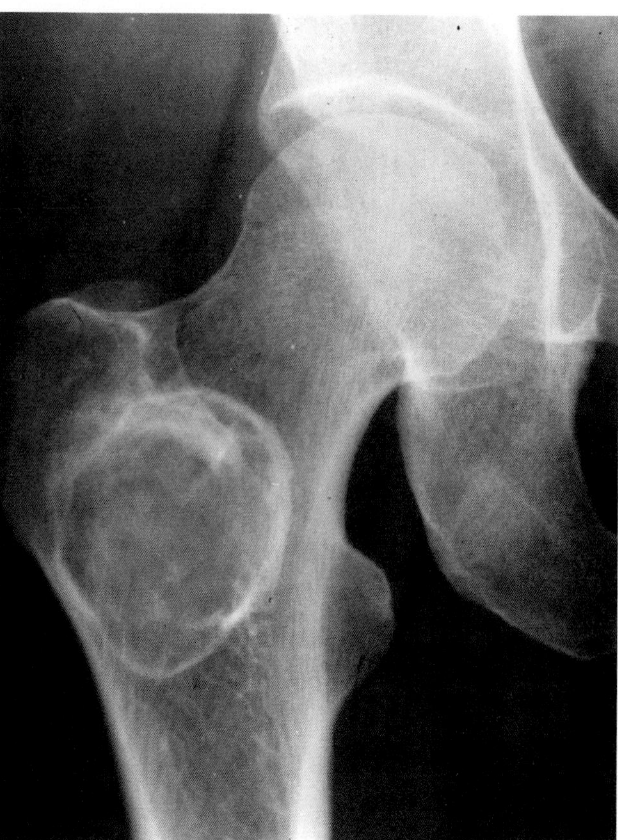

FIGURE 55.3. Fibrous Dysplasia. This patient has a well-defined lytic lesion with a hazy, ground-glass appearance in the neck of the right femur. The pelvis was uninvolved. It is not unusual for monostotic fibrous dysplasia to involve the proximal femur and spare the pelvis.

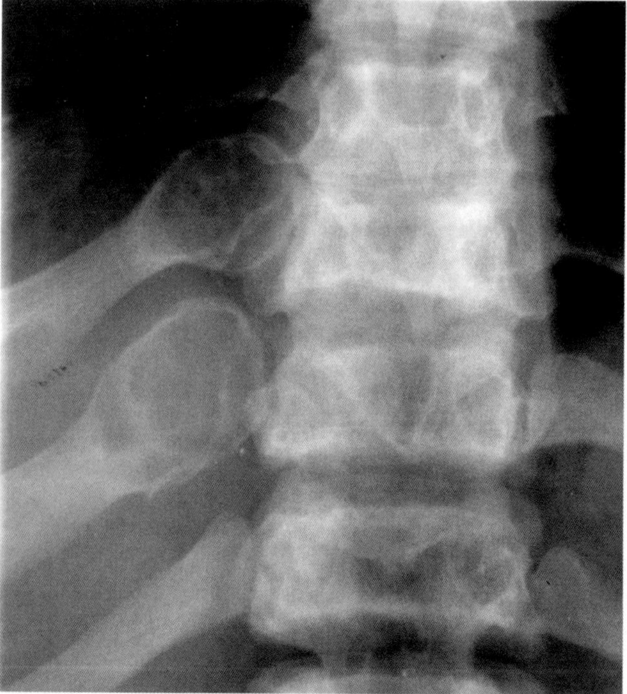

FIGURE 55.4. Fibrous Dysplasia. When fibrous dysplasia affects the ribs, the posterior ribs often demonstrate a lytic expansile appearance, as in this example. When the anterior ribs are involved, they are most often sclerotic in appearance. Note also the involvement of the thoracic spine.

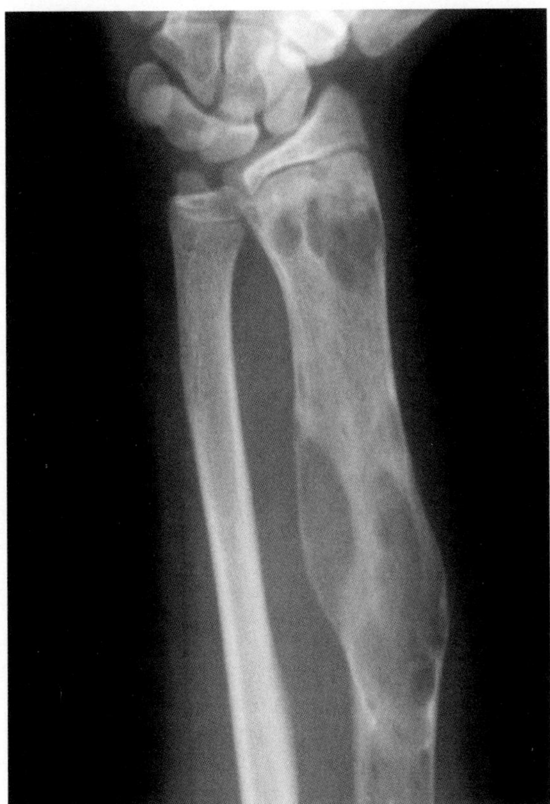

FIGURE 55.5. **Fibrous Dysplasia.** Polyostotic fibrous dysplasia is seen in the radius in this child. Parts of this lesion have a hazy, ground-glass appearance, whereas others are more lytic appearing. A hazy, ground-glass appearance is often present in fibrous dysplasia, but just as often, the appearance can be purely lytic or even sclerotic.

FIGURE 55.6. **Adamantinoma.** This mixed lytic and sclerotic process in the midshaft of the tibia is characteristic of fibrous dysplasia. An adamantinoma has an identical appearance and should be considered in any tibial lesion that resembles fibrous dysplasia. Biopsy showed this to be an adamantinoma.

one may choose not to include it in the differential—a misdiagnosis will not occur more than once or twice in a lifetime.

McCune Albright Syndrome. Polyostotic fibrous dysplasia occasionally occurs in association with cafe au lait spots on the skin (flat pigmented skin lesions) and precocious puberty. This complex is called McCune–Albright syndrome. The bony lesions in this syndrome, and even in the simple polyostotic form, often occur unilaterally, that is, throughout one-half of the body. This does not happen often enough to be of any diagnostic use in differentiating fibrous dysplasia from other lesions.

The presence of multiple lesions of fibrous dysplasia in the jaw has been termed cherubism. This is from the physical appearance of the child with puffed-out cheeks having an angelic look. The jaw lesions in cherubism regress in adulthood.

Discriminator. No periosteal reaction.

ENCHONDROMA

Enchondromas occur in any bone formed from cartilage and may be central, eccentric, expansile, or nonexpansile. They invariably contain calcified chondroid matrix except when in the phalanges of the hands and feet. An enchondroma is the most common benign lytic lesion in the phalanges (Fig. 55.7). If a lytic lesion is present without calcified chondroid matrix anywhere except in the phalanges, I do not include enchondroma in my differential.

Occasionally, it is difficult to differentiate between an enchondroma and a bone infarct. An infarct usually has a well-defined, densely sclerotic, serpiginous border (Fig. 55.8), whereas an enchondroma does not (Fig. 55.9). An enchondroma often causes mild endosteal scalloping, whereas a bone infarct will not. Although these criteria are helpful in separating an infarct from an enchondroma, they are not foolproof.

It is difficult, if not impossible, to differentiate an enchondroma from a chondrosarcoma. Clinical findings (primarily pain) serve as a better indicator than radiographic findings, and indeed pain in an apparent enchondroma should warrant surgical investigation. Cortical destruction and periostitis should not be seen in an enchondroma either. Trying to differentiate histologically an enchondroma from a chondrosarcoma is also difficult, if not impossible, at times. Biopsy of an apparent enchondroma should not be performed routinely for histologic differentiation.

Since benign enchondromas are often misdiagnosed by experienced pathologists, radiologists should not mention the possibility of a chondroid lesion being a chondrosarcoma or use phrases such as "chondrosarcoma cannot be excluded" as this will invariably lead to a biopsy, which can then result in unnecessary radical or extensive surgery. It is better to simply say "no aggressive features noted." The surgeon is then more likely to follow it with imaging and clinical correlation for the presence of pain referable to the lesion.

Multiple enchondromas occur on occasion; this condition has been termed Ollier disease (Fig. 55.10). It is not hereditary and carries a low risk of malignant degeneration. The

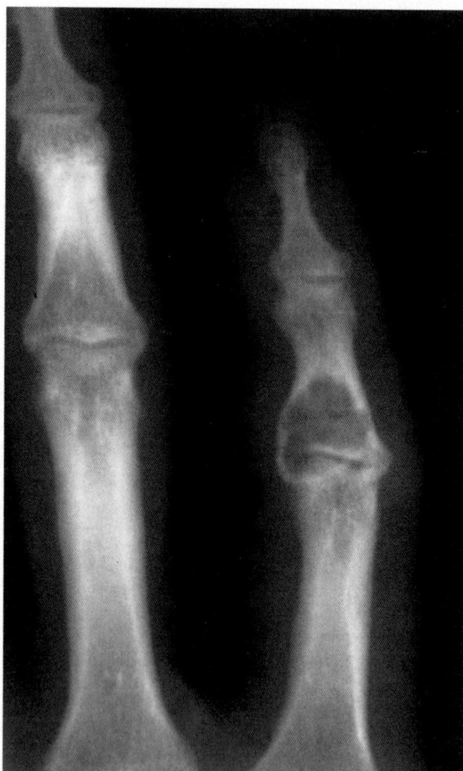

FIGURE 55.7. **Enchondroma.** A lytic lesion in the phalanges is most commonly an enchondroma. This is the only location in the skeleton where an enchondroma does not contain calcified chondroid matrix. These most often present with pathologic fractures, as in this example.

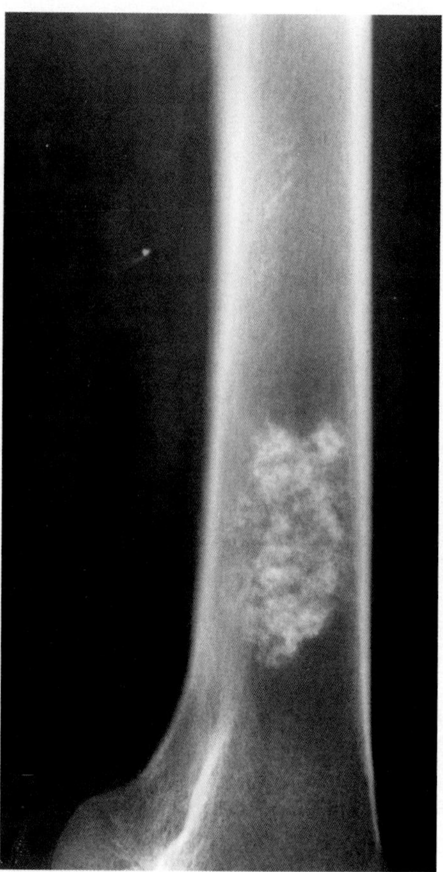

FIGURE 55.9. **Enchondroma.** This lesion in the distal right femur shows the stippled punctate calcification typical of chondroid matrix seen in an enchondroma.

presence of multiple enchondromas associated with soft tissue hemangiomas is known as Maffucci syndrome (Fig. 55.11). This syndrome also is not hereditary, is quite rare, and carries a higher risk of malignant degeneration of both the enchondromas and the hemangiomas, as well as an increased risk for developing other malignancies.

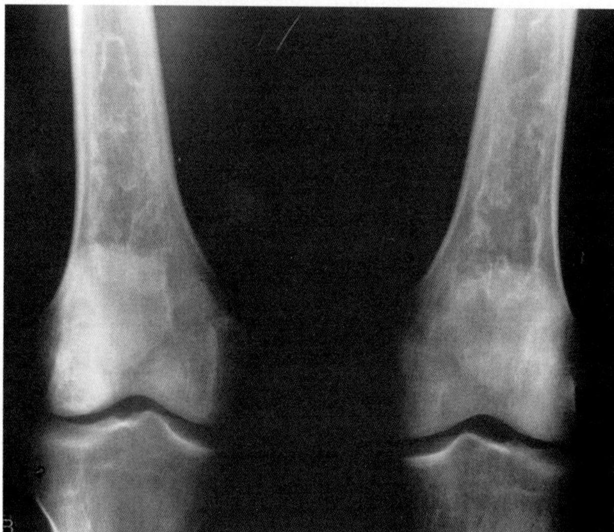

FIGURE 55.8. **Bone Infarct.** These lytic lesions in the distal femurs with calcified, serpiginous borders are typical of bone infarcts. Occasionally, differentiating between a bone infarct and an enchondroma can be difficult on radiographs; however, in this example, infarcts are easily diagnosed.

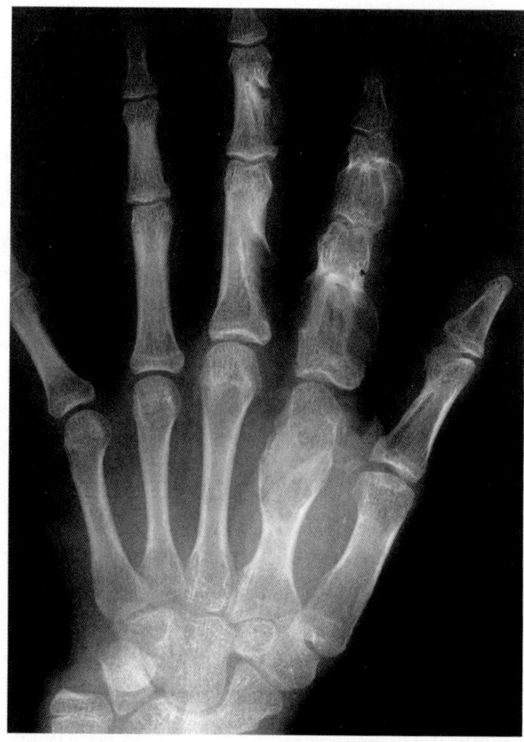

FIGURE 55.10. **Ollier Disease.** Multiple enchondromas are present throughout the hand. This is a typical example of Ollier disease.

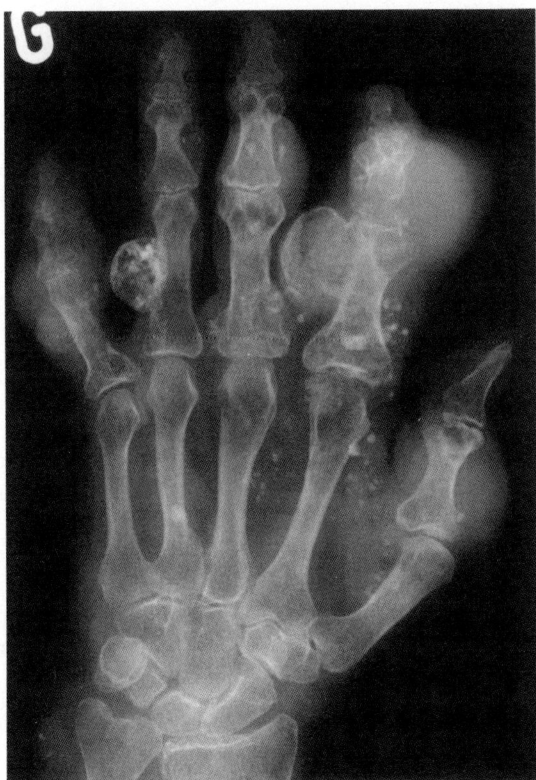

FIGURE 55.11. **Maffucci Syndrome.** Multiple enchondromas in the phalanges are associated with soft tissue phleboliths. This combination of findings invariably represents hemangiomas and enchondromas in Maffucci syndrome.

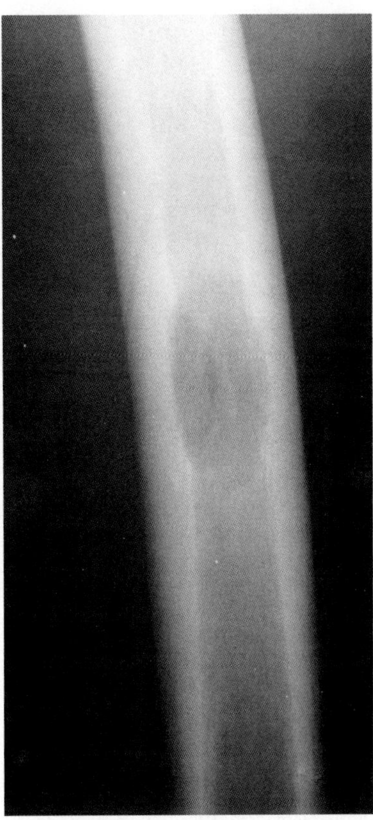

FIGURE 55.12. **Eosinophilic Granuloma (EG).** A well-defined lytic lesion is seen involving the mid-femur in this 20-year-old patient. Biopsy showed this to be EG.

Discriminators. (1) Must have calcification (except in phalanges), (2) No periostitis or pain.

EOSINOPHILIC GRANULOMA

Eosinophilic granuloma (also known as *LCH of bone*) is the most common and least severe form of Langerhans cell histiocytosis, the other forms being Letterer–Siwe disease and Hand–Schuller–Christian disease. Although these forms may be merely different phases of the same disease, most investigators categorize them separately. The bony manifestations of all three disorders are similar and are discussed in this review simply as EG.

Eosinophilic granuloma, unfortunately for radiologists, has many appearances. It can be lytic or sclerotic; it may be well defined or ill defined; it might or might not have a sclerotic border; and it might or might not elicit a periosteal response. The periostitis, when present, is typically benign in appearance (thick, uniform, wavy) but can be lamellated or amorphous. Eosinophilic granuloma can mimic Ewing sarcoma and present as a permeative (multiple small holes) lesion.

How, then, can one distinguish EG from any of the other lytic lesions in this differential? Remember that it is difficult to exclude EG from almost any differential of a bony lesion, be it benign or malignant. Eosinophilic granuloma occurs almost exclusively in patients less than the age of 30 years (usually <20 years); therefore, the patient's age is the best criterion. I recommend mentioning EG as a differential possibility for any lesion in a patient less than the age of 30 years. Because EG can look like anything, so long as the radiograph is not of an arthritide or trauma, EG can be mentioned without even looking at the radiograph!

Eosinophilic granuloma is most often monostotic (Fig. 55.12), but it can be polyostotic (Fig. 55.13) and, thus, has to be included

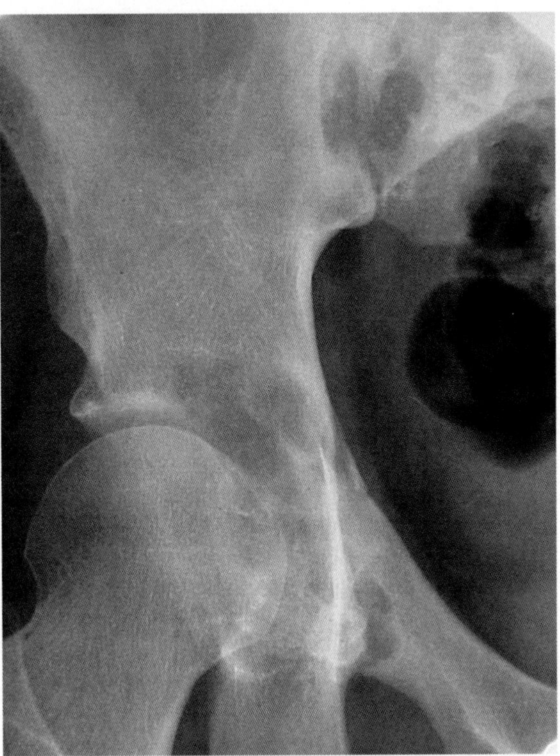

FIGURE 55.13. **Eosinophilic Granuloma (EG).** Well-defined lytic lesions are present throughout the pelvis in this 24-year-old patient. In addition to the lesion around the right hip, a lesion is seen at the right sacroiliac joint. Biopsy showed this to be EG.

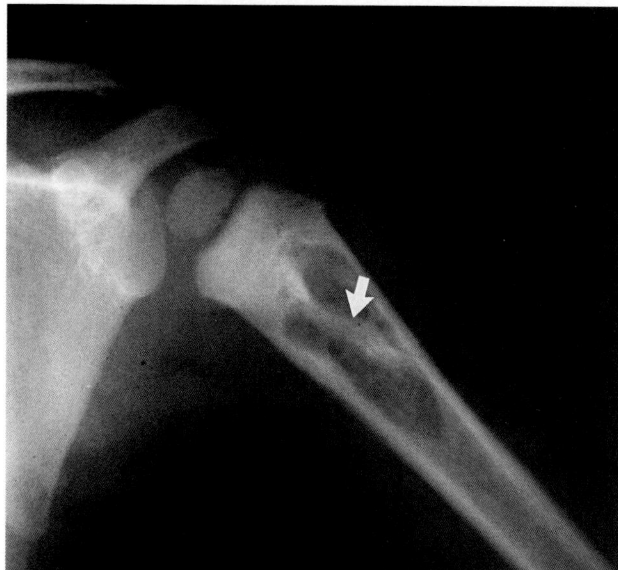

FIGURE 55.14. Eosinophilic Granuloma (EG). This well-defined lytic lesion contains a bony sequestrum (*arrow*), which is typical of osteomyelitis or EG. Biopsy revealed this to be EG.

whenever multiple lesions are present in a patient younger than the age of 30 years.

Eosinophilic granuloma might or might not have a soft tissue mass associated, so the presence or absence of a soft tissue mass will not help in the differential diagnosis. It is important to note the presence of a soft tissue mass (or its absence), but it will usually do little to narrow the differential diagnosis.

Most radiologists are inept at evaluating the soft tissues because they are difficult to see, and CT and MR have made it unnecessary in most cases to rely on plain radiographs for the soft tissues. Fortunately, in most cases, the presence or absence of a soft tissue mass will not alter the differential diagnosis. The treating physician will undoubtedly want to know whether the soft tissues are involved and to what extent; this can be satisfactorily demonstrated with MR.

Eosinophilic granuloma occasionally has a bony sequestrum (Fig. 55.14). Only a few other entities have been described that on occasion have bony sequestra—osteomyelitis, lymphoma, and fibrosarcoma; therefore, when a sequestrum is identified, EG, osteomyelitis, lymphoma, and fibrosarcoma should be considered. As discussed in Chapter 61, an osteoid osteoma will often give an appearance of a sequestration when the nidus is partially calcified.

Clinically, EG might or might not be associated with pain; therefore, clinical history is noncontributory for the most part.

Discriminator: Must be less than age 30 years.

GIANT CELL TUMOR

Giant cell tumor is an uncommon tumor found almost exclusively in adults in the ends of long bones and in flat bones.

It is important to realize that one is unable to tell whether a giant cell tumor is benign or malignant, regardless of its radiographic appearance. Histologically, a giant cell tumor cannot be divided into either a benign or a malignant category. Most surgeons curettage and pack the lesions and consider them benign unless they recur. Even then, they can still be benign and recur a second or third time. About 15% of giant cell tumors are thought to be malignant on the basis of their recurrence rate. When malignant, they can metastasize to the lungs, but they do so rarely.

Four classic radiographic criteria for diagnosing giant cell tumors exist. If any of these criteria are not met when looking at a lesion, giant cell tumor can be eliminated from the differential diagnosis.

1. Giant cell tumor occurs only in patients with closed physes; this is valid at least 98% to 99% of the time and is extremely useful. I will not entertain the diagnosis of giant cell tumor in a patient with open physes.
2. The lesion must be epiphyseal and abut the articular surface (Fig. 55.15). There is disagreement as to whether giant cell tumors begin in the epiphyses or metaphyses or from the physeal plate itself; however, except for rare cases, when radiologists see the lesions, they are epiphyseal and are flush against the articular surface. The metaphysis also has some of the tumor in it because the lesions are generally very large. When one sees a giant cell tumor, it will be epiphyseal. Perhaps more importantly, it should be flush against the articular surface of the joint. This occurs in 98% to 99% of giant cell tumors; therefore, if I have a lesion that is separated from the articular surface by a definite margin of normal bone, I will not include giant cell tumor in the diagnosis. This rule does not apply in flat bones, such as in the pelvis or in the apophyses (Fig. 55.16), which have no articular surfaces.
3. Giant cell tumors are said to be eccentrically located in the bone, as opposed to being centrally placed in the medullary cavity. When a bony lesion is quite large, it can be difficult to tell whether it is central or eccentric. I do not find this to be a terribly useful description, but it is one of the classic "rules" of a giant cell tumor.
4. The lesion must have a sharply defined zone of transition (border) that is not sclerotic. This is a very helpful finding in giant cell tumor. The only places this does not apply is in flat bones, such as the pelvis (Fig. 55.17) and the calcaneus.

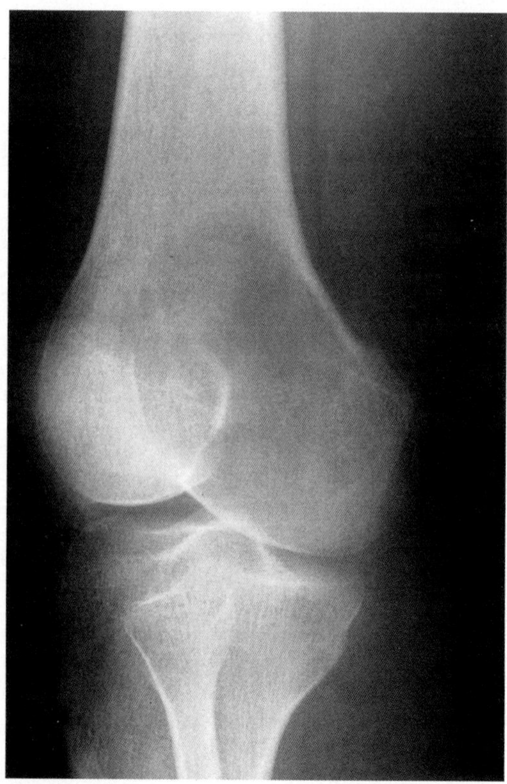

FIGURE 55.15. Giant Cell Tumor. A well-defined lytic lesion without a sclerotic margin is seen abutting the articular surface of the distal femur in a patient who has closed epiphyses. These are all characteristics of a giant cell tumor.

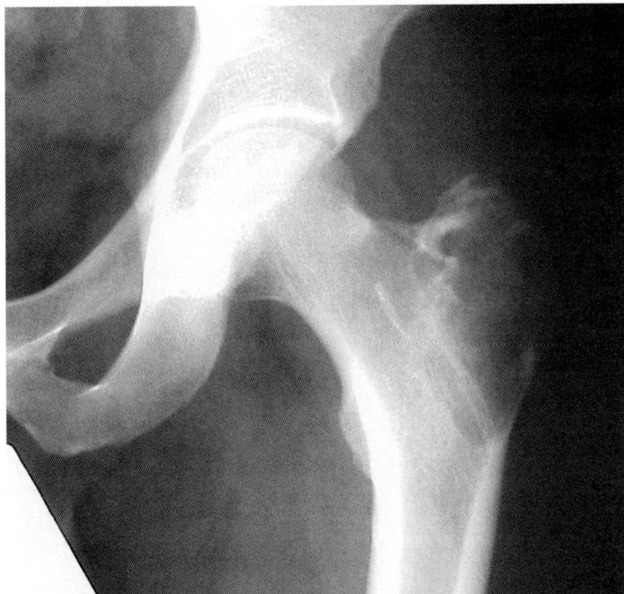

FIGURE 55.16. **Giant Cell Tumor.** This well-defined lytic lesion that does not have a sclerotic margin completely involves the greater trochanter. The apophyses have the same differential diagnosis as lesions in the epiphyses, which makes giant cell tumor a strong possibility in this example. Biopsy showed this to be a giant cell tumor.

It is important to realize that the four criteria for a giant cell tumor apply only to giant cell tumors and not to any other lesion. For instance, I know of no other lesion that depends on whether the physes are open or closed. No other lesion in any of my lists use as a diagnostic factor whether the zone of transition is sclerotic or not (many lesions, such as nonossifying fibromas [NOFs], will usually have a sclerotic margin, but it does not occur enough to include as a discriminator). No other lesion must always abut the articular surface, and no other lesion has the classic description of being eccentrically placed (although several lesions, including NOF and chondromyxoid fibroma, are eccentric most of the time).

Thus, while these four criteria apply well for giant cell tumor, they do not apply at all for any other lesions. Residents have a tendency to apply these criteria to every lucent bone lesion encountered for the simple reason that they have learned the four criteria.

Once one of the criteria is violated, the remainder do not even have to be used to eliminate a giant cell tumor. For instance, if a lytic lesion is found in the middiaphysis of a bone, giant cell tumor can be excluded. There is no need to check further to see whether it is eccentric, whether it has a nonsclerotic margin, or whether the physes are closed.

Again, these rules will be greater than 95% effective and, in my experience, close to 99% effective. It should be emphasized that these criteria only apply to giant cell tumors of long bones. They would not work, for instance, in the sacrum, pelvis, or the calcaneus, three locations where giant cell tumors often occur. If a case is found that does not fit the criteria, another pathologist should review the slides. Many pathologists refer to aneurysmal bone cysts (ABCs) as giant cell tumors; hence, they have giant cell tumors that do not obey any of the criteria. These pathologists may be correct, but they are not in the mainstream of what most people use for giant cell tumor criteria, both radiographically and histologically.

Discriminators. (1) Physes must be closed, (2) Must abut the articular surface, (3) Must be well defined with a nonsclerotic margin, (4) Must be eccentric.

NONOSSIFYING FIBROMA

An NOF (also known as a fibroxanthoma) is probably the most common bone lesion encountered by radiologists. It reportedly occurs in up to 20% of children and usually spontaneously regresses so as to be seen only rarely after the age of 30. "Fibrous cortical defect" is a common synonym, although some people divide the two lesions on the basis of size, with a fibrous cortical defect being smaller than 2 cm in length (Fig. 55.18) and an NOF being larger than 2 cm (Fig. 55.19).

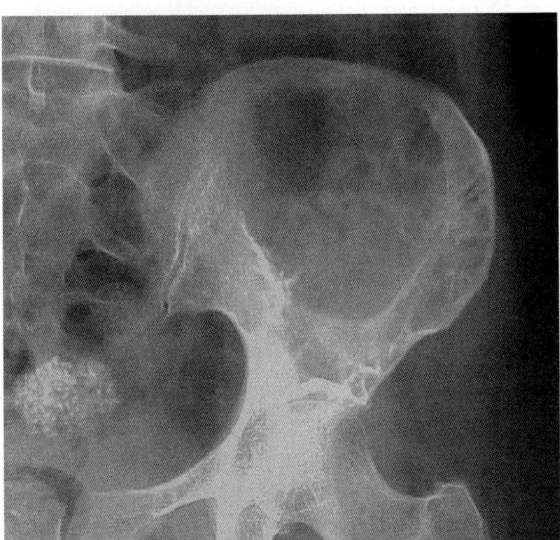

FIGURE 55.17. **Giant Cell Tumor.** A large, well-defined lytic lesion in the iliac wing is seen, which does contain a sclerotic margin and does not appear to abut any articular surface. The pelvis is a good location for giant cell tumor, which this proved to be at biopsy. The usual rules for giant cell tumors such as the presence of a nonsclerotic margin do not apply in flat bones.

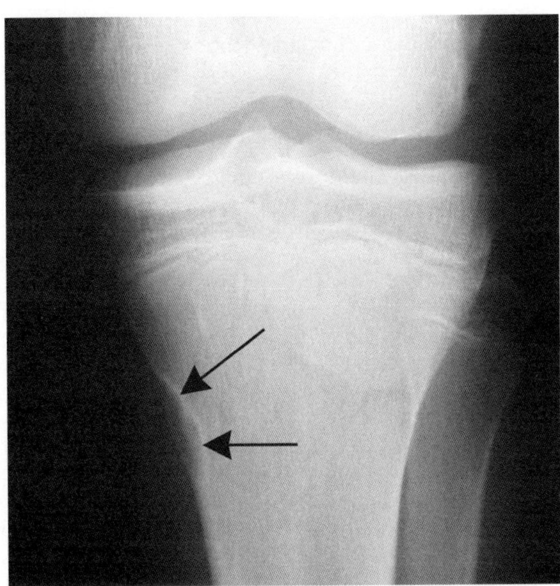

FIGURE 55.18. **Fibrous Cortical Defect.** A well-defined lytic lesion is seen in the medial metaphysis of this tibia (*arrows*), which is typical of a fibrous cortical defect.

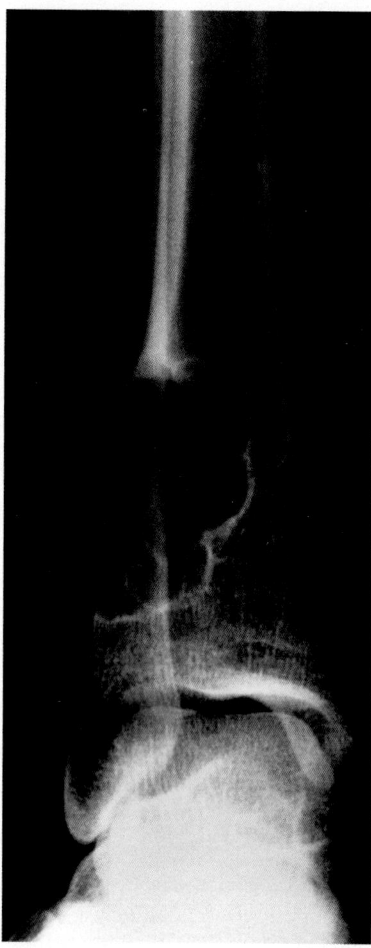

FIGURE 55.19. Nonossifying Fibroma (NOF). A large, well-defined lytic lesion, which is slightly expansile with scalloped sclerotic margins, is seen in the distal tibia in this young patient. This is a characteristic appearance of an NOF. The examination was obtained for a sprained ankle and not for this asymptomatic lesion.

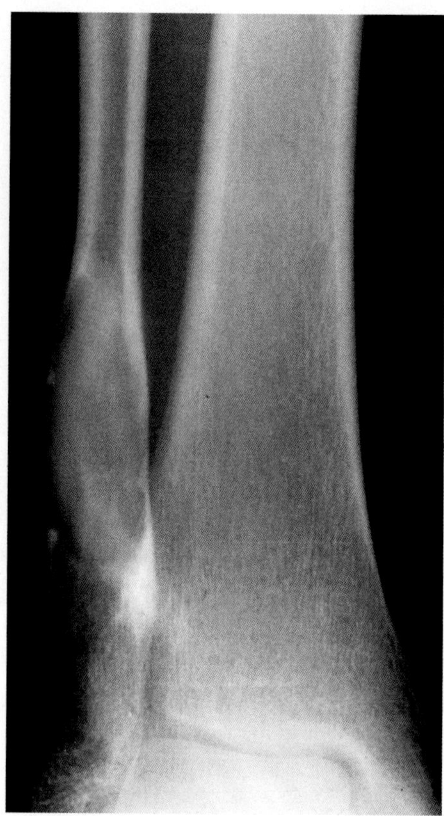

FIGURE 55.20. Nonossifying Fibroma (NOF). A well-defined, expansile lytic lesion in the distal fibula is noted in this asymptomatic patient, which is characteristic of an NOF.

Histologically, these lesions are identical; therefore, it seems appropriate to refer to them all as NOFs rather than to subdivide them by their size.

NOFs are benign, asymptomatic lesions that typically occur in the metaphysis of a long bone, emanating from the cortex. They classically have a thin, sclerotic border that is scalloped and slightly expansile (Fig. 55.20); however, this is a general description that probably applies to only 75% of the lesions and could equally apply to most of the lesions in FEGNOMASHIC. They do not have to have expansion or a scalloped or sclerotic border and are not limited to the metaphyses. Then how are they best recognized? The best way is to familiarize oneself with their general appearance by looking at examples in textbooks. That can be done in 15 minutes. It is important to recognize these lesions because they are what I call "don't touch" lesions (see Chapter 60); that is, the radiologist's diagnosis should be the final word and thereby supplant a biopsy. These lesions are so characteristic that no differential diagnosis should be entertained, although a few entities can indeed occasionally simulate them.

If a CT or MR is obtained of an NOF, there will often appear to be interruption of the cortex, which can be misinterpreted as cortical destruction (Fig. 55.21). This merely represents cortical replacement by benign fibrous tissue and should not warrant further investigation.

If the patient is older than 30 years of age, NOF should not be included in the differential diagnosis. NOFs must be asymptomatic and exhibit no periostitis, unless there is a history of antecedent trauma. They routinely "heal" with sclerosis and eventually disappear (Fig. 55.22), usually around the ages of 20 to 30 years. During this healing period, they can appear hot on a radionuclide bone scan because there is osteoblastic activity. These lesions can occasionally get quite large (Fig. 55.23); therefore, growth or change in size should not alter the diagnosis. They are most commonly seen about the knee but can occur in any long bone. Occasionally, multiple NOFs are seen about the knee, each of which is characteristic in appearance.

Discriminators. (1) Must be younger than age 30 years, (2) No periostitis or pain.

OSTEOBLASTOMA

Osteoblastomas are rare lesions that could justifiably be excluded from this differential without the fear of missing a diagnosis more than once in a lifetime. Why, then, include them? The mnemonic FEGNOMASHIC would not have nearly the same ring without the extra vowel, so osteoblastoma remains.

Osteoblastomas have two appearances: (1) They look like large osteoid osteomas and are often called giant osteoid osteomas. Because osteoid osteomas are primarily sclerotic lesions due to reactive bone formation and do not resemble bubbly lucent lesions, this is not the type of osteoblastoma we are concerned with in this differential; (2) They simulate ABCs. They are expansile, often having a soap bubble appearance. If an

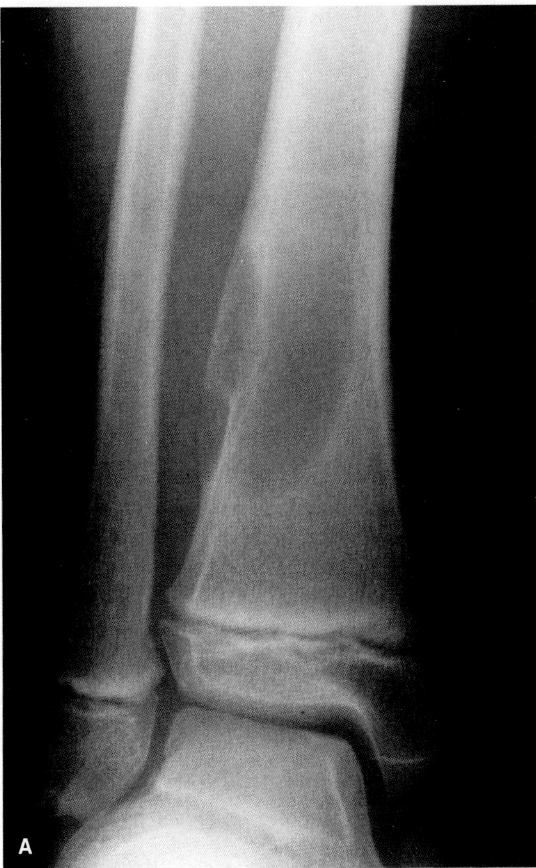

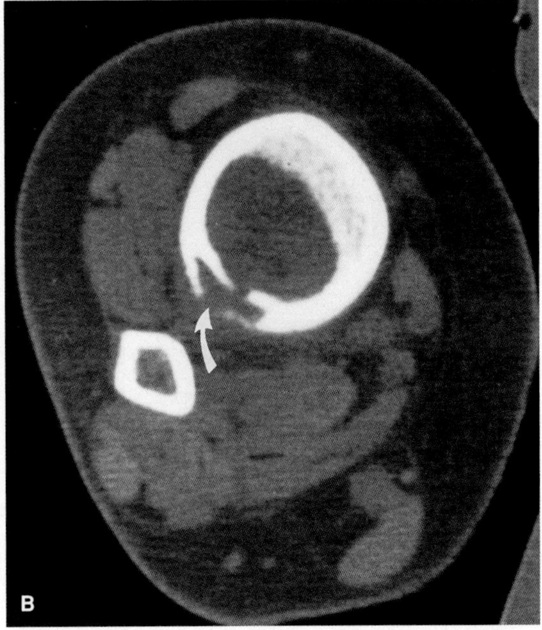

FIGURE 55.21. Nonossifying Fibroma. A: A well-defined, lytic lesion that is minimally expansile is seen in the distal tibia in this child who was examined for a sprained ankle. **B:** A CT examination showed apparent cortical destruction (*arrow*), which was believed to be suggestive of an aggressive lesion. Biopsy showed this to be a nonossifying fibroma. Both CT and MR will often show apparent cortical destruction, which is merely cortical replacement by benign fibrous tissue.

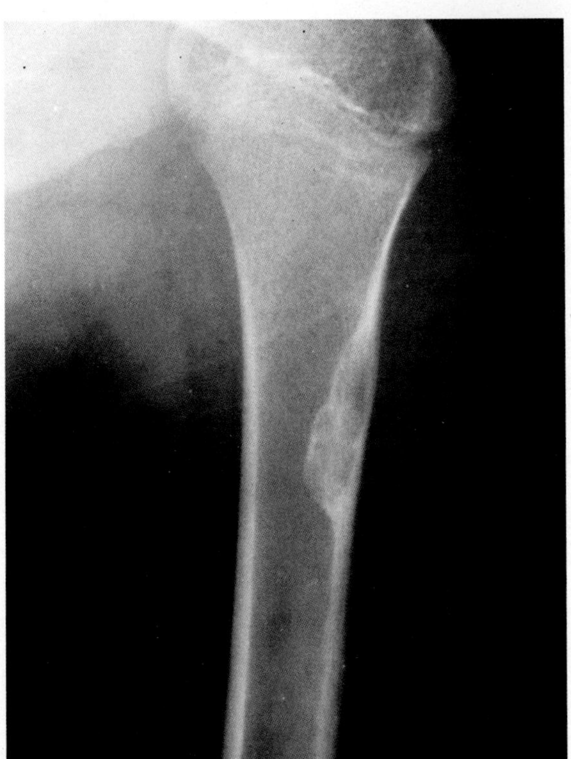

FIGURE 55.22. Healing Nonossifying Fibroma (NOF). A predominantly sclerotic lesion, which is minimally expansile and well defined, is seen in the proximal humerus in this child who is asymptomatic. This is a typical appearance of a disappearing or healing NOF. With time, this lesion will melt into the normal bone and essentially disappear.

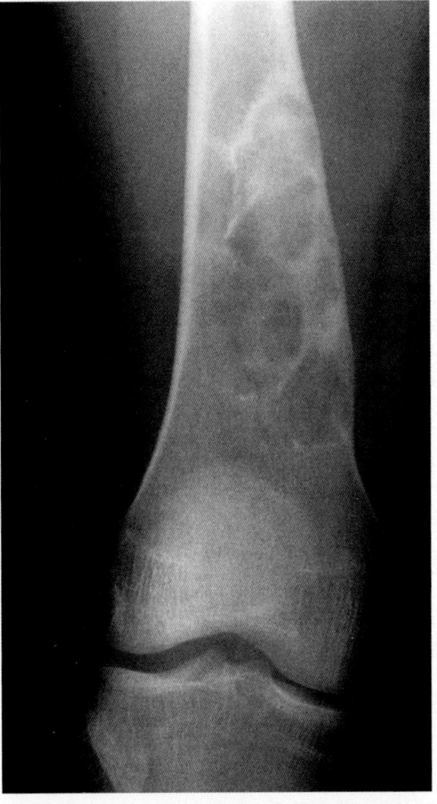

FIGURE 55.23. Nonossifying Fibroma (NOF). This large, well-defined lytic lesion with faint sclerotic margins is seen in the distal femur. Because of its size, many thought it was not an NOF. The lesion underwent biopsy and was found to be an NOF.

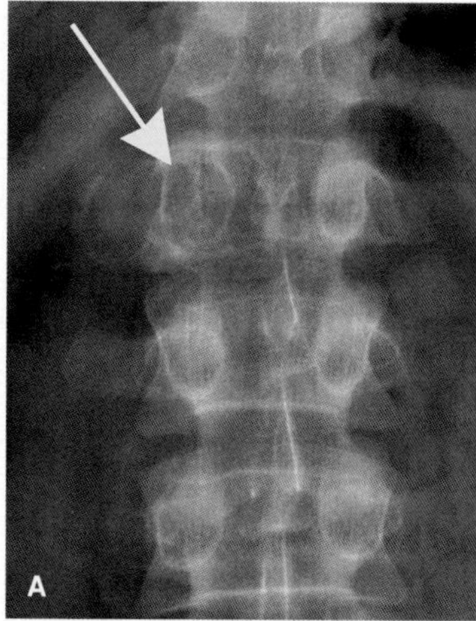

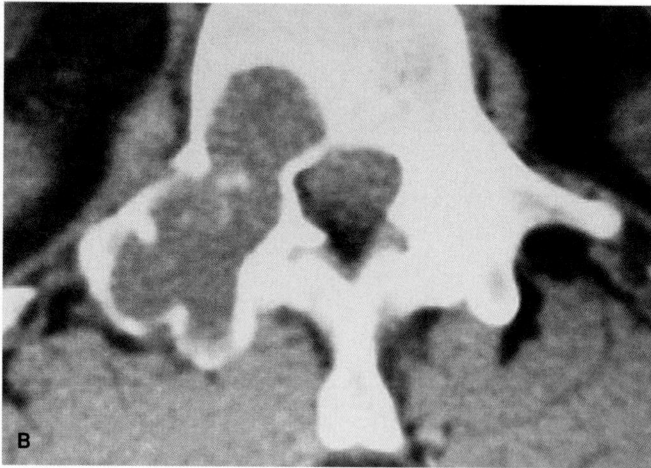

FIGURE 55.24. Osteoblastoma. A lytic expansile lesion involving the right T-12 pedicle (*arrow*) and transverse process is seen on this anteroposterior radiograph in (**A**) which is seen on the CT scan (**B**) to extend into the vertebral body. It has intact cortices and contains some calcified matrix. This is a classic example of an osteoblastoma of the spine.

ABC is being considered, so should an osteoblastoma. Osteoblastomas commonly occur in the posterior elements of the vertebral bodies, and about half of the cases demonstrate speckled calcifications (Fig. 55.24). A classic radiology differential is that of an expansile lytic lesion of the posterior elements of the spine, which includes osteoblastoma, ABC, and tuberculosis.

Discriminator. Mentioned when ABC is mentioned (especially in the posterior elements of the spine).

METASTATIC DISEASE AND MYELOMA

Metastatic disease should be considered for any lytic lesion—benign or aggressive in appearance—in a patient more than 40 years of age. Metastatic disease can appear perfectly benign radiographically (Fig. 55.25), so it is not valid to say, "Because this lesion looks benign, it should not be a metastasis." Most metastatic disease has an aggressive appearance and will not be in the FEGNOMASHIC differential, but a significant number appear benign. In fact, metastases can have any radiographic appearance; therefore, any bone lesion in a patient older than the age of 40 years should have metastatic disease as a consideration, unless trauma or arthritis is the primary concern.

For statistical purposes, I do not mention metastatic disease in a patient younger than the age of 40 years. I will be correct more than 99% of the time using 40 as a cut-off age. Otherwise, metastatic diseases would have to be mentioned in every single case of a lytic lesion, and I prefer to limit the list of differential possibilities. I am not claiming that metastatic disease does not occur in patients younger than the age of 40 years, only that I consider it acceptable to miss it (unless given a history of a known primary neoplasm).

Although myeloma most commonly presents as a diffuse permeative process in the skeleton (Fig. 55.26), it can present as either a solitary lesion (Fig. 55.27) or multiple lytic lesions. Bubbly, lytic bone lesions of myeloma are more correctly called plasmacytomas. I mention plasmacytoma separately from metastatic disease because it can occur in a slightly younger population (age greater than 35 years is my cut-off) and can precede clinical or hematologic evidence of myeloma by 3 to 5 years. In general, there is no harm in lumping all metastatic disease, including myeloma, into one group and using greater than age 40 as the limiting factor.

Virtually any metastatic process can present as a lytic, benign-appearing lesion; therefore, it serves no purpose to try to guess the source of the metastatic disease from its appearance. In general, lytic expansile metastatic diseases tend to come from thyroid and renal tumors (Fig. 55.28). The only metastatic lesion that is said to always be lytic is renal cell carcinoma.

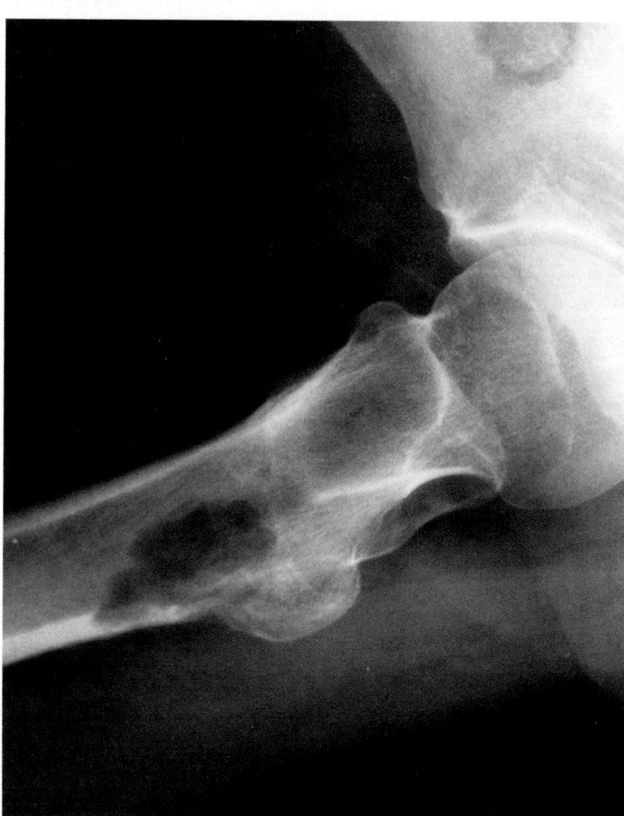

FIGURE 55.25. Metastatic Disease. A well-defined lytic lesion is seen in the proximal femur in this 50-year-old patient who has pain associated with this lesion. Biopsy showed this to be a renal metastasis. A significant number of metastatic lesions can have a completely benign appearance, as in this example.

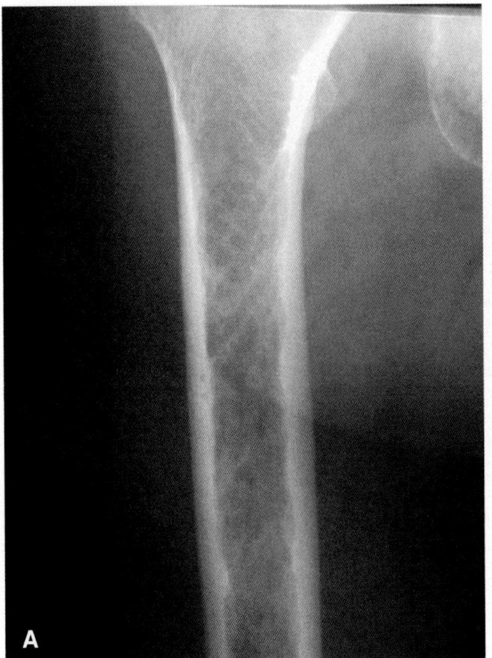

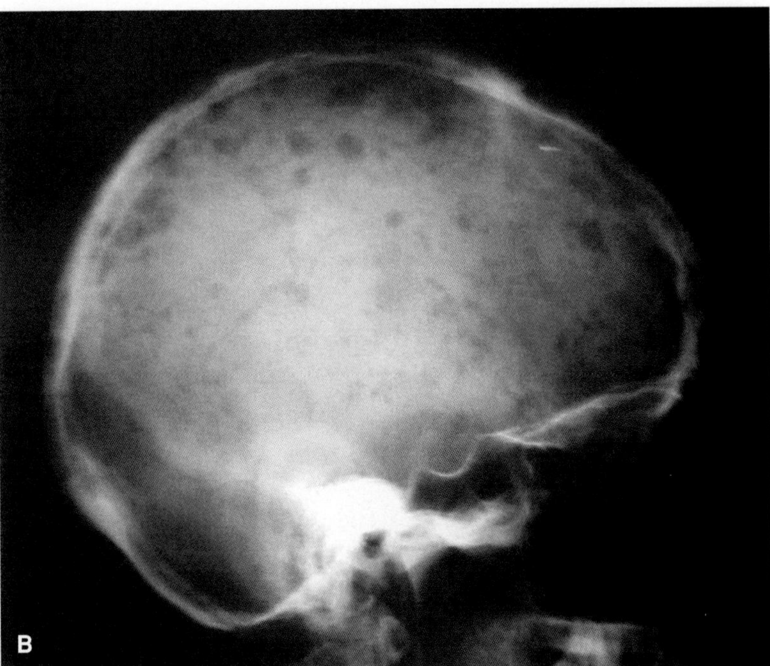

FIGURE 55.26. **Multiple Myeloma. A:** A diffuse permeative pattern is present throughout the femur in this patient with multiple myeloma. **B:** A lateral skull radiograph shows a typical presentation of multiple myeloma in the skull with multiple small well-defined lucent lesions throughout the calvarium.

Plasmacytomas involving a vertebral body often have a characteristic appearance on CT and MRI called a "mini-brain" (Fig. 55.29). Unlike metastatic disease, lymphoma, and infection, when plasmacytomas involve a vertebral body they tend to spare some of the bone; struts of cortical bone persist, giving the appearance of a cut brain specimen we are familiar with from our neuroanatomy classes. This finding is virtually pathognomonic of a plasmacytoma.

Discriminator. Must be older than age 40 years.

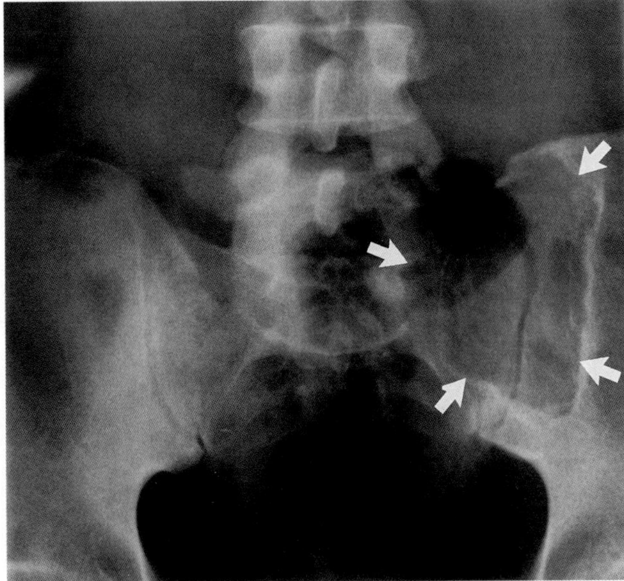

FIGURE 55.27. **Plasmacytoma.** A large, well-defined lytic lesion is seen in the left ilium (*arrows*) in this patient with multiple myeloma. This is a common location for a plasmacytoma. Like metastases, plasmacytomas often have a completely benign appearance.

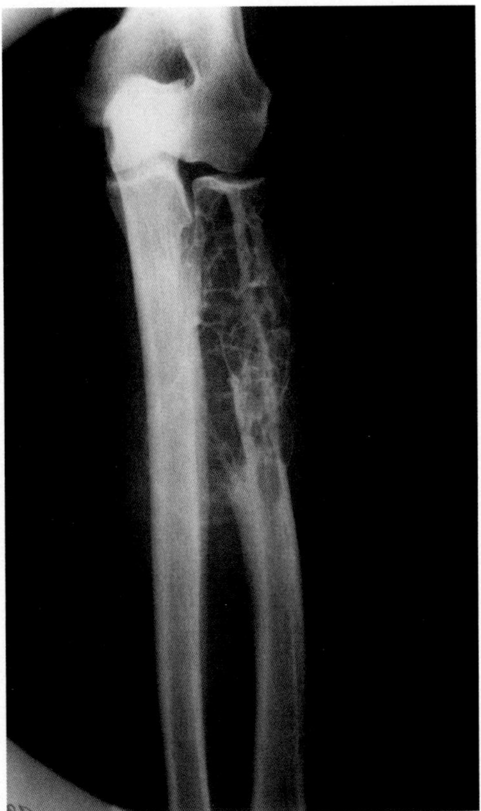

FIGURE 55.28. **Metastatic Disease.** An expansile lesion with a soap-bubble appearance is present in the proximal radius in a patient with renal cell carcinoma. An expansile lytic lesion is a common finding with renal or thyroid metastatic disease.

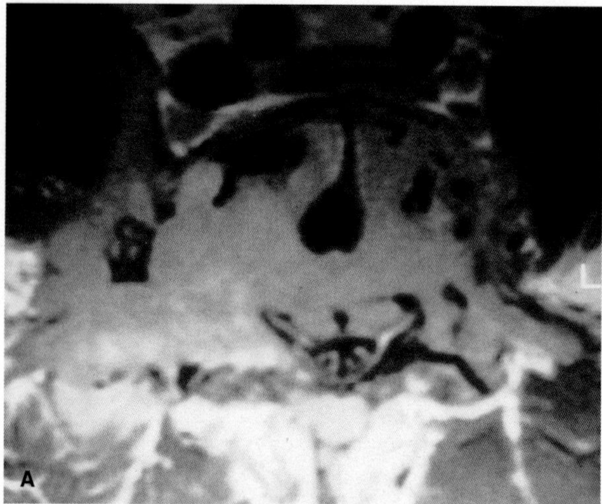

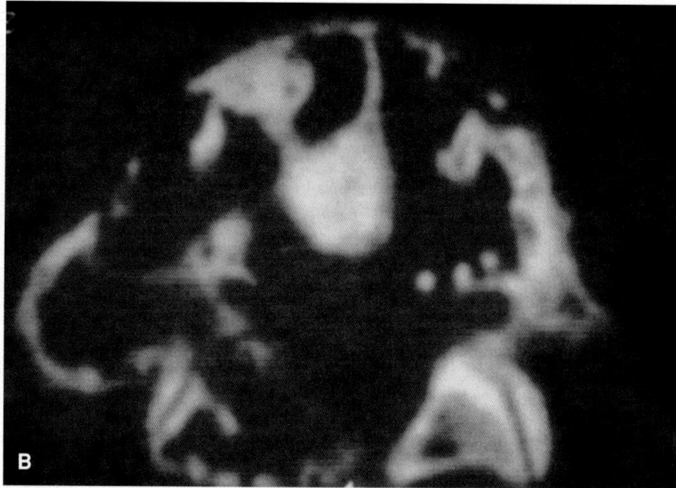

FIGURE 55.29. **Plasmacytoma. A:** An axial MRI and (**B**) a CT through the L5 vertebral body reveal a "mini-brain" appearance, with the remaining bony struts resembling cerebral gyri and sulci in an anatomic cut brain section. This is characteristic of a plasmacytoma.

ANEURYSMAL BONE CYST

ABCs are the only lesions I know of that are named for their radiographic appearance. They are virtually always aneurysmal or expansile (Figs. 55.30 and 55.31). Rarely, an ABC will present before it is expansile, but that is unusual enough not to worry about. ABCs primarily occur in patients who are less than the age of 30 years, although occasionally one will be encountered in older patients. I use bony expansion and age of less than 30 years as fairly rigid guidelines and seldom miss the diagnosis of ABC. They often have fluid/fluid levels on CT or MRI (Fig. 55.32), although this is a nonspecific finding as many other lesions can have fluid/fluid levels.

There are apparently two types of ABCs: a primary type and a secondary type. The secondary type occurs in conjunction with another lesion or from trauma, whereas a primary ABC has no known cause or association with other lesions. Secondary ABCs have been said to occur with giant cell tumors, osteosarcomas, and many other lesions. As to occurring after

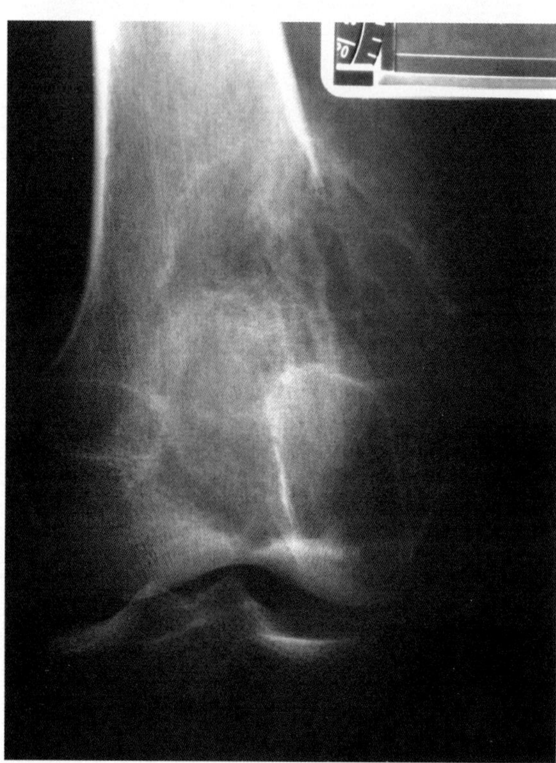

FIGURE 55.30. **Aneurysmal Bone Cyst (ABC).** An expansile lytic lesion is present in the distal femur in this 24-year-old patient who presents with pain. This is a fairly typical appearance of an ABC.

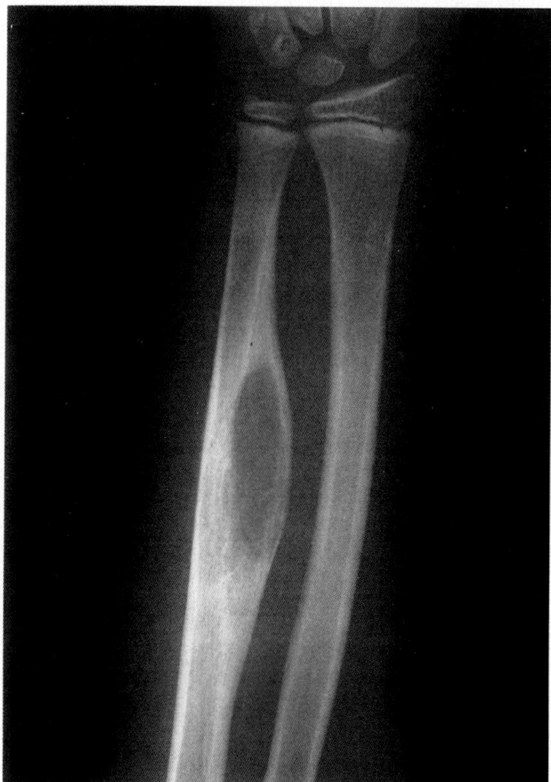

FIGURE 55.31. **Aneurysmal Bone Cyst (ABC).** A well-defined expansile lesion is seen in the midshaft of the ulna in a child who presents with pain in this region. This is a characteristic appearance of an ABC.

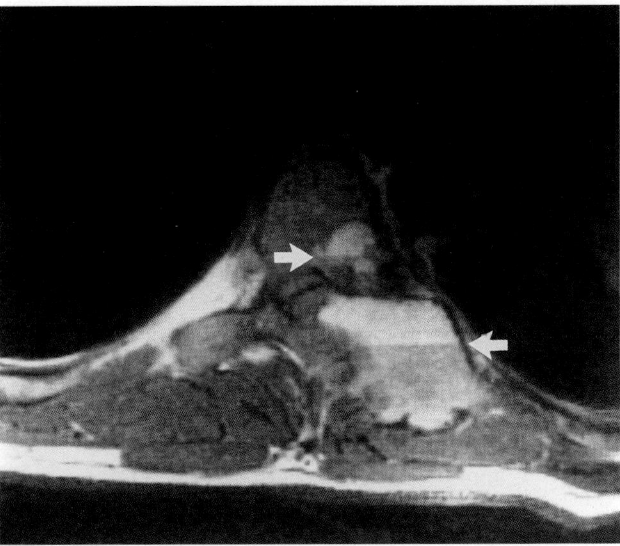

FIGURE 55.32. **Aneurysmal Bone Cyst (ABC).** An axial T2-weighted image through a thoracic vertebral body shows an expansile lesion involving the posterior elements which has several fluid/fluid levels (*arrows*). This is a typical appearance of an ABC.

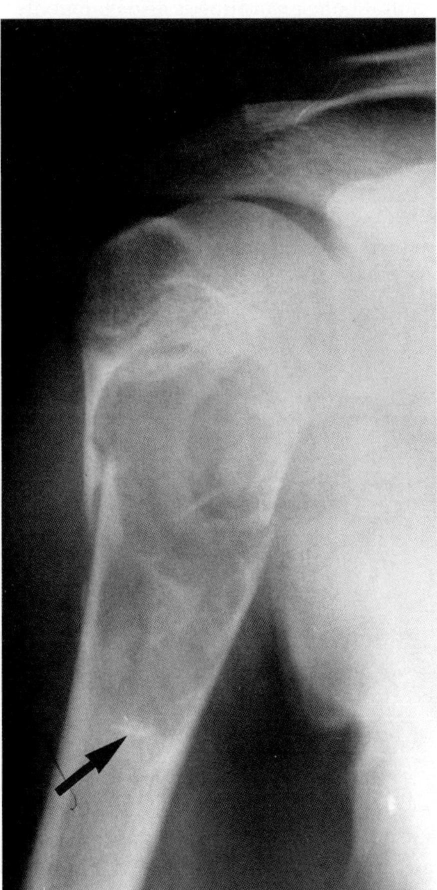

FIGURE 55.33. **Solitary Bone Cyst.** A well-defined lytic lesion is present in the proximal humerus in this child who suffered a fracture through the lesion. The location and central appearance, as well as the age of the patient, are characteristic of a solitary bone cyst. A piece of cortical bone has broken off and descended through the serous fluid contained within the lesion and can be seen in the dependent portion of the lesion (*arrow*) as a fallen fragment sign. A fallen fragment sign is said to be pathognomonic for a unicameral bone cyst.

trauma, I do not understand why they would be age limited if trauma were causative. Also, malignant tumors were once thought to occur after trauma because of the frequent association of a history of antecedent trauma with malignant bone tumors. This is not seriously considered today and is thought to be coincidental. I suspect that ABCs and trauma are also coincidental, but this is mere speculation.

ABCs typically present because of pain. They can occur anywhere in the skeleton, and there is no location that would make them more highly ranked in the differential diagnosis. As with osteoblastoma, they often occur in the posterior elements of the spine.

Discriminators. (1) Must be expansile, (2) Must be younger than age 30 years.

SOLITARY BONE CYST

Solitary bone cysts are also called simple bone cysts or unicameral bone cysts. They are not necessarily unicameral (one compartment), however. This is the only lesion in FEGNOMASHIC that is always central in location. Many of the other lesions may be central, but a solitary bone cyst can be excluded if it is not. It is one of the few lesions that does not occur most commonly around the knees. Two-thirds to three-fourths of these lesions occur in the proximal humerus (Fig. 55.33) and proximal femur (Fig. 55.34). Applying this rule by itself is not that helpful, or one-third to one-fourth of the lesions would be missed.

Solitary bone cysts are usually asymptomatic unless fractured, which is a common occurrence. Even when pathologic fractures occur, they rarely form periostitis. A classic

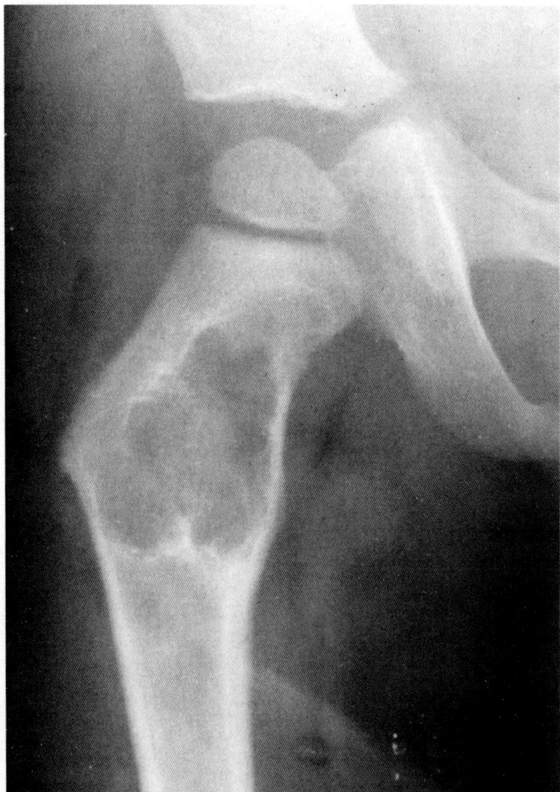

FIGURE 55.34. **Solitary Bone Cyst.** A well-defined lytic lesion, which is central in location, is seen in the proximal femur in this child. This is characteristic of a solitary bone cyst.

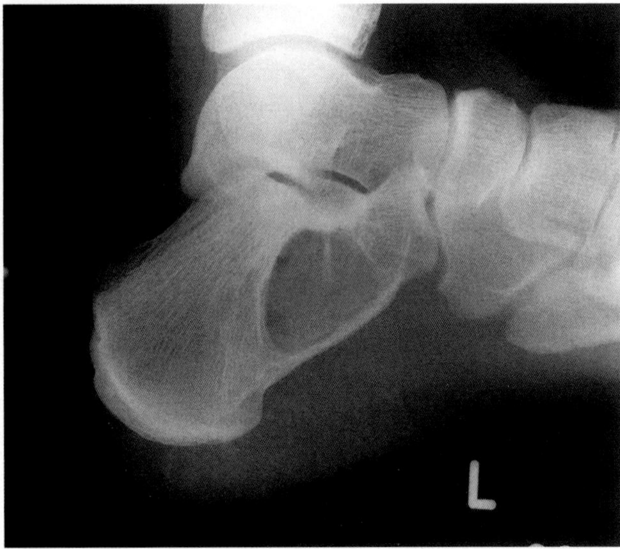

FIGURE 55.35. **Solitary Bone Cyst.** A well-defined lytic lesion is seen in the calcaneus abutting the inferior surface, which is typical in location and appearance for a solitary bone cyst. A solitary bone cyst in the calcaneus occurs almost exclusively in this location and is not subject to pathologic fracture as readily as when one occurs in the proximal femur and humerus.

radiographic finding for a solitary bone cyst is the fallen fragment sign (see Fig. 55.33). This occurs when a piece of cortex breaks off after a fracture in a solitary bone cyst, and the piece of cortical bone sinks to the gravity-dependent portion of the lesion. This has not been described in any other lesion and indicates a fluid-filled, single cavity cystic lesion, rather than a lesion filled with matrix. It is a very uncommon finding.

Solitary bone cysts occur almost exclusively in young patients (<30 years of age). Although long bones are most commonly involved, solitary bone cysts have been described in almost every bone in the body. They begin at the physeal plate in long bones and grow into the shaft of the bone; therefore, they are not epiphyseal lesions. They can, however, extend up into an epiphysis after the plate closes, but this is unusual. A fairly common location is in the calcaneus, where they have a characteristic location adjacent to the inferior surface of the calcaneus (Fig. 55.35).

Discriminators. (1) Must be central, (2) Must be younger than age 30 years.

HYPERPARATHYROIDISM (BROWN TUMORS)

Brown tumors of hyperparathyroidism (HPT) can have almost any appearance, from a purely lytic lesion (Fig. 55.36) to a sclerotic process. In general, when the patient's HPT is treated, the brown tumor undergoes sclerosis and will eventually disappear. If a brown tumor is going to be considered in the differential diagnosis, additional radiographic findings of HPT should be seen. Subperiosteal bone resorption is pathognomonic for HPT and should be searched for in the phalanges (particularly in the radial aspect of the middle phalanges) (Fig. 55.36) and medial aspect of the proximal tibias; subchondral bone resorption is also commonly seen, such as in the distal clavicles and sacroiliac joints. If the physes are open, they should have a frayed, ragged appearance, as in rickets, owing to the effect of parathormone. Osteoporosis or osteosclerosis might suggest that renal osteodystrophy with secondary HPT is present, but subperiosteal resorption must be present, or brown tumor can be safely excluded from the differential.

We seldom encounter brown tumors today, likely due to the more aggressive and successful treatment of renal disease than was seen 30 years ago.

Discriminator. Must have other evidence of HPT.

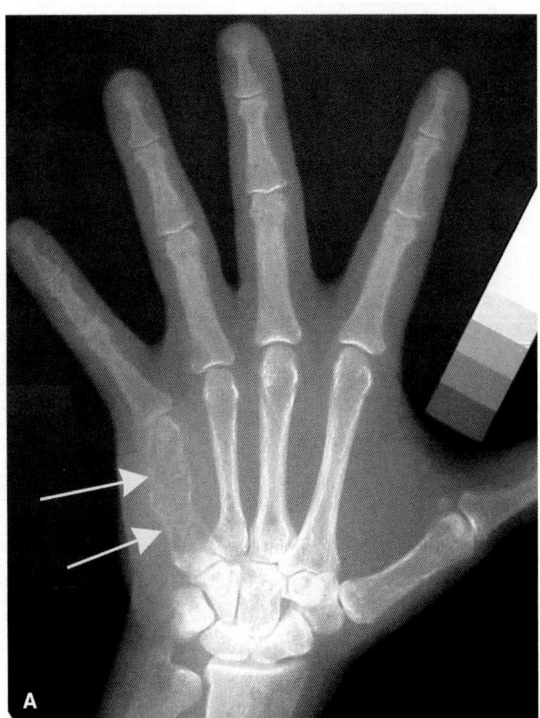

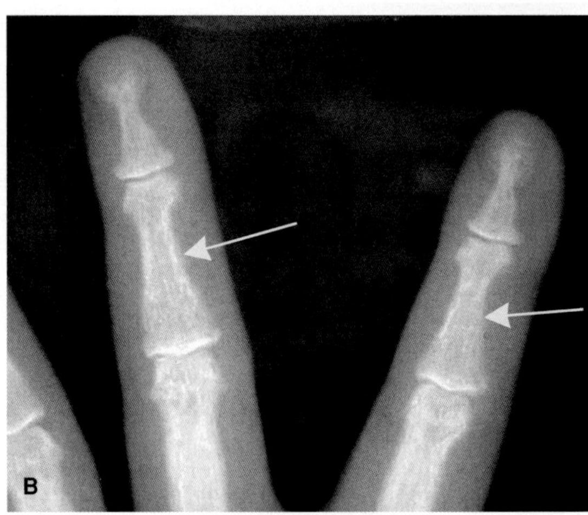

FIGURE 55.36. **Brown Tumor. A:** An expansile lytic lesion is seen in the fifth metacarpal (*arrows*), and a second, smaller lytic lesion is seen in the proximal portion of the fourth proximal phalanx. This patient can be noted to have subperiosteal bone resorption, best seen in the radial aspect of the middle phalanges (**B**) (*arrows*) as indistinct, interrupted cortex. This makes the diagnosis of hyperparathyroidism with multiple brown tumors most likely.

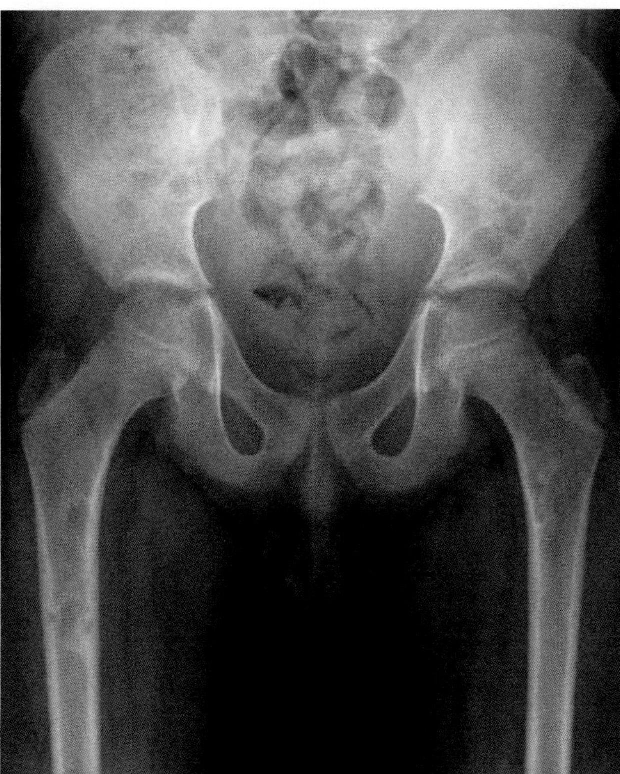

FIGURE 55.37. **Cystic Angiomatosis.** Multiple lytic lesions are seen in the pelvis and femurs in this asymptomatic young woman. These were found to be hemangiomas.

HEMANGIOMAS

Multiple hemangiomas, also known as cystic angiomatosis or cystic lymphangiomatosis, while uncommon, are seen more frequently than brown tumors and should probably replace them as the "H" in FEGNOMASHIC. Cystic angiomatosis is usually an incidental finding of multiple lytic lesions throughout the skeleton (Fig. 55.37). Although they are incidental, some feel they are in a similar category to Gorham disease (massive osteolysis or disappearing bone disease), but without the destructive potential. Cystic angiomatosis should be considered when multiple lytic lesions are encountered which are asymptomatic.

Discriminator. Multiple lesions.

INFECTION

Unfortunately, there is no reliable way radiographically to exclude a focus of osteomyelitis. It has a protean radiographic appearance and can occur at any location and in a patient of any age. It might or might not be expansile, have a sclerotic or nonsclerotic border, or have associated periostitis. Therefore, infection will be in almost every differential diagnosis of a lytic lesion, which is acceptable, as it is one of the most common lesions encountered. Soft tissue findings such as obliteration of adjacent fat planes are notoriously unreliable and even misleading, as tumors and EG can do the same thing.

When osteomyelitis occurs near a joint, if the articular surface is abutted, invariably the joint will be involved and show either cartilage loss or an effusion (Fig. 55.38), or both. This finding is not particularly helpful, as any lesion can cause an effusion, but it is occasionally useful in ruling out osteomyelitis when no effusion is present and the lesion abuts the articular surface.

If a bony sequestrum is present, osteomyelitis should be strongly considered (Fig. 55.39). As mentioned previously, the only lesions described that demonstrate sequestra are infection, EG, lymphoma, and fibrosarcoma, with osteoid osteoma sometimes mimicking a sequestrum. The finding of a sequestrum in osteomyelitis can be significant for treatment in that it usually requires surgical removal rather than antibiotics alone because a sequestrum is a focus of devitalized bone that does not have a blood supply and will not be effectively treated

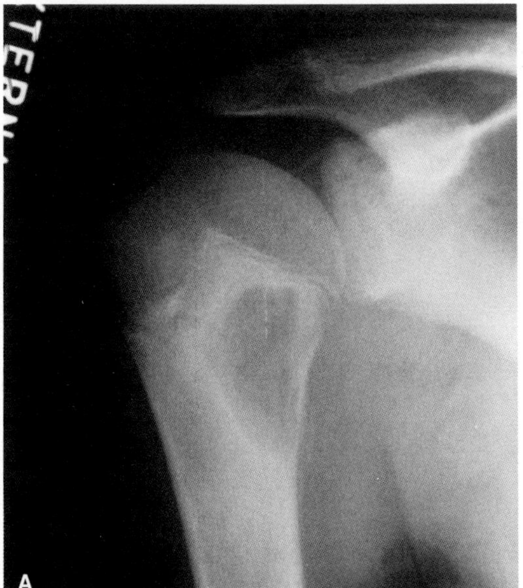

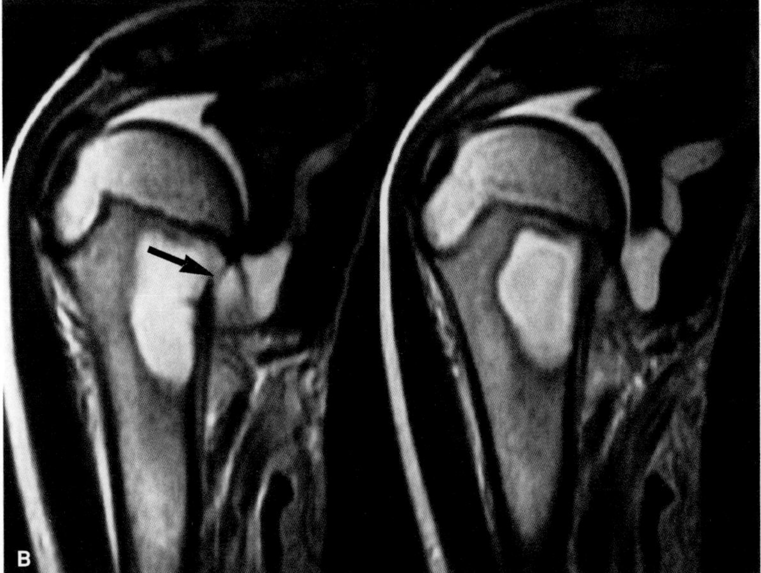

FIGURE 55.38. **Brodie Abscess. A:** A radiograph of the proximal humerus in this child with shoulder pain reveals a well-defined lytic lesion in the medial metaphysis. **B:** A T2-weighted MR of the humerus shows the lesion to have high signal and an associated joint effusion. The probable site of connection to the joint can be seen (*arrow*), which likely represents a draining abscess. Aspiration of the joint fluid revealed pus. This is a large focus of osteomyelitis or Brodie abscess.

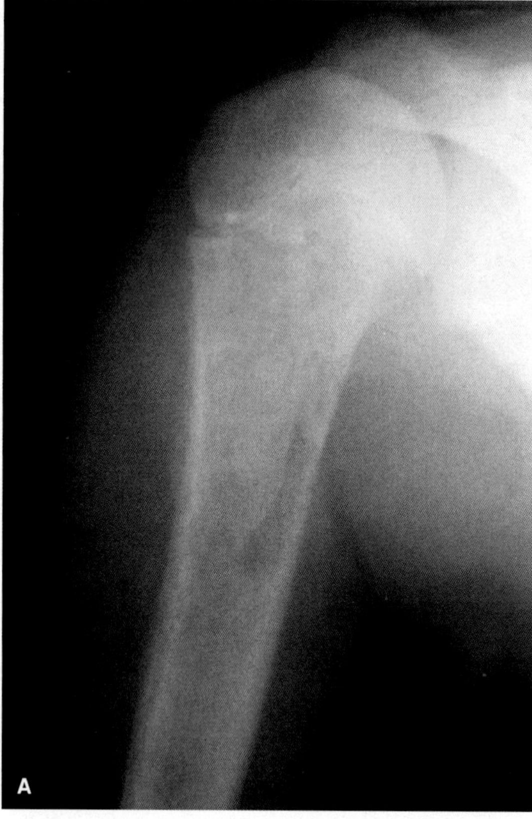

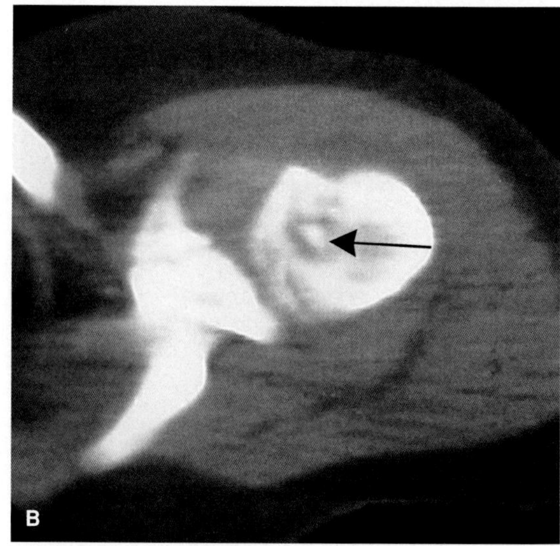

FIGURE 55.39. **Osteomyelitis. A:** A lytic lesion is present in the proximal humerus, which has some associated periostitis laterally. **B:** A CT scan through this area reveals a lytic lesion that contains a calcific density within (*arrow*), which is a bony sequestrum. This is an area of osteomyelitis with a bony sequestration.

with parenteral medication. For this reason, CT is routinely recommended when osteomyelitis is considered.

Discriminator: None.

CHONDROBLASTOMA

Chondroblastomas are rare lesions but are among the easiest lesions for radiologists to deal with because they occur only in the epiphyses (Fig. 55.40) (a handful of cases have been reported in the metaphyses but this is rare) and they occur almost exclusively in patients younger than the age of 30 years. From 40% to 60% demonstrate calcification, so absence of calcification is not helpful. Presence of calcification is helpful as long as it is certain that it is not detritus or sequestra from infection or EG, both of which can occur in the epiphyses.

The differential diagnosis of a lytic lesion in the epiphysis of a patient less than 30 years of age is simple: (1) infection (most common), (2) chondroblastoma, and (3) giant cell tumor (it has its own diagnostic criteria, so it can usually be definitely ruled out or in). This is an old, classic differential and probably encompasses 98% of epiphyseal lesions.

A caveat on epiphyseal lesions is to consider always the possibility of a subchondral cyst or geode (Fig. 55.41), which has been described in four disease processes: (1) degenerative joint disease (must have joint space narrowing, sclerosis, and osteophytes), (2) rheumatoid arthritis, (3) calcium pyrophosphate dihydrate crystal disposition disease or pseudogout, and (4) avascular necrosis. Be certain no joint pathology that might indicate one of these processes is present, or an unnecessary biopsy of a geode might be performed on the basis of the differential of an epiphyseal lesion.

Apophyses are identical to epiphyses as far as the differential diagnosis of lytic lesions, with the exception of geodes, which only occur adjacent to articular surfaces. The carpal bones, the tarsal bones, and the patella have a tendency to behave like epiphyses in their differential diagnosis of lesions. Therefore, a lytic lesion in these areas has a similar differential diagnosis as an epiphyseal lesion.

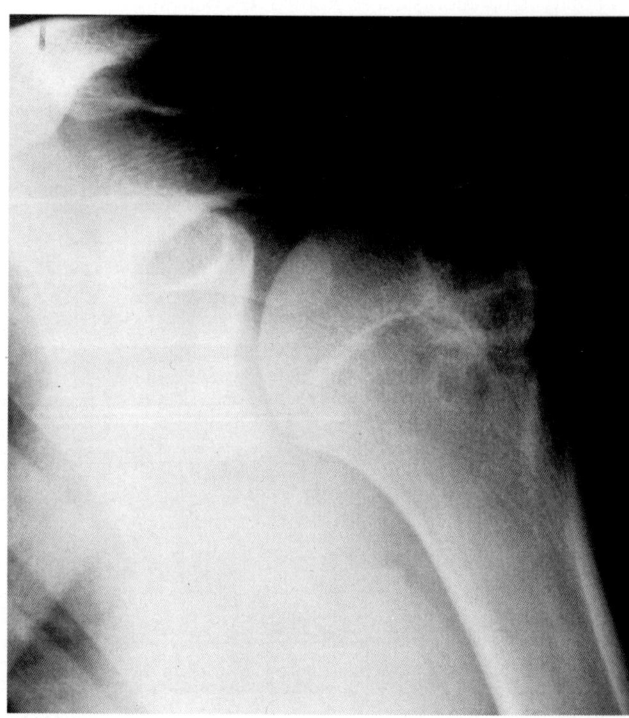

FIGURE 55.40. **Chondroblastoma.** A radiograph in this young patient shows a well-defined lytic lesion in the greater tuberosity of the humerus. Biopsy showed this to be a chondroblastoma.

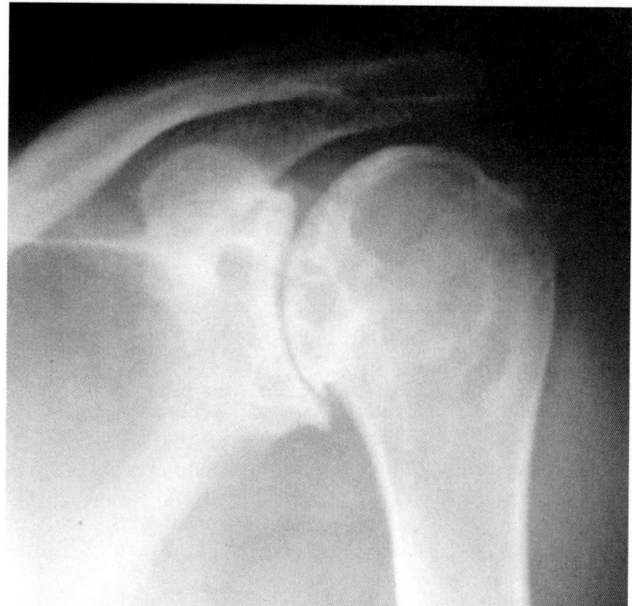

FIGURE 55.41. Geode. A large, well-defined lytic lesion in the proximal humerus is present, which is associated with marked degenerative disease of the glenohumeral joint. When definite degenerative joint disease is present and associated with a lytic lesion, the lytic lesion should be considered to be a geode. A biopsy was performed, which confirmed this to be a geode, or subchondral cyst; however, the biopsy could have been avoided.

Discriminators. (1) Must be less than 30 years of age, (2) Must be epiphyseal.

CHONDROMYXOID FIBROMA

Like the osteoblastoma, the chondromyxoid fibroma is such a rare lesion that failure to mention it is probably not going to result in missing more than one in a lifetime. Why include it then? I recommend not including it, but it is part of the classic FEGNOMASHIC differential. If it is mentioned, at least know what it looks like. Basically, chondromyxoid fibromas resemble NOFs. Unlike NOFs, however, they can be seen in a patient of any age. Chondromyxoid fibromas often extend into the epiphyses (Fig. 55.42), whereas NOFs rarely do. They can present with pain, also, which will not occur with an NOF. Even though chondromyxoid fibromas are cartilaginous lesions, calcified cartilage matrix is virtually never seen radiographically.

Discriminators. (1) Mention when an NOF is mentioned, (2) No calcified matrix.

SUMMARY

That, in essence, is the differential diagnosis for a benign-appearing lucent lesion of bone. It is probably, 98% accurate, which is good enough for most radiologists. To increase the accuracy to 99%, it would be necessary to add many uncommon or rare lesions, and the whole process would become too confusing for most radiologists to learn and apply. If you have a favorite lesion that is not on this list, by all means add it. Likewise, if the list is already too cumbersome, forget about osteoblastoma, brown tumors, hemangiomas, and chondromyxoid fibroma. I am unable to make it much simpler than that and still be reasonably accurate.

Some of the lesions I have purposefully omitted are intraosseous ganglion, pseudotumor of hemophilia, hemangioendothelioma, ossifying fibroma, intraosseous lipoma, glomus tumor, neurofibroma, plasma cell granuloma, and schwannoma. Others could be added to this list, of course, but are best left to the pathologist—not the radiologist—for the diagnosis.

There are several features that are somewhat useful in separating the various lesions in FEGNOMASHIC. For instance, if the patient is younger than the age of 30 years, be sure to consider EG, chondroblastoma, NOF, solitary bone cyst, and ABC (Table 55.2). If the patient is more than 30 years of age, those five lesions can be excluded. Note that this is not a differential diagnosis for lesions in patients less than the age of 30 years; it simply means these entities should not be

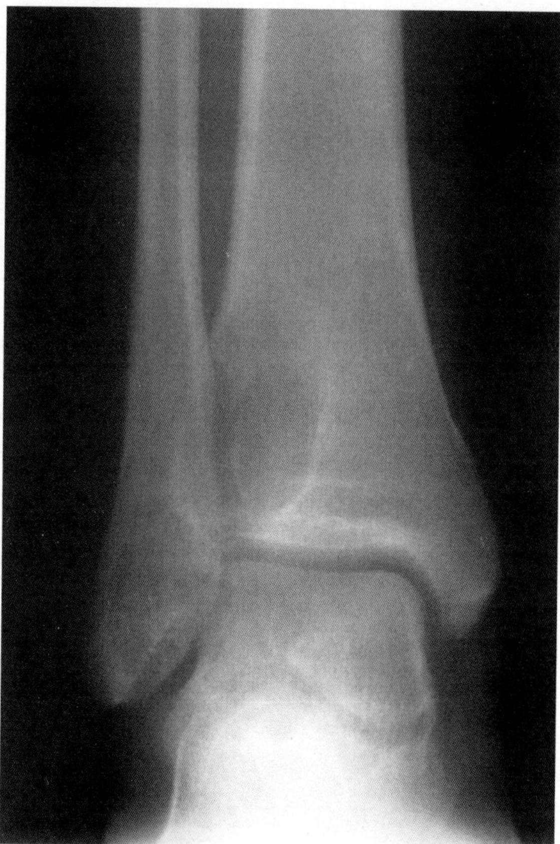

FIGURE 55.42. Chondromyxoid Fibroma. A well-defined lytic lesion in the distal tibia that extends slightly into the epiphysis is noted on this anteroposterior radiograph. A nonossifying fibroma (NOF) could certainly have this appearance; however, this underwent biopsy and was found to be a chondromyxoid fibroma. Chondromyxoid fibromas often will extend into the epiphysis, as in this example, whereas NOFs usually will not.

TABLE 55.2

LESIONS IN PATIENTS YOUNGER THAN 30 YEARS OF AGE

Lesion
EG
ABC
NOF
Chondroblastoma
Solitary bone cyst

EG, eosinophilic granuloma; ABC, aneurysmal bone cyst; NOF, nonossifying fibroma.

TABLE 55.3

AUTOMATICS

Younger than age 30
Infection
EG
Older than age 40
Infection
Metastatic disease and myeloma

EG, eosinophilic granuloma.

TABLE 55.4

LESIONS THAT HAVE NO PAIN OR PERIOSTITIS

Fibrous dysplasia
Enchondroma
NOF
Solitary bone cyst

NOF, nonossifying fibroma.

TABLE 55.5

EPIPHYSEAL LESIONS

Infection
Giant cell tumor
Chondroblastoma
Geode

TABLE 55.6

DIFFERENTIAL FOR RIB LESIONS (FAME)

Fibrous dysplasia
ABC
Metastatic disease and myeloma
Enchondroma and EG

ABC, aneurysmal bone cyst; EG, eosinophilic granuloma.

TABLE 55.7

MULTIPLE LESIONS (FEEMHI)

Fibrous dysplasia
EG
Enchondroma
Metastatic disease and myeloma
Hyperparathyroidism (brown tumors)
Hemangiomas
Infection

EG, eosinophilic granuloma.

mentioned in older patients. For those younger than the age of 30 years, other lesions such as fibrous dysplasia and infection must also be mentioned.

There are a few lytic lesions that have no good discriminators other than age and, therefore, must be mentioned routinely. I call these lesions "automatics" because one should automatically mention them regardless of the location or appearance of the lesion. *Infection* and *EG* must be mentioned for those younger than the age of 30 years, whereas *metastatic disease* and *infection* must be included in any differential in a patient older than the age of 40 years (Table 55.3). These lesions have a protean radiographic appearance and should be mentioned not only in the benign, cystic differential, but also for an aggressive lesion.

If periostitis or pain is present (assuming no trauma, which can be a foolhardy assumption), you can exclude *fibrous dysplasia*, *solitary bone cyst*, *NOF*, and *enchondroma* (Table 55.4). If the lesion is epiphyseal, the differential is *infection*, *giant cell tumor*, *chondroblastoma* (and do not forget *geodes*) (Table 55.5). If the patient is more than 40 years of age, add metastatic disease and myeloma and remove chondroblastoma from the epiphyseal list.

The epiphyseal differential tends to apply also to the tarsal bones (especially the calcaneus), the carpal bones, and the patella. In the calcaneus, a unicameral bone cyst should also be considered and has a characteristic appearance and location (see Fig. 55.35). Apophyses are "epiphyseal equivalents" and have the same differential as epiphyses. The difference between an epiphysis and an apophysis is that epiphyses contribute to the length of a bone, whereas apophyses serve as tendon and ligament attachment sites.

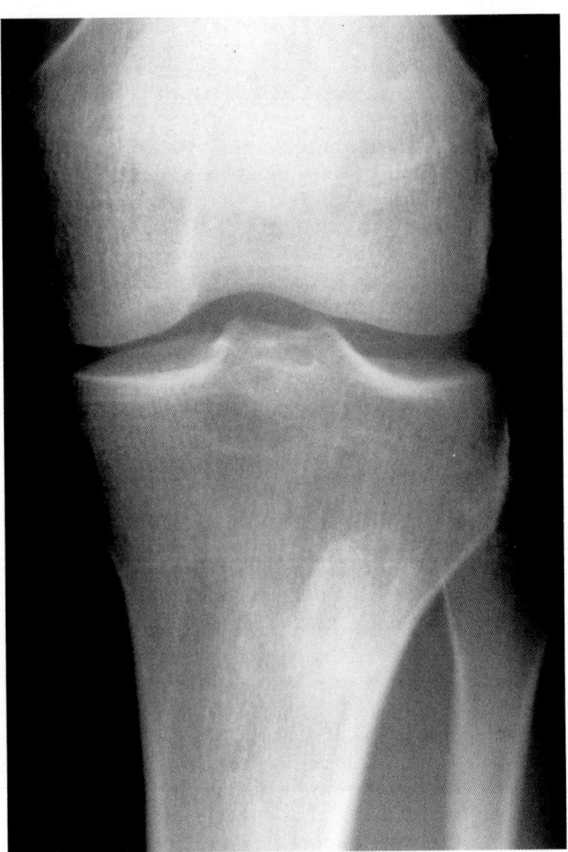

FIGURE 55.43. **Healing Nonossifying Fibroma.** A radiograph of the knee in this 25-year-old patient reveals a sclerotic lesion in the proximal tibia which is a healing or resolving nonossifying fibroma.

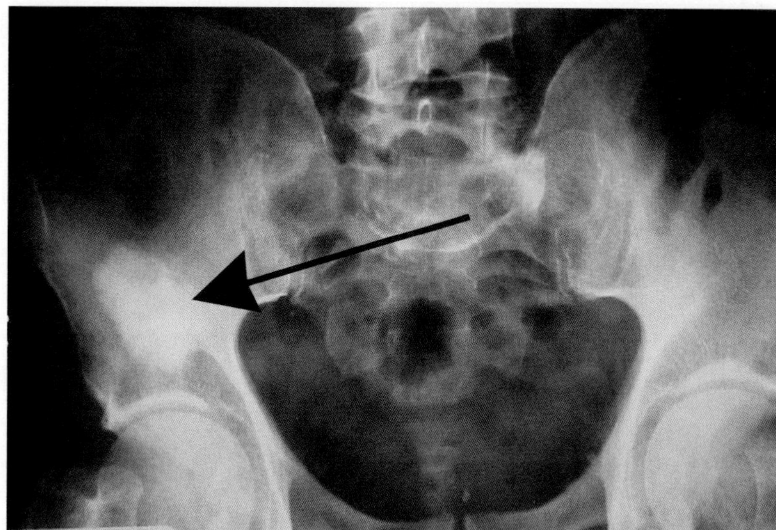

FIGURE 55.44. **Giant Bone Island.** A large sclerotic lesion is present in the right supra-acetabular region of the ilium (*arrow*), which represents a giant bone island. The slightly feathered margins of the trabeculae blending in with the normal bone, and the long axis of the lesion being in the direction of primary weight bearing, are characteristic for a bone island.

A classic differential for benign, lytic rib lesions is the mnemonic FAME, in which F = *fibrous dysplasia*, A = *ABC*, M = *metastatic diseases* and *myeloma*, and E = *enchondroma* and *EG* (Table 55.6).

If there are multiple lytic lesions present, FEEMHI is a useful mnemonic of the lesions in FEGNOMASHIC which can be multiple. F = *fibrous dysplasia*, E = *enchondroma*, E = *EG*, M = *metastatic disease* and *myeloma*, H = *hyperparathyroidism* (brown tumors) and *hemangiomas*, and I = *infection* (Table 55.7).

A few findings that just do not seem to narrow the differential diagnosis are presence or absence of a soft tissue mass, expansion of the bone (except it must be present in an ABC), a sclerotic or nonsclerotic border (except it must be nonsclerotic in giant cell tumor), presence or absence of bony struts or compartments in the lesion, and size of the lesion.

If calcified matrix is identified in a lesion, it is tempting to narrow the differential to either the osteoid series or the chondroid series of lesions, depending on the character of the matrix. Be careful of this. Very few radiologists can reliably differentiate chondroid from osteoid matrix. Routine calcification of a lesion or debris, detritus, or sequestrations in osteomyelitis can mimic chondroid or osteoid calcification and be misleading. The only lesion that must exhibit calcified matrix is the enchondroma (except in the phalanges). Chondroblastomas and osteoblastomas demonstrate calcified matrix about half the time, and chondromyxoid fibromas never have radiographically demonstrable calcified matrix.

DIFFERENTIAL DIAGNOSIS OF A SCLEROTIC LESION

Many lucent bone lesions spontaneously regress and are not usually seen in patients more than 30 years of age. When these lesions regress, they often fill in with new bone and have a sclerotic or blastic appearance. Therefore, when a sclerotic focus is identified in a 20- to 40-year-old patient, especially if it is an asymptomatic, incidental finding, the following lesions should be considered: NOF (Fig. 55.43), EG, ABC, solitary bone cyst, and chondroblastoma. Several other lesions should be included that can also appear sclerotic: fibrous dysplasia, osteoid osteoma, infection, brown tumor (healing), and perhaps a giant bone island (Fig. 55.44). In any patient older than the age of 40 years, the number one possibility should be metastatic disease.

Suggested Readings

Dahlin DC. Giant cell tumor of bone: highlights of 407 cases. *AJR Am J Roentgenol* 1985;144:955–960.

David R, Oria RA, Kumar R, et al. Radiologic features of eosinophilic granuloma of bone. *AJR Am J Roentgenol* 1989;153:1021–1026.

Gold RH, Hawkins RA, Katz RD. Bacterial osteomyelitis: findings on plain radiography, CT, MR, and scintigraphy. *AJR Am J Roentgenol* 1991;157:365–370.

Skeletal Lesions Interobserver Correlation Among Expert Diagnosticians (SLICED) Study Group. Reliability of histopathologic and radiologic grading of cartilaginous neoplasms in long bones. *J Bone Joint Surg Am* 2007;89:2113–2123.

CHAPTER 56 ■ MALIGNANT BONE AND SOFT TISSUE TUMORS

CLYDE A. HELMS AND EMILY N. VINSON

RADIOGRAPHIC FINDINGS

Malignant bone tumors, thankfully, are not very common. Nevertheless, every radiologist should be able to recognize them and give a useful differential diagnosis. First, how does one recognize a malignant tumor and differentiate it from a benign process? This can be difficult and often impossible. Recognizing that it is *aggressive* is usually easy, but stating that it is *malignant* is another matter altogether. Processes such as infection and eosinophilic granuloma can mimic malignant tumors and are, of course, benign. They will often be included in the differential diagnosis of an aggressive lesion along with malignant tumors. What radiographic criteria are useful for determining malignant versus benign? Standard textbooks give four aspects of a lesion to be examined: (1) cortical destruction, (2) periostitis, (3) orientation or axis of the lesion, and (4) zone of transition. Let me discuss each of these criteria and show why only the last one—the zone of transition—is accurate to a 90% plus rate. It is important to recognize that these are "plain film" (radiographic) criteria and do not apply to CT or MR imaging in many instances.

Cortical Destruction

Benign fibro-osseous lesions and cartilaginous lesions often have part of their noncalcified matrix (fibrous matrix or chondroid matrix, both of which are radiolucent on plain radiographs) replacing cortical bone, which can give the false impression of cortical destruction on radiographs (Fig. 56.1) or CT. Also, benign processes such as infection and eosinophilic granuloma can cause extensive cortical destruction and mimic a malignant tumor. It is well known that aneurysmal bone cysts cause such thinning of the cortex as to make the cortex radiographically undetectable (Fig. 56.2). For these reasons, cortical destruction can occasionally be misleading. Cortical destruction always makes one think of a malignant lesion when using the "gestalt approach," but the lesion must also have other criteria for a malignant process, such as a wide zone of transition.

Periostitis

Periosteal reaction occurs in a nonspecific manner whenever the periosteum is irritated, whether it is irritated by a malignant tumor, a benign tumor, infection, or trauma. Callus formation in a fracture is actually just periosteal reaction of the most benign type. Periosteal reaction occurs in two types: benign or aggressive, based more on the timing of the irritation than on whether it is a malignant or benign process causing the periostitis. For example, a slow-growing benign tumor will cause thick, wavy, uniform, or dense periostitis (Fig. 56.3A) because it is a low-grade chronic irritation that gives the periosteum time to lay down thick new bone and remodel into more normal cortex. A malignant tumor causes a periosteal reaction that is high grade and more acute; hence, the periosteum does not have time to consolidate. It appears lamellated (onion-skinned) (Fig. 56.3B) or amorphous or even sunburst-like. If the irritation stops or diminishes, the aggressive periostitis will solidify and appear benign. Therefore, when periostitis is seen, the radiologist should try to characterize it into either a benign (thick, dense, wavy) type or an aggressive (lamellated, amorphous, sunburst) type. Unfortunately, judging the lesion by its periostitis can be very misleading. First, it takes considerable experience to characterize periostitis accurately because many times the reaction is not clearly benign or aggressive. Second, many benign lesions can cause aggressive periostitis, such as infection, eosinophilic granuloma, aneurysmal bone cysts, osteoid osteomas, and even trauma. Seeing *benign* periostitis, however, can be very helpful because malignant lesions

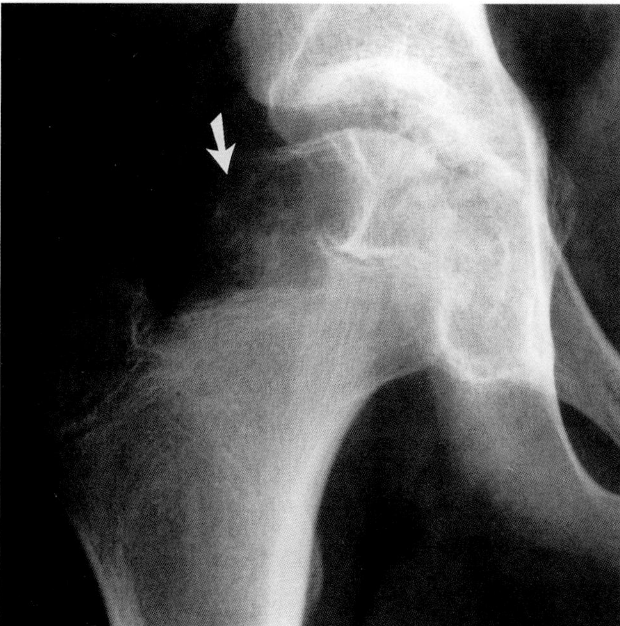

FIGURE 56.1. **Apparent Cortical Destruction.** This benign chondroblastoma has noncalcified chondroid tissue replacing cortical bone in the proximal femur (*arrow*), which gives this lesion a destructive appearance. This is an example of cortical replacement, rather than cortical destruction, which can be very confusing if one uses cortical destruction as an aggressive or malignant key. Note in this example that the zone of transition is narrow as one would expect in a benign lesion such as this.

will not cause benign periostitis. Some investigators with great experience in dealing with malignant bone tumors state that the only way benign periostitis can occur in a malignant lesion is if there is a concomitant fracture or infection. Exceptions to this are extremely uncommon.

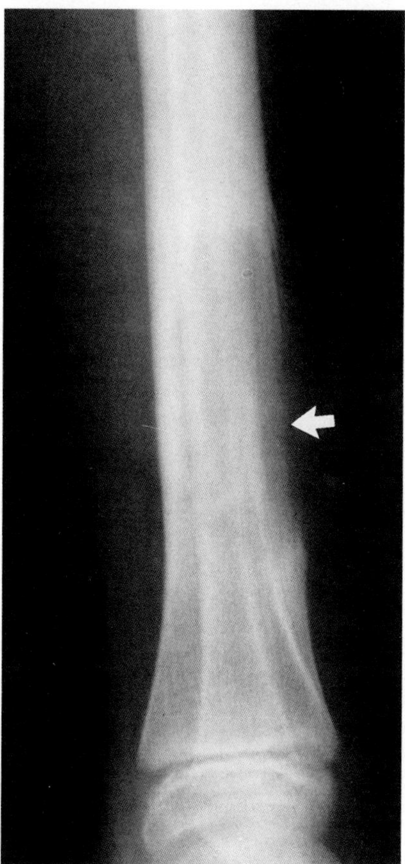

FIGURE 56.2. **Aneurysmal Bone Cyst.** This benign lesion has thinned the cortex to such a degree as to make it imperceptible (*arrow*). As in Figure 56.1, this could be misconstrued as cortical destruction, giving the false impression of a malignant or very aggressive lesion.

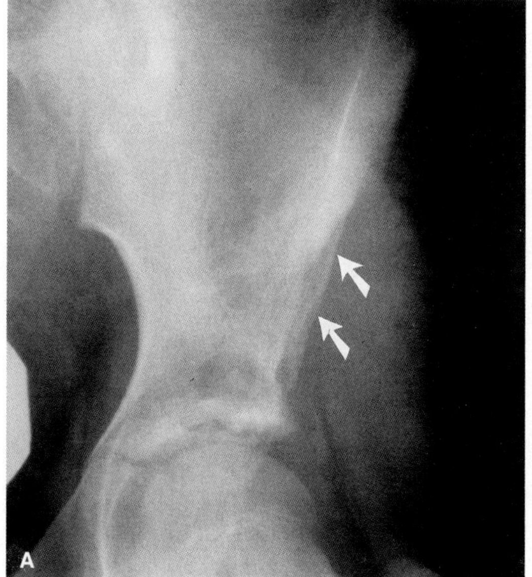

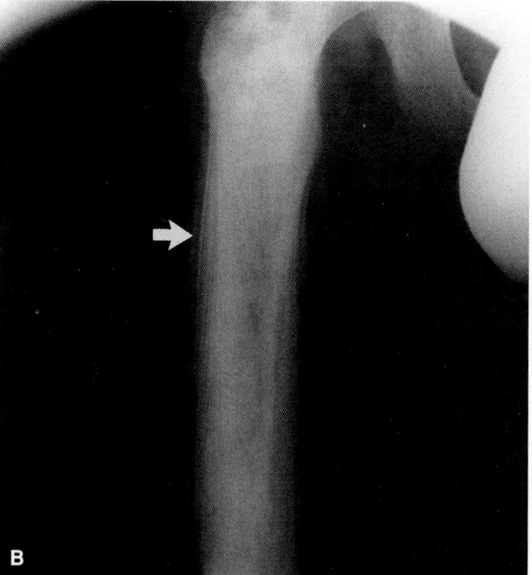

FIGURE 56.3. **Periostitis. A:** Benign periostitis. Thick, wavy periostitis (*arrows*) along the ilium in a child with a permeative lesion in the pelvis is characteristic for infection or eosinophilic granuloma. Ewing sarcoma was initially considered in the differential; however, the benign periostitis would make a malignant lesion very unlikely. Biopsy showed this lesion to be eosinophilic granuloma. **B:** Aggressive periostitis. Lamellated or onion-skin periostitis (*arrow*) is characteristic of an aggressive process such as in this patient with Ewing sarcoma of the femur. Again, this aggressive type of periostitis could conceivably occur in a benign process such as infection or eosinophilic granuloma.

Orientation or Axis of the Lesion

This is a very poor determinant of benign versus aggressive lesions and rarely helps to determine into which category the lesion should be placed. It has been said that if a lesion grows in the long axis of a long bone, rather than being circular, it is benign. There are simply too many exceptions for this to be helpful. For example, Ewing sarcoma, an extremely malignant lesion, usually has its axis along the shaft of a long bone. Conversely, many fibrous cortical defects are circular, yet totally benign. Thus, the axis of the lesion is not helpful in assessing benignity versus malignancy.

Zone of Transition

This is without question the most reliable radiographic indicator for benign versus malignant lesions. Unfortunately, it also has some drawbacks. The zone of transition is the border of the lesion with the normal bone. It is said to be "narrow" if it is so well defined that it can be drawn with a fine-point pen (Fig. 56.4). If it is imperceptible and cannot be clearly drawn at all, it is said to be "wide" (Fig. 56.5). Obviously, all shades of gray lie in between, but most lesions can be characterized as having either a narrow or wide zone of transition. If the lesion has a sclerotic border, it, of course, has a narrow zone of transition. If a lesion has a narrow zone of transition, a benign process should be considered as the most likely possibility.

The exceptions to this are uncommon. If a lesion has a wide zone of transition, it is aggressive, although not necessarily malignant. As with aggressive periostitis, many benign lesions as well as malignant lesions can cause a wide zone of transition. A few of the same processes that can cause aggressive periostitis and thereby mimic a malignant tumor can have a wide zone of transition (i.e., infection and eosinophilic granuloma). They are aggressive in their radiographic appearance because they are usually fast-acting, aggressive lesions. The zone of transition is usually easier to characterize than the periostitis, plus it is always present to evaluate, whereas many lesions, benign or malignant, have no periostitis. For these reasons, the zone of transition is the most useful indicator of whether a lesion is benign or malignant.

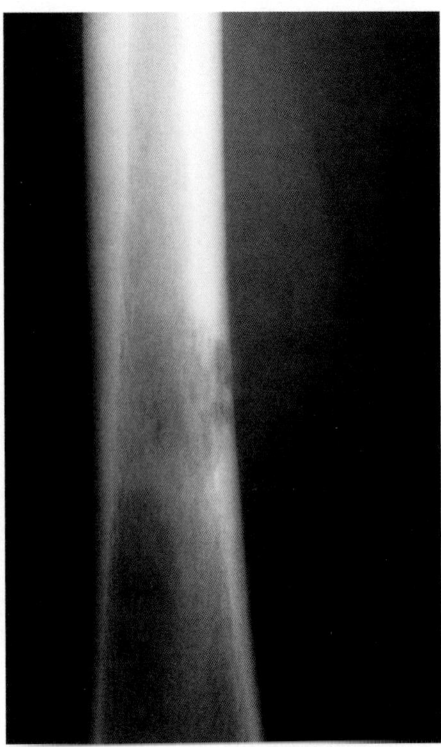

FIGURE 56.5. **Wide Zone of Transition.** A lytic, permeative process is seen in the midshaft of the femur in this patient that on biopsy was found to be a malignant fibrous histiocytoma. The zone of transition in this lesion is said to be wide, as it cannot be easily drawn with a fine-point pen. A permeative lesion such as this, by definition, has a wide zone of transition.

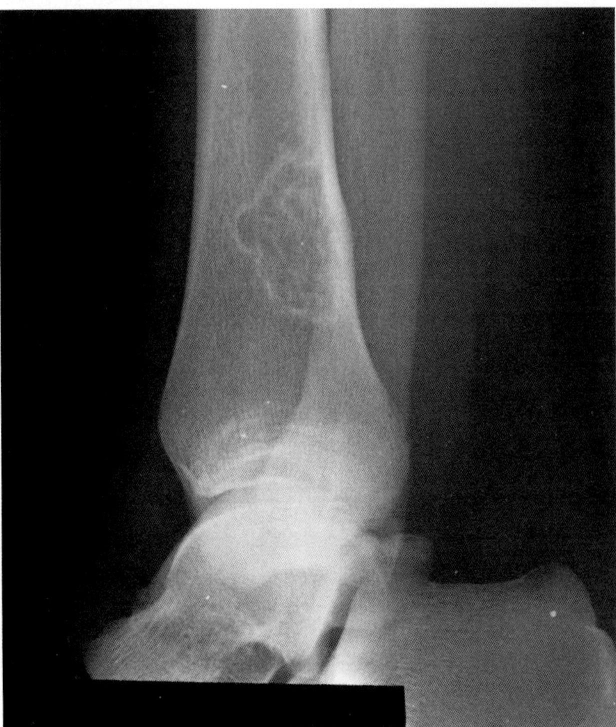

FIGURE 56.4. **Narrow Zone of Transition.** When the margins of a lesion can be drawn with a fine-point pen, as in this example, it is said to be a narrow zone of transition, which is characteristic of a benign lesion. A narrow zone of transition might or might not have a sclerotic border. This is a nonossifying fibroma.

A lesion consisting of multiple small holes is said to be "permeative" (see Chapter 59 for discussion of the difference between a permeative lesion and a pseudopermeative lesion). It has no perceptible border and therefore has a wide zone of transition. Round cell tumors such as multiple myeloma, primary lymphoma of bone (reticulum cell sarcoma), and Ewing sarcoma are typical of this type of lesion. Infection and eosinophilic granuloma also can have this same appearance.

Once it is decided that a particular lesion is most likely malignant, the differential is fairly straightforward. First, the list of malignant tumors is relatively short, and second, most tumors follow somewhat strict age groupings. Jack Edeiken, one of the pre-eminent bone radiologists of our era, evaluated 4,000 malignant bone tumors and found that they could be diagnosed correctly 80% of the time just by using the patient's age. He basically divides the tumors into decades of when they usually affect a patient. For example, osteosarcoma and Ewing sarcoma are the only childhood primary malignant tumors of bone, and after the age of 40, only metastatic disease, myeloma, and chondrosarcoma are common (Table 56.1). Although there are certainly outliers that are uncommon, these age guidelines are extremely useful. It is inappropriate to mention Ewing sarcoma in a 40-year-old patient or metastatic

TABLE 56.1

AGE OF PATIENTS WITH MALIGNANT BONE TUMORS

1–30	Ewing sarcoma, osteogenic sarcoma
30–40	Giant cell tumor, parosteal sarcoma, malignant fibrous histiocytoma, first-degree lymphoma of bone
Over 40	Chondrosarcoma, metastatic disease, myeloma

disease in a 15-year-old patient, unless there is a known primary tumor. In fact, any bone lesion, regardless of its appearance, could be a metastatic lesion and would be suspicious in a patient with a known primary tumor.

Magnetic Resonance Imaging

Although plain radiographs are the best modality for characterizing a bony lesion—that is, being able to distinguish benign from malignant and generating a differential diagnosis—MR is without question the imaging procedure of choice for determining the extent of a lesion, both in the skeleton and in the soft tissues.

In assessing benignity versus malignancy, MR is somewhat controversial. Benign lesions tend to be well marginated, to have uniform and homogeneous signal, not to encase neurovascular structures, and not to invade bone. Malignant lesions tend to have irregular margins, inhomogeneous signal, and may encase neurovascular structures or invade bone.

Although almost all tumors will have low signal on T1-weighted images, which become very high in signal intensity with T2 weighting (as will fluid collections), there are a few exceptions. Malignant fibrous histiocytomas (MFHs, now commonly referred to by the more general term *pleomorphic undifferentiated sarcoma*) and desmoid tumors can occasionally demonstrate low signal on both T1-weighted and T2-weighted sequences. Any tumor with calcification will be low in signal on both T1 and T2 sequences.

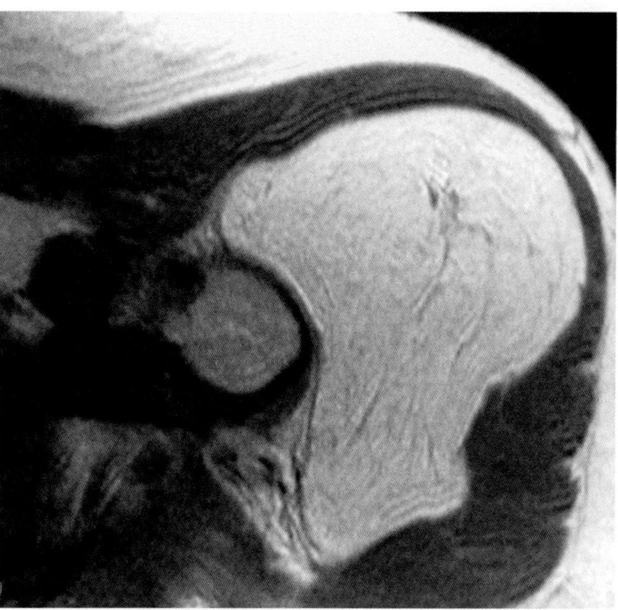

FIGURE 56.6. **Lipoma.** This axial proton-density image through the pelvis shows a large mass lateral to the femur, which has sharp margins and signal characteristics similar to the subcutaneous fat. This is a lipoma. Lipomas will usually contain a small amount of low-signal linear tissue, as in this example, which should not be a cause to consider this lesion malignant.

In some instances, MR will characterize the lesion better than radiographs and enable a specific diagnosis to be made. Lipomas are easily diagnosed with MR by their homogeneous high signal on T1-weighted images and sharp margins, whether they are intraosseous or in the soft tissues (Fig. 56.6). Hemangiomas and arteriovenous malformations most commonly have mixed high and low signals on both sequences because of the combination of fatty elements and blood (Fig. 56.7). They characteristically have low-signal serpiginous vessels visible.

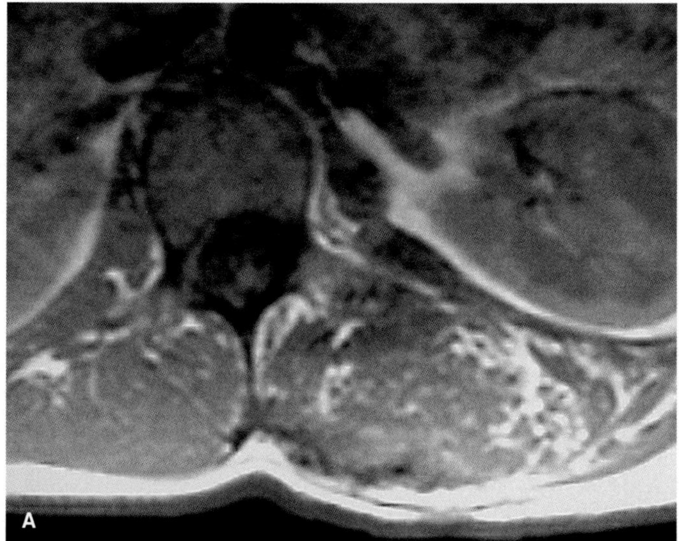

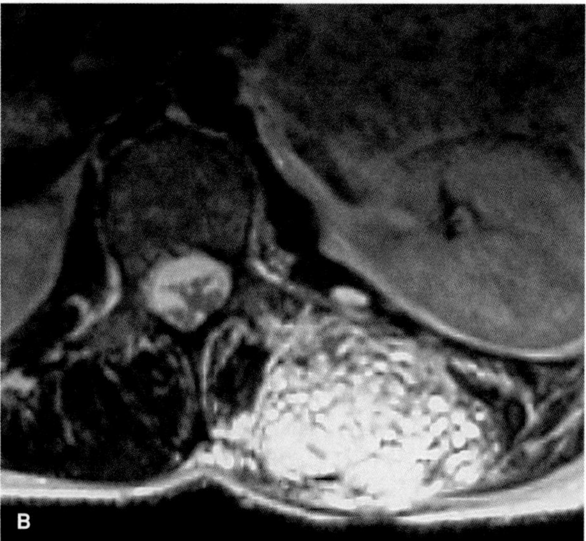

FIGURE 56.7. **Hemangioma. A:** A T1-weighted axial image through the midback in a 30-year-old patient with a mass shows a predominantly low-signal mass with stippled areas of high signal representing fat around numerous vessels. **B:** An FSE T2-weighted axial image reveals inhomogeneous high signal with punctate areas of very bright signal representing vessels. Hemangiomas typically have mixed fatty and vascular tissue, which gives high signal on both T1 and T2 sequences.

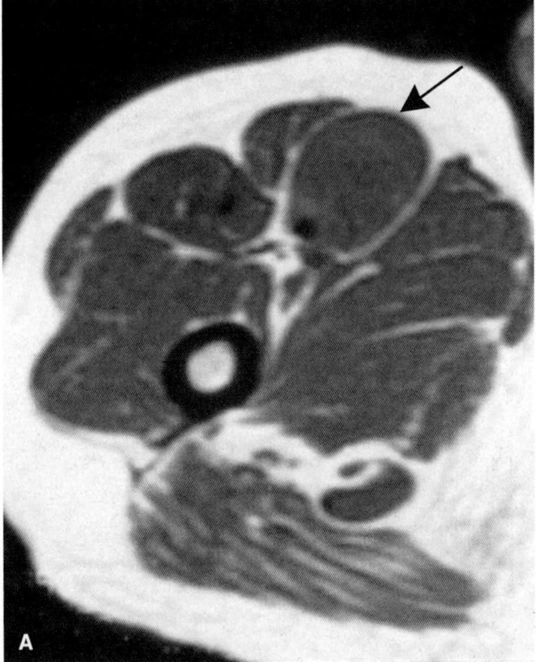

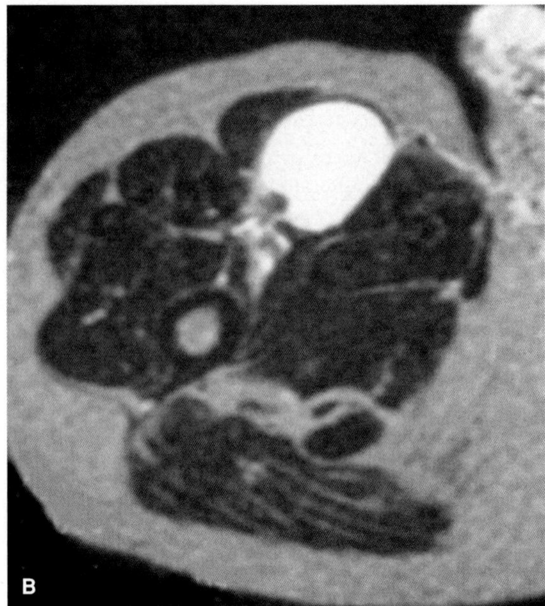

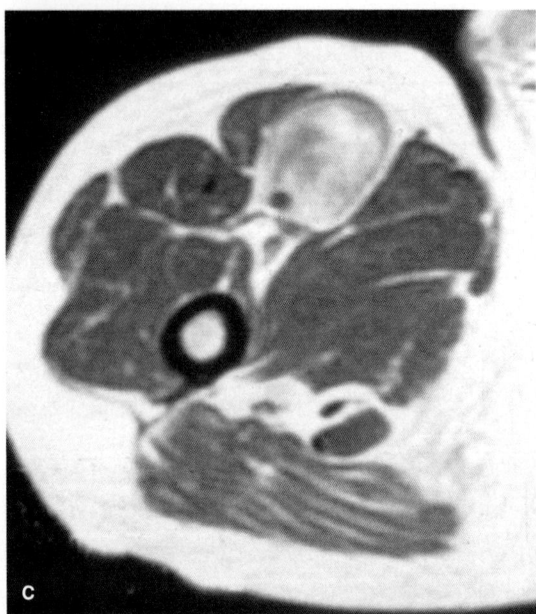

FIGURE 56.8. Schwannoma. A: A T1-weighted axial image shows a mass (*arrow*) in the anterior thigh. **B:** A T2-weighted image shows homogeneous high signal identical to that seen in a fluid collection. **C:** A T1-weighted image taken after administration of gadolinium shows diffuse enhancement of the mass, indicating that this is a solid tumor. Biopsy revealed this to be a schwannoma.

The finding of a low-signal mass on T1-weighted images that is high in signal on T2-weighted images is suspicious for a tumor, but this is a very nonspecific finding and needs to be correlated clinically. Intramuscular injection sites can mimic soft tissue tumors, as can any area of soft tissue trauma. Many malignant tumors exhibit high signal radiating from involved bone, which is soft tissue edema and virtually indistinguishable from tumor spread.

Intravenous gadolinium contrast should be routinely given when a presumed fluid collection is found, which is not an obvious ganglion or bursa, to differentiate a solid mass (which will diffusely enhance with contrast) from a fluid collection (which will have rim enhancement) (Fig. 56.8). Otherwise, gadolinium administration need not be routinely employed when imaging a tumor. All solid tumors will enhance with the exception of myxoid or necrotic areas or foci of matrix (osteoid or cartilaginous). Therefore, gadolinium often adds nothing to the workup of a tumor. In postop cases, gadolinium can be used to differentiate a seroma from a solid mass but is otherwise not useful—scar tissue from the surgery and residual or recurrent tumor both enhance. Once it has been decided to give gadolinium (and, I repeat, it is seldom necessary in tumor imaging), there is no need to do postcontrast imaging in multiple planes. A single axial sequence will suffice to see if the mass enhances or not. Additional planes of imaging are a waste of time. Finally, the postcontrast images should not be fat suppressed unless the precontrast T1 images are fat suppressed. If gadolinium and fat suppression are both used on the postcontrast images, two variables have been changed compared to the precontrast images; any increased signal in the mass could be either due to enhancement from the gadolinium or from the effect of the fat suppression (Fig. 56.9).

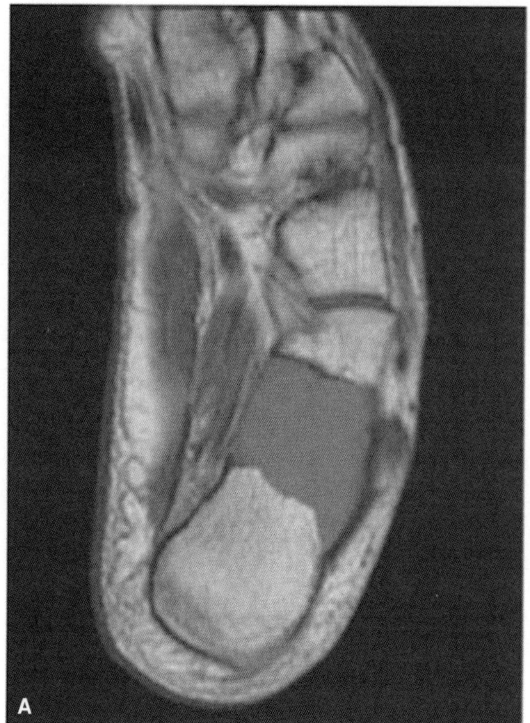

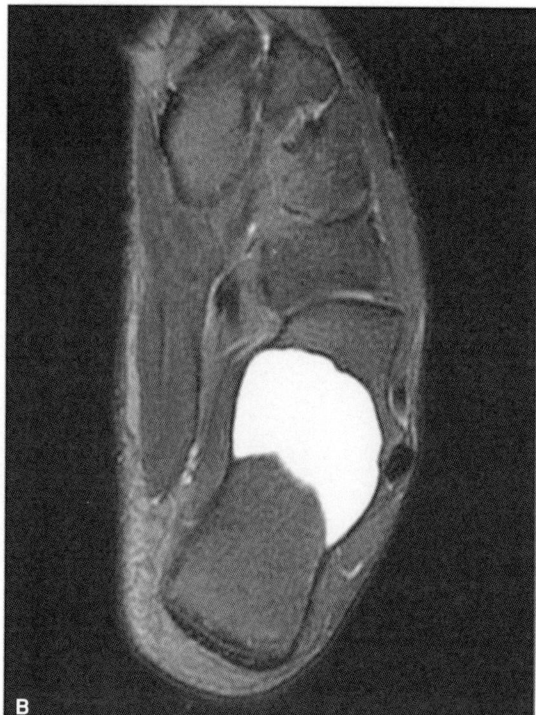

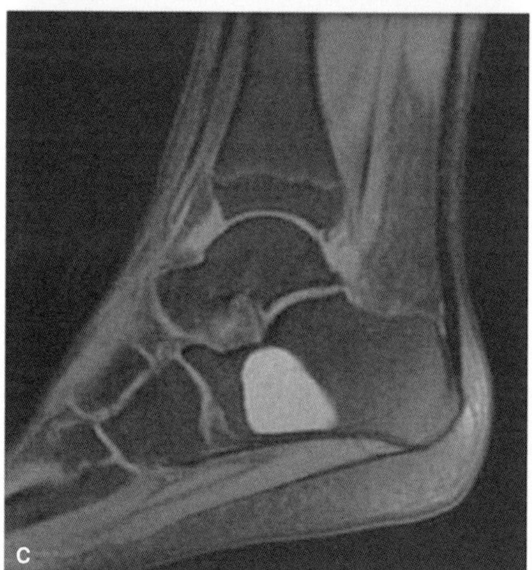

FIGURE 56.9. Effect of Fat Suppression. A: An axial T1-weighted image through the calcaneus shows a low-signal mass that is homogeneously high signal on T2-weighted image. **B:** This is the typical appearance of a unicameral bone cyst, which is a fluid-filled benign bone tumor. **C:** A sagittal T1-weighted image with fat suppression shows the lesion to be uniformly increased in signal. Had gadolinium been administered, one might wrongly assume this is an enhancing, solid tumor and not a unicameral bone cyst. As no contrast was given, the apparent increased signal is due to the effect of fat suppression.

TUMORS

Osteosarcoma

Osteosarcoma is the most common malignant primary bone tumor. These occur almost exclusively in children and young adults (<30 years old). Some texts describe a second peak of osteosarcoma around the sixth decade, but this is probably because of secondary osteosarcoma in Paget disease and because of prior radiation. Although osteosarcoma typically occurs toward the end of a long bone, it may occur anywhere in the skeleton with enough frequency that location is not a helpful discriminator. These lesions are usually destructive, with obvious sclerosis present from either tumor, new bone formation, or reactive sclerosis (Figs. 56.10 and 56.11); however, on occasion, an osteosarcoma can be entirely lytic. These are usually telangiectatic osteosarcomas. There are many different types and classifications of osteosarcomas, but it serves little purpose for the radiologist to try to distinguish between most of them. MR of an osteosarcoma generally reveals a large soft tissue component with heterogeneous high and low signal intensities on both T1-weighted and T2-weighted images (Fig. 56.10).

Parosteal Osteosarcoma

A type of osteosarcoma that should be distinguished from the central osteosarcoma is the parosteal osteosarcoma. A parosteal osteosarcoma originates from the periosteum of the bone and grows outside the bone (Fig. 56.12). It often wraps around the diaphysis without breaking through the cortex at all. It occurs in an older age group than the central

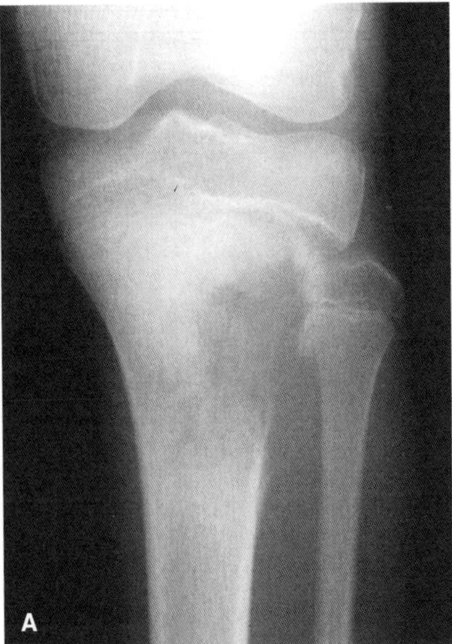

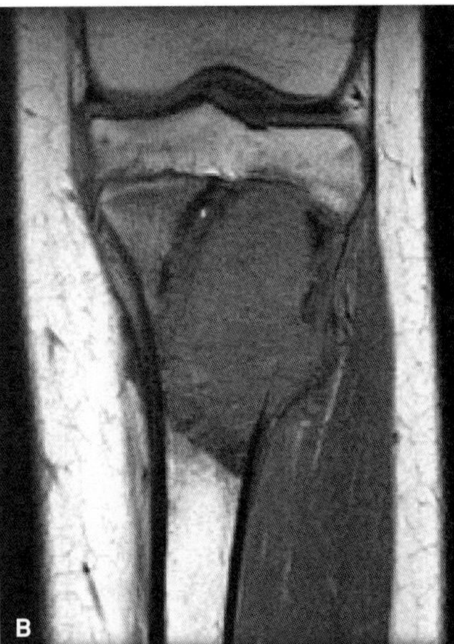

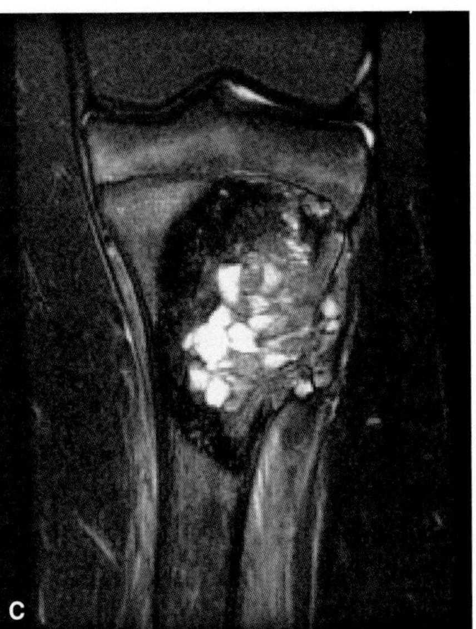

FIGURE 56.10. **Osteosarcoma. A:** A mixed lytic and sclerotic lesion in the proximal tibia of a child is noted, which is characteristic for an osteogenic sarcoma. **B:** A coronal T1-weighted image shows the full extent of the lesion with some soft tissue extension. **C:** These findings are also observed on the T2-weighted image.

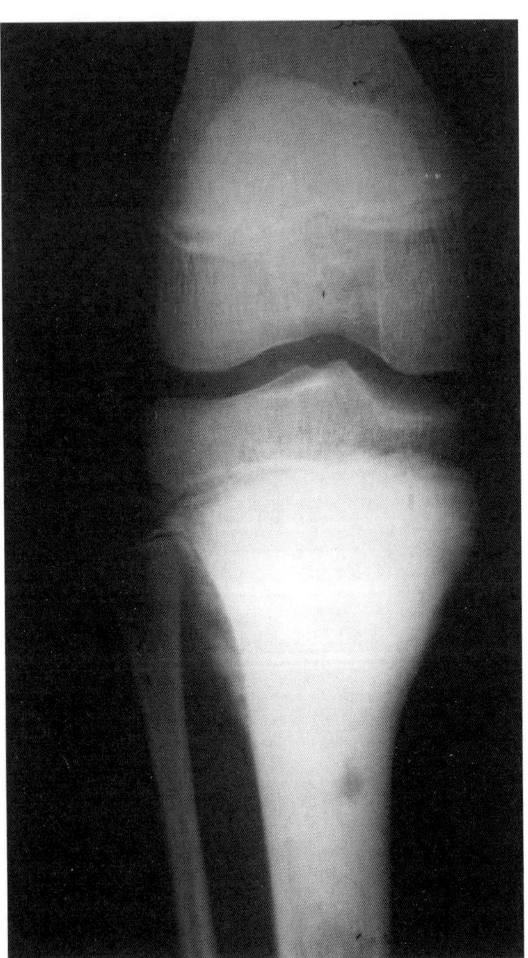

FIGURE 56.11. **Osteosarcoma.** A densely sclerotic lesion in the proximal tibia of a child is seen, which is characteristic for an osteosarcoma.

osteosarcomas and is not as aggressive or as deadly as long as it has not extended into the medullary portion of the bone. Treatment used to consist of merely shaving the tumor off the bone from which it was arising; however, recurrence rates were so high that now wide bloc excisions are performed. Once a parosteal osteosarcoma violates the cortex of the adjacent bone, it is considered to be as aggressive as a central osteosarcoma and is treated in a similar fashion—that is, by radical excision. The radiologist needs to evaluate the lesion for invasion of the adjacent cortex to help determine treatment and prognosis. This is best done with CT or MR (Fig. 56.13). A common location from which parosteal osteosarcomas arise is the posterior femur, near the knee.

A lesion that can mimic an early parosteal osteosarcoma in this location is a cortical desmoid. A cortical desmoid is an avulsion injury that is totally benign but can appear somewhat aggressive. Unfortunately, it can appear malignant histologically, so biopsy can lead to disastrous consequences. Amputations for benign cortical desmoids that were confused with malignancies have occurred.

Another lesion that can be confused with a parosteal osteosarcoma is an area of myositis ossificans. Like cortical desmoids, areas of myositis ossificans can be histologically confused for malignancies with disastrous consequences. Differentiation is, of course, vital. Fortunately, differentiation between parosteal osteosarcoma and myositis ossificans is usually easily done radiographically (see Chapter 60 for discussion of differential points between parosteal osteosarcoma and myositis ossificans and cortical desmoids).

Ewing Sarcoma

The classic Ewing sarcoma is a permeative (multiple small holes) lesion in the diaphysis of a long bone in a child (see Fig. 56.3B). Only about 40% of these tumors occur in the diaphysis, however, with the remainder being metaphyseal, diametaphyseal, and in flat bones. They do tend to be primarily in children and adolescents, although a significant number occur in patients in their 20s, especially in flat bones. Although most often permeative in appearance, they can elicit

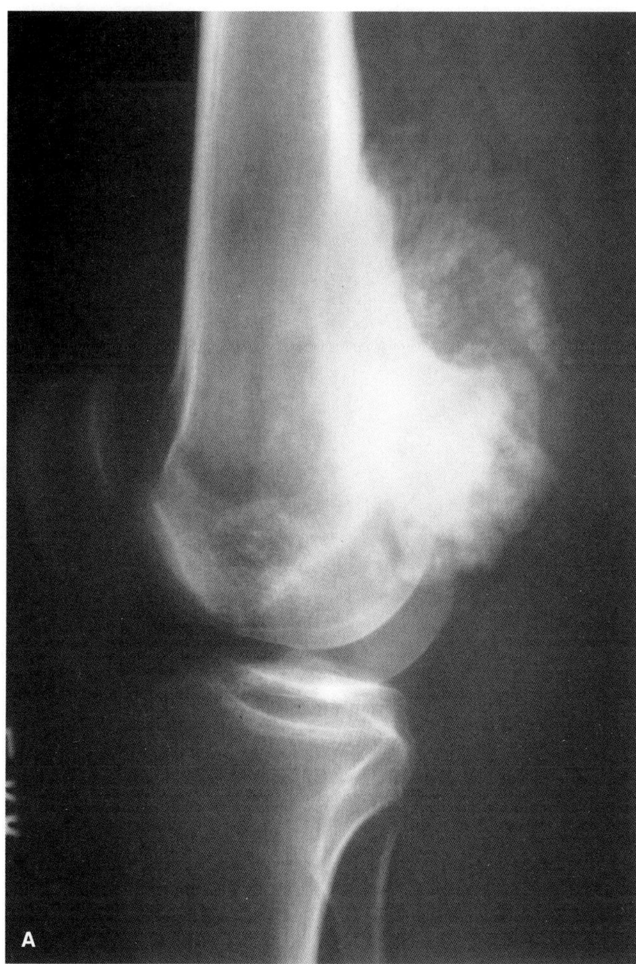

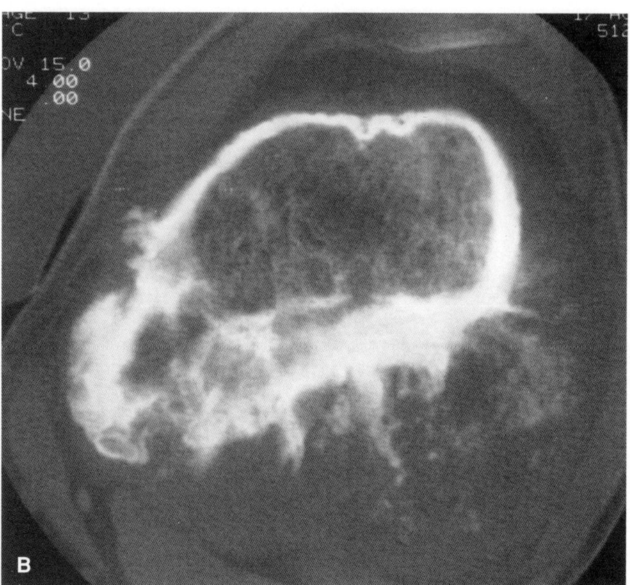

FIGURE 56.12. **Parosteal Osteosarcoma. A:** A lateral radiograph of the knee shows a bony lesion emanating from the posterior cortex of the distal femur with a large, calcified soft tissue mass. Note that the densest calcification is central and the periphery is only faintly calcified, characteristics that are typical for a parosteal osteosarcoma. **B:** A CT through the lesion reveals the tumor to be invading the medullary portion of the bone. This is a poor prognostic sign and is an essential information to the surgeon.

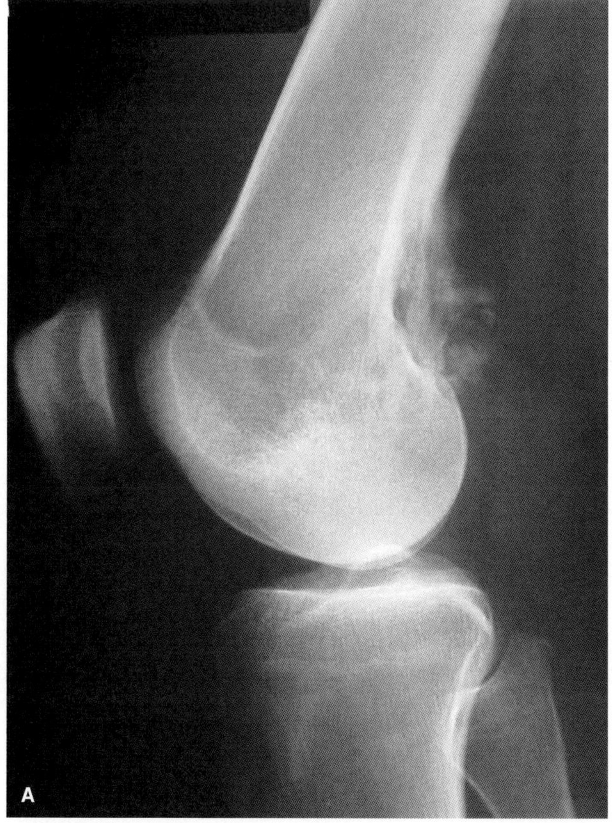

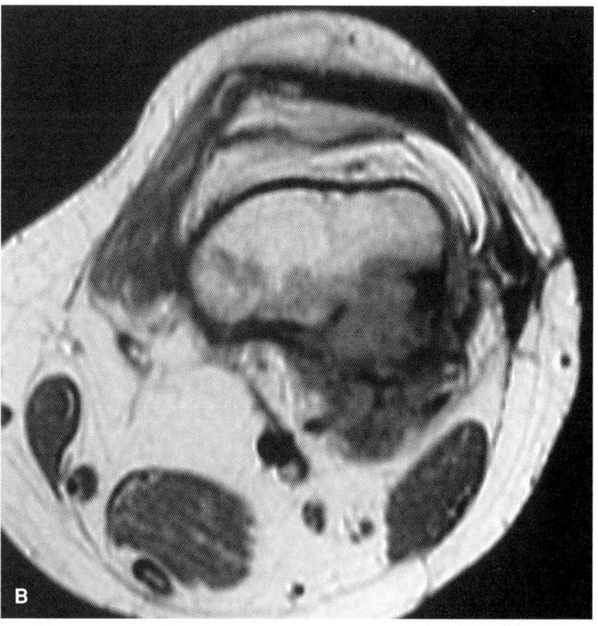

FIGURE 56.13. **Parosteal Osteosarcoma. A:** A lateral radiograph in a different patient with a parosteal osteosarcoma shows soft tissue calcification extending from the posterior femur. **B:** A proton-density axial image reveals considerable bony involvement.

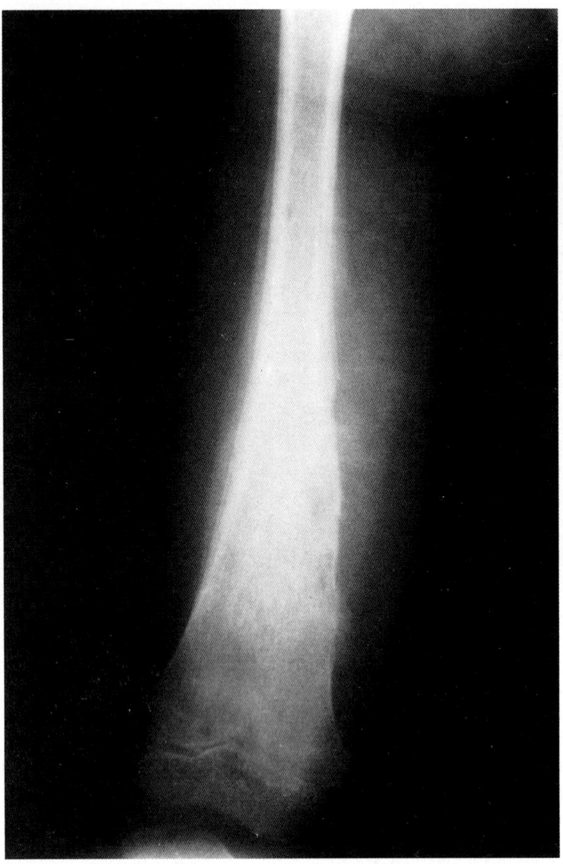

FIGURE 56.14. **Ewing Sarcoma.** An anteroposterior radiograph of the femur of a child shows a predominantly sclerotic process with large amounts of sunburst periostitis in the diaphysis, which on biopsy was found to be Ewing sarcoma.

reactive new bone that can give the lesion a partially sclerotic or "patchy" appearance. Ewing sarcomas often have an onion-skin type of periostitis, but they can also have periostitis that is sunburst or amorphous in character (Fig. 56.14). Rarely, if ever, will a Ewing sarcoma have benign-appearing periostitis (thick, uniform, or wavy).

If benign periostitis is present, other lesions should be considered instead, such as infection and eosinophilic granuloma. The classic differential diagnosis for a permeative lesion in a child is Ewing sarcoma, infection, and eosinophilic granuloma. These three entities can appear radiologically identical. Ewing sarcoma should be removed from the differential diagnosis if definite benign periostitis or a sequestration is present. The presence or absence of a soft tissue mass is not helpful in distinguishing between these three lesions. The presence of symptoms is not helpful, as all three entities can be symptomatic.

Chondrosarcoma

Chondrosarcomas have a protean appearance that makes it difficult, at times, to make the diagnosis with any assurance. They most commonly occur in patients older than the age of 40 years. Chondrosarcoma rarely occurs in children, although occasionally one will be encountered from malignant degeneration of an osteochondroma. It can be extremely difficult to differentiate histologically a low-grade chondrosarcoma from an enchondroma. The diagnosis of chondrosarcoma usually

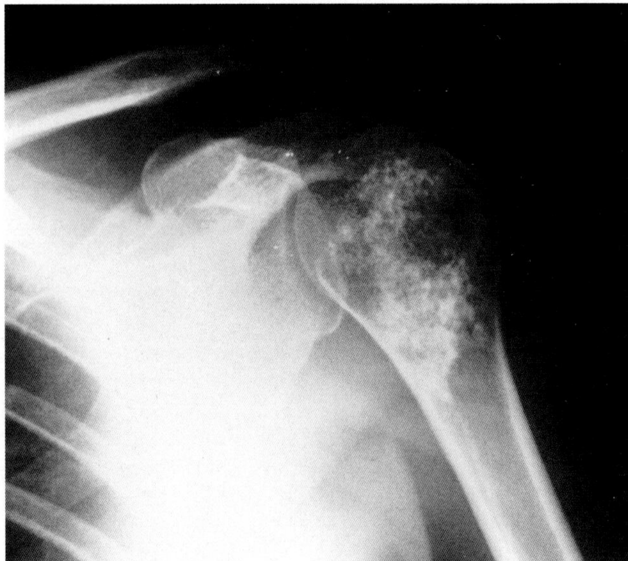

FIGURE 56.15. **Chondrosarcoma.** Typical snowflake or popcorn-like amorphous calcification in the proximal humerus is seen, which is typical of an enchondroma. This patient, however, had pain associated with this lesion, and on biopsy, this was found to be a chondrosarcoma.

initiates radical excision and therapy, although it is debatable (and somewhat controversial) whether a low-grade chondrosarcoma is even a malignant tumor. For these reasons, the diagnosis of "possible chondrosarcoma" should be reserved for those lesions that are painful (Fig. 56.15) or that show definite aggressive characteristics such as periostitis and cortical destruction. The truth of the matter is neither radiologists nor pathologists can reliably distinguish between enchondromas and low-grade chondrosarcomas. MRI can be very useful in distinguishing a benign enchondroma from a chondrosarcoma. If a soft tissue mass or edema is present, it is unlikely to be an enchondroma.

Chondrosarcoma should be considered in the diagnosis any time there is a bony or soft tissue mass with amorphous, snowflake calcification in an older patient (>40 years) (Fig. 56.16). Without the presence of calcified chondroid matrix, the lesion is indistinguishable from any other aggressive lytic lesion such

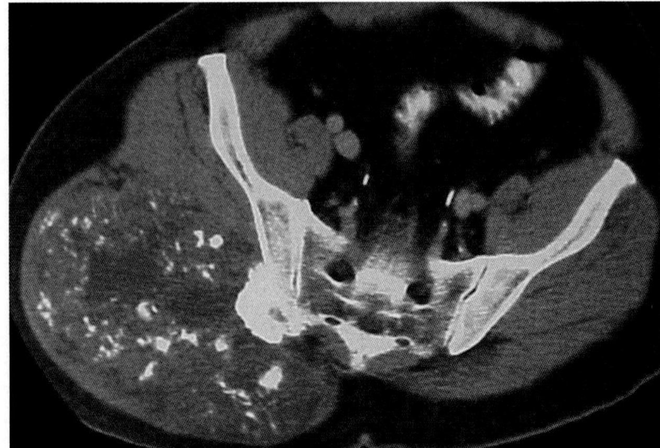

FIGURE 56.16. **Chondrosarcoma.** A large soft tissue mass with amorphous, irregular calcification is seen in a lesion arising from the ilium on this CT of the pelvis. This is typical for a chondrosarcoma.

as metastatic disease, plasmacytoma, or infection. Usually the radiologist can only give a long differential diagnosis such as this, which is entirely acceptable. The lesion will have to undergo biopsy at any rate, and therefore, it is not necessary for the radiologist to make the diagnosis. This is the case for most malignant tumors.

Malignant Giant Cell Tumor

It is said that approximately 15% of giant cell tumors are malignant; however, this is based on their rate of recurrence rather than on the presence of metastatic disease, which is rare. Unfortunately, there does not seem to be any way to predict which giant cell tumor will become malignant. Radiologically, the benign and malignant giant cell tumors appear identical. Histologically, the benign and the malignant giant cell tumors can appear similar. If metastases (usually to the lung) occur, the tumor is considered by most oncologists to be malignant. This is quite rare. Malignant giant cell tumors tend to occur primarily in the fourth decade of life.

Malignant Fibrous Histiocytoma—Formerly Called Fibrosarcoma

MFHs are lytic malignant tumors that do not produce osteoid or chondroid matrix. They usually do not cause reactive new bone and, therefore, are almost always lytic in appearance. This lytic appearance may take any form, from permeative (Fig. 56.17) to moth-eaten to a fairly well-defined area of lysis

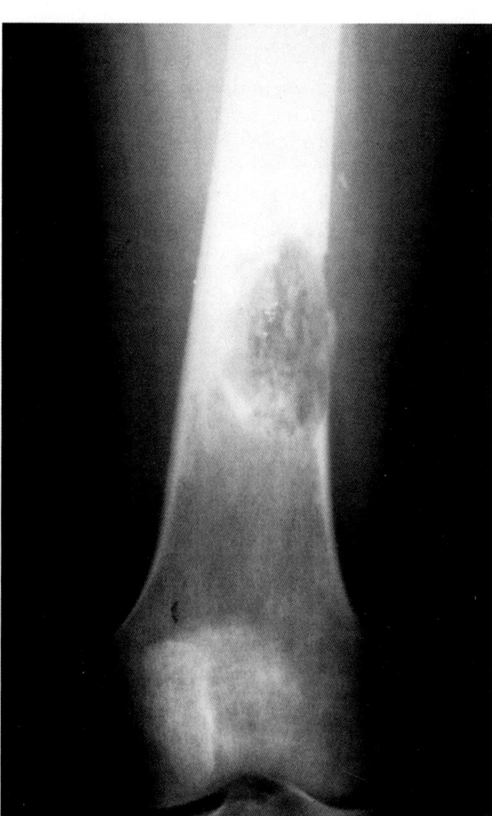

FIGURE 56.17. **Malignant Fibrous Histiocytoma (MFH) of Bone.** An ill-defined lytic lesion that is permeative or moth-eaten in appearance is seen in the diaphysis of the femur that on biopsy was shown to be an MFH.

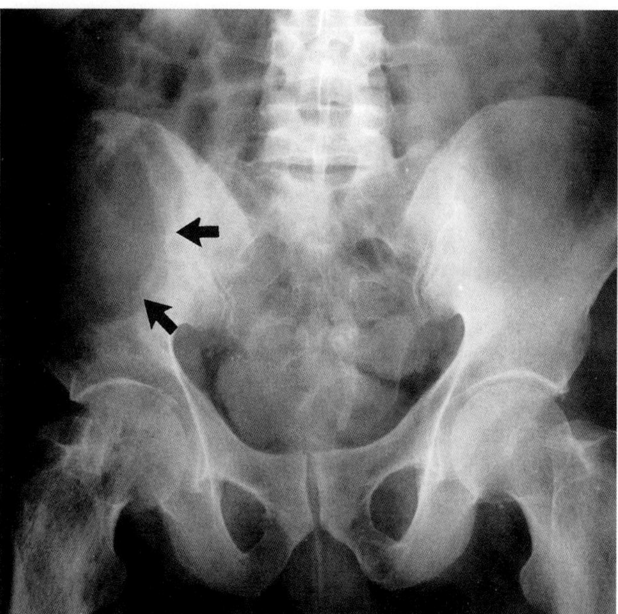

FIGURE 56.18. **Malignant Fibrous Histiocytoma (MFH) of Bone.** A large, lytic, destructive process of the entire right iliac wing (*arrows*) is noted, which is fairly well defined. On biopsy, this was shown to be an MFH. MFHs can be very slow growing and will occasionally have a narrow zone of transition such as this.

(Fig. 56.18). The age range for fibrosarcoma is quite broad, but they tend to predominate in the fourth decade. This is one of the few malignant tumors that can, on occasion, have a bony sequestrum.

Desmoid Tumor

A desmoid tumor (not to be confused with a cortical desmoid; see Chapter 60) is a half-grade fibrosarcoma. It has also been called a desmoplastic fibroma or aggressive fibromatosis. They most commonly arise in the soft tissues and are uncommon in the bony skeleton. These lesions, when in bone, are lytic but are usually fairly well defined because of their slow growth. They often have benign periostitis present that has thick spicules or "spikes." They usually have a multilocular appearance with thick bony septa (Fig. 56.19). They are slow growing and do not metastasize, but they can exhibit inexorable tumor extension into surrounding soft tissues with devastating results.

Primary Lymphoma of Bone (Formerly Called Reticulum Cell Sarcoma)

This is a neoplasm that has a radiologic appearance identical to Ewing sarcoma—that is, a permeative or moth-eaten pattern (Fig. 56.20). Primary lymphoma of bone tends to occur in an older age group than Ewing sarcoma, and whereas Ewing sarcomas are typically systemically symptomatic, patients with primary lymphoma of bone are often asymptomatic. It is said to be the only malignant tumor that can involve a large amount of bone while the patient is asymptomatic.

Metastatic Disease

Metastatic lesions must be included in any differential diagnosis of a bone lesion in a patient greater than the age of

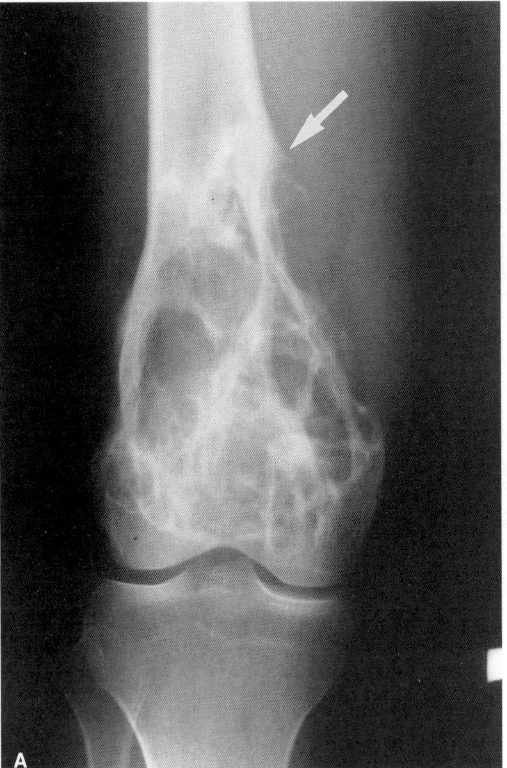

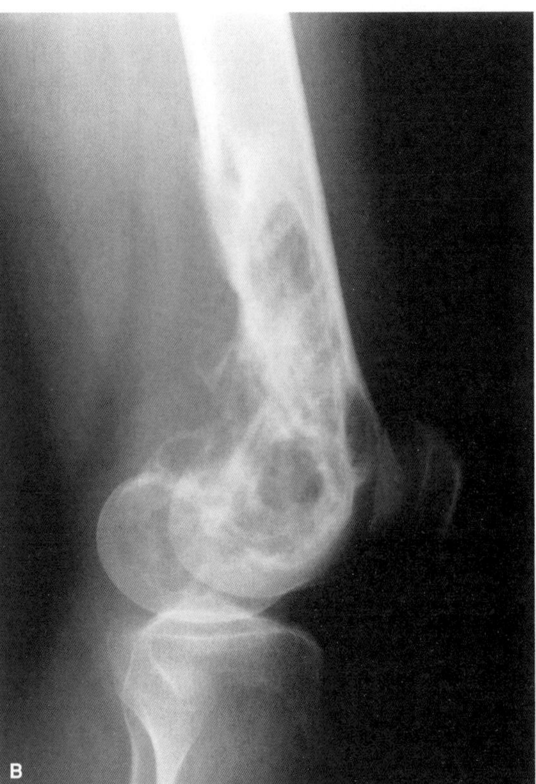

FIGURE 56.19. Desmoid Tumor of Bone. A multilocular, heavily septated, destructive, lytic lesion of the distal femur is noted in these anteroposterior (**A**) and lateral (**B**) radiographs of the femur, which is fairly characteristic for a desmoid tumor. The thick septa and narrow zone of transition are characteristic of a benign process, whereas the Codman triangle (*arrow*) and large amount of bony destruction indicate an aggressive process.

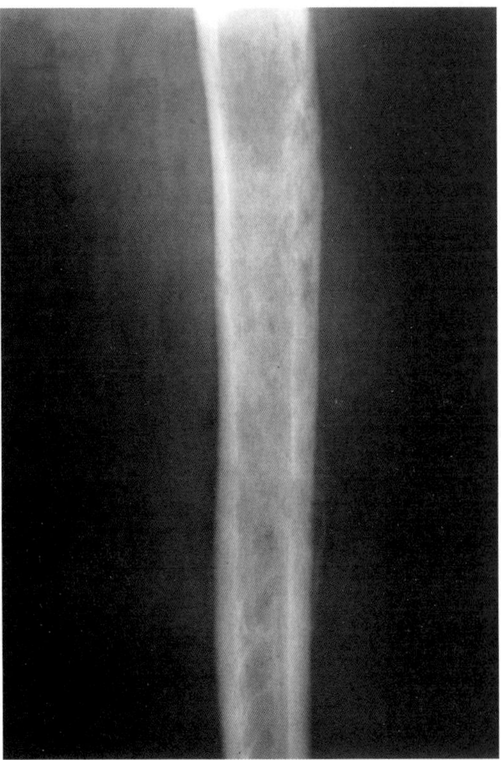

FIGURE 56.20. Primary Lymphoma of Bone. A diffuse permeative pattern is seen throughout the humerus in this 35-year-old patient that is characteristic of primary lymphoma of bone.

40 years. They can have virtually any appearance. They can mimic a benign lesion or an aggressive primary bone tumor. It can be difficult, if not impossible, to judge the origin of the tumor from the appearance of the metastatic focus, although some appearances are fairly characteristic. For instance, multiple sclerotic foci in a man are most likely prostatic metastases (Fig. 56.21), although lung, bowel, or almost any

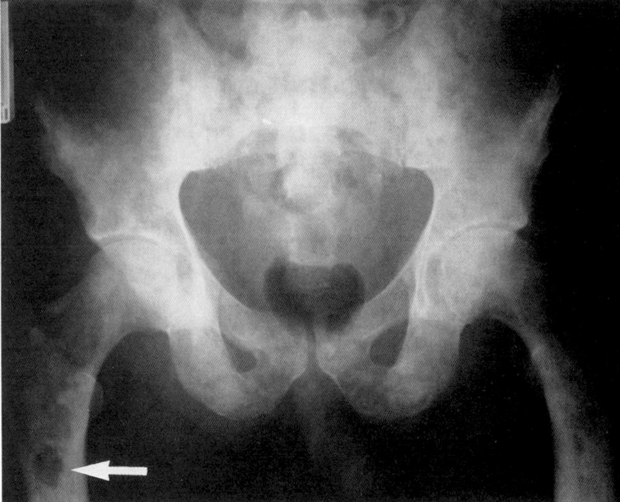

FIGURE 56.21. Metastatic Prostate Carcinoma. Diffuse blastic metastases are seen throughout the pelvis and proximal femurs with a lytic, destructive lesion seen in the right proximal femur (*arrow*). Prostate metastases tend to be blastic but can occasionally be lytic.

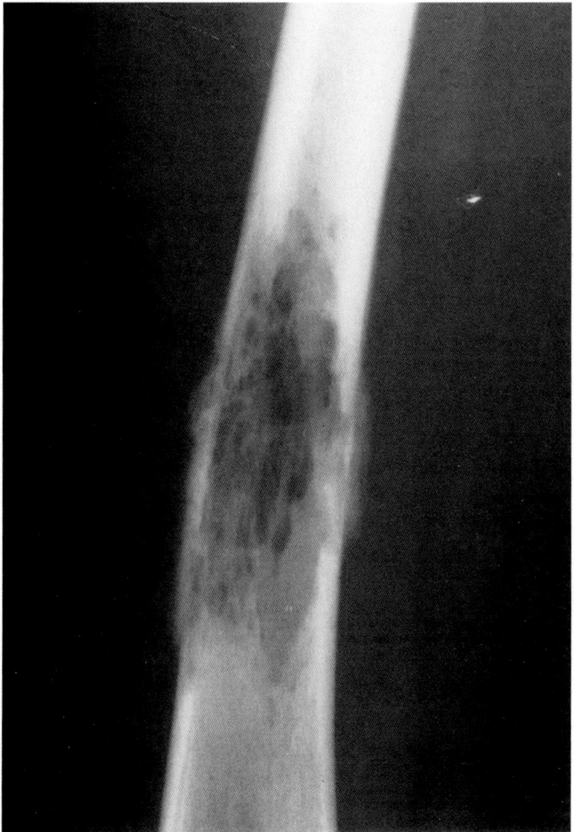

FIGURE 56.22. **Metastatic Renal Cell Carcinoma.** A lytic lesion in the diaphysis of the femur is noted, which is typical for renal cell carcinoma. As many as one-third of renal cell carcinomas present initially with a bony metastasis. Renal cell carcinoma virtually never presents with a blastic metastatic focus.

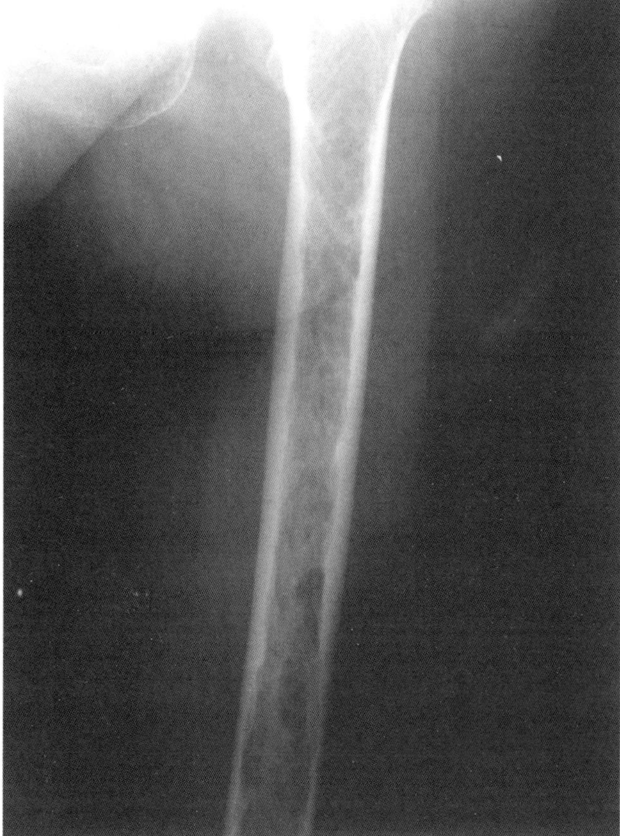

FIGURE 56.23. **Multiple Myeloma.** A diffuse, moth-eaten pattern is seen throughout the diaphysis of the femur in this 45-year-old patient that is characteristic for myeloma. Primary lymphoma of bone could have a similar appearance.

other metastatic tumor could present like this. In a woman, the same picture would most likely be from breast metastases. Although nearly every metastatic bone lesion can be either lytic or blastic, the only primary tumor that virtually never presents with blastic metastatic disease is renal cell carcinoma. The classic differential diagnosis for an expansile, lytic metastasis is renal cell or thyroid carcinoma (Fig. 56.22).

Myeloma

Like metastases, myeloma should only be considered in a patient older than the age of 40 years, although some radiologists use age 35 for the lower limits of myeloma. Myeloma typically has a diffuse permeative appearance (Fig. 56.23) that can mimic a Ewing sarcoma or primary lymphoma of bone. Because of the age criteria, Ewing sarcoma and myeloma are not in the same differential, however. Myeloma frequently involves the calvarium (Fig. 56.24). Rarely, myeloma can present with multiple sclerotic foci resembling diffuse metastatic disease. Myeloma is one of the only lesions that is not characteristically hot on a radionuclide bone scan; therefore, radiologic "bone surveys" are performed in place of radionuclide bone scans when evidence of myeloma is found clinically. Occasionally, myeloma will present with a lytic bone lesion called a plasmacytoma. This lesion can mimic any lytic bone lesion, benign or aggressive, in its appearance; it can precede other evidence of myeloma by up to 5 years. A plasmacytoma in a vertebral body has a characteristic appearance called a "mini-brain" (see Chapter 55, Fig. 55.29).

Soft Tissue Tumors

Pleomorphic Undifferentiated Sarcomas. There is no concise, useful differential diagnosis for soft tissue tumors, whether or not there is calcification, bony destruction, fat

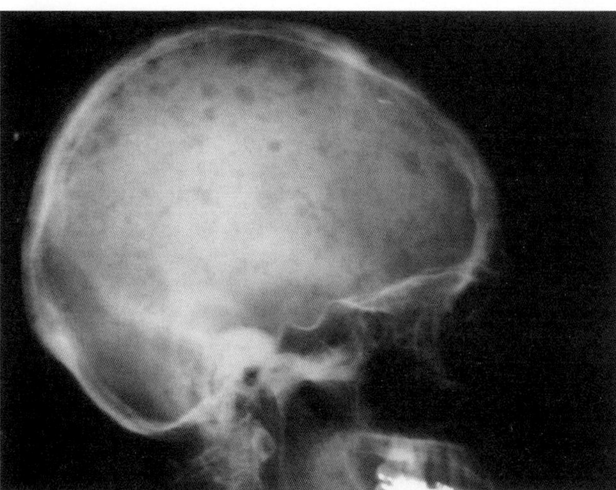

FIGURE 56.24. **Multiple Myeloma.** A lateral view of the skull shows multiple lytic lesions in the calvarium, which is a characteristic appearance of multiple myeloma.

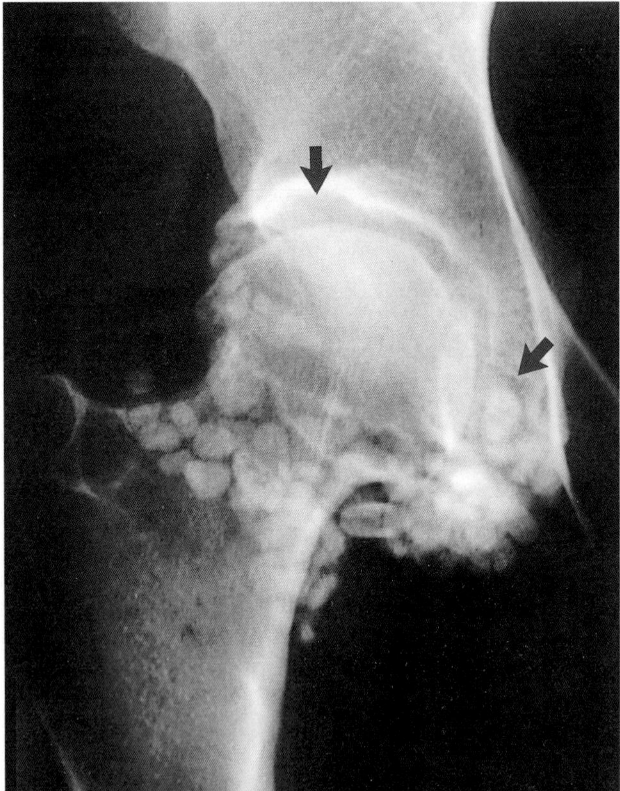

FIGURE 56.25. Synovial Osteochondromatosis. Multiple calcific loose bodies in a hip joint, as in this example, are virtually pathognomonic for synovial osteochondromatosis. Notice the erosions in the acetabulum (*arrows*). In up to 20% of cases, the loose bodies are nonossified; in such cases, this process is indistinguishable from pigmented villonodular synovitis.

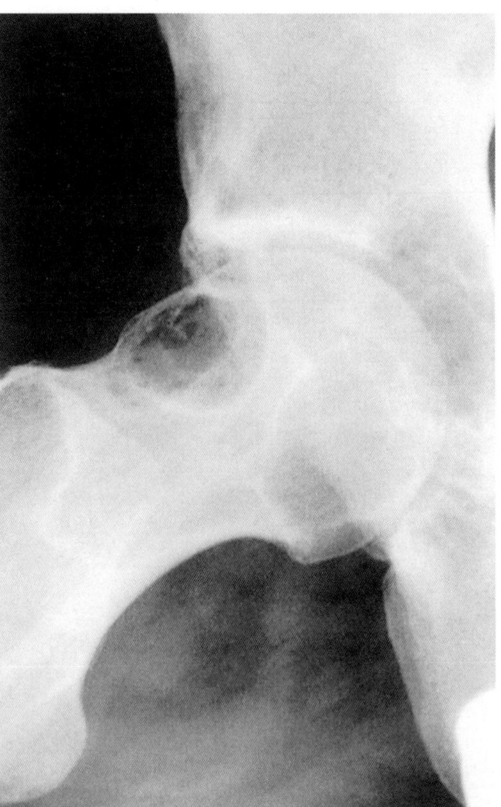

FIGURE 56.26. Pigmented Villonodular Synovitis (PVNS). Large erosions in the femoral head and acetabulum are characteristic for PVNS; however, nonossified synovial osteochondromatosis could present similarly.

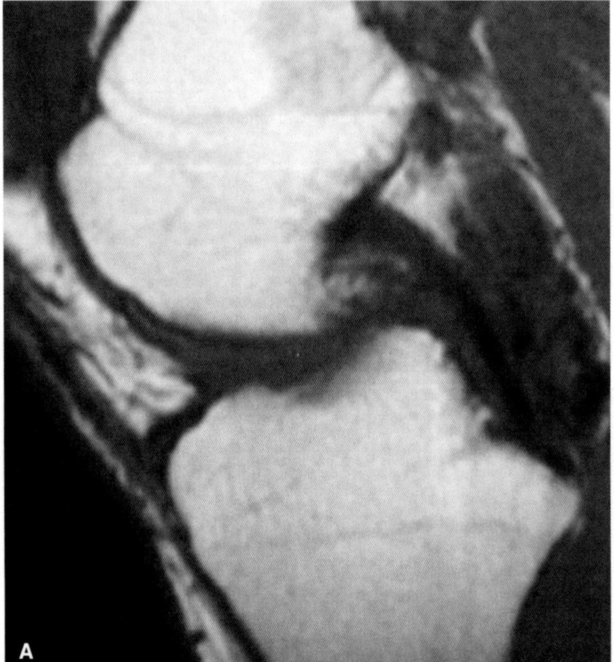

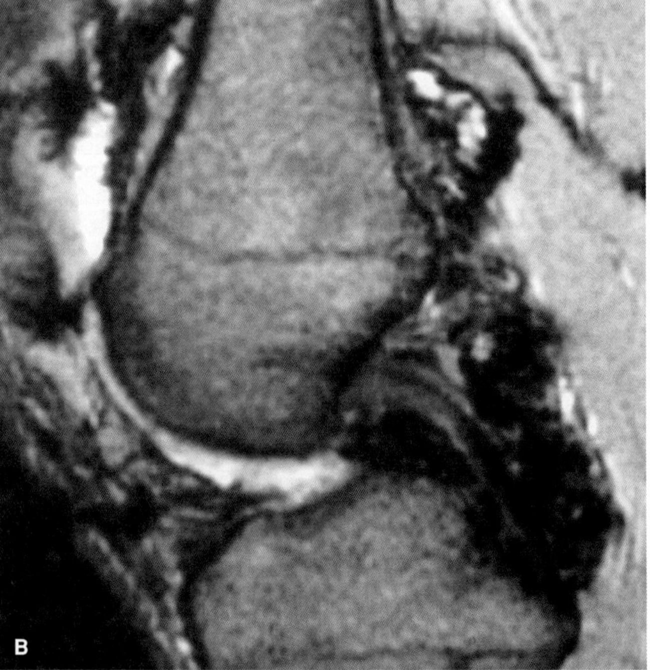

FIGURE 56.27. Pigmented Villonodular Synovitis (PVNS). Proton-density (**A**) and T2-weighted (**B**) sagittal images of the knee in this patient with painful swelling show diffuse low signal throughout the synovium. The low signal on both T1- and T2-weighted images is typical for hemosiderin deposits in PVNS.

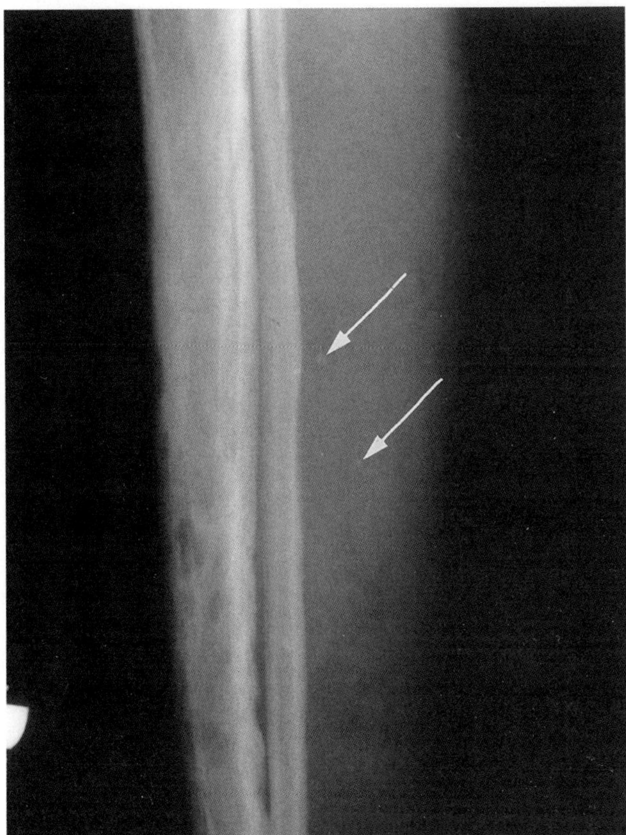

FIGURE 56.28. Hemangioma. Multiple irregular lytic lesions, predominantly cortical in nature, are seen in the tibia in this patient with a soft tissue mass. Cortical holes such as this occur almost exclusively in radiation and soft tissue hemangioma. Note the phleboliths in the posterior soft tissues (*arrows*) that are often seen in hemangioma and make this an easy diagnosis.

plane involvement, and so forth. The two most common soft tissue tumors, ***MFH*** and ***liposarcoma***, have recently been reclassified by pathologists under a single heading called pleomorphic undifferentiated sarcomas. This is because, when high grade, they are virtually indistinguishable histologically. For radiologists, it is just as well because we never could tell an MFH from a liposarcoma anyway. Liposarcomas seldom display fatty elements on MRI, and both tumors often have hemorrhage, which can resemble fat on T1-weighted images. Some pathologists still separate out MFH from liposarcoma, but most do not. A lipoma, obviously, can be separated out by the appearance of fat, but a liposarcoma might or might not have fat present. Therefore, one is generally left to giving descriptions of size and extent of the tumor and letting the pathologist determine the diagnosis.

Synovial sarcomas (formerly called synoviomas) only very rarely originate in a joint. They are often adjacent to joints. There are no malignant tumors that routinely need to be considered in the differential diagnosis of joint lesions. Synovial sarcomas are one of two types of tumors (along with neural tumors) that are typically homogeneously bright on T2-weighted images—to the extent that they can be mistaken for a fluid collection. As mentioned previously, whenever a mass is found on MRI that resembles a fluid collection in a location that is atypical for a ganglion or bursa, contrast must be given to determine if it is indeed fluid or a solid mass.

Synovial osteochondromatosis is a benign joint lesion that occurs from metaplasia of the synovium and leads to multiple calcific loose bodies in a joint. This can histologically mimic a chondrosarcoma and therefore is best diagnosed radiographically, as it has a pathognomonic radiographic appearance (Fig. 56.25). Up to 30% of the time, the loose bodies do not calcify, however, and the osteochondromatosis then can mimic pigmented villonodular synovitis (PVNS).

Pigmented villonodular synovitis is a benign synovial soft tissue process that causes joint swelling and pain and occasionally, periarticular erosions (Fig. 56.26). It virtually never has calcifications associated with it. The MR appearance of PVNS is characteristic. Marked low signal intensity lining the synovium is seen on T1- and T2-weighted images because of the hemosiderin deposits (Fig. 56.27).

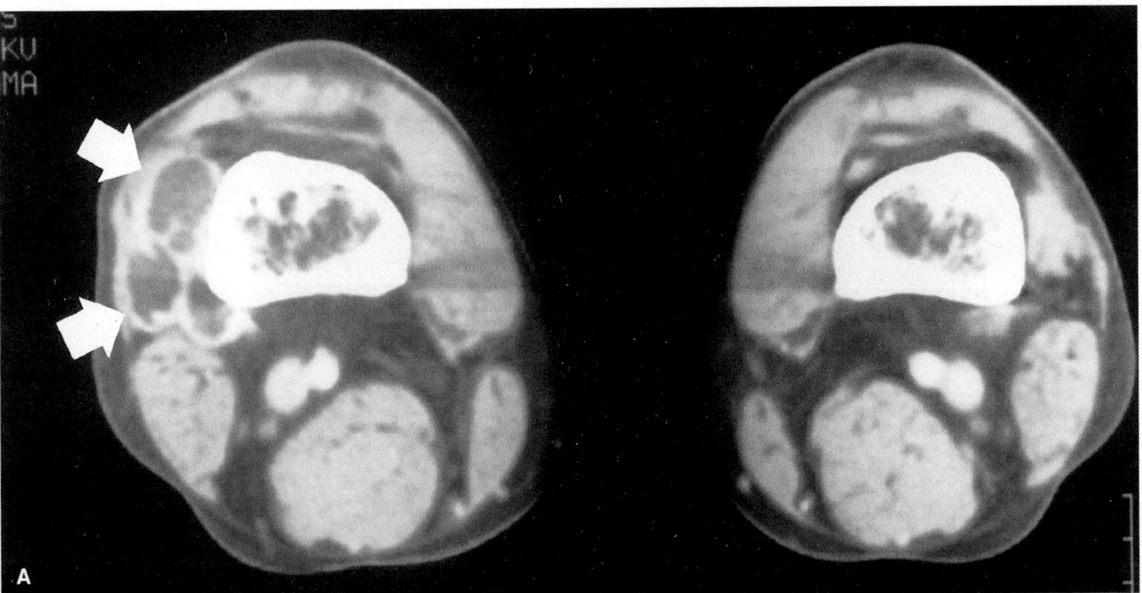

FIGURE 56.29. Atypical Synovial Cyst. A: A CT scan through the distal femurs in a patient with a soft tissue mass around the right knee shows a multilocular soft tissue mass adjacent to the distal right femur (*arrows*). (*continued*)

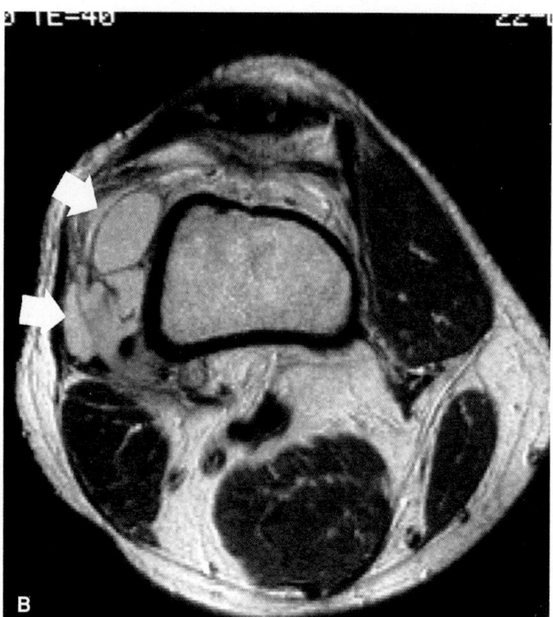

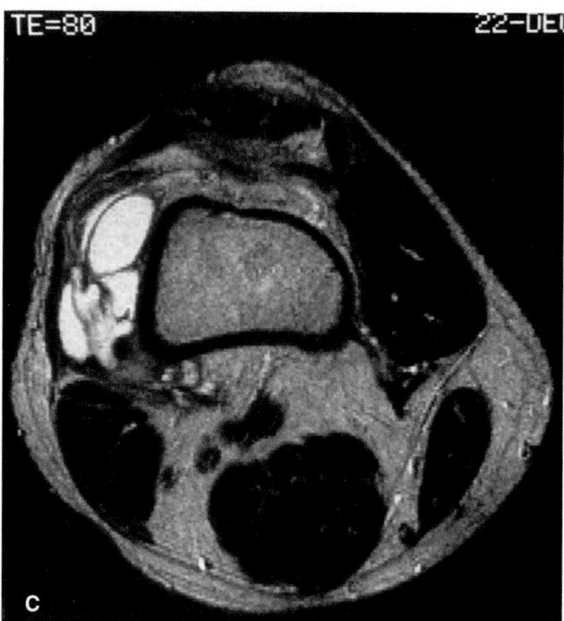

FIGURE 56.29. (*Continued*) **B:** A proton-density MR through the same area shows intermediate intensity signal in a homogeneous multilocular soft tissue mass (*arrows*). **C:** A T2-weighted image shows high-intensity signal in the lesion, which is typical for fluid, although a tumor could have these signal characteristics. This was an atypical synovial cyst arising from the knee joint.

Chronic bleeding into a joint, the so-called hemosiderotic arthritis, could have a similar appearance but is encountered uncommonly.

Hemangiomas will often have phleboliths associated with them and often cause cortical holes in adjacent bone that can mimic a permeative or moth-eaten pattern (Fig. 56.28), a pseudopermeative pattern. The true permeative pattern of round cell lesions occurs in the intramedullary or endosteal part of the bone and can be differentiated from a pseudopermeative pattern by the intact cortex.

Atypical synovial cysts, such as Baker cysts around the knee, can present as a soft tissue mass and result in an unnecessary biopsy. On CT, these lesions may not be appreciated as fluid-filled lesions and their association with a joint can be easily overlooked. MR will demonstrate a very high signal intensity with T2 weighting that is very homogeneous and often septated (Fig. 56.29). Gadolinium should be given to determine if it is truly a fluid collection or a solid mass. As mentioned previously, synovial sarcomas and neural tumors often mimic fluid collections on T2-weighted images.

Suggested Readings

Berquist T, Ehman R, King B, Hodgman CG, Ilstrup DM. Value of MR imaging in differentiating benign from malignant soft-tissue masses: study of 95 lesions. *AJR Am J Roentgenol* 1990;155(6):1251–1255.

Brien EW, Mirra JM, Kerr R. Benign and malignant cartilage tumors of bone and joint: their anatomic and theoretical basis with an emphasis on radiology, pathology and clinical biology. I. The intramedullary cartilage tumors. *Skeletal Radiol* 1997;26(6):325–353.

CHAPTER 57 ■ SKELETAL TRAUMA

CLYDE A. HELMS AND EMILY N. VINSON

Most of the differential diagnoses in skeletal radiology that I use are geared to be 95% inclusive—that is, the correct diagnosis will be mentioned 95% of the time. The yield can be increased by lengthening the list, but if the list gets too long, it can be unwieldy and less useful for the clinician. In trauma cases, however, being right 95% of the time is not good enough. Missing the correct diagnosis 5% of the time is unacceptable. Fractures simply should not be missed.

Before starting with specific examples, a few key points should be kept in mind concerning radiology of trauma. First, have a high index of suspicion. Every radiologist in the world has missed fractures on radiographs because they were not sufficiently attuned to the possible presence of a fracture. Often, the history is either nonexistent or misleading, and the anatomic area of concern is therefore overlooked. When in doubt, examine the patient. Orthopedic surgeons rarely miss seeing fractures on radiographs because they have examined the patient, they know where the patient hurts, and they have a high index of suspicion. Second, always get two radiographs at 90 degrees to each other in every trauma case. A high percentage of fractures are seen only on one view (the anteroposterior or the lateral) and will therefore be missed unless two views are routinely obtained. Third, once a fracture is identified, do not forget to look at the rest of the radiograph. About 10% of all cases have a second finding that often is as significant as or even more so than the initial finding. Many fractures have associated dislocation, foreign bodies, or additional fractures, so be sure to examine the entire image.

Finally, do not hesitate to obtain a CT scan or an MR study if the radiographs fail to confirm what is believed to be present clinically. MR imaging is being used more frequently as a primary imaging tool for trauma, replacing CT or radionuclide studies in cases in which the plain radiographs are negative or equivocal. Make sure that an expensive examination such as CT or MR is truly going to affect patient care rather than just show an abnormality and then have the same treatment whether positive or negative. For example, there is no reason to do a CT scan or an MR study to find a subtle or occult fracture of the radial head in the elbow because the patient is going to have a posterior splint regardless of the results of the advanced study (assuming the patient had trauma to the elbow, has pain, and the radiograph shows a displaced fat pad indicative of fluid in the joint). On the contrary, an elderly patient who has hip pain after a fall and has a negative radiograph would benefit from an MR study because his treatment will depend on whether or not an occult fracture is present.

SPINE

The cervical spine is one of the most commonly radiographed parts of the body in a busy emergency department and can be one of the most difficult examinations to interpret. One of the most important pieces of information for the radiologist to have is the clinical history. If the patient has been involved in an automobile accident and has no neck pain, it is extremely unlikely that a fracture is present. The so-called precautionary radiographs are not justified. On the contrary, if the radiographs are negative in a trauma victim who has neck pain or neurologic deficits, obtain a CT scan.

Usually, a cross-table lateral view of the C-spine is obtained first to avoid unduly moving the patient who might have a cervical fracture. If the lateral C-spine appears normal, the remainder of the C-spine series, including flexion and extension views (if the patient can cooperate), may be obtained, though in many trauma centers a noncontrast CT scan of the cervical spine with sagittal and coronal reformations is performed, either in addition to or instead of cervical spine radiographs. What does one look for on the lateral C-spine? First, make certain that all seven cervical vertebral bodies can be visualized. A large number of fractures are missed because the shoulders obscure the lower C-spine levels (Fig. 57.1). If the entire cervical spine is not visualized, repeat the radiograph with the shoulders lowered.

Next, evaluate five parallel (more or less) lines for step-offs or discontinuity as follows (Fig. 57.2):

Line 1 is the prevertebral soft tissue and extends down the posterior aspect of the airway; it should be several millimeters from the first three or four vertebral bodies and then moves farther away at the laryngeal cartilage. It should be less than one vertebral body width from the anterior vertebral bodies from C3 or C4 to C7, and it should be smooth in its contour.

Line 2 follows the anterior vertebral bodies and should be smooth and uninterrupted. Anterior osteophytes can encroach on this line and extend beyond it and should therefore be ignored in drawing this line. Interruption of the anterior vertebral body line is a sign of a serious injury (Fig. 57.1B).

Line 3 is similar to the anterior vertebral body line (line 2) except that it connects the posterior vertebral bodies. Like line 2, it should be smooth and uninterrupted, and any disruption signifies a serious injury.

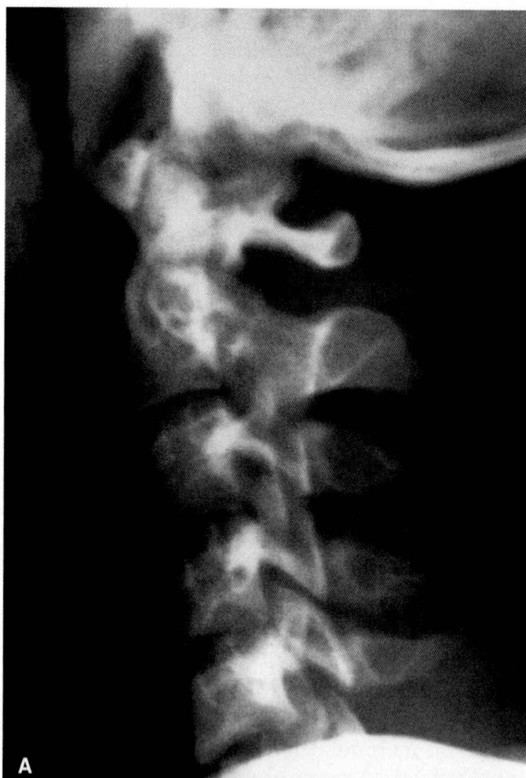

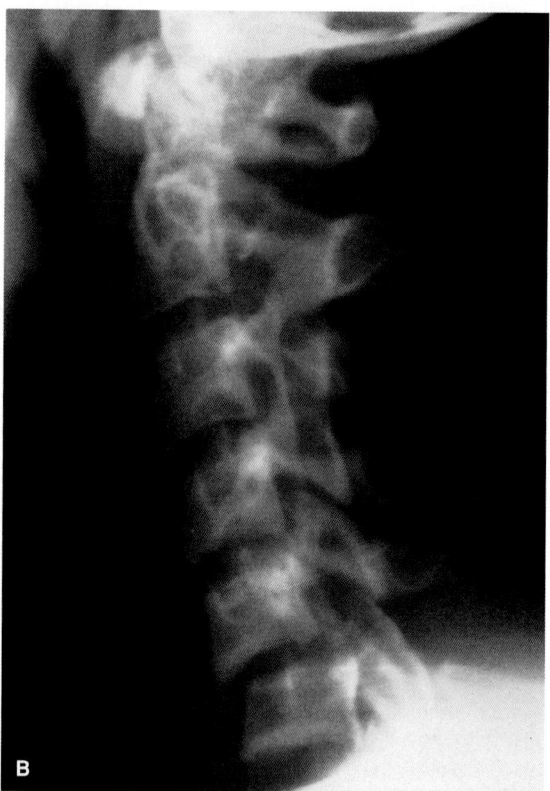

FIGURE 57.1. **Shoulders Obscuring C5–C6 Dislocation.** This patient presented to the emergency department after an injury suffered while diving into a shallow swimming pool. He had neck pain but no neurologic deficits. **A:** The initial radiograph of the C-spine obtained was interpreted as within normal limits. Only five cervical vertebrae are visible, however, because of high-riding shoulders. **B:** A repeat examination with the shoulders lowered reveals a dislocation of C5 on C6. To visualize C7, the shoulders were lowered even further. The C7 vertebral body must be visualized on every lateral C-spine examination in a trauma setting.

Line 4 connects the posterior junction of the lamina with the spinous processes and is called the spinolaminar line. The spinal cord lies between lines 3 and 4; therefore, any offset of either of these lines could mean a bony structure is impinging the cord. It takes very little force against the cord to cause severe neurologic deficits, and any bony structure lying on the cord must be recognized as soon as possible.

Line 5 is not really a line so much as a collection of points—the points being the posterior tips of the spinous processes. The spinous processes themselves are quite variable in their size and appearance, although that of C7 is consistently the largest. A fracture of one of the spinous processes, by itself, is not a serious injury, but it occasionally heralds other, more serious injuries.

After visually inspecting these five lines on the lateral C-spine, then inspect the C1–C2 area a little more closely. Make certain that the anterior arch of C1 is no greater than 2.5 mm from the dens (Fig. 57.3). Any greater separation than this (except in children, for whom up to 5 mm can be normal) is suspicious for disruption of the transverse ligament between C1 and C2 (Fig. 57.4).

The disc spaces are examined next to see that there is no inordinate widening or narrowing, either of which could indicate an acute traumatic injury. If a disc space is narrowed, it will usually be secondary to degenerative disease but make certain that associated osteophytosis and sclerosis are present before diagnosing degenerative disease.

The examination of the lateral C-spine as described here can be done in less than 1 minute. If it is normal, then the remainder of the examination can be completed, including flexion and extension views. It is imperative that the patient initiate the flexion and extension without help from the technician or anyone else. A patient, if conscious and alert, will not injure himself or herself with voluntary flexion and extension and will have muscle guarding preventing motion if there is an injury present. Even gentle pressure to aid in flexion or extension can cause severe injury if a fracture or dislocation is present. A few examples of fractures, dislocations, and other abnormalities are illustrated in the following paragraphs.

Jefferson Fracture. A blow to the top of the head, such as when an object falls directly on the apex of the skull, can cause the lateral masses of C1 to slide apart, splitting the bony ring of C1. This is called a Jefferson fracture as shown in Figure 57.5. It nicely illustrates how a bony ring will not break in just one place but must break in several places. This is a rule that is seldom violated. All the vertebral rings, when fractured, must fracture in two or more places. The bony rings of the pelvis behave similarly.

CT is excellent at demonstrating the complete bony ring of C1 and shows the fractures as well as any associated soft tissue mass, much better than radiographs do. In diagnosing a Jefferson fracture on radiographs, the lateral masses of C1 must extend beyond the margins of the C2 body (Fig. 57.5A). Just seeing asymmetry of the spaces on either side of the dens is not enough to make the diagnosis, as this can be normally asymmetrical with positional rotation or with rotatory fixation of the atlantoaxial joint.

"Clay-Shoveler's" Fracture. A relatively innocuous injury is a fracture of the C6 or C7 spinous process called a "clay-shoveler's" fracture. Supposedly, workers shoveling sticky clay

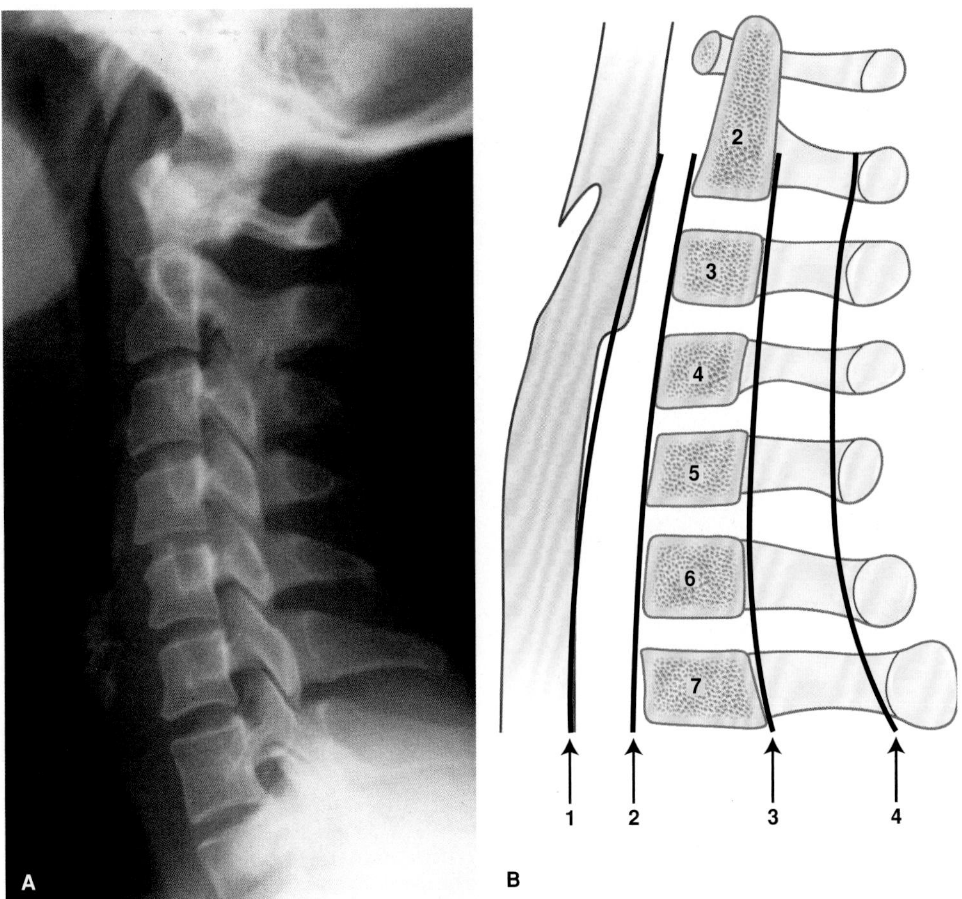

FIGURE 57.2. **Normal Lateral Cervical Spine. A:** Lateral radiograph of a normal cervical spine. **B:** Diagrammatic representation of a lateral C-spine showing four parallel lines that should be observed in every lateral C-spine examination. Line 1 is the soft tissue line that is closely applied to the posterior border of the airway through the first four or five vertebral body segments and then widens around the laryngeal cartilage and runs parallel to the remainder of the cervical vertebrae. Line 2 demarcates the anterior border of the cervical vertebral bodies. Line 3 is the posterior border of the cervical vertebral bodies. Line 4 is drawn by connecting the junction of the lamina at the spinous process, which is called the spinolaminar line. It represents the posterior extent of the central canal that contains the spinal cord itself. These lines should be generally smooth and parallel with no abrupt step-offs.

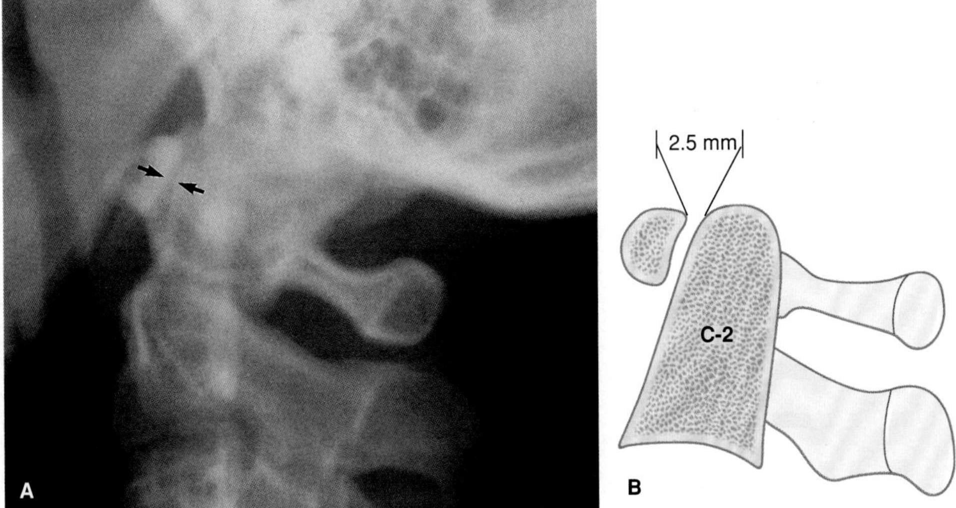

FIGURE 57.3. **Normal C1 and C2.** A lateral radiograph (**A**) and drawing (**B**) of the upper cervical spine showing the normal distance of the anterior arch of C1 less than 2.5 mm in distance from the odontoid process (dens) of C2 (*arrows*).

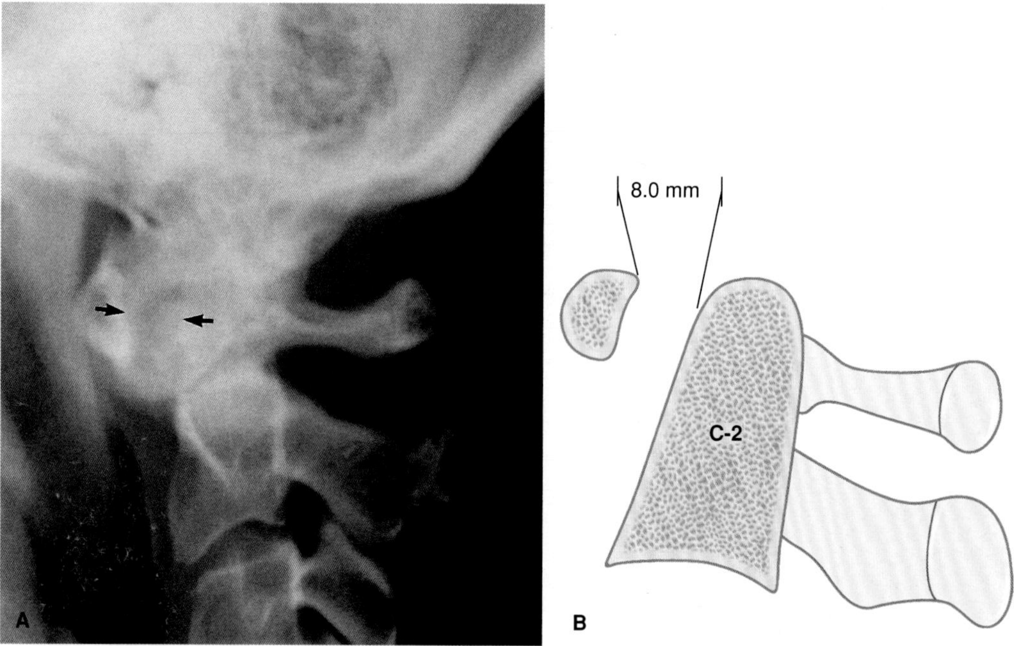

FIGURE 57.4. **C1–C2 Dislocation.** A lateral radiograph (**A**) and drawing (**B**) of the upper cervical spine in a patient who suffered trauma to the neck shows the anterior arch of C1 is 8 mm anterior to the odontoid process of C2 (*arrows*). This is diagnostic of a dislocation of C1 on C2 and indicates rupture of the transverse ligaments that normally hold these vertebral segments together.

would toss the shovel full of clay over their shoulders; once in a while, the clay would stick to the shovel, causing the ligaments attached to the spinous processes (supraspinous ligaments) to undergo a tremendous force pulling on the spinous process and avulsing it. This can occur at any of the lower cervical spinous processes (Fig. 57.6).

"Hangman's" Fracture. A "hangman's" fracture is an unstable, serious fracture of the upper cervical spine that is caused by hyperextension and distraction (such as hitting one's head on a dashboard). This is a fracture of the posterior elements of C2 and, usually, displacement of the C2 body anterior to C3 (Fig. 57.7). These patients actually do better than one might

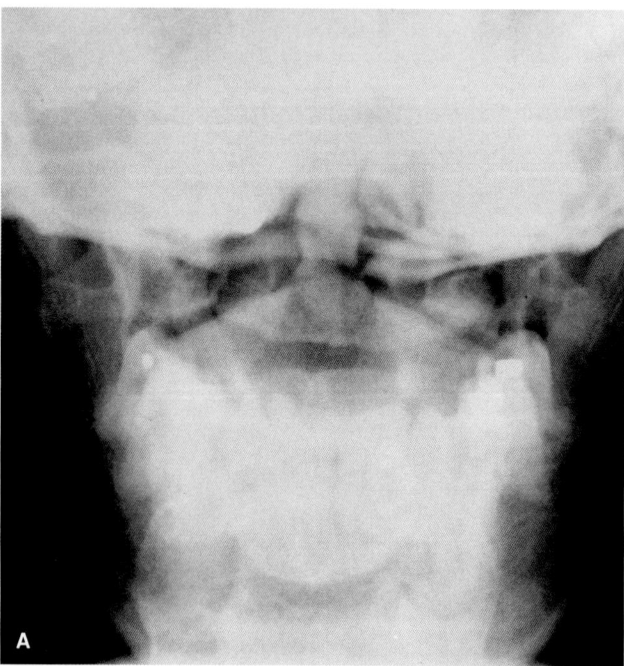

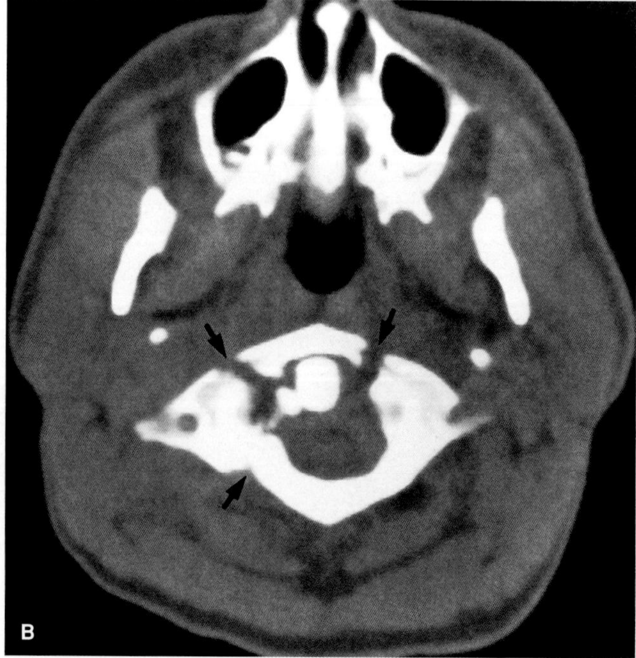

FIGURE 57.5. **Jefferson Fracture. A:** An AP open-mouth odontoid view is suspicious for the lateral masses of C1 being laterally displaced on the body of C2. Because of overlying structures, however, this is difficult to appreciate. **B:** A CT examination was obtained and shows multiple fracture sites in the C1 ring (*arrows*). This is called a Jefferson fracture. CT should be routinely used in spinal trauma because of frequent shortcomings of plain radiographs.

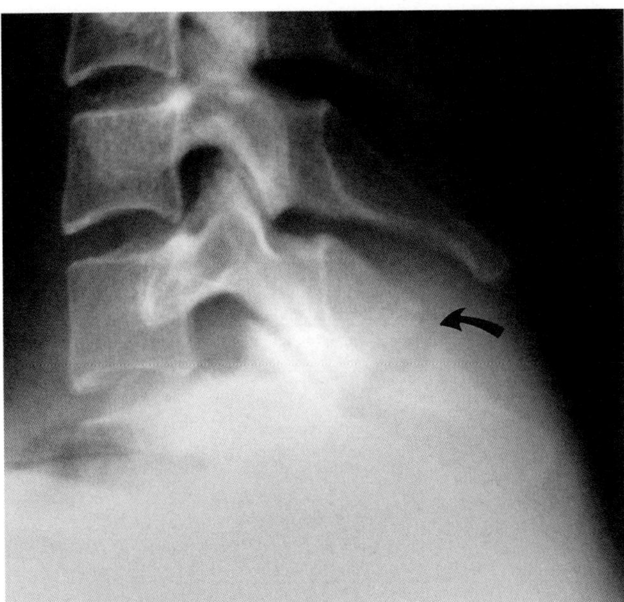

FIGURE 57.6. **Clay-Shoveler's Fracture.** A nondisplaced fracture of the C7 spinous process (*arrow*) is noted, which is diagnostic of a clay-shoveler's fracture.

think. They often escape neurologic impairment because of the fractured posterior elements of C2 that, in effect, causes a decompression and takes pressure off the injured area.

Flexion Teardrop Fracture. Severe flexion of the cervical spine can cause a disruption of the posterior ligaments with anterior compression of a vertebral body. This is called a flexion "teardrop" fracture (Fig. 57.8). A teardrop fracture is usually associated with spinal cord injury, often from the posterior portion of the vertebral body being displaced into the central canal.

Unilateral Locked Facets. Severe flexion associated with some rotation can result in rupture of the apophyseal joint ligaments and facet joint dislocation. This can result in locking of the facets in an overriding position that, in effect, causes some stabilization to protect against further injury. This is called unilateral locked facets (Fig. 57.9). It occasionally occurs bilaterally.

"Seatbelt Injury." "Seatbelt injury" is seen secondary to hyperflexion at the waist (as occurs in an automobile accident while restrained by a lap belt). This causes distraction of the posterior elements and ligaments and anterior compression of the vertebral body. It usually involves the T12, L1, or L2 level. Several variations of this injury can occur: a fracture of the posterior body is called a Smith fracture and a fracture through the spinous process is called a Chance fracture. Horizontal fractures of the pedicles, laminae, and transverse processes can also occur (Fig. 57.10).

Spondylolysis. A somewhat controversial spinal abnormality that may or may not be caused by trauma is spondylolysis. Spondylolysis is a break or defect in the pars interarticularis portion of the lamina (Fig. 57.11). On oblique views, the posterior elements form the figure of a "Scottie dog," with the transverse process being the nose, the pedicle forming the eye, the inferior articular facet being the front leg, the superior articular facet representing the ear, and the pars interarticularis (the portion of the lamina that lies between the facets) equivalent to the neck of the dog. If a spondylolysis is present, the pars interarticularis, or the neck of the dog, will have a defect or break. It often looks as if the Scottie dog has a collar around the neck.

The cause of a spondylolysis is controversial but thought to be congenital and/or posttraumatic. Many believe this is a stress-related injury from infancy that develops when toddlers

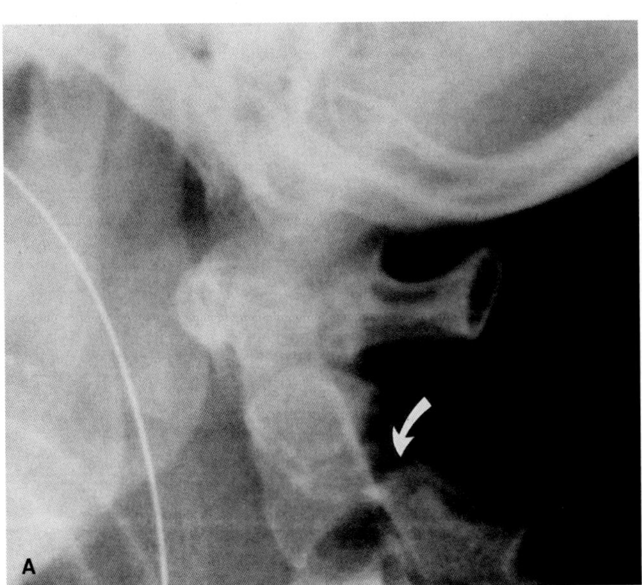

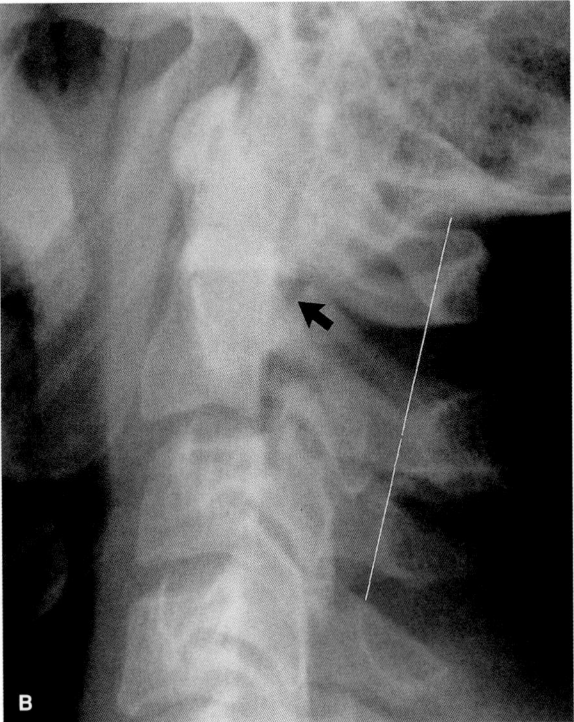

FIGURE 57.7. **Hangman's Fracture. A:** Lateral radiograph of a patient with a hangman's fracture shows an obvious example of the posterior elements of the CT vertebral body fractured and displaced inferiorly (*arrow*). **B:** This view shows a very subtle fracture through the posterior elements of C2 (*arrow*) in another patient. A line drawn through the spinolaminar lines of the posterior elements shows the C2 spinolaminar line to be offset posteriorly in this example.

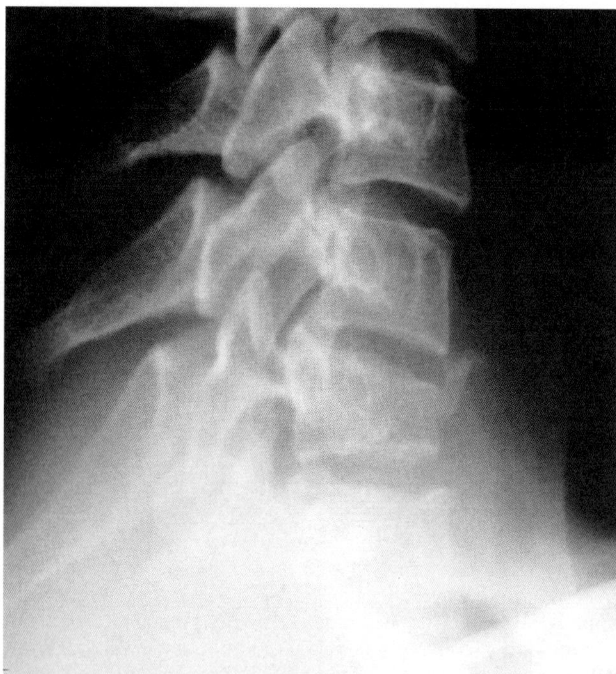

FIGURE 57.8. **Flexion Teardrop Fracture.** This patient suffered a hyperflexion injury in an automobile accident and presented to the emergency department with severe neurologic deficits. A lateral radiograph of the lower cervical spine shows wedging anteriorly of the C7 vertebral body with some displacement of the posterior vertebral line at C7 into the spinal canal. A small avulsion fracture off of the anterior body is also noted.

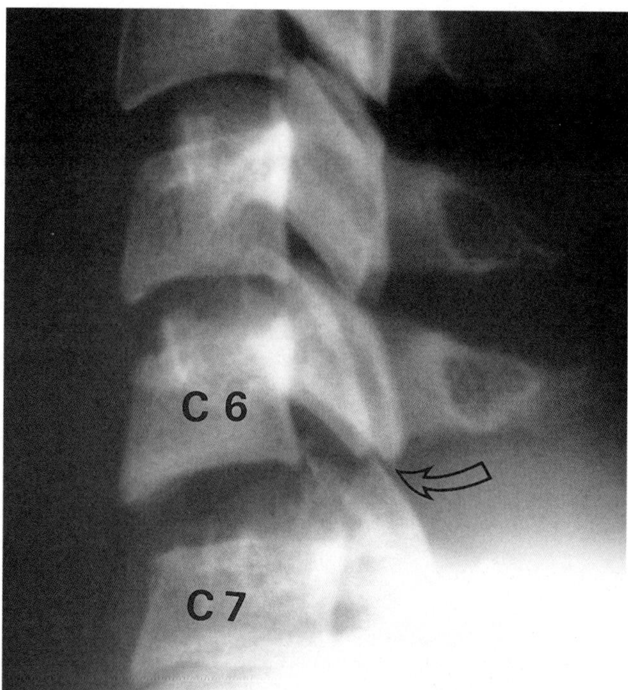

FIGURE 57.9. **Unilateral Locked Facets.** The C6–C7 disc space is abnormally widened, and the C7 vertebra is posteriorly located in relation to C6. Also note the C7 facets, which are dislocated and locked on the C6 facets (*arrow*). When the facets are perched in this manner, it is termed locked facets, which are unilateral in this example.

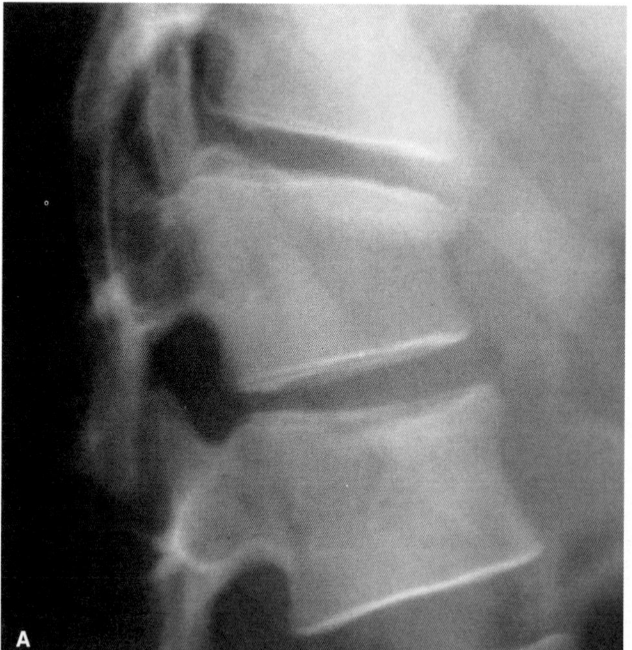

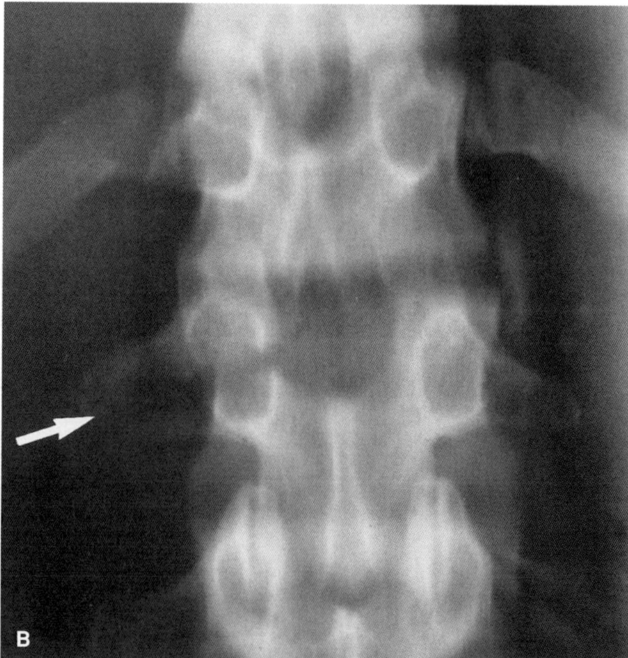

FIGURE 57.10. **Seatbelt Fracture.** Hyperflexion at the waist can cause anterior wedging of the vertebral body in the lower thoracic or upper lumbar region as shown in (**A**). By itself, although painful, it is somewhat innocuous; however, (**B**) shows a horizontal fracture through the right transverse process and pedicle (*arrow*) because of extreme traction during the flexion injury. When fracture of the posterior elements occurs, this injury is considered to be unstable and potentially debilitating. Any anterior wedging injury to a vertebral body should have the posterior elements of that level closely inspected.

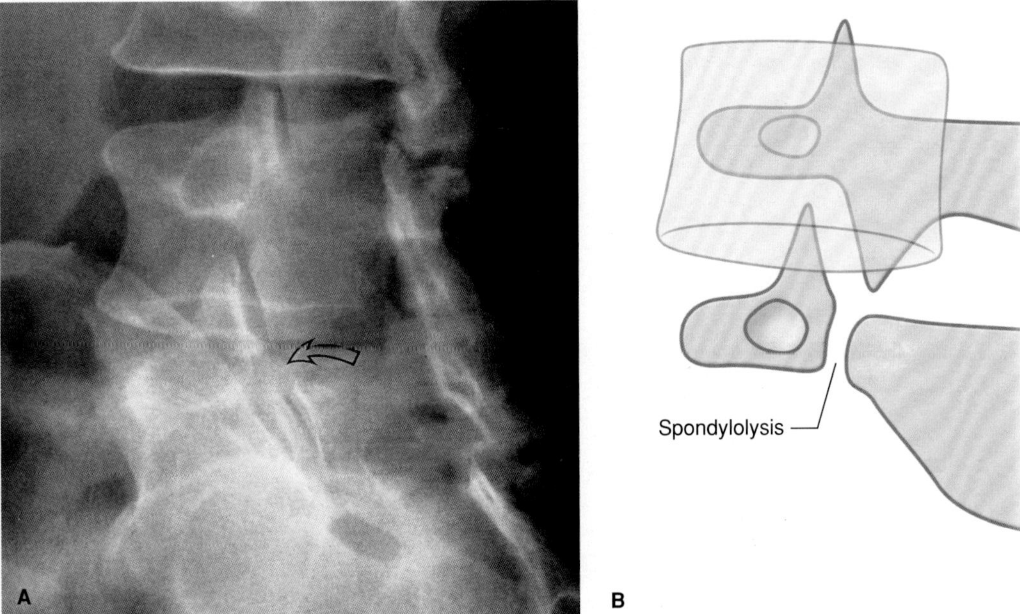

FIGURE 57.11. Spondylolysis. A: An oblique radiograph of the lumbar spine shows a defect in the neck of the "Scottie dog" at L5 (*arrow*), which is diagnostic of a spondylolysis. **B:** A drawing of an oblique view of the lumbar spine shows how a spondylolysis appears as a "collar" around the Scottie dog's neck.

try to walk and repeatedly fall on their buttocks, sending stress to their lower lumbar spine. The significance of spondylolysis is just as controversial as its etiology. More and more clinicians are coming to the viewpoint that a spondylolysis is an incidental finding with no clinical significance in most cases. It has been reported in up to 10% of the asymptomatic population. Certainly, some patients have pain related to a spondylolysis and get relief after rest or immobilization and some with surgical stabilization. It is important to identify spondylolysis preoperatively in patients undergoing lumbar discectomy, so

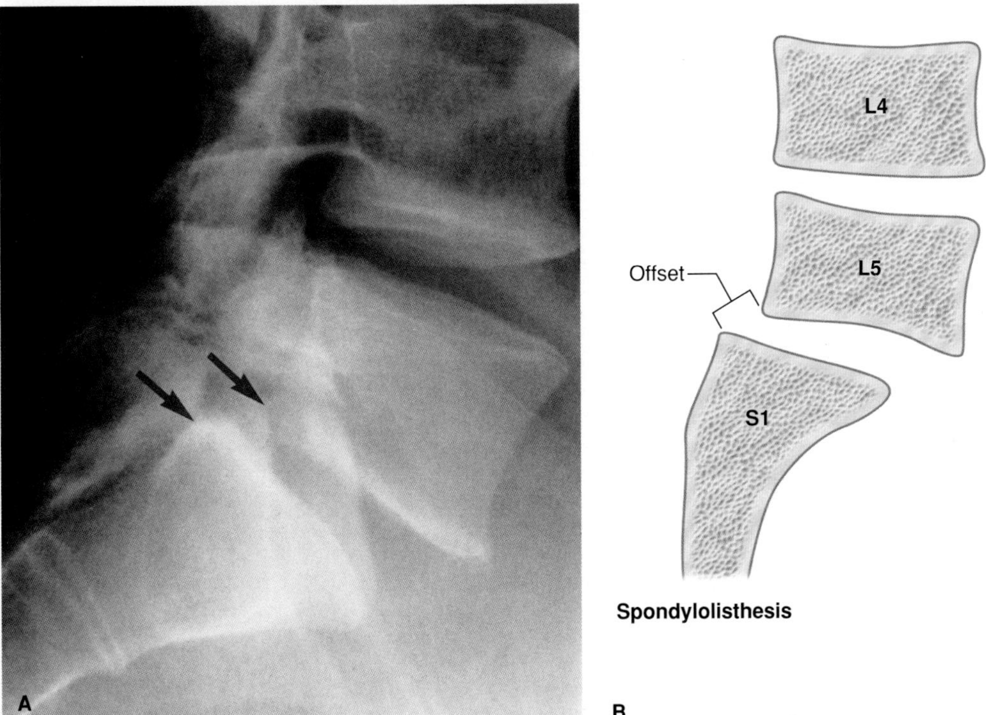

FIGURE 57.12. Spondylolisthesis. A: A lateral radiograph of the lumbar spine shows that the L5 vertebral body is slightly anteriorly offset on the S1 body as noted by the posterior margins (*arrows*). **B:** The drawing illustrates this more clearly. Because this offset is less than 25% as measured by the length of the S1 endplate, it is termed a grade 1 spondylolisthesis. A grade 2 offset is more than 25% but less than 50% of the length of the S1 endplate.

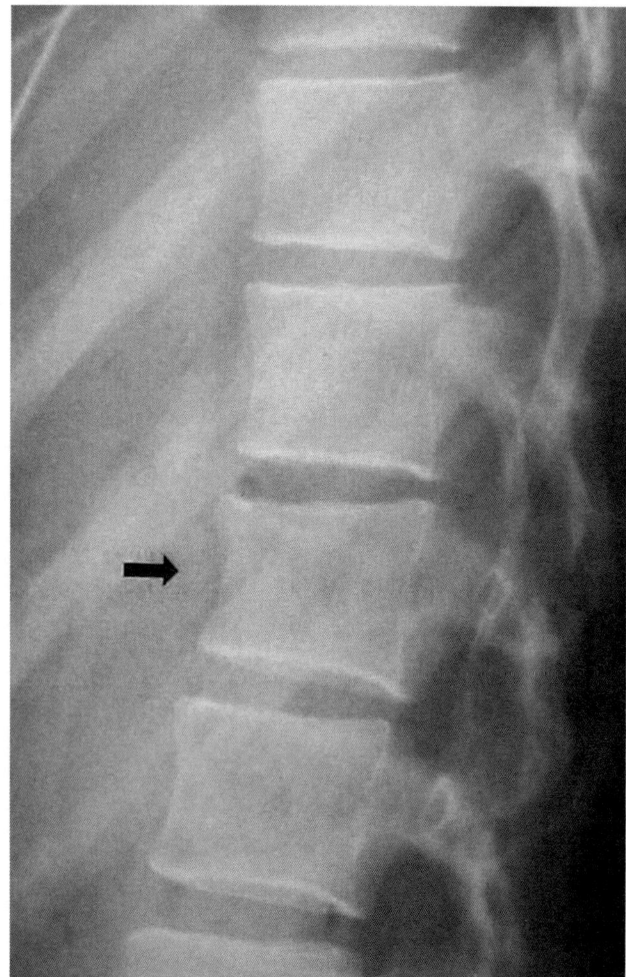

FIGURE 57.13. **Anterior Wedge Compression Fracture.** Anterior compression of this lower T spine vertebral body (*arrow*) is present, which may or may not be acute. If the patient has pain in this area, it is most likely acute and must be protected with a back brace until the symptoms abate.

that the possibility of clinical symptoms from the spondylolysis that can mimic disc symptoms can be evaluated. Although radiographs can usually show spondylolysis, CT will show it to better advantage as well as demonstrate any associated disc disease. MR will also show spondylolysis, but it can be difficult to see and is easily overlooked.

If spondylolysis is bilateral and the vertebral body in the more cephalad position slips forward on the more caudal body, spondylolisthesis is said to be present (Fig. 57.12). Spondylolisthesis may or may not be symptomatic. If severe, it can cause neuroforaminal stenosis and can impinge on the nerve roots in the spinal canal. If it is symptomatic, it can be stabilized surgically.

Anterior wedge-type compression fractures of the spine are commonly seen (Fig. 57.13), especially at the thoracolumbar junction, due to an old injury; they are passed off by the radiologist, if they are mentioned at all, as incidental findings. The problem with this is you cannot tell from a radiograph if the fracture is old or new, even if degenerative changes are present (which are often not related to the fracture). If acute and left unprotected, a wedge compression fracture can proceed to delayed further collapse with resulting severe neurologic deficits (Fig. 57.14). This is called Kummell disease and typically occurs 1 to 2 weeks after the initial trauma. Multiple

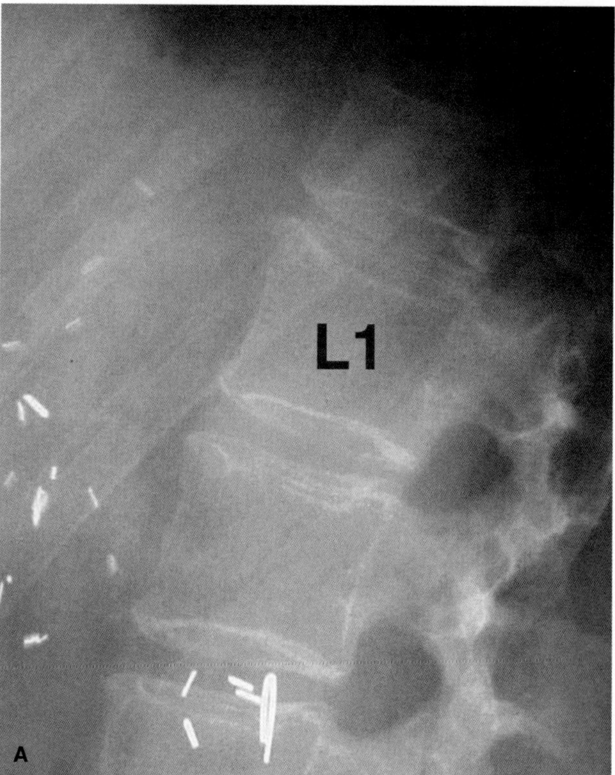

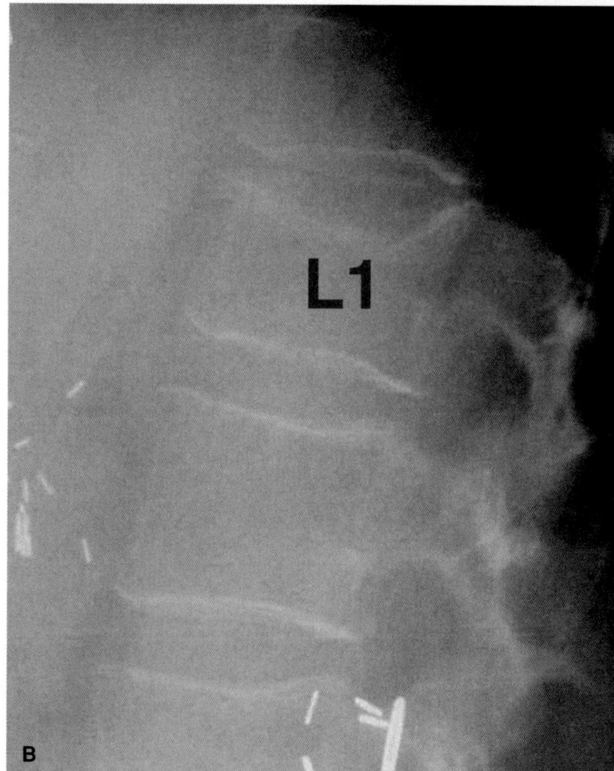

FIGURE 57.14. **Kummel Disease. A:** Very minimal anterior wedging of the L1 vertebral body is noted by comparing the height of the anterior body versus the posterior height. This patient had been in an auto accident and complained of back pain. No treatment for his back was given. **B:** After several weeks of continuing pain, he presents with leg weakness, which proceeded to paraplegia. A spine radiograph now shows progression of the vertebral body collapse of L1. This almost certainly could have been avoided with simple bracing of the spine after the initial injury.

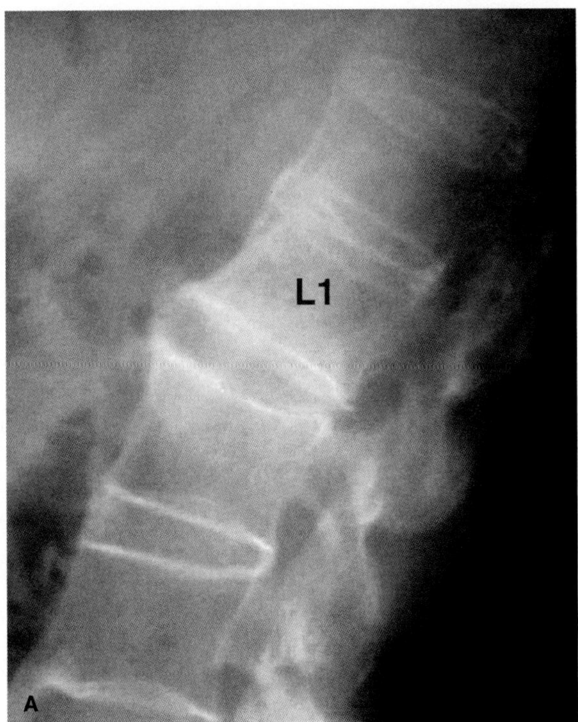

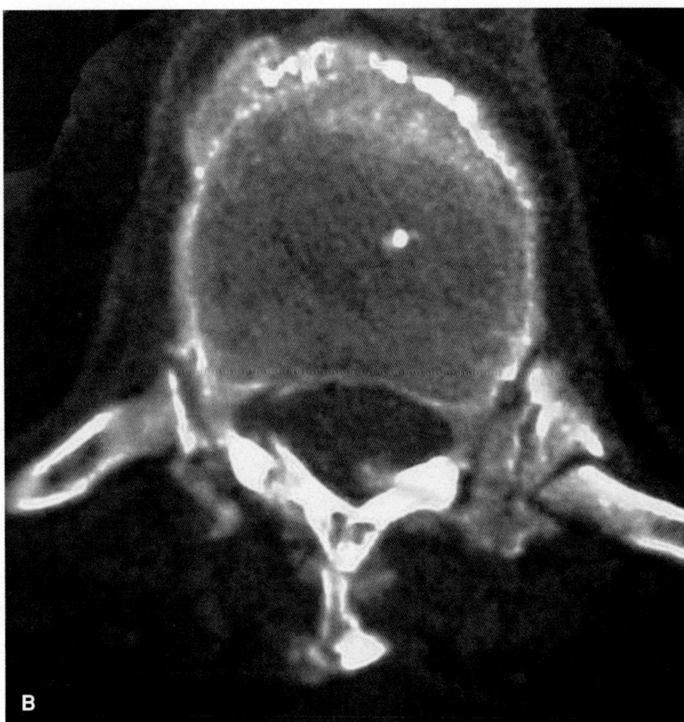

FIGURE 57.15. **Spine Fracture in Ankylosing Spondylitis. A:** A lateral radiograph following trauma shows fusion of the spine anteriorly, which was secondary to ankylosing spondylitis. Minimal anterior wedging of the L1 vertebral body is present, which was overlooked. **B:** Two weeks later, a CT of the spine was performed because of the sudden onset of paralysis. This axial image through L1 shows a fracture of the posterior elements, which was undoubtedly present on the initial visit to the emergency room. Patients with ankylosing spondylitis need to be examined closely for any back pain following trauma and imaged with CT or MRI if any pain is present.

lawsuits have been filed against radiologists who failed to mention minor anterior wedging of a vertebral body, which went on to further collapse with associated paraplegia. All that needs to be mentioned is that a fracture is present, which is of indeterminate age and requires clinical correlation. If the patient has pain in that location, a back brace needs to be worn until they are pain free. Old imaging studies, if available, can help determine if it is an old fracture. If no pain is present on physical exam, it can be safely assumed to be an old fracture. It is not necessary to obtain a CT or MRI even if pain is present because the treatment will be the same regardless of what the CT or MRI reveal. No spine surgeon will operate on a stable spine fracture without kyphosis or neurologic deficits, so the CT or MRI adds nothing but time and expense.

Patients who have fusion of their spine from ankylosing spondylitis and, to a lesser extent, from diffuse idiopathic skeletal hyperostosis (DISH) are at a very high risk of spinal fractures from even relatively minor trauma. Patients with ankylosing spondylitis typically have marked osteoporosis that further magnifies their risk of fracture. A fused spine is more likely to fracture than a normal spine in a manner similar to a long glass pipette breaking more easily than a short one because it has a long lever arm. A small force at one end is greatly magnified further down the lever arm. For that reason, a patient with ankylosing spondylitis should be treated as though a spinal fracture is present if they have back pain following trauma. CT and/or MRI are mandatory if radiographs are negative (Fig. 57.15).

HAND AND WRIST

Several seemingly innocuous fractures in the hand require surgical fixation rather than just casting and, therefore, should be recognized by the radiologist as serious injuries.

Bennett Fracture. One such fracture is a fracture at the base of the thumb into the carpometacarpal joint, a Bennett fracture (Fig. 57.16). Because of the insertion of the strong thumb adductors at the base of the thumb, it is almost impossible to keep the metacarpal from sliding off its proper alignment. It almost always requires internal fixation. The radiologist occasionally has to remind a nonorthopedic practitioner of this, as well as closely examine the alignment of a Bennett fracture in plaster that has not been internally fixed with wires.

A comminuted fracture of the base of the thumb that extends into the joint has been termed a Rolando fracture (Fig. 57.17), and a fracture of the base of the thumb that does not involve the joint has been called a pseudo-Bennett fracture.

Mallet finger or baseball finger is an avulsion injury at the base of the distal phalanx (Fig. 57.18) where the extensor digitorum tendon inserts. With the extensor tendon inoperative, the distal phalanx flexes without opposition, which can result in a flexion deformity and inability to extend the distal phalanx if not properly treated.

A fracture at the volar aspect of the base of the interphalangeal and metacarpophalangeal joints from an avulsion of the volar plate can appear innocent but often requires surgical intervention. The volar plate is a dense fibrocartilaginous band that covers the joint on the volar aspect and can get interposed in the joint once it is torn, often requiring surgical removal.

"Gamekeeper's Thumb." Another innocent-appearing fracture that often requires internal fixation is an avulsion on the ulnar aspect of the first metacarpophalangeal joint (Fig. 57.19); this is where the ulnar collateral ligament of the thumb inserts. If the ulnar collateral ligament is torn, normal function of the thumb can be impaired, and this can have a serious result if not properly treated. While the avulsion can be purely ligamentous, if a small piece of bone is avulsed with the ligament, the injury

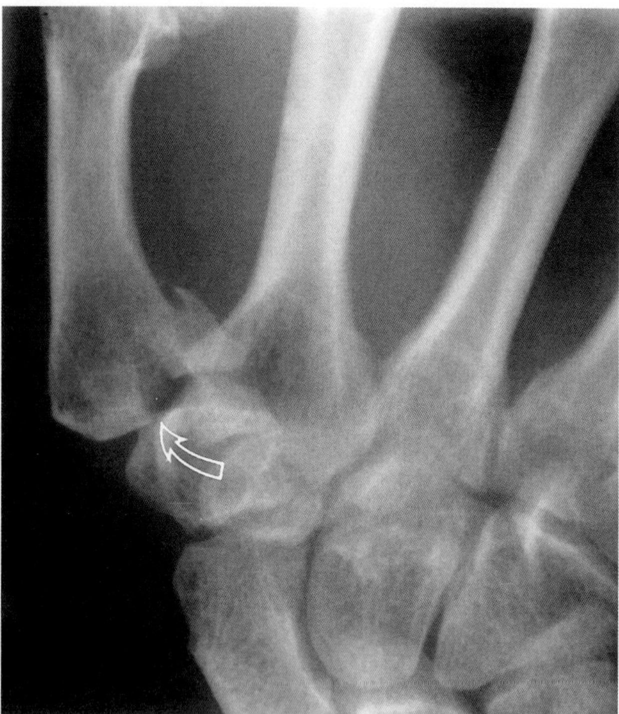

FIGURE 57.16. **Bennett Fracture.** A small corner fracture of the base of the thumb is noted, which involves the articular surface of the base of the thumb (*arrow*); this is a serious injury that almost always requires internal fixation.

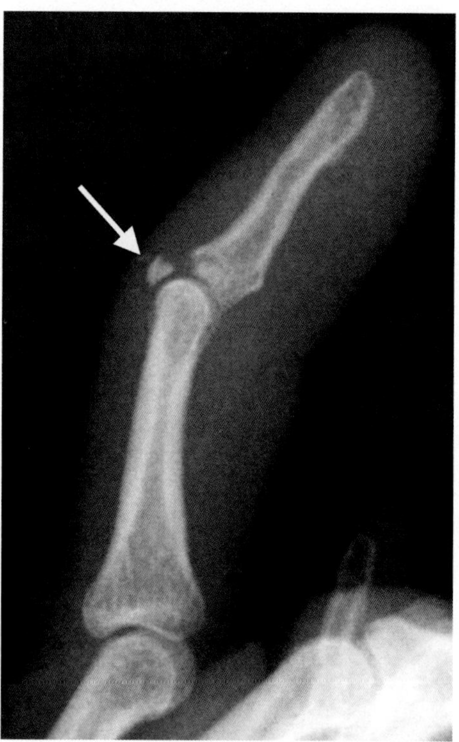

FIGURE 57.18. **Mallet Finger.** A small avulsion injury is noted at the dorsal aspect of the base of the distal phalanx (*arrow*), which is where the extensor digitorum tendon inserts. This is termed a mallet finger or baseball finger because it is often caused by a baseball striking the distal phalanx and causing the avulsion.

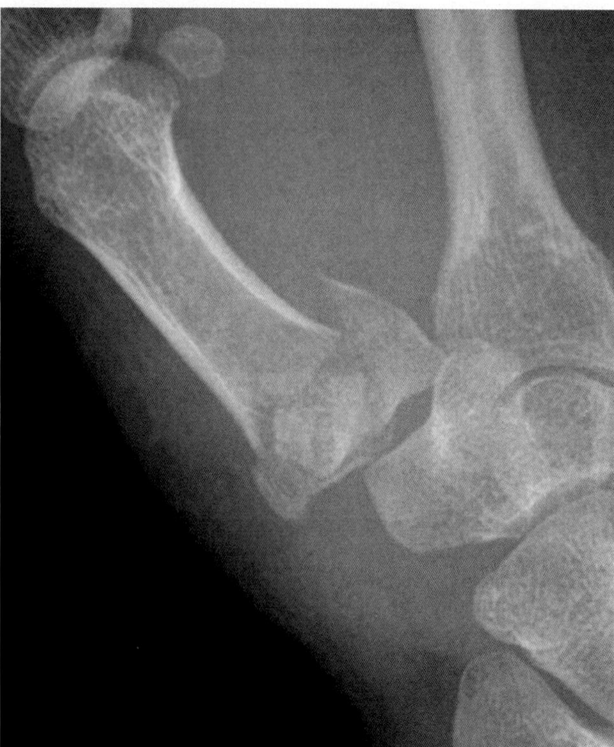

FIGURE 57.17. **Rolando Fracture.** A comminuted fracture of the base of the thumb that extends into the articular surface is a more serious type of Bennett fracture, which has been termed a Rolando fracture.

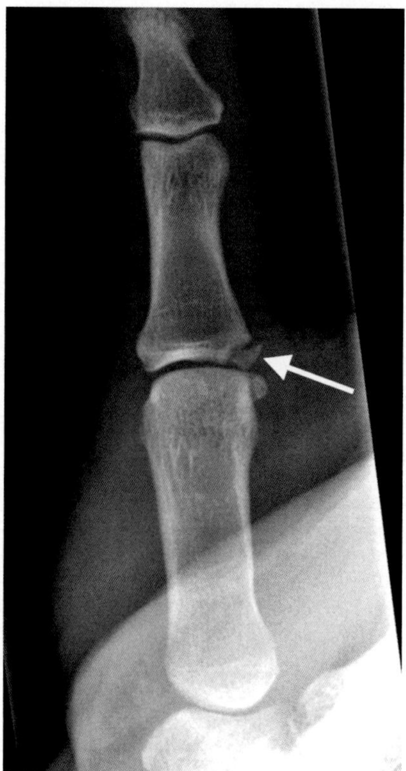

FIGURE 57.19. **Gamekeeper's Thumb.** A small avulsion injury on the ulnar aspect of the first metacarpophalangeal joint (*arrow*) is diagnostic of a gamekeeper's thumb. This is the insertion site for the ulnar collateral ligament and usually requires internal fixation.

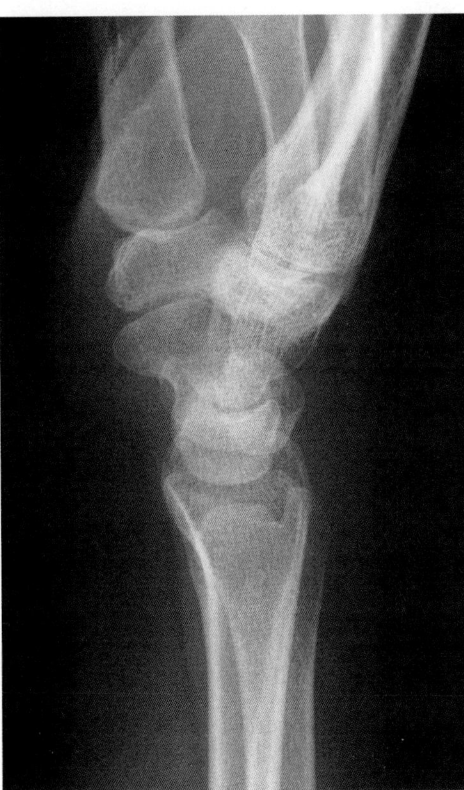

FIGURE 57.20. **Normal Lateral Radiograph of the Wrist.** The normal lateral view should show the lunate seated in the distal radius and the capitate seated in the lunate. A line drawn up through the radius should connect all three structures. Compare this radiograph with the drawing in Figure 57.21A.

can be seen on radiographs. This injury is called a "gamekeeper's thumb" because of the propensity of English game wardens to acquire it from breaking rabbits' necks between their thumb and forefinger. A more current scenario is falling on a ski pole and having the pole jam into the webbing between the thumb and the index finger. This avulsion injury usually requires pinning to fix the ligament securely.

Lunate/Perilunate Dislocation. A fall on an outstretched arm can result in any number of wrist fractures and dislocations. One such serious injury is the lunate/perilunate dislocation. This occurs when the ligaments between the capitate and the lunate are disrupted, allowing the capitate to dislocate from the cup-shaped articulation of the lunate. This is best seen on lateral views. Ordinarily, on the lateral view, the capitate should be seen seated in the cup-shaped lunate (Figs. 57.20 and 57.21A). In a dorsal dislocation (the capitate occasionally dislocates volarly, but this is uncommon), the capitate and all of its surrounding bones, including the metacarpals, come to lie dorsal to a line drawn through the radius and the lunate (Figs. 57.21B and 57.22). If the capitate then pushes the lunate volarly and tips it over, the line drawn up through the radius shows the lunate volarly displaced and the line goes through the capitate. This has been termed a lunate dislocation (Figs. 57.21C and 57.22). Failure to diagnose and treat this disorder can result in permanent median nerve impairment, as it can get impinged by the volarly displaced lunate.

A lunate or perilunate dislocation can be diagnosed on an anteroposterior (AP) view of the wrist by noting a triangular or pie-shaped lunate (Fig. 57.23B). Ordinarily, the lunate has a rhomboid shape on the AP view, with the upper and lower borders parallel.

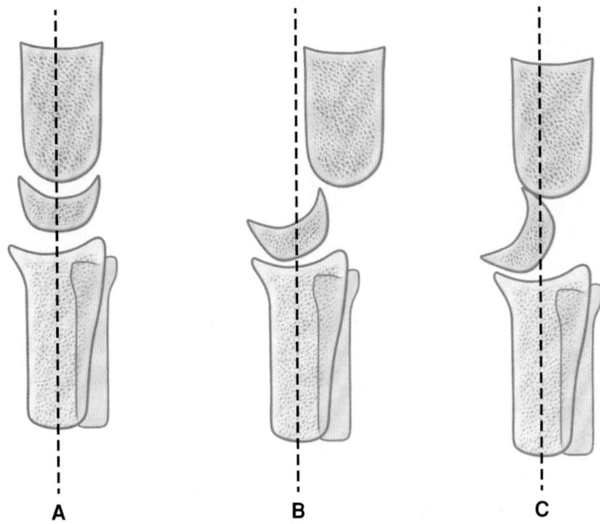

FIGURE 57.21. **Perilunate and Lunate Dislocations.** Schematic depiction of normal lateral wrist (**A**), perilunate dislocation (**B**), and lunate dislocation (**C**) (dorsal is to the right).

Several fractures are known to be associated with a perilunate dislocation, the most common of which is a transscaphoid fracture. The capitate, radial styloid, and triquetrum are also known to fracture frequently when a perilunate dislocation occurs.

Hook of the Hamate Fracture. One of the most difficult wrist fractures to identify radiologically is a fracture of the hook of the hamate. A special view, the carpal tunnel view,

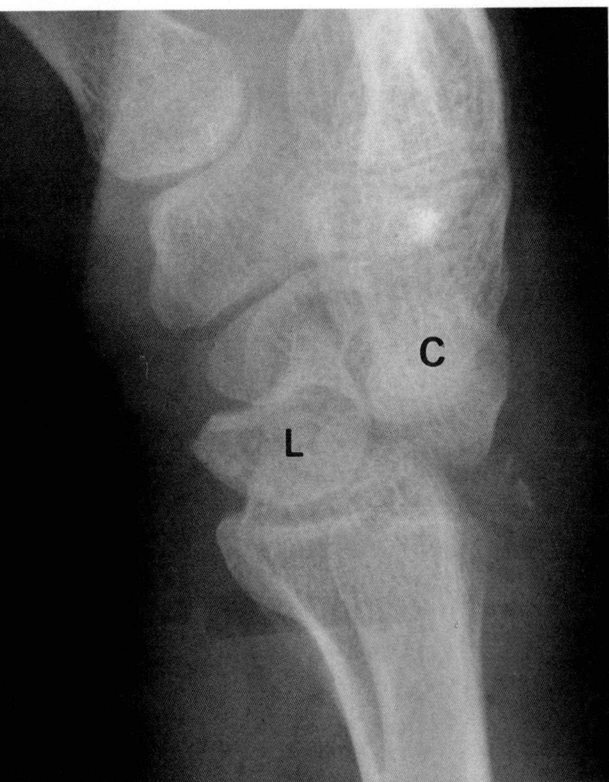

FIGURE 57.22. **Perilunate Dislocation.** Although the lunate (*L*) is normal in relation to the distal radius, the capitate (*C*) and the remainder of the wrist are dorsally displaced in relation to the lunate. Compare this radiograph with the drawing in Figure 57.21B.

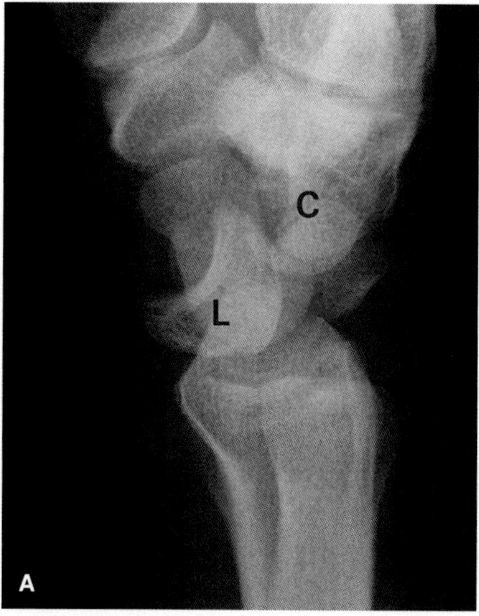

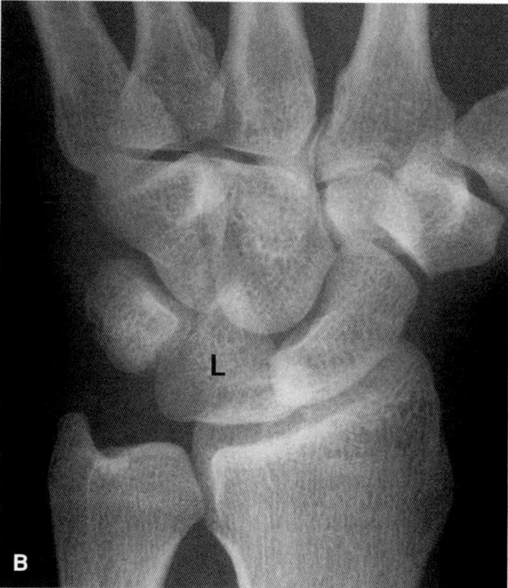

FIGURE 57.23. **Lunate Dislocation. A:** The lateral radiograph of the wrist shows the lunate (*L*) tipped off of the distal radius, whereas the capitate (C) seems to be normally aligned in relation to the radius, yet is dislocated from the lunate. Compare this with the drawing in Figure 57.21C. The anteroposterior (AP) view shows a pie-shaped lunate (**B**) (*L*) rather than a lunate with a more rhomboid shape. A pie-shaped lunate on the AP view is diagnostic of a perilunate or lunate dislocation.

should be obtained when trying to see the hook of the hamate. This view is obtained with the wrist (palm down) flat on the image detector plate and the fingers pulled dorsally. The x-ray beam is angled about 45 degrees parallel to the palm of the hand so that the carpal tunnel is in profile. The hook of the hamate is seen as a bony protuberance off the hamate on the ulnar aspect of the carpal tunnel. A fractured hook of the hamate is often identified with the carpal tunnel view (Fig. 57.24) but can occasionally be very difficult to visualize. A CT scan will often show an obvious fracture that the radiograph does not (Fig. 57.25) and should be considered in any possible carpal fracture when plain radiographs are not diagnostic.

A fracture of the hook of the hamate most commonly occurs from a fall on the outstretched hand. A clinical setting that has gained attention in sports medicine circles is that of a professional athlete who participates in an activity in which the butt of a club, bat, or racket is held in the palm of the hand. Overswinging can result in the butt of the club levering off the hook of the hamate. This has been seen in professional baseball players, tennis players, and golfers. It is not seen as often in amateurs because they usually are not strong enough to exert enough force to lever the hook off and, if they do, will usually terminate that activity, allowing healing, whereas a professional will continue participation, which can lead to a nonunion of the fracture.

Rotary subluxation of the scaphoid is another wrist injury seen after a fall onto the outstretched hand. This results from rupture of the scapholunate ligament, which allows the scaphoid to rotate volarly and the lunate to tilt dorsally. On an AP wrist radiograph, a space is seen between the scaphoid and the lunate (Fig. 57.26) where ordinarily they are closely opposed. This has been called the "Terry Thomas" sign after a famous British actor (circa 1950s) with a gap between his two front teeth.

Scaphoid Fracture. A fracture of the scaphoid is a potentially serious injury because of the high rate of avascular necrosis that occurs with this injury. When avascular necrosis occurs, it usually requires surgical intervention with a metallic screw

FIGURE 57.24. **Carpal Tunnel View of a Fractured Hamate.** A carpal tunnel view of the wrist in this patient shows a faint lucency surrounded by sclerosis in the left hamate (*arrow*), which represents a fracture through the base of the hook of the hamate with moderate reactive sclerosis.

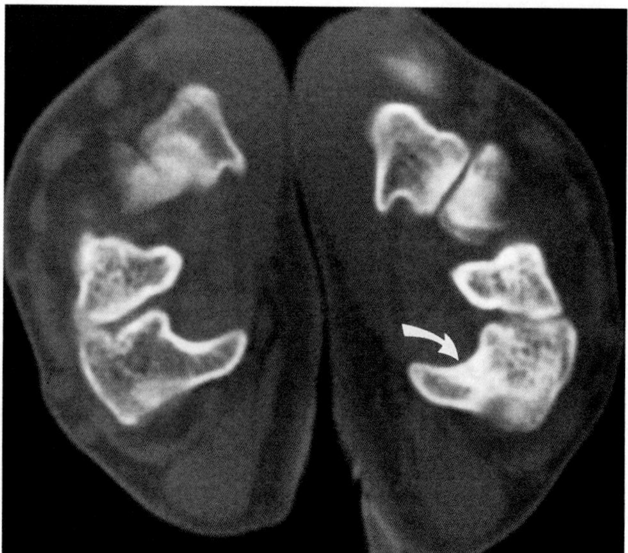

FIGURE 57.25. **CT of a Fractured Hook of the Hamate.** A CT scan through the wrist in this patient shows sclerosis in the left hook of the hamate (*arrow*), which represents a healing fracture. Compare this with the opposite hamate. This could not be seen on the radiographs, even in retrospect.

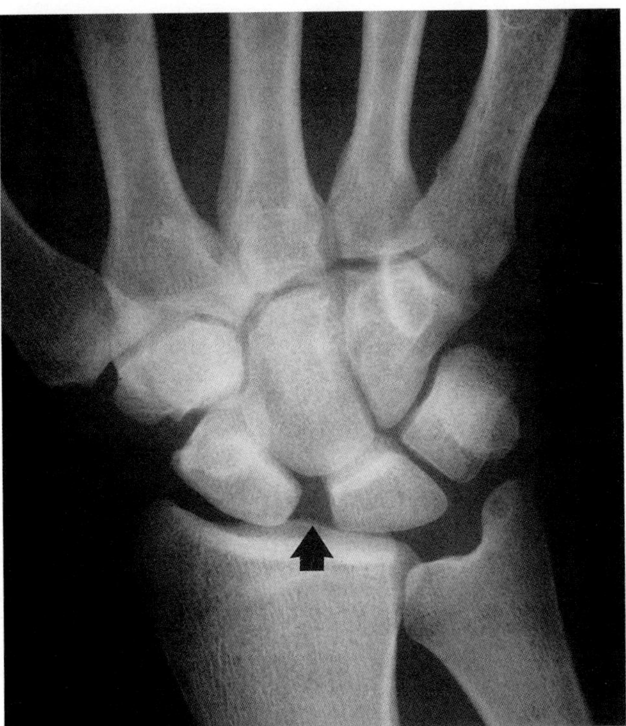

FIGURE 57.26. **Rotatory Subluxation of the Scaphoid.** An AP view of the wrist shows a gap or space between the scaphoid and the lunate (*arrow*). This is abnormal and represents the "Terry Thomas" sign, which means the scapholunate ligament is ruptured. This is diagnostic of a rotatory subluxation of the navicular.

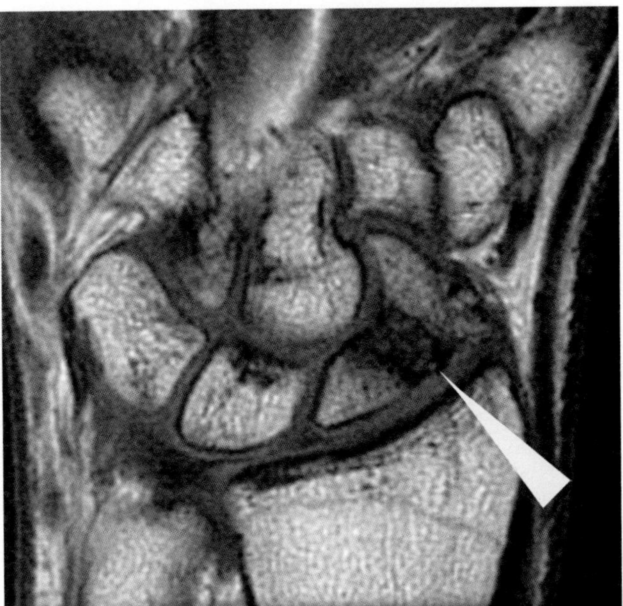

FIGURE 57.27. **Scaphoid Fracture.** A coronal T1-weighted image of the wrist in a patient with snuffbox tenderness and a normal radiograph shows a fracture of the mid-waist of the scaphoid (*arrowhead*).

and bone grafting to obtain healing. This fracture can be very difficult to detect initially; therefore, whenever a fracture of the scaphoid is clinically suspected (trauma with pain over the snuffbox of the wrist), the wrist should be casted and repeat radiographs obtained in 1 week. Often, the fracture is then visualized because of the disuse osteoporosis and hyperemia around the fracture site. Thus, in the acute setting, a negative radiograph does not exclude a fractured scaphoid. Instead of casting the wrist and repeating the radiographs in a week, many patients now get immediate MRI to determine if a fracture is present (Fig. 57.27). This has been shown to be less expensive overall than having the patient casted and reexamined in a week.

If avascular necrosis of the scaphoid develops, it is the proximal fragment that undergoes necrosis because the blood supply to the scaphoid begins distally and runs proximally. A fracture with disruption of the blood supply thus leaves the proximal pole without a vascular supply, and hence, it dies. Avascular necrosis is diagnosed by noting increased density of the proximal pole of the scaphoid compared with the remainder of the carpal bones (Fig. 57.28).

Avascular necrosis can occur in other carpal bones, most commonly the lunate. This is called Kienböck malacia and is most often caused by trauma; however, it is also thought to be idiopathic. It is diagnosed by noting the increased density in the lunate, which may or may not go on to collapse and fragmentation (Fig. 57.29). It often requires surgical bone grafting and occasionally removal or proximal carpal row fusion. It has a high association with a discrepancy between the length of the radius and the ulna as seen at the radiocarpal joint. If the ulna is shorter than the radius, it is termed negative ulnar variance and there is an increased incidence of Kienböck malacia (Fig. 57.29). If the ulna is longer than the radius, it is termed positive ulnar variance and there is an increased incidence of triangular fibrocartilage tears.

A common avulsion fracture in the wrist is a triquetral fracture. It is best seen on a lateral radiograph, which shows a small chip of bone off the dorsum of the wrist (Fig. 57.30). This is virtually pathognomonic of an avulsion from the triquetrum.

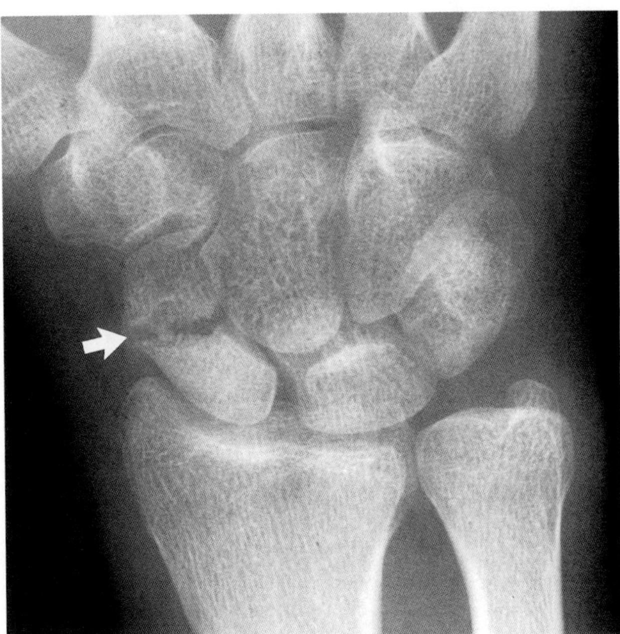

FIGURE 57.28. **Avascular Necrosis of the Scaphoid.** An AP view of the wrist shows a fracture through the waist of the scaphoid (*arrow*). The proximal half of the navicular is slightly sclerotic in relation to the remainder of the carpal bones, which indicates avascular necrosis of the proximal half.

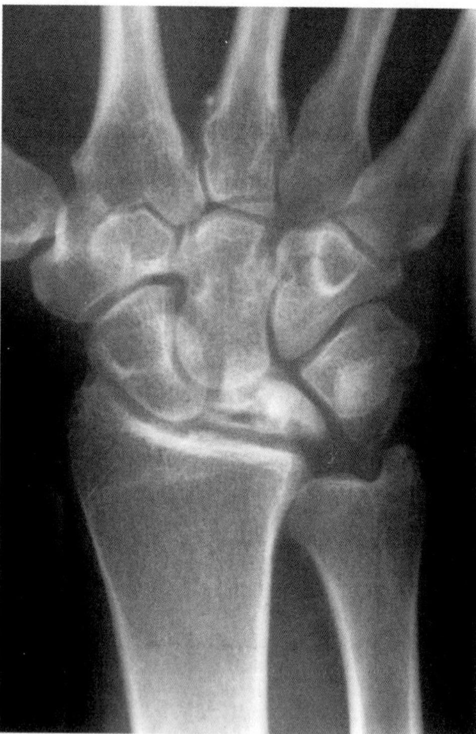

FIGURE 57.29. **Kienböck Malacia.** An AP view of the wrist reveals the lunate to be sclerotic and abnormal in shape. The lunate has collapsed because of aseptic necrosis. This is known as Kienböck malacia. Note that the ulna is shorter than the radius; this is termed negative ulnar variance, which is often associated with Kienböck malacia.

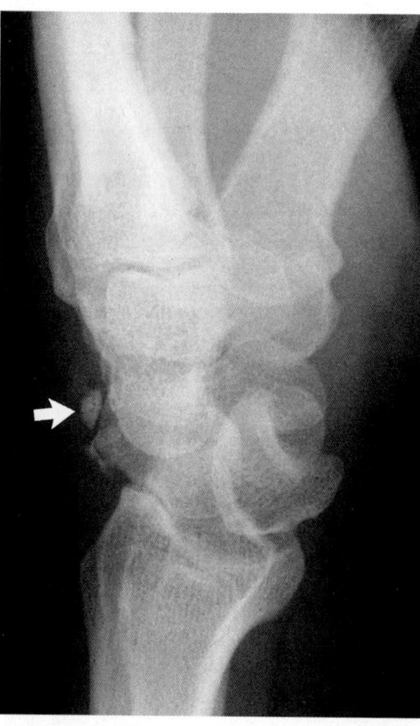

FIGURE 57.30. **Triquetral Fracture and Perilunate Dislocation.** A perilunate or lunate dislocation is present (it is difficult to classify exactly which has occurred because both the lunate and the capitate are out of their normal positions). A small avulsion fragment is seen on the dorsum of the wrist (*arrow*), which is virtually diagnostic of an avulsion off the triquetrum. It is often associated with a lunate or perilunate dislocation.

ARM

Colles Fracture. One of the most common fractures of the forearm is a fracture of the distal radius and ulna after a fall on an outstretched arm. This results in a dorsal angulation of the distal forearm and wrist and is called a Colles fracture (Fig. 57.31). When the fracture angulates volarly, it is called a Smith fracture (Fig. 57.32). A Smith fracture is a much less common occurrence than a Colles fracture. Sometimes, the radius and ulna suffer a traumatic insult, and the force on the bones causes bending instead of a frank fracture. This has been termed a plastic bowing deformity of the forearm (Fig. 57.33) and is often treated by breaking the bones with the patient under anesthesia and resetting them. Left untreated, a plastic bowing deformity can result in reduced supination and pronation.

Monteggia Fracture. The forearm is a two-bone system that has some of the same properties as a ringbone. As mentioned previously, a solid ring cannot break in only a single place; it must break in at least two points. In the forearm, a fracture of one bone should be accompanied by a fracture of the other. If the second fracture is not present, a dislocation of the nonfractured bone usually occurs. The most common example of this is a fracture of the ulna with a dislocation of the proximal radius (Fig. 57.34). This is called a Monteggia fracture. The dislocated radial head can be missed clinically and develop into avascular necrosis with subsequent elbow dysfunction. Whenever the forearm is fractured, the elbow must be examined to exclude a dislocation.

Galeazzi Fracture. A fracture of the radius with dislocation of the distal ulna is called a Galeazzi fracture (Fig. 57.35). This is less common than a Monteggia fracture.

Elbow Fractures. A helpful indicator of a fracture about the elbow is a displaced posterior fat pad. Ordinarily, the posterior fat pad is not visible on a lateral view of the elbow because it is tucked away in the olecranon fossa of the distal humerus.

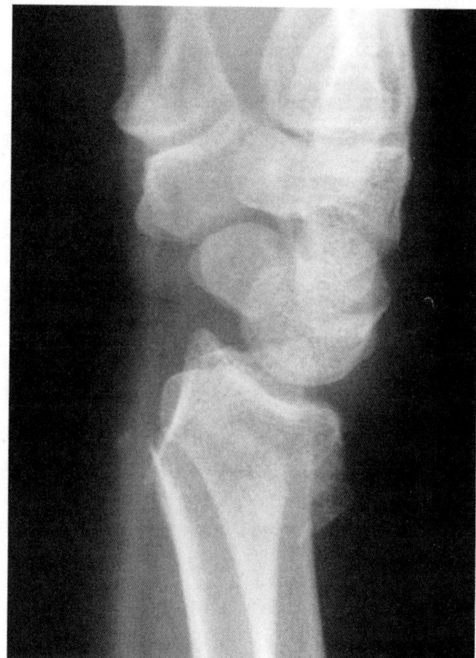

FIGURE 57.31. **Colles Fracture.** A fracture of the distal radius with dorsal angulation is noted, which has been termed a Colles fracture.

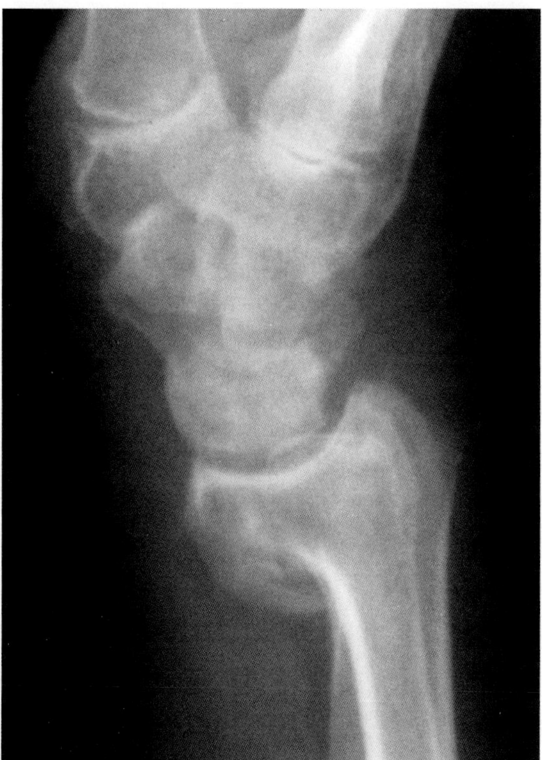

FIGURE 57.32. **Smith Fracture.** A fracture of the distal radius with volar angulation such as this is called a Smith fracture. This is a much less common injury than the Colles fracture, shown in Figure 57.31.

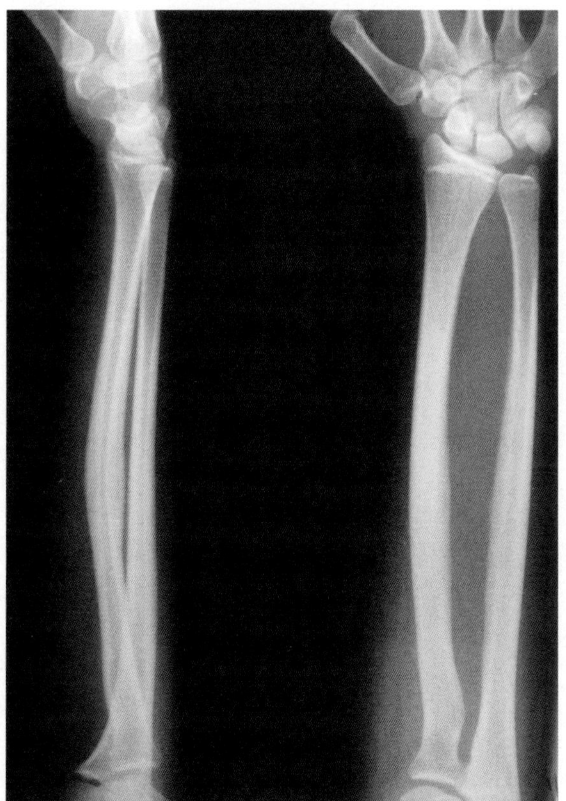

FIGURE 57.33. **Plastic Bowing Deformity of the Forearm.** These AP and lateral views of the forearm of a child show the radius to be abnormally bowed anteriorly. This has been termed a plastic bowing deformity of the forearm and occurs only in children.

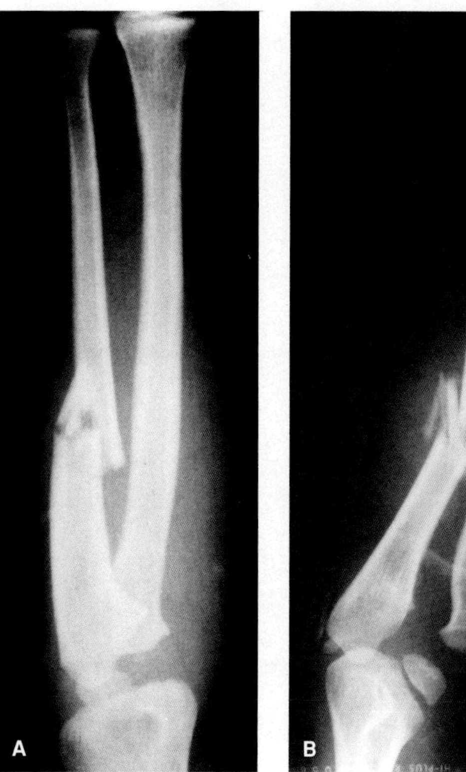

FIGURE 57.34. **Monteggia Fracture.** A blow to the forearm such as with a policeperson's nightstick can result in a fracture of the ulna (**A**). Although the head of the radius appears normally placed in (**A**), the lateral examination shown in (**B**) reveals the head of the radius to be dislocated. Failure to recognize this abnormality can result in death of the radial head, with subsequent elbow dysfunction. This illustrates the importance of always obtaining two views of a bone after trauma.

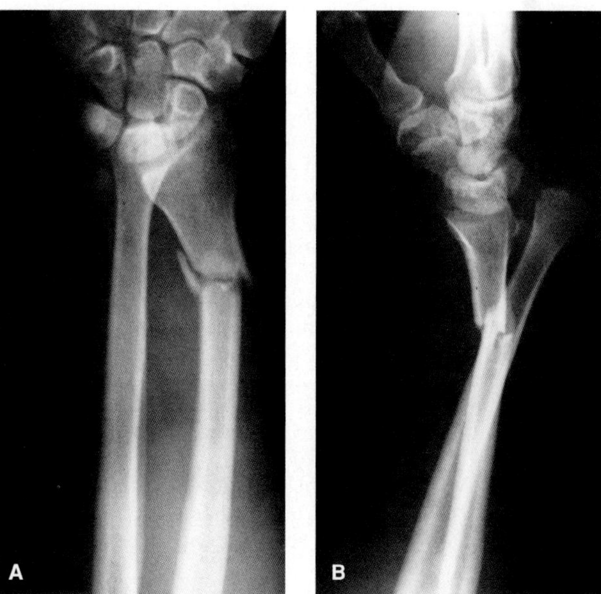

FIGURE 57.35. **Galeazzi Fracture. A:** A fracture of the distal radius in this patient is seen on the AP view without a definite fracture of the ulna. **B:** This view shows an obvious dislocation of the distal ulna, which would almost certainly not be missed clinically. This has been termed a Galeazzi fracture and is much less common than the Monteggia fracture.

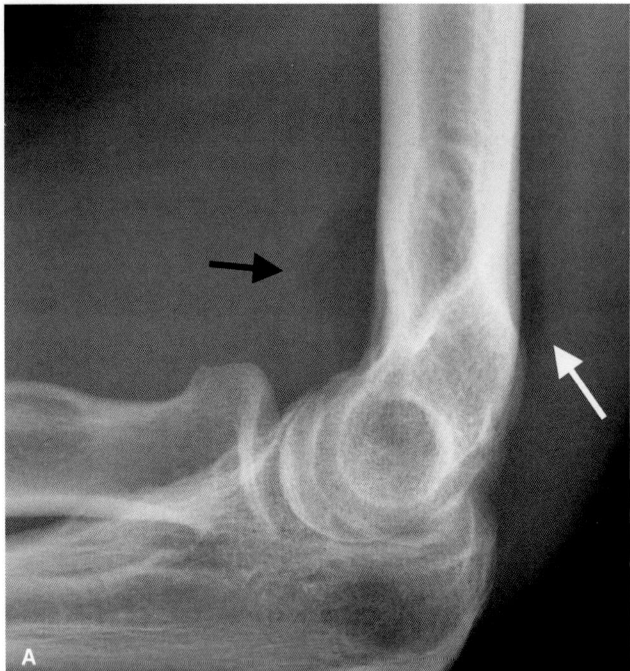

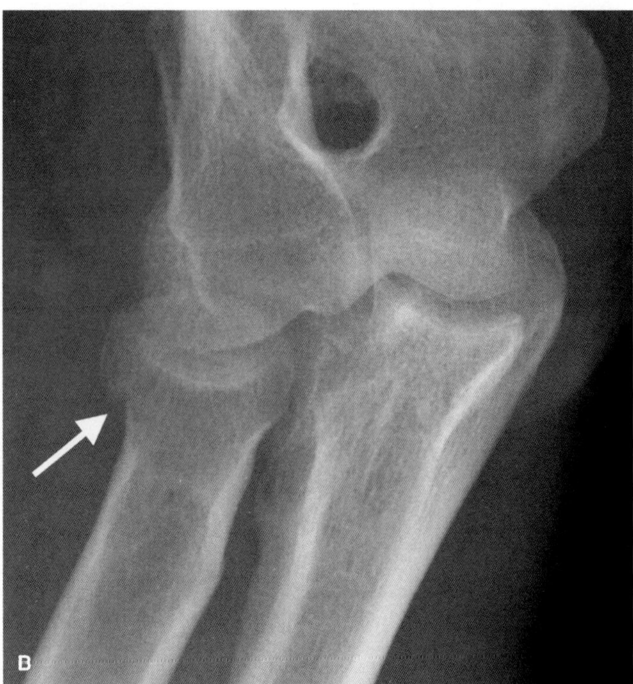

FIGURE 57.36. **Displaced Elbow Fat Pads.** **A:** On the lateral view of this elbow, the posterior fat pad is faintly visible (*white arrow*) and the anterior fat pad is elevated and anteriorly displaced (*black arrow*), consistent with a joint effusion. These findings indicate a fracture about the elbow that in an adult should be in the radial head. **B:** An oblique view shows the fracture of the radial head (*arrow*). Even without seeing the fracture on the radiographs, it should be surmised to be present when the posterior fat pad is visualized in the setting of trauma. The elevated and displaced anterior fat pad has been termed a sail sign.

When the joint becomes distended with blood secondary to a fracture, the posterior fat pad is displaced out of the olecranon fossa and is visible on the lateral view (Fig. 57.36A). Therefore, in the setting of trauma, a visible posterior fat pad indicates a fracture. In an adult (physes closed), the fracture site is almost always the radial head (Fig. 57.36B). In a child (physes open), it is usually indicative of a supracondylar fracture (Fig. 57.37).

Often, the fracture itself is not visualized, and extraordinary steps are taken by clinicians and radiologists alike to demonstrate the fracture. These steps include oblique views, special radial head views, tomograms, and even CT scans or MR studies. These are absurd attempts to document pathology that will be treated identically whether or not it is radiographically recorded. As long as there is no obvious deformity or loose body, it does not matter whether the fracture is definitely identified or not in a patient with a posttraumatic painful elbow and a visible posterior fat pad. An infection, an arthritide, or any elbow effusion could cause a joint effusion and a displaced posterior fat pad, but the clinical setting would not be to rule out a fracture.

The anterior fat pad also gets displaced with a joint effusion. Ordinarily it is visible as a small triangle just anterior to the distal humeral diaphysis on a lateral view (Fig. 57.38). With an effusion, it gets displaced superiorly and outward from the humerus and has been called a "sail sign" because it resembles a spinnaker sail (see Figs. 57.36 and 57.37).

Shoulder dislocations are generally easily diagnosed, both clinically and radiographically. The most common shoulder dislocation is the anterior dislocation. It is at least 10 times more common than a posterior dislocation. For all practical purposes, anterior and posterior dislocations are the only two types of shoulder dislocations about which to be concerned.

An anterior dislocation occurs when the arm is forcibly externally rotated and abducted. This is commonly seen when football players "arm tackle," when kayakers "brace" with the paddle above their heads and allow their arms

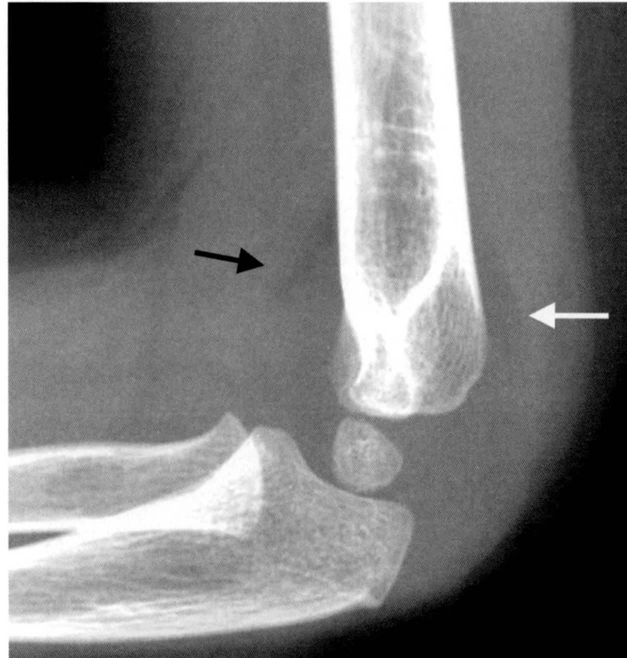

FIGURE 57.37. **Displaced Elbow Fat Pads.** A lateral view of the elbow in this child shows a posterior fat pad (*white arrow*) and a sail sign anteriorly (*black arrow*). This is indicative of a fracture about the elbow, which in a child (physes are open) usually means a supracondylar fracture.

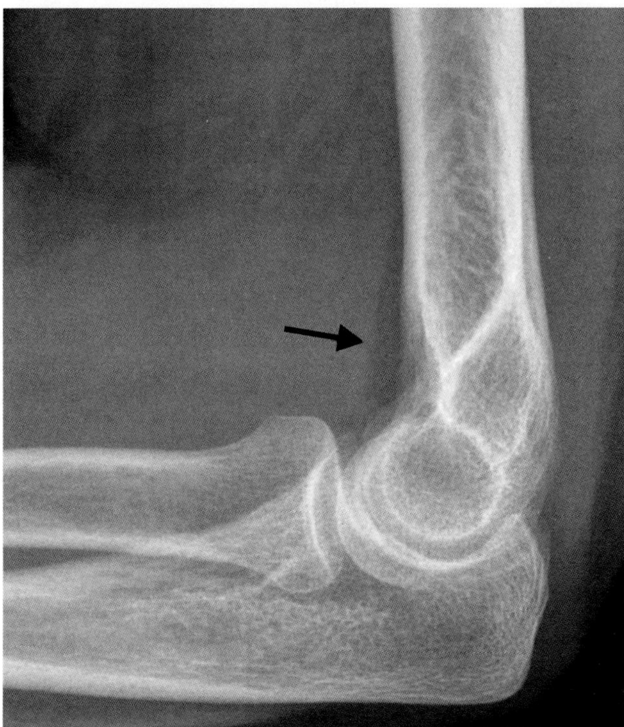

FIGURE 57.38. **Normal Anterior Fat Pad of the Elbow.** Note the normal fat pad lucency just anterior to the humerus of this normal elbow (*arrow*) and compare this with the sail sign of the abnormal displaced anterior fat pads in Figures 57.36 and 57.37.

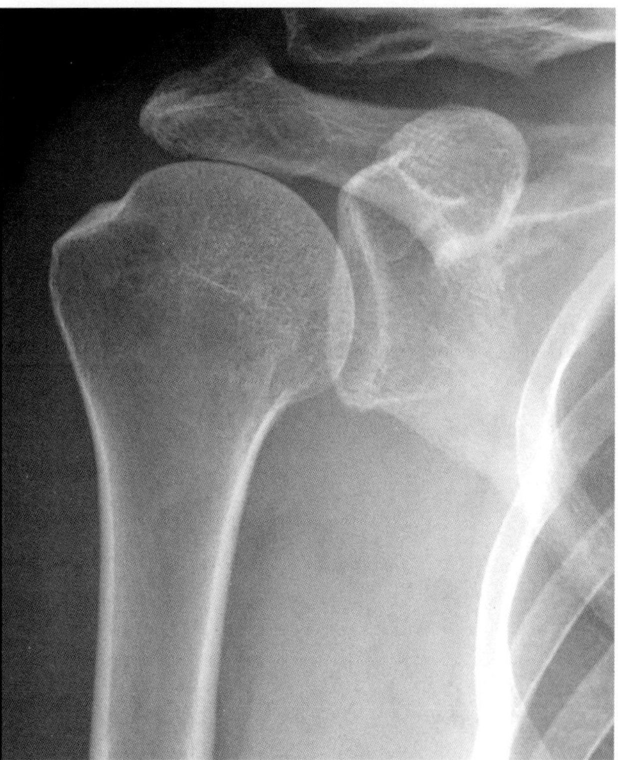

FIGURE 57.40. **Normal AP View of the Shoulder.** Note in this example of a normal shoulder that the humeral head slightly overlaps the glenoid, which has been termed the crescent sign.

to get too far posterior, when skiers plant their uphill pole and get it stuck, and from other similar athletic positions. Radiographically, the diagnosis is easily made on an AP shoulder radiograph: the humeral head is seen to lie inferiorly and medial to the glenoid (Fig. 57.39). The humeral head often impacts on the inferior lip of the glenoid causing an indentation on the posterosuperior portion of the humeral head; this is called a Hill–Sachs deformity. The presence of a Hill–Sachs deformity is said to indicate a greater likelihood of recurrent dislocation, and some surgeons use it as an indicator to intervene surgically to prevent a recurrence. A bony irregularity or fragment off the inferior glenoid, which occurs from the same mechanism as the Hill–Sachs deformity, is called a Bankart deformity. It is not seen radiographically as often as the Hill–Sachs deformity.

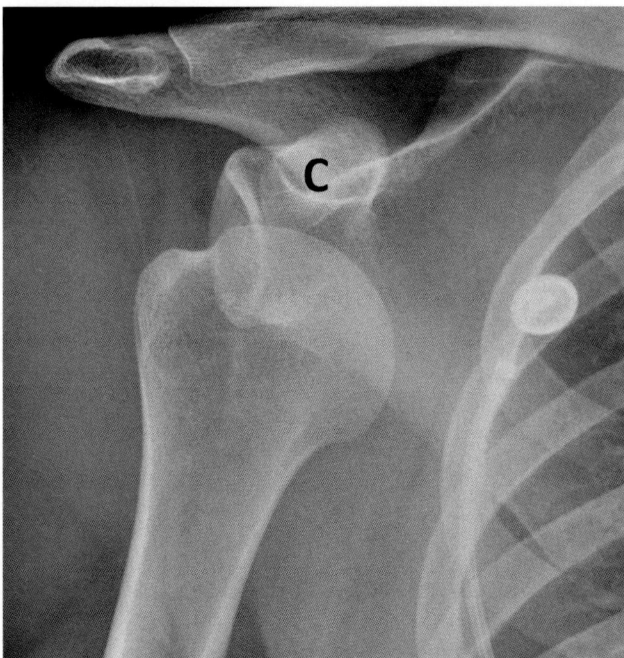

FIGURE 57.39. **Anterior Shoulder Dislocation.** An AP view of the right shoulder shows the humeral head to lie medial to the glenoid and inferior to the coracoid process (C). This is diagnostic of an anterior dislocation of the shoulder.

A posterior dislocation can be a difficult diagnosis to make, both clinically and radiographically. An AP view may look completely normal, or nearly so. On the AP view of a normal shoulder, the humeral head should slightly overlap the glenoid (Fig. 57.40), forming what has been called a "crescent sign." In a patient with a posterior dislocation, this crescent of bony overlap is usually absent and a small space may be seen between the glenoid and the humeral head (Fig. 57.41). The posteriorly dislocated humeral head is positioned in internal rotation and is often "perched" on the posterior rim of the glenoid; though the malalignment may not be immediately apparent, the impaction fracture on the anterior portion of the humeral head (reverse Hill–Sachs lesion or trough sign) may be evident (Fig. 57.42A). If a posterior dislocation is suspected but cannot be confirmed radiographically, CT scanning can provide a definitive diagnosis (Fig. 57.42B). The most common cause of a posterior shoulder dislocation is a seizure, and the injury is occasionally seen bilaterally.

The best way to unequivocally diagnose a dislocated shoulder radiographically is to obtain a transscapular view (also called a "scapular-Y" view). An axillary view will show basically the same thing but requires the patient to move the arm and shoulder, which can be painful and may

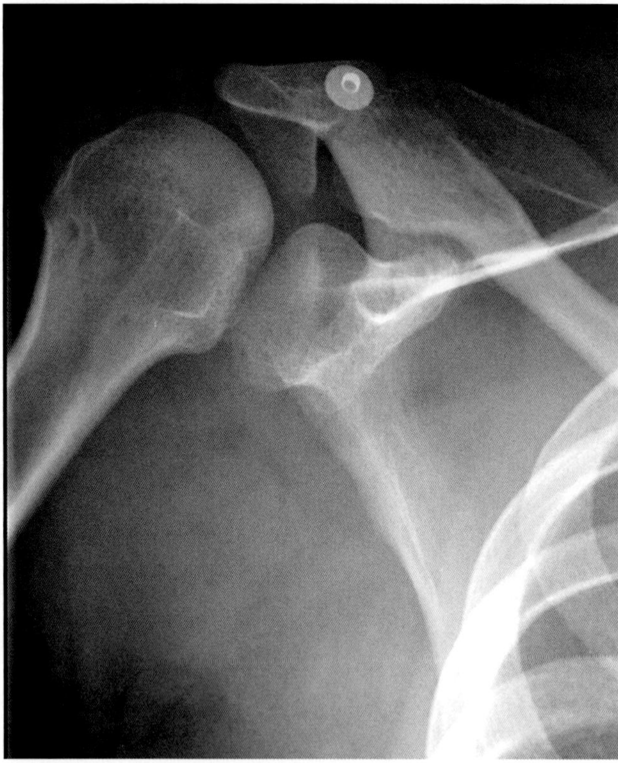

FIGURE 57.41. Posterior Shoulder Dislocation. Note that the humeral head in this patient is slightly displaced from the glenoid on the AP view. This is termed absence of the crescent sign and is often seen with a posterior dislocation. Compare this with the normal shoulder in Figure 57.40.

even redislocate the shoulder if it has spontaneously reduced itself. The transscapular view is obtained by angling the x-ray beam across the shoulder in the same plane as the blade of the scapula. This gives an en face view of the glenoid, and the humeral head can easily be related to it as either normal, anterior (Fig. 57.43A), or posterior (Fig. 57.43B). Because of frequently overlapping ribs and clavicles, the exact anatomy is often difficult to discern on the transscapular view. To find the glenoid, one has to find the coracoid, the spine of the acromion, and the blade of the scapula. These three structures all lead to the glenoid and form a "Y" around it. All that is necessary to find the center of the glenoid is to find two of those bony landmarks, usually the coracoid and the blade of the scapula. The humeral head can then be found and its position determined. Posterior dislocations can occasionally be difficult to diagnose even on the transscapular view, however, and in some cases CT is needed to confirm (or exclude) the diagnosis.

An entity that can be mistaken for a dislocated shoulder is a traumatic hemarthrosis, which displaces the humeral head inferolaterally on the AP radiograph (Fig. 57.44). Because the anterior dislocation displaces inferomedially, it should not be confused with this. The posterior dislocation will easily be excluded by looking at a transscapular view or by noting that the humerus is not internally rotated on the AP view. This has been termed a pseudodislocation. It should be recognized so that attempts to "reduce" the "dislocation" are not made. Also, it can suggest a subtle or occult humeral head fracture.

If a fracture is suspected about the shoulder and the radiographs are negative or equivocal, a CT scan should be performed. A complex joint such as the shoulder or hip is best examined with CT scanning when the full extent of the fracture needs to be identified (Fig. 57.45).

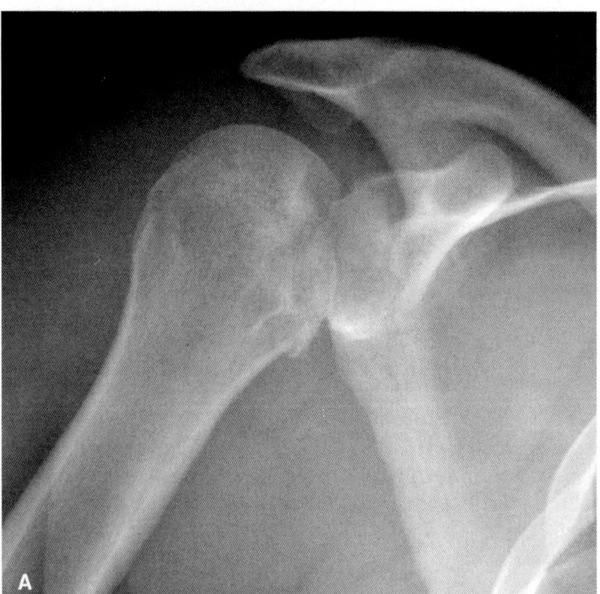

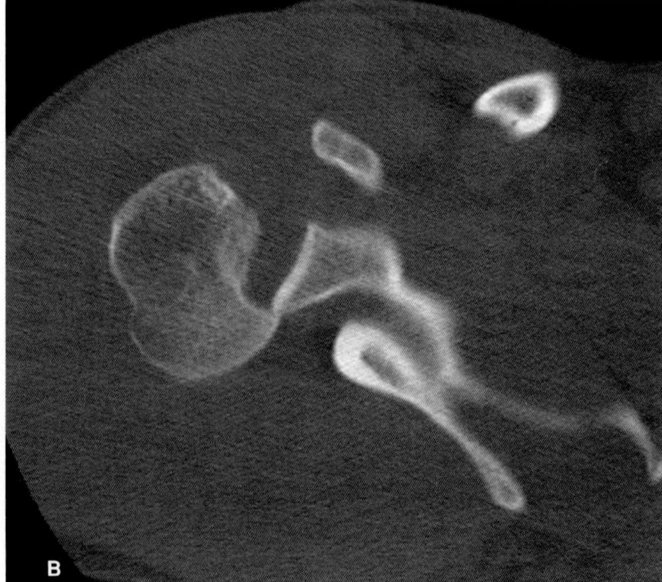

FIGURE 57.42. Posterior Shoulder Dislocation. A: An AP view of the right shoulder shows the humeral head to be internally rotated, and an impaction fracture (reverse Hill–Sachs lesion) is noted of the anterior medial humeral head. **B:** Axial CT image shows the large trough-like defect caused by the impaction lesion of the humeral head, the edge of which is perched upon and locked on the posterior glenoid rim.

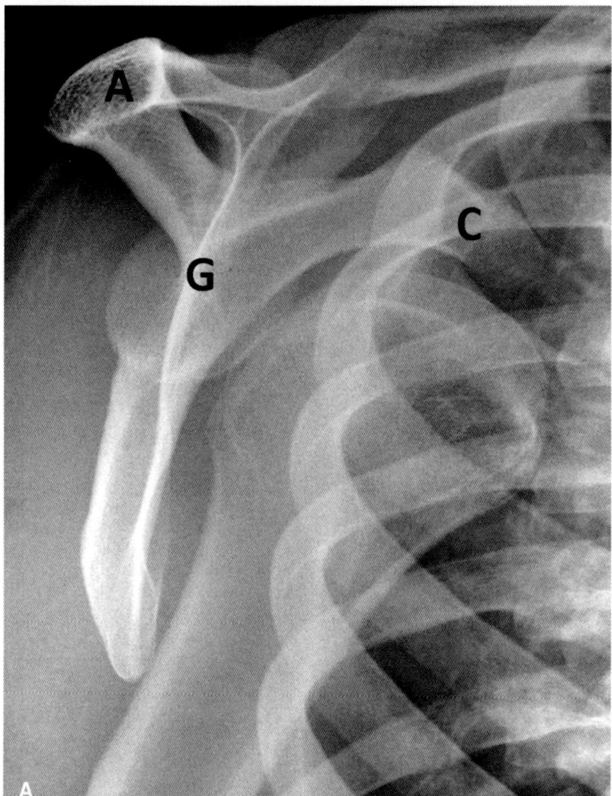

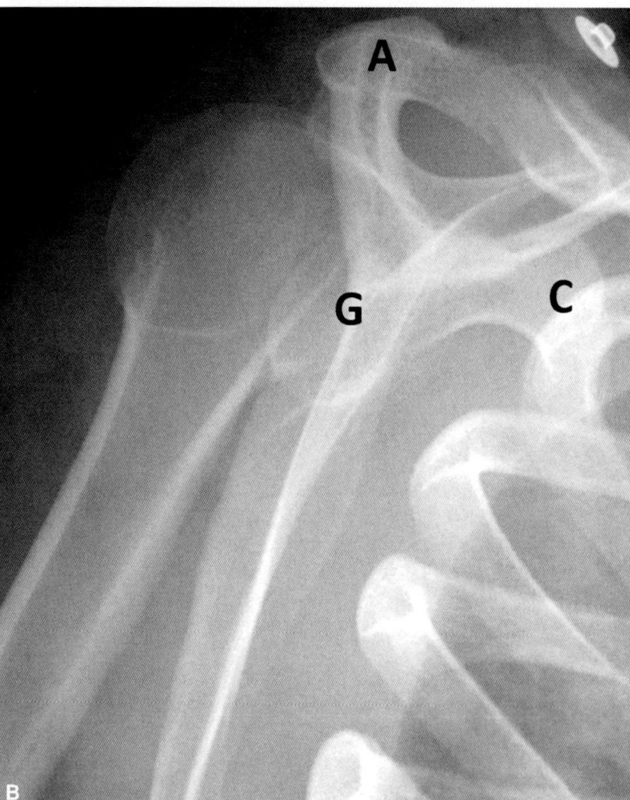

FIGURE 57.43. Transscapular Views of Anterior and Posterior Dislocations. These transscapular views of the shoulder are obtained by aiming the x-ray beam parallel to the shoulder blade. The coracoid process (*C*) can be seen anteriorly and the spine of the acromion (*A*) can be seen posteriorly. Both of these structures extend inwardly and meet at the glenoid (*G*). **A:** The humeral head is seen in this example to lie anterior to the glenoid. **B:** The humeral head is seen in this example to lie posterior to the glenoid.

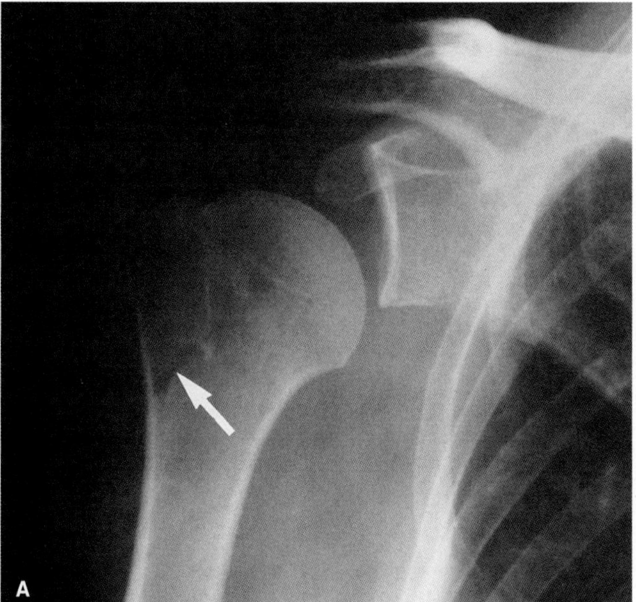

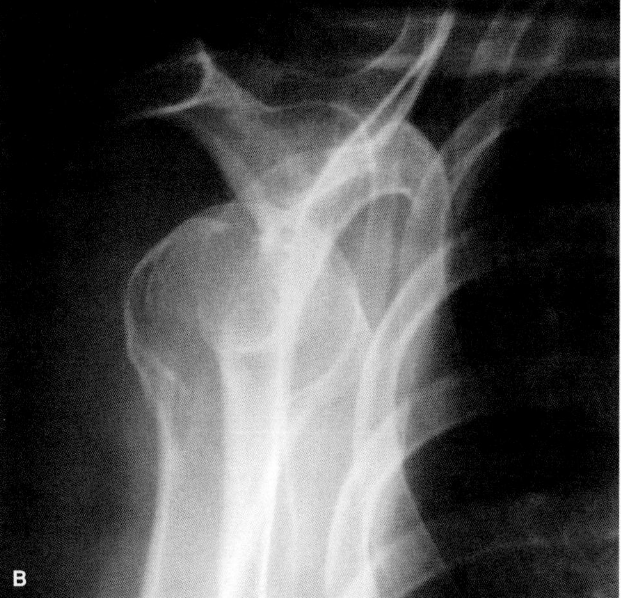

FIGURE 57.44. Pseudodislocation of the Shoulder. A: An AP view of the shoulder in this patient who had trauma to the shoulder shows the humeral head to be inferiorly placed in relation to the glenoid with absence of the normal crescent sign. A dislocation was suspected. **B:** The transscapular lateral view, however, reveals the humeral head to be normally placed over the glenoid. This is a pseudodislocation owing to a hemarthrosis. A search for an occult fracture should be made. In this case, a fracture can be seen in (**A**) (*arrow*), which caused bleeding into the joint.

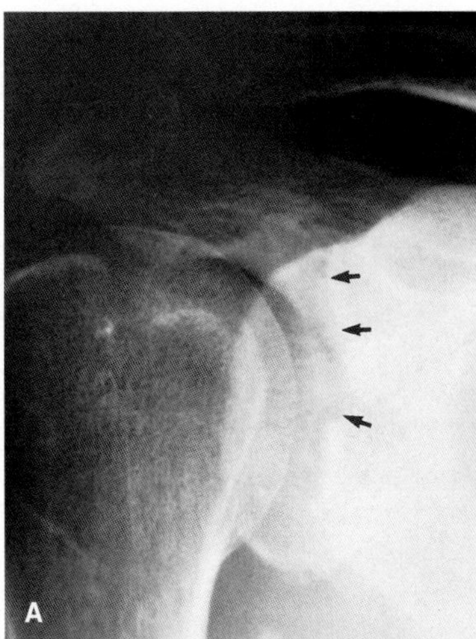

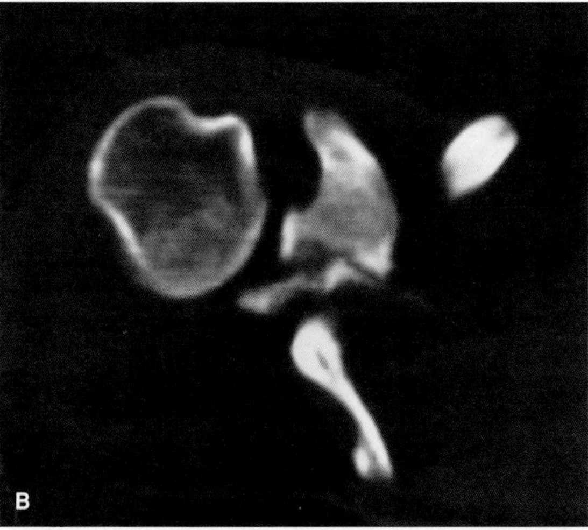

FIGURE 57.45. **Fracture of the Glenoid. A:** An AP view of the shoulder demonstrates a faint lucency indicative of a fracture of the glenoid (*arrows*) with a fragment of bone seen inferior to the joint. **B:** The full extent of the fracture cannot be appreciated until the CT is examined. On the CT scan, the fracture can be seen to extend fully through the scapula and is seen to be slightly displaced in the articular portion.

PELVIS

Fractures of the pelvis, and especially those involving the acetabulum, can be difficult to evaluate completely with radiographs alone. CT scanning should be considered in almost all acetabular fractures because of the possibility of free fragments and subtle fractures that plain radiographs do not show (Fig. 57.46).

Sacral fractures are said to occur in half the cases that have pelvic fractures. They can be difficult to see on even the best of radiographs because the sacrum is often hidden by bowel gas. In looking for sacral fractures, one should examine the arcuate lines of the sacrum bilaterally to see whether they are intact. Fractures often interrupt these lines and because of the side-to-side asymmetry can therefore be easily identified (Fig. 57.47).

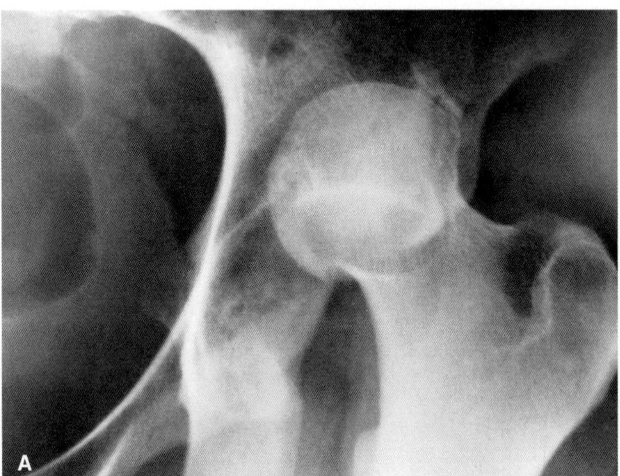

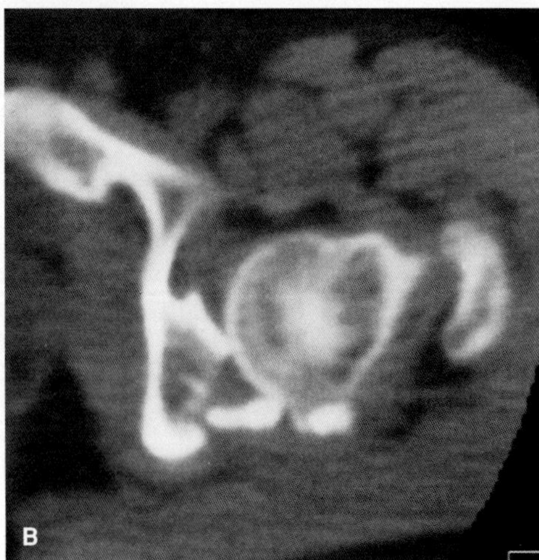

FIGURE 57.46. **Dislocation of the Hip. A:** An AP radiograph of the left hip shows dislocation of the femoral head, which lies slightly superior to the acetabulum. **B:** Fractures are easily identified on the CT scan. A cortical break through the articular surface of the posterior acetabulum as well as the dislocation is identified.

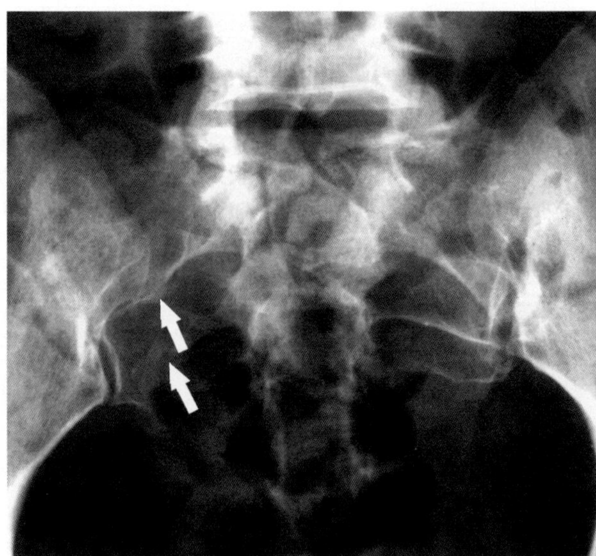

FIGURE 57.47. **Fracture of the Sacrum.** An AP view of the sacrum in this patient shows normal arcuate lines on the left side of the sacrum that are interrupted on the right side (*arrows*). Interruption of these lines indicates a fracture through this portion of the sacrum.

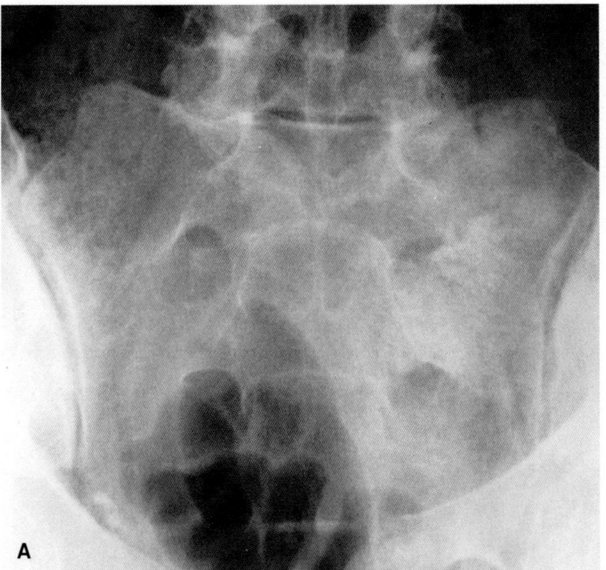

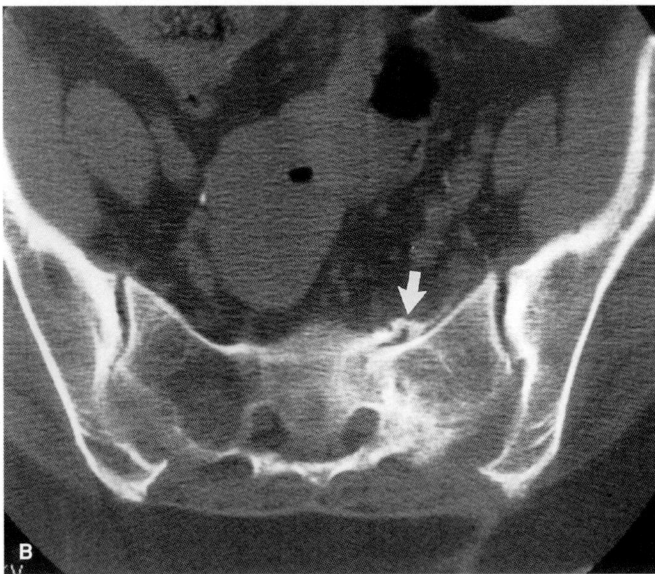

FIGURE 57.48. **Sacral Stress Fracture. A:** Faint sclerosis is noted in the left part of the sacrum as compared with the right in this patient complaining of pelvic pain. A radionuclide bone scan showed increased isotope uptake on the left half of the sacrum, and metastatic disease was postulated. **B:** A CT scan through this region that demonstrates a cortical disruption (*arrow*) indicative of a fracture. This is a characteristic radiographic and CT appearance of a stress fracture of the sacrum.

Sacral stress fractures in patients who are osteoporotic or who have undergone radiation therapy can present as patchy or linear sclerosis on the sacral ala that may or may not show cortical disruption on plain radiographs (Fig. 57.48A). These should be differentiated from metastatic disease because of their characteristic location, appearance, and history of prior radiation and by seeing a cortical break. CT will usually, but not always, demonstrate cortical disruption (Fig. 57.48B). These fractures have a characteristic appearance on radionuclide bone scans (Fig. 57.49A), termed the Honda sign because of the similar appearance to the car logo. The Honda sign is seen only with bilateral stress fractures; unilateral fractures will have increased radionuclide uptake throughout one sacral ala. MR will demonstrate an area of diffuse low signal on T1-weighted images corresponding to the area of involvement (Fig. 57.49B). Sacral stress fractures have also been termed insufficiency fractures, indicating that the underlying bone is abnormal, similar to a pathologic fracture.

Avulsion injuries affect the pelvis quite often and should be easily recognized by radiologists. On occasion, an avulsion injury can have an aggressive appearance, and if not diagnosed radiographically, a biopsy might be performed. This can be calamitous, as avulsion injuries have been known to mimic

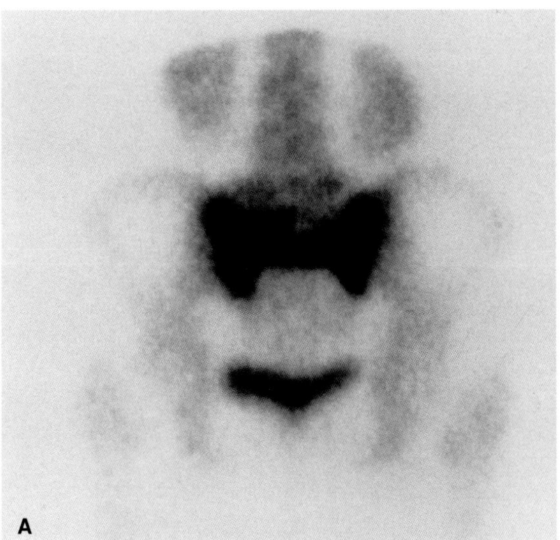

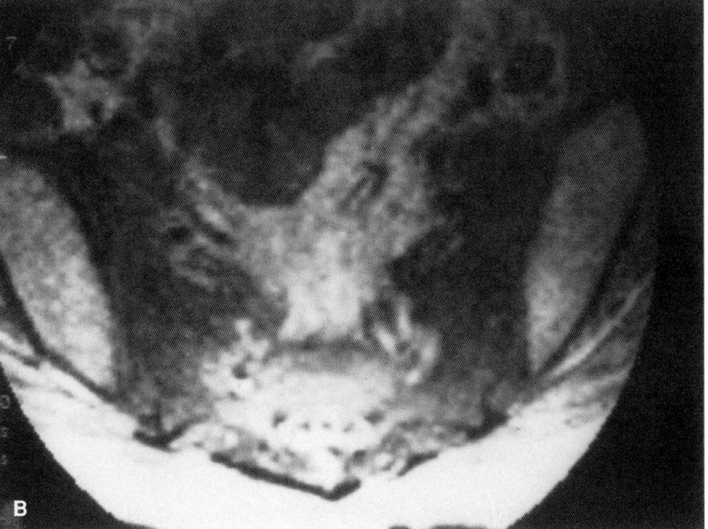

FIGURE 57.49. **Sacral Stress Fracture. A:** A radionuclide bone scan in an osteoporotic patient with pelvic pain shows a classic "Honda sign" seen with bilateral sacral stress fractures. **B:** A T1-weighted coronal MR in this patient shows diffuse low signal throughout the sacrum adjacent to the sacroiliac joints bilaterally. This represents edema and hemorrhage in the fractures and corresponds to the bone scan Honda sign.

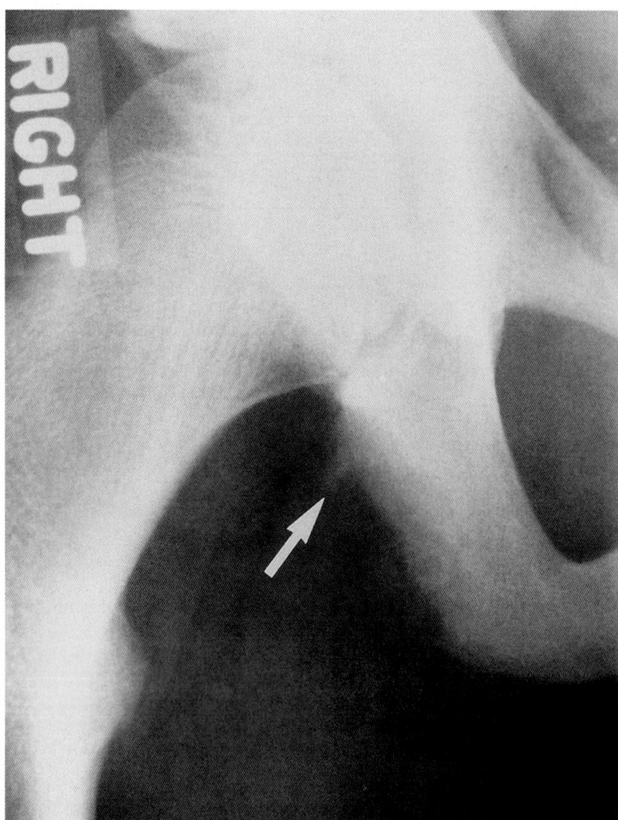

FIGURE 57.50. **Avulsion Off the Ischium.** An AP view of the pelvis shows an area of cortical disruption and periostitis at the right ischium (*arrow*) in a patient complaining of pain at this site. These findings are characteristic for an ischial avulsion and should not undergo biopsy.

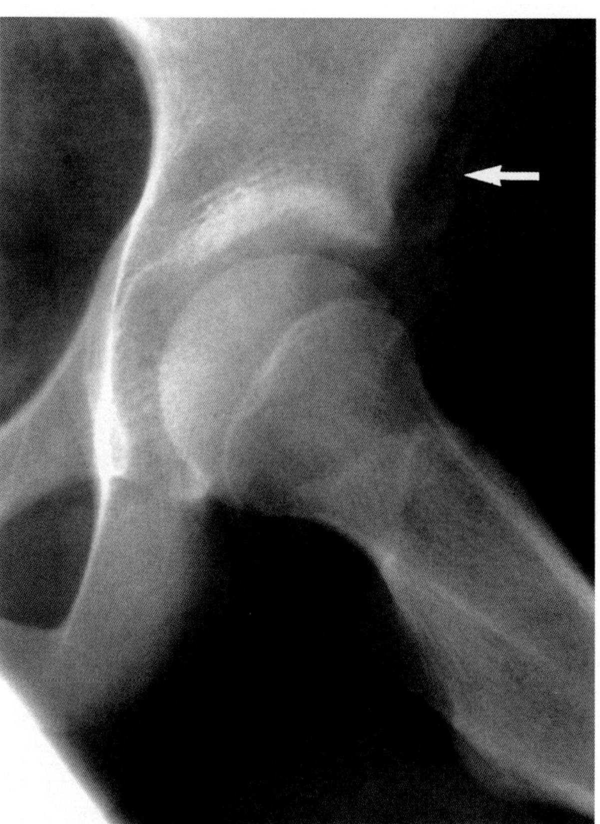

FIGURE 57.51. **Rectus Femoris Avulsion.** An AP view of the left hip shows a faint calcific density superior to the acetabulum (*arrow*), which is characteristic for an avulsion of the rectus femoris muscle from the anterior inferior iliac spine.

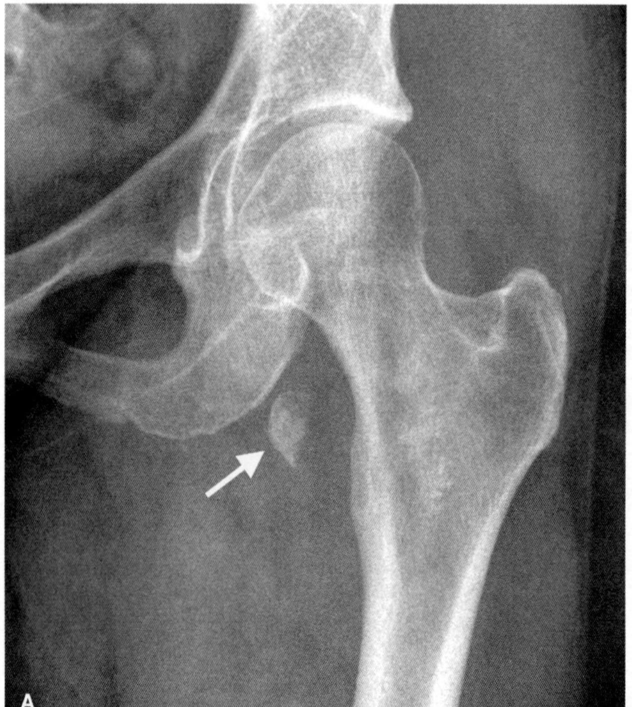

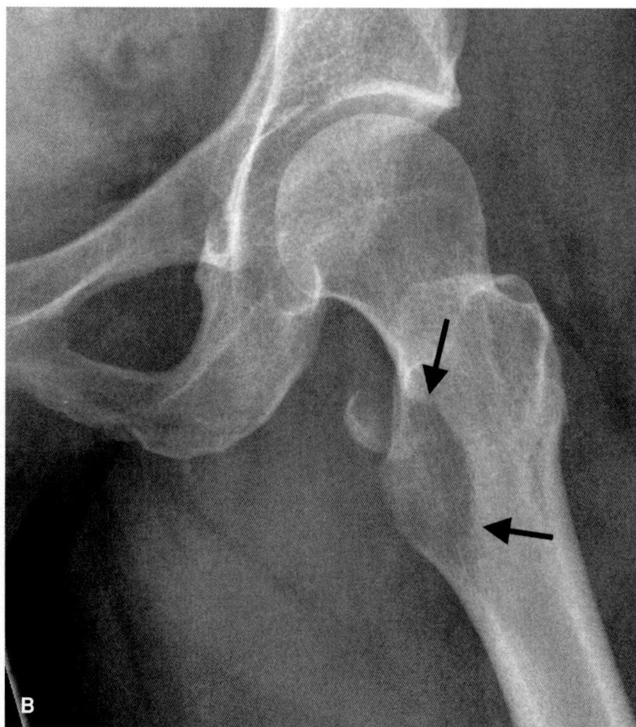

FIGURE 57.52. **Pathologic Avulsion Fracture of the Lesser Trochanter. A:** An AP view of the left hip shows an isolated avulsion fracture of the lesser trochanter (*white arrow*), which occurred during walking; in an adult, an isolated avulsion in this location is suspicious for a pathologic fracture. **B:** The frog-leg lateral view reveals an underlying lucency in the femur (*black arrows*), which in this case is a lytic metastatic lesion from a renal cell carcinoma.

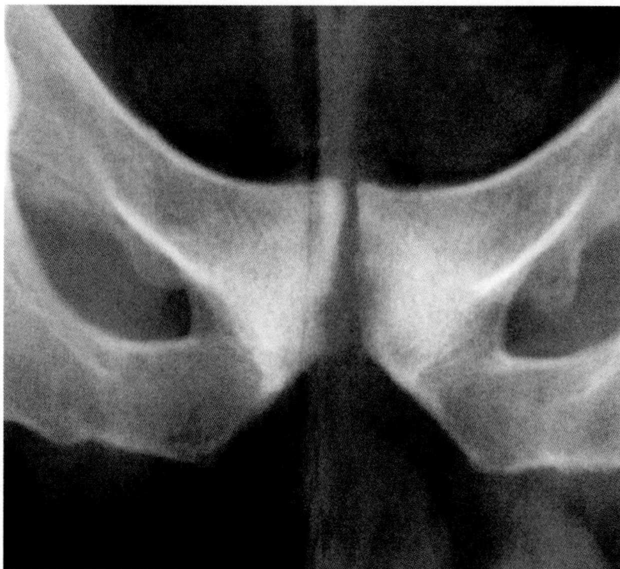

FIGURE 57.53. **Osteoarthritis of the Symphysis Pubis.** Sclerosis with erosion is noted at the symphysis in this ultramarathoner complaining of severe pubic pain. This is characteristic of degenerative joint disease (DJD) or osteoarthritis at this site in such an overuse setting. Erosions are ordinarily not seen in DJD, except in certain joints such as the symphysis pubis, sacroiliac, and the acromioclavicular.

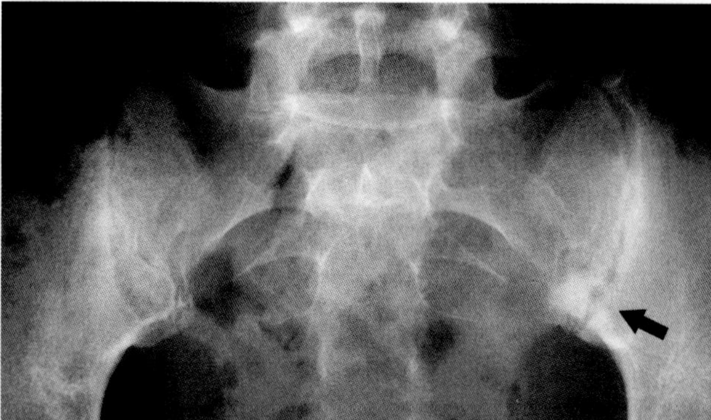

FIGURE 57.54. **Osteoarthritis of the Sacroiliac Joint.** Sclerosis and erosions (*arrow*) are seen in the left sacroiliac joint in this young professional dancer. Although this has the appearance of an inflammatory arthritis, this is also seen in degenerative joint disease or osteoarthritis secondary to overuse.

malignant lesions histologically, with a misdiagnosis leading to radical treatment (Fig. 57.50). Therefore, when an avulsion injury is a consideration, it becomes a "do not touch" lesion (see Chapter 60). Common sites for pelvic avulsions include the ischium, the superior and inferior anterior iliac spines (Fig. 57.51), and the iliac crest. These injuries are said to be fairly common in long jumpers, sprinters, hurdlers, gymnasts, and cheerleaders.

An avulsion fracture that deserves special mention is that of the lesser trochanter of the proximal femur; in children and adolescents, these avulsions typically occur as the result of an athletic injury and are benign. In adults, however, isolated avulsion fractures of the lesser trochanter usually only occur in the setting of an underlying bone lesion, such as a metastasis, and should prompt inspection for an underlying lesion and further investigation for a site of primary malignancy (Fig. 57.52). Lesser trochanter fractures are much more commonly seen in the setting of comminuted intertrochanteric hip fractures and in that setting are not necessarily associated with underlying malignancy.

Another area in the pelvis that can demonstrate radiologic findings as a result of stress is the symphysis pubis. In ultramarathoners, cross-country skiers, soccer players, and other athletes, the symphysis can be affected by degenerative joint disease (DJD) or osteoarthritis (Fig. 57.53). The hallmarks of DJD are sclerosis, joint space narrowing, and osteophytosis. In certain joints, however, erosions can occur as a result of DJD. These joints include the temporomandibular joint, the acromioclavicular joint, the symphysis pubis, and the sacroiliac joint.

When the sacroiliac joints are involved with DJD, this can closely resemble a human leukocyte antigen B27 (HLA-B27) spondyloarthropathy (Fig. 57.54) and lead to erroneous diagnosis and treatment. Large osteophytes can develop across the sacroiliac joints and mimic sclerosis or even a tumor (Fig. 57.55).

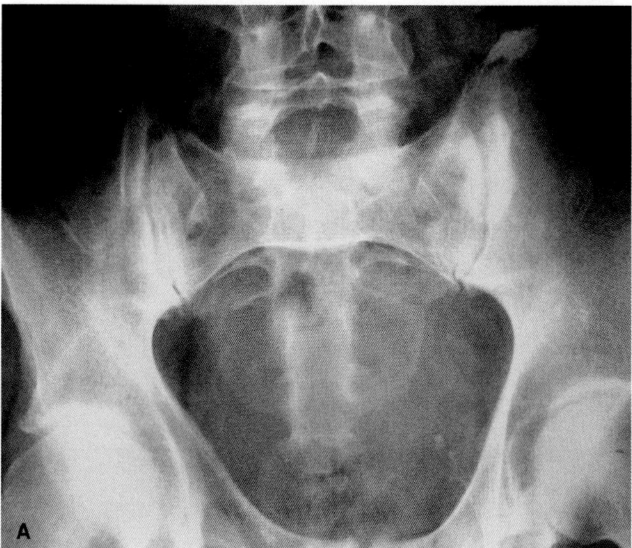

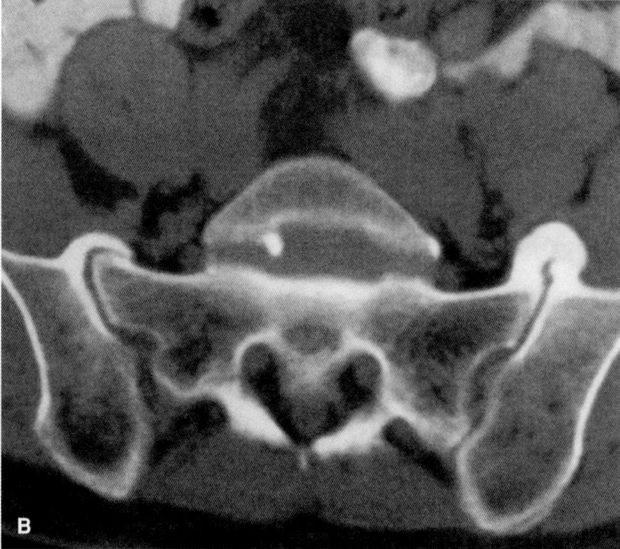

FIGURE 57.55. **Sacroiliac Osteophytes. A:** An AP view of the pelvis in this marathoner shows dense sclerosis over both sacroiliac joints. **B:** A CT through this area demonstrates dense, bridging osteophytes, characteristic of degenerative joint disease.

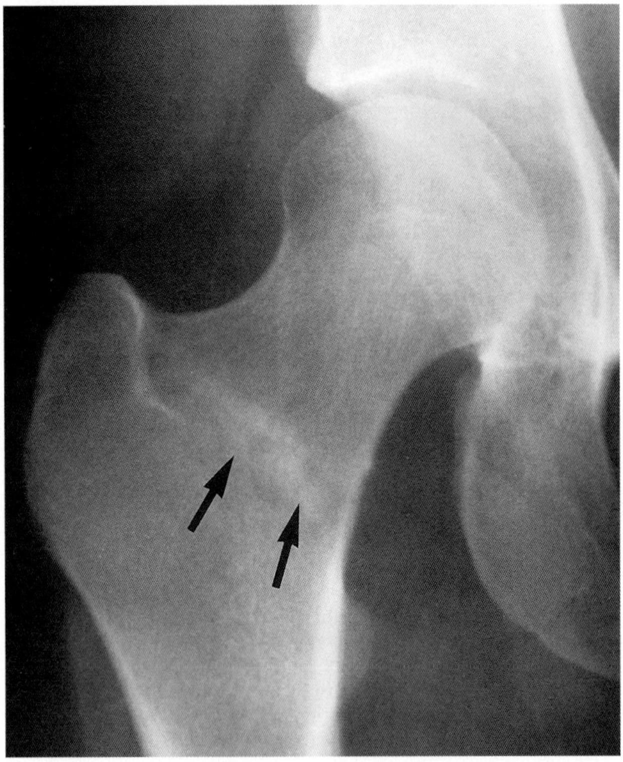

FIGURE 57.56. **Stress Fracture of the Femoral Neck.** An area of linear sclerosis (*arrows*) is seen at the base of the femoral neck in a runner with hip pain. This is diagnostic of a stress fracture of the femur.

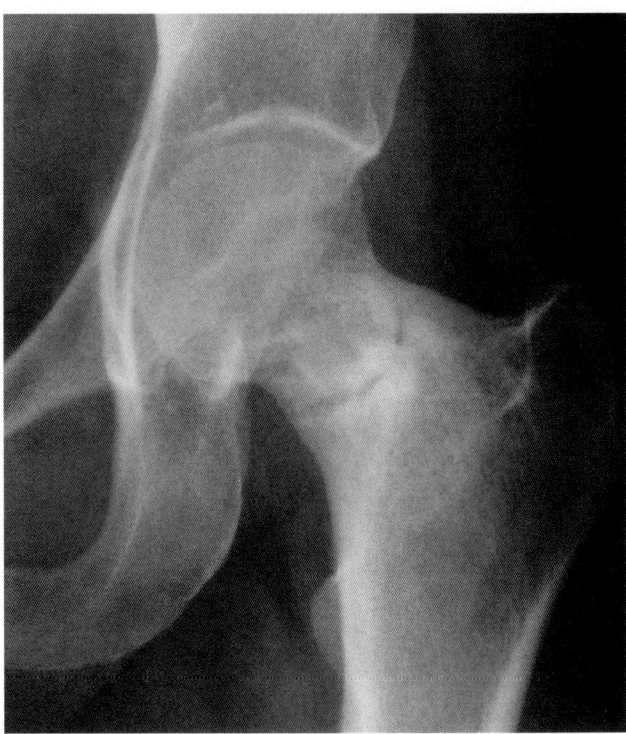

FIGURE 57.57. **Femoral Stress Fracture.** A linear lucency with surrounding sclerosis is seen in the femoral neck in this jogger with hip pain. This is a severe femoral neck stress fracture.

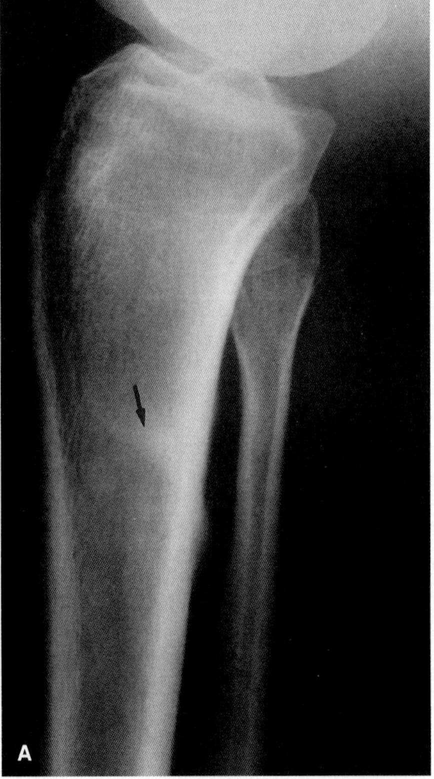

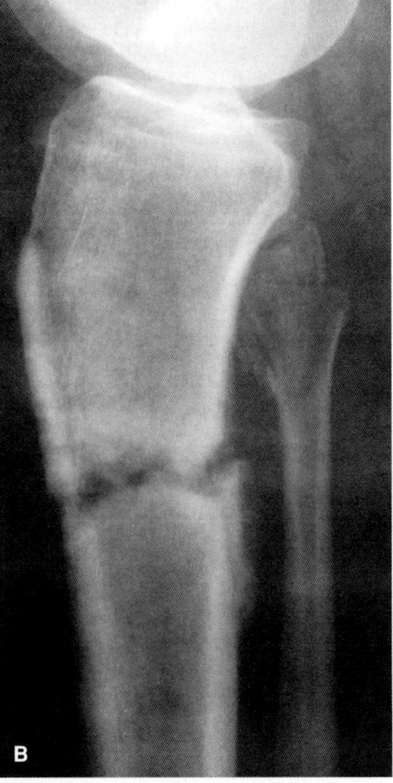

FIGURE 57.58. **Stress Fracture of the Proximal Tibia. A:** A faint linear sclerotic area (*arrow*) is seen, which is characteristic for a stress fracture of the proximal tibia. **B:** This view shows the result of continued exercise in this patient: a complete fracture of the tibia and the proximal fibula.

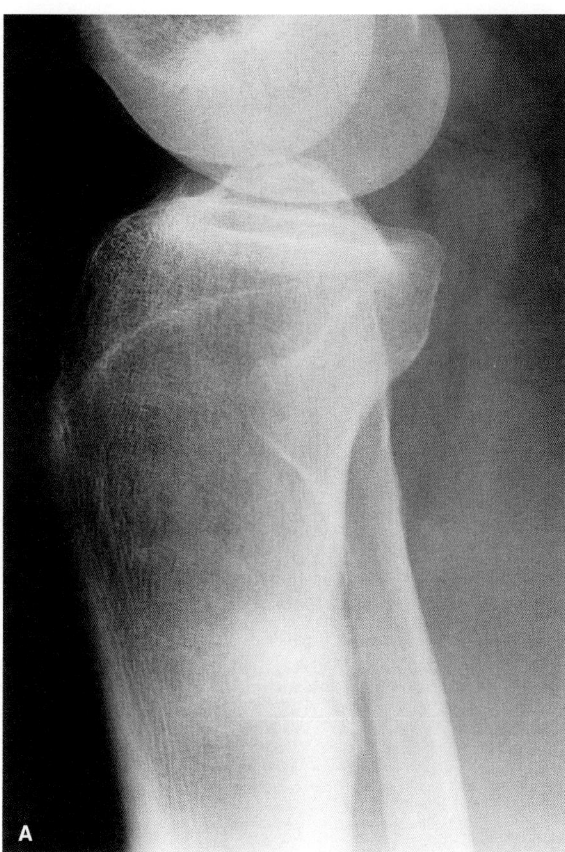

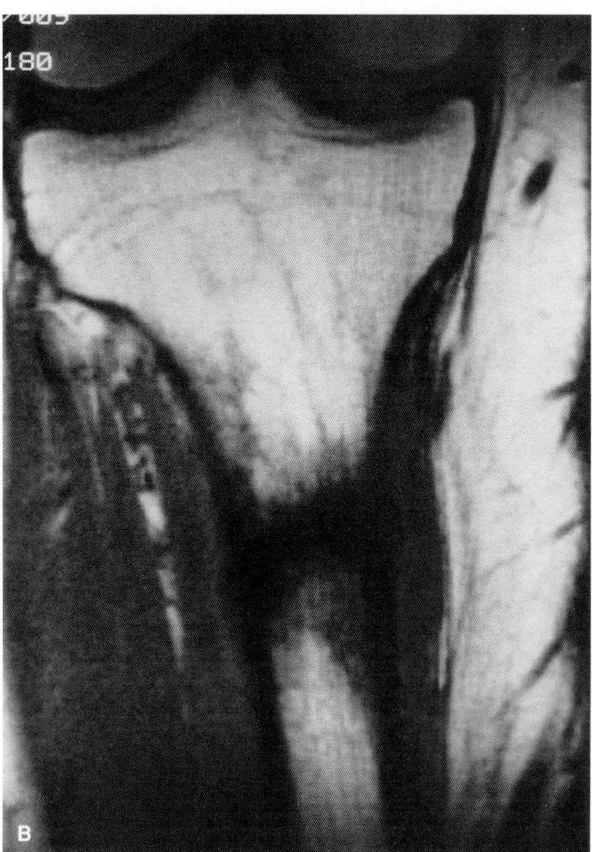

FIGURE 57.59. **Stress Fracture of the Tibia. A:** An irregular focus of sclerosis is seen in the posterior proximal tibia with adjacent periostitis. There was concern that this might represent a primary bone tumor, and the surgeons recommended a biopsy. **B:** An MR scan was performed, however, which shows a linear low-signal area running obliquely across the tibia on this T1-weighted coronal image, which is characteristic for a stress fracture. No significant soft tissue mass was found. The patient's recent history included an increase in his jogging. A stress fracture was diagnosed on the basis of these images.

LEG

Overt fractures in the femur and the lower leg are, for the most part, straightforward and deserve no special radiologic treatment for fear of missing subtle abnormalities.

Stress fractures, however, need to be considered in anyone with hip or leg pain, as overlooking the diagnosis can lead to a complete fracture. The most serious stress fracture, and fortunately one of the rarest, is the femoral neck stress fracture (Fig. 57.56). Rarely, these progress to complete fractures (Fig. 57.57) that, with continued weight bearing, can displace; these are very serious lesions.

Stress fractures also occur in the distal diaphysis of the femur and in the proximal, middle, and distal thirds of the tibia. All of these stress fractures need to be treated with utmost caution because complete fractures are not uncommon with continued stress (Fig. 57.58). Sclerosis in a weight-bearing bone that has a horizontal or oblique linear pattern should be considered a stress fracture until proved otherwise. A history of repetitive stress is not always obtained, and therefore, the diagnosis should not depend solely on the history. A stress fracture occasionally will appear somewhat aggressive, with aggressive periostitis and no definite linearity to the sclerosis (Fig. 57.59A). If this is mistaken for a tumor and undergoes biopsy, it can be confused with a malignancy, with subsequent radical therapy. These should, therefore, not undergo biopsy under any circumstance. If the clinical presentation is unusual for a stress fracture and the radiographs are not diagnostic, take additional radiographs 1 or 2 weeks later. CT and MR sometimes will better delineate the lesion (Fig. 57.59B). Stress fractures can be difficult to diagnose radiologically early on but should be straightforward after several weeks.

In patients on long-term medications affecting bone turnover, insufficiency fractures can on rare occasions develop in the lateral cortex of the proximal to midfemoral diaphysis (Fig. 57.60); these are sometimes referred to as "atypical" femoral fractures because most stress and insufficiency fractures develop on the compressive, or medial, side of the femur. Focal lateral cortical thickening, with or without a lucent fracture line, is seen. These fractures are important to diagnose as they can easily progress to complete fractures and they are, therefore, often prophylactically internally fixated; they are also often bilateral, so recognition should prompt imaging of the contralateral femur.

One final stress fracture that deserves mention because it is frequently misdiagnosed clinically and overlooked radiographically is the calcaneal stress fracture (Fig. 57.61). It is often clinically misdiagnosed as a "heel spur" or plantar fasciitis and can be a somewhat subtle radiographic finding.

Hip Fracture. Overt fractures in the lower extremity are uncommonly missed on radiographs; however, a few exceptions should be noted. Hip fractures in the elderly population can be very difficult to detect (Fig. 57.62), and a high index of suspicion should be maintained. A negative radiograph in an elderly

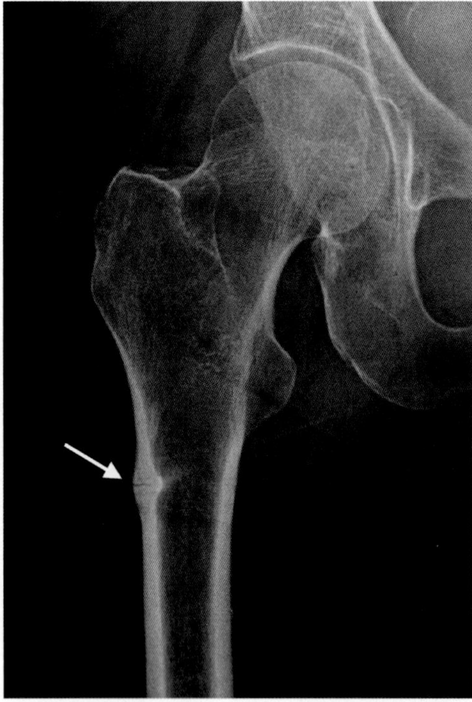

FIGURE 57.60. **Atypical Femoral Fracture.** Focal lucency with surrounding cortical thickening is seen in the lateral cortex of the proximal femoral diaphysis (*arrow*) in this osteoporotic patient on long-term therapy with an osteoclast-inhibiting agent, consistent with an atypical femoral insufficiency fracture.

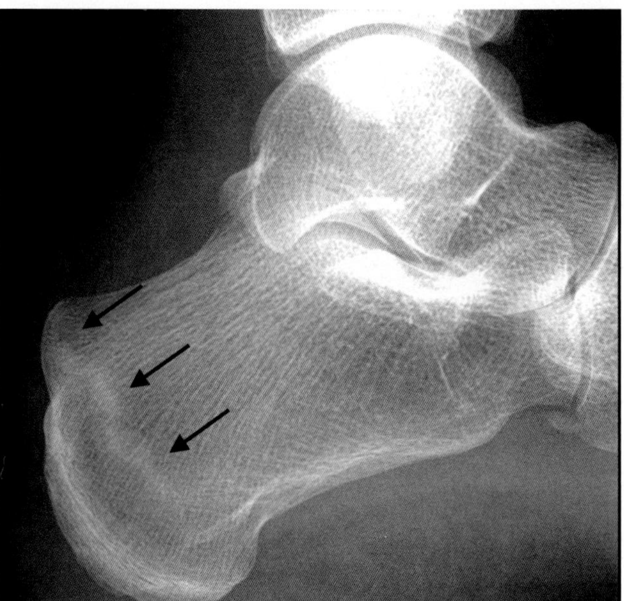

FIGURE 57.61. **Calcaneal Stress Fracture.** A curvilinear band of sclerosis is seen in the posterior calcaneus (*arrows*), which is diagnostic for a stress fracture of the calcaneus.

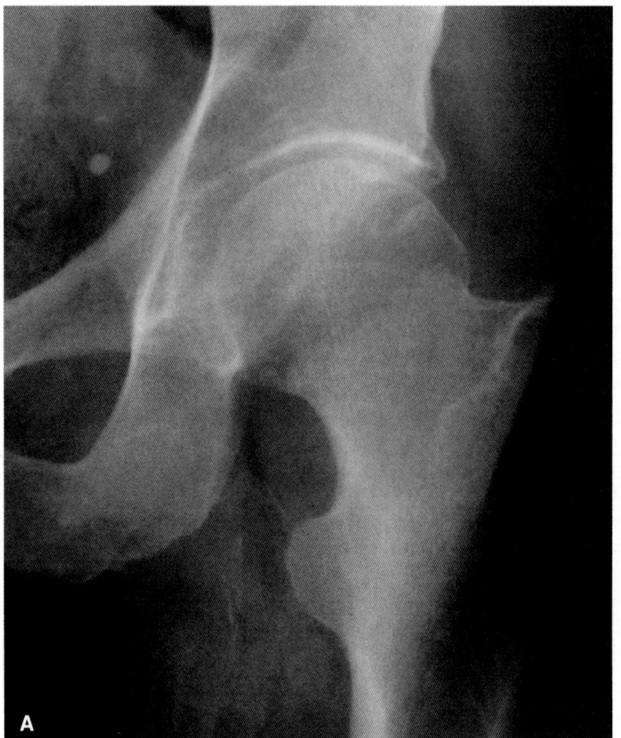

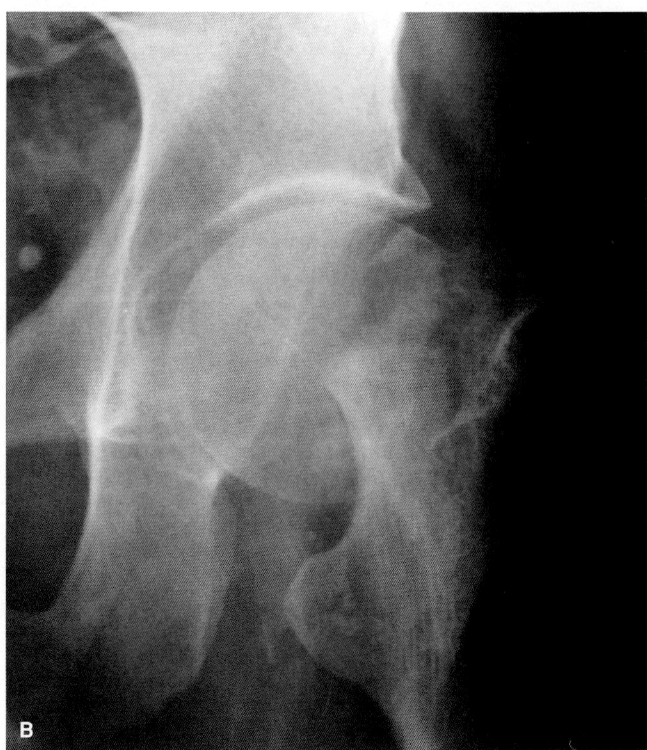

FIGURE 57.62. **Fracture of the Hip. A:** An AP view of the hip was obtained in an elderly man following a fall. It was interpreted as normal, and the patient was dismissed from the emergency department. Two weeks later, the patient returned to the emergency department unable to walk and another radiograph (**B**) was obtained. It shows a complete fracture through the femoral neck. In retrospect, the fracture can be faintly seen in (**A**) and should have been picked up initially. Fractures of the hip in the elderly can be very difficult to see and should be diligently searched for with additional views when the clinical setting is appropriate.

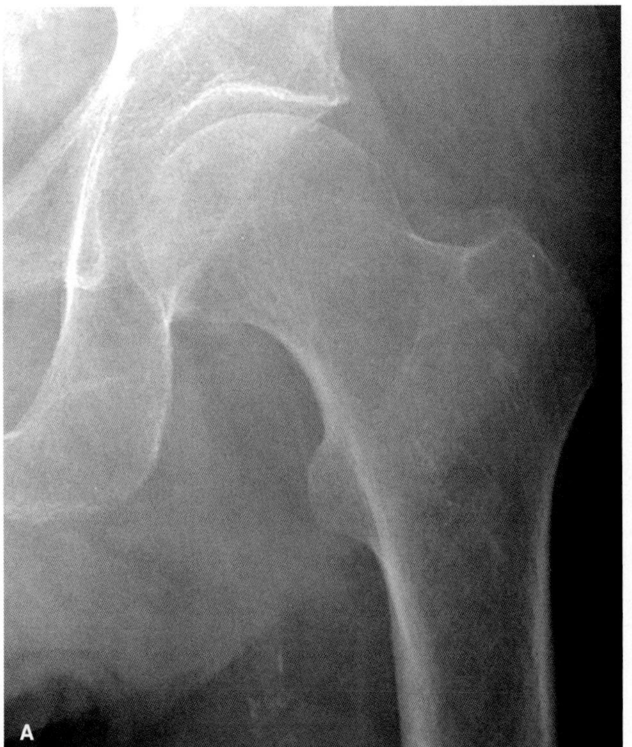

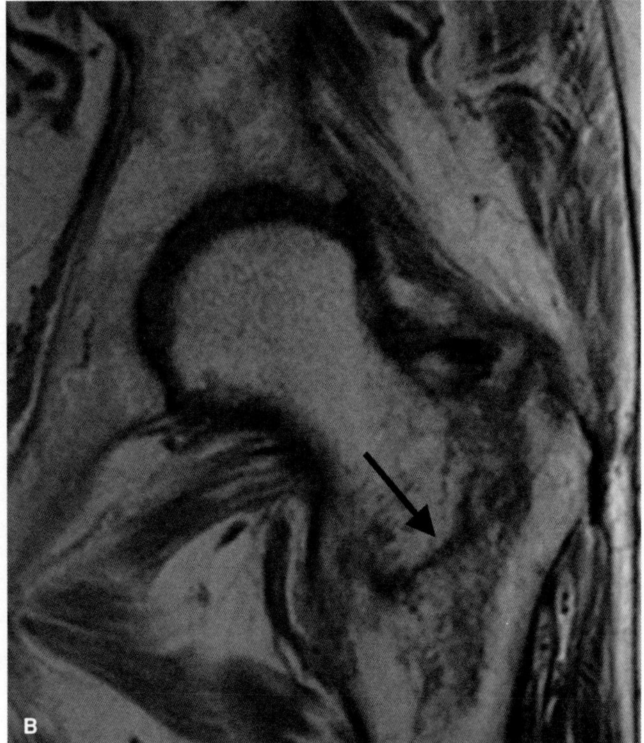

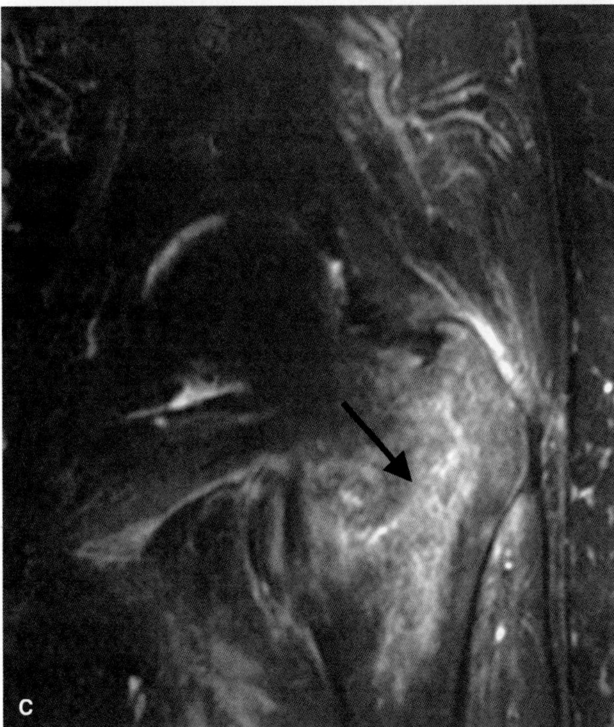

FIGURE 57.63. Occult Fracture of the Hip. A: An AP radiograph in an elderly patient with hip pain after a fall appears normal. **B, C:** An MR was obtained because of clinical suspicion of a fracture. Coronal T1-weighted (**A**) and T2-weighted (**B**) images show curvilinear signal abnormality with surrounding edema in the intertrochanteric region (*arrows*), confirming the fracture.

patient with hip pain after trauma (even relatively mild trauma) does not exclude a femoral neck fracture. MR has been shown to be very useful in demonstrating femoral neck fractures that are occult (Fig. 57.63).

Tibial Plateau Fracture. Another fracture that can be difficult to exclude on routine radiographs is a tibial plateau fracture. A cross-table lateral radiograph should be obtained in cases of knee trauma to look for a fat–fluid level (Fig. 57.64); this indicates a fracture that allows fatty marrow to leak into the knee joint. In the appropriate clinical setting, MRI or CT may be necessary to make the diagnosis.

Lisfranc Fracture. A serious fracture in the foot that can be missed radiographically when little or no displacement occurs is the Lisfranc fracture (Fig. 57.65). It is named after a surgeon in Napoleon's army who would do forefoot amputations in patients with gangrenous toes as a result of frostbite. The

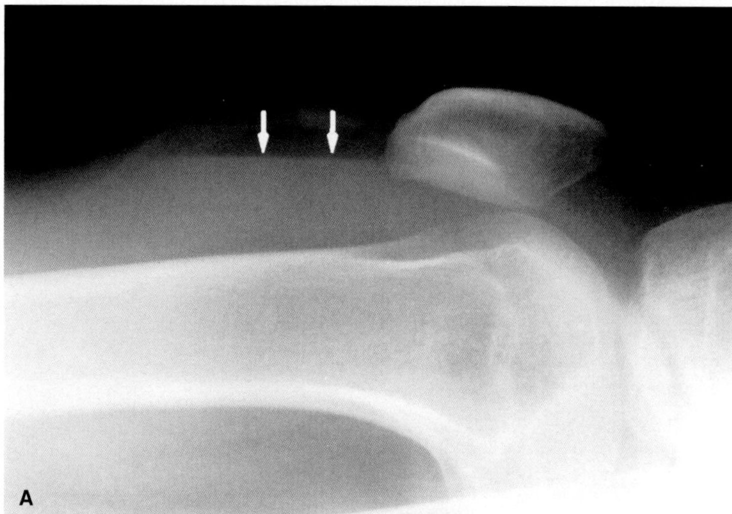

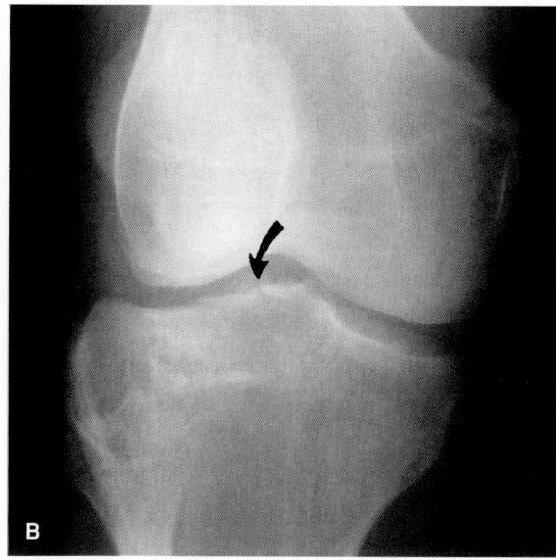

FIGURE 57.64. **Tibial Plateau Fracture. A:** A cross-table lateral radiograph of the knee reveals a fat–fluid level (*arrows*), which indicates a fracture with fatty marrow leaking into the joint. **B:** An AP view shows a barely discernible fracture (*arrow*) near the tibial spines, indicative of a tibial plateau fracture.

Lisfranc fracture is a fracture–dislocation of the tarsometatarsals. If the dislocation is slight—which it often is, especially on non–weight-bearing radiographs—it can be easily overlooked. A key to normal alignment is that the medial border of the second metatarsal should always line up with the medial border of the second (middle) cuneiform. If it does not, a Lisfranc fracture–dislocation should be suspected. This fracture is seen most commonly in patients who catch the forefoot in something such as a hole in the ground or a horseback rider falling and hanging by the forefoot in the stirrups. It is also commonly seen as a neurotrophic or Charcot joint in diabetics.

Fracture of the calcaneus can be difficult to appreciate on routine radiographs. Böhler angle is a normal anatomic landmark that should be looked for in every lateral foot radiograph when trauma has occurred (Fig. 57.66). If this angle is narrower than 20 degrees, it indicates a compression of the calcaneus, as seen in jumping injuries (Fig. 57.67).

This chapter is a fairly simplified overview of some commonly overlooked fractures and dislocations and should not be interpreted as a substitute for the more complete texts listed in the references.

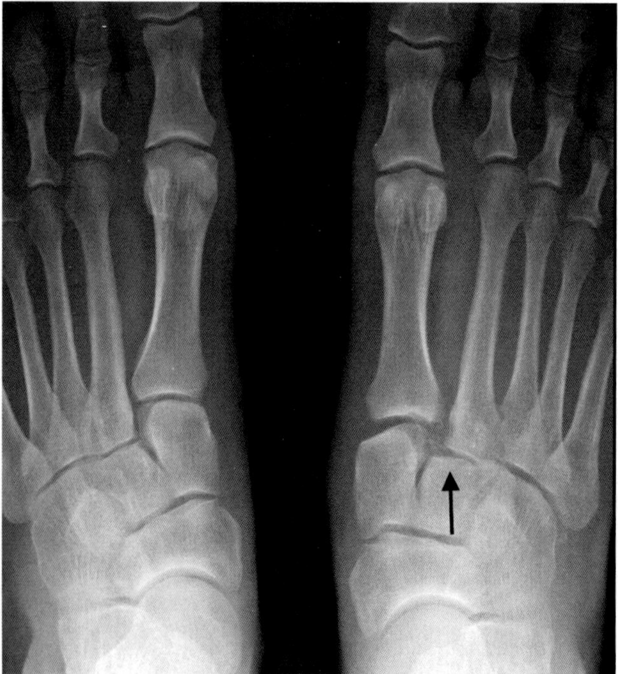

FIGURE 57.65. **Lisfranc Fracture.** A standing AP view of the feet in this patient with a right foot injury shows a widened space between the right first and second metatarsals with the base of the right second metatarsal displaced off the second cuneiform (*arrow*); the normal left foot is included for comparison. This is indicative of a Lisfranc fracture–dislocation.

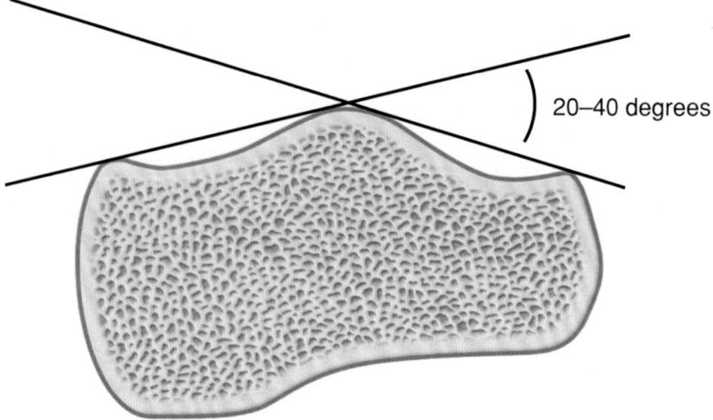

FIGURE 57.66. **Böhler Angle in a Normal Calcaneus.** This drawing depicts the normal calcaneus with a line across the anterior process extending to the apex of the calcaneus intersecting with a line from the posterior portion of the calcaneus to the apex. This is termed Böhler angle, and when it becomes flattened or less than 20 degrees, a calcaneal fracture should be diagnosed.

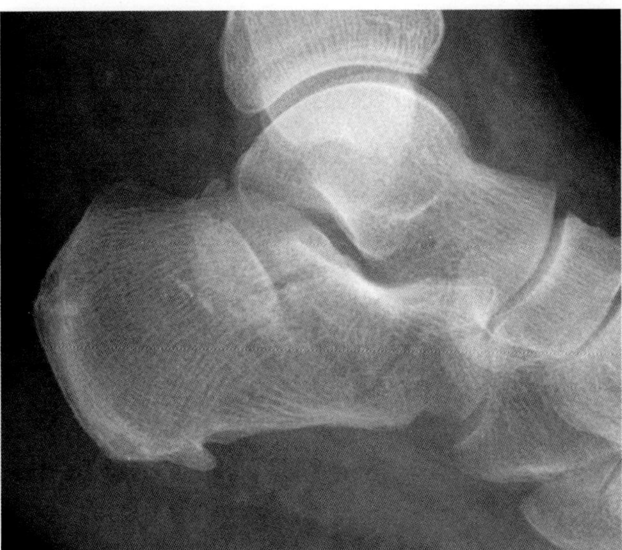

FIGURE 57.67. **Calcaneal Fracture.** Böhler angle in this calcaneus is less than 20 degrees, which is indicative of a fracture of the calcaneus.

Suggested Readings

Dorsay TA, Major NM, Helms CA. Cost-effectiveness of immediate MR imaging versus traditional follow-up for revealing radiographically occult scaphoid fractures. *AJR Am J Roentgenol* 2001;177:1257–1263.

Harris JH Jr, Harris WH. *The Radiology of Emergency Medicine*. 4th ed. Baltimore, MD: Lippincott Williams & Wilkins; 2000.

Mirvis SE, Diaconis JN, Chirico PA, Reiner BI, Joslyn JN, Militello P. Protocol-driven radiologic evaluation of suspected cervical spine injury: efficacy study. *Radiology* 1989;170:831–834.

Rockwood CA Jr, Green DP. *Fractures in Adults*. 5th ed. Philadelphia, PA: Lippincott Williams & Wilkins; 2001.

Rogers LF. *Radiology of Skeletal Trauma*. 3rd ed. New York: Churchill Livingstone; 2002.

CHAPTER 58 ■ ARTHRITIS

CLYDE A. HELMS AND EMILY N. VINSON

OSTEOARTHRITIS

Osteoarthritis, or degenerative joint disease (DJD), is the most common arthritide. It is believed to be caused by trauma—either overt or as an accumulation of microtrauma over years—although there is also a hereditary form called primary osteoarthritis that occurs primarily in middle-aged women. The hallmarks of DJD are ***joint space narrowing***, ***sclerosis***, and ***osteophytosis*** (Table 58.1 and Fig. 58.1). If all three of these findings are not present on the radiograph, another diagnosis should be considered. Joint space narrowing is the least specific finding of the three; yet, it is virtually always present in DJD. Unfortunately, joint space narrowing is also seen in almost every other joint abnormality.

Sclerosis should be present in varying amounts in all cases of DJD unless severe osteoporosis is present. Osteoporosis will cause the sclerosis to be diminished. For instance, in long-standing rheumatoid arthritis in which the cartilage has been destroyed, DJD often occurs with very little sclerosis. Osteophytosis will be diminished in the setting of osteoporosis also. Otherwise, sclerosis and osteophytosis should be prominent in DJD.

The only disorder that will cause osteophytes without sclerosis or joint space narrowing is diffuse idiopathic skeletal hyperostosis. This is a common bone-forming disorder that at first glance resembles DJD, except that there is no joint space narrowing (or disc space narrowing in the spine) and there is no sclerosis (Fig. 58.2). Diffuse idiopathic skeletal hyperostosis is not believed to be caused by trauma or stress as is DJD and is not painful or disabling as DJD can be. Millions of dollars per year are awarded to federal employees at retirement, representing "disability" payments for supposed DJD acquired during their employment, when, in fact, these retirees have diffuse idiopathic skeletal hyperostosis and have been misdiagnosed.

Osteoarthritis is divided into two types: primary and secondary. Secondary osteoarthritis is what radiologists refer to when speaking of DJD. It is, as mentioned, secondary to trauma of some sort. It can occur in any joint in the body but is particularly common in the hands, knees, hips, and spine.

Primary osteoarthritis is a familial arthritis that affects middle-aged women almost exclusively and is seen only in the hands. It affects the distal interphalangeal joints, the proximal interphalangeal joints, and the base of the thumb in a bilaterally symmetrical fashion (Fig. 58.3). If it is not bilaterally symmetrical, the diagnosis of primary osteoarthritis should be questioned.

A type of primary osteoarthritis that can be very painful and debilitating is erosive osteoarthritis. It has the identical distribution mentioned for primary osteoarthritis but is associated with osteoporosis of the hands, as well as erosions. It is uncommon, and radiologists generally see little of this disorder. It is also called Kellgren arthritis.

There are a few exceptions to the classic triad of findings seen in DJD (sclerosis, joint space narrowing, and osteophytes). Several joints may also exhibit erosions as a manifestation of DJD: the ***temporomandibular joint***, the ***acromioclavicular joint***, the ***sacroiliac (SI) joints***, and the ***symphysis pubis*** (Table 58.2). When erosions are seen in one of these joints, DJD must be considered or inappropriate treatment may be instituted (Fig. 58.4).

A subchondral cyst or geode (taken from the geologic term used when a volcanic rock has a gas pocket that leaves a large cavity in the rock) is often found in joints affected with DJD. Geodes are cystic formations that occur around joints in various disorders, including, in addition to ***DJD***, ***rheumatoid arthritis***, ***calcium pyrophosphate dihydrate crystal deposition disease (CPPD)***, and ***avascular necrosis (AVN)*** (Table 58.3). Presumably, one method of geode formation is that synovial fluid is forced into the subchondral bone, causing a cystic collection of joint fluid. Another etiology is following a bone contusion in which the contused bone forms a cyst. They rarely cause problems by themselves but are often misdiagnosed as something more sinister (Fig. 58.5).

TABLE 58.1

HALLMARKS OF DEGENERATIVE JOINT DISEASE

Joint space narrowing
Sclerosis
Osteophytes

RHEUMATOID ARTHRITIS

Rheumatoid arthritis is an autoimmune connective tissue disorder of unknown etiology that can affect any synovial joint in the body. The radiographic hallmarks are ***soft tissue swelling***, ***osteoporosis***, ***joint space narrowing***, and ***marginal erosions***. In the hands, it is classically a ***proximal*** process that is ***bilaterally symmetrical*** (Table 58.4 and Fig. 58.6). There are so many exceptions to these rules, however, that I have come to regard them as no better than 80% accurate. Rheumatoid arthritis has a large variety of appearances, and from its radiographic appearance alone, it can be very difficult to diagnose with any degree of assurance.

Rheumatoid arthritis in large joints is fairly characteristic in that it causes marked joint space narrowing and is associated with osteoporosis. Erosions might or might not be present and tend to be marginal—that is, away from the weight-bearing portion of the joint. In the hip, the femoral head tends to migrate axially, whereas in osteoarthritis, it tends to migrate superolaterally (Figs. 58.7 and 58.8). In the shoulder, the humeral head tends to be "high-riding" (Fig. 58.9). Other things to think of when confronted with a high-riding shoulder are a torn rotator cuff and CPPD (Table 58.5).

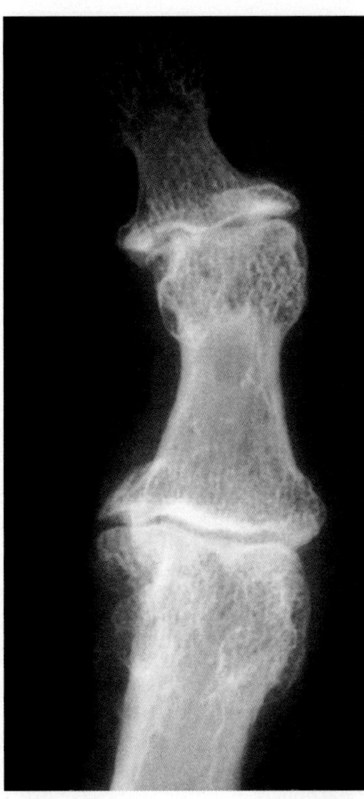

FIGURE 58.1. Osteoarthritis (DJD). A radiograph of a finger with osteoarthritis (DJD) of the distal and proximal interphalangeal joints. Both joints demonstrate joint space narrowing, subchondral sclerosis, and osteophytosis, which are hallmarks of degenerative joint disease.

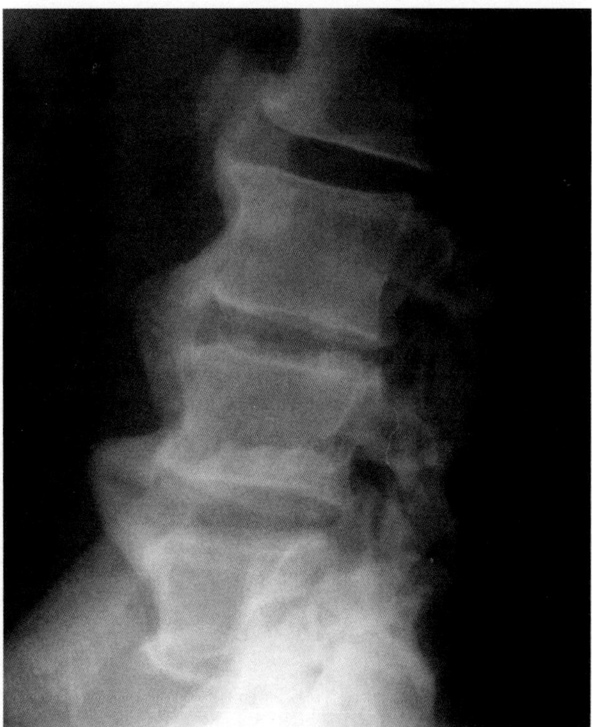

FIGURE 58.2. Diffuse Idiopathic Skeletal Hyperostosis. A lateral view of the lumbar spine shows extensive osteophytosis without significant disc space narrowing or sclerosis. This is a classic picture for diffuse idiopathic skeletal hyperostosis.

TABLE 58.2

JOINTS THAT HAVE EROSIONS AS A FEATURE OF DEGENERATIVE JOINT DISEASE

Sacroiliac
Acromioclavicular
Temporomandibular
Symphysis pubis

TABLE 58.3

DISEASES IN WHICH GEODES ARE FOUND

Degenerative joint disease
Rheumatoid arthritis
CPPD
Avascular necrosis

TABLE 58.4

HALLMARKS OF RHEUMATOID ARTHRITIS

Soft tissue swelling
Osteoporosis
Joint space narrowing
Marginal erosions
Proximal distribution (hands)
Bilaterally symmetric

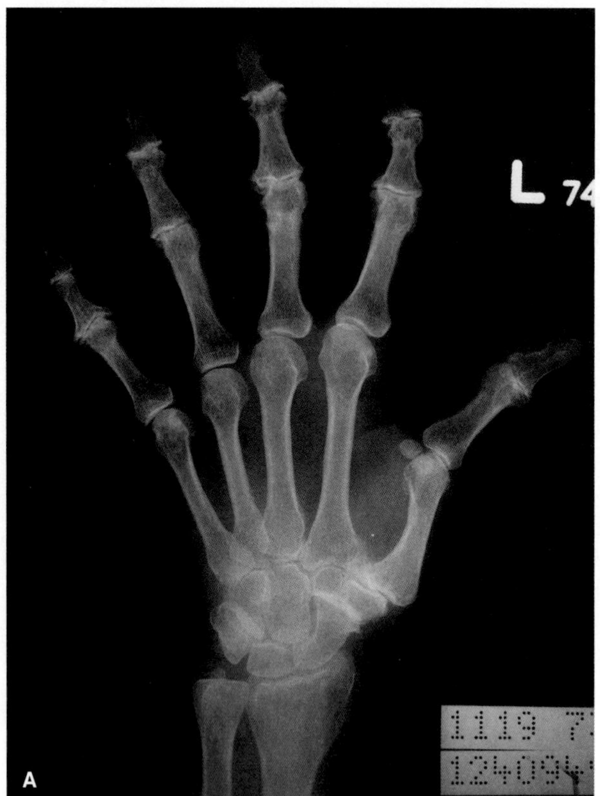

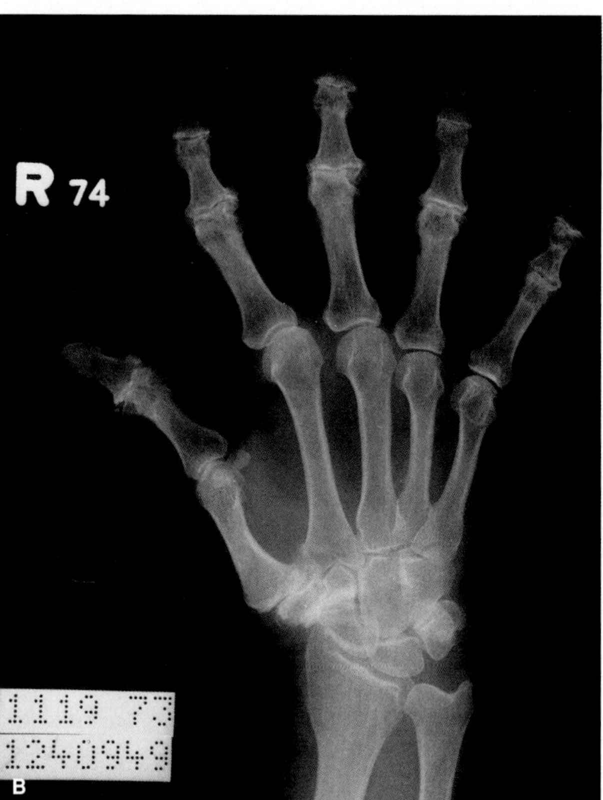

FIGURE 58.3. **Primary Osteoarthritis.** Bilateral hand radiographs (**A** and **B**) in a patient with primary osteoarthritis. Present are classic findings of osteophytosis, joint space narrowing, and sclerosis at the distal interphalangeal joints, the proximal interphalangeal joints, and at the base of the thumb. This is bilaterally symmetrical, which is typical for primary osteoarthritis.

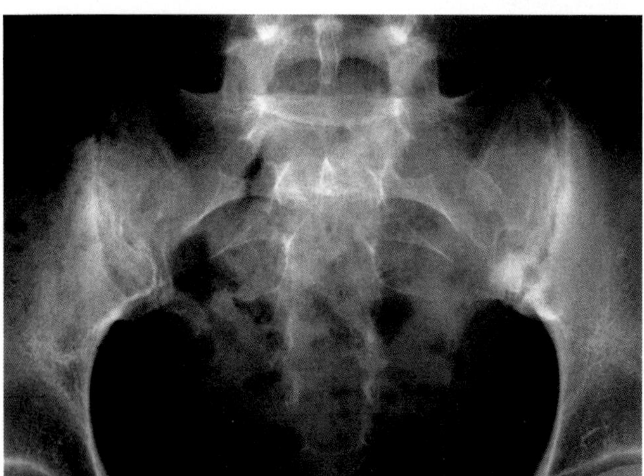

FIGURE 58.4. **Osteoarthritis of the Sacroiliac (SI) Joint.** A young woman who is a professional dancer complained of left-sided hip pain. An AP view of the pelvis demonstrated left SI joint sclerosis, joint irregularity, and erosions. A complete workup to rule out a human leukocyte antigen (HLA)-B27 spondyloarthropathy was negative, and no laboratory or clinical evidence for infection was found. Her clinical history pointed to this being completely occupation related, and an aspiration biopsy to rule out infection was therefore not performed. This is not an unusual appearance for DJD of the SI joints.

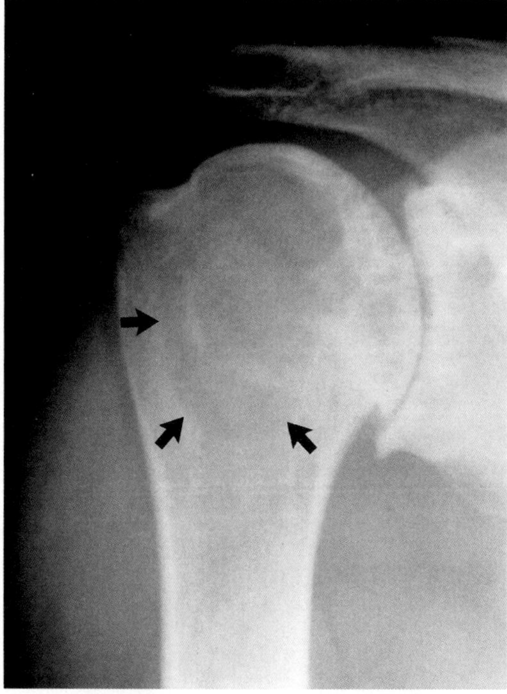

FIGURE 58.5. **Subchondral Cyst or Geode of the Shoulder.** This patient has marked degenerative joint disease (DJD) of the shoulder with joint space narrowing, sclerosis, and osteophytosis. A large lytic process (*arrows*) is seen in the humeral head, which is a subchondral cyst or geode often seen in association with DJD. Because of the DJD in the shoulder, a biopsy to rule out a more sinister lesion in the humeral head should be avoided.

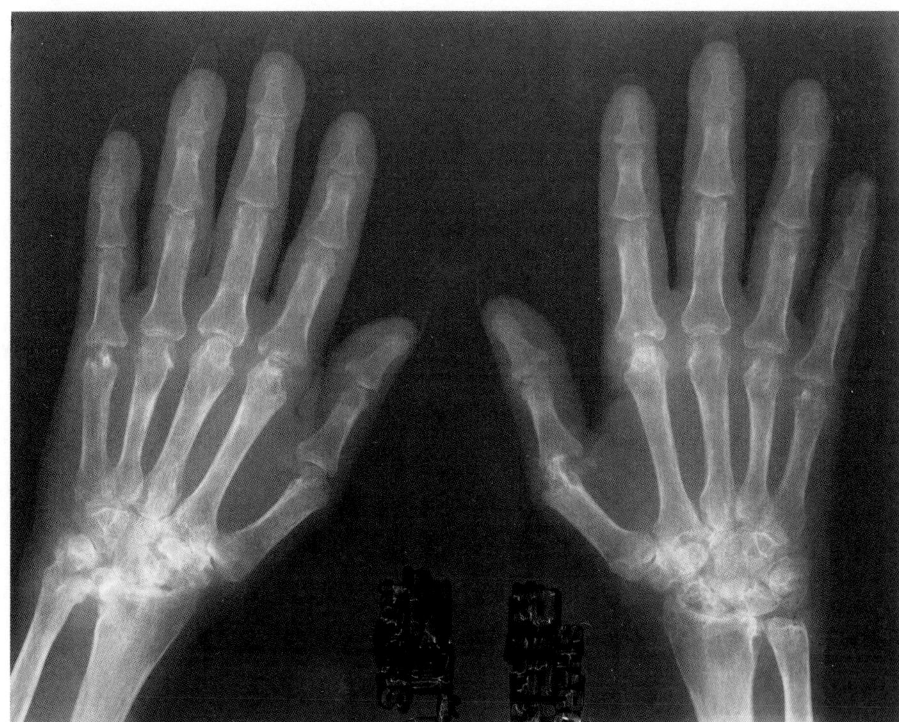

FIGURE 58.6. Rheumatoid Arthritis. An erosive arthritis affecting primarily the carpal bones and the metacarpophalangeal joints is seen, which has associated osteoporosis and soft tissue swelling (note the soft tissue over the ulnar styloid processes). It is a bilaterally symmetrical process in this patient, which is classic.

TABLE 58.5

CAUSES OF HIGH-RIDING SHOULDER

Rheumatoid arthritis
CPPD
Torn rotator cuff

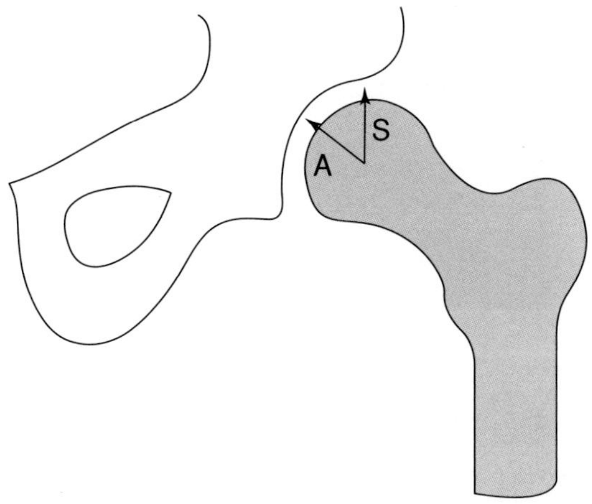

FIGURE 58.7. Migration of the Femoral Head. A drawing of the hip showing routes of migration of the femoral head. Osteoarthritis of the hip tends to cause superior (*S*) migration of the femoral head in relation to the acetabulum, whereas rheumatoid arthritis tends to cause axial (*A*) migration of the femoral head in relation to the acetabulum.

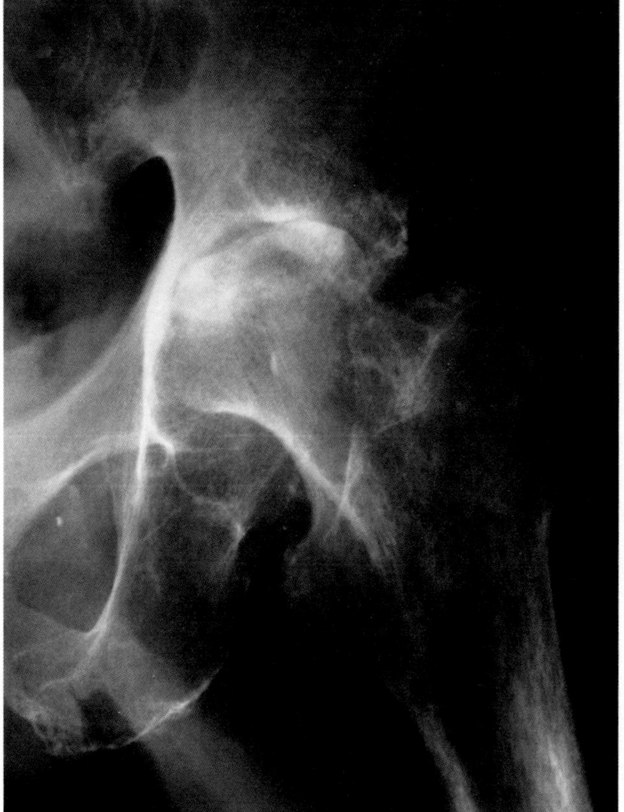

FIGURE 58.8. Rheumatoid Arthritis of the Hip. Note the severe joint space narrowing in this patient with rheumatoid arthritis. The femoral head has migrated in an axial direction with fairly concentric joint space narrowing. Minimal secondary degenerative changes have occurred as noted by the sclerosis in the superior portion of the joint; however, these have been diminished somewhat by the osteoporosis that usually accompanies rheumatoid arthritis.

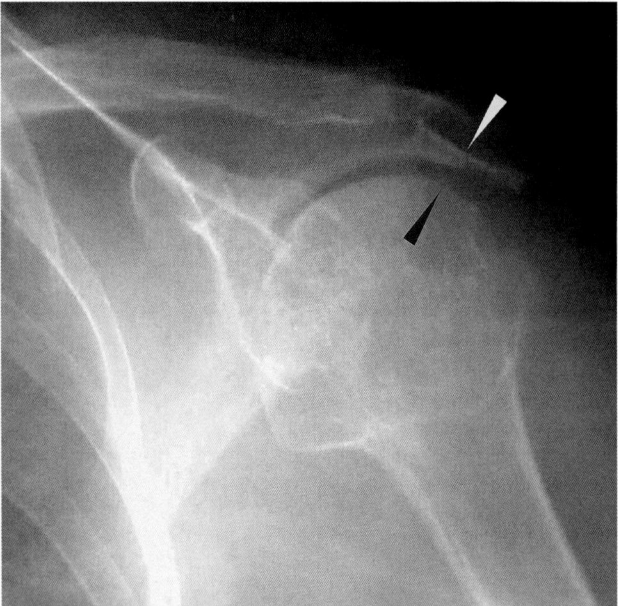

FIGURE 58.9. **Rheumatoid Arthritis in the Shoulder.** An AP view of the shoulder in this patient with rheumatoid arthritis shows that the distance between the acromion and the humeral head is diminished (*arrows*). Ordinarily, this space is about 1 cm in width to allow the rotator cuff to pass freely beneath the acromion. This is a common finding in rheumatoid arthritis as well as in CPPD.

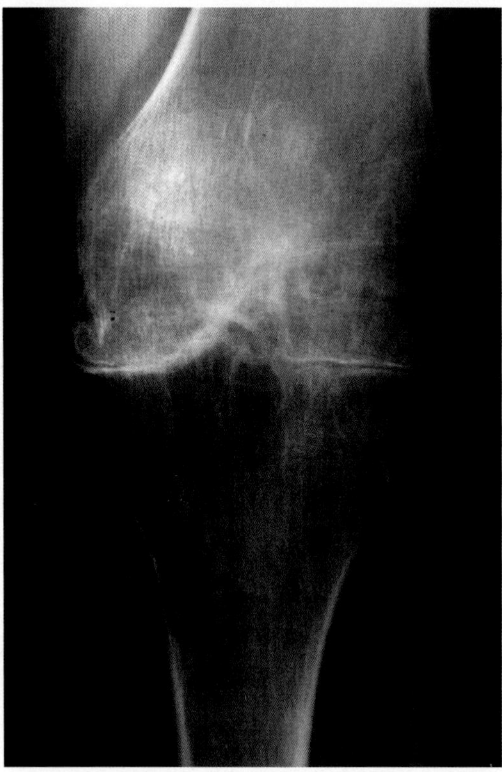

FIGURE 58.10. **Secondary Degenerative Joint Disease (DJD) in the Knee in a Patient With Rheumatoid Arthritis.** This patient has a history of long-standing rheumatoid arthritis. An AP view of the knee shows severe osteoporosis and joint space narrowing. Secondary DJD is occurring, as evidenced by the sclerosis and osteophytosis; however, these findings are out of proportion to the severe joint space narrowing. When DJD narrows a joint to this extent, the osteophytosis and the sclerosis are invariably much more pronounced.

When rheumatoid arthritis is long standing, it is not unusual for secondary DJD to superimpose itself on the findings one would expect with rheumatoid arthritis. This picture of DJD differs somewhat from that usually seen, in that the sclerosis and the osteophytes are considerably diminished in severity as compared with the joint space narrowing (Fig. 58.10).

HLA-B27 SPONDYLOARTHROPATHIES

A group of diseases that was formerly known as rheumatoid variants is now known as the seronegative, human leukocyte antigen B27 (HLA-B27)–positive spondyloarthropathies. These disorders are all linked to the HLA-B27 histocompatibility antigen. Included in this group of diseases are ankylosing spondylitis, inflammatory bowel disease, psoriatic arthritis, and reactive arthritis (previously called Reiter syndrome). They are characterized by bony ankylosis, proliferative new bone formation, and predominantly axial (spinal) involvement.

One of the more characteristic findings in these disorders is that of syndesmophytes in the spine. A syndesmophyte is a paravertebral ossification that resembles an osteophyte, except that it runs vertically, whereas an osteophyte has its orientation in a horizontal axis. Sometimes it can be difficult to decide whether a particular paravertebral ossification is an osteophyte or a syndesmophyte based on its orientation alone (Fig. 58.11).

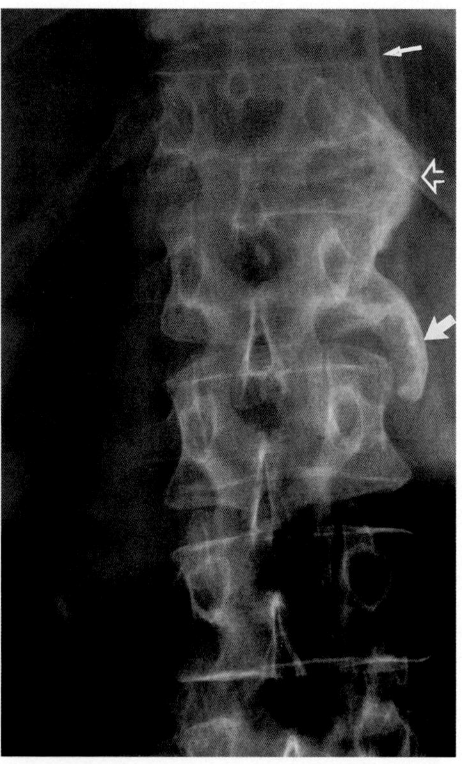

FIGURE 58.11. **Psoriasis With Syndesmophytes.** The large paravertebral ossification on the left side of the T12–LI disc space (*open arrow*) is difficult to differentiate between an osteophyte and a syndesmophyte. Either could have this appearance. The paravertebral ossification at the left LI–L2 disc space (*large solid arrow*) definitely has a vertical rather than a horizontal orientation, however, as does the faint ossification seen at the T11–T12 disc space (*small solid arrow*). These definitely represent syndesmophytes. It makes sense, therefore, to assume that the ossification at the T12–LI disc space is almost certainly a syndesmophyte as well. This patient has large nonmarginal, asymmetrical syndesmophytes, which are typical of psoriatic arthritis or reactive arthritis. This patient has psoriasis.

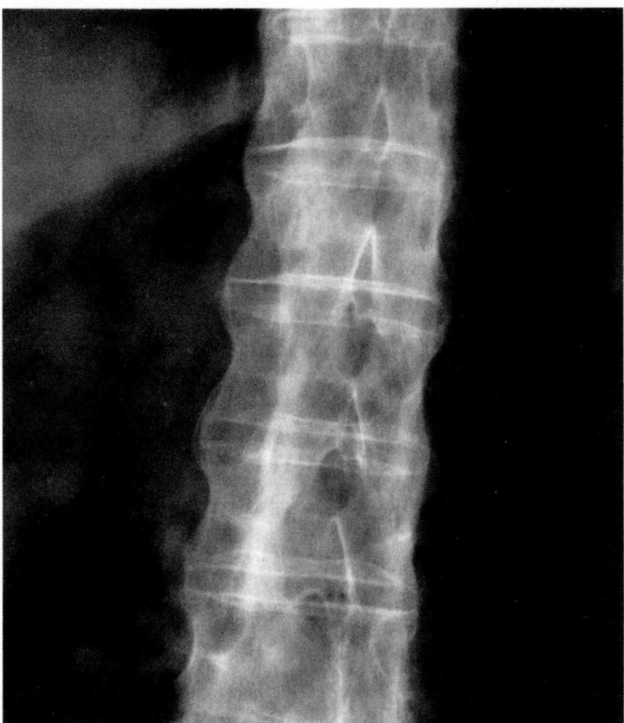

FIGURE 58.12. **Marginal, Symmetrical Syndesmophytes in Ankylosing Spondylitis.** Bilateral marginal syndesmophytes are seen bridging the disc spaces throughout the lumbar spine in this patient. This is a so-called bamboo spine and is classic for ankylosing spondylitis and inflammatory bowel disease.

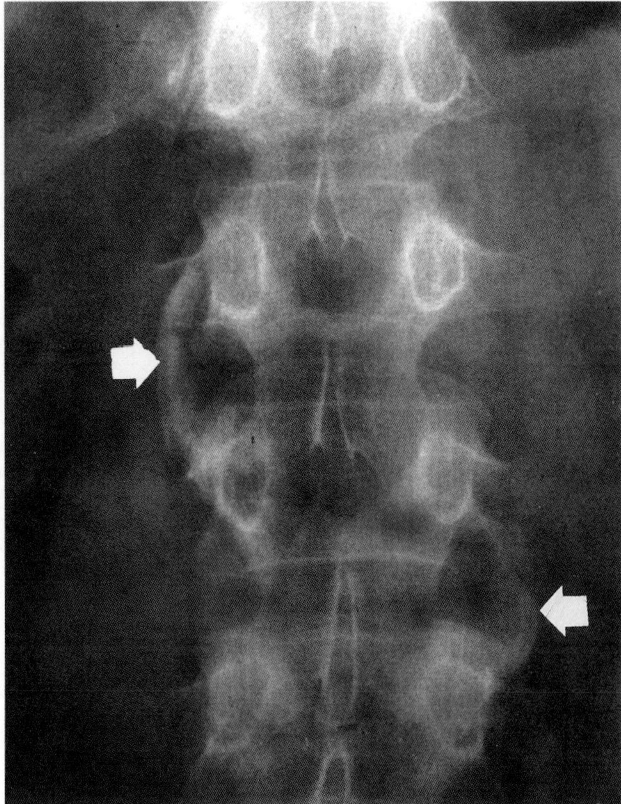

FIGURE 58.13. **Syndesmophytes in Psoriatic Arthritis.** Large, bulky, nonmarginal, asymmetrical syndesmophytes (*arrows*) are seen in this patient with psoriatic arthritis.

Bridging osteophytes and large syndesmophytes can have a similar appearance, with both having an orientation halfway between vertical and horizontal. How should one evaluate those cases? Look at the other vertebral bodies and use the ossifications on them to determine whether they are osteophytes or syndesmophytes. If no other level is involved, one might not be able to tell one from the other.

Syndesmophytes are classified as to whether they are marginal and symmetrical or nonmarginal and asymmetrical. A marginal syndesmophyte has its origin at the edge or margin of a vertebral body and extends to the margin of the adjacent vertebral body. They are invariably bilaterally symmetrical as viewed on an AP spine radiograph. Ankylosing spondylitis classically has marginal, symmetrical syndesmophytes (Fig. 58.12). Inflammatory bowel disease has an identical appearance when the spine is involved. Nonmarginal, asymmetrical syndesmophytes

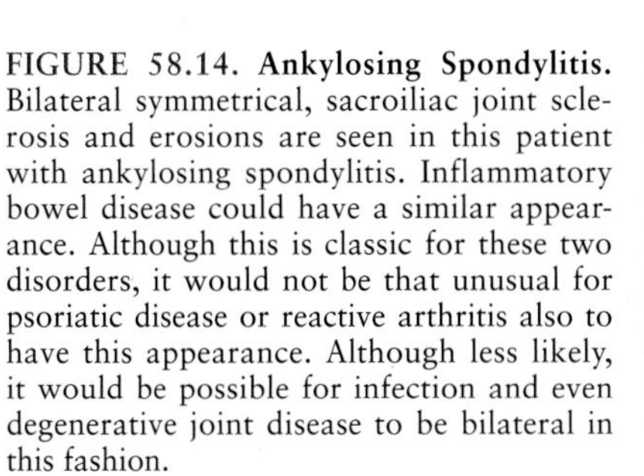

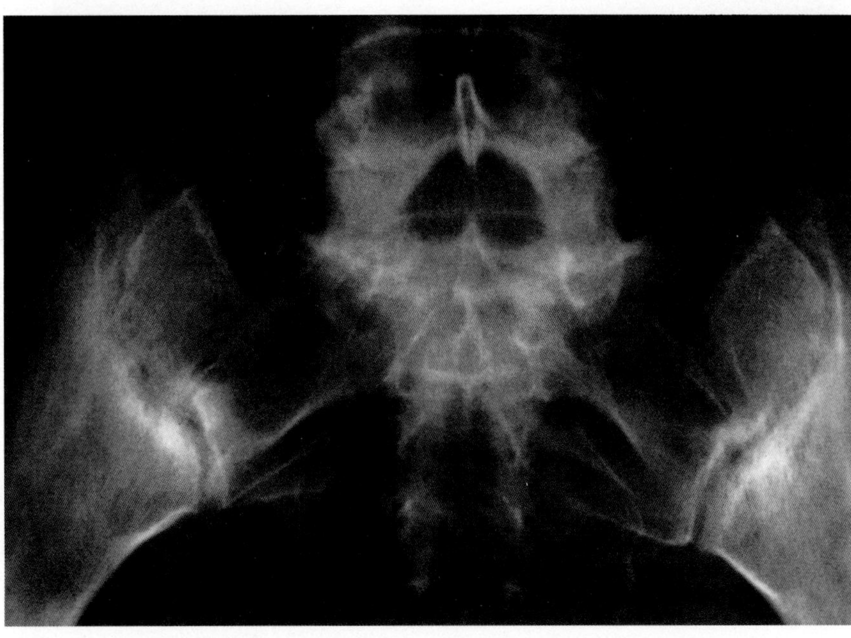

FIGURE 58.14. **Ankylosing Spondylitis.** Bilateral symmetrical, sacroiliac joint sclerosis and erosions are seen in this patient with ankylosing spondylitis. Inflammatory bowel disease could have a similar appearance. Although this is classic for these two disorders, it would not be that unusual for psoriatic disease or reactive arthritis also to have this appearance. Although less likely, it would be possible for infection and even degenerative joint disease to be bilateral in this fashion.

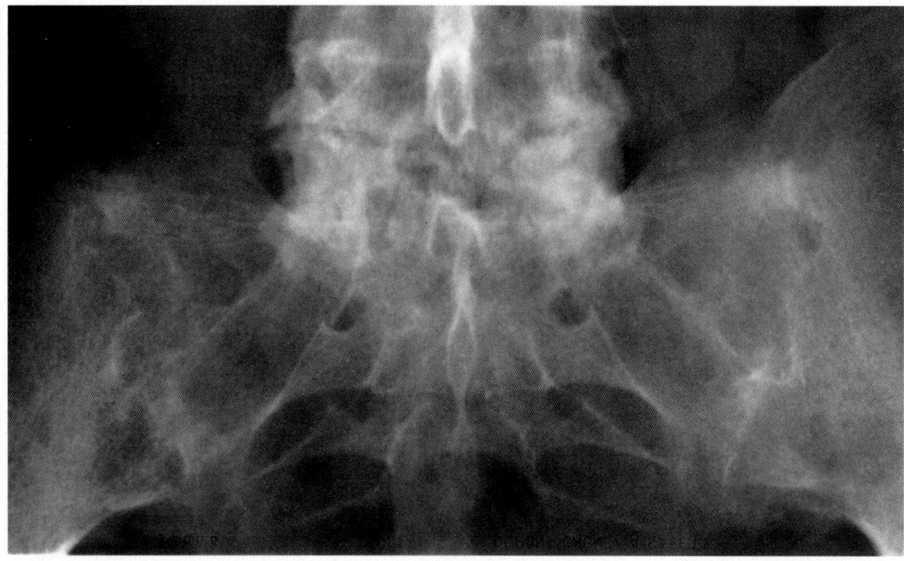

FIGURE 58.15. Fusion of the Sacroiliac (SI) Joints in Ankylosing Spondylitis. Bilateral complete fusion of the SI joints in this patient with ankylosing spondylitis makes the SI joints totally indistinguishable. Inflammatory bowel disease could have a similar appearance.

are generally large and bulky. They emanate from the vertebral body away from the endplate or margin and are unilateral or asymmetrical as viewed on an AP spine radiograph (Figs. 58.11 and 58.13). Psoriatic arthritis and reactive arthritis classically have this type of syndesmophyte.

Involvement of the SI joints is common in the HLA-B27 spondyloarthropathies. The patterns of involvement, like the patterns of involvement of the spine, are somewhat typical for each disorder. Ankylosing spondylitis and inflammatory bowel disease typically cause bilaterally symmetrical SI joint disease, which is initially erosive in nature and progresses to sclerosis and fusion (Figs. 58.14 and 58.15). It is extremely unusual to have asymmetrical or unilateral SI joint disease in these two disorders.

Reactive arthritis and psoriatic arthritis can exhibit unilateral or bilateral SI joint involvement. It seems that it is bilateral about 50% of the time. It is often asymmetrical when it is bilateral, but exact symmetry can be difficult to assess; therefore, when it is definitely bilateral and not clearly asymmetrical, consider the SI joints to be in the bilateral symmetrical category. This means that if there is bilateral, symmetrical SI joint disease, it could be caused by any of the four HLA-B27 spondyloarthropathies. If there is unilateral (or clearly asymmetrical) SI joint involvement, one can exclude ankylosing spondylitis and inflammatory bowel disease and consider reactive arthritis or psoriatic disease. In this latter example, one would also have to consider infection and DJD (remember that DJD can cause erosions in the SI joints). Although seen less commonly, gout can also affect the SI joints unilaterally (Table 58.6 and Figs. 58.4 and 58.16).

Computed tomography can be very helpful in examining the SI joints and is considered by many to be the diagnostic procedure of choice because of the unobstructed view of the entire joint (Fig. 58.17).

Large joint involvement with the HLA-B27 spondyloarthropathies is uncommon (except for ankylosing spondylitis),

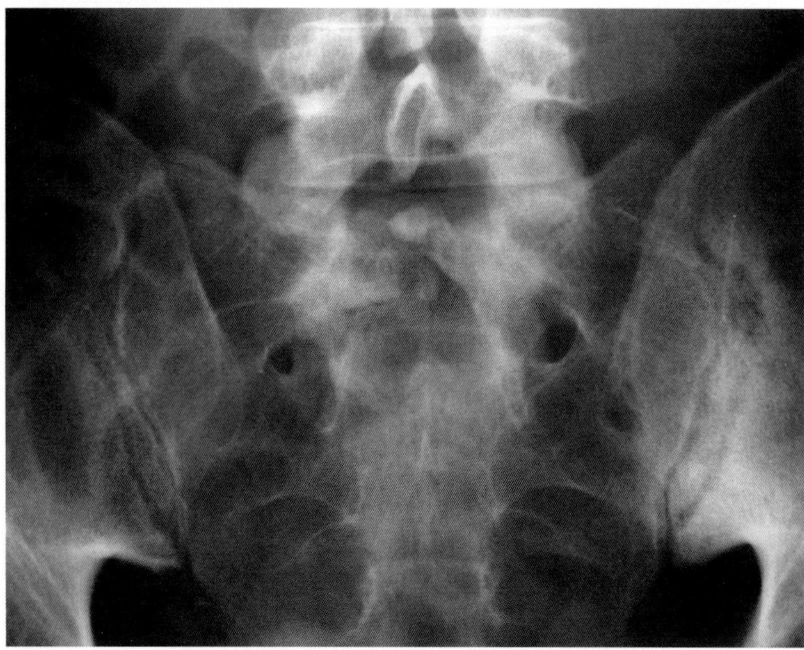

FIGURE 58.16. Psoriasis With Sacroiliac (SI) Joint Disease. Unilateral SI sclerosis and erosions are seen in this patient with psoriasis. Ankylosing spondylitis and inflammatory bowel disease virtually never have this appearance.

TABLE 58.6

CAUSES OF SACROILIAC JOINT DISEASE

Ankylosing spondylitis
Inflammatory bowel disease
Psoriasis
Reactive arthritis
Infection
Degenerative joint disease (DJD)
Gout

but when it does occur, the arthropathy will resemble rheumatoid arthritis (Fig. 58.18). The hips are involved in up to 50% of the patients with ankylosing spondylitis.

Small joint involvement, specifically in the hands and the feet, is not common in ankylosing spondylitis and inflammatory bowel disease. Psoriasis causes a distinctive arthropathy that is characterized by its ***distal*** predominance, ***proliferative erosions***, ***soft tissue swelling***, and ***periostitis***. Proliferative erosions are different from the clean-cut, sharply marginated erosions seen in all other erosive arthritides in that they have fuzzy margins with wisps of periostitis emanating from them (Fig. 58.19A). The severe forms are often associated with bony ankylosis across joints (Fig. 58.19B) and arthritis mutilans deformities. A fairly common finding is a calcaneal heel spur that has fuzzy margins as opposed to the well-corticated heel spur seen in DJD or post trauma (Fig. 58.20).

Reactive arthritis causes identical changes in every respect to psoriasis, with the exception that the hands are not as commonly involved as the feet and reactive arthritis occurs almost exclusively in men. The interphalangeal joint of the great toe is a commonly affected location in reactive arthritis (Fig. 58.21).

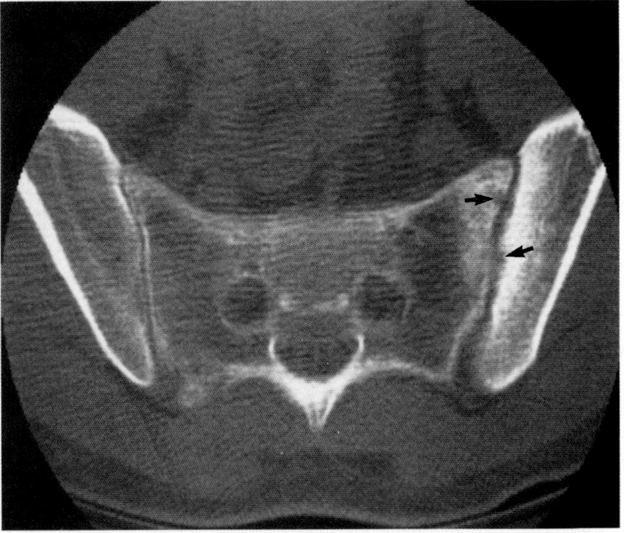

FIGURE 58.17. **CT of the Sacroiliac (SI) Joints in Psoriasis.** A CT scan through the SI joints in this patient with psoriasis shows unilateral SI joint sclerosis and erosions (*arrows*), typical for psoriasis or reactive arthritis. Infection could have a similar appearance.

CRYSTAL-INDUCED ARTHRITIS

The crystal-induced arthritides include primarily gout and pseudogout (CPPD). Ochronosis and Wilson disease are so rare that they are not covered in this chapter.

Gout

Gout is a metabolic disorder that results in hyperuricemia and leads to monosodium urate crystals being deposited in various

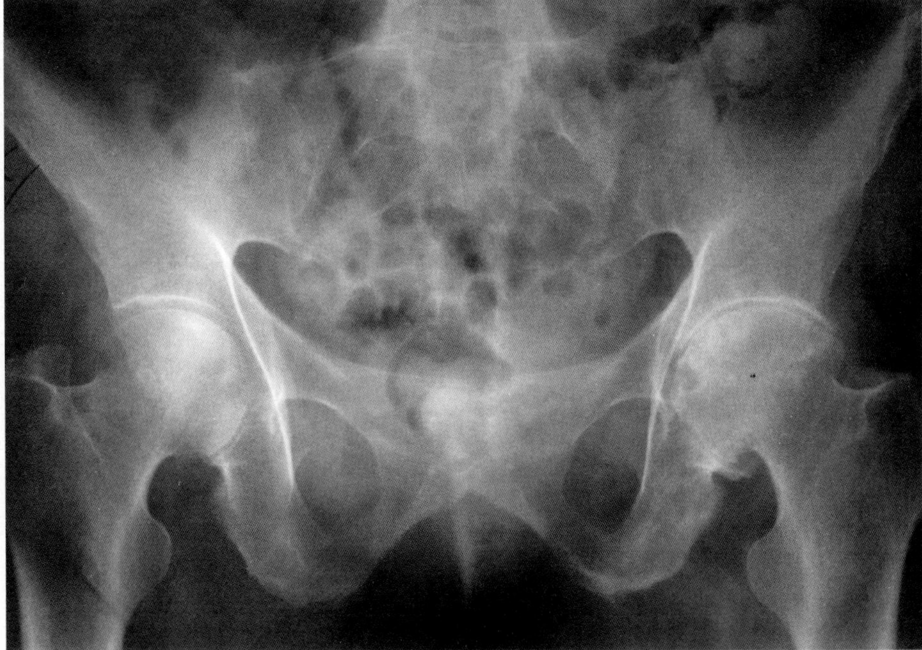

FIGURE 58.18. **Ankylosing Spondylitis With Hip Disease.** An anteroposterior view of the pelvis in this patient with ankylosing spondylitis shows bilateral complete fusion of the sacroiliac (SI) joints. Concentric left hip joint narrowing is present with axial migration of the femoral head. This would be a typical finding in rheumatoid arthritis; however, the SI joint changes make this typical for ankylosing spondylitis. Note the secondary degenerative joint disease changes in the left hip as well.

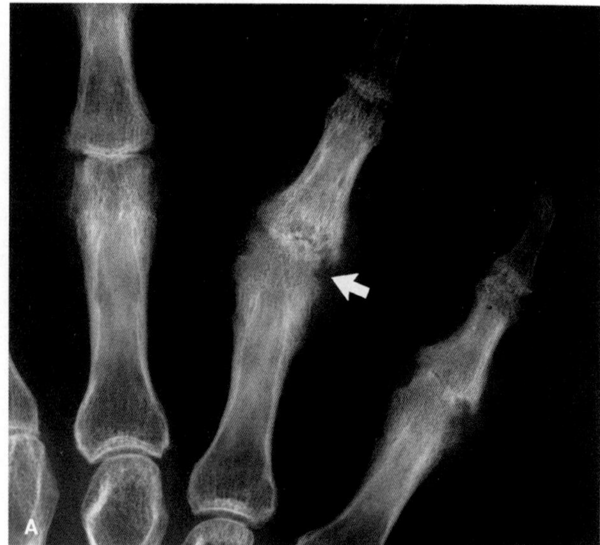

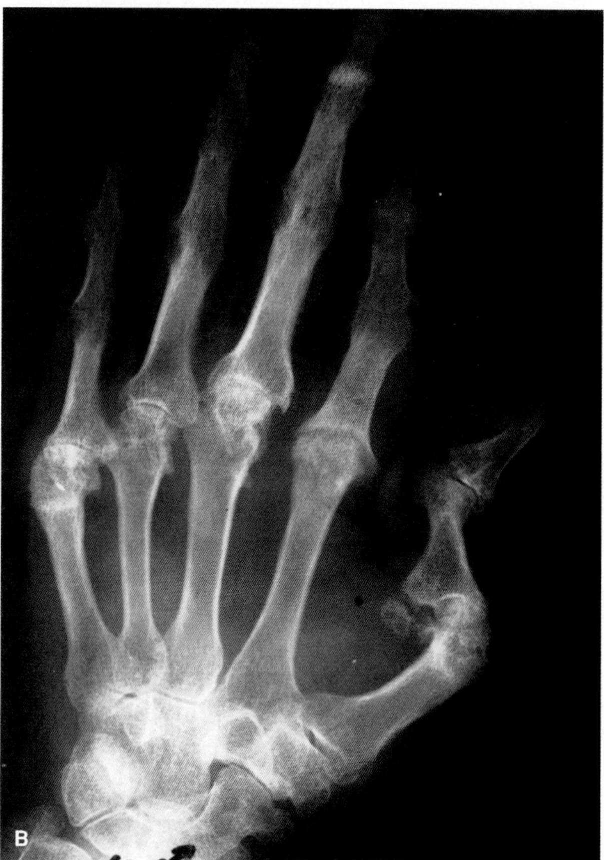

FIGURE 58.19. Psoriatic Arthritis. A: Cartilage loss at the proximal interphalangeal joints of the third, fourth, and fifth digits in this hand is apparent, with erosions noted most prominently in the fourth digit (*arrow*). These erosions are not sharply demarcated but are covered with fluffy new bone. These are termed proliferative erosions. Note also the periostitis along the shafts of each of the proximal phalanges. **B:** Advanced psoriatic arthritis. Fusion or ankylosis is apparent across the proximal interphalangeal joints of the second through the fifth digits. Several of the distal interphalangeal joints are also ankylosed. Severe joint space narrowing at the metacarpophalangeal joints is noted. This distal distribution is typical for psoriatic arthritis in advanced stages.

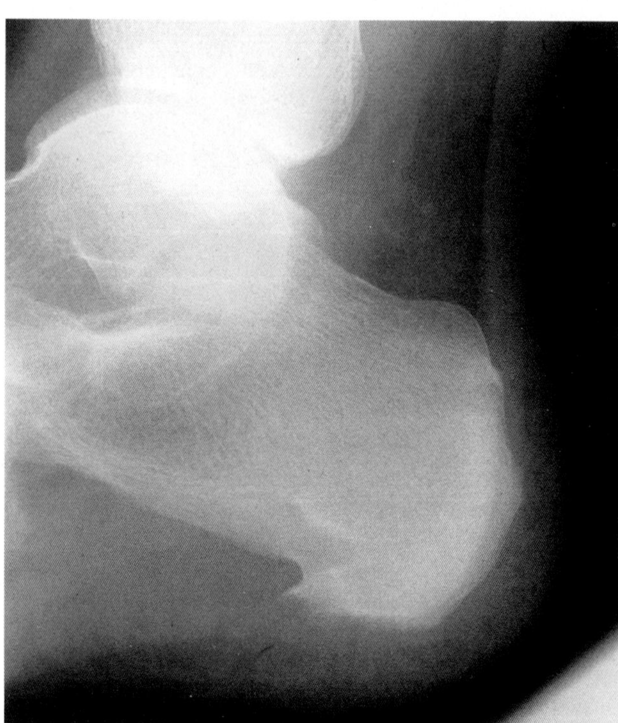

FIGURE 58.20. Reactive Arthritis. A lateral view of a calcaneus in a patient with reactive arthritis shows poorly defined new bone on the posteroinferior margin of the calcaneus with a calcaneal spur, which is also poorly defined. This is typical of psoriatic or reactive arthritis as opposed to the well-formed calcaneal spur in degenerative joint disease.

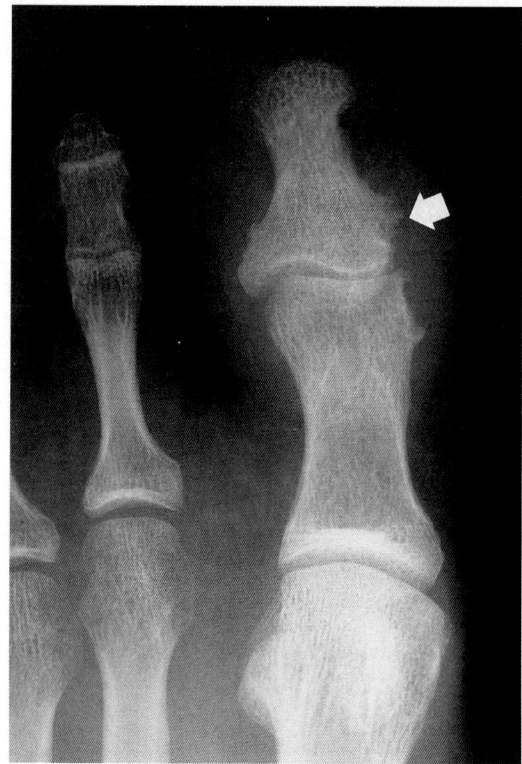

FIGURE 58.21. Reactive Arthritis. An AP view of the large toe in a patient with reactive arthritis shows fluffy periostitis (*arrow*) in the erosions adjacent to the interphalangeal joint of the great toe. Marked soft tissue swelling is also present throughout the great toe. These changes are typical in appearance and location for reactive arthritis or psoriasis.

TABLE 58.7

HALLMARKS OF GOUT

Well-defined erosions (sclerotic margins)
Soft tissue nodules
Random distribution
No osteoporosis

sites in the body, especially joints. The actual causes of the hyperuricemia are myriad and include heredity.

The arthropathy caused by gout is very characteristic radiographically. It takes 4 to 6 years for gout to cause radiographically evident disease, and most patients are treated successfully long before the destructive arthropathy occurs; therefore, gouty arthritis is not commonly encountered.

The classic radiographic findings in gout are ***well-defined erosions***, often with sclerotic borders or overhanging edges; ***soft tissue nodules*** that calcify in the presence of renal failure; and a ***random distribution*** in the hands ***without marked osteoporosis*** (Table 58.7 and Fig. 58.22). Even though erosions with overhanging edges occur with gout, they can occur in other disorders as well and are by no means pathognomonic. The sclerotic margins of the erosions are rarely seen in any other arthritide; therefore, this is a very useful differential point. Gout typically affects the metatarsophalangeal joint of the great toe (Fig. 58.23). In the advanced stages, it can be very deforming (Fig. 58.24). Patients with gout often have chondrocalcinosis because they have a predisposition for CPPD; as many as 40% of patients with gout concomitantly have CPPD.

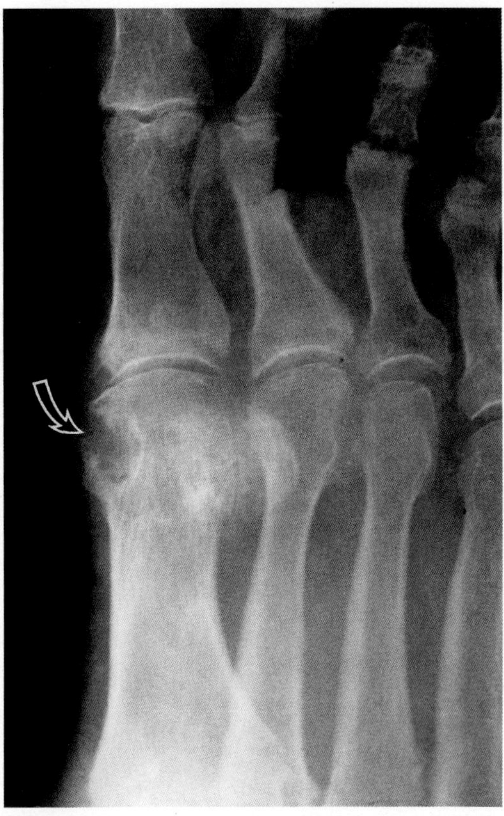

FIGURE 58.23. Gout. A sharply marginated erosion with an overhanging edge (*arrow*) and a sclerotic margin is seen in the first metatarsal head in this patient with gout. This appearance and location are classic for gout, whereas psoriasis and reactive arthritis usually involve the interphalangeal joint and do not have erosions that are this sharply marginated.

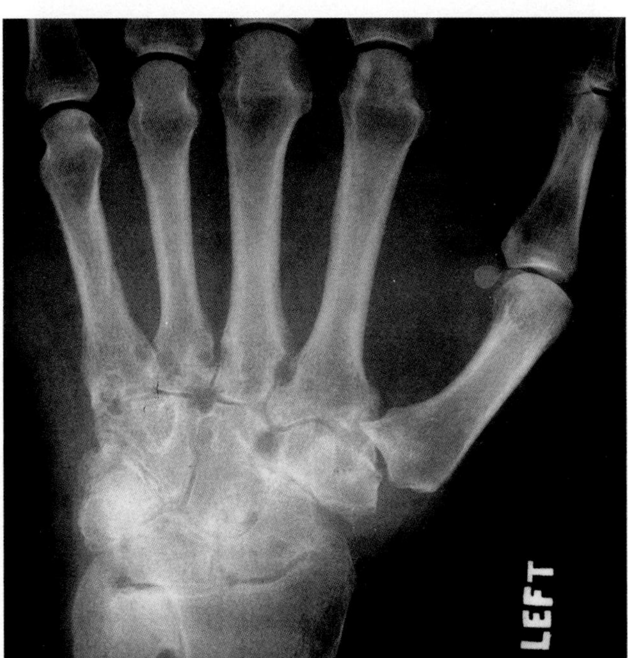

FIGURE 58.22. Gout. Sharply marginated erosions, some with a sclerotic margin, are noted throughout the carpus and proximal metacarpals. These erosions are classic in gout. Note the absence of marked demineralization.

Pseudogout (Calcium Pyrophosphate Dihydrate Crystal Deposition Disease—CPPD)

CPPD has a classic triad: pain, cartilage calcification, and joint destruction. The patient may have any combination of one or more of this triad at any one time. Each of these is addressed individually in some detail in this chapter, but note that two of the three are radiographic findings. This is a disorder that is best diagnosed radiographically.

The pain of CPPD is nonspecific. It can mimic that of gout (hence the term "pseudogout"), infection, or just about any arthritis. It is typically intermittent for a large number of years until DJD occurs and becomes the main cause of pain.

TABLE 58.8

MOST COMMON LOCATION OF CHONDROCALCINOSIS IN CPPD

Knee
Triangular fibrocartilage of wrist
Symphysis pubis

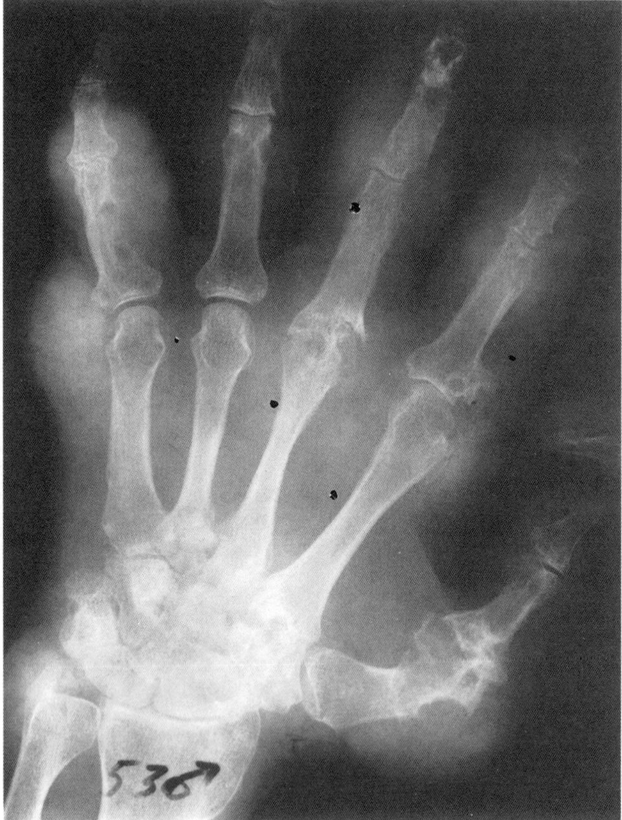

FIGURE 58.24. Advanced Gout. Marked diffuse and focal soft tissue swelling is present throughout the hand and the wrist in this patient with long-standing gout. Destructive, large, well-marginated erosions, some with overhanging edges, are noted near multiple joints. The focal areas of soft tissue swelling are called tophi, some of which are calcified. These only calcify with coexistent renal disease.

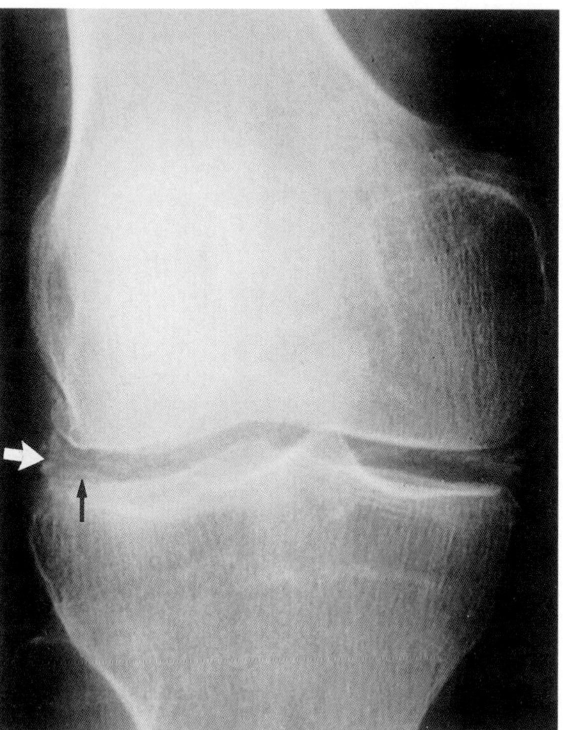

FIGURE 58.25. Chondrocalcinosis in the Knee. Cartilage calcification known as chondrocalcinosis is seen in the fibrocartilage (*white arrow*) and in the hyaline articular cartilage (*black arrow*) in this patient with CPPD.

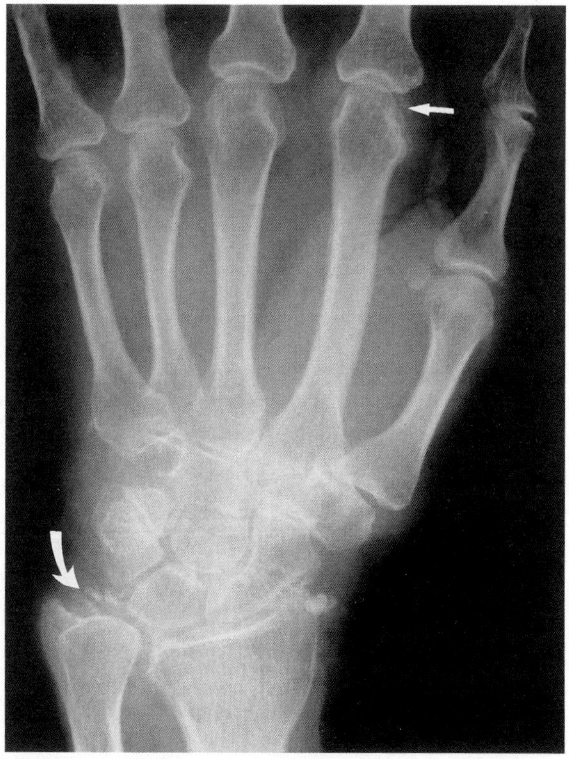

FIGURE 58.26. Chondrocalcinosis in the Wrist. This patient with CPPD exhibits chondrocalcinosis in the triangular fibrocartilage of the wrist (*curved arrow*). A small amount of chondrocalcinosis is also seen in the second metacarpophalangeal joint (*small arrow*). Triangular fibrocartilage calcification is one of the more common locations for chondrocalcinosis to occur.

Cartilage calcification, known as chondrocalcinosis, can occur in any joint but tends to affect a few select sites in most patients. These are the medial and lateral compartments of the ***knee*** (Fig. 58.25), ***the triangular fibrocartilage of the wrist*** (Fig. 58.26), and the ***symphysis pubis*** (Table 58.8). Chondrocalcinosis in these areas is virtually diagnostic of CPPD. When CPPD crystals occur in the soft tissues, such as in the rotator cuff of the shoulder, a radiograph cannot differentiate between CPPD and calcium hydroxyapatite, which occurs in calcific tendinitis. Calcium hydroxyapatite does not occur in the joint cartilage except in extremely unusual cases; therefore, all chondrocalcinosis can be considered to be secondary to CPPD.

The joint destruction or arthropathy is virtually indistinguishable from DJD. In fact, it is DJD. It is caused by CPPD crystals eroding the cartilage. There are a few features of the DJD caused by CPPD that will help distinguish it from DJD caused by trauma or overuse, however. The main difference is one of location. The DJD of CPPD has a proclivity for the ***shoulder***, the ***elbow*** (Fig. 58.27), the ***radiocarpal joint*** in the wrist (Fig. 58.28), the ***patellofemoral joint*** of the knee, and the ***metacarpophalangeal (MCP) joints*** in the hand (Table 58.9). These are areas not normally involved by DJD of wear and tear (such as in the distal interphalangeal joints of the hands, the hips, and the medial compartments of the knees). When DJD is seen in the joints that CPPD tends to involve, a search for chondrocalcinosis should be made. If necessary, a joint aspiration for CPPD crystals may be required to confirm the diagnosis.

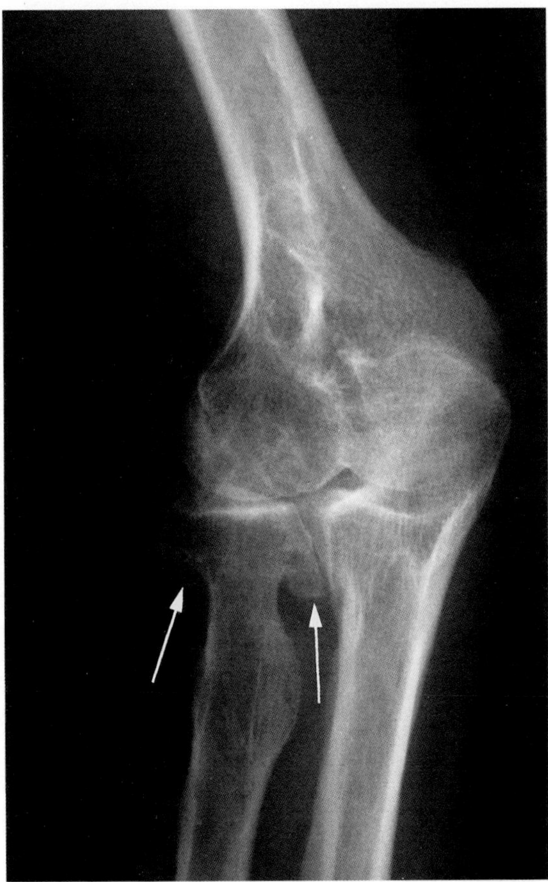

FIGURE 58.27. **Calcium Pyrophosphate Dihydrate Crystal Deposition Disease Arthropathy.** Degenerative joint disease (DJD) of the elbow is seen in this patient with CPPD. Note the joint space narrowing with minimal sclerosis and large osteophytes (*arrows*). Osteophytes of this nature are termed drooping osteophytes and are often seen in CPPD. The elbow is an unusual place for DJD to occur except in the setting of CPPD or trauma.

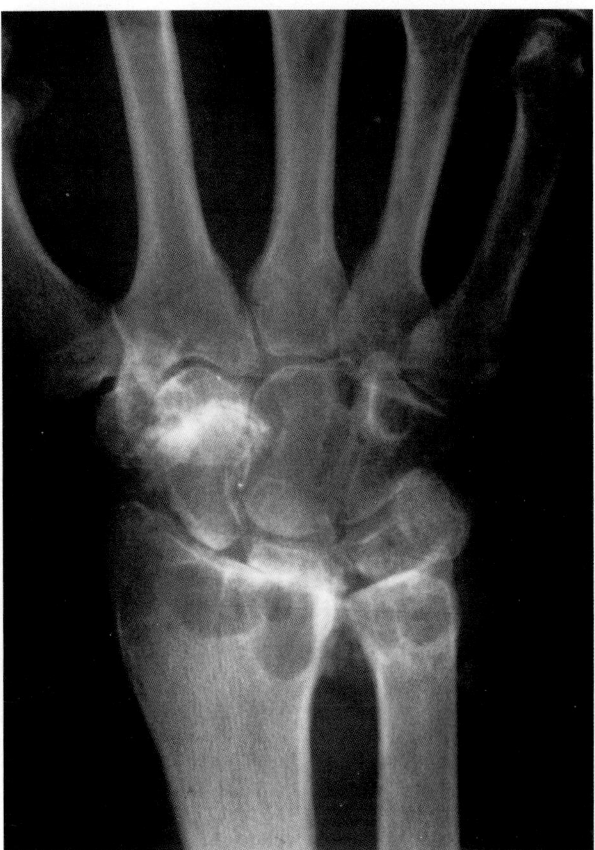

FIGURE 58.28. **Calcium Pyrophosphate Dihydrate Crystal Deposition Disease Arthropathy.** Marked degenerative joint disease (DJD) at the radiocarpal joint is seen in this patient with CPPD. Severe joint space narrowing and sclerosis with large subchondral cysts or geodes are all hallmarks of DJD. This is an unusual location for DJD except in the setting of CPPD or trauma.

Occasionally, the arthropathy of CPPD causes such severe destruction that a neuropathic or Charcot joint is mimicked on the radiograph. This has been termed a pseudo-Charcot joint. It is not a true Charcot joint because of the presence of sensation.

There are three diseases that have a high degree of association with CPPD. These are ***primary hyperparathyroidism***, ***gout***, and ***hemochromatosis*** (Table 58.10). This is not a differential diagnosis for chondrocalcinosis. These are diseases that tend to occur at the same time that CPPD occurs. If the patient has one of these three disorders, he or she is more likely to have CPPD than is a nonaffected person. There is probably no good reason to work up every patient with chondrocalcinosis for one of the three associated diseases because they are so uncommon and CPPD is extremely common.

TABLE 58.9

MOST COMMON LOCATION OF ARTHROPATHY IN CPPD

Shoulder
Radiocarpal joint
Patellofemoral joint
Elbow
MCP joints in hand

COLLAGEN VASCULAR DISEASES

Scleroderma, systemic lupus erythematosus, dermatomyositis, and mixed connective tissue disease are all grouped together as collagen vascular diseases. The striking abnormality in the hands in each of these disorders is osteoporosis and soft tissue wasting. Systemic lupus erythematosus characteristically has severe ulnar deviation of the phalanges (Fig. 58.29). Erosions are generally not a feature of these disorders. Soft tissue calcifications are typically present in scleroderma (Fig. 58.30) and dermatomyositis. The calcifications in scleroderma are

TABLE 58.10

DISEASES WITH HIGH ASSOCIATION WITH CPPD

Primary hyperparathyroidism
Gout
Hemochromatosis

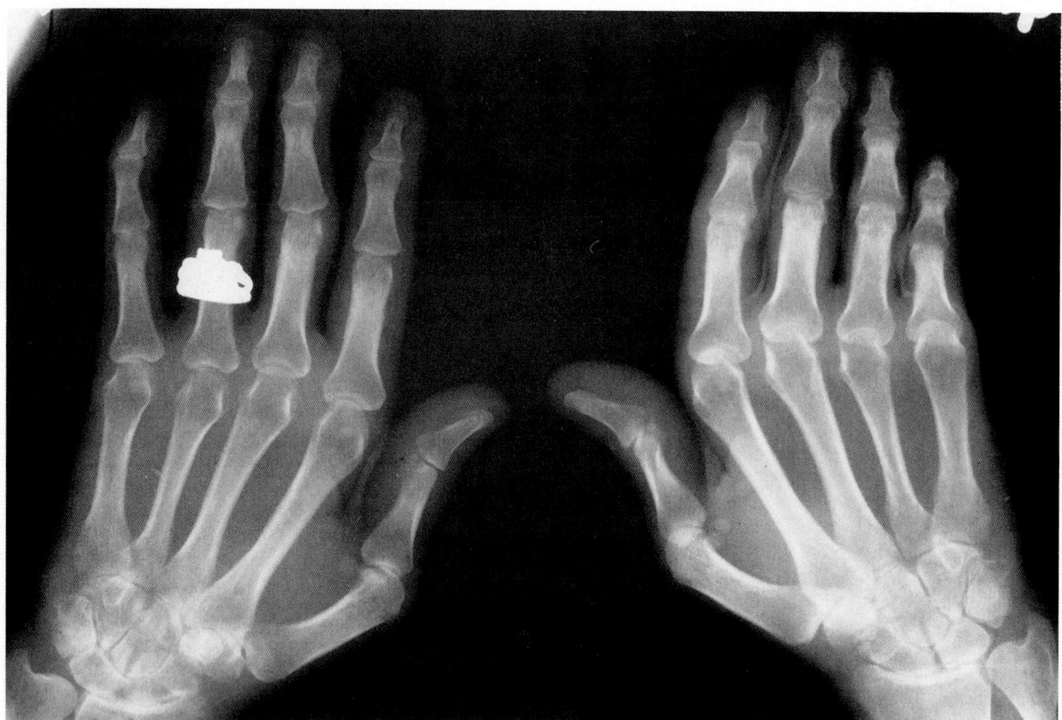

FIGURE 58.29. **Systemic Lupus Erythematosus.** Marked soft tissue wasting, as noted by the concavity in the hypothenar eminence, with ulnar deviation of the phalanges, seen primarily in the right hand, are hallmarks of systemic lupus erythematosus.

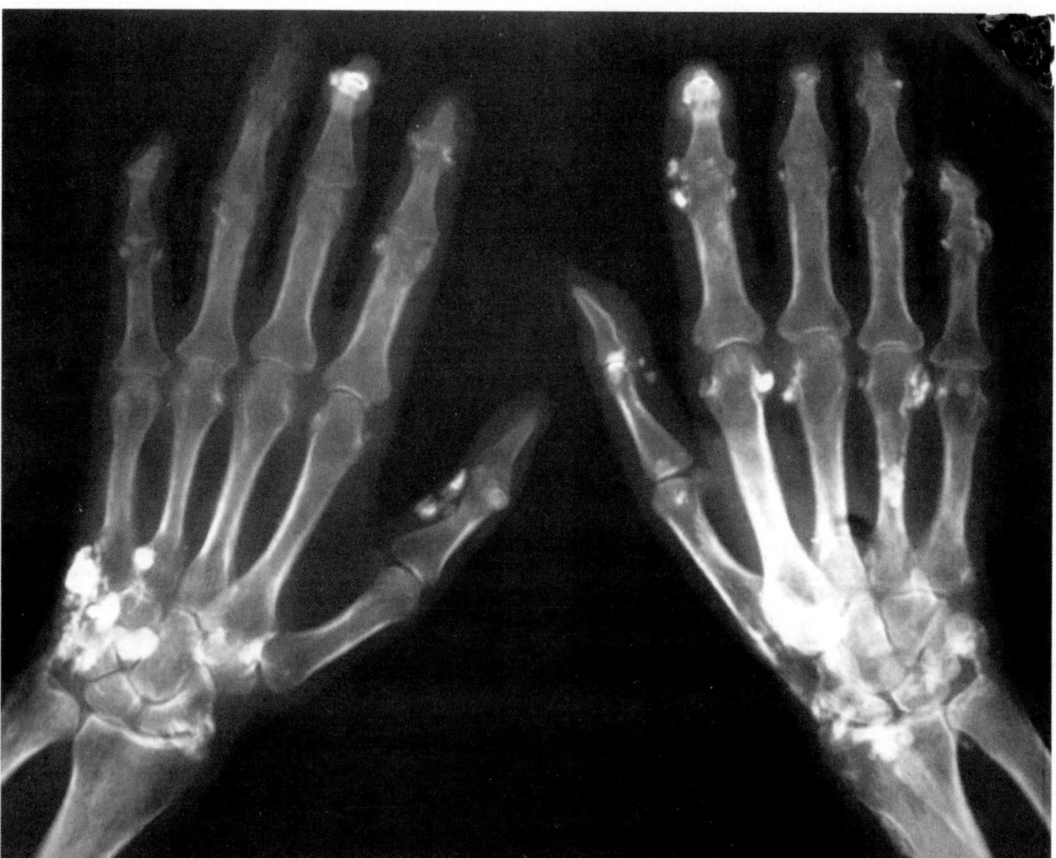

FIGURE 58.30. **Scleroderma.** Diffuse subcutaneous soft tissue calcification is seen throughout the hands and wrists in this patient with scleroderma. Soft tissue wasting and osteoporosis are also present, as well as bone loss in multiple distal phalanges secondary to the vascular abnormalities often present in this disease.

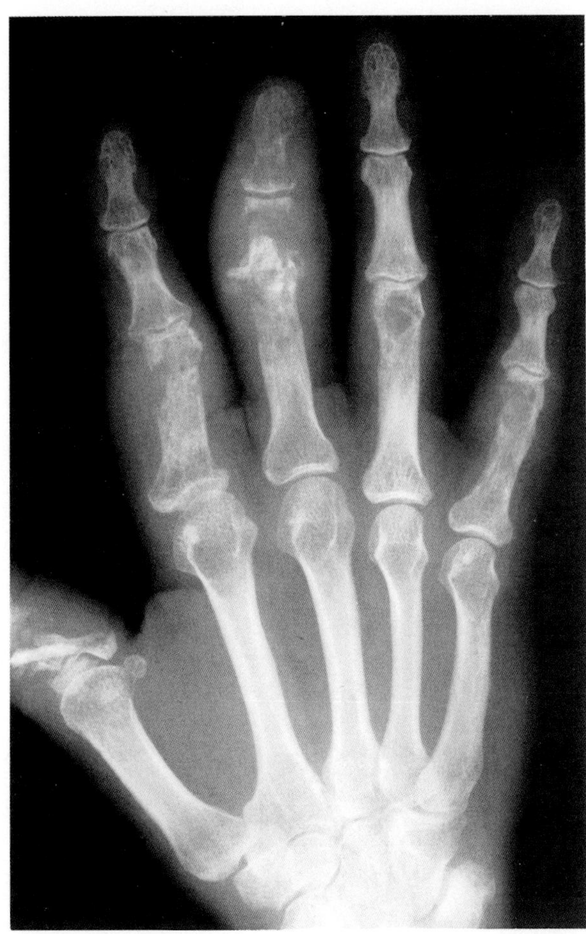

FIGURE 58.31. **Sarcoid.** An AP view of the hand in this patient with sarcoid demonstrates classic changes of bony involvement with this granulomatous process. Note the lace-like pattern of destruction seen most prominently in the proximal phalanges and in the distal third phalanx. Soft tissue swelling and some areas of severe bony dissolution are also noted, which occur in more advanced patterns of sarcoid. These changes are typically limited to the hands but can rarely occur in other parts of the skeleton.

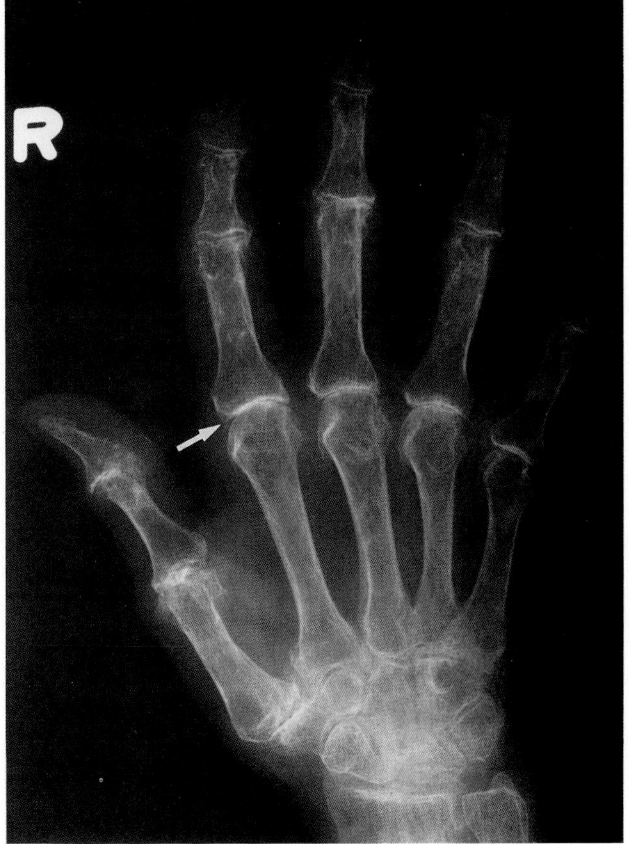

FIGURE 58.32. **Hemochromatosis.** An AP view of the hand in this patient with hemochromatosis shows severe joint space narrowing throughout the hand, which is most marked at the metacarpophalangeal joints. Associated sclerosis at the metacarpophalangeal joints with large osteophytes seen off the metacarpal heads suggests degenerative joint disease (DJD). These are very unusual joints for DJD to occur in; yet, this is the classic appearance of hemochromatosis. No chondrocalcinosis is seen in the triangular cartilage in this patient; however, a small amount of chondrocalcinosis can be seen at the second metacarpophalangeal joint (*arrow*). Fifty percent of patients with hemochromatosis also have CPPD.

typically subcutaneous, whereas in dermatomyositis, they are intramuscular in location. Mixed connective tissue disease is an overlap of scleroderma, systemic lupus erythematosus, polymyositis, and rheumatoid arthritis. It has a myriad of radiographic findings.

SARCOIDOSIS

Sarcoidosis is a disease that causes deposition of granulomatous tissue in the body, primarily in the lungs, but also in the bones. In the skeletal system, it has a predilection for the hands, where it causes lytic destructive lesions in the cortex. These often have a so-called lace-like appearance, which is characteristic (Fig. 58.31). It can have associated skin nodules in the hands.

HEMOCHROMATOSIS

Hemochromatosis is a disease of excess iron deposition in tissues throughout the body leading to fibrosis and eventual organ failure. Twenty to 50% of patients with hemochromatosis have a characteristic arthropathy in the hands that should suggest the diagnosis. The classic radiographic changes are essentially DJD, which involves the second through the fourth MCP joints (Fig. 58.32). Up to 50% of the patients with hemochromatosis also have CPPD; therefore, a search should be made for chondrocalcinosis. Another finding that is often seen in hemochromatosis is called squaring of the metacarpal heads. They appear enlarged and block-like as a result of the large osteophytes commonly seen in this disorder. The osteophytes are often said to be "drooping" because of the unusual way they hang off the joint margin.

NEUROPATHIC OR CHARCOT JOINT

The radiographic findings for a Charcot joint are characteristic and almost pathognomonic. A classic triad has been described that consists of ***joint destruction***, ***dislocation***, and ***heterotopic new bone*** (Table 58.11 and Fig. 58.33).

TABLE 58.11

HALLMARKS OF A NEUROPATHIC JOINT

Joint destruction
Dislocation
Heterotopic new bone formation

Joint destruction is seen in every type of arthritis and therefore seems very nonspecific; however, nothing causes as severe destruction in a joint as a Charcot joint. Progressive joint destruction occurs in a neuropathic joint because the joint is rendered unstable by inaccurate muscle action and is unprotected by intact nerve reflexes. Early in the development of a Charcot joint, the joint destruction may merely appear to be joint space narrowing. It is extremely difficult to make the diagnosis this early. In the spine, instead of joint space destruction, there is disc space destruction (Fig. 58.34).

Dislocation, like joint destruction, can be present in varying degrees. Early on, the joint may have subluxation instead of dislocation.

Heterotopic new bone has also been termed debris or detritus and consists of soft tissue calcification or clumps of ossification adjacent to the joint. It too can be present in varying amounts.

The most commonly seen Charcot joint today is in the foot of a patient with diabetes mellitus. The disease typically affects the first and second tarsometatarsal joints in a fashion similar to a Lisfranc fracture–dislocation (Fig. 58.35).

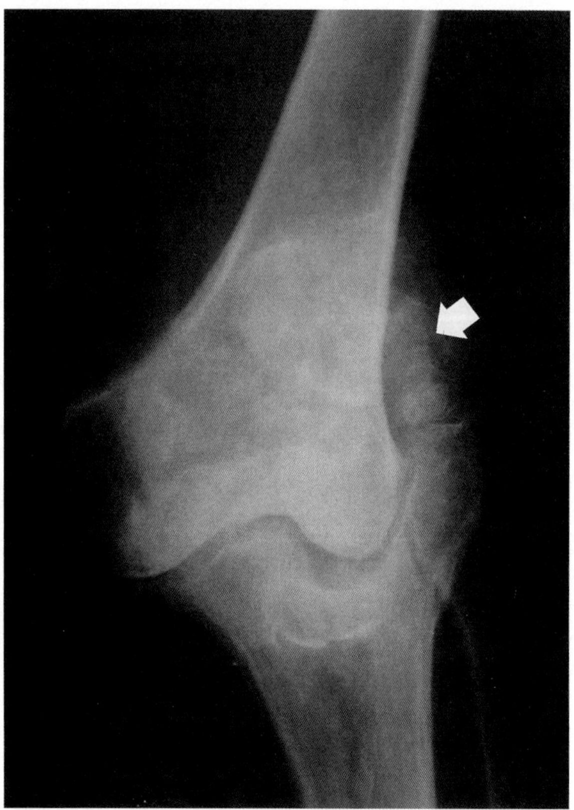

FIGURE 58.33. **Charcot Joint.** An AP view of the knee in this patient with tabes dorsalis shows the classic changes of a neuropathic or Charcot joint. Note the severe joint destruction, the subluxation, and the heterotopic new bone (*arrow*).

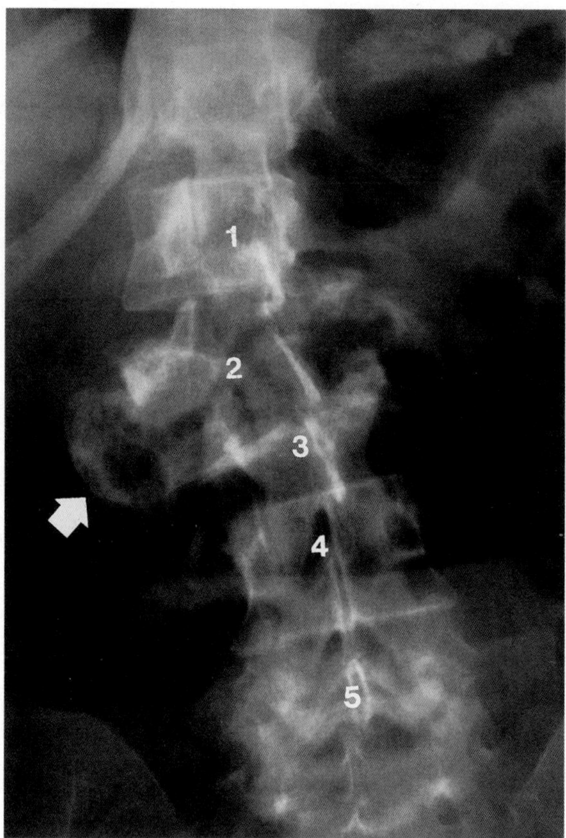

FIGURE 58.34. **Charcot Spine.** An AP view of the spine in this paraplegic patient shows severe destruction of the L2 and L3 vertebral bodies and the intervening disc space, heterotopic new bone (*arrow*), and malalignment or dislocation. *Numbers* indicate lumbar vertebrae.

Tabes dorsalis from syphilis is rarely seen today. More commonly seen is a Charcot joint in a patient with paralysis who continues to use the affected limb for support. A Charcot joint that is also seen on occasion is the so-called pseudo-Charcot joint in CPPD.

HEMOPHILIA, JUVENILE RHEUMATOID ARTHRITIS, AND PARALYSIS

Why would clinically disparate entities like paralysis, juvenile rheumatoid arthritis (JRA), and hemophilia be covered in the same section? Because they are usually radiographically indistinguishable.

The classic findings for JRA and hemophilia are ***overgrowth of the ends of the bones*** (epiphyseal enlargement) associated with ***gracile diaphyses*** (Fig. 58.36). Joint destruction might or might not be present. A finding that is purported to be classic for JRA and hemophilia is widening of the intercondylar notch of the knee. This sign can be quite variable and difficult to use. It is rarely present when the other classic signs are also not present and obvious.

Another process that can mimic the findings in JRA and hemophilia is a joint that has undergone disuse from paralysis (Fig. 58.37). It has always been said that the reason the epiphyses are overgrown in JRA and hemophilia is because of the hyperemia; however, many other things cause hyperemia without affecting the size of the epiphyses (such as rheumatoid

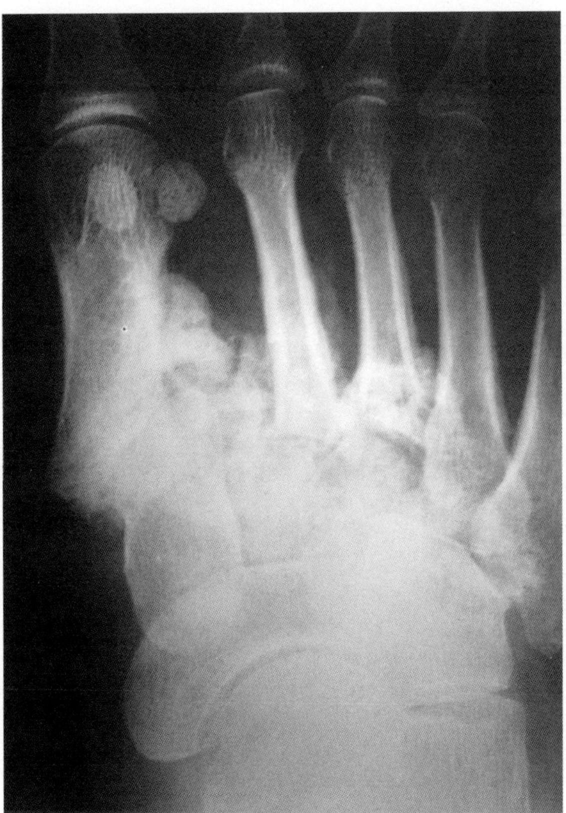

FIGURE 58.35. **Lisfranc Charcot Joint.** Dislocation of the second and third metatarsals along with joint destruction and large amounts of heterotopic new bone are present in the foot of this diabetic patient. These findings are classic for a Charcot joint, which has been termed a Lisfranc fracture–dislocation. It is most commonly seen secondary to trauma rather than as a Charcot joint but is the most common neuropathic joint seen today.

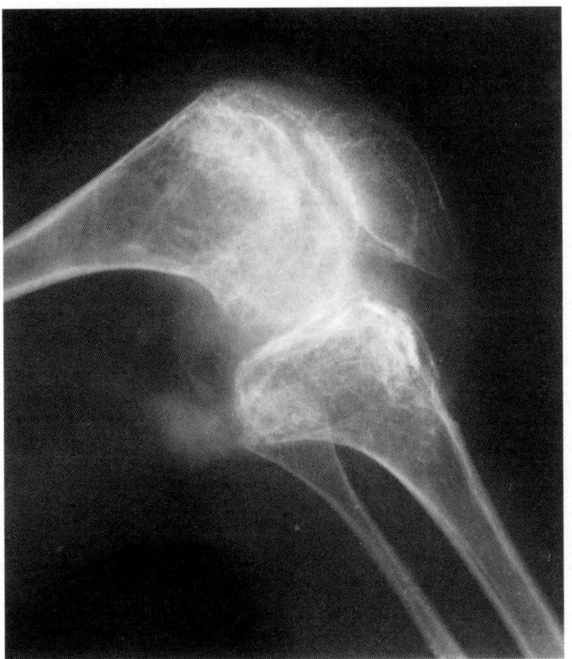

FIGURE 58.36. **Juvenile Rheumatoid Arthritis (JRA).** A lateral view of the knee in this patient with JRA shows the classic findings of overgrowth of the ends of the bones and associated gracile diaphyses. These changes can also be seen in patients with hemophilia or paralysis.

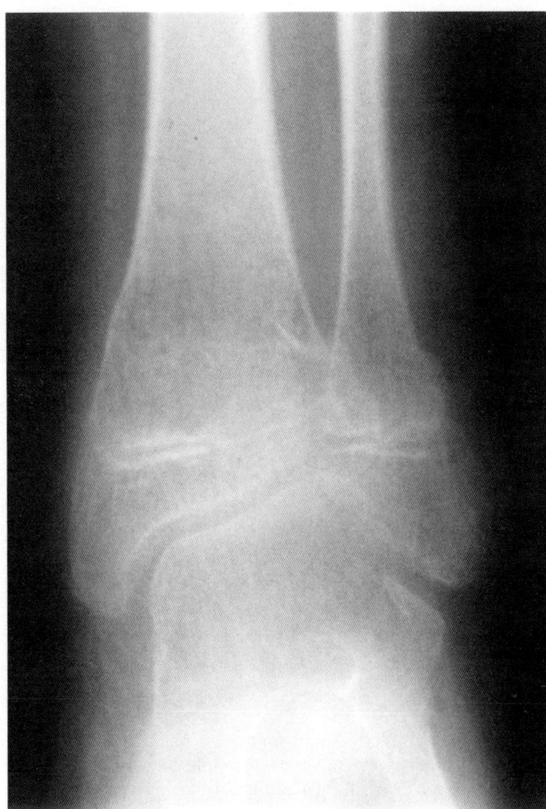

FIGURE 58.37. **Muscular Dystrophy Simulating Juvenile Rheumatoid Arthritis (JRA) or Hemophilia.** An AP view of the ankle in this patient with muscular dystrophy shows subtle changes of overgrowth of the distal tibia and the fibular epiphyses. Marked tibiotalar slant, which can also be present in JRA or hemophilia, is also present.

arthritis and infection). The common denominator shared by JRA, hemophilia, and paralysis is disuse. This is most likely what causes the overgrowth of the ends of the bones seen in all three of these disorders.

SYNOVIAL CHONDROMATOSIS

Synovial chondromatosis is a relatively common disorder caused by a benign neoplasia of the synovium, resulting in deposition of nodules of cartilage in the joint. Most of the time, these cartilaginous deposits calcify and are readily seen on a radiograph (Fig. 58.38). It is most commonly seen in the knee, hip, and elbow. Up to 30% of the time, the cartilaginous deposits do not calcify. In these cases, all that is seen on the radiograph is a joint effusion, unless erosions or joint destruction occur (Fig. 58.39).

The chondral nodules begin in the synovium and then tend to shed into the joint, where they can cause symptoms of free fragments or "joint mice." They then embed into the synovium and tend not to be free in the joint after a while. It is usually necessary to perform a complete synovectomy to relieve the symptoms; recurrences are not uncommon.

An uncommon presentation that can lead to diagnostic confusion is when the loose bodies are tightly packed in a joint, giving it the appearance on MRI of a tumor (Fig. 58.40). This has been termed tumefactive synovial chondromatosis. If a biopsy is performed, it can get interpreted as a chondrosarcoma with resultant radical surgery. As no malignant tumors arise in joints, this should not present a problem in diagnosis.

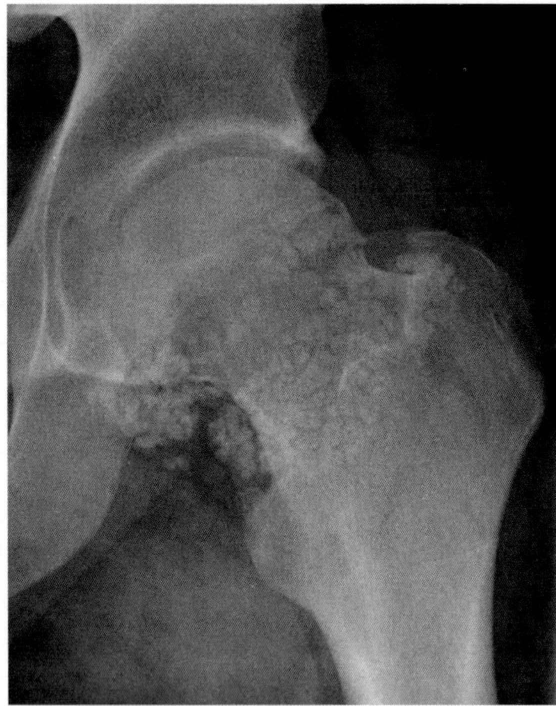

FIGURE 58.38. **Synovial Chondromatosis.** An AP view of the hip in this patient with left hip pain shows multiple calcified loose bodies in the hip joint, which is virtually diagnostic of synovial chondromatosis.

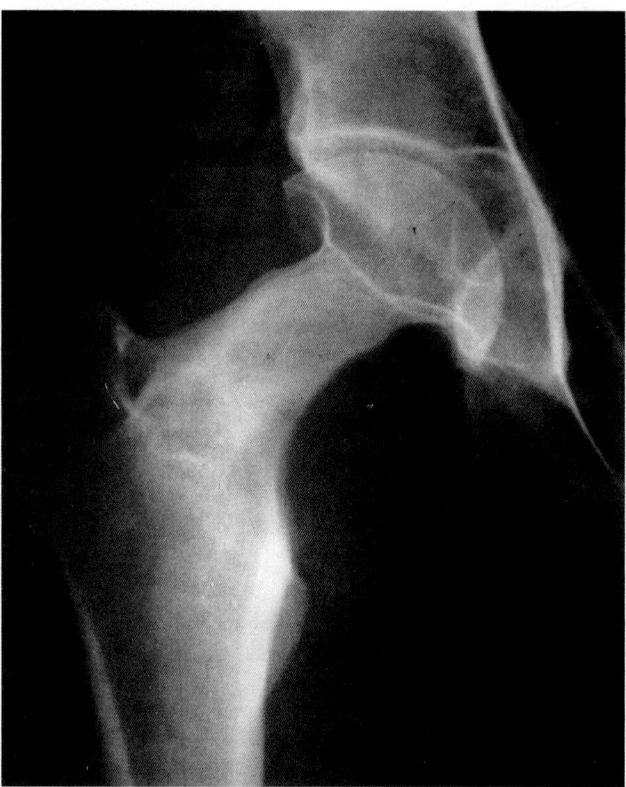

FIGURE 58.39. **Synovial Chondromatosis Without Calcification.** An AP view of the hip in this patient shows the femoral neck to be eroded, having an "apple core" appearance. This has occurred from the pressure erosion of multiple nonossified chondral bodies in the joint. This is nonossified synovial chondromatosis. It usually does not cause this degree of bony erosion and is indistinguishable from pigmented villonodular synovitis.

PIGMENTED VILLONODULAR SYNOVITIS

Pigmented villonodular synovitis (PVNS) is an uncommon, chronic, inflammatory process of the synovium that causes

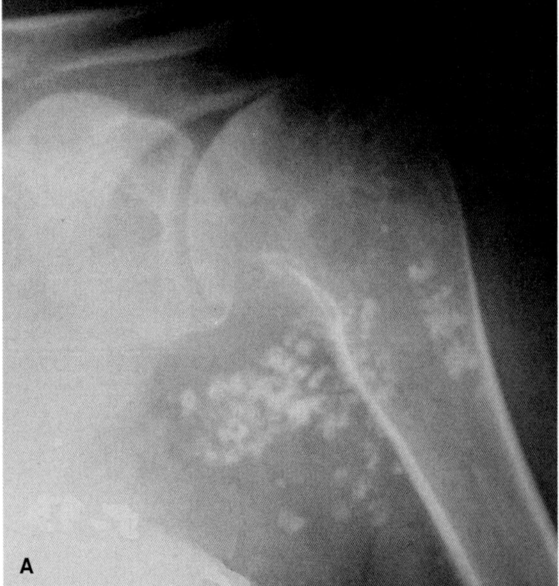

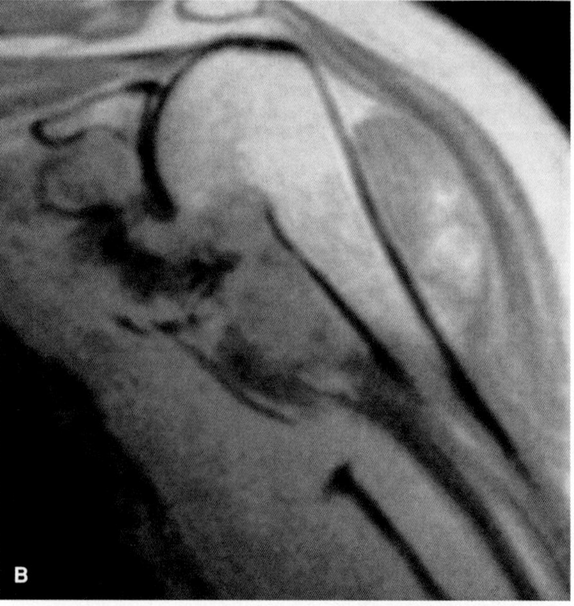

FIGURE 58.40. **Tumefactive Synovial Osteochondromatosis. A:** A radiograph of the shoulder shows a partially calcified mass that is eroding the medial aspect of the humerus. Coronal proton-density (**B**) and T2-weighted (**C**) images of the shoulder reveal a large mass encircling the humeral head that was interpreted as a sarcoma. A biopsy was performed and called "chondrosarcoma," which resulted in a forequarter amputation. The intra-articular nature of the mass was not appreciated until after the radical surgery, when it was correctly recognized as synovial chondromatosis.

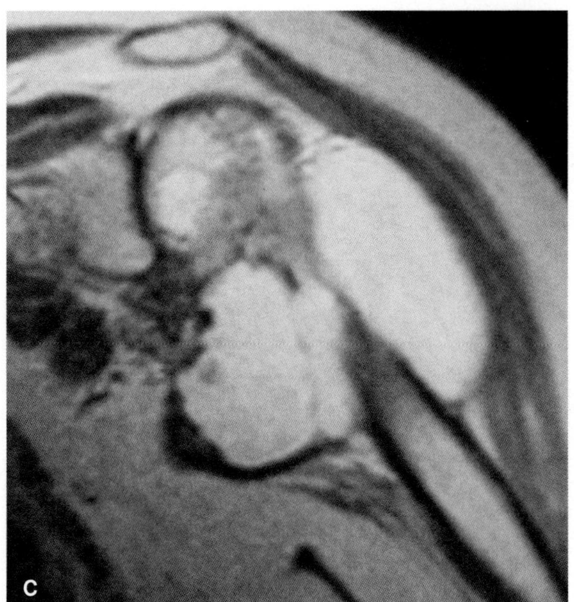

FIGURE 58.40. (*Continued*)

synovial proliferation. A swollen joint with lobular masses of synovium occurs and causes pain and joint destruction (Fig. 58.41). It rarely, if ever, calcifies. It has been termed giant cell tumor of tendon sheath and tendon sheath xanthoma when it occurs in a tendon sheath, which is not unusual. Joints with PVNS look radiographically identical to noncalcified synovial chondromatosis, yet they are much less common. Therefore, whenever PVNS is a consideration, synovial chondromatosis should be mentioned. PVNS has a characteristic appearance on MR with low–signal intensity hemosiderin seen lining the synovium on both T1- and T2-weighted images (Fig. 58.42).

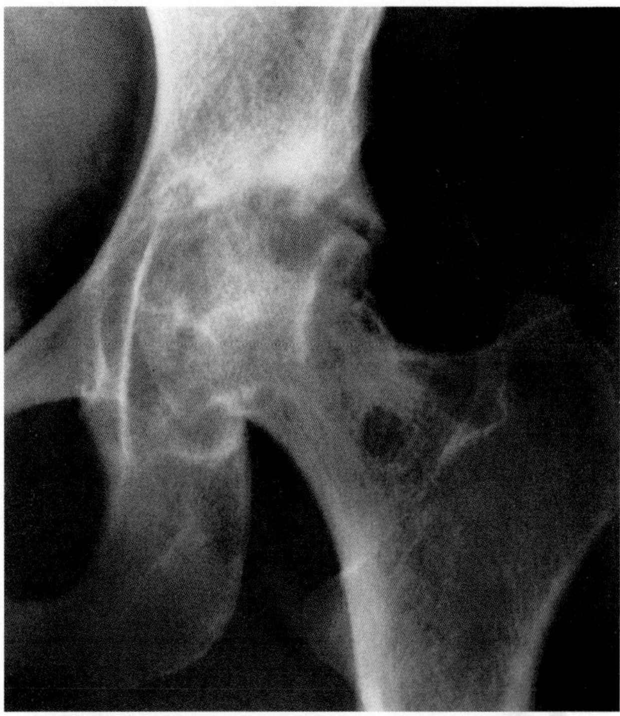

FIGURE 58.41. **Pigmented Villonodular Synovitis.** An AP view of the hip in this patient shows joint space destruction and bony erosions throughout the femoral head and neck. Pigmented villonodular synovitis or synovial chondromatosis could have this appearance.

SUDECK ATROPHY

Also known as shoulder–hand syndrome, reflex sympathetic dystrophy, and chronic regional pain syndrome, Sudeck atrophy

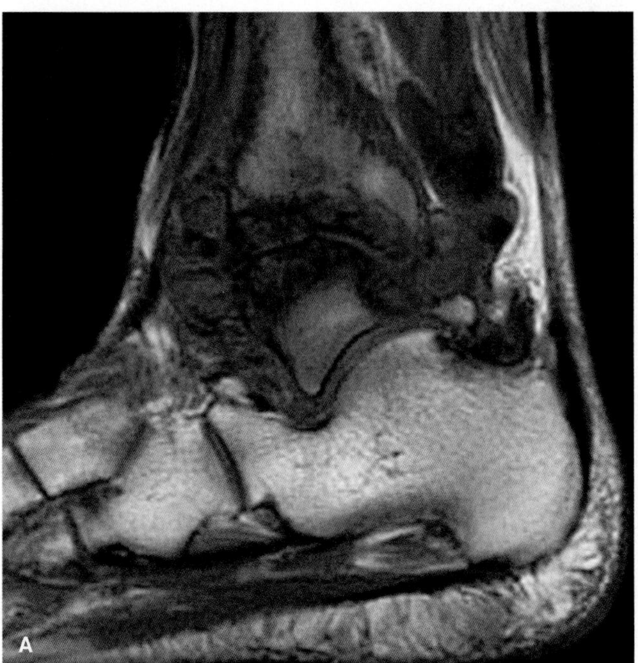

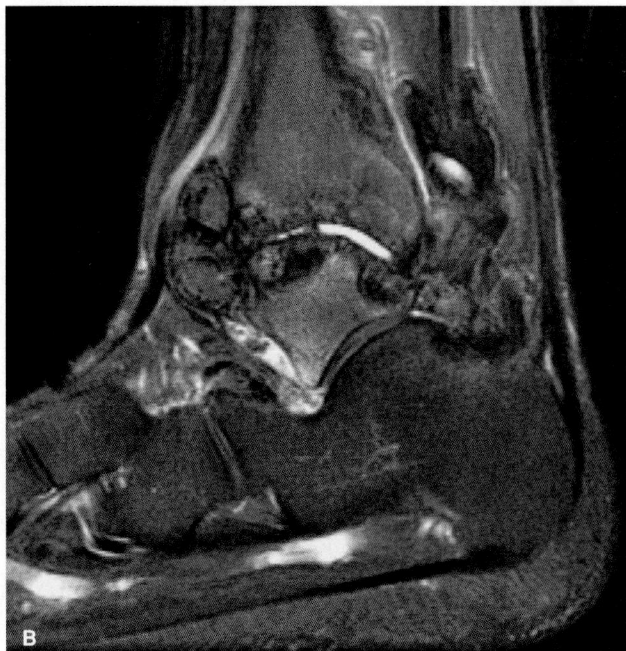

FIGURE 58.42. **Pigmented Villonodular Synovitis (PVNS).** Sagittal T1-weighted (**A**) and fat-suppressed T2-weighted (**B**) images of an ankle with PVNS show a soft tissue mass emanating from the ankle joint, which is low signal on both sequences and has very–low-signal hemosiderin lining parts of the synovium, which is characteristic for PVNS.

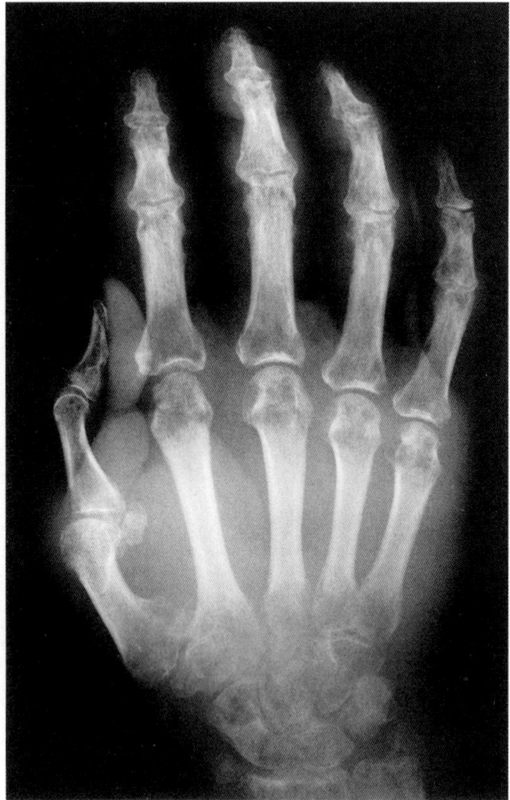

FIGURE 58.43. **Sudeck Atrophy.** Diffuse soft tissue swelling and marked osteoporosis that is so aggressive that it has a spotty or permeative appearance is noted around all of the joints in the hand. This patient has severe hand pain and dysfunction following minor trauma. This is characteristic of Sudeck atrophy.

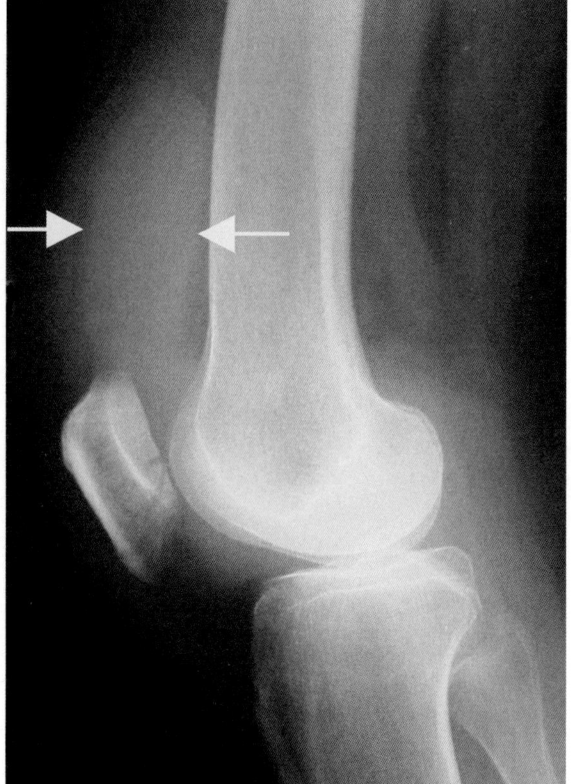

FIGURE 58.44. **Knee Joint Effusion.** This patient has joint fluid in the knee, with widely displaced fat pads. The suprapatellar fat pad (*left arrow*) is more than 5 mm from the anterior suprafemoral fat pad (*right arrow*), which indicates a joint effusion. The patella is fractured.

is a poorly understood joint affliction that typically occurs after minor trauma to an extremity, resulting in pain, swelling, and dysfunction. Severe patchy osteoporosis and soft tissue swelling are seen radiographically (Fig. 58.43). It typically affects the distal part of an extremity such as a hand or foot; yet, intermediate joints such as the knee and the hip are believed by some to be occasionally involved. The pain usually subsides, but the osteoporosis may persist. The swelling, with time, will subside and the skin may become atrophic. It is important for the radiologist to recognize the aggressive osteoporosis in this disorder and differentiate it from disuse osteoporosis so that the treating physician can begin aggressive physical therapy.

JOINT EFFUSIONS

Most joint effusions are clinically obvious and do not require radiographic validation. The elbow is an exception. In the setting of trauma to the elbow, an effusion indicates a fracture. The radiographic signs of an elbow effusion are generally clearly seen (displaced fat pads, as described in Chapter 57) and have proved to be valid. Clinical determination of an elbow effusion can be difficult; therefore, the radiologist can be very helpful in this area.

Clinical determination of a hip effusion is also very difficult. The presence of a hip effusion can be valuable in certain clinical settings. For instance, a patient with pain in the hip and an effusion should have the joint aspirated to rule out an infection. If only pain was present, an aspiration would probably not be performed. The radiology literature mentions displacement of the fat stripes about the hip as being an indicator for an effusion, but this has been proved to be unfounded. The only fat pad around the hip that gets displaced with an effusion is the obturator internus, and it is uncommonly seen.

The radiographic sign for a knee effusion that seems to be the most reliable is the measurement of the distance between the suprapatellar fat pad and the anterior femoral fat pad (Fig. 58.44). A distance between these two fat pads of more than 10 mm is definite evidence for an effusion. A distance of less than 5 mm is normal. A distance of 5 to 10 mm is equivocal. It does not make any difference if there is an effusion in the knee—regardless, the patient gets treated the same. If it were vital to the patient, one could aspirate the joint or perform an MR study to find out. I should point out that an MR should never be performed just to see whether there is fluid in the joint.

Shoulder effusions are very difficult to detect unless they are massive enough to displace the humeral head inferiorly, as with a fracture and hemarthrosis (see Chapter 57). Fortunately, as with most other joints, treatment is not based solely on the presence or absence of an effusion, so it hardly matters. The same is true in the ankle, wrist, and smaller joints.

AVASCULAR NECROSIS

Avascular necrosis (AVN), or osteonecrosis, can occur around almost any joint for a host of reasons including steroids, trauma, various underlying disease states, and even idiopathically. It is often seen in renal transplant patients.

The hallmark of AVN is increased bone density at an otherwise normal joint. Increased density at a narrowed joint usually

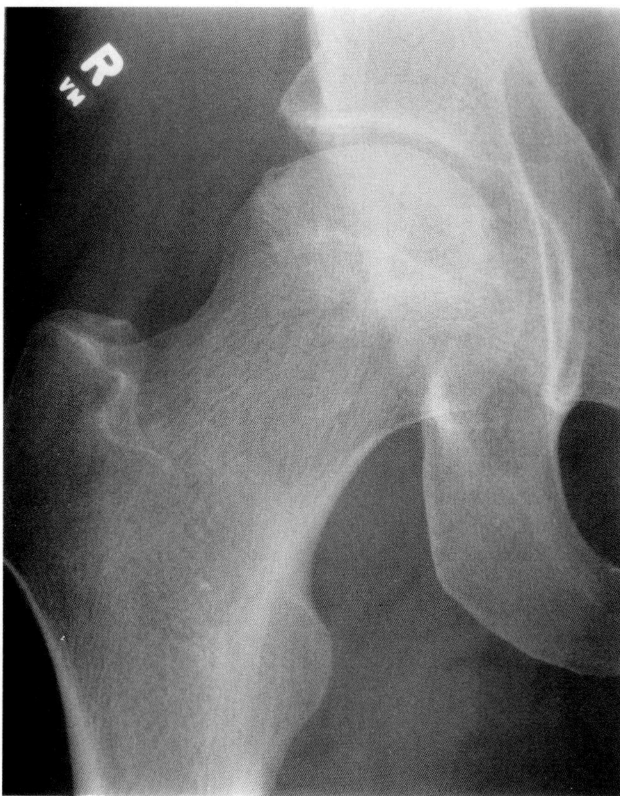

FIGURE 58.45. **Early Avascular Necrosis of the Hip.** Patchy sclerosis is present in the femoral head in this patient with a renal transplant and avascular necrosis of the right hip. No subchondral lucency or articular surface irregularity in the weight-bearing region is yet present, with the exception of a small cortical irregularity seen laterally.

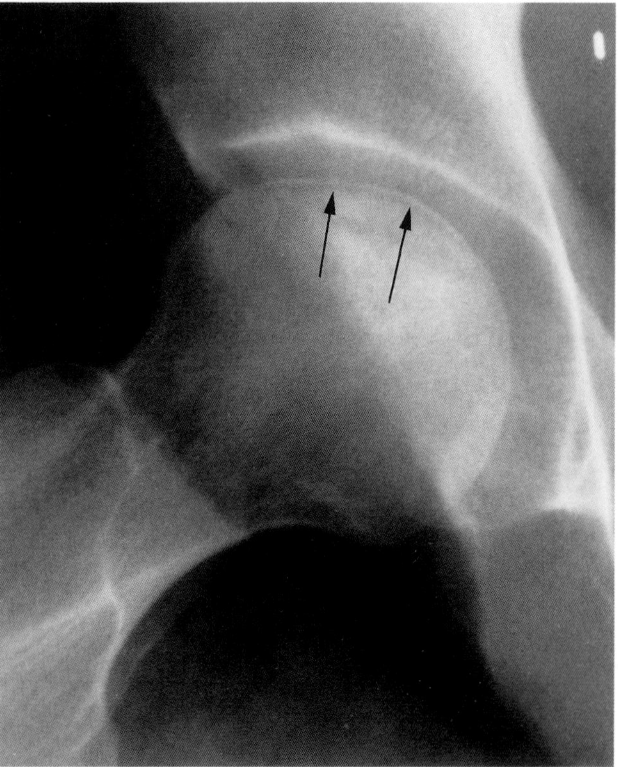

FIGURE 58.46. **Avascular Necrosis (AVN) of the Hip.** A subchondral lucency (*arrows*) is seen in the weight-bearing portion of this hip with AVN. Patchy sclerosis throughout the femoral head is also noted.

indicates DJD; however, if either osteophytes or joint space narrowing are absent, another disorder should be considered.

The earliest sign of AVN is a joint effusion. This often is not visible radiographically or is so nonspecific that it does not help with the diagnosis unless the clinical setting had already raised suspicion for AVN. The next sign for AVN is a patchy or mottled density (Fig. 58.45). In the knee, this density increase can occur throughout an entire condyle, whereas in the hip, it often involves the entire femoral head. Next, a subchondral lucency often develops that forms a thin line along the articular surface (Fig. 58.46). This lucent line has been described as being an early indicator for AVN, whereas, in fact, it is a late finding. Also, the lucent line stage is often not present in the evolution of AVN. Therefore, using the lucent line as one of the main criteria for AVN can lead to missing early findings in some cases and missing the diagnosis completely in others.

The final sign in AVN is collapse of the articular surface and joint fragmentation (Fig. 58.47). I must stress that these changes all occur on only one side of a joint, which makes for an easy diagnosis because almost everything else around the joints involves both sides of the joint.

MR is extremely useful in evaluating AVN. It is the most sensitive imaging study available, often showing AVN when radiographs or radionuclide scans are normal. In the hip, AVN typically has an area of low or mixed signal intensity on T1-weighted images, which is located in the anterosuperior portion of the femoral head and which has a serpiginous margin (Figs. 58.48 and 58.49). If the anterior portion of the femoral head is not involved, the diagnosis of AVN should be questioned, as it is uncommon to present otherwise. Posterior femoral head AVN can occasionally be found after posterior

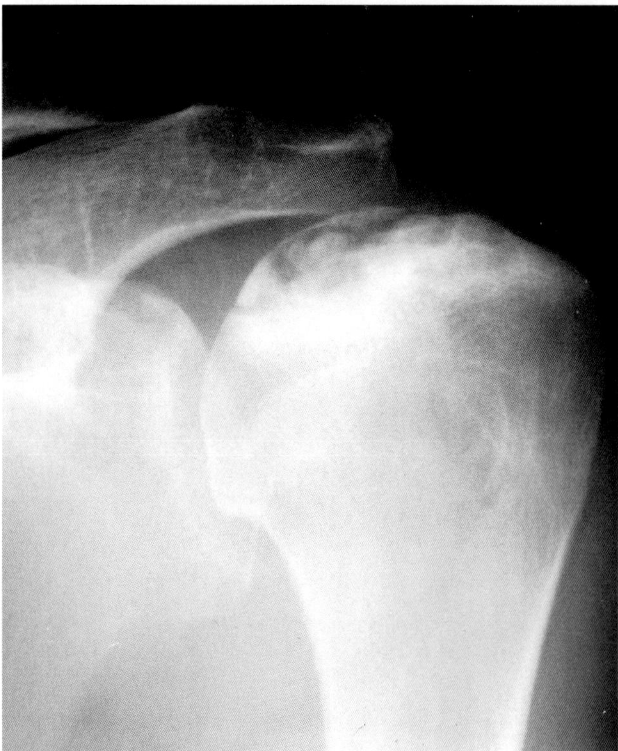

FIGURE 58.47. **Avascular Necrosis (AVN) of the Shoulder.** Articular surface collapse is present in this shoulder with long-standing AVN. Dense bony sclerosis is also present.

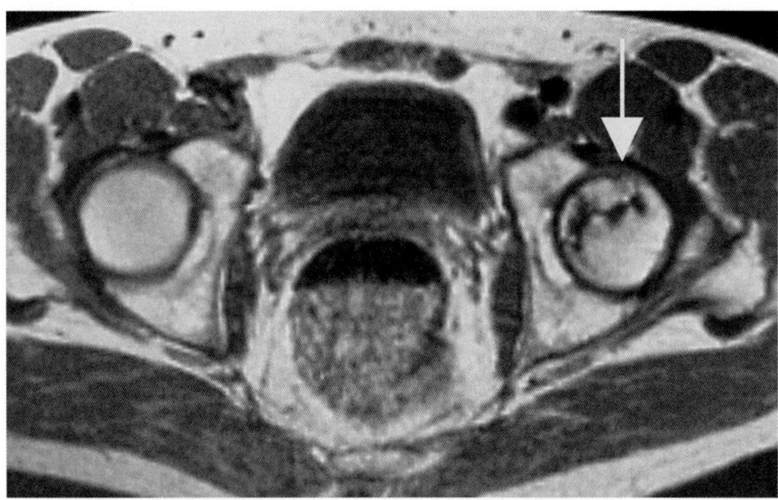

FIGURE 58.48. **Avascular Necrosis (AVN) of the Hip.** An axial T1-weighted image of the hips shows a focal area of abnormality in the left femoral head (*arrow*), which is characteristic for AVN. The low-signal serpiginous border is a typical finding, as is the anterior location.

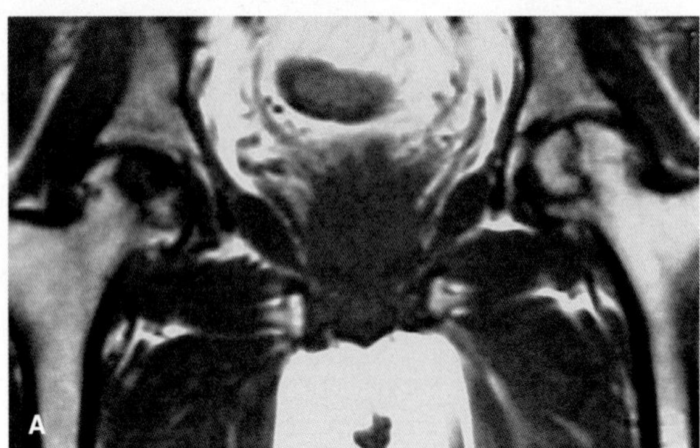

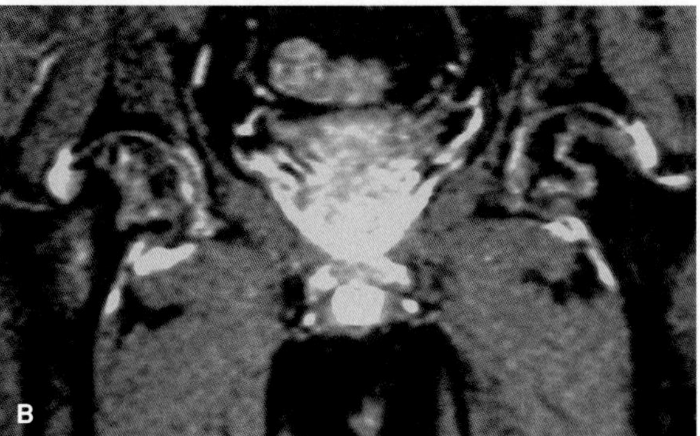

FIGURE 58.49. **Avascular Necrosis (AVN) of the Hip.** Coronal T1-weighted (**A**) and STIR (**B**) images show bilateral AVN.

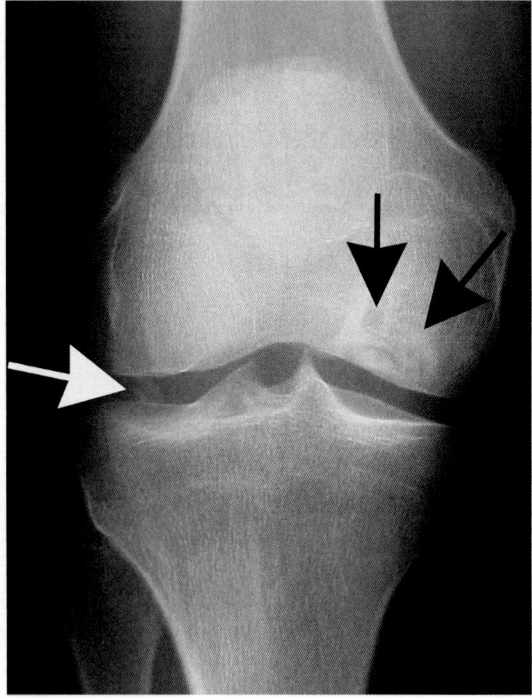

FIGURE 58.50. **Osteochondritis Dissecans.** A small focal area of avascular necrosis (AVN) in the medial condyle of the femur (*black arrows*) is present, which is an area of osteochondritis dissecans. Part of the area of AVN has shed an osteochondral fragment (*white arrow*) into the joint.

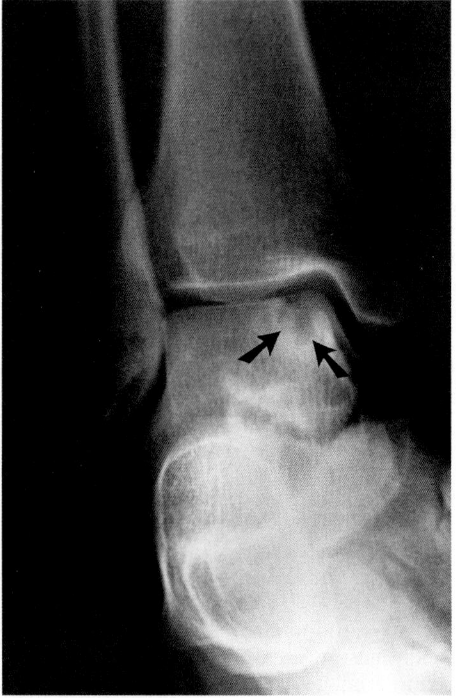

FIGURE 58.51. **Osteochondritis Dissecans of the Talus.** A focal area of avascular necrosis in the talus as seen here (*arrows*) is called osteochondritis dissecans. The talus is the second most common site after the knee and, as in the knee, can cause a loose body in the joint.

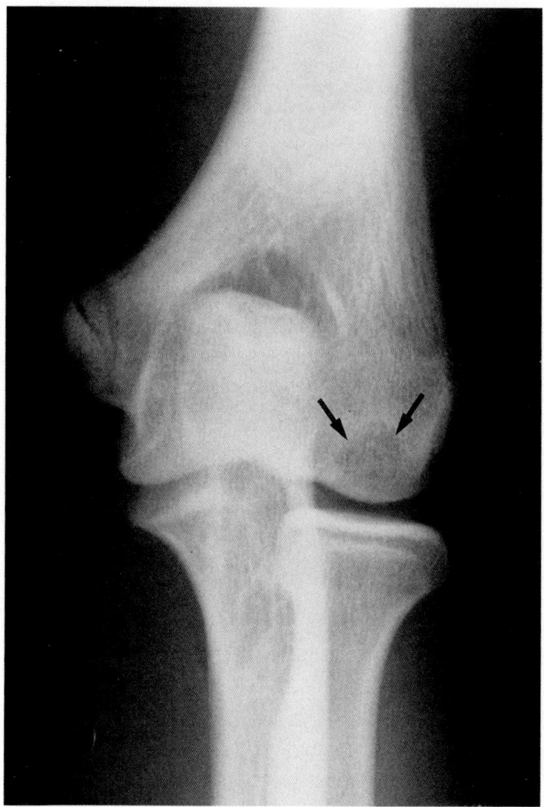

FIGURE 58.52. **Osteochondritis Dissecans of the Elbow.** The third most common site for osteochondritis dissecans is in the capitellum of the elbow. The faint lucency seen in this capitellum (*arrows*) was at first believed to be a chondroblastoma or an area of infection.

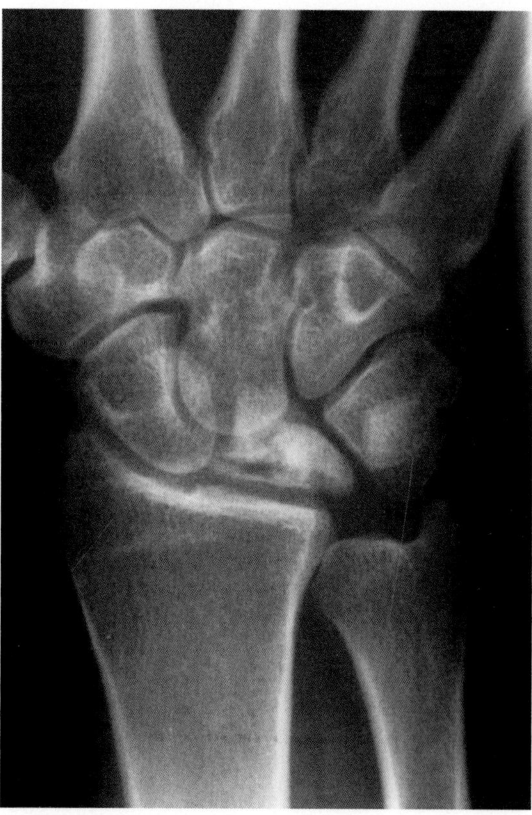

FIGURE 58.54. **Kienböck Malacia.** Avascular necrosis (AVN) of the lunate, Kienböck malacia, is demonstrated in this patient's wrist. The increased density and partial fragmentation of the lunate are characteristic for AVN. Also, note the slightly shortened ulna (in comparison with the radius), which is called negative ulnar variance. Negative ulnar variance is said to have a high association with Kienböck malacia.

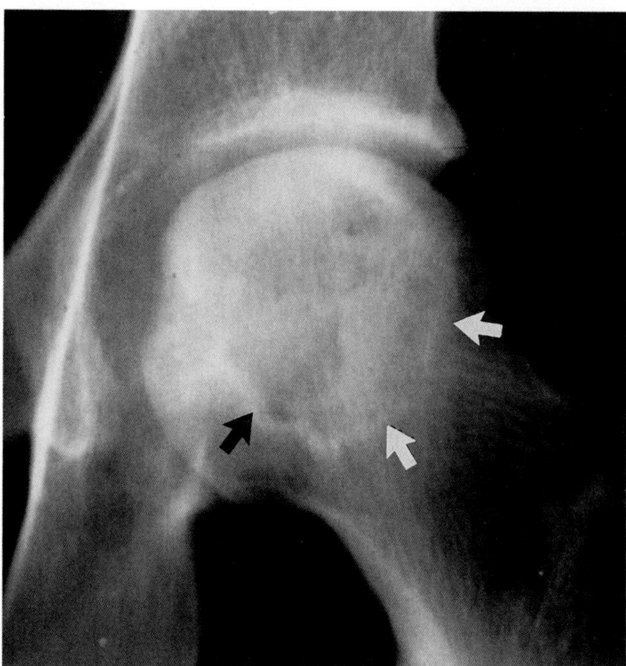

FIGURE 58.53. **Geode in the Hip.** A large cystic lesion (*arrows*) is seen in this patient with avascular necrosis (AVN) of the hip. Note the adjacent patchy sclerosis, indicative of AVN. A subchondral cyst or geode should be considered any time a lytic lesion is found around a joint.

dislocation of the hip because of the impaction of the femoral head on the posterior column of the acetabulum.

A form of AVN that is smaller and more focal than that just described is osteochondritis dissecans. It is most likely caused by trauma; however, this is controversial, with one school of thought believing the cause is idiopathic. It occurs most often in the knee at the medial epicondyle (Fig. 58.50). It also is frequently seen in the dome of the talus (Fig. 58.51) and occasionally in the capitellum (Fig. 58.52). Osteochondritis dissecans frequently leads to a small fragment of bone being sloughed off and becoming a free fragment in the joint, a "joint mouse" (see Fig. 58.50).

AVN is one of the disorders around joints in which subchondral cysts or geodes can occur. It is the only one of the four disorders (rheumatoid arthritis, DJD, and CPPD being the others) that can have an essentially normal joint and have a geode (Fig. 58.53). The other disorders will have any or a combination of joint space narrowing, osteophytes, osteoporosis, chondrocalcinosis, or other findings.

A host of names have been ascribed to certain bones with AVN, usually with the eponym being the first person to describe the disorder. These have been called osteochondroses. They are believed to be idiopathic for the most part but can also occur secondary to trauma. A few of the more common epiphyses involved are the following: the carpal lunate, Kienböck malacia (Figs. 58.54 and 58.58); the tarsal navicular, Köhler disease (Fig. 58.55); the metatarsal heads, Freiberg infraction (Fig. 58.56); the femoral head, Legg–Perthes disease; the ring epiphyses of the spine, Scheuermann disease (Fig. 58.57); and the tibial tubercle, Osgood–Schlatter

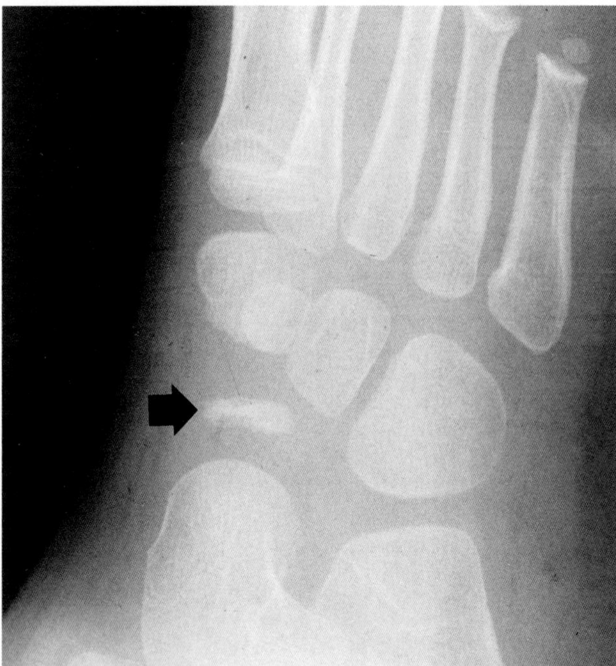

FIGURE 58.55. **Köhler Disease.** Flattening and sclerosis of the tarsal navicular (*arrow*) in children is thought by many to be avascular necrosis and is called Köhler disease. Others have found this to be an asymptomatic normal variant and believe that it is an incidental finding.

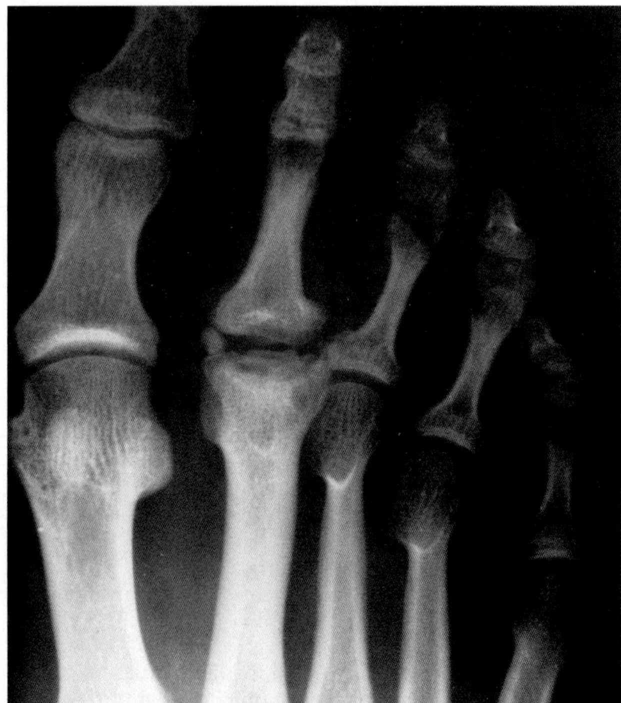

FIGURE 58.56. **Freiberg Infraction.** Flattening, collapse, and sclerosis of the second metatarsal head, as seen in this patient, are typical of avascular necrosis or Freiberg infraction. It can also involve the third or fourth metatarsal heads. Note the compensatory hypertrophy of the cortex of the second metatarsal, which is often found with this disorder.

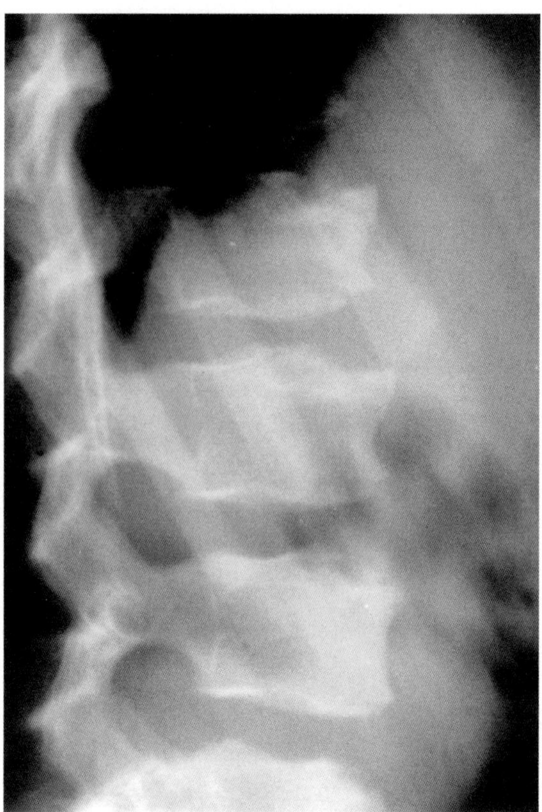

FIGURE 58.57. **Scheuermann Disease.** Avascular necrosis of the apophyseal rings of the vertebral bodies is called Scheuermann disease. He originally described a painful kyphosis with multiple vertebral bodies involved. It is most commonly seen without kyphosis or pain and with only a few vertebral bodies involved.

disease, also called surfer knees. MR can be very useful in identifying AVN in these sites. It shows diffuse low signal on T1-weighted images, which involves the entire area of AVN (Fig. 58.58).

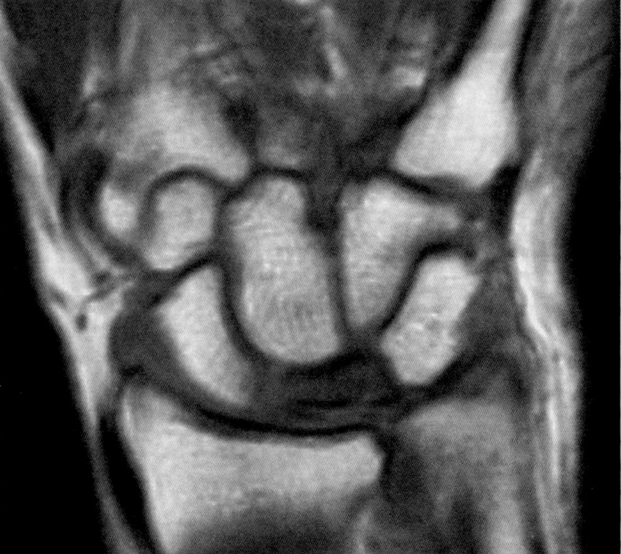

FIGURE 58.58. **Kienböck Malacia.** A coronal T1-weighted image of the wrist shows low signal throughout the lunate, which is characteristic for avascular necrosis of the lunate or Kienböck malacia.

Suggested Readings

Helms CA, Chapman GS, Wild JH. Charcot-like joints in calcium pyrophosphate dihydrate deposition disease. *Skeletal Radiol* 1981;7:55–58.

Mitchell DG, Kressel HY, Arger PH, Dalinka M, Spritzer CE, Steinberg ME. Avascular necrosis of the femoral head: morphologic assessment by MR imaging, with CT correlation. *Radiology* 1986;161:739–742.

Resnick D, Niwayama G, Coutts R. Subchondral cysts (geodes) in arthritic disorders: pathologic and radiographic appearance of the hip joint. *AJR Am J Roentgenol* 1977;128:799–806.

Resnick D, Niwayama G, Goergen TG, et al. Clinical, radiographic and pathologic abnormalities in calcium pyrophosphate dihydrate deposition disease (CPPD): pseudogout. *Radiology* 1977;122:1–15.

Resnick D, Shaul SR, Robins JM. Diffuse idiopathic skeletal hyperostosis with extraspinal manifestations. *Radiology* 1975;115:513–524.

CHAPTER 59 ■ METABOLIC BONE DISEASE

CLYDE A. HELMS AND EMILY N. VINSON

OSTEOPOROSIS

Osteoporosis is defined as diminished bone *quantity* in which the bone is otherwise normal. This contrasts to osteomalacia in which the bone quantity is normal but the *quality* of the bone is abnormal in that it is not normally mineralized. Osteomalacia results in excess nonmineralized osteoid. It is not possible in many cases to distinguish between osteoporosis and osteomalacia on radiographs; hence, many prefer the term "osteopenia" for the radiographic finding of diminished mineralization.

There are myriad causes of osteoporosis, the most common of which is primary osteoporosis (the so-called senile osteoporosis or osteoporosis of aging). This is seen most commonly in postmenopausal women and is a major health concern because of the increase of vertebral body and hip fractures in this patient population.

Secondary osteoporosis implies that an underlying disorder, such as thyrotoxicosis or renal disease, has caused the osteoporosis. Only about 5% of the cases of osteoporosis are of the secondary type. The differential diagnosis for secondary osteoporosis is quite long and probably should not be memorized. One cannot even be sure whether it is osteoporosis or osteomalacia on the basis of the radiographs; therefore, the differential for presumed osteoporosis would have to include the causes of osteomalacia.

The main radiographic finding in osteoporosis is thinning of the cortex. Although this can be seen in any bone, it is most reliably demonstrated in the second metacarpal at the mid-diaphysis. The normal metacarpal cortical thickening should be approximately one-fourth to one-third the thickness of the metacarpal (Fig. 59.1). In osteoporosis, this cortical thickness is decreased (Fig. 59.2). The metacarpal cortex (and all bony cortices, for that matter) decreases in thickness normally with age and is thinner in females than in males of the same age. Several tables have been published that give the normal metacarpal cortical measurement that have age and sex adjustments to allow the determination of normal. Unfortunately, these only determine the mineralization of the peripheral skeleton and do not seem to relate to whether vertebral body or hip fractures will occur.

Measurement of bone mineral content for the purposes of predicting fracture risk and monitoring response to therapy is usually done by means of dual-energy x-ray absorptiometry (DXA), which compares a patient's bone mineral density of the spine and hip with that of a healthy 30-year-old adult.

Exercise and proper diet seem to help delay the onset of primary osteoporosis. Calcium additives have not been shown to reverse the process of primary osteoporosis. Estrogen clearly plays a role in alleviating postmenopausal osteoporosis, yet its use in a widespread manner is somewhat controversial. Bisphosphonate drugs inhibit osteoclastic activity and thus slow bone loss and are commonly prescribed to treat osteoporosis and to prevent bony complications related to osseous metastatic disease, as they reduce fracture risk. Rarely, patients on long-term bisphosphonate therapy may develop unusual fractures of the femur which occur in atypical locations relative to the typical sites of femoral insufficiency fractures (see Chapter 57).

A type of osteoporosis that can be seen in a patient of any age is disuse osteoporosis. It results from immobilization from any cause, most commonly following the treatment of a fracture. The radiographic appearance of disuse osteoporosis is different from primary osteoporosis in that it occurs somewhat more rapidly and gives the bone a patchy appearance (Fig. 59.3). This is from osteoclastic resorption in the cortex causing intracortical holes. If allowed to continue with disuse, the bone would resemble any bone with marked osteoporosis—that is, severe cortical thinning.

Occasionally, aggressive osteoporosis from disuse can mimic a permeative lesion such as an Ewing sarcoma or multiple myeloma because of the multiple cortical holes that project over the medullary space, thus resembling a medullary permeative process (Fig. 59.4). The way to differentiate a true intramedullary permeative process from an intracortical process such as osteoporosis is to observe the cortex and see whether it is solid or riddled with holes (Fig. 59.5). If the cortex is

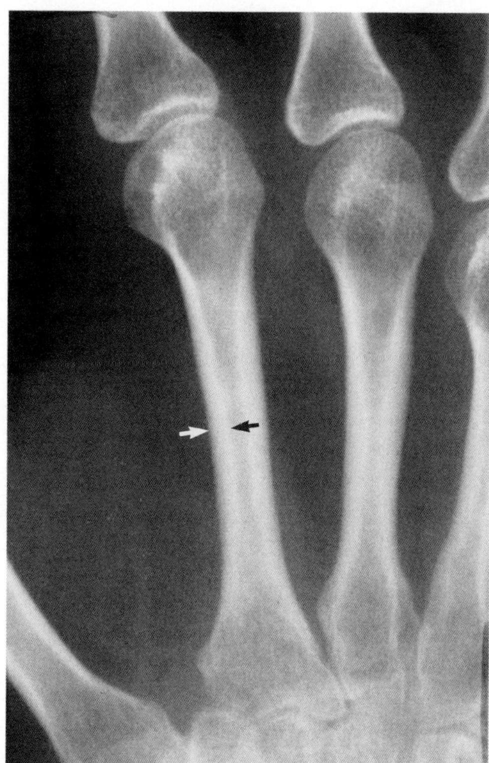

FIGURE 59.1. **Normal Mineralization.** The cortical width (*arrows*) at the midsecond metacarpal in this patient with normal mineralization is greater than one-third of the total width of the metacarpal.

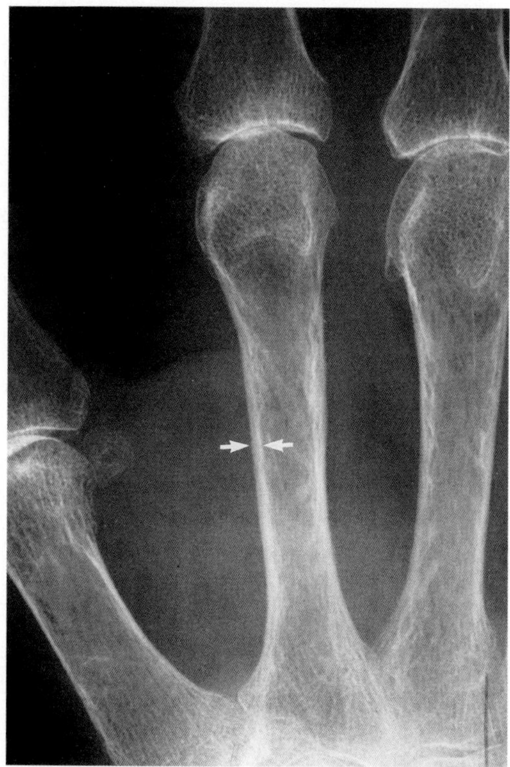

FIGURE 59.2. **Osteoporosis.** Severe cortical narrowing (*arrows*) at the midsecond metacarpal cortex is seen in this patient with severe osteoporosis. Note the intracortical tunneling that occurs in more aggressive forms of osteoporosis.

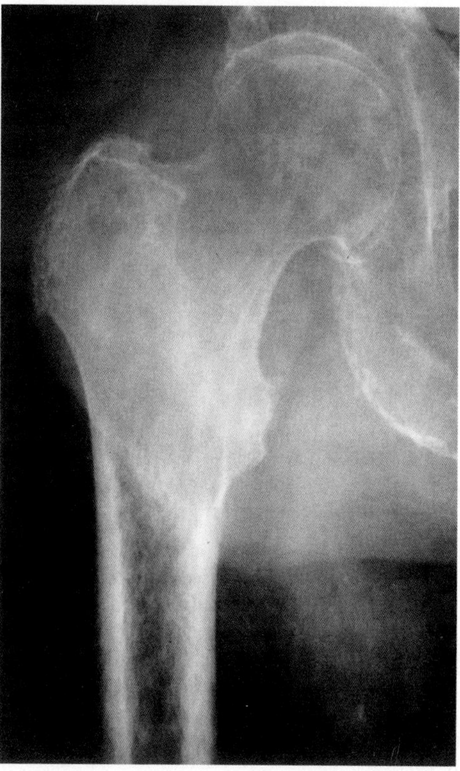

FIGURE 59.3. **Disuse Osteoporosis.** A mottled, patchy appearance is present in the proximal right femur in this patient with aggressive disuse osteoporosis secondary to an amputation. Note the mottled, irregular cortex seen in the femoral shaft, which is representative of cortical holes that can be seen in aggressive osteoporosis.

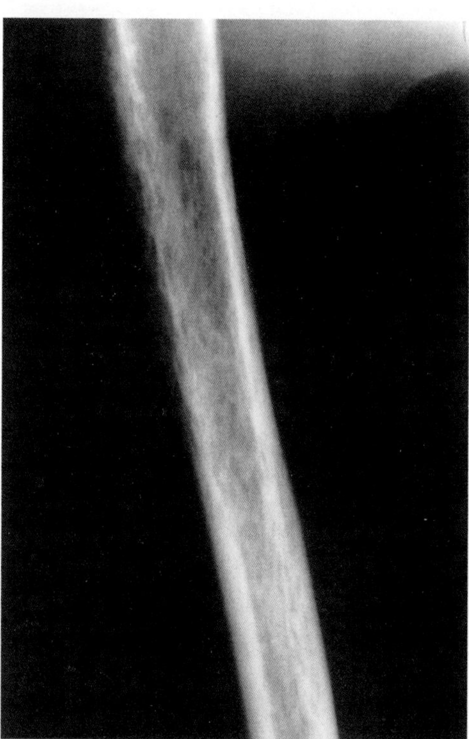

FIGURE 59.4. **Aggressive Osteoporosis.** Multiple small holes are seen in the cortex and overlying the medullary space in the proximal humerus of this patient who has suffered a stroke. This represents aggressive osteoporosis from disuse and is mimicking an aggressive permeative process. These holes are, however, almost entirely within the cortex of the bone.

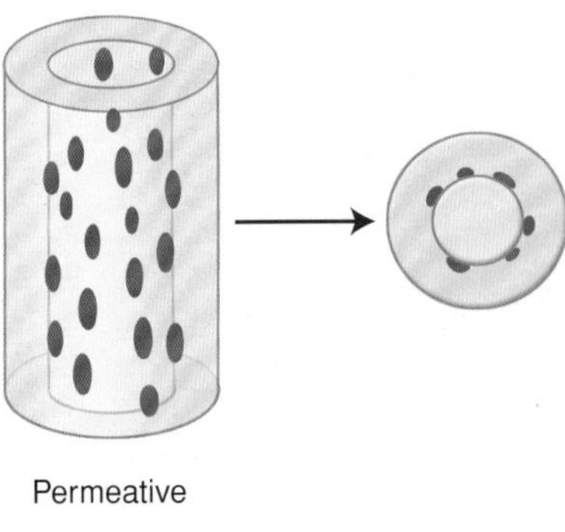

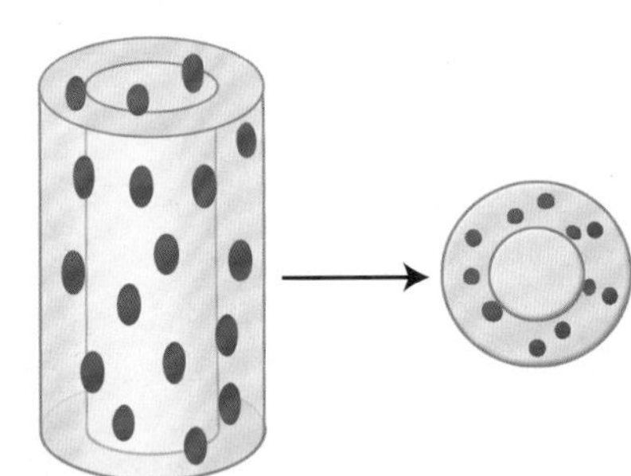

FIGURE 59.5. **Differentiation of Permeative Process. A:** Schematic of a permeative lesion. A true permeative process has multiple small holes secondary to endosteal involvement with sparing of the cortex. This represents a marrow process. **B:** Schematic of a pseudopermeative process. A pseudopermeative process such as osteoporosis has multiple small cortical holes that are then superimposed over the marrow, giving a similar appearance to a permeative process.

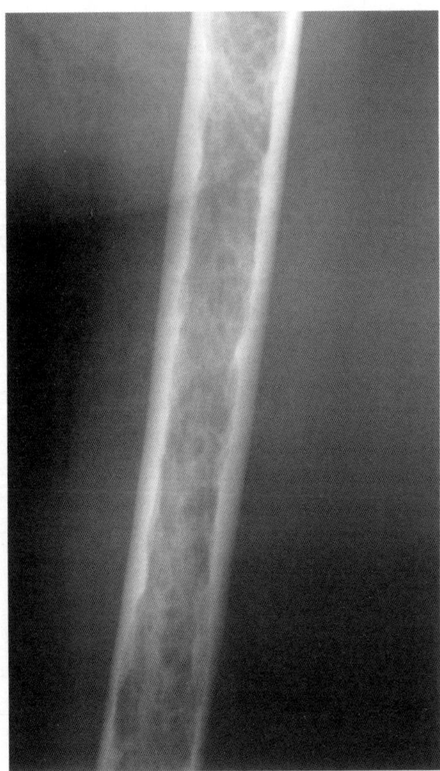

FIGURE 59.6. **Myeloma Causing a Permeative Process.** A diffuse permeative process throughout the femur is seen in this patient with myeloma. Note that the cortex is solid, although the endosteum has some scalloping. This is a true permeative process.

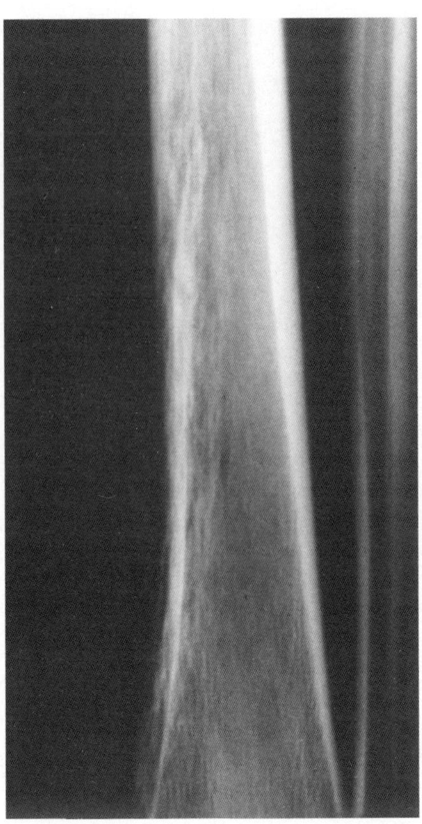

FIGURE 59.7. **Pseudopermeative Process Secondary to Hemangioma.** A permeative pattern is seen in the distal tibia in this patient with pain and swelling. It was thought to represent an Ewing sarcoma, and a biopsy was performed with subsequent heavy loss of blood. This was found to be a hemangioma. An examination of the cortex demonstrates that the medial aspect is diffusely riddled with cortical holes compared with the lateral aspect. The endosteum laterally also is completely spared, making a marrow process very unlikely. Hemangioma, radiation, and osteoporosis can cause a pseudopermeative process, although in this example, osteoporosis and radiation would be unlikely because of its focal nature.

solid, one can assume the permeative process is emanating from the medullary space (Fig. 59.6); if the cortex has multiple small holes, assume the permeative pattern is from the cortical process. I call a permeative appearance that is secondary to cortical holes a "pseudopermeative" process to distinguish it from a true permeative process.

Other causes for a pseudopermeative process include hemangioma and radiation. A hemangioma can cause cortical holes in two ways: from focal hyperemia causing focal osteoporosis or by the blood vessels themselves tunneling through the cortex (Fig. 59.7). Radiation can cause cortical holes in bone and mimic a permeative pattern because of the death of cortical osteocytes, which can result in large lacunae in the cortex (Fig. 59.8). The cortical holes from radiation can be large, in which case they would not be confused with a true permeative process, but they can also be small and resemble an aggressive lesion.

If a permeative lesion is found, the differential diagnosis is usually an aggressive process such as Ewing sarcoma, infection, or eosinophilic granuloma in a young person (<30 years of age) or multiple myeloma, metastatic carcinomatosis, or primary lymphoma of bone in an older patient. If, however, the permeative pattern is a result of cortical holes—that is, a pseudopermeative pattern—the differential diagnosis is considerably less sinister: *aggressive osteoporosis*, *hemangioma*, or *radiation changes*. This differential diagnosis does not arise often but is very useful when it does (Table 59.1).

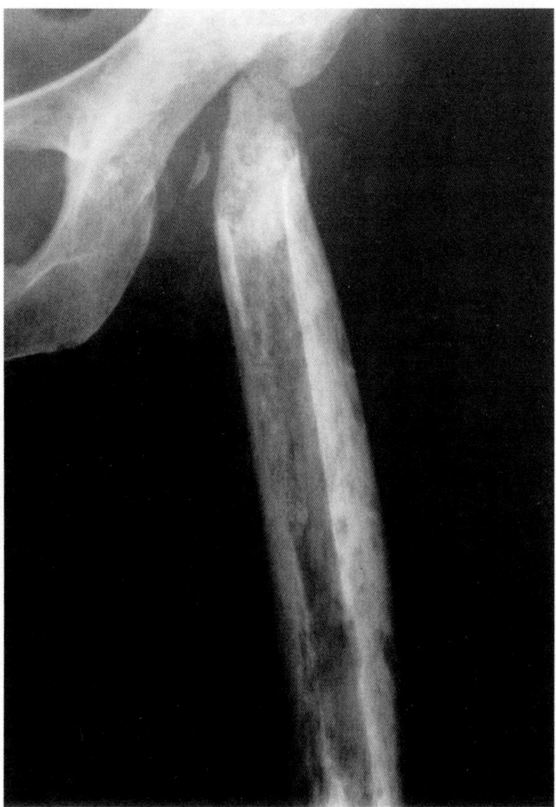

FIGURE 59.8. **Pseudopermeative Pattern Secondary to Radiation.** This patient had a fibrosarcoma treated with excision of the femoral head and subsequent radiation. A follow-up radiograph shows a diffuse permeative pattern throughout the proximal femur. Because the cortex is riddled with holes, it was thought that this was secondary to radiation rather than tumor recurrence. This is a pseudopermeative appearance secondary to radiation.

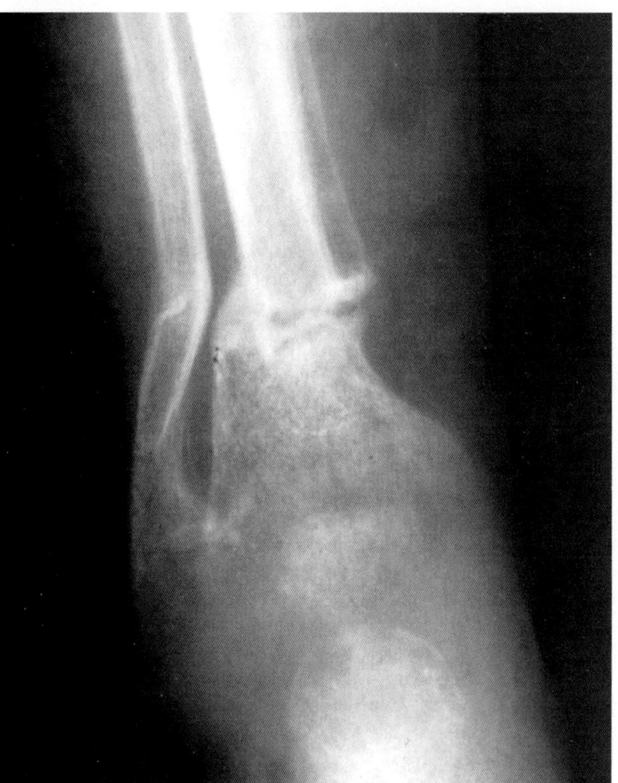

FIGURE 59.9. **Looser Fractures in Osteomalacia.** A horizontal fracture of the tibia and the fibula is present in this child with osteomalacia (rickets). Fractures of this type are called Looser fractures and are virtually pathognomonic for osteomalacia; however, they are rarely seen.

OSTEOMALACIA

Osteomalacia is the result of too much nonmineralized osteoid. The most common cause is renal osteodystrophy. The radiographic findings are almost identical to those of osteoporosis, and for the most part, the two disorders are indistinguishable. The only finding that is pathognomonic for osteomalacia is a Looser fracture (also called Looser zone), which is a fracture through large osteoid seams (Fig. 59.9). They are extremely uncommon but tend to occur in the femur, pelvis, and scapula.

In children, osteomalacia is called rickets. It causes the epiphyseal plates to become flared and irregular and the long bones to undergo bending from the bone softening (Fig. 59.10). As in adults, the most common cause is renal disease, although other causes such as biliary disease and dietary insufficiencies are occasionally seen.

TABLE 59.1

DIFFERENTIAL DIAGNOSIS OF PSEUDOPERMEATIVE PATTERN

Aggressive osteoporosis
Hemangioma
Radiation

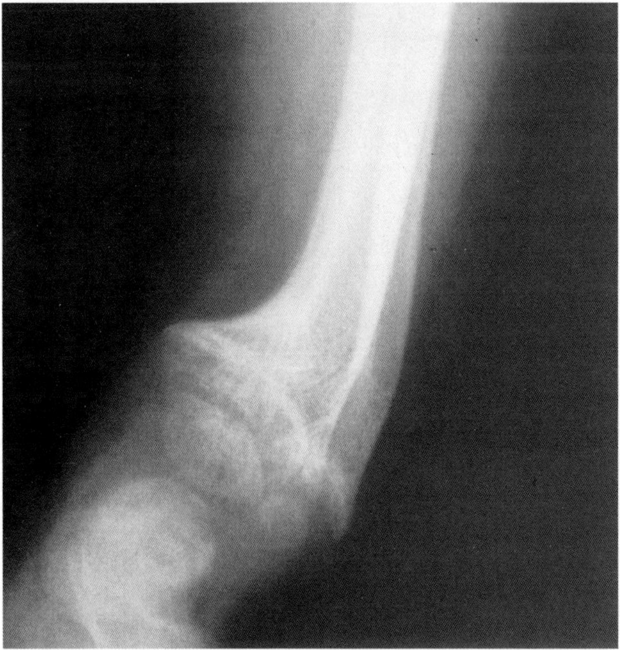

FIGURE 59.10. **Rickets.** Osteomalacia in children is called rickets and is identified by fraying and splaying of the physes as well as bending of the bone secondary to softening. This patient had renal osteodystrophy.

HYPERPARATHYROIDISM

Hyperparathyroidism occurs from excess parathyroid hormone. Parathyroid hormone causes osteoclastic resorption in bone, which leads to osteoporosis and osteomalacia. Primary HPT is caused by parathyroid adenomas and hyperplasia. Up to 40% of patients with primary HPT will demonstrate skeletal abnormalities radiographically. The most common cause of HPT is from renal disease, which leads to secondary HPT. Secondary HPT is the result of the parathyroid glands secreting excess PTH in response to the hypocalcemia that occurs.

The radiographic sign that is pathognomonic for HPT is subperiosteal bone resorption. It is seen most commonly on the radial aspect of the middle phalanges of the hand (Fig. 59.11), but it can be seen in any long bone in the body. It is commonly seen on the medial aspect of the proximal tibia, and subchondral bone resorption may be seen at the sacroiliac joints (Fig. 59.12) and in the distal clavicle.

Other radiographic findings include osteosclerosis, usually diffuse, but often involving the spine in a manner resembling the stripes on rugby jerseys; hence, the name "rugger jersey spine" (Fig. 59.13). Brown tumors are cystic lesions that are often expansile and aggressive in appearance (Fig. 59.14). They were once said to be more common in primary HPT but are seen more commonly associated with secondary HPT today because of the overwhelming preponderance of patients with secondary disease compared with primary disease. A brown tumor can have a variety of appearances, so the only thing characteristic about it is that it is associated with subperiosteal bone resorption. If the underlying HPT is treated, the subperiosteal resorption may disappear before the brown tumor does. This is not commonly seen, however.

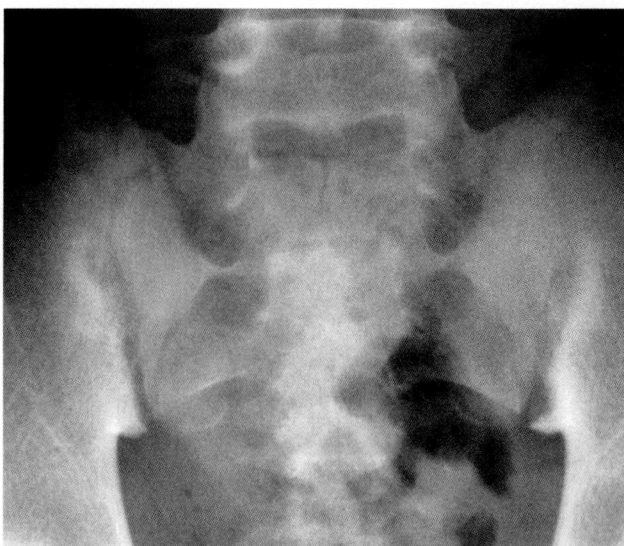

FIGURE 59.12. Hyperparathyroidism (HPT). Bilateral sacroiliac joint erosive changes with sclerosis are present in this patient with renal osteodystrophy and secondary hyperparathyroidism. Bilateral sacroiliac joint changes such as these are often seen with HPT.

Metabolic bone surveys (radiographs of the hands, spine, and long bones) were once routinely obtained in patients to look for subperiosteal bone resorption, brown tumors, osteosclerosis, calcifications, and Looser fractures. They are no longer recommended, however, as the yield of positive findings

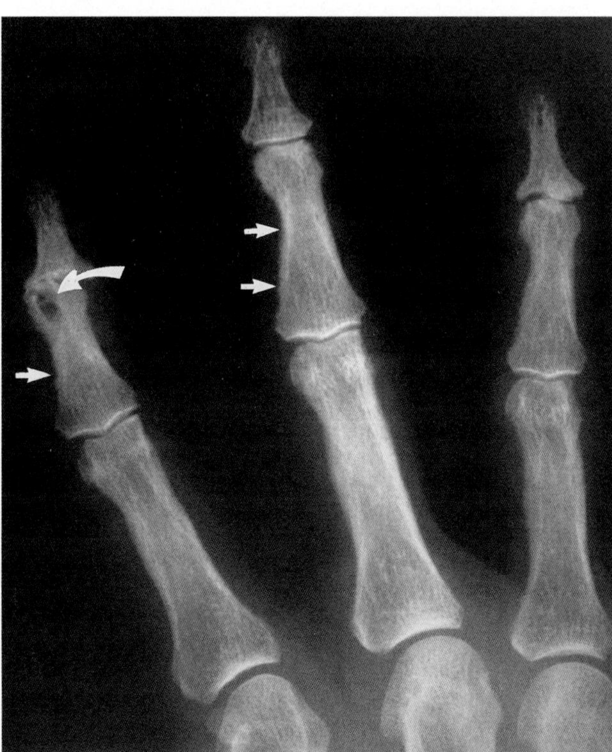

FIGURE 59.11. Hyperparathyroidism (HPT). Subperiosteal bone resorption can be seen at the radial aspect of the middle phalanges (*straight arrows*), which is pathognomonic for HPT. The lytic lesion seen in the distal middle phalanx (*curved arrow*) may be a small brown tumor.

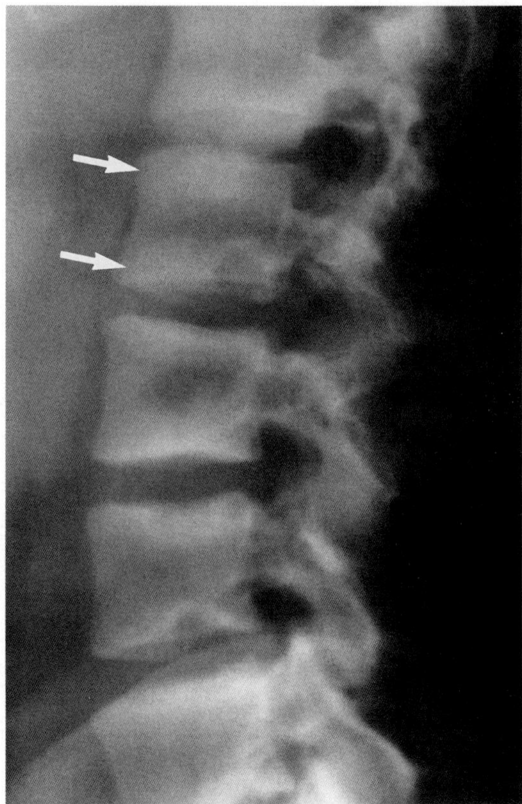

FIGURE 59.13. Hyperparathyroidism (HPT). Sclerotic bands present at the vertebral body endplates (*arrows*) are characteristic of a rugger jersey spine. This is seen in HPT.

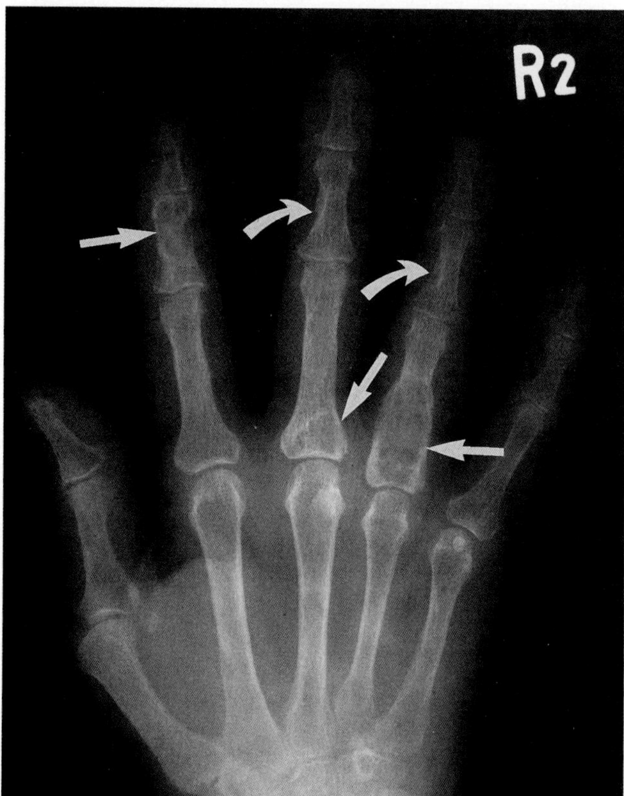

FIGURE 59.14. Brown Tumors in Hyperparathyroidism (HPT). Several lytic lesions are present in the phalanges (*straight arrows*) in this patient with HPT; these are brown tumors. Note the subperiosteal bone resorption in the radial aspect of the middle phalanges (*curved arrows*), which is pathognomonic for HPT.

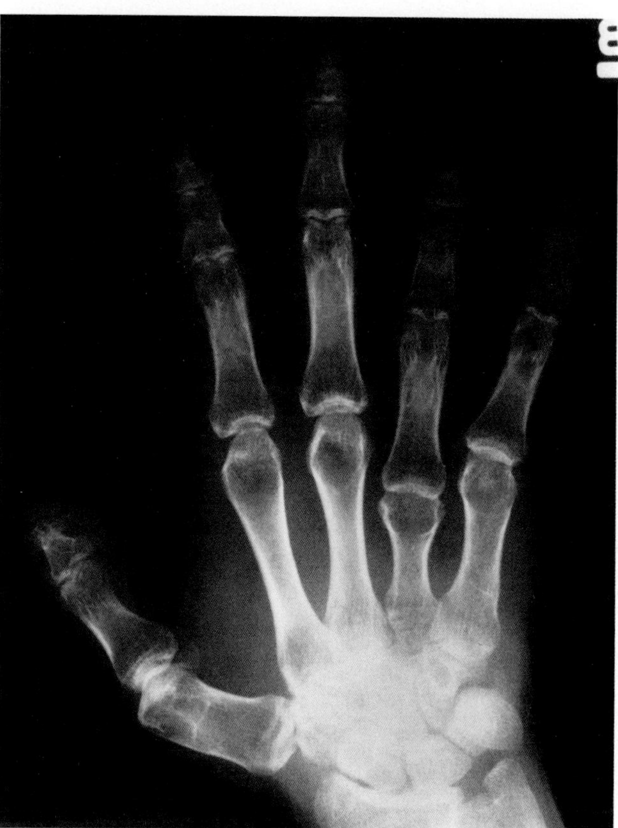

FIGURE 59.15. Pseudohypoparathyroidism. Brachydactyly is present in several of the metacarpals in this patient with pseudohypoparathyroidism. A short fourth metacarpal as seen here is a frequent finding in this entity.

is extremely low and rarely will a positive finding affect treatment. In place of the metabolic bone survey, it is now recommended that radiographs of the hands be obtained to look for subperiosteal resorption. A radionuclide bone scan can be obtained in selected cases, which will show increased radionuclide uptake by brown tumors and Looser fractures. Also, investigation of causes of hypercalcemia, which can be caused by metastatic disease or metabolic bone disease, should include a bone scan.

HYPOPARATHYROIDISM

Hypoparathyroidism occurs because of a deficiency of the parathyroid glands to secrete normal amounts of PTH. Few skeletal changes occur in hypoparathyroidism. The calvarium on occasion will show thickening, and calcification in the basal ganglia of the brain has been described.

PSEUDOHYPOPARATHYROIDISM AND PSEUDOPSEUDOHYPOPARATHYROIDISM

Pseudohypoparathyroidism is caused by a congenital failure of tissues to respond to PTH. The parathyroid glands are normal in these cases. Treating these patients with PTH is of no help because the problem lies in the end organs, not the parathyroid glands. A characteristic appearance is seen in these patients: obesity, round facies, short stature, and brachydactyly (Fig. 59.15). The tubular bones of the hands and feet are often all short. In pseudopseudohypoparathyroidism, there is no parathyroid abnormality and no end-organ problem; these patients merely resemble patients with pseudohypoparathyroidism. In summary, hypoparathyroidism is a parathyroid gland problem, pseudohypoparathyroidism is an end-organ problem, and pseudopseudohypoparathyroidism is a mimicker of pseudohypoparathyroidism morphologically.

PITUITARY GLAND HYPERFUNCTION

A secreting adenoma or hyperplasia of the anterior lobe of the pituitary gland will result in accelerated bone growth. If it occurs before the physes close, it causes gigantism. If it occurs after the physes are closed, the result is acromegaly.

Acromegaly has several characteristic radiographic features in the skeletal system. The skull radiograph invariably shows calvarial thickening, enlarged sinuses, and an enlarged sella turcica. The jaw is prognathic. The terminal tufts of the distal phalanges become hypertrophied and have a so-called spade appearance (an appearance not unlike a spade or shovel) (Fig. 59.16). The joint spaces are occasionally minimally enlarged because of hypertrophy of the hyaline articular cartilage. Early degenerative joint disease ensues because the cartilage itself is abnormal. The soft tissues also hypertrophy, with various measurements of soft tissue thickening used by some as an indicator for acromegaly. For instance, thickening of the heel pad adjacent to the calcaneus has been used as a sign of acromegaly.

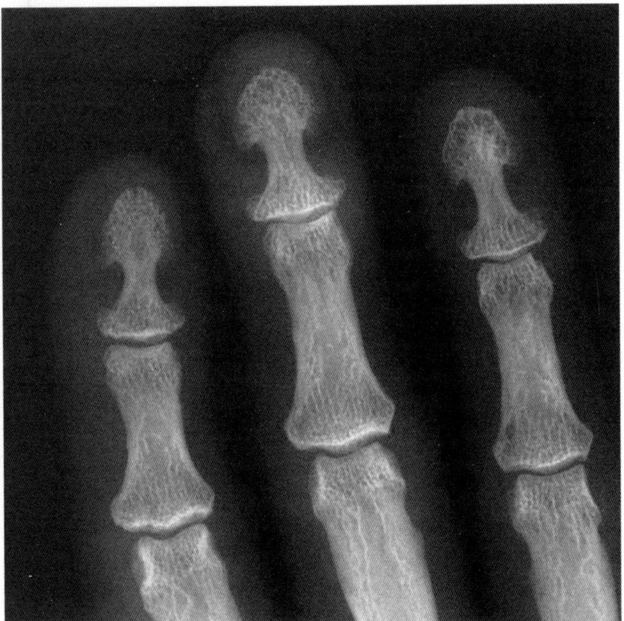

FIGURE 59.16. **Acromegaly.** Enlargement of the distal tufts in the phalanges (the so-called spade tufts) are characteristic of acromegaly.

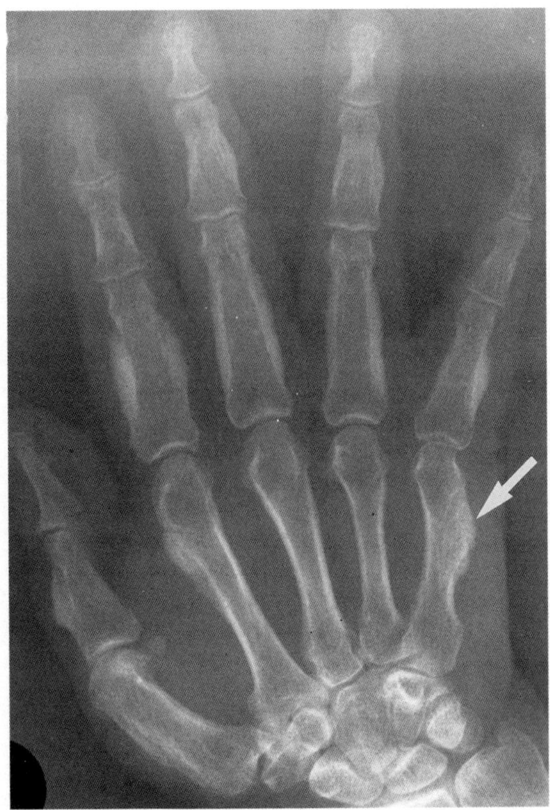

FIGURE 59.17. **Thyroid Acropachy.** Extensive periostitis is noted in the metacarpals and phalanges in this patient with thyroid acropachy. It is characteristic to have marked involvement of the ulnar aspect of the fifth metacarpal (*arrow*) in this entity.

THYROID GLAND HYPERFUNCTION

In children, hyperthyroidism can result in increased skeletal maturation; however, this is seldom marked. A rare manifestation of hyperthyroidism in adults is thyroid acropachy. This occurs only after prior thyroidectomy and the cause is unknown. A characteristic appearing periostitis occurs in the metacarpals and phalanges of the hands and feet (Fig. 59.17). It invariably involves the ulnar aspect of the fifth metacarpal, a useful differential point that can be used to tell thyroid acropachy from other causes of diffuse periostitis such as hypertrophic pulmonary osteoarthropathy and pachydermoperiostosis, a rare form of idiopathic periostitis and skin thickening.

THYROID GLAND HYPOFUNCTION

Decreased thyroid secretion, or cretinism, results in delayed skeletal maturation in children. Delay in ossification of epiphyseal centers with occasional appearance of "stippled" epiphyses is seen. A delay in physeal closure also occurs, in some instances with failure of physeal closure noted in the third and fourth decades.

OSTEOSCLEROSIS

The radiographic finding of diffuse increased bone density, osteosclerosis, is somewhat uncommon, yet every radiologist must have a differential diagnosis for this process. Fortunately, it is a rather short differential and there are criteria to narrow down the list of possibilities.

The list of diseases that can cause diffuse osteosclerosis is quite long, but a list that includes 95% to 98% of the pathologic processes is all that is really necessary. The entities I include in the differential diagnosis of diffuse osteosclerosis are listed in Table 59.2.

The mnemonic I use to remember them is "*R*egular *S*ex *M*akes *O*ccasional *P*erversions *M*uch *M*ore *P*leasurable *A*nd *F*antastic." I will cover each of these topics in generalities, trying to point out the features of each that should be looked for to allow inclusion or exclusion from the differential.

Renal Osteodystrophy

Anything that causes HPT can cause osteosclerosis, but renal disease is by far the most common disease in which osteosclerosis

TABLE 59.2

DIFFERENTIAL DIAGNOSIS OF DIFFUSE BONY SCLEROSIS (DENSE BONES)

Renal osteodystrophy
Sickle cell disease
Myelofibrosis
Osteopetrosis
Pyknodysostosis
Metastatic carcinoma
Mastocytosis
Paget's disease
Athletes
Fluorosis

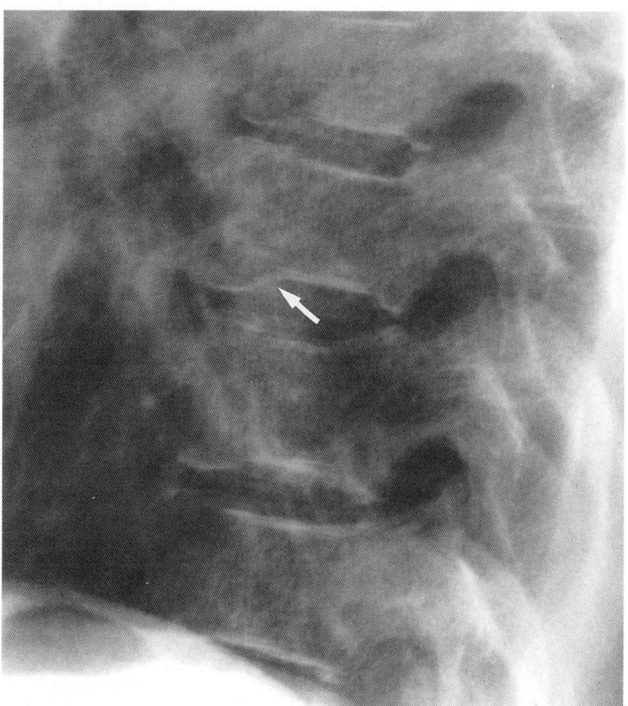

FIGURE 59.18. **Sickle Cell Disease.** Step-off deformities (*arrow*) are seen in the endplates of several vertebral bodies in this patient with sickle cell disease. They are also called fish vertebrae.

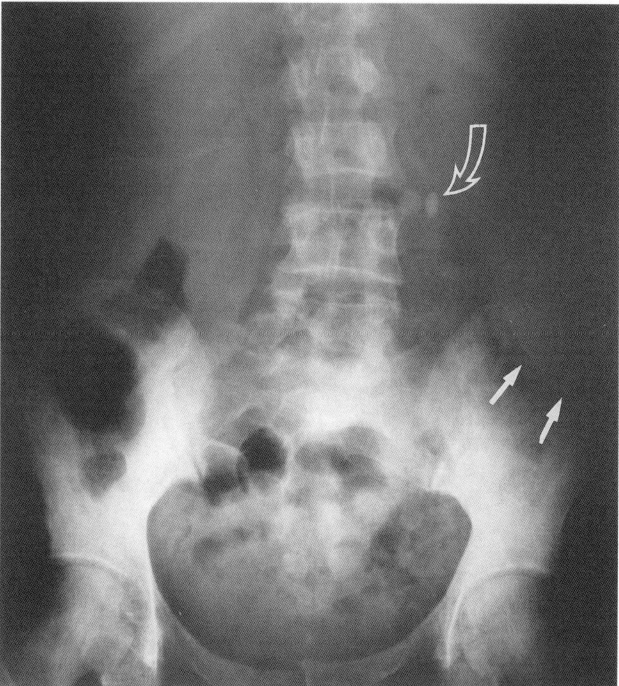

FIGURE 59.19. **Myelofibrosis.** Diffuse increased bone density is seen throughout the pelvis and spine in this patient with myelofibrosis. The spleen is markedly enlarged (*straight arrows*), and opaque iron tablets (*curved arrow*) can be seen, which were taken for the anemia that is often found in this disorder.

is seen. Although the most common presentation of renal osteodystrophy is osteopenia, about 10% to 20% of the patients with renal osteodystrophy will exhibit osteosclerosis, and the reasons for it are unknown. As mentioned previously, the sine qua non of renal osteodystrophy is subperiosteal bone resorption, seen earliest and most reliably at the radial aspect of the middle phalanges of the hands. Subperiosteal bone resorption is not seen nearly as frequently today as it was 30 years ago, likely due to better and earlier treatment of renal disease.

Sickle Cell Disease

Like renal osteodystrophy, the underlying cause of dense bones in sickle cell disease is unknown. It only occurs in a small percentage of patients. Additional signs to look for are bone infarcts and step-off deformities of the vertebral body endplates (Fig. 59.18). These are also called "fish" vertebrae after their appearance like the vertebrae found in fish. Avascular necrosis of the hip is frequently an accompanying finding.

Myelofibrosis

Also called agnogenic myeloid metaplasia, myelofibrosis is a disease caused by progressive fibrosis of the marrow in patients older than 50 years of age. It leads to anemia with marked splenomegaly and extramedullary hematopoiesis. Whenever osteosclerosis is seen in a patient older than 50 years of age, a search should be made for a large spleen and extramedullary hematopoiesis (Fig. 59.19).

Osteopetrosis

This is a hereditary abnormality that results in extremely dense bones throughout the skeleton (Fig. 59.20). There are congenita and tarda forms, with different degrees of severity in each. The congenita form occurs at birth and can be lethal. Anemia, jaundice, hepatosplenomegaly, and infections are often present in this form. The tarda form is seen in older children and adults and has milder clinical problems. The tarda form may be so mild that it has no clinical findings. Although uncommon, it is not so rare that one will never see a case; therefore, it should be included in this differential diagnosis.

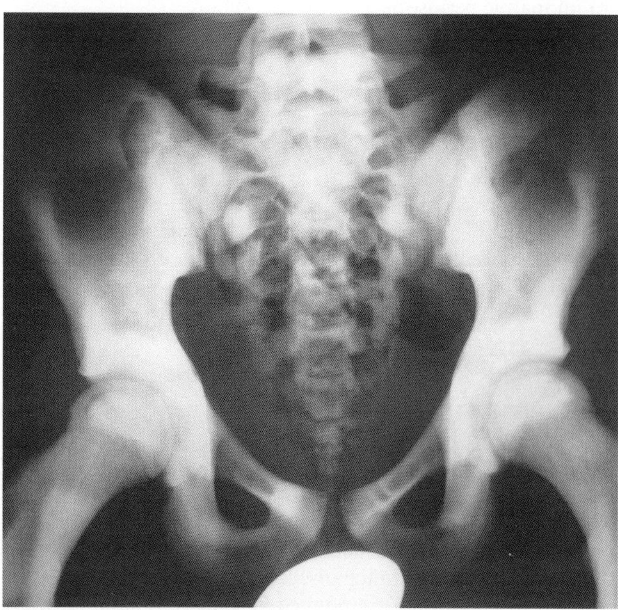

FIGURE 59.20. **Osteopetrosis.** Marked, diffuse bony sclerosis is seen throughout the skeleton in this patient with osteopetrosis.

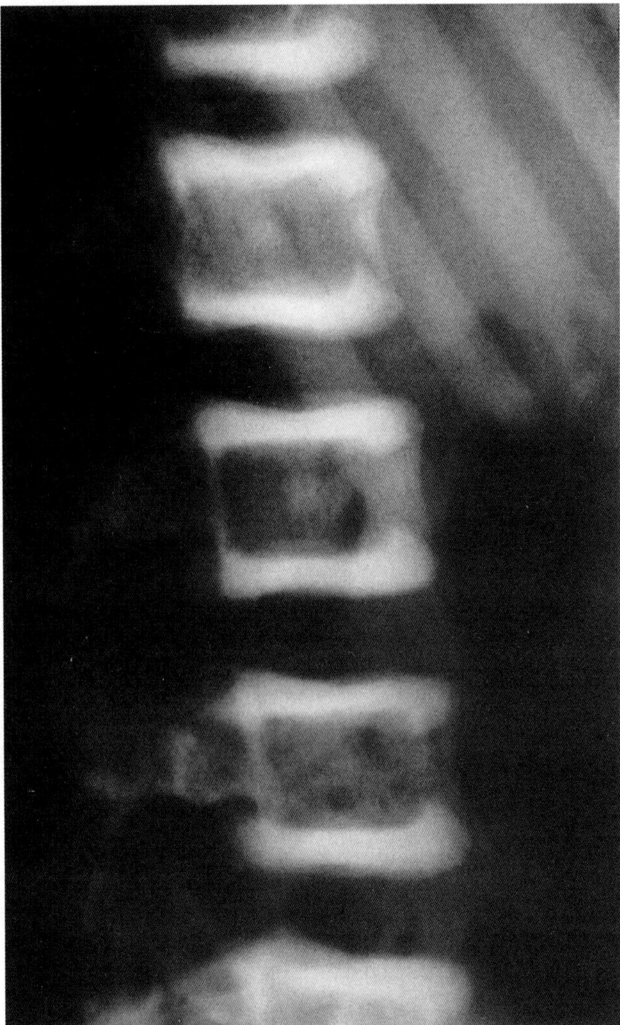

FIGURE 59.21. Sandwich Vertebrae. Dense bands of sclerosis parallel to the endplates are seen in this patient with osteopetrosis. These are called sandwich vertebrae, which are much more distinct than the dense bands of sclerosis seen in a rugger jersey spine (see Fig. 59.13).

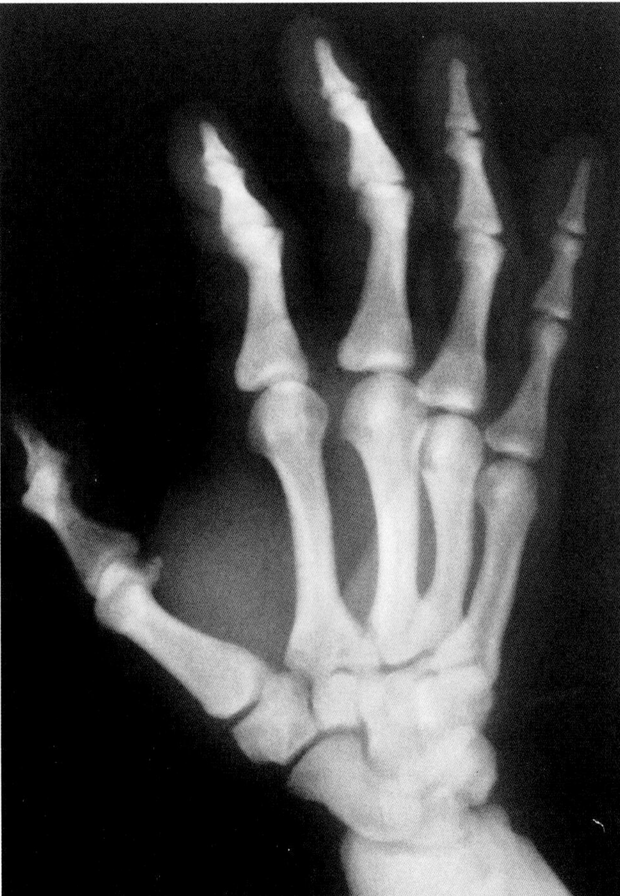

FIGURE 59.22. Pyknodysostosis. Diffuse, dense sclerosis is seen throughout the hand and wrist in this patient with pyknodysostosis. Note the absent distal phalangeal tufts that appear pointed and sclerotic, which is virtually pathognomonic for pyknodysostosis.

A characteristic finding is the so-called bone-in-bone appearance often seen in the vertebral bodies in which the vertebrae have a small replica of the vertebral body inside the normal one. Also characteristic are the "sandwich vertebrae" in which the endplates are densely sclerotic, giving the appearance of a sandwich (Fig. 59.21). The sandwich vertebrae appearance resembles a rugger jersey spine but can be differentiated by being much denser and more sharply defined.

Pyknodysostosis

This is the other congenital abnormality with dense bones that should be considered in the differential diagnosis of osteosclerosis. It is seen less commonly than osteopetrosis. These patients are typically short and have hypoplastic mandibles. The distinguishing radiographic finding that is essentially pathognomonic is acroosteolysis with sclerosis. The distal phalanges often have the appearance of chalk that has been put into a pencil sharpener: they are pointed and dense (Fig. 59.22). No other disease process has this appearance. Another name for this disorder is Toulouse–Lautrec syndrome, named for the famous artist who was afflicted with pyknodysostosis.

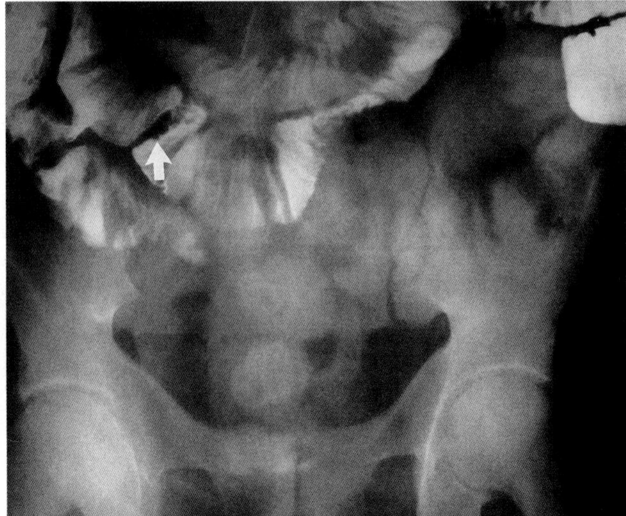

FIGURE 59.23. Mastocytosis. Uniform increased bone density is seen throughout the pelvis in this patient with mastocytosis. Small bowel thickened folds with nodules (*arrow*) can be seen in this barium study; these are often found in mastocytosis.

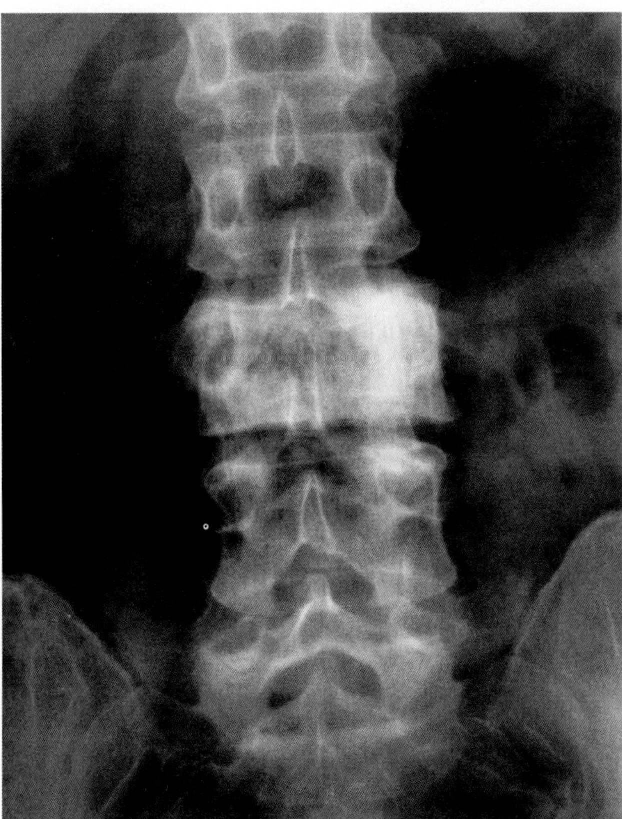

FIGURE 59.24. **Paget's Disease.** Dense, bony sclerosis with overgrowth of the vertebral body is seen at the L3 vertebra in this patient with Paget's disease. The left L3 pedicle is markedly dense and enlarged.

Metastatic Carcinoma

Only rarely will diffuse metastatic carcinoma cause a problem in diagnosis. I have seen only a handful of cases in which diffuse metastatic carcinoma mimicked diffuse osteosclerosis, and in every case, the primary tumor was either prostate or breast carcinoma. If cortical destruction or a lytic component is present, it simplifies the differential diagnosis, so a search should be made for these.

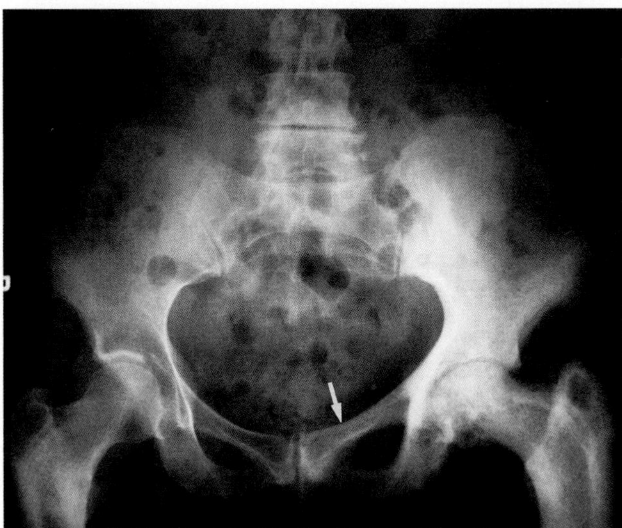

FIGURE 59.25. **Paget's Disease.** Bony sclerosis with some bony enlargement is seen in the left pelvis and proximal femur of this patient and is characteristic of Paget's disease. Note the cortical thickening of the left superior pubic ramus (*arrow*), which is called thickening of the iliopectineal line and is commonly seen in Paget's disease.

Mastocytosis

This is another rare disorder that can cause uniformly increased bone density. Unfortunately, there are no other radiographic findings that might help with the diagnosis. Patients with this disease have thickened small bowel folds with nodules, but of course, to see them, an upper GI contrast study must be performed (Fig. 59.23). Urticaria pigmentosa is a characteristic skin lesion found in these patients.

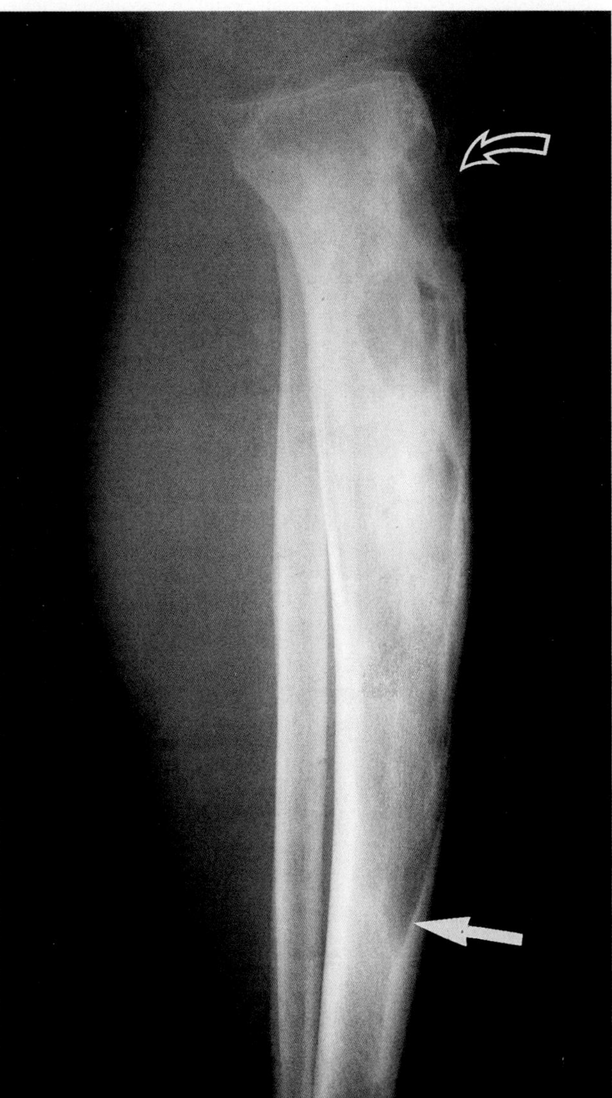

FIGURE 59.26. **Paget's Disease.** A lytic process involving the proximal two-thirds of the tibia is noted and has a blade of grass or flame-shaped leading edge (*straight arrow*), which is characteristic of Paget's disease. This represents the lytic phase of the Paget's disease. The sclerotic phase of the Paget's disease can be seen in the midportion of this lesion, and an area of probable sarcomatous degeneration can be seen in the proximal tibia (*curved arrow*), where apparent cortical destruction is noted. This represents all three phases or stages of Paget's disease.

Paget's Disease

Diffuse Paget's disease that could be confused with one of the other diseases in the differential diagnosis of generalized osteosclerosis is very rare. Paget's disease classically causes bony enlargement (Fig. 59.24), but this is not always present. It occurs most commonly in the pelvis (Fig. 59.25), where it has been said that the iliopectineal line on the pelvic brim must be thickened if Paget's disease is present. In fact, the iliopectineal line is usually, but not always, thickened. Paget's disease can occur in any bone in the body, including the smaller bones of the hands and feet.

Paget's disease has three distinct phases visible radiographically: a lytic phase, a sclerotic phase, and a mixed lytic–sclerotic phase. The lytic phase often has a sharp leading edge called a flame-shaped or blade-of-grass leading edge (Fig. 59.26). In a long bone, with the sole exception being the tibia, Paget's disease always starts at the end of the bone; therefore, if a lesion is present in the middle of a long bone and does not extend to either end, one can safely exclude Paget's disease.

Athletes

Radiographs of professional athletes quite often demonstrate increased cortical thickness and apparent diffuse osteosclerosis to the point of appearing pathologic. Undoubtedly, increased stress causes hypertrophy of bone as well as muscle. The increased density in these otherwise normal subjects is occasionally misinterpreted as abnormal, with extensive workups and even bone biopsy resulting.

Fluorosis

This is a rare disorder that is usually a result of chronic intake of fluoride in certain geographic areas where large amounts of fluoride are present in the drinking water. It can also be a result of long-term therapy with sodium fluoride for osteoporosis.

A radiographic finding that patients with fluorosis often have is ligamentous calcification. Calcification of the sacrotuberous ligament is said to be characteristic of fluorosis.

SUMMARY

There are other categories of disease that could be covered in a chapter on metabolic bone disease, but most of the remaining disorders are exceedingly rare and not likely to be seen by most radiologists on a routine basis.

Suggested Readings

Cooper KL. Radiology of metabolic bone disease. *Endocrinol Metab Clin North Am* 1989;18:955–976.

Helms CA, Munk PL. Pseudopermeative skeletal lesions. *Br J Radiol* 1990;63: 461–467.

McAfee JG. Radionuclide imaging in metabolic and systemic skeletal diseases. *Semin Nucl Med* 1987;17:334–349.

CHAPTER 60 ■ SKELETAL "DON'T TOUCH" LESIONS

CLYDE A. HELMS AND EMILY N. VINSON

Skeletal "don't touch" lesions are those processes that are so radiographically characteristic that a biopsy or additional diagnostic tests are unnecessary. Not only does the biopsy result in unnecessary morbidity and cost, but in some instances, as is discussed in this chapter, a biopsy can also be frankly misleading and lead to additional unnecessary surgery.

Most radiology training stresses giving a differential diagnosis of a lesion, leaving it up to the clinician to decide between the various entities. For the "don't touch" lesions, however, a differential list is inappropriate as that often makes the next step in the decision-making process a biopsy. Because these lesions do not need to undergo biopsy for a final diagnosis, a radiologic diagnosis should be made without a list of differential possibilities. These lesions can be classified into three categories: (1) posttraumatic lesions, (2) normal variants, and (3) lesions that are real but obviously benign.

POSTTRAUMATIC LESIONS

Myositis ossificans is an example of a lesion that should not undergo biopsy because its aggressive histologic appearance can often mimic a sarcoma. Unfortunately, radical surgery has been performed based on the histologic appearance of myositis ossificans when the radiologic appearance was diagnostic. The typical radiologic appearance of myositis ossificans is circumferential peripheral calcification with a lucent center (Fig. 60.1). This is often best appreciated on a computed tomographic scan. A malignant tumor that mimics myositis ossificans has an ill-defined periphery and a calcified or ossific center (Fig. 60.2). Periosteal reaction can be seen with myositis ossificans or with a tumor. Occasionally, the peripheral calcification of myositis ossificans can be too faint to appreciate; in these cases, a computed tomographic scan should help or else delayed radiographs 1 or 2 weeks later are recommended. Biopsy should be avoided when myositis ossificans is a clinical consideration. MRI can be misleading because the peripheral calcification is not as well seen, and edema in the soft tissues can extend beyond the calcific rim (Fig. 60.3).

Avulsion Injury. Another posttraumatic entity in which a biopsy can be misleading is any avulsion injury. These injuries can have an aggressive radiographic appearance, but because of their characteristic location at ligament and tendon insertion sites (e.g., anterior-inferior iliac spine or ischial tuberosity), they should be recognized as benign (Figs. 60.4 and 60.5). As with myositis ossificans, delayed radiographs of several weeks will usually allow the problem case to become more radiographically clear. Biopsy can lead to the mistaken diagnosis of a sarcoma and should therefore be avoided. Any area undergoing healing can have a high nuclear-to-chromatin ratio and a high mitotic figure count, thereby occasionally simulating a malignancy histologically. ***Cortical desmoid*** is a process on the medial supracondylar ridge of the distal femur that is considered by many to be the result of an avulsion of the adductor magnus muscle. It occasionally simulates an aggressive lesion radiographically, and histologically, it can look malignant. In many instances, biopsy has led to amputation for this benign, radiographically characteristic lesion (Figs. 60.6 and 60.7). Cortical desmoids occur only on the posteromedial condyle of the femur. They might or might not be associated with pain and can have increased radionuclide uptake on a bone scan. They might or might not exhibit periosteal new bone and usually occur in young people. Biopsy should be avoided in all cases. Painful cortical desmoids should become asymptomatic with rest. They are often seen as an incidental finding on MRI of the knee and have a characteristic appearance (Fig. 60.8).

Trauma can lead to large, cystic geodes or subchondral cysts near joints and can be mistaken for other lesions, resulting in a biopsy being ordered. Although the biopsy specimen is not likely to mimic a malignant process, it is nevertheless avoidable. Because geodes from degenerative disease almost always are associated with additional findings such as joint space narrowing, sclerosis, and osteophytes, a diagnosis should be made radiographically (Fig. 60.9). On occasion, however, the additional findings are subtle and can be missed (Fig. 60.10). Geodes can also occur in the setting of calcium pyrophosphate dihydrate crystal disease, rheumatoid arthritis, and avascular necrosis.

Discogenic Vertebral Sclerosis. An entity that is often confused for metastatic disease to the spine is discogenic vertebral disease. It can mimic metastatic disease very closely, and unless the radiologist is familiar with this process, it can lead to an unnecessary biopsy. Discogenic vertebral disease most often is sclerotic and focal (Fig. 60.11). It is always adjacent to the endplate and the associated disc space should be narrow. Osteophytosis is invariably present. It really is a variant of a Schmorl node and should not be confused with a metastatic focus. On occasion, it can be lytic or even mixed lytic–sclerotic. The typical clinical setting is a middle-aged woman with chronic low back pain. Old radiographs often confirm the benign nature of this process. In the setting of disc space

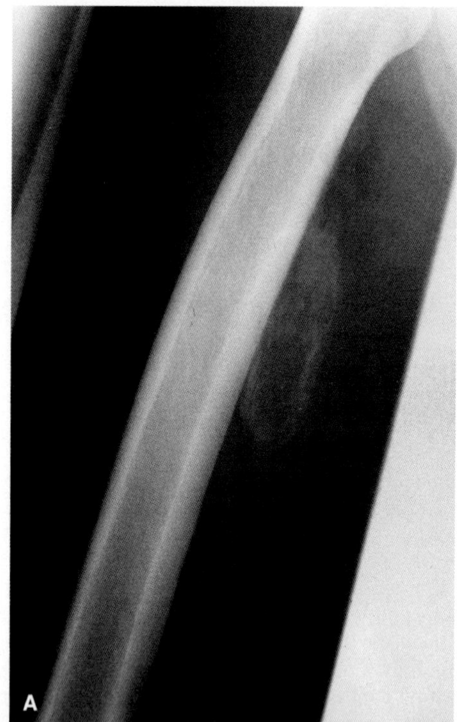

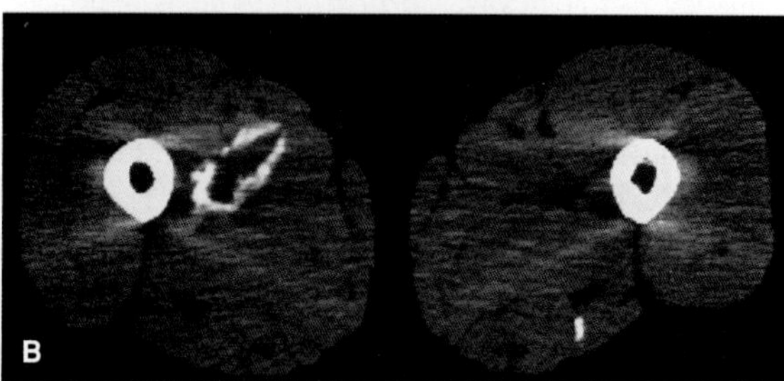

FIGURE 60.1. **Myositis Ossificans. A:** A radiograph of the femur in this patient who presented with a soft tissue mass shows a calcific density adjacent to the posterior cortex of the femur, which is calcified primarily in its periphery. If it is difficult on the radiograph alone to state definitely that this is peripheral circumferential calcification, a computed tomographic scan, as shown in (**B**), can be helpful in showing that the calcification is unequivocally peripheral in nature. This is virtually diagnostic of myositis ossificans.

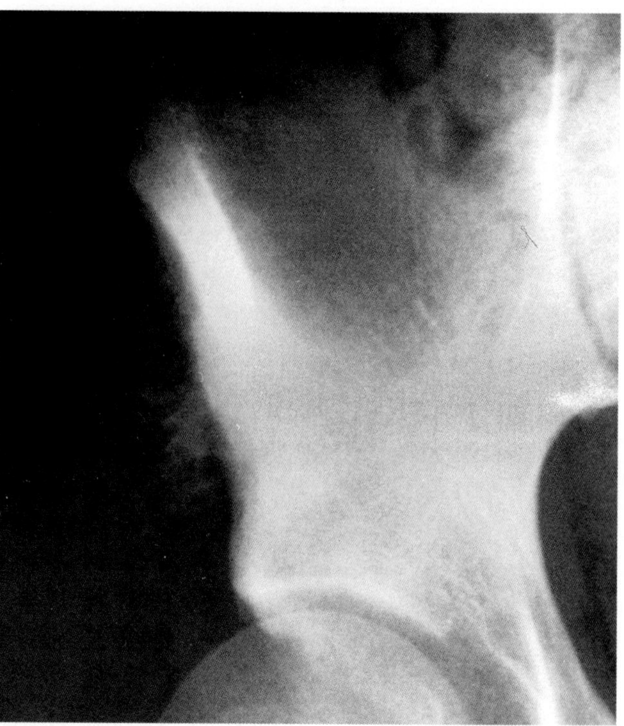

FIGURE 60.2. **Osteogenic Sarcoma.** Hazy, ill-defined calcification is seen adjacent to the iliac wing in this patient, which can be ascertained from the radiograph as definitely not being circumferential in nature. Even though a prior history of trauma was obtained in this case, myositis ossificans is not a consideration with this appearance of calcification. Biopsy showed this to be an osteogenic sarcoma.

narrowing and osteophytosis, focal sclerosis adjacent to an endplate should not undergo biopsy.

Fracture. Occasionally, a fracture will be the cause of extensive osteosclerosis and periostitis, which can mimic a primary bone tumor (Fig. 60.12). Lack of immobilization can result in exuberant callus, which can be misinterpreted as aggressive periostitis or even new tumor bone. Results of a biopsy in such a case might resemble a malignant lesion; therefore, any case associated with trauma should be carefully reviewed for a fracture.

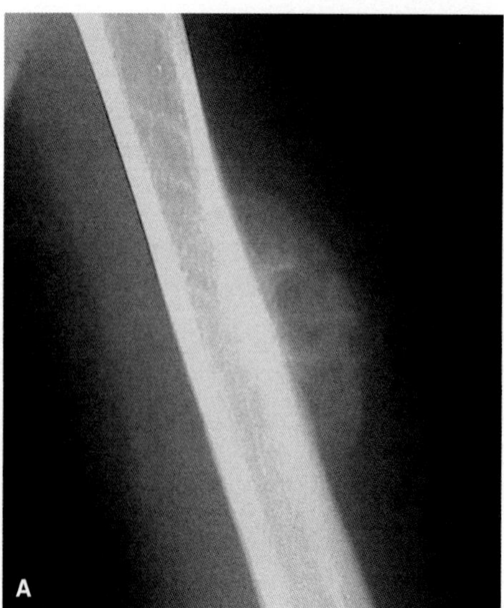

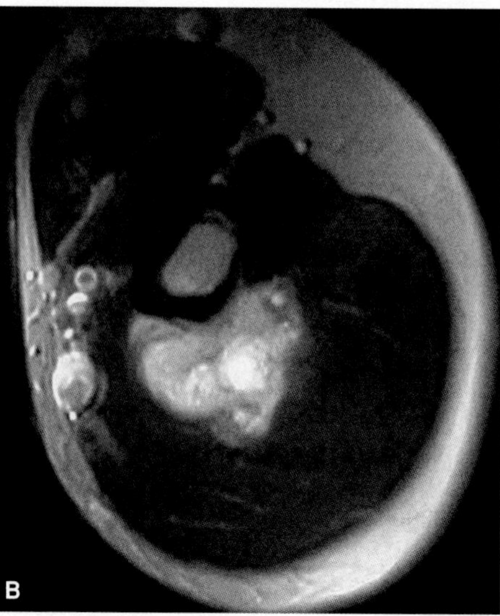

FIGURE 60.3. **Myositis Ossificans. A:** A radiograph of the humerus in this 30-year-old man shows a calcific mass adjacent to the diaphysis of the humerus. The calcification is not clearly peripheral in nature, although the central portion is less well mineralized. **B:** An axial T2-weighted image through the mass shows only a high–signal-intensity mass without evidence of calcification.

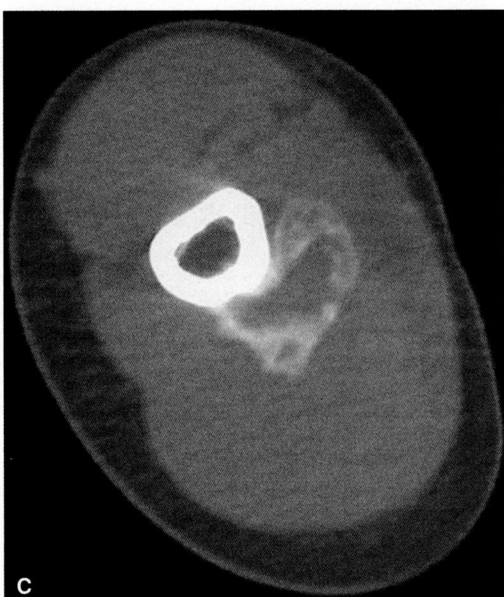

FIGURE 60.3. (*Continued*) C: A CT scan through the mass demonstrates the typical peripheral calcification which is virtually pathognomonic for myositis ossificans.

Pseudodislocation of the Humerus. Another traumatic process that can be misdiagnosed radiologically, leading to inappropriate treatment and morbidity, is a pseudodislocation of the humerus (Fig. 60.13). This results from a fracture with hemarthrosis, which causes distention of the joint and migration of the humeral head inferiorly. An axial or transscapular view shows it is not anteriorly or posteriorly dislocated (the usual forms of shoulder dislocation) but merely inferiorly subluxated. On an anteroposterior view, it can mimic a posterior dislocation in that the normal superimposition of the humeral head and the glenoid is missing. Often, attempts are made to "relocate" the humeral head, which, of course, are both fruitless (because it is not dislocated) and painful. A fracture is invariably present, and if not seen on the initial radiographs, it should be sought after with additional views. The transscapular or the axial view is the key to making the diagnosis

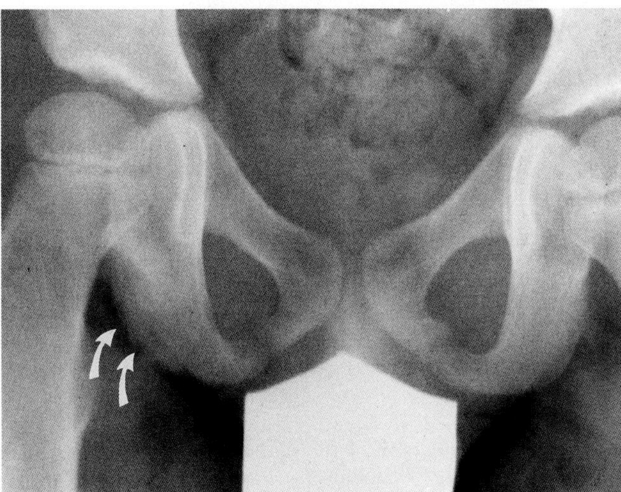

FIGURE 60.4. **Avulsion Injury.** Cortical irregularity (*arrows*) at the ischial tuberosity in this patient with pain over this region raises the question of possible tumor. This is a classic appearance, however, for an avulsion injury from this region, and a biopsy should be avoided.

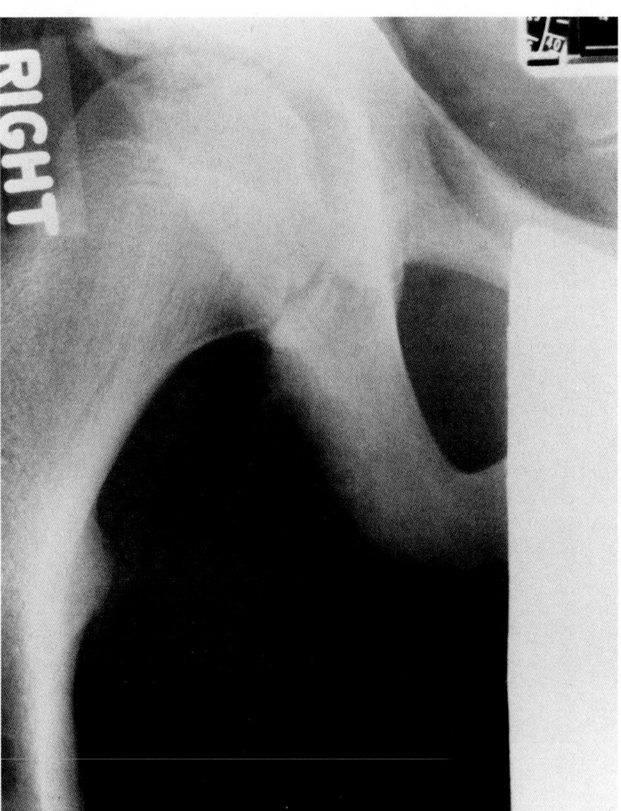

FIGURE 60.5. **Avulsion Injury.** Cortical irregularity with a Codman triangle of periostitis is seen along the ischial tuberosity that was at first thought to represent a malignancy. Because of the characteristic location, an avulsion injury was considered and the lesion was observed. It healed without sequelae.

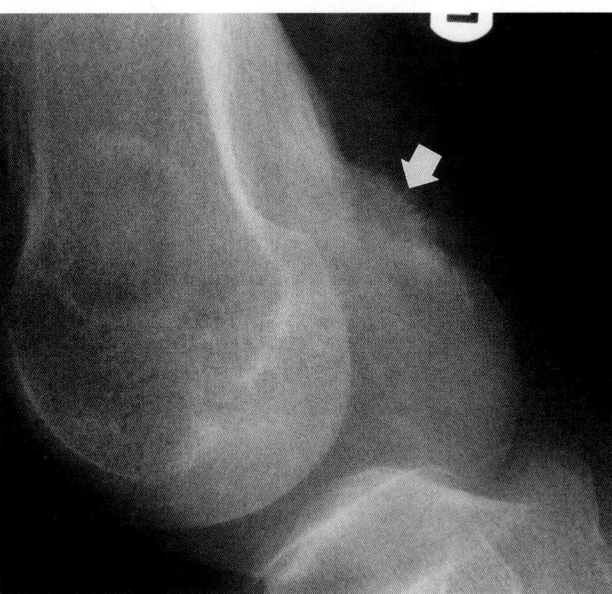

FIGURE 60.6. **Cortical Desmoid.** A focal cortical irregularity in this patient is seen in the posterior aspect of the femur (*arrow*) with adjacent periostitis noted. Although a tumor such as an early parosteal osteosarcoma could perhaps have this appearance, this is a characteristic location and appearance for a cortical desmoid and should not undergo biopsy. Pain will disappear with rest.

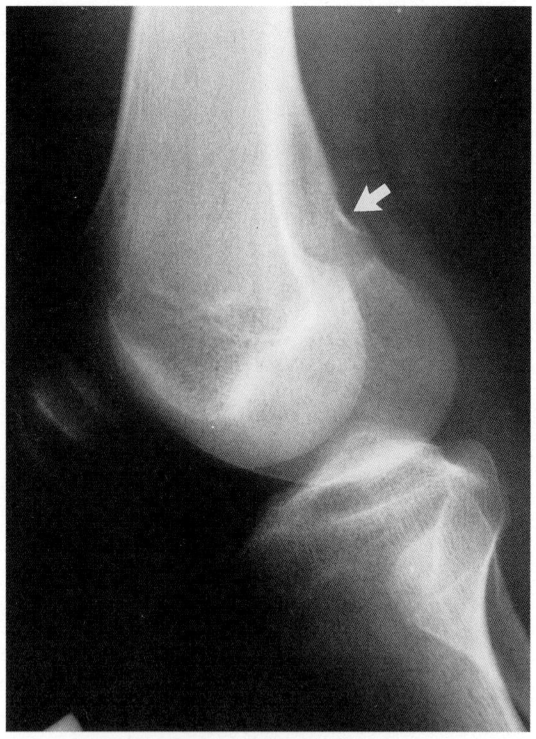

FIGURE 60.7. **Cortical Desmoid.** A well-defined cortical defect is seen in the posterior distal femur (*arrow*), which is a common appearance for a fairly well-healed cortical desmoid.

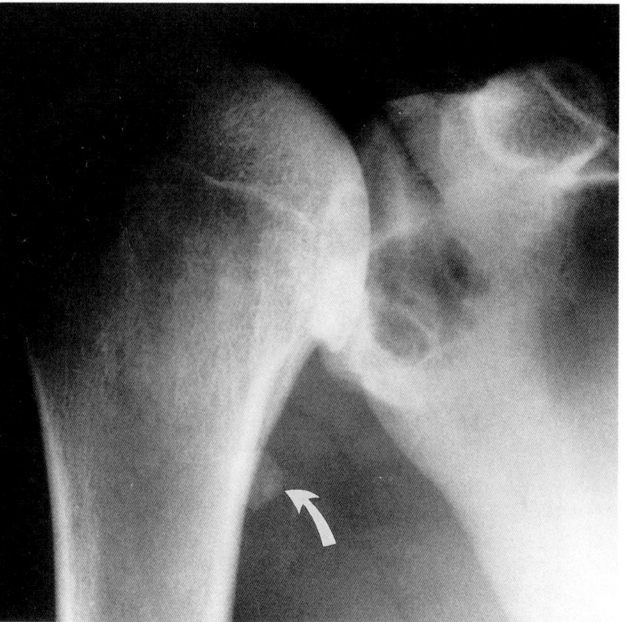

FIGURE 60.9. **Geode.** A large cystic lesion was found in the shoulder in this middle-aged weight lifter, and the possibility of a metastatic process was considered. Because the humeral head has sclerosis and osteophytosis as well as a loose body in the joint (*arrow*), degenerative disease of the shoulder was diagnosed; this makes the cystic lesion almost certainly a geode or subchondral cyst.

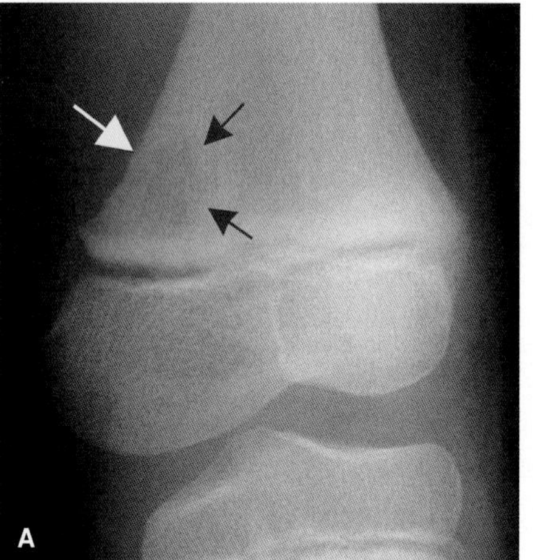

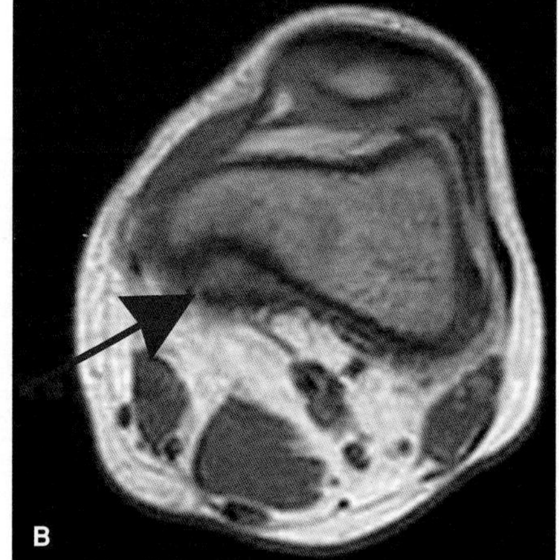

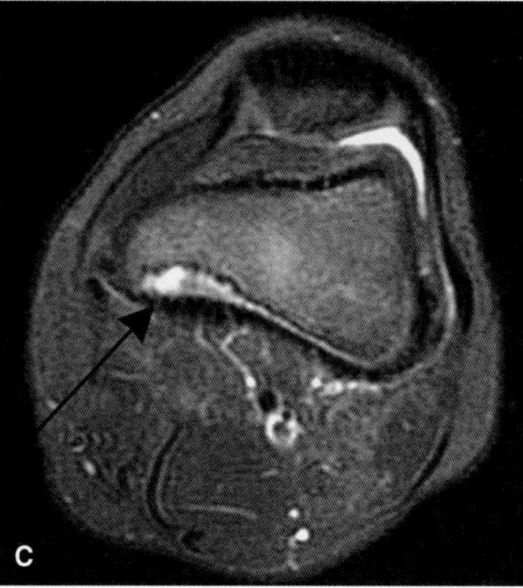

FIGURE 60.8. **Cortical Desmoid. A:** An anteroposterior radiograph of the knee in a child shows a faint lytic lesion (*arrows*) in the medial aspect of the distal femur. Axial T1- (**B**) and T2-weighted (**C**) images through the lesion show a cortically based process (*arrows*) in the medial supracondylar ridge which is characteristic of a cortical desmoid.

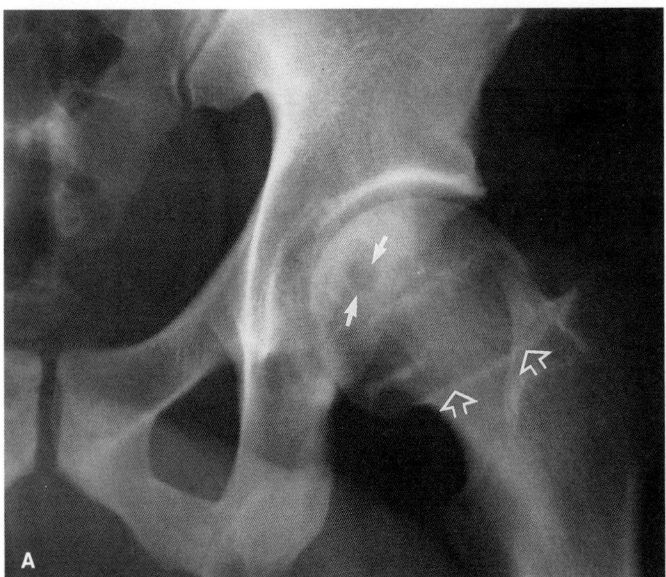

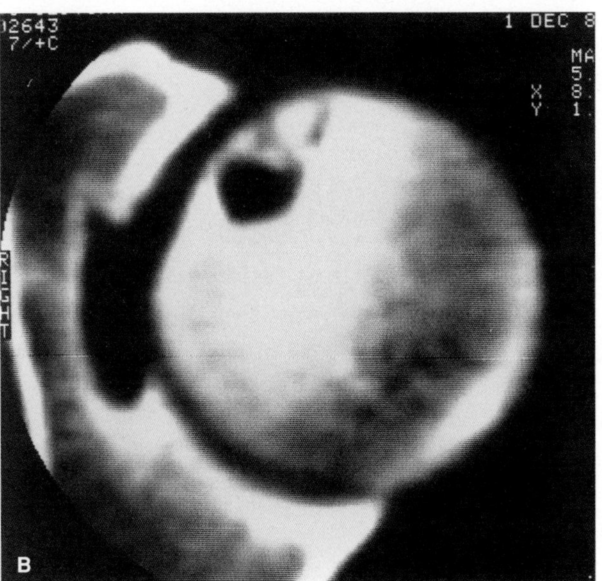

FIGURE 60.10. **Geode. A:** A cystic lesion was noted in the femoral head (*arrows*) of a young man with a painful hip. **B:** A computed tomographic scan through this area shows the subarticular nature and adjacent sclerosis. The differential diagnosis of infection, eosinophilic granuloma, and chondroblastoma was given. A ring of osteophytes (*open arrowheads*) was noted in retrospect on the radiograph (**A**) in the subcapital region, which indicates degenerative disease of the hip. Degenerative joint disease is extremely unusual in a 20-year-old healthy man; however, it makes the lytic lesion in the femoral head almost certainly a subchondral cyst or geode. This was an active soccer player who had been playing with pain in his hip for several years following an injury that had caused the degenerative disease. Unfortunately, a biopsy was performed anyway, and a subchondral cyst or geode was confirmed.

of a pseudodislocation. If necessary, the joint can be aspirated to confirm the presence of a bloody effusion and to show the normal position of the humeral head when fluid has been removed from the joint.

FIGURE 60.11. **Discogenic Vertebral Sclerosis.** This patient has sclerosis on the inferior portion of the L4 vertebral body associated with minimal osteophytosis and joint space narrowing at the adjacent disc space. This is the classic appearance for discogenic vertebral sclerosis, and a biopsy to rule out metastatic disease should not be performed.

NORMAL VARIANTS

Dorsal Defect of the Patella. A normal variant that has been described in the patella that can be mistaken for a pathologic process is a lytic defect in the upper outer quadrant called a dorsal defect of the patella (Fig. 60.14). It can mimic a focus of infection or osteochondritis dissecans. It is a normal developmental anomaly, however, and because of its characteristic location, it should not undergo biopsy. On MR, it will have an appearance similar to many other bony lesions—that is, low signal on T1-weighted images and high signal on T2-weighted images (Fig. 60.15).

Pseudocyst of the Humerus. Another entity often confused for a lytic pathologic lesion is a pseudocyst of the humerus (Fig. 60.16). This is merely an anatomic variant caused by the increased cancellous bone in the region of the greater tuberosity of the humerus that gives this region a more lucent appearance on radiographs. With hyperemia and disuse caused by rotator cuff problems or any other shoulder disorder, this area of lucency may appear strikingly more lucent and mimic a lytic lesion. Many of these have mistakenly undergone biopsy, and several have even had repeat biopsies after the initial pathology report stated "normal bone, no lesion in specimen." Because of the associated hyperemia from the shoulder disorder (be it rotator cuff injury or whatever), a bone scan can show increased radionuclide uptake and thus sway the surgeon to perform a biopsy of this normal variant. It is radiographically characteristic in its location and appearance and should not undergo biopsy. Although other lesions such as a chondroblastoma, giant cell tumor, infection, or even a metastatic focus could occur in a similar location, they do not have quite the same appearance as a pseudocyst of the humerus.

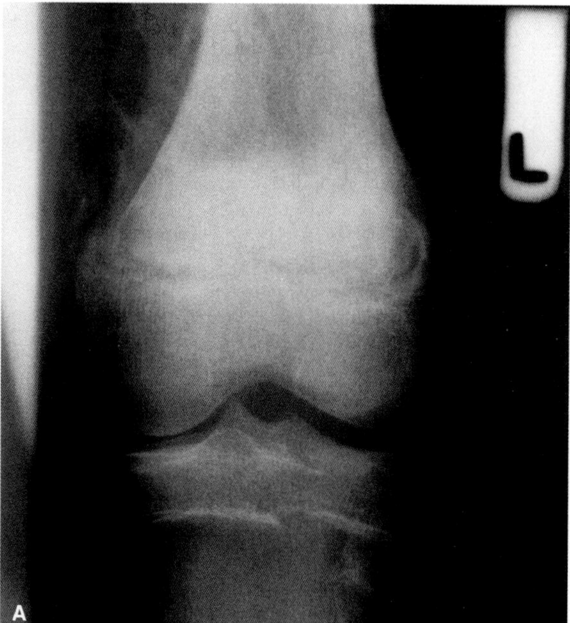

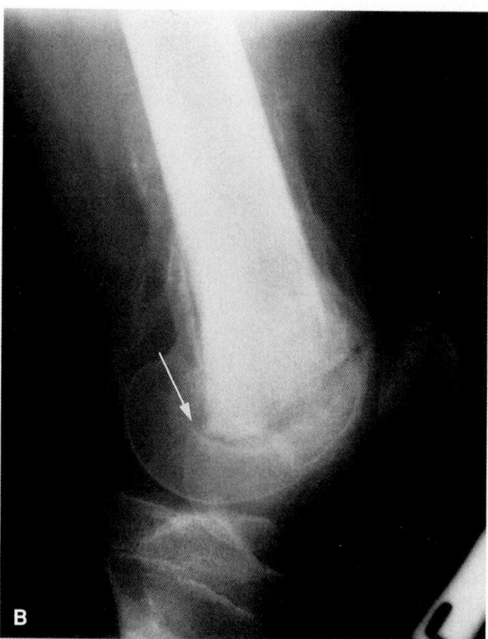

FIGURE 60.12. Fracture Mimicking Osteosarcoma. A: This 16-year-old patient had experienced pain around the knee for 2 weeks before these radiographs. The knee radiographs showed diffuse sclerosis and extensive periostitis about the distal femur, which is thought to be characteristic of an osteogenic sarcoma. The periosteal reaction, however, was thought to be much too thick, dense, and wavy to represent malignant type of periostitis. **B:** A small offset of the epiphysis can be seen (*arrow*), which indicates an epiphyseal slippage consistent with a Salter epiphyseal fracture. This teenager had fallen off a bicycle and fractured the femur, yet continued to be active. The lack of immobility caused exuberant periostitis or callus with a large amount of reactive sclerosis, all of which mimicked an osteogenic sarcoma.

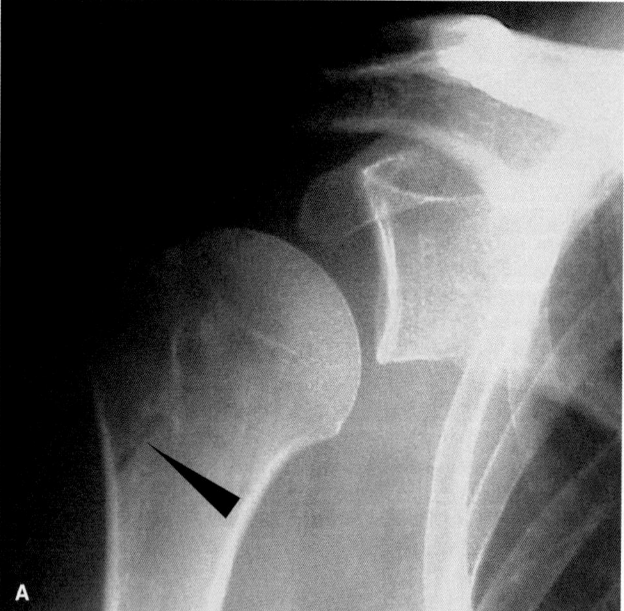

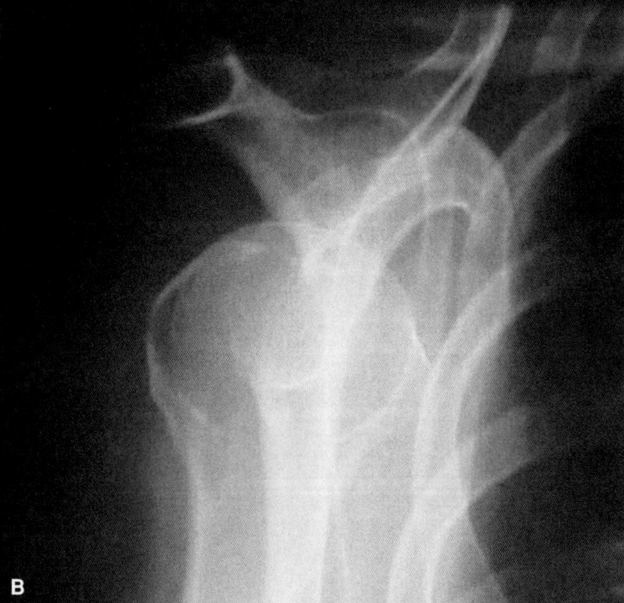

FIGURE 60.13. Pseudodislocation of the Shoulder. A: This patient experienced trauma to the shoulder with resultant pain and immobility and was thought to have a dislocation of the shoulder after the anteroposterior radiograph was seen. The humeral head is inferiorly placed in relation to the glenoid; however, this is not the characteristic location of an anterior or posterior dislocation. **B:** The transscapular view shows the humeral head to be situated normally over the glenoid without anterior or posterior dislocation. These findings are characteristic of a pseudodislocation caused by hemarthrosis or blood in the joint, which allows the shoulder to be subluxed rather than dislocated. When a pseudodislocation is seen, as in this example, search for an occult fracture should ensue. In this case as seen on (**A**), a fracture (*arrowhead*) was initially missed.

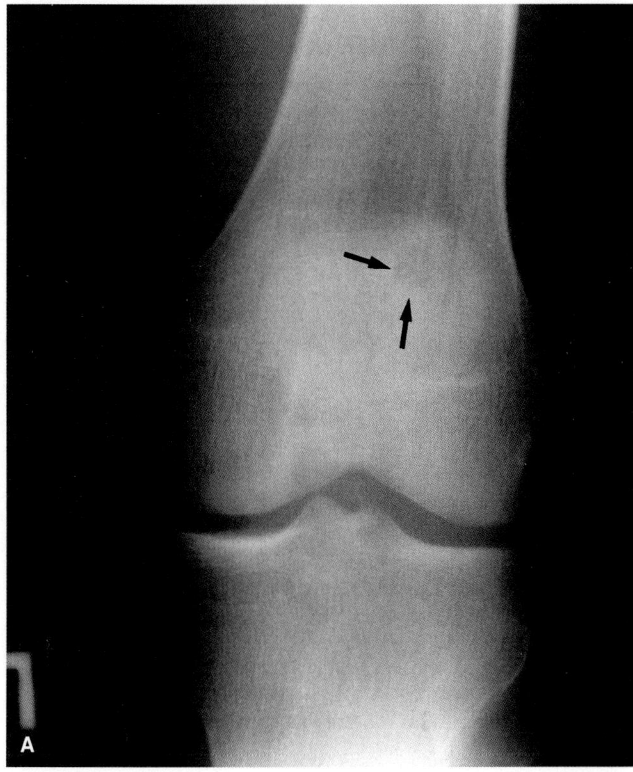

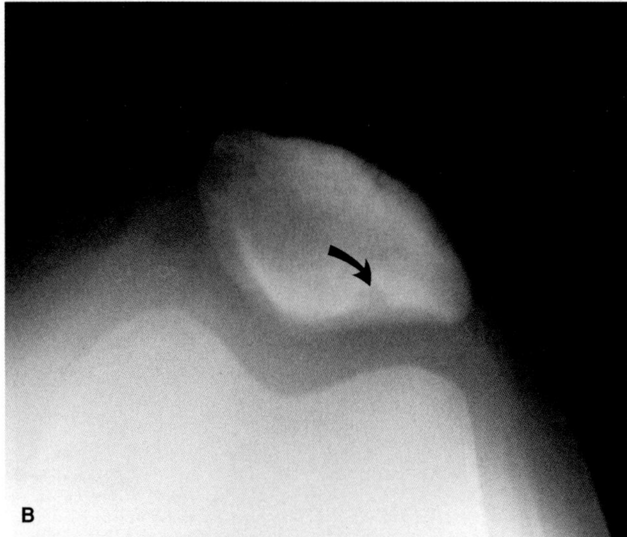

FIGURE 60.14. **Dorsal Defect of the Patella.** A lytic defect in the upper outer quadrant of the patella was seen in this patient on the AP radiograph (**A**) and the axial or sunrise view (**B**) (*arrows*), which is characteristic of a normal variant called dorsal defect of the patella. It occurs only in the upper outer quadrant and should be asymptomatic.

Os Odontoideum. A normal variant of the cervical spine that may, in fact, be posttraumatic is an os odontoideum. It is an unfused dens that may move anterior to the C2 body with flexion and can mimic a fractured dens (Fig. 60.17). Many of these require surgical fixation; some surgeons fuse every case believing that they are all unstable. Radiologists should recognize that this process is not acute and, thus, save the patient halo fixation and possible immediate surgical intervention. Most of these cases are seen after trauma, and if no neurologic deficits are present, these patients can be seen electively and spared the morbidity associated with treatment of the acutely fractured cervical spine. The radiologic signs for recognizing an os odontoideum are the smooth, often well-corticated, inferior border of the dens and the hypertrophied, densely corticated anterior arch of C1. This latter finding presumably represents compensatory hypertrophy and indicates a longstanding condition.

OBVIOUSLY BENIGN LESIONS

Multiple real lesions exist that should be recognized radiographically as benign and left alone. These are lesions that should be diagnosed by the radiologist, not the pathologist.

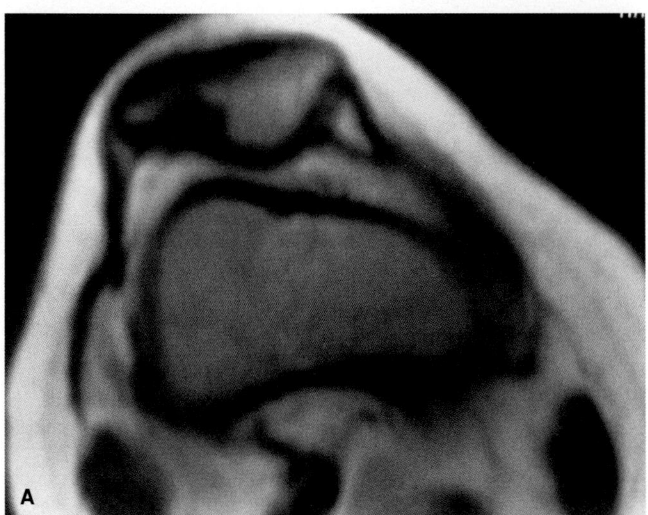

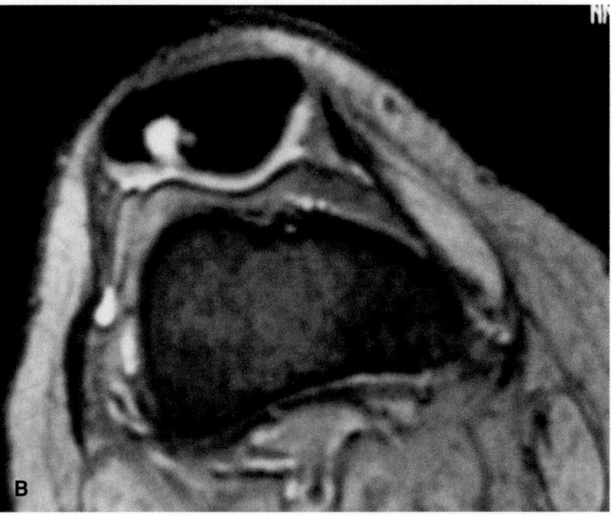

FIGURE 60.15. **Dorsal Defect of the Patella. A:** An axial T1-weighted MR shows a focal area of low signal in the patella in a subarticular location in the lateral facet of the patella. **B:** The axial T2-weighted image shows high signal in the lesion. This is typical in location and appearance of a dorsal defect of the patella.

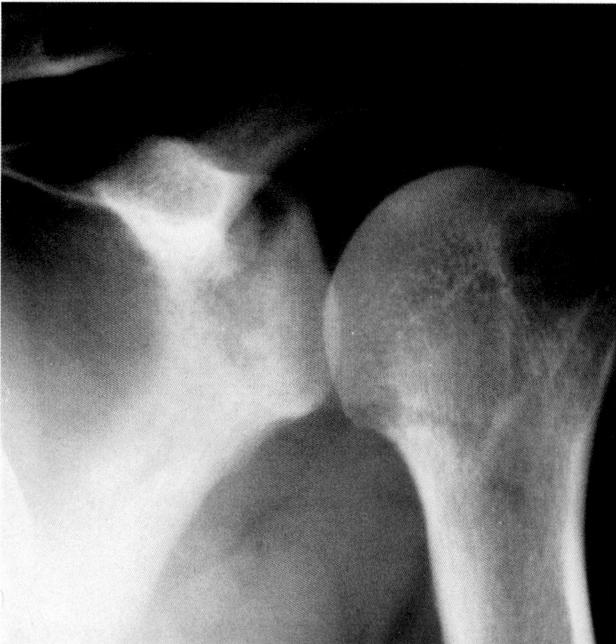

FIGURE 60.16. **Pseudocyst of the Humerus.** A well-defined lucency is seen in the greater tuberosity, which was thought to represent a lytic lesion. This patient was symptomatic and had increased radionuclide uptake on isotope bone scan. This is a characteristic location and appearance, however, for a pseudocyst of the humerus, which merely represents decreased cortical bone in this region. This becomes more pronounced when pain in the shoulder is present and hyperemia or disuse osteoporosis occurs.

Listing a differential in these cases often spurs the surgeon to a biopsy, when, in fact, no biopsy should be necessary.

Nonossifying Fibroma. Perhaps the most often encountered lesion in this category is the nonossifying fibroma. Nonossifying fibroma is identical to a fibrous cortical defect, but the term is usually reserved for defects larger than 2 cm. They are, classically, lucent lesions located in the cortex of the metaphysis of a long bone and have a well-defined, often sclerotic, scalloped border with slight cortical expansion (Fig. 60.18). They are almost exclusively found in patients younger than the age of 30 years; hence, the natural history of the lesion is involution. As they involute, they fill in with new bone, giving it a sclerotic appearance (Fig. 60.19); thus, they can have some increased radionuclide activity on bone scans. They are most often mistaken for an area of infection, eosinophilic granuloma, fibrous dysplasia, or aneurysmal bone cyst. They are asymptomatic and have never been reported to be associated with malignant degeneration. On occasion, a pathologic fracture can occur through these lesions, but most surgeons do not advocate prophylactic curettage to prevent fracture, as with unicameral bone cysts. Nonossifying fibromas can be quite large but invariably have a benign appearance (Fig. 60.20) and biopsy should be avoided. The asymptomatic nature should help differentiate them from most of the other lesions in the differential diagnosis and thereby preclude even giving a differential diagnosis. On occasion, they are found to be multiple, yet each lesion is so characteristic that they should be easily diagnosed.

Bone islands are not a radiographic dilemma when they are 1 cm or less in size. Occasionally, however, they grow to golf ball size or larger and mimic sclerotic metastases (Fig. 60.21). They are always asymptomatic. Radiographically, two signs can be found to help distinguish giant bone islands from

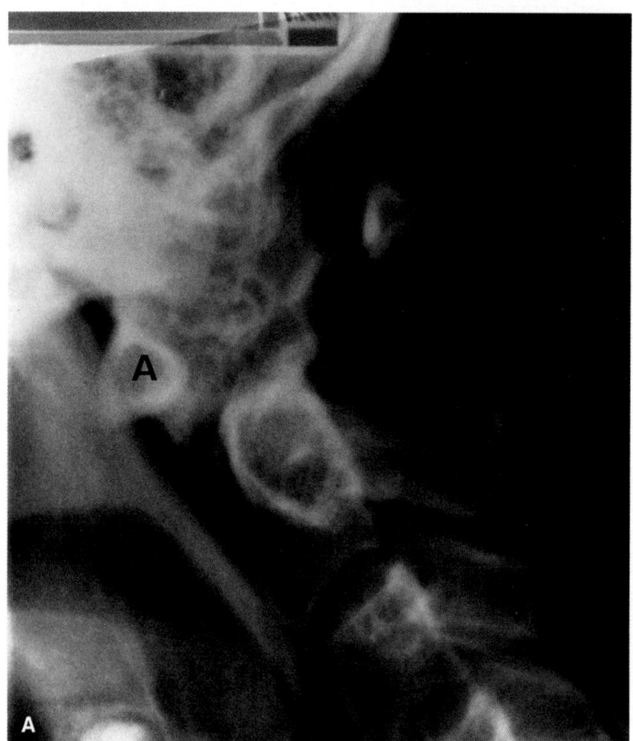

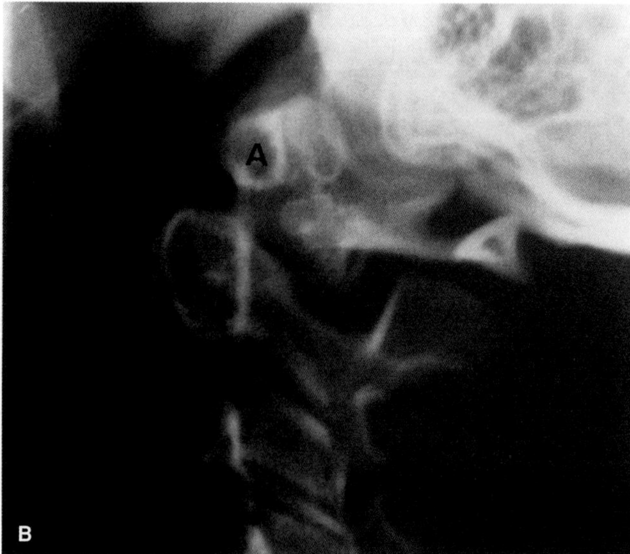

FIGURE 60.17 **Os Odontoideum.** Flexion (**A**) and extension (**B**) views show the anterior arch (*A*) of the C1 vertebrae has moved markedly anterior in relation to the body of C2 in flexion. The odontoid or dens is difficult to see but appears to be separated from the body of C2. Because of the smooth borders of the separated dens and because of the cortical hypertrophy of the anterior arch of C1, this can safely be called an os odontoideum, which is a congenital or long-standing posttraumatic abnormality rather than an acute fracture. Obviously, patients with this condition should have no neurologic problems, yet in many instances are still believed to be unstable and undergo surgical fusion. This, however, can be done on an elective basis.

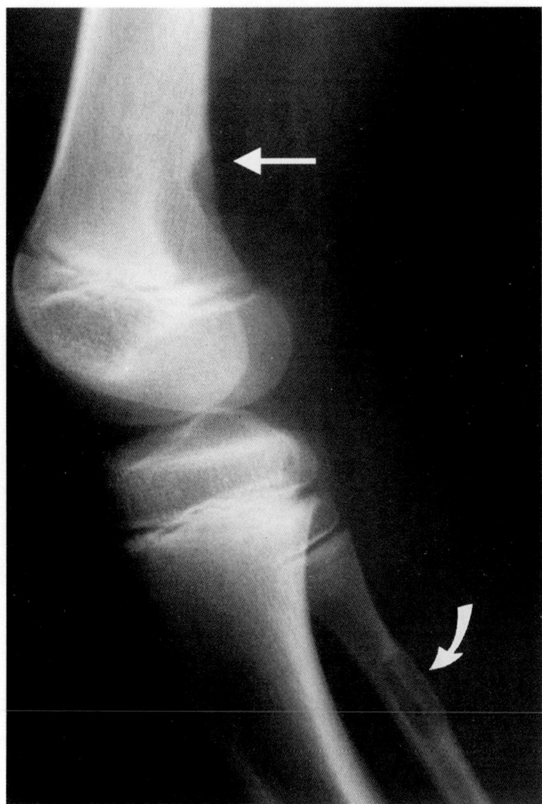

FIGURE 60.18. **Nonossifying Fibroma (NOF).** A well-defined, slightly expansile, lucent lesion is seen in the fibula (*lower curved arrow*); this is characteristic of a nonossifying fibroma. A second lucent lesion is seen in the posterior distal femur (*upper straight arrow*), which is also typical in appearance of a nonossifying fibroma.

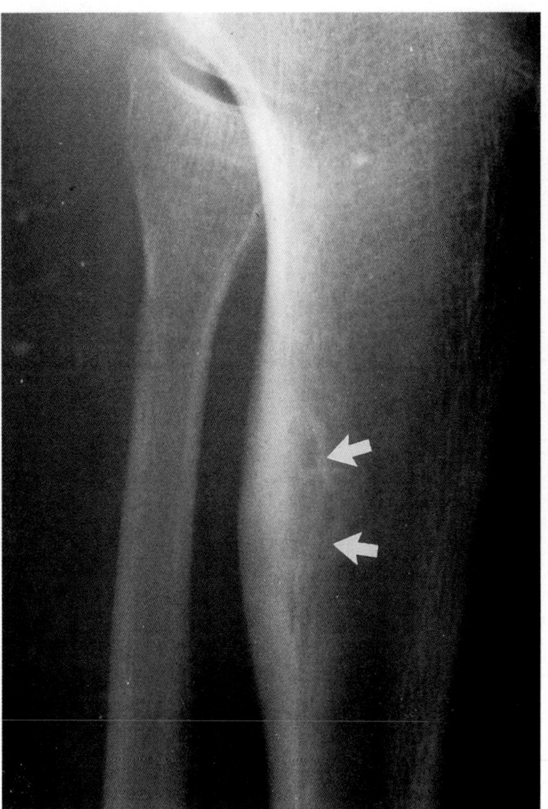

FIGURE 60.19. **Healing Nonossifying Fibroma.** A minimally sclerotic process is seen in the proximal tibia (*arrows*), which was thought by the surgeons to represent a focus of infection or an osteoid osteoma, even though the patient was asymptomatic. This is a characteristic appearance for a disappearing or healing nonossifying fibroma and should not undergo biopsy.

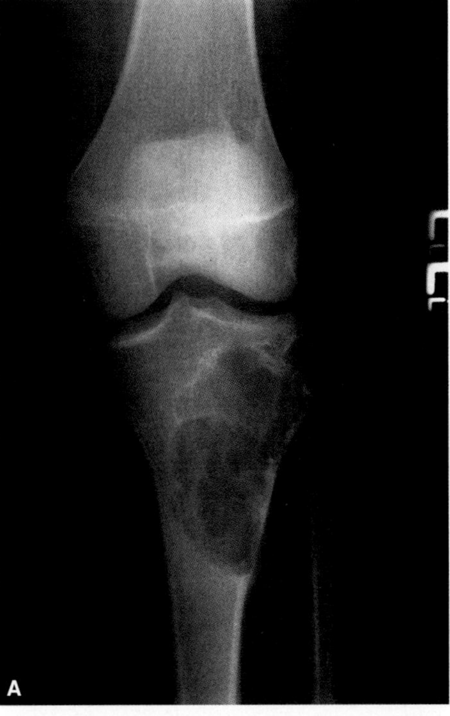

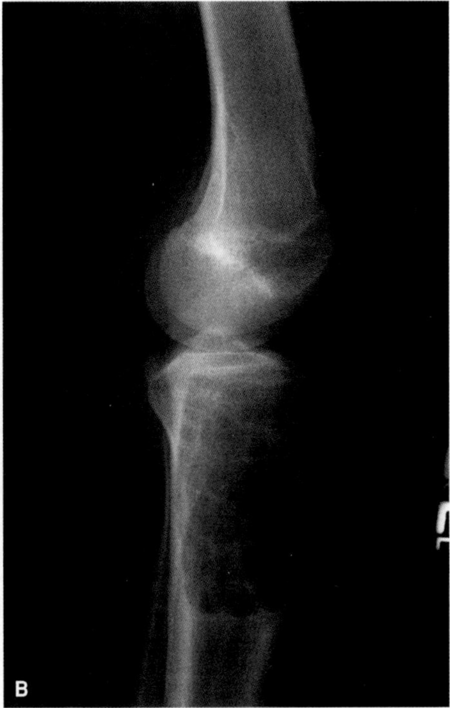

FIGURE 60.20. **Nonossifying Fibroma.** AP (**A**) and lateral (**B**) radiographs of the tibia show a large, well-defined, minimally expansile lytic lesion of the proximal tibia, which is characteristic of a nonossifying fibroma. Even though the patient was asymptomatic, biopsy was performed and the diagnosis confirmed. A second nonossifying fibroma can be seen in the femur just superior to the patella.

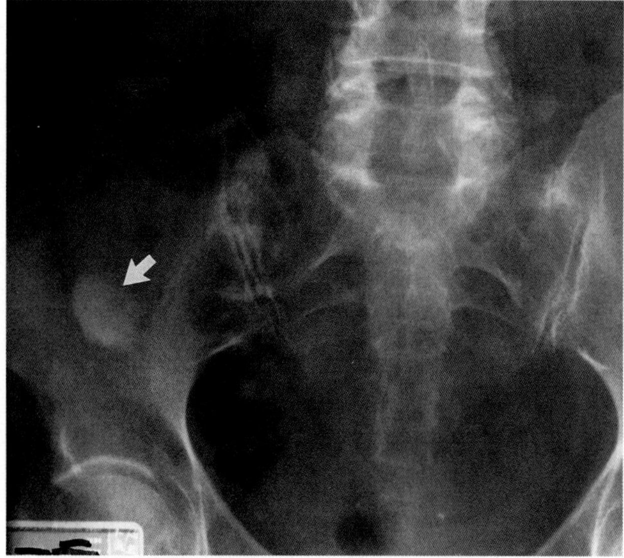

FIGURE 60.21. **Giant Bone Island.** A large sclerotic focus is seen in the right iliac wing (*arrow*). Note how the lesion is somewhat spherical or oblong in the lines of trabecular stress, which is characteristic of a bone island. This patient was asymptomatic and had no evidence of a primary carcinoma.

metastases. First, bone islands usually are oblong with their long axis in the axis of stress on the bone—for example, in a long bone they align themselves along the axis of the diaphysis. Second, the margins of a bone island, if examined closely, will show bony trabeculae extending from the lesion into the normal bone in a spiculated fashion. This is characteristic of a bone island and helpful in differentiating it from a more aggressive process.

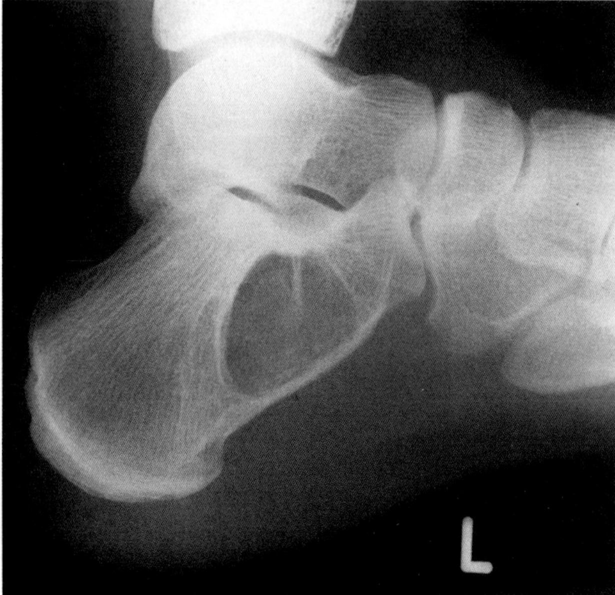

FIGURE 60.22. **Unicameral Bone Cyst.** A well-defined lytic lesion on the anterior-inferior portion on the calcaneus, as in this example, is virtually pathognomonic for a unicameral bone cyst or simple bone cyst. Because this is an area of diminished stress, it is thought not to be necessary to curettage and pack this lesion prophylactically in an effort to avoid a pathologic bone fracture, which is often done in the femur and humerus with unicameral bone cysts.

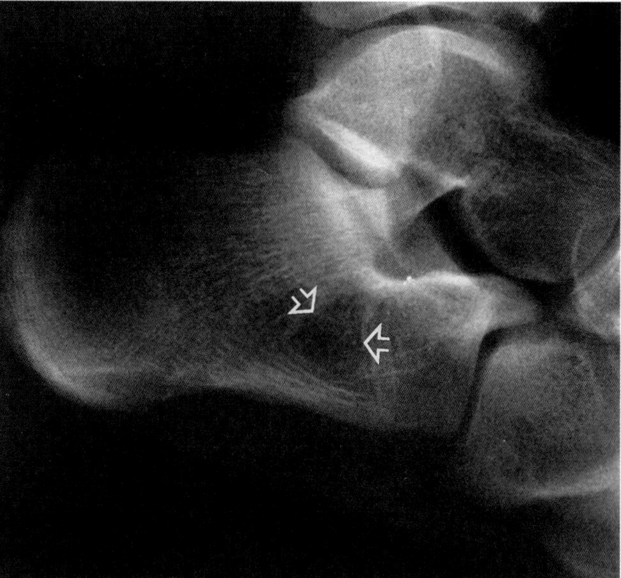

FIGURE 60.23. **Pseudocyst of the Calcaneus.** An area of radiolucency is seen on the anterior-inferior portion of the calcaneus (*arrows*) similar to the example in Figure 60.22 but not as well defined. This is a pseudocyst similar to the pseudocyst of the humerus that results from diminished stress through this region.

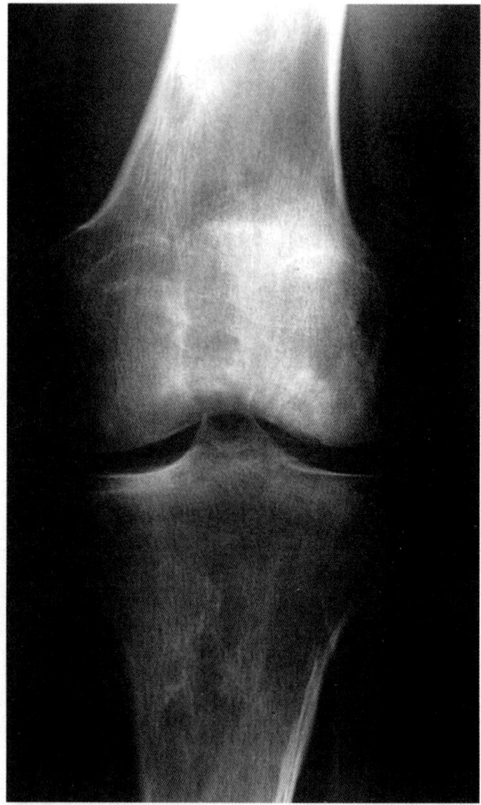

FIGURE 60.24. **Early Bone Infarct.** Patchy demineralization is seen in the distal femur and proximal tibia in this patient with systemic lupus erythematosus. The opposite leg was similarly involved. This is characteristic for early bone infarcts and should not be confused with infection or metastatic disease.

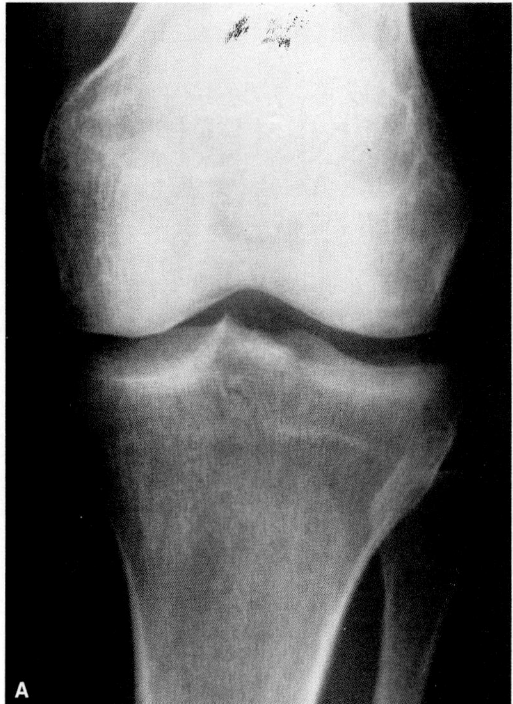

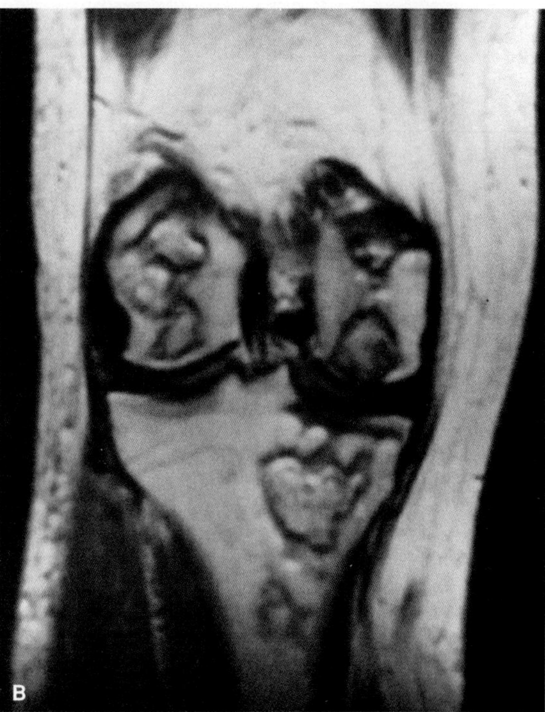

FIGURE 60.25. **Bone Infarct. A:** A radiograph of the knee shows a permeative pattern in the proximal tibia, which was at first thought to be infection or a primary tumor. **B:** A T1-weighted coronal MR image shows the characteristic serpiginous border seen with bone infarct in the tibia and in the femur. MR can on occasion better characterize the ill-defined early bone infarct, as in this example. This patient has systemic lupus erythematosus.

Unicameral bone cysts are often prophylactically curettaged and packed so as to prevent fracture with subsequent deformity. When these cysts occur in the calcaneus, however, they should be left alone. They always occur in the anterior-inferior portion of the calcaneus (Fig. 60.22), an area that does not receive undue stress. In fact, a pseudotumor of the calcaneus is seen in the identical position because of the absence of stress and the resulting atrophy of bony trabeculae (Fig. 60.23). These lesions are asymptomatic, only rarely fracture, and should not suffer the same fate as their counterparts in long bones—that is, surgical removal.

Bone Infarction. Early in the course of its development, a bone infarct can have a patchy or a mixed lytic–sclerotic pattern or even resemble a permeative process (Fig. 60.24). In a patient with bone pain and a permeative bone lesion, many aggressive disorders head the differential list and a biopsy soon ensues. If this process can be noted to be multiple and in the diametaphyseal region of a long bone, especially if the patient has an underlying disorder such as sickle cell anemia or systemic lupus erythematosus, areas of early bone infarction should be considered. In some cases, the characteristic MR appearance of an infarct may save a patient from biopsy when the radiographs are equivocal (Fig. 60.25).

CONCLUSION

These are but a few of the many examples in skeletal radiology in which the well-trained radiologist can be of invaluable assistance to the clinician and the patient by helping avert a needless biopsy. Dozens of other examples are nicely shown in normal variant textbooks, which are widely available. Because of the potential harm in performing a needless biopsy, the examples described in this chapter are stressed. When these lesions are encountered by the radiologist, a differential diagnosis should not be offered, as it will often lead the surgeon to a biopsy in an attempt to get a diagnosis. A biopsy in many of these entities is not only unnecessary but can be misleading.

Suggested Readings

Barnes GR Jr, Gwinn JL. Distal irregularities of the femur simulating malignancy. *Am J Roentgenol Radium Ther Nucl Med* 1974;122:180–185.

Helms C. Pseudocyst of the humerus. *AJR Am J Roentgenol* 1978;131:287–292.

Helms C, Richmond B, Sims R. Pseudodislocation of the shoulder: a sign of an occult fracture. *Emerg Med* 1986;18:237–241.

Holt RG, Helms CA, Munk PL, Gillespy T 3rd. Hypertrophy of C-1 anterior arch: useful sign to distinguish os odontoideum from acute dens fracture. *Radiology* 1989;173:207–209.

Johnson JF, Brogdon BG. Dorsal effect of the patella: incidence and distribution. *AJR Am J Roentgenol* 1982;139:339–340.

Lipson S. Discogenic vertebral sclerosis with calcified disc. *New Engl J Med* 1991;325:794–799.

Martel W, Seeger J, Wicks J, Washburn RL. Traumatic lesions of the discovertebral junction in the lumbar spine. *AJR Am J Roentgenol* 1976;127:457–464.

Minderhoud J, Braakman R, Penning L. Os odontoideum: clinical, radiological, and therapeutic aspects. *J Neurol Sci* 1969;8:521–544.

Munk PL, Helms CA, Holt RG. Immature bone infarcts: findings on plain radiographs and MR scans. *AJR Am J Roentgenol* 1989;152:547–549.

Murray R, Jacobson H. *The Radiology of Skeletal Disorders.* 2nd ed. New York: Churchill Livingstone; 1977:603.

Onitsuka H. Roentgenologic aspects of bone islands. *Radiology* 1977;123: 607–612.

Ostlere SJ, Seeger LL, Eckardt JJ. Subchondral cysts of the tibia secondary to osteoarthritis of the knee. *Skeletal Radiol* 1990;19:287–289.

Resnick D, Cone RO 3rd. The nature of humeral pseudocysts. *Radiology* 1984;150:27–28.

Resnick D, Niwayama G, Coutts RD. Subchondral cysts (geodes) in arthritic disorders: pathologic and radiographic appearance of the hip joint. *AJR Am J Roentgenol* 1977;128:799–806.

Schneider R, Kaye J, Ghelman B. Adductor avulsive injuries near the symphysis pubis. *Radiology* 1976;120:567–569.

Wootton JR, Cross MJ, Holt KW. Avulsion of the ischial apophysis. The case for open reduction and internal fixation. *J Bone Joint Surg* 1990;72(7): 625–627.

CHAPTER 61 ■ MISCELLANEOUS BONE LESIONS

CLYDE A. HELMS AND EMILY N. VINSON

There are a host of bony conditions, diseases, and syndromes that do not fit conveniently into any of the preceding chapters yet should be given some mention in an attempted overview of musculoskeletal radiology. These are listed alphabetically for lack of a more scientific basis.

ACHONDROPLASIA

The most common cause of dwarfism is achondroplasia, a congenital, hereditary disease of failure of endochondral bone formation. The femurs and humeri are more profoundly affected than the other long bones, although the entire skeleton is abnormal. A characteristic finding is that the spine typically has narrowing of the interpedicular distances in a caudal direction (Fig. 61.1), the opposite of normal, in which the interpedicular distances get progressively wider as one proceeds down the spine. The long bones are short but have normal width, giving them a thick appearance.

AVASCULAR NECROSIS (OSTEONECROSIS)

The term "avascular necrosis" (AVN) or osteonecrosis refers to the lack of blood supply with subsequent bone death and ensuing bony collapse in an articular surface. The etiology of AVN is an extensive differential that most commonly includes *trauma*, *steroids*, *aspirin*, *renal disease*, *collagen vascular diseases*, *alcoholism*, and *idiopathic* causes (Table 61.1). The radiographic appearance ranges from patchy sclerosis (Fig. 61.2A) to articular surface collapse and fragmentation (Fig. 61.3). Just before collapse, a subchondral lucency is occasionally seen (Fig. 61.4); however, this is a late and inconstant sign of AVN. MR is extremely valuable in demonstrating the presence and extent of AVN (Fig. 61.2B), even when radiographs are apparently normal. MR is currently considered to be the most efficacious way to evaluate a joint for AVN. It is useful not only in AVN of the hip but also in the knee, wrist, foot, and ankle.

HYPERTROPHIC PULMONARY OSTEOARTHROPATHY

Hypertrophic osteoarthropathy is manifested by clubbing of the fingers and periostitis, usually in the upper and lower extremities (Fig. 61.5), which might or might not be associated with bone pain. It is most commonly seen in patients with lung cancer or other lung disease (in which case it is referred to as *hypertrophic pulmonary osteoarthropathy*) but many other etiologies have been reported, including GI disorders and liver disease. The actual mechanism of formation of periostitis secondary to a distant malignancy or other process is unknown. The differential diagnosis for periostitis in a long bone without an underlying bony abnormality would include *hypertrophic osteoarthropathy*, *venous stasis*, *thyroid acropachy*, *pachydermoperiostosis*, and *trauma* (Table 61.2).

MELORHEOSTOSIS

Melorheostosis is a rare, idiopathic disorder characterized by thickened cortical new bone that accumulates near the ends of long bones, usually only on one side of the bone, and has an appearance likened to "dripping candle wax" (Fig. 61.6). It can affect several adjacent bones and can be symptomatic.

MUCOPOLYSACCHARIDOSES (MORQUIO, HURLER, AND HUNTER SYNDROMES)

The mucopolysaccharidoses are a group of inherited lysosomal storage diseases characterized by the abnormal accumulation of various mucopolysaccharides such as keratan sulfate (Morquio) and heparan sulfate (Hurler and Hunter). These patients have short stature, primarily from shortened spines, and characteristic radiographic findings. In the spine, patients

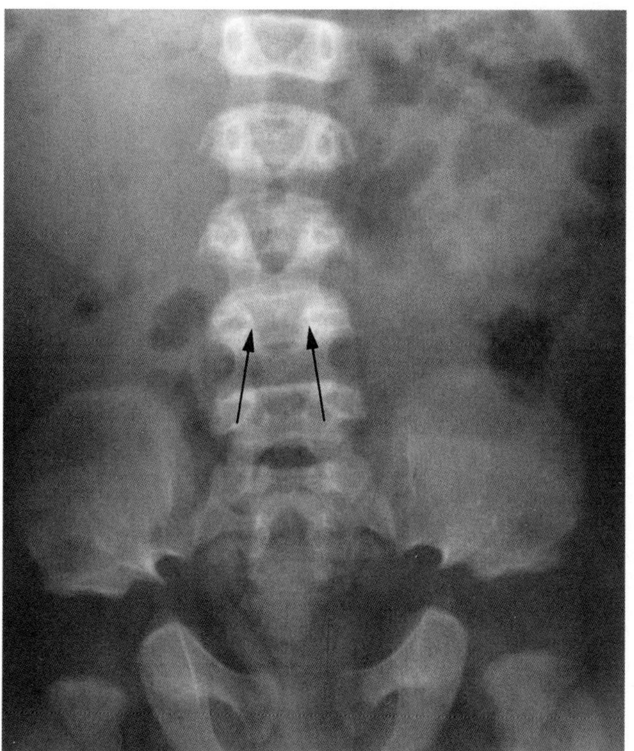

FIGURE 61.1. **Achondroplasia.** An anteroposterior radiograph of the spine in this patient with achondroplasia demonstrates narrowing of the interpedicular distance (*arrows*) in a caudal direction, which is characteristic of this disorder. Ordinarily, the interpedicular distance widens in each vertebra in a caudal direction.

with Morquio have platyspondyly (generalized flattening of the vertebral bodies) with a central anterior projection or "beak" off the vertebral body, as viewed on a lateral radiograph (Fig. 61.7). Hurler and Hunter show platyspondyly with a beak that is anteroinferiorly positioned (Fig. 61.8). The pelvis in these disorders is similar in appearance to that of achondroplastics, with wide, flared iliac wings and broad femoral necks. A characteristic finding in the hands is a pointed proximal fifth metacarpal base that has a notched appearance to the ulnar aspect (Fig. 61.9).

TABLE 61.1

COMMON CAUSES OF AVASCULAR NECROSIS

Trauma
Steroids
Renal disease
Collagen vascular diseases
Alcoholism
Idiopathic causes

MULTIPLE HEREDITARY EXOSTOSES

Also known as diaphyseal aclasis, this is a not uncommon hereditary disorder that seems to affect multiple members of a family with multiple osteochondromas or exostoses. An osteochondroma is a cartilage-capped bone outgrowth that may be pedunculated or sessile in appearance. In the multiple hereditary form, the knees are virtually always involved (Fig. 61.10). Undertubulation (a widened diameter of the bone) is invariably present at the site of the exostosis. The incidence of malignant degeneration in this population has been reported to be as high as 20%, but this is a gross overestimation, with malignant degeneration being extremely rare. As with solitary osteochondromas, the more axially situated lesions are more prone to undergo malignant degeneration, whereas the more peripheral appendicular lesions are less likely to do so. The proximal femurs are frequently involved and have a characteristic appearance (Fig. 61.11).

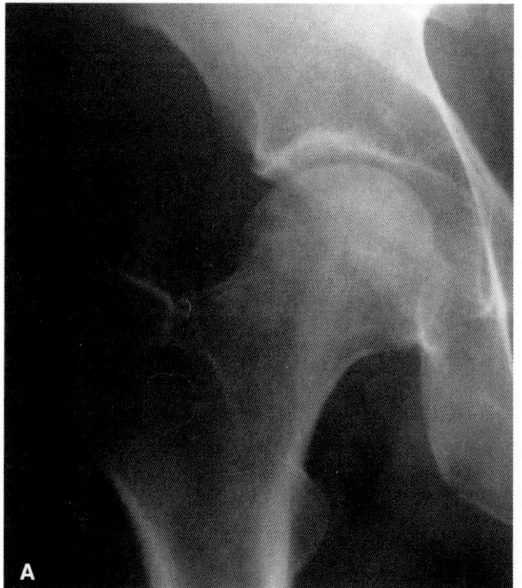

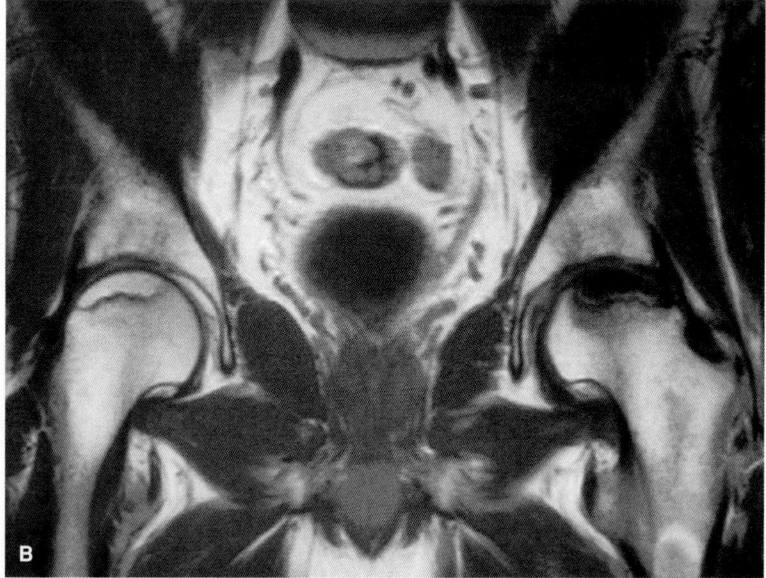

FIGURE 61.2. **Avascular Necrosis (AVN). A:** A radiograph of the hip in this patient with AVN shows faint, patchy sclerosis throughout the femoral head. This is a relatively early radiographic finding for AVN. **B:** Coronal T1-weighted MR image shows typical findings in AVN. Diffuse low signal in the left hip is noted, which has more extensive involvement than the right. The right hip has a low-signal serpiginous rim which is characteristic of AVN.

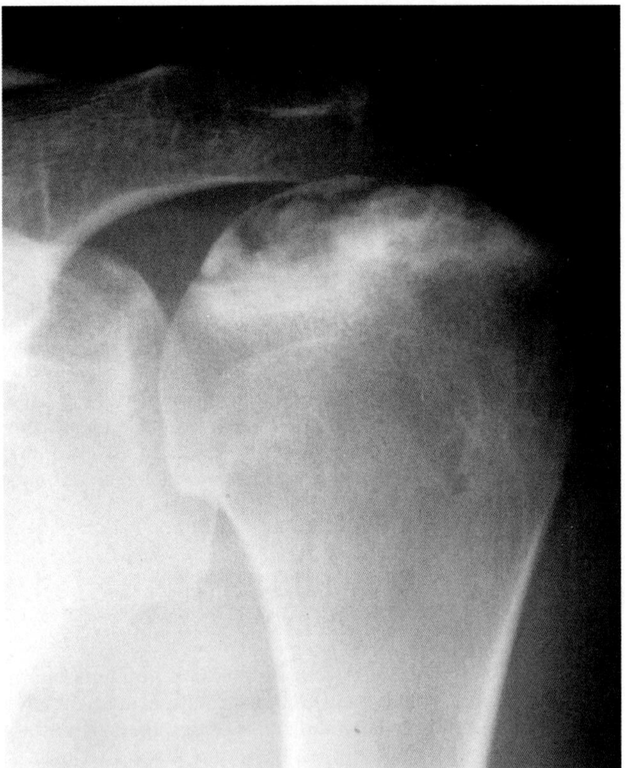

FIGURE 61.3. **Avascular Necrosis (AVN).** An AP radiograph of the shoulder reveals articular surface collapse in this patient who was treated with steroids for systemic lupus erythematosus. This is an advanced stage of AVN.

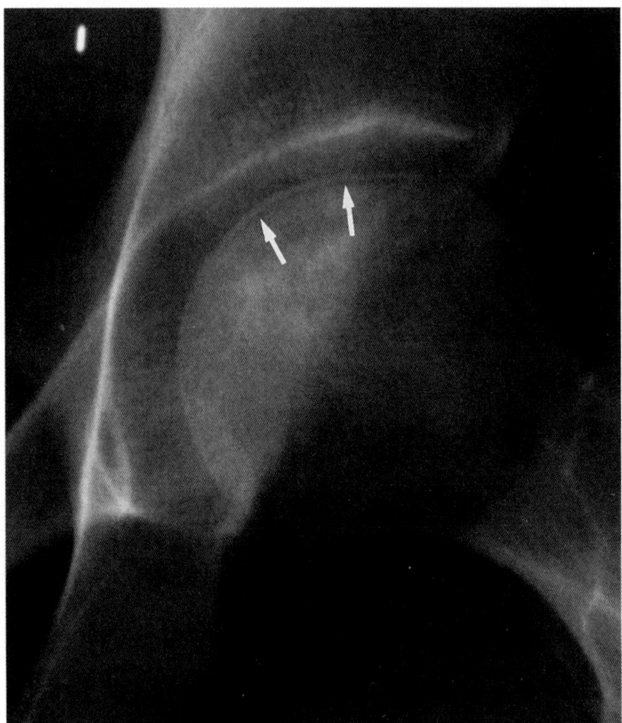

FIGURE 61.4. **Avascular Necrosis (AVN).** A frog-leg lateral view of the hip in this patient with sickle cell disease shows a subchondral lucency (*arrows*) and patchy sclerosis in the femoral head, indicative of AVN. This is a relatively advanced stage of AVN. The subchondral lucency is often better demonstrated with the frog-leg lateral view.

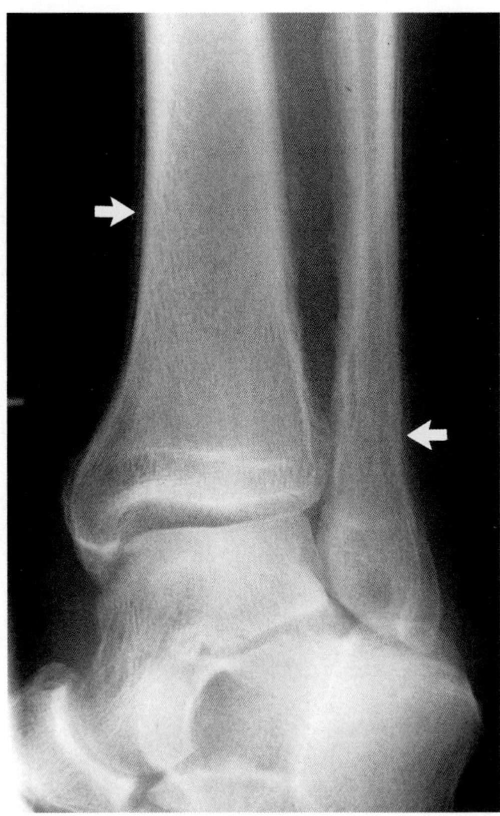

FIGURE 61.5. **Hypertrophic Pulmonary Osteoarthropathy.** Periostitis can be seen along the shafts of the distal tibia and fibula (*arrows*) in this patient with bronchogenic carcinoma and leg pain. This is characteristic of hypertrophic pulmonary osteoarthropathy.

OSTEOID OSTEOMA

The etiology of osteoid osteoma is unknown. It is a painful lesion that occurs almost exclusively in patients less than 30 years of age and is treated successfully with surgical excision or thermal ablation.

Radiographically, an osteoid osteoma is said to have a classic appearance, but it has several different appearances, which can make diagnosis difficult. The classically described radiographic appearance is a cortically based sclerotic lesion in a long bone that has a small lucency within it that is called the nidus (Fig. 61.12A). It is the nidus that causes the pain and the surrounding reactive sclerosis. If the nidus is surgically removed or thermally ablated, complete cessation of pain is the rule. CT is often very helpful in demonstrating the exact location of the nidus (Fig. 61.12B).

If the nidus of an osteoid osteoma is located in the medullary rather than the cortical portion of a bone, or if it is located in a joint, there is much less reactive sclerosis present.

TABLE 61.2

PERIOSTITIS WITHOUT UNDERLYING BONY LESIONS

Trauma
Hypertrophic pulmonary osteoarthropathy
Venous stasis
Thyroid acropachy
Pachydermoperiostosis

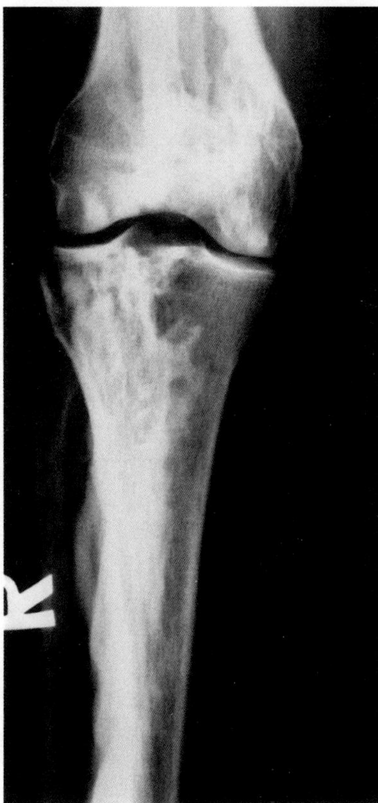

FIGURE 61.6. **Melorheostosis.** Dense, wavy new bone is seen adjacent to the lateral tibial cortex, which has a dripping candle wax appearance, which is classic for melorheostosis. A similar pattern can be seen in the medial aspect of the distal femur.

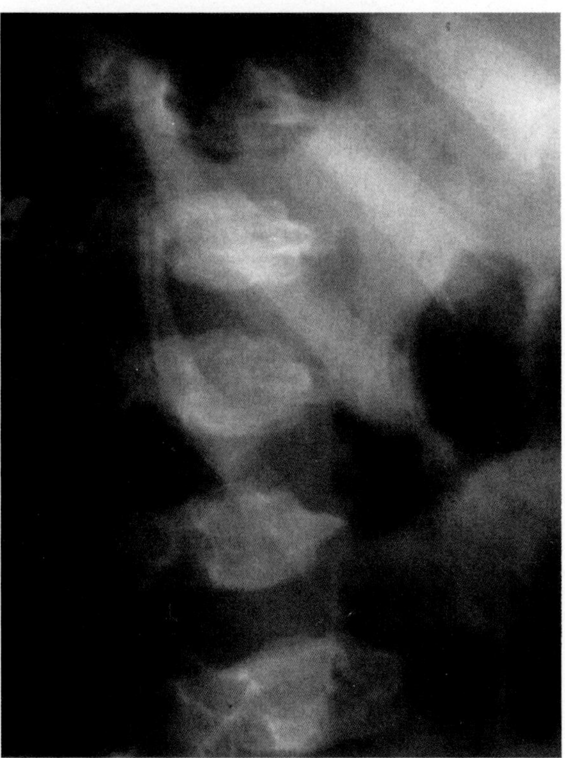

FIGURE 61.7. **Morquio Syndrome.** A lateral radiograph of the spine reveals a central beak or anterior bony projection off the vertebral bodies in this patient with Morquio syndrome.

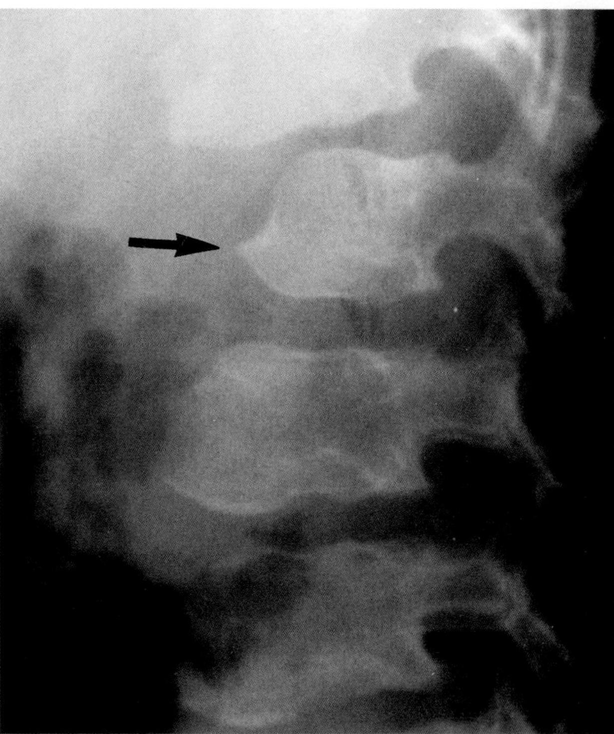

FIGURE 61.8. **Hurler Syndrome.** A lateral radiograph of the spine in this patient with Hurler syndrome shows an inferiorly placed bony projection extending anteriorly off the vertebral bodies (*arrow*).

This gives the lesion a different overall appearance than the more common cortical lesion in that it does not appear as sclerotic. Up to 80% of osteoid osteomas are located intracortically, with the remainder being in the intramedullary part of a bone. Rarely, an osteoid osteoma will be present in the periosteum, causing exuberant periostitis.

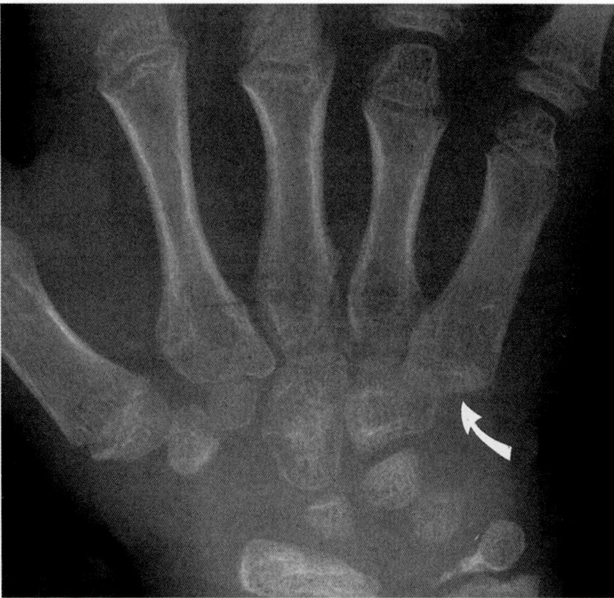

FIGURE 61.9. **Hurler Syndrome.** An anteroposterior radiograph of the hand in this patient with Hurler syndrome shows a notch (*arrow*) at the base of the fifth metacarpal, which is a characteristic finding in all of the mucopolysaccharidoses.

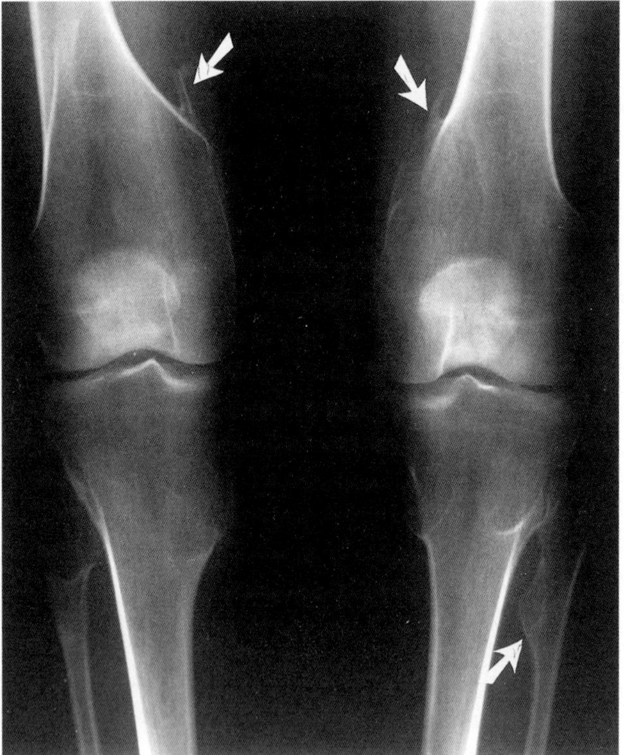

FIGURE 61.10. **Multiple Hereditary Exostoses.** The knees are involved in virtually every case of multiple hereditary exostoses. They typically show not only multiple exostoses (*arrows*) but marked undertubulation in the metaphyses.

The nidus itself is usually lucent but often develops some calcification within it. It then has the appearance of a sequestrum, as is seen in osteomyelitis. If the nidus calcifies completely, it blends in with the surrounding sclerosis and cannot be seen on most radiographs. Therefore, the diagnosis of an osteoid osteoma in no way depends on seeing a nidus.

Because an osteoid osteoma resembles osteomyelitis, regardless of the appearance of the nidus, it can be difficult to differentiate the two radiographically. It cannot be reliably done with radiographs, CT, or MR. However, because the nidus is extremely vascular, it avidly accumulates radiopharmaceutical bone-scanning agents. An osteoid osteoma will have an area of increased uptake corresponding to the area of reactive sclerosis but, in addition, will demonstrate a second area of increased uptake corresponding to the nidus (Fig. 61.13). This has been termed the double-density sign. In contrast, osteomyelitis has a central photopenic area corresponding to the radiographic lucency that represents an avascular focus of purulent material,

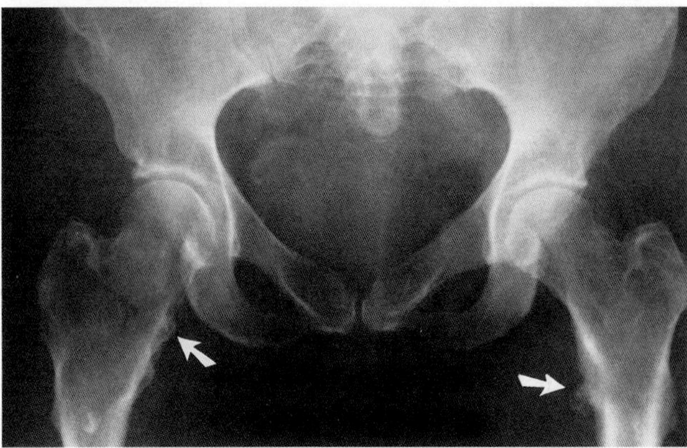

FIGURE 61.11. **Multiple Hereditary Exostoses.** The femoral necks are often involved in multiple hereditary exostoses. They will show undertubulation, as in this example, and usually have one or more exostoses (*arrows*).

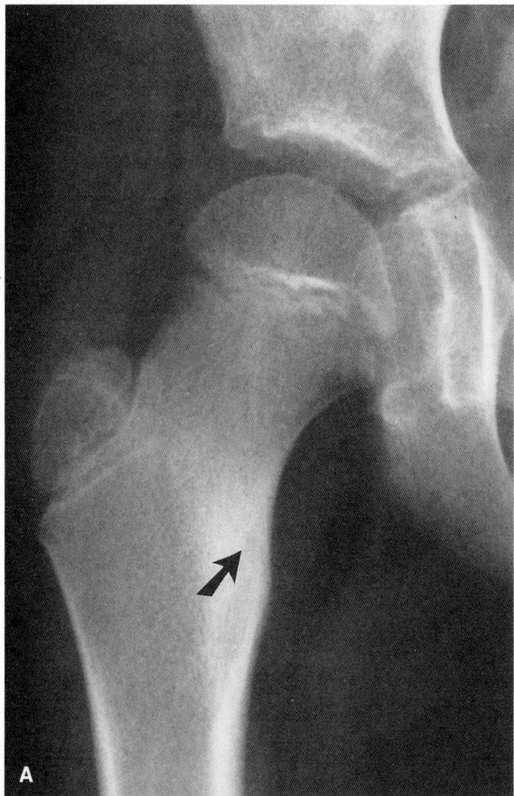

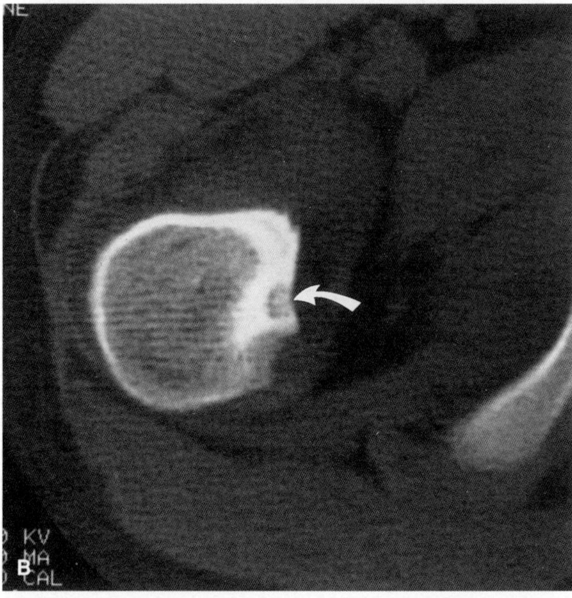

FIGURE 61.12. **Osteoid Osteoma. A:** An AP radiograph of the femur in a child with hip pain shows an area of sclerosis medially near the lesser trochanter with a small lucency (*arrow*), which is the nidus of an osteoid osteoma. Osteomyelitis could have this identical appearance. **B:** A CT scan of the femur shows the sclerosis medially and the lucent nidus (*arrow*) to better advantage. The CT scan gives the surgeon a more precise anatomic location of the nidus than the radiograph.

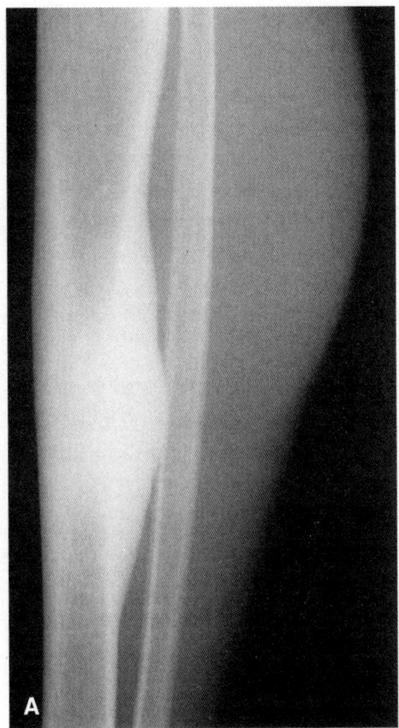

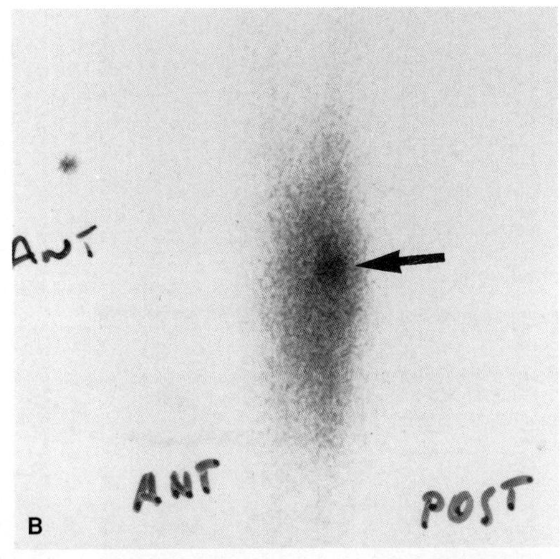

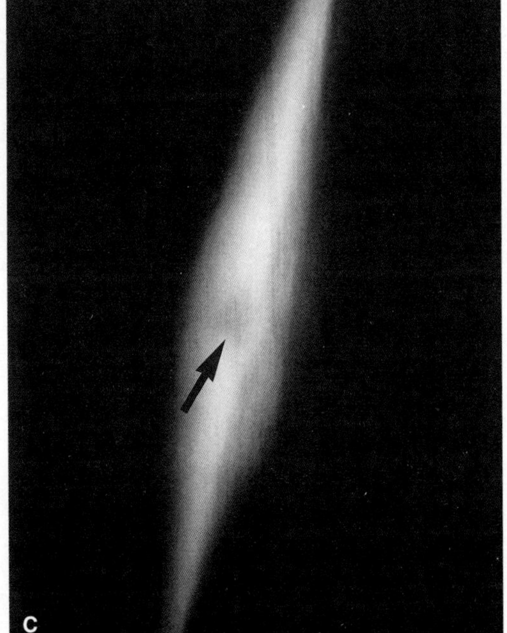

FIGURE 61.13. Osteoid Osteoma. A: A lateral radiograph of the tibia in this child with leg pain shows cortical thickening in the posterior diaphysis. No lucency in the sclerotic area could be identified. **B:** A radionuclide bone scan reveals uptake corresponding to the area of sclerosis in the tibia, with a more marked area of uptake centrally (*arrow*), which is the double-density sign of an osteoid osteoma. **C:** The surgical specimen shows the nidus (*arrow*) as a faint lucency within the sclerotic bone.

often surrounded by increased uptake due to reactive sclerosis. The natural history of an osteoid osteoma is presumed to be spontaneous regression, as they are rarely seen in patients older than the age of 30.

OSTEOPATHIA STRIATA

Also known as Voorhoeve disease, this disorder is manifested by multiple 2- to 3-mm-thick linear bands of sclerotic bone aligned parallel to the long axis of a bone (Fig. 61.14). It usually affects multiple long bones and is asymptomatic; hence, it is usually an incidental finding.

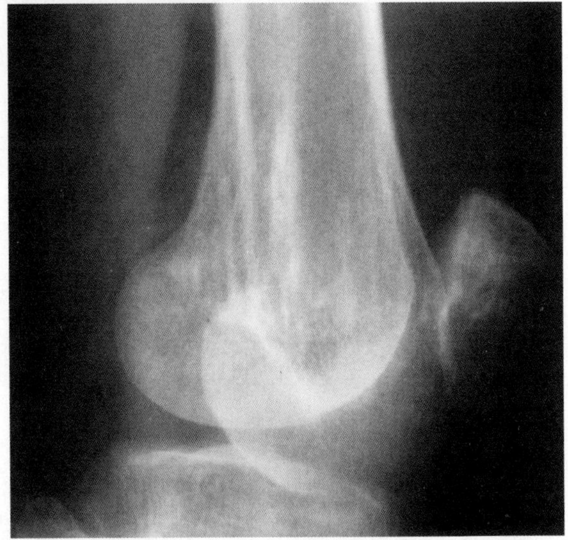

FIGURE 61.14. Osteopathia Striata. Multiple linear dense streaks are seen in the distal femur, which are characteristic of osteopathia striata.

OSTEOPOIKILOSIS

Osteopoikilosis is a hereditary, asymptomatic disorder that is usually an incidental finding of multiple small (3 to 10 mm) sclerotic bony densities affecting primarily the ends of long bones and the pelvis (Fig. 61.15). It has no clinical significance other than that it can be confused for diffuse osteoblastic metastases.

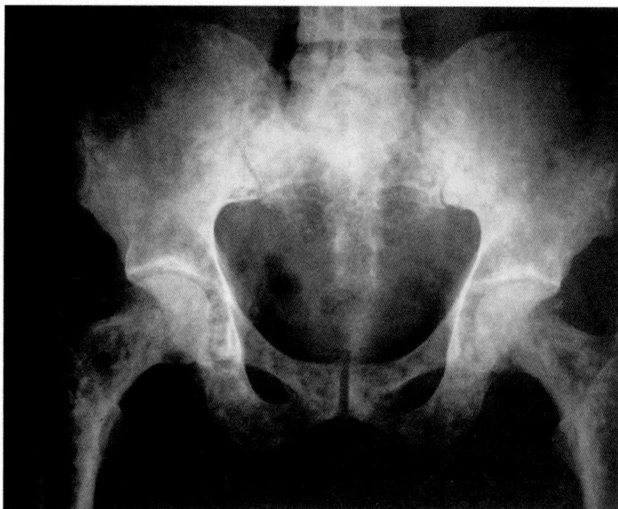

FIGURE 61.15. **Osteopoikilosis.** An AP view of the pelvis reveals multiple small, round sclerotic foci throughout the pelvis and femurs. These are diagnostic of osteopoikilosis. This is occasionally mistaken for metastatic disease.

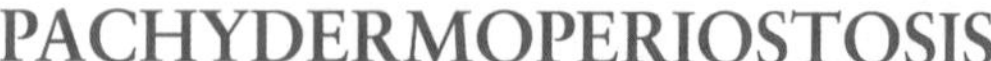

PACHYDERMOPERIOSTOSIS

Pachydermoperiostosis or primary hypertrophic osteoarthropathy is a rare, familial disease that is manifested by thickening of the skin of the extremities and face, clubbing of the fingers, and widespread periostitis. The periosteal reaction is similar to that of hypertrophic pulmonary osteoarthropathy, but pachydermoperiostosis is only occasionally painful.

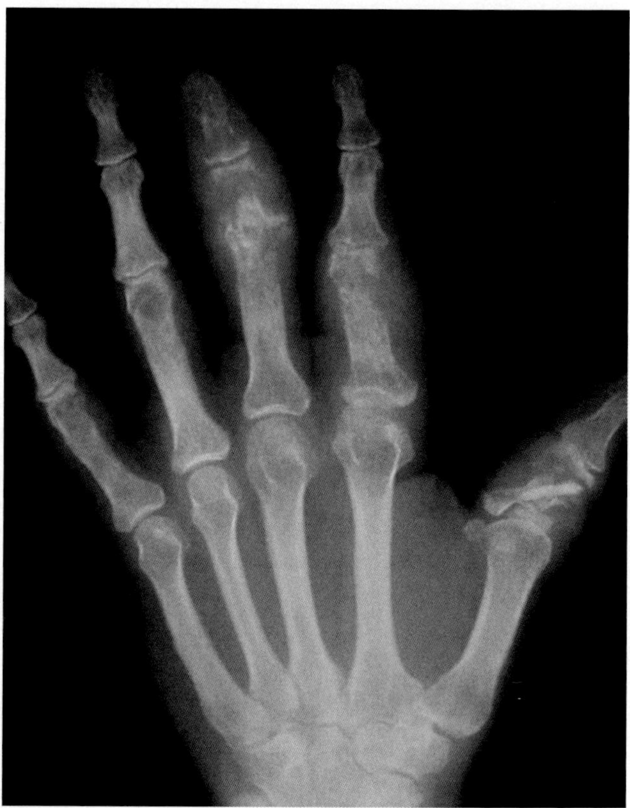

FIGURE 61.16. **Sarcoid.** An AP radiograph of a hand in a patient with sarcoidosis shows multiple lytic and destructive lesions, many of which demonstrate a lacelike pattern.

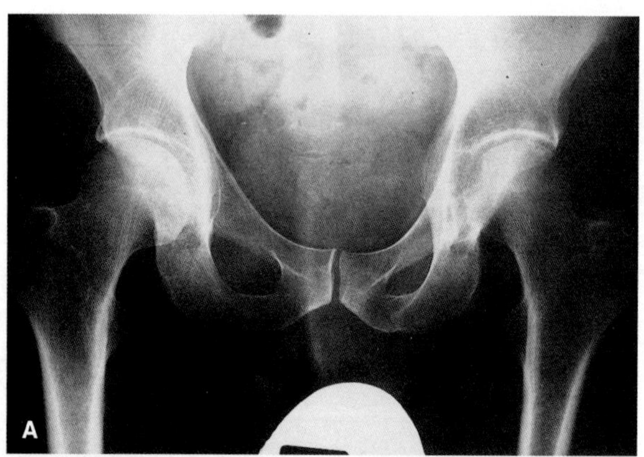

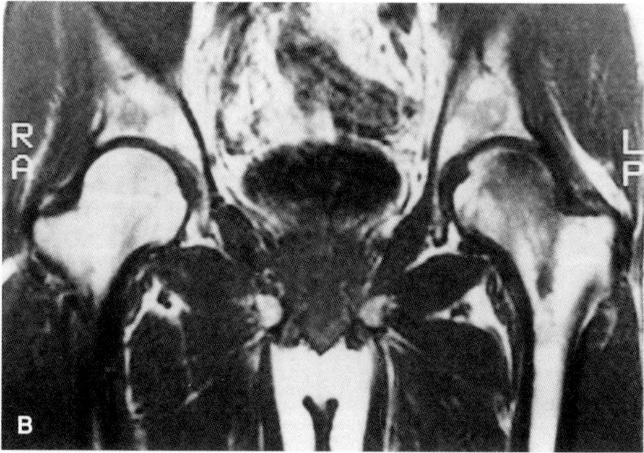

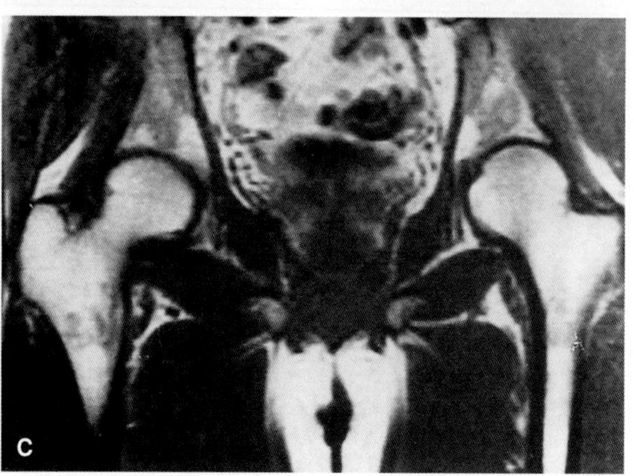

FIGURE 61.17. **Idiopathic Transient Osteoporosis of the Hip.** **A:** A radiograph of a 40-year-old man with left hip pain shows osteoporosis involving the left hip, with no other abnormalities seen. **B:** A T1-weighted coronal MR done at the same time as the radiograph shows low signal in the superior portion of the left femoral head. This is a characteristic appearance of avascular necrosis (AVN) but is a nonspecific finding. Clinically, this patient had no underlying causes for AVN, and he was treated conservatively. **C:** Seven months later, after near total cessation of the hip pain, a repeat MR shows no abnormality in the hip. This is consistent with idiopathic transient osteoporosis of the hip.

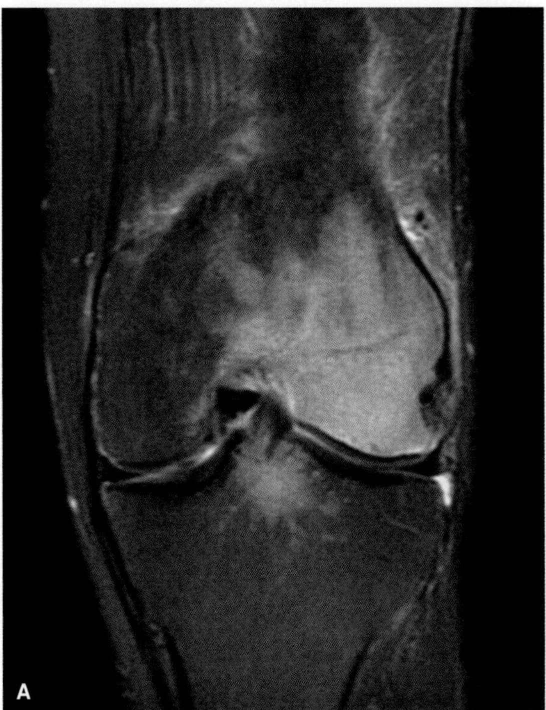

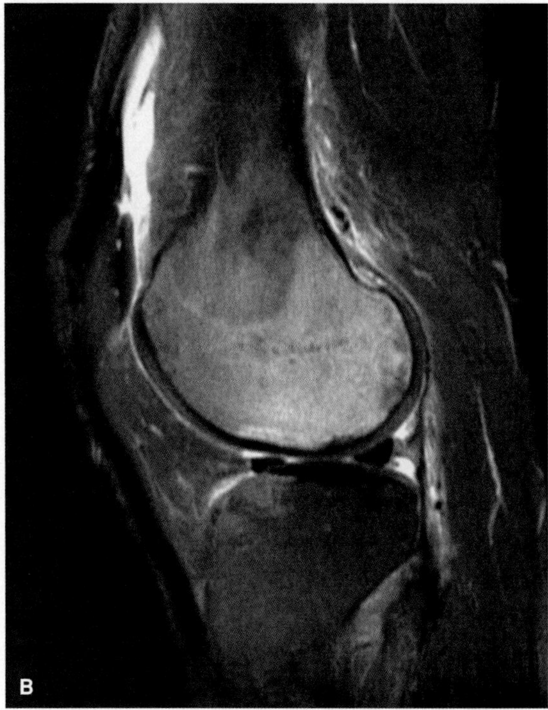

FIGURE 61.18. **Painful Bone Marrow Edema of the Knee.** Coronal (**A**) and sagittal (**B**) T2-weighted images with fat suppression show marked high signal in the lateral condyle in a middle-aged woman with sudden onset of pain. The pain resolved over a 6-month period. This is typical of painful bone marrow edema syndrome.

SARCOIDOSIS

Sarcoidosis is a noncaseating granulomatous disease that primarily affects the lungs. When the musculoskeletal system is involved, the hands are mainly affected, with the spine and long bones only infrequently involved. Sarcoid causes a characteristic lacelike pattern of bony destruction in the hands (Fig. 61.16). Multiple phalanges are typically affected in either one or both hands. It is so radiographically characteristic that there is almost no differential diagnosis for this pattern.

TRANSIENT OSTEOPOROSIS OF THE HIP

Also known as idiopathic transient osteoporosis of the hip (ITOH), this poorly understood disorder is an idiopathic process that begins with a painful hip with no underlying disorder or other findings other than osteoporosis, which is limited to the painful hip. Its appearance on MR is similar to early AVN, in that low signal on T1-weighted images and high signal on T2-weighted images are seen throughout the femoral head and neck (Fig. 61.17); however, the edema is typically greater than with AVN and no well-demarcated margin is present. Transient osteoporosis of the hip invariably is self-limited with full resolution, though subarticular insufficiency fractures may occur during the period of osteoporosis. It tends to occur more often in middle-aged men, though women may also be affected, particularly during the third trimester of pregnancy or in the early postpartum period.

A similar process occurs in the knee which has been called painful bone marrow syndrome (Fig. 61.18A,B). It is seen most commonly in the medial femoral condyle but can occur laterally or in the proximal tibia adjacent to the joint. Protected weight bearing is recommended to prevent insufficiency fractures. Painful bone marrow edema has been reported in the hip (ITOH), knee, distal clavicle, and ankle. It can occur in several different locations over time or simultaneously and then is called regional migratory osteoporosis. As with ITOH, these all are self-limited and are treated simply with pain management and protected weight bearing.

Suggested Readings

Helms CA, Hattner RS, Vogler JB, 3rd. Osteoid osteoma: radionuclide diagnosis. *Radiology* 1984;151:779–784.

Korompilias AV, Karantanas AH, Lykissas MG, Beris AE. Bone marrow edema syndrome. *Skeletal Radiol* 2009;38:425–436.

Mankin HJ. Nontraumatic necrosis of bone (osteonecrosis). *N Engl J Med* 1992;326:1473–1479.

Marcove RC, Heelan RT, Huvos AG, Healey J, Lindeque BG. Osteoid osteoma. Diagnosis, localization, and treatment. *Clin Orthop Relat Res* 1991;(267):197–201.

Mitchell DG, Kressel HY, Arger PH, Dalinka M, Spritzer CE, Steinberg ME. Avascular necrosis of the femoral head: morphologic assessment by MR imaging, with CT correlation. *Radiology* 1986;161:739–742.

Takatori Y, Kokubo T, Ninomiya S, Nakamura T, Okutsu I, Kamogawa M. Transient osteoporosis of the hip. Magnetic resonance imaging. *Clin Orthop Relat Res* 1991;271:190–194.

CHAPTER 62 ■ MAGNETIC RESONANCE IMAGING OF THE KNEE

CLYDE A. HELMS AND EMILY N. VINSON

MR of the knee has developed into one of the most frequently requested examinations in radiology. This is because of its inherent accuracy in depicting internal derangements and its ability to allow orthopedic surgeons to use it as a road map for subsequent therapeutic arthroscopic procedures. Also, MR has a very–high-negative predictive value; therefore, a normal MR knee examination is highly accurate in excluding an internal derangement.

TECHNIQUE

The proper imaging protocol is essential for a high diagnostic accuracy rate. If the appropriate sequences are obtained, an accuracy of 90% to 95% can be expected. A sagittal T1-weighted (or proton density–weighted) sequence is essential for examining the menisci, and 4- or 5-mm-thick slices with a relatively small field of view and at least a 256 × 192 matrix are recommended. The knee should be imaged using a dedicated knee coil and externally rotated about 5 to 10 degrees (should not exceed 10 degrees) to put the anterior cruciate ligament (ACL) in the plane of imaging. Fast spin echo (FSE, also called turbo spin echo) T2-weighted or T2* GRASS (gradient-recalled acquisition in the steady state) sagittal images are obtained primarily to examine the cruciate ligaments and cartilage.

FSE sequences are particularly poor for examining the menisci. Even when performed as fast proton-density images with a short echo train length, they have too much blurring to provide an accurate demonstration of meniscal tears. Conventional spin-echo images have consistently given a sensitivity for meniscal tears in the 90% to 95% range, whereas FSE proton–density sequences have been reported in multiple papers to be only around 80% sensitive for meniscal tears.

Coronal images are obtained to examine the collateral ligaments and cartilage and to look for meniscocapsular separations. These abnormalities can generally only be seen with T2-weighted images. Coronal T1-weighted images are therefore a waste of time, because nothing can be seen on these images that cannot be seen equally as well on the sagittal images or the T2 or T2* coronal images. The coronal images are useful for confirming a meniscal tear that is seen on the sagittal images, especially radial tears. It is rare to see a linear tear solely on the coronal images; therefore, coronal meniscus–sensitive sequences are typically not necessary.

Axial images are used for viewing the patellofemoral cartilage, identifying bursal fluid collections, and for a second look at the cruciate and collateral ligaments. As for the coronal images, to afford an opportunity to see any pathology, T2-weighted images must be obtained.

MENISCI

The normal meniscus is a fibrocartilaginous, C-shaped structure that is uniformly low in signal on both T1- and T2-weighted images. Many centers have found that the menisci are more easily examined if they fat-suppress the T1- or proton density–weighted sequences (Fig. 62.1). With T2* sequences, the menisci will usually demonstrate some internal signal. With T1-weighted sequences, any signal within the meniscus is abnormal, except in children, in whom some signal is normal and represents normal vascularity.

Meniscal Degeneration. Meniscal signal that does not disrupt an articular surface is representative of intrasubstance degeneration (Fig. 62.2), which is myxoid degeneration of the fibrocartilage. It most likely represents aging and normal wear and tear. It is not thought to be symptomatic and cannot be diagnosed clinically or with arthroscopy. Some choose, therefore, not to mention intrasubstance degeneration in the radiology interpretation.

Meniscal Tear. When high signal in a meniscus disrupts the superior or inferior articular surface, a meniscal tear is diagnosed. Meniscal tears have many different configurations and locations; an oblique horizontal tear extending to the inferior surface of the posterior horn of the medial meniscus is the most common type (Fig. 62.3). A fairly common meniscus tear is a parrot beak or radial tear. This tear occurs along a plane perpendicular to the long axis of the meniscus and involves

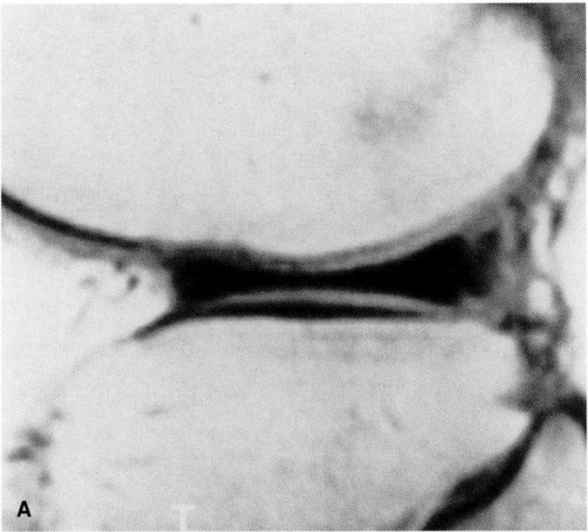

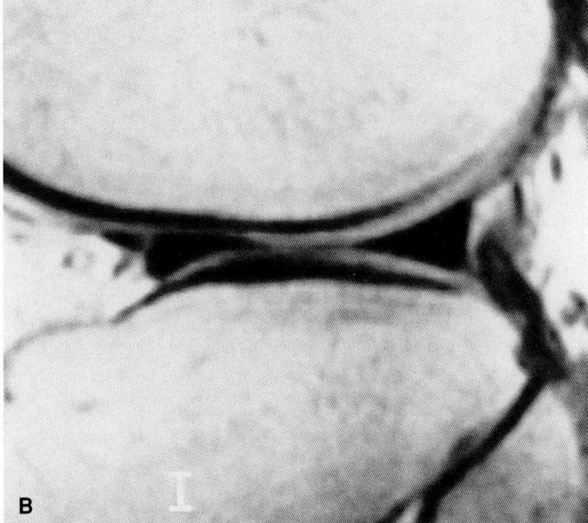

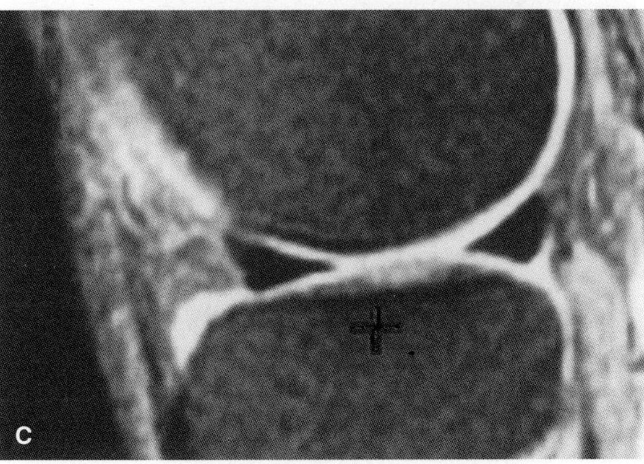

FIGURE 62.1. **Normal Meniscus. A:** A sagittal T1-weighted image through a normal lateral meniscus demonstrates uniform low signal in the meniscus. This is a section through the body of the meniscus, as it has a bow-tie configuration. With 4- or 5-mm-thick slices, two sections of the body should be seen in each meniscus. **B:** In the same sequence, this sagittal image demonstrates uniform low signal in the anterior and posterior horns of this normal lateral meniscus. **C:** This sagittal proton-density image shows how fat suppression accentuates the menisci.

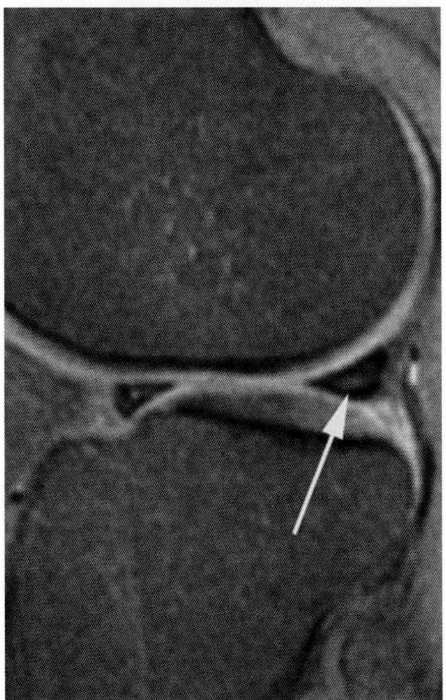

FIGURE 62.2. **Intrasubstance Degeneration.** Faint intermediate signal can be seen in the posterior horn of this meniscus (*arrow*) that does not disrupt the articular surface of the meniscus. This is intrasubstance degeneration.

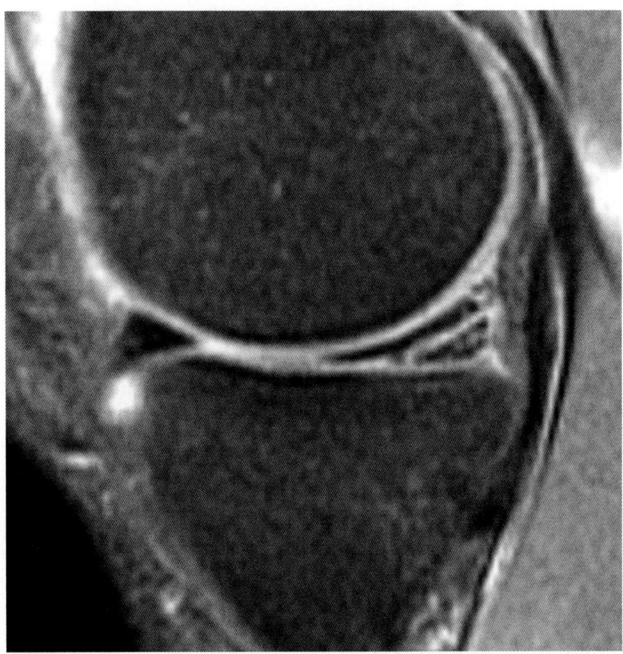

FIGURE 62.3. **Meniscal Tear.** This sagittal fat-suppressed proton-density image shows linear high signal in the posterior horn of the meniscus that disrupts the inferior articular surface. This is the appearance of a meniscal tear.

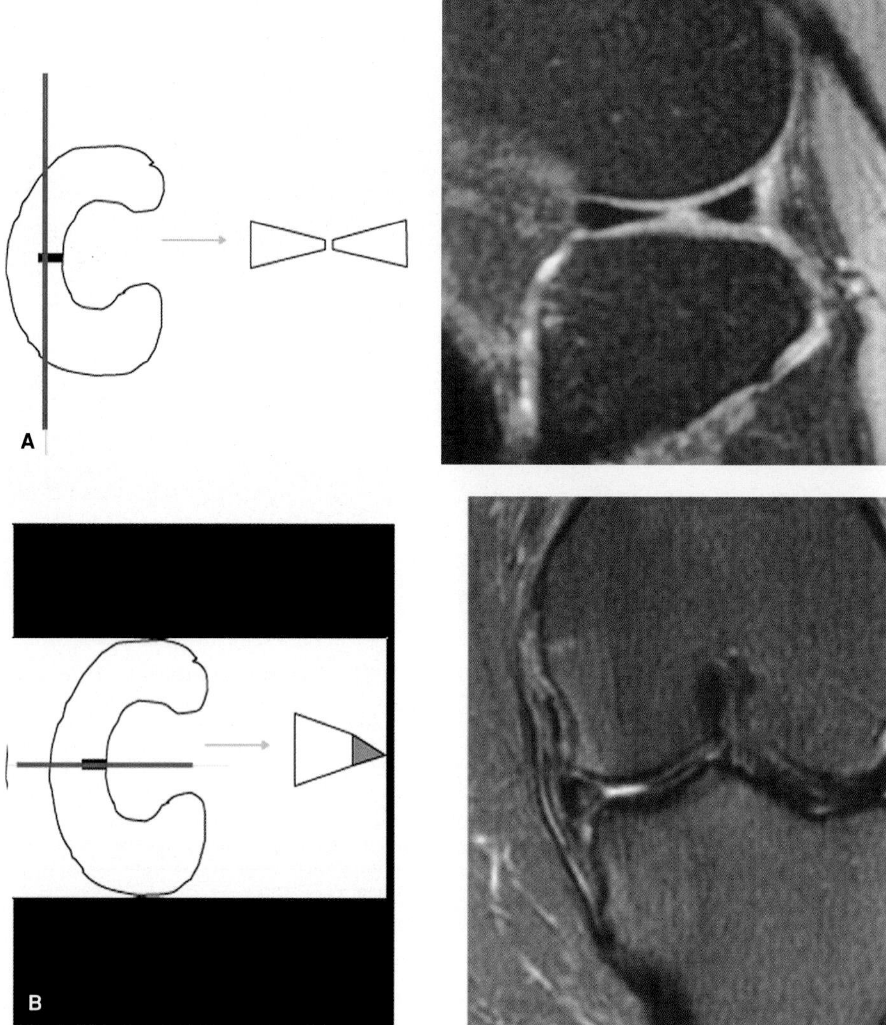

FIGURE 62.4. **Radial Tear. A:** A drawing of a mid-body radial tear with a sagittal image. The tear is depicted as a cleft in the bow-tie. **B:** A drawing of the same tear with a coronal image. The tear is depicted as a truncated triangle.

at least the inner free edge portion of the meniscus; if large, a radial tear may extend across the full width of the meniscus. Its appearance on MR is dependent on the location of the tear relative to the imaging plane. If the tear involves the mid-body of the meniscus, a sagittal plane image shows a cleft (Fig. 62.4A), whereas the same tear on a coronal image is shown as a truncated meniscus (Fig. 62.4B).

It has been shown that MR imaging sensitivity for meniscal tears decreases significantly when the ACL is torn. These frequently overlooked tears occur in the periphery of the menisci and in the posterior horn of the lateral meniscus. Hence, great care must be used in examining these areas of the menisci in patients with ACL tears.

Bucket-Handle Tear. A common meniscal tear is a bucket-handle tear, reported in up to 10% of some series. When a longitudinally-oriented tear of the meniscus results in the inner free edge of the meniscus becoming displaced towards the intercondylar notch, it is termed a bucket-handle tear (Fig. 62.5). It is most easily recognized by observing on the sagittal images that only one image is present that has the bow-tie appearance of the body segment of the meniscus (Fig. 62.6). Normally, two contiguous sagittal images with a bow-tie shape are seen, because the normal meniscus is 9- to 12-mm wide and the sagittal

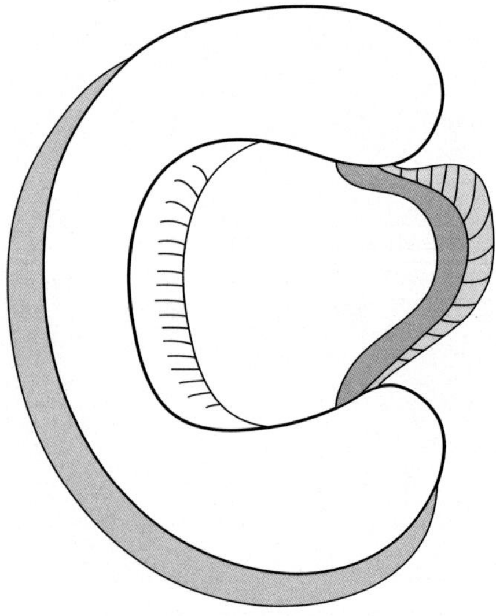

FIGURE 62.5. **Bucket-Handle Tear.** This drawing illustrates a bucket-handle tear, with the torn free edge of the meniscus displaced as the handle of the bucket.

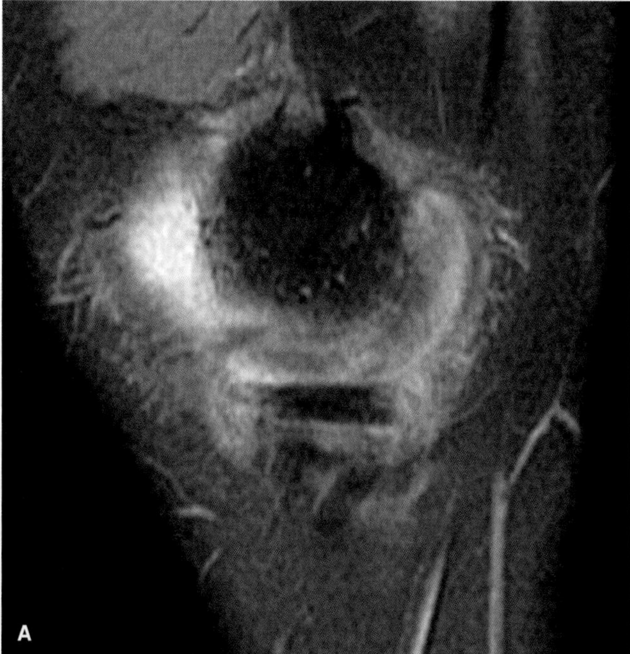
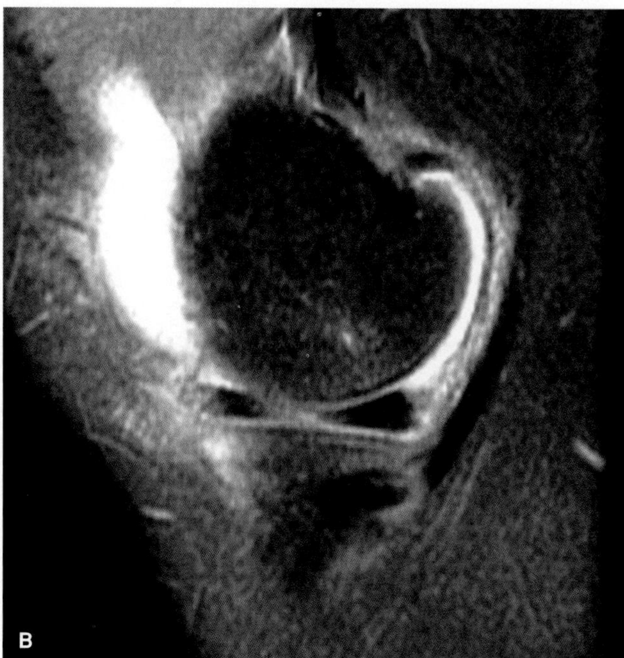

FIGURE 62.6. **Bucket-Handle Tear.** Sagittal proton-density images through the medial meniscus at its most medial aspect reveal one bow-tie, indicative of the body of the meniscus (**A**), with the adjacent image (**B**) showing apparently normal anterior and posterior horns. However, since there should be two consecutive sagittal images with a bow-tie configuration, this suggests a tear involving the inner margin of the meniscus, such as a bucket-handle tear.

images are 4 to 5 mm in thickness. On the coronal images, a bucket-handle tear may reveal the meniscus to be shortened and truncated; however, the torn meniscus often remodels and truncation cannot be appreciated. The displaced inner edge of the meniscus (the "handle" of the bucket) should be seen in the intercondylar notch on sagittal or coronal views (Fig. 62.7A and B).

Discoid Meniscus. A discoid meniscus is a large meniscus that can have many different shapes: lens shaped, wedged, flat, and others. Whether it is congenital or acquired is not known. It is seen in the lateral meniscus in up to 3% of the population, with a discoid medial meniscus being much less common. A discoid meniscus is thought to be more prone to tear than a normal meniscus, and it can be symptomatic even without being torn. Although they are easily identified on coronal images by noting extension of meniscal tissue into the tibial spines at the intercondylar notch (Fig. 62.8), they are most reliably diagnosed by noting more than two consecutive sagittal images that show the meniscus with a bow-tie appearance (Fig. 62.9).

Meniscal Cysts. Meniscal cysts occur in about 5% of cases and can cause pain even if the meniscus is not torn to the articular surface. The etiology is unknown. They occur more frequently in discoid menisci. If the meniscus is not torn, the surgical approach used by some is percutaneous decompression and packing, whereas if a meniscal tear is associated with the cyst,

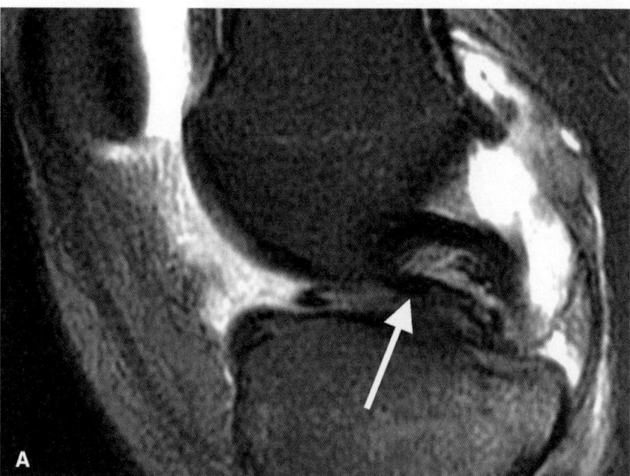
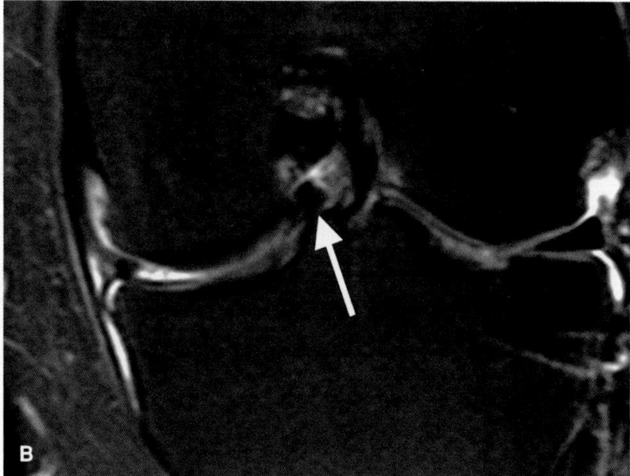

FIGURE 62.7. **Displaced Fragment in Bucket-Handle Tear. A:** A sagittal fat-suppressed T2-weighted image through the intercondylar notch in a patient with a bucket-handle tear reveals the displaced free fragment or handle (*arrow*) just inferior to the posterior cruciate ligament, sometimes called the "*double PCL sign.*" **B:** A coronal fat-suppressed T2-weighted image in a different patient with a bucket-handle tear shows the displaced fragment in the intercondylar notch (*arrow*).

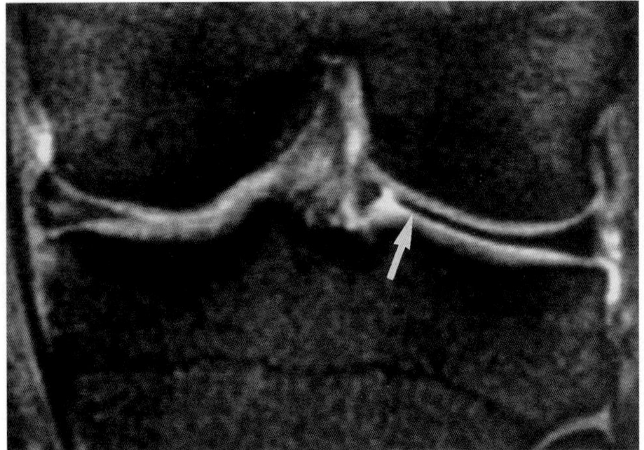

FIGURE 62.8. **Discoid Lateral Meniscus.** A coronal gradient-echo image through the intercondylar notch shows a large lateral meniscus, with meniscal tissue extending into the notch medially (*arrow*).

it is approached intra-articularly. Hence, accurate diagnosis of a tear is imperative. The intrameniscal portion of the cyst typically does not get as bright as fluid in signal on T2 sequences (Fig. 62.10), which has misled many radiologists into discounting the presence of a cyst. A meniscal cyst will enlarge the meniscus and give it a swollen appearance, unless it decompresses into the adjacent soft tissues (called a parameniscal cyst) or into the joint via a meniscal tear. Decompression peripherally into a parameniscal cyst does not indicate a meniscal tear. A meniscal tear, by definition, has to disrupt the articular surface of the meniscus.

Transverse Ligament. The lateral meniscus often has what appears to be a tear on the anterior horn near its upper margin, which is a pseudotear from the insertion of the transverse ligament (Fig. 62.11). This can easily be differentiated from a real tear by following it medially across the knee in the Hoffa fat pad, where it inserts into the anterior horn of the medial meniscus.

CRUCIATE LIGAMENTS

Anterior Cruciate Ligament. The normal ACL is seen in the intercondylar notch as a linear, predominantly low-signal structure on T1-weighted images; it often shows some linear striations near its insertion onto the medial tibial spine when viewed on sagittal images (Fig. 62.12). When torn, the ACL is most often simply not visualized, although sometimes the actual disruption will be seen (Fig. 62.13). T2-weighted images are imperative for obtaining the highest accuracy in diagnosing ACL tears, because fluid and hemorrhage will often obscure the ligament on T1-weighted images. Partial tears or sprains of the ACL are manifested by high signal and/or laxity within an otherwise intact ligament. MR is highly accurate in diagnosing a torn ACL, with sensitivities reported in the literature approaching 100%.

Posterior Cruciate Ligament. The normal posterior cruciate ligament (PCL) is a gently curved, homogeneously low-signal

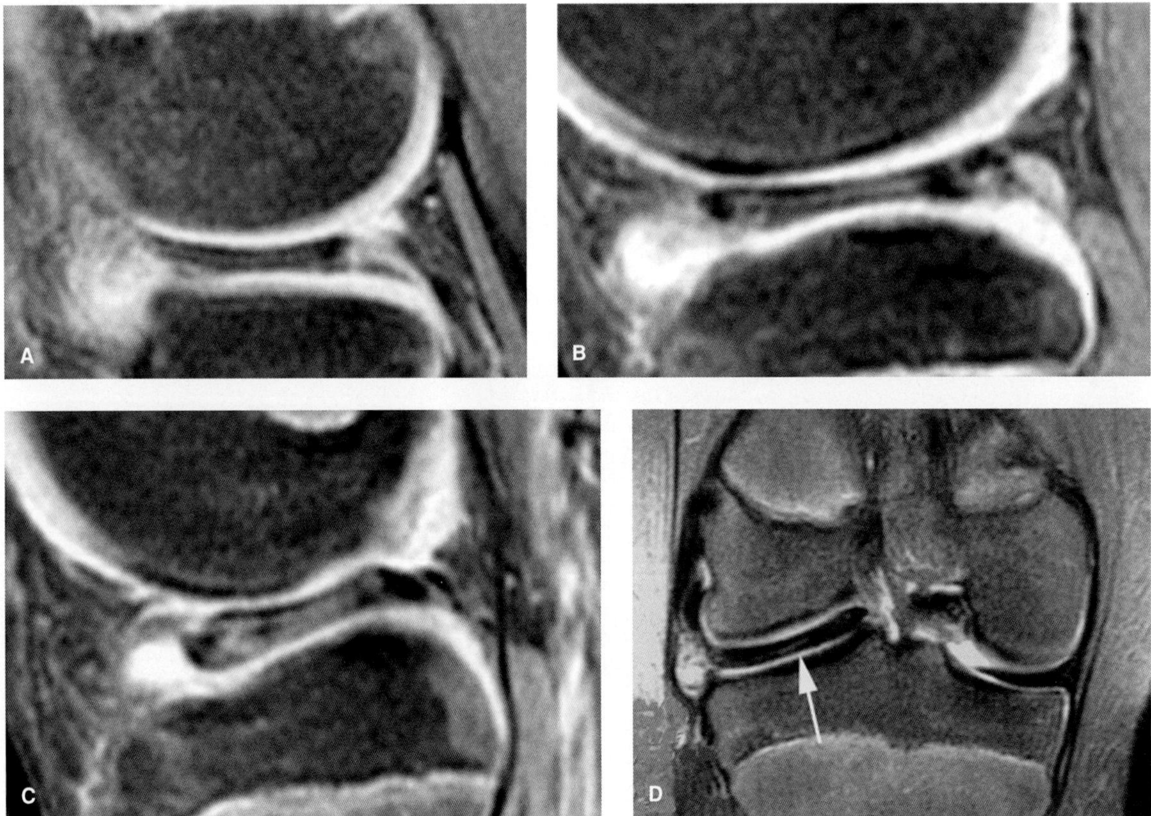

FIGURE 62.9. **Discoid Lateral Meniscus.** Three consecutive 4-mm-thick proton-density images through the lateral meniscus, beginning with the most lateral (**A**) and extending medially (**B, C**), each showing the meniscus to have a bow-tie configuration. Because only two images should have a bow-tie shape, indicative of the body of the meniscus, this is diagnostic of a discoid lateral meniscus. **D:** A coronal T2-weighted image shows the discoid lateral meniscus (*arrow*) to be much larger than the medial meniscus and extends into the intercondylar notch.

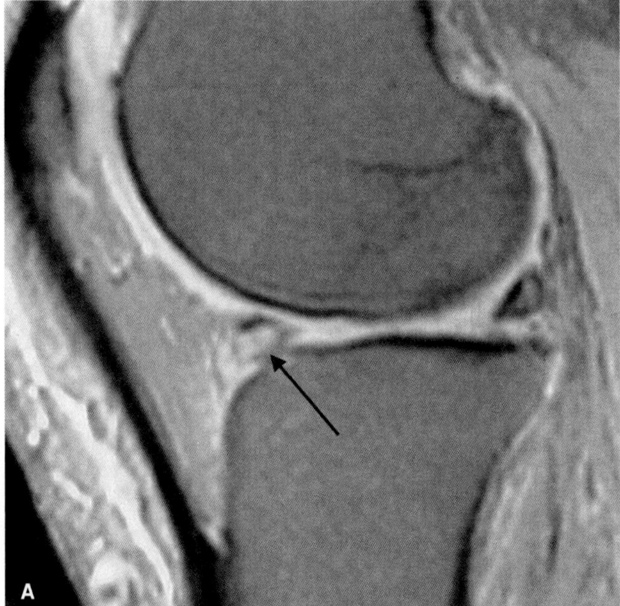

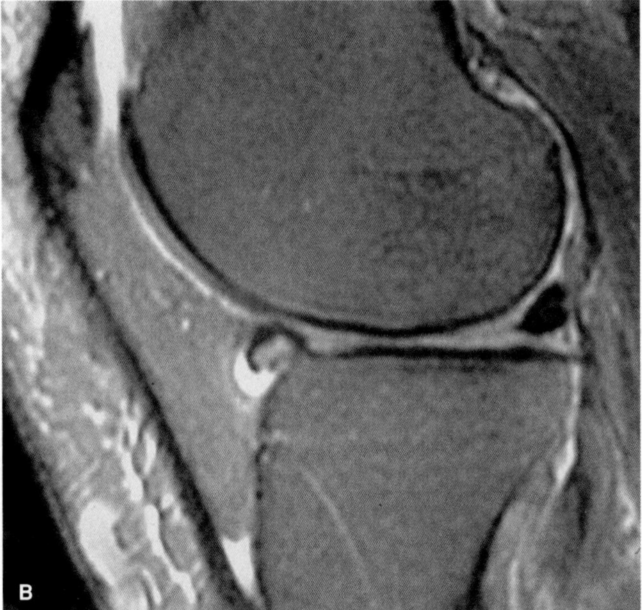

FIGURE 62.10. Meniscal Cyst. A sagittal proton density–weighted image (**A**) through the medial meniscus shows a swollen anterior horn filled with increased signal (*arrow*). A T2-weighted image (**B**) shows high signal similar to fluid in the parameniscal portion, whereas the intrameniscal signal is only intermediate.

structure (Fig. 62.14) that is infrequently torn and even less frequently repaired by surgeons. When torn, it appears thickened and it has diffuse intermediate signal throughout (Fig. 62.15). This increased signal usually does not get brighter with T2-weighted images and is therefore often overlooked. The normal PCL is 6 mm or less in diameter as measured on sagittal images. When torn, it is almost always thicker than 7 mm. Most orthopedic surgeons do not even inspect the PCL at arthroscopy and do not repair it when torn in isolation, because it is rarely a cause of instability.

Meniscofemoral Ligament. A low-signal, round structure is often seen just anterior or posterior to the PCL, as seen in the sagittal views. A loose body or a displaced fragment of a piece of torn meniscus can have this appearance (Fig. 62.16), but it is most commonly caused by a meniscofemoral ligament that extends obliquely across the knee from the medial femoral condyle to the posterior horn of the lateral meniscus. If it passes in front of the PCL, it is called the ligament of Humphrey, and if it passes behind the PCL, it is called the ligament of Wrisberg (Fig. 62.17). Either one of these ligaments is present in up to 72% of all knees.

The insertion of the ligament of Humphrey or Wrisberg onto the lateral meniscus can produce a pseudotear similar to that caused by the transverse ligament on the anterior horn of the lateral meniscus (Fig. 62.18). Prior to diagnosing a tear

FIGURE 62.11. Pseudotear From a Transverse Ligament. A sagittal T1-weighted image through the lateral meniscus shows linear high signal through the upper anterior horn (*arrow*), which resembles a tear. This is the insertion of the transverse ligament onto the meniscus.

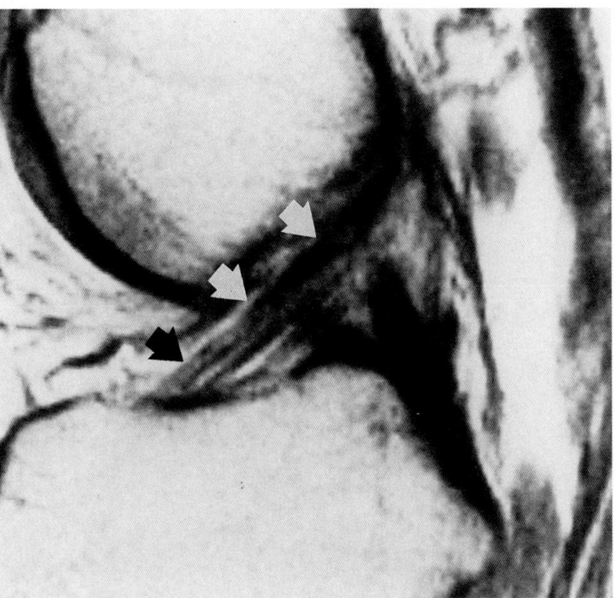

FIGURE 62.12. Normal Anterior Cruciate Ligament (ACL). A sagittal T1-weighted image through the intercondylar notch shows the normal appearance of the ACL (*arrows*).

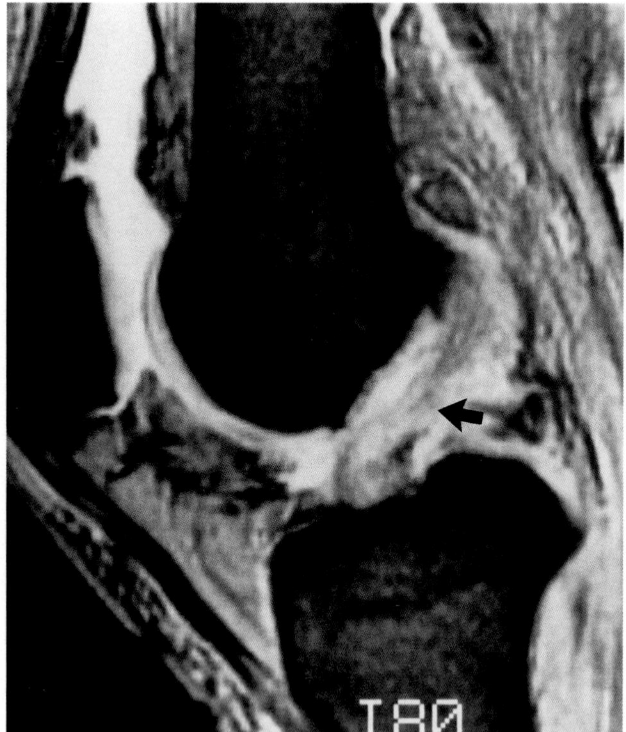

FIGURE 62.13. **Torn Anterior Cruciate Ligament (ACL).** A sagittal T2-weighted image through the intercondylar notch shows fibers of the ACL that are disrupted centrally (*arrow*). This is a common MR appearance of a torn ACL.

on the upper aspect of the posterior horn of the lateral meniscus, care must be taken to look for a meniscofemoral ligament to be certain it is not a pseudotear from the ligament's insertion. Similarly, prior to diagnosing a loose body in front of or behind the PCL, care must be taken to try and follow the structure across to the lateral meniscus to determine whether it is a meniscofemoral ligament.

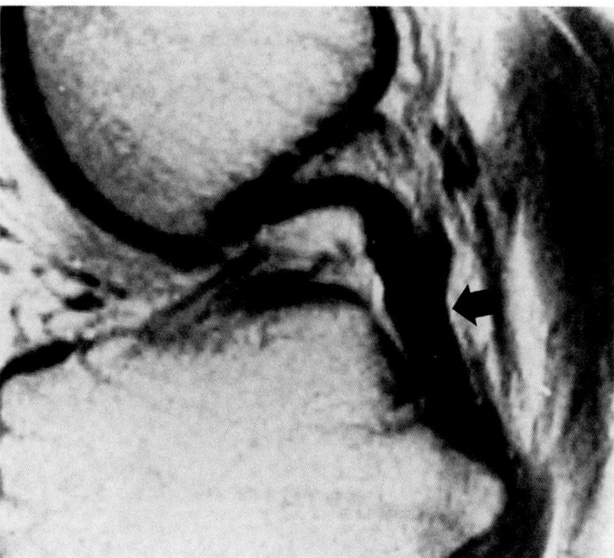

FIGURE 62.14. **Normal Posterior Cruciate Ligament (PCL).** A sagittal T1-weighted image through the intercondylar notch shows the appearance of the normal PCL, with its characteristic uniform low signal (*arrow*).

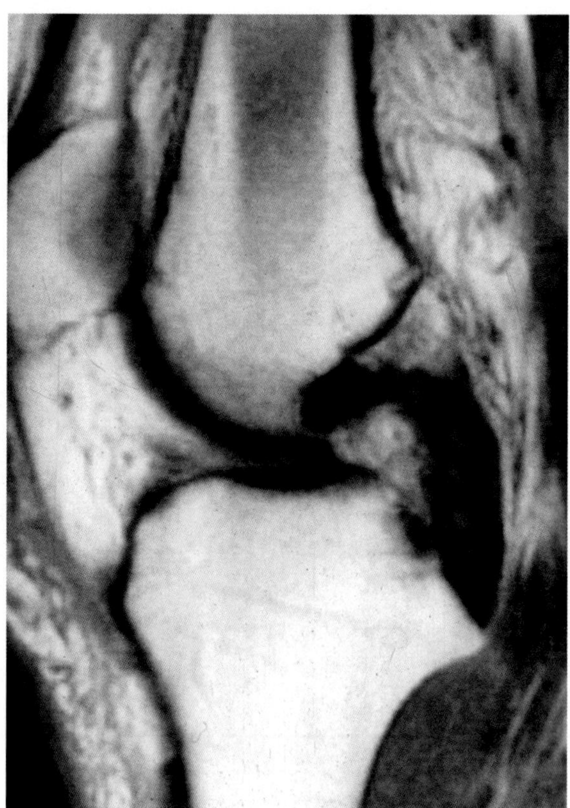

FIGURE 62.15. **Torn Posterior Cruciate Ligament (PCL).** A sagittal through the intercondylar notch reveals the PCL to have diffuse intermediate signal throughout and is thicker than normal. This is typical of a torn PCL.

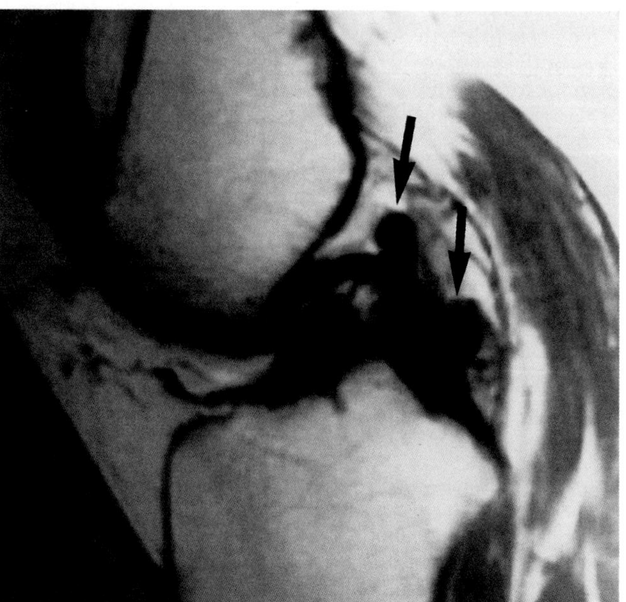

FIGURE 62.16. **Loose Bodies.** A sagittal T1-weighted image through the intercondylar notch in this patient shows two rounded, low-signal structures (*arrows*) that are loose, intra-articular bodies. A meniscofemoral ligament of Wrisberg could have the appearance of either of these loose bodies.

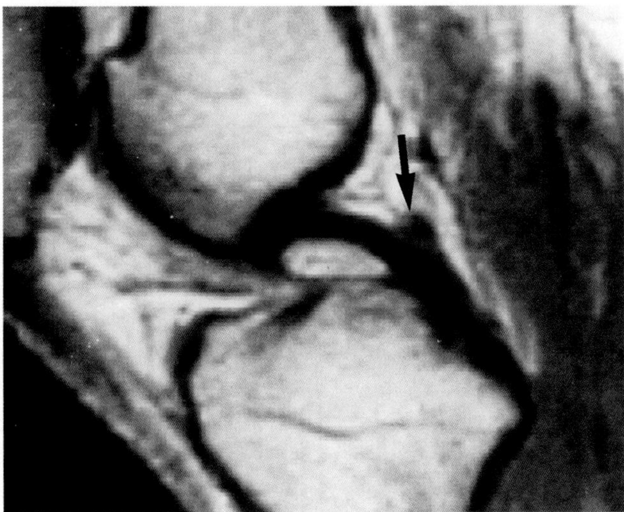

FIGURE 62.17. **Ligament of Wrisberg.** A sagittal through the intercondylar notch shows a rounded, low-signal structure posterior to the posterior cruciate ligament, which is the meniscofemoral ligament of Wrisberg (*arrow*).

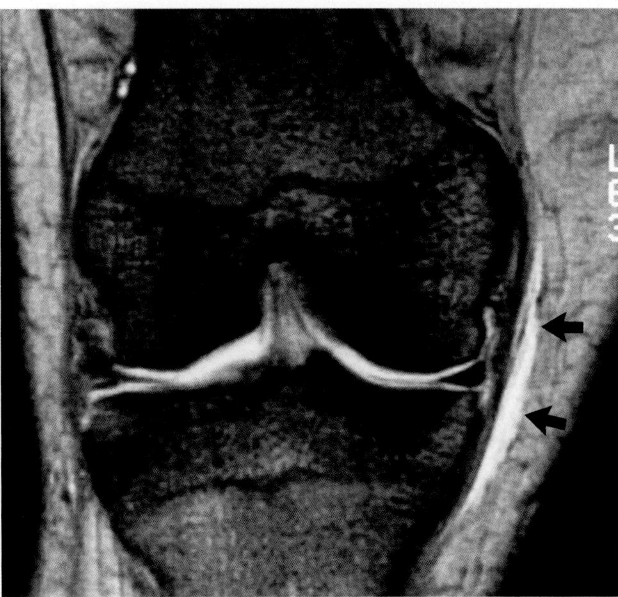

FIGURE 62.19. **Grade 1 Sprain of the Medial Collateral Ligament (MCL).** A gradient-recalled echo coronal image reveals high signal adjacent to the MCL (*arrows*), which represents edema and hemorrhage from a sprain of the MCL. The MCL is clearly intact; hence, a complete tear is easily excluded.

COLLATERAL LIGAMENTS

Medial Collateral Ligament. The medial collateral ligament (MCL) originates on the medial femoral condyle and inserts on the tibia. It is closely applied to the joint and is intimately associated with the medial joint capsule and the medial meniscus. The MCL is uniformly low in signal on T1 and T2 or T2* sequences. Injuries to the MCL usually occur from a valgus stress to the lateral part of the knee (such as a "clipping" injury in football). A grade 1 injury represents a mild sprain and is diagnosed on MR by the presence of fluid or hemorrhage in the soft tissues medial to the MCL. The ligament is otherwise normal (Fig. 62.19). A grade 2 injury is a partial tear and is seen as high signal in and around the MCL on T2 or T2* coronal sequences. The ligament is intact, although the deep or superficial fibers may show minimal disruption. A grade 3 injury is a complete disruption of the MCL. It is best appreciated on T2 or T2* images (Fig. 62.20).

A meniscocapsular separation occurs when the medial meniscus is torn from its attachment to the joint capsule. This occurs most commonly at the site of the MCL and often occurs concomitantly with an MCL injury. It is easily recognized on a T2 or T2* coronal image by noting joint fluid extending between the medial meniscus and the capsule (Fig. 62.21). It is essential to use T2 or T2* sequences, as a T1-weighted sequence will not detect the fluid between the meniscus and the capsule.

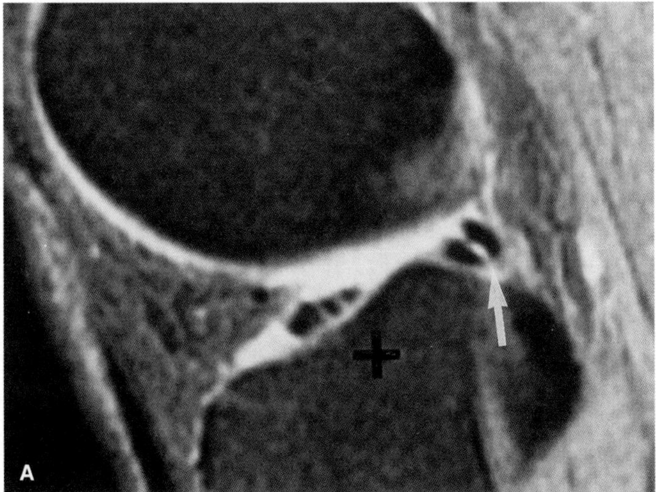

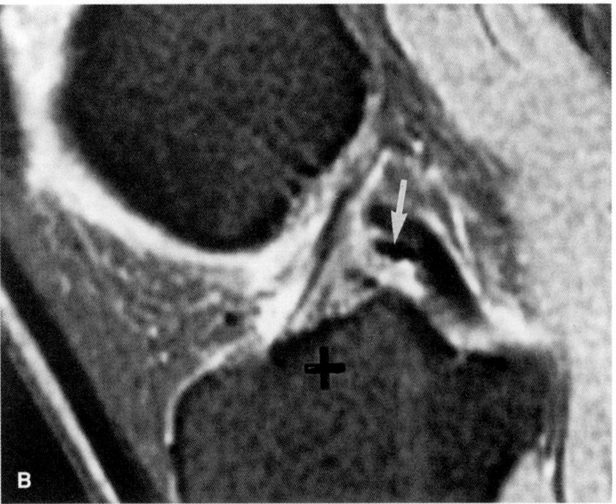

FIGURE 62.18. **Pseudotear From the Ligament of Humphrey Insertion. A:** A sagittal proton-density fat-suppressed image through the lateral meniscus reveals an apparent tear of the posterior horn (*arrow*) which is the insertion of the ligament of Humphrey onto the meniscus. (The "speckled" appearance in the anterior horn of the lateral meniscus is a frequently seen normal variant and should not be confused for a torn meniscus.) **B:** On the image through the intercondylar notch, a ligament of Humphrey (*arrow*) is seen anterior to the posterior cruciate ligament (PCL). The ligament of Humphrey could be followed on adjacent images, from anterior to the PCL to its insertion on the posterior horn of the lateral meniscus.

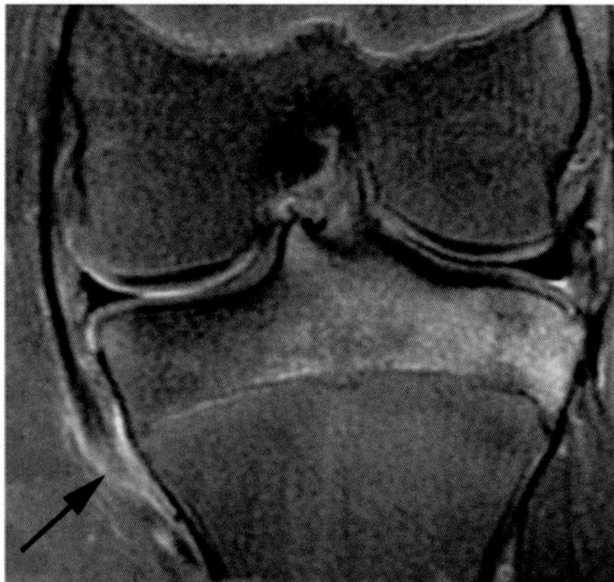

FIGURE 62.20. **Torn Medial Collateral Ligament (MCL).** A coronal T2-weighted image shows the MCL disrupted distally (*arrow*).

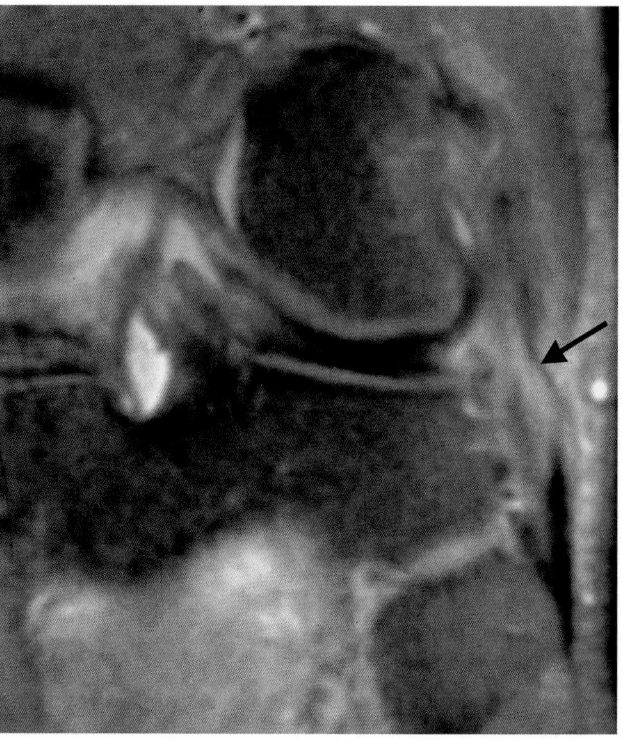

FIGURE 62.22. **Lateral Collateral Ligament Tear.** A coronal fat-suppressed T2-weighted image reveals a tear of the lateral collateral ligament (fibular collateral ligament) (*arrow*). The normal ligament should be a low-signal structure between the femur and the fibula.

Lateral Collateral Ligament. The lateral collateral ligament (LCL) consists of three parts. The most posterior structure is the tendon of the biceps femoris, which inserts onto the head of the fibula. Next, anterior to the biceps, is the true LCL, also called the fibular collateral ligament, which extends from the lateral femoral condyle to the head of the fibula. The biceps and the fibular collateral ligament usually join and insert onto the head of the fibula in a conjoined fashion. Anterior to the fibular collateral ligament is the iliotibial band, which extends into the fascia more anteriorly and inserts onto Gerdy tubercle on the tibia. The LCL is torn infrequently in comparison to the MCL, but a tear can require surgery if instability is present. A torn LCL is seen as disruption of the ligamentous fibers on coronal images (Fig. 62.22).

PATELLA

Chondromalacia Patella. The patellar cartilage commonly undergoes degeneration, causing exquisite pain and tenderness. This is called chondromalacia patella. It can be diagnosed on sagittal images but is more easily identified on axial images. Chondromalacia patella begins with focal swelling and degeneration of the cartilage. This can be seen as high-signal foci in

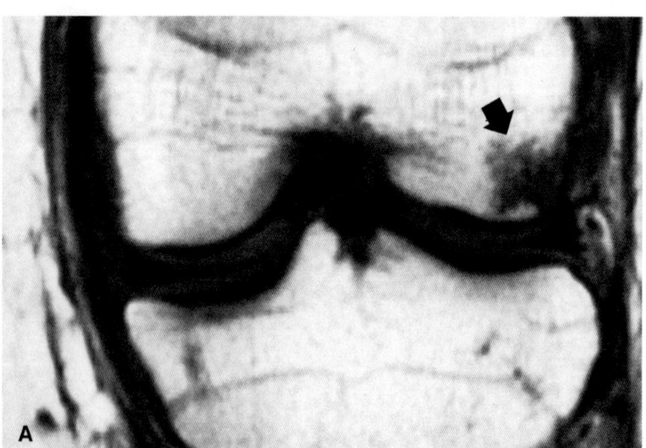

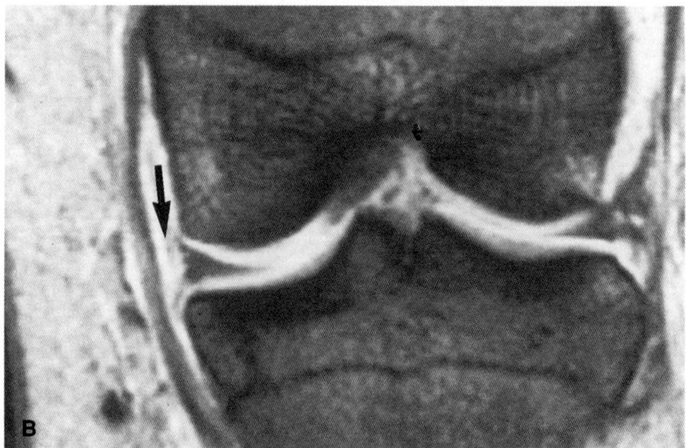

FIGURE 62.21. **Meniscocapsular Separation. A:** A T1-weighted coronal image reveals a contusion of the lateral femoral condyle (*arrow*), indicative of a valgus strain, which is often associated with a medial collateral ligament (MCL) tear. The MCL appears normal on this image; however, the linear low signal in the soft tissues just adjacent to the MCL is suggestive of fluid. This would indicate a partial tear or sprain of the MCL. **B:** A coronal gradient-echo image in the same knee reveals fluid between the medial meniscus and the MCL (*arrow*), which is diagnostic for a meniscocapsular separation. Faint high signal in the MCL and adjacent to it indicates a partial tear. A T2-weighted or T2* sequence in the coronal plane is necessary to see these abnormalities.

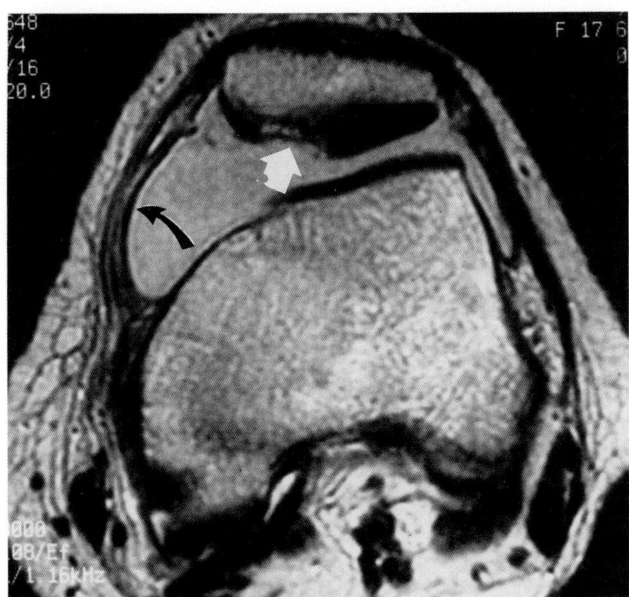

FIGURE 62.23. **Chondral Defect in Patella.** An axial fast spin-echo T2-weighted image through the patella shows a large cartilage defect on the apex and medial facet of the patella (*white arrow*) in this patient who suffered a dislocated patella. Note the high signal throughout the medial retinaculum (*curved arrow*), a frequent finding after a patella dislocation.

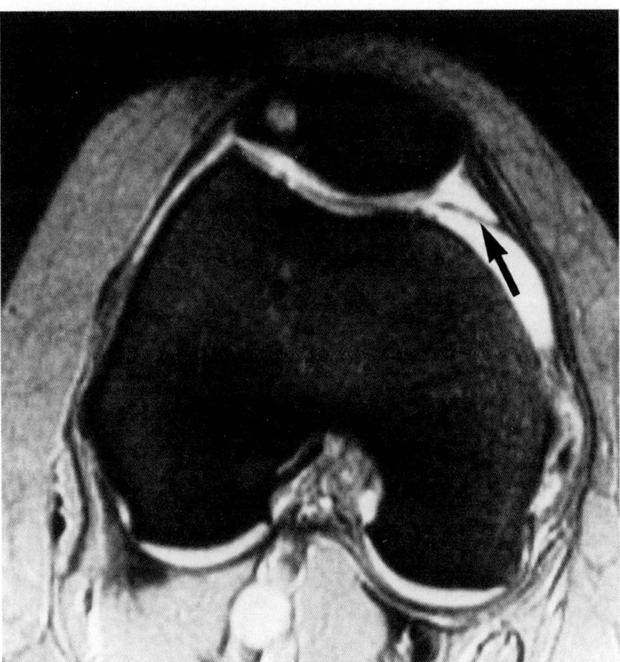

FIGURE 62.24. **Plica.** An axial gradient-echo image through the patella shows a low-signal linear structure (*arrow*) extending from the medial capsule toward the medial facet of the patella. This is a medial patellar plica that is not abnormally thickened. Without the joint effusion or the T2 weighting, the plica would not be visualized.

the cartilage. Its progression causes thinning and irregularity of the articular surface of the cartilage; finally, the underlying bone is exposed. This final stage occurs more commonly from trauma than from wear and tear. A frequent cause of a patellar cartilage defect is dislocation of the patella, in which the patella strikes the lateral femoral condyle and displaces a piece of patellar articular cartilage (Fig. 62.23). The lateral femoral condyle invariably has a contusion following a dislocated patella.

Patellar Plica. A normal structure seen in over half of the population is the medial patellar plica. It is an embryologic remnant from when the knee was divided into three compartments. It is a thin, fibrous band that extends from the medial capsule toward the medial facet of the patella (Fig. 62.24). Supra- and infrapatellar plicae also exist. The medial patellar plica can, on rare occasions, thicken and cause clinical symptoms that are indistinguishable from those of a torn meniscus; this has been termed "plica syndrome." An abnormal plica can be removed arthroscopically quite easily.

BONY ABNORMALITIES

Contusions. The most frequently encountered bony abnormality seen with MR is a contusion. A contusion represents microfractures from trauma. They are also called bone bruises. They are easily identified on T1-weighted images as subarticular areas of inhomogeneous low signal. With T2 weighting, a contusion will show increased signal for several weeks, depending on its severity (Fig. 62.25). Visualization of increased signal with T2* images can be difficult because of the susceptibility artifacts of the bone seen with T2* images. Contusions can progress to osteochondritis dissecans if they are not treated with decreased weight bearing; hence, an isolated bone contusion, with no other internal derangement, is a serious finding that requires protection.

A commonly seen contusion is one that occurs on the posterior part of the lateral tibial plateau with an associated

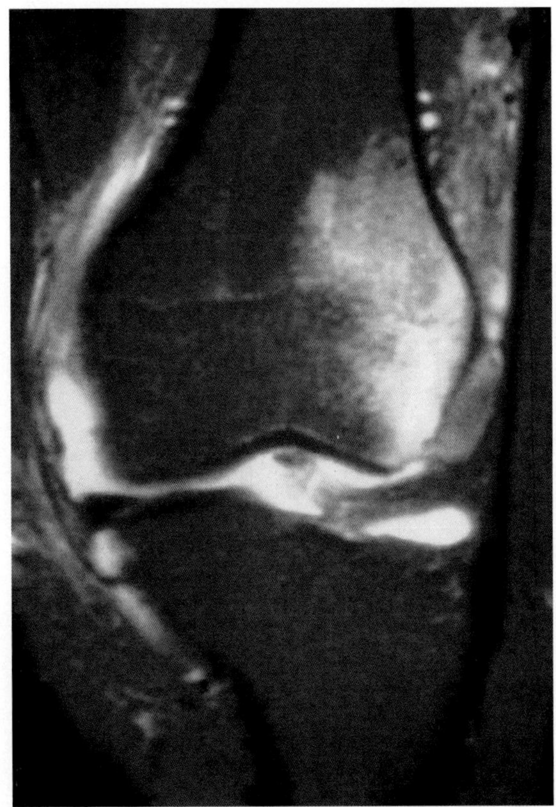

FIGURE 62.25. **Contusion.** A coronal fat-suppressed T2-weighted image shows a focus of high signal in the lateral femoral condyle, which is a characteristic appearance of a severe bone contusion. This occurred from a patella dislocation.

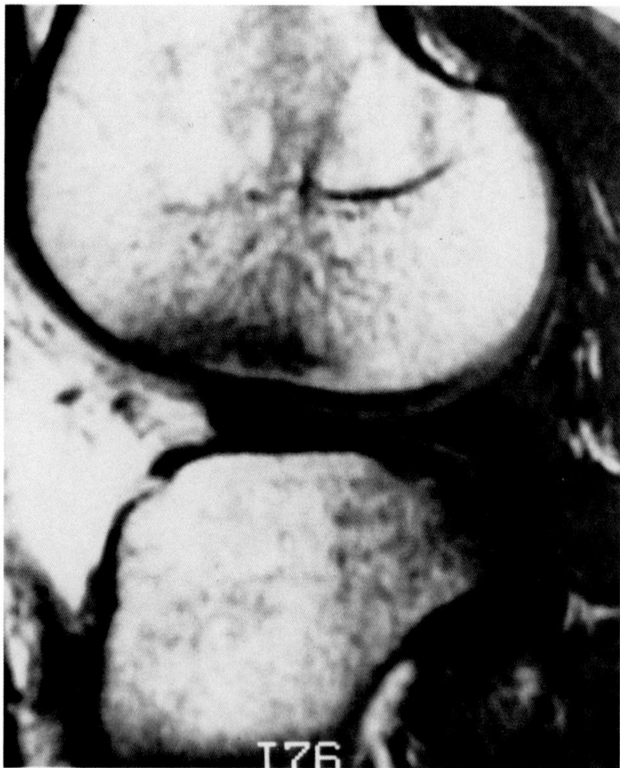

FIGURE 62.26. **Contusion.** A sagittal T1-weighted image through the lateral compartment shows irregular low signal in a subarticular location of the posterior tibial plateau and in the anterior part of the lateral femoral condyle. These findings are characteristic of bone contusions. This distribution of contusions in the posterior lateral tibial plateau and anterior in the lateral femoral condyle is almost always associated with a torn anterior cruciate ligament.

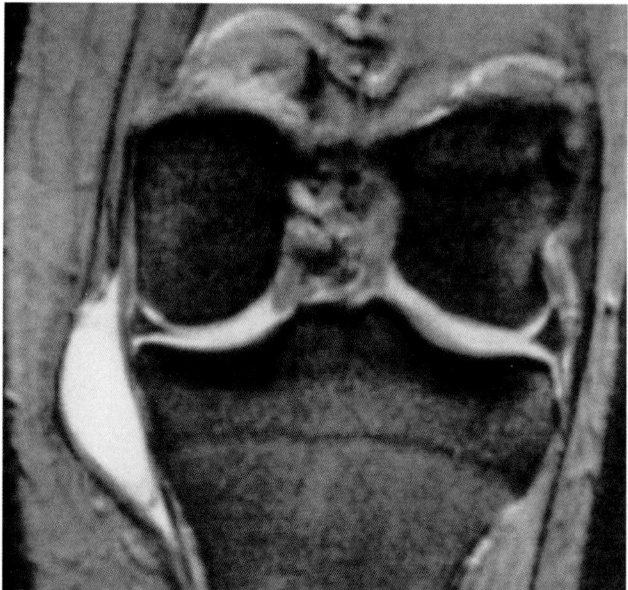

FIGURE 62.27. **Pes Anserinus Bursitis.** A coronal T2* gradient-echo image shows a fluid collection below the medial joint line near the insertion of the pes anserinus tendons. This is pes anserinus bursitis.

"kissing" contusion in the central to anterior lateral femoral condyle (Fig. 62.26). This has been called a "pivot-shift" contusion pattern. It is invariably associated with a torn ACL. Acute ACL tears have been reported to have this type of contusion in over 90% of cases.

Fractures. MR is useful in examining fractures about the knee. Tibial plateau fractures can be imaged precisely with CT; however, MR allows the soft tissues to be seen in addition to any bony abnormalities. A fracture that is almost always associated with an internal derangement is the Segond fracture. A small, bony fragment pulled off the lateral tibial joint line by an avulsion of the lateral joint capsule, it is almost always

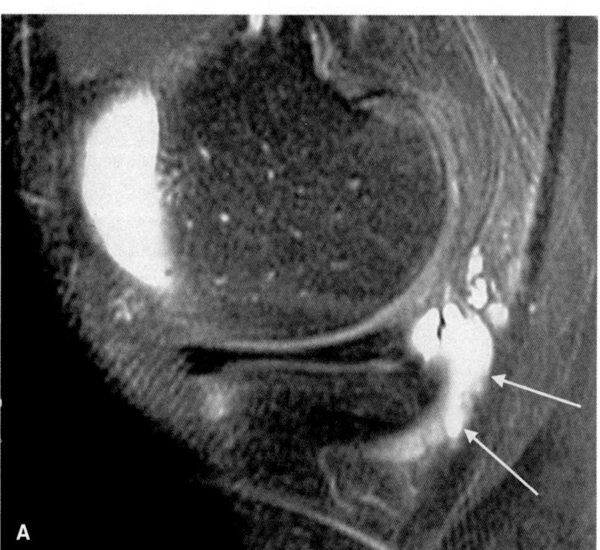

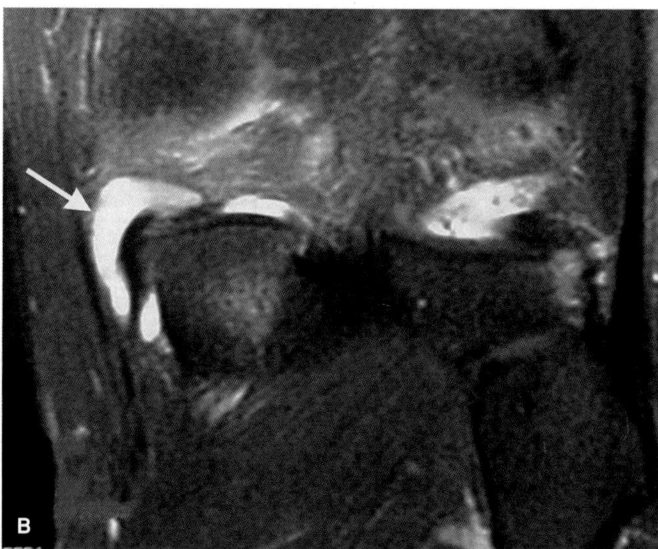

FIGURE 62.28. **Semimembranosus Tibial Collateral Ligament Bursa. A:** A sagittal fat-suppressed T2-weighted image through the medial aspect of the knee shows a fluid collection (*arrows*) at the joint line that is adjacent to the posterior horn of the medial meniscus. This is characteristic of a semimembranosus medial collateral ligament bursa. **B:** A coronal fat-suppressed T2-weighted image shows that this bursa has a comma-shaped appearance at the joint line (*arrow*).

associated with an ACL tear. Because of its small size, a Segond fracture is often more easily seen on radiographs than on MR.

BURSAE

An abnormality that can cause joint pain and clinically mimic plica syndrome or a torn meniscus is bursitis. Two bursae typically are identified medially that can become symptomatic. The first is the pes anserine bursa, which is somewhat uncommon. Three tendons—the sartorius, the gracilis, and the semitendinosus—insert onto the anteromedial aspect of the tibia in a fan-shaped manner that has been likened to a goose's foot, hence the name pes anserinus. A bursa lies beneath the insertion site, which can become inflamed and cause medial joint line or patellar pain; this can be confused clinically with a torn medial meniscus (Fig. 62.27). A second and much more common medial bursa is the semimembranosus tibial collateral ligament bursa. It occurs at the medial joint line and often mimics a meniscal cyst. It has a characteristic comma shape as it drapes over the semimembranosus tendon (Fig. 62.28). Making the diagnosis of pes anserinus or semimembranosus tibial collateral ligament bursitis with MR imaging can prevent an unnecessary arthroscopy procedure—one in which the bursae would be overlooked, since they are extracapsular structures.

Suggested Readings

Crues JV 3rd, Mink J, Levy TL, Lotysch M, Stoller DW. Meniscal tears of the knee: accuracy of MR imaging. *Radiology* 1987;164:445–448.

De Smet AA, Graf BK. Meniscal tears missed on MR imaging: relationship to meniscal tear patterns and anterior cruciate ligament tears. *AJR Am J Roentgenol* 1994;162:905–911.

Helms CA, Laorr A, Cannon WD Jr. The absent bow tie sign in bucket-handle tears of the menisci in the knee. *AJR Am J Roentgenol* 1998;170:57–61.

Mink JH, Deutsch AL. Magnetic resonance imaging of the knee. *Clin Orthop Relat Res* 1989;244:29–47.

Mink JH, Deutsch AL. Occult cartilage and bone injuries of the knee: detection, classification, and assessment with MR imaging. *Radiology* 1989;170: 823–829.

Murphy BJ, Smith RL, Uribe JW, Janecki CJ, Hechtman KS, Mangasarian RA. Bone signal abnormalities in the posterolateral tibia and lateral femoral condyle in complete tears of the anterior cruciate ligament: a specific sign? *Radiology* 1992;182:221–224.

Rodriguez W Jr, Vinson EN, Helms CA, Toth AP. MRI appearance of posterior cruciate ligament tears. *AJR Am J Roentgenol* 2008;191:1031.

Silverman JM, Mink JH, Deutsch AL. Discoid menisci of the knee: MR imaging appearance. *Radiology* 1989;173:351–354.

CHAPTER 63 ■ MAGNETIC RESONANCE IMAGING OF THE SHOULDER

CLYDE A. HELMS AND EMILY N. VINSON

MR of the shoulder is well accepted for its diagnostic utility for abnormalities of the rotator cuff and the glenoid labrum. It has been shown to have a high degree of accuracy. MR of the shoulder can be performed following instillation of gadolinium and saline or without arthrography, with some controversy as to which technique is superior.

ANATOMY

The rotator cuff is composed of the tendons of four muscles that converge on the greater and lesser tuberosities of the humerus: the supraspinatus, infraspinatus, subscapularis, and teres minor (Fig. 63.1). Of these, the supraspinatus most commonly causes clinically significant problems and is the one that is most commonly surgically treated. The supraspinatus tendon lies just superior to the scapula and inferior to the acromioclavicular (AC) joint and acromion. It inserts onto the greater tuberosity of the humerus. Two to three centimeters proximal to its insertion is a section of the tendon called the "critical zone." This area is reported to have decreased vascularity and is therefore less likely to heal following trauma. The critical zone of the supraspinatus tendon is a common location for rotator cuff tears. Most cuff tears, however, begin distal to this at the bone/tendon interface on the greater tuberosity.

The glenoid labrum is a fibrocartilaginous ring that surrounds the periphery of the bony glenoid of the scapula. It serves as an attachment site for the capsule and broadens the base of the glenohumeral joint to allow increased stability. Tears or detachments of the glenoid labrum most commonly occur from, and result in, dislocations or instability of the humerus.

ROTATOR CUFF

The etiology of rotator cuff disease has for decades thought to be due to impingement, or wear and tear on the cuff due to entrapment from the acromion and AC joint osteophytes. Coracoacromial arch decompression was one of the most common procedures for shoulder pain whereby the coracoacromial ligament was cut, the anterolateral portion of the acromion was removed, and AC joint osteophytes were resected. More recently coracoacromial arch decompression has largely been abandoned, with most shoulder specialists agreeing that impingement is not a true entity, and that intrinsic degeneration is the most likely source of most rotator cuff problems. Treating intrinsic degeneration requires debriding the abnormal tissue and repairing the cuff.

The rotator cuff is best seen on oblique coronal images that are aligned parallel to the supraspinatus muscle (Fig. 63.2) and on the oblique sagittal images (Fig. 63.3). Both T1- (or proton density) and T2-weighted sequences are typically performed, although little diagnostic information is present on the T1-weighted images and they are not obtained by many radiologists. Multiple acceptable variations of imaging sequences are available to demonstrate the normal and abnormal structures that can be seen. A fat-suppressed fast spin-echo T2-weighted oblique coronal sequence is gaining popularity as the primary sequence for imaging the rotator cuff in many imaging centers. The slice thickness should be no greater than 5 mm, and 3 mm is preferable. As with most joint imaging, a small field of view (16 to 20 cm) is recommended. A dedicated shoulder coil or a surface coil placed anteriorly over the shoulder is necessary.

When a joint effusion is present, the intra-articular structures, such as the labrum, biceps, and articular surface of the cuff, are more easily evaluated. Therefore, many feel an MR following an arthrogram is superior to a non-arthrogram MR. An MR arthrogram is typically performed by injecting 10 to 15 mL of a saline/gadolinium mixture and then obtaining T1-weighted sequences with fat suppression, in addition to T2-weighted sequences, in multiple planes. This can be a time-consuming examination; hence, some centers have begun injecting 10 to 15 mL of saline for joint distension and omitting the gadolinium. This means the fat-suppressed T1-weighted sequences can be eliminated, which saves considerable imaging time. High-quality T2-weighted sequences with fat suppression are very close to the quality of images obtained with T1-weighting (they suffer minimally from a decreased signal-to-noise ratio).

In examining the rotator cuff, the most anterior oblique coronal images will show the supraspinatus tendon. A useful landmark for noting the anterior portion of the supraspinatus tendon is the bicipital groove, with the anterior most fibers of the supraspinatus found immediately posterolateral to the groove. This is where most cuff tears begin and can be overlooked if the patient's shoulder is internally rotated, which is common (Fig. 63.4).

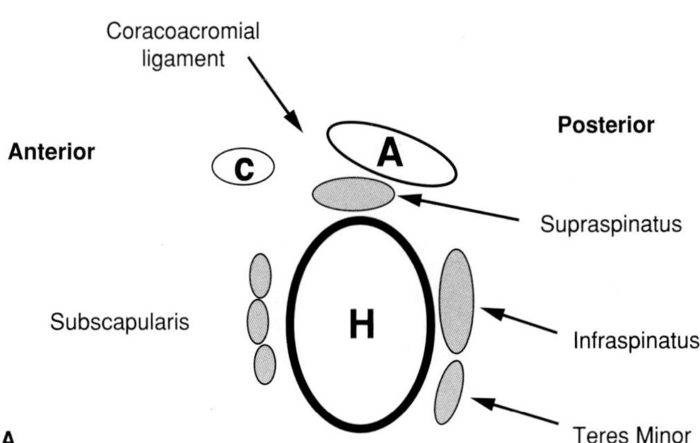

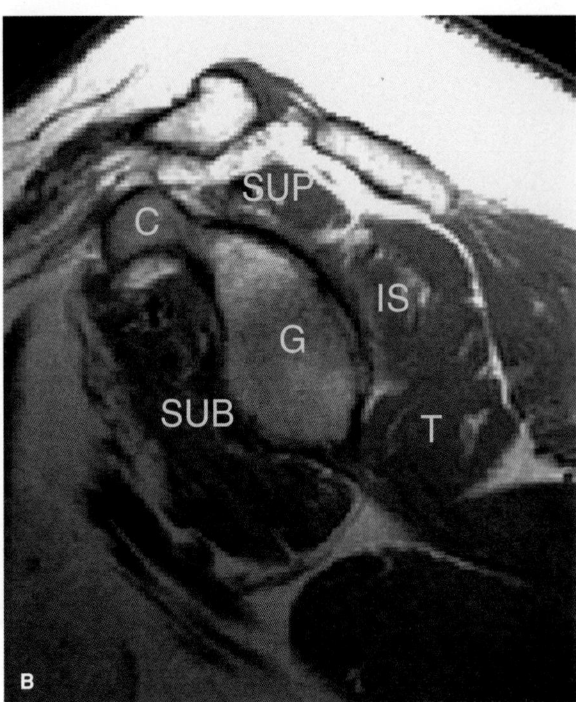

FIGURE 63.1. **Normal Shoulder Anatomy. A:** This drawing shows the rotator cuff muscles in a sagittal plane (anterior is on the left). *C*, coracoid; *A*, acromion; *H*, humeral head. **B:** This sagittal T1-weighted image through the glenoid shows the normal cuff musculature (*SUB*, subscapularis; *SUP*, supraspinatus; *IS*, infraspinatus; *T*, teres minor; *C*, coracoid process; *G*, glenoid).

The normal supraspinatus tendon is said to be uniformly low in signal on all pulse sequences. Unfortunately, this is not always the case. In fact, it often has some intermediate to high signal in the tendon, which causes much confusion. If the signal in the tendon gets brighter on the T2-weighted images, it is

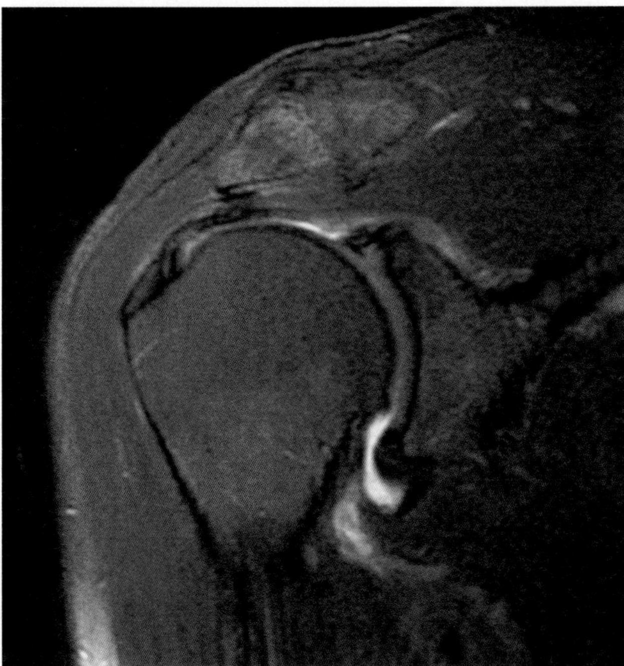

FIGURE 63.2. **Oblique Coronal Image of Normal Rotator Cuff.** This oblique coronal image fat-suppressed T2-weighted image through the supraspinatus shows a normal supraspinatus with a broad footprint where the tendon inserts onto the greater tuberosity.

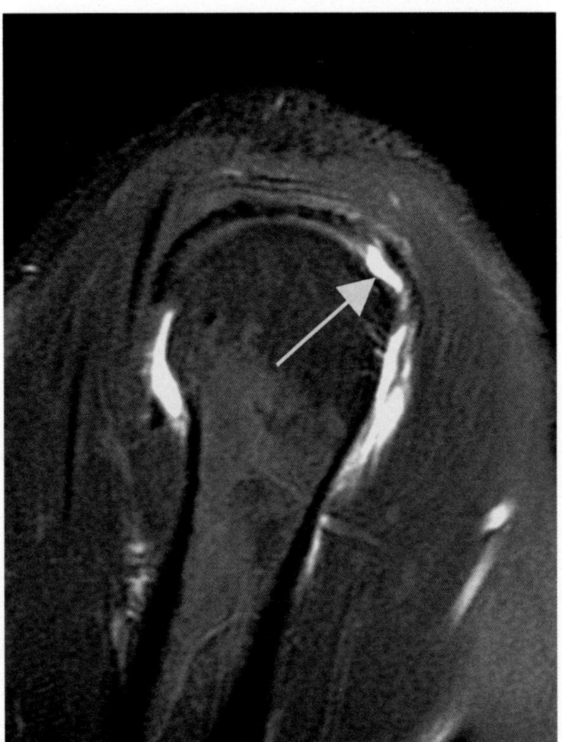

FIGURE 63.3. **Oblique Sagittal Image of a Torn Rotator Cuff.** An oblique coronal fat-suppressed T2-weighted image shows the rotator cuff inserting onto the greater tuberosity in a normal fashion except at the far anterior portion (*arrow*). This indicates a partial tear of the articular surface fibers of the cuff.

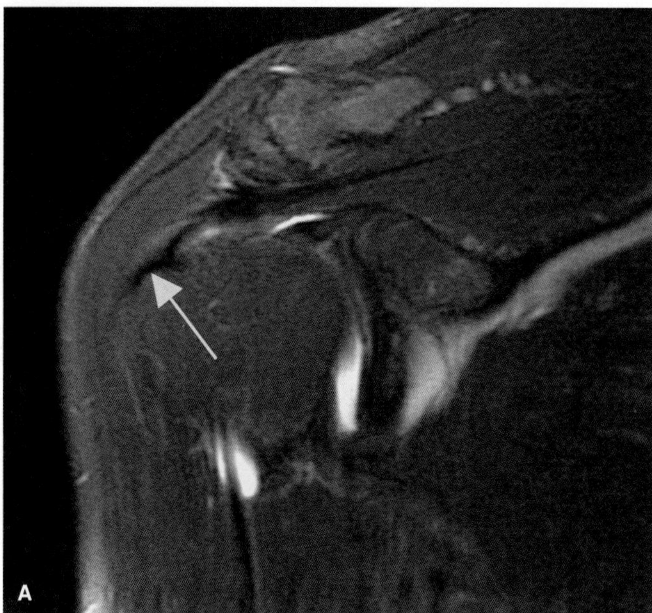

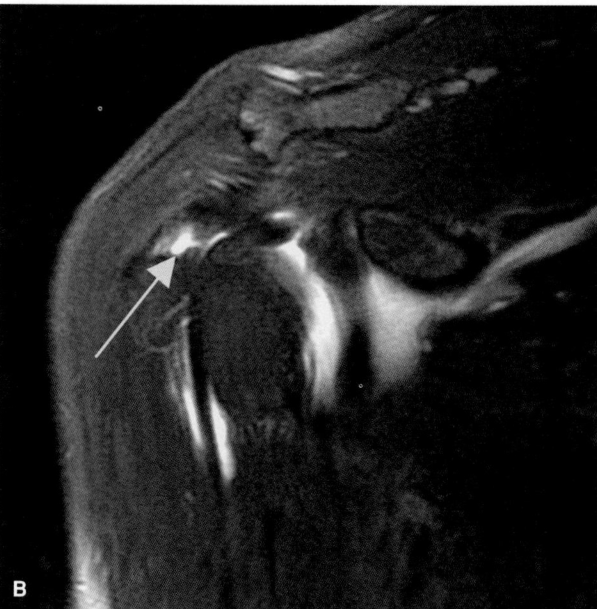

FIGURE 63.4. **Internal Rotation Hiding Partial Tear of the Supraspinatus Tendon. A:** An oblique coronal fat-suppressed T2-weighted image shows an apparent normal supraspinatus inserting onto the greater tuberosity (*arrow*). **B:** One slice more anteriorly the bicipital groove can be identified with the fibers of the supraspinatus just lateral to the groove lifted off of the greater tuberosity (*arrow*). This is a partial tear of the rotator cuff at its anterior most portion.

abnormal and represents either tendinitis (most investigators prefer the term "tendinosis" or "tendinopathy" over tendinitis, as no inflammatory cells are found histologically) or a partial-thickness tear. A partial tear can be diagnosed by noting thinning of the tendon itself (Fig. 63.5).

Myxoid and fibrillar degeneration of the supraspinatus tendon are commonly found in autopsy specimens in older patients. The majority of asymptomatic shoulders in patients over the age of 50 are believed to have some tendon degeneration in the supraspinatus; this has been termed "tendinosis." This is seen as high signal in the critical zone on T1-weighted images that does not increase with T2 weighting. Many reserve the term myxoid degeneration for those cuffs that display intermediate signal as well as some thickening (Fig. 63.6).

Myxoid degeneration is felt by many surgeons to be more significant than anatomic impingement as a source of cuff pathology. Rather than decompressing the coracoacromial arch by removing bony structures and the coracoacromial ligament, which might be sources of impingement, these surgeons resect the areas of myxoid degeneration in the cuff tendons and repair the cuff.

Tendon degeneration (tendinosis) can be seen in asymptomatic shoulders of all ages; hence, it needs to be correlated with the clinical picture. If the signal gets brighter on T2-weighted images, it must be considered pathologic—either tendinosis or a partial tear.

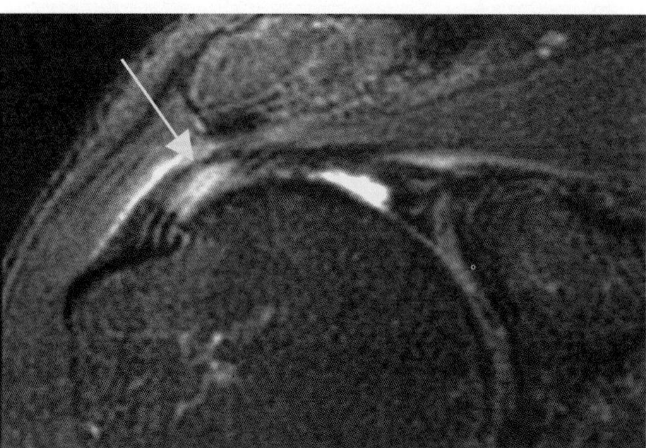

FIGURE 63.5. **Partial Cuff Tear.** An oblique coronal fat-suppressed T2-weighted image shows thinning of the supraspinatus tendon (*arrow*), which is a partial tear of the articular side of the cuff.

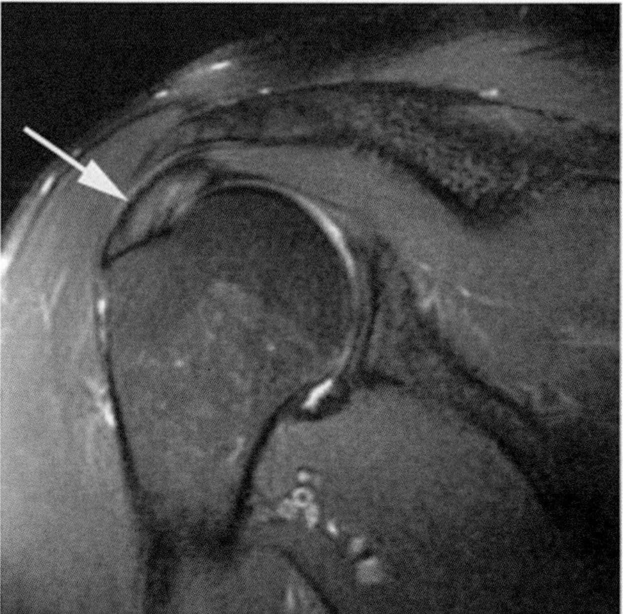

FIGURE 63.6. **Myxoid Degeneration.** An oblique coronal fat-suppressed T2-weighted image shows intermediate signal in a thickened supraspinatus tendon (*arrow*), which indicates myxoid degeneration.

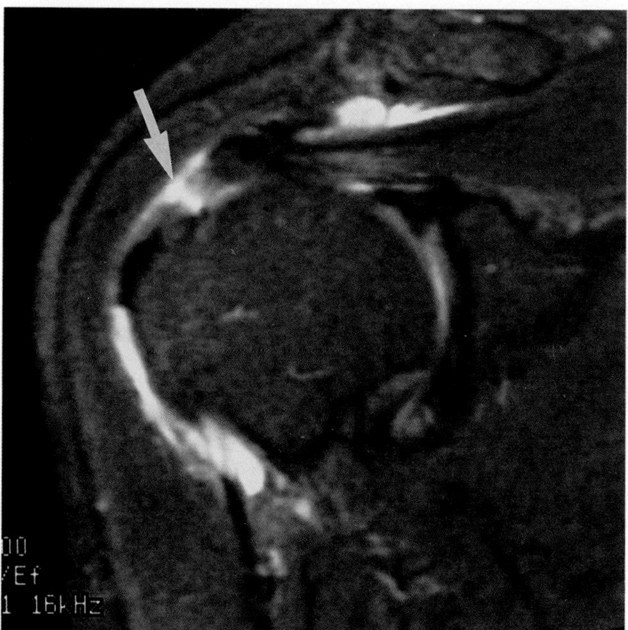

FIGURE 63.7. **Complete Tear of the Supraspinatus Tendon.** An oblique coronal fat-suppressed T2-weighted image shows disruption of the supraspinatus tendon (*arrow*) with fluid in the torn tendon.

If disruption of the supraspinatus tendon is seen, obviously, a full-thickness tear is present. In these cases, fluid is invariably present in the subacromial bursa (Fig. 63.7). It should be noted that fluid in the subacromial bursa can also occur from isolated subacromial bursitis or for several days following a therapeutic injection into the bursa. In the setting of a full-thickness tendon tear, care should be made to look for retraction of the supraspinatus muscle, as marked retraction will obviate some types of surgery.

Partial-thickness cuff tears have marked clinical significance because most agree that they will not heal on their own if they are greater than 25% of the cuff thickness. Although we generally cannot be so precise as to what percentage of the cuff is involved, we can usually identify partial cuff tears. Although partial cuff tears can involve either the bursal side of the cuff or the articular side (Figs. 63.3 and 63.5), the vast majority of partial tears occur on the articular side.

A particular type of articular-sided partial tear has been described, which is commonly seen. This has been termed a rim-rent tear (Fig. 63.8). It occurs at the insertion of the fibers of the cuff onto the greater tuberosity. It most commonly occurs anteriorly at the insertion of the supraspinatus and, as mentioned previously, can be easily overlooked if the patient's arm is internally rotated. This is the most commonly seen cuff tear on MRI.

BONY ABNORMALITIES

Abnormalities of the humeral head include sclerosis and cystic changes about the greater tuberosity, which are commonly present in patients with impingement syndrome and rotator cuff tears. Bony impaction on the posterosuperior aspect of the humeral head can be seen in patients with anterior instability of the glenohumeral joint. This is called a Hill–Sachs lesion and is best identified on the superior most two or three axial images (Fig. 63.9). A Hill–Sachs lesion almost always indicates that the anteroinferior labrum will be torn or detached (a Bankart lesion). The normal humeral head should be round on the superior slices.

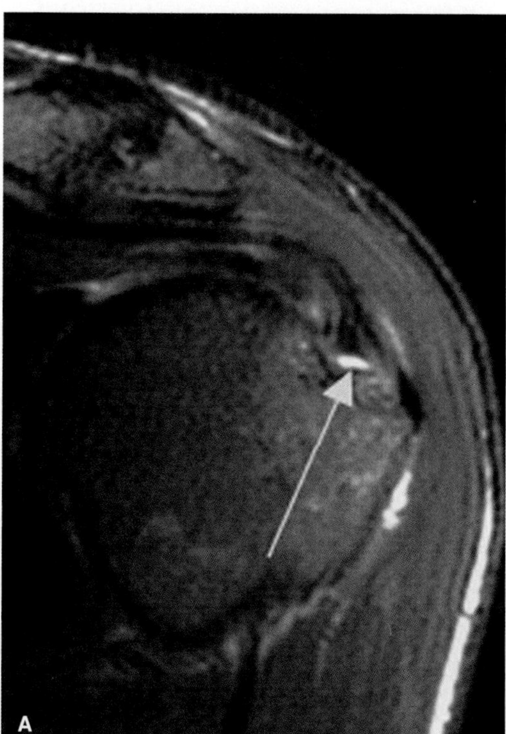

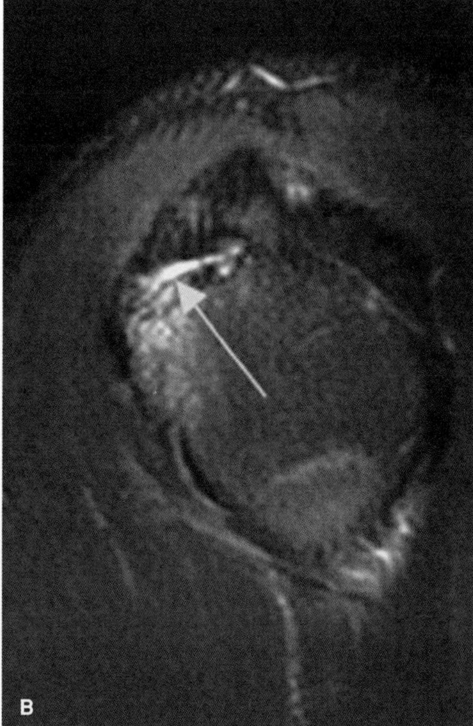

FIGURE 63.8. **Rim-Rent Tear. A:** An oblique coronal fat-suppressed T2-weighted image shows increased signal at the insertion of the supraspinatus onto the greater tuberosity (*arrow*). **B:** An oblique sagittal image shows linear high signal anteriorly between the cuff fibers and the greater tuberosity (*arrow*). This is an articular-sided partial tear called a rim-rent tear.

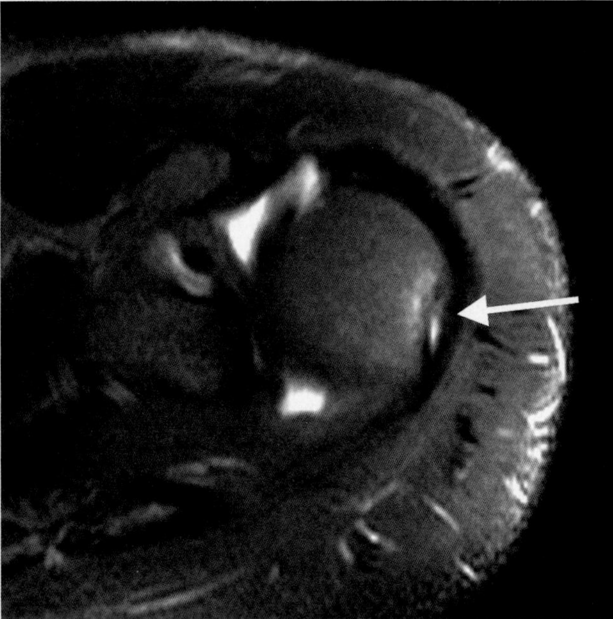

FIGURE 63.9. **Hill–Sachs Lesion.** An axial fat-suppressed T2-weighted image through the superior portion of the humeral head shows a posterior impaction (*arrow*) caused by the glenoid during an anterior dislocation of the humerus. This has been termed a Hill–Sachs lesion.

GLENOID LABRUM

Tears or detachments of the glenoid labrum cause glenohumeral joint instability. They are commonly caused by dislocations, but less traumatic episodes, such as repeated trauma from throwing, can result in labral tears. Torn or detached labra are often repaired arthroscopically with good results.

The glenoid labrum is best imaged on axial T1- or T2*-weighted sequences. T1-weighted axial images are not necessary to diagnose labral abnormalities and can be omitted from the shoulder protocol. Fluid in the joint makes for easier assessment of the labrum; hence, MR arthrography has evolved into a routine examination in many centers.

The normal labrum is a triangular-shaped low-signal structure as viewed on an axial image, with the anterior labrum usually larger than the posterior labrum (Fig. 63.10). The superior labrum is evaluated on the oblique coronal views.

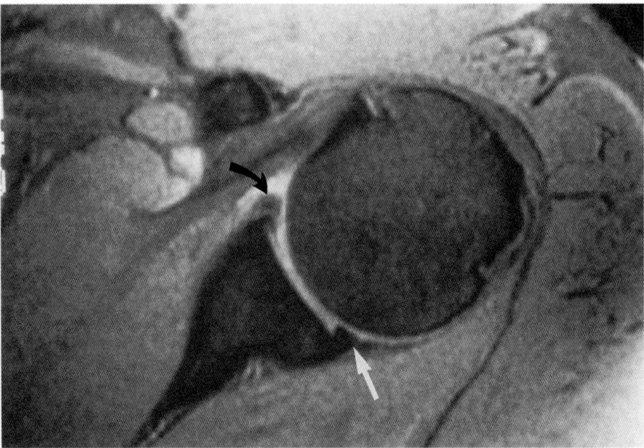

FIGURE 63.10. **Normal Labrum.** An axial T2* image shows a normal anterior (*black arrow*) and posterior (*white arrow*) glenoid labrum. The anterior labrum is usually larger than the posterior labrum.

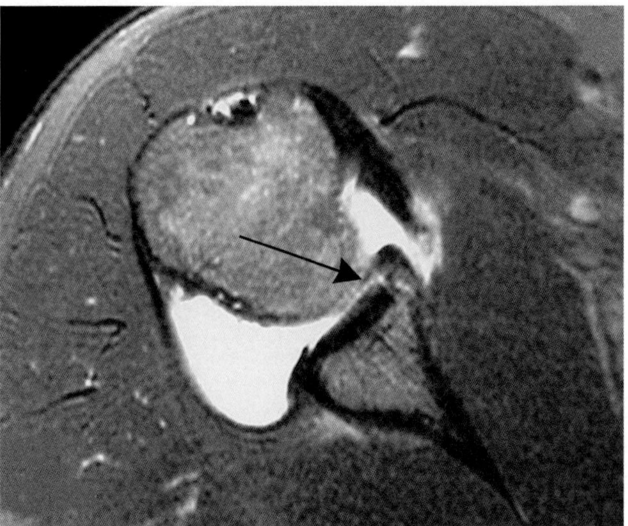

FIGURE 63.11. **Torn Labrum.** An axial fat-suppressed T2-weighted image shows a tear of the anterior labrum (*arrow*).

If no joint effusion is present, a labral tear can be difficult to see unless it is quite severe. If joint fluid extends between the bony glenoid and the base of the labrum, a detached labrum is present. Tears or detachments of the labrum are diagnosed by noting fluid extending between the labrum and the bony glenoid or by truncation of the labrum (Fig. 63.11). Superior labral tears are called Superior Labrum Anterior to Posterior (SLAP) lesions (Fig. 63.12). They are often seen in throwing athletes secondary to the pull of the long head of the biceps that inserts on the superior labrum. They are also seen in older patients in association with cuff tears.

Several normal variants in the labrum that can mimic a torn or detached labrum have been described. Two occur solely in the anterosuperior portion of the labrum, an area where tears are uncommon. The first is a sublabral foramen, which is an opening beneath the anterosuperior labrum and the bony glenoid that mimics a detachment (Fig. 63.13). This is seen in up

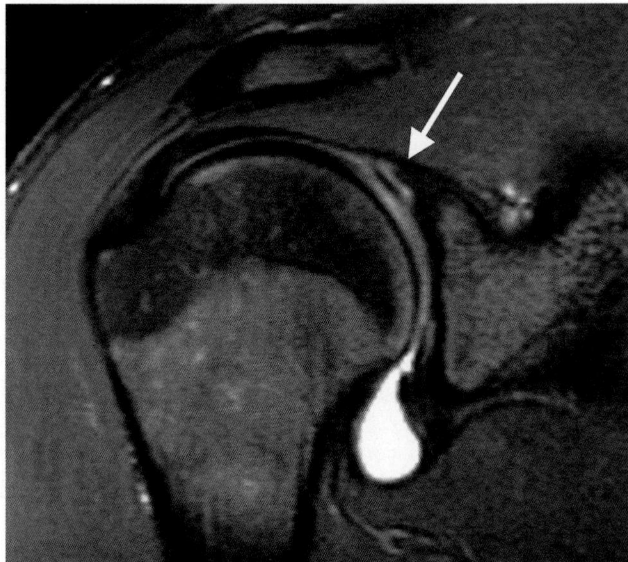

FIGURE 63.12. **Superior Labrum Anterior to Posterior (SLAP) Lesion.** An oblique coronal fat-suppressed T2-weighted image following arthrography shows a torn superior labrum (*arrow*).

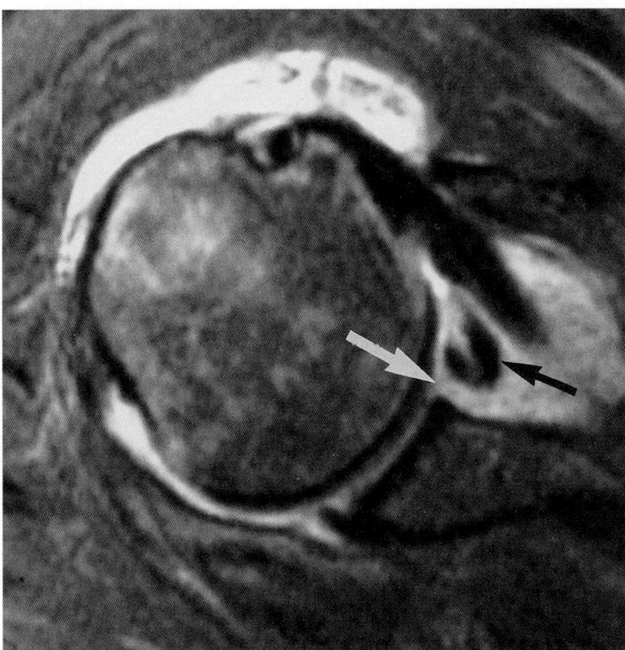

FIGURE 63.13. Sublabral Foramen. This axial fat-suppressed T2-weighted image reveals fluid between the glenoid and the anterior labrum (*white arrow*), which is the appearance of a detached labrum; however, this is a sublabral foramen that is a normal variant seen only in the anterosuperior labrum. Note the normal middle glenohumeral ligament (*black arrow*) anterior to the labrum.

to 20% of the population. A second variant is called a Buford complex. It consists of an absent anterosuperior labrum in association with a thickened "cord-like" middle glenohumeral ligament. This is seen in about 3% of the population. A sublabral recess is often seen on the oblique coronal images that can mimic a SLAP tear. It is found in up to 70% of shoulders. A sublabral recess should be seen only on the anterior part of the superior labrum and should be thin and smooth (Fig. 63.14)

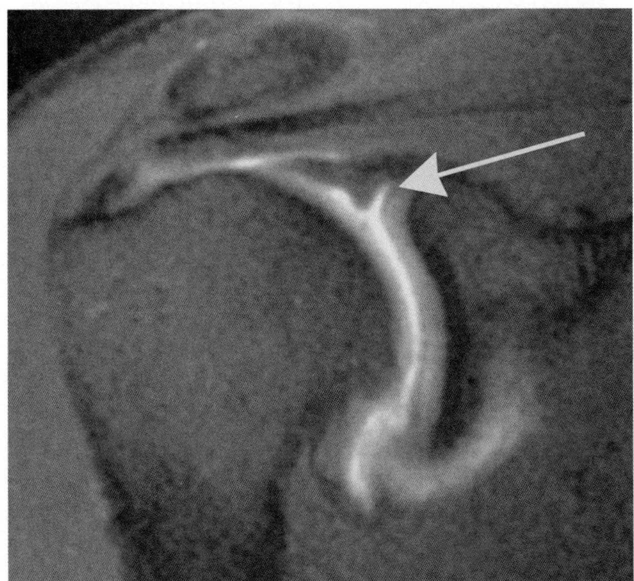

FIGURE 63.14. Sublabral Recess. An oblique coronal fat-suppressed T1-weighted image following arthrography shows fluid between the superior labrum and the cartilage of the bony glenoid (*arrow*), which is thin and smooth. This is a sublabral recess.

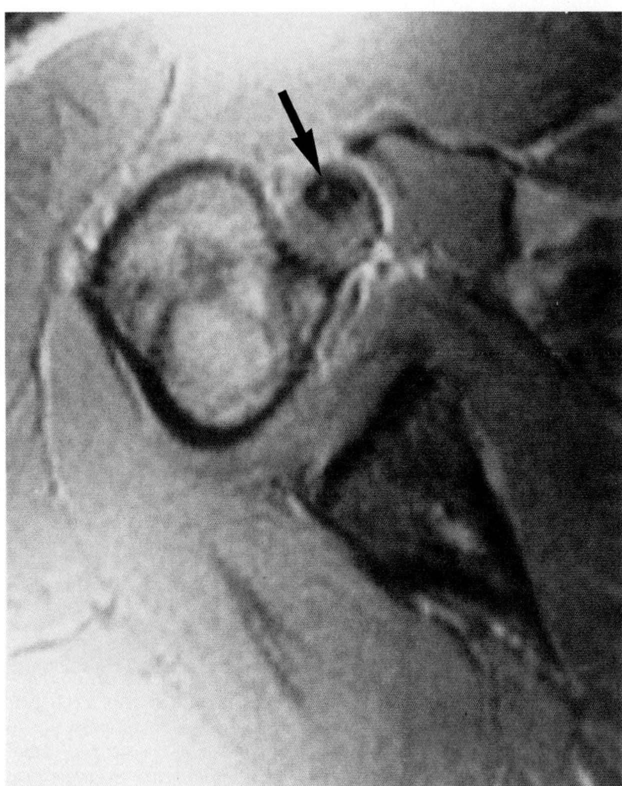

FIGURE 63.15. Biceps Tendinosis. An axial T2* GRASS image shows the biceps tendon (*arrow*) to be swollen and filled with high signal, indicating tendinosis.

and extends medially, whereas a SLAP tear is typically more irregular and extends superiorly or laterally.

BICEPS TENDON

The long head of the biceps tendon runs in the bicipital groove between the greater and the lesser tuberosities and inserts onto the superior labrum. In tenosynovitis, fluid can be seen in the tendon sheath surrounding an otherwise normal tendon. Because fluid in the glenohumeral joint can normally fill the biceps tendon sheath, this diagnosis is difficult to make with MR alone. If the tendon is enlarged and/or has signal within it, tendinosis or a partial tear is present (Fig. 63.15). If the tendon is not seen on one or more of the axial images, it is disrupted or dislocated. Dislocation is uncommon, but when it occurs, the tendon can be seen to lie anteromedial to the joint. A subscapularis tear must be present if the biceps is dislocated.

SUPRASCAPULAR NERVE ENTRAPMENT

The suprascapular nerve is made up of branches from the C4, C5, and C6 roots of the brachial plexus. It runs superior to the scapula, from anterior to posterior, just medial to the coracoid process. It gives off a branch that innervates the supraspinatus muscle as it courses posteriorly in the suprascapular notch and then innervates the infraspinatus muscle after it runs through the spinoglenoid notch in the posterior scapula. A fairly common finding is a ganglion in the spinoglenoid notch

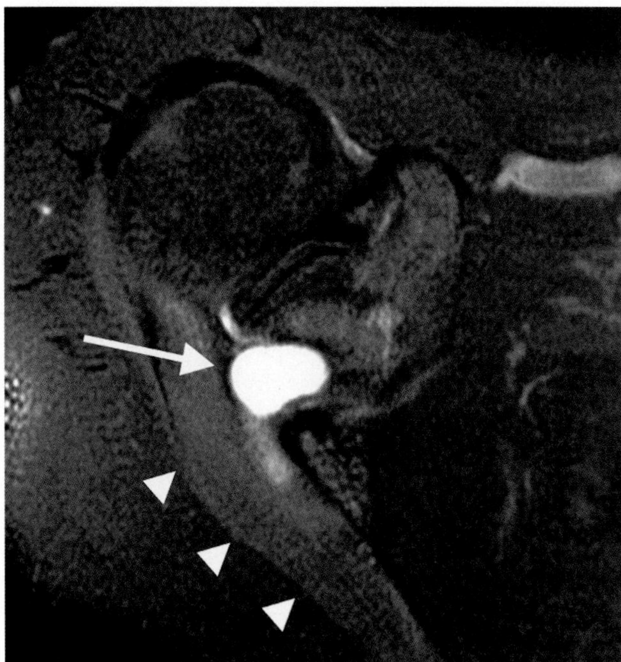

FIGURE 63.16. **Ganglion in Spinoglenoid Notch.** An axial fat-suppressed T2-weighted image reveals a high-signal mass posterior to the scapula in the spinoglenoid notch (*arrow*). This is a ganglion emanating from a tear of the posterior superior labrum that has impressed the suprascapular nerve causing edema in the infraspinatus muscle (*arrowheads*) and shoulder pain.

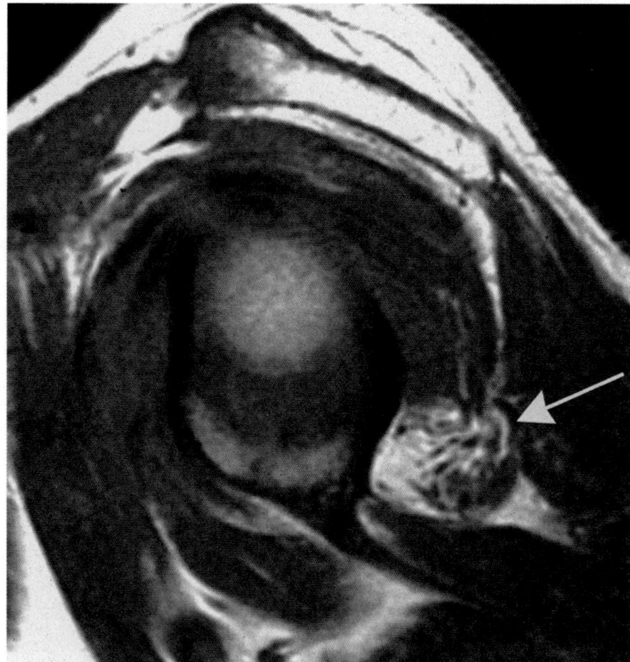

FIGURE 63.17. **Quadrilateral Space Syndrome.** This oblique sagittal T1-weighted image shows fatty atrophy of the teres minor muscle (*arrow*), which is diagnostic of quadrilateral space syndrome.

that impresses the infraspinatus portion of the nerve with resultant pain and atrophy of the infraspinatus muscle (Fig. 63.16). This syndrome is most commonly seen in males who are athletic, particularly weight lifters, and in this population is almost always associated with a tear of the superior and/or posterior labrum and the subsequent formation of a paralabral ganglion in the spinoglenoid notch. The ganglion can be percutaneously drained with CT guidance or surgically removed, however, may recur if the associated labral tear is not addressed. It can also spontaneously rupture, which results in cessation of symptoms. Clinically these patients can mimic having a rotator cuff tear; hence, MR is critical in making this diagnosis.

QUADRILATERAL SPACE SYNDROME

The oblique sagittal T1-weighted images are useful to look for fatty atrophy in any of the cuff muscles. If the infraspinatus is smaller than the other muscles and/or has fatty infiltration, the aforementioned suprascapular nerve entrapment secondary to a ganglion in the spinoglenoid notch is the likely diagnosis. If the teres minor has fatty atrophy (Fig. 63.17), the diagnosis is quadrilateral space syndrome. This most commonly occurs from fibrous bands or scar tissue in the quadrilateral space impinging on the axillary nerve. The quadrilateral space lies between the teres minor superiorly, the teres major inferiorly, the long head of the triceps medially, and the diaphysis of the humerus laterally. The axillary nerve traverses the quadrilateral space and innervates the teres minor and deltoid muscles; however, the deltoid is never involved in quadrilateral space syndrome. Quadrilateral space syndrome is found in about 1% of shoulder MR examinations. These patients present clinically similar to a rotator cuff tear, and many patients have had needless surgery for presumed cuff pathology when the real problem was quadrilateral space syndrome. Generally, no surgery is necessary as physical therapy is usually successful in breaking up the fibrous bands or scar tissues that cause this entity.

PARSONAGE–TURNER SYNDROME

The oblique sagittal fat-suppressed T2-weighted images are useful for identifying muscle edema. In about 1% of cases,

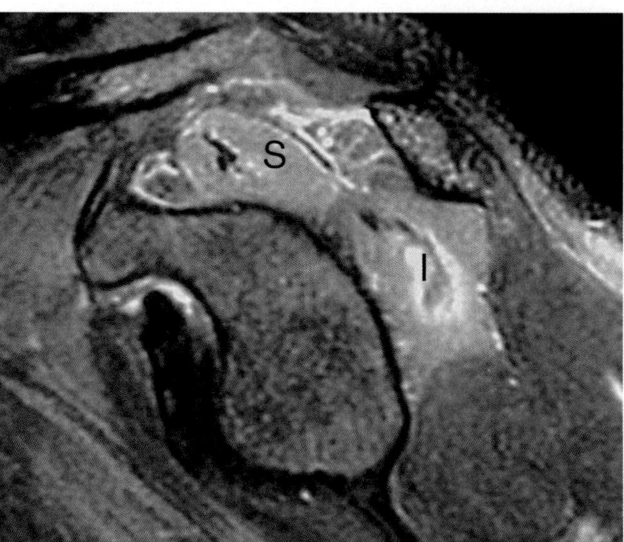

FIGURE 63.18. **Parsonage–Turner Syndrome.** An oblique sagittal fat-suppressed T2-weighted image shows edema in the supraspinatus (*S*) and the infraspinatus (*I*) muscles consistent with involvement of the suprascapular nerve. The sudden onset with no history of trauma is characteristic for Parsonage–Turner syndrome.

neurogenic edema is found in muscle groups that correspond to a particular nerve distribution (i.e., supraspinatus/infraspinatus, suprascapular nerve; teres minor/deltoid, axillary nerve). This is characteristic for Parsonage–Turner syndrome (Fig. 63.18). It is not pathognomonic because a traumatic nerve injury (such as a brachial plexus injury) could have a similar appearance. It becomes pathognomonic once the clinical presentation is provided. If there is no history of trauma, and the onset is sudden, with severe pain, followed in a day or two with profound weakness, the edema pattern is virtually pathognomonic for Parsonage–Turner syndrome.

The etiology of Parsonage–Turner syndrome is unknown, but it seems to have an association with prior vaccinations, viral illness, or general anesthesia in about one-third of cases. It is bilateral in about 10% to 15% of cases. It affects all ages of both sexes and is self-limited. It can affect either the axillary or suprascapular nerve, or both simultaneously. Unnecessary shoulder, brachial plexus, and cervical spine surgery have been performed on patients with Parsonage–Turner syndrome before the correct diagnosis was made.

Parsonage–Turner syndrome was first described in the radiology literature in 1998, indicating we all missed it on MR for over 15 years. That is because we did not routinely fat suppress our shoulder MR images until the early 1990s, and the edema in the muscles was not conspicuous enough to be picked up on non–fat-suppressed sequences.

References and Suggested Readings

Budoff JE, Nirschl RP, Guidi EJ. Débridement of partial-thickness tears of the rotator cuff without acromioplasty. Long-term follow-up and review of the literature. *J Bone Joint Surg Am* 1998;80(5):733–748.

Carroll KW, Helms CA. Magnetic resonance imaging of the shoulder: a review of potential sources of diagnostic errors. *Skeletal Radiol* 2002;31(7):373–383.

Fritz RC, Helms CA, Steinbach LS, Genant HK. Suprascapular nerve entrapment: evaluation with MR imaging. *Radiology* 1992;182(2):437–444.

Fukuda H. The management of partial-thickness tears of the rotator cuff. *J Bone Joint Surg Br* 2003;85(1):3–11.

Helms CA, Martinez S, Speer KP. Acute brachial neuritis (Parsonage–Turner syndrome): MR imaging appearance—report of three cases. *Radiology* 1998;207(1):255–259.

Helms CA, McGonegle SJ, Vinson EN, Whiteside MB. Magnetic resonance arthrography of the shoulder: accuracy of gadolinium versus saline for rotator cuff and labral pathology. *Skeletal Radiol* 2011;40(2):197–203.

Kjellin I, Ho CP, Cervilla V, et al. Alterations in the supraspinatus tendon at MR imaging: correlation with histopathologic findings in cadavers. *Radiology* 1991;181(3):837–841.

Palmer WE, Brown JH, Rosenthal DI. Rotator cuff: evaluation with fat-suppressed MR arthrography. *Radiology* 1993;188(3):683–687.

Papadonikolakis A, McKenna M, Warme W, Martin BI, Matsen FA 3rd. Published evidence relevant to the diagnosis of impingement syndrome of the shoulder. *J Bone Joint Surg Am* 2011;93(19):1827–1832.

Rafii M, Firooznia H, Sherman O, et al. Rotator cuff lesions: signal patterns at MR imaging. *Radiology* 1990;177(3):817–823.

Singson RD, Hoang T, Dan S, Friedman M. MR evaluation of rotator cuff pathology using T2-weighted fast spin-echo technique with and without fat suppression. *AJR Am J Roentgenol* 1996;166(5):1061–1065.

Vinson EN, Helms CA, Higgins LD. Rim-rent tear of the rotator cuff: a common and easily overlooked partial tear. *AJR Am J Roentgenol* 2007;189(4):943–946.

CHAPTER 64 ■ MAGNETIC RESONANCE IMAGING OF THE FOOT AND ANKLE

CLYDE A. HELMS AND EMILY N. VINSON

Magnetic resonance imaging (MRI) is playing an increasingly important role in the examination of the foot and ankle. Orthopedic surgeons and podiatrists are learning that critical diagnostic information can be obtained in no other way and are relying on MR for many therapeutic decisions.

TENDONS

One of the more common reasons to perform MR of the foot and ankle is to examine the tendons. Although multiple tendons course through the ankle, only a few are routinely affected pathologically. These are primarily the flexor tendons, located posteriorly in the ankle. The extensor tendons, located anteriorly, are rarely abnormal. Only those tendons that are more commonly seen to be abnormal will be discussed in detail.

Tendons can be directly traumatized or be injured from overuse. Either etiology can result in *tenosynovitis*, which is seen on MR as fluid in the tendon sheath with the underlying tendon appearing normal; *tendinosis*, which is seen as an increased signal within a tendon that does not get fluid-bright on T2-weighted images and represents myxoid degeneration. The tendon may or may not demonstrate focal or fusiform swelling; *a partial tear*, which has a fluid signal within the tendon on T2-weighted images or is attenuated in its diameter; and, *tendon rupture*, which is best identified on axial images by noting the absence of a tendon on one or more images. Complete tendon disruption can be difficult to see on sagittal or coronal images because of the tendency for tendons to run oblique to the plane of imaging. An exception to this is the Achilles tendon, which is usually best seen on a sagittal image.

It is important to distinguish between a partial tear and a complete disruption because surgical repair is often warranted for the latter and not for the former. Making the distinction clinically is often difficult.

Achilles Tendon

The Achilles tendon does not have a sheath associated with it; therefore, tenosynovitis does not occur. Tendinosis and partial tears are commonly seen in the Achilles tendon. Because complete disruption is such an easy clinical diagnosis, MR is usually not necessary. Complete disruption is commonly seen in athletes and in males who are approximately 40 years of age. It is also commonly associated with other systemic disorders that cause tendon weakening, such as rheumatoid arthritis, collagen vascular diseases, crystal deposition diseases, and hyperparathyroidism.

Achilles tendon disruption can be treated surgically or by placing the patient in a cast with equinus positioning (marked plantar flexion) for several months. Which treatment is superior is a controversial issue, with both methods of treatment seemingly working well. MR is being used by many surgeons to help decide if surgery should be performed. If a large gap is present (Fig. 64.1), some surgeons feel surgery should be performed for reapposition of the torn ends of the tendon; on the contrary, if the ends of the tendon are not retracted, nonsurgical treatment is preferred. No published papers have shown that this is, in fact, valid.

Posterior Tibial Tendon

The flexor tendons are easily remembered and identified by using the mnemonic "Tom, Dick, and Harry," with Tom representing the posterior tibial tendon (PTT), Dick the flexor digitorum longus tendon, and Harry the flexor hallucis longus (FHL) tendon. The PTT is the most medial and the largest, except for the Achilles, of the flexor tendons (Fig. 64.2). The PTT inserts onto the navicular, second and third cuneiforms, and the bases of the second to fourth metatarsals. As it sweeps under the foot, it provides some support for the longitudinal arch; hence, problems in the arch or plantar fascia can sometimes lead to stress on the PTT with resulting tendinitis or even rupture. Posterior tibial tendinosis and rupture are commonly encountered in patients with rheumatoid arthritis.

Differentiation of partial tears from tendon rupture can be difficult, and MR has become very valuable for making this distinction. Most surgeons will operate on a disrupted PTT; however, nonoperative therapy is usually preferred for tendinosis and partial tears.

Posterior tibial tendinosis is seen on axial T1-weighted images as swelling and/or signal within the normally low-signal tendon on one or more images (Fig. 64.3). T2-weighted images show the signal in the tendon getting brighter but not

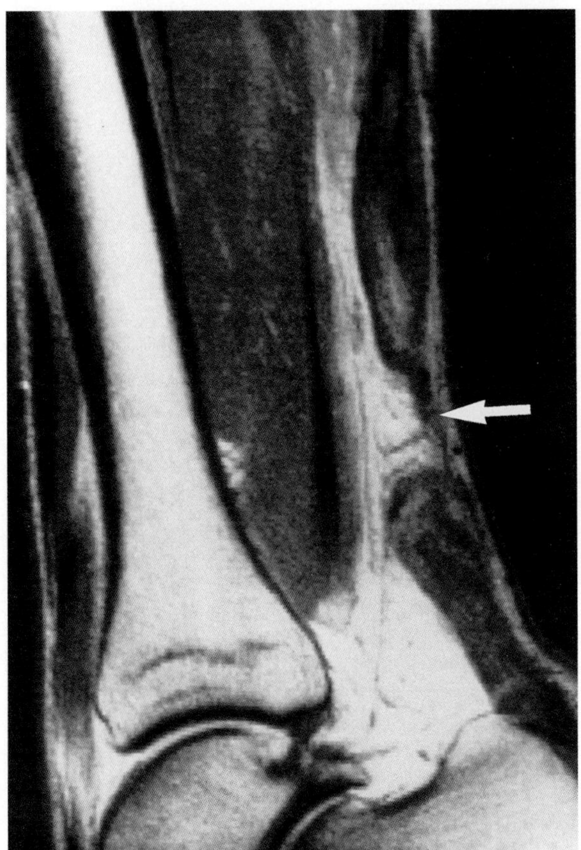

FIGURE 64.1. **Torn Achilles Tendon.** A sagittal T1-weighted image reveals the Achilles tendon to be torn with a 2-cm gap. Only a thin remnant of the tendon remains intact across the gap (*arrow*). Note the high signal in the swollen ends of the separated tendon, indicative of hemorrhage.

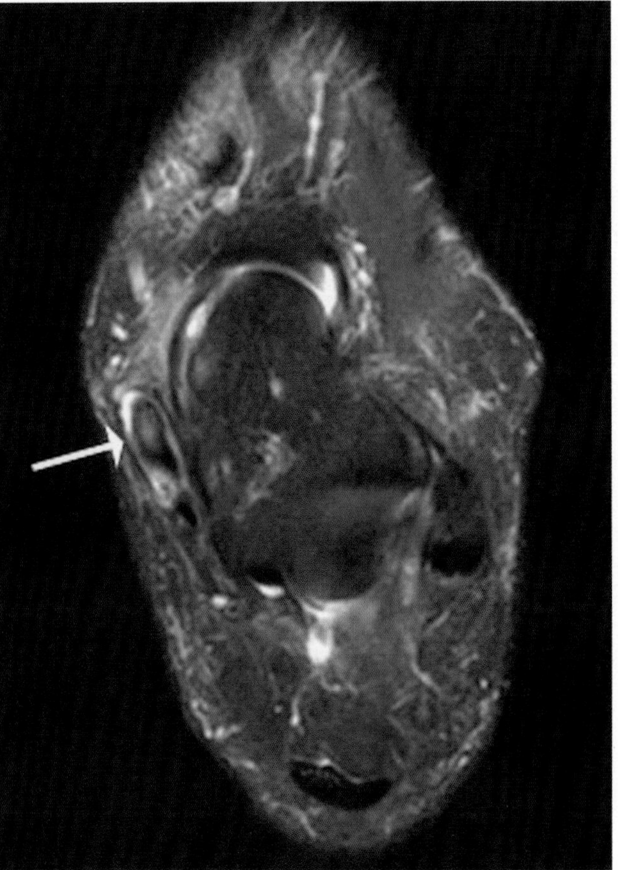

FIGURE 64.3. **Posterior Tibial Tendon Tendinosis.** An axial fat-suppressed T2-weighted image through the ankle at the level of the midcalcaneus shows the posterior tibial tendon (*arrow*) swollen and containing intermediate signal intensity. This is the appearance of tendinosis.

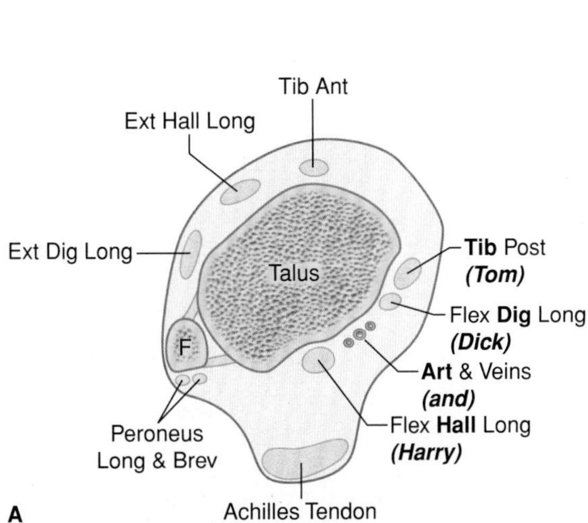

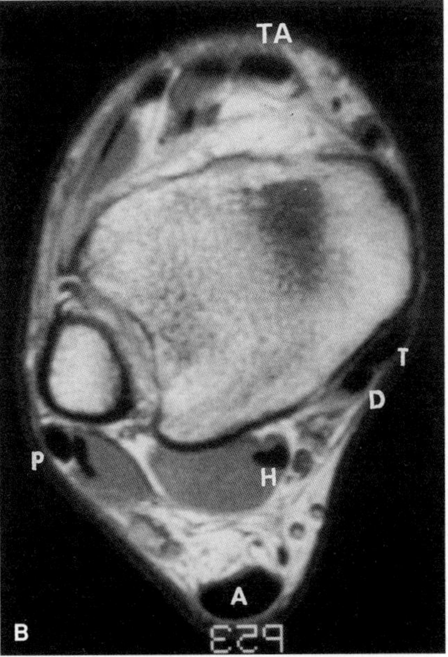

FIGURE 64.2. **Normal Ankle Anatomy. A:** This drawing of the tendons around the ankle at the level of the tibiotalar joint shows the relationship of the flexor tendons posteriorly and the extensor tendons anteriorly. **B:** An axial T1-weighted image through the ankle just above the tibiotalar joint shows the normal anatomy. *A*, Achilles tendon; *T*, posterior tibial tendon; *D*, flexor digitorum tendon; *H*, flexor hallucis tendon; *P*, peroneal tendons; *TA*, tibialis anterior tendon.

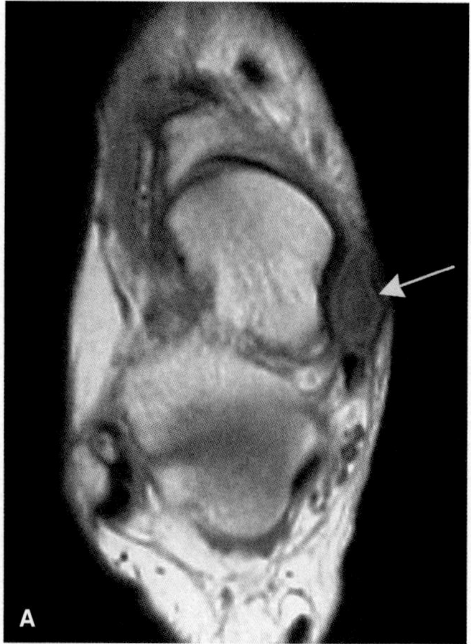

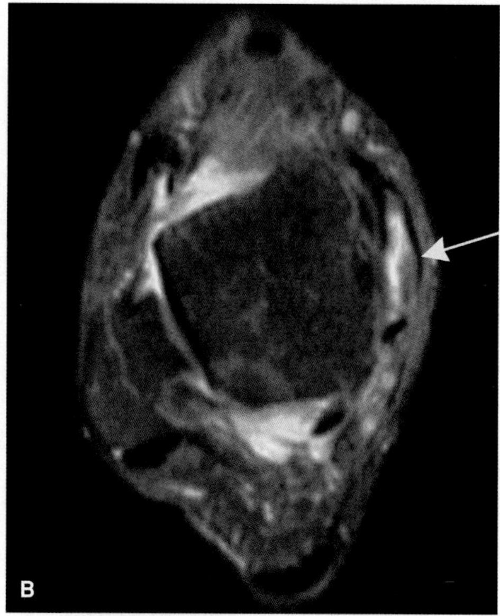

FIGURE 64.4. Torn Posterior Tibial Tendon. Axial T1- (**A**) and T2-weighted (**B**) images through the ankle in this patient with chronic pain reveal a distended posterior tibial tendon sheath (*arrows*) with no low-signal tendon identified within. This is a tear of the posterior tibial tendon.

fluid-bright. Tendon disruption is diagnosed by noting the absence of the tendon on one or more axial images (Fig. 64.4). This typically occurs just at or above the level of the tibiotalar joint.

Rupture of the PTT results clinically in a flat foot due to the loss of arch support given by this tendon. The spring ligament runs just deep to the PTT and then goes underneath the neck of the talus, which it supports in a sling-like fashion. When the PTT tears, the stress is then placed on the spring ligament to support the talus and the arch. The spring ligament has a high incidence of disruption when the PTT tears. The spring ligament is identified on axial and coronal images just deep to the PTT. When it is stressed, it typically gets scarred and thickened (Fig. 64.5). A tear can be diagnosed by noting a gap in the ligament.

After the PTT and the spring ligament tear, the next structures to fail are the subtalar joint ligaments in the sinus tarsi. In a report of 20 patients with PTT tears, it was found that 92% of the cases had abnormal spring ligaments (thickened or torn), and 75% had an abnormal sinus tarsi. It is clear these structures are linked, and injury or stress to one can affect the others.

Flexor Hallucis Longus Tendon

The FHL tendon is easily identified near the tibiotalar joint because it is usually the only tendon at that distal level that has muscle still attached. In the foot, the FHL can be seen beneath the sustentaculum tali, which it uses as a pulley to plantar flex the foot.

The FHL is known as the Achilles tendon of the foot in ballet dancers because of the extreme flexion positions they employ. Ballet dancers often will have tenosynovitis of the FHL, seen on MR as fluid in the sheath surrounding the tendon. Care must be taken to have clinical correlation because fluid can be seen in the FHL tendon sheath from a joint effusion, because the FHL tendon sheath communicates with the tibiotalar joint in as many as 20% of normal patients. Rupture of the FHL is rare.

Peroneal Tendons

The peroneus longus and the peroneus brevis tendons can be seen posterior to the distal fibula, to which they are bound by a thin fibrous structure, the superior peroneal retinaculum.

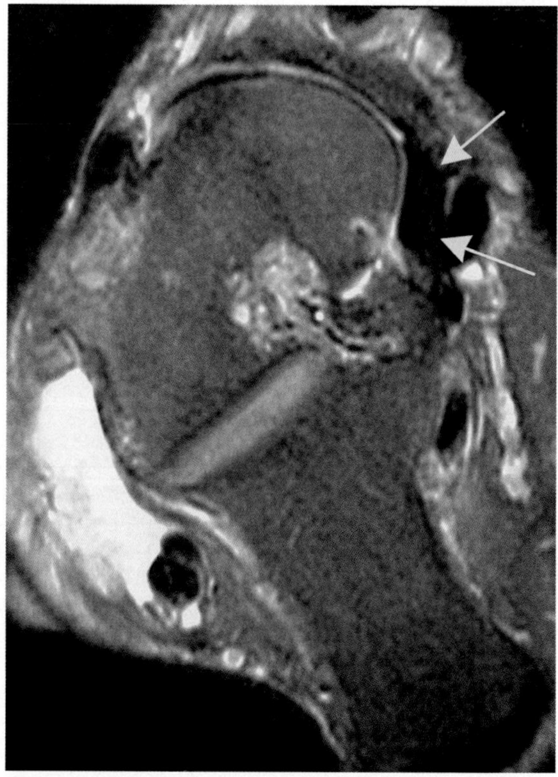

FIGURE 64.5. Abnormal Spring Ligament. An axial T2-weighted image through the ankle shows a thickened spring ligament (*arrows*) just deep to the posterior tibial tendon.

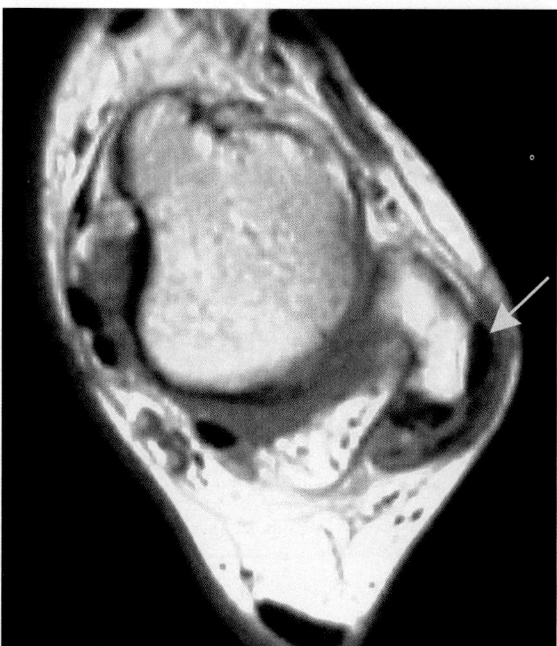

FIGURE 64.6. **Dislocated Peroneus Longus Tendon.** An axial T1-weighted image in this rock climber who injured his ankle in a fall shows a low-signal rounded structure (*arrow*) lateral to the lateral malleolus. This is a dislocated peroneus longus tendon.

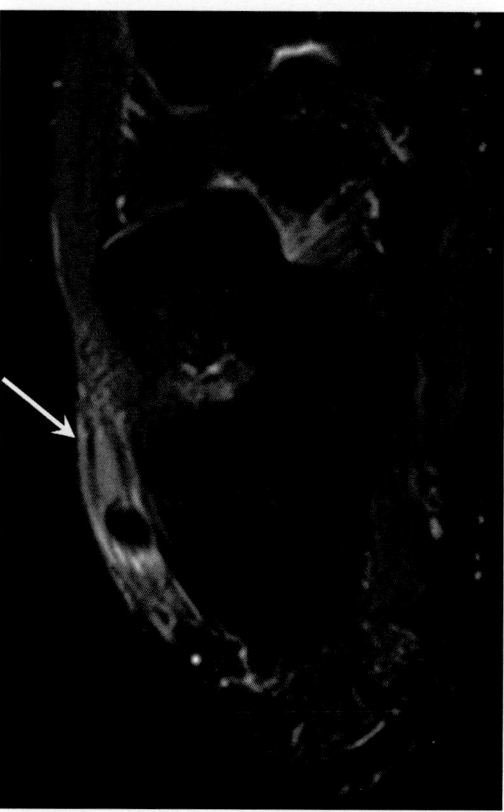

FIGURE 64.7. **Longitudinal Split Tear of the Peroneus Brevis.** This axial fat-suppressed T2-weighted image shows the peroneus brevis (*arrow*) with a "V" or chevron shape with fluid separating the two limbs, which is characteristic for a longitudinal split tear of the brevis.

The fibula serves as a pulley for the tendons to work as the principal evertor of the foot. The tendons course close together adjacent to the lateral aspect of the calcaneus until a few centimeters below the lateral malleolus where they separate, with the peroneus brevis tendon inserting onto the base of the fifth metatarsal and the peroneus longus tendon crossing under the foot to the base of the first metatarsal.

Disruption of the superior peroneal retinaculum, often seen in skiing accidents, can result in lateral displacement of the peroneus tendons (Fig. 64.6) and must be surgically corrected. It sometimes occurs with a small bony avulsion, called a flake fracture, off the fibula.

Entrapment of the peroneal tendons in a fractured calcaneus or fibula can occur and is easily diagnosed with MR or CT. This can be a difficult diagnosis to make clinically. Complete disruption of the peroneal tendons is uncommon but is easily noted with MR.

Longitudinal split tears of the peroneus brevis are commonly seen in patients following an inversion ankle sprain with associated dorsiflexion. The peroneus brevis gets trapped against the fibula by the peroneus longus and a longitudinal split tear of the peroneus brevis results. These patients have chronic lateral ankle pain, often associated with ankle instability due to the lateral collateral ligament disruption that also occurs with the inversion trauma. A split tear of the peroneus brevis is easily identified on MRI by noting either a chevron or "V" shape to the tendon distal to the fibula (Fig. 64.7), or noting a division of the tendon into two parts. There is an 80% association with lateral ligament tears, and therefore, close attention should be paid to the ligaments when a split tear of the peroneus brevis is found.

AVASCULAR NECROSIS

Avascular necrosis commonly occurs in the foot and ankle. The talar dome is the second most common location of an osteochondral lesion (OCL, formerly called osteochondritis dissecans—the knee is the most common site). MR is useful in identifying and staging an OCL. Even when not apparent on radiographs, MR can show an OCL as a focal area of low signal in the subarticular portion of the talar dome on T1-weighted images. On T2-weighted images, if high signal is seen surrounding the dissecans fragment in the bone at the bed of the fragment or throughout the fragment (Fig. 64.8), the fragment is most likely unstable. This seems to be more valid in adults than in adolescents for the knee, and this is likely true in the talus. If the fragment has become displaced and lies in the joint as a loose body, MR can sometimes be useful to localize it; however, loose bodies in any joint can be exceedingly difficult to find.

Diffuse low signal throughout a tarsal bone on T1- and T2-weighted images is typical for avascular necrosis. If the signal is increased on T2-weighted images, it may or may not be reversible. This process occasionally occurs in the tarsal navicular bone (Fig. 64.9). MR can be useful in making this diagnosis when radiographs are normal or equivocal.

TUMORS

A few tumors have a predilection for the foot and ankle. Up to 16% of synovial sarcomas occur in the foot. Desmoid tumors are commonly seen in the foot. Giant cell tumors of tendon sheath are often found in the tendon sheaths of the foot and ankle (Fig. 64.10). They are characterized by marked low signal in the synovial lining and in the tendons on T1- and T2-weighted images, just as pigmented villonodular synovitis appears in a joint.

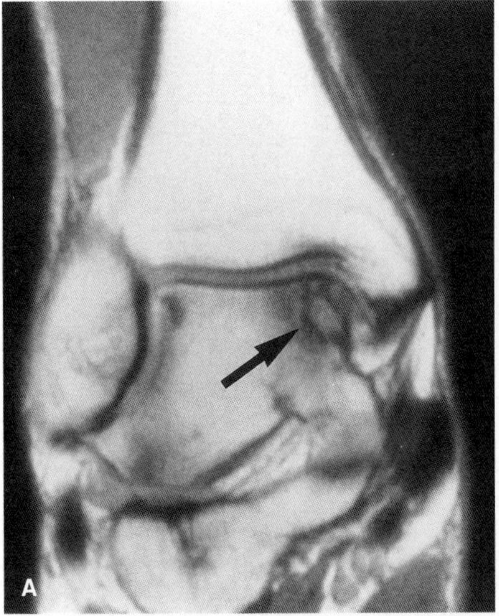

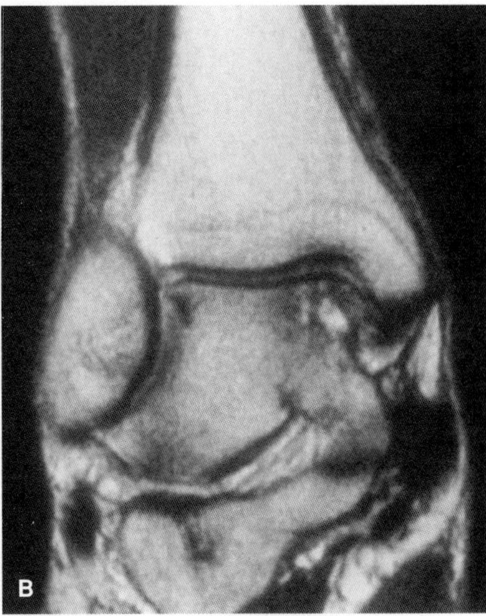

FIGURE 64.8. **Unstable Osteochondritis Dissecans of the Talus. A:** Coronal proton density image through the talus shows a focus of low signal in the medial subarticular part of the talus (*arrow*). This is a characteristic appearance for osteochondritis dissecans. **B:** A T2-weighted image shows high signal throughout the focus of osteochondritis dissecans, which indicates an unstable fragment.

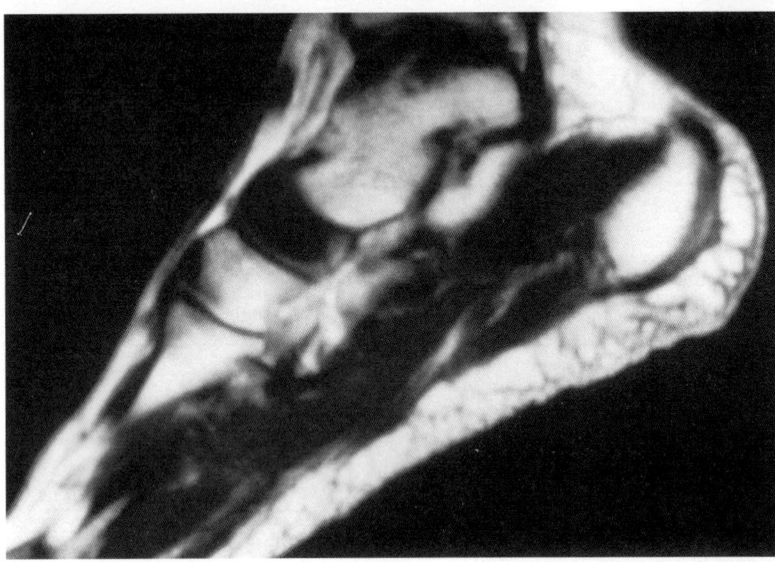

FIGURE 64.9. **Avascular Necrosis of the Tarsal Navicular.** A T1-weighted sagittal image of the ankle in this patient with pain on the dorsum of the foot shows diffuse low signal throughout the tarsal navicular. This is a characteristic appearance for avascular necrosis and will often precede any radiographic findings.

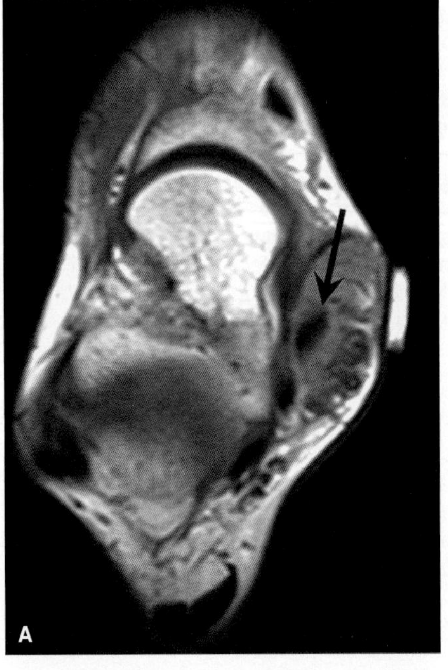

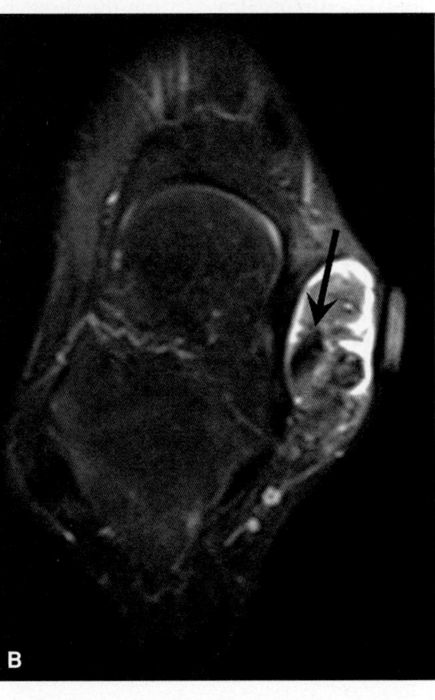

FIGURE 64.10. **Giant Cell Tumor of Tendon Sheath.** Axial T1- (**A**) and T2-weighted (**B**) images reveal a mass surrounding the posterior tibial tendon (*arrows*), which is confined by the tendon sheath. Although high-signal fluid is present, low-signal material is also present within and lining the distended tendon sheath. This low signal is hemosiderin, which is typically found in a giant cell tendon of tendon sheath. Pigmented villonodular synovitis in a joint has an identical appearance.

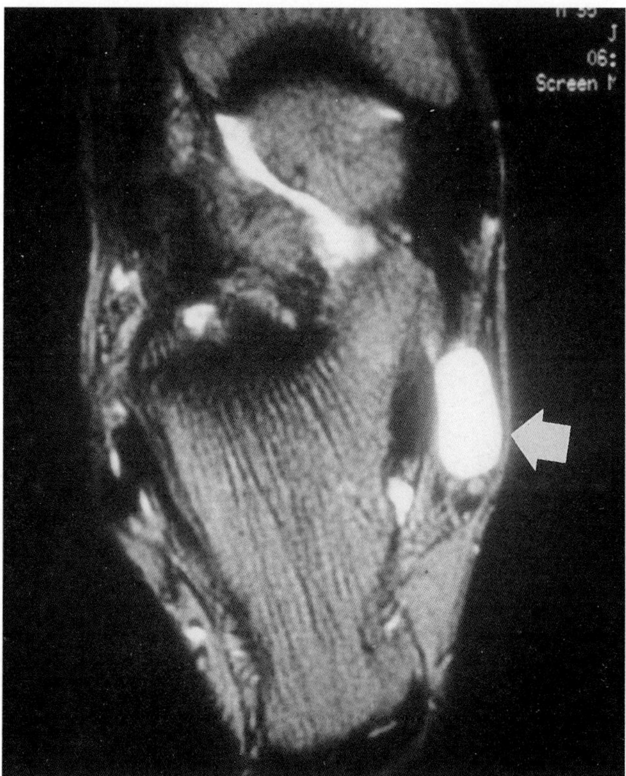

FIGURE 64.11. Ganglion-Causing Tarsal Tunnel Syndrome. A fat-suppressed T2-weighted axial image of the ankle in a patient complaining of pain and paresthesia on the plantar aspect of the foot shows a homogeneous high-signal mass (*arrow*) lying adjacent to the flexor hallucis longus tendon. This is the position of tarsal tunnel that contains the tibial nerve that can be impinged by a mass, such as in this case, resulting in tarsal tunnel syndrome. This was a ganglion.

The differential diagnosis for calcaneal tumors is similar to that of the epiphyses—giant cell tumor, chondroblastoma, and infection—with a unicameral bone cyst added. While that differential diagnosis works over 95% of the time in the epiphyses, it may be less than 50% inclusive in the calcaneus, but it is a good starting point.

Soft tissue tumors in the medial aspect of the foot and ankle can press on the posterior tibial nerve, resulting in tarsal tunnel syndrome. Clinically, patients with tarsal tunnel syndrome present with pain and paresthesia in the plantar aspect of the foot. In the aforementioned mnemonic, "Tom, Dick, and Harry," the "and" is for artery, nerve, and vein; the nerve referred to is the posterior tibial nerve. The nerve is easily compressed in the tarsal tunnel, which is bounded medially by the flexor retinaculum, a strong fibrous band that extends across the medial ankle joint for approximately 5 to 7 cm in a superior to inferior direction. Ganglions and neural tumors, both of which can look similar on T1- and T2-weighted images, often lie in the tarsal tunnel (Fig. 64.11) and compress the posterior tibial nerve, resulting in pain and paresthesia on the plantar aspect of the foot extending into the toes. Tarsal tunnel syndrome often occurs secondary to trauma or fibrosis or it can occur idiopathically. Regardless, this syndrome may not respond to surgical intervention; hence, MR is valuable in delineating a treatable lesion in many cases.

Anomalous muscles in the foot or the ankle are reported to be present in up to 6% of the population. These can be mistaken for a tumor, and biopsy may be performed unnecessarily. MR will show these "tumors" to have imaging characteristics identical to normal muscle (Fig. 64.12) and to be sharply circumscribed. Accessory soleus and peroneus brevis muscles are the most common accessory muscles encountered around the foot and ankle.

LIGAMENTS

MR is not the best way to diagnose acute ankle ligament abnormalities. The clinical evaluation is usually straightforward and no diagnostic imaging of any type is necessary. Nevertheless, in clinically equivocal cases or when the examination is ordered for other reasons, the ligaments can be clearly evaluated with high-quality MR in most instances.

The deltoid ligament lies medially as a broad band beneath the tendons. Although often seen on coronal images deep to the PTT, it has a variable anatomic appearance. Injury to the deltoid ligament accounts for only 5% to 10% of ankle ligament sprains.

The lateral ligaments are injured in over 90% of ankle sprains. The lateral complex is made up of two parts: a superior group, the anterior and the posterior tibiofibular ligaments that make up part of the syndesmosis (Fig. 64.13), and

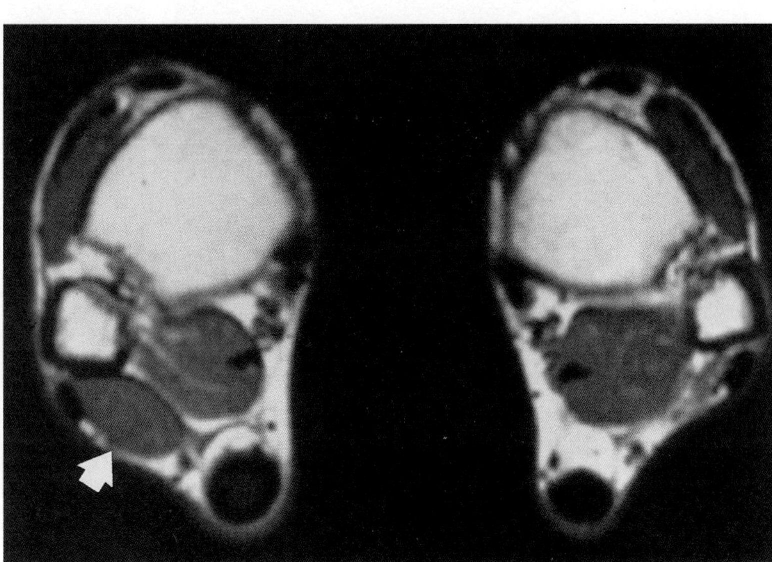

FIGURE 64.12. Anomalous Muscle. An axial T1-weighted image of both ankles in this patient complaining of a mass in the right ankle shows an anomalous muscle (*arrow*) lateral to the flexor hallucis longus muscle that is responsible for the mass the patient feels. This is a peroneus quartus muscle.

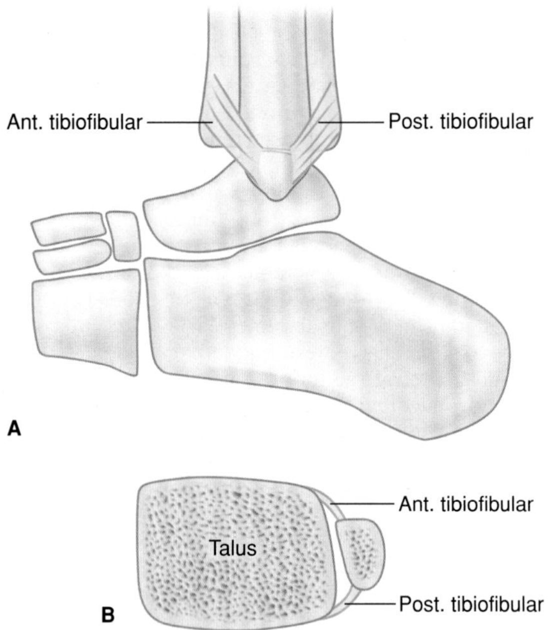

FIGURE 64.13. **Schematic of Lateral Collateral Ligaments. A:** This drawing of the ankle in a lateral view shows how the anterior and the posterior tibiofibular (*tib-fib*) ligaments extend off the fibula and course superiorly to the tibia. **B:** A drawing in the axial plane shows that the fibula has a flat or convex surface at the origin of these ligaments.

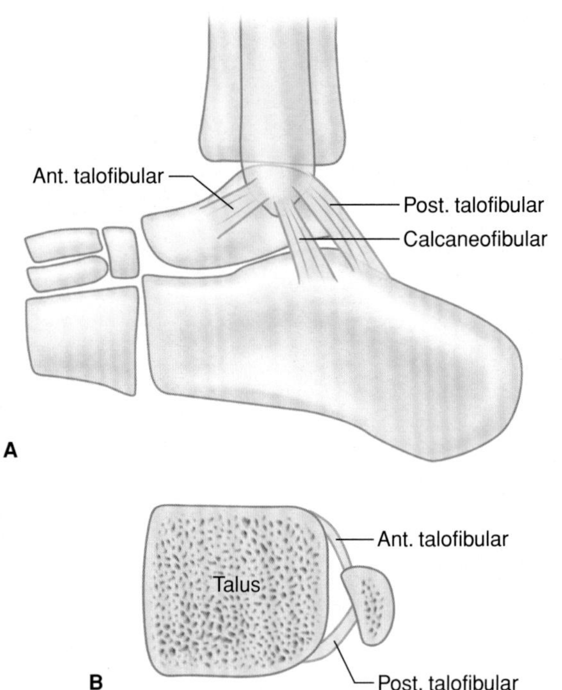

FIGURE 64.14. **Schematic of Lateral Collateral Ligaments. A:** This drawing of the ankle in a lateral view shows how the anterior and the posterior talofibular ligaments, and the calcaneofibular ligament extend off the fibula and course inferiorly. These ligaments arise off of the fibula more distally than the anterior and the posterior tibiofibular ligaments. **B:** A drawing in the axial plane shows that the anterior and the posterior talofibular ligaments arise from the level of the distal fibula, which has a concave medial surface, the malleolar fossa.

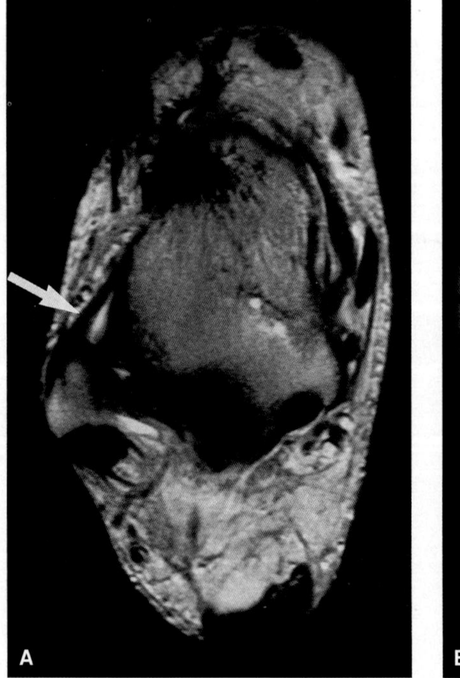

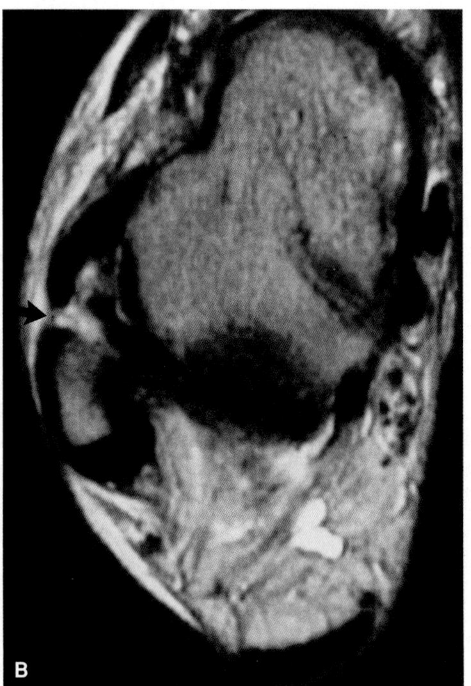

FIGURE 64.15. **Anterior Talofibular Ligament. A:** An axial T2-weighted image through the distal fibula at the level of the malleolar fossa (the concave medial surface of the fibula) shows an intact anterior talofibular ligament (*arrow*) that makes up part of the joint capsule at this level. Note the high-signal joint fluid adjacent to the ligament. **B:** This axial T2-weighted image at the level of the malleolar fossa reveals a thickened anterior talofibular ligament that has a disruption (*arrow*). The marked thickening of the ligament indicates a chronic process.

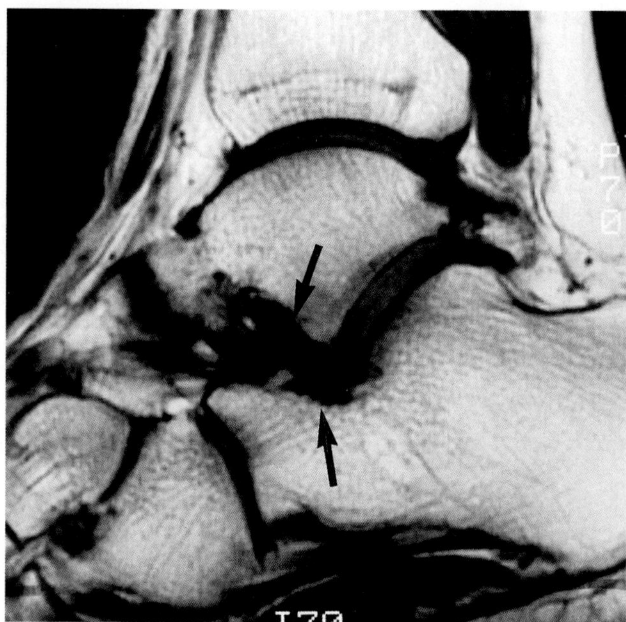

FIGURE 64.16. **Sinus Tarsi Syndrome.** A sagittal T1-weighted image in a patient with chronic lateral ankle pain shows absence of the normal fat in the sinus tarsi (*arrows*). This is virtually diagnostic of sinus tarsi syndrome except in the setting of an acute ankle sprain.

an inferior group, the anterior and the posterior talofibular ligaments and the calcaneofibular ligament (Fig. 64.14). The anterior and the posterior tibiofibular ligaments can be seen on axial images at or slightly below the tibiotalar joint. The anterior and the posterior talofibular ligaments are seen on the axial images just below the tibiotalar joint and emanate from a concavity in the distal fibula called the malleolar fossa (Fig. 64.14B). The most commonly torn ankle ligament is the anterior talofibular ligament. It is easily identified when a joint effusion is present because it makes up the anterior capsule of the joint (Fig. 64.15). The anterior talofibular ligament is usually torn without other ligaments being involved; however, if the injury is severe enough, the next ligament to tear is the calcaneofibular ligament. Even with very severe trauma, the posterior talofibular ligament will rarely tear.

Several entities have a high association with chronic tears of the lateral ligaments. These include chronic lateral ankle instability, sinus tarsi syndrome, split tears of the peroneus brevis, and anterolateral impingement syndrome.

Patients with sinus tarsi syndrome present with lateral ankle pain and tenderness and a perception of hindfoot instability. The sinus tarsi is the cone-shaped space between the talus and the calcaneus that opens up laterally. It is a fat-filled space through which traverse several important ligaments that provide subtalar stability. In sinus tarsi syndrome, these ligaments are torn and the fat is replaced with granulation tissue or scar tissue. Hence, on T2-weighted images, there may be high (granulation tissue) or low (scar) signal, but on T1-weighted images, there is low signal in the sinus tarsi (Fig. 64.16). In the acutely sprained ankle, the sinus tarsi may have replacement of the fat due to hemorrhage and edema, which will, in most cases, resolve.

Anterolateral impingement syndrome results from hypertrophy and scarring of the synovium in the lateral gutter of the ankle. The lateral gutter is the space between the tibia and the fibula and is bound by the lateral ankle ligaments. Patients with anterolateral impingement syndrome present with lateral ankle pain and inability to dorsiflex normally. They often

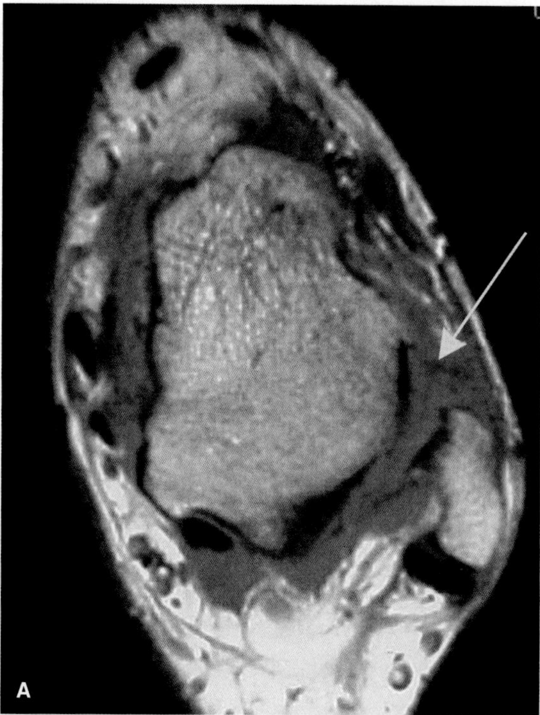

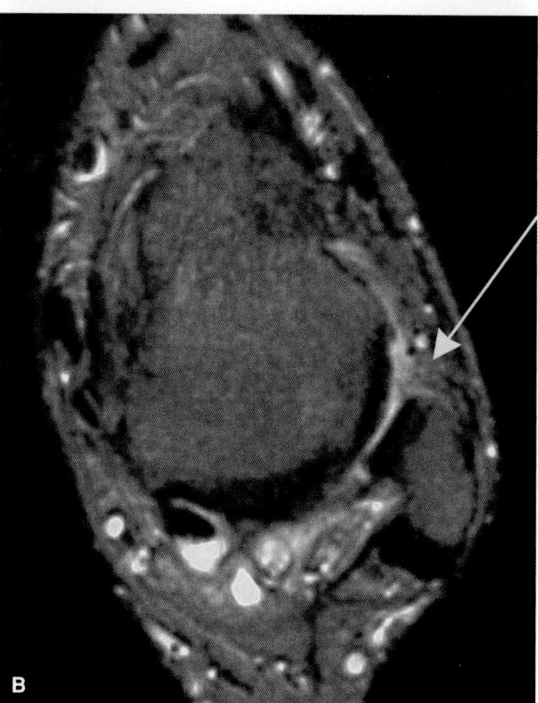

FIGURE 64.17. **Anterolateral Impingement Syndrome.** This axial T1-weighted image through the ankle (**A**) reveals absence of the anterior talofibular ligament (*arrow*). The corresponding T2-weighted image (**B**) shows low-signal scar tissue deep to the expected location of the anterior talofibular ligament (*arrow*), which indicates anterolateral impingement syndrome.

have a click on dorsiflexion. Arthroscopic resection of the scar tissue has been reported with good results. MR images show low-signal tissue in the lateral gutter on T1- and T2-weighted images (Fig. 64.17). The anterior talofibular ligament is commonly torn or fibrosed in this condition.

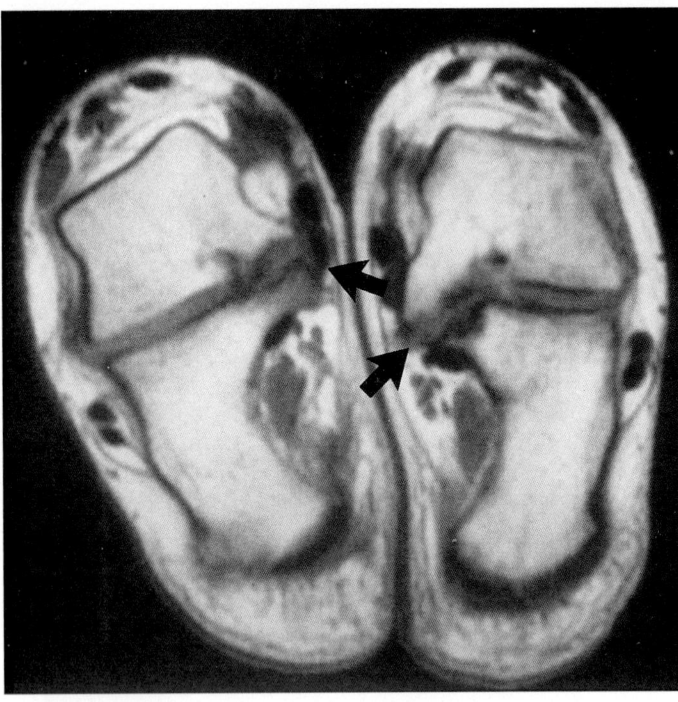

FIGURE 64.18. **Tarsal Coalition.** An axial T1-weighted image in a patient with painful flat feet shows bilateral talocalcaneal coalition (*arrows*), which is primarily fibrous. The normal joint space is irregular and widened bilaterally. In cases of suspected coalition, both ankles should be imaged as coalition often occurs bilaterally.

BONY ABNORMALITIES

Tarsal coalition is a common cause of a painful flat foot. It occurs most commonly at the calcaneonavicular joint and the middle facet of the talocalcaneal joint (Fig. 64.18). Up to 80% of patients with tarsal coalition have bilateral coalition. It can be difficult (or impossible) to see the coalition on radiographs; however, CT and MR will show bony coalition with a high degree of accuracy. The coalition is most commonly fibrous or cartilaginous. In these cases, secondary findings, such as joint space irregularity at the affected joint or degenerative joint disease at nearby joints that are subjected to accentuated stress, can be seen.

Fractures of the foot and ankle are usually well documented with radiographs. Stress fractures, however, can be difficult to radiographically or clinically diagnose, and they can mimic more sinister abnormalities. MR will show stress fractures as linear low signal on T1-weighted images with high-signal intensity edema on T2-weighted images (Fig. 64.19).

MR has had mixed reviews when used for diagnosing osteomyelitis in the foot. In diabetic patients with foot infections, diagnosing osteomyelitis is important because the treatment is often much more aggressive—including amputation—than if the bone is not involved. If the marrow appears normal, MR is highly accurate in predicting no osteomyelitis; however, if low-signal intensity is present in the marrow around a joint on

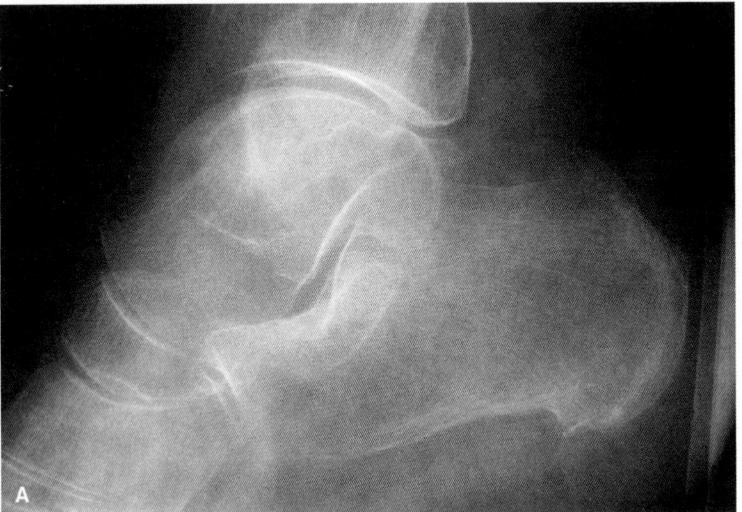

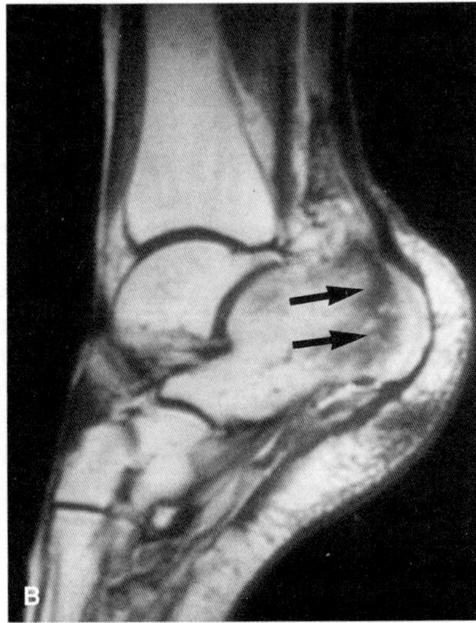

FIGURE 64.19. **Calcaneal Stress Fracture.** A 70-year-old patient with a prior history of lung cancer presented with heel pain and a normal radiograph (**A**). A bone scan showed diffuse increased radionuclide uptake throughout the posterior calcaneus. A sagittal T1-weighted image (**B**) revealed a linear area of low signal (*arrows*), which is characteristic for a stress fracture. Metastatic disease would not have this appearance.

T1-weighted images, osteomyelitis may or may not be present. Marrow signal abnormality can be caused by edema or hyperemia without infection. The only definitive MR findings for osteomyelitis are cortical disruption, a bony abscess (not a common finding), or a sinus track (an even less common finding). MR is therefore very sensitive but not very specific in diagnosing osteomyelitis in the foot and ankle.

References and Suggested Readings

Anzilotti K Jr, Schweitzer ME, Hecht P, Wapner K, Kahn M, Ross M. Effect of foot and ankle MR imaging on clinical decision making. *Radiology* 1996;201:515–517.

Balen PF, Helms CA. Association of posterior tibial tendon injury with spring ligament injury, sinus tarsi abnormality, and plantar fasciitis on MR imaging. *AJR Am J Roentgenol* 2001;176:1137–1143.

Erdman W, Tamburro F, Jayson HT, Weatherall PT, Ferry KB, Peshock RM. Osteomyelitis: characteristics and pitfalls of diagnosis with MR imaging. *Radiology* 1991;180:533–539.

Erickson SJ, Quinn SF, Kneeland JB, et al. MR imaging of the tarsal tunnel and related spaces: normal and abnormal findings with anatomic correlation. *AJR Am J Roentgenol* 1990;155:323–328.

Erickson SJ, Smith JW, Ruiz ME, et al. MR imaging of the lateral collateral ligament of the ankle. *AJR Am J Roentgenol* 1991;156:131–136.

Keigley BA, Haggar AM, Gaba A, Ellis BI, Froelich JW, Wu KK. Primary tumors of the foot: MR imaging. *Radiology* 1989;171:755–759.

Kijowski R, Blankenbaker DG, Shinki K, Fine JP, Graf BK, De Smet AA. Juvenile versus adult osteochondritis dissecans of the knee: appropriate MR imaging criteria for instability. *Radiology* 2008;248:571–578.

Oden RR. Tendon injuries about the ankle resulting from skiing. *Clin Orthop Relat Res* 1987;216:63–69.

Quinn SF, Murray WT, Clark RA, Cochran CF. Achilles tendon: MR imaging at 1.5 T. *Radiology* 1987;164:767–770.

Rosenberg ZS, Cheung Y, Jahss MH, Noto AM, Norman A, Leeds NE. Rupture of posterior tibial tendon: CT and MR imaging with surgical correlation. *Radiology* 1988;169:229–235.

SECTION XI

PEDIATRIC RADIOLOGY

SECTION EDITORS: Andrew T. Trout and Alan S. Brody

CHAPTER 65 ■ IMAGING CHILDREN—WHAT YOU NEED TO KNOW

ANDREW T. TROUT AND ALAN S. BRODY

Don't skip this section. It would be easy to do so, as it's an introductory chapter, there are no images, and your radiology faculty probably won't ask you about this stuff in conference or at the workstation. This chapter is key though—we are sharing pearls and clearing up misconceptions that will make you a better radiologist, a better doctor, and might help you answer one of those dreaded medical questions that come up at parties. So please, read on . . . it will be worth it.

WORKING WITH CHILDREN IN THE RADIOLOGY DEPARTMENT

You can't just use radiology techniques and equipment designed for adults and expect to get good images of children. Children are small, move more, and cooperate less than adults. In addition, working with children usually means working with parents as well. Parents are often more concerned and more demanding about their children's care than they are about their own. This includes concerns about radiation exposure and anything that might be done, or administered, to their children.

Positive interactions with children require a special set of skills. In many ways, however, techniques that work well with children work well with anyone, and so these skills and techniques will be applicable to most of what you do in radiology. The hospital can be a frightening place for anyone (child or adult). Calm, quiet, and simple directions and explanations will go far to decrease fear and improve cooperation. Once children begin talking, they can understand much of what is said to them. Children as young as 2 years old can follow simple directions. Children should be addressed directly, rather than through their parents or caretakers. Kneeling to provide a face-to-face position, using simple words, and explaining honestly what to expect can dramatically improve cooperation. Begin every encounter by introducing yourself and briefly describing your role. Be clear about what you plan to do, and describe things in simple terms. Do not give options that aren't real. "Are you ready for us to start?" suggests that you are willing to wait as long as needed until the child is ready. "We're going to start now." is more honest and unlikely to be misunderstood. Remember that children (and even some adults) often take things literally. Telling a child that you will "shoot a picture" suggests either a gun or a syringe, either one a good reason to be frightened and stop cooperating. In any situation where more than one person is involved, a single voice should be chosen to speak to the child.

Infants cannot follow directions but respond well to calm and quiet. Bundling/swaddling infants is a useful technique that often provides comfort and reduces agitation (for both the child and the parent[s]). Plus, learning to swaddle is a skill that will serve you well outside of radiology, if you have to care for children. Feeding a baby will almost always result in a child ready for sleep. If the baby doesn't need to be NPO for the procedure, this can calm the child and get them to lie still. A recently fed infant, swaddled and warm can even make it through an MRI (with hearing protection, or course).

For any young child, painful procedures such as IV placement should be completed well before imaging, if possible. The best approach to a painful procedure depends on the child. Some want to be told everything, others don't want the details and just want to get the procedure done. While keeping the child involved, interacting with the family is an important part of providing the best experience. Parents can be very helpful in tasks such as holding and feeding their child. Parents are often good guides to what will and what won't work with their child.

Child life practitioners are increasingly being employed in pediatric centers. Child life practitioners have a background in child development and behavior and can help children understand their imaging studies and help them cooperate and cope, sometimes reducing or eliminating the need for sedation. If you are fortunate enough to have child life practitioners in your radiology department, you already know how important their input and assistance can be.

RADIATION RISK

Concern about the risk of radiation from diagnostic imaging peaked in 2001 with the publication of a paper that calculated the long-term risk of cancer from CT scanning based on the radiation dose used for imaging at that time and from data from atomic bomb studies. Read that last sentence again and think about all of the assumptions that went into those calculations . . .

When that paper was written in 2001, it was common to use a single CT technique for patients regardless of age (or size), with the dose for young children many times the dose necessary for diagnostic image quality. This is no longer the practice in the vast majority of the American medical system. Following publication of that work and others, efforts began to reduce radiation dose for medical imaging studies. Efforts were focused on CT but expanded to all modalities employing ionizing radiation, and in many institutions, adult doses were decreased by 50% without losing diagnostic quality. In young children, doses were decreased by up to 90% in some cases.

While it was worthwhile to look at techniques and optimize them for the indication and patient being imaged, the effort had important unintended consequences. The emphasis on childhood cancer deaths generated a one-sided fear of radiation exposure and specifically of CT scanning that is still pervasive today. Parents concerned about radiation exposure began to refuse indicated CT scans, and less appropriate or less accurate modalities were often substituted, simply because they were "radiation free." Parents weren't the only ones that got caught up in radiation fear. Referring physicians became reluctant to order a CT scan even when it was the most appropriate study. Radiologists even got caught up in the emphasis on radiation dose, emphasizing, sometimes singularly, targeting radiation doses that were ALARA (As Low As Reasonably Achievable). A focus on ALARA and dose reduction had the unintended consequence of an increase in nondiagnostic CT scans due to unacceptable image noise. One study found that 6% of CT scans performed at major children's hospitals were nondiagnostic. ALARA is an outdated term that ignores both the benefit of the imaging examination and the important issue of image quality. Indeed, the medical physicist Louis K. Wagner has suggested that instead, we should think in terms of benefit/risk ratios and we should use the term AHARA (As High As Reasonably Achievable), always working toward providing the greatest benefit at the lowest risk.

What's the point of talking about this here? The point is: risks should always be placed in context. In the case of imaging modalities, that context needs to include risk of cancer (which is to the general population, rather than the individual patient), the benefit that comes from the knowledge obtained from the imaging study, efficacy of potential alternatives, and increasingly cost to the patient and society. Importantly, the decision to perform a CT scan or other diagnostic study using ionizing radiation is a choice with an extremely small or, possibly, no risk. Contrast this with the sporadic risk of cancer to the population which is high. Over our lifetimes, each of us has a risk of 40% of developing cancer. Of those cancers, 50% will be fatal; meaning each of us has a 20% risk of dying of cancer, unrelated to specific radiation exposure. One of the reasons that there remains doubt about the real risk of diagnostic imaging is that the background risk of cancer in the population is so high, and the risk of cancer attributable to diagnostic imaging is so small. It is now generally accepted that it is impossible to accurately quantify the risk of ionizing radiation in the range used for a CT scan and fivefold variations in calculated values are common. If we assume the risk is at the higher end of published estimates that equates to a 1/4,000 risk of a fatal cancer from a CT scan. This is the same as stating that CT scanning is 99.975% safe. It is hard to imagine avoiding a 99.975% safe test when there is even a small chance of a health benefit.

SEDATION AND ANESTHESIA

Young children may have difficulty lying still for longer imaging examinations (e.g., MRI or FDG-PET) and may not be able to hold their breath for the duration required to acquire some images (e.g., CT or MRI). As such, use of sedation or anesthesia is more common in the pediatric population than in the adult population and becomes an additional variable to consider in the benefit/risk calculation as it relates to imaging of the child. While sedation/anesthesia can generally be accomplished without difficulty or significant risk, particularly by dedicated pediatric practitioners, sedation events are not risk free. Typical risks include prolonged recovery time and risks of vomiting and aspiration. There is increasing data that suggest possible neurotoxic effects of anesthesia but this remains an area of uncertainty.

Sedation/anesthesia should absolutely be used when it helps acquire needed images (another case of not letting fear of small risks overwhelm potential benefit). That said, alternatives and advancements exist, and continue to be developed, that can obviate the need for sedation in some cases. For example, ultrasound (US) may be sufficient to provide an initial assessment of a soft tissue abnormality. Modern CT systems can now acquire images so fast as to freeze motion. MR sequences are being developed that can either be acquired more quickly (e.g., compressed sensing) or that can be acquired free breathing (e.g., radial/propeller sequences).

Distraction techniques can also reduce the need for sedation or anesthesia. Video goggles in MRI, DVD players in US, and tablets in fluoroscopy can all be very effective. Involvement of child life practitioners plays a significant role as well.

CONTRAST MATERIAL CONSIDERATIONS

Contrast materials are utilized in pediatric imaging for CT, MRI, fluoroscopy, and increasingly US. Contrast materials bring diagnostic value to imaging of children for many of the same reasons they do in adults. That said, the role of these agents is continually being re-evaluated as the evidence related to risks and benefits evolves. Take, for example, the growing body of data related to gadolinium deposition. While deleterious effects have yet to be demonstrated, there is a push to optimize (use in a way that balances risk and benefit rather than just blanket avoidance) utilization of gadolinium-based contrast materials in pediatric imaging, particularly given the potential long lifespan of the patient being imaged.

In all cases, it is reasonable to consider whether contrast material brings value to the imaging examination being performed. If there is anticipated value in administering contrast material, then many of the considerations that apply to adults apply to children, including:

- Risk for, treatment of and prophylaxis against, allergic-like contrast reactions
- Issues of nephrotoxicity and nephroprotection
- Risk for nephrogenic systemic fibrosis
- Etc.

If contrast material isn't anticipated to add value or might pose undo risk, then avoidance is warranted. In children, this has the potential added advantage of avoiding a painful needle stick (for intravenous contrast materials).

Most contrast materials for pediatric imaging are administered on a weight-based basis. In some cases, this means very small volumes are being administered, which means automated/power injection may not be possible and careful technique is required to adequately time imaging.

One factor somewhat unique to pediatric imaging is that patients may be less willing to consume oral contrast materials due to taste or texture. In these cases, flavorings can help mask or improve the taste of the contrast material and are used liberally in many pediatric practices. In general, flavorings cause no imaging artifacts.

MODALITY-SPECIFIC SPECIAL CONSIDERATIONS FOR PEDIATRIC IMAGING

Radiographs

While radiographs have much lower radiation doses than CT scans, many more radiographs are performed in the pediatric population and it is worth optimizing dose and image quality to maintain the highest benefit/risk ratio. Using dose charts based on the thickness of the body part to be imaged is a way to provide an appropriate image quality/dose ratio with children of different sizes.

Probably the biggest difference when it comes to obtaining radiographs in children versus adults is that different patient position and beam direction are used in order to provide the best images and to maximize detection of abnormalities. Some of those differences include:

Chest Radiographs. CXRs in young children can be performed AP in the supine position. Devices that hold the child in an upright position exist (the much maligned Pigg-O-Stat—look it up, it's worth it) but are not necessary. If inspiratory/expiratory chest radiographs are required for assessment of air trapping, these are best performed using bilateral decubitus radiographs to avoid issues related to cooperation. When evaluating young infants for pneumothorax, upright films are not necessary. Decubitus radiographs are possible in all but the sickest infants and are much easier to interpret than cross-table laterals.

Abdominal Radiographs. In infants, it is usually not possible to distinguish small and large bowel on radiographs. Bowel dilation should only be divided into proximal when there are few loops and distal when there are many. Young children in particular may have little gas intermixed with their stool, making stool-filled distal bowel difficult to distinguish from collapsed bowel.

Measuring bowel loops to determine the presence of dilation is silly—normal bowel changes caliber dramatically throughout childhood. Two-view abdominal radiographs are better performed with supine and decubitus views (vs. upright in adults). Left lateral decubitus views require less cooperation and have the benefit of increasing the amount of gas in the right lower quadrant which is helpful when appendicitis is a consideration (a common occurrence).

Musculoskeletal Radiographs. Evaluation of the musculoskeletal system requires small field-of-view images for diagnostic image quality in most cases. It is tempting to fit all of both lower extremities on a single image. This may be adequate for gross evaluations such as the presence or absence of a bone dysplasia or evaluation of limb length, but for trauma, suspected bone lesions, and especially for suspected child abuse, dedicated views of each area are essential and obtaining multiple projections (frontal and lateral) is critical for detection of abnormalities. In some cases, this means obtaining a large number of images. At least 20 separate radiographs are required for a skeletal survey for child abuse (radiation risk is not even a consideration here due to the risk to the child from missed abuse and the benefit of diagnosis.

Fluoroscopy

Fluoroscopy plays a role throughout childhood in imaging disorders of the gastrointestinal (GI) and genitourinary tracts. Of particular importance are assessment for malrotation with volvulus, fluoroscopic reduction of intussusception, and assessment for vesicoureteral reflux. Nearly all fluoroscopic studies can be achieved with the child awake, with sedation required only in exceptional cases. Key to technique is the use of pulsed, intermittent fluoroscopy and appropriate field of view to optimize radiation dose and image quality.

One key difference between adult and pediatric fluoroscopic studies is that double-contrast GI studies are rarely performed in children who either cannot tolerate the distention or may not be able to maintain the gas. This isn't really a problem, as mucosal processes are rarely in question and instead, most questions relate to plumbing (rotation, reflux) and flow.

Ultrasound

US is the workhorse of pediatric imaging. It is the first study for the initial evaluation of the abdomen, with the exception of trauma. Indications elsewhere in the body are similar to adults, with the addition of head US performed in young infants. Motion, including respiratory motion, can make ultrasound challenging, but techniques including color and spectral Doppler and elastography can be performed in children with excellent results. High-frequency, small-footprint transducers should be used in small children. Most ultrasound machines have pediatric settings that are a good starting point for many examinations. Sedation is almost never required, and distraction techniques such as showing movies are very effective. At all ages, the ultrasound technologist is probably the most important factor in obtaining high-quality images. Find a technologist who works well with children, learn from him or her, and encourage him or her to teach others.

Nuclear Medicine

The practice of pediatric nuclear medicine is highly variable between institutions in terms of the type and number of procedures performed. Basic nuclear medicine studies including diuretic renal scans (for urinary tract obstruction), hepatobiliary (e.g., HIDA) scans (for biliary atresia), and cystograms (for vesicoureteral reflux) are still the backbone of a pediatric nuclear medicine practice. 18-F FDG-PET is increasingly being used, however, for the staging and follow-up of pediatric malignancies such as lymphoma and sarcomas (bone and soft tissue). The ^{123}I-MIBG scan is an examination that is almost unique to pediatrics and is still extensively used for the diagnosis, staging, and follow-up of neuroblastoma.

Details of nuclear medicine imaging technique and protocols are beyond the scope of this text but the reader should be aware of the North American Consensus Guidelines for Pediatric Administered Radiopharmaceutical Activities which provide recommended activities for commonly used radiopharmaceuticals. This can be an invaluable resource when you are in practice and are asked to do a nuclear medicine study on a child.

MRI

MRI is a dominant imaging modality in pediatrics, in part due to the fact that images can be obtained without use of ionizing radiation. This benefit has very likely been given greater weight than it deserves, but MRI has other advantages as well, including high soft tissue contrast and the ability to acquire images with multiple types of contrast (T1 weighting, T2 weighting, diffusion weighting, etc.). MRI also has disadvantages though as it relates to imaging the child, including long examinations and the need for breath holds (thus requiring sedation/anesthesia), as well as issues with cost and availability.

The role of MRI continues to increase in pediatrics with increasing use in the emergency department and increasing availability of quantitative techniques (e.g., elastography).

Vendors are still working to optimize protocols and hardware (e.g., coils) for pediatric imaging, as systems have largely been designed for imaging adults. This is further complicated by the fact that children come in sizes from the tiny premature neonate to the obese young adult.

Rapid and motion robust sequences play a significant role in optimizing MR imaging of the child and are becoming increasingly available. Respiratory triggering and navigation can also be helpful to acquire quality images. In general, attention to keeping protocols short will facilitate the successful imaging of a child of any age (adults would probably benefit from this philosophy as well).

CT

CT technique should be optimized to image children of a variety of sizes, requiring adjustments of field of view and technique (kVp, mAs, etc.). In the era of pediatric-specific protocols, maximizing the benefit/risk ratio for CT scanning should emphasize obtaining diagnostic quality images over further reductions in radiation exposure. One mistake not to make—HRCTs should be acquired using volume acquisition in both inspiration and expiration. One millimeter every 10-mm interval scanning for high-resolution chest CT has little or no dose savings compared to a scan of the entire chest and only serves to hide portions of the lung from view.

Chest CT is particularly challenging in young children as respiratory motion (which may obscure small structures) must be balanced with the risk of sedation or anesthesia and the frequent associated occurrence of large areas of atelectasis. In the absence of dedicated pediatric practitioners who have skill in maintaining lung aeration, it is probably better to deal with motion rather than large areas of atelectasis.

Evaluation of the mediastinum and hila is made much easier with intravenous contrast. Even experienced pediatric radiologists struggle with the lack of fat in the mediastinum and the size of the hila at different ages. With the exception of CTPA and dedicated cardiac CT, routine contrast chest technique usually provides all the information needed even when evaluation of the vessels is required. Contrast timing, tenuous IVs, increased risk of motion with a rapid injection, and artifact from a dense contrast stream can all be avoided by performing chest CTA only when necessary.

Abdominopelvic CT can also be challenging as many children have very little intraperitoneal fat which makes interpreting abdominal CT more difficult. This can be exacerbated by reduced radiation doses which can further obscure subtle pathology. Intravenous contrast material is required for the vast majority of abdominopelvic CT examinations except for CTs done for renal stones. Oral contrast material can help by separating bowel from other structures but is not necessary when evaluating for appendicitis or trauma. Multiphase (e.g., arterial and portal venous phase) CTs are rarely done in children, simply due to the pathology being imaged.

Suggested Readings

Brenner D, Elliston C, Hall E, Berdon W. Estimated risks of radiation-induced fatal cancer from pediatric CT. *AJR Am J Roentgenol* 2001;176(2):289–296.

Brody AS, Guillerman RP. Don't let radiation scare trump patient care: 10 ways you can harm your patients by fear of radiation-induced cancer from diagnostic imaging. *Thorax* 2014;69(8):782–784.

Garcia Guerra G, Robertson CM, Alton GY, et al; Western Canadian Complex Pediatric Therapies Follow-up Group. Neurotoxicity of sedative and analgesia drugs in young infants with congenital heart disease: 4-year follow-up. *Paediatr Anaesth* 2014;24(3):257–265.

Goske MJ, Strauss KJ, Coombs LP, et al. Diagnostic reference ranges for pediatric abdominal CT. *Radiology* 2013;268(1):208–218.

Podberesky DJ, Angel E, Yoshizumi TT, et al. Comparison of radiation dose estimates and scan performance in pediatric high-resolution thoracic CT for volumetric 320-detector row, helical 64-detector row, and noncontiguous axial scan acquisitions. *Acad Radiol* 2013;20(9):1152–1161.

Treves ST, Gelfand MJ, Fahey FH, Parisi MT. 2016 Update of the North American Consensus Guidelines for Pediatric Administered Radiopharmaceutical Activities. *J Nucl Med* 2016;57(12):15N–18N.

Wagner LK. Should risk from medical imaging be assessed in the absence of benefit and vice versa? *Pediatr Radiol* 2014;44(Suppl 3):414–417.

CHAPTER 66 ■ PEDIATRIC NEURORADIOLOGY

USHA D. NAGARAJ, BLAISE V. JONES, AND CAMILLA E. LINDAN

INTRODUCTION

Although often treated as dramatically disparate entities, pediatric and adult neuroradiology are in fact complementary to each other. An understanding of the developing brain adds insight to the comprehension of neuropathology in the adult, just as familiarity of the response of the adult brain to insult informs and illuminates the assessment of the pediatric patient.

Many of the abnormalities encountered in adult neuroradiology are lesions that develop over time as a consequence of chronic repetitive minor insults. Because of the length of time required to develop such lesions, they are decidedly uncommon in pediatric patients. For example, degenerative disc disease is one of the most common pathologies encountered by an adult neuroradiologist, but it is extremely rare in children. Therefore, when a solitary abnormal disc is identified on radiographs in a child, it is much more likely to reflect focal infectious/inflammatory disease.

There are equally dramatic differences in the ability of the brain to respond to insults as a result of its degree of development and maturation. Accordingly identical injuries can manifest in dramatically different ways, both on physical examination and imaging, depending upon the degree of CNS maturation. An understanding of the normal pace and pattern of brain development and its varying ability to respond to insults is essential for the appropriate assessment and interpretation of findings on neuroimaging studies.

A number of pediatric pathologies are covered in detail in other chapters in this text, such as neoplasms and traumatic injuries of the brain and spine, and congenital head and neck malformations. In this chapter, we will focus on normal brain development in the fetal and neonatal period, and a variety of pathologies that are unique to pediatrics, such as congenital malformations, neonatal encephalopathy, and the phakomatoses. We will also review some spinal pathologies that are more frequently encountered in pediatrics, such as scoliosis and syringomyelia.

NORMAL DEVELOPMENT

One of the most challenging concepts in pediatric neuroimaging is establishing a foundation for what is normal, especially in the fetus and very young infant. Whether it is a fetal or infant brain MRI, knowing the postconceptual age at the time of imaging is essential, and having an atlas of normal brain development to reference can be extremely helpful in order to recognize milestones of development (Fig. 66.1). Some of these milestones are outlined in Table 66.1.

Myelination begins in the 5th fetal month and continues throughout life. The fatty structure of lipoprotein causes T1 shortening wherever myelin is deposited, but the T2 hypointensity of myelin reflects the displacement of interstitial water by the progressive thickening of the myelin sheath on axons, and thus appears later. In a normal infant myelination appears complete on conventional T1-weighted images (T1WI) by around 12 months, on T2-weighted images (T2WI) by 24 months, and on FLAIR images by 40 months of age. For this reason we rely on T1WI for myelin evaluation in the first year of life and T2WI in the second year.

In the term neonate we should see T1 hyperintense myelin in the deep cerebellar white matter, dorsal brainstem, and posterior limbs of the internal capsules (Fig. 66.2). The genu and splenium of the corpus callosum are myelinated by 6 months of age, and by 1 year of age the appearance of white matter myelination in T1 is similar to that of an adult. T2WI beyond a year of life show progressive myelination of the white matter of the cerebral hemispheres marked by T2 hypointense signal. Ill-defined symmetric FLAIR hyperintensity in the peritrigonal regions (so-called "terminal zones of myelination") reflects the greater concentration of interstitial fluid in these regions, and persists through the first several years of life.

Mild delays in sulcation and myelination can often be attributed to in-utero or perinatal stress, but more profound delays should raise concern for inborn errors of metabolism and leukodystrophies.

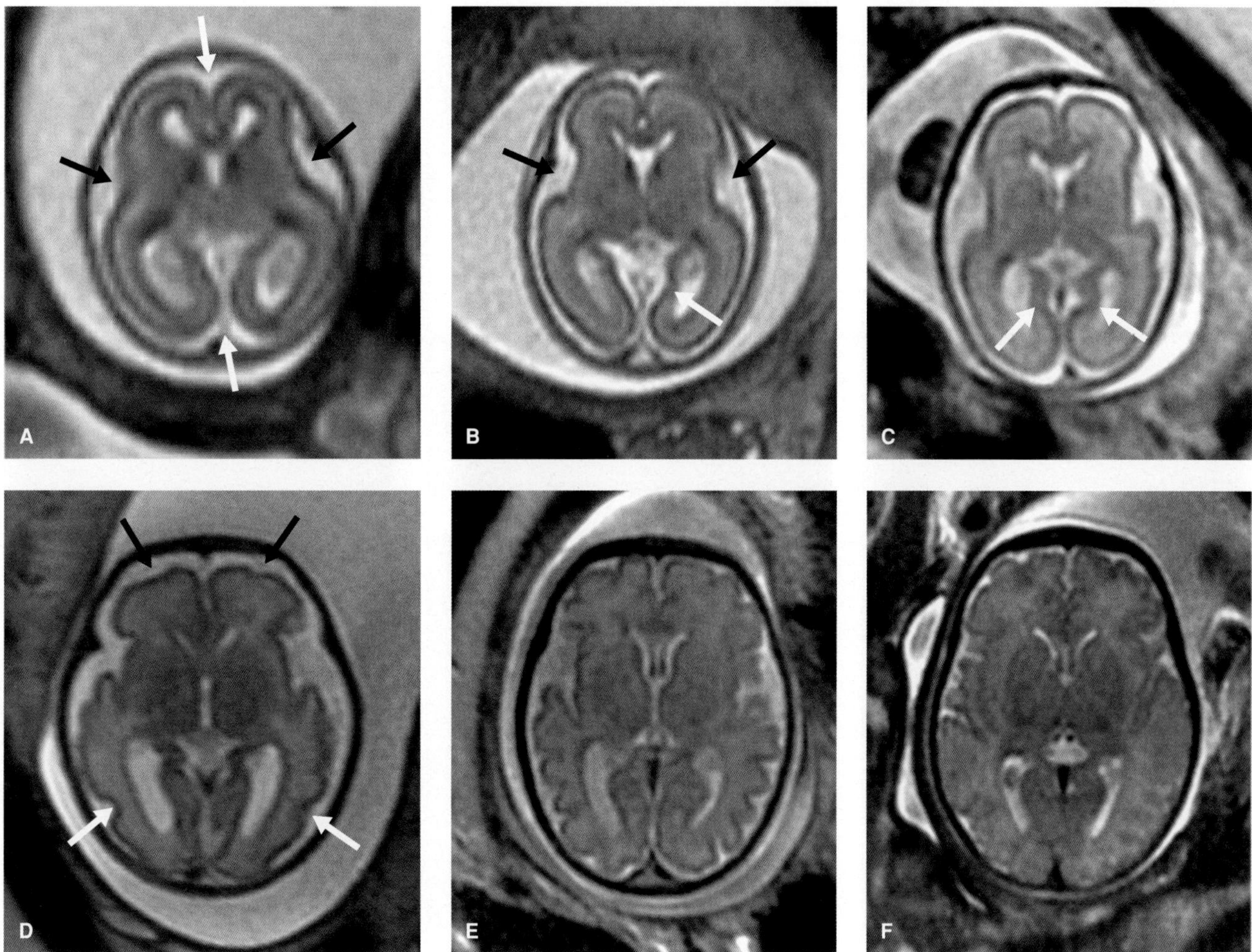

FIGURE 66.1. **Axial T2 SSFSE images through the normal fetal brain at 18 (A), 22 (B), 26 (C), 30 (D), 34 (E), and 38 (F) weeks gestational age.** At 18 weeks (**A**) we have the interhemispheric (*white arrows*) and broad sylvian fissures (*black arrows*) present. At 22 weeks (**B**) there is more operculization of the sylvian fissures (*black arrows*) and the calcarine fissures start to form (*white arrow*). By 26 weeks (**C**) the calcarine fissures (*white arrows*) are well-formed. By 30 weeks (**D**) the temporal (*white arrows*) and frontal sulci (*black arrows*) are formed or forming. By 34 weeks (**E**) all of the primary sulci have formed. By 38 weeks (**F**) the appearance is similar to a term infant brain.

TABLE 66.1

PRENATAL BRAIN DEVELOPMENTAL MILESTONES

■ GESTATIONAL AGE (WEEKS)	■ STRUCTURE VISIBILITY
16–18	Sylvian Fissure
20–22	Parieto-occipital Fissure
22–23	Calcarine fissure and Callosal sulcus
24–25	Central sulcus and Cingular sulcus
26	Precentral sulcus
27	Postcentral sulcus and superior temporal sulcus
29	Superior and inferior frontal sulci
33	Inferior temporal sulcus
34	All primary sulci and most secondary sulci

ABNORMALITIES OF MIDLINE DEVELOPMENT

While the normal neonatal corpus callosum can appear quite thin, the splenium should be at least as thick as the genu by 1 year of age. Developmental abnormalities of the corpus callosum are referred to as ***dysgenesis* of the corpus callosum**, a spectrum that ranges from complete agenesis through partial agenesis to hypoplasia of the corpus callosum. In complete agenesis of the corpus callosum, the lateral ventricles have a parallel orientation, with posterior dilation termed *colpocephaly*. The axons that would normally have crossed the midline instead line up in an anterior to posterior configuration along the medial aspect of each lateral ventricle; these tracts are called *Probst bundles*. Coronal images demonstrate upturned anterior horns of the lateral ventricles, absence of the cingulate sulcus allows the interhemispheric sulci to extend all the way to the third ventricular margin, and there is usually underrotation of the hippocampi (Fig. 66.3).

Partial agenesis or hypogenesis of the corpus callosum is usually seen as truncation of the anterior–posterior dimension,

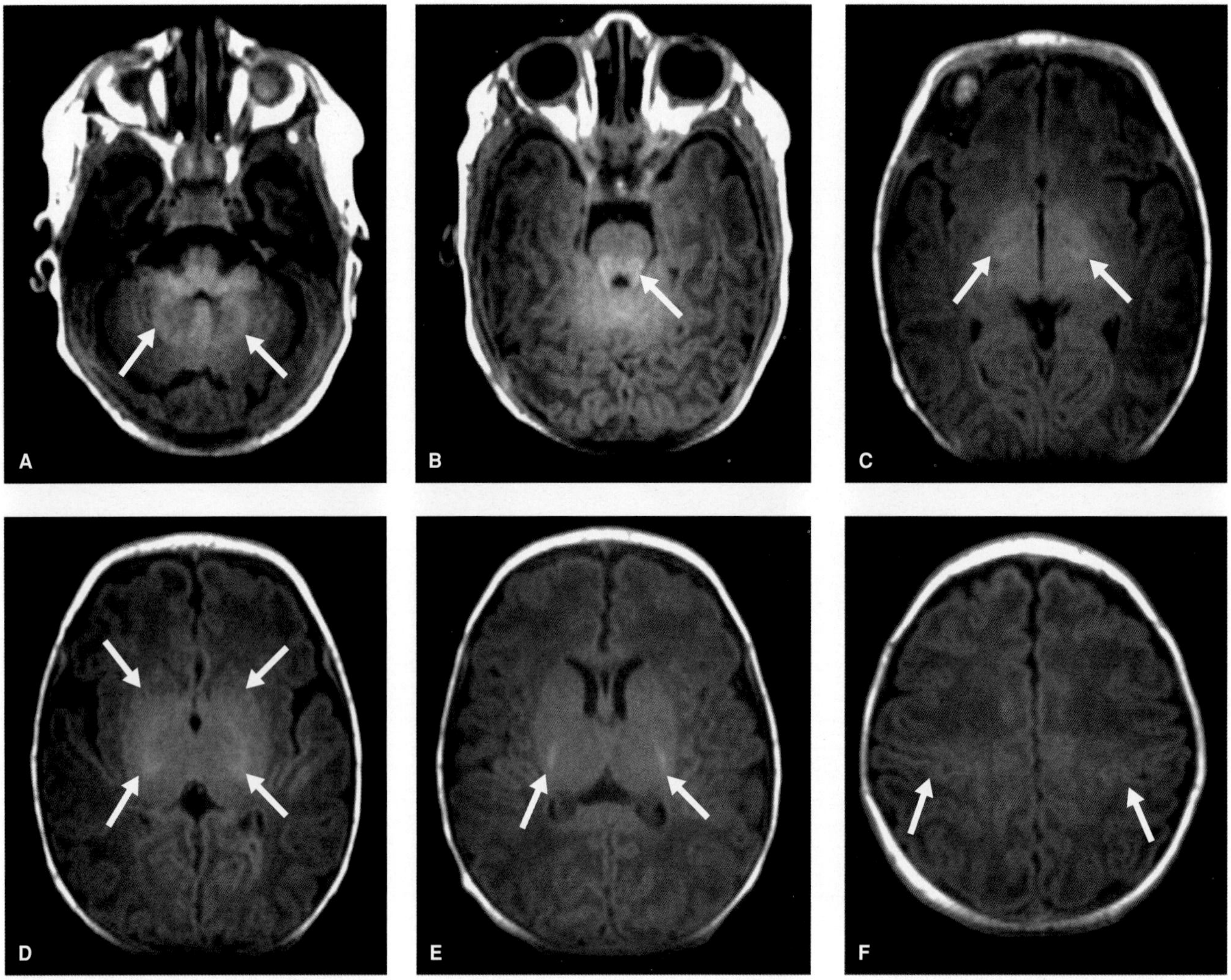

FIGURE 66.2. **Axial T1 3D SPGR Images Through the Brain in a Normal Term Neonate.** There is T1 hyperintense myelination (*white arrows*) in the deep cerebellar white matter (**A**), dorsal brain stem (**B**), subthalamic nuclei (**C**), ventrolateral thalami and basal ganglia (**D**), posterior limbs of the internal capsules (**E**), and perirolandic cortex (**F**).

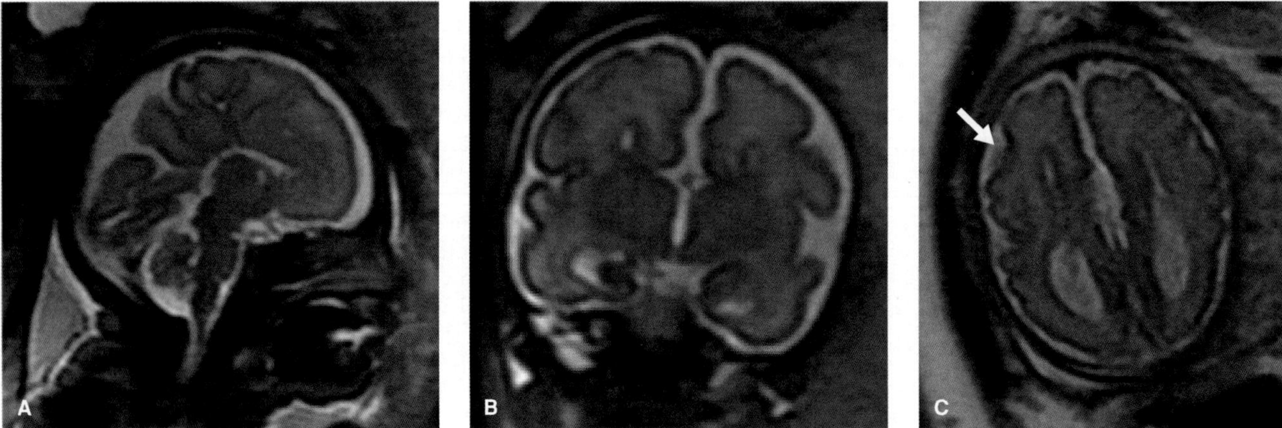

FIGURE 66.3. **T2-SSFSE Images From Fetal MRI of a 31-Week 6-Day Gestational Age Fetus With Complete Agenesis of the Corpus Callosum.** On midline sagittal (**A**) image there is absence of the cingulate sulcus with sulci radiating up to the third ventricular margin. On coronal (**B**) image one can see the "Texas longhorn" appearance of the lateral ventricles. On axial (**C**) image there is colpocephaly and parallel configuration of the lateral ventricles. There is also suspected cortical malformation in the right frontal lobe (*arrow*).

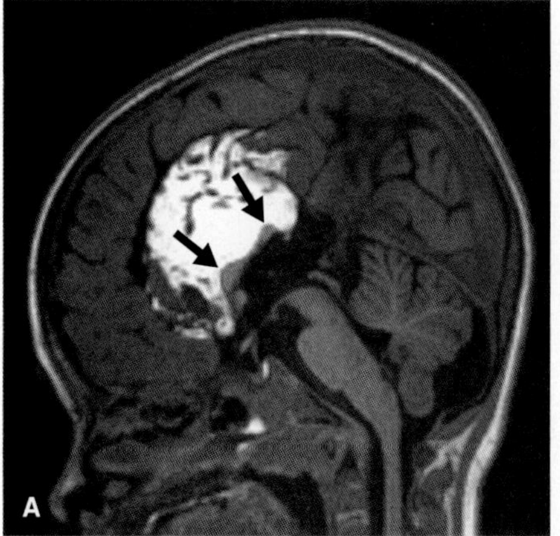

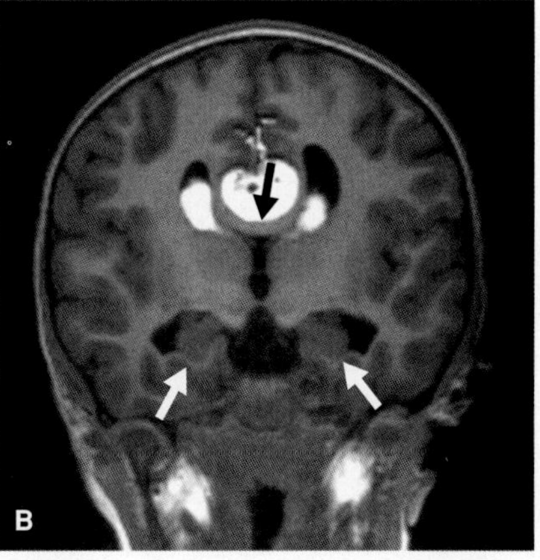

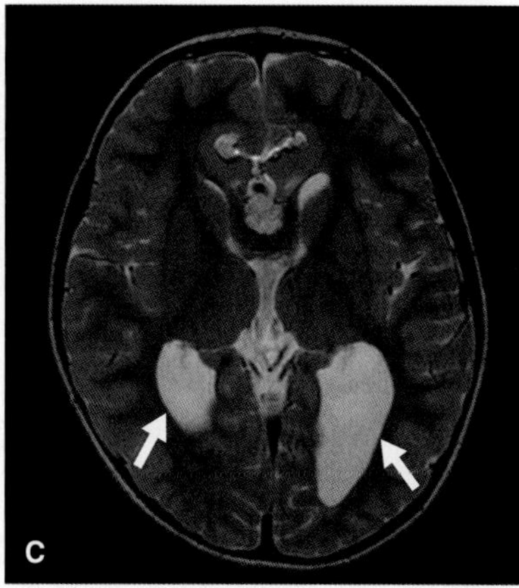

FIGURE 66.4. **A 5-Year-Old Male With Dysgenesis of the Corpus Callosum With an Interhemispheric Lipoma.** On sagittal (**A**) and coronal (**B**) T1 SPGR images there is a large T1 hyperintense interhemispheric lipoma which extends into the lateral ventricles. The corpus callosum is hypogenetic with only small portions of the genu and splenium present (*black arrows*). The hippocampi (*white arrows*) are underrotated giving them a globular appearance. Axial T2-weighted image (**C**) shows associated colpocephaly (*white arrows*).

though it can also be segmental, with the callosum appearing as two separate commissures. They are frequently associated with interhemispheric cysts or lipomas (Fig. 66.4). Regional gliosis or encephalomalacia in the brain can cause focal atrophy of the corpus callosum as well secondary to axonal injury.

The term **septo-optic dysplasia** was first used by de Morsier in 1956 to describe the postmortem findings of optic nerve hypoplasia and agenesis of the septum pellucidum. With the advent of MR imaging, a broad diversity of findings have been identified in association with optic nerve hypoplasia: partial or complete absence of the septum pellucidum, dysgenesis of the corpus callosum, anomalies of the hypothalamic–pituitary axis, and malformations of cortical development, most notably schizencephaly (Fig. 66.5). Optic nerve hypoplasia is more reliably diagnosed on ophthalmologic examination, as only 50% of affected patients have appreciable optic nerve hypoplasia on MRI.

Holoprosencephaly encompasses a spectrum of malformations caused by abnormalities of differentiation and midline cleavage of the prosencephalon during the 5th gestational week. The imaging hallmark is abnormal communication of gray and/or white matter across midline; facial dysmorphism is seen in up to 80% of cases and includes hypotelorism, cyclopia, ethmocephaly, cebocephaly, and midline cleft lip/palate.

Alobar holoprosencephaly implies complete absence of cleavage with anterior displacement of the cerebral tissue into a "pancake" configuration and a large monoventricle that expands posteriorly into a dorsal cyst. There is a greater degree of cleavage with ***semilobar holoprosencephaly***, where some differentiation of the posterior lateral ventricles is evident, and the anterior falx cerebri can be partially present in ***lobar holoprosencephaly***, *though differentiation between the*

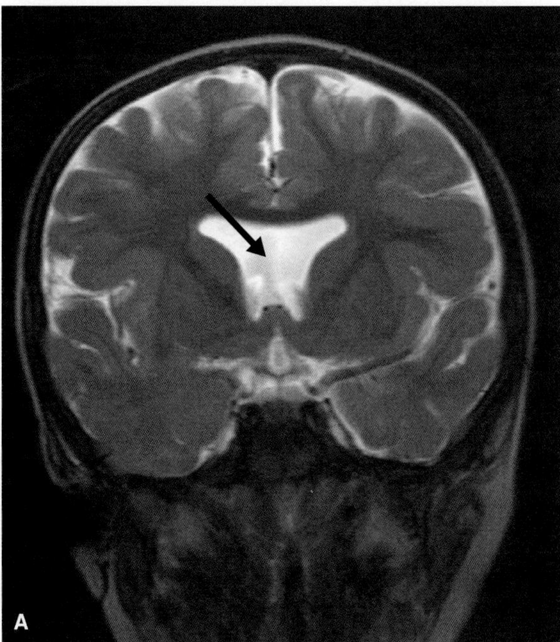

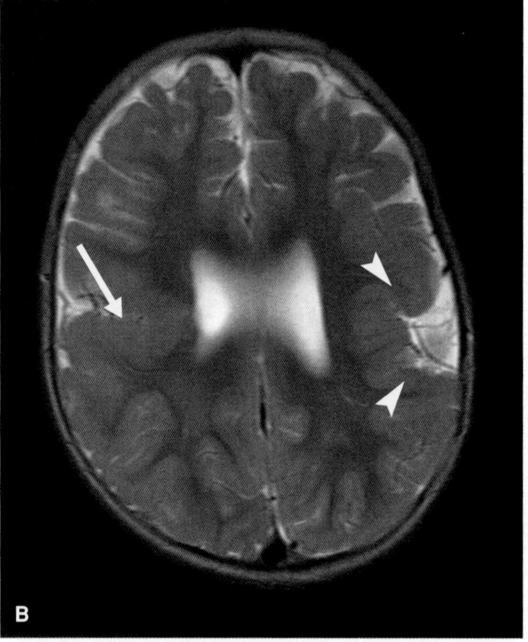

FIGURE 66.5. **A 2-Year-Old Male With Hypoplastic Optic Nerves on Ophthalmologic Examination.** Coronal T2-weighted image (**A**) demonstrates absence of the septum pellucidum (*arrow*). **B**: Axial T2-weighted image shows right perisylvian closed-lip schizencephaly (*white arrow*) lined by dysplastic cortex. There is also left perisylvian polymicrogyria (*arrowheads*).

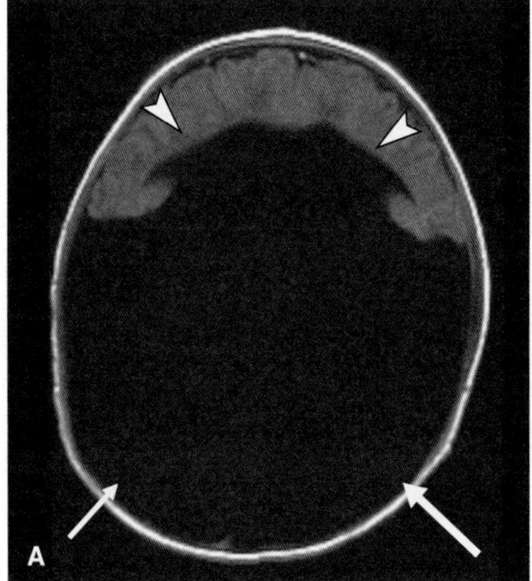

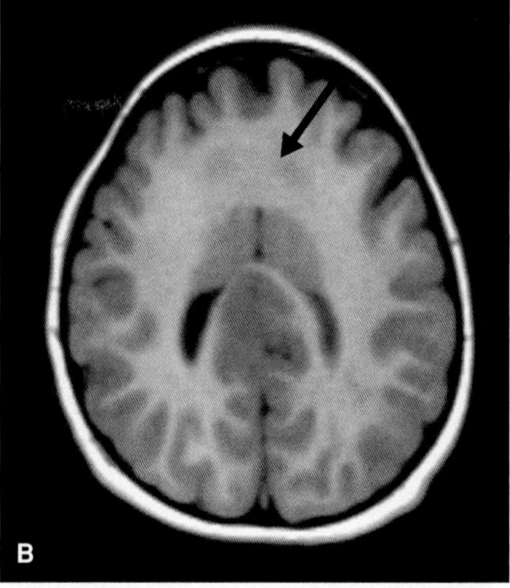

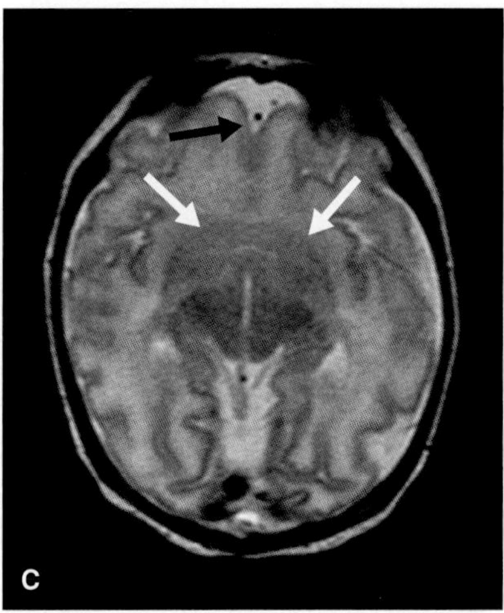

FIGURE 66.6. **Holoprosencephaly spectrum.** Axial T1-weighted image (A) of a different patient at 6 days of age with alobar holoprosencephaly. There is anterior flattening (a.k.a "pancake") of cerebral tissue (*arrowheads*) with a crescent-shaped monoventricle communicating with a dorsal cyst (*arrows*). Axial (**B**) T1-weighted 3D SPGR image of a 3-year-old female with semilobar holoprosencephaly. There is absence of the anterior corpus callosum with incomplete separation of the frontal lobes (*black arrow*). Axial T2 FSE (**C**) image from a 3 day old with lobar holoprosencephaly. There is incomplete separation of the basal ganglia (*white arrows*) and partial separation of the frontal lobes with an azygos anterior cerebral artery present (*black arrow*).

two is somewhat arbitrary. In the middle interhemispheric variant of holoprosencephaly, also known as ***syntelencephaly***, there is lack of separation of the posterior frontal and parietal regions with cleavage of the anterior frontal and occipital lobes (Fig. 66.6).

POSTERIOR FOSSA MALFORMATIONS

The majority of posterior fossa malformations can be categorized as one of the Chiari malformations, or a cystic malformation of the Dandy–Walker continuum. Less frequently encountered are the so-called molar tooth malformations and rhombencephalosynapsis.

Hans Chiari first described three subtypes of posterior fossa malformations associated with hydrocephalus in 1891. The Chiari III malformation is rare and is characterized by a cervico-occipital encephalocele containing posterior fossa contents, and many others have described various posterior fossa abnormalities using the Chiari designation, such as Chiari 0, Chiari 1.5, and Chiari IV. However, Chiari I and Chiari II are the most commonly encountered.

The **Chiari I** malformation is characterized by cerebellar tonsillar protrusion below the foramen magnum in the absence of an open spinal dysraphism or intracranial mass effect. While there is no absolute consensus on the degree of tonsillar descent necessary for the diagnosis, many use a position of the tonsil ≥5 mm below a line drawn from the basion to opisthion (McRae line) as the criterion. The classic clinical presentation is an occipital headache induced or exacerbated by a Valsalva maneuver, but up to 14% of cases identified on imaging are asymptomatic. Associated imaging findings include abnormal pointed morphology of the cerebellar tonsils, dorsal tilt of the dens, basilar invagination, platybasia, and effacement of the CSF spaces at the foramen magnum. Associated syringomyelia is an important finding as this is one of the main causes of neurologic symptoms and deficits (Fig. 66.7). Hydrocephalus, though reported, is relatively uncommon in this population. Posterior fossa decompression is the surgical treatment with suboccipital craniectomy and C1 laminectomy alone, or with the addition of duraplasty, cerebellar tonsil cautery, and CSF shunting in certain cases.

The **Chiari II** malformation comprises a constellation of imaging findings in the brain associated with an open spinal dysraphism (either a myelomeningocele or myelocele). The malformation can be identified on prenatal ultrasound by bifrontal concavity of the calvarium ("lemon" sign) and a flattened cerebellum wrapping around the brainstem ("banana sign"). Postnatal imaging findings include small posterior cranial fossa with a downward sloping tentorium and herniation

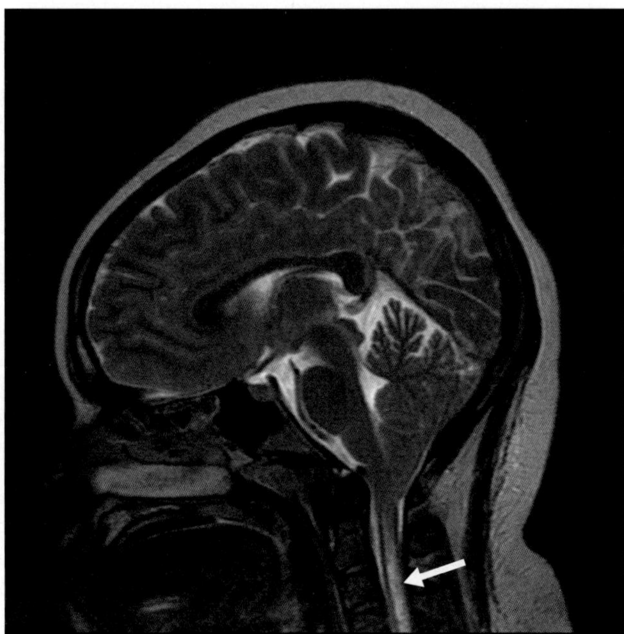

FIGURE 66.7. **Sagittal T2WI From a 16-Year-Old Female With Chiari I Malformation.** The cerebellar tonsils are pointed and extend down into the upper cervical spinal canal. There is a partially imaged syrinx of the upper cervical spinal cord (*white arrow*).

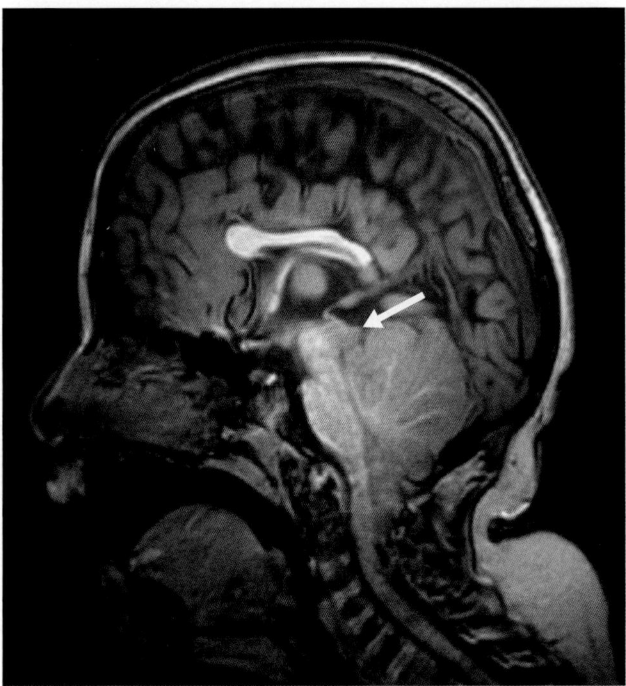

FIGURE 66.8. **Sagittal T1WI From a 6-Year-Old Male With Chiari II Malformation.** In addition to posterior fossa crowding and hindbrain herniation there is hypogenesis of the corpus callosum and tectal beaking (*white arrow*).

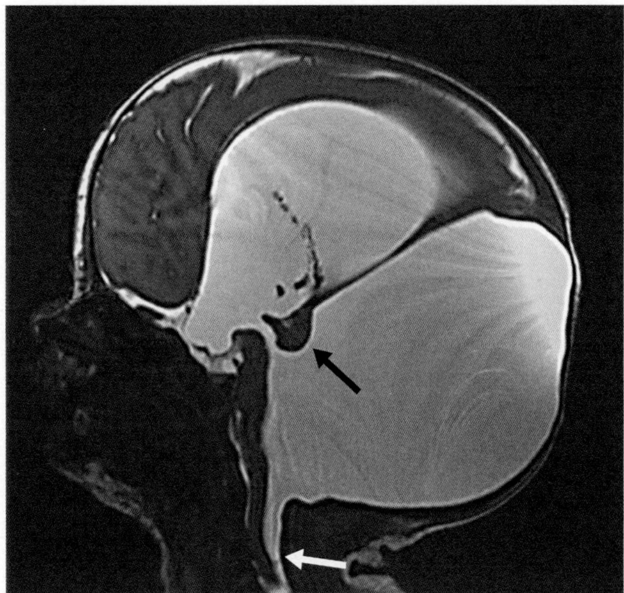

FIGURE 66.9. **Sagittal FIESTA Image From a 1-Day-Old Female With Classic Dandy–Walker Malformation.** There is a torcular–lambdoid inversion with an upward-sloping tentorium, hypoplastic rotated vermis (*black arrow*), and enlarged posterior fossa. A portion of the Blake pouch remnant is seen in the upper cervical spinal canal (*white arrow*) at the level of obstruction.

of cerebellar tissue into the cervical canal, a medullary "kink" dorsal to the upper cervical spinal cord, tectal beaking, and falx insufficiency (marked by interdigitating hemispheric sulci). Many cases will also exhibit stenogyria (gyri that are abnormally numerous and small), subependymal gray matter heterotopia, and hypogenesis of the corpus callosum (Fig. 66.8). Some of these manifestations, most notably the herniation of cerebellar tissue into the cervical canal, can be improved by prenatal repair of the myelomeningocele.

Dandy–Walker Continuum

This group of posterior fossa malformations includes a number of abnormalities characterized by varying degrees of vermian hypoplasia and malposition in association with posterior fossa cysts. One theory is that these abnormalities are all developmental anomalies of the rhombencephalic vesicle roof, but the terminology and classification are controversial and not universally agreed upon. Thus the ideal approach systematically focuses on the size of the posterior fossa, the size, morphology, and orientation of the vermis, and the size of the cisterna magna (Table 66.2).

The classic ***Dandy–Walker malformation*** is a triad of complete or partial agenesis of the vermis, cystic dilation of fourth ventricle, and an enlarged posterior fossa with upward displacement of the tentorium. The elevation of the tentorium places the torcula herophili above the lambdoid sutures, an angiographic finding key to the diagnosis prior to the advent of cross-sectional imaging, termed "torcular–lambdoid inversion." Obstructive hydrocephalus is a common complication but is not a part of the malformation itself (Fig. 66.9).

A hypoplastic vermis is often rotated counterclockwise such that the tegmento-vermian angle, formed by lines drawn along the brainstem and ventral vermis, is >18 degrees. The presence of this finding without enlargement of the posterior fossa has been termed "Dandy–Walker variant" by some, but this term is variably applied and imprecise. Children with isolated vermian hypoplasia often have normal neurodevelopmental outcomes. In the postnatal period the height of the vermis should be roughly equal to the distance between the midbrain tectum and obex.

Blake pouch is an embryonic structure that perforates in the first trimester to form the foramen of Magendie and foramina of Luschka. When this perforation is delayed or incomplete, it can result in a ***Blake pouch remnant*** or cyst causing upward

TABLE 66.2

"DANDY–WALKER CONTINUUM" FEATURES

■ STRUCTURE	■ "CLASSIC" DANDY–WALKER MALFORMATION	■ VERMIAN HYPOPLASIA	■ BLAKE POUCH REMNANT	■ MEGA CISTERNA MAGNA
Posterior fossa size	Large	Normal	Normal	Normal
Vermis size	Hypoplastic	Hypoplastic	Normal	Normal
T–V angle	>18 degrees	>18 degrees	>18 degrees	Normal

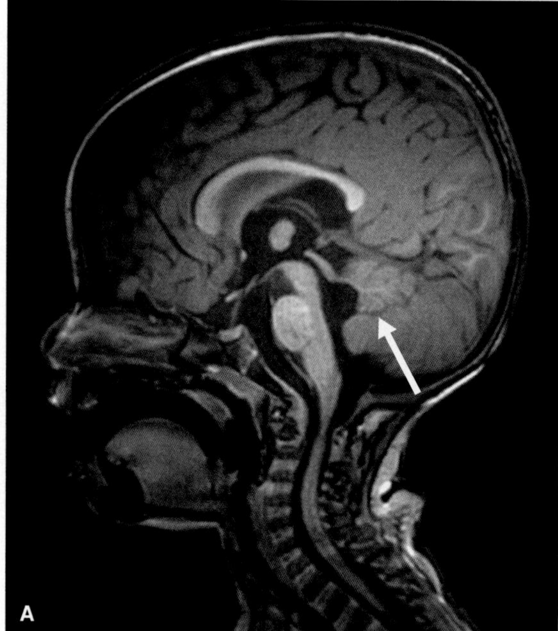

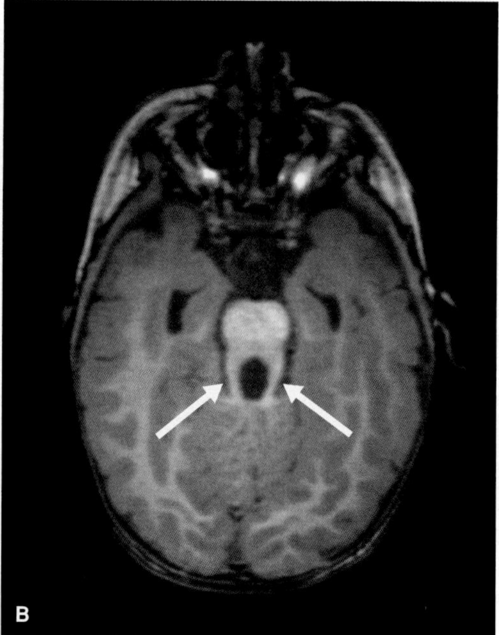

FIGURE 66.10. Sagittal T1WI (A) and axial T1WI (B) of a 15-month-old female with JSRD. A: The vermis (*white arrow*) is hypoplastic. **B:** The superior cerebellar peduncles (*white arrows*) are elongated in a "molar tooth" configuration.

displacement of an otherwise normally formed cerebellar vermis. The vermis is normal in size and morphology in this entity, but the tegmento-vermian angle is increased. Considered normal up to 20 weeks gestational age, Blake pouch remnant can be seen in isolation or can be associated with other anomalies and, depending on the degree of nonperforation, can result in obstructive hydrocephalus. ***Mega cisterna magna*** is believed to be the result of delayed fenestration of Blake pouch; it is defined as isolated enlargement of the cisterna magna (>10 mm) with a normal tegmento-vermian angle and is considered a normal variant.

Joubert Syndrome and Related Disorders (JSRD) is a heterogeneous group of disorders mostly resulting from mutations of genes encoding ciliary proteins. Clinically these patients are described to have episodes of irregular breathing during infancy ("panting" or "laughing" respirations) with oculomotor apraxia. The classic neuroimaging findings include vermian hypoplasia and the "molar tooth sign," where the thickening and elongation of the superior cerebellar peduncles resemble the root of an extracted molar tooth on axial MR images (Fig. 66.10). There can be hypoplasia or even absence of some of the lower brainstem nuclei. Additional associated anomalies include polydactyly, colobomas, and polycystic kidneys.

Rhombencephalosynapsis is the incomplete separation of the cerebellar hemispheres in association with partial or complete absence of the vermis. MR imaging can uniquely demonstrate the transversely oriented continuous folia (Fig. 66.11), and the flattened fastigial recess caused by at least partial absence

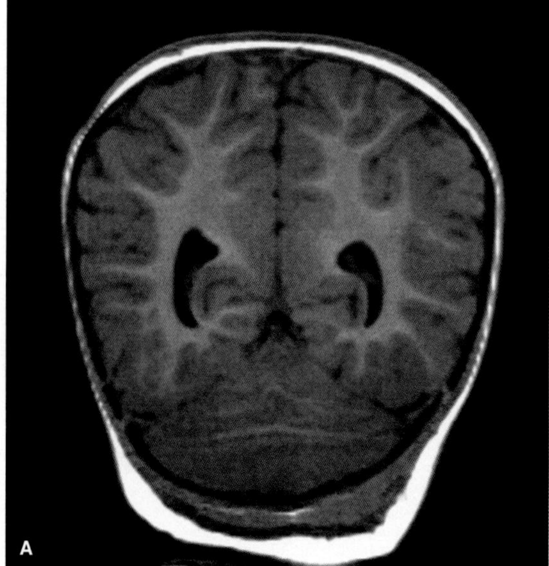

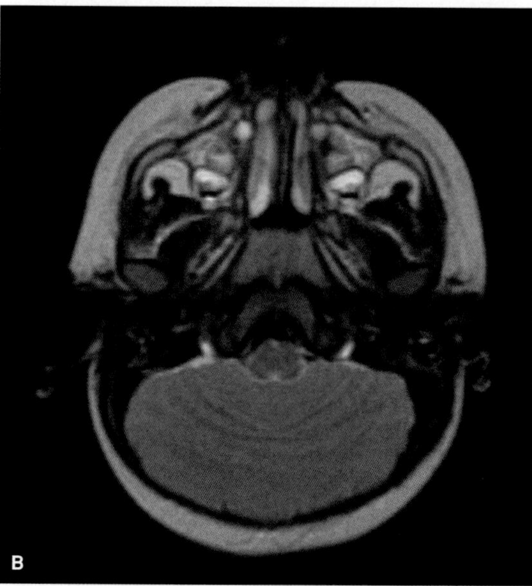

FIGURE 66.11. Coronal T1WI (A) and axial T2WI (B) in an 11-month-old female with rhombencephalosynapsis.

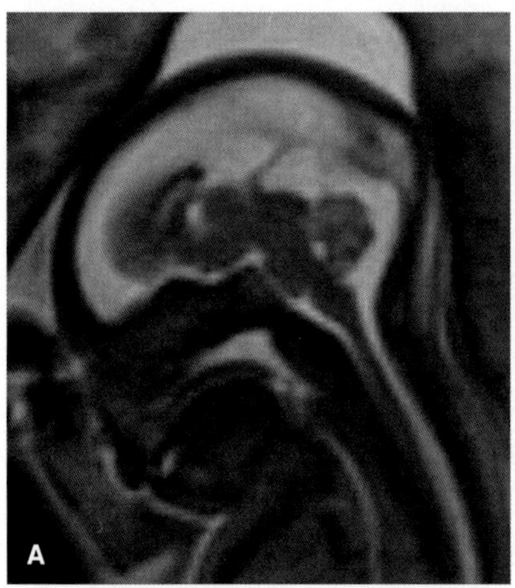

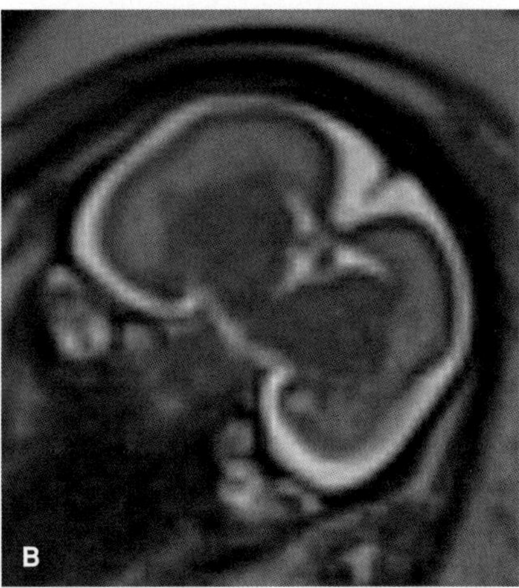

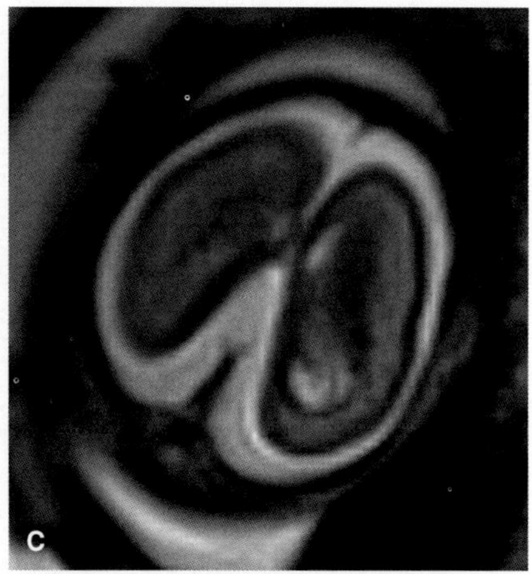

FIGURE 66.12. Sagittal (A), coronal (B), and axial (C) T2 SSFSE images from fetal MRI of the brain of a 25-week 2-day gestational age fetus. **A:** There is microcephaly marked by a decreased craniofacial ratio. **B, C:** There is absence of the normal gyral–sulcal pattern and even the sylvian fissures have not formed. Findings are compatible with microlissencephaly.

of the cerebellar vermis. Up to 65% of these patients have coexisting aqueductal stenosis. Other associated syndromes include Gomez–Lopez-Hernandez syndrome and VACTERL.

MALFORMATIONS OF CORTICAL DEVELOPMENT

These brain malformations are thought to result from disturbances of cellular proliferation, cellular migration, and/or cortical organization, and there is often evidence for disturbance of all three components.

Microlissencephaly is the most severe manifestation of *decreased* cellular proliferation, in which there is near-complete absence of the sulci and gyri with marked microcephaly (Fig. 66.12). ***Microcephaly with simplified gyral pattern*** is a milder phenotype where the brain is smaller than normal, with a reduced number of simple-appearing gyri.

The most extreme manifestation of *increased* cellular proliferation is ***hemimegalencephaly***, a hamartomatous overgrowth of part or all of a cerebral hemisphere. Unchecked proliferation and abnormal differentiation result in a bizarre appearance of the affected hemisphere, with a paradoxically enlarged lateral ventricle, thickened and ill-defined cortical ribbon, and mineralization and neuronal heterotopia causing the "white matter" to appear prematurely myelinated (Fig. 66.13). It is vital to closely evaluate the contralateral hemisphere to exclude additional abnormalities, as functional hemispherotomy (surgical disconnection of the entire affected

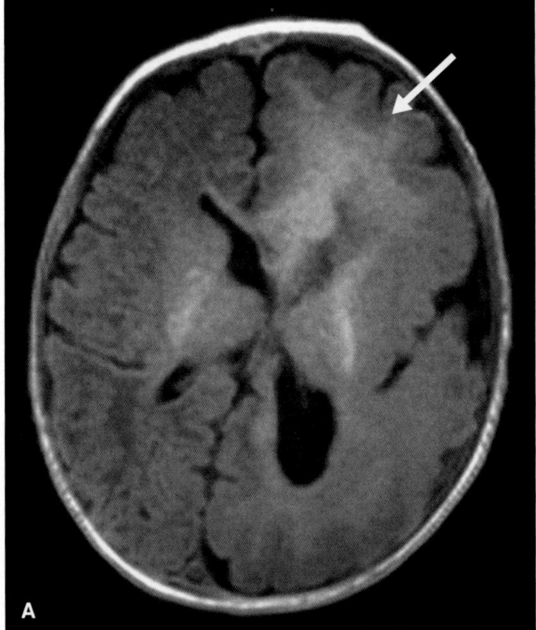

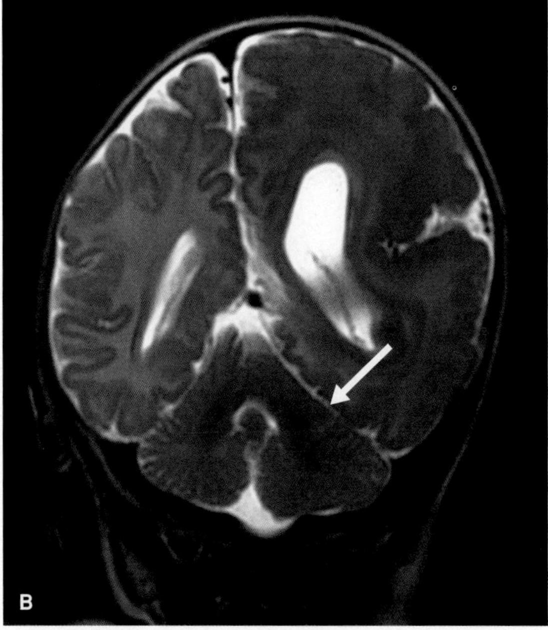

FIGURE 66.13. Axial T1-weighted (A) and coronal T2-weighted (B) images of the brain in a 2-month-old male with left hemimegalencephaly and CLOVES syndrome with lipomatous overgrowth of the right lower extremity. **A:** There is enlargement and dysplasia of the left cerebral hemisphere with the appearance of asymmetric accelerated myelination (*arrow*) and left unilateral ventriculomegaly. **B:** There is also mild enlargement of the left cerebellar hemisphere (*arrow*).

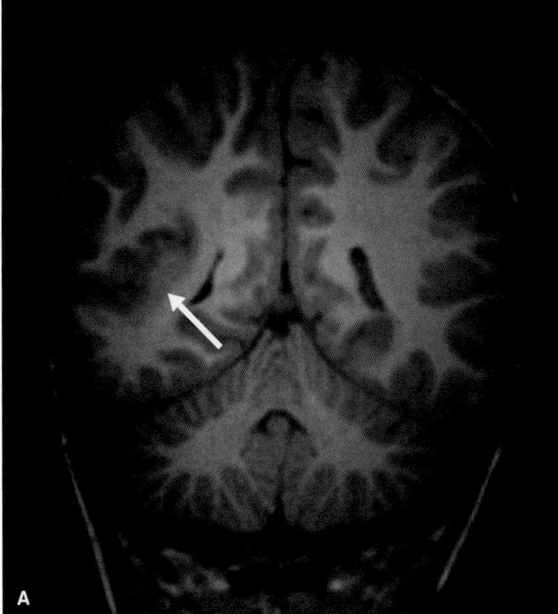

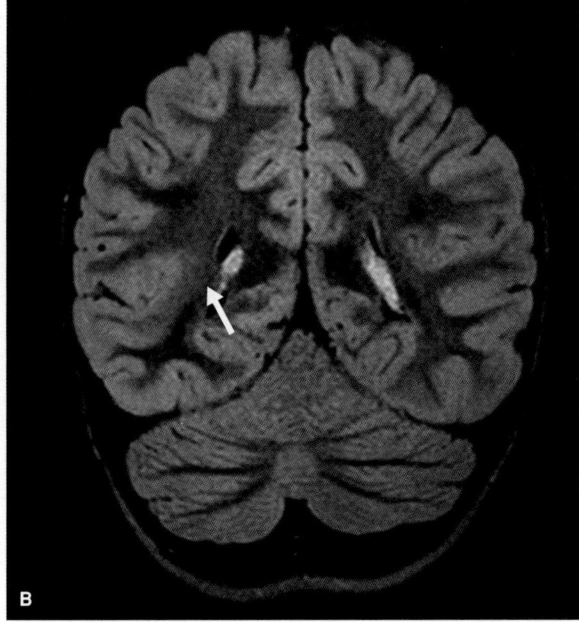

FIGURE 66.14. Coronal T1 SPGR (A) and coronal Cube FLAIR (B) images from MRI of the brain in a 6-year-old male with epilepsy. A: There is subtle blurring of the gray–white matter junction in the right posterior temporal region (*arrow*). **B:** There is also "funnel-shaped" extension of FLAIR hyperintense signal abnormality toward the ventricle (*arrow*). The patient underwent surgical resection and pathology was consistent with focal cortical dysplasia type IIb.

hemisphere) is the treatment of choice for this condition. Contralateral malformations may make such surgery moot.

A less dramatic and more localized increase in proliferation in association with abnormal cellular differentiation can result in type II focal cortical dysplasia (FCDII), a leading cause of medically refractory epilepsy in children. These lesions can be very subtle on imaging, with focal cortical thickening, blurring of the gray–white matter junction, and a funnel-shaped white matter signal abnormality extending from the subcortical region toward the ventricle (Fig. 66.14).

Gray matter heterotopia is the result of arrest of the radial migration of neurons from the germinal matrix along the walls of the ventricles to the developing cerebral cortex during the migrational phase. On imaging we see nodules of tissue that parallel normal gray matter in signal intensity on all pulse sequences (Fig. 66.15). ***Band heterotopia*** is a genetically driven migrational arrest that typically appears as smooth symmetric bands of gray matter found between the ventricular surface and cerebral cortex. The overlying cortex is either normal or along the lissencephaly/pachygyria

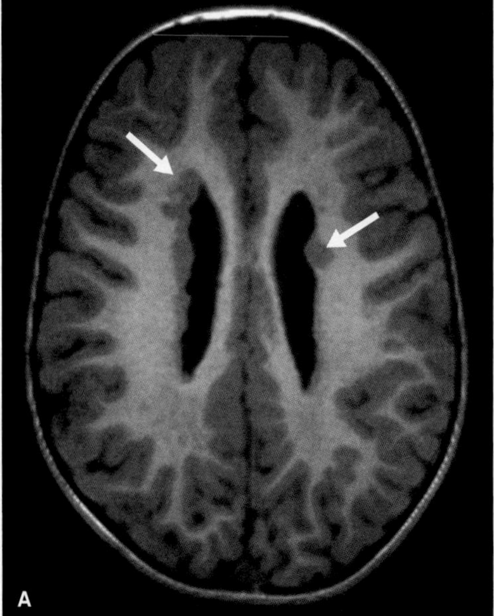

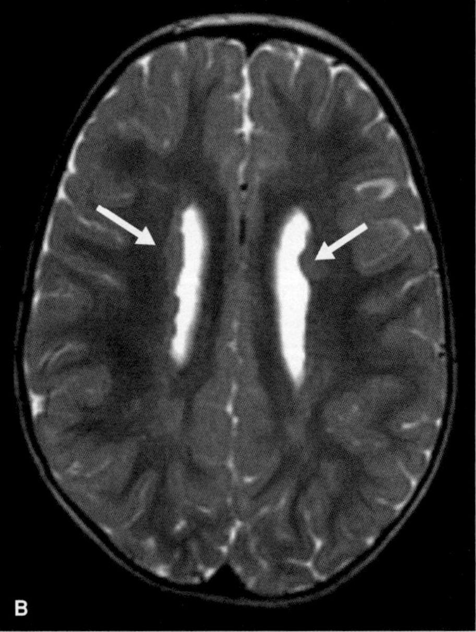

FIGURE 66.15. Axial T1-weighted (A) and axial T2-weighted (B) images of the brain in a 21-month-old male with numerous subependymal and periventricular gray matter heterotopias (*arrows*) lining the lateral ventricles. It can be noted that these nodules parallel gray matter signal on all pulse sequences. Associated dysmorphology of the ventricular system is a common finding in these patients.

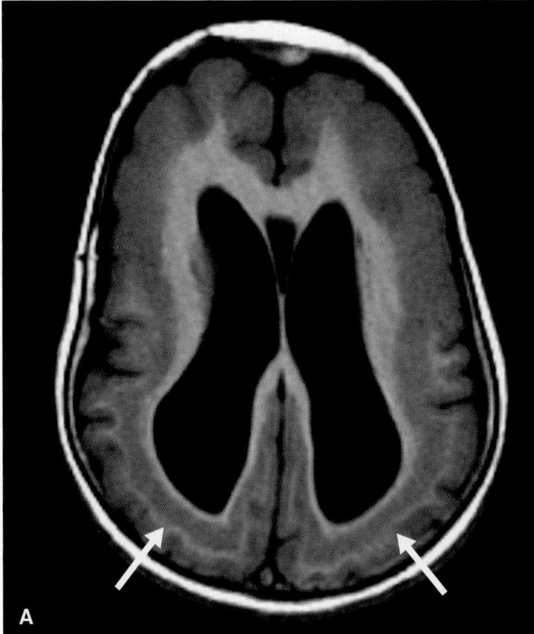

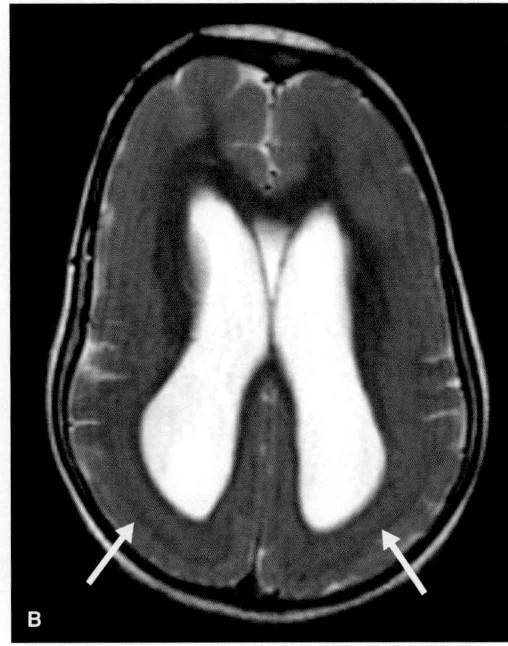

FIGURE 66.16. **Axial T1-weighted (A) and axial T2-weighted (B) images from MRI of the brain in a 9-year-old female with pachygyria with posterior band heterotopia.** A smooth band of signal that parallels gray matter signal (*arrows*) is seen in the parieto-occipital lobes and is separated from the overlying undulating cortex by white matter.

spectrum and nearly all affected patients are female (Fig. 66.16).

Lissencephaly/Pachygyria. Lissencephaly is the result of arrested neuronal migration resulting in an abnormally thickened cortex and absence of the normal gyral–sulcal pattern. In the complete form (agyria) there is complete absence of gyri/sulci, with an "hour-glass" or "figure-of-8" appearance due to broad and shallow sylvian fissures. In pachygyria, the gyri are present but abnormally broad, with shallow sulci. A characteristic feature is the cell-sparse zone, a very thin band of white matter signal separating a thin outer cortical layer from a thick inner cortical layer (Fig. 66.17).

Polymicrogyria results from abnormalities of late neuronal migration and cortical organization, causing an increased number of abnormally small gyri. In the fetus and neonate, polymicrogyria has the appearance of increased or decreased gyral/sulcal

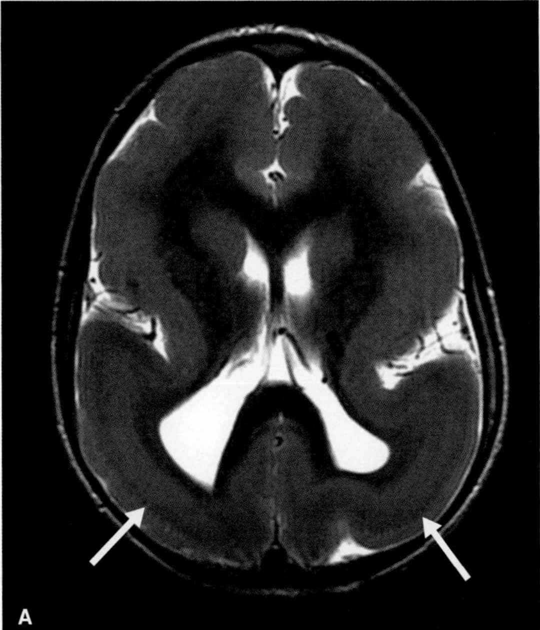

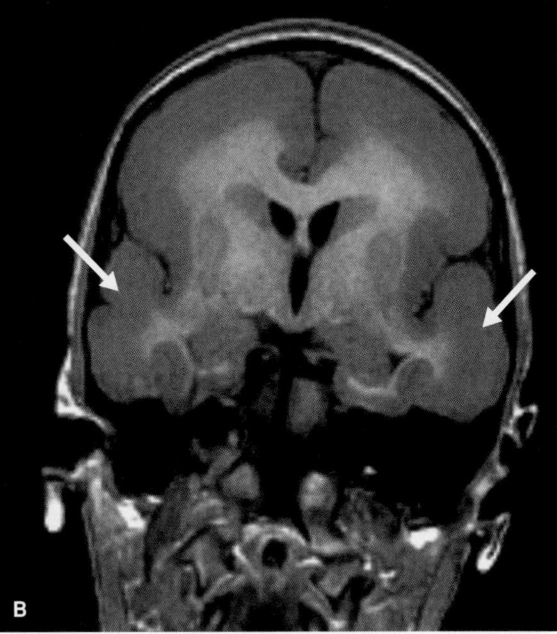

FIGURE 66.17. **Axial T2-weighted (A) and coronal T1-weighted (B) images from MRI of the brain in an 8-year-old female with lissencephaly.** There is near-complete agyria with bilateral frontotemporal pachygyria. Axial image (**A**) demonstrates the hour-glass appearance of the brain as a result of vertically oriented sylvian fissures. The cell-sparse zone (*arrows*) is seen as a thin line in the outer aspect of the thickened cortex of the occipitotemporal lobes that parallels white matter signal.

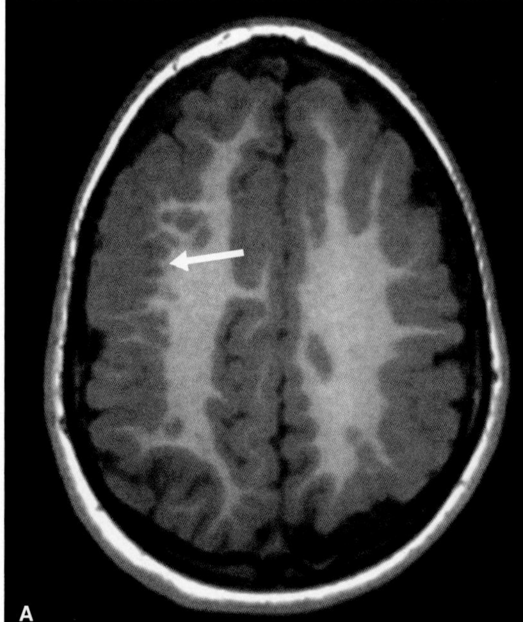

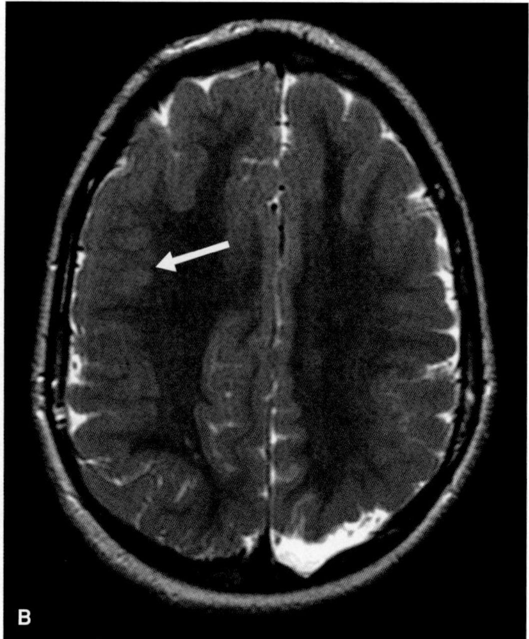

FIGURE 66.18. Axial T1-weighted (A) and axial T2-weighted (B) images from MRI of the brain in a 6-year-old female with extensive bilateral polymicrogyria, most severely affecting the right (*arrows*) greater than left perisylvian regions with relative sparing of the posterior parieto-occipital lobes.

development pattern, focal or diffuse. Once myelination is complete, the lesion has the appearance of cortical thickening with irregularity of the gray–white matter junction. Polymicrogyria can be focal or diffuse and can occur anywhere in the brain, though it is most commonly perisylvian (Fig. 66.18).

Schizencephaly is believed to reflect a prevention of neuronal migration from the germinal matrix outward, resulting in a transmantle cleft lined by dysplastic gray matter extending from the ependyma to the pial surface. In closed-lip schizencephaly, the cortices of the cleft are immediately apposed, while in open-lip schizencephaly, CSF communicates between the ventricle and the overlying subarachnoid space. Schizencephaly is bilateral in up to 50% of cases, and contralateral polymicrogyria is common in unilateral cases (Fig. 66.19).

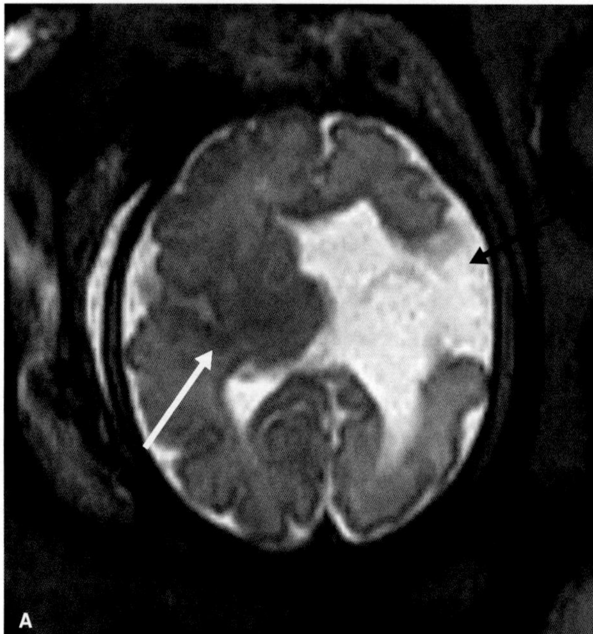

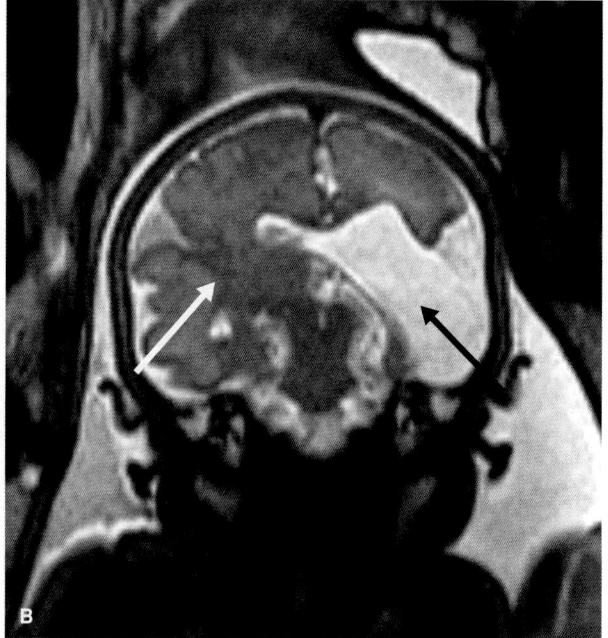

FIGURE 66.19. Axial (A) and coronal (B) T2 SSFSE images from fetal MRI of the brain of a 35 week 6-day gestational age fetus. Readily apparent is the left frontoparietotemporal (*black arrow*) open-lip schizencephaly. Closer inspection reveals the right perisylvian closed-lip schizencephaly (*white arrow*) with surrounding polymicrogyria.

NEONATAL ENCEPHALOPATHY

The WHO classifies infants born prior to 28 weeks of gestation as "extremely preterm," those between 28 and 32 weeks as "very preterm," and those born between 32 and 37 weeks as "moderate to late preterm." This *term*inology reflects the dramatic impact that the time of delivery has on overall survival and morbidity, but the focus on the time of *delivery* can be misleading in regard to response to injury. Severe hypoxia can have a similar effect on the 26-week gestation infant whether they are in the womb or an NICU incubator, and the wise clinician will not ignore the likelihood that pathologies evident after birth may have started well prior to delivery.

In the interpretation of imaging studies of the injured neonatal brain there is a great temptation to propose theories of the nature of insult based upon the regions of the brain injured and the imaging features of the injury. Unfortunately there is a great deal of overlap between patterns of injury and instigating insults, such that the level of accuracy in making such "back projections" is typically less than can be clinically relied upon. A clear understanding of how the developing brain responds to injury is of great value however, so that contradictions between clinical expectations and imaging findings can be recognized and explored, which can lead to more directed and effective treatment strategies.

Malformations

Although neuronal migration continues to occur throughout gestation and beyond delivery, a majority occurs between 12 and 24 weeks. Accordingly, injuries occurring prior to 24 weeks of gestation that disrupt this process often result in fetal demise or severe global brain malformations. The most obvious of these is hydranencephaly (Fig. 66.20), a severe in-utero brain injury generally attributed to bilateral internal carotid artery occlusion. This attribution is a result of the fact that the surviving brain in infants with hydranencephaly is supplied exclusively by the posterior circulation or meningeal branches of the external carotid arteries. Less severe or localized insults may manifest as specific migrational abnormalities like schizencephaly.

Periventricular Leukomalacia

Periventricular leukomalacia (PVL) is a distinct pattern of white matter injury that affects the developing brain between 24 and 34 weeks of gestational age, caused by damage to oligodendrocyte precursor cells (pre-oligodendrocytes, oligodendrocyte progenitor cells [OPCs]). The damage is thought to be a result of hypoxia and ischemia superimposed upon preexisting inflammatory factors. There is a strong correlation of maternal infection and placental inflammation in infants with PVL, and it is thought that the periventricular white matter represents a "watershed zone" of cerebral blood flow in the immature brain, with poor autoregulation. PVL is a pattern of injury that is seen in many children diagnosed with cerebral palsy; symmetric loss of periventricular white matter surrounding the trigones of the lateral ventricles, with a characteristic angular morphology of the adjacent lateral ventricles as they expand into the vacated parenchyma (Fig. 66.21C). The ability of the brain to mount a reparative response to injury is markedly limited prior to 34 weeks of gestation; as a result there is little or no gliosis. The pattern of injury has also been called "white matter injury of prematurity (WMOP)," acknowledging the high frequency in which it is detected in children born prematurely. However, it should be recognized that the injury can and does occur in utero.

This injury can be recognized by transcranial US, where the injured white matter may appear abnormally hyperechoic (Fig. 66.21A). Sensitivity of US and CT for the detection of PVL is relatively low in the early stages, but MR imaging

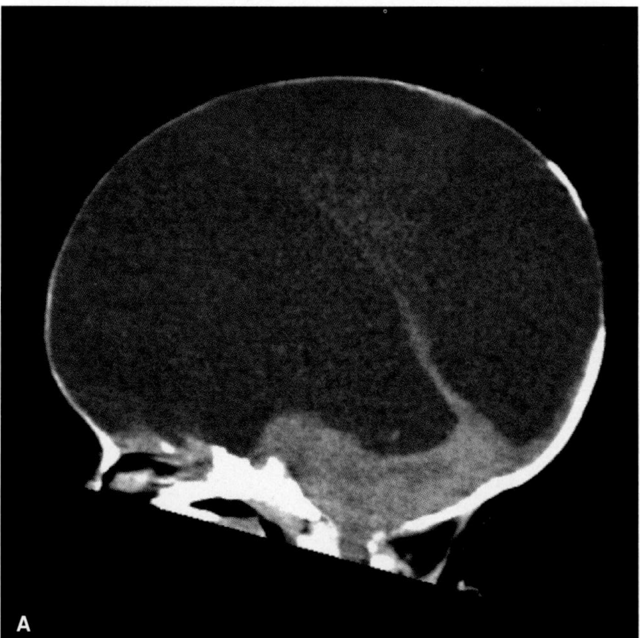

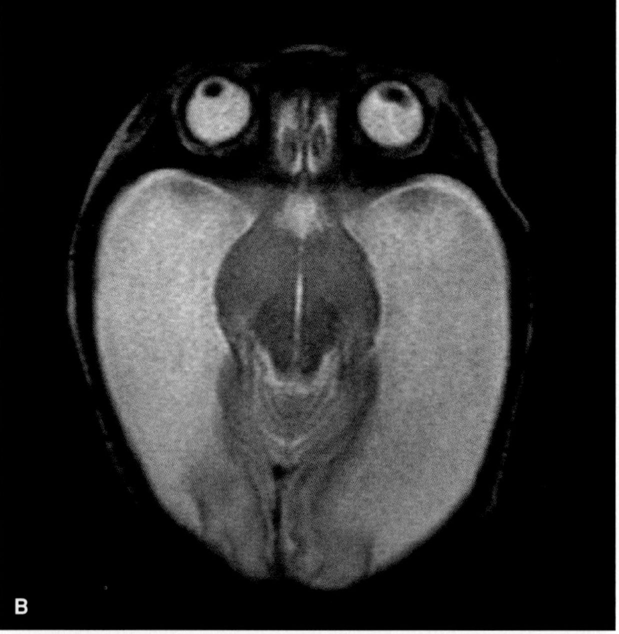

FIGURE 66.20. Hydranencephaly. Sagittal CT (**A**) and axial (**B**) T2-weighted MR images of a neonate with hydranencephaly show absence of all brain parenchyma supplied by the carotid arteries, with preservation of the posterior fossa structures and medial temporal lobes. Sometimes meningeal branches of the external carotid artery will preserve some additional cortex in this condition, but that is uncommon. Macrocrania is typical, as CSF is still generated but in the absence of the cerebral hemispheres cannot be effectively resorbed. CSF diversion with a ventricular shunt is usually performed as a palliative measure.

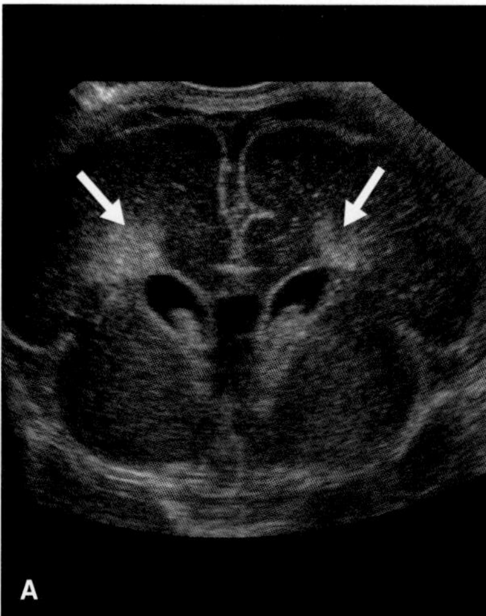

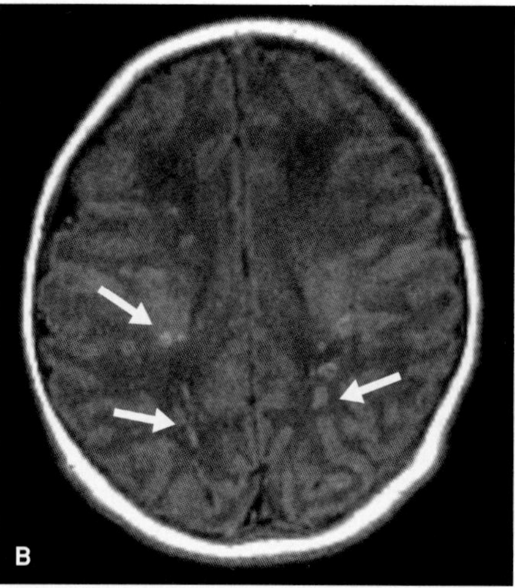

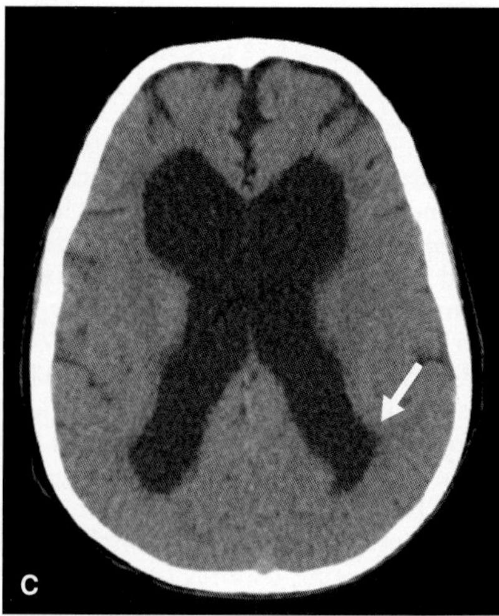

FIGURE 66.21. **Periventricular Leukomalacia (PVL).** Coronal head US image obtained through the anterior fontanelle (**A**) shows abnormal increased echogenicity in the white matter bordering the bodies of the lateral ventricles (*arrows*), an early finding of periventricular injury in the neonate. Axial T1-weighted MR image (**B**) shows multiple small foci of hyperintense signal in the periventricular white matter (*arrows*). These foci exhibit diffusion restriction. If an infant is stable enough to tolerate MR imaging, it is the study of choice to diagnose ischemic injury. Axial noncontrast CT image through the lateral ventricles in a 6 year old with cerebral palsy (**C**) shows the chronic sequelae of PVL, with enlargement and angular morphology (*arrow*) of the lateral ventricles resulting from loss of periventricular white matter.

will show punctate foci of abnormal hyperintensity in the periventricular white matter on T1WI (Fig. 66.21B). As the injury evolves, cystic changes can be identified with any of these modalities, and as the walls of these cysts break down, the characteristic angular pattern of ventricular expansion becomes manifest.

After 34 weeks, the population of mature oligodendrocytes is sufficient to provide a much greater resistance to white matter injury in the face of similar insult. At this stage there is also an ability to mount an astrocyte-mediated gliotic response to injury. Inflammatory/hypoxic injury extending beyond 34 weeks gestational age may therefore result in a white matter injury with more extensive surrounding gliosis.

Deep Nuclear Injury

In more severe hypoxic/ischemic injury, a primary factor in the pattern and propagation of injury is the presence of excitatory synapses that rely on the neurotransmitter glutamate and are populated by *N*-methyl-d-aspartate (NMDA) receptors. These receptors are overexpressed in the developing brain and are concentrated in the thalamic and subthalamic nuclei. Hypoxia and/or ischemia can cause these receptors to remain open, causing an influx of calcium and subsequent neuronal death. This excitatory neurotoxicity is not limited to neonates, but does result in a characteristic pattern of injury seen most commonly after severe hypoxia (Fig. 66.22A).

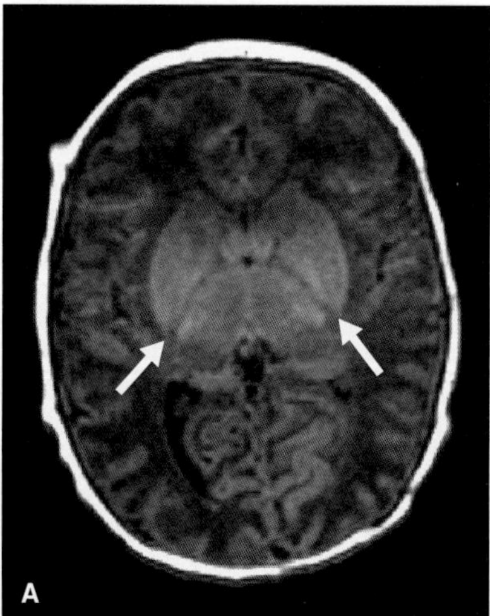

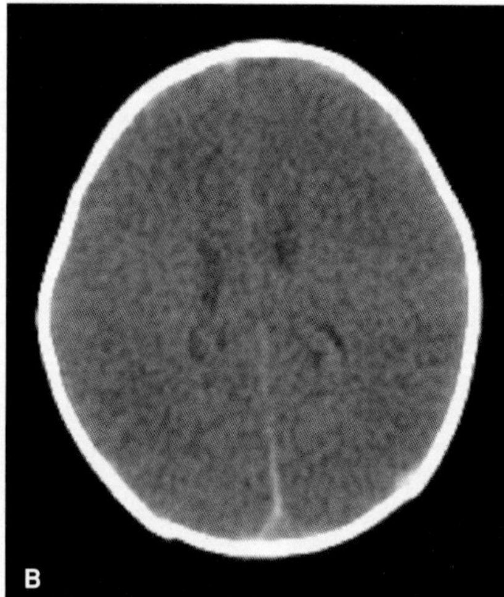

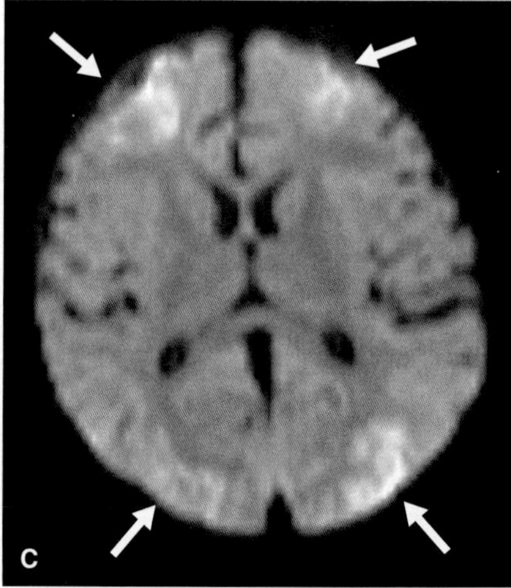

FIGURE 66.22. **Patterns of Diffuse Ischemic Injury.** Axial T1-weighted (**A**) image in a 3 day old with a deep nuclear pattern of hypoxic–ischemic injury shows abnormal hyperintense signal in the ventrolateral thalami and adjacent basal ganglia. Note the hypointense appearance of the posterior limb of the internal capsule (PLIC) on each side (*arrows*). In the normal neonate this structure appears hyperintense on T1-weighted images (Figure 66.2E) due to the presence of myelin, but the abnormal signal in the adjacent structures overwhelms the signal in this child. **B:** Axial CT in a neonate with congenital heart disease and prolonged arrest demonstrates the diffuse pattern of cerebral injury, with global loss of gray–white differentiation and sulcal effacement. Axial diffusion image in an infant with liver failure (**C**) shows restricted diffusion at the junction of the anterior and middle cerebral artery territories on each side (*arrows*), a "watershed" distribution indicating poor perfusion pressure to the entire cerebrum.

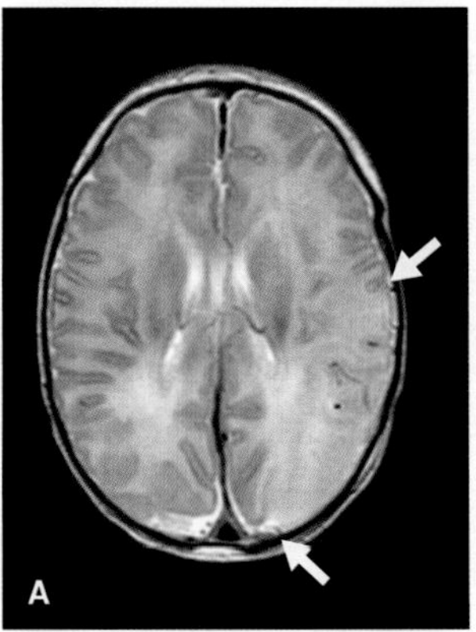

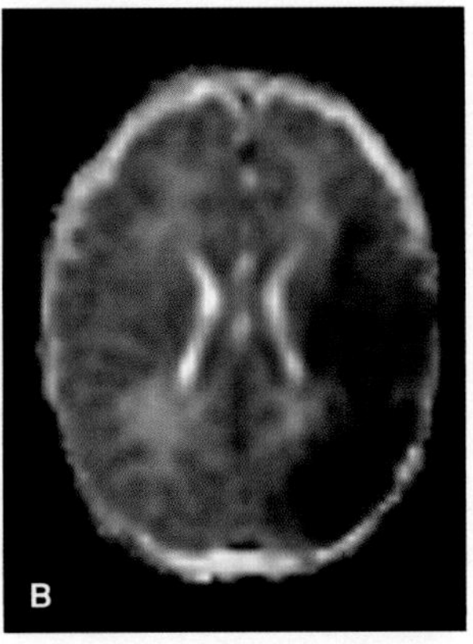

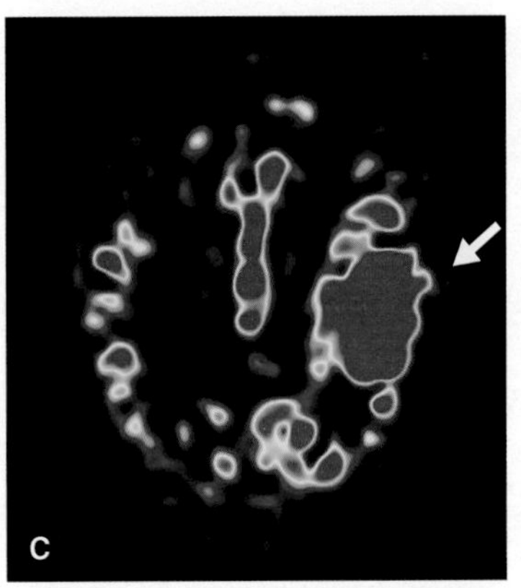

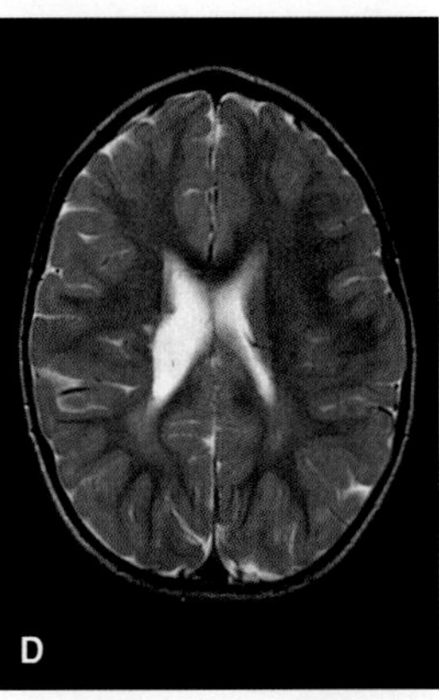

FIGURE 66.23. **Focal Arterial Ischemic Injury.** Axial T2-weighted image (**A**) in a 2 day old with seizures shows loss of the cortical ribbon in the left middle cerebral artery territory (*arrows*), confirmed by marked diffusion restriction on the ADC map (**B**). ASL perfusion imaging (**C**) shows corresponding hyperperfusion (*arrow*), reflecting expansion of the capillary bed and decreased transit time in response to the infarction (luxury perfusion). Seizures are a very common presenting symptom in the neonate with acute ischemic injury. Axial T2-weighted image in an infant with early left-hand preference (**D**) shows gliosis and volume loss in the right periventricular white matter from a remote "silent" infarction in the proximal right MCA.

Diffuse and Peripheral Injury

In the neonate at term, the response to hypoxic–ischemic insult is similar to the older child or adult. Severe global hypoperfusion can result in a diffuse injury, with complete loss of gray and white matter differentiation (Fig. 66.22B). More limited hypoperfusion injuries may affect only the familiar "watershed" or boarder zones between the anterior and middle, and middle and posterior cerebral artery territories (Fig. 66.22C). Focal arterial occlusion will result in classic infarction patterns, just as seen in adults (Fig. 66.23A–C). One common clinical scenario is the infant demonstrating early hand preference; normally hand preference should not be evident prior to 18 months of age. Imaging often reveals a periventricular injury in these infants, likely the result of transient proximal middle cerebral artery occlusion with infarction in the distribution of the perforating lenticulostriate arteries (Fig. 66.23D).

THE PHAKOMATOSES

Neurocutaneous disorders, also known as phakomatoses, are hereditary syndromes that are grouped together because they primarily affect structures of ectodermal origin, that is, the nervous system and skin.

Neurofibromatosis types 1 and 2 are forever historically linked on the basis of their original clinical description. Although they share some similar features, they are clinically and genetically distinct disorders. Both are autosomal dominant, resulting from abnormalities of different tumor suppression genes (Table 66.3).

Neurofibromatosis type 1 (von Recklinghausen disease, NF-1) is the most common of the phakomatoses. Located on chromosome 17, the NF-1 gene codes for neurofibromin, which has numerous functions including tumor suppression, myelination, and neuronal and astrocytic development. Its expression in osteoblasts and vascular endothelium results in additional manifestations. Patients with NF-1 develop multiple cutaneous lesions (café au lait spots, axillary freckling, cutaneous neurofibromas, and Lisch nodules) and for this reason NF-1 was termed "peripheral neurofibromatosis." Clinical criteria for the diagnosis of NF-1 are noted in Table 66.4.

On brain MRI, characteristic foci of T2 hyperintensity are seen in more than 75% of children with NF-1 (Fig. 66.24). Most common in the basal ganglia, thalami, deep cerebral white matter, and cerebellum, these do not exhibit mass effect or enhancement, and they may overlap gray and white matter structures. They are dynamic, typically absent in young infants, increasing in frequency until around age 10, decreasing

TABLE 66.3

NEUROFIBROMATOSIS: NF-1 VERSUS NF-2

■ FEATURES	■ NF-1	■ NF-2[a]
Epidemiology		
Incidence	1 in 4,000	1 in 50,000
Age at presentation	Childhood	Young adult
Affected chromosome	17	22[a]
CNS Findings		
Brain T2 hyperintensities	Yes	No
Optic gliomas	Yes	No
CN (vestibular) schwannomas	No	Yes[a]
Meningiomas	No	Yes
Dural ectasia	Yes	No
Spinal glial tumors	Rare	Yes
Nerve sheath tumors (NST)	Neurofibromas	Schwannomas
Malignant degeneration of NST	Yes	No
Plexiform neurofibromas	Yes	No
Skeletal Findings		
Scoliosis	Common	Uncommon
Sphenoid dysplasia	Yes	No
Thinning long bone cortex (ribbon ribs)	Yes	No
Vascular dysplasia	Yes	No

For NF-2, use the number 2 as your mnemonic: NF-2 patients typically have 2 (bilateral) acoustic schwannomas and an abnormal chromosome 22.

TABLE 66.4

NEUROFIBROMATOSIS TYPE 1: DIAGNOSTIC CRITERIA

■ DIAGNOSIS REQUIRES 2 OR MORE OF THE FOLLOWING:
Six or more café au lait macules (>5 mm prepubertal, >15 mm postpubertal)
Two or more neurofibromas or one plexiform neurofibroma
Freckling: axillary or inguinal
Optic pathway glioma
Distinctive bony lesion (sphenoid dysplasia, long bone cortical thickening +/- pseudoarthrosis)
First-degree relative with NF-1

National Institutes of Health Consensus Development Conference, 1988.

after puberty, and rarely seen in adulthood. On pathology they are characterized by spongiform changes due to abnormal myelin vacuolization, and their subsequent resolution is presumed due to myelin repair. Although benign in and of themselves, they can make identification of adjacent neoplastic lesions more difficult.

Optic pathway gliomas (OPG) are a common feature of NF-1 and most are pilocytic astrocytomas. Unlike sporadic tumors, OPG in patients with NF-1 generally have an indolent course, and asymptomatic tumors are frequently followed. They are recognized on MR imaging as fusiform enlargement of the optic nerves with variable enhancement, and extension to optic chiasm (Fig. 66.25A,B), and may also spread dorsally into the optic tracts and adjacent brain.

Glial neoplasms develop in the brain with frequency in NF-1, but like the OPG are often indolent and may even spontaneously regress. Their behavior may be difficult to predict from imaging (Fig. 66.25C) and surveillance with contrast-enhanced MRI is required. Signal abnormalities in the brain that are discrete, in atypical locations or enhance should raise the possibility of low grade glioma and may require closer interval follow-up depending on size and location. Treatment is usually reserved for those causing neurologic symptoms or showing rapid progression. Other cranial abnormalities in NF-1 include macrocephaly, vascular dysplasia/stenosis, and bony dysplasias, most frequently in the sphenoid wing. The latter are invariably associated with adjacent neurofibromas.

The most common spinal lesions in NF-1 are neurofibromas of the exiting nerve roots, glial cord tumors, and scoliosis due to bony dysplasia and dural ectasia (Fig. 66.26A). Peripheral nerve tumors may grow to a large size, discovered when they cause mass effect or pain (Fig. 66.26B).

Much less common than NF-1, ***neurofibromatosis type 2 (NF-2)*** results from a mutation on chromosome 22 which affects the tumor suppressor gene merlin (also known as schwannomin). Historically termed "central neurofibromatosis," NF-2 is essentially a multiple neoplasm syndrome with few cutaneous manifestations. People with NF-2 develop schwannomas on multiple cranial and peripheral nerves; bilateral vestibular schwannomas are diagnostic of this syndrome (Fig. 66.27A). Meningiomas are also common, identified in 60% of patients. The most frequent spine tumors are schwannomas arising from the dorsal nerve roots. These often have a "dumbbell" configuration as they pass through the neural foramina, with their medial component impinging upon the spinal cord. Intramedullary ependymomas are common, but often slow growing. Progressive neurologic impairment due to compression of the brain and cord (Fig. 66.27B,C) is inevitable. A useful mnemonic for this syndrome is **MISME**: Multiple, Inherited, Schwannomas, Meningiomas, Ependymomas.

Tuberous sclerosis (TS) is an autosomal dominant disorder caused by mutations in the TSC1 and/or TSC2 genes, which encode for hamartin and tuberin, respectively. The syndrome is characterized by dysplastic tumor-like lesions in the brain, lungs, skin, kidneys, and heart. Epilepsy is often the presenting neurologic symptom and is present in up to 90% of patients.

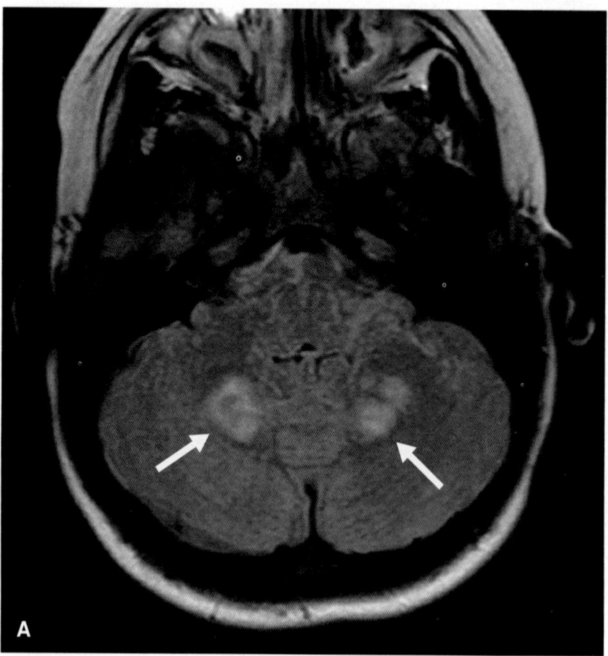

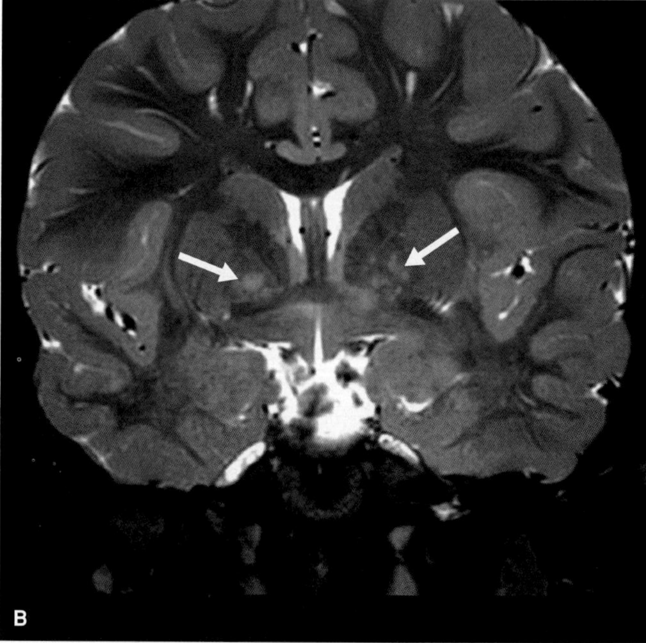

FIGURE 66.24. **T2/FLAIR Hyperintense Lesions.** Axial FLAIR (**A**) and coronal T2 (**B**) images demonstrate multiple foci of hyperintensity in the cerebellar white matter, basal ganglia, and hypothalamus (*arrows*) typical of NF-1. Pathologically they are comprised of areas of myelin vacuolization and glial proliferation, and they typically do not enhance nor cause mass effect. They decrease during adolescence and resolve by adulthood.

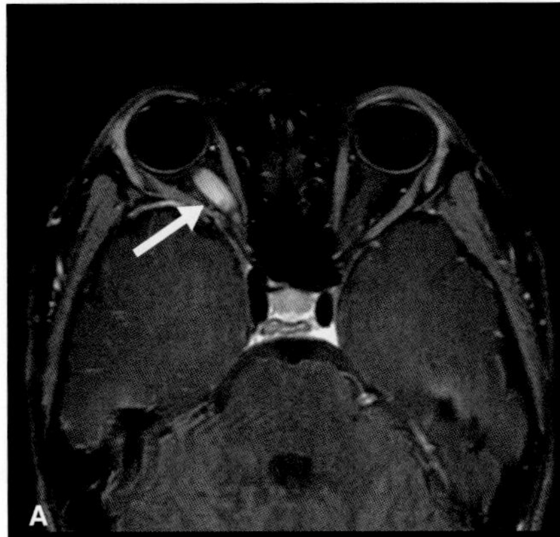

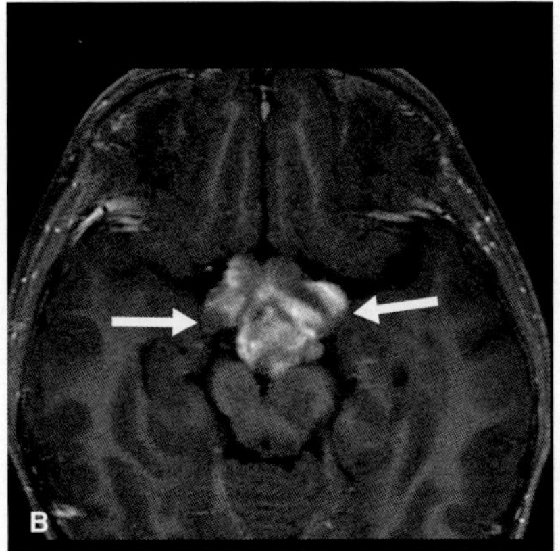

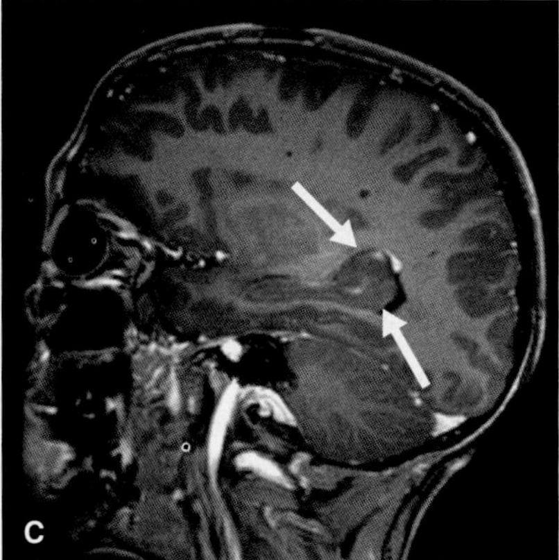

FIGURE 66.25. **Glial Tumors in NF-1.** Axial T1-weighted image with contrast (**A**) in a 5 year old with NF-1 shows isolated abnormal enhancement of the right intraorbital optic nerve (*arrow*). Gliomas of the visual pathways are diagnosed in nearly 20% of children with NF-1. An axial image through the suprasellar cistern (**B**) in a 6 year old shows a much larger and more diffuse lesion in the chiasm, with heterogeneous enhancement (*arrows*). Parasagittal contrast-enhanced image in a 10 year old with NF-1 (**C**) shows a glial tumor projecting into the lateral ventricle from the right temporal lobe (*arrows*). Glial tumors in the patient population are frequently indolent, and treatment is often delayed until lesions become overtly symptomatic.

Fifty percent of patients are cognitively impaired. Cutaneous lesions include angiofibromas and depigmented nevi (also known as ash-leaf spots).

Brain MRI demonstrates abnormalities in 95% of children with TS. The characteristic peripheral TS signal abnormality is the cortical–subcortical dysplastic lesion or "tuber." Individual patients may have only one or up to several dozen. Characterized by expanded broad polygonal gyri overlying abnormal subcortical white matter, their appearance on MRI alters with myelination. In neonates the abnormal gyri appear hyperintense on T1WI and hypointense on T2WI. In contrast, once myelination is completed, these lesions are best visualized on T2-weighted sequences, where they are hyperintense relative to normal white matter (Fig. 66.28). With time the subcortical component may become cystic, and some lesions may develop calcifications. Enhancement is uncommon but when present is not clinically significant.

The most characteristic brain lesions seen in patients with TS are subependymal nodules (SEN) that protrude inward from the outer walls of the lateral ventricles. Like the peripheral tubers, these are hyperintense on T1WI and hypointense on T2WI in infants, but become more isointense to white matter with age. SEN begin to calcify after the first year of life, and show variable enhancement (Fig. 66.29A–D).

Both SEN and peripheral tubers contain dysplastic neurons and balloon cells, but SEN near the caudothalamic groove may develop proliferation of the balloon cells and become subependymal giant cell astrocytomas (SEGA). Occurring in 5% of patients with TS, these benign neoplasms can enlarge to obstruct the foramen of Monro and cause hydrocephalus.

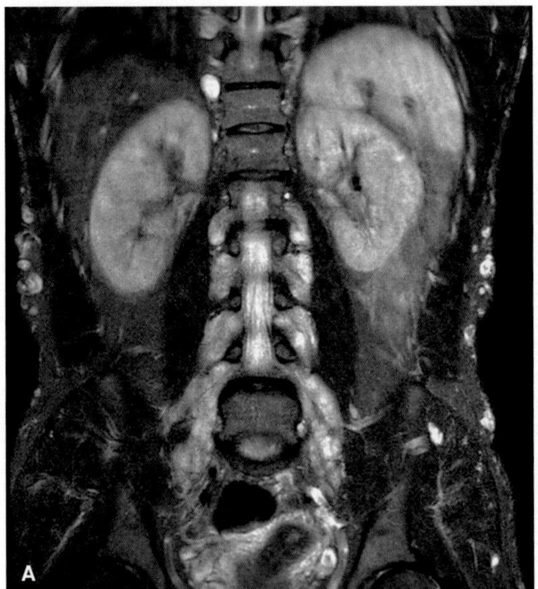

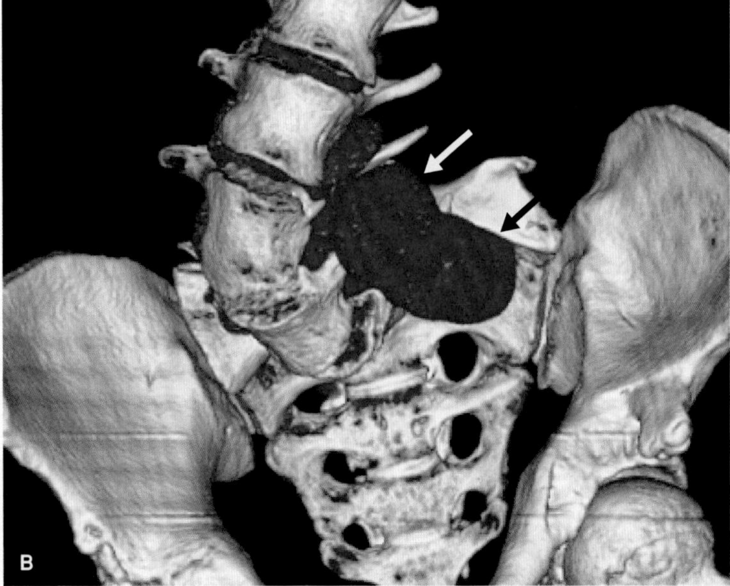

FIGURE 66.26. **Spinal Lesions in NF-1.** Coronal STIR image of the lumbar spine in a 10 year old with NF-1 (**A**) shows large plexiform neurofibromas arising from every lumbar and sacral nerve root, as well as innumerable small subcutaneous neurofibromas. Volume-rendered reconstruction from a CT myelogram in a teenager with NF-1 (**B**) shows severe dural ectasia (*arrows*) and kyphoscoliosis, with complete slip of L5 relative to S1.

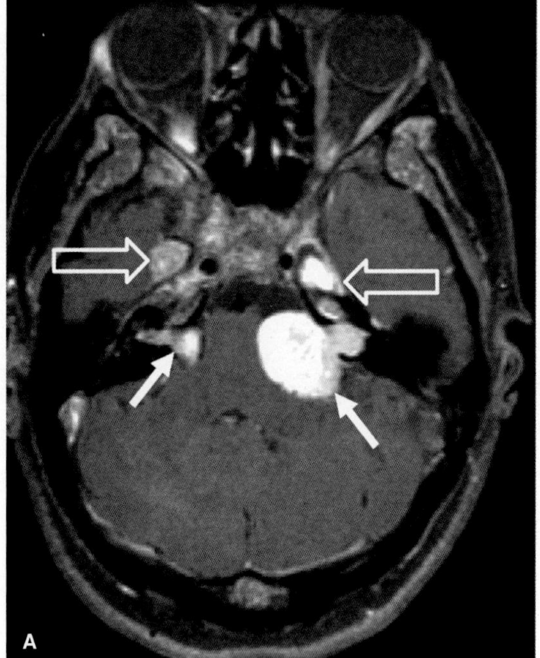

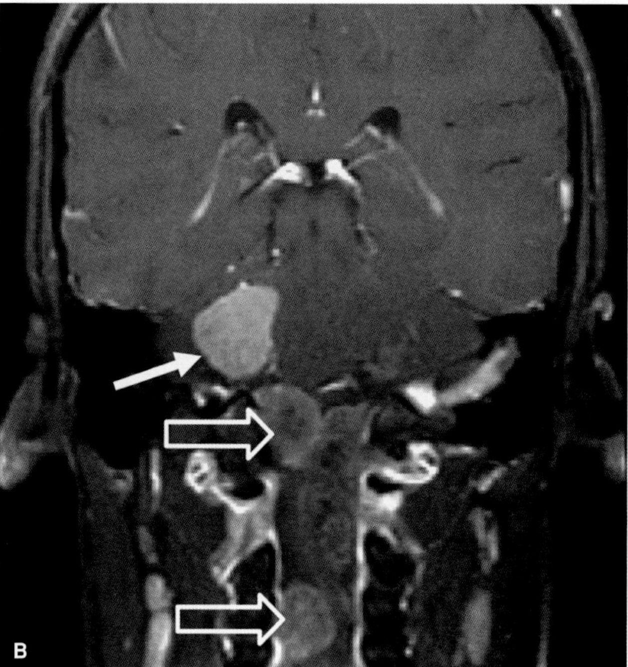

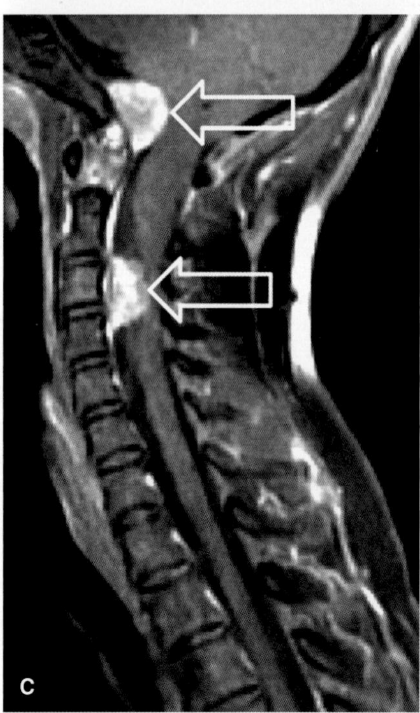

FIGURE 66.27. **Axial T1-weighted image with contrast demonstrates multiple cranial nerve tumors in this patient with NF-2 (A).** Bilateral vestibular or "acoustic" schwannomas (*arrows*) are diagnostic, but numerous other cranial nerves are often affected and must be meticulously evaluated (*open arrows*). Coronal and sagittal T1-weighted images of the cervical spine with contrast (**B, C**) show several large extramedullary tumors impinging upon the medullar and cervical cord. The tumors in this example were not associated with nerve roots and thus are meningiomas. Note the large right vestibular schwannoma (*arrow* in **B**).

This is why evaluation for developing SEGAs is the primary reason for imaging follow-up in patients with TS.

Most patients with TS will have curvilinear white matter lesions that extend from the ventricular margin toward the peripheral tubers, reflecting tracts of disordered neuronal migration caused by the mutation of the tuberin gene. Other less common CNS manifestations of TS include benign gliomas of the retina (giant optic drusen or retinal astrocytoma) and giant aneurysms.

The disordered proliferation causing lesions in TS is directed by the mTOR pathway. Agents that inhibit this cellular metabolic pathway can halt the progression of TS lesions, and cause regression. Renal and pulmonary lesions can also be a significant source of morbidity in TS, and imaging plays a prominent role in surveillance for all manifestations of this condition.

Unlike the classic phakomatoses, the ***Sturge–Weber syndrome (encephalotrigeminal angiomatosis)*** is not an inherited condition, but rather a consequence of failure of development of venous structures draining cerebral cortex, eye, and skin. In the face this results in a cutaneous capillary malformation called a port-wine nevus. The primitive venous drainage of the cerebrum is termed a pial angioma, and cannot adequately drain the underlying brain, resulting in chronic venous insufficiency with ischemia, and leading to subcortical calcification, gyral atrophy, and gliosis. In the eye the lesion is a choroidal hemangioma and can result in glaucoma and exudative retinal detachment. MR with contrast administration can reveal the full extent of pial angiomatosis and is helpful in cases where calcific atrophic changes have not yet occurred. Primitive venous drainage (developmental venous anomalies [DVAs])

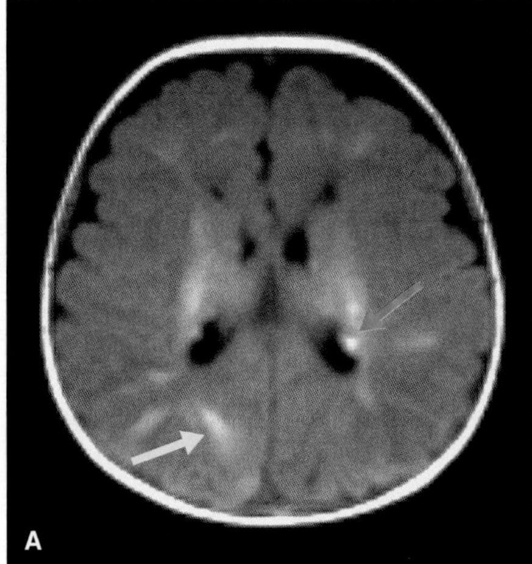

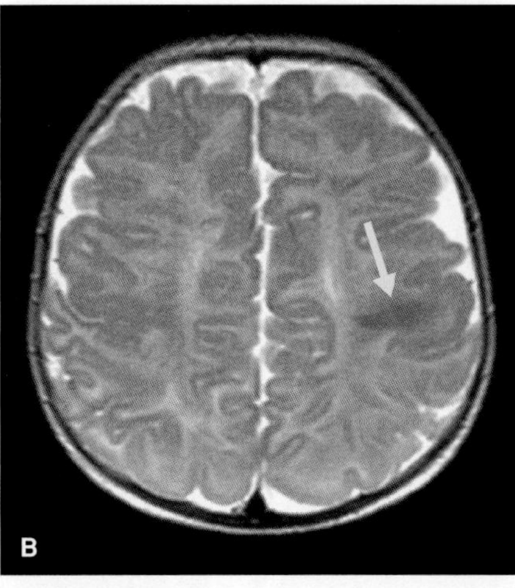

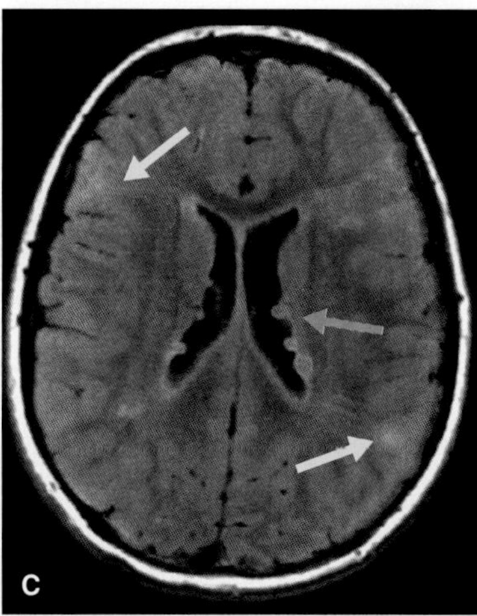

FIGURE 66.28. **Tuberous Sclerosis Lesions.** Axial T1-weighted image (**A**) in a 2 month old with tuberous sclerosis demonstrates multiple central (*orange arrow*) and peripheral (*yellow arrow*) lesions of TS, all of which appear hyperintense relative to the surrounding unmyelinated white matter. For the same reasons the infiltrating dysplastic cells of these lesions are hypointense (*yellow arrow*) on T2-weighted images in infants (**B**). However, as the brain matures, the peripheral lesions become evident as regions of subcortical hyperintensity (*yellow arrows*) with widening of the overlying gyri, as shown on this FLAIR image in a teenager with TS (**C**).

and ipsilateral choroid plexus hypertrophy is another feature of this entity (Fig. 66.30).

von Hippel– Lindau syndrome (CNS angiomatosis) is an autosomal dominant disorder consisting of retinal, cerebellar and spinal hemangioblastomas. Other features include renal cell carcinoma, pheochromocytoma, cysts in the kidneys, liver, and pancreas. It typically manifests in the second and third decades.

Hemangioblastomas develop in 50% of patients, and although considered benign neoplasms they are a common source of symptoms and have a high postsurgical recurrence rate. These vascular lesions are prone to sudden spontaneous hemorrhage. Characteristic features of hemangioblastomas include a well-circumscribed cystic lesion with an enhancing mural nodule (Fig. 66.31). Other appearances include a solid enhancing mass, solid tumors with central cysts, or an isolated cystic lesion. A helpful finding suggesting the diagnosis is a large blood vessel leading to the enhancing nodule.

PEDIATRIC SPINE

The typical adult neuroradiology practice is dominated by spine imaging, a consequence of the ubiquitous nature of back pain and degenerative conditions. Degenerative disease is relatively uncommon in pediatrics, and trauma, infection, and tumors of the spine and cord are covered in other chapters, so this section will focus on congenital malformations, syringomyelia, and scoliosis.

Congenital Spinal Malformations

At the beginning of the 3rd week of gestation, the dorsal aspect of the embryo develops a neural plate made up of neural ectoderm, which is continuous on either side with cutaneous ectoderm. In a process called neurulation, the neural ectoderm folds inward and forms a tube, with the center of the tube becoming the ventricles and the central canal of the spinal cord. In order for this process to complete, the neural ectoderm must detach from the adjacent cutaneous ectoderm, which then comes together to completely cover the neural tube. This process, takes place between 24 and 27 days of gestation, closing earlier toward the head. Many congenital spine malformations can be linked to a disruption of this complex and vital process.

Myelomeningocele and Myelocele

If the infolding neural plate fails to detach from the adjacent cutaneous ectoderm the neural tube will not close, and the central canal of the spinal cord will communicate with the amniotic sac. This exposed neural tissue is referred to as the neural placode; if it projects beyond the plane of the back the malformation is called a myelomeningocele (Fig. 66.32), and if it lays flat relative to the rest of the back it is the less common myelocele. These are the two open spinal dysraphisms, sometimes categorized as spina bifida aperta.

Located in the lumbar region in the vast majority of cases, the failure of neural tube closure results in a cascade of "upstream" malformations that together comprise the Chiari II malformation. These malformations are typically diagnosed prenatally by US, and often further imaged with fetal MR imaging. When diagnosed in utero the malformation can be repaired prenatally, markedly reducing the incidence and severity of the associated posterior fossa malformations.

Lipomyelomeningocele, Lipomyelocele, and Intradural Lipoma

If the infolding neural plate successfully detaches from the cutaneous ectoderm but mesodermal tissue becomes trapped between the two edges, this will also prevent closure of the neural tube, with intact skin covering the defect. The interspersed mesodermal tissue prevents the normal development of the posterior bony elements and differentiates into fat, which is contiguous with the subcutaneous fat and tethers the cord at the site of the malformation (Fig. 66.33). The lesion, called a lipomyelomeningocele (or lipomyelocele if the placode does not project beyond the posterior laminar line), may be inapparent at delivery and go undiagnosed until years later when the child presents with bladder or bowel dysfunction.

If the mesodermal tissue completely separates from the overlying mesoderm, the posterior elements of the bony canal can close, and the result is an intradural lipoma.

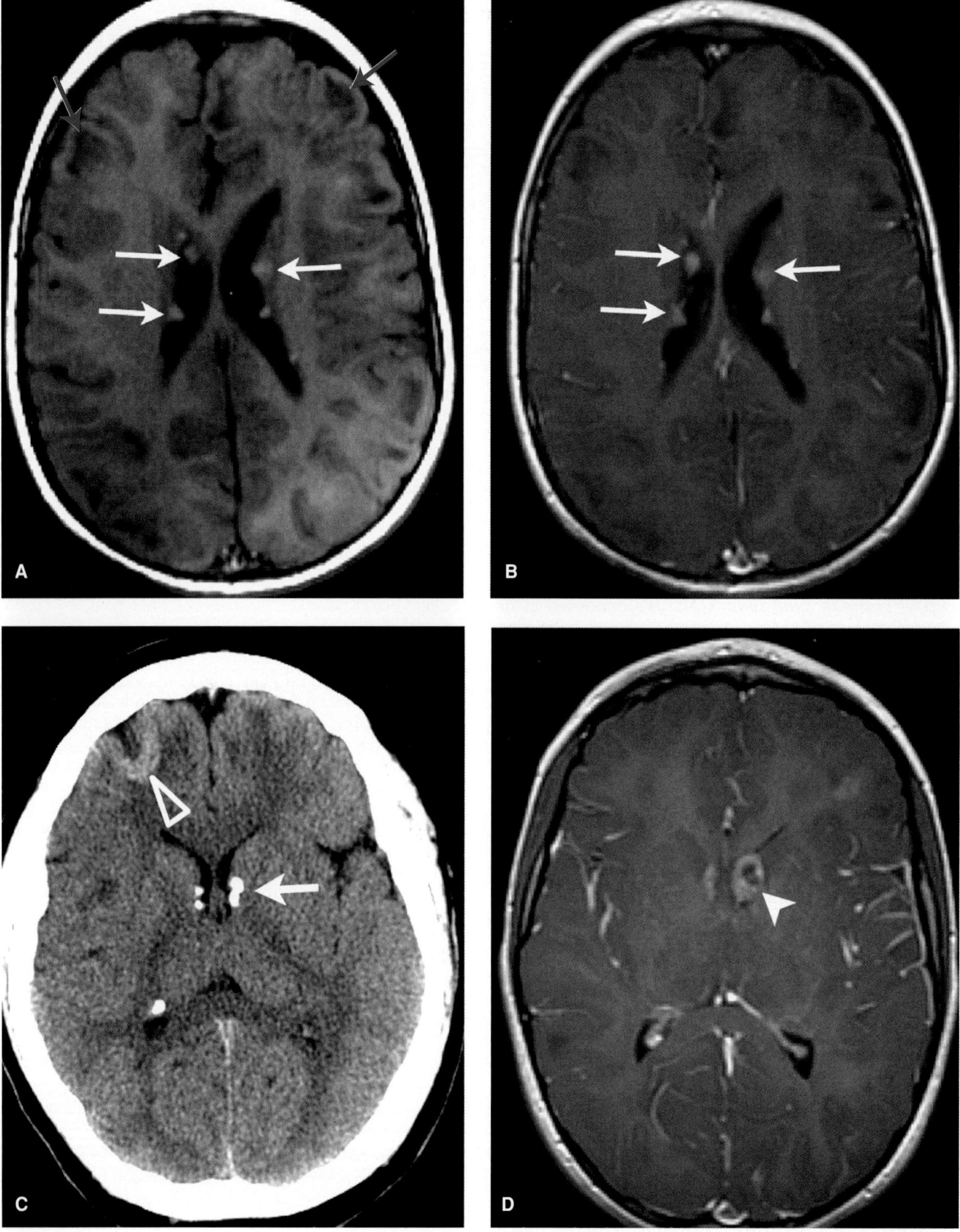

FIGURE 66.29. **Tuberous Sclerosis.** T1WI (**A**), postcontrast T1WI (**B**), CT image (**C**), and postcontrast T1WI (**D**). Numerous subcortical tubers (*red arrows* in **A**) and subependymal nodules (*white arrows* in **A**) are evident on precontrast T1WI. The subependymal nodules enhance mildly (*arrows* in **B**). Enhancement of these benign lesions is common and does not reflect malignancy. Subependymal nodules (*arrow* in **C**) and subcortical tubers (*arrowhead* in **C**) may calcify, best appreciated on CT. Subependymal nodules on MRI may be most conspicuous on gradient echo and T2-weighted imaging, as the lesions are low signal intensity in stark contrast to the high signal intensity CSF within the ventricles. Enhancing nodules in the region of the foramen of Monro (*arrowhead* in **D**) may enlarge, leading to hydrocephalus and are termed subependymal giant cell astrocytoma or "subependymal giant cell astrocytoma (SEGA)."

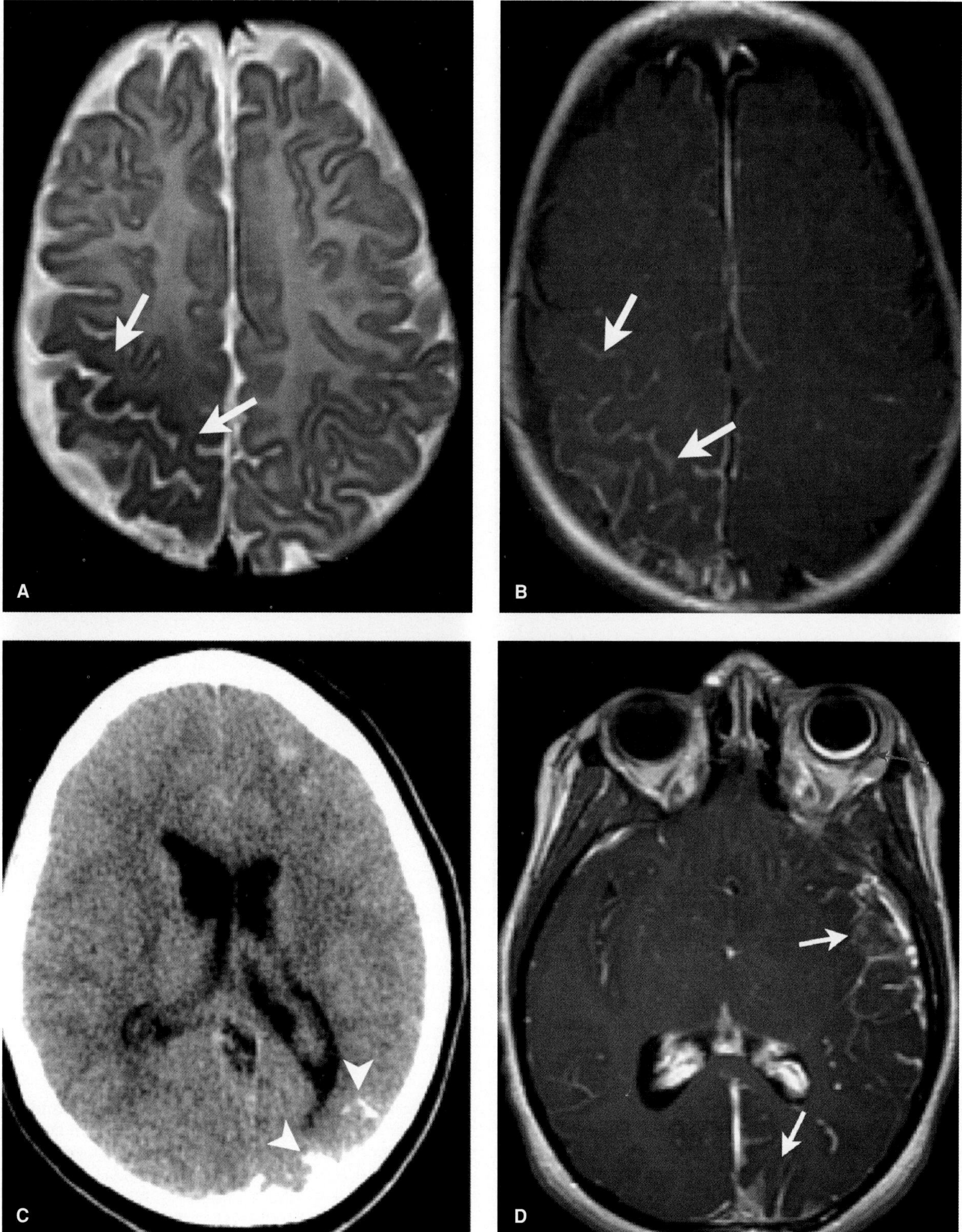

FIGURE 66.30. **Sturge–Weber Syndrome.** T2WI (**A**) and postcontrast T1WI (**B**) in a 3 month old with a port-wine stain. CT image (**C**) and postcontrast T1WI (**D**) from a different patient with Sturge–Weber syndrome. The pathologic condition of the brain is called pial angiomatosis, which is best recognized by contrast enhancement of the cortex and leptomeninges (*arrows* in **B** and **D**). These pial angiomas undergo age-dependent calcification and appear as gyral calcifications on CT (*arrowheads* in **C**) and T2 shortening on MR (*arrows* in **A**). Ipsilateral choroid plexus hypertrophy and choroidal angiomas (*red arrow* in **D**) are other features of this entity.

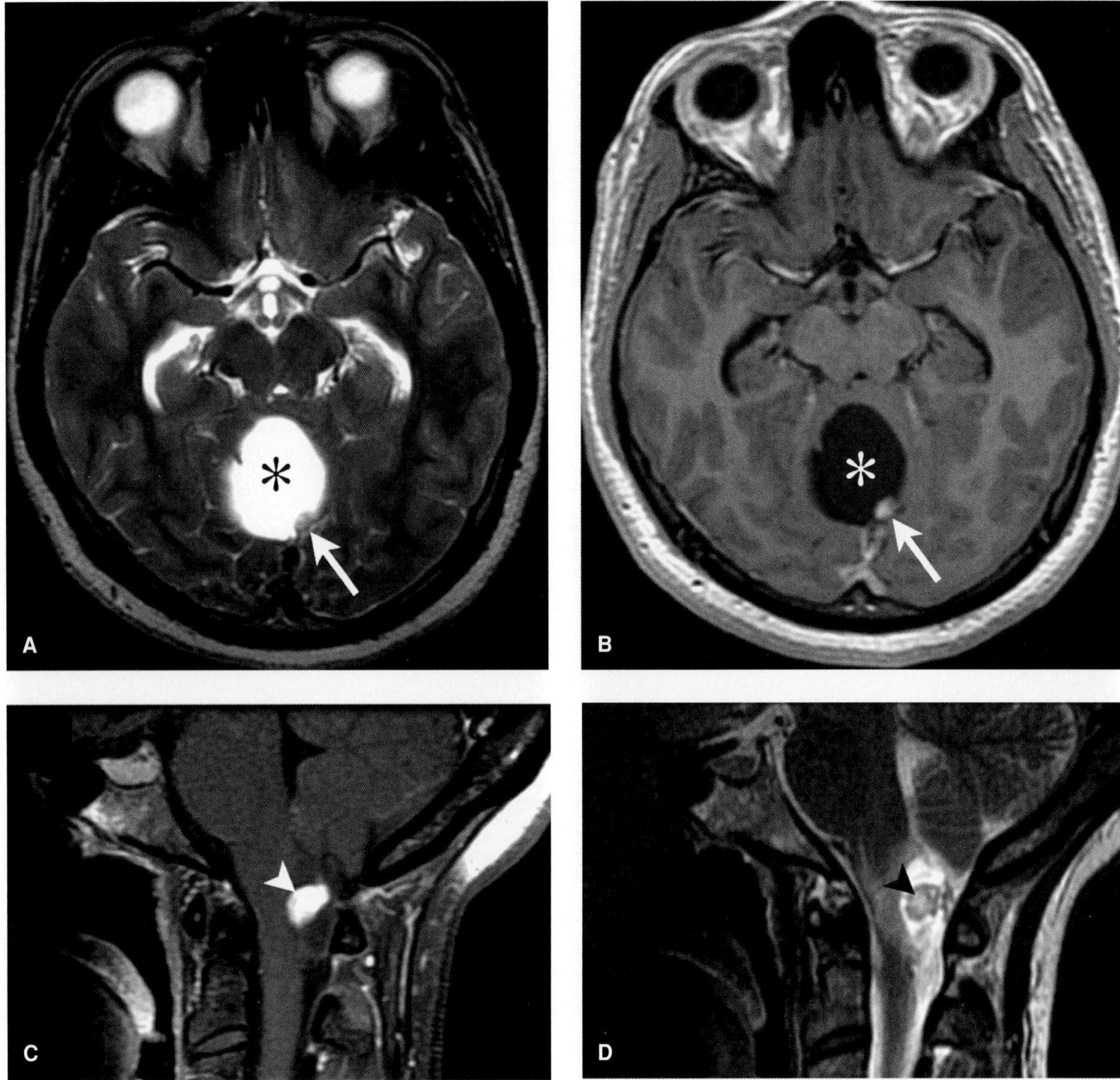

FIGURE 66.31. **von Hippel–Lindau Syndrome.** T2-weighted images (**A**, **D**) and postcontrast T1-weighted images (**B**, **C**). The large cystic lesion (*) with a contrast enhancing mural nodule (*arrows* in **A** and **B**) is classic for cerebellar hemangioblastoma. Often a vascular flow void may be noted associated with the nodule, providing further support for the diagnosis of a vascular neoplasm. The syndrome of von Hippel–Lindau also includes retinal hemangioblastomas; spinal hemangioblastomas (*arrowheads* in **C** and **D**); renal cell carcinoma; pheochromocytoma; renal, hepatic, and pancreatic cysts.

Dorsal Dermal Sinus

Rarely the neural tube will successfully separate from the cutaneous ectoderm and close but a defect in the skin will persist, with a tract that descends into the subcutaneous tissues or spinal canal called a dorsal dermal sinus. There may be an inclusion of skin tissue at the base of the tract, consisting of squamous epithelium alone (epidermoid) or multiple skin elements (dermoid). If unrecognized, a dorsal dermal sinus may present with catastrophic infection, as the tract can provide easy entry of pathogens into the CNS (Fig. 66.34).

Caudal Regression Syndrome

Also known as caudal agenesis, *caudal regression syndrome* is characterized by agenesis of a portion of the caudal spine usually in association with spinal cord, anorectal and/or genitourinary anomalies. While most cases are sporadic infants of diabetic mothers are known to have a higher risk. There are two groups described based on morphology. Group 1 patients have a high (L1 or higher) blunted conus with separation of the anterior and posterior nerve roots in a "double-bundle" configuration. Group 2 have a low-lying tethered cord and may have an additional closed spinal dysraphism such as an intradural lipoma or lipomyelomeningocele.

Myelocystocele

The embryologic basis of this lesion remains uncertain, but instead of a persistent connection with the cutaneous ectoderm, the major abnormality in myelocystocele is a focal dilation of the central canal that causes the cord to protrude

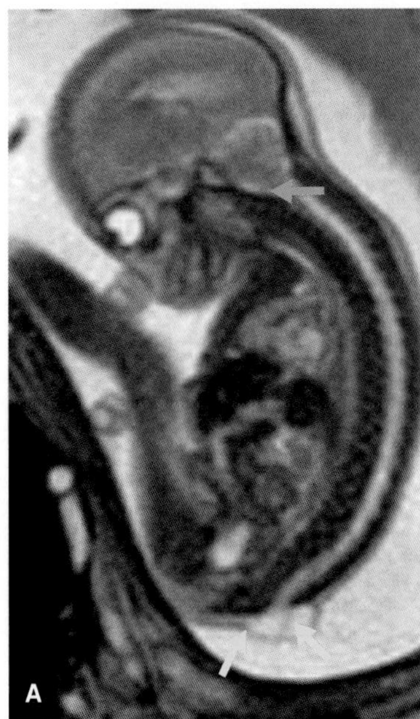

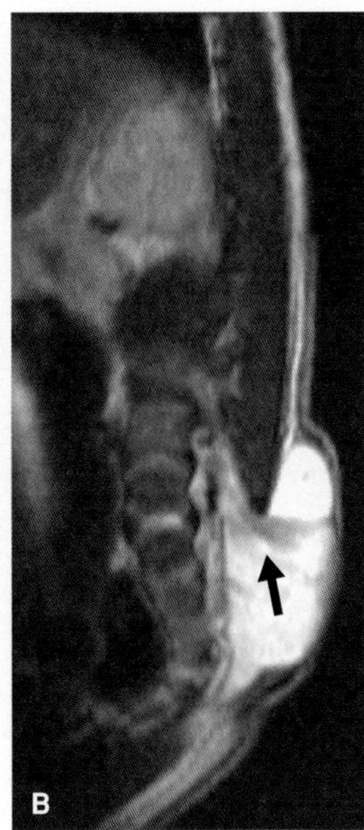

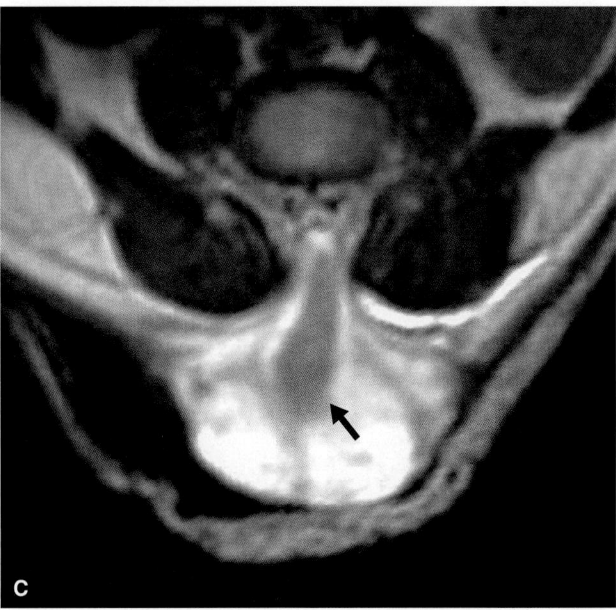

FIGURE 66.32. **Myelomeningocele.** Sagittal T2-weighted image from a fetal MRI (**A**) shows a focal defect in the posterior elements at the lumbosacral junction with the distal cord exposed to the amniotic sac (*yellow arrows*). Note the Chiari II malformation at the craniocervical junction (*blue arrow*). Sagittal (**B**) and axial (**C**) images from a 1 day old with an unrepaired myelomeningocele show the dorsal extension of the spinal cord outside of the canal (*black arrows*). The material dorsal to the lesion is a bandage; the examination was performed with the infant prone.

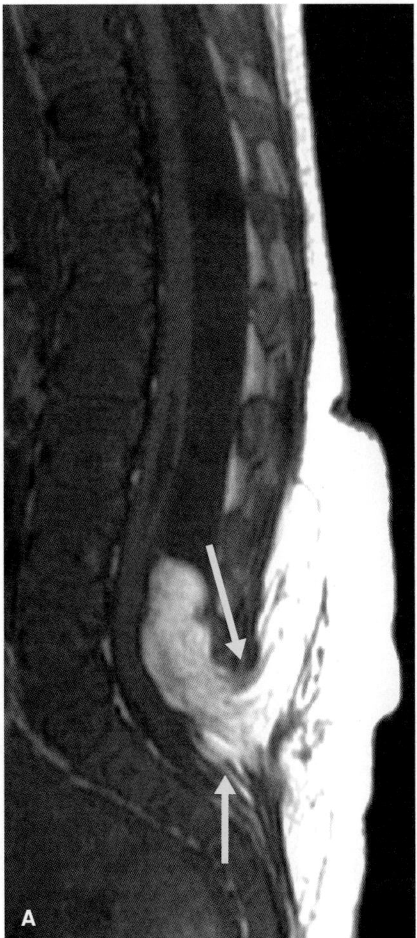

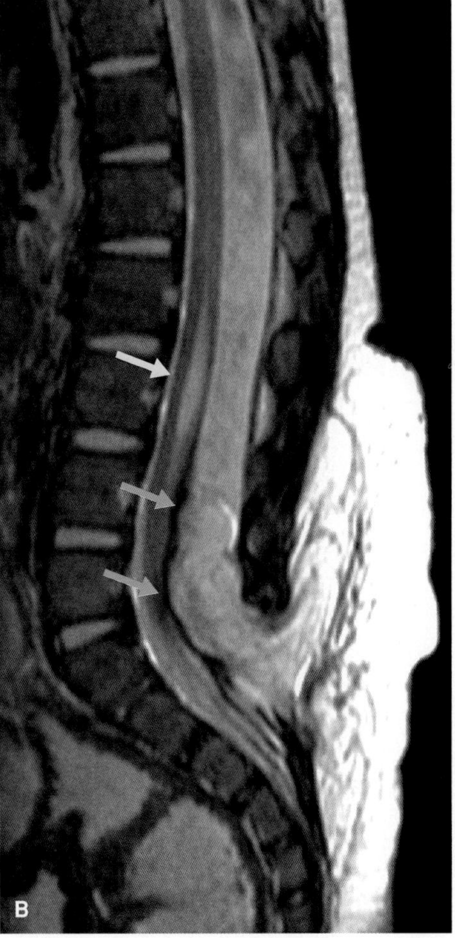

FIGURE 66.33. **Lipomyelocele.** Sagittal T1- (**A**) and T2-weighted (**B**) images of a 3 year old with a lipomyelocele show fatty tissue extending through a large defect in the posterior elements at the lumbosacral junction (*yellow arrow*) into the spinal canal to directly adhere to the dorsal aspect of the spinal cord (placode-lipoma interface). The cord is tethered by the lesion, and there is a small syrinx just cranial to the lipoma (*yellow arrow* in **B**). Note the chemical shift artifact along the dorsal aspect of the cord where the lipoma attaches (*blue arrows*).

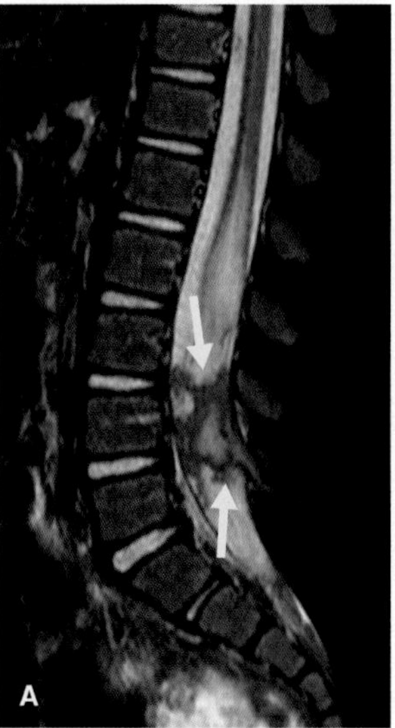

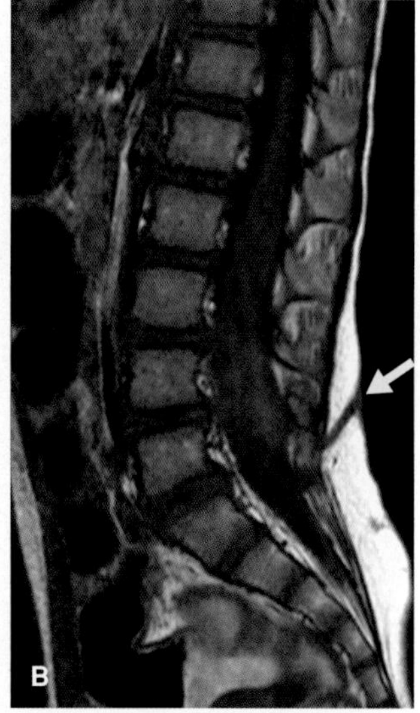

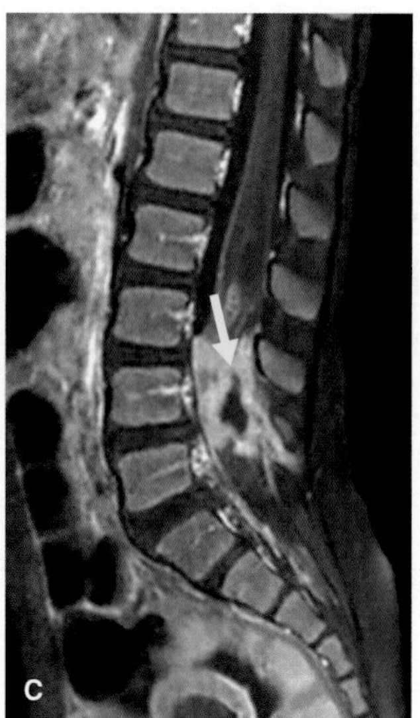

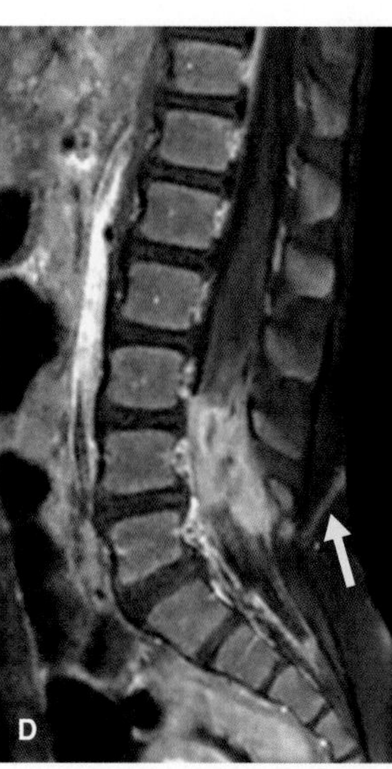

FIGURE 66.34. **Infected Dorsal Dermal Sinus.** Sagittal T2-weighted image (**A**) from a 2 year old with fever and lower extremity weakness shows a heterogeneous mass (arrows) in the spinal canal dorsal to L4, with a tract extending between the L4 and L5 spinous processes. Sagittal T1-weighted image without contrast (**B**) shows the tract extending through the subcutaneous fat to the skin surface (*arrow*). Post-contrast T1-weighted images (**C, D**) show marked enhancement of the intraspinal abscess, with a central region of non-enhancing purulent material (*arrow* in **C**). The tract also enhances (*arrow* in **D**).

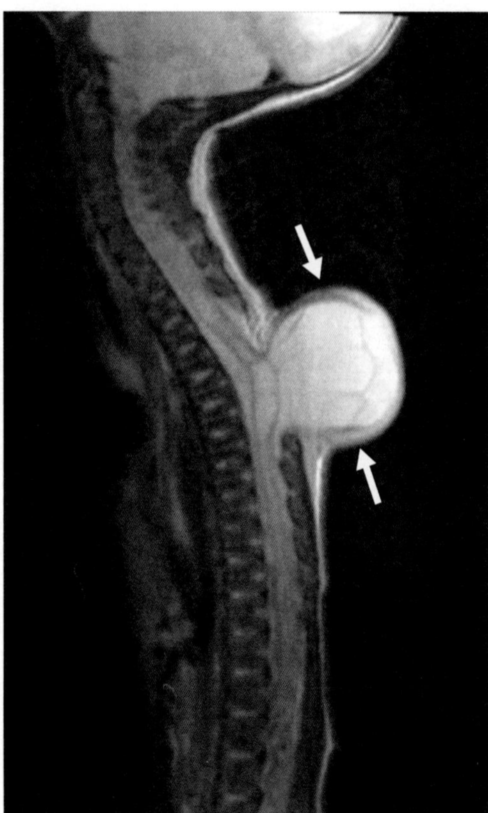

FIGURE 66.35. **Nonterminal Myelocystocele.** Sagittal T2-weighted image of a neonate with an upper thoracic mass shows a skin-covered sac containing a cyst that is surrounded by neural tissue (*arrows*). There is a syrinx in the adjacent thoracic cord and a large defect in the posterior elements. Because the lesion is skin covered it cannot be a myelomeningocele, and because the cystic structure within it is surrounded by neural tissue, it fits the criteria for a nonterminal myelocystocele.

through a defect in the dorsal elements (Fig. 66.35). Skin-covered lesions, myelocystoceles are usually lumbar or lumbosacral (terminal myelocystocele), but can occur in the cervical or thoracic spine (nonterminal myelocystocele), as can any of the congenital spine malformations. Unlike other closed (skin-covered) spinal dysraphisms, myelocystoceles can be associated with hindbrain herniation.

Split Cord Malformations

It is thought that the development of the neural plate and subsequent infolding to form the neural tube is induced by the notochord, a streak of cells situated between the ectoderm and endoderm. If the notochord is divided, two separate neural tubes may form, resulting in two hemicords, called diastematomyelia or split cord malformation (SCM). The two hemicords can each have their own dural sac (Type 1 SCM), in which case they may be separated by a bony spur (Fig. 66.36), or they may reside within a single dural sac (Type 2 SCM). SCMs are frequently "tandem" lesions, found in association with another malformation such as myelomeningocele. This is why it is important to look for additional lesions when a spinal malformation is diagnosed.

Tethered Cord Syndrome

The tethered cord syndrome is a clinical diagnosis based upon the constellation of pain, gait abnormalities, sensory disturbances, and/or lower extremity weakness, in association with a structural abnormality of the distal cord that could be a cause of increased tension or restricted mobility of the conus medullaris. The major congenital spinal malformations listed above all have tethering effects on the distal cord, but some children may have the symptom complex with much less obvious abnormalities, such as thickening or fatty infiltration of the filum terminale (fibrolipoma of the filum). However, these can also be incidental findings in asymptomatic children and adults. Prone

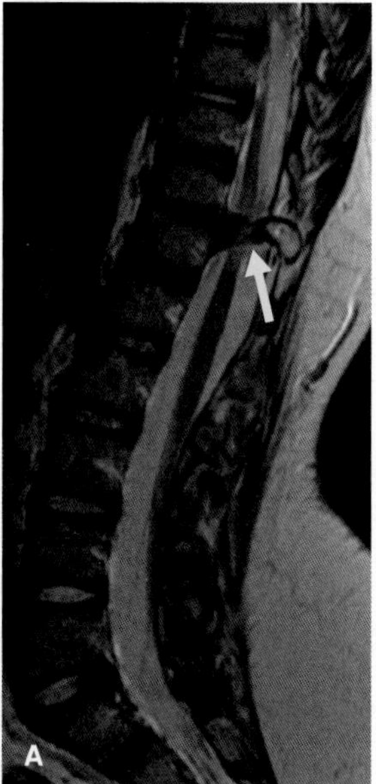

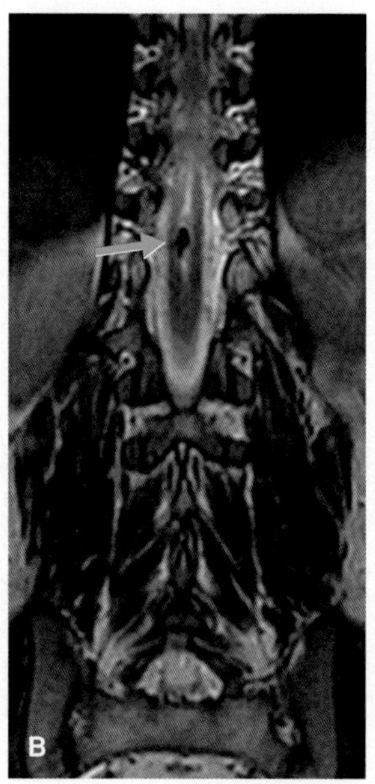

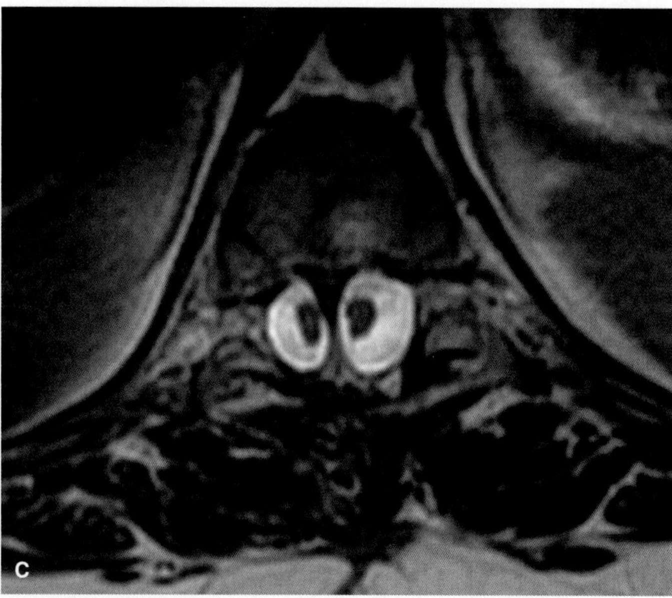

FIGURE 66.36. Type 1 Split Cord Malformation. Sagittal T2-weighted image (**A**) shows a large bony spur (*yellow arrow*) arising from the T11 and T12 vertebrae and extending to the posterior elements. The splitting of the cord into two hemicords, each within its own dural tube, is clearly demonstrated by both the coronal (**B**) and axial (**C**) images at that level. This spur (*blue arrow*) will cause tethering if the two hemicords re-fuse, as they do in this case, with symptoms worsening as the patient grows. Also called diastematomyelia, these malformations are often associated with other congenital spinal abnormalities, so a thorough evaluation of the entire spinal axis is necessary when they are discovered.

or cine imaging demonstrating reduced mobility of the conus may be helpful in clinical decision making (Fig. 66.37).

Syringomyelia

From the same root word as syringe, syringomyelia or syrinx is the term used to describe a cystic cavity within the spinal cord, usually representing the dilated central canal (Fig. 66.38). In that sense it is analogous to hydrocephalus in the brain, in that there is enlargement of a space normally occupied by CSF. Cystic myelomalacia can also be appropriately termed syrinx, but typically communicates with the central canal regardless.

Most syrinxes are the result of congenital hindbrain malformations such as the Chiari I or Chiari II malformation. Obstruction of both the obex and the subarachnoid space

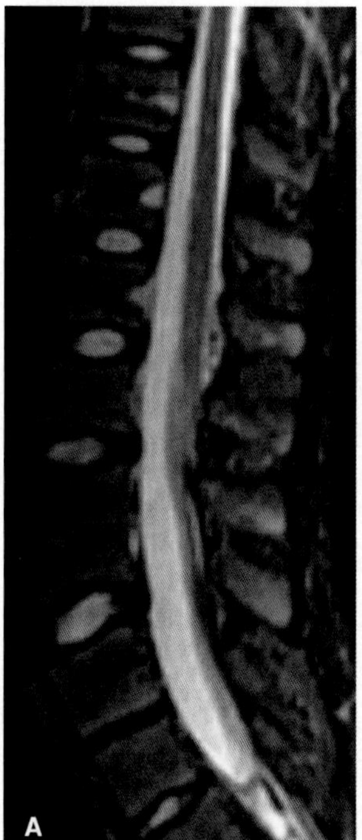

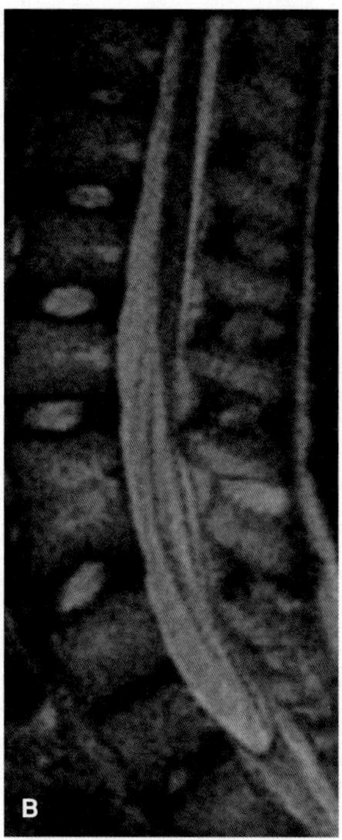

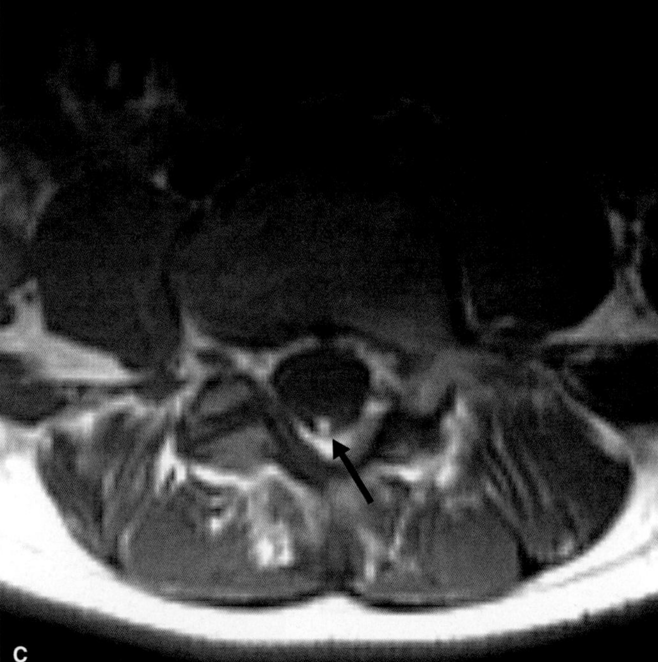

FIGURE 66.37. Fatty Filum Terminale With Tethered Cord. Sagittal STIR image (**A**) in a 12 year of with an anorectal malformation shows a low-normal position of the conus medullaris at L2-3 and a segmentation anomaly of L4 and L5, and to a lesser degree S1/2. An image obtained with the patient prone (**B**) shows no change in position of the cord; normally the conus will fall toward the anterior margin of the spinal canal. Axial T1-weighted image (**C**) in the same patient shows thickening and fatty infiltration of the filum terminale (*arrow*), sometimes called a fibrolipoma of the filum.

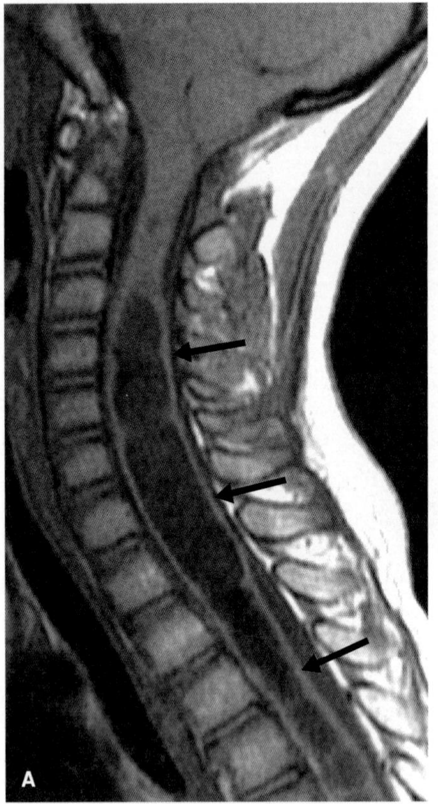

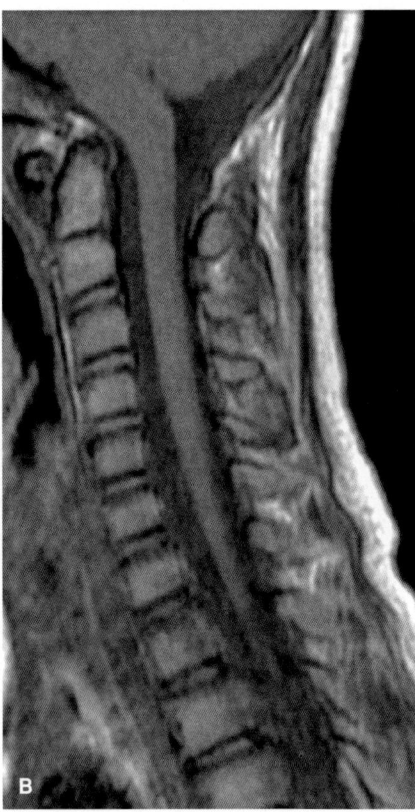

FIGURE 66.38. **Syringomyelia and Chiari I.** Sagittal T1-weighted image (**A**) shows marked crowding at the craniocervical junction caused by an abnormally low position of the cerebellar tonsils, with a large syrinx expanding the spinal cord (*arrows*). Repeat imaging (**B**) in the same patient 5 years after suboccipital decompression and resection of the dysplastic cerebellar tonsils shows collapse of the syrinx cavity.

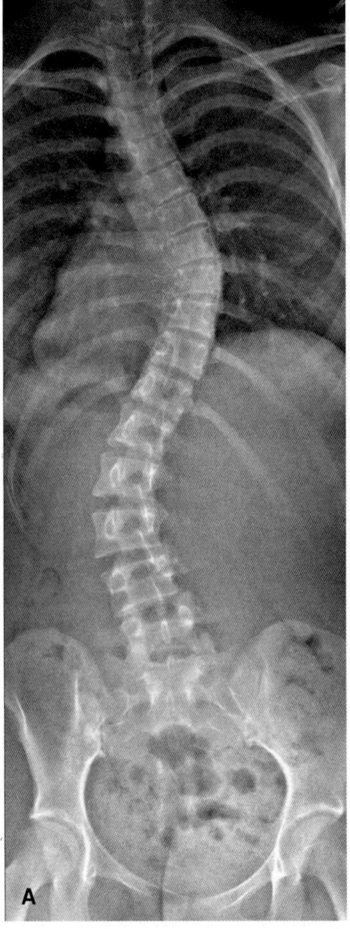

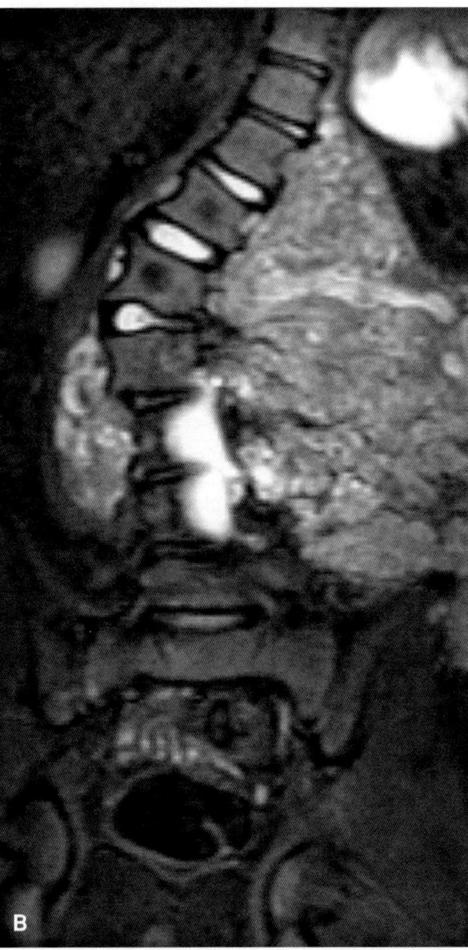

FIGURE 66.39. **Idiopathic and Syndromic Scoliosis.** PA radiograph in a teenager with idiopathic scoliosis (**A**), displayed with the heart to the left side of the image by orthopedic convention. **B:** Coronal STIR image in a teenager with NF-1 and acute lumbar scoliosis shows a large burden of plexiform neurofibroma associated with the curvature.

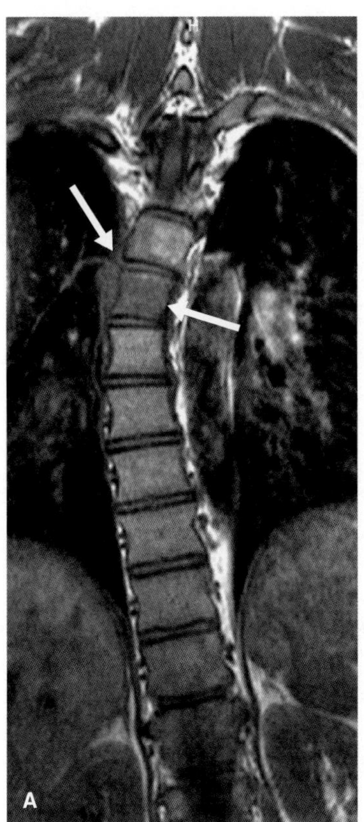

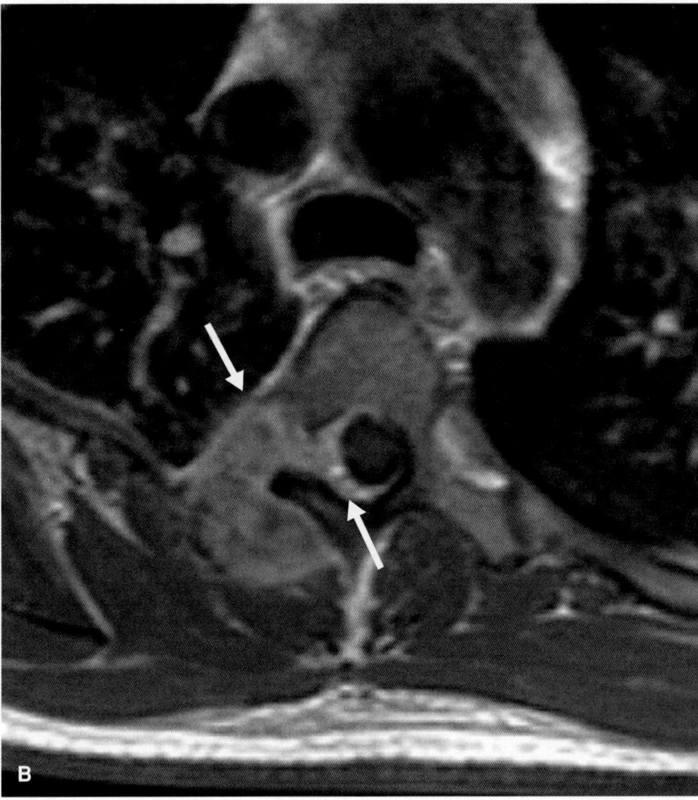

FIGURE 66.40. **Pathologic Scoliosis.** Coronal T1-weighted image of the thoracic spine in a teenager with an acute painful scoliosis (**A**) shows infiltration of the T4 vertebral body and a paraspinal soft tissue mass (*arrows*). Axial T1-weighted image with contrast (**B**) shows the osteosarcoma to enhance diffusely and erode the pedicle and vertebra and invade the spinal canal (*arrows*). Atypical clinical presentation of scoliosis should prompt further investigation with imaging.

at the foramen magnum results in entrapment of CSF within the central canal and progressive dilation. These cases can be successfully treated by surgical decompression of the foramen magnum, relieving the obstruction. Less commonly, syringomyelia can be caused by an obstructing tumor, or adhesions resulting from infection. The normal central canal is frequently visible on MR imaging, and diameters of up to 3 mm are likely of no significance. If a syrinx cavity is identified, careful review of the entire spinal column, with special attention to the craniocervical junction, is required.

Scoliosis

The majority of scoliotic deformities in children (80%) are idiopathic, and are divided into infantile, juvenile, and adolescent types. The adolescent form (age 10 to 18) is the most frequent, with a female preponderance and typically presenting with a primary thoracolumbar curve convex to the right (dextroscoliosis). Scoliosis is defined as any lateral spinal curvature >10 degrees. By convention, the Cobb angle is measured from a 2D radiograph obtained with the patient standing, the orientation of which is horizontally reversed from the conventional display, as if viewing the patient from the back (Fig. 66.39A). Progression is most common in the juvenile form of idiopathic scoliosis and may accelerate during growth spurts. CT with 3D reconstructions is helpful to demonstrate bony anomalies and to display complex curvatures for surgical planning. Nonidiopathic scoliosis may be due to vertebral anomalies such as hemivertebrae or neural anomalies such as SCM or syrinx. Scoliosis may also develop during childhood secondary to neuromuscular conditions such as cerebral palsy and muscular dystrophy. Syndromic etiologies include neurofibromatosis type 1 in which bony dysplasia causes short segment angulation (Fig. 66.39B).

Children may also present with scoliosis secondary to a serious underlying pathology such as tumor or infection. Any new atypical scoliosis, rapidly progressive or painful scoliosis, or neurologic deterioration are indications for urgent imaging (Fig. 66.40). MRI is the imaging modality of choice to evaluate the cord and bone marrow for an underlying condition such as infection, syrinx, cord tethering, or neoplasm.

Suggested Readings

Abdel Razek AA, Kandell AY, Elsorogy LG, Elmongy A, Basett AA. Disorders of cortical formation: MR imaging features. *Am J Neuroradiol* 2009;30(1):4–11.

Barkovich AJ, Guerrini R, Kuzniecky RI, Jackson GD, Dobyns WB. A developmental and genetic classification for malformations of cortical development: Update 2012. *Brain* 2012;135(5):1348–1369.

Barkovich AJ, Millen KJ, Dobyns WB. A developmental and genetic classification for midbrain-hindbrain malformations. *Brain* 2009;132(12):3199–3230.

Garel C, Chantrel E, Brisse H, et al. Fetal cerebral cortex: Normal gestational landmarks identified using prenatal MR imaging. *Am J Neuroradiol* 2001; 22(1):184–189.

Groenendaal F, de Vries LS. Fifty years of brain imaging in neonatal encephalopathy following perinatal asphyxia. *Pediatr Res* 2017;81(1–2):150–155.

Jones BV. Cord cystic cavities: Syringomyelia and prominent central canal. *Semin Ultrasound CT MR* 2017;38(2):98–104.

Manoukian SB, Kowal DJ. Comprehensive imaging manifestations of tuberous sclerosis. *AJR Am J Roentgenol* 2015;204(5):933–943.

Merhar SL, Chau V. Neuroimaging and other neurodiagnostic tests in neonatal encephalopathy. *Clin Perinatol* 2016;43(3):511–527.

Raybaud C. The corpus callosum, the other great forebrain commissures, and the septum pellucidum: Anatomy, development, and malformation. *Neuroradiology* 2010;52(6):447–477.

Robinson AJ. Inferior vermian hypoplasia—Preconception, misconception. *Ultrasound Obstet Gynecol* 2014;43(2):123–136.

Rufener SL, Ibrahim M, Raybaud CA, Parmar HA. Congenital spine and spinal cord malformations—Pictorial review. *AJR Am J Roentgenol* 2010;194(3 Suppl):S26–S37.

Ryabets-Lienhard A, Stewart C, Borchert M, Geffner ME. The optic nerve hypoplasia spectrum: Review of the literature and clinical guidelines. *Adv Pediatr* 2016;63(1):127–146.

Singhal R, Perry DC, Prasad S, Davidson NT, Bruce CE. The use of routine preoperative magnetic resonance imaging in identifying intraspinal anomalies in patients with idiopathic scoliosis: a 10-year review. *Eur Spine J* 2013;22(2):355–359.

Tortori-Donati P, Rossi A, Cama A. Spinal dysraphism: A review of neuroradiological features with embryological correlations and proposal for a new classification. *Neuroradiology* 2000;42(7):471–491.

Vézina G. Neuroimaging of phakomatoses: overview and advances. *Pediatr Radiol* 2015;45 Suppl 3:S433–S442.

Welker KM, Patton A. Assessment of normal myelination with magnetic resonance imaging. *Semin Neurol* 2012;32(1):15–28.

Winter TC, Kennedy AM, Woodward PJ. Holoprosencephaly: a survey of the entity, with embryology and fetal imaging. *Radiographics* 2015;35(1):275–290.

CHAPTER 67 ■ PEDIATRIC CHEST

ALAN S. BRODY

INTRODUCTION

Pediatricians and pediatric radiologists are fond of saying that children are not small adults. This is true, but let's be real here, they're closely related. Much of what you need to know about the pediatric chest will come from your study of the adult chest. In this chapter I will try to emphasize disease processes that are not seen in adults, and the situations where not realizing that children differ from adults will lead you to make mistakes.

THE PEDIATRIC CHEST RADIOGRAPH

The most difficult aspect of imaging the chest in children is probably separating normal from abnormal. In general, the younger the child the larger the heart, the wider the chest relative to the height, and the less well-defined the lung markings, particularly the pulmonary vascularity. Adding difficulty is the frequent lack of cooperation in young children. Chest radiographs (CXRs) cannot be expected to have been obtained at full inflation in all cases, and rotation or otherwise suboptimal positioning may be difficult to avoid (Fig. 67.1).

Single-view CXRs are commonly obtained in children, particularly in infants, but the lateral CXR can add useful information. The lateral provides a second chance to evaluate an uncooperative child. Abnormal lung volume seen only on the frontal view may be due to the level of inspiration, not lung pathology. Heart size is better evaluated with two views. Important tracheal abnormalities may be seen only on lateral view.

Repeating imaging studies is discouraged, particularly in children. In the case of the CXR this may be a false economy. There is no detectable risk from the radiation exposure from a second CXR, and risks from additional imaging or other diagnostic testing can be avoided if a question is answered by obtaining a better CXR.

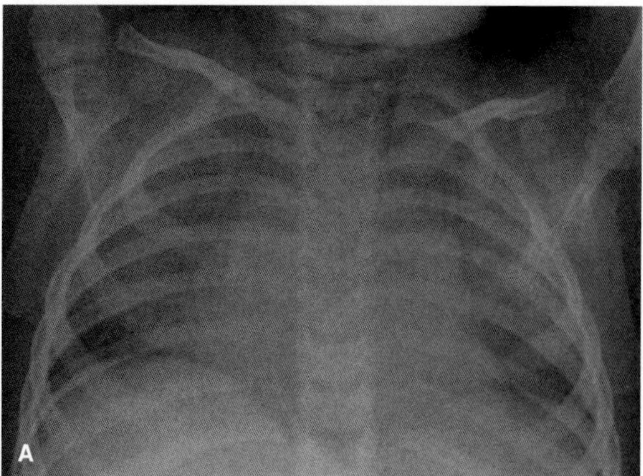

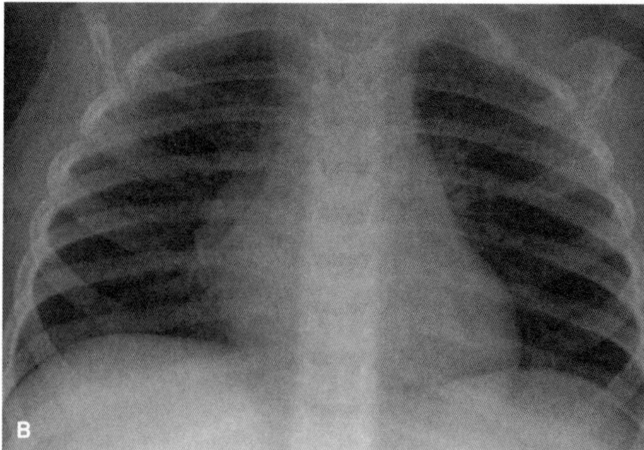

FIGURE 67.1. **Always Carefully Assess the Quality of CXRs, and Have a Low Threshold for Repeating Limited Studies That Suggest Pathology.** Initial chest radiograph (**A**) obtained at expiration could be interpreted as showing cardiomegaly, pulmonary edema, or bilateral ill-defined infiltrates. A repeat CXR a few minutes later (**B**) is normal.

The Heart

In a newborn infant, the transverse cardiac diameter may be up to 60% of the transverse dimension of the chest measured between the inner rib margins. The cardiothoracic ratio decreases as the child grows older, and should be less than 50%, with the heart appearing similar to an adult, by the second decade.

It is widely accepted that the frontal radiograph is more likely to falsely suggest cardiomegaly than the lateral CXR. A guide for normal heart size is that a line drawn along the posterior tracheal wall on the lateral CXR should pass posterior to the heart. While this is a useful guide, comparisons with cross-sectional imaging have shown that heart size on CXR does not correlate well with true chamber volumes.

Cardiac configuration, particularly in congenital heart disease, has been used to suggest specific types of heart disease for many years, but with very little success. Congenital heart disease occurs in about 1% of the population, and the heart will appear normal in many or most of these. An appearance suggesting a "boot-shaped heart" or "egg on a string" is probably more likely due to normal variation than to the malformation classically associated with that description.

The right margin of the left atrium is visible in one-third of normal children. When well seen this can simulate a mediastinal mass.

The aortic knob is often difficult to see in the first several months of life. See below for tracheal findings of aortic arch abnormalities. The ascending aorta is never prominent in normal children. The location of the descending aorta may be suggested by increased attenuation of the pedicles on the side of the overlying aorta.

The Thymus

The thymus is the "elephant in the room" when evaluating the chest in young children. The thymus is proportionately largest at birth, but continues to grow, more slowly than the child, until puberty, when it is reaches its maximum size. The thymus then atrophies, but can still be seen as well-defined anterior mediastinal soft tissue through young adulthood. In the first year of life, the thymus can be the dominant structure in the chest, sometimes as prominent as the heart (Fig. 67.2). It widens the superior mediastinum, often obscures the aortic

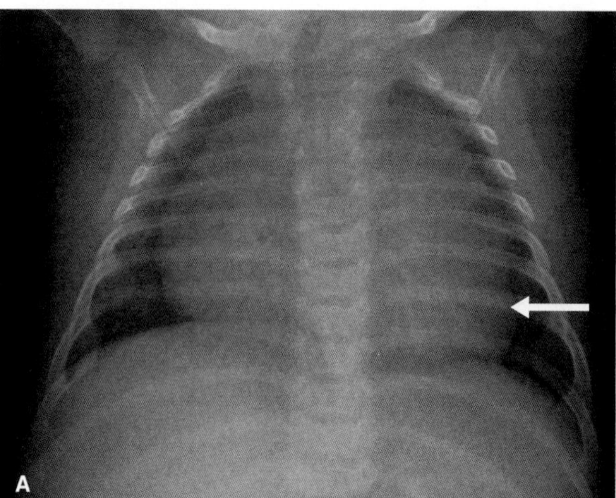

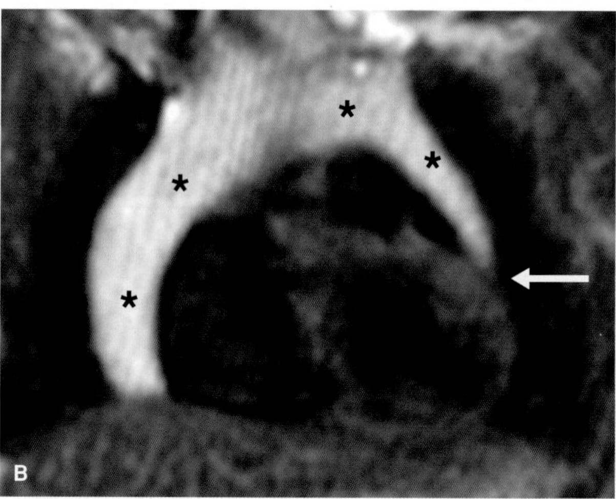

FIGURE 67.2. **Thymus on CXR (A) and MRI (B).** Nearly the entire cardiomediastinal silhouette is formed by the thymus (*). The right lobe forms the entire right cardiomediastinal border. A left-sided thymic notch indicates the lower edge of the left lobe of the thymus with only a small portion of the cardiac silhouette below.

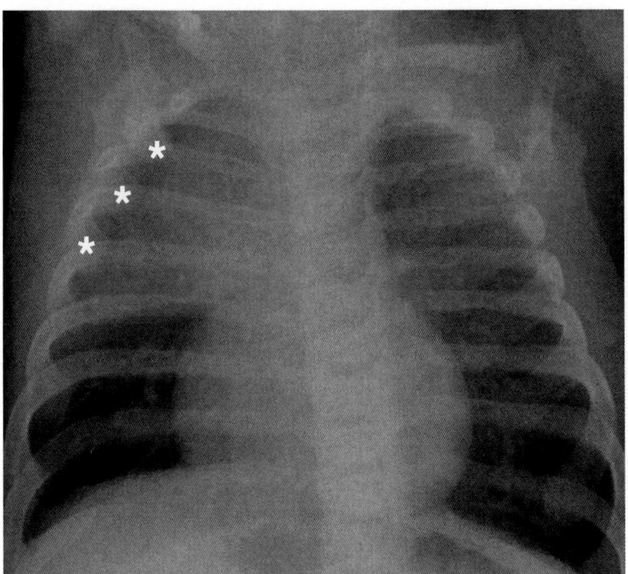

FIGURE 67.3. **Large Normal Right Lobe of the Thymus.** The anterior rib ends (*) indent the soft thymus causing the "wave sign."

arch, and can extend along the right cardiac border to the diaphragm and simulate cardiomegaly. This apparent enlargement of the heart is only seen on the frontal view; one reason that the lateral view is regarded as more reliable than the frontal view when evaluating heart size.

The thymus is soft, so it does not narrow or displace vessels or other structures. Anterior rib end impressions cause a wavy edge laterally (the thymic wave sign) (Fig. 67.3) that is often better seen on shallow oblique views. On the lateral view, the thymus is denser anteriorly, and often along the minor fissure. A thymic notch can often be seen on frontal view marking the transition between the inferior border of the thymus and the cardiac margin.

In newborns the thymus can involute in response to physiologic stress within 6 hours. The thymus can also grow following recovery from a period of stress, although this takes weeks or months. This "thymic rebound" is most often seen after the completion of chemotherapy, and can be seen in other situations of prolonged physiologic stress such as of multiple stage cardiac surgeries (Fig. 67.4).

Additional information on the thymus is included in the section on the mediastinum.

The Lungs

Lung volume is an important aspect of CXR interpretation in children. Low lung volumes simulate cardiomegaly and pulmonary edema (Fig. 67.1). Hyperinflation is the primary finding in asthma, and is much more common in viral than in bacterial pneumonia. Unfortunately there are no simple measurements that have been shown to correlate highly with lung volume. Counting ribs provides a rough assessment of lung volume. The top of the hemidiaphragm is closer to the anterior than the posterior ribs supporting the use of an anterior rib count. The 6th anterior rib should be the first to cross the diaphragm. An inspiration of less than 5 or more than 7 ribs is very likely to be abnormal. It is a good rule to count ribs before suggesting cardiomegaly, a hazy appearance of the parenchyma, or hyperinflation. The appearance of the diaphragm should also be considered, as a flattened diaphragm suggests hyperinflated lungs.

If lung attenuation is asymmetric, it may be difficult to determine which lung is abnormal. A useful guide is that the lung with the more normal appearance of the pulmonary vasculature is usually the normal lung (Fig. 67.5). An expiratory CXR to evaluate for air trapping, as would be seen with an obstructing foreign body, can be useful. In children who can't follow instructions, bilateral decubitus radiographs are usually easier to obtain and interpret (Fig. 67.5). In this context, gravity is relied upon to create expiration and to demonstrate air trapping in a lung that fails to compress when on the downward side. Obliterative bronchiolitis, also called Swyer–James–MacLeod syndrome when asymmetric will cause one lung to

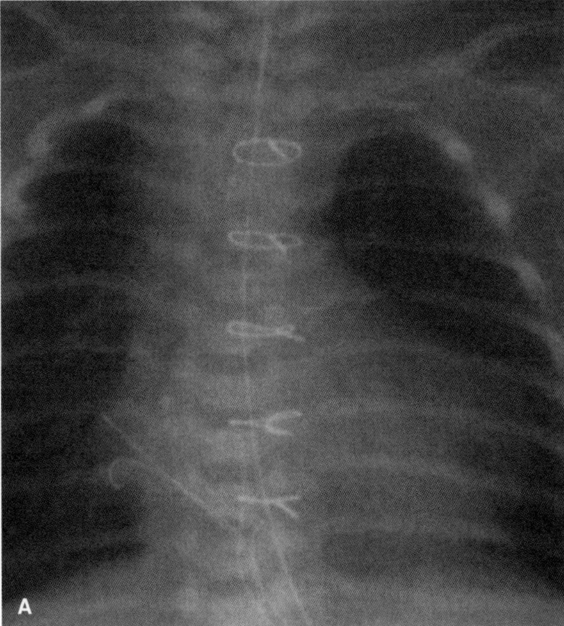

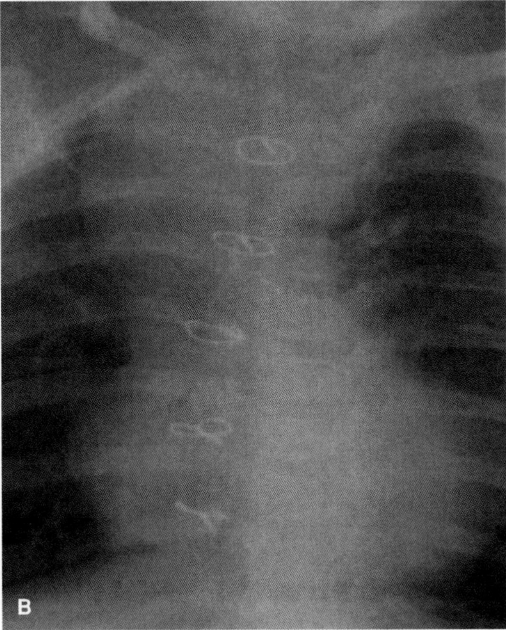

FIGURE 67.4. **Rebound (Asymmetric) Enlargement of the Thymus. A:** Early postoperative CXR shows a normal mediastinal contour. **B:** Four months later a large right paratracheal mass has developed. *(continued)*

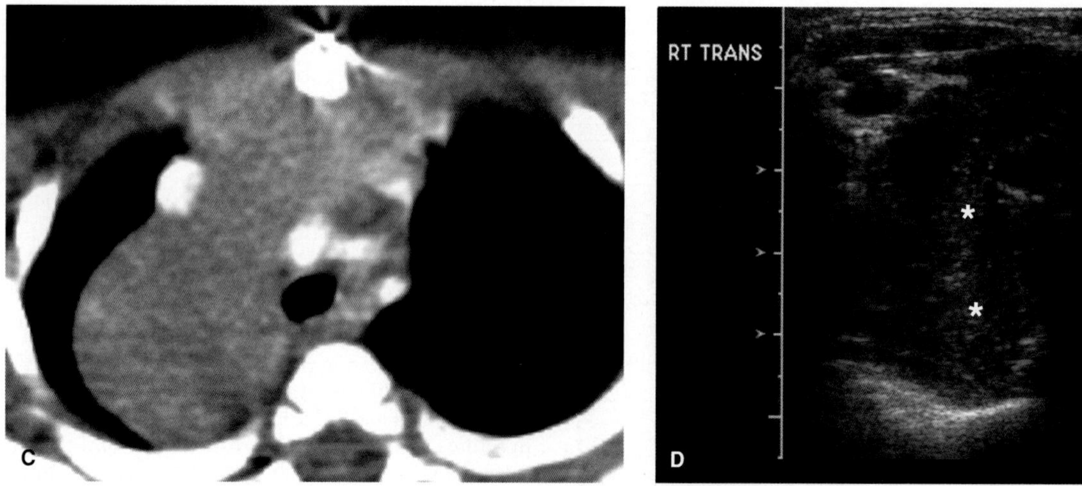

FIGURE 67.4. (*Continued*) An aneurysm was suspected but CT (**C**) and US (**D**) demonstrate normal thymic tissue (*). The "dot-dash" appearance of the thymus is very useful for distinguishing normal thymus from other tissues.

be hyperlucent (Fig. 67.6). Asymmetric pulmonary vascularity or mild hypoplasia may result in a hyperdense lung.

The Trachea

The normal trachea is round, and similar in size from the thoracic inlet to the carina. An anterior impression at the level of the brachiocephalic (innominate) artery crossing is a common finding in children when it is mild, narrowing the tracheal diameter less than 50%. A greater degree of narrowing may be associated with symptoms. A decrease in the anteroposterior size of the trachea otherwise suggests tracheomalacia or extrinsic compression. The tracheal air column is particularly valuable as an indicator of aortic arch abnormalities. On a frontal expiratory CXR the trachea often buckles, at times dramatically (Fig. 67.7). The trachea always buckles in the direction opposite to the location of the aortic arch.

The normal trachea lies slightly to the right of the midline, due to the position of the aortic arch. A true midline trachea is abnormal, and a sign of a double aortic arch although this is rarely appreciated prospectively. Often more useful than the position of the arch, which is affected by rotation, is the presence of an impression on the tracheal air column. A focal right-sided impression on the trachea is almost always due to a right arch (Fig. 67.8). Bilateral impressions, right higher than left are classically seen with a double arch. Patients with symptomatic vascular rings have been reported to have tracheal abnormalities in all cases. The abnormality, typically an impression on the tracheal air column, may be seen only on the lateral view.

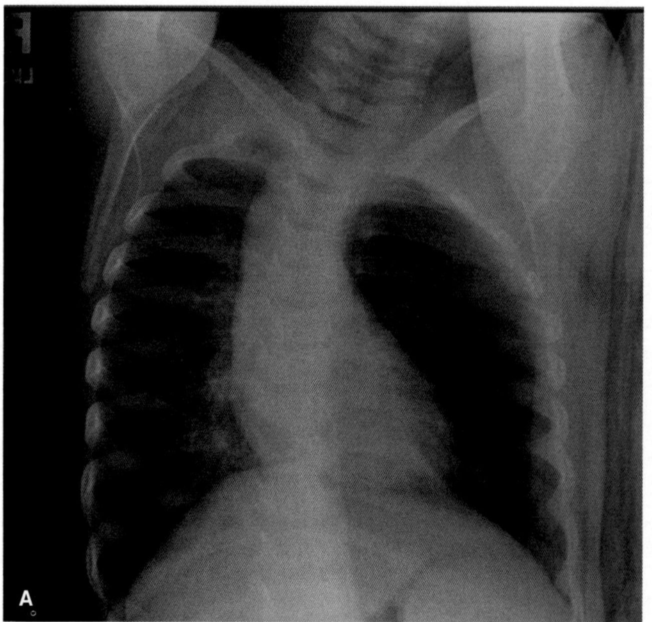

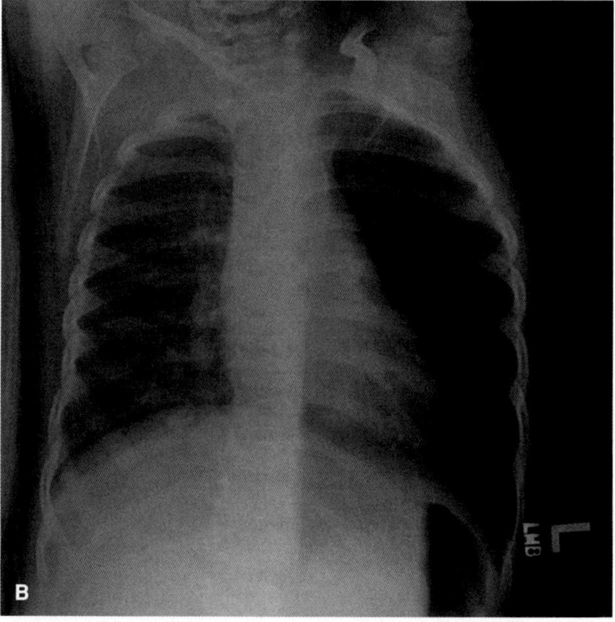

FIGURE 67.5. Air Trapping due to a Foreign Body. A right lateral decubitus image (**A**) demonstrates the normal collapse of the "down" lung and the hyperinflation of the "up" lung. Left lateral decubitus image (**B**) demonstrates persistent hyperinflation of the "down" lung. A single decubitus image may be sufficient, but in subtle cases comparing both decubitus images is very helpful.

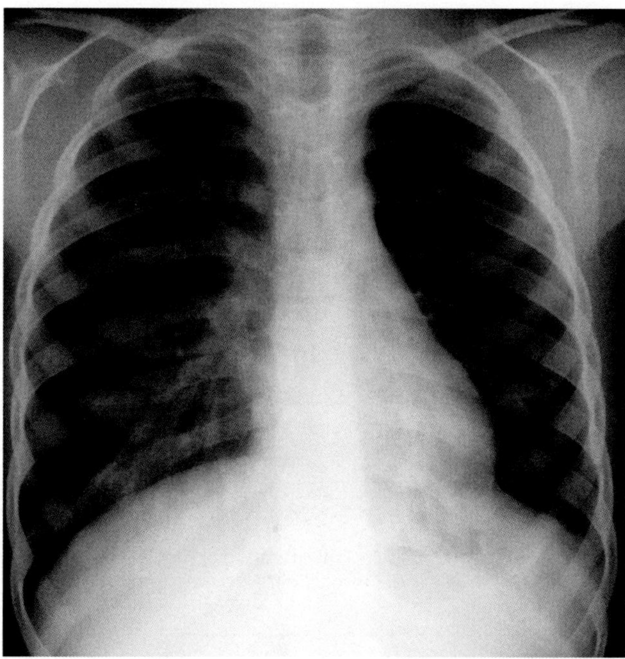

FIGURE 67.6. **Swyer–James Syndrome (Bronchiolitis Obliterans).** The left lung is small and relatively hyperlucent when compared with the right lung. The left pulmonary vascularity is decreased. Lung volume can be increased, normal, or decreased in Swyer–James syndrome. Air trapping due to a foreign body will usually have increased lung volume, and should not have decreased lung volume in the absence of atelectasis.

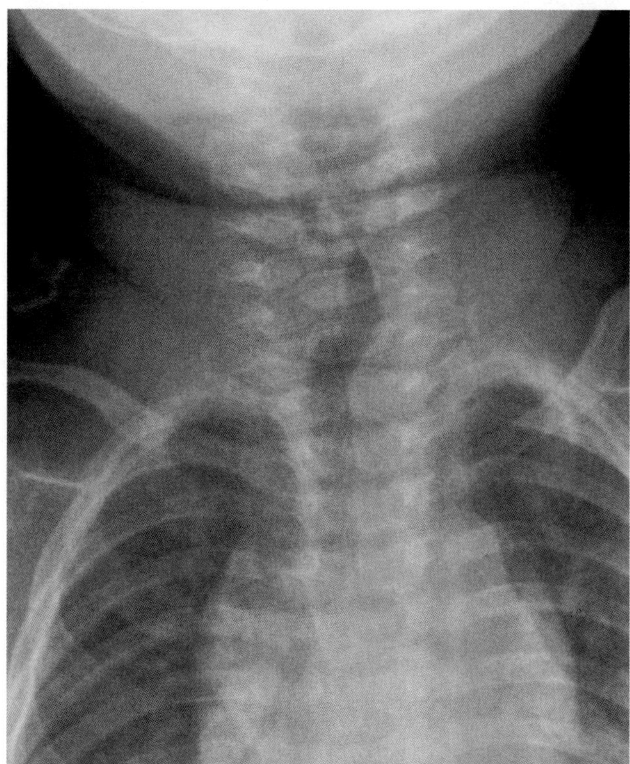

FIGURE 67.7. **Normal Tracheal Buckling.** The sharp angles of the buckled trachea are very different from the more rounded displacement seen with masses. The preserved tracheal diameter is also a clue to normal buckling. Remember, the trachea always buckles away from the aortic arch.

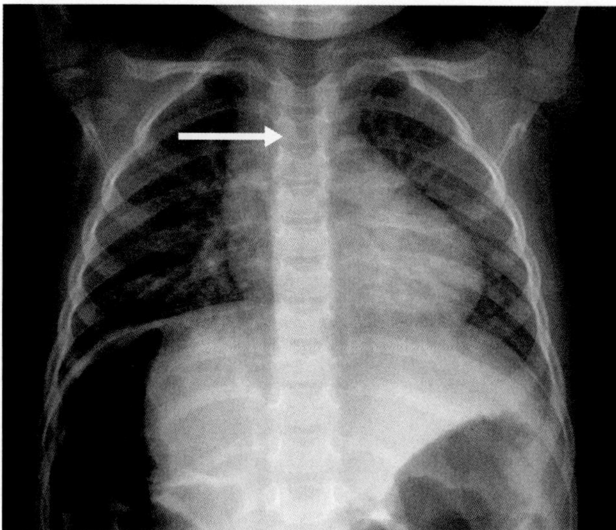

FIGURE 67.8. **Right-Sided Impression on the Trachea in a Patient With a Right Aortic Arch (and Chilaiditi's).**

THE NEONATAL CHEST

This section, and most on the subject, discusses neonatal lung disease separately from heart disease. This is reasonable as the presence of heart disease is usually suspected clinically and determined quickly. Without history, however, increased pulmonary vascularity and parenchymal changes of pulmonary edema can be difficult or impossible to distinguish from lung disease. The different types of neonatal lung disease have patterns that can be recognized, but the most important things to recognize are positions of lines and tubes, and complications of care, particularly air leaks.

Neonatal Lung Disease

Four patterns of chest radiographic abnormality can provide a framework for identifying the different types of lung disease seen in the first week of life.

Diffuse ground-glass opacity suggests neonatal surfactant deficiency. Hyaline membrane disease and infant respiratory distress syndrome are common synonyms. The ground-glass appearance is granular, not hazy, and should be very evenly distributed throughout the lungs (Fig. 67.9A). This differentiation requires experience, which can be difficult to obtain as surfactant deficiency is treated early with exogenous surfactant and the findings of surfactant deficiency resolve almost immediately (Fig. 67.9B). There should be no findings suggesting pleural fluid. Either asymmetry or fluid suggests the possibility of Group B streptococcal pneumonia which can closely simulate the appearance of surfactant deficiency. Exogenous surfactant is administered by endotracheal tube and it may be distributed unevenly, and then can cause a heterogeneous appearance.

Bilaterally symmetrical coarse linear and branching opacities suggest meconium aspiration (Fig. 67.10). In near term or term infants stress in the immediate prenatal period can cause the fetus to pass meconium into the amniotic fluid. Aspirated meconium-stained fluid causes mechanical and chemical airway trauma due to its particulate nature and the presence of irritants including bile. The result is areas of atelectasis and inflammation alternating with areas of hyperinflation. The lungs are usually hyperinflated. While the mechanism

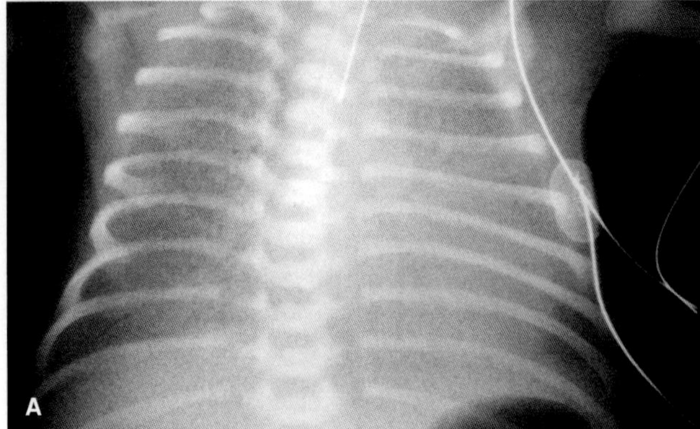

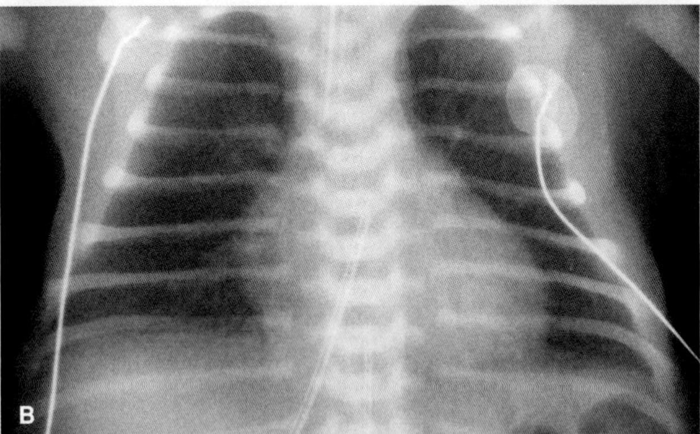

FIGURE 67.9. **Surfactant Deficiency Disease. A:** Shortly after birth, the lung volumes are low with granular diffusely increased attenuation. There are no pleural effusions and the opacity is evenly distributed throughout both lungs. These features help to distinguish surfactant deficiency from other causes of diffuse opacity. Air bronchograms, as seen in this child, may or may not be present. **B:** After treatment with endotracheal surfactant, lung volumes have dramatically improved and lung opacity has virtually disappeared.

is different, the appearance can be very similar to old BPD (see below). In meconium aspiration, the CXR abnormality appears almost immediately and improves over time. Age and clinical information therefore allow easy differentiation.

Linear opacities, central greater than peripheral particularly when radiating from the hila, suggest retained lung fluid, also called transient tachypnea of the newborn (Fig. 67.11A).

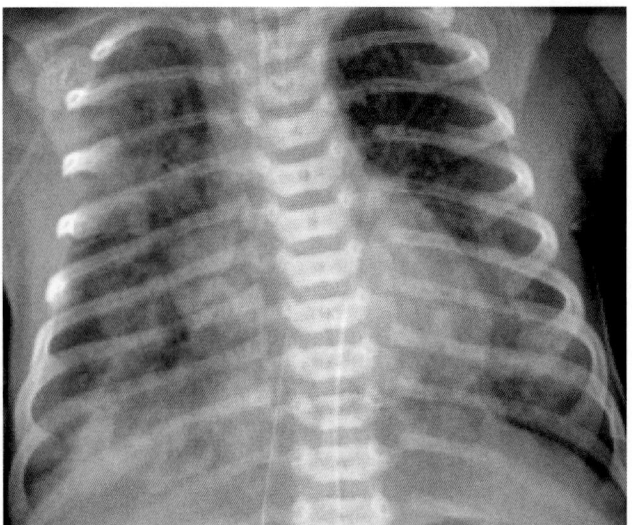

FIGURE 67.10. **Meconium Aspiration.** Hyperinflation and coarse linear and nodular opacities throughout both lungs is typical of meconium aspiration.

This occurs when fetal lung fluid is not fully cleared at the time of birth, and is then absorbed from the alveoli and cleared through lymphatics. In addition to the linear opacities reflecting distended lymphatics there is commonly pleural fluid. Lack of normal thoracic compression during vaginal birth as may occur in precipitous delivery or Cesarean section has been suggested as the mechanism although this is an area of dispute. Retained lung fluid resolves both clinically and radiographically by 72 hours (Fig. 67.11B) and should not be suggested in older infants.

The presence of ill-defined asymmetric opacities is much less specific than the above patterns, but neonatal pneumonia (Fig. 67.12) and pulmonary hemorrhage are possible causes of this pattern. Pulmonary hemorrhage in newborns, unlike in older children or adults is symptomatic, presenting with blood in the endotracheal tube. It is very unlikely that a radiologist will be the first to suggest this possibility. Neonatal pneumonia is very difficult to diagnose by any means, and there are no data that allow assessment of the accuracy of CXRs in identifying neonatal pneumonia. Suggesting the possibility of pneumonia on a chest radiograph is also unlikely to affect clinical

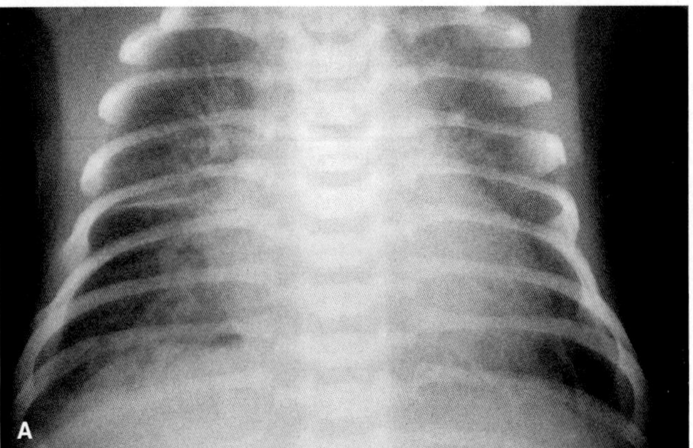

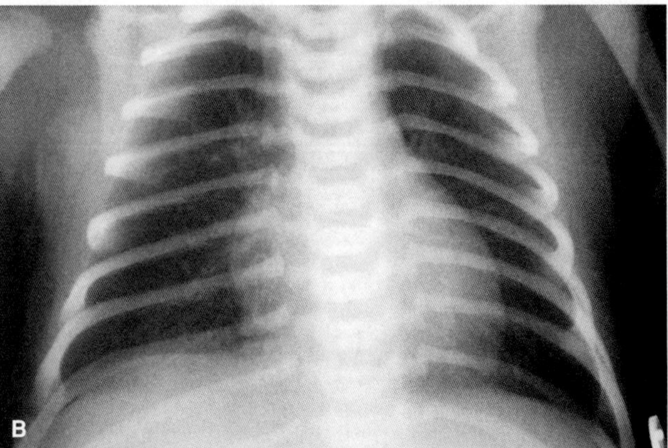

FIGURE 67.11. **Retained Lung Fluid. A:** On the first day of life, the lungs of this term newborn show diffuse haziness, streaky parahilar opacities, and bilateral pleural effusions. **B:** The following day, all the abnormalities have resolved, which is the typical sequence of events in an infant with retained lung fluid. Retained lung fluid is a diagnosis of exclusion. Do not suggest this diagnosis in a child more than 72 hours old!

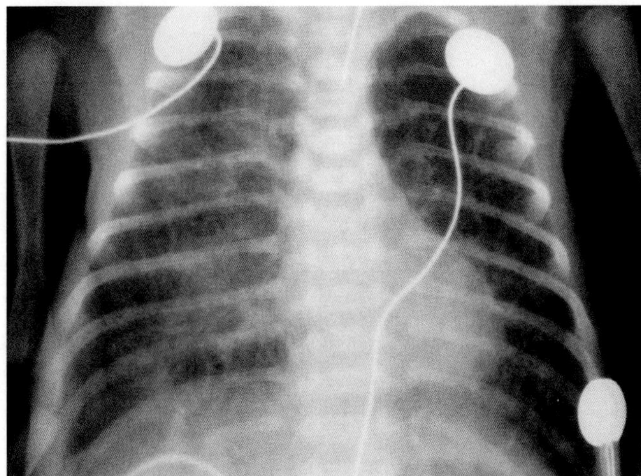

FIGURE 67.12. **Neonatal Pneumonia.** The appearance of neonatal pneumonia is nonspecific. An asymmetric appearance with confluent opacities should raise concern for pneumonia. Neonatal pneumonia is rare, and other causes including pulmonary hemorrhage can produce this appearance.

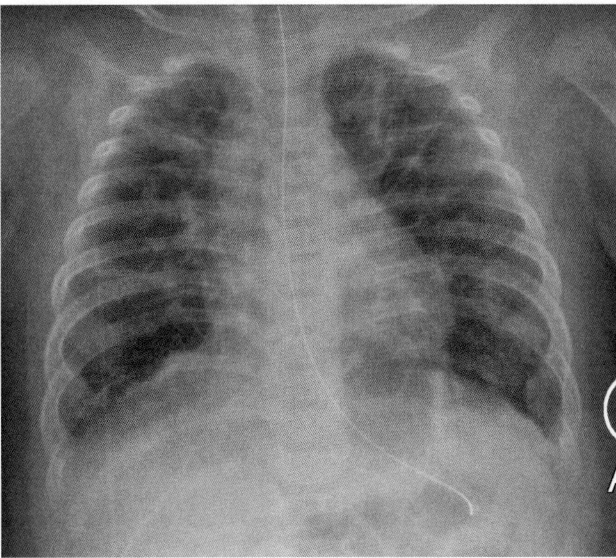

FIGURE 67.14. **"Old BPD" Coarse Linear and Reticular Opacities Are Distributed Throughout the Lungs.** The lungs are hyperinflated.

care as most newborn infants in the NICU will be on antibiotics with closely observed respiratory status. This information is included for completeness and because atelectasis causing persistent asymmetric opacities seems to be uncommon in newborn infants and so asymmetric opacities may be more likely to reflect a true abnormality than in older children or adults.

Pneumonia due to Group B streptococcus (GBS) has a different appearance than pneumonias caused by other organisms. GBS is more likely to present with diffuse ground-glass opacities which can simulate surfactant deficiency (Fig. 67.13). The appearance may be indistinguishable from surfactant deficiency, but the presence of pleural fluid suggests infection rather than uncomplicated surfactant deficiency. In the immediate neonatal period, GBS usually causes pneumonia, later in early infancy GBS is more likely to cause meningitis.

Chronic lung disease becomes the most common cause of lung abnormalities in older infants in the neonatal ICU. Bronchopulmonary dysplasia (BPD), is the term used for this chronic lung disease. BPD was initially described in the 1960s, but the disease described at that time was largely secondary to barotrauma and oxygen toxicity, related to treatment. The pathophysiology of classic BPD was described in the 1960s as areas of hyperinflation alternating with opacities due to atelectatic lung that is due to inflammation earlier in the course that progresses to fibrosis. This appearance still occurs, and is often referred to as "old BPD" (Fig. 67.14). Current treatment results in less trauma and now BPD often has a relatively homogeneous hazy appearance (Fig. 67.15). This has been called "new BPD." The pathophysiology that has been suggested is diffuse capillary leak.

Airleak

Pneumothorax. The appearance of pneumothorax in neonates differs from older children and adults. Neonatal CXRs are generally obtained supine, and the large abdomen of the

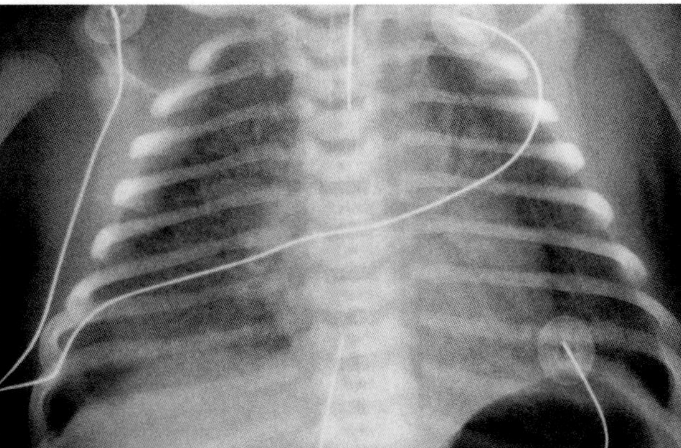

FIGURE 67.13. **Neonatal Pneumonia due to Group B Beta Streptococcus, Unlike Other Causes of Pneumonia GBS Can Simulate Surfactant Deficiency.** The lungs are diffusely hazy, with a granular appearance that is similar to that seen with hyaline membrane disease. More heterogeneous opacity and the presence of pleural effusions can suggest the diagnosis, especially in a term or near term infant. Remember that pneumonia is rare, and that surfactant deficiency is common in premature infants.

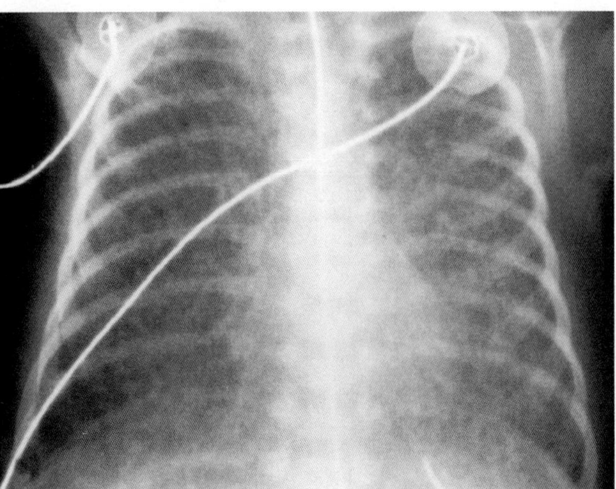

FIGURE 67.15. **"New BPD."** The diffuse hazy opacity is thought to reflect capillary leak.

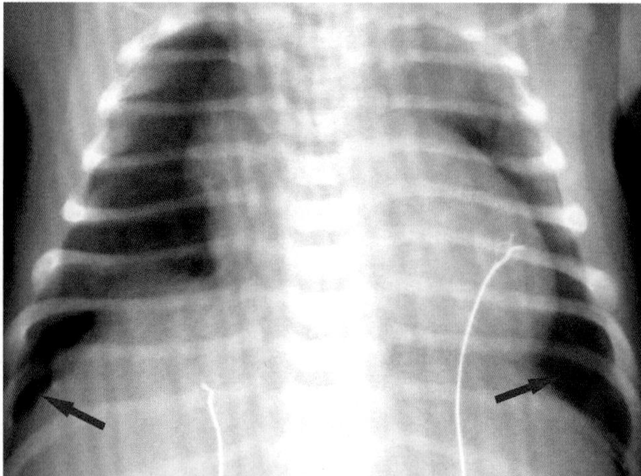

FIGURE 67.16. **Bilateral Pneumothoraces in a Neonate.** In a supine infant the anterior pneumothoraces (*arrows*) cause increased radiolucency and sharpened definition along the mediastinum on the right and the heart border on the left. The costophrenic angles are deepened and sharply defined.

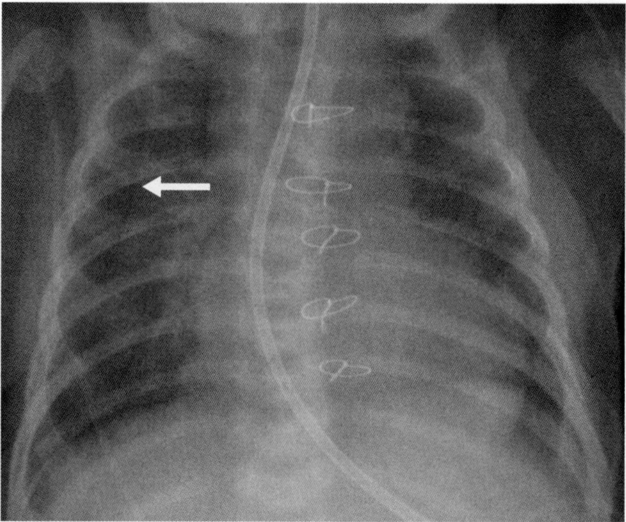

FIGURE 67.18. **A Skin Fold (*arrow*) Simulates a Right-Sided Pneumothorax.** Unlike a pneumothorax, there is no pleural line defining the interface between the lung and the "pneumothorax." The peripheral lucency disappears inferiorly rather than extending to a pleural surface. If this were a pneumothorax this amount of air would not be limited to the lateral upper lung but would extend to the lung base, the highest point in a supine infant. Not sure? Get a decubitus view!

newborn makes the pleural space at the lung bases higher than the apices. Basal pneumothoraces, particularly medially located, are more common than apical pneumothoraces. These basal pneumothoraces are seen as lucency adjacent to the cardiomediastinal silhouette with a sharply defined cardiac or diaphragmatic margin much more often than with a pleural line (Fig. 67.16). The lungs are usually very stiff in infants with neonatal lung disease. Even with a tension pneumothorax, the lung rarely collapses (Fig. 67.17). Watch out for skin folds. A skin fold can be easily mistaken for a pneumothorax. Signs that you are dealing with a skin fold and not a pneumothorax include the absence of the thin white pleural line at the interface between the central higher attenuation and the peripheral lower attenuation, a line that ends in the middle of the lung instead of extending to a pleural surface, and a "pneumothorax" in a dependent portion of the lung, such as the lateral pleura adjacent to the upper lobe in a supine infant (Fig. 67.18). If in doubt, don't spend time guessing, get a decubitus view of the chest.

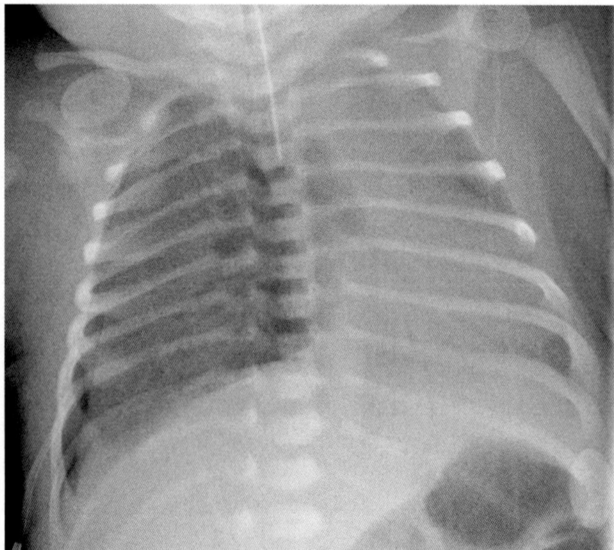

FIGURE 67.17. **There Is a Large Right-Sided Pneumothorax With Shift of the Midline to the Left, but the Lung Has Not Collapsed.** The lung is abnormally stiff in this infant with surfactant deficiency and the lung remains almost normal in size.

Pneumomediastinum. The best sign of a pneumomediastinum in a neonate is elevation of the thymus from the rest of the mediastinum (Fig. 67.19). Subcutaneous emphysema in the neck is much less common than in older people, while air dissecting into the peritoneum is more common. Tension pneumomediastinum is extremely rare and isolated pneumomediastinum almost never requires drainage.

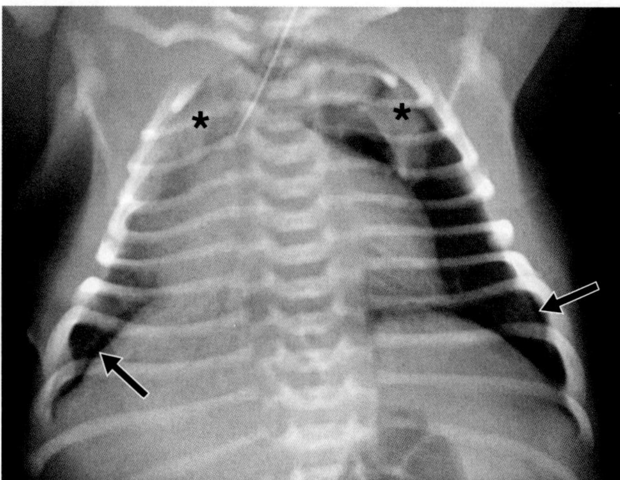

FIGURE 67.19. **Pneumomediastinum.** Air in the mediastinum has elevated both lobes of the thymus (*), separating them from the remaining mediastinal structures. Bilateral pneumothoraces are present as well (*arrows*).

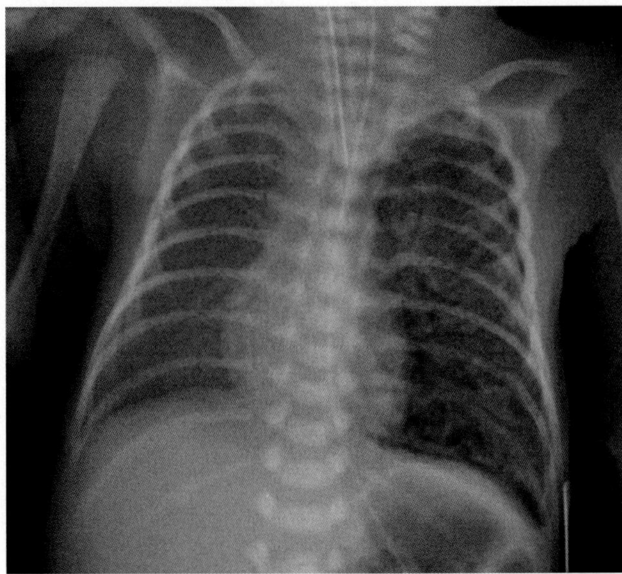

FIGURE 67.20. **Pulmonary Interstitial Emphysema.** The left lung shows round and rod-like lucencies throughout. The right lung shows the much finer and regularly distributed granular opacities of surfactant deficiency. A left pneumothorax is present as well.

Pneumopericardium. Pneumopericardium is best distinguished from pneumomediastinum by air surrounding the entire cardiac silhouette, particularly superiorly. A lateral radiograph frequently makes the distinction easier. Pneumopericardium is rare, but tension pneumopericardium can occur and can require drainage.

Pulmonary Interstitial Emphysema. Pulmonary Interstitial Emphysema (PIE) is a complication of barotrauma that occurs when alveolar tears allow air to enter the pulmonary interstitium and lymphatics. This extra-alveolar air stiffens the lung, often resulting in progression of focal disease, and the development of pneumomediastinum or pneumothorax. The CXR appearance of PIE is one of small round and rod-like lucencies superimposed on a background of higher attenuation lung (Fig. 67.20). This can be difficult to distinguish from other forms of heterogeneous opacity including air bronchograms. Clues include rapid onset and a distribution involving the peripheral as much as the central lung. PIE usually resolves quickly, but there is an entity of persistent PIE that can persist for months.

Support Equipment in Neonates

Endotracheal tube position should be assessed by relative position rather than a specific measurement. Tip positioning midway between the thoracic inlet and the carina can be considered satisfactory in all neonates and infants.

The umbilical arteries and umbilical vein provide access to the central circulation in newborn infants. The two types of catheters are distinguished by their course. The umbilical venous catheter (UVC) extends cephalad from the umbilicus with a straight or gently curving course (Fig. 67.21), while the umbilical arterial catheter (UAC) first extends caudad and then turns and extends cephalad (Fig. 67.21). The turning point forms an acute angle that usually lies close to the bottom of the sacroiliac joint. On lateral radiographs, the catheters are even easier to distinguish as the UVC remains anterior and the UAC passes posteriorly to the posteriorly located aorta and overlies the spine. Because one is located far anteriorly and the other far posteriorly, slight rotation on a frontal radiograph will alter the relative position of the catheters. For this reason, location to the right or left side of the spine is not a reliable way to identify the catheter location, or to suggest malposition.

The UAC enters the umbilical artery that connects to the internal iliacartery and to the aorta. Incorrectly positioned UACs are almost always within the aorta, with the catheter tip either too high or too low. There are two accepted placements, both of which avoid positioning near the origins of the visceral or anterior spinal arteries; high placement, with the catheter tip between T6 and T9, and low placement with the catheter tip ideally at the bottom of L3. Neither has been shown to be better and the choice is one of local or personal preference.

The course of a UVC is more complex, and there are multiple opportunities for malposition. The catheter enters the umbilical vein which extends cephalad from the umbilicus and connects to the left portal vein. The UVC then passes through the ductus venosus into the inferior vena cava (IVC). The ductus venosus enters the IVC just below the hepatic veins. At the level of the diaphragm, the tip of the UVC is in the IVC. There is a risk of important complications if the catheter tip is within the liver, so a "slightly low" position of the UVC should not be ignored. UVC catheters advanced into the upper right atrium frequently cross the foramen ovale and enter the left

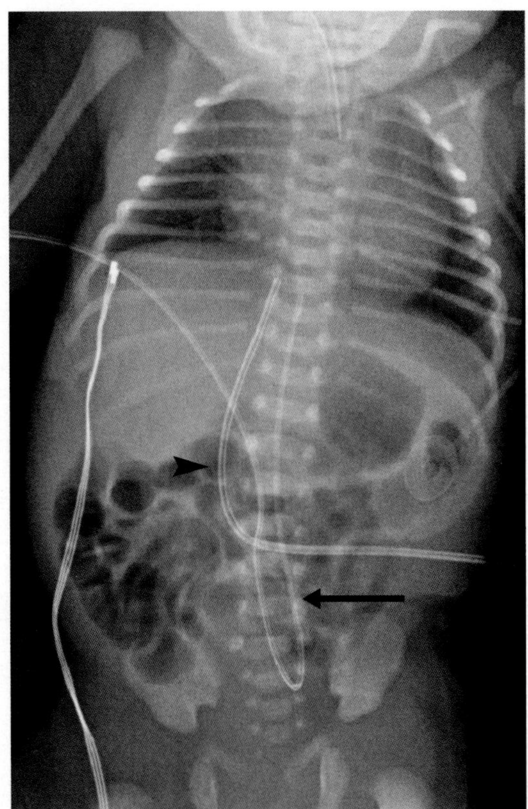

FIGURE 67.21. Umbilical venous catheter (*arrowhead*) enters at the umbilicus and extends cephalad, while the umbilical arterial catheter (*arrow*) extends caudal and then makes an acute angle and extends cephalad.

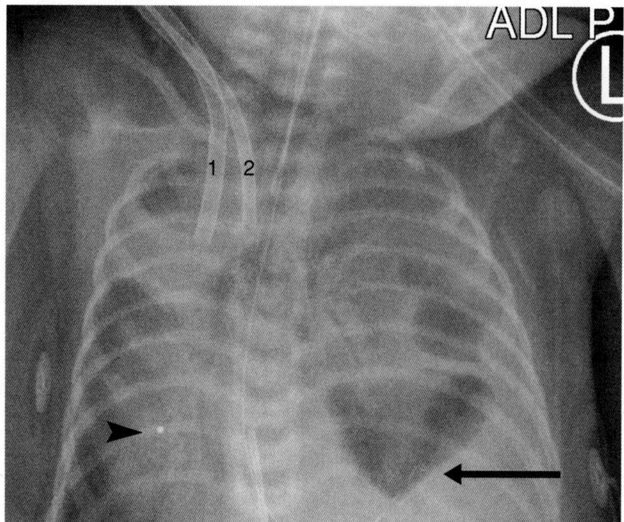

FIGURE 67.22. Extracorporeal Membrane Oxygenation (ECMO) Catheters in a Newborn With a Left Diaphragmatic Hernia. The venous catheter (1) enters the internal jugular vein and extends through the SVC into the right atrium. The tip of this catheter is marked by the small radiodense marker (*arrowhead*), not the end of the wire spiral that strengthens the proximal catheter. The arterial catheter (2) enters the common carotid artery and ends just above the aortic arch. The tip of the patient's orogastric tube (*arrow*) is in the lower left hemithorax, indicating that the stomach has herniated into the left chest.

atrium. This can cause confusion when a blood gas obtained through a UVC is reported as arterial when the tip is in the well-oxygenated blood of the left atrium.

Extracorporeal membrane oxygenation (ECMO) can be performed through a single catheter, which usually ends in the right atrium but can be placed in any large vein. This type of ECMO does not allow full bypass of the heart. Full bypass requires two catheters that allow blood to enter the ECMO circuit from the right atrium and return to the child through a carotid artery and into the aorta. Similar to Fontan physiology, blood can flow passively through the right heart so no right-sided support is required. The right atrial catheter is conventionally placed. One widely used catheter is opaque proximally but not distally. The tip is indicated by an easily missed 1 to 2 mm radiodense marker. If missed, position may be incorrectly reported causing consternation among the surgeons, often followed by wrath. Access to the aorta is provided by placing the second catheter into a carotid artery. Blood flow in the carotid is reversed from the normal situation and enters the aorta (Fig. 67.22). A list of useful measurements for catheter position is provided in Table 67.1.

TABLE 67.1

USEFUL MEASUREMENTS FOR CATHETER TIP POSITION IN CHILDREN

Umbilical arterial catheter (UAC)	T6–T9 or top of L3
Umbilical venous catheter (UVC)	Diaphragm
Upper extremity PICC	carina to two vertebral bodies (including interspaces) below carina
Lower extremity PICC	at diaphragm
Venous extracorporeal membrane oxygenation (ECMO) catheter	low right atrium
Arterial ECMO catheter	above aortic arch

CONGENITAL LUNG MALFORMATIONS

Congenital lung malformations (CLMs) are a heterogeneous group of focal lesions that vary widely in appearance, from air-filled cysts to solid soft tissue masses and from sharply circumscribed lesions to those diffusely involving a portion of the lung. These lesions are described as separate entities, but different malformations can be seen in the same patient, and different histologic appearances can be found in a single lesion. The term "hybrid lesion" for example, is used specifically when histologic features of both a sequestration and a congenital pulmonary airway malformation (CPAM) are found in one lesion. The use of categories such as bronchopulmonary foregut malformations is inconsistent in the literature and is often more confusing than useful. The origin of CLM is debated, with abnormal lung budding and airway obstruction at some stage of development two possible causes.

CLMs are now more commonly identified prenatally than after birth. These lesions are well seen on fetal US and fetal MRI as areas of abnormal signal, and by the presence of mass effect (Fig. 67.23). The natural history of most congenital lung lesions is to decrease in size relative to the fetus during gestation. While they decrease in size, most do not completely resolve. They are frequently occult on CXR but can be seen on postnatal CT scans. Most children with these lesions will be asymptomatic at birth, and because any surgery will usually be delayed until 3 to 4 months of age, initial imaging is usually limited to a CXR. In the absence of an unexpectedly large abnormality on CXR or the development of symptoms, CT scanning is usually performed close to the time when resection

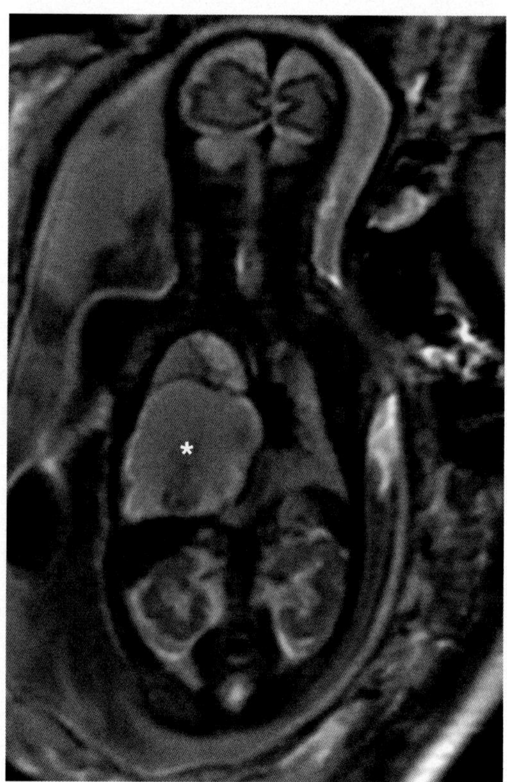

FIGURE 67.23. Fetal MRI Showing a Large Right-Sided Type 1 Congenital Pulmonary Airway Malformation (CPAM). A dominant cyst is present (*) as well as several smaller cysts. It is common for CPAMs to decrease in relative size during late gestation. (Courtesy of Usha Nagaraj, MD.)

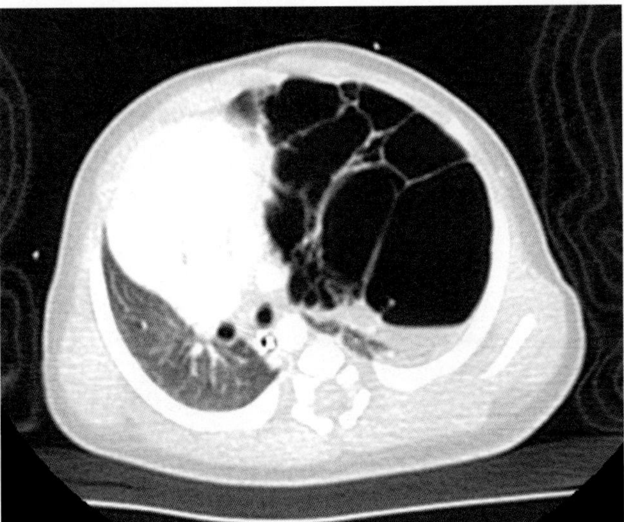

FIGURE 67.24. **Type 1 Congenital Pulmonary Airway Malformation (CPAM).** Contrast-enhanced CT in a 1 day old shows a lesion with multiple large cysts. There is mediastinal shift and a fluid level in one of the cysts. Type 1 CPAMs contain one or more cysts greater than 2 cm and make up about half of CPAMs. CPAMs were previously called congenital cystic adenomatoid malformations (CCAM).

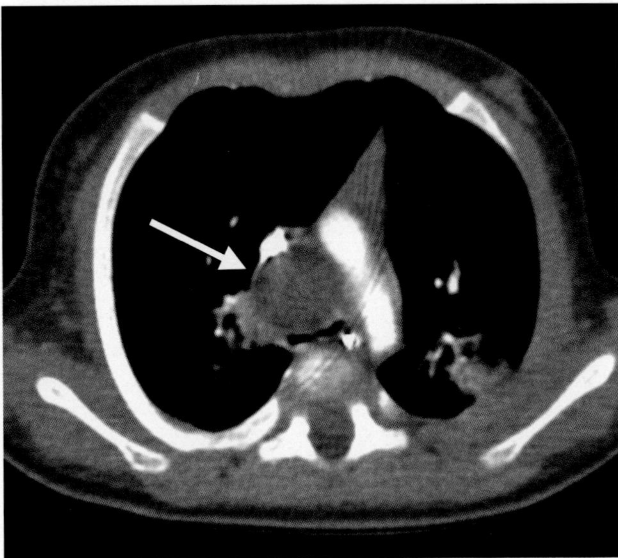

FIGURE 67.25. **Mediastinal Bronchogenic Cyst in a 3-Month-Old Infant.** CT shows a well-circumscribed low-attenuation lesion in the middle mediastinum (*arrow*). The lesion causes local mass effect without surrounding other structures and does not enhance.

is planned. Most are resected although the need for resection is debated.

The single most important feature to identify on imaging is the presence or absence of a feeding vessel (artery) supplying the lesion. A feeding vessel identifies the lesion as a sequestration, or at least one containing histologic features of sequestration. In addition to providing a specific diagnosis, these vessels arise from the aorta and must be identified at surgery to avoid life threatening bleeding. The origin of the vessel may be from the abdominal aorta as well as the thoracic aorta, so the upper abdomen should be included on a CT scan when a lower lobe lesion is suspected.

Congenital Pulmonary Airway Malformation

CPAM, previously called a congenital cystic adenomatoid malformation, is the most common malformation, making up about ¼ to ½ of lung lesions diagnosed prenatally. CPAMs are usually solitary, and most contain both solid tissue and air-filled cysts (Fig. 67.24). CPAMs are classified into five types. Type 1 if there is at least 1 cyst ≥2 cm in size; Type 2 if there are multiple smaller cysts; and Type 3 if all cysts are <5 mm. Type 3 lesions are larger, usually affecting an entire lobe. Type 3 lesions are associated with hydrops and a poor prognosis. Sixty to 70% are Type 1, while Type 3 lesions are rare (about 10%). Type 0 and 4 lesions are extremely rare.

Sequestration

A pulmonary sequestration is a mass of nonfunctioning lung tissue that does not connect to the rest of the tracheobronchial tree. Intralobar sequestrations are within the visceral pleura and aerate from collateral ventilation. Extralobar sequestrations have their own pleura and cannot become aerated. Intralobar sequestrations can be solid or cystic and usually contain both components. Arterial and venous drainage is variable, but is most commonly from the aorta and to a pulmonary vein. The radiographic feature that best identifies a sequestration is the presence of the abnormal feeding artery that supplies the tissue (Fig. 67.25). Both types are most common in the lower lobes, left more common than right.

Foregut Duplication Cysts

These include bronchogenic cysts (BCs), esophageal duplication cysts, and neurenteric cysts. BCs are round, well-defined masses that can occur in mediastinum or in the lung, usually centrally (Fig. 67.26). Aberrant budding of the bronchopulmonary foregut is thought to result in a cyst lined with respiratory epithelium and filled with fluid or mucus. BCs do not communicate with the tracheobronchial tree and air

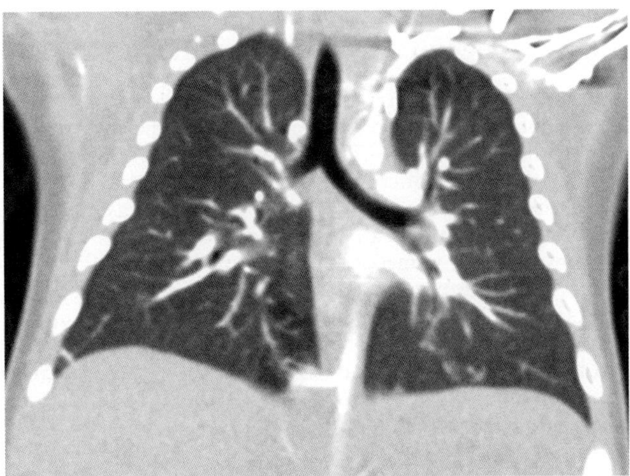

FIGURE 67.26. **Intralobar Sequestration.** The most important feature to identify in a congenital lung lesion is the presence of a feeding vessel. A feeding vessel indicates a sequestration. Lesions containing elements of more than one congenital lesion occur, particularly hybrid lesions with elements of sequestration and CPAM, so the appearance of the parenchymal abnormality may vary. Air within the abnormal area indicates an intralobar sequestration.

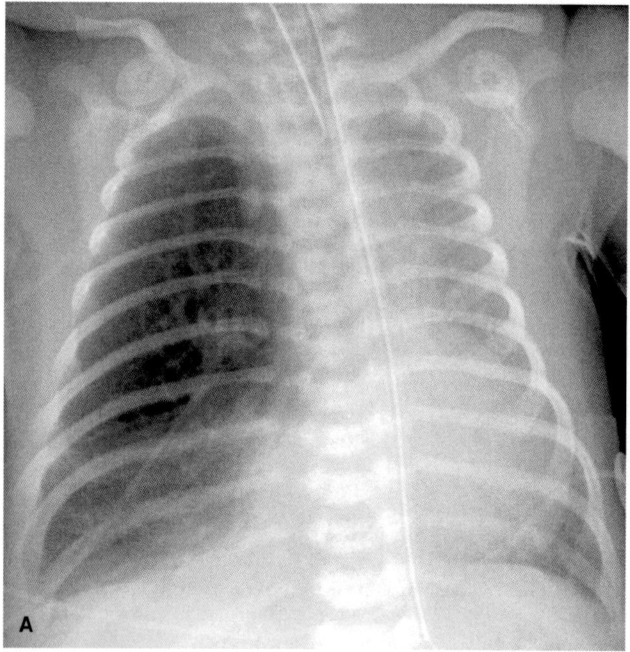

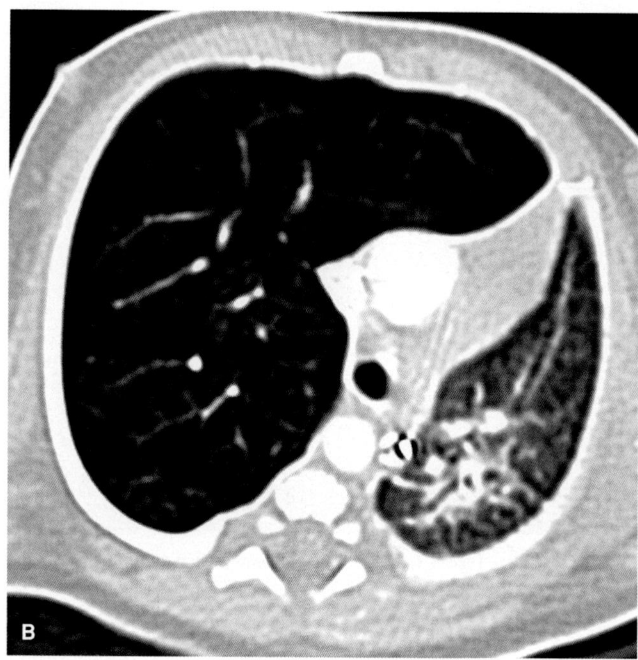

FIGURE 67.27. **Fourteen-Day-Old Infant With Congenital Lobar Overinflation.** CXR (**A**) shows marked hyperinflation in the right upper lobe with compression of the right middle lobe, right lower lobe, and the left lung. CT (**B**) shows marked hyperinflation of the left upper lobe. The lung markings are maintained and there are no cystic or solid areas.

within one suggests infection. On CT, BCs are homogeneous in attenuation and commonly have greater than water level attenuation, thought to be due to highly proteinaceous mucus. They can simulate a solid mass, but will show either absent enhancement or enhancement limited to the wall and/or a mural nodule. Esophageal duplication cysts occur adjacent to the esophagus and appear similar to mediastinal BCs. Neurenteric cysts are very rare, occur in the posterior mediastinum, and can be associated with vertebral body anomalies. The purpose of imaging foregut cysts is to confirm the diagnosis, identify their relationship to adjacent structures, and assess for associated abnormalities.

Congenital Lobar Overinflation

Congenital Lobar Overinflation (CLO), also called congenital lobar emphysema, is a developmental abnormality that results in overinflation of a lobe (Fig. 67.27). An airway abnormality, particularly abnormal cartilage and airway malacia resulting in a check-valve mechanism, has been suggested as the etiology, but in half of the cases, no anatomic cause is found. CLO can present in the immediate newborn period as a solid mass due to slow clearance of fetal lung fluid. Hyperinflation develops rapidly. CLO occurs most commonly in the left upper, right upper, and middle lobes. Lower lobe involvement and involvement of more than one lobe are both rare, probably occurring in less than 5% of cases.

Other Congenital Parenchymal Abnormalities

Abnormalities affecting the entire lung include pulmonary agenesis, where no bronchus is present; pulmonary atresia where a short, blind-ending bronchus is present, and pulmonary hypoplasia where the size of the lung and/or the number of bronchopulmonary segments are decreased. Unlike surgical resections, in which the abnormal cardiac position often causes both vascular and airway complications, the congenital abnormalities are commonly asymptomatic and may not be identified until later in life.

Pulmonary venolobar, or scimitar, syndrome affects both the lung and the pulmonary vascularity. There is abnormal drainage of a lobe to the IVC, hepatic vein, or left atrium. The configuration of the abnormal vein has been likened to a scimitar sword. The affected lobe is small. There is often abnormal arterial supply from the aorta as well. This does not indicate a coexisting sequestration. The scimitar vein is impressive when seen, but is not identified prospectively in most cases (Fig. 67.28).

Congenital Anomalies of the Trachea and Bronchi

Bronchial atresia occurs when there is focal interruption of a bronchus during lung development. The cause is unknown, but there is normal development of the bronchial tree distal to the interruption suggesting a prenatal traumatic event. The airway distal to the occlusion produces mucus that collects behind the occlusion. This mucocele is seen in nearly all cases of bronchial atresia and may be round or branching (Fig. 67.29). The lung distal to the occluded airway is aerated by collateral ventilation. Air trapping in this portion of the lung is characteristic of bronchial atresia. A soft tissue nodule associated with focal air trapping will almost always be due to bronchial atresia.

The tracheal bronchus spectrum is the same as in adults. Smaller size and patient motion may make correct identification of anomalous bronchi more difficult than in adults, but the anomalies are the same.

Pulmonary situs needs to be determined in children with situs anomalies or heterotaxy syndromes. Bronchial branching patterns can be atypical, unreliable, and sometimes difficult to define. As such, defining the relationship of the main bronchi (right and left) to the pulmonary arteries is the best way to define pulmonary situs. An eparterial bronchus arises above the

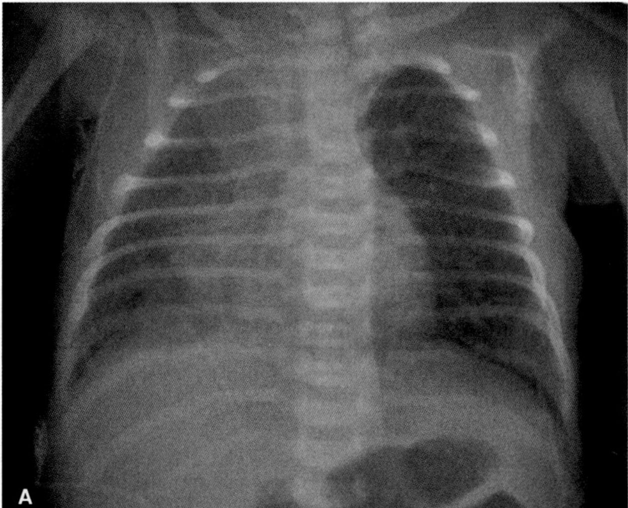

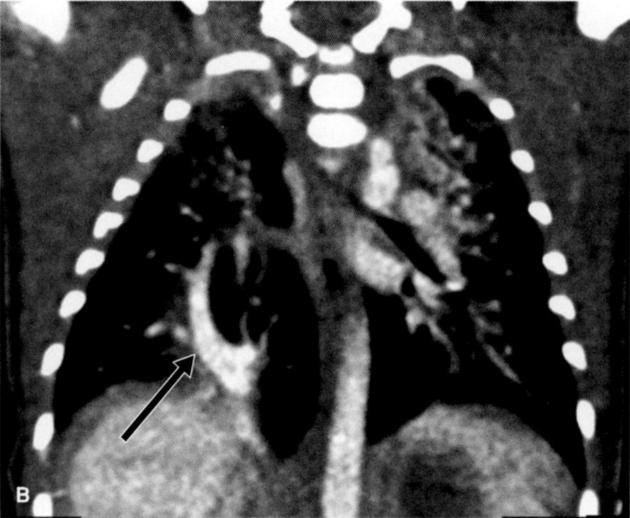

FIGURE 67.28. **Scimitar or Hypogenetic Lung Syndrome.** CXR (**A**) shows shift of the heart and mediastinum to the right due to a smaller right lung. There is ill-defined increased attenuation centrally and in the lung base. The appearance is nonspecific, as is most commonly the case in children with scimitar syndrome. Coronal CT image (**B**) demonstrates the scimitar vein (*arrow*). This vein could be easily followed to its connection to the IVC. The entire drainage of the left lung was through this vessel.

level where the pulmonary artery crosses the central bronchus; a hyparterial bronchus arises below this level. Normally the right upper lobe bronchus is eparterial, all others are hyparterial.

Tracheal stenosis can be focal or diffuse. Focal tracheal stenosis is often due to airway trauma such as repeated suctioning or prolonged intubation. Diffuse stenosis is usually congenital and the trachea may be equally narrow throughout its length, or may have a carrot shape, tapering from normal size below the vocal cords to small at the carina. Complete tracheal rings, where there is no membranous posterior trachea, causes focal tracheal stenosis and can be identified by a small, perfectly round tracheal lumen (Fig. 67.30). Tracheal stenosis associated with congenital heart disease is often due to complete tracheal rings. Most children do not outgrow complete tracheal rings and then surgery is the only treatment.

Esophageal bronchi can occur, with the most severe form associated with tracheal agenesis where a distal fistula connects a carina to the esophagus. The main bronchi are horizontal in these cases.

PULMONARY INFECTION

Pneumonia in Children

Infection of the lower respiratory tract is the most common infectious disease of children. The diagnosis is usually made

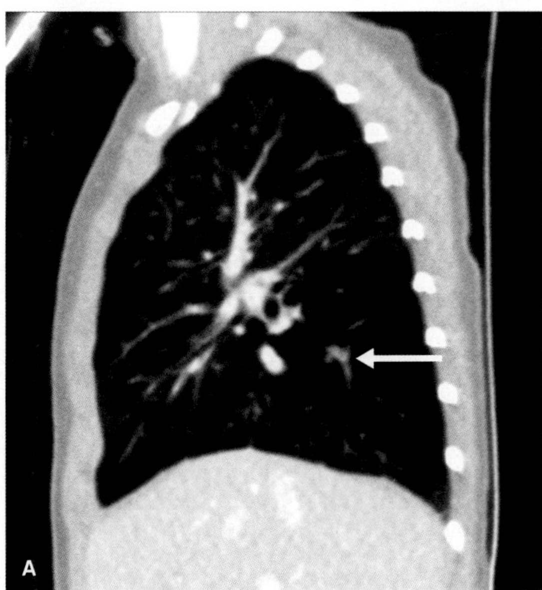

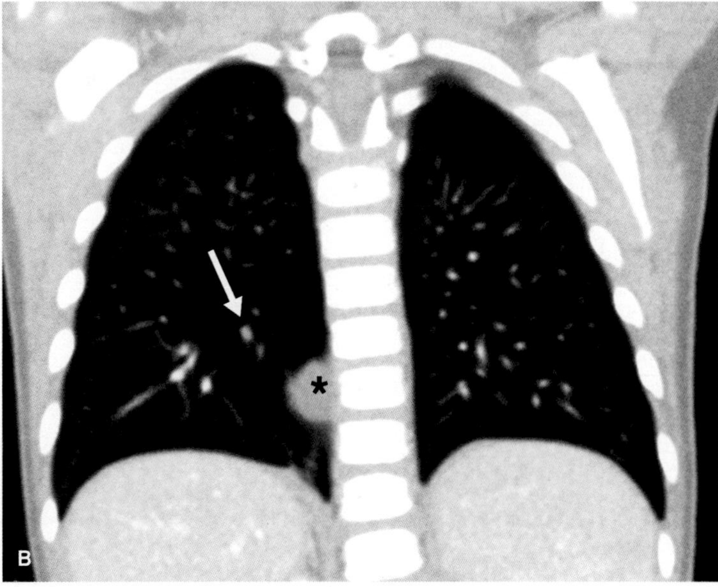

FIGURE 67.29. **Bronchial Atresia and a Bronchogenic Cyst in a 20-Month-Old Infant.** Sagittal (**A**) and coronal (**B**) CT images show a well-defined area of decreased parenchymal attenuation with a central linear structure (*arrows*), lower in attenuation than the contrast-enhanced vessels caused by mucus in the obstructed airway. On the coronal image a second lesion is seen (*). This was resected and found to be an unrelated bronchogenic cyst. It is not rare to find more than one separate congenital lesion in a child.

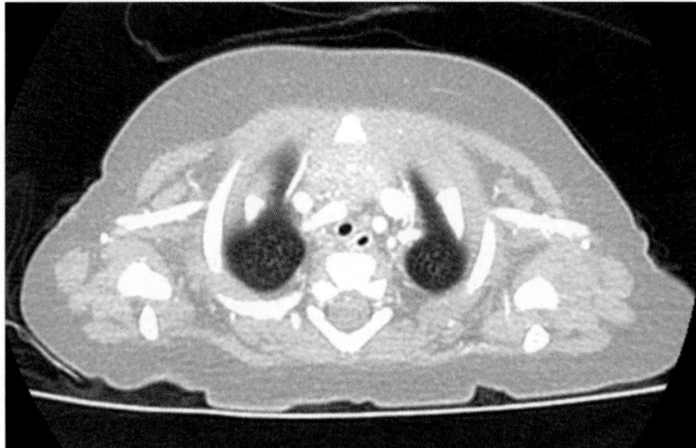

FIGURE 67.30. **Complete Tracheal Rings.** Single image from a CT scan at the level of the innominate artery shows a small airway with an almost round appearance, rather than the flattened appearance of extrinsic compression or the D-shaped appearance of the normal trachea. There is no tracheal membrane forming the posterior trachea; instead the wall is entirely surrounded by the cartilaginous tracheal ring. This usually requires surgical correction, and is often associated with congenital heart disease.

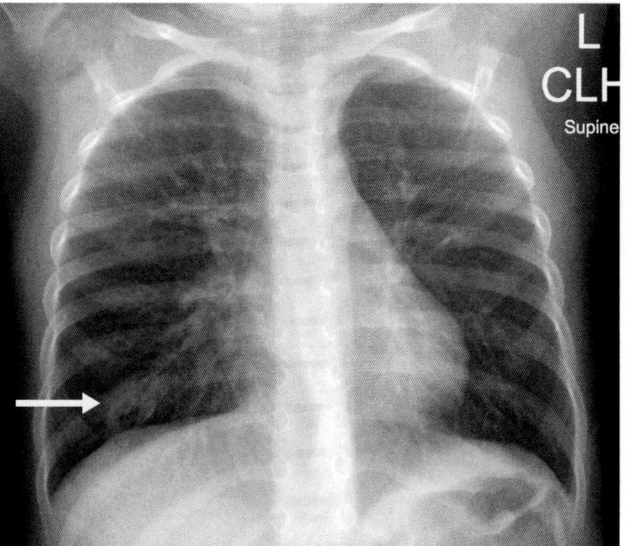

FIGURE 67.31. **The "Airways Disease" Pattern on CXR in a 3-Year-Old Child.** The lungs are hyperinflated, with a flat diaphragm and the 8th rib the first rib crossing the diaphragm. Central lung markings are prominent with peribronchial thickening. Small focal opacities (*arrow*) are common in children with airways disease and are far more likely to represent atelectasis than pneumonia.

by history and physical examination. A chest radiograph is not needed to make a diagnosis of pneumonia, and children are routinely treated for pneumonia on clinical grounds alone. Because of the variability of clinical, laboratory, and imaging findings in children with pneumonia, a CXR is still obtained frequently. The CXR is particularly useful in excluding pneumonia when the CXR is normal, resolving conflicting clinical and laboratory findings, and identifying other causes of respiratory distress.

Probably the most common reason given for obtaining a CXR is to determine whether a bacterial pneumonia is present, in order to decide whether to administer antibiotics. The "viral" and "bacterial" description of the CXR is widely used, despite general agreement that these two patterns do not reliably distinguish between the different causes of pneumonia. It is also important to recognize that the "viral" pattern includes the atypical pneumonias such as mycoplasma pneumoniae.

The "viral" CXR is characterized by hyperinflation and a relatively symmetrical appearance with peribronchial thickening, particularly centrally; and ill-defined perihilar opacities. Scattered subsegmental opacities representing atelectasis are common and can be prominent (Fig. 67.31). There should be no pleural effusion, and no segmental or larger confluent opacities. Authors have pointed out that in infants and very young children the most common response to lower respiratory tract infection of any etiology is inflammation of the airways and increased mucus production. With the small size of the airways, hyperinflation and areas of atelectasis result, causing a "viral" CXR even when the infection is bacterial. Newborn infants with documented bacterial infection almost never have a well-defined lobar infiltrate.

The bacterial pattern is characterized by normal lung volumes and an asymmetrical appearance with one or more dominant opacities in the mid or peripheral lung. These opacities are well-defined and limited to a lobe or segment(s) and may contain air bronchograms. Pleural effusion is the best predictor of bacterial infection, but is not present in the majority of cases (Fig. 67.32).

Studies have evaluated the ability of the CXR to identify a viral or bacterial etiology for pneumonia. Overall correlation is poor between the CXR appearance and serologic or culture evidence of a bacterial or viral infection. In one study, however, the authors reported that a viral pattern correlated well with the absence of bacterial infection, while the bacterial pattern correlated poorly with the presence of bacterial infection. This finding is consistent with anecdotal but wide experience that it is rare to see a patient with a viral pattern have a bacterial etiology identified, while it is not uncommon to see well-defined opacities that suggest bacterial infection to resolve within days; much more quickly than expected with a true bacterial pneumonia.

The child's age is probably the most important predictor of the infectious agent. In the newborn period, maternal immunity provides protection from viral infection, while bacterial infection may be transmitted at birth from the mother, both factors increasing the likelihood of bacterial infection. GBS and gram-negative enteric bacteria are the most common causes of pneumonia in the first month of life. *Chlamydia trachomatis* can also be transmitted during birth and chlamydia pneumonia is a cause of a "viral" appearance in 6- to 12-week-old infants (Fig. 67.33). Between 1 and 3 months, *Streptococcus pneumoniae* is the most common etiology. From a few months of age to a few years, viral infections predominate. In older children, bacterial infections become increasingly common. Table 67.2 lists common causes of community acquired pneumonia.

Specific Etiologies of Pneumonia in Children

Respiratory syncytial virus (RSV) is the most common etiology of pulmonary infection in infants and young children, and the most common cause of bronchiolitis. Bronchiolitis is clinically defined as a disease of wheezing and respiratory distress in children less than 2 years old. It is a seasonal disease, occurring in the winter months. About 20% of children will experience bronchiolitis in their first year, and 10% of these will require hospitalization. The CXR shows the classic viral appearance, often with prominent areas of atelectasis that change rapidly ("wandering" or "shifting" atelectasis).

Mycoplasma pneumonia is the most common cause of pneumonia in children, responsible for 40% or more of pediatric pneumonia. Mycoplasma primarily affects children from school age through adolescence. The CXR commonly shows a "viral" pattern, with hilar adenopathy and small pleural

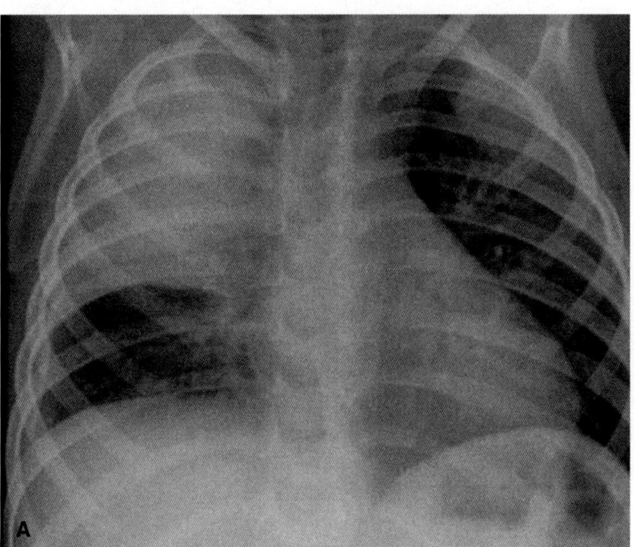

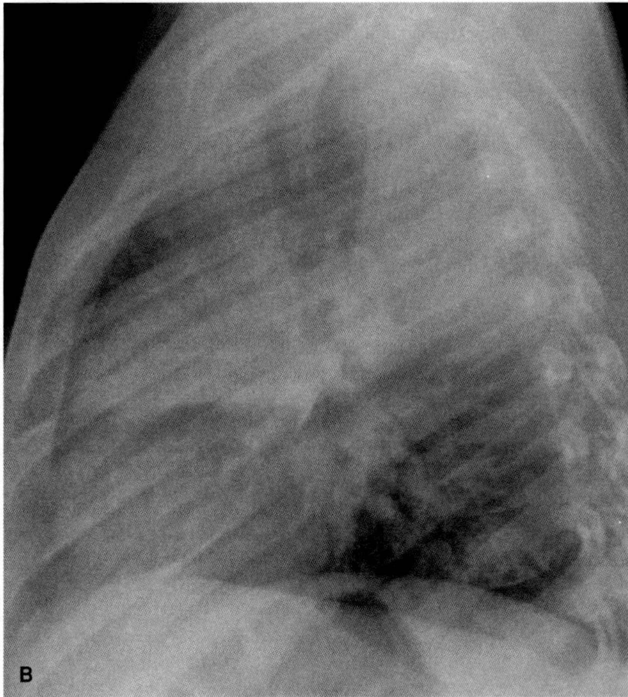

FIGURE 67.32. **Bacterial Pneumonia. A:** Frontal view. **B:** Lateral view. A typical alveolar consolidation in the right upper lobe. Note that the fissures are not displaced, indicating that there is little volume loss. A right pleural effusion is also present.

effusions seen in some cases. Focal disease has been reported, but this is complicated by the fact that mycoplasma can occur in a mixed infection, particularly with pneumococcus.

S. pneumoniae is the most common cause of bacterial pneumonia in children after the neonatal period. Routine immunization has reduced the incidence of pneumococcal pneumonia by 60% to 70%, but these infections remain a common cause of pneumonia. Pneumococcus produces the classic "bacterial" CXR, usually with a single well-defined infiltrate. Round pneumonia is a manifestation of streptococcal pneumonia with a strikingly mass-like appearance. Round pneumonia occurs in the lower lobes in children less than 8 years old (Fig. 67.34). The first step in separating round pneumonia from a mass is to evaluate the chest for associated abnormalities of the chest wall,

FIGURE 67.33. **Chlamydia Pneumonia.** There are prominent bilateral, central, and peribronchial opacities with scattered opacities particularly in the lung bases. The appearance is similar to that seen with viral infections. In a 6 to 12 week old with cough and a "viral" CXR, chlamydia pneumonia should be considered.

TABLE 67.2

SOME OF THE COMMON ORGANISMS CAUSING COMMUNITY-ACQUIRED PNEUMONIA IN CHILDREN

- First month
  - Gram-negative rods
  - Group B streptococcus
  - *Listeria* (esp. premature infants)
- 1 month–6 months
  - *Chlamydia trachomatis*
  - *Streptococcus pneumoniae*
  - Adenovirus
  - Respiratory syncytial virus
  - Influenza and parainfluenza
- 6 months–5 years
  - RSV
  - Parainfluenza
  - Influenza
  - Rhinovirus
  - Adenovirus
  - *S. pneumoniae*
  - *Mycoplasma pneumoniae*
  - *Chlamydia pneumoniae*
- Over 5 years
  - *M. pneumoniae*
  - *C. pneumoniae*
  - *S. pneumoniae*
  - Rhinovirus
  - Adenovirus
  - Influenza

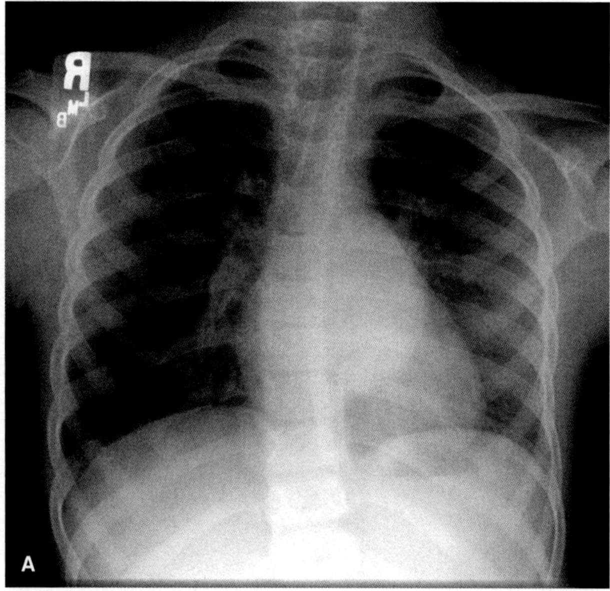

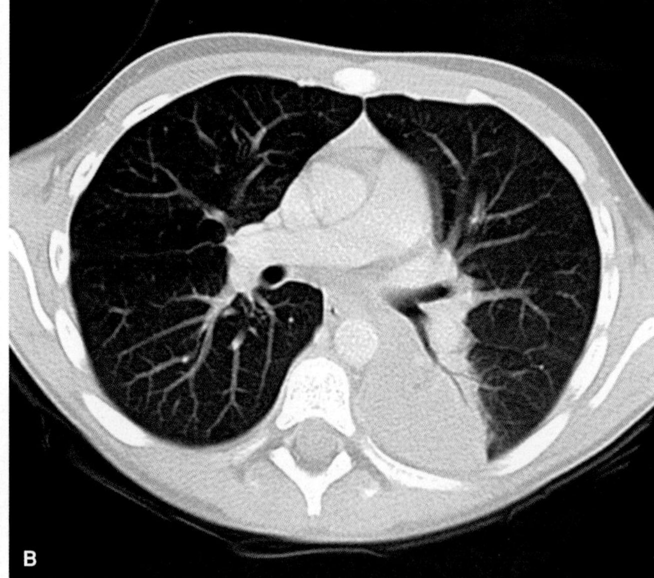

FIGURE 67.34. Round Pneumonia in a 7-Year-Old Boy. CXR (**A**) shows an apparent retrocardiac mass. There are no rib changes and the patient presented with fever, cough, and leukocytosis. An axial CT image (**B**) shows an air bronchogram within the mass, identifying it as a round pneumonia. With this CXR and a presentation suggesting pneumonia, a short term follow-up CXR would be a reasonable plan.

which would indicate a mass. If the chest wall is normal, the least invasive way to distinguish round pneumonia from a mass is by the clinical presentation. A child younger than 8 years old who presents with symptoms of pneumonia and a lower lobe "mass" is far more likely to have a round pneumonia than a neoplasm. A follow-up CXR in 1 to 2 weeks provides confirmation, as the sharply defined round shape does not persist for long. It is not necessary to see resolution; the change in appearance tells you that this is not a mass. A CT scan will distinguish pneumonia from a mass, but is not necessary in most cases.

Mycobacterium Tuberculosis

Childhood tuberculosis (TB) is most often pulmonary primary disease until the age of puberty, after which adult type reactivation disease becomes more common. Primary pulmonary TB occurs when inhaled *Mycobacterium tuberculosis* bacilli cause focal pulmonary inflammation, called the primary focus. Bacilli then spread to local lymph nodes causing lymphadenopathy. The primary focus and lymphadenopathy form the primary tuberculous (Ghon) complex.

Signs and symptoms of TB in children are less specific than in older patients, and children are less likely to have positive cultures. Childhood TB is more likely to progress and to disseminate to areas outside the lung. Because children rarely produce sputum, and because children are less likely to be culture positive, child-to-child transmission is extremely rare. Childhood infection is regarded as a sentinel event reflecting recent infection from an adult.

Unlike reactivation disease that usually occurs as apical disease, the most common finding in primary TB is adenopathy. Parenchymal disease is also common, and the classic appearance of primary TB is a nonspecific infiltrate associated with hilar or mediastinal lymphadenopathy (Fig. 67.35). The infiltrate can occur in any location, but is most often peripheral and in the mid or lower lung. There is usually a single primary focus, but there can be multiple foci. Hilar adenopathy occurs on the side opposite to the infiltrate in up to one-third of the cases.

For screening, a frontal view of the chest is sufficient. When TB is suspected, a lateral view is recommended to improve detection of hilar adenopathy. CT scanning increases detection of adenopathy and may show a subtle infiltrate that is not seen on chest radiograph, but is usually limited to complicated cases. Resolution of radiographic findings is slow, up to 2 years for CXRs.

LUNG MASSES

The most common lung mass in a child is a pseudomass, most commonly a round pneumonia. Metastases are the most common neoplasms in the pediatric chest; at least 10 times more common than primary neoplasms. Metastases in the lungs of children behave and appear no different than those in the lungs of adults.

The most common true lung mass in children is inflammatory myofibroblastic tumor (IMT), also called plasma cell granuloma and xanthogranuloma. IMT has been classified as both a benign and a very low-grade malignant tumor. IMT usually presents as a solid mass that abuts the pleural or mediastinal surface. IMT may be invasive, and can be difficult to distinguish from more aggressive tumors.

Among the neoplasms of pulmonary origin, benign lesions are more common than malignant. Pulmonary hamartoma is the most common primary benign neoplasm. It usually presents as a solitary, noncalcified lobular mass. Next most common are pulmonary chondroma and respiratory papillomatosis.

Endobronchial carcinoid and pleuropulmonary blastoma (PPB) are the most common primary malignant pulmonary lesions. PPB usually occurs in children younger than 6 years old. PPB can begin as a cystic lesion that progresses to a solid one. Cystic PPB in neonates can be radiographically indistinguishable from a CPAM. Clues to the presence of PPB in a neonate are pneumothorax, multiple lesions, and family history (DICER1).

Lung Nodules and Cysts

Nodules are a common finding on pediatric CT scans, seen in 40% of children with chest trauma. Unlike adults, malignancy is rarely the cause, except in the case of metastases. Again, unlike adults, it is extremely rare to have metastatic disease with an

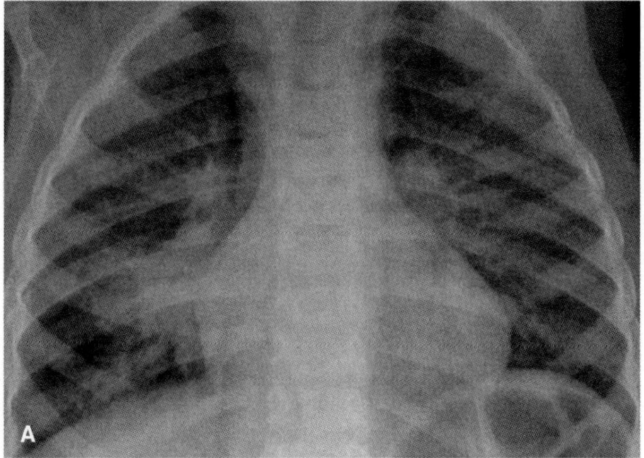

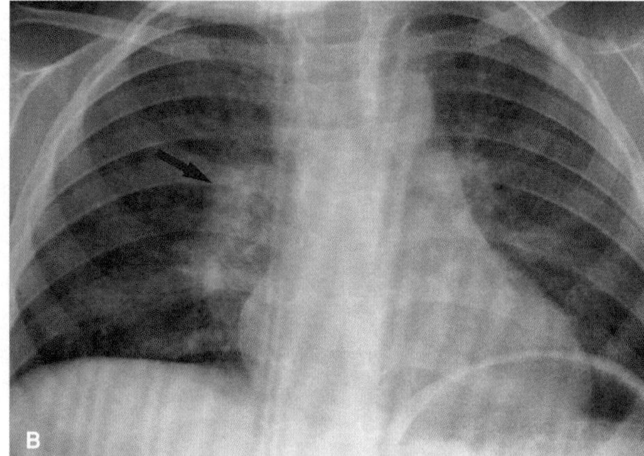

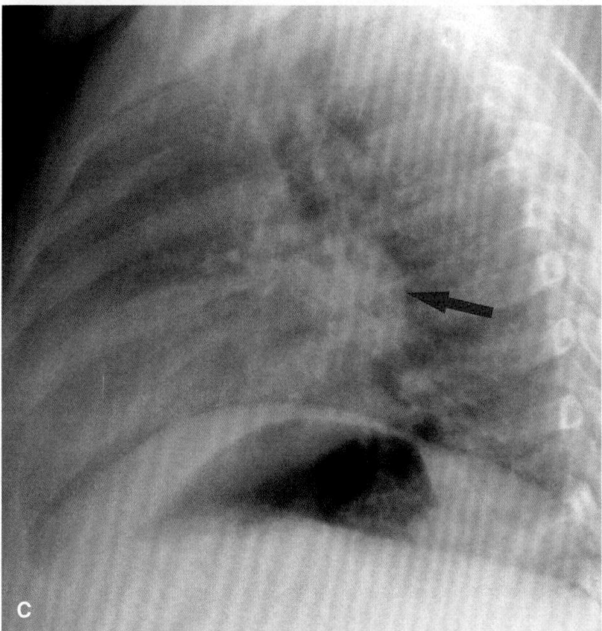

FIGURE 67.35. Primary Tuberculosis. A: The initial radiograph of this child showed an area of consolidation with fullness in the right hilar region. **B** and **C:** After 2 weeks of therapy, the consolidation has resolved, but right hilar lymphadenopathy persists (*arrows*). Note how nonspecific this appearance is. It may be impossible to suggest the diagnosis initially without a suggestive history. Persistent adenopathy after treatment for pneumonia should raise concern for other etiologies than community-acquired pneumonia, including tuberculosis.

unknown primary, further decreasing the concern for neoplasm when lung nodules are detected. Remember that the Fleischner criteria for lung nodule follow-up apply to adults older than 35 years. They have no relevance for pediatric patients.

Adult appearances of emphysema are very rarely seen in children, so emphysema should not be suggested as a cause of lung cysts. Lymphangioleiomyomatosis is very rare in children, but can be a cause of thin-walled cysts. Langerhans cell histiocytosis (LCH) occurs in children and may present with irregularly shaped cysts. It is not related to smoking, and unlike in adults, the cysts do not spare the lung bases. When lung nodules are associated with cysts, pulmonary involvement by respiratory papillomatosis and LCH should be considered.

Mediastinal Lesions

Several schemes have been used to describe mediastinal anatomy. In children, a line drawn along the anterior vertebral bodies and a line from the top of the sternum parallel to the vertebral line can be used to divide the mediastinum into anterior, middle, and posterior divisions. It is important to remember that these are arbitrary divisions, with no fascial planes or other structures to limit lesions or processes to a specific division.

The thymus is the largest normal structure in the anterior mediastinum. The thymic contour is rounded in infants, and is more rectangular than triangular. By school age, the borders straighten and the thymus becomes triangular. The thymus is homogeneous on imaging with no mass effect and smooth contours. Small vessels are commonly seen within the thymus. On CT or MRI, a normal appearance of the thymus is usually sufficient to exclude the presence of tumor or other lesion. The thymus has a very characteristic "dot-dash" appearance on ultrasound that can be used to confirm the presence of normal thymus and so exclude other causes of an anterior mediastinal process.

The middle mediastinum includes the heart and vascular structures. A several millimeter round or linear calcification is often seen at the site of the closed ductus arteriosus, between the aorta and pulmonary artery. This should not be mistaken for pathologic calcification.

Table 67.3 lists some of the causes of mediastinal lesions. Lymphoma is the most common anterior mediastinal mass in children. It is usually easily distinguished from the thymus by features including an irregular contour, heterogeneous attenuation, and mass effect. Teratomas may be immature malignant or mature benign lesions. The presence of fat, fluid, and calcification are essentially diagnostic of a teratoma, but are not present in the majority of cases. Calcification, for example, is seen in about ¼. The term lymphatic malformation is preferable to lymphangioma or cystic hygroma. Prior hemorrhage or infection may result in a complex appearance. Neurogenic tumors make up 90% of posterior mediastinal tumors with most being neuroblastomas (Fig. 67.36).

TABLE 67.3

MEDIASTINAL LESIONS IN CHILDREN

Any Division
Thymus
Lymphoma/leukemia
Adenopathy
Mediastinitis
Hematoma
Anterior
Teratoma
Thyroid (rare)
Thymoma (rare)
Middle
Bronchopulmonary foregut malformations
Hiatal hernia
Esophageal lesions
Cardiac/pericardial lesions
Great vessel anomalies
Posterior
Neuroblastoma
Other neurogenic tumors
Neurenteric cyst
Spinal tumors and infection
Aortic or azygos anomalies
Extramedullary hematopoesis

CHEST WALL

The most important thing to know about the child's chest wall is that children with asymptomatic palpable anterior chest wall lesions should have a CXR, and if the CXR is normal no further evaluation. This axiom was based on a study that included a relatively small number of subjects, but at one of the largest children's hospitals in the United States no exception has been seen in 20 years. This does not apply to the posterior chest! Table 67.4 lists some of the chest wall lesions in children.

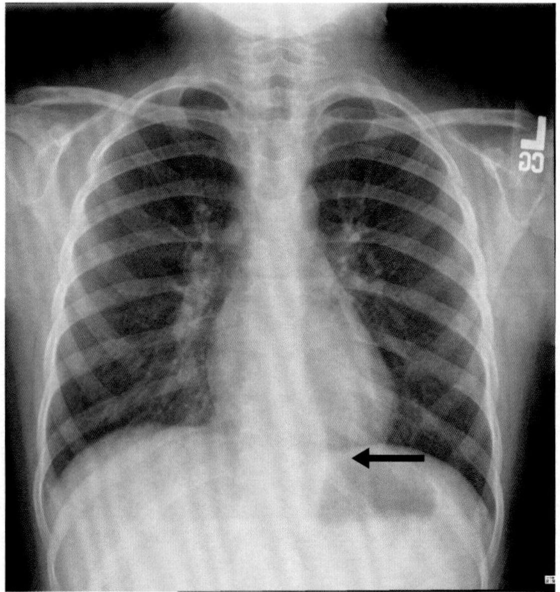

FIGURE 67.36. **Left Paraspinal Widening due to Neuroblastoma** (*arrow*). The paraspinal stripe should never have a convex margin, and should not be wider than the width of the pedicle.

TABLE 67.4

CHEST WALL LESIONS IN CHILDREN

Developmental
Asymmetry
Costal cartilage
Pectus excavatum and carinatum
Infection
Fungal
Bacterial
Neoplasm
Benign
Osteochondroma
Fibrous dysplasia
Malignant
Metastases
Rhabdomyosarcoma
Askin tumor (Ewing family)
Trauma
Postsurgical
Blunt trauma
Child abuse

DIFFUSE (INTERSTITIAL) LUNG DISEASE

As in adults, "interstitial" lung disease in the child affects more than the lung interstitium. Also like adults, the term interstitial lung disease is too widely used to insist on the more correct "diffuse lung disease." Among pediatric pulmonologists, these diseases are described as childhood interstitial lung disease and the acronym chILD is popular. Enough said. For the general radiologist there are two things to know about chILD. First, interstitial lung disease does occur in children as well as adults. Second, these are a confusing group of diseases that occur in difficult to image patients. Referral to a pediatric pulmonologist and/or pediatric thoracic radiologist should be made as soon as possible. The author finds these diseases fascinating, and for those who share a bit of that interest, here are some additional thoughts.

The causes of chILD are different from the causes of adult ILD (Table 67.5). Idiopathic pulmonary fibrosis is by far the most common cause of ILD in adults, while chILD is made up of a diverse group of diseases without a predominant disease. In fact, idiopathic pulmonary fibrosis, does not occur in children. In addition, there are diseases seen in children that are not seen in adults. As in adult ILD, the CT appearance is frequently nonspecific. The findings in this group often overlap, and it is frequently impossible to make a specific diagnosis. There are several CT appearances, however, that suggest a specific diagnosis.

Neuroendocrine hyperplasia of infancy is a relatively common form of chILD that frequently has a very specific CT appearance, and a typical clinical presentation. In a child with hypoxia and a gradual onset of symptoms, who presents in the first two years of life, and a CXR that is normal or "viral" NEHI should be high on the differential. The classic imaging appearance of NEHI is ground-glass opacities most marked in the right middle lobe and lingula, and otherwise distributed predominantly in a perimediastinal location (Fig. 67.37).

Surfactant protein mutations often present in infancy with an alveolar proteinosis pattern. While there is a differential for "crazy paving," in the newborn infant with respiratory distress, a surfactant protein mutation is by far the most likely cause (Fig. 67.38).

Alveolar growth abnormality results from a prenatal or perinatal lung insult and is a common form of chILD in infants. This is the pathologic appearance seen in infants with

TABLE 67.5

CAUSES OF DIFFUSE (INTERSTITIAL) LUNG DISEASE IN CHILDREN

Diffuse developmental disorders[a]	Arrested development at pre-alveolar stages of lung maturation, or abnormal vascular development	Acinar/alveolar dysgenesis, congenital alveolar dysplasia, alveolar capillary dysplasia with misalignment of the pulmonary veins
Disorders of lung structure associated with specific mutations[a]	Diverse disorders where a specific genetic defect is known (excludes surfactant dysfunction disorders)	Filamin A (FLNA), forkhead box F1 (FOXF1), coatomer protein complex subunit alpha (COPA), stimulator of interferon (STING)
Alveolar growth abnormalities[a]	Abnormal alveolar development, simplified lung structure, large airspaces	Bronchopulmonary dysplasia, lung hypoplasia, associated with Trisomy 21 or other chromosomal disorder
Specific conditions of undefined etiology[a]	2 unrelated disorders with well- defined pathologic criteria	Neuroendocrine hyperplasia of infancy, pulmonary interstitial glycogenosis
Surfactant dysfunction disorders[a]	Due to ineffective surfactant or abnormal regulation of surfactant metabolism	SP-B, SP-C, ABCA3, thyroid transcription factor 1, GMCSF receptor deficiency, lysinuric protein intolerance
Lymphatic disorders	Can present at any age, severe variations present at or near birth	Lymphangiectasia, lymphangiectasis
Disorders of the otherwise normal child	Acute, short duration episodes are excluded	Obliterative bronchiolitis, aspiration, pulmonary hemorrhage, hypersensitivity pneumonitis, eosinophilic pneumonia
Disorders of the immunocompromised child	Primary or related to transplantation/rejection	Opportunistic infections, related to therapeutic intervention, LIP
Disorders related to systemic disease	Respiratory disease may precede other symptoms, but usually do not present initially as respiratory disease	Autoimmune, rheumatoid, metabolic disease, Langerhans cell histiocytosis

[a]Most common in children less than two years old.

BPD, in pulmonary hypoplasia due to oligohydramnios, and it can also be seen in association with cardiac and chromosomal abnormalities such as trisomy 21. The classic CT appearance consists of ground-glass opacity, cysts, and distorted secondary pulmonary lobular architecture with the secondary lobules varying in size and attenuation (Fig. 67.39).

An increasing number of disorders of lung structure associated with specific genetic mutations are being identified. This group does not have a unifying underlying physiology, unlike the surfactant disorders that also have specific genetic mutations. As new genetic disorders are identified, recognition of disparate appearing changes in different systems due to a single mutation will almost certainly increase.

SYSTEMIC CONDITIONS AFFECTING THE LUNG

Immunodeficiencies

Primary immunodeficiency (PrID) can be classified by the affected component of the immune system: Humoral (B cell), cellular (T cell), combined B and T cell, complement, and phagocyte. Bacterial infections are more common in humoral PrID; viral and opportunistic infection more common in cellular PrID. Newborn testing is now performed in most states for severe combined immunodeficiency and DiGeorge syndrome.

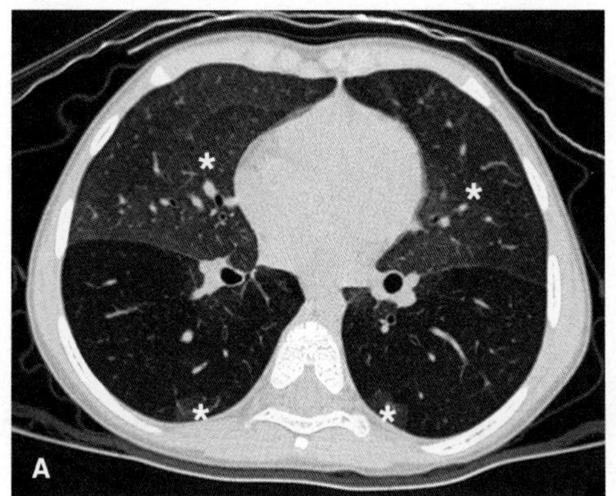

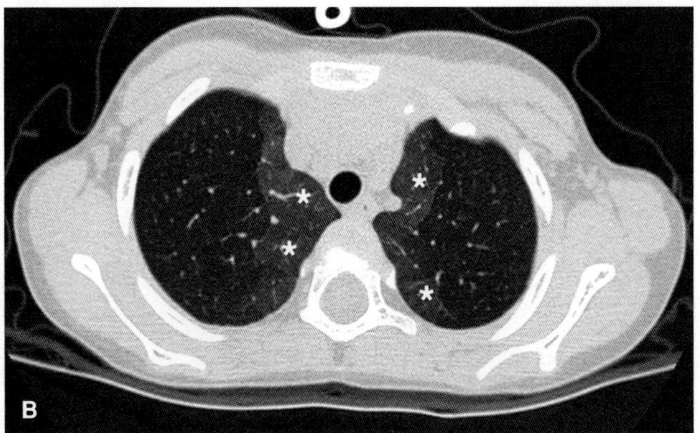

FIGURE 67.37. **Two Images of a 2 Year Old With Neuroendocrine Cell Hyperplasia of Infancy (NEHI).** Geographic areas of ground-glass opacity (*) with otherwise normal appearing lung is the hallmark of NEHI. Ground glass is most marked in the middle lobe and lingua (**A**). Additional areas of ground glass are often present in the perimediastinal lung (**B**) and less commonly in the subpleural lung (**A**).

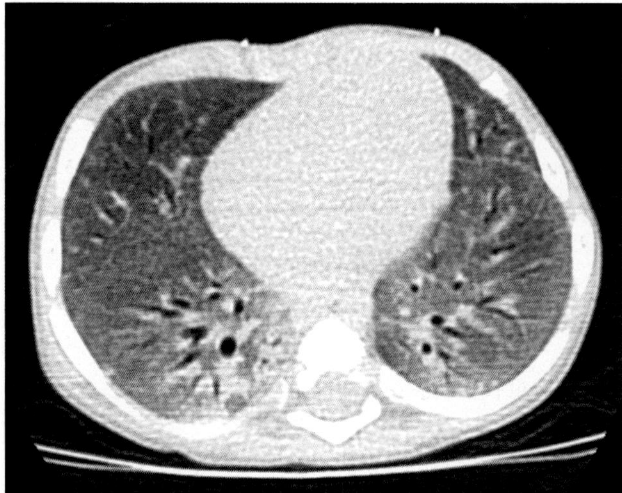

FIGURE 67.38. **10 Month Old With Tachypnea Since Birth and Worsening Respiratory Distress.** A diagnosis of surfactant protein ABCA3 mutation was made by a blood test for genetic analysis. Biopsy was not necessary. The classical appearance of "crazy paving" is often seen in these infants, but the septal thickening is variable and may be far less striking than the diffuse ground-glass opacity.

There are no screening tests for the majority of PrIDs, so the diagnosis is usually made when frequent or unusual infections occur. Small or absent thymus, adenoids, or tonsils are a feature of several PrIDs, and their presence or absence can be useful in the differential diagnosis. A broad range of genetic defects are associated with PrIDs and genetic testing will likely be a primary diagnostic tool in the future.

Cystic Fibrosis

Cystic fibrosis (CF) is caused by a defect in a cell membrane chloride channel called the cystic fibrosis transmembrane regulator (CFTR). There are over 3,000 mutations that result in defective CFTR. Newborn screening for CF is performed in all states in the United States and is widely performed worldwide. Almost all cases of CF are now identified by newborn screening. CXRs in children with CF are either normal or show findings of mild airways disease in the great majority of children with CF. CT scans most often are either normal or show mild bronchiectasis and bronchial wall thickening with some mucous plugging. The cystic bronchiectasis and major mucous plugging once characteristic of children with CF are now seen in a small minority of cases. New drug therapies, called CFTR modulators, can correct the basic defect of CF and are likely to further decrease the severity of CF lung disease in the future.

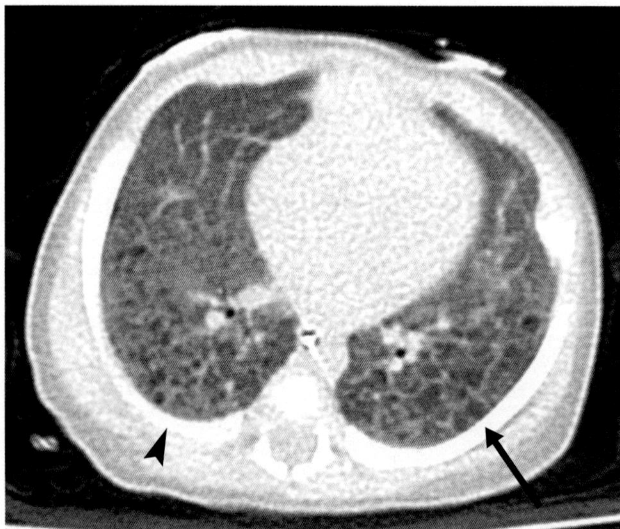

FIGURE 67.39. **Alveolar Growth Abnormality.** A 2 month old born at 30 weeks intubated at birth for respiratory distress. The appearance of an alveolar growth abnormality is nonspecific. The distinguishing features include distorted secondary lobular architecture with lobules of varying size and attenuation (*arrow*). Cysts (*arrowhead*) and ground-glass opacity also suggest the diagnosis.

Sickle Cell Disease

The most common chest finding in children with sickle cell disease is cardiomegaly, usually mild. The most common pulmonary manifestation is the acute chest syndrome. ACS is defined similarly in adults and children. In children, a cause of ACS is identified less than 15% of the time. Rib infarcts and associated pain have been suggested to be a common etiology, and pain management and incentive spirometry have been suggested to be useful in speeding the resolution of ACS.

Rheumatoid/Collagen Vascular Disease

Diffuse lung disease is the most common pulmonary manifestation of these diseases. Band-like or focal peripheral areas of "reticular ground-glass" areas which have both characteristics, suggest this etiology and may precede a clinical diagnosis (Fig. 67.40).

LUNG TRAUMA

Spontaneous pneumothorax (SP) in children occurs primarily in teenage boys. Apical blebs are commonly found in patients with SP, and abnormal collagen has been suggested as an etiology. SP can be divided into primary, in which there is no associated respiratory disease; and secondary in which respiratory disease such as asthma is present. Primary is more common than secondary, and both are much more common

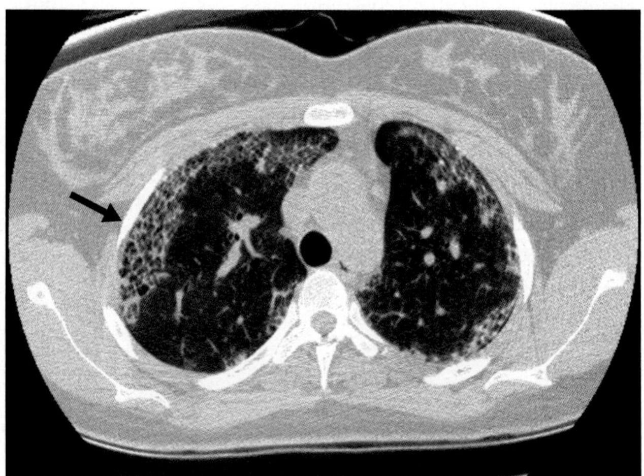

FIGURE 67.40. **17 Year Old With Polymyositis.** The peripheral opacities have been described as "reticular ground glass." When these changes are marked (*arrow*) the appearance can be similar to idiopathic pulmonary fibrosis, but the distribution is different, with frequent upper lobe involvement and without a basilar predominance. It is important to remember that idiopathic pulmonary fibrosis does not occur in children.

in males than in females. One study found that all CT abnormalities in patients with SP were located in the apices and suggested that CT can be limited to the upper lungs.

Pneumomediastinum

Most commonly no etiology is identified in otherwise well children with pneumomediastinum. When an etiology is identified, asthma is the most common, with foreign body aspiration an important cause rarely seen in adults. Unlike adults, pneumomediastinum is rarely due to esophageal trauma in children and an esophagram is not routinely required.

Blunt Force Trauma

Blunt force trauma makes up about ¾ of chest trauma in children. Pulmonary contusions are the most common injury. A sign that may distinguish contusion from atelectasis is the presence of subpleural sparing. Pulmonary lacerations are rare, occurring in less than 2% of significant chest trauma. Aortic and tracheal injury is rare, but does occur. CXRs are usually abnormal in aortic injury with an indistinct aortic knob seen in 94% in one study. Children's ribs are more flexible than those of adults and substantial lung injury can be seen without rib fractures.

In one study, more than 98% of significant chest injuries were identified on abdominal CT, supporting focused CT rather than "pan scanning."

THE UPPER AIRWAY

Evaluating the Upper Airway

In school age and older children, the airway is similar to the adult airway and the normal structures are usually well seen. In infants and young children a short neck, redundant soft tissues, and limited cooperation make airway evaluation more challenging. Several techniques may be useful in addressing these challenges. If there is concern for an acute airway abnormality frontal and lateral views should be obtained. A single lateral view can be used if a study is requested only to evaluate the size of the tonsils and adenoids. Images should be obtained during inspiration to avoid buckling of the airway and normal airway collapse. Extension of the neck is very helpful, particularly when evaluating the retropharyngeal soft tissues.

The trachea is not normally a midline structure, but is located slightly off-midline, on the side opposite to the aortic arch. When the trachea buckles in expiration it buckles away from the aortic arch so should normally buckle to the right. Buckling can be striking. The sharp angulations of the buckled trachea distinguish this normal appearance from the bowed appearance of the trachea when there is a neck mass (Fig. 67.7).

Upper Airway Infection

Croup. Croup, also called laryngotracheobronchitis, is a viral infection that affects the upper and lower airways, particularly the subglottic trachea. Croup is the most common infectious disease of the upper airway. Parainfluenza virus is the most common pathogen, but many other viruses and even mycoplasma can cause croup. Croup has a gradual onset, often with low-grade fever. Patients classically develop a barking cough and frequently stridor. Croup has a seasonal pattern, occurring most often in the fall. Children 6 months to 3 years are most commonly affected.

Frontal radiographs show symmetrical narrowing of the subglottic airway with a configuration that is described as a pencil point or church steeple (Fig. 67.41A). On lateral view, the subglottic airway may be narrowed and often has a hazy appearance reflecting the tapering seen on frontal view (Fig. 67.41B). The epiglottis and aryepiglottic folds are normal, distinguishing croup from epiglottitis.

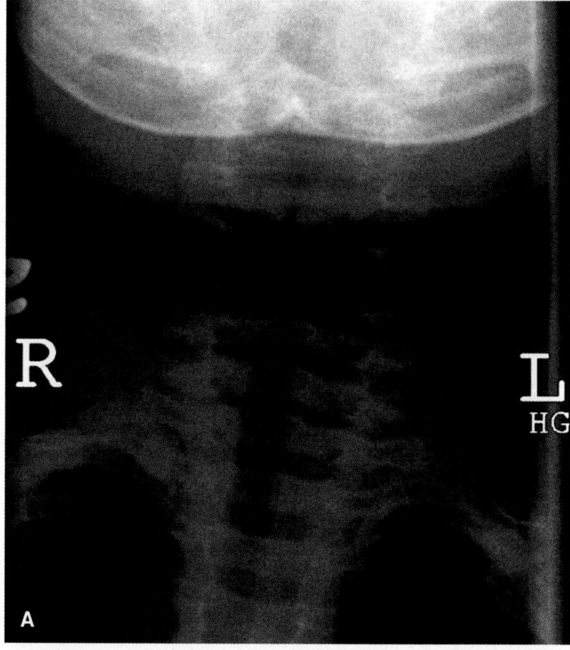

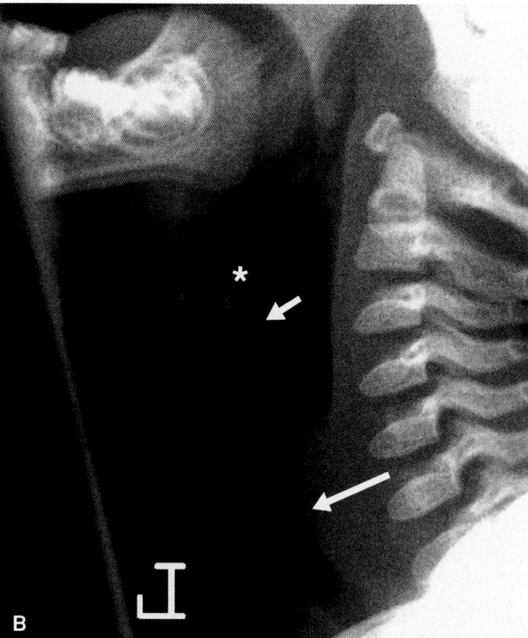

FIGURE 67.41. **Croup.** In the AP view (**A**) symmetrical subglottic narrowing causes loss of the normal "shoulders" of the subglottic airway. This has been called the steeple or pencil point sign. On the lateral view (**B**) the subglottic airway blurs below the vocal cords reflecting the narrowing seen on frontal view (*arrow*). The epiglottis (*) is normal. It's mildly broad appearance reflects a U-shaped or omega epiglottis. More important than the shape of the epiglottis in distinguishing croup from epiglottitis is the appearance of the aryepiglottic folds (*arrowhead*) which should be thin.

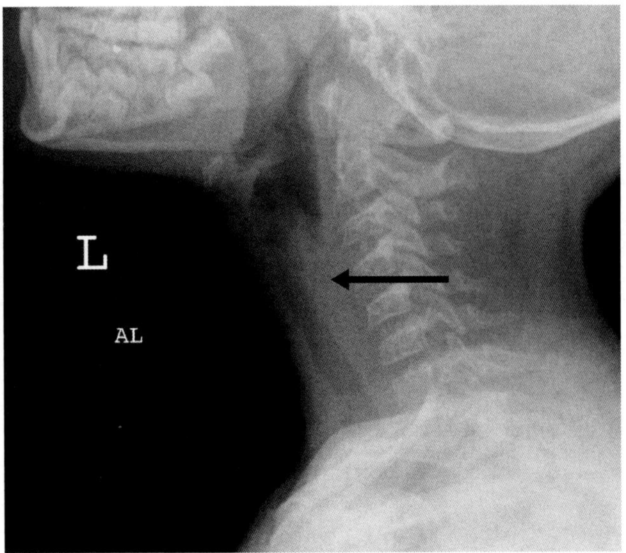

FIGURE 67.42. **Bacterial Tracheitis in a 6 Year Old.** The tracheal wall is irregular and there is an intraluminal filling defect (*arrow*).

Bacterial Tracheitis

Bacterial tracheitis, also called bacterial croup and membranous croup also affects the subglottic airway, but is a much more virulent infection. Onset is sudden and high fever is common. Bacterial tracheitis often affects older children. Mucopurulent exudates form on the airway wall and can detach and obstruct the airway. *Moraxella catarrhalis* and *Staphylococcus aureus* are the most common pathogens.

Identification of an intraluminal filling defect, representing a sloughed membrane, is a specific but not sensitive sign on airway radiographs (Fig. 67.42). Other findings include an irregular airway wall and asymmetric narrowing, but these do not reliably distinguish viral croup from bacterial tracheitis. Airway endoscopy with direct visualization of the exudate is the most reliable diagnostic method.

Epiglottitis

Since the widespread use of *Haemophilus influenzae* vaccine, epiglottitis has become a rare cause of upper airway disease. Although now very rare, epiglottitis still occurs and is a life-threatening infection. Epiglottitis has also been called supraglottitis. This is an appropriate term as inflammation is not limited to the epiglottis. The term supraglottitis is a useful one as it reminds us that swelling involves the aryepiglottic folds as well as the epiglottis and the swollen folds are as important as the swollen epiglottis in causing airway obstruction (Fig. 67.43).

Retropharyngeal Abscess

The retropharyngeal space lies posterior to the airway from the skull base to the tracheal carina. The retropharyngeal space contains lymph nodes that are prominent in children but regress after puberty. The spread of oropharyngeal flora to these lymph nodes is thought to be the most common mechanism of retropharyngeal abscess. Polymicrobial infections are common with Group A streptococcus, the most common single organism. Widening of the retropharyngeal soft tissues on a lateral neck radiograph is the most common finding. Be careful, though. Redundant soft tissue causing retropharyngeal soft tissue widening is very common and can be easily mistaken for pathologic widening.

Laryngomalacia

Laryngomalacia is a congenital softening of the soft tissues of the pharynx that leads to airway collapse with inspiration. It is the most common cause of noisy breathing in infants and is the most common congenital abnormality of the larynx. Children with laryngomalacia usually present in the first month of life and may be symptomatic at birth. Improvement is usually seen by 6 months with resolution of symptoms by 18 months. Treatment is rarely needed, with 90% of cases of laryngomalacia resolving spontaneously.

Obstructive Sleep Apnea

Obstructive sleep apnea (OSA) does occur in children and can be an important cause of respiratory and CNS issues. The first step in treatment is usually tonsillectomy and adenoidectomy, and weight loss if appropriate. If this is unsuccessful, multiple treatments are available. A lateral neck radiograph can be used to evaluate adenoid size. When necessary, MRI performed under sedation to simulate sleep provides the most complete evaluation. Expertise is required to interpret these studies, and careful interpretation is required, as the results will often influence the type of surgery performed.

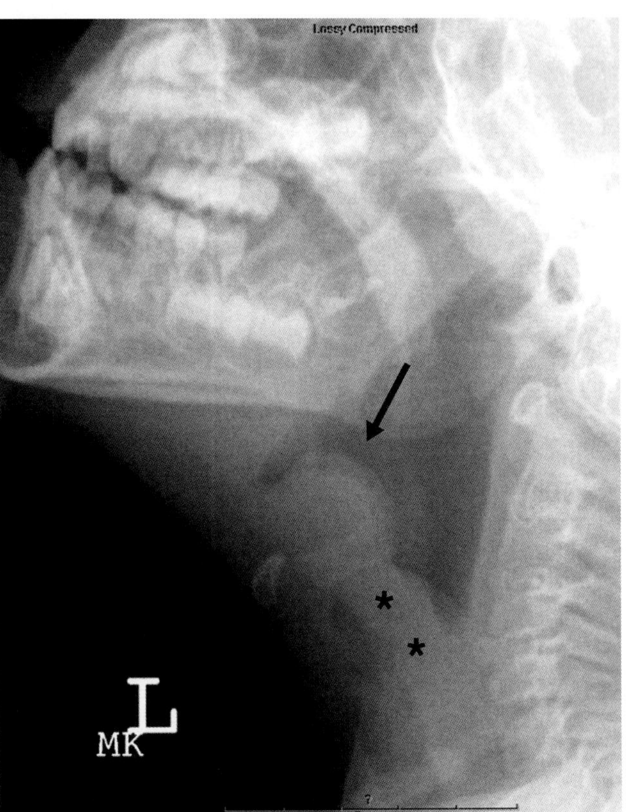

FIGURE 67.43. **Epiglottitis.** The epiglottis (*arrow*) is broad and short. The aryepiglottic folds are thickened (*). Note that the attenuation of the aryepiglottic folds is similar to the surrounding soft tissues of the neck reflecting almost complete obliteration of the airway. This image shows that the obstruction is due to the thickened folds as much or more than to the swollen epiglottis.

Suggested Readings

Agrons GA, Courtney SE, Stocker JT, Markowitz RI. From the archives of the AFIP: lung disease in premature neonates: radiologic-pathologic correlation. *Radiographics* 2005;25(4):1047–1073.

Ampofo K, Bender J, Sheng X, et al. Seasonal invasive pneumococcal disease in children: role of preceding respiratory viral infection. *Pediatrics* 2008;122(2):229–237.

Baez JC, Lee EY, Restrepo R, Eisenberg RL. Chest wall lesions in children. *AJR Am J Roentgenol* 2013;200(5):W402–W419.

Bano S, Chaudhary V, Narula MK, et al. Pulmonary Langerhans cell histiocytosis in children: a spectrum of radiologic findings. *Eur J Radiol* 2014;83(1):47–56.

Berrocal T, Madrid C, Novo S, Gutiérrez J, Arjonilla A, Gómez-León N. Congenital anomalies of the tracheobronchial tree, lung, and mediastinum: embryology, radiology, and pathology. *Radiographics* 2004;24(1):e17.

Bettenay FA, de Campo JF, McCrossin DB. Differentiating bacterial from viral pneumonias in children. *Pediatr Radiol* 1988;18(6):453–454.

Breen M, Zurakowski D, Lee EY. Clinical significance of pulmonary nodules detected on abdominal CT in pediatric patients. *Pediatr Radiol* 2015;45(12):1753–1760.

Bullaro FM, Bartoletti SC. Spontaneous pneumomediastinum in children: a literature review. *Pediatr Emerg Care* 2007;23(1):28–30.

Chang AB, Masel JP, Masters B. Post-infectious bronchiolitis obliterans: clinical, radiological and pulmonary function sequelae. *Pediatr Radiol* 1998;28(1):23–29.

Cruz AT, Starke JR. Pediatric tuberculosis. *Pediatr Rev* 2010;31(1):13–25; quiz 25–26.

Daltro P, Fricke BL, Kuroki I, Domingues R, Donnelly LF. CT of congenital lung lesions in pediatric patients. *AJR Am J Roentgenol* 2004;183(5):1497–1506.

Deutsch GH, Young LR, Deterding RR, et al. Diffuse lung disease in young children: application of a novel classification scheme. *Am J Respir Crit Care Med* 2007;176(11):1120–1128.

Dishop MK, Kuruvilla S. Primary and metastatic lung tumors in the pediatric population: a review and 25-year experience at a large children's hospital. *Arch Pathol Lab Med* 2008;132(7):1079–1103.

Donnelly LF. Maximizing the usefulness of imaging in children with community-acquired pneumonia. *AJR Am J Roentgenol* 1999;172(2):505–512.

Donnelly LF. Magnetic resonance sleep studies in the evaluation of children with obstructive sleep apnea. *Semin Ultrasound CT MR* 2010;31(2):107–115.

Donnelly LF, Lucaya J, Ozelame V, et al. CT findings and temporal course of persistent pulmonary interstitial emphysema in neonates: a multiinstitutional study. *AJR Am J Roentgenol* 2003;180(4):1129–1133.

Edwards DK, Higgins CB, Gilpin EA. The cardiothoracic ratio in newborn infants. *AJR Am J Roentgenol* 1981;136(5):907–913.

Epelman M, Kreiger PA, Servaes S, Victoria T, Hellinger JC. Current imaging of prenatally diagnosed congenital lung lesions. *Semin Ultrasound CT MR* 2010;31(2):141–157.

Eslamy HK, Newman B. Pneumonia in normal and immunocompromised children: an overview and update. *Radiol Clin North Am* 2011;49(5):895–920.

Esposito S, Bosis S, Cavagna R, et al. Characteristics of Streptococcus pneumoniae and atypical bacterial infections in children 2–5 years of age with community-acquired pneumonia. *Clin Infect Dis* 2002;35(11):1345–1352.

Ferwerda A, Moll HA, de Groot R. Respiratory tract infections by Mycoplasma pneumoniae in children: a review of diagnostic and therapeutic measures. *Eur J Pediatr* 2001;160(8):483–491.

Garcia-Garcia ML, Calvo C, Pozo F, Villadangos PA, Pérez-Breña P, Casas I. Spectrum of respiratory viruses in children with community-acquired pneumonia. *Pediatr Infect Dis J* 2012;31(8):808–813.

Giuseppucci C, Reusmann A, Giubergia V, et al. Primary lung tumors in children: 24 years of experience at a referral center. *Pediatr Surg Int* 2016;32(5):451–457.

Guimaraes CV, Donnelly LF, Warner BW. CT findings for blebs and bullae in children with spontaneous pneumothorax and comparison with findings in normal age-matched controls. *Pediatr Radiol* 2007;37(9):879–884.

Guo W, Wang J, Sheng M, Zhou M, Fang L. Radiological findings in 210 paediatric patients with viral pneumonia: a retrospective case study. *Br J Radiol* 2012;85(1018):1385–1389.

Hudak ML, Martin DJ, Egan EA, et al. A multicenter randomized masked comparison trial of synthetic surfactant versus calf lung surfactant extract in the prevention of neonatal respiratory distress syndrome. *Pediatrics* 1997;100(1):39–50.

Jesenak M, Banovcin P, Jesenakova B, Babusikova E. Pulmonary manifestations of primary immunodeficiency disorders in children. *Front Pediatr* 2014;2:77.

Kaneko M, Suzuki K, Furui H, Takagi K, Satake T. Comparison of theophylline and enprofylline effects on human neutrophil superoxide production. *Clin Exp Pharmacol Physiol* 1990;17(12):849–859.

Kim YW, Donnelly LF. Round pneumonia: imaging findings in a large series of children. *Pediatr Radiol* 2007;37(12):1235–1240.

Langston C. New concepts in the pathology of congenital lung malformations. *Semin Pediatr Surg* 2003;12(1):17–37.

Laya BF, Goske MJ, Morrison S, et al. The accuracy of chest radiographs in the detection of congenital heart disease and in the diagnosis of specific congenital cardiac lesions. *Pediatr Radiol* 2006;36(7):677–681.

Leung AN, Müller NL, Pineda PR, FitzGerald JM. Primary tuberculosis in childhood: radiographic manifestations. *Radiology* 1992;182(1):87–91.

Maldonado JA, Henry T, Gutierrez FR. Congenital thoracic vascular anomalies. *Radiol Clin North Am* 2010;48(1):85–115.

Manchanda, S., Bhalla AS, Jana M, Gupta AK. Imaging of the pediatric thymus: Clinicoradiologic approach. *World J Clin Pediatr* 2017;6(1):10–23.

McIntosh K. Community-acquired pneumonia in children. *N Engl J Med* 2002; 346(6):429–437.

Menashe A, Atzaba-Poria N. Parent-child interaction: Does parental language matter? *Br J Dev Psychol* 2016;34(4):518–537.

Michelow IC, Olsen K, Lozano J, et al. Epidemiology and clinical characteristics of community-acquired pneumonia in hospitalized children. *Pediatrics* 2004; 113(4):701–707.

Neuman MI, Monuteaux MC, Scully KJ, Bachur RG. Prediction of pneumonia in a pediatric emergency department. *Pediatrics* 2011;128(2):246–253.

Newman B. Thoracic neoplasms in children. *Radiol Clin North Am* 2011; 49(4):633–664, v.

Nissen MD. Congenital and neonatal pneumonia. *Paediatr Respir Rev* 2007; 8(3):195–203.

Olarte L, Barson WJ, Barson RM, et al. Pneumococcal pneumonia requiring hospitalization in US children in the 13-valent pneumococcal conjugate vaccine era. *Clin Infect Dis* 2017;64(12):1699–1704.

Oymar K, Skjerven HO, Mikalsen IB. Acute bronchiolitis in infants, a review. *Scand J Trauma Resusc Emerg Med* 2014;22:23.

Pabon-Ramos WM, Williams DM, Strouse PJ. Radiologic evaluation of blunt thoracic aortic injury in pediatric patients. *AJR Am J Roentgenol* 2010;194(5):1197–1203.

Pauze DR, Pauze DK. Emergency management of blunt chest trauma in children: an evidence-based approach. *Pediatr Emerg Med Pract* 2013;10(11):1–22; quiz 22–23.

Perez-Velez CM, Marais BJ. Tuberculosis in children. *N Engl J Med* 2012; 367(4):348–361.

Pickhardt PJ, Siegel MJ, Gutierrez FR. Vascular rings in symptomatic children: frequency of chest radiographic findings. *Radiology* 1997;203(2):423–426.

Ranganath SH, Lee EY, Restrepo R, Eisenberg RL. Mediastinal masses in children. *AJR Am J Roentgenol* 2012;198(3):W197–W216.

Sandu K, Monnier P. Congenital tracheal anomalies. *Otolaryngol Clin North Am* 2007;40(1):193–217, viii.

Satou GM, Lacro RV, Chung T, Gauvreau K, Jenkins KJ. Heart size on chest x-ray as a predictor of cardiac enlargement by echocardiography in children. *Pediatr Cardiol* 2001;22(3):218–222.

Schlesinger AE, Braverman RM, DiPietro MA. Pictorial essay. Neonates and umbilical venous catheters: normal appearance, anomalous positions, complications, and potential aid to diagnosis. *AJR Am J Roentgenol* 2003;180(4):1147–1153.

Semple T, Akhtar MR, Owens CM. Imaging bronchopulmonary dysplasia—a multimodality update. *Front Med (Lausanne)* 2017;4:88.

Soudack M, Plotkin S, Ben-Shlush A, et al. The added value of the lateral chest radiograph for Diagnosing Community Acquired Pneumonia in the Pediatric Emergency Department. *Isr Med Assoc J* 2018;1(20):5–8.

Stuckey-Schrock K, Hayes BL, George CM. Community-acquired pneumonia in children. *Am Fam Physician* 2012;86(7):661–667.

Wahlgren H, Mortensson W, Eriksson M, Finkel Y, Forsgren M, Leinonen M. Radiological findings in children with acute pneumonia: age more important than infectious agent. *Acta Radiol* 2005;46(4):431–436.

Wasilewska E, Lee EY, Eisenberg RL. Unilateral hyperlucent lung in children. *AJR Am J Roentgenol* 2012;198(5):W400–W414.

Zorc JJ, Hall CB. Bronchiolitis: recent evidence on diagnosis and management. *Pediatrics* 2010;125(2):342–349.

CHAPTER 68 ■ CONGENITAL AND PEDIATRIC HEART DISEASE

ROBERT J. FLECK, Jr.

Pediatric radiologists have played a role in the diagnosis of congenital heart disease (CHD) since the advent of the chest x-ray, and their role has evolved as more modalities have become available for diagnosis and evaluation of CHD, both prior to and after palliation. Currently, many pregnancies in the developed world are evaluated by prenatal ultrasound which affords a good opportunity to diagnose many CHD conditions prior to birth and leads to fetal echocardiography with prenatal care and delivery in a center capable of caring for children born with heart lesions. Many congenital heart lesions present relatively early in life and result in a chest x-ray and/or echocardiography. Chest x-ray is sometimes helpful but often not specific for anatomic delineation of the structural lesion; whereas echocardiography is often diagnostic and outlines the anatomy of the heart, valves, great arteries, and veins in great detail during infancy. The radiologist's contribution to the diagnosis of CHD with a chest x-ray is still important in modern medicine, but more difficult in that we must now recognize certain abnormalities when children present with undiagnosed CHD.

CT and MRI have become the imaging modality of choice for evaluating the many diseases that affect the heart in children. CT angiography can provide a complete evaluation of the chest including the great arteries, coronary arteries, pulmonary arteries (PAs) and veins, the airways and lungs, all of which may have clinically important findings prior to or after surgery. MRI provides unique information about the myocardium, chamber function, vessel flow, and the mediastinum and soon will be capable of providing structural information about the lungs, lung perfusion, and ventilation. MRI plays a huge role in the assessment of palliated CHD, and in the diagnosis and assessment of cardiomyopathy.

Due to space and time constraints, this chapter will begin with a framework for assessment of the chest x-ray and include more of the advanced imaging for illustrating the chest x-ray findings and points of discussion about the use of MRI and CT as "teasers" to provide for further in-depth learning about imaging of the heart.

PULMONARY VASCULARITY

In the assessment of CHD, the pulmonary vascularity assessment is very important, yet, difficult to master. There are four types of patterns: (1) increased pulmonary vascularity due to increased flow of blood through the lungs (active congestion); (2) increased pulmonary vascularity due to elevated pulmonary venous pressure (passive congestion); (3) decreased pulmonary vascularity due to obstruction of blood flow through the PA; (4) normal pulmonary vascularity (Table 68.1). Importantly, studies have shown that radiologists have good sensitivity and specificity for detecting normal or increased pulmonary vascularity but poor sensitivity for identifying decreased vascularity. However, the specificity for decreased vascularity was good; therefore, when decreased vascularity is recognized, it is most likely present. This is not to minimize the importance of classifying vascularity but to encourage careful attention and calibration of the eye, so that pulmonary vascularity can be properly noted when it is abnormal because this is where we can still make a difference in undiagnosed CHD when shunt vascularity, passive congestion, or decreased pulmonary vascularity are present in a child presenting with relatively nonspecific symptoms of respiratory distress.

Active congestion, or increased flow through the pulmonary vasculature, is the most commonly encountered, undiagnosed CHD vascular flow pattern encountered by routine chest x-ray. This appearance is seen when a systemic to pulmonary, left-to-right shunt is occurring that is large enough to detect on a chest x-ray. This usually requires pulmonary flow 2 to 2.5 times that of the left ventricle (LV) cardiac output. This amount of increased blood flow is in the range that needs clinical attention. In this situation, the main pulmonary artery (MPA) segment of the mediastinal silhouette and pulmonary vessels becomes enlarged. A rule of thumb is that if the descending PA on the right is as large as the trachea diameter and other vessels are increased in diameter and appear somewhat torturous, then pulmonary vascularity is increased

TABLE 68.1

PULMONARY VASCULAR PATTERNS

Increased vascularity (active) without cyanosis
- Atrial septal defect
- Ventricular septal defect
- Patent ductus arteriosus
- Aortopulmonary window
- Ruptured aneurysm of sinus of Valsalva
- Coronary artery fistula
- Partial anomalous pulmonary venous return

Increased vascularity (active) with cyanosis
- Total anomalous pulmonary venous return (types 1, 2)
- Persistent truncus arteriosus
- Complete endocardial cushion defect
- Transposition of the great vessels complex
- Single ventricle (without pulmonary stenosis)

Increased vascularity (passive)
- Total anomalous pulmonary venous return (type 3)
- Pulmonary vein atresia
- Hypoplastic left heart syndrome (in failure)
- Cor triatriatum

Decreased vascularity
- Tetralogy of Fallot
- Pseudotruncus arteriosus
- Hypoplastic right heart syndrome (right-to-left shunt)
    - Tricuspid atresia
    - Pulmonary atresia
    - Tricuspid stenosis
    - Hypoplastic RV
- Ebstein anomaly
- Uhl anomaly
- Trilogy of Fallot
- Single ventricle or transposition of great vessels with pulmonary stenosis or atresia
- Tricuspid or pulmonary insufficiency with right-to-left shunt

Normal vascularity
- Left heart lesions
    - Coarctation of the aorta
    - Interrupted aortic arch
    - Hypoplastic left heart syndrome (before failure develops)
    - Endocardial fibroelastosis
    - Cardiomyopathy
    - Aberrant left coronary artery
    - Mitral stenosis and insufficiency
    - Aortic stenosis and insufficiency
    - Cor triatriatum
- Right heart lesions (without right-to-left shunt)
    - Pulmonary stenosis or insufficiency
    - Tricuspid insufficiency

(Fig. 68.1). The margins of the vessels are sharply defined if there is no component of passive congestion. Often there is a mixed pattern of active and passive congestion and the margins of the vessels appear indistinct due to interstitial fullness and the lungs are frequently hyperinflated due to small-airway obstruction.

Passive congestion occurs when there is elevation of the pulmonary venous pressure. Causes include abnormalities of the LV, mitral valve, right atrium (RA) (cor triatriatum), or obstruction of pulmonary venous return (total anomalous pulmonary venous return [TAPVR] or pulmonary vein stenosis). The pulmonary veins enlarge and become ill-defined due to fluid leaking into the interstitial tissues of the lungs (Fig. 68.2).

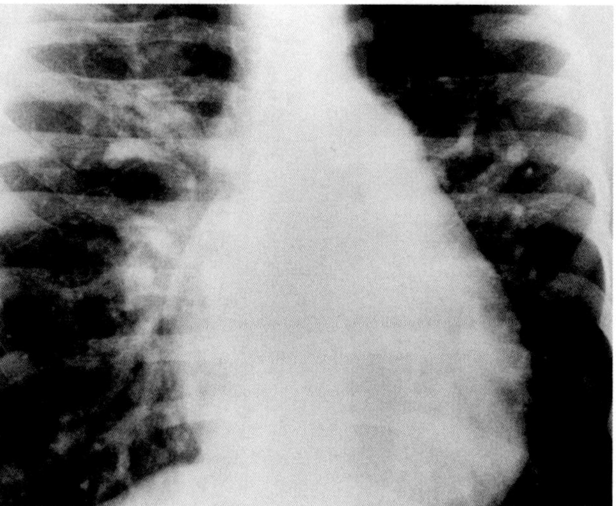

FIGURE 68.1. Active Congestion. Large but distinct pulmonary vessels extend into the periphery of the lung as the result of left-to-right shunting in a patient with a large ventricular septal defect.

There is often compensation for this by increased lymphatic flow, but depending on the pulmonary venous pressure and the time course, interstitial edema can leak into the alveoli to become alveolar pulmonary edema and into the pleural spaces, creating pleural effusion.

Decreased pulmonary vascularity is caused by substantially decreased blood flow to the pulmonary vascular bed usually due to obstruction of the right ventricular outflow at the infundibulum, pulmonary valve, or main PA. The diminished flow to the lungs causes the lungs to appear symmetrically hyperlucent with thin, small vessels and often a concave main PA segment (Fig. 68.3).

Normal pulmonary vascularity is commonly seen even in the presence of congenital heart lesions that would be expected to cause decreased pulmonary vascularity and in situations where the alteration of blood flow is not large enough to

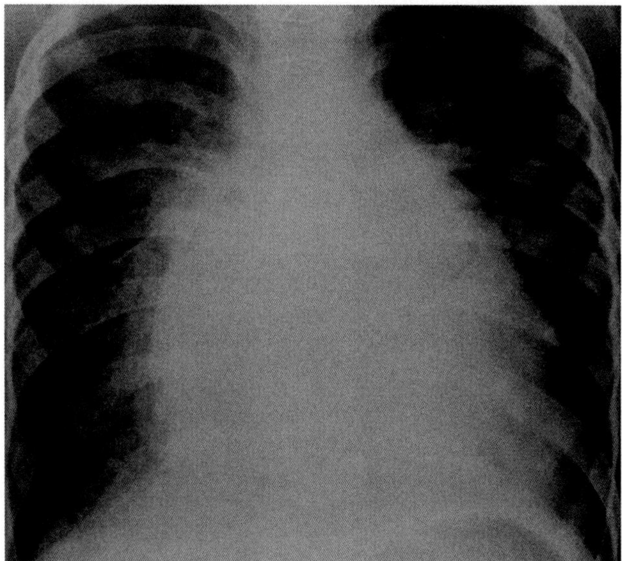

FIGURE 68.2. Passive Congestion. Passive vascular congestion is caused by mitral insufficiency and results in indistinctness of the pulmonary vascular markings.

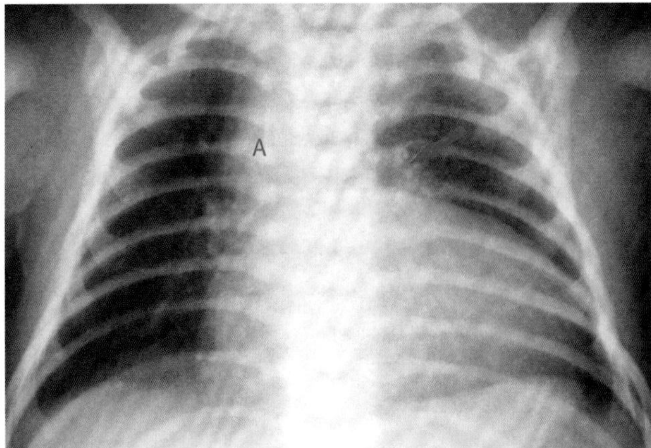

FIGURE 68.3. Decreased Vascularity Is Evident in a Patient With Tetralogy of Fallot. Note the right aortic arch (*A*), concave pulmonary artery segment (*arrow*), and the characteristic "boot" configuration of the heart caused by right ventricular hypertrophy.

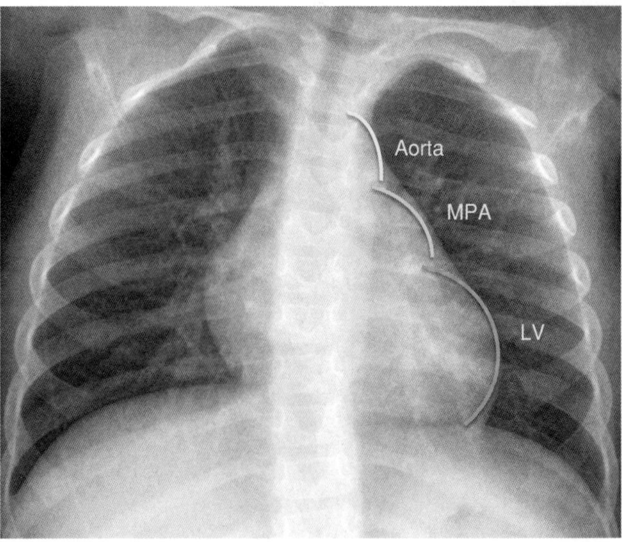

FIGURE 68.4. Chest X-Ray in a Typical 3 Year Old. The *yellow* contour is the transverse aortic knob. The *green* contour represents the main pulmonary artery (*MPA*) segment which is usually gently convex in normal patients. The *blue* contour is the left ventricle (*LV*).

cause a perceptible change in caliber of the pulmonary vessels. Uncomplicated valvular diseases, coarctation of the aorta, and early cardiomyopathy have normal blood flow and so normal pulmonary vascularity.

Asymmetric pulmonary blood flow bears mentioning because it is often present in CHD, especially in tetralogy of Fallot (TOF), truncus arteriosus, pulmonic stenosis, and postoperative patients. Asymmetric pulmonary blood flow can be due to focal pulmonary arterial stenosis (William syndrome) or underlying lung abnormality (prematurity, congenital diaphragmatic hernia).

Cardiac and Mediastinal Contours

One of my mentors used to say, "A normal chest x-ray does not rule out CHD, but careful analysis of chest x-ray abnormalities can provide very good clues to underlying pathophysiology!"

The trachea is a lucent column of air and provides important information about adjacent structures. The most important of these structures is the aortic arch. The location of the aortic arch is an important clue in evaluating CHD, and the aortic knob is often difficult to see in young children. If the tracheal air column is visible, it is generally positioned slightly to the opposite side of midline from the aorta. There is frequently a slight, rounded impression into the air column on the side of the aorta. The presence of a right aortic arch often causes trachea displacement to the left and indentation on the right side of the trachea (Fig. 68.3). A right aortic arch can be seen in TOF, truncus arteriosus, double aortic arch, and right aortic arch with an aberrant left subclavian artery.

There are three contours along the left cardiomediastinal silhouette. The first contour visible along the normal mediastinum is from the transverse aortic "knob" which, when visible, can be assessed for size, position, and morphology (Fig. 68.4). The most commonly encountered contour abnormality is seen in coarctation of the aorta which can be associated with aortic valvar abnormality (see below) (Fig. 68.5).

The second contour visible along the normal mediastinum is the main PA segment. If the main PA is small, this segment is concave and the pulmonary vascularity is usually decreased, such as is seen in TOF (Fig. 68.3). This contour can be large due to a left-to-right shunt, poststenotic dilation from pulmonary valvar stenosis, pulmonary valvular insufficiency, or pulmonary hypertension (Fig. 68.6).

The most inferior mediastinal contour is the heart and pericardium. On the left this is usually the LV and on the right it is usually the RA. Assessing the heart size in pediatric patients is fraught with peril, but some guidelines are helpful. First, the cardiothoracic ratio changes rapidly with age from about 65% of the transverse dimension of the chest to the normal adult ratio of less than 50%. Second, the size of

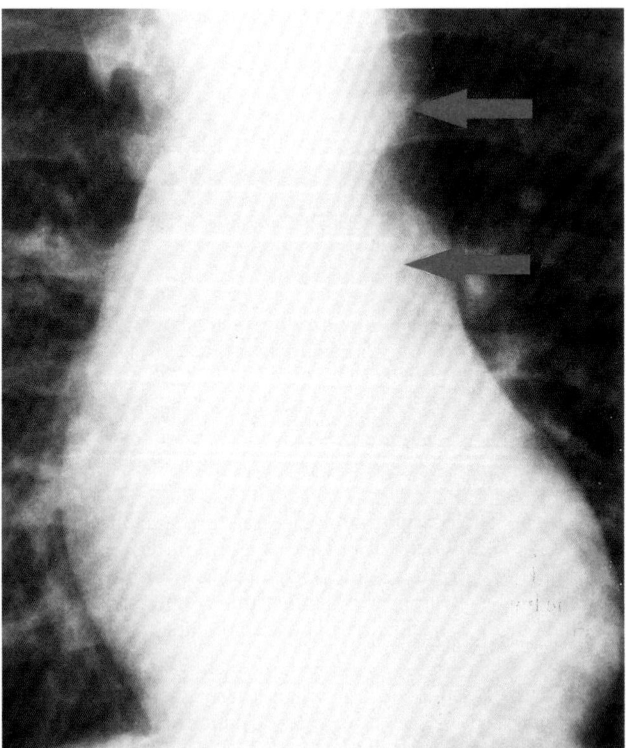

FIGURE 68.5. Coarctation of the Aorta. Prestenotic and poststenotic dilation of the aorta creates the characteristic "figure-3" sign (*arrows*).

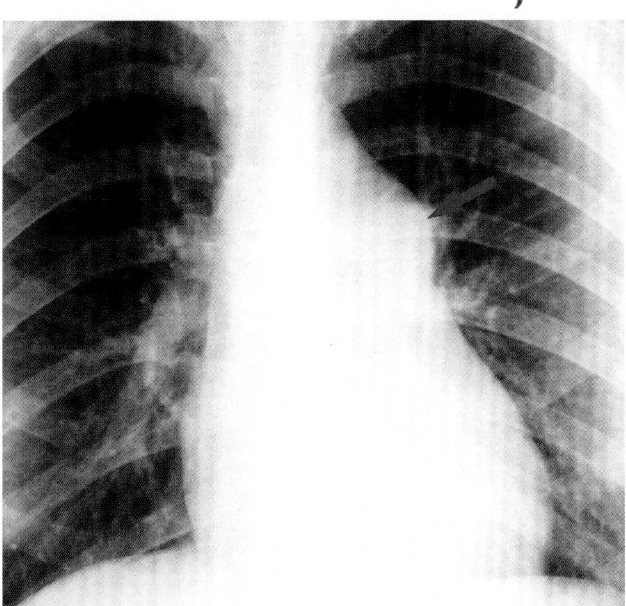

FIGURE 68.6. **Pulmonary Artery Enlargement.** Poststenotic dilation of the pulmonary artery is seen in this patient with valvular pulmonic stenosis (*arrow*).

the heart in young children relative to the transverse diameter of the chest depends greatly on their degree of inspiration (at low inspiration, the heart appears large). Therefore, it is important to assess the degree of pulmonary inflation prior to suggesting that the heart is large or small. Six anterior rib ends above the diaphragmatic shadow are normal. If there is a lateral chest x-ray available, then this can be used to assess for cardiomegaly by tracing a line down the anterior trachea. If the posterior aspect of the heart doesn't extend beyond this line, then it is unlikely that cardiomegaly is present. The other major confounder of cardiac size in children is thymic tissue, which can be quite prominent. When considering cardiomegaly, keep in mind that it may be pericardial effusion resulting in the enlarged pericardial silhouette. Generally, a pericardial effusion has a more globular, saggy appearance (Fig. 68.7A), but it can be difficult to determine. Echocardiography is indicated for both cardiomegaly and pericardial effusions, so it is usually the arbiter of truth (Fig. 68.7B). There are many causes of pericardial effusions because they can accompany viral infections, Kawasaki disease, renal failure, collagen vascular disease, rheumatic fever, malignancies, and many others. Noncardiac etiologies of cardiac enlargement include arteriovenous fistulas (vein of Galen aneurysm, infantile hemangioma of the liver), chronic anemias such as sickle cell disease and thalassemia, and hyperparathyroidism.

ACYANOTIC HEART DISEASE WITH INCREASED PULMONARY VASCULARITY

This is one of the most commonly encountered undiagnosed CHD found by chest x-ray in day-to-day practice. A left-to-right shunt causes an increase in the size of the heart, PAs, and the main PA segment. Most common causes include atrial septal defect (ASD), patent ductus arteriosus (PDA), or ventricular septal defect (VSD). If a left-to-right shunt is large enough, the pulmonary pressures will eventually increase and the shunt will reverse because of pulmonary hypertension, a phenomenon called Eisenmenger physiology.

Ventricular septal defect is the most common congenital heart anomaly and can be isolated or associated with more complex CHD. Perimembranous defects are both the most common and the most likely to be symptomatic. These occur where the membranous and muscular septum fuse. Muscular VSDs are often small, multiple, less hemodynamically significant, and tend to close over time. Conal VSDs are uncommon (5%) and occur due to an abnormal development of the conus portion of the truncus during cardiac development. They are most commonly seen in TOF or truncus arteriosus.

A VSD is usually not evident either clinically or radiographically in the newborn due to the high pulmonary vascular resistance at birth. Without a pressure gradient between the ventricles, little blood will shunt left to right. As pulmonary vascular resistance drops, the left-to-right shunt increases and a murmur may become clinically evident. The symptoms and presentation depend on the size of the defect and hemodynamics of the patient. A moderate to large VSD usually results in symptomatic presentation in the first 2 years of life. Small defects often close or remain asymptomatic. Radiographic features (in addition to increased vascularity) that can suggest a VSD include a prominent LV, main PA segment

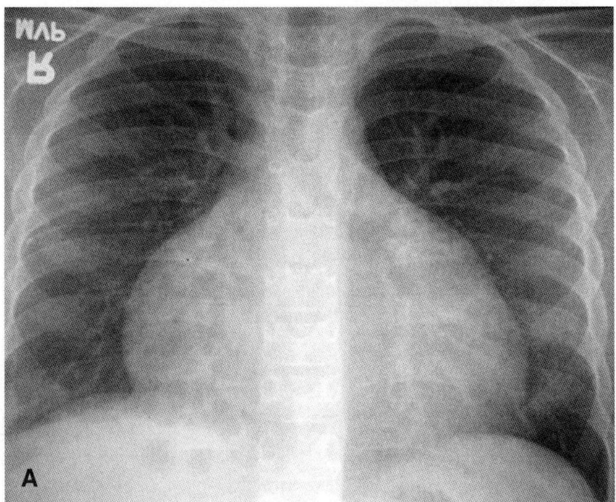

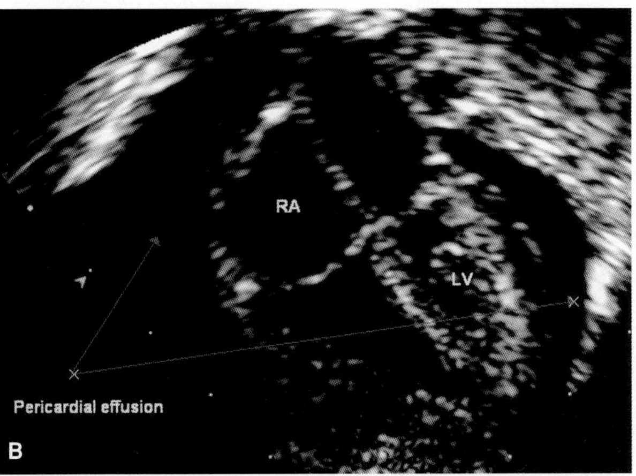

FIGURE 68.7. **Pericardial Effusion. A:** The cardiac silhouette is markedly enlarged and has a rounded, globular appearance caused by a pericardial effusion that developed secondary to bacterial endocarditis. **B:** US is the best method for verifying a pericardial effusion seen as anechoic fluid surrounding the heart. *RA*, right atrium; *LV*, left ventricle.

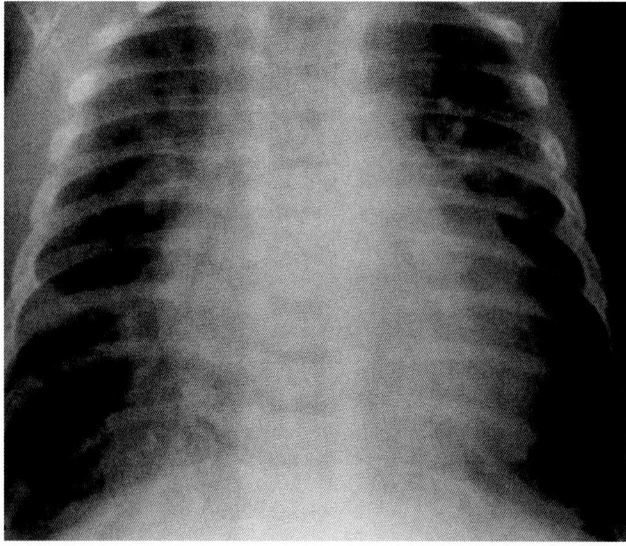

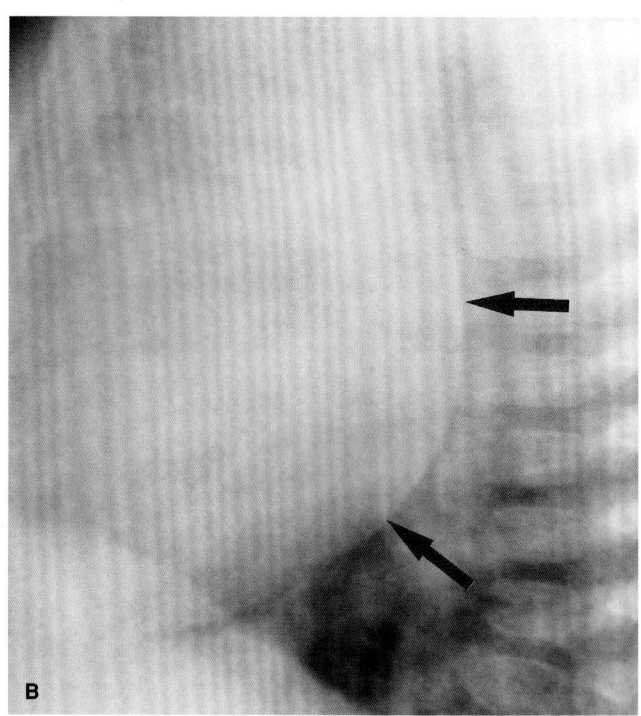

FIGURE 68.8. **Ventricular Septal Defect (VSD). A:** Cardiac enlargement that is predominantly left sided and increased pulmonary vascularity are characteristic of a VSD. **B:** Lateral view demonstrates left atrial enlargement (*arrows*).

enlargement (Fig. 68.8A), and enlargement of the left atrium (Fig. 68.8B).

Atrial septal defect is the cardiac defect most commonly missed in infancy because it is a low-pressure left-to-right shunt that increases as the pulmonary resistance decreases after birth. If the shunt is large enough, the pulmonary vascularity will be increased on the chest x-ray and this is how it is detected radiologically, often on a chest x-ray to rule out pneumonia. Clues to the presence of an ASD (in addition to increased vascularity) include an enlarged or prominent right heart border due to RA enlargement (Fig. 68.9A) (the LA does not enlarge because it acts much like a passive conduit for the blood shunted from the LA to the RA). The RV may extend into the retrosternal space on the lateral view (Fig. 68.9B). However, the best clue is the increased pulmonary vascularity.

Patent Ductus Arteriosus. During fetal life, the right ventricular blood flow is shunted away from the developing lungs via the ductus arteriosus and into the aorta. Immediately after birth, the ductus arteriosus starts to close. Concurrently, the pulmonary vascular resistance rapidly decreases. If the ductus arteriosus remains open, blood shunts from the aorta into the

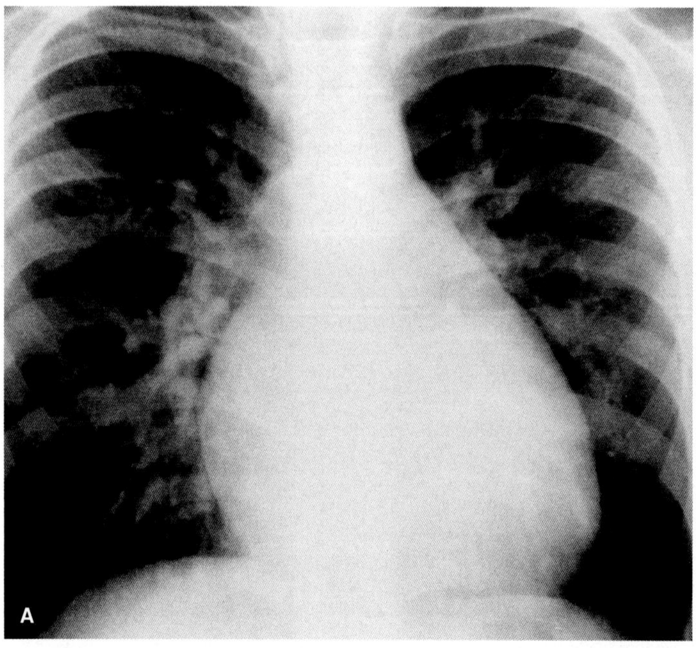

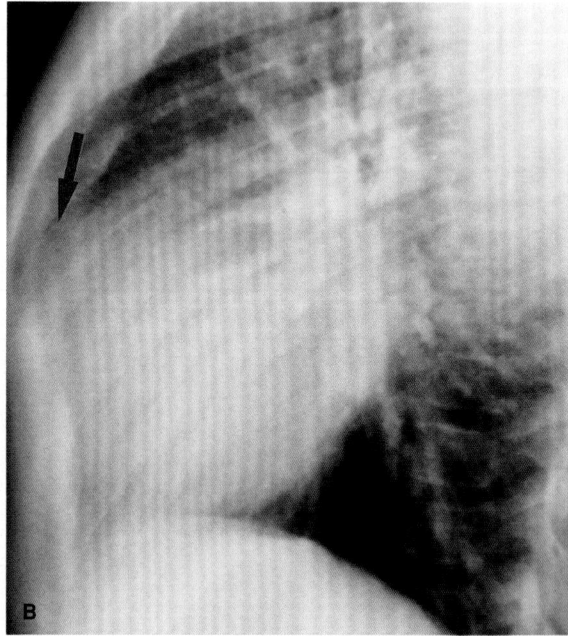

FIGURE 68.9. **Atrial Septal Defect (ASD). A:** Cardiomegaly, mild right atrial enlargement, and increased pulmonary vascularity are characteristic of an ASD. **B:** Lateral view shows a normal LA and fullness in the retrosternal region (*arrow*) caused by right ventricular enlargement.

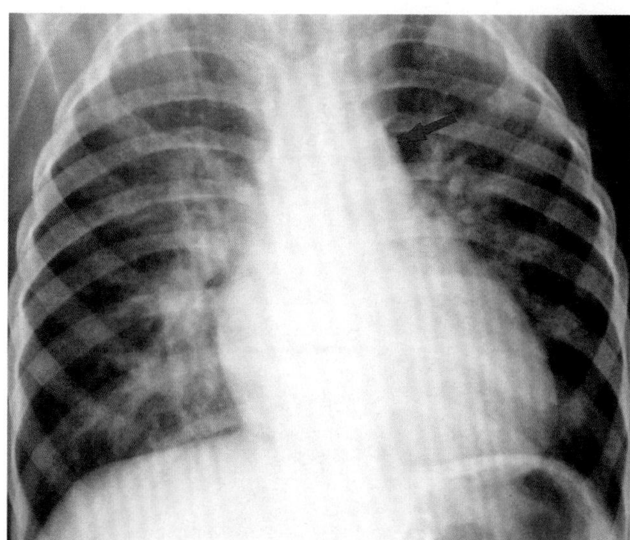

FIGURE 68.10. **Patent Ductus Arteriosus (PDA).** The heart is enlarged, with left-sided prominence and increased pulmonary vascularity. Note the prominent aorta (*arrow*).

lower-resistance pulmonary vascular bed and causes increased vascularity. The consequence of a PDA is that the left side of the heart dilates. Subsequently, the aorta, LA, LV, and PA become enlarged if the shunt is especially large. On chest x-ray, these findings may be difficult to identify and increased pulmonary vascularity is a more reliable finding (Fig. 68.10). The diagnosis is confirmed with transthoracic echocardiography and these are often closed by device placement via angiography. The premature infant complications of lung immaturity may cause prolonged patency of the ductus arteriosus. It is important to remember that some cardiac anomalies are "ductal dependent" for systemic blood flow, especially hypoplastic left heart or an interrupted aortic arch. These anomalies may not be identified until the ductus closes.

An aortopulmonary window is a rare condition that develops when there is incomplete division of the primitive truncus arteriosus and there is absence of a wall between the aorta and PA immediately above the valves. This results in shunting of blood into the low-resistance pulmonary circulation. The physiology is the same as that of a PDA. Another rare cause of left-to-right shunting of blood is a coronary artery fistula which can shunt blood from the aorta to the right cardiac chambers, coronary sinus, or PA.

CYANOTIC HEART DISEASE WITH INCREASED PULMONARY VASCULARITY

When encountering a chest x-ray with increased pulmonary vascularity, it is important to know if the patient is cyanotic. If the patient is cyanotic, the cyanosis implies that there is deoxygenated blood mixing with oxygenated blood. These are the so-called "admixture" cardiac lesions and indicate complex CHD.

The classic and most common CHD resulting in this pattern is **complete transposition of the great vessels** (D-transposition). In this condition the systemic veins, pulmonary venous flow, and atrioventricular connections are normally connected, but the origin of the PA and aorta are reversed (aorta arises from RV, PA arises from LV) resulting in ventriculoarterial discordance. This creates a circuit of blood that returns from the body and is then pumped back to the body, and a second circuit in which blood returns from the lungs and is then pumped back to the lungs, which is incompatible with life unless there is mixing of the two circuits at some level. This mixing is typically a VSD, ASD, or PDA. Due to advances in prenatal diagnosis, these lesions are rarely unknown.

The "classic" chest x-ray appearance of **complete transposition of the great vessels** with increased vascularity is not common due to prenatal diagnosis and early intervention. Other signs that may be present include an oval heart shape with a prominent apex and variable cardiomegaly and a narrow upper mediastinum due to superimposition of the aorta and main pulmonary artery in the anterior–posterior plane. These findings, combined with thymic atrophy (due to stress) can create an "egg-on-a-string" appearance (Fig. 68.11).

Once the diagnosis is confirmed, the patient will be taken to catheterization and a balloon atrial septostomy (Rashkind procedure) will be performed to allow free mixing of oxygenated and deoxygenated blood until the definitive repair can be performed.

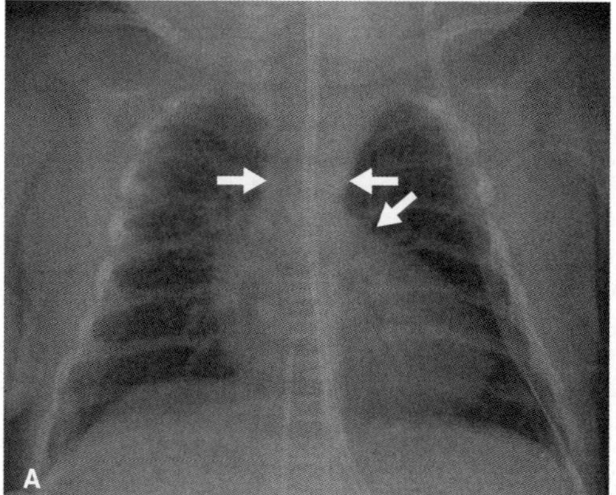

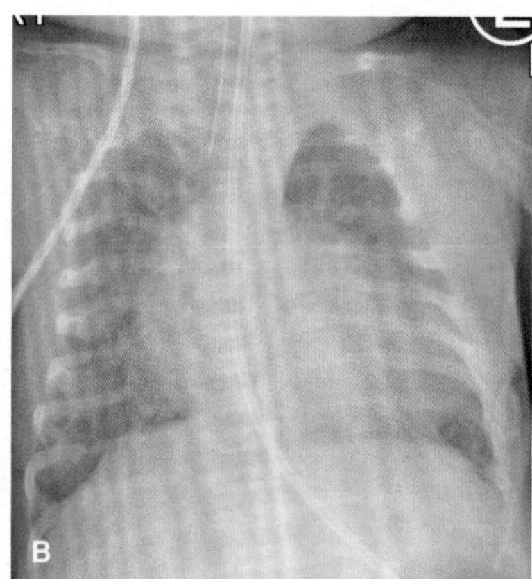

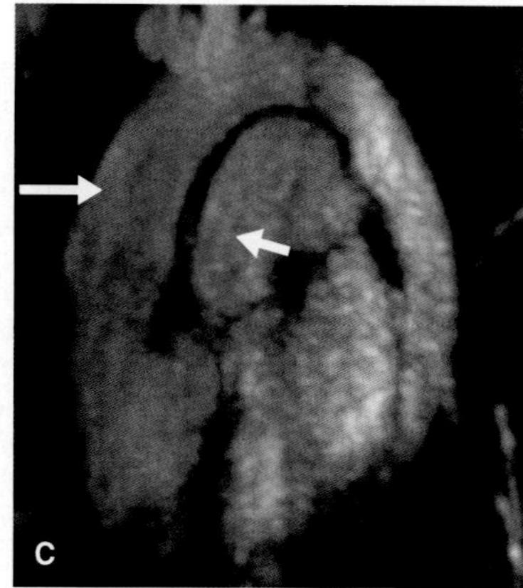

FIGURE 68.11. **D-Transposition of the Great Arteries. A:** Portable chest x-ray on day-of-life 2 showing the oval-shaped cardiac silhouette, narrow superior mediastinum (*horizontal paired arrows*) and the concave main pulmonary artery segment. This constellation of findings has been coined "the egg-on-a-string." Note that the pulmonary vascularity is normal to decreased. **B:** Day-of-life 14 demonstrates how the pulmonary vascularity and cardiac silhouette have increased due to decreasing pulmonary vascular resistance. **C:** Sagittal contrast angiography shows the parallel, superimposed course of the aorta and pulmonary arteries. The aorta (*long arrow*) arises from the anterior (**right**) ventricle and the pulmonary artery (*short arrow*) arises from the posterior (**left**) ventricle.

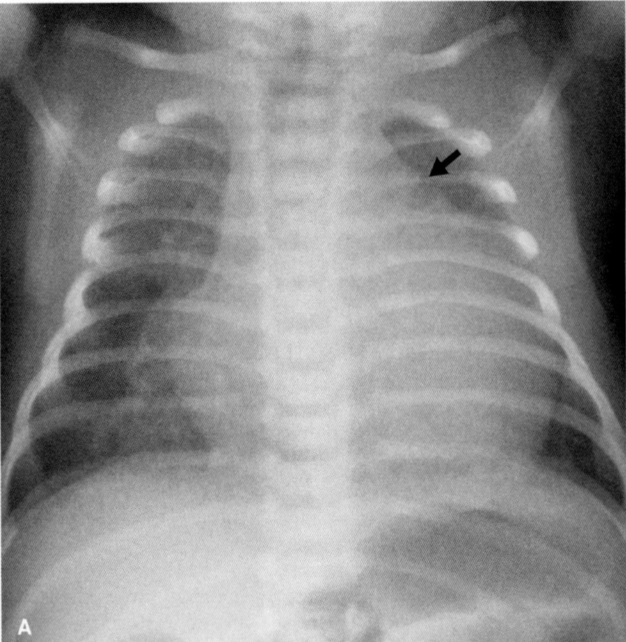

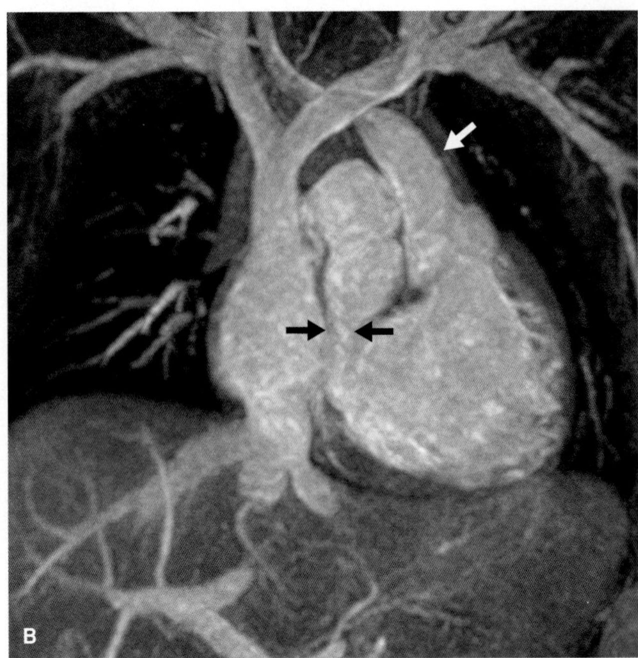

FIGURE 68.12. L-Transposition of the Great Arteries ("Corrected Transposition"). A: Portable chest x-ray of an infant with L-TGA showing the cardiomegaly and increased pulmonary vascularity. The *arrow* is pointing out the upper mediastinal border which creates the heart border in l-TGA. B: A noncontrast cardiac- and respiratory-gated whole-heart image correlates nicely with the radiograph showing the aorta as border forming (*arrow*). This image also shows how development of right ventricular outflow narrowing (*paired arrows*) led to a decrease in pulmonary vascularity.

Corrected transposition (L-Transposition) is much less common and much more variable in presentation and could be initially detected by chest x-ray in an adult or child. In this condition, the ventricles are also inverted such that the morphologic LV is attached to the RA and the morphologic RV is attached to the left atrium. Since the pulmonary artery and aorta are also transposed, the flow through the heart is "corrected." Systemic venous blood flows into the RA to LV to PA to the pulmonary circulation and returns to the heart through the pulmonary veins into the LA to the RV to the aorta and body. Usually there is a coexisting cardiac defect such as a VSD allowing systemic-to-pulmonary shunting. Due to the associated abnormalities, most patients are symptomatic and present in the first month of life.

The chest x-ray appearance of pulmonary vascularity in corrected transposition can be variable. If a large VSD is present and there is no pulmonary outflow restriction, the pulmonary vascularity will be increased (Fig. 68.12A). The ascending aorta becomes border forming along the left side of the heart on chest x-ray due to the aorta arising from the leftward and posterior RV (Fig. 68.12B). This is a very characteristic finding on chest x-ray that can suggest the diagnosis in the absence of increased pulmonary vascularity.

Double-outlet right ventricle is another CHD that can have variable vascularity. The presenting vascular pattern will be increased without the presence of pulmonic stenosis. As the name implies, both arteries arise from the RV and the only outlet from the LV is a VSD (Fig. 68.13).

The clinical presentation of double-outlet right ventricle (DORV) can vary from mild to marked cyanosis. If there is no pulmonic stenosis, the presentation is often congestive heart failure. The chest x-ray appearance of DORV is variable and depends on the relative flow to the PA versus the aorta. Absence of pulmonary stenosis results in a large main PA segment, increased vascularity, and moderate cardiomegaly. Severe pulmonic stenosis results in a concave PA segment and decreased vascularity with mild cardiomegaly.

Total anomalous pulmonary venous return (TAPVR) is present when all the blood returning from the lungs returns to the right side of the heart. Typically, all the pulmonary veins come to a single confluence and then empty into an anomalous site such as a systemic vein (supracardiac is most common [Fig. 68.14]), coronary sinus, or RA. Drainage into a vein below the heart (portal vein, IVC, hepatic veins, or ductus venosus) often has associated obstruction to pulmonary venous return and presents on chest x-ray as pulmonary edema with a normal size heart.

The blood flow physiology requires an ASD, patent foramen ovale (PFO), or VSD to allow shunting of blood from the right heart to the systemic circulation. Therefore, the right heart and PA are enlarged and there is increased blood flow to the lungs. Children born with this condition often have mild cyanosis at birth, which can be missed. If obstruction to pulmonary venous return develops, these patients can present with progressive cyanosis and metabolic acidosis. This is one condition that often presents to emergency in which the radiologist can quickly make the diagnosis from the chest x-ray and immediately communicate the findings to the physicians caring for the patient. The appearance of obstructive TAPVR is a normal heart size with severe interstitial or alveolar pulmonary edema (Fig. 68.15). This pattern has a short differential diagnosis list: TAPVR with obstruction, hypoplastic left heart, and pulmonary vein atresia. BAM! Home Run!! The "snowman" is a radiologic classic but rarely encountered (Fig. 68.14).

However, this only occurs when the vertical vein empties into the brachiocephalic vein. If the drainage is into one of the other veins, such as the azygos, the appearance will not be of the "snowman." Overload of the right side of the heart and pulmonary congestion usually present in the first few days of life and may present on chest x-ray.

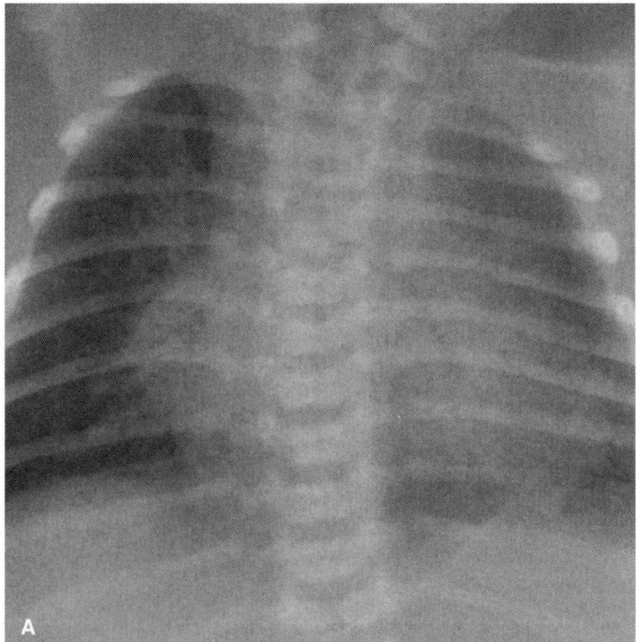

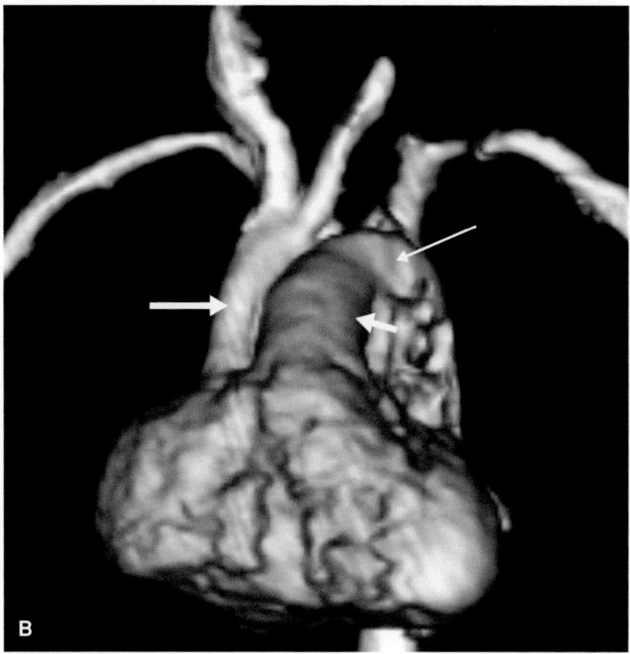

FIGURE 68.13. **Double-Outlet Right Ventricle (DORV). A:** Portable chest x-ray of an infant with DORV showing the cardiomegaly and increased pulmonary vascularity. **B:** A 3D surface rendering of a contrast MRA shows the side-by-side relationship of the great arteries. These great arteries are malpositioned because the aorta (*long arrow*) is to the right of the pulmonary artery (*short arrow*) and a large ductus arteriosus (*long thin arrow*) supplies the descending aorta because of interruption of the aorta distal to the left common carotid.

Cor triatriatum is a rare anomaly that also presents in early infancy with pulmonary venous obstruction. In this anomaly, the pulmonary veins empty into a common confluence separated from the LA by a partial membrane causing obstruction to return of the pulmonary venous flow to the left heart. This results in passive pulmonary edema, usually cardiomegaly. The name, cor triatriatum, derives from the appearance of an extra "atrium" posterior to the LA (Fig. 68.16).

Truncus arteriosus is a rare anomaly and only represents about 1% of CHD. It occurs when there is failure of the primitive truncus to divide correctly into the aorta and PA. The truncus overrides a large VSD. The chest x-ray presents with cardiomegaly and active pulmonary congestion. If a right arch is present, the diagnosis is highly likely (Fig. 68.17). Another clue can be concavity of the MPA segment.

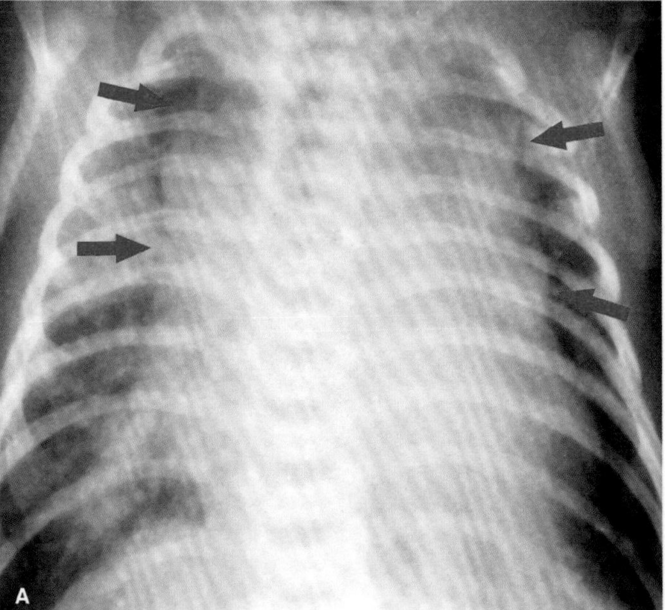

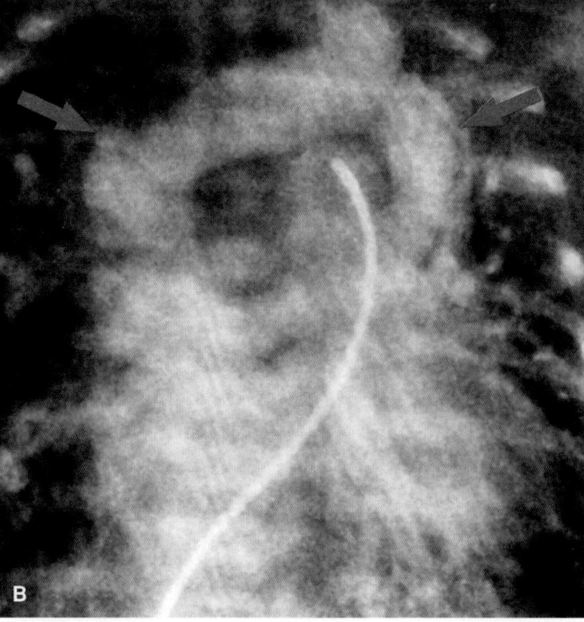

FIGURE 68.14. **Total Anomalous Pulmonary Venous Return, Type 1. A:** The characteristic snowman (*arrows*) or figure-8 configuration results from cardiomegaly combined with prominence of the superior mediastinum because of the anomalous pulmonary vein. **B:** Cardioangiogram demonstrates the inverted, U-shaped vessel (*arrows*), which constitutes the upper portion of the snowman.

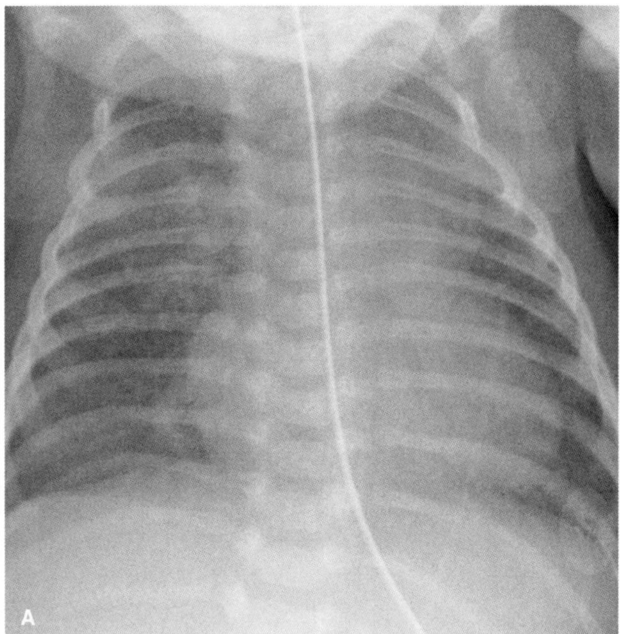

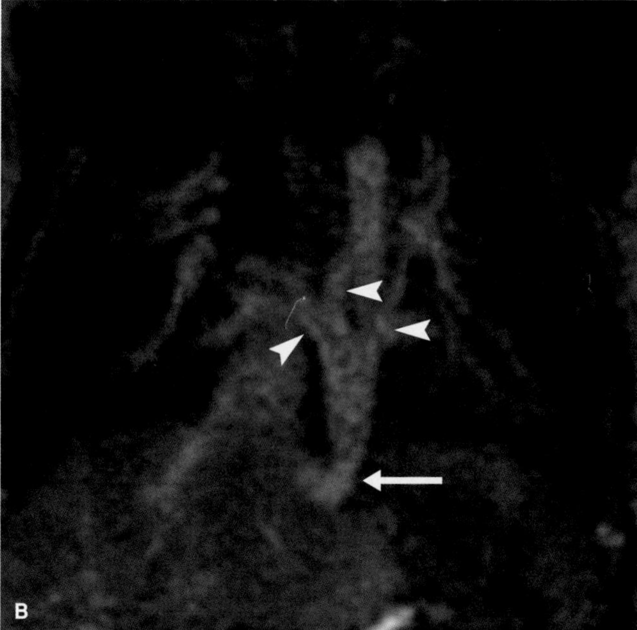

FIGURE 68.15. **Total Anomalous Pulmonary Venous Return. A:** Portable chest x-ray of a 16-day-old male who presented cyanotic to the emergency department. The increased pulmonary vascularity with passive congestion and relatively normal heart suggested TAPVR with obstruction or hypoplastic left heart. Immediate echocardiography demonstrated TAPVR. **B:** A 3D maximum intensity projection from a contrast MRA shows the confluence of the pulmonary veins (*small arrowheads*) into a vertical draining vein to the IVC.

DECREASED PULMONARY VASCULARITY

This group of conditions that presents with decreased pulmonary vascularity usually has obstruction on the right side of the heart and an intracardiac right-to-left shunt. As stated in the beginning of this section, the sensitivity for detecting decreased pulmonary vascularity is poor but the specificity is good. Therefore, chest x-ray is specific for decrease vascularity.

FIGURE 68.16. **Cor Triatriatum.** Sagittal MR image reveals the membrane (*arrow*) within the left atrium into which the common pulmonary vein enters, resulting in pulmonary venous obstruction.

Tetralogy of Fallot is the most common cyanotic CHD, accounting for 6% of CHDs overall. Although four components were originally described (perimembranous VSD, pulmonic stenosis, right ventricular hypertrophy, and an aorta that overrides the VSD), it is really the components of the right ventricular outflow tract (RVOT) obstruction and a

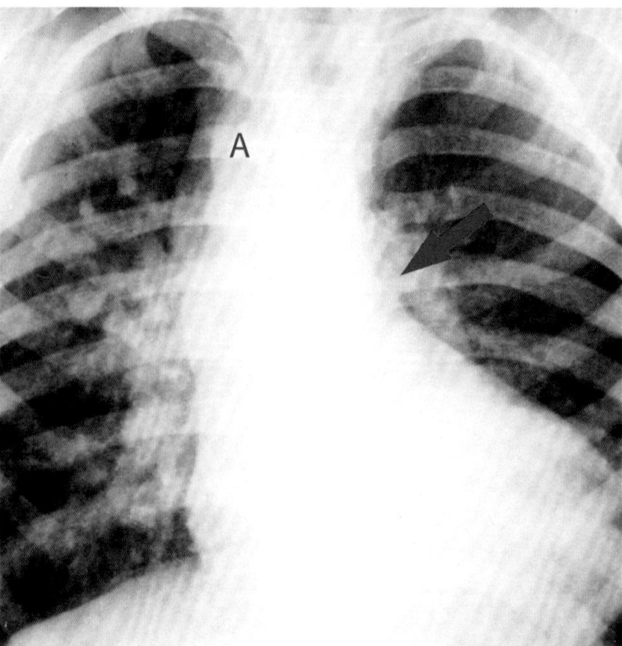

FIGURE 68.17. **Persistent Truncus Arteriosus.** Note oval cardiomegaly, increased pulmonary vascularity, a concave pulmonary artery segment (*arrow*), and a right aortic arch (*A*).

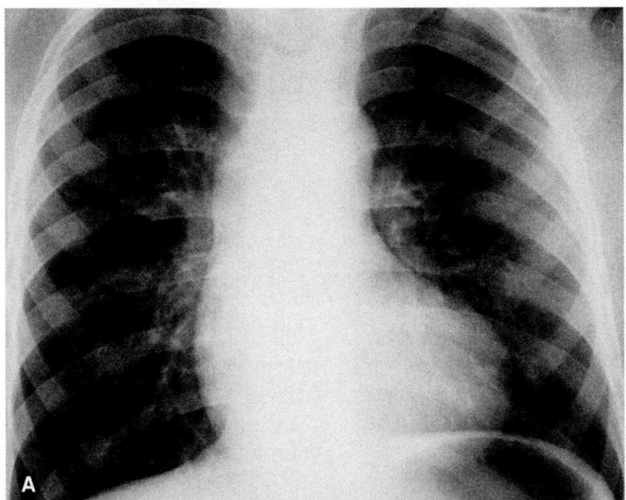

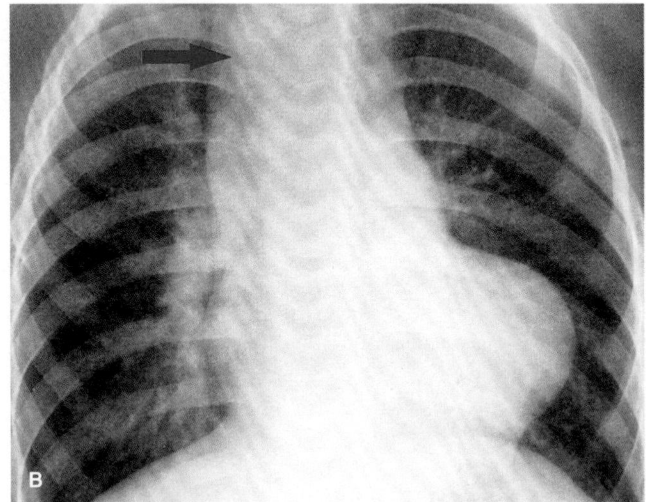

FIGURE 68.18. **Tetralogy of Fallot. A:** The upwardly displaced cardiac apex caused by right ventricular hypertrophy and the concave pulmonary artery shadow are characteristic of the tetralogy of Fallot. **B:** Another child with the characteristic "boot-shaped" heart but more normal pulmonary vascularity, because of less severe pulmonary stenosis. Note the right-sided aortic arch (*arrow*).

large perimembranous VSD that dominate the physiology. The aortic arch is right sided in 25% of cases and even more frequently right sided in pulmonary atresia. The right aortic arch can also have a retroaortic innominate vein present.

The clinical presentation depends largely on the severity of pulmonary outflow obstruction because greater right-to-left shunting results in greater cyanosis. Less severe RVOT obstruction can result in very mild disease and it is often referred to as a "pink" TOF.

The chest x-ray appearance can mimic the clinical presentation and can range from normal to "classic" in appearance. The classic appearance is an uplifted apex due to the RV hypertrophy and a concave main PA segment with decreased pulmonary vascularity (Fig. 68.18). In addition, 25% will have a right aortic arch. The uplifted apex and the concave MPA segment results in the "boot-shaped heart" or "coeur en sabot," as described in the original paper by Fallot.

The current approach to treatment is complete surgical repair which results in excellent long-term survival and good quality of life. However, over time, the pulmonary valve can become insufficient or stenotic and require surgical replacement.

The most severe form of TOF is that in which the pulmonary valve is atretic because the flow to the lungs relies on either a ductus arteriosus or systemic collaterals from the aorta or other systemic vessels. Cardiac CTA and MRI have an important role in evaluating the anatomy prior to surgery because they can show the blood supply to the PAs, the origins and course of aortopulmonary collaterals, and whether the PAs are continuous or discontinuous. All are important in the surgical repair.

Tricuspid atresia, without TGA, typically presents with a chest x-ray that has decreased vascularity, and the patient has cyanosis on the first day of life. The right atrial border can be prominent and the MPA segment concave (Fig. 68.19). The physiology of this stems from complete atresia of the tricuspid valve, allowing no communication of blood from the RA to the RV. Therefore, an atrial-level shunt is required and in 80% of cases, this is a patent foramen ovale. Typically, the RV is hypoplastic, but the size of the RV and the RVOT depends on the size of the VSD, allowing forward flow of blood from the LV to the RV. Flow to the PA is dependent on a ductus arteriosus. Since most of the systemic blood is shunted to the left side, patients present with cyanosis.

Immediate needs of the patient are aimed at increasing pulmonary blood flow by keeping the ductus arteriosus open, performing a modified Blalock–Taussig shunt or a superior cavopulmonary anastomosis (bidirectional Glenn) and eventually a total cavopulmonary anastomosis (Fontan).

Ebstein anomaly is a rare condition that can be variable in its clinical and chest x-ray presentation. The underlying abnormality is a redundant tricuspid valve that balloons into the RV and is adherent to the RV myocardium. Physiologically, the heart has difficulty getting blood from the RA to the RV to perfuse the lungs. Since blood has difficulty passing from the RA to the RV, it instead passes from the RA to the LA via a patent foramen ovale or ASD, causing variable cyanosis. The most severely affected subjects have extreme cardiomegaly and decreased pulmonary vascularity with clinical cyanosis (Fig. 68.20).

NORMAL PULMONARY VASCULARITY

As discussed in the beginning of this section, recognizing normal pulmonary vascularity is something we are very good at doing. Unfortunately, it doesn't really help that much to narrow the differential diagnosis, and many CHD lesions have variable vascularity. This is where the observed contours of the heart and mediastinum can be especially helpful.

Pulmonic valvar stenosis is the third most common CHD after VSD and ASD. Clinically, patients are often asymptomatic and the disease is first suspected when a systolic heart murmur is noted. Chest x-ray can range from normal to having an enlarged MPA segment (Fig. 68.6). The left PA is usually normal size. RV hypertrophy can cause uplifting of the cardiac apex and fullness of the retrosternal space. The most common cause is commissural fusion (90%) and a dysplastic valve is much less common, but can be seen in the Noonan syndrome.

Aortic valvar stenosis is relatively common but actually less common than TOF as a pediatric heart lesion. However, aortic valvar abnormalities are the most common congenital abnormality of the heart because of bicuspid aortic valves. Aortic valvar stenosis presenting early in life is often critical and accounts for perhaps 10% of the presentations. The remainder, like pulmonic valvar stenosis, presents as an

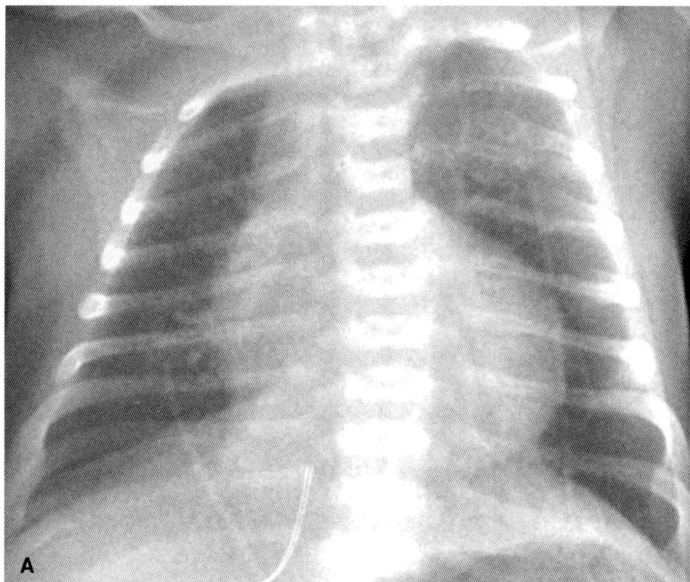

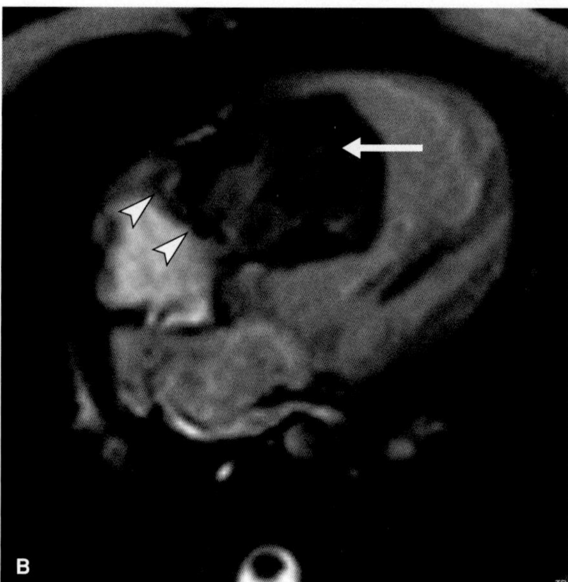

FIGURE 68.19. **Tricuspid Atresia. A:** Portable chest x-ray of newborn with prenatal diagnosis of tricuspid atresia. The decreased pulmonary vascularity, prominent right atrial border, and concave MPA segment are relatively characteristic. **B:** One image from a four-chamber SSFP cine MR shows the plate-like atresia (*arrowheads*) and the small right ventricle with the hypertrophied muscle (*short arrow*). Due to the small size of the VSD, there was little forward flow through the RV, resulting in a very small pulmonary artery.

asymptomatic systolic ejection murmur later in childhood or in adult life. The leaflets are usually bicuspid due to commissural fusion, thickened and rigid, and the stenosis is progressive with time. Probably the best clue on a chest x-ray is a prominent ascending aortic shadow along the right mediastinum just above the heart, and with age and elongation of the aorta, the transverse segment becomes conspicuous (Fig. 68.21). LV hypertrophy may also occur but the heart doesn't enlarge unless heart failure is present.

Coarctation of the aorta is one of the congenital heart lesions that can present later in life with signs first recognized from a chest x-ray or a renal ultrasound performed to evaluate hypertension. On the chest x-ray, the dilation of the ascending and transverse aorta and poststenotic dilation of the descending aorta, coupled with the inward pinching of the aorta form the "figure-3" sign (Fig. 68.5). If there are well-developed collaterals, usually not until age 8, there may be rib notching (Fig. 68.22) or an undulating density in the retrosternal area representing dilated intercostal arteries or mammary arteries, respectively, but this is not often seen. Clinically, the patients may have bounding upper-extremity pulses or have upper-extremity hypertension relative to the lower extremities. When

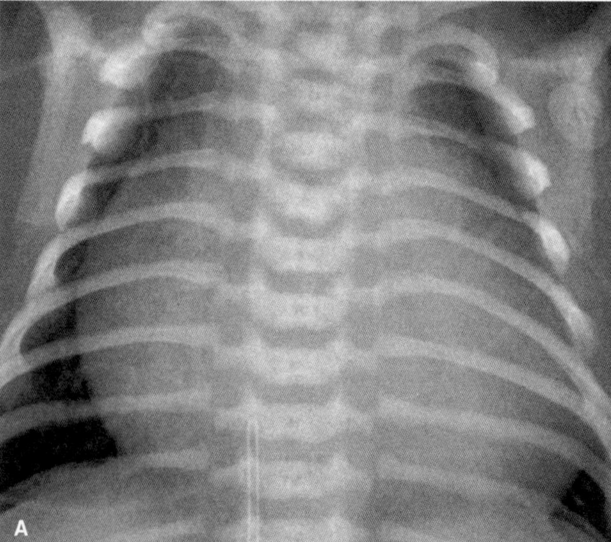

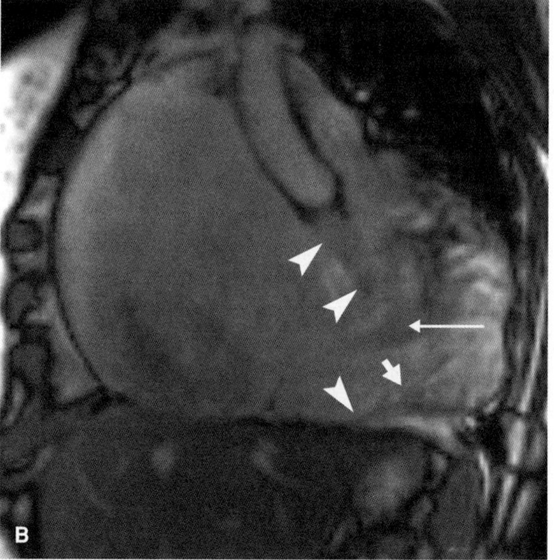

FIGURE 68.20. **Ebstein Anomaly. A:** Ebstein anomaly. Note the severe cardiomegaly with marked right atrial enlargement. Pulmonary vascularity typically is decreased. **B:** Unrepaired Ebstein anomaly in an adult. Coronal oblique SSFP cine MR shows the redundant tricuspid valve (*arrowheads*) "atrializing" a good portion of the RV inflow, a huge right atrium, and the tricuspid regurgitation (*thin arrow*).

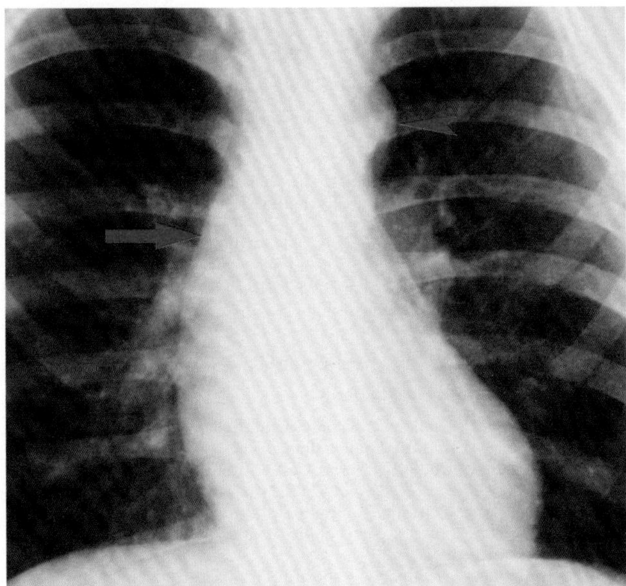

FIGURE 68.21. **Aortic Valve Stenosis.** The ascending aorta (*arrow*) and aortic arch (*arrowhead*) are prominent in this 5-year-old child with congenital aortic stenosis.

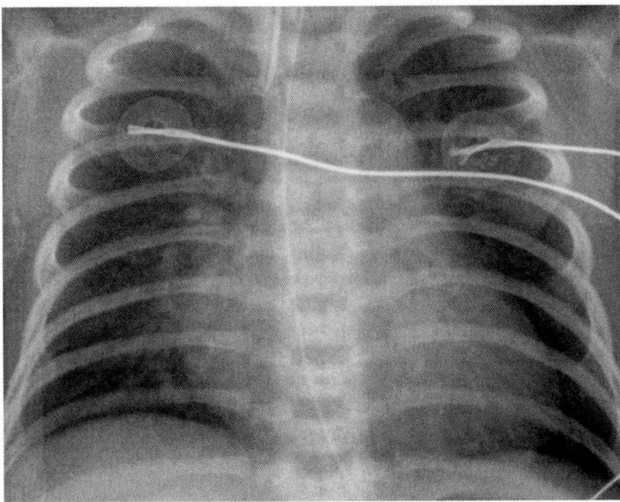

FIGURE 68.23. **Hypoplastic Left Heart Syndrome.** Cardiomegaly and passive pulmonary vascular congestion usually develop within the first few days of life.

performing renal Doppler ultrasound for hypertension, it is important to assess the descending aorta pulse profile. If tardus parvus is present in the aorta, the patient probably has coarctation of the aorta. There are two main types of coarctation of the aorta: localized and diffuse. The diffuse type, termed "infantile" because of its early presentation, is associated with VSD, ASD, and mitral valve abnormalities in many cases. The localized is often termed juxtaductal and the narrowing lies at or just distal to the ductus arteriosus. Both types are associated with bicuspid aortic valves.

Hypoplastic left heart syndrome is a type of single-ventricle heart disease that occurs as a spectrum of underdevelopment of left-sided heart structures (aorta, aortic valve, LV, mitral valve, and left atrium). They are usually diagnosed by prenatal screening ultrasound because of inability to obtain a "four-chamber view" and then sent for fetal echocardiography and appropriately referred for care, but can present without prior knowledge at birth. They are dependent on an atrial-level shunting of blood from the left to the right atrium and on a large ductus arteriosus to provide blood flow to the brain and body. If patients are undiagnosed and discharged, they will present in cardiac extremus due to closing of the ductus arteriosus. Chest x-ray often shows a normal heart and pulmonary vascularity that can range from normal to pulmonary interstitial edema (Fig. 68.23). Often, the clinical presentation is severe and out of proportion to the chest x-ray, which appears relatively normal. Fortunately, many cases are recognized prenatally or early after birth, and survival has become the norm since the Norwood procedure was developed in the early 1980s. This two-stage procedure, and its new modifications, now allows survival in greater than 80% of patients, but is only palliative and not a cure because of many long-term morbidities and eventual failure of the systemic RV.

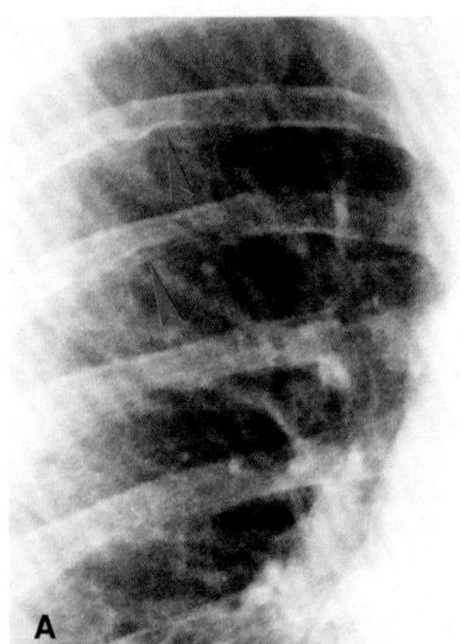

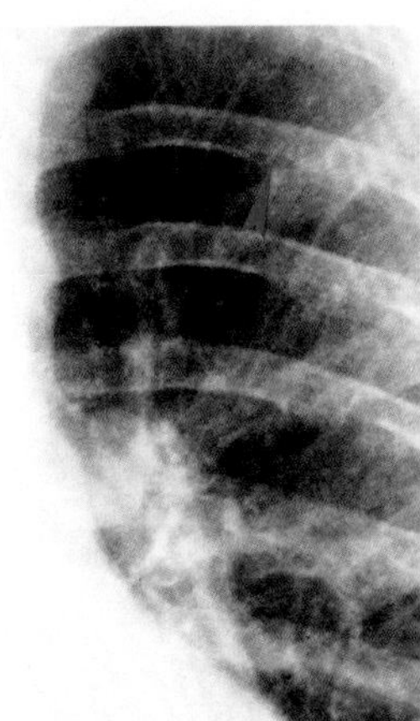

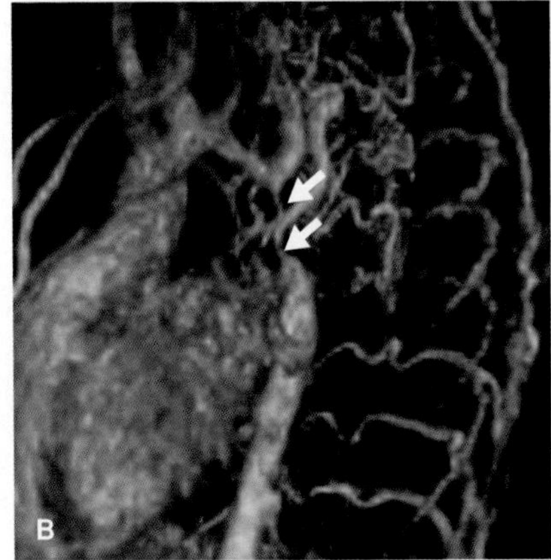

FIGURE 68.22. **Coarctation With Rib Notching. A:** The small notches (*arrowheads*) along the inferior edges of some of the upper ribs bilaterally are caused by enlarged collateral vessels. **B:** An 11-year-old male presented with upper extremity hypertension. MRA shows a long segment of coarctation (*arrows*) and a large number of dilated intercostal collaterals.

CARDIAC MALPOSITIONS

The relationship between thoracic and abdominal viscera is described in terms of situs. Situs of the atria, bronchopulmonary system, and abdominal organs should be designated separately. Situs solitus is the normal configuration of the thoracoabdominal viscera with the cardiac apex, the stomach, and spleen on the left and the liver on the right. Situs inversus totalis is a complete mirror image of the thoracoabdominal viscera. Every other configuration is a heterotaxy syndrome.

Assuming there is not an extracardiac cause of "malposition," the position of the heart is described as levocardia, dextrocardia, or mesocardia. Levocardia is when the apex and the bulk of the heart are to the left. Dextrocardia is when the apex of the heart is to the right and the bulk of the heart is on the right. Mesocardia should be used when the heart is in the center and the laterality of the bulk of the heart is indeterminate. If possible, the laterality of the apex should be described when the heart is mesocardiac. For example, "mesocardia is with the apex to the right," but sometimes the direction of the apex cannot be determined on a chest x-ray alone.

When heterotaxy is suggested, clues can help define the relationships of the thoracoabdominal viscera. In the chest, the best indicator of the two major groups of atrial isomerism on chest x-ray is the relationship of the upper lobe bronchus to the PA. If there are bilateral eparterial bronchi, right atrial isomerism and asplenia are very likely to be present. Bilateral trilobed lungs and a liver that spans the abdomen are usually present as well. Polysplenia syndromes typically have hyparterial bronchi and bilobed lungs, with an asymmetric liver with its bulk on the left or right.

SUMMARY

Diagnosing specific abnormalities of CHD and getting everything correct based on a chest x-ray is an unreasonable expectation. Being able to accurately determine the pulmonary vascularity and recognize cardiac enlargement and cardiomediastinal abnormalities, so that you can suggest further consultation with a cardiologist, is invaluable. Always speak with the ordering physician when suspicious because additional clinical information (e.g., cyanosis or acyanosis) can be very helpful and there is no better way to communicate your concern. Generally, avoid recommendations of echocardiography and instead first recommend cardiology consultation. Let the cardiologist put all the historical, clinical, and physical examination data together and be the arbitrator of the next steps.

Suggested Readings

Chest X-Ray in the Evaluation of Congenital Heart Disease

Fonseca B, Chang R, Senac M, Knight G, Sklansky MS. Chest radiography and the evaluation of the neonate for congenital heart disease. *Pediatr Cardiol* 2005;26:367–372.

Laya BF, Goske MJ, Morrison S, et al. The accuracy of chest radiographs in the detection of congenital heart disease and in the diagnosis of specific congenital cardiac lesions. *Pediatr Cardiol* 2006;36:677–681.

Teele SA, Emani SM, Thiagarajan RR, Teele RL. Catheters, wires, tubes and drains on postoperative radiographs of pediatric cardiac patients: the whys and wherefores. *Pediatr Cardiol* 2008;36:1041–1053.

Tumkosit M, Yingyong N, Mahayosnond A, Choo KS, Goo HW. Accuracy of chest radiography for evaluating abnormal pulmonary vascularity in children with congenital heart disease. *Int J Cardiovasc Imaging* 2012;28:69–75.

Repair of Congenital Heart Disease

Gaca AM, Jaggers JJ, Dudley LT, Bisset GS 3rd. Repair of congenital heart disease: a primer—part 1. *Radiology* 2008;247:617–631.

Gaca AM, Jaggers JJ, Dudley LT, Bisset GS 3rd. Repair of congenital heart disease: a primer—part 2. *Radiology* 2008;248:44–60.

Rodríguez E, Soler R, Fernández R, Raposo I. Postoperative imaging in cyanotic congenital heart diseases: part 1, normal findings. *AJR Am J Roentgenol* 2007;189:1353–1360.

Soler R, Rodríguez E, Alvarez M, Raposo I. Postoperative imaging in cyanotic congenital heart diseases: part 2, complications. *AJR Am J Roentgenol* 2007;189:1361–1369.

MRI in Congenital Heart Disease

Caro-Dominguez P, Yoo SJ, Seed M, Grosse-Wortmann L. Magnetic resonance imaging of cardiovascular thrombi in children. *Pediatr Radiol* 2018;48:722–731.

Fratz S, Chung T, Greil GF, et al. Guidelines and protocols for cardiovascular magnetic resonance in children and adults with congenital heart disease: SCMR expert consensus group on congenital heart disease. *J Cardiovasc Magn Reson* 2013;15:51.

Lu JC, Dorfman A, Attili AK, Mahani MG, Dillman MD, Agarwal PP. Evaluation with cardiovascular MR imaging of baffles and conduits used in palliation or repair of congenital heart disease. *Radiographics* 2012;32:E107–E127.

Woodard PK, Ho VB, Akers SR. ACR Appropriateness Criteria® known or suspected congenital heart disease in the adult. *J Am Coll Radiol* 2017;14:S166–S176.

Specific Congenital Heart Disease

Geva T. Repaired tetralogy of Fallot: the roles of cardiovascular magnetic resonance in evaluating pathophysiology and for pulmonary valve replacement decision support. *J Cardiovasc Magn Reson* 2011;13:9.

Geva T, Martins JD, Wald RM. Atrial septal defects. *Lancet* 2014;383:1921–1932.

Hanneman K, Newman B, Chan F. Congenital variants and anomalies of the aortic arch. *Radiographics* 2017;37:32–51.

Visceroatrial Situs

Ghosh S, Yarmish G, Godelman A, Haramati LB, Sindola-Franco H. Anomalies of visceroatrial situs. *AJR Am J Roentgenol* 2009;193:1107–1117.

Lapierre C, Déry J, Guérin R, Viremouneix L, Dubois J, Garel L. Segmental approach to imaging of congenital heart disease. *Radiographics* 2010;30:397–411.

Other

Anwar S, Singh GK, Miller J, et al. 3D printing is a transformative technology in congenital heart disease. *JACC: Basic to Translational Science* 2018;3:294–312.

CHAPTER 69 ■ ABDOMEN

ETHAN A. SMITH AND ANDREW T. TROUT

OBSTRUCTION—GENERAL

Suspected gastrointestinal (GI) tract obstruction is a relatively common reason for a child to be referred for imaging. Patients typically present with vomiting, abdominal distention, feeding intolerance, and, in older children, abdominal pain. GI tract obstructions can be due to congenital and acquired causes, and the differential diagnosis is initially quite broad. However, by considering the patient's age and a few clinical factors, the differential diagnosis can often be narrowed to a shorter list of possibilities and the imaging approach can be tailored accordingly. For example, a suspected obstruction in a neonate is much more likely to be due to a congenital cause such as bowel atresia, while an obstruction in a previously healthy teenage patient is more likely to be due to an acquired infectious or inflammatory disorder like appendicitis. Similarly, clinical factors, such as the presence of bilious versus nonbilious emesis, allow the differential diagnosis to be shortened by defining the likely site of obstruction as either proximal (nonbilious) or distal (bilious), relative to the ampulla of Vater. The goal of imaging in children with suspected obstruction is to determine the most likely cause of the obstruction and to appropriately triage patients to either surgical or nonsurgical management.

OBSTRUCTION—CONGENITAL

Esophageal Atresia and Tracheoesophageal Fistula

Esophageal atresia is the most common cause of congenital esophageal obstruction. This condition is the result of abnormal development of the foregut early in gestation, which leads to discontinuity of the esophagus and frequently an associated fistulous connection between the esophagus and the trachea (tracheoesophageal fistula [TEF]). There are several subtypes of esophageal atresia/TEF, the most common being a complete esophageal atresia with a blind-ending esophageal pouch and distal fistulous connection between the lower portion of the trachea and the distal segment of the esophagus. The site of the atresia is most commonly the proximal third of the esophagus, usually just above the level of the carina. Other, less common, types of esophageal atresia/TEF are detailed in Figure 69.1. Esophageal atresia/TEF can be associated with other congenital abnormalities, including vertebral anomalies, congenital heart disease, anorectal malformations, and other features of the VACTRL (V, vertebral; A, anal; C, cardiac; T, tracheoesophageal; R, renal; L, limb) association.

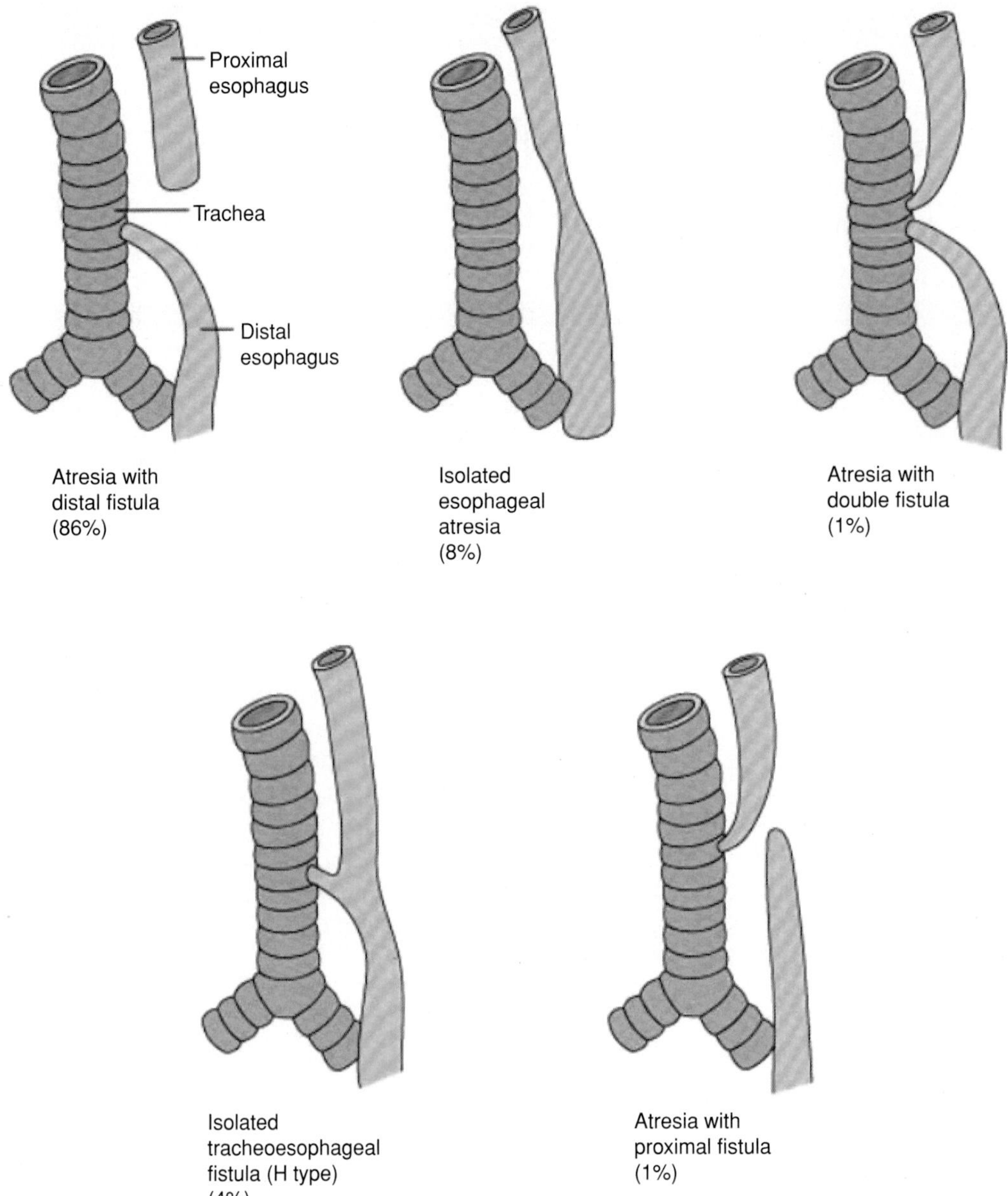

FIGURE 69.1. **Diagrammatic Representation of the Spectrum of Esophageal Atresia and Tracheoesophageal Fistulae.** The most common form is complete esophageal atresia with a distal tracheoesophageal fistula. Symptoms and imaging findings depend on the specific malformation. Any connection of the proximal esophagus to the trachea allows for aspiration. A connection between the trachea and distal esophagus (or continuity of the esophagus) is required for gas to be present in the bowel.

Pregnancies complicated by esophageal atresia may have polyhydramnios, as the discontinuity of the esophagus prevents normal swallowing of amniotic fluid. If the diagnosis of esophageal atresia/TEF is not made on prenatal imaging, the abnormality typically becomes evident within the first few hours of life when the neonate is unable to tolerate feeding. Inability to place a nasogastric or orogastric tube often leads to further clinical suspicion of the diagnosis.

The most common initial imaging test in a patient with suspected esophageal atresia/TEF is a chest radiograph. An air-filled, blind-ending esophageal pouch is often visible and if nasogastric tube placement has been attempted, the tube will be coiled in the atretic proximal esophagus (Fig. 69.2). The presence or absence of gas in the stomach and small bowel further helps define the type of esophageal atresia/TEF. If there is gas in the stomach and small bowel, then a distal fistula must be present. The lack of gas in the stomach and small bowel indicates the lack of a distal fistula.

Frequently, a chest radiograph is the only imaging test needed to define the abnormality in esophageal atresia/TEF. Occasionally, surgeons may request that the radiologist inject contrast into the pouch (the so-called "pouchogram") to further define the anatomy. Most frequently, this is done to exclude the possibility of a rare proximal fistula between the esophageal pouch and the trachea that would need to be addressed at surgery (Fig. 69.3). There are a few important technical considerations when performing a "pouchogram" in these patients. First, it is imperative to obtain a true lateral view which is most likely to demonstrate the presence of a proximal TEF. Second, as the pouch is often quite short, reflux

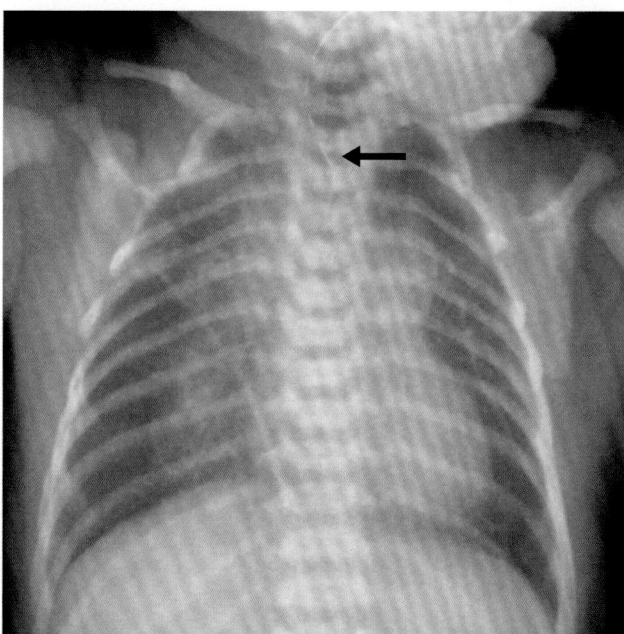

FIGURE 69.2. **Esophageal Atresia and Tracheoesophageal Fistula.** AP chest radiograph shows a nasogastric tube curled in the blind-ending esophageal pouch (*arrow*).

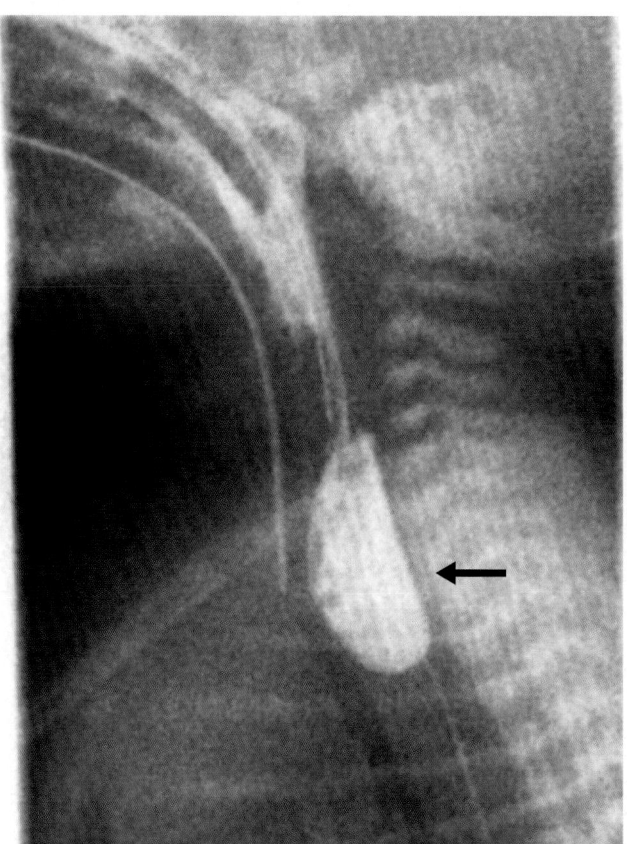

FIGURE 69.3. **Esophageal Atresia and Tracheoesophageal Fistula.** Lateral fluoroscopic image showing the blind-ending esophageal pouch distended with contrast material (*arrow*). This study was performed to delineate the anatomy prior to surgery and to exclude the presence of a proximal tracheoesophageal fistula.

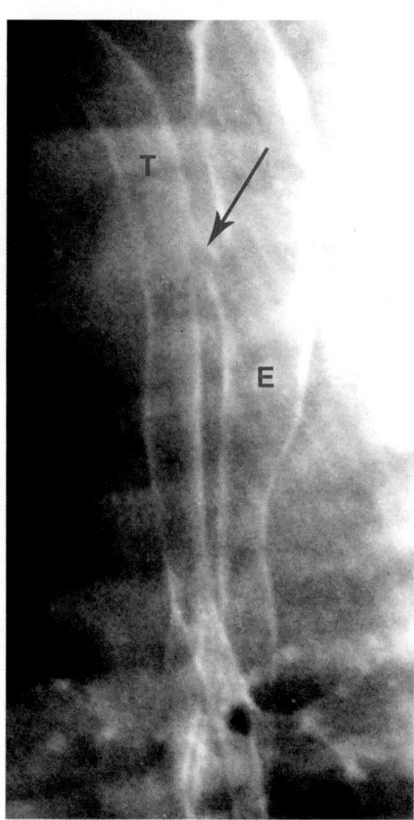

FIGURE 69.4. **Tracheoesophageal Fistula.** The trachea (*T*) and esophagus (*E*) are connected by a fistula (*arrow*).

of contrast into the hypopharynx often occurs and aspiration of small amounts of contrast is common. As such, either inert (barium sulfate) or iso-osmolar contrast should be used to avoid chemical pneumonitis, if aspiration occurs. The use of a catheter with only an end hole may help to limit the amount of reflux into the hypopharynx. Finally, it is advisable to include the hypopharynx in all images while injecting contrast, so that if any contrast is seen in the trachea it can be determined whether it came from aspiration versus a small proximal TEF.

Although rare, TEF without esophageal atresia (H-type fistula) merits special consideration. Patients with isolated TEF may present later in childhood, as they do not have feeding intolerance and may present with coughing with feeding or with recurrent pneumonia due to aspiration via the H-type TEF. H-type fistulae may not be visible on endoscopy due to dynamic collapse, and an esophagram may be needed to demonstrate the fistula (Fig. 69.4). As with the pouchogram, care must be taken to obtain a true lateral view to visualize the fistula. Other signs of a potential H-type fistula on esophagram include subtle tethering of the esophagus toward the lower trachea and visualization of ingested contrast material in the trachea/airways.

Duodenal Obstruction

Malrotation and Midgut Volvulus. Malrotation occurs due to failure of the normal sequence of rotation of the bowel and mesentery during development (Fig. 69.5). Normally, the ligament of Treitz is relatively fixed in the left upper quadrant, and the cecum is fixed in the right lower quadrant, giving a broad base to the mesentery, which prevents twisting. In malrotation, the base of the mesentery is relatively short and is thus prone to twisting (volvulus). It is important to distinguish between malrotation and midgut volvulus. Malrotation is the

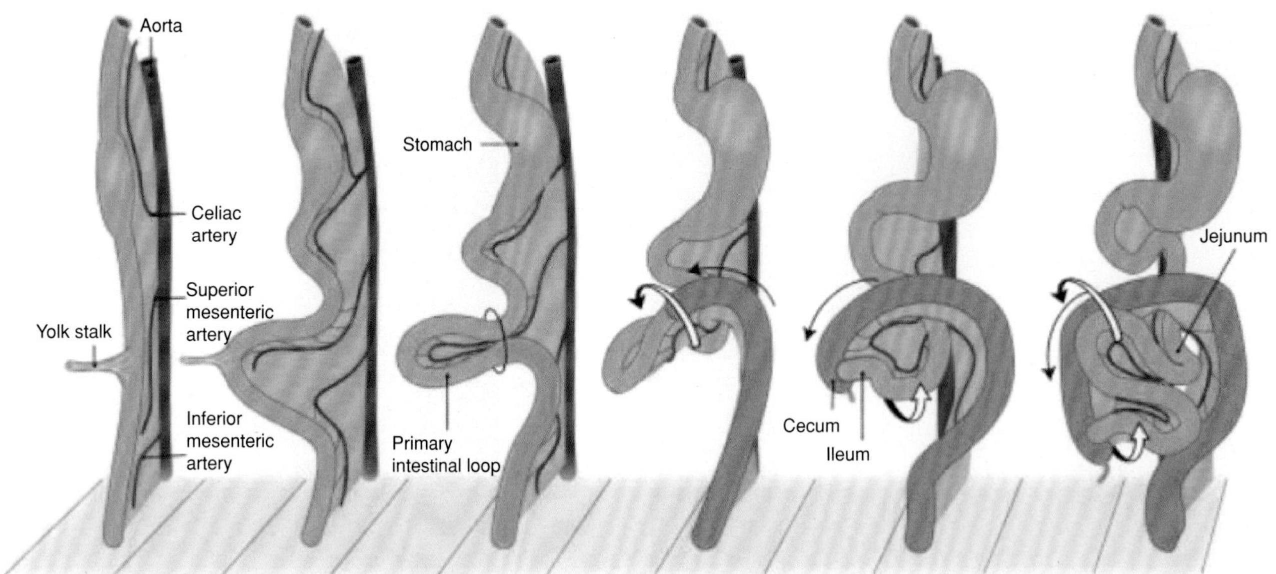

FIGURE 69.5. **Diagrammatic Representation of the Normal Process of Intestinal Rotation During Development.** In this process, the gut herniates outside of the abdomen, rotates, and then moves back into the abdomen where it becomes fixed. Failure of this process results in "malrotation" which can predispose to midgut volvulus.

anatomic abnormality that predisposes to midgut volvulus, but a patient can be malrotated without having a midgut volvulus. If volvulus occurs, the resulting obstruction is typically seen in the third portion of the duodenum. Midgut volvulus can be catastrophic as it involves the mesenteric vessels and can result in venous and arterial ischemia of the bowel.

The most common clinical presentation of midgut volvulus is bilious emesis (due to obstruction distal to the ampulla of Vater). Most patients with malrotation and midgut volvulus present in the first month of life. However, malrotation with midgut volvulus can present at any age and cases have been reported late into adulthood.

Malrotation may be identified fluoroscopically but may also be incidentally detected on cross-sectional imaging. The diagnosis of volvulus, however, is most frequently made with a fluoroscopic upper GI series, and suspicion for volvulus is an indication for urgent upper GI. To confirm normal rotation, or to diagnose malrotation by upper GI, both lateral and anteroposterior (AP) projection images of the duodenum are required. In the normal state, the third portion of the duodenum should be posterior in location, just in front of the spine, on the lateral view and should cross midline on the AP view (Fig. 69.6). The ligament of Treitz should be to the left of midline, at similar level as the duodenal bulb. In malrotation, the third portion

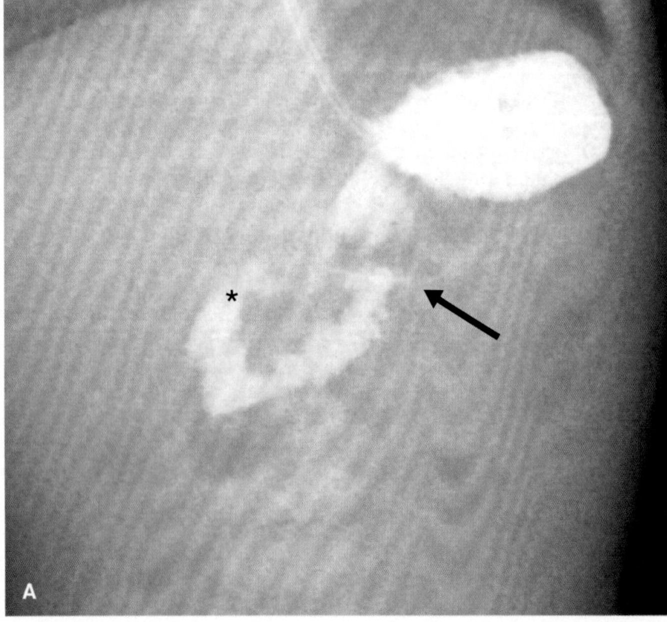

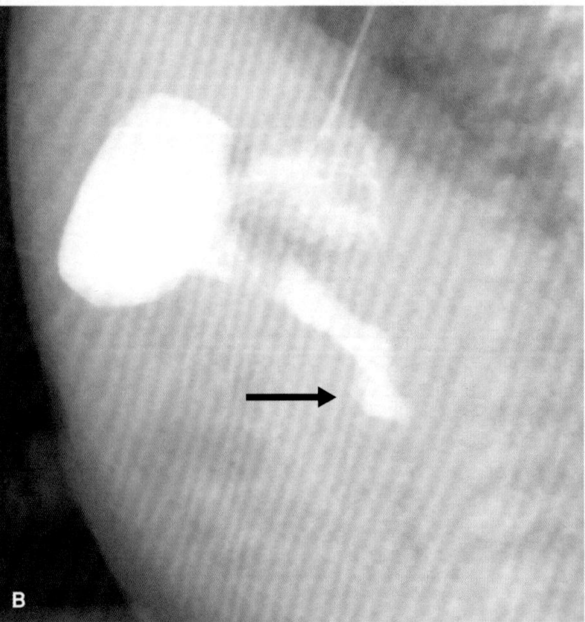

FIGURE 69.6. **Normal Duodenum on Upper GI Series. A:** AP image demonstrating a normal duodenal course with normal positioning of the ligament of Treitz. The duodenum should cross to the left of midline and then ascend, with the ligament of Treitz (*arrow*) located at a similar level as the duodenal bulb (*). **B:** Lateral image showing that the third portion of the duodenum (*arrow*) is located posteriorly, just in front of the spine, confirming a retroperitoneal location. Both AP and lateral views are required to confirm normal rotation.

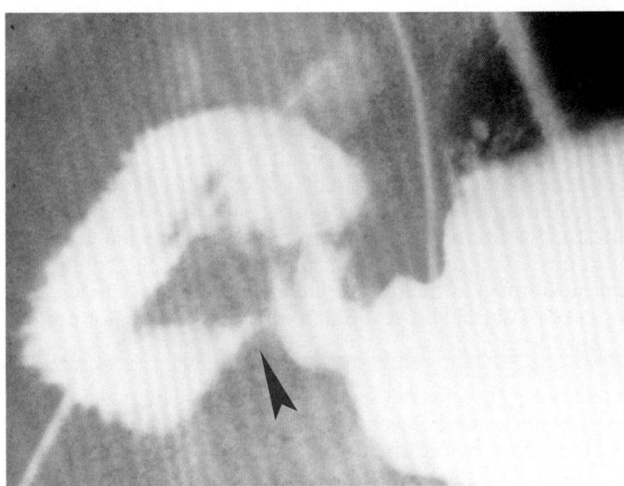

FIGURE 69.7. **Midgut Volvulus.** Fluoroscopic imaging in a child with midgut volvulus shows a tapered beak (*arrowhead*) at the site of obstruction in the third portion of the duodenum.

of the duodenum frequently does not cross midline and may extend anteriorly in the lateral view. The ligament of Treitz may be to the right of midline, or may be abnormally low. The cecum is frequently abnormal in position as well, either in the midline or high in the right upper quadrant. Malrotation on computed tomography (CT), magnetic resonance imaging (MRI), or ultrasound manifests as the third portion of the duodenum not passing between the superior mesenteric artery (SMA) and the aorta. Small bowel loops may be primarily located in the right side of the abdomen, and the colon may be only on the left side. The relationship between the SMA and superior mesenteric vein (SMV) may be reversed with the SMA to the right and the SMV to the left (normally, the position of the SMA and SMV mirrors the aorta and the inferior vena cava [IVC]).

The diagnosis of midgut volvulus depends on seeing varying degrees of duodenal obstruction, often with twisting or a "corkscrew" appearance of the third portion of the duodenum. If obstructed, there is often "beaking" of the third portion of the duodenum, as the lumen is obstructed by the twisting (Fig. 69.7).

Malrotation with midgut volvulus is a surgical emergency, with prompt surgical intervention required to avoid catastrophic bowel ischemia. The corrective surgical procedure is called a "Ladd procedure," during which adhesive bands are lysed and the bowel is untwisted, with the small bowel placed in the right abdomen and the colon in the left. Importantly, the procedure reduces the likelihood of recurrent volvulus, but does not "correct" the malrotation, so subsequent imaging studies will still show an abnormal course of the duodenum and abnormal position of the small bowel and colon.

Duodenal Atresia. Duodenal atresia has a strong association with trisomy 21. During normal embryologic development of the duodenum, the lumen undergoes a sequence of occlusion by normal cellular proliferation and subsequent recanalization. Failure of this normal recanalization results in duodenal atresia, with the obstruction occurring in the second portion of the duodenum. Patients typically present with feeding intolerance early in neonatal life. Vomiting may be bilious or nonbilious, depending on the exact level of the atresia relative to the ampulla of Vater. Radiographs classically demonstrate a "double bubble" sign, caused by gaseous distention of the stomach and duodenal bulb, with no distal bowel gas (Fig. 69.8). However, this classic appearance will be absent when an enteric tube has been placed for decompression. When the classic double bubble is present, no further imaging is needed. If an upper GI is done, the contrast will be confined to the dilated stomach and duodenal bulb and will not extend distally. Duodenal atresia is treated surgically with a duodeno-duodenostomy bypassing the atretic segment.

Annular Pancreas. Development of the pancreas occurs in two parts, with the dorsal and ventral pancreatic buds arising on either side of the second portion of the duodenum. During normal development, the ventral bud rotates around the duodenum and fuses with the dorsal bud in the normal anatomic position. If this rotation proceeds abnormally, pancreatic tissue can circumferentially surround the duodenum and cause narrowing or obstruction. Depending on the degree of obstruction, patients may present early in life with feeding intolerance or may not present until later in childhood or even adulthood. An upper GI series will demonstrate circumferential narrowing of the second portion of the duodenum due to extrinsic compression from the pancreatic tissue. CT or MRI may be useful to demonstrate the abnormal pancreatic tissue surrounding the duodenum. Treatment of annular pancreas is surgical, typically with bypass of the narrowed segment of the duodenum.

Duodenal Web. Redundancy of the duodenal mucosa may result in a circumferential area of relative narrowing or a pouch-like structure ("windsock deformity") that can cause partial duodenal obstruction. An upper GI series may demonstrate relative luminal narrowing or a filling defect caused by the redundant tissue. The treatment of duodenal webs is surgical, with resection of the redundant tissue or rarely bypass of the involved segment. Occasionally, endoscopic balloon dilation or resection of the web may be attempted.

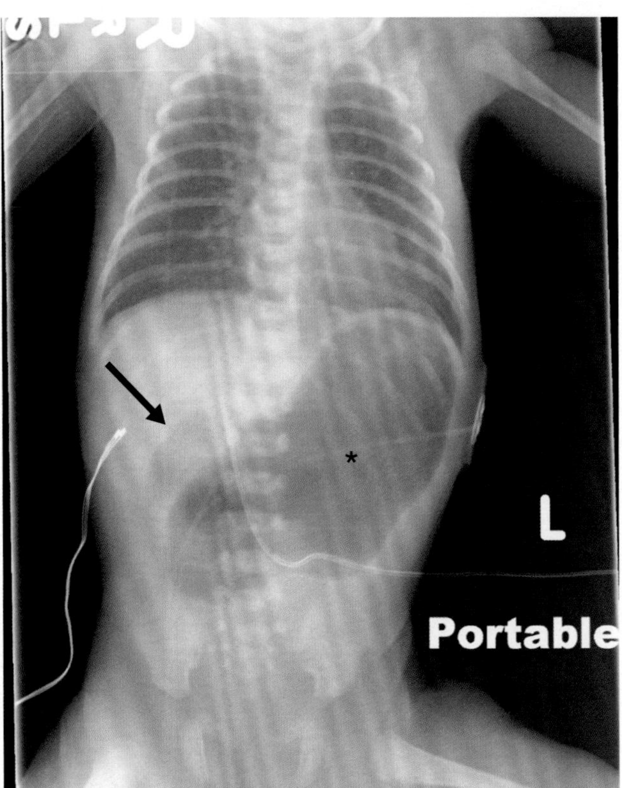

FIGURE 69.8. **Duodenal Atresia.** Abdominal radiograph obtained shortly after birth demonstrates a gas-filled, dilated stomach (*) and duodenal bulb (*arrow*). This represents the so-called "double bubble" sign, diagnostic of duodenal atresia.

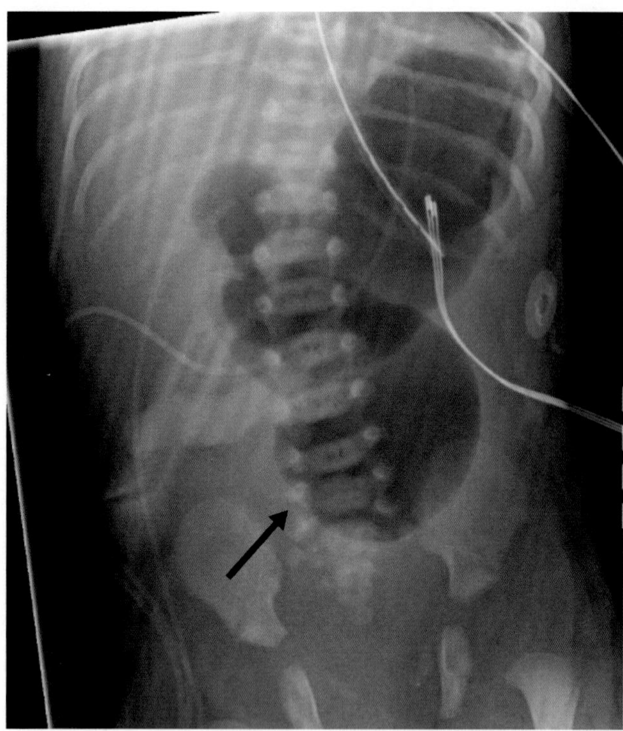

FIGURE 69.9. **Jejunal Atresia.** Abdominal radiograph in a newborn male shows a dilated stomach and duodenum, with an additional dilated loop of bowel representing the dilated proximal jejunum (*arrow*). This appearance has been called the "triple bubble" sign.

Small Bowel Obstruction

Jejunal and Ileal Atresia. Small bowel atresia can occur at any level of the jejunum or ileum. Commonly, there is a single short atretic segment; but, cases with multiple atretic segments do occur. Small bowel atresia is most likely due to a vascular insult in fetal life, resulting in ischemia and scarring, a theory supported by the frequent finding of a wedge-shaped mesenteric defect associated with the atretic segment of small bowel.

Neonates with small bowel atresia typically present early in life with feeding intolerance, bilious vomiting (obstruction distal to the ampulla of Vater), and varying degrees of abdominal distention. The radiographic appearance depends on the location of the atresia. In patients with very proximal jejunal atresia, a "triple bubble" sign may be present, with dilation of the stomach, the duodenum, and the short segment of the jejunum proximal to the atresia (Fig. 69.9). In patients with more distal jejunal atresia, and with ileal atresia, multiple dilated small bowel loops are typically present. A very dilated bowel segment is said to be characteristic of small bowel atresia but is not always seen. An additional sign that can be encountered on radiographs is the presence of peritoneal calcifications (Fig. 69.10). This finding indicates that there has been an in utero bowel perforation, with spillage of meconium into the peritoneal cavity, resulting in inflammation and resultant calcification ("meconium peritonitis"). Occasionally, a discrete peripherally calcified cystic mass, called a meconium pseudocyst, may be present.

Depending on the number of dilated loops and the suspected site of obstruction, an upper GI series (for suspected more proximal obstruction) or a contrast enema (for suspected distal obstruction) may be performed. Sometimes both studies are required to fully characterize an abnormality. If an upper GI series is performed, contrast will fill the dilated bowel loops but will not extend distal to the site of the atresia. If a contrast enema is performed, attempts should be made to reflux the contrast material as far as possible retrograde into the small bowel, approaching the dilated loops. The appearance of the colon on enema for small bowel atresia depends on the site of the atresia. For example, in a distal ileal atresia, the colon is typically diffusely small in caliber ("microcolon"), as the lack of contiguity of the GI tract in utero prevents normal colonic development by obstructing the normal flow of intestinal secretions into the colon. However, if the atresia is more proximal (jejunum or proximal ileum), the colon may appear normal, as intestinal secretions from the relatively long segment of normal bowel distal to the atresia allow for normal colonic development.

Treatment of small bowel atresias is with surgical bypass or resection of the affected segment. Care must be taken during surgery to examine the entire small bowel, as additional sites of atresia may be present.

Meconium Ileus. Neonatal obstruction of the distal ileum by retained meconium is termed meconium ileus. This condition is strongly associated with cystic fibrosis, and is likely secondary to abnormally viscous intestinal secretions and meconium, resulting in obstruction at the ileocecal valve. Patients present with failure to pass meconium, abdominal distention, feeding intolerance, and vomiting. Radiographs demonstrate a distal obstructive pattern, with multiple dilated bowel loops. Calcifications related to in utero perforation and meconium peritonitis may be present. A contrast enema with water-soluble contrast is both diagnostic and therapeutic. Typically, the contrast enema will demonstrate a diffuse microcolon, with contrast refluxing into a dilated terminal/distal ileum containing multiple filling defects representing the retained meconium (Fig. 69.11). Although refluxing contrast into the terminal ileum is important, the enema should

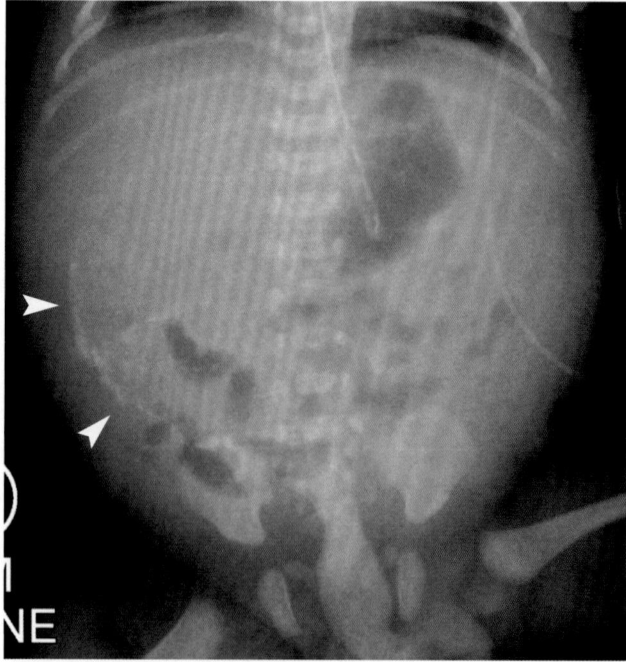

FIGURE 69.10. **Meconium Peritonitis.** Abdominal radiograph in a neonate with abdominal distention showing curvilinear calcifications in the right abdomen (*arrowheads*), typical of meconium peritonitis. There is mass effect on the adjacent gas-filled bowel loops, suggesting the presence of a meconium pseudocyst as well, later confirmed at ultrasound.

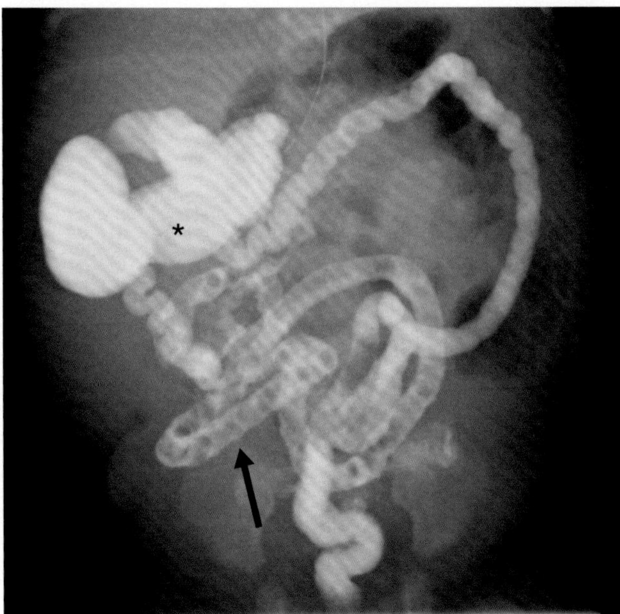

FIGURE 69.11. **Meconium Ileus.** Image from a contrast enema showing a diffusely small-caliber colon consistent with a microcolon. There are multiple filling defects in the terminal ileum, representing meconium (*arrow*). Contrast could be refluxed all the way back to the dilated distal small bowel (*). The finding of meconium ileus should prompt further workup for cystic fibrosis.

be performed carefully due to the relatively increased risk of perforation of a microcolon. The hyperosmotic water-soluble contrast causes shift of water into the bowel lumen, loosening up the tenacious meconium and allowing it to pass through the colon. These fluid shifts also have the potential to result in dehydration in a neonate that is not taking much by mouth or that is not appropriately monitored. Additional enemas may be required to completely clear the meconium. Occasionally, surgical intervention is required. When findings consistent with meconium ileus are encountered, a comprehensive workup for cystic fibrosis should be initiated.

Colonic Obstruction

Small Left Colon. This condition, which is also called "functional immaturity of the colon" and "meconium plug syndrome," occurs in infants of diabetic mothers and in infants whose mothers received tocolytics (e.g., magnesium sulfate) during pregnancy. Radiographs will demonstrate a distal obstructive pattern. Water-soluble contrast enema is the diagnostic test of choice. As the name implies, small left colon syndrome manifests as a dilated proximal colon with an abrupt caliber change, usually at the splenic flexure, and diffusely small caliber of the more distal colon (Fig. 69.12). Filling defects in the more proximal dilated colon represent retained meconium. The contrast enema is generally therapeutic and the obstruction resolves with passage of the meconium. Surgery is not typically necessary. Unlike meconium ileus, this condition does not have an association with cystic fibrosis, despite the confusing nomenclature ("meconium plug syndrome").

Colonic Atresia. Colonic atresia is much less common than small bowel atresias, probably due to the redundant blood supply to the colon. The etiology is most likely an ischemic event. The atretic segment is most commonly located at the junction of the descending colon and sigmoid colon. Patients typically present shortly after birth with abdominal distention and vomiting, and radiographs will demonstrate a distal obstructive pattern. Contrast enema will show a small-caliber distal colon which ends abruptly, and contrast will not reflux into the dilated proximal bowel loops. The treatment for colonic atresia is surgery.

Hirschsprung Disease. Hirschsprung disease occurs due to lack of normal ganglion cells innervating the colon. This leads to abnormal colonic peristalsis and varying degrees of obstruction. The rectum is always involved, and the extent of proximal involvement varies. Involvement is typically contiguous from the rectum proximally. The clinical presentation in patients with Hirschsprung disease can vary, depending on the length of the involved segment and the degree of obstruction. Some patients will present with findings of frank colonic obstruction in a neonate with abdominal distention, failure to pass meconium, and vomiting. In some patients, the condition may not be diagnosed until later in life when the child undergoes evaluation for chronic, refractory constipation.

Depending on the degree of obstruction, the radiographic appearance of Hirschsprung disease can range from findings of a distal bowel obstruction with multiple dilated bowel loops to a nearly normal bowel gas pattern, often with evidence of constipation. The contrast enema is the imaging test of choice in evaluation of patients with suspected Hirschsprung disease. The imaging appearance can vary, but typically the affected segment is contracted (smaller caliber) compared to the more proximal unaffected colon (Fig. 69.13). The "recto-sigmoid ratio" is often described as a diagnostic measure for Hirschsprung disease. In normal colon, the rectum is larger in diameter than the more proximal colon (e.g., sigmoid and descending colon). However, in Hirschsprung disease, the rectum (and the full length of colon involved by Hirschsprung

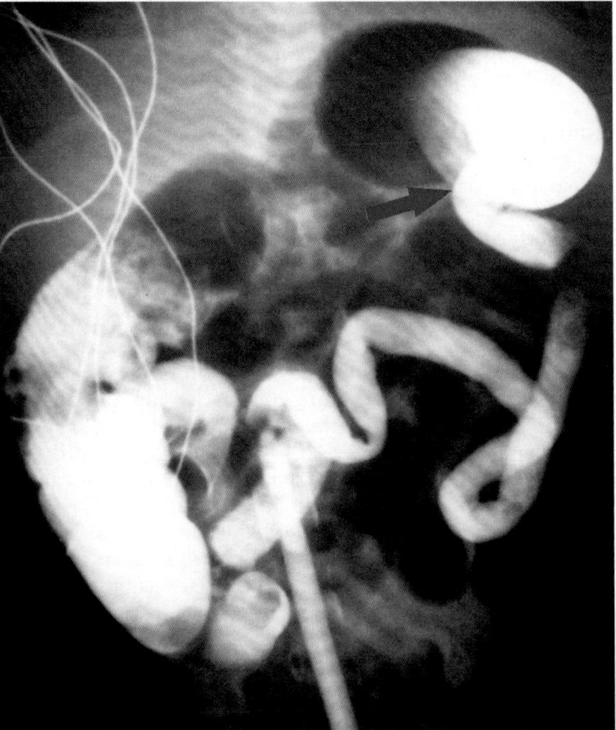

FIGURE 69.12. **Meconium Plug Syndrome (Small Left Colon Syndrome).** Contrast enema demonstrates a small left colon with the characteristic transition zone (*arrow*). These findings mimic those of Hirschsprung disease.

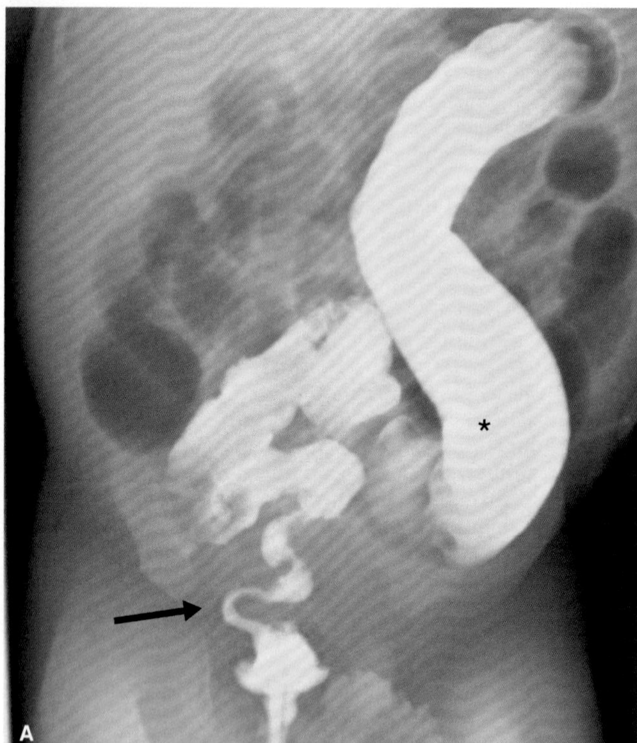

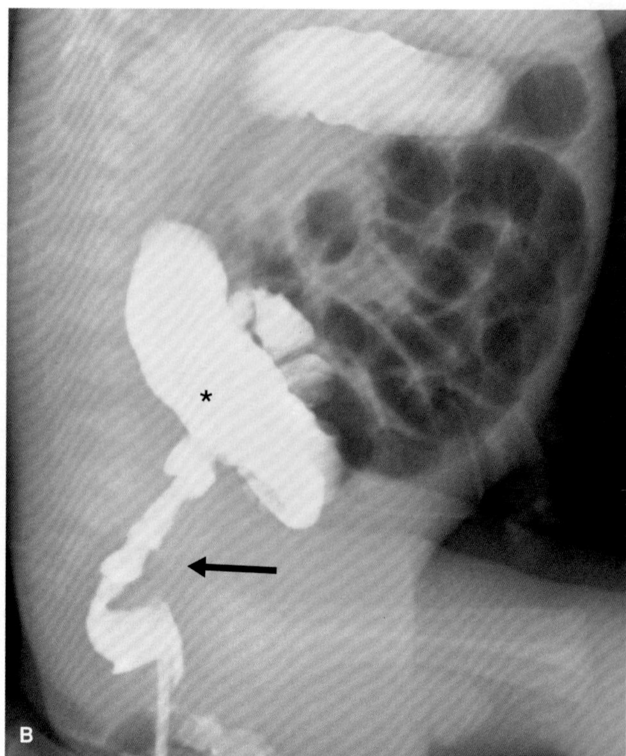

FIGURE 69.13. **Hirschsprung Disease. A:** AP view from a contrast enema demonstrates a small-caliber rectum and distal sigmoid colon (*arrow*) and dilated colon more proximally (*). This represents an abnormal "rectosigmoid ratio" highly suggestive of Hirschsprung disease. **B:** The lateral view confirms the findings, with a small-caliber rectum (*arrow*) and dilated more proximal colon (*).

disease) is contracted and will typically be smaller in caliber than the more proximal, unaffected colon (Fig. 69.13). It is important to obtain a true lateral view with complete distention of the rectum, to avoid false positives caused by underdistention. An additional finding that may be helpful is visualization of an irregular "sawtooth" appearance of the rectal wall on the lateral view, caused by abnormal peristalsis and spasm. In general, the role of the contrast enema is to make the diagnosis if possible, determine the approximate location of the transition zone (the transition between dilated and contracted colon), and to exclude other causes of colonic obstruction. Importantly, the radiographic transition zone may not correlate well with the transition zone at pathology, but estimating the level of obstruction is helpful for surgical planning nonetheless.

Total colonic aganglionosis is a rare form of Hirschsprung disease that involves the entire colon. The lack of ganglion cells can rarely extend into the proximal small bowel as well. In total colonic aganglionosis, the colon can appear diffusely small in caliber ("microcolon") or may be normal in caliber, with or without associated small bowel dilation.

The contrast enema is not always diagnostic, and in some cases can be completely normal, in Hirschsprung disease. For this reason, most patients will also undergo rectal suction biopsy for definitive diagnosis. A normal-appearing colon may occur in two settings, either a very short-segment Hirschsprung disease involving only the rectum, or rarely in total colonic aganglionosis.

Imperforate Anus/Anorectal Malformation. Failure of normal development of the hindgut can lead to anorectal malformation and/or imperforate anus, resulting in a distal colonic obstruction. The condition is usually clinically apparent, with absence of an anal opening on physical examination. Frequently, there is a fistulous connection that develops between the distal colon and the urinary tract, or rarely the perineum. In boys, this typically manifests as a rectovesical or rectourethral fistula. In girls, a more complex malformation involving the rectum and genitourinary system, called a cloaca, may be present. Anorectal malformations are often accompanied by other anomalies as part of the VACTRL association.

Radiographs in patients with anorectal malformation will typically demonstrate a distal obstructive pattern (Fig. 69.14). A prone, cross-table lateral view may be helpful to distend the distal colon/rectum with gas and better demonstrate the level of obstruction. Traditionally, these malformations have been classified as "high" or "low," depending on the site of obstruction relative to the pubococcygeal line. These malformations are often associated with skeletal abnormalities, including dysplasia/hypoplasia of the sacrum. Determination of the "sacral ratio" has been shown to have prognostic value in terms of bowel function after surgical repair.

Patients with imperforate anus are treated surgically, often with a colostomy shortly after birth to relieve the obstruction, followed by definitive surgical correction several months later. Prior to definitive surgical correction, a fluoroscopic distal colostogram may be performed, with injection of contrast through the mucous fistula distending the distal colon to identify the presence of a fistula (typically between the rectum and the urinary tract) and to define the length of the distal segment for surgical planning (Fig. 69.15).

OBSTRUCTION—ACQUIRED

Esophageal Obstruction

Acquired esophageal obstructions are rare in children. Older children and young adults can develop primary achalasia

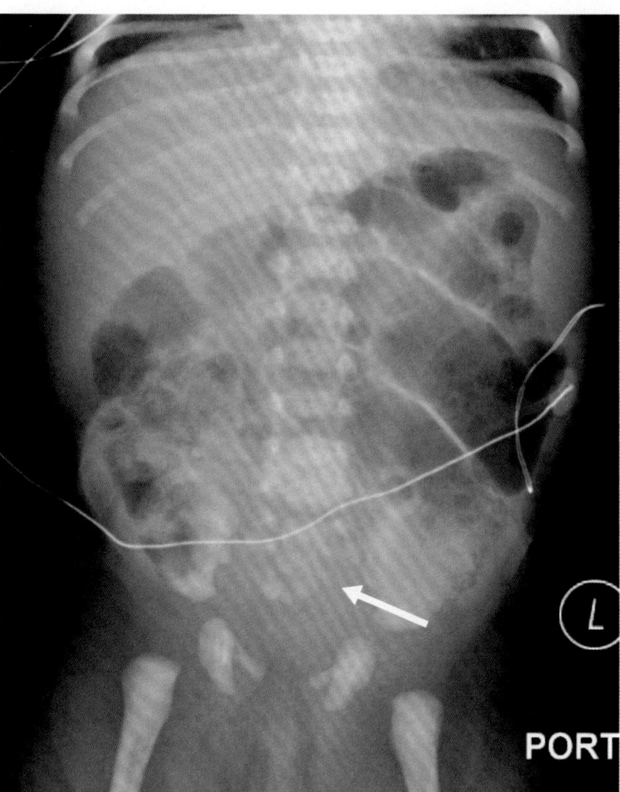

FIGURE 69.14. **Anorectal Malformation.** Abdominal radiograph in a neonate showing dilated loops of bowel due to obstruction from an anorectal malformation and imperforate anus. Note the dysplastic appearance of the sacrum (*arrow*).

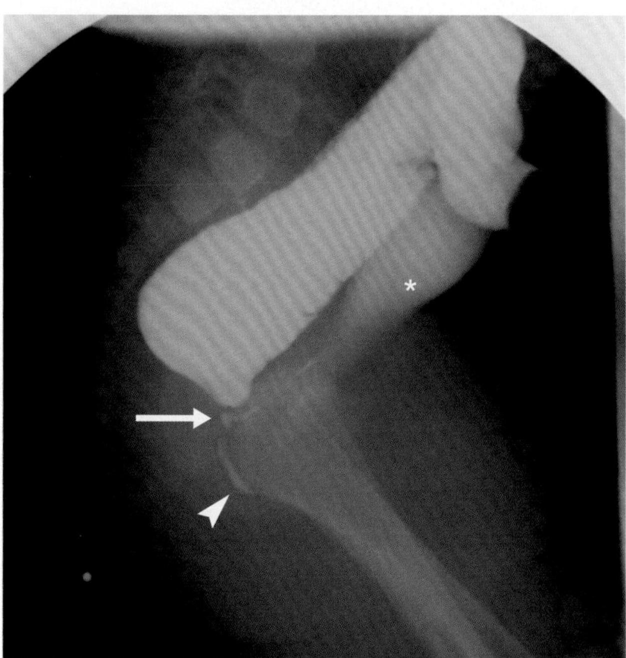

FIGURE 69.15. **Anorectal Malformation in a Different Patient.** High-pressure colostogram, with contrast being injected through an ostomy and distending the distal colon. The colon terminates in a rectourethral fistula (*arrow*) connecting the rectum and the posterior urethra. Contrast refluxes back into the bladder (*) and is also present in the membranous portion of the urethra (*arrowhead*). A fistula between the rectum and the urinary tract or perineum is present in most patients with an anorectal malformation.

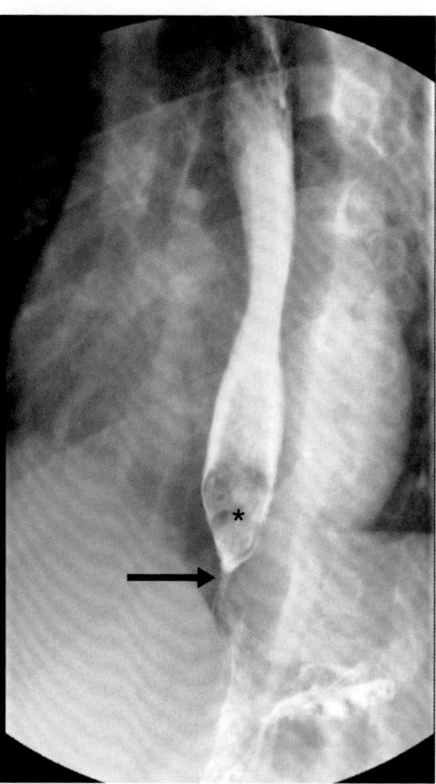

FIGURE 69.16. **Eosinophilic Esophagitis and Stricture.** Fluoroscopic image from an esophagram in a patient with a sensation of a retained food bolus. There is a tight stricture of the distal esophagus (*arrow*). Just above this, a filling defect (*) is present, representing an impacted food bolus that is too large to get past the stricture.

and strictures related to gastroesophageal reflux disease, just like in adults, but these are relatively infrequent. One cause of acquired esophageal obstruction that warrants specific mention is eosinophilic esophagitis (EoE). EoE is an allergic inflammatory condition that occurs in susceptible patients, often in patients with asthma and other forms of atopy. The resultant inflammatory response can cause esophageal dysmotility, focal strictures, or diffuse esophageal narrowing. Patients may present with varying clinical symptoms, from dysphagia to food bolus impaction. Undiagnosed EoE is the most common cause of new-onset food bolus impaction in children and young adults. An esophagram may show focal strictures, which are typically located relatively high in the esophagus (Fig. 69.16). Alternatively, the entire esophagus may be diffusely small in caliber or may be entirely normal fluoroscopically. In the setting of clinical suspicion for EoE, even if imaging is normal, patients should undergo endoscopy and esophageal biopsy. Treatment is with medical therapy and occasionally endoscopic balloon dilation if focal strictures are present.

Hypertrophic Pyloric Stenosis

Hypertrophic pyloric stenosis (HPS) is caused by abnormal hypertrophy of the pyloric muscle, resulting in gastric outlet obstruction. The exact etiology is not known but may be related to abnormal innervation or nitric oxide synthase activity, leading to prolonged pylorospasm and ultimately hypertrophy of the muscle and gastric outlet obstruction. HPS is considered an acquired condition, as patients are normal at birth but progress to development of the disorder typically between 2 and 12 weeks of age. The condition is more common in males and has some familial inheritance with incomplete penetrance. The typical clinical presentation is that of recurrent nonbilious emesis, which is often forceful (projectile vomiting).

Ultrasound is the imaging test of choice and should be the first-line imaging modality if HPS is suspected clinically. Ultrasound allows direct assessment of the morphology of the pylorus, including the length of the pyloric channel and thickness of the wall. Images should be obtained in both the longitudinal and transverse planes, relative to the pylorus. The diagnosis is made based on identification of an abnormally elongated and thickened pylorus (Fig. 69.17). Diagnostic cutoffs for measurements vary, but in general, a pyloric wall thickness of greater than 3 mm and a pyloric channel length of greater than 14 mm are sufficient to make the diagnosis. Hypertrophied muscle and mucosa may cause a convex margin between the pylorus and the fluid-filled gastric antrum and duodenal bulb. Importantly, the examination should be carried out over the course of several minutes to exclude false-positive studies due to transient collapse of the gastric antrum or pylorospasm. If needed, the patient can be fed during the examination and turned right side down to ensure maximum distention of the antrum with fluid. A small amount of fluid passing through the pylorus during imaging does not exclude the diagnosis of HPS and is, in fact, frequently present. It is important to remember that the diagnosis of HPS depends on the persistent abnormal morphology of the pylorus, not whether contents pass through the pylorus during imaging. It is also important to understand that HPS is a progressive process and depending on the timing of presentation and imaging, varying degrees of obstruction may be present.

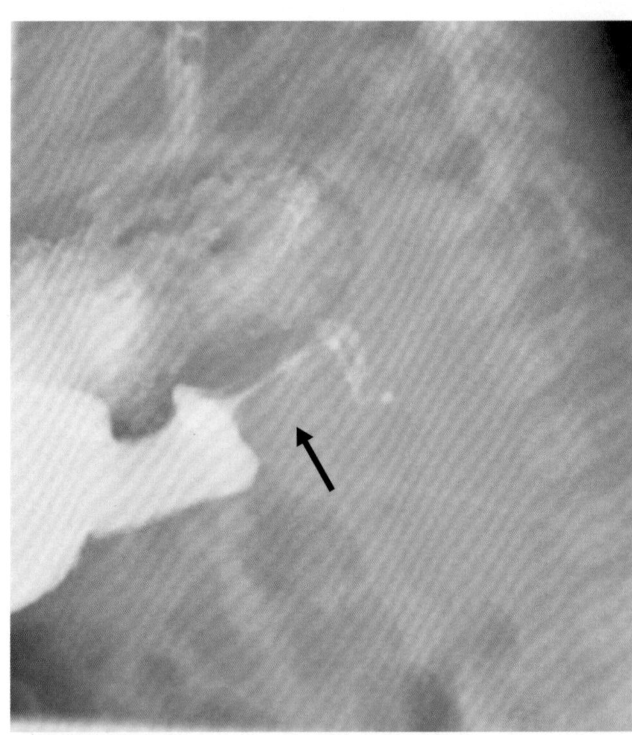

FIGURE 69.18. Hypertrophic Pyloric Stenosis. Fluoroscopic image from an upper GI study showing an elongated, thin pyloric channel (*arrow*) consistent with hypertrophic pyloric stenosis.

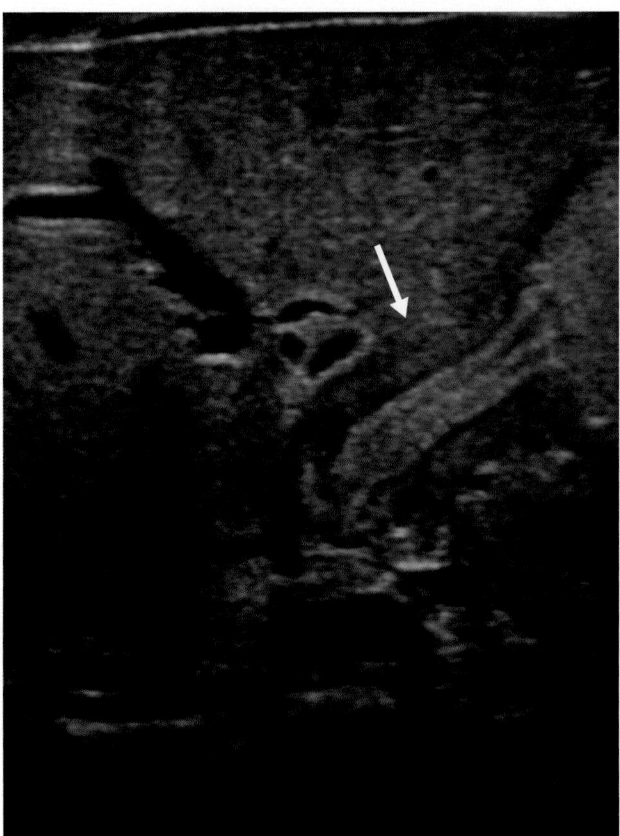

FIGURE 69.17. Hypertrophic Pyloric Stenosis. Transverse ultrasound image showing an elongated and thickened pylorus (*arrow*). The abnormal morphology of the pylorus remained present throughout the study consistent with hypertrophic pyloric stenosis (as opposed to transient pylorospasm).

If radiographs are obtained due to vomiting, they may show varying degrees of gastric distention, although distention of the stomach may depend on how recently the patient vomited. The bowel gas pattern distal to the stomach is typically normal. If a UGI series is obtained, the stomach may be dilated and contain debris. There is frequently an extrinsic impression in the gastric antrum caused by the hypertrophied muscle ("umbrella" or "mushroom" signs). Gastric emptying is commonly delayed. When the stomach does empty, the pyloric channel is elongated and thin, often with a "tram-track" appearance (Fig. 69.18). Similar to the appearance of the gastric antrum, the hypertrophied pylorus frequently causes extrinsic compression on the duodenal bulb.

The treatment of HPS is typically surgical. The hypertrophied pylorus is incised longitudinally to disrupt the contiguity of the muscle and alleviate the obstruction (called a "pyloromyotomy").

Small Bowel Obstruction

Small bowel obstructions in children can occur from a variety of causes, both mechanical and inflammatory. The patient's age and clinical history can often guide the differential diagnosis. The basic differential diagnosis for a pediatric small bowel obstruction can be remembered using the mnemonic AAIIMM; Adhesions, Appendicitis, Inguinal hernia, Intussusception, Midgut volvulus, Meckel diverticulum. The list can then be narrowed by using the age and clinical presentation, allowing for appropriate imaging to make the definitive diagnosis. For example, appendicitis is rare in very young children and would be an uncommon cause of small bowel obstruction in a 1 year old; however, appendicitis is high on the list

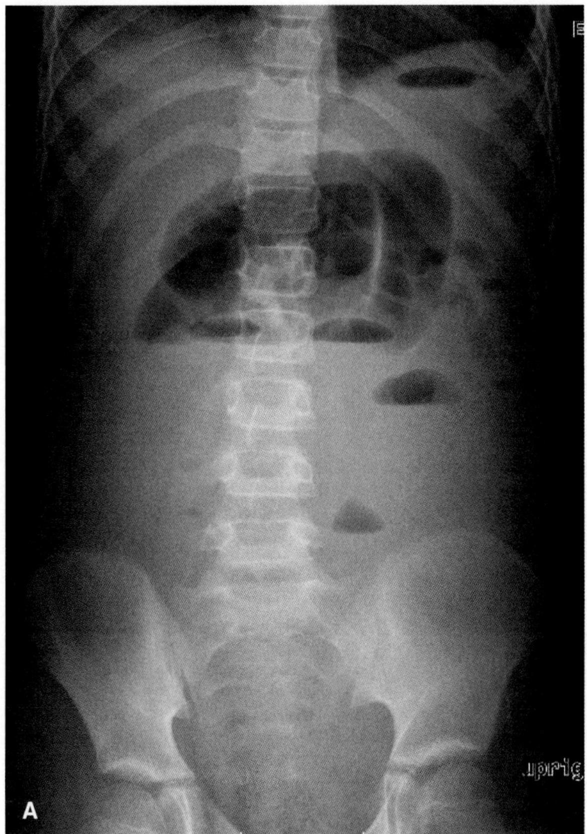

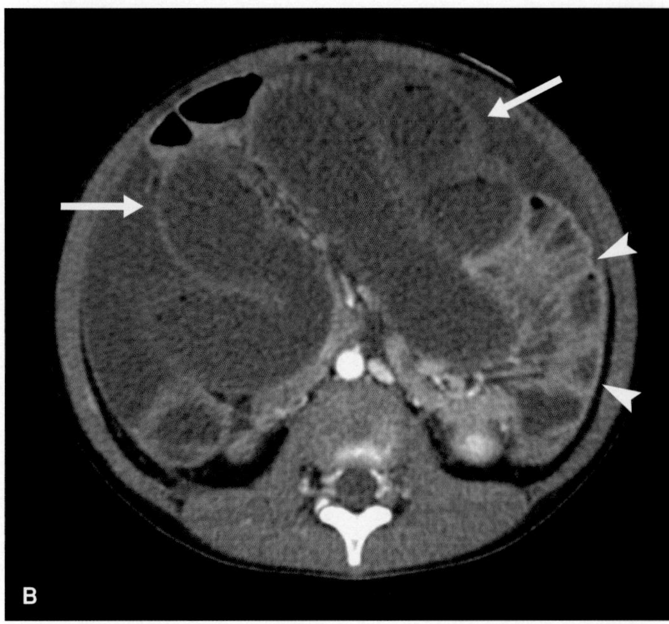

FIGURE 69.19. **Closed Loop Small Bowel Obstruction. A:** Upright abdominal radiograph in a patient with abdominal pain and vomiting showing dilated small bowel loops with multiple air–fluid levels. There is a paucity of colonic bowel gas. **B:** Contrast-enhanced axial CT image showing dilated, fluid-filled small bowel loops (*arrows*) and decompressed distal small bowel (*arrowheads*) consistent with a small bowel obstruction. The dilated loops demonstrate relative hypoenhancement of the bowel wall, suspicious for ischemia. At surgery, the patient was found to have a closed-loop obstruction with necrotic bowel due to an adhesion from prior appendectomy.

of differential diagnoses in a previously healthy teenager presenting with abdominal pain and bowel obstruction. Abdominal radiographs are often the first imaging study obtained and will show varying patterns of obstruction, typically with dilated small bowel loops and differential air–fluid levels (Fig. 69.19). The next imaging test depends on the differential diagnosis and may include ultrasound, fluoroscopy, CT, or rarely MRI.

Adhesions. As in adults, pediatric patients who have had previous abdominal surgery are at risk for developing adhesions, and these adhesive bands can lead to obstruction anywhere along the bowel. Adhesions can also develop in patients with prior intra-abdominal infections or other inflammatory processes, or in patients with omphalomesenteric duct remnants. In the setting of suspected acute small bowel obstruction, abdominal radiographs followed by contrast-enhanced CT are the most common imaging modalities. The actual adhesive band is typically not visible by imaging. Instead, the typical findings are multiple dilated small bowel loops, usually with an abrupt transition point to decompressed distal bowel. It is important to evaluate for signs of bowel ischemia, including decreased mural enhancement, bowel wall thickening, pneumatosis, and extensive mesenteric edema/ascites, as these findings should direct the patient to emergent surgical management (Fig. 69.19).

Appendicitis. Appendicitis, and most commonly perforated appendicitis, is one of the most common causes of bowel obstruction in a previously healthy older child. This may be the result of a true mechanical obstruction, or more typically, an ileus caused by the extensive inflammation associated with appendiceal rupture and peritonitis. Details of appendicitis imaging will be discussed in a later section.

Incarcerated Inguinal Hernia. Inguinal hernias are relatively common in infants under 6 months of age and are more common in boys. Indirect hernias are most common, caused by failure of the normal closure of the processus vaginalis, resulting in persistent communication between the peritoneal cavity and the scrotum. Bowel loops, most commonly distal small bowel loops, can become trapped or incarcerated within the hernia, resulting in obstruction and, in some cases, ischemic necrosis. Radiographs will typically show a distal obstruction pattern, and gas-filled bowel loops may be visible in the inguinal regions or even within the scrotum (Fig. 69.20). Often, additional imaging is not required because the entity is clinically evident. US may occasionally be obtained, demonstrating dilated and thick-walled bowel loops in the inguinal canal or scrotum, often with associated free fluid. The treatment for incarcerated inguinal hernia may include initial attempts at manual reduction, but ultimately surgical intervention is often required.

Ileocolic Intussusception. After 6 months of age, ileocolic intussusception becomes an increasingly common cause of bowel obstruction. Intussusception occurs when a segment of proximal bowel, most commonly the terminal

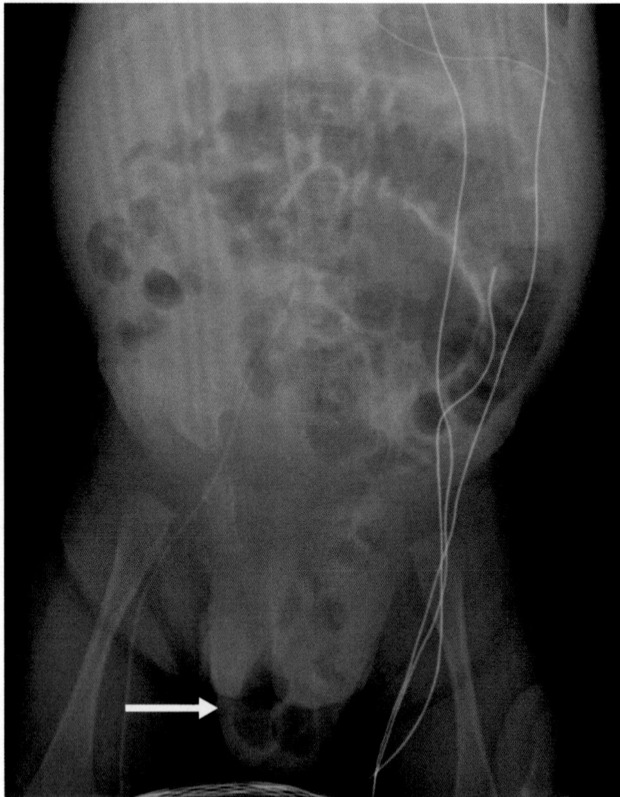

FIGURE 69.20. **Inguinal Hernia.** Abdominal radiograph in an infant obtained for line placement shows nondilated, gas-filled loops of bowel within the scrotum (*arrow*), diagnostic of an indirect inguinal hernia.

ileum, telescopes into a more distal bowel segment. Most intussusceptions in children are ileocolic and the cause is idiopathic, but likely related to reactive lymph nodes. Idiopathic intussusception is rarer in children over 6 years of age; and in older children and those with repeated intussusceptions, a lead point is more likely to be present. Pathologic lead points include tumors, polyps, diverticula, or inflammatory bowel wall thickening as can be seen in Henoch–Schönlein purpura.

Radiographs may demonstrate a distal obstructive pattern. Occasionally, a soft tissue mass, representing the intussusception itself, will be visible, often in the right upper quadrant. If the colon contains gas, one may see the intussusceptum outlined by colonic gas, appearing as a rounded soft tissue/gas interface (Fig. 69.21). Ultrasound (US) is the imaging test of choice in suspected intussusception, due to its high specificity and high negative predictive value. A typical US protocol for imaging for intussusception includes images of all four quadrants of the abdomen, tracing along the expected course of the colon. The intussusception typically appears as a soft tissue mass which has concentric layers ("target" appearance) in the transverse plane, representing the multiple layers of bowel wall and intervening mesentery (Fig. 69.21). When imaged in the longitudinal plane, the proximal loop of bowel extending into the intussusception is often visible, and the intussusception can have a reniform appearance (the "pseudokidney sign"). With color Doppler, the abnormal bowel loops may demonstrate any pattern from hyperemia to lack of blood flow due to venous ischemia. If there is diminished blood flow, this implies that the intussusception may have been present for a longer time and may be more difficult to reduce. Trapped fluid between the layers of bowel wall in the intussusception is another sonographic sign that the intussusception may be more difficult to reduce.

Most cases of intussusception are treated with fluoroscopic air enema reduction (Fig. 69.22). This works by increasing the intraluminal pressure, forcing the intussusceptum

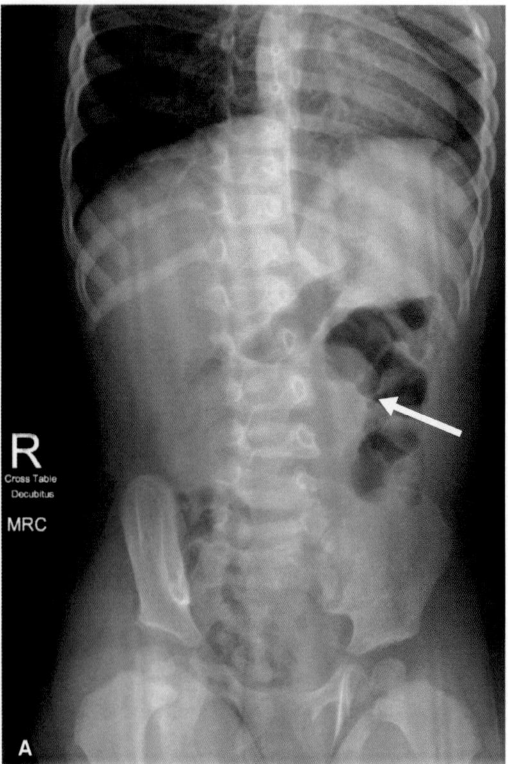

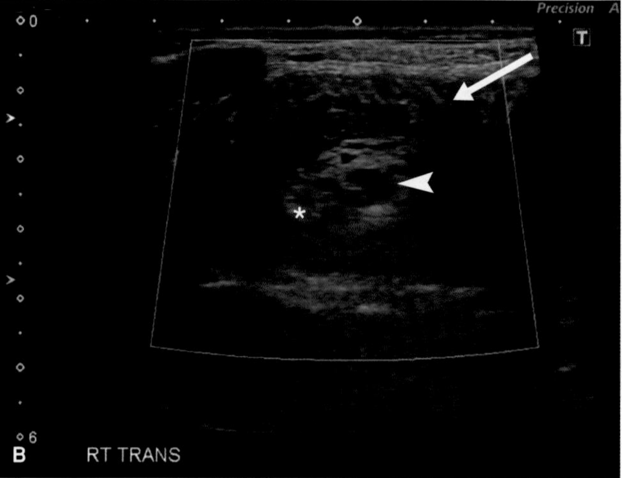

FIGURE 69.21. **Ileocolic Intussusception. A:** Abdominal radiograph in a child with abdominal pain showing a soft tissue mass partially outlined by air in the colon (*arrow*). **B:** Ultrasound image in the same child showing a rounded mass with concentric rings ("target appearance"), typical of an intussusception (*arrow*). Note the hyperechoic fat within the intussusception (*) and the hypoechoic lymph node within the mesenteric fat (*arrowhead*). Mesenteric fat and lymph nodes within the intussusception are common findings in ileocolic intussusception.

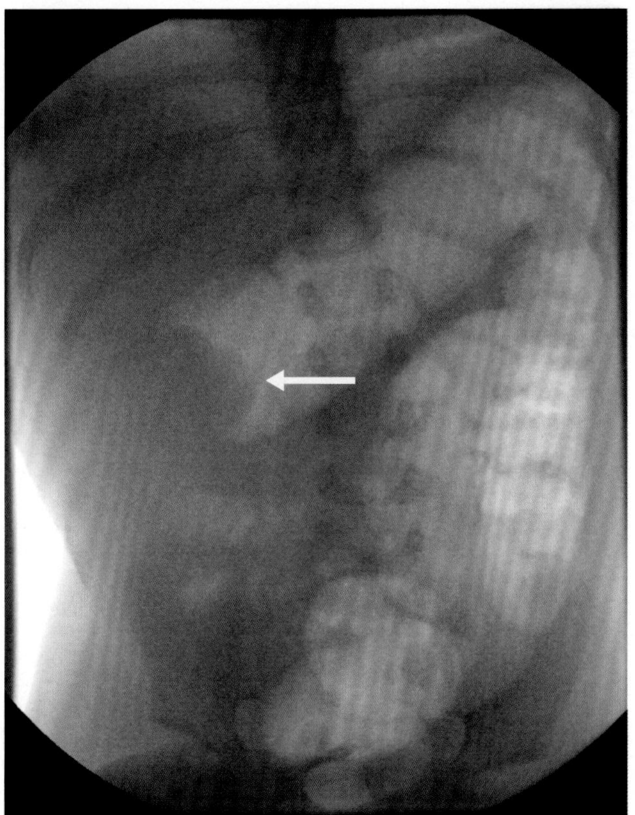

FIGURE 69.22. **Air Enema Reduction of Intussusception.** Fluoroscopic image during an air enema showing the intussusception outlined by gas in the proximal transverse colon (*arrow*). The majority of uncomplicated ileocolic intussusceptions can be successfully reduced by air enema.

back to its normal position. Contraindications to attempted enema reduction include pneumoperitoneum and peritoneal signs. The most important potential complication of enema reduction is bowel perforation, and care must be taken during the reduction to maintain intraluminal pressures below 120 mm Hg. Using air enema, successful reduction can be achieved in approximately 80% of cases. In those cases that are refractory to enema reduction, surgical reduction is performed.

Malrotation With Midgut Volvulus. Although most common in neonates under 1 month of age, malrotation with volvulus can occur at any age. This entity should be considered in the differential diagnosis of a patient with bilious emesis and a proximal obstructive pattern on radiographs. Detailed imaging findings were described in an earlier section.

Meckel Diverticulum. Meckel diverticulum results from persistence of a normal embryologic structure, the vitelline duct. This results in varying degrees of abnormality from a fibrous band connecting the umbilicus to the distal ileum (omphalomesenteric band) to a true diverticulum arising from the distal ileum, typically located approximately 2 ft (60.96 cm) from the ileocecal valve. Obstruction can result from inflammation, similar to that of appendicitis (Meckel diverticulitis), from twisting due to a persistent connection between the diverticulum and the mesentery, or related to bowel loops becoming entrapped by fibrous band(s). The actual Meckel diverticulum may be visible at US or CT if it is inflamed; however, often the diverticulum and/or band is occult by imaging and the diagnosis is inferred based on the finding of an obstruction and/or inflammation centered in the right lower quadrant but not involving the appendix. Treatment is surgical, with resection of the diverticulum and/or band to relieve the obstruction.

INFECTION AND INFLAMMATION

Necrotizing Enterocolitis

Necrotizing enterocolitis (NEC) is an inflammatory process of the small and large bowel seen in infants that were born prematurely, or in infants with a history of underlying congenital heart disease. The pathophysiology is unclear, but most likely the condition is caused by relative hypoperfusion of the bowel, resulting in inflammation and susceptibility to infection. The end result is bowel wall inflammation and increased risk for bowel wall ischemia and perforation. Infants typically present between 2 weeks and 4 months of life with abdominal distention, feeding intolerance, and bloody stools. NEC is most commonly identified in infants who have been hospitalized for much of their life. The earliest radiographic finding in NEC is a nonspecific ileus, often with associated bowel wall thickening visible as separation of bowel loops and an elongated, tubular appearance of the bowel lumen. Later findings of NEC include pneumatosis, which manifests as linear and bubbly lucencies in the bowel wall, and portal venous gas, branching lucencies overlying the liver (Figs. 69.23 and 69.24). The diagnosis of NEC is often made clinically, and the purpose of serial radiographs is to identify findings supporting the clinical diagnosis (pneumatosis and portal venous gas), as well as to evaluate for pneumoperitoneum, which indicates bowel perforation. Pneumoperitoneum is an indication for emergent intervention, either with

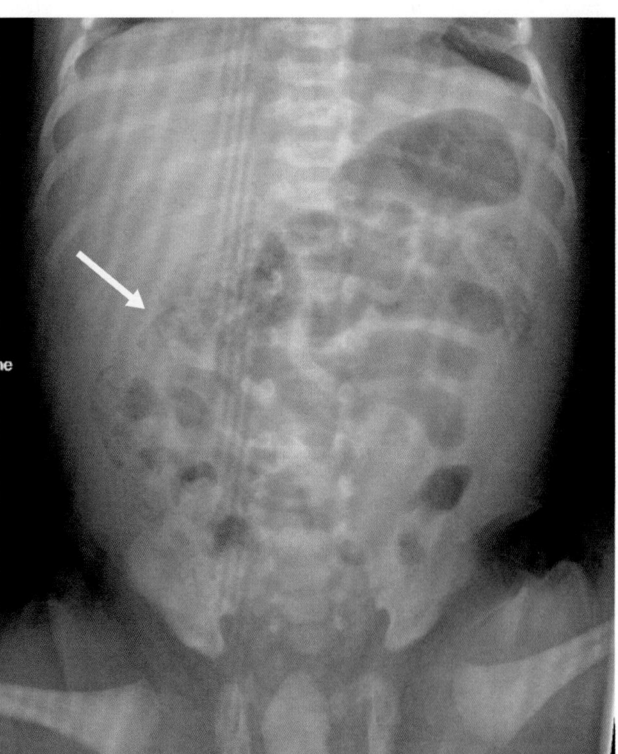

FIGURE 69.23. **Pneumatosis Intestinalis.** Supine radiograph in an infant with suspected necrotizing enterocolitis showing linear lucencies along the bowel wall (*arrow*) consistent with pneumatosis.

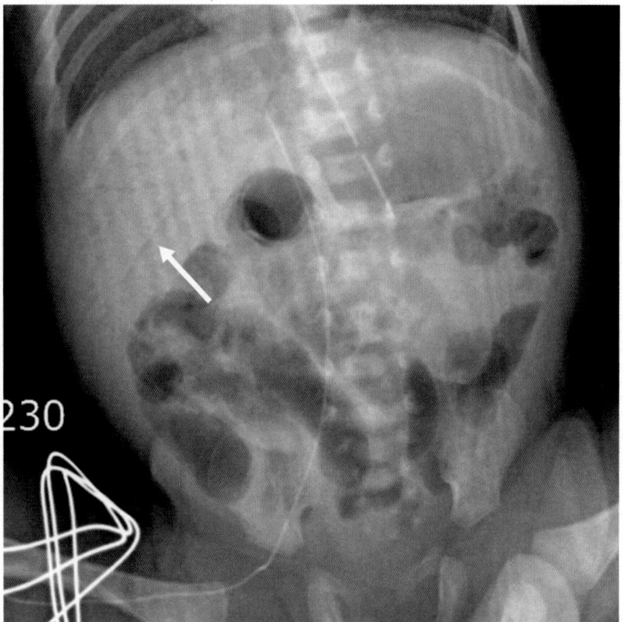

FIGURE 69.24. **Portal Venous Gas.** Supine radiograph in another infant with necrotizing enterocolitis showing branching linear lucencies over the liver (*arrow*) consistent with portal venous gas.

surgery or with percutaneous drain placement. If perforation is not suspected, NEC is treated medically with bowel rest and antibiotics.

Appendicitis

Acute appendicitis is the most common indication for abdominal surgery in children. Appendicitis occurs when the appendiceal lumen is occluded, often by fecal contents (fecalith or calcified appendicolith), resulting in obstruction and secondary infection. If left untreated, this can ultimately result in appendiceal perforation and abscess formation. Appendicitis is relatively rare in very young children and becomes more common after approximately 2 years of age. Patients typically present with abdominal pain, often localized to the right lower quadrant. Fevers and other signs of infection may or may not be present. Traditionally, a diagnosis of appendicitis was made based on clinical and physical examination findings, with an accepted negative laparotomy rate of 20% to 30%. Modern practice, however, relies heavily on imaging to confirm the diagnosis of acute appendicitis prior to surgery, with a corresponding reduction in the negative appendectomy rate. Imaging is also important to preoperatively identify cases of perforated appendicitis that may benefit from initial nonoperative treatment with antibiotics and drain placement.

Radiographs are often the first imaging test obtained, as the patients may present with more generalized abdominal pain. Findings on radiographs may vary from a frankly obstructed bowel gas pattern to completely normal. It is important to scrutinize the right lower quadrant to look for a calcified fecalith. Free air identifiable on radiographs is extremely rare, even in the setting of perforation.

Ultrasound is the initial diagnostic test of choice in suspected acute, uncomplicated appendicitis, regardless of patient size. Images should be obtained with graded compression (progressively increasing pressure), to displace bowel gas. The highest frequency transducer that allows adequate penetration should be used. Imaging should include the right lower quadrant and pelvis to identify the occasional appendix that extends deep into the pelvis. Occasionally, imaging from a posterior or lateral approach can be helpful to identify a retrocecal appendix. The normal appendix on ultrasound is a vermiform, tubular structure with easily visible mural layers and a compressible lumen. In the setting of appendicitis, the appendix often becomes dilated over 6 mm in diameter, although size alone is not adequate to make the diagnosis. The normal layers of the appendiceal wall often become poorly defined and the lumen becomes noncompressible due to distention by purulent fluid. Increased echogenicity and bulk of the periappendiceal fat, indicating inflammation, has been shown to be the most reliable sign of acute appendicitis (Fig. 69.25). Occasionally, a

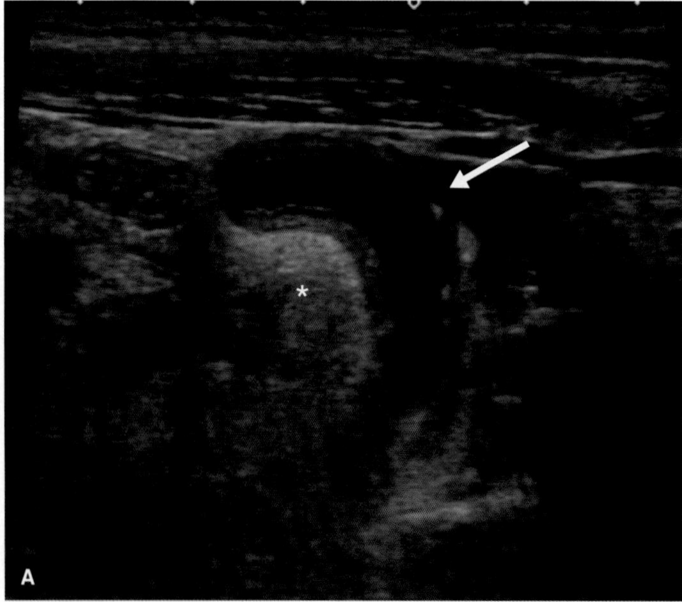

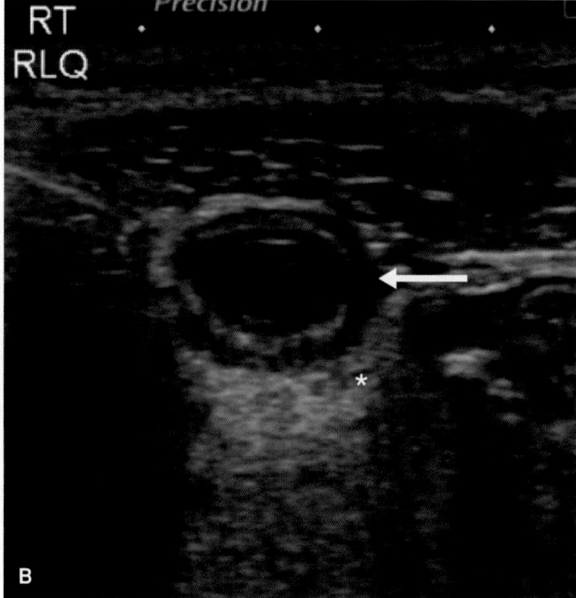

FIGURE 69.25. **Acute Appendicitis on Ultrasound.** Longitudinal (**A**) and transverse (**B**) sonographic images of the right lower quadrant showing a dilated appendix (*arrows*) with increased echogenicity of the adjacent periappendiceal fat (*), indicating inflammation.

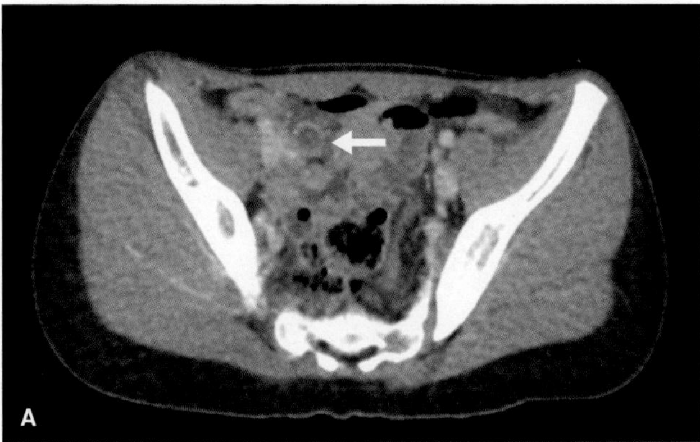

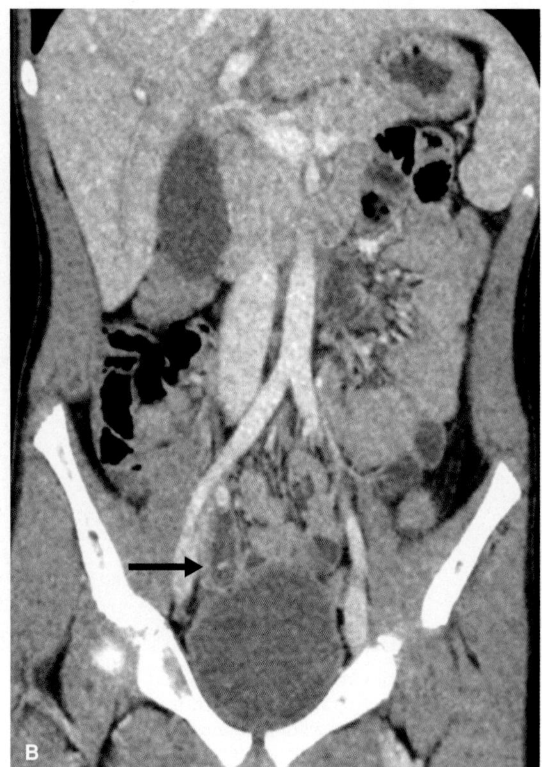

FIGURE 69.26. **Acute Appendicitis on CT.** **A:** Axial contrast-enhanced CT image showing a dilated appendix (*arrow*) with adjacent inflammatory fat stranding consistent with acute appendicitis. **B:** Coronal contrast-enhanced CT image in a different patient with acute appendicitis showing a dilated fluid-filled appendix with a small intraluminal calcification consistent with an appendicolith (*arrow*).

calcified fecalith may be seen within the appendiceal lumen as a shadowing, echogenic structure. While ultrasound is not sensitive for perforation, specific signs of appendiceal perforation in the context of an abnormal appendix include identification of an abscess, visualization of a defect in the appendiceal wall, or extensive inflammation throughout the right lower quadrant and pelvis, not localized to the appendix.

CT also plays an important role in the diagnosis of acute appendicitis. In some centers with limited ultrasound experience or resources, CT is the first-line imaging test in acute appendicitis. In most pediatric centers, CT is reserved for cases where the appendix is not visible at US but there is high clinical suspicion for appendicitis, or for cases where perforated appendicitis is suspected. CT findings in acute, uncomplicated appendicitis include dilation of the appendix, periappendiceal fat stranding, and a calcified appendicolith (Fig. 69.26). In the setting of suspected perforated appendicitis, the main purpose of CT is to identify a discrete abscess that may require surgical or percutaneous drainage and to identify extraluminal appendicolith(s) that need to be removed at surgery.

MRI is being increasingly used in the setting of suspected acute appendicitis, to avoid the ionizing radiation exposure associated with CT. A typical MRI protocol relies mostly on T2-weighted (T2W) sequences to identify fluid and inflammation in the right lower quadrant (Fig. 69.27). The actual appendix may or may not be visualized.

Inflammatory Bowel Disease

Crohn disease (CD), ulcerative colitis (UC), and indeterminate colitis are all forms of inflammatory bowel disease (IBD) that occur in both children and in adults. While these conditions are much more common in older children, rarely IBD may occur in young children, as early as the first few years of life. The goal of imaging in IBD is to aid in the diagnosis, establish the disease burden at baseline, quantify response to medical therapy, identify complications that may require surgical intervention (e.g., strictures or abscesses), and to assess for associated abnormalities (e.g., sclerosing cholangitis, autoimmune pancreatitis, gallstones, etc.).

Crohn Disease. CD causes transmural inflammation and can affect any portion of the GI tract from the mouth to the anus and can affect the skin of the perineum and perioral region. Younger patients with CD often present with more extensive proximal small bowel disease, affecting the jejunum, while older children typically present with involvement of the terminal ileum and/or colon.

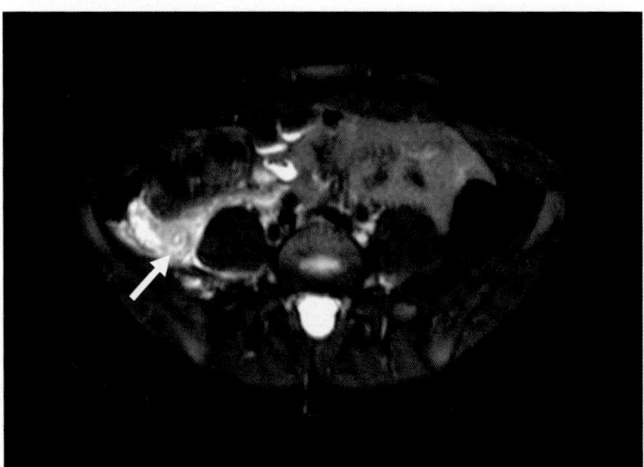

FIGURE 69.27. **Acute Appendicitis on MRI.** Axial T2W image with fat saturation demonstrating hyperintense signal consistent with edema and inflammation surrounding the mildly dilated appendix (*arrow*). Note that the appendiceal wall is also thickened and demonstrates T2W hyperintense signal consistent with edema.

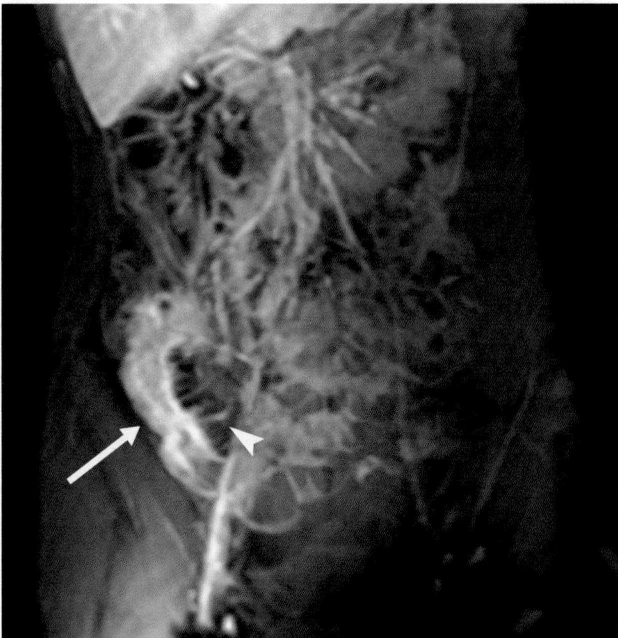

FIGURE 69.28. **Active Crohn Disease.** Coronal T1W postcontrast image from an MR enterography demonstrates wall thickening and mural hyperenhancement of a long segment of distal and terminal ileum (*arrow*). Note the engorged vasa recta (*arrowhead*), a secondary sign of active inflammation.

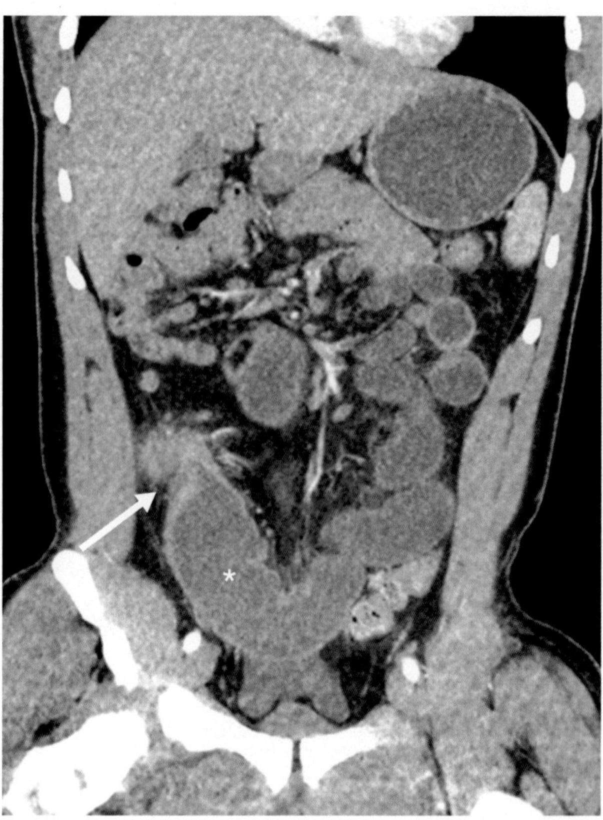

FIGURE 69.29. **Crohn Disease With Terminal Ileal Stricture.** Coronal image from a CT enterography shows wall thickening and inflammation of a short segment of the terminal ileum (*arrow*). The bowel proximal to the inflamed segment is dilated (*) as the result of a stricture. Strictures in Crohn disease usually have a combination of active inflammation and fibrosis.

CT enterography (CTE) and MR enterography (MRE) are the imaging modalities of choice when evaluating known or suspected CD. There are some data suggesting that CTE is slightly more sensitive in pediatric patients, but in clinical practice, both are essentially equivalent. Imaging findings of active CD include inflammation involving the bowel wall, typically bowel wall thickening and hyperenhancement (Fig. 69.28). At MRE, the bowel wall may be T2W hyperintense, indicating edema and inflammation. Involvement in CD may be discontinuous, with normal intervening bowel between inflamed segments. Other findings associated with CD include fibrofatty proliferation, engorgement of vasa recta, ulceration of the bowel wall, and localized bowel wall thinning (pseudosacculation). When evaluating patients with CD, it is important to look for evidence of strictures and penetrating disease which alter therapy. Strictures manifest as fixed luminal narrowing with upstream dilation (often over 3 cm in diameter) (Fig. 69.29). Penetrating disease includes both fistulae and sinus tracts. Fistulae connect two epithelialized surfaces (e.g., bowel lumen to bowel lumen or bowel lumen to skin surface) and typically manifest as tethering of the affected bowel loops, often with associated enhancement of the fistula tract and the involved bowel loop(s). A sinus tract does not connect two epithelialized surfaces and typically appears as a linear enhancement arising from the bowel wall, extending into the adjacent fat. Both fistulae and sinus tracts are associated with the development of intra-abdominal abscesses. MRE is superior to CTE in the evaluation of perianal fistulous disease (Fig. 69.30).

CD may be detected by ultrasound in a child presenting with abdominal pain. Ultrasound has also been used as a modality to evaluate known CD. Affected bowel segments are typically markedly thickened and hyperemic, with thickening and increased echogenicity of adjacent fat, indicating inflammation. Ultrasound does have limited sensitivity, as it is somewhat difficult and time consuming to evaluate the entire small and large bowel.

Ulcerative Colitis. UC is an inflammatory process that involves the colon in a contiguous fashion. CTE and MRE are often ordered at diagnosis to exclude the presence of small bowel disease. At imaging, the colon typically demonstrates

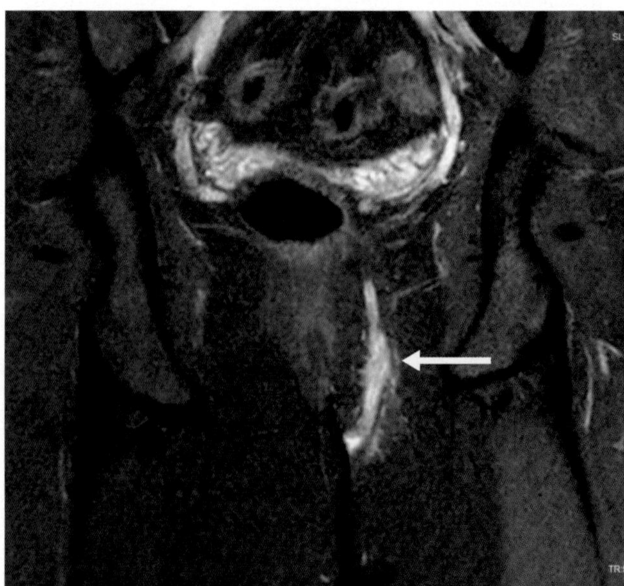

FIGURE 69.30. **Perianal Fistula in the Setting of Crohn Disease.** Coronal STIR image showing a linear hyperintense tract from rectum to the skin surface (*arrow*) consistent with an intersphincteric fistula.

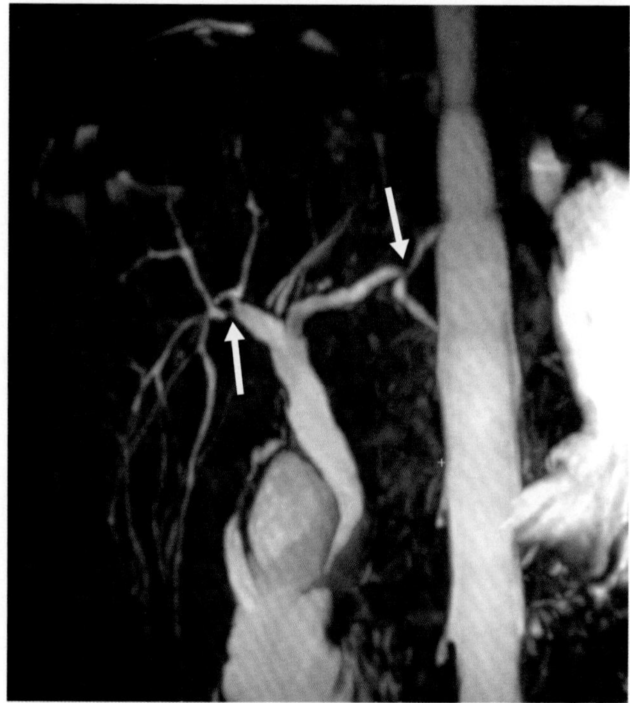

FIGURE 69.31. **Sclerosing Cholangitis.** Coronal oblique maximum-intensity projection from an MRCP showing mildly dilated extrahepatic bile ducts and irregularity of the intrahepatic bile ducts, with multiple areas of narrowing consistent with strictures (*arrows*).

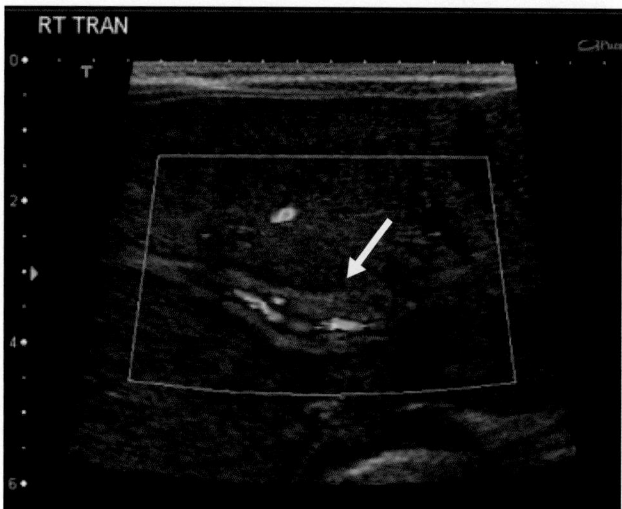

FIGURE 69.32. **Biliary Atresia.** Transverse ultrasound image of the porta hepatis demonstrating the lack of a visible common hepatic duct. Instead, there is a triangular echogenic tissue (*arrow*), the so-called "triangular cord" sign.

wall thickening and adjacent inflammation, although the degree of wall thickening may be relatively mild. Occasionally, the colon may appear normal at imaging. In the setting of pancolitis, there may be mild thickening and hyperenhancement of the terminal ileum due to reflux of inflammatory secretions from the cecum (so-called "backwash ileitis"). If present, this type of inflammation is typically mild and only involves the distal portion of the terminal ileum.

One important association with UC is the increased frequency of sclerosing cholangitis in these patients. Sclerosing cholangitis can affect patients with both CD and UC, but is more commonly associated with UC. Sclerosing cholangitis typically manifests as irregular biliary dilation, with beading of the bile ducts, representing areas of alternating strictures and dilation (Fig. 69.31).

Indeterminate Colitis. In some patients, especially in younger children, despite imaging, endoscopy and biopsy, distinction between CD and UC is not possible. These patients are often given a diagnosis of indeterminate colitis. Many of these patients end up manifesting features of CD later in their disease course.

HEPATOBILIARY

Congenital Hepatobiliary Disorders

Biliary Atresia. Biliary atresia is the most common cause of neonatal cholestasis, and is the result of an obliterative cholangiopathy in which the central intrahepatic bile ducts and extrahepatic bile ducts become atretic due to a poorly understood inflammatory process. The end result is cholestasis, and patients present with jaundice and acholic stools at the time of birth or shortly thereafter. If the condition is left untreated, the cholestasis causes progressive liver disease, fibrosis, and ultimately cirrhosis. Treatment involves restoring biliary drainage from the liver via a Kasai procedure or portoenterostomy, where a loop of bowel is brought up to the liver and anastomosed to the liver hilum, with resection of more distal bile ducts. Even with appropriate surgical treatment, a significant number of patients go on to end-stage liver disease and require liver transplantation.

Ultrasound is often the first imaging test in a neonate with cholestasis. The liver parenchyma can vary in appearance from normal to heterogeneous and nodular due to progressive fibrosis, even early in life. Normal extrahepatic bile ducts will not be present. Instead, there may be triangular hyperechoic tissue near the bifurcation of the main portal vein, representing fibrosis of the common hepatic duct, the so-called "triangular cord sign" (Fig. 69.32). This finding has high specificity but relatively low sensitivity for biliary atresia. The gallbladder may be completely absent, or may be small and irregular. Intrahepatic biliary dilation is typically not present.

Further workup for suspected biliary atresia may involve hepatobiliary scintigraphy. Patients are typically pretreated for several days with phenobarbital. Lack of pretreatment can result in a false-positive result. Hepatocyte uptake of the tracer occurs in biliary atresia, but there is no biliary excretion (Fig. 69.33). The diagnosis depends on the lack of any radiotracer activity excreted into the bowel on delayed (~24-hour) images.

Choledochal Cysts. Choledochal cysts are characterized by focal or diffuse dilation of intra- and/or extrahepatic bile ducts. The most widely accepted theory for the etiology of choledochal cysts is that an anomalous pancreaticobiliary junction, with a common channel draining the common bile duct and the pancreatic duct, allows for reflux of pancreatic enzymes into the common bile duct and causes inflammation and mural damage. The Todani classification is the most widely accepted classification system for choledochal cysts but erroneously includes Caroli disease which has a different etiopathogenesis (Fig. 69.34). Type I choledochal cyst, with diffuse dilation of the extrahepatic bile ducts, is the most common but can be difficult to distinguish from type IV (Fig. 69.35).

FIGURE 69.33. **Biliary Atresia.** Planar image from a HIDA scan showing uptake of tracer in the liver (*), but no excretion of tracer into the bowel.

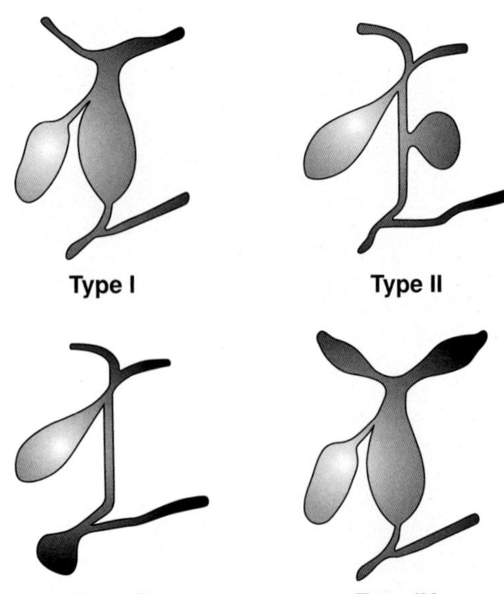

FIGURE 69.34. **Diagrammatic Representation of the Subtypes of Choledochal Cysts.** Type I—fusiform dilation of the common bile (+/– common hepatic) duct. Type II—saccular diverticulum from the common bile duct. Type III—saccular dilation (choledochocele) that herniates into the duodenum. Type IV—fusiform dilation of both intra- and extrahepatic bile ducts. In clinical practice, there is often overlap of types I and IV.

Clinically, choledochal cysts typically present before age 10 years—with jaundice, abdominal pain, and rarely a palpable abdominal mass. Ultrasound will show varying degrees of dilation of the bile ducts, which can sometimes be massively dilated. MRI with MRCP is the imaging modality of choice to fully characterize a suspected choledochal cyst and identify an anomalous pancreaticobiliary junction (Fig. 69.36). Choledocholithiasis can occur in association with choledochal cysts.

Treatment of choledochal cysts involves surgical resection. This is done not only to improve biliary drainage but also to reduce the risk of development of cholangiocarcinoma in adulthood.

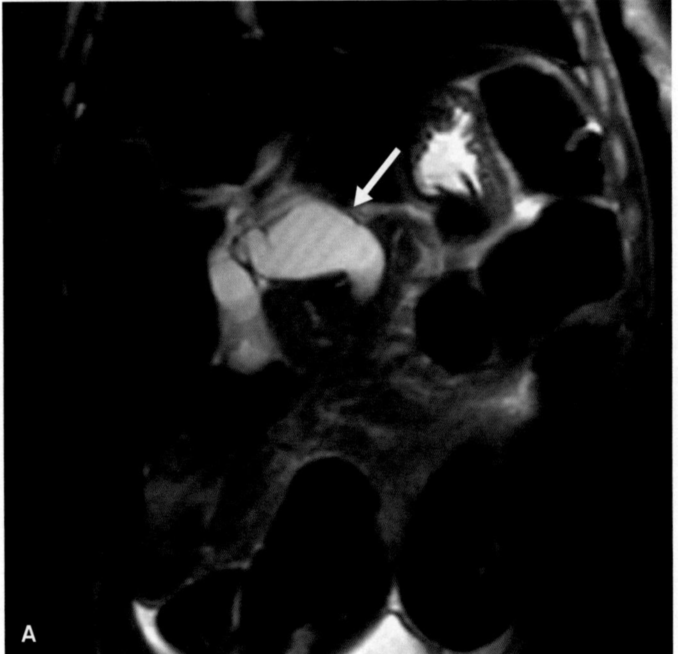

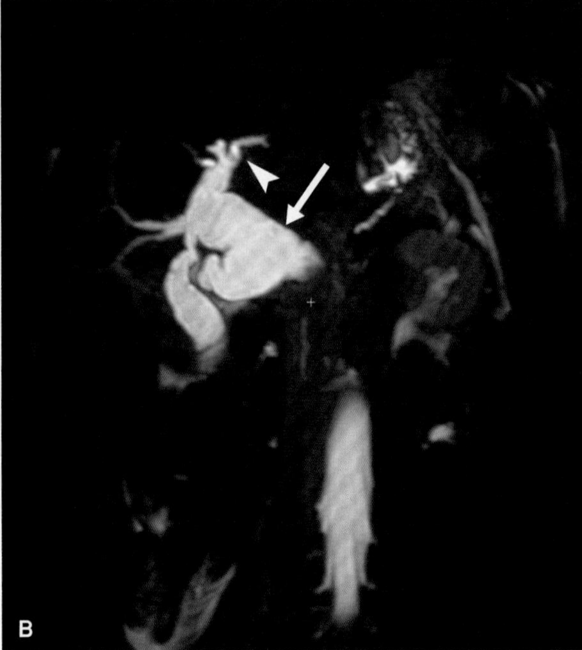

FIGURE 69.35. **Choledochal Cysts in Two Different Patients. A:** Coronal T2W image in a young child showing marked dilation of the extrahepatic bile ducts (*arrow*) consistent with a type I choledochal cyst. **B:** Coronal maximum-intensity projection image from an MRCP in a different child showing dilation of both the intrahepatic (*arrowhead*) and extrahepatic bile ducts (*arrow*) consistent with a type IV choledochal cyst.

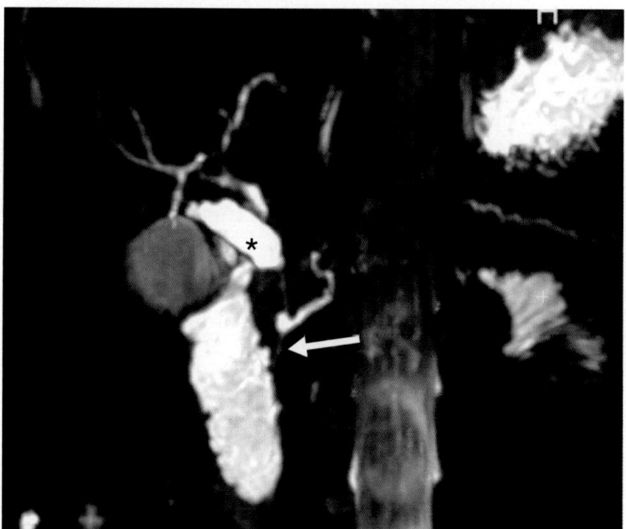

FIGURE 69.36. **Choledochal Cyst.** Coronal oblique maximum-intensity projection image from an MRCP showing focal dilation of a portion of the common hepatic duct and common bile duct (*). The pancreatic duct inserts into the common bile duct proximal to the ampulla of Vater, a so-called "long common channel" (*arrow*), which is an anatomic finding associated with the development of choledochal cysts.

Caroli Disease. Caroli disease has previously been classified as a type V choledochal cyst, but is a distinct entity caused by a congenital ductal plate malformation involving the intrahepatic bile ducts. The end result is cystic dilation of multiple intrahepatic biliary ducts. The extrahepatic bile ducts are typically normal. Involvement can be diffuse throughout the liver or can be segmental. US, CT, and MRI will all show the "central dot sign," which represents a portal vein branch completely surrounded by the dilated intrahepatic bile duct (Fig. 69.37). Caroli disease can be associated with other manifestations of ciliopathies, including polycystic kidney disease.

GENITOURINARY

Renal Fusion and Migration Anomalies

The spectrum of renal fusion and migration anomalies, including horseshoe kidney, cross-fused ectopia, lump/pancake kidney, and pelvic kidney is not unique to pediatrics. These developmental abnormalities may be detected prenatally or may be detected during imaging for other abnormalities at any point during life. The importance of these anomalies relates to increased susceptibility to trauma and the potential for complications including stone formation, collecting system obstruction, and rarely, development of tumors. Fused renal moieties may be difficult to fully assess by ultrasound and thus cross-sectional imaging, including CT and MR urography (MRU), plays a greater role in these patients (Fig. 69.38).

Multicystic Dysplastic Kidney

Multicystic dysplastic kidney (MCDK) reflects complete or segmental renal dysplasia as a result of abnormal development of the kidney. Postnatally, the dysplastic kidney will often be diffusely or segmentally small, but can rarely be enlarged. The renal parenchyma will be replaced by multiple cysts of varying sizes (Fig. 69.39), with little or no recognizable renal tissue. Intervening parenchyma, where present, is abnormal, appearing echogenic by ultrasound. MCDK is not typically a diagnostic dilemma, though occasionally a cluster of large cysts can mimic a very dilated collecting system. The key to differentiating the two is that the cysts of MCDK do not communicate (vs. dilated calyces).

MCDK may be unilateral or bilateral, the latter of which is associated with oligohydramnios and its associated effects (Potter sequence: specific facies, pulmonary hypoplasia, clubbed feet) and is often incompatible with life. Unilateral renal dysplasia is often asymptomatic and is generally associated with compensatory hypertrophy of the contralateral kidney. Importantly, MCDK can be associated with abnormalities of the contralateral kidney, including vesicoureteral

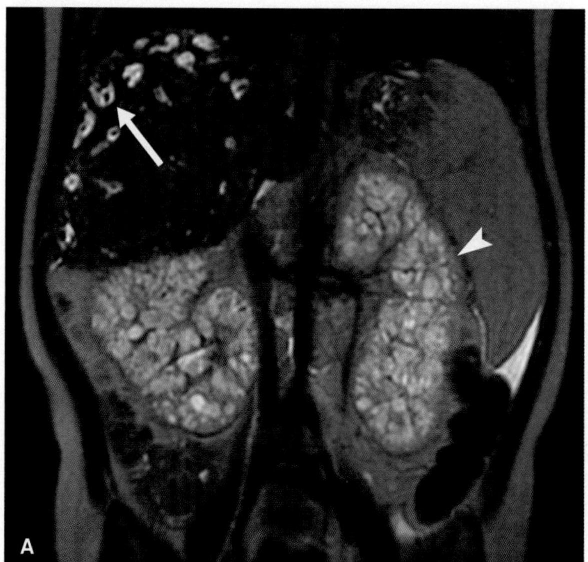

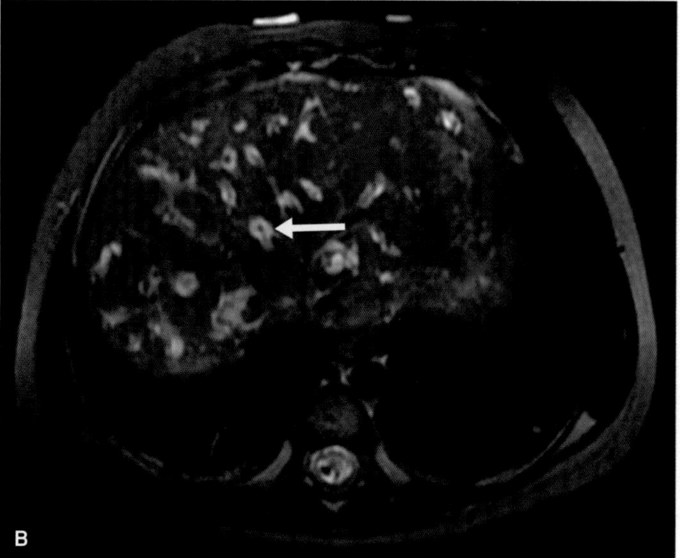

FIGURE 69.37. **Caroli Disease.** Coronal (**A**) and axial (**B**) T2W images in an adolescent boy showing cystic dilation of intrahepatic bile ducts with a "central dot" sign (*arrows*). Note the patient also has innumerable renal cysts (*arrowhead*) consistent with polycystic kidney disease. Both Caroli disease and polycystic kidney disease are due to congenital abnormalities of the primary cilia ("ciliopathies").

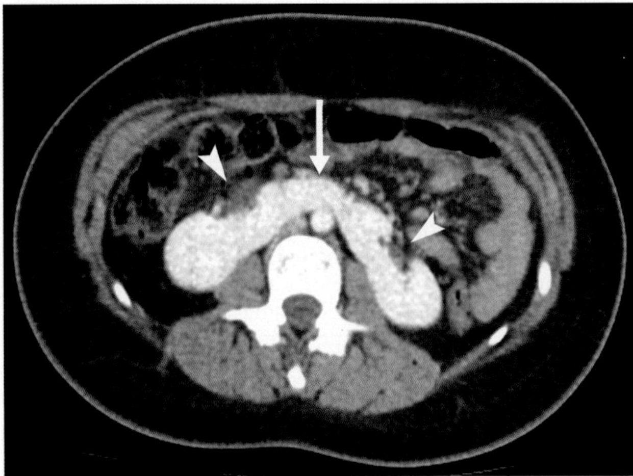

FIGURE 69.38. **Horseshoe Kidney.** Axial CT image with intravenous contrast shows a bridge of renal tissue connecting the kidneys across midline (*arrow*). The renal pelves of both kidneys are oriented anteriorly (*arrowheads*). In horseshoe kidney, renal moieties are present on both sides of the spine, with either a parenchymal or fibrous bridge across midline. This is different than cross-fused ectopia, in which one kidney is orthotopic (in its renal fossa or relatively close) and the other kidney is heterotopic (out of its normal location) and is fused to the orthotopic kidney. This results in both kidneys being located on one side of the abdomen.

reflux (VUR) and ureteropelvic junction obstruction, both of which have greater significance in a solitary-functioning kidney. Imaging serves to assess the dysplastic kidney (ultrasound for anatomy, scintigraphy for function) and to rule out abnormalities of the contralateral kidney (ultrasound, voiding cystourethrography, or nuclear cystography). A proportion of MCDK spontaneously regresses, while others remain present throughout life. Previously, MCDK was either surgically resected or followed serially with ultrasound to ensure regression. This is no longer routine practice and imaging is generally reserved for complications that may develop, such as infection or hypertension.

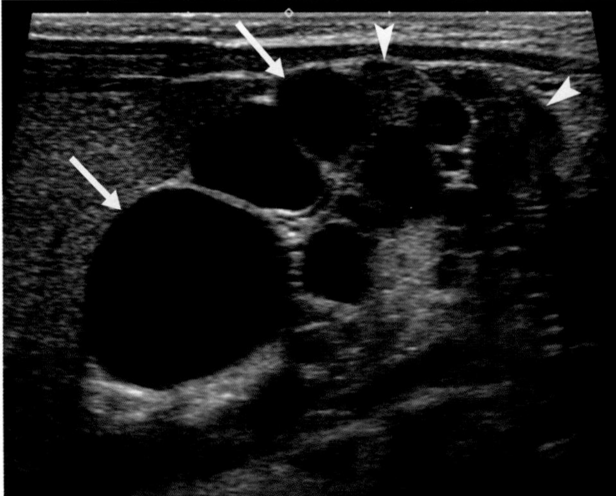

FIGURE 69.39. **Multicystic Dysplastic Kidney.** Longitudinal ultrasound image of the right kidney shows multiple renal cysts (some indicated by *arrows*) replacing much of the kidney with some residual, abnormally echogenic lower pole renal parenchyma (*arrowheads*). Multiple large cysts and a very dilated renal collecting system can sometimes appear similar but are distinguished by the fact that cysts should not communicate/connect.

Duplex Kidney and Collecting System Duplication

Renal collecting system duplication occurs early in renal development due to splitting of the renal precursor tissue (metanephric blastema and ureteric bud), which results in separate drainage systems for different portions of the kidney (typically upper and lower poles). This can range from a bifid renal pelvis separated by a prominent column of Bertin but drained by a single ureter to full duplication with two (or more) renal moieties, each with its own ureter to the level of the bladder (Fig. 69.40). Some degree of renal collecting system duplication is not an uncommon finding. In systems with multiple moieties, the relative size of each moiety is variable. The most common finding in collecting system duplication of any type is asymmetry in renal size. A difference of 1 cm or more in renal length side to side suggests either duplication of one kidney or global scarring of the other.

Some cases of collecting system duplication are completely asymptomatic and are detected incidentally on imaging performed for other reasons. Other cases may be complicated by obstruction or VUR. The classic association of complications is described by the Weigert–Meyer rule which states: in a duplicated collecting system, the upper-moiety collecting system is typically obstructed with ectopic insertion of the draining ureter which terminates in a ureterocele (Fig. 69.41). The lower-moiety ureter typically inserts orthotopically but allows VUR. Not all ureters in the context of collecting system duplication insert into the bladder. In a small number of cases, the ectopic ureter can insert into the bladder neck, urethra, or vagina, resulting in persistent wetting due to urine leakage.

Imaging plays a role in the identification of a duplicated collecting system and in defining anatomy and the associated complications. Ultrasound is the usual starting point and can generally define the renal anomalies and degree of scarring and dysplasia related to obstruction. However, ultrasound is limited in its ability to define complex ureteral anatomy. MRU can provide exquisite anatomic detail of these complex duplicated collecting systems, is the test of choice for identification of distant ectopic ureters, and can assist in surgical planning (Fig. 69.40). Cystography of some form (voiding or nuclear) can be used to document reflux to the lower moiety (Fig. 69.40). Both MRU and scintigraphy can be used to define relative split function of the renal moieties and the degree of collecting system obstruction, both of which are important for surgical planning.

Antenatal/Perinatal Hydronephrosis

Prenatally identified hydronephrosis (dilation of the renal pelvis and calyces) is a common indication for postnatal ultrasound. The purpose of postnatal ultrasound is to determine whether the hydronephrosis has resolved and to assess the renal parenchyma. Relative dehydration in the immediate postnatal period may cause underestimation of the degree of hydronephrosis, and imaging is typically deferred until approximately 1 week after birth. Hydronephrosis that persists after birth suggests either collecting system obstruction, most commonly ureteropelvic junction obstruction, or VUR, both of which require further evaluation and potentially intervention.

The urinary tract dilation (UTD) classification system provides a common, standardized language to classify the severity of urinary tract abnormality based on the anteroposterior renal pelvic diameter (measured in the kidney, NOT in an extrarenal pelvis), calyceal dilation, renal parenchymal

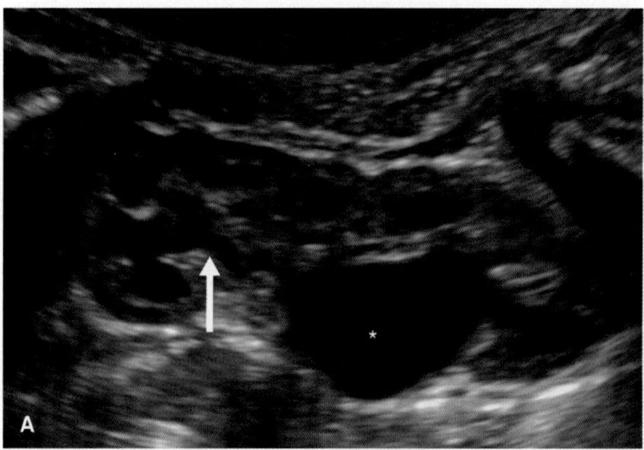

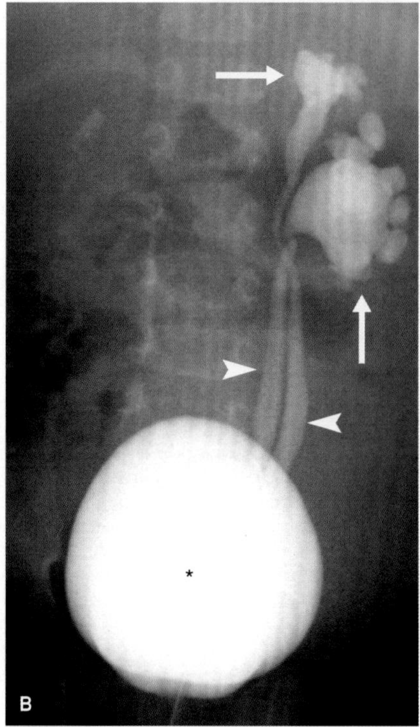

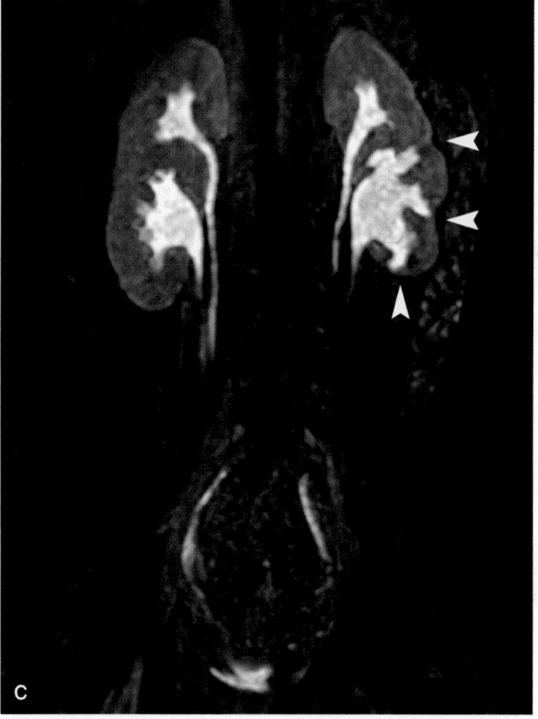

FIGURE 69.40. Renal Duplication. A: Longitudinal ultrasound image of the kidney shows a dilated lower-moiety collecting system (*asterisk*) and a nondilated upper-moiety collecting system (*arrow*). **B:** Coronal fluoroscopic spot image from a voiding cystourethrogram (VCUG) in a different child shows two separate renal pelves (*arrows*) with two separate ureters (*arrowheads*) to the level of the bladder (*asterisk*). The presence of contrast in the ureters and collecting systems reflects reflux to both moieties. The renal pelves and calyces are dilated. **C:** Coronal MIP T1-weighted post-contrast image from an MR urogram in a different child shows bilaterally duplicated kidneys, each with two renal pelves and two ureters. There is multifocal scarring involving the lower moiety on the left (*arrowheads*).

thickness and appearance, bladder abnormalities, and ureteral abnormalities (Table 69.1; Fig. 69.42). An important definition for this classification system is that central calyces are those that are directly connected to the renal pelvis, while peripheral calyces cup the medullary pyramids and drain to the central calyces (Fig. 69.42).

Febrile Urinary Tract Infection

VUR reflects incompetence of the ureterovesical junction (UVJ), allowing retrograde flow of urine from the bladder into the ureters and up to the kidney. VUR is likely the result of an abnormally perpendicular ureteral insertion angle, which allows the UVJ to remain open during bladder contraction and voiding. Repeated episodes of infection and inflammation related to VUR-induced pyelonephritis can lead to renal scarring and ultimately renal insufficiency.

The purpose of imaging in the child with febrile UTI is to assess for anatomic abnormalities, to document the presence or absence of VUR, and to assess for uncommon complications (e.g., renal abscess). The primary imaging modalities utilized in the assessment of the child with febrile UTI are ultrasound, voiding cystourethrography (fluoroscopic or sonographic), nuclear cystography, and potentially renal cortical scintigraphy.

The purpose of ultrasound is not to diagnose pyelonephritis (which is a clinical diagnosis), though findings of pyelonephritis including segmental or geographic areas of increased echogenicity and decreased perfusion (by Doppler) can be apparent by ultrasound (Fig. 69.43). Instead, the purpose of

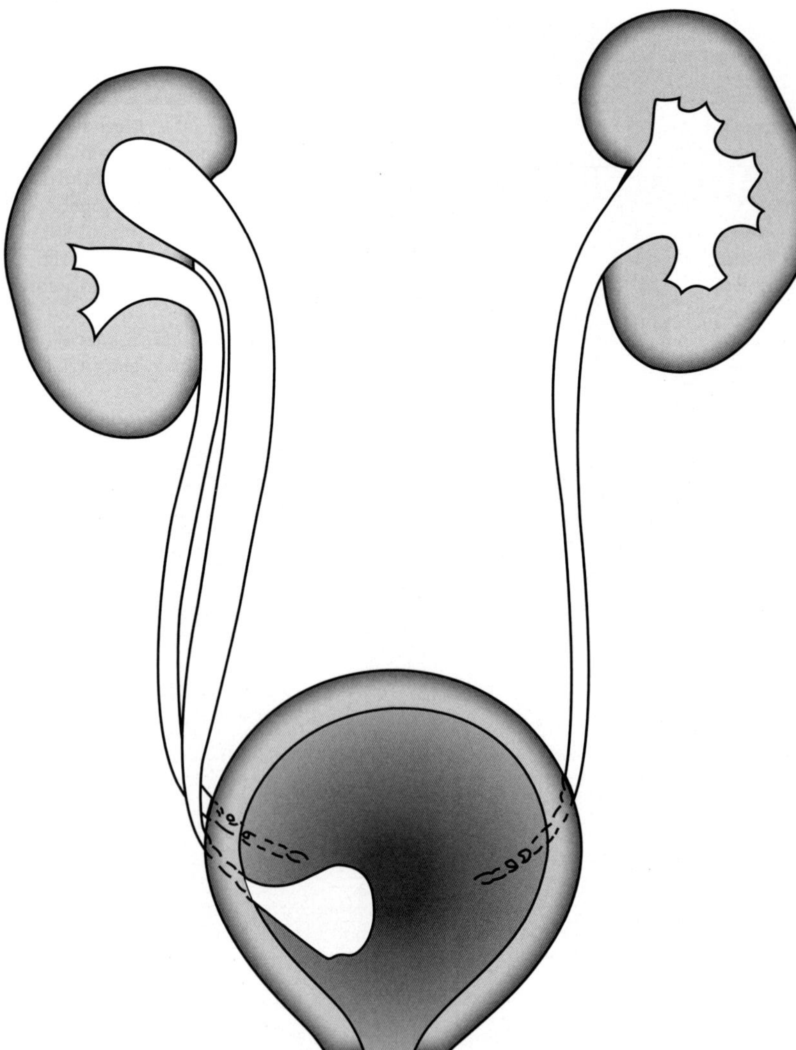

FIGURE 69.41. **Weigert–Meyer Rule.** While not all renal duplication anomalies are symptomatic, the classic association of complications related to collecting system duplication is shown here. There is obstruction of the upper-moiety collecting system with ectopic insertion of the draining ureter which terminates in a ureterocele. The lower-moiety ureter inserts orthotopically and allows vesicoureteral reflux.

TABLE 69.1

URINARY TRACT DILATION (UTD) CLASSIFICATION SYSTEM

■ UTD CLASSIFICATION	■ FINDINGS
P1	Anteroposterior renal pelvis diameter 10–15 mm *OR* Central calyceal dilation
P2	Anteroposterior renal pelvis diameter ≥15 mm *OR* Peripheral calyceal dilation (cupping medullary pyramids) *OR* Persistent ureteral dilation with any P1 or P2 finding
P3	Anteroposterior renal pelvis diameter ≥10 mm *AND* Abnormal renal parenchyma (thinning, echogenicity, cysts) *OR* Abnormal bladder

Anteroposterior renal pelvis diameter is measured on a transverse image, preferably prone, and must be measured in the kidney (not in the extrarenal portion of the renal pelvis). There is no specific cutoff for ureteral dilation.

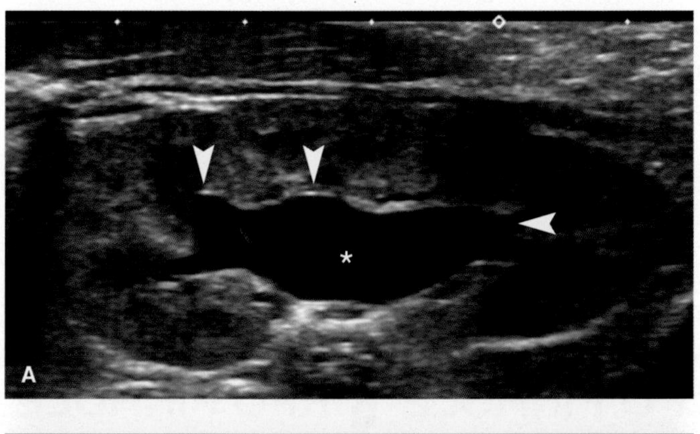

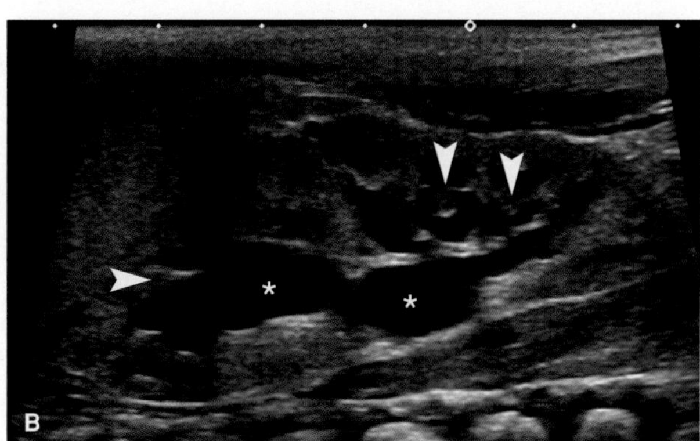

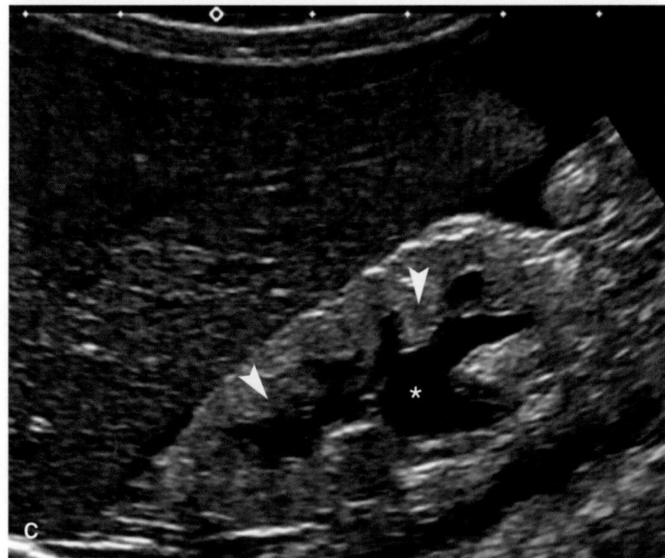

FIGURE 69.42. Urinary Tract Dilation (UTD) Classification System. A: UTD P1. Longitudinal ultrasound image of P1 dilation showing dilation of the renal pelvis (*asterisk*) and central calyces (*arrowheads*). **B:** UTD P2. Longitudinal ultrasound image of P2 dilation in a different child showing dilation of the renal pelvis (*asterisks*) and peripheral calyces which cup the medullary pyramids (*arrowheads*). **C:** UTD P3. Longitudinal ultrasound image of P3 dilation in a different child showing dilation of the renal pelvis (*asterisk*) and peripheral calyces which cup the medullary pyramids (*arrowheads*). The renal parenchyma is also diffusely abnormal with diffusely increased echogenicity.

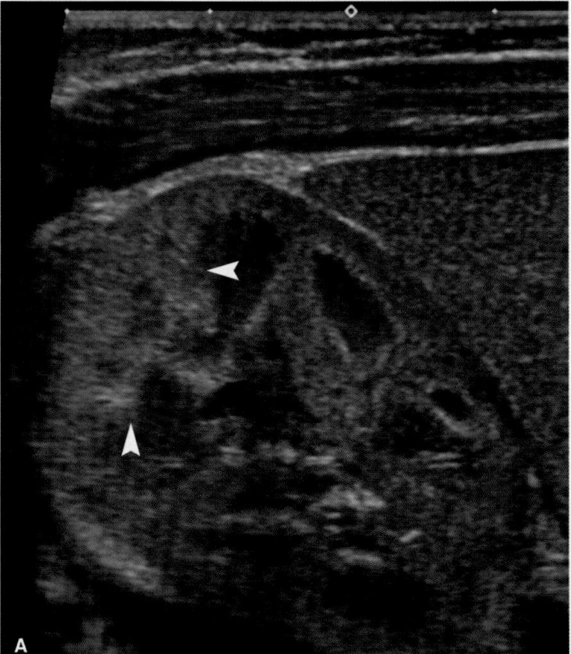

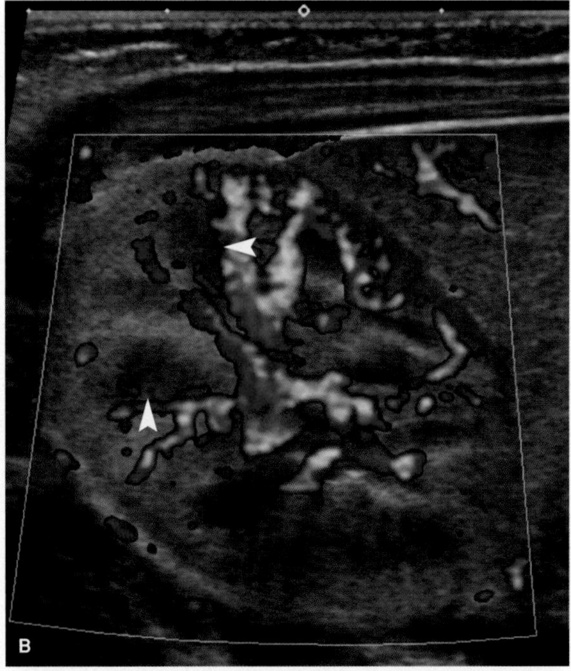

FIGURE 69.43. Pyelonephritis. A: Transverse ultrasound image shows a wedge-shaped area of increased echogenicity (*arrowheads*) with loss of corticomedullary differentiation. There is preserved corticomedullary differentiation elsewhere in the kidney, with the medullary pyramids appearing relatively hypoechoic compared to the overlying renal cortex. **B:** Transverse color Doppler ultrasound image in the same patient shows decreased blood flow in the area of abnormal echogenicity (*arrowheads*). There is preserved blood flow elsewhere in the kidney.

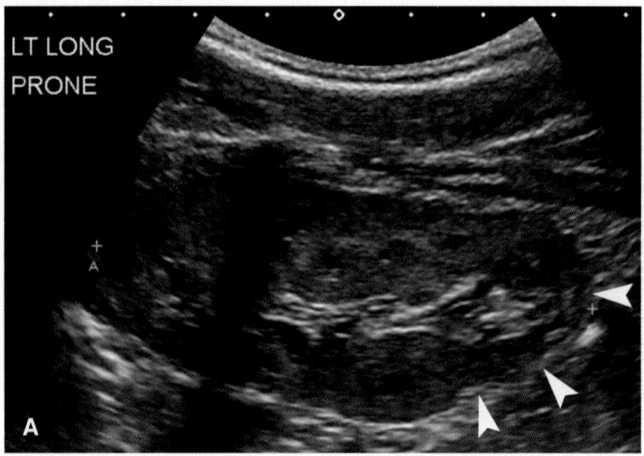

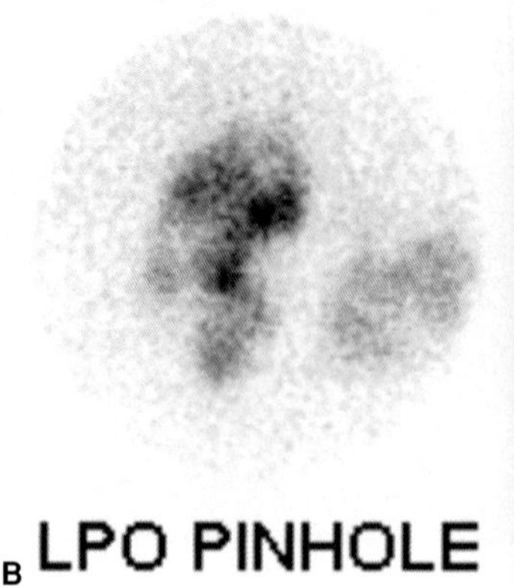

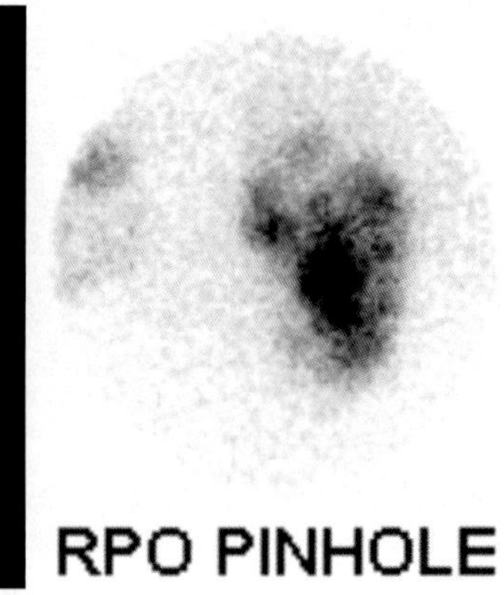

FIGURE 69.44. **Renal Scarring. A:** Longitudinal ultrasound image shows multiple small parenchymal defects in the lower pole of the kidney reflective of scarring (*arrowheads*). Normally, the renal contour should be relatively smooth as it is in the upper pole. **B:** Pinhole images from Tc-99m dimercaptosuccinic acid (DMSA) scan in the same patient show multifocal parenchymal defects in both kidneys manifest as areas of photopenia. Defects by DMSA can reflect either active pyelonephritis, due to decreased perfusion, or can reflect scarring, due to parenchymal loss. Distinction of pyelonephritis from scarring depends on clinical history with parenchymal defects persisting for more than 6 months after infection reflective of scarring. In this case, both scarring and active pyelonephritis were present.

ultrasound in the child with febrile UTI is to assess for anatomic and morphologic abnormalities including duplication of the collecting system, ureteral or collecting system dilation, and renal scarring (reflective of prior episodes of pyelonephritis). Renal scarring can manifest as focal parenchymal defects, geographic or global parenchymal thinning, or diffuse atrophy (Fig. 69.44). More than 1-cm difference in renal length side to side, in the absence of a duplicated collecting system, raises the possibility of global scarring/volume loss. Thickening of the urothelium may also be apparent but is a nonspecific finding and the sensitivity and specificity of this finding for infection are not well established. Ultrasound can also detect stones, which can serve as a nidus for infection, and ultrasound can be used to assess for rare complications of pyelonephritis including renal or perinephric abscess.

Fluoroscopic and sonographic voiding cystourethrography allow direct visualization of VUR based on instillation of contrast material (iodinated contrast or ultrasound contrast) into the bladder. The images performed during these examinations include prefilling images of the pelvis and renal fossae to assess for calculi or anatomic abnormalities; an early filling image of the bladder to assess for ureterocele (Fig. 69.45); right and left lateral oblique images at maximal bladder filling targeted at the UVJ to assess for grade 1 VUR and to define the anatomy of the UVJ if reflux is identified (Fig. 69.45); an image of the urethra during voiding (frontal for girls, oblique for boys) to assess urethral anatomy (Fig. 69.45); and a postvoid image of the bladder and renal fossae to asses for postvoid residual and reflux during voiding (Fig. 69.45). Further images may be obtained, as needed, to further characterize VUR.

Any retrograde flow of contrast into the ureters or renal collecting system during voiding cystourethrography is considered abnormal. Systems exist for the grading of fluoroscopically detected VUR (Fig. 69.46) and these systems have been extrapolated to ultrasound. Nuclear cystography is similar, in that radiotracer is instilled into the bladder and images are obtained to assess for reflux into the renal collecting systems.

All three methods of assessment for VUR are effective but each has advantages and disadvantages. Fluoroscopic VCUG provides the best assessment of anatomy and is the initial test of choice in boys with febrile UTI, due to the need to assess the anatomy of the male urethra. The main limitation of fluoroscopy is that imaging is intermittent (to maintain low radiation dose) and thus intermittent episodes of lower-grade reflux may not be detected. Voiding urosonography is limited by a smaller field of view and a short half-life of the contrast material, which may mean intermittent, lower-grade reflux is missed. Nuclear cystography allows continuous monitoring for VUR and consequently has higher sensitivity, but anatomic detail is limited and grade 1 VUR cannot be diagnosed by this technique due to the significant activity in the bladder. Nuclear cystography is acceptable as a first test in a girl with febrile UTI but otherwise is primarily used for follow-up of children with previously identified VUR in whom anatomic assessment is no longer necessary.

Renal cortical scintigraphy may be used to assess for acute pyelonephritis, or renal scarring as sequelae of VUR, and repeated episodes of pyelonephritis. Both appear as photopenic defects in the kidney (Fig. 69.44).

Posterior Urethral Valves

Posterior urethral valve is an important differential diagnosis in male infants and neonates with renal collecting system dilation. A thin membrane of tissue at the level of the prostatic urethra partially or completely obstructs the outflow of the urinary tract, leading to upstream dilation. Posterior urethral valves often result in significant renal injury and ultimately renal failure requiring renal replacement. Treatment of the valves is relatively straightforward, involving ablation of the valve tissue to relieve the obstruction. However, extensive damage to the kidneys and bladder may have already occurred in utero, and additional medical and surgical treatment is often required to manage these patients.

Because posterior urethral valves obstruct the entire urinary tract, they are typically suspected based on fetal imaging findings of oligohydramnios and bilateral collecting system dilation in a male infant (Fig. 69.47). Partial or incomplete posterior urethral valves, causing less complete obstruction, do exist, accounting for delayed or less severe presentation, but are less common.

Ultrasound and voiding cystourethrography are the two studies that are generally performed in the setting of suspected posterior urethral valves. Findings on ultrasound include hydroureteronephrosis (typically bilateral), bladder wall thickening and trabeculation (due to outlet obstruction), bladder wall diverticula, and varying degrees of renal dysplasia (Fig. 69.47). Findings of dysplasia include any or all of the following: decreased size of the kidney(s), increased cortical

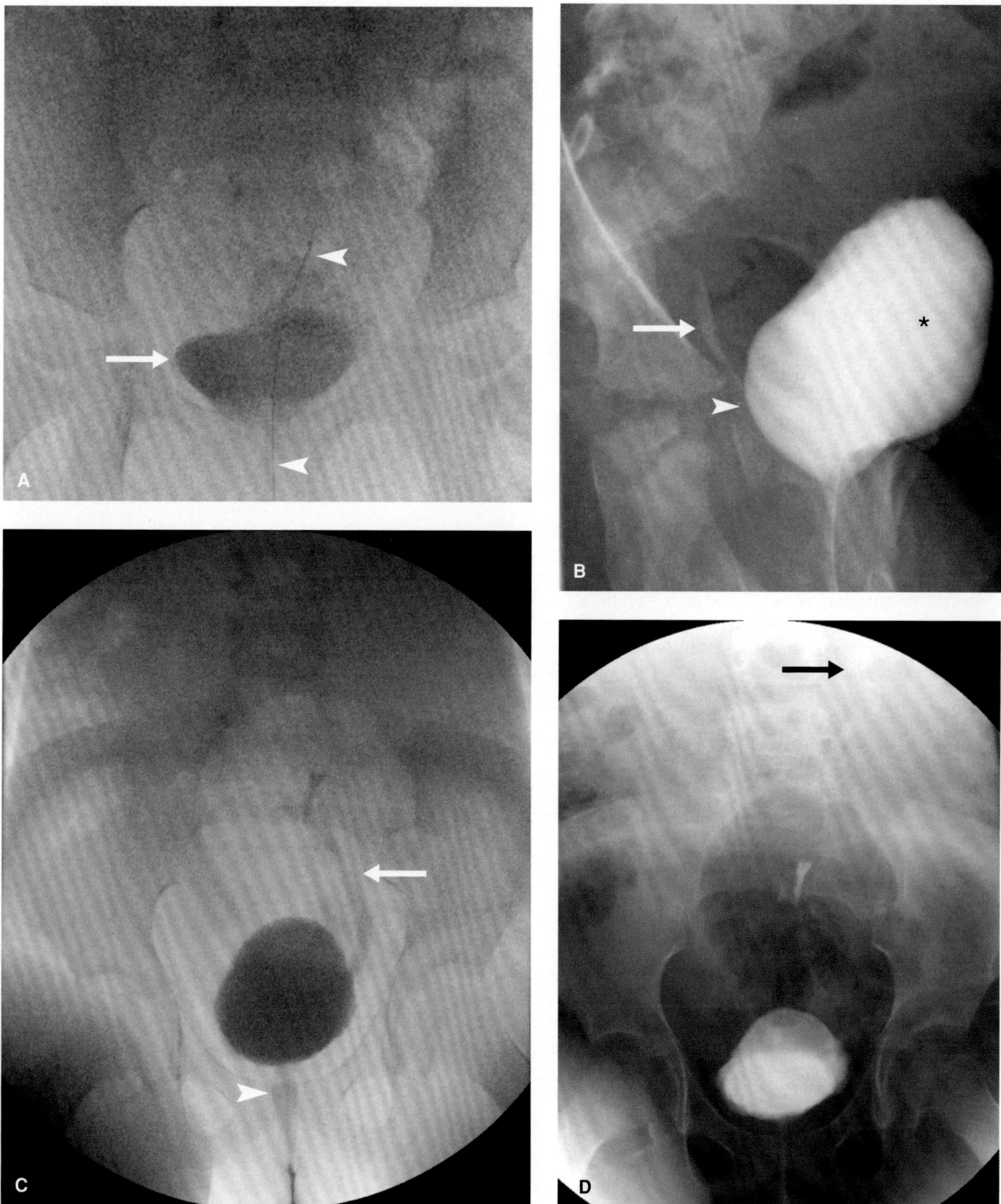

FIGURE 69.45. **Fluoroscopic Voiding Cystourethrography (VCUG).** **A:** Early filling image of bladder. Fluoroscopic image hold shows a bladder catheter (*arrowheads*) and partial contrast filling of the bladder (*arrow*). The early filling image is the first image obtained as part of a fluoroscopic VCUG after the prefilling images. The purpose of this image is to look for filling defects in the contrast pool that suggest the presence of a ureterocele. Images obtained after further filling of the bladder may not show a ureterocele which can be compressed or everted as bladder pressure increases. **B:** Grade 1 vesicoureteral reflux (VUR). Oblique fluoroscopic spot image obtained at maximal bladder filling and targeted at the vesicoureteral junction in a different child shows reflux of contrast material in a normal-caliber distal right ureter (*arrow*). The ureter is seen to the level of its insertion to the bladder at the vesicoureteral junction (*arrowhead*). Bilateral oblique images are a key element of a complete fluoroscopic voiding cystourethrogram because grade 1 VUR may be obscured by the contrast-filled bladder (*asterisk*) when the patient is supine and because it is important to define the insertion of the ureter to exclude ectopic insertion. **C:** Left VUR during voiding. Fluoroscopic image hold obtained during voiding as part of a VCUG in a different child shows reflux of contrast material in a normal-caliber left ureter (*arrow*). The female urethra is normal (*arrowhead*). Some cases of VUR may only manifest during voiding when bladder pressure is further increased. **D:** Left grade 2 VUR. Fluoroscopic spot image obtained after voiding in the same patient shows refluxed contrast material extending to the level of the left renal pelvis (*arrow*). Small amounts of contrast material reaching the renal pelvis may only be apparent on a spot image (and not apparent on a fluoroscopic image hold).

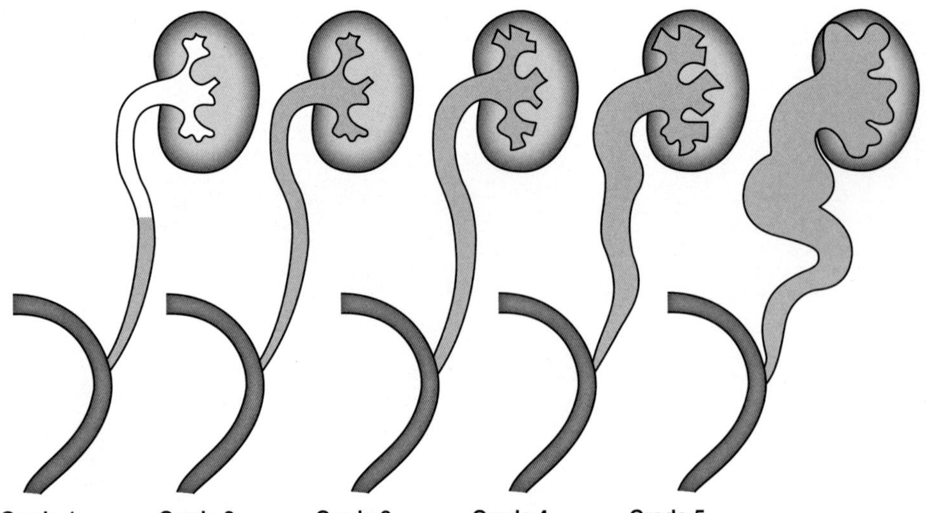

FIGURE 69.46. Diagrammatic representation of fluoroscopic grading of vesicoureteral reflux. Grade 1-reflux to the level of the ureter only. Grade 2-reflux to the level of the kidney without pelvicalyceal dilation. Grade 3-reflux to the level of the kidney with mild pelvic dilation and blunting of the fornices. Grade 4-reflux to the level of the kidney with ureteral dilation and tortuosity. Grade 5-reflux to the level of the kidney with severe dilation of the renal pelvis and calyces and the ureter.

echogenicity or loss of corticomedullary differentiation, and parenchymal cysts. The dilated posterior urethra may be visible by ultrasound and the appearance of the bladder and dilated posterior urethra has been likened to a "keyhole."

Voiding cystourethrography will typically show a small bladder with trabeculation, wall thickening, and sometimes diverticula and generally will show reflux into the dilated renal collecting systems to the level of the kidneys. On voiding, the posterior urethra is dilated and a thin membrane of tissue can be seen at the level of the valves in the prostatic urethra (Fig. 69.47).

Other imaging modalities including MRI and scintigraphy can be used to assess the degree of renal dysplasia and residual function.

Gonadal Torsion

Acute gonadal torsion (testicle or ovary) is considered a surgical emergency. As with ischemia of any organ, time is tissue and time to surgery is directly linked to salvageability of the gonad. Torsion occurs when there is inadequate fixation of the gonad, allowing the gonad to twist on its vascular pedicle. This twisting initially results in impaired venous drainage and progresses to compromised arterial flow as the number of twists increases.

Acute Testicular Torsion. Ultrasound is the imaging test of choice for confirmation of clinically suspected testicular torsion. Decreased or absent blood flow to the affected testicle is the most specific diagnostic finding (Fig. 69.48). In acute torsion, the affected testicle may be larger than the unaffected testicle and may appear more heterogeneous. Swirling/twisting of the spermatic cord is an important associated finding, manifesting as what is referred to as a "spermatic cord knot" above the level of the testicle (Fig. 69.48).

Acute Ovarian Torsion. Assessment of blood flow is not as helpful in evaluating ovarian torsion. Blood flow can still be detected in a torsed ovary, and blood flow can occasionally be difficult to detect even in the normal pediatric ovary, especially in prepubertal girls. As such, size discrepancy and ovarian morphology are more useful imaging features. The torsed ovary is generally much larger than the unaffected side and the affected ovary may appear abnormal with increased heterogeneity and peripheral follicles (Fig. 69.49). Occasionally, the torsed ovary can be so large that it is confused for a pelvic neoplasm. Cutoffs of 20-mL ovarian volume and a 15× size discrepancy side to side have been suggested to be specific findings of torsion. Swirling/twisting of the adnexal vessels may be seen but should not be relied on for the diagnosis.

ABDOMINOPELVIC TUMORS

Neuroblastoma

Neuroblastoma, a tumor of neural crest origin, is one of the two most common abdominal tumors in children. The adrenal gland is the most common site of origin but tumors can arise anywhere along the sympathetic chain, from the skull base to the pelvis. The growth pattern of neuroblastoma is frequently more infiltrative than the other common abdominal tumor (Wilms tumor), with tumors commonly encasing vessels and capable of invading adjacent solid organs and extending into the spinal canal (Fig. 69.50). The appearance of neuroblastoma is highly variable from small masses that can be asymptomatic, to large tumors occupying substantial portions of the abdomen and exerting substantial mass effect. Metastatic disease is common at diagnosis and most commonly involves the bone marrow (Fig. 69.50). Lung metastases from neuroblastoma are rare.

While neuroblastoma can be detected by radiography or ultrasound, full evaluation and staging require CT or MRI of the primary tumor to quantify tumor size and to identify image-defined risk factors (IDRFs)—a specific set of findings that are associated with more difficult surgical resection. Tumors are generally heterogeneous by all imaging modalities, with calcifications present in some tumors at diagnosis and becoming more prevalent through therapy.

Assessment for metastatic neuroblastoma is via radioiodine (^{123}I is preferred over ^{131}I) labeled metaiodobenzylguanidine (MIBG) scanning. Any uptake beyond the normal biodistribution, and particularly any uptake in bone, reflects metastatic disease (Fig. 69.50). Most neuroblastomas are also 18F-FDG avid and can also be imaged by PET scan.

Unless the tumor is small and resectable, treatment of neuroblastoma involves chemotherapy followed by surgical resection and further chemotherapy. Follow-up imaging, generally both cross-sectional imaging (CT/MRI) and MIBG scanning, is performed during therapy. Tumors typically shrink, become more fibrotic, and some will calcify during chemotherapy.

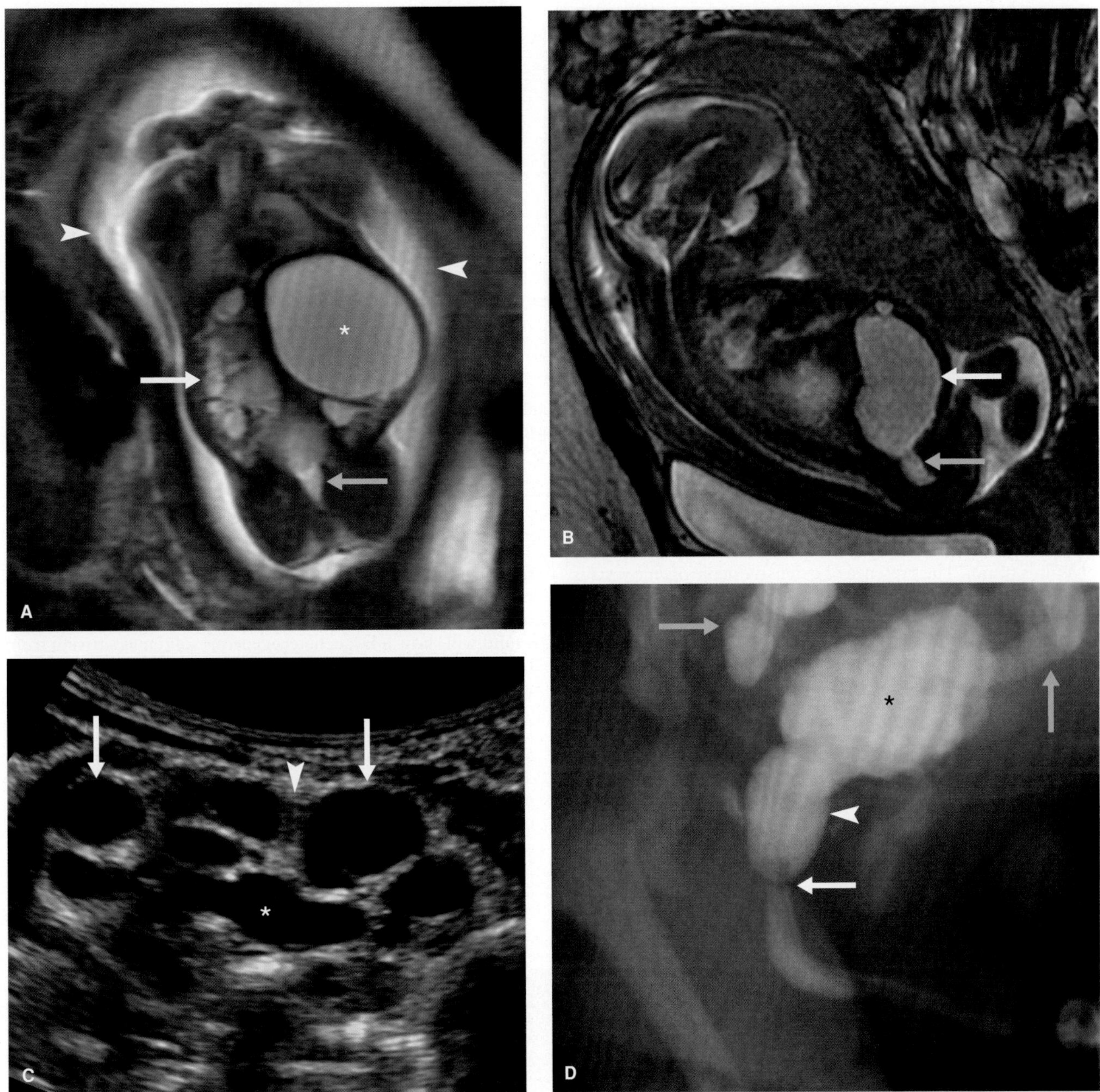

FIGURE 69.47. **Posterior Urethral Valves. A:** Coronal T2-weighted image from a fetal MRI shows massive dilation of one renal collecting system (*asterisk*) and dilation of the other renal collecting system with cystic renal dysplasia (*arrow*). The dilated posterior urethra is partially visualized (*blue arrow*). Amniotic fluid (*arrowheads*) is decreased in volume reflective of oligohydramnios. **B:** Sagittal T2-weighted image from the same fetal MRI shows bladder dilation (*arrow*) with dilation of the posterior urethra (*blue arrow*), giving a "keyhole" appearance. **C:** Dysplastic kidney in a different boy with posterior urethral valves. Longitudinal ultrasound image shows a small kidney with dilation of the renal pelvis (*asterisk*) and multiple renal cysts (*arrows*). Intervening renal parenchyma (*arrowhead*) is abnormal, with increased echogenicity and decreased corticomedullary differentiation. These are all findings of obstructive uropathy. **D:** Oblique fluoroscopic spot image of the urethra and bladder (*asterisk*) in the same boy during VCUG, as the ultrasound shows dilation of the posterior urethra (*arrowhead*) above the level of a thin membrane of tissue (*arrow*) reflecting posterior urethral valves. The bladder is small and trabeculated and there is bilateral vesicoureteral reflux (*blue arrows*).

Ganglioneuroma (benign) and ganglioneuroblastoma (malignant, but less aggressive than neuroblastoma) are other variants of neural crest tumors that can also develop in the adrenal gland and along the sympathetic chain. These tumors may occur in older children more frequently than neuroblastoma and are generally smaller and more well defined; however, these tumors often cannot be distinguished from neuroblastoma by imaging.

Renal Tumors

Wilms Tumor. Wilms tumor is the most common primary renal mass in children. The tumor arises from persistent immature metanephric blastemas, which are embryologic precursors to normal renal tissue. The presence of metanephric blastema in neonates is relatively common. If the tissue persists beyond 4 months of age, the lesions are termed "nephrogenic rests."

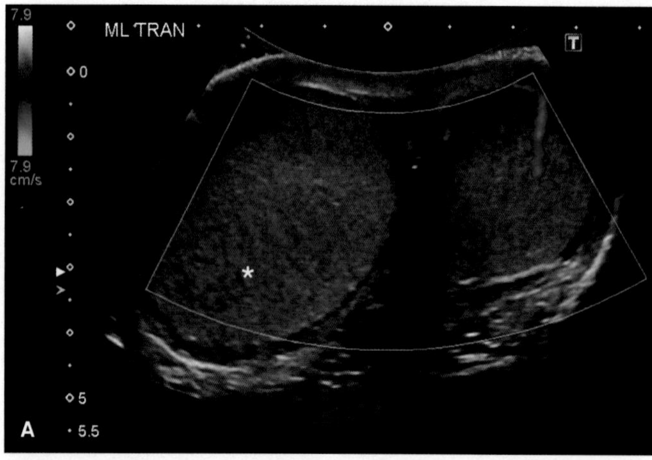

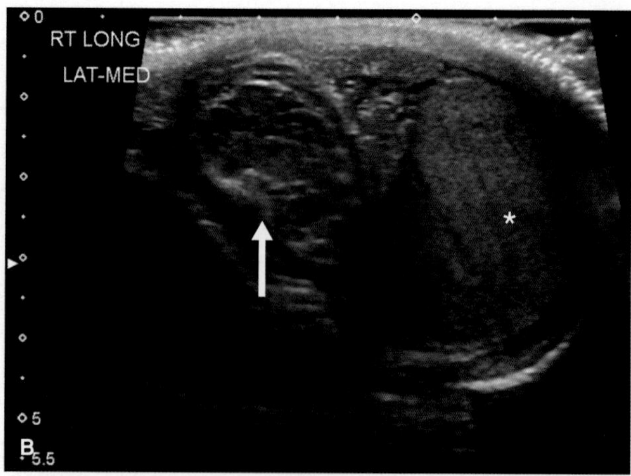

FIGURE 69.48. **Testicular Torsion. A:** Transverse color Doppler ultrasound image shows absence of flow to the right testicle (*asterisk*) with preserved flow to the left testicle. The right testicle is homogeneous in echotexture in this case. In cases where detection of torsion is more delayed, the testicle may become heterogeneous in echotexture. **B:** Longitudinal gray scale image in the same patient shows a twisted spermatic cord (*arrow*) above the testicle (*asterisk*). The testicle has a transverse lie.

The presence of these rests increases the risk for development of Wilms tumor. The presence of extensive nephrogenic rests is termed "nephroblastomatosis" (Fig. 69.51).

Wilms tumor typically presents in children between 1 and 6 years of age, although the tumor has been reported in all age groups, including adults. The most common clinical presentation is a palpable abdominal mass. Hematuria is relatively rare. The tumors are typically large at presentation. Local spread is to the retroperitoneal lymph nodes and contiguous tumor extension into blood vessels, including the renal vein and IVC (Fig. 69.52). Metastases are most commonly to the lungs, but can also involve the liver. Metastatic disease to bone is rare, except in very advanced cases. The staging of Wilms tumor depends on local extent, the integrity of the tumor capsule, locoregional spread, and metastatic disease (Table 69.2). In general, Wilms tumor has a good prognosis, with over 90% 5-year survival rates.

Abdominal radiographs may be the first imaging test obtained and frequently demonstrate a large soft tissue mass, usually displacing bowel loops (Fig. 69.52). Calcifications are uncommon, occurring in about 10% of Wilms tumors. Ultrasound will show a large, heterogeneous solid mass arising from the kidney (Fig. 69.52). Frequently, there is a "claw" of normal renal tissue surrounding the mass. Evaluation for tumor thrombus in the renal vein and IVC should be performed using Doppler. CT or MRI is typically used for definitive staging evaluation (Fig. 69.52). The primary tumor is typically large and heterogeneous, but in general demonstrates hypoenhancement relative to normal renal parenchyma. CT is the preferred modality to evaluate for pulmonary metastatic disease, which manifests as solid, noncalcified pulmonary nodules. CT and MRI have been shown to have equivalent accuracy for the identification of locoregional spread and abdominal metastatic disease. Both multifocal and bilateral Wilms tumors occur, so

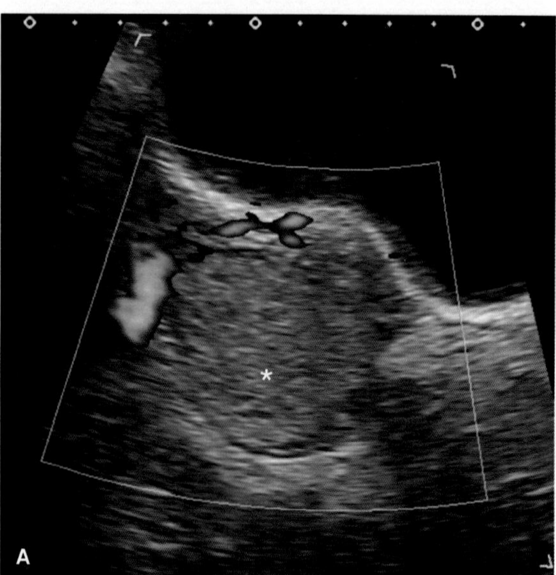

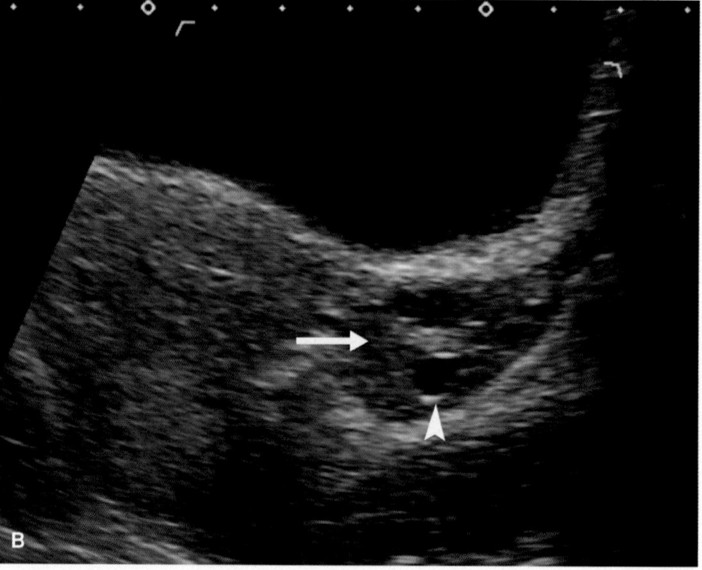

FIGURE 69.49. **Ovarian Torsion. A:** Ovarian torsion. Power Doppler image of the right ovary shows the ovary to be enlarged and relatively uniformly hyperechoic, with no visible normal ovarian follicles (*asterisk*). There is no detectable blood flow in the ovary. **B:** Grayscale image of the normal left ovary for comparison shows the ovary (*arrow*) to be normal in size and echotexture, with normal-appearing ovarian follicles (*arrowhead*).

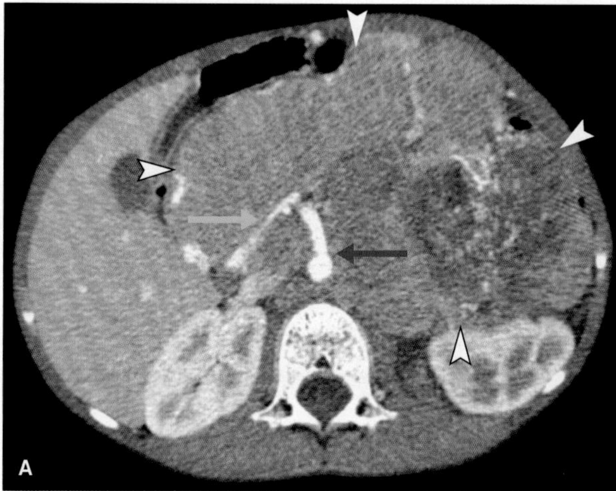

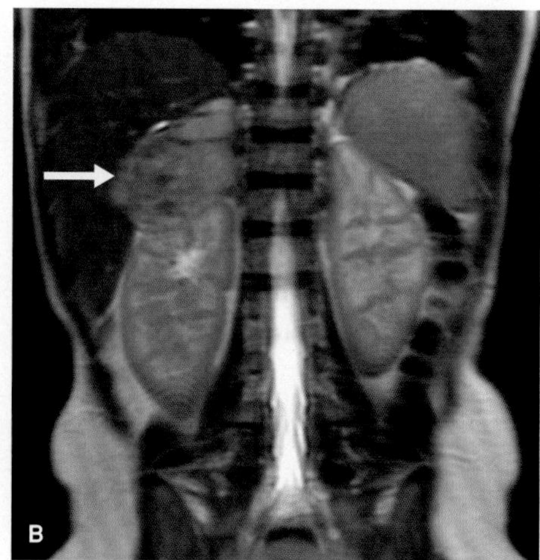

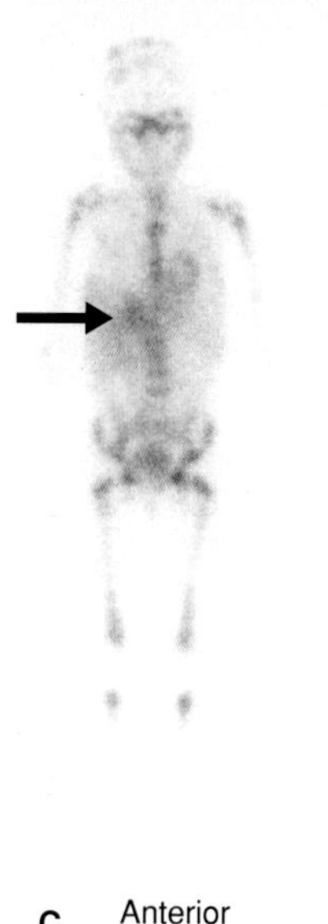

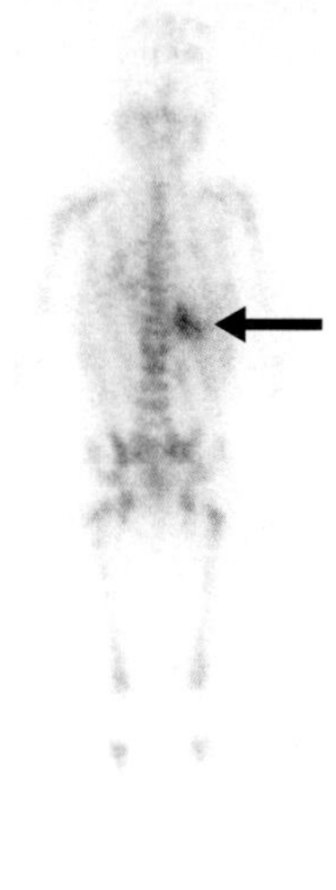

FIGURE 69.50. **Neuroblastoma. A:** Axial image from a CT with intravenous contrast material shows a large, heterogeneous mass (*arrowheads*) that exerts significant mass effect and encases the aorta and superior mesenteric artery (*white arrow*) as well as the portal vein (*blue arrow*). **B:** Neuroblastoma in a different patient. Coronal T2-weighted MR image shows a right suprarenal mass (*arrow*) that exerts mild mass effect on the upper pole of the right kidney. **C:** I-123 MIBG scan in the same patient shows the right suprarenal mass to be MIBG avid (*arrows*). There is widespread abnormal uptake of MIBG in the bones of the axial and appendicular skeleton reflective of metastatic disease. The normal biodistribution of MIBG includes the salivary glands, thyroid (if not blocked), heart, liver, urinary tract (excretion), and low-level soft tissue activity. Any uptake in bone is abnormal and reflects metastatic disease.

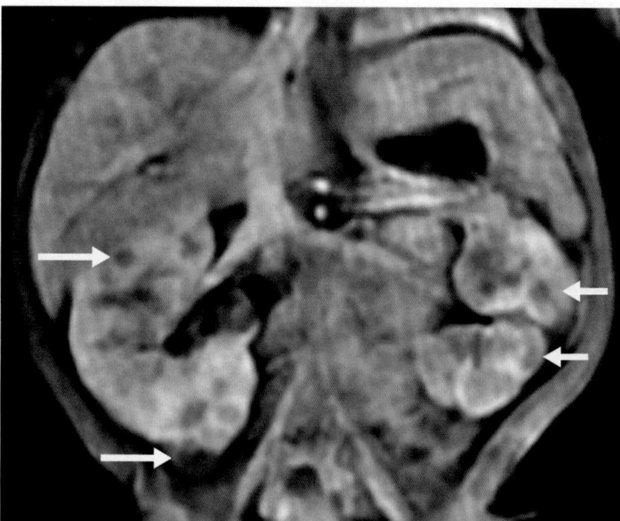

FIGURE 69.51. **Nephroblastomatosis.** Coronal T1-weighted, fat-saturated MR image following gadolinium-based contrast material administration shows multiple hypoenhancing masses in both kidneys (some indicated by *arrows*) in this child with a history of Wilms tumor. Nephrogenic rests are generally hypoenhancing compared to normal renal cortex.

it is critical to evaluate the contralateral kidney for masses, as the presence of bilateral disease will change treatment.

Mesoblastic Nephroma. Congenital mesoblastic nephroma is the most common solid renal mass in children under 6 months of age. This is a hamartomatous lesion that can appear identical to Wilms tumor at imaging. Surgical excision is typically curative and the prognosis is excellent.

Renal Cell Carcinoma. Renal cell carcinoma (RCC) typically occurs in older children. Unlike in adults, pediatric RCC is often associated with genetic translocations, most commonly the Xp11 translocation (20% to 40%). Pediatric RCC typically presents with hematuria, abdominal pain, and occasionally a palpable abdominal mass. RCC is often smaller at presentation than Wilms tumor. Metastatic disease is to locoregional lymph nodes, lungs, and bone. At imaging, pediatric RCC appears similar to adult RCC, with a heterogeneously enhancing renal mass, typically without calcifications (Fig. 69.53).

Other Renal Masses. Several other types of renal malignancies can present in children. Clear cell sarcoma occurs in the same age group as Wilms tumor and appears identical to Wilms tumor at imaging, with the exception that calcifications and bone metastases are relatively more frequent. Rhabdoid

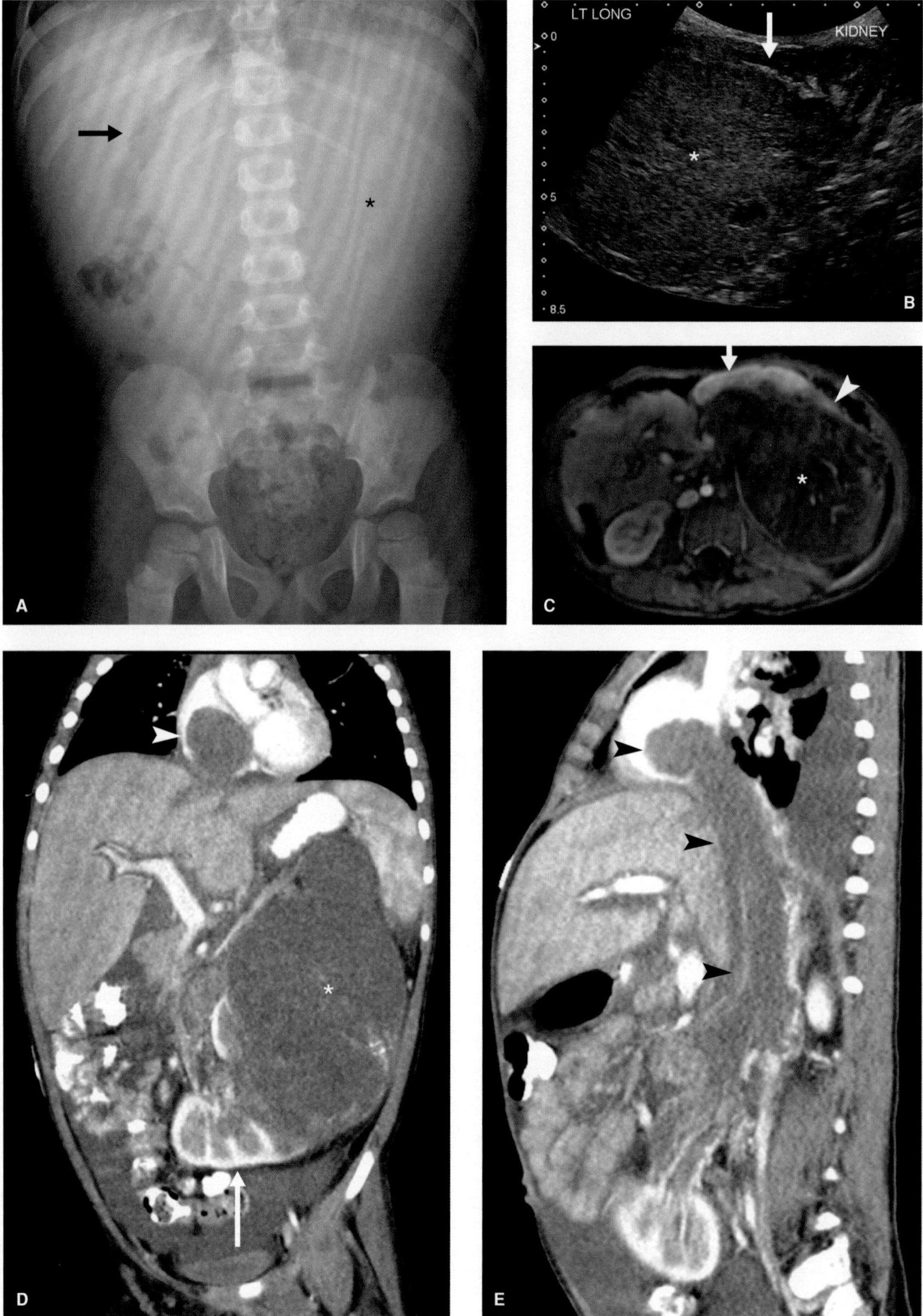

FIGURE 69.52. **Wilms Tumor. A:** Frontal radiograph of the abdomen shows a paucity of bowel gas in the left upper quadrant (*asterisk*), with mass effect displacing bowel loops and the stomach into the right hemiabdomen (*arrow*). There are no calcifications to suggest that this reflects neuroblastoma. **B:** Longitudinal ultrasound image in the same patient shows a large mass (*asterisk*) arising from the upper pole of the kidney. A claw of renal tissue (*arrow*) is present at the interface between the tumor and kidney. **C:** Axial T1-weighted, fat-saturated MR image in the same patient shows a large, hypoenhancing mass arising from the left kidney (*asterisk*). The remainder of the kidney is displaced anteriorly and to the right (*arrow*) and there is a claw of renal tissue at the interface between the tumor and the kidney (*arrowhead*). **D:** Coronal CT image with intravenous contrast in a different patient with Wilms tumor shows a large mass (*asterisk*) arising from the upper pole of the left kidney (*arrow*). Note the claw of renal tissue at the interface between the tumor and the kidney. A filling defect is present in the right atrium (*arrowhead*) reflective of tumor thrombus. **E:** Sagittal CT image with intravenous contrast in the same patient shows contiguous extent of tumor thrombus (*arrowheads*) through the IVC to the right atrium. Distention of the IVC is a clue that this is tumor thrombus rather than bland thrombus.

TABLE 69.2

WILMS TUMOR STAGING

■ STAGE	■ FINDINGS
Stage I	Tumor confined to the kidney without capsular or vascular invasion No biopsy or rupture Completely removed at surgery
Stage II	Tumor extends beyond renal capsule, +/– vascular invasion No biopsy or rupture Completely removed at surgery Negative retroperitoneal lymph nodes
Stage III	Tumor not completely removed at surgery Positive retroperitoneal lymph nodes Preoperative biopsy or rupture
Stage IV	Metastatic disease
Stage V	Bilateral tumors at diagnosis

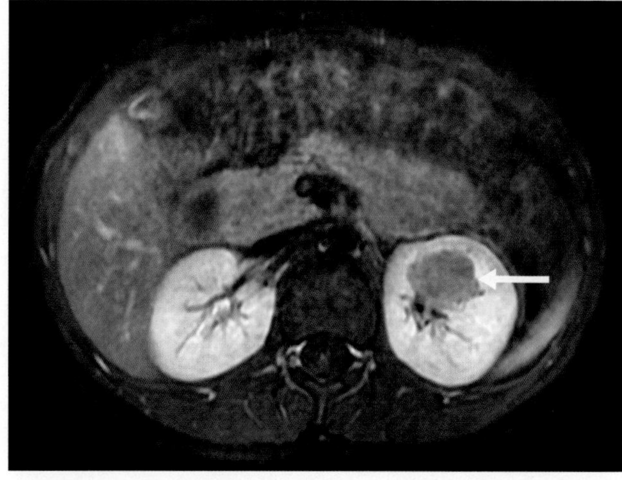

FIGURE 69.53. **Renal Cell Carcinoma.** Axial T1-weighted, fat-saturated MR image following administration of a gadolinium-based contrast material shows a hypoenhancing mass in the left kidney.

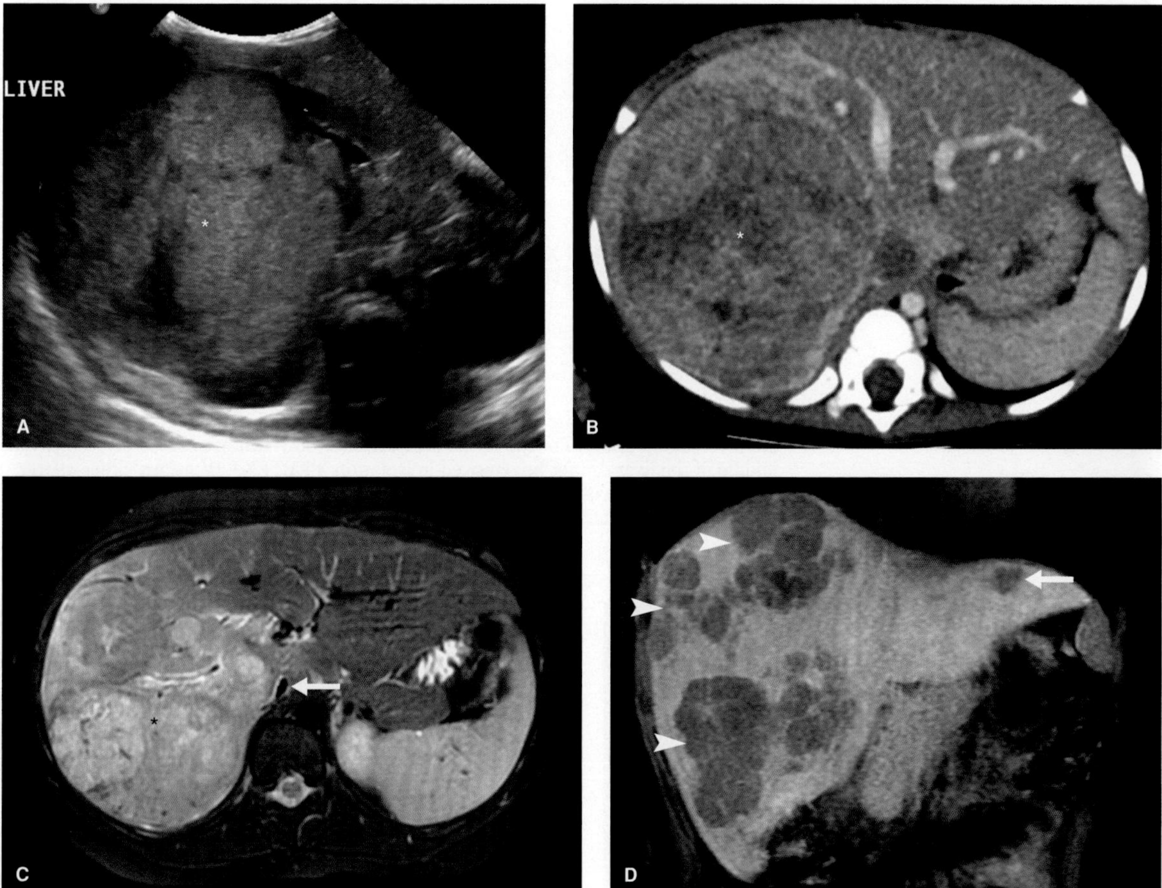

FIGURE 69.54. **Hepatoblastoma. A:** Transverse ultrasound image shows a large, heterogeneous mass arising from the right hepatic lobe (*asterisk*). Determining the origin of a mass of this size on ultrasound can be difficult. **B:** Axial CT image with intravenous contrast in the same patient shows a large, heterogeneous mass arising from the right hepatic lobe (*asterisk*). It is critically important to define the relationship of the tumor to the liver veins (portal and hepatic), as this defines staging and is important for planning resection. Calcifications are not present in this case but hepatoblastomas are known to calcify. **C:** Axial T2-weighted, fat-saturated MR image in the same patient shows a heterogeneously T2-weighted hyperintense mass in the right hepatic lobe (*asterisk*). The inferior vena cava (*arrow*) is narrowed due to mass effect but is patent without tumor thrombus. **D:** Coronal T1-weighted, fat-saturated MR image following administration of a gadolinium-based contrast material in a different patient with multifocal hepatoblastoma shows multiple hypoenhancing masses in the right lobe of the liver (*arrowheads*) as well as a tumor deposit in the left hepatic lobe (*arrow*). Defining the extent of disease, in this case PRETEXT IV, is critical to tumor staging and therapy planning.

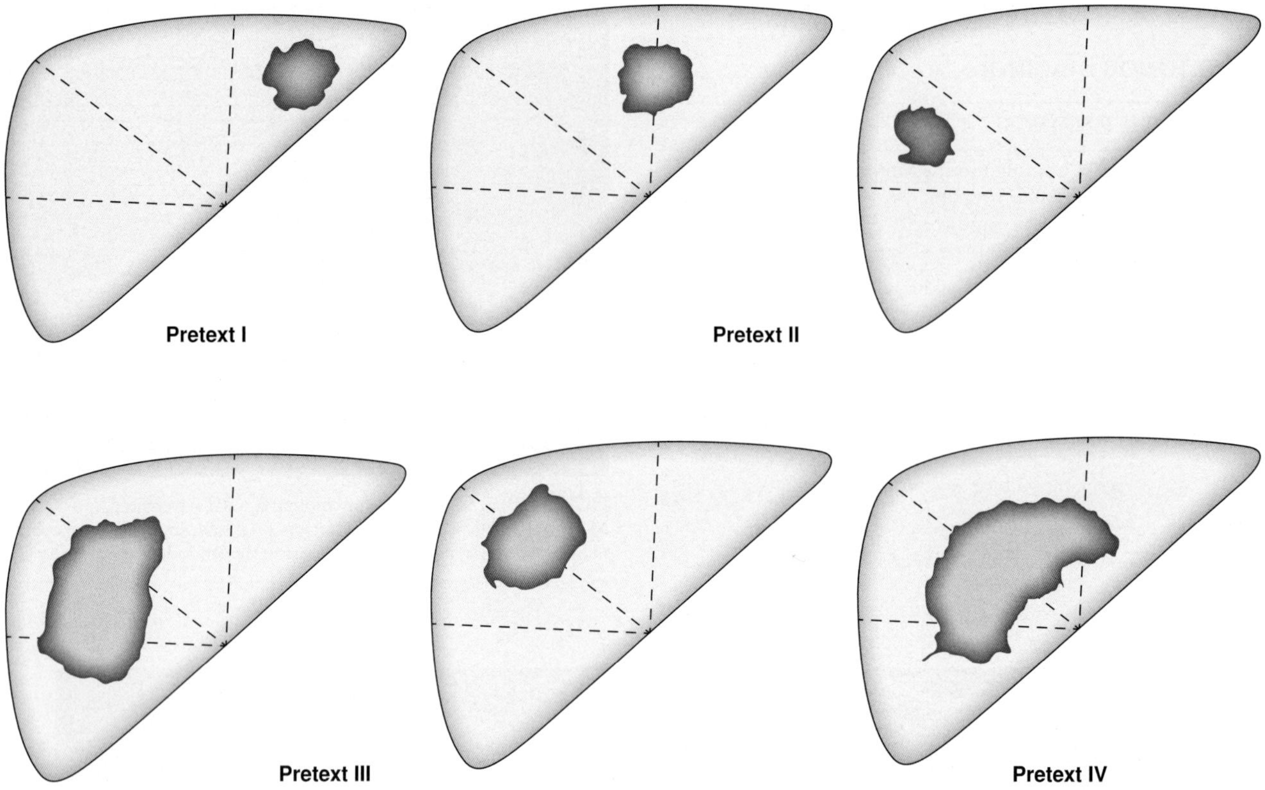

Pretext I

Pretext II

Pretext III

Pretext IV

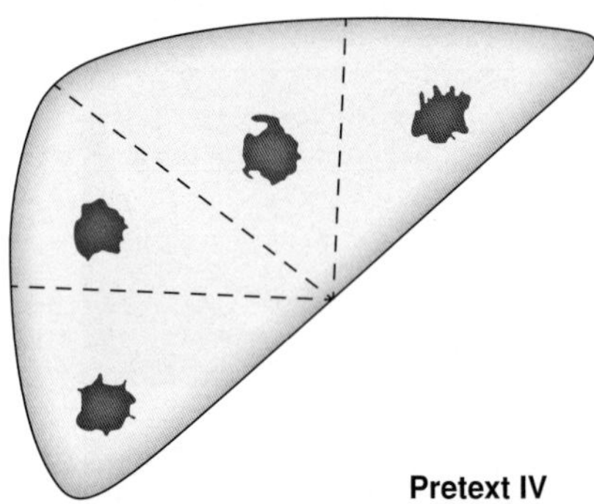

FIGURE 69.55. **PRETEXT Staging of Hepatoblastoma.** Local extent of hepatoblastoma is described using the PRETEXT system, which is a way of telling the surgeon how many contiguous liver sections (the liver is composed of four sections: right posterior, right anterior, left medial, and left lateral) will need to be removed to fully resect the tumor. PRETEXT I means either the left lateral or right posterior sections are involved by tumor. PRETEXT II means either the right anterior or left medial sections are involved by tumor and half of the liver (entire right lobe or entire left lobe) will need to be resected. PRETEXT III means either three adjacent sections are all involved by tumor or the right anterior and left medial sections are involved by tumor. For the latter, a trisectionectomy will need to be performed since the middle of the liver cannot be removed in isolation. PRETEXT IV means either a large tumor involves all sections of the liver or multifocal tumor involves all sections.

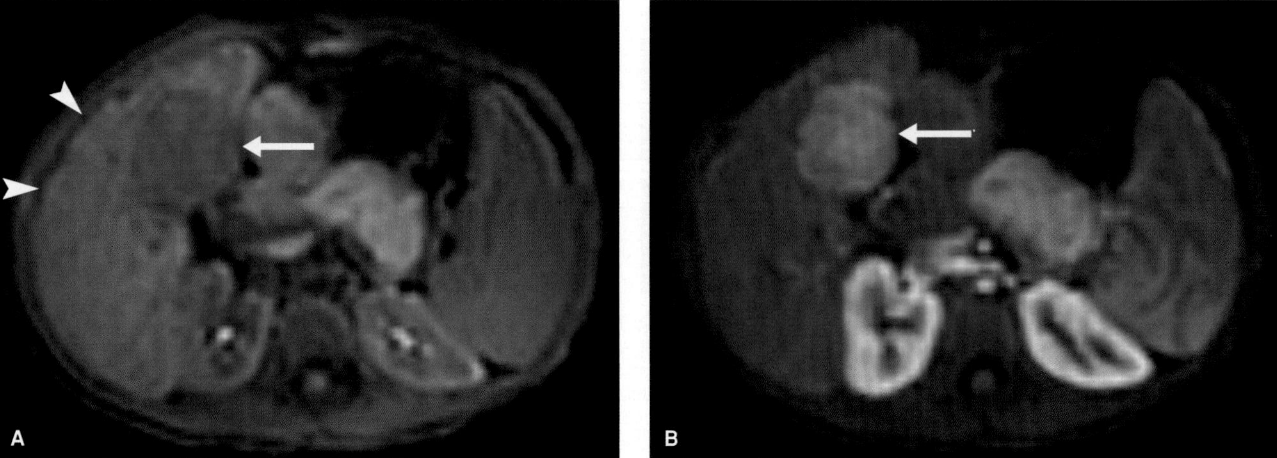

FIGURE 69.56. **Hepatocellular Carcinoma (HCC). A:** Precontrast T1-weighted, fat-saturated MR image shows a hypointense mass (*arrow*) arising from the liver with macronodular surface contour (*arrowheads*) related to fibrosis and regeneration in a child with Alagille syndrome. **B:** In the arterial phase following administration of a gadolinium-based contrast material, the tumor enhances heterogeneously (*arrow*).

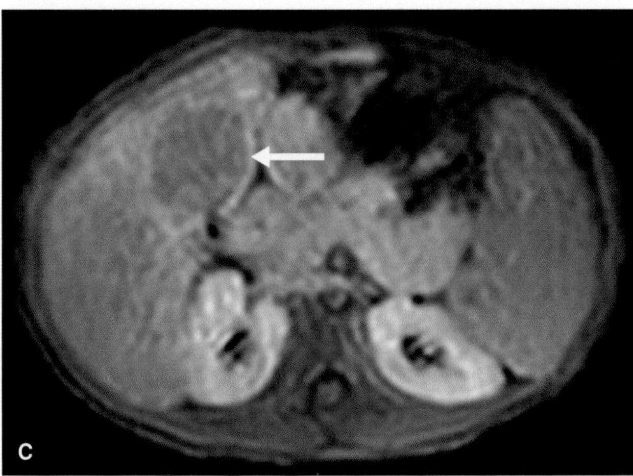

FIGURE 69.56. (*Continued*) **C:** In the late venous phase, the tumor (*arrow*) washes out relative to background liver. A thin rim of enhancement is present, suggestive of a capsule. Arterial enhancement, portal venous phase washout, and the presence of a capsule are all features of hepatocellular carcinoma. Classical HCC (like this) occurs in the context of underlying liver disease (Alagille syndrome in this case), in contrast to fibrolamellar HCC, which occurs in a normal background liver.

tumor is an aggressive renal neoplasm with a poor prognosis that typically occurs in younger children. At imaging, the tumor manifests as a large, aggressive-appearing mass. Crescentic subcapsular fluid is a characteristic, but not always present, finding. There is an association between rhabdoid tumor and synchronous brain tumors, often in the posterior fossa. Renal medullary carcinoma is an aggressive neoplasm with a very poor prognosis that occurs in teenagers and young adults with sickle cell trait.

Liver Tumors

Hepatoblastoma. Hepatoblastoma is the most common primary liver tumor in young children. There is an increased incidence of hepatoblastoma in children with a history of being born premature. The tumor most commonly occurs between the ages of 6 months and 4 years. Hepatoblastoma typically presents as a palpable abdominal mass which is otherwise asymptomatic. Patients may occasionally have abdominal pain related to the large size of the tumor. Serum α fetoprotein (AFP) is typically markedly elevated. Patients may also have increased platelets as a paraneoplastic effect. Metastatic disease is relatively rare at diagnosis (10%) and is typically to the

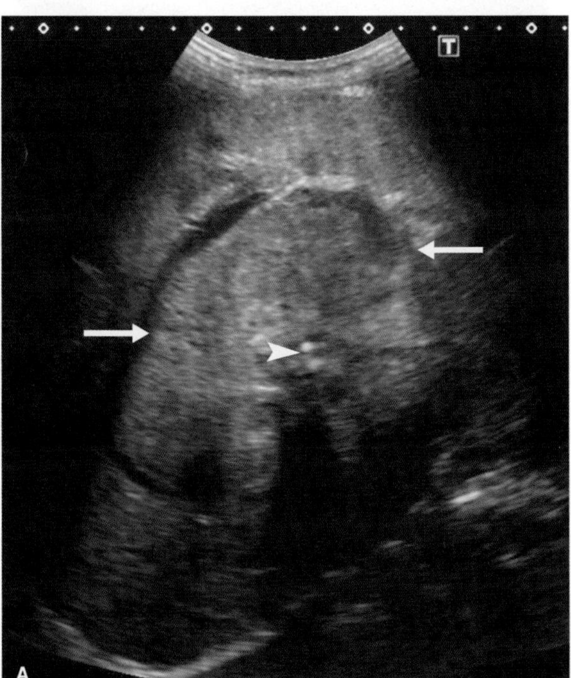

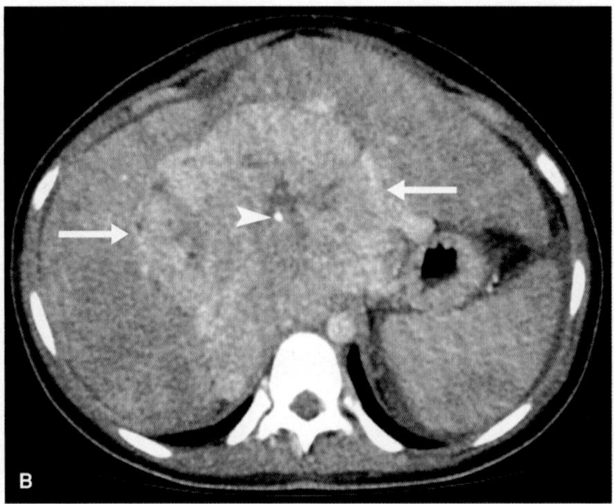

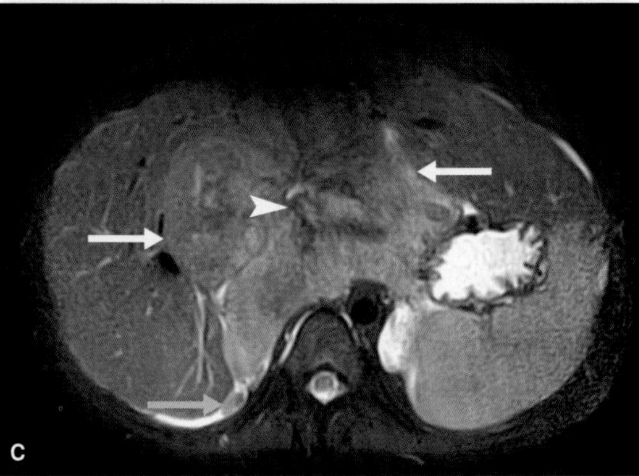

FIGURE 69.57. **Fibrolamellar Hepatocellular Carcinoma. A:** Transverse ultrasound image shows a large heterogeneous mass arising from the liver (*arrows*) with central calcification (*arrowhead*). **B:** Axial CT image with intravenous contrast in the same patient shows a heterogeneously enhancing mass in the central liver (*arrows*) with central hypoenhancement and calcification (*arrowhead*) reflective of a large central scar. **C:** Axial T2-weighted MR image in the same patient shows a large heterogeneously T2-hyperintense mass (*arrows*) with central irregular low signal reflective of scar (*arrowhead*). A subdiaphragmatic tumor implant (*blue arrow*) reflects metastatic disease.

lungs. Multifocal hepatoblastoma occurs, so it is important to evaluate the entire liver for additional masses.

Tumors may initially be identified by ultrasound, most commonly appearing as a large, heterogeneous mass arising from the liver (Fig. 69.54). CT and MRI are required to define the local extent of disease, as well as the overall stage of the patient. At CT and MRI, hepatoblastoma typically appears as a large, heterogeneous mass, generally hypoenhancing relative to the normal liver (Fig. 69.54). Areas of hemorrhage and dystrophic calcifications are not uncommon. The tumor also has a propensity for vascular invasion, often into the hepatic veins and IVC, but also into the portal vein. MRI is more sensitive than CT for multifocal liver tumor. Sensitivity can be further increased with the use of hepatocyte-specific MR contrast agents. Local extent of disease is described using the PRETEXT system (Fig. 69.55). Overall stage is determined based on locoregional and metastatic spread.

Treatment for hepatoblastoma is with neoadjuvant chemotherapy and subsequent surgical resection, if possible. If the disease is multifocal and unresectable, patients may require liver transplantation for local control of disease.

Hepatocellular Carcinoma. Hepatocellular carcinoma (HCC) tends to occur in older children and in children with underlying liver disease. In contrast to at-risk adults who are often screened for the disease, in children, HCC is often relatively large at presentation. Multifocal disease also occurs. Staging depends on local extent of disease, including vascular invasion and metastatic spread, which typically occurs to the lungs. Hepatocyte-specific gadolinium-based contrast agents may increase sensitivity for multifocal disease.

At MRI, HCC can be of variable size. The tumor typically becomes more heterogeneous as the size increases. Similar features to adult HCC may be present, including loss of signal on out-of-phase images indicating intracellular lipid, mild T2 hyperintensity, and restricted diffusion. The tumors typically arterially enhance and demonstrate venous phase washout (Fig. 69.56). A capsule may also be visible during the venous

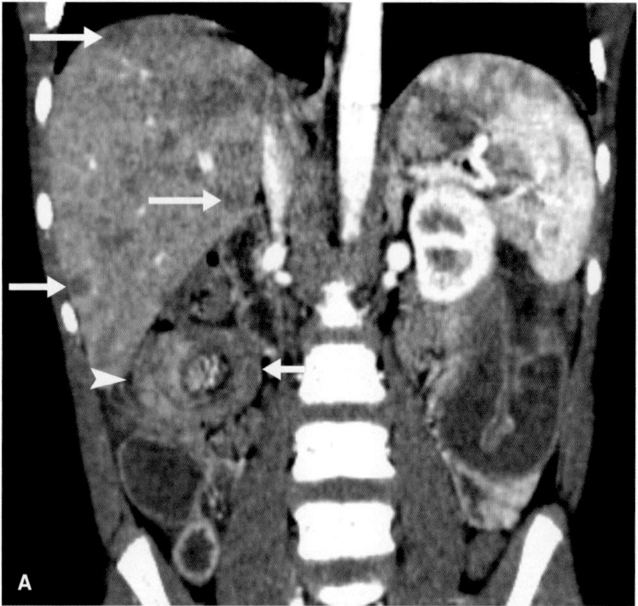

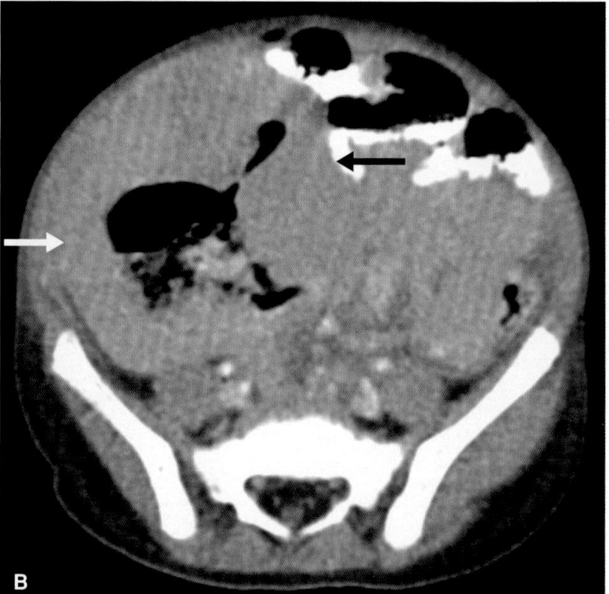

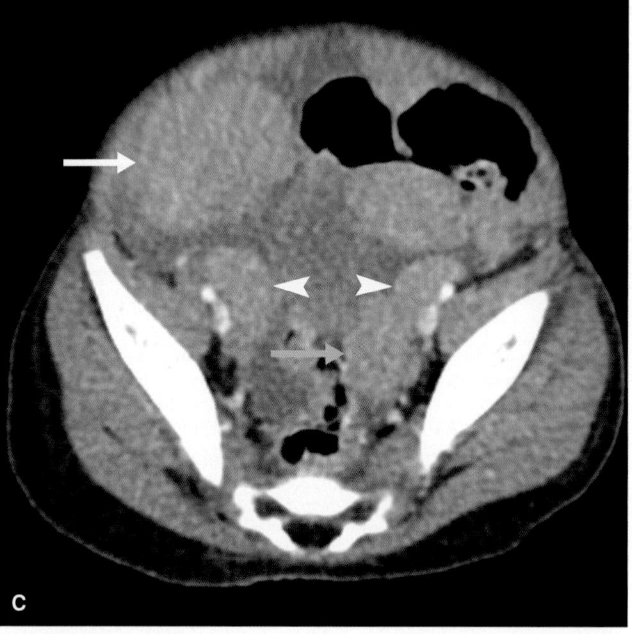

FIGURE 69.58. **Burkitt Lymphoma.** **A:** Coronal CT image with intravenous contrast shows a right abdominal intussusception (*arrow*). There is heterogeneous enhancement and asymmetric thickening of one wall of the intussusception (*arrowhead*). While in this case, this reflects involvement by Burkitt lymphoma, heterogeneous enhancement is common in intussusceptions and should not be overinterpreted. A clue to the fact that this reflects tumor causing intussusception is the presence of multiple hypoenhancing tumor implants in the liver (*blue arrows*). **B:** Axial CT image with intravenous and oral contrast in a different patient with Burkitt lymphoma shows aneurysmal dilation of a bowel segment in the right lower quadrant, with significant wall thickening (*arrow*). This appearance is characteristic of Burkitt lymphoma. **C:** Additional axial CT image in the same patient, lower down in the abdomen/pelvis, shows the caudal aspect of the tumor-involved bowel loop (*arrow*) as well as large iliac chain lymph nodes (*arrowheads*) and peritoneal tumor implant (*blue arrow*). Burkitt lymphoma is one of the tumors in children that is known to spread to the peritoneum.

phase. In general, the tumors are hypoenhancing relative to the rest of the liver on the hepatocyte phase, if a hepatocyte-specific contrast agent is used.

Treatment of pediatric HCC involves a combination of chemotherapy and surgery. In cases of extensive or multifocal disease, liver transplantation may be considered. In rare cases, percutaneous ablation or transarterial chemoembolization (TACE) may be considered.

Fibrolamellar HCC. The fibrolamellar variant of HCC occurs in older children and young adults. The masses are typically large at presentation and patients usually present with a palpable mass and nonspecific constitutional symptoms. The tumors are often well circumscribed and have exuberant fibrosis, interspersed with parallel sheets of tumors cells. The tumors do not produce or excrete AFP.

Ultrasound will demonstrate a large, heterogeneous liver mass (Fig. 69.57). At CT, the tumor is large and demonstrates a central fibrous scar (Fig. 69.57). Calcifications may be present. MRI will show a large mass with a central scar that is hypointense on all sequences (Fig. 69.57). Fibrolamellar HCC typically demonstrates heterogeneous arterial enhancement and iso- to hyperenhancement to the liver on the venous and delayed phases, with variable delayed hyperenhancement of the fibrous central scar.

The prognosis for fibrolamellar HCC is similar to that of classical HCC. Aggressive surgical resection has the best chance for long-term survival, but local recurrence rates are relatively high. Unresectable tumors have a poor prognosis.

Lymphoma

Non-Hodgkin lymphoma is more common than Hodgkin lymphoma in children, and Burkitt lymphoma is the most common type of non-Hodgkin lymphoma in children. The abdomen is one of the more common locations for non-Hodgkin lymphoma to present in children. Presentations include nodular implants in solid organs (liver, spleen, and kidney) but also intestinal, mesenteric, and omental/peritoneal masses (Fig. 69.58). Tumor masses are comprised of generally relatively homogeneous soft tissue, can be quite large, and are typically infiltrative in appearance. Intestinal masses can present with intussusception, either outside of the typical age range or that recurs or fails to reduce (Fig. 69.58). Burkitt lymphoma is highly FDG avid and thus 18F-FDG PET is typically used in staging and follow-up. Importantly, doubling times of Burkitt lymphoma can be as short as 24 hours, meaning these masses can grow rapidly, causing acute symptoms. Treatment is by chemotherapy with surgical resection reserved for tumors causing intestinal obstruction.

Suggested Readings

Adeb M, Darge K, Dillman JR, Carr M, Epelman M. Magnetic resonance urography in evaluation of duplicated renal collecting systems. *Magn Reson Imaging Clin N Am* 2013;21(4):717–730.

Alamo L, Meyrat BJ, Meuwly JY, Meuli RA, Gudinchet F. Anorectal malformations: finding the pathway out of the labyrinth. *Radiographics* 2013;33(2):491–512.

Al-Hussaini A, AboZeid A, Hai A. How does esophagus look on barium esophagram in pediatric eosinophilic esophagitis? *Abdom Radiol (NY)* 2016; 41(8):1466–1473.

Alkhori NA, Barth RA. Pediatric scrotal ultrasound: review and update. *Pediatr Radiol* 2017;47(9):1125–1133.

Bagade S, Khanna G. Imaging of omphalomesenteric duct remnants and related pathologies in children. *Curr Probl Diagn Radiol* 2015;44(3):246–255.

Berrocal T, Lamas M, Gutieérrez J, Torres I, Prieto C, del Hoyo ML. Congenital anomalies of the small intestine, colon, and rectum. *Radiographics* 1999; 19(5):1219–1236.

Berrocal T, Madrid C, Novo S, Gutiérrez J, Arjonilla A, Gómez-León N. Congenital anomalies of the tracheobronchial tree, lung, and mediastinum: embryology, radiology, and pathology. *Radiographics* 2004;24(1):e17.

Chavhan GB, Babyn PS, Manson D, Vidarsson L. Pediatric MR cholangiopancreatography: principles, technique, and clinical applications. *Radiographics* 2008;28(7):1951–1962.

Chow JS, Koning JL, Back SJ, Nguyen HT, Phelps A, Darge K. Classification of pediatric urinary tract dilation: the new language. *Pediatr Radiol* 2017;47(9):1109–1115.

Chung EM, Conran RM, Schroeder JW, Rohena-Quinquilla IR, Rooks VJ. From the radiologic pathology archives: pediatric polycystic kidney disease and other ciliopathies: radiologic-pathologic correlation. *Radiographics* 2014;34(1):155–178.

Chung EM, Cube R, Lewis RB, Conran RM. From the archives of the AFIP: Pediatric liver masses: radiologic-pathologic correlation part 1. Benign tumors. *Radiographics* 2010;30(3):801–826.

Chung EM, Graeber AR, Conran RM. Renal tumors of childhood: radiologic-athologic correlation part 1. The 1st decade: from the radiologic pathology archives. *Radiographics* 2016;36(2):499–522.

Chung EM, Lattin GE Jr, Cube R, et al. From the archives of the AFIP: pediatric liver masses: radiologic-pathologic correlation. Part 2. Malignant tumors. *Radiographics* 2011;31(2):483–507.

Chung EM, Lattin GE Jr, Fagen KE, et al. Renal tumors of childhood: radiologic-pathologic correlation part 2. The 2nd decade: from the radiologic pathology archives. *Radiographics* 2017;37(5):1538–1558.

Chung EM, Pavio M. Pediatric extranodal lymphoma. *Radiol Clin North Am* 2016;54(4):727–746.

Chung EM, Soderlund KA, Fagen KE. Imaging of the pediatric urinary system. *Radiol Clin North Am* 2017;55(2):337–357.

Cogley JR, O'Connor SC, Houshyar R, Al Dulaimy K. Emergent pediatric US: what every radiologist should know. *Radiographics* 2012;32(3):651–665.

Decter RM. Renal duplication and fusion anomalies. *Pediatr Clin North Am* 1997;44(5):1323–1341.

Derinkuyu BE, Boyunağa Ö, Öztunalı Ç. Imaging features of Burkitt lymphoma in pediatric patients. *Diagn Interv Radiol* 2016;22(1):95–100.

Dillman JR, Adler J, Zimmermann EM, Strouse PJ. CT enterography of pediatric Crohn disease. *Pediatr Radiol* 2010;40(1):97–105.

Edwards EA, Pigg N, Courtier J, Zapala MA, MacKenzie JD, Phelps AS. Intussusception: past, present and future. *Pediatr Radiol* 2017;47(9):1101–1108.

Esposito F, Mamone R, Di Serafino M, et al. Diagnostic imaging features of necrotizing enterocolitis: a narrative review. *Quant Imaging Med Surg* 2017;7(3):336–344.

Gongidi P, Bellah RD. Ultrasound of the pediatric appendix. *Pediatr Radiol* 2017;47(9):1091–1100.

Govindarajan KK. Biliary atresia: where do we stand now? *World J Hepatol* 2016;8(36):1593–1601.

Hains DS, Bates CM, Ingraham S, Schwaderer AL. Management and etiology of the unilateral multicystic dysplastic kidney: a review. *Pediatr Nephrol* 2009;24(2):233–241.

Hochart V, Lahoche A, Priso RH, et al. Posterior urethral valves: are neonatal imaging findings predictive of renal function during early childhood? *Pediatr Radiol* 2016;46(10):1418–1423.

Hwang SM, Jeon TY, Yoo SY, Choe YH, Lee SK, Kim JH. Early US findings of biliary atresia in infants younger than 30 days. *Eur Radiol* 2018;28(4): 1771–1777.

Kumar P, Kumar C, Pandey PR, Sarin YK. Congenital duodenal obstruction in neonates: over 13 years' experience from a single centre. *J Neonatal Surg* 2016;5(4):50.

Kurtz MP, Chow JS, Johnson EK, Rosoklija I, Logvinenko T, Nelson CP. Imaging after urinary tract infection in older children and adolescents. *J Uro* 2015;193(5 Suppl):1778–1782.

Langer JC. Intestinal rotation abnormalities and midgut volvulus. *Surg Clin North Am* 2017;97(1):147–159.

Linam LE, Darolia R, Naffaa LN, et al. US findings of adnexal torsion in children and adolescents: size really does matter. *Pediatr Radiol* 2007;37(10):1013–1019.

Long FR, Kramer SS, Markowitz RI, Taylor GE. Radiographic patterns of intestinal malrotation in children. *Radiographics* 1996;16(3):547–556; discussion 556–560.

Mollard BJ, Smith EA, Dillman JR. Pediatric MR enterography: technique and approach to interpretation-how we do it. *Radiology* 2015;274(1):29–43.

Mortelé KJ, Rocha TC, Streeter JL, Taylor AJ. Multimodality imaging of pancreatic and biliary congenital anomalies. *Radiographics* 2006;26(3):715–731.

Ngo AV, Stanescu AL, Phillips GS. Neonatal bowel disorders: practical imaging algorithm for trainees and general radiologists. *AJR Am J Roentgenol* 2018;210(5):976–988.

Nour-Eldin NE, Abdelmonem O, Tawfik AM. Pediatric primary and metastatic neuroblastoma: MRI findings: pictorial review. *Magn Reson Imaging* 2012;30(7):893–906.

O'Donovan AN, Habra G, Somers S, Malone DE, Rees A, Winthrop AL. Diagnosis of Hirschsprung's disease. *AJR Am J Roentgenol* 1996;167(2): 517–520.

Piepsz A. Antenatally detected hydronephrosis. *Semin Nucl Med* 2007;37(4): 249–260.

Putnam LR, John SD, Greenfield SA, et al. The utility of the contrast enema in neonates with suspected Hirschsprung disease. *J Pediatr Surg* 2015;50(6):963–966.

Riccabona M. Imaging in childhood urinary tract infection. *Radiol Med* 2016;121(5):391–401.

Rodriguez MM. Congenital anomalies of the kidney and the urinary tract (CAKUT). *Fetal Pediatr Pathol* 2014;33(5–6):293–320.

Sarhan OM, Alghanbar M, Alsulaihim A, Alharbi B, Alotay A, Nakshabandi Z. Multicystic dysplastic kidney: impact of imaging modality selection on the initial management and prognosis. *J Pediatr Urol* 2014;10(4):645–649.

Sharp SE, Parisi MT, Gelfand MJ, Yanik GA, Shulkin BL. Functional-metabolic imaging of neuroblastoma. *Q J Nucl Med Mol Imaging* 2013;57(1):6–20.

Siegel MJ, Chung EM. Wilms' tumor and other pediatric renal masses. *Magn Reson Imaging Clin N Am* 2008;16(3):479–497.

Sivit CJ, Siegel MJ, Applegate KE, Newman KD. When appendicitis is suspected in children. *Radiographics* 2001;21(1):247–262.

Stanescu AL, Liszewski MC, Lee EY, Phillips GS. Neonatal gastrointestinal emergencies: step-by-step approach. *Radiol Clin North Am* 2017;55(4):717–739.

Swift CC, Eklund MJ, Kraveka JM, Alazraki AL. Updates in diagnosis, management, and treatment of neuroblastoma. *Radiographics* 2018;38(2): 566–580.

CHAPTER 70 ■ PEDIATRIC MSK

NANCY A. CHAUVIN AND ASEF KHWAJA

INTRODUCTION

The musculoskeletal system in children differs significantly from adults. Bone composition in the young child is dramatically different than adult bone. The anatomy and physiology of children makes them vulnerable to unique injuries as well as varied manifestations of infection and inflammatory conditions. In addition, children are at risk for specific bone lesions and soft tissue tumors that are not seen in adults. Congenital and developmental osseous disorders are common and imaging plays an important role in their diagnosis and management. The focus of this chapter is to describe the growth and development of the immature skeleton, highlighting pathology that is unique to children.

GROWTH AND DEVELOPMENT OF THE IMMATURE SKELETON

Bone Composition

In children, the structure of the long bone consists of epiphyses, located at the ends of most bones which are separated from the metaphysis by the primary physis or growth plate. The shaft of the tubular bone is the diaphysis. The epiphyses are initially cartilaginous, converting to bone with the development of the secondary ossification center. The primary physis is responsible for the longitudinal growth of the bone while the secondary physis is responsible for the spherical growth of the epiphysis.

Pediatric bones are less dense, more porous, and have a lower mineral content compared with adult bones. This makes young bones much more elastic and pliable and able to undergo a greater degree of deformation before breaking, making greenstick and torus (buckle) fractures very common in the pediatric population. The increased porosity also inhibits fracture propagation; thus comminuted fractures are relatively uncommon in children.

MR Appearance of Bone

In the newborn, the bone marrow is entirely hematopoietic (red marrow). Bone marrow transformation to fatty (yellow) marrow begins within the first year of life and occurs in a predictable pattern. In the body as a whole, marrow transformation begins in the periphery, first occurring in the phalanges of the fingers and toes and progressing centrally. By skeletal maturity, fatty marrow conversion in the appendicular skeleton is typically complete with conversion within the axial skeleton occurring at a slower pace throughout life. Marrow transformation within the individual long bones also occurs in a predictable pattern. The epiphyses are the first to convert to fatty marrow, occurring within 6 months of the radiologic appearance of the secondary ossification center. Transformation continues within the diaphysis, followed by the metaphyses, with the proximal metaphysis the last to convert.

Hematopoietic marrow on MR, due to the low fat content, is of low signal intensity (SI) on T1-weighted sequences and is of high SI on water-sensitive images. Typically, hematopoietic marrow T1-weighted signal is isointense or hyperintense relative to skeletal muscle, except in the newborn period due to high number of red blood cells where it can appear T1-weighted hypointense relative to skeletal muscle. Beyond the neonatal period, marrow that is hypointense relative to muscle on T1-weighted imaging is considered suspicious for marrow disease.

On MR, the physis has a trilaminar appearance comprising the zone of cartilage which contains active chondrocytes; zone of provisional calcification where the cartilage matrix becomes calcified; and the primary spongiosa, the region where woven bone is formed. The cartilaginous zone demonstrates intermediate to high SI on water-sensitive images. The zone of provisional calcification has low SI on all sequences, while the primary spongiosa is of high SI on water-sensitive sequences (Fig. 70.1). The physis thickness should be uniform and as skeletal maturity approaches will become thin and eventually disappear, leaving a physeal scar. The perichondrium is the fibrocartilaginous structure that surrounds the physeal cartilage and is of low signal on all sequences. This is tightly tethered to the physis and acts as a barrier to disease. The periosteum is a thin, low SI structure that parallels the bone cortex and is loosely attached to the shaft and tightly attached to the perichondrium. Deep to the periosteum is a rich, vascular network that helps to feed the growing metaphyses.

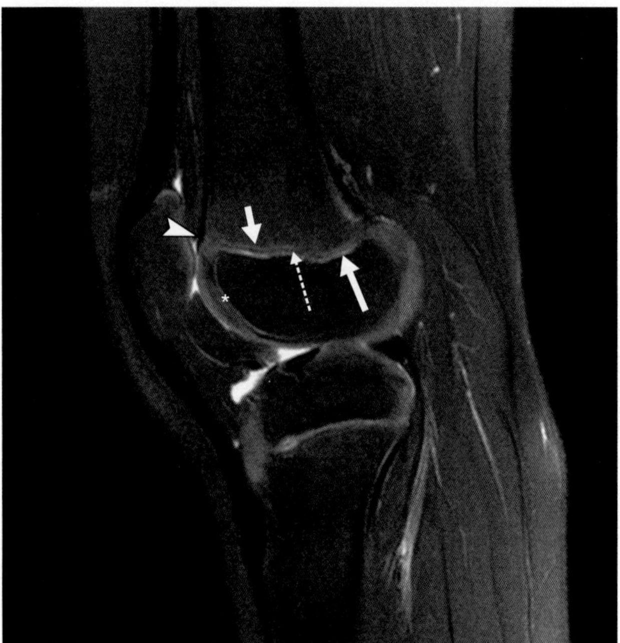

FIGURE 70.1. **Normal Knee MRI.** Sagittal T2-weighted fat-saturated MR image of a 6-year-old girl. Trilaminar appearance of the primary physis with zone of cartilage (*long arrow*), zone of provisional calcification (*dashed arrow*), and primary spongiosa (*short arrow*). This is surrounded by the perichondrium (*arrowhead*). The primary physis is responsible for the longitudinal growth of the bone. The same layers are present in the secondary physis (*) which is responsible for the spherical growth of the epiphysis. In children, the metaphyses will demonstrate increased SI compared to the epiphyses as the epiphyses have more fatty marrow.

ACCIDENTAL TRAUMA

Fractures

Types of injury in children vary with age due to the structural changes in the growing skeleton. Five common fracture patterns are seen in children which are dependent on the degree of force imposed on the bone; plastic deformation, buckle fractures, greenstick (unicortical) fractures, complete fractures, and physeal injuries. Plastic deformation occurs from longitudinal stress and results in bowing of the bones, with an intact periosteum. These injuries are common within the forearm, tibia, and fibula. No fracture line is depicted on radiographs and periosteal reaction is seen on follow-up imaging. Buckle or torus fractures result from axial loading on an extremity, occurring at the metaphysis or metadiaphysis. There is acute angulation of the cortex opposite the bending force (Fig. 70.2). At the site of fracture, the cortex is compressed and bulges without extension of the fracture to the cortex. Buckle fractures represent 50% of pediatric wrist fractures and typically can be managed by primary care physicians. Greenstick fractures are incomplete fractures resulting from perpendicular forces that break one cortex, the side opposite the site of stress. Complete fractures propagate completely through a bone and can be spiral, oblique, or transverse. Physeal injuries are described below.

Acute Physeal Trauma. Physeal cartilage is prone to injury as it is weaker than both bone and ligaments. Cartilage is most vulnerable to injury during periods of active growth, such as during early adolescence. The weakest portion is the zone of provisional calcification, the region between the physeal cartilage and the metaphyseal bone. The Salter–Harris classification defines the type of physeal injury and in general, the higher the numerical type, the greater the risk of consequent growth arrest (Table 70.1). Injuries to the physis have an important effect on the potential longitudinal growth of the bone and may create growth arrest and angular deformities. Notably, Salter–Harris I fractures are rare, often subtle, and may be occult.

Chronic Physeal Trauma. Sports training of significant intensity and duration that results in repetitive loading can alter metaphyseal perfusion and interfere with the mineralization of hypertrophied chondrocytes leading to chronic physeal injuries. Classic chronic physeal injuries occur in the knees of athletes who participate in high-intensity running, in the proximal humerus of baseball players ("little league shoulder") (Fig. 70.3), and in the distal radius in gymnasts ("gymnast wrist") (Fig. 70.4). Chronic physeal trauma manifests radiographically as widening of the primary physis, often with sclerosis at the margins of the adjacent metaphysis. On MR, the affected physis will become wider and irregular, demonstrating increased SI on water-sensitive images. Prompt cessation of the activity is imperative to prevent permanent physeal damage and physeal bar development.

Physeal Bars. A subset of physeal injuries (either sequela of trauma, infection, or ischemia) can lead to cellular disruption and ischemia, giving rise to the development of an abnormal osseous connection (a "bone bridge" or "bone bar") between the epiphysis and metaphysis. These bone bars can result in limb length discrepancy, angular deformity, or altered joint mechanics that may cause significant long-term morbidity. Approximately 15% of all fractures in childhood involve the physis; however, less than 10% of those injuries result in physeal bars and significant growth arrest. The incidence of physeal bar formation is higher after injuries to the distal femur,

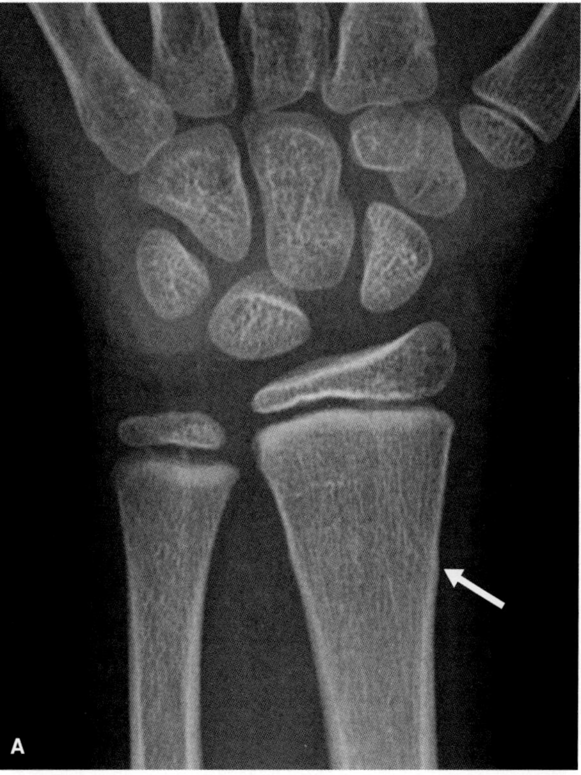

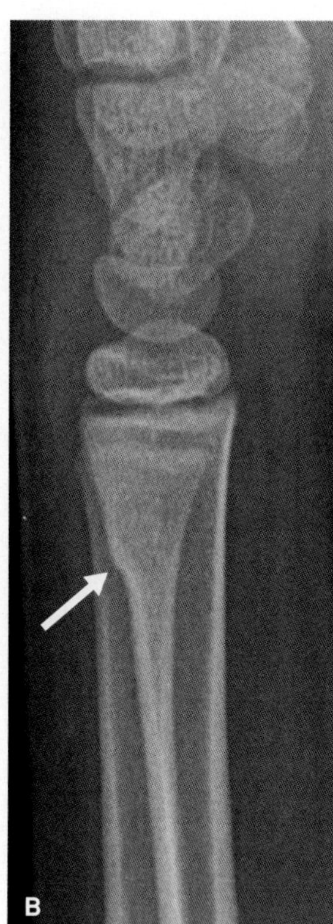

FIGURE 70.2. **Buckle Fracture.** AP (**A**) and lateral (**B**) radiographs of the wrist in an 8-year-old girl who fell on her outstretched hand. **A:** There is subtle cortical buckling of the distal radial diametaphysis (*arrow*). This is more conspicuous on the lateral view where there is cortical obliquity of the dorsal aspect of the distal radius (*arrow*). Minimal soft tissue swelling is present. Careful evaluation should be made to discern if the fracture extends to the physis, as Salter II fractures are managed differently.

proximal tibia, and distal tibia. It is important to note that the distal femur and proximal tibial physes contribute to the greatest proportion of limb growth, and therefore, bars in these regions have the biggest impact on limb length discrepancies.

When a physis is injured and a physeal bar forms in the periphery or eccentrically in the bone, the bar will result in tethering which will give rise to an angular deformity. If the central portion of the physis is affected, there will be central tethering with overall shortening of the affected bone (Fig. 70.5). The larger a physeal bar is, the greater impact it will have on growth of the bone. Physeal bars may begin to form 1 to 2 months after injury but may not become clinically apparent until years later during adolescent growth spurts. Young children with complex physeal fractures should be followed until skeletal maturity. On conventional radiographs, a physeal bar may appear as partial osseous bridging of the radiolucent growth plate with a sclerotic bridge of bone. Alternatively, indirect signs may be apparent such as asymmetry of growth recovery lines or tethering at the bridge. MR imaging can detect early fibrous bars and established bone bars. Isovoxel gradient echo sequences are excellent in determining the location and size of the bar. Treatment is determined by the location and size of the bone bridge, extent of the deformity, and the estimated future growth potential of the child.

Apophyseal Injuries. Apophyses are growth centers that serve as attachment sites for tendons and have a physis at its

TABLE 70.1

DESCRIPTION OF THE SALTER–HARRIS FRACTURE CLASSIFICATION, TYPES I–V

■ TYPE	■ CHARACTERISTICS OF SALTER–HARRIS FRACTURE
I	Separation through the physis, usually through areas of hypertrophic and degenerating cartilage cell columns
II	Fracture through a portion of the physis that extends through the metaphyses
III	Fracture through a portion of the physis that extends through the epiphysis
IV	Fracture across the metaphysis, physis, and epiphysis
V	Crush injury to the physis

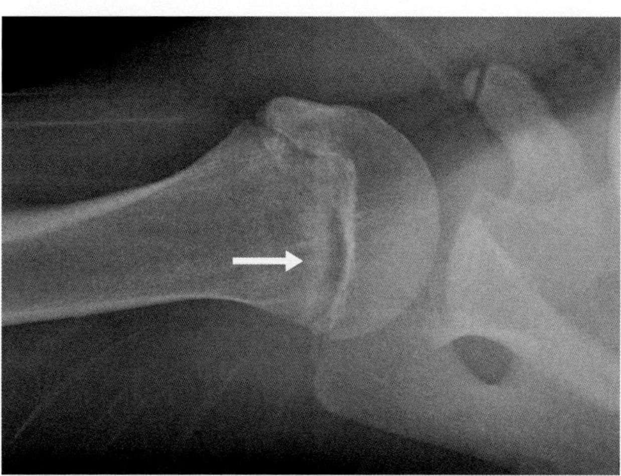

FIGURE 70.3. **Little League Shoulder.** Axillary radiograph of the right shoulder of a 15-year-old baseball pitcher. There is abnormal widening of the medial aspect of the proximal humeral physis with adjacent metaphyseal sclerosis (*arrow*) due to chronic trauma sustained in repetitive overhead motion. Comparison views with the asymptomatic shoulder may be useful in challenging cases.

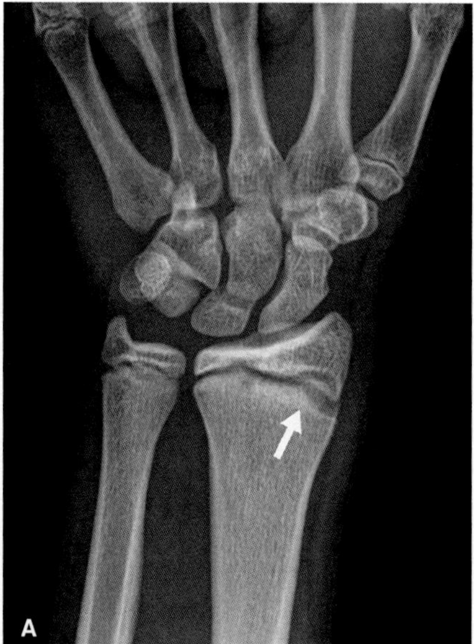

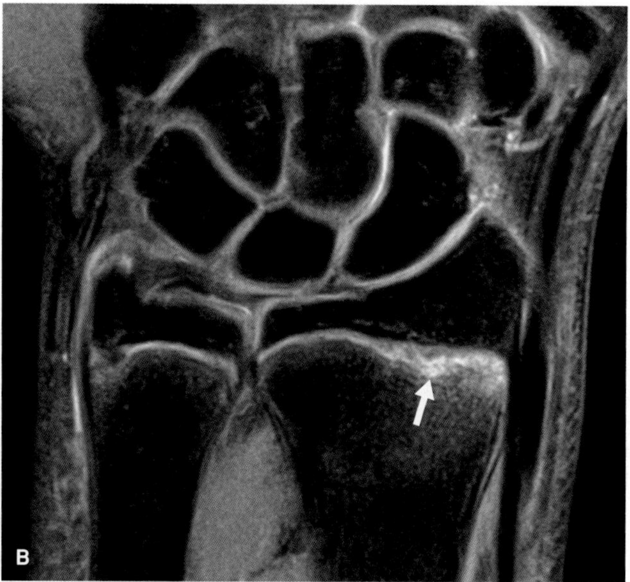

FIGURE 70.4. Gymnast Wrist. A 13-year-old female competitive gymnast with wrist pain. **A:** AP wrist radiograph demonstrates abnormal lateral distal radial physeal widening (*arrow*). On (**B**) coronal intermediate-weighted fat-saturated MR imaging, there is abnormal widening of the lateral aspect of the distal radial physis with widening of the zone of cartilage (*arrow*) due to repetitive trauma and interference with bone mineralization. Mild bone marrow edema is seen within the adjacent metaphysis.

bone interface. Apophyseal injuries are either due to repetitive submaximal stress on an apophysis ("traction apophysitis") or if a large force is placed on an apophysis, it may displace acutely, termed an apophyseal avulsion fracture.

Traction apophysitis causes microavulsions at the chondro-osseous junction with resultant secondary inflammatory changes that attempt to repair the physis leading to overgrowth. Common sites of apophysitis within the extremities and the pelvis are listed in (Tables 70.2 and 70.3). Traction apophysitis typically manifests radiographically as widening and irregularity at the physis (Fig. 70.6). Over time, irregular ossification/overgrowth can form at the tendinous insertion due to chronic stress injury at the chondro-osseous junction. On MR, there is often marrow edema within the apophysis with widening of the apophyseal physis. Adjacent soft tissue edema or bursal fluid is common.

Acute apophyseal injuries are common in active adolescents due to the inherent weakness of the apophyseal cartilage. They result from extreme, unbalanced, and often eccentric muscular

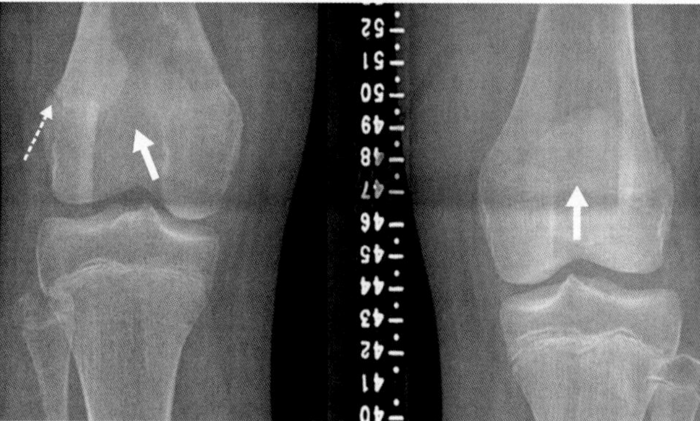

FIGURE 70.5 Bone Bar. AP scanogram radiographs of the knees in a 13-year-old girl with healed osteomyelitis of the right distal femur with injury to the distal femoral physis. There is a large bone bar within the central aspect of the distal right femur (*solid arrow*) with a small portion of open physis laterally (*dashed arrow*). The left knee is normal with visible distal femoral physis (*arrow*). There is associated foreshortening of the right femur compared with the normal left femur.

TABLE 70.2

COMMON SITES AND MECHANISM FOR TRACTION APOPHYSITIS WITHIN THE EXTREMITIES

■ LOCATION	■ TRACTION APPLIED
Medial epicondyle of the elbow	"Little League elbow" due to chronic valgus stress applied to the medial epicondylar apophysis in young baseball pitchers which causes medial elbow pain
Inferior patellar pole	"Sinding–Larsen–Johansson" syndrome resulting from excessive force exerted by the patellar tendon on the lower pole of the patella. Overuse syndrome in athletes which causes anterior knee pain
Tibial tuberosity	"Osgood–Schlatter" disease, pain at the anterior tibial tuberosity due to repetitive traction of the distal patellar tendon on the maturing anterior tibial tubercle
Base of the fifth metatarsal	"Iselin disease," traction of the peroneus brevis tendon on the base of the fifth metatarsal apophysis which presents with lateral foot pain
Calcaneus	"Sever disease," excessive traction of the Achilles tendon onto the calcaneal apophysis causing heal pain

TABLE 70.3

PELVIC SITES OF CHRONIC APOPHYSITIS AND ACUTE APOPHYSEAL INJURIES

■ LOCATION	■ MUSCLE/TENDON ATTACHMENT
Iliac crest	Abdominal musculature
Anterior superior iliac spine (ASIS)	Sartorius, tensor fasciae latae
Anterior inferior iliac spine (AIIS)	Rectus femoris muscle
Greater trochanter	Hip rotators
Lesser trochanter	Iliopsoas muscle
Ischial tuberosity	Hamstrings

contractions that result in severe pain and loss of function. Pelvic avulsion injuries occur at six sites (Table 70.3). The ischial tuberosity is the most common site, at the origin of the hamstring muscle group. In the acute setting, radiographs will typically demonstrate the sharply marginated piece of avulsed bone adjacent to its origin. MR may be needed to evaluate the degree of displacement of the avulsion fragment. It is not unusual for subacute/healing avulsion fractures to have an aggressive appearance on radiographs and MR and mimic processes such as tumor and infection, making history invaluable in the diagnosis.

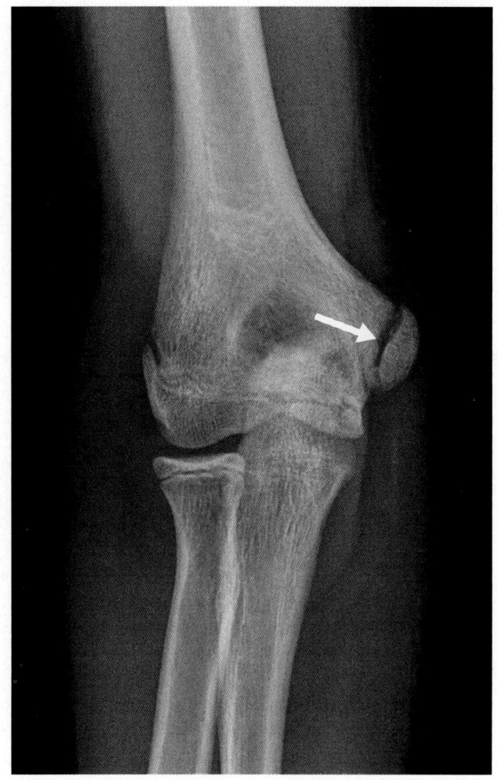

FIGURE 70.6. Medial Epicondylar Apophysitis. AP radiograph of the right elbow in a 13-year-old baseball pitcher with medial elbow pain. There is widening and irregularity of the physis adjacent to the medial epicondylar apophysis (*arrow*) consistent with trauma due to repetitive valgus stress.

Fractures Unique to Children

Upper Extremity. Clavicle fractures are the most common of all pediatric fractures. They may be seen in newborns as a result from birth trauma. The vast majority occur in the middle one-third of the bone. In children less than 13 years of age, direct impact to the shoulder may lead to a physeal fracture of the lateral clavicle, known as a "periosteal sleeve" fracture. In skeletally mature patients, this type of injury may cause separation of the acromioclavicular joint. Salter I and II fractures can also occur in the medial clavicle and must be distinguished from clavicular head dislocations. If clavicular head dislocation is suspected, CT scanning allows evaluation of displacement and assessment of vascular or other soft tissue injury.

Humerus fractures, not including injuries at the elbow, peak during adolescence secondary to increased sports participation and are most commonly Salter II fractures. Fractures typically heal well with immobilization by a sling. In the absence of significant trauma, one should consider pathologic fracture as the humerus is a common site for bone cysts and other benign lesions.

Elbow fractures represent approximately 10% of all fractures in children. In order to accurately diagnose injuries in the elbow, one must be familiar with the predictable pattern of normal elbow ossification (appearance of the ossification centers) which can be remembered with the mnemonic "CRITOE" (Table 70.4). The age of closure of the ossification centers is less predictable with estimated ages also provided in the table. In young children, supracondylar fractures are

TABLE 70.4

"CRITOE." AGE OF THE APPEARANCE AND PHYSEAL CLOSURE OF THE OSSIFICATION CENTERS OF THE ELBOW

■ OSSIFICATION CENTER	■ AGE OF APPEARANCE (IN YEARS)	■ AGE AT CLOSURE (IN YEARS)
C = capitellum	1	14
R = radial head	3	16
I = internal (medial) epicondyle	5	15
T = trochlea	7	14
O = olecranon	9	14
E = external (lateral) epicondyle	11	16

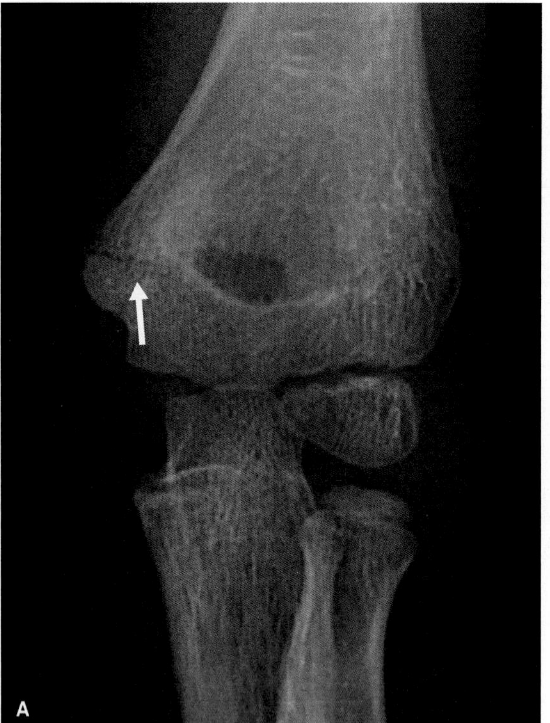

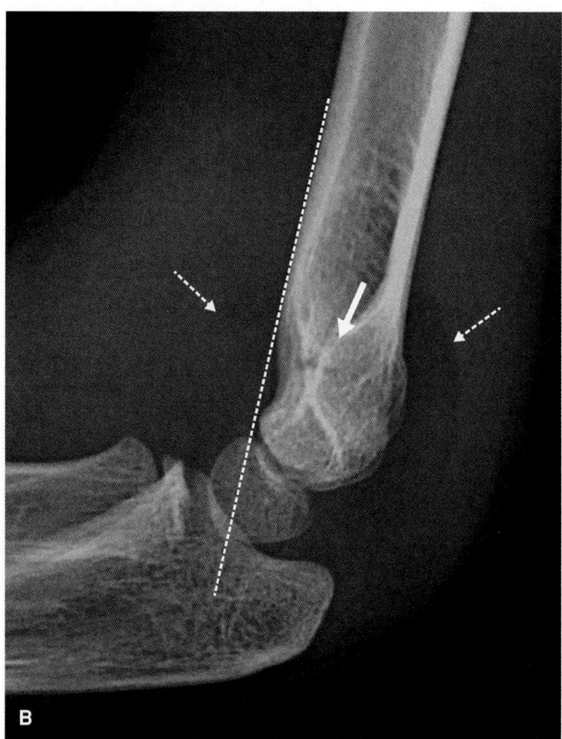

FIGURE 70.7. **Supracondylar Fracture.** AP (**A**) and lateral (**B**) radiographs of the elbow in a 7-year-old boy with elbow pain after falling backward onto his outstretched arm. **A:** There is incomplete fracture lucency seen within the distal humeral metaphysis (*arrow*). On the lateral view (**B**), the fracture is evident (*arrow*) along with elevation of the anterior and posterior fat pads consistent with posttraumatic hemarthrosis (*dashed arrows*). There is adjacent soft tissue swelling. The anterior humeral line (*dashed line*) is not displaced. The radiocapitellar alignment is maintained.

the predominant injury with a peak incidence at around 5 to 7 years. The most common mechanism is a FOOSH injury and the hyperextension load (e.g., fall from monkey bars) which causes the olecranon to be displaced posteriorly, causing stress on the thin and flimsy bone plate of the distal humerus. On a lateral radiograph, the classic figure-of-8 appearance of the distal humerus and the anterior humeral line should always be assessed and a joint effusion should be sought by looking for the "fat pad sign." In addition, in the normal elbow, the anterior humeral line (line drawn along the anterior cortex of the distal humerus) should bisect the middle third of the capitellum. In the setting of a supracondylar fracture, the capitellum is displaced posterior to the anterior humeral line (Fig. 70.7). In the setting of trauma and elbow pain, if no fracture is seen but a hemarthrosis is present ("fat pad sign" which reflects elevation of the fat pads that are displaced by fluid or blood products within the joint), conservative management is recommended with follow-up radiographs to evaluate healing of an occult fracture. The presence of a posterior fat pad is a stronger indicator of an occult fracture about the elbow compared to just uplifting of the anterior fat pad. Of note, occult fractures are seen in approximately 30% of patients on follow-up imaging. Supracondylar fractures have the highest rate of complications among upper extremity fractures. Complications include neurovascular compromise, compartment syndrome, Volkmann ischemic contractures, and cubitus varus.

Lateral condylar fractures traverse the intra-articular portion of the lateral condyle and extend to some degree into the nonossified epiphyseal cartilage of the lateral trochlear and intercondylar region or capitellum, making the extent of the injury greater than is radiographically seen. A lateral condylar fracture can be difficult to depict on AP view and may be better seen on external oblique view (Fig. 70.8). The degree of

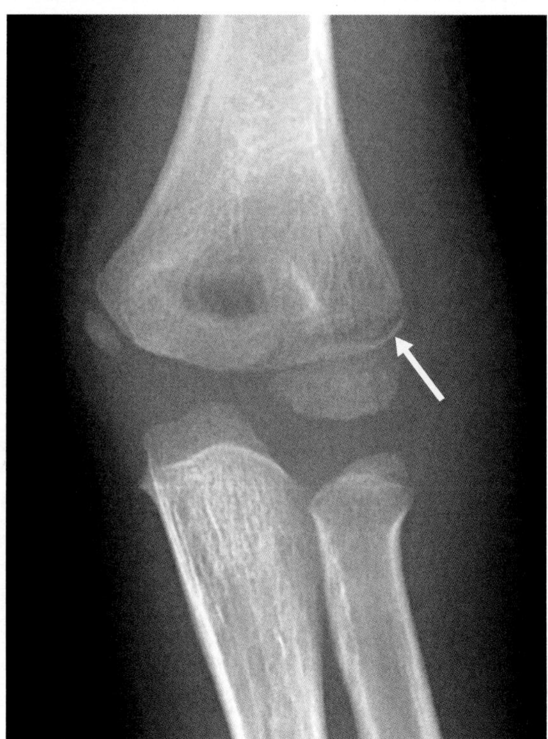

FIGURE 70.8. **Lateral Condylar Fracture.** Oblique radiograph of the elbow in a 6-year-old girl with elbow pain after a fall. There is a minimally displaced fracture involving the lateral condyle (*arrow*). Since the fracture was minimally displaced, the patient was treated with casting.

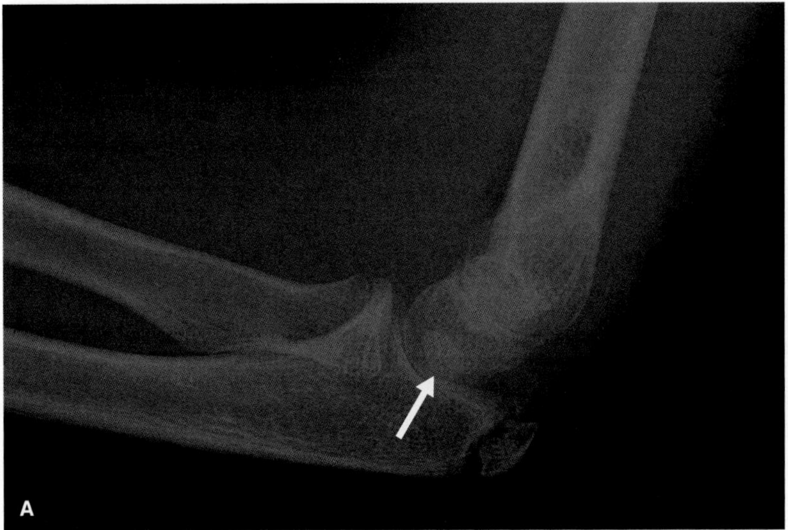

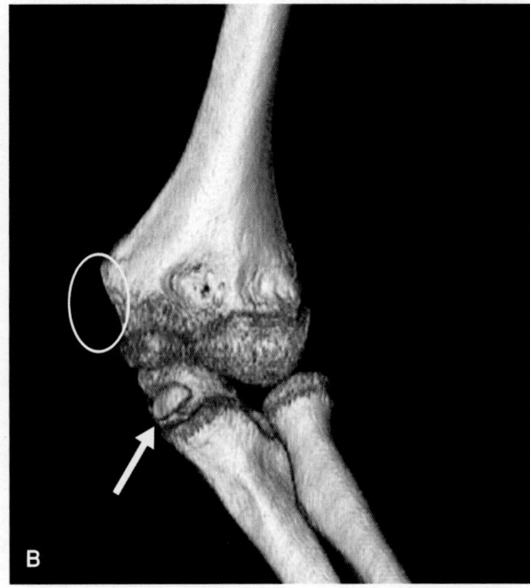

FIGURE 70.9. **Entrapped Medial Epicondylar Apophysis.** A 12-year-old boy with dislocation of the elbow and persistent pain. **A:** Lateral radiograph of the elbow demonstrates the entrapped epicondylar apophysis within the humeroulnar joint (*arrow*). **B:** 3D reconstructed CT image (obtained for surgical planning) demonstrates an absent medial epicondyle in the expected location (*oval*). The displaced apophysis is located within the ulnohumeral joint (*arrow*). The patient underwent open reduction and internal fixation.

displacement should be noted as this will impact the operative technique (i.e., open vs. closed reduction). In very young children, MR can be useful to assess fracture extension in unossified cartilage.

Acute medial condylar fractures make up about one-fifth of all elbow fractures and slightly more than half occur in the setting of elbow dislocation. Radiographs usually demonstrate a mildly displaced apophysis with variable degrees of physeal widening and epicondylar rotation. In challenging cases, comparison views may be useful. In the setting of elbow dislocation, the apophysis may become entrapped within the humeroulnar joint (Fig. 70.9). If a medial epicondylar apophysis is not seen in a child older than 6 to 7 years of age, close inspection of the elbow joint is needed. If the medial epicondyle is displaced greater than 5 mm, fractures require surgical fixation.

Less common fractures of the elbow include olecranon fractures and proximal radial metaphyseal fractures. Olecranon fractures are the most commonly missed elbow fractures. Proximal radial metaphyseal fractures are usually Salter–Harris II fractures that occur from a FOOSH mechanism with the elbow in extension and valgus.

Childhood forearm fractures are very common, comprising 40% to 50% of all fractures in children. The majority of fractures are located in the distal aspect of the forearm. As in adults, forearm fracture–dislocation injuries also occur: Monteggia and Galeazzi fractures with fracture of the ulna and dislocation of the radial head and radial fracture with disruption of the distal radioulnar joint, respectively.

Acute injuries to the wrist usually occur by a FOOSH injury. Since the carpal bones are largely cartilaginous, injuries typically result in fractures of the distal forearm. In older children, the most common carpal bone fracture is a scaphoid fracture which is important to recognize due to the risk of avascular necrosis (AVN) and is treated similarly to adults. Hand injuries are common but seldom complicated. One common injury is a phalangeal buckle fracture which may be subtle and oblique radiographs are often useful.

Lower Extremity. Slipped capital femoral epiphysis (SCFE) is a physeal injury of the proximal femur in which the femoral metaphysis displaces anteriorly, superiorly, and laterally with respect to the epiphysis. Patients report hip pain, medial thigh pain, and/or knee pain with an insidious onset of limp and decreased range of hip motion. It is more common in boys and mainly occurs between 10 and 16 years of age. Additional risk factors include obesity, hypothyroidism, low growth hormone levels, trisomy 21, and other endocrine disorders. Approximately 20% of patients have bilateral involvement at the time of presentation and an additional 20% to 40% will progress to asynchronous slips within 18 months of the initial SCFE. Therefore, radiographs should include the entire pelvis in both the frontal (AP) and frog-leg lateral positions.

The frog-leg lateral is the most sensitive radiographic projection, as the slipped epiphysis moves posteriorly and to a lesser extent, more medially. Typical radiographic signs of SCFE may include widening and irregularity of the proximal femoral physis, relative loss of height of the epiphysis on the AP projection, loss of the anterior concavity of the femoral neck, the metaphyseal "blanch sign" (crescent-shaped area of increased density at the proximal and medial femoral neck as a result of the projection of the posterior portion of the femoral head), and metaphyseal cystic change in chronic cases. "Kline's line" is drawn along the superior margin of the femoral neck. In normal hips, this line will intersect the lateral aspect of the epiphysis. In SCFE, the epiphysis is displaced medially and Kline's line does not intersect the epiphysis or intersects more laterally compared with the asymptomatic side (Fig. 70.10). In patients with equivocal radiographs, MR can be useful, particularly in "preslip" SCFE in which there is imminent slip as demonstrated by widening of the physis and periphyseal bone marrow edema. This is often associated with a joint effusion and reactive synovitis.

In cases of mild or moderate SCFE, in situ pinning is performed. Depending on the patient's age and risk factors, the asymptomatic hip may be prophylactically pinned due to increased risk of slippage. In more severe cases of SCFE, patients may undergo open reduction with gentle manipulation of the head of the femur back into its normal anatomic location, followed by screw fixation. The most common complications following SCFE are AVN and chondrolysis. Continued follow-up radiographic evaluation is necessary as evidence of AVN may not be depicted for up to 12 months following surgery.

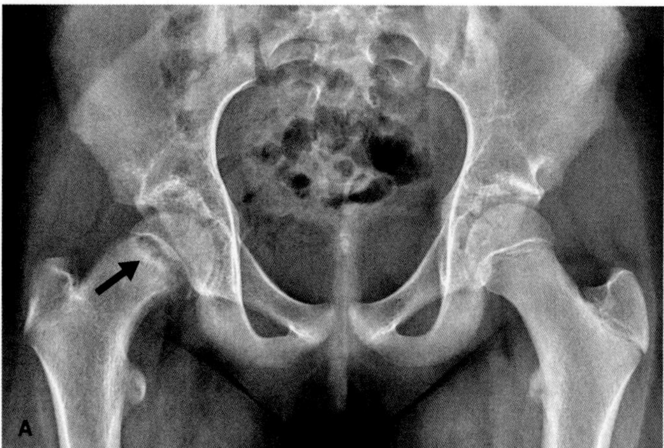

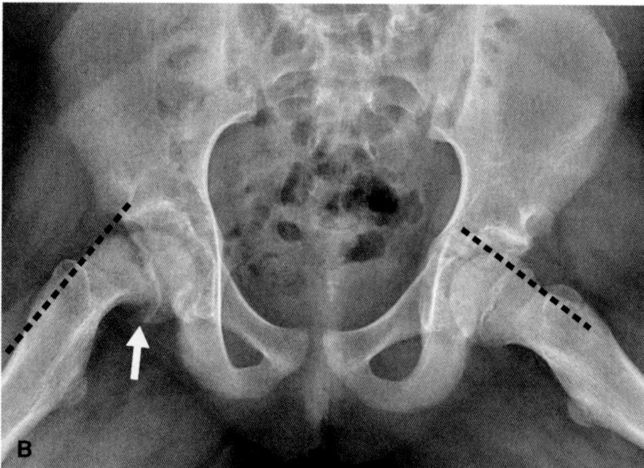

FIGURE 70.10. **Slipped Capital Femoral Epiphysis.** AP (**A**) and frog-leg lateral (**B**) radiographs of the hips in an obese 11-year-old girl with right hip pain. **A:** There is abnormal widening and lucency of the right proximal femoral physis (*arrow*) with adjacent metaphyseal sclerosis, as compared with the normal, asymptomatic left hip. There is relative loss of height of the right proximal femoral epiphysis as compared with the left. On the frog-leg view (**B**), the right hip demonstrates medial (and posterior) slippage of the proximal femoral epiphysis with respect to the metaphysis (*arrow*). The Kline's line (*dashed lines*) does not intersect the epiphysis on the right; however, intersects the lateral aspect of the epiphysis in the normal left hip. The patient underwent in situ pinning of the right hip with prophylactic pinning of the asymptomatic left hip.

Patellar sleeve fractures occur when the cartilage of the inferior pole of the patella is pulled off from the inferior patellar pole, often with a small avulsed osseous fragment. Radiographs may show a small bone fragment inferior to the lower pole of the patella, patella alta, and a joint effusion. The extent of cartilaginous and soft tissue injury is often severely underestimated; thus MR is generally obtained to evaluate the full extent of injury (Fig. 70.11).

Tibial spine avulsion fractures or tibial eminence fractures are seen in children 8 to 13 years of age and are usually sports-related injuries occurring especially during cycling or skiing. The cause is thought to be due to relative weakness of the incompletely ossified tibial eminence compared to the stronger anterior cruciate ligament (ACL) fibers. During hyperextension injuries, traction forces along the ACL cause avulsion of the tibial spine. AP and lateral radiographs of the knee are useful in depicting the fracture fragment and the degree of displacement. Notch views can supplement in challenging cases. In skeletally immature patients, the actual size of the fragment may be significantly larger than what it appears to be on radiographs due to the presence of cartilage in the fragment. MRI is useful in evaluating the nonosseous concomitant injuries as well as assessing obstacles for reduction such as entrapment of the transverse intrameniscal ligament (Fig. 70.12). Treatment is based on the amount of displacement and the presence of additional intra-articular injuries.

Tibial tubercle fractures are most commonly seen in teenage boys and the injury usually involves active extension of the knee with vigorous contraction of the quadriceps muscles, typically in jumping sports. Clinical history and physical examination findings are often useful in distinguishing an acute injury from a chronic repetitive injury (i.e., Osgood–Schlatter disease). Radiographs are usually adequate to determine if just the tubercle is involved or if there is fracture extension into the epiphysis as well as the degree of displacement and comminution (Table 70.5). Fractures confined to the tubercle can be managed conservatively; however, fractures that extend into the epiphysis require surgical fixation.

Fractures of the proximal tibial metaphysis can occur due to axial loading injuries sustained by young children jumping on trampolines or in similar environments such as bounce houses, generally with another larger child/adult. These fractures, termed "trampoline fractures," are usually a nondisplaced and nonangulated linear or buckle fracture of the proximal tibial metaphysis and can be quite subtle (Fig. 70.13).

The tibial "toddler's fracture" is a nondisplaced oblique fracture of the distal tibia that typically presents in children

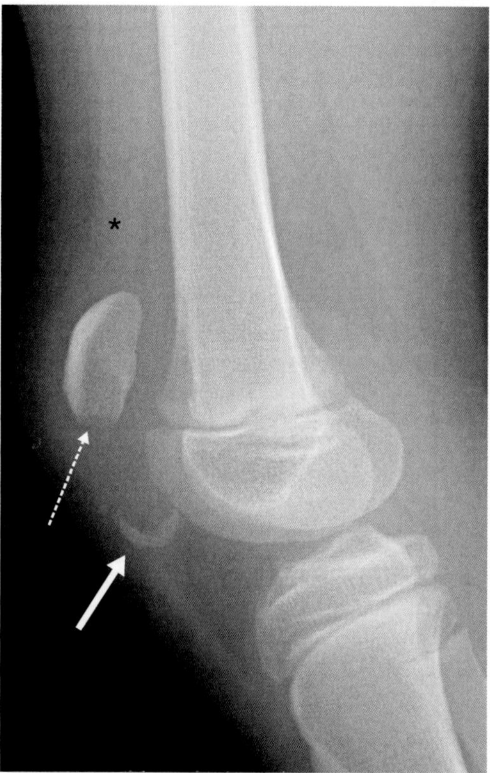

FIGURE 70.11. **Patellar Sleeve Fracture.** An 8-year-old boy with knee pain and swelling after soccer injury with inability to bear weight. Lateral radiograph of the knee demonstrates a displaced osseous avulsion injury of the inferior patellar pole (*arrow*) with adjacent soft tissue edema. Donor site of the inferior patella (*dashed arrow*). The patella is high riding with redundancy of the quadriceps tendon (*). The patient underwent open reduction and internal fixation.

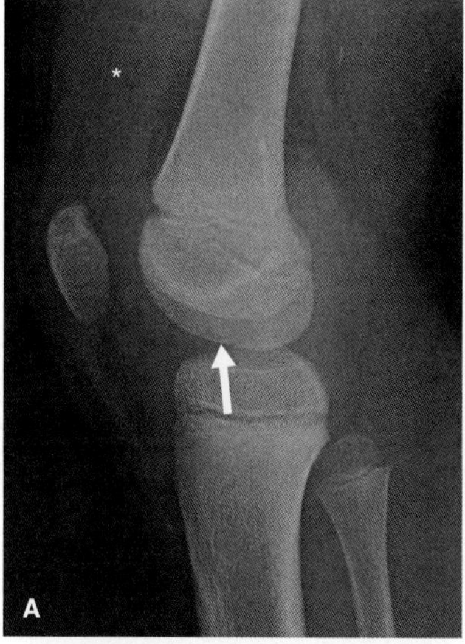

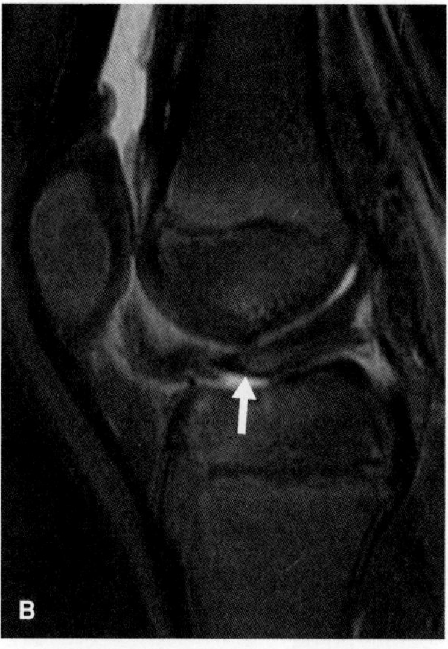

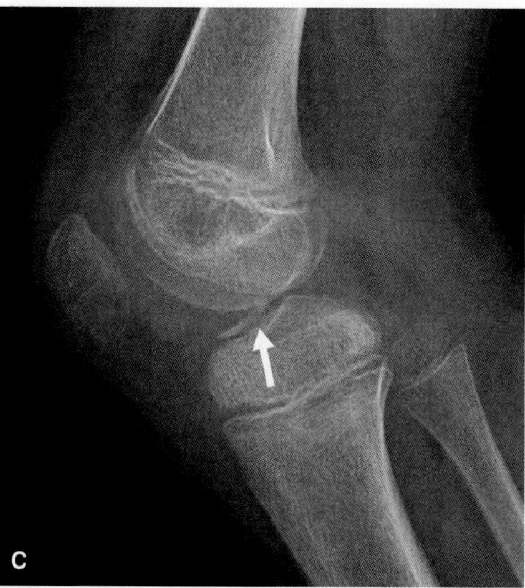

FIGURE 70.12. **Tibial Spine Avulsion Fracture.** An 8-year-old boy with knee pain immediately after being tackled from behind while playing football, who sustained a hyperextension knee injury. **A:** Initial lateral knee radiograph demonstrates a joint effusion (*) with a subtle linear density superior to the tibial epiphysis (*arrow*) in keeping with an avulsion fracture of the tibial spine. **B:** Sagittal T2-weighted fat-saturated MR image obtained 2 days later better demonstrates the avulsion of the cortex of the tibial spine, at the ACL attachment (*arrow*). There is adjacent bone marrow edema and no interposed structures between the fracture fragment and fracture bed. **C:** The child was treated conservatively with casting, and follow-up radiograph of the knee obtained 3 weeks later shows increased ossification of the fracture fragment with early bridging (*arrow*). The joint effusion has decreased and there is interval disuse demineralization.

between 1 and 4 years of age. The nature of the trauma is usually mild, such as twisting injury from tripping while walking or running or fall from a modest height. Since children at this age are often unable to provide a history, it is common that no history of trauma can be elicited. Often, there is no bruising or focal tenderness and children are nonweight bearing. Conventional radiographic findings are often subtle with a faint oblique line crossing the distal tibial shaft, terminating medially (Fig. 70.14). An oblique projection is more sensitive in depicting the fracture line. Radiographs, however, can be normal. Young children with an acute onset of limp, refusal to bear weight and normal radiographs should be casted with follow-up radiographic examination to evaluate for signs of healing. Much less commonly, these injuries can affect the fibula.

TABLE 70.5

CLASSIFICATION OF TIBIAL TUBERCLE FRACTURES ACCORDING TO THE OGDEN CLASSIFICATION (WITH MODIFICATION)

■ TYPE	■ DESCRIPTION
Ia	Fracture of the distal aspect of the tibial tubercle near the patellar tendon insertion
Ib	The fragment is displaced anteriorly and proximally
IIa	Fracture extends through the junction of the ossification of the proximal end of the tibia and the tubercle
IIb	Tubercle fragment is comminuted
IIIa	Fracture extends to the joint and is associated with discontinuity of the joint surface
IIIb	Tubercle fragment is comminuted

Distal tibial transitional fractures, the triplane and Tillaux fractures, are the second most common physeal injuries in children. They are only seen in adolescents, generally between 10 and 16 years of age, when the physis closes in an asymmetric pattern. The distal tibial physeal closure begins centrally and then proceeds in an anteromedial direction, then posteromedially, and finally laterally, which predicts the specific injury pattern.

Triplane fractures are Salter IV fractures and have sagittal, transverse, and coronal components traversing the physis. AP radiographs will show the epiphyseal component and the lateral radiograph will demonstrate the metaphyseal component (Fig. 70.15). Juvenile Tillaux fractures are isolated to the anterolateral portion of the distal tibial epiphysis, a Salter III injury. Tillaux fractures are seen in teenagers nearing skeletal maturity, affecting the only remaining portion of the distal tibial physis. AP radiographs demonstrate a vertical fracture line within the distal tibial epiphysis extending laterally. The lateral radiograph will show an avulsed fragment displaced anteriorly (Fig. 70.16). Triplane and Tillaux fractures that are displaced more than 2 mm typically need surgical reduction and CT is often used for presurgical planning.

Stress fractures or fatigue fractures from repetitive stress injury can be seen within the tibia and fibula in children. Tibial stress fractures usually involve the proximal third of the bone and are more common posteriorly. Stress fractures may involve any part of the diaphysis. Occasionally, cortical disruption with linear lucency may be seen in the setting of repetitive trauma. Periosteal reaction, or focal cortical thickening, of the long bone may be indicative of a healing stress reaction. As in adults, MR is a more sensitive modality for assessing stress injuries, particularly in the acute setting. Insufficiency fractures are uncommon in active young children; however, can be seen in adolescents with the so-called "female athlete triad": osteoporosis, amenorrhea, and eating disorders.

Metatarsal and tarsal bones injuries are an important cause of foot pain in the young child. Impaction injuries of the hindfoot in toddlers can cause nondisplaced or buckle-type fractures of the talus or calcaneus. Nondisplaced cuboid fractures

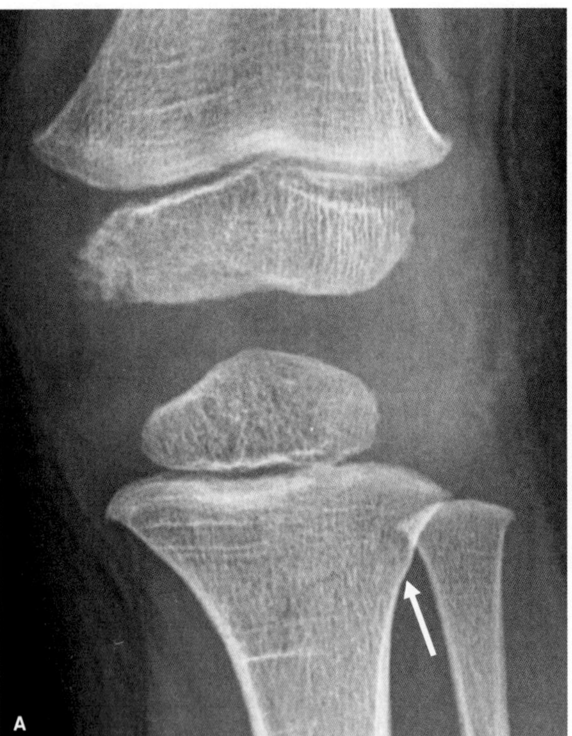

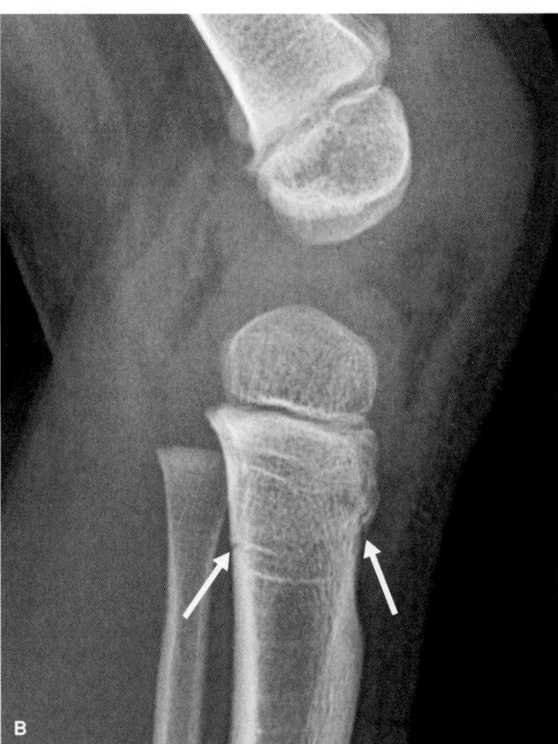

FIGURE 70.13. **Trampoline Fracture.** A 3-year-old with inability to bear weight on the left leg after playing on a trampoline. **A:** AP radiograph of the knee demonstrates a subtle buckle fracture along the lateral aspect of the proximal tibial metaphysis (*arrow*). **B:** Lateral radiograph demonstrates a transverse, nondisplaced fracture of the proximal tibial metaphysis with adjacent soft tissue swelling (*arrows*). This is a common location for lower extremity axial loading injuries in children.

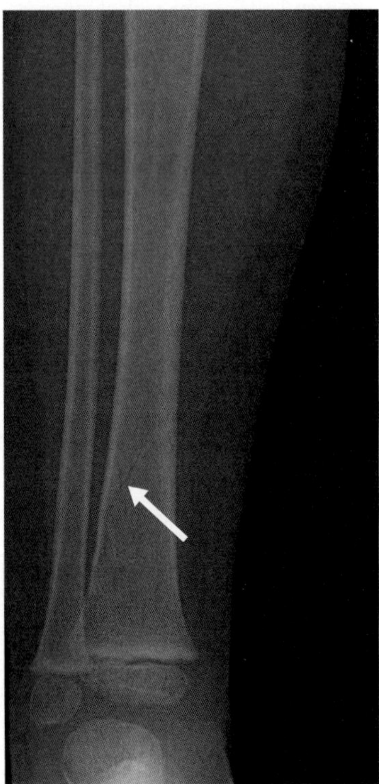

FIGURE 70.14. **Toddler's Fracture.** A 4-year-old boy with limp after sliding down a playground slide while seated on his mom's lap. There is a nondisplaced fracture of the distal tibial diametaphysis (*arrow*). The mechanism of injury was likely that the child's leg was caught and twisted along the side of the slide as weight of the parent was applied to the child's leg.

may occur in young children with forced plantar flexion of the foot, with compression of the cuboid and the fourth and fifth metatarsals. While the initial radiographs are typically normal, follow-up radiographs will demonstrate linear sclerosis along the base or distal aspect of the cuboid (Fig. 70.17). Metatarsal fractures are common and can result from either impaction injuries or when twisting forces are applied to the foot. A common fracture is a first metatarsal fracture or "bunk bed fracture" which is sustained when a child falls or jumps from a height (vertical loading with plantar flexion) and there is buckle injury of the proximal aspect of the metatarsal.

Osteochondral Injuries

Ostoechondral lesions (OCLs) are caused by an acute injury or repetitive microtrauma that leads to thinning of the articular cartilage, fragmentation of the subchondral bone, and occasionally, loose bodies. The most common locations for OCLs are the weight-bearing regions of the femoral condyles, the capitellum of the elbow in the throwing athlete and gymnasts, and the ankle (Table 70.6). Affected children frequently complain of pain, swelling, and locking. Conventional radiographs typically demonstrate a radiolucent region in the subchondral bone with or without fragmentation. Associated findings include joint effusion and loose bodies. Radiographs alone are unable to evaluate the stability of the fragment and the presence of loose cartilaginous fragments. MR imaging is the preferred modality. Ancillary MR imaging findings of instability in adults are less reliable in children with a rim of high SI surrounding the fragment on T2-weighted images, sensitive but not specific; fracture of the articular cartilage overlying the lesion, moderately sensitive and specific; and the presence of associated cysts or a fluid-filled defect beneath the fragment,

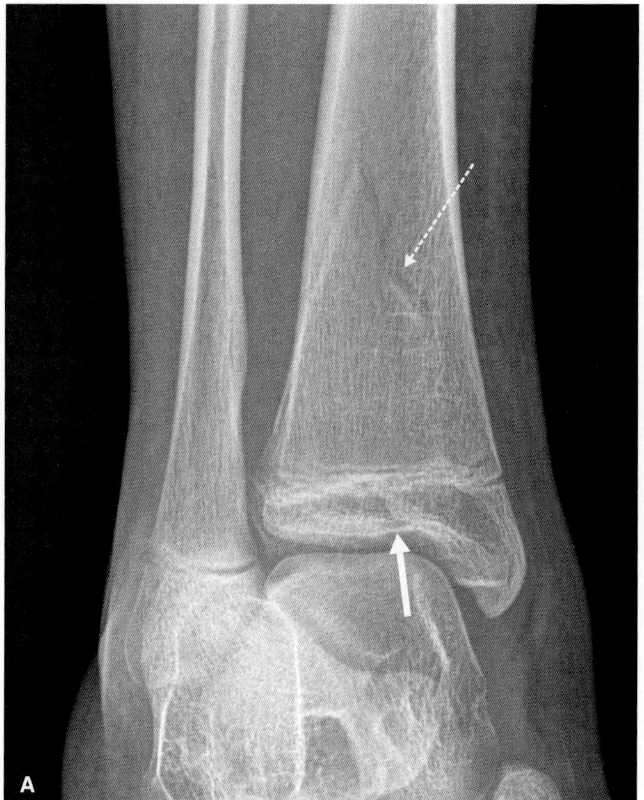
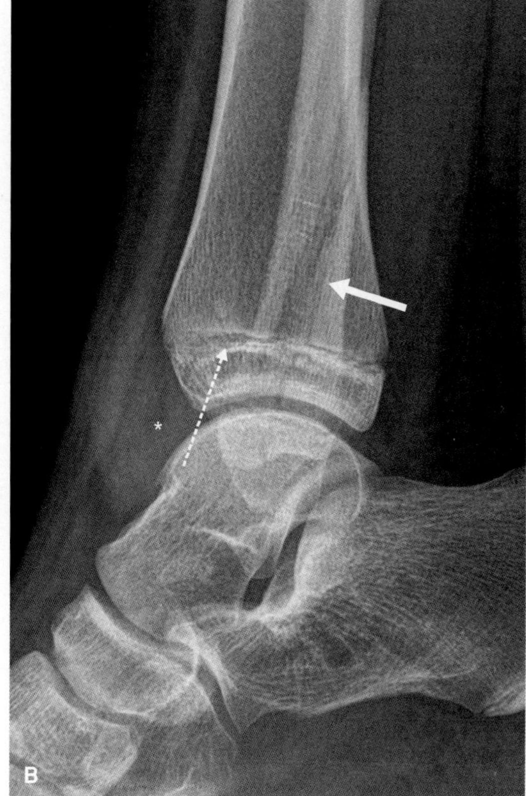
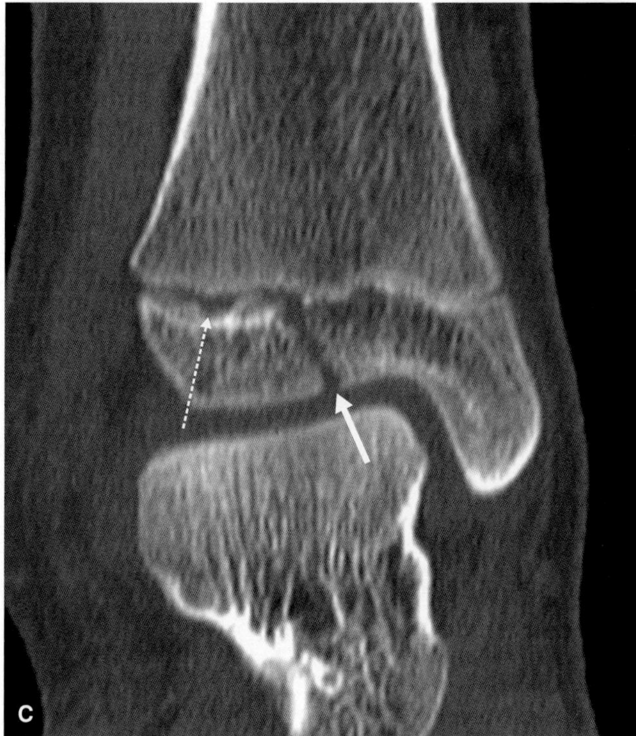

FIGURE 70.15. **Triplane Fracture.** A 12-year-old girl with ankle pain and swelling after softball injury. **A:** AP radiograph of the ankle shows a subtle Salter III fracture of the distal tibial epiphysis (*solid arrow*) with fracture lucency within the distal tibial metaphysis in the coronal plane (*dashed arrow*). **B:** Lateral radiograph of the ankle demonstrates that the metaphyseal fracture is a Salter II fracture (*solid arrow*) with widening of the distal tibial physis anteriorly (*dashed arrow*). There is a joint effusion (*). **C:** Coronal reformatted CT of the ankle better demonstrates the Salter III component (*solid arrow*) as well as the lateral physeal extension (*dashed arrow*).

insensitive but highly specific. Recent OCL studies in skeletally immature patients show that a high rim SI surrounding a lesion predicts instability of the fragment if it is associated with an outer rim of low T2 SI, prominent fragmentation of the subchondral bone, or if the SI is similar to that of joint fluid. Also, cysts surrounding the osteochondral fragment predict instability if they are numerous or large (Fig. 70.18).

Osteochondroses

Osteochondroses or "bone-cartilage conditions" are common in the young children and comprise a heterogeneous group of injuries to the epiphyses, physis, and apophyses. Osteochondroses result from a disturbance in endochondral ossification and are typically self-limited. Rapid growth, genetics,

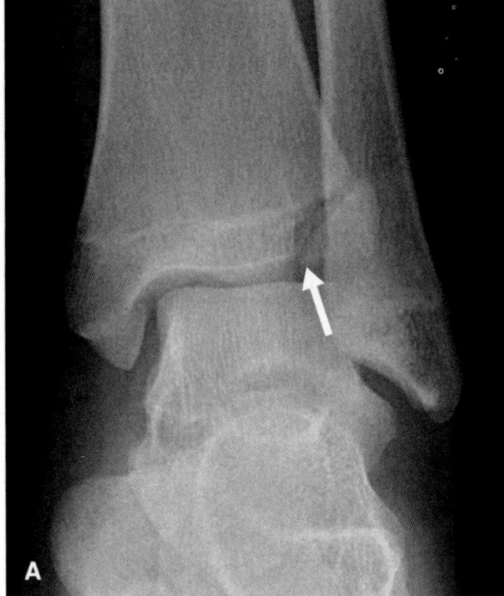

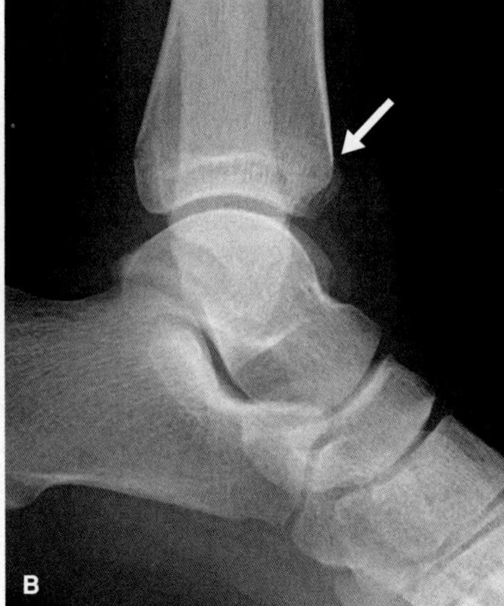

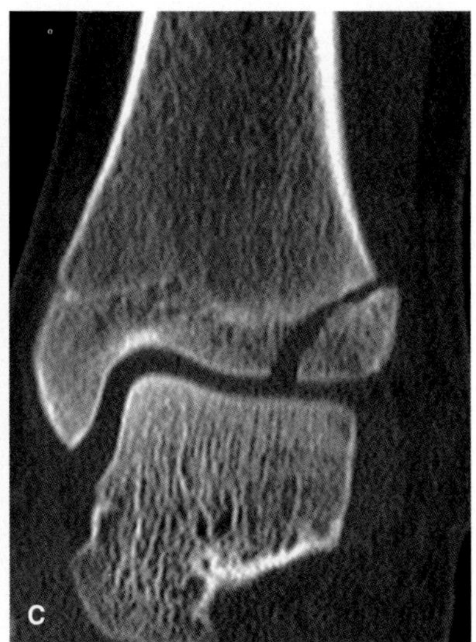

FIGURE 70.16. **Tillaux Fracture.** A 12-year-old female cheerleader with ankle injury after a fall. **A:** AP radiograph of the ankle shows a Salter III fracture of the lateral aspect of the distal tibial epiphysis with mild lateral displacement (*arrow*). The central, medial aspect of the physis has already closed. **B:** Lateral ankle radiograph demonstrates mild anterior displacement of the fracture fragment (*arrow*). There is an associated joint effusion. **C:** Coronal CT reformatted image more accurately demonstrates the degree of fracture displacement (5 mm) and the patient underwent screw fixation.

anatomic considerations, trauma, diet, and a defect in vascular supply are proposed etiologies. Osteochondroses follow a unique series of events: necrosis of the bone, revascularization, reorganization with granulation tissue formation and invasion, osteoclast resorption of necrotic segments, and ultimately osteoid replacement with mature lamellar bone formed.

FIGURE 70.17. **Cuboid Fracture.** A 6-year-old boy with persistent limp after falling down steps 1 week prior. AP radiograph of the foot demonstrates linear sclerosis at the base of the cuboid (*arrow*), in keeping with healing nondisplaced cuboid fracture. This type of fracture can also be seen along the distal aspect of the cuboid.

Legg–Calvé–Perthes Disease. Legg–Calvé–Perthes disease is an osteochondrosis of the femoral head and is a common cause of hip pain and limp in preadolescent children. There is a peak age of 5 to 6 years and it is five times more common in boys. This entity is idiopathic and most cases are unilateral with approximately 15% occurring bilaterally. When both hips are affected, it is usually an asynchronous course. Early in the course of disease, radiographs may demonstrate widening of the medial joint space (indicative of a joint effusion) and asymmetrically smaller femoral epiphysis of the affected side with sclerosis. The physis may become indistinct. Lucency may be seen within the femoral metaphysis. Over time, the epiphysis may begin to fragment and flatten (Fig. 70.19). Coxa magna of the femoral neck develops. MRI is used to evaluate the extent of disease and assess for revascularization of the femoral head. Early reperfusion of the lateral column is associated with improved prognosis. Prognostic indicators include the extent of osteonecrosis, amount of lateral extrusion, physeal involvement, and metaphyseal abnormalities. Physeal abnormalities and metaphyseal lucencies are

TABLE 70.6

LOCATIONS FOR OSTEOCHONDRAL LESIONS IN CHILDREN

LOCATION	COMMON OCL LOCATIONS
Knee	Lateral aspect of the medial femoral condyle, weight-bearing surface of the medial or lateral femoral condyle, patella, trochlea
Elbow	Capitellum, lateral aspect of the trochlea
Ankle/foot	Medial aspect of the talus, lateral aspect of the talus, central talar dome, distal tibia, subtalar facet, talar head

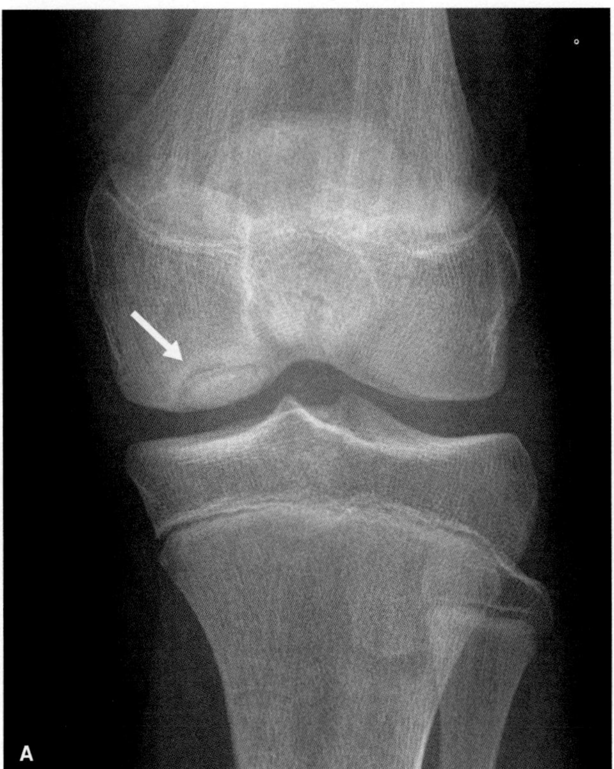

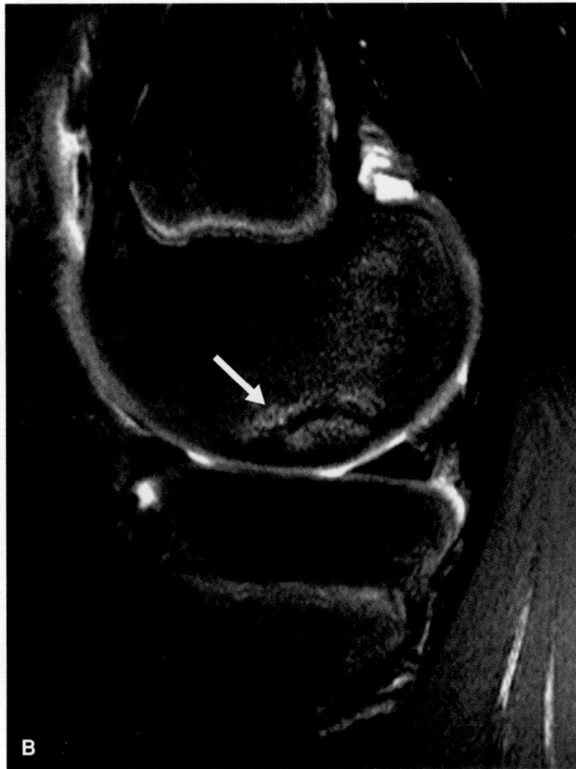

FIGURE 70.18. **Juvenile Osteochondral Lesion of the Knee.** A 14-year-old boy with knee pain. **A:** AP radiograph of the knee demonstrates an osteochondral lesion within the lateral aspect of the medial femoral condyle which is surrounded by lucency and mild amount of reactive sclerosis within the adjacent parent bone (*arrow*). **B:** Sagittal fluid-sensitive MR image of the knee shows the osteochondral lesion with adjacent marrow edema within the parent bone (*arrow*). The overlying cartilage is intact; there is no fluid signal undercutting the lesion nor are there "cystic" changes within the parent bone. The lesion can be classified as a "stable lesion."

indicative of subsequent growth disturbance. The younger the age at presentation, the more benign the course.

Panner Disease. Panner disease is a self-limiting osteochondrosis of the developing capitellum that affects children younger than 12 years. This is most commonly seen in baseball pitchers and falls into the spectrum of "little leaguers elbow." The cause is presumed to be repetitive chronic impaction injury to the tenuous blood supply of the capitellum. The entire capitellum is typically involved as opposed to osteochondral lesions of the capitellum seen in adolescents. Children typically present with dull elbow pain and stiffness. Conventional radiographs will demonstrate demineralization of the capitellum with loss of the normally sharp cortical margins, followed by sclerosis and loss of volume and ultimately progressing to frank fragmentation. On MR, the capitellum will demonstrate abnormal, low T1-weighted signal with variable T2-weighted signal depending on the stage of disease. The overlying articular cartilage is not affected and lesions typically heal with rest (Fig. 70.20). Unlike OCLs of the capitellum, Panner disease has an excellent prognosis.

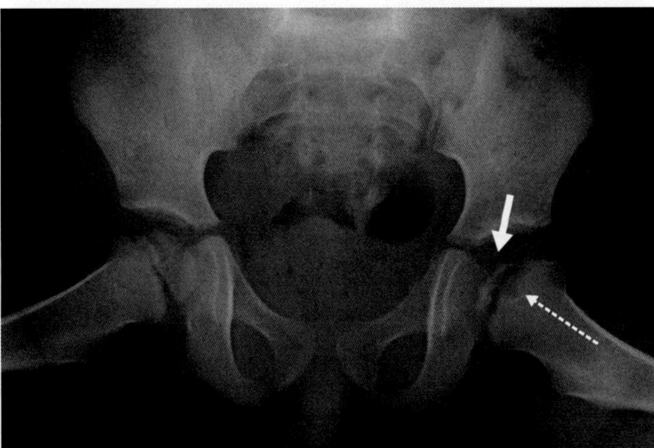

FIGURE 70.19. **Legg–Calvé–Perthes Disease.** AP frog-leg radiograph of the pelvis in a 6-year-old boy with left hip pain. There is fragmentation and severe flattening of the left proximal femoral epiphysis (*arrow*) with associated broadening of the metaphysis and metaphyseal lucency (*dashed arrow*). Lucency in the metaphysis represents tongues of cartilage from physeal damage and is associated with a poor outcome with increased risk of early physeal closure. The right hip is normal.

Köhler Disease. Köhler disease is an osteochondrosis of the tarsal navicular bone which occurs between 4 and 9 years of age with a higher prevalence in boys (6:1 ratio of boys to girls). Kohler disease may be bilateral in 25% of cases. This entity presents with midfoot pain and limp and symptoms usually increase with weight bearing and increased activity. Radiographs are diagnostic in the correct clinical setting and demonstrate sclerosis and narrowing/flattening of the tarsal navicular bone. Of note, this appearance can also be seen in asymptomatic children. MRI will demonstrate abnormal marrow signal within the navicular bone with T1-weighted low SI and either low or increased SI on fluid-sensitive sequences depending on the stage. Cortical irregularity, fragmentation, and adjacent soft tissue edema may be present and correlation with symptoms and site of pain is imperative. Most cases are treated conservatively with rest, ice, and analgesics.

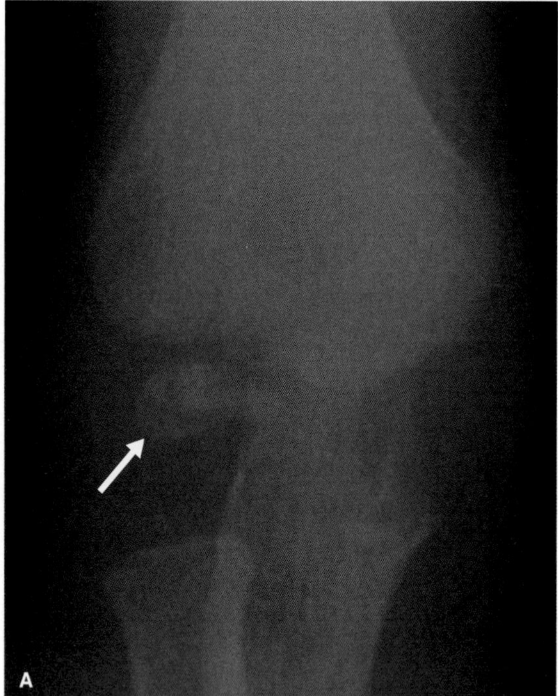

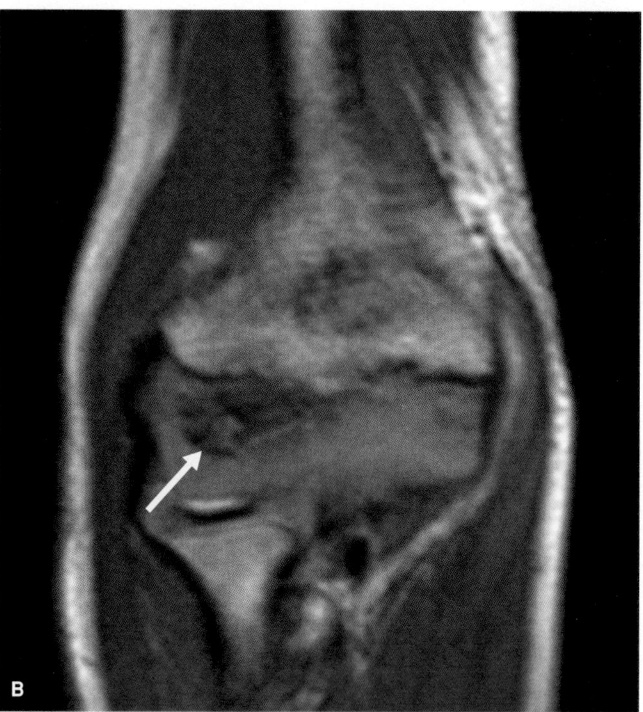

FIGURE 70.20. **Panner Disease.** A 7-year-old male baseball player with right elbow pain. **A:** AP radiograph of the elbow shows sclerosis and fragmentation of the capitellum (*arrow*). The cortical borders of the capitellum are not discrete. **B:** Coronal proton-density MR image demonstrates loss of the expected fat signal within the capitellum with areas of sclerosis (*arrow*). The articular cartilage is intact.

Freiberg's Infraction. Freiberg's infraction is an osteochondrosis of the metatarsal head and most commonly affects the second metatarsal head, followed by the third metatarsal head. Freiberg's infraction is most prevalent in athletic adolescent girls. Radiographs demonstrate widening of the metatarsophalangeal (MTP) joint with collapse and sclerosis of the metatarsal head. This may be associated with loose body formation, dorsal spurring, and consequent thickening of the metatarsal shaft, and CT may be useful for presurgical planning (Fig. 70.21). Treatment is usually symptomatic with avoidance of activities that load the foot or casting.

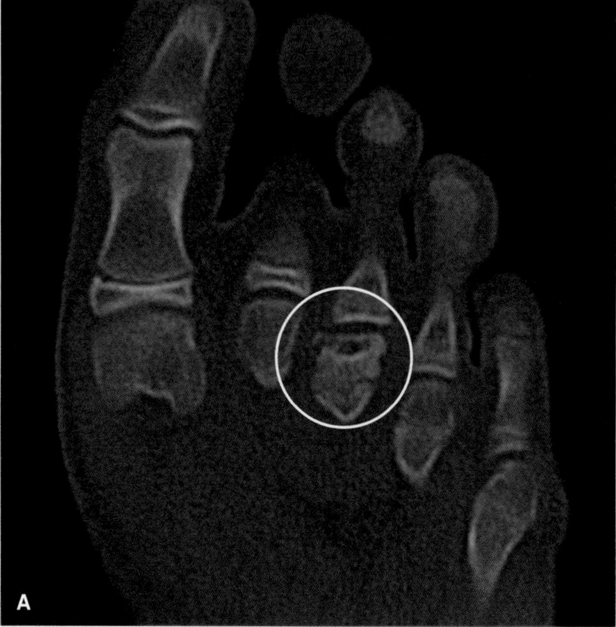

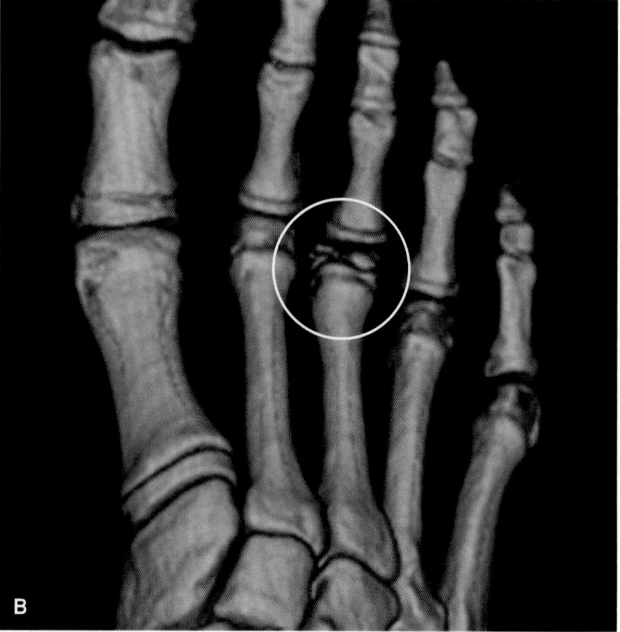

FIGURE 70.21. **Freiberg's infraction.** A 12-year-old male football kicker presents with tender bony lesion at the distal third metatarsal. **A:** Axial CT image and (**B**) 3D CT image of the forefoot demonstrate subchondral collapse of the third metatarsal with sclerosis and fragmentation (*circle*) with widening of the third MTP joint compatible with Freiberg's infraction.

NONACCIDENTAL TRAUMA

Almost 1 million children are harmed or endangered annually in the United States which results in 1,200 fatalities each year. The majority of children are less than 5 years of age, with almost half being less than 1 year old. Additional risk factors for abuse include multiple births, boys, stepchildren, prematurity, physical disability, low birth weight, and low socioeconomic status.

The clinical presentation of nonaccidental trauma (NAT) is often nonspecific. Imaging studies are crucial in the evaluation, particularly when the history of trauma is not given. Although skeletal injuries rarely pose a threat to the life of an abused child, they are the most common abuse-related injury aside from pure soft tissue injuries and are often the strongest radiologic indicator of abuse. Common patterns of injury can be seen at different stages of life. In infancy, skull fractures, rib fractures, and displaced metaphyseal injuries predominate. After 1 year of age, long bone injuries predominate. Fractures with a high specificity for abuse include classic metaphyseal lesions (CMLs); rib fractures, especially posterior; scapular fractures; spinous process fractures; and sternal fractures. Low-specificity, common radiographic findings include subperiosteal new bone formation, clavicular fractures, long bone shaft fractures, and linear skull fractures. At any age, multiple fractures seen in varied stages of healing, particularly with inconsistent histories, are highly suggestive of NAT. Underlying conditions such as metabolic bone disease, Caffey disease, osteogenesis imperfecta (OI), rickets, and bone fragility secondary to prematurity should be considered in the differential diagnosis.

The initial radiologic work-up in suspected child abuse should include a full skeletal survey with additional brain imaging as indicated (discussed elsewhere). Surveys should adhere to the American College of Radiology "Practice Guidelines for Skeletal Surveys in Children." Each anatomic region should be imaged with a separate radiologic exposure using high-detail imaging systems.

The most specific skeletal injury in the evaluation of child abuse is the "classic metaphyseal lesion" (CML). CMLs are also known as "corner fractures" or "bucket handle" fractures because of their distinct appearance. They are the most frequently encountered long bone injury in abused children and are commonly seen in the distal femora, proximal and distal tibiae, and the proximal humeri. They typically occur in children less than 2 year of age and are incurred by excessive traction and torsional forces. On frontal radiographs, the metaphyseal fragment will appear as a discrete triangular bony fragment ("corner fracture"). If the image is obtained in an angulated projection, curvilinear density will be evident, with separation of the peripheral margin of the metaphyseal fragment ("bucket handle") (Fig. 70.22). While there may be associated soft tissue swelling, bruising is often absent.

CMLs may heal without significant callus or subperiosteal new bone formation which makes dating assessment difficult. As CMLs heal, the fracture line becomes indistinct and there may be associated sclerosis or cortical thickening. After 4 weeks, CMLs will become inconspicuous and long-term sequelae are minimal. This warrants the need for follow-up skeletal surveys 2 weeks after the initial survey, as this will increase the sensitivity of depicting subtle or occult fractures.

Inflicted rib fractures are most commonly seen in infants and are often multiple and bilateral. The posterior or axillary portions of the rib are typically involved as the chest is squeezed during violent shaking of the infant. When force is placed in the AP dimension, stress is delivered to the ventral cortex of the posterior aspect of the rib which articulates with the transverse process, leading to a fulcrum effect and fracture.

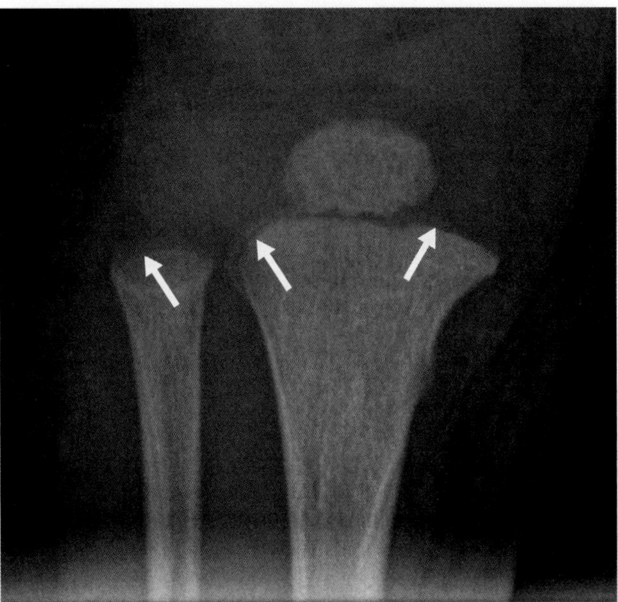

FIGURE 70.22. Nonaccidental Trauma, Classic Metaphyseal Fracture. A 2-month-old boy presenting with fever and displaced midshaft femur fracture. Skeletal survey was performed to evaluate for additional fractures. AP radiograph of the knee demonstrates bucket handle fractures of the proximal tibia and fibula with the metaphyseal fractures oriented along the plane of the physes (*arrows*). Since the image was obtained in an angulated projection, the peripheral margins of the metaphyseal fragments are evident giving rise to a handle-like appearance.

This stress also causes fractures along the lateral aspects of the ribs as the chest is being crushed (Fig. 70.23). Due to the inherit plasticity of ribs in children, rib fractures are not typically associated with cardiopulmonary resuscitation. In the acute setting, rib fractures may be difficult to depict, particularly if they are incomplete, nondisplaced, and oblique to the incident x-ray beam or involve the costovertebral junction. Oblique chest radiographs increase sensitivity for fracture depiction. Since rib fractures heal with sclerosis and callus formation, follow-up skeletal surveys become very important.

Diaphyseal fractures are abusive injuries commonly seen in the femur, humerus, and tibia. Long bone fractures result from direct trauma and are typically transverse. Spiral leg fractures in nonambulating patients are quite suggestive of NAT.

Vertebral fractures are rare in child abuse. Compression vertebral fractures are mainly caused by hyperextension and hyperflexion injuries incurred during shaking followed by direct impact against a hard surface. Common sites include injury at the thoracolumbar junction and lumbar spine. If vertebral fractures are suspected, injuries can be associated with paraspinal ligamentous and/or spinal cord injury and MR imaging should be obtained.

Skull fractures are common in both accidental and nonaccidental trauma, and unfortunately, there is no pattern of skull fracture that is specific for abuse. Features that are suggestive of NAT include bilateral fractures; fracture diastasis; fractures that cross sutures; stellate and depressed skull fractures, especially of the occiput (Fig. 70.23). Skull fractures typically do not heal with periosteal reaction or callus, which makes dating fractures difficult. The presence of a scalp hematoma may be useful as most will disappear after 3 to 4 days. However, it should be stressed that lack of scalp hematoma does not exclude a fracture and the absence of fracture is not predictive of intracranial injury.

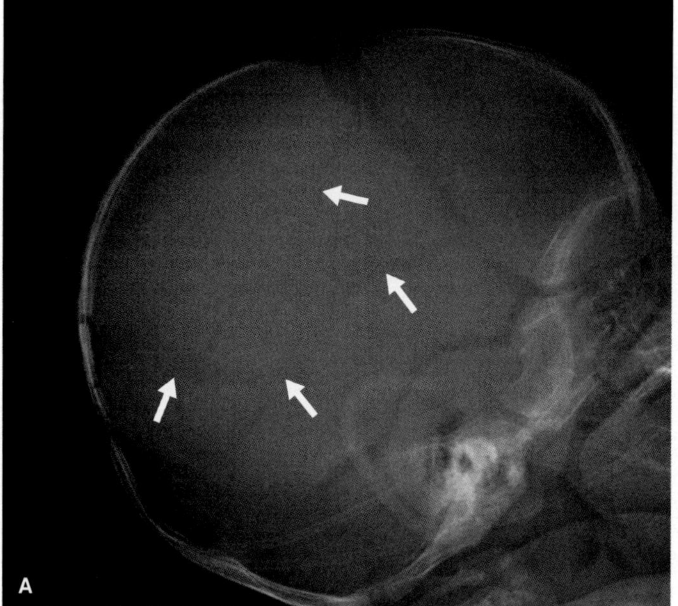

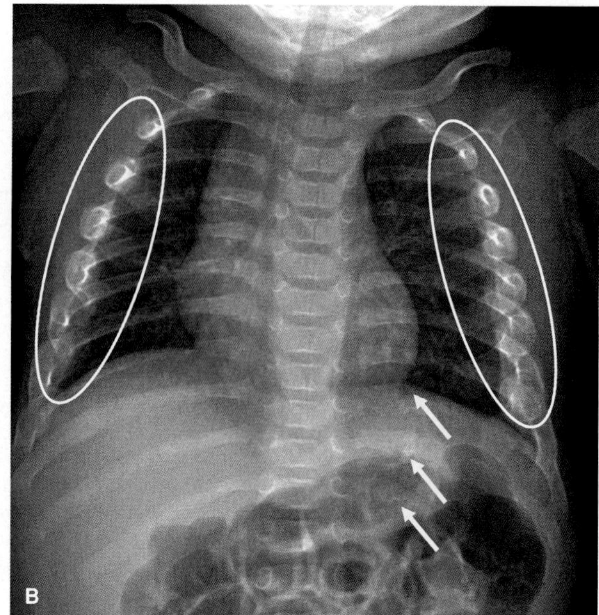

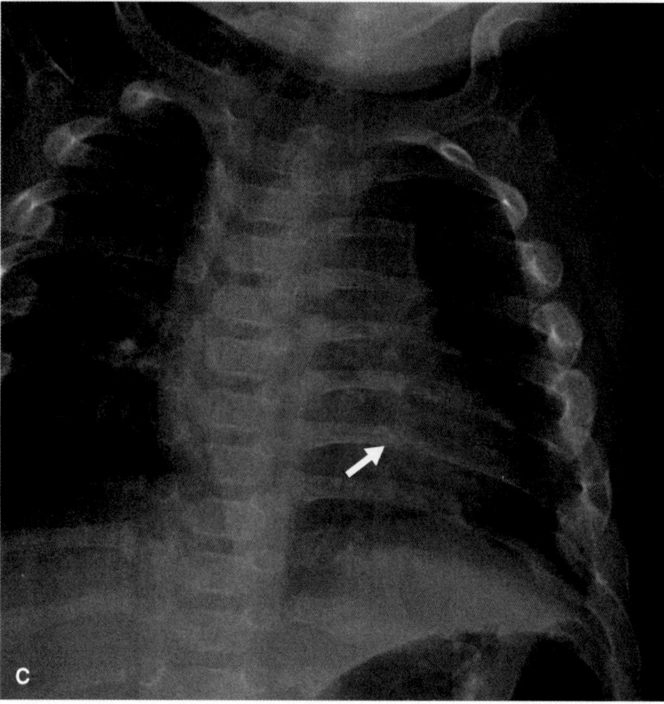

FIGURE 70.23. **Nonaccidental Trauma.** A 3-month-old girl presenting with seizures. **A:** Lateral radiograph of the skull demonstrates a comminuted left parietal fracture with displacement and extension into the left temporal and occipital bones (*arrows*) with an adjacent large scalp hematoma. **B:** Frontal view of the chest shows multiple healing bilateral lateral rib fractures with abundant callus (*ovals*) with adjacent pleural thickening as well as left posterior rib fractures (*arrows*). **C:** Oblique radiograph show the healing fractures along with an acute fracture of the left 7th posterior rib (*arrow*).

INFECTION

Acute Osteomyelitis

Infection involving the bone occurs by three major pathways: hematogenous, direct inoculation from trauma, and via extension from adjacent soft tissue infections. In children, acute osteomyelitis is most commonly acquired hematogenously with the most common organisms being *Staphylococcus aureus*, *β-hemolytic streptococcus* and *Streptococcus pneumoniae*, *Escherichia coli*, and *Pseudomonas aeruginosa*. In Europe, *Kingella kingae* has become a frequent organism in children less than 4 years of age.

Acute hematogenous osteomyelitis primarily involves the metaphyses of the long bones or metaphyseal equivalents (osseous regions adjacent to a physis) where organisms flourish in the slow-flowing venous sinusoids. This yields an exudative inflammatory response resulting in increased intraosseous pressure, edema, stasis of blood flow, and small vessel thrombosis which results in bone necrosis and absorption. Left untreated, this inflammatory process will perforate the cortex and uplift the periosteum, as it is loosely attached to bone, yielding subperiosteal abscesses and ultimately dissecting into the adjacent soft tissues. While it has been described that pyogenic metaphyseal osteomyelitis infrequently crosses the growth plate into the epiphysis beyond 2 years of age due to the obliteration of vascular channels crossing the physis, current literature demonstrates that transphyseal osteomyelitis is quite common in all age groups (Fig. 70.24).

Imaging plays a crucial role in diagnosis and management. Diagnosis is often delayed and multifocal involvement

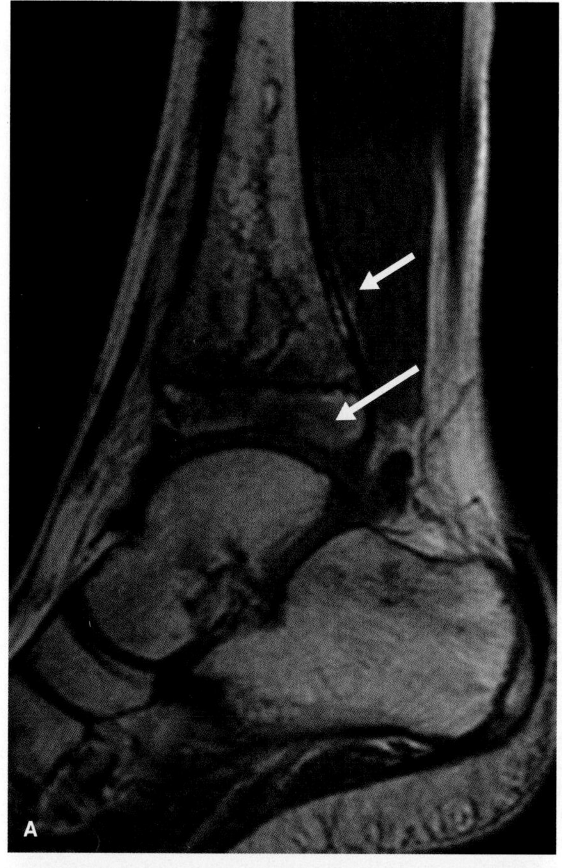

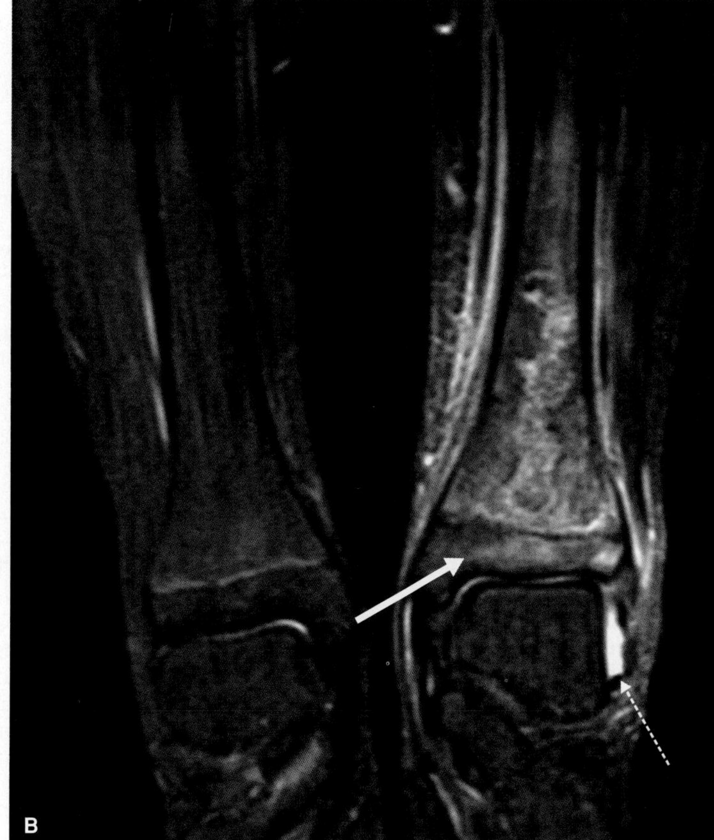

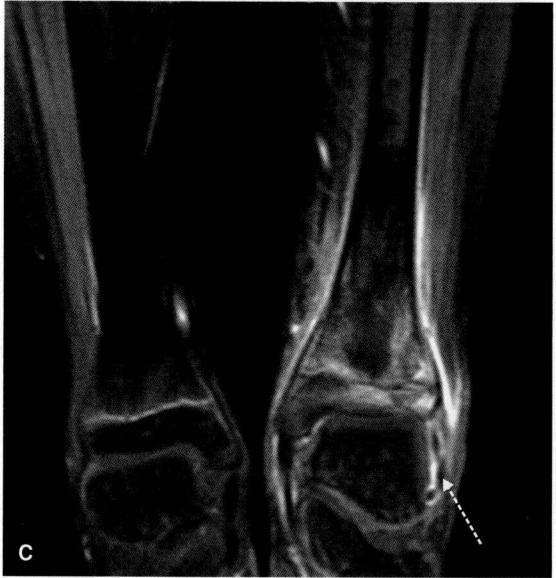

FIGURE 70.24. **Osteomyelitis.** A 10-year-old boy with ankle pain and swelling. **A:** Sagittal T1-weighted MR image of the left ankle and (**B**) coronal fluid-sensitive MR image of the ankles demonstrate patchy, abnormal low SI within the distal tibial metaphysis with adjacent soft tissue edema compatible with osteomyelitis with transphyseal extension (*long arrows*). There is mild uplifting of the periosteum of the posterior distal tibial metaphysis (*short arrow*) and a small ankle effusion (*dashed arrow*). **C:** Coronal T1-weighted fat-saturated postcontrast image of the ankles shows corresponding abnormal enhancement with mild synovitis (*dashed arrow*). The right ankle is normal for comparison.

is frequent. On conventional radiography, affected bones are typically normal early in the course of infection; however, radiographs may demonstrate obliteration of the fat planes, suggestive of deep soft tissue swelling. When using MR in children, large field of view coronal fluid-sensitive imaging can be useful as an initial survey sequence in children who cannot accurately locate their symptoms. Infected marrow will demonstrate hypointense signal on T1-weighted images and hyperintense signal on fluid-sensitive imaging. Post gadolinium, T1-weighted fat-suppressed imaging is useful in depicting intramedullary, subperiosteal, and soft tissue abscesses including pyomyositis. MR with contrast also plays an important role in imaging the neonate or young infant, as the epiphyseal cartilage can be infected with or without involvement of the adjacent bone. Without the use of gadolinium, infection isolated to epiphyseal cartilage may be undetectable. Most cases of epiphyseal osteomyelitis or chondritis occur in children younger than 4 years of age and are best demonstrated as avascular/nonenhancing regions of affected cartilage.

Complications of acute osteomyelitis include thrombophlebitis, which can be seen in up to 30% of cases and is typically associated with methicillin-resistant *S. aureus* (MRSA). Septic emboli to the lungs and brain can occur. Delayed complications include growth arrest due to bone bar formation, pathologic fracture, and chronic osteomyelitis.

Septic Arthritis and Toxic Synovitis

Septic arthritis may be caused by hematogenous bacterial seeding or by direct extension into the joint space in the setting of osteomyelitis or adjacent soft tissue infection. In the very young infant, multifocal involvement is common with the hip being the most frequent site. Ultrasound is a valuable screening tool to depict abnormal joint fluid; however, MRI is often used to evaluate for concomitant osteomyelitis. Imaging cannot reliably differentiate a reactive effusion (toxic synovitis) from septic arthritis. If there is clinical suspicion for an infected joint (elevated white blood count [WBC], elevated inflammatory markers, restricted motion or non-weight bearing, fever), emergent drainage and concomitant antibiotics are necessary.

Toxic synovitis, or transient/reactive synovitis, is a self-limited disease with no known long-term sequela. It is a common entity, particularly involving the hip in young children between 3 and 10 years of age. Children appear nontoxic and present with pain and limp and are usually afebrile with normal to marginally elevated WBC and inflammatory markers. Parents often report a preceding viral or bacterial upper respiratory or gastrointestinal illness (within 4 to 5 weeks). Ultrasound can confirm the presence of a joint effusion and give an indication of the complexity of the fluid and the severity of synovial thickening. Patients suspected of toxic synovitis are treated with rest and analgesics and symptoms begin to resolve within 24 to 48 hours. Joint aspiration is performed if there is concern for septic arthritis.

BONE LESIONS

Benign Bone Lesions

It is important to recognize the typical appearance of benign bone tumors in an effort to avoid unnecessary procedures. Many of the benign bone lesions found in children are described in the adult musculoskeletal sections of this text.

Osteochondroma. Osteochondromas are a very common benign tumor/tumor-like lesion of bone and occur in approximately 1% to 2% of the population. Osteochondromas are thought to represent a developmental defect of bone growth secondary to an injury to the perichondrium, rather than a true tumor. Physeal cartilage herniates through this defect and growth results in an osseous excrescence with continuity to the underlying medullary canal and cortex, with an overlying cartilaginous cap. The long bones of the lower extremity are the most commonly affected, with many found about the knee. Most osteochondromas are asymptomatic and found incidentally or with cosmetic deformity from the slowly growing lesion. Symptoms depend on the location of the lesion and relate to irritation of adjacent muscles, nerves, tendons, blood vessels, and even bones. Some can develop overlying adventitial bursa which may subsequently become inflamed, infected, or hemorrhagic. Although pain can occur with fracture of the osteochondroma, pain secondary to malignant degeneration is rare in children.

The radiographic hallmark of an osteochondroma is an osseous excrescence with continuity of the cortex and medullary space from the underlying bone into the osteochondroma. The shape of osteochondromas varies and they can be sessile with a broad area of continuity to the underlying bone or pedunculated with a narrow stalk. When pedunculated, the lesion usually points away from the nearest joint. Radiographs are usually diagnostic; however, CT and MRI can be used to confirm the diagnosis. MRI is particularly useful in confirming marrow continuity with the lesion and evaluating the effects on adjacent soft tissues, size of the cartilage cap, and to evaluate for bursa development. If the cartilaginous cap is more than 1.5 cm in thickness, the very rare transformation to chondrosarcoma should be considered. Treatment of osteochondromas involves resection of large and symptomatic lesions.

Multiple osteochondromas are seen in patients with hereditary multiple exostoses (HME), also known as familial osteochondromatosis or diaphyseal aclasis (Fig. 70.25). HME is autosomal dominant and usually manifests by 10 years of age.

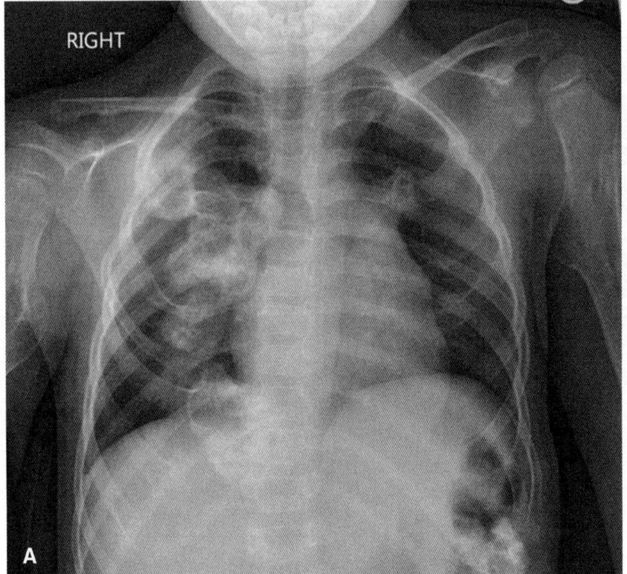

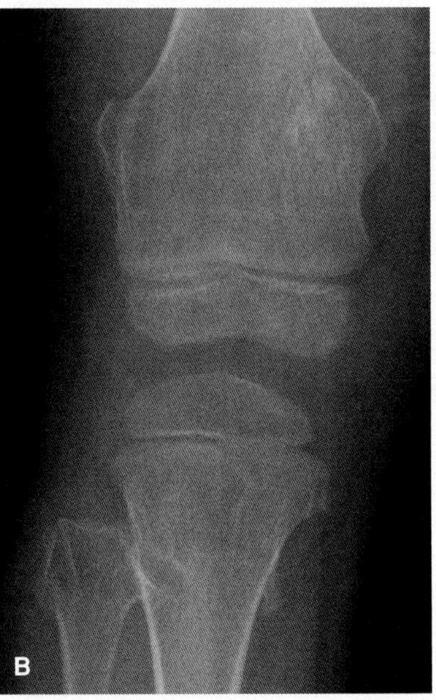

FIGURE 70.25. **Multiple Hereditary Exostoses.** A 4-year-old girl with multiple sessile and pedunculated osteochondromas. **A:** Frontal radiograph of the chest with sessile osteochondromas about both proximal humeri as well as multiple lesions seen along the anterior ribs. **B:** AP radiograph of the knee demonstrating additional osteochondromas seen about the distal femur and proximal tibial metaphyses.

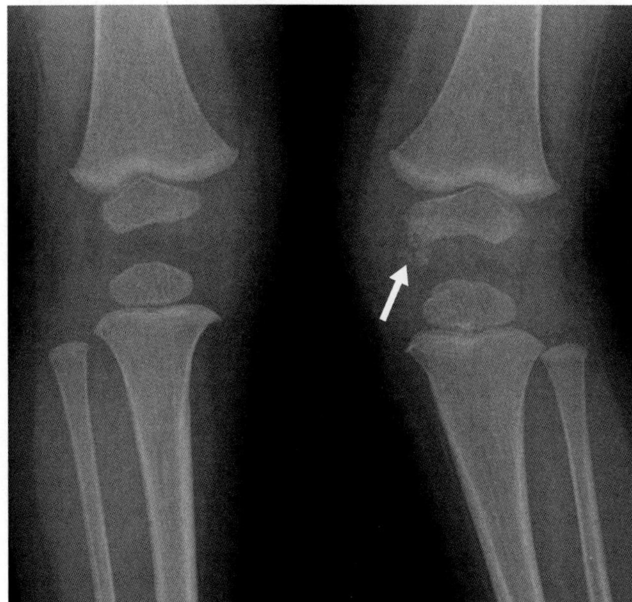

FIGURE 70.26. **Trevor Disease.** A 2-year-old girl with acquired genu valgum of the left leg. AP standing radiograph of the knees demonstrates mild genu valgum of the left knee with asymmetric enlargement of the distal femoral epiphysis with abnormal ossification along the medial aspect (*arrow*) giving rise to an irregular joint surface and angular deformity. The associated cartilage abnormality is not well appreciated radiographically.

Trevor Disease. Dysplasia epiphysealis hemimelica, also known as Trevor disease, is a distinct disorder secondary to osteochondroma development from an epiphysis that predominantly affects the lower extremities. On radiographs, there is eccentric, asymmetric enlargement of the epiphysis with early appearance of the ossification center (Fig. 70.26). Skeletal survey is indicated in patients to assess for involvement of other joints.

Chondroblastoma. Chondroblastomas are uncommon benign cartilaginous neoplasms that characteristically arise eccentrically in the epiphyses or apophyses of children, with 70% occurring in the humerus, femur, and tibia. Patients usually present with joint pain, muscle wasting, and swelling. On radiographs, chondroblastomas are well-defined lucent lesions with smooth or lobulated borders and a thin sclerotic rim with perhaps endosteal scalloping. Internal calcifications can be seen within half of the cases, and it is not uncommon to have prominent adjacent periosteal reaction. CT can be used to evaluate the cartilaginous matrix and potential cortical breach. MR is best suited for transphyseal or transcortical extension and typically demonstrates a much wider area of involvement than appreciated on radiographs. Lesions typically have cartilage signal with low or intermediate T1W signal and increased SI on T2-weighted imaging. There is typically adjacent bone marrow edema, periosteal reaction, and soft tissue reaction which may falsely suggest a more aggressive tumor or infection (Fig. 70.27). Treatment includes curettage and packing of the lesion or radiofrequency ablation. Recurrence rates are higher when the lesion is in close proximity to the physis, as complete excision is difficult. Rarely, chondroblastomas may undergo malignant transformation and metastasize to the lungs.

Langerhans Cell Histiocytosis. Langerhans cell histiocytosis (LCH) is a disorder resulting from the proliferation and accumulation of the Langerhans cell, a histiocyte. The cause is unknown although some studies suggest abnormal immune regulation as the underlying factor and others consider it a neoplastic process. LCH manifests in a variety of ways, ranging from a single osseous lesion to disseminated disease involving multiple organ systems.

The localized form of LCH usually presents in children 10 to 12 years of age. Solitary lesions can present with pain, tenderness, and mass. LCH can involve any bone; however, there is a predilection for flat bones and more than half of the lesions in localized LCH occur in the skull, mandible, pelvis, and ribs. When there is long bone involvement, LCH usually occurs within the diaphysis with the femur being the most common long bone site.

Radiographic appearance depends on location and phase of disease. Early-phase lesions usually have poorly defined margins and a permeative pattern and can be confused with Ewing sarcoma or infection. Lesions may progress and demonstrate cortical erosion, periosteal reaction, and soft tissue production. Later-phase lesions in the long bones are usually well-defined lytic lesions that are mildly expansile with a sclerotic margin. Skull lesions have a lytic, punched-out appearance with well-defined margins, and the unequal involvement of the inner and outer table gives rise to the characteristic beveled edge (Fig. 70.28). If there are multiple skull lesions, they may coalesce giving a "geographic" appearance. Mandibular involvement may lead to a "floating tooth" appearance due to the destruction of alveolar bone. When in the spine, LCH tends to involve the vertebral bodies of the thoracic spine and can present with painful scoliosis. There is invariably loss of vertebral body height which may only be some mild wedge deformity or result in marked height loss and the characteristic "vertebra plana" appearance (Fig. 70.29).

CT is helpful to define the bony anatomy and involvement, particularly in the skull base. As with other lesions, MRI is superior to CT in evaluating for bone marrow involvement and for any soft tissue masses. MRI is particularly helpful in evaluating calvarial lesions where it can show extension into the dura matter or brain parenchyma and in the spine where preservation of the adjacent disc spaces helps to differentiate LCH from infection as well as to evaluate for epidural soft tissue extension. The lytic lesion of LCH seen on radiographs will appear as low signal on T1-weighted images and increased SI on T2-weighted images. There is often perilesional edema in early-stage lesions. Both the osseous lesion and any soft tissue components usually enhance after intravenous contrast administration. As lesions heal, they show decreased T2 SI secondary to ossification and decreased edema.

Nuclear medicine bone scintigraphy and skeletal survey may both be used to evaluate for multifocality, as some lesions on one modality are missed on the other. More recently, both whole-body MRI and FDG-PET scans have been reported as alternative for following and assessing for multifocal disease. FDG PET may also be helpful in differentiating active versus healed lesions and to assess therapeutic response.

Solitary bone lesions are usually followed until spontaneous involution. However, depending on location and symptoms, more aggressive therapy may be warranted. Directed therapy includes curettage, ablative techniques, and direct intralesional methylprednisolone injection, while more disseminated disease may be treated with steroids and chemotherapy.

Malignant Bone Tumors

Osteosarcoma. Osteosarcoma is the most common malignant primary bone tumor in children and young adults. There is a slight male predominance with a peak incidence in patients between 15 and 25 years of age. Patients usually present with pain and/or swelling which persists over weeks to months. There are multiple types of osteosarcoma including

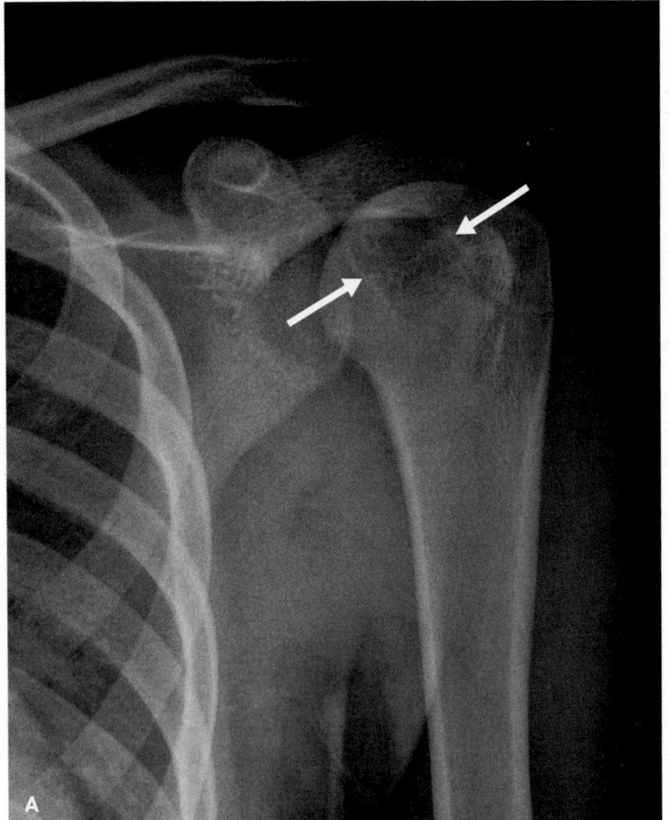

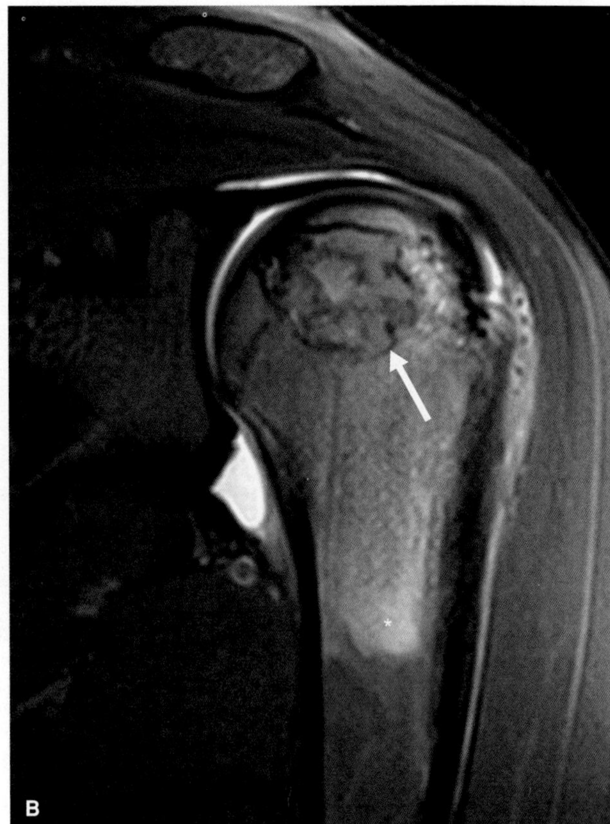

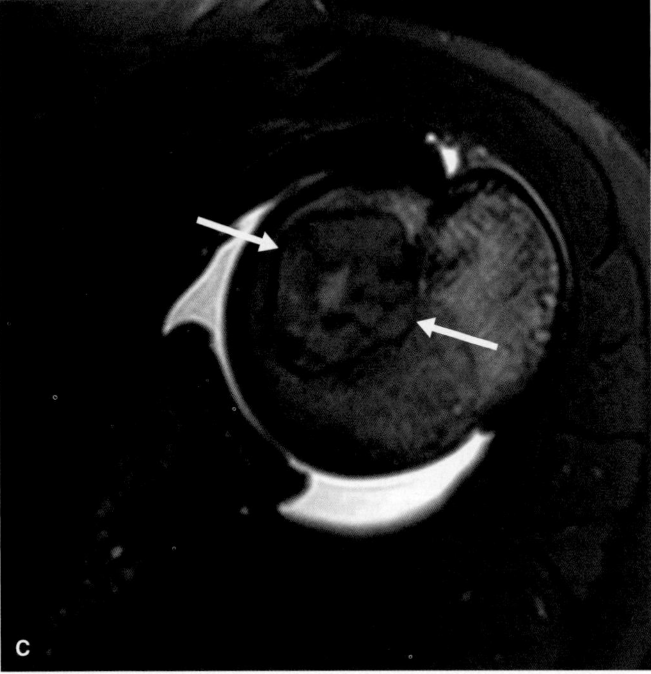

FIGURE 70.27. **Chondroblastoma.** A 16-year-old girl, nearly skeletally mature, with left shoulder pain for several weeks. **A:** AP radiograph of the left shoulder demonstrates a well-demarcated lucent lesion with a narrow zone of transition centered within the proximal humeral epiphysis which crosses the physis into the proximal metaphysis (*arrows*). **B:** Axial and (**C**) coronal proton density fat-saturated MR images of the shoulder show a lesion centered in the epiphysis with transphyseal spread (*arrow*). There is a thin sclerotic border and internal chondroid matrix. There is extensive surrounding marrow edema involving the proximal humeral diametaphysis (*) with a reactive joint effusion and mild adjacent soft tissue edema.

intramedullary (high-grade, telangiectatic, low-grade, small cell, osteosarcomatosis, and gnathic), surface (parosteal, periosteal, intracortical, and high-grade surface), extraskeletal, and secondary osteosarcoma. The extraskeletal and secondary types are rare in children. Osteosarcomas are defined histologically by the presence of tumor cells that produce osteoid matrix. However, other tissue types may be present and conventional osteosarcomas are further classified histologically into osteoblastic, chondroblastic, and fibroblastic varieties.

The high-grade intramedullary type is most common and is referred to as "conventional osteosarcoma." These osteosarcomas arise from the medullary cavity of the metaphysis of long bones, most commonly in the distal femur and proximal tibia. On radiographs, conventional osteosarcoma typically appears as a mass that contains fluffy, cloudlike opacity which represents osteoid matrix production. Lesions usually have a mixed lytic and sclerotic appearance with cortical erosion and destruction. Given the aggressive growth pattern, there

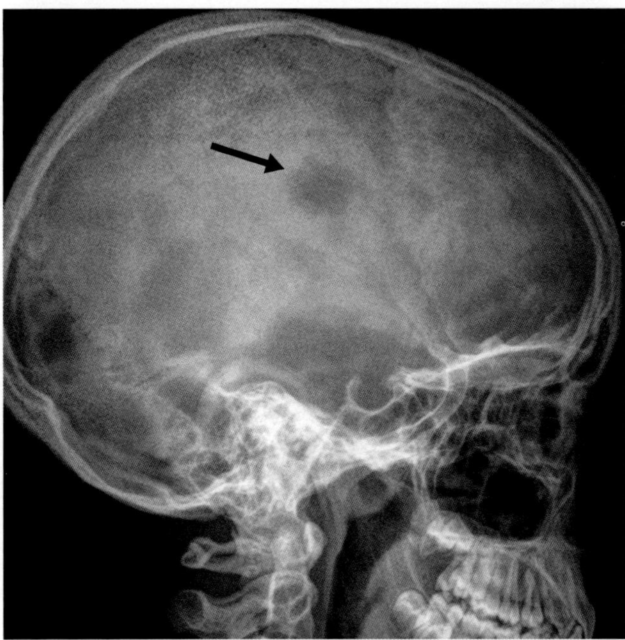

FIGURE 70.28. **Eosinophilic Granulomatosis.** A 12-year-old boy with scalp swelling. Lateral skull radiograph shows a lucent lesion with beveled edge or "hole in hole" appearance (*arrow*) due to unequal involvement of the inner and outer table of the calvarium.

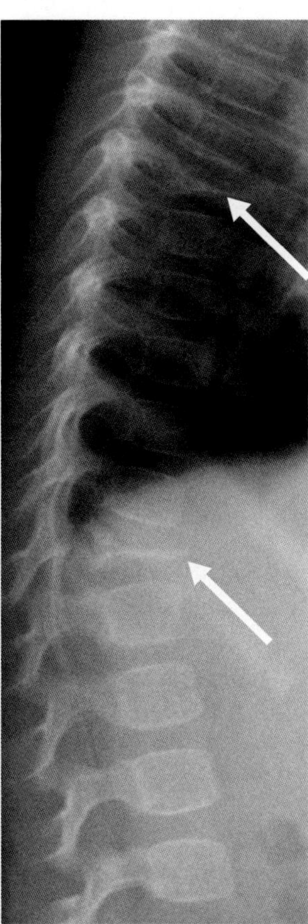

FIGURE 70.29. **Eosinophilic Granulomatosis.** A 2-year-old girl with back pain. Lateral view of the spine shows marked height loss in the T6 and T12 vertebral bodies, the so-called "vertebra plana" (*arrows*). There is mild associated focal kyphosis at these regions.

is often spiculated (sunburst) periosteal new bone and periosteal elevation is frequently seen resulting in Codman triangles (Fig. 70.30). However, depending on the histologic subtype, osteosarcomas can also appear as predominantly lytic lesions with little or no periosteal reaction. MRI allows for the evaluation of extent of marrow involvement and to evaluate for skip lesions. With this in mind, it is important to obtain longitudinal images of the entire bone, from joint to joint, in order to adequately stage and assess the patient. Marrow involvement is seen as abnormal low SI on T1-weighted images with increased SI on T2-weighted images. Soft tissue extension is well delineated on MRI and usually has a heterogeneous appearance and will enhance after administration of intravenous gadolinium contrast along with the osseous component. Fat-suppressed T1-weighted images after intravenous gadolinium administration are also helpful in evaluating for joint involvement in the presence of an effusion. About 10% to 20% of patients will have metastatic disease at the time of presentation with the lung being the most common site. Chest CT should be performed for staging of patients with osteosarcoma. As with the primary tumor, pulmonary metastatic disease can calcify. Furthermore, lesions based on the pleural surface can lead to a pneumothorax, hemothorax, or malignant pleural effusion. While MRI is the modality of choice in assessing the local extent of the primary lesion for surgical planning, FDG PET-CT is typically used for assessment of metastatic disease and may allow the noninvasive estimation of the histologic grade of the primary tumor. In addition, FDG PET-CT is useful in detecting recurrence at both the primary site and distant sites, often complementary to other imaging modalities.

Telangiectatic osteosarcoma is an uncommon subtype of intramedullary osteosarcoma but deserves mention given it is often confused with aneurysmal bone cysts (ABC). Telangiectatic osteosarcomas tend to occur around the knee and contain large cystic cavities filled with blood or necrotic tumor, and the walls/septations contain malignant cells that produce osteoid. The classic radiographic appearance is a lytic lesion with a wide zone of transition and endosteal scalloping. The overlying cortex tends to undergo expansile remodeling rather than destruction. MRI and CT are both helpful in further characterization and in helping to differentiate a telangiectatic osteosarcoma from an aneurysmal bone cyst as they demonstrate an osteoid matrix with enhancing peripheral nodular/septal soft tissue components.

The two most common surface osteosarcomas are the parosteal and periosteal subtypes. The parosteal subtype is most common and tends to occur in an older patient population. Periosteal osteosarcomas are intermediate-grade lesions which are thought to arise from the deep layers of the periosteum and arise in patients of the same age as conventional osteosarcoma. They tend to arise in the diaphysis with the femur and tibia representing the most common location. On radiographs, they appear as a thickened, scalloped cortex with adjacent periosteal reaction. There is often little ossification as they are usually chondroblastic. CT and MRI are helpful in surface osteosarcomas to evaluate for soft tissue components and involvement of adjacent structures.

Treatment of osteosarcoma involves a combination of chemotherapy and surgery. MRI is critical to surgical planning as a variety of techniques can be used depending on the location and spread of the primary tumor. Of note, osteosarcoma is not radiosensitive. Also, chest CT is important for follow-up as 80% of relapses occur only in the lung.

Ewing Sarcoma Family of Tumors. Ewing sarcoma is a small, round blue cell tumor of childhood and belongs to the family of tumors including extraosseous Ewing sarcoma, Askin tumor, and primitive neuroectodermal tumors (PNET). It is the second most common primary malignant bone tumor

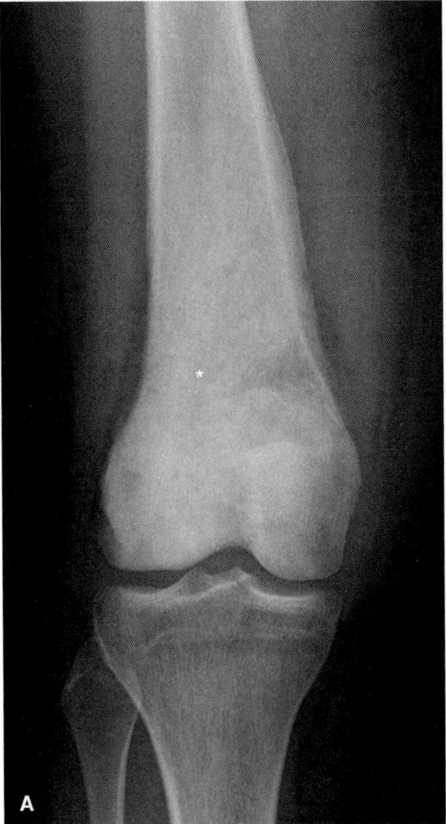

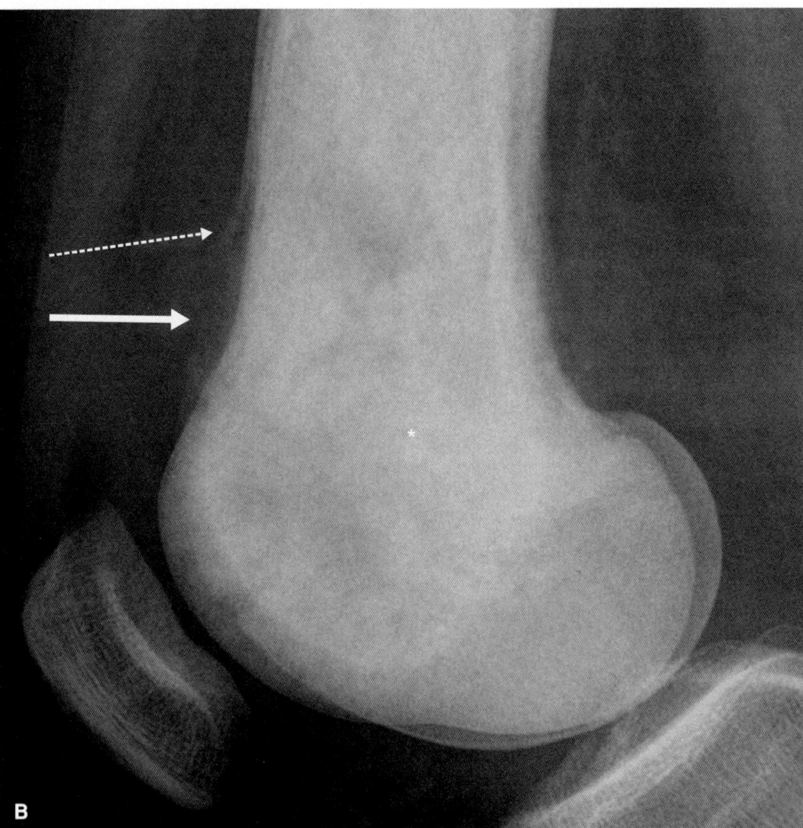

FIGURE 70.30. **Osteosarcoma.** A 17-year-old boy with knee pain. **A:** AP and (**B**) lateral radiographs of the right knee show a sclerotic lesion centered in the distal femoral metaphysis (*). On the lateral view, there is spiculated periosteal reaction in a "sunburst" pattern (*arrow*) and with periosteal reaction resulting in a "Codman triangle" appearance (*dashed arrow*).

in children and adolescents with an annual incidence of approximately 200 cases. Ewing sarcoma is most frequent in the first three decades of life, with a peak between 10 and 20 years of age. There is a slight male predominance and it is rare in African-American and Asian populations. The presentation of Ewing sarcoma is nonspecific and usually consists of pain, mass, or swelling. Patients can also have fever, elevated erythrocyte sedimentation rate, and raised white blood cell count mimicking osteomyelitis.

Ewing sarcoma most commonly occurs in the extremities, the ribs, and the pelvis. The femur is the most commonly involved bone and lesions in long bones typically arise in the metadiaphysis and diaphysis. On radiographs, Ewing sarcomas typically have an aggressive appearance with bone destruction leading to a moth-eaten or permeative pattern. There is usually periosteal reaction which may appear lamellated (onion skin-like). They also have a wide zone of transition with poor margination. An associated soft tissue mass is also a common finding and the mass tends to be much larger in size in comparison to the amount of underlying bone destruction (Fig. 70.31). The soft tissue component may be missed on radiographs as Ewing sarcomas do not undergo ossification and CT and MRI can show the extent of the lesion with greater detail. Ewing sarcoma is usually homogeneous and low to isointense SI to muscle on T1-weighted images and intermediate to high SI on T2-weighted images. As lesion size increases, heterogeneity in the lesion becomes more common and may represent necrosis or hemorrhage. Ewing sarcoma will enhance after the administration of intravenous contrast material and is usually either diffuse or peripheral/nodular in appearance. Given that a substantial number of patients have metastatic disease, proper staging of patients is required. This entails a multimodality approach and may include FDG PET-CT, MRI of the primary tumor, and chest CT owing to the frequency of metastatic lung disease. MRI and FDG PET-CT are often obtained for follow-up. In particular, MRI plays a key role as decrease in primary tumor size on MRI has been correlated to a favorable histologic response to chemotherapy. The treatment of Ewing sarcoma requires a multimodality approach and involves chemotherapy along with surgery and, possibly, radiotherapy.

Leukemia. Acute leukemia is the most common malignancy of children. The most common type is acute lymphoblastic leukemia (ALL) with a peak incidence at 2 to 3 years of age. Children will often present with skeletal manifestations including limp, pain, swelling, and tenderness along with hepatosplenomegaly, lymph node enlargement, and fever.

On radiographs, the most common skeletal finding is diffuse demineralization. This may lead to pathologic fractures, including vertebral compression fractures. Transverse lucent metaphyseal bands, the so-called "leukemic lines," are seen in up to about 50% of patients with skeletal findings. These are nonspecific and seen as a uniform and regular lucency across the width of the metaphysis in those bones associated with rapid growth such as the distal femurs, proximal tibiae/humeri, vertebral bodies, and iliac crests (Fig. 70.32A). Patients may also have lytic lesions and the bone can often have a "moth-eaten" pattern. MRI shows an infiltration of the bone marrow with homogeneous decreased SI on T1-weighted images and increased SI on fluid-sensitive images. The abnormal marrow will enhance after the administration of intravenous

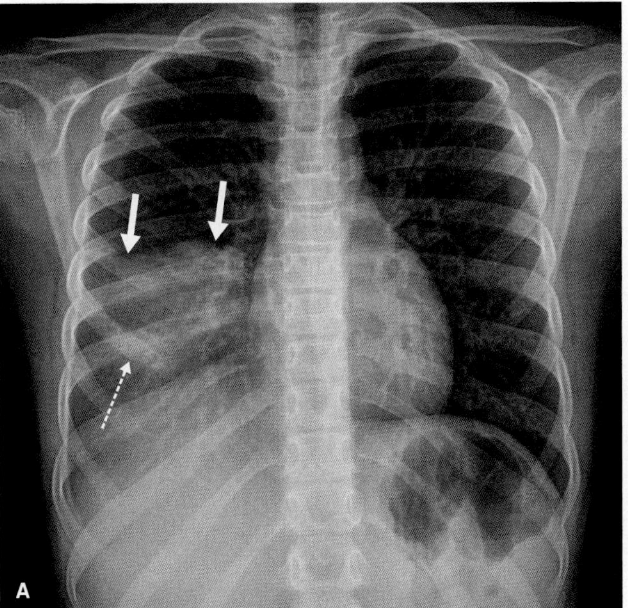

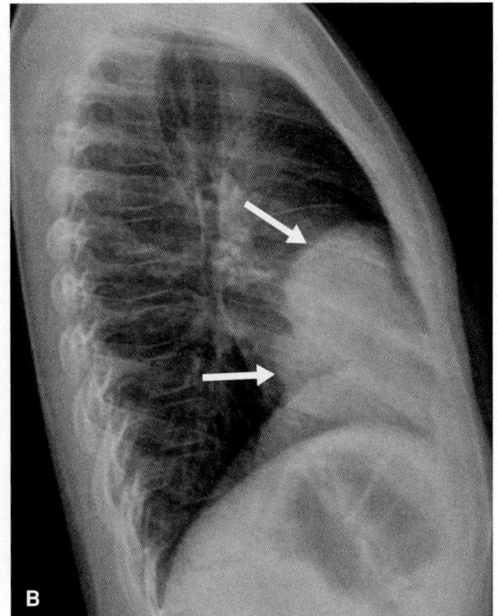

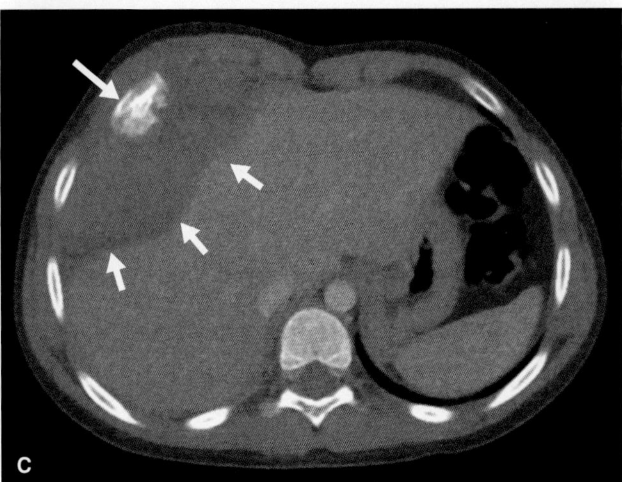

FIGURE 70.31. **Ewing Sarcoma.** A 9-year-old boy with chest pain, fever, and cough. **A:** PA and (**B**) lateral chest radiographs demonstrate an opacity within the inferior, anterior right hemithorax (*arrows*). There is sclerosis and irregularity of the distal aspect of the right 6th rib (*dashed arrow*). On the lateral view, this has a lobulated, mass-like appearance. **C:** Axial CT of the chest after intravenous contrast demonstrates sclerosis, cortical destruction, and periosteal reaction of the anterior aspect of the 6th rib (*long arrow*) with an adjacent large soft tissue mass (*short arrows*) with resultant mass effect on the liver.

gadolinium contrast. Marrow replacement may be so complete so as to include all the bones and resulting in the "flip-flop" sign with an inversion of the normal appearance of bone marrow on MRI (i.e., hypointense on T1-weighted sequences and hyperintense on fluid-sensitive sequences) (Fig. 70.32B,C).

SOFT TISSUE LESIONS

Hemangiomas

Hemangiomas are benign vascular tumors and are classified according to the International Society for the Study of Vascular Anomalies (ISSVA). The infantile hemangioma is the most common vascular tumor of infancy. Infantile hemangiomas follow a characteristic clinical pattern. They are not present at birth, although sometimes a precursor lesion such as discoloration or macule may be present. There is rapid growth after birth during the proliferative phase, with a peak at about 1 year of age. An involuting phase follows with spontaneous regression and decrease in size over many years. The final stage is a fibrotic stage with small residual fibrofatty tissue remaining for life. Infantile hemangiomas can be superficial or deep and most commonly involve the skin, followed by the liver. The superficial lesions are usually diagnosed clinically and are classically described as a "strawberry mark." Deep lesions may be more difficult to diagnose clinically and may require imaging.

A few scenarios warrant further evaluation with imaging. If patients have five or more lesions, screening is often done to evaluate for liver involvement. Lesions surrounding the orbit are evaluated with MRI, as growth could create vision problems depending on extent of the lesion. Similarly, those in a bearded distribution could involve the airway. When present over the lumbar spine, there may be associated spinal cord abnormalities and screening is often performed. Infantile hemangiomas are associated with PHACE syndrome (Posterior fossa brain malformations; Hemangiomas of the face, neck, or scalp; Arterial anomalies; Coarctation of the aorta and Cardiac defects; and Eye abnormalities) and LUMBAR syndrome (Lower body infantile hemangiomas, Urogenital anomalies, Ulceration, Myelopathy, Bony deformities, Anorectal malformations, Arterial anomalies, and Renal anomalies). Congenital hemangiomas can be distinguished from infantile hemangiomas clinically as they are present at birth because the proliferative phase occurs in utero.

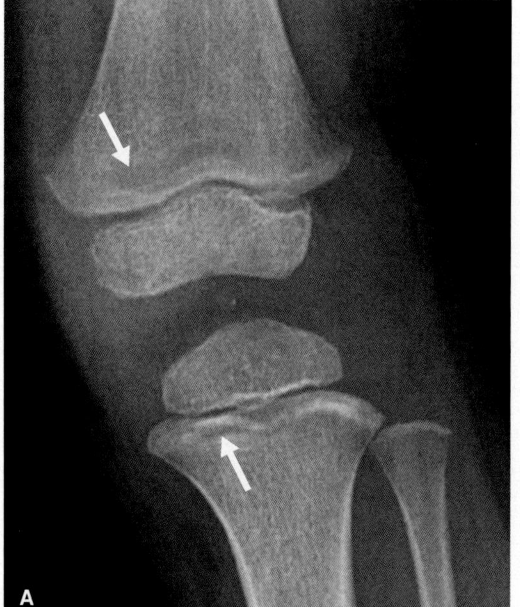

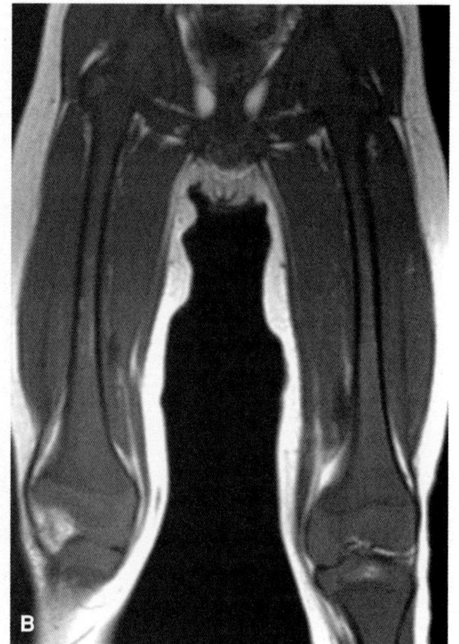

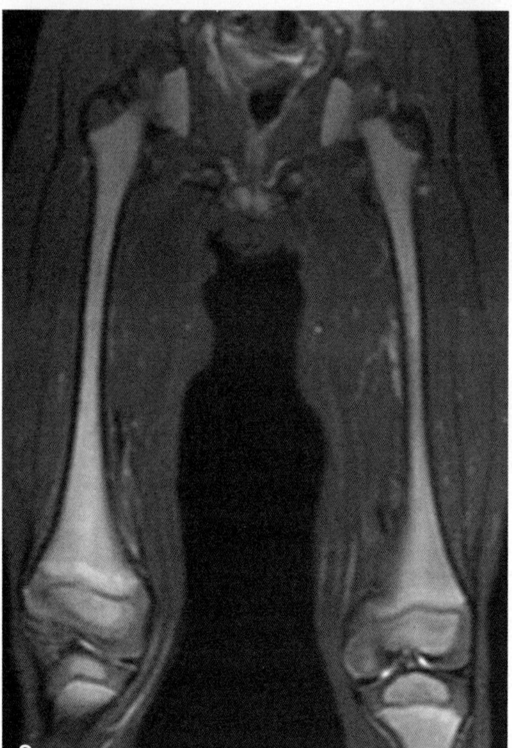

FIGURE 70.32. **Leukemia.** An 8-year-old boy with left leg pain and limp. **A:** Frontal radiograph of the left knee demonstrates metaphyseal lucent bands compatible with leukemic lines. Coronal (**B**) T1-weighted and (**C**) fluid-sensitive MR images show the MR "flip flop" sign. There is diffusely low, abnormal SI within all the bones on the T1-weighted image with loss of the expected fat signal within the epiphyses and diaphyses in this 8-year-old boy. There is diffuse, abnormally high SI within the bones on the fluid-sensitive image.

Ultrasound is the primary diagnostic imaging modality for hemangiomas and should be performed with color and spectral Doppler imaging. On ultrasound, infantile hemangiomas are well-defined, lobular/ovoid soft tissue lesions with heterogeneous echogenicity. Individual vessels are not discretely seen on gray scale imaging but there is marked vascularity on color Doppler imaging with five or more vessels per square centimeter. Spectral Doppler shows low-resistance arterial waveforms (Fig. 70.33). As the lesion involutes, it will show decreased vascularity and increased echogenicity. MRI of infantile hemangiomas shows a well-defined lesion with increased SI on T2-weighted images and intermediate SI on T1-weighted images. Flow voids may be present and there is early intense and uniform enhancement after injection of intravenous gadolinium contrast material. The lesions become more heterogeneous as they involute. Of note, there should be no perilesional edema and other etiologies should be considered if present.

Treatment is not usually required as the lesions involute. However, in cases where there may be secondary loss of function or cosmetic issues, medical treatment with propranolol and, possibly, embolization or surgery may be performed.

Fibromatosis Colli

Fibromatosis colli, also known as "pseudotumor of infancy" or "sternomastoid pseudotumor," is a form of infantile

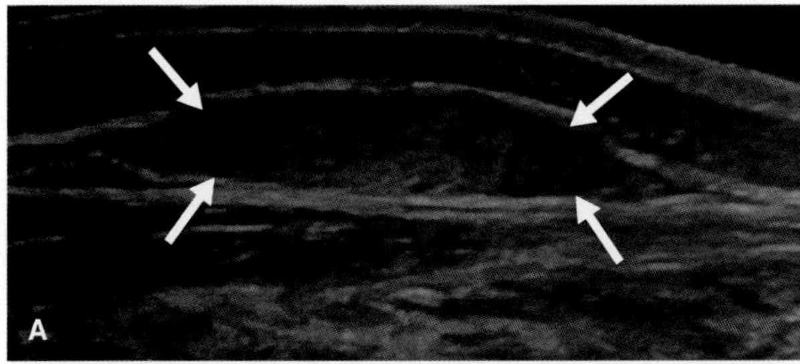
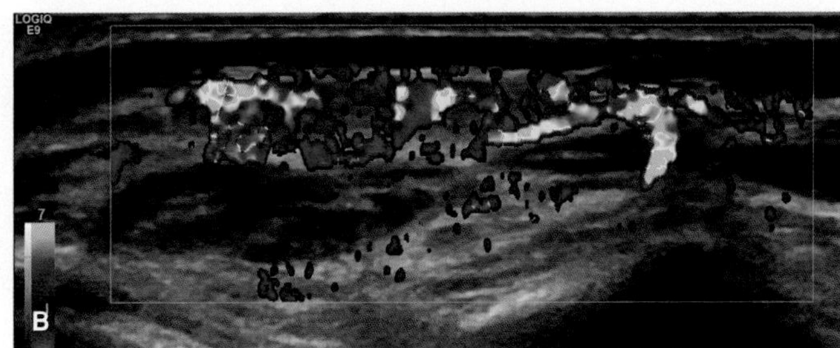
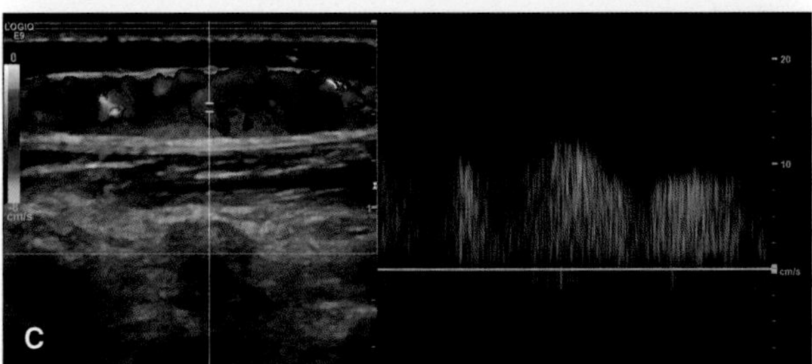

FIGURE 70.33. **Hemangioma.** A 3-month-old girl with palpable lump on her back. **A:** Sagittal gray scale image of her upper back, in the region of interest, shows a well-demarcated, heterogeneous, ovoid mass within the subcutaneous tissues, deep to the fatty layer (*arrows*). No calcifications or cysts. **B:** On color Doppler, there is increased vessel density. **C:** Spectral display demonstrates low-resistance arterial waveforms along with venous flow (not shown). Given that the lesion was not present at birth, findings are consistent with an infantile hemangioma.

fibromatosis in the sternocleidomastoid muscle. It is a benign condition that usually manifests at about 2 weeks of life with a palpable mass in the sternocleidomastoid muscle. Fibromatosis colli is usually unilateral, with right-sided involvement more common, and can cause torticollis. The exact cause is unknown, but the majority of cases resolve by 2 years of age.

Ultrasound is the imaging modality of choice. Findings vary and can show a homogeneous enlarged sternocleidomastoid muscle with a fusiform appearance and maintained muscle fibers or even a discrete hypoechoic mass within the sternocleidomastoid muscle itself (Fig. 70.34). Features such as irregular margins, loss of fascial planes, or extension beyond the sternocleidomastoid muscle are atypical and should raise concern for other etiologies. MR is suggested if there are atypical findings on ultrasound, symptoms do not resolve after 12 months, or there are symptoms/physical findings that are not typical. On MRI, there is diffuse enlargement of the sternocleidomastoid muscle without discrete mass and with clear surrounding fascial planes. The enlarged muscle shows abnormal, increased SI on T2-weighted images. Treatment is conservative with stretching and physical therapy.

CONSTITUTIONAL DISORDERS OF BONE

Skeletal Dysplasias

Skeletal dysplasias represent a heterogeneous group of disorders which are characterized by abnormal bone and cartilage growth.

The prevalence of any individual dysplasia is rare. Some are lethal in the perinatal period, while nonlethal dysplasias usually present in infancy or early childhood due to growth disturbances. The diagnosis of a particular dysplasia can be

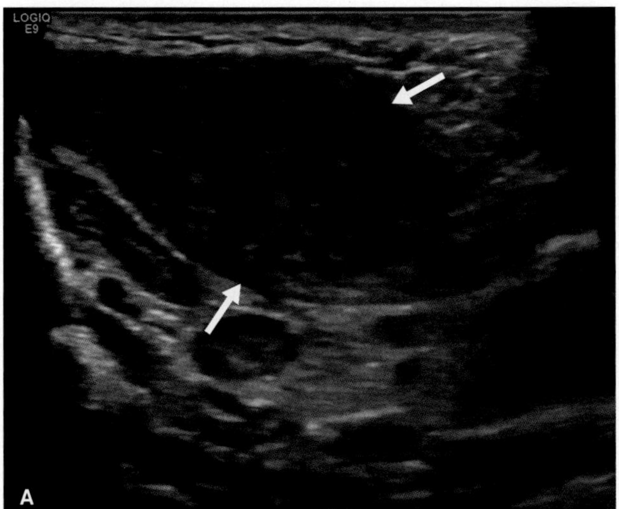
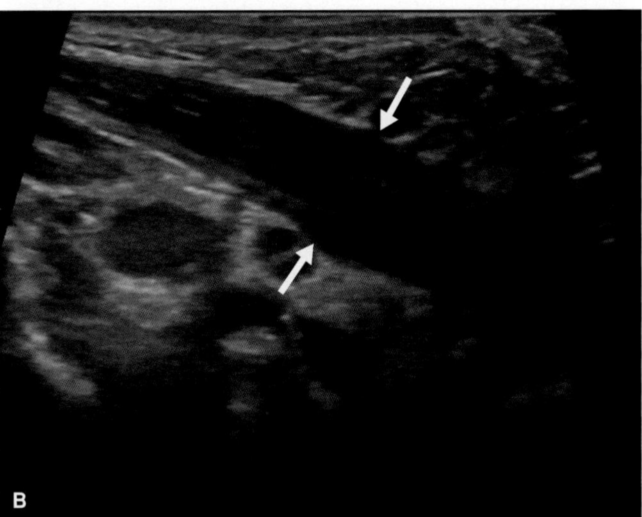

FIGURE 70.34. **Fibromatosis Colli.** A 4-week-old girl with torticollis and firmness along the right aspect of her neck. Sagittal ultrasound images of the right (**A**) and left (**B**) sternocleidomastoid (SCM) muscles (*arrows*). There is fusiform thickening of the right SCM; however, the muscle fibers remain visible. The margins are discrete and there is no extension beyond the muscle. Findings are compatible with fibromatosis colli. The left SCM (*arrows*) is normal.

TABLE 70.7

TYPICAL SKELETAL RADIOLOGIC FEATURES TO EVALUATE IN ASSESSING FOR A SKELETAL DYSPLASIA

■ ANATOMIC LOCATION	■ RADIOLOGIC FINDINGS IN SKELETAL DYSPLASIAS
Skull	■ Cranial sutures—craniosynostoses ■ Wormian bones ■ Frontal bossing ■ Midface/mandibular hypoplasia and retrognathia ■ J-shaped sella
Chest	■ Ribs—shortened, gracile, thickened, fusion ■ Absent/hypoplastic clavicles ■ Cardiac silhouette size for associated cardiac abnormalities
Spine	■ Alignment—scoliosis, kyphosis/gibbus deformity, accentuated lordotic curvature. Craniocervical alignment and development ■ Vertebral body shape—flattened (platyspondyly), coronal cleft, interpediculate distance, posterior scalloping, anterior beaking ■ Segmentation/fusion anomalies
Pelvis	■ Delayed ossification ■ Short iliac bones with narrow sacroiliac notches ■ Steep or flat acetabular roof ■ Delayed or irregular femoral head ossification
Long bones	■ Epiphysis—delayed ossification, irregular or flat appearance ■ Metaphysis—widened, irregular ■ Diaphysis—cortical thinning or thickening, bowing ■ Phalanges—cone shaped

quite difficult and requires the assimilation of family and clinical history, physical examination, radiologic examination, and molecular and genetic tests. Comparison to textbooks is helpful with *Taybi and Lachman's Radiology of Syndromes, Metabolic Disorders and Skeletal Dysplasias* one of the more commonly used books.

Radiologic assessment is integral to many of the dysplasias and begins with a complete skeletal survey. Skeletal surveys performed for evaluation of a syndrome or metabolic disorder consist of less images compared with a survey for NAT. For skeletal dysplasias, the entire arms and legs can be exposed on a single film when the size of the child permits. In addition, whole-body AP and lateral radiographs will likely suffice instead of imaging the spine and trunk separately. Two views (AP and lateral) of the skull are typically sufficient and oblique radiographs of the ribs are not necessary. Having an ordered approach can be helpful in assessment and many are described in the literature. In general, one must assess the relative size, shape, and proportions of each bone. For the long bones, dysplasias may affect the proximal portions of the extremities (rhizomelia), the middle portion (mesomelia), or the distal portion (acromelia). Shortening of the entire extremity is micromelia. Assessment of the extremities, skull, chest, spine, and pelvis is important, with notable findings shown in Table 70.7 and can also help assist the radiologist into a specific diagnosis.

Achondroplasia. Achondroplasia is the most common nonlethal skeletal dysplasia and patients have normal mentation and life span. On radiographs, patients have rhizomelia. The skull is enlarged with frontal bossing and a small/narrow foramen magnum is seen on cross-sectional imaging. The thorax is small with shortened ribs. There is narrowing of the interpedicular distance, particularly in the more caudal segments of the lumbar spine, and there is posterior vertebral body scalloping and gibbus deformity. The iliac wings are rounded with flat acetabular roofs, narrow sacrosciatic notches, and a champagne glass–shaped pelvic inlet. The hands show brachydactyly with trident configuration. In the lower extremities, the proximal femurs show a scooped-out appearance in infancy while the distal femur has a deep notch in the central growth plate (chevron deformity) and there is fibular overgrowth (Fig. 70.35).

Thanatophoric Dwarfism. Thanatophoric dwarfism is one of the most common lethal skeletal dysplasias. Typical imaging features include "cloverleaf skull" due to craniosynostosis, curved long bones including "French telephone receiver" appearance to the femurs, platyspondyly, short ribs and handlebar clavicles, and micromelia. In particular, the presence of platyspondyly can help to distinguish thanatophoric dwarfism from other forms of dwarfism.

Mucopolysaccharidoses. The mucopolysaccharidoses are a group of metabolic disorders that involve defective activity of the lysosomal enzymes which blocks degradation of mucopolysaccharides. Long chains of sugar carbohydrates occur within the cells that help build bone, cartilage, tendons, corneas, skin, and connective tissue. There is a wide range of clinical features and severity depending on subtypes. The most common subtypes include Hunter, Hurler, Sanfilippo, and Morquio syndromes. Common osseous features include an enlarged skull with J-shaped sella, paddle or oar-shaped ribs, and beaking of the thoracolumbar vertebral bodies sometimes with gibbus deformity. The iliac wings are flared and small with inferior tapering and steep acetabular roofs. The metacarpals show proximal tapering (Fig. 70.36).

Osteogenesis Imperfecta. OI is an inherited disorder of connective tissue characterized by increased bone fragility and low bone mass. Other clinical findings include blue sclera, dentinogenesis imperfecta, skin hyperlaxity, and joint

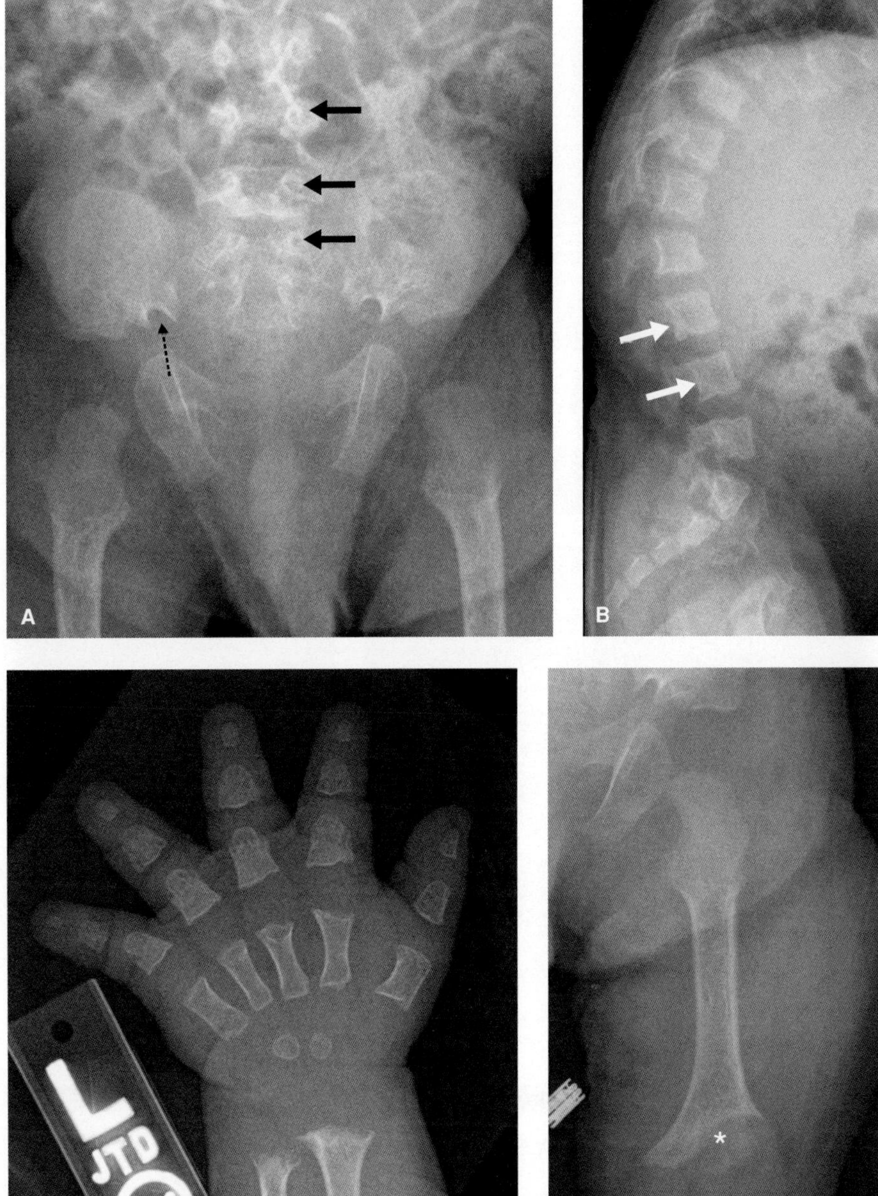

FIGURE 70.35. **Achondroplasia.** A 1-month-old male with achondroplasia. **A:** AP radiograph of the pelvis shows rounded iliac wings with flattened acetabular roofs and narrow sacrosciatic notches (*dashed arrow*). There is narrowing of the interpedicular distance in the lumbar spine (*arrows*). **B:** Lateral view of the lower spine shows shortened vertebral bodies (in AP dimension) with mild posterior vertebral body scalloping (*arrows*). **C:** Frontal radiograph of the left hand shows short and thickened appearance of the bones. There is wide separation of the second and third digits, "trident" configuration. **D:** AP radiograph of the left femur shows scooped-out appearance to the proximal femur. There is a flared appearance to the distal femoral metaphysis with notch in the central aspect of the distal physis (*).

hypermobility. Classification is based on clinical findings and disease severity with eight types currently recognized (Table 70.8). There is wide variation in the radiographic presentation of patients with OI, ranging from normal or near normal to severe abnormalities. Also, patients with some forms of OI may not have blue sclera, and the lack of this clinical finding does not exclude the diagnosis of OI. The most common type is the more mild type 1 disease.

The main radiographic features are diffuse demineralization, fractures, and deformities. Fractures typically involve the long bones and the spine. The skull will often show an abnormal number of wormian bones (Fig. 70.37). Popcorn calcifications are also described at the metaphysis/epiphysis which are secondary to ossification of the displaced and fragmented physis. Importantly, the diagnosis of OI can be difficult and cases may be confused with NAT, especially in those younger than 2 years of age and without a family history of OI. Knowledge of those fractures that is highly specific for child abuse can be helpful.

Osteopetrosis. Osteopetrosis is a rare bone disease that results from a failure of osteoclasts to resorb bone. Decreased osteoclastic activity leads to decreased elasticity of bone, impaired repair functions, and increased risk of fracture. Patients are also at greater risk for postsurgical complications such as infection and delayed union.

The hallmark of osteopetrosis is increased density in the medullary portion of the bone with relative sparing of the cortices. The autosomal dominant form of osteopetrosis has two phenotypic variants. Type 1 has uniform sclerosis of the long bones, skull and spine. Type 2 has the "bone-within-bone" appearance and sclerosis of the skull base. In the spine, the "bone-within-bone" appearance is also known as the "sandwich vertebra" or "picture frame" vertebral bodies (Fig. 70.38).

Cleidocranial Dysplasia. Cleidocranial dysplasia is a relatively common dysplasia and findings include: wide sutures and numerous wormian bones, absence/hypoplasia of the clavicles and pubic bones, posterior wedging of thoracic vertebral

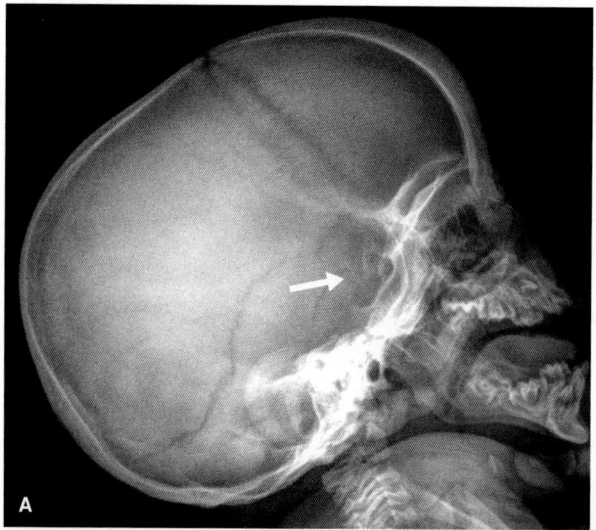

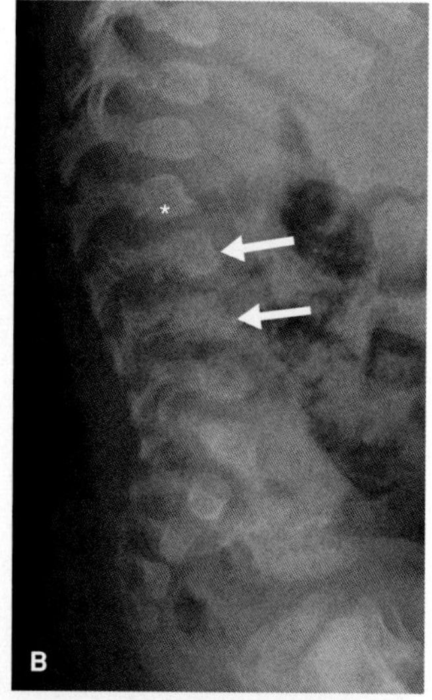

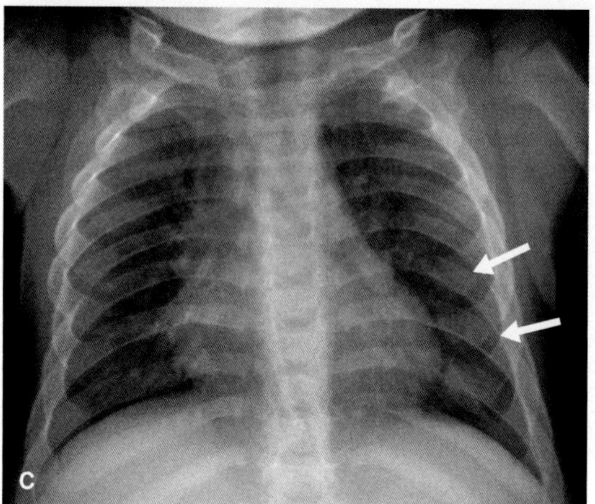

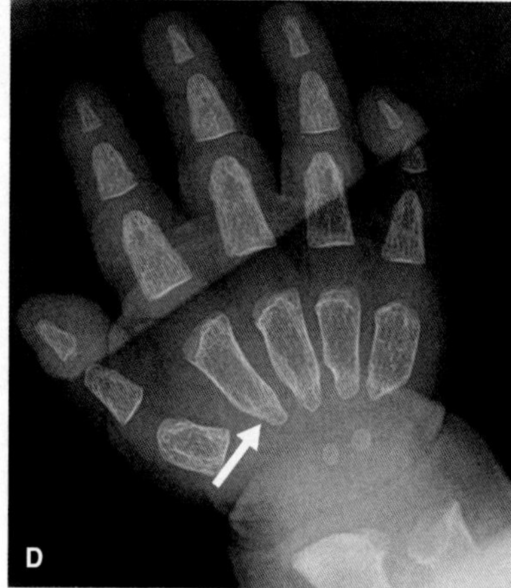

FIGURE 70.36. **Mucopolysaccharidoses.** A 1-year-old girl with Hurler syndrome. **A:** Lateral radiograph of the skull shows J-shaped sella (*arrow*). **B:** Lateral radiograph of the lower spine shows anterior vertebral body beaking (*arrows*) and focal kyphosis at the thoracolumbar junction with a hypoplastic L1 vertebral body (*). **C:** AP radiograph of the chest shows paddle-shaped ribs (*arrows*). The clavicles are broadened and the scapulae appear small with dysplastic appearance of the glenoid. **D:** PA view of the right hand shows proximal tapering of the metacarpals (*arrow*).

TABLE 70.8

OSTEOGENESIS IMPERFECTA SUBTYPES

TYPE	CLINICAL SEVERITY	TYPICAL FEATURES	INHERITANCE
I	Mild nondeforming	Normal height or mild short stature; blue sclera; no dentinogenesis imperfecta	Autosomal dominant
II	Perinatal lethal	Multiple rib and long bone fractures at birth; marked deformities; broad long bones; low density of skull bones on x-rays; dark sclerae	Autosomal dominant, rarely autosomal recessive
III	Severely deforming	Very short; triangular face; severe scoliosis; grayish sclerae; dentinogenesis imperfecta	Autosomal dominant
IV	Moderately deforming	Moderately short; mild to moderate scoliosis; grayish or white sclera; dentinogenesis imperfecta	Autosomal dominant
V	Moderately deforming	Mild to moderate short stature; dislocation of radial head; mineralized interosseous membrane; hyperplastic callus; white sclera; no dentinogenesis imperfecta	Autosomal dominant
VI	Moderately to severely deforming	Moderately short; scoliosis; accumulation of osteoid in bone tissue, fish-scale pattern of bone lamellation; white sclera; no dentinogenesis imperfecta	Autosomal recessive
VII	Moderately deforming	Mild short stature; short humeri and femora; coxa vara; white sclera; no dentinogenesis imperfecta	Autosomal recessive

Adapted from Glorieux FH. Osteogenesis imperfecta. *Best Pract Res Clin Rheumatol* 2008;22(1):85–100.

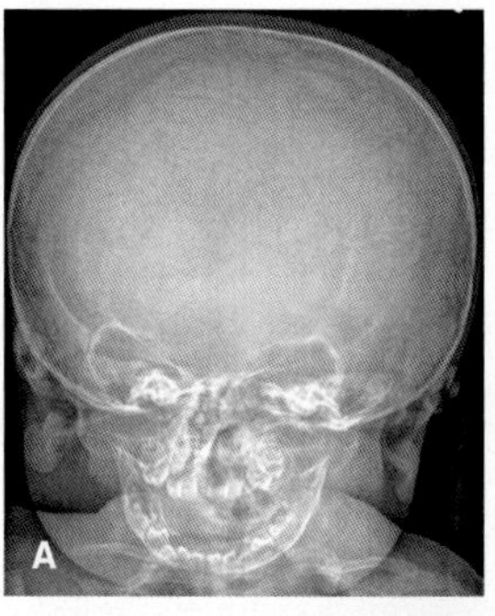

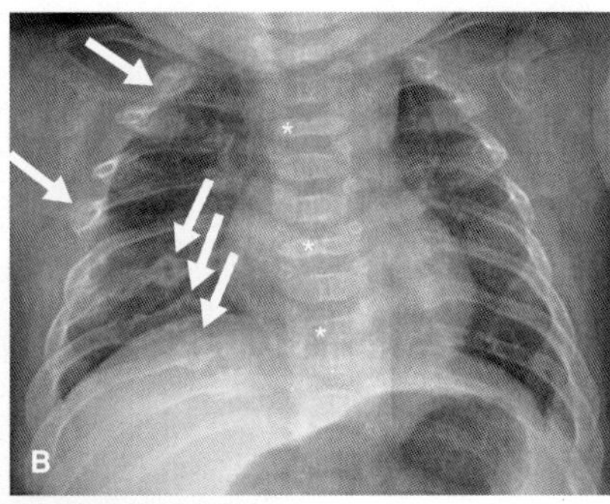

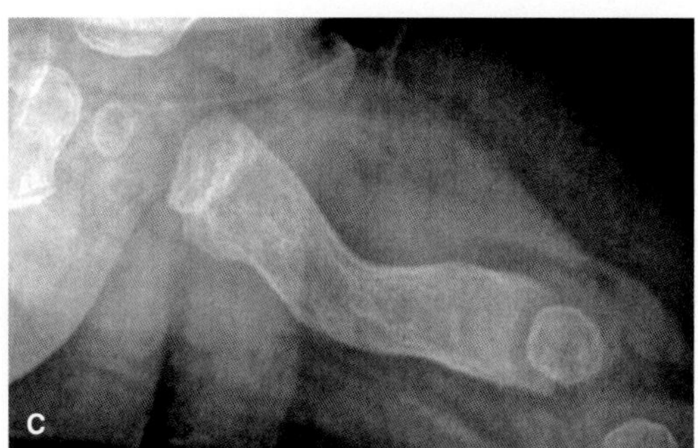

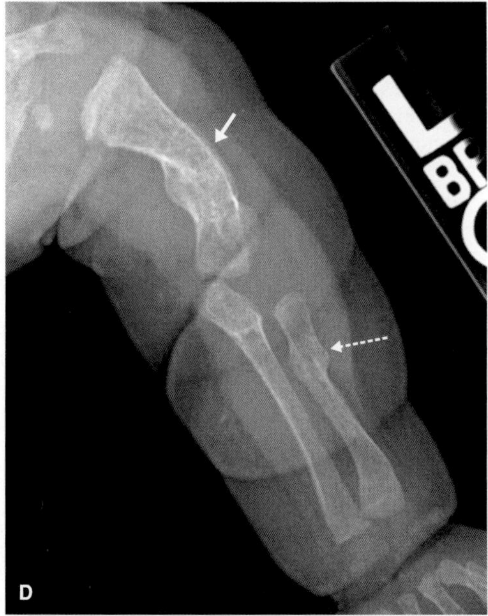

FIGURE 70.37. **Osteogenesis Imperfecta.** A 4-month-old male with osteogenesis imperfecta. **A:** AP radiograph of the skull shows thinned calvarium with numerous wormian bones. **B:** AP radiograph of the chest shows diffuse bone demineralization with numerous healing rib fractures (*arrows*). There is height loss in many of the thoracic vertebral bodies, compatible with compression fractures (*). **C:** Lateral radiograph of the left femur shows bowing deformity of the diaphysis. **D:** AP radiograph of the left arm shows a healing fracture of the mid diaphysis of the humerus with bowing deformity (*solid arrow*). There is also a healing fracture of the proximal diaphysis of the radius (*dashed arrow*).

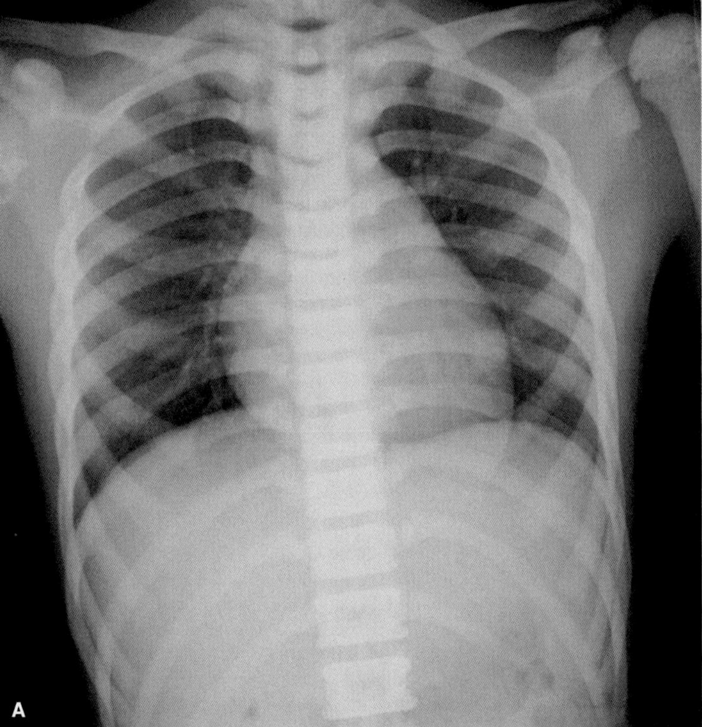

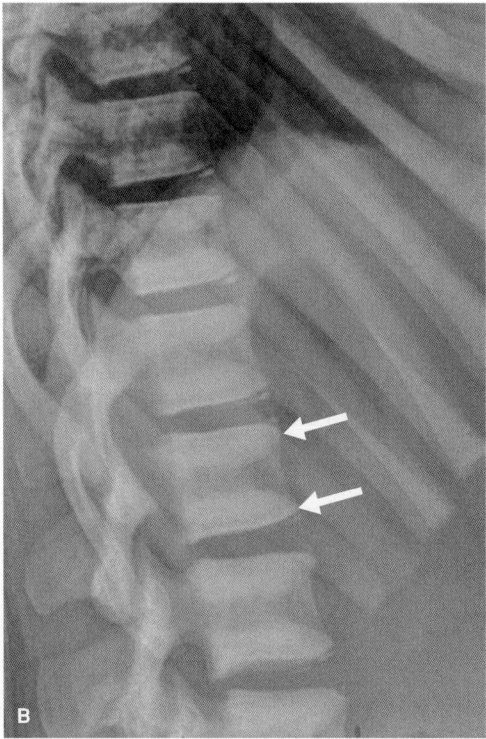

FIGURE 70.38. **Osteopetrosis.** A 10-year-old boy with osteopetrosis. **A:** AP radiograph of the chest shows diffusely increased bone density. **B:** Lateral radiograph of the lower thoracic and upper lumbar spine shows sclerosis at the superior and inferior endplates of the vertebral body resulting in the "sandwich vertebra" appearance (*arrows*).

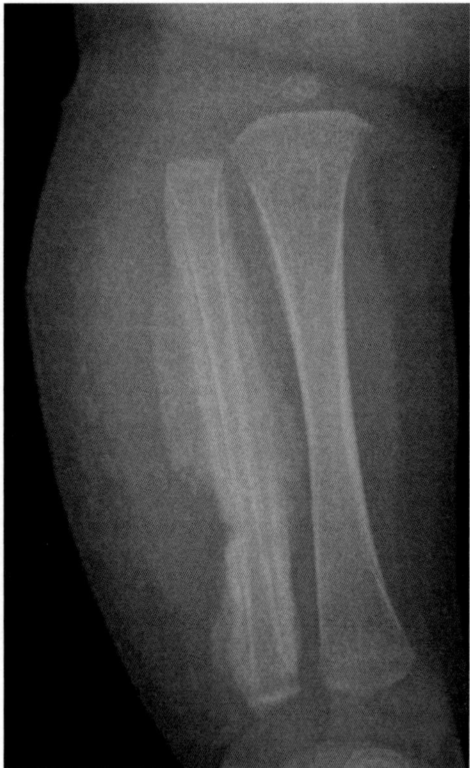

FIGURE 70.39. Caffey Disease. A 2-month-old girl with right lower leg swelling. No fever. AP radiograph of the distal right lower leg shows soft tissue swelling laterally with diffuse periosteal reaction and cortical thickening involving the entire fibular shaft, most pronounced in the diaphysis. The tibia is normal. Bone biopsy was consistent with Caffey disease and no other lesions were seen on the follow-up skeletal survey.

bodies, numerous pseudoepiphyses of the metacarpals, and tapered distal phalanges.

Caffey Disease

Caffey disease is also called infantile cortical hyperostosis and is characterized by presentation before the 5th month of life, hyperirritability, soft tissue swelling, and bone lesions, particularly mandible involvement. It is an inherited disorder, with autosomal dominant or recessive inheritance. The long bones, clavicle, scapulae, and ribs can also be involved and demonstrate diaphyseal new bone formation sparing the epiphyses and metaphyses (Fig. 70.39). Radiographs demonstrate diffuse cortical thickening of the mandible due to subperiosteal new bone formation. Babies may also have swelling of the adjacent joints and soft tissues. This is typically a self-limiting process with bone remodeling and resorption occurring by age 2. Occasionally, long bones of the distal extremities may fuse, which may cause growth problems, or if ribs are involved, scoliosis and thoracic cage deformity.

Neurofibromatosis

Neurofibromatosis type I (NF1), also known as von Recklinghausen disease, is an autosomal dominant disorder due to mutation or deletion of the *NF1* gene on chromosome 17. NF1 is characterized by the formation of neurofibromas and abnormalities related to mesodermal dysplasia. While this phakomatosis (congenital neurocutaneous disorder) affects multiple organ systems, skeletal abnormalities are seen in up to 50% of patients.

Discrete neurofibromas occur before puberty and may deform adjacent bones due to mass effect and pressure-induced changes. Spinal deformities are common, with

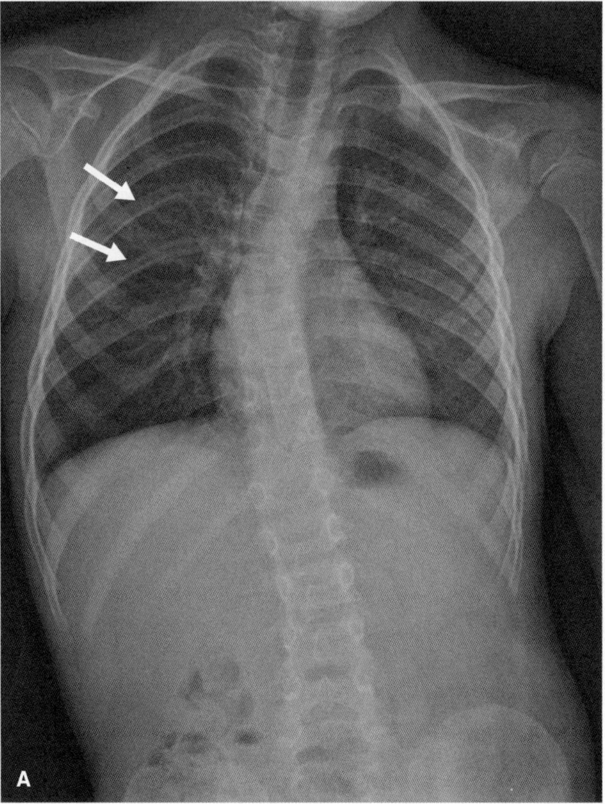

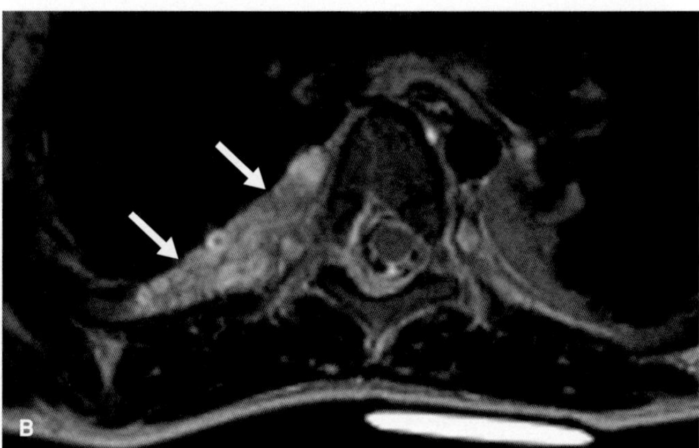

FIGURE 70.40. Neurofibromatosis With Dystrophic Scoliosis. An 11-year-old boy with dextroscoliosis. **A:** AP radiograph of the thoracolumbar spine shows the focal dextroscoliosis centered at T5. There is thinning of the right 6th and 7th posterior ribs (*arrows*) with associated increased intercostal distance. **B:** Axial fluid-sensitive MR image of the posterior aspect of the chest at the T6 level demonstrates a plexiform neurofibroma within the right T6–T7 interspace (*arrow*) which resulted in pressure remodeling of the undersurface of the right 6th rib. There is mild neuroforaminal involvement and resultant scoliosis.

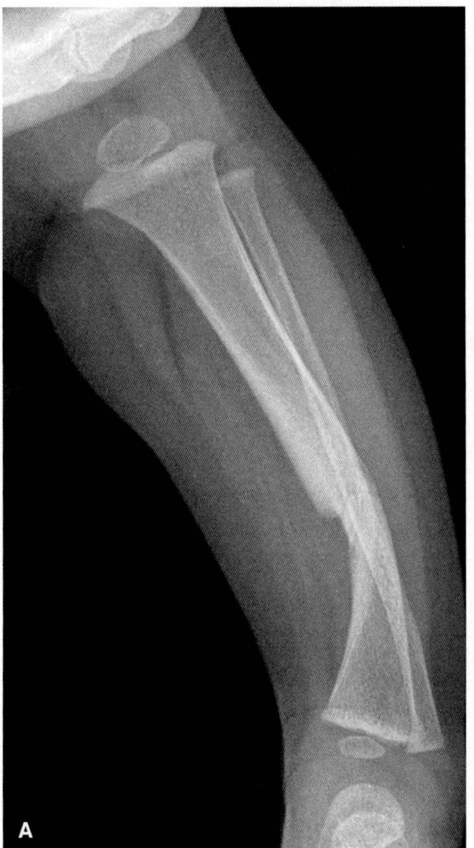

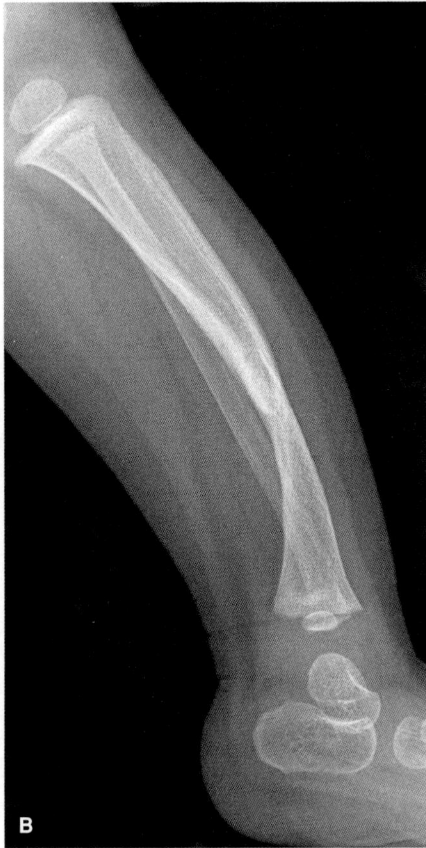

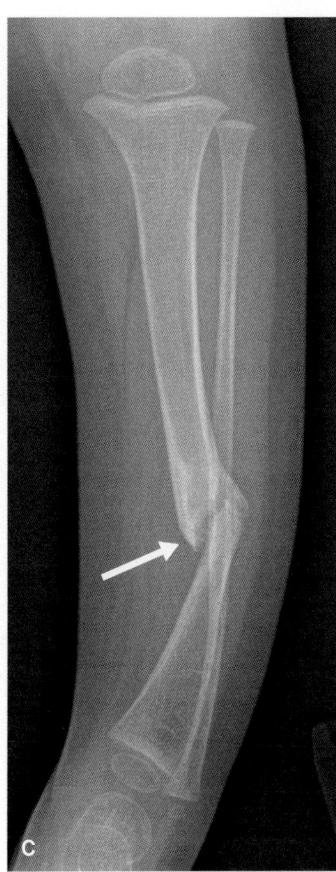

FIGURE 70.41. **Neurofibromatosis and Tibial Pseudoarthrosis.** A 1-year-old boy with NF1 and deformity of the left lower leg. **A:** Frontal and (**B**) lateral radiographs of the left tibia and fibula demonstrate anterior and lateral bowing with deformity of the diaphysis of the tibia, centered at the distal diaphysis. **C:** Frontal radiograph of the tibia at the age of 3 years; the tibia fractured and developed a pseudoarthrosis (*arrow*).

scoliosis being the most common complication (21% of all patients). Dystrophic scoliosis occurs due to bony changes related to neurofibromas affecting the spine. Kyphosis often predominates over scoliosis, with sharply angulated segments of four to six vertebrae. More rapid progression is indicative of a poorer prognosis. Imaging characteristics include vertebral scalloping, neuroforaminal widening (expanded due to dumbbell neurofibromas), transverse process spindling, and rib penciling (underlying mesodermal dysplasia and bony remodeling from adjacent neurofibroma giving rise to thin ribs) (Fig. 70.40). Posterior vertebral scalloping is due to bone weakness and circumferential dilation of the dural sac (dural ectasia). This can lead to spinal instability and angular deformity. Posterior vertebral scalloping can also be seen in Marfan syndrome, achondroplasia, and associated with spinal tumors.

Additional osseous findings related to the effects of mesodermal dysplasia that can be seen in the pectoral and pelvic girdles as well as the long bones include regions of cortical thinning, erosive defects, periosteal proliferation, sclerosis, and cyst-like lesions. Multiple, symmetric bilateral lower extremity nonossifying fibromas may also be seen in NF1. Bowing and pseudoarthrosis can affect a variety of bones but is most common in the tibia. Tibial bowing may be one of the earliest manifestations of the NF1, typically presenting within the first few years of life. The bowing is usually anterolateral (as opposed to benign positional bowing in infants which is posteromedial) and tends to involve the distal diaphysis, resulting in limb shortening (Fig. 70.41). Fractures in this region typically occur before age 3 with pseudoarthrosis development.

METABOLIC BONE DISEASE

Rickets

Rickets is a disorder characterized by impaired mineralization and ossification of cartilage and osteoid and delayed endochondral ossification in children. This results in the excessive physeal cartilage, growth failure, and skeletal deformities. There are many causes, but most cases of rickets are caused by a deficiency of vitamin D. Although rickets has decreased in incidence since the discovery of vitamin D and food fortification, there are still populations at risk including exclusively breast-fed infants and African Americans (due to the pigmentation reducing vitamin D production in the skin). Clinically, patients with rickets manifest short stature, failure to thrive, weakness, and bowing deformities.

The earliest manifestation of rickets is that of demineralization; however, this can be difficult to determine on radiographs. The most diagnostic radiographic finding is due to disordered mineralization and ossification at the growth plate and metaphysis. These findings are most prominent in the metaphyses of bones with the greatest growth: the distal radius and ulna, distal femur, proximal tibia, proximal humerus, and the anterior rib ends. One of the earliest changes at the physis is the loss of the zone of provisional calcification. Widening, fraying, and cupping of the metaphysis are seen due to the accumulation of unossified cartilage (Fig. 70.42). When evaluating the wrist, it is important to know that the distal ulnar metaphysis may normally appear cupped and

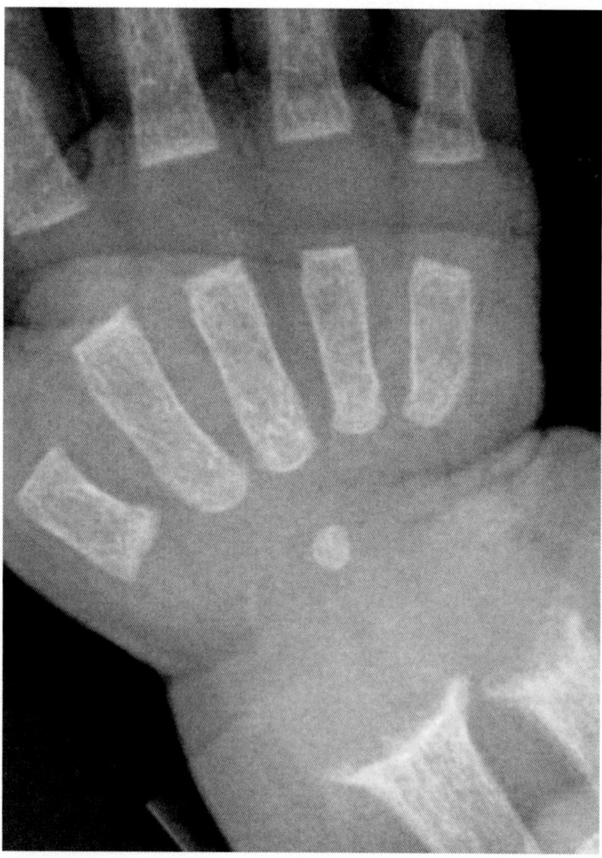

FIGURE 70.42. **Rickets.** A 7-month-old girl who is exclusively breastfed without vitamin D supplementation. Frontal radiograph of the right wrist shows fraying and "cupped" appearance to the distal radial and ulnar metaphyses. There is loss of definition of the zone of provisional calcification with osseous demineralization.

should not be mistaken for rickets if the distal radial metaphysis appears normal. The ossification centers in the epiphysis and in the small bones of the hands and feet are also affected with delayed development and demineralization, although the findings are not as pronounced due to a slower growth rate. The skull may also show poor ossification with indistinct margins and apparently widened sutures. Diaphyseal findings are thought to represent effects of secondary hyperparathyroidism: subperiosteal resorption, cortical thinning, intracortical tunneling, and endosteal resorption. Due to the abnormal bone, weight-bearing patients may have insufficiency fractures or bowing deformity as well.

Treatment of nutritional rickets relies on vitamin D supplementation. Changes of healing can be seen on radiographs within 2 to 3 months with mineralization of the zone of provisional calcification representing one of the earliest findings. Vitamin D supplementation is helpful in preventing nutritional rickets.

Scurvy

Scurvy is due to a chronic deficiency of vitamin C, also known as ascorbic acid which is required for the proper biosynthesis of collagen. Abnormal collagen production leads to vascular fragility along with abnormal bone matrix which occurs in the same areas of greatest bone growth as seen in rickets. Scurvy may go unrecognized clinically and there is often a delay in diagnosis. Therefore, it is important to recognize the findings on radiologic studies in at-risk populations in order to facilitate the diagnosis.

The bones are diffusely demineralized on radiographs with cortical thinning. In addition, there are many "classic" signs of scurvy. The growth plate is irregular with a dense band along the metaphyseal side at the zone of provisional calcification known as the Frankel line. Peripheral extension of this line results in a pointed, "beaked" contour of the metaphysis. A lucent line adjacent to the Frankel line, more diaphyseal

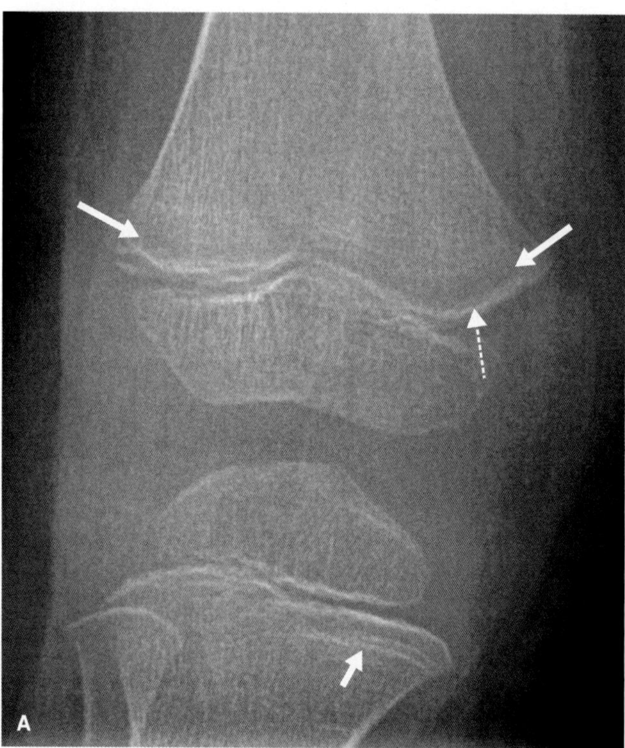

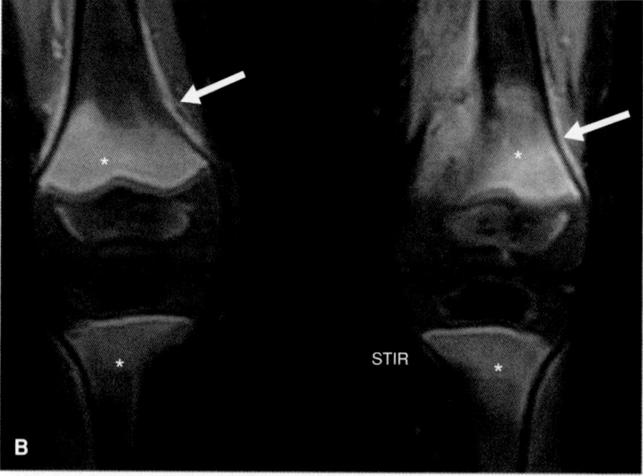

FIGURE 70.43. **Scurvy.** A 4-year-old autistic boy with limp and refusal to bear weight. **A:** Frontal radiograph of the right knee shows diffuse bone demineralization. There is lucency in the distal femoral metaphysis and the Trümmerfeld zone (*long solid arrows*) and increased conspicuity of the zone of provisional calcification, Frankel line (*dashed arrow*). Growth recovery lines are also present, most notable in the proximal tibial metaphysis (*short arrow*). **B:** Coronal fluid-sensitive MR image at the level of the knees shows symmetric increased signal intensity in the metaphyses of the distal femur and proximal tibia (*) as well as ill-defined increased periosseous signal intensity (*arrows*).

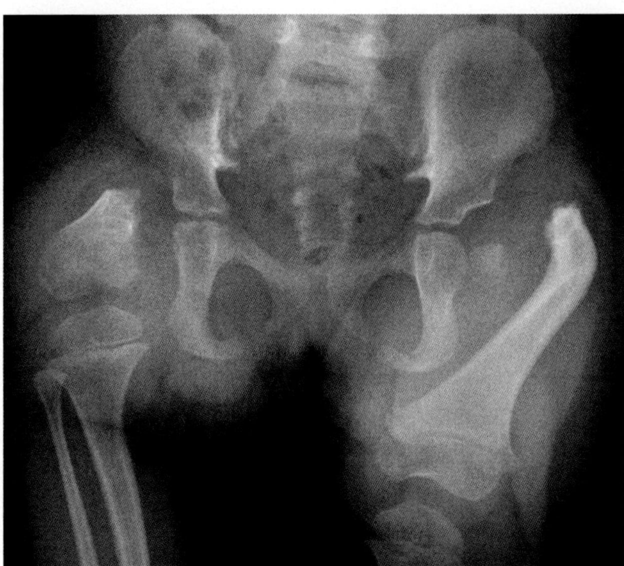

FIGURE 70.44. **Proximal Focal Femoral Deficiency.** A 4-year-old girl with bilateral lower extremity deformities. Frontal radiograph of the pelvis shows hypoplasia of both femurs and bilateral acetabular dysplasia, right worse than left. The right femoral head ossification center is absent.

in location, is known as the Trummerfeld zone or scurvy line and represents accumulated hemorrhage (Fig. 70.43A). Pelkan spur is a healing metaphyseal pathologic fracture seen as a density adjacent to the metaphysis. The Wimberger ring sign is a thin sclerotic cortex surrounding a lucent epiphysis. Due to vascular fragility, subperiosteal hemorrhage can occur and results in periosteal elevation and reaction.

On MRI, patients will have increased T2W SI and decreased T1W SI in the metaphyseal marrow in the long bones, particularly in the bones about the knee. Periosteal elevation can be seen with subperiosteal hemorrhage showing increased T1W and T2W SI. Edema is often seen in the adjacent soft tissues (Fig. 70.43B). Although findings are nonspecific, diffuse symmetric bilateral metaphyseal changes with adjacent soft tissue edema and periosteal reaction should raise suspicion for scurvy. Treatment is with exogenous vitamin C.

Lead Poisoning

Childhood lead poisoning has decreased substantially since the removal of lead from paint and gasoline but it remains the most common form of heavy metal poisoning. Cases of lead poisoning today result from exposure to dust and paint chips from homes that were painted with lead-based paint. At-risk populations include non-Hispanic blacks, Mexican Americans, children from households below the federal poverty level, and those living in areas with high prevalence of lead poisoning. Most children are asymptomatic but children can present with abdominal pain, encephalopathy, neuropathy, and anemia.

Lead poisoning in children can lead to dense metaphyseal bands, the so-called "lead lines." However, dense metaphyseal bands can be seen in many diseases, with the most common cause being normal variation. In lead poisoning, the dense band is due to lead ion deposition in the zone of provisional calcification. It is not the lead itself which causes the density. Lead inhibits osteoclastic remodeling but does not affect osteoblasts and results in increased thickness and trabeculae. One helpful sign occurs with growth of the patient. Lead lines can be distinguished clearly from the zone of provisional calcification once interval growth has occurred, whereas normal variant dense metaphyseal bands are always contiguous with the zone of provisional calcification. Also, evaluation of the proximal fibula is helpful. In patients with normal variant dense metaphyseal band, the proximal fibula will not have a similar dense band, while those with lead poisoning have similar-appearing dense metaphyseal bands in both the tibial and fibular metaphyses. Abdominal radiographs may also show ingested lead fragments within the bowel.

CONGENITAL AND DEVELOPMENTAL BONE AND JOINT DISORDERS

Lower Limb

Proximal Focal Femoral Deficiency. Proximal focal femoral deficiency is a congenital disorder which ranges from hypoplasia to complete absence of the proximal femur. Up to 15% of cases will have bilateral involvement. PFFD is associated with deformities in the ipsilateral limb including: fibular hemimelia (up to 80% of cases), shortened tibia, hypoplastic patella, agenesis of the cruciate ligaments, deficiency of the lateral rays of the foot, talocalcaneal coalition, and equinovalgus or equinovarus deformity. Radiographs are the mainstay of diagnosis and help guide treatment. Given associated ipsilateral limb deformities and leg length abnormalities, it is imperative to image both lower extremities in total. The initial configuration of the proximal femoral shaft has a high correlation with the severity of deformity in PFFD (Fig. 70.44). MRI and US can be used for additional evaluation when the femoral head or connection between the femoral head and femoral shaft is not seen on radiographs. This can help avoid incorrect classification.

Blount Disease. Blount disease is a condition with excessive medial bowing of the tibia, tibia vara. It is thought to occur as a result of abnormal stresses on the posteromedial proximal tibial physis, leading to delayed endochondral ossification at the medial physis. This results in asymmetric growth and varus angulation. There are three types based on age at presentation: infantile (early onset), juvenile (late onset), and adolescent. Infantile is the most common type and is diagnosed before the age of 4 years. There is an association between increased body weight and Blount disease.

The diagnosis is made on standing radiographs of the lower extremities. Genu varum is present as measured by the angle of intersection of lines along the midshaft of the femur and tibia. Additionally, there is depression, irregularity, fragmentation, and beaking of the proximal medial tibial metaphysis and deficiency of the medial proximal tibial epiphysis (Fig. 70.45). It is important to distinguish Blount disease from physiologic bowing. Blount disease is usually unilateral and asymmetric. MRI can be performed to evaluate the proximal tibial physis as well as to assess the structures of the knee joint and is helpful in preoperative planning. Treatment is surgical with hemiepiphysiodesis and guided growth with osteotomy.

Tarsal Coalition. Tarsal coalition is an abnormal fibrous, cartilaginous, or bony connection between two of the tarsal bones. Patients present with chronic pain, often as adolescents. The most common coalitions are talocalcaneal and calcaneonavicular. Tarsal coalition is common and estimated to

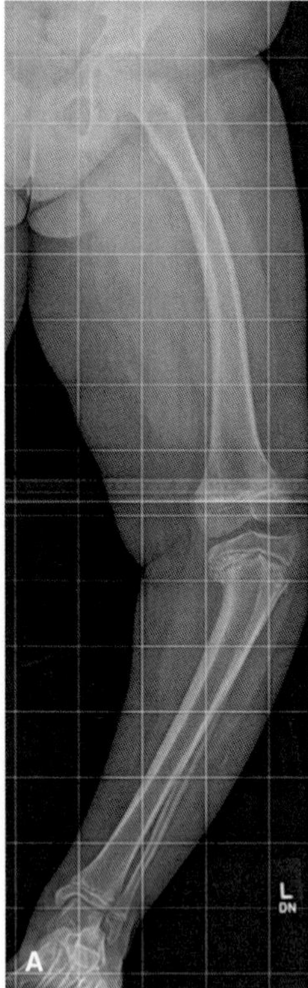

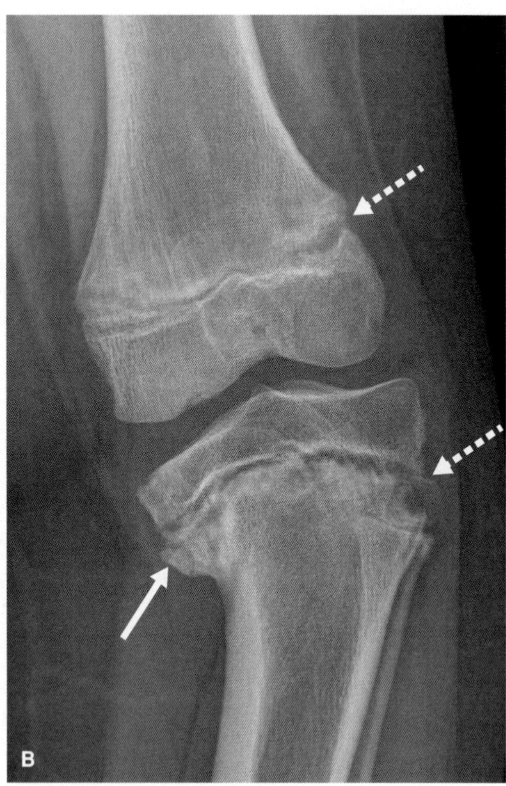

FIGURE 70.45. Blount Disease. A 9-year-old boy with genu varus. **A:** Standing AP radiograph of the left lower extremity shows genu varus. **B:** Frontal radiograph of the knee shows depression, irregularity, beaking, and fragmentation at the proximal medial tibial metaphysis (*solid arrow*) with increased tibiofibular angle. There is resultant widening of the lateral aspect of the distal femoral physis and proximal tibial physis (*dashed arrows*).

affect 1% to 2% of the population with bilateral involvement in approximately 50% of cases.

On radiographs, calcaneonavicular coalitions are best seen on the oblique view of the foot. Direct, bony connection may be seen in osseous coalition. In cases of fibrous or cartilaginous coalition, there is close approximation of the calcaneus and navicular with irregularity at the joint margin. The lateral view of the foot shows associated findings

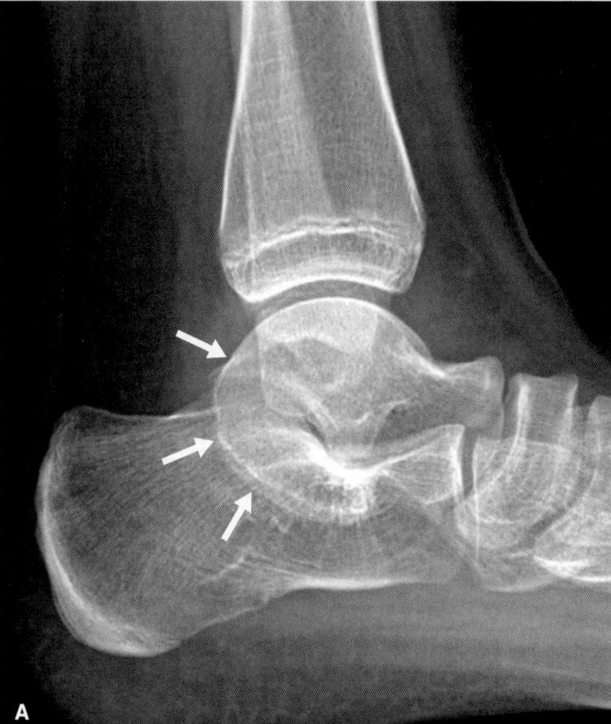

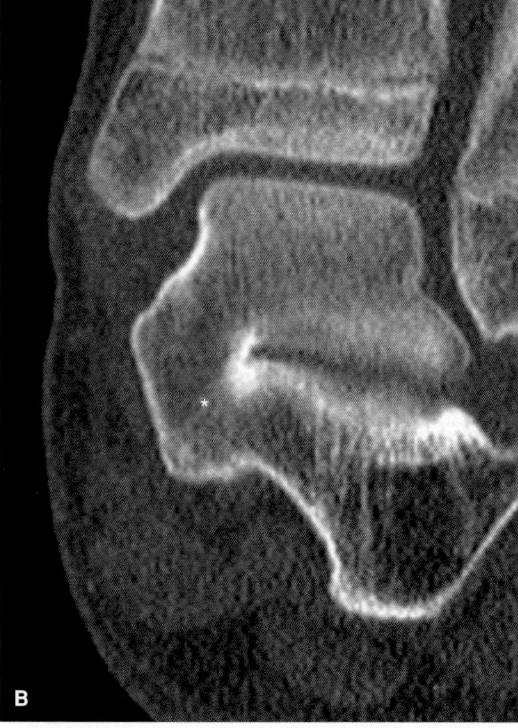

FIGURE 70.46. Talocalcaneal Coalition. A 14-year-old boy with chronic left ankle pain. **A:** Lateral radiograph of the left ankle shows a continuous "C sign" following the contour of the talar dome to the sustentaculum tali (*arrows*). **B:** Coronal reformatted CT image of the left foot shows osseous talocalcaneal coalition at the middle talocalcaneal joint (*).

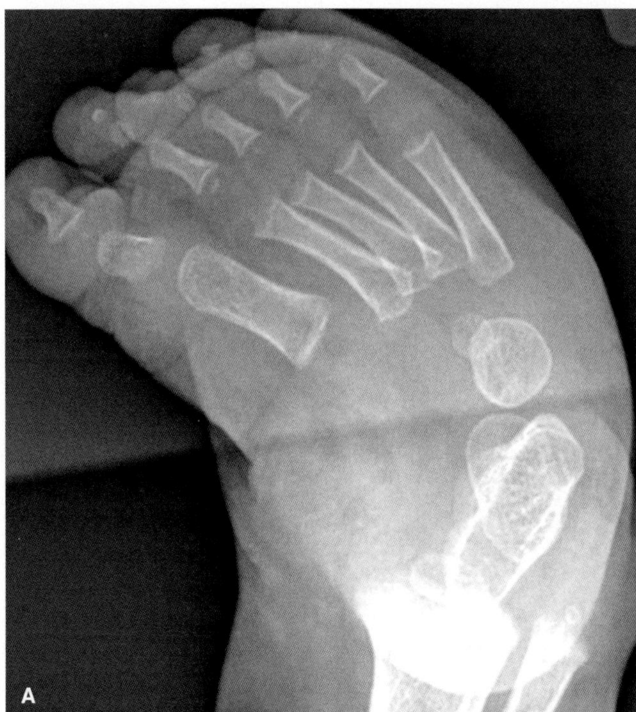

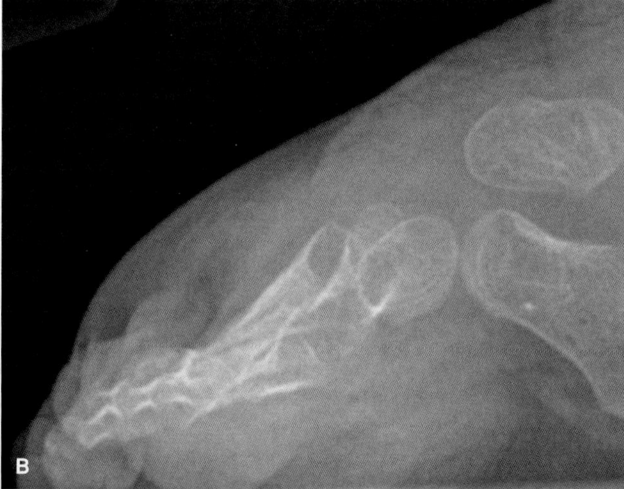

FIGURE 70.47. **Congenital Talipes Equinovarus.** An 8-month-old boy with fixed foot deformity (adduction, supination, and varus). **A:** Frontal and (**B**) lateral radiographs of the foot with simulated weight bearing show a near-parallel configuration of the talus and calcaneus with decreased talocalcaneal angle. There is adduction and varus deformity of the forefoot.

including an elongated appearance to the anterior–superior calcaneus extending toward the navicular, the so-called "anteater's nose."

Findings of talocalcaneal coalition include talar beaking, poor visualization of the talocalcaneal joint space, rounding of the lateral talar process, and lack of depiction of the middle facet on lateral radiographs. The "C sign" can be seen on lateral radiographs as well with a C-shaped line that outlines the medial talar dome and posterior–inferior sustentaculum (Fig. 70.46).

CT is invaluable in the diagnosis and surgical planning of tarsal coalition, especially talocalcaneal coalition which is not as easily depicted on radiographs. As with radiographs, a direct bony connection may be seen or narrowing, irregularity, and sclerosis may be seen in the setting of a nonosseous coalition. Both feet should be imaged due to the high occurrence of bilateral involvement. MRI has been shown to be equally as effective as CT for diagnosis of tarsal coalition. In addition to findings similar to CT, fluid-sensitive sequences may show bone marrow edema at the site of fused articulation. Treatment is conservative initially and includes casting, physical therapy, orthotics, and anti-inflammatory medication. Those that fail conservative therapy go on to surgical resection.

Congenital Talipes Equinovarus (Clubfoot). Congenital talipes equinovarus or "clubfoot" is a common developmental disorder of the lower limb. The foot is fixed in adduction, supination, and in varus. The calcaneus, navicular, and cuboid bones are medially rotated relative to the talus. The forefoot is pronated in relation to the hindfoot which gives rise to pes cavus. The ligaments and tendons of the foot tightly hold the foot in a fixed deformity.

Weight-bearing radiographs will demonstrate four features: hindfoot equinus with a lateral talocalcaneal angle less than 35 degrees, hindfoot varus on AP radiographs with a talocalcaneal angle less than 20 degrees, metatarsus adductus with adduction and varus deformity of the forefoot and talus to first metatarsal angle greater than 15 degrees, as well as medial subluxation of the navicular on the talus. On the lateral view, there is a near-parallel arrangement of the talus and calcaneus (Fig. 70.47). Many patients require orthopedic intervention and options range from serial casting to surgical release.

Developmental Dysplasia of the Hip. Developmental dysplasia of the hip (DDH) includes a spectrum of abnormalities ranging from mild to markedly abnormal development of the femoral head and acetabulum. The reported incidence of DDH ranges from 1.5 to 30 per 1,000 births. Although the exact etiology is unknown, normal hip development requires close association and congruency of the acetabulum with the femoral head. Multiple risk factors are described including breech position in utero, oligohydramnios, family history, female gender, and first born. Other conditions associated with fetal motion constraint such as club foot, molding deformity of the skull, and sternocleidomastoid torticollis have an increased association with DDH. The left hip is more commonly involved than the right. Physical examination can reveal a hip click or clunk with upward force and abduction at the hip (Ortolani test) or with downward force and adduction (Barlow test) in young infants. Asymmetric skinfolds and leg length discrepancies can also be seen on examination.

Ultrasound is the primary imaging modality in screening for and evaluating DDH in children younger than 6 months of age. After 6 months of age, the femoral head ossification center obscures acetabular evaluation and radiographs are utilized. On US, both static and dynamic images of the hips are taken in transverse and coronal planes to evaluate both the morphology of the acetabulum and positioning of the femoral head. On static US images, measurements and assessment focus on a standard coronal image of the hip at the level of the mid acetabulum. A normally positioned femoral head is more than 50% covered by the acetabulum (Fig. 70.48A,B). The Graf alpha angle can be measured and is the angle formed

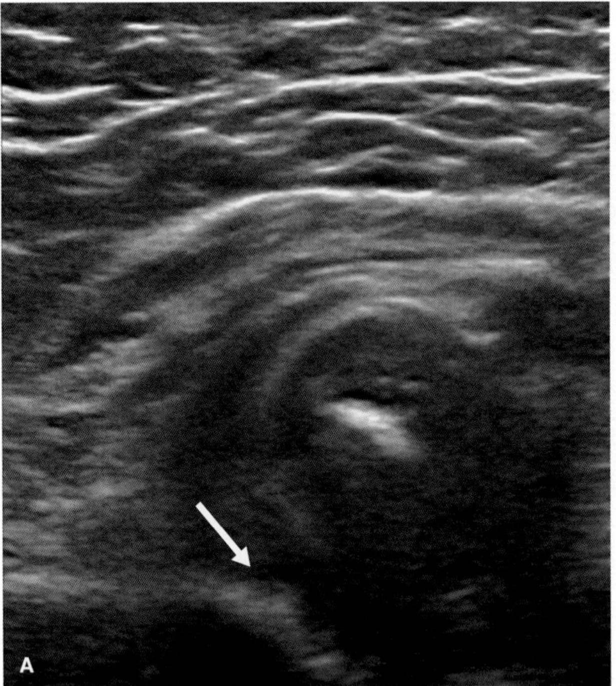

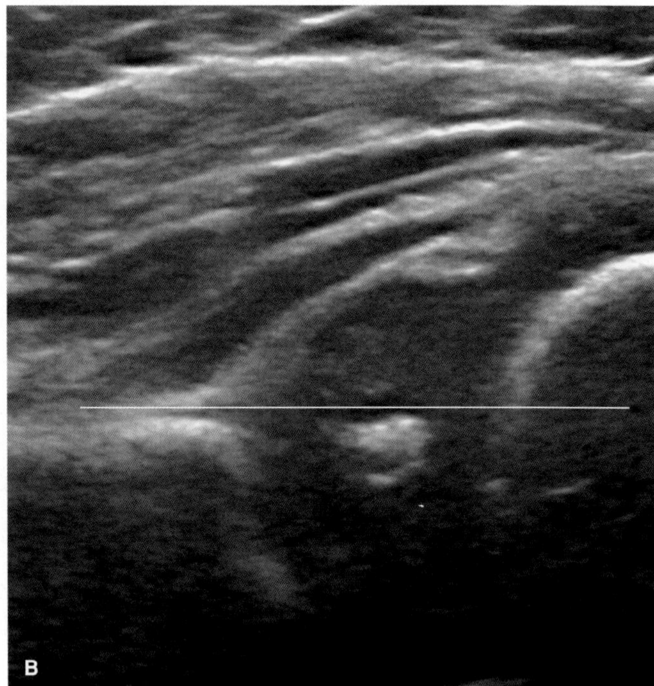

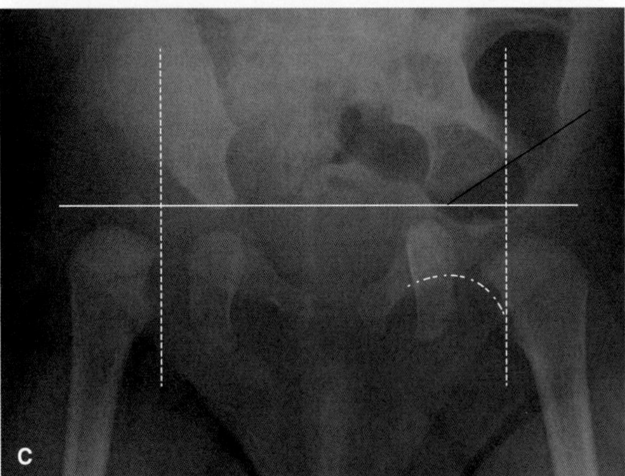

FIGURE 70.48. **Developmental Hip Dysplasia.** A 6-month-old girl with right developmental hip dysplasia and normal left hip. **A:** US of the right hip in the coronal neutral position shows dislocation of the right proximal femoral epiphysis relative to the iliac bone (*arrow*). **B:** US of the left hip in the coronal neutral position for comparison shows normal alignment of the left femoral head to the acetabulum. There is greater than 50% coverage of the femoral head as measured using a line drawn along the iliac bone. **C:** AP radiograph of the pelvis in the same patient shows delayed ossification of the proximal right femoral ossification center relative to the left with shallow right acetabulum. The horizontal Hilgenreiner line (*solid line*) and vertical Perkin line are drawn (*dashed line*). The left femoral head is normally located in the medial inferior quadrant of the intersecting lines while the right femoral head is abnormal in the lateral superior quadrant corresponding to the findings on US and indicative of dislocation. The acetabular angle is shown on the left with a line along the acetabular roof (*solid black arrow*) intersecting the Hilgenreiner line. A normal Shenton line is drawn on the left (*curved dashed line*).

by the cortex of the ilium and the acetabular roof. An alpha angle less than 60 degrees is abnormal. Stress is also applied to evaluate for laxity.

In the older infant, an anteroposterior radiograph of the pelvis in neutral position allows for morphologic assessment of the hips, while a frog-leg lateral view can help determine whether a subluxated hip reduces. Findings include delayed femoral head ossification, a shallow acetabulum, and abnormal position of the femoral head relative to the acetabulum (Fig. 70.48C). There are many lines and angles which can be drawn to help assess for DDH on radiographs (Table 70.9).

Treatment is determined by the age at diagnosis. When treated early, there is greater success and lower incidence of residual dysplasia and long-term complications. In patients up to 6 months, closed reduction with a Pavlik harness is the treatment of choice. If unsuccessful or in older infants, closed surgical reduction with hip spica casting is performed. Open reduction followed by spica casting is reserved for cases where the hip is irreducible by closed means.

After reduction and casting, proper location of the femoral head in the acetabulum should be confirmed. This is important as excessive abduction is postulated to lead to AVN. MRI may show obstacles such as labral inversion, limbus formation, ligamentous hypertrophy, and enlargement of the pulvinar. The administration of intravenous gadolinium contrast is used by some institutions to assess femoral head perfusion.

Upper Limb

Shoulder Dysplasia. Developmental shoulder dysplasia is usually caused by traction injury during birth leading to brachial plexus palsy. Risk factors include shoulder dystocia, breech presentation, forceps delivery, and fetal macrosomia.

Radiographs are useful once the proximal humeral epiphyses develop as one can see an asymmetrically small, aspherical, and flattened humeral head. The glenoid will appear

TABLE 70.9

RADIOGRAPHIC EVALUATION FOR DEVELOPMENTAL DYSPLASIA OF THE HIP ON AN AP PELVIS RADIOGRAPH

■ DEMARCATION	■ LOCATION	■ SIGNIFICANCE
Hilgenreiner line	Horizontal line through both triradiate cartilages	Normal femoral head should lie within the inferior medial quadrant of the acetabulum as defined by the intersection of Perkins and Hilgenreiner lines
Perkins line	Vertical line intersecting the lateral rim of the acetabular roof, drawn perpendicular to Hilgenreiner line	
Shenton line	C-shaped line along the inferior aspect of the pubic ramus and continuing to the inferior border of the femoral neck	Normal hip, this should be a smooth line
Acetabular angle (index)	Angle formed by a line through the acetabular roof and the Hilgenreiner line	In neonates, acetabular angle should be less than 30 degrees and decreased, as the patient ages, to less than 22 degrees at 1 year of age and older
Anterior center-edge angle	Angle formed from a vertical line through the center of the ossified femoral head and line along the lateral margin of the acetabular roof	Center-edge angle less than 20 degrees is indicative of DDH

dysplastic with a hypoplastic scapula and there is glenoid retroversion. US and MRI are increasingly being used in infants and very young children to better depict and quantify these and other abnormalities such as differences in relative muscle bulk (vs. the contralateral shoulder) and nerve root avulsion.

Treatment depends heavily on imaging findings. Those with early findings of dysplasia can be treated with physical therapy and botulinum toxin injection or closed reduction. Older children and those with greater findings of dysplasia may require surgery, and nerve grafting may be performed in those with multiple nerve root avulsions.

Amniotic Band Syndrome

Amniotic band syndrome (also known as constriction band syndrome) comprises a wide range of congenital anomalies where fetal parts get entrapped with fibrous bands of disrupted amnion which typically leads to limb and digital amputations and constriction rings (Fig. 70.49). Maldevelopment is caused by a vascular insult that occurs during early embryogenesis. Uncommonly, major abnormalities may also occur in the craniofacial region and body wall (body wall complex). This is usually diagnosed prenatally and treatment is dependent on the body part and severity of the constriction. If blood flow is demonstrated within the distal limb, fetoscopic release may be attempted. Postnatally, radiographs are obtained to evaluate the osseous structures involved in order to provide prognostic information and possible surgical planning.

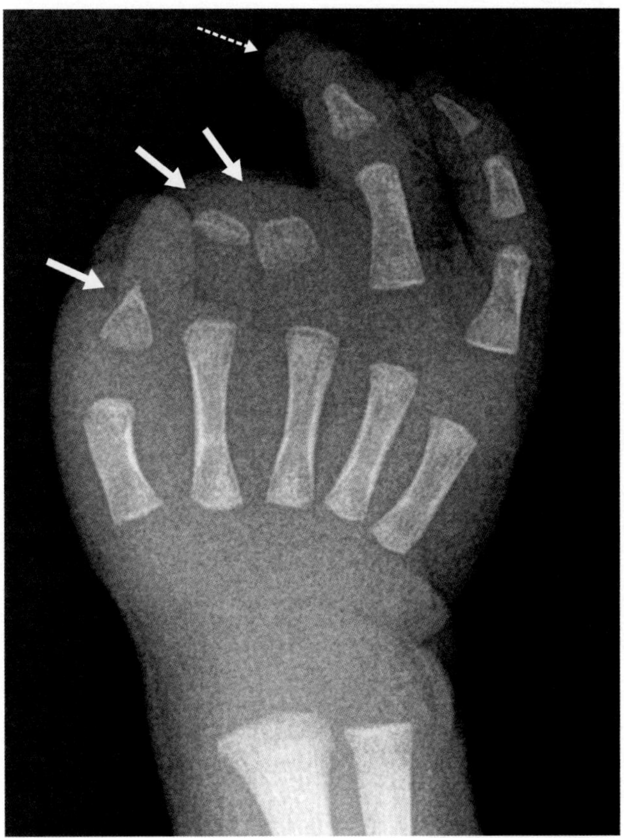

FIGURE 70.49. Amniotic Band Syndrome. An 8-month-old girl with congenital left hand deformity and no other abnormalities. Frontal radiograph of the hand shows partial amputation of the first through fourth fingers with truncated and tapered proximal phalanges in the first through third fingers (*solid arrows*) and absent distal phalanx in the fourth finger (*dashed arrow*). There is soft tissue syndactyly of the second and third fingers. Findings are due to a constrictive amniotic band which causes ischemia and amputation.

INFLAMMATORY CONDITIONS

Juvenile Idiopathic Arthritis

Juvenile idiopathic arthritis (JIA) is an umbrella term that encompasses all forms of inflammatory arthritis that begin before the age of 16, persist for more than 6 weeks, and are of unknown etiology. It is the most common childhood rheumatic entity and the exact etiology is not fully understood but is thought to include both environmental and genetic factors.

The hallmark feature of all subtypes of JIA is joint inflammation. This typically begins as inflammation of the synovial lining. If left untreated, synovial inflammation progresses to synovial hyperplasia with increased vascularity, resulting in a highly cellular inflammatory pannus. The pannus will eventually erode into the overlying cartilage and bone as a result of antibody deposition and degradative enzymes, leading to articular destruction. In children, inflammation may also cause growth disturbances, both systemically and locally in affected joints.

Radiographs have poor sensitivity in depicting early active arthritis and show erosive change late in the disease course as articular and epiphyseal cartilage must be eroded before any osseous manifestations can been seen. Radiographic findings early on in the disease course are often nonspecific and include soft tissue swelling, joint effusions, and osseous demineralization (both periarticular and generalized demineralization). As the disease progresses, localized hyperemia of the joint may result in epiphyseal enlargement, accelerated maturation, and osseous overgrowth. Initially, this may lead to increased length of the affected limb; however, in long-standing disease, accelerated maturation leads to premature physeal fusion and resultant limb shortening or joint malalignment. For weight-bearing joints, standing radiographs are recommended.

The use of US and MRI has been steadily increasing as these modalities can reliably assess abnormalities within the synovium, cartilage, and bone (US can assess the bone surface while MRI can assess for bone marrow edema). US allows for a rapid and inexpensive method for evaluating synovial proliferation, joint fluid, cartilage thickness, cortical erosions, tenosynovitis, and enthesitis. Multiple joints can be assessed at one visit without the need for sedation. If synovial thickening is present on gray scale imaging, it is important to use color or power Doppler to evaluate for increased synovial vascularization which would be compatible with synovitis.

MRI is the best noninvasive imaging modality to evaluate for inflammation of the joints, tendons, and entheses. It is useful for the depiction of bone marrow edema as well as assessment of intra-articular structures that cannot be accessed with an ultrasound probe. Multiple planar pulse sequences include T1-weighted, cartilage-specific, fluid-sensitive as well as post-gadolinium sequences. Postcontrast imaging should be obtained in the early phase (<5 minutes) after injection to provide optimal discrimination of enhancing synovium from more slowly enhancing effusion. Active arthritis is seen as pathologic enhancement of thickened synovium (Fig. 70.50). The goal of intervention is to suppress synovial and entheseal inflammation in order to prevent cartilage and bone damage. Treatments include both systemic therapy as well as direct medicinal joint injections.

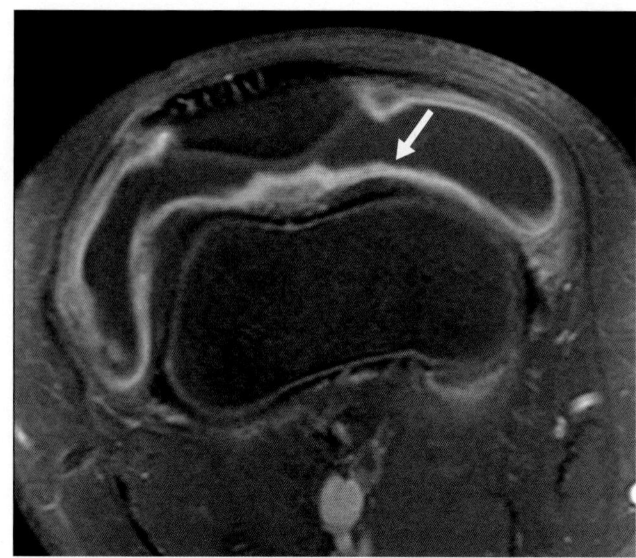

FIGURE 70.50. JIA. A 12-year-old boy with knee swelling for several weeks. Axial T1-weighted fat-saturated MR image after intravenous contrast administration shows diffuse synovial thickening and enhancement (*arrow*). A moderate knee joint effusion is present. Laboratory work revealed a normal white blood cell count, elevated sedimentation rate, and positive antinuclear antibody (ANA) test. The patient had anterior uveitis on slit-lamp examination.

Hemophilic Arthropathy

Hemophilia A and B are X-linked congenital bleeding disorders caused by the absence or decrease of clotting factor VIII or factor IX, respectively. Joint bleeding is the most frequent manifestation of the disease and repeated hemarthroses may lead to hemophilic arthropathy which can have a significant negative impact on mobility and quality of life. Synovitis is one of the earliest complications of hemarthrosis which is characterized by synovial hypertrophy and inflammation with neoangiogenesis and subsequent bleeding. The pathogenic mechanisms and molecular pathways by which blood in the joint causes articular and bone damage is not fully known.

Large joints are most commonly involved in the following order: knee, elbow, ankle, hip, and shoulder. It is not uncommon for the same joint to be repeatedly involved. In the knee, classic findings include a widened intercondylar notch, squared margins of the patella, and bulbous femoral condyles with flattened surfaces. Repeated bleeds into the elbow joint lead to enlargement of the radial head with a widened trochlear notch. Ankle deformity may arise due to undergrowth of the lateral aspect of the distal tibial epiphysis. MRI is optimal for early disease. Gradient sequences may be useful to assess for hemosiderin, and gadolinium is useful for the depiction of synovitis. Cartilage sequences should be utilized to assess for chronicity, including cartilage thinning and erosive changes.

Chronic Recurrent Multifocal Osteomyelitis

Chronic recurrent multifocal osteomyelitis (CRMO) is an idiopathic inflammatory disorder of children and young adults that is characterized by exacerbations and remissions of nonbacterial osteomyelitis. CRMO may also be seen in conjunction with other inflammatory disorders such as psoriasis and inflammatory bowel disease and lesions are treated with anti-inflammatory therapies. Since there is no laboratory confirmation test, CRMO remains a disease of exclusion. Biopsy may be performed in challenging cases which in early cases show nonspecific inflammation with granulocytic infiltration, with or without multinucleated giant cells. As the lesion progresses, plasma cells and histiocytes may be present. Imaging plays an important role in the diagnosis and management.

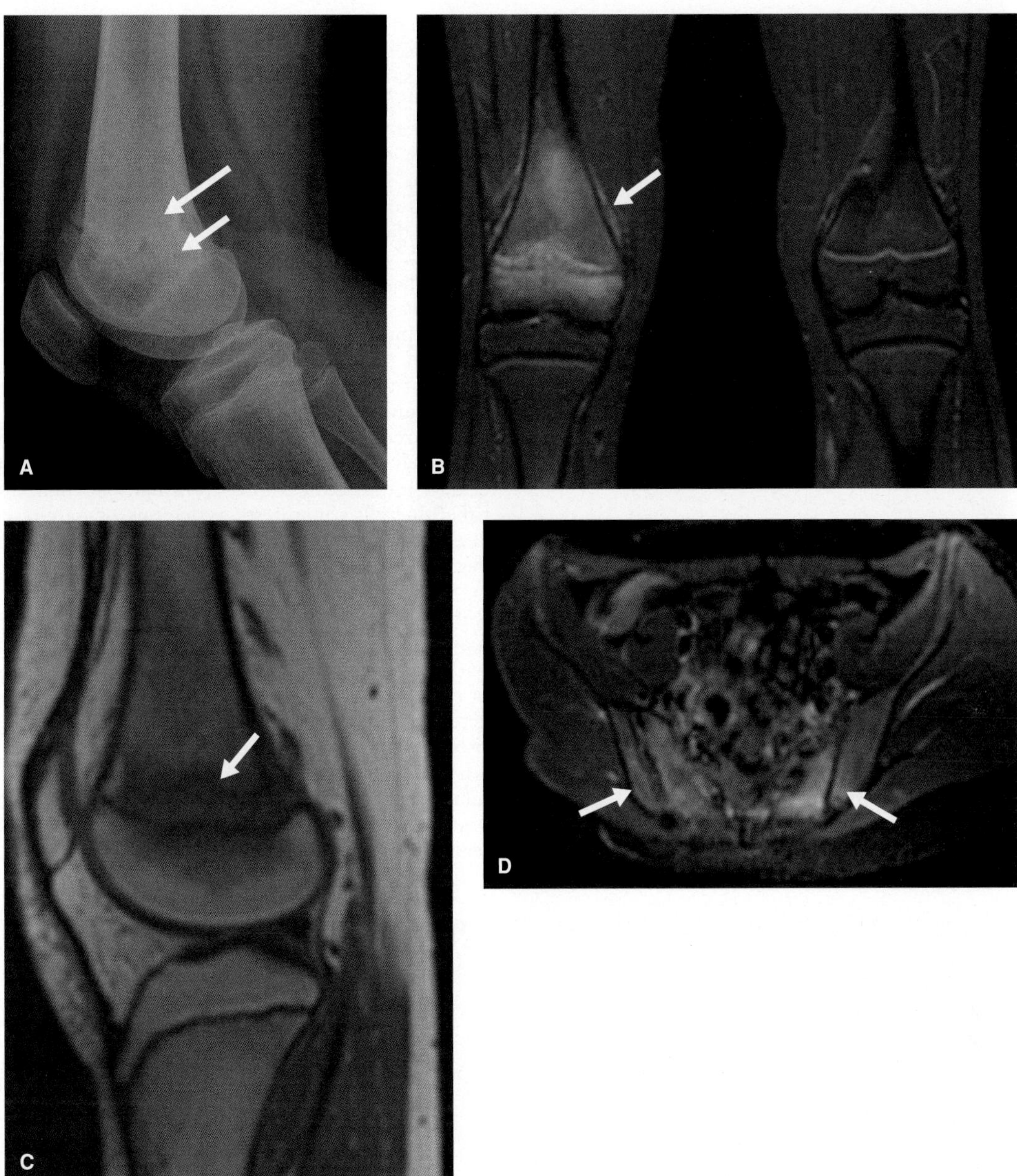

FIGURE 70.51. CRMO. A 12-year-old girl with right knee pain for several months and no known trauma. No fevers and her white blood cell count and inflammatory markers were normal. **A:** Lateral radiograph of the right knee shows sclerosis in the distal femoral metaphysis (*long arrow*) and subphyseal pyramidal-shaped lucencies (*short arrow*). There is no periosteal reaction or soft tissue mass. Mild sclerosis is also seen within the epiphysis. **B:** Coronal fluid-sensitive MRI of the knees shows increased SI in the distal right femoral metaphysis and epiphysis with widened and irregular distal femoral physis. Mild adjacent soft tissue edema is seen along the distal femoral metaphysis (*arrow*). **C:** Sagittal T1-weighted image of the right knee shows low SI in the distal right femur corresponding to the radiographic findings (follow-up imaging 2 years later demonstrated a bony bar [not shown]). **D:** WB-MRI was performed for additional lesions. Axial fluid-sensitive MR of the pelvis at the level of the sacroiliac joints shows increased SI around both sacroiliac joints (*arrows*) compatible with sacroiliitis. Symptoms improved with NSAIDs.

Patients typically present with nonspecific complaints such as pain, tenderness, swelling, or limited range of motion at one or more sites. Fever, weight loss, or other systemic features are usually absent. The onset may be insidious, with symptoms present for months to years before diagnosis. Characteristic locations include the mandible and medial aspect of the clavicle (an uncommon site for hematogenous infectious osteomyelitis). Long bone lesions are most commonly seen in the metaphyses of the lower extremities. Rib, vertebral, sacroiliac joint, and pelvic (metaphyseal equivalents) involvement is common.

Imaging should begin with conventional radiographs of the symptomatic sites. Initially, radiographs demonstrate an osteolytic lesion adjacent to the growth plate in the metaphysis. Over time, there is progressive sclerosis around the lytic regions. Inflammation can disrupt the physis and extend to the adjacent epiphysis (Fig. 70.51A). Periosteal reaction and soft tissue swelling may be present. MR imaging is useful for determining the local extent of disease and for surveillance. In active inflammatory lesions, there are typical findings of bone marrow edema with or without adjacent soft tissue edema and periostitis. Transphyseal disease seen on MR is typically underestimated on conventional radiographs. Joint effusions and synovial inflammation may be seen in the adjacent joint. Imaging of CRMO patients typically involves whole-body imaging (e.g., whole-body MRI or bone scan) to evaluate multiple involved sites as well as to depict clinically occult sites of inflammation (Fig. 70.51B–D).

HEMOGLOBINOPATHIES

Hemoglobinopathies are a group of genetic disorders that possess an abnormality within the hemoglobin molecule. The two most clinically relevant conditions within the pediatric population are sickle cell disease and β-thalassemia. Both have variable courses, and osseous manifestations can vary greatly even within the same disease and depending on therapeutic interventions.

Sickle Cell Disease

Sickle cell disease and its variants result from a single point mutation in the β-chain of the hemoglobin molecule. This causes the hemoglobin molecules to become "sticky" with abnormal polymerization, deforming the red blood cells into the classic sickle shape. This results in microvascular occlusion and ischemic events. Sickle cell patients maintain red marrow in the majority of the axial and appendicular skeleton, including the ankles and wrists. Red marrow persistence may cause widened medullary spaces, thinned cortices, demineralization, and a coarsened trabecular pattern. This is commonly recognized within the skull with widening of the diploic space of the calvarium and thinning of the inner or outer calvarial table, giving rise to the classic "hair on end" pattern.

The same bony remodeling occurs within the spine. Progressive cortical thinning and smooth biconcavity may develop in the vertebral bodies due to weakened bone and pressure effect from the adjacent disc and is referred to as "codfish" vertebrae. Sharper depressions can occur in the central portions of the endplates due to focal infarction, producing the classic "Lincoln log" or "H-shaped" vertebral bodies (Fig. 70.52). Diffuse sclerosis may also be seen in the spine from repetitive infarctions.

Sickle cell dactylitis or "hand-foot" syndrome will affect approximately 50% of pediatric patients, the majority between 6 months and 2 years of age. The small tubular bones of the hands and feet are particularly prone to infarction resulting in painful crises. In these bones, the transformation of red marrow to yellow marrow occurs much later in sickle cell patients, making episodes uncommon after 6 years of age. Initial radiographs are usually normal; however, over time, dactylitis manifests as regions of patchy lucency with periosteal reaction. More severe cases will demonstrate bony destruction and deformity.

Sickle cell osteonecrosis is also seen within the long bones. Radiographs are relatively insensitive for acute infarction but may demonstrate later stages with sclerosis or osteolysis. MRI with fluid-sensitive sequences depicts acute changes as areas of increased fluid SI representing marrow-like edema. A characteristic serpiginous "double line" is described which consists of a hyperintense inner line (inflammatory response) and a hypointense outer border (reactive bone interface). Cortical infarctions can also occur, resulting in cortical thickening or "bone-in-bone" appearance secondary to layered subperiosteal new bone formation.

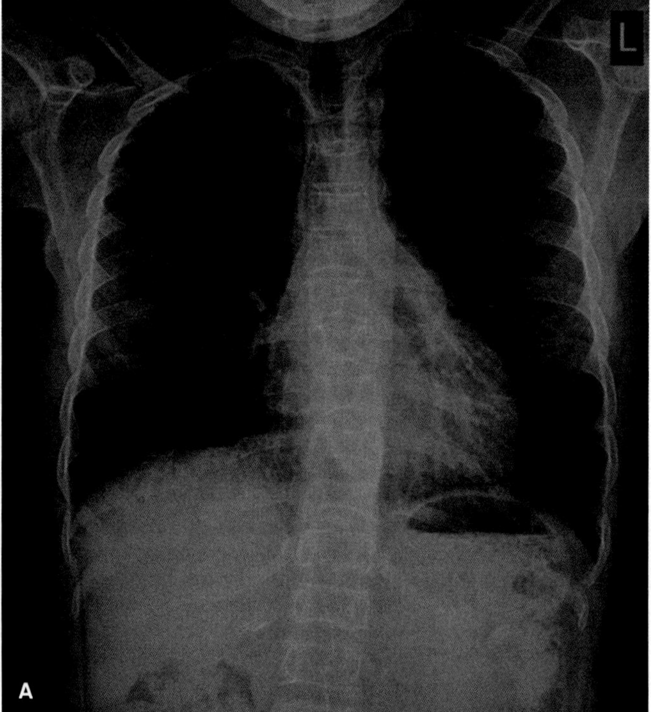

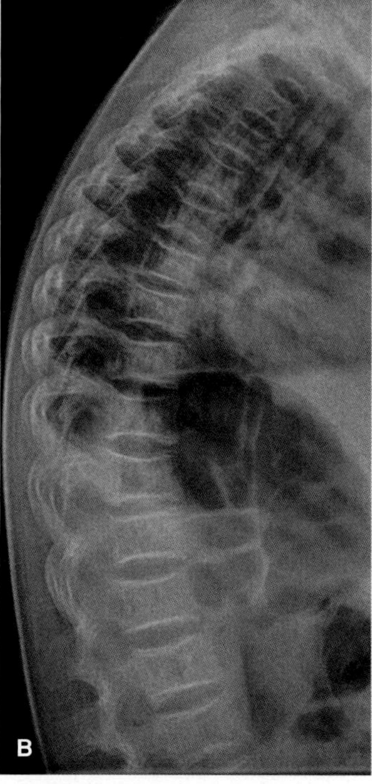

FIGURE 70.52. **Sickle Cell Disease.** A 14-year-old girl with cough. **A:** AP and (**B**) lateral radiographs of the chest demonstrate no acute cardiopulmonary process; however, demonstrate sickle cell osteopathy of the spine. There is demineralization with coarsening of the trabecular pattern. Multilevel vertebral abnormalities are present with "codfish vertebrae" due to pressure of the adjacent disc in the setting of weakened bone. There is an absent splenic shadow (secondary to autoinfarction), postsurgical changes of cholecystectomy, and a mildly prominent cardiac silhouette.

Sickle cell–related epiphyseal osteonecrosis is most common in the humeral and femoral heads and often bilateral. Radiographic findings of later-stage epiphyseal infarction include crescentic subchondral lucency and articular irregularity and subchondral collapse and fragmentation. This is often more pronounced in the weight-bearing joints, such as the hip, where articular deformity may lead to secondary degenerative changes. MRI is most sensitive for depiction of epiphyseal osteonecrosis. Coronal and sagittal imaging planes are utilized to evaluate for loss of epiphyseal sphericity. Early closure of the physes may occur secondary to osteonecrosis or subsequent transphyseal revascularization of the femoral head, resulting in foreshortened bones and compensatory metaphyseal cupping.

Osteomyelitis in sickle cell patients is usually due to *Salmonella* or other gram-negative organisms such as *Escherichia coli* and is a challenging diagnostic problem, as the spectrum of bone crises and bone infection overlap and both may present with pain, fevers, abnormal inflammatory markers, and soft tissue swelling of the affected region. Blood cultures can be useful but are generally positive in only half of the cases. Features of osteomyelitis and osteonecrosis will overlap by imaging, and biopsy or aspiration is often needed for definitive diagnosis, noting both may demonstrate an infiltrate of neutrophils, macrophages, and necrotic tissue.

β-Thalassemia

The β-thalassemias are genetic disorders affecting the β-globin gene that result in reduced or absent synthesis of β-globin chains, ultimately affecting erythropoiesis and red cell lifespans. As a result, anemia, hepatosplenomegaly, cardiomegaly with congestive heart failure, and significant marrow expansion with secondary osseous deformities occur. Osseous imaging findings in this disorder are related to extramedullary hematopoiesis as well as a result of iron chelation therapy which is distinctly different compared with sickle cell disease. Many of the classically described skeletal findings have become less apparent due to improved therapies and decreased degrees of marrow expansion.

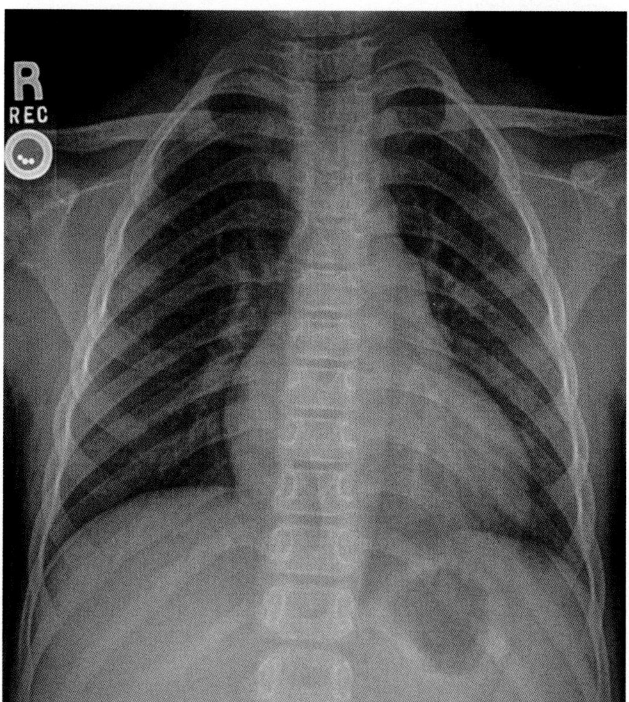

FIGURE 70.53. **β-Thalassemia.** An 11-year-old boy with β-thalassemia and cough. Frontal radiograph of the chest without an acute process. There is expansion of the proximal aspects of multiple contiguous ribs due to increased bone marrow production in the setting of high red blood cell turnover.

Osseous changes occur due to severe anemia and a massive, increased demand for red blood cells which produce diffuse marrow expansion of the calvarium, spine, pelvis, and nearly all tubular bones. This results in cortical thinning and resorption of cancellous bone with coarsening of the trabecular markings. Ribs are commonly involved as demonstrated by expansion of the head and neck of the ribs (Fig. 70.53).

Calvarial thickening is most prominent within the frontal bones with thinning of the outer table and prominent subperiosteal spicules, creating the "hair on end" appearance. In addition, the marked marrow expansion results in diminished pneumatization of the paranasal sinuses. Marrow expansion in the maxillary bones may ventrally displace the central incisors and laterally displaces the orbits which give rise to the pathognomonic facial appearance of thalassemia, the so-called "rodent facies."

Thalassemia patients who have not undergone transfusion therapy demonstrate an infantile marrow distribution. In patients receiving transfusions without iron chelation therapy, there is a mix of hematopoietic marrow and iron deposition throughout the majority of the skeleton. Patients receiving transfusions along with chelation therapy will show iron deposition predominately within the axial skeleton with hematopoietic marrow in the remainder.

Suggested Readings

Ablin DS, Greenspan A, Reinhart M, Grix A. Differentiation of child abuse from osteogenesis imperfecta. *AJR Am J Roentgenol* 1990;154(5):1035–1046.

Ablin DS, Jain K, Howell L, West DC. Ultrasound and MR imaging of fibromatosis colli (sternomastoid tumor of infancy). *Pediatr Radiol* 1998;28(4):230–233.

Ackman J, Altiok H, Flanagan A, et al. Long-term follow-up of Van Nes rotationplasty in patients with congenital proximal focal femoral deficiency. *Bone Joint J* 2013;95-B(2):192–198.

ACR–AIUM–SPR–SRU Practice Parameter for the Performance of the Ultrasound Examination for Detection and Assessment of Developmental Dysplasia of the Hip. Revised 2013.

Aitken GT. Proximal femoral deficiency—definition, classification, and management. In: Aitken GT, ed. *Proximal Femoral Focal Deficiency: A Congenital Anomaly*. Washington, DC: National Academy of Sciences; 1969:1–22.

Almeida A, Roberts I. Bone involvement in sickle cell disease. *Br J Haematol* 2005; 129(4):482–490.

Arnold WD, Hilgartner MW. Hemophilic arthropathy. Current concepts of pathogenesis and management. *J Bone Joint Surg Am* 1977;59(3):287–305.

Arora R, Fichadia U, Hartwig E, Kannikeswaran N. Pediatric upper-extremity fractures. *Pediatr Ann* 2014;43(5):196–204.

Azouz EM, Saigal G, Rodriguez MM, Podda A. Langerhans' cell histiocytosis: pathology, imaging and treatment of skeletal involvement. *Pediatr Radiol* 2005;35(2):103–115.

Azouz EM, Slomic AM, Marton D, Rigault P, Finidori G. The variable manifestations of dysplasia epiphysealis hemimelica. *Pediatr Radiol* 1985;15:44–49.

Babhulkar SS, Pande K, Babhulkar S. The hand-foot syndrome in sickle-cell haemoglobinopathy. *J Bone Joint Surg Br* 1995;77(2):310–312.

Baron JH. Sailors' scurvy before and after James Lind—a reassessment. *Nutr Rev* 2009;67:315–332.

Bedoya MA, Chauvin NA, Jaramillo D, Davidson R, Horn BD, Ho-Fung V. Common patterns of congenital lower extremity shortening: diagnosis, classification, and follow-up. *Radiographics* 2015;35(4):1191–1207.

Bedoya MA, Jaramillo D, Chauvin NA. Overuse injuries in children. *Top Magn Reson Imaging* 2015;24(2):67–81.

Beltran LS, Rosenberg ZS, Mayo JD, et al. Imaging evaluation of developmental hip dysplasia in the young adult. *AJR Am J Roentgenol* 2013;200:1077–1088

Bernard EJ, Nicholls WD, Howman-Giles RB, Kellie SJ, Uren RF. Patterns of abnormality on bone scans in acute childhood leukemia. *J Nucl Med* 1998;39(11):1983–1986.

Bernard SM, McGeehin MA. Prevalence of blood lead levels > or = 5 micro g/dL among US children 1 to 5 years of age and socioeconomic and demographic factors associated with blood of lead levels 5 to 10 micro g/dL, Third National Health and Nutrition Examination Survey, 1988–1994. *Pediatrics* 2003;112(6 pt 1):1308–1313.

Berry DH, Gresik MV, Humphrey GB, et al. Natural history of histiocytosis X: a pediatric oncology group study. *Med Pediatr Oncol* 1986;14:1–5.
Binkovitz LA, Olshefski RS, Adler BH. Coincidence FDG-PET in the evaluation of Langerhans cell histiocytosis: preliminary findings. *Pediatr Radiol* 2003;33:598–602.
Blickman JG, van Die CE, de Rooy JW. Current imaging concepts in pediatric osteomyelitis. *Eur Radiol* 2004;14(Suppl 4):L55–L64.
Blickman JG, Wilkinson RH, Graef JW. The radiologic "lead band" revisited. *AJR Am J Roentgenol* 1986;146(2):245–247.
Bodnar LM, Simhan HN, Powers RW, Frank MP, Cooperstein E, Roberts JM. High prevalence of vitamin D insufficiency in black and white pregnant women residing in the northern United States and their neonates. *J Nutr* 2007;137:447–452.
Boles CA, el-Khoury GY. Slipped capital femoral epiphysis. *Radiographics* 1997;17:809–823.
Bonafe L, Cormier-Daire V, Hall C, et al. Nosology and classification of genetic skeletal disorders: 2015 revision. *Am J Med Genet A* 2015;167A:2869–2892.
Burnett MW, Bass JW, Cook BA. Etiology of osteomyelitis complicating sickle cell disease. *Pediatrics* 1998;101(2):296–297.
Campanacci M, Picci P, Gherlinzoni F, Guerra A, Bertoni F, Neff JR. Parosteal osteosarcoma. *J Bone Joint Surg Br* 1984;66:313–321.
Carter R, Anslow P. Imaging of the calvarium. *Semin Ultrasound CT MR* 2009;30(6):465–491.
Centers for Disease Control and Prevention (CDC). Blood lead levels—United States, 1999-2002. *MMWR Morb Mortal Wkly Rep* 2005;54(20):513–516.
Chambers HG. Ankle and foot disorders in skeletally immature athletes. *Orthop Clin North Am* 2003;34(3):445–459.
Chambers HG, Shea KG, Carey JL. AAOS Clinical Practice Guideline: diagnosis and treatment of osteochondritis dissecans. *J Am Acad Orthop Surg* 2011;19(5):307–309.
Chang CY, Rosenthal DI, Mitchell DM, Handa A, Kattapuram SV, Huang AJ. Imaging findings of metabolic bone disease. *Radiographics* 2016;36(6):1871–1887.
Chauvin NA, Jaimes C, Laor T, Jaramillo D. Magnetic resonance imaging of the pediatric shoulder. *Magn Reson Imaging Clin N Am* 2012;20(2):327–347.
Chauvin NA, Khwaja A. Imaging of inflammatory arthritis in children: status and perspectives on the use of ultrasound, radiographs, and magnetic resonance imaging. *Rheum Dis Clin North Am* 2016;42:587–606.
Cheema JI, Grissom LE, Harcke HT. Radiographic characteristics of lower-extremity bowing in children. *Radiographics* 2003;23(4):871–80.
Chesney RW. Rickets: the third wave. *Clin Pediatr (Phila)* 2002;41:137–139.
Chesney RW. Rickets: an old form for a new century. *Pediatr Int* 2003;45:509–511.
Crawford SC, Harnsberger HR, Johnson L, Aoki JR, Giley J. Fibromatosis colli of infancy: CT and sonographic findings. *AJR Am J Roentgenol* 1988; 151(6):1183–1184.
Crim JR, Kjeldsberg KM. Radiographic diagnosis of tarsal coalition. *AJR Am J Roentgenol* 2004;182(2):323–328.
Daffner RH, Lupetin AR, Dash N, Deeb ZL, Sefczek RJ, Schapiro RL. MRI in the detection of malignant infiltration of bone marrow. *AJR Am J Roentgenol* 1986;146:353–358.
Daldrup-Link HE, Steinbach L. MR imaging of pediatric arthritis. *Magn Reson Imaging Clin N Am* 2009;17(3):451–467, vi.
De Smet AA, Ilahi OA, Graf BK. Reassessment of the MR criteria for stability of osteochondritis dissecans in the knee and ankle. *Skeletal Radiol* 1996;25(2):159–163.
De Smet AA, Ilahi OA, Graf BK. Untreated osteochondritis dissecans of the femoral condyles: prediction of patient outcome using radiographic and MR findings. *Skeletal Radiol* 1997;26(8):463–467.
de Vernejoul MC. Sclerosing bone disorders. *Best Pract Res Clin Rheumatol* 2008;22(1):71–83.
Delgado J, Jaramillo D, Chauvin NA. Imaging the injured pediatric athlete: upper extremity. *Radiographics* 2016;36(6):1672–1687.
DeLuca HF. Overview of general physiological features and functions of vitamin D. *Am J Clin Nutr* 2004;80:1689S–1696S.
Discepola F, Powell TI, Nahal A. Telangiectatic osteosarcoma: radiologic and pathologic findings. *Radiographics* 2009;29(2):380–383.
Donnelly LF. Toddler's fracture of the fibula. *AJR Am J Roentgenol* 2000; 175(3):922.
Donnelly LF. Developmental dysplasia of the hip. In: Donnelly LF. *Pediatric Imaging: The Fundamentals*. Philadelphia, PA: Elsevier; 2009:188–191.
Dugan LO, Meyer SJ, Chua GT. General case of the day. Acute lymphoblastic leukemia. *Radiographics* 1993;13(1):221–223.
Dunbar JS, Owen HF, Nogrady MB, et al. Obscure tibial fracture of infants—the toddler's fracture. *J Can Assoc Radiol* 1964;15:136–144.
Dupuis CS, Westra SJ, Makris J, Wallace EC. Injuries and conditions of the extensor mechanism of the pediatric knee. *Radiographics* 2009;29:877–886.
Dwek JR, Chung CB. A systematic method for evaluation of pediatric sports injuries of the elbow. *Pediatr Radiol* 2013;43 Suppl 1:S120–S128.
Ecklund K, Jaramillo D. Patterns of premature physeal arrest: MR imaging of 111 children. *AJR Am J Roentgenol* 2002;178(4):967–972.
Eggert P, Viemann M. Physiological bowlegs or infantile Blount's disease. Some new aspects on an old problem. *Pediatr Radiol* 1996;26(5):349–352.
Ejindu VC, Hine AL, Mashayekhi M, Shorvon PJ, Misra RR. Musculoskeletal manifestations of sickle cell disease. *Radiographics* 2007;27(4):1005–1021.
Emery KH, Bisset GS 3rd, Johnson ND, Nunan PJ. Tarsal coalition: a blinded comparison of MRI and CT. *Pediatr Radiol* 1998;28(8):612–616.
Emery KH, Zingula SN, Anton CG, Salisbury SR, Tamai J. Pediatric elbow fractures: a new angle on an old topic. *Pediatr Radiol* 2016;46(1):61–66.
Favara BE, Feller AC, Pauli M. Contemporary classification of histiocytic disorders. The WHO Committee on histiocytic/reticulum cell proliferations. Reclassification Working Group of the Histiocyte Society. *Med Pediatr Oncol* 1997;29:157–166.
Fernandez-Latorre F, Menor-Serrano F, Alonso-Charterina S, Arenas-Jiménez J. Langerhans cell histiocytosis of the temporal bone in pediatric patients: imaging and follow-up. *AJR* 2000;174:217–221.
Flors L, Leiva-Salinas C, Maged IM, et al. MR imaging of soft-tissue vascular malformations: diagnosis, classification, and therapy follow-up. *Radiographics* 2011;31(5):1321–1340; discussion 1340–1341.
Foad SL, Mehlman CT, Ying J. The epidemiology of neonatal brachial plexus palsy in the United States. *J Bone Joint Surg Am* 2008;90(6):1258–1264.
Gilbertson-Dahdal D, Wright JE, Krupinski E, McCurdy WE, Taljanovic MS. Transphyseal involvement of pyogenic osteomyelitis is considerably more common than classically taught. *AJR Am J Roentgenol* 2014;203:190–195.
Gillespie H. Osteochondroses and apophyseal injuries of the foot in the young athlete. *Curr Sports Med Rep* 2010;9(5):265–268.
Glorieux FH. Osteogenesis imperfecta *Best Pract Res Clin Rheumatol* 2008; 22(1):85–100.
Golriz F, Donnelly LF, Devaraj S, Krishnamurthy R. Modern American scurvy—experience with vitamin C deficiency at a large children's hospital. *Pediatr Radiol* 2017;47(2):214–220.
Goo HW, Yang DH, Ra YS, et al. Whole-body MRI of Langerhans cell histiocytosis: comparison with radiography and bone scintigraphy. *Pediatr Radiol* 2006;36(10):1019–1031.
Greenspan A. Sclerosing bone dysplasias: a target-site approach. *Skeletal Radiol* 1991;20(8):561–583.
Grissom L, Harcke HT, Thacker M. Imaging in the surgical management of developmental dislocation of the hip. *Clin Orthop Relat Res* 2008;466(4):791–801.
Gulko E, Collins LK, Murphy RC, Thornhill BA, Taragin BH. MRI findings in pediatric patients with scurvy. *Skeletal Radiol* 2015;44(2):291–297.
Gurney JG, Severson RK, Davis S, Robison LL. Incidence of cancer in children in the United States. Sex-, race-, and 1-year age-specific rates by histologic type. *Cancer* 1995;75(8):2186–2195.
Hall CM. International nosology and classification of constitutional disorders of bone (2001). *Am J Med Genet* 2002;113:65–77.
Haque S, Bilal Shafi BB, Kaleem M. Imaging of torticollis in children. *Radiographics* 2012;32(2):557–571.
Harper GD, Dicks-Mireaux C, Leiper AD. Total body irradiation-induced osteochondromata. *J Pediatr Orthop* 1998;18:356–358.
Hartkamp MJ, Babyn PS, Olivieri F. Spinal deformities in deferoxamine-treated homozygous beta-thalassemia major patients. *Pediatr Radiol* 1993; 23(7):525–528.
Helix-Giordanino M, Randier E, Frey S, Piclet B; French association of foot surgery (AFCP). Treatment of Freiberg's disease by Gauthier's dorsal cuneiform osteotomy: retrospective study of 30 cases. *Orthop Traumatol Surg Res* 2015;101(6 Suppl):S221–S225.
Hesper T, Zilkens C, Bittersohl B, Krauspe R. Imaging modalities in patients with slipped capital femoral epiphysis. *J Child Orthop* 2017;11:99–106.
Heywood CS, Benke MT, Brindle K, Fine KM. Correlation of magnetic resonance imaging to arthroscopic findings of stability in juvenile osteochondritis dissecans. *Arthroscopy* 2011;27(2):194–199.
Hillmann JS, Mesgarzadeh M, Revesz G, Bonakdarpour A, Clancy M, Betz RR. Proximal femoral focal deficiency: radiologic analysis of 49 cases. *Radiology* 1987;165(3):769–773.
Ho-Fung V, Jaimes C, Delgado J, Davidson RS, Jaramillo D. MRI evaluation of the knee in children with infantile Blount disease: tibial and extra-tibial findings. *Pediatr Radiol* 2013;43(10):1316–1326.
ISSVA Classification of Vascular Anomalies ©2014 International Society for the Study of Vascular Anomalies. Available from www.issva.org/classification. Accessed March 14, 2018.
Iyer RS, Thapa MM. MR imaging of the paediatric foot and ankle. *Pediatr Radiol* 2013;43 Suppl 1:S107–S119.
Jaimes C, Chauvin NA, Delgado J, Jaramillo D. MR imaging of normal epiphyseal development and common epiphyseal disorders. *Radiographics* 2014; 34(2):449–471.
Jaramillo D, Dormans JP, Delgado J, Laor T, St Geme JW 3rd. Hematogenous osteomyelitis in infants and children: imaging of a changing disease. *Radiology* 2017;283(3):629–643.
Jaramillo D, Shapiro F. Musculoskeletal trauma in children. *Magn Reson Imaging Clin N Am* 1998;6(3):521–536.
John SD, Moorthy CS, Swishuck LE. Expanding the concept of the toddler's fracture. *Radiographics* 1997;17:367–376.
Johnson CM, Navarro OM. Clinical and sonographic features of pediatric soft-tissue vascular anomalies part 1: classification, sonographic approach and vascular tumors. *Pediatr Radiol* 2017;47(9):1184–1195.
Kakel R. Trampoline fracture of the proximal tibial metaphysis in children may not progress into valgus: A report of seven cases and brief review. *Orthop Traumatol Surg Res* 2012;98(4):446–449.
Kalayjian BS, Herbut PA, Erf LA. The bone changes of leukemia in children. *Radiology* 1946;47:223–233.
Kan JH, Hernanz-Schulman M, Frangoul HA, Connolly SA. MRI diagnosis of bone marrow relapse in children with ALL. *Pediatr Radiol* 2008;38(1):76–81.

Karasick D, Schweitzer ME, Eschelman DJ. Symptomatic osteochondromas: imaging features. *AJR Am J Roentgenol* 1997;168:1507–1512.

Keats TE, Riddervold HO, Michaelis LL. Thanatophoric dwarfism. *Am J Roentgenol Radium Ther Nucl Med* 1970;108(3):473–480.

Keith A. Studies on the anatomical changes which accompany certain growth disorders of the human body: 1. The Nature of the Structural Alterations in the Disorder known as Multiple Exostoses. *J Anat* 1920;54:101–115.

Khana G, Sato TSP, Ferguson P. Imaging of chronic recurrent multifocal osteomyelitis. *Radiographics* 2009;29:1159–1177.

Kijowski R, Blankenbaker DG, Shinki K, Fine JP, Graf BK, De Smet AA. Juvenile versus adult osteochondritis dissecans of the knee: appropriate MR imaging criteria for instability. *Radiology* 2008;248(2):571–578.

Kim HJ, Chalmers PN, Morris CD. Pediatric osteogenic sarcoma. *Curr Opin Pediatr* 2010;22(1):61–66.

Kleinman PK. Problems in the diagnosis of metaphyseal fractures: *Pediatr Radiol* 2008;38 Suppl 3:S388–S394.

Kocher MS, Mandiga R, Zurakowski D, Barnewolt C, Kasser JR. Validation of a clinical prediction rule for the differentiation between septic arthritis and transient synovitis of the hip in children. *J Bone Joint Surg Am* 2004; 86-A(8):1629–1635.

Kollipara R, Dinneen L, Rentas KE, et al. Current classification and terminology of pediatric vascular anomalies. *AJR Am J Roentgenol* 2013;201(5): 1124–1135.

Kooy A, de Heide LJ, ten Tije AJ, et al. Vertebral bone destruction in sickle cell disease: infection, infarction or both. *Neth J Med* 1996;48(6):227–231.

Koskimies E, Syvänen J, Nietosvaara Y, Mäkitie O, Pakkasjärvi N. Congenital constriction band syndrome with limb defects. *J Pediatr Orthop* 2015;35(1):100–103.

Kozlowski K, Grigor WG. Probably congenital histiocytosis X with unusual radiographic finding in a 7-week-old infant. *Pediatr Radiol* 1980;9:45–47.

Kransdorf MJ, Smith SE. Lesions of unknown histogenesis: Langerhans cell histiocytosis and Ewing sarcoma. *Semin Musculoskelet Radiol* 2000;4(1): 113–125.

Kwack KS, Cho JH, Lee JH, Cho JH, Oh KK, Kim SY. Septic arthritis versus transient synovitis of the hip: gadolinium-enhanced MRI finding of decreased perfusion at the femoral epiphysis. *AJR Am J Roentgenol* 2007; 189:437–445.

LaFrance RM, Giordano B, Goldblatt J, Voloshin I, Maloney M. Pediatric tibial eminence fractures: evaluation and management. *J Am Acad Orthop Surg* 2010;18(7):395–405.

Langer LO Jr, Baumann PA, Gorlin RJ. Achondroplasia. *Am J Roentgenol Radium Ther Nucl Med* 1967;100(1):12–26.

Laor T, Jaramillo D. MR imaging insights into skeletal maturation: what is normal? *Radiology* 2009;250(1):28–38.

Laor T. Musculoskeletal imaging: evaluation of congenital anomalies. *Pediatr Radiol* 2008;38 Suppl 2:S246–S250.

Lateur LM, Van Hoe LR, Van Ghillewe KV, Gryspeerdt SS, Baert AL, Dereymaeker GE. Subtalar coalition: diagnosis with the C sign on lateral radiographs of the ankle. *Radiology* 1994;193:847–851.

Laval-Jeantet M, Balmain N, Juster M, Bernard J. Relations of the perichondral ring to the cartilage in normal and pathologic growth. *Ann Radiol (Paris)* 1968; 11:327–335.

Lawrence DA, Rolen MF, Haims AH, Zayour Z, Moukaddam HA. Tarsal coalitions: radiographic, CT, and MR imaging findings. *HSS J* 2014;10(2): 153–66.

Leone AJ Jr. On lead lines. *Am J Roentgenol Radium Ther Nucl Med* 1968; 103:165–167.

Letts M, Davidson D, Ahmer A. Osteochondritis dissecans of the talus in children. *J Pediatr Orthop* 2003;23(5):617–625.

Levin TL, Sheth SS, Ruzal-Shapiro C, Abramson S, Piomelli S, Berdon WE. MRI marrow observations in thalassemia: the effects of the primary disease, transfusional therapy, and chelation. *Pediatr Radiol* 1995;25(8):607–613.

Lonergan GF, Baker AM, Morey MK, Boos SC. From the archives of the AFIP. Child abuse: radiologic-pathologic correlation. *Radiographics* 2003;23: 811–845.

Lonergan GJ, Cline DB, Abbondanzo SL. Sickle cell anemia. *Radiographics* 2001;21(4):971–994.

Maheshwari AV, Cheng EY. Ewing sarcoma family of tumors. *J Am Acad Orthop Surg* 2010;18(2):94–107.

Malanga GA, Ramirez-Del Toro JA. Common injuries of the foot and ankle in the child and adolescent athlete. *Phys Med Rehabil Clin N Am* 2008;19(2):347–371, ix.

Malghem J, Vande Berg B, Noel H, Maldague B. Benign osteochondromas and exostotic chondrosarcomas: evaluation of cartilage cap thickness by ultrasound. *Skeletal Radiol* 1992;21:33–37.

Mar WA, Taljanovic MS, Bagatell R, et al. Update on imaging and treatment of Ewing sarcoma family tumors: what the radiologist needs to know. *J Comput Assist Tomogr* 2008;32(1):108–118.

Markowitz RI, Zackai E. A pragmatic approach to the radiologic diagnosis of pediatric syndromes and skeletal dysplasias. *Radiol Clin North Am* 2001;39(4):791–802, xi.

Mckie J, Radomisli T. Congenital vertical talus: A review. *Clin Podiatr Med Sug* 2010;27:145–156.

Melchiorre D, Manetti M, Matucci-Cerinic M. Pathophysiology of hemophilic arthropathy. *J Clin Med* 2017;6(7):63.

Menapace D, Mitkov M, Towbin R, Hogeling M. The changing face of complicated infantile hemangioma treatment. *Pediatr Radiol* 2016;46(11):1494–1506.

Menashe SJ, Tse R, Nixon JN, et al. Brachial plexus birth palsy: multimodality imaging of spine and shoulder abnormalities in children. *AJR Am J Roentgenol* 2015;204(2):W199–W206.

Merrow AC, Gupta A, Patel MN, Adams DM. 2014 revised classification of vascular lesions from the International Society for the Study of Vascular Anomalies: radiologic-pathologic update. *Radiographics* 2016;36(5):1494–1516.

Meyer JS, Harty MP, Mahboubi S, et al. Langerhans cell histiocytosis: presentation and evolution of radiologic findings with clinical correlation. *Radiographics* 1995;15:1135–1146.

Miedzybrodzka Z. Congenital talipes equinovarus (clubfoot): a disorder of the foot but not the hand. *J Anat* 2003;202:37–42.

Milgram JW. The origins of osteochondromas and enchondromas: a histopathologic study. *Clin Orthop Relat Res* 1983;174:264–284.

Mirbey J, Besancenot J, Chambers RT, Durey A, Vichard P. Avulsion fractures of the tibial tuberosity in the adolescent athlete: risk factors, mechanism of injury, and treatment. *Am J Sports Med* 1988;16(4):336–340.

Mitnick JS, Pinto RS. Computed tomography in the diagnosis of eosinophilic granuloma. *J Comput Assist Tomogr* 1980;4:791–793.

Morrissy R. *Lovell and Winter's Pediatric Orthopaedics*. 5th ed. Philadelphia, PA: Lippincott Williams & Wilkins; 2001:1218–1247.

Munns CF, Shaw N, Kiely M, et al. Global consensus recommendations on prevention and management of nutritional rickets. *J Clin Endocrinol Metab* 2016;101(2):394–415.

Murphey MD, Choi JJ, Kransdorf MJ, Flemming DJ, Gannon FH. Imaging of osteochondroma: variants and complications with radiologic-pathologic correlation. *Radiographics* 2000;20(5):1407–1434.

Murphey MD, Robbin MR, McRae GA, Flemming DJ, Temple HT, Kransdorf MJ. The many faces of osteosarcoma. *Radiographics* 1997;17: 1205–1231.

Murphey MD, Senchak LT, Mambalam PK, Logie CI, Klassen-Fischer MK, Kransdorf MJ. From the radiologic pathology archives: Ewing sarcoma family of tumors: radiologic-pathologic correlation. *Radiographics* 2013;33(3): 803–831.

Murphey MD, wan Jaovisidha S, Temple HT, Gannon FH, Jelinek JS, Malawer MM. Telangiectatic osteosarcoma: radiologic-pathologic comparison. *Radiology* 2003;229(2):545–553.

Navarro SM, Matcuk GR, Patel DB, et al. Musculoskeletal imaging findings of hematologic malignancies. *Radiographics* 2017;37:881–900.

Neuhauser EB, Wittenborg MH, Berman CZ, Cohen J. Irradiation effects of roentgen therapy on the growing spine. *Radiology* 1952;59:637–650.

Newman JS, Newberg AH. Congenital tarsal coalition: multimodality evaluation with emphasis on CT and MR imaging. *Radiographics* 2000;20(2):321–332; quiz 526–527, 532.

Nimkin K, Kleinman PK. Imaging of child abuse. *Radiol Clin North Am* 2001;39:843–864.

Oestreich AE, Ahmad BS. The periphysis and its effect on the metaphysis. II. Application to rickets and other abnormalities. *Skeletal Radiol* 1933; 22:115–119.

Oestreich AE. The acrophysis: a unifying concept for enchondral bone growth and its disorders. 1. Normal growth. *Skeletal Radiol* 2003;32:121–127.

Oliveira JC, Abreu MS, Gomes FM. Sternocleidomastoid tumour in neonate: fibromatosis colli. *BMJ Case Rep* 2018;2018. pii: bcr-2017-223543. doi: 10.1136/bcr-2017-223543.

Onikul E, Fletcher BD, Parham DM, Chen G. Accuracy of MR imaging for estimating intraosseous extent of osteosarcoma. *AJR Am J Roentgenol* 1996; 167:1211–1215.

Ording Muller LS, Humphries P, Rosendahl K. The joints in juvenile idiopathic arthritis. *Insights Imaging* 2015;6(3):275–284.

Palmucci S, Attinà G, Lanza ML, et al. Imaging findings of mucopolysaccharidoses: a pictorial review. *Insights Imaging* 2013;4(4):443–459.

Panda A, Gamanagatti S, Jana M, Gupta AK. Skeletal dysplasias: a radiographic approach and review of common non-lethal skeletal dysplasias. *World J Radiol* 2014;6(10):808–825.

Parnell SE, Phillips GS. Neonatal skeletal dysplasias. *Pediatr Radiol* 2012;42 Suppl 1:S150–S157.

Patel CV. The foot and ankle: MR imaging of uniquely pediatric disorders. *Magn Reson Imaging Clin N Am* 2009;17(3):539–547, vii.

Patel NB, Stacy GS. Musculoskeletal manifestations of neurofibromatosis type 1. *AJR AJR Am J Roentgenol* 2012;199:W99–W106.

Perez-Rossello JM, Feldman HA, Kleinman PK, et al. Rachitic changes, demineralization, and fracture risk in healthy infants and toddlers with vitamin D deficiency. *Radiology* 2012;262(1):234–241.

Piehl FC, Davis RJ, Prugh SI. Osteomyelitis in sickle cell disease. *J Pediatr Orthop* 1993;13(2):225–227.

Pirkle JL, Brody DJ, Gunter EW, et al. The decline in blood lead levels in the United States. The National Health and Nutrition Examination Surveys (NHANES). *JAMA* 1994;272(4):284–291.

Polat AV, Bekci T, Say F, Bolukbas E, Selcuk MB. Osteoskeletal manifestations of scurvy: MRI and ultrasound findings. *Skelet Radiol* 2015;44: 1161–1164.

Pontell D, Hallivis R, Dollard MD. Sports injuries in the pediatric and adolescent foot and ankle: common overuse and acute presentations. *Clin Podiatr Med Surg* 2006;23(1):209–231, x.

Pöyhiä TH, Lamminen AE, Peltonen JI, Kirjavainen MO, Willamo PJ, Nietosvaara Y. Brachial plexus birth injury: US screening for glenohumeral joint instability. *Radiology* 2010;254(1):253–260.

Prakken B, Albani S, Martini A. Juvenile idiopathic arthritis. *Lancet* 2011; 377(9783):2138–2149.

Raber SA. The dense metaphyseal band sign. *Radiology* 1999;211(3):773–774.

Rao P, Carty H. Non-accidental injury: review of the radiology. *Clin Radiol* 1999;54:11–24.

Rauch F, Glorieux FH. Osteogenesis imperfecta. *Lancet* 2004;363:1377–1385.

Reinus WR, Gilula LA. Radiology of Ewing's sarcoma: Intergroup Ewing's Sarcoma Study (IESS). *Radiographics* 1984;4(6):929–944.

Renaud A, Aucourt J, Weill J, et al. Radiographic features of osteogenesis imperfecta. *Insights Imaging* 2013;4(4):417–429.

Restrepo R, Palani R, Cervantes LF, Duarte AM, Amjad I, Altman NR. Hemangiomas revisited: the useful, the unusual and the new. Part 2: endangering hemangiomas and treatment. *Pediatr Radiol* 2011;41(7):905–915.

Restrepo R, Palani R, Cervantes LF, Duarte AM, Amjad I, Altman NR. Hemangiomas revisited: the useful, the unusual and the new. Part 1: overview and clinical and imaging characteristics. *Pediatr Radiol* 2011;41(7):895–904.

Rexroad JT, Moser RP III, Georgia JD. "Fish" or "fish mouth" vertebrae? AJR *Am J Roentgenol* 2003;181(3):886–887.

Robbin MR, Murphey MD, Temple HT, Kransdorf MJ, Choi JJ. Imaging of musculoskeletal fibromatosis. *Radiographics* 2001;21(3):585–600.

Rosenbaum DG, Servaes S, Bogner EA, Jaramillo D, Mintz DN. MR Imaging in postreduction assessment of developmental dysplasia of the hip: goals and obstacles. *Radiographics* 2016;36(3):840–854.

Ruzal-Shapiro C, Berdon WE, Cohen MD, Abramson SJ. MR imaging of diffuse bone marrow replacement in pediatric patients with cancer. *Radiology* 1991;181(2):587–589.

Sabharwal S. Blount disease. *J Bone Joint Surg Am* 2009;91(7):1758–1776.

Sabharwal S. Blount disease: an update. *Orthop Clin North Am* 2015;46(1):37–47.

Sachs HK. The evolution of the radiologic lead line. *Radiology* 1981;139(1):81–85.

Samet JD, Rusinak D, Grant T. Case 174: Hunter Syndrome. *Radiology* 2011;261:321–324.

Schima W, Amann G, Stiglbauer R, et al. Preoperative staging of osteosarcoma: efficacy of MR imaging in detecting joint involvement. *AJR Am J Roentgenol* 1994;163:1171–1175.

Shore RM, Chesney RW. Rickets: Part II. *Pediatr Radiol.* 2013;43(2):152–172.

Shore RM, Chesney RW. Rickets: Part I. *Pediatr Radiol* 2013;43(2):140–151.

Sinigaglia R, Gigante C, Bisinella G, Varotto S, Zanesco L, Turra S. Musculoskeletal manifestations in pediatric acute leukemia. *J Pediatr Orthop* 2008;28(1):20–28.

Smith JA. Bone disorders in sickle cell disease. *Hematol/ Oncol Clin North Am* 1996;10(6):1345–1356.

Smith SE, Murphey MD, Jelinek JS, Torop AH, Mulligan ME, Flemming DJ. Imaging of Ewing sarcoma and primitive neuroectodermal tumor of bone with pathologic correlation and emphasis on CT and MRI [abstr]. *Radiology* 1998;209(P):420.

Soldado F, Aguirre M, Peiró JL, et al. Fetoscopic release of extremity amniotic bands with risk of amputation. *J Pediatr Orthop* 2009;29(3):290–293.

Starr V, Ha BY. Imaging update on developmental dysplasia of the hip with the role of MRI. *AJR Am J Roentgenol* 2014;203(6):1324–1335.

Steinbach HL, Noetzli M. Roentgen appearance of the skeleton in osteomalacia and rickets. *Am J R Roentgenol Radium Ther Nucl Med* 1964;91: 955–972.

Stevens MA, El-Khoury GY, Kathol MH, Brandser EA, Chow S. Imaging features of avulsion injuries. *Radiographs* 1999;19:655–672.

Storer SK, Skaggs DL. Developmental dysplasia of the hip. *Am Fam Physician* 2006;74(8):1310–1316.

Tenenbein M, Reed MH, Black GB. The toddler's fracture revisited. *Am J Emerg Med* 1990;8(3):208–211.

Thapa MM, Iyer RS, Gross JA. Pictorial essay of pediatric upper extremity trauma: normal variants and unique injuries. *Can Assoc Radiol J* 2013; 64(2):101–107.

Theppeang K, Glass TA, Bandeen-Roche K, Todd AC, Rohde CA, Schwartz BS. Gender and race/ethnicity differences in lead dose biomarkers. *Am J Public Health* 2008;98(7):1248–1255.

Tiderius C, Jaramillo D, Connolly S, et al. Post-closed reduction perfusion magnetic resonance imaging as a predictor of avascular necrosis in developmental hip dysplasia: a preliminary report. *J Pediatr Orthop* 2009;29(1):14–20.

Tigges S, Nance EP. Skeletal case of the day. Radiation-induced osteochondroma. *AJR Am J Roentgenol* 1992;158:1368–1369.

Torres MFL, DiPietro MA. Developmental dysplasia of the hip. *Ultrasound Clinics* 2009;4(4):445–455.

Tunaci M, Tunaci A, Engin G, et al. Imaging features of thalassemia. *Eur Radiol* 1999;9(9):1804–1809.

Tyler PA, Madani G, Chaudhuri R, Wilson LF, Dick EA. The radiological appearances of thalassaemia. *Clin Radiol* 2006;61(1):40–52.

Vanhoenacker FM, De Beuckeleer LH, Van Hul W, et al. Sclerosing bone dysplasias: genetic and radioclinical features. *Eur Radiol* 2000;10(9):1423–1433.

Vanhoenacker FM, Van Hul W, Wuyts W, Willems PJ, De Schepper AM. Hereditary multiple exostoses: from genetics to clinical syndrome and complications. *Eur J Radiol* 2001;40:208–217.

Warniment C, Tsang K, Galazka SS. Lead poisoning in children. *Am Fam Physician* 2010;81(6):751–757.

Waters PM, Smith GR, Jaramillo D. Glenohumeral deformity secondary to brachial plexus birth palsy. *J Bone Joint Surg Am* 1998;80:668–677.

Weinstein M, Babyn P, Zlotkin S. An orange a day keeps the doctor away: scurvy in the year 2000. *Pediatrics* 2001;108:e55.

Windebank K, Nanduri V. Langerhans cell histiocytosis. *Arch Dis Child* 2009; 94:904–908.

Worch J, Matthay KK, Neuhaus J, Goldsby R, DuBois SG. Ethnic and racial differences in patients with Ewing sarcoma. *Cancer* 2010;116(4):983–988.

Yarmish G, Klein MJ, Landa J, Lefkowitz RA, Hwang S. Imaging characteristics of primary osteosarcoma: nonconventional subtypes. *Radiographics* 2010;30(6):1653–1672.

Zhu G, Wu X, Zhang X, Wu M, Zeng Q, Li X. Clinical and imaging findings in thalassemia patients with extramedullary hematopoiesis. *Clin Imaging* 2012;36(5):475–482.

SECTION XII

NUCLEAR RADIOLOGY

SECTION EDITOR: Brett J. Mollard

CHAPTER 71A ■ INTRODUCTION TO NUCLEAR MEDICINE

BRETT J. MOLLARD

INTRODUCTION

Nuclear medicine encompasses both therapeutic and diagnostic modalities that remain among the most cost effective for the diagnosis, management, and treatment of a variety of diseases. Radiographic, ultrasound, computed tomography (CT), and magnetic resonance imaging (MRI) studies provide high spatial resolution and important anatomic or structural information from which pathologic processes are inferred. **Nuclear medicine studies, on the other hand, directly assess physiologic and functional information.** Anatomic imaging can provide the dimensions of a lesion and assess for changes in size, whereas nuclear medicine scintigraphy can assess if a lesion is functionally or metabolically active (Fig. 71A.1). Positron emission tomography (PET)/CT and SPECT/CT have become commonplace and have improved the sensitivity and specificity for neural, cardiac, and oncologic imaging. PET/CT has greatly improved patient throughput, tumor staging, and evaluation of tumor response to therapy (Fig. 71A.2). Molecular medicine/imaging promises to bring applications of genomics and protein messaging quickly into the clinical arena. We now have the ability to follow gene therapy as well as stem cell therapy through their introduction into the patient. Lymphoscintigraphy assists surgeons to better stage melanoma and breast cancer intraoperatively and has significantly decreased patient morbidity following nodal staging procedures by decreasing the number of complications (such as lymphedema) from unnecessary radical lymph node dissections. Handheld probes allow better localization of sentinel nodes as well as small and difficult lesions identified on fluorine-18 fluorodeoxyglucose (F-18 FDG)/PET scans. Current therapeutic options include antibody therapy for lymphoma, I-131 MIBG and yttrium (Y-90)-labeled octreotide for several different neuroendocrine tumors, various options for skeletal metastatic disease (strontium [Sr-89], samarium [Sa-153], radium [Ra-223]), and research is ongoing for new therapeutic agents.

The material in this section is intended to provide an overview of the specialty and to prepare residents for the core examination.

IMAGING PRINCIPLES

The basic principles of diagnostic nuclear radiology are simple to grasp, yet somehow seem to elude first-year residents as they are overwhelmed with information at the outset of their training. Nuclear medicine scintigraphy provides maps of the biodistribution of radiotracers that have been administered to a patient. The knowledge of the normal patterns of uptake, distribution, and excretion allows us to determine the presence or absence of disease.

Sometimes a radionuclide or radioisotope of a naturally occurring element essential to normal biologic function (e.g., iodine-123) or an analog (e.g., technetium-99m pertechnetate [Tc-99m-O_4]) is used without additional chemical alteration (Fig. 71A.3). More commonly, a radioactive isotope is combined with a physiologically "active" compound to create a radiopharmaceutical which can be administered intravenously, orally, or via direct injection. Thus, Tc-99m-O_4 (the form that technetium is eluted in from a generator) may be combined with a diphosphonate compound for skeletal imaging (e.g., T-99m MDP). If the same radioisotope is combined with an iminodiacetic acid derivative, the biologic distribution reflected by the images will be that of a biliary scan (transformed into a HIDA agent). This simple concept is the foundation for imaging the biodistribution of radiolabeled blood cells, monoclonal antibodies, peptides, and energy substrates such as glucose and fatty acids. If this unifying principle can be kept in mind while reading the various sections on nuclear imaging, the diverse number and types of studies may seem somewhat less bewildering.

RADIOTHERAPY

Radiotherapy is an extremely important arm of nuclear medicine and is critical to several areas of clinical medicine. The distinguishing feature of therapeutic radioisotopes and radiopharmaceuticals from diagnostic agents is that they are particulate emitters (i.e., emit particles), with beta minus (β^-) emitters (electron emitters) being utilized much more

The editors wish to thank Dr. David K. Shelton for his work in the 4th edition establishing the foundation for this chapter.

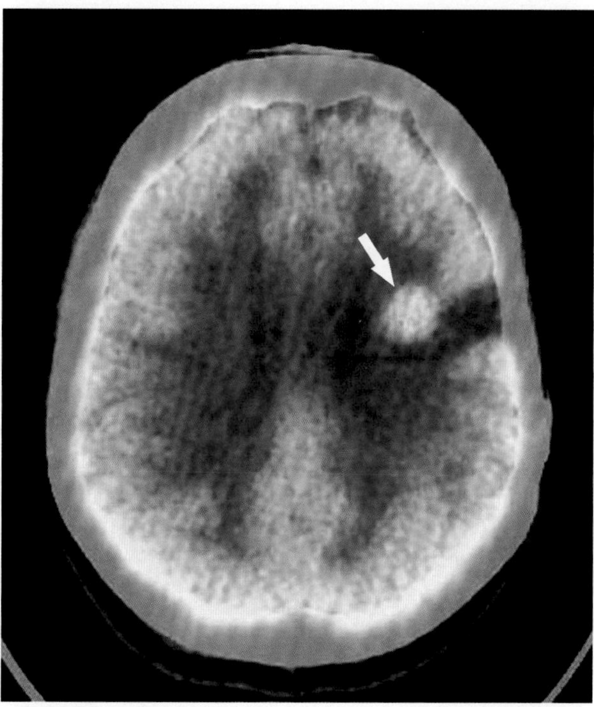

FIGURE 71A.1. **PET/CT Scan of Brain.** Fused FDG PET/CT image demonstrating increased metabolic activity within the left frontal lobe (*arrow*), confirming the recurrence of glioblastoma after previous surgery and radiotherapy.

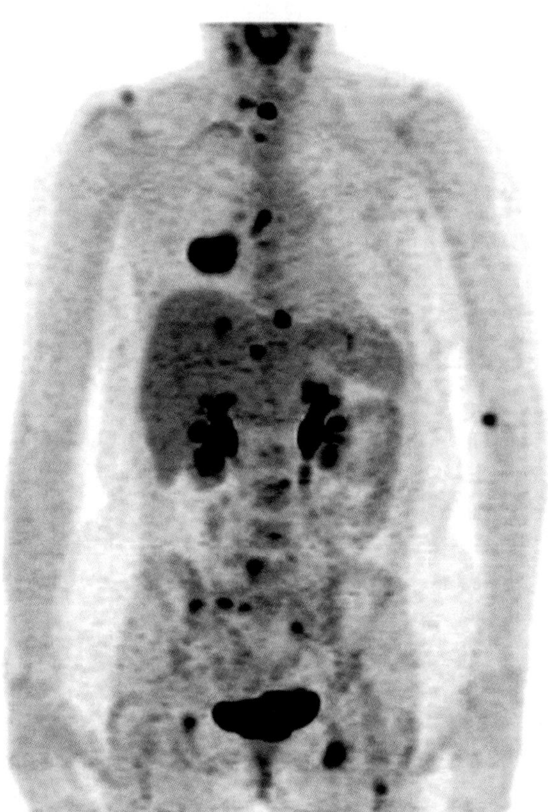

FIGURE 71A.2. **Maximum Intensity Projection (MIP) Image From Whole-Body PET FDG Scan.** Whole-body PET/CT scan was done for initial staging in a breast cancer patient with multiple areas of abnormal hypermetabolic foci consistent with diffuse metastatic breast cancer.

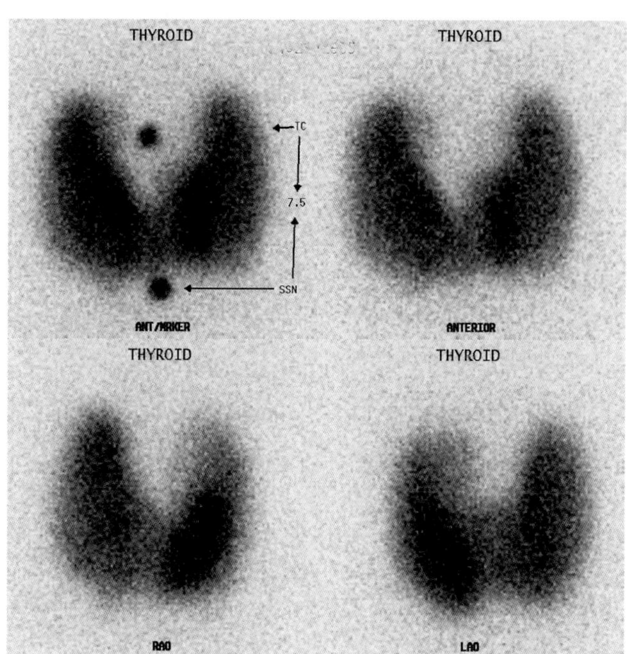

FIGURE 71A.3. **Iodine-123 Thyroid Scan.** The patient presented with symptoms and laboratory findings of hyperthyroidism. The scan shows diffuse, homogeneous enlargement of the thyroid gland with an increased uptake of 77%, consistent with Graves disease. She was subsequently successfully treated with oral I-131.

commonly than alpha (α) emitters (helium nuclei emitters). β^- particles (electrons) only travel a short distance through tissues, depositing most of their energy within a couple of millimeters, and resulting in tumor cell damage and death. I-131, for example, is utilized for benign thyroid conditions such as Graves disease, toxic adenoma, and Plummer disease or toxic multinodular goiter (Fig. 71A.3). I-131 is also the primary treatment of choice for thyroid remnant ablation following thyroidectomy and for treating thyroid cancer metastases. I-131 can be used in a similar manner to treat other malignancies when coupled to a variety of targeting agents, including MIBG, antibody agents, etc.

Radioimmunotherapy (RIT) with monoclonal antibodies is now being utilized for refractory lymphoma treatment with ibritumomab tiuxetan (yttrium-90 Zevalin©) and formerly tositumomab (I-131 Bexxar©) (Fig. 71A.4). RIT is also being studied for refractory metastatic breast cancer. Radioembolotherapy (RET) is used in the treatment of unresectable hepatocellular carcinoma and metastatic liver disease by injecting Y-90–coated microspheres directly into the hepatic artery branches feeding the respective tumors. The Y-90 microspheres are injected by interventional radiologists after careful planning and dosimetry calculations to minimize radiation toxicity to nontarget tissue.

AN APPROACH TO IMAGE INTERPRETATION

A basic fund of anatomic, physiologic, and nuclear imaging knowledge is necessary in order to make intelligent diagnoses and differential diagnoses based on nuclear medicine images.

When preparing to discuss a case, it is first important to determine the radiopharmaceutical and, therefore, the type of study which may be as simple as reviewing the film margins or paperwork for textual information. It is poor form to ask,

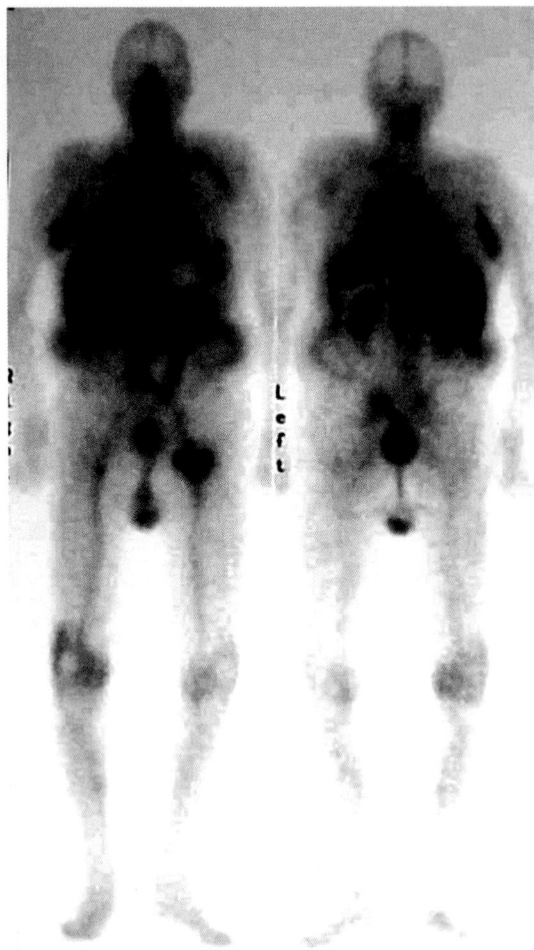

FIGURE 71A.4. **Indium-111 Zevalin© Antibody Diagnostic Scan.** Whole-body scan demonstrates normal biodistribution of the antibody agent and multiple foci of increased uptake, consistent with known B-cell lymphoma. The patient was then successfully treated with Y-90 Zevalin© radioimmunotherapy with good clinical and CT response.

"What type of study is this?" when the information is readily at hand. At the same time, one may also glean important information about the age and sex of the patient, the site of injection, the temporal sequence when multiple images are present, the type of images (planar or tomographic, static or dynamic), and patient orientation during imaging (right/left, oblique, posterior, upright/supine, etc.).

Several methods can be utilized to determine the type of radiopharmaceutical when not provided on the images. Relative count density may help distinguish radiotracer type as medium- and high-energy isotopes (indium-111, gallium-67, iodine-131, etc.) have lower count density based on longer half-lives and therefore lower administered doses. This results in noisier images compared to high count density isotopes such as Tc-99m. Dynamic acquisitions and flow studies using Tc-99m agents will also be noisy given the short acquisition times (typically 1 to 5 s/frame).

The number and type of images presented and the type of acquisition (e.g., PET, SPECT, or planar) are very helpful. If a series of frames is provided, the study is either a dynamic acquisition with the typical timing of seconds or minutes per frame or possibly a series of SPECT image slices that will usually have more counts and appear somewhat smoothed because of the processing algorithms employed.

The biodistribution of activity is often sufficient to determine the radiopharmaceutical in use. Is there evidence of cardiac or great vessel blood pool activity? Is skeletal activity present? What organs or structures are visualized? Are there obvious focal abnormalities? From a knowledge of the biodistribution evident on the images and a reasonable assumption about the likely radioisotope, one may make some conjecture as to the most likely radiopharmaceutical in use.

After determining the radiopharmaceutical and the type of study, proceeding with the rest of the analysis is fairly straightforward. There are two common errors that continue to cause problems for each new generation of residents. First, it is extremely difficult to "see what is not there." Always "take attendance" and be certain that all organs and structures that should be "present" on a given study are visualized with their normal pattern and relative uptake of radiopharmaceutical. Next, frequently more than one finding of importance will exist. It is easy to suffer from "satisfaction of search" and quit looking for additional abnormalities after one is found. A rigid approach to image analysis is required to prevent both of these errors.

When studying dynamic series such as arterial flow studies, Tc-99m–labeled red blood cell studies for GI hemorrhage localization, renal function images, and so forth, it is important to note the time per frame because you will need to make comments concerning the timing of the arrival of the radiopharmaceutical in various structures. This information may be critical to image interpretation and is frequently overlooked. Identifying changes from one frame to the next may be difficult. One approach to enhance and speed the detection of abnormalities and asymmetries is to directly compare the first and last frames of a study, where differences will be most obvious. This will allow you to direct your attention to areas of change and define the correct timing of events. It is helpful to "back through" the images from last to first after identifying any abnormalities on the later images. With this approach, the anatomic location and temporal appearance of pathologies such as a GI bleed can be rapidly assessed and characterized.

An orderly approach to image analysis for static images is also required but will vary based on the type of study in question. Here are specific techniques for some common studies that may be helpful.

Skeletal Imaging. Review the images provided with a "top–down" approach, addressing skeletal structures first on the anterior view, then on the posterior view (Fig. 71A.5). Note areas of increased or decreased activity without attaching strong clinical significance to them initially. Always comment on the renal activity that should normally be present and use this as a reminder to evaluate soft tissue activity for abnormal increases, decreases, and asymmetry. This type of approach works well with many of the whole-body imaging studies, although the biodistribution will vary.

SPECT Myocardial Perfusion Imaging. Always view the raw data images first, if available, and evaluate for quality control (QC) issues, artifacts, and ancillary or incidental findings (breast attenuation, motion, pacemaker artifact, pulmonary uptake, breast tumor, etc.). Always review the exercise data to confirm adequacy of stress or determine what, if any, pharmacologic agent was employed. Next review the short-axis slices, then the vertical long-axis slices, and finally the horizontal long-axis slices. Note the presence or absence of areas of decreased perfusion and whether they appear fixed or seem to change between stress and rest images. Note the chamber sizes and whether or not the left ventricle becomes more dilated at stress relative to rest (transient ischemic dilation [TID]). Attempt to confirm the presence of any defects in two planes. Then evaluate the wall motion, brightening, and thickening. Check the

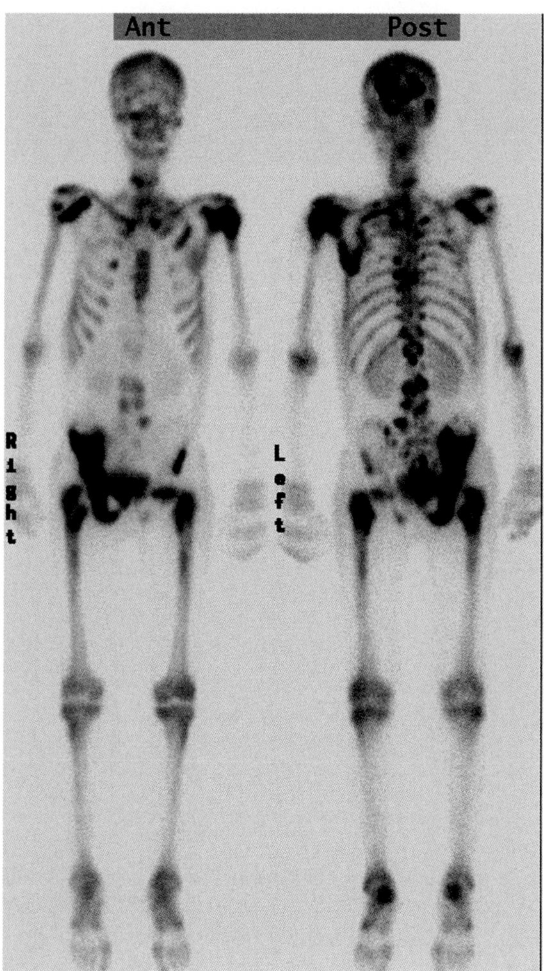

FIGURE 71A.5. **Whole-Body Bone Scan With Tc-99m Methylene Diphosphonate (MDP).** The scan demonstrates multiple areas of increased uptake due to diffuse osseous metastatic disease in this patient with prostate cancer.

end-diastolic and end-systolic volumes. Evaluate the stress and rest data including the ejection fractions. Is the study normal or does it demonstrate reversible changes of ischemia? Does it demonstrate a fixed defect consistent with infarction or hibernating myocardium? Does it demonstrate poststress dilatation or decreased LVEF after stress?

Ventilation–Perfusion Imaging for Pulmonary Embolus. Always review the chest radiograph or chest CT first, if provided. If not initially available, comment that review of the radiograph is essential prior to making a definitive statement about the likelihood of pulmonary embolus. Review the perfusion study in its entirety first. Note the presence of any defects, their relative sizes (lobar, segmental, and subsegmental), and their locations. Attempt to confirm the findings on more than one view. Once the number and location of the defects are known, attempt to match these defects in the corresponding areas on the ventilation study. Summarize the findings and segmental anatomy, verbally reciting the number and size of matched and mismatched defects. State that there is no evidence of pulmonary embolism (normal study) or offer a probability of pulmonary embolus based on the findings. Then determine if another study such as CT angiography may be needed.

Hepatobiliary Imaging. For this and any other study where flow studies and dynamic imaging are performed, studying the images in the order in which they were acquired is best: flow study first, then dynamic images using the approach outlined previously, and finally static images (right lateral or left anterior oblique views would be typical) when obtained. Note the temporal sequence of the arrival of the arterial bolus in the kidneys, spleen, and finally liver if an arterial flow study of the abdomen is provided. With approximately 80% of hepatic blood flow arriving via the portal system, the liver should appear later than the other organs—if it does not, portal hypertension may be present. Early flow to the gallbladder fossa implies significant inflammation. On the dynamic series, note the appearance of the early images, then study the later images: Are gallbladder activity and bowel activity present? If so, "back through" the images and note their first appearance. Is activity visualized in the normal sequence of intrahepatic ducts, common hepatic duct, gallbladder, common bile duct, and duodenum? Is there activity in any areas other than expected—stomach, esophagus, or free spill into the peritoneum? Are there any focal accumulations of labeled bile in the liver, gallbladder fossa, or elsewhere? Are there any photopenic defects within the liver?

For a situation in which a finding has been made but no explanation is readily apparent, it is helpful to contemplate the finding while considering a standard list of generic causes as well as mechanisms that might lead to the finding. One such generic list uses the mnemonic VINDICATE: Vascular (any cause of increased/decreased blood flow, collagen vascular diseases); Infectious (always include TB, fungal, HIV); Neoplastic (benign or malignant, primary or metastatic); Drug-induced (radiopharmaceutical preparation and QC, recent prior radiopharmaceutical administration or contrast study, thyroid hormone ingestion); Idiopathic (sarcoidosis, amyloidosis); Congenital; Artifact (related to patient, clothing, imaging equipment, computer processing, or film processing); Trauma; or Endocrine/metabolic (Paget disease, hyperparathyroidism, etc.).

If the physiologic mechanisms of radiopharmaceutical localization are understood, then mechanistic explanations for findings allow another route to a solution. Thus, from a mechanistic standpoint, increased activity on a bone scan is caused by either increased delivery of radiopharmaceutical to the bone or increased incorporation due to either increased osteoblastic activity or increased dwell time for extraction by normally functioning osteoblasts. Reasons for increased delivery include the following: arterial injection, arteriovenous malformation, infection, tumor, localized inflammation due to trauma, increased use of a limb, neurologic reflex-related increased flow, and apparent increased uptake with actual reduced uptake in the contralateral body part. Reasons for increased osteoblastic activity include the following: normal growth in epiphyseal bone and enhanced repair in response to fracture, infection, and benign or malignant tumors. Increased dwell time may be caused by constricting clothing, tourniquets, venous obstruction, and lymphatic obstruction.

When analyzing a case, it is best to follow your initial comments concerning the findings with a final image review as you verbally summarize what you believe to be pertinent to the diagnosis. It is not uncommon to realize only as the summary is presented aloud that a specific diagnosis is indicated or that the findings significantly limit the differential diagnosis.

The foregoing discussion is not meant to be all-encompassing and does not do justice to the entire spectrum of studies and diseases that will be encountered. However, it should provide a starting point for development of one's own approach to image analysis and case-discussion skills. Consider using the images in each of the subsequent chapters as sample unknown cases and attempt to analyze them before reading the captions. This sort of practice will undoubtedly enhance one's ability to take unknown cases with greater confidence and accuracy.

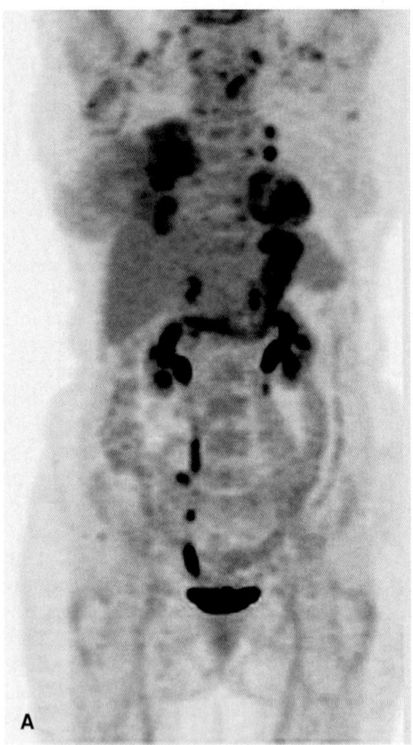

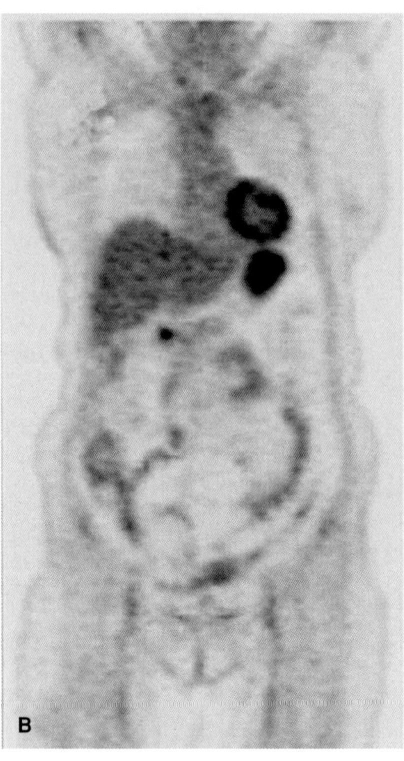

FIGURE 71A.6. **Response to Therapy Demonstrated on Whole-Body PET FDG Maximum Intensity Projection Scans. A:** Baseline scan shows extensive and metastatic disease in a patient with inflammatory breast cancer. **B:** Follow-up scan after two cycles of chemotherapy shows excellent early response to therapy which is a predictor of how the patient will ultimately respond.

SECTION OVERVIEW

As you will see in the following chapters, nuclear medicine offers several distinct advantages over traditional anatomically oriented imaging techniques. There is *whole-body* detection of disease with bone, WBC, I-131, I-123 MIBG, In-111 octreotide, and F-18 FDG PET/CT scans. It can provide ***functional evaluation*** with computer analysis such as with radionuclide ventriculography, gated cardiac SPECT, renal scintigraphy, gallbladder ejection fraction, gastric emptying, esophageal transit, and thyroid uptake. ***Split function*** analysis can be done for kidneys, lungs, and brain. ***Diagnostic evaluation*** is done with I-123 for thyroid nodules, F-18 FDG PET for pulmonary nodules and numerous malignancies, diuretic renography for ureteral obstruction, and Tc-99m RBC for hepatic hemangioma and GI bleed.

Response to therapy can be assessed for various malignancies utilizing malignancy-specific radiopharmaceuticals such as In-111 pentetreotide for carcinoid, I-123 MIBG for neuroblastoma, I-123/I-131 for thyroid cancer, Tc-99m MDP for both primary and secondary (metastatic) osseous malignancies, and F-18 FDG PET for classically hypermetabolic malignancies such as lung cancer, breast cancer, and lymphoma (Fig. 71A.6).

Single-photon (non-positron emitters such as Tc-99m) and dual-photon (positron emitters) emitting radiopharmaceuticals are used in ***molecular imaging***, including agents such as F-18 FDG, C-11 choline, F-18 fluorothymidine, and F-18 dopamine, many of which are currently experimental. Radiotracer techniques are commonly utilized for stem cell tracking and in studying genomics and proteomics. ***Targeted radiotherapy*** techniques are current areas of interest with the ability to deliver therapeutic agents directly to target cells, minimizing systemic effects of therapy.

CHAPTER 71B ■ ESSENTIAL SCIENCE OF NUCLEAR MEDICINE

BRETT J. MOLLARD

RELEVANT ASPECTS OF RADIATION PHYSICS

Types of Radiation in Nuclear Medicine. The electromagnetic spectrum of radiation can be divided into nonionizing and ionizing radiation. Nonionizing radiation includes commonly encountered forms of electromagnetic radiation such as visible light, microwave, and radiofrequencies (used in radio transmissions and in MRI). **The ionizing radiation used in diagnostic medical imaging includes x-rays, γ-rays, and annihilation radiation.** *The difference between these forms of radiation lies in their origin.* **X-rays** are produced by bombarding a metal target with electrons. In diagnostic radiology, this is achieved by bombarding a metal target with high-energy electrons within an x-ray tube, producing a spectrum of x-ray energies. **γ-Rays** are produced from within the atomic nucleus as unstable nuclei transition to a more stable state. In nuclear medicine, γ-ray energies for single-photon emitters (non-PET agents) lie typically in the 80 to 350 keV range (Table 71B.1).

Annihilation radiation is produced when a particle and its antiparticle interact and annihilate each other—this is the type of radiation detected in PET. When positrons annihilate electrons, the mass of each β-particle (positron and electron) is converted into two photons with fixed energy (the energy equivalent of the mass of each β-particle is determined by the equation $E = mc^2$ [511 keV for a β-particle]). The photons created are emitted in opposite directions (conservation of momentum).

Ionizing radiation comes in two forms: electromagnetic radiation (photons) and particulate matter (β-particles, α-particles, neutrons, etc.). The particle of most common medical interest is the **β-particle**, which may take the form of an ***electron (beta minus particle [β^-])*** or ***positron (beta plus particle [β^+])***, both of which originate from the decay of an unstable nucleus (neutron → electron; proton → positron). β-Particles, unlike x-rays and γ-rays, readily interact with matter and transfer energy to the surrounding tissues. This produces a high radiation dose within a short range of a few millimeters. Electron-emitting radionuclides (β^--particles) such as iodine-131 (I-131), yttrium-90 (Y-90), and lutetium-177 (Lu-177) can be used for therapeutic purposes (radiotherapy) when administered at high doses (curie range) for treatment of benign conditions such as Graves disease and various malignancies (thyroid cancer, lymphoma, bone metastases, etc.).

Bremsstrahlung, or "braking radiation," is a form of radiation that is rarely of interest in the imaging portion of nuclear medicine (contrary to radiography where bremsstrahlung is the primary component of x-ray beam generation), though does play a minor role in radiation safety. Bremsstrahlung radiation is generated when high-energy electrons interact with an atomic nucleus and generate x-rays. The probability of bremsstrahlung events occurring increases as particle energy and atomic number (Z) of the atom increases and, therefore, infrequently occur within soft tissue (low Z material). Surrounding a β-emitting source with a low-density material such as plastic (low Z material) will stop the β-particles and decrease the radiation received to technologists handling the source. If necessary, additional photon radiation (γ-rays) can be reduced by surrounding the plastic shielding layer with a denser material such as lead or tungsten (used to block 511-keV photons). Occasionally, bremsstrahlung imaging with a gamma camera may be used to validate dose distribution after the administration of β-particle–emitting therapeutics such as Y-90–coated microspheres. The spatial resolution of the resulting images is very poor.

Photon Interactions With Matter. Photoelectric and Compton interactions are the primary interactions of photons with matter (i.e., the patient) in nuclear medicine. In a **photoelectric interaction**, also known as the **"photoelectric effect,"** an incident photon interacts with an inner shell (k-shell) orbital electron of an atom and transfers all its energy to the inner k-shell electron, resulting in ejection of the electron (known as a photoelectron) and ionization of the atom (Fig. 71B.1). Photon energy exceeding that of the k-shell electron binding energy is converted into electron kinetic energy (velocity of the ejected electron). The ejected electron may have sufficient energy

The editors wish to thanks Dr. Ramsey D. Badawi, Dr. Jerome T. Bushberg, and Linda Kroger for their works in the 4th edition establishing the foundation for this chapter.

TABLE 71B.1

RADIONUCLIDES

RADIONUCLIDE (SYMBOL)	METHOD OF PRODUCTION	MODE OF DECAY (%)	PRINCIPAL IMAGING PHOTONS keV (ABUNDANCE)	*T*½	COMMENTS
Chromium-51 (Cr-51)	Nuclear reactor (neutron activation)	EC (100)	320 (9)	27.8 days	Used for in vivo red cell mass determinations, not for imaging; samples counted in sodium iodide well-counter
Cobalt-57 (Co-57)	Cyclotron	EC (100)	122 (86) 136 (11)	271 days	Primarily used as a uniform flood field source for gamma camera quality control
Fluorine-18 (F-18)	Cyclotron	β^+ (97) EC (3)	511 (AR)	110 minutes	This radionuclide accounts for more than 80% of all clinical PET use; typically used to label fluorodeoxyglucose (FDG).
Gallium-67 (Ga-67)	Cyclotron	EC (100)	93 (40) 184 (20) 300 (17) 393 (4)	78 hours	In practice, the 93-, 184-, and 300-keV photons are used for imaging.
Indium-111 (In-111)	Cyclotron	EC (100)	171 (900) 245 (94)	2.8 days (67.2 hours)	Principally utilized when optimal imaging occurs more than 24 hours after injection; both photons are used in imaging
Iodine-123 (I-123)	Cyclotron	EC (100)	159 (83)	13.2 hours	Replaced I-131 for most diagnostic imaging applications to reduce radiation dose
Iodine-125 (I-125)	Nuclear reactor (neutron activation)	EC (100)	35 (6) 27 (39) 28 (76) 31 (20)	60.2 days	Used as I-125 albumin for in vivo blood/plasma volume determinations; not utilized for imaging, samples counted in well-counter
Iodine-131 (I-131)	Nuclear reactor (U-235 fission)	β^- (100)	284 (6) 364 (81) 637 (7)	8.0 days	Typical use now reserved for therapeutic applications; imaging is limited by high-energy photon (364 keV) and high patient dosimetry mostly from β-particles.
Krypton-81 m (Kr-81 m)	Generator product	IT (100)	190 (67)	13 seconds	Ultrashort-lived parent (Rb-81, 4.6 hours) and high expense limit the use of this agent.
Molybdenum-99 (Mo-99)	Nuclear reactor (U-235 fission)	β^- (100)	181 (16) 740 (12) 780 (4)	67 hours	The source (parent) for Mo/Tc generators; not used directly; 740- and 780-keV photons used to identify the contamination of Tc-99m elution as "moly breakthrough."
Phosphorus-32 (P-32)	Nuclear reactor (neutron activation)	β^- (100)		14.3 days	Used in the treatment of polycythemia vera, metastatic bone disease, and serous effusions
Samarium-153 (Sm-153)	Nuclear reactor (U-235 fission)	β^- (100)	103 (28)	46 h	Used for palliative treatment of metastatic bone pain
Strontium-89 (Sr-89)	Nuclear reactor (U-235 fission)	β^- (100)	910 (0.02)	50.5 days	Used for palliative treatment of metastatic bone pain
Technetium-99m (Tc-99m)	Generator product	IT (100)	140 (90)	6.02 hours	This radionuclide, typically in kit form, accounts for more than 70% of all imaging studies.
Thallium-201 (Tl-201)	Cyclotron	EC (100)	69–80 (94) 167 (10)	73.1 hours	Majority of photons are low-energy x-rays (69–80 keV) from mercury 201 (Hg-201), the daughter of Tl-201
Xenon-133 (Xe-133)	Nuclear reactor (U-235 fission)	β^- (100)	81 (37)	5.3 days	Xe-133 is a heavier than air gas; low abundance and energy of photon reduces image resolution.

β^-, beta minus decay; β^+, beta plus decay; EC, electron capture; IT, isomeric transition (i.e., gamma ray emission).

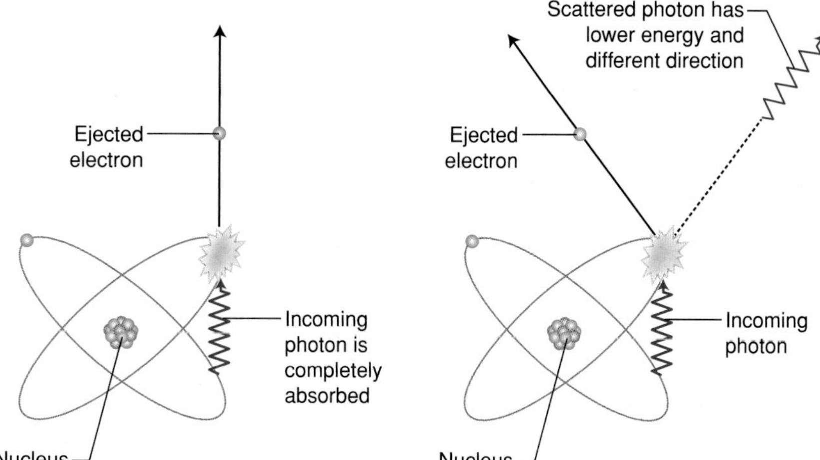

FIGURE 71B.1. Relevant Photon Interactions With Matter. Left: Photoelectric interaction. **Right:** Compton scatter.

to ionize additional atoms. In a **Compton interaction**, also known as **"Compton scatter,"** the incident photon imparts a portion of its energy to an outer shell (valence) electron resulting in ejection of the outer shell electron and emission of a new, lower-energy photon at an angle to the initial incident photon trajectory (Fig. 71B.1) equal to the kinetic energy lost by the incident photon and dependent on the angle of interaction. In essence, the photon is deflected (scattered) and slows down in the process. Small angles are associated with small transfers of energy to the electron and larger angles are associated with larger transfers of energy with the maximum energy transfer occurring at 180 degrees (photon deflected backward, resulting in backscatter).

When a photon interacts with an atom, the likelihood of a photoelectric or Compton interaction is dependent on the photon energy and on the electron density of the target. Compton scatter is the most prevalent soft tissue interaction for typical nuclear medicine photon energies, especially with higher-energy radionuclides such as gallium-67 and PET radiotracers. Photoelectric interactions occur with higher frequency within the detector (high Z material) though Compton scatter remains the dominant interaction.

Units. Various units have been established to describe radiation and its effects. Because the scientific community in the United States is in transition between conventional units and the Système Internationale (SI), a table of both units with their conversion factors is provided in Table 71B.2. **Activity** is used to describe the quantity of the radionuclide being administered and represents the rate of **nuclear decays per second,** denoted by *curies* (Ci) in conventional units and *becquerels* (Bq) in SI units. The *roentgen* (R) is a conventional unit used to express **radiation exposure** and is a **measure of the ionization of a volume of air by x-rays and γ-rays** (coulombs/kg in SI units). Radiation exposure can be used for a rough estimate of absorbed radiation dose to a patient. **Absorbed dose** is the **amount of energy deposited by ionizing radiation per unit mass in joules/kg;** the conventional unit is the radiation absorbed dose (*rad*) and the SI unit is the *gray* (Gy).

Because certain types of radiation are more biologically damaging than others, a **radiation weighting factor** (also called **quality factor,** W_R) is multiplied by the absorbed dose based on the type of incident ionizing radiation (x/γ-rays, β-particles, α-particles, neutrons, etc.) to yield the **equivalent dose,** which is measured in *rem* (roentgen equivalent man) in conventional

TABLE 71B.2

CONVENTIONAL AND SI RADIOLOGIC UNITS AND CONVERSION FACTORS

	CONVENTIONAL UNITS		MULTIPLY BY THE CONVENTIONAL UNITS TO OBTAIN SI UNITS	SI UNITS		
QUANTITY	NAME	SYMBOL		NAME	SYMBOL	EXAMPLE
Activity	Curie	Ci	3.7×10^{10}	Becquerel[a]	Bq	10 mCi = 370 MBq
Exposure	Roentgen	R	2.58×10^{-4}	Coulombs per kilogram	C/kg	
Absorbed dose	Radiation-absorbed dose	rad[b] (acronym)	10^{-2}	Gray[c]	Gy	100 rad = 1 Gy
Equivalent dose	Roentgen-equivalent man	rem (acronym)	10^{-2}	Sievert	Sv	100 rem = 1 Sv
Effective dose	Roentgen-equivalent man	rem (acronym)	10^{-2}	Sievert	Sv	100 rem = 1 Sv

[a] 1 Bq = 1 disintegration/s.
[b] 1 rad = 0.01 J/kg.
[c] 1 gray = 1 J/kg.

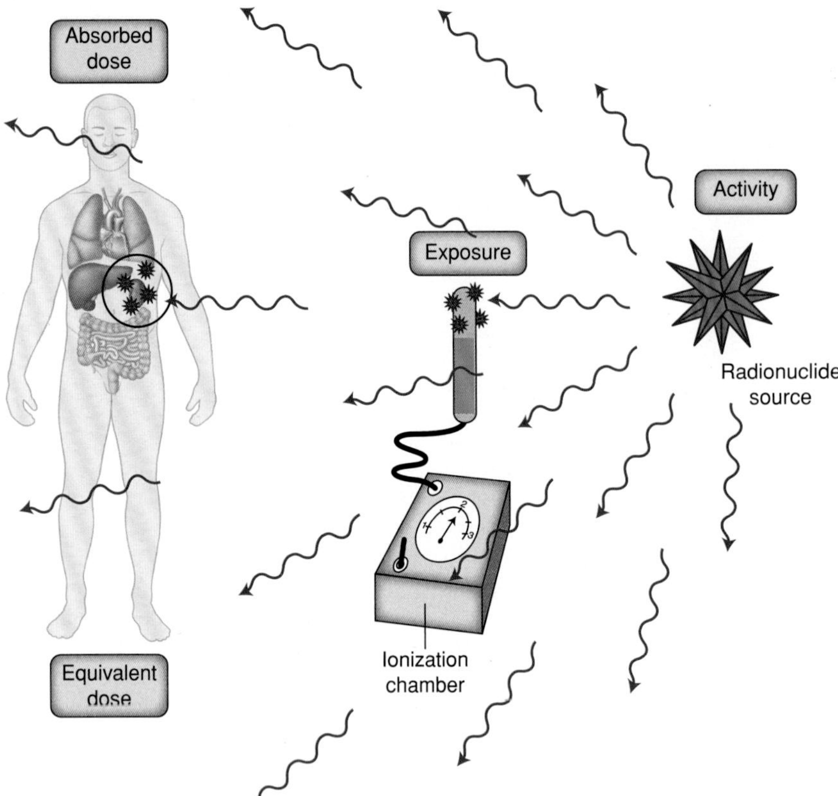

FIGURE 71B.2. **Graphical Representation of Radiation Units.** Activity (either inside or outside of the body) relates to the number of disintegrations per second and is a property of the radioactive source (units: becquerel/curie). Exposure is a measure of the ionization caused as radiation transits the air and can be measured with an ionization chamber (units: coulombs/kg or R). Absorbed dose is a measure of the energy per unit mass deposited by radiation in tissue (units: gray/rad). Dose equivalent (sievert/rem) measures the biologic effects on tissue of radiation and is the product of the absorbed dose and the quality factor. The quality factor for photons and β-particles is 1. For neutrons, it is between 5 and 20, depending on the energy. For α-particles, it is 20.

units and the *sievert* (Sv) in SI units. The quality factor is equal to one for photons and electrons, and therefore, 1 roentgen approximately equals 1 rad in the diagnostic energy range for soft tissue, which approximately equals 1 rem (Fig. 71B.2). That is, 1 R ≈ 1 rad (0.01 Gy) ≈ 1 rem (0.01 Sv).

A dimensionless **tissue weighting factor** (W_T) is used to take into account the different sensitivity of various organs to radiation and convert the mean equivalent dose (H_T), which only takes into account the type of incident radiation, to the **effective dose**, which factors in relative organ sensitivity to radiation. The tissue weighting factor for a particular tissue or organ represents the fraction of the total radiation detriment to the whole body attributed to that tissue when the whole body is irradiated uniformly. The tissue weighting factors have been developed from a reference population for both sexes and a wide range of ages and should not be used to calculate the dose to a specific patient for the purpose of assigning risk. The W_T values are: 0.01 for bone surface, brain, salivary gland, and skin; 0.04 for bladder, esophagus, liver, and thyroid; 0.08 for gonads[a]; 0.12 for breast, bone marrow, colon, lung, stomach, and the remainder tissues[b]. The effective dose[c] (E) is calculated as $E = \Sigma W_T \times H_T$, where $\Sigma W_T = 1$. The primary concerns are the development of radiation-induced fatal cancers and severe inheritable genetic mutations (stochastic/random effects).

- **Activity:** Rate of nuclear decays per second – amount of radiation produced (Bq or Ci)
- **Radiation exposure:** Measure of the ionization of air by radiation (coulombs/kg or R)
- **Absorbed dose:** Measure of energy deposited within a unit of mass (Gy or rad)
- **Equivalent dose:** Measure of radiation dose to tissue factoring in energy and type of radiation (Sv or rem)
- **Effective dose:** Measure of patient radiation dose factoring in both energy/type of radiation and organ/tissue sensitivity (Sv or rem)

RADIATION SAFETY

Radiation Exposure to the Worker. X-ray technologists receive an average annual exposure (equivalent dose) of 0.5 to 1 mSv (50 to 100 mrem), whereas a nuclear medicine technologist receives 2 to 3 mSv (200 to 300 mrem). Occupational exposure to nuclear medicine technologists performing PET procedures can be four to five times higher due to the high-energy gamma rays (511 keV). The majority of whole-body radiation to the nuclear medicine worker comes from exposure to the patient during dose administration, while setting the patient up for imaging, and from radiopharmaceutical preparation and injection.

The **Nuclear Regulatory Commission (NRC)** limits for radiation exposure (total effective equivalent dose) are 50 mSv/yr (5 rem/yr) for designated occupationally exposed workers and 1 mSv/yr (100 mrem/yr) for members of the public.

- **Annual occupational dose limit:** 50 mSv/yr (5 rem/yr)
- **Annual public dose limit:** 1 mSv/yr (100 mrem/yr)

The primary risk of radiation exposure is an increased lifetime risk of cancer (stochastic effect). For each additional sievert of radiation exposure (effective dose), the lifetime risk of cancer increases by approximately 5% (5×10^{-4}/rem). The cancer risk in the general population is approximately 40%.

[a]The W_T for gonads is applied to the mean of the doses to testes and ovaries. [b]Shared by remainder tissues (14 in total, 13 in each sex) which are adrenals, extrathoracic tissue, gallbladder, heart, kidneys, lymphatic nodes, muscle, oral mucosa, pancreas, prostate (male), small intestine, spleen, thymus, and uterus/cervix (female). [c]See ICRP Publication 103, The 2007 Recommendations of the International Commission on Radiological Protection. Ann. ICRP37 (2–4), Elsevier, 2008, for a more complete discussion of the concept of effective dose.

Therefore, a lifetime occupational whole-body dose of 50 mSv (5 rem)—for example, 2.5 mSv/yr × 20 years—will increase the risk of developing cancer from 40% to 40.25% and a 2-mSv dose from a ventilation/perfusion increase lifetime cancer risk from 40% to 40.01%. With these numbers, several caveats to radiation exposure need to be remembered: Any increased risk is spread over a lifetime; increased risks from exposure are additive; and the minimum latency of cancer is 4 to 8 years with the mean for solid tissue tumors being closer to 20 to 25 years.

- **Estimated 5% increased lifetime risk of cancer per 1-Sv effective dose received**
- **A 2-mSv ventilation/perfusion increase lifetime cancer risk from approximately 40% to 40.01%**

Contamination poses another potential source of occupational radiation exposure within the workplace. The following guidelines exist to minimize radiation exposure from contamination:

(1) Follow standard precautions by wearing protective clothing
(2) Use plastic-backed absorbent to restrict any spills
(3) Wash hands frequently
(4) Use covers over collimators that can be discarded if contaminated
(5) Monitor and wipe test frequently (see below)
(6) Avoid eating or drinking when handling radioactivity

Radiation Exposure to the General Population and Patient. The average annual per capita effective dose to the population in the United States is 6.2 mSv/yr (620 mrem/yr). Natural background radiation from atmospheric and terrestrial sources contributes 3.1 mSv/yr (310 mrem/yr) (~50%), while man-made sources, almost entirely from medical procedures, provide the other 3.1 mSv/yr (~50%). Nuclear medicine examinations account for ~26% of the dose from medical procedures with the largest contribution coming from Tc-99m and Tl-201 myocardial perfusion imaging, though Tl-201 use is on the decline.

Radionuclides and radiopharmaceuticals have variable biodistributions within the human body, and therefore, dosimetric considerations take into effect the initial activity administered, the biodistribution, the physical and biologic half-lives, as well as possible pathologic processes. The **physical half-life** (T_P) is defined as the time required for the number of radioactive atoms in a sample to decrease by one-half, while the **biologic half-life** (T_B) is the time required for half of the radionuclide to be eliminated by biologic processes (primarily via renal and hepatic/GI clearance). These half-lives can be combined into an **effective half-life** (T_E) by the relationship $\frac{1}{T_E} = \frac{1}{T_P} + \frac{1}{T_B}$, which designates the time for an amount of radiopharmaceutical distributed in tissues and organs to decrease by one-half. The effective whole-body dose from most nuclear medicine diagnostic procedures is equivalent to one-half to six times the average annual per capita effective dose from natural background (~2 mSv for a Tc-99m MAA lung perfusion study to 20 mSv for a tumor imaging study with 185 MBq of Ga-67 citrate). Patients receive additional radiation when CT is added to PET or SPECT imaging. There are currently no standard scanner parameters for the CT component of PET/CT or SPECT/CT examinations, which range from low-dose CT images for attenuation correction and anatomic localization to full diagnostic examinations. This results in a widely variable dose from the CT component.

The **critical organ** designates the organ or tissue that receives the largest dose of radiation or that has the highest radiosensitivity to a radiopharmaceutical. The dose to the critical organ depends on the radionuclide concentration by the organ, geometric factors, the effective retention in that organ, and the relative radiosensitivity of the organ. Interestingly, in many cases, the dose to any organ (the target organ) comes as much from the organ itself as it does from the surrounding tissue (the source).

Nuclear medicine scintigraphy requires special consideration when imaging the pregnant patient. Radiotherapy and diagnostic I-131 imaging are the only absolute contraindications for nuclear medicine scintigraphy in pregnancy. A risk-versus-benefit analysis is necessary to assess the appropriateness of the examination. Modalities without ionizing radiation (MRI or ultrasound) and delay of imaging until after delivery should be considered when possible. When nuclear medicine scintigraphy is performed, measures should be taken to minimize the radiation dose to the patient, such as halving the normal adult dose while doubling the imaging time and increasing hydration to enhance radiotracer excretion. For PET/CT scans, the CT tube current may be reduced to 20 mA without significantly impacting the PET portion of the study, though will compromise the quality of the CT images.

Lactating females that receive a radiopharmaceutical require counseling regarding breast-feeding as many radiopharmaceuticals may be excreted into breast milk. Breast-feeding cessation guidelines are based on the physical and biologic half-lives of the radiopharmaceuticals to predict when the breast milk is safe to drink. The recommended times for successions of breast-feeding are listed in Table 71B.3. If the radiopharmaceutical is not listed in Table 71B.3, refer to the package insert provided by the radiopharmaceutical manufacturer for their recommendation.

Radiation Safety in the Workplace—General Guidelines. The goals of radiation safety are to minimize exposure to radiation to workers, patients, and the public. Three basic principles exist to minimize one's radiation exposure: **time, distance, and shielding.**

- **Minimize time of exposure** to radioactive source
- **Maximize distance** from radioactive source
  - **Inverse square law**: Exposure will decrease by a factor of 100 by moving 10 ft away (**radiation dose** $\propto \frac{1}{d^2}$, where d is the distance between the individual and the radioactive source)
- **Use shielding** (lead aprons, syringe and vial shields, etc.) whenever possible

Regulations. The U.S. NRC governs nuclear material and its by-products as well as accelerator-produced radioactive materials. By-products include reactor-produced radionuclides such as molybdenum-99 and iodine-131. The NRC licenses users (individuals or institutions) and governs many aspects of nuclear medicine operations including the standards for protection against radiation (radiation protection program), waste disposal, granting licenses, surveys, instrumentation, and training requirements. Many states have become "agreement states" by accepting the responsibility to regulate radioactive materials. These states are responsible for licensing users and enforcing regulations comparable with those of the NRC.

The central objective of all radiation protection programs promotes efforts to keep radiation exposures *as low as reasonably achievable (ALARA)*. The NRC requires an ALARA program that represents an administrative philosophy to encourage, enforce, teach, and observe all reasonable ways to minimize radiation doses and exposure. The ALARA program extends into personnel exposure (worker), medical events (patient), and environmental releases (general public) to achieve this dose minimization goal.

TABLE 71B.3

RECOMMENDATIONS FOR CESSATION OF BREAST-FEEDING AFTER ADMINISTRATION OF RADIOPHARMACEUTICALS TO MOTHERS

RADIOPHARMACEUTICAL	ADMINISTERED ACTIVITY	IMAGING PROCEDURE	RECOMMENDED DURATION OF INTERRUPTION OF BREAST-FEEDING[a]
Tc-99m sodium pertechnetate	1110 MBq (30 mCi)	Thyroid scan and Meckel scan	24 hours
Tc-99m kits (general rule)	185–935 MBq (5–25 mCi)		24 hours
Tc-99m DTPA	370–555 MBq (10–15 mCi)	All renal scan	None
Tc-99m MAA	111–185 MBq (3–5 mCi)	Lung perfusion scan	12 hours
Tc-99m SC	185 kBq (5 μCi)	Liver spleen scan	6 hours
Tc-99m MDP	555–935 MBq (15–25 mCi)	Bone scan	None
Tc-99m sestamibi/tetrofosmin[b]	370–1110 MBq (10–30 mCi)	Cardiac studies	None
F-18 FDG	370–740 MBq (10–20 mCi)	Tumor, neuro, or cardiac PET scan	12 hours
Ga-67 citrate	222–370 MBq (6–10 mCi)	Infection and tumor scans	4 weeks
Tl-201 chloride	111 MBq (3 mCi)	Myocardial perfusion	2 weeks
Sodium I-123	1.11 MBq (30 μCi)	Thyroid uptake only	None
Sodium I-123	7.4–14.8 MBq (200–400 μCi)	Thyroid scan	None
Sodium I-131	185 kBq (5 μCi)	Thyroid uptake	Discontinue[c]
Sodium I-131	370 MBq (10 mCi)	Thyroid cancer Metascan or Graves therapy	Discontinue[c]
Sodium I-131	1,221 MBq (33 mCi)	Outpatient therapy for hyperfunctioning nodule	Discontinue[c]
Sodium I-131	3.7 GBq (100 mCi) or more	Thyroid cancer treatment (ablation)	Discontinue[c]

[a]Adapted from NRC Regulatory Guide 8.39, 1997. See Romney BM, et al. for derivation of milk concentration values for radiopharmaceuticals.
[b]Minimal F-18 FDG in breast milk (*J Nucl Med* 42:1238–1242, 2001). Waiting 6 half-lives (12 hours) lowers the exposure to the infant from the mother.
[c]Discontinuance is based not only on the excessive time recommended for cessation of breast-feeding but also on the high dose the breasts themselves would receive during the radiopharmaceutical breast transit.
DTPA, diethylenetriaminepentaacetic acid; FDG, fluorodeoxyglucose; MAA, macroaggregated albumin; MDP, methylene diphosphonate; SC, sulfur colloid.

The NRC regulations that cover nuclear medicine are found in the Code of Federal Regulations parts 19, 20, and 35. Part 19 covers the rights and responsibilities of workers to maintain a safe environment and employers to educate their workers. Part 20 covers regulations of radiation protection for facilities to include dose limits for personnel and the environment. Part 35 focuses on medical utilization of radiation sources, listing medical event definitions (formerly referred to as misadministrations and discussed in more detail later in this chapter), and training requirements for authorized users. Board certification in diagnostic radiology or nuclear medicine suffices to qualify the individual as an authorized user under most circumstances.

Radiation Safety Instruments. Two types of radiation detectors are commonly used for radiation safety in the Nuclear Medicine Department. The **Geiger–Müller (GM) detector** is a *gas-filled survey meter* that measures radiation in counts per minute. The GM meter is a **very sensitive** radiation detector that is useful for localizing very small quantities of activity but does not typically provide an accurate exposure rate. Its primary use is as a laboratory survey instrument looking for contamination. The **ion chamber**, another *gas-filled detector*, is used to **accurately measure radiation exposure**, especially at high levels. The ion chamber has several uses that include quantifying exposure levels, assaying doses prior to administration (dose calibrator, see later discussion), and checking packages for compliance with transportation regulations.

- **GM detector:** Very sensitive gas-filled detector used as a survey instrument to detect contamination
- **Ion chamber:** Gas-filled detector that accurately detects exposure rates—used to quantify exposure levels, assay doses prior to administration, and check packages for compliance with transportation regulations

Radiopharmaceutical Possession and Handling. In general, compliance regulations require "cradle to grave" documentation of all radioactive substances. These requirements begin with an authorized individual ordering the radiopharmaceuticals, then setting standards for packaging and shipping, followed by procedures for the receipt of the package, and finally demonstrating documentation of its use (patient or research) and disposal. Meticulous records of each step are imperative for adequate documentation of the "life" of a radioactive substance.

Radiation Monitoring. In a personnel monitoring program, designated workers exposed to radiation wear dosimetry badges, typically a thermoluminescent dosimeter (TLD) or an optically stimulated luminescence dosimeter (OSLD). TLD and OSLD both exist in badge form to estimate whole body exposure. TLDs also exist in ring form to estimate hand exposure for technologists, given direct and frequent handling of unit doses during radiopharmaceutical administration.

- **TLD:** Radiation excites electrons within the TLD material.
  - **Badge reading:** Electrons return to ground state following heating and emit light proportional to the amount of radiation dose received.
- **OSLD:** Radiation exposure traps electrons within specific areas of a crystalline structure.
  - **Badge reading:** Visible light exposure causes emission of stored energy in the form of light proportional to the amount of radiation dose received.

The nuclear medicine workplace requires frequent monitoring for contamination. A typical monitoring program is as follows:

Daily. A GM survey meter is used to check over all work surfaces and trash. As a general rule, if any reading is greater than two times background, then the area should be decontaminated (wash area) and resampled until readings are less than twice background. In an unrestricted area (general public area), all readings should be less than two times background. Label all contaminated trash as radioactive and store for decay. The parameters for a **decay-in-storage** program will be specified in the institution's radioactive materials license. Most licenses specify that waste be held for **10 physical half-lives.**

Weekly. Perform a radiation field survey using an **ion chamber** to survey controlled areas within the workplace. Dose rates in **unrestricted areas** must be **less than 20 μSv** (2 mrem) in any 1 hour **and less than 1 mSv** (100 mrem); however, all potential exposures should be kept ALARA.

Weekly. Wipe test multiple sample areas of the workplace. Count in a NaI (Tl) gamma counter using a wide energy window for 1 minute. An acceptable threshold is 200 disintegrations/min per 100 cm^2 of surface area. If exceeded, then decontaminate and resample until within limits.

RADIOPHARMACEUTICALS

Mechanism of Localization of Radiopharmaceuticals. A radiopharmaceutical (which in an imaging context may be known as a radiolabeled tracer or radiotracer) is a specific compound containing a radionuclide. The compound determines the biodistribution of the radiopharmaceutical. Many radiopharmaceuticals act like analogs of natural biologic compounds and localize by means of a physiologic process. For example, Tc-99m-pertechnetate is analogous to the iodide molecule and distributes to the thyroid, salivary glands, stomach, and kidneys. Technetium-99m sulfur colloid acts like a colloid particle of approximately 1 micron and distributes throughout the reticuloendothelial system (liver, spleen, and bone marrow). Substituted iminodiacetic acid Tc-99m agents (HIDA) are analogous to bilirubin and are actively transported into hepatocytes and excreted into the biliary tree. F-18 FDG acts as a glucose analog that is transported into the cell, phosphorylated, and subsequently physiologically trapped within the cell. The concentration of F-18 FDG within tissues following an uptake period of 45 to 90 minutes correlates with glucose utilization (see Table 71B.4 for other examples).

Generation of Radiopharmaceuticals. An ideal radiotracer consists of a tracer with a desired physiologic mechanism (such as entering the biliary system) labeled with a radionuclide that has a physical half-life long enough to allow for radiotracer localization and imaging, though not too long in order to limit unnecessary patient irradiation. Thus, radiotracers cannot be stored long term and must be generated daily for immediate use, either by cyclotrons or generators.

Cyclotron-produced radionuclides are shipped to a nuclear medicine pharmacy (local or third-party nuclear pharmacy) for radiopharmaceutical production. Radiopharmaceuticals are typically sold and distributed as unit doses from a third-party nuclear pharmacy unless the hospital facility has an on-site cyclotron (usually large academic centers). Cyclotron-produced radionuclides can be found in Table 71B.1 and include radionuclides such as F-18 and I-123.

Generators are widely used and contain a parent radionuclide that decays into a desired daughter radionuclide at a predictable rate. Generators can be kept on-site, allowing for instant access to radionuclide for both routine scheduled examinations and unexpected add-on inpatient and emergency exams such as ventilation/perfusion lung scans and hepatobiliary scans. Common generators include molybdenum-99/technetium-99m (Moly generator) and strontium-82/rubidium-82 (used for cardiac PET perfusion imaging) generators. The most common radionuclide in nuclear medicine procedures is Tc-99m and the generation of this radionuclide is described in detail below.

Moly Generator. Mo-99 undergoes β^- and γ decay with high-energy γ-rays (740 and 780 keV) and a physical half-life ($T_{1/2}$) of 67 hours, while Tc-99m decays with a $T_{1/2}$ of 6 hours via 140-keV γ-rays (Fig. 71B.3). The **Mo-99 is adsorbed to an alumina column where it decays into Tc-99m pertechnetate** (**$^{99m}TcO_4^-$**). The Tc-99m pertechnetate can be removed from the alumina column via a process known as **elution.** Normal saline (sodium chloride) passes over the alumina column and chloride ions are exchanged for Tc-99m pertechnetate ions ($^{99m}TcO_4^-$). The resulting solution, known as the **eluate,** can be removed from the generator in the form of sodium pertechnetate ($Na^{99m}TcO_4$) (Fig. 71B.4).

After eluting (also referred to as "milking") the Moly generator, the shorter-lived daughter Tc-99m begins immediately reaccumulating on the column at a predictable rate, entering a state of **transient equilibrium** (Fig. 71B.5). The percent yield of Tc-99m from elution can be determined based on the time from last elution with maximal Tc-99m yield at approximately 23 hours. This allows daily elution every 24 hours that is both convenient and efficacious with respect to yield.

Moly generators undergo **quality control** following each elution to assess for two sources of contamination: Mo-99 (moly) and aluminum ion (Al^{3+}) breakthrough. This refers to Mo-99 or aluminum ions inadvertently leaving the alumina column and entering the eluate solution that is used to label tracers for patient administration.

Moly breakthrough results in an unnecessary exposure of patients and technologists to the damaging β^- particles and high-energy γ-rays from Mo-99 decay. This is a form of **radionuclidic impurity** (wrong radionuclide within the eluate). The assay for Moly breakthrough looks for the very high-energy photons (740 and 780 keV) emitted by Mo-99. The entire eluate is placed in a lead container, called a Moly pig, which absorbs the majority of the 140-keV Tc-99m photons but allows most of the higher-energy Mo-99 photons to pass through. The pig is then assayed in a dose calibrator with the Mo-99 button selected to detect the 740- and 780-keV Mo-99 γ-rays. The **NRC limit is 0.15 μCi of Mo-99 per mCi of Tc-99m** at the time of administration.

Aluminum breakthrough causes flocculation of particles within Tc-99m kits into colloid that results in image degradation. These colloid particles cause increased lung uptake on sulfur colloid liver–spleen scans and increased liver uptake on bone scans. This is a form of **chemical impurity** (incorrect chemical within the eluate, correct radionuclide/radiotracer). The QC procedure to check for aluminum breakthrough is

TABLE 71B.4

BIODISTRIBUTION: MECHANISM OF LOCALIZATION OF RADIOPHARMACEUTICALS

■ IMAGING PROCEDURE	■ RADIOPHARMA-CEUTICALS	■ MECHANISM OF LOCALIZATION	■ CLOSEST BIOCHEMICAL ANALOG	■ CRITICAL ORGAN (GRAY)
Lung perfusion scan	Tc-99m macroaggregated albumin	Capillary blockade	Thromboembolus	Lungs (1.5–4.8 mGy)
Lung ventilation scan	Xe-133 gas	Compartment localization	Air	Trachea (6.4 mGy)
Bone scan	Tc-99m methylene diphos-phonate	Chemical adsorption onto bone crystal	Phosphate	Bladder (1–3 mGy)
Hepatobiliary scan	Tc-99m iminodiacetic acid	Active hepatocyte cellular transport	Bilirubin	Gallbladder (1.2–1.8 mGy)
Myocardial perfusion scan	Tl-201 Chloride	ATP transport system	Potassium	Kidneys (4–9 mGy)
Labeled WBC scan	In-111 WBC Tc-99m HMPAO	Active migration of leuko-cyte to the site of infec-tion or inflammation after binding of radionuclide to intracellular component	Migratory leuko-cyte	Spleen (84–180 mGy) (7.9 mGy)
Renal scan	Tc-99m DTPA Tc-99m MAG3 (mertiatide)	Glomerular filtration Glomerular filtration and tubular secretion	Inulin p-aminohippurate	Bladder (0.7–6 mGy)
Thyroid	I-123	Active transport	Iodine	Thyroid (110–200 mGy)
Brain scan	Tc-99m HMPAO (hexamethylpropylene amine oxime)	Lipophilic passive transport	Fatty acid	Lachrymal gland (51.6 mGy)
Gated equilibrium blood pool scan	Tc-99m–labeled RBCs	Compartment localization of RBC after Tc-99m binds to intracellular hemoglobin	RBC	Spleen (22 mGy)
Tumor imaging	F-18 fluorodeoxyglucose (FDG)	Cellular uptake via glucose transporters followed by metabolic trapping of FDG-6-phosphate	Glucose	Bladder (4 mGy)
	Ga-67 citrate	Unknown, iron receptor theory	Ferric ion	Colon (6–9 mGy)
	In-111 OncoScint monoclo-nal antibody (satumomab pendetide)	Antibody–antigen complex	Antibody	Spleen (32 mGy)
Meckel scan	Tc-99m pertechnetate	Active ion transport	Iodide	Thyroid (1.2–1.8 mGy)
Liver spleen scan	Tc-99m colloid	Reticuloendothelial phagocytosis	Colloid particle	Liver (2–4 mGy)

ATP, adenosine triphosphate; WBC, white blood cell; HMPAO, hexametazime; DTPA, diethylenetriaminepentaacetic acid; MAG3, mertiatide; RBCs, red blood cells; Tc, technetium.

the **colorimetric spot test** where a drop of eluate is placed on the colorimetric paper and compared with a standard. **The maximum permissible amount of aluminum is 10 μg/mL of the eluate.**

Radiopharmaceutical Production. Many of the Tc-99m–based radiopharmaceuticals are produced by adding the generator eluate, the "free" or unbound Tc-99m pertechnetate ($^{99m}TcO_4^-$), to a "cold" kit containing the chelate (e.g., MDP,

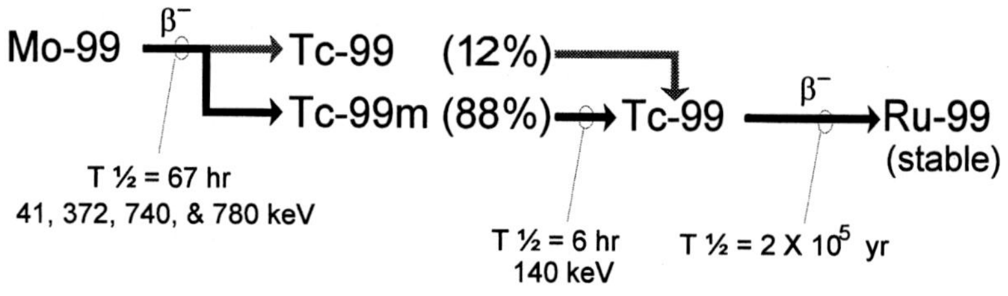

FIGURE 71B.3. **Mo-99/Tc-99m Decay Scheme.** The Mo-99 decays with both high-energy photons and β-particles (electrons). Twelve percent of Mo-99 decays directly to Tc-99, while the other 88% produces metastable Tc-99m. Tc-99m gives up its 140-keV photon and reaches Tc-99.

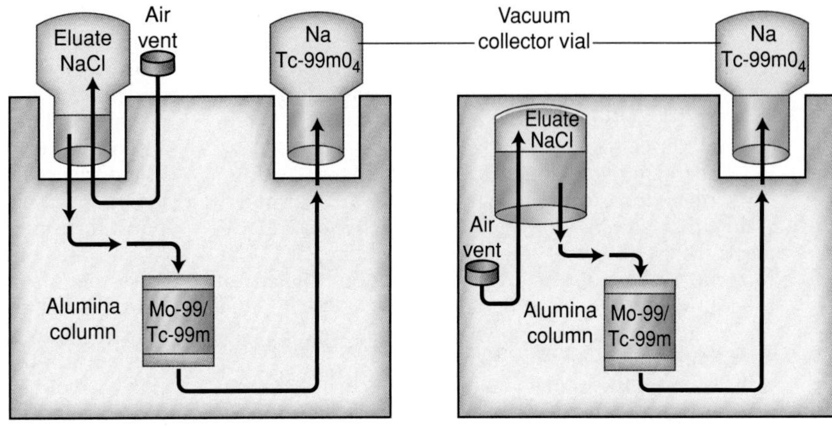

FIGURE 71B.4. **Wet/Dry Generators.** Both dry and wet generators use a vacuum collection vial; the difference is in the source of the NaCl eluate. The dry generator has a replaceable vial while the wet generator has a fixed one. Both types of generators use the alumina column and are, therefore, susceptible to aluminum and Mo-99 (Moly) breakthrough. The end product is also the same: sodium pertechnetate (Na Tc-99mO_4). Dry generators are now very rarely used and are primarily of historical interest.

DTPA, DISIDA) and a reducing agent, usually stannous chloride ($SnCl_2$). The stannous chloride reduces the Tc-99m from the stable valence state of +7 to the less stable/more reactive +3 and +4 states necessary for chelation with most kit tracers. Some kits, including sulfur colloid and MAG3, require heat to allow for the chelation to occur. The introduction of air or water during kit preparation can lead to the production of **radiopharmaceutical impurities** (correct radionuclide, wrong radiopharmaceutical). Introduced air may cause oxidation of stannous ions (Sn^{+2} to Sn^{+4}), which inhibits the reduction of Tc-99m and prevents complexation with the tracer. Excess water will hydrolyze stannous chloride to stannous hydroxide, a colloid. **Hydrolyzed-reduced Tc-99m,** also known as Tc-99m dioxide ($^{99m}TcO_2$), is another impurity that may form during radiopharmaceutical preparation and result in liver and spleen uptake secondary to colloid formation.

Radiochemical purity is defined as the percentage of the total radioactivity in a source that is present in the form of the desired chemical (i.e., the radiopharmaceutical). The **Food and Drug Administration (FDA)** mandates the testing

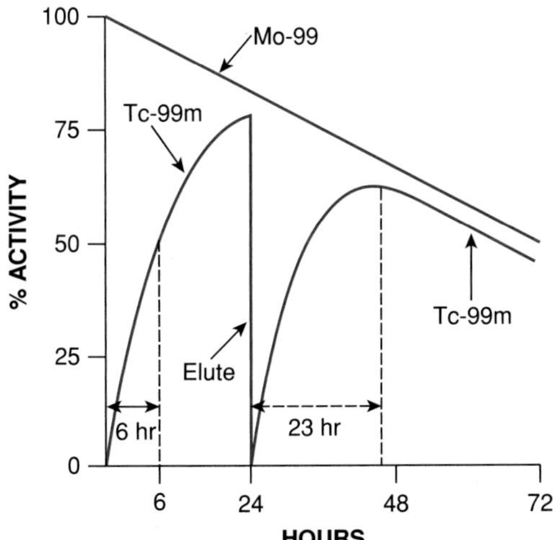

FIGURE 71B.5. **Mo-99/Tc-99m Generator Elution Curves.** The regrowth of the daughter (Tc-99m) on the column takes a predictable course after each elution. Inspection of the curves reveals that approximately 50% of the activity will be present 6 hours after an elution and that maximum activity is achieved at 23 hours after elution. This is convenient for a daily morning-scheduled elution and allows for an unplanned elution by midday if needed.

of radiopharmaceuticals for radiochemical purity prior to commercial release of a new product. **The procedure to test for impurities involves separating the different species based on solubility using appropriate solvents.** Various solvents and media are used in the separation method, but the **most common method is thin-layer chromatography** (**TLC**), which consists of glass fiber strips impregnated with silica gel. After placing a drop of the radiopharmaceutical on the end (origin) of a TLC strip, the strip is placed origin end down in a shallow pool of solvent until the solvent front reaches the top. Because free Tc-99m is soluble in acetone and saline, it migrates with the solvent front, leaving behind the insoluble species for that particular solvent. **In saline,** both Tc-99m dioxide (hydrolyzed-reduced Tc-99m) and Tc-99m tin colloid are insoluble and remain at the origin, while the Tc-99m radiopharmaceutical migrates with any free Tc-99m to the top. **In acetone,** only the free Tc-99m migrates to the top, leaving behind all other species. By cutting the strips into an origin half and a solvent front half, each part of the strip can be counted in a gamma counter. The total value of radiochemical impurities is calculated by subtracting from 100% the sum of the percentage of the various impurities present (free Tc-99m, Tc-99m tin colloid, and Tc-99m dioxide). No NRC limits are set for radiochemical purity, but the U.S. Pharmacopoeia, which sets standards for pharmacies, defines the lower limit of acceptability for purity for most radiopharmaceuticals as 90%, with a few exceptions. The manufacturer's package insert will provide specific information for each radiopharmaceutical.

- **Saline:** Radiopharmaceutical moves up column, hydrolyzed-reduced Tc-99m and Tc-99m sulfur colloid remain at bottom
- **Acetone:** Only free Tc-99m pertechnetate moves up column

Medical Events. The NRC defines certain errors in the administration of radiopharmaceuticals as **medical events.** Medical events were formerly called "misadministrations." The **current NRC definition of a medical event** is as follows:

A. The administration of a by-product material that results in one of the following conditions (1 or 2) unless its occurrence was as the direct result of patient intervention (e.g., I-131 therapy patient takes only half of the prescribed dose, then refuses to take the balance):
   a. A dose that differs from the prescribed dose by more than 0.05-Sv (5 rem) effective dose equivalent, 0.5 Sv (50 rem) to an organ or tissue, or 0.5-Sv (50 rem) shallow dose equivalent to the skin; and one of the following conditions had also occurred.
      i. The total dose delivered differs from the prescribed dose by 20% or more.

ii. The total dosage delivered differs from the prescribed dosage by 20% or more or falls outside the prescribed dosage range for a given procedure that has been established by the licensee (e.g., 370 to 1,100 MBq [10 to 30 mCi] Tc-99m-MDP for an adult bone scan).
iii. The fractionated dose delivered differs from the prescribed dose, for a single fraction, by 50% or more.

b. A dose that exceeds 0.05-Sv (5 rem) effective dose equivalent, 0.5 Sv (50 rem) to an organ or tissue, or 0.5-Sv (50 rem) shallow dose equivalent to the skin from any of the following:
i. An administration of a wrong radioactive drug containing the by-product material
ii. An administration of a radioactive drug containing the by-product material by the wrong route of administration
iii. An administration of a dose or dosage to the wrong individual or human research subject
iv. An administration of a dose or dosage delivered by the wrong mode of treatment
v. A leaking sealed source

B. Any event resulting from intervention of a patient or human research subject in which the administration of a by-product material results or will result in unintended permanent functional damage to an organ or a physiologic system, as determined by a physician. Patient intervention means actions by the patient, whether intentional or not, which affect the radiopharmaceutical administration.

Federal law requires that medical events be reported to the NRC no later than the next calendar day after the discovery of the event. This must be **followed by a written report within 15 days** that details a number of items including the cause of the medical event, the effect (if any) on the individual involved, and proposed corrective actions. Other reporting requirements can be found in 10CFR35. It should be noted that Agreement States may have different, and possibly more restrictive, definitions of medical events (misadministrations) and reporting requirements.

IMAGING SYSTEMS AND RADIATION DETECTORS

Image Content. Most x-ray, MR, and US images carry a predominance of anatomic information (although this is less true for Doppler US and dynamic flow MRI). For nuclear medicine images, anatomic information is secondary to the functional content. Currently, there is an increasing tendency to interpret nuclear medicine images in correlation with roughly contemporaneous anatomic images thanks to the development of combined imaging modalities such as PET/CT or SPECT/CT. In the absence of combined scanning devices, functional and anatomic images may be digitally reoriented or coregistered ("fused") with each other prior to display and interpretation; this process is becoming increasingly common in clinical practice, particularly in neuroimaging.

Nuclear medicine images reflect not only the biodistribution of the radiopharmaceutical but also the anatomic, pathologic, and artifact overlays present at the time of imaging. Thus, their interpretation must be tempered with a knowledge of not only the patterns of the normal and pathologic processes but also with a knowledge of the influence of the individual patient's physiology, habitus, and positioning, as well as with the technical aspects of the examination. Taking all of these variables together will enable the interpreting physician to avoid erroneous diagnoses made from the interplay of physiologic, anatomic, and technical factors.

Scintillation Detectors. Almost all nuclear medicine imaging devices available today are based on scintillation detector technology. Such detectors consist of a scintillating crystal that emits visible light photons on interaction with a γ-ray or annihilation photon. These visible light photons are then converted into an electrical signal by photomultiplier tubes (PMTs) optically coupled to the scintillation crystal (Fig. 71B.6). In most imaging systems, a scintillation crystal is coupled to an array of PMTs. When an incoming photon interacts with the crystal, the resulting light distribution is most intense nearest to the interaction point and falls off with distance. By examining the ratio of signals from the PMT array, it is therefore possible to determine the point of interaction to within a few millimeters (Fig. 71B.7). The earliest form of such an imaging detector was called the Anger camera after its inventor, Hal Anger. **Gamma cameras** are the modern-day equivalent of Anger cameras and are the most widely used imaging tools in nuclear medicine today.

The faces of the PMTs in the array cover a significant portion of the crystal in order to maximize light collection. Direct readout of the PMT signals would generate a distorted distribution of events because PMTs do not have a perfectly linear response with respect to the distance from their center. The signals are therefore adjusted by means of a stored correction matrix. This correction matrix is dependent on the energy of the incoming photons and may also vary with time, as the PMT gains drift or as the crystal ages. An important part of imaging scintillation detector QC is to ensure that this correction matrix is kept accurate. This is particularly true for rotating gamma cameras, where a fault in one part of the detector can affect a large fraction of the final image and may produce **ring artifacts.** The correction matrix may consist of several components—these may include uniformity, energy, and linearity.

The thickness of the scintillator material is an important design consideration. **Thicker crystals** are more likely to stop the incoming photons, resulting in **greater sensitivity**. This is crucial in high-energy applications such as PET imaging. However, there is more light spreading in thicker crystals, thus

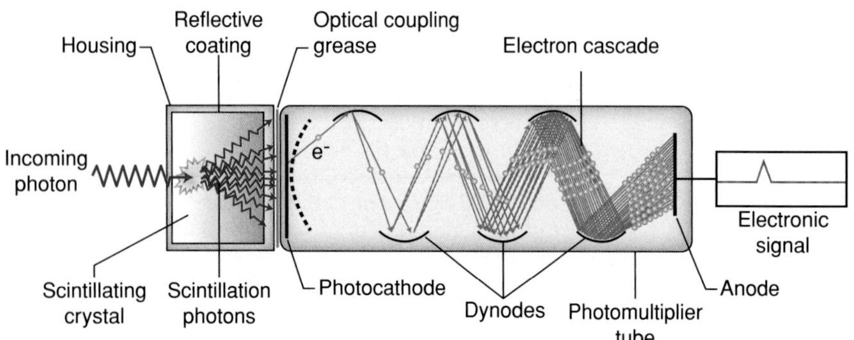

FIGURE 71B.6. **Components of a Scintillation Detector.**

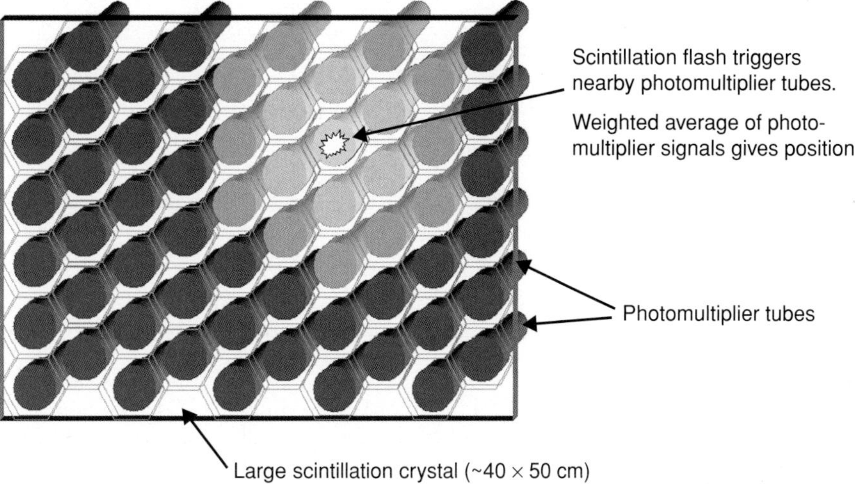

FIGURE 71B.7. Components of a Gamma Camera Detector.

reducing spatial resolution. Thinner crystals are preferred for low-energy photon imaging.

- **Thick crystals:** Higher sensitivity, lower spatial resolution (e.g., PET imaging)
- **Thinner crystals:** Lower sensitivity, higher spatial resolution (e.g., thyroid imaging)

The optimal scintillator material is also dependent on the application. Important material parameters are stopping power, scintillation light output, speed of scintillation light decay, and cost. Sodium iodide (NaI) is cheap and produces numerous scintillation light photons for a given amount of deposited interaction energy, making it ideal for single-photon imaging with gamma cameras. For PET applications, the high-energy annihilation photons require materials of greater stopping power. As will be explained below, PET detectors must operate at very high data rates, so the speed of scintillation light decay is also important. Current materials of choice include lutetium oxyorthosilicate (LSO) and its variants, bismuth germinate (BGO), lutetium–yttrium orthosilicate (LYSO), and gadolinium silicate (GSO). BGO and LYSO have the greatest stopping power, but LSO and GSO produce scintillation light more quickly and can operate at higher data rates.

Collimation. Determination of the interaction point alone is insufficient to generate an image. It is also necessary to determine the direction from which the incoming photon impinges upon the detector. In an optical imaging device, such as a photographic camera, this is achieved with a lens. In nuclear medicine, where the photon wavelengths are too short for lens-based refraction to be effective, this is achieved either with an absorbing collimator in the case of single-photon imaging or with coincidence circuitry (also known as "electronic collimation") in the case of PET imaging.

Pinhole Collimators. The simplest form of an absorbing collimator is the pinhole collimator made of a hollow cone of lead or tungsten with a small hole at the apex (Fig. 71B.8, pinhole collimator). This results in a low-sensitivity device since the object allows passage of a very small solid angle of light at the detector face. Sensitivity can be increased by enlarging the collimator hole, but this reduces the spatial resolution of the image. A pinhole collimator has the property that objects that are closer to the pinhole than the detector are magnified in the image. The degree of magnification is given simply by the ratio of the distances from the pinhole to the object and from the pinhole to the detector. This magnification property renders it particularly useful for imaging small structures such as the thyroid or focal areas of the skeleton. In sequential studies, care must be taken to ensure that the pinhole–organ distance is constant or else variations in the degree of magnification will render size comparisons impossible. The geometry of pinhole collimators results in inversion of the imaged object, which is corrected through image postprocessing.

- **Pinhole collimators create magnified images (high spatial resolution) that are inverted.**

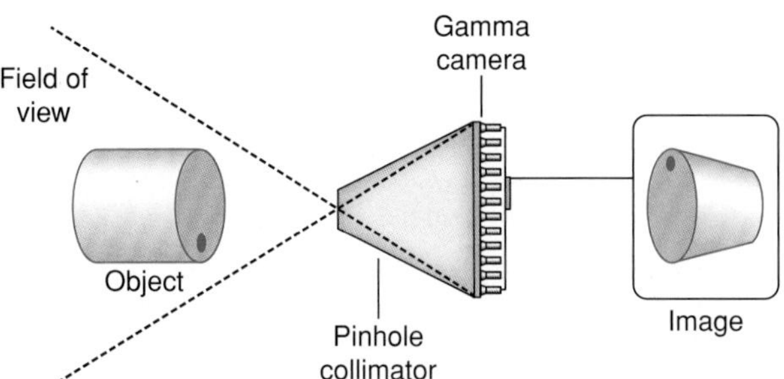

FIGURE 71B.8. **Pinhole Collimation.** The image is inverted and since the magnification increases as the distance to the pinhole decreases, it is distorted.

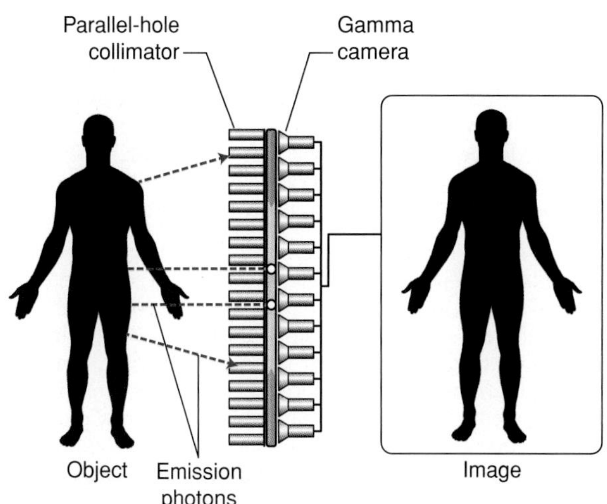

FIGURE 71B.9. **Parallel-Hole Collimation.** Only photons traveling parallel to the collimator holes may hit the detector. The image is not inverted, and there is no magnification.

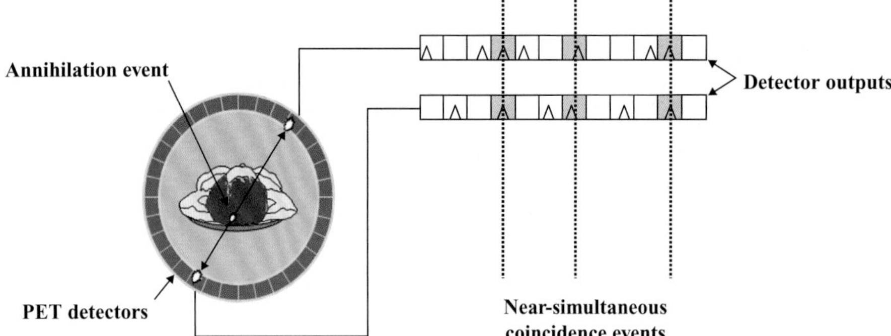

FIGURE 71B.10. **The Principle of Coincidence Detection.** When pulses from separate detector elements occur together in a short space of time, it is assumed that the photons that gave rise to those pulses arose from a single annihilation event.

Parallel-hole collimators consist of a lattice of lead or tungsten constructed to form an array of closely spaced small parallel holes (Fig. 71B.9). Placing such a device in front of a scintillation camera prevents photons that are not parallel to the holes from reaching the crystal, absorbing scattered/deflected photons. As a result, only γ-rays traveling in a straight line parallel to the collimator holes will hit the detector and contribute to image creation. There is no image magnification or minification. Image spatial resolution falls off as the distance from the object to the collimator face increases, and therefore, it is important to have the collimator as close to the patient as possible.

The absorbing lattice forms what are known as the collimator "septa" and the geometry of the septa has important effects on the image created. The primary parameters are septal length, septal thickness, and hole diameter. Longer septa and narrower holes result in an increase in spatial resolution at the expense of a decrease in sensitivity as a larger number of photons are absorbed by the septa. This results in fewer photons hitting the detector to contribute to image creation and results in noisier images. Collimator parameters are chosen to optimize imaging and are dependent on the size of anatomy being imaged and γ-ray energy of the radionuclide being imaged. For Ga-67 imaging (maximum photon energy 300 keV), high-energy collimators with longer, thicker septa should be utilized as higher-energy photons can penetrate short and thin lead septa. **Low-energy high-resolution collimators are used for most single-photon emitters such as Tc-99m.** In some circumstances, greater sensitivity is desired and low-energy general purpose collimators might be chosen. Inappropriate use of low-energy high-resolution collimators with high-energy photon emitters results in degraded images with a smudgy appearance.

Converging and Diverging Collimators. A **converging collimator** can be used to **obtain a magnified image** with greater sensitivity than a pinhole collimator. Reversing the orientation of such a device results in a **diverging collimator.** This **minifies the image** but results in a larger field of view, allowing more of the body to be imaged without moving the patient.

Electronic Collimation or Coincidence Detection. Specially designed ultra–high-energy collimators are used to detect the 511-keV γ-rays created from positron–electron annihilation events. There is no adequate septal design that can achieve an appropriate trade-off between septal penetration, sensitivity, and resolution for the high-energy 511-keV photons. This can be overcome by employing **coincidence detection.** Coincidence detection takes advantage of the fact that each annihilation event results in two annihilation photons traveling in almost exactly opposite directions. It takes approximately 3 ns for a photon to travel about 1 m, which is approximately the distance between the opposing coincidence detector elements in modern PET/CT machines. If two opposing detectors are set up to measure the time of arrival of the photons as well as their position, it is possible to examine the data for pairs of detection events that occur within such a short time window—that is, for pairs of an event that are "coincident." These can then be considered to have arisen from the same annihilation event that must have occurred along the line connecting the locations of the two detection events ("line of sight"). Current PET systems consider events to be coincident if they occur within 4 to 12 ns of each other. In this way, the flight direction of the photons can be constrained without the use of an absorbing collimator (i.e., there is no physical collimator/septa), and images can be generated from the resulting data. This process is known as **electronic collimation** or, more commonly, as coincidence detection (Fig. 71B.10).

False or "random" coincidences can be detected if two photons from unrelated annihilation events happen to interact with the detectors within the coincidence time window and register as a true event. Random coincidences can be corrected for but always result in increased noise in the image. The rate of random coincidences increases roughly in proportion to the square of the activity in the field of view. This places an upper limit on the activity concentration within the patient at the time of imaging to prevent excessive image noise (i.e., there is an upper dose limit for administered radioactivity).

Removal of the absorbing collimators results in a significant increase in sensitivity as γ-rays are no longer absorbed by the collimator septa. The coincidence detectors must be capable of operating at very high data rates to account for the increased number of photons reaching the detector. Most PET scanners achieve a high-rate capability by detector segmentation—that is, the scanner consists of an array of small detectors (typically 100 to 300), rather than a small number of large detectors (typically 2 or 3 in a collimated design). Thus, if one small detector is busy processing a signal, the others are free to continue obtaining data. Unfortunately, this design option increases the complexity and cost of the resulting scanner. A typical PET "block" detector is shown in Figure 71B.11.

Time-of-Flight-Assisted PET. Recent advancements in detector physics and electronics have allowed the development of sensitive PET detectors with very fast response times of 500 ps or less. These fast response times allow new detectors to generate constraints on the possible position of the originating annihilation event between the two detectors, increasing spatial resolution by more accurately determining the point of annihilation. This approach is known as **"time-of-flight"** PET and appears to be particularly beneficial for imaging obese patients.

Energy Analysis. Although each radionuclide has one or more imaging photon energies (Table 71B.1), Compton interactions between the original photon, patient, and camera produce a wide range of energies that may be detected (Fig. 71B.12). These various energies can be displayed by most gamma cameras using a **multichannel analyzer function**, which plots frequency of event against photon energy. The desired photon energy range is that which contains those events where the

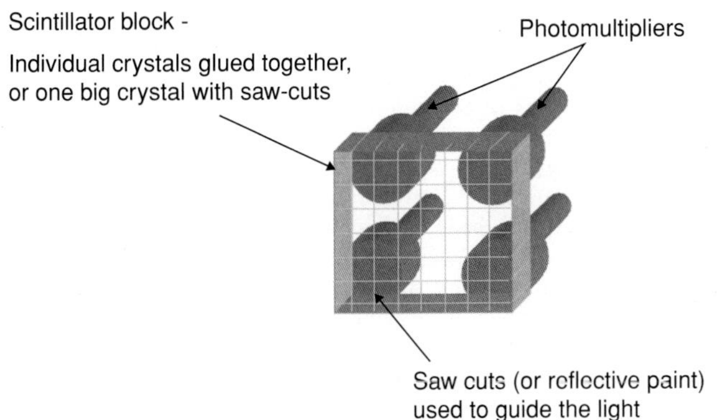

FIGURE 71B.11. **A Block Detector for PET Imaging.**

incident photons deposit all their energy and is known as the **full-energy peak or photopeak**. The energies outside the photopeak arise from Compton scattering events, either within the patient or within the detector itself.

- Radionuclides can be identified via photopeak recognition on multichannel analyzer plots (e.g., data spike at 140 keV for Tc-99m).

The multichannel analyzer function is used to select an energy "window" of acceptance of ± 10% around the photopeak of the radionuclide being imaged (e.g., 126 to 154 keV for Tc-99m), excluding most scattered photons from the image. Multiple windows can be simultaneously acquired for radionuclides such as gallium-67 (93, 184, and 300 keV) and indium-111 (172 and 245 keV). PET scanners have poorer energy resolution than gamma cameras and compensate by using a larger energy window of ± 15% to 30% of the 511-keV photopeak at the expense of increased scatter, particularly when imaging large patients.

Planar and Tomographic Imaging. A gamma camera with a parallel-hole collimator collects data as sets of projections from γ-rays through the patient within a straight line as the collimator septa absorb the majority of deflected/scattered photons prior to reaching the detector. A computer algorithm converts the intensity of radiation behind each collimator hole to a map of radiation intensity and a planar scintigraphic (photons "scintillate" within the crystals) image is obtained, a process referred to as **planar imaging**. This is analogous to digital radiography except that the photons originate from within the patient rather than from an x-ray tube. Think of the patient as a walking x-ray machine.

A disadvantage of planar imaging is that overlapping structures cannot be differentiated from one another as they lie along the same line of sight—there is no depth perception with planar imaging. This can be compensated for by taking planar images from additional angles (i.e., multiplanar imaging). This allows two or more structures within a line to be separated from one another as the structures will not overlap on all lines of sight. If a sufficiently large number of views are acquired, the entire three-dimensional structure can be recovered and converted into a series of parallel planar images (i.e., a stack of images) via CT in a similar manner as x-ray CT. In nuclear medicine, this is performed using a set of rotating gamma cameras for single-photon emitting agents (SPECT) and the higher-energy dual-photon emitting agents in PET. Both modalities can be paired with x-ray CT for anatomic localization and attenuation correction purposes (SPECT/CT and PET/CT).

PET scanners typically consist of a complete ring of detectors that simultaneously acquire all projections necessary for image reconstruction. Most SPECT gamma camera setups consist of one, two, or three flat detectors that rotate around

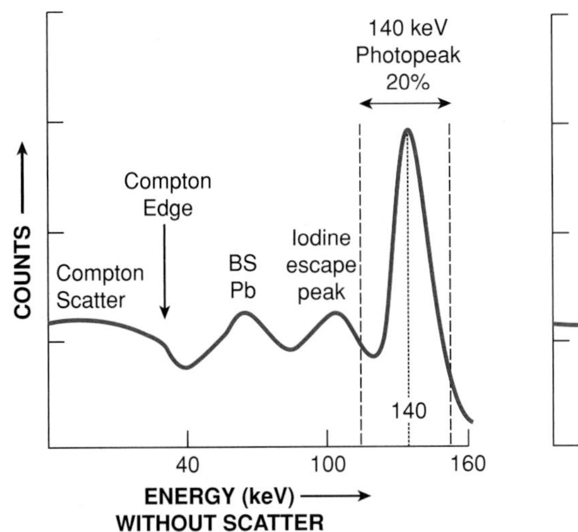

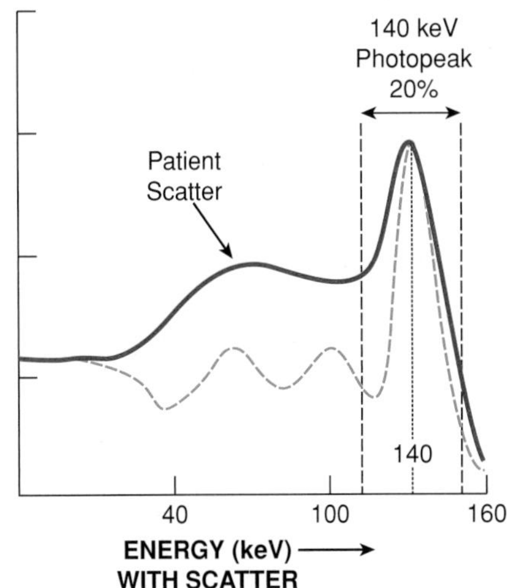

FIGURE 71B.12. **Tc-99m Photospectra.** The left photospectrum describes the energies present from the radionuclide imaged by itself (without scatter), while the right photospectrum is from the radionuclide imaged from inside a patient (with scatter). The primary energies of the curve include (1) Compton scatter (0 to 50 keV); (2) Compton edge at 50 keV—note that in the patient, scatter contributes to a broad increase in the 90 to 140 keV level; (3) backscatter (BS)—primary gamma undergoes 180-degree scatter from behind the crystal and upon reentering the crystal they are completely absorbed; (4) lead x-ray peak (Pb)—photoelectric absorption in lead shielding of camera housing causes 75- to 90-keV x-ray photons; (5) iodine escape peak (112 keV)—iodine K-shell electrons escape the sodium iodide crystal with an energy of 28 keV, and therefore an incoming gamma of say 140 keV would lose this much energy before it was registered by the PM tubes (140 – 28 = 112 keV); (6) photopeak—for imaging purposes, a 20% window over the 140-keV photopeak defines the limits of acceptance of detected energies. Note that some of the scatter photons from the patient are accepted, contributing to decreased image quality (loss of resolution).

the patient to acquire the necessary projection sets for SPECT imaging. Early SPECT systems resulted in an increase in the average distance between the patient and the collimator compared to planar imaging and resulted in a decrease in spatial resolution, though this was offset by the much-improved depth information gained (e.g., being able to differentiate vascular territories in cardiac SPECT). Some cameras are capable of noncircular orbits to reduce the average distance to the patient and thus improve spatial resolution.

A typical SPECT study might consist of 60 stops or projection angles with each stop consisting of 5 seconds of acquisition time. Increasing the acquisition time results in a larger number of counts but also increases the likelihood of patient discomfort and motion. This trade-off between total signal intensity and patient motion must also be made in PET imaging. SPECT data are usually reconstructed into a 64 × 64 image matrix—if the data are very rich in counts, this may be increased to 128 × 128 for images with higher spatial resolution (larger matrix = smaller pixels for a given field of view). PET data are acquired with between roughly 100 and 250 projection angles (depending on the system design) and are usually reconstructed on a 128 × 128 image matrix. Pixel sizes for PET images would typically be approximately 5 × 5 mm for body imaging and 2 × 2 mm for brain imaging.

Image Reconstruction. There are a range of ways to reconstruct an image volume from a set of projections. Filtered backprojection is an analytic approach that will generate an exact replica of the object in the limit of an infinite number of projection angles and noise-free data and was the main reconstruction algorithm used in nuclear medicine until the end of the 20th century. The major disadvantage of filtered backprojection is that it gives equal weight to all projections in the raw data, even those with very few counts, and which are statistically untrustworthy. This results in streak artifact in the image. **Iterative reconstruction** is a commonly used method that applies weighting factors to the data based on statistical considerations. These can be very computationally intensive, but accelerated methods that approximate the full algorithms have been introduced. Currently, the most popular of these is the **ordered subsets-expectation-maximization (OSEM)** method. These iterative methods are more robust to noisy data, but when the number of acquired counts is low, they will tend to produce mottled or "blobby" images, which can render image interpretation difficult.

Image properties are dependent not just on the quality of the acquired data but also on the choice of reconstruction parameters. The relationship is complex, but loosely speaking, **more iterations and/or subsets will result in higher spatial resolution but noisier images.** Too few iterations and/or subsets will result in poor spatial resolution and will interfere with the detection of small lesions and anatomy. All images, regardless of reconstruction method, can be filtered to reduce noise. Many different filters are available and filter optimization is an extremely complex and task-dependent problem. Choice of reconstruction method is often guided by the manufacturer. **Filtration reduces noise at the expense of spatial resolution.**

Attenuation Correction. In nuclear medicine and radiology, photons (γ-rays and x-rays) interact with molecules and particles as they travel through patients and air prior to reaching the detector. The photons transfer kinetic energy to the surrounding matter during this process resulting in a loss of energy. This loss of energy is known as **attenuation**. The amount of attenuation a photon experiences is dependent on the initial energy of the incident photon, the type of matter being traversed, and the depth of travel through the material.

The **mass attenuation coefficient** (μ, m^2/kg) of a material is an indicator of the ability of a material to **absorb and scatter (i.e., attenuate)** incident radiation. The mass attenuation coefficient is largely dependent on the density and atomic number of the material and increases with increasing material density. This is why lead is often used in shielding material.

The thickness of the material required to reduce the intensity of a narrow beam of radiation by 50% is known as the **half-value layer (HVL)**. The HVL gives you information on the intensity/quality of an x-ray beam in radiography and the source radiation within a patient for nuclear medicine. This plays an important factor in determining acceptable dosage ranges for various radiopharmaceuticals by ensuring that a sufficient number of γ-rays reach the detector to create an image of diagnostic quality. The HVL for high-energy 511-keV photons in soft tissue for PET imaging is approximately 7 cm, and the HVL for lower-energy 140-keV photons in soft tissue for Tc-99m imaging is approximately 4.6 cm.

- **Cardiac perfusion example:** A patient measuring 35 cm in AP thickness will require approximately twice the dose for a Tc-99m–labeled radiotracer than a patient measuring 25 cm in AP thickness undergoing the same examination (radioactivity emitted from roughly the center of the patient traversing through an extra 5 cm of patient). Large patient size can lead to attenuation artifacts that mimic myocardial defects, with diaphragmatic attenuation causing apparent inferior wall defects and breast attenuation causing apparent anterior or lateral wall defects.
- **Shielding example:** Tc-99m 140-keV photons have an HVL of 0.027 cm within lead, making lead an excellent ingredient for creating shielding material. Lead can be incorporated into walls, clothing, and even glass.

In planar imaging, attenuation can sometimes be helpful as it reduces the amount of interference from overlying organs along a line of sight. In tomographic imaging (SPECT and PET), however, it introduces significant image distortions. In particular, deep structures are poorly visualized while superficial structures are overly intense. The lungs are less dense and therefore less attenuating than soft tissue and can also be represented with falsely elevated intensity. This may sometimes help with lesion detection in the lung, but in general, attenuation effects render images more difficult to interpret and interfere with lesion detection.

Several methods have been developed to correct for radiation attenuation by the patient by creating an attenuation map of the patient. The most common methods include transmission scanning and addition of low-dose CT. Transmission scanning creates an attenuation map of the patient by rotating a radioactive source with a similar photon energy to the radionuclide being imaged around the patient to mirror the radionuclide being used. Low-dose CT has become the attenuation correction method of choice following the development of SPECT/CT and PET/CT devices and creates an attenuation map similar to transmission scanning. CT transmission scans are usually much faster than radionuclide transmission scans and allow for shorter scan times. They also have the added benefit of providing anatomic correlation by allowing fusion of scintigraphic and CT images.

There are several inherent limitations with transmission CT.

- CT acquires a snapshot of lung motion, whereas emission imaging represents a time average of tidal lung motion as imaging is acquired over a period of several minutes rather than seconds with CT. The resulting mismatch between the emission and transmission data very frequently leads to image artifacts and misregistrations at the lung/liver boundary.
- CT contrast can lead to erroneous estimates of attenuation factors and can result in artifacts in the emission image that may mimic lesions. This is particularly true for PET, where the disparity between the emission photon energy (511 keV)

and the transmission photon energy (70 to 140 keV for CT) is very large.

- Foreign metallic material such as prostheses, surgical clips, and foreign bodies such as bullet fragments can lead to erroneous focal artifacts in the emission data. Review of non–attenuation-corrected images is helpful in identifying these artifacts.

When attenuation correction is applied, data should also be corrected for scattered photons that erroneously fall within the accepted energy window. Failure to account for scatter prior to attenuation correction can lead to focal artifacts in dense regions and will interfere with quantitative measurements. Scatter correction can also be helpful in planar imaging.

Imaging Moving Organs. Radionuclide imaging takes place over several minutes, which creates a challenge when trying to image organs that move on the timescale of seconds or less. Thus, both cardiac and respiratory motions result in blurring of images. While respiratory motion itself is not of particular clinical interest, cardiac motion is, and this has led to innovative methods for imaging it. Such methods include cardiac "gating," where ECG signals are used to trigger acquisition. This allows the computer to sort the incoming data into several bins, each one corresponding to a particular part of the cardiac cycle. Over many cycles, enough data are collected to allow each bin to be reconstructed separately and a movie of the cardiac motion can be constructed.

Similar methods may be applied to respiratory motion, although this is more problematic since respiratory motion is not as regular as cardiac motion. Respiratory gating may be employed to reduce motion blurring (which can be very significant at the lung base) and thus enhance detection of small lesions and quantification of tracer uptake.

Quality Control for Imaging Systems. The QC program of a nuclear medicine department must cover instrumentation (Table 71B.5) as well as radiopharmaceutical preparation. The goal of the QC of a gamma camera is to assure both the uniform response of the detectors and the correct location of the scintillation events occurring in the crystal. An additional goal for PET camera QC is to confirm adequate calibration for quantitative accuracy (accurate SUV calculation).

In addition to the specific procedures described below, total imaging performance may be assessed using commercially available phantoms. These phantoms are filled by the operator with an appropriate radionuclide in aqueous solution and are designed so that areas of cold and hot activity are present in varying dimensions. A subsequent acquisition, reconstruction, and display of the phantom can test the contrast, resolution, field uniformity, and attenuation correction of the imaging system.

Gamma Camera Quality Control

Intrinsic Flood. The quickest and easiest check of a gamma camera is by the **daily** acquisition of an **intrinsic (no collimator)** flood image. An intrinsic flood field image is obtained by exposing the entire crystal to either a uniform source of radioactivity, typically from a point source of Tc-99m or a commercially prepared sheet source of Co-57. **Extrinsic (with collimator)** flood images can also be obtained, which factor in nonuniformities associated with the collimator (see Collimator Quality Control below). Sources must deliver count rates with less than 1% variation across the surface of the crystal. This is accomplished by positioning the point source at least 4-collimator crystal widths from the detector. The sheet source, which is placed on the detector face during the acquisition of the flood, is purchased with the manufacturer's guarantee that there is less than 1% inherent variation. A visual inspection of the flood will give an adequate qualitative assessment of nonuniformities. The human eye can detect significant nonuniformities of 5% or more, and computer analysis performed with flood field-specific software can detect subtle changes over time. If the pattern is abnormal, remedies include reloading correction matrices, replacing PMTs, and addressing other electronic or mechanical problems (Fig. 71B.13).

In a similar vein, a quantitative value of general camera performance can be obtained by comparing the uniformity flood field image acquired with and without the uniformity correction. This difference value, termed "data loss," represents additional processing time imposed by the correction circuits to reach a set number of counts. Using a 1 to 2 million count flood, the data loss can be calculated as the percentage difference between the time required to obtain an intrinsic flood with and without the uniformity correction turned on. Typically, differences under 15% are normal for most recent

TABLE 71B.5

PLANAR AND SPECT CAMERA RECOMMENDED QUALITY-CONTROL PROCEDURES

PROCEDURE	FREQUENCY	CAMERA SYSTEM	COMMENT
Flood field	Daily	Planar	Intrinsically or extrinsically; intrinsic flood is acquired for 1–2 million counts with and without uniformity correction; percent difference should be less than 15% for most systems
Sensitivity	Weekly	Planar	Intrinsically or extrinsically; result is in counts per minute per μCi
Spatial resolution	Weekly	Planar	Intrinsic or extrinsic; use bar phantom
Linearity	Weekly	Planar	Bar phantom or multihole phantom
High-count collimator flood	Weekly	SPECT	30 million counts for 64 × 64 matrix; 90 million counts for 128 × 128 matrix
Center of rotation	Weekly	SPECT	Corrected to less than 0.5 pixel for 64 × 64 matrix to less than 1.0 pixel for 128 × 128 matrix
Pixel calibration	Monthly	SPECT	Measurement of pixel size in both X and Y directions; used for attenuation correction
Jaszczak or Carlson phantom	Quarterly	SPECT	Commercially available phantoms that test total system performance

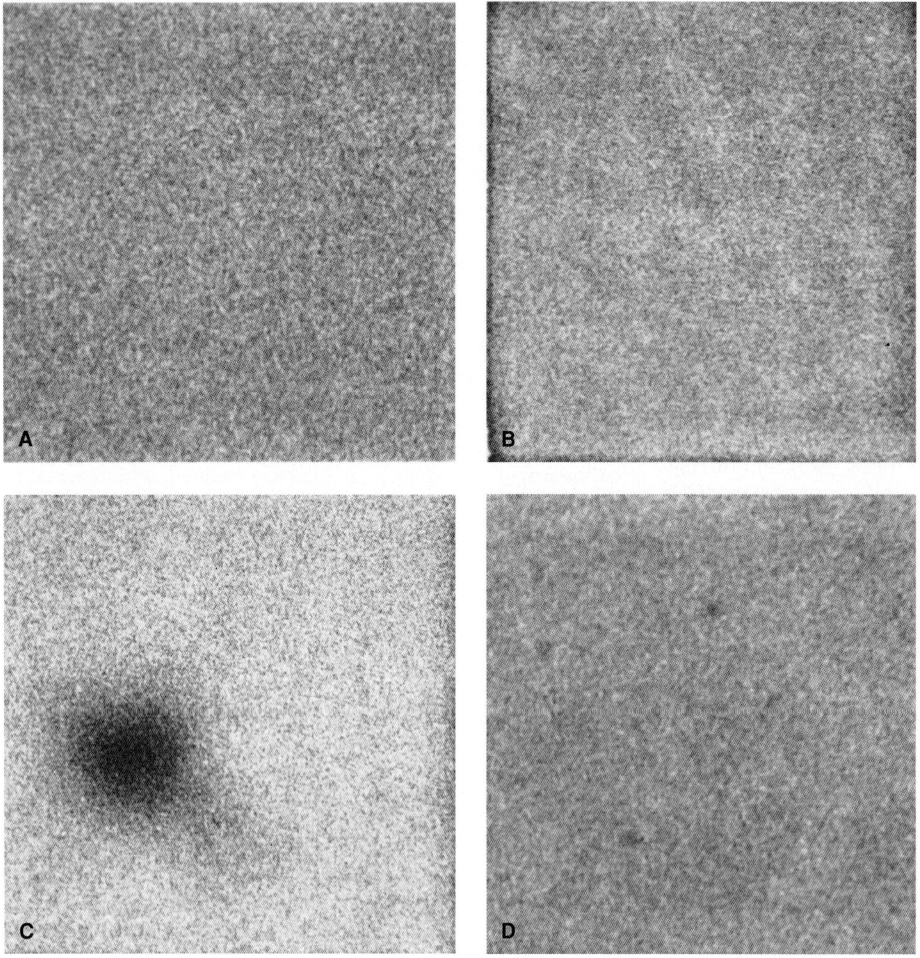

FIGURE 71B.13. **Intrinsic Floods.** **A:** Normal uniform flood, with correction matrices applied. **B:** Same camera as in (**A**) but with the correction matrices turned off. The correction matrices are able to compensate sometimes for striking nonuniformities in the flood field. These corrections are acceptable as long as they do not represent too great a data loss and prolong imaging times. **C:** Uncorrectable off-peak PM tube. The photopeak for this PM tube had drifted down and was accepting more counts than its neighboring PM tubes. **D:** Uncorrectable crystal hydration ("measles"). The *dark spots* are areas in the crystal where water has breached the manufacturer's watertight seal to gain access to a hygroscopic sodium iodide crystal. The expensive crystal had to be replaced.

gamma camera systems. Greater differences significantly prolong the imaging times and require either a reacquisition of the uniformity or other correction matrix or implicate a hardware electronic problem requiring a service call.

Resolution and Linearity. Two basic QC procedures performed to assure correct positioning of events are **spatial resolution** and **linearity** (Fig. 71B.14). These are generally performed **weekly** by acquiring a flood with a specially designed phantom sandwiched between a Co-57 sheet source and the camera, with (extrinsic) or without (intrinsic) the collimator. Alternatively, a Tc-99m point source at 4-collimator distance can be substituted for the sheet source. Several commercial bar phantoms, such as PLES (parallel lines equally spaced) and four quadrant, are available to assess spatial resolution using a series of equally spaced lead bars. Linearity can also be assessed by the visual inspection of any of these straight bar phantoms or can be individually assessed by a dedicated phantom such as an orthogonal (perpendicular to crystal) hole phantom. In general, inspection of these types of floods will reveal any **linearity distortion** such as **pincushion** or **barreling**.

Collimator Quality Control. The QC for collimators is directed at assessing the integrity of the collimator. Imperfections from

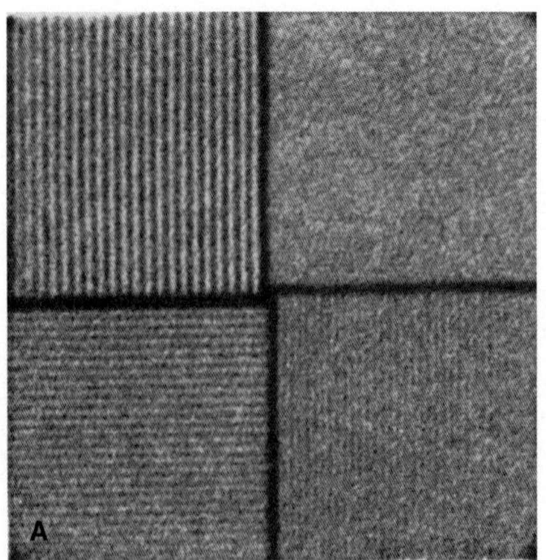

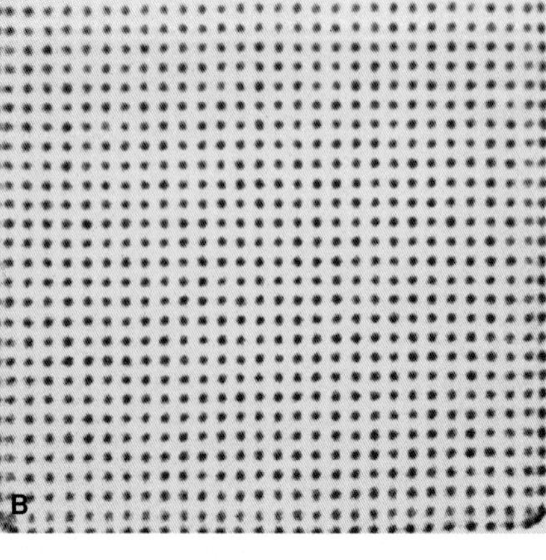

FIGURE 71B.14. **Spatial Resolution and Linearity of a Gamma Camera.** Both of these floods were acquired without the collimator using a Co-57 sheet source over the phantom. **A:** Four-quadrant bar phantom. The distance between the bars is equal within a quadrant but progressively diminishes between quadrants. This bar flood demonstrates the lack of visibility of the bars in the quadrant with the narrowest bars. Rotating the bars 90 degrees will allow the entire crystal to be checked. Linearity can also be assessed with this phantom. **B:** Orthogonal hole phantom. Pincushion (inward) and barrel (outward) distortion can easily be evaluated by visual inspection of this flood. Both are absent here.

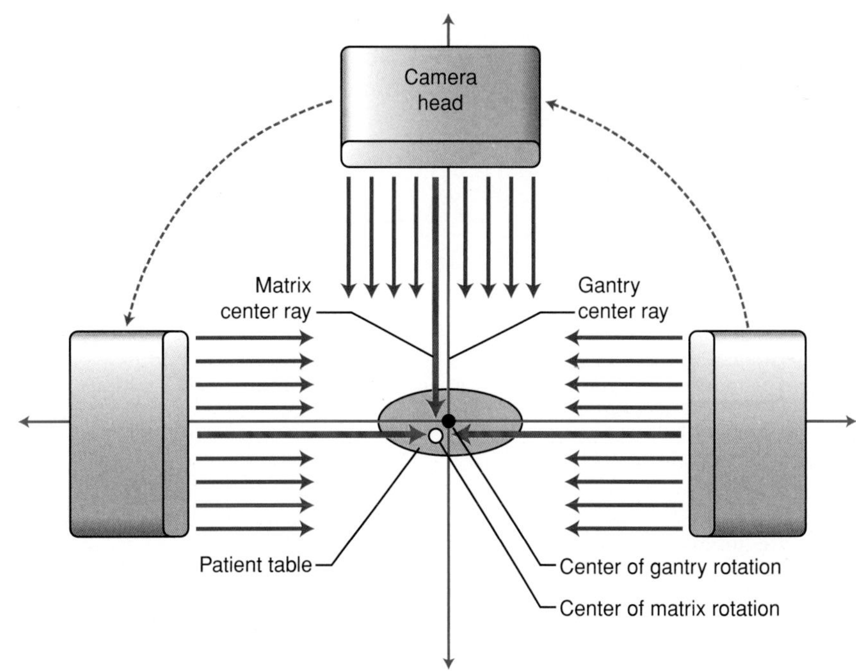

FIGURE 71B.15. Center of Rotation (COR). This illustration is diagrammatically exaggerated for clarity. The COR represents the difference between mechanical center of rotation (*black dashed arrow/black dot*) and the center of the projected image matrix (*gray dashed arrow/black circle*). This difference must be adjusted to less than 0.5 pixel for a 64 × 64 matrix and 1 pixel for a 128 × 128 matrix, to avoid SPECT reconstruction defects.

damaged septa in the collimator will introduce nonuniformities causing image degradation. The effect of these collimator imperfections can be minimized by mathematically applying a statistically high-count extrinsic collimator flood to each individual raw planar image prior to reconstruction. This extrinsic collimator flood is acquired using a Co-57 sheet source for 30 million counts when using a 64 × 64 matrix and for 90 million counts when using a 128 × 128 matrix.

Center of Rotation. In addition to the routine planar camera QC, there are several **SPECT-specific QC** procedures that are necessary to minimize artifacts (Table 71B.5). The most important of these relates to the camera's mechanical center of rotation (COR), which must be calibrated with the center of the computer's matrix as it is projected from the face of the crystal (Fig. 71B.15). For various mechanical and electronic reasons, these are not perfectly aligned. An offset greater than half a pixel for a 64 × 64 matrix will result in loss of contrast, loss of spatial resolution, and distortion in the tomographic images. The COR calibration is performed by imaging a point or line source at multiple opposing intervals over 360 degrees. The COR is then calculated by averaging the difference in the sets of offset of the source from the matrix center as seen by the opposing pairs of images. The COR value is stored by the computer for use during the ensuing reconstruction of the three-dimensional images. When this calibration factor is applied during reconstruction, the matrix centers are shifted to align with the mechanical COR. This COR calibration must be performed for each collimator, zoom factor, and matrix size used for SPECT acquisitions.

Pixel-size calibration prior to attenuation correction is a necessary QC procedure to match the matrix size with the physical dimensions of the body part being imaged. Pixel calibration is easily performed by acquiring two-point or line sources separated by a known distance. The computer calculates and stores the pixels per millimeter calibration factor for subsequent attenuation corrections.

PET Scanner Quality Control

Most PET scanners consist of a full ring of detectors, obviating the need for rotation. This changes the way that detector nonuniformities manifest in the images. For example, a problem with a single detector is unlikely to reinforce and create ring artifacts. Additionally, since there are many detectors in a system, the impact of a single detector failure may not be so great that imaging must cease until repair, as with planar and SPECT imaging. However, since there are so many detectors in a system, the chance of a component failure becomes statistically greater. There are also downstream components that can impact large numbers of detectors at once if they fail, producing an immediate impact on image quality. The segmented nature of most PET detectors removes the need for pixel-size calibration, but it is necessary to check the alignment of the PET and CT components for combined PET/CT systems. In addition, the CT component of a PET/CT system requires all the QC procedures that a standalone CT scanner would.

Daily Check. Every day the detectors are illuminated by a rotating source of high-energy photons (usually a positron emitter) and the results are compared with a high-quality reference scan. The comparison is usually automated and examines the data both for overall drift and for specific variations for detector performance, such as failed or failing detectors.

Timing Alignment and PMT Gain Adjustment. In a PET scanner, timing signals from the detectors must be well-synchronized or coincidence sensitivity will be compromised. PMTs have a tendency to drift, similar to gamma cameras, and gains must be adjusted to keep the responses in range. The frequency with which these adjustments are carried out is dependent on the hardware; some manufacturers recommend weekly updates, whereas others design the system so that these procedures are carried out at normalization time (see following).

Normalization and Calibration. The sensitivity of detectors in a PET system is quite variable. In addition, geometric considerations mean that there are systematic variations in sensitivity across the field of view. To account for these, a high-count density acquisition using a rotating radioactive source is performed and a sensitivity correction matrix is computed from it. This process is known as **detector normalization.** It is usually supplemented with a scan of a cylindrical source containing a known amount of activity. The source concentration

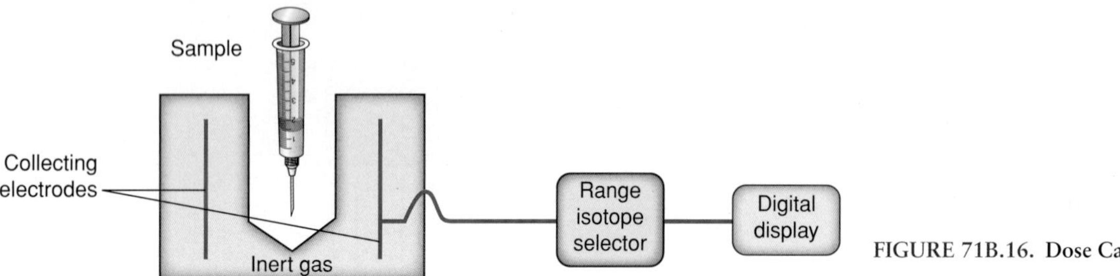

FIGURE 71B.16. **Dose Calibrator.**

is determined using the dose calibrator used for measuring patient unit doses, allowing the scanner to be calibrated appropriately for accurate quantitative measurements (SUV). Care must be taken to ensure that the cylindrical source is placed centrally in the field of view with no additional attenuating material obscuring the detectors. Depending on the implementation of the software, placing the source off-center or with additional attenuating media can negatively impact the normalization.

Normalization should be performed not less frequently than **once per quarter**—once per month is common. In addition, **normalization should be performed after system repair or modification.** After normalization, the baseline reference scan is set and a QC check will be performed **daily**.

Phantoms and Acceptance Testing. Total imaging performance may be assessed using commercially available phantoms. Examples of these include the Derenzo phantom, the Jaszczak phantom, the Rollo phantom, the Hoffman brain phantom, and the IEC chest phantom. These phantoms are filled by the operator with an appropriate radionuclide in aqueous solution and are designed so that areas of cold and hot activity are present in varying dimensions. A subsequent acquisition, reconstruction, and display of the phantom can test the imaging system's contrast, resolution, field uniformity, and attenuation correction. The National Equipment Manufacturer's Association (NEMA) has issued standard performance tests for nuclear medicine imaging equipment, and these are frequently used as part of acceptance testing of new scanners (see the reading list for full details).

Nonimaging Detector Systems

Dose Calibrator. As a mandatory requirement by the NRC, all diagnostic and therapeutic doses must be calibrated prior to administration (see section on Medical Events for prescription limits). The dose calibrator is an ionization chamber, not a sodium iodide crystal. It is a cylinder that holds a defined volume of inert gas (typically argon) and a cylindrical collecting electrode (Fig. 71B.16). A voltage applied across the electrodes will not pass current until the gas is ionized by radiation emitted from a radiopharmaceutical in the well. The measurement of the current is proportional to the activity for a given radionuclide. By calibrating to known radionuclides and known amounts of activity, the current can be equated to dose activity. A series of buttons imprinted with the radionuclide names reside on the face of the control unit. A calibration factor is assigned to each button, unique for that particular radionuclide, to adjust the correct proportionality between current and activity. **The dose calibrator will read activity with any button selected, but it is only accurate for the isotope for which the button has been calibrated.** As opposed to the well-counter, which measures only in the microcurie range (great assay for contamination), the dose calibrator is capable of measuring quantities in the curie, millicurie, and microcurie ranges. The well-counter, therefore, cannot act as a substitute for a dose calibration.

- Ionization chamber
- Current generated is proportional to radioactivity and used to estimate the sample activity
- MUST select the radionuclide being analyzed to get an accurate reading
- Excellent for assaying unit doses (µCi to Ci range)

The **QC for the dose calibrator** consists of periodic checks on its performance.

- **Constancy measures the activity of long-lived reference sources to look for deviations from expected values** and is performed **daily**. Isotopes with long physical half-lives such as Co-57 (120 keV) in the Tc-99m channel and Cs-137 (662 keV) in the molybdenum-99 (Mo-99) channel are assayed and the measured activity must agree with the calculated activity by ±5%.
- **Linearity assesses the accuracy of measurements over a wide range of activity**, usually from 10 µCi to around 200 mCi (maximum administered dose) and is performed **quarterly**. With a high-activity Tc-99m source, a series of measurements is collected either over a 48-hour period or by using commercially available simulated decay (leaded) cylinders. These measurements are compared with calculated measurements (using decay factors) and should agree within ±10%.
- **Accuracy** measures certified sources of different photon energies, typically Co-57 and Cs-137, obtained from the National Institute of Standards and Technology (formerly the National Bureau of Standards) and is performed **annually**. The measurements must agree with the known source activity within ±10%.
- **Geometry** is evaluated to compensate for measurements made of sources in different volume dilutions or in different containers. This is performed **at installation and after repairs**. Glass and plastic syringes can affect readings significantly. The operator applies these calculated correction factors to activity measurements (e.g., 2% is added for volumes greater than 20 mL).

Sodium Iodide Well-Counter. The **sodium iodide well-counter** is used to quantify small amounts of activity in examinations

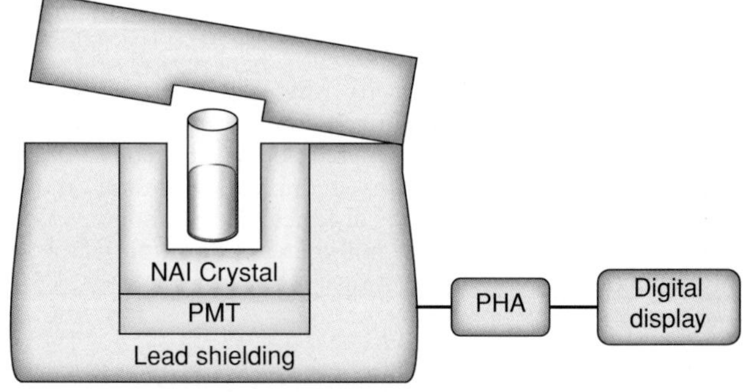

FIGURE 71B.17. **Sodium Iodide Well-Counter.** PMT, photomultiplier tube; NAI, sodium iodide; PHA, pulse height analyzer.

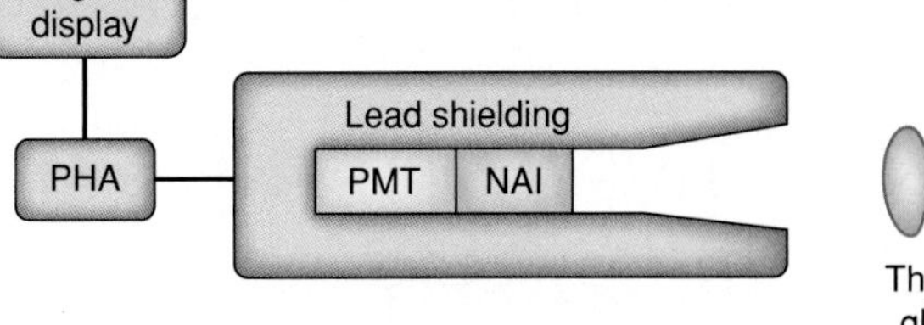

FIGURE 71B.18. **Thyroid Uptake Probe.** PMT, photomultiplier tube; NAI, sodium iodide; PHA, pulse height analyzer.

such as an in vitro Schilling test or **survey wipe tests.** It consists of a sodium iodide crystal in the shape of a cylinder with a hole drilled within the center and sits on top of a single PMT. This design provides for **excellent geometric and detection efficiency** (Fig. 71B.17).

The **QC** for the sodium iodide well-counter consists of **daily assessment of the high voltage and sensitivity.** In addition, **resolution and chi-square are checked quarterly.**

Thyroid Uptake Probe. The **thyroid uptake probe** is used to quantitate the percentage of radioactive iodine taken up by the patient's thyroid and to survey workers (called bioassay) for possible radioiodine contamination. This is commonly performed after radioiodine therapeutic administrations that may have resulted in some of the radioiodine entering the body (called internal contamination). The probe consists of a single 2- or 3-in-thick sodium iodide crystal, 5 cm in diameter, juxtaposed to a single PMT. The field of view is defined by a cone-shaped flat-field collimator (Fig. 71B.18). No imaging is performed with this probe; only quantitative count measurements are performed at a fixed crystal-to-patient distance. The **quality control** for the thyroid uptake probe is **identical to that of the sodium iodide well-counter.**

Suggested Readings

Bushberg JT, Seibert JA, Leidholdt EM, Boone JM. *The Essential Physics of Medical Imaging*. 3rd ed. Philadelphia, PA: Lippincott Williams & Wilkins; 2012.

Cherry SR, Sorensen JA, Phelps ME. *Physics in Nuclear Medicine*. 4th ed. Philadelphia, PA: Elsevier Saunders; 2012.

Kowalsky RJ, Falen S. *Radiopharmaceuticals in Nuclear Pharmacy & Nuclear Medicine*. 2nd ed. Washington, DC: APhA Publications; 2004.

Mettler FA, Guiberteau MJ. *Essentials of Nuclear Medicine Imaging*. 6th ed. Philadelphia, PA: WB Saunders Co; 2012.

National Electrical Manufacturers Association. *NEMA Standards Publication NU-2 2007. Performance Measurements for Positron Emission Tomographs*. Rosslyn, VA: National Electrical Manufacturers Association; 2007.

Saha GB. *Fundamentals of Nuclear Pharmacy*. 5th ed. New York: Springer-Verlag; 2004.

Valk PE, Bailey DL, Townsend DW, Maisey MN, eds. *Positron Emission Tomography—Basic Science and Clinical Practice*. London: Springer-Verlag; 2003.

Vallabhajosula S. *Molecular Imaging: Radiopharmaceuticals for PET and SPECT*. New York: Springer; 2009.

Zanzonico P. Routine quality control of clinical nuclear medicine instrumentation: a brief review. *J Nucl Med* 2008;49:1114–1131.

CHAPTER 72A ■ GASTROINTESTINAL, LIVER–SPLEEN, AND HEPATOBILIARY SCINTIGRAPHY

BRADLEY FEHRENBACH

GASTROINTESTINAL STUDIES

Nuclear medicine imaging studies can provide considerable information in the functional evaluation of the gastrointestinal (GI) system. Routine studies include hepatobiliary, GI bleeding studies, and gastric-emptying measurements. Other examinations that are less frequently ordered, such as a Meckel scan, provide clinically valuable information.

ESOPHAGEAL IMAGING

The esophageal transit study, performed with swallowed solutions or with solid boluses labeled with Tc-99m sulfur colloid (SC), is an examination which can be done in lieu of esophageal manometry. It has been reported to detect esophageal dysmotility in 50% of symptomatic patients with an otherwise normal evaluation for dysphagia.

In the supine or upright position with a gamma-camera imaging in the anterior projection, the patient swallows a radiolabeled bolus while dynamic data are obtained via a computer. The esophagus is divided into three regions of interest (ROIs): upper, middle, and lower. Transit times are then calculated from time–activity curves representing the ROIs. The normal esophagus demonstrates sequential activity from proximal to distal with no visualized esophageal activity remaining after 10 seconds. Regional analysis may differentiate between achalasia and scleroderma. It is important to remember that esophageal scintigraphy is functional and does not provide detailed anatomic information. Barium or endoscopic evaluation is necessary to exclude the possibility of neoplasm or infection as the cause of impaired esophageal function (Fig. 72A.1).

GASTROESOPHAGEAL REFLUX

The evaluation of heartburn and atypical chest pain in the adult commonly raises the clinical question of gastroesophageal reflux disease (GERD). In the pediatric population, failure to thrive and recurrent pneumonia also raise concern for significant GERD. A common diagnostic tool currently used in the diagnosis of GERD is acid reflux monitoring. This examination unfortunately requires nasoesophageal intubation and 24-hour continuous recording. It is invasive and unwieldy, especially in pediatric patients.

Gastroesophageal reflux scintigraphy is performed with acidified orange juice mixed with Tc-99m SC. The acid decreases the lower esophageal sphincter pressure and delays gastric emptying. ROIs are established via computer to correspond to the stomach and the segments (upper, middle, and lower) of the esophagus. In the pediatric population, ROIs over the lungs detect aspiration by the end of the study or on delayed imaging 1 to 3 hours later. Images may be recorded in adults with an abdominal binder that increases abdominal pressure sequentially in 10-mm Hg increments to a maximum of 100 mm Hg. Normal patients have no detectable esophageal activity. This examination is reported to have 90% sensitivity in the detection of GERD (Fig. 72A.2).

GASTRIC EMPTYING

Gastric emptying is a complex physiologic process directed not only by neuroendocrine processes but also by a host of local factors. Food type, pH, and fat content as well as food osmolality affect the rate of gastric emptying. Impaired gastric emptying has many causes, for example, diabetes mellitus, electrolyte disturbances, postvagotomy syndromes, and some medications.

Excluding mechanical obstruction is important in diagnosing the cause of the patient's symptoms. Endoscopy or barium studies are superior in the detection of gastric ulcers, tumors, or bezoars. Gastric-emptying scintigraphy has become the gold standard in the clinical evaluation of gastric motility. It is a simple test to perform, though interpretation is based on complicated mathematical models. Solid food, liquids, or both are labeled with a radiotracer and consumed by the patient. Digital images of the stomach are acquired and a time–activity curve is generated for the graphic analysis of the rate of emptying (Fig. 72A.3).

The normal half-emptying time ($T_{1/2}$) of radioactive solids and liquids varies with the technique employed. In general, the normal $T_{1/2}$ is less than 90 minutes for solids and less than 60 minutes for liquids. If possible, each laboratory should establish its own normal $T_{1/2}$ values. Liquid gastric emptying

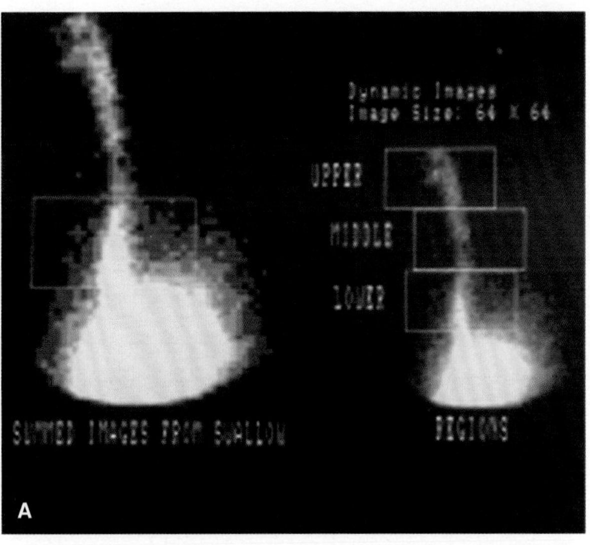

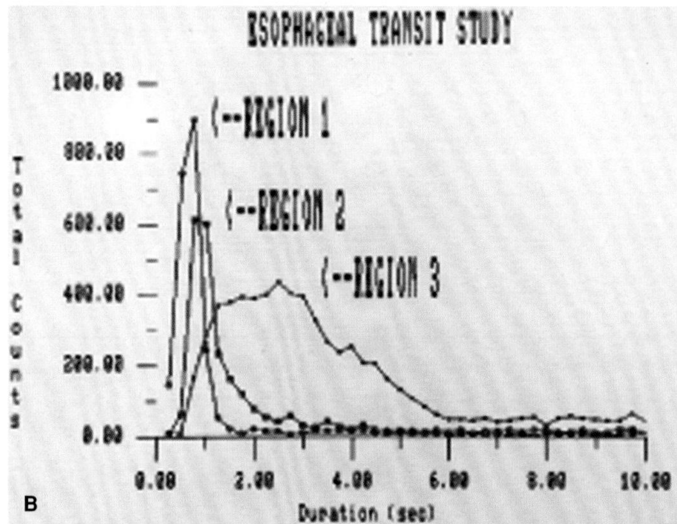

FIGURE 72A.1. **Normal Esophageal Transit Study. A:** A composite image of the esophagus and stomach is used to generate regions of interests around the upper, middle, and lower esophagus. **B:** Time–activity curves for each region are displayed for 10 seconds after the swallow. Inspection of the curves allows the calculation of the transit time.

usually follows an exponential curve, whereas solid emptying is biphasic with an initial lag phase followed by a linear curve. To evaluate gastric emptying, gastric-emptying scintigraphy can be performed with liquid, solid, or both (by using two different radiopharmaceuticals and a dual-energy camera). However, the medical literature states that solid gastric-emptying studies are more sensitive for the detection of gastroparesis than are liquid studies. *Visual interpretation of the stomach images is invaluable in understanding the "number" generated for* $T_{1/2}$.

The standard protocol for gastric-emptying scintigraphy is to calculate gastric-emptying rate at 30 minutes, 1 hour, 2 hours, 3 hours, and 4 hours after the consumption of 4-oz egg whites labeled with 1-mCi Tc-99m SC, along with 2 pieces of toast, 1 packet of jelly, and 4 oz of water (Fig. 72A.4).

Normal gastric emptying parameters according to the SNMMI guidelines are given in Table 72A.1.

The gastric-emptying technique can be extended using bowel transit times to evaluate and to time the transit between the stomach and colon, colonic transit, and to characterize the disorders of the bowel's smooth muscle or enteric nervous system, though this is not commonly used.

FIGURE 72A.2. **Abnormal Gastroesophageal Reflux Study.** Three regions of interests (ROIs) are established over the esophagus. A time–activity curve corresponding to the upper ROI for 60 minutes shows refluxed activity after 3 minutes, which continues for about 30 minutes.

GASTROINTESTINAL BLEEDING SCINTIGRAPHY

Patients who present with clinically suspected upper GI bleeding are usually evaluated and concurrently treated by endoscopy, which is sufficient in the vast majority of cases. GI bleeding scintigraphy is typically reserved for cases where upper or lower endoscopy is unable to identify the source of a GI bleed. In this setting, GI bleeding scintigraphy with in vitro Tc-99m–tagged red blood cells is very sensitive and can locate the bleeding site. Continuous 1-minute dynamic frames are acquired over the abdomen and pelvis in the anterior projection for at least 60 minutes or until the patient has bled enough to locate the source of hemorrhage. Scintigraphy can detect bleeding rates as low as 0.1 mL/min versus contrast angiography, which detects 1 mL/min of GI bleeding. The study should be done emergently during the clinical period of suspected active bleeding, especially if percutaneous embolization by interventional radiology is being considered. Repeated imaging can be done at any time up to 24 hours after red cell labeling, but care should be taken because blood may have moved into the colon rather than originated from the colon.

Accurate hemorrhage localization is required for the treatment of a bleeding site. If angiographic therapy for a bleeding site is proposed, the more sensitive GI bleeding study should be done first to confirm the presence of a bleed. The GI bleeding

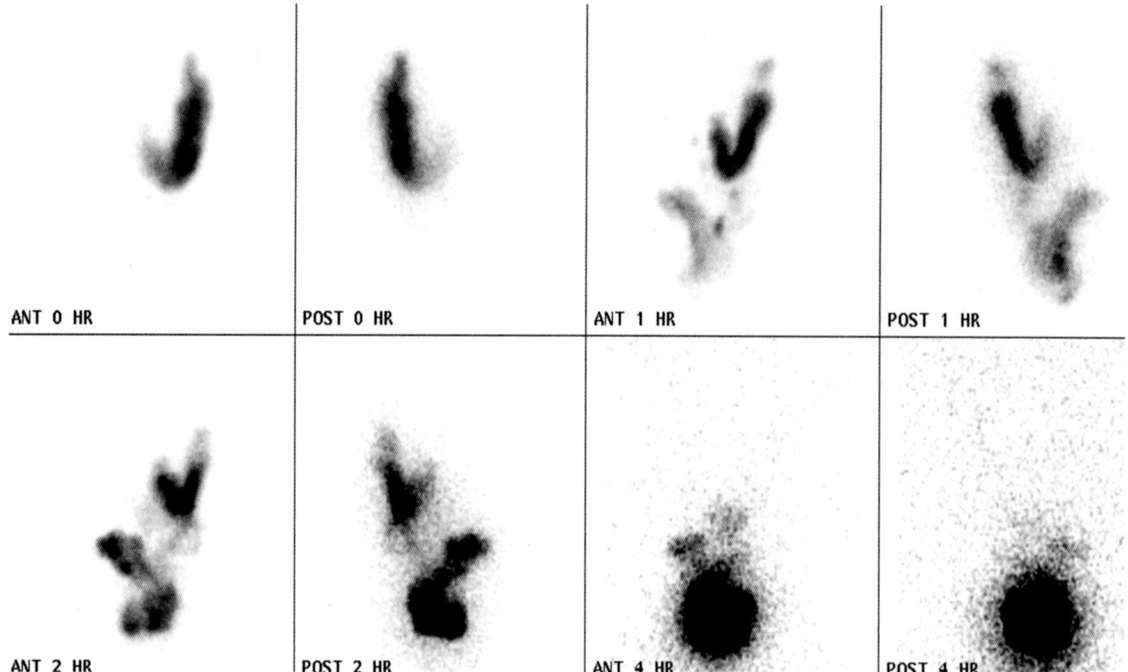

FIGURE 72A.3. **Normal Gastric Emptying.** Using the geometric means of activity within corresponding anterior and posterior images, this study shows normal gastric emptying at 2 hours (55%) and 4 hours (100%).

study will guide the selection of appropriate vessels for embolization or infusion of vasoreactive drugs. Positive GI bleeding studies demonstrate three cardinal findings:

1. An abnormal focus of radiotracer arises from "out of nowhere" as it enters the bowel lumen.
2. Activity persists and may increase with time.
3. Activity moves with peristalsis antegrade, retrograde, or in both directions (Figs. 72A.5 to 72A.7).

Intraluminal extravasated radiotracer may follow a serpentine path through the abdomen when it arises from the small bowel or follow the normal course of the colon if it arises from the large bowel. To interpret the images, one should be aware of false positives such as bladder or genital activity, which can be identified by obtaining postvoid and lateral pelvic views.

MECKEL SCAN

A Meckel diverticulum is a congenital malformation of the GI tract that occurs in 2% to 4% of the population. Approximately 20% to 57% of Meckel diverticula contain ectopic

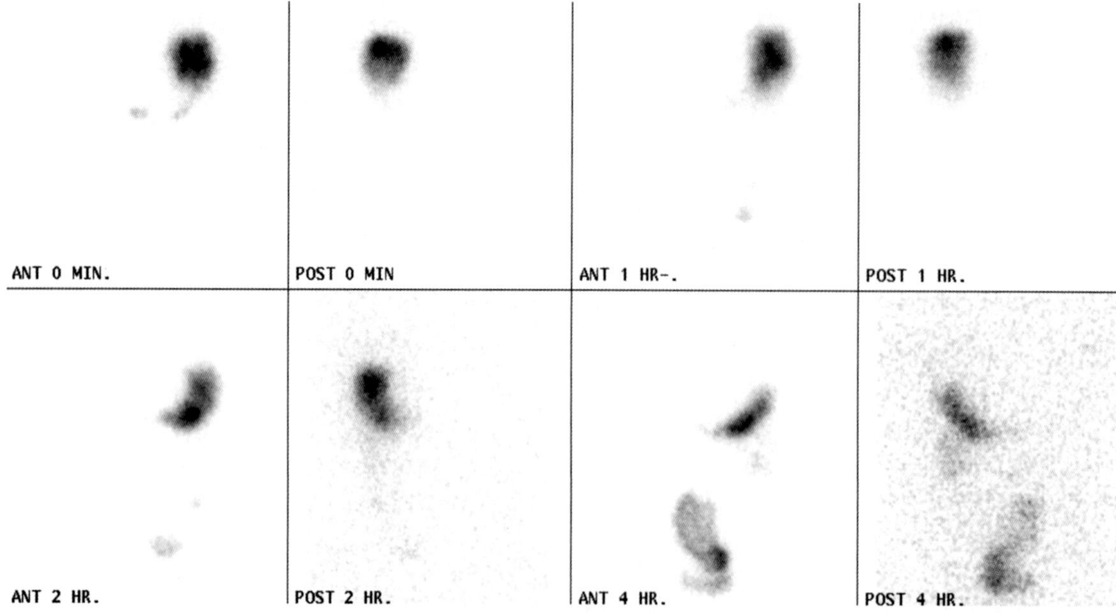

FIGURE 72A.4. **Gastroparesis.** Delayed gastric emptying at 2 hours (18%) and 4 hours (72%).

TABLE 72A.1

NORMAL LIMITS FOR GASTRIC RETENTION

TIME POINT (h)	LOWER LIMIT (%) (A LOWER VALUE SUGGESTS ABNORMALLY RAPID GASTRIC EMPTYING)	UPPER LIMIT (%) (A GREATER VALUE SUGGESTS ABNORMALLY DELAYED GASTRIC EMPTYING)
0.5	70	
1.0	30	90
2.0		60
3.0		30
4.0		10

Reprinted with permission from Donohoe KJ, Maurer AH, Ziessman HA, et al. Procedure guideline for adult solid-meal gastric-emptying study 3.0. *J Nucl Med Technol* 2009;37(3):196–200.

gastric mucosa, which may ulcerate and bleed. Tc-99m-O_4 is given intravenously and dynamic imaging of the abdomen is performed immediately following injection for 1 hour. Tc-99m-O_4 localizes in the gastric mucosa and can be used to detect the acid-producing mucosa in the diverticulum, with a focus of activity accumulating within the middle or right lower quadrant of the abdomen as the ectopic gastric mucosa concentrates the Tc-99m-O_4 in synchrony with the stomach. Detection may be enhanced by the use of pentagastrin to stimulate uptake or cimetidine to block the outflow of Tc-99m-O_4 from the diverticulum (Fig. 72A.8).

LIVER AND SPLEEN STUDIES

Liver/Spleen Scan

Liver/spleen scanning is performed by intravenous injection of Tc-99m–radiolabeled SC. Colloid imaging provides information on the basis of organ perfusion and the distribution of reticuloendothelial cells which phagocytize the colloid particles (Kupffer cells in the liver and reticuloendothelial cells in the spleen). Reticuloendothelial cells in the bone marrow

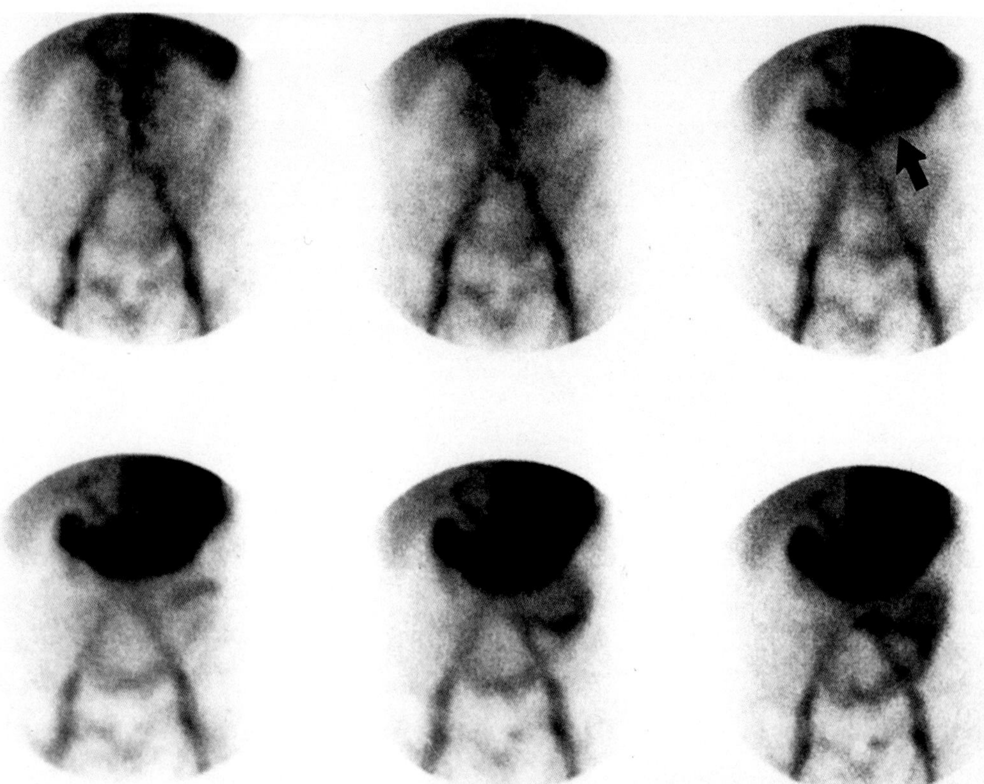

FIGURE 72A.5. Upper Gastrointestinal Bleeding Because of Gastric Varices. Sequential 5-minute images of the abdomen, in a patient with negative endoscopy, show tagged red cells filling the lumen of the stomach (*arrow*). This diagnosis cannot be made if there is free Tc-99m-O_4 mixed with the red cells; Tc-99m-O_4 is excreted physiologically in the stomach. The tagged red blood cells used had no free Tc-99m-O_4.

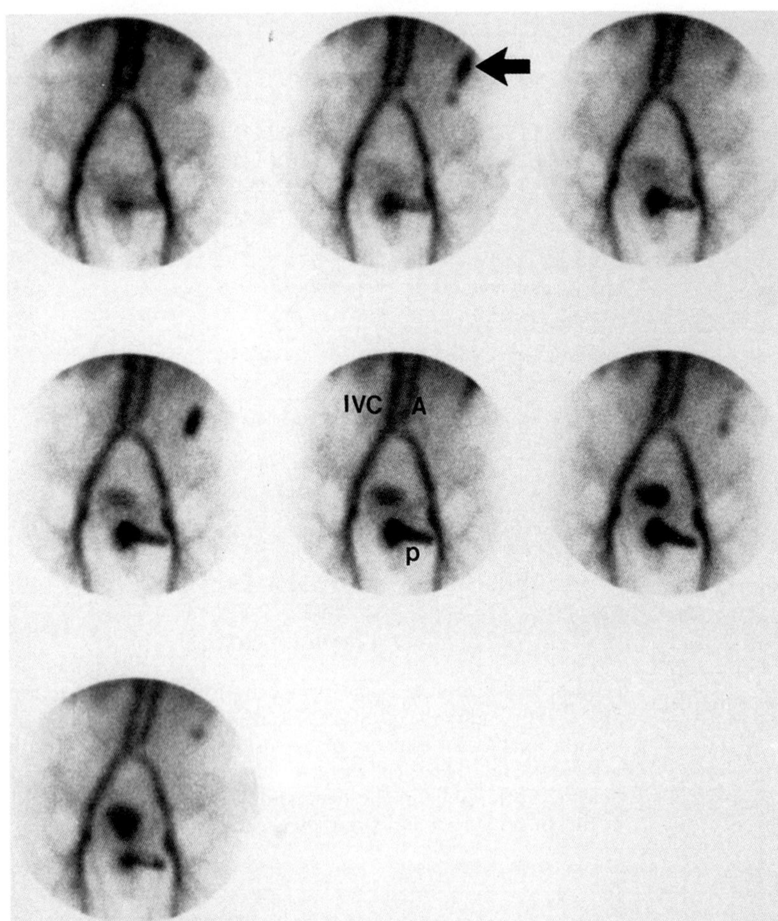

FIGURE 72A.6. Splenic Flexure Bleeding in the Colon Because of Diverticular Disease. Sequential 5-minute images show a small focus of bleeding (*arrow*) in the left upper quadrant that varies with the intensity as it accumulates and moves through the colon. Note that the patient has a large, static blood pool in the penis. Unchanging blood pools such as the aorta (*A*), the inferior vena cava (*IVC*), and penis (*p*) should not be misinterpreted as hemorrhage.

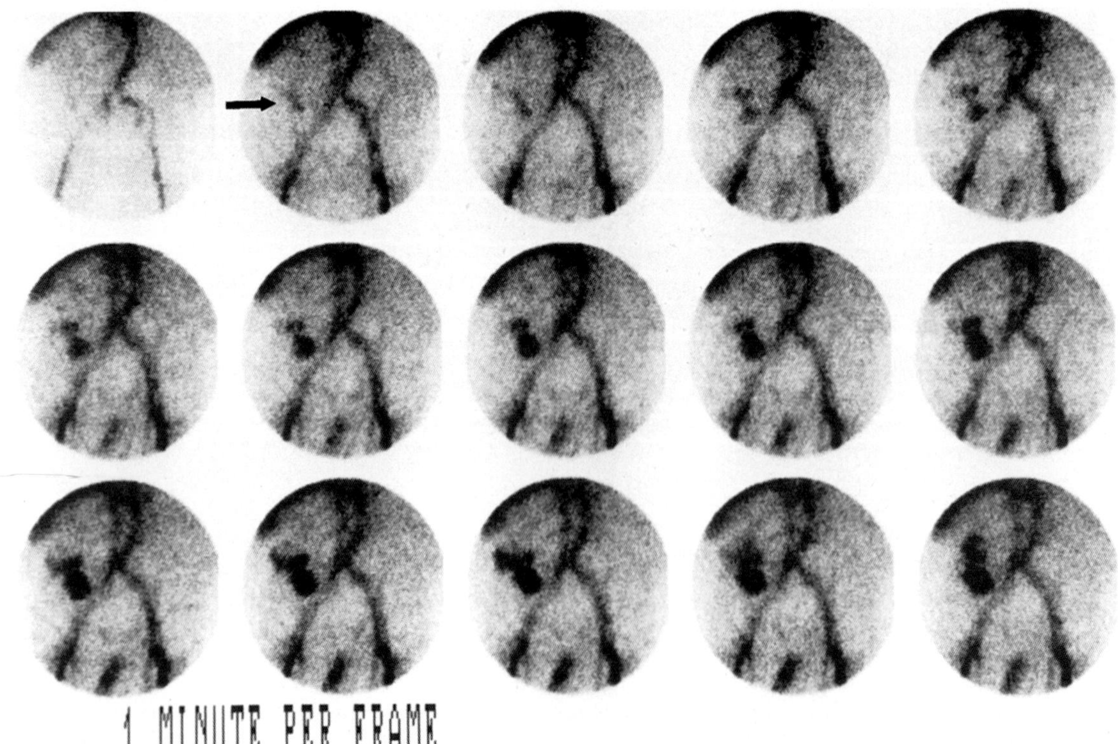

FIGURE 72A.7. Cecal Bleeding Because of Angiodysplasia. Images show a right lower quadrant hemorrhage (*arrow*).

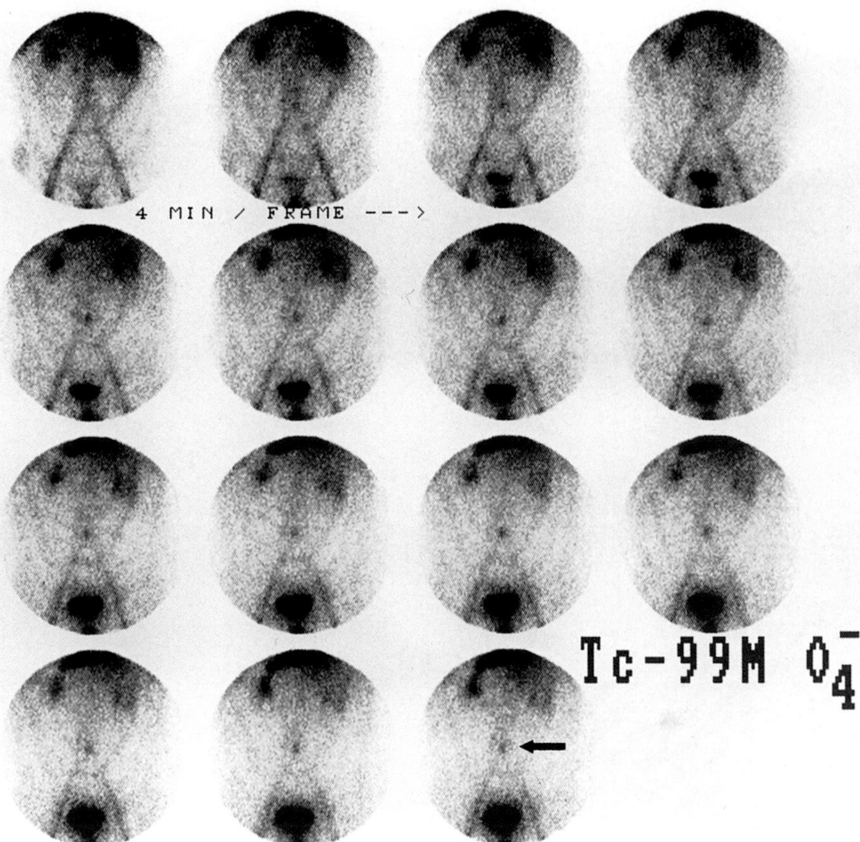

FIGURE 72A.8. **Meckel Diverticulum.** A small focus (*arrow*) of Tc-99m-O_4 uptake gradually becomes visible in the ectopic gastric mucosa of a Meckel diverticulum in the mid-abdomen.

are minimally seen. The liver/spleen scan is an inexpensive and easy means to evaluate for focal or diffuse hepatic disease, but it lacks disease specificity. Radiotracer uptake may be abnormal in a multitude of diseases. To make matters worse, hepatic lesions less than 1 cm in diameter are routinely not visible, even with SPECT. MR, CT, and US have better spatial resolution for hepatic masses and are the mainstay in the evaluation of indeterminate hepatic masses. Tc-99m SC liver SPECT, however, can be very specific in diagnosing focal nodular hyperplasia (FNH), a benign lesion consisting of focal hepatocyte proliferation in response to an arteriovenous malformation. Lesions which are large enough to be identified on SPECT and are isointense or more intense than liver parenchyma on uptake may be confidently diagnosed as FNH. This is due to the presence or increased concentration of reticuloendothelial cells within the lesion. Tc-99m SC can also be useful in diagnosing masses outside of the liver as myelolipomas or extramedullary hematopoiesis.

Liver/spleen radionuclide imaging remains accurate and easy for the evaluation of liver and spleen size, configuration, and position. This helps in the evaluation of suspected hepatomegaly in patients with obstructive lung disease, causing diaphragmatic flattening or in patients with anatomic variants such as large left liver lobe or a Riedel lobe on the right. A normal study is shown in Figure 72A.9.

Alterations in perfusion and reticuloendothelial system function caused by cirrhosis and hepatitis are seen as a "shift" of activity to the spleen, bone marrow, and lungs. The liver/spleen scan provides information that helps monitor the disease process and the efficacy of therapy (Fig. 72A.10).

Liver/spleen scans can be "subtracted" from other nuclear medicine studies to provide spatial information about the liver or the spleen in relation to a suspected abnormality. Indium-111 (In-111) leukocyte scans (for infection), gallium-67 scans (for inflammation, lymphoma, or hepatoma), In-111 octreotide scans (for neuroendocrine tumors), and labeled-antibody scans have physiologic uptake in the liver and/or the spleen. Subtracting the liver/spleen scan from any of these scans confirms "hot" abnormalities adjacent to the liver or the spleen (Fig. 72A.11). This may be particularly useful in cirrhotic livers with regenerating nodules.

Heat-Damaged Red Blood Cell Scan for Splenic Tissue

Tc-99m–labeled red blood cells that have been damaged by heating are preferentially extracted from the circulation by splenic tissue. Applications include diagnosis of polysplenia, splenosis, and confirmation of accessory splenic tissue. Acquiring CT and SPECT can help better detection and localization of these lesions (Fig. 72A.12).

HEPATOBILIARY IMAGING

Nuclear medicine imaging of the gallbladder and the biliary system is easily performed with Tc-99m–labeled iminodiacetic acid compounds. Only two of the numerous iminodiacetic acid radiotracers that have been developed are still commercially available, disofenin and mebrofenin. HIDA (lidofenin) is actually no longer commercially available. These radiopharmaceuticals are excreted unchanged into the biliary system and work even in the presence of elevated serum bilirubin, though higher radiopharmaceutical doses may be necessary.

Acute Cholecystitis. Hepatobiliary scans are most commonly used to evaluate for suspected acute cholecystitis. A minimum of 2-hour fasting is recommended in the preparation for this scan. The anterior dynamic images of normal hepatobiliary

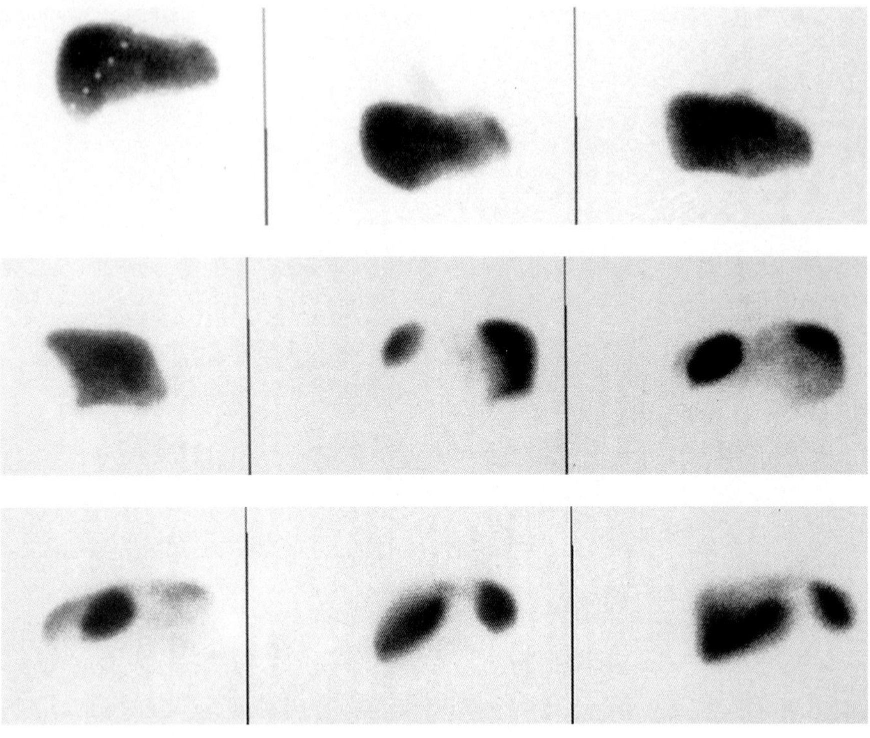

FIGURE 72A.9. **Normal Liver/Spleen Scan.** Sequential images begin with an anterior projection with a lead marker (row of cold dots) on the right costal margin. Subsequent images are anterior, right anterior oblique, right lateral, right posterior oblique, posterior, left posterior oblique, left lateral, and left anterior oblique from left to right, top to bottom. Note the homogeneous labeling of the liver and the spleen and the relative size and position of these two organs in various projections.

scans show a prompt and homogeneous uptake of the radiopharmaceutical by the liver. The liver activity decreases progressively as the radiotracer is excreted into the biliary system and drains into the small bowel. The activity should be seen in the major extrahepatic ducts, gallbladder, and the small bowel within 1 hour (Fig. 72A.13). Most patients with acute cholecystitis have a stone or stones obstructing the cystic duct. A small minority of patients, usually the chronically ill, have acalculous cholecystitis. The hallmark of acute cholecystitis by cholescintigraphy is the nonvisualization of the gallbladder at both 1- and 4-hour intervals after IV injection of the biliary agent, or 30 minutes after morphine administration. **Chronic cholecystitis** is suggested when the gallbladder is not visualized at 1 hour but is seen by 4 hours (without morphine augmentation). When properly done, the nuclear medicine hepatobiliary examination has a sensitivity and specificity of 98% and greater than 95% accuracy rate in the diagnosis of acute cholecystitis. Small doses of IV morphine (typically 2 mg) can be administered during the examination to cause sphincter of Oddi contraction, which increases pressure within the biliary tree and preferentially fills

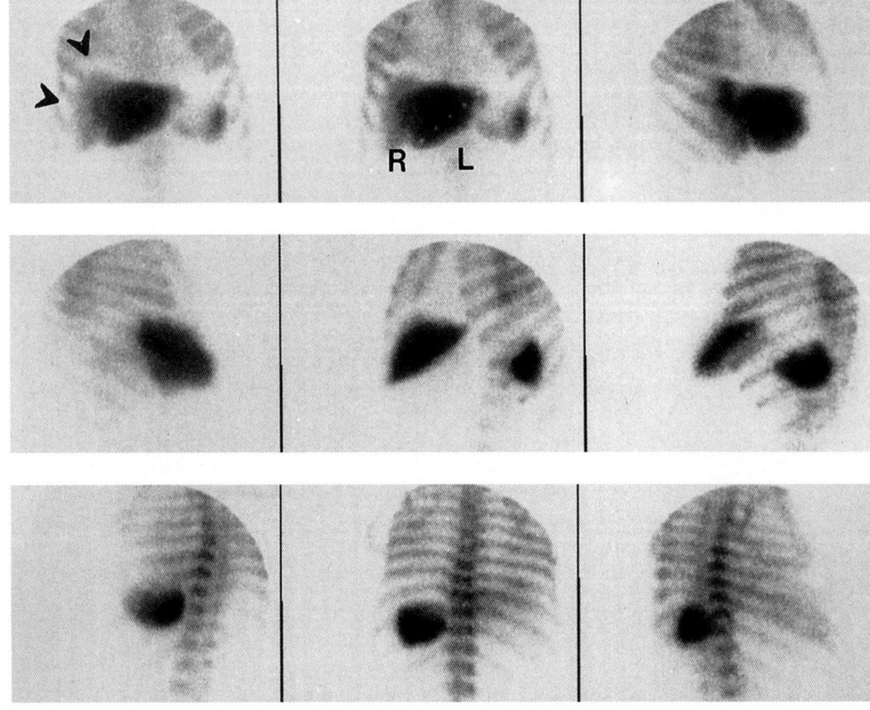

FIGURE 72A.10. **Abnormal Liver/Spleen Scan in a Patient With Cirrhosis.** The liver is small and labels poorly. The left lobe of the liver (*L*) is better seen than the right lobe (*R*). Note the "colloid" shift of the radiopharmaceutical to the bone marrow and the spleen. Ascites separate the liver from the right ribs (*arrowheads*). Compare this figure with Figure 72A.9.

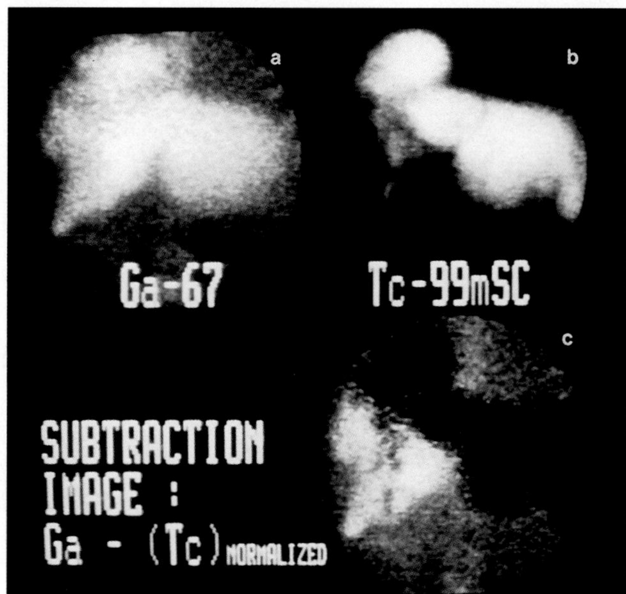

FIGURE 72A.11. **Liver/Spleen Subtraction From a Gallium-67 Scan in a Patient With a Hepatoma. A:** Image of Ga-67 distribution in the anterior projection at 48 hours. **B:** Matched image of colloid distribution. Careful selection of the gamma camera energy windows allows simultaneous imaging of the two radiopharmaceuticals. The subtraction image (**C**) shows the gallium-avid hepatoma, which does not label with the colloid.

the gallbladder. It is a useful way to speed up a "normal scan" because the diagnosis of acute cholecystitis is excluded as soon as the gallbladder is seen and expedites patient care. Morphine administration may also allow true-negative scans to be performed in patients who have stimulated their gallbladders to contract by eating before the scan.

Increased blood flow on radionuclide angiograms of the gallbladder fossa aids in the diagnosis of acute cholecystitis. A **"rim sign"** on the hepatobiliary scan images is seen as a curved band of increased activity around the gallbladder fossa, which represents poor excretion of radiotracer from inflamed hepatocytes. The rim sign is usually associated with gangrenous cholecystitis (Fig. 72A.14).

A pitfall in the interpretation of acute cholecystitis may be caused by prolonged fasting, resulting in a distended, atonic high-pressure gallbladder. This can be avoided by pretreating the patient with analogs of cholecystokinin (CCK), a short-acting natural hormone that causes prompt gallbladder contraction and allows the gallbladder to refill. A false-positive diagnosis of acute cholecystitis may also occur with previous cholecystectomy, tumor obstructing the cystic duct, and agenesis of the gallbladder. **Mirizzi syndrome** can be suspected when there is evidence of acute cholecystitis (nonvisualization of gallbladder) and common bile duct obstruction.

Acalculous biliary disease includes chronic acalculous cholecystitis, cystic duct syndrome, and gallbladder dyskinesis. These patients present with similar complaints of right upper quadrant pain, fatty-food intolerance, and epigastric distress. Routine cholescintigraphy and US may be normal. CCK-assisted cholescintigraphy in acalculous biliary disease demonstrates

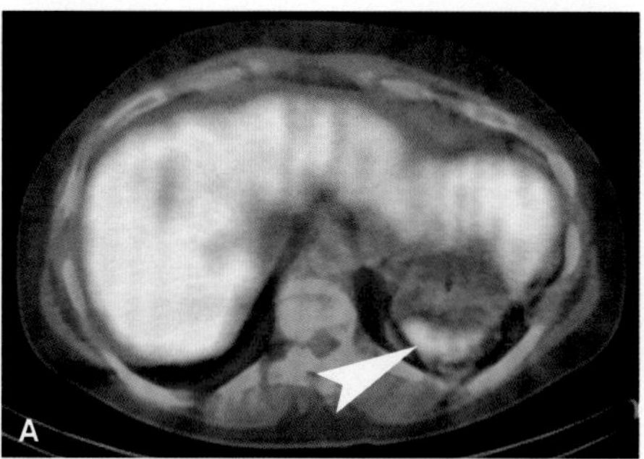

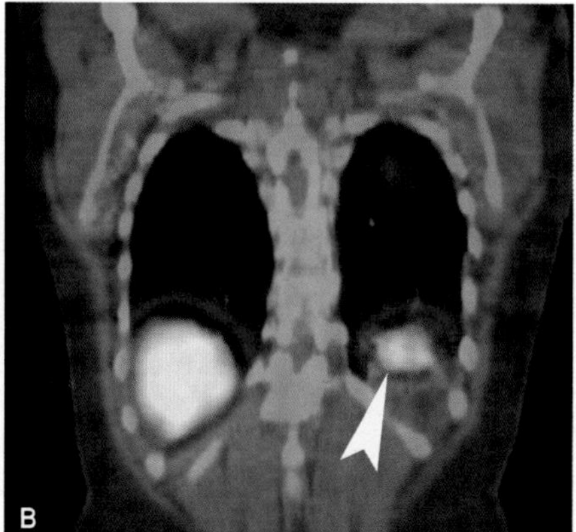

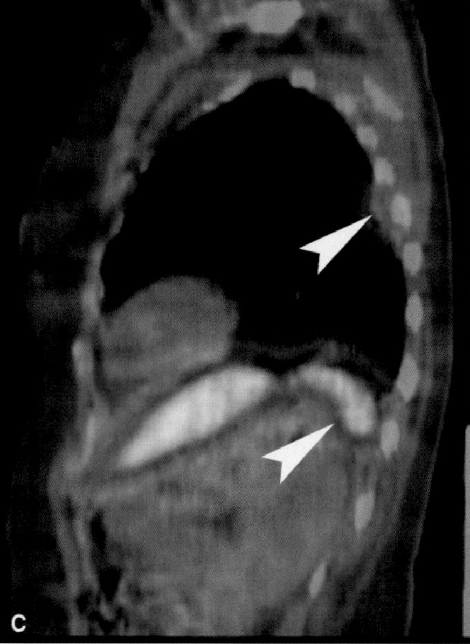

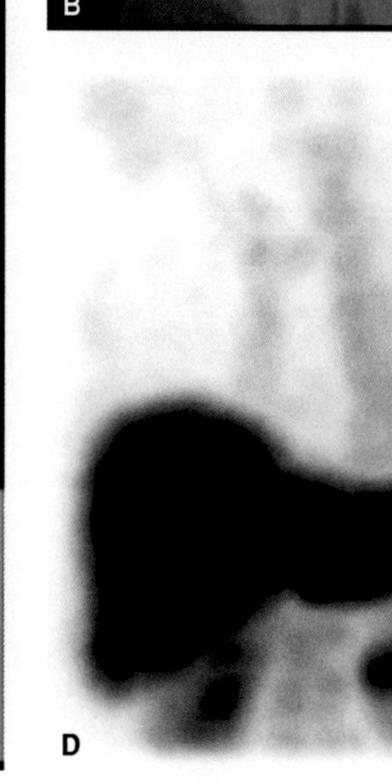

FIGURE 72A.12. **SPECT-CT Demonstrating Splenosis.** Heat-damaged Tc-RBC scan with SPECT/CT shows intrathoracic and intra-abdominal splenosis (*arrowheads*). Fusion SPECT/CT: Axial (**A**), coronal (**B**), sagittal (**C**) fusion SPECT/CT, and coronal planar SPECT (**D**).

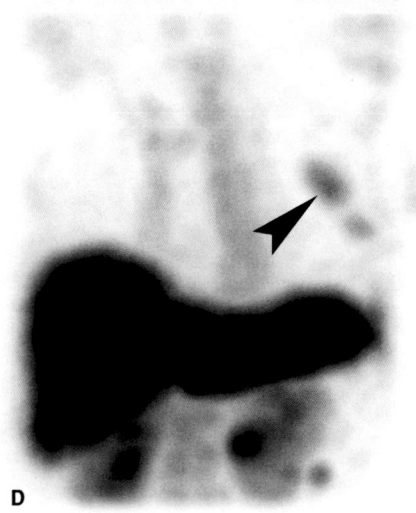

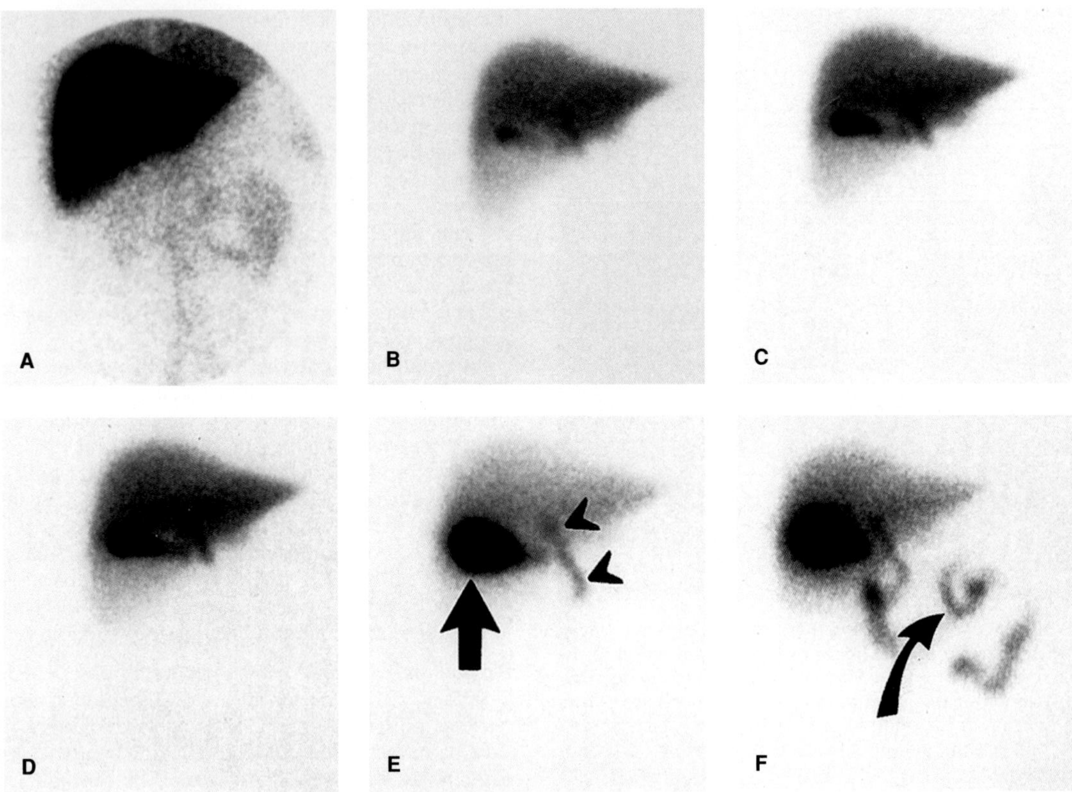

FIGURE 72A.13. **Normal Hepatobiliary Scan.** Images of the liver immediately after injection (**A**) and at subsequent 5-minute intervals (**B–F**) show rapid clearance of the blood pool followed promptly by the central biliary duct and gallbladder (*arrow*) activity. Activity continues to fill the common bile duct (*arrowheads*) at 20 minutes (**E**) and the small bowel (*curved arrow*) at 25 minutes (**F**).

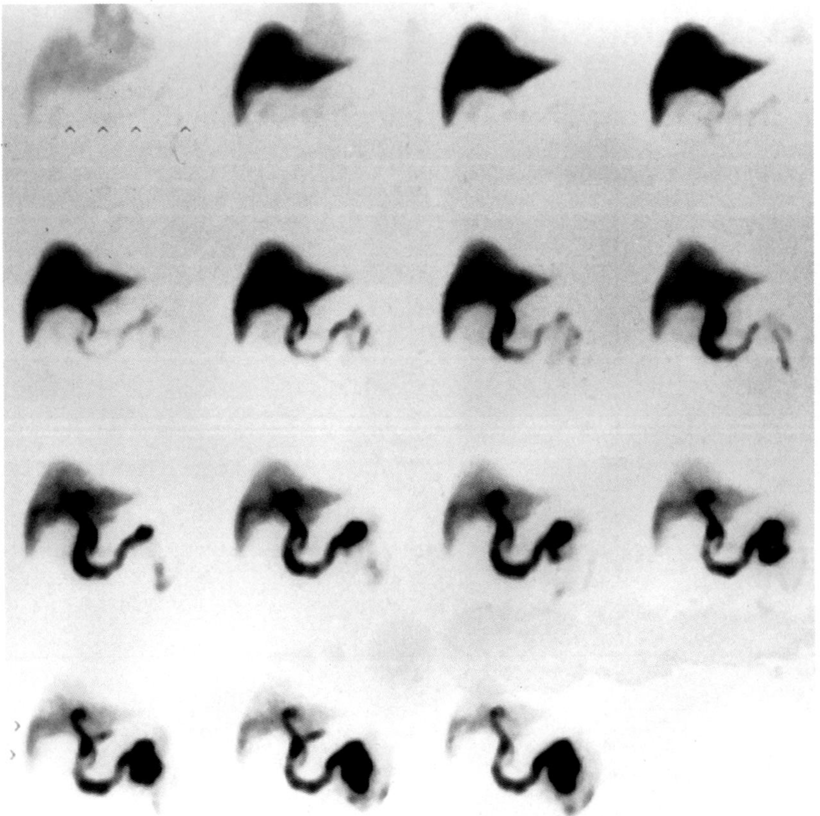

FIGURE 72A.14. **Acute Cholecystitis Diagnosed by Hepatobiliary Scan.** The first hepatobiliary scan in this patient was positive for acute cholecystitis, but the referring service did not believe the diagnosis. The scan was repeated on the next day. In it, the first image shows radioisotope left over from that first scan. A dim line of activity in the transverse colon is marked. Cholecystokinin (CCK) was used as a pretreatment for the second scan. Starting with the second image, the dose is rapidly concentrated and excreted by the liver into bile ducts and small bowel. The gallbladder never fills. As the liver clears, a "hot rim" of activity is seen around the gallbladder fossa, *which* indicates inflammation caused by the severe acute cholecystitis.

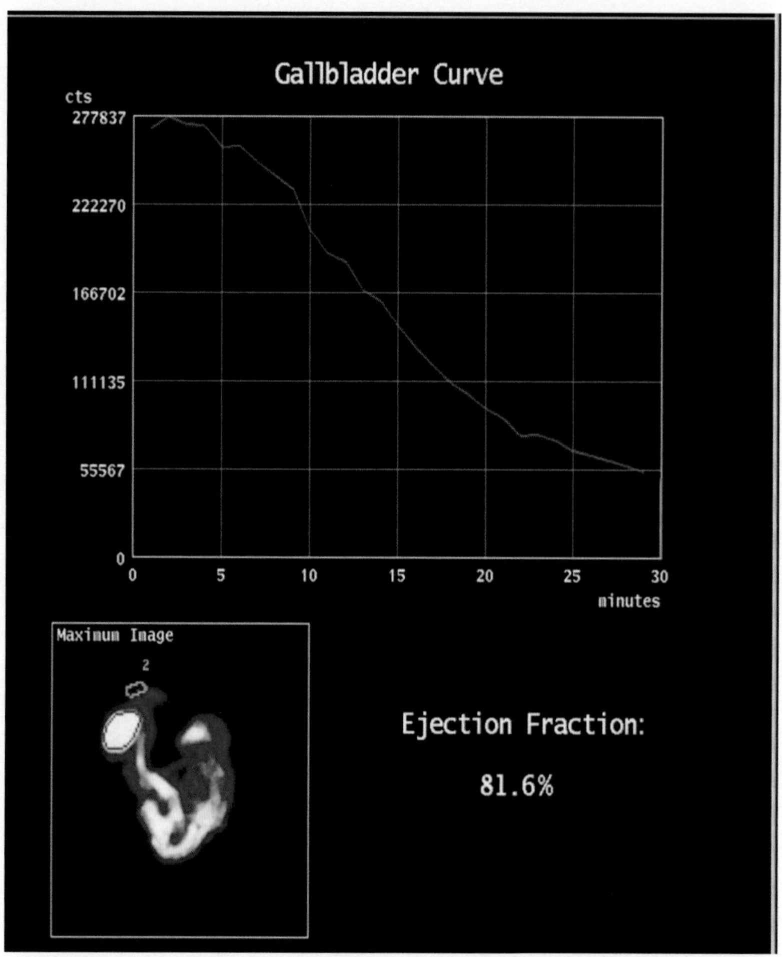

FIGURE 72A.15. **Normal Gallbladder Ejection Fraction (GBEF).** HIDA scan demonstrates normal gallbladder filling, followed by cholecystokinin infusion and a normal GBEF (normal >30%).

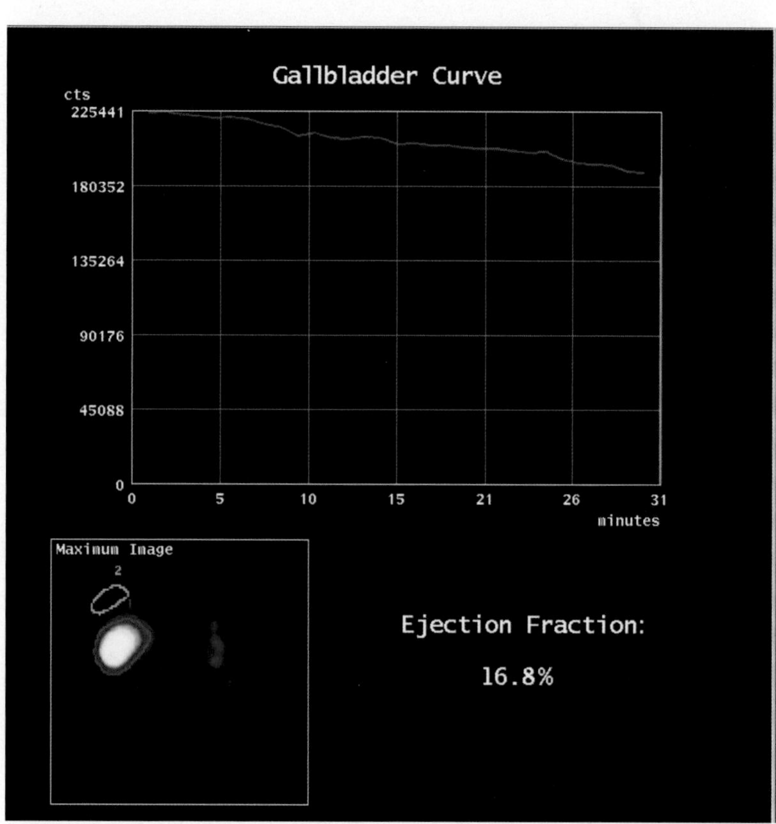

FIGURE 72A.16. **Abnormal Gallbladder Ejection Fraction (GBEF).** The gallbladder has filled normally (excluding acute cholecystitis) but there is a decreased GBEF (16.8%) following cholecystokinin infusion, consistent with chronic cholecystitis (normal >30%).

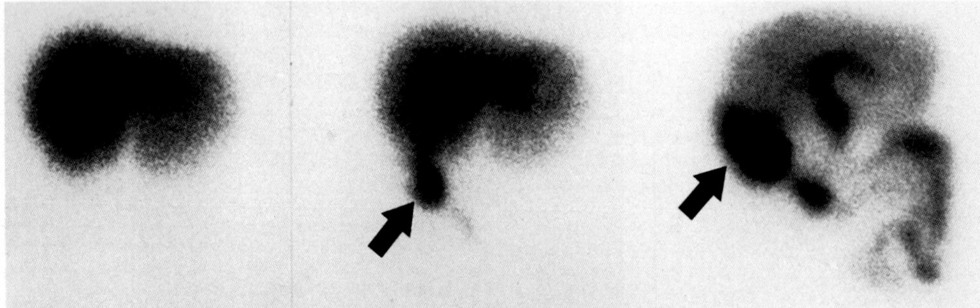

FIGURE 72A.17. **Biliary Leak After Cholecystectomy Detected by a Hepatobiliary Scan.** Images (**left** to **right**) obtained immediately, 30 minutes, and 1 hour after administration of the biliary agent show accumulation of bile in the area around the right lobe of the liver (*arrows*).

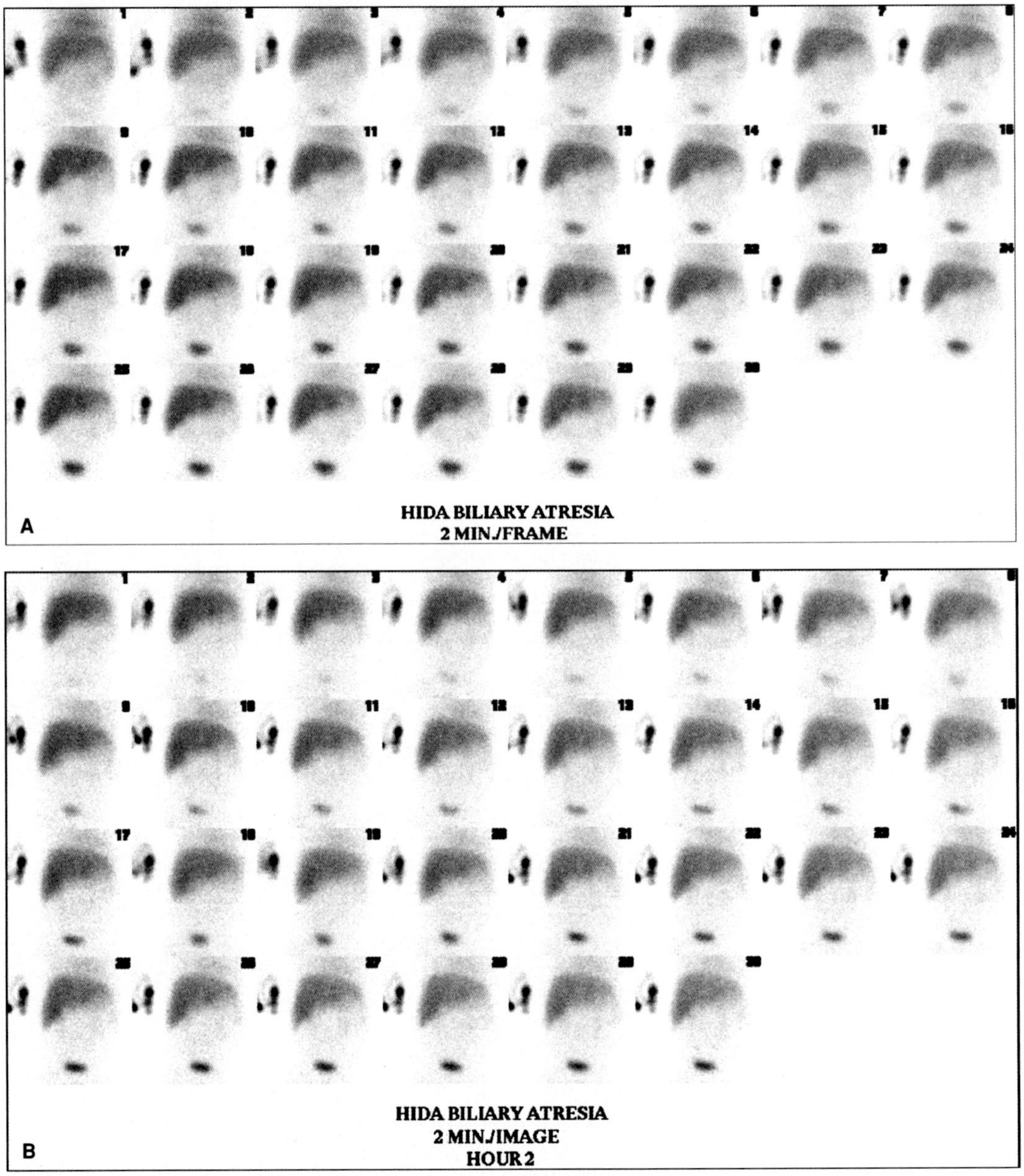

A

HIDA BILIARY ATRESIA
2 MIN./FRAME

B

HIDA BILIARY ATRESIA
2 MIN./IMAGE
HOUR 2

FIGURE 72A.18. **Biliary Atresia on HIDA Scan. A:** First-hour images. **B:** Second-hour images. No scintigraphic evidence of biliary excretion into the bowel or gallbladder is seen within 2 hours after injection of Tc-99m-mebrofenin, consistent with biliary atresia.

decreased gallbladder contraction and decreased gallbladder ejection fraction. A commonly recommended and clinically useful method to calculate gallbladder ejection fraction is to administer IV CCK 1 hour after the injection of biliary radiotracer and when the gallbladder is well visualized. Slow CCK infusion is preferable because it is more physiologic, results in more complete emptying, and has fewer side effects. If 0.02 mcg/kg of CCK is infused over 30 minutes, then a gallbladder ejection fraction of greater than 30% is considered normal (Fig. 72A.15). Abnormal or low gallbladder ejection fraction is consistent with gallbladder dyskinesia or chronic cholecystitis (Fig. 72A.16).

Other uses for the hepatobiliary scan include the detection of postoperative complications and bile leaks in trauma (Fig. 72A.17). The excretion phase of the scan is important in evaluating hepatic and common bile duct patency. A delay in the visualization of the bile ducts of more than 1 hour suggests obstruction. Caution must be exercised to differentiate severe hepatocellular disease from obstruction, as both present with delays in biliary visualization though severe hepatocellular disease will result in delayed clearance of radiotracer from the blood pool (e.g., persistent cardiac uptake). The hepatobiliary scan maintains a niche in differentiating neonatal hepatitis from **biliary atresia** (Fig. 72A.18). In the latter case, the radiolabeled bile will never enter the bowel or the gallbladder. Unfortunately, if the hepatitis is bad enough, the radiopharmaceutical may not leave the liver. If bowel activity is seen (and this may take 4 to 24 hours), the diagnosis of biliary atresia is excluded.

HEPATIC BLOOD POOL SCINTIGRAPHY

Cavernous hemangioma is the most common benign hepatic tumor and the second most common hepatic tumor, second to metastatic disease. Frequently subcapsular in location, these tumors are often found incidentally by US, CT, or MR. Although there are specific criteria for the diagnosis of hepatic hemangioma by these techniques, no study is 100% specific. Cavernous hemangiomas have a significant risk of hemorrhage with biopsy and therefore a noninvasive diagnostic approach is preferred. Scintigraphy with Tc-99m–labeled red blood cells using an in vitro labeling technique has proved both sensitive and specific for cavernous hemangioma. A flow study should be performed initially and will demonstrate normal or decreased early uptake if the suspected lesion is a hemangioma. Tumors and inflammatory lesions tend to have increased arterial flow. Subsequent delayed SPECT imaging will reveal foci of increased activity within the liver that are hotter than the surrounding parenchyma. Sensitivity decreases with lesions smaller than 1.5 cm, greater organ depth, and with single-detector SPECT as opposed to multidetector SPECT. Specificity is generally high, although isolated cases of increased activity on delayed imaging with both colon and lung carcinoma metastases have been reported. In general, if two of the four imaging techniques demonstrate the characteristic features of cavernous hemangioma, no further evaluation is warranted (Fig. 72A.19).

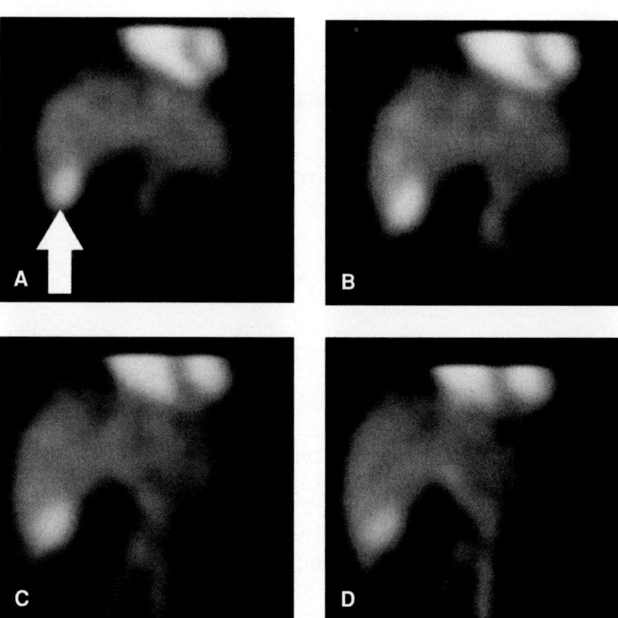

FIGURE 72A.19. **Hepatic Hemangioma.** At first glance, this study (**A–D**) could be confused with a biliary scan. However, note the vascular blood pool and that these are four coronal slices from a SPECT study of the liver performed 1 hour after the injection of 25 mCi of Tc-99m-O_4–labeled red blood cells. The area of increased activity (*arrow*), *which simulates a gallbladder*, is actually a hemangioma in the liver of this hepatic transplant recipient.

Suggested Readings

Balon HR, Fink-Bennett DM, Brill DR, et al. Procedure guideline for hepatobiliary scintigraphy. Society of Nuclear Medicine. *J Nucl Med* 1997;38(10):1654–1657.

Chamarthy M, Freeman LM. Hepatobiliary scan findings in chronic cholecystitis. *Clin Nucl Med* 2010;35:244–251.

Charron M. Pediatric inflammatory bowel disease imaged with Tc-99m white blood cells. *Clin Nucl Med* 2000;25(9):708–715.

Charron M, Di Lorenzo C, Kocoshis S. CT and 99mTc-WBC vs colonoscopy in the evaluation of inflammation and complications of inflammatory bowel diseases. *J Gastroenterol* 2002;37(1):874–875.

Chatziioannou SN, Moore WH, Ford PV, Dhekne RD. Hepatobiliary scintigraphy is superior to abdominal ultrasonography in suspected acute cholecystitis. *Surgery* 2000;127(6):609–613.

Connolly LP, Treves ST, Bozorgi F, O'Connor SC. Meckel's diverticulum: demonstration of heterotopic gastric mucosa with technetium-99m-pertechnetate SPECT. *J Nucl Med* 1998;39(8):1458–1460.

Donohoe KJ, Maurer AH, Ziessman HA, Urbain JL, Royal HD. Procedure guideline for gastric emptying and motility. Society of Nuclear Medicine. *J Nucl Med* 1999;40(7):1236–1239.

Ford PV, Bartold SP, Fink-Bennett DM, et al. Procedure guideline for gastrointestinal bleeding and Meckel's diverticulum scintigraphy. Society of Nuclear Medicine. *J Nucl Med 1999*:40(7):1226–1232.

Hustinx R. PET imaging in assessing gastrointestinal tumors. *Radiol Clin North Am* 2004;42(6):1123–1139, ix.

Kamel EM, Thumshirn M, Truninger K, et al. Significance of incidental 18F-FDG accumulations in the gastrointestinal tract in PET/CT: correlation with endoscopic and histopathologic results. *J Nucl Med* 2004;45(11):1804–1810.

Klein HA. Esophageal transit scintigraphy. *Semin Nucl Med* 1995;25(4):306–317.

Klingensmith WC 3rd, Lawrence SP. The gastric emptying study: protocol design considerations. *J Nucl Med Technol* 2008;36(4):195–199.

Krishnamurthy S, Krishnamurthy GT. Cholecystokinin and morphine pharmacological intervention during 99mTc-HIDA cholescintigraphy: a rational approach. *Semin Nucl Med* 1996;26(1):16–24.

Mariani G, Boni G, Barreca M, et al. Radionuclide gastroesophageal motor studies. *J Nucl Med* 2004;45(6):1004–1028.

Maurer AH. Gastrointestinal bleeding and cine-scintigraphy. *Semin Nucl Med* 1996;26(1):43–50.

Maurer AH, Krevsky B. Whole-gut transit scintigraphy in the evaluation of small-bowel and colon transit disorders. *Semin Nucl Med* 1995;25(4):326–338.

Nadel HR. Hepatobiliary scintigraphy in children. *Semin Nucl Med* 1996;26(1):25–42.

Szepes A, Bertalan V, Várkonyi T, Pávics L, Lonovics J, Madácsy L. Diagnosis of gallbladder dyskinesia by quantitative hepatobiliary scintigraphy. *Clin Nucl Med* 2005;30(5):302–307.

Tripathi M, Chandrashekar N, Kumar R, et al. Hepatobiliary scintigraphy: an effective tool in the management of bile leak following laparoscopic cholecystectomy. *Clin Imaging* 2004;28(1):40–43.

Urbain JL, Charkes ND. Recent advances in gastric emptying scintigraphy. *Semin Nucl Med* 1995;25(4):318–325.

Ziessman HA, Fahey FH, Hixson DJ. Calculation of a gallbladder ejection fraction: advantage of continuous Sincalide infusion over the three-minute infusion method. *J Nucl Med* 1992;33(4):537–541.

Zuckier LS, Freeman LM. Selective role of nuclear medicine in evaluating the acute abdomen. *Radiol Clin North Am* 2003;41(6):1275–1288.

CHAPTER 72B ■ PULMONARY SCINTIGRAPHY

BRADLEY FEHRENBACH

Although CT angiography (CTA) has taken the primary role in diagnosing pulmonary embolism (PE), ventilation–perfusion (V/Q) scans remain an important imaging test. A scintigraphic lung scan is a physiologic map that evaluates the primary functions of the lung, pulmonary vasculature perfusion, and segmental bronchioalveolar tree ventilation. Most commonly, V/Q scans are used to evaluate patients suspected of having pulmonary emboli. In an attempt to provide more accurate results, the criteria for interpreting V/Q studies have been periodically revised. Different approaches that compare defects on the perfusion scan with those found on the ventilation scan and/or chest x-ray (CXR) have been developed in order to estimate the probability of PE. This chapter describes radiopharmaceuticals used, examination techniques, imaging protocols, and criteria for the interpretation of V/Q scans.

ANATOMY AND PHYSIOLOGY

Understanding the segmental anatomy of the lungs (Fig. 72B.1) is vital to the interpretation of lung scans. The three-dimensional location of ventilation or perfusion defects must be individually determined and correlated with the segmental or subsegmental anatomy of the lung. Pulmonary emboli will have a segmental or a subsegmental distribution pattern, usually peripheral and wedge shaped.

Although pulmonary ventilation occurs primarily via the branching bronchial tree, other pathways exist by which distal alveoli can be aerated. The pores of Kohn connect adjacent alveoli and the canals of Lambert connect alveoli with respiratory, terminal, and preterminal bronchioles. These canals and pores permit collateral ventilation of alveoli whose conducting airways are blocked. Collateral air drift is dynamic and is mediated by neurohormonal control mechanisms that can be altered by pathologic events, atmospheric/alveolar gas tension, and drugs.

Both ventilation and pulmonary blood flow demonstrate significant variation due to gravity. When a patient is in an upright posture, the gradient for blood flow is from the apices to the lung bases; the apices receive only one-third of the blood volume that the bases receive. A corresponding ventilation gradient exists when the patient sits upright. Since the intrapleural pressure is greater at the bases, the differential negative intrapleural pressure at the apices causes the alveoli at the apices to remain more open at expiration than the alveoli at the lung bases. Therefore, the basilar alveoli undergo greater changes in size over the respiratory cycle. This results in greater gas exchange occurring in the bases and greater oxygen tension in the apices. On average, ventilation at the base is 1.5 to 2 times that of the apex. When a patient is supine, the ventilation gradient shifts from superoinferior to anteroposterior and perfusion is increased to the dependent posterior portions of the lungs.

Normally, capillary perfusion and alveolar ventilation are matched in order to maximize gas exchange. Diseases that produce localized hypoxia invoke autoregulatory mechanisms that divert blood flow away from the hypoventilated pulmonary segments. These dynamic changes prevent nonventilated lung segments from being perfused. Conversely, localized hypoperfusion rarely induces localized bronchoconstriction. Primary vascular disorders such as PE, if unassociated with parenchymal consolidation or pulmonary infarction, usually have normal ventilation. Thus, an anatomic perfusion defect with normal ventilation is referred to as a V/Q mismatch and is the hallmark of PE diagnosis.

VENTILATION LUNG SCAN

Radiopharmaceuticals

Xenon-133. Xe-133 is a radioisotope used to perform ventilation lung scans. It is a noble gas produced by fission of U-235 in a nuclear reactor with a half-life of approximately 5.3 days. Xe-133 undergoes γ-decay and β^--decay (i.e., electrons). The principal photon energy is 81 keV, resulting in significant attenuation by soft tissues. Xe-133 ventilation scans should be performed before perfusion lung scans because Compton scatter from the higher-energy Tc-99m macroaggregated albumin (MAA) (140 keV) down-scatters into the region of the 81-keV photopeak of the Xe-133 and would interfere with ventilation images. The usual adult dose of Xe-133 for a ventilation scan is 10 to 20 mCi (370 to 740 MBq).

Xenon-127. Xe-127 is a cyclotron-produced isotope with a physical half-life of 36.4 days and principal photon energies of 203 keV, 172 keV, and 365 keV. Because it has higher-energy photons, Xe-127 ventilation scans can be performed, if needed

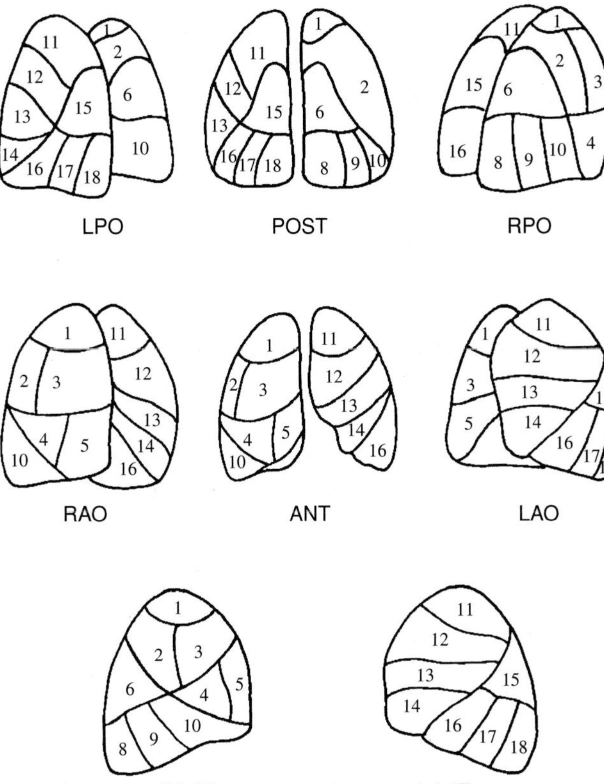

FIGURE 72B.1. **Pulmonary Segment Anatomy.** Bronchopulmonary segments of the right lung: (*1*) apical; (*2*) posterior; (*3*) anterior; (*4*) lateral; (*5*) medial; (*6*) superior; (*7*) medial basal; (*8*) posterior basal; (*9*) lateral basal; and (*10*) anterior basal. Bronchopulmonary segments of the left lung: (*11*) apical posterior; (*12*) anterior; (*13*) superior lingual; (*14*) inferior lingual; (*15*) superior; (*16*) anterior medial basal; (*17*) lateral basal; and (*18*) posterior basal. *LPO*, left posterior oblique; *POST*, posterior; *RPO*, right posterior oblique; *RAO*, right anterior oblique; *ANT*, anterior; *LAO*, left anterior oblique; *RLAT*, right lateral; *LLAT*, left lateral. (Adapted with minor modifications from Sostman HD, Gottschalk A. *Diagnostic Nuclear Medicine*. 2nd ed. Baltimore, MD: Lippincott Williams & Wilkins; 1988:513.)

after the perfusion scan, since down-scatter image deterioration is not a significant problem. Unfortunately, because Xe-127 is cyclotron produced, it is both expensive and of limited availability. The usual adult dose is 8 to 15 mCi (296 to 555 MBq).

Krypton-81m. Kr-81m is another noble gas used for ventilation scans. It has an extremely short half-life of only 13 seconds and is produced from an Rb-81 generator. Kr-81m decays by isomeric transition (similar to Tc-99m) and has a photon energy of 191 keV. The higher energy allows the ventilation scan to be acquired, if needed, after an abnormal perfusion scan. Unfortunately, the generator is expensive and therefore Kr-81m is limited in use. The usual adult dose is 10 to 20 mCi (370 to 740 MBq).

Technetium-99m Aerosols. Ventilation scans can be performed using aerosolized rather than gaseous agents. Radioisotope-labeled aerosols are produced by nebulizing radiopharmaceuticals into a fine mist that is inhaled. Tc-99m diethylenetriaminepentaacetic acid (DTPA) is the most commonly used radioaerosol. The advantages of Tc-99m aerosols are that they are widely available, inexpensive, and have a 140-keV photopeak ideal for gamma camera imaging. The nebulizer-produced mist is passed through a settling bag, which traps larger particles. The mist is delivered to the patient via a nonrebreather valve and is inhaled. The process is inefficient; only 2% to 10% of the aerosolized radioisotope is deposited within the lungs. Of the typical 30 mCi of nebulized Tc-99m DTPA given, only 1 to 2 mCi are actually deposited within the lungs.

The site of deposition of the aerosolized particles depends on the size of the inhaled particle. The larger the particle, the greater the gravitational effect, which results in more central deposition. Particles larger than 2 μm localize in the trachea and pharynx. Current aerosol nebulizers can produce microaerosols of less than 0.5 μm. Thus, microaerosol particles are small enough to reach the distal tracheobronchial tree and reflect regional ventilation. Patients with narrowed airways caused by asthma, bronchitis, or chronic obstructive pulmonary disease (COPD) have more central deposition of the particles than normal patients due to airway turbulence. This results in poor visualization of the peripheral lungs. The deposited Tc-99m DTPA is absorbed across the alveolar membrane with a clearance half-life of 60 to 90 minutes. The half-life is approximately 20 minutes shorter in tobacco smokers due to their increased alveolar permeability.

Dosimetry. The critical organ for Xe-133 is the trachea, which receives a dose of 0.64 rad/mCi. The lung dose is 0.01 to 0.04 rad/mCi, whereas the whole-body absorbed dose is 0.001 rad/mCi.

For Tc-99m aerosols, the lungs receive an absorbed dose of 0.1 rad/mCi, the bladder wall a dose of 0.18 rad/mCi, and the entire body a dose of 0.01 rad/mCi.

Ventilation Scan Technique

Ventilation scanning using radioactive gases requires special equipment to prevent leakage of the gas into the imaging room and beyond. Gas delivery systems consist of a shielded spirometer, oxygen delivery system, and a xenon charcoal trap to capture most of the exhaled xenon. Because xenon is heavier than air, loose xenon pools at floor level and can be collected by utilizing negative pressure ventilation with floor vents to trap the Xe-133.

Xenon-133 Ventilation Scanning. The patient is initially fitted with an airtight face mask. While the patient takes a maximal inspiration, Xe-133 is injected into the mask intake tubing. The patient is instructed to hold his or her breath as long as possible. A 100,000-count first-breath posterior projection image of the lungs is then obtained. The ventilation system is then switched so that the patient rebreathes the air–Xe-133 mixture. After 5 minutes of rebreathing, a posterior 100,000-count equilibrium image is obtained. The distribution of Xe-133 activity on the equilibrium image represents aerated lung volume. The ventilation system is then readjusted so that the patient breathes in fresh air and exhales the Xe-133 mixture into the trap. Serial posterior 30-second washout images are obtained over a 5-minute interval. The Xe-133 normally washes out of the lungs within 3 to 4 minutes. Because the lung bases are better ventilated than the apices, the Xe-133 washes out of the bases faster than at the apices in a normal patient. If possible, all images should be performed with the patient in an upright position.

Xenon-127 ventilation scanning is performed in the same manner as Xe-133 ventilation lung scans. The Xe-127 ventilation scan needs to be performed only if the perfusion scan is abnormal.

Krypton-81m Ventilation Scanning. The high-photon energy of Kr-81m allows ventilation scans to follow perfusion scans. Immediately after each perfusion image and without moving, the patient inhales Kr-81m and the corresponding ventilation image is obtained. This process is repeated until ventilation and perfusion images are obtained in all six matching positions.

Technetium-99m Aerosol Ventilation Scanning. The patient inhales the nebulized aerosol while in the supine position to avoid the normal apex to base gravity gradient. After inhaling the Tc-99m aerosol for 3 to 5 minutes, the patient sits upright and is imaged in the same projections as for the perfusion lung scan. The exhaled aerosol is trapped in a filter that is stored until decay is sufficient for safe disposal.

A Tc-99m aerosol ventilation lung scan can be performed either before or after the perfusion lung scan. If the perfusion scan is performed first, a small dose (0.5 mCi) of Tc-99m MAA is used with a large dose (30 mCi) of Tc-99m DTPA. If the ventilation scan is performed first, 5 to 10 mCi of Tc-99m DTPA and 5 mCi of Tc-99m MAA are administered.

PERFUSION LUNG SCAN

Radiopharmaceuticals

Perfusion lung scanning is based on the principle of capillary blockade. Particles slightly larger than the pulmonary capillaries (>8 μm) are injected intravenously and travel to the right heart where venous blood is uniformly mixed. Radiolabeled particles in the pulmonary arterial blood then pass into the distal pulmonary circulation. Because the radioactive particles are larger than the capillaries, they lodge in the precapillary arterioles. Their distribution in the lung reflects the relative blood flow to pulmonary segments. Pulmonary segments with decreased or absent blood flow have less activity within.

Tc-99m macroaggregated albumin (MAA) is the radiopharmaceutical used to perform most perfusion lung scans. MAA is prepared by heat denaturation of human serum albumin. The MAA particles are irregularly shaped molecules, but the size range and number of particles in commercially available kits are tightly controlled. Most particles are in the 20- to 40-micron size range, with 90% of the particles between 10 and 90 μm. Particles larger than 150 μm should not be injected because they can obstruct more proximal arterioles. The size and number of particles in a kit are checked by counting a sample volume in a light microscopy hemocytometer. Tc-99m MAA is prepared by adding Tc-99m pertechnetate (Tc-99mO_4) to the MAA kit. The MAA is cleared from the lungs by breaking down into smaller particles that pass through the alveolar capillaries into the systemic circulation where they are removed by the reticuloendothelial system. The biologic half-life of MAA particles in the lung is 2 to 9 hours. The physical half-life of Tc-99m MAA is 6 hours.

A minimum of 60,000 Tc-99m MAA particles must be injected to ensure reliable count statistics and image quality. Typically, 200,000 to 500,000 particles are injected and less than 0.1% of capillaries are temporarily and safely occluded. However, several types of patients should receive a reduced number of particles during a perfusion scan. Patients with pulmonary hypertension and right to left shunts should be given only 100,000 particles. Children should also be injected with only 100,000 particles because they have fewer pulmonary arterioles. To perform reduced count imaging, each perfusion view is imaged for a longer time interval, allowing for nearly equivalent count statistics. Alternatively, the kit can be reconstituted with higher than usual Tc-99m activity per particle; the normal 5-mCi dose can be administered but with fewer particles. Contraindications to perfusion lung scanning include severe pulmonary hypertension and allergy to human serum albumin products.

Dosimetry. The normal adult dose is 3 to 5 mCi (111 to 185 MBq). The lung is the critical organ and receives an absorbed dose of 0.15 to 0.5 rad/mCi. The whole-body and gonadal-absorbed doses are both 0.15 rad/mCi.

Perfusion Scan Technique

The syringe containing the Tc-99m MAA should be gently agitated prior to injection to resuspend all particles. The patient is injected in the supine position while taking slow, deep breaths to minimize the pulmonary perfusion gravitational gradient. Blood should not be drawn into the syringe because aspirated blood may form clots, which become labeled by the Tc-99m MAA. Injection of clumped Tc-99m MAA particles or labeled clot can result in multiple small focal "hot spots" scattered through the lungs.

The patient is usually imaged in the upright position using a large field of view, high-resolution gamma camera. Images (500,000 counts) are obtained in the anterior, posterior, right lateral, left lateral, right posterior oblique, left posterior oblique, right anterior oblique, and left anterior oblique positions. If needed, supplemental or decubitus views can be added to clarify findings on the standard views.

V/Q SCANS

Indications. The most common indication for V/Q scans is the diagnosis of suspected PE. However, the examination has also been used to monitor pulmonary function of lung transplants, to provide preoperative estimates of lung function in lung carcinoma patients in whom partial or complete pneumonectomy is planned (split lung function study), and to evaluate right to left shunts. A chest radiograph (CXR) should be obtained within 24 hours prior to obtaining a V/Q scan. Airspace disease, effusions, pulmonary edema, or pneumothorax may explain sudden respiratory deterioration and eliminate the need for a V/Q scan.

CT Angiography Versus Ventilation/Perfusion Scans. There are situations in which V/Q scan should be the first option to diagnose PE and times when CTA should be the first option. The sensitivity and accuracy of CTA have increased with the use of thin-cut helical CT and multidetector CT (MDCT) (Fig. 72B.2). CT pulmonary angiogram should be considered when the patient is in the ICU, has an abnormal CXR, high clinical probability for PE, or a relative contraindication for anticoagulation. CT angiogram also has the benefit of showing additional abnormities not detected or underestimated on CXR. V/Q scan is highly sensitive and avoids the use of iodinated contrast. It should be considered when the clinical probability is low, the CXR is normal, and when the patient has a contraindication for iodinated contrast.

Physiologic changes in pregnancy often mimic PE, making clinical diagnosis unreliable and resulting in diagnostic imaging. Both V/Q and CTA expose the mother and fetus to radiation and potential latent carcinogenic risk. However, the risks of undiagnosed PE or inappropriate anticoagulation generally outweigh the potential risk from diagnostic imaging. The fetus' radiation dose is higher from V/Q scan (640 to 800 μGy) than from CTA (3 to 131 μGy) according to some authors, whereas other authors estimate that the fetal dose is comparable. There is no consensus regarding which study is the first choice during pregnancy, and thus the clinician should consider clinical and CXR findings, radiation dose, and patient concerns when deciding on the appropriate diagnostic imaging. However, a common recommendation is to key in on the CXR. If the CXR is normal, one can start with the V/Q scan. If the CXR is abnormal, CTA should be the first choice.

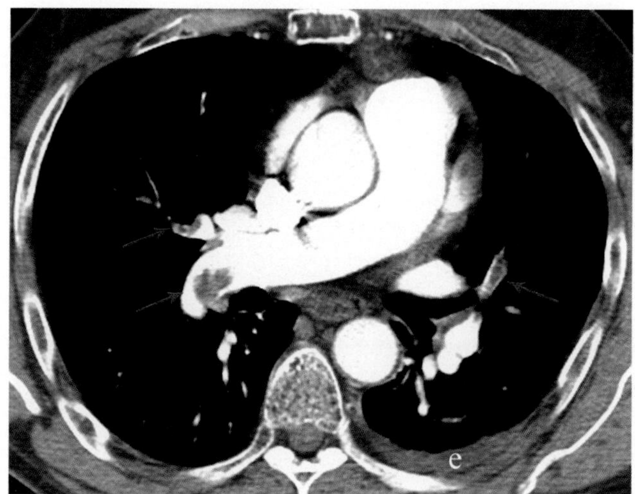

FIGURE 72B.2. **CT Pulmonary Angiogram With MDCT.** Scan demonstrates multiple, bilateral pulmonary emboli (*arrows*), and a left pleural effusion.

Regarding radiation dose to the breast, a typical CT PE examination will deliver 20 to 60 mSv. For 64-slice CT, the breast radiation dose is 50 to 80 mSv. For V/Q scan, the breast radiation is 0.28 to 0.9 mSv. Thus, the radiation dose to the breast is 65 to 250 times higher for CTA than for V/Q scan.

Normal ventilation scans (Fig. 72B.3A) have homogeneous radiopharmaceutical distribution throughout all lung fields on all three phases of the scan: initial breath, equilibrium, and washout. A subtle base to apex gradient may be seen because there is more lung parenchyma at the base than at the apex. The first-breath Xe-133 image is often grainy because it has relatively poor count statistics. However, it still reflects regional lung volume. The equilibrium images have greater activity and will fill in areas of restrictive lung disease. The washout phase of the study demonstrates rapid clearance of the Xe-133 from the lungs. Normal half-time for xenon washout is less than 1 minute. Washout is complete within 3 minutes. Retention (trapping) of xenon in the lungs in a focal or in a diffuse pattern is an indication of obstructive lung disease (Fig. 72B.4).

Normal Tc-99m DTPA aerosol scans resemble normal Tc-99m MAA perfusion scans. However, activity is frequently present within the trachea and the mainstem bronchi, especially in smokers. Swallowed Tc-99m DTPA aerosol is sometimes seen within the esophagus and the stomach.

Normal perfusion scans show well-defined margins of both lungs on all views with sharply defined costophrenic angles. A mild base to apex count activity gradient is present due to the physical difference in lung thickness of the base compared with the apex. Tracer distribution should otherwise be homogeneous (Fig. 72B.3B).

The heart causes a smoothly defined defect along the left medial lung border that is curvilinear in all projections. A prominent, focal triangular margin suggests the presence of a perfusion defect abutting the heart. The hila are usually seen, even in normal patients. Focal asymmetric perihilar perfusion defects are abnormal. Cardiomegaly, tortuosity of the aorta, and mediastinal or hilar enlargement cause defects along the medial border of the lung, associated with less well-defined corresponding defects on the ventilation scan. The size and shape of any mediastinal structure on the V/Q scan should match its appearance on the CXR.

Abnormal Scans. Focal defects or inhomogeneous tracer distribution is abnormal on either ventilation or perfusion scans. Focal perfusion defects should be compared with the corresponding areas on the ventilation scan and vice versa. The relative size and shape of V/Q defects should then be correlated with the corresponding areas on a recent CXR. Ideally, the correlative CXR should have been performed no more than 6 to 12 hours (certainly no more than 24 hours) prior to the V/Q scan since acute findings may change rapidly.

Ventilation scans are abnormal if areas of delayed xenon wash-in or washout are present. Restrictive changes or defects on the single-breath image may disappear on the equilibrium images when xenon bypasses obstructed pulmonary bronchioles through the pores of Kohn and canals of Lambert (see Fig. 72B.12). Movement by collateral air drift occurs more slowly than through the bronchioles, resulting in delayed wash-in and washout. Focal areas of abnormal retention therefore suggest obstructive lung disease (Figs. 72B.4 and 72B.5).

PULMONARY EMBOLISM

PE is a common cause of death in the United States. Dahlen and Alpert estimated that 30% of untreated patients with PE die as a consequence of their emboli, in comparison to 10% to 16% mortality for patients treated with anticoagulant therapy. Anticoagulants, however, place patients at significant risk for life-threatening bleeding and should not be prescribed without high probability for the diagnosis of venous thrombosis or PE.

Pulmonary emboli usually originate from thrombi within the deep venous system of the legs and pelvis. Predisposing factors include prolonged immobilization, surgery (particularly intrapelvic or hip surgery), history of prior PE, pre-existing cardiac disease, estrogen therapy, smoking, hypercoagulable states (such as with cancer), and congenital defects of thrombolysis.

PE can be difficult to diagnose clinically. In 70% of patients who survive pulmonary emboli, the emboli may not be clinically suspected. The classic triad of dyspnea, hemoptysis, and pleuritic chest pain occurs in less than 20% of patients with pulmonary emboli. Larger emboli increase the likelihood of symptoms. Symptoms associated with PE, however, are nonspecific. Pulmonary infection or inflammation, pneumothorax, cancer, edema, heart failure, and myriad other causes may produce similar symptoms. An electrocardiogram should be performed in patients suspected of having PE to detect cardiac causes for chest pain or dyspnea. If a patient develops acute cor pulmonale because of pulmonary emboli, the electrocardiogram may show signs of right heart strain.

Radiographic Findings of PE. The CXR is normal in 12% of patients with PE. Patients with an abnormal CXR are more likely to have intermediate lung scan interpretation compared with patients with a normal CXR, decreasing the utility of performing a V/Q scan.

The classic radiographic findings are a wedge-shaped, pleural-based infarct (Hampton hump), or a wedge-shaped area of oligemia (Westermark sign). The most common but nonspecific CXR finding of PE is atelectasis or opacities in the region with emboli. An elevated diaphragm, small pleural effusion, or prominent hilum are also frequently seen.

Both CT and MRI have been used to diagnose pulmonary emboli. The sensitivity of CT is 73% to 95% with a specificity of 87% to 97%. Spiral CT and MR accurately detect emboli in the segmental or larger pulmonary arteries, but more peripheral emboli may not be apparent.

Acute PE on CTA appears as an intraluminal filling defect, which partially or completely occludes the PA, or as an abrupt vessel cutoff. Commonly, mild vascular distention is present within the affected vessel at the thrombus site.

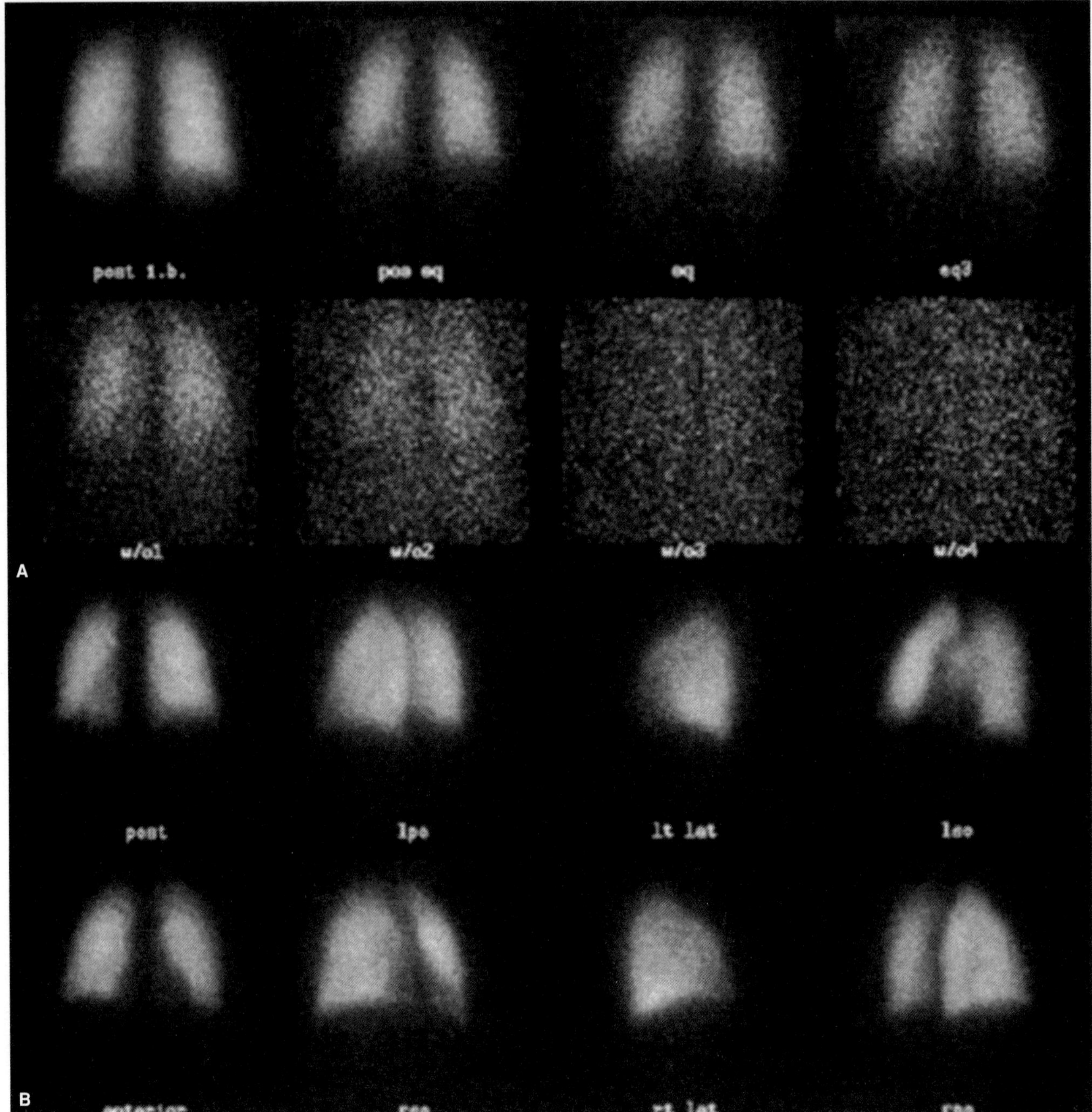

FIGURE 72B.3. **Normal V/Q Scan. A:** Normal Xe-133 ventilation lung scan (**top two rows**). *post ib*, posterior initial breath; *pos eq*, posterior equilibrium; *eq*, equilibrium; *eq3*, equilibrium after 3 minutes; *wo/1*, 1 minute after start of washout; *wo/2*, 2-minute washout; *wo/3*, 3-minute washout; *wo/4*, 4-minute washout. **B:** Normal Tc-99m MAA perfusion lung scan (**bottom two rows**). *post*, posterior; *lpo*, left posterior oblique; *lt lat*, left lateral; *lao*, left anterior oblique; *rao*, right anterior oblique; *rt lat*, right lateral; *rpo*, right posterior oblique.

Other indirect signs suggesting PE include dilated central PA, dilated RA, or wedge-shaped consolidation. Misdiagnosis of PE by CT can be due to artifacts related to respiratory motion, image noise, PA catheter, blood flow, and image reconstruction. Pathologic factors, such as mucus plugging or perivascular edema, can also lead to misdiagnosis of PE on CT.

CT Findings of DVT. Since inadequately treated DVT is associated with recurrent PE, protocols have been developed to depict PE and lower-extremity DVT when lower-extremity Doppler US is not available. This technique has been referred to as combined CT pulmonary angiography and indirect CT venography. No additional contrast agent is necessary to perform indirect CT venography after a patient undergoes a CT pulmonary angiogram. Not only does the addition of indirect CT venography provide alternative diagnoses for the patient's presentation but CT venography also increases the diagnosis of thromboembolic disease by 20%, compared with CT pulmonary angiogram alone.

V/Q Scan Interpretation

Multiple, bilateral perfusion defects with a normal ventilation scan are the classic diagnostic findings of PE (Fig. 72B.6).

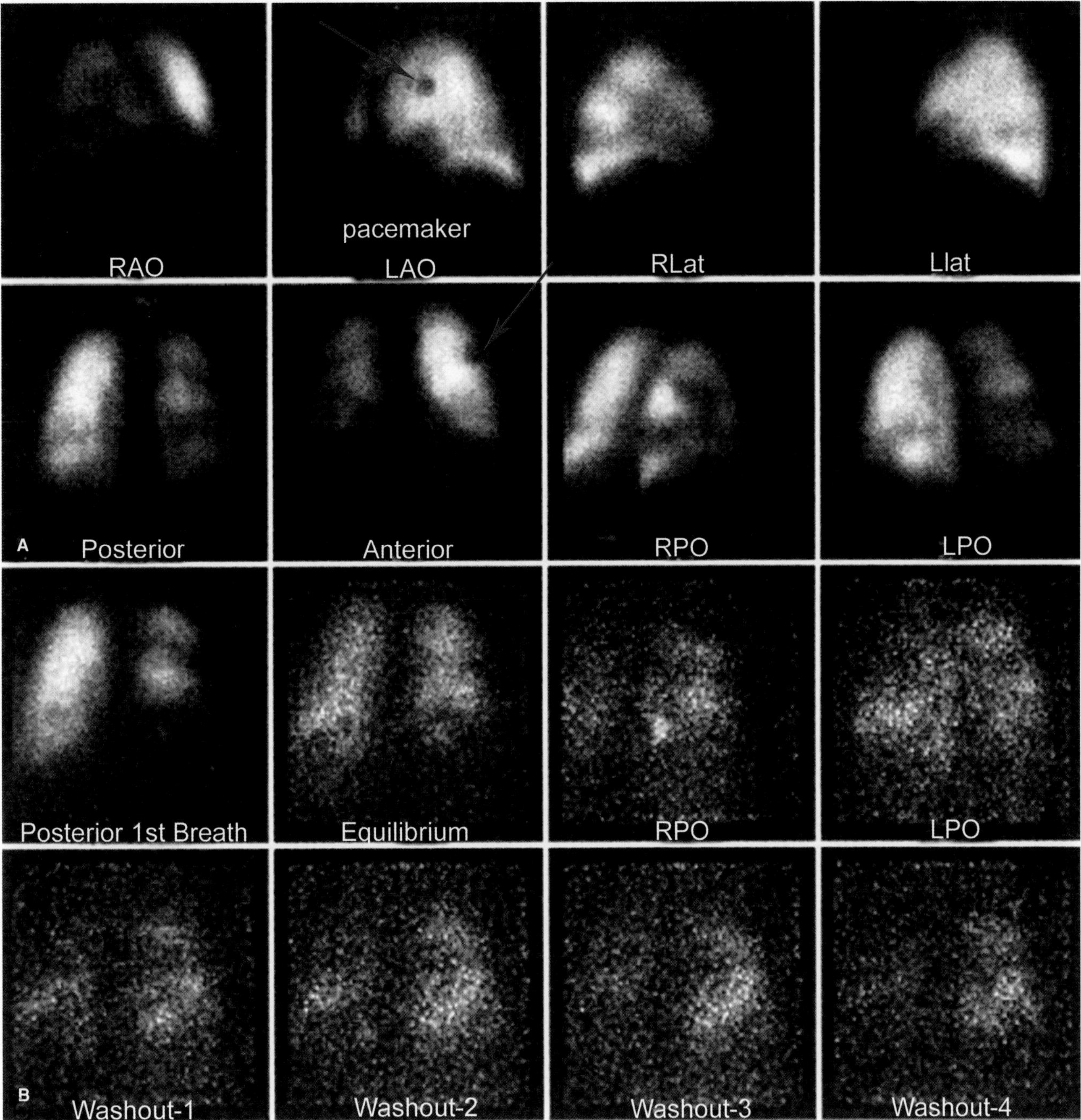

FIGURE 72B.4. **Chronic Obstructive Pulmonary Disease. A:** Tc-99m MAA perfusion (**top two rows**). Moderate to large bilateral perfusion defects match the ventilation scan defects. A nonsegmental defect is also present over the left upper lobe, representing an artifact secondary to a cardiac pacemaker (*arrow*). **B:** Xe-133 ventilation scan (**bottom two rows**). Patchy defects are seen in the mid and lower lung zones on the right on the initial breath image. The defects partially fill in on the equilibrium images (*equilibrium, RPO, LPO*). Persistent retention of Xe-133 is seen in these same regions on the washout images *1* to *4*. Labeling is the same as in Figure 72B.1.

Pulmonary emboli that occlude pulmonary arteries produce segmental perfusion defects that extend to the pleural surface. However, pneumonia, COPD, tumors, and prior infarcts may also produce perfusion defects. The ventilation scan is performed to improve the low specificity of the perfusion scan. As the bronchial tree is unaffected by intravascular emboli, the ventilation of the embolized region remains normal. Most nonembolic lung diseases have both ventilation and perfusion abnormalities, which are typically matched defects. Pulmonary emboli are more common in the lower lobes, because more pulmonary blood flow goes to the basilar pulmonary segments.

Criteria have been developed to categorize V/Q scan findings according to the likelihood that emboli will be demonstrated on pulmonary angiography. All interpretation schemes are based on carefully analyzing perfusion scan defects to determine whether they correspond to the anatomic segments or the subsegments of the lung. An understanding of the segmental anatomy of the lung is essential. The shape, location, and size of any defect are analyzed for fit to a specific pulmonary segment on all views.

Size of segmental defect must be assessed. By definition, a defect of less than 25% of a pulmonary segment is a small

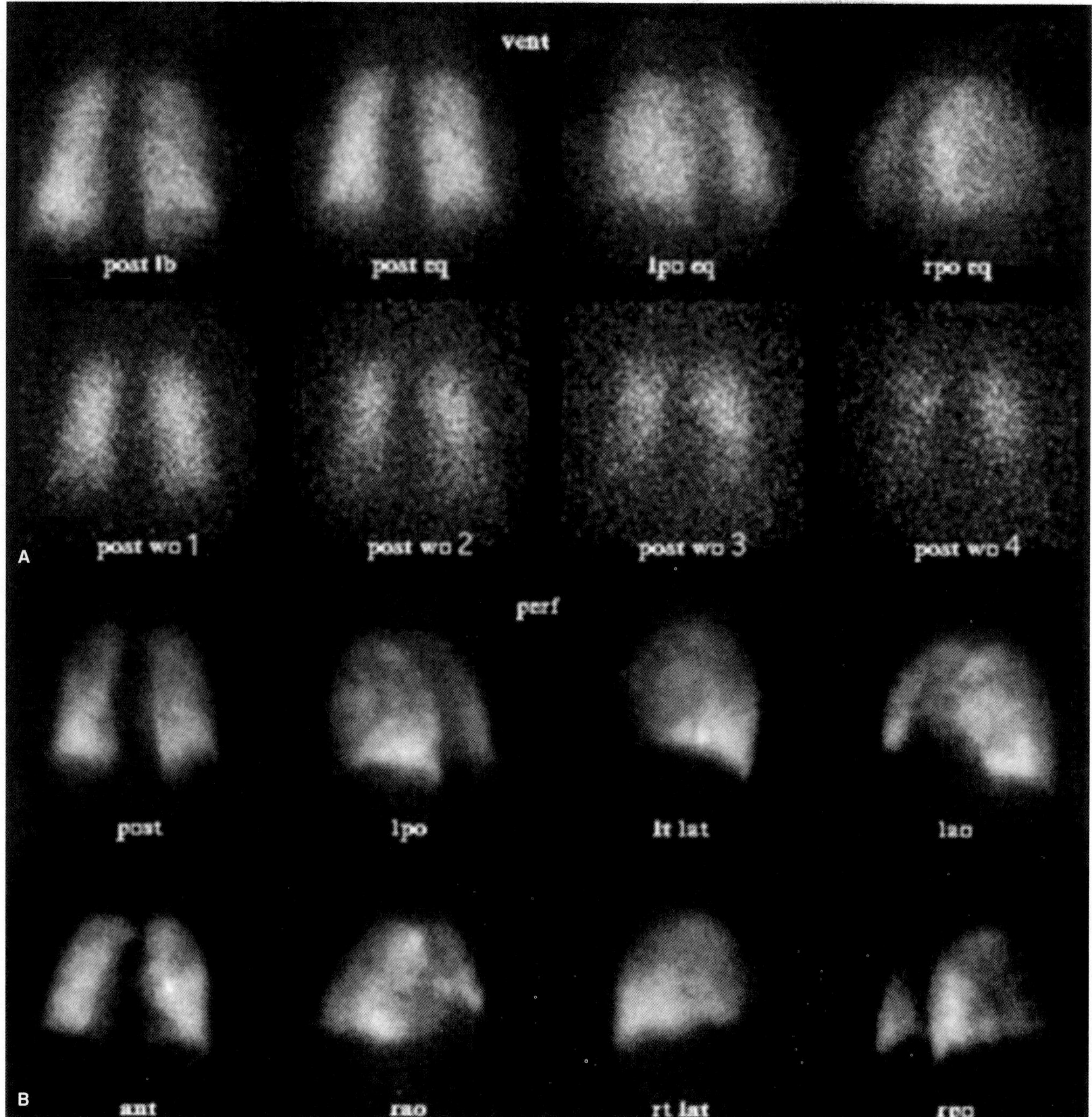

FIGURE 72B.5. **Chronic Obstructive Pulmonary Disease. A:** Ventilation scan, posterior projection (**top two rows**). Obstructive changes in the middle and upper lobes cause the retention of Xe-133 on a 4-minute washout image (*post wo/4*). *post ib*, posterior initial breath; *post eq*, posterior equilibrium; *lpo eq*, left posterior oblique equilibrium; *rpo eq*, right posterior oblique equilibrium; second row, postwashout images 1 to 4 minutes. **B:** Tc-99m MAA perfusion scan (**bottom two rows**), labeling is the same as in Figure 72B.1. Patchy, inhomogeneous uptake is seen primarily in the middle and upper lung zones. Perfusion defects match those seen on initial breath image of the ventilation scan.

defect, 25% to 75% a moderate defect, and greater than 75% a large defect. Subsegmental defects are summed to constitute full segment equivalents. Two moderate or four small perfusion defects are equivalent to a full segment defect. Even experienced readers tend to underestimate the size of segmental defects.

Interpretation schemes compare defects visualized on the perfusion scan with the corresponding regions of the ventilation scan and CXR. A perfusion defect that corresponds with normal ventilation is termed a *mismatched defect.* A perfusion defect the same size and location as a ventilation defect is called a *matched defect*. Perfusion defects that match ventilation and CXR abnormalities in size and location are called *triple matched defects*. The size and number of matched and/or mismatched segmental defects are used to estimate the likelihood that the defects represent pulmonary emboli.

Nonsegmental defects should be compared to CXRs to determine whether a mass, effusion, or mediastinal or hilar structure is responsible for the perfusion scan finding. Non-wedge-shaped defects, or wedge-shaped defects that do not correspond to segmental anatomy, are usually not due to pulmonary emboli. Common nonsegmental defects include

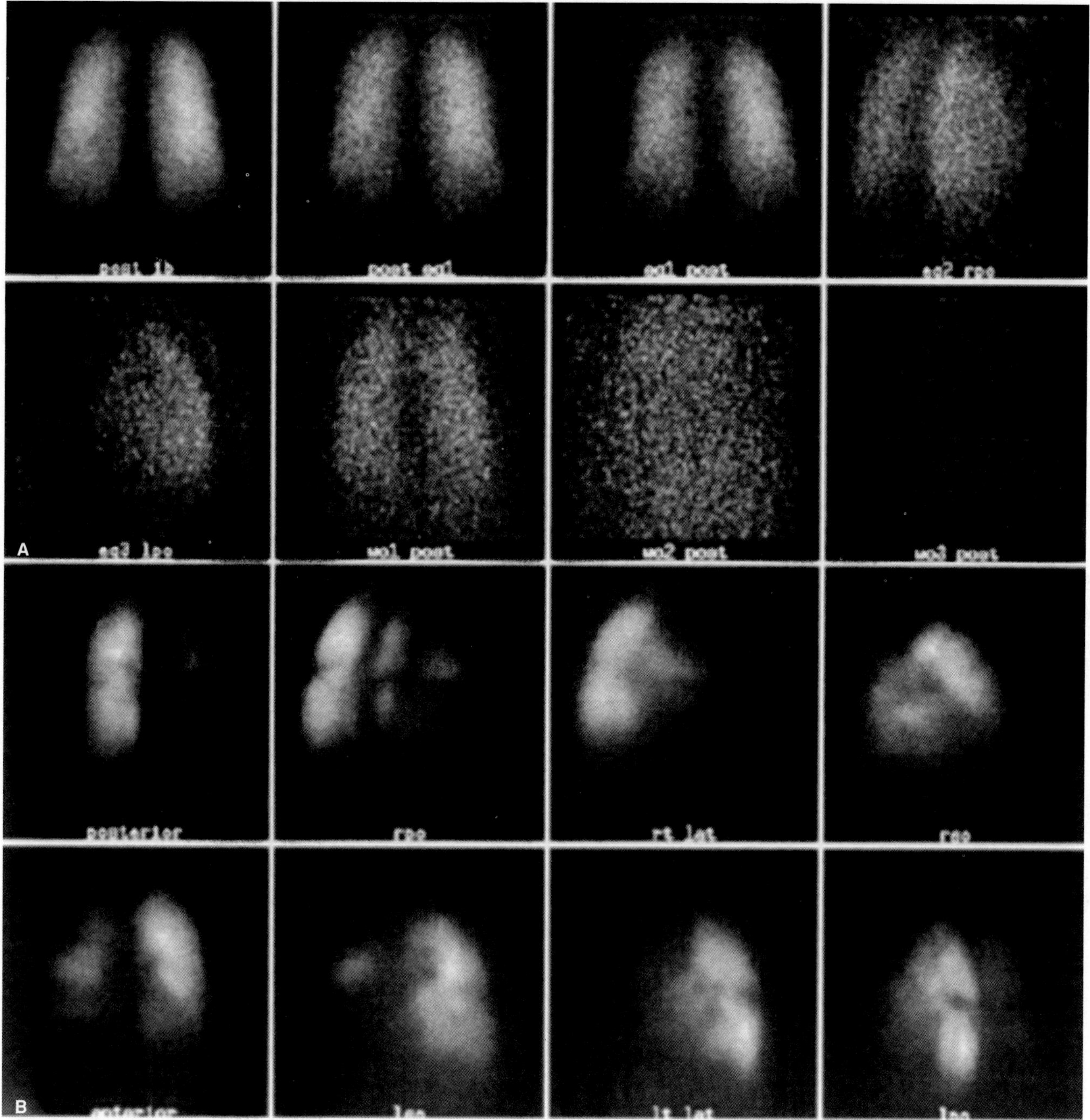

FIGURE 72B.6. **High-Probability V/Q Scan. A:** Xe-133 ventilation scan (**top two rows**) is normal. **B:** Tc-99m MAA perfusion scan (**bottom two rows**). Perfusion scan demonstrates the absence of perfusion to most segments of the right lung with multiple subsegmental defects in the left lung. Labeling is the same as in Figure 72B.3.

cardiomegaly, pleural effusions (Fig. 72B.7), adenopathy, hilar and parenchymal masses, cardiac pacemakers (Fig. 72B.5), pneumonia, large bullae, atelectasis, pulmonary hemorrhage, and aortic aneurysm or tortuosity.

Diagnostic Criteria. Biello criteria originally categorized V/Q scans as normal, low probability, intermediate, or high probability. The PIOPED study used a modified Biello criteria with more detailed categorizations of V/Q scan patterns. The PIOPED classification has undergone several revisions after retrospective analysis of the data pointed out the subcategories of incorrectly classified scan patterns. The amended PIOPED criteria are listed in Table 72B.1 (Figs. 72B.3, 72B.4, 72B.7, and 72B.8).

Stripe and Fissure Signs. Two types of perfusion defects not listed in either the original PIOPED or the Biello criteria have been found to strongly correlate with a normal pulmonary angiogram.

Central perfusion defects that have a rim or a stripe of increased activity around them have a less than 10% probability of being caused by PE. The defect as seen in different views does not extend to the pleural surface. The surrounding stripe of perfused lung is called the *stripe sign*. Pulmonary emboli perfusion defects extend to the pleural surface and have no overlying stripe of perfused lung.

Perfusion defects that match the location and shape of the major or minor fissures of the lung usually represent pleural

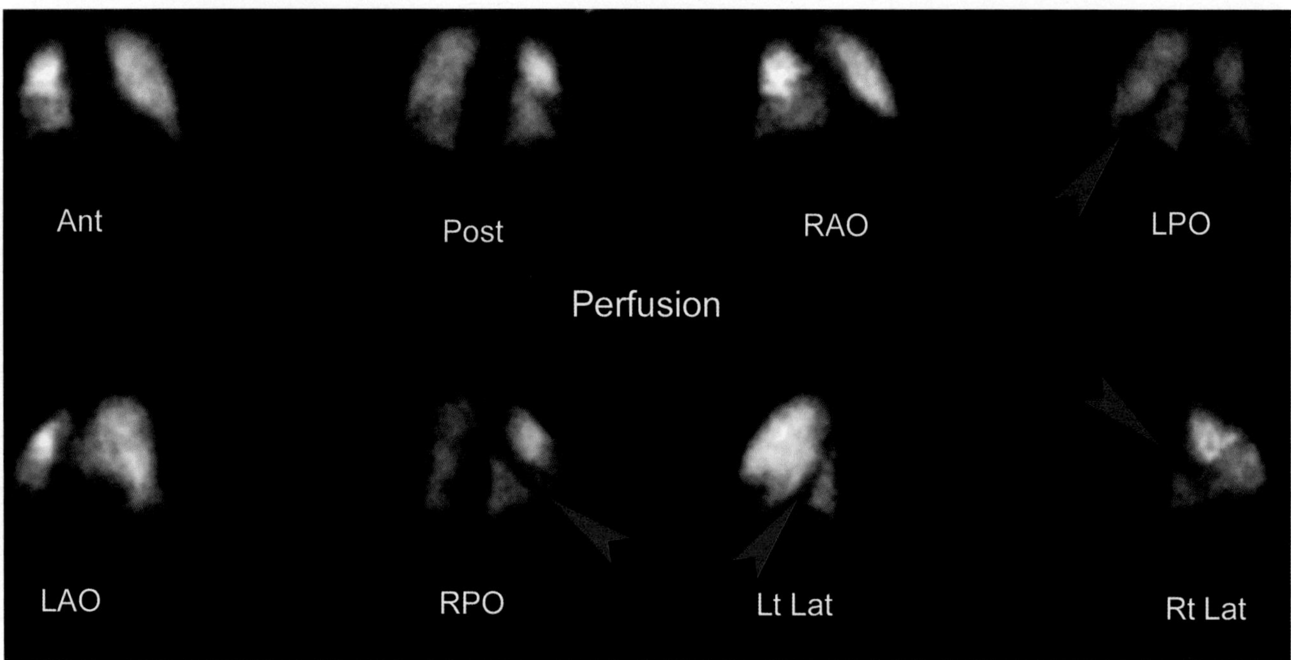

FIGURE 72B.7. **Low-Probability Perfusion Scan With Bilateral Pleural Effusions.** Scan demonstrates bilateral wedge-shaped defects that correspond to pleural effusions (*arrowheads*) within the major fissures bilaterally and the minor fissure on the right. Labeling is the same as in Figure 72B.1.

TABLE 72B.1

AMENDED PIOPED CRITERIA

V/Q SCAN CATEGORY	CRITERIA	LIKELIHOOD OF PE (%)	PREVALENCE OF PE (%)
High	Two or more mismatched perfusion segments or segmental equivalents without corresponding ventilation or CXR abnormalities: a. ≥2 large segmental perfusion defects b. One large and two moderate segmental defects c. ≥4 moderate segmental defects	≥80	87
Intermediate	1. One moderate to ≤2 large mismatched segments or segmental equivalents without corresponding ventilation or CXR abnormalities 2. Triple matched defects in the lower lung zone 3. Single moderate matched V/Q defects with normal CXR 4. Corresponding V/Q defects and small pleural effusion 5. Findings difficult to classify as normal, high, or low	20–79	35
Low	1. Multiple matched V/Q defects with a normal CXR 2. Corresponding V/Q defects and CXR opacities (triple matched defects) in the middle or upper lung zones 3. Corresponding V/Q defects and large pleural effusions (more than one-third of the hemithorax) 4. Any perfusion defect with substantially larger CXR abnormality 5. Any defect with a rim of surrounding normally perfused lung (stripe sign) 6. >3 small perfusion defects with normal CXR 7. Nonsegmental perfusion defects	≤19	12
Very low	<3 small perfusion defects with a normal CXR		2.5
Normal	No defects present on the perfusion scan or they exactly match the shape of the lungs on CXR		0

PE, pulmonary embolism; V/Q, ventilation/perfusion.

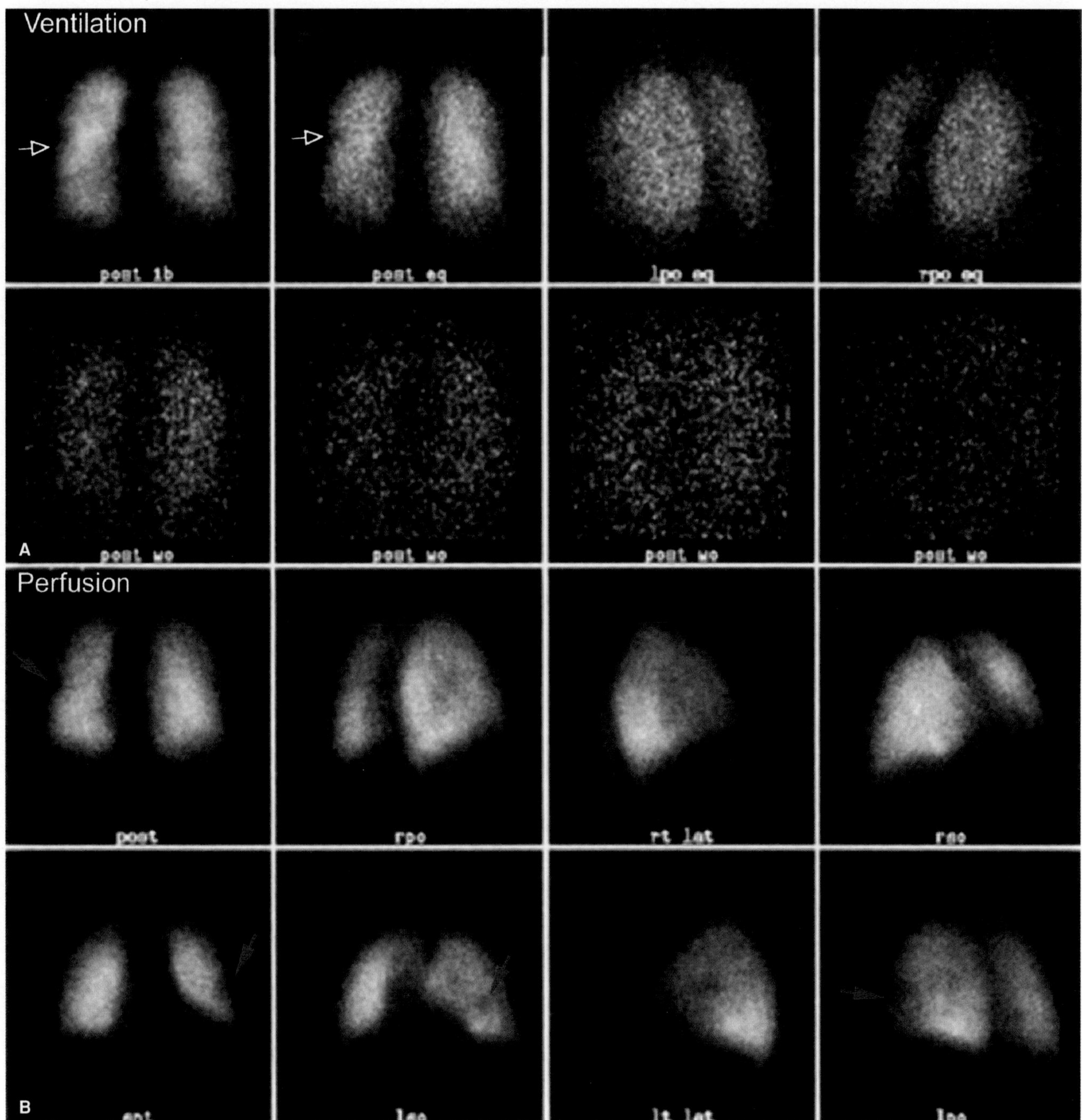

FIGURE 72B.8. Intermediate-Probability V/Q Scan. A: Xe-133 ventilation scan (**top two rows**) demonstrates a moderate-sized defect in the anterior medial basal segment of the left lower lobe (*open arrows*). **B:** Tc-99m macroaggregated albumin perfusion lung scan (**bottom two rows**). A single, moderate-sized matched perfusion defect is seen in the anterior medial basal segment of the left lower lobe (*arrows*). Labeling is the same as in Figure 72B.1. *wo*, washout.

effusions tracking into the fissures (Fig. 72B.7). When this type of defect is seen, the lateral view can be repeated with the patient in the supine or decubitus position to demonstrate layering of the fluid. The *fissure sign* usually correlates with the presence of a pleural effusion on CXR.

PIOPED Findings. The PIOPED study was designed to evaluate the usefulness of V/Q scans for diagnosing acute PE. In the original study, 13% of patients had high-probability V/Q scans, 39% intermediate, 34% low, and 14% normal or near-normal scans. The interobserver agreement in classifying scans was very good (92% to 95%) for normal/near-normal scans and high-probability scans but was significantly worse for low and intermediate scans (25% to 30%). The prevalence of thromboembolism in patients who underwent angiography was 33%. The sensitivity of a high-probability scan was 41% with a specificity of 97%.

The positive predictive value for a high-probability scan was 91% in patients with no prior history of PE but fell to 74% in those who had previously documented pulmonary emboli. Prior PE may leave residual perfusion defects that cannot be distinguished from acute emboli unless comparison

TABLE 72B.2

WELLS CRITERIA FOR OBJECTIVE CLINICAL ASSESSMENT OF PE[a]

CLINICAL FEATURES	SCORE (POINTS)
Clinical signs and symptoms of DVT (objectively measured leg swelling and pain with palpation in deep vein system)	3.0
Heart rate >100 beats/min	1.5
Immobilization >3 consecutive days (bed rest except to access bathroom) or surgery in previous 4 weeks	1.5
Previously objectively diagnosed PE or DVT	1.5
Hemoptysis	1.0
Malignancy (cancer patients receiving treatment within 6 months or receiving palliative treatment)	1.0
PE as likely or more likely than alternative diagnosis (based on history, physical examination, chest radiograph, ECG, and blood tests)	3.0

[a]Based on Wells PS, Anderson DR, Rodger M, et al. Excluding pulmonary embolism at the bedside without diagnostic imaging: management of patients with suspected pulmonary embolism presenting to the emergency department by using a simple clinical model and d-dimer. *Ann Intern Med* 2001;135:98–107; and van Belle A, Büller HR, Huisman MV, et al. Effectiveness of managing suspected pulmonary embolism using an algorithm combining clinical probability, D-dimer testing, and computed tomography. *JAMA* 2006;295:172–179.

Score: ≤4 = low probability, ≥4.5 = high probability.

PE, pulmonary embolism; DVT, deep venous thrombosis.

scans are available. Use of two segmental equivalents as the criteria for high probability yielded a likelihood for PE of 71%. Use of 2.5 segmental equivalent mismatched defects was 100% predictive of PE.

The negative predictive value of a normal or near-normal scan was 91% to 96%, while that of a low-probability scan was 84% to 88%. Patients with normal or nearly normal V/Q scans are highly unlikely to have clinically significant pulmonary emboli.

Clinical Assessment and V/Q Scan Interpretation. The V/Q scan should not be interpreted in a clinical vacuum. The PIOPED study demonstrated that adding the clinical assessment, such as Wells criteria (Table 72B.2), to V/Q scan interpretation improved the chance of correctly evaluating the patient's risk of having PE. An increased D-dimer level is not specific for venous thromboembolism and may occur in disseminated intravascular coagulation, infections, sepsis, recent trauma, and postoperative states. Thus, the Wells criteria in association with the D-dimer test are also often used by clinicians to determine who needs further evaluation for PE.

Of patients with high-probability scans and a high clinical suspicion, 96% had emboli on pulmonary angiography. Of patients with low-probability scans and low clinical suspicion, 96% had no evidence of PE on angiography. Patients with high-probability scans but intermediate clinical suspicion had an 88%-positive PE rate, while those with high-probability scans and low clinical suspicion had a 56%-positive PE rate. Patients with high-probability scans and high or intermediate clinical suspicion have a high risk of having pulmonary emboli that justifies treatment with anticoagulants. Patients with low-probability scans and low clinical suspicion have a very low chance of having PE.

V/Q Scans and Pulmonary Angiography. Patients with intermediate-probability scans have a significant risk of having PE. However, the V/Q scan alone is insufficient in determining which of these require anticoagulation therapy. Patients with intermediate-probability scans (Fig. 72B.9) and multiple risk factors or clinical findings suggestive of DVT should undergo another examination such as Doppler US or CTA. If DVT is diagnosed, the patient can be placed on anticoagulants that would treat the DVT and PE, if present. If the noninvasive search for DVT is negative, then CTA or pulmonary angiography should be performed. The location of mismatched defects on the perfusion scan would be the most likely site for PE. CTA or pulmonary angiogram should also be strongly considered to confirm the diagnosis of PE in patients with high-probability scans when anticoagulation is risky. It may also be indicated in patients with low-probability scans but high clinical suspicion for having PE.

V/Q Scans With SPECT and Low-Dose CT. Both V/Q SPECT and CTA have higher diagnostic accuracy versus V/Q alone (Fig. 72B.10). Recently, hybrid gamma camera/CTA systems have been introduced to allow for simultaneous V/Q SPECT and CTA, which may be used for diagnosing PE.

A prospective study by Gutte et al. in 2009 used a hybrid camera to compare the diagnostic ability of V/Q SPECT, V/Q SPECT combined with low-dose CT without intravenous contrast, and CTA for diagnosing PE. V/Q SPECT alone and V/Q SPECT combined with low-dose CT had a high sensitivity, higher than that of CTA. Both V/Q SPECT with low-dose CT and CTA had 100% specificity whereas V/Q SPECT alone had a lower specificity. Moreover, perfusion SPECT with low-dose CT had a high sensitivity and a low specificity.

Low-dose CT eliminates the need for CXR and increases sensitivity, specificity, and accuracy compared with CXR for alternative diagnosis. With combined scanners, V/Q SPECT with low-dose CT not only reduces radiation exposure but also gives a higher sensitivity and specificity for PE compared with CTA.

Follow-Up V/Q Scans Post Anticoagulation. Most patients with PE show a gradual reduction in the size of perfusion defects with normalization of their scans within 3 months. Defects still present after 3 months of anticoagulation will usually remain as permanent abnormalities. The larger the initial defect, the less likely it is to completely resolve. Perfusion scan defects are thought to last longer than filling defects detectable on CT and pulmonary angiographies.

Follow-up scans done within 2 weeks of the initiation of anticoagulation therapy may show new defects that do not

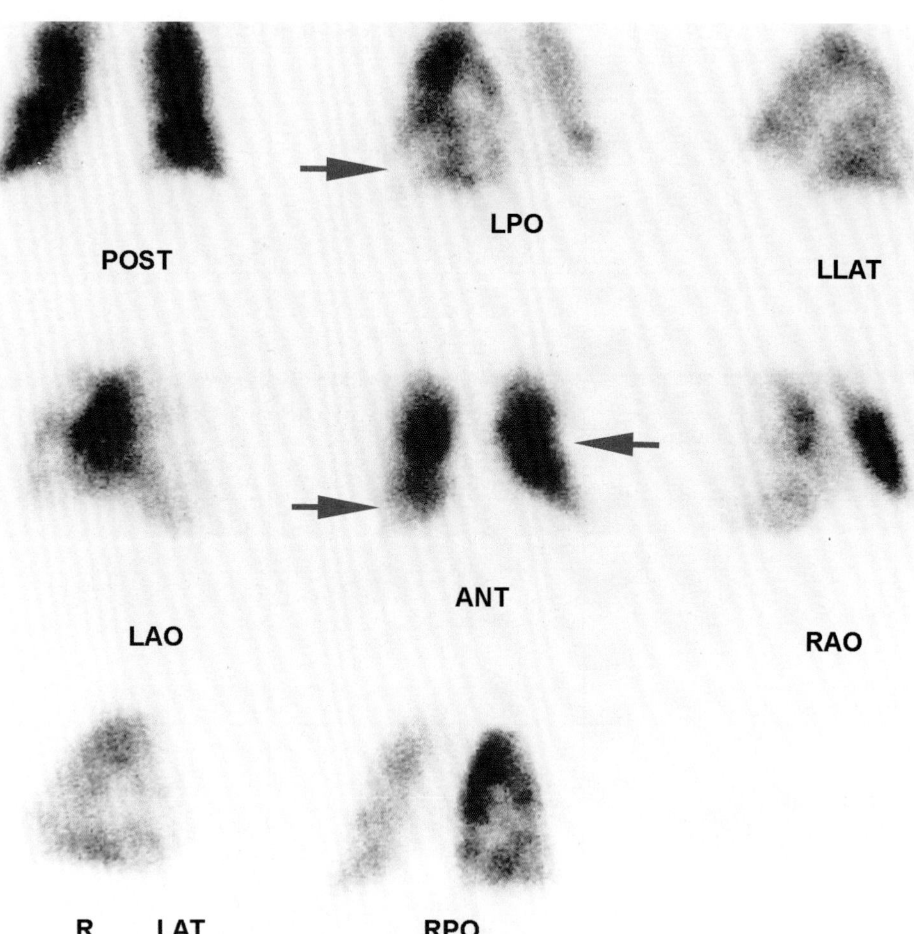

FIGURE 72B.9. **Intermediate-Probability V/Q Scan.** Tc-99m MAA perfusion scan demonstrates multiple bilateral small and moderate defects (*arrows*). The Xe-133 ventilation scan was normal. Labeling is the same as in Figure 72B.1.

represent recurrent emboli. Large central thrombi may fragment and produce small distal thrombi. Thus, emboli that were previously nonocclusive may become obstructive and show as new defects. The diagnosis of recurrent PE is more likely if multiple new large or moderate defects are present in areas that were previously normal (Fig. 72B.11).

False-Positive V/Q Scans. Mismatched perfusion defects can represent chronic pulmonary emboli in patients with a remote history of PE. Follow-up V/Q scans after patients have been placed on oral anticoagulants are useful as baselines in this patient population. If old scans are available, it is possible to determine which emboli are old and which are new. Patients with a history of PE are at higher risk of having a PE than patients without such a history. Mismatched perfusion defects can also be produced by extrinsic compression of the pulmonary vessels such as masses or adenopathy. The pulmonary vessels may also become obstructed by mediastinal fibrosis, intraluminal metastases, sarcomas, and lymphangitic carcinomatosis. Radiation therapy and vasculitis, such as Takayasu arteritis and systemic lupus erythematosus, can also cause false-positive scans.

False-Negative V/Q Scans. V/Q scans may be falsely negative if the emboli are only partially occlusive. Very small emboli may produce perfusion defects too small to be visualized on a perfusion scan, but are thought to be clinically insignificant.

Nonthromboembolic Pulmonary Disease

Asthma produces bronchospastic narrowing of the airways, resulting in decreased ventilation. Focal segmental or subsegmental ventilation defects are present on the first-breath image during an acute asthma attack. These defects may wash in on the equilibrium images. Defects associated with mucus plugs may persist. Bronchospasm induces localized hypoxia, which in turn produces localized vasoconstriction and perfusion scan defects that match the ventilation defects. This can result in an intermediate or a low-probability scan. Most V/Q defects caused by asthma will resolve within 24 hours of bronchodilator therapy.

Lung neoplasms may produce V/Q scan abnormalities. Focal parenchymal masses and extrinsic mediastinal or chest wall tumors that displace lung parenchyma tend to produce matching V/Q defects, which correspond to the size and shape of the mass on CXR.

The V/Q defects do not correspond to segmental anatomy unless the mass has invaded or compressed a local branch of the bronchovascular tree. This may result in a perfusion defect, a ventilation defect, or a matched defect.

Quantitative Perfusion Lung Scan. Perfusion lung scans are useful in preoperatively estimating a lung carcinoma patient's postsurgical pulmonary function. The quantitative perfusion scan is performed in the same manner as that of a regular perfusion lung scan except that a single posterior image is obtained. Regions of interest are drawn around each lung and the counts over each lung are obtained. Often, each lung is split into three regions of interest: upper, middle, and lower. The percentage of the total count that each lung contributes is calculated (Fig. 72B.12). The postoperative forced expiratory volume in 1 second (FEV1) is estimated by multiplying the preoperative FEV1 by the percent perfusion going to the lung that will remain after pneumonectomy. With SPECT

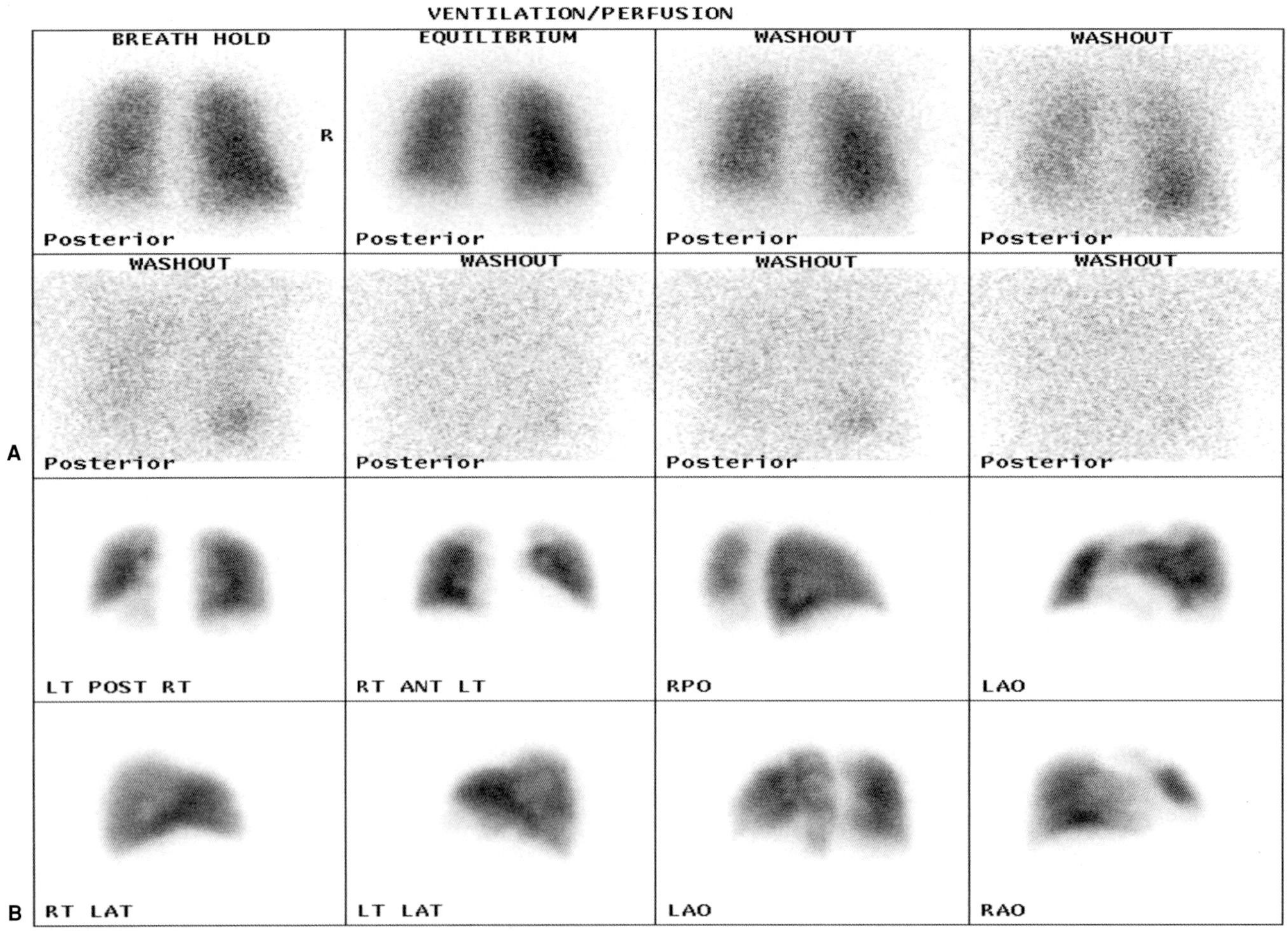

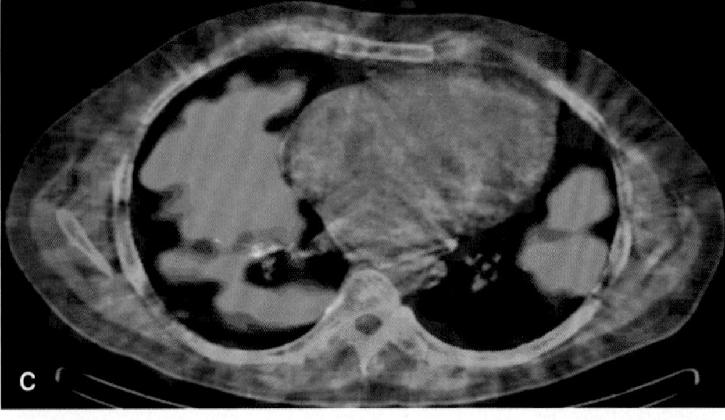

FIGURE 72B.10. **High-Probability Ventilation/Perfusion Scan With SPECT. A:** Xenon-133 ventilation scan (**top two rows**) demonstrates normal ventilation on the breath-hold and wash-in images but moderate retention in the right lower lobe. **B:** Technetium-99m macroaggregated albumin perfusion scan (**bottom two rows**) demonstrates small to moderate unmatched perfusion defects in the left apical posterior and left apical segments, large unmatched perfusion defect in the lateral basal segment of the left lower lobe, small unmatched defect in the medial basal segment of the left lower lobe, and small nonsegmental matched perfusion defect in the right lung base. **C:** SPECT of thorax demonstrates multiple perfusion defects consistent with high probability for pulmonary embolism. Labeling is the same as in Figure 72B.1.

acquisition or a lateral projection, outcomes for an upper or a lower lobectomy could also be estimated. A patient needs to have a postoperative FEV1 of 800 to 1,000 mL to have adequate lung function.

Chronic Obstructive Pulmonary Disease. The narrowed airways associated with COPD reduce ventilation. Xenon scans demonstrate delayed wash-in and delayed washout. First-breath images may have defects that gradually fill in on the equilibrium phase. Xenon washes out of the affected area more slowly than the rest of the lung and may still be visible on images more than 3 minutes after the patient is switched to breathing room air.

Perfusion lung scans are also frequently abnormal. Localized hypoxia in the lung induces localized vasoconstriction. Destruction of lung and inflammatory narrowing of blood vessels produce areas of reduced perfusion. Regions of the lung that demonstrate obstructive changes on the ventilation scan usually have corresponding abnormalities on the perfusion scan (Figs. 72B.4 and 72B.5). When the ventilatory changes are widespread, the perfusion scan has a mottled appearance. Perfusion scans may be normal if the ventilatory obstructive changes produce little hypoxia or vascular damage. Since COPD tends to affect the lung apices more than the bases, V/Q abnormalities are usually more pronounced at the apices. However, α-1-antitrypsin deficiency produces more pronounced emphysematous changes in the lower lobes, which are reflected on the V/Q scan.

Inflammatory/Infectious Disease of the Lung. Areas of consolidation on CXR will be abnormal on a V/Q scan. Consolidated areas do not ventilate well and produce defects on ventilation scans. The resulting local hypoxia produces reflex vasoconstriction and may cause perfusion defects in the consolidated region. Perfusion defects which are significantly smaller than the consolidated region on CXR are of low probability for PE. Perfusion defects which are significantly larger than the CXR abnormality are of high probability for PE.

Tc-99m aerosol clearance from the lung has also been used to evaluate inflammatory diseases of the lung. Normals have a Tc-99m aerosol lung clearance half-life of approximately 60 minutes. Increased permeability of inflamed pulmonary epithelium shortens the clearance time. Alveolitis and acute respiratory distress syndrome have rapid Tc-99m aerosol lung clearance. Smokers also have faster than normal aerosol clearance. Conversely, processes that thicken the alveolar membranes or cause fibrosis will have prolonged Tc-99m aerosol clearance. Abnormal aerosol clearance is a very sensitive but nonspecific indicator of inflammation.

Smoke Inhalation. Many patients with serious burns also have inhalation injury of the lungs. Of patients admitted to a hospital for burns, 20% to 30% develop pulmonary complications and 70% to 75% of these patients die. Smoke consists of a mixture of toxic gases and particles. Inhalation of these toxins combines with thermal injury to produce severe pulmonary damage. A CXR is insensitive in detecting early inhalation injury with a lag period of 12 to 48 hours before the CXR

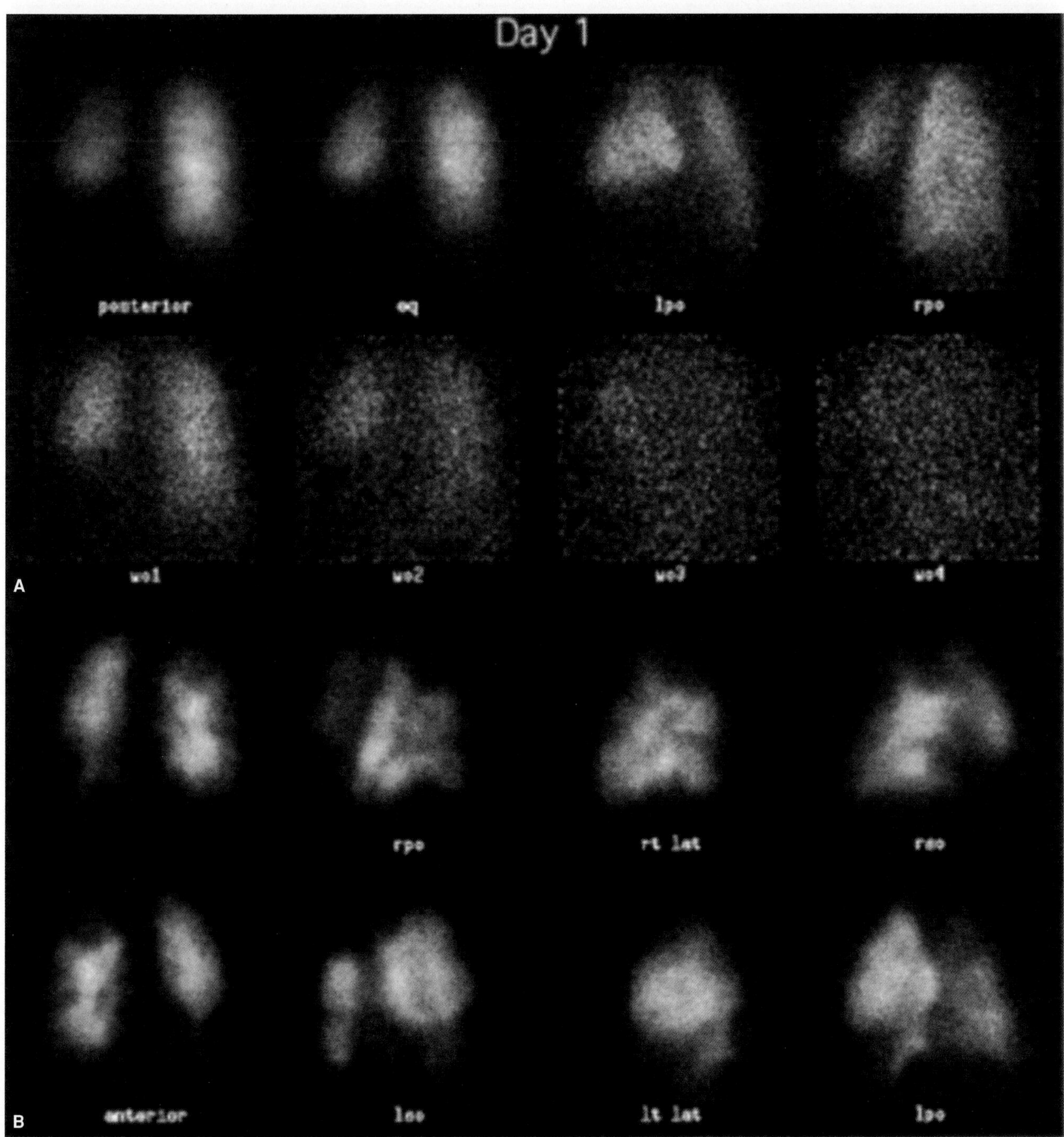

FIGURE 72B.11. **Recurrent Pulmonary Emboli. A:** Xe-133 ventilation scan (**top two rows**) demonstrates lack of ventilation of most of the left lower lobe due to a pleural effusion. **B:** Tc-99m macroaggregated albumin (MAA) perfusion scan (**third and fourth rows**) demonstrates multiple moderate and large mismatched perfusion defects in the right lung. (*continued*)

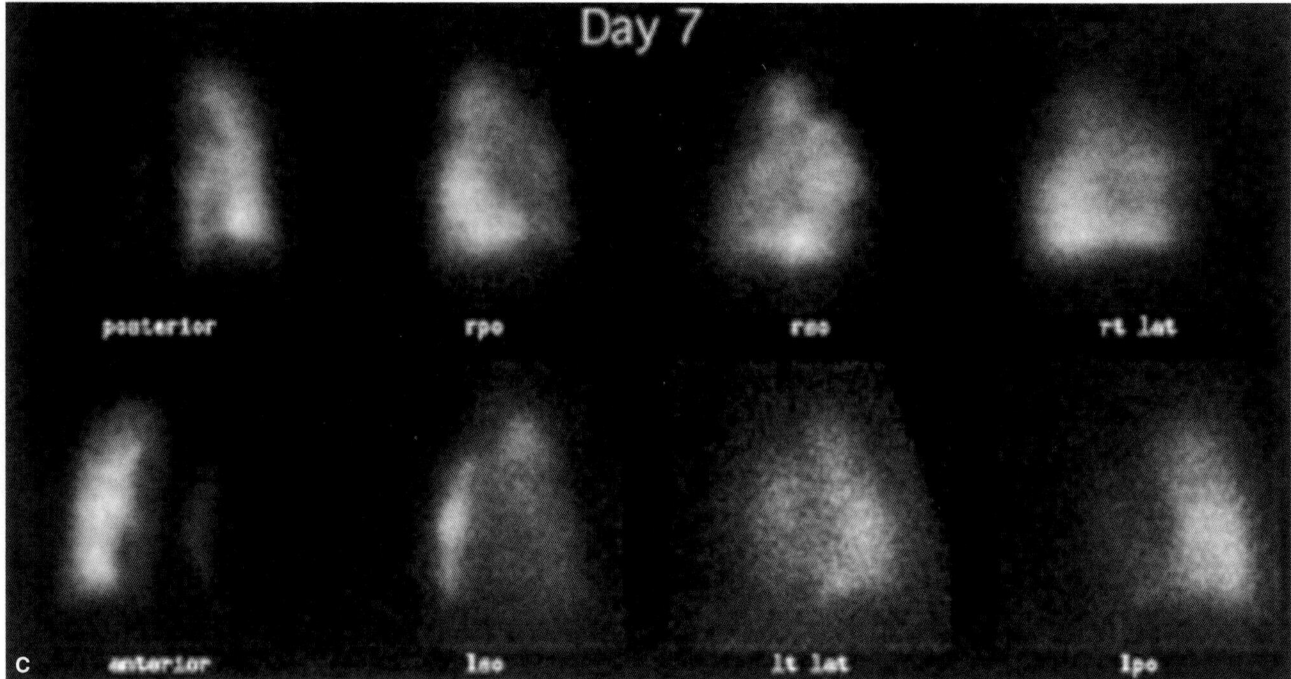

FIGURE 72B.11. (*Continued*) **C:** Repeat Tc-99m MAA perfusion scan was performed 1 week later. Patient had recurrent symptoms while being treated with heparin. Marked improvement seen in the perfusion defects previously noted in the right lung indicates the resolution of some of the emboli with therapy. The left lung on the new scan shows almost complete absence of perfusion indicative of new emboli to the lungs despite anticoagulation.

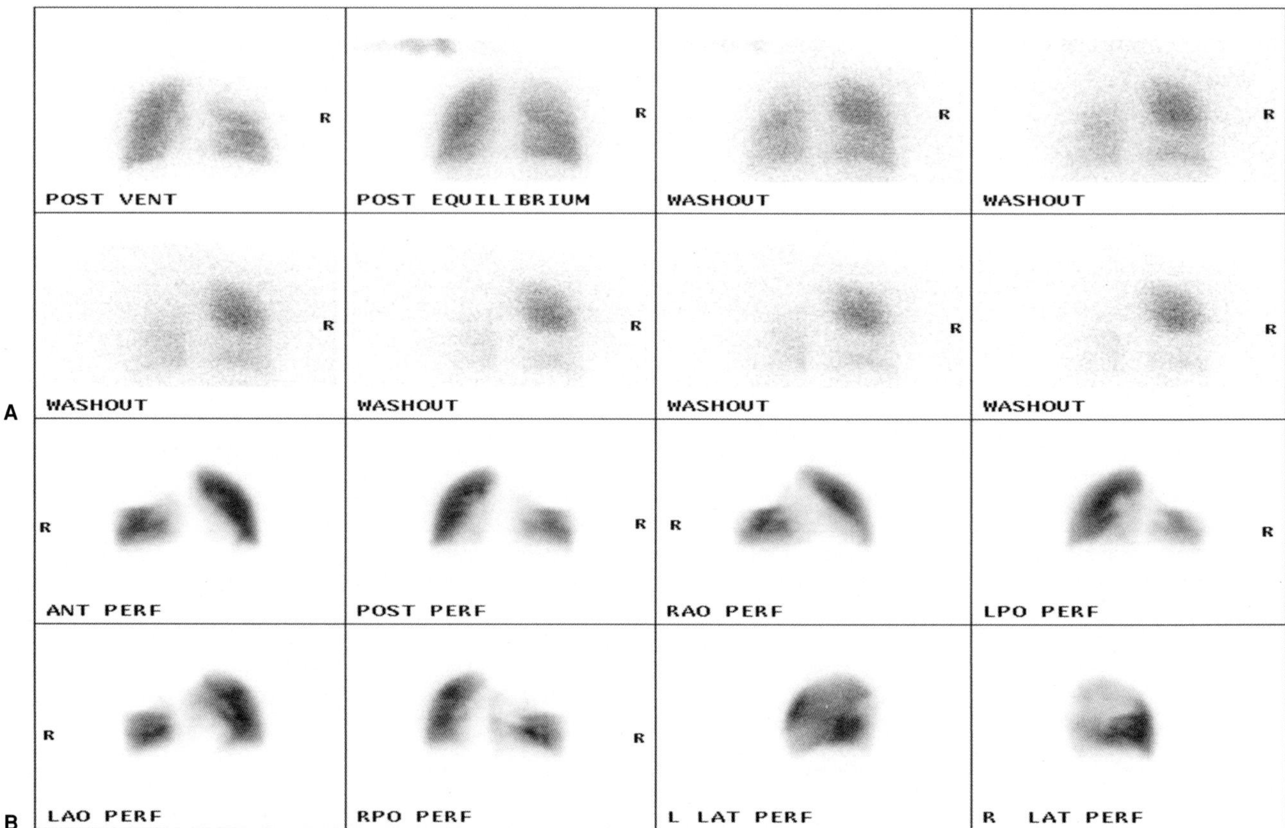

FIGURE 72B.12. **Quantitative Tc-99m Macroaggregated Albumin Perfusion Scan. A:** Xenon-133 ventilation scan (**top two rows**) demonstrates asymmetric ventilation with delayed uptake within the right upper lobe consistent with a restrictive process. There is significant xenon retention within the right upper lobe on the washout images consistent with an obstructive process. **B:** Technetium-99m macroaggregated albumin perfusion scan (**bottom two rows**) demonstrates a markedly diminished perfusion to the right upper lobe, which is matched.

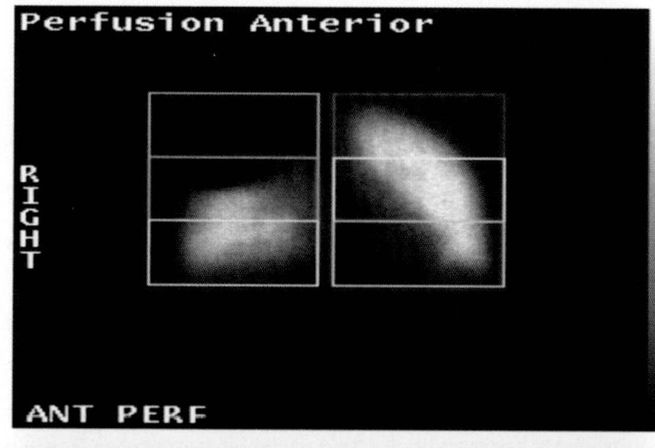

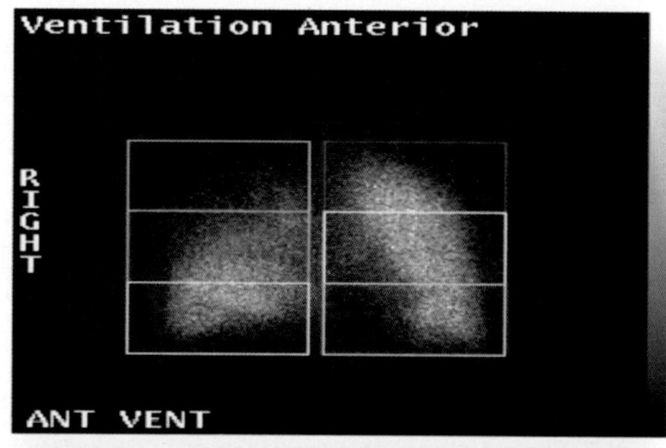

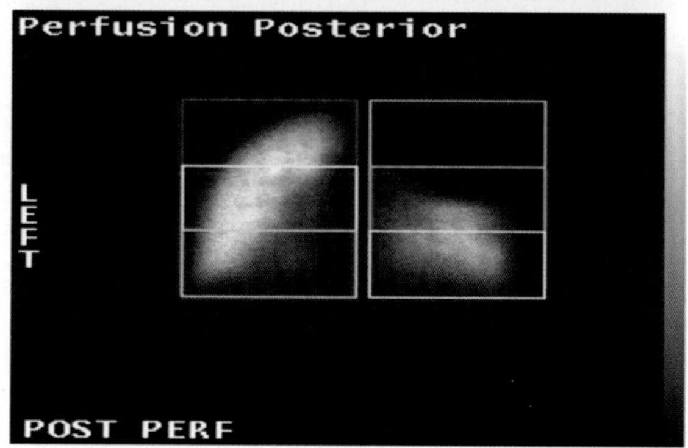

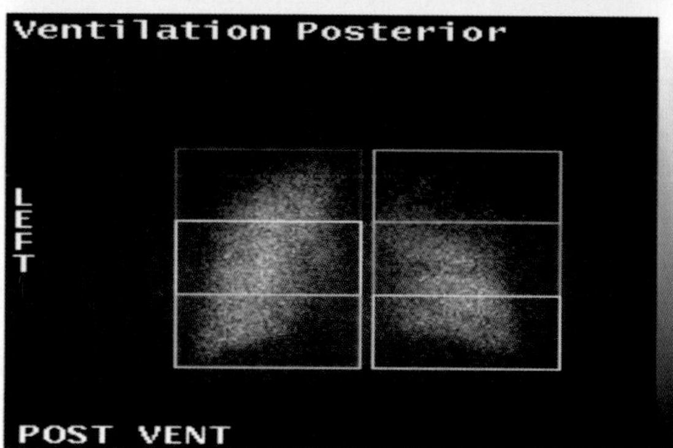

C

	Perfusion% Geometric Mean		Ventilation% Geometric Mean	
	Right	Left	Right	Left
Upper	1.1	18.0	5.3	14.5
Middle	13.2	32.6	20.0	27.3
Lower	19.8	15.2	17.1	15.9
Total	34.2	65.8	42.4	57.6

FIGURE 72B.12. (*Continued*) C: Quantitative ventilation and perfusion. The percentage of the pulmonary perfusion to each lung is calculated based on the relative counts over each lung on the posterior image.

becomes abnormal. Xenon-in-saline ventilation scans have proven useful in detecting inhalation lung injury. Xenon-133 under pressure will dissolve in saline. When injected intravenously, the xenon remains in solution until it reaches the lungs. In the alveolar capillaries, the xenon diffuses across the capillary membrane into the alveoli and is exhaled. Normally, the xenon washes out of the lungs in less than 2 minutes. Areas of inhalational injury demonstrate the retention of xenon. The xenon in saline study is 92% accurate in detecting lung injury.

Suggested Readings

Bell WR, Simon TL, DeMets DL. The clinical features of submassive and massive pulmonary emboli. *Am J Med* 1977;62:355–360.

Biello DR, Mattar AG, McKnight RC, Siegel BA. Ventilation–perfusion studies in suspected pulmonary embolism. *AJR Am J Roentgenol* 1979;133:1033–1037.

Cham MD, Yankelevitz DF, Henschke CI. Thromboembolic disease detection at indirect CT venography versus CT pulmonary angiography. *Radiology* 2005;234:591–594.

Dahlen JE, Alpert JS. Natural history of pulmonary embolism. *Prog Cardiovasc Dis* 1975;17:259–270.

De Faucal P, Peltier P, Planchon B, et al. Evaluation of indium-111-labeled antifibrin monoclonal antibody for the diagnosis of venous thrombotic disease. *J Nucl Med* 1991;32:785–791.

Elgazzar AH, Silberstein EB, Hughes J. Perfusion and ventilation scans in patients with extensive obstructive airways disease: utility of single-breath (washin) xenon-133. *J Nucl Med* 1995;36:64–67.

Eng J, Krishnah JA, Segal JB, et al. Accuracy of CT in the diagnosis of pulmonary embolism: a systematic literature review. *AJR Am J Roentgenol* 2004;183:1819–1827.

Fraser RS, Muller NL, Coleman N, Pare PD. *Diagnosis of Diseases of the Chest.* 4th ed. Philadelphia, PA: WB Saunders; 1999.

Freeman LM, Stein EG, Sprayregen S, Chamarthy M, Haramati LB. The current and continuing important role of ventilation–perfusion scintigraphy in evaluating patients with suspected pulmonary embolism. *Semin Nucl Med* 2008;38:432–440.

Goldberg SN, Richardson DD, Palmer EL, Scott JA. Pleural effusion and ventilation/perfusion scan interpretation for acute pulmonary embolus. *J Nucl Med* 1996;37:1310–1313.

Gottschalk A, Sostman HD, Coleman RE, et al. Ventilation–perfusion scintigraphy in the PIOPED study. Part II. Evaluation of the scintigraphic criteria and interpretations. *J Nucl Med* 1993;34:1119–1126.

Gottschalk A, Stein PD, Henry JW, Relyea B. Matched ventilation, perfusion and chest radiographic abnormalities in acute pulmonary embolism. *J Nucl Med* 1996;37:1636–1638.

Groves AM, Yates SJ, Win T, et al. CT pulmonary angiography versus ventilation–perfusion scintigraphy in pregnancy: implications from a UK survey of doctors' knowledge of radiation exposure. *Radiology* 2006;240: 765–770.

Gutte H, Mortensen J, Jensen C, von der Recke P, Kristoffersen US, Kjaer A. Added value of combined simultaneous lung ventilation-perfusion single-photon emission computed tomography/multi-slice-computed tomography angiography in two patients suspected of having acute pulmonary embolism. *Clin Respir J* 2007;1:52–55.

Gutte H, Mortensen J, Jensen CV, et al. Detection of pulmonary embolism with combined ventilation-perfusion SPECT and low-dose CT: head-to-head comparison with multidetector CT angiography. *J Nucl Med* 2009;50: 1987–1992.

Henry JW, Stein PD, Gottschalk A, Raskob GE. Pulmonary embolism among patients with a nearly normal ventilation/perfusion lung scan. *Chest* 1996;110:395–398.

Juni JE, Alavi A. Lung scanning in the diagnosis of pulmonary embolism: the emperor redressed. *Semin Nucl Med* 1991;21:281–296.

Kipper MS, Moser KM, Kortman KE, Ashburn WL. Longterm follow-up of patients with suspected pulmonary embolism and a normal lung scan. Perfusion scans in embolic suspects. *Chest* 1982;82:411–415.

Leung AN, Bull TM, Jaeschke R, et al; ATS/STR Committee on Pulmonary Embolism in Pregnancy. American Thoracic Society documents: an official American Thoracic Society/Society of Thoracic Radiology clinical practice guideline—evaluation of suspected pulmonary embolism in Pregnancy. *Radiology* 2012;262(2):635–646.

Line BR. Scintigraphic studies of inflammation in diffuse lung disease. *Radiol Clin North Am* 1991;29:1095–1114.

Lull RJ, Anderson JH, Telepak RJ, Brown JM, Utz JA. Radionuclide imaging in the assessment of lung injury. *Semin Nucl Med* 1980;10:302–310.

Morrell NW, Nijran KS, Jones BE, Biggs T, Seed WA. The underestimation of segmental defect size in radionuclide lung scanning. *J Nucl Med* 1993;34:370–374.

Muto P, Lastoria S, Varrella P, et al. Detecting deep venous thrombosis with technetium-99m-labeled synthetic peptide P280. *J Nucl Med* 1995;36:1384–1391.

Palevsky HI. The problems of the clinical and laboratory diagnosis of pulmonary embolism. *Semin Nucl Med* 1991;21:276–280.

Parker JA, Coleman RE, Siegel BA, Sostman HD, McKusick KA, Royal HD. Procedure guideline for lung scintigraphy: 1.0. Society of Nuclear Medicine. *J Nucl Med* 1996;37:1906–1910.

PIOPED Investigators. Value of the ventilation/perfusion scan in acute pulmonary embolism. Results of the prospective investigation of pulmonary embolism diagnosis (PIOPED). *JAMA* 1990;263:2753–2759.

Robinson PJ. Ventilation-perfusion lung scanning and spiral computed tomography of the lungs: competing or complementary modalities? *Eur J Nucl Med* 1996;23:1547–1553.

Schaible TF, Alavi A. Antifibrin scintigraphy in the diagnostic evaluation of acute deep venous thrombosis. *Semin Nucl Med* 1991;21:313–324.

Sostman HD, Coleman RE, DeLong DM, Newman GE, Paine S. Evaluation of revised criteria for ventilation–perfusion scintigraphy in patients with suspected pulmonary embolism. *Radiology* 1994;193:103–107.

Sostman HD, Gottschalk A. The stripe sign: a new sign for diagnosis of nonembolic defects on pulmonary perfusion scintigraphy. *Radiology* 1982;142:737–741.

Sostman HD, Gottschalk A. Prospective validation of the stripe sign in ventilation-perfusion scintigraphy. *Radiology* 1992;184:455–459.

Sostman HD, Layish DT, Tapson VF, et al. Prospective comparison of helical CT and MR imaging in clinically suspected acute pulmonary embolism. *J Magn Reson Imaging* 1996;6:275–281.

Susskind H. Technetium-99m-DTPA aerosol to measure alveolar-capillary membrane permeability. *J Nucl Med* 1994;35:207–209.

van Belle A, Buller HR, Huissman MV, et al. Effectiveness of managing suspected pulmonary embolism using an algorithm combining clinical probability, D-dimer testing, and computed tomography. *JAMA* 2006;295:172–179.

van Rossum AB, Treurniet FE, Kieft GJ, Smith SJ, Schepers-Bok R. Role of spiral volumetric computed tomographic scanning in the assessment of patients with clinical suspicion of pulmonary embolism and an abnormal ventilation/perfusion scan. *Thorax* 1996;51:23–28.

Wells PS, Anderson DR, Rodger M, et al. Excluding pulmonary embolism at the bedside without diagnostic imaging: management of patients with suspected pulmonary embolism presenting to the emergency department by using a simple clinical model and d-dimer. *Ann Intern Med* 2001;135:98–107.

Wittram C, Maher MM, Yoo AJ, Kalra MK, Shepard JA, McLoud TC. CT angiography of pulmonary embolism: diagnostic criteria and causes of misdiagnosis. *Radiographics* 2004;24:1219–1238.

Worsley DF, Alavi A. Comprehensive analysis of the results of the PIOPED study. Prospective Investigation of Pulmonary Embolism Diagnosis Study. *J Nucl Med* 1995;36:2380–2387.

Worsley DF, Alavi A. Radionuclide imaging of acute pulmonary embolism. *Radiol Clin North Am* 2001;39:1035–1052.

CHAPTER 72C ■ SKELETAL SYSTEM SCINTIGRAPHY

BRETT J. MOLLARD

TECHNIQUE

Musculoskeletal imaging studies performed with gamma cameras and technetium-99m (Tc-99m) labeled diphosphonates are a staple of nuclear medicine. The bone scan is a map of osteoblastic activity that occurs in response to various benign and malignant conditions. It is an excellent complement to anatomic studies of the skeletal system and is usually far more sensitive in detecting bony abnormalities such as osteomyelitis and osseous metastatic disease. After intravenous injection, blood flow is required to deliver the radiopharmaceutical to the extracellular space around functioning osteoblasts. Within minutes, osteoblasts begin to assemble labeled diphosphonates into the hydration shell of hydroxyapatite crystals as they are formed and modified. Osteoclastic function is not measured by this technique.

Radiopharmaceuticals. Technetium-based diphosphonates, primarily Tc-99m MDP, are the primary radiopharmaceuticals used for skeletal scintigraphy. Tc-99m has a physical half-life of 6 hours and a gamma-ray energy of 140 keV (Table 72C.1). The usual adult dose is approximately 20 mCi intravenously; however, up to 30 mCi may be used in heavy patients or for better detail.

Fluorine-18 sodium fluoride (NaF) is a positron-emitting radionuclide used for PET (and PET-CT) bone scans. A dose of 5 to 15 mCi is given intravenously and imaging is performed as early as 30 minutes (axial skeleton) and as late as 120 minutes (appendicular skeleton) following administration. Attenuation correction with CT is typically unnecessary given the high intrinsic image quality. Fluorine-18 has an energy of 511 keV and half-life of 120 minutes.

Three common radionuclides are used for internal radiotherapy of painful osseous metastatic disease: strontium-89, samarium-153, and radium-223.

- **Strontium-89 (Metastron)** is a **pure β emitter** with an energy of 1.46 MeV and a 50.5-day half-life. It is given intravenously with a typical dose of 2 to 4 mCi.
- **Samarium-153 (Quadramet)** is a **β emitter** with 0.81 MeV and has a gamma photon of 103 keV, which can be used for imaging. The usual dose is 1 mCi/kg intravenously and it has a half-life of 1.9 days.
- **Radium-223 (Xofigo)** is an **α emitter** with an energy range of 5 to 7.5 MeV and a half-life of 11.4 days. The recommended dose is 1.35 μCi/kg.

Biodistribution and Physiology. Tc-99m MDP is administered intravenously and delivered to the skeletal system based on vascular distribution. Vigorous osteoblastic activity in the growth plates of juvenile skeletons, healing fractures, pathologic conditions stimulating skeletal blood flow, and bone repair increase the frequency of bone labeling. The technetium agents are excreted by the kidneys. In a normal subject, 50% is excreted by 4 hours and up to 80% of the injected diphosphonate will be excreted by 24 hours. Normal renal function clears soft tissue activity thus improving the quality of bone images because of improved target to background ratios. Decreased renal function for any reason degrades image quality. Waiting 3 to 4 hours before delayed skeletal imaging is a compromise between radiotracer decay and the clearance of background activity around the skeleton. Three- and four-phase skeletal scintigraphy have proven clinically useful in determining the vascular nature of lesions as well as in separating soft tissue injury or infection such as cellulitis from a focal skeletal disease such as osteomyelitis. ***Phase 1*** is the dynamically acquired **arterial phase.** ***Phase 2*** is a set of static images, which can be acquired in multiple views, representing the **blood pool and soft tissue phase.** ***Phase 3*** is acquired 3 to 4 hours later and represents the **delayed skeletal uptake.** ***Phase 4*** can be acquired the following morning **if better skeletal detail is needed**, usually reserved for patients with poor renal function, such as in patients with a diabetic foot.

The mechanism of Tc-99m MDP tracer localization is by **chem-adsorption** to the mineral phase of bone, primarily in the areas of increased osteogenic activity. The **bladder is the critical organ** for Tc-99m MDP with 26 mGy/20 mCi and the whole-body radiation absorbed dose is 1.3 mGy/20 mCi. Fluorine-18 (hydroxyl analog), strontium-89 (calcium analog), and radium-223 (calcium analog) avidly bind to hydroxyapatite crystals in bone. The mechanism of action of samarium-153 is unknown.

F-18-fluorodeoxyglucose (FDG) is a glucose analog radiopharmaceutical that acts as a glucose analog and is trapped inside hypermetabolic tumor cells and is therefore also capable of identifying malignant tumors and osseous metastatic disease.

Technical Issues. Skeletal scintigraphy has a resolution of about 5 mm in the best conditions. Adult IV doses of 20 mCi (740 MBq) or more Tc-99m MDP are usually adequate for static imaging 3 to 4 hours after injection. Flow images are typically acquired in the anterior and posterior planes or plantar and palmar views of the area of concern. Blood pool

The editors wish to thanks Dr. Amir Kashefi and Dr. David K. Shelton for their works in the 4th edition establishing the foundation for this chapter.

TABLE 72C.1

RADIONUCLIDES USED IN SKELETAL SCINTIGRAPHY

RADIONUCLIDE	USE DOSAGE	HALF-LIFE	ENERGY	DECAY
Tc-pyrophosphate	15–25 mCi	6 hours	140 keV	Isomeric transition
Tc-MDP	20–30 mCi	6 hours	140 keV	Isomeric transition
Fluorine-18	5–15 mCi	110 minutes	511 keV	Positron
Strontium-89	2–4 mCi	50.5 days	1.46 MeV	β only
Samarium-153	1 mCi/kg	1.9 days	0.81 MeV 103 keV	β and γ

images can be obtained in multiple views similar to "spot-view" images. Whole-body delayed images are typically acquired in the anterior and posterior planes with oblique, lateral, or other spot views as needed. The static "spot views" usually have better resolution than the whole-body images (smaller field of view allows for smaller pixel size). **High-resolution, low-energy collimation** is most commonly used to obtain high-quality images. Ultra–high-resolution collimation will produce a minor improvement in image quality but at the expense of prolonged imaging time. A pinhole collimator can be used to produce higher-resolution images of small body regions such as the wrist. SPECT imaging may be used for improved contrast resolution and better anatomic depiction in areas such as the spine, skull, knees, or ankles.

Combining SPECT with CT improves attenuation correction in SPECT and improves accuracy in identifying the anatomical site and extent of disease. Application of SPECT-CT improves sensitivity and specificity of skeletal scintigraphy.

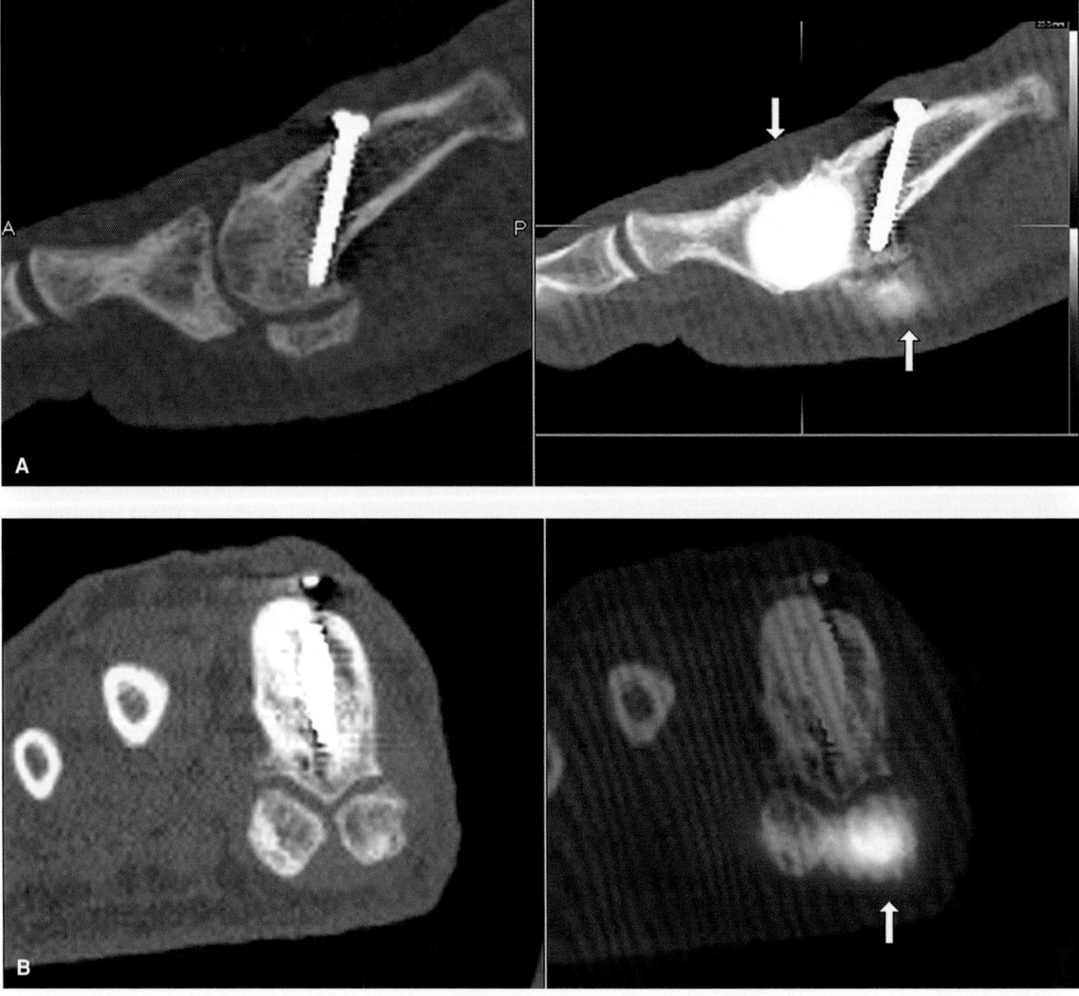

FIGURE 72C.1. **SPECT-CT of the Foot. A:** Sagittal SPECT-CT. **B:** Coronal SPECT-CT. This patient with history of screw in the foot and severe pain was referred to evaluate for hardware loosening. SPECT-CT of the foot revealed that screw is not loose and two main causes of the pain are (1) severe osteoarthritis of the first metatarsal-phalangeal (MTP) joint (*arrow*); and (2) tibial sesamoiditis (*arrow*). (Images courtesy of John Bauman, Valley Radiologists, Federal Way, WA.)

The clinical benefits of SPECT-CT in benign orthopedic conditions are also promising. Adding the low-dose multislice CT to SPECT has been found critical to correctly diagnose 59% of lesions in nononcologic patients with inconclusive Tc-99m MDP bone scans (Fig. 72C.1). In patients with extremity pain without a history of cancer that underwent both three-phase bone scintigraphy and SPECT-CT, the SPECT-CT findings led to revision of the diagnostic category in 32% of patients.

INTERPRETATION

Normal Skeletal Scintigram. In the normal adult, skeletal radiotracer uptake is uniform and symmetrical. Uptake is greater in the axial skeleton (pelvis and spine) than in the appendicular skeleton (skull and extremities). Low levels of background soft tissue uptake are typically present. The kidneys should appear slightly more intense than soft tissue background and relatively symmetric. The renal collecting system, ureters, and bladder activity appear very intense due to renal clearance of radiotracer. Children will demonstrate intense, symmetrical activity in their growth plates, which should be evaluated carefully.

Trauma to the skeleton may be undetectable on standard radiographic examinations, particularly stress fractures (overuse of a normal bone) and insufficiency fractures (normal use of a weakened/osteopenic bone). Scintigraphic remodeling from trauma precedes radiographically detectable fracture healing by approximately 10 days. Decreased or normal osteoblastic activity is seen at the fracture site in the first phase of repair. The subsequent osteoblastic activity then shows as a "hot spot," weeks before the calcified callus appears on a radiograph (Figs. 72C.2 and 72C.3). In an uncomplicated fracture, repaired bone returns to normal scintigraphic appearance as the callus at the fracture site remodels over a period of months (Fig. 72C.4). Healing of a complicated fracture in a weight-bearing bone (including healing with angulation) may take many years to return to normal activity on bone scans and some fractures may show remodeling on bone scans for

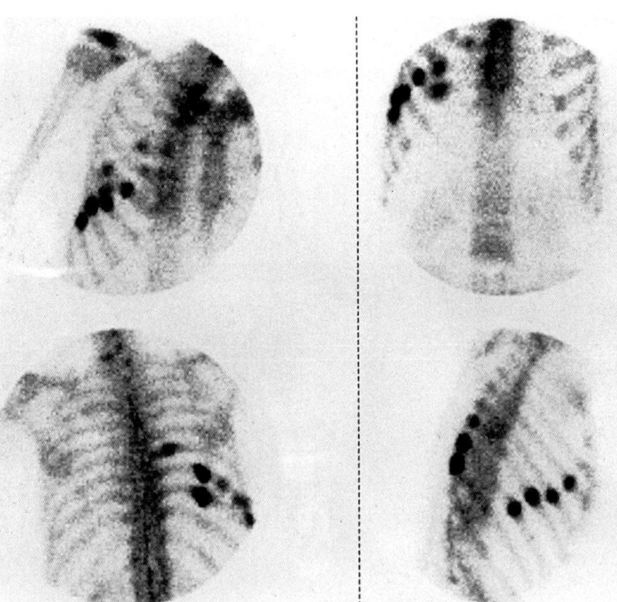

FIGURE 72C.2. **Multiple Rib Fractures.** Vigorous osteoblastic repair activity is seen in two rows of fractures, which were not visible on radiographs. Note the "linear array" distribution not seen with the metastases in scans of Figures 72C.13 and 72C.14.

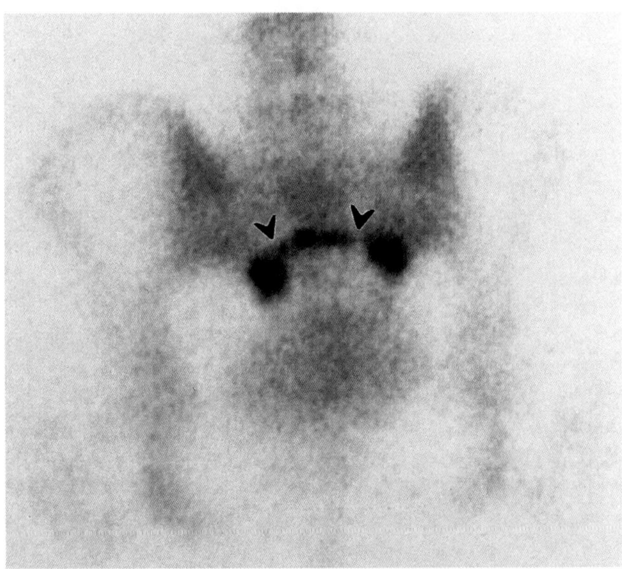

FIGURE 72C.3. **Occult Sacral Fracture.** A posterior image of the pelvis shows a horizontal line of increased uptake (*arrowheads*) across the sacrum, which marks healing along a painful fracture that is invisible on radiographs. This can take the shape of an "H," called the **Honda sign.**

life. Bone scans or SPECT of the spine are frequently useful in osteoporotic vertebral fractures prior to vertebroplasty. The scan evaluates for a metastatic pattern and for the acuity and level of the fracture.

The three-phase bone scan can accurately diagnose shin splints and discriminate them from stress fractures. ***Shin splints*** demonstrate **superficial, vertically oriented uptake in the tibia,** usually **posteromedially.** ***Stress fractures*** **are more localized and run horizontally.** Recent studies have shown that pinhole bone scan is more sensitive than plain film or CT for scaphoid and other fractures of the wrist, as is MRI. Whole-body bone scans are useful in detecting unsuspected fractures following severe cases of multitrauma.

Prosthetic joint replacements may loosen and/or become infected. Bone surrounding a hip joint prosthesis is expected to have increased osteoblastic activity for up to 6 months. Thereafter, increased labeling correlates with infection, loosening, and heterotopic bone formation, depending on the pattern of localization. The ***toggle sign*** is indicative of **prosthetic loosening** and refers to a hot spot at the tip of a prosthesis and two areas of increased uptake at the proximal end, like a toggle switch. Radiographs and occasionally radiolabeled white blood cell scans may be required to further diagnose abnormal findings (Fig. 72C.5). A Tc-99m sulfur colloid scan can be performed to differentiate expanded marrow space (matched uptake on WBC and sulfur colloid scan) from infection (uptake on WBC scan without matching uptake on sulfur colloid scan) in cases with increased uptake on both Indium-111–tagged WBC scans and bone scans.

Arthropathies and Arthritides. Inflammation of a joint creates increased blood flow and increases the amount of radiotracer supplied to those portions of the bone bounded by the synovial capsule. Increased bone labeling is seen in toxic synovitis, septic joints, inflammation associated with early degenerative conditions, and connective tissue arthropathies. In early osteoarthrosis, high-resolution bone scan images detect increased subchondral bone labeling long before there are radiographic findings. Intense, abnormal labeling is also seen

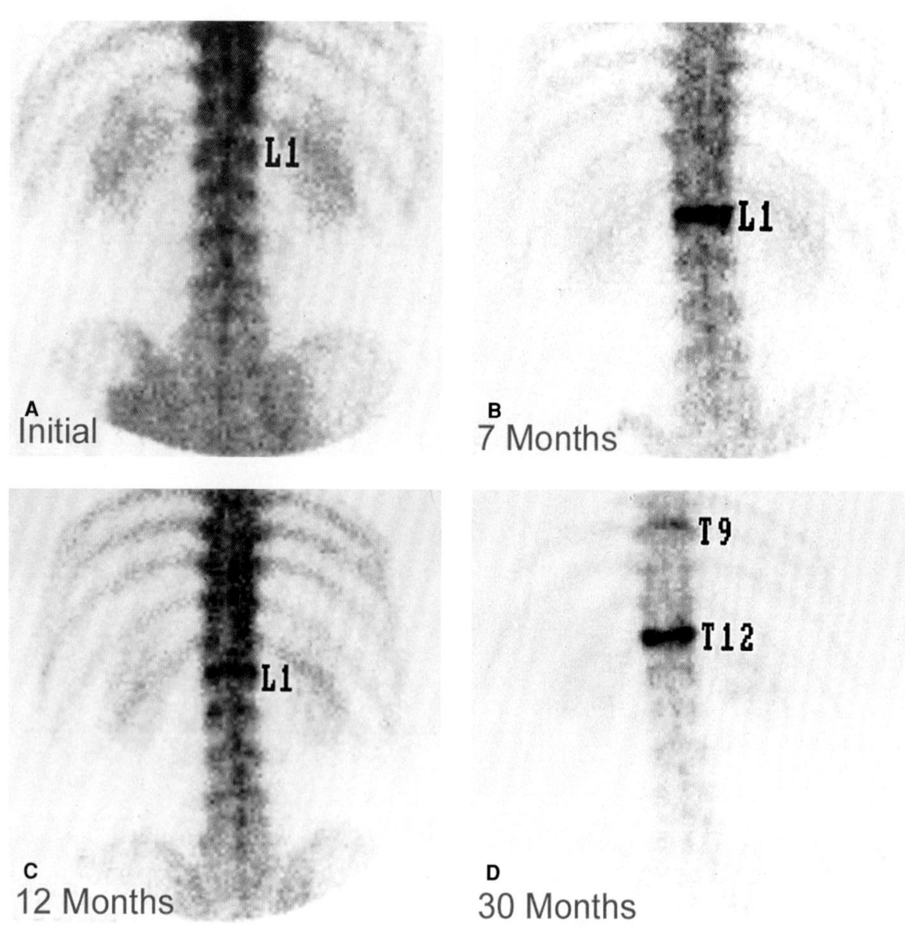

FIGURE 72C.4. **Fracture Healing.** Serial bone scans of the lower thoracic and lumbar spine at intervals of months listed show a normal spine (**A**) followed by a compression fracture of *L1* (**B**), which gradually heals (**C**) only to be replaced by new fractures at *T9* and *T12* (**D**). Note the horizontal, linear pattern of a simple vertebral compression fracture.

in neuropathic joints long before the abnormality is detected by radiographs (Fig. 72C.6).

Osteomyelitis can be diagnosed with high sensitivity and specificity within the first several days of symptoms on three-phase bone scan ("hot" on all three phases) and MRI while radiographic manifestations may not be seen for 10 to 14 days. Interpretation becomes increasingly difficult and specificity declines when the target is small (e.g., bones of the foot) though conspicuity can be improved with higher-resolution gamma cameras (Figs. 72C.7 and 72C.8). False-negative examinations have been reported in children when the duration of clinical illness is brief.

Cellulitis adjacent to bone is seen as a soft tissue area of increased activity on the arterial and immediate blood pool phases with little or no focally increased activity in the bone on the third phase. In the peripheral skeleton where bones are small, it is frequently more difficult to tell the difference between an infection adjacent to a bone with increased soft tissue and increased periosteal labeling from an infection within the bone. Bone scans may take months to normalize after infections of bone are sterilized and thus a WBC scan may be useful for follow-up.

Vascular Phenomena. There is a strong vascular influence on the labeling of bones. Increased blood flow stimulates

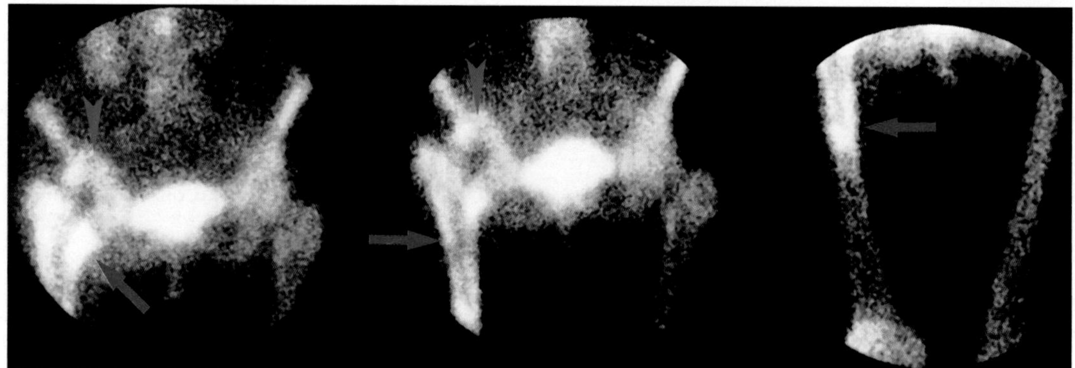

FIGURE 72C.5. **Hip Prosthesis Loosening.** Anterior images of the pelvis, hips, and femurs show intense labeling around the femoral (*arrows*) and acetabular (*arrowheads*) components of a 2-year-old total hip arthroplasty. Both had loosened without infection.

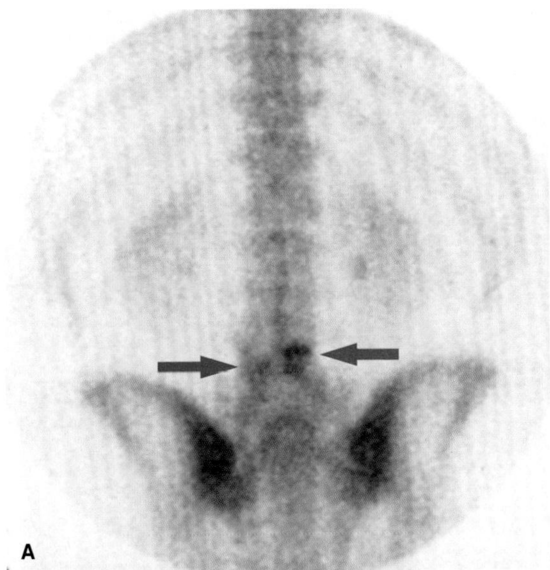

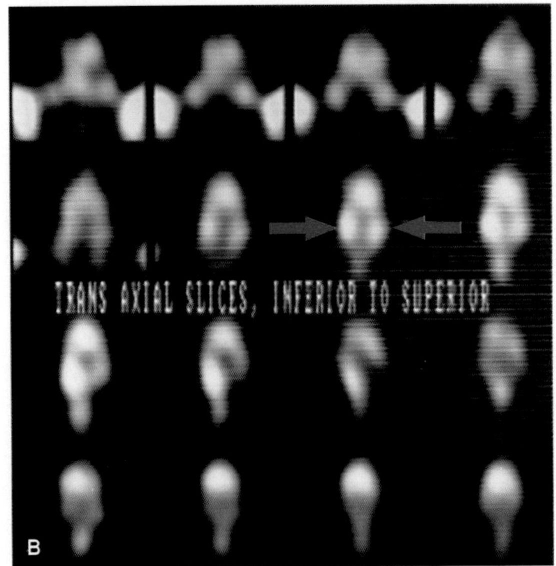

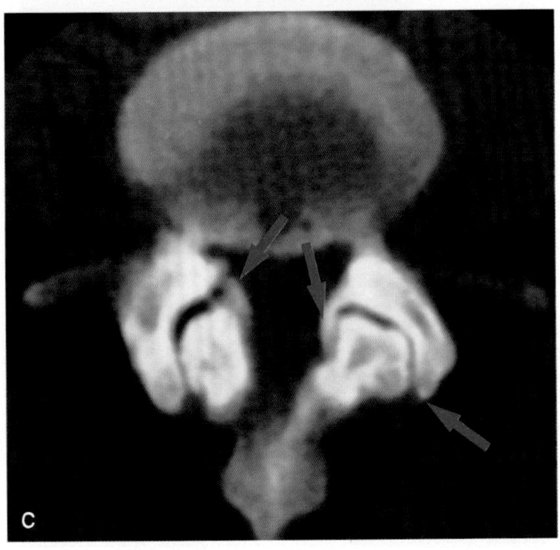

FIGURE 72C.6. L4–L5 Facet Degenerative Arthropathy. A: A planar, posterior image of the lumbar spine shows small areas of increased activity (*arrows*) in the lower lumbar spine in a patient with chronic low back pain. **B:** Transaxial SPECT images of the same lumbar spine start at the L5–S1 facet joint level and continue up to the L3–L4 level. Note the conspicuity of the abnormality. Areas of increased bone labeling at the L4–L5 facet joints are marked by *arrows*. **C:** The CT of the same level shows hypertrophic spurs (*arrows*) embracing the facet joints.

FIGURE 72C.7. Osteomyelitis of the Second Toe and Metatarsal and Septic Second Metatarsal Phalangeal Joint. A: A plantar bone scan shows increased activity in the second proximal phalanx (*long arrow*), metatarsal phalangeal joint (*fat arrow*), and second metatarsal (*arrowhead*) indicating reactive bone stimulated by the infection. Decreased activity in the distal toe corresponds with necrotic tissue. **B:** A radiograph shows destructive changes in the second proximal phalanx (*arrow*) but appears normal in the second metatarsal phalangeal joint and metatarsal phalangeal shaft. Note the bone destruction (*arrowhead*) of the middle and distal phalanges of the second toe.

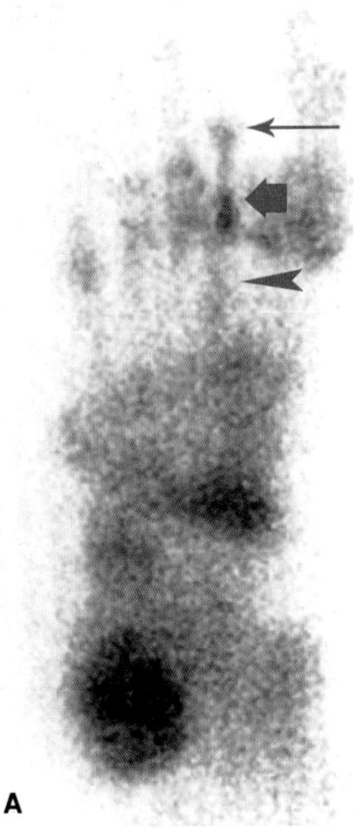

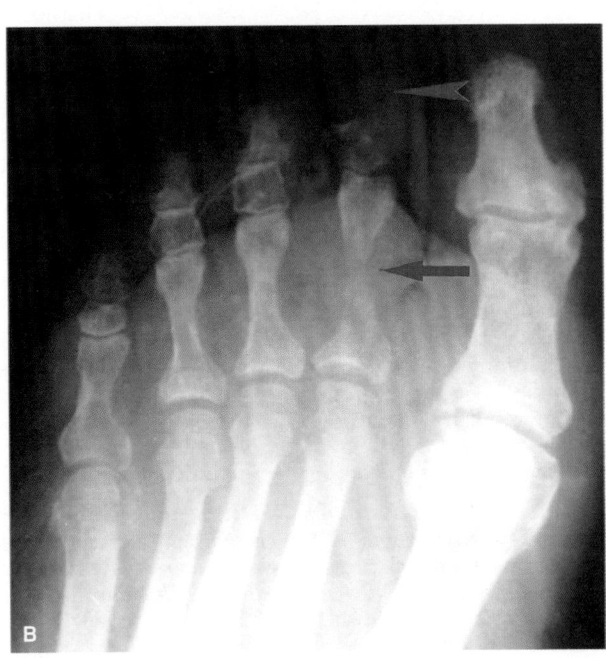

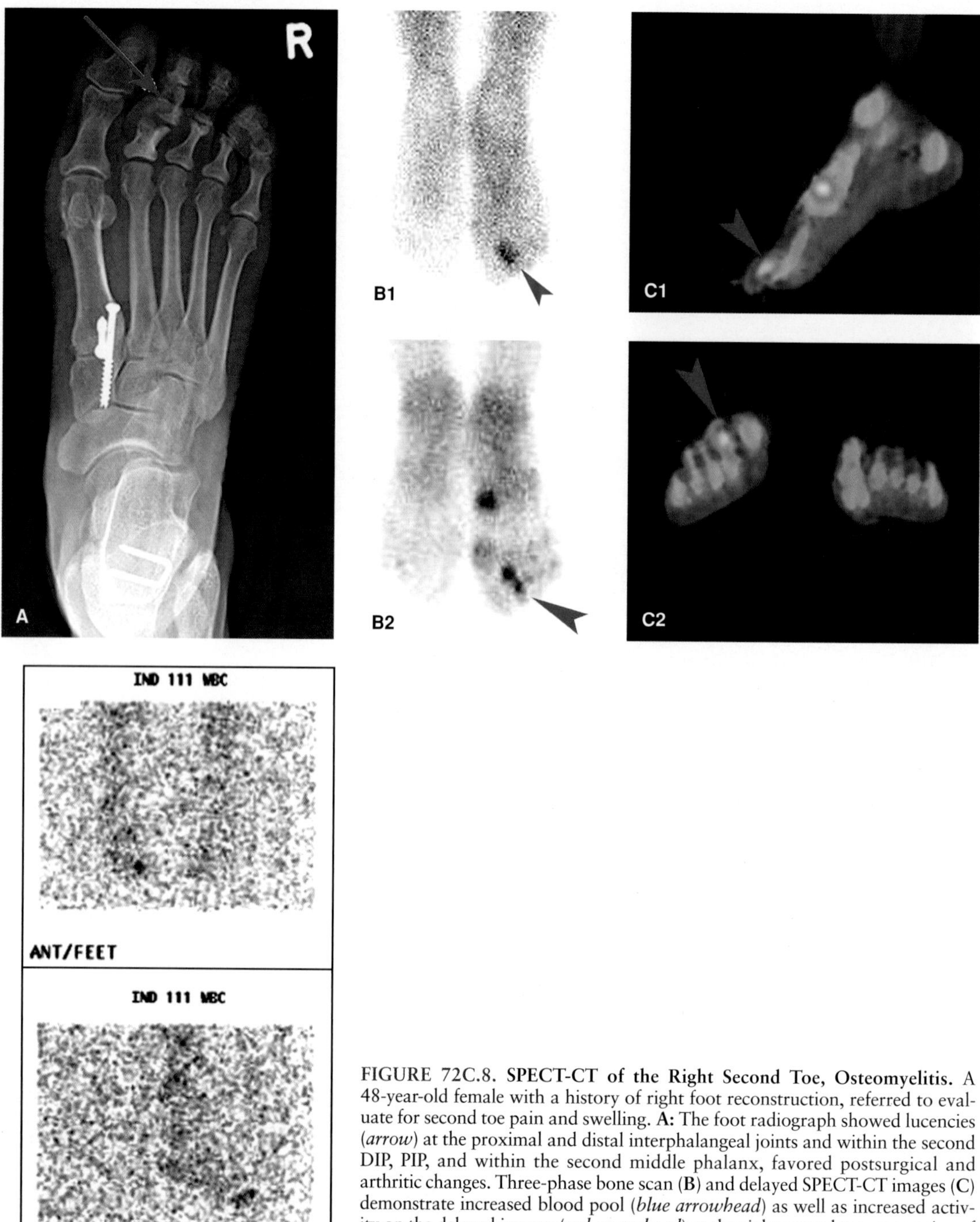

FIGURE 72C.8. **SPECT-CT of the Right Second Toe, Osteomyelitis.** A 48-year-old female with a history of right foot reconstruction, referred to evaluate for second toe pain and swelling. **A:** The foot radiograph showed lucencies (*arrow*) at the proximal and distal interphalangeal joints and within the second DIP, PIP, and within the second middle phalanx, favored postsurgical and arthritic changes. Three-phase bone scan (**B**) and delayed SPECT-CT images (**C**) demonstrate increased blood pool (*blue arrowhead*) as well as increased activity on the delayed images (*red arrowhead*) at the right second toe, suggestive of osteomyelitis. **D:** Indium-111 white blood cell study confirmed osteomyelitis of the right second toe.

increased osteoblastic and osteoclastic activities. Increased flow and presence of radiotracer usually results in increased radiotracer deposition. Common pathologic conditions, such as tumor and trauma, cause hyperemia and increased blood pooling with increased delivery of radiopharmaceuticals to the osteoblasts. This is an appropriate response to injury.

Reflex sympathetic dystrophy (RSD, also known as complex regional pain syndrome—CRPS) is an example of an inappropriate excessive vascular response where the affected extremity will usually be "hotter" than the unaffected extremity due to the release of sympathetic vascular tone causing the feeding arteries to dilate (Fig. 72C.9), increasing perfusion. However, "***Atypical RSD***" occurs in about **10% of cases** and demonstrates vasospasm with decreased flow and **decreased uptake** on the affected side. A bone scan is also a simple test of the vascular status of a bone or bone graft. If osteoblasts are labeled, the blood supply must be intact. ***Acute avascular necrosis (AVN)*** shows no labeling of the affected bone, but in later phases will be "hot." Bone subjected to radiation therapy may lose blood supply and osteoblastic activity. Square-edged radiation portals produce typical areas of decreased labeling (Fig. 72C.10).

Abnormal Soft Tissue Uptake. Areas of increased soft tissue uptake may be seen with tumors such as breast carcinoma or as normal symmetrical, physiologic breast uptake.

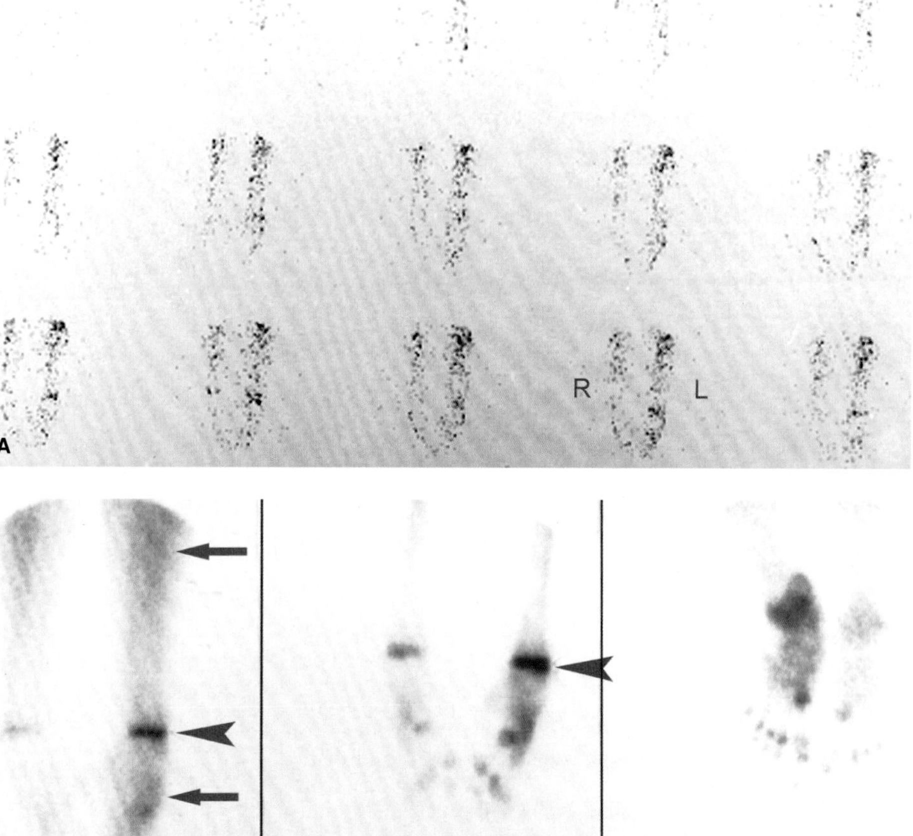

FIGURE 72C.9. **Reflex Sympathetic Dystrophy.** Three-phase bone scan of a 13-year-old boy with a painful left ankle and foot. **A:** The initial bolus, filmed at 1 second per frame in the anterior projection with heels together, arrives in the left foot (*L*) and ankle earlier than the right foot (*R*). **B:** The early blood pool image (**left**) shows greater blood pooling (*arrows*) in the same area. The 3-hour delayed images (**center** and **right**, anterior and plantar projections, respectively) show a generalized increase in bone labeling. Note the preferential labeling of the physeal plates (*arrowheads*), which is expected in a juvenile patient.

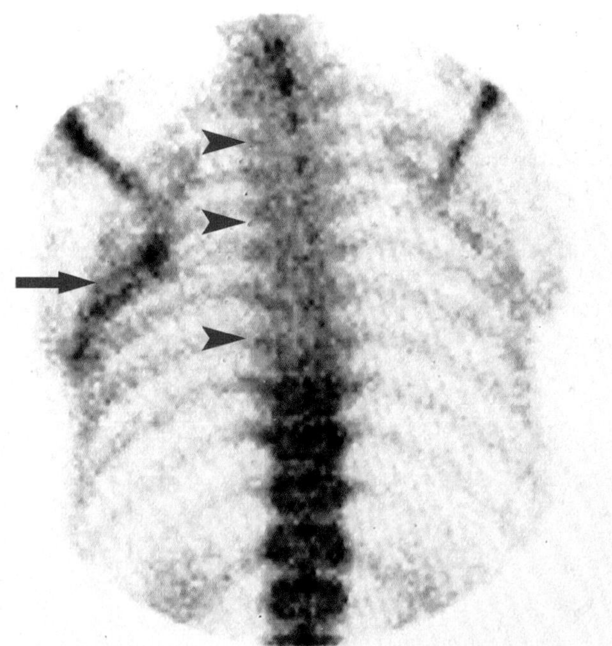

FIGURE 72C.10. **Radiation Therapy Changes.** Decreased uptake is seen in the thoracic spine (*arrowheads*) within the radiotherapy portal. Note the reactive changes in the lateral left ribs (*arrow*) where a lateral thoracotomy was performed in this patient with bronchogenic carcinoma of the lung.

Atherosclerotic uptake can be seen in the femoral and carotid arteries. Diffuse liver uptake may be seen with diffuse liver disease or with technical problems such as colloid formation in the radiotracer due to aluminum contamination. Focal abnormal uptake in the liver is usually seen with mucinous metastatic disease such as colon or breast cancer. Soft tissue trauma, cellulitis, bursitis, and rhabdomyolysis will also demonstrate abnormal soft tissue uptake.

Heterotopic Bone. Repair of soft tissue injuries sometimes leads to the formation of heterotopic bone. Histologically, normal bone may form from differentiating fibroblasts after trauma. Muscle crush injuries healing with the formation of heterotopic bone (myositis ossificans) are readily labeled on bone scans, occurring weeks before the plain film shows signs of calcification. The heterotopic bone may be safely resected after the blood pool phase becomes inactive, otherwise there is an increased risk of recurrence. Soft tissues around joint prostheses, in paralyzed limbs, and in burn injuries are common sites of heterotopic bone formation.

Metabolic Conditions. Increased parathormone levels (or the presence of tumor-produced parathormone-like substances) simultaneously increase serum calcium and phosphate. Hyperparathyroidism causes calcium phosphate complexes to precipitate in the lungs and the stomach. This "metastatic calcification" is rarely seen on radiographs but is routinely visible as increased uptake on bone scans. Other generalized skeletal abnormalities such as tumoral calcinosis, hypertrophic osteoarthropathy (usually seen with pulmonary disease such as bronchogenic carcinoma), systemic mastocytosis, and many other diseases with

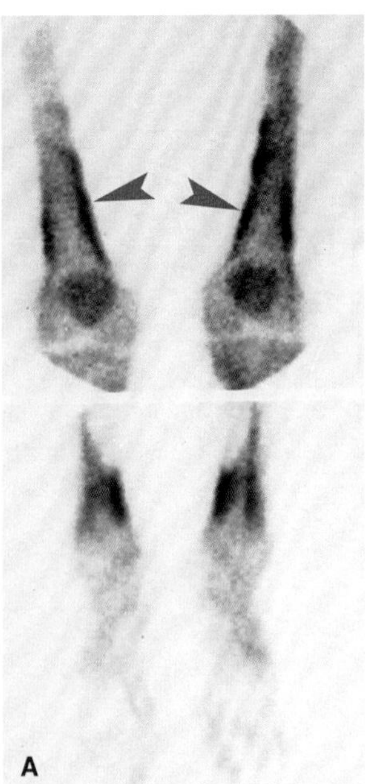

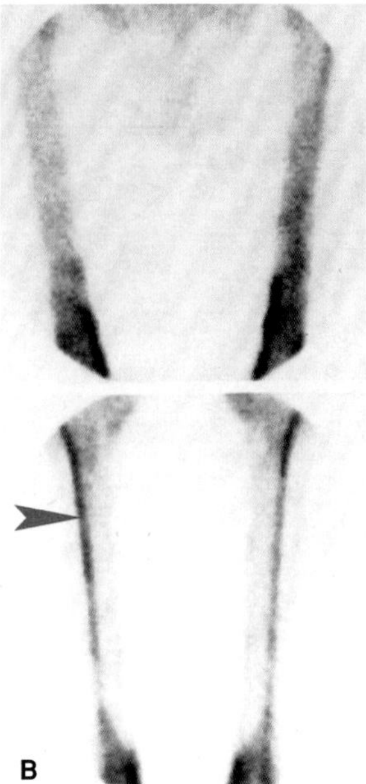

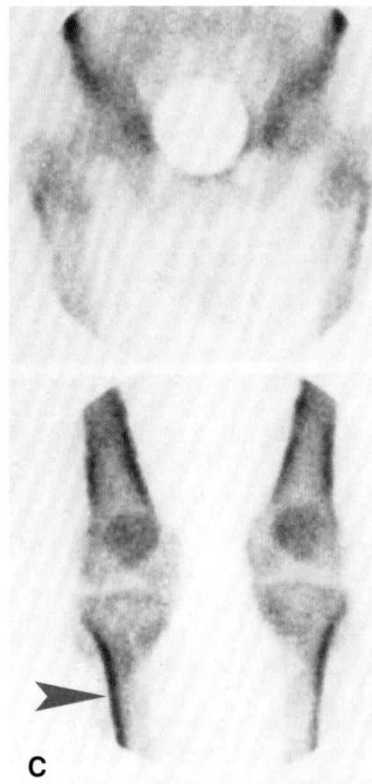

FIGURE 72C.11. **Hypertrophic Osteoarthropathy.** A bone scan performed to detect metastases in a patient with carcinoma of the lung shows increased periosteal labeling (*arrowheads*), principally in the metaphyses of the lower extremity. The patient does not have metastases. **A:** Distal femurs and distal tibias. **B:** Mid-femurs and mid-tibias. **C:** Proximal femurs and tibias.

calcification or ossification of tissues may be shown with bone scans (Fig. 72C.11).

Bone Dysplasias. Benign bone dysplasias frequently show the expected increase in labeling on bone scans. Paget disease of bone, fibrous dysplasia, enchondromas, exostoses, and many other benign conditions of bone are detected by bone scan. Comparison with skeletal radiographs will clarify these multicentric diagnoses. An efficient way to screen the whole skeleton for polyostotic disease is the bone scan. In the osteolytic phase of Paget disease of bone, the radiographic changes are accompanied by marked increases in bone labeling. This repair continues with increased labeling during the radiographic stage of sclerotic, expansile pagetic bone. The increased activity on bone scans may eventually disappear, as repair is complete (Fig. 72C.12). Fibrous dysplasia is a benign condition of bone that may also be polyostotic. It is readily detected by bone scans because of its intense bone labeling.

Primary Bone Tumors. There are two principal ways in which bone tumors are detected by bone scans. Osteosarcomas and chondrosarcomas may have abnormal osteoblastic or chondroblastic activity associated with the production of abnormal tumor calcification. This is a malignant process with the tumor itself being "hot" (Figs. 72C.13 and 72C.14). Metastases from calcifying or ossifying primary tumors to other nonskeletal sites may also take up Tc-99m diphosphonates directly, making them readily detected by scintigraphy. The Tc-99m diphosphonate may also be avidly concentrated by the normal osteoblasts reacting to the destructive presence of the primary tumor. This process makes the bone adjacent to tumors much more intense than the surrounding bone. Some malignancies may arise in the soft tissues adjacent to bone and invade through periosteum into the bone. In either case, the resulting reactive osteoblastic changes show the extent of invasion without showing the tumor itself. An extremely destructive bone tumor may destroy bone more quickly than repair can be effected. Thus, a "cold" defect in a bone with a primary malignancy is an indication of a very aggressive tumor. High-grade sarcomas usually show this phenomenon.

Bone scan may also be useful in benign bone tumors. **Osteomas** (bone islands) may be neutral or not seen on bone scan even though they appear sclerotic on radiographs. **Osteoid osteomas** are typically very hot and will show the "double-density" sign on bone scan because of the very hot nidus.

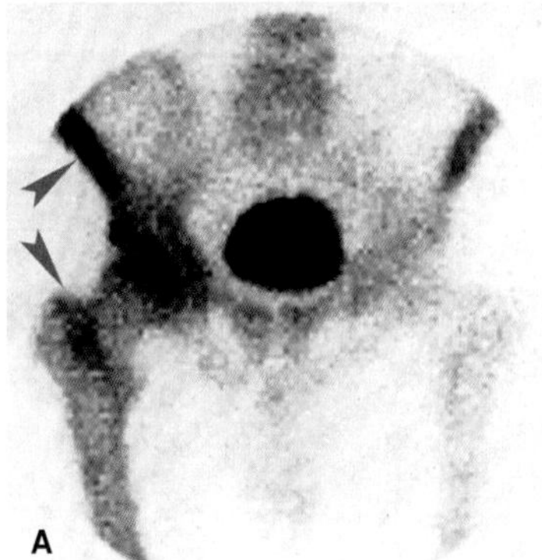

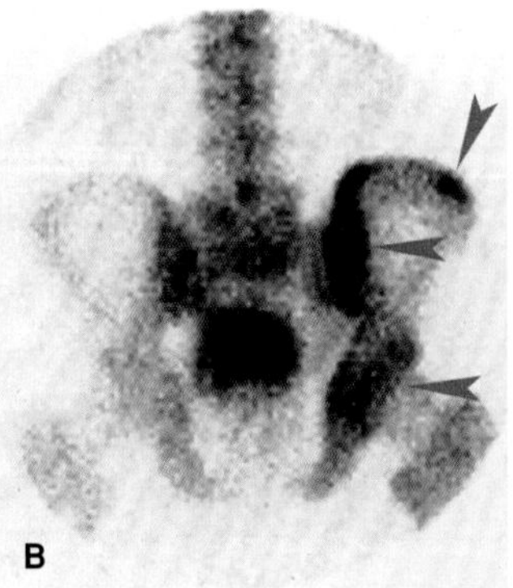

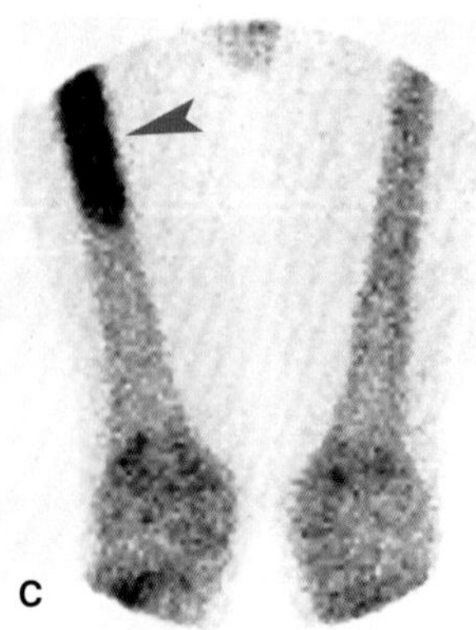

FIGURE 72C.12. **Paget Disease of Bone.** Images of the pelvis and femurs of a 60-year-old man with carcinoma of the prostate. There is abnormal, increased uptake in the right hemipelvis and proximal right femur (*arrowheads*), which is characteristic of pagetic bone. Note the distal "flame edge" of the pagetic portion of the femur. The patient does not have bony metastatic disease. **A:** Anterior pelvis. **B:** Posterior pelvis. **C:** Anterior view of distal femurs.

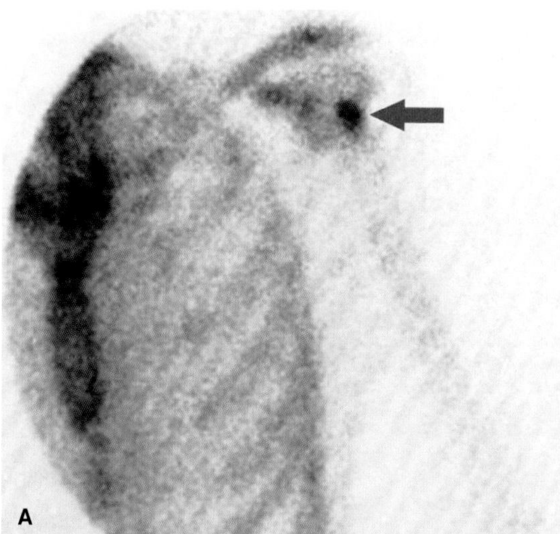

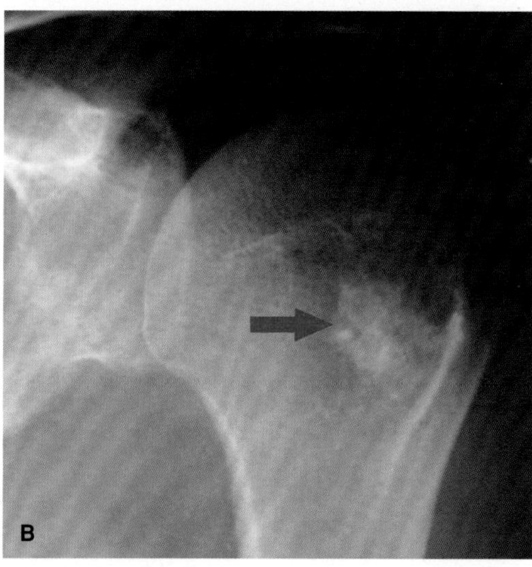

FIGURE 72C.13. **Low-Grade Chondrosarcoma. A:** An area of reactive bone (*arrow*) is seen in the proximal left humeral metaphysis. **B:** A radiograph shows the calcified cartilaginous matrix (*arrow*) of this tumor.

Metastatic Bone Disease. The most common use of the bone scan is for the detection and monitoring of metastatic tumor involving the skeleton. The tumors monitored include prostate, lung, breast, thyroid, and renal cell carcinoma among many others. **The majority of metastases arise within the axial skeleton in a pattern that reflects the distribution of the erythropoietic marrow.** The likelihood of a metastasis peripheral to erythropoietic marrow is low. Most metastases are multiple at the time of discovery. Thus, a solitary hot spot in the skull or a rib has a low probability (<10%) of being a metastatic lesion. Comparison bone scans at intervals of 3 to 6 months allow an accurate assessment of tumor spread (Fig. 72C.15). Because of its high sensitivity, bone scan can be used when a cancer patient has new back pain or bone pain. Likewise, bone scan is helpful when an indeterminate sclerotic lesion (e.g., bone island) or a lytic lesion (e.g., venous lake in skull) is seen on an anatomic study.

Knowledge of a given primary tumor's propensity to metastasize to the skeleton is helpful for scan interpretation. Confusion arises if an inexperienced observer cannot distinguish between common degenerative or posttraumatic changes and metastases. Merely counting the hot spots is of little value.

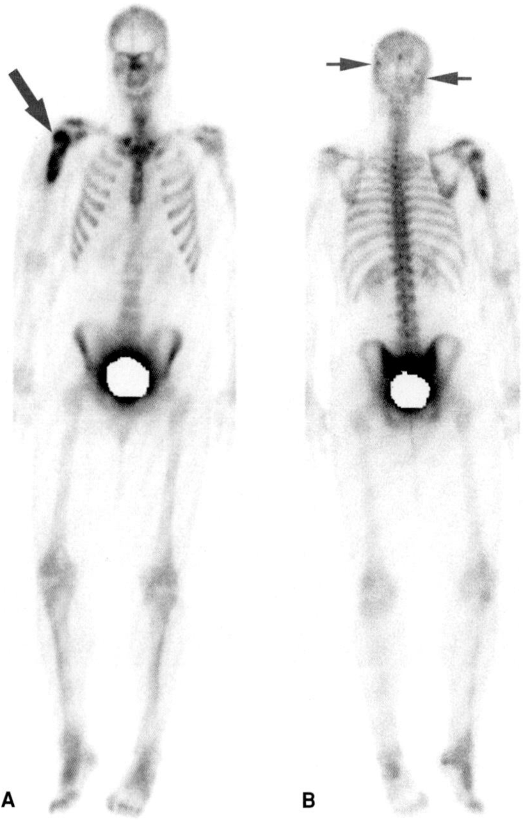

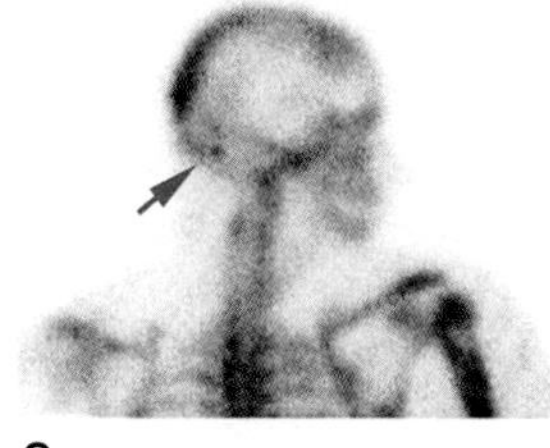

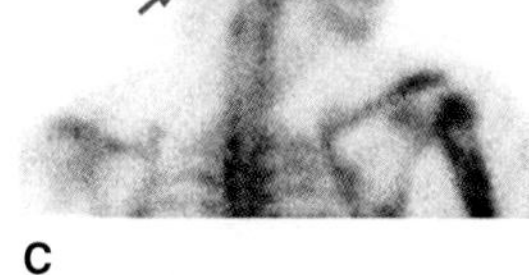

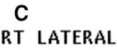

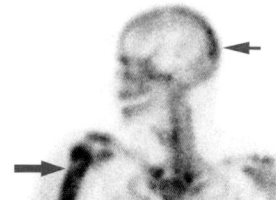

FIGURE 72C.14. **Osteogenic Sarcoma and Metastases.** A 26-year-old man with a large primary tumor (*large arrows*) in the proximal half of the humerus and several punctate foci of increased uptake (*small arrows*) in the posterior calvarium, consistent with metastases. **A:** Anterior whole-body view. **B:** Posterior whole body. **C:** Right lateral skull and neck. **D:** Left lateral skull and neck.

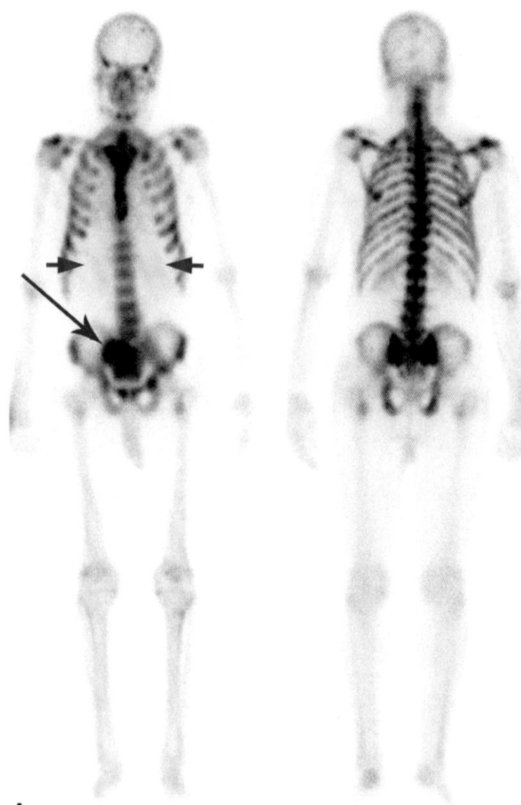

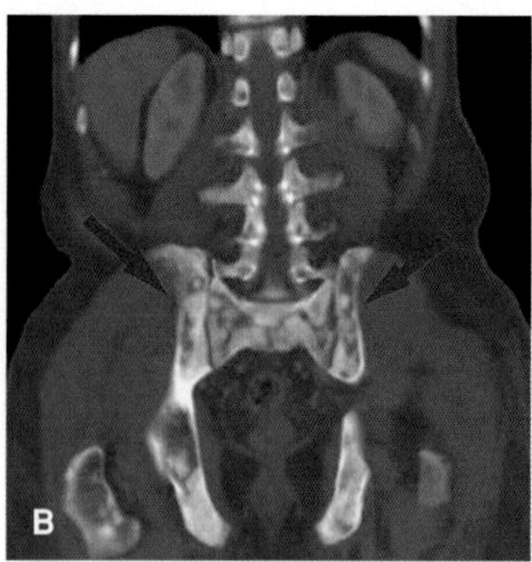

FIGURE 72C.15. **Superscan. A:** Numerous prostate cancer metastases produce almost uniform "hot spots" of intense isotope accumulation that leave little or none of the radiopharmaceutical for renal excretion (*short arrows*) or soft tissue uptake. Intense activity in the pelvis (*long arrow*) is because of multiple metastatic lesions to the pelvic bones and is not bladder activity. **B:** Coronal CT image of the pelvis confirmed multiple metastases to the pelvis (*arrows*).

Experience is necessary to judge metastatic disease in the skeleton. Changes in labeling reflect the status of bone repair and not the status of the metastases. Increased numbers and size of individual lesions usually indicate that the tumor load of the skeleton is expanding. Increased intensity of the individual lesions (in the absence of new lesions) frequently means that the tumor has become static and that the osteoblasts around it are engaged in vigorous repair. This ***"flare" response*** early after institution of chemotherapy is usually a good indicator of tumor response to therapy (e.g., treated disease) and should not be misinterpreted as worsening metastatic disease.

Aggressive metastases may destroy bone so quickly that there is little to no repair (Fig. 72C.16). Identifying these metastases in critical, weight-bearing bones such as the femur is important since the detection and treatment can prevent pathologic fractures. The bone scan can also guide biopsy in cases in which pathologic diagnosis of a bone lesion is required (Fig. 72C.17).

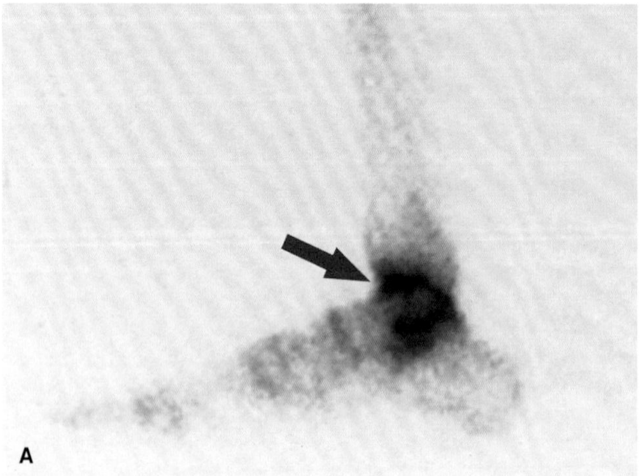

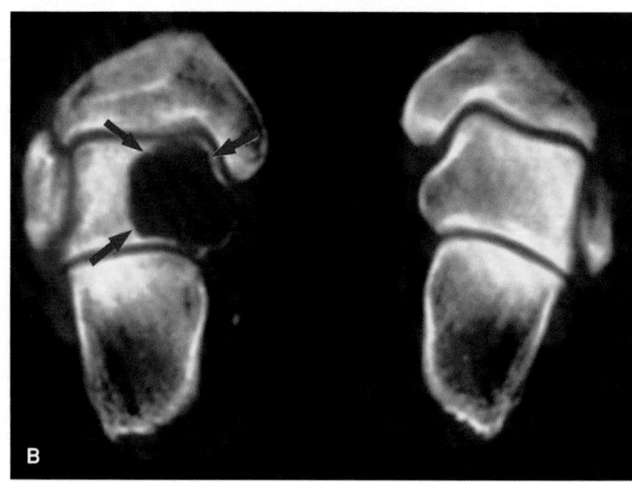

FIGURE 72C.16. **Aggressive Metastasis. A:** A medial projection bone scan of the ankle and foot of a patient with renal cell carcinoma shows a halo of increased activity (*arrow*) around the ankle joint. **B:** A CT scan of the ankle shows a scooped out lesion (*arrows*) of the right talus where the metastasis has destroyed bone so fast that bone repair has no chance to form. The talus does not show a hot spot. The bone scan is abnormal because of hemarthrosis irritation of the synovium. Inflammation of the synovium causes increased synovial perfusion and increased delivery of radiopharmaceutical to all of the bones of the corresponding joint.

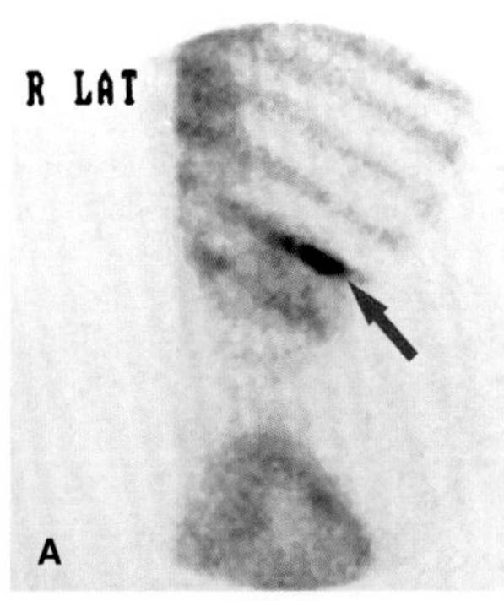

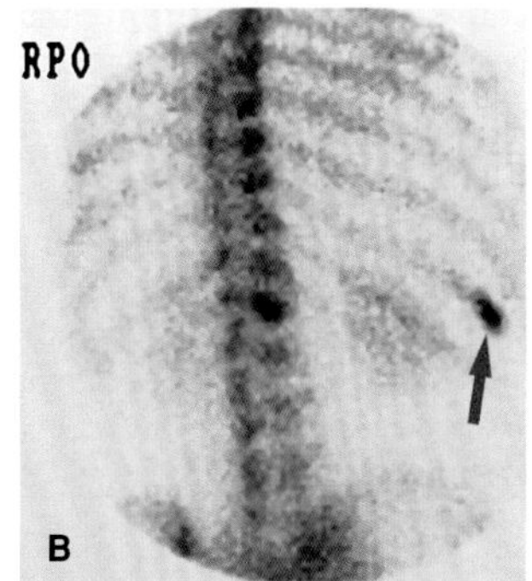

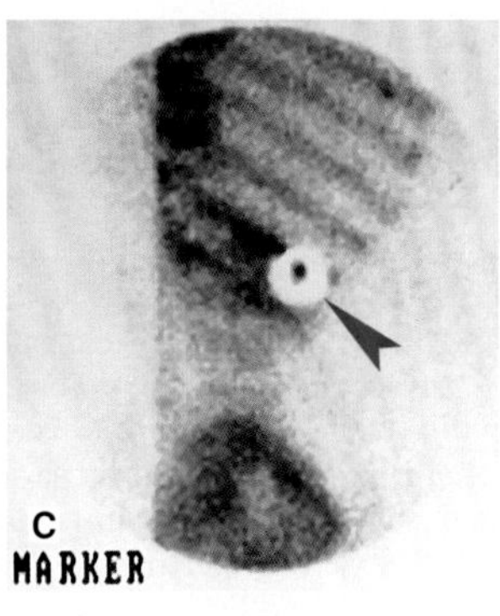

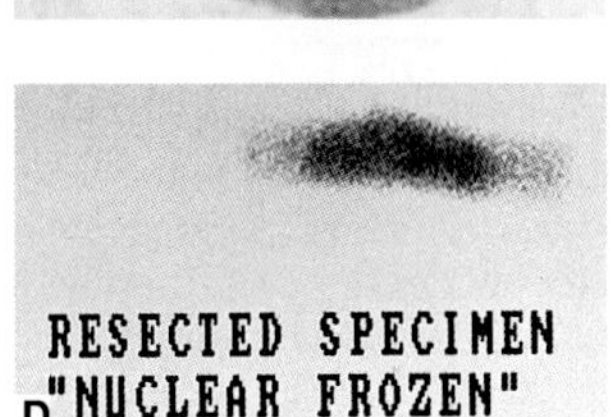

FIGURE 72C.17. **Resection of a Solitary Metastasis.** Rib images (**A, B**) from a bone scan show a solitary metastasis (*arrows*), from an adenocarcinoma of unknown origin, is located with a "cold" lead ring (*arrowhead*) (**C**) maneuvered over the right lateral rib lesion before surgery to locate the correct rib for resection. On the way to the surgical pathologist, the resected rib was imaged (**D**) to confirm that the correct rib had been resected.

Particle Disease. Most commonly occurs in 1 to 5 years after arthroplasty, secondary to microabrasive wear and shedding of tiny particles of the prosthesis material. The foreign materials activate an inflammatory process via a granulomatous response and giant cell (histiocytes) migration. This cascade causes an increase in osteoclastic activity and therefore increases radiotracer activity along the periphery of the bone scan and F-18 NaF PET-CT (Fig. 72C.18).

F-18 NaF PET-CT

F-18 labeled NaF is poised to become the future radiotracer of choice for skeletal scintigraphy due to highly specific bone uptake, rapid clearance from the blood pool (minimal protein binding), and dosimetry similar to that of Tc-99m MDP.

Numerous studies in the past decade have proved that F-18 NaF PET-CT is superior to planar and SPECT imaging with Tc-99m MDP for localizing and characterizing both malignant and benign bone lesions (Fig. 72C.18). In addition, imaging can be performed in less than 1 hour after F-18 NaF administration, resulting in a faster, more convenient study for the patient compared with Tc-99m MDP scintigraphy. F-18 NaF PET, however, is unable to yield an equivalent to a three-phase bone scan, maintaining a role for Tc-99m MDP.

SYSTEMIC RADIONUCLIDE PALLIATIVE PAIN THERAPY

Approximately 65% of patients with prostate or breast cancer and 35% of those with advanced lung, thyroid, and kidney cancers will have bone pain due to skeletal metastases, which significantly decreases the patient's quality of life. Management of bone pain is extremely difficult and usually involves different approaches such as analgesics, hormone therapies, bisphosphonates, external beam radiation, and systemic radiopharmaceuticals. Systemic radionuclide therapy has successfully relieved the pain in approximately 80% (60% to 92%) of patients with bone metastases. Patients generally

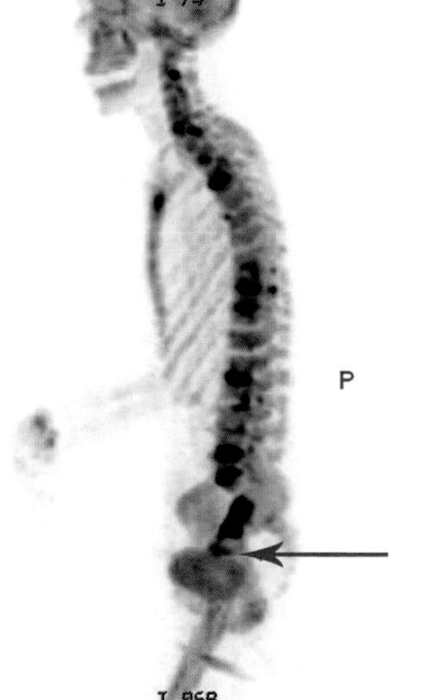

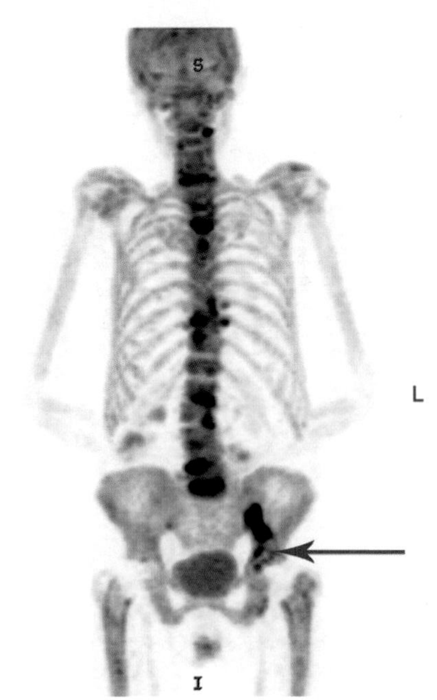

FIGURE 72C.18. **^{18}F-Fluoride PET-CT.** Maximum intensity projection of ^{18}F-fluoride PET-CT in a patient with history of bilateral hip arthroplasties and breast cancer shows increased activity at the roof of left acetabulum, compatible with particle disease (*arrows*) and multiple joint centered foci of increased activity in the axial and appendicular skeleton, compatible with arthropathic changes. **A**, anterior; **P**, posterior; **R**, right; **L**, left.

have better results when systemic radionuclide therapy is considered in the earlier stages of the metastatic disease.

Radioactive isotopes of P-32 and Sr-89 were the first bone-seeking radiopharmaceuticals approved for the treatment of painful bone metastases. Sm-153, Sr-89, Re-186, Re-188, and Ra-223 are β^--emitting bone-seeking radioisotopes, and of these only Sm-153, Sr-89, and Ra-223 have been approved for use in the United States. Although these radioisotopes have different physical properties, they have very similar clinical efficacy for pain palliative therapy. Ra-223 is a FDA-approved α emitter used to help treat bone pain in patients with metastatic prostate cancer. Ra-223 is a calcium mimetic that binds to hydroxyapatite in areas of bone turnover. The high-energy α particles create double-strand DNA that breaks in surrounding cells, including cancer cells, leading to cell death. Bone marrow cells are relatively spared due to the short distance traveled by α particles. Moreover, Ra-223 has been shown to prolong survival by approximately 3 months compared to placebo.

How to select the patients and what are the contraindications of systemic radionuclide therapy? The best candidates are patients with severe bone pain despite analgesics or the ones who cannot tolerate analgesic side effects and have had bone scintigraphy within 8 weeks, demonstrating osteoblastic lesions. External beam therapy is not a contraindication and can be used as an adjunct for limited areas. Patients should have a life expectancy of more than 4 weeks and, due to myelotoxicity effects, patients should be off chemotherapy and large-field radiation therapy within the past 4 to 12 weeks.

Pregnancy, breastfeeding, acute kidney injury, and chronic kidney disease stage IV or V (glomerular filtration rate [GFR] <30 mL/min/1.73 m^2, or on dialysis) are absolute contraindications for therapy. Relative contraindications include hemoglobin <9 mg/dL, white blood cell count <3,500/dL, absolute neutrophil count <1,500/dL, platelet count <100,000/dL, and GFR 30 to 50 mL/min/1.73 m^2. Transfusions can be given if blood counts fall below a critical level. Patients with extensive bone marrow involvement (low blood counts or "superscan") due to severe myelotoxicity should not be treated with radiopharmaceuticals.

BONE MINERAL DENSITOMETRY

Bone mineral densitometry is a screening test used to accurately diagnose and follow patients after institution of therapy for osteoporosis or osteopenia. Dual-energy x-ray absorptiometry (DEXA) uses two x-ray energies with different attenuation coefficients for dense bone, muscle, and fat. DEXA is typically performed over the lumbar spine (L1–L4) and the bilateral femoral necks. Vertebral bodies and femurs may be excluded due to the presence of sclerosis, lytic or blastic lesions, cement, or hardware as these entities will artificially affect the observed bone mineral density. The wrist or ankle can be used as a surrogate under these circumstances. The measured bone mineral density is compared to a database of patients with normal bone mineral density for age and sex to give a **Z score** (Fig. 72C.19). The Z score is stated in standard deviations above or below the normal average for a patient's age and sex. The **T score** compares the individual against peak young normals of the same sex, in standard deviations. A T score between −1 and −2.5 is considered **osteopenia.** A T score

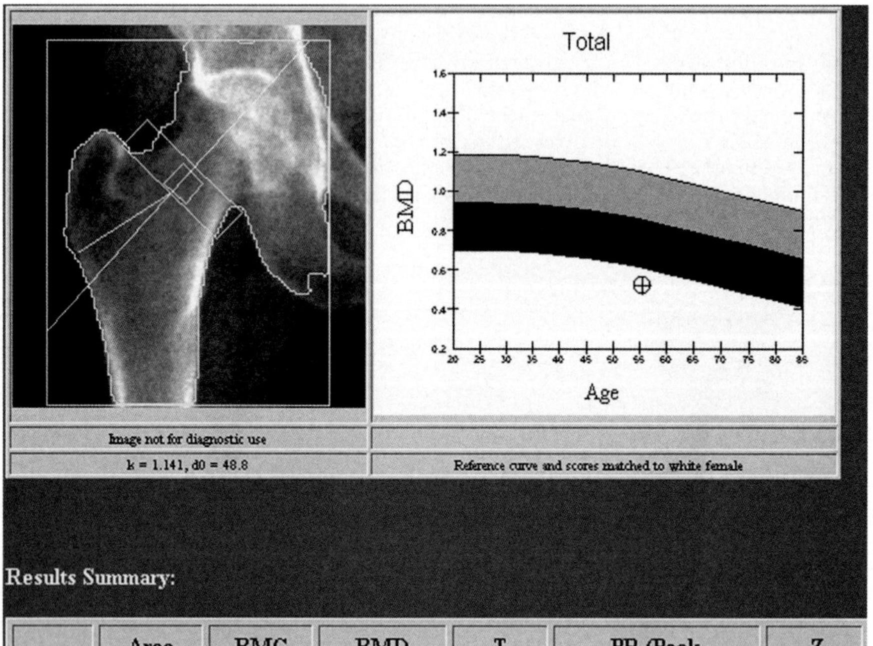

Region	Area [cm²]	BMC [(g)]	BMD [g/cm²]	T Score	PR (Peak Reference)	Z Score
Neck	5.04	1.93	0.382	-4.2	45	-3.1
Troch	9.81	3.70	0.377	-3.2	54	-2.5
Inter	24.09	14.70	0.610	-3.2	55	-2.7
Total	**38.94**	**20.33**	**0.522**	**-3.4**	**55**	**-2.7**
Ward's	1.06	0.25	0.238	-4.2	32	-2.5

FIGURE 72C.19. **Bone Mineral Densitometry (BMD) With DEXA Scan.** DEXA scan of the right hip in a 55-year-old woman demonstrates low BMD, low Z scores, and low T scores, consistent with significant osteoporosis. Her spine showed similar changes, indicating high-fracture risk.

of −2.5 or worse is defined as **osteoporosis**. A T score of −1 or better is considered normal. For each T score standard deviation below normal, the fracture risk is increased by approximately a factor of 3. Bone mineral densitometry can also be measured using CT.

Suggested Readings

Batt ME, Ugalde V, Anderson MW, Shelton DK. A prospective controlled study of diagnostic imaging for acute shin splints. *Med Sci Sports Exerc* 1998;30:1564–1571.

Brown ML, Collier BD, Fogelman I. Bone scintigraphy: Part I. Oncology and infection. *J Nucl Med* 1993;34:2236–2240.

Brunader R, Shelton DK. Radiologic bone assessment in the evaluation of osteoporosis. *Am Fam Physician* 2002;65:1357–1364.

Collier BD, Fogelman I, Brown ML. Bone scintigraphy: Part 2. Orthopedic bone scanning. *J Nucl Med* 1993;34:2241–2246.

Collier BD, Fogelman I, Rosenthal I, eds. *Skeletal Nuclear Medicine*. St. Louis, MO: Mosby; 1996.

Collier BD, Hellman RS, Krasnow AZ. Bone SPECT. *Semin Nucl Med* 1987;17:247–266.

Connolly LP, Connolly SA. Skeletal scintigraphy in the multimodality assessment of young children with acute skeletal symptoms. *Clin Nucl Med* 2003;28:746–754.

Corcoran RJ, Thrall JH, Kyle RW, Kaminski RJ, Johnson MC. Solitary abnormalities in bone scans of patients with extraosseous malignancies. *Radiology* 1976;121:663–667.

Cummings SR, Black DM, Nevitt MC, et al. Bone density at various sites for prediction of hip fractures. The study of Osteoporotic Fractures Research Group. *Lancet* 1993;341:72–75.

De Maeseneer M, Lenchik L, Everaert H, et al. Evaluation of lower back pain with bone scintigraphy and SPECT. *Radiographics* 1999;19:901–912.

Evan-Sapir E. Imaging of malignant bone involvement by morphologic, scintigraphic, and hybrid modalities. *J Nucl Med* 2005;46:1356–1367.

Freeman LM, Blaufox MD, eds. Metabolic bone disease. *Semin Nucl Med* 1997; 27:195–305.

Freeman LM, Blaufox MD, eds. Orthopedic nuclear medicine (Part I). *Semin Nucl Med* 1997;27:307–389.

Freeman LM, Blaufox MD, eds. Orthopedic nuclear medicine (Part II). *Semin Nucl Med* 1998;28:1–131.

Grant FD, Fahey FH, Packard AB, Davis RT, Alavi A, Treves ST. Skeletal PET with 18F-fluoride: applying new technology to an old tracer. *J Nucl Med* 2008;49:68–78.

Groves AM, Cheow H, Balan K, Courtney H, Bearcroft P, Dixon A. 16-MDCT in the detection of occult wrist fractures: a comparison with skeletal scintigraphy. *AJR Am J Roentgenol* 2005;184:1470–1474.

Helyar V, Mohan HK, Barwick T, et al. The added value of multislice SPECT/CT in patients with equivocal bony metastasis from carcinoma of the prostate. *Eur J Nucl Med Mol Imaging* 2010;37:706–713.

Kozin F, Soin JS, Ryan LM, Carrera GF, Wortmann RL. Bone scintigraphy in the reflex sympathetic dystrophy syndrome. *Radiology* 1981;138:437–443.

Langsteger W, Heinisch M, Fogelman I. The role of fluorodeoxyglucose, 18F-dihydroxyphenylalanine, 18F-choline, and 18F-fluoride in bone imaging with emphasis on prostate and breast. *Semin Nucl Med* 2006;36:73–92.

Linke R, Kuwert T, Uder M, Forst R, Wuest W. Skeletal SPECT/CT of the peripheral extremities. *AJR Am J Roentgenol* 2010;194:W329–W335.

Matin P. Bone scintigraphy in the diagnosis and management of traumatic injury. *Semin Nucl Med* 1983;13:104–122.

McNeil BJ. Value of bone scanning in neoplastic disease. *Semin Nucl Med* 1984;14:277–286.

Merkow RL, Lane JM. Current concepts of Paget's disease of bone. *Orthop Clin North Am* 1984;15:747–763.

Orzel JA, Rudd TG. Heterotopic bone formation: clinical, laboratory, and imaging correlation. *J Nucl Med* 1985;26:125–132.

Paes FM, Serafini AN. Systemic metabolic radiopharmaceutical therapy in the treatment of metastatic bone pain. *Semin Nucl Med* 2010;40:89–104.

Palestro CJ. Nuclear medicine and the failed joint replacement: past, present, and future. *World J Radiol* 2014;6(7):446–458.

Pandit-Taskar N, Batraki M, Divgi CR. Radiopharmaceutical therapy for palliation of bone pain from osseous metastases. *J Nucl Med* 2004;45:1358–1365.

Renzulli JF, Collins J, Mega A. Radium-223 dichloride: illustrating the benefits of a multidisciplinary approach for patients with metastatic castration-resistant prostate cancer. *J Multidiscip Healthc* 2015;8:279–286.

Rosenthal DI, Chandler HL, Azizi F, Schneider PB. Uptake of bone imaging agents by diffuse pulmonary metastatic calcifications. *AJR Am J Roentgenol* 1977;129:871–874.

Ryu JS, Kim JS, Moon DH, et al. Bone SPECT is more sensitive than MRI in the detection of early osteonecrosis of femoral head after renal transplantation. *J Nucl Med* 2002;43:1006–1011.

Savelli G, Maffioli L, Maccauro M, De Deckere E, Bombardieri E. Bone scintigraphy and the added value of SPECT (single photon emission tomography) in detecting skeletal lesions. *Q J Nucl Med* 2001;45:27–37.

Schauwecker DS. The scintigraphic diagnosis of osteomyelitis. *AJR Am J Roentgenol* 1992;158:9–18.

Schirrmeister H, Glatting G, Hetzel J, et al. Prospective evaluation of the clinical values of planar bone scans, SPECT, and (18)F-labeled NaF PET in newly diagnosed lung cancer. *J Nucl Med* 2001;42:1800–1804.

Shehab D, Elgazzar AH, Collier BD. Heterotopic ossification. *J Nucl Med* 2002;43:346–353.

Stevenson JS, Bright RW, Dunson GL, Nelson FR. Technetium-99m phosphate bone imaging: a method for assessing bone graft healing. *Radiology* 1974;110:391–394.

Sutter CW, Shelton DK. Three-phase bone scan in osteomyelitis and other musculoskeletal disorders. *Am Fam Physician* 1996;54:1639–1647.

Treves ST, ed. *Pediatric Nuclear Medicine and Molecular Imaging*. New York: Springer; 2014.

Vande Streek P, Carretta RF, Weiland FL, Shelton DK. Upper extremity radionuclide bone imaging: the wrist and hand. *Semin Nucl Med* 1998;28:14–24.

Weiss PE, Mall JC, Hoffer PB, Murray WR, Rodrigo JJ, Genant HK. 99mTc-methylene diphosphonate bone imaging in the evaluation of total hip prosthesis. *Radiology* 1979;133:727–729.

CHAPTER 72D ■ ENDOCRINE GLAND SCINTIGRAPHY

MARC G. COTE AND BRETT J. MOLLARD

THYROID

Imaging Methods. Diagnosis and treatment of thyroid disease requires the evaluation of thyroid function, anatomy, and tissue characterization of thyroid lesions. Radionuclide scintigraphy and measurement of radioiodine uptake form the basis of functional assessment of the thyroid. Functional imaging combined with serologic serum levels of thyroid hormones allows for the determination and classification of thyroid disease. Ultrasound (US) is the modality of choice for anatomic assessment of the thyroid gland and in the evaluation of thyroid nodules. Thyroid nodules are frequently incidentally identified on CT scans, which lack specificity in nodule characterization relative to US. Nodules smaller than 1 cm are typically below the spatial resolution of scintigraphy and therefore not diagnostically assessed.

Radionuclide scintigraphy is used to assess the physiologic function of the gland and to determine the presence or the functional status of thyroid nodules following fine-needle aspiration (FNA). Thyroid imaging is most commonly indicated to evaluate hyperthyroidism. Solitary thyroid nodules are best evaluated initially with US and subsequently with FNA, depending on the presence of various suspicious features (size, shape, echogenicity, microcalcifications, etc.). The rise of single-photon emission computed tomography with computed tomography (SPECT-CT) has allowed for a better localization of focal radioiodine uptake in patients with iodine-avid thyroid cancer. Dual-photon positron emission tomography with computed tomography (PET-CT) utilizing F-18 fluorodeoxyglucose (FDG) has emerged as a useful adjunct to iodine scintigraphy when evaluating for the recurrence of poorly differentiated non–iodine-avid thyroid cancer.

Normal thyroid parenchyma appears relatively homogeneous with technetium-99m pertechnetate (Tc-99mO_4) or iodine-123 (I-123) scintigraphy. Iodine is trapped via active transport and organified onto the tyrosine contained in the intrathyroidal thyroglobulin within the thyroid follicles. Tc-99mO_4 is only trapped and will subsequently wash out of the gland since it is not organified. I-123 is the radiopharmaceutical of choice for thyroid imaging, particularly, when imaging nodules (Table 72D.1). Tc-99mO_4 is best reserved for imaging hyperthyroid patients in conjunction with an iodine-131 (I-131)-radioactive iodine uptake (RAIU—the percentage of the administered dose present in the thyroid gland at a specific time after oral administration, usually obtained at 4 and 24 hours).

The functional status of a thyroid nodule may be categorized as hyperfunctioning ("hot"), hypofunctioning ("cold"), or indeterminate (sometimes called "warm") relative to the normal parenchymal uptake of radioiodine. The term "warm" is misleading to clinicians and should not be used. Hot nodules usually represent hyperfunctioning adenomatous tissue and are rarely malignant. Although solitary cold nodules are hypofunctioning adenomatous tissue in approximately 40% of cases, they may harbor malignancy in up to 15% of cases. Indeterminate nodules have the same significance as that of cold nodules. The term "warm" should be avoided since it is easily misunderstood by the referring health care provider to have the same clinical significance as that of a "hot" nodule. Indeterminate nodules are due to normal activity overlying or surrounding a hypofunctioning cold nodule.

Tc-99mO_4 is inexpensive but has the disadvantages of a lower target-to-background ratio and inability to exclude discordant nodules, which requires an additional I-123 study for discordant nodule exclusion. **A discordant nodule demonstrates increased Tc-99mO_4 uptake but decreased I-123 uptake and therefore may harbor malignancy.** Physiologically, discordant nodules can still trap Tc-99mO_4 but have lost their ability to organify and retain iodine. Since pertechnetate imaging is performed 4 to 6 hours after administration, initial trapping of the radiopharmaceutical may reveal uptake that is isointense or increased relative to normal parenchyma. I-123 imaging is performed 18 to 24 hours after administration, allowing sufficient time for trapped iodine to wash out and reveal the true nature of the nodule.

Historically, RAIU served as a measure of thyroid function for many years prior to the development of laboratory assays. The development of accurate serologic methods of measuring serum levels of thyroid hormones and ultrasensitive third- and fourth-generation thyroid stimulating hormone (TSH) assays provides a superior method of evaluating thyroid function. Serum TSH is the single best test for screening thyroid function. Only in cases of suspected pituitary or hypothalamic disease is the TSH alone insufficient for screening the thyroid

TABLE 72D.1

RADIOPHARMACEUTICALS USED FOR THYROID IMAGING

ISOTOPE	HALF-LIFE	PRINCIPAL GAMMA RAY (keV)	ADVANTAGES	DISADVANTAGES	COMMENTS
I-123	13 hours	159	Physiologic Good organ-to-background ratio Same dose can be used for imaging and uptake	Expensive Image 4 hours after administration	
I-131	8 days	364	Inexpensive Widely available Long half-life	High-radiation dose per mCi High-energy photon Unsuitable for gamma-camera imaging	Whole-body scans used for the evaluation of residual thyroid and metastatic disease in patients with thyroid cancer
Tc-99m	6 hours	140	Inexpensive Excellent imaging qualities	Requires separate dose of I-123 or I-131 for uptake measurements Must repeat imaging with I-123 if hot nodule found	
F-18 FDG	110 minutes	511	Excellent imaging qualities Usefulness limited to non–iodine-avid thyroid tumors with thyroglobulin level >10 ng/mL	Expensive High-energy photon Requires a PET-CT camera	Whole-body scans used for evaluation of residual non–iodine-avid thyroid and metastatic disease in patients with thyroid cancer

functional status. Measurement of the RAIU is usually indicated for one of the three reasons:

1. Differentiating Graves disease (uptake high, usually >35% at 24 hours) from subacute or factitious hyperthyroidism (uptake usually <2%)
2. Assisting in the calculation of radioactive iodine dose for the treatment of Graves disease
3. Assessing suspected toxic multinodular goiters

If the 24-hour RAIU is to be performed using I-131, 5 to 10 μCi is administered orally but no imaging is possible at this RAIU dose. Alternately, I-123 administered orally may be used to perform both the imaging and the uptake studies using a dose of 200 to 400 μCi. For the RAIU uptake, a nonimaging uptake probe is used to obtain counts in a neck-phantom standard. At 24 hours, counts are obtained from the patient's neck for thyroid counts and counts are obtained from the thigh to determine the background activity. Many laboratories also count the patient at 4 to 6 hours so that markedly hyperthyroid rapid turnover patients are not missed. Rapid turnover patients show a markedly elevated 4- to 6-hour RAIU (25% to 50%) but a lower, if not normal, 24-hour RAIU. Rapid turnover is seen in the setting of marked Graves disease when the small dose of radioactive iodine is rapidly organified and released into the bloodstream as thyroid hormone and subtracted with the thigh background counts.

$$\%\text{Uptake} = \frac{\text{Neck} - \text{thigh cpm} \times 100}{\text{Standard} - \text{background cpm}}$$

where cpm = counts per minute. Normal = 10% to 30% at 24 hours (highly dependent on iodine intake).

Embryology, Anatomy, and Physiology. The thyroid gland initially arises from the foramen cecum of the base of the tongue and the floor of the pharynx as midline thickening. It then descends into the lower neck where the thyroid gland forms as two lobes of approximately equal size (5 × 2 cm) positioned on either side of the trachea and connected across the midline by the thin thyroid isthmus inferiorly (Fig. 72D.1). The midline pharyngeal thickening persists as the thyroglossal duct, extending from the tongue base to the isthmus. The inferior aspect of the thyroglossal duct persists as the pyramidal lobe (midline extension cranially of the isthmus or left lobe) in approximately 40% of patients. Failure of the thyroid to descend may result in a lingual thyroid. Pediatric patients with a lingual thyroid are at high risk of developing hypothyroidism, with an estimated risk of approximately 30%. Thyroglossal duct persistence beyond the second gestational month of the thyroid's descent may occur and result in a persistent thyroglossal duct.

Histologically, the thyroid gland is composed of the thyroid hormone–secreting follicular cells arranged in acini, with central collections of colloid. Parafollicular cells ("C cells"), which produce calcitonin, comprise a small proportion of the cell population and are predominantly located in the superior two-thirds of the gland. Parafollicular "C" cells reside in the connective tissue adjacent to the follicular cells. Parafollicular "C" cells that undergo malignant degeneration are the anatomic origin of medullary thyroid cancer.

The role of the thyroid gland is the production, storage, and release of thyroid hormones. TSH, produced by the anterior portion of the pituitary gland, regulates the thyroid's production and release of thyroid hormones. TSH secretion is regulated by hypothalamic thyrotropin-releasing hormone (TRH) and suppressed by circulating thyroxine (T4) and triiodothyronine (T3). Iodine is absorbed within the stomach and small bowel from dietary sources with approximately 25% of absorbed iodine organified within the thyroid and

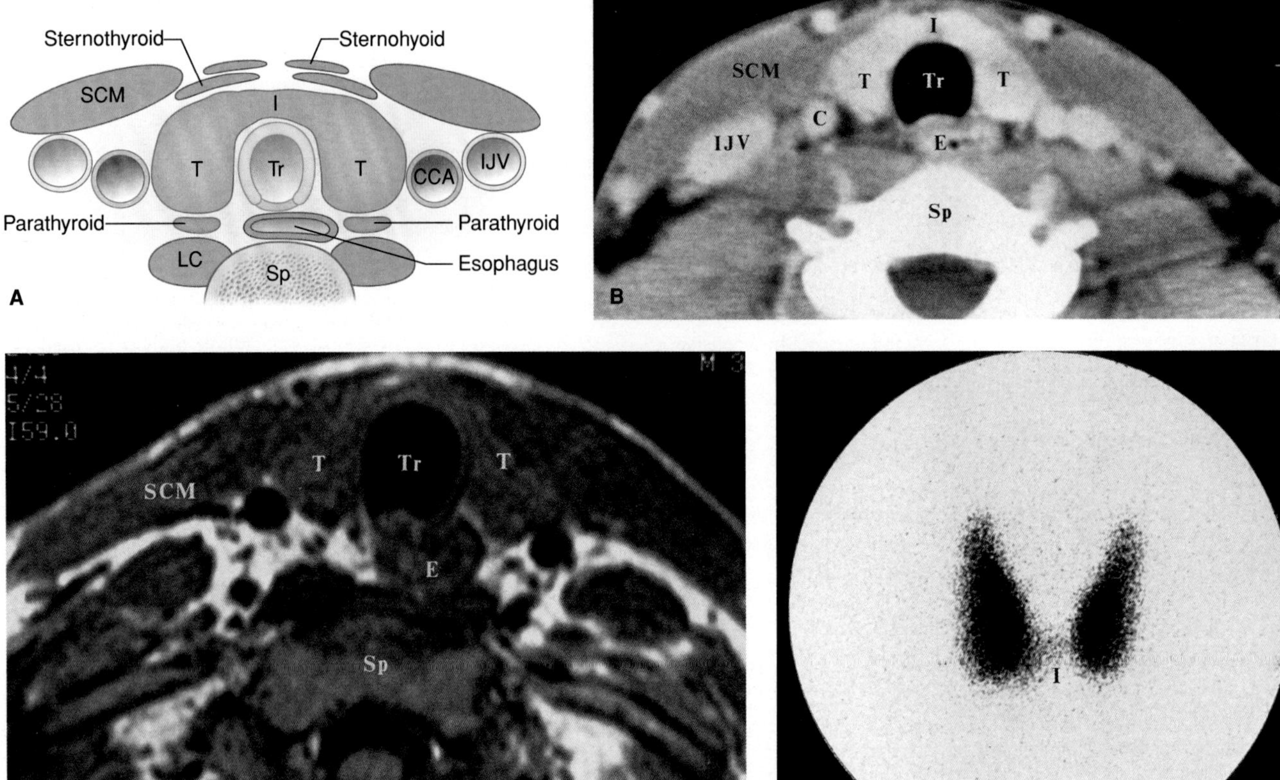

FIGURE 72D.1. **Normal Thyroid.** Diagram (**A**), CT image (**B**), and T1-weighted MR image (**C**) of the thyroid gland in cross-section. **D:** Normal I-123 thyroid scan. *T*, thyroid gland; *I*, isthmus of thyroid gland; *Tr*, trachea; *CCA*, common carotid artery; *IJV*, internal jugular vein; *E*, esophagus; *SCM*, sternocleidomastoid muscle; *LC*, longus colli muscle; *Sp*, spine.

the remaining 75% excreted in the urine. Recommended daily adult allowance for iodine is 100 to 150 mg. Developed countries typically fortify certain foods with iodine and exceed the recommended dose, though iodine deficiency is still endemic in certain parts of the world.

Hypothyroidism. In iodine-deficient endemic areas, hypothyroidism is usually caused by dietary iodine deficiency with a pathognomonic concomitant goiter (enlarged gland). Chronic thyroiditis (Hashimoto disease) is the most common noniatrogenic cause of hypothyroidism in iodine-replete areas, and a goiter is usually clinically evident. Prior treatment of hyperthyroidism with radioactive I-131 is another common cause (without goiter). Neonatal hypothyroidism is due to thyroid dysgenesis (agenesis, hypoplasia, or ectopia). Pediatric lingual thyroid has a 30% chance of developing hypothyroidism with potential consequences to brain development if hypothyroidism is not diagnosed early and treated. Clinical features of hypothyroidism include weight gain, cold intolerance, sluggishness, fatigue, and dry skin. Laboratory findings include elevated serum TSH and low serum T4.

Hyperthyroidism. Graves disease is the most common cause of hyperthyroidism. Other causes include subacute or painless thyroiditis, toxic nodular goiter, early phase of postpartum thyroiditis (thyrotoxicosis precedes the subsequent development of transient hypothyroidism), and factitious hyperthyroidism due to ingestion of thyroid hormone tablets. Clinical features of hyperthyroidism include weight loss, increased appetite, tremor, heat intolerance, palpitations, muscle weakness, goiter, exophthalmos, and mood changes or irritability. Laboratory findings include a markedly decreased (suppressed) serum TSH and an elevated serum T4.

Goiter refers to the clinical finding of generalized thyroid enlargement. Goiter may be associated with increased, decreased, or normal thyroid-hormonal function. Thyroid enlargement may be suspected by physical examination and confirmed with thyroid US. Goiters extending into the thorax (substernal goiter) may be incidentally detected by anatomic imaging and verified with I-123 scintigraphy. Tc-99mO_4 is not useful with substernal goiter due to the large amount of blood pool activity within the chest.

Multinodular goiter is a commonly used clinical term for adenomatous hyperplasia. Imaging studies reveal a diffusely abnormal enlarged nodular gland with a heterogeneous uptake of the radiopharmaceutical, or a pattern of multiple discrete hot nodules on a background of normal or "cool" parenchyma. Photopenic regions should be palpated and dominant palpable nodules should be marked to assure that they do not represent a dominant cold nodule. A 4.1% rate of malignancy occurs in patients with a dominant palpable cold nodule in the setting of multinodular goiter. The hot nodules represent autonomously functioning thyroid adenomas, which are usually benign (Fig. 72D.2).

Nontoxic goiter may be related to iodine deficiency, excessive consumption of goitrogens in the diet (cooking deactivates goitrogens), medications, or a thyroid enzyme deficiency. The

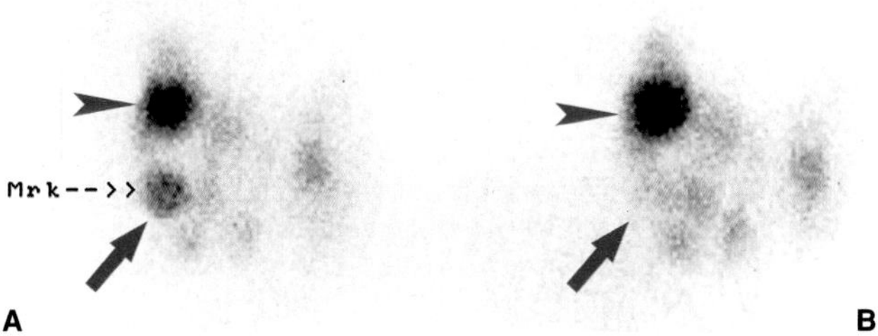

FIGURE 72D.2. **Thyroid Nodules.** Two images from an I-123 thyroid scan. **A:** A radioactive marker was placed over a 2-cm palpable nodule (*arrow*) in the right thyroid lobe. **B:** The image on the right, without the marker, demonstrates the palpable nodule (*arrow*) to be cold. The second palpable nodule in the right upper lobe (*arrowhead*) is shown to be hot. Biopsy confirmed the cold palpable nodule to be papillary thyroid cancer with multinodular goiter. This case illustrates the importance of palpating and marking nodules.

gland is usually soft and symmetric but may appear multinodular with age.

Thyroiditis. All types of thyroiditis are characterized by a rapid asymmetric glandular enlargement, with or without nodularity. Infection of the thyroid gland may be acute and suppurative because of gram-positive bacteria or subacute because of viral infection, which may involve only a portion of the gland. Subacute viral infection usually causes focal edematous enlargement of the gland. Subacute viral infection may have a protean presentation that mimics some of the clinical features of Graves disease because of the release of all preformed thyroid hormone as a response to the inflammation. The RAIU allows for the differentiation of this syndrome from Graves disease. Subacute viral thyroiditis has a very low RAIU and scintigraphy is rarely indicated. The majority of patients with subacute thyroiditis will resolve and return to a euthyroid state after a transient period of hypothyroidism and elevation of RAIU as the gland returns to normal.

Graves disease is the most common cause of hyperthyroidism. It is an autoimmune disorder in which thyroid-stimulating antibodies cause hyperplasia and hyperfunction of the thyroid gland. The gland is usually enlarged two- to threefold, homogeneous on thyroid scan, without palpable nodules, and with elevated RAIU (Fig. 72D.3). The treatment of choice for non-pregnant, non–breast-feeding adults with Graves disease is oral I-131 in conjunction with ß-blockers such as propranolol, to control symptoms during therapy. Treatment options include subtotal thyroidectomy or antithyroid drugs such as propylthiouracil, methimazole, and carbimazole.

I-131 in the form of sodium iodide has been in use for many years. It is given by mouth either as a capsule or as a liquid. After uptake by the gland, the high-energy β particles (mean energy of 0.19 MeV) deliver an average of 0.01 Sv/mCi (1 rad/mCi) to the thyroid cells. Surrounding structures are relatively spared, given the average range of the β particles is 0.8 to 1.0 mm in soft tissue. Most patients will become euthyroid or hypothyroid after a single dose and 10% to 20% of patients require a second or third dose. Patients generally become euthyroid by 10 to 12 weeks after therapy and frequently become hypothyroid by 6 to 12 months. Estimation of the dose of I-131 is empiric. A commonly used formula is:

$$\text{Dose in mCi} = \frac{100 - 150 \text{ uCi/g} \times \text{wt of the gland in grams}}{\text{24-hr RAIU\% uptake} \times 10}$$

resulting in a typically administered oral dose of approximately 5 to 20 mCi of I-131. The higher the dose, the quicker the response and the sooner the patient becomes hypothyroid. The smaller the dose, the longer it takes to become euthyroid and the later the development of hypothyroidism. However, it appears that hypothyroidism cannot be avoided, merely delayed by using small doses of I-131. Therefore, it has become a common policy in many centers to give larger doses of I-131 in the range of 15 to 25 mCi, with the understanding that hypothyroidism is inevitable and is easily treated with daily replacement levothyroxine. It is important to document with laboratory testing that females of childbearing age are not pregnant prior to treatment with radioactive iodine, since iodine crosses the placental barrier and will damage the fetal thyroid. The physician should ascertain that the woman is not breast-feeding, since human milk concentrates iodine and the I-131 in her milk would result in exposure to her infant. Many recommend waiting 4 to 6 weeks or more after cessation of breast-feeding, to allow the breast tissue to involute and decrease breast tissue exposure to I-131.

Complications are uncommon. Transient worsening of thyrotoxicosis is, however, fairly common. It occurs a few days to 2 to 3 weeks after treatment and is due to the release of preformed thyroid hormone from disrupted follicles. Occasionally, patients develop symptoms of subacute thyroiditis, with pain and tenderness in the thyroid often radiating to the ears or the jaw. Temporary hypoparathyroidism and recurrent laryngeal nerve damage have been reported after radioactive iodine treatment, but both are exceedingly rare. Though serious and life threatening, thyroid storm is a very rare complication, more often seen after surgery in inadequately prepared patients. The patient's risk of genetic damage is no greater than their baseline pretreatment risk, provided they wait 6 months prior to conception. Carcinogenesis is not statistically increased. All forms of thyroiditis may be mistaken for tumor because of rapid asymmetric enlargement and nodularity.

Acute (suppurative) thyroiditis is secondary to bacterial infections caused by *Streptococcus*, *Staphylococcus*, or *Pneumococcus*. The condition presents with fever, severe sore throat, and asymmetric swelling, and may result in sepsis from hematogenous spread or extend into the mediastinum via fascial planes.

Subacute (viral) thyroiditis has many eponyms but is commonly known as de Quervain or granulomatous thyroiditis. Subacute thyroiditis presents with thyroid pain and hyperthyroidism

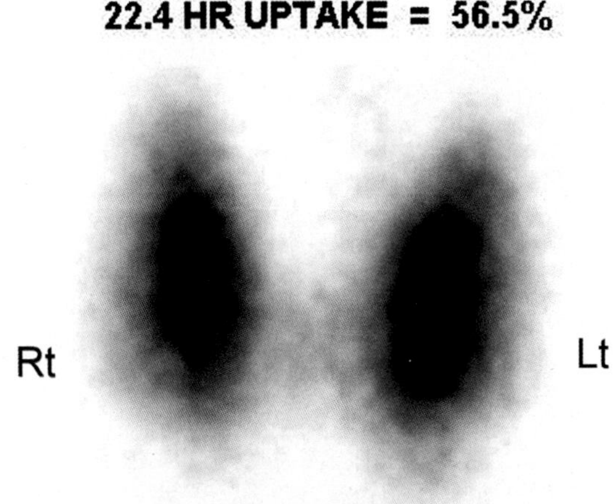

FIGURE 72D.3. **Graves Disease.** This I-123 scan demonstrates diffuse intense thyroid uptake without cold nodules. Elevated radioiodine uptake is present at 4 hours, 38.4%, and at 24 hours, 56.5%.

following an upper respiratory infection. Inflammation of the thyroid gland results in release of thyroid hormone into the bloodstream. Iodine uptake is usually decreased or is absent in the acute stages. The disease runs a subacute course of a few weeks to a few months before returning back to a euthyroid state.

Postpartum thyroiditis typically presents in months 2 to 6 postpartum as a result of nonpainful inflammatory changes. Women at risk of developing postpartum thyroiditis include those with autoimmune disorders, positive antithyroid antibodies, or previous history of postpartum thyroiditis. Clinically, the early phase manifests as hyperthyroid symptoms with subsequent development of hypothyroid symptoms in the later stage. The majority of patients will return to a euthyroid state within a year with a minority requiring lifelong thyroid hormone replacement treatment.

Hashimoto thyroiditis is the most common cause of goiter and primary hypothyroidism in adults in developed countries. It is an autoimmune disorder with circulating antithyroid antibodies. Histology demonstrates diffuse lymphocytic infiltration of the gland. The thyroid is diffusely enlarged with a rubbery palpable texture. Its early phase is a hyperthyroid-like picture that subsequently evolves into its final hypothyroid sine qua non. Diffuse homogeneous hypermetabolism is seen on F-18 FDG PET-CT due to the preferential utilization of glucose by intrathyroidal lymphocytes.

Riedel thyroiditis is a rare inflammatory fibrosing process that involves the thyroid and commonly extends into the neck. Radionuclide uptake is absent (cold) in the involved areas.

Secondary hyperthyroidism may develop in patients with hydatidiform moles or choriocarcinoma. A subunit of the human chorionic gonadotropin (hCG) produced by these conditions demonstrates considerable similarity to TSH, thereby directly stimulating the thyroid. Clinical history and serum determination of hCG should be performed if this is a consideration.

Thyroid Nodules

Thyroid nodules are extremely common, while thyroid cancer is relatively rare. Nodules can be palpated in 4% to 7% of American adults who are asymptomatic for thyroid disease. Autopsy studies demonstrate thyroid nodules in 50% of patients with clinically normal thyroid glands. US studies can detect thyroid nodules in 36% to 41% of middle-aged adults, with some studies reporting even higher rates of 67%. Thyroid cancer, on the other hand, affects only 0.1% of the population. The incidence of thyroid cancer has increased to 53,990 new cases each year (40,900 women and 13,090 men) per the American Cancer Society as of 2018. Thyroid cancer represents less than 1% of all cancer and is responsible for less than 0.5% of all cancer deaths. The challenge of clinical evaluation and imaging studies is to establish the likelihood of malignancy and to select for surgery, only those patients at a high risk for thyroid malignancy. Recent consensus panels have developed algorithms for the workup and management of thyroid nodules.

US is highly sensitive for the detection of thyroid nodules but the specificity for determining malignancy is low. Recent consensus panels have discouraged the routine use of US for screening. Neither MR nor CT improves specificity. This is not surprising since the histologic differentiation of a benign follicular adenoma from a well-differentiated follicular carcinoma is based solely on the identification of vascular invasion.

I-123 and Tc-99mO_4 uptake in nodules may be classified as hypofunctioning (cold) (Fig. 72D.4), hyperfunctioning (hot) (Fig. 72D.5), or indeterminate relative to the rest of the gland. In a patient with a nodular goiter, the main concern is whether or not thyroid carcinoma is present. Single cold nodules have a 10% to 15% incidence of malignancy, while malignancy is exceedingly rare in hot nodules. A multinodular gland with one or more cold nodules may harbor cancer in up to 5% of patients. Hot nodules identified on Tc-99mO_4 imaging must be confirmed with I-123 as thyroid carcinoma may occasionally trap Tc-99mO_4, resulting in a hot nodule. These nodules are cold on I-123 and are called ***discordant thyroid nodules***.

The differential diagnosis of thyroid nodules is as follows:

Follicular adenoma is the most common benign neoplasm of the thyroid and represents about 20% of thyroid nodules. There are many subtypes based on the histologic criteria, including Hürthle cell adenoma, colloid adenoma, and others. Most are solitary, round or oval, and well encapsulated. Regressive changes are extremely common and greatly affect a nodule's imaging appearance. These include focal necrosis, hemorrhage, edema, infarction, fibrosis, and calcification.

Adenomatous hyperplasia is responsible for up to 50% of thyroid nodules. Adenomatous nodules, also called colloid

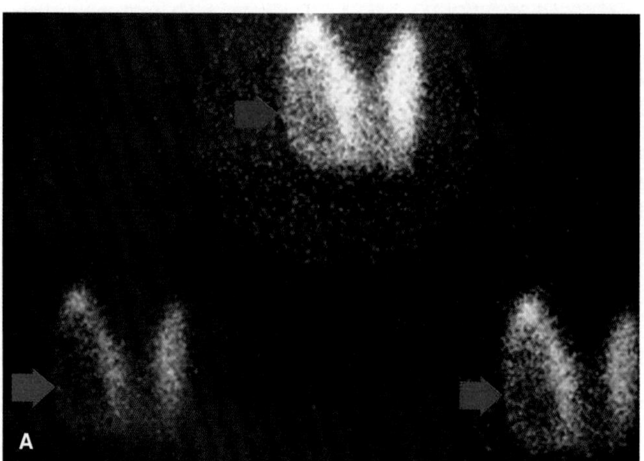

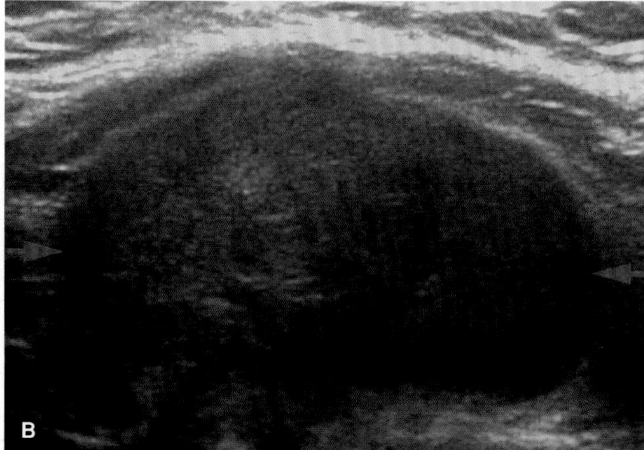

FIGURE 72D.4. **Cold Nodule—Follicular Adenoma. A:** I-123 scan photographed at three different intensities demonstrates a large hypofunctioning nodule (*arrows*) in the right thyroid lobe. **B:** Longitudinal US image of the right thyroid lobe reveals a well-defined solid nodule (*arrows*) with a hypoechoic rim.

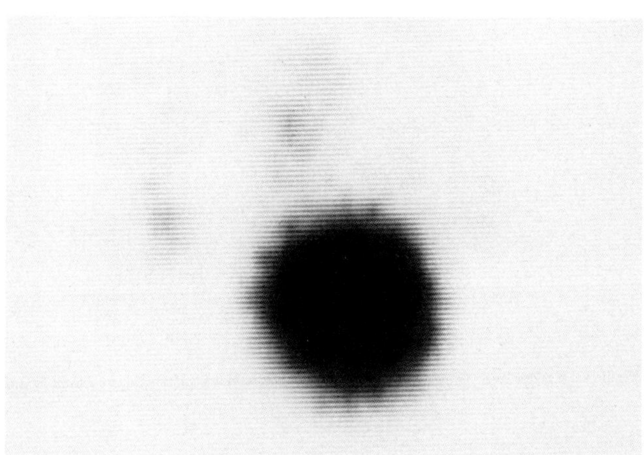

FIGURE 72D.5. **Hot Nodule.** A hyperfunctioning adenoma demonstrates intense radionuclide activity with the suppression of the function of the remainder of the gland.

nodules, are not true neoplasms but are the result of cycles of hyperplasia and involution of a thyroid lobule. They are frequently multiple but one nodule may be dominant. Regressive changes are common including necrosis, hemorrhage, cystic degeneration, and calcification.

Thyroid cysts are extremely rare. Most cystic nodules found in the thyroid are actually cystic degeneration of an adenomatous nodule or a follicular adenoma. The incidence of malignancy within a thyroid cyst is reported to be in the range of 0.5% to 3.0%. Therefore, fluid should be submitted for cytology and the area aspirated should have adequate sampling.

Hemorrhagic cysts also usually represent hemorrhage into an adenomatous nodule or a follicular adenoma. Hemorrhage into normal parenchyma may also produce a hemorrhagic cyst.

Thyroid Cancer

Thyroid Cancer. It is estimated that 53,990 new thyroid cancer cases occur each year (American Cancer Society estimates for 2018), resulting in more than 2,060 deaths per year in the United States. Thyroid cancer's annual incidence has increased to approximately 14.2/100,000 population (per 2010 to 2014 data), felt to be secondary to the increased detection of subclinical disease while survival has improved to 98%. Thyroid cancer may precede the development of other primary carcinomas since recent longitudinal studies suggest that thyroid cancer survivors have a 30% increased incidence of a second primary carcinoma. Malignant nodules cannot be reliably differentiated from benign nodules by any imaging method. FNA with good sampling technique and good cytologic support is essential in every suspicious case. Malignant cytology by FNA has been found in 5.3% to 12.6% of thyroid nodules, with rates differing based on nodule size and patient age and gender. While specificity by imaging is fairly low, a number of criteria can be used to assess the relative risk of malignancy (Tables 72D.2 and 72D.3). Every assessment of thyroid nodules must consider all clinical and imaging features. A nodule that is hot on radioiodine scan is extremely unlikely to be malignant. A nodule that is solitary and cold on scintigraphy has a 6% to 10% chance of being malignant. A history of neck irradiation, particularly in childhood, increases the risk of malignancy by 5- to 10-fold (0.3 to 12.5/10,000 person-years). Nodules with extensive cystic component (>50% cystic) or well-defined peripheral calcification as seen in US are unlikely to be malignant. Regression of nodule size following thyroid hormone therapy is a sign of a benign nodule. Large, predominantly solid nodules with irregular contour and poor margination on US examination are likely to be malignant. Five-year survival rates with treatment are approximately 90% to 95%. The histologic types of thyroid malignancy are as follows:

TABLE 72D.2

SIGNS SUGGESTING BENIGN ETIOLOGY

Extensive cystic component
Multiple nodules
Hot on radionuclide scan
Peripheral calcification
Shrinkage in size following LT4 suppression hormone therapy
Sudden onset
Female gender
Older patient

Papillary carcinoma is the most common type accounting for 75% of cases and can be imaged with iodine imaging. Patients are predominantly female (female:male = 4:1), with an average age of 45. The major route of spread is from lymphatic to regional nodes, followed by hematogenous dissemination to the lung and the bone (Figs. 72D.6 to 72D.8).

Follicular carcinoma represents 15% of thyroid cancer cases, is more common in females, and amenable to iodine imaging. The primary route of spread is hematogenous to the lung and the bone. Prognosis is not as good as that of papillary carcinoma.

Medullary carcinoma arises from parafollicular cells (C cells) and is associated with multiple endocrine neoplasia (MEN II) in some cases. Calcitonin is a useful tumor marker. Prognosis is worse than for papillary or follicular carcinoma. The tumor spreads by both lymphatic and hematogenous routes. Although the tumor does not concentrate I-131 or I-123, metastases can be detected by thallium-201 (Tl-201), Tc-99m(V) DMSA (dimercaptosuccinic acid, pentavalent form), and I-123/131-MIBG (meta-iodo-benzyl-guanidine). Indium-111 (In-111)

TABLE 72D.3

SIGNS SUGGESTING MALIGNANCY

Imaging
Solid nodule
Cold on radionuclide scan
Irregular contour
Poor margination
Presence of microcalcifications
Size >4–5 cm
Clinical
Hard on palpation
History of neck irradiation
Age <20 years
Male
Neck pain
Hoarseness/voice changes
Cervical adenopathy
Familial history of thyroid cancer

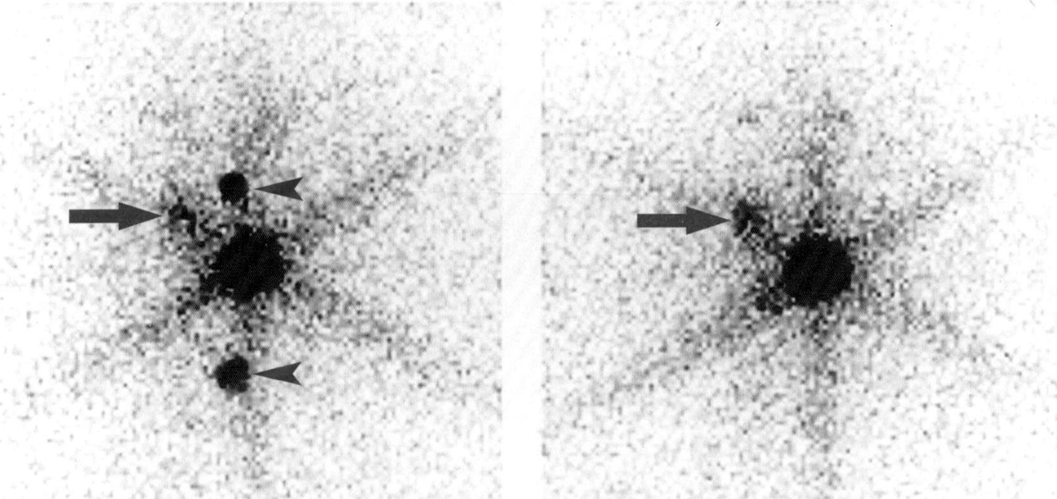

FIGURE 72D.6. **Thyroid Cancer Metastasis.** I-131 scan of the neck in a patient who has undergone near-total thyroidectomy for thyroid cancer. *Arrowheads* indicate radioactive markers of the chin and suprasternal notch. The large star artifact is due to septal penetration of the collimator. The center of the star represents the original thyroid bed. A lymph-node metastasis is evident in the right upper neck (*arrows*).

pentetreotide scintigraphy has a sensitivity of 65% to 70% as well. F-18 FDG PET-CT in a retrospective study showed a sensitivity of 85.7% and a specificity of 83.3%. I-131 MIBG has also been used for the treatment, if the tumor displays avidity on the diagnostic scan for I-123 or I-131 MIBG.

Anaplastic carcinoma is an extremely lethal malignancy generally occurring in an older population with no effective treatment since it no longer takes up iodine either for imaging or for treatment. Five-year survival rate is less than 4%. The tumor demonstrates very aggressive local invasion and spreads early to distant sites.

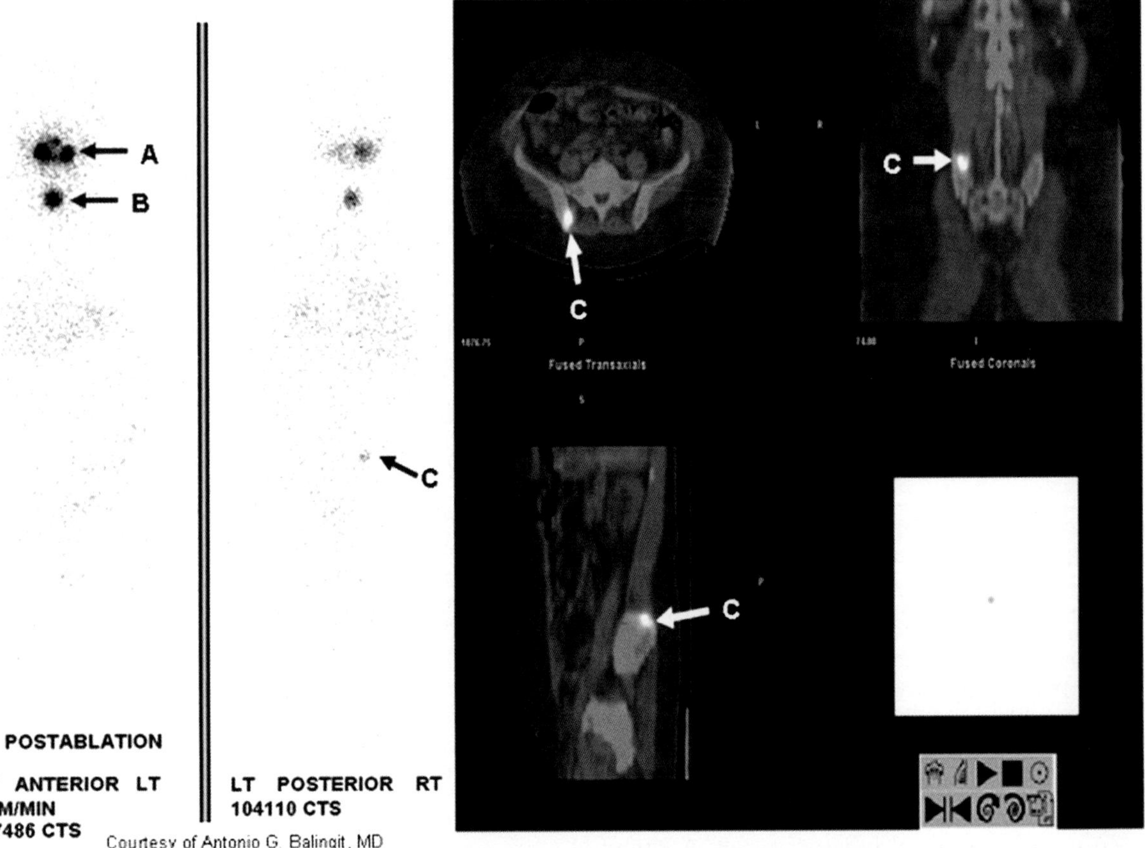

FIGURE 72D.7. **Thyroid Follicular Cancer Pelvic Metastasis With SPECT.** The I-123 planar body scan (**left**) shows parotid gland uptake (*arrow* A) and residual thyroid bed uptake (*arrow* B). A faint focus of activity is seen (*arrow* C) on the planar image. SPECT-CT (**right**) localizes the focal activity in the right iliac wing as a bony metastasis (*arrow* C).

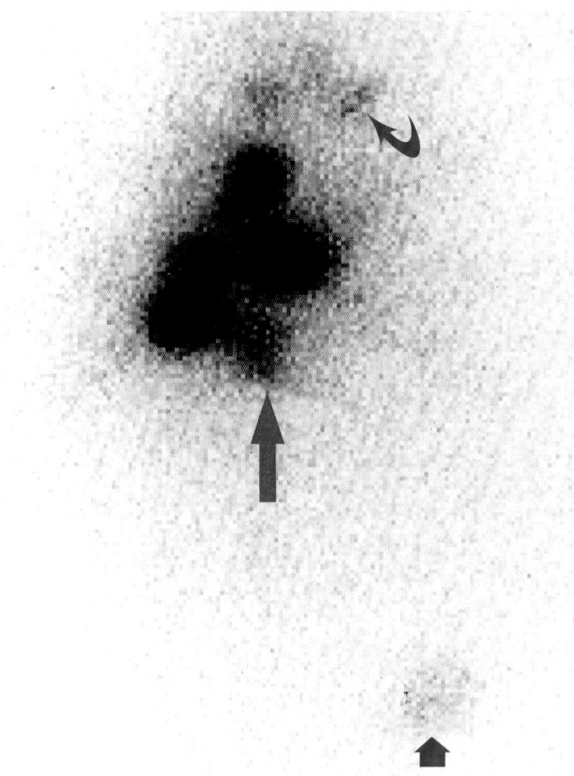

FIGURE 72D.8. **Thyroid Cancer Recurrence With Lymph-Node Metastases.** I-131 whole-body scan postthyroidectomy shows intense radionuclide activity in papillary carcinoma lymph-node metastases in the neck (*long red arrow*). Normal activity is present in the stomach (*short blue arrow*) and submandibular salivary glands (*curved blue arrow*).

Thyroid Cancer Imaging and Therapy. Historically, initial postthyroidectomy I-131 whole-body scan with its 72-hour RAIU was used exclusively with the surgical pathology report of the thyroid tumor, its size, the presence or absence of contralateral lobe involvement, and lymph-node status determination. Over the years, I-123 has gained acceptance for imaging thyroid cancer due to the improved count statistics and avoidance of potential stunning of cancer cells from I-131 β particles that could theoretically blunt treatment response from a subsequent therapeutic I-131 dose. The selection of I-131 or I-123 remains controversial for pretreatment scintigraphy, with some recent data supporting use of I-123 scintigraphy.

Diagnostic I-131 or I-123 scans of the whole body, neck, and chest are performed to determine the completeness of surgery, staging, and to evaluate the response to treatment. Radioiodine uptake in the thyroid bed frequently represents residual thyroid tissue. Salivary, stomach, bowel, bladder, and breast activity represents physiologic traces of iodine distribution. Nasal secretions may contain radioiodine, which may act as a source of contamination and should not be confused with metastatic disease. Whole-body radionuclide scans using I-131 or I-123 are effective in demonstrating thyroid metastases and tumor recurrence following thyroidectomy for papillary carcinoma (Fig. 72D.8). **Focal uptake in the lungs, skeleton, or in the neck remote from the thyroid bed is pathologic.** Several recent studies advocate for the addition of SPECT-CT of the neck in either the immediate postablation setting or combination pre- and postablation SPECT-CT for more accurate staging. Preablation or postablation SPECT-CT have demonstrated significant changes in management in 11% to 58% of cases. F-18 FDG PET-CT is reserved for non–iodine-avid tumors including medullary and anaplastic carcinoma and in the setting of biochemical evidence of recurrence (i.e., elevated serum thyroglobulin) with a negative radioiodine whole-body scan. F-18 FDG PET-CT imaging has demonstrated a sensitivity of 60% to 89% and a specificity of 60% to 89% in non–iodine-avid recurrence. Tl-201, Tc-99m-sestamibi (Tc-99m MIBI), and Tc-99m-tetrofosmin have shown some utility in imaging non–iodine-avid thyroid cancer, but evaluation has largely been replaced by F-18 FDG PET-CT. Hürthle cell carcinoma has similarities to follicular cell carcinoma since Hürthle cell is well differentiated, but Hürthle cell carcinoma has a lower avidity for iodine. Hürthle cell carcinoma typically follows an aggressive course with a higher mortality compared with the other differentiated thyroid cancers. A recent study demonstrated a 95% sensitivity with F-18 FDG in detecting remnant or metastatic Hürthle cells.

Lymph-node involvement on anatomic imaging (US, CT, MRI) is determined primarily by size criteria with subsequent pathologic confirmation. Normal lymph nodes in the neck are less than 10 mm in short axis.

Postablation Imaging of Thyroid Cancer Patients. The use of recombinant human thyroid-stimulating hormone (rhTSH) treatment to image postablation patients for follow-up screening is an option that does not require withdrawal of levothyroxine replacement that maintains a better quality of life for patients. Studies comparing the efficacy of levothyroxine withdrawal versus the use of the traditional withdrawal method indicate an 88% success rate in ablation. Serum thyroglobulin is a sensitive serum marker of recurrent differentiated thyroid cancer. On day 1, baseline serum thyroglobulin levels are obtained and an intramuscular injection of 0.9 mg of rhTSH is administered on days 1 and 2. Serum thyroglobulin levels are obtained on days 3 and 5. Low or undetectable baseline Tg levels that are ≥2 ng/mL following rhTSH stimulation are suggestive of a recurrent thyroid cancer. I-131 or I-123 is given 24 hours after the second rhTSH dose and imaging can be performed at 48 hours after I-131 administration or at 24 hours for I-123.

Radioiodine Therapy. Most authorities agree with postthyroidectomy ablation in primary thyroid tumors larger than 1.5 cm. Some disagreement now exists in the literature on the treatment of patients with I-131 if primary tumor size is smaller than 1 cm.

According to the Nuclear Regulatory Commission, NUREG-1556, Vol. 9, patients receiving 33 mCi or more of I-131 require hospitalization until the residual amount of I-131 falls below 33 mCi or a rate-meter reading of less than 7 mR/hr at 1 m, unless it can be shown that it is unlikely that releasing the patient would result in a member of the public receiving a dose greater than 5 mSv (500 mrem). Doses up to 33-mCi I-131 are frequently administered on an outpatient basis to ablate residual thyroid tissue status postthyroidectomy. Revised NRC rules for doses greater than 33-mCi I-131 as an outpatient require extensive regulatory documentation and calculations. Some authors advocate larger I-131 doses on the grounds that 33 mCi I-131 is inadequate to ablate thyroid cancer and may cause a stunning effect that makes the thyroid more radioresistant on subsequent treatment. Doses of 100- to 200-mCi I-131 are frequently used depending on the tumor cytology, size, and the presence of capsular, vascular, or lymph-node involvement. Recent studies compared high- versus low-dose I-131 and postthyroidectomy I-131 ablation dosing. Some clinics, depending on the tumor size and presence or absence of distant metastases, will use dosimetry calculations to determine the I-131 dose to maximize the dose delivered to the tumor burden but limit marrow exposure to the I-131. Elderly patients are at increased risk of overexposure.

Conventional treatment with I-131 used thyroid hormone withdrawal to achieve pretreatment hypothyroidism (serum

TSH greater than 35 to 40 IU/mL) prior to whole-body I-131 imaging or ablation since elevated TSH results in active transport of the iodine into the thyroid cell. This is to ensure maximal stimulation of residual thyroid and/or thyroid cancer and thereby promote appropriate localization of the radioiodine. Iodine-rich foods such as shellfish, bread, and kelp should be avoided at least 2 to 4 weeks prior to therapy. Dairy products should also be limited since these are a rich source of "cold" iodine that can inhibit the uptake of I-131. A radiographic study with iodinated contrast will delay therapy by at least 2 to 3 months, unless clinical maneuvers to deplete the patient of the exogenous iodine are performed. Iodine depletion can be ascertained with a 24-hour iodine urine collection assay. rTSH injections stimulate iodine uptake with subsequent I-131 dosing. This technique avoids the hypothyroid withdrawal state and is finding greater acceptance as a treatment option in patients.

The frequency of side effects varies directly with the dose of radioiodine administered. Doses greater than 100 mCi may cause sialadenitis, which may lead to permanent xerostomia. For this reason, patients should be strongly encouraged to drink copious amounts of water and suck on sialogogues such as lemon drops or sour candy for 3 to 7 days posttherapy. Pulmonary fibrosis has been reported in patients who have had multiple doses of radioiodine therapy for extensive pulmonary disease. Leukemia has been reported in patients who have received cumulative doses in excess of 600 to 800 mCi.

Metastases to the thyroid gland are rare. The most common primary tumors that metastasize to the thyroid are breast, lung, kidney, malignant melanoma, and lymphoma.

PARATHYROID

Parathyroid disorders are classified in terms of function: excessive parathyroid hormone (PTH) production (hyperparathyroidism) and insufficient PTH production (hypoparathyroidism). Parathyroid scintigraphy is performed to localize parathyroid abnormalities such as hyperplasia, adenomas, and carcinoma in patients with clinical evidence of hyperparathyroidism. There is no role for imaging in hypoparathyroidism. The causes of hyperparathyroidism are listed in Table 72D.4.

Imaging Methods. Approximately 80% to 85% of abnormal parathyroid glands are located near the thyroid. Ectopic locations for abnormal parathyroid tissue include thymus (10% to 15%), posterior mediastinum (5%), retroesophageal (1%), within the carotid sheath (1%), and parapharyngeal (0.5%). US, scintigraphy with Tl-201, Tc-99m MIBI, CT, or MR have various sensitivities and specificities that depend on whether or not the patient has had prior surgery. The use of SPECT-CT cameras has improved the localization of hyperfunctioning parathyroid glands, especially ectopic parathyroids (Fig. 72D.9). At centers with very experienced surgeons, surgery is curative in 92% to 98% of patients with previously unoperated hyperparathyroidism, but reoperation success decreases to 62% in patients who require a repeat surgery. Localization procedures are indicated in patients who are surgical failures requiring a second surgery and may be helpful prior to a first operation when the local surgical experience is limited.

TABLE 72D.4

CAUSES OF HYPERPARATHYROIDISM

Primary hyperparathyroidism
Solitary parathyroid adenoma, 85%
Parathyroid hyperplasia, 10%
Multiple parathyroid adenomas, 4%
Parathyroid carcinoma, 1%
Secondary hyperparathyroidism
Diffuse or adenomatous parathyroid hyperplasia due to calcium-losing renal disease
Tertiary hyperparathyroidism
Autonomous parathyroid function resulting from long-standing secondary hyperparathyroidism
Paraneoplastic syndromes
Ectopic parathormone production
Bronchogenic carcinoma
Renal cell carcinoma

Radionuclide subtraction imaging (Fig. 72D.10) has been used to detect parathyroid adenomas with a sensitivity of about 75% and a specificity of 90%. Tc-99mO_4/Tl-201 or Tc-99m MIBI/I-123 subtraction techniques are in use today by a minority of laboratories, with the washout method having gained favor over the difficulty of the subtraction method. Thyroid tissue concentrates Tc-99mO_4, Tl-201, and Tc-99m MIBI (Fig. 72D.11). Parathyroid adenomas take up Tl-201 but not Tc-99mO_4, which is the basis for dual-isotope imaging with Tl-201 and Tc-99mO_4. Tl-201 images are first acquired and then, without moving the patient, Tc-99mO_4 is administered and imaging at the technetium peak is performed. The Tc-99mO_4 images are subtracted from the Tl-201 images and any residual foci of activity are indicative of parathyroid adenoma(s). False-positive results can be seen as a result of patient movement between studies or with Tl-201 uptake in thyroid nodules, sarcoid-containing lymph nodes, or metastases to the neck as the technique is predicated on the presence of an underlying normal thyroid gland.

Tc-99m MIBI and Tc-99m Tetrofosmin Imaging. Tc-99m MIBI is superior to Tl-201 and the radiopharmaceutical of choice. While a few clinics still use the subtraction imaging techniques, Tc-99m MIBI has virtually replaced Tc-99mO_4/Tl-201 subtraction imaging at most centers. Tc-99m MIBI and Tc-99m-tetrofosmin were thought to have similar sensitivities and specificities to other imaging methods, but Tc-99m MIBI is now felt to be the radiopharmaceutical of choice. Tc-99m isonitriles use the differential washout rate between thyroid cells and abnormal parathyroids. Attention to radiochemical purity and preparation of Tc-99m MIBI affects the washout rates. When Tc-99m MIBI or Tc-99m-tetrofosmin is used for parathyroid imaging, immediate and delayed images of the neck and mediastinum are performed. Parathyroid adenomas may or may not be visualized on initial imaging but tend to retain the radiopharmaceutical on delayed (1 to 2 hours) images while the normal thyroid gland washes out (Fig. 72D.11). Retention occurs in the mitochondria-rich cells of adenomas. False negatives may be seen in clear cell adenomas, which histologically contain a paucity of mitochondria. The emergence of SPECT-CT has improved the localization of ectopic parathyroids (Fig. 72D.9).

Anatomy. Most people (80%) have four parathyroid glands, two superior and two inferior. However, autopsy studies have demonstrated that 20% of individuals have three, five, or, six parathyroid glands. The superior parathyroid glands arise from the fourth branchial pouch along with the thyroid gland and are seldom ectopic. The inferior parathyroid glands arise from the third branchial pouch along with the thymus and are more commonly ectopic, usually in the mediastinum. Normal glands measure 5 × 3 × 1 mm in size and average 10 to 80 mg and are not usually demonstrated by any imaging method. The normally located parathyroid glands are found posterior to the thyroid lobes superficial to the longus colli muscles (Fig. 72D.1) and between the trachea and the carotid sheath.

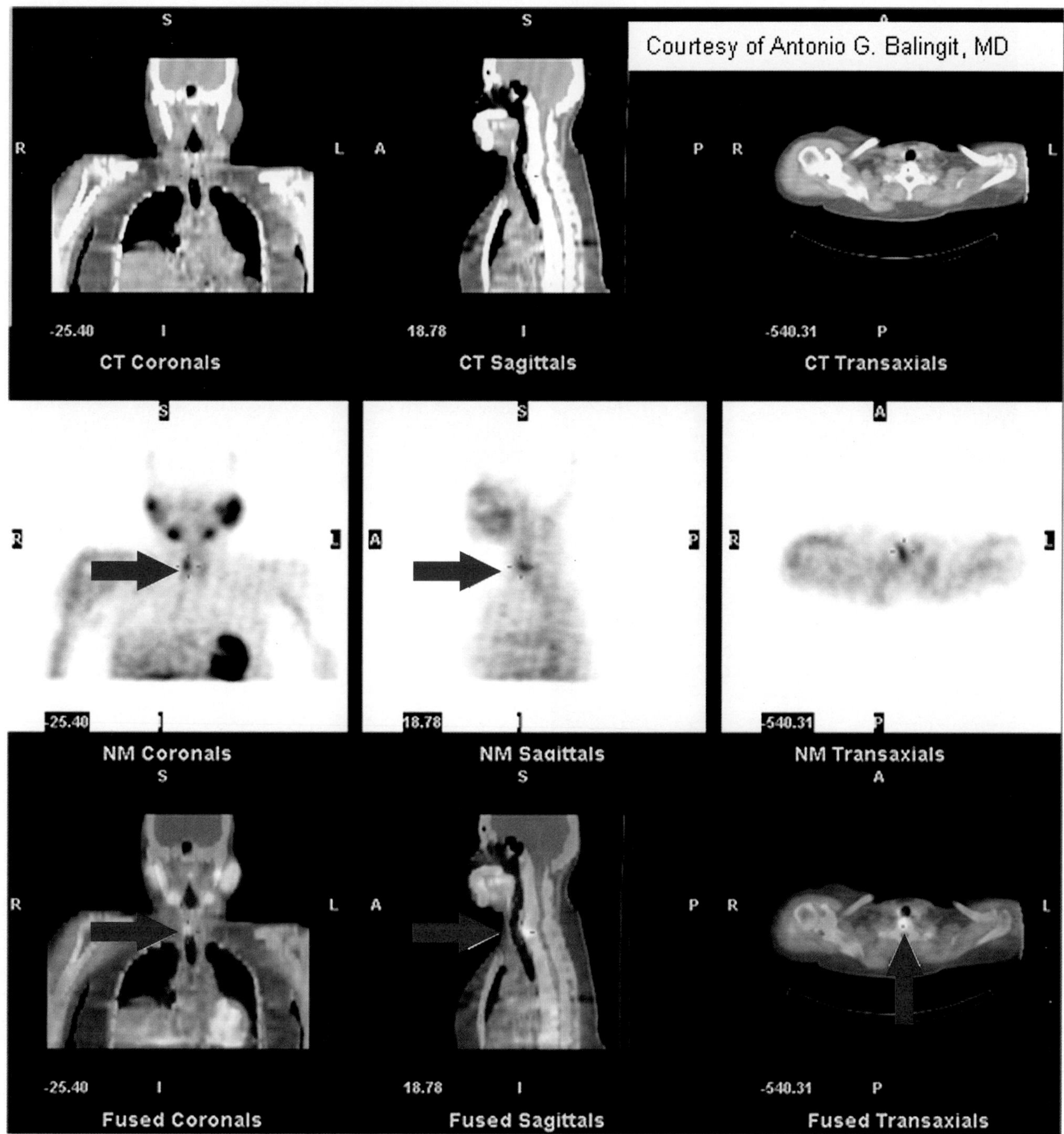

FIGURE 72D.9. **Parathyroid Adenoma: Technetium Sestamibi SPECT-CT Scan.** *Arrows* indicate the parathyroid adenoma with various SPECT coronal, sagittal, and transaxial images. Surgery confirmed a parathyroid adenoma.

Parathyroid adenomas are characteristically oval in shape and 8 to 15 mm in greatest diameter. Their cellularity is homogeneous, giving a uniform internal appearance on all imaging modalities.

Multiple Gland Disease. Parathyroid hyperplasia cannot be differentiated from multiple parathyroid adenomas by imaging methods. Hyperplasia affects all of the parathyroid glands but is frequently asymmetric. The individual glands have the same imaging appearance as parathyroid adenomas.

Parathyroid carcinomas are usually larger than adenomas (at least 2 cm in size). The internal architecture is much more heterogeneous and may demonstrate cystic degeneration. Invasion of adjacent muscle or vessels may be demonstrated. The differentiation of parathyroid carcinoma from a large adenoma can usually be made only histologically.

Ectopic parathyroids are most common in the anterosuperior mediastinum or low in the neck. Immediate and delayed imaging of the neck and mediastinum with Tc-99m MIBI or Tc-99m tetrofosmin has a diagnostic sensitivity of 75%. CT, MR, and scintigraphy have all reported sensitivities of approximately 75%. SPECT-CT using Tc-99m MIBI has allowed for better localization (Fig. 72D.9).

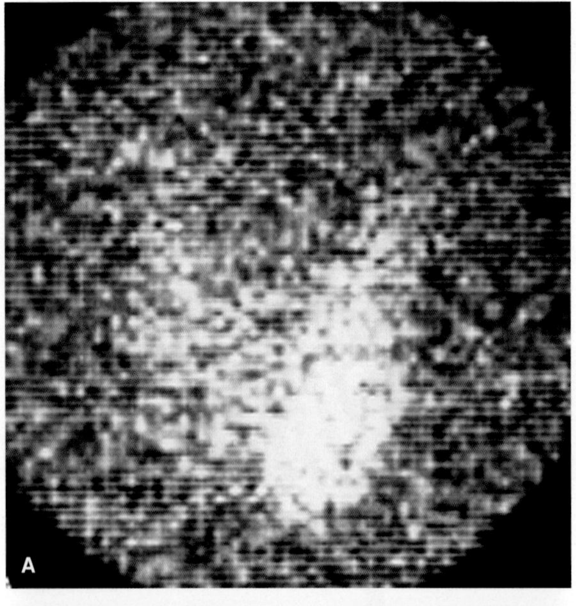

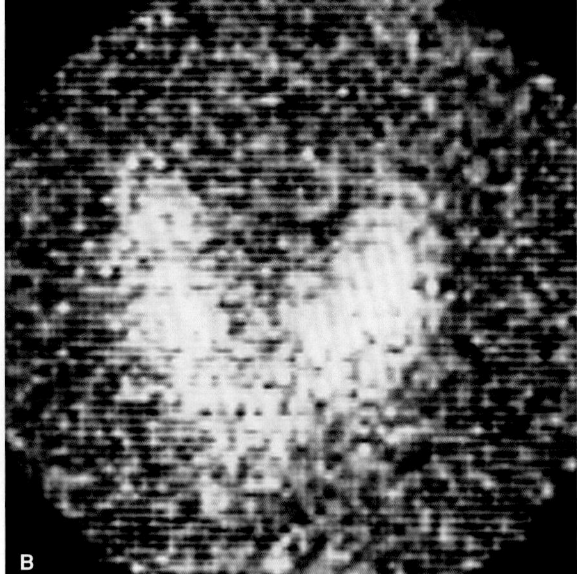

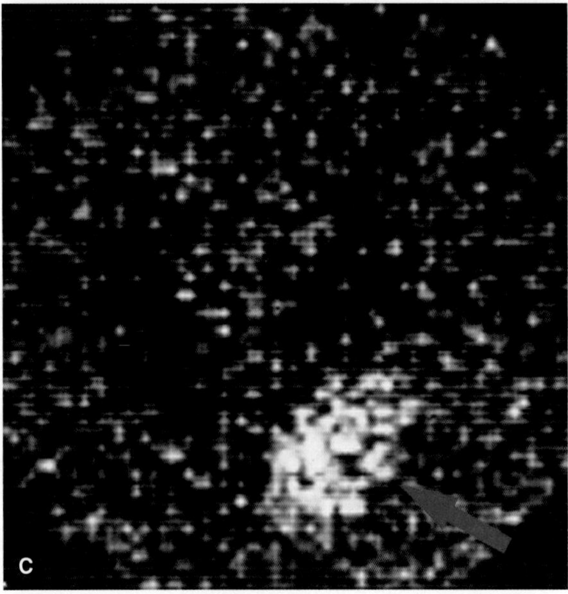

FIGURE 72D.10. **Parathyroid Adenoma: Technetium–Thallium Subtraction Technique. A:** Thallium image demonstrates radionuclide activity in both the thyroid gland and the parathyroid adenoma. **B:** Tc-99mO_4 image shows the uptake in the thyroid gland but not in the parathyroid adenoma. **C:** Subtraction image shows a residual focus of activity, identifying a parathyroid adenoma at the lower pole of the left thyroid lobe (*arrow*).

ADRENAL

High-resolution anatomic imaging of the adrenal glands is performed with CT or MRI and is discussed in Chapters 47 and 50. Incidental indeterminate adrenal lesions are commonly identified on CT and MRI of the abdomen, though are unable to identify if these lesions are clinically significant or not. Functional imaging of hyperplastic or neoplastic adrenal masses can be performed with I-131 6-β-iodomethyl-19-norcholesterol (NP 59) or I-131/I-123 MIBG (meta-iodo-benzyl-guanidine), with MIBG as the agent of choice. MIBG is taken up by cells of adrenal medullary origin (i.e., a norepinephrine analog) including lesions such as pheochromocytoma and tumors of neural crest origin such as neuroblastoma and medullary thyroid cancer, which often concentrate MIBG. MIBG is the first-line functional imaging agent for neuroblastoma and detects primary neuroblastoma and metastases in more than 90% of cases with a sensitivity of 88% to 93% and specificity of 83% to 92%. MIBG can be used in treating malignant lesions that are MIBG avid when labeled with I-131(72). PET-CT using F-18 FDG in a small cohort of patients has shown promise in imaging malignant adrenal tumors with a sensitivity of 100% and a specificity of 100%.

NEUROENDOCRINE

Neuroendocrine tumors such as pheochromocytomas, paragangliomas, and neuroblastomas can be imaged with I-123 MIBG (Fig. 72D.12) or with In-111 pentetreotide (Octreoscan).

In-111 pentetreotide is a synthetic somatostatin analog but with a longer plasma half-life than native somatostatin and is the preferred imaging agent by many clinics for imaging neuroendocrine tumors (listed in Table 72D.5) and is the radiopharmaceutical of choice when imaging carcinoid tumors (Fig. 72D.13). It has an overall sensitivity of approximately 86% to 95% and is more sensitive and specific than CT or MRI. SPECT-CT increases the sensitivity in visualizing lesions and aids in the anatomic localization of the tumor

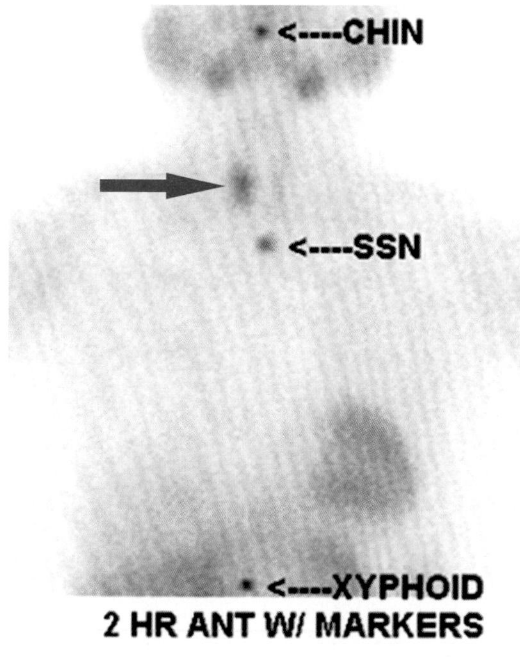

FIGURE 72D.11. **Parathyroid Adenoma: Technetium Sestamibi Planar Scan.** *Red arrow* indicates the delayed imaging, which is the focus of radionuclide activity in the lower pole of the right lobe of the thyroid. Surgery confirmed a parathyroid adenoma.

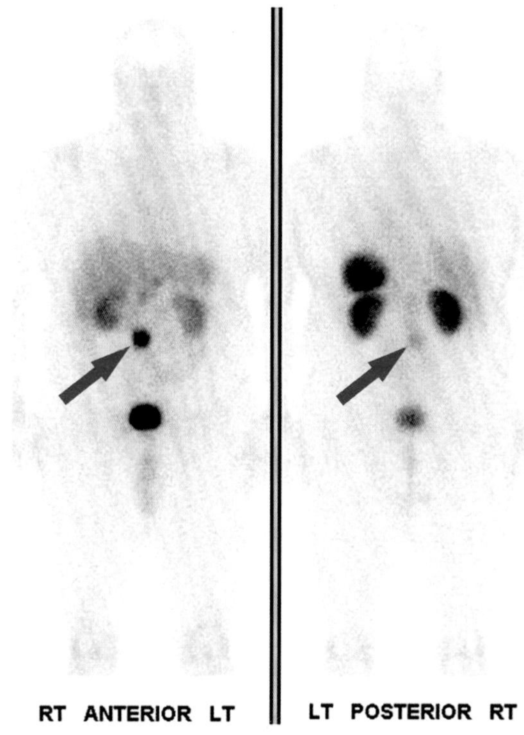

FIGURE 72D.13. **Carcinoid: In-111 Pentetreotide Planar Scan.** The planar image shows a distinct intense focus of activity (*arrows*) confirmed to be carcinoid at surgery.

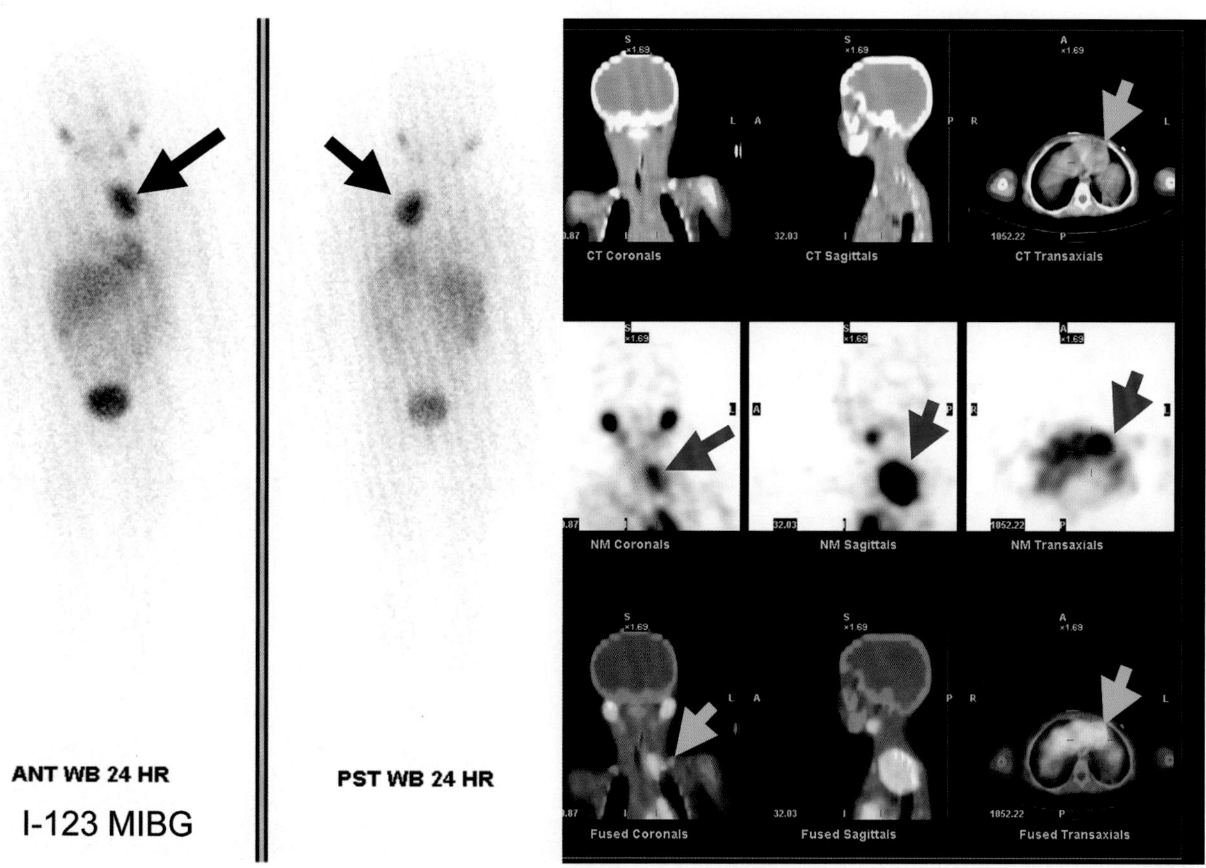

FIGURE 72D.12. **I-123 MIBG Scan in Pediatric Patient With Neuroblastoma.** The whole-body I-123 MIBG planar scan (**left two images**) shows abnormal intense uptake of I-123 MIBG (*black arrows*). The SPECT-CT scan from the same day (**right nine images**) better depicts the mass (*green and blue arrows*).

TABLE 72D.5

TUMORS THAT MAY BE IMAGED WITH INDIUM-111 PENTETREOTIDE

■ ISOTOPE	■ HALF-LIFE	■ PRINCIPAL GAMMA RAY (keV)	■ TUMORS AMENABLE TO IMAGING
In-111	67.9 hours	171 and 245	▪ Adrenal medullary tumors: pheochromocytoma, neuroblastoma, ganglioneuroma ▪ Carcinoid tumors (high sensitivity) ▪ Gastroenteropancreatic (GEP) tumors: for example, gastrinoma, insulinoma, glucagonoma, vasoactive intestinal polypeptide-secreting tumor (VIPoma) ▪ Medullary thyroid carcinoma ▪ Merkel cell tumor of the skin ▪ Paraganglioma ▪ Pituitary adenomas

(Fig. 72D.14). Sensitivities vary according to tumor type with carcinoid and paraganglioma having fairly high sensitivities.

I-123 MIBG may be used in the evaluation of pheochromocytoma, paraganglioma, and medullary thyroid cancer though is predominantly used in the evaluation of nonmetastatic adrenal pheochromocytoma. CT and MRI have a high sensitivity of 93% to 100% in detecting pheochromocytomas and a variable specificity ranging from 50% to 90%. A meta-analysis of 15 I-123 MIBG studies demonstrated a sensitivity of 92% and specificity of approximately 94%. I-131 MIBG is currently under investigation as a therapeutic agent in I-123 MIBG positive cases. New promising PET radiotracers are currently under investigation and include 68-gallium (Ga) DOTA-NOC, 68-Ga DOTA-NOC, 68-Ga DOTA-TOC, and 6-18-F fluorodopamine.

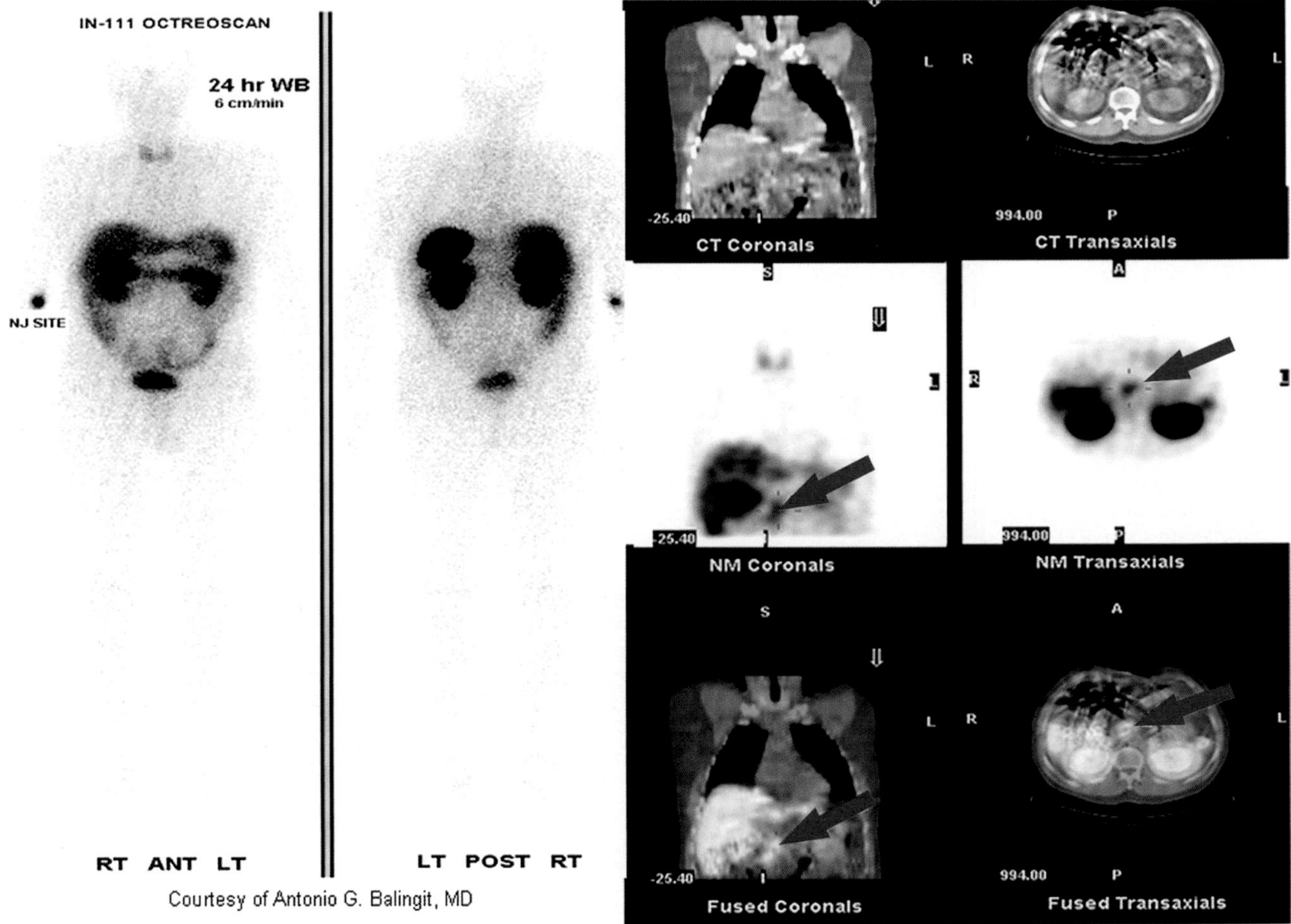

FIGURE 72D.14. **Insulinoma: In-111 Pentetreotide (Octreoscan) Planar and SPECT-CT Scan.** The planar image shows no clear focus of activity with diffuse activity in the bowel. The *arrows* on the SPECT-CT indicate the focus of activity later confirmed at exploratory laparotomy to be the insulinoma.

Suggested Readings

Akslen LA, Haldorsen T, Thoresen SO, Glattre E. Survival and causes of death in thyroid cancer: a population-based study of 2479 cases from Norway. *Cancer Res* 1991;51:1234–1241.

American Cancer Society. *Cancer Facts & Figures 2009*. Atlanta, GA: American Cancer Society; 2018.

Avram AM. Radioiodine scintigraphy with SPECT/CT: an important diagnostic tool for thyroid cancer staging and risk stratification. *J Nucl Med* 2012;53:754–764.

Bal CS, Kumar A, Pant GS. Radioiodine dose for remnant ablation in differentiated thyroid carcinoma: a randomized clinical trial in 509 patients. *J Clin Endocrinol Metab* 2004;89:1666–1673.

Ballinger JR, Cooper MS. Increasing the radiochemical purity of 99mTc-sestamibi commercial preparations results in improved sensitivity of dual-phase planar parathyroid scintigraphy. *Nucl Med Commun* 2006;27:543–544.

Barbaro D, Boni G, Meucci G, et al. Radioiodine treatment with 30 mCi after recombinant human thyrotropin stimulation in thyroid cancer: effectiveness for postsurgical remnants ablation and possible role of iodine content in L-thyroxine in the outcome of ablation. *J Clin Endocrinol Metab* 2003;88:4110–4115.

Baudin E, Habra MA, Deschamps F, et al. Therapy of endocrine disease: treatment of malignant pheochromocytoma and paraganglioma. *Eur J Endocrinol* 2014;171:R111–R122.

Belfiore A, La Rose GL, La Porta GA, et al. Cancer risk in patients with cold thyroid nodules: relevance of iodine intake, sex, age and multinodularity. *Am J Med* 1992;93:363–369.

Bénard F, Lefebvre B, Beuvon F, Langlois MF, Bisson G. Rapid washout of technetium-99m-MIBI from a large parathyroid adenoma. *J Nucl Med* 1995; 36:241–243.

Bergenfelz A, Tennvall J, Valdermarsson S, Lindblom P, Tibblin S. Sestamibi versus thallium subtraction scintigraphy in parathyroid localization: a prospective comparative study in patients with predominantly mild primary hyperparathyroidism. *Surgery* 1997;121:601–605.

Berna L, Chico A, Matías Guiu X, et al. Use of somatostatin analogue scintigraphy in the localization of recurrent medullary thyroid carcinoma. *Eur J Nucl Med* 1998;25:1482–1488.

Berthe E, Henry-Amar M, Michels JJ, et al. Risk of second primary cancer following differentiated thyroid cancer. *Eur J Nucl Med Mol Imaging* 2004;31:685–691.

Bessey LJ, Lai NB, Coorough NE, Chen H, Sippel RS. The incidence of thyroid cancer by fine needle aspiration varies by age and gender. *J Surg Res* 2013; 184:761–765.

Brander A, Viikinkoski P, Nickels J, Kivisaari L. Thyroid gland: US screening in a random adult population. *Radiology* 1991;181:683–687.

Chen MK, Yasrebi M, Samii J, Staib LH, Doddamane I, Cheng DW. The utility of I-123 pretherapy scan in I-131 radioiodine therapy for thyroid cancer. *Thyroid* 2012;22:304–309.

Cooper DS, Doherty GM, Haugen BR, et al. Revised American Thyroid Association management guidelines for patients with thyroid nodules and differentiated thyroid cancer. *Thyroid* 2009;19:1167–1214.

Dadparvar S, Krishna L, Brady LW, et al. The role of iodine-131 and thallium-201 imaging and serum thyroglobulin in the management of differentiated thyroid carcinoma. *Cancer* 1993;71:3767–3773.

David A, Blotta A, Bondanelli M, et al. Serum thyroglobulin concentrations and (131)I whole-body scan results in patients with differentiated thyroid carcinoma after administration of recombinant human thyroid-stimulating hormone. *J Nucl Med* 2001;42:1470–1475.

Davies L, Welch HG. Increasing incidence of thyroid cancer in the United States, 1973–2002. *JAMA* 2006;295:2164–2167.

Eslamy HK, Ziessman HA. Parathyroid scintigraphy in patients with primary hyperparathyroidism: 99mTc sestamibi SPECT and SPECT/CT. *Radiographics* 2008;28:1461–1476.

Ezzat S, Sarti DA, Cain DR, Braunstein GD. Thyroid incidentalomas: prevalence by palpation and ultrasonography. *Arch Intern Med* 1994;154:1838–1840.

Fjeld JG, Erichsen K, Pfeffer PF, Clausen OP, Rootwelt K. Technetium-99m-tetrofosmin for parathyroid scintigraphy: a comparison with sestamibi. *J Nucl Med* 1997;38:831–834.

Flynn MB, Tarter J, Lyons K, Ragsdale T. Frequency and experience with carcinoma of the thyroid at a private, a Veterans Administration, and a university hospital. *J Surg Oncol* 1991;48:164–170.

Freitas JE, Freitas AE. Thyroid and parathyroid imaging. *Semin Nucl Med* 1994;24:234–245.

Hall P, Boice JD Jr, Berg G, et al. Leukaemia incidence after iodine-131 exposure. *Lancet* 1992;340:1–4.

Hall P, Holm LE, Lundell G, et al. Cancer risks in thyroid cancer patients. *Br J Cancer* 1991;64:159–163.

Hassan FU, Mohan HK. Clinical utility of SPECT/CT imaging post-radioiodine therapy: does it enhance patient management in thyroid cancer? *Eur Thyroid J* 2015;4:239–245.

Haugen BR, Pacini F, Reiners C, et al. A comparison of recombinant human thyrotropin and thyroid hormone withdrawal for the detection of thyroid remnant or cancer. *J Clin Endocrinol Metab* 1999;84:3877–3885.

Hoefnagel CA, Delprat CC, Zanin D, van der Schoot JB. New radionuclide tracers for the diagnosis and therapy of medullary thyroid carcinoma. *Clin Nucl Med* 1988;13:159–165.

Iagaru A, Kalinyak JE, McDougall IR. F-18 FDG PET/CT in the management of thyroid cancer. *Clin Nucl Med* 2007;32:690–695.

Iagaru A, Masamed R, Singer PA, Conti PS. Detection of occult medullary thyroid cancer recurrence with 2-deoxy-2-[F-18]fluoro-D-glucose-PET and PET/CT. *Mol Imaging Biol* 2007;9:72–77.

Ilias I, Chen CC, Carrasquillo JA, et al. Comparison of 6–18F-fluorodopamine PET with 123I-metaiodobenzylguanidine and 111In-pentetreotide scintigraphy in localization of nonmetastatic and metastatic pheochromocytoma. *J Nucl Med* 2008;49:1613–1619.

Ilias I, Divgi C, Pacak K. Current role of metaiodobenzylguanidine in the diagnosis of pheochromocytoma and medullary thyroid cancer. *Semin Nucl Med* 2011;41:364–368.

Jacobson AF, Deng H, Lombard J, Lessig HJ, Black RR. 123I-metaiodobenzylguanidine scintigraphy for the detection of neuroblastoma and pheochromocytoma: results of a meta-analysis. *J Clin Endocrinol Metab* 2010;95:2596–2606.

Johnson NA, Tublin ME. Postoperative surveillance of differentiated thyroid carcinoma: rationale, techniques, and controversies. *Radiology* 2008;249:429–444.

Kamran SC, Marqusee E, Kim MI, et al. Thyroid nodule size and prediction of cancer. *J Clin Endocrinol Metab* 2013;98:564–570.

Krenning EP, Kwekkeboom DJ, Bakker WH, et al. Somatostatin receptor scintigraphy with [111In-DTPA-D-Phe1] and [123I-Try3]-octreotide: the Rotterdam experience with more than 1000 patients. *Eur J Nucl Med* 1993;20:716–731.

Lee J, Yun MJ, Nam KH, Chung WY, Soh EY, Park CS. Quality of life and effectiveness comparisons of thyroxine withdrawal, triiodothyronine withdrawal, and recombinant thyroid-stimulating hormone administration for low-dose radioiodine remnant ablation of differentiated thyroid carcinoma. *Thyroid* 2010;20:173–179.

Lind P, Gallowitsch HJ, Langsteger W, Kresnik E, Mikosch P, Gomez I. Technetium-99m tetrofosmin whole body scintigraphy in the follow-up of differentiated thyroid carcinoma. *J Nucl Med* 1997;38:348–352.

Luigi S, Charboneau JW, Osti V, et al. The thyroid gland. In: Rumack CM, Wilson SR, Charboneau JW, Johnson JM, eds. *Diagnostic Ultrasound*. 3rd ed. St. Louis, MO: Elsevier Mosby; 2005:735–794.

Maurea S, Klain M, Mainolfi C, Ziviello M, Salvatore M. The diagnostic role of radionuclide imaging in evaluation of patients with nonhypersecreting adrenal masses. *J Nucl Med* 2001;42:884–892.

Maurea S, Mainolfi C, Bazzicalupo L, et al. Imaging of adrenal tumors using FDG PET: comparison of benign and malignant lesions. *AJR Am J Roentgenol* 1999;173:25–29.

Maxon HR 3rd, Englaro EE, Thomas SR, et al. Radioiodine-131 therapy for well-differentiated thyroid cancer—a quantitative radiation dosimetric approach: outcome and validation in 85 patients. *J Nucl Med* 1992;33:1132–1136.

McBiles M, Lambert AT, Cote MG, Kim SY. Sestamibi parathyroid imaging. *Semin Nucl Med* 1995;25:221–234.

McDougall IR. *Thyroid Diseases in Clinical Practice*. New York: Oxford University Press; 1992.

McEwan AJ, Shapiro B, Sisson JC, Beierwaltes WH, Ackery DM. Radio-iodobenzylguanidine for the scintigraphic location and therapy of adrenergic tumors. *Semin Nucl Med* 1985;15:132–153.

Meier DA, Dworkin HJ. The autonomously functioning thyroid nodule. *J Nucl Med* 1991;32:30–32.

Miyamoto S, Kasagi K, Misaki T, Alam MS, Konishi J. Evaluation of technetium-99m MIBI scintigraphy in metastatic differentiated thyroid carcinoma. *J Nucl Med* 1997;38:352–356.

Mortenson JD, Woolner LB, Bennett WA. Gross and microscopic findings in clinically normal thyroid glands. *J Clin Endocrinol Metab* 1955;15:1270–1280.

Pacini F, Ladenson PW, Schlumberger M, et al. Radioiodine ablation of thyroid remnants after preparation with recombinant human thyrotropin in differentiated thyroid carcinoma: results of an international, randomized, controlled study. *J Clin Endocrinol Metab* 2006;91:926–932.

Palestro CJ, Tomas MB, Tronco GG. Radionuclide imaging of the parathyroid glands. *Semin Nucl Med* 2005;35:266–276.

Palmedo H, Bucerius J, Joe A, et al. Integrated PET/CT in differentiated thyroid cancer: diagnostic accuracy and impact on patient management. *J Nucl Med* 2006;47:616–624.

Paltiel HJ, Gelfand MJ, Elgazzer AH, et al. Neural crest tumors: I-123 MIBG imaging in children. *Radiology* 1994;190:117–121.

Park HM, Perkins OW, Edmondson JW, Schnute RB, Manatunga A. Influence of diagnostic radioiodines on the uptake of ablative dose of iodine-131. *Thyroid* 1994;4:49–54.

Pryma D, Schöder H, Gönen M, Robbins RJ, Larson SM, Yeung HW. Diagnostic accuracy and prognostic value of 18F-FDG PET in Hürthle cell thyroid cancer patients. *J Nucl Med* 2006;47:1260–1266.

Rojeski MT, Gharib H. Nodular thyroid disease. Evaluation and management. *N Engl J Med* 1985;313:428–436.

Ron E, Modan B, Preston D, Alfandary E, Stovall M, Boice JD Jr. Thyroid neoplasia following low-dose radiation in childhood. *Radiat Res* 1989; 120:516–531.

Rufini V, Calcagni ML, Baum RP. Imaging of neuroendocrine tumors. *Semin Nucl Med* 2006;36:228–247.

Sandeep TC, Strachan MW, Reynolds RM, et al. Second primary cancers in thyroid cancer patients: a multinational record linkage study. *J Clin Endocrinol Metab* 2006;91:1819–1825.

Sandler MP, Patton JA, Gross MD, et al. *Endocrine Imaging*. Norwalk, CT: Appleton & Lange; 1992.

Sarkar SD, Kalapparambath TP, Palestro CJ. Comparison of (123)I and (131)I for whole body imaging in thyroid cancer. *J Nucl Med* 2002;43: 632–634.

Schlumberger M, Ricard M, De Pouvourville G, Pacini F. How the availability of recombinant human TSH has changed the management of patients who have thyroid cancer. *Nat Clin Pract Endocrinol Metab* 2007;3:641–650.

Schluter B, Bohuslavizki KH, Beyer W, Plotkin M, Buchert R, Clausen M. Impact of FDG PET on patients with differentiated thyroid cancer who present with elevated thyroglobulin and negative 131I scan. *J Nucl Med* 2001;42:71–76.

Schmidt D, Szikszai A, Linke R, Bautz W, Kuwert T. Impact of 131I SPECT/spiral CT on nodal staging of differentiated thyroid carcinoma at the first radioablation. *J Nucl Med* 2009;50:18–23.

Schteingart DE. Management approaches to adrenal incidentalomas. A view from Ann Arbor, Michigan. *Endocrinol Metab Clin North Am* 2000;29: 127–139.

Shammas A, Degirmenci B, Mountz JM, McCook BM, Branstetter B, Bencherif B, Joyce JM, Carty SE, Kuffner HA, Avril N, et al. 18F-FDG PET/CT in patients with suspected recurrent or metastatic well-differentiated thyroid cancer. *J Nucl Med* 2007;48:221–226.

Shankar LK, Yamamoto AJ, Alavi A, Mandel SJ. Comparison of 123I scintigraphy at 5 and 24 hours in patients with differentiated thyroid cancer. *J Nucl Med* 2002;43:72–76.

Sharma P, Singh H, Bal C, Kumar R. PET/CT imaging of neuroendocrine tumors with (68)Gallium-labeled somatostatin analogues: an overview and single institutional experience from India. *Indian J Nucl Med* 2014;29:2–12.

Sharp SE, Trout AT, Weiss BD, Gelfand MJ. MIBG in neuroblastoma diagnostic imaging and therapy. *Radiographics* 2016;36:258–278.

Shi W, Johnston CF, Buchanan KD, et al. Localization of neuroendocrine tumors with [111In] DTPA-octreotide scintigraphy (Octreoscan): a comparative study with CT and MR imaging. *QJM* 1998;91:295–301.

Shore RE, Hildreth N, Dvoretsky P, Andresen E, Moseson M, Pasternack B. Thyroid cancer among persons given x-ray treatment in infancy for an enlarged thymus gland. *Am J Epidemiol* 1993;137:1068–1080.

Siddiqi A, Foley RR, Britton KE, et al. The role of 123I diagnostic imaging in the follow-up of patients with differentiated thyroid carcinoma as compared to 131I scanning: avoidance of negative therapeutic uptake due to stunning. *Clin Endocrinol* 2001;55:515–521.

Spencer CA, Schwartzbein D, Guttler RB, LoPresti JS, Nicoloff JT. Thyrotropin (TSH)-releasing hormone stimulation test responses employing third and fourth generation TSH assays. *J Clin Endocrinol Metab* 1993;76:494–498.

Tessler FN, Middleton WD, Grant EG, et al. ACR thyroid imaging, reporting and data system (TI-RADS): white paper of the ACR TI-RADS committee. *J Am Coll Radiol* 2017;14:587–595.

Thompson NW. Localization studies in patients with primary hyperparathyroidism. *Br J Surg* 1988;75:97–98.

Tucker MA, Jones PH, Boice JD Jr, et al. Therapeutic radiation at a young age is linked to secondary thyroid cancer. The Late Effects Study Group. *Cancer Res* 1991;51:2885–2888.

Tuttle M, Leboeuf R, Robbins RJ, Qualey R. Empiric radioactive iodine dosing regimens frequently exceed maximum tolerated activity levels in elderly patients with thyroid cancer. *J Nucl Med* 2006;47:1587–1591.

Tuttle RM, Lopez N, Leboeuf R, et al. Radioactive iodine administered for thyroid remnant ablation following recombinant human thyroid stimulating hormone preparation also has an important adjuvant therapy function. *Thyroid* 2010;20:257–263.

United States Nuclear Regulatory Commission. Title 10 Code of Federal Regulations Part 35, Subpart C, Section 35.75, August 2007.

Wilson NM, Gaunt J, Nunan TO, Coakley AJ, Collins RE, Young AE. Role of thallium-201/technetium-99m subtraction scanning in persistent or recurrent hypercalcaemia following parathyroidectomy. *Br J Surg* 1990;77:794–795.

Zoller M, Kohlfuerst S, Igerc I, et al. Combined PET/CT in the follow-up of differentiated thyroid carcinoma: what is the impact of each modality? *Eur J Nucl Med Mol Imaging* 2007;34:487–495.

CHAPTER 73 ■ CARDIOVASCULAR SYSTEM SCINTIGRAPHY

ARPIT GANDHI

Nuclear medicine applications in the cardiovascular system include myocardial perfusion imaging (MPI), myocardial viability imaging, gated ventricular blood pool studies, and detection and quantitation of intracardiac shunts.

MYOCARDIAL PERFUSION SCANS

Technique

Exercise on a treadmill, or simulation of exercise by administration of pharmacologic agents, is used in conjunction with perfusion agents. Cardiac stress improves the sensitivity of the examination and allows detection of lesser degrees of coronary stenosis. Under conditions of stress, normal coronary arteries vasodilate and flow increases. The stenotic vessels are unable to dilate normally and will appear to have relatively decreased perfusion on stress images.

Step-wise increases in physical exercise are monitored by sequential electrocardiogram (ECG), blood pressure, and pulse measurements while the patient is queried for symptoms of angina. The radiopharmaceutical is injected under conditions of maximal exercise (at least 85% of maximum predicted heart rate [MPHR]), which is continued for 30 to 60 seconds after injection to obtain optimal mapping of stress perfusion. Exercise should reach at least 85% of the MPHR in order to achieve adequate stress. Exercise may be stopped in the presence of chest pain with ischemic changes on the ECG.

One method for calculating MPHR is: *MPHR = 220 – age*. Adequacy of the exercise challenge can be more thoroughly estimated from a calculation of the "double product" (DP) (systolic pressure × heart rate = DP). For exercise to be judged as adequate, the DP should at least double from rest to peak exercise and should rise to above 20,000.

For those patients who cannot perform sufficient physical exercise, pharmacologic agents (vasodilatory and inotropic agents) can be used to simulate cardiac stress. Vasodilatory agents such as adenosine, dipyridamole, and regadenoson increase coronary blood flow in normal vessels by three to five times. Adenosine has a short half-life of 30 seconds and does not require a reversal agent. Dipyridamole blocks the reuptake of adenosine, thereby increasing its endogenous levels. Regadenoson is a selective adenosine receptor. Unlike adenosine and dipyridamole, which are given as infusions, regadenoson is given as a fixed intravenous bolus. Aminophylline may be used to reverse side effects from dipyridamole and regadenoson. Dobutamine is an adrenergic agent that can be used when vasodilators are contraindicated, such as in severe asthma or recent caffeine use. Dobutamine has direct inotropic and chronotropic effects, which result in increased coronary blood flow, simulating exercise. Diseased coronary arteries with greater than 50% stenoses are unable to dilate and demonstrate decreased myocardial perfusion during the stress acquisition relative to the rest acquisition.

Image Acquisition. Planar imaging has largely been replaced by SPECT imaging with reconstruction of the LV myocardium into short axis, vertical long axis, and horizontal long axis planes. A 180-degree acquisition is generally preferred over a 360-degree acquisition because of the asymmetry of the heart in the thorax and because of spine attenuation effects in the posterior projections. ECG-gated acquisitions allow evaluation of wall motion and thickening. Functional data may be obtained including end-diastolic volume (EDV), end-systolic volume (ESV), and left ventricular ejection fraction (LVEF).

Prone imaging may be performed after the standard supine acquisition and may help reduce false-positive examinations because of breast or diaphragm attenuation, subdiaphragmatic activity, or motion artifact. However, new hybrid SPECT/CT cameras use the CT anatomic data to provide accurate attenuation correction, thus reducing artifacts. The SPECT camera itself can be a single-, dual-, or triple-headed camera.

Radiopharmaceuticals

Thallium-201 (Tl-201) is a potassium analog that is delivered to the myocardium proportional to blood flow. It is actively transported into viable cells by the sodium/potassium (Na^+/K^+) adenosine triphosphatase pump. It decays by electron capture and emits low-energy, poorly penetrating photons (69 to 83 keV) that are susceptible to attenuation artifact from chest wall soft tissues. Other disadvantages of Tl-201 include requirement of an on-site cyclotron for radioisotope production, relatively high absorbed dose (0.24 rad/mCi whole body at the usual dose of 2 to 5 mCi), and long physical half-life of

The editors wish to thank Dr. David K. Shelton for his work in the 4th edition establishing the foundation for this chapter.

73 hours, which necessitates the administration of low doses to minimize the absorbed dose and results in poor image counts.

Stress imaging using Tl-201 may be performed with exercise stress or a pharmacologic challenge. Images may be acquired immediately after injection or after waiting 5 to 10 minutes to allow the exercised patient's heart rate and respiratory rate to decrease in order to minimize motion artifact.

Rest or redistribution imaging is usually performed 3 to 4 hours after the stress injection. Tl-201 undergoes a complex "redistribution" within the myocardium governed by cellular washout, radiotracer re-extraction, and renal excretion. Ischemic myocardium undergoes delayed extraction and washout compared to normal myocardium, appearing as a defect on initial stress images and subsequently normalizes or "fills in" on rest images. In contrast, scar will show a perfusion defect that persists on redistribution imaging.

In addition, the initial Tl-201 images of the chest and heart may help assess the heart's performance. High lung activity immediately after exercise usually indicates that left ventricular failure occurred during exercise. Poststress dilation of the heart compared with resting images is an indicator of significant multivessel disease. Both immediate high lung activity and poststress dilation of the heart infer a poor prognosis with an increased risk of subsequent cardiac events (angina, infarction, arrhythmia, and sudden death) (Fig. 73.1).

Technetium-99m (Tc-99m) is used to label two commercially available myocardial perfusion agents: sestamibi and tetrofosmin.

Tc-99m sestamibi (trade name Cardiolite) is taken up by the perfused myocardium by passive diffusion and is bound in the myocyte within myocardial mitochondria. Sestamibi is fixed in the myocardium and does not undergo significant redistribution or washout. Imaging is delayed for 15 minutes to 1 hour after stress to allow for biliary and background clearance. Because there is neither redistribution nor significant washout of Tc-99m sestamibi, a repeat injection for resting images is commonly performed on a different day. With this *2-day protocol,* stress imaging is usually done first. An alternative *1-day protocol* uses a small dose (8 mCi) for the initial rest scan, followed 4 hours later by the stress scan with a larger dose, typically threefold higher than the rest dose (about 20 to 25 mCi). The higher dose is used for stress imaging to maximize stress imaging quality (improved signal-to-noise ratio).

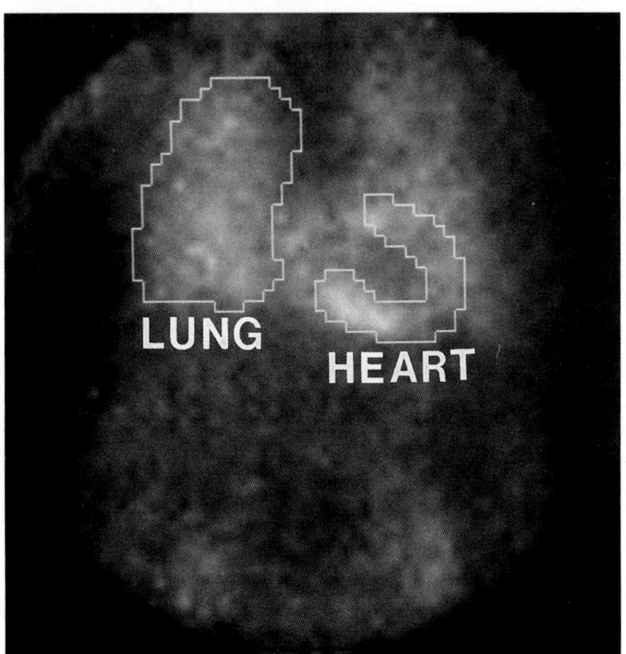

FIGURE 73.1. **Abnormal Tl-201 Lung/Heart Ratio.** This frame is an anterior projection acquired immediately after the start of a stress SPECT study. The lung:heart ratio of 0.77 is markedly elevated, indicating that the patient experienced heart failure during exercise.

Tc-99m tetrofosmin (trade name Myoview) is rapidly extracted from the blood by perfused myocardium in a fashion that resembles Tc-99m sestamibi. The two agents have proven to act clinically in a very similar manner but availability and pricing make important considerations. Tc-99m tetrofosmin has slower hepatobiliary clearance compared to Tc-99m sestamibi and is generally used for the rest portion of a *1-day protocol* stress test.

Both the Tc-99m labeled agents are easy to image with good soft tissue penetration (140-keV gamma energy), high photon flux from typical doses of 8 to 25 mCi, and offer an opportunity to perform gated imaging, which can be used to evaluate wall motion and left ventricular functional parameters such as LVEF.

Dual Isotope Myocardial Scans. An alternative way to maximize the logistical patient throughput involves the use of a Tl-201 and a Tc-99m agent for sequential scans. The most widely used dual isotope scan technique uses a resting Tl-201 scan, which can be immediately or subsequently followed by a Tc-99m (sestamibi or tetrofosmin) stress scan. Because the energy and photon flux of the subsequent Tc-99m scan is higher than the Tl-201 scan, there is no problem with cross talk between the rest and stress images. Excellent scan quality can be obtained with this *1-day protocol.* When needed, a delayed 24-hour redistribution thallium scan can be obtained to evaluate a "fixed defect" for viability.

Interpretation

Myocardial Ischemia. MPI demonstrates relative regional myocardial perfusion. Areas of myocardium with poor blood supply, usually due to coronary atherosclerosis, fail to increase radiotracer uptake during the stress component as the diseased vessels are unable to appropriately vasodilate in response to exercise or pharmacologic stress. **Reversible ischemia** refers to an area of decreased perfusion or uptake at stress that improves or is normal at rest. Reversible changes detected by either exercise or pharmacologic dilation of normal vessels usually correspond with coronary stenoses greater than 50%. Revascularization by angioplasty or coronary artery bypass surgery corrects the underlying disease process (atherosclerosis), restoring perfusion to the affected myocardium. Another frequent location of ischemic tissue can be seen immediately adjacent to an area of infarct. This is called **periinfarct ischemia.**

Short axis summary presentations of myocardial perfusion are often presented in a 2D "polar map" or "bull's-eye" format (Fig. 73.2). The circumferential profile of isotope distribution is compared with a normal database for age and gender as an aid in interpretation. Depending on the statistical assumptions used and the population studied, the sensitivity and specificity for detecting myocardial ischemia range from the high 80s to the low 90s. It is important to remember that according to Bayes theorem, the positive and negative predictive values of a test will vary according to the prevalence of disease in the population being tested.

In addition, many computer programs will present the perfusion data in a semiquantitative method. One such program uses a 20-segment model, which divides the short axis bull's-eye into 20 segments and grades each segment on a scale of

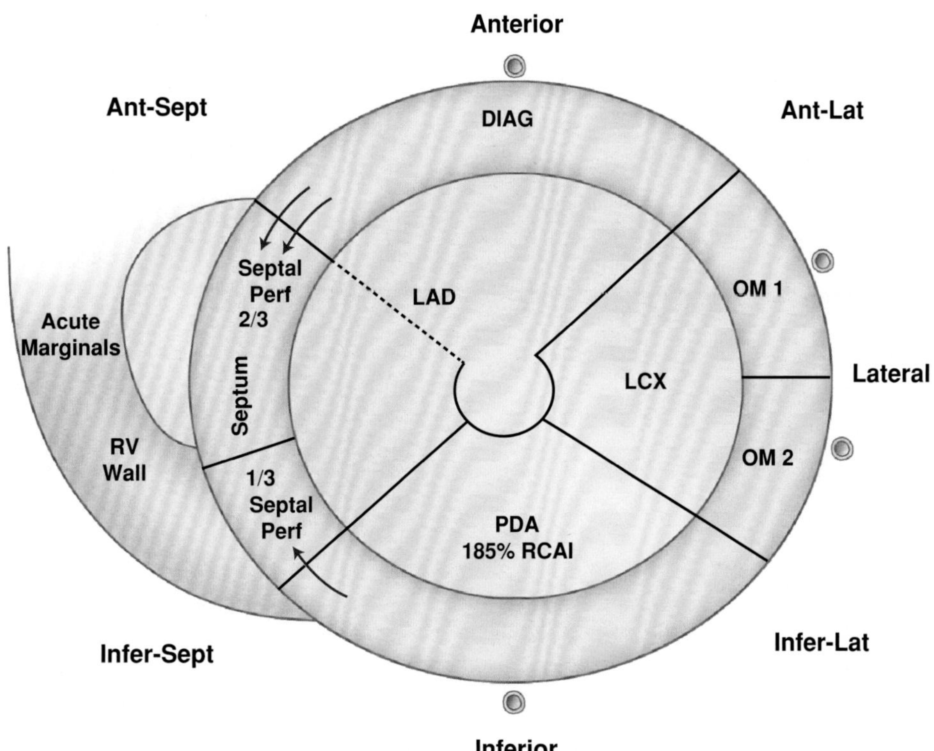

FIGURE 73.2. **LV Short Axis Vascular Distributions and Wall Names.** The schematic diagram locates the expected position of the principle coronary arteries. The left anterior descending artery (*LAD*) usually serves the apex. The names of the wall segments are listed in a clockwise fashion as *Anterior, Anterior–Lateral, Lateral, Inferior–Lateral, Inferior, Inferior–Septal, Septal,* and *Anterior–Septal.* The LAD sends diagonal vessels (numbered with digits in the order with which they leave the LAD; e.g., D1, D2, etc.) onto the anterior and anterior–lateral walls and septal perforators down into the septum. The left circumflex (*LCX*) sends obtuse marginal (*OM*) branches along the free wall numbered in their sequence (*OM1, OM2,* etc.). The posterior descending artery (*PDA*), which arises from the right coronary artery (*RCA*) 85% of the time, serves the inferior wall and the inferior–septal wall.

0 to 4. In this method, 0 is normal, 1 is mildly reduced, 2 is moderately reduced, 3 is severely reduced, and 4 is absence of activity. A ***summed stress score (SSS)*** is then calculated for the stress data as a whole. In a similar fashion, a ***summed rest score (SRS)*** and then a ***summed difference score (SDS)*** are calculated. While not infallible, the SSS is a very good, objective method to quantify the severity of the ischemia and to communicate with clinicians. An SSS of less than 4 is normal, 4 to 8 is mild, 9 to 13 is moderate, and more than 13 is severe.

The presence and severity of ischemic myocardium correlates strongly with the prognosis for adverse cardiac events including angina and cardiac death (Fig. 73.3). The myocardial perfusion scan can also detect causes of ischemia, which cannot be seen on coronary arteriography. These include capillary disease in diabetics, left bundle branch block, vasospasm, vasculitis, or cardiomyopathy, which may produce ischemic myocardium even with normal arteries. Conversely, ischemia may not be detected if there is inadequate exercise, inadequate pharmacologic challenge, or balanced triple vessel disease. Fortunately, it is uncommon for all three coronary arteries to be hemodynamically compromised equally, and poststress dilation (transient ischemic dilatation [TID]) or decrease in LVEF will usually be present.

Hibernating Myocardium. Severe ischemia leads to a phenomenon known as ***hibernating myocardium.*** Under these conditions, the myocytes have sufficient metabolic activity to maintain cellular viability but not contractility. Hibernating myocardium simulates infarction and demonstrates both decreased blood flow and contractility. It is important to differentiate from infarction because it represents viable myocardium which will return to normal function after revascularization (Fig. 73.4).

Rest-injected Tl-201 with delayed imaging may be performed to detect hibernating myocardium. Severely ischemic myocardium has slow radiotracer uptake, clearance, and redistribution. Therefore, delayed imaging up to 24 hours may be necessary. Tl-201 is reinjected at the delayed time point to improve image quality.

Hibernating myocardium can also be evaluated with F-18 fluorodeoxyglucose (FDG) PET/CT or contrast-enhanced MRI. Hibernating myocardium demonstrates preserved F-18 FDG metabolism on PET imaging and normal gadolinium washout on delayed-enhancement MRI sequences (i.e., lacks delayed enhancement that is indicative of scar).

Myocardial infarction produces layers of nonperfused scar tissue which are detected as areas of thin myocardium with decreased radiotracer uptake at ***both stress and rest*** imaging. The extent of an infarct, from subendocardial to transmural, is reflected by the size and degree of the perfusion defect (Fig. 73.5).

Breast tissue, poorly positioned arms, and subdiaphragmatic structures interposed between the heart and gamma camera absorb gamma rays as they travel from the heart to the gamma camera, which can result in perceived perfusion defects (attenuation artifacts) on planar or SPECT images. Intense subdiaphragmatic radioactivity adjacent to the heart (radioactivity within the liver and GI tract) may cause an increase in apparent perfusion of the inferior wall of the heart secondary to scatter radiation and volume averaging or cause a paradoxical decrease in apparent inferior wall perfusion due to an attempt to limit star artifact during filtered backprojection (FBP) reconstruction. Failing to recognize these artifacts can lead to false-positive interpretations of ischemia or infarction.

Several techniques exist to reduce these artifacts. ***Repeat stress imaging with the patient in the prone position*** changes the position of the heart, breasts, diaphragm, and subdiaphragmatic organ, removing the attenuation artifacts and correcting apparent perfusion defects. Repeat prone positioning may also help with motion artifacts. Unfortunately, some obese patients in whom there is plenty of breast or subdiaphragmatic

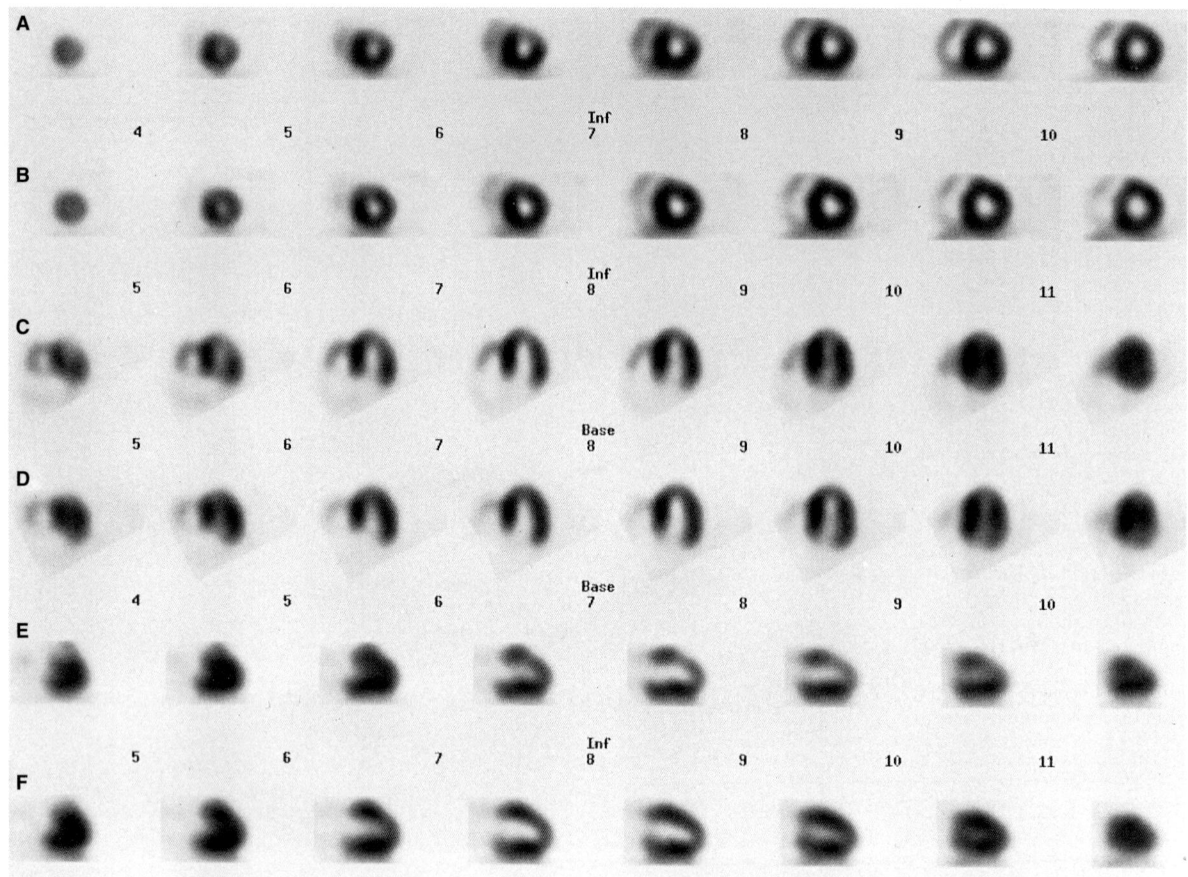

FIGURE 73.3. **SPECT of Left Anterior Descending Artery Reversible Ischemia.** The row of short axis stress images (**A**) has a perfusion defect in the anterior wall which perfuses normally in the rest of the short axis images (**B**). This is also visible in the horizontal long axis stress (**C**) and vertical long axis stress images (**E**) which have the same perfusion defect. At rest, the matched images (**D, E,** and **F**) show normal perfusion.

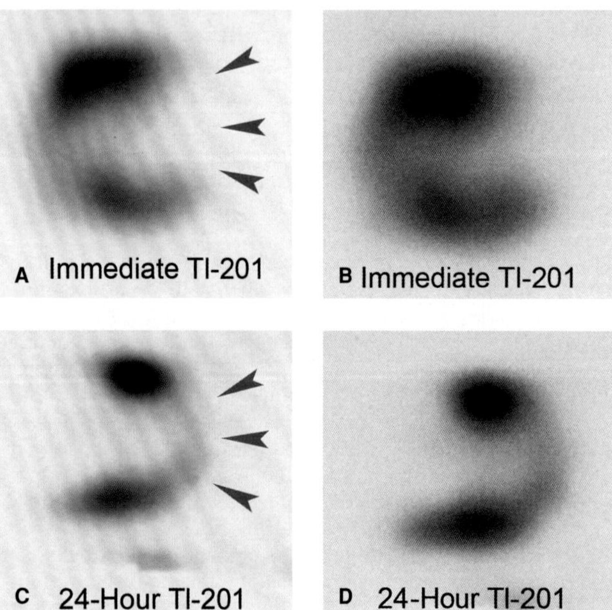

FIGURE 73.4. **Hibernating Myocardium.** Two vertical long axis Tl-201 images at rest (**A** and **B**) are compared with matched images at 24 hours (**C** and **D**). The large anteroapical defect (*arrowheads*) partly fills in over time, indicating that some hibernating (viable) myocardium is present in the midst of what looked initially to be infarcted tissue.

attenuation may not be able to lay prone for the duration of the study (Fig. 73.6). ***Gated acquisitions*** provide cine clips of cardiac wall motion that allow correlation of wall motion with perfusion abnormalities. The normal wall moves inward during systole, thickens as it contracts, and becomes brighter on the display. Myocardium with normal wall motion, brightening, and thickening is likely not ischemic, infarcted, or hibernating. ***Software attenuation correction algorithms*** on combination SPECT/CT cameras can reduce attenuation artifacts by utilizing the transmission CT (attenuation map) to correct for emission photons lost due to absorption by excessive patient soft tissue between the heart and gamma camera (Fig. 73.7).

Stunned Myocardium. Delayed recovery of myocardial function following reperfusion after a period of severe ischemia is known as ***stunned myocardium***. Stunned myocardium may remain hypokinetic or akinetic following reperfusion but will demonstrate redistribution on Tl-201 redistribution imaging and preserved F-18 FDG metabolism on PET. Myocardial wall motion will improve with time, unlike in infarct. Stress-induced transient ischemic dilation (TID) may be a manifestation of stunned myocardium.

Infarct Avid Scans. Acute infarcts may also be detected with Tc-99m–labeled pyrophosphate. Ionized calcium released from myocytes forms dystrophic calcifications with phosphates and a "hot spot" is formed, marking the infarcted tissue. Antimyosin antibodies labeled with Tc-99m or indium-111 (In-111) also localize on the fringes of acute infarctions. The need for

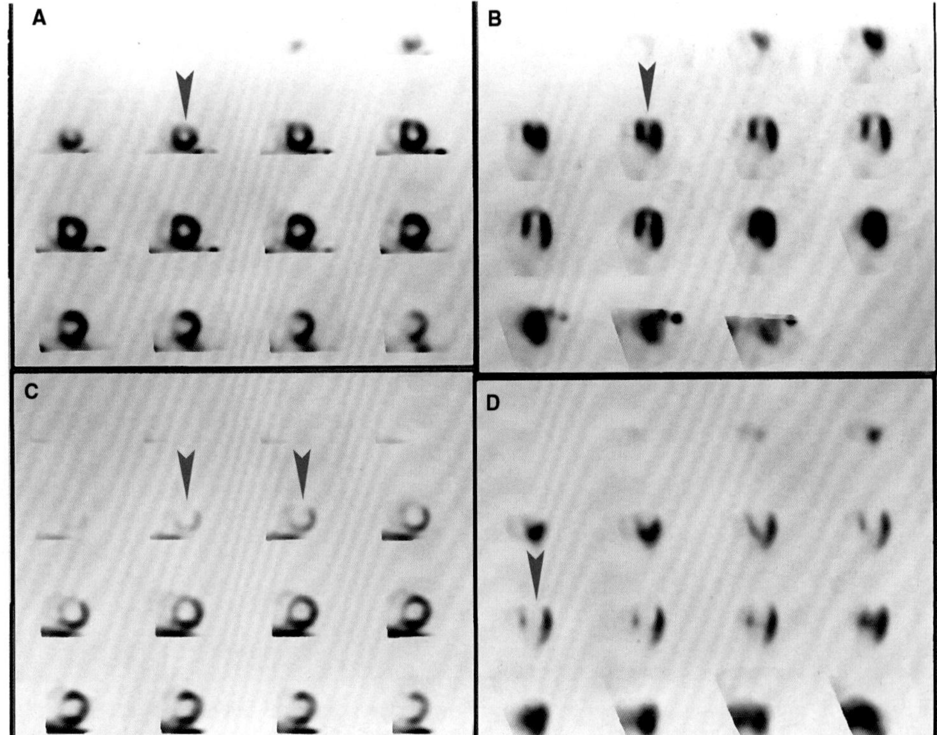

FIGURE 73.5. **Resting Images of Infarcts in Left Anterior Descending Artery (LAD) Distribution.** Short axis (**A**) and horizontal long axis (**B**) SPECT images show a small anterior LAD infarct (*arrowheads*). This is compared with another patient who has a much larger LAD infarct (**C** and **D**) in the same vascular distribution (*arrowheads*). Note that the second patient's infarct extends from the anterolateral wall to the septum. The ventricle is also dilated at rest.

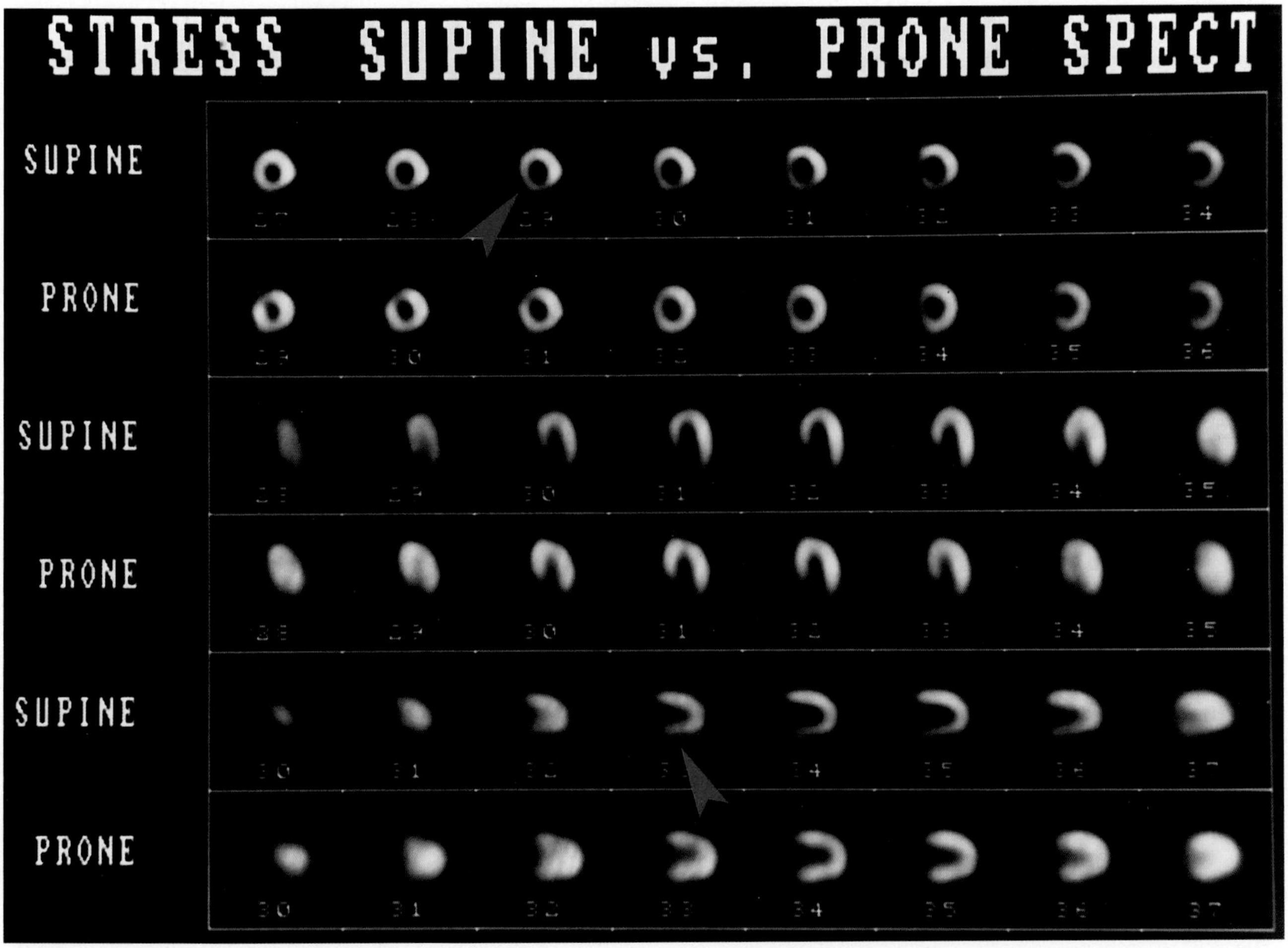

FIGURE 73.6. **Stress Versus Prone Imaging.** Tc-99m sestamibi imaging with a single-headed SPECT camera shows a defect in the inferior wall during stress imaging (*arrowheads*) which is not present when the patient is reimaged in the prone position.

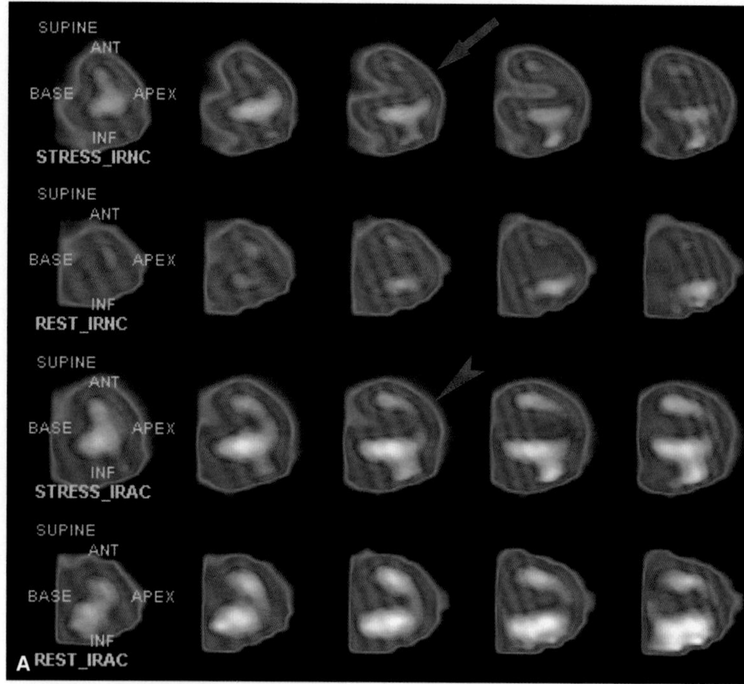

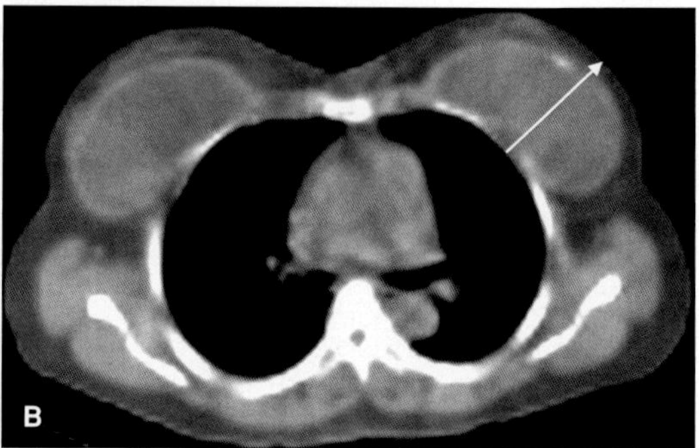

FIGURE 73.7. **Attenuation Correction. A:** An anterior wall defect caused by attenuation secondary to large breasts is corrected by simultaneous transmission (CT) and emission (SPECT) scans. A noncorrected vertical long axis scan (*IRNC*—top two rows) shows an apparent anterior wall defect (*arrow*), which disappears when the transmission scan (**B**) is used to correct for the asymmetric attenuation (*IRAC*—bottom two rows). The anterior wall (*arrowhead*) is normal. **B:** The CT transmission scan shows the large breasts (*arrow* on the left side) with implants, which are causing the attenuation artifact. The anterior wall (*arrowhead*) is normal. *IRNC*, iterative reconstruction noncorrected; *IRAC*, iterative reconstruction attenuation-corrected.

imaging of acute infarction is rare. Contused myocardium is also detected with these techniques.

Emergency Department (ED) Infarct Screening. Many EDs use MPI SPECT to safely and cost-effectively screen patients for acute myocardial infarction or acute coronary syndrome (ACS). The patient is injected in the ED with a myocardial perfusion tracer. If the perfusion scan is negative for ischemia, the patient can be safely discharged home. If a reversible perfusion defect is identified, the patient will typically be admitted for evaluation of ACS and often will undergo heart catheterization and/or coronary artery bypass grafting (CABG) to correct or bypass the obstructive coronary lesion(s).

Positron Emission Tomography (PET)

Technique. PET is more expensive than standard MPI but offers the advantages of coincidence imaging, higher-energy photons, efficient attenuation correction, and different radiopharmaceuticals. PET scanning with coincidence detection allows high photon flux since collimators are not required. PET scans have higher spatial resolution and less attenuation artifacts than standard SPECT MPI. Thus, PET scans may eventually become the gold standard for MPI.

Radiopharmaceuticals. PET perfusion imaging agents include rubidium-82 (Rb-82) and ammonia-13 (N-13 NH_3). Rest images are compared with stress images as in standard MPI. Both PET tracers have the advantage of short half-lives, which permit administration of higher activities with lower overall radiation exposure. The short half-lives preclude the use of exercise stress. Pharmacologic stress is used instead. Rb-82 is a potassium analog and is eluted from a Strontium-82 generator on site. It has a 76-second half-life. Altogether, an Rb-82 study takes less than an hour (Fig. 73.8). N-13 NH_3 has a 10-minute half-life and is produced from a cyclotron. Because its positron energy is lower, it offers higher-resolution images than Rb-82.

F-18 FDG PET can be used to assess viability. As in oncologic imaging, F-18 FDG uptake corresponds to glucose metabolism. FDG has a 110-minute half-life and produces lower-energy positrons resulting in higher spatial resolution. Viable myocardium will demonstrate glucose metabolism under a glucose loading protocol (to prime the myocardium to preferentially metabolize glucose) whereas infarcted myocytes have lost the ability to metabolize glucose and therefore lack F-18 FDG avidity. Resting injection F-18 FDG PET is compared to a defect seen on a rest MPI scan to evaluate for viability (Fig. 73.9).

Interpretation. Defects on stress imaging that reverse on rest imaging are indicative of coronary stenosis (see Fig. 73.8). Fixed defects on stress and rest identify infarcted or hibernating myocardium. With FDG imaging, ***hibernating myocardium*** will show normal or even relatively increased FDG uptake compared with the rest scan. This is due to a shift from free fatty acid (FFA) metabolism to glucose metabolism in hibernating myocardium, particularly when primed with glucose loading (see Fig. 73.9). True infarction will show no significant FDG uptake.

GATED BLOOD POOL SCANS

The radionuclide ventriculogram (RNV) or multigated acquisition scan (MUGA) is a timed (gated) study that uses cardiac blood pool images to calculate the LVEF. It uses Tc-99m–labeled red blood cells. Other characteristics of the left ventricle (LV) can also be assessed including size, wall motion, rate of systolic emptying, and diastolic filling. Right ventricle (RV)

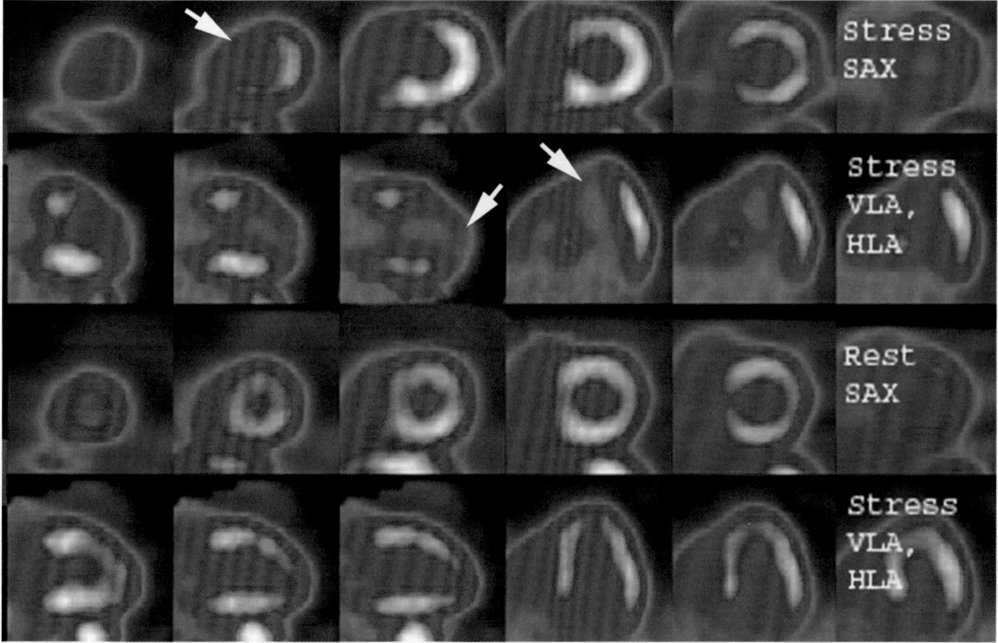

FIGURE 73.8. **Rubidium-82 PET Myocardial Perfusion Scan.** *SAX* (short axis), *VLA* (vertical long axis), and *HLA* (horizontal long axis) views are shown for stress and rest. The large, reversible defect (*short arrows*) in the anterior and septal walls is demonstrative of ischemia in the left anterior descending artery distribution.

evaluation is better accomplished by the first-pass study, to be discussed later.

Technique

The red blood cells are labeled with Tc-99m, using one of several techniques. Doses of 20 to 30 mCi are commonly used for typical adult patients. Electrocardiographic (ECG) leads are placed to obtain a suitable gating signal (the R wave) for the computer. Using the ECG as a measure of the cardiac cycle's length, the cardiac cycle is divided into a minimum of 16 frames for the analysis of systolic function. Higher temporal resolution of 32 frames per cardiac cycle is required for good measurement of diastolic function. The result of this acquisition is a composite, "averaged" series of images representing the patient's cardiac cycle. Data from an adequate number of cardiac cycles (several hundred) must be obtained to make the images statistically significant for analysis. Typical acquisition time is 5 to 20 minutes per view (Fig. 73.10).

Analysis of the functional parameters of the LV is most accurate from images obtained in the "best septal" left anterior oblique (LAO) view. This view produces the greatest separation of the activity of the LV from that of the RV.

Computer processing of the image data is performed by spatial and temporal smoothing algorithms. The edge of the ventricular blood pool is outlined using computerized edge detection methods. The volume curve is generated by plotting the number of counts in the ventricle versus time during the cardiac cycle (Fig. 73.11). The LVEF is calculated as follows:

(End-diastolic counts – end-systolic counts)/
(End-diastolic counts – background)

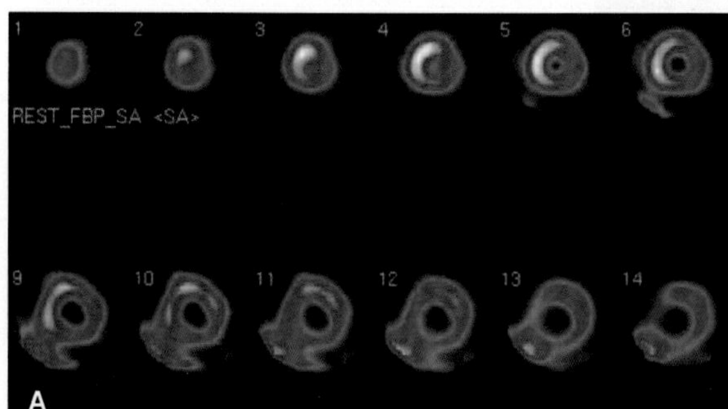

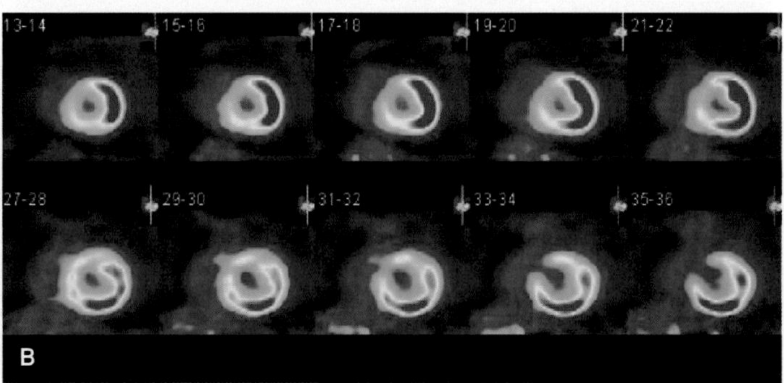

FIGURE 73.9. **FDG PET Myocardial Viability Scan.** Rb-82 resting scan (**A**) shows defects in the lateral wall. F-18 FDG resting PET scan (**B**) demonstrates normal uptake consistent with fully viable, hibernating myocardium.

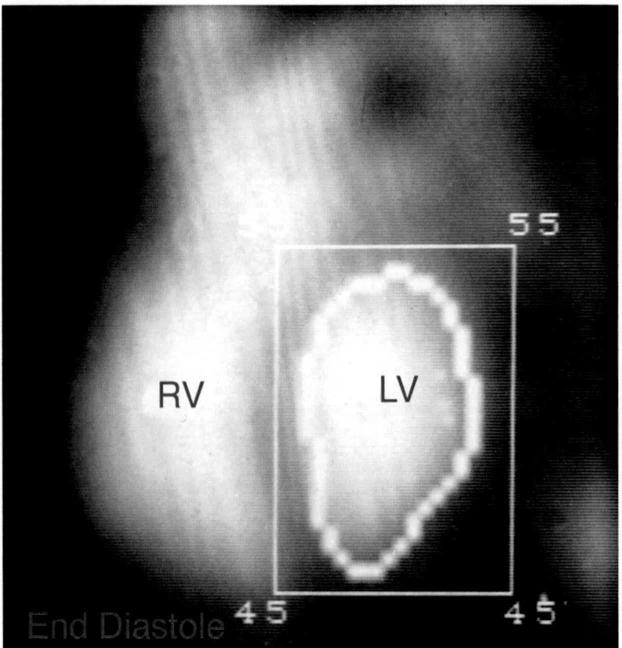

FIGURE 73.10. **Normal-Gated Blood Pool Image.** An end-diastolic image is shown with a computer-generated region of interest around the left ventricle (*LV*) blood pool. The right ventricle (*RV*) is adjacent.

Background correction cancels out in the numerator. The background activity affects the calculated LVEF. High background falsely elevates the LVEF. Low background will falsely lower the LVEF.

Arrhythmias such as frequent premature beats and atrial fibrillation tend to falsely lower the LVEF. The R–R (R-wave) interval histogram from the ECG can demonstrate the presence of arrhythmias. Most nuclear medicine computer systems allow the analysis of selected populations of beats of the same R–R interval to yield a more accurate LVEF.

Cardiac output (CO) in liters per minute may be calculated if the heart rate, LVEF, and left ventricular end-diastolic volume (LVEDV) are known. The product of all three is the CO. The LVEDV can be measured by comparing the count rate of a blood sample of known volume with the count rate of the ventricle at end diastole and end systole.

The normal resting LVEF typically ranges from 50% to 75%. The exact range of normal calculated by radionuclide ventriculography (RNV) will depend on multiple factors, such as number of frames acquired, counts within each image, and methods of background correction and edge detection.

Interpretation

Left Ventricular Ejection Fraction. A common application of RNV is monitoring the LVEF in patients on cardiotoxic drugs. The accuracy of LVEF calculated by RNV is considered superior to most non–nuclear-based techniques because it is volume based. The number of counts is proportional to the volume.

End-Diastolic Volume. The relative end-diastolic size and shape of the RV and LV chambers (RVEDV and LVEDV) should always be noted. Though they appear roughly equal in a normal "best septal" LAO view, the RVEDV is normally greater than the LVEDV. The stroke volumes of the ventricles are equal because the RV ejection fraction (RVEF) is smaller than the LVEF. As the LV fails for any reason, it dilates and usually becomes rounder in shape.

Wall motion of various regions of the LV is best evaluated by visually observing a cine display of the beating heart in orthogonal views. The LAO ("best septal") view is the critical view but the anterior and left posterior oblique views are complementary.

As the ventricular wall is damaged or infarcted, the progression of wall motion abnormality is from normal to hypokinetic to akinetic. If an aneurysm forms, the wall will become dyskinetic and demonstrate paradoxical motion. This analysis is true for gated SPECT as well as for RNV. To determine the degree of abnormality, it is important to concentrate on the margins of the LV chamber, which is the interface of the endocardial surface and blood.

Fourier phase analysis provides powerful additional information on the amount of motion (amplitude) of various LV wall segments and their relative timing (phase). The amplitude image is especially useful for confirming areas suspected

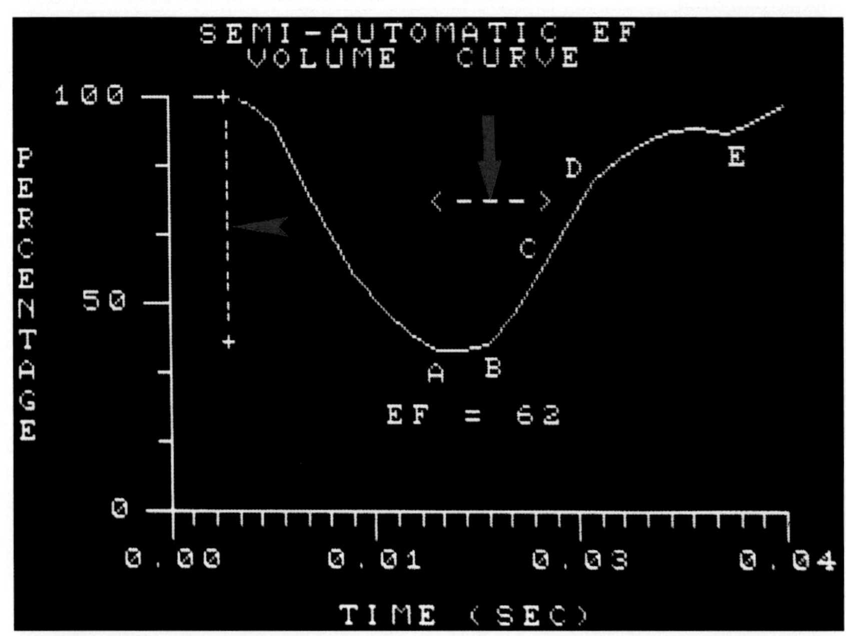

FIGURE 73.11. **Left Ventricular Time Activity Curve.** The graph (from the patient in Fig. 73.9) shows a curve that displays relative volume of the ventricles during the cardiac cycle. The vertical *dashed line* (*arrowhead*) represents the relative stroke volume expressed as an ejection fraction (*EF*) of 62%. The curve begins at end diastole, A marks end systole, B marks the start of diastolic filling, C marks the peak filling rate, D the end of rapid filling, and E the beginning of atrial contraction. The horizontal *dashed line* (*arrow*) shows the interval of the first third of diastole during which more than half of the stroke volume is recovered.

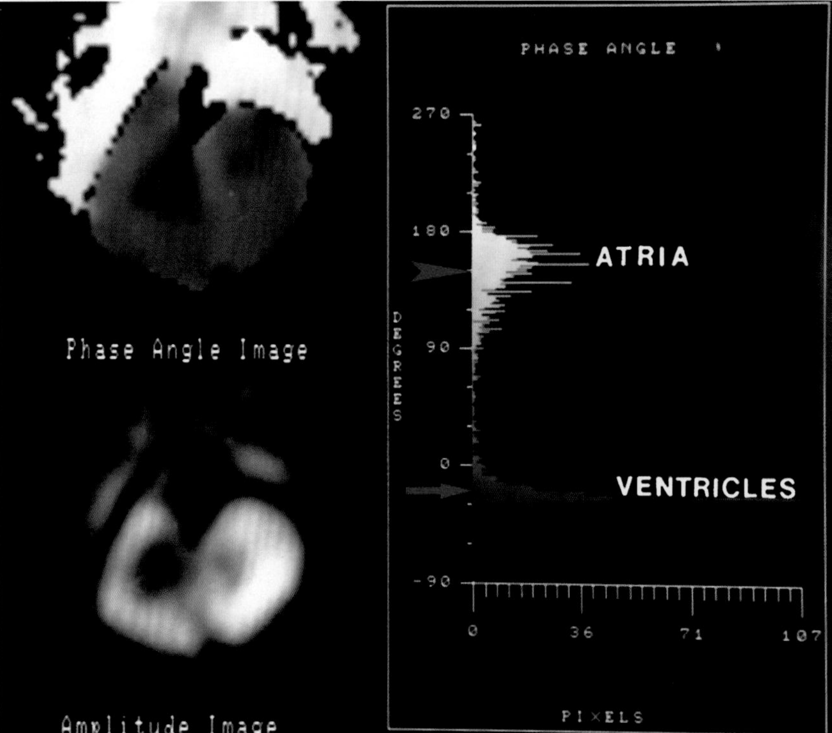

FIGURE 73.12. **Normal Fourier Phase and Amplitude Images.** The lower (Amplitude) image (from the same patient in Figs. 73.9 and 73.10) shows the relative displacement of blood in each chamber of the heart. The pixel brightness depicts the relative degree of motion. The upper (Phase Angle) image shows the relative timing of contraction of each chamber. The histogram summarizes the number of pixels with a given phase angle. The cardiac cycle is represented on an arbitrary scale of –90 to 270 degrees. Note that the gray pixels (*arrow*) representing ventricular motion are tightly grouped around –30 degrees, indicating synchronous contraction. Approximately 180 degrees up the time scale, there is a cluster of white pixels (*arrowhead*) corresponding to atrial motion.

to be hypokinetic or akinetic on the cine display. Damaged areas of myocardium contract with less vigor than normal areas. The phase display may help detect such areas because damaged areas contract slowly. A dyskinetic aneurysmal area will demonstrate wall motion of the segment on the amplitude image but in the opposite direction (180 degrees out of phase, i.e., paradoxical) compared with undamaged areas (Figs. 73.12 and 73.13).

Valvular Regurgitation. The severity of aortic or mitral regurgitation correlates with the ratio of the LV to RV stroke volumes. In normal individuals, the LV and RV stroke

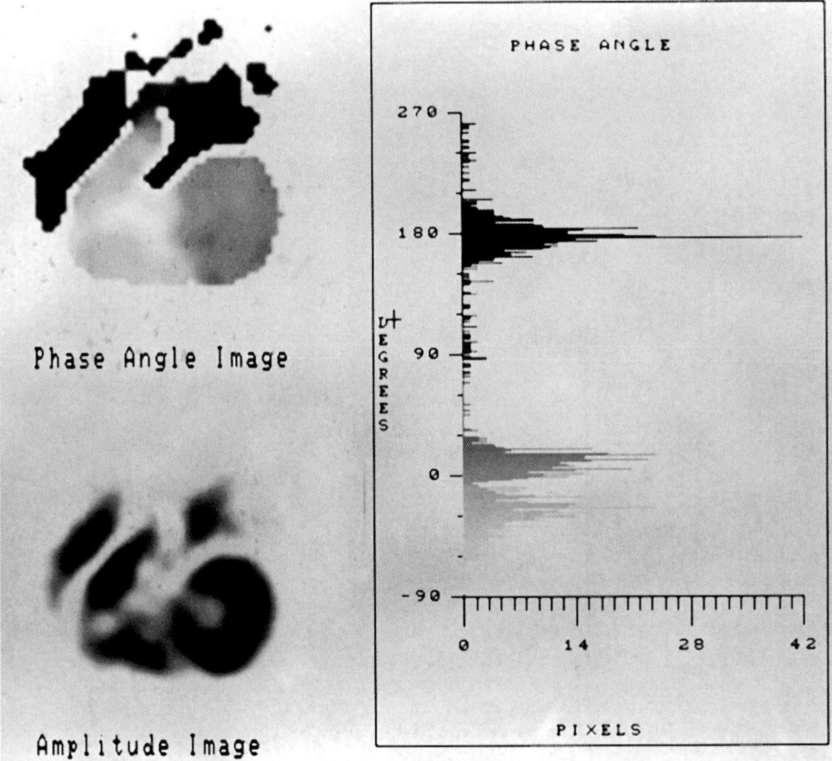

FIGURE 73.13. **Fourier Phase and Amplitude in Left Bundle Branch Block.** Two separate populations of phase values are seen in the RV and LV. The lighter colored RV contracts before the darker colored LV. This is much easier to see in color. LV, left ventricle; RV, right ventricle.

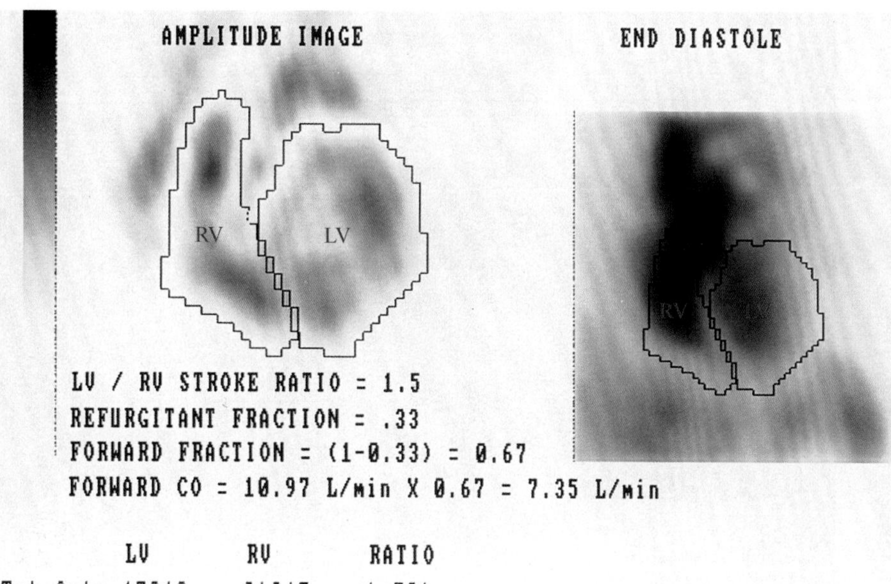

FIGURE 73.14. **Mitral Regurgitation Calculated From a Fourier Amplitude Image.** The total counts in the LV and RV regions of interest yield a 1.5 to 1 LV/RV stroke ratio with a 0.33 regurgitant fraction. The global cardiac output (CO) of 10.97 is multiplied by the complement of the regurgitant fraction (0.67) to generate a forward CO of 7.35 L/min. LV, left ventricle; RV, right ventricle.

volumes are assumed to be equal. In individuals with regurgitant lesions, the LV has to pump blood from the RV, in addition to the regurgitant blood. Therefore, the ratio of the LV to RV stroke volume is increased. The regurgitant fraction can be calculated as follows:

(LV stroke counts – RV stroke counts)/LV stroke counts

This method works only when there are regurgitant valves on one side of the septum. It cannot differentiate aortic regurgitation from mitral regurgitation; however, the suspect valve is usually known (Fig. 73.14).

Exercise Radionuclide Ventriculogram. The RNV study can also be done while the patient is exercising to monitor cardiac functional response to exercise. Normal patients should be able to augment or increase their LVEF at least 5% at each stage of exercise. Patients with regurgitant valves, significant coronary disease, or congestive cardiomyopathy will usually experience a drop in their LVEF as exercise increases.

RIGHT VENTRICULAR STUDIES

First-Pass Function Studies

Right ventricular function is more difficult to assess by the RNV study than LV function. This is because labeled activity in the RV cannot be isolated as well from other chambers as can LV activity. RV function is best assessed by analyzing images from the first pass of a radionuclide bolus through the right-sided chambers and lungs before the overlapping

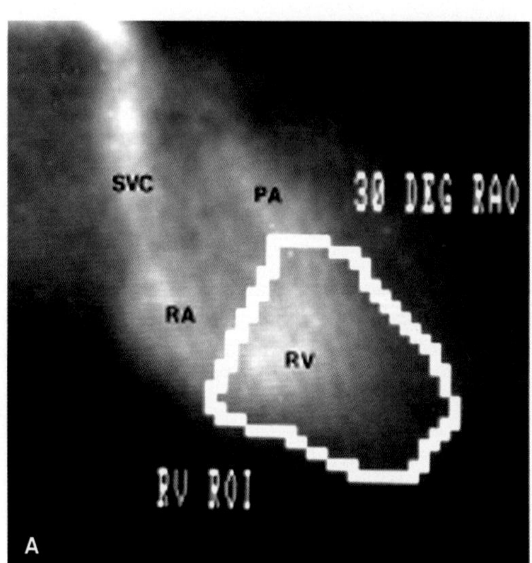

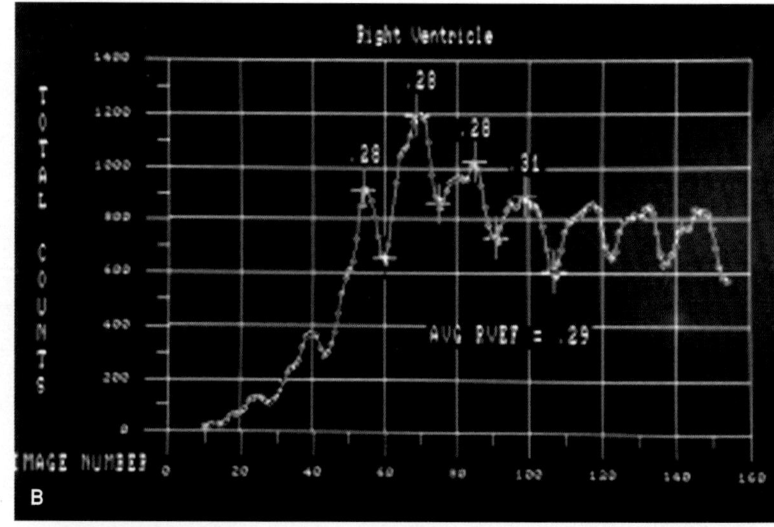

FIGURE 73.15. **Right Ventricular First-Pass Function Study. A:** Fast dynamic right ventricular ejection fraction by first pass. The acquisition totaled 512 frames taken at 40-millisecond intervals in the right anterior oblique (*RAO*) projection as a radioactive bolus traversed the right atrium (*RA*) and ventricle (*RV*). An image of the *RV* is made by summing dozens of individual frames. A fixed region of interest (*ROI*) is drawn around the RV. **B:** A time–activity curve from the ROI in (**A**) shows the relative volume of the ventricle rising and falling with diastole and systole. Peaks and valleys in the curve are flagged and beat-by-beat ejection fractions are averaged. SVC, superior vena cava; PA, pulmonary artery.

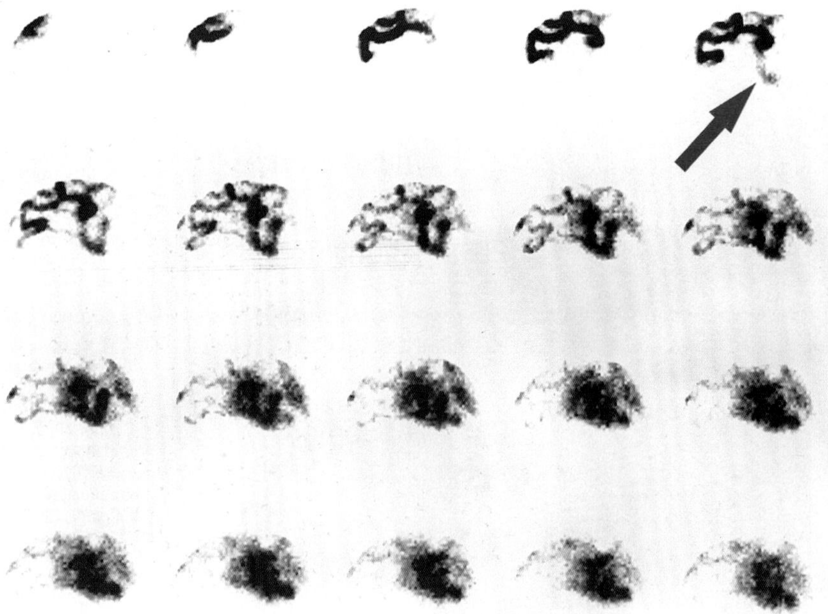

FIGURE 73.16. **Superior Vena Cava (SVC) Obstruction.** A first-pass study with a 1-second frame is shown in the anterior projection after injection in the right antecubital vein. Serpiginous collateral veins on the chest wall probably communicate with the intercostal and azygos veins. Very little flow courses through the SVC into the RA and ventricle (*arrow*). The patient required stenting of the SVC to relieve obstruction caused by encircling tumor.

left-sided chambers are seen. The patient is usually imaged in the right anterior oblique (RAO) projection. A bolus of high specific activity isotope is rapidly injected, followed immediately by a nonradioactive flush dose. This activity will pass through the RV in three to eight heartbeats. A region of interest (ROI) is established around the RV and an average RVEF is then calculated (Fig. 73.15). The RVEF is normally lower than LVEF with a normal range of 32% to 52%.

First-Pass Flow Studies

The first-pass study in an anterior projection can also be used to detect abnormalities of blood flow to one lung compared with the other. The effect of extrinsic compression on the pulmonary artery by a mediastinal or hilar mass can be easily detected. Abnormal blood flow to a lung segment such as that seen in pulmonary sequestration can be detected. Obstruction of the superior vena cava is also easily diagnosed (Fig. 73.16).

Left-to-right intracardiac shunts can be detected and quantified using a first-pass imaging technique. Instead of using an ROI over the RV for analysis, an area of lung is used. In a normal person, the bolus of activity passes into and out of the lung exponentially in a way that can be mathematically described by a gamma function. If a left-to-right shunt is present, some blood that has gone through the lungs to the left side of the heart reenters the right side of the heart and is pumped back

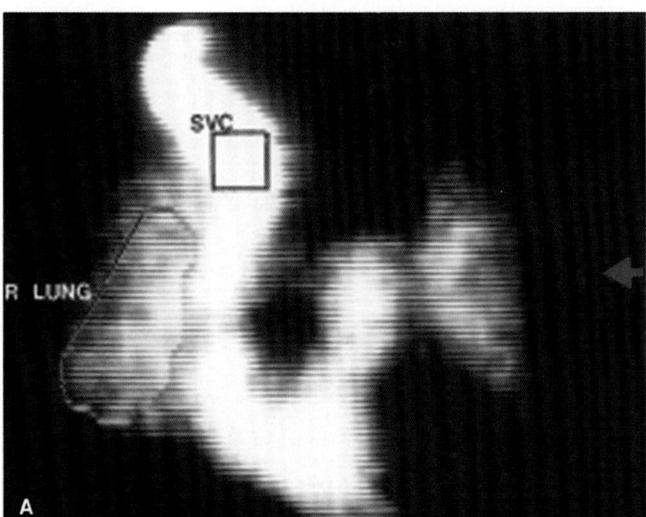

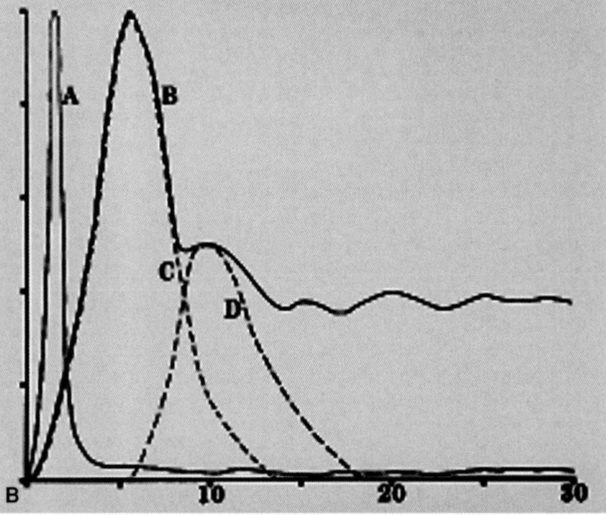

FIGURE 73.17. **Abnormal Left-to-Right Shunt Study. A:** Regions of interest are drawn around the superior vena cava (*SVC, square box*) and the right lung (*R lung*) on image data from a first-pass flow study. Note the lack of activity in the LV (*arrow*) in this summary of images from the dextrophase of the flow. **B:** Graph shows time–activity curve of the activity within the two regions shown in (**A**). *A* is the sharp bolus injection passing through the SVC. *B* is the right lung time–activity curve, which rises exponentially but does not follow the fitted gamma variate curve (*C*) on the way down. This indicates early recirculation because of a left-to-right shunt. The shunt is quantified by comparing the area under C with the area under the fitted recirculation gamma variate (*D*).

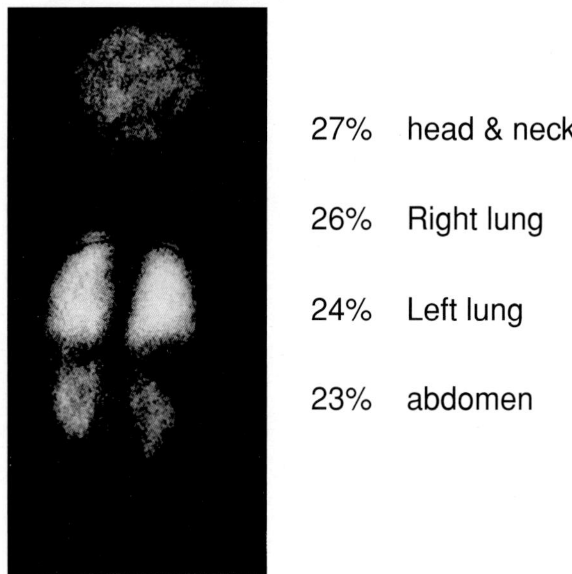

FIGURE 73.18. **Abnormal Right-to-Left Shunt Study.** A significant portion of the injected Tc-99m macroaggregated albumin (*MAA*) particles are seen in capillary beds outside the lungs in the brain and kidneys. This indicates and measures the amount of shunted blood.

into the lungs. This causes a prolongation of the washout of activity from the lung ROI. A mathematical method can then be used to detect and quantify the amount of the left-to-right shunt and is sensitive enough to detect shunts with a ratio as low as 1.2:1, far below the 2:1 shunt that can be detected by chest radiograph (Fig. 73.17).

Right-to-left shunts can be detected by using an IV injection of macroaggregated albumin particles. In a normal person, less than 10% of the injected dose should pass through normal arteriovenous shunts in the lungs and be found in the systemic circulation. After injection, static images of the patient's whole body are performed. Regions of interest are taken over the lungs, head, neck, abdomen, and extremities. The amount of radioactivity outside the lungs in the systemic circulation is then quantified and correlates with shunt severity. Cerebral cortex uptake is diagnostic, though uptake in organs such as the kidney and thyroid gland may be due to free Tc-99m pertechnetate. The study can be repeated at a later date to evaluate for progression (Fig. 73.18).

Suggested Readings

Allman KC. 18F-FDG PET and myocardial viability assessment: trials and tribulations. *J Nucl Med* 2010;51:505–506.

Anagnostopoulos C, Harbinson M, Kelion A, et al. Procedure guidelines for radionuclide myocardial perfusion imaging. *Heart* 2004;90:i1–i10.

Bax JJ, Cornell JH, Visser FC, et al. Comparison of fluorine-18-FDG with rest-redistribution thallium-201 SPECT to delineate viable myocardium and predict functional recovery after revascularization. *J Nucl Med* 1998; 39:1481–1486.

Bax JJ, Patton JA, Poldermans D, Elhendy A, Sandler MP. 18-Fluorodeoxyglucose imaging with positron emission tomography and single photon emission computed tomography: cardiac applications. *Semin Nucl Med* 2000; 30:281–298.

Beller GA. First annual Mario S. Verani, MD, Memorial lecture: clinical value of myocardial perfusion imaging in coronary artery disease. *J Nucl Cardiol* 2003;10:529–542.

Camici PG, Prasad SK, Rimoldi OE. Stunning, hibernation, and assessment of myocardial viability. *Circulation* 2008;117:103–114.

Crean A, Dutka D, Coulder R. Cardiac imaging using nuclear medicine and positron emission tomography. *Radiol Clin North Am* 2004;42:619–634.

DePuey EG, Berman DS, Garcia EV. *Cardiac SPECT Imaging*. 2nd ed. Philadelphia, PA: Lippincott Williams & Wilkins, 2001.

Di Carli MF, Dorbala S, Meserve J, El Fakhri G, Sitek A, Moore SC. Clinical myocardial perfusion PET/CT. *J Nucl Med* 2007;48:783–793.

Dilsizian V, Arrighi JA, Diodati JG, et al. Myocardial viability in patients with chronic coronary artery disease. Comparison of 99mTc-sestamibi with thallium reinjection and [18F] fluorodeoxyglucose. *Circulation* 1995;91(12): 3026.

Germano G, Berman DS. *Clinical Gated Cardiac SPECT*. Malden, MA: Blackwell Publishing, 2006.

Gibbons RJ, Balady GJ, Bricker JT, et al. ACC/AHA 2002 guidelines update for exercise testing: summary article. A report of the American College of Cardiology/American Heart Association Task Force on Practice Guidelines (Committee to Update the 1997 Exercise Testing Guidelines). *J Am Coll Cardiol* 2002;40(8):1531–1540. Available from http://www.acc.org/clinical/guidelines/exercise/dirIndex.htm.

Hayes SW, De Lorenzo A, Hachamovitch R, et al. Prognostic implications of combined prone and supine acquisitions in patients with equivocal or abnormal supine myocardial perfusion SPECT. *J Nucl Med* 2003;44:1633–1640.

Heller G, Hendel R. *Nuclear Cardiology: Practical Applications*. 2nd ed. New York: McGraw-Hill, 2010.

Iskandrian AE, Garcia EV. *Nuclear Cardiac Imaging: Principles and Applications*. New York: Oxford University Press, 2008.

Kapur A, Latus KA, Davies G, et al. A comparison of three radionuclide myocardial perfusion tracers in clinical practice: the ROBUST study. *Eur J Nucl Med Mol Imaging* 2002;29:1608–1616.

Leppo JA. Dipyridamole myocardial perfusion imaging. *J Nucl Med* 1994; 35:730–733.

Loong CY, Anagnostopoulos C. Diagnosis of coronary artery disease by radionuclide myocardial perfusion imaging. *Heart* 2004;90(Suppl 5):v2–v9.

Mahmarian JJ, Cerqueira MD, Iskandrian AE, et al. Ragadenoson induces comparable left ventricular perfusion defects as adenosine: a quantitative analysis from the ADVANCE MPI 2 trial. *JACC Cardiovasc Imaging* 2009;2:959–968.

Masood Y, Lia YH, Depuey G, et al. Clinical validation of SPECT attenuation correction using x-ray computed tomography-derived attenuation maps: multicenter clinical trial with angiographic correlation. *J Nucl Cardiol* 2005;12:676–686.

Miller DD, Younis LT, Chaitman BR, Stratmann H. Diagnostic accuracy of dipyridamole technetium 99m-labeled sestamibi myocardial tomography for detection of coronary artery disease. *J Nucl Cardiol* 1997;4:18–24.

Robinson VJ, Corley JH, Marks DS, et al. Causes of transient dilatation of the left ventricle during myocardial perfusion imaging. *AJR Am J Roentgenol* 2000;174:1349–1352.

Santoro GM, Sciagra R, Buonamici P, et al. Head-to-head comparison of exercise stress testing, pharmacologic stress echocardiography, and perfusion tomography as first-line examination for chest pain in patients without history of coronary artery disease. *J Nucl Cardiol* 1998;5:19–27.

Sharir T, Germano G, Kavanagh PB, et al. Incremental prognostic value of post-stress left ventricular ejection fraction and volume by gated myocardial perfusion single photon emission computed tomography. *Circulation* 1999;100:1035–1042.

Sinusas AJ. Multimodality cardiovascular molecular imaging: an overview. *J Nucl Med* 2010;51:1S–2S.

Slomka PJ, Nishima H, Berman DS, et al. Automated quantification of myocardial perfusion SPECT using simplified normal limits. *J Nucl Cardiol* 2005;12:66–77.

Tamaki N, Ohtani H, Yamashita K, et al. Metabolic activity in the areas of new fill-in after thallium-201 reinjection: comparison with positron emission tomography using fluorine-18-deoxyglucose. *J Nucl Med* 1991;32:673–678.

Tamaki N, Takahashi N, Kawamoto M, et al. Myocardial tomography using technetium-99m-tetrofosmin to evaluate coronary artery disease. *J Nucl Med* 1994;35:594–600.

Van Train KF, Garcia EV, Maddahi J, et al. Multicenter trial validation for quantitative analysis of same-day rest–stress technetium-99m-sestamibi myocardial tomograms. *J Nucl Med* 1994;35:609–618.

Watanabe K, Sekiya M, Ikeda S, Miyagawa M, Kinoshita M, Kumano S. Comparison of adenosine triphosphate and dipyridamole in diagnosis by thallium-201 myocardial scintigraphy. *J Nucl Med* 1997;38:577–581.

Wijns W, Vatner SF, Camici PG. Hibernating myocardium. *N Engl J Med* 1998; 339:173–181.

Yamagishi H, Shirai N, Yoshiyama M, et al. Incremental value of left ventricular ejection fraction for detection of multivessel coronary artery disease in exercise (201)Tl gated myocardial perfusion imaging. *J Nucl Med* 2002;43: 131–139.

Zaret BL, Beller GA. *Clinical Nuclear Cardiology*. 4th ed. Philadelphia, PA: Mosby Elsevier, 2010.

CHAPTER 74 ■ NUCLEAR BRAIN IMAGING

JASON J. BAILEY AND RICHARD K. J. BROWN

POSITRON EMISSION TOMOGRAPHY AND SINGLE-PHOTON EMISSION COMPUTED TOMOGRAPHY

F-18 fluorodeoxyglucose (FDG) is used for positron emission tomography (PET) as it crosses the blood–brain barrier (BBB) and, as a glucose analog, typically demonstrates uptake throughout the brain parenchyma.

Technetium-99m (Tc-99m) hexamethylpropyleneamine oxime (HMPAO) and Tc-99m ethyl cysteinate dimer (ECD) can be used for single-photon emission computed tomography (SPECT) imaging after crossing the BBB and being irreversibly trapped within the brain parenchyma; however, the superior resolution and increasing availability of PET imaging has led to decreased usage of brain SPECT for many indications.

There is a large overlap of clinical indications for SPECT and PET brain imaging, including dementia, epilepsy, stroke, tumors, and trauma.

Radiopharmaceuticals: Tc-99m HMPAO, Tc-99m ECD, and F-18 FDG

Technique. In preparation for a brain FDG PET scan, patients should fast for at least 4 hours prior to injection of 5 to 10 mCi of FDG as elevated serum glucose levels can interfere with FDG uptake in the brain. Scanning is typically performed 60 to 90 minutes after injection of 8 mCi of FDG with the patient lying calmly on the scanning table with eyes open. If the patient's eyes are closed, this may result in artificially decreased metabolism in the occipital lobe, which can suggest a diagnosis of Alzheimer disease instead of dementia with Lewy bodies, as discussed below. Brain FDG-PET scans are typically interpreted with the assistance of a normal age-matched databank, which is typically fused onto the study being reviewed. Areas of parenchyma that demonstrate greater than two standard deviations lower than the metabolism seen in the normal databank are displayed with certain colors to objectively identify areas of decreased brain metabolism.

Brain perfusion SPECT scans are performed with a multidetector rotating camera with high-resolution collimators to achieve three-dimensional images of the brain. The scanning agent, typically 15 to 30 mCi of either Tc-99m HMPAO or Tc-99m ECD, is injected with a patient in a controlled resting state, typically in supine position with eyes closed in a quiet room. Scanning should be performed at least 60 minutes post-injection (Fig. 74.1).

For ictal SPECT scanning performed to identify an active seizure focus, radiotracer must be injected during seizure activity. For ictal scanning, the patient must be carefully and continuously monitored with an IV catheter in place and agent readily available nearby, with injection occurring immediately after seizure onset.

Interpretation

Dementia. The most important use for brain SPECT and PET imaging in the workup of the dementia patient is to differentiate **Alzheimer's disease** (**AD**) from other dementia types. **Patients with AD demonstrate decreased perfusion to the parietal and temporal lobes bilaterally, with sparing of the occipital lobes** (Figs. 74.2 and 74.3; see Fig. 74.1). More specific features of AD include sparing of the anterior tips of the temporal lobes, hypometabolism in the precuneus, and hypometabolism in the posterior cingulate gyrus. Posterior cingulate gyrus hypometabolism is frequently the earliest metabolic abnormality detectable in AD. Hypometabolic defects in AD are typically bilateral and asymmetric, and in advanced cases can extend to the frontal lobe. Detection of AD with PET has a sensitivity of 78% to 83% and specificity of 78% to 94%. In patients with AD of varying severity, the magnitude and extent of hypometabolism correlate with the severity of the dementia symptoms.

Dementia with Lewy bodies (**DLB**), which is characterized by visual hallucinations, cognitive decline, and parkinsonian symptoms, demonstrates temporoparietal hypoperfusion

The editors wish to thanks Dr. David H. Lewis and Dr. Jon Umlauf for their works in the 4th edition establishing the foundation for this chapter.

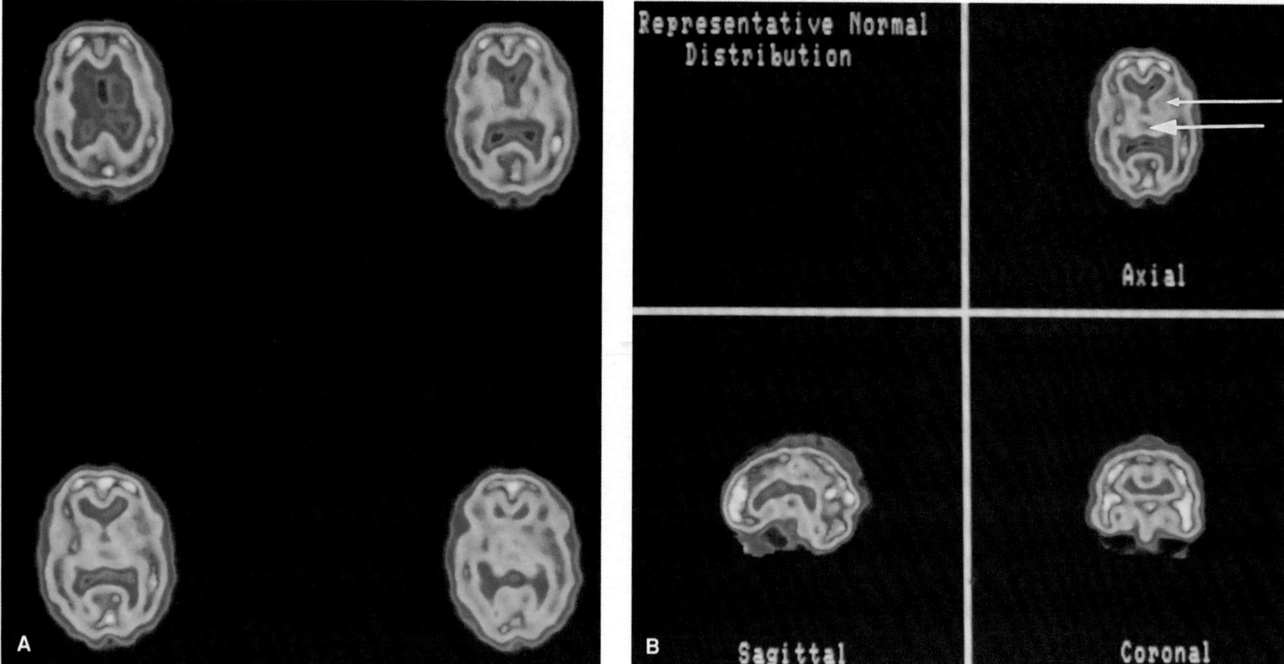

FIGURE 74.1. **Normal Hexamethylpropyleneamine Oxime (HMPAO) Study.** Selected images from a normal Tc-99m HMPAO study. **A:** Axial images. **B:** Representative central images in three standard planes (axial, sagittal, and coronal to long axis of brain). *Large arrow* indicates the brainstem; *small arrow* indicates the basal ganglia. With modern equipment, it should be possible to routinely obtain scans that resolve gyri, basal ganglia, and brainstem. Interpreters should consult an atlas to familiarize themselves with the normal distribution of radiotracer in the brain structures.

on brain SPECT, similar to AD. **DLB, however, also involves hypoperfusion of the occipital lobe, including the primary visual cortices, differentiating it from AD.** Primary visual cortex hypometabolism, if present, is highly specific for DLB. Sparing of the posterior aspect of the cingulate gyrus (the cingulate island sign) has been described as a finding that helps differentiate DLB from AD; however this finding has not been proven to be specific for DLB and remains controversial.

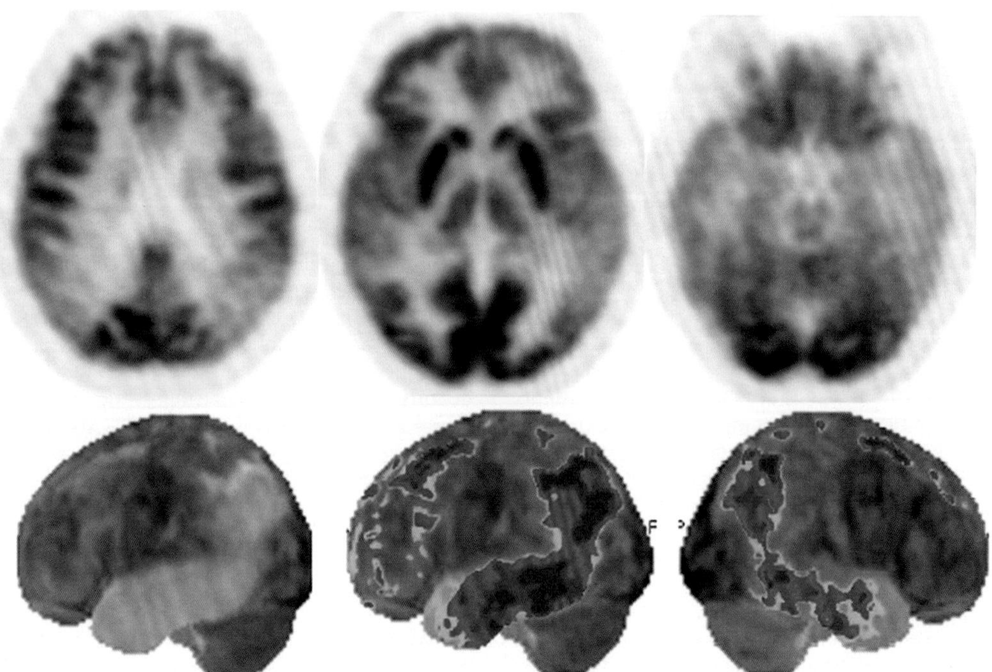

FIGURE 74.2. **PET in Alzheimer Disease.** Transaxial plane from FDG-PET scan in Alzheimer disease. Note preservation of metabolism in sensorimotor cortex, visual cortex, basal ganglia, thalami, and cerebellum. Note deficit of metabolic activity in temporoparietal association cortex bilaterally. (Image courtesy of Satoshi Minoshima, MD, PhD.)

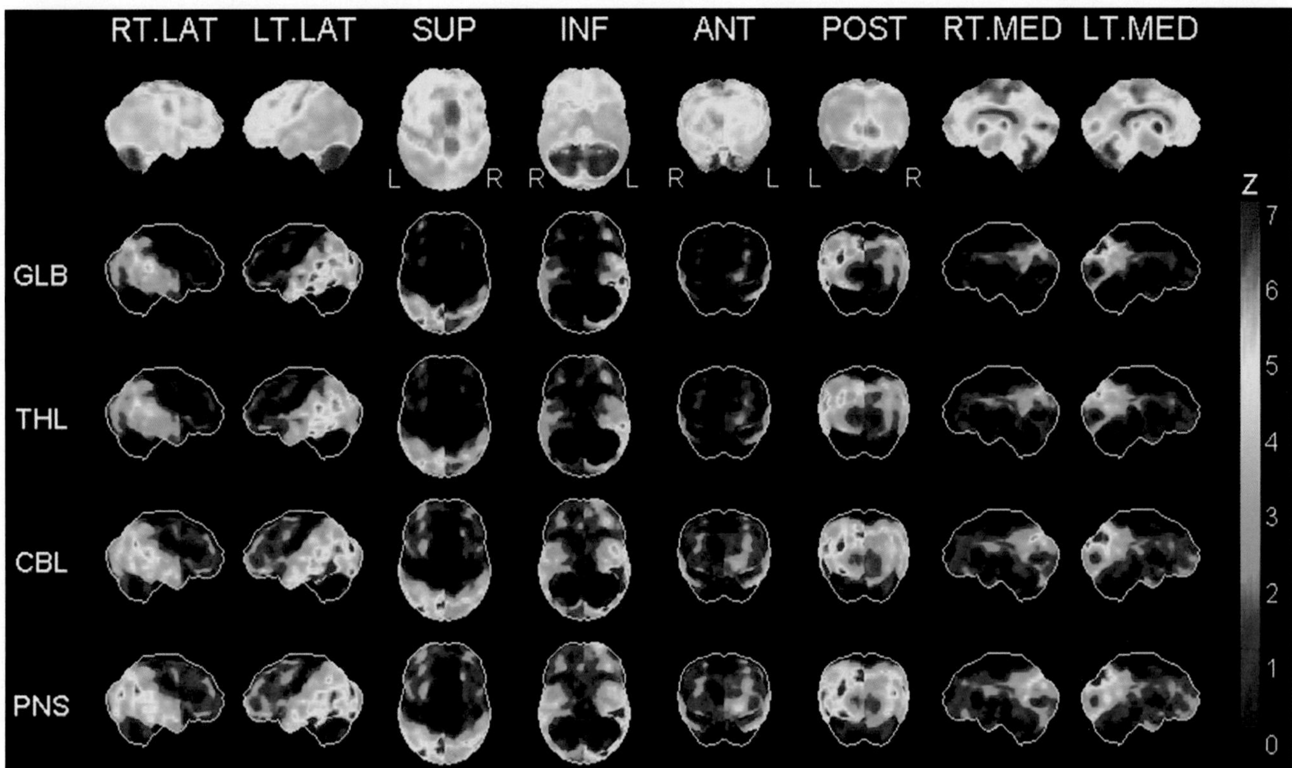

FIGURE 74.3. **Three-Dimensional SSP Display of SPECT in Alzheimer Disease.** Stereotactic three-dimensional surface projection display of z-scores in brain SPECT in Alzheimer disease showing statistically significant decreases in perfusion in bilateral temporoparietal association cortices and also in posterior cingulate. GLB, THL, CBL, and PNS indicate that each corresponding row is normalized to global, thalamic, cerebellar, and pons uptake, respectively.

Frontotemporal dementia (FTD) demonstrates hypometabolism in the frontal and anterior temporal lobes. The anterior cingulate gyrus is also typically involved. **Involvement of the anterior aspect of the temporal lobes helps differentiate FTD from AD, which spares the anterior tips of the temporal lobes.** FTD also can present as a frontal-predominant variant, which spares the temporal lobes and typically presents with behavioral changes as well as a temporal-predominant variant (semantic dementia) that spares the frontal lobes and typically presents with language and word-finding difficulty.

Vascular dementia results in defects in a random distribution and can coexist with Alzheimer disease in a proportion of the elderly. Vascular dementia is generally suspected based on clinical history and CT or MRI findings and rarely requires PET imaging for diagnosis. Vascular dementia typically demonstrates multiple areas of hypometabolism with abrupt margins in vascular distributions.

Seizures. Temporal lobe syndrome with typical complex partial seizures is typically evaluated with electroencephalography (EEG), MRI, and continuous video monitoring. If these modalities are concordant and suggestive of a seizure focus, patients may be offered temporal lobectomy without SPECT or PET imaging. In patients with complex partial seizures with discordant EEG, MRI, and clinical findings, however, ictal and interictal brain SPECT and interictal brain PET imaging can help localize a seizure focus prior to surgery. In mesial temporal lobe epilepsy, up to 85% of patients can be cured surgically if the focus of abnormal brain tissue is limited to a single temporal lobe.

During interictal scanning, seizure foci tend to have decreased activity. During ictal scanning, a seizure focus typically demonstrates increased perfusion (Fig. 74.4). Ictal SPECT may identify seizure foci and is especially useful in epileptogenic cortical developmental disorders where MRI and EEG often fail to find the epileptogenic focus. An ictal SPECT study showing an area of increased regional blood flow, which may correspond to an area of decreased regional blood flow on interictal SPECT, is strong evidence for an epileptogenic lesion. Ictal SPECT is reported to be greater than 90% accurate, more accurate than interictal SPECT and PET.

FDG scanning must be performed interictally in seizure patients, as the 110-minute half-life of F-18 does not allow the radiotracer to be made available for ictal scanning at bedside. **Interictally, the seizure focus is usually hypometabolic.** This is now thought to be due to interruptions with adjacent neurons, which reduce neural activity and thus metabolism. Loss of neural connections can also result in decreased metabolism in connected and more distant sites (diaschisis). Sites of temporal epilepsy are identified as hypometabolic foci in 70% to 85% of interictal scans with a false-positive rate of only 5%.

Stroke and Ischemia. On both brain SPECT and PET scanning, acute stroke appears as an area of decreased perfusion in a vascular distribution. The extent of stroke can be determined a short time after its occurrence with functional brain scanning (Figs. 74.5 and 74.6). For example, Tc-99m ECD has been shown to have a specificity of 98% and sensitivity of 86% for acute stroke localization. Given the need for immediate diagnosis and exclusion of intracerebral hemorrhage, clinical findings combined with noncontrast head CT are typically the initial workup for stroke prior to emergent tissue plasminogen activator (tPA) administration with diffusion-weighted

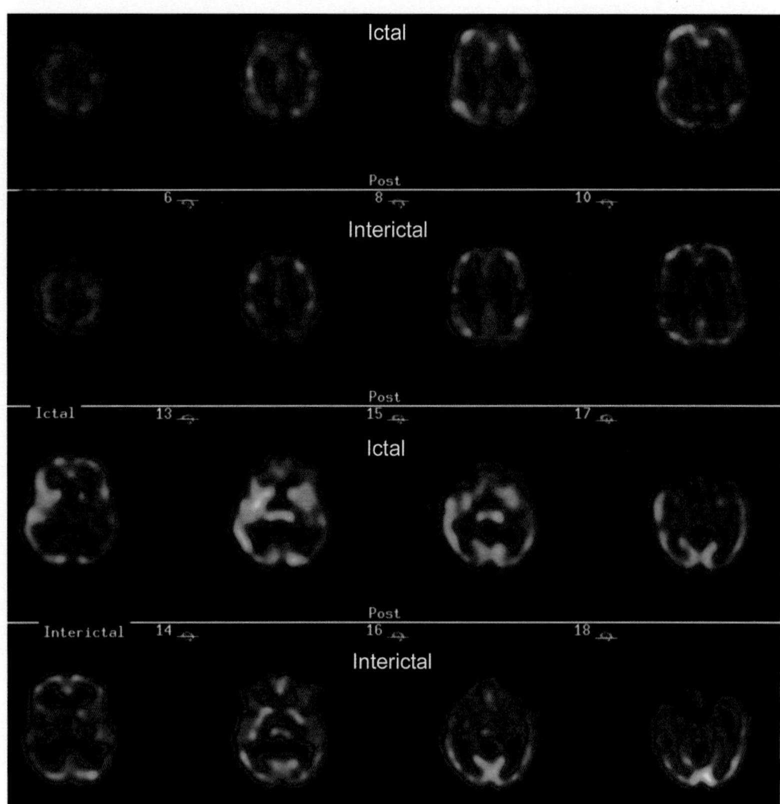

FIGURE 74.4. **Ictal and Interictal SPECT Scans in Complex Partial Epilepsy.** Transverse axial images of Tc-99m ECD injected with seizure ictus on rows 1 and 3 and also injected during interictal time period on rows 2 and 4. Ictal imaging shows increased uptake in right hemisphere, which is predominantly in right temporal lobe. Interictal imaging shows relatively decreased uptake in right temporal lobe.

MRI used occasionally for its high accuracy early in the disease course. Functional imaging has not been widely employed because of the potential to delay therapy when stroke has already been confirmed clinically.

Brain SPECT and PET can also be used to evaluate for ischemia related to vasospasm after subarachnoid hemorrhage, which occurs in 30% of patients with subarachnoid hemorrhage (Fig. 74.7). Functional brain imaging in association with neurologic examination and transcranial Doppler (TCD) artery narrowing assessment allows effective noninvasive monitoring and early intervention. Brain SPECT has been shown to have a similar sensitivity and specificity of TCD in vasospasm.

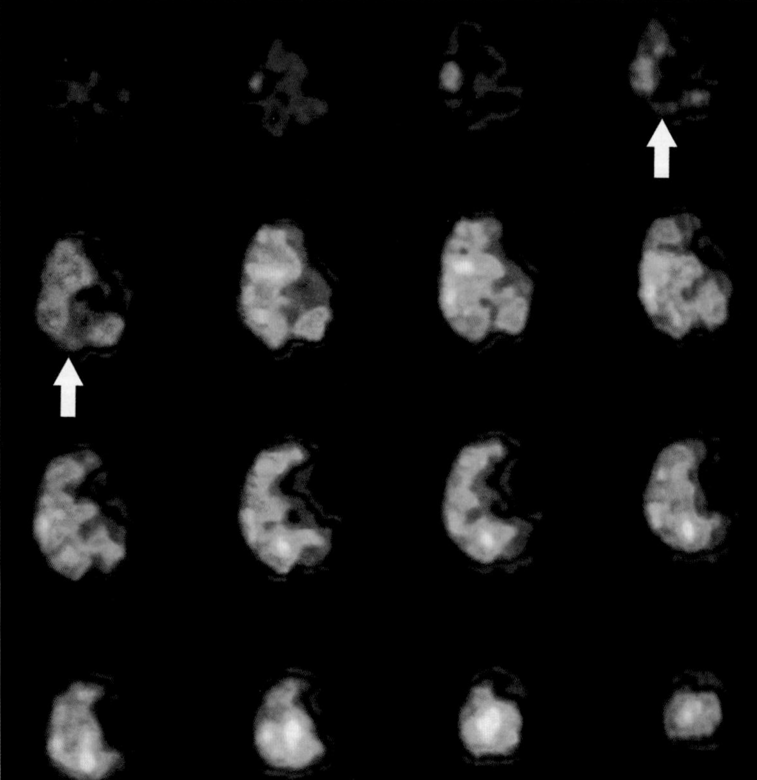

FIGURE 74.5. **Cerebral Infarction.** Transaxial images reformatted into the plane of the orbitomeatal line (standard CT format) from an I-123 iofetamine scan show a large region of absent perfusion (*arrows*) in the distribution of the left middle cerebral artery after cerebral infarction. Note the decreased cerebellar activity on the side opposite the infarct (*arrow*), an example of crossed cerebellar diaschisis. This phenomenon results from decreased right cerebellar metabolism due to decreased neuronal communication between the right cerebellum and the infarcted portion of the left cerebral hemisphere. (All iofetamine images in this chapter were obtained during phase III trials of the agent under approved protocol. Modern equipment allow significant improvement in resolution.)

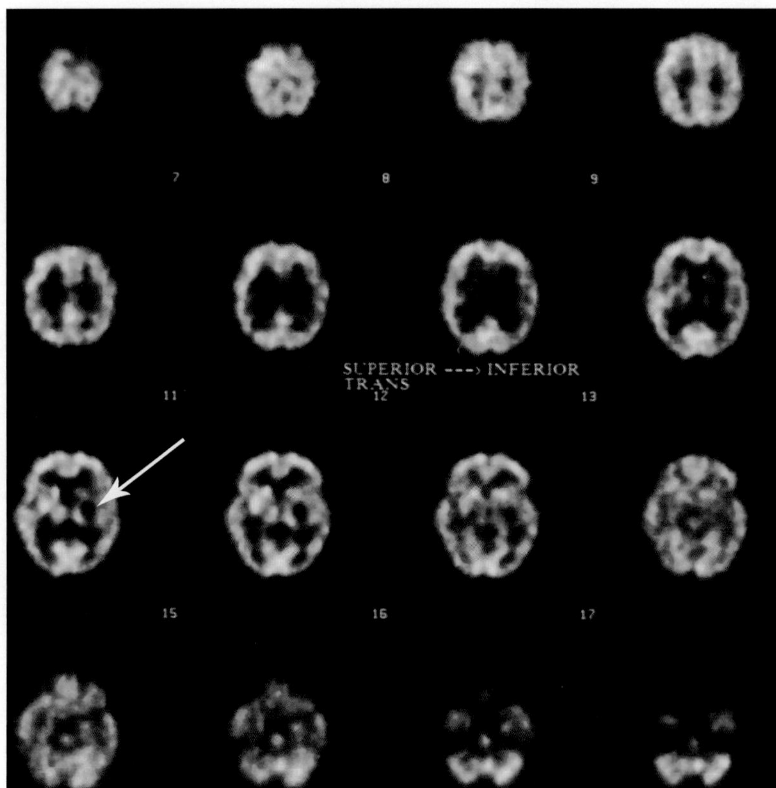

FIGURE 74.6. **Subcortical Cerebral Infarct.** Transverse axial images of Tc-99m ECD in a patient with acute stroke shows absence of uptake in the left lenticular nucleus (*arrow*).

After a cerebral infarction, there is decreased demand for oxygen metabolism within infarcted brain tissue but persistent compensatory vasodilation, leading to luxury perfusion. As revascularization occurs, blood flow to the region increases and the infarcted area typically remains in a state of luxury perfusion for days to weeks, presenting as increased perfusion on both SPECT and PET imaging.

It is possible to perform the equivalent of pharmacologic coronary stress imaging for cerebral vessels using acetazolamide to test vasodilatory reserve. Studies with and without acetazolamide may provide information on the mechanism of ischemia. These studies may also be useful in presurgical planning when carotid surgery or intracranial/extracranial bypass surgery is contemplated because they can indicate the physiologic significance of an anatomic vascular lesion. Interpretation of these studies depends on identification of a significant area of relatively decreased perfusion (actually indicating increased perfusion in the unaffected portions of the brain) after stimulation, which was not present in the study without stimulation, which would indicate impaired vasodilatory reserve (Fig. 74.8). This is exactly analogous to evaluation of coronary artery reserve with dipyridamole or adenosine stress imaging as discussed elsewhere.

Brain Tumors. PET can play an important role in the evaluation and management of patients with brain tumors, including the grading of tumors, prognostication, and differentiation of recurrent tumor from radiation necrosis. The sensitivity for making the determination of radiation necrosis versus tumor recurrence may be as high as 86% with a specificity of 56%. FDG studies have concluded that high-grade tumors are hypermetabolic, whereas low-grade tumors can be hypometabolic. One distinction from this typology is juvenile pilocytic astrocytomas, which typically have a high-glucose metabolism despite their benign nature. It should be noted that PET may not differentiate between primary lymphomas of the CNS, brain metastases, or malignant gliomas because all of these may be hypermetabolic.

Brain Trauma. SPECT brain imaging has been proposed to confirm the presence of a focal or diffuse injury in patients with persistent symptoms after trauma despite normal or nondiagnostic anatomic imaging studies. The increased sensitivity of functional SPECT relative to CT or MR favors this use and is supported by ACR Practice Guidelines on brain perfusion SPECT (2007). In addition, recent studies in mild traumatic brain injury patients have shown important abnormalities in cerebellar function and its relationship to the cerebral cortex with both SPECT and PET studies.

Parkinson disease (PD) can be evaluated using SPECT brain imaging using the cocaine analogs I-123 β-CIT (2β-carboxymethoxy-3β-4-iodophenyl tropane) (DOPASCAN) and I-123 FP-CIT (fluoropropyl-2β-carbomethoxy-3β-4-iodophenyl nortropane) (DaTscan). PD is a clinical diagnosis based on classic motor dysfunction including bradykinesia, rigidity, and rest tremor. The main neuropathologic feature is severe degeneration of the dopaminergic neurons in the substantia nigra. In 10% to 20% of cases, there is ambiguity in the clinical diagnosis, and additional testing can improve diagnostic accuracy. Specifically, testing can differentiate essential tremor from parkinsonian syndromes.

DOPASCAN and DaTscan bind with high affinity to the dopamine transporter that degenerates in the setting of PD. Before administering the radiopharmaceutical, the thyroid should be protected with an appropriate dose of sodium perchlorate (at least 200 mg, 60 minutes before injection).

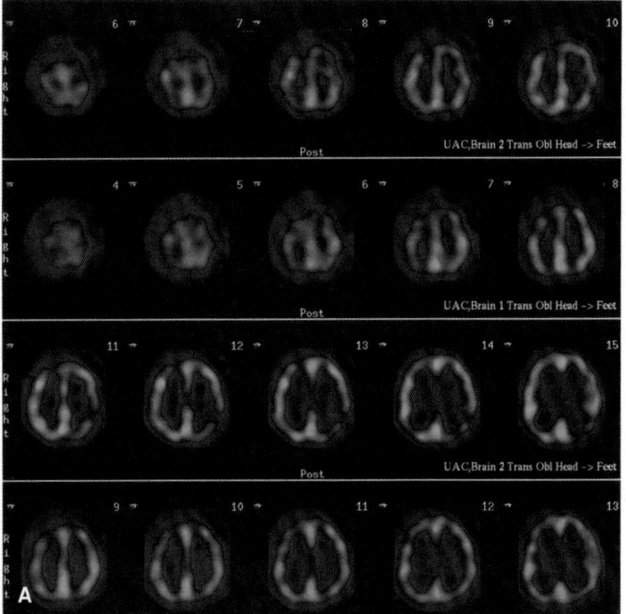

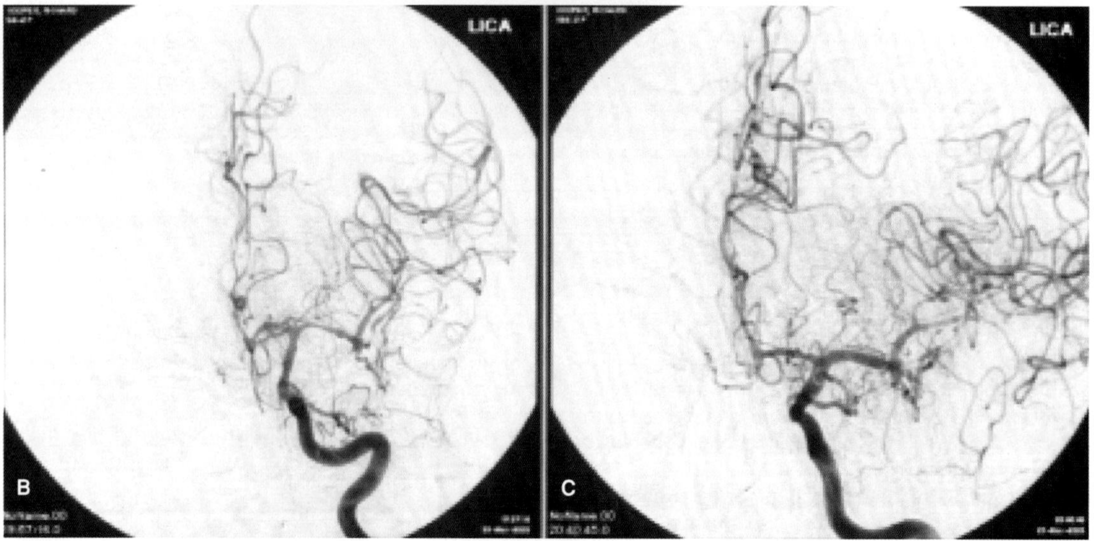

FIGURE 74.7. **Subarachnoid Hemorrhage and Cerebral Vasospasm. A:** Transverse axial images of Tc-99m ECD show baseline scan on rows 2 and 4 and scan during vasospasm on rows 1 and 3. New defect is seen in left hemisphere in posterior frontoparietal cortex corresponding to ischemia from vasospasm. **B:** Left internal carotid angiogram shows vasospasm in midportion of left middle cerebral artery. **C:** Later angiogram of left internal carotid artery shows resolution of vasospasm after percutaneous transluminal microballoon angioplasty.

The radiopharmaceutical is injected slowly over 20 minutes. The patient is imaged 18 to 24 hours postinjection with DOPASCAN and 3 to 6 hours postinjection with DaTscan. Because the radiopharmaceuticals affect presynaptic uptake of dopamine, patients can continue their therapeutic dopamine prior to imaging. Because these tracers are cocaine analogs, however, cocaine itself can interfere with the study.

The normal appearance of the striatum, including the caudate and putamen, should be a crescentic region of radiotracer uptake, which can be described as resembling a comma. **The abnormal appearance of the striatum seen in PD involves degeneration of its posterior aspect and can be described as resembling a period (Fig. 74.9).** Visual and semi-quantitative assessment of the striatum can be aided by fusion techniques with the patient's own brain MRI and with a normal age-matched control database.

CEREBRAL PERFUSION IMAGING

Tc-99m HMPAO and Tc-99m ECD are lipophilic radiotracers that can cross the intact BBB by passive diffusion with nearly complete first pass extraction and therefore can be used to assess parenchymal cerebral perfusion via planar brain imaging. HMPAO and ECD have largely replaced traditional planar brain imaging with diethylenetriaminepentaacetic acid (DTPA) and glucoheptonate (GH) for the evaluation of brain death.

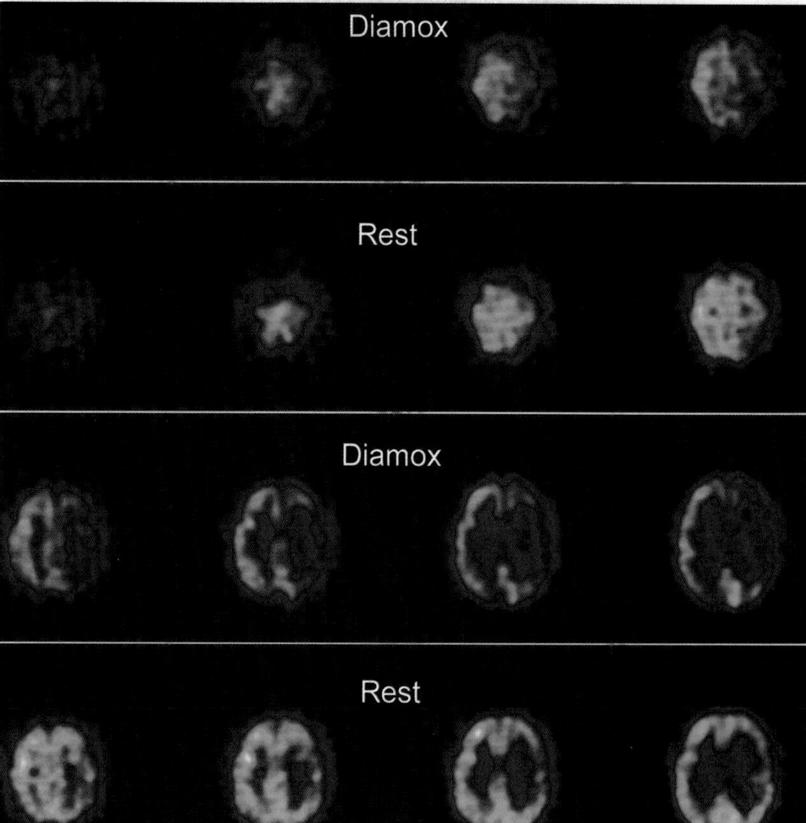

FIGURE 74.8. Acetazolamide Vascular Reserve Testing in Occlusive Carotid Disease. Transverse axial images of Tc-99m ECD with acetazolamide on rows 1 and 3 and at rest on rows 2 and 4. Images show decreased uptake in left hemisphere with acetazolamide that improves largely at rest. This finding indicates exhausted vasodilatory reserve in left hemisphere corresponding to the left internal carotid artery occlusion.

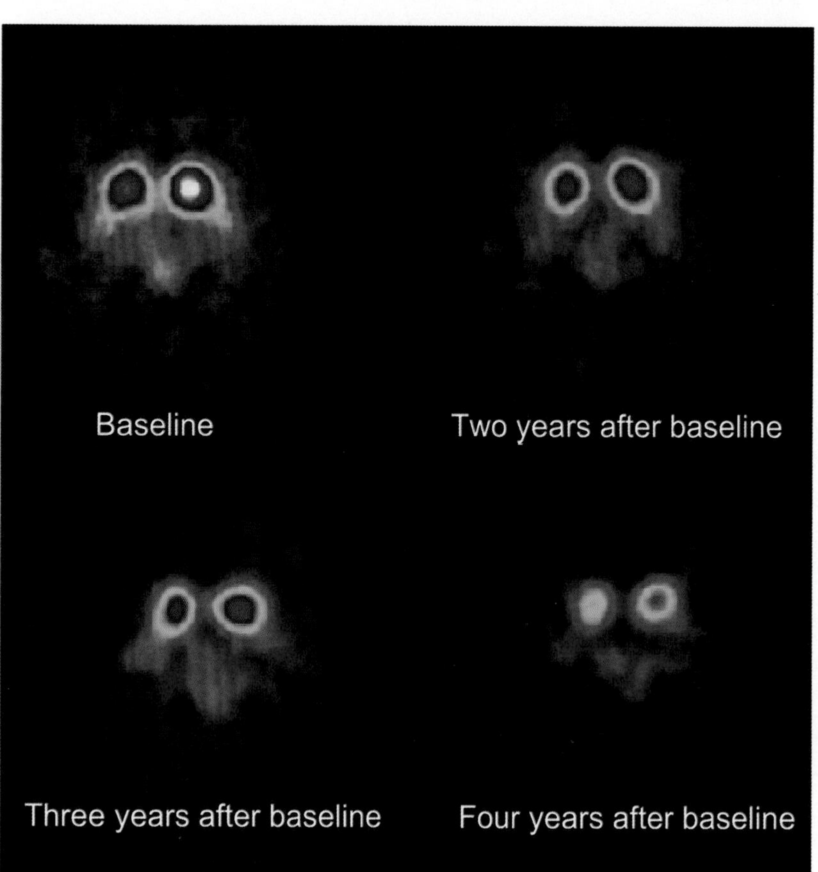

FIGURE 74.9. I-123 Ioflupane (FP-CIT) SPECT. I-123 ioflupane SPECT images at level of basal ganglia over time in a patient with Parkinson disease show progressive decline in uptake, reflecting loss of dopaminergic function.

Radiopharmaceutical. Tc-99m HMPAO; Tc-99m ECD.

Technique. The technique for cerebral perfusion imaging is similar to that of traditional planar brain imaging. A dose of 30 mCi of Tc-99m HMPAO or ECD is injected intravenously. Flow images are typically obtained at a rate of 1 image every 3 seconds for 60 seconds with the camera anterior to the head. Immediate and delayed static images in anterior, posterior, and lateral projections are obtained.

Interpretation. For the evaluation of brain death, complete absence of brain activity, including in the cerebellum, is consistent with brain death. This must be seen in the presence of prompt common carotid artery and scalp flow in order to confirm that absence of cerebral perfusion is not related to something other than brain death such as extravasation of radiotracer during injection. Absence of brain perfusion during cerebral imaging is one of the supportive criteria used to diagnose brain death according to the Uniform Determination of Death Act (*National Conference of Commissioners on Uniform State Laws*, 1981). **A perfusion scan consistent with brain death does not diagnose but only supports a clinical diagnosis of brain death.** It is also important to note that imaging of the injection site should be performed to confirm proper injection. Newer brain perfusion agents have advantages over conventional agents such as Tc-99m GH or Tc-99m DTPA for diagnosing brain death as they are not as dependent on the quality of bolus injection, are easier to interpret, and allow for evaluation of posterior fossa blood flow.

For the evaluation of other intracranial pathology, increased radiotracer uptake can indicate vascular malformations, high-grade or vascular brain tumors, or an inflammatory process, whereas decreased radiotracer uptake can indicate low-grade or benign tumors, areas of encephalomalacia or edema, or an occlusive vascular process. **Complete absence of brain activity including the cerebellum in the presence of prompt common carotid and scalp flow is consistent with brain death.**

PLANAR BRAIN IMAGING

Radiopharmaceuticals traditionally used for planar brain imaging do not cross the intact BBB, such as Tc-99m DTPA and Tc-99m GH, and therefore can be used to detect BBB breakdown.

Radiopharmaceutical. Tc-99m DTPA; Tc-99m GH.

Technique. A dose of 15 to 20 mCi of Tc-99m DTPA or GH is injected intravenously. Flow images are typically obtained at a rate of 1 image every 3 seconds for 60 seconds with the camera anterior to the head. Immediate and delayed static images in anterior, posterior, and lateral projections are obtained. Immediate static images are useful to evaluate blood pool abnormalities, whereas delayed static images after clearance of the background activity are used to detect breakdown of the BBB.

Interpretation. Interpretation of the static images depends primarily on detecting or excluding radiopharmaceutical localization within the brain parenchyma. Some activity is invariably present within the soft tissues of the scalp and intracerebral blood vessels. Increased uptake or asymmetric localization indicates breakdown of the BBB, although these findings are nonspecific and the differential diagnosis of intracerebral radiotracer includes cerebral infarction, primary or metastatic tumor, and CNS infection. For this reason, clinical information is essential for interpretation.

In the presence of brain death, the radioactive bolus stops at the base of the skull because of increased intracranial pressure that exceeds cerebral perfusion pressure. It is important to have a good bolus injection and if distinct activity is not identified in the common carotid artery, the injection should be repeated. Absence of intracerebral arterial flow and nonvisualization of major venous sinuses on subsequent static images support a diagnosis of brain death (Fig. 74.10). The "hot nose sign," due to increased collateral blood flow in the

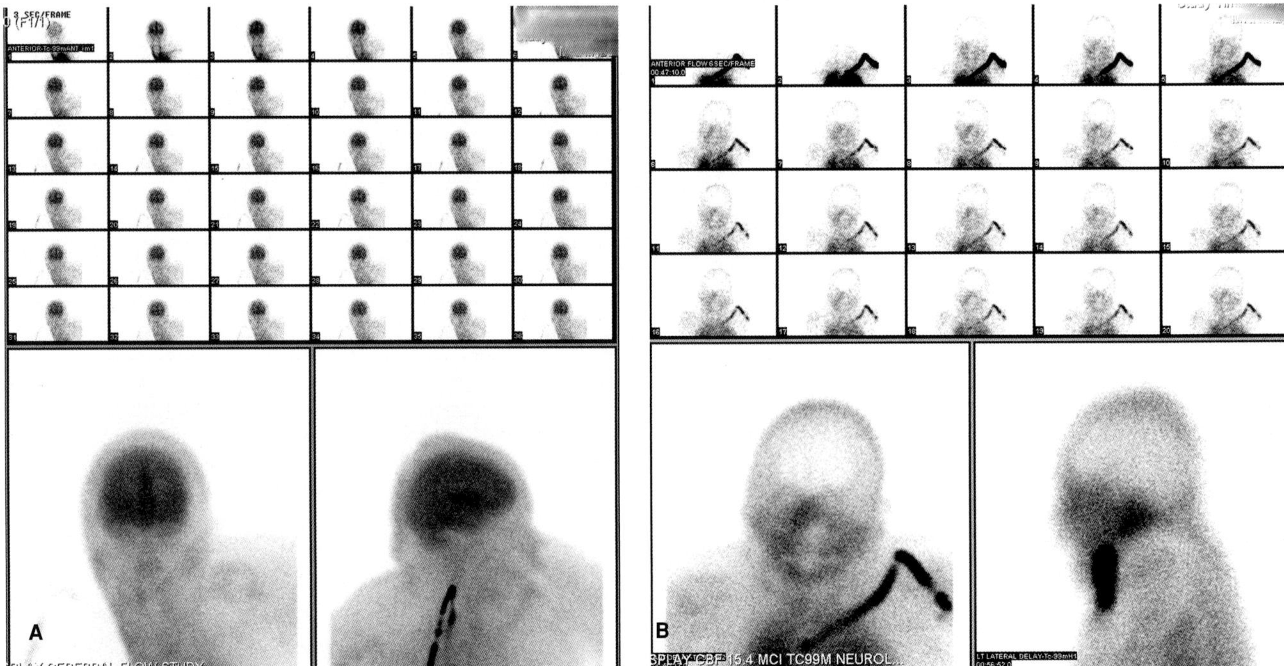

FIGURE 74.10. **Brain Perfusion Planar Scans for Brain Death. A:** Planar scan demonstrates uptake in brain parenchyma and therefore does not meet nuclear medicine criteria for the corroboration of the clinical impression of brain death. **B:** Absence of radiotracer uptake in brain meets criteria for the corroboration of the clinical impression of brain death by total absence of cerebral blood flow.

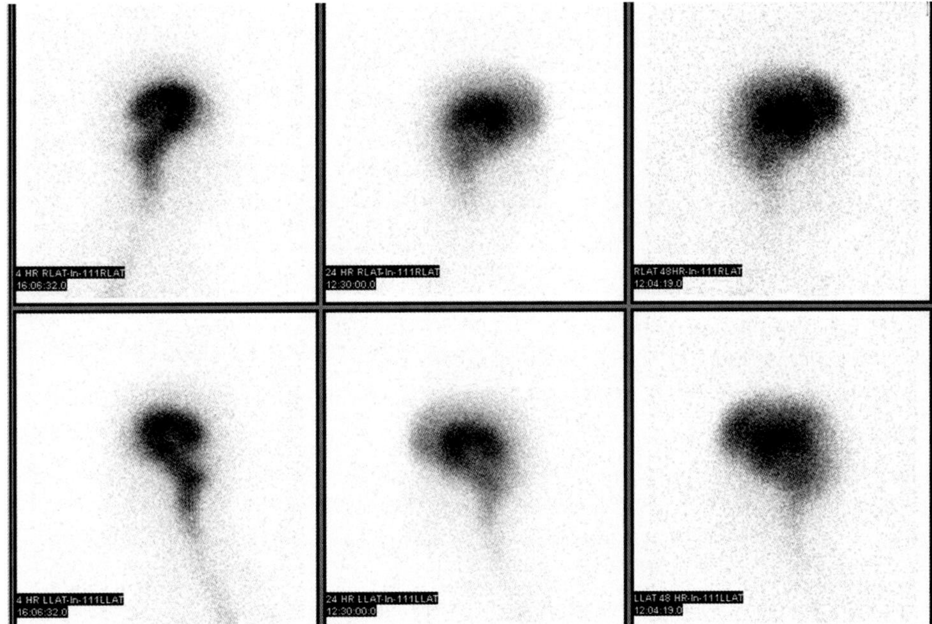

FIGURE 74.11. **Normal Pressure Hydrocephalus on Cisternogram.** Selected images from an In-111 DTPA cisternogram in lateral views shown at 4 to 6 hours, 24 hours, and 48 hours. Abnormal uptake is seen in lateral ventricles, which persists through 48 hours.

nasal area via the external carotid artery, is a nonspecific secondary sign of brain death.

CEREBROSPINAL FLUID STUDIES

Cerebrospinal fluid (CSF) is formed in the choroid plexus as an ultrafiltrate of plasma. It flows from the ventricles through the foramina of the fourth ventricle and ascends over the convexities of the brain to be absorbed by the arachnoid villi. Processes that impede flow over the convexities or absorption of the fluid by the villi result in communicating hydrocephalus. Tracer techniques are ideal for imaging of this process because they are injected in small amounts and do not alter the CSF flow. Patency and flow in therapeutic shunts and reservoirs can also easily be evaluated by injecting the tracer directly into the device.

Radiopharmaceuticals: In-111 DTPA, Tc-99m DTPA, and Tc-99m Pertechnetate

Hydrocephalus. The standard cisternogram is performed by intrathecal injection of 0.5 mCi of Indium-111 (In-111) DTPA. Initial images may be obtained to ensure intrathecal injection. Subsequently, the radiopharmaceutical ascends to the basilar cisterns in approximately 4 hours and flows over the convexities within 24 hours in a normal individual. Images of the basal cisterns are obtained at 4 to 6 hours. If images at 24 hours show ascent over the convexities with activity in the interhemispheric fissure and relative clearance of the basilar cisterns, imaging may be terminated. Otherwise, images should be obtained at 48 and 72 hours.

Standard cisternography performed for hydrocephalus is intended to evaluate for normal pressure hydrocephalus (NPH), a poorly understood form of communicating hydrocephalus clinically associated with ataxia, dementia, and urinary incontinence. In the presence of NPH, cisternography demonstrates early localization of activity within the lateral ventricles that persists beyond 24 hours and demonstrates delayed clearance over the convexities (Fig. 74.11). Although these findings indicate an increased likelihood of a clinical response to shunting, they are not univariate predictors of outcome.

CSF Leak. Cisternography can also be used to evaluate for CSF leak with high sensitivity. Imaging is performed between 1 and 3 hours after intrathecal injection and at 24 hours and sometimes 48 hours. Patient and camera position are chosen to maximize the likelihood of detection with lateral views for CSF rhinorrhea and anterior views for CSF otorrhea. Cotton pledgets should be placed in the nostrils after intrathecal injection of radiotracer and are placed in a well counter 4 to 6 hours later to evaluate for the presence of radiotracer. A serum sample from peripheral blood drawn concurrently is also counted. A pledget activity exceeding 1.5 times the serum concentration is highly suggestive of CSF rhinorrhea.

Shunts and Reservoirs. CSF shunt and reservoir studies are performed by direct injection of radiotracer into the device. In-111 DTPA, Tc-99m DTPA, and Tc-99m pertechnetate can all be used for assessing shunts and reservoirs. A small volume of radiopharmaceutical such as 0.1 to 0.2 mCi Tc-99m pertechnetate in 0.1 mL of normal saline is typically injected. Dynamic gamma camera imaging for 10 minutes is usually first performed in the supine position. If radiotracer drains from the reservoir, images of the downstream tip of the catheter are obtained.

Shunts are evaluated primarily for patency. If the proximal portion is occluded manually (or contains a check valve), flow through the distal limb can be evaluated. The tracer should flow freely into the peritoneum (for ventriculoperitoneal shunts). Delayed flow or persistent activity at the shunt tip suggests malfunction. If the CSF flow is disturbed and opening pressure is low, the blockage is in the proximal limb. If opening pressure is high (more than 20 cm H_2O), the obstruction is distal to the reservoir.

Overshunting is also described when the opening pressure is low and $T_{1/2}$ in the supine position is less than 1 minute. Overshunting may be an indication for shunt valve adjustment or possibly shunt revision. Typically, patients with overshunting have headache that progresses in severity from morning to evening.

Suggested Readings

Alberts MJ, Faulstich ME, Gray L. Stroke with negative brain magnetic resonance imaging. *Stroke* 1992;23(5):663–667.

Alexandrov AV, Black SE, Ehrlich LE, et al. Simple visual analysis of brain perfusion on HMPAO SPECT predicts early outcome in acute stroke. *Stroke* 1996;27(9):1537–1542.

Assessment of brain SPECT. Report of the Therapeutics and Technology Assessment Subcommittee of the American Academy of Neurology. *Neurology* 1996;46(1):278–285.

Bogousslavsky J, Delaloye-Bischof A, Regli F, Delaloye B. Prolonged hypoperfusion and early stroke after transient ischemic attack. *Stroke* 1990;21(1):40–46.

Bonte FJ, Harris TS, Roney CA, Hynan LS. Differential diagnosis between Alzheimer's and frontotemporal disease by the posterior cingulate sign. *J Nucl Med* 2004;45(5):771–774.

Booij J, Tissingh G, Boer GJ, et al. [123I]FP-CIT SPECT shows a pronounced decline of striatal dopamine transporter labeling in early and advanced Parkinson's disease. *J Neurol Neurosurg Psychiatry* 1997;62(2):133–140.

Borghesani PR, DeMers SM, Manchanda V, Pruthi S, Lewis DH, Borson S. Neuroimaging in the clinical diagnosis of dementia: observations from a memory disorders clinic. *J Am Geriatr Soc* 2010;58(8):1453–1458.

Bose A, Pacia SV, Fayad P, Smith EO, Brass LM, Hoffer P. Cerebral blood flow (CBF) imaging compared to CT during the initial 24 hours of cerebral infarction. *Neurology* 1990;40(Suppl 1):190.

Brass LM, Walovitch RC, Joseph JL, et al. The role of single photon emission computed tomography brain imaging with 99m Tc-bicisate in the localization and definition of mechanism of ischemic stroke. *J Cereb Blood Flow Metab* 1994;14(Suppl 1):S91–S98.

Brown RK, Bohnen NI, Wong KK, Minoshima S, Frey KA. Brain PET in suspected dementia: patterns in altered FDG metabolism. *RadioGraphics* 2014;34(3):684–701.

Brun A, Englund B, Gustafson L, et al. Clinical and neuropathological criteria for frontotemporal dementia. The Lund and Manchester Groups. *J Neurol Neurosurg Psychiatry* 1994;57(4):416–418.

Chollet F, Celsis P, Clanet M, Guiraud-Chaumeil B, Rascol A, Marc-Vergnes JP. SPECT study of cerebral blood flow reactivity after acetazolamide in patients with transient ischemic attacks. *Stroke* 1989;20(4):458–464.

Cooke D, Koppula B, Seiler D, et al. Semiquantitative software SPECT analysis in aneurysmal subarachnoid hemorrhage-related vasospasm. *Nucl Med Commun* 2010;31(1):53–58.

Darcourt J, Booji J, Tatsch K, et al. EANM procedure guidelines for brain neurotransmission SPECT using (123)I-labelled dopamine transporter ligands, version 2. *Eur J Nucl Med Mol Imaging* 2010;37(2):443–450.

Davis SM, Andrews JT, Lichtenstein M, Rossiter SC, Kaye AH, Hopper J. Correlations between cerebral arterial velocities, blood flow, and delayed ischemia after subarachnoid hemorrhage. *Stroke* 1992;23(4):492–497.

Di Chiro G, Ommaya AK, Ashburn WL, Briner WH. Isotope cisternography in the diagnosis and follow up of cerebrospinal fluid rhinorrhea. *J Neurosurg* 1968;28(6):522–529.

Drzezga A, Arnold S, Minoshima S, et al. 18F-FDG PET studies in patients with extratemporal and temporal epilepsy: evaluation of an observer-independent analysis. *J Nucl Med* 1999;40(5):737–746.

Haense C, Herholz K, Jagust WJ, Heiss WD. Performance of FDG PET for detection of Alzheimer's disease in two independent multicenter samples (NEST-DD and ADNI). *Dement Geriatr Cogn Disord* 2009;28(3):259–266.

Hammers A, Koepp MJ, Labbe C, et al. Neocortical abnormalities of [11C]-flumazenil PET in mesial temporal lobe epilepsy. *Neurology* 2001;56(7):897–906.

Harbert JC. Radionuclide cisternography. *Semin Nucl Med* 1971;1(1):90–106.

Hartshorne ME. Positron emission tomography. In: Orrison WW, Lewine JD, Sanders JA, Hartshorne MF, eds. *Functional Brain Imaging*. St. Louis, MO: Mosby; 1995:187–212.

Hattori N, Swan M, Stobbe GA, et al. Differential SPECT activation patterns associated with PASAT performance may indicate frontocerebellar functional dissociation in chronic mild traumatic brain injury. *J Nucl Med* 2009;50(7):1054–1061.

Ho SS, Berkovic SF, Berlangieri SU, et al. Comparison of ictal SPECT and interictal PET in the presurgical evaluation of temporal lobe epilepsy. *Ann Neurol* 1995;37(6):738–745.

Holman BL, Johnson KA, Gerada B, Carvalho PA, Satlin A. The scintigraphic appearance of Alzheimer's disease: a prospective study using technetium-99m-HMPAO SPECT. *J Nucl Med* 1992;33(2):181–185.

Hughes CP, Siegel BA, Coxe WS, et al. Adult idiopathic communicating hydrocephalus with and without shunting. *J Neurol Neurosurg Psychiatry* 1978;41(11):961–971.

Hustinx R, Pourdehnad M, Kaschten B, Alavi A. PET imaging for differentiating recurrent brain tumor from radiation necrosis. *Radiol Clin North Am* 2005;43(1):35–47.

Idea RJ, Lewis DH. Timely diagnosis of brain death in an emergency trauma center. *AJR Am J Roentgenol* 1994;163(4):927–928.

Infield B, Davis SM, Donnan GA, et al. Streptokinase increases luxury perfusion after stroke. *Stroke* 1996;27(9):1524–1529.

Jeffery PJ, Monsein LH, Szabo Z, et al. Mapping the distribution of amobarbital sodium in the intracarotid Wada test by use of Tc-99m HMPAO with SPECT. *Radiology* 1991;178(3):847–850.

Kagi G, Bhatia KP, Tolosa E. The role of DAT-SPECT in movement disorders. *J Neurol Neurosurg Psychiatry* 2010;81(1):5–12.

Kim HJ, Karp JS, Mozley PD, et al. Simulating technetium-99m cerebral perfusion studies with a three-dimensional Hoffman brain phantom: collimator and filter selection in SPECT neuroimaging. *Ann Nucl Med* 1996;10(1):153–160.

Krishnanathan R, Minoshima S, Lewis D. Tc-99m ECD neuro-SPECT and diffusion weighted MRI in the detection of the anatomical extent of subacute stroke: a cautionary note regarding reperfusion hyperemia. *Clin Nucl Med* 2007;32(9):700–702.

Kuzniecky R, Mountz JM, Wheatley G, Morawetz R. Ictal single-photon emission computed tomography demonstrates localized epileptogenesis in cortical dysplasia. *Ann Neurol* 1993;34(4):627–631.

la Fougère C, Rominger A, Förster S, Geisler J, Bartenstein P. PET and SPECT in epilepsy: a critical review. *Epilepsy Behav* 2009;15(1):50–55.

Launes J, Nikkinen P, Lindroth L, Brownell AL, Liewendahl K, Iivanainen M. Diagnosis of acute herpes simplex encephalitis by brain perfusion single photon emission computed tomography. *Lancet* 1988;1(8596):1188–1191.

Laurin NR, Driedger AA, Hurwitz GA, et al. Cerebral perfusion imaging with technitium-99m HM-PAO in brain death and severe central nervous system injury. *J Nucl Med* 1989;30(10):1627–1635.

LeBihan D. Molecular diffusion nuclear magnetic resonance imaging. *Magn Reson Q* 1991;7(1):1–30.

Leveille J, Demonceau G, Walovitch RC. Intrasubject comparison between technetium-99m-ECD and technetium-99m-HMPAO in healthy human subjects. *J Nucl Med* 1992;33(4):480–484.

Lewis DH, Hsu S, Eskridge J, et al. Brain SPECT and transcranial Doppler ultrasound in vasospasm-induced delayed cerebral ischemia after subarachnoid hemorrhage. *J Stroke Cerebrovasc Dis* 1992;2(1):12–21.

Lipton AM, Benavides R, Hynan LS, et al. Lateralization on neuroimaging does not differentiate frontotemporal lobar degeneration from Alzheimer's disease. *Dement Geriatr Cogn Disord* 2004;17(4):324–327.

Masdeu JC, Abdel-Dayem H, Van Heertum RL. Head trauma: use of SPECT. *J Neuroimaging* 1995;5(Suppl 1):S53–S57.

Matsuda H, Higashi S, Asli IN, et al. Evaluation of cerebral collateral circulation by technetium-99m HM-PAO brain SPECT during Matas test: report of three cases. *J Nucl Med* 1988;29(10):1724–1729.

McKusick KA, Malmud LS, Kordela A, Wagner HN Jr. Radionuclide cisternography: normal values for nasal secretion of intrathecally injected 111-In-DTPA. *J Nucl Med* 1973;14(12):933–934.

Messa C, Fazio F, Costa DC, Ell PJ. Clinical brain radionuclide imaging studies. *Semin Nucl Med* 1995;15(2):111–143.

Minoshima S, Foster NL, Kuhl DE. Posterior cingulate cortex in Alzheimer's disease. *Lancet* 1994;344(8926):895.

Minoshima S, Foster NL, Sima AA, Frey KA, Albin RL, Kuhl DE. Alzheimer's disease versus dementia with Lewy bodies: cerebral metabolic distinction with autopsy confirmation. *Ann Neurol* 2001;50(3):358–365.

Monsein LH, Jeffery PJ, van Heerden BB, et al. Assessing adequacy of collateral circulation during balloon test occlusion of the internal carotid artery with 99mTc-HMPAO SPECT. *AJNR Am J Neuroradiol* 1991;12(6):1045–1051.

Moretti JL, Caglar M, Weinmann P. Cerebral perfusion imaging tracers for SPECT: which one to choose? *J Nucl Med* 1995;36(3):359–363.

Mrhac L, Zakko S, Parikh Y. Brain death: the evaluation of semi-quantitative parameters and other signs in HMPAO scintigraphy. *Nucl Med Commun* 1995;16(12):1016–1020.

National Institute of Neurological Disorders and Stroke rt–PA Stroke Study Group. Tissue plasminogen activator for acute ischemic stroke. *N Engl J Med* 1995;333(24):1581–1587.

O'Brien DF, Taylor M, Park TS, Ojemann JG. A critical analysis of "normal" radionucleotide shuntograms in patients subsequently requiring surgery. *Childs Nerv Syst* 2003;19(5–6):337–341.

O'Connell RA. Psychiatric disorders. In: Van Heertum RL, Tikofsky RS, eds. *Cerebral SPECT Imaging*. 2nd ed. New York: Raven Press; 1995.

Palmini A, Andermann F, Olivier A, et al. Focal neuronal migration disorders and intractable partial epilepsy: a study of 30 patients. *Ann Neurol* 1991;30(6):741–749.

Peterman SB, Taylor A Jr, Hoffman JC Jr. Improved detection of cerebral hypoperfusion with internal carotid balloon occlusion and 99mTc–HMPAO cerebral perfusion SPECT imaging. *AJNR Am J Neuroradiol* 1991;12(6):1035–1041.

Pietrzyk U, Herholz K, Schuster A, von Stockhausen HM, Lucht H, Heiss WD. Clinical applications of registration and fusion of multimodality brain images from PET, SPECT, CT, and MRI. *Eur J Radiol* 1996;21(3):174–182.

Ramsay SC, Yeates MG, Lord RS, et al. Use of technetium-HMPAO to demonstrate changes in cerebral blood flow reserve following carotid endarterectomy. *J Nucl Med* 1991;32(7):1382–1386.

Reid RH, Gulenchyn K, Ballinger JR. Clinical use of technetium-99m HM-PAO for determination of brain death. *J Nucl Med* 1989;30(10):1621–1626.

Rudd TG, Shurtleff DB, Loeser JD, Nelp WB. Radionuclide assessment of cerebrospinal fluid shunt function in children. *J Nucl Med* 1973;14(9):683–686.
Shishido F, Uemura K, Inugami A, et al. Discrepant 99mTc-ECD images of CBF in patients with subacute cerebral infarction: a comparison of CBF, CMRO2 and 99mTc-HMPAO imaging. *Ann Nucl Med* 1995;9(3):161–169.
Silverman DH. Brain 18F-FDG PET in the diagnosis of neurodegenerative dementias: comparison with perfusion SPECT and with clinical evaluations lacking nuclear imaging. *J Nucl Med* 2004;45(4):594–607.
Silverman DH, Small GW, Chang CY, et al. Positron emission tomography in evaluation of dementia: Regional brain metabolism and long-term outcome. *JAMA* 2001;286(17):2120–2127.
Society of Nuclear Medicine Brain Imaging Council. Ethical clinical practice of functional brain imaging. *J Nucl Med* 1996;37(7):1256–1259.
Soucy JP, McNamara D, Mohr G, Lamoureux F, Lamoureux J, Danais S. Evaluation of vasospasm secondary to subarachnoid hemorrhage with technetium-99m-hexamethyl-propyleneamine oxime (HM-PAO) tomoscintigraphy. *J Nucl Med* 1990;31(6):972–977.
Suess E, Malessa S, Ungersbock K, et al. Technetium-99m-d,1-hexamethylpropyleneamine oxime (HMPAO) uptake and glutathione content in brain tumors. *J Nucl Med* 1991;32(9):1675–1681.
Tatsch K. Imaging of the dopaminergic system in parkinsonism with SPECT. *Nucl Med Commun* 2001;22(7):819–827.

CHAPTER 75 ■ SCINTIGRAPHIC DIAGNOSIS OF INFLAMMATION AND INFECTION

JEFFREY P. LIN

In clinical practice, nuclear medicine evaluation of patients with suspected inflammatory or infectious conditions plays multiple important roles. As such patients are often first evaluated with anatomic imaging modalities (as such techniques are faster and readily available), nuclear medicine techniques are used for further evaluation of abnormalities identified on such studies. In other situations, nuclear medicine studies assume a primary role in diagnosis when anatomic examinations are inconclusive, unrevealing, or otherwise unable to be performed—for example, in the patient with suspected osteomyelitis with a normal-appearing radiograph or who is unable to receive a magnetic resonance imaging (MRI) scan because of an implanted metallic device.

Scintigraphic evaluation of infection and inflammation is extremely broad in scope, encompassing numerous radiopharmaceuticals, imaging techniques, and diseases. In addition to discussing the roles of Gallium-67 (^{67}Ga) citrate and in vitro radiolabeled leukocytes (white blood cells [WBCs]), this chapter also discusses the potential of fluorine-18-fluorodeoxyglucose positron emission tomography (^{18}F-FDG PET) for imaging inflammation and infection.

GALLIUM-67

^{67}Ga accumulates at sites of infection and inflammation through nonspecific mechanisms, which likely differ from uptake in neoplasms (see Chapter 76). Most circulating ^{67}Ga is bound to transferrin, and increased blood flow and vascular membrane permeability at sites of inflammation result in increased delivery and accumulation. ^{67}Ga also binds to lactoferrin, which is taken up by leukocytes at inflammatory foci. Bacteria may directly take up ^{67}Ga, and bacteria-produced siderophores form a complex with ^{67}Ga which is presumably transported into the bacterium (and then eventually phagocytosed by macrophages). Although some ^{67}Ga may be transported bound to leukocytes, it also accumulates at sites of inflammation and infection even when circulating leukocytes are absent, unlike radiolabeled leukocytes discussed later.

^{67}Ga decays by electron capture and has a physical half-life of 78.3 hours. With principal photon energies of 93, 184, and 296 keV used for imaging but a poor photon yield per disintegration, ^{67}Ga is a suboptimal imaging agent. Imaging is usually performed 18 to 72 hours after intravenous injection of 185- to 370-MBq (5- to 10-mCi) ^{67}Ga citrate, utilizing a gamma camera equipped with a medium-energy collimator and capable of imaging multiple energy peaks. Normal biodistribution of ^{67}Ga is variable and includes bone, bone marrow, liver, gastrointestinal (GI) tract, urinary tract, and soft tissues. Prominent uptake may sometimes be seen in nasopharynx, lacrimal glands, thymus, breasts, and spleen (Fig. 75.1).

Although labeled leukocyte imaging is the radionuclide test of choice for imaging inflammation and infection in immunocompetent patients, ^{67}Ga imaging remains useful for multiple indications, which include the following:

Fever of Undetermined Origin. Fever of undetermined origin (FUO) is defined as greater than 3-week duration of several episodes of fever exceeding 38.3°C without a defined diagnosis after appropriate inpatient or outpatient evaluation. Etiologies of FUO are numerous; the most common causes are infections, malignancy, and collagen vascular disease. Less frequent etiologies include granulomatous diseases, pulmonary emboli, cerebrovascular accidents, drug fever, and factitious fever. Radionuclide imaging is typically employed when other imaging tests fail to localize the source of the fever. Because nearly 80% of FUOs are due to an entity other than infection, ^{67}Ga is often preferred over WBC imaging for this indication because it can identify sites of infection, inflammation, and tumor (Fig. 75.2).

Spinal Osteomyelitis. Radiolabeled leukocyte imaging is preferred for imaging osteomyelitis in most parts of the skeleton. However, ^{67}Ga remains the radionuclide procedure of choice for diagnosing spinal osteomyelitis. This is because radiolabeled leukocytes have a high rate of false negativity for this indication. ^{67}Ga imaging is frequently performed in conjunction with bone scintigraphy, and the combined studies are interpreted as follows:

- *Positive for osteomyelitis:* (a) ^{67}Ga uptake without bone scan uptake (spatially incongruent), or (b) ^{67}Ga and bone scan uptake at same location (spatially congruent) but ^{67}Ga uptake is **more** intense than bone scan uptake (Fig. 75.3).
- *Equivocal for osteomyelitis:* ^{67}Ga and bone scan uptake are spatially congruent and demonstrate similar intensities (Fig. 75.4).

The editors wish to thank Dr. Christopher J. Palestro for his work in the 4th edition establishing the foundation for this chapter.

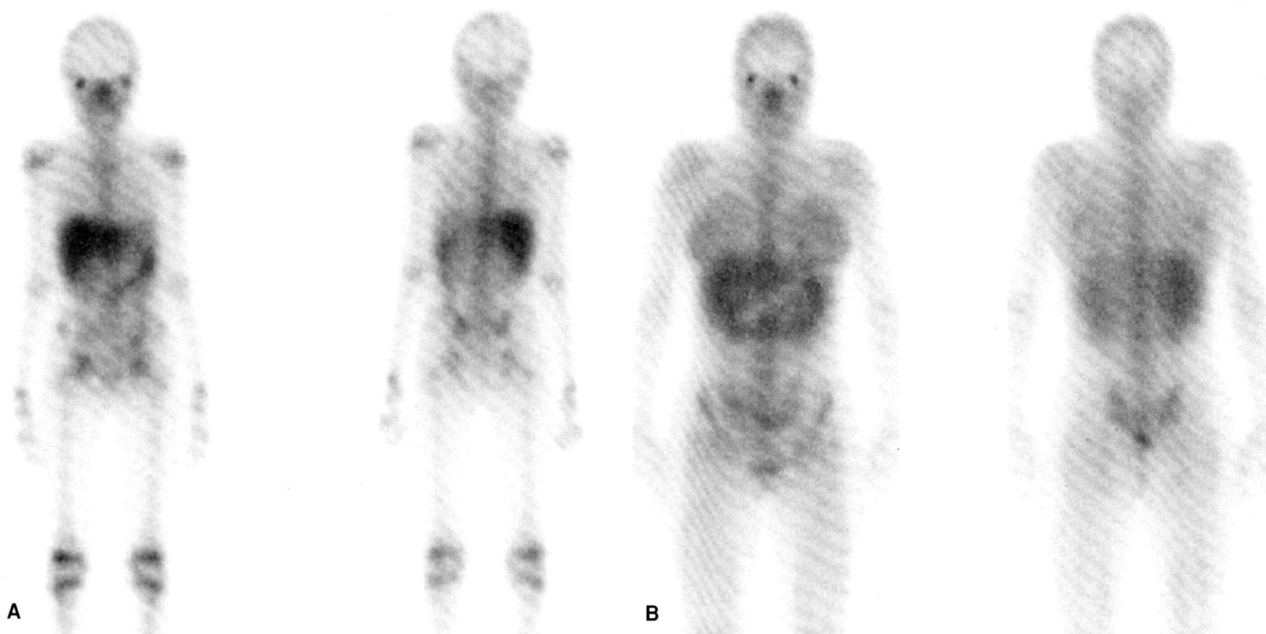

FIGURE 75.1. **Normal Gallium-67 Studies. A:** Pediatric patient: Anterior and posterior whole-body ^{67}Ga images performed on an 11-year-old child. Prominent skeletal uptake is normal in children. The distal femoral and proximal tibial growth plates are easily identified. **B:** Adult patient: Anterior and posterior whole-body ^{67}Ga images performed on a 20-year-old woman. Note more soft tissue and less skeletal activity than in the pediatric patient illustrated in (**A**). There is physiologic breast activity, which can be confused with abnormal pulmonary uptake, but may be resolved by performing oblique and lateral views or SPECT.

- *Negative for osteomyelitis:* (a) ^{67}Ga images are normal, regardless of bone scan findings, or (b) ^{67}Ga and bone scan uptake are spatially congruent but ^{67}Ga uptake is <u>less</u> intense than bone scan uptake (Fig. 75.5).

Opportunistic Infection. Because localization of ^{67}Ga does not require a leukocyte response, it is the radionuclide procedure of choice for identifying infections in immunocompromised patients. Many opportunistic infections affect the lungs,

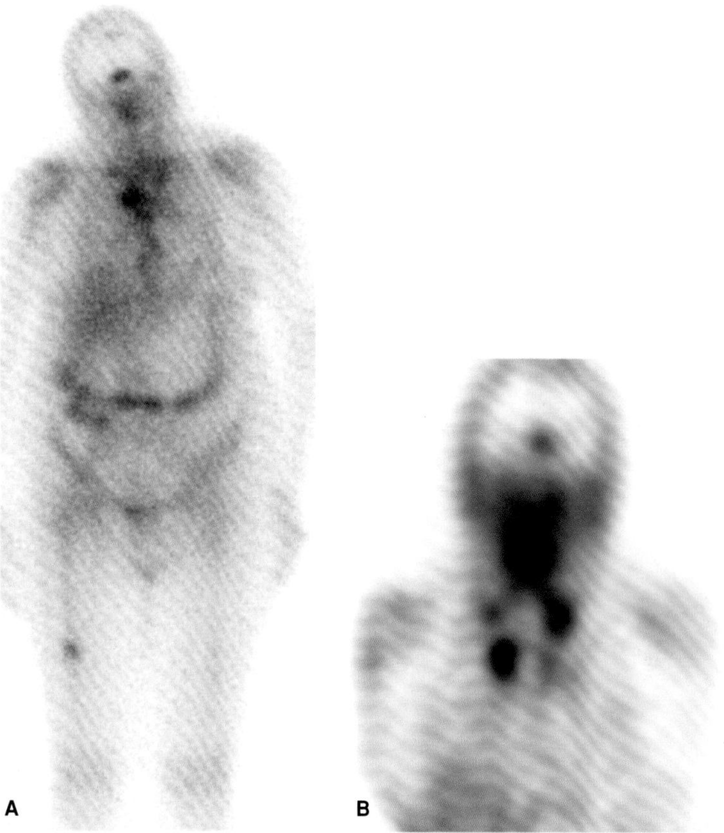

FIGURE 75.2. **Metastatic Renal Cell Carcinoma in a Patient With Fever of Undetermined Origin.** Anterior whole-body (**A**) and coronal SPECT (**B**) images from a ^{67}Ga study performed in an 81-year-old woman with persistent fevers and a history of renal cell carcinoma demonstrate focally increased activity in the brain, left supraclavicular region, mediastinum, and distal right femur. Mediastinal lymph node biopsy confirmed involvement by metastatic renal cell carcinoma. Brain and femoral metastases were radiographically confirmed.

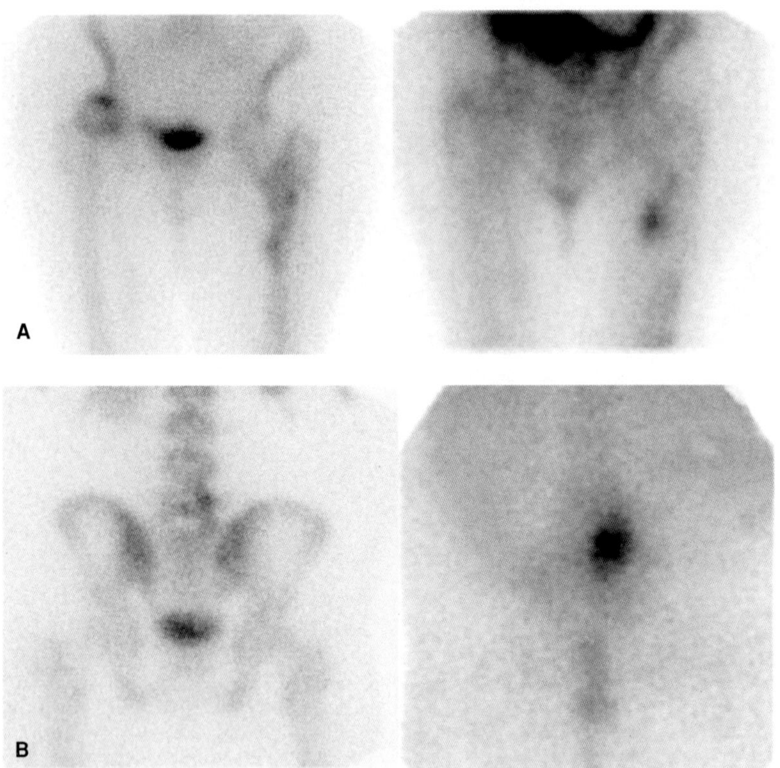

FIGURE 75.3. **Positive Bone/^{67}Ga Study. A:** Bone scan (**left**) and ^{67}Ga (**right**) images demonstrate irregularly increased activity in the proximal left femur on the bone scan, whereas the abnormal ^{67}Ga activity occupies a much smaller area (spatially incongruent). **B:** Bone scan (**left**) and ^{67}Ga (**right**) images demonstrate increased uptake at the right L5 pedicular region on both studies (spatially congruent) BUT which is more intense on the ^{67}Ga study than on the bone scan.

and a normal ^{67}Ga scan of the chest excludes infection with a high degree of certainty. Focal or localized ^{67}Ga uptake in the pulmonary parenchyma may indicate bacterial pneumonia (even in immunocompetent patients). In HIV-positive patients, diffuse uptake may be seen with *Pneumocystis jirovecii* pneumonia (Fig. 75.6), and lymph node uptake of ^{67}Ga is often associated with mycobacterial disease or lymphoma. ^{67}Ga may also help diagnose abdominal infections, such as abscesses or colitis. Lastly, some disease entities are known for not being ^{67}Ga-avid, including Kaposi sarcoma, a malignancy often found in AIDS patients. Therefore, this diagnosis is suggested in such patients who have focal abnormalities on radiographs without corresponding ^{67}Ga uptake.

Other Pulmonary Infections. ^{67}Ga is a sensitive indicator of pulmonary inflammation and also shows uptake in sarcoidosis, interstitial pneumonitis, drug reactions, collagen vascular disease, and pneumoconioses. However, the intensity and pattern of uptake are not usually diagnostic of specific illnesses.

In sarcoidosis, pulmonary uptake of ^{67}Ga correlates with disease activity and can be used to monitor response to therapy. ^{67}Ga scintigraphy is reportedly up to 97% sensitive for detection of active sarcoidosis at both pulmonary and extrapulmonary sites (Fig. 75.7).

Interstitial Nephritis. Interstitial nephritis is a well-recognized cause of acute renal failure. Although biopsy is required for definitive diagnosis, ^{67}Ga can suggest the diagnosis by showing renal uptake that is more intense than lumbar spine uptake, in contrast with acute tubular necrosis which is characterized by little or no renal uptake (Fig. 75.8).

RADIOLABELED LEUKOCYTES

Although a variety of in vitro leukocyte labeling techniques have been developed, the only approved methods in the United States employ the lipophilic compounds ^{111}In-oxyquinoline and ^{99m}Tc-exametazime (HMPAO). The labeling procedure requires withdrawing whole blood from the patient, separating the leukocytes from erythrocytes and platelets, incubating with radiolabel, and reinjecting into the patient.

^{111}Indium-Labeled Leukocytes. ^{111}In decays by electron capture with a half-life of 67 hours. It has photopeaks of 173 and 247 keV, and has imaging characteristics superior to ^{67}Ga. Imaging is performed using a gamma camera with a medium-energy collimator and windows centered on both

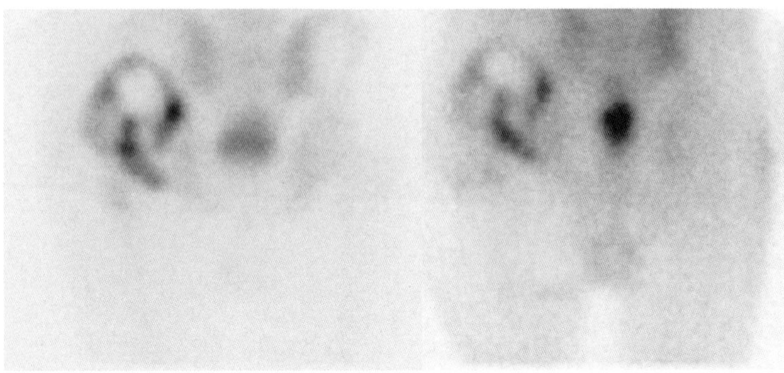

FIGURE 75.4. **Equivocal Bone/^{67}Ga Study.** Posterior bone (**left**) and ^{67}Ga (**right**) images from a study performed on a patient with a failed left hip arthroplasty. The spatial distribution and intensity of uptake of both radiotracers are virtually identical, and hence, this study is equivocal for infection.

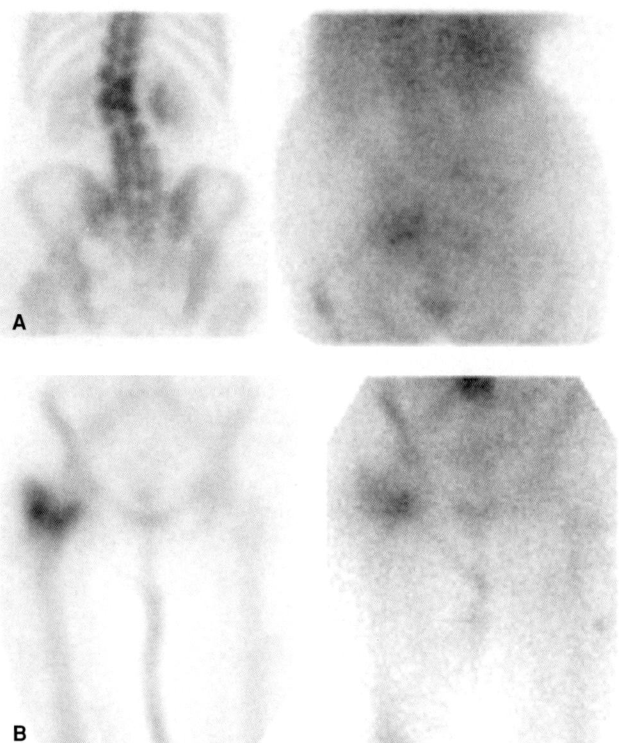

FIGURE 75.5. **Negative Bone/^{67}Ga Study. A:** Bone scan (**left**) and ^{67}Ga (**right**) images demonstrate increased activity at lower thoracic/upper lumbar vertebrae on the bone scan, but normal on ^{67}Ga image. **B:** Bone scan (**left**) and ^{67}Ga (**right**) images demonstrate increased activity in the intertrochanteric region on both studies (spatially congruent) BUT which is less intense on the ^{67}Ga study than on the bone scan.

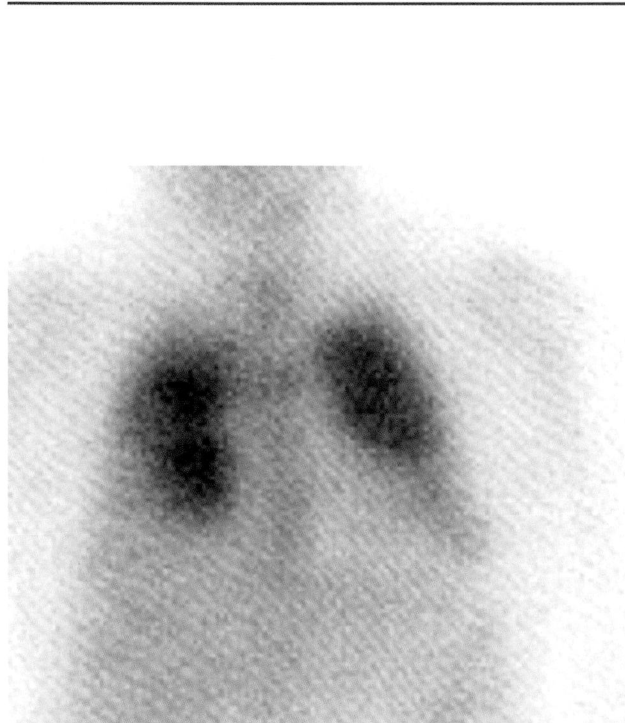

FIGURE 75.6. ***Pneumocystis jirovecii* Pneumonia.** ^{67}Ga image of the chest demonstrates intense, diffuse bilateral pulmonary activity, which in an AIDS patient with a normal chest radiograph, strongly suggests pneumocystis pneumonia.

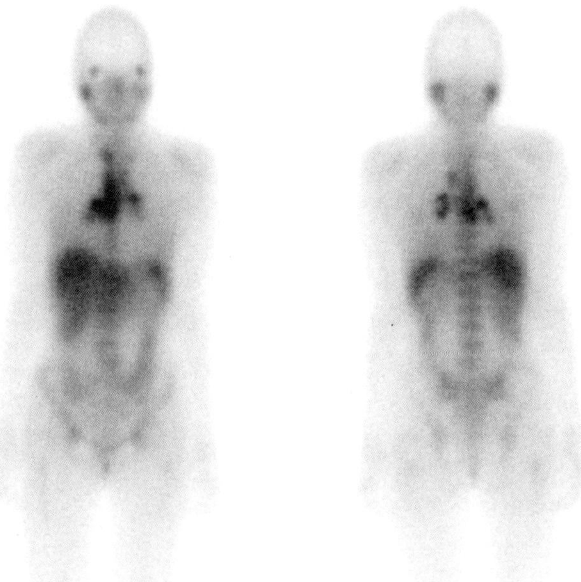

FIGURE 75.7. **Sarcoidosis.** Anterior and posterior whole-body ^{67}Ga images demonstrate bilateral hilar and mediastinal activity, a pattern characteristic of sarcoidosis. Prominent parotid and submandibular gland activity is often seen in sarcoidosis as well. Moderately intense activity in the descending colon is normal.

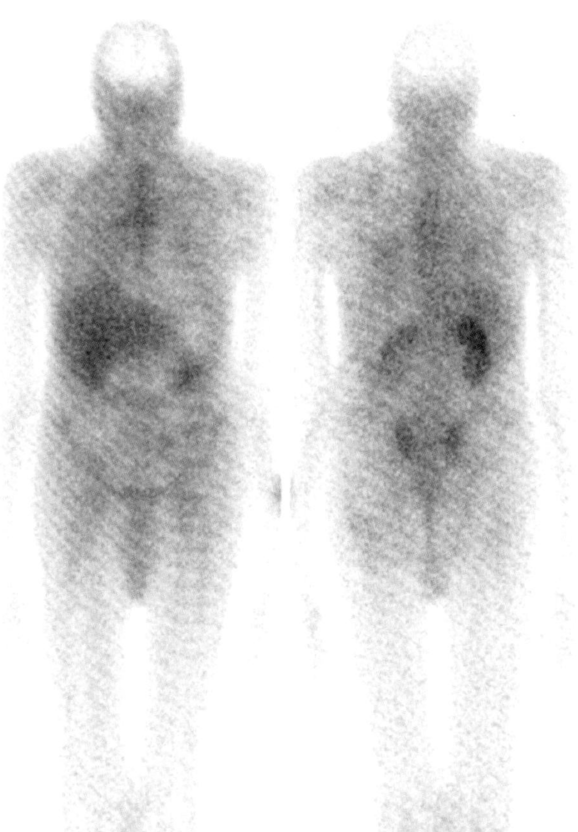

FIGURE 75.8. **Interstitial Nephritis.** Anterior and posterior whole-body ^{67}Ga images demonstrate renal activity which is more intense than adjacent lumbar spine activity, a pattern typical of interstitial nephritis.

photopeaks. The spleen is the critical organ for radiation dosage, limiting the adult dose to about 18.5 MBq (500 μCi).

High target (infection) to background ratios provide excellent image contrast. Images obtained shortly after injection show intense pulmonary activity, probably because of leukocyte activation during the labeling process. This resolves by 24 hours after injection, the usual imaging time for ^{111}In-WBCs, at which time the normal distribution is limited to liver, spleen, and bone marrow.

Advantages of the ^{111}In label include its virtually constant normal distribution, label stability, and 67-hour physical half-life enabling delayed imaging (particularly valuable for musculoskeletal infections).

^{99m}Technetium-Labeled Leukocytes. For ^{99m}Tc-WBC studies, imaging is performed using a gamma camera with a low-energy parallel hole collimator with a window centered on the 140-keV photopeak of ^{99m}Tc. The usual adult dose is 185 to 370 MBq (5 to 10 mCi), which is higher than the dose for ^{111}In-WBCs.

The normal biodistribution of ^{99m}Tc-WBCs is more variable than that of ^{111}In-WBCs. Both agents show early pulmonary activity and uptake in the reticuloendothelial system (liver, spleen, and bone marrow). However, ^{99m}Tc-WBC activity is also seen in the blood pool, occasionally in the gallbladder, and excreted into the urinary tract and GI tract (Fig. 75.9). Imaging is usually performed within a few hours after injection of ^{99m}Tc-WBCs, which is earlier than with ^{111}In-WBCs.

Advantages of ^{99m}Tc-WBCs include a photon energy that is optimal for imaging, a high-photon flux, and the ability to detect abnormalities within a few hours after injection. Disadvantages include urinary tract activity, which appears shortly after injection, and colonic activity, which appears by 4 hours after injection, as these can limit evaluation of adjacent pathology. The instability of the label and the 6-hour half-life of ^{99m}Tc limit its use when 24-hour delayed imaging is required, such as for indolent infections.

Mechanism of Accumulation. Radiolabeled leukocytes accumulate at sites of leukocytic immune response, which include

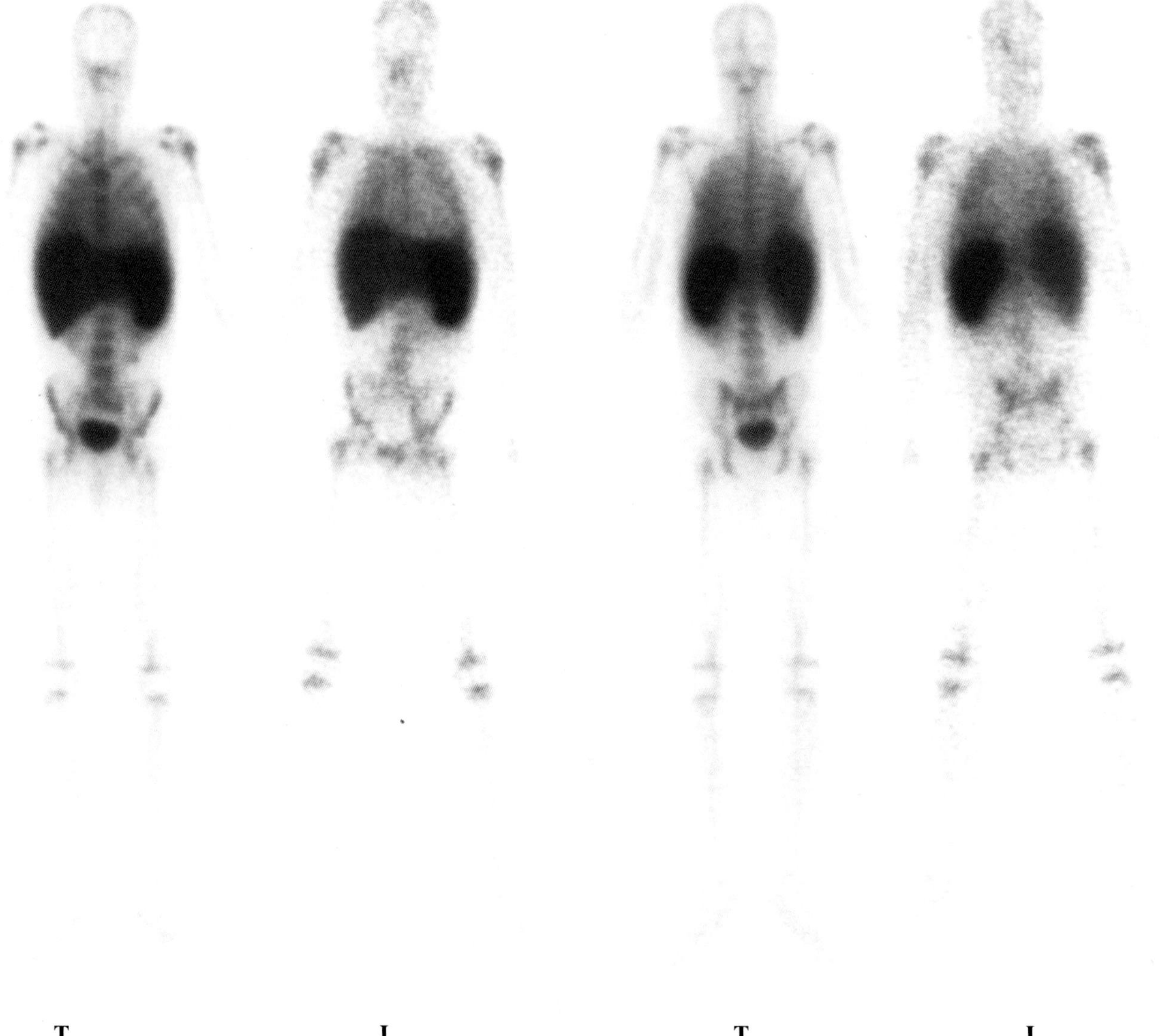

FIGURE 75.9. **Normal White Blood Cell (WBC) Studies in the Same Adolescent Male Patient, Approximately 2 Weeks Apart.** Anterior images on the left and posterior images on the right. Compare the biodistribution of ^{99m}Tc-WBCs at 90 minutes post injection with that of ^{111}In-WBCs at 18 hours post injection. Note the cardiac, femoral vessel, renal, and bladder activity on the ^{99m}Tc-WBC images, which is not present on the ^{111}In-WBC. Faint early intestinal activity is superimposed on the sacrum in the anterior ^{99m}Tc-WBC image. Physeal plate marrow activity on both studies is normal for the patient's age. T, ^{99m}Tc-WBC; I, ^{111}In-WBC.

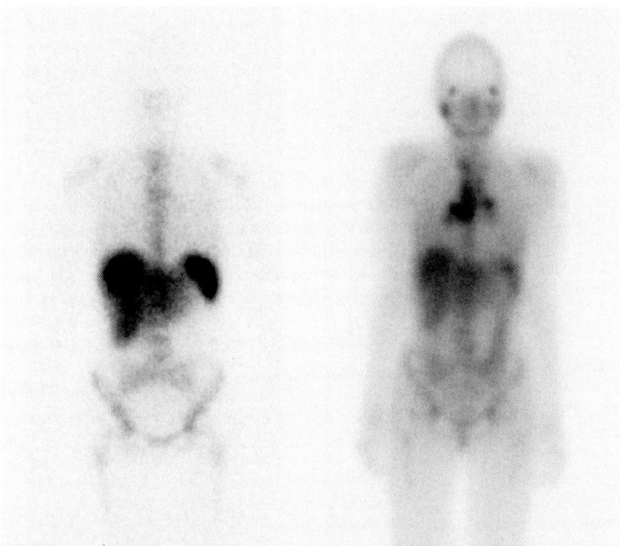

FIGURE 75.10. **Sarcoidosis.** Anterior ^{111}In-WBC (**left**) and ^{67}Ga (**right**) whole-body images of a patient with sarcoid (same patient as illustrated in Fig. 75.7). Compare the normal ^{111}In-WBC image to the obviously abnormal ^{67}Ga image. Radiolabeled WBC studies are not useful for detecting inflammation and infections in which neutrophils are not the predominant cellular response.

areas of inflammation regardless of whether infection is also present. Uptake depends on intact chemotaxis, which is not affected by the labeling procedure. The number and types of cells labeled are also important, requiring patients to have an adequate granulocyte count (>3 × 10^6 cells/mL) in order to supply enough cells for labeling. Lastly, uptake depends on the cellular components of a particular inflammatory response. Since the majority of leukocytes labeled are neutrophils, this procedure is most useful for identifying neutrophil-mediated inflammatory processes such as bacterial infections. The procedure is less useful for illnesses in which the predominant cellular response is not neutrophilic, such as opportunistic infections, tuberculosis, and sarcoidosis (Fig. 75.10). Indications for radiolabeled leukocyte imaging include the following:

Fever of Undetermined Origin. As mentioned previously, ^{67}Ga may be the preferred radionuclide test for FUO because of its ability to image many diverse etiologies. However, there are some data to suggest that ^{111}In-WBC imaging is more sensitive early in the course of an illness, whereas ^{67}Ga is more sensitive later in the illness; thus, the selection of the procedure might be governed by the duration of the illness.

Osteomyelitis. Three-phase bone scintigraphy is the radionuclide procedure of choice for diagnosing osteomyelitis in bones not affected by underlying conditions. Focal hyperperfusion, focal hyperemia, and focally increased bony uptake on delayed images are the classical presentation of osteomyelitis. However, bone scans are not specific (reflecting areas of new bone formation in general) and may also show abnormalities at sites of fractures, orthopedic hardware, and neuropathic joints even in the absence of infection. In such situations, often called "complicating osteomyelitis," the bone scan is nonspecific.

While WBC scintigraphy is the procedure of choice for diagnosing complicating osteomyelitis at nearly all sites in the skeleton, the spine represents an important exception. Although increased WBC uptake in the spine is virtually diagnostic of osteomyelitis, more than 50% of cases of vertebral osteomyelitis present as decreased activity on WBC images,

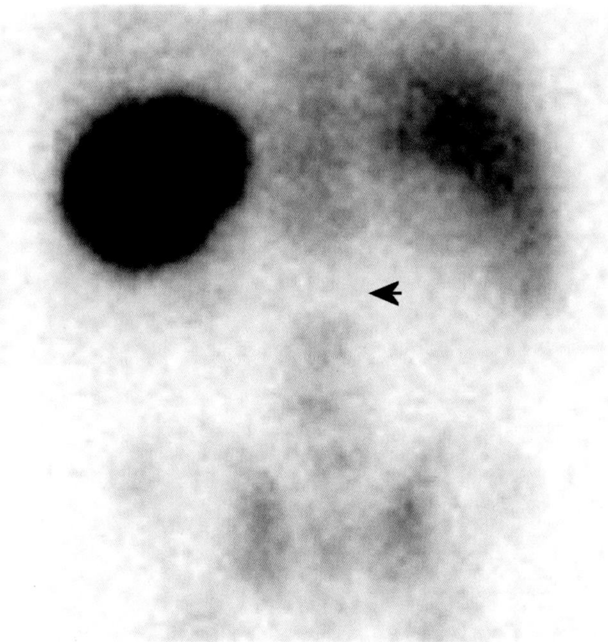

FIGURE 75.11. **Spinal Osteomyelitis.** Posterior ^{111}In-WBC image of the abdomen demonstrates absent activity in the midlumbar spine (*arrow*). Photopenia is seen in more than 50% of all cases of spinal osteomyelitis. Although decreased activity on WBC images may be consistent with spinal osteomyelitis, the finding is not specific and may represent other causes.

for reasons which are poorly understood. Furthermore, this photopenia is not specific for vertebral osteomyelitis and can be seen with other entities such as tumor, infarction, and Paget disease (Fig. 75.11).

An important unique advantage of ^{111}In-labeled WBCs (as opposed to ^{99m}Tc-WBCs) is the ability to perform a bone scintigraphy examination concurrently: dual-isotope imaging permits simultaneous detection of and distinction between ^{111}In-labeled WBCs and ^{99m}Tc-tagged bone scan agent. These images can then be precisely compared (and even overlaid) to determine whether the ^{111}In-labeled WBC uptake colocalizes to the site of bone scan uptake (osteomyelitis), within adjacent soft tissue (cellulitis), or both. In contrast, ^{99m}Tc-WBCs cannot be distinguished from ^{99m}Tc-based bone agent by simultaneous imaging, requiring the two studies to be performed sequentially. This makes precise comparisons between two studies difficult, and also requires a delay of at least 48 to 72 hours between the tests.

To maximize accuracy, WBC scintigraphy is frequently performed in conjunction with ^{99m}Tc sulfur colloid, which images the bone marrow. Labeled WBCs accumulate at both areas of infection and within the hematopoietically active bone marrow. However, the "normal" distribution of hematopoietically active bone marrow is variable, and may be altered by systemic diseases (such as sickle cell disease and Gaucher disease) or local insults (such as fractures, orthopedic hardware, and neuropathic joint). Further, the normal distribution of hematopoietically active marrow in children changes with age. Consequently, it may not be possible to determine if an area of activity on a WBC image represents infection or marrow. Performing complementary bone marrow imaging with ^{99m}Tc sulfur colloid overcomes this problem. The overall accuracy of combined WBC/marrow imaging is approximately 90%.

These combined studies are interpreted as follows:

- *Positive for osteomyelitis:* WBC activity without corresponding uptake on the sulfur colloid bone marrow image (i.e., WBC

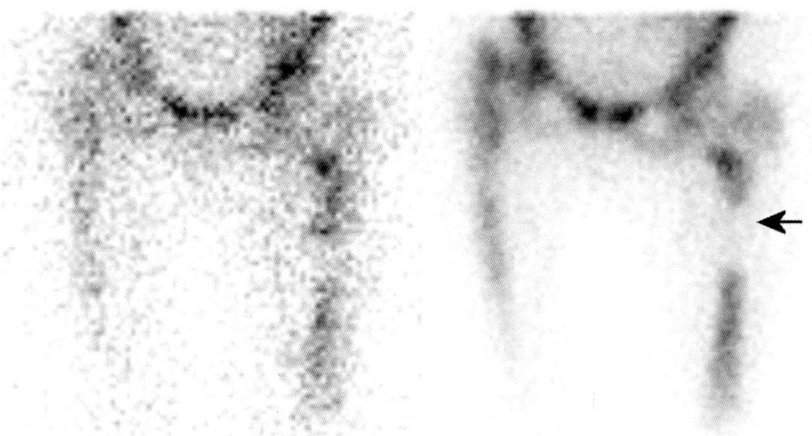

FIGURE 75.12. **Infected Orthopedic Hardware.** ^{111}In-WBC image (**left**) on a patient with an intramedullary rod in the left femur shows slightly increased left femoral activity. ^{99m}Tc sulfur colloid bone marrow image (**right**) obtained concurrently shows photopenic area (*arrow*) at a site of increased ^{111}In-WBC activity, and this study is positive for infection. Notice that most of the remaining left femoral activity on the ^{111}In-WBC image has corresponding uptake on ^{99m}Tc sulfur colloid and is therefore due to bone marrow, not infection.

accumulation not due to bone marrow distribution but because of infection) (Fig. 75.12).

- *Negative for osteomyelitis:* Any other patterns of WBC and sulfur colloid findings (Fig. 75.13).

Postoperative Infection. Radionuclide tests complement anatomic imaging modalities and facilitate the differentiation of abscess from other fluid collections, normal postoperative changes, and tumor (Fig. 75.14). ^{67}Ga may detect intra-abdominal infection, but may be obscured by colonic activity and limited by the need to wait 48 hours or more between radiotracer injection and imaging. Furthermore, ^{67}Ga accumulates at normally healing surgical incisions. In contrast, radiolabeled WBCs do not accumulate in normally healing surgical wounds, and the presence of uptake indicates infection. For these reasons, WBC imaging is the preferred radionuclide study for the evaluation of postoperative infection (Fig. 75.15). However, certain sites may show intense activity on WBC images without infection, including granulating wounds such as "ostomies" (tracheostomies, ileostomies, feeding gastrostomies, etc.) and skin grafts (Fig. 75.16). Vascular access lines, dialysis catheters, and even lumbar puncture sites can also provide false-positive results.

Cardiovascular Infections. Bacterial endocarditis is usually diagnosed by echocardiography, and radionuclide methods play a very limited role in the diagnostic workup. However, both ^{67}Ga and WBC imaging are more sensitive than echocardiography in detecting myocardial abscesses, which are serious complications of infective endocarditis. WBC imaging is the radionuclide procedure of choice for diagnosing prosthetic vascular graft infection with a sensitivity of more than 90% and a specificity ranging from 53% to 100% (Fig. 75.17). Causes of false-positive results include perigraft hematoma, bleeding, graft thrombosis, pseudoaneurysms, and graft endothelialization, which occur within the first 2 weeks after placement.

Central Nervous System Infections. The differential diagnosis of a contrast-enhancing brain lesion identified on CT or MRI includes abscess, tumor, cerebrovascular accident, and even multiple sclerosis. WBC imaging provides valuable information about contrast-enhancing brain lesions. A positive study is usually most consistent with infection; a negative result rules out infection with a high degree of certainty. Faint uptake has been observed in brain tumors, and false-negative results have been reported in patients receiving high-dose steroids.

Pulmonary Imaging. Although pulmonary uptake of WBCs is a normal physiologic event during the first few hours after injection, such uptake at 24 hours is abnormal. Focal, segmental, or lobar pulmonary uptake may represent bacterial pneumonia (Fig. 75.18), but may also be seen in patients with cystic fibrosis due to WBC accumulation in pooled secretions at regions of bronchiectasis. Nonsegmental focal pulmonary

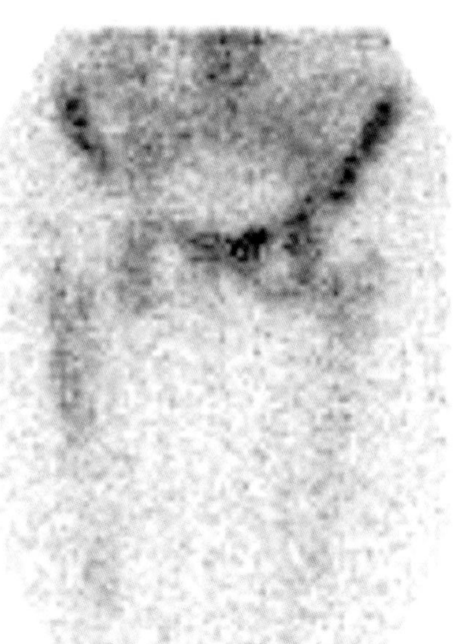

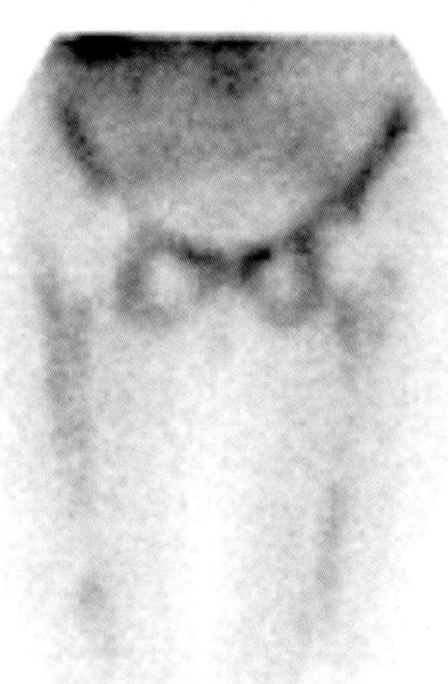

FIGURE 75.13. **Aseptically Loosened Right Total Hip Replacement.** ^{111}In-WBC image (**left**) demonstrates increased activity around the femoral component of a right total hip replacement, and infection cannot be excluded. ^{99m}Tc sulfur colloid bone marrow image (**right**) shows that bone marrow distribution accounts for the increased activity on the ^{111}In-WBC study. Therefore, the combined study is negative for infection.

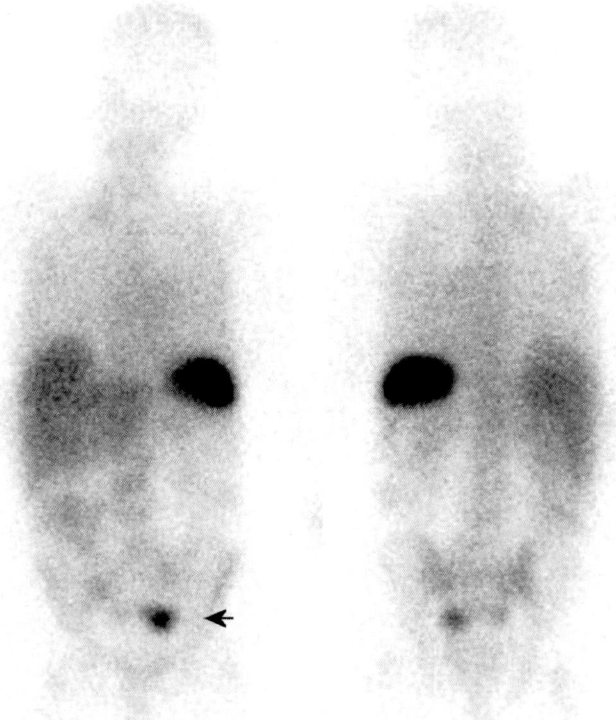

FIGURE 75.14. **Pelvic Abscess in a Patient With Fever of Undetermined Origin (FUO).** Anterior and posterior whole-body ^{111}In-WBC images demonstrate a focus of intense activity in the left lower quadrant of the abdomen (*arrow*). Subsequent CT scan (not shown) confirmed a pelvic abscess. Faint ascending and transverse colonic activity was attributed to antibiotic-associated colitis.

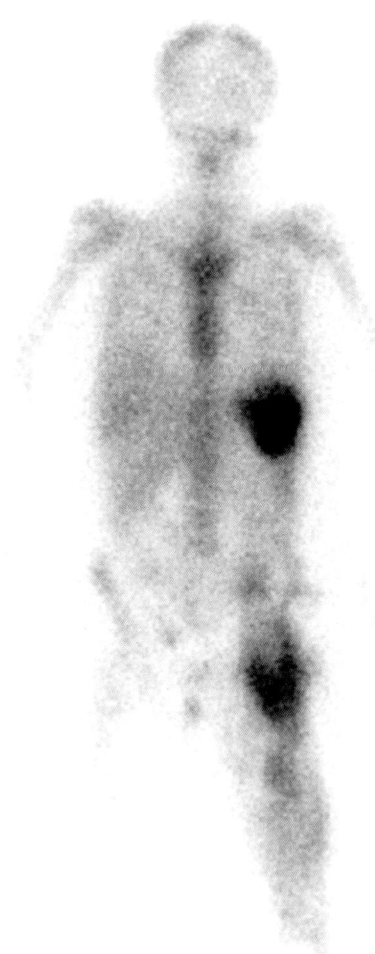

FIGURE 75.15. **Postoperative Infection.** Patient with a history of multiple abdominal surgeries was noted to have a mass-like collection on CT scan of the abdomen and pelvis (not shown). Differential diagnosis included postoperative changes and tumor. On this anterior whole-body ^{111}In-WBC image, abnormal accumulation of labeled leukocytes extends from the left abdomen into the thigh. Multiple abscesses were subsequently drained.

uptake is usually caused by technical problems during labeling or reinfusion and is not associated with infection.

Diffuse pulmonary uptake on images obtained more than 4 hours after reinjection of labeled cells may be seen with pulmonary edema, opportunistic infection, radiation pneumonitis, pulmonary drug toxicity, and adult respiratory distress syndrome (Fig. 75.19). However, the pattern may also be seen in septic patients who have normal chest radiographs and no clinical evidence of respiratory tract inflammation or infection, possibly due to cytokine activation.

Inflammatory Bowel Disease. ^{111}In-WBCs do not accumulate in a normal bowel. Such activity is abnormal and may be seen with infectious colitis (including antibiotic-associated or pseudomembranous colitis), inflammatory bowel disease, ischemic colitis, and GI bleeding (Fig. 75.20). However, ^{99m}Tc-WBC imaging is now considered the radionuclide study of choice for inflammatory bowel disease, a group of idiopathic, chronic disorders that include Crohn disease and ulcerative colitis. Imaging findings supporting a diagnosis of Crohn disease include skip areas of activity in the colon or the presence of small bowel activity (Fig. 75.21). ^{99m}Tc-WBC imaging can be a sensitive screening test for detecting inflammatory bowel disease. In patients with known inflammatory bowel disease, ^{99m}Tc-WBC imaging may be used to help distinguish active inflammation from scarring. Serial studies can also be used to monitor effectiveness of the therapy.

SPECT-CT

Single photon emission computed tomography (SPECT) is a nuclear-medicine imaging technique which provides three-dimensional analysis of radiotracer activity. A gamma camera rotates over the patient (often in a 360-degree arc), and the data are reconstructed by computer. SPECT-CT scanners incorporate a conventional CT scanner, and the two sets of images are combined for analysis. This permits the functional information provided by radiotracers (such as ^{67}Ga, ^{111}In-WBCs, and ^{99m}Tc-WBCs) to be integrated with the anatomic detail provided by the CT images, and can vastly improve diagnostic confidence and accuracy. In patients being evaluated for osteomyelitis, SPECT-CT is especially useful for distinguishing whether radiotracer accumulation corresponds to a site in the skeleton, soft tissues, or both (Fig. 75.22).

FLUORINE-18-FLUORODEOXY-GLUCOSE POSITRON EMISSION TOMOGRAPHY

PET/CT imaging with the glucose analog ^{18}F-FDG is more typically used to image neoplasms, as discussed in Chapter 76. However, ^{18}F-FDG PET also detects sites of active inflammation. ^{18}F-FDG is therefore similar to ^{67}Ga in its nonspecific nature,

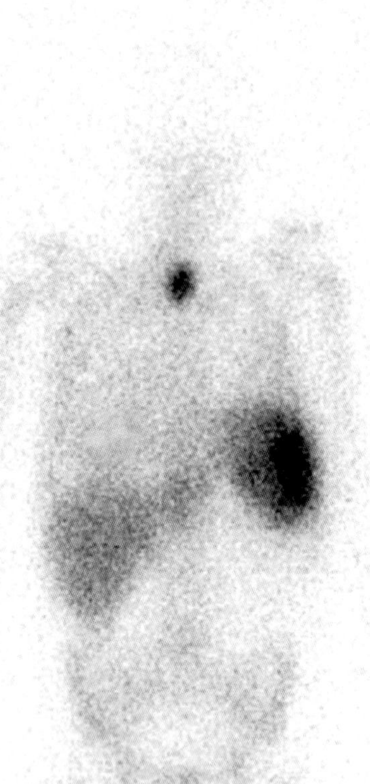

FIGURE 75.16. **White Blood Cell (WBC) Activity at a Tracheostomy Site.** Anterior whole-body ^{111}In-WBC image shows focally increased activity at a tracheostomy site. "Ostomies" are granulating wounds and can show intense uptake.

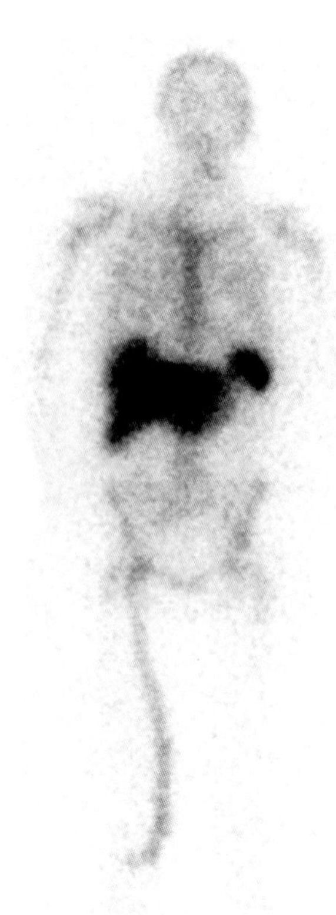

FIGURE 75.17. **Prosthetic Vascular Graft Infection.** ^{111}In-WBC study demonstrates linearly increased activity along the medial aspect of the right thigh from the groin to knee, along the course of an infected prosthetic femoral popliteal graft.

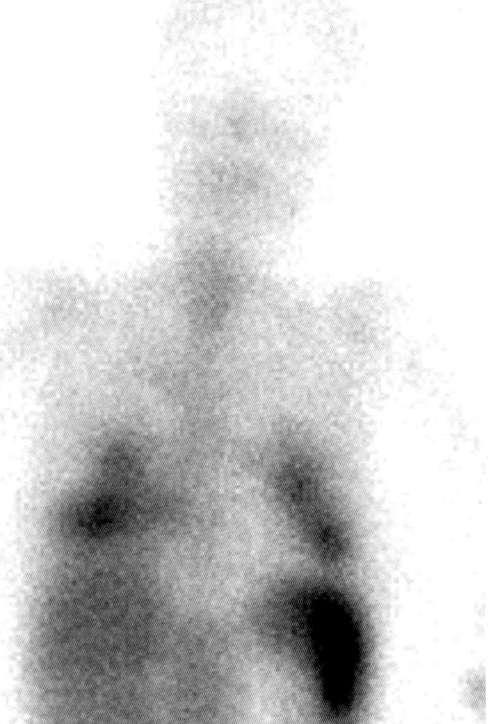

FIGURE 75.18. **Focal White Blood Cell (WBC) Pulmonary Activity.** Focal pulmonary activity that is segmental or lobar in appearance, as shown in this ^{111}In-WBC image, usually associated with bacterial pneumonia.

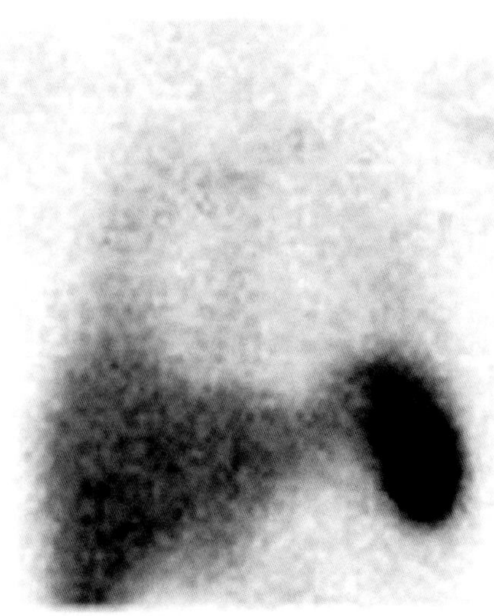

FIGURE 75.19. **Diffuse White Blood Cell (WBC) Pulmonary Activity.** ^{111}In-WBC image demonstrates mild, diffuse bilateral pulmonary activity. While this is a normal finding on images performed shortly after injection, this is abnormal on later images and is associated with many entities, but not bacterial pneumonia.

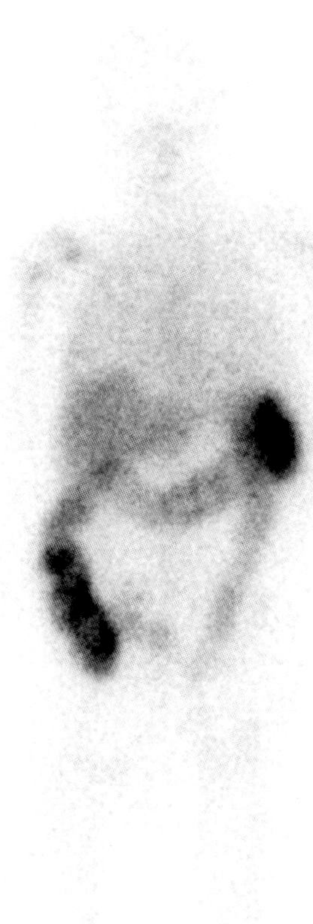

FIGURE 75.20. **Colitis.** Anterior whole-body ^{111}In-WBC image demonstrates pancolonic activity, most pronounced at the ascending colon.

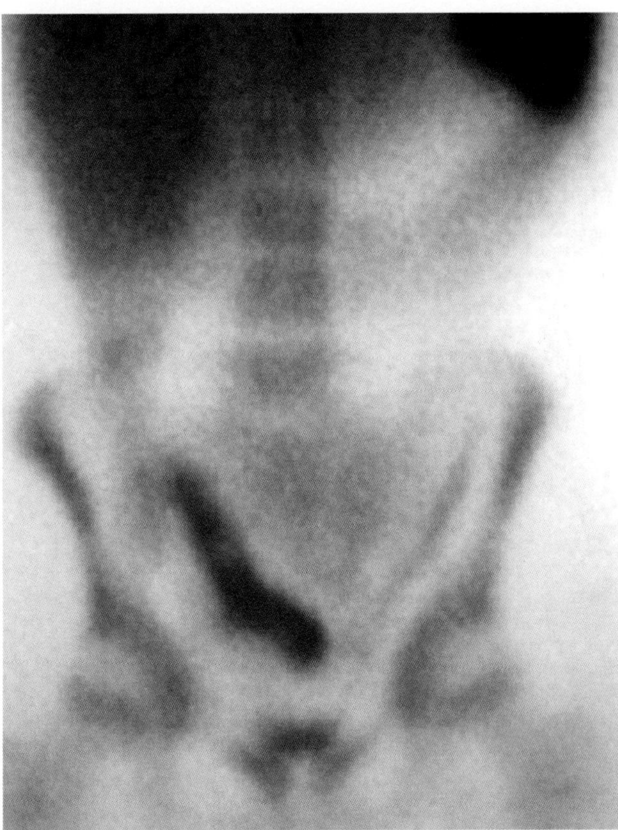

FIGURE 75.21. **Crohn Disease.** On this ^{99m}Tc-WBC image, activity is present in the distal jejunum, proximal and distal ileum, and colon (and most intense in the ileum). Small bowel activity in a patient with colitis supports the diagnosis of Crohn disease. (Courtesy of Dr. Martin Charron.)

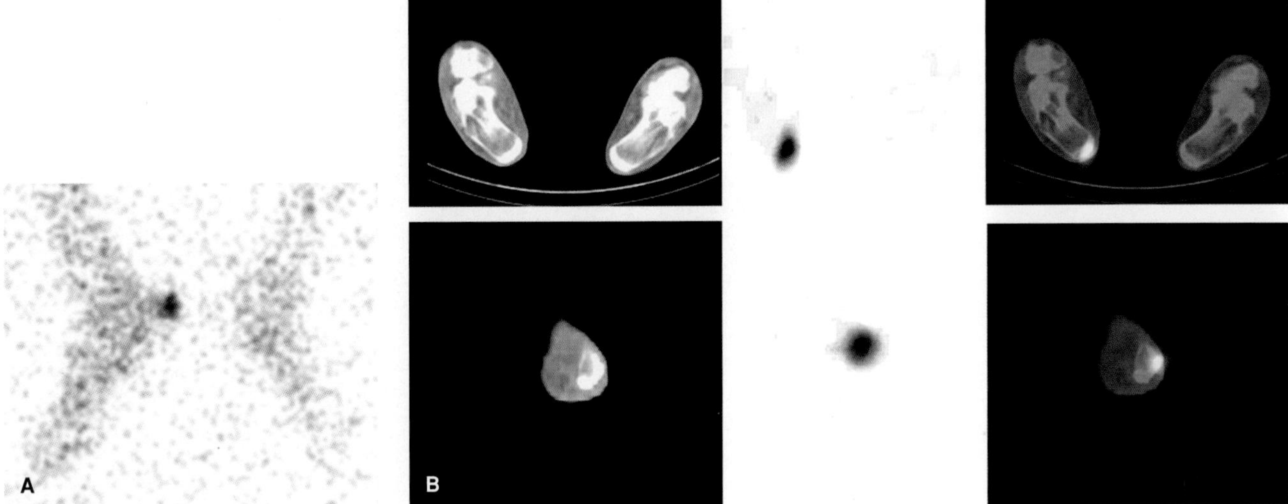

FIGURE 75.22. **Right Calcaneal Osteomyelitis. A:** Twenty-four-hour planar ^{111}In-WBC image shows focally increased activity along the posterior aspect of the right heel. It is not possible to determine whether this focus extends into the bone or is confined to the soft tissues. **B:** On the axial and sagittal SPECT/CT images, the ^{111}In-WBC activity clearly extends into the bone. (Reproduced with permission from Kwee TC, Kwee RM, Alavi A. ^{18}F-FDG PET for diagnosing prosthetic joint infection: Systematic review and met analysis. *Eur J Nucl Med Mol Imaging* 2008;35:2122–2132.)

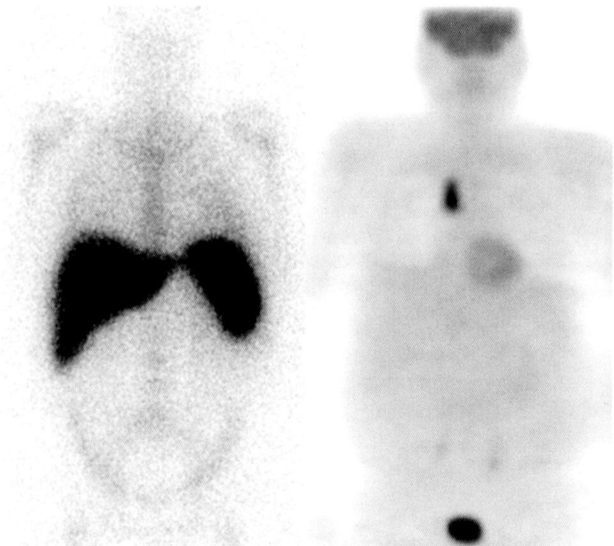

FIGURE 75.23. **Recurrent Lung Carcinoma in a Patient With Fever of Undetermined Origin (FUO).** An 81-year-old man with chronic lymphocytic leukemia and a remote history of lung carcinoma, with unexplained fever and an elevated leukocyte count. The ^{111}In-WBC study (**left**) was negative. ^{18}F-FDG PET (**right**) demonstrated focal hypermetabolism in the right paratracheal region, corresponding to lymph nodes on CT (not shown). The final diagnosis was recurrent lung carcinoma.

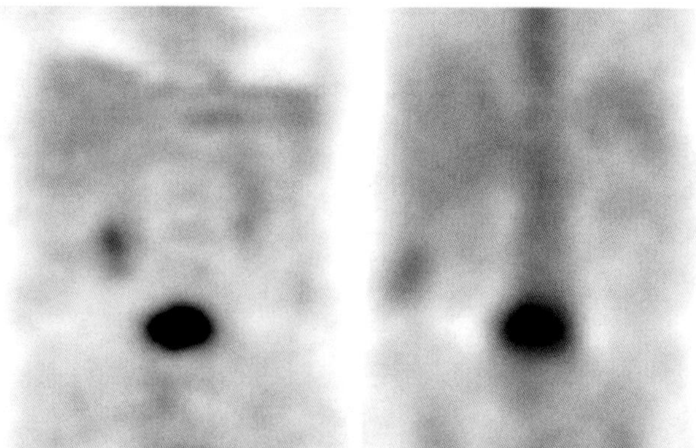

FIGURE 75.25. **Spinal Osteomyelitis.** ^{18}F-FDG PET (**left**) and ^{67}Ga SPECT images (**right**) both show intense radiotracer accumulation in the lower lumbar spine of a patient with spinal osteomyelitis. (Reproduced with permission from Love C, Tomas MB, Tronco GG, Palestro CJ. ^{18}F-FDG PET of infection and inflammation. *Radiographics* 2005;25:1357–1368.)

but is also exquisitely sensitive to diverse etiologies. Therefore, it represents an exciting alternative for evaluation of FUO, many cases of which are due to causes other than infection (Fig. 75.23).

Although not approved in the United States for evaluation of inflammation and infection, published literature indicates that ^{18}F-FDG PET is also useful in various other conditions, including sarcoidosis (Fig. 75.24), peripheral osteomyelitis, vertebral osteomyelitis (Fig. 75.25), and vasculitis (such as giant cell arteritis), among others.

CONCLUSION

Radionuclide imaging can be critical in the diagnosis of infection and inflammation by complementing anatomic imaging, and in many cases, provides functional information not available by other imaging modalities. The choice of specific nuclear medicine test requires careful consideration of the patient's clinical situation and indications for the study.

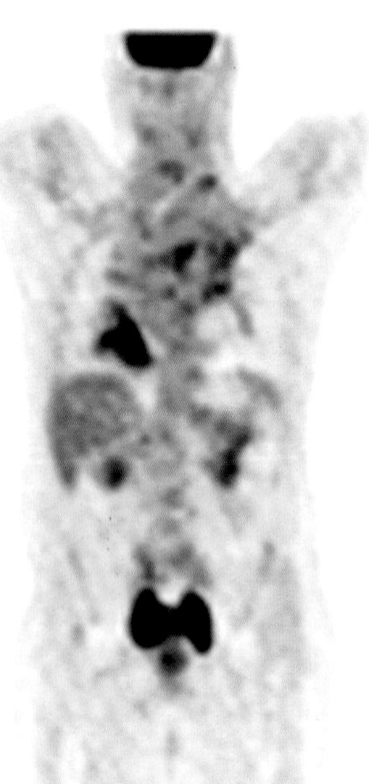

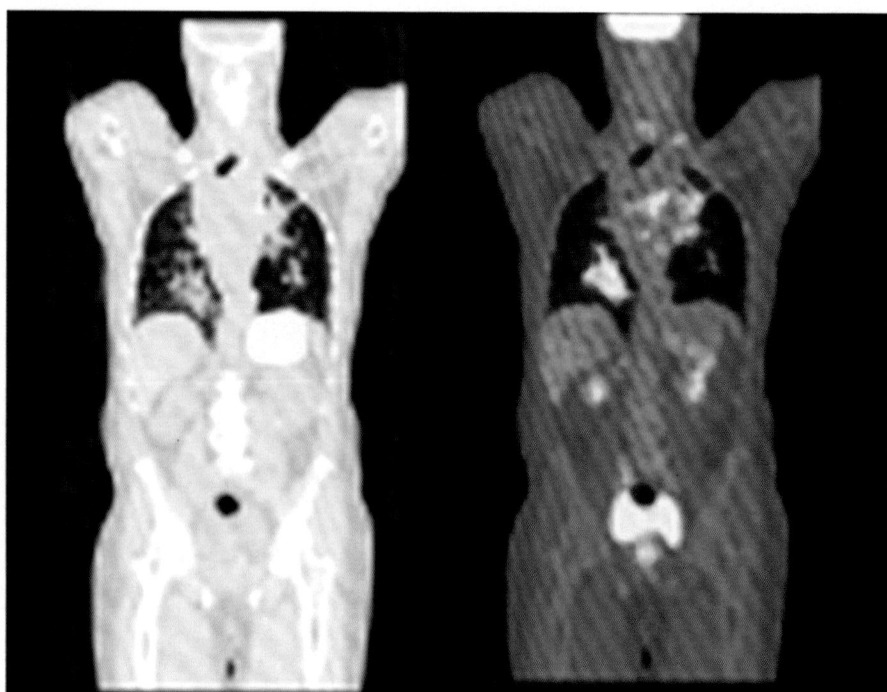

FIGURE 75.24. **Sarcoidosis.** Coronal ^{18}F-FDG PET/CT images demonstrate hypermetabolism in mediastinal lymph nodes and in the right lower lung of a 71-year-old male with active sarcoidosis.

Suggested Readings

Bar-Shalom R, Yefremov N, Guralnik L, et al. SPECT/CT using 67Ga and 111In-labeled leukocyte scintigraphy for diagnosis of infection. *J Nucl Med* 2006;47:587–594.

Bleeker-Rovers CP, van der Meer JW, Oyen WJ. Fever of unknown origin. *Semin Nucl Med* 2009;39:81–87.

Charron M. Pediatric inflammatory bowel disease imaged with Tc-99m white blood cells. *Clin Nucl Med* 2000;25:708–715.

Filippi L, Schillaci O. Usefulness of hybrid SPECT/CT in 99mTc-HMPAO-labeled leukocyte scintigraphy for bone and joint infections. *J Nucl Med* 2006;47:1908–1913.

Fineman DS, Palestro CJ, Kim CK, et al. Detection of abnormalities in febrile AIDS patients with In-111-labeled leukocyte and Ga-67 scintigraphy. *Radiology* 1989;170:677–680.

Granquist L, Chapman SC, Hvidsten S, Murphy MS. Evaluation of 99mTc-HMPAO leukocyte scintigraphy in the investigation of pediatric inflammatory bowel disease. *J Pediatr* 2003;143:48–53.

Jamar F, Buscombe J, Chiti A, et al. EANM/SNMMI guideline for 18F-FDG use in inflammation and infection. *J Nucl Med* 2013;54:647–658.

Kramer EL, Divgi CR. Pulmonary applications of nuclear medicine. *Clin Chest Med* 1991;12:55–75.

Kwee TC, Kwee RM, Alavi A. FDG-PET for diagnosing prosthetic joint infection: Systematic review and met analysis. *Eur J Nucl Med Mol Imaging* 2008;35: 2122–2132.

Love C, Opoku-Agyemang P, Tomas MB, Pugliese PV, Bhargava KK, Palestro CJ. Pulmonary activity on labeled leukocyte images: physiologic, pathologic, and imaging correlation. *Radiographics* 2002;22:1385–1393.

Love C, Tomas MB, Tronco GG, Palestro CJ. FDG PET of infection and inflammation. *Radiographics* 2005;25:1357–1368.

Martin-Comin J, Prats E. Clinical applications of radiolabeled blood elements in inflammatory bowel disease. *Q J Nucl Med* 1999;43:74–82.

Palestro CJ, Goldsmith SJ. The role of gallium and labeled leukocyte scintigraphy in the AIDS patient. *Q J Nucl Med* 1995;39:221–230.

Palestro CJ, Kim CK, Swyer AJ, Vallabhajosula S, Goldsmith SJ. Radionuclide diagnosis of vertebral osteomyelitis: indium-111-leukocyte and technetium-99m-methylene diphosphonate bone scintigraphy. *J Nucl Med* 1991;32:1861–1865.

Palestro CJ, Love C. Radionuclide imaging of musculoskeletal infection: conventional agents. *Semin Musculoskelet Radiol* 2007;11:335–352.

Palestro CJ, Love C, Bhargava KK. Labeled leukocyte imaging: current status and future directions. *Q J Nucl Med Mol Imaging* 2009;53:105–123.

Palestro CJ, Love C, Tronco GG, Tomas MB. Role of radionuclide imaging in the diagnosis of postoperative infection. *Radiographics* 2000;20:1649–1660.

Palestro CJ, Swyer AJ, Kim CK, Muzinic M, Goldsmith SJ. Role of In-111 labeled-leukocyte scintigraphy in the diagnosis of intracerebral lesions. *Clin Nucl Med* 1991;16:305–308.

Palestro CJ, Torres MA. Radionuclide imaging of nonosseous infection. *Q J Nucl Med* 1999;43:46–60.

Schmidt KG, Rasmussen JW, Frederiksen PB, Kock-Jensen C, Pedersen NT. Indium-111-granulocyte scintigraphy in brain abscess diagnosis: limitations and pitfalls. *J Nucl Med* 1990;31:1121–1127.

CHAPTER 76 ■ POSITRON EMISSION TOMOGRAPHY

ROBERT R. FLAVELL AND SPENCER BEHR

INTRODUCTION

Positron emission tomography (PET) imaging is a vital part of molecular imaging in today's clinical workplace. With the combination of anatomic and molecular imaging into one machine, PET/CT, and more recently PET/MR, these systems have become a critical part of routine patient care. Clinical applications have and will continue to grow into the foreseeable future, especially with the expanding library of clinical PET agents.

PET Instrumentation. PET imaging is possible in only a subset of isotopes that undergo beta plus (positron) decay. These positron-emitting radionuclides are unstable atoms that become stable when a proton within the nucleus decays into a neutron by emission of a positron. Positrons have the same mass as an electron but are positively charged. Within milliseconds of emission, the positron is annihilated by colliding with a nearby electron. This event results in the release of two high-energy (511 keV; the energy equivalent of the mass of a beta particle [$E = mc^2$]) γ-ray photons that travel in opposite directions (at nearly a 180-degree angle, conserving momentum). These high-energy photons are highly penetrative in soft tissue and therefore leave the body with limited absorption or deflection. It is these photons that are generate the images in PET systems.

The most common positron-emitting radionuclides include gallium-68 (Ga-68), fluorine-18 (F-18), nitrogen-13 (N-13), oxygen-15 (O-15), carbon-11 (C-11), and rubidium-82 (Rb-82). There are two methods of generating radionuclides—generators and cyclotron. The bulk of current clinical PET imaging is based on F-18, an unstable radioisotope with a half-life of 109 minutes that is produced in a cyclotron. While F-18 can be produced at distribution centers and shipped to imaging facilities, other positron emitters with shorter half-lives (75 seconds to 20 minutes) must be made via onsite cyclotrons within minutes of their use. In cases like Rb-82, the generator sits next to the scanner itself.

It should be noted that the distance the positron travels away from the parent atom prior to annihilation is ***directly proportional*** to the energy of the parent atom. Therefore, higher-energy parent atoms such as Rb-82 will have a higher "positron travel" than lower-energy parent atoms such as F-18 and will impact image spatial resolution. Positrons generated from low-energy parent atoms will travel shorter distances and result in improved spatial resolution.

PET cameras consist of a ring of scintillation detectors set to detect ***coincident*** photons. A coincident event occurs when two 511-keV photons are simultaneously detected by two detectors, indicating that an annihilation event has occurred somewhere in the column of space between the two detectors (i.e., line of coincidence). Noncoincident photons are usually due to scatter and mostly rejected during data reconstruction. These raw data projections are reconstructed into cross-sectional images by algorithms similar to those used in CT and MR. The spatial resolution of most commercial PET systems is 4 to 5 mm, though some time-of-flight (TOF) systems have resolution down to 2 mm. These TOF systems utilize the timestamp of when each photon of a matched coincident pair reaches the detector to narrow down a smaller segment along the line of coincidence where the annihilation event occurred. This improves image spatial resolution and lesion detection.

PET scans viewed alone provide limited morphologic detail and can be difficult to interpret. Hybrid instruments combine two imaging technologies into one system and include PET/CT, SPECT/CT, and more recently PET/MR. CT provides excellent anatomic detail but lacks functional information and PET provides functional (metabolic) information but lacks precise morphology. The union of PET and multidetector CT (MDCT) allows for correlation of complementary findings into a single comprehensive examination. Therefore, PET/CT scanners have now virtually supplanted all stand-alone PET systems. The typical PET/CT scanner consists of a PET scanner immediately adjacent to an MDCT scanner. A patient table, accurately calibrated for position, runs through both scanning assemblies. Computer software is used to fuse the two sets of images into composite images.

Over the past few years, a new hybrid technology has been emerging—PET/MR. While the concept of PET/MR was introduced before PET/CT, the technologic challenges of performing PET acquisition in the high magnetic field of MR delayed its implementation. However, the emergence of newer magnetic-insensitive PET photodiodes has made PET/MR a reality.

As photons travel through the body, they can be absorbed or attenuated, resulting in the loss of detection of true coincidence events. This loss of photon counts results in image artifacts and noise. Photon attenuation is increased when the origin of the photons is from deep within the body because of the greater thickness of intervening soft tissues. Attenuation is less in the thorax because of the air-filled lungs than in the abdomen or pelvis. To account for this attenuation,

attenuation correction must be applied to all PET images. The CT transmission data is used to create an attenuation map that is applied to the PET images to compensate for attenuation defects. For PET-only systems, the attenuation map is generated using an external source of germanium-68/Ga-68. The attenuation correction process increases sensitivity for detection of positron activity, but it may introduce artifacts into the images such as misregistration between the PET and CT data sets. Therefore, optimal interpretation of PET images includes viewing of both attenuation-corrected and attenuation-uncorrected PET images.

Performing PET/CT. In the case of F 18 FDG scans, patients fast for 4 to 6 hours prior to the scan to limit metabolic activity with the GI tract and limit the amount of circulating insulin within the blood stream. Blood glucose should be under good control (<150 mg/dL) to limit the competition for FDG uptake by glucose. Insulin administration and oral diabetic medication should be held prior to FDG injection to prevent shifting uptake into muscle tissue. The timing of the last insulin dose varies by the route of administration and the type of insulin being used. Strenuous activity should be limited for 24 hours prior to and immediately following radionuclide administration to limit muscle uptake of FDG. Speech should be minimized after injection, especially in patients being studied for head and neck malignancy to limit FDG uptake in the muscles of the head, neck, and larynx. The bladder is emptied by voiding or catheterization just prior to scanning. Manual or continuous irrigation of the bladder with saline and scanning the pelvis first is helpful in limiting bladder activity that may obscure disease activity in the uterus, ovaries, or pelvic lymph nodes. Alternatively, diuretics such as furosemide can be administered to accelerate clearance of urinary activity. The usual dose is 10 to 20 mCi (0.22 mCi/kg body weight) given by IV injection. Pediatric patient dose is determined by the patient's weight with a lower limit of 2 mCi.

Scans are performed approximately 60 minutes after IV injection of FDG to allow time for cellular uptake of FDG, which decreases background and clearance of FDG from the blood pool. The patient lies supine on the scanning table with arms overhead or at the sides. The arms-at-side position is preferred for head and neck scanning, whereas holding the arms overhead is best for body scanning. Patients scanned with the arms at the sides also may generate beam-hardening artifacts (see Fig. 76.5). Whole-body CT scans from the vertex or base of the skull to midthigh is usually without IV administration of CT contrast agents. Some institutions prep the bowel with oral contrast as part of patient preparation. While administration of IV and/or oral-iodinated or barium-containing contrast agents would improve CT diagnostic quality, it would introduce artifacts in attenuation correction for the PET images and alter standardized uptake value (SUV) calculation. MDCT scanning generally takes less than 2 minutes. PET scanning is performed over 10 to 30 minutes, depending upon the area covered, number of acquisitions, and scanner speed. CT and PET images are reconstructed separately and then fused into composite images utilizing image readout software.

PET/CT Interpretation. Axial, coronal, and sagittal reformatted CT, attenuation-corrected PET, attenuation-uncorrected PET, and fused PET/CT images are viewed interactively on a workstation. Software allows the rotation of maximum intensity projection (MIP) images to aid in the localization of tracer activity. Window width and level settings are optimized interactively. Assessment of normal and pathologic radiotracer uptake is made by visual inspection, by the SUV, and by glucose metabolic rate calculation.

F-18 FDG is currently the most widely used and applicable tracer in PET/CT imaging. Understanding its properties is fundamental for interpreting the majority of PET/CT scans. F-18 is the radioisotope in the radiotracer molecule 2-[F-18] fluoro-2 deoxy-D-glucose (FDG). FDG is an analog of glucose—therefore it distributes and tends to concentrate in areas of high metabolic activity in the human body by active glucose transport through the cell membrane like regular glucose. Tumor cells with a high rate of mitosis are typically highly metabolically active and have an increased number of glucose transporters and therefore concentrate FDG in higher concentrations than normal tissue. FDG is subsequently phosphorylated into F-18 FDG-6-phosphate. Unlike glucose, F-18 FDG-6-phosphate cannot be further metabolized and is thus trapped in most tissues. The liver is the major exception, where concentrated phosphatase enzymes can dephosphorylate FDG-6-phosphate and clear it from the liver.

FDG accumulation depends on both the blood supply to the tissue as well as the level of its glycolytic metabolic activity. Organs with higher metabolic activity, like the brain, will accumulate more FDG. In addition, multiple factors can affect the biodistribution of FDG such as blood-sugar level, blood-insulin level, and muscular activity. FDG is excreted mainly in the urine, like glucose. However, in contrast to glucose, FDG cannot be reabsorbed, which results in intense activity within the ureters and bladder. Variable activity of the GI tract, liver, thymus, breast, salivary glands, and bone marrow is also commonly seen. The uptake by myocardium largely depends on the metabolic state of the heart at the time of the injection. Accumulation of FDG is also seen in interstitial body fluids including pleural, peritoneal, and synovial fluids. Variable excretion from lacrimal, salivary, and sweat glands needs to

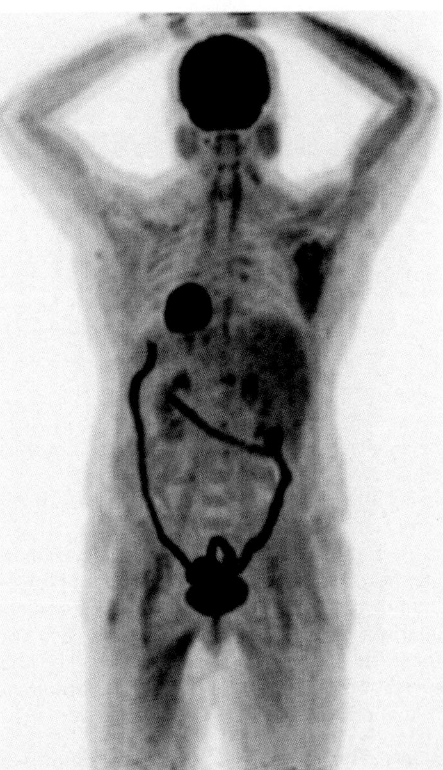

FIGURE 76.1. **Whole-Body FDG Maximum Intensity Project (MIP) PET Imaging Demonstrating Abnormal Physiologic FDG-PET Biodistribution With Intense Musculoskeletal and Colonic Uptake.** Patient was found to be on the medication, metformin, which is the likely reason for the colonic uptake. In addition, upon questioning, the patient was found to have eaten French fries prior to radiotracer injection. Postprandial scans commonly demonstrate intense musculoskeletal and cardiac hypermetabolism.

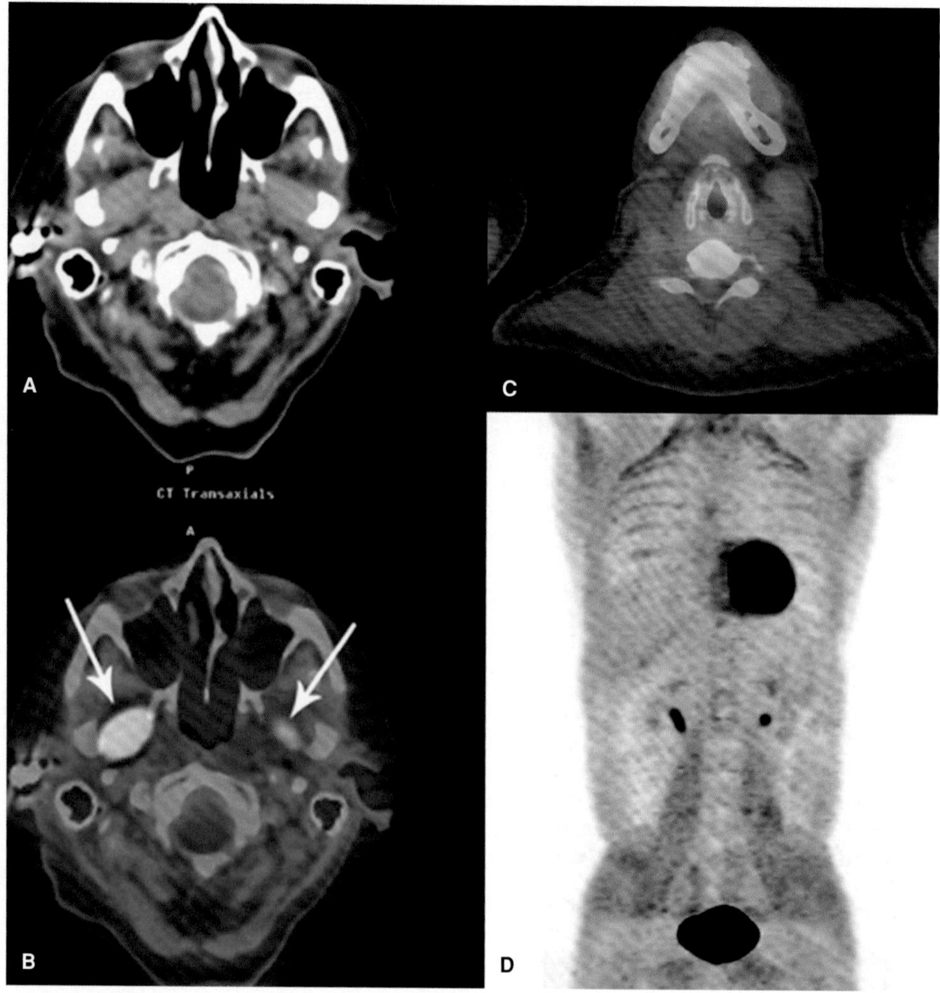

FIGURE 76.2. **Physiologic Fluorodeoxyglucose (FDG) Activity in Muscle.** Axial CT (**A**) and fused PET/CT images (**B**) demonstrate avid uptake of FDG by the greater pterygoid muscles (*arrows*). This activity is physiologic and is caused by talking and mastication. It should not be confused with malignant lesions. **C:** Axial fused PET/CT images of the larynx demonstrate increased activity in the vocal chords secondary to phonation during uptake phase. This can be problematic for the evaluation of laryngeal carcinomas if activity is excessive. **D:** PET MIP image demonstrating diffuse symmetric muscle activity in a patient who performed strenuous exercise within 12 hours prior to FDG injection.

be recognized as variants on PET images and not mistaken for hypermetabolic lesions.

FDG is an indiscriminate identifier of foci of high metabolic activity within the body. Its usefulness is based on the fact that most malignant tumors are more metabolically active and take up more glucose than normal tissues. However, some nonmalignant pathologic processes including infections, foci of inflammation, and benign neoplasms can also concentrate FDG on the basis of their metabolic activity. The challenge to PET interpretation is the differentiation of pathologic activity from normal and normal variant FDG activity.

Skeletal muscle FDG uptake is dependent on muscle activity and insulin levels. In a resting state, muscle uptake of FDG is negligible. Heavy muscle activity in the 24 hours prior to imaging may result in high FDG uptake. Patients should minimize activity following FDG injection to minimize uptake by skeletal muscles. Patients with breathing difficulty may show prominent uptake in the muscles of the chest wall and diaphragm. Insulin injection by diabetics increases skeletal muscle FDG uptake similar to nonfasting patients (Fig. 76.1). Eye movement increases uptake in the ocular muscles and talking increases uptake in the vocal cords and the muscles of mastication (Fig. 76.2).

Brain uptake of FDG should always be prominent as the brain uses glucose as its primary energy source (Fig. 76.3). Normal gray matter uptake is particularly avid and difficult to differentiate from malignant brain lesions. Focal low-level activity may be seen in areas that have been radiated or resected. Nonfasting studies can result in diffuse low-level activity.

Cardiac muscle uptake is particularly intense after eating. Fasting for 4 to 6 hours prior to FDG scanning decreases FDG uptake as the myocardium switches to fatty acid metabolism and this uptake can be further reduced by adhering to a high-fat, low-carbohydrate diet for the 24 hours preceding the scan. Most patients show variable and nonuniform myocardial FDG activity, even after a fast, caused by nonuniform transition to fatty acid metabolism by the myocardium. Hibernating myocardium will preferentially use glucose for metabolism and thus will have high uptake of FDG. FDG activity is most variable at the base of the left ventricle (Fig. 76.4).

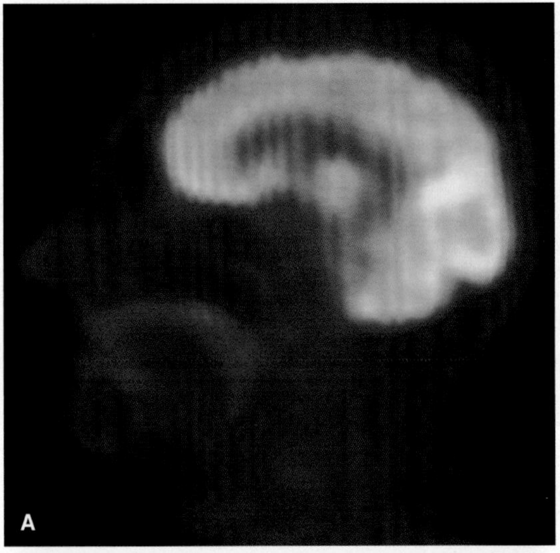

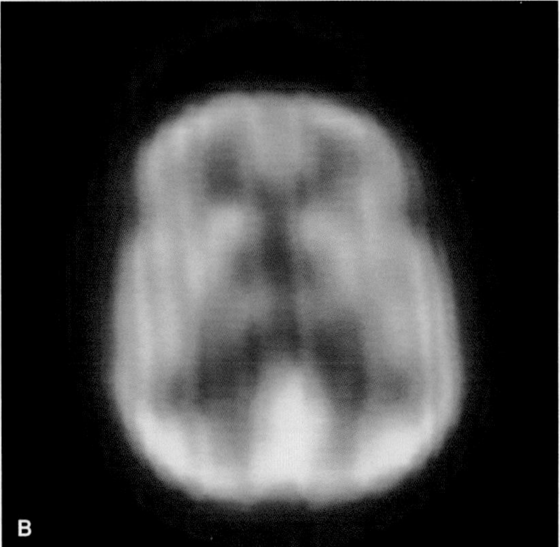

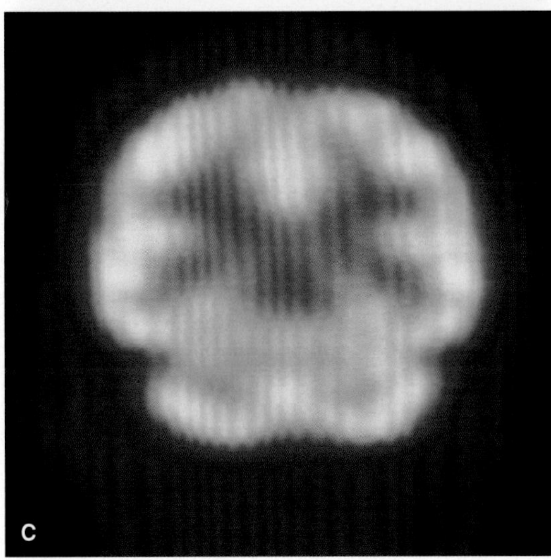

FIGURE 76.3. **Physiologic Fluorodeoxyglucose (FDG) Activity in the Brain.** PET images of the brain in sagittal (**A**), axial (**B**), and coronal (**C**) planes demonstrate diffuse brain uptake of FDG most prominent in the gray matter. FDG activity reflects the use of glucose as a primary energy source for the brain.

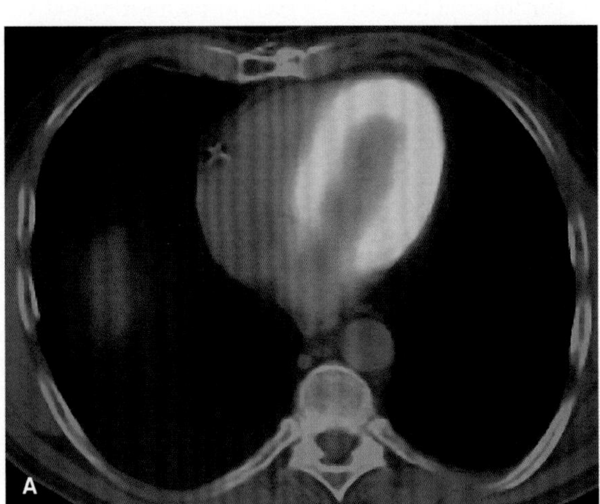

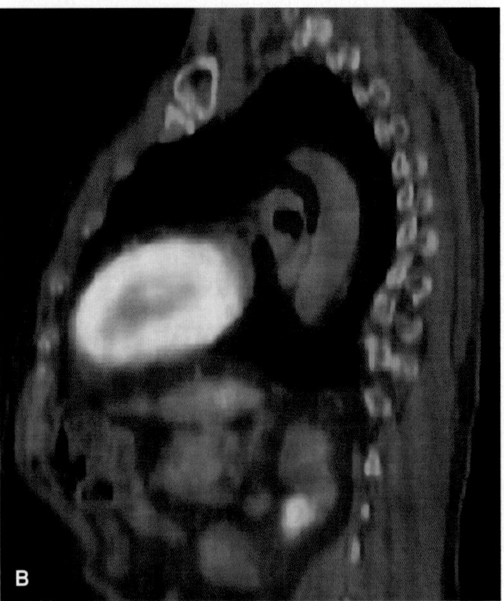

FIGURE 76.4. **Physiologic Fluorodeoxyglucose Activity in the Heart.** Fused PET/CT images in axial (**A**) and sagittal (**B**) planes demonstrate normal prominent myocardial uptake by the LV.

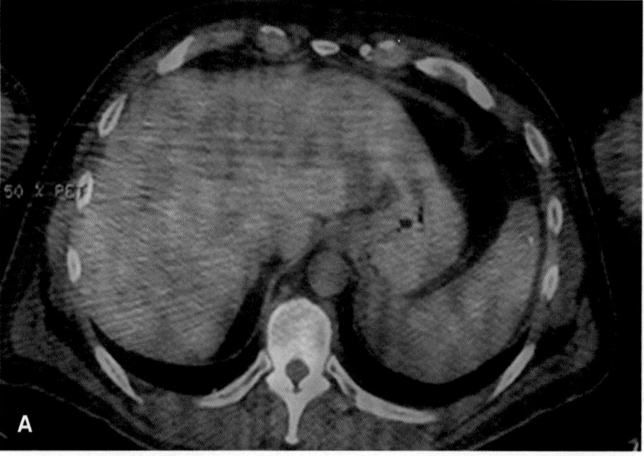

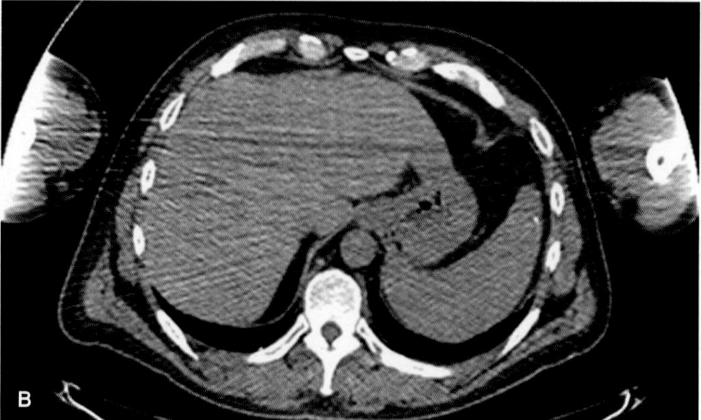

FIGURE 76.5. **Physiologic Fluorodeoxyglucose (FDG) Activity in the Liver. A:** FDG activity is strikingly heterogeneous but normal on the fused PET/CT image. High metabolic activity within the liver combined with variable clearance of FDG from hepatocytes results in this heterogeneous pattern, which makes the detection of hepatic masses somewhat difficult. **B:** The corresponding CT image demonstrates the streaks of beam-hardening artifact resulting from the patient being in arms-at-side position. This artifact can also decrease FDG activity seen on attenuation-corrected images as seen in the anterior portion of the right and left hepatic lobes as compared to the posterior portions of (**A**).

Liver. The entire liver demonstrates low-level FDG activity in nearly all patients. Hepatic uptake of FDG is not surprising because the liver is a major site of carbohydrate metabolism, glycolysis, and glycogen storage. However, hepatocytes also have high levels of FDG-6-phosphatase, which acts to clear FDG from hepatocytes. Uptake in the liver can appear heterogeneous and mimic the appearance of multiple small metastases (Fig. 76.5).

Gallbladder activity is rarely seen. FDG activity in the gallbladder bed suggests acute or chronic cholecystitis, gallbladder cancer, or adjacent liver tumor.

Spleen activity is usually slightly greater than blood pool but normally less than liver. Spleen uptake is substantially increased by the activation of extramedullary hematopoiesis and can also be seen in the setting of postchemotherapy or immunotherapy treatments.

Bone marrow uptake is mild to moderate, diffuse, and symmetric within the spine, pelvis, ribs, sternum, and proximal femurs. Asymmetric or heterogeneous uptake is caused by skeletal metastases, old fractures, and effects of radiation therapy. Diffuse homogeneous FDG uptake can be seen in bone marrow activation of hematopoiesis by severe anemia and marrow rebound following chemotherapy with or without marrow-stimulating medications.

Stomach activity is usually low level and best recognized on axial images by its characteristic position and shape. FDG activity is accentuated by stomach muscle contraction. Foci of uptake in the lower thorax may represent inflammation within a hiatal hernia or in the distal esophagus related to reflux.

Colon activity is highly variable and usually more intense than in the small bowel. Intense FDG uptake makes the recognition of pathologic sites in the abdomen difficult (Fig. 76.6). Colon activity varies with colon muscle contraction, mucosal inflammation, amount of lymphoid tissue in the colon wall, and possibly uptake by colonic bacteria. Multifocal or segmental activity suggests inflammatory bowel disease, while intense focal activity suggests colon carcinoma, malignant peritoneal implants, or adjacent lymph node metastases. Focal activity can also be seen in benign entities such as hyperplastic polyps. Patients on metformin can demonstrate intense uptake in the distal small bowel and right colon, which can mimic enterocolitis. The CT can be helpful in these situations as the colon and small bowel will look normal.

Urinary Tract. FDG is excreted by glomerular filtration without significant renal tubular reabsorption. This results in concentrated radionuclide activity in the urine (Fig. 76.7). The bladder should be emptied prior to PET imaging. Good hydration facilitates FDG clearance and decreases collecting system activity. High (but normal) renal collecting system activity impairs the detection of small renal lesions. Partial filling of the ureters resulting from normal peristalsis may show focal high FDG activity anywhere along the course of the ureters. Bladder diverticula commonly retain urine with FDG even after bladder emptying.

Uterus. The endometrium commonly demonstrates intense FDG uptake during active menstruation. Activity may also be seen in vaginal tampons. Fibroids may also have variable, focal FDG uptake. However, a pelvic US or MRI should be obtained in situations in which the CT features are not classic for a uterine fibroid and in postmenopausal females to exclude malignancy.

Ovaries can have focal uptake in corpus luteal cysts (Fig. 76.8), but this should only be seen in premenopausal women. Any uptake in a postmenopausal female is pathologic and should be worked up with an ultrasound or MRI.

Salivary gland uptake is normally minimal to low. Radiation therapy, infection, and inflammation increase FDG activity.

Thyroid gland uptake is normally diffuse and low level. Intense diffuse activity is associated with Graves disease and thyroiditis. An asymmetric focus of activity suggests possible thyroid cancer and warrants US evaluation and consideration of biopsy.

Brown Fat. A pattern of symmetric uptake in the paraspinal regions, mediastinum, neck, and supraclavicular areas may be localized on the CT images as coming from fat (Fig. 76.9). Brown fat can have an atypical presentation including in the interatrial septum of the heart and adjacent to the adrenal glands. When a patient is cold or anxious, increased levels of catecholamines increase glycolytic activity in brown fat. This may be very difficult to differentiate from lymphadenopathy. Keeping the scan room warm and sedating anxious patients may diminish this activity.

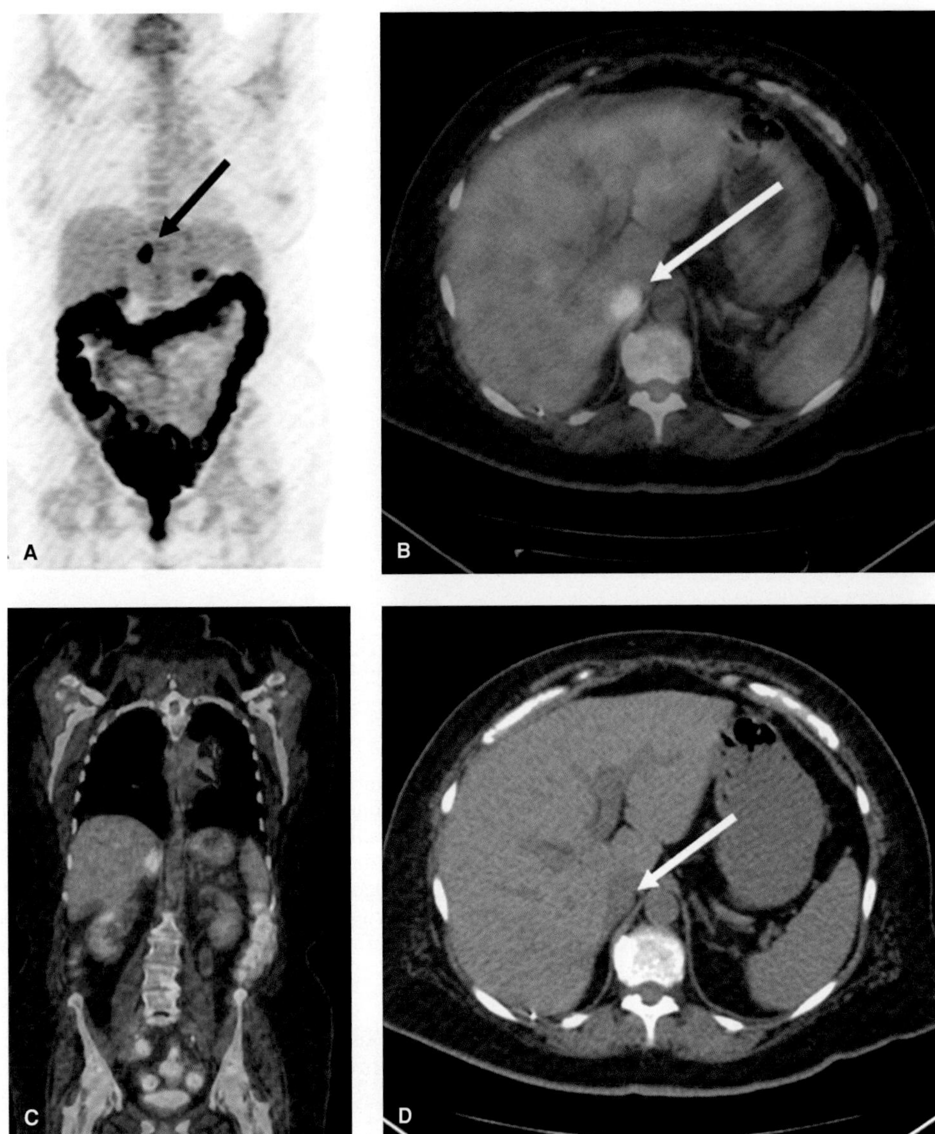

FIGURE 76.6. **Massive Physiologic Colon Activity.** PET MIP image (**A**) and a fused PET/CT coronal image (**C**) show massive colon activity, which can make the evaluation of the abdomen challenging. Note again the normal heterogeneous fluorodeoxyglucose activity in the liver. Also, note the focal activity above the right kidney is a focal adrenal (*arrows* in **A, B, D**) metastasis.

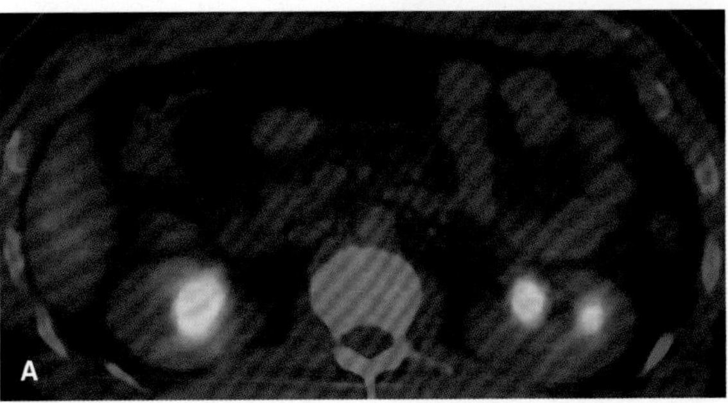

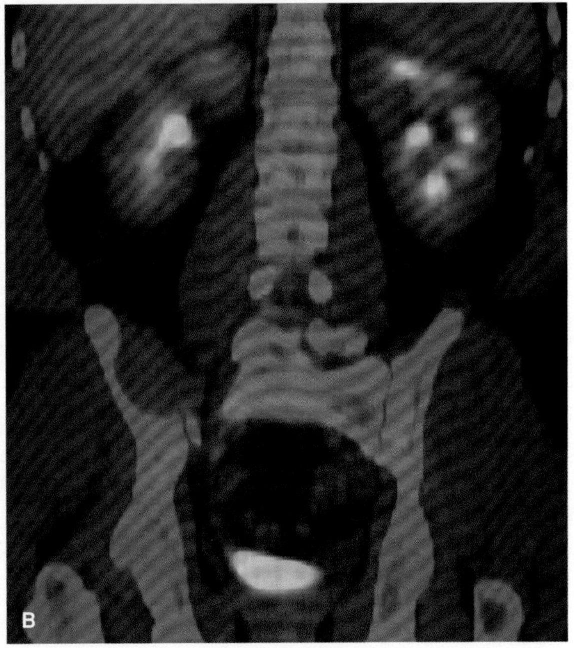

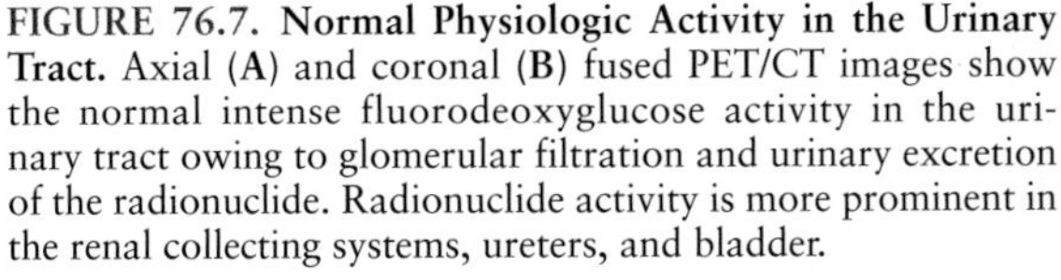

FIGURE 76.7. **Normal Physiologic Activity in the Urinary Tract.** Axial (**A**) and coronal (**B**) fused PET/CT images show the normal intense fluorodeoxyglucose activity in the urinary tract owing to glomerular filtration and urinary excretion of the radionuclide. Radionuclide activity is more prominent in the renal collecting systems, ureters, and bladder.

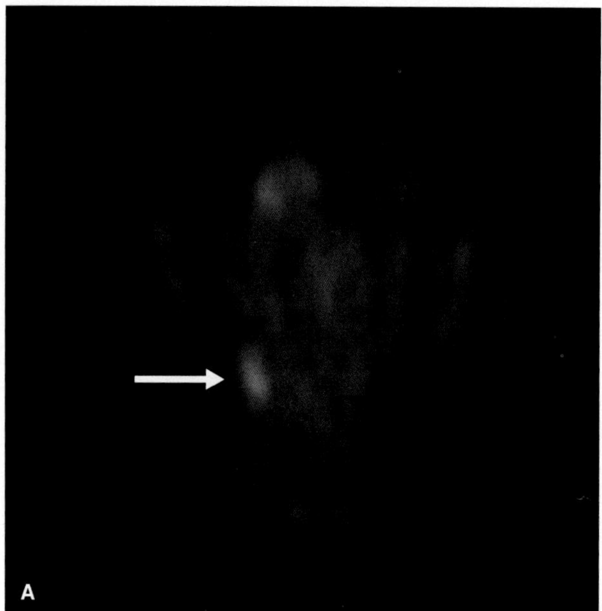

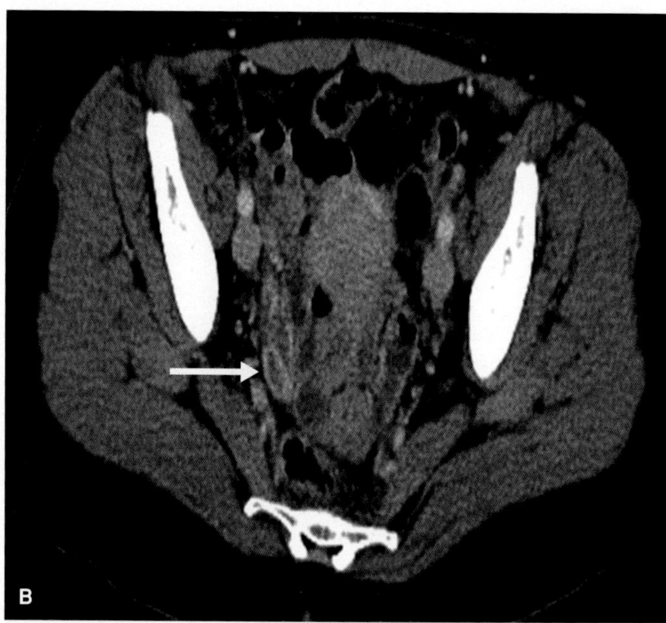

FIGURE 76.8. **FDG Uptake in a Corpus Luteum Cyst.** Focal FDG uptake in the right ovary seen on an FDG PET (*arrow* in **A**) in a 46-year-old female for restaging examination that has classic findings on corresponding CT (*arrow* in **B**). **A:** Axial FDG PET. **B:** Axial postcontrast CT.

Standard Uptake Values. In an attempt to semiquantitatively assess the uptake of radiotracer, SUVs were introduced to take into consideration the weight of the patient as well as the administered dose. Software to calculate SUVs is available with most imaging systems. An SUV is calculated by placing a region of interest over the area to measure tracer activity in microcuries/cubic centimeter (μCi/cm^3). This value is obtained by dividing the administered dose (in microcuries) by the patient's body weight (in grams).

$$\text{SUV} = \frac{\text{Tracer activity in focus}}{\text{Administered dose/Patient's body weight}}$$

Most malignant tumors have an SUV greater than 2.5 to 3.0, while physiologic activity usually ranges from 0.5 to 2.5

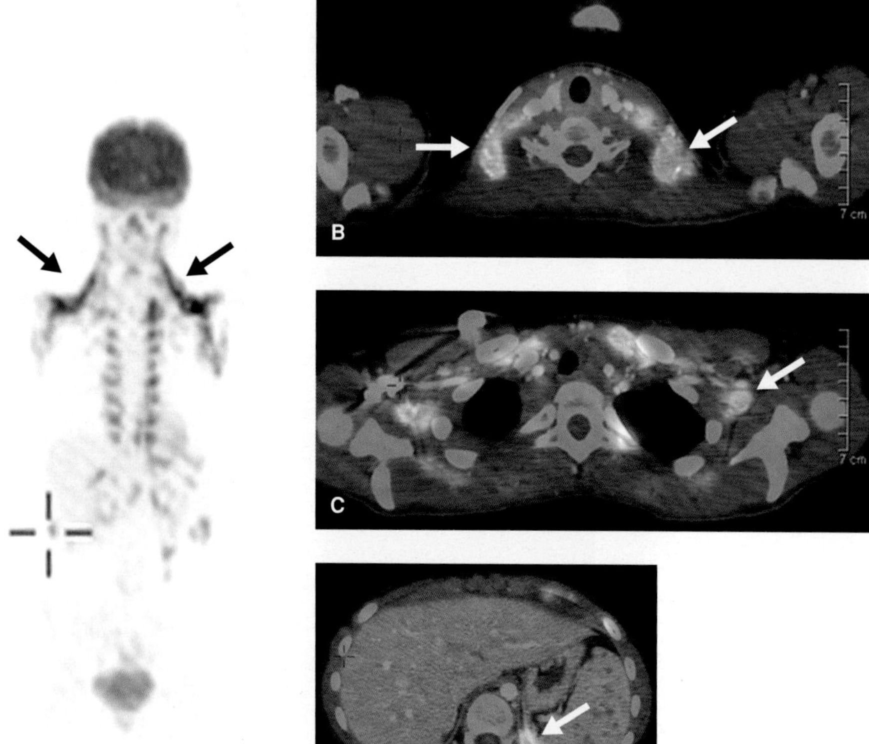

FIGURE 76.9. **Extensive Brown Fat Hypermetabolism.** Whole-body MIP from FDG PET (**A**) demonstrates extensive hypermetabolism in the neck, paramediastinal, and upper abdominal regions (*black arrows*). PET/CT fusion images (**B**, **C**, and **D**) demonstrate that in all cases the hypermetabolism is associated with areas of normal-appearing fat (*white arrow*).

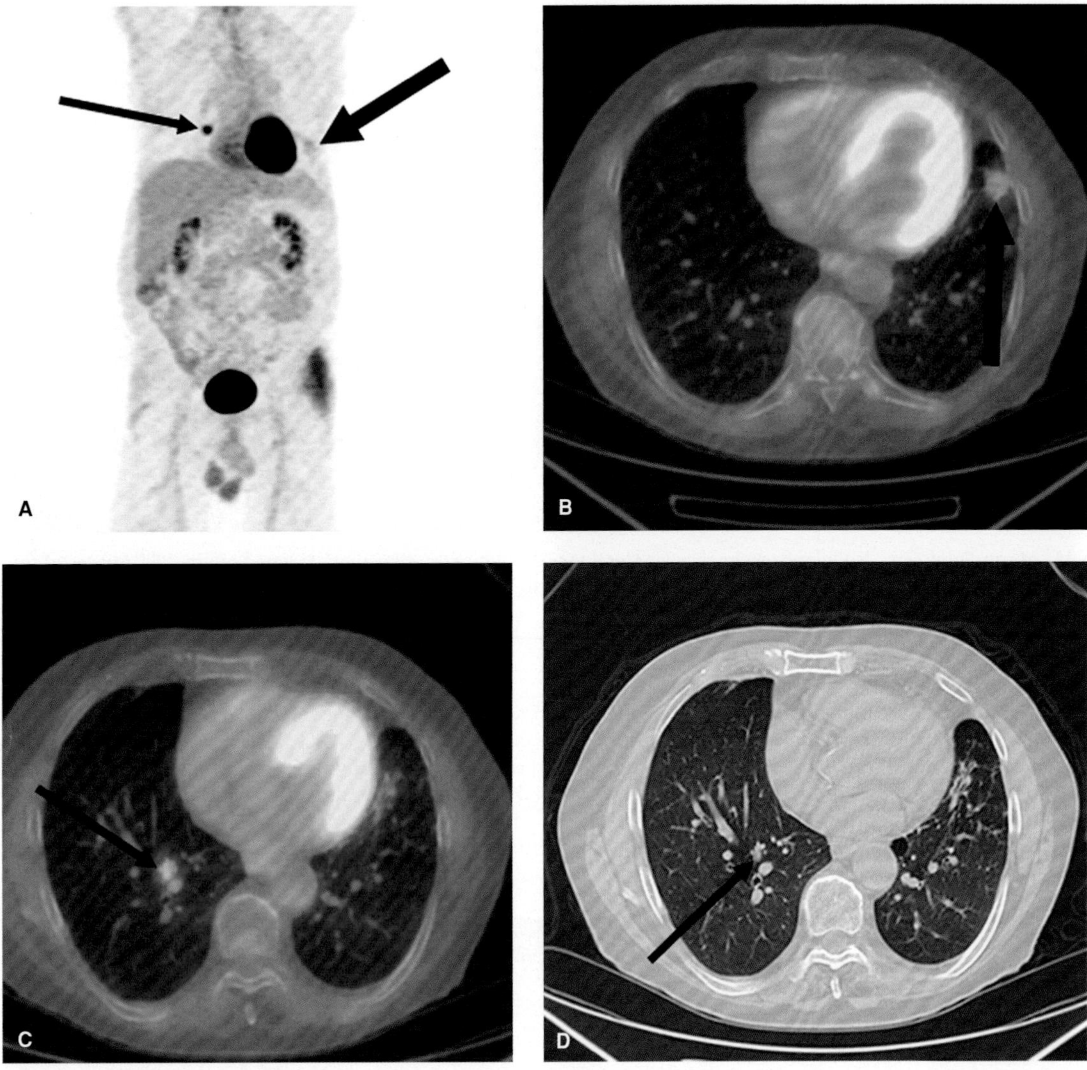

FIGURE 76.10. **Hot Pulmonary Nodule: Incidental Carcinoma.** Focal hypermetabolic pulmonary lesion incidentally discovered in the right lung (*thin arrows* in **A**, **C**, **D**) while evaluating larger density in the lingula (*large arrows* in **A**, **B**). Note the limited FDG activity in the substantially larger lingular lesion which is indicative of an inflammatory lesion. **A:** PET MIP image. **B:** Fused PET/CT image of lingular lesion. **C:** Fused PET/CT image of right lung incidental carcinoma. **D:** Noncontrast CT of right lung pulmonary nodule (carcinoma).

depending on the organ system. However, relying on SUV has limitations as FDG uptake can vary greatly with tumor types. For example, adenocarcinoma in situ of the lung can have near-physiologic SUVs. In addition, many factors can affect the uptake of FDG including lean body weight, state of hydration, insulin level, blood-sugar level, distribution of nontarget organs and space, etc. Taking into consideration only body weight limits the accurate assessment of the accumulated activity, especially for purposes of comparison; however, it does have advantages over pure visual evaluation.

ONCOLOGIC PET IMAGING

Currently PET is utilized in oncology for three major indications: ***initial staging***, ***evaluation of response to treatment***, and ***assessment for recurrence***. Recent literature also cites emerging application of PET for predicting the prognosis of some malignancies based on uptake values. In addition, primary assessment of single pulmonary nodules by PET is an acceptable next step in the evaluation of malignancy for nodules greater than 8 mm in size (Fig. 76.10). Although there are a few hypometabolic malignancies causing false-negative PET cases, the majority of common cancers are highly metabolically active and glucose avid (Fig. 76.11). In addition, there are a few nonmalignant processes with high metabolic activity, which should be recognized to avoid false-positive results. These include infectious and inflammatory conditions as well as a few benign neoplastic processes.

Lung Cancer. Traditionally, lung cancer has been classified into small cell lung cancer (15%) and nonsmall cell lung cancer (85%). The majority of lung cancers are intensely hypermetabolic and PET has proven to be significantly more sensitive and specific for the detection of sites of metastatic disease than CT. Broadly speaking, PET has found value in initial characterization of the solitary pulmonary nodule, presurgical staging (Fig. 76.12), detecting recurrence, and monitoring response to therapy.

Solitary Pulmonary Nodule. PET plays an important role in characterizing solitary pulmonary nodules. Primary lung cancers are commonly hypermetabolic on PET. Conversely, benign

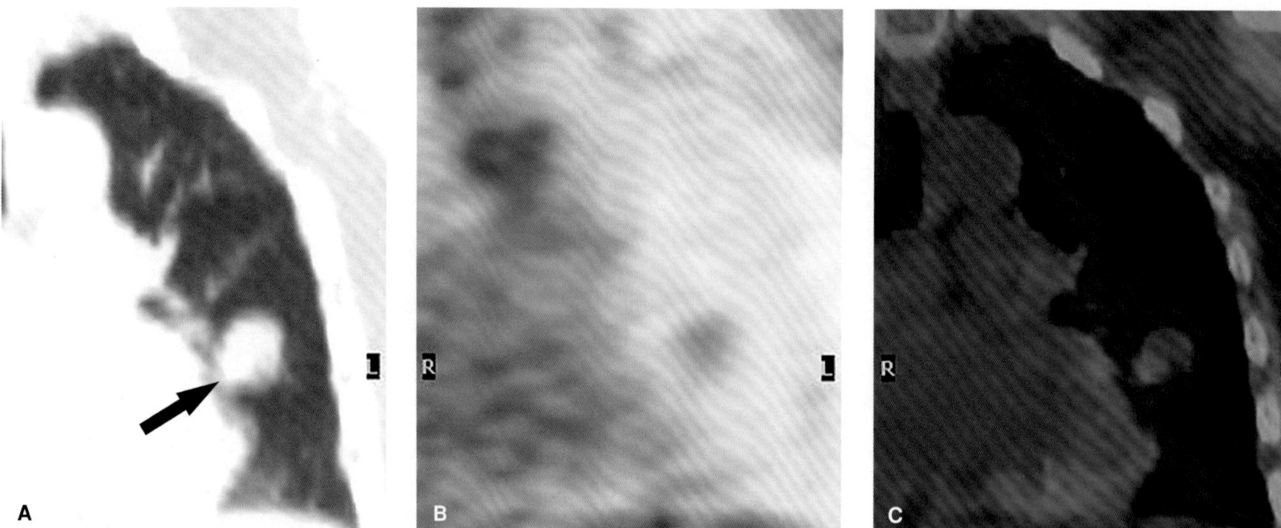

FIGURE 76.11. **Warm Pulmonary Nodule: Bronchoalveolar Carcinoma.** Mild increased activity is noted on the PET images of this bronchoalveolar cell carcinoma of the lung (*arrow*). Mild activity is compatible with either an inflammatory or a neoplastic process. **A:** CT. **B:** Corrected PET. **C:** Fused PET/CT.

lesions such as granulomas, scarring, and hamartomas accumulate less FDG and appear photopenic on PET imaging. PET is highly sensitive for cancer in the solitary pulmonary nodule (greater than 90%) while the specificity is variable, as low as 75% in some studies. For this reason, the absence of hypermetabolism in a solitary pulmonary nodule permits a conservative surveillance management strategy, for example, with serial CT surveillance. In contrast, increased uptake in the tumor is not definitive for malignancy and should be confirmed with biopsy. False-positive results occur with tuberculosis, fungal infections, and sarcoidosis. Furthermore, if a solitary pulmonary nodule is a metastasis, PET can potentially detect the extrapulmonary

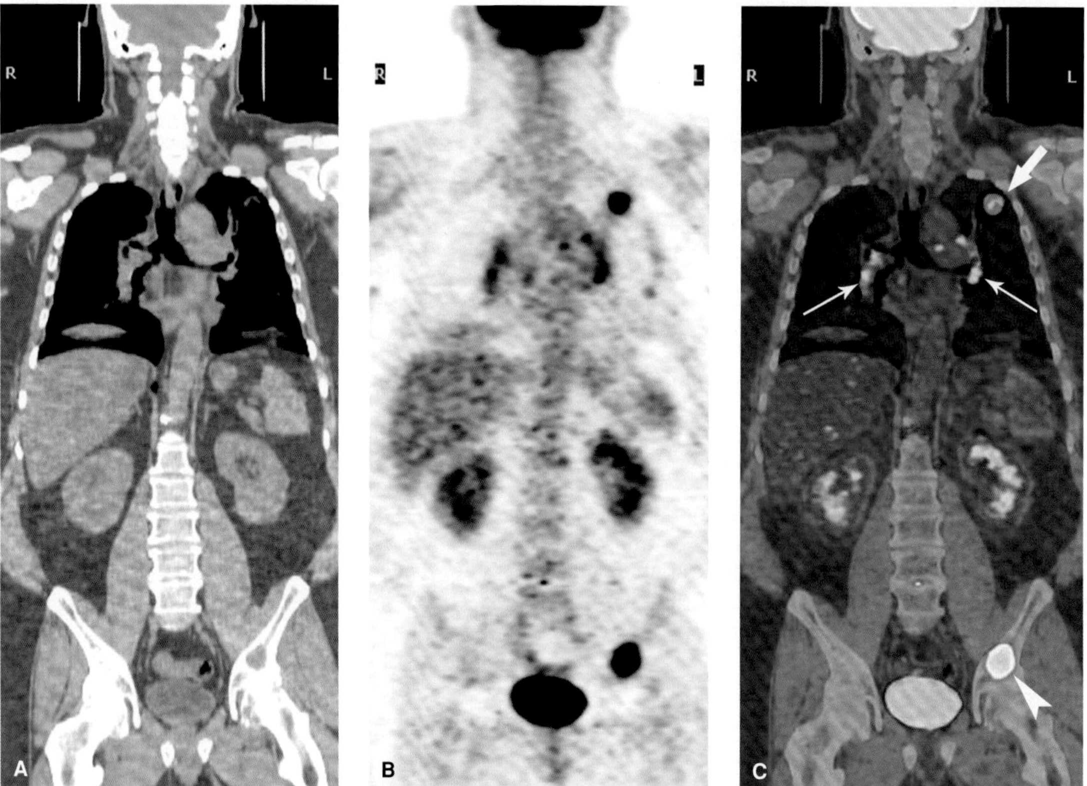

FIGURE 76.12. **Lung Cancer Staging.** PET/CT in coronal plane demonstrates FDG hyperactivity in the primary lung cancer (*wide arrow*) as well as within hilar lymph nodes (*thin arrows*) and the left acetabulum (*arrowhead*), indicating widespread metastatic disease. Heterogeneous activity in the liver, spine, bowel, both kidneys, and bladder is normal. **A:** CT. **B:** Corrected PET. **C:** Fused PET/CT.

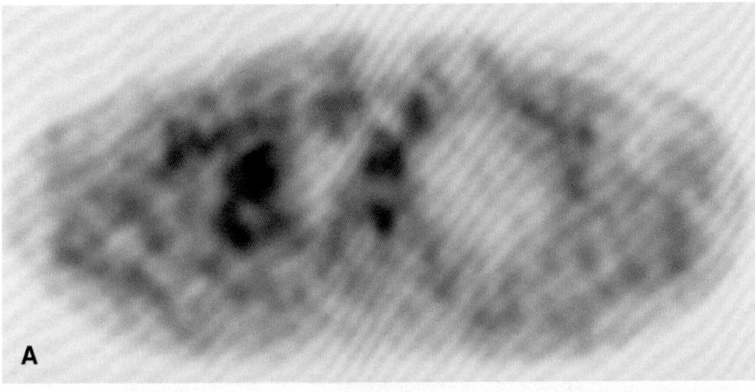

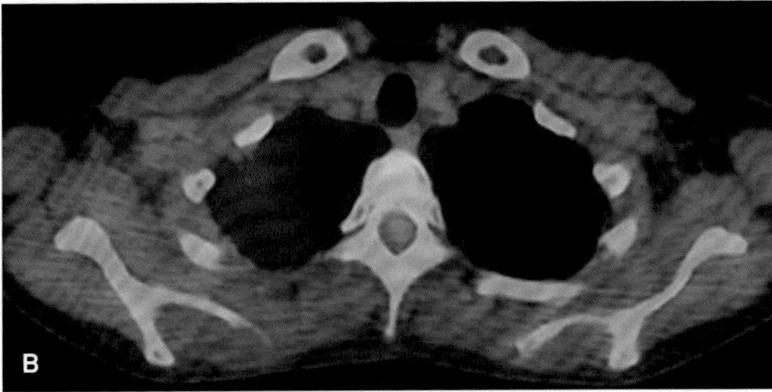

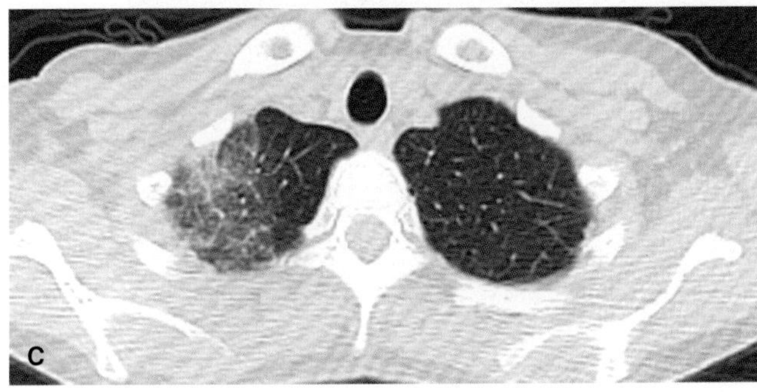

FIGURE 76.13. **Postradiation Pneumonitis.** Axial PET/CT images show high FDG activity in the right upper lobe in a patient who has undergone radiation therapy in the previous 4 months. Focal hyperactivity during this time frame is nonspecific and compatible with either postradiation pneumonitis or tumor recurrence. **A:** Attenuation-corrected PET. **B:** Fused PET/CT. **C:** Noncontrast CT.

primary cancer in the same study. While the SUV is an imperfect parameter, many authors have suggested using a cutoff of 2.5 or greater as suspicious for malignancy. However, values less than 2.5 may indicate malignancy in nodules under 1 cm due to volume averaging. In these cases, the qualitative perception of increased hypermetabolism should raise suspicion. An additional important exception to this rule is subsolid (ground glass) nodules, which commonly demonstrate minimal or no hypermetabolism. PET therefore has limited utility in the workup of a primarily ground glass nodule.

Staging. Initial presurgical staging is a critical role of PET in lung cancer imaging. Importantly, lymph nodes that are normal by CT size criteria can still harbor metabolically active malignant cells, which may be detectable by PET. For this reason, PET significantly lowers the rate of futile thoracotomies in lung cancer patients. PET/CT is significantly more sensitive and specific than CT alone for hilar and mediastinal lymph node involvement in lung cancer. However, false-positive hypermetabolism can be found due to inflammatory or infectious lymph nodes. PET also aids in the detection of distant metastases, including contralateral lung, pleural, adrenal, bone, or liver. Furthermore, PET can help delineate the presence of tumor within larger regions of atelectasis or consolidation.

Detecting Recurrence and Monitoring Response to Therapy. Unfortunately, recurrent disease is common in lung cancer patients treated with either surgery or radiation. PET is useful in detecting recurrence. However, on initial baseline postsurgical or postradiation studies (Fig. 76.13), it is often difficult to discriminate posttreatment changes from recurrence. In particular, radiation pneumonitis can be metabolically active in the 6 months following radiation therapy.

Lymphoma. Staging in lymphoma is based on the presence of disease above or below the diaphragm, involvement of single or multiple nodal basins, and confinement to lymph nodes or spread to extranodal tissues with disease stage used to ultimately guide management (Fig. 76.14). FDG PET is more sensitive and specific than CT in lymphoma staging (86% vs. 81% sensitive and 96% vs. 41% specific) due to its ability to detect metabolically avid disease in nodes that are not enlarged. In addition, FDG uptake correlates with histologic grade and the degree of the proliferative activity of the lymphomatous tissue. However, not all malignant lymphomas are highly metabolically active and therefore can produce a false-negative result on PET. Low-grade lymphomas show little to no FDG uptake and mucosal-associated lymphoid tissue (MALT) lymphomas are easily overlooked because of the background activity of the GI tract. There are many potential false-positive FDG-PET scans such as sarcoidosis, tuberculosis, pyogenic abscesses, histoplasmosis and other fungal infections, and discitis. In practice, hypermetabolic lymph nodes are considered malignant until proven benign, usually by biopsy.

Initial Staging. FDG PET is an excellent modality for the initial assessment of Hodgkin disease and aggressive non–Hodgkin lymphoma (NHL) but is less useful for low-grade follicular NHL. FDG PET is superior to CT for nodal disease in the thorax and abdomen. FDG PET is also excellent for extranodal disease, which is present in 40% of lymphoma patients, but has inherent limitations. Diffuse lymphomatous involvement of the spleen is a challenge for all imaging modalities, including PET. Diffuse splenic activity greater than that of liver activity is consistent with diffuse lymphomatous infiltration of the spleen. Focal hyperactivity in the spleen suggests focal lymphoma, whether or not a corresponding mass is shown on CT (Fig. 76.15). Bone marrow assessment is also limited as a variable degree of activity is always present in normal marrow spaces. However, focal FDG uptake can guide the choice of bone marrow biopsy to increase the yield of marrow biopsy. Diffuse hyperactive marrow on PET images could be caused by hyperplasia of normal marrow after chemotherapy rather than representing lymphomatous tissue. Increased activity in the spleen usually accompanies hyperplasia of the marrow and may provide a clue to the correct diagnosis. An osteolytic bone lesion in NHL as well as other malignancies may be a photopenic on Tc-99m MDP radionuclide bone scans. FDG PET can demonstrate significant metabolic activity in these cold osteolytic lesions characterizing them accurately as aggressive disease.

Early Assessment of Treatment Response. Interim FDG PET can provide important prognostic information. Patients

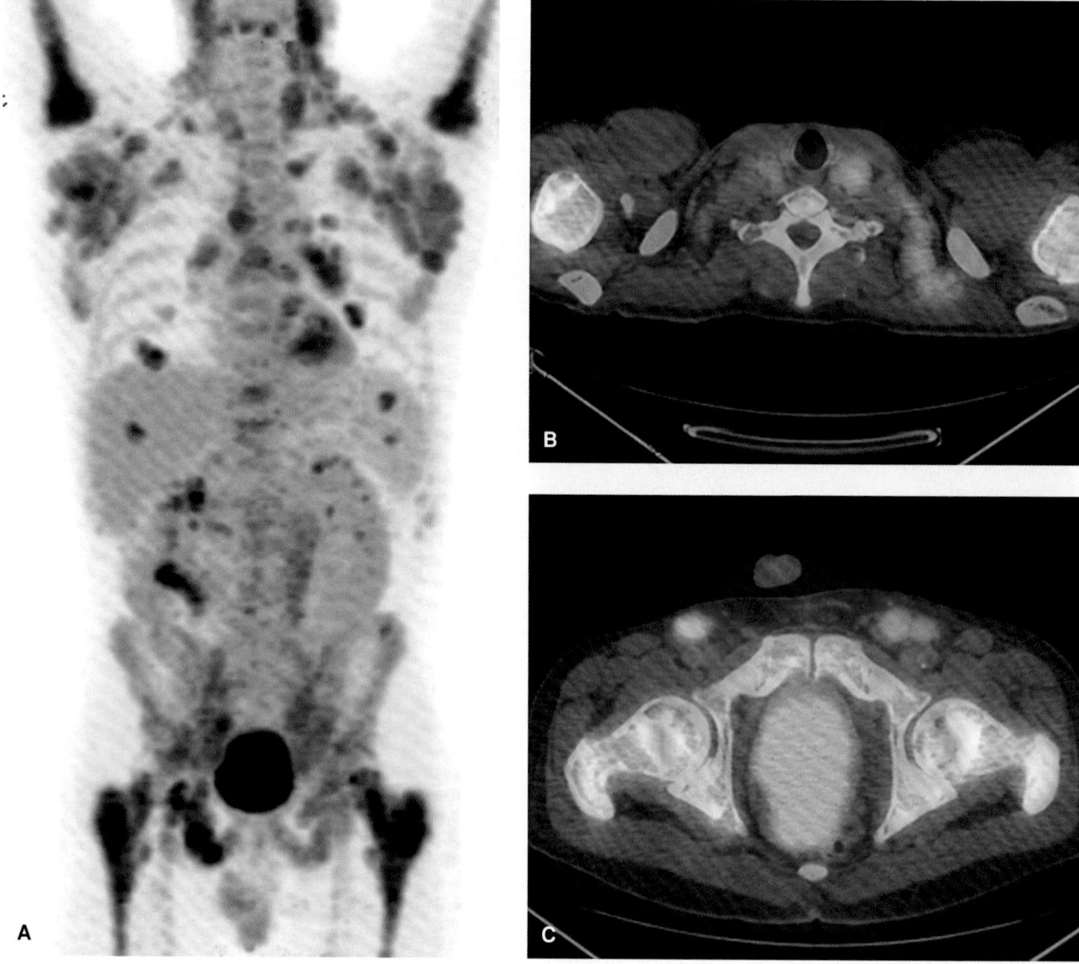

FIGURE 76.14. **Lymphoma Staging.** PET/CT demonstrates extensive adenopathy and multiple bony lesions in a patient with lymphoma. Whole-body scanning indicated that detectable disease was above and below the diaphragm. **A:** Attenuation-corrected PET MIP. **B:** Fused PET/CT axial view through the humeral heads. **C:** Fused PET/CT axial view through the femoral heads.

who do not have any residual FDG avid disease for both HL and NHL have an excellent chance of disease-free survival (Fig. 76.16). SUV measurements before, during, and after treatment provide semiquantitative measurements of the response to therapy.

Posttherapy Residual Mass. If no residual activity is detected on PET after the completion of the course of treatment, it can be concluded that the patient is in remission with a favorable prognosis. Lack of FDG uptake in residual soft tissue masses on CT is highly suggestive of no residual viable tumor. However, any focal FDG uptake needs to be interpreted with caution as it may represent either residual hypermetabolic neoplastic tissue or active inflammation with ongoing necrosis. These cases may require biopsy or short-term repeat FDG-PET imaging to confirm the diagnosis.

Detection of Recurrence. Periodic PET scanning is reliable for the assessment of continuing remission. Comparison with initial (pretherapy) and posttherapy PET and CT scans is of utmost importance. FDG activity is highly indicative of active tumor, whereas the absence of FDG activity indicates continued remission. Sources of error in the use of PET for staging and follow-up of lymphoma include infection, drug toxicity, effects of radiation therapy and surgery, and physiologic activity. Infections are common in bone marrow–suppressed patients, especially in the respiratory and GI tracts. Active infection and inflammation show PET activity that may be mistaken for lymphomatous involvement. Drugs, such as bleomycin, may injure the lungs and result in diffuse FDG lung activity. Granulocyte colony–stimulating factor therapy used to stimulate proliferation of granulocytes may cause focal marrow activity, mimicking lymphoma involvement. Inflammatory response and healing induced by radiation therapy or surgical procedures cause PET hypermetabolism. False-positive FDG uptake in the thymus tissue may be seen with thymic rebound, which commonly occurs in children and young adults undergoing treatment for lymphoma.

Melanoma. Early-stage melanoma (85% of patients) is curable by surgery, whereas 15% of patients have advanced local disease or metastases. Diagnosis is usually made by physical examination and biopsy. While primary melanoma lesions can be seen on FDG PET, other cutaneous processes can also show FDG uptake such as acne and carbuncles, which may mimic melanomas or skin metastases. Although FDG PET is highly specific (97%), it is relatively insensitive for these regional node metastases (as low as 17% sensitivity) as regional lymph nodes can have a microscopic volume of the disease. Sentinel lymph node biopsy is therefore required to evaluate regional lymph nodes. FDG PET is primarily used in melanoma patients with stage T3a or worse disease. It is highly useful

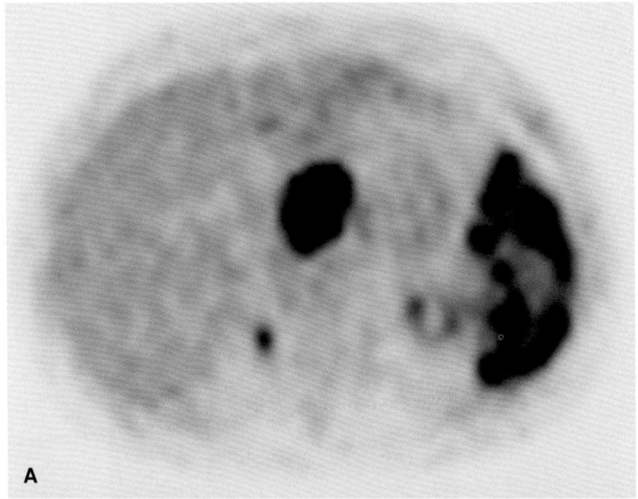

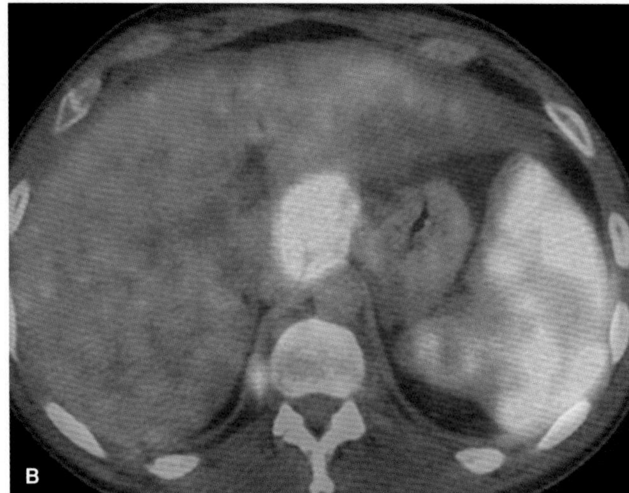

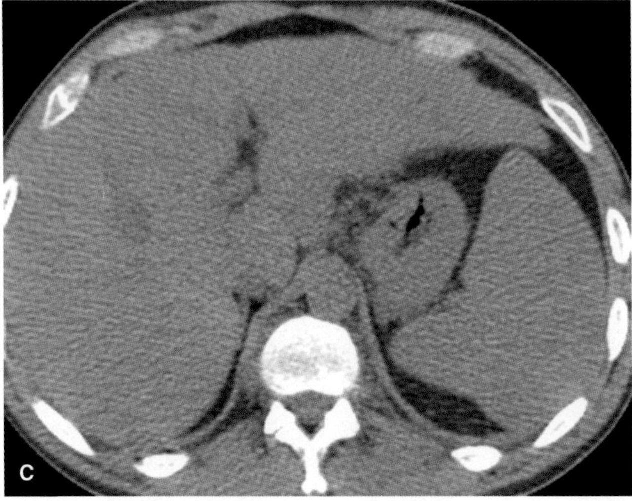

FIGURE 76.15. **Spleen Lymphoma.** PET reveals a multifocal hypermetabolic lesion in the spleen caused by lymphoma. The lesions are not apparent on noncontrast CT. Large periportal and retrocrural nodal metastases are also seen (**B**). **A:** Attenuation-corrected PET axial image. **B:** Fused PET-CT. **C:** Noncontrast CT.

in the demonstration of distant metastases, which occur most commonly in the lungs, liver, adrenal glands, GI tract, and bone, as well as in unusual sites such as the spleen, thyroid, gallbladder, pancreas, and skin. Whole-body PET is 92% sensitive and 90% specific in the detection of distant metastases. Limitations are small lung metastases that are too small to be detected by PET and brain metastases due to the high physiologic background.

Melanoma may recur many years after apparent cure and is often widespread before detection. Whole-body FDG PET is useful for surveillance, with detection rates for recurrence similar to those of initial staging for distant metastases.

Esophageal Cancer. PET has found routine use in initial staging and in monitoring of response to therapy in esophageal cancer. PET can detect sites of distant metastases in approximately 20% of patients prior to surgical resection. PET is the most accurate imaging modality for following response to neoadjuvant chemotherapy prior to surgical resection. Patients with little decrease in hypermetabolism in the primary lesion have substantially poorer prognosis. In determining the extent of disease, it is important to consider that inflammatory changes are common in the esophagus, particularly at the gastroesophageal junction where reflux esophagitis is a common finding. In general, inflammatory changes will be segmental and have no associated mass on CT imaging.

Recurrent disease following definitive surgical or radiation therapy can be detected using PET. PET is highly sensitive for detecting recurrence in the surgical bed; however, the specificity is lower owing to the common finding of postsurgical hypermetabolism. In this scenario, PET is highly sensitive (95%) and somewhat specific (80%). For these reasons, PET/CT has become the standard of care in initial staging, monitoring response to therapy, and in detection of recurrence in patients with esophageal cancer.

Gastric Cancer. Primary gastric neoplasms are difficult to detect on both CT and PET imaging as the stomach is typically decompressed and the gastric mucosa routinely demonstrates physiologic and inflammatory uptake. The sensitivity for lymph node metastases is low (approximately 40%), while specificity of locoregional hypermetabolic lymph nodes for metastatic disease is high (95%). Common sites of metastatic disease for gastric cancer include liver, peritoneum, and bones, which in many cases are as easily detected by CT or MRI. For this reason, the benefit of PET/CT in gastric cancer is less compared to that in other neoplasms such as lung cancer or lymphoma.

Pancreatic Cancer. Due to the lack of anatomic details with PET imaging such as vascular involvement, local staging is best accomplished by either contrast-enhanced CT or MRI. FDG PET is useful in the differentiation of chronic pancreatitis from pancreatic cancer and can be highly valuable in the detection of distant metastases. In addition, FDG PET provides useful prognostic markers such as total lesion glycolysis and mean tumor volume as well the ability to reliably assess

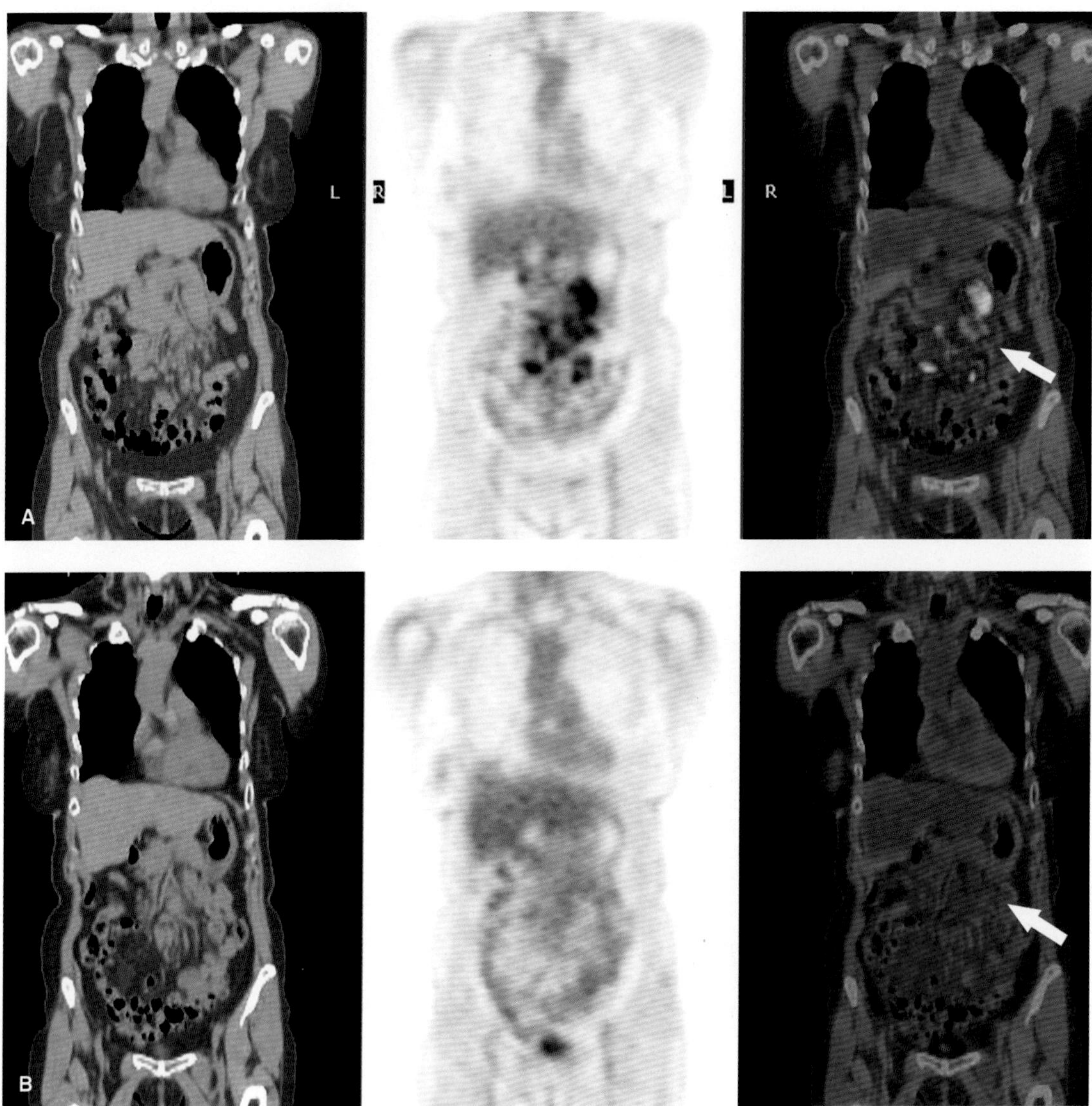

FIGURE 76.16. **Lymphoma: Early Response to Therapy.** Before an appreciable change in size is detectable by CT, FDG PET shows an early, favorable response to chemotherapy. **A:** Coronal-plane PET/CT shows hypermetabolic activity in mesenteric adenopathy (*arrow*), indicating involvement by lymphoma. **B:** Follow-up scan obtained after the first course of chemotherapy shows a lack of FDG activity within the mesenteric adenopathy (*arrow*) that is not changed on CT.

treatment response. Persistent high activity on postradiation cases suggests very poor prognosis.

Colorectal Cancer. Most (95%) colon cancers are FDG-avid adenocarcinomas. Currently FDG PET is widely utilized for staging and restaging of patients and for the assessment of response to treatment. In about 40% of cases, clinical staging is modified by PET results with approximately 20% of patients found to have metastatic disease at the time of diagnosis. Since accurate upstaging by PET can prevent unnecessary surgery in patients with advanced disease, FDG PET can provide one-stop accurate assessment for whole-body staging at the time of initial diagnosis (Fig. 76.17). PET is currently not widely employed for early detection or colon cancer screening though some groups are using hybrid PET/CT with virtual colonoscopy to offer functional and anatomic imaging for early detection of adenomatous polyps and small colon cancers. Nonspecific colonic activity can be a source of false-positives (Fig. 76.6). Diffuse activity is usually physiologic, especially in the descending and sigmoid colon. Benign conditions, including sigmoid diverticulitis, inflammatory polyps, and fecal material, can accumulate FDG. Any focal activity in the colon should be further evaluated. The bladder should be emptied immediately prior to imaging and scanning should begin in the pelvis and proceed superiorly to limit obscuration of the rectum by excreted bladder radioactivity.

FDG PET has low sensitivity (29%) for regional node metastases because involved nodes are often small, have a limited number of tumor cells, and are located close to and masked by bowel activity. When pericolic nodes are FDG-positive, specificity for malignancy is high (96%). PET sensitivity is equal to or slightly better than CT alone in the detection of hepatic metastases, and PET/CT specificity for hepatic metastases approaches 100%. Small lesions (<1 cm) are often not detected on PET, and anatomic localization of lesions within the liver by PET alone is not precise enough for surgical planning of resection of hepatic metastases. However, PET demonstration of extrahepatic metastases (11% to 23% of patients) precludes hepatic resection for cure. The major role of PET is in the detection of distant metastases, which

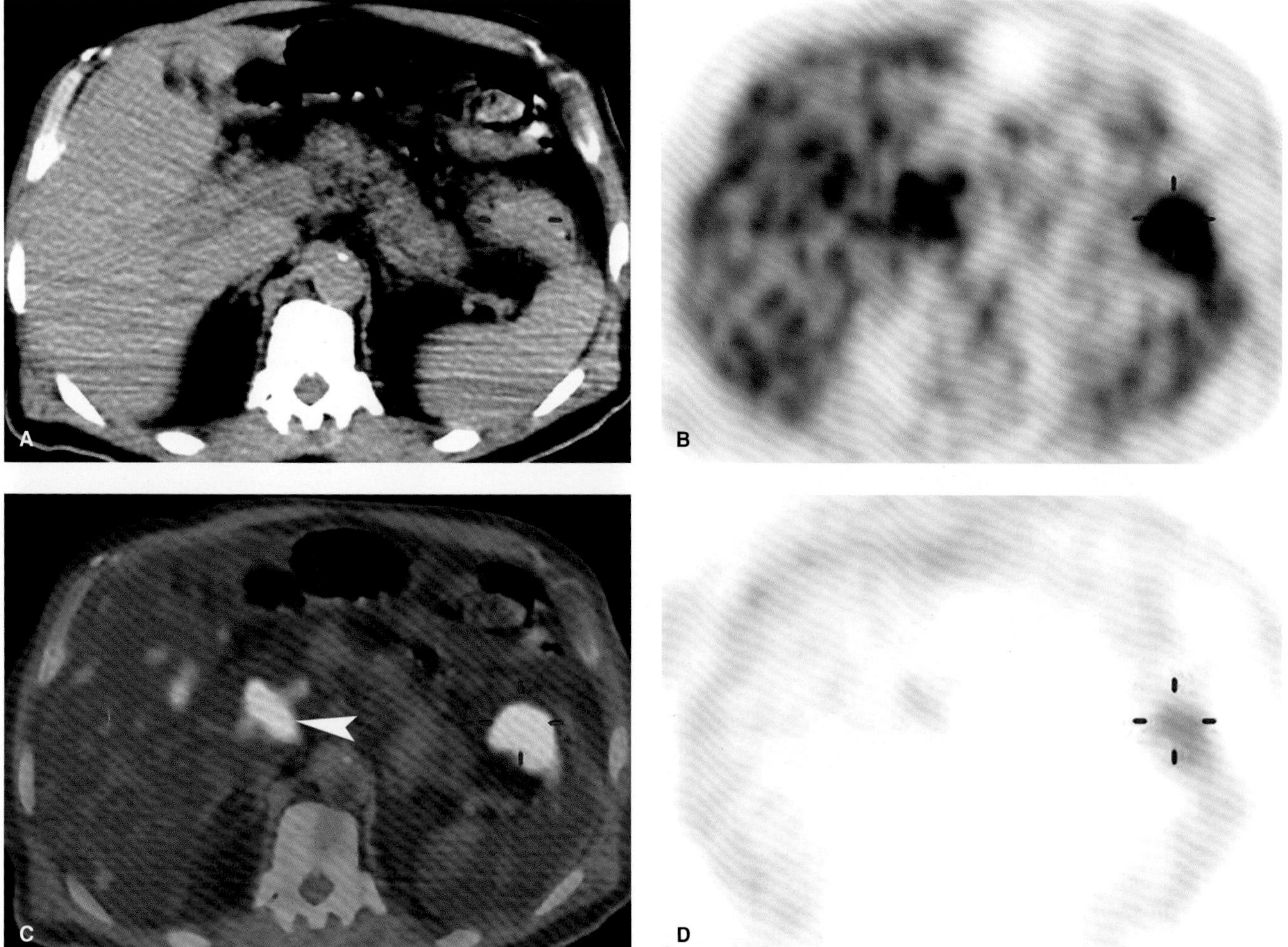

FIGURE 76.17. **Colon Cancer Staging.** A colon cancer (between *cursors*) in the splenic flexure is hypermetabolic on PET/CT as is metastatic adenopathy in the porta hepatis (*arrowhead*). **A:** CT. **B:** Corrected PET. **C:** Fused PET/CT. **D:** Uncorrected PET.

precludes surgery for cure. FDG PET is 97% sensitive and 76% specific in assessing for metastatic disease.

Recurrence of colon cancer can occur at the anastomotic site, surgical bed, or at distant sites, usually liver or lung. Activity at the anastomotic site needs to be interpreted with caution as healing and active granulation tissue present soon after surgery can avidly accumulate FDG (Fig. 76.18). Correlation with CT findings, the time of surgery, and/or radiation therapy is also helpful. Chronic scarring at the surgical site commonly produces nonspecific soft tissue density on CT. In assessing for recurrence more than 6 months after surgery or radiotherapy, focal FDG uptake with a corresponding soft tissue nodule on CT is indicative of tumor recurrence, whereas surgical scarring is not hypermetabolic.

Hepatic Malignancies. The combination of heterogeneous uptake and relatively high physiologic background of metabolic activity of the hepatic parenchyma can make detection of small hypermetabolic foci challenging. In addition, FDG uptake by hepatocellular carcinoma (HCC) is inversely related to the degree of tumor differentiation, so well-differentiated HCC only shows low FDG accumulation. Therefore, one should be cautious in utilizing FDG as the primary evaluation for HCC. However, once the diagnosis is established, FDG can provide valuable regional as well as whole-body assessment of the stage of HCC. The overall sensitivity of FDG for the detection of primary HCC is around 70%; specificity is limited. Nonmalignant hepatic lesions such as hepatic adenoma may show increased activity and contribute to false-positive results.

The sensitivity of FDG for the detection of cholangiocarcinoma mainly depends on its morphologic appearance. The nodular (focal) subtype can be detected up to 80% of the time, whereas detection of the infiltrative subtype is below 20%. Inflammation associated with biliary obstruction causes false-positive results. FDG PET is not a first-line modality for the detection of cholangiocarcinoma, although it can be used for staging of the extrahepatic disease and in detection of recurrence.

Hepatic Metastases. PET is most accurate for metastases in the liver that are larger than 1 cm (Fig. 76.19). Demonstration of smaller lesions is limited by PET resolution and physiologic liver background activity. Background FDG activity is commonly heterogeneous in the liver, so focal activity must be interpreted with caution. Metastases appear as discrete foci of increased activity, often multiple and varying in size. Large metastases with necrotic centers may appear as rings of increased activity (Fig. 76.20). Occasionally, metastatic lesions, even large ones, do not show increased FDG activity. In patients with colorectal carcinoma, PET may show only 70% of the liver lesions evident on resection specimens.

Gallbladder cancer shows high affinity for FDG and is detected with high sensitivity. Local invasion of liver is more accurately evaluated by CT or MR. FDG PET provides regional

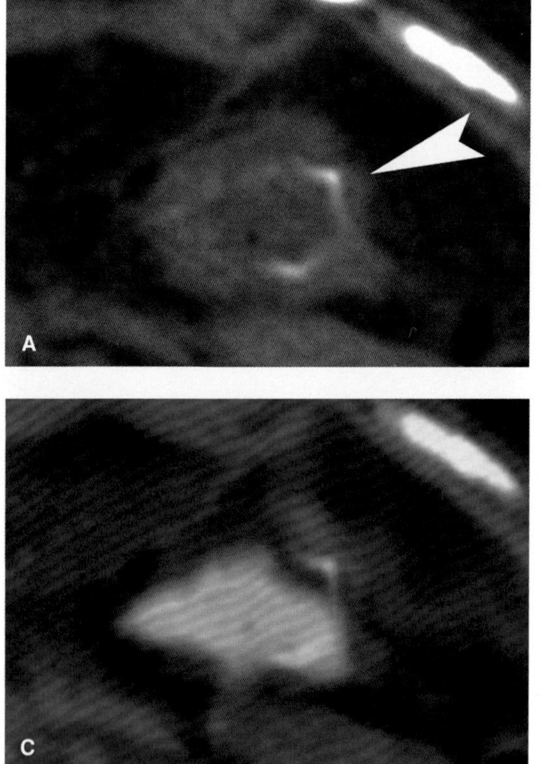

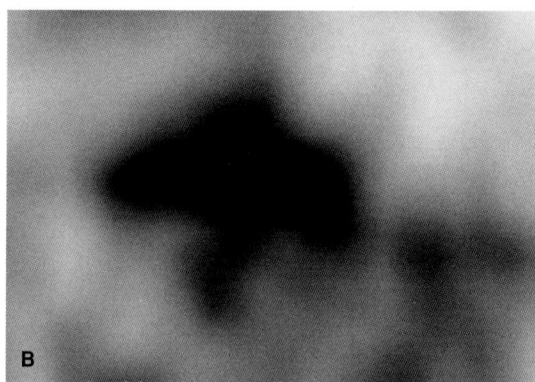

FIGURE 76.18. **Colon Cancer: Anastomosis Activity.** **A:** CT shows mass effect at the colonic anastomotic site (*arrowhead*) following recent colon cancer resection. Note the metallic bowel anastomosis sutures. PET (**B**) and fused PET/CT (**C**) images of the same area show marked hypermetabolic activity caused by postoperative inflammation. Recurrent tumor may have a similar appearance.

and whole-body staging of gallbladder cancers. Hypermetabolic activity in the gallbladder bed is more commonly caused by inflammatory diseases of the gallbladder than by malignancy (Fig. 76.21). Correlation with CT, MR, or US is of great value in minimizing false-positive results. Active hepatic foci near the gallbladder fossa can be misinterpreted as a gallbladder focus. Multiplanar assessment improves the accuracy of localization and should be employed routinely.

Breast Cancer. FDG PET is reliable for the assessment of breast lesions larger than 15 to 20 mm (Fig. 76.22). While symmetric, diffuse uptake of FDG can be seen in lactation (Fig. 76.23), focal uptake is suspicious. Detection of microscopic cancers is typically below the current threshold of PET. Overall, the uptake of FDG in breast cancer is less than that of lung cancer. An SUV above 2.0 suggests malignancy. False-positive uptake occurs with inflammatory breast disease as

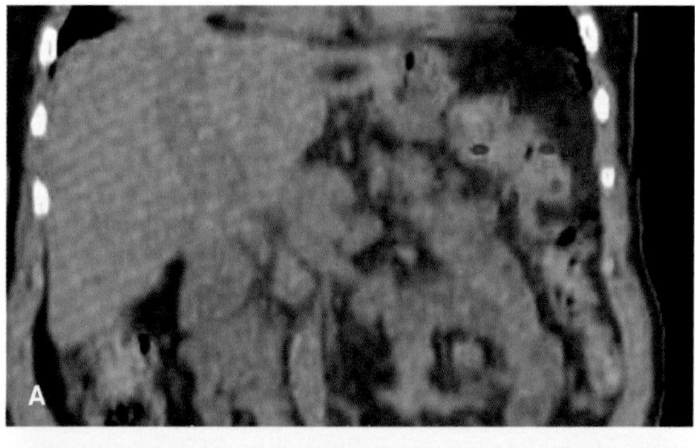

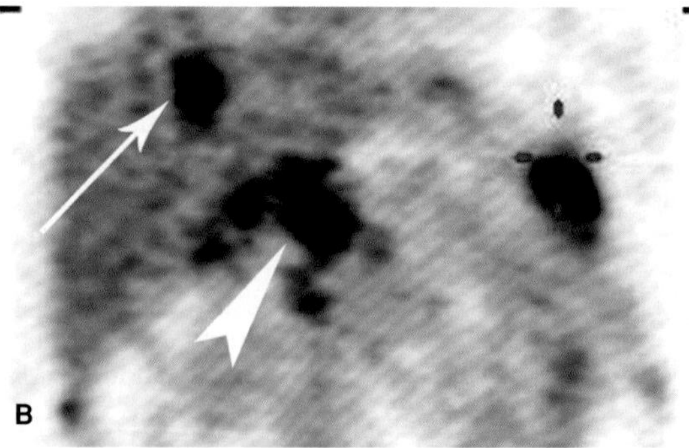

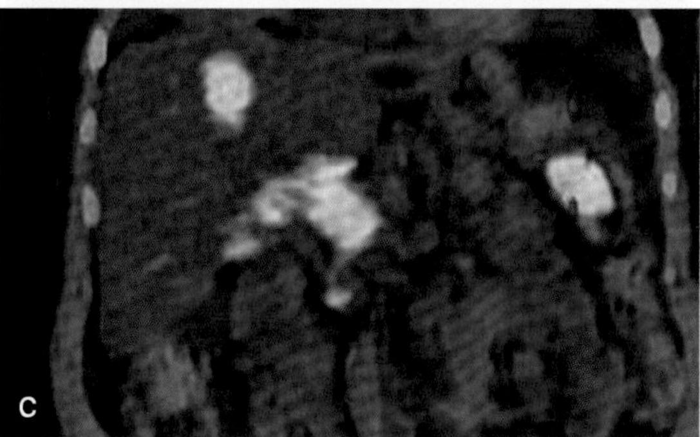

FIGURE 76.19. **Hepatic Metastasis: Colon Cancer.** Coronal PET images in the same patient shown in Figure 76.17 reveal a hepatic metastasis (*arrow*) that is barely visible on the corresponding noncontrast CT. Hypermetabolic activity is also evident in metastatic lymph nodes in the porta hepatic (*arrowhead*) and in the primary cancer in the splenic flexure of the colon (between *cursors*). **A:** CT without contrast. **B:** Corrected PET. **C:** Fused PET/CT.

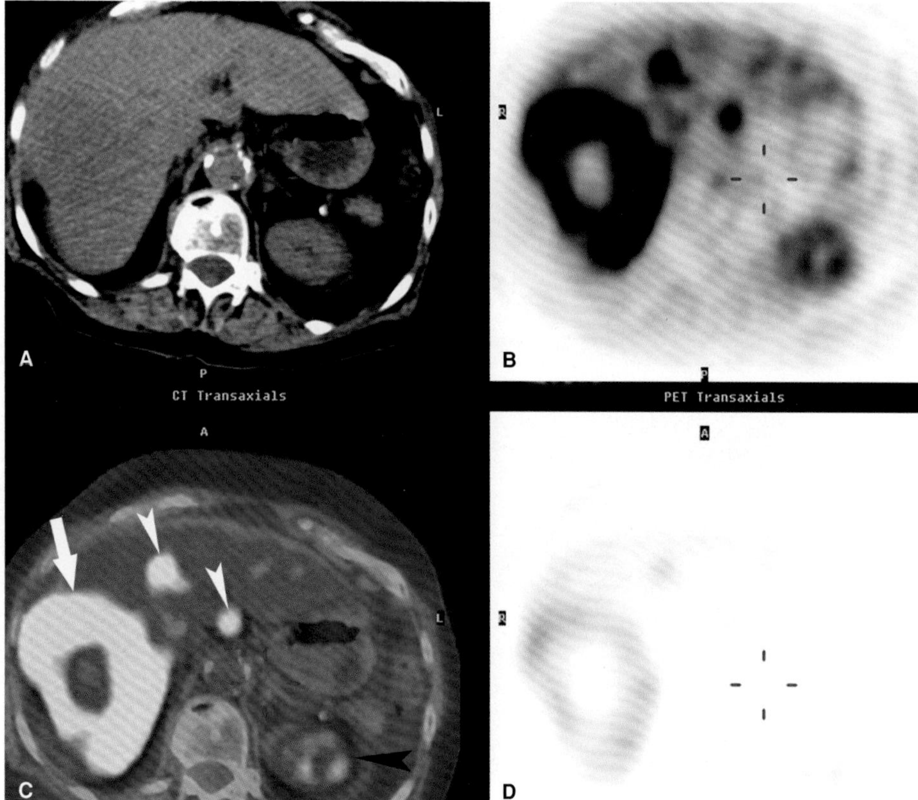

FIGURE 76.20. **Necrotic Hepatic Metastasis.** PET/CT shows a very large liver metastasis with central necrosis (*arrow*) in a patient with a history of colon cancer and poor response to chemotherapy. Two additional smaller metastases (*white arrowheads*) are also evident. Normal physiologic activity is seen in the left kidney (*black arrowhead*). **A:** CT. **B:** Corrected PET. **C:** Fused PET/CT. **D:** Uncorrected PET.

well as fibroadenomas. False-negative rates of up to 60% for invasive lobular cancers and up to 24% for invasive ductal cancers have been reported. As with melanoma staging, sentinel node lymphoscintigraphy is very valuable and exceeds PET capabilities in preoperative staging of the axillary nodes. However, FDG PET is very accurate in whole-body staging, can reliably assess the response to treatment, and is widely used in the detection of recurrence.

Fasting is a must for PET assessment of breast cancer patients because of the relatively low avidity of breast cancer tissue for FDG. In addition, the radiotracer should be injected on the side contralateral to the side of the primary. This is done to minimize the rate of false positives on the ipsilateral side as extravasated radiotracer can be taken in the lymphatics, resulting in intense uptake of FDG on the side of the injection. Detailed assessment of axillary and internal mammary

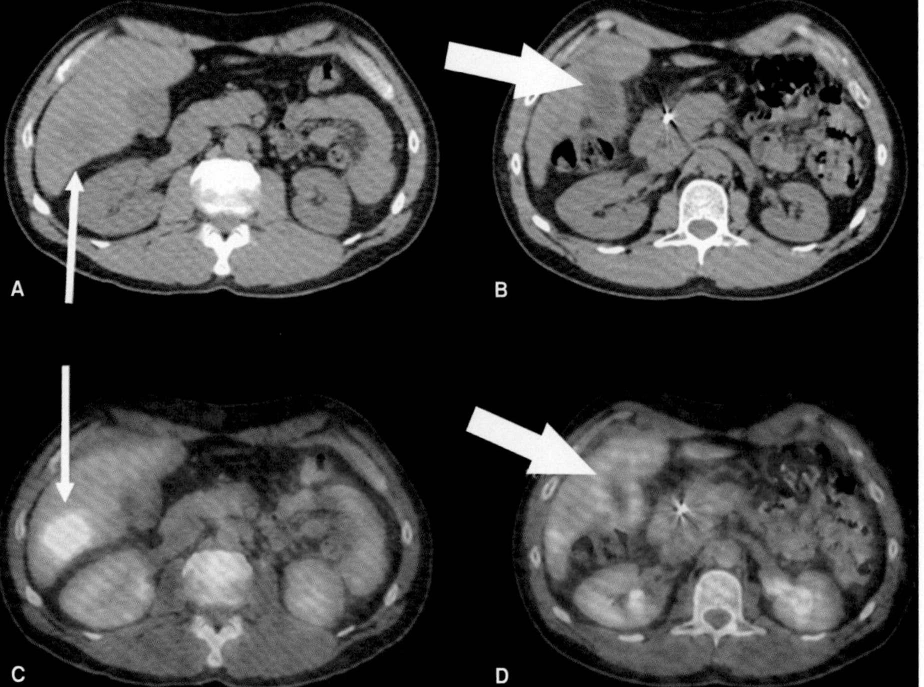

FIGURE 76.21. **Cholecystitis.** High metabolic activity in the gallbladder wall (*large arrow* in **B, D**) in a patient with asymptomatic cholecystitis 6 weeks after treatment for metastatic colon cancer to the liver (*small arrow* in **A, C**) with Y-90 microsphere embolization. Gallbladder uptake of fluorodeoxyglucose may represent inflammation or tumor. Physiologic activity is seen in the bilateral renal pelvis. Metallic artifact seen in **B, D** from coil embolization of the right gastric artery. **A:** CT. **B:** CT. **C:** Fused PET-CT at the same level as **A. D:** Fused PET-CT at the same level as **B.**

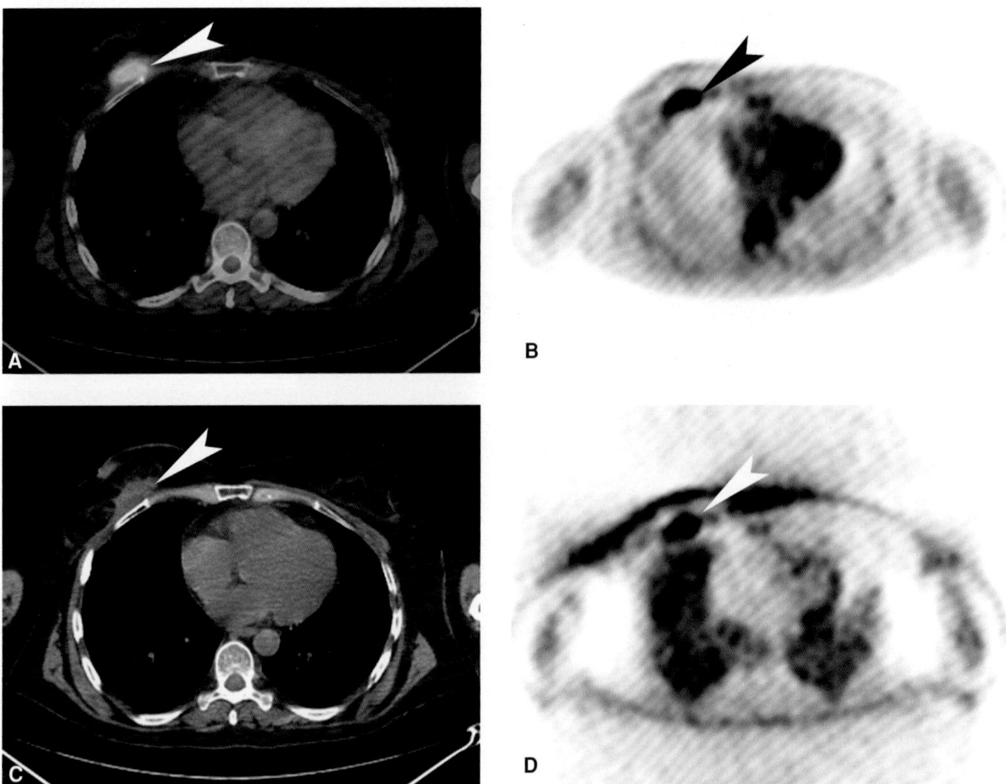

FIGURE 76.22. **Breast Cancer PET/CT.** Axial images through the thorax demonstrate marked fluorodeoxyglucose (FDG) activity within a carcinoma (*arrowhead*) in the right breast. Normal myocardial FDG activity is seen in the heart and vertebral body. **A:** Fused PET/CT. **B:** PET with attenuation correction. **C:** Noncontrast CT. **D:** PET without attenuation correction. FDG activity on the PET with attenuation correction and on the fused PET/CT images is confirmed by identifying activity in the same focus on the PET image without attenuation correction.

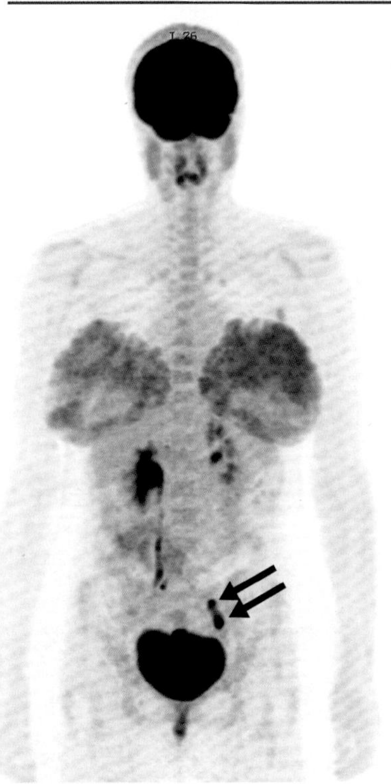

FIGURE 76.23. **Diffuse Breast Uptake on FDG PET.** A 32-year-old woman with a diagnosis of endometrial cancer underwent FDG PET. In addition to metastatic adenopathy (*arrows*) in the pelvis, intense diffuse breast uptake was seen, consistent with lactation as the patient had recently given birth.

nodal chains in coronal and sagittal planes is essential on both PET and CT images (Figs. 76.24 and 76.25). The opposite breast is assessed for bilateral disease. Postoperative muscle flaps may contain hypermetabolic muscle tissue. Postradiation pneumonitis can mimic transthoracic extension of breast cancer. Knowledge of the site and time of radiation therapy, as well as correlation with radiographic findings, are essential for correct interpretation. FDG PET may detect bone metastases not evident on radionuclide bone scans.

Cervical Cancer. FDG PET is clearly superior to CT and US in regional node assessment at the time of cervical cancer diagnosis, while MR is still the modality of choice for local tumor staging. FDG PET has been successfully employed for the evaluation of response to treatment and is the modality of choice for restaging and detection of recurrence. Some institutions administer furosemide or perform urinary bladder irrigation with a Foley prior to scanning or employing continuous irrigation to reduce bladder activity, which may obscure subtle disease activity.

Uterine Cancer. FDG PET has limited value in primary detection and in assessing the depth of invasion of endometrial cancer. However, similar to cervical cancer and other gynecologic malignancies, FDG PET is valuable for the assessment of regional nodes and the peritoneal cavity, for whole-body screening for distant metastases, and for the detection of recurrent tumor (Fig. 76.26). Special attention should be focused on the peritoneal surface to detect subtle peritoneal seeding. Section-by-section correlation with CT is crucial. Uterine fibroids and periovulatory hypermetabolism of the ovary may cause interpretation difficulties.

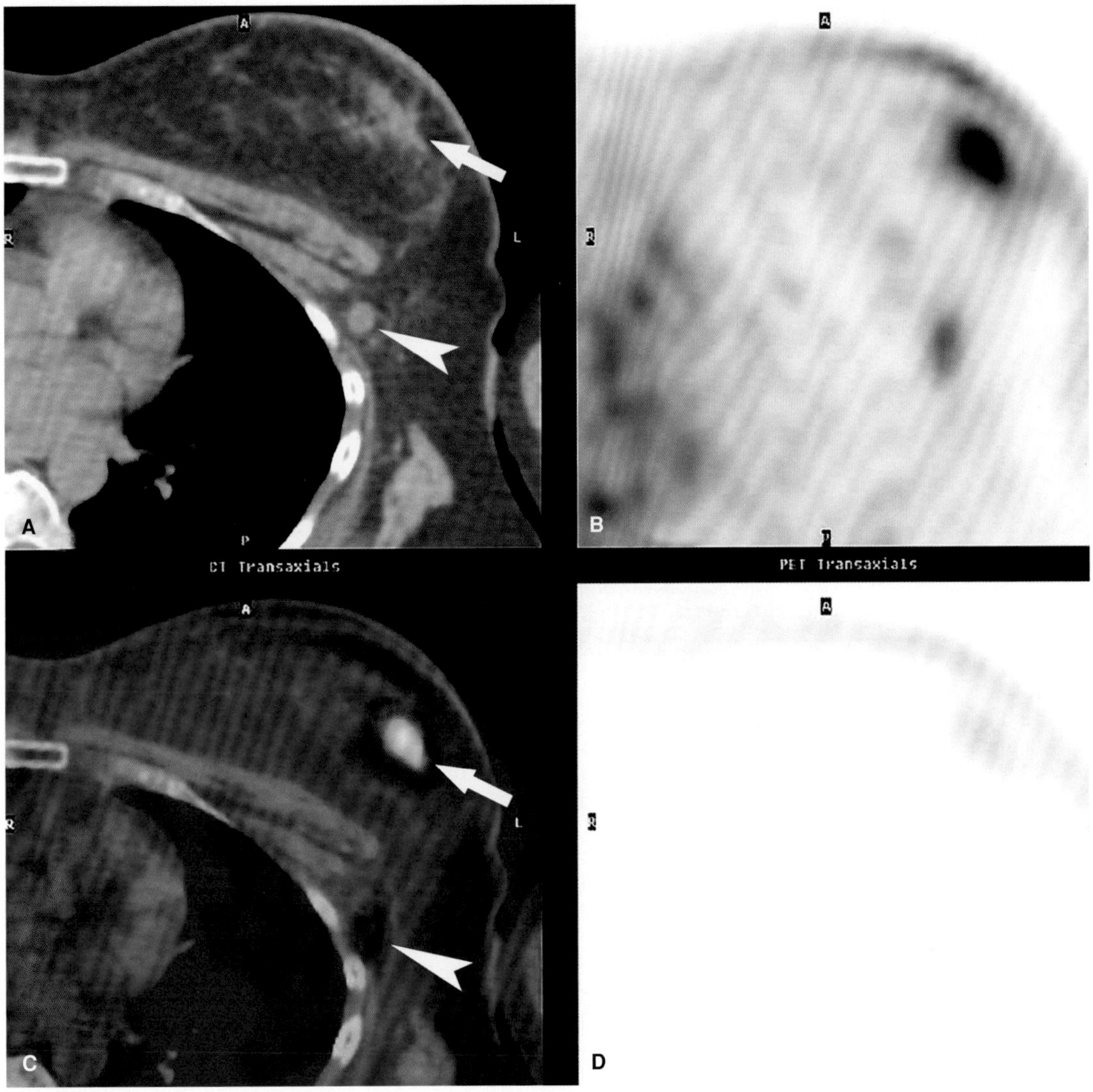

FIGURE 76.24. **Breast Cancer: Axillary Node Metastasis.** Axial images from PET/CT demonstrate hypermetabolic activity in the cancer (*arrows*) within the left breast and within an axillary lymph node (*arrowheads*) that would be considered benign by CT size criteria. **A:** CT. **B:** Corrected PET. **C:** Fused PET/CT. **D:** Uncorrected PET.

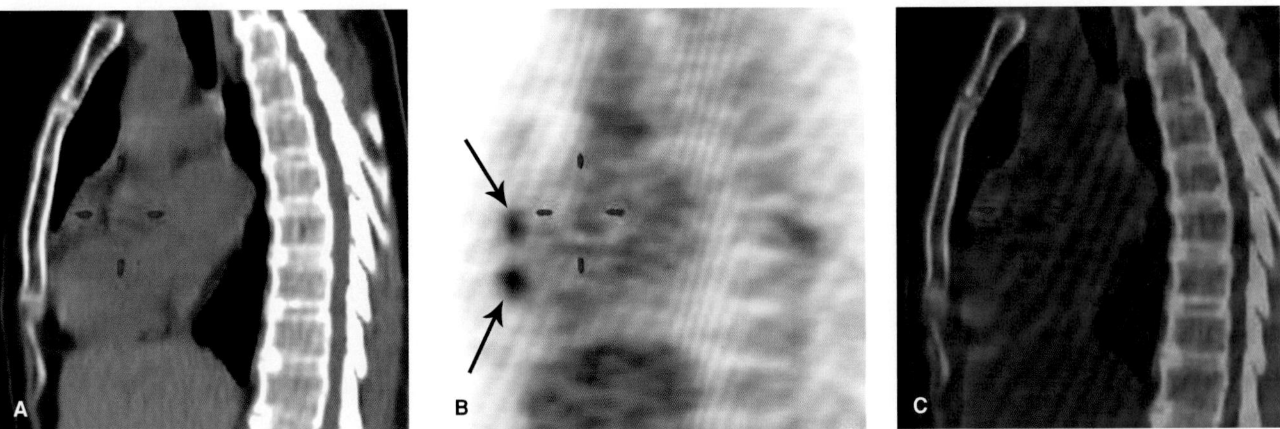

FIGURE 76.25. **Breast Cancer: Internal Mammary Node Metastases.** Sagittal images from PET/CT in a woman with breast cancer reveal breast cancer recurrence in internal mammary lymph nodes (*arrows*). **A:** CT without contrast. **B:** Corrected PET. **C:** Fused PET/CT.

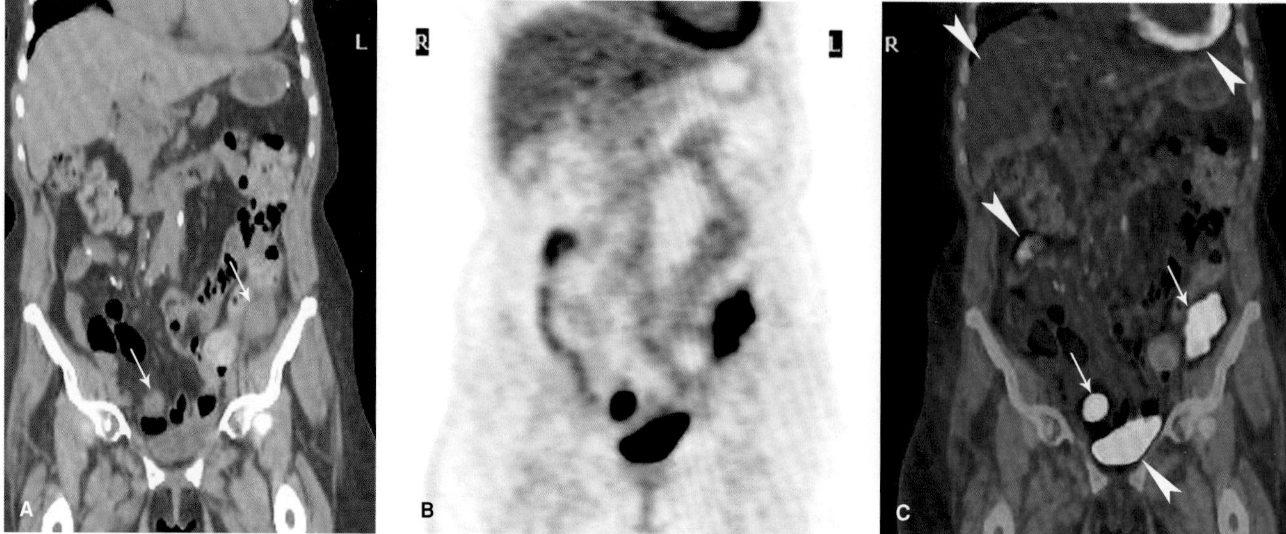

FIGURE 76.26. **Uterine Cancer Recurrence.** PET/CT images in a woman post total abdominal hysterectomy and bilateral oophorectomy for uterine cancer reveals recurrence of tumor in two locations (*arrows*). Physiologic activity (*arrowheads*) is seen in the bladder, liver, heart, and bowel. **A:** CT without contrast. **B:** Corrected PET. **C:** Fused PET/CT.

Ovarian Cancer. Hybrid PET-CT imaging is superior to CT or PET alone in staging and detecting recurrence of ovarian cancer (Fig. 76.27). However, small peritoneal metastases (<5 mm) can be missed with PET-CT without dedicated abdominal reconstructions. In addition, FDG PET provides whole-body screening for recurrent disease in patients with elevated cancer antigen 125. Focal ovarian uptake can be normal in premenstrual woman due to corpus luteal cysts. However, any focal ovarian uptake in a postmenopausal woman is considered abnormal and ultrasound should be performed. Multiplanar assessment is useful to follow the track of distal ureters in the pelvis to avoid mistaking ureteral activity for nodal metastases.

Renal Malignancies. Owing to high physiologic activity in the renal parenchyma and in the urinary collecting system, detection of hypermetabolic lesions in the genitourinary tract is challenging. The efficacy of FDG for further characterization of renal lesions detected by other modalities is expectedly low. However, FDG is outstanding in the detection of extrarenal involvement by renal carcinoma. FDG is used for the detection of normal-sized nodes that harbor malignancy as well as metastatic osseous foci. FDG PET is superior to Tc-99m methylene diphosphonate (MDP) bone scans in detection of lytic lesions, which may be cold on bone scan. FDG PET can also be used to detect recurrence in patients after nephrectomy.

Ureter and Urinary Bladder Malignancies. Limitations of FDG in the detection of bladder tumors are mainly caused by the presence of intense urinary FDG activity in the bladder (Fig. 76.28). However, FDG readily detects extravesical involvement. FDG PET is superior to CT and MR for the accurate detection of involved regional nodes and whole-body staging. Aggressive hydration, frequent voiding, and rinsing the bladder prior to PET scanning have been employed with limited success; however, continuous irrigation does demonstrate improved detection. If there is an obstructed nonfunctional kidney, a primary ureteral mass can be seen on FDG PET due to lack of excreted radiotracer in the collecting system.

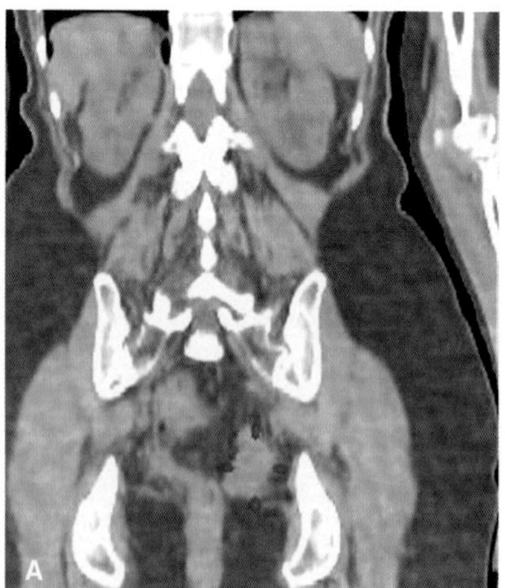

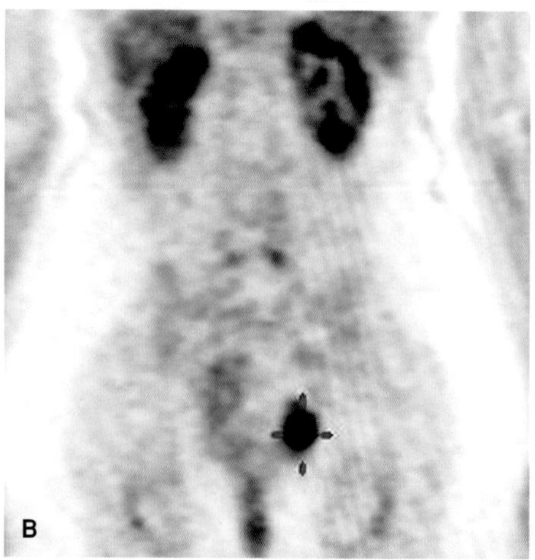

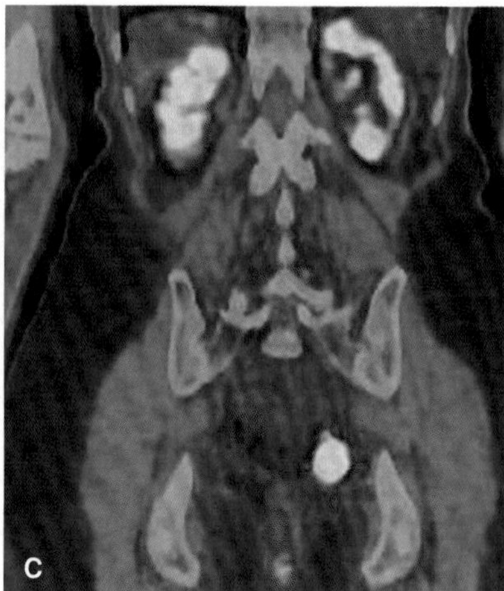

FIGURE 76.27. **Ovarian Cancer, Stage 1.** PET/CT shows a hypermetabolic focus in the left ovary (between *cursors*). Further evaluation confirmed an ovarian cancer confined to the ovary. Similar FDG activity may be seen in physiologic ovarian cysts. **A:** CT. **B:** Corrected PET. **C:** Fused PET/CT.

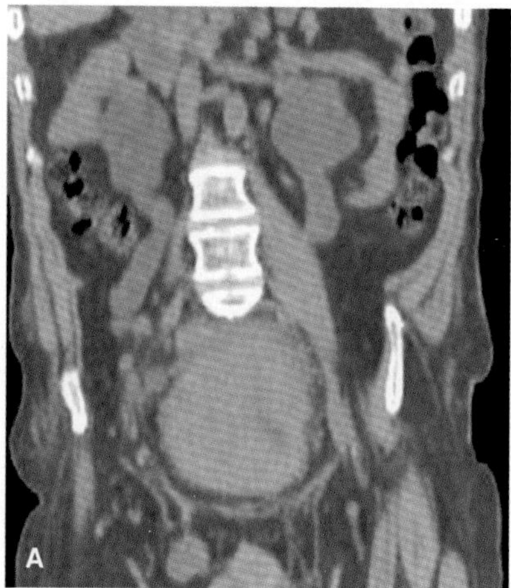

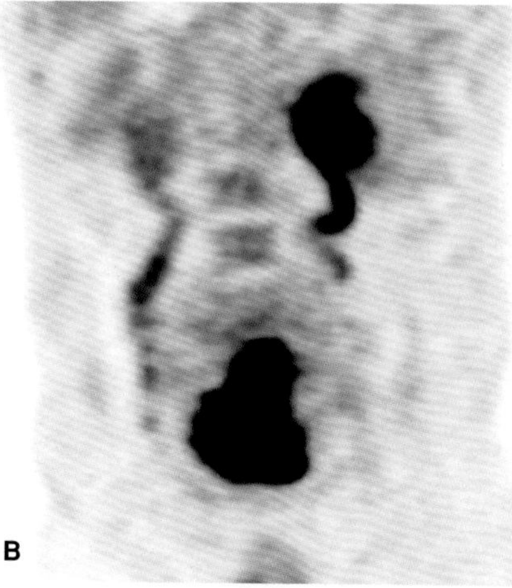

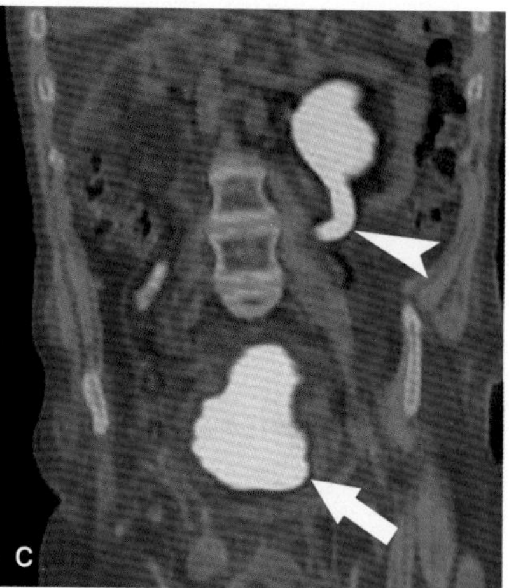

FIGURE 76.28. **Transitional Cell Carcinoma of the Bladder.** A large bladder tumor (*arrow*) shows fluorodeoxyglucose hyperactivity. Hydronephrosis of the left renal collecting system (*arrowhead*) caused by the obstructing bladder tumor is apparent. **A:** CT. **B:** Corrected PET. **C:** Fused PET/CT.

Adrenal Malignancy. Limited studies have shown some benefit to FDG PET in differentiating benign from malignant adrenal lesions (Figs. 76.29 and 76.30). CT and MR remain the imaging methods of choice to differentiate the common benign adrenal adenoma from adrenal metastases (see Chapter 48). FDG activity above vascular blood pool levels should be followed especially in the setting of a nodule by CT or MR. FDG activity above that of the liver is worrisome for malignant involvement.

Testicular Malignancies. PET is superb in the detection of testicular cancer metastatic deposits throughout the body, but it is difficult within the testis due to high physiologic activity that persists in men until old age. Seminoma is usually more FDG avid than nonseminoma, but PET is successfully used for both subtypes. Postoperative changes can pose difficulty in the interpretation of PET images. Also, urinary bladder activity can overshadow the pelvis, therefore some institutions give diuretics prior to imaging and have the patient void to clear FDG from the collective systems. Correlation with corresponding CT images is imperative for initial staging as well as for assessment for recurrence.

Prostate Cancer. FDG uptake is low in most prostate cancers, especially when the tumor is well differentiated. Because of its variable uptake, the value of FDG in the evaluation of prostate cancer has not been established. FDG has low sensitivity for the detection of osseous metastases caused by prostate cancer. Diffuse uptake within the prostate may be an indication of prostatitis whereas focal asymmetric uptake may indicate a high-grade malignancy versus focal prostatitis and should be followed with physical examination, serologic evaluation, and possible biopsy if indicated. However, there is great promise in PET imaging with new novel targeted agents, such as choline, fluciclovine, and PSMA-directed agents in prostate cancer (see below).

Head and Neck Malignancies. Common malignancies of the head and neck including squamous cell cancer of the mucosal surfaces and adenocarcinoma of salivary and lacrimal glands are well evaluated by PET, as these are among the most intensely hypermetabolic malignancies (Fig. 76.31). PET/CT is extremely sensitive and specific for the detection of disease, with a sensitivity of 98%, specificity of 92%, and an accuracy of 94%. PET/CT is highly sensitive for not only the lymph node metastases in these cases, but also in the detection of occult primary malignancy as well as metastatic disease (Fig. 76.32).

In comparison with other anatomic regions, PET evaluation of the head and neck is challenging owing to common intense physiologic uptake in areas including the brain, extraocular and facial muscles, tonsils, vocal cords, and in brown fat. Furthermore, mildly hypermetabolic reactive lymphadenopathy in the head and neck is a common finding. PET is excellent for the detection of recurrence, but interpretation of postoperative and postradiation changes is challenging. Because inflammation in the treatment bed causes PET activity, posttreatment PET scans are best delayed for 2 to 3 months after therapy.

Sarcomas and Osseous Malignancies. PET has become the standard of care in staging and restaging many types of soft tissue sarcomas and primary bony tumors. Oligometastatic disease is common in these patients, which can be treated with locoregional therapies including radiation and surgery. In considering the likelihood of metastatic disease, the distribution of hypermetabolism should be carefully considered. In particular, periarticular osseous hypermetabolism is generally more likely to represent arthritis (Fig. 76.33). In addition, diffuse skeletal uptake can be seen with bone marrow stimulation (Fig. 76.34). Multifocal FDG uptake and/or CT is helpful to differentiate this from diffuse osseous metastases (Fig. 76.35).

In considering the role of PET in evaluating for osseous metastatic disease (Figs. 76.36 and 76.37), the underlying primary malignancy should be considered. While PET is highly sensitive in many diseases including breast cancer and myeloma, in other diseases, most notably prostate cancer, bone scintigraphy is a better examination.

Neuroendocrine Tumors. Neuroendocrine tumors most commonly arise from the pancreas or midgut and are best evaluated by nuclear imaging techniques. In general, low-grade neuroendocrine tumors are better evaluated using somatostatin receptor–directed agents such as In-111 pentetreotide or Ga-68 DOTATATE (Fig. 76.38). Conversely, in high-grade tumors, evaluation with FDG PET is more sensitive. Importantly, high- and low-grade tumors can coexist in the same patient. Therefore, both imaging techniques are considered important in these cases, for detection of metastatic disease as well as selection of appropriate therapy. One emerging application of this technique is in the field of theranostics, where uptake of a somatostatin receptor–directed nuclear imaging agent can be used to predict the response of a therapeutic agent such as Lu-177 DOTATATE.

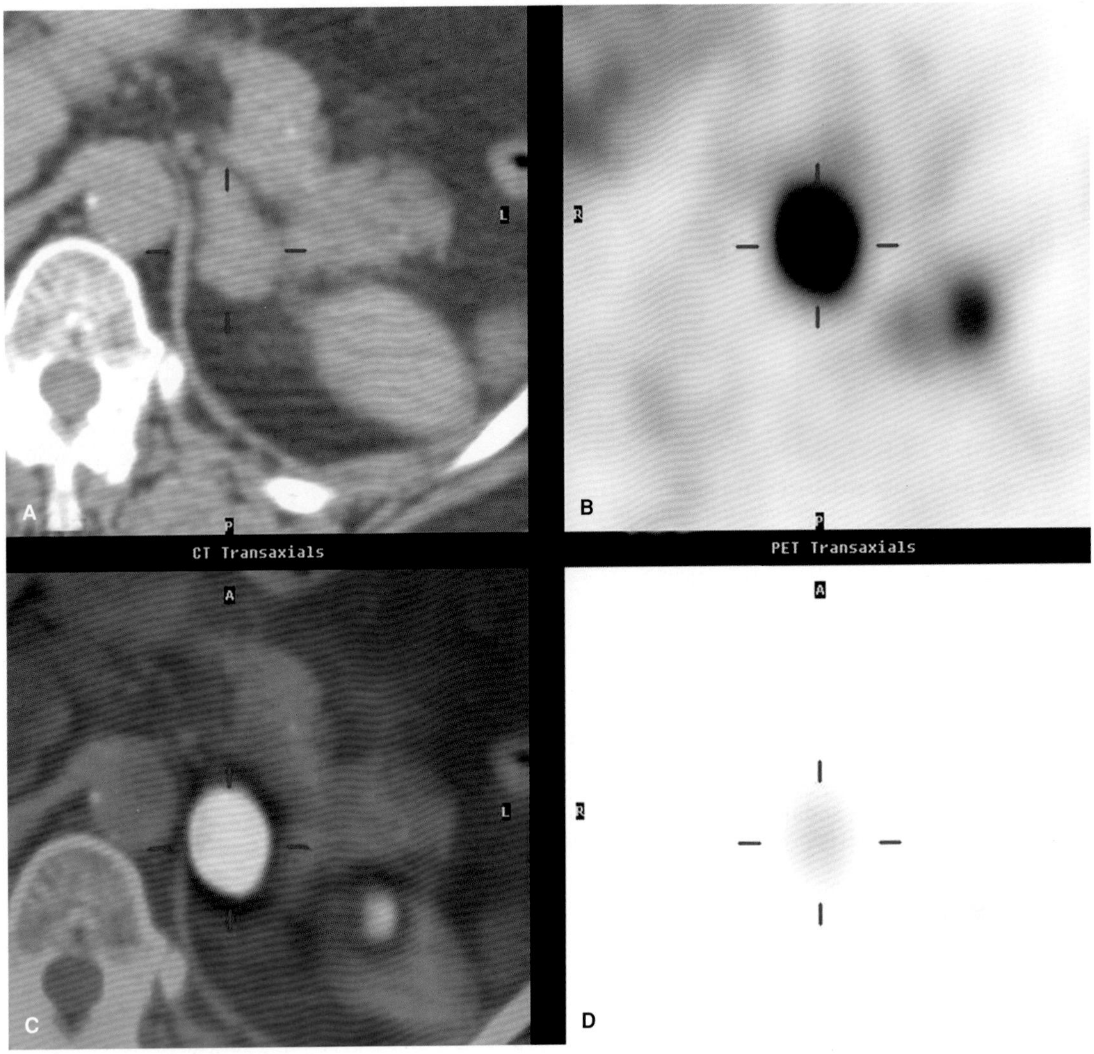

FIGURE 76.29. **Adrenal Metastasis.** PET/CT of a patient with a history of lung cancer shows a focus of FDG activity in the left adrenal gland (between *cursors*). Biopsy confirmed metastatic disease. This was the only site of disease recurrence in this patient. **A:** CT. **B:** Corrected PET. **C:** Fused PET/CT. **D:** Uncorrected PET.

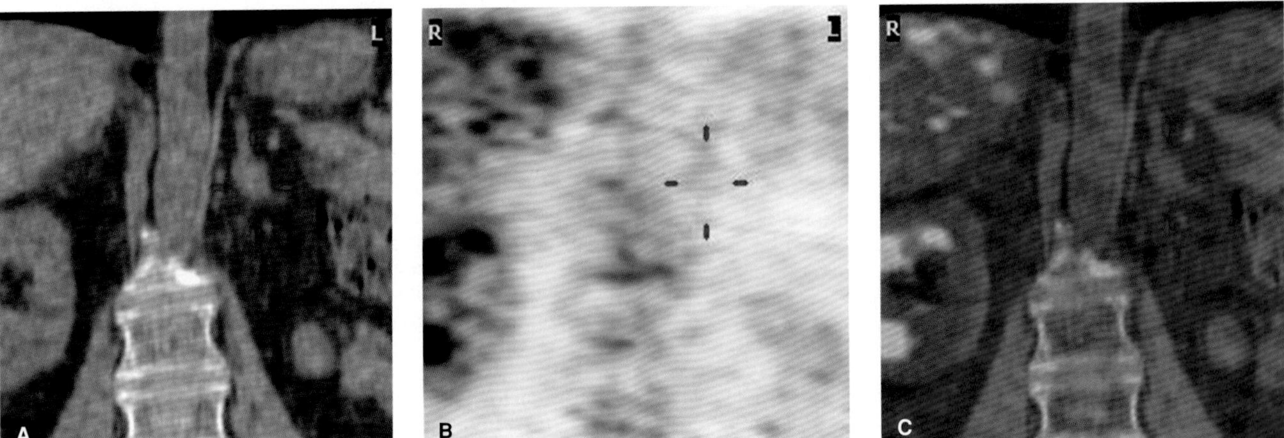

FIGURE 76.30. **Benign Adrenal Adenoma.** PET-CT of a patient with a history of colon cancer reveals enlargement of the left adrenal gland (between *cursors*). PET shows a hypometabolic lesion compatible with benign adrenal adenoma. Adrenal protocol CT was confirmatory. **A:** CT. **B:** Corrected PET. **C:** Fused PET-CT.

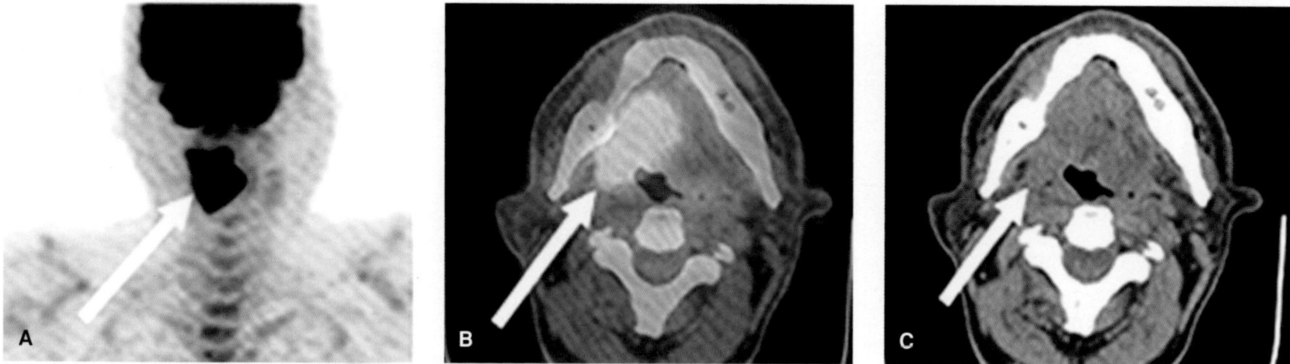

FIGURE 76.31. **Squamous Cell Carcinoma of the Tongue.** PET-CT shows that the tumor is localized to the primary site (*arrows*) on the right base of the tongue without evidence of metastatic disease. **A:** PET MIPS. **B:** Fused PET-CT. **C:** Noncontrast CT.

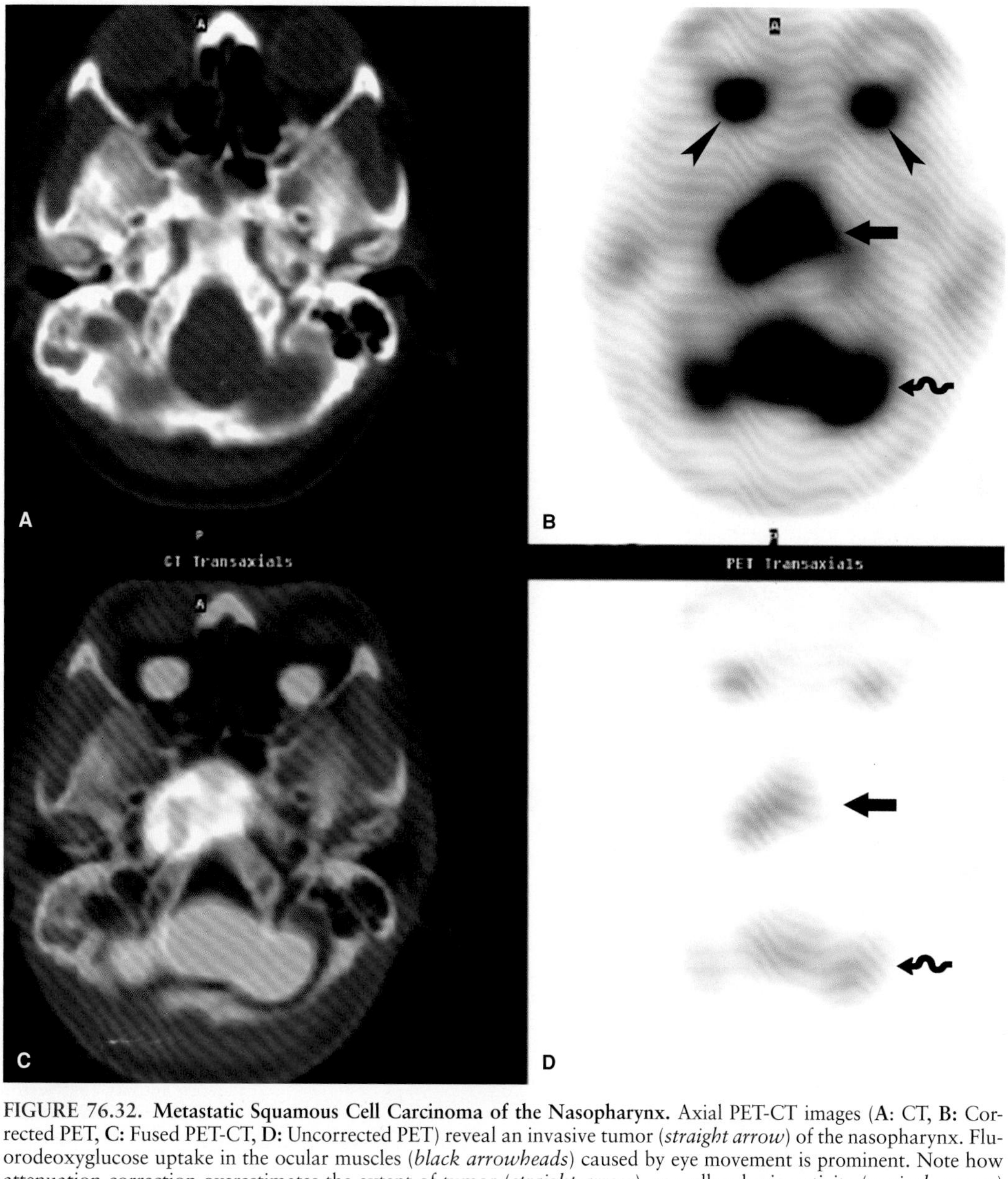

FIGURE 76.32. **Metastatic Squamous Cell Carcinoma of the Nasopharynx.** Axial PET-CT images (**A:** CT, **B:** Corrected PET, **C:** Fused PET-CT, **D:** Uncorrected PET) reveal an invasive tumor (*straight arrow*) of the nasopharynx. Fluorodeoxyglucose uptake in the ocular muscles (*black arrowheads*) caused by eye movement is prominent. Note how attenuation correction overestimates the extent of tumor (*straight arrow*), as well as brain activity (*squiggly arrow*) in **B** and **C** as compared to the uncorrected PET image (**D**). Careful correlation with CT and other imaging studies is needed for accurate interpretation. (*continued*)

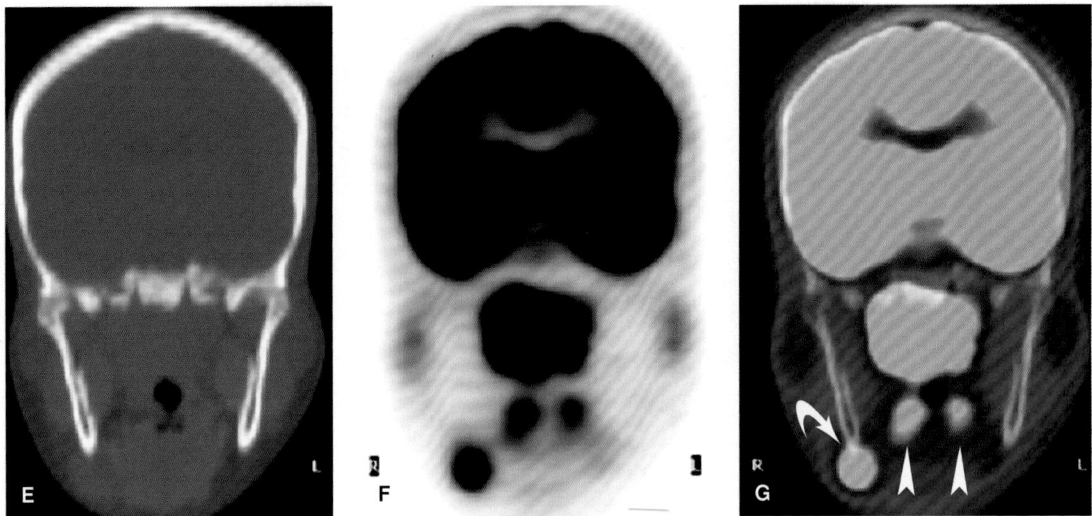

FIGURE 76.32. (*Continued*) Coronal-plane PET-CT images (**E:** CT, **F:** Corrected PET, **G:** Fused PET-CT) show metastatic spread of tumor to the nasopharyngeal lymph nodes (*white arrowheads*) and the mandible (*curved arrow*).

PET IMAGING IN INFLAMMATION AND INFECTION

Since hypermetabolism on PET is not specific to tumors and is seen in inflammatory and infectious conditions, it can be used for detection of these orders as well.

Fever of unknown origin (FUO) is defined as recurrent fevers without apparent cause recurring over a period of at least 3 weeks. This condition carries a wide differential diagnosis including both infectious and neoplastic causes. Whole-body PET is a useful examination in detecting both of these causes.

Sarcoidosis is a relatively common inflammatory disorder involving many sites of disease including skin, lungs, lymph nodes,

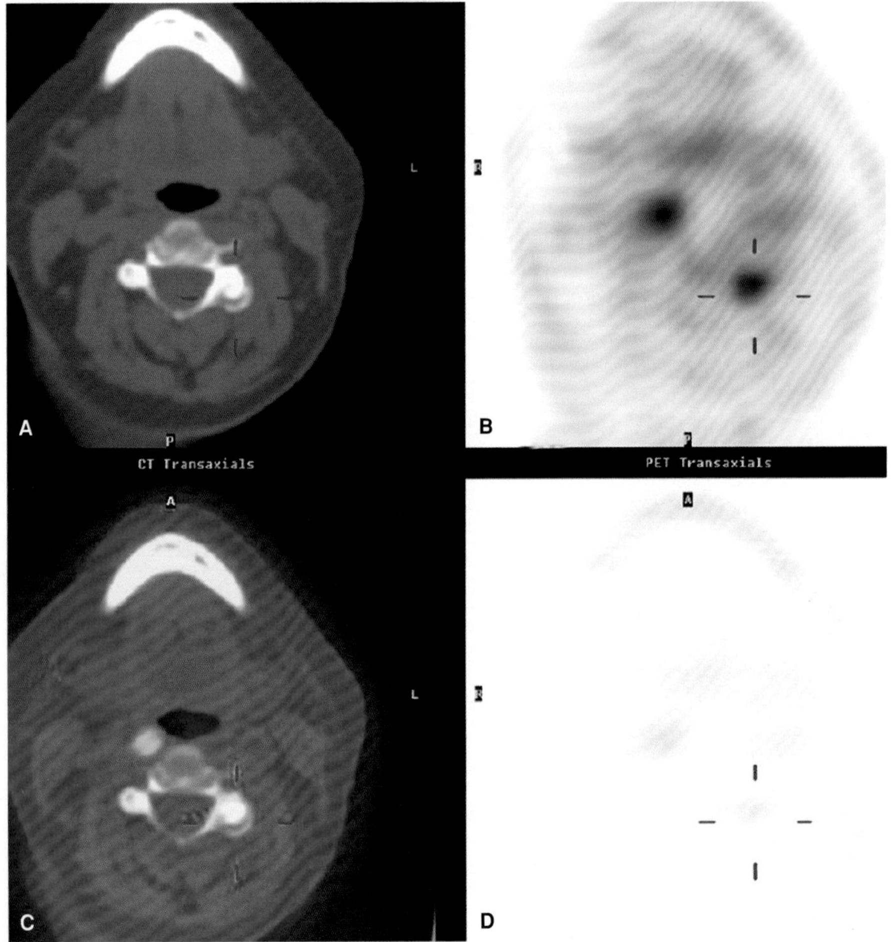

FIGURE 76.33. **Facet Hypertrophy, Not Metastasis.** PET-CT in a patient with breast cancer demonstrates focal fluorodeoxyglucose activity (between *cursors*) in the cervical spine. Correlation of PET with CT confirms that the activity represents benign inflammation associated with degenerative disease in the facet joint. **A:** CT. **B:** Corrected PET. **C:** Fused PET-CT. **D:** Uncorrected PET.

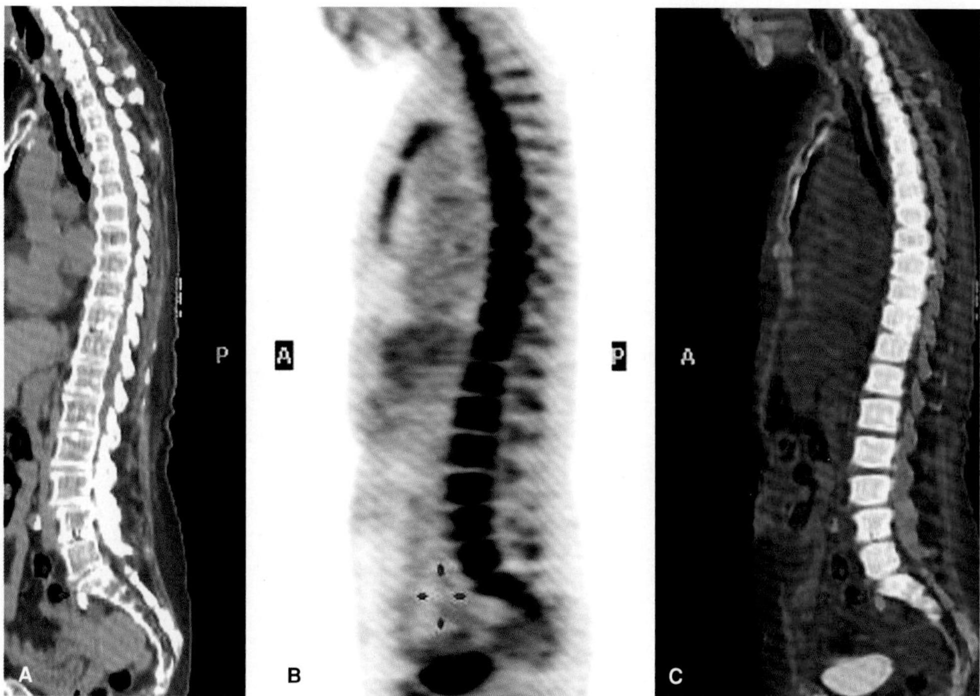

FIGURE 76.34. **Benign Hypermetabolic Bone Marrow.** Marked diffuse fluorodeoxyglucose uptake is seen throughout the spine on PET in a patient with colon cancer. Correlation with the CT scan shows no evidence of metastatic disease. These findings are indicative of diffuse marrow stimulation related to recovery from chemotherapy or marrow-stimulating drugs. **A:** CT. **B:** Corrected PET. **C:** Fused PET-CT.

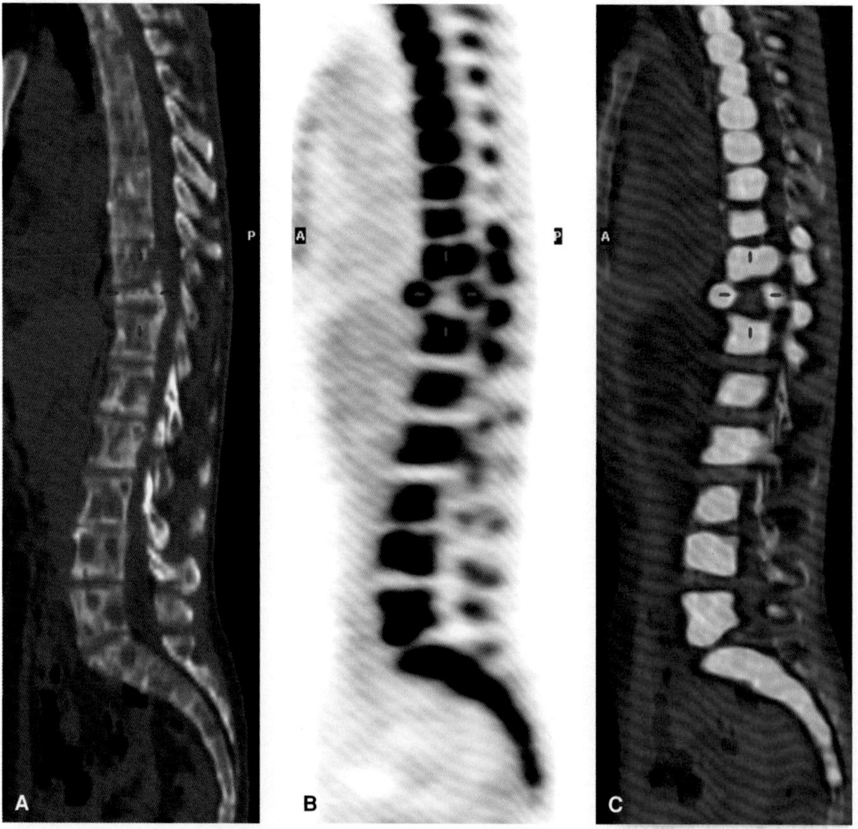

FIGURE 76.35. **Diffuse Metastatic Disease With Hypermetabolic Bone Marrow.** Compare with Figure 76.34. In this patient with breast cancer, advanced lytic destructive change is evident throughout the spine on CT. PET shows diffuse marrow hyperactivity, representing both hypermetabolic marrow stimulation and osseous metastatic disease. **A:** CT. **B:** Corrected PET. **C:** Fused PET-CT. Crosshairs highlight a pathologic compression deformity of the thoracic vertebral body.

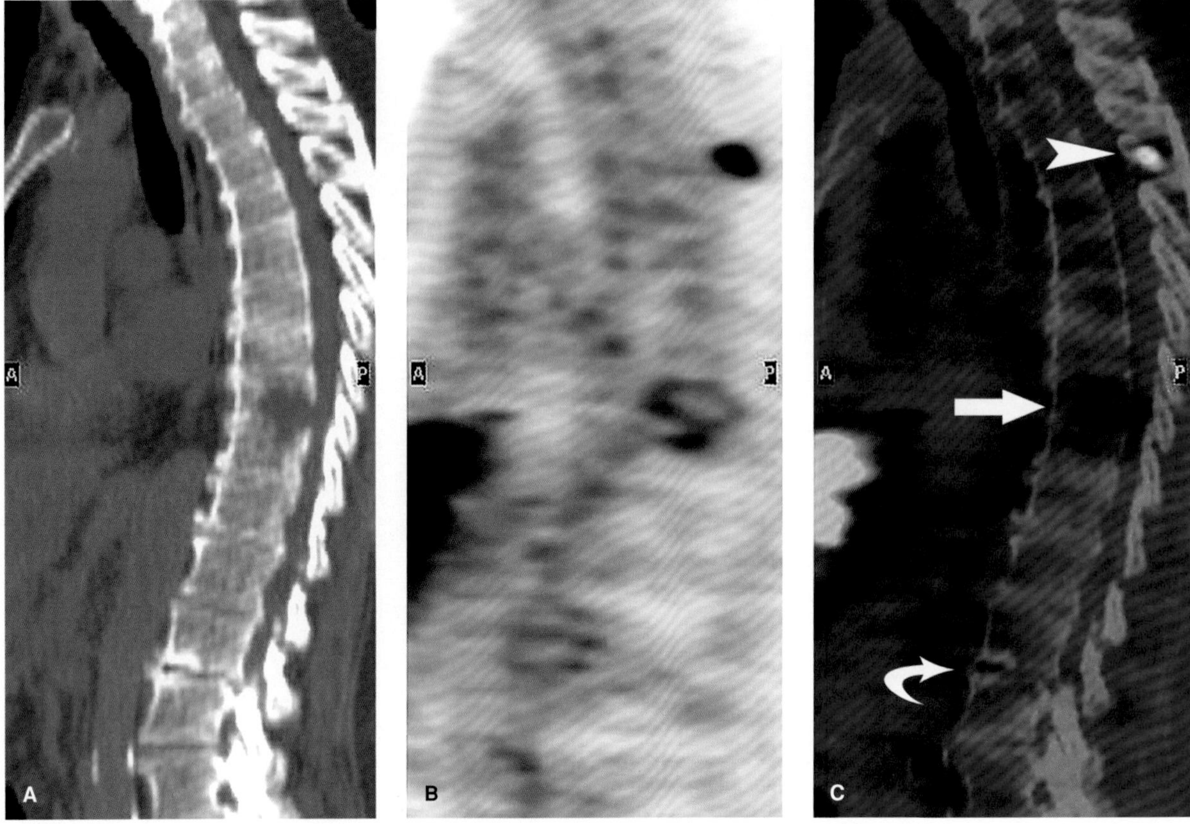

FIGURE 76.36. **"Hot" and "Cold" Osseous Metastases.** PET-CT of the spine in another patient with breast cancer reveals an osseous metastasis with high fluorodeoxyglucose (FDG) activity (*arrowhead*), a metastasis that is obviously destructive on CT but hypometabolic on PET (*straight arrow*), and degenerative change (*curved arrow*) that shows no FDG uptake. **A:** CT. **B:** Corrected PET. **C:** Fused PET-CT.

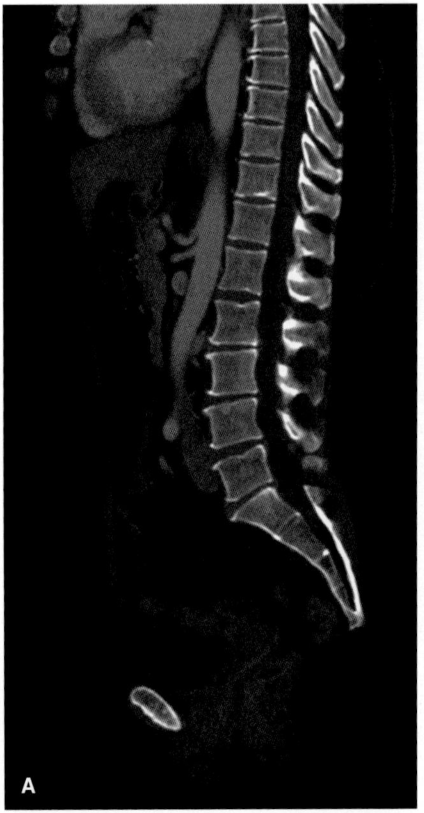

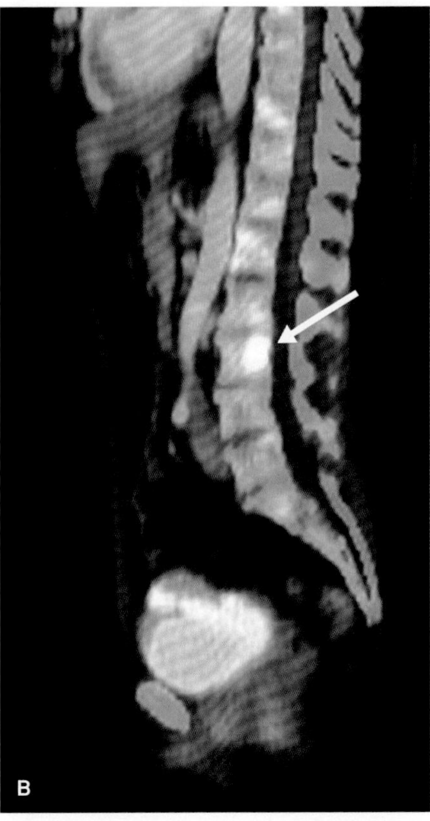

FIGURE 76.37. **FDG avid osseous metastasis.** A 43-year-old woman with new diagnosis of breast cancer. Sagittal CT scan through the lumbar spine (**A**) disclosed no evidence of metastatic disease. PET/CT (**B**) demonstrates a hypermetabolic metastasis (*arrow*) at the posterior aspect of the L3 vertebral body.

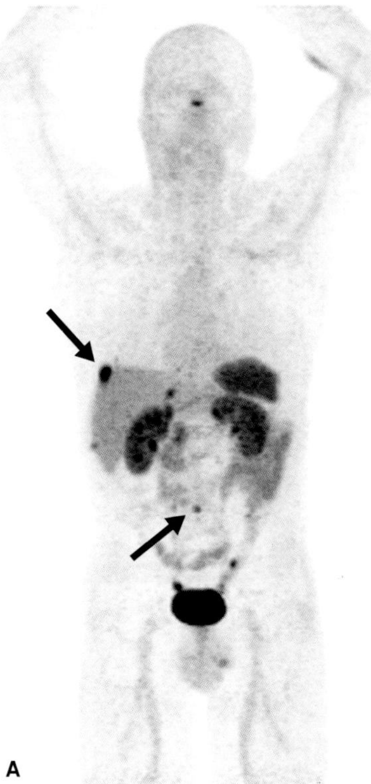

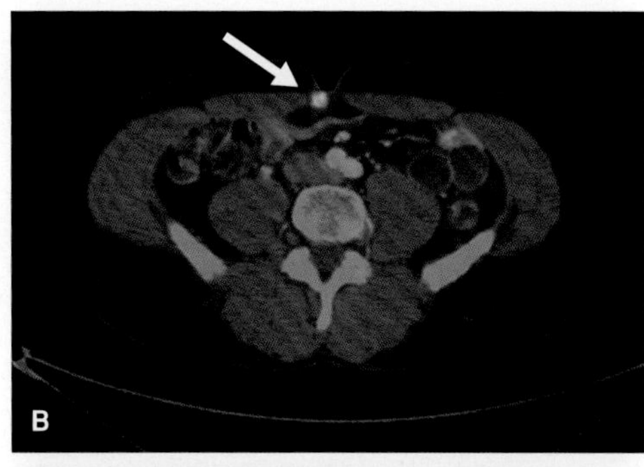

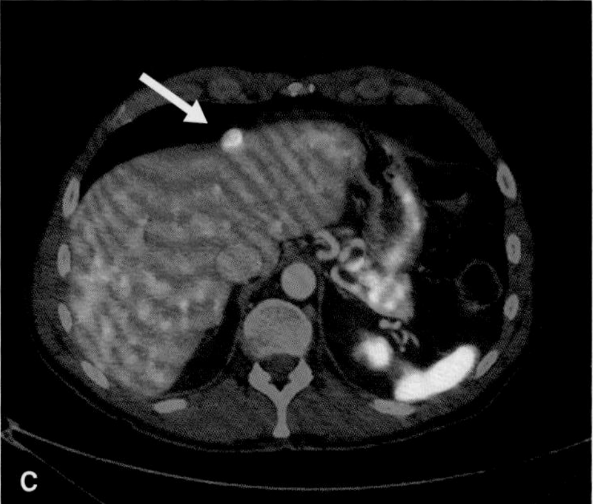

FIGURE 76.38. **Somatostatin Receptor Avid Metastases.** A 61-year-old man with history of carcinoid. ^{68}Ga-DOTATOC PET/CT maximum intensity projection (**A**) demonstrates multiple areas (*black arrows*) of uptake scattered throughout the abdomen, in addition to the normal physiologic uptake in the pituitary and adrenal glands, spleen, liver, kidneys, and bladder. PET/CT fusion images (**B**, **C**) demonstrate that the abnormal areas of uptake correspond with peritoneal nodules and are therefore consistent with peritoneal metastatic disease (*white arrows*).

and the heart. FDG uptake correlates with disease activity and thus can be used to determine the extent of disease, if and when treatment is indicated, and the response to treatment in patients with known sarcoidosis. One area where PET has proven particularly useful is in monitoring cardiac involvement (Fig. 76.39), which is relatively uncommon but often life-threatening due to the arrhythmias that are caused. In these cases, FDG-PET imaging is compared with myocardial perfusion images, with active sites of disease often manifesting as intense hypermetabolism with a matching perfusion defect. In these cases, proper dietary preparation with a high-fat, low-carbohydrate diet is essential to minimize false-positive cardiac uptake.

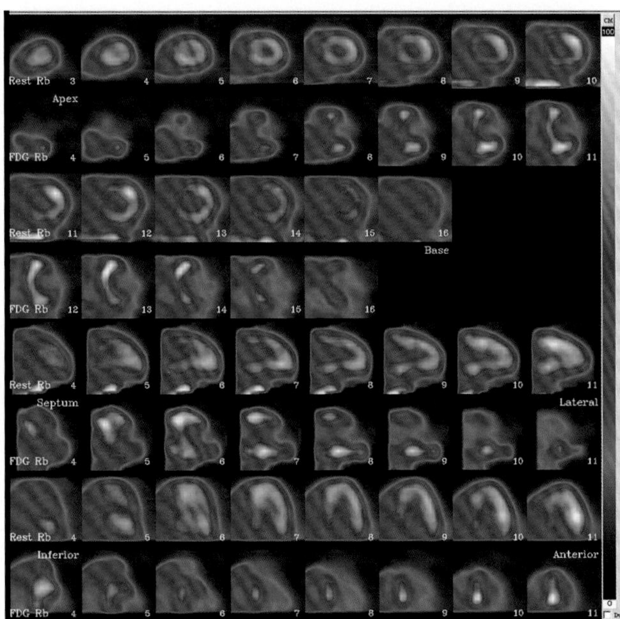

FIGURE 76.39. **Cardiac Sarcoidosis.** A 46-year-old man presented with ventricular tachycardia and normal cardiac catheterization. A cardiac sarcoid protocol PET study demonstrated perfusion defects at the base of the interventricular septum and inferior wall (*top row*), with matching areas of increased hypermetabolism (*bottom row*). A subsequent biopsy confirmed cardiac sarcoid.

PITFALLS IN PET CT

Physiologic activity, reflecting normal glucose metabolism, is seen in numerous organs and muscles as described previously (Figs. 76.2 to 76.7). Any focus of FDG activity must be scrutinized as a possible site of normal physiologic activity.

Brown Fat. It is critical to match any FDG uptake on the PET to the CT, especially in patients at risk for nodal lesions such as lymphoma and breast cancer (see Fig. 76.9). While the typical appearance is symmetric neck, supraspinatus, and paraspinous in the distribution, one should be aware of the atypical presentations including intraatrial and paraadrenal.

Inflammatory processes result in increased glucose metabolism and therefore will have increased FDG uptake. Therefore, infection and inflammatory processes must be considered in the differential diagnosis of any hypermetabolic lesions (Fig. 76.21). Correlation with clinical history and CT findings is essential for recognition. Arthritis is a common cause of uptake in the hips, knees, and shoulders (Fig. 76.40) and in the sternoclavicular, acromioclavicular, and spinal facet joints (Fig. 76.33). Pneumonia and radiation pneumonitis show variable FDG activity in the lungs (Fig. 76.13). Sarcoidosis is associated with heterogeneous uptake in areas of involvement. Hemorrhoid uptake is related to acute inflammation. Patients receiving chemotherapy are immunosuppressed and may develop infections in unusual sites.

Immunotherapy has emerged as a key therapeutic modality in many cancers, most notably in melanoma. These therapies

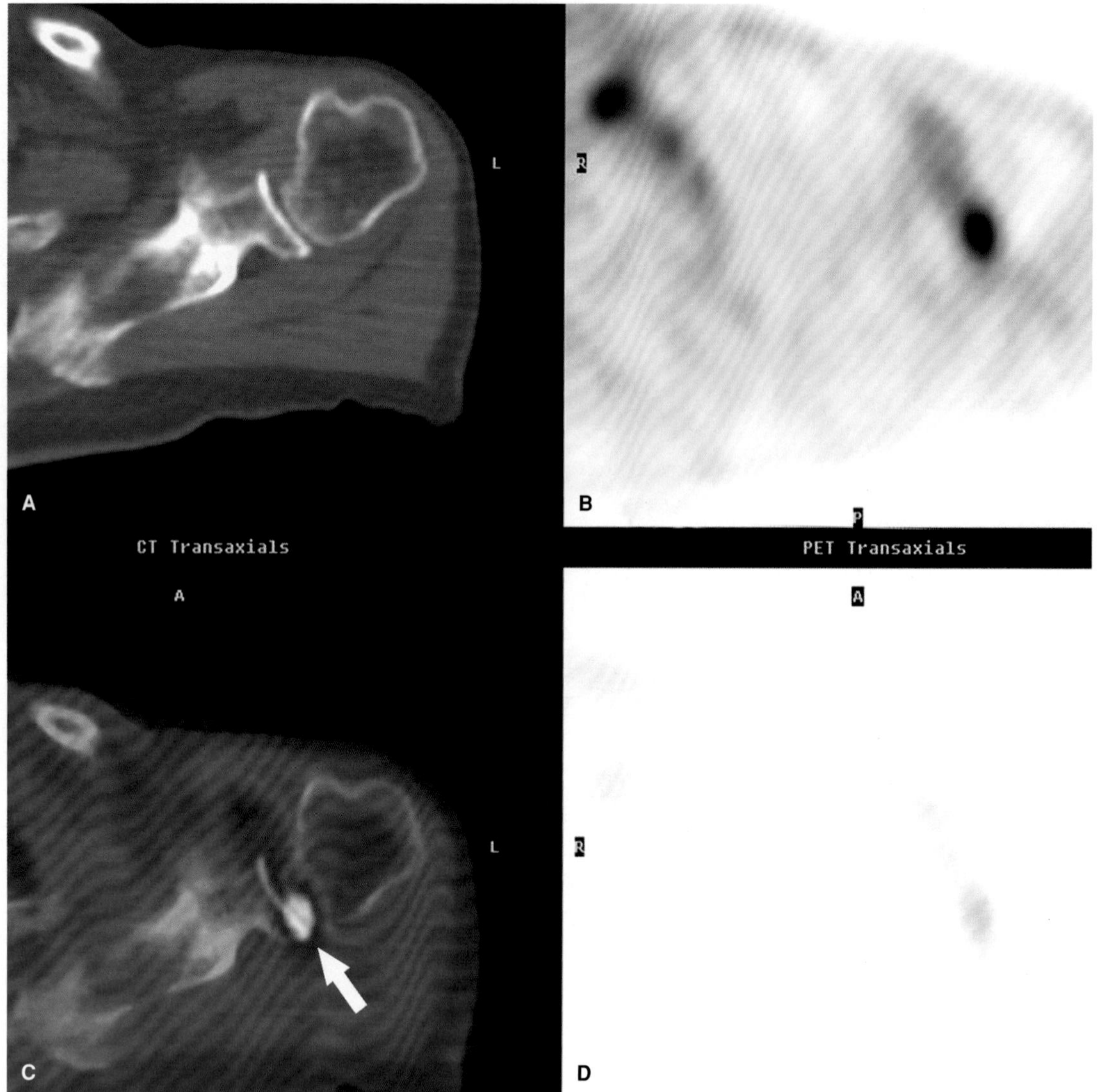

FIGURE 76.40. **Shoulder Arthritis.** PET-CT shows intense fluorodeoxyglucose activity (*arrow*) confined to the shoulder joint, indicative of inflammation rather than metastatic disease. **A:** CT. **B:** Corrected PET. **C:** Fused PET-CT. **D:** Uncorrected PET.

can produce a very complex imaging pattern and in these cases it can be difficult to distinguish true progression of disease from treatment-related effects. For example, extensive hypermetabolic lymphadenopathy and sarcoid-like reactions are common and can be difficult or impossible to distinguish confidently from metastatic disease. Other inflammatory side effects are commonly seen, including hypophysitis, adrenalitis, colitis (Fig. 76.41), and synovitis. These side effects are commonly seen on scans immediately after initiation of immunotherapy.

Benign tumors may also concentrate on FDG. FDG hyperactivity is not specific for malignant neoplasia. Examples of benign FDG avid tumors include hibernoma and fibroelastomas.

Recent Surgery. Any trauma can result in FDG uptake, including healing surgical sites. This uptake is related to increased metabolism and inflammatory response associated with tissue repair. Surgical sites such as tracheotomies, sternotomies (activity persists for 6 months), and joint prosthesis healing (which must be differentiated from infection) can be challenging to assess on FDG PET.

Fractures can demonstrate FDG uptake for weeks while fracture healing occurs (Fig. 76.42). Uptake is related to the hematoma evolution along with the granulation tissue and callous formation. Correlation with CT reviewed on bone windows is usually diagnostic.

Low Uptake by Malignant Tumors. A number of malignant lesions show little to no FDG activity and may be missed on PET scans. These include lobular carcinoma of the breast, low-grade lymphoma, salivary gland neoplasms, many prostate cancers, adenocarcinoma in situ of the lung, carcinoid tumors, and extensively necrotic primary tumors and lymph nodes.

Attenuation correction artifacts appear as artifactual foci of apparently increased PET activity on attenuation-corrected PET images. These are induced by any highly attenuating object, including metallic joint prostheses, fracture fixation rods, vertebroplasty sites, cardiac pacemakers, dental devices, concentrations of oral contrast, and contrast-enhanced blood vessels. Attenuation-correction software overcorrects photopenic areas seen on CT adjacent to the highly attenuating objects. The artifact is accentuated when the patient moves between the

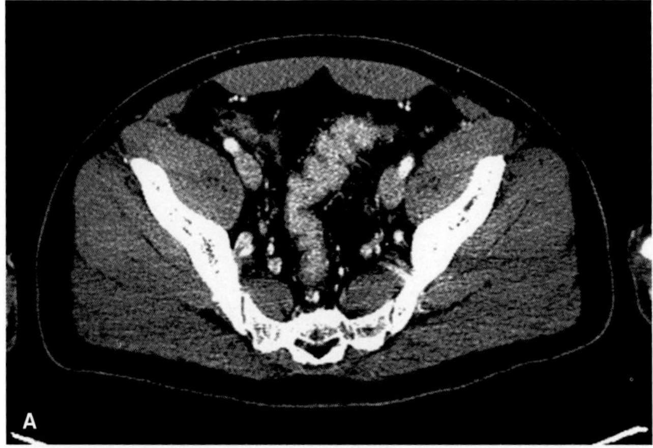

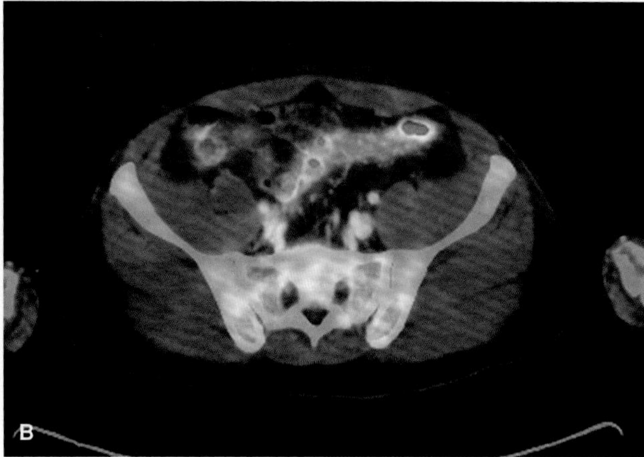

FIGURE 76.41. **FDG-PET/CT Immunotherapy-Associated Colitis.** The patient was under treatment with pembrolizumab and had been experiencing diarrhea since initiation of therapy. CT (**A**) and PET/CT fusion (**B**) demonstrate hypermetabolic sigmoid colon wall thickening and hypermetabolism, consistent with immunotherapy-induced colitis.

emission (PET) and transmission (CT) scans. This artifact is recognized by identifying that the high-activity focus appears adjacent to a high-attenuation object shown on the CT scan. Attenuation-uncorrected PET images show a photopenic defect in the same area. The artifact is limited by attenuation-weighted iterative reconstruction algorithms used on some systems.

Misregistration. Since the CT and PET are acquired at separate time points, misregistration of the PET findings with the CT should always be considered. The most common etiologies of misregistration is seen in the lung and bowel. Misregistration of bowel activity occurs when peristalsis displaces bowel contents between the PET scan and the CT scan. Artefactual foci of increased or decreased activity are seen adjacent to bowel on PET images. This pitfall is recognized by carefully correlating the CT images with the PET images. Patient movement between the CT and PET acquisitions causes misregistration of FDG activity on the fusion images. This is also commonly seen with breathing misregistration between the CT and PET data sets. Since the PET can take up to 2 to 3 minutes in most instances, there will be some degree of misregistration in the lung bases and upper abdomen compared to the CT. When one encounters a focus of uptake on the PET, they should always carefully inspect the CT images both above and below the suspected area for any CT correlate including lesions in the upper abdomen.

CT truncation artifacts occur as a result of objects outside the CT field of view. These appear as a series of dark lines on the attenuation-corrected PET images. This artifact is most commonly seen in obese patients or those who move their arms or legs during the long PET-CT scan time. The attenuation-correction algorithm does not correct for attenuation of CT x-rays by objects or tissues outside the field of view.

Thymic Rebound. The normal thymus regresses during adolescence, becoming diffusely fatty infiltrated. Thymic cell death may be induced by chemotherapy or corticosteroids. Following cessation of therapy, the thymus commonly rebounds, returning to soft tissue density on CT and demonstrating moderate-to-high FDG activity (Fig. 76.43). This phenomenon should not be confused with lymphoma or nodal metastatic disease.

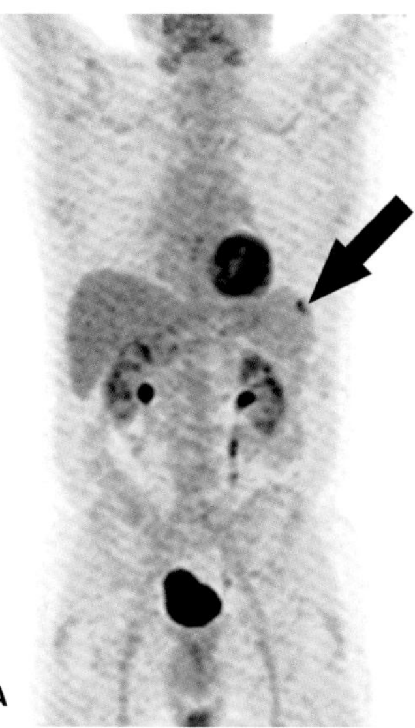

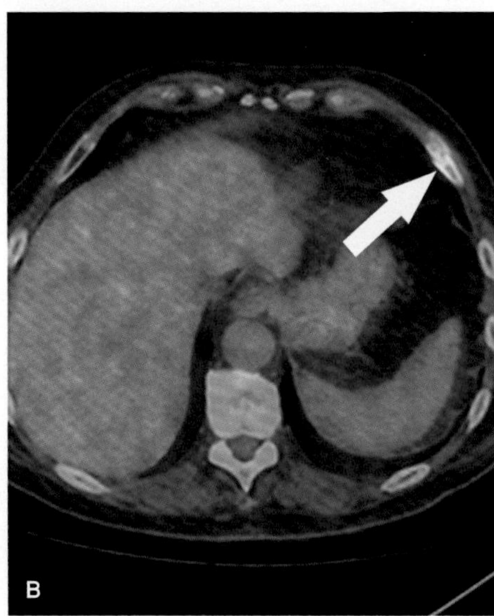

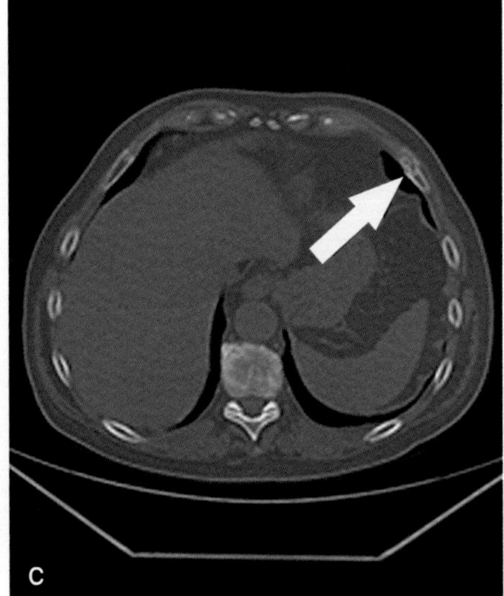

FIGURE 76.42. **Rib Fracture. A:** PET MIPS. **B:** Fused PET-CT. **C:** CT. Images show a focus of hyperactivity (*arrow*) in a left rib.

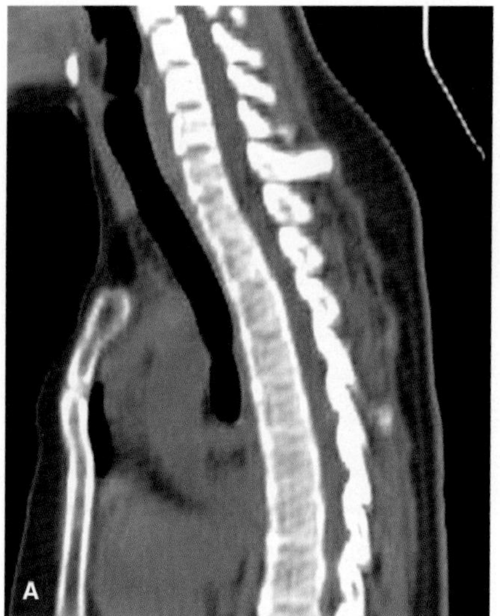

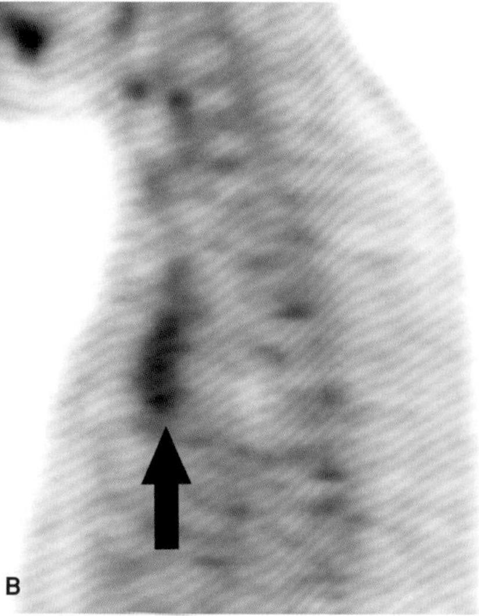

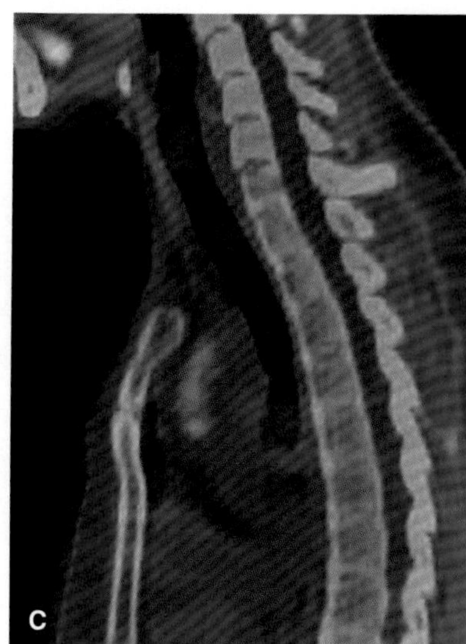

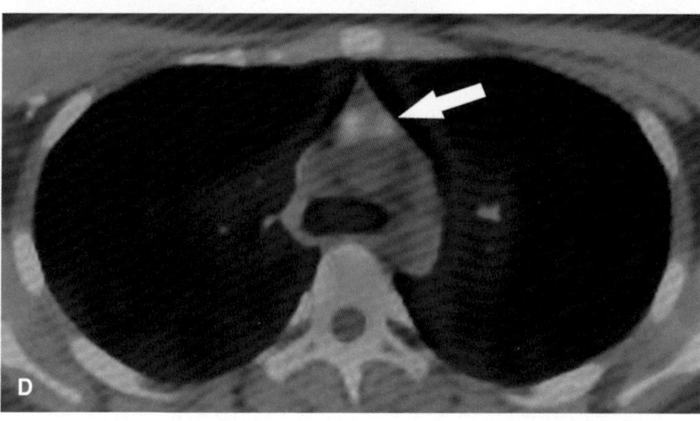

FIGURE 76.43. **Thymic Rebound.** On this follow-up scan of a patient examined following the completion of chemotherapy for colon carcinoma, the thymus (*arrows*) shows fluorodeoxyglucose hyperactivity and has become soft tissue density on CT. This is a common event following chemotherapy. **A:** Sagittal CT. **B:** Sagittal PET, corrected. **C:** Sagittal fused PET-CT. **D:** Axial fused PET-CT.

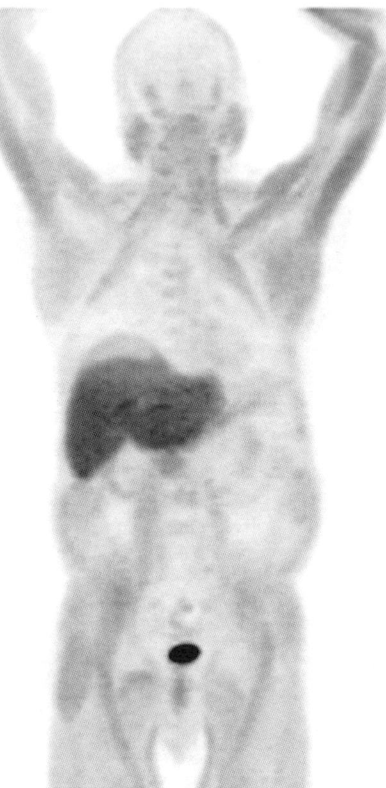

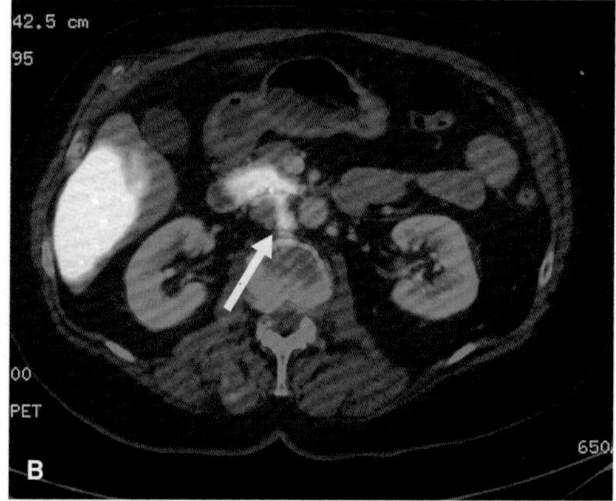

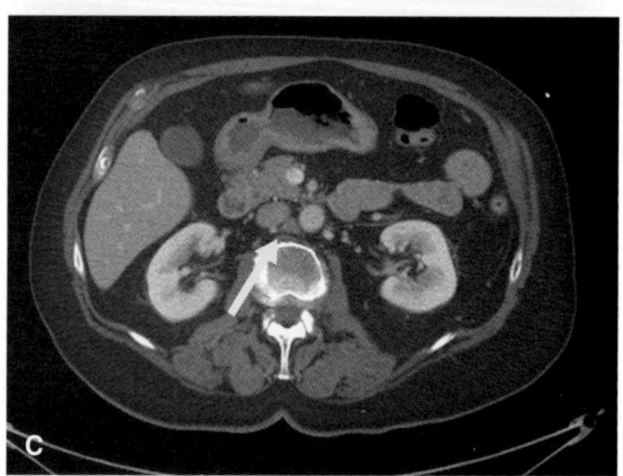

FIGURE 76.44. **F-18 Fluciclovine, PET/CT.** A 73-year-old man with biochemical recurrence of prostate cancer after radical prostatectomy underwent ^{18}F-fluciclovine PET/CT. Whole-body maximum intensity projection (**A**) demonstrates normal biodistribution including muscle, bladder, liver, and pancreas. However, close inspection of PET/CT fusion (**B**) and CT images (**C**) demonstrates radiotracer uptake within a borderline enlarged retroperitoneal lymph node (*arrow*), therefore consistent with metastatic disease.

Osteophytes develop in the vertebral column and from joints. They may be metabolically active and take up FDG, mimicking paravertebral adenopathy.

Injection Leakage. FDG uptake may be seen at the injection site or within lymph nodes that drain the injection site if skin infiltration occurs during FDG injection or if thrombus is present at the tip of an indwelling catheter.

Medications. Some medications can alter the distribution of FDG uptake. For example, metformin can lead to prominent FDG uptake in the right lower quadrant bowel, which can mimic enterocolitis.

EMERGING TRACERS

Currently, the yardstick of PET imaging is measured against FDG and for good reason. F-18 FDG has tremendous versatility in imaging for diagnosis, pretreatment, and posttreatment scenarios. However, FDG is not the perfect tracer for all disorders and as such, it does have its limitations. For example, FDG is limited in the evaluation of well-differentiated neuroendocrine tumors, and for these lesions somatostatin receptor–targeting agents such as Ga-68 DOTATATE are far more sensitive (see section Neuroendocrine Tumor). Furthermore, in prostate cancer, FDG PET is insensitive and for this reason, other tracers such as choline, fluciclovine, and prostate-specific membrane antigen–binding derivatives have emerged.

Fluciclovine. F-18 fluciclovine, also known as anti-1-amino-3-F-18-fluorocyclobutane-1-carboxylic acid (FACBC), is a leucine analog, which is primarily taken up by amino acid transporters. This compound was recently approved for imaging in prostate cancer, and has an advantage of having little or no genitourinary clearance at the early time points typically used for imaging. Normal biodistribution includes muscle, liver, and pancreas (Fig. 76.44). The primary use of this tracer is in patients with new diagnosis of high-risk prostate cancer, and those with biochemical relapse after definitive therapy. In the latter case, detection of sites of disease allows for delivery of locoregional therapy such as radiation treatment.

Prostate-Specific Membrane Antigen (PSMA). There are several forms of PSMA-based PET imaging agents with both Ga-68 and F-18 radionucleotides. Preliminary studies with these agents have shown great promise in imaging all phases of prostate cancer staging. While it is primarily been investigated in prostate cancer, PSMA expression is seen in other benign and malignant processes such as fibrous dysplasia, lymphoma, and squamous cell carcinoma of the head and neck.

Suggested Readings

Basu S, Hess S, Nielsen Braad PE, Olsen BB, Inglev S, Høilund-Carlsen PF. The basic principles of FDG-PET/CT imaging. *PET Clin* 2014;9(4):355–370.

Blodgett TM, Fufui MB, Snyderman CH, et al. Combined PET-CT in the head and neck: part 1. Physiologic, altered physiologic, and artifactual FDG uptake. *Radiographics* 2005a;25(4):897–912.

Blodgett TM, Fufui MB, Snyderman CH, et al. Combined PET-CT in the head and neck: part 2. Diagnostic uses and pitfalls of oncologic imaging. *Radiographics* 2005b;25(4):913–930.

Bouchelouche K, Choyke PL. PET/computed tomography in renal, bladder and testicular cancer. *PET Clin* 2015;10(3):361–374.

Cheson BD. PET/CT in lymphoma: Current overview and future directions. *Semin Nucl Med* 2018;48(1):76–81.

Deroose CM, Hindié E, Kebebew E, et al. Molecular imaging of gastroenteropancreatic neuroendocrine tumors: current status and future directions. *J Nucl Med* 2016;57(12):1949–1956.

Dibble EH, Yoo DC, Noto RB. Role of PET/CT in workup of fever without a source. *Radiographics* 2016;36(4):1166–1177.

Dunphy MP, Lewis JS. Radiopharmaceuticals in preclinical and clinical development for monitoring of therapy by PET. *J Nucl Med* 2009;50(Suppl 1):106S–121S.

Eubank WB, Mankoff DA, Takasugi J, et al. 18Fluorodeoxyglucose positron emission tomography to detect mediastinal or internal mammary metastases in breast cancer. *J Clin Oncol* 2001;19(15):3516–3523.

Flavell RR, Naeger DM, Aparici CM, Hawkins RA, Pampaloni MH, Behr SC. Malignancies with Low Fluorodeoxyglucose Uptake at PET/CT: Pitfalls and prognostic importance: Resident and fellow education feature. *Radiographics* 2016;36(1):293–294.

Flechsig P, Mehndiratta A, Haberkorn U, Kratochwil C, Giesel FL. PET/MRI and PET/CT in lung lesions and thoracic malignancies. *Semin Nucl Med* 2015;45(4):268–281.

Fogelman I, Cook G, Israel O, Van Der Wall H. Positron emission tomography and bone metastases. *Semin Nucl Med* 2005;35(2):135–142.

Garg G, Benchekroun MT, Abraham T. FDG-PET/CT in the postoperative period: Utility, expected findings, complications, and pitfalls. *Semin Nucl Med* 2017;47(6):579–594.

Goldberg MA, Mayo-Smith WW, Papanicolaou M, Fischman AJ, Lee MJ. FDG PET characterization of renal masses: preliminary experience. *Clin Radiol* 1997;52(7):510–515.

Groheux D, Cochet A, Humbert O, Alberini JL, Hindié E, Mankoff D. 18F-FDG PET/CT for staging and restaging of breast cancer. *J Nucl Med* 2016;57(Suppl 1):17S–26S.

Himeno S, Yasuda S, Shimada H, Tajima T, Makuuchi H. Evaluation of esophageal cancer by positron emission tomography. *Jpn J Clin Oncol* 2002;32(9):340–346.

Hofman MS, Hicks RJ, Maurer T, Eiber M. Prostate-specific membrane antigen PET: clinical utility in prostate cancer, normal patterns, pearls, and pitfalls. *Radiographics* 2018;38(1):200–217.

Kapoor V, Fukui MB, McCook BM. Role of 18F-FDG PET/CT in the treatment of head and neck cancers: posttherapy evaluation and pitfalls. *AJR Am J Roentgenol* 2005a;184:589–597.

Kapoor V, Fukui MB, McCook BM. Role of 18F-FDG PET/CT in the treatment of head and neck cancers: principles, technique, normal distribution, initial staging. *AJR Am J Roentgenol* 2005b;184(2):579–587.

Kapoor V, McCook BM, Torok FS. An introduction to PET-CT imaging. *Radiographics* 2004;24(2):523–543.

Koga H, Sasaki M, Kuwabara Y, et al. An analysis of the physiological FDG uptake pattern in the stomach. *Ann Nucl Med* 2003;17(8):733–738.

Kostakoglu L, Hardoff R, Mirtcheva R, Goldsmith SJ. PET-CT fusion imaging in differentiating physiologic from pathologic FDG uptake. *Radiographics* 2004;24(5):1411–1431.

Kwee RM, Marcus C, Sheikhbahaie S, Subramaniam RM. PET with fluorodeoxyglucose F-18/computed tomography in the clinical management and patient outcomes of esophageal cancer. *PET Clin* 2015;10(2):197–205.

Lakhani A, Khan SR, Bharwani N, et al. FDG PET/CT pitfalls in gynecologic and genitourinary oncologic imaging. *Radiographics* 2017;37(2):577–594.

Lakhman Y, Nougaret S, Miccò M, et al. Role of MR imaging and FDG PET/CT in selection and follow-up of pelvic exenteration for gynecologic malignancies. *Radiographics* 2015;35(4):1295–1313.

Laurens ST, Oyen WJ. Impact of fluorodeoxyglucose PET/computed tomography on the management of patients with colorectal cancer. *PET Clin* 2015;10(3):345–360.

Lee SI, Catalano OA, Dehdashti F. Evaluation of gynecologic cancer with MR imaging, 18F-FDG PET/CT, and PET/MR imaging. *J Nucl Med* 2015;56(3):436–443.

Lerut T, Flamen P, Ectors N, et al. Histopathologic validation of lymph node staging with FDG-PET scan in cancer of the esophagus and gastroesophageal junction: a prospective study based on primary surgery with extensive lymphadenectomy. *Ann Surg* 2000;232(6):743–752.

Liu Y. Role of FDG PET-CT in evaluation of locoregional nodal disease for initial staging of breast cancer. *World J Clin Oncol* 2014;5(5):982–989.

Love C, Tomas MB, Tronco GG, Palestro CJ. FDG PET of infection and inflammation. *Radiographics* 2005;25(5):1357–1368.

MacMahon H, Naidich DP, Goo JM, et al. Guidelines for management of incidental pulmonary nodules detected on CT images: from the Fleischner Society 2017. *Radiology* 2017;284(1):228–243.

Maurer AH, Burshteyn M, Adler LP, Steiner RM. Utility of FDG PET/CT in inflammatory cardiovascular disease. *Radiographics* 2011;31(5):1271–1286.

Meller J, Sahlmann CO, Scheel AK. 18F-FDG PET and PET/CT in fever of unknown origin. *J Nucl Med* 2007;48(1):35–45.

Paes FM, Singer AD, Checkver AN, Palmquist RA, De La Vega G, Sidani C. Perineural spread in head and neck malignancies: clinical significance and evaluation with 18F-FDG PET/CT. *Radiographics* 2013;33(6):1717–1736.

Perng P, Marcus C, Subramaniam RM. (18)F-FDG PET/CT and melanoma: staging, immune modulation and mutation-targeted therapy assessment, and prognosis. *AJR Am J Roentgenol* 2015;205(2):259–270.

Rajadhyaksha CD, Parker JA, Barbaras L, Gerbaudo VH. Normal and benign pathologic findings in 18-FDG-PET and PET-CT. An interactive web-based image atlas. Joint Program in Nuclear Medicine, Harvard Medical School, 2005. Available from http://www.jpnm.org

Ruilong Z, Daohai X, Li G, Xiaohong W, Chunjie W, Lei T. Diagnostic value of 18F-FDG-PET/CT for the evaluation of solitary pulmonary nodules: a systematic review and meta-analysis. *Nucl Med Commun* 2017;38(1):67–75.

Stafford SE, Gralow JR, Schubert EK, et al. Use of serial FDG PET to measure the response of bone-dominant breast cancer to therapy. *Acad Radiol* 2002;9(8):913–921.

Sugawara Y, Zasadny KR, Kison PV, Baker LH, Wahl RL. Splenic fluorodeoxyglucose uptake increased by granulocyte colony-stimulating factor therapy: PET imaging results. *J Nucl Med* 1999;40(9):1456–1462.

Szyszko TA, Cook GJR. PET/CT and PET/MRI in head and neck malignancy. *Clin Radiol* 2018;73(1):60–69.

Wahl RL, Siegel BA, Coleman RE, Gatsonis CG. Prospective multicenter study of axillary nodal staging by positron emission tomography in breast cancer: a report of the staging breast cancer with PET study group. *J Clin Oncol* 2004; 22(2):277–285.

Wallitt KL, Khan SR, Dubash S, et al. Clinical PET imaging in prostate cancer. *Radiographics* 2017;37(5):1512–1536.

Wang HY, Ding HJ, Chen JH, et al. Meta-analysis of the diagnostic performance of [18F]FDG-PET and PET/CT in renal cell carcinoma. *Cancer Imaging* 2012;12(3):464–474.

Wimber AG, Burger IA, Sala E, Hricak H, Weber WA, Vargas HA. Molecular imaging of prostate cancer. *Radiographics* 2016;36(1):142–215.

Wong ANM, McArthur GA, Hofman MS, Hicks RJ. The advantages and challenges of using FDG PET/CT for response assessment in melanoma in the era of targeted agents and immunotherapy. *Eur J Nucl Med Mol Imaging* 2017;44(Suppl 1):67–77.

Yau YY, Chan WS, Tam YM, et al. Application of intravenous contrast in PET/CT: does it really introduce significant attenuation correction error? *J Nucl Med* 2005;46(2):283–291.

Ziai P, Hayeri MR, Salei A, et al. Role of optimal quantification of FDG PET imaging in the clinical practice of radiology. *Radiographics* 2016;36(2):481–496.

INDEX

Note: Page number followed by f indicates figure only.

E

G

J

K

O

CCS0918